Fourteenth Edition

TEXTBOOK
OF
MEDICINE

Edited by

PAUL B. BEESON, M.D.

Distinguished Physician, United States Veterans Administration,
University of Washington School of Medicine;
Formerly Nuffield Professor of Clinical Medicine, University of Oxford

WALSH McDERMOTT, M.D.

Professor of Public Affairs in Medicine, Cornell University Medical College;
Attending Physician, The New York Hospital; Special Advisor to the
President, Robert Wood Johnson Foundation

W. B. SAUNDERS COMPANY · Philadelphia · London · Toronto

W. B. Saunders Company: West Washington Square
Philadelphia, PA 19105

12 Dyott Street
London WC1A 1DB

833 Oxford Street
Toronto, Ontario M8Z 5T9, Canada

Library of Congress Cataloging in Publication Data

Main entry under title:

Textbook of medicine.

First–13th editions by R. L. Cecil.

Includes index.

1. Internal medicine.   I. Beeson, Paul B.   II. McDermott,
    Walsh, 1909–   III. Cecil, Russell La Fayette, 1881–1965.
    Textbook of medicine. [DNLM: 1. Medicine. WB100 T354]

RC46.C4 1975   616   74–4553

ISBN 0–7216–1660–7

Listed here are the latest translated editions of this book, together with
the language of the translation and the publisher:

Portuguese (13th Edition)—Editoria Guanabara Koogan,
                      Rio de Janeiro, Brazil
Serbo-Croat (11th Edition)—Medicinska Knjiga, Belgrade, Yugoslavia
Spanish (13th Edition)—Nueva Editorial Interamericana S.A., de C.V.,
              Mexico

Textbook of Medicine

Single Vol: ISBN 0-7216-1660-7
Vol I: ISBN 0-7216-1661-5
Vol II: ISBN 0-7216-1662-3

Last digit is the print number: 9   8   7   6   5   4   3   2

Preface

This fourteenth edition of the Textbook of Medicine is dedicated in warm and respectful affection to the memory of Russell L. Cecil and Robert F. Loeb. Their influence goes on in the essential character created and maintained by them for the book and in the long-range effects they have had as teachers and editors. Although their names no longer appear on the title page, the book still carries their imprint throughout.

Each played a different yet essential part in the development of this textbook. In the mid-1920's, Dr. Cecil had the wisdom to perceive that a single-authored text in medicine would no longer suffice and created the first multiauthored textbook of medicine. Twenty years later he had the further wisdom to perceive that the scientific base of medicine had so enlarged that his own background in science was no longer sufficiently contemporary. Hence he invited Dr. Loeb to join him as coeditor. This marriage of the private physician–professor and the full-time academic professor was a very happy one; each complemented the other perfectly. Both were dedicated to the idea of getting the key concepts and useful practices of the specialist and the scientist into a form that could be employed by physicians and medical students. Under the coeditorship of Dr. Loeb the textbook changed subtly. It became less the repository of established doctrine and more the expression of advanced, ongoing ideas in medicine.

Dr. Cecil tended to worry more about the physician and Dr. Loeb about the medical student; yet each was deeply interested in both. Each had ample claims to distinction quite aside from the book, and in the course of their long careers, each benefited many people. It was their joint editorial venture, however, that allowed them to exert a healing influence on the many thousands of patients they never got to see and a learning influence on the many thousands of students who could not know personally their extraordinary dedication to teaching. This lengthened shadow is a very real part of their memorial and our legacy.

It is appropriate at this time to mention others who have shared editorial responsibilities of the textbook throughout its 14 editions. There has always been an Associate Editor responsible for the section on Diseases of the Nervous System. In the first seven editions Foster Kennedy served in that capacity. Harold Wolff took over for the eighth through eleventh editions and has been followed by Fred Plum. Walsh McDermott served as Associate Editor from the sixth edition, and in the eighth edition Alexander Gutman also joined in that role.

By its tenth edition (1959) when this textbook had attained world recognition and probably the widest use of any English language textbook of medicine, Cecil and Loeb retired from academic medicine and from their joint editorship. The W. B. Saunders Company invited us to succeed them as coeditors, and we gladly accepted with the goal of striving to maintain the high standards set by our predecessors. We invited four others to serve with Dr. Plum as Associate Editors. They were Alexander Bearn, Hereditary Diseases; Philip Bondy, Endocrine and Metabolic Diseases; Carl Moore, Hematologic and Hematopoietic Diseases; and Marvin Sleisenger, Gastrointestinal Diseases. At the time of preparing the twelfth edition, Dr. Bondy had to withdraw because of other responsibilities and was succeeded by Nicholas Christy.

When the planning for the present edition was just getting under way, Carl Moore died suddenly, to be mourned by friends and students everywhere. He had contributed powerfully to the development of his section on Hematologic and Hematopoietic Diseases, and because of his great experience and breadth of understanding had been able to write about one quarter of that section himself. We believe that his Introduction to Hematologic Diseases in the eleventh to thirteenth editions deserves to rank with another Cecil "classic," Fuller Albright's Introduction to the Endocrine section, which appeared in the seventh to tenth editions. We prized Moore's association with the book not only for the standard of his own section but also for his advice about organization of the entire work.

We welcome to the present edition a new colleague, Ralph Nachman, as Associate Editor for Hematologic and Hematopoietic Diseases. Thus the Cornell Medical Center tradition in editorship of this book and the Moore tradition of excellence in editorship of Hematology remains strong.

There are 200 contributors to the present edition, of whom 72 are making contributions for the first time. In addition, a considerable number of contributors to previous editions have elected to rewrite rather than simply revise, so that fully half the present edition is assembled from new manuscripts. As Editors, we have accepted responsibility for maintaining reasonable balance in the length and style of contributions. In consultation with the expert editorial staff of the Saunders Company, we have again given special attention to the headings of sections, chapters, and paragraphs in order to make the book as easy to use as possible. In the Table of Contents we have reverted to a style employed in some of the earlier editions, which we think makes for easier use than that in some more recent editions. We have also introduced a system of cross-reference by chapter, which is made easier by printing the chapter number in the running head of each right-hand page.

A major goal in this edition has been to give as much information as practical about therapy. Each contributor has been specially requested to pay attention to this point. Furthermore, we have introduced five new chapters solely about treatment: Antimicrobial Therapy, Cytotoxic and Immunosuppressive Agents, Medical Treatment of Hormone-Dependent Cancers, Respiratory Failure and Its Management, and Diet Therapy in Acute and Chronic Disease. A new essay appears in Part I, dealing with Care of the Patient with Terminal Illness. Various other areas in which treatment is complex have been given additional space, e.g., management of renal insufficiency, management of shock and heart failure, use of anticonvulsant drugs, treatment of pain, and the problems of drug intoxications and addictions.

We view seriously our responsibility as custodians of what has become a classic medical text during the past half century; yet we realize full well that for the expert quality of the substance, it is the contributors who must be thanked. We do this with gratitude.

But contributors and editors acting alone would not make a book; there are others we must thank. We should like to acknowledge the help and dedication of our secre-taries, Miss Phyl Woolford and Mrs. Irma Sway. We are deeply indebted to our editorial assistant, Mrs. Helen Miller of New York, who for four editions has served as the major link between contributors, the publisher, and ourselves and has carried out the task faultlessly. We continue to find it a pleasure to work with all the people of the Saunders Company and especially wish to thank David Kilmer for his careful editing.

As this is the last edition that will have the benefit of his experience and wisdom, we insist, despite his protest, on paying homage to John Dusseau, Editor and Vice-President. In the finest tradition of the book publisher's role, he has continuously served as confidant, friend, sensitive critic, and counselor. To work with him has been our great good fortune.

PAUL B. BEESON
WALSH McDERMOTT

Contributors

ALBERT J. AGUAYO, M.D.

Mechanical Lesions of the Nerve Roots and Spinal Cord

Associate Professor of Neurology and Neurosurgery, McGill University. Associate Physician, The Montreal General Hospital, Montreal, Quebec, Canada.

MARGARET J. ALBRINK, M.D.

Obesity

Professor of Medicine, West Virginia University School of Medicine. Member of Medical Staff, West Virginia University Hospital, Morgantown, West Virginia.

THOMAS P. ALMY, M.D.

Disorders of Motility

Third Century Professor of Medicine, Dartmouth Medical School. Staff Member, Mary Hitchcock Memorial Hospital, Hanover, New Hampshire; Consultant in Medicine, Veterans Administration Center, White River Junction, Vermont.

GERALD D. AURBACH, M.D.

Parathyroid

Chief, Metabolic Diseases Branch, National Institute of Arthritis, Metabolism, and Digestive Diseases, National Institutes of Health, Bethesda, Maryland.

K. FRANK AUSTEN, M.D.

*Connective Tissue Diseases ("Collagen Diseases")
Other Than Rheumatoid Arthritis: Introduction;
Periarteritis Nodosa*

Theorore B. Bayles Professor of Medicine, Harvard Medical School. Physician-in-Chief, Robert B. Brigham Hospital, Boston, Massachusetts.

J. RICHARD BARINGER, M.D.

Herpes Simplex Encephalitis

Associate Professor (in Residence) and Vice-Chairman, Department of Neurology, University of California, San Francisco. Chief, Neurology Service, Veterans Administration Hospital, San Francisco, California.

ALEXANDER G. BEARN, M.D.

*Genetic Principles: Introduction; Pedigree Analysis in
Inherited Disease; Inborn Errors of Metabolism and
Molecular Disease; Polygenic and Multifactorial Inheritance;
Pharmacogenetics; Population Genetics; Heredity and
Environment; Congenital Malformations; Prevention and
Management of Genetic Disease; Acatalasia; Albinism;
Dysautonomia; Laurence-Moon Syndrome; Lipoatrophic
Diabetes; Lipoid Proteinosis; Marfan's Syndrome; The
Mucopolysaccharidoses; Wilson's Disease; Werner's Syndrome*

Professor and Chairman, Department of Medicine, Cornell University Medical College. Physician-in-Chief, The New York Hospital, New York, New York.

MARGARET R. BECKLAKE, M.D., F.R.C.P.

Physical and Chemical Irritants

Professor, Departments of Experimental Medicine and of Epidemiology and Health, McGill University. Associate Physician, Royal Victoria Hospital, Montreal, Quebec, Canada.

PAUL B. BEESON, M.D.

*On Becoming a Clinician; Granulomatous Diseases of
Unproved Etiology; Introduction; Polymyalgia Rheumatica
and Cranial Arteritis; Lethal Midline Granuloma; Wegener's
Granulomatosis; Weber-Christian Disease; Fibrosing
Syndromes; Eosinophilic Syndromes; Viral Diseases
(Presumptive); Infective Endocarditis; Familial
Mediterranean Fever*

Distinguished Physician, United States Veterans Administration, University of Washington School of Medicine, Seattle, Washington. Formerly Nuffield Professor of Clinical Medicine, University of Oxford, England.

ABRAM S. BENENSON, M.D.

Typhoid Fever

Professor and Chairman, Department of Community Medicine, University of Kentucky College of Medicine, Lexington, Kentucky.

JOHN E. BENNETT, M.D.

*Nocardiosis; Cryptococcosis; Mucormycosis;
Aspergillosis; Candidiasis*

Head, Clinical Mycology Section, Laboratory of Clinical Investigation, National Institute of Allergy and Infectious Diseases, Bethesda, Maryland.

ERNEST BEUTLER, M.D.

Galactosemia

Clinical Professor of Medicine, University of Southern California. Chairman, Division of Medicine, City of Hope Medical Center, Duarte, California.

CHARLES E. BILLINGS, M.D.

Electric Shock

Professor of Preventive Medicine, The Ohio State University College of Medicine. Attending Physician, University Hospitals, Columbus, Ohio.

PHILIP K. BONDY, M.D.

Medical Treatment of Hormone-Dependent Cancers

Cancer Research Campaign Professor of Medicine and Consultant in Medicine, Ludwig Institute of Cancer Research, Sutton. Honorary Consultant, Royal Marsden Hospital, Sutton, Surrey, England.

THOMAS H. BOTHWELL, M.D., D.Sc., F.R.C.P.

Hemochromatosis

Professor of Internal Medicine, University of the Witwatersrand Medical School. Chief Physician, Johannesburg Hospital, Johannesburg, South Africa.

MICHAEL C. BRAIN, D.M.

The Anemias: Introduction; Aplastic Anemia; Sideroblastic Anemia; Myelophthisic Anemia

Professor of Medicine, McMaster University. Physician, McMaster University Medical Centre and Civic Hospitals, Hamilton, Ontario, Canada.

LLOYD L. BRANDBORG, M.D.

Neoplastic Diseases of the Alimentary Tract: Introduction; Neoplasms of the Esophagus; Malignant Neoplasms of the Stomach; Benign Neoplasms of the Stomach

Clinical Professor of Medicine, University of California, San Francisco. Chief, Gastroenterology Section, Veterans Administration Hospital, San Francisco; Consultant, Letterman General Hospital, Oakland Naval Hospital, U.S. Public Health Service Hospital, San Francisco, David Grant Air Force Base, California, and William Beaumont General Hospital, El Paso, Texas.

NEAL S. BRICKER, M.D.

Acute Renal Failure

Professor and Chairman, Department of Medicine, Albert Einstein College of Medicine, Bronx, New York.

WALLACE BRIGDEN, M.D., F.R.C.P.

Disease of the Myocardium

Lecturer in the London Hospital Medical School and the Institute of Cardiology. Consultant Physician to the London Hospital and Physician to the Cardiac Department; Physician to the National Heart Hospital, London, England.

ELMER B. BROWN, M.D.

Acute Hemorrhagic Anemia; Anemia Associated with Infection and Chronic Systemic Diseases; Hypochromic Anemias

Professor of Medicine, Washington University School of Medicine. Associate Physician, Barnes Hospital, St. Louis, Missouri.

ANTHONY D. M. BRYCESON, M.D., F.R.C.P.E., D.T.M.&H.

Leishmaniasis

Senior Lecturer, London School of Hygiene and Tropical Medicine. Consultant Physician, Hospital for Tropical Diseases, London, England.

GEORGE F. CAHILL, Jr., M.D.

Diabetes Mellitus

Professor of Medicine, Harvard Medical School. Director, Joslin Research Laboratories; Harvard Physician, Peter Bent Brigham Hospital, Boston, Massachusetts.

PAUL CALABRESI, M.D.

Cytotoxic and Immunosuppressive Agents

Professor and Chairman, Department of Medicine, Brown University. Physician-in-Chief, Roger Williams General Hospital and Women's and Infants' Hospital of Rhode Island, Providence; Consultant, Rhode Island Hospital, Providence Veterans Administration Hospital, and The Miriam Hospital, Providence, and The Memorial Hospital, Pawtucket, Rhode Island.

PAUL P. CARBONE, M.D.

Lymphoreticular Neoplasms: Introduction; Lymphocytic and Histiocytic Lymphomas; Burkitt's Lymphoma

Associate Director for Medical Oncology, National Cancer Institute, Bethesda, Maryland.

HUGH CHAPLIN, Jr., M.D.

Hemoglobinuria; Transfusion Reactions

Professor of Medicine and Preventive Medicine, Washington University School of Medicine. Associate Physician, Barnes Hospital, St. Louis, Missouri.

CHARLES L. CHRISTIAN, M.D.

Diseases of the Joints

Professor of Medicine, Cornell University Medical College. Physician-in-Chief, Hospital for Special Surgery, New York, New York.

NICHOLAS P. CHRISTY, M.D.

Diseases of Metabolism: Introduction; Diseases of the Endocrine System: Introduction; The Anterior Pituitary; Endocrine Syndromes Associated with Cancer

Professor of Medicine, Columbia University College of Physicians and Surgeons. Director, Medical Service, The Roosevelt Hospital; Visiting Physician, Francis Delafield Hospital; Associate Attending Physician, The Presbyterian Hospital, New York, New York.

LEIGHTON E. CLUFF, M.D.

Shigellosis; Cholera; Diseases Caused by Malleomyces; Anthrax; Listeriosis; Erysipeloid of Rosenbach

Professor of Internal Medicine, University of Florida. Chairman, Department of Medicine, University of Florida Teaching Hospitals, Gainesville, Florida.

JAY D. COFFMAN, M.D.

Diseases of the Peripheral Vessels

Professor of Medicine, Boston University School of Medicine. Section Head, Peripheral Vascular Department, University Hospital, Boston, Massachusetts.

C. LOCKARD CONLEY, M.D.

Hemoglobin, the Hemoglobinopathies, and the Thalassemias

Professor of Medicine, The Johns Hopkins University School of Medicine. Head, Hematology Division, The Johns Hopkins University and Hospital, Baltimore, Maryland.

REX B. CONN, M.D.

Normal Laboratory Values of Clinical Importance

Professor of Laboratory Medicine, The Johns Hopkins University. Director, Department of Laboratory Medicine, The Johns Hopkins Hospital, Baltimore, Maryland.

ROBERT B. COUCH, M.D.

Mycoplasmal Diseases

Professor of Microbiology and Immunology and Medicine, Baylor College of Medicine. Attending Physician, The Methodist Hospital, Houston; Attending Physician in Medicine, Ben Taub Hospital, Houston, Texas.

ALEXANDER CRAMPTON SMITH, M.A., M.B., Ch.B., F.F.A.R.C.S.

Tetanus

Nuffield Professor of Anaesthetics, University of Oxford, England. Consultant Anaesthetist (Honorary), Oxfordshire Area Health Authority (Teaching).

ANTHONY N. DAMATO, M.D.

Cardiac Arrhythmia

U.S. Public Health Service Hospital, Staten Island, New York.

LESLIE J. DeGROOT, M.D.

The Thyroid

Professor of Medicine, University of Chicago School of Medicine, Chicago, Illinois.

ROGER M. DES PREZ, M.D.

Tuberculosis; Extrapulmonary Tuberculosis

Professor of Medicine, Vanderbilt University School of Medicine. Chief, Medical Service, Veterans Administration Hospital, Nashville. Visiting Staff, Vanderbilt University Hospital, Nashville, Tennessee.

BERTRAM D. DINMAN, M.D., Sc.D.

Carbon Monoxide Poisoning

Non-resident lecturer, University of Michigan School of Public Health. Medical Director, Aluminum Company of America, Pittsburgh, Pennsylvania.

PHILIP R. DODGE, M.D.

Infections and Inflammatory Diseases of the Central Nervous System and Its Coverings: Introduction; Aids to Diagnosis in Intracranial and Intraspinal Inflammatory Disease; Spinal Epidural Infections; Transverse Myelitis or Myelopathy; Syphilitic Infections of the Central Nervous System

Professor of Pediatrics and Neurology and Head, Edward Mallinkrodt Department of Pediatrics, Washington University School of Medicine. Medical Director, St. Louis Children's Hospital; Pediatrician-in-Chief, Barnes Hospital, St. Louis, Missouri.

WILBUR G. DOWNS, M.D.

Yellow Fever

Clinical Professor of Epidemiology, Yale University School of Medicine, New Haven, Connecticut.

DAVID A. DRACHMAN, M.D.

Dizziness and Vertigo

Professor of Neurology, Northwestern University School of Medicine. Attending Physician and Chief of Neurology, Passavant Pavilion, Northwestern Memorial Hospital, Chicago, Illinois.

PIERRE M. DREYFUS, M.D.

Nutritional Disorders of the Nervous System

Professor of Neurology, University of California, Davis. Chief of Neurology, Sacramento Medical Center, Sacramento, California.

PETER JAMES DYCK, M.D.

Diseases of the Peripheral Nervous System

Professor of Neurology, Mayo Medical School, Rochester, Minnesota.

DAVID L. EARNEST, M.D.

Other Diseases of the Colon, Rectum, and Anus

Assistant Professor of Medicine, University of California School of Medicine, San Francisco. Staff Gastroenterologist, San Francisco General Hospital, San Francisco, California.

RICHARD V. EBERT, M.D.

Abnormal Air Spaces; Diffuse Lung Disease

Professor of Internal Medicine, University of Minnesota Medical School, Minneapolis, Minnesota.

HAROLD V. ELLINGSON, M.D., Ph.D., M.P.H.

Motion Sickness and Problems of Air Travel

Professor and Chairman, Department of Preventive Medicine, Ohio State University College of Medicine, Columbus, Ohio.

KARL ENGELMAN, M.D.

The Adrenal Medulla and Sympathetic Nervous System; The Carcinoid Syndrome

Associate Professor of Medicine and Pharmacology, University of Pennsylvania School of Medicine. Chief, Hypertension and Clinical Pharmacology Section, and Director, Clinical Research Center, Hospital of the University of Pennsylvania, Philadelphia; Attending Physician, Veterans Administration Hospital, Philadelphia General Hospital, and Children's Hospital of Philadelphia, Pennsylvania.

ALVAN R. FEINSTEIN, M.D.

Science, Clinical Medicine, and the Spectrum of Disease; Neoplasms of the Lung

Professor of Medicine and Epidemiology and Director, Johnson Clinical Scholar Program, Yale University School of Medicine. Attending Physician, Yale–New Haven Hospital, New Haven; Chief, Clinical Biostatistics, West Haven Veterans Administration Hospital, West Haven, Connecticut.

F. ROBERT FEKETY, Jr., M.D.

Staphylococcal Infections

Professor of Internal Medicine, University of Michigan Medical School. Attending Physician, University Hospital, Ann Arbor, Michigan.

HARRY A. FELDMAN, M.D.

Meningococcal Disease

Professor and Chairman, Department of Preventive Medicine, State University of New York, Upstate Medical Center. Attending Physician, State University and Silverman Hospitals; Consultant, Syracuse Psychiatric Hospital, Syracuse, New York.

PHILIP FELIG, M.D.

Nutritional Maintenance and Diet Therapy in Acute and Chronic Disease

Professor of Medicine and Vice Chairman, Department of Medicine, Yale University School of Medicine. Attending Physician, Yale–New Haven Hospital, New Haven; Consultant in Metabolism and Endocrinology, Veterans Administration Hospital, West Haven, Connecticut.

THOMAS F. FERRIS, M.D.

Renal Disease in Pregnancy

Professor of Medicine, Ohio State University. Director, Division of Renal Diseases, Ohio State University Hospitals, Columbus, Ohio.

SYDNEY M. FINEGOLD, M.D.

Disease Due to Nonsporeforming Anaerobic Bacteria

Professor of Medicine, Department of Medicine, UCLA School of Medicine. Chief, Infectious Disease Section, Veterans Administration Wadsworth Hospital Center, Los Angeles, California.

ALFRED P. FISHMAN, M.D.

Heart Failure; Shock

William Maul Measey Professor of Medicine, University of Pennsylvania School of Medicine. Director of Cardiovascular-Pulmonary Division, Hospital of the University of Pennsylvania; Attending Physician, Philadelphia General Hospital, Philadelphia, Pennsylvania.

ROBERT A. FISHMAN, M.D.

Intracranial Tumors and States Causing Increased Intracranial Pressure

Professor and Chairman, Department of Neurology, School of Medicine, University of California, San Francisco. Attending Neurologist, Veterans Administration Hospital, Fort Miley, San Francisco General Hospital, and Letterman General Hospital, Presidio, San Francisco, California.

EDMUND B. FLINK, M.D., Ph.D.

Heavy Metal Poisoning

Professor and Chairman, Department of Medicine, West Virginia University School of Medicine. Chief, Medical Service, West Virginia University Hospital, Morgantown, West Virginia.

DONALD S. FREDRICKSON, M.D.

Lipid Storage Disorders

President, Institute of Medicine, National Academy of Sciences, Washington, D.C.

NORBERT FREINKEL, M.D.

Hypoglycemic Disorders

Kettering Professor of Medicine, Professor of Biochemistry, and Director, Center for Endocrinology, Metabolism and Nutrition, Northwestern University Medical School. Director, Endocrine-Metabolic Clinics, Northwestern University Medical School; Attending Physician, Northwestern Memorial Hospital, Chicago; Consultant in Endocrinology, Veterans Administration Research Hospital, Chicago, Illinois.

PARK S. GERALD, M.D.

Chromosomes and Their Disorders

Professor of Pediatrics, Harvard Medical School. Chief, Clinical Genetics Division, Children's Hospital Medical Center, Boston, Massachusetts.

NORMAN GESCHWIND, M.D.

Focal Disturbances of Higher Nervous Function

James Jackson Putnam Professor of Neurology, Harvard Medical School. Director, Neurological Unit, Boston City Hospital, Boston, Massachusetts.

GILBERT H. GLASER, M.D., Med.Sc.D.

The Epilepsies

Professor of Neurology and Chairman, Department of Neurology, Yale University School of Medicine. Neurologist-in-Chief, Yale–New Haven Hospital, New Haven; Consultant Neurologist, Veterans Administration Hospital, West Haven, Connecticut.

ROBERT A. GOOD, Ph.D., M.D.

The Primary Immunodeficiency Diseases

Professor of Medicine and Pediatrics, Cornell University Medical College. President and Director, Sloan-Kettering Institute for Cancer Research. Attending Physician and Director of Research, Memorial Hospital for Cancer and Allied Diseases, New York, New York.

ROBERT A. GOODWIN, Jr., M.D.

Pulmonary Tuberculosis; Diseases Due to Mycobacteria Other Than M. tuberculosis and M. leprae

Professor of Medicine, Vanderbilt University School of Medicine. Chief, Pulmonary Disease Section, Veterans Administration Hospital, Nashville; Visiting Staff, Vanderbilt University Hospital, Nashville, Tennessee.

MORTON I. GROSSMAN, M.D., Ph.D.

Peptic Ulcer: Pathogenesis and Pathology

Professor of Medicine and Physiology, UCLA School of Medicine. Senior Medical Investigator, Wadsworth Veterans Administration Hospital, Los Angeles, California.

THORSTEIN GUTHE, M.D., M.P.H.

Treponemal Diseases; Relapsing Fevers; Phagedenic Tropical Ulcer; The Rat-Bite Fevers

Head, Medical Department, Elkem-Spigerverket, Oslo, Norway. Former Chief Medical Officer, Venereal Diseases and Treponematoses, World Health Organization, Geneva, Switzerland.

ROBERT J. HAGGERTY, M.D.

Common Accidental Poisoning

Professor and Chairman, Department of Pediatrics, University of Rochester School of Medicine and Dentistry. Pediatrician-in-Chief, Strong Memorial Hospital; Consulting Pediatrician, Genesee Hospital and Rochester General Hospital, Rochester, New York.

CONSTANTINE L. HAMPERS, M.D.

Dialysis

Assistant Clinical Professor of Medicine, Harvard Medical School. Senior Associate in Medicine, Peter Bent Brigham Hospital, Boston, Massachusetts.

JAMES B. HANSHAW, M.D.

Cytomegalovirus Infections

Professor of Pediatrics and Microbiology, University of Rochester School of Medicine. Pediatrician-in-Chief, The Genesee Hospital, Rochester, New York.

EDWARD D. HARRIS, Jr., M.D.

Systemic Sclerosis

Associate Professor of Medicine, Dartmouth Medical School. Staff Physician, Mary Hitchcock Memorial Hospital, Hanover; Chief, Connective Tissue Disease Section, Dartmouth/Hitchcock Medical Center, Hanover, New Hampshire.

RICHARD J. HAVEL, M.D.

Disorders of Lipid Metabolism

Professor of Medicine and Director, Cardiovascular Research Institute, University of California School of Medicine. Attending Physician, University of California Hospitals, San Francisco, California.

ROBERT P. HEANEY, M.D.

Bone Physiology and Calcium Homeostasis; The Osteoporoses; The Osteomalacias; Osteitis Fibrosa; Bone Intoxications

Professor of Medicine, Creighton University School of Medicine. Vice President for Health Sciences, Creighton University, Omaha, Nebraska.

VICTOR HERBERT, M.D., J.D.

Megaloblastic Anemias

Clinical Professor of Pathology and Clinical Professor of Medicine, Columbia University College of Physicians and Surgeons. Medical Investigator and Director of the Hematology and Nutrition Laboratory, Veterans Administration Hospital, Bronx, New York.

ALBERT HEYMAN, M.D.

Syncope; Hyperventilation

Professor of Neurology, Duke University Medical Center. Attending Neurologist, Duke University Medical School and Durham Veterans Administration Hospital, Durham, North Carolina.

HOWARD H. HIATT, M.D.

Man and His Environment

Dean, Harvard School of Public Health, and Professor of Medicine, Harvard Medical School. Board of Consultation in Medicine, Beth Israel Hospital; Consultant, Peter Bent Brigham Hospital and Children's Hospital, Boston, Massachusetts.

PATRICK J. HOGAN, M.D.

Pericarditis

Instructor of Internal Medicine, Baylor College of Medicine. Staff, Methodist Hospital, Houston, Texas.

JAMES F. HOLLAND, M.D.

The Acute Leukemias

Professor and Chairman, Department of Neoplastic Diseases, and Professor of Medicine, Mt. Sinai School of Medicine of the City University of New York. Director, The Cancer Center, and Attending Physician, Mt. Sinai Hospital, New York, New York.

EDWARD W. HOOK, M.D.

Pneumococcal Pneumonia; Salmonella Infections Other Than Typhoid Fever

Henry B. Mulholland Professor and Chairman, Department of Medicine, University of Virginia School of Medicine. Physician-in-Chief, University of Virginia Hospital, Charlottesville, Virginia.

DOROTHY M. HORSTMANN, M.D.

Mumps; Viral Meningitis and Encephalitis

Professor of Epidemiology and Pediatrics, Yale University School of Medicine. Attending Pediatrician, Yale–New Haven Hospital, New Haven, Connecticut.

JOHN BERNARD LLOYD HOWELL, M.D., Ph.D.

The Diaphragm; The Chest Wall; Chronic Obstructive Lung Disease: Introduction; Chronic Bronchitis; Bronchiectasis; Asthma: Acute Reversible Airway Obstruction; Chronic Airway Obstruction; Localized Airway Obstruction

Professor of Medicine, University of Southampton Medical School. Consultant Physician, Southampton University Hospitals Group, Southampton, England.

CHARLES M. HUGULEY, Jr., M.D.

The Chronic Leukemias

Professor of Medicine, Emory University School of Medicine. Attending Hematologist and Oncologist, Emory University Hospital and Grady Memorial Hospital, Atlanta, Georgia.

J. WILLIS HURST, M.D.

Diseases of the Aorta

Professor and Chairman, Department of Medicine, Emory University School of Medicine, Atlanta, Georgia.

JON I. ISENBERG, M.D.

Peptic Ulcer: Diagnostic Studies and Medical Treatment

Associate Professor of Medicine, University of California at Los Angeles. Chief, Gastroenterology Section, Wadsworth Veterans Administration Hospital, Los Angeles, California.

GEORGE GEE JACKSON, M.D.

The Common Cold; Rhinoviral Respiratory Disease; Viral Pharyngitis, Laryngitis, Croup, and Bronchitis; Adenoviral Infections; Respiratory Syncytial Viral Disease; Parainfluenza Viral Diseases

Professor of Medicine and Chief, Section of Infectious Diseases, Abraham Lincoln School of Medicine, University of Illinois College of Medicine. Attending Physician, University of Illinois Hospital, Chicago; Consultant in Infectious Diseases, Westside Veterans Administration Hospital, Chicago, Illinois.

ERNST R. JAFFÉ, M.D.

Methemoglobinemia and Sulfhemoglobinemia

Professor of Medicine and Head, Division of Hematology, Albert Einstein College of Medicine. Attending Physician (Medicine), Bronx Municipal Hospital Center, Hospital of the Albert Einstein College of Medicine, and Lincoln Hospital, Bronx, New York.

DAVID GERAINT JAMES, M.A., M.D. (Cambridge), F.R.C.P.

Sarcoidosis

Dean, Royal Northern Hospital, London, England; Consultant Ophthalmic Physician, St. Thomas' Hospital, London. Clinical Professor of Medicine, University of Miami, Florida. Consulting Physician, Sydney Hospital, Sydney, Australia.

HENRY D. JANOWITZ, M.D.

Chronic Inflammatory Diseases of the Intestine

Clinical Professor of Medicine, Mount Sinai School of Medicine. Head, Division of Gastroenterology, Mount Sinai Hospital, New York, New York.

ERNEST JAWETZ, M.D., Ph.D.

Trachoma and Inclusion Conjunctivitis; Lymphogranuloma Venereum

Professor of Microbiology and Medicine, University of California Medical Center, San Francisco, California.

GRAHAM H. JEFFRIES, M.B., Ch.B. (N.Z.), D.Phil. (Oxon.)

Diseases of the Liver

Professor and Chairman, Department of Medicine, The Milton S. Hershey Medical Center, Pennsylvania State University College of Medicine. Chief, Medical Service, The Milton S. Hershey Medical Center Hospital, Hershey, Pennsylvania.

KARL M. JOHNSON, M.D.

Arthropod-Borne Viral Fevers, Viral Encephalitides, and Viral Hemorrhagic Fevers: Introduction; Dengue; West Nile Fever; Fevers Caused by Group A Arboviruses: Chikungunya, O'nyong-nyong, Mayaro, and Ross River; Rift Valley Fever; Sandfly Fever; Arthropod-Borne Viral Encephalitides; Viral Hemorrhagic Fevers: Introduction; Hemorrhagic Fever Caused by Dengue Viruses; Crimean Hemorrhagic Fever; Hemorrhagic Diseases Caused by Arenaviruses: Argentine and Bolivian Hemorrhagic Fevers and Lassa Fever; Epidemic Hemorrhagic Fever: Hemorrhagic Nephrosonephritis

Director, Middle America Research Unit, National Institute of Allergy and Infectious Diseases, National Institutes of Health, U.S. Public Health Service, Balboa Heights, Canal Zone.

RICHARD T. JOHNSON, M.D.

Viral Infections of the Nervous System: Introduction; Herpes Zoster; Slow Infections of the Nervous System

Professor of Neurology and Associate Professor of Microbiology, The Johns Hopkins University School of Medicine. Neurologist, The Johns Hopkins Hospital, Baltimore, Maryland.

ROBERT L. JOHNSON, M.D.

Alterations in Atmospheric Pressure

Deputy Chief, Biomedical Research Division, Life Sciences Directorate, Lyndon B. Johnson Space Center, Houston, Texas.

THOMAS C. JONES, M.D.

Malaria; Pneumocystosis; Trichomoniasis; Toxoplasmosis

Assistant Professor of Medicine and Public Health, Cornell University Medical College. Assistant Attending Physician, The New York Hospital, New York, New York.

FRED S. KANTOR, M.D.

Serum Sickness; Drug Allergy; Allergic Rhinitis; Vasomotor Rhinitis; Urticaria; Angioneurotic Edema; Insect Stings

Professor of Medicine, Yale University School of Medicine. Attending Physician, Yale–New Haven Hospital, New Haven, Connecticut.

ALBERT Z. KAPIKIAN, M.D.

Enteroviral Diseases

Head, Epidemiology Section, Laboratory of Infectious Diseases, National Institute of Allergy and Infectious Diseases, National Institutes of Health, Bethesda, Maryland.

NATHAN G. KASE, M.D.

The Ovaries

Professor and Chairman, Obstetrics and Gynecology, Yale University School of Medicine. Chief of Service, Yale–New Haven Hospital, New Haven, Connecticut.

DONALD KAYE, M.D.

Gonococcal Disease

Professor and Chairman, Department of Medicine, The Medical College of Pennsylvania. Chief of Medicine, Hospital of the Medical College of Pennsylvania, Philadelphia; Consultant in Medicine, Veterans Administration Hospital, Philadelphia, Pennsylvania.

C. HENRY KEMPE, M.D.

Variola and Vaccinia

Professor of Pediatrics, University of Colorado Medical Center. Consultant, Colorado General Hospital, Children's Hospital, Fitzsimons Army Hospital, and Veterans Administration Hospital, Denver, Colorado.

DAVID N. S. KERR, M.S., F.R.C.P.

Role of the Kidney in Health and Disease; Investigation of Renal Function; Chronic Renal Failure

Professor of Medicine, University of Newcastle upon Tyne. Consultant Physician, Royal Victoria Infirmary, Newcastle upon Tyne, England.

EDWIN D. KILBOURNE, M.D.

Introduction to Viral Diseases; Influenza; Measles; Rubella; Exanthemata Associated with Enteroviral Infections

Professor and Chairman, Department of Microbiology, Mount Sinai School of Medicine of the City University of New York, New York.

THOMAS KILLIP, M.D.

Coronary Artery Disease

Professor of Medicine, Northwestern University Medical School. Chairman, Department of Medicine, Evanston Hospital, Evanston, Illinois.

PRISCILLA KINCAID-SMITH, M.D., F.R.A.C.P., F.R.C.P., D.C.P.

Treatment of Irreversible Renal Failure by Transplantation and Dialysis: Introduction; Renal Transplantation

Reader in Medicine, University of Melbourne. Physician-in-Charge, Department of Nephrology, Royal Melbourne Hospital, Melbourne, Australia.

SEYMOUR J. KLEBANOFF, M.D., Ph.D.

Neutrophil Function; Neutrophil Dysfunction Syndromes

Professor of Medicine, University of Washington School of Medicine, Seattle, Washington.

RICHARD KNIGHT, M.B., B.Chir., M.R.C.P., D.T.M.&H.

Amebiasis

Lecturer, Liverpool School of Tropical Medicine, Liverpool, England. Clinical Assistant to Tropical Unit, United Liverpool Visiting Fellow, and Physician, Department of Clinical Sciences, University of Papua, New Guinea.

VERNON KNIGHT, M.D.

Brucellosis

Professor of Medicine and Professor and Chairman, Microbiology and Immunology, Baylor College of Medicine. Senior Attending Physician, The Methodist Hospital, Houston; Attending Physician, Ben Taub General Hospital, Houston, Texas.

HILARY KOPROWSKI, M.D.

Rabies

Director, The Wistar Institute, Philadelphia, Pennsylvania.

O. DHODANAND KOWLESSAR, M.D.

Diseases of the Pancreas

Professor of Medicine, Thomas Jefferson University, Jefferson Medical College. Director, Division of Gastroenterology, and Director, Clinical Research Center, Jefferson Medical College and Thomas Jefferson University Hospital, Philadelphia, Pennsylvania.

RICHARD M. KRAUSE, M.D.

Rheumatic Fever

Professor and Senior Physician, Rockefeller University, New York, New York.

CALVIN M. KUNIN, M.D.

Enteric Bacterial Infections; Urinary Tract Infections and Pyelonephritis

Professor of Internal Medicine, University of Wisconsin School of Medicine. Chief, Medical Service, Veterans Administration Hospital, Madison, Wisconsin.

HENRY G. KUNKEL, M.D.

Immune Disease: Introduction

Professor, Rockefeller University. Adjunct Professor of Medicine, Cornell University Medical School, New York, New York.

HAROLD P. LAMBERT, M.D., F.R.C.P.

Food Poisoning

Professor of Microbial Diseases, St. George's Hospital Medical School, University of London. Consultant Physician, St. George's Hospital, London, England.

DAVID H. LAW, M.D.

Gastrointestinal Bleeding

Professor of Medicine (Vice-Chairman), University of New Mexico School of Medicine. Chief, Medical Service, Albuquerque Veterans Administration Hospital, Albuquerque, New Mexico.

ALEXANDER LEAF, M.D.

Posterior Pituitary

Jackson Professor of Clinical Medicine, Harvard Medical School. Chief, Medical Services, Massachusetts General Hospital, Boston, Massachusetts.

AARON B. LERNER, M.D.

Disorders of Melanin Pigmentation

Professor of Dermatology, Yale University School of Medicine. Professor and Chairman, Department of Dermatology, Yale–New Haven Hospital, New Haven, Connecticut.

HERBERT L. LEY, Jr., M.D., M.P.H.

Rocky Mountain Spotted Fever; Tick-Borne Rickettsioses of the Eastern Hemisphere; Rickettsialpox; Scrub Typhus; Trench Fever; Q Fever; Bartonellosis

Medical consultant in foods and drugs, Bethesda, Maryland.

GRANT W. LIDDLE, M.D.

Adrenal Cortex

Professor and Chairman, Department of Medicine, Vanderbilt University. Physician-in-Chief, Vanderbilt University Hospital, Nashville, Tennessee.

PHILIP H. LIEBERMAN, M.D.

Eosinophilic Granuloma and Related Syndromes

Associate Professor of Pathology, Cornell University Medical

School. Chief, Surgical Pathology Service, Memorial Hospital for Cancer and Allied Diseases, New York, New York.

HAROLD I. LIEF, M.D.

Medical Aspects of Sexuality

Professor of Psychiatry, School of Medicine, University of Pennsylvania. Director, Division of Family Study, Marriage Council of Philadelphia, and Center for the Study of Sex Education in Medicine, all affiliates of the School of Medicine of the University of Pennsylvania, Philadelphia, Pennsylvania.

MORTIMER B. LIPSETT, M.D.

The Testis

Professor of Medicine, Case Western Reserve School of Medicine. Director, The Cancer Center, Cleveland, Ohio.

JOHN N. LOEB, M.D.

Mode of Action of Hormones

Associate Professor of Medicine, College of Physicians and Surgeons, Columbia University; Adjunct Assistant Professor, Rockefeller University. Associate Attending Physician, Presbyterian Hospital, New York, New York.

DANIEL S. LUKAS, M.D.

Pulmonary Hypertension

Associate Professor of Medicine, Cornell University Medical College. Chief, Cardiopulmonary Service, and Attending Physician, Memorial Hospital for Cancer and Allied Diseases; Associate Attending Physician, The New York Hospital, New York, New York.

PHILIP D. MARSDEN, M.D.

Leeches as Agents of Disease; Arthropoda of Medical Importance; Venomous Arthropods; Protozoan and Helminthic Diseases: Introduction; Protozoan Diseases: Introduction; Other Protozoan Diseases: Introduction; Giardiasis; Balantidiasis; Coccidiosis; Primary Amebic Meningoencephalitis; Helminthic Diseases: Introduction; The Cestodes; Hermaphroditic Flukes; The Nematodes; Tropical Pyomyositis; Eosinophilia in Relation to Helminthic Infections

Visiting Professor of Tropical Medicine, University of Brasilia. Physician, General Medical Service, Sobradinmo Hospital. Visiting Professor of Public Health, Cornell University Medical College. Senior Lecturer, Department of Clinical Tropical Medicine, London School of Hygiene and Tropical Medicine. Physician, Hospital for Tropical Diseases, London, England.

JOHN H. McCLEMENT, M.D.

Diseases of the Pleura

Professor of Medicine, New York University School of Medicine. Director, Chest Service, Bellevue Hospital, New York; Attending Physician, University Hospital, New York, New York.

FRED R. McCRUMB, Jr., M.D.

Plague

Special Assistant to the Director, Fogarty International Center, National Institutes of Health, Bethesda, Maryland.

WALSH McDERMOTT, M.D.

Medicine in Modern Society; Chemical Contamination of Water and Air; Introduction to Microbial Diseases; Foot-and-

Mouth Disease; Bacterial Diseases: Introduction; Pneumonia: Introduction; Hemophilus influenzae Infections; Granuloma Inguinale; Drugs and Microbes

Professor of Public Affairs in Medicine, Cornell University Medical College. Attending Physician, The New York Hospital, New York, New York. Special Advisor to the President, Robert Wood Johnson Foundation, Princeton, New Jersey.

FLETCHER H. McDOWELL, M.D.

Cerebrovascular Diseases

Professor of Neurology, Cornell University Medical College. Attending Neurologist, The New York Hospital; Medical Director, Burke Rehabilitation Hospital, New York, New York.

PAUL R. McHUGH, M.D.

Dementia; Psychologic Illness in Medical Practice; Psychologic Testing in Clinical Medicine

Professor of Psychiatry and Chairman, Department of Psychiatry, University of Oregon Medical School, Portland, Oregon.

GORDON MEIKLEJOHN, M.D.

Colorado Tick Fever

Professor and Chairman, Department of Medicine, University of Colorado Medical School. Staff, Colorado General Hospital, Denver General Hospital, Veterans Administration Hospital, and Fitzsimons Army General Hospital, Denver, Colorado.

JACK H. MENDELSON, M.D.

Alcohol Abuse and Alcohol-Related Illness

Professor of Psychiatry, Harvard Medical School. Director, Alcohol and Drug Abuse Research Center, McLean Hospital, Belmont, Massachusetts.

JAMES H. MEYER, M.D.

Peptic Ulcer: Complications and Surgical Treatment

Assistant Professor of Medicine, University of California, San Francisco. Staff, Veterans Administration Hospital, San Francisco, California.

ROBERT B. MILLMAN, M.D.

Drug Abuse, Addiction, and Intoxication: Introduction; The Opiates; Central Nervous System Depressants; Central Nervous System Stimulants; Cannabis; Psychedelics; Miscellaneous Inhalants

Assistant Professor of Public Health, Cornell University Medical College; Adjunct Assistant Professor, Rockefeller University. Director, Adolescent Development Program, The New York Hospital–Cornell Medical Center and Rockefeller University, New York, New York.

SHERMAN A. MINTON, Jr., M.D.

Snakebite; Marine Venoms

Professor of Microbiology, Indiana University School of Medicine, Indianapolis, Indiana.

STEPHEN I. MORSE, M.D.

Whooping Cough

Professor and Chairman, Microbiology and Immunology, State University of New York, Downstate Medical Center, Brooklyn, New York.

ARNO G. MOTULSKY, M.D.

Genetic Counseling

Professor of Medicine and Genetics, University of Washington. Attending Physician, University Hospital, Seattle, Washington.

FRANCIS P. MULDOWNEY, M.D., F.R.C.P.

Obstructive Nephropathy

Research Professor of Medicine, University College, Dublin. Physician in Charge, Metabolic and Renal Unit, St. Vincent's Hospital and National Maternity Hospital, Dublin, Ireland.

EDWARD S. MURRAY, M.D., M.P.H.

Rickettsial Diseases: Introduction; The Typhus Group

Professor of Microbiology, Harvard School of Public Health, Cambridge, Massachusetts.

W. P. LAIRD MYERS, M.D.

The Care of the Patient with Terminal Illness

Professor of Internal Medicine, Cornell University Medical College. Chairman, Department of Medicine, and Attending Physician, Memorial Sloan-Kettering Cancer Center; Member, Sloan-Kettering Institute for Cancer Research; Attending Physician, The New York Hospital, New York, New York.

RALPH L. NACHMAN, M.D.

Hematologic and Hematopoietic Diseases: Introduction; Hemorrhagic Disorders: Disorders of Primary Hemostasis

Professor of Medicine, Cornell University Medical College. Attending Physician, The New York Hospital, New York, New York.

JAMES R. NELSON, M.D.

Hearing Loss

Adjunct Associate Professor of Neurosciences, University of California School of Medicine, La Jolla. Attending Neurologist, University Hospital of San Diego County, San Diego, and Veterans Administration Hospital, La Jolla, California.

THOMAS F. O'BRIEN, Jr., M.D.

Neoplasms of the Small Intestine; Neoplasms of the Large Intestine

Associate Professor of Medicine, Bowman Gray School of Medicine. Chief, Gastroenterology Section, North Carolina Baptist Hospital, Winston-Salem; Member, Courtesy Staff, Forsyth Memorial Hospital, Winston-Salem, North Carolina.

ROBERT K. OCKNER, M.D.

Vascular Diseases of the Intestine; Diseases of the Peritoneum

Associate Professor of Medicine, University of California School of Medicine, San Francisco. Attending Physician, University of California–Moffitt Hospitals, Ft. Miley Veterans Administration Hospital, and San Francisco General Hospital, San Francisco, California.

W. E. ORMEROD, M.A., D.Sc., D.M.

African Trypanosomiases

Reader in Medical Protozoology, London School of Hygiene and Tropical Medicine, London, England.

ELLIOTT F. OSSERMAN, M.D.

Plasma Cell Dyscrasias

American Cancer Society Professor of Medicine and Associate Director, Institute of Cancer Research, Columbia University College of Physicians and Surgeons. Visiting Physician, Francis Delafield Hospital, New York; Attending Physician, Presbyterian Hospital, New York, New York.

DEMOSTHENES PAPPAGIANIS, M.D., Ph.D.

Coccidioidomycosis

Professor and Chairman, Department of Medical Microbiology, School of Medicine, University of California, Davis, California.

SOLOMON PAPPER, M.D.

Chronic Pyelonephritis

Distinguished Professor of Medicine, University of Oklahoma College of Medicine. Distinguished Physician, Oklahoma City Veterans Administration Hospital, Oklahoma City, Oklahoma.

RUSSEL H. PATTERSON, Jr., M.D.

Injuries of the Head and Spine

Professor of Surgery (Neurosurgery), Cornell University Medical College. Attending Surgeon-in-Charge, The New York Hospital, New York, New York.

WILLIAM STANLEY PEART, M.D., F.R.C.P., F.R.S.

Arterial Hypertension

Professor of Medicine, St. Mary's Hospital Medical School (University of London), London, England.

JOSEPH K. PERLOFF, M.D.

Congenital Heart Disease

Professor of Medicine and Pediatrics, University of Pennsylvania. Chief, Cardiovascular Section, University of Pennsylvania School of Medicine, Philadelphia, Pennsylvania.

ROBERT G. PETERSDORF, M.D.

Bacterial Meningitis

Professor and Chairman, Department of Medicine, University of Washington School of Medicine. Physician-in-Chief, University of Washington Hospital, Seattle, Washington.

FRED PLUM, M.D.

Disorders of the Nervous System and Behavior: Introduction; Consciousness and Its Disturbances: Introduction; The Pathogenesis of Stupor and Coma; Sleep and Its Disorders; Acute Drug Poisoning; Headache; Idiopathic Autonomic Insufficiency; Acute Anterior Poliomyelitis; Abnormalities in Respiratory Control

Ann Parrish Titzell Professor of Neurology, Cornell University Medical College. Neurologist-in-Chief, The New York Hospital, New York, New York.

JEROME B. POSNER, M.D.

Delirium and Exogenous Metabolic Brain Disease; Pain; Nonmetastatic Effects of Cancer on the Nervous System

Professor of Neurology, Cornell University Medical College. Chief, Neuropsychiatric Service, Memorial Sloan-Kettering Cancer Center; Attending Neurologist, The New York Hospital, New York, New York.

OSCAR D. RATNOFF, M.D.

Hemorrhagic Disorders: Coagulation Defects

Professor of Medicine, Case Western Reserve University School of Medicine. Career Investigator of the American Heart Association; Visiting Physician, University Hospitals of Cleveland, Cleveland, Ohio.

SEYMOUR REICHLIN, M.D., Ph.D.

The Control of Anterior Pituitary Secretion; The Pineal

Professor of Medicine, Tufts University School of Medicine. Senior Physician and Chief, Division of Endocrinology, Tufts–New England Medical Center, Boston, Massachusetts.

EDWARD H. REINHARD, M.D.

Polycythemia

Professor of Medicine, Washington University School of Medicine. Associate Physician and Director of the Blue Medical Service, Barnes Hospital, St. Louis; Member of Consulting Staff, Jewish Hospital and Veterans Administration Hospital, St. Louis, Missouri.

DONALD J. REIS, M.D.

Degenerative and Heredofamilial Diseases of the Central Nervous System

Professor of Neurology, Cornell University Medical College. Attending in Neurology, The New York Hospital, New York, New York.

RICHARD B. ROBERTS, M.D.

Antimicrobial Therapy

Associated Professor of Medicine and Head, Division of Infectious Diseases, Cornell University Medical College. Associate Attending Physician, The New York Hospital and Memorial Sloan-Kettering Cancer Center, New York, New York.

HEONIR ROCHA, M.D.

Diphtheria; Chagas' Disease

Professor and Chairman, Department of Medicine, University of Bahia School of Medicine, Bahia, Brazil.

DAVID E. ROGERS, M.D.

Psittacosis

President, The Robert Wood Johnson Foundation, Princeton, New Jersey.

SAUL A. ROSENBERG, M.D.

Hodgkin's Disease

Professor of Medicine and Radiology, Stanford University School of Medicine. Chief, Division of Oncology, Stanford University Hospital, Stanford, California.

JOHN ROSS, Jr., M.D.

Acquired Valvular Heart Disease

Professor of Medicine and Head, Cardiology Division, Department of Medicine, University of California, San Diego, School of Medicine. Attending Physician, University Hospital, San Diego County, La Jolla, California.

WENDELL F. ROSSE, M.D.

Hemolytic Disorders: Extracorpuscular Mechanisms

Professor of Medicine, Duke University Medical Center.

Chief of Medical Service, Veterans Administration Hospital, Durham, North Carolina.

LEWIS P. ROWLAND, M.D.

Diseases of Muscle and Neuromuscular Junction

Henry L. and Lucy Moses Professor of Neurology, College of Physicians and Surgeons, Columbia University. Director, Department of Neurology, Neurological Institute, Presbyterian Hospital, New York, New York.

GERALD F. M. RUSSELL, M.D., F.R.C.P., F.R.C.P.Ed., F.R.C.Psych.

Anorexia Nervosa

Professor of Psychiatry, Royal Free Hospital School of Medicine, University of London. Consultant Psychiatrist, Royal Free Hospital, London, England.

JAY P. SANFORD, M.D.

Hospital-Associated Infections: Endogenous Microbial Disease; Klebsiella and Other Gram-Negative Bacterial Pneumonias; Leptospirosis

Professor of Internal Medicine, University of Texas Southwestern Medical School. Chief, Infectious Disease Service and Microbiology Laboratory, Parkland Memorial Hospital, Dallas; Consultant in Internal Medicine, Dallas and Temple, Texas, Veterans Administration Hospitals, Brooke General Hospital, and Wilford Hall USAF Hospital, San Antonio; Attending Physician, Parkland Memorial, Presbyterian, and St. Paul Hospitals, Dallas, Texas.

PAUL D. SAVILLE, M.D., F.R.C.P.

Osteomyelitis; Osteonecrosis; Congenital and/or Hereditary Disorders Involving Bone; Paget's Disease of Bone: Osteitis Deformans; Fibrous Dysplasia; Hypertrophic Osteoarthropathy; Tumors of Bone

Professor of Medicine, Creighton University and University of Nebraska. Director, Metabolic Research Laboratory, and Chief, Rheumatology Service, Creighton University; Chief of Rheumatology, University of Nebraska, Omaha, Nebraska.

LABE C. SCHEINBERG, M.D.

The Demyelinating Diseases

Professor of Neurology, Albert Einstein College of Medicine. Director of Neurology, St. Barnabas Hospital, Bronx, New York.

RUDI SCHMID, M.D., Ph.D.

Porphyria

Professor of Internal Medicine, University of California, San Francisco, School of Medicine. Attending Physician, Moffitt-University Hospital, San Francisco, California.

RICHARD P. SCHMIDT, M.D.

Neurologic Diagnostic Procedures

Dean, College of Medicine, and Professor of Neurology, State University of New York, Upstate Medical Center. Attending Neurologist, University Hospital, Syracuse; Consultant, Veterans Administration Hospital, Syracuse, New York.

GEORGE E. SCHREINER, M.D.

Toxic Nephropathy; Cysts of the Kidney; Tumors of the Kidney; Miscellaneous Renal Disorders

Professor of Medicine, Georgetown University School of Medicine. Director, Nephrology Division, Georgetown University Hospital, Washington, D. C.

PETER H. SCHUR, M.D.

Systemic Lupus Erythematosus

Associate Professor of Medicine, Harvard Medical School. Physician, Robert B. Brigham Hospital, Boston; Senior Associate in Medicine, Peter Bent Brigham Hospital, Boston, Massachusetts.

WILLIAM B. SCHWARTZ, M.D.

The Nephropathy of Potassium Depletion; The Nephropathy of Hypercalcemia; Renal Tubular Acidosis; The Nephropathy of Acute Hyperuricemia; Balkan Nephritis; Analgesic Nephropathy; Disorders of Fluid, Electrolyte, and Acid-Base Balance

Endicott Professor of Internal Medicine, Tufts University School of Medicine. Physician-in-Chief, Tufts–New England Medical Center Hospital, Boston, Massachusetts.

NEVIN S. SCRIMSHAW, Ph.D., M.D.

Nutrient Requirements; Assessment of Nutritional Status; Nutrition and Infection; Kwashiorkor, Marasmus, and Intermediate Forms of Protein-Calorie Malnutrition; Undernutrition, Starvation, and Hunger Edema; Deficiencies of Individual Nutrients: Vitamin Diseases

Professor of Human Nutrition and Head, Department of Nutrition and Food Science, Massachusetts Institute of Technology, Cambridge, Massachusetts.

CHARLES R. SCRIVER, M.D., C.M., F.R.S.C.

Inborn Errors of Amino Acid Metabolism

Professor of Pediatrics and Associate Professor of Biology, McGill University. Physician, Montreal Children's Hospital; Director, DeBelle Laboratory for Biochemical Genetics, McGill University–Montreal Children's Hospital Research Institute, Montreal, Quebec, Canada; Co-Director, MRC Genetics Group.

SOL SHERRY, M.D.

Thromboembolic Diseases

Professor and Chairman, Department of Medicine, Temple University School of Medicine. Physician-in-Chief, Temple University Hospital, Philadelphia, Pennsylvania.

JAMES B. SIDBURY, Jr., M.D.

Glycogen Storage Disease; Pentosuria; Fructosuria and Hereditary Fructose Intolerance

Professor of Pediatrics, Duke University School of Medicine, Durham, North Carolina.

DONALD H. SILBERBERG, M.D.

Encephalitic Complications of Viral Infections and Vaccines

Professor of Neurology, School of Medicine, University of Pennsylvania. Neurologist, Hospital of the University of Pennsylvania; Consultant in Neurology, Veterans Administration Hospital, Philadelphia, Pennsylvania.

RICHARD T. SILVER, M.D.

Leukemoid Reactions; Myeloproliferative Disorders

Professor of Clinical Medicine, Cornell University Medical College. Attending Physician, The New York Hospital, New York, New York.

MARVIN H. SLEISENGER, M.D.

Diseases of the Digestive System: Introduction; Diseases of Malabsorption; Other Inflammatory Diseases of the Intestine

Professor and Vice Chairman, Department of Medicine, University of California, San Francisco. Chief, Medical Service, Ft. Miley Veterans Administration Hospital, San Francisco, California.

JAMES P. SMITH, M.D.

Respiratory Failure and Its Management

Clinical Associate Professor of Medicine, Cornell University Medical College. Associate Attending Physician and Head, Respiratory Care Unit, The New York Hospital, New York, New York.

LLOYD H. SMITH, Jr., M.D.

Primary Hyperoxaluria; Disorders of Purine Metabolism; Disorders of Pyrimidine Metabolism

Professor and Chairman, Department of Medicine, School of Medicine, University of California, San Francisco, California.

CHARLES J. STAHL, M.D.

Drowning

Professorial Lecturer in Forensic Science, Graduate School of Arts and Sciences, The George Washington University. Captain, Medical Corps, United States Navy. Chief, Forensic Sciences Division, and Registrar, Registry of Forensic Pathology, Armed Forces Institute of Pathology, Washington, D.C.; Consultant in Forensic Pathology, Professional Division, Bureau of Medicine and Surgery, Department of the Navy, Washington, D.C.

GENE H. STOLLERMAN, M.D.

Streptococcal Diseases: Introduction; Group A Streptococcal Infection; Clinical Syndromes of Group A Streptococcal Infection; Treatment of Group A Streptococcal Infection and Chemoprophylaxis of Nonsuppurative Complications; Prophylaxis of Streptococcal Infection

Professor and Chairman, Department of Medicine, University of Tennessee College of Medicine. Physician-in-Chief, City of Memphis Hospital, Memphis, Tennessee.

MORTON N. SWARTZ, M.D.

Parameningeal Infections

Professor of Medicine, Harvard Medical School. Chief, Infectious Disease Unit, Massachusetts General Hospital, Boston, Massachusetts.

WILLIAM C. THOMAS, Jr., M.D.

Renal Calculi

Professor of Medicine, University of Florida College of Medicine. Associate Chief of Staff for Research, Veterans Administration Hospital, Gainesville, Florida.

H. RICHARD TYLER, M.D.

Polymyositis and Dermatomyositis

Associate Professor of Neurology, Harvard University. Physician and Head, Section of Neurology, Peter Bent Brigham Hospital, Boston; Consultant in Neurology, Children's Hospital Medical Center, Beth Israel, Hospital for Women, Robert B. Brigham Hospital and West Roxbury Veterans Administration Hospital, Boston, Massachusetts.

JOHN P. UTZ, M.D.

Actinomycosis; The Mycoses: Introduction; Histoplasmosis;

Blastomycosis; Paracoccidioidomycosis; Maduromycosis; Chromomycosis; Sporotrichosis

Professor of Medicine, School of Medicine, Georgetown University, Washington, D.C.

WILLIAM N. VALENTINE, M.D.

The Leukopenic State and Agranulocytosis; Infectious Mononucleosis

Professor of Medicine, University of California at Los Angeles. Senior Attending Physician, Veterans Administration Center, Los Angeles, California.

NIEL WALD, M.D.

Radiation Injury

Professor and Chairman, Department of Radiation Health, and Professor of Radiology, Graduate School of Public Health and School of Medicine, University of Pittsburgh. Active Medical Staff (Radiology) and Director, Radiation Medicine Department, Presbyterian-University Hospital, Pittsburgh; Consultant Staff, Children's Hospital of Pittsburgh, Pittsburgh, and Aliquippa Hospital, Aliquippa, Pennsylvania.

JOHN H. WALSH, M.D.

Peptic Ulcer: Clinical and Endocrine Aspects

Associate Professor of Medicine, University of California, Los Angeles, California.

KENNETH S. WARREN, M.D.

Schistosomiasis

Associate Professor of Medicine, Case Western Reserve University School of Medicine. Assistant Physician, University Hospitals, Cleveland, Ohio.

M. F. R. WATERS, M.A., M.B., M.R.C.Path., F.R.C.P.

Leprosy

Member of the Senior Scientific Staff, British Medical Research Council. Director, Leprosy Research Unit, National Leprosy Control Centre, Sungei Buloh, Selangor, Malaysia.

LAWRENCE W. WAY, M.D.

Diseases of the Gallbladder and Bile Ducts

Associate Professor of Surgery, University of California School of Medicine, San Francisco. Chief of Surgery, Ft. Miley Veterans Administration Hospital, San Francisco, California.

PAUL WEBB, M.D.

Disorders Due to Heat and Cold

Principal Associate, Webb Associates, Yellow Springs, Ohio. Associate Professor of Preventive Medicine, The Ohio State University.

ROBERT I. WEED, M.D.

Diseases of the Spleen

Professor of Medicine and of Radiation Biology and Biophysics, University of Rochester School of Medicine and Dentistry. Staff, Strong Memorial Hospital, Rochester, New York.

CLAYTON E. WHEELER, Jr., M.D.

Orf; Molluscum Contagiosum; Certain Cutaneous Diseases with Significant Systemic Manifestations: Introduction;

Cutaneous Manifestations of Internal Malignancy; Erythemas; Contact Dermatitis; Behçet's Disease; Pemphigus; Acanthosis Nigricans; Mast Cell Disease; Lethal Cutaneous and Gastrointestinal Arteriolar Thrombosis; Angiokeratoma Corporis Diffusum; Incontinentia Pigmenti; Hereditary Anhidrotic Ectodermal Defect; Neurofibromatosis of von Recklinghausen; Ainhum; Toxic Epidermal Necrolysis; Ehlers-Danlos Syndrome; Pseudoxanthoma Elasticum

Professor of Dermatology, University of North Carolina School of Medicine. Chairman, Department of Dermatology, North Carolina Memorial Hospital, Chapel Hill, North Carolina.

M. HENRY WILLIAMS, Jr., M.D.

Respiratory Disease: Introduction; Pulmonary Structure and Function: Introduction; Ventilatory Function; Conducting Airways; Alveolar Structure and Function; Pulmonary Circulation; Disability Evaluation; Hypoxemia

Professor of Medicine, Albert Einstein College of Medicine. Director, Chest Service, Bronx Municipal Hospital Center, Bronx, New York.

EMANUEL WOLINSKY, M.D.

Clostridial Diseases: Introduction; Clostridial Myonecrosis; Other Clostridial Diseases; Clostridial Gastroenteritis

Professor of Medicine, Case Western Reserve University School of Medicine. Chief, Division of Infectious Diseases, and Director of Microbiology, Cleveland Metropolitan General Hospital, Cleveland, Ohio.

THEODORE E. WOODWARD, M.D.

Tularemia

Professor of Medicine, University of Maryland School of

Medicine. Physician-in-Chief, University of Maryland Hospital, Baltimore, Maryland.

OLIVER M. WRONG, D.M., F.R.C.P.

Glomerular Disease

Professor of Medicine, University College Hospital Medical School, London. Consultant Physician, University College Hospital, London, England.

JAMES B. WYNGAARDEN, M.D.

The Use and Interpretation of Laboratory-Derived Data

Professor and Chairman, Department of Medicine, Duke University Medical School, Durham, North Carolina.

MELVIN D. YAHR, M.D.

The Extrapyramidal Disorders: Introduction; The Parkinsonian Syndrome; Essential Tremor; Senile Tremor; The Choreas; Tics; Athetosis; Dystonia Musculorum Deformans; Spasmodic Torticollis; Hemiballism

Henry P. and Georgette Goldschmidt Professor of Neurology and Chairman, Department of Neurology, Mt. Sinai Hospital. Neurologist-in-Chief, Department of Neurology, Mt. Sinai Medical Center, New York, New York.

LAWRENCE E. YOUNG, M.D.

Hemolytic Disorders: Introduction; Intracorpuscular Abnormalities

Alumni Distinguished Service Professor of Medicine, University of Rochester School of Medicine and Dentistry. Director, University of Rochester Associated Hospitals Program in Internal Medicine, Rochester, New York.

Contents

PART VII. GRANULOMATOUS DISEASES OF UNPROVED ETIOLOGY

PART VIII. MICROBIAL DISEASES

SECTION ONE.   VIRAL DISEASES, 182

Viral (and Filter-Passing Microbial) Infections of the Respiratory Tract, 184

PART X. DISORDERS OF THE NERVOUS SYSTEM AND BEHAVIOR

PART XI.   RESPIRATORY DISEASE

SECTION ONE.   STRUCTURE AND FUNCTION, 808

SECTION TWO.   THE DIAPHRAGM, *J. B. L. Howell*, 816

SECTION THREE.   THE CHEST WALL, *J. B. L. Howell*, 817

SECTION FOUR.   AIRWAY OBSTRUCTION, 821

Generalized Airway Obstruction: Chronic Obstructive Lung Disease, 821

VOLUME II

PART XII.   CARDIOVASCULAR DISEASES

PART XIII.   RENAL DISEASES

PART XIV. DISEASES OF THE DIGESTIVE SYSTEM

PART XV.   DISEASES OF NUTRITION

PART XVI.   HEMATOLOGIC AND HEMATOPOIETIC DISEASES

SECTION ONE.   THE ANEMIAS, 1399

SECTION TWO.   HEMOLYTIC DISORDERS, 1434

PART XVIII. DISEASES OF THE ENDOCRINE SYSTEM

PART XIX. DISEASES OF BONE

PART XX. CERTAIN CUTANEOUS DISEASES WITH SIGNIFICANT SYSTEMIC MANIFESTATIONS

PART XXI. MISCELLANEOUS HEREDITARY DISORDERS AFFECTING MULTIPLE ORGAN SYSTEMS

PART XXII. NORMAL LABORATORY VALUES OF CLINICAL IMPORTANCE

SUMMARY OF CONTENTS

Part I
THE NATURE OF MEDICINE

1. ON BECOMING A CLINICIAN

Paul B. Beeson

This essay is addressed to the student entering upon the study of clinical medicine. To leaf through a modern medical textbook for the first time must be a daunting experience for you. How can anyone hope to master so much scientific and technical information? The task *is* difficult, indeed impossible. Nevertheless, some encouragement should come from observing that senior medical students and young doctors on the hospital staff appear to have made a satisfactory adjustment to the challenge. Furthermore, as your acquaintance with clinical teachers grows, you will observe that although each of them has special knowledge and experience in some area of clinical medicine, he makes no pretense of knowing it all. You will also find that clinicians frequently disagree, and that each of them comes to wrong conclusions from time to time. Clinical teachers must in fact appear to be very different from those under whom your preclinical work was done. Biochemists and pharmacologists have "hard" facts to propound. We, on the other hand, deal with such commodities as pain and nausea. We must accept any kind of problem. We cannot insist on working with inbred strains of people, we cannot control the environment from which they come, we know that their recollection of past events is faulty, and we cannot reduce them to subcellular fractions in order to determine what is going on. We must even question the opinions of our colleagues. We live, therefore, in an atmosphere of doubt and uncertainty, and make our decisions and take our actions on the basis of probabilities. You will have the same handicaps, and you too will make mistakes. Simply try to ensure that each mistake constitutes a learning experience which leaves you a better doctor.

A word of encouragement can be inserted here. Students as a rule accommodate to clinical medicine with astonishing speed. I never cease to be surprised at the progress they make during the first few years. They learn by their own study and practice, by attending lectures and conferences, by observing senior people at work, and by informal discussions with fellow students and housemen in ward offices, corridors, and dining rooms. Good-natured arguments facilitate the process, because debate tends to fix the information that emerges. In that connection you will find it helpful to adopt a habit of offering your point of view tentatively rather than in the form of a positive assertion.

But how should you *begin* the study of clinical medicine? I have not found it helpful (except as an editor!) to read a book like this in systematic cover-to-cover fashion. In my judgment, you should use it the way the mature clinician does, as a place in which information can be obtained about problems being dealt with at the time. Inasmuch as common disorders occur commonly, this practice will in good time ensure that you will have read and thought about such frequently encountered disorders as peptic ulcer, angina pectoris, and urinary tract infection. Furthermore, although at first glance a medical text seems to be a sort of dictionary describing hundreds of unrelated entities, you will find that knowledge of one helps the study of another, because there often are dovetailing aspects or useful contrasts. You should make it a rule to examine the references which accompany the discussions, and to consult some of them. That is the kind of study doctors must carry on for themselves throughout life. Reading in connection with specific clinical problems is likely to provide knowledge that sticks.

What about the many uncommon maladies described in textbooks? The student of any age really needs only to know how to find out about them. One test of a good doctor is whether he can come to a correct diagnosis even though he has never met the disease before.

Medical knowledge and practice are continually changing. In order to incorporate the steady flow of new information, a textbook must be extensively rewritten every few years. Let me illustrate this by citing an example of changes that have taken place during my own clinical career. The third edition of this book, which appeared in 1933, the year I graduated from medical school, contained a chapter on nephritis by H. A. Christian, Professor of Medicine at Harvard and Physician-in-Chief to the Peter Bent Brigham Hospital. Christian had been a leader in American medicine since early in the century and had made important contributions to a wide range of subjects. His name is still attached to the Hand-Schüller-Christian and Weber-Christian syndromes. His chapter on nephritis employed this classification:

1. Acute and subacute nephritis
    (a) With renal edema (nephrosis syndrome)
    (b) Hemorrhagic nephritis
2. Chronic nephritis
    (a) With renal edema
    (b) Without renal edema
3. Essential hypertension progressing into chronic nephritis
4. Renal arteriosclerosis progressing into chronic nephritis

His approach to renal disease was based on history, physical examination, blood pressure, urinalysis, and observation of the clinical course. Most of today's "routine" biochemical determinations were not available to him, though he knew of course that elevated blood urea and acidosis are characteristic of renal failure. His treatment of all forms of nephritis was mainly rest and diet. Now compare that perspective of kidney disease with the discussions in the current edition, in chapters on Investigation of Renal Function, Glomerular Disease, Acute Tubular Necrosis, Nephrotic Syndrome, Arterial Hypertension, Chronic Pyelonephritis, Renal Disease in Pregnancy, the Nephropathy of Potassium Depletion, Hypercalcemia and Hyperuricemia, and Disorders of Fluid and Electrolyte Balance. You will note that the trend in terminology has shifted from purely descriptive to pathogenetic. Our current concepts and management have resulted from intensive study of renal diseases by clinicians who have specialized in the field and have been able to apply new biochemical, physiologic, and immunologic approaches, using sophisticated clinical chemistry, renal biopsy, electron microscopy, immunofluorescence, and similar procedures. Today's management makes use of a variety of effective pharmacologic preparations: diuretics, antimicrobials, corticosteroids, antihypertensives, and cytotoxic agents. Our understanding of fluid and electrolyte dynamics is based upon ready availability of good clinical biochemical methods. Our ultimate forms of treatment—hemodialysis and renal transplantation—involve scientific and technical developments scarcely imaginable in Christian's day.

The example cited is in no way unusual. Similar advances characterize every branch of general medicine. This kind of progress has been achieved largely by full-time clinical scientists working in medical schools and research institutes all over the world. They have concentrated on specific problems and have been greatly aided by new knowledge and techniques developed by other workers in biologic and physical sciences. Such investigation-in-depth is essential to the advancement of clinical medicine. We have for all time departed from the era of clinical "giants" like Christian who could be looked upon as authorities in many aspects of internal medicine. That is why a modern textbook must be compiled from the writings of scores of contributors.

The medical student should be aware that our exciting advances in medicine have *created* some serious new problems. Our therapy now makes use of powerful drugs, all of which can do harm. Few hospital patients receive less than half a dozen different medications. In addition to intrinsic toxicity these can interact with each other to produce unwanted effects. A substantial part of hospital medicine today is in fact devoted to overcoming untoward effects of therapy. Knowing when to stop a certain treatment is as important as knowing when to bring it into use. There are risks too in many of our present diagnostic procedures, e.g., a 1 per cent incidence of death or serious complication from coronary or cerebral angiography. We must acknowledge that the recent scientific and technologic explosion in clinical medicine has created its own kind of "pollution."

Having recognized the essential role of the specialist investigator in bringing about what are really immense advances in clinical medicine, we should give some consideration to the impact of this on trends in the practice of medicine as well as the training of future doctors. Does it follow, because we owe our advances in medical sciences to specialists, that the best medical care must be given by specialists? Shall we say to young people now entering the profession that the age of specialization is here, and advise each of them to select a narrow field for his or her medical practice?

I believe that in the actual provision of medical care there is still need for the generalist. Diseases do not always present themselves in pure culture, and in fact the perspective of the clinical scientist can sometimes be skewed. It seems fair to say, for example, that a good family doctor (now, alas, in short supply in America) can deal effectively with the great majority of episodes for which patients seek a doctor's help. When we focus on internal medicine, the field with which this book is concerned, it can be said with assurance that the well-trained internist, e.g., one who has been certified by the American Board of Internal Medicine or has attained Membership of the Royal College of Physicians, is capable of dealing with most medical illnesses, including those for which hospital care is required. To do that in exemplary fashion is, however, a full-time job, which does not permit substantial parts of the doctor's time and effort to be devoted to research. Inasmuch as a major re-

sponsibility of a university is acquisition of new knowledge, the funds available for salaries in medical school departments go mainly to doctors who are active investigators. Consequently, the medical student and the house officer in a teaching hospital may need to be reminded that outside the medical school orbit much excellent medical care is provided by generalist physicians. In the setting of a teaching hospital the clinical investigator can be a superb teacher of undergraduate and graduate medical students, and can, by combining forces with many other specialists in the institution, provide sophisticated medical service for the patients. This, however, is an expensive and somewhat inefficient way of offering medical care which, though well suited to the diverse functions of a teaching institution, does not make a realistic pattern for professional care in the larger community. Specialized skill, although essential to any good system of medical care, is not needed in the proportion found among the members of medical school faculties.

Can we have it both ways, even in our teaching centers? I think this is possible and desirable. Pressure from within and without will probably dictate some revising of present medical school priorities, though the schools must always support a high proportion of specialist investigators. But even today one finds occasional excellent generalists in medical schools, people who like the environment but do not wish to engage personally in research. They are likely to be the doctors who take care of their colleagues and their colleagues' families. They find satisfaction in dealing with a broad range of clinical problems and are willing to devote all their energies to clinical practice. They are confident of their ability to deal with most of the problems that come to them, yet have no hesitation about calling for specialist advice when they need it. They exercise some discrimination in their diagnostic approach and know when to cut corners.

One of the most important qualities needed by today's physician is ability to restrain his curiosity. He must constantly remind himself that a potentially injurious diagnostic procedure should only be carried out when possible benefit to the patient justifies the risk. A diagnostic test should never be done just for the sake of "thoroughness," that is to say, before someone else suggests that it be done, or because a specialist feels he must do it to protect his own reputation, "just in case. . . ."

Let us speculate on how a good doctor would go about the care of an elderly patient who has recently developed obstructive jaundice. The *probability* is that this patient has neoplastic disease not amenable to surgery or chemotherapy. There is, however, the possibility that the biliary obstruction is caused by some other lesion such as stone or nonmalignant tumor. The doctor has many options. He can make use of a variety of remarkably accurate diagnostic procedures: barium x-ray studies, isotopic scan of the liver or pancreas, laparoscopy, needle biopsy of the liver, celiac angiography, or endoscopic probing of the duodenum (for cytology, or for cannulation and retrograde visualization of the biliary or pancreatic ducts). It is tempting to proceed with some or all of these procedures, because a precise diagnosis may well be achieved. But that may not be in the patient's interest in view of high probability of incurable disease. The doctor in charge can discuss with colleagues the chances of curative surgery or chemotherapy. Or he can do nothing further, feeling that the sensible option is to allow the disease to run its course, and spare the patient the discomfort, dangers, and expense of elaborate study. He may, however, choose a compromise: calling on a surgeon to operate without further delay, while the patient's general condition is still good, in order to treat definitively a nonmalignant lesion if there be one; or, if the obstruction is due to cancer, to divert the flow of bile into the intestine. This course would be likely at least to give the patient some months of comfortable life, even though the cancer is not treated. The good doctor will then "stay with" the patient, meeting problems as they come, as described so well by Dr. Myers in Ch. 3.

I close by offering a few precepts: (1) Each patient must be given *enough of your time.* Sit down; listen to him; ask thoughtful questions; examine him carefully; go back and do it again. So many medical mistakes are simply due to failure of the doctor to give enough time. (2) Work to develop your *ability to study* about your patient's clinical problems. (3) Train yourself to *concentrate on each problem to the exclusion of all else.* Here is the way Trotter, a great English neurosurgeon, put it:

... As long as medicine is an art, its chief and characteristic instrument must be human faculty. We come therefore to the very practical question of what aspects of human faculty it is necessary for the good doctor to cultivate. ... The first to be named must always be the power of attention, of giving one's whole mind to the patient without the interposition of oneself. It sounds simple but only the very greatest doctors ever fully attain it. It is an active process and not either mere resigned listening or even politely waiting until you can interrupt. Disease often tells its secrets in a casual parenthesis. ...

If you will give each patient the time he deserves, if you will learn to concentrate, and if you can then study appropriately, you will have much of what it takes to care for people, even in today's world.

2. SCIENCE, CLINICAL MEDICINE, AND THE SPECTRUM OF DISEASE

Alvan R. Feinstein

A textbook of medicine contains concepts and data for at least two distinctly different types of clinical decisions. With *explicatory** decisions, doctors choose names, causes, and mechanisms that provide intellectual explanations for the ailments observed in patients. With *interventional* decisions, doctors choose therapeutic strategies intended to prevent or to remedy the ailments.

The explicatory decisions are often regarded as the main scientific activity of clinical medicine. For diagnostic selections, modern technology has allowed diseases to be identified more precisely than ever before. The morphologic abnormalities that formerly could be demonstrated only at necropsy are now often revealed during life with the aid of roentgenography, biopsy, cytology, or surgical exploration; and many other ailments that cannot be depicted morphologically are identified with the aid of chemical, microbial, electrophysiologic, or other laboratory procedures. For ideas about causes and mechanisms of disease, doctors have received scientific confirmation both from the diagnostic tests performed in individual patients and from the many experimental models

*The word *explicatory* is used here to refer to diagnostic citations or pathogenetic explanations or both.

that have been tested during clinical investigation. The explicatory decisions thus enable doctors to apply at the bedside the major advances that laboratory research has brought to diagnostic medical science.

A doctor's interventional decisions, on the other hand, are often regarded mainly as art. The pharmaceutical, surgical, and other agents used for therapeutic intervention are highly developed scientifically, but the decisions themselves are still often made as acts of judgment, generally unsupported by the type of scientific evidence that sustains the explicatory activities. The available evidence to prove the value of a treatment may be quantitatively defective, consisting mainly of anecdotal reports of clinical experiences that have not been thoroughly enumerated; or the evidence may seem qualitatively unappealing, depending on such "soft" data as a patient's pain, a family's anxiety, or an employer's forbearance.

With medical activities demarcated into explicatory science and interventional art, a medical student (or a practicing clinician) often develops the belief that the purely clinical work of patient care does not present any scientific challenges. According to this belief, a clinician's principal science is contained in the "workup" that reveals diagnostic names and pathogenetic mechanisms. Once this challenge is completed, no further scientific thinking may seem necessary. After choosing a therapeutic agent according to the established diagnosis, the clinician would need only the arts of human perception and communication for telling the patient what is wrong and what is planned.

Despite popular acceptance, this demarcation of art and science in clinical work has at least three major inaccuracies. The demarcation is based on the idea that science consists only of explication, but science contains another major component: prediction. In dealing with a sick patient, a clinician is scientifically challenged not merely to explain what is wrong and how it went wrong, but also to predict what may happen and how its occurrence can be altered. To perform these predictions, a clinician must make the type of interventional decisions with which prognosis is estimated, therapy chosen, and results evaluated. A second conceptual error arises from the belief that the choice of treatment depends almost entirely on a diagnostic citation. Although diagnosis is usually an important first step, the scientific selection and appraisal of therapy require analysis of data much more intricate than the mere identification of a disease. The most cogent information often includes symptoms, signs, and other clinical phenomena rather than a diagnostic title alone. A third misconception is the idea that important clinical phenomena cannot be expressed in "hard" scientific terms because the descriptions usually contain verbal categories rather than measured dimensions. The fallacy here is that "hard" information must be precise and reproducible, but it need not be dimensional. Some of the outstanding accomplishments of biologic science—including the work of Darwin, Virchow, and modern geneticists and electron microscopists—have been based on precise, reproducible, but nondimensional descriptions. With better standards of observation and classification, the verbal categories of "soft" clinical data could readily be improved into "hard" scientific quality.

Even when these attributes of clinical work are recognized, they may be regarded as scientifically unimportant because ordinary medical practice does not provide the experimental challenges offered by laboratory research. This belief is also inappropriate, however, because every act of clinical therapy is constructed in the same architectural sequence used for an experiment: a prepared entity is exposed to a planned maneuver and undergoes an observed response. This basic construction of an experiment can be used to outline all of a doctor's interventional decisions in clinical practice.

Despite similar challenges in the applicability of scientific methods, the "experiments" of the laboratory and bedside contain major differences in goals, reasoning, and procedures. In motive, the laboratory investigator seeks to understand how nature works and what it does; the clinician wants to change what nature has done or to thwart what it might do. In hypothesis, the laboratory investigator is innovative, wanting to test a new idea; the clinician is repetitive, wanting to reproduce the successful result achieved with the therapy used in a similar situation of the past. In cause-effect comparisons, the laboratory investigator can contrast the results of a concurrent "control group"; the clinician often relies on the "historical controls" of previous experience. In choice of data, the laboratory investigator can confine his observations only to the immediate events that seem most pertinent; the clinician must note all phenomena that can indicate a change in the patient's medical condition and way of life. These major differences in orientation require different strategies for the scientific methods used in the experiments of laboratory explication or clinical intervention, but both sets of activities offer the intellectual challenges of planning and evaluating an experiment.

In contemporary medicine, however, the methods used for acquiring and analyzing clinical data are not yet as scientifically well developed as the techniques that have been employed in laboratory research. Consequently, a doctor's explicatory decisions are often supported by excellent scientific evidence, but the interventional decisions are not. The purely clinical activities of contemporary medicine may thus seem more like art than science. The scientific improvement of this clinical art offers a prime target for future research, but in the meantime the reader of any compendium of clinical knowledge must deal with the state of the art in its existing form. The rest of this chapter will be concerned with certain caveats to help warn about some of the imperfections, and with a few suggestions to help resolve some of the difficulties.

One of the principal problems arises from the complex clinical spectrum associated with a disease. With increasing frequency in modern medicine, diseases are diagnostically identified as abnormalities not in a patient's clinical state (such as fever, jaundice, or chest pain), but in a paraclinical entity. The paraclinical abnormalities of disease can be diagnostically cited in such terms as morphologic structure *(coronary artery disease, carcinoma),* biochemical function *(diabetes mellitus, hyperthyroidism),* physiologic function *(atrial fibrillation, malabsorption)* or microbial invasion *(viral infection, meningococcemia).* Although the aid of modern diagnostic technology allows these paraclinical abnormalities to be diagnosed with unprecedented specificity and consistency, the principal "lesion" of each such paraclinical disease has an associated spectrum of diverse clinical manifestations that may not always occur specifically or consistently.

Some of the clinical manifestations represent the primary effects of the disease's principal abnormality, whereas other manifestations can be regarded as secondary effects or complications. In coronary artery disease, for example, angina pectoris is a primary effect and congestive heart failure is secondary. In peptic ulcer, pain is a primary effect and pyloric obstruction is secondary. Since different primary and secondary manifestations can appear alone or in various overlapping combinations, the disease in a particular patient may occur with some, all, or none of the possible clinical manifestations. An illustration of the diverse clinical spectrum that can be associated with a single disease is shown in the Venn diagram for lung cancer in Ch. 540. Certain patients with lung cancer may be wholly asymptomatic; others can have primary features, such as hemoptysis; others can have the secondary features of systemic or metastatic manifestations; and yet others may have various combinations of these primary and secondary elements. The complexity of a disease's spectrum will thus produce subsets of patients who have the same diagnosis but different clinical manifestations, and who may also differ in prognosis and therapy.

The existence of these different subsets creates important defects in any "textbook picture of disease." Since the author can seldom describe all the diverse possibilities, the "classic" textbook description is usually based on the most common or pathognomonic manifestations. The reader who expects that the disease will always occur in this classic manner may then be surprised, perplexed, or dismayed by the many occasions in which a patient appears from a less common subset. A quantitative example of subset distributions is shown in the disease spectrum shown in Ch. 540. The most common single subset in the 1032 instances of lung cancer consisted of 340 patients with the concurrence of pulmonic and systemic manifestations; but 70 patients were wholly asymptomatic, and 34 had metastatic features only. Similarly, coronary artery disease can occur without angina pectoris in certain patients who have no symptoms or in others with manifestations only of congestive heart failure; hepatitis may first be found as advanced cirrhosis in a patient who never had jaundice.

The occurrence of an asymptomatic subset in a disease's spectrum is responsible for the frequent practice of "screening" in modern medicine. The purpose of the screening tests is to find the disease in circumstances in which it has produced no overt manifestations to arouse diagnostic suspicion. The occurrence of the many diverse subsets in a disease's spectrum is also responsible for some of the major current difficulties in evaluating prognosis and therapy. Despite similarity in diagnosis, the patients in the different subsets may have striking differences in prognosis. For example, Table 1 in Ch. 540 shows that the six-month survival rate for patients with lung cancer was 44 per cent, but the rate ranged from 84 per cent in the localized asymptomatic subset to 14 per cent in the worst of the metastatic subsets. In acute myocardial infarction, a patient with only chest pain has a much better prognosis than a patient with shock and pulmonary edema.

These natural prognostic distinctions will substantially affect the selection and appraisal of therapy. Since the "experiments" of routine clinical treatment are based on a repetitive hypothesis, a doctor chooses treatment for an individual patient by reviewing previous clinical experience, recalling the patients with similar manifestations, noting the outcomes of the therapy given to the "resemblance group," ascertaining which treatment gave the best result, and trying to reproduce that success in the current patient. To select the appropriate resemblance group, the doctor must have data for suitably demarcated subsets of patients.

Such data may not always be available. The results of previous treatment are often reported for all patients with the same disease, regardless of subsets; or the subsets distinguished in the reported results may be different from the particular one in which a subsequent patient is encountered. The absence of these details often creates difficulty in choice of treatment for an individual patient and arouses controversy in comparative evaluations of treated groups. One physician, treating diabetes mellitus with Regimen X, may have had a group of patients whose prognostic expectations were substantially different from those of another physician's patients treated with Regimen Y. One surgeon's Stage I cancer patients may be predominantly asymptomatic, whereas another surgeon's Stage I patients may have a high proportion of weight loss and fatigue. During arguments about the merits of the compared therapy, the clinicians may not realize that some of the crucial post-therapeutic differences arose not from different methods of treatment, but from prognostic differences in the subsets who constituted the treated groups.

To this complexity of clinical subsets for a single disease is added the further complexity introduced by co-morbidity and demography. Since an individual patient may have more than one disease, the presence of associated ailments will create extra subsets in the spectrum of the "principal" disease, and may produce pathologic effects that alter prognosis and treatment in those subsets. The number of potential subsets for a disease becomes even larger when the cited clinical and co-morbid demarcations are augmented by such demographic features as age, race, sex, and occupation.

This enormous variability of individual patients and diseases would pose insurmountable problems in clinical decisions if each decision depended on determining a unique subset for that patient and on having adequate background information for previous experience with that subset. Fortunately, many small subsets can be combined into larger "determinant" groups for which therapeutic decisions can be based on satisfactory amounts of previous data or experience. For example, a patient with acute rheumatic fever is usually treated with salicylate if there is no clinical evidence of carditis, and with steroids if severe carditis is present. In this decision, the *no carditis* and *severe carditis* groups act as therapeutically determinant subsets, regardless of the many smaller subgroups into which the patients could be classified by virtue of demography or other clinical phenomena. The selection of therapeutically determinant "super" subsets has traditionally been a fundamental decision in clinical judgment. With the availability of electronic data processing and computers to help in the analysis of previous experience, future judgments can be supported with an improved quantification in both subsets and data.

A different type of therapeutic intervention is aimed not at a disease or a determinant subset, but at a specific clinical manifestation, such as pain, constipation, or insomnia. Thus a patient may receive an antimicrobial drug for the disease pneumococcal pneumonia, but codeine for the associated symptom of pleuritic pain; radiation or chemotherapy may be given for Hodgkin's disease and blood transfusions for the associated weakness and anemia. For patients with acute myocardial infarction, the only treatment directed at the disease itself is bed rest. All other treatments are chosen according to the associated clinical manifestations: e.g., narcotics or analgesics for pain, diuretics or digitalis for congestive heart failure, and appropriate agents for arrhythmia.

For the many minor ailments encountered in primary medical care or family practice, a specific disease may not be diagnosed and treatment may be intended only to relieve symptoms. Encountering such ailments as an upper respiratory infection, a sprained muscle, or a gastrointestinal upset, the practitioner may decide prognostically that the ailment is self-limited and does not require more extensive diagnostic or therapeutic efforts. Another common event in general medical practice is a temporary, acute exacerbation of a chronic major ailment that has been relatively stable. In these events, which may occur in such conditions as chronic alcoholism, irritable colon syndrome, or neurotic anxiety, patients are also often treated for symptoms only.

In all the circumstances just described, the clinician's scientific challenges in interventional decisions were to determine the target(s) to be treated and to choose the best mode(s) of therapy. A different set of challenges consists of evaluating the patient's condition afterward to decide what the treatment accomplished and whether it has been successful. For this purpose, the clinician again often uses individual manifestations, rather than a disease diagnosis, as an index of accomplishment. Furthermore, the evaluation of a particular response may depend on graded subsets composed of changes in clinical manifestations. Thus the effect of treatment on congestive heart failure may be called *excellent* if both dyspnea and edema disappear; *fair* if one disappears while the other remains; and *poor* if both remain.

The data used to identify transitions in clinical state often require additional details that may not have been necessary for decisions about diagnosis, prognosis, and therapy. For example, a description of substernal chest pain provoked by exertion and relieved by rest will often suffice for a clinical diagnosis of coronary artery disease, but the evaluation of response of the angina to treatment will usually depend on further information about its frequency and the associated amounts of exertion or rest. Similarly, the amount of jaundice may not be crucial for a diagnosis of hepatitis, but may be a valuable index of therapeutic response. Other examples of clinical details that are sometimes diagnostically unimportant but therapeutically valuable are the patient's weight (in treatment of edematous congestive heart failure), the size of a massive spleen (in treatment of chronic monocytic leukemia), the frequency of bowel movements (in treatment of various gastrointestinal disorders), and the frequency of urination (in treatment of cystitis or prostatitis).

The challenges of directly communicating with patients are often regarded as a nonscientific form of clinical art, mainly because the contents of the communications, which are much more complex than any of the complexities already cited, create diverse data and subsets that are even more difficult to specify. Nevertheless, many of the decisions made during these communications require the intellectual discipline used by a scientist to select suitable information, organize data, recapitulate previous experience, and evaluate responses. The discipline of scientific reasoning may not contribute to a clinician's creative insight and artful perception in dealing with the personal attributes of people, but without such reasoning the insight and perception will often be used ineffectually.

Whether a practicing doctor is involved in decisions of communication, explication, or intervention, clinical medicine will always contain and unite elements of both art and science. The complexity of people and human ailments will demand many artful judgments that cannot be expressed in scientific terms, but a scientific discipline is required for the optimal use of modern technology in identifying, explaining, preventing, or treating the ailments. To be properly adapted to its human recipients, this scientific discipline must contain suitable provision for the important personal and clinical information that is not perceived with "scientific" equipment or expressed in "scientific" dimensions. The art and science of clinical medicine are intermingled, symbiotic, and inseparable. Without the art, there can be no data for the science. Without the science, there can be no reason for the art.

3. THE CARE OF THE PATIENT WITH TERMINAL ILLNESS

W. P. L. Myers

There is perhaps no more controversial medical issue of our time than that dealing with the care of the patient with terminal illness. Endless articles in the lay press dealing with death and dying, death with dignity, a patient's right to die, euthanasia, and so forth are testimony to the enormous interest and concern of the public and to the confusion that abounds. It is not the intent of this chapter to sort out these conflicting attitudes and beliefs, but rather to provide an approach to the problem for the student of medicine. Final answers cannot be written, but the reader will find an approach that is based on long personal experience with terminal illness and on the premise that it is the individual that matters. It is necessary to understand this at the outset, because an entirely different approach could be adopted if one proceeded on the premise that it is the greatest good for the greatest number of people that matters.

The Hippocratic oath demands of each of us that we practice our art for the benefit of our patients. Implicit in this charge is the preservation of life. Nowhere in the original or in its modern version does the word "prolong" appear, with respect to a patient's life. "Prolong" is a word that has come to mean the unnecessary continuation of life in a setting in which, usually in the eyes of a patient's family, recovery is impossible. It is a word most used by the laity because, in general, physicians do not view their efforts in these terms. They are more likely to take the long view and consider that their efforts should be to preserve life, since such efforts are in the main to be equated with what is beneficial for the patient. Therapeutic efforts in a seemingly hopeless situation can be viewed by the patient's family as needless efforts to prolong life, whereas the physician, from his vantage point of seeing a disease in perspective, may regard the same efforts as fully justifiable in terms of his obligation to the patient. The dilemma that arises, however, is that there are those who reasonably question preservation of life as the sole objective of treatment. The physician must always act in his patient's interests, but undoubtedly there are situations in which these are not best served by endless efforts to preserve life. Where does the physician draw the line? How is he to tell when to pursue treatment aggressively and when not to? Are there any guideposts?

MEDICAL ANALYSIS OF TERMINAL ILLNESS

It is important at the outset to define "terminal illness," because an accurate medical analysis of a given situation is the keystone for all future considerations, both medical and humanitarian. How can we tell if a patient is terminally ill? This determination may tax all the skills a physician can muster, and yet he may end up defining a patient as terminally ill who would not be so regarded by another doctor. We must begin somewhere, however, and there is no better place to begin than to be sure that the medical details have been set forth and have been analyzed in the fullest. It has been said that all problems could be solved if one only knew the right questions to ask. One approach to the matter of determining whether a patient is, in fact, terminally ill is for the physician to ask himself a few brief questions. The seven questions listed below are presented with a cancer patient in mind, but they can serve as a model for this approach to other diseases as well:

1. Has the patient had a complete history and physical examination?
2. Is there histologic evidence of cancer, and where is the primary site?
3. Is the presenting problem caused by a second primary cancer?
4. What is the extent of the disease?
5. What medical complications, both those caused by the tumor and those unrelated to the tumor, exist?
6. What was the previous treatment, and was it adequate?
7. Is the disease process active and progressive or chronic and stable?

The answers to these questions are fundamental to the proper assessment of a patient's illness, all the more so if he has been categorized as terminally ill. The questions are considered in greater detail as follows:

Question 1: Has the patient had a complete history and physical examination? It is almost embarrassing to include such a question in a list of this sort, but many patients have been improperly designated as being terminally ill because of what *appears* to be, without the benefit of a complete history and physical examination. Unfortunately the reason for this is that such patients frequently are seen initially by those who lack interest or who are guided by an attitude of hopelessness, especially when it comes to cancer. The following case will serve to emphasize the importance of a complete history and physical examination:

The patient was a 62-year-old white man from Central America who had had mild intermittent diarrhea for several years. Six months before admission he had been treated for malignant lymphoma, histiocytic type, of the stomach. He did well subsequently, but in the week prior to admission he developed anorexia followed by watery diarrhea and rectal bleeding. He had been treated with prednisone, 30 mg daily, for five days before admission. On admission he was found to be febrile and his abdomen was distended and tender, but there was no rebound tenderness. His stool was positive for blood. There was no peripheral lymphadenopathy. It was assumed that he had recurrent intra-abdominal malignant lymphoma, and when he went into shock the day after admission, he was considered to be terminally ill. He responded briefly to medical measures, but shock recurred and he died on the third day after admission. Autopsy disclosed diffuse colonic amebiasis with perforation and peritonitis. There was no evidence of recurrent malignant lymphoma.

In retrospect, further inquiry into the patient's history of intermittent diarrhea should have been made, especially in view of the fact that he came from Central America. The presence of fever, abdominal distention, and rectal bleeding, even without overt signs of perforation at the time of admission, should have led to a more careful examination, in particular a proctoscopic examination, to establish the correct diagnosis. Even so, the patient might not have recovered, but at least he would have had treatment directed against the correct disease, which in this instance was non-neoplastic.

Question 2: Is there histologic evidence of cancer, and where is the primary site? Consignment of patients to the ranks of the "terminally ill" has occurred all too often without histologic evidence of cancer and especially without attempts to define a primary site, if a histologic diagnosis of cancer has been made. The latter does not always have a therapeutic implication, but often it does, notably in those instances in which tumors originate in the breast, prostate, and thyroid. The following is a case in point:

The patient was a 50-year-old man seen in the clinic because of abdominal complaints and back pain. Evidences of tumor were noted intra-abdominally as well as in the lungs and left supraclavicular area. The impression was that he had metastatic carcinoma probably of gastrointestinal tract origin, despite negative gastrointestinal x-rays. A subsequent biopsy of the left supraclavicular lymph node was interpreted as "metastatic carcinoma." The hopeless attitude expressed by one of the patient's attending physicians was brought out by the following note he entered in the patient's record:
"This unfortunate patient has hopeless cancer as evidenced by left supraclavicular nodes. Biopsy shows metastatic adenocarcinoma. The exact site of primary is not apparent. This is now a purely academic question. He has hopeless cancer originating in the upper abdomen and is suitable only for terminal care."

Fortunately, other physicians did not share this opinion, and, in the attempt to discover a primary site, an acid phosphatase was obtained. This proved to be markedly elevated, indicating a diagnosis of metastatic carcinoma of the prostate. After orchiectomy and estrogen therapy, a chest film showed regression of mediastinal disease, and the patient remained alive with his disease in remission for many months. He finally died about three and a half years after having been regarded by one physician as being suitable only for terminal care.

Question 3: Is the presenting problem caused by a second primary cancer? It is difficult for a patient, once treated for cancer, not to have all subsequent clinical disease interpreted as manifestations of the original cancer. A patient previously treated for cancer of the pancreas may now have advanced metastatic disease and correctly be considered terminally ill. But if the metastatic disease is, in fact, caused by a second primary cancer such as carcinoma of the breast, the patient may respond dramatically to hormonal treatment and be anything but terminally ill. This possibility must always be kept in mind, particularly when there has been an appreciable time interval between the diagnosis of the original tumor and the appearance of metastatic disease.

Question 4: What is the extent of the disease? The accurate assessment of the extent of a cancer is the major determinant of treatment. In general, surgery and radiotherapy are utilized for localized and regional disease, whereas systemic treatment is applied to disseminated disease. Patients whose extent of disease is incorrectly evaluated may receive the wrong treatment or may inap-

propriately be considered to be terminally ill. Obviously, jaundice in a patient with known cancer may or may not represent metastatic disease. Only by judging each manifestation on its own merits can a correct assessment of the extent of disease be made. Again, a case report will serve to emphasize this point:

A 41-year-old man was admitted to the hospital because of suspected recurrent islet cell cancer of the pancreas. He had undergone a subtotal pancreatectomy and splenectomy elsewhere, and although the operation was thought to have been curative, the patient subsequently developed recurrent hypoglycemia. He was referred for chemotherapy. Examination revealed slight hepatomegaly but no intra-abdominal masses. Although a celiac arteriogram and a liver scan suggested that a large metastasis was present in the right lobe of the liver, it was *not assumed* that the patient had nonresectable cancer. At operation, it was established that, contrary to the preoperative laboratory data, no metastasis existed in the liver and it was possible to resect a residual tumor in the head of the pancreas by means of a Whipple procedure. The patient is alive some three years later and is without evidence of recurrent disease.

In this case, an accurate appraisal of the extent of disease, as determined at surgery, led to definitive and hopefully curative treatment. Had the extent of disease been *assumed* to be nonresectable, the patient would have been subjected to noncurative forms of treatment.

Question 5: What medical complications, both those caused by the tumor and those unrelated to the tumor, exist? This question is really a corollary to the last one but deserves special emphasis because a metabolic or infectious complication may be more life-threatening than the underlying cancer, and often if properly identified and treated, the patient may not needlessly lose his life. The following case is illustrative:

A 64-year-old woman was admitted to the hospital with a diagnosis of mammary carcinoma metastatic to the brain. Two years previously she had undergone a left radical mastectomy for infiltrating duct carcinoma of the breast. She had had positive axillary nodes and received postoperative radiation therapy. She remained well until seven weeks before admission when she developed double vision and dysphagia. On examination she had bilateral ptosis and motor weakness of cranial nerve V bilaterally without sensory impairment. Shortly after admission she underwent emergency tracheostomy for severe stridor, and radiation therapy to the brain was begun. At this point a resident physician, unwilling to assume that everything was caused by metastatic cancer, observed: "This lady really has little evidence for spread of her breast carcinoma. . . . I am hard put to assign her neurologic signs to an anatomic lesion, especially bilateral jaw weakness without any impairment of the sensory component of cranial nerve V. Right now she has marked ptosis bilaterally and paresis of gaze in all directions—without any pupillary abnormalities! The quick fatigue in the jaw muscles brings up myasthenia gravis which could explain all her signs."

A test with edrophonium chloride confirmed the resident's suspicions and a diagnosis of myasthenia gravis was made. The radiation therapy to the brain was stopped and the patient has done very well on medical management of her myasthenia and has had no demonstrable recurrence of breast cancer during these past four years.

Question 6: What was the previous treatment, and was it adequate? Corollary: Was previous treatment in any way responsible for the patient's present problems? At times "terminal" situations arise because patients have not received adequate treatment. No patient should be so regarded without a careful review of the type and adequacy of prior treatment, including treatment of coexistent diseases unrelated to the primary one. Of course previous treatment may also cause problems which can be misinterpreted as manifestations of the underlying malignancy. For example, a rare but remarkable complication of radiotherapy, that of radiation nephritis, is illustrated by the following case:

The patient, a 63-year-old man, was admitted to the hospital for what ultimately proved to be a spindle and giant cell sarcoma of the duodenum which was treated by radiotherapy to the upper abdomen. Two months later, the patient was re-explored and radon seeds were inserted throughout the residual tumor mass. Six months later and during the ensuing 18 months the patient's course was marked by the gradual appearance of recurrent fluid accumulation (peripheral, peritoneal, pleural), hypertension, anemia, thrombopenia, albuminuria, and azotemia. He eventually succumbed to renal failure some 26 months after the initial radiotherapy had been given.

From a clinical viewpoint, the patient had been regarded as having had recurrent intra-abdominal cancer on the basis of a cytologic examination of the peritoneal fluid which was reported to have revealed malignant cells. However, at autopsy none of the organs or tissues showed evidence of residual tumor or metastases. The kidneys presented the classic picture of radiation nephritis, and in retrospect it was apparent that this lesion was responsible for the clinical findings. Had it been recognized that the patient did not have recurrent cancer but rather the renal complications of radiation therapy, it is possible that more aggressive measures directed at his renal failure might have altered the outcome.

Question 7: Is the disease process active and progressive or chronic and stable? There are many so-called terminal diseases, metastatic cancer among them, that pursue a chronic course. A patient may have metastases from a cancer for which we have no specific therapy and he may therefore be "written off" as terminally ill. However, the natural history of the cancer in that patient may not be progressive, and the physician should take this into account when forming his own appraisal of a patient with an incurable illness. In addition, rare but clearly documented, inexplicable remissions of advanced cancer have occurred, and these serve to remind us of the incompleteness of our knowledge and the fallibility of our judgments.

THE TRULY "TERMINAL" PATIENT

If the physician has asked the aforementioned questions and has satisfied himself that, in fact, his patient is nearing death from an illness which is progressive, unrelenting, and disseminated and which cannot be arrested or reversed in our present state of knowledge (or perhaps more accurately, ignorance), how then should he manage the problem? Here again, he should have an approach or way of thinking about the over-all problem and should use the technique of asking himself some further critical questions. The principal questions are these:

1. What does the patient know about his situation?
2. What is the patient's attitude regarding the prospect of death?
3. Does he have pain and, if so, is it being relieved?
4. Is the patient being comforted physically, mentally, and spiritually?
5. Is the physician prepared to give of himself to the patient and "go down to the wire" with him? As a corollary, is the physician willing to continue to think about the problems his patient presents until the end?
6. What is the attitude of the patient's family, and how is it being dealt with?
7. Is the patient undergoing experimental study, and, if so, are humanitarian principles being observed or compromised?

There may be other questions one could ask, but these will serve most situations, and they should be considered in some depth.

Question 1: What does the patient know about his situation? Too often the physician fails to ask this question and, if he does, he does not record it on the patient's chart, so there is no general knowledge of this among the various personnel caring for the patient. This, in turn, leads to a lack of coordination in treatment efforts. The care of a patient can be improved substantially if his understanding of his illness is brought to light and recorded in a manner that will permit all medical and nursing personnel involved to know and act accordingly.

By asking a patient what he understands about his illness, the physician provides an opportunity for the patient to tell the physician, directly or indirectly, how much he wants to know. Some patients are quite content to leave it all to the doctor, but usually, if given the opportunity, they will ask questions. There is no standard answer to a patient's question, but the physician should be truthful insofar as his answer goes. *Truth can always be supported by hope;* an outlook with a grave prognosis can be coupled, in a compassionate manner, with a positive statement regarding what the physician plans to do and how other patients have responded under similar circumstances. Although this approach is not uniformly followed by the medical profession, it is increasingly so, because doctors have come to know that the erosion of trust between themselves and their patients, created by a failure to tell a patient as much truth as the doctor believes the patient seeks to know, is a more severe blow to the patient than dealing with the truth. There is no need, however, to tell the patient all the details, particularly in view of the fact that our fallibility could lead us to tell a patient more than we know. In addition, by seeking to know what the patient understands, the physician can correct misconceptions which are often the basis of fear and anxiety. Relief of these major burdens of a terminally ill patient should be of primary concern to the physician.

Attempts by a patient's family to persuade the physician to go along with an outright lie regarding the patient's illness should never be acceded to. Good intentions were never more misplaced; the lie creates further problems and is an insult to the patient. In addition, seriously ill patients usually know they are seriously ill, and explanations that do not seem likely create fear that the patient's doctor does not know the real diagnosis. This torment can be worse than the knowledge of the primary illness.

Question 2: What is the patient's attitude regarding the prospect of death? Attitudes toward death and dying are being more openly discussed and analyzed than ever before. The patient stricken with a fatal illness has been noted as going through various stages which have been categorized, progressively, as denial, anger, bargaining, depression, and, ultimately, acceptance (Kübler-Ross). This dissection is useful because it can form a basis for a physician's approach to his patient. For example, understanding that a patient's anger (which may be directed at the physician) is part of the unfolding reaction to his illness permits the physician to deal with this in a helpful rather than defensive manner. Learning about a patient's attitude takes time which a physician may be unwilling or unable to spend. In addition, a physician may be at a loss as to how to broach the subject, although usually this only requires that one give a patient the realization that he will be listened to. This obviously entails choosing a proper time, such as returning to see the patient after regular rounds. The press of time may not always permit this, and under these and other circumstances, the physician would do well to enlist the help of a clergyman or rabbi, preferably the patient's, or if he doesn't have one, the hospital chaplain or rabbi.

There are times when a patient will feel freer to discuss his or her attitude about death with the spiritual adviser than with the physician, and the adviser can be of enormous help in these situations. The fear of death is a human emotion widely considered in any discussion of death and dying, but the fear of *not* dying has received little attention. Patients may seek assurances from a clergyman that death is imminent, believing that the physician will not provide such assurances because doing so would be a denial of his role in preserving life.

Those who have had experience in the care of dying patients will not have failed to be impressed with the peace that patients experience when they have become convinced of the inevitability of their own death. Rhoads has written of this penultimate moment: "It was as if tearing away the veil of uncertainty at the same time released him from fear. He became calm, gentle, considerate of those about him, assuming a new dignity, as if he had already partly crossed the threshold."

Question 3: Does the patient have pain, and, if so, is it being relieved? The specter of death being painful is firmly rooted in the lay mind, and there is no doubt that osseous metastases, nerve root compression or infiltration, ischemic neuritis, and so forth can cause great pain. Yet pain as a major feature of terminal illness is uncommon. When it occurs it is essential that it be relieved; there is no excuse for a terminal illness being marked by uncontrolled pain except that the physician has not fully analyzed the cause of the patient's pain and utilized those measures available to him for control.

The skillful use of narcotics, radiotherapy, nerve blocks, and, rarely, cordotomy can all be applied individually and together to achieve control. Clearly, however, relief of pain will best be achieved by a careful analysis of its cause and by measures directed against the cause. Thus pain in the thigh in a patient with metastatic cancer may be referred pain or it may represent metastases in the femur. Radiotherapy directed to the wrong area will not relieve pain, and it is the primary physician's responsibility to see to it that treatment is directed against the cause.

In a terminal illness narcotics should not be withheld for fear of addiction, assuming the physician has made an accurate determination that the illness is in its terminal stages. Often doctors achieve less than satisfactory results because they fail to adjust the dose of the narcotic to fit the situation. There are no rigid rules of dose and time intervals, but rather these must be adapted to each patient's need. Oral administration of narcotics will usually suffice in all but the most serious pain problems if the dose and time intervals have been carefully adjusted. At times, physicians worry too much about the development of tolerance. Of course, the risk of tolerance will increase with increasing doses of a narcotic, but cross-tolerance between narcotics is incomplete and substitution of one narcotic for another may often be helpful if tolerance does become a problem. Also the combination of non-narcotic analgesics with narcotics may permit adequate pain relief with lower doses of narcotics and hence a lower risk of developing tolerance. The guiding principle, then, is to be flexible in adopting a program that is suitable for each individual patient and not to be too concerned with standardized regimens.

The subject of pain and its management is considered in Ch. 349.

Question 4: Is the patient being comforted physically, mentally, and spiritually? It is important to draw a distinction between measures undertaken as primary treatment for a disease and those undertaken for the patient's comfort. The latter are often misinterpreted by the laity as needless efforts to prolong life, whereas in the terminally ill patient they are only intended for the relief of discomfort. These measures might include antimicrobial drugs to relieve high fever and drenching sweats caused by infection, oxygen to relieve air hunger, an indwelling catheter to prevent decubitus ulcers secondary to incontinence, and intravenous fluids to relieve thirst and dehydration. These measures do not prolong the life of a dying patient; they, like the relief of pain, merely make more tolerable the period of dying. Yet they have become the targets of those who do not understand and who therefore accuse the medical profession of preventing patients from "dying with dignity." Departing this life in a dignified manner is a noble objective and is often achieved, but in many instances it is not. Dignity is defined in one dictionary as "the presence of poise and self-respect in one's deportment to a degree that inspires respect." This is a reasonable definition; but in those instances in which dignity is lost, it is the illness that is responsible, not the physician, unless through the *injudicious* ordering of drugs, he renders his patient incompetent and robs him of his chance to meet his final hour with courage and character.

Dignity is a quality of human character that is a consequence of what lies within the soul. It is not something that can be taken away by another person. It may lie dormant only to appear under adverse circumstances, such as the prospect of death, or it may be in evidence in all that a person does. Those who have had experience in the treatment of dying patients have often been struck by their fortitude of character and spirit. The medical profession is privileged to go through life with this particular view of humanity, which may only rarely be revealed to people in other walks of life.

Having attended to the patient's physical comfort, the concerned physician will see to it that, to the best of his ability, he brings about mental comfort to the patient. Fear and anxiety are too often left unattended. Narcotics may be useful in allaying both, but even more important is the understanding that physicians can bring to their patients by listening and by giving a patient the realization that his burden is shared by the physician: these, plus a careful interpretation to the patient concerning what is happening to him. Fear can often be counteracted with knowledge and understanding better than with any drug in the pharmacopeia. Lewis Thomas has alluded to the observations of Osler and his own experience that there appears to be no such thing as the agony of death. Regarding the ultimate moment of death he has cited observations that there may be a physiologic mechanism which somehow relieves the patient of all fear and anguish. As we learn more about the pathophysiology of dying, we will undoubtedly come to understand more about such a possible mechanism.

Finally, is the patient being comforted spiritually? A visit by a clergyman is not necessarily synonymous with spiritual comfort, because some patients do not experience comfort under these circumstances, despite the best efforts of the clergyman. It all depends on the patient's background, and this must be known to his physician. Spiritual comfort can come in many forms, and the doctor who really cares about his patient will see to this aspect of his needs. Usually, however, the clergyman is indispensable in providing spiritual comfort. The physician and clergyman need each other, and the patient needs them both. It has been observed that what a physician can provide a patient in these circumstances will depend upon his own beliefs and his coming to terms with his own mortality. If he views life as simply a biologic accident, one in which consciousness dies with the flesh, and one in which there is no divinity in each person, he will be in no position to help his patient in a spiritual sense. If, on the other hand, he views life as a continuum and divine guidance as something operative in all lives, his manner, compassion, gentleness, and understanding will not be lost on the patient seeking spiritual solace. In considering the question of consciousness and what happens to it, Thomas has written: ". . . there is still that permanent vanishing of consciousness to be accounted for. Are we to be stuck forever with this problem? Where on earth does it go? Is it simply stopped dead in its tracks, lost in humus, wasted? Considering the tendency of nature to find uses for complex and intricate mechanisms, this seems to me unnatural. I prefer to think of it as somehow separated off at the filaments of its attachment and then drawn like an easy breath back into the membrane of its origin, a fresh memory for a biospherical nervous system, but I have no data on the matter."

Question 5: Is the physician prepared to give of himself to the patient and "go down to the wire" with him? As a corollary, is the physician willing to continue to think about the problems his patient presents until the end? The phrase "dying a little with each patient" perhaps sounds trite, but it is a useful way of indicating the eventuality of real commitment to a patient. There is no substitute for making sure that your patient never once worries about being abandoned. Of course, no true physician would ever really abandon his patient, but I am speaking of a greater commitment: one that makes the patient know that you are there at all times, at the very least in spirit. Most people face illness with courage, hope, a willingness to place their trust in others, and a capacity to endure. They do this quietly, not seeking praise but simply because this is the way they are made. For a doctor to abandon a fellow human being at such times, through some well-meant but misguided effort to hurry him out of the world, is breaking the faith that he has pledged to all patients.

Now, any position that one takes can be pushed to absurdity, and clearly certain judgments must be taken every day as part of a doctor's life in determining what should or should not be done for a patient. If a patient with far-advanced cancer, whose disease has been resistant to treatment, has a cardiac arrest, he obviously should not be resuscitated. Likewise, one does not transfuse such a patient to maintain a normal hemoglobin, and so on. Therapeutic intervention need *not* be undertaken just because it *can* be undertaken. Nevertheless, these judgments are thinking judgments, and are made in the context of the earlier remarks. There is often a lot of living that has still to be "lived through" between the diagnosis of a terminal illness and death, and it is the quality of that living which should concern a physician. Helping a patient out of this world usually demands more skill, and certainly more understanding, than helping him into the world. Nevertheless, this can be done without abandoning the principles that guide physicians

throughout their lives; if they will but continue to think, they will make decisions as nearly right as they can be.

A. E. Clark-Kennedy has written the following about the moral problem of preserving life: "According to Christian teaching, life is a gift, and the doctor is under a moral obligation to keep his patient alive as long as he can by means put into his hands. . . . A man has been given his life and it is not for him to opt out of it. But even Roman Catholic moralists hold that a doctor is only under an obligation to keep his patient alive as long as life can be reasonably maintained. Further, he need only use ordinary methods. These are those easily available." The key words are "reasonably," "ordinary," and "easily available." Obviously what is reasonable, ordinary, and easily available in a big university hospital will differ from what those terms would mean in a remote hospital in Africa. Further, these terms are also subject to the individual physician's interpretation. In this connection, this same author goes on to identify as "extraordinary" methods of treatment: "palliative surgery such as . . . oophorectomy, adrenalectomy, and even hypophysectomy in carcinoma of the breast." These surgical procedures are certainly available in many countries, but he has chosen to identify them as "extraordinary"; in the United States they would not generally be so regarded. Remissions of metastatic breast cancer have at times been so striking after endocrine surgery (in one recent case report, as long as 25 years after oophorectomy) that there is little doubt as to the value of these procedures in some patients.

One must also consider the thought that physicians may persist in their efforts to preserve life in the realization that they see and know only in part and that some unforeseen event may occur to alter an outcome which the physician, in his fallibility, has come to expect. Further, a patient is less apt to be fearful that his doctor will try to sustain his life than he is that the doctor will give up, notwithstanding the popular idea that healthy persons, contemplating terminal illness, usually express the wish to be allowed to die quickly. Recently, formalized documents have been executed as "living wills," and, although they are not legally binding, they are supposed to give some indication as to what a person wants in a terminal illness. These wills state, in part, that the signer "be allowed to die and not be kept alive by artificial means or heroic measures." As noted, these pronouncements are generally made by people who are healthy. Sick people do not usually express these sentiments, perhaps because of denial or because, facing death, they want to live. There is, of course, a middle ground which responsible physicians should take. They should not, on the one hand, aggressively resuscitate a patient who has had prolonged cerebral anoxia after cardiac arrest, or, on the other hand, consign a terminally ill patient to a state of stupor with morphine just to be relieved of the awesome burden of caring for him.

One attempt to articulate the middle ground has been as follows: "When, in the opinion of the attending physicians, measures to prolong life which have no realistic hope of effecting significant improvement will cause further pain and suffering to the patient and the family, we support conservative, passive medical care in place of heroic measures in the management of a patient afflicted with a terminal illness" (New York Academy of Medicine, 1973). Although the word "prolong" appears in this statement, it is qualified by referring to measures which have "no realistic hope of effecting significant improvement," and in this sense it does not conflict with earlier statements about the use, or misuse, of the word "prolong." This statement puts the burden of these decisions squarely on the attending physicians, where it belongs. This burden implies that a doctor will continue to try to analyze what is happening to his patient, but that what action he takes will be dictated by the over-all circumstances. Note also the reference to "physicians," to indicate that decisions to stop active medical care are usually best taken in consultation with one's colleagues.

Question 6: What is the attitude of the patient's family, and how is it being dealt with? Failure of the medical profession to explain to families what is happening to their terminally ill relatives is the cause of many of the articles published in newspapers and magazines about the increasing insensitivity of doctors. One hears repeatedly from families that "no one tells them anything." It is imperative that at least one member of the family, usually the next of kin, be fully informed of the patient's illness by the responsible physician. This should not be a single session but should be reviewed several times during the course of the patient's illness so that members of the family may have as complete an understanding as is possible for laymen to have. This does not mean that the physician has to have individual sessions with every member of the family; his time obligations must be respected. If a number of relatives are involved, it may be useful to meet with them together, because the physician's explanations, relayed by one member to others in the family, are subject to wide distortions.

It is wise to tell the family what you are doing and why, so that they will not harbor misconceptions. If you are giving fluids, antimicrobials, or oxygen, explain that these are designed for the patient's comfort. If members of a family understand, they will be more helpful and supportive to the patient; but if they are kept in the dark, they may sublimate their anxiety into hostility toward everyone and everything connected with their dying relative.

Further, physicians should give families an opportunity to express their own feelings. Guilt, frustration, and fear are all intermingled with grief, and someone must let the family know that their feelings are normal, that such feelings happen to everyone, and that those caring for the patient understand. No one can do this better than the responsible physician, and he should not delegate this to someone else.

The family also needs to have some reasonable projection as to the patient's life expectancy, but it is unwise to be too specific. Only the inexperienced claim such clairvoyance. Also they should know what to expect in terms of new developments in the patient's course. If the natural history of the disease permits some projections, this information should be shared. Finally, it is important not to engage in speculations as to what might have been had this or that been done or not done earlier in the patient's illness. The family likewise should be discouraged from making such speculations themselves, because they serve no useful purpose and may needlessly promote anxiety and bitterness.

Question 7: Is the patient undergoing experimental study, and, if so, are humanitarian principles being observed or compromised? Although this chapter is not concerned primarily with human experimentation, it is necessary to give this important subject some consideration in the context of the care of the terminally ill, because

often new procedures or treatments are undertaken for the first time in humans with a limited life expectancy. Under these circumstances the approach of the physician to the terminally ill patient must, of necessity, be modified. In his quest for new knowledge, however, he must be prepared to see to it that the rules under which human experimentation is carried out are strictly observed.

Some have proposed that experiments done not for the immediate good of the patient but for the general welfare of mankind should be carried out by those who do not simultaneously have responsibility for the clinical care of the subject. Thus patients who are the subjects of such experiments would have two physicians: a physician-friend and a physician-investigator. Such a system would avoid the subtle alterations of reasoning that may take place when one physician tries to be both. However, if an investigator is true to himself, to his patient, and to the ethical principles which should guide his professional life, it is quite feasible for the same physician to be both friend and investigator. This relationship between investigator and investigatee has been defined by Guttentag as ". . . a partnership between the two, resulting from the fact of their being fellow human beings. . . ." He characterizes this relationship as one of "mutual trust and confidence, of openness between experimenter and subject." In the last analysis, then, the ethics of human experimentation arise from those of the individual investigator and from his perceptions and integrity in dealing with another human being. The essence of experimentation by one human being on another has been captured in this quotation from Paul Tillich:

Man becomes man in personal encounters. Only by meeting a "thou" does man realize he is an "ego." No natural object within the whole universe can do this to him. Man can transcend himself in all directions in knowledge and control. He can use everything for his purposes. Nobody can say where the final limits of human power lie. In his encounter with the universe, man is able to transcend any imaginable limit. But there is a limit for man which is definite and which he always encounters, the other man. The other one, the "thou," is like a wall which cannot be removed or penetrated or used. He who tries to do so, destroys himself.

All human experimentation is based upon the integrity of the individual investigator and the obtaining of informed consent, freely given. Various codes have been developed, beginning with the Nuremberg Code in 1947, and in one form or another they contain the following provisions:

1. Prior voluntary consent must be obtained from all subjects.
2. The study must hold promise of results for the good of society unprocurable by other means.
3. The study must be based on animal experimentation.
4. It must avoid all unnecessary physical and mental suffering.
5. The degree of risk must never exceed that determined by the humanitarian importance of the problem.
6. It must be conducted only by scientifically qualified persons.
7. The human subject must always be at liberty to withdraw.
8. The scientist must be prepared to terminate the study if the subject is endangered to the point of disability or death.

Informed consent is still the most difficult thing to achieve, and the physician, in obtaining this, must keep in mind the following additional principles as outlined by the Board of Regents of the University of the State of New York:

(1) ... it is the patient, and not the physician, who has the right to decide what factors are or are not relevant to his consent, regardless of the rationality of his assessment.... A physician has no right to withhold from a prospective volunteer any fact which he knows may influence the decision.

(2) ... the physician, when he is acting as experimenter, has no claim to the doctor-patient relationship, that, in a therapeutic situation, would give him the generally acknowledged right to withhold information if he judged it in the best interest of the patient.

(3) No person can be said to have volunteered for an experiment unless he had first understood what he was volunteering for. Any matter which might influence him in giving or withholding consent is material. Deliberate nondisclosure of the material fact is no different from deliberate misrepresentation of such a fact.

Physicians dealing with terminal patients who are the subjects of experimentation must assure themselves that all these principles are being observed.

In conclusion, there is no greater test of the qualities of a physician than that imposed by the care of the terminally ill. It calls upon the doctor to exercise medical skill and at the same time to become involved with a fellow human being in the most trying and yet most ennobling of human relationships. How his patient fares will be determined in large part by how the physician meets this test.

Clark-Kennedy, A. E.: Man, Medicine and Morality. Hamden, Conn., Shoe String Press, 1970, pp. 196, 200.

Kübler-Ross, E.: On Death and Dying. New York, The Macmillan Company, 1969.

New York Academy of Medicine: Statement on Measures Employed to Prolong Life in Terminal Illness. Bull. N.Y. Acad. Med., 49 (2nd ser.):349, 1973.

Rhoads, P. S.: Management of the patient with terminal illness. J.A.M.A., 192:661, 1965.

Thomas, L.: The long habit. N. Engl. J. Med., 286:825, 1972.

Tillich, P.: Love, Power and Justice: Ontological Analyses and Ethical Applications. New York, Oxford University Press, 1960, p. 78.

4. MEDICINE IN MODERN SOCIETY

Walsh McDermott

Medicine is not a science but a learned profession deeply rooted in a number of sciences and charged with the obligation to apply them for man's benefit. So complex a process could hardly be reduced to a neat symmetrical design and fitted within the covers of a book. Yet this subject, the beneficial uses of medical science, is not without any design at all—it has a conceptual base on which all medical teaching and all medical books should rest. To consider this base, or certain aspects of it, seems proper at the start of a textbook of medicine. Although the book itself is addressed to medical students and graduate physicians of all ages, this essay is presented mainly for those now entering the profession.

One part of the conceptual base is set forth above in the opening sentence that ends ". . . to apply them for man's benefit." Traditionally this applying is made with compassion and in accord with a widely recognized moral and ethical code. The responsibilities of medicine are thus threefold: to generate scientific knowledge and to teach it to others; to use the knowledge for the health of an individual or a whole community; and to judge the moral and ethical propriety of each medical act that directly affects another human being. These three areas of responsibility command the efforts of individuals from a wide range of scientific disciplines and professions. The

physicians who actually apply the knowledge, however, are of two sorts: those who deal through a personal encounter with one patient at a time and those who deal with people as groups.

The activities of both sorts of physicians are based on the concept that each disease entity has its own pathogenic chain—the whole series of events that determine its causation and maintenance—and that understanding this chain for a particular disease not only permits clearer recognition of its clinical manifestations, but reveals any weak links that might be exploited for prevention or therapy.

Approach to the body of knowledge organized in this way (both in books and elsewhere) is made from one of two viewpoints. The physician in public health or community medicine is constantly reaching for ways in which pathogenic chains can be broken by some continuing intervention that affects a number of people at once, e.g., to reduce the incidence of goiter by putting iodine in table salt. By contrast, physicians acting through the personal encounter system will search the same knowledge sectors and with educated discrimination will extract those elements appropriate for the solution of a problem in an individual. The viewpoints from which the knowledge is scrutinized are different, but the body of knowledge about each disease is the same. Textbooks about diseases and their pathogenic chains serve both these viewpoints and form important instruments for this process of the beneficial uses of science.

The physician who treats one patient at a time and the physician who deals with a community as a whole both exert compassion, but it is of two quite different sorts. The compassion exercised by the physician who treats individuals takes the form of a cultivated instinct to lend support and comfort to a particular fellow human being. By contrast, the "group" compassion of the public health or community physician necessarily takes the form of what the writer has previously termed "statistical compassion." By this is meant an imaginative compassion for people whom one never gets to see as individuals and, indeed, can know only as data on a graph. This compassion—the deep-seated instinct to try to help those whom one never gets to see—is a characteristic form of motivation for political leaders and other social activists, and "statistical" successes bring them major satisfactions. Such is really not the case with most physicians, who usually do not derive as much satisfaction from seeing improvement on a graph as they do from seeing improvement in an individual. *Indeed, part of the self-selection in choosing medicine as a career seems to be a self-image of a person whose professional activities are to relate directly with individuals rather than with groups.* Thus the system of public health or community medicine —based on physicians *not* seeing patients as individuals —runs contrary to most medical instincts. Yet until we have significant numbers of physicians for whom "statistical compassion" is as rewarding as it is to the leaders in certain other walks of life, we will fail as a society to derive the full measure of the benefits of our medical science.

The scientific basis of medicine had been building up throughout the whole nineteenth century, but the *uses* of that science in the sense of decisively altering or preventing disease were largely accomplished through the public health or "community" physicians who dealt with people as groups. Chlorination of water supplies and the pasteurization of milk are cases in point. It was not until the discovery of insulin in 1921, and not really until the advent of the modern antimicrobial era 40 years ago, that the clinical physicians had much in the way of decisive therapies or preventives derived from science. Since that time most of the practical uses of biomedical science and technology have been of a nature fitted to the clinical or personal system, and, despite recent efforts, the other system has been allowed to languish. Indeed, the evolution of the highly complex and extraordinarily effective instrument that is today's university-based medical center has been almost exclusively devoted to the one system—the personal encounter system of one patient at a time.

We could tolerate this so long as what medicine had to offer was technologically simple and physicians were spread out across the whole of society much more evenly than they are now. But the coincidence of massive scientific innovation and wide social change has created a situation in which the application of medical science for man's benefit can no longer be managed by just one of the two systems—we desperately need both.

For there are two critically different populations involved, each of which is the primary responsibility of one of the systems. These two populations are the *constituency* and the *community*. The members of the constituency represent a progressively selected group, in part self-selected, and the selection is based on the presence of a medical problem, frequently one that is quite complex. Each member, in effect, has *voted* to obtain the services of a physician (or center or medical group) and has cast this vote as an individual without reference to others. The constituency is thus a collection of individuals who share in common only the fact that each has perceived a self-problem of illness or disease. It is the group known familiarly as the physician's "practice." The community, by contrast, is made up of people distinguished by the possession in common of some factor not directly related to disease. Usually, but not invariably, this common factor is a domicile located within some geographically defined boundary. In health terms, therefore, the community is a wholly unselected group, and at any one point in time many more of its members are well than are sick. *The community and the constituency thus differ strikingly in the prevalence of significant illness and disease. Because of this difference, an institutional form appropriate to meet the needs of one group would be markedly different from the form appropriate for the other.* Our challenge today is to develop such a two-type institutional form so that the needs of both groups may be equally served.

What the community needs is recognition of weakness in pathogenic chains that may be exploited in the prevention of disease. For nonpreventable disease the community needs straightforward medical care close to home, safeguarded by continuous mechanisms for identifying those who need care in the first place and mechanisms for sifting the few who need complex care from the many who do not. These few join the constituency—that self-selected group of people derived from a much larger population base than could be satisfactorily served by a single personal encounter physician. What the properly sifted members of the constituency need is an institution that can offer a complete array of talents appropriate for the solution of any currently solvable medical problem, no matter how rarely occurring or complicated it might be. Whether for the community or for the constituency, the actual provision of the care is the responsibility of

the personal encounter physician. Community medicine (or the larger public health system of which it is a part) is thus responsible *not* for the delivery of personal health services to the members of a community, but for ensuring that the community receives the proper health services of all sorts. And prominent among these are the invention of better mechanisms than we have now for both the continuous community scan of who needs care at any moment and appropriate entry points for the care of those identified. Neither of these two systems is inherently of greater social value than the other, but in the course of developing the personal encounter system to its present high point of technologic effectiveness for the individual, we have failed to mount a comparable effort for the nourishment of the other system responsible for the medical welfare of every member of the group. Without such a healthy watchdog we have allowed the personal encounter system to become unevenly distributed throughout our population. The speedy correction of this imbalance is the critical challenge facing medicine today, and how well we meet it will determine the role of the physician in society. For the imbalance of the two systems affects our efforts for the beneficial uses of science not only at the level of medical care for the community and the constituency, but in those even larger matters that have to do with how the developing individual can be aided in his or her continuous interaction with the environment.

It is not possible to do justice to all these issues in this book, although some are indeed considered. For others, certain key references to the valuable literature that has been developing in recent years are set forth below. There remain a few, however, that are so vital to the conceptual base forming the theme of this chapter that they deserve special mention.

Moral judgments must be made by the physician engaged in individual patient care, but they are to be made on his own professional acts and those of his colleagues, not on the actions of those who sought his care. Any moral judgments he might make on his patients' behavior are private matters to be kept within himself; he must not permit them to influence his own professional acts. This has long been the medical tradition, and it is important that it not be forgotten in the tumult of today's world of clashing value systems. The prospect of moral and ethical problems of an essentially new type is also now emerging before us. There is general awareness that advances in medical science are leading to various ethical conflicts that have to be faced by the personal encounter physician. What is less well recognized, however, is that this situation will also become socially serious for the nonclinical system, whether it be called public health or community medicine. Critical phenomena in human development formerly thought to represent the hand of fate are now found to be, at least in part, environmentally determined, and hence manipulable—such matters as the full expansion of an individual's intelligence or perhaps his or her degree of educability. If we develop the power to significantly influence such critical matters—and scientifically we are getting closer to it every day—we may find ourselves faced with seeking to protect the "interests" of an unborn or newborn child in the receipt of a particular intervention against the "rights" of its parents to be free from outside interference. And this question of how to ensure the best opportunity for the individual without destroying family structure in the process will not be an ethical problem to be faced by medicine in rare instances, but one that will involve whole societies. Yet we cannot run away from such questions, for it is the wise application of our science and technology, made with either form of compassion, that allows us to approach one of our major goals — that of ensuring that every child born into the world has the maximal chance to make his run through life's most productive years.

Finally, we must heed a concept of medicine that is ageless. In the life of an individual there ultimately may come a time when all the knowledge so carefully presented by the contributors to this book no longer has usefulness, yet life must go on, at least for a time. Whenever this happens, and it happens every day, it is up to each of us to follow to the fullest measure the charge laid down long ago for "the physician to become himself the treatment."

Beeson, P. B.: Some good features of the British National Health Service. Arch. Intern. Med., 133:708, 1974.

Dubos, R.: So Human an Animal. New York, Charles Scribner's Sons, 1969.

McDermott, W.: Demography, culture, and economics and the evolutionary stages of medicine. *In* Kilbourne, E. D., and Smillie, W. G. (eds.): Human Ecology and Public Health. 4th ed. New York, The Macmillan Company, 1969.

Morison, R. S.: Where is biology taking us? Science, 155:429, 1967.

Rogers, D. E.: The doctor must himself become the treatment. Lecture given at the University of North Carolina. February 20, 1974. The Pharos (to be published).

Part II
GENETIC PRINCIPLES

5. INTRODUCTION

Alexander G. Bearn

It is a convenient if misleading abstraction to consider that all diseases of man are due either to the action of environmental agents or to hereditary influences. This simplistic view has been nurtured by innumerable studies that relegate a disease into one or the other category. It is more correct, however, as well as more rewarding, to consider that both environmental and hereditary influences play a role in the etiology of disease. In some conditions genetic influences are clearly decisive, whereas in others the disease appears to be independent of the genetic constitution of the patient. In most diseases, both genetic and environmental factors play a detectably influential role. The science of human genetics is concerned primarily with the recognition of hereditary variations in man. Most of these variations are not harmful; indeed they are beneficial, for they confer on the species the capacity to adapt to an ever-changing environment. But when these variations are extreme and are associated with clinical disease, they come within the realm of the physician. Since medical genetics is an applied science, certain general genetic principles will be discussed before considering in detail the direct application of genetics to clinical medicine.

After the establishment of the principle of genetic transmission by Gregor Mendel, Johannsen, in 1909, introduced the word *gene* to denote a unit of heredity. A structural gene is now defined, operationally, as a functional unit of inheritance situated on a chromosome and responsible for the synthesis of a specific polypeptide. It has been estimated that there are probably no less than 100,000 genes in man. Since the number of well documented examples of genetic variability is of the order of 1000, it is apparent that despite the acceleration in discovery of new genetic entities 99 per cent of the human genome remains to be discovered.

The chemical nature of a gene was unrecognized until 1944, when a soluble extract derived from pneumococci of one genotype was found to effect a stable heritable change when added to a growing culture of pneumococci of another genotype. The prompt identification of the transforming substance present in the extract as deoxyribonucleic acid (DNA) launched the present era of molecular biology. The genetic information encoded in the DNA that determines polypeptide structure is transcribed through the synthesis of another macromolecule, ribonucleic acid (RNA). Part of this RNA is termed *messenger RNA* (mRNA), and the linear amino acid sequences in the polypeptide chain are precisely determined by the linear sequences of the coding units ("*codons*"—see below) in the mRNA. These relationships are often referred to as the central dogma of molecular biology, and can be depicted schematically:

$$DNA \xrightarrow{transcription} RNA \xrightarrow{translation} polypeptide$$

The universality of this biologic truth was momentarily shaken by the discovery in 1970 that several RNA animal tumor viruses contain polymerase activity (reverse transcriptase) which uses RNA as a template for the synthesis of double-stranded DNA and thus reverses the familiar direction of genetic transcription. This discovery raised the possibility that an RNA-dependent DNA polymerase might indicate the presence of an oncogenic virus. Although this enzyme has now been detected in certain nononcogenic viruses as well, the function of viral reverse transcriptase remains a question of central biologic importance in the problem of neoplasia.

Deoxyribonucleic Acid (DNA). Deoxyribonucleic acid is constructed from three essential components: the five-carbon sugar 2-deoxy-D-ribose; phosphoric acid, which confers on DNA its acidic properties; and nitrogenous bases. Two of the bases are purines, adenine (A) and guanine (G), and two are pyrimidines, thymine (T) and cytosine (C). In 1953 Watson and Crick assembled the available physical and chemical data on DNA into the present model for the structure of DNA. Two polynucleotide chains are twisted together to form a double helix. The two chains are held together by hydrogen bonds between the bases which face inward forming the core, and the phosphate-sugar groups form an external helical backbone. Adenine must always pair with thymine (A-T), and guanine with cytosine (G-C). The result of this pairing leads to a precise complementary relationship between the bases on the two chains. Thus, if part of the base sequence were TTGCC, the corresponding portion of the complementary strand would read AACGG.

Replication of DNA. One of the chief attractions of the Watson-Crick model for DNA is that it contains a built-in system for self-replication. As the double helix of a parent molecule unwinds, the sequence of bases in each strand acts as a template for the synthesis of a new strand of DNA in two daughter molecules. The replication is catalyzed by the enzyme DNA polymerase and has been termed *semiconservative,* because both parental strands are conserved in the next generation, each now paired with a newly synthesized complementary partner.

Ribonucleic Acid (RNA). Ribonucleic acid differs from deoxyribonucleic acid in three important ways. (1) The sugar D-ribose replaces the 2-deoxy-D-ribose of DNA. (2) The pyrimidine base uracil (U) replaces the thymine of DNA. (3) RNA is a single-stranded polymer in contrast to double-stranded DNA.

Messenger Ribonucleic Acid (mRNA). Messenger RNA is formed by the transcription of one of the strands of DNA and is catalyzed by the specific enzyme RNA polymerase (transcriptase). The sequence of bases in mRNA is identical to that in the corresponding uncopied strand of DNA except that uracil replaces thymine. In this way single-stranded RNA carries into the cytoplasm the genetic information originally encoded in nuclear DNA. In bacteria, mRNA has a half-life of about two minutes, and it has been calculated that during this time 10 to 20 molecules of protein can be synthesized. In cells of higher organisms the bulk of mRNA appears to be much more stable, and may remain functional for two to three days and direct the synthesis of several thousand molecules of protein.

Transfer RNA (tRNA).   Before amino acids are assembled into polypeptide chains they must first be "activated." This activation is accomplished by the enzyme amino-acyl-tRNA synthetase which attaches the phosphate group of adenine to the carboxyl group of an amino acid to form amino-acyl-adenylate. The activated amino acid is now joined to another type of RNA called transfer RNA. Mammalian cells contain more than 20 different transfer RNA's, and at least one transfer RNA is specific for each of the amino acids. Each transfer RNA molecule is folded into a cloverleaf pattern and has two recognition sites. One site binds the "activated" amino acid, whereas the second, often called the anticodon, recognizes the codon in the mRNA. Thus the fidelity of translation is assured by the specific binding of the amino acid, with the tRNA catalyzed by the specific activating enzyme and by complementary pairing of the anticodon of tRNA with the codon of the mRNA.

Ribosomal RNA (rRNA).   More than 80 per cent of the RNA of most cells is found in small cytoplasmic particles, closely associated with the endoplasmic reticulum, called ribosomes. These ribosomal particles represent the protein synthetic machinery of the cell and consist of about half protein and half RNA. There are some 50 different proteins in a single ribosome; the RNA does not contain any genetic information, and its function is unknown. Mammalian ribosomes have a diameter of approximately 200 Å and a sedimentation coefficient of 80 S, and dissociate into 60 S and 40 S subunits in low concentrations of magnesium ion. Messenger RNA, bearing the instructions for protein synthesis, must become attached to the ribosomes on which the polypeptide is synthesized. In bacteria, mRNA contains several "sticky points" which enable it to adhere to the smaller ribosomal subunit. When this has occurred, the larger ribosomal subunit becomes attached to form the final functional ribosome, and the sequential assembly of amino acids into protein begins.

Protein Synthesis.   Translation is initiated as soon as mRNA becomes bound to the ribosomes. In bacteria the initiation of translation is effected by the codon, AUG, which binds a specific tRNA, n-formylmethionyl-tRNA, to the ribosome complex. The second codon then recognizes its specific tRNA, and the second amino acid in sequence is brought into alignment. A peptide bond is formed between the two amino acids, and the ribosome moves along the mRNA so that the third codon, recognizing its tRNA, brings the third amino acid into position with further elongation of the peptide chain (Fig. 1). The information that a polypeptide chain is completed and that its synthesis must be terminated is specified by a special chain-terminating codon. A ribosome takes about ten seconds to read an entire mRNA molecule of average length, and a single mRNA molecule may move over the surfaces of several ribosomes simultaneously. This explains why a cell needs relatively little mRNA to synthesize a great deal of protein. A molecule of mRNA attached to several ribosomes simultaneously is called a polyribosome; polyribosomes synthesizing hemoglobin (a protein of molecular weight 64,500), on the average, contain four to six ribosomes.

Codons.   Because most proteins normally contain 20 different amino acids and because DNA has only four different nucleotide bases, it is evident that more than one base is required to prescribe for a particular amino acid. It is now known that a sequence of three bases (a codon) is needed to code for each amino acid, and that the code is nonoverlapping. Thus a gene with 1500 nucleotide pairs would determine the sequence of a polypeptide chain consisting of 500 amino acids. Since the four-letter code is triplet in nature, there are 64 ($4 \times 4 \times 4$) possible codons, of which 61 have been shown to code for one of the 20 amino acids. The three remaining codons represent signals that the polypeptide chain is completed and are called chain-terminating codons. Two codons serve to initiate polypeptide synthesis as well as to insert amino acids and are sometimes designated chain-initiating codons. One of the unresolved problems of eukaryotic organisms such as man is that they possess more DNA in their genome than is needed for genetic information. Multiple copies of structural genes almost certainly occur and may account for much of the redundancy. The genetic code is said to be *universal* in the sense that all plant and animal species have thus far been found to use the same genetic code, and *degenerate* because certain amino acids can be specified by more than one triplet.

Certain acridine dyes induce mutations in bacteriophage by inserting an extra nucleotide into the pre-existing (normal) sequence. Because of this extra nucleotide, the reading frame becomes altered distal to the point of insertion and results in a disruption of normal protein synthesis. The correct reading frame of the code can be restored by a deletion of another nucleotide (or by the insertion of an additional two extra nucleotides) distal to the insertion. This model makes the prediction that a double mutant, consisting of an insertion followed by a deletion, will result in a polypeptide chain with an altered amino acid sequence between the two mutations. If the segment of DNA between the two mutations is short, and does not code for amino acids vital for functional specificity, a protein with a normal function may still be produced. A mutation in the codon which terminates the reading of the code is referred to as a terminator mutation. Three variant hemoglobins (Hb Constant Spring, Hb Tak, and Hb Wayne) have been reported in which either the α or β chain has been elongated. In Hb Constant Spring and Hb Tak the increased length of the molecule is due to a terminator mutation, whereas in Hb Wayne the increased chain length is caused by a frame-shift mutation.

Structural Genes, Control Genes, and the Structure-Rate Hypothesis.   The most extensive understanding of genetic regulatory mechanisms has stemmed from the investigations of the β-galactosidase enzyme system in *Escherichia coli*. These studies have led to the formulation of new concepts of regulation in bacteria, according to which a hierarchy of control genes and structural genes has been established. Thus, whereas certain genes (structural genes) are responsible for the actual synthesis of specific protein and enzymes, and contain the DNA code which specifies their amino acid sequences, other genes (control genes) are responsible for the regulation of the production of these proteins. Although the distinction between a control gene mutation and a structural gene mutation can be resolved in microorganisms by tracing the mutation to a locus within or outside the structural gene, techniques for a similar analysis in man are not yet available. It is increasingly clear, however, that the regulation of gene function in man is far more complex than in bacteria, and the application of the Jacob-Monod model is undoubtedly a misleading oversimplification.

A dramatic example of a structural gene mutation in man was most clearly demonstrated when Ingram re-

Figure 1. A schematic diagram of the genetic control of protein synthesis. A=adenine, T=thymine, G=guanine, C=cytosine, U= uracil. The codons indicated represent code words for the amino acids indicated. The messenger RNA (mRNA) moves across the ribosomes in the direction of the arrow. tRNA=transfer RNA; rRNA=ribosomal RNA. (For details see text.)

ported in 1956 that sickle cell hemoglobin differed from normal hemoglobin in a single amino acid substitution. Since that time a very large number of structural mutants have been identified in man, and in many instances the precise amino acid substitution has been identified. The question of whether, in man, there are also control gene mutations which so drastically affect synthesis that only very small quantities of a structurally normal protein are formed has been less easy to document.

Although many of the hereditary diseases studied by Garrod are characterized by the synthesis of a decreased quantity of an enzyme of apparently normal structure, rigorous structural studies have seldom been performed. The apparent absence of a specific protein in certain genetic disorders may be due to a structural gene mutation that has resulted in the synthesis of a modified protein which has become immunologically, enzymatically, and chemically unrecognizable. The growing concept that the gene controlling the structure of a protein also influences the amount of protein synthesized has been termed the structure-rate hypothesis. In most instances the mutational event leads to decreased synthesis; rarely, however, an increased synthesis of the mutant protein may occur. An increased enzymatic activity has been ob-

served in G6PD Hektoen, a structural mutant in the glucose-6-phosphate dehydrogenase system, and in a pseudocholinesterase mutant designated Cynthiana (see Ch. 740). In certain inherited diseases the primary biochemical abnormality probably resides in a decreased or defective synthesis of messenger RNA. In thalassemia a decreased synthesis of the β globulin chain of normal hemoglobin is associated with a deficiency of functional mRNA for globin chains. In those rare forms of thalassemia in which β chain synthesis is totally absent, a deletion of the DNA sequences coding for the β chain mRNA is responsible for the lack of globin synthesis.

Watson, J. D.: Molecular Biology of the Gene. 2nd ed. New York, Benjamin, 1970.

6. PEDIGREE ANALYSIS IN INHERITED DISEASE

Alexander G. Bearn

Inspection and analysis of human pedigrees form the basis for an understanding of the application of the laws of Mendel to human disease. Analysis of a pedigree begins with the affected individual, who is referred to as the propositus, proband, or index case. Using the propositus as the point of departure, a pedigree is constructed, and the pattern of the pedigree is analyzed. It is worth emphasizing, however, that the construction of human pedigrees beyond first- and second-degree relatives is an occupation more likely to please the physician than to provide a deeper genetic understanding of the patient's disease. Human memories are notoriously untrustworthy, and great care must be exercised when very large pedigrees are compiled and recorded.

Autosomal Inheritance. When there are two alleles, A and a, at a locus, three possible genotypes exist, which can be represented AA, Aa, and aa. The genotypes AA and aa are called *homozygotes*; Aa is a *heterozygote*. A gene can be recognized only by the effect it produces; thus in the strictest sense it is incorrect to speak of dominant or recessive genes, but only of dominant or recessive effects. If the phenotype Aa cannot be easily distinguished from the phenotype AA, but is clearly different from aa, the effect of gene A is said to be dominant over the effect of gene a. In this circumstance there are only two phenotypes corresponding to the three genotypes AA, Aa, aa. However, the failure to detect a phenotypic difference between the genotypes AA and Aa is usually testimony to the insensitivity of the methods employed. If the gene product of A and a can both be detected in the heterozygote Aa, the genes are said to exert an effect which is *co-dominant*. In many ways it would be preferable to discard the terms "dominant" and "recessive" and instead to state whether the genes concerned are phenotypically expressed in a single or double dose; for the sake of convenience, however, the terms are often retained.

Autosomal Dominant Traits. Autosomal genes are those genes situated on chromosomes other than the X and Y. Dominant traits are defined as those traits that are fully manifested by the presence of a gene in the heterozygous state. Thus far, approximately 1000 well established autosomal dominant traits have been identified in man. Satisfactory examples of dominant traits are those responsible for the formation of certain blood group antigens. In the ABO system, the genes controlling the formation of A and B substances are dominant over O. Thus it is not ordinarily possible to distinguish serologically AA from AO individuals, or BB from BO individuals. However, heterozygous individuals of type AB can be recognized because the product of genes A and B can be detected.

An autosomal dominant trait can be recognized in human pedigrees by its transmission from one generation to the next. Except for sporadic cases in which a fresh mutation in the germ cell has arisen in either the father or the mother, and provided illegitimacy can be excluded, every affected individual has at least one affected parent and may have affected offspring and sibs (Fig. 2). The more severe the condition, the larger is the proportion of sporadic cases caused by fresh mutation. According to mendelian laws, a heterozygous affected individual married to a normal homozygote will, on the average, transmit the trait to half his offspring, both sexes being equally affected. Neurofibromatosis, Huntington's chorea, and achondroplastic dwarfism are examples of dominant traits of clinical significance.

In contrast to recessive disorders, most dominant traits in man frequently exert only mild effects, and marked variation in the expression of the trait is the

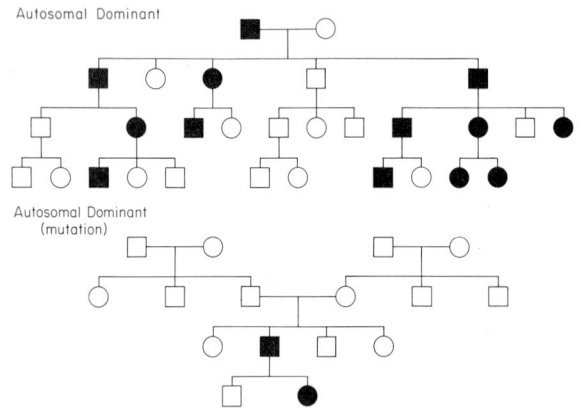

Figure 2. Pedigrees of autosomal dominant traits. In the lower pedigree the normal parents of the affected individual suggest the possibility of a new mutation. (For details see text.)

rule. In some instances the expression of the abnormal gene may be so weak that a generation appears to be skipped because the carrier of the abnormal gene is clinically normal. When a gene that can be clinically expressed in the heterozygous condition occurs in the homozygous state, the effect is usually more severe and may be lethal. Although examples are common in species in which experimental matings can be constructed, such examples are exceptional in man, because marriage of two clinically affected heterozygotes is rare. An increased paternal age effect has been demonstrated among parents of sporadic cases of achondroplastic dwarfism, Marfan's syndrome (see Ch. 933), and certain other dominantly inherited disorders.

The molecular basis for the more than 1000 genetically dominant diseases now known is quite obscure. It is of interest that in contrast to recessively inherited diseases in which an impairment of enzyme function is the rule, defective enzymes are only rarely found in dominant diseases. A deficiency of the inhibitor of the first component of complement, *C1-esterase inhibitor,* in hereditary angioneurotic edema and a deficiency of *uroporphyrinogen-1-synthetase* in porphyria are exceptions to this general rule (see Ch. 76 and 942). It appears that in most dominantly inherited disorders the abnormal gene determines a protein with a structural rather than an enzymatic function. Several hemolytic disorders are due to the presence of a single unstable mutant hemoglobin (see Ch. 746 to 751). The presence of one of these abnormal hemoglobin genes is sufficient to shorten the life of the red cells.

Autosomal Recessive Traits. In an autosomal recessive trait, the father and the mother of the affected individual are usually normal, as are more distant ancestors. On the average, one fourth of the brothers and sisters of the index case will be affected. If the trait is rare, an increased consanguinity will be observed among the parents of those affected. According to mendelian laws, two normal parents, both heterozygous for a recessive trait, will produce offspring of whom, on the average, one quarter will be homozygous for the normal allele, one quarter homozygous for the abnormal allele and thus affected, and one half heterozygous for the abnormal allele, like the parents. Affected individuals usually have phenotypically normal offspring who are all carriers of the abnormal gene. If an affected individual marries an individual heterozygous for the same gene, one half of the offspring will be affected and one half will be heterozygous carriers (Fig. 3). Approximately 800 well established recessive traits have been identified in man.

Certain aspects of the segregation ratio in autosomal recessive conditions must be emphasized. Because of the small size of families and because ascertainment of the family is usually through an affected member, the mean observed proportion of affected individuals will be greater than expected. Only when the size of the sibships is large will the expected ratio of one affected to three unaffected be realized in pooled data. Thus the analysis of the expected ratio in families of various sizes requires a correction factor whose magnitude depends on the number of children in the sibship. The simplest correction is to subtract in each family the index case from the total number of affected individuals and then determine the proportion of affected children among the remaining sibs.

The disadvantage of the term "recessive" is emphasized by the increasing number of instances in which refined biochemical observations enable the recognition of the trait in the clinically normal heterozygote. Indeed, because of its importance in genetic counseling, the detection of healthy heterozygous carriers of genes that in the homozygous condition cause overt disease is becoming one of the most significant aspects of medical genetics. In recent years, the biochemical detection of heterozygotes for autosomal recessive diseases has been greatly facilitated by the development of techniques to culture skin fibroblasts. Although the culturing of human fibroblasts has been relatively uninformative in dominant disorders, in approximately 25 per cent of all autosomal recessive diseases the precise biochemical defect can be detected in cultured fibroblasts derived from a simple skin biopsy.

X-Linked Inheritance. *Dominant X-Linked Traits.* This mode of inheritance is uncommon. Heterozygous affected females will transmit the trait to both sexes with a frequency of 50 per cent. Affected males will transmit the trait to all their daughters, but to none of their sons (Fig. 4). This rule of X-linked dominant inheritance enables critical distinction from traits inherited in an autosomal dominant fashion, in which an affected male transmits the trait to both sons and daughters. The variability of expression of an X-linked dominant trait is less in males than in females. If the trait is uncommon, the incidence in females is roughly twice that in males. The erythrocyte antigen Xgᵃ and vitamin D resistant rickets (hypophosphatemic rickets) are inherited as X-linked dominant traits. Approximately 100 loci have been identified on the human X chromosome.

Autosomal Recessive

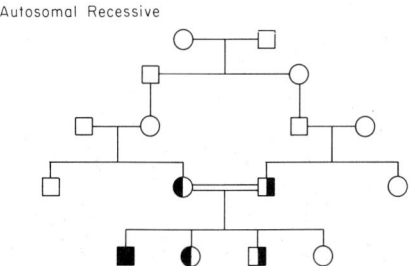

Figure 3. Pedigree of autosomal recessive trait. Note: both parents are heterozygous. One sib is affected, two are carriers, and one is normal. Double line (⹀) indicates that parents are related by descent (first cousins).

X-linked Dominant

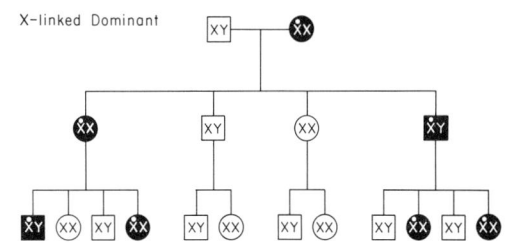

Figure 4. Pedigree of dominant X-linked trait. The X chromosome bearing the abnormal gene is designated by a small white dot.

Recessive X-Linked Traits. Recessive X-linked traits are relatively common. On the average, half the sons of normal heterozygous females will be normal, and half will be affected. If the trait is rare, parents and relatives will be normal except for male relatives in the female line; for instance, on the average, one half of the maternal uncles will be affected. An affected male married to a normal female will have normal offspring. All their daughters will be carriers, and they, in turn, can transmit the trait to the next generation. The rare event of an affected male married to a carrier female will result in equal proportions of affected male and female offspring. The unaffected males will be genotypically normal; the unaffected females, however, will be heterozygous carriers (Fig. 5). The common red-green color blindness is inherited as an X-linked recessive trait; other, less common traits include hemophilia (see Ch. 797), pseudohypertrophic muscular dystrophy (see Ch. 476), congenital agammaglobulinemia (Bruton) (see Ch. 62), and the Wiskott-Aldrich syndrome (see Ch. 69). In the general population the frequency of affected females will be roughly the square of the frequency of affected males.

The Lyon Hypothesis. Since the human female bears two X chromosomes, it might have been expected that the concentration of proteins determined by genes on the X chromosome would be twice that observed in males who have only one chromosome. Thus it might have been expected that the concentration of factor VIII (antihemophilic factor) in females would be twice that found in males. This is not the case, and the explanation is provided by a hypothesis first advanced by Mary Lyon.

In all adult females only one of the two X chromosomes is genetically active. Early in differentiation one of the X chromosomes becomes inactive and forms the Barr body. Inactivation is random; but once one of the two X chromosomes in any cell is inactivated, the same X chromosome remains inactive during all its subsequent cell divisions. For example, in X-linked hemophilia, on the average, only half the X chromosomes are genetically active and synthesizing antihemophilic globulin, and thus the amount of antihemophilic globulin synthesis is approximately the same in males and females. Greater variability in expression of an X-linked trait is a natural consequence of the Lyon hypothesis. The number of cells determining a specific function at the time of inactivation is small, and thus chance alone could influence the number of such cells inactivated.

Y-Linked Inheritance. If a trait is determined by a gene in the Y chromosome, it will be transmitted through the father to all his sons and none of his daughters. Thus far, the only genes that have been shown to be located in the Y chromosome are those that determine "maleness." (See also XYY Syndrome in Ch. 859.)

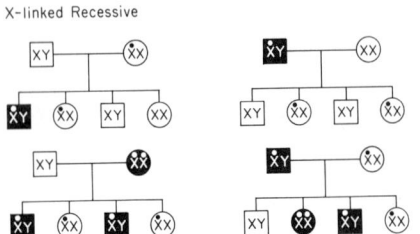

Figure 5. Pedigrees of recessive X-linked trait. The X chromosome bearing the abnormal gene is designated by a small white dot.

Sex Limitation. Autosomal genes that are expressed only in males may mimic sex-linkage but can be formally distinguished if affected individuals reproduce. If a gene is on an autosome, affected males can transmit the trait to their sons; if the gene is on the X chromosome, they cannot.

Modification of Gene Expression. The manifestation of an abnormal gene is influenced not only by its normal allele, but also by alleles at other loci, and by environment. The terms expressivity and penetrance have been employed to describe the variable manifestation of a gene. These vague words are usually best avoided unless they can be used with precision, e.g., it would be precise but cumbersome to say that the gene for Huntington's chorea is 0 per cent penetrant at the age of 10 and 95 per cent penetrant at 65. Some genetically determined traits such as those determining the blood antigens are present at birth, whereas others such as Huntington's chorea appear only in adult life. A negative correlation between the age of onset of a trait in parents and sibs suggests that the expression of a gene may be influenced by the type of normal allele present. The effect can be seen in certain dominant diseases such as the nail-patella syndrome and in the dominant form of muscular dystrophy. The concept of anticipation, which asserts that hereditary diseases tend to have a progressively earlier age of onset with successive generations, is a statistical artifact which is based on a bias of ascertainment.

Consanguinity. It is mandatory in taking a family history to inquire whether there is parental consanguinity. When confronted with a patient, particularly a child, whose disorder does not fit any clear-cut diagnosis, the history of consanguinity in the parents is often the first clue that the patient is suffering from a rare, recessively inherited disorder. In all autosomal recessive disorders the affected individual has inherited one abnormal gene from each parent. It is thus evident that an individual will be more likely to inherit the same allele from each parent if the two parents have genes inherited from a common ancestor. First cousins have, on the average, one eighth of their genes derived from a common ancestor. When the two first cousins marry, their offspring will have, on the average, one sixteenth of their genes derived from the common ancestor. It is frequently of interest to calculate the expected frequency of first-cousin marriages among parents of those with rare autosomal recessive disorders. Providing that the frequency of the disease in the population can be estimated and the frequency of first-cousin marriages in the general population is known, the calculation can be made according to the following formula. If k is the frequency of first-cousin marriages in a rare recessive disease, then as a first approximation $k = c/16q$, where c is the frequency of first-cousin marriages in the general population and q is the frequency of the abnormal gene. The frequency of cousin marriages is variable. In some isolated populations a frequency of as high as 30 per cent has been recorded, whereas in the United States in an urban population the frequency may be as low as 0.05 per cent. Let us suppose a recessively inherited disease has a frequency in the population of 1 in 10,000 (q^2); then the frequency of the gene, which in double dose causes the disease, is 1 in 100 (q). If the frequency of consanguinity in the general population is 0.5 per cent, then k, the parental consanguinity, is 3 per cent, a six-fold increase over normal. If the disease is much rarer, 1 in 100,000, then 10 per cent of the individuals affected by the disease will have parents who are first cousins. As the frequency of c increases, the expected frequency of parents who are first cousins will also increase. In some geographically isolated populations c may reach as high as 2 per cent. If a recessively inherited disease in such an isolate has a frequency of 1 in 100,000, 40 per cent of the parents of the affected individuals will be first cousins.

It is important to realize that an increased frequency of consanguinity will not be observed if the recessive disease is common. Thus in cystic fibrosis of the pancreas, which has a frequency of approximately 1 in 2500, no increase in parental consanguinity can be detected. Although the frequency of albinism in the general population is approximately 1 per 20,000, the unexpectedly high consanguinity in the parents (k = 20 per cent) of some patients is due to the existence of more than one gene for this condition. No increase in consanguinity would be expected in dominant or X-linked traits.

Although in most populations the consanguinity rate is approximately 1 per cent or less, and in general is decreasing, certain geographic and cultural isolates remain in which there is a high coefficient of inbreeding. These isolates may shelter rare genes which because of the high consanguinity rate are likely to become manifest. More than 90 per cent of patients described with the Ellis–van Creveld syndrome have been found in the Old Order Amish living in Pennsylvania, Ohio, Indiana, and Ontario. Other rare recessive diseases found within this genetic isolate include pyruvate kinase deficiency, a form of dwarfism associated with hypoplasia of the cartilage and hair, and a form of limb-girdle muscular dystrophy. It is worth remembering that, in general, the offspring of first-cousin marriages are slightly more likely to have congenital malformations, as well as mental and physical defects, than are children from unrelated parents.

Association. The occurrence of two traits in the same person more often than would be expected by chance is called association. A consistent positive association between blood group A and carcinoma of the stomach, and between duodenal ulceration and blood group O, has long been recognized. Such an association may be due to many causes, and does not indicate that the genes controlling blood group antigens are on the same chromosome as those associated with the development of duodenal ulceration. If an association is found between two characters in the general population, it is important to determine whether the association persists when the two characters are examined in sibships. If geographic or social stratification is the cause of the association, the correlation will disappear. If, for example, a mixed population of Africans and Europeans is examined, a positive association between cDe Rhesus blood group (common in African populations) and dark skin color would be found. This association would disappear if individual sibships were examined.

Sometimes two characters are associated because they are due to the action of a single gene. Thus clouding of the cornea and mental retardation are two traits that are associated in Hurler's syndrome. The two traits are not caused by two genes, but are due to a single gene with a so-called pleiotropic effect. When a gene causes a pleiotropic effect, the association found in the general population persists when sibships are examined. Pleiotropic effects of genes are common, and may be of clinical importance. Familial intestinal polyposis (see Ch. 669) is an early consequence of the effect of a gene that later commonly leads to carcinoma of the colon.

Autosomal Linkage. The site of a gene on a chromosome is termed a *locus*. Alternative forms of genes which occupy corresponding sites on homologous chromosomes are called alleles. Applied to human genetics, Mendel's law of independent assortment states that traits controlled by two or more pairs of allelic genes will be transmitted to the children of the next generation, either together or separately, by chance alone. The law holds only for genes situated on different chromosomes or at widely separated loci on the same chromosome. However, if two genes occupy closely adjacent sites on the same chromosome, they tend to segregate together and are said to be linked. The occasional segregation of linked genes is due to crossing over at meiosis. The frequency of crossing over gives an estimate of closeness of the linkage. It is important to remember that even if two genes are present on the same chromosomes, they will appear unlinked if they are so far apart that free (50 per cent) recombination between two loci can take place.

The application of somatic cell genetics as well as the development of more discriminating methods for chromosome identification has enabled the assigment of specific loci to individual autosomes. Structural loci can already be assigned to 19 of the 22 autosomes. In many instances more than one genetic locus can be assigned to a particular chromosome. Chromosome 1 has 15 loci assigned, including the Rh locus. Chromosomes 3, 8, and 9 still await the assignment of specific loci.

Linkage of two genes, that is, close enough proximity of their loci on the chromosome that crossing over between the two loci is insufficient to lead to independent segregation, does not cause association of the two characters in the general population. In any one sibship the two characters may be associated, in which case the genes are on the same chromosome and are said to be linked in coupling (cis configuration). If the characters are dissociated, the genes responsible are distributed on each of the two homologous chromosomes and are described as being linked in repulsion (trans configuration). A common error is to suppose that the association of two characters in the single sibship implies genetic linkage. If true linkage exists and sufficient pedigrees are collected, an equal number of sibships will be found in which the two characters are not in repulsion. There are several known instances of autosomal linkage in man, including the ABO blood group locus and the locus for the nail-patella syndrome; the Rh blood groups and one form of elliptocytosis; and Lutheran blood group and the secretor locus (which determines whether soluble ABO blood substances are present in saliva and other body fluids). The loci determining the β and δ chains of hemoglobin are also very closely linked (see Ch. 746). The mathematical procedures devised to detect linkage have been greatly aided by the development of computer techniques.

Linkage has one important practical consequence for clinical medicine. If a mutant causing a serious inherited disease is closely linked to one causing a common trait, healthy carriers of the disease may be detected in unaffected members of the family by the presence or absence of the common trait. It would, of course, be important to know whether the two linked genes in the family under investigation were in the coupling or repulsion phase. Accurate information regarding the phase can be obtained by studying the distribution of the two traits in three generations.

The Histocompatibility Locus and Susceptibility to Disease. It is increasingly evident that much of clinical medicine in the coming decades will be concerned with the identification of those individuals who have an enhanced susceptibility to a particular disease. Smoking and lung cancer is the classic example of an environmental determinant of a human disease, whereas a deficiency of serum alpha-1-antitrypsin is an example of a genetic determinant in pulmonary emphysema.

In recent years the major histocompatibility locus (HL-A) has emerged as an important locus which can determine increased susceptibility to disease. There is a high degree of polymorphism at this locus, and a particular allele may determine a particular disease susceptibility.

Acute anterior uveitis, Reiter's syndrome, and ankylosing spondylitis occur in an increased frequency among patients carrying HL-A27. The data on classic ankylosing spondylitis are particularly impressive. In some series, 95 per cent of patients with the disease and 50 per cent of their first-degree relatives possess the antigen. Since the HL-A27 antigen is present in approximately 5 per cent of the normal white population, it can be calculated that ankylosing spondylitis is 20 times more likely to occur in individuals who possess this antigen. Gluten-sensitive enteropathy occurs in a high frequency among patients expressing the histocompatibility antigen HL-A8, and psoriasis among those expressing HL-A13.

The reasons for these associations are not clear; in some instances the HL-A antigen may be related to an antigen of the infecting organism. It is also possible that because of linkage disequilibrium certain alleles at adjacent loci are maintained in coupling. In this way the genes influencing the manifestations of ankylosing spondylitis could remain closely associated with a particular allele at the HL-A locus. The possibility that specific immunoresponse genes may play a decisive role in the etiology of certain diseases has been raised by these observations.

McKusick, V. A.: Human Genetics. 2nd ed. Englewood Cliffs, N. J., Prentice-Hall, 1969.
McKusick, V. A., and Claiborne, R. (eds.): Medical Genetics. New York, HP Publishing Company, 1973.
Nora, J. J., and Fraser, F. C.: Medical Genetics: Principles and Practice. Philadelphia, Lea & Febiger, 1974.
Stern, C.: Principles of Human Genetics. 3rd ed. San Francisco, W. H. Freeman, 1973.

7. INBORN ERRORS OF METABOLISM AND MOLECULAR DISEASE

Alexander G. Bearn

Development of the concept of an inborn error of metabolism by Archibald Garrod in the first decade of this century was one of the most brilliant insights in the history of genetics, for it introduced the seminal hypothesis that the primary action of a gene is to control the synthesis of a specific enzyme. Subsequent work has fully substantiated Garrod's belief that the block in a metabolic pathway arises from an inherited deficiency of a specific enzyme. More recently the term inborn error of metabolism has been extended to include hereditary alterations in proteins that have no enzymatic functions.

The development of precise chemical methods that enable a comparison to be made between normal and genetically altered proteins led to the introduction of the term *molecular disease,* to emphasize that the difference between a normal and an affected individual might reside in the substitution of a single amino acid residue in the primary sequence of a protein molecule. Although the metabolic block may affect protein, carbohydrate, lipid, nucleic acid, porphyrin, or pigment metabolism, the *primary* abnormality invariably lies in the genetic specification of the synthesis of a protein.

In some inborn errors of metabolism the mutational event simply affects the active site of the enzyme. In these instances, although the enzyme will be functionally altered, the presence of cross-reacting material can be detected by immunologic methods. In other instances the mutation results in a protein which is functionally inert, and no cross-reacting material can be detected immunologically. Using the terminology of microbial genetics, the former class of mutants is frequently termed CRM (cross-reacting material) (+) and the latter CRM (−). At the pseudocholinesterase locus, for instance, 17 CRM (+) mutants and 18 CRM (−) mutants have been recognized. In the Lesch-Nyhan syndrome there are 21 CRM (+) mutants, and no CRM (−) have been described. Even when there is no apparent cross-reacting material detectable by immunologic methods, the protein, although no longer recognizable by antisera developed against the normal protein, may be present.

Some of the clinical conditions for which a demonstrated abnormality in a specific protein has been observed are listed in Table 1. In most of these a deficiency in a specific enzymatic activity is demonstrable, whereas in others a normal quantity of a structurally abnormal nonenzymic protein is synthesized. The classic example of a "molecular disease" affecting a nonenzyme is sickle cell anemia, in which the only difference between normal and sickle cell hemoglobin is the substitution of a valine for a glutamic acid in the β chain of hemoglobin.

It is increasingly being recognized that many of the inborn variations in metabolism are unassociated with clinical disease (Table 2). These biochemical variations represent the more conspicuous examples of the importance of human biochemical diversity. In some instances they provide a critical genetic background for the expression of an environmentally controlled disorder; in others the physiologic effect of the genetic variation is not apparent.

Genetic Heterogeneity. It is becoming increasingly axiomatic that identical or closely similar clinical syndromes may be determined by different mutant genes. In some instances, the mutations may be at different loci (nonallelic genes) (Table 3), whereas in others they occur at the same locus (allelic genes). In an individual cistron, genes may be allelic at the same codon (eualleles) or at a different codon (heteroalleles). In hemoglobins S and C the mutations occur at the same codon and are thus examples of eualleles. Hurler's and Scheie's syndromes are examples of heteroalleles, for in these instances the mutations occur at different codons but in the same cistron (see Ch. 934 and 935).

Even before the syndromes of recessive albinism yielded to biochemical probes, it was evident that the two clinical syndromes must be caused by genes at different loci, because it was well known that two albinos may marry and produce normally pigmented offspring. Indeed, it is a safe generalization to assume that the majority of inherited diseases presently regarded as homogeneous entities represent the clinical effects of different mutant genes.

Genetic heterogeneity can be detected at several different levels of biologic organization. Although Hurler's and Hunter's syndromes appear clinically similar, genetic heterogeneity is evident, because family studies indicate that Hurler's syndrome is controlled by a gene on an autosome, whereas in Hunter's syndrome the disease is X-linked. Similar variations exist among the spastic paraplegias: some pedigrees indicate autosomal inheritance, whereas others are clearly X-linked. Genetic heterogeneity can be demonstrated in recessive deaf mutism, and nonallelism can be definitely inferred, because marriage between deaf mutes, as with marriage between albinos, can result in normal offspring. Sometimes genetic heterogeneity can be strongly suspected from examining the clinical spectrum of a disease, as is the case in the various inherited mucopolysaccharidoses. When the syndromes associated with nonspherocytic anemias are examined biochemically, it is evident that they are due to a number of different genes. Heterogeneity among the X-linked hemophilias is strongly suggested as a result of functional and immunologic studies of factor VIII in different families. Heterogeneity is also evident in families exhibiting C'3 esterase deficiency. In some instances "genetic compounds" result in additional phenotypic variation. These genetic compounds arise when the individual carries two different mutant alleles. Hemoglobins S and C are controlled by euallelic genes, and individuals who have hemoglobin SC disease can thus be said to illustrate the phenotypic consequences of a genetic compound (euallelic homozygotes).

Now that it is firmly established that genes control the specificity of particular proteins, genetic heterogeneity can also be detected by techniques that discriminate between closely similar protein molecules. The application of electrophoretic techniques to serum protein and red cell enzymes has disclosed a surprising degree of heterogeneity in normal persons. However, any estimate of genetic heterogeneity based on the application of electrophoretic techniques will be too low, because it seems that less than half the mutational events leading to a specific amino acid substitution will result in an altered net charge of the protein.

Screening for Inborn Errors of Metabolism. The central purpose of any screening program is the detection of in-

TABLE 1. Inborn Errors of Metabolism

Disorder	Primary Defect	Carrier Detection	Prenatal Diagnosis
Amino acid metabolism:			
Phenylketonuria	Phenylalanine hydroxylase	+	
Albinism I	Tyrosinase		
II	?		
Tyrosinemia	p-Hydroxyphenylpyruvate oxidase		
Tyrosinosis	Tyrosine transaminase		
Homocystinuria	Cystathionine synthetase	+	(+)
(a) Pyridoxine responsive			
(b) Pyridoxine unresponsive			
Cystathioninuria	Cystathionase	+	(+)
Alcaptonuria	Homogentisic acid oxidase		
Maple syrup urine disease	Oxidative decarboxylase of branched chain ketoacids	+	+
Intermittent branched-chain ketoaciduria	Oxidative decarboxylase of branched chain ketoacids		(+)
Hypervalinemia	Valine transaminase	+	(+)
Isovaleric acidemia	Isovaleryl-CoA-oxidase		
Beta-hydroxyisovaleric aciduria	Beta-methylcrotonyl-CoA-carboxylase	+	
Methylmalonic aciduria			+
(a) Vitamin B_{12} responsive	Deoxyadenosyl transferase		
(b) Vitamin B_{12} unresponsive	Methylmalonyl-CoA-mutase		
Hyperammonemia I	Carbamyl phosphate synthetase		(+)
II	Ornithine transcarbamylase	+	(+)
Citrullinemia	Argininosuccinic acid synthetase	+	(+)
Argininosuccinicaciduria	Argininosuccinase	+	(+)
Hyperargininemia	Arginase	+	(+)
Hyperlysinemia	Lysine-ketoglutarate reductase		
Saccharopinuria	Aminoadipic semialdehyde–glutamate reductase		
Histidinemia	Histidase	+	
Hyperprolinemia I	Proline oxidase	+	
II	Δ'-pyrroline-5-carboxylate dehydrogenase	+	
Hydroxyprolinemia	Hydroxyproline oxidase (?)		
Glycylprolinuria	?		
Ketotic hyperglycinemia	Propionyl-CoA-carboxylase	+	(+)
Nonketotic hyperglycinemia	Glycine decarboxylase (?)		
Hyper-beta-alaninemia	Beta-alanine-alpha-ketoglutarate amino transferase		
Carnosinemia	Carnosinase		
Hypersarcosinemia	Sarcosine dehydrogenase	+	
Cystinosis	?	+	(+)
Hartnup disease	Tubular reabsorption of monoamino-monocarboxylic acids	+	
Cystinuria (three types)	Transepithelial transport of cystine and dibasic amino acids	+	
Iminoglycinuria	Transport of imino acids and glycine	+	
Carbohydrate metabolism:			
Pentosuria	Xylitol dehydrogenase	+	
Fructosuria	Liver fructokinase		
Fructose intolerance	Fructose-1-phosphate aldolase		
Fructose-1,6-diphosphatase deficiency	Fructose-1,6-diphosphatase	+	
Glycogenosis I	Glucose-6-phosphatase	+	
II	Alpha-1,4-glucosidase	+	+
III	Amylo-1,6-glucosidase	+	(+)
IV	Amylo(1-4 to 1-6)-transglucosidase	+	(+)
V	Muscle phosphorylase		
VI	Liver phosphorylase	+	
VII	Muscle phosphofructokinase	+	
VIII	Liver phosphorylasekinase	+	
Galactosemia	Galactose-1-phosphate uridyl transferase	+	+
Galactokinase deficiency	Galactokinase	+	
Hyperoxaluria I	Alpha-ketoglutarate:glyoxalate carboligase		
II	D-Glyceric dehydrogenase		
Renal glycosuria	?		
Pyruvate decarboxylase deficiency	Pyruvate decarboxylase	+	(+)
Lactase deficiency	Lactase		
Sucrase-isomaltase deficiency	Sucrase, isomaltase		
Glucose-galactose malabsorption	?	+	
Hurler's syndrome	Alpha-L-iduronidase	+	(+)
Hunter's syndrome	Sulfoiduronate sulfatase	+	(+)
Sanfilippo's syndrome A	Heparan sulfate sulfatase		
B	N-acetyl-alpha-glucosaminidase		
Morquio's syndrome	?		
Scheie's syndrome	Alpha-L-iduronidase		
Maroteaux-Lamy syndrome	?		
I-cell disease	?		
Mannosidosis	Alpha-mannosidase		(+)
Fucosidosis	Alpha-1-fucosidase		(+)
Gaucher's disease (three types)	Glucocerebrosidase	+	+
Globoid cell leukodystrophy	Galactocerebroside Beta-galactosidase	+	+

(*Table continues on following page.*)

TABLE 1. Inborn Errors of Metabolism (*Continued*)

Disorder	Primary Defect	Carrier Detection	Prenatal Diagnosis
Lipid metabolism:			
Hyperlipoproteinemia	Lipoprotein lipase	+	
Hypercholesterolemia	?		
Hypertriglyceridemia	?		
Combined hyperlipidemia	?		
Abetalipoproteinemia	Betalipoproteins		
Hypobetalipoproteinemia	Low density lipoproteins		
Tangier disease	Alpha lipoproteins	+	
Norum disease	Lecithin:cholesterol acetyl transferase		
Gangliosidosis GM$_1$ (types I and II)	Beta galactosidase	+	+
Gangliosidosis GM$_2$ (Tay-Sachs)	Hexosaminidase A	+	+
Gangliosidosis GM$_2$ (Sandhoff)	Hexosaminidase A and B	+	+
Fabry's disease	Ceramide trihexosidase	+	+
Metachromatic leukodystrophy I	Arylsulfatase A	+	+
II	Arylsulfatase A, B, C, and steroid sulfatase	+	
Lactosylceramidosis	Lactosylceramidase		
Niemann-Pick disease	Sphingomyelinase		+
Wolman's disease	Acid lipase		
Cholesterylester storage disease	?		
Cerebrotendinous xanthomatosis	?		
Refsum's disease	Phytanic acid alpha hydroxylase	+	(+)
Nucleic acid metabolism:			
Gout	?		
Lesch-Nyhan syndrome	Hypoxanthine-guanine phosphoribosyl transferase		+
Hyperuricemia	Adenine phosphoribosyl transferase	+	
Xanthinuria	Xanthine oxidase		
Xanthurenic aciduria	Kynureninase		
Orotic aciduria I	Orotidylic pyrophosphorylase and decarboxylase	+	(+)
II	Orotidylic decarboxylase		
Xeroderma pigmentosum	UV-specific endonuclease		
Porphyrin and heme metabolism:			
Erythropoietic porphyria	Uroporphyrinogen-III cosynthetase	+	(+)
Acute intermittent porphyria	Uroporphyrinogen-I synthetase	+	
Porphyria variegata	?		
Coproporphyria	?		
Porphyria cutanea tarda	?		
Protoporphyria	?		
Crigler-Najjar syndrome (two types)	Glucuronyltransferase		
Gilbert's syndrome	Bilirubin uptake		
Dubin-Johnson syndrome	Bilirubin excretion		
Erythrocyte metabolism:			
Hemolytic anemia	Pyruvate kinase	+	
	Hexokinase	+	
	Glucosephosphate isomerase	+	
	Triosephosphate isomerase	+	
	2,3-Diphosphoglyceromutase	+	
	Phosphoglycerate kinase	+	
	Glucose-6-phosphate dehydrogenase	+	(+)
	6-Phosphogluconate dehydrogenase		
	Glutathione reductase		
	Glutathione peroxidase		
	Glutathione synthetase		
Methemoglobinemia	NADH-methemoglobin reductase	+	
Leukocyte metabolism:			
Myeloperoxidase deficiency	Myeloperoxidase	+	
Chronic granulomatous disease	?	+	
Chédiak-Higashi syndrome	?	+	

(Table continues on opposite page.)

dividuals in whom it is likely that a specific hereditary disease will develop and against which preventive or therapeutic measures are potentially available. Screening for genetic diseases can be performed at three principal phenotypic levels. In many instances the recognition of overt clinical disease represents the only phenotypic level at which the inborn error can be recognized. Thus in Huntington's chorea no biochemical abnormality has been found to be characteristic of the disease, and early recognition of signs and symptoms represents the only means to arrive at a diagnosis. Early diagnosis of polyposis of the colon is important because of the frequency of malignant transformation. The recognition of genital abnormalities at birth in females may aid in early detection of the adrenogenital syndrome. Inborn errors can also be recognized by the presence of an abnormal metabolite in physiologic fluids. The enzymatic deficiency may lead to an accumulation of the substrate

TABLE 1. Inborn Errors of Metabolism (*Continued*)

Disorder	Primary Defect	Carrier Detection	Prenatal Diagnosis
Abnormalities of plasma proteins:			
Analbuminemia	Albumin		
Atransferrinemia	Transferrin		
Afibrinogenemia	Fibrinogen		
Alpha₁-antitrypsin deficiency	Alpha₁-antitrypsin	+	
Acatalasia	Catalase	+	(+)
Suxamethonium sensitivity	Pseudocholinesterase		
Hereditary angioedema	C1̄-inhibitor		
C1q deficiency	C1q		
C1r deficiency	C1r		
C2 deficiency	C2		
C3 deficiency	C3		
X-linked agammaglobulinemia	?		
Severe combined immunodeficiency	Adenosine deaminase (?)		
Selective IgA deficiency	?		
X-linked immunodeficiency with increased IgM	?		
Hemophilia A	Factor VIII	+	
Hemophilia B	Factor IX	+	
von Willebrand's disease	?		
Hageman trait	Factor XII	+	
PTA deficiency	Factor XI	+	
Parahemophilia	Factor V	+	
Hypoprothrombinemia	Factor II	+	
Factor VII deficiency	Factor VII	+	
Factor X deficiency	Factor X	+	
Fibrin-stabilizing factor deficiency	Factor XIII	+	
Hormone and vitamin metabolism:			
Adrenogenital syndrome	21-Hydroxylase		+
	11-Hydroxylase		
	3-Beta-hydroxysteroiddehydrogenase		
	17-Hydroxylase		
	Desmolase		
Aldosterone deficiency	18-Hydroxylase		
Familial goiter	Iodide transport		
	Peroxidase		
	Iodotyrosine coupling		
	Iodotyrosine deiodinase		
	Thyroglobulin synthesis		
Renal diabetes insipidus	?	+	
Vitamin D dependent rickets	25-Hydroxycholecalciferol-1-hydroxylase		
Formiminotransferase deficiency	Formiminotransferase		
Miscellaneous:			
Cystic fibrosis	?		
Wilson's disease	?	+	
Hemochromatosis	?		
Menkes' kinky hair syndrome	Intestinal copper absorption		
Sulfite oxidase deficiency	Sulfite oxidase deficiency		
Hypophosphatasia	Alkaline phosphatase (?)		
Lysosomal acid phosphatase deficiency	Acid phosphatase	+	+
Renal tubular acidosis I	Gradient defect		
II	Bicarbonate wastage		

(+) = Prenatal diagnosis may prove to be possible, because the defect is expressed in cell culture.

for the reaction catalyzed by the normal enzyme and to a deficiency of the product. An increased level of blood galactose in galactosemia and of phenylalanine in phenylketonuria are examples in which the disturbance of the normal metabolic relationships leads to detection of disease.

Since genes control the synthesis of proteins, the most direct way of identifying an inborn error is to utilize a screening program which detects a qualitative change in the structure of the protein, e.g., electrophoretically, or by its altered enzymatic or immunologic activity. Mass screening for inborn errors of metabolism in the general population is expensive and time consuming, and a careful estimate of the cost of such a program must be balanced against the potential gains. When this is done, the cost for most countries would seem to be prohibitive. For the moment it seems wiser to focus on those families and populations who are particularly at risk and for whom effective therapy for the inborn errors of metabolism is available. Screening for Tay-Sachs disease among Ashkenazic Jews and sickle cell hemoglobin among black populations are examples of screening programs which, when carefully carried out, can be of undoubted benefit. Amniocentesis and expanding usefulness of cultured fibroblasts to identify certain inborn errors of metabolism before birth can be expected to increase sharply in the years ahead and will increase the usefulness of screening programs.

TABLE 2. A Selection of Common Inherited Polymorphisms

Blood groups, e.g., ABO, MNS, Rh
Leukocyte groups
Platelet groups
Histocompatibility antigens (HL-A system)
Hemoglobin (α, β, γ, δ-chains)
Myoglobin
Serum proteins:
    Albumin
    Alpha$_1$-antitrypsin
    Group-specific component (Gc)
    Haptoglobin (α, β-chains)
    Ceruloplasmin
    Alpha$_2$-macroglobulin (Xm)
    Complement (C3, C4)
    Beta-lipoprotein (Ag-, Ld-, Lp- types)
    Transferrin
    Fibrinogen
    Immunoglobulins (Am, Gm, InV)
Enzymes:
    Glucose-6-phosphate dehydrogenase
    Phosphoglucomutase (PGM 1, 2, 3)
    Phosphohexoseisomerase
    Lactate dehydrogenase
    Adenine phosphoribosyl transferase
    Hypoxanthine-guanine phosphoribosyl transferase
    Peptidases (A, B, C, D, E)
    Pseudocholinesterase (E1, E2)
    Amylase
Phenylthiocarbamide testing
Beta-aminoisobutyric aciduria
Color blindness

TABLE 3. Some Illustrative Examples of Genetic Diseases Showing Nonallelic Heterogeneity

Albinism
Cystic fibrosis
Deafness
Diabetes insipidus, neurohypophyseal type
Osteogenesis imperfecta
Pituitary dwarfism
Retinitis pigmentosa
Sanfilippo's syndrome A and B

Harris, H.: The Principles of Human Biochemical Genetics. *In* Neuberger, A., and Tatum, E. L. (eds.): Frontiers of Biology. Vol. 19. New York, American Elsevier Publishing Company, 1970.
McKusick, V. A.: Mendelian Inheritance in Man: Catalogs of Autosomal Dominant, Autosomal Recessive, and X-linked Phenotypes. 4th ed. Baltimore. The Johns Hopkins Press, 1975.

8. POLYGENIC AND MULTIFACTORIAL INHERITANCE

Alexander G. Bearn

Traits determined by the collaboration of many genes at different loci are called polygenic, in contrast to those traits which are determined by a single gene (monogenic). Most of the differences among normal people are determined by the interaction of many genetic and environmental factors (multifactorial inheritance).

Polygenic inheritance, in which many genes each contribute a minor effect, is best established for those traits which show continuous variation in the form of a "normal" distribution curve. Height is an example of a polygenic (and multifactorial) trait in which the extremes

of the normal distribution are not considered abnormal. The degree of resemblance among relatives can be deduced from the number of genes they share in common. Dizygotic twins, however, will have 50 per cent of their genes in common, as will all sibs. Parents and children also have 50 per cent of their genes in common. Thus it would be expected that if one parent is 6'0" and the other 5'6", all the children, on the average, would be 5'9". Polygenic models have been advanced for inheritance of high blood pressure, diabetes mellitus, and rheumatoid arthritis, as well as a variety of congenital defects.

In clinical medicine polygenic and multifactorial inheritance should be suspected when the disease under consideration is "known to run in families," and when, in addition, examination of the affected and unaffected sibs in any sibship does not support inheritance in a simple dominant or recessive fashion. When this occurs, it is reasonable to suspect that within such families a large number of "risk genes" are present. "Risk genes" are of course present in the normal population, but in low frequency. If in any one individual there is a particularly large number of high "risk genes," the latent disorder becomes overt. This phenomenon is known as the "threshold effect" (Fig. 6). When examining a pedigree for a possible polygenic inheritance pattern, it is worth remembering that polygenic inheritance becomes more likely if in the empiric risk figure for the disease the frequency of affected sibs increases with the number of affected sibs already born. This latter fact is particularly important in genetic counseling. The elegance and complexity of the mathematical models advanced for polygenic-multifactorial disease should not obscure the fact that each of the "risk genes" has, like any other gene, a specific biochemical consequence. Eventually,

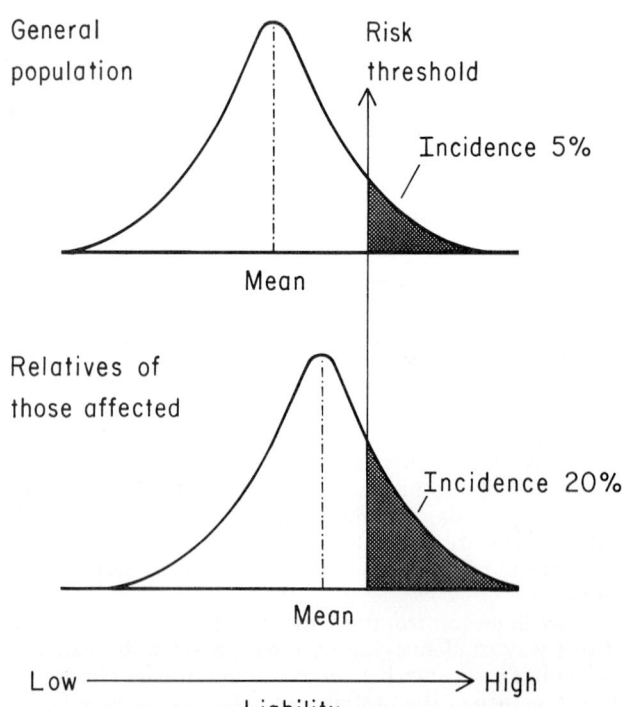

Figure 6. Diseases which conform to a polygenic multifactorial model of inheritance lead to an increased incidence of disease among the relatives of affected individuals. This increased incidence is related to the lowering of the "risk threshold" and is most evident among close relatives (sibs, uncle-niece, first cousins).

the vague concept of genetic susceptibility of polygenic inheritance must yield to the central dogma that genes control the synthesis of specific proteins each of which has specific enzymatic functions.

Carter, C. O.: Genetics of common disorders. Br. Med. Bull., 25:52, 1969.

9. PHARMACOGENETICS

Alexander G. Bearn

It has long been recognized that certain people respond unusually to the administration of specific drugs. In some instances the altered reaction has an immunologic basis, in others it appears to be idiosyncratic without obvious cause; and in some the difference appears to be contingent on the genetic constitution of the host. Pharmacogenetics is concerned with those deviant responses to specific drugs that are genetically determined. The breakdown and disposal of drugs in the body are usually dependent on a series of specific gene-controlled enzymatic reactions. Mutant genes in the population that alter these reactions can result in serious clinical consequences.

Inherited Diseases Discovered or Precipitated by the Use of Drugs. Several diseases have been disclosed or precipitated as a direct result of the administration of drugs which for their proper metabolic disposal require an intact enzyme system. In the absence of pharmacologic overload, the defective enzyme system does not cause disease.

Glucose-6-Phosphate Dehydrogenase Deficiency. A severe hemolytic anemia (favism) may be produced by the ingestion of the broad bean *Vicia fava.* The anemia is due to deficiency of the X-linked enzyme glucose-6-phosphate dehydrogenase in the erythrocytes of susceptible subjects (see Glucose-6-Phosphate Dehydrogenase in Ch. 740). It is of interest that a deficiency of the enzyme is a necessary but not sufficient cause for the anemia that follows ingestion of fava beans. Additional genetic factors, presently poorly identified, are also required if the disease is to be manifest. Severe neonatal jaundice in the Mediterranean basin and Far East may occasionally be associated with glucose-6-phosphate dehydrogenase deficiency.

Persons with glucose-6-phosphate dehydrogenase deficiency are particularly susceptible to hemolytic reactions after administration of the antimalarial drug primaquine and certain other drugs, including aspirin and phenacetin. The mutation in the black population is characterized by a mean enzyme activity of 10 to 20 per cent of normal, and the increased susceptibility to hemolysis is restricted to the older red cells. The risk of hemolysis is significantly less than in the Mediterranean type of glucose-6-phosphate dehydrogenase deficiency in which the residual enzymatic activity is less than 5 per cent of normal and increased susceptibility to hemolysis occurs in young as well as old cells. Interestingly, a severe hemolytic anemia may occur during the course of acute viral hepatitis and infectious mononucleosis in individuals with deficiency of glucose-6-phosphate dehydrogenase. The trait is present in about 10 per cent of blacks in the United States and may reach as high as 35 per cent in certain African and Mediterranean popula-

tions. The deficiency provides some protection against falciparum malaria and accounts for the persistence of the gene at a very high level in these populations. The relationship of glucose-6-phosphate dehydrogenase deficiency and resistance to falciparum malaria affords one of the better examples of a balanced polymorphism in which a heterozygous advantage can be clearly demonstrated.

Isoniazid. When a group of individuals is given a standard dose of the antituberculosis drug isoniazid (INH), two subpopulations can be identified. In one group the blood level of isoniazid is high and very little acetylated INH is excreted in the urine (slow inactivators), whereas in the second group the blood isoniazid is considerably lower and acetylated INH appears in the urine in large quantities (rapid inactivators). Twin studies show a similar metabolic response in monozygotic twins, whereas notable differences are apparent in dizygotic twins. Pedigree analysis indicates that the capacity to acetylate isoniazid is inherited as a simple recessive trait. The "slow inactivators" lack the liver enzyme N-acetyltransferase present in "rapid inactivators." Although it is clinically reassuring that rapid acetylators show an impairment of the antituberculosis effect of the drug, slow acetylators are more likely to encounter undesirable side effects such as peripheral neuropathy, a mischance which can be avoided if pyridoxine is administered concomitantly. It is of some clinical importance that the absence of the acetylating enzyme also makes more likely the toxic effects of the antiepileptic drug phenelzine and the antihypertensive agent hydralazine, because both these agents are acetylated by N-acetyltransferase.

The gene determining N-acetyltransferase deficiency occurs in 60 per cent of the black and white populations, but in only 10 per cent of Eskimo and Japanese populations. This polymorphism is of particular interest, because the aberrant gene has no clinical effect unless drugs which require acetylation for their metabolism are administered.

Suxamethonium (Succinylcholine). Suxamethonium is a commonly employed short-acting muscle relaxant. Its short action is due to the rapidly inactivating influence of the serum enzyme cholinesterase. Genetic variants of the enzyme are known which fail to hydrolyze suxamethonium and as a consequence cause a prolonged, but fortunately rarely fatal, apnea. This increased sensitivity to suxamethonium occurs in about 1 in 3000 patients and can be caused by a large number of different alleles at the pseudocholinesterase locus.

Hemoglobin Zürich and Other Drug-Sensitive Hemoglobins. The red cells from patients with the unstable hemoglobins (Zürich, Shepherd's Bush, and Torino) exhibit an unusual tendency to hemolysis when exposed to certain drugs. The sulfonamides are particular offenders, but all drugs which cause hemolysis in patients with glucose-6-phosphate deficiency may be potentially harmful.

Anticoagulant Resistance. Two families have been reported in which some members are extremely resistant to warfarin and other coumarin congeners. Approximately ten times the usual dose of warfarin was needed to increase the prothrombin time to an expected level. This provides an example in which resistance to a drug is genetically determined. The frequency of the trait is undoubtedly rare.

Glaucoma. Repeated instillation of glucocorticoids

into the eye is followed by an increase in intraocular pressure. The ocular response is controlled by a pair of allelic genes. Those individuals, perhaps 5 per cent of the population, who have an unusually brisk response to the instillation of glucocorticoids are particularly liable to develop glaucoma.

Porphyria. The well known sensitivity of individuals with porphyria to barbiturates, particularly the short-acting compound thiopental (thiopentone), is a classic example of a genetically determined altered response to a drug.

Malignant Hyperthermia. This is an autosomal dominantly inherited condition causing a frequently fatal hyperthermia associated with muscle rigidity that may follow the administration of anesthetic agents such as halothane, succinylcholine, or methoxyflurane. It is particularly important to inform affected individuals that half of their first-degree relatives are at a similar risk. This condition occurs in 1 out of 20,000 anesthetized patients.

Vesell, E. S.: Advances in pharmacogenetics. *In* Steinberg, A. G., and Bearn, A. G. (eds.): Progress in Medical Genetics. Vol. 9. New York, Grune & Stratton, 1973, p. 291.

10. POPULATION GENETICS

Alexander G. Bearn

Gene Frequency. Although genes are expressed in individuals, it is often of interest to consider the distribution of mutant genes in the general population. The basis of population genetics is the Hardy-Weinberg law, which was formulated in a context of concern that a dominant trait would eventually displace a normal trait in the population. In particular, it arose in response to the fallacious assertion that if brachydactyly is a dominant trait, then "in the course of time, one would expect in the absence of counteracting factors to get three brachydactylous persons to one normal."

If the frequency of a particular gene A is p, then its alternate allele a is $(1-p)=q$; the population will consist of individuals of three genotypes: those who are homozygous AA, those who are heterozygous Aa, and those who are homozygous aa. The frequency of these genotypes in a randomly mating population will be in the proportion p^2 (AA), 2pq (Aa), and q^2 (aa). One important consequence of this formulation is that whatever the initial frequency of the genes A and a in the population, the proportion of the three genotypes will tend to remain constant during succeeding generations, providing that the three genotypes are equally fertile. If the mating in the population is not random or if there is not equal viability of the three genotypes, the frequency calculations require considerable adjustment, and in small populations substantial changes in gene frequency may occur simply as a matter of chance.

The Hardy-Weinberg law has a very useful practical consequence. If the frequency of a recessive disease in a particular population is known, the frequency of heterozygous carriers as well as the frequency of the abnormal gene can be calculated. Thus for a recessively inherited disease aa (q^2) with a frequency of 1 per 10,000, the

frequency of the gene a (q) will be the square root of 1/10,000 or 1/100. The frequency of heterozygous carriers will be $2 \times p \times q = 2 \times 99/100 \times 1/100$ or approximately 1/50. Thus for this particular inherited disease there will be 200 clinically unaffected carriers of the abnormal gene in the population for every affected individual. Cystic fibrosis of the pancreas, the most frequent recessively inherited disease in the white population, has a frequency of approximately 1 in 2500 (q^2); thus the frequency of heterozygous carriers is approximately 1 in 25 (2pq).

Mutation and Selection. A mutation is a stable heritable change in the genetic material. This change may affect a single locus, or it may consist of chromosome breakage with loss or rearrangement of the fragments. In molecular terms a point mutation can be regarded as an alteration, addition, or deletion of one of the bases of the DNA molecule. The simplest mutational event is the substitution of one nucleotide for another in the DNA sequence. Although this usually results in the substitution of one amino acid for another in the polypeptide chain (e.g., glutamic acid at position 6 of the beta polypeptide chain is replaced by valine in hemoglobin S), it is not invariable, because several different triplets can code for the same amino acid. Mutations which either insert or delete nucleotide into the genetic code usually cause more extensive substitutions in the polypeptide synthesis than single nucleotide substitutions. It will be recalled that the genetic code is read as successive triplets; an insertion or deletion will upset the regularity of the triplets, and the translation of the code into amino acids distal to the point of insertion or deletion will be altered. From what is known about the genetic code, about 75 per cent of mutations will result in a single base change, resulting in the substitution of one amino acid for another; about 20 per cent of the mutations will be synonymous, in which the base change in the codon does not change the amino acid specified; and in about 5 per cent the base triplet change will result in a nonsense triplet, leading to a chain termination and the synthesis of a polypeptide lacking a variable portion of its carboxyl terminal amino acid sequence. The effect of a mutation in a somatic cell is restricted to the life of an individual, whereas mutation in the germ line can be transmitted to future generations. The natural mutation rate can be greatly increased by x-rays, ultraviolet rays, increased temperature, and various chemical mutagens such as nitrogen mustard, ethylene sulfonate, and 5-bromouracil. Chemical mutagens are thought to achieve their effects by direct structural modification of a purine or pyrimidine base, or by substitution of a base analogue for one of the normal bases.

The germinal mutation rate is usually expressed as the number of mutations per locus per generation. The average spontaneous mutation rate is usually expressed as the number of mutations per locus per generation. The average spontaneous mutation rate for a number of autosomal, recessive, and X-linked traits is 3×10^{-5}. One common, often unavoidable, error in estimating mutation rates in man is the failure to recognize that indistinguishable clinical syndromes can be caused by different genes (see Genetic Heterogeneity in Ch. 7). Thus the frequencies deduced by the elegant studies of Haldane on mutation rate for hemophilia must be revised downward, because Christmas disease, another bleeding disorder determined by a gene on the X chromosome, had not been discovered when the original calculations were made. Since heterogeneity appears to be the rule in inherited disease, all estimates of mutation rate are likely to be high. Nonhereditary conditions which mimic mutations are termed phenocopies and will also lead to overestimation of mutation rates. Spontaneous mutation rates tend to increase with advancing age. The occurrence of new mutations for chondrodystrophy is almost linearly related to paternal age. It is approximately three times more likely for a chondrodystrophic child to be born of unaffected parents if the father is 45 years of age or older than if he is 25 years old.

The frequency of most genes in the population is relatively stable. When a gene is rare and severely disadvantageous, the mutation rate is balanced by the elimination of the disadvantageous gene by natural selection. The frequency of the disadvantageous gene, however, can be stabilized at a high level if the heterozygotes are slightly favored and leave a greater number of progeny than either homozygote. The concept of *balanced polymorphism* has been defined as the existence of two or more discontinuous forms of a species in such proportion that the rarest of them cannot be maintained at its frequency in the population by recurrent mutation. As a general proposition, if the rarer of the two allelic forms occurs in a frequency that is greater than 1 per cent, the existence of balanced polymorphism should be entertained. An example of such a balanced polymorphism is the increased resistance of individuals heterozygous for sickle cell trait to falciparum malaria. Although patients with sickle cell disease (homozygotes) usually die before they can reproduce and thus cannot transmit the gene to the next generation, the incidence of the sickle cell trait may reach 40 per cent in certain West African populations. Theoretically, the high frequency of the sickle cell gene could be maintained if the heterozygote were 25 per cent more fit than the so-called normal homozygote. It has now been shown unequivocally that death from falciparum malaria is much less frequent in carriers of the sickle cell trait than in noncarriers, and thus the heterozygote does have an advantage. How much of the advantage is due to differential mortality and how much to differential fertility is uncertain, but this example serves to emphasize that the effect of genes can be assessed only in relation to a particular environment. It is, however, being slowly appreciated that the example of balanced polymorphism provided by the advantage to individuals heterozygous for the sickle cell trait may be atypical. In most instances a distinct advantage for the heterozygote cannot be demonstrated, and the possibility that certain polymorphic traits are genetically neutral is becoming increasingly discussed.

Muller introduced the term *genetic load* to describe the total genetic disability of a population. It is composed of the *mutational load,* the load caused by recurrent mutations from a normal to a lethal or sublethal gene, and the *segregational load,* which is due to the segregation of harmful genes from favorable heterozygotes. The sickle cell gene is maintained in the population because of its heterozygous advantage, and thus contributes to the segregational load. It has been estimated that, on the average, each person has three to six genes which, if homozygous instead of heterozygous, would be lethal. The relative contribution of the segregational and mutational loads to the total load is unsettled.

Stern, C.: Principles of Human Genetics. 3rd ed. San Francisco, W. H. Freeman and Company, 1973.

11. HEREDITY AND ENVIRONMENT

Alexander G. Bearn

To disentangle the relative importance of genetic and environmental influences in the causation of disease is an important but frequently difficult undertaking. In many diseases, the genetic influences are major and environmental influences are trivial, whereas in others the environment plays a major role and the genetic constitution is unimportant. For example, the genetic constitution is solely responsible for the appearance of erythrocyte antigens, the environment being without detectable influence. Many of the inborn errors of metabolism are determined by a single gene that is necessary for their expression. However, the phenotypic expression of genetic diseases such as phenylketonuria and galactosemia can be impressively influenced by alteration of the diet.

Paradoxically, the greatest difficulty in assessing relative roles of genetic and environmental influences is encountered with the common diseases of man. In disorders such as essential hypertension, coronary artery disease, and schizophrenia several genes influence the disease, but environmental factors are also highly relevant. It is important to recognize that a familial concentration of cases will be expected even when the trait is multifactorially inherited. If the frequency of a multifactorially determined trait is n, it can be shown that the frequency of the trait in first-degree relatives (parents and sibs) will be approximately $\sqrt{n}$. Although in many infections the environmental agent is crucial, the importance of the genotype of the host should not be discounted. It seems likely that, in the past, infectious diseases were powerful selective agents, and the ability to survive epidemic disasters was probably dependent, at least in part, on the individual's genotype.

Comparative studies of identical and nonidentical twins, although traditionally regarded as being of great pertinence, have not enabled sharp distinctions between hereditary and environmental influences to be drawn. Even when identical twins are reared apart, they have shared a similar environment before birth, and dogmatic conclusions are treacherous. Nevertheless, with proper regard for their limitations, studies on twins are frequently informative.

More recently, the traditional if somewhat specious nature-nurture polemic has been illuminated by fundamental studies on gene regulation. Evidence has now accumulated which suggests that, at any given time, as much as 80 per cent of the genetic material in the cells of higher organisms is inactive. This inactivation can be reversed by certain environmental influences, and the previously inactive genes can be restored to activity. Certain steroid hormones possess the capacity to influence gene activity, and a number of these have now been shown to influence directly the synthesis of mRNA and tRNA. Indeed, the administration of estrogen to a rooster can activate genes in the rooster's liver cells so that they synthesize egg yolk proteins—proteins more useful to the molecular biologist than to the rooster.

McKusick, V. A.: Human Genetics, 2nd ed. Englewood Cliffs, N. J., Prentice-Hall, 1969.

Stern, C.: Principles of Human Genetics. 3rd ed. San Francisco, W. H. Freeman and Company, 1973.

12. CONGENITAL MALFORMATIONS

Alexander G. Bearn

The term congenital malformation is usually applied to important structural defects present at birth that are not caused by a birth injury. The relative importance of congenital malformation has increased as more effective control has been exercised over the environmental agents of disease. In 1900, in the United States, approximately 3.3 per cent of the total infant mortality could be ascribed to congenital malformations, whereas in 1964 congenital malformations accounted for 25 per cent of the total infant mortality. During the first 15 years of life congenital malformations are responsible for approximately 15 per cent of the annual death rate. It has also been estimated that 7 per cent of children have a congenital malformation of consequence recognizable by the age of one year, yet only 43 per cent of such malformations are detectable at birth. In most malformations no major etiologic factor can be identified, and it must be presumed that their existence depends on complicated interactions of genetic and environmental influences or on particular genetic combinations. The frequency of many congenital malformations is compatible with a polygenic model with a threshold beyond which there is a risk of malformation. First-degree relatives (sibs and children) of an individual with a congenital malformation are at greater risk than members of the general population. This is because first-degree relatives will have a curve of distribution of high risk genes approximately halfway between the general population and those affected. The first-degree relatives of a patient with cleft lip and cleft palate are approximately 40 times more likely to develop the malformation than the population at large. The approximate frequency and sex ratio of the major malformations per 1000 births are illustrated in Table 4.

Genetic Factors. With the exception of mongolism (trisomy 21), relatively few congenital malformations can be ascribed to specific genes or autosomal chromosomal abnormalities. Congenital hydrocephalus is occasionally inherited in an X-linked fashion. Congenital pyloric stenosis is five times more frequent in males, and hare lip and cleft palate twice as common. Congenital dislocation of the hip and spina bifida are more frequent in females. Twin studies and pedigree patterns seldom provide any useful genetic information in the common malformations. The offspring of consanguineous marriages show a slight increase in the frequency of congenital malformations.

Environmental Factors. Contrary to popular belief, there is little direct evidence that environmental factors such as viral diseases, maternal ingestion of drugs, or maternal irradiation makes a significant contribution to the *common* malformations, although each of these factors materially increases the frequency of certain *specific* malformations. Recent evidence suggests that approximately 70 per cent of mothers exposed to rubella during the first trimester give birth to children with severe congenital defects, including cataracts, deafness, heart disease, and neonatal thrombocytopenic purpura.

Some evidence indicates that first-born children are more likely to have a congenital defect than later children. This is particularly true of anencephaly, congenital dislocation of the hip, talipes equinovarus, and pyloric stenosis. Striking regional differences in the incidence of congenital defects have been recognized, and have been well documented for anencephaly and spina bifida. An increased frequency of congenital dislocation of the hip in Lapps and certain American Indians is well recognized. An inexplicable but marked seasonal variation in the incidence of certain malformations has also been reported. It has been estimated that nearly one third of the pregnancies complicated by hydramnios result in congenital malformations.

The risk that a congenital malformation will recur with subsequent pregnancies depends on the specific abnormality and its cause. For the three most common neurologic malformations, anencephaly, hydrocephalus, and spina bifida, the recurrence rate in subsequent children is approximately 4 per cent after the first malformation, but much higher after two malformations. If it is recalled that the recurrence rate for a simple recessively inherited disease is 25 per cent, the role of genetic factors in congenital malformation can be put in perspective.

Drug-Induced Embryopathy. Fetal malformations can be regarded as the consequence of developmental unpunctuality, and are liable to follow environmental insults during the first three months of fetal life. There is growing evidence that errors in embryonic development are particularly likely to arise between the sixth and eighth weeks. It is therefore clearly prudent to minimize frivolous medication during the first three months of pregnancy. The importance of drugs as possible etiologic agents in congenital malformations has been emphasized, and perhaps overemphasized, by the thalidomide tragedy. Indeed, it is virtually impossible to specify a drug that will *not* result in an increased frequency of congenital malformations when administered to a sufficiently large panel of different laboratory animals. To assume that a drug that causes a congenital malformation in one species will necessarily cause one in man is as misguided as to assume that if a drug is harmless in animals, it will be harmless in man. It is certainly worth emphasizing that had thalidomide merely increased the frequency of a common malformation, such as cleft lip or cleft palate, rather than the strikingly tragic malformation of phocomelia ("seal extremities"), the causal association might still be unrecognized. During the two- to three-year period during which thalidomide (alphaphthalimidoglutarimide) was freely available, approximately 7000 infants throughout the world were born

TABLE 4. Approximate Frequency and Sex Ratio of Common Congenital Malformations

Malformation	Frequency/1000 Births (Range)*	M:F
Congenital heart disease	4.5 (1.0–10.0)	1:1
Pyloric stenosis	4.0 (0.5–4.0)	4:1
Talipes equinovarus	1.8 (0.6–6.8)	2:1
Myelomeningocele	1.5 (0.5–4.4)	1:1
Down's syndrome (mongolism)	1.6	1:1
Hydrocephalus†	1.2 (0.3–4.2)	1:1‡
Anencephaly	1.0 (0.1–7.0)	1:2
Congenital dislocated hip	1.0 (0.5–60.0)	1:6
Cleft lip ± cleft palate	1.0 (0.5–4.0)	2:1
Klinefelter's syndrome	1.0	1:0

*Reported range in various studies and populations.
†Without spina bifida.
‡Excluding X-linked recessive hydrocephalus.

with thalidomide-induced deformities. Only thalidomide, the antitumor drug aminopterin (4-aminopteroyl glutamate), and progesterone, administered during pregnancy, have been reported to be definitely teratogenic to man.

Warkany, J.: Congenital Malformations. Chicago, Year Book Medical Publishers, 1971.

CHROMOSOMES AND THEIR DISORDERS

Park Gerald

13. INTRODUCTION

Modern human cytogenetics began in 1956, when Tjio and Levan employed techniques that had been created for use with other organisms to demonstrate the presence of 46 chromosomes (23 pairs) in cultured human fibroblasts. The field became of major medical importance with the observation in 1959 that an additional chromosome was present in patients with Down's syndrome (mongolism). It was soon thereafter brought to clinical maturity when simple means were discovered for obtaining chromosome preparations with cultured leukocytes from peripheral blood.

Modern cytogenetics entered its second and present period of growth with the introduction of a fluorescent stain which permitted identification of each of the 22 pairs of non-sex chromosomes (autosomes) as well as the 2 sex chromosomes (XX in the female and XY in the male). Additional staining procedures have since been developed which provide further evidence for the uniqueness of each chromosome pair and even of individual regions within chromosomes.

Frequency of Chromosomal Abnormalities. Chromosomal abnormalities occur with greatly different frequencies at various times in life. The highest frequency and the greatest variety are found among spontaneous abortuses, 30 to 40 per cent of whom have a major chromosomal defect. Among liveborn infants, about 6 per 1000 have a chromosomal defect sufficiently severe to cause disability at some time in their lives. About half of these abnormalities involve the autosomes, whereas the remainder are sex chromosomal disorders. Among adults in the general population, the abnormalities are largely confined to the sex chromosomal disorders.

There are clinically definable subgroups within these population segments that have an increased risk for a chromosomal disorder. Infants with multiple congenital defects, for example, have a 5 to 10 per cent probability of possessing a major autosomal abnormality. The occurrence in a family of individuals with a similar group of congenital malformations is often the result of an inheritable chromosomal disorder. Such families may also have an increased number of spontaneous abortions. Sex chromosomal disorders occur with increased frequency among infertile males and among women with primary amenorrhea. They are also found to be unusually frequent among males incarcerated in penal institutions.

Preparation of Cells for Chromosomal Analysis. The chromosomes in the nondividing (interphase) cell are so extended and intertwined that they cannot be individually distinguished. During cell division (mitosis), however, they become greatly condensed and are then visible as separate entities. Dividing cells can be arrested in that phase of mitosis (metaphase) at which the chromosomes are most contracted by treatment with colchicine. By the use of colchicine and by swelling the cells in hypotonic solution to increase the separation of the chromosomes, preparations can be produced in which each chromosome is clearly visible.

Dividing cells can be obtained directly from bone marrow or by culturing a small piece of skin. The procedure required for obtaining either of these specimens, however, is unpleasant for the patient. In addition, skin cells must be cultured for several weeks before a sufficient number of dividing cells is present. Fortunately, the normally nondividing leukocyte from peripheral blood can be stimulated to divide when exposed to phytohemagglutinin (PHA). PHA appears to act only on lymphocytes (specifically, thymus-dependent lymphocytes). Stimulated lymphocytes undergo a transient wave of mitosis that reaches a peak in three to four days. By a combination of PHA, colchicine, and hypotonic treatments, suitable chromosome preparations can be obtained from a few drops of capillary blood.

In view of the simplicity of the procedure, most chromosomal analyses are now carried out with peripheral blood specimens. Bone marrow cells may nonetheless be used in the study of diseases, such as myelogenous leukemia, which are confined to these cells. Skin cells may be examined when a difference between the skin cell and lymphocyte chromosome complement is suspected, or when blood samples cannot be obtained, as in abortuses.

Amniocentesis. The amniotic fluid comprises a special source of fetal cells which has attained great practical importance in recent years. Ten to 20 ml of fluid can be withdrawn with apparent safety as early as the fourteenth to fifteenth week of gestation. The amniotic cells may be examined directly for sex determination by staining for the Barr body (sex chromatin mass) or for the Y body, as will be described later. More commonly, they are cultured and the dividing cells are treated to obtain metaphase preparations by the methods previously mentioned. Amniotic cells are unusual in that tetraploid cells (cells with two complete chromosomal complements) occur with significant frequency even when the fetus is cytologically normal. This may indicate that amniotic cells may arise in part from the fetal membranes and may not be totally representative of the fetus proper. Chromosomal examination of the fetus may alter in the future if attempts to obtain fetal blood or skin biopsies through an amnioscope are successful.

Amniocentesis for chromosomal analysis can be considered for those pregnancies in which the risk of a chromosomally abnormal fetus is thought to be significantly greater than the risk of damage to the fetus from the amniocentesis procedure itself (see Ch. 18).

Methods of Chromosome Identification. The chromosomes present in metaphase have replicated but have not yet longitudinally divided, as would have occurred if mitosis had proceeded further. The unseparated parts are known as *sister chromatids,* or *chromatids,* and remain attached together at the centromere (Fig. 1). This leads to an X-like or inverted V configuration. The portions of a chromatid extending above and below the centromere are the chromosome arms. Chromosomes are

Figure 1. Schematic representation of human metaphase chromosomes and the terms commonly used to describe their gross morphologic features.

described as metacentric, submetacentric, or acrocentric, according to the position of the centromere (Fig. 1). The acrocentric chromosomes frequently possess a small

amount of chromosomal material, called a satellite, connected to the short arm by a constricted region (the secondary constriction). Secondary constrictions are also found near the centromere on the long arms of chromosomes 1, 9, and 16.

When conventional stains are used, the chromosomes display no longitudinal features other than the centromere and secondary constrictions (Fig. 1). When certain fluorescent stains, such as quinacrine mustard, are applied directly or when Giemsa stain is used after various pretreatments (e.g., trypsin, urea, heat), the chromosomes display a characteristic banded appearance (Fig. 2). The location and morphology of the individual bands in each chromosome are sufficiently constant that a system of nomenclature for each band has been devised (Fig. 3). This is becoming of great importance, because it is now possible to associate a particular gene with a par-

Figure 2. Karyotype of a normal male cell stained by the trypsin-Giemsa banding technique. Each chromosome pair can be identified and is given a specific number. The group designation (A, B, C, etc.), used before identification of individual chromosomes was possible, is also shown. The X chromosome in that system was classified in the C group, and the Y was frequently included in the G group. (Constructed from a karyotype kindly provided by Dr. K. Hirschhorn.)

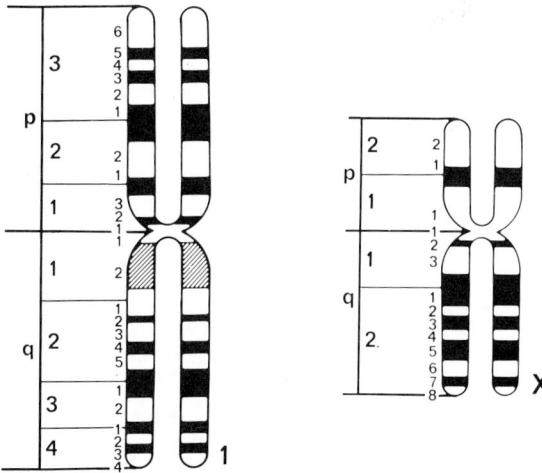

Figure 3. Schematic representation of human chromosomes 1 and X, showing their standardized banding patterns. A numbering system for the individual bands was adopted at the Paris conference (1971) on Standardization in Human Cytogenetics (Birth Defects Original Article Series, 8:1, 1972). The Rh blood group locus is in chromosome 1 near band 34 on the short arm. The loci for the following enzymes have been tentatively localized to regions in the long arm of the X: phosphoglycerate kinase (near band 13), hypoxanthine-guanine phosphoribosyl transferase (near band 26), and glucose-6-phosphate dehydrogenase (near band 28).

ticular band by such techniques as somatic cell hybridization.

The chromosomes from a single metaphase are customarily arranged in a standardized format, known as a *karyotype* (Fig. 2). Conventionally, the chromosomes are arranged in pairs and are ordered on the basis of decreasing length. Since the chromosome pairs could not be individually identified when the first karyotypes were prepared, chromosomes with similar morphology were originally classified into groups (A to G). Now that each pair can be recognized, the autosomes are numbered from 1 to 22, and the sex chromosomes are identified as X and Y (Fig. 2).

Nomenclature for Chromosomal Abnormalities. In the shorthand notation now generally used to describe the chromosome complement of an individual, the number of chromosomes is specified first, followed by the listing of the sex chromosomes. In this notation the normal female karyotype is 46,XX and the normal male is 46,XY. Any deviations from the normal karyotype are written after the sex chromosome listing. An individual autosome is referred to by number, its upper (shorter) arm by p and its lower arm by q. A plus or a minus sign written *after* the p or q indicates an increase (+) or decrease (−) in length of the arm. When written before a designated chromosome, the sign indicates that the chromosome is extra (+) or missing (−). (Examples: 46,XY,18q− describes a male with 46 chromosomes, including one chromosome 18 whose long arm is diminished in length; 47,XX,+21 describes a female with 47 chromosomes, including an extra chromosome 21 in addition to the 46 chromosomes of the normal karyotype.)

The Barr Body and the Y Body. Despite the detail revealed by the various banding techniques, none is able to distinguish between the two X chromosomes of the normal female. It is known that only one X chromosome is active in any cell; each X chromosome in excess of one condenses to form a sex chromatin mass (Barr body) visible at the periphery of the nucleus. The number of X

chromosomes may be indirectly determined by examination of buccal mucosal cells for the number of Barr bodies.

Condensed, inactive X chromosomes are also delayed in the timing of their DNA synthesis, relative to the active X chromosome. The late-replicating X chromosome can be identified by autoradiography using tritiated thymidine.

In over 99 per cent of males, the distal part of the long arm of the Y chromosome fluoresces brilliantly after staining with quinacrine. The intensity is sufficiently great that this region can be seen as a spot of fluorescence, the Y body, in the interphase nucleus. Y-bearing cells can thereby be recognized in cells from blood, hair follicles, and tissue sections, and even in sperm.

Polymorphic Variations in the Human Karyotype. In addition to those alterations in the karyotype which are directly or potentially associated with disease, some variations are known which are apparently without consequence to the individual who possesses them or to his progeny. These polymorphic variations, as they are called, may represent changes in the DNA sequence of the chromosomal region concerned. They are transmitted to progeny as part of the chromosome which contains them. The more commonly recognized variations of this type occur in the length of the short arms of the acrocentric chromosomes, the size of their satellites, the length of the fluorescent segment in the long arm of the Y, and the length of the secondary constrictions of 1, 9, and 16.

14.   MEIOTIC AND MITOTIC NONDISJUNCTION

Meiotic Nondisjunction. Since gametes (sperm or ova) contain only half as much genetic material as a somatic cell, the behavior of the chromosomes during their formation is obviously a unique process, to which the term meiosis is applied. Of the many steps involved in meiosis, those of concern here are only the steps that lead to a reduction in the chromosome number from 46 in the precursor cell to 23 in the gamete. Meiosis consists of two successive stages or divisions (Fig. 4). During first meiotic division, each replicated chromosome pairs with its identical partner. Next, each member of a pair enters one of the two new daughter cells formed. During second meiotic division, sister chromatids separate at the cen-

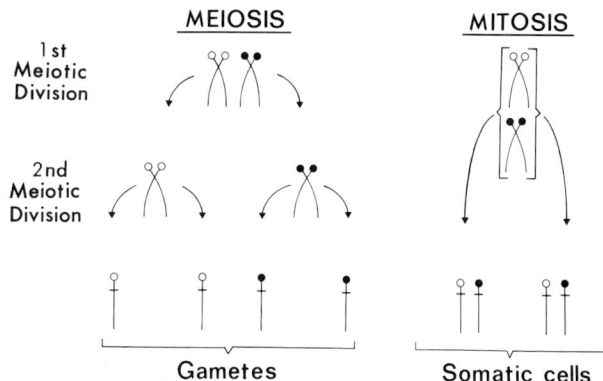

Figure 4. Schematic representation of the behavior during meiosis of a single pair of acrocentric chromosomes, contrasted with their behavior during mitosis. The round bodies on the short arms represent the satellites which are characteristically present on acrocentric chromosomes.

tromere, analogous to their behavior in mitosis, and the two new chromosomes enter the two daughter cells produced at this state (Fig. 4). Of the four cells formed from a gonadal precursor cell, each contains one chromosome from every autosomal pair and one sex chromosome (either an X or Y). (In the formation of the female sex cell, only one of the four cells becomes a functional ovum. In the male, all four cells become spermatozoa.)

Maintenance of the normal chromosome number in the gametes requires the separation of the paired chromosomes at first meiotic division and the separation of sister chromatids at second meiotic division. The failure to disjoin properly (nondisjunction) at either first or second meiotic division will produce gametes with abnormal numbers of chromosomes (Fig. 5). This will result in formation of an individual with an abnormal number of chromosomes in each cell. By using marker genes or polymorphic variations (Fig. 5), it is sometimes possible to identify the parent in whom the nondisjunction occurred and even to distinguish between first and second meiotic division nondisjunction. It is now known that nondisjunction can occur during gametogenesis in either the male or the female and during either first or second meiotic division. Some types of meiotic errors, however, are more likely to be associated with certain kinds of chromosomal abnormalities than with others (see below).

Mitotic Nondisjunction. Mitosis resembles second meiotic division in that sister chromatids become separated, with one of the two newly formed chromosomes going to each of the daughter cells. Failure of separation (mitotic nondisjunction) of the chromatids may occur and lead to creation of two cell lines, one with 47 chromosomes and one with 45 chromosomes. If mitotic nondisjunction occurs at the first cleavage division of the zygote (the cell formed by union of ovum and sperm), an individual with two cell lines (if both cell lines are viable), neither of which is normal in karyotype, will result. If mitotic nondisjunction occurs subsequent to the first cleavage division, a third and normal cell line will be present.

GAMETES PRODUCED BY
NONDISJUNCTION

Figure 5. Production of gametes with an altered number of chromosomes by the two types of meiotic nondisjunction. When polymorphic variation in the satellites of acrocentric chromosomes occurs, a distinction may be made between first and second meiotic nondisjunction of these chromosomes.

Individuals with two or more chromosomally distinct cell types are referred to as mosaics. Mosaicism usually results from mitotic nondisjunction or anaphase lag loss. In the latter, sister chromatids separate properly at mitosis, but one of the newly formed chromosomes fails to be incorporated in a daughter cell. This leads to creation of a new cell line with one chromosome less than the main cell line.

15. CHANGES IN CHROMOSOME NUMBER

Chromosomal abnormalities limited to a change in chromosome number are usually the consequence of nondisjunctional errors. This abnormality is much more common than the group of disorders which result from change in chromosomal structure. The presence of an ad-

Clinical and Cytogenetic Characteristics of Common Syndromes Associated with Change in Chromosome Number

Autosomal Abnormalities	Common Name	Approximate Frequency among Liveborn Infants	Mechanism of Origin	Major Clinical Findings
47, +21	Trisomy 21 or Down's syndrome	1:1000	Material first meiotic division nondisjunction	Mental retardation, abnormal brain development (microgyria), characteristic facies, marked hypotonia
47, +18	Trisomy 18 or Edwards' syndrome	1:11,000	Probably maternal meiotic nondisjunction	Mental retardation, severe failure to thrive, periarticular limitation of motion of distal interphalangeal joints
47, +13	Trisomy 13 or Patau's syndrome	1:15,000	Probably maternal meiotic nondisjunction	Mental retardation, abnormal brain development (arrhinencephaly), cleft palate (and cleft lip), ocular colobomata, postaxial polydactyly
Sex Chromosomal Abnormalities				
45, X (45, XO)	Turner's syndrome	1:6000	Maternal (22%) or paternal (78%) meiotic nondisjunction	Short stature, failure of secondary sexual development, pterygium colli, neonatal edema of hands and feet
47, XXX	Triple X syndrome	1:2000	Possibly maternal meiotic nondisjunction	Usually clinically normal; may be mentally retarded and deficient in secondary sexual development
47, XXY	Klinefelter's syndrome	1:2000	Maternal (61%) or paternal (39%) meiotic nondisjunction	Mild increase in stature, micro-orchidism, infertility, gynecomastia, behavioral changes
47, XYY	XYY syndrome	1:2000	Paternal second meiotic division nondisjunction	Significantly increased stature, behavioral changes

ditional autosome (trisomy) occurs with reasonable frequency, whereas the absence of an autosome is almost never found among liveborn individuals.

A change in the number of sex chromosomes is less deleterious than a change in the number of autosomes. Individuals with as many as three extra sex chromosomes are able to survive, although they are usually mentally defective and congenitally malformed. Individuals with a single sex chromosome (one X chromosome) are, surprisingly, only moderately affected. Individuals with only Y chromosomes, that is, without any X chromosome, have never been found.

The clinical features associated with the more frequently encountered changes in chromosome number are given in the accompanying table. Each type of chromosomal aberration is associated with a relatively characteristic group of clinical findings. It is therefore highly probable that the clinical findings associated with each chromosomal aberration are at least in part determined by the specific genes present on the chromosome involved.

16. CHANGES IN CHROMOSOMAL STRUCTURE

Chromosomal Breakage. Changes in chromosomal structure are largely the consequence of chromosomal breakage. The constancy of the human karyotype from cell to cell and from individual to individual conceals the true frequency with which the continuity of the genetic material is interrupted. In most instances, a break in a chromosome is quickly repaired, with restoration of the normal chromosome structure and without harmful consequences. The exceptions to this are of two kinds and include, on the one hand, the production of chromosomal rearrangements and, on the other hand, diseases characterized by the presence of unrepaired chromosomal breaks.

Chromosomal Rearrangements; Reciprocal Translocations. If two or more chromosomal breaks occur simultaneously in the same cell, the repair process occasionally may unite the chromosomal fragments incorrectly, with production of a chromosomal rearrangement (Fig. 6). One of the most common rearrangements encountered is that which is produced by an exchange of terminal chromosomal segments between two different chromosomes, with formation of a reciprocal translocation (Fig. 6A). A reciprocal translocation occurring between two acrocentrics, with the chromosomal breakpoints in each being located very near to the centromere, is given the special name of *centric fusion translocation* (Fig. 6B). The two most common rearrangements observed in man are centric fusions between chromosomes 14 and 21 and between chromosomes 13 and 14. The minute chromosome produced during a centric fusion translocation (Fig. 6B) is usually lost so that a cell with only 45 chromosomes results. The minute chromosome appears to have little essential genetic material, because its loss has no effect on the cell or the individual.

The types of rearrangement illustrated in Figure 6 apparently produce no change in the amount of genetic material in the cells in which they occur. Such rearrangements are described as *balanced rearrangements,* and the individuals who possess them are carriers of the balanced rearrangement.

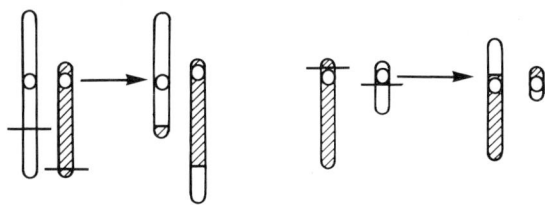

A. Reciprocal Translocation   B. Reciprocal Translocation, Centric Fusion Type

C. Inversion (Pericentric)   D. Inversion (Paracentric)

Figure 6. Schematic representation of the mechanisms underlying some type of chromosomal rearrangements. The horizontal lines represent the points of chromosomal breakage and reunion. The chromosomes are depicted as having single chromatids (i.e., they are unreplicated). It is not known, however, whether rearrangements usually occur before or after replication.

Transmission of a Reciprocal Translocation. When meiosis occurs in a reciprocal translocation carrier, the translocated chromosomes will pair with each other, as well as with their untranslocated partners. Separation of the individual members of this pairing group is often quite abnormal, with any one, two, three, or four chromosomes being incorporated in a single gamete. Since gross amounts of genetic imbalance are poorly tolerated, only a few of the possible abnormal types of progeny will be liveborn. The remaining abnormal types may appear as abortuses or may not be detected at all (because the embryo expires before implantation).

The variety of liveborn progeny expected depends dramatically upon the specific reciprocal translocation. A carrier of a centric fusion translocation between chromosomes 14 and 21, for example, will produce equal numbers of children with the balanced rearrangement and children who are chromosomally normal. A smaller number will have the genetic equivalent of an extra chromosome 21 (and have Down's syndrome), the only type of abnormal progeny produced by this rearrangement able to survive until birth.

Individuals with balanced or unbalanced reciprocal translocation may also be born of chromosomally normal parents. In this case the reciprocal translocation is assumed to have originated during gametogenesis.

Occasionally, a somatic cell may develop a chromosomal rearrangement which may then be passed on to its cellular descendants. This has been observed particularly in some forms of leukemia and in some solid tumors. Chronic myelogenous leukemia, for example, is characterized by a rearrangement (probably a reciprocal translocation) occurring in the leukemic cells which involves chromosome 22 and another autosome, usually chromosome 9. One chromosome 22 in this case has the appearance of a 22q− and is referred to as the Philadelphia chromosome (Ph[1]) (see Ch. 764).

Chromosomal Rearrangements; Deletions. A chromosome may undergo breakage so that an interstitial or a terminal segment of one arm is lost. These abnormalities are known as *chromosomal deletions*. In general they are sporadic, because the abnormality is not present in the ancestors of the affected individual. The loss of genetic material leads to production of multiple congenital malformations if an autosome is involved or to abnormal sexual development if a sex chromosome is affected. The most commonly encountered autosomal chromosomal deletion syndromes have the karyotypes 46,XX or XY,5p− (the cri du chat syndrome) and 46,XX or XY, 18q−.

Diseases Associated with Unrepaired Chromosomal Breaks. There are three diseases (Bloom's syndrome, Fanconi's anemia, and ataxia telangiectasia) now known in which unrepaired chromosomal breakage commonly occurs with several times the frequency observed in normal individuals. Each of these diseases is inherited as an autosomal recessive condition. In addition to the unrepaired breaks, other cytogenetic abnormalities are present with an abnormally high frequency. These include chromosomal rearrangements, deletions, "fusion figures," and endoreduplication (in Fanconi's anemia). The fusion figures appear to result from a break in a single chromatid in each of two chromosomes, followed by union of the ends from nonsister chromatids. Endoreduplication is a different type of cytogenetic abnormality and results when two cycles of chromosomal replication occur without an intervening cell division—each metaphase chromosome possesses four juxtaposed sister chromatids instead of the normal two. Although chromosomal breaks and rearrangements as well as fusion figures are perhaps likely consequences of an abnormality in the DNA repair process, it is not yet possible to visualize a rational connection of this with endoreduplication.

Clinically, these three syndromes are also associated with congenital malformations and a predisposition to malignancy. Cultured fibroblasts from patients with Fanconi's anemia are unusually likely to undergo transformation (a change which superficially at least resembles the development of malignancy) when exposed to the SV-40 virus. This increase in frequency of transformation is also observed with fibroblasts from Fanconi's heterozygotes.

Ford, E. H. R.: Human Chromosomes. New York, Academic Press, 1973.
Levine, H.: Clinical Cytogenetics. Boston, Little, Brown & Company, 1971.
Miller, O. J., Miller, D. A., and Warburton, D.: Application of new staining techniques to the study of human chromosomes. Prog. Med. Genet., 9:1, 1973.

17. PREVENTION AND MANAGEMENT OF GENETIC DISEASE

Alexander G. Bearn

The cardinal principles underlying the prevention and management of disease are similar, whether the disease is determined primarily by environmental agents or by genetic influences, and in both instances accurate diagnosis is a prerequisite. Treatment of the patient with inherited disease must not depend exclusively on alleviation of the metabolic defect; symptomatic treatment is often of great value, and the need for sympathetic handling of a patient with a disease that is inherited, and which may be transmitted to subsequent generations, is paramount.

Although in this chapter considerable emphasis is placed on specific, individually rare, genetic syndromes, it must be realized that the magnitude of the genetic component in the causation of all disease must be assessed if control and treatment of the disease are to be optimal. Indeed, it has been a tragic misconception, too long held, that in contrast to disease caused by environmental agents, there is no effective prevention or treatment for inherited diseases. This misguided view is quickly drained of validity when it is remembered that the expression of a disease process requires the interaction of environmental and genetic influences. Realization that 20 per cent of the hyperlipidemic survivors of a myocardial infarct occurring under the age of 60 suffer from a monogenic inherited hyperlipidemic disorder suggests that it is prudent to investigate the first-degree relatives of such individuals to ascertain those particularly at risk. Moreover, an understanding of the genetic aspects of such common diseases as obesity, hypertension, and emphysema is necessary for a comprehensive approach to prevention and management. Furthermore, an awareness of genetic influences in the metabolism of many drugs will increase the effectiveness of a physician confronted with a variety of puzzling clinical syndromes.

In the balance of this chapter attention is drawn, in particular, to those specific modalities of treatment which can be applied to inherited disease, and which stem from an understanding of the nature of the primary molecular defect. Therapeutic manipulation of the cellular environment in which the gene must act and display its nature is an approach more tractable and less perilous than direct interference with the genetic material itself.

Restriction of Substrate. General dietary restriction is often an effective way to reduce the excessive substrate that accumulates behind an inherited metabolic block. A general reduction in protein intake will improve the clinical manifestations of a number of rare inherited diseases affecting the urea cycle, including arginosuccinicaciduria, citrullinemia, and hyperammonemia. In some rather more common diseases, such as phenylketonuria and galactosemia, specific dietary restrictions are needed. The elimination of phenylalanine from the diet of phenylketonuric infants, if instituted before two years of age, is increasingly recognized as effective therapy. Similarly, elimination of galactose in the neonatal period for patients with galactosemia has resulted in an increased mental alertness, as well as the prevention of cataracts in those individuals who have a recessively inherited galactokinase deficiency. Defective oxidation of phytanic acid is the specific inherited defect in Refsum's disease; dietary restriction of this lipid will significantly ameliorate the symptoms of this disorder.

Provision of the Biologically Active End-Product. An inherited enzymatic defect will lead not only to an accumulation of the substrate on which the enzyme normally acts but also to a decrease in the end-product. When the end-product is of key biological importance, simple replacement will overcome the consequences of the metabolic block. Many instances of familial goiter associated with a deficiency of a specific enzyme can be effectively prevented by the administration of thyroid hormone. Human growth hormone is effective treatment of the recessively inherited form of pituitary dwarfism, and the ill effects of X-linked diabetes insipidus can be prevented by supplying antidiuretic hormone. Oroticaciduria, in which there is an inherited deficiency of enzymes that transform orotic acid to uridine, can be effectively circumvented by providing the uridine-starved cells with exogenous dietary uridine. Dietary phosphorus will overcome the excessive urinary loss of phosphate in X-linked hypophosphatemic rickets, and administration of dietary copper will effectively combat the inherited copper deficiency of Menkes' syndrome.

Removal of a "Toxic Product." In some hereditary diseases the accumulation of a "toxic product" may be responsible for the manifestations of the disease, and removal of the excess material may reverse the phenotypic consequences of the abnormal gene. Removal of the increased tissue copper in Wilson's disease by penicillamine is a particularly striking example of the effectiveness of this form of treatment. Similarly, removal of iron in hemochromatosis by phlebotomy is another example of therapy designed to remove accumulated toxic material.

Augmentation of Enzymatic Activity. Active efforts are being directed toward increasing the residual enzymatic activity that is usually present in patients with autosomal recessively inherited diseases. The administration of barbiturates, for example, to patients with the Crigler-Najjar syndrome has been found to increase the activity of the enzyme glucuronyl transferase, and simultaneously to decrease the serum bilirubin level.

Many biologically important enzymes require essential cofactors for their activity. In some inborn errors of metabolism the mutational event affects the ability of the enzyme to combine with cofactor. Pyridoxine (vitamin B_6) is a cofactor for the enzyme cystathionine synthetase. In more than half the patients with cystathioninuria, in whom there is a decrease in activity of this enzyme, the defect can be overcome by administration of large doses of pyridoxine. Similarly, the metabolic ketoacidosis of some patients with methylmalonic aciduria can be overcome by the administration of pharmacologic doses of the cofactor vitamin B_{12}.

Enzyme Replacement. Direct replacement of the missing enzyme is an attractive and direct approach to the treatment of recessively inherited disease, and although there are a number of substantial obstacles to this simple concept, progress is being made. It should be emphasized, however, that to be effective the enzyme must not only retain its biologic activity when administered to the patient, but must also gain access to the organs and cellular organelles in which excessive substrate has accumulated. Moreover, since the infused enzyme will have a finite half-life, continuous administration or gradual release from an implanted "depot store" must be achieved. Enzyme infusions have been attempted in the mucopolysaccharidoses, in which their therapeutic effect is still unproved, and in metachromatic leukodystrophy, in which the effect is rather more promising.

Surgical Treatment. Numerous examples of the application of surgery to the treatment of inherited disease could be cited. This is particularly likely to be effective in diseases transmitted in a mendelian dominant fashion. The prevention of neoplastic transformation in polyposis of the colon and the removal of the spleen in hereditary spherocytosis are examples of inherited diseases in which surgery can play an important therapeutic role. It should not be overlooked that surgery is a quick and permanent cure for polydactyly as well as for certain other dominantly inherited defects.

Allotransplantation of the organ in which the deficient enzyme is normally synthesized has been attempted in a variety of inherited diseases. Renal transplantation has been performed in patients with Fabry's disease and in cystinosis. In Fabry's disease renal transplantation appears to ameliorate the manifestations; in cystinosis allotransplantation is effective in overcoming uremic nephropathy but does not affect the disease itself. Although in general the results are encouraging, considerably more work will be needed before organ transplantation can be recommended as a routine therapeutic measure in any inborn error of metabolism. Bone marrow transplantation is presently the only effective therapy in patients with severe combined immunodeficiency disease.

18. GENETIC COUNSELING

Arno G. Motulsky

Genetic counseling provides information concerning the risks of occurrence of genetic disorders and the reproductive options available to prospective parents. Since genetic factors play an etiologic role in many different diseases, genetic counseling has become an important component of patient management. If there is a significant risk that a given disease will recur in future children, physicians should provide or arrange for genetic counseling even if the patient or parents do not specifically request such advice. Genetic counseling not only gives factual information but also adapts the communication process to the needs of the individual patient and his family. Alleviation of guilt and explanations regarding the nature and severity of the disease under study are always required. The natural history of the disease, including its variability from patient to patient as well as the potential personal, medical, and social burden, must be conveyed.

Diagnosis. Accurate diagnosis is a prerequisite for genetic counseling. Similar-appearing diseases may be inherited by different modes of transmission (heterogeneity) or may not be genetic at all. Accurate diagnosis requires a carefully obtained family history which is best denoted by conventional pedigree symbols. Information about relatives regarding age, onset of a given disease, health status, and cause of death is obtained. Knowledge of the ethnic origin of the family may be helpful in considering certain genetic diseases; Tay-Sachs disease is common in Jews of European origin, and cystic fibrosis is rare in blacks. Advanced maternal age is a predisposing factor to chromosomal errors such as Down's and Klinefelter's syndromes. Advanced paternal age may be found when new mutations for autosomal dominant diseases such as Marfan's disease or achondroplasia are suspected. Historic data on the immediate family are more accurate than information regarding more remote relatives. Occasionally, physicians' and hospital records have to be obtained for documentation of suspected diseases. Genetic diseases manifesting anomalies of stature or a characteristic physiognomy can sometimes be recognized in photographs of family members. If the parents are related, or if both the father's and mother's ancestors originated from a restricted rural area, autosomal recessive inheritance should be considered as the possible cause for an obscure disease. The mode of inheritance together with the clinical and laboratory findings of a given patient may be helpful in defining various subtypes of clinically similar-appearing genetic disorders such as Hurler's (autosomal recessive) and Hunter's (X-linked recessive) disease, or Marfan's disease (autosomal dominant) and homocystinuria (autosomal recessive). Diagnosis and appropriate counseling for the majority of genetic diseases require knowledge of the clinical and genetic features of the disease rather than special "genetic tests." Suitable cytogenetic and enzymatic tests should be available in the investigation of some conditions. However, because chromosomal aberrations usually are sporadic events and do not run in families, chromosomal analyses are not helpful for counseling in most genetic diseases.

Recurrence Risks. If a disease is transmitted by a mendelian or monogenic pattern, recurrence risks can be well defined. Lack of clinical manifestation (diminished penetrance) or variable expression is particularly frequent in autosomal dominant disorders. In addition to the information that a given gene will be transmitted with a certain probability, the actual recurrence risk of the clinical symptomatology and the risk for severe manifestations associated with that gene must be communicated to the patient. As an example, only 10 to 20 per cent of the gene carriers for Waardenburg's syndrome (autosomal dominant) are deaf. Deafness, rather than the pigmentary and eye anomalies associated with that condition, is disabling, and the problems and recurrence risks of deafness must be stressed during genetic counseling. Some genetic diseases transmitted by an autosomal dominant mechanism, such as polycystic kidneys and Huntington's chorea, only express themselves clinically in the middle-aged. The risk for unaffected offspring of patients, which is 50 per cent at birth, becomes progressively less as a person remains unaffected beyond the age at which these diseases first manifest. Curves plotting the age of onset can be used to quantitate these risks. McKusick's catalogue of mendelian disorders gives helpful short descriptions and literature citations for the known mendelian genetic diseases.

Since in polygenic conditions the number of genes and their relative contributions are unknown, genetic theory does not allow prediction of genetic risks, and so-called empiric risk figures must be relied on for counseling. Similarly, the transmission of viable chromosomal aberrations, such as translocations, does not usually follow mendelian principles, and counseling must also be based on empirically derived risk figures. Empiric risk figures are obtained from observing the frequency of recurrence of the disease in many affected families. Fortunately, recurrence risks for polygenic diseases are rarely higher than 5 per cent. Because empiric risks are derived from genetically heterogeneous families, they do not have the scientific precision of recurrence risks for mendelian disease. Risk assessment requires recognition of the occasional monogenic variant among the broad category of a common disease by careful consideration of the family history and possible differentiating clinical and laboratory features. For instance, autosomal dominant familial hypercholesterolemia is found in 5 per cent of patients who have a myocardial infarction at or below age 60.

Absolute recurrence risks are more meaningful to a family than relative risks. A 1000-fold increase in recurrence risk for a certain disease in a family appears frightening. However, for a condition which occurs in 1 of 100,000 births, a 1000-fold increase means that the absolute or actual risk of recurrence is only 1 per cent – a rather low risk. In mendelian diseases the recurrence risk is fixed (e.g., 25 per cent for autosomal recessive disease), whether several or no affected children preceded. In polygenic diseases, if several sibs are affected in a given family, more disease-producing genes are operative in that sibship, and the risk for future offspring becomes higher.

The meaning of genetic risks must be conveyed in terms understandable to patients. Qualitative terms such as "high" for 50 per cent risks, "substantial" for 25 per cent risks, and "low" for risks of 5 per cent or less may be helpful for optimal communication. The probability that approximately 3 per cent of all children of normal couples will develop serious birth defects, genetic disease, or mental retardation should be communicated as a measure against which the additional risks can be gauged.

Once the significance of the recurrence risk and the contribution of heredity to the disorder have been considered, reproductive alternatives which are meaningful within the social, emotional, and religious framework of the particular family must be discussed. Occasionally, it may be appropriate to give firm and directive advice. More generally, genetic counseling should be nondirective and should provide the necessary information to allow a couple to make their own decisions regarding future reproduction. A genetic counselor should not force his values on those who seek his advice. On the other hand, a scientifically cool and aloof stance is not sufficient, and a sympathetic discussion of the many problems faced by the family is required.

Heterozygote Detection. Heterozygote detection is particularly important in sisters of males affected with X-linked recessive diseases such as hemophilia and Duchenne type muscular dystrophy, because regardless of their husband's genetic constitution, there is a 50 per cent risk that the sons of female carriers will be affected. In contrast, autosomal recessive disease becomes evident only when *both* parents are carriers, and a heterozygote sib of an affected patient must mate with another heterozygote for the disease to occur. The chance that an unrelated mate will be a carrier is usually quite low. Specialized laboratory tests for carrier detection (such as creatine phosphokinase enzyme assays in Duchenne muscular dystrophy) may be helpful but must be carefully standardized on normal subjects and known heterozygotes before applying them for individual carrier identification. Detection of carriers is relatively simple in the hemoglobinopathies, and an increasing number of heterozygote states for various enzyme deficiencies such as Tay-Sachs disease can be recognized.

Reproductive Options. Fragmentary data suggest that couples who sought genetic counseling have had fewer children if the genetic risk was more than 10 per cent. If a couple decides that the risks for further reproduction are too high, several options besides contraception sometimes must be discussed. Adoption is becoming less practicable because fewer babies are available. Sterilization of either husband or wife may be considered, but it must be emphasized that this is an irreversible procedure. Thus sterilization is undesirable for prevention of autosomal recessive conditions, because remarriage after possible divorce or death could eliminate the genetic risks almost entirely. Artificial insemination by a donor other than the husband may be acceptable to occasional couples to prevent autosomal recessive disease or autosomal dominant disease contributed by the husband.

Intrauterine Diagnosis. Amniocentesis performed during the fourteenth to sixteenth week of pregnancy allows the diagnosis of genetic disease in fetuses. When performed by a trained gynecologist, the procedure has proved safe to mother and fetus. During amniocentesis amniotic fluid containing cells of fetal origin is aspirated transabdominally. After a 10- to 20-day period of cell culture, chromosomes can be visualized to ascertain fetal sex and to detect various chromosomal aberrations. Many enzyme deficiencies can be detected by suitable assays. An increased level of α-fetoprotein is frequently observed in spina bifida and other neural tube malformations. Amniocentesis is therefore indicated in the following conditions: (1) chromosomal aberrations, (2) detection of male fetuses who have a 50 per cent risk of being affected with serious X-linked diseases, (3) inborn errors of metabolism which can be detected by amniotic cell assay, and (4) spina bifida and anencephaly. Most amniocenteses are performed in pregnant women over 38 to 40 years of age who have a significant chance of carrying babies with Down's syndrome or in women who had a previous child with that disorder. In both situations the recurrence risk is 1 to 2 per cent; this risk becomes significantly higher if either parent is a translocation carrier for Down's syndrome (5 per cent for male carriers and 20 per cent for female carriers).

Intrauterine diagnosis provides a definite diagnosis and replaces statistical likelihood with certainty. Parents may select abortion if the fetus is affected and, with monitoring of future pregnancies by amniocentesis, may be assured unaffected children.

Detection of Genetic Disease in Relatives. Optimal genetic counseling in some diseases includes the testing of relatives at risk. In some conditions the detection of latent disease in sibs and other relatives, if followed by suitable therapy, may be lifesaving. A sib of a patient with Wilson's disease (autosomal recessive) has a 25 per cent chance of being affected but may be too young to exhibit overt symptoms. Sibs of patients with hereditary polyposis of the colon (autosomal dominant) have a 50 per cent chance of being affected and therefore carry the certain risk of developing malignant transformation of one of the many polyps. In general, vigorous attempts should be made to examine relatives, using appropriate tests, when a genetic condition causes serious preventable or treatable disease. Possible carriers for serious X-linked diseases (such as hemophilia) and for chromosomal carrier status (such as Down's syndrome associated

with translocation) should be sought in families for prevention by intrauterine diagnosis and possible abortion.

Genetic Screening. Genetic counseling has usually been retrospective and has followed the advent of a sick child or relative. In prospective counseling, advice is given before a sick person is born. Such an approach is possible for common autosomal recessive diseases such as sickle cell anemia, thalassemia major, and Tay-Sachs disease in populations with high frequencies of these genes. Eight per cent of the American black population are carriers of the sickling gene, and 4 per cent of the American Jewish population of European extraction are carriers of the Tay-Sachs gene. Mass screening for heterozygote detection followed by suitable genetic counseling has been proposed.

Identification of the sickle cell trait before reproduction permits the prevention of sickle cell anemia if carriers refrain from mating with each other or if those already married have no children. Such programs raise many ethical and social problems, and it is doubtful whether mating and reproductive choices which are logical from the points of view of medicine, genetics, and public health would actually be made. Unfortunately, many sickling screening programs have been established without adequate counseling. Often the mistaken notion has been promoted that the sickle cell trait represents a mild form of sickle cell disease. Needless anxiety and occupational discrimination against sickle cell trait carriers have resulted. Screening programs for Tay-Sachs disease have been more successful because intrauterine detection of this condition is possible.

With the present tendency for couples to have smaller families, there is greater concern that children should be healthy, and thus genetic counseling will become more important. The principles of genetic counseling are simple and should be mastered by every physician. Although for complex genetic problems referral to a genetics clinic in a medical center is necessary, increased education in the principles of human genetics will enable genetic counseling to be undertaken by primary care physicians in many instances.

Clow, C. L., Fraser, F. C., Laberge, C., and Scriver, C. R.: On the application of knowledge to the patient with genetic disease. *In* Steinberg, A. G., and Bearn, A. G. (eds.): Progress in Medical Genetics. Vol. IX. New York, Grune & Stratton, 1973.
McKusick, V. A.: Mendelian Inheritance in Man. Baltimore, The Johns Hopkins Press, 1971.
Nora, J. J., and Fraser, F. C.: Medical Genetics: Principles and Practice. Philadelphia, Lea & Febiger, 1974.

Part III
ENVIRONMENTAL FACTORS IN DISEASE

19. MAN AND HIS ENVIRONMENT

Howard H. Hiatt

All disturbances in health reflect the interplay of environmental and genetically determined host factors. In that sense a textbook of medicine is concerned in its entirety with a consideration of man and his environment. However, the complexity of environmental factors affecting health makes it appropriate to offer a few introductory generalizations about them. Further, attention to how alteration of environmental factors can prevent or ameliorate disease is particularly urgent at this time of justifiable concern with the limitations and economic costs of therapeutic medicine.

The dimensions of man's environment are suggested when we consider that it encompasses everything that impinges on man other than the genes of the germ cell. Indeed, studies in other forms indicate that the genetic apparatus itself often includes material that was once "environment." For example, a bacterial cell may become resistant to an antimicrobial drug as a result of infection with a virus containing the information necessary for the synthesis of enzymes that inactivate the drug. Not only is the bacterium thus able to make the enzymes in question, but because viral nucleic acid may become a part of the genetic apparatus of the cell, the cell can pass on to its progeny the capacity to inactivate the drug. A related phenomenon may explain the presence of tumor viral nucleic acid in certain animal cells. The expression of the nucleic acid in terms of tumor production may require one or more further environmental exposures—for example, to x-rays or to a chemical. This multifactorial etiology is characteristic of all diseases, and the complex interaction of causes has been likened by MacMahon and Pugh to a "web" of causation. Fortunately, effective action does not require complete unraveling of such webs—the disruption of any one thread may be sufficient to induce a favorable change in health status.

DETERMINANTS OF RESPONSE TO ENVIRONMENTAL FACTORS

It has long been recognized that many environmental substances are harmful only to individuals of a specific genetic constitution. Individuals with genetic defects in metabolic pathways may be poisoned by substances that are readily tolerated by most people. An example is the damage done by the muscle relaxant drug suxamethonium to people with abnormal forms of the enzyme pseudocholinesterase. A diet containing "normal" amounts of phenylalanine will be profoundly damaging to persons homozygous for a particular gene. People unable to convert certain dietary constituents to biologically active forms, such as those with vitamin D resistant rickets, will manifest deficiency states even when receiving the substance in amounts adequate for "normal" individuals. Such conditions are worthy of special emphasis, for although they are infrequent, they are but recognized manifestations of individual variations that are ubiquitous. Responses to drugs, chemicals, microorganisms, stress, and other environmental factors, particularly at low doses, reflect in part the genetically determined constitution of the person exposed. Differences from the "normal" in lipoprotein profiles have already been well documented in the families of patients with complications of atherosclerosis; thus genetic predisposition probably makes the cardiovascular system of certain people more susceptible to the ravages of such known potentially harmful factors as hypertension, obesity, and too little exercise. Similarly, individual susceptibility likely explains in part why many but not all cigarette smokers develop lung cancer. Critical to preventive medicine is the development of methods for identifying people for whom specific environmental factors are hazardous, so that appropriate measures can be directed at those at risk.

Response to environmental factors is greatly affected by other environmental conditions prevailing at the time of exposure. One example is a drug the administration of which leads to altered metabolism of, and thereby to altered action of, a second drug. Another is the effect of nutritional status on the response to infectious agents; malnutrition may explain at least in large part why the fatality rate from measles is so much greater in rural Guatemala than in the United States. An individual with compromised function as a result of earlier exposure to one environmental factor may be particularly prone to the effects of another; for example, people with pneumoconiosis are sensitive to carbon monoxide and those with coronary artery disease to carbon disulfide.

Timing of exposure may also be important, particularly during prenatal life. A few of the known congenital malformations and spontaneous abortions have thus far been traced to identified environmental insults, but over 80 per cent are of unknown cause. Drugs, other chemicals, viruses, bacteria, carbon monoxide, and ionizing radiation are among factors known to cause congenital malformations, but only if exposure occurs during the first trimester of pregnancy. Thalidomide, for example, given to a pregnant woman can cause serious anomalies in the offspring. Exposure early in the sensitive period leads to ear anomaly, later to arm deformity, and later yet to leg deformity. Exposures after the first trimester produce no anomalies.

Environmental factors may affect the incidence or the course of a disease, or both; the condition of the host at the time of exposure helps determine which. For example, in mice, x-rays may activate a pre-existing tumor virus, thereby producing cancer. However, even in the absence of latent oncogenic viral DNA, x-rays may themselves lead to cancer by inducing a mutation of cellular DNA. Finally, by their lethal effects on cells, x-rays may be used to destroy cancer, and thus are used therapeutically. Similarly, diethylstilbestrol will produce temporary remissions of breast cancer in some patients; however, it is also known to lead to the appearance of cancer, and some young women have developed cancer of the vagina after exposure to diethylstilbestrol during intrauterine life 20 years earlier. Since many environmental factors cause disease only after latent periods measured in decades, alertness and continued monitoring of potential hazards are required.

CLASSIFICATION OF ENVIRONMENTAL FACTORS

In considering the variety of environmental factors known to be harmful to health, it must be emphasized that the field is in a state of flux, and there are few broadly accepted organizing principles. In developing countries the environmental influences of principal importance are naturally occurring, whereas in Europe and North America, where many of these have been controlled, attention is now focused increasingly on the health hazards of environmental conditions created by man. Some factors are detrimental to health when present in excess, and others when deficient; many lead to problems under either circumstance. Many and probably most environmental factors injurious to health have yet to be identified, and new ones are constantly appearing as a result of increased population, increased affluence, and technologic advances.

A prevailing classification breaks down the principal environmental factors into chemical, physical, biologic, and social. A few examples of each follow.

Chemical Factors. The role of chemicals in inducing human disease is variable and complicated. No chemical can be considered completely nontoxic, even though many are required in small amounts for physiologic processes. For example, the benefits of small amounts of fluoride on tooth development are now accepted. Studies of disease patterns in areas of hard and soft water supply suggest that one or more trace metals may offer some protection against atherosclerosis. Lead, arsenic, mercury, cadmium, cobalt, selenium, tin, manganese, and other metals can produce acute poisoning and may be introduced by contaminated food or water. Polychlorinated biphenyls, organochlorine, and organophosphorus insecticides may gain access via the same route. A variety of chemicals, including silica, asbestos, lead, and many solvents, may be present in toxic amounts in the air, particularly in and near industrial plants.

Over 10,000 synthetic compounds are now in commercial production in amounts between 500 and 1 million kilograms per year. Some are carcinogenic, some mutagenic, and some teratogenic. Because the long-term effects of a substance cannot be known with certainty for decades, testing for chronic as well as acute effects should be carried out before widespread human exposure is permitted. However, since it is impossible to test comprehensively all new compounds, it is particularly important to pay attention to those structurally related to other substances known to be toxic. In many instances in which relation between cancer and environmental exposure is well established, the specific chemicals responsible remain to be identified, as for example the carcinogenic constituents of cigarette smoke.

Physical Factors. Home accidents account for 1 to 2 per cent of all deaths in the United States and Europe, and automobile accidents cause 150,000 deaths and 6 million injured per year in those two areas. Modern transportation has had detrimental effects on health in addition to the loss of life and limb caused by automobile accidents; there is evidence that one factor contributing to coronary artery disease is lack of exercise.

Excessive heat, cold, and noise are harmful, as are both nonionizing and ionizing radiation. Less than 2 per cent of our total exposure to ionizing radiation comes from occupational sources and fallout consequent to nuclear weapons testing and nuclear power development. Almost one third of our exposure is from medical diagnostic procedures, and two thirds from natural sources. However, with increasing dependence on nuclear power certain in the years ahead, this could change significantly. The effect of ionizing radiation on the gene pool is cumulative. The most important somatic effect is carcinogenesis. Whether radiation effects contribute to mortality from causes other than cancer is uncertain.

Biological Factors. Man may be exposed to pathogenic bacteria, viruses, and parasites through inspired air, ingested food and water, and skin contact. The soil is a common source of pathogenic microorganisms and parasites, and many occupations have special biologic hazards, such as anthrax and brucellosis. Many infectious agents produce both acute and chronic disease. Some virus-induced conditions, such as kuru, become manifest only after a latent period of years. Although there have been many claims and much speculation, no unequivocal evidence yet exists for a microbiologic agent as a cause of cancer in man. However, it is likely that at least some forms of human cancer are viral in origin.

Social Factors. Social factors, including economic, psychologic, and cultural factors, all affect health. There is evidence that schizophrenia, crime, suicide, alcoholism, and drug abuse have higher rates in impoverished and crowded areas. Infant mortality is as much as three times higher in the poverty sectors than in more affluent parts of the same cities. Pasamanick and Knobloch (1962) have shown that although black and white infants manifest no differences in developmental tests at 40 weeks of age, by three years the performance of black children is significantly behind that of the white. Whether poverty itself, poor housing, inadequate diet, less education, a combination of these, or other factors are responsible is yet to be established. However urgent the need for more knowledge in this area, existing information is sufficient to provide strong incentive for improving conditions.

Examination of mortality data reveals that major improvements in health have resulted to a much greater extent from changes in a variety of environmental factors than from medical measures. This is particularly apparent in studies of deaths from infectious diseases in the preantimicrobial era (see accompanying figure). Although precise explanations for the dramatic health improvements in the eighteenth, nineteenth, and early twentieth centuries are not available, there is reason to believe that they resulted from better nutrition, removal of hazards from the physical environment by improved water supply and sewage disposal, and a decrease in the birth rate. Other factors may also have contributed, including changes in the virulence of some of the microorganisms, notably the streptococci.

A, Respiratory tuberculosis: mean annual death rate, England and Wales. *B*, Scarlet fever: mean annual death rate of children under 15, England and Wales. (From McKeown, T., and Lowe, C. R.: An Introduction to Social Medicine. Oxford, Blackwell, 1974.)

BEHAVIORAL CHANGE

It was earlier pointed out that in order to prevent or alter an illness we do not always require an understanding of the mechanism whereby an environmental factor contributes to it, and often not even a precise identification of the specific offending factor. On the other hand, however difficult it may be to establish a cause-and-effect relationship between environmental factor and disease, it may be far more difficult to exploit such knowledge. Consider, for example, our failures to achieve the attitudinal and behavioral changes required to take advantage of the knowledge that gonorrhea is transmitted sexually and that a variety of pulmonary and cardiac diseases are aggravated by cigarette smoking. One important step is, of course, behavioral change in the physician. It is unlikely that even the most enlightened patient will be appropriately moved by statistics relating cigarettes, obesity, or lack of exercise to disease if those statistics are offered by his physician who himself pays them no heed. Further, just as the physician who has diagnosed a condition that requires penicillin must en-

sure that the drug is received, so he must do everything possible to achieve the environmental changes that he feels are dictated by his patient's health.

Much of the health benefit resulting from a recognition of responsible environmental factors and their alteration can be achieved only through action directed at population groups. Here the responsibilities of the physician include participation with other members of society in those actions necessary to achieve the desired ends.

CONCLUSIONS

An examination of the present state of knowledge of the relationships of environmental factors and health leads to certain conclusions. First, there is great need for careful and extensive data collection and analysis. The paucity and unreliability of available data and the complexity of the problems that confront us have led too often in this chapter and in this book to the use of such expressions as "is believed to," "may," "conflicting reports exist," and so on, and undoubtedly even more often to our overlooking associations. Better patient records and information systems are required to help correlate data concerning illness, drugs, chemicals, and physical, nutritional, social, and other environmental factors that affect health in order to alert society to dangers as early as possible. However, even these will never replace the contribution of the astute physician who regards every patient not only as a human being in need of attention and devotion, but also as one presenting a problem in need of a solution. It is relevant to recall that rubella and thalidomide were recognized as teratogens not in a research laboratory or by a computerized medical record system, but by astute clinicians in the course of their practice.

The most sophisticated techniques of modern science will help demonstrate mutagenic, carcinogenic, teratogenic, and other effects of environmental factors on human cells and test organisms. Modern technology can contribute greatly needed quantification to environmental health studies. We require methods for assessing the effects of a variety of factors on human behavior and emotions and on other mental functions, although precise methodology in this area is likely to be a long way in the future. Cost-benefit studies, both medical and economic, are necessary for the physician to make enlightened decisions concerning the risks to which diagnosis and treatment inevitably expose his patient. The risk of anaphylaxis to penicillin is surely worth taking in the individual with pneumococcal pneumonia who has never had the drug previously. The risk of thromboembolic disease from oral contraceptives now seems reasonable in the young woman seeking birth control. (Whether this will continue to be the case when all their health effects are uncovered remains uncertain.) Many other more difficult choices exist, and with the growing medical armamentarium and increasing information concerning the effects of drugs, chemicals, and procedures, many more difficult decisions are placed daily before the physician in his practice.

In recent decades there have been no major improvements in over-all mortality rates from the principal killers, cardiovascular disease and cancer.* More than 80 per cent of cases of cancer in the United States are thought to be the result of potentially controllable environmental factors. Similarly, a variety of environmental factors are known to aggravate cardiovascular disease. These and related facts make mandatory increased attention to preventive measures. The exciting implications of the application of our rapidly growing understanding of biology and chemistry to medical problems are widely recognized, and fundamental and clinical research has been and must continue to be encouraged. However, it is at least equally important that we address the present neglect of the benefits that can be achieved from available knowledge. Social and individual action could surely lead to the prevention or amelioration of many diseases, including several that are occupationally related. In this area the physician is often in a unique position to help identify problems and contribute to campaigns to alter responsible conditions.

Gregg, N. M.: Congenital cataract following German measles in mother. Trans. Ophthalmol. Soc. Australia, 3:35, 1942.

---

*However, some changes, including a marked increase in survival of children with acute leukemia and a decline in age-adjusted death rates from coronary heart disease, are not reflected in the over-all data.

Health Hazards of the Human Environment. Geneva, World Health Organization, 1972.

MacMahon, B., and Pugh, T. P.: Epidemiology: Principles and Methods. Boston, Little, Brown & Company, 1970.

McBride, W. G.: Thalidomide and congenital abnormalities. Lancet, 2:1358, 1961.

McKeown, T., and Lowe, C. R.: An Introduction to Social Medicine. 2nd ed. Oxford, Blackwell, 1974.

20. CHEMICAL CONTAMINATION OF WATER AND AIR

Walsh McDermott

Chemical contamination may occur in one's own special environment, notably in one's work-place, such as factory or kitchen, or it may occur in the environment we share with the community at large. Both types of contamination stem in large measure from our skill in manipulating chemicals. As the use of this skill continues, new chemical threats are constantly being introduced. This occurs at a considerably faster rate in the special environments of small clusters of people than it does in the environment at large. Within these small groups the effects of a particular chemical contamination can be quite serious and may even be fatal. Once the presence of a particular chemical is identified as a threat to health, however, its dangers can be neutralized in some way, or its use in the process or the product can be abandoned. It is the *initial* identification that may be quite difficult. For the health damage produced by a particular chemical may take the form of a well known disease entity — asthma or primary carcinoma of the liver, to mention two actual examples. To detect a correlation between one or only a few instances of a well known disease and some one of the many chemicals in a particular "occupational" environment is obviously difficult. Yet the feat must be accomplished early; otherwise conceivably large numbers of people might be seriously harmed. A constant vigilance and a keen epidemiologic sensitivity must be a prominent part of the skill of clinicians engaged in occupational medicine. In a sense these are the pioneers at the outermost frontier of the subject of environmental contamination. Likewise, the physician not engaged in occupational medicine should be quick to consult the medical staff of his patient's work-place when some disease arises in a setting that might be viewed as representing something of a surprise.

Some of the more common chemical offenders are discussed in the chapters that follow and in Ch. 535 to 537. Because the chemical nature of occupational environments is ever changing, however, for comprehensive coverage the practitioner or student must consult the periodical literature or textbooks in occupational medicine. Of necessity, therefore, the present discussion is limited to chemicals in our larger environment, particularly chemicals in the water or air.

Like so many problems in medicine today, the one presented by chemical contamination of our air and water is only partly medical. The effects of contaminants on an individual would be medical; yet the forces that expose the individual to the contaminants would be technologic, economic, or cultural. As modulation of these forces requires social action on a broad scale, the physician's role has to be chiefly one of educator and counselor for those of his patients who are concerned citizen activists and for the public authorities. But the physician is frequently "a concerned citizen" too. It is imperative, therefore, that while serving as counselor or educator he be able to distinguish between his advice given as a physician based on scientific and professional evidence relating to *human health*, and his advice given as a concerned citizen—albeit one with a fairly broad background in biology.

The crux of the matter is that with a very few exceptions (see below) the risks to health posed by chemical contamination of our air or water are not tangible disease realities of the sort with which the physician is accustomed to deal. Instead the fact that there are health risks at all is an intellectual judgment based mainly on biologic analogies rather than on evidence established by direct medical observations. To be sure, the physician is well schooled in making judgments among offsetting risks, but he is usually dealing with risks all of which loom for the immediate future of his patient. In weighing chemical threats from the environment, however, he must frequently offset health gains that are clear and immediate against health risks that are far off and theoretical, and indeed might become a problem only for some future generation.

A splendid example of such offsetting threats may be seen in the chemical contamination of our streams and lakes, some of which serve as community water supplies. The availability of this water made it possible to build the United States as an urbanized society, but to do so required the development of a technology whereby the water could be decontaminated of its threats to health. These threats were all actual disease-producing agents. Because they were living organisms they had the property of death and dissolution, and a highly effective technology was based on these biologic properties. For the past 50 years or so, however, on an increasing scale, we have been contaminating the water not only with our microbes but with the direct or indirect products of our chemical industry. Whereas our microbes are biodegradable, many of these chemicals are not; indeed some are not simplified at all, either by biologic degradation or by any other process of decay. Technologic solutions for this part of the problem are to be expected in the form of substituting more readily degradable pesticides and detergents. The over-all problem, however, cannot be solved purely through technologic means. For the chemical contamination, like that by man's microbes, is part of his aura and is derived from his presence and way of life. To change the aura significantly would require major changes in the way of life; yet it is only the microbial part of his aura that can be clearly incriminated as producers of disease.

Microbes, however, can contribute to the process by more ways than one. The methylation of inorganic mercury in large bodies of water appears to take place through microbial action. This microbial process is of the greatest importance; it converts a form of mercury of rather low toxicity for man into one that is quite dangerous, because, unlike inorganic mercury, methyl mercury is readily absorbed and distributed throughout the tissues of man. Strictly speaking, the *demonstrable* dangerous contamination is in the food chain, i.e., the fish; but as fish cannot methylate inorganic mercury, it is clearly a contaminant of the water. Indeed two outbreaks in Japan (the Minamata Bay and River and the Agono

River) of serious disease from methyl mercury acquired through this *microbe to water to fish to man* route represent one of the few solid examples of human disease from chemical contamination of a large body of water.*

The many offsetting factors that must be weighed in a judgment on the health risks of chemical contamination of water in general are well illustrated by the story of chlorophenothane (DDT). Indeed the DDT situation may be regarded as a fine prototype of the whole problem. As a pesticide this chlorinated hydrocarbon has been marvelously effective in enhancing agricultural productivity; unfortunately it is relatively stable chemically over a wide range of conditions and thus persists for long periods in the environment. Here it produces a number of unsought ecologic effects. These include critically harmful disturbances of the calcium metabolism of predatory birds; interference with various forms of marine life; and persistence in the food chain whereby it can accumulate in the tissues of a number of organisms, including man. All these effects are reason enough for insisting on strict controls on the use of DDT and on an intensive effort to develop less stable but comparably effective substitutes. Moreover, the property of accumulation in human tissue is obviously disquieting from the standpoint of human health. Thus far, however, there is no evidence that this accumulation has led to recognizable disease in humans. The World Health Organization in a 20-year experiment involving more than 200,000 DDT spraymen has received no reports of toxic effect except from accidental swallowing, and even that caused no deaths. No adverse effects were observed in a clinical study of chronic low-grade exposure in which a group of volunteers received daily for 18 months a dosage 200 times the estimated usual exposure from food (Hayes, W. S., et al., 1956).

The physician must offset the theoretic risk that these accumulations might ultimately lead to human disease against the demonstrable health gains from controlling some of the world's major diseases such as malaria (or filariasis) and those caused by arboviruses and rickettsia. And at the present time, there is no wholly satisfactory substitute for DDT in disease control. Faced with this choice between the clear and present danger of vector-borne diseases and the theoretic risk that tissue accumulation of low concentrations of DDT might lead to disease a few decades hence, the physician has no choice but to opt for continued use of DDT under proper control. Yet in making this choice—and the DDT situation can be viewed as the prototype of many more—he must be keenly aware of the critical nature of the factors it was *not* possible to include in the decision.

For to say that low-grade continued exposure to DDT has produced no recognizable disease in man is not to say that it exerts no *physiologic effects*. On the contrary, it is a potent inducer of the microsomal enzyme system of the liver. As this system plays a critical role in the metabolism of drugs and other chemicals introduced to the body from the outside, it serves as a major protective mechanism against chemical threats from the environment, and hence consideration of its workings is appropriate.

The activity of the microsomal enzyme system is minimal at birth and in early life but increases steadily

---

*The current problem concerning contamination of the environment by mercury is not limited to, or even principally, one of contamination of water, but has to do with the presence of methyl mercury in foodstuffs (see references at end of chapter).

throughout adulthood. It is inducible; and the buildup of enzymatic capability as the individual grows older is thought to be a reflection of increasing experience with chemicals from the environment acting as inducers. Activity of the system induced by one chemical may also be effective on another. Consequently when more than one drug (or adventitious chemical) are being taken into the body simultaneously, the metabolic disposition of one of the drugs can be significantly altered by the presence and inducing capabilities of the other drug or adventitious chemical. Such "cross-over" effects have obvious implications for multiple drug therapies and conceivably might also attain significance when one of the chemical compounds was an environmental contaminant. The only endogenous materials metabolized via the hepatic microsomal system are the steroid hormones, and their hydroxylation can be considerably enhanced when the system is induced. In theory, therefore, it could be imagined that the presence of DDT with its known potency as an inducer of the hepatic microsomal system could lead to an increased demand for the synthesis of some hormone. There is no evidence that such a DDT phenomenon with steroid hormones actually occurs. But the postulated phenomenon can serve as an imaginary example of how an adventitious chemical in the environment could alter the course of bodily metabolic activities *through an adaptive hepatic system that is known to exist.*

The question arises whether the decades-long stimulation of such an adaptive mechanism in an individual carries with it a risk to the total organism or whether, on balance, such continued stimulation is a good thing. In general, the many bodily systems that work toward homeostasis are regarded as normal processes whose continued operation is not harmful in itself. But some of these systems require the synthesis of protein, and this requires an allocative process involving protein precursors. In effect, therefore, as emphasized by V. R. Potter, there is a "physiologic cost" involved in each of these adaptive enzymatic processes in the sense that one is accomplished at some cost to all possible others. When the "triggering" of the system comes chiefly from the external environment, as in the hepatic microsomal system, the long-continued engagement with a wealth of chemical stimuli conceivably might result in "physiologic costs" that would be harmful to the organism. This could be so; conversely, as our knowledge advances, the notion may prove to have been ridiculously naïve. Our current state of knowledge simply does not permit judgment of the question at this time. It is really the fact that we are dealing with so many "unknowns" that serves to temper any tendency to complacency based on the present absence of detectable disease resulting from chemical contamination of water. For any situation in which a variety of chemicals pass through a series of living systems that at some stage may include the human body is bound to be not only complex but a situation that is continuously subject to change. It is this fact—that the door is wide open for trouble rather than that trouble has already occurred—that characterizes our present situation with respect to possible adverse effects on health from chemical contaminants of our water.

One expressed fear about pesticides in the water also concerns contamination of the air, specifically that the world's newly released oxygen content might be undergoing subtle reduction. Approximately 60 per cent of the world's newly released oxygen each year comes from the activity of oceanic plant life which it was feared might be harmed by the pesticide pollution of the oceans. However, careful studies of Machta and Hughes (1970) have revealed that there has been no change in the world atmosphere's content of oxygen in the 60-year period from 1910 to 1970. Their "negative" data can now serve as a baseline for monitoring this question throughout the future. Fears of reduction in the global oxygen supply from combustion on land can be set completely to rest by examining the quantitative aspects of the question.

With respect to chemical contamination of the air, the challenge to the physician is the same as with water, namely, he must learn to distinguish at any one point in time between what are presently demonstrable health hazards and what are *current stimuli* that conceivably might be generating health effects to be recognized only several decades later. In broad terms two distinct types of widespread chemical contamination exist: a "London type," composed principally of sulfur compounds from burning coal or certain grades of oil, and a "Los Angeles" type, composed mainly of petroleum products introduced into the atmosphere principally from automobiles, and consisting chiefly of carbon monoxide, carbon dioxide, oxides of nitrogen, lead, and unburned or partially oxidized hydrocarbons. None of these chemicals are present in concentrations sufficiently high in themselves to produce acute toxicity in man. In the Los Angeles type of contamination the visible and palpable "smog" is a result of *sunlight* acting on certain of these discharged chemicals to produce more reactive chemicals, whereas in London it frequently results from *fog* physically trapping the sulfur compounds from the coal. Both types exist in both countries, but in the United States it is the hydrocarbon type that is our basic problem. It is overlaid in certain localities by the sulfur type, for the use of coal varies considerably from region to region. It is highly probable that with both types, one of the important end-results—irritation of certain body and plant cells—is much the same.

In terms of presently demonstrable effects on health the evidence is convincing that the irritation from chemicals in the air is definitely harmful to persons who have sustained damage to their cardiovascular or bronchopulmonary systems, notably that apparently enlarging number of patients with chronic obstructive pulmonary disease (see Ch. 502 to 507). The physician is on quite solid ground in attempting to protect his patients with damaged lungs or bronchi from the aggravating effects of chemically polluted urban air. Sometimes this can be accomplished by emigration, sometimes by window fans with filters. Often, however, particularly among urban poverty groups, it cannot be accomplished at all. For these unfortunates, and indeed for the majority of those with chronic pulmonary disease in all socioeconomic groups, protection, if it is to come, will have to come from the community efforts now in progress in many localities to reduce chemical contamination of the air.

In terms of presently demonstrable effects it must be appreciated that virtually the entire "health case" for reducing the chemical contamination of the air rests on the protection of this population with damaged cardiopulmonary systems. For no convincing case has yet been assembled to the effect that bronchopulmonary disease with its frequent cardiac sequels can be *initiated* by continued exposure to the chemical contamination of urban air. This is not to say there is no medical case at all for continued efforts to minimize contamination of the air for the sake of the far larger population with undamaged bronchopulmonary structures. On the contrary, such a case does exist. The physician must recognize clearly, however, that the case for action to protect the population at large is of quite a different nature from that for action to protect those already damaged. For those damaged the evidence is of a conventional medical sort, i.e., it is based on systematic clinical, laboratory, and epidemiologic observations. For the population at large, however, the case is not derived from actual scientific observations. On the contrary, *as in the case of chemical contamination of the water*, the argument for decontaminating the air can be no more than an intellectual judgment based mainly on biologic analogies.

There is one difference between the problems with air and with water. As mentioned previously, at present there is no recognized disease of unknown pathogenesis that seems to have any relationship to widespread chemical contamination of water. By contrast, in the disease complex of bronchitis and emphysema (chronic obstructive pulmonary disease), there *is* a commonly occurring disease grouping of unknown pathogenesis that starts in early middle age, is clearly aggravated by chemicals in the air, and hence might also be *initiated* by them. But to demonstrate convincingly that such a causative relationship exists is a difficult task that has not yet been accomplished despite careful and intensive studies of laboratory animals and man. The epidemiologic problems involved have to do with the great difficulties in separating for analysis the various factors of conceivable relevance such as cigarette smoking and degree of exposure to particular chemicals in the air. After the first five years of planned long-term studies in The Netherlands (Vlagtwedde/Vlaardingen), it was not possible to demonstrate that residence in areas of high air pollution was associated with an unusual incidence of bronchopulmonary abnormalities. The factor of age seemed to produce a far greater decrease of pulmonary function than smoking or living in a polluted area. Conceivably the *impact* of the chemicals that led ultimately to disease might be something that occurs relatively early in life. Studies in young children in the United Kingdom suggest that continued exposure to high levels of pollution increases the risk of serious respiratory disease in children (Colley and Reid, 1970).

But the major problem is how to study what are in effect "water dripping on stone" effects. The chemicals now contaminating the air, taken singly or collectively, are not present in quantities that produce detectable bronchopulmonary damage in the short run. Thus if the "current stimuli" represented by these chemicals play a significant role in the pathogenesis of such a major disease grouping as chronic bronchopulmonary disease, the effects presumably would take the form of steady but individually minute episodes of damage that ultimately fail to heal completely and emerge to significance only when accumulated over decades. Questions of this type, i.e., 30- to 40-year effects in humans, are far more difficult to answer than questions of the role of environmental contaminants on plant life or other elements of the nonhuman ecology.

To be sure, the physician in his role of public educator and counselor should support well organized efforts to develop the new methods and new research institutional arrangements necessary for the productive study of these medical questions of this essentially new type. But he should also not fail to stress that because of the very nature of these questions as they apply to *human health,* it seems highly unlikely that answers concerning air pollution as an initiator of disease will be forthcoming in the near future. Whatever action is to be taken, therefore, must be based on the medical information that is available now. From the standpoint of health, therefore, we are left with the following dilemma. On the one hand, most of the actions necessary to abolish air pollution as a potential danger to health are costly and likely to prove quite disruptive to the economy and the whole style of life. To campaign for these actions in the name of health without a convincing scientific case that the evils to be corrected represent a widespread danger to health might be unwise. On the other hand, if, a few decades hence, it were shown convincingly that long-continued chemical contamination of the air *of the present sort* did have the property of initiating chronic bronchopulmonary disease, the proportion of the population of any industrialized country that would by then have been irreversibly affected would be large indeed.

There seems to be no obvious solution for this dilemma so long as the major case for minimizing air pollution is viewed as being primarily a "health matter" and health is considered principally in terms of detectable disease. But there are more subtle aspects to health than definable disease, including even definable mental disease. There is the whole affect involved in one's response to one's environment. The intense love of their city shown by so many Leningraders when it was under siege in World War II is a case in point. These are not the kinds of phenomena that lend themselves readily to comparative weighing in the scale against the major economic factors that might be disrupted in "air reform." Nevertheless, they deserve attention too.

What it comes down to is that, except for those already afflicted with cardiopulmonary disease, the present chemical pollution of urban air is not really a health problem in the orthodox sense; it is a widespread *social* evil that is quite unacceptable on a number of counts, of which the possible health effects are only one (Dubos, 1970). Viewed in this way it becomes the physician's role to characterize continuously what is known or seems highly probable about the health aspects of the matter. Included should be encouragement of attempts to develop more sensitive methods for the essentially permanent monitoring of the possible effects of long-continued chemical stimuli. The physician presents this knowledge not as a determining reason in itself for air control, but as only one portion of a total argument for cleansing this part of our external environment. Once the medical contribution can be regarded as but one contribution to a much larger total effort, the physician can escape from the trap of seeming to be minimizing the significances of a particular form of contamination of the air on the grounds that it is not a *known* danger to health. For the physician to operate in such a cooperative professional-social role is not new; most of the impressive twentieth century accomplishments of medicine in extending life expectancy from birth were made in exactly this way.

Burns, J. J.: Interaction of environmental agents and drugs. Environ. Res., 2:352, 1969.
Conney, A. H., et al.: Effects of pesticides on drugs and steroid metabolism. Clin. Pharmacol. Ther., 8:2, 1967.
Dubos, R.: Reason Awake! Science for Man. New York, Columbia University Press, 1970.
Goodman, L. S., and Gilman, A.: The Pharmacological Basis of Therapeutics. New York, The Macmillan Company, 1965.

Keil, J. E., Sandifer, S. H., Finklea, J. H., and Priester, L. E.: Serum vitamin A elevation in DDT-exposed volunteers. Bull. Environ. Contam. Toxicol., 9:317, 1972.

Lu, F. C., Berteau, P. E., and Clegg, D. J.: *In* FAO/IAEA/ILO/WHO: Mercury contamination in man and his environment. IAEA Techn. Rep. Ser. No. 137, 1972, p. 67.

Machta, L., and Hughes, E.: Atmospheric oxygen in 1967 to 1970. Science, 168:1582, 1970.

Royal College of Physicians: Air Pollution and Health. London, Pitman Medical and Scientific Publishing Company, Ltd., 1970.

Sweden, National Institute of Public Health. Nord. Hyg. T. Suppl. 4, 1971.

FOOD POISONING

Harold P. Lambert

21. INTRODUCTION

Food may cause illness in three ways. The most common varieties are produced by *contamination with microorganisms or their products*. Although the gastrointestinal tract is an important mode of entry for many viral, bacterial, and parasitic agents of disease, the term "food poisoning" is conventionally restricted to two main types of syndromes: various forms of acute gastroenteritis caused by bacteria or their products in food; and neurologic syndromes such as botulism or paralytic shellfish poisoning caused by the toxic products of microorganisms. Second, food may be *contaminated by poisonous chemicals*. Examples include heavy metal poisoning by mercury, antimony, cadmium, arsenic, or zinc; poisoning by simple salts such as sodium fluoride or potassium chlorate; and poisoning by organic compounds such as insecticides and orthotricresyl phosphate. Third, *poisonous plants or animals may be eaten in error*. The material may be inherently poisonous, as are some species of mushroom and many other plants; or it may have become secondarily poisonous by incorporating a substance toxic to man during its own food cycle, as in certain forms of shellfish and fish poisoning.

22. BACTERIAL FOOD POISONING

The infectious type of bacterial food poisoning requires the ingestion of living organisms, albeit often in very large numbers, and their subsequent multiplication in the gastrointestinal tract. The most important example of this type of illness is Salmonella gastroenteritis, which is dealt with in Ch. 213. Shigella species may give rise to very similar syndromes, but these are not conventionally classified as episodes of food poisoning, although water- or food-borne outbreaks of Shigella infection do sometimes occur. In the toxin type of bacterial food poisoning, such as that associated with staphylococci, the illness is caused by toxin formed in food before its ingestion, and does not depend on the ingestion of living organisms. Although a generally useful concept, the distinction between the "infection" and "toxin" types of food poisoning has become less rigid than formerly with the demonstration and partial identification of a number of enterotoxins produced by bacterial gut pathogens, including those which produce disease only when ingested as living organisms.

STAPHYLOCOCCAL FOOD POISONING

Etiology and Epidemiology. This common form of food poisoning is caused by the multiplication of an enterotoxin-forming strain of Staphylococcus in the food before ingestion. Contamination of food with staphylococci is extremely common, because the organism can be grown from the hands of about 50 per cent of people. Heavy growth may often be obtained from apparently noninfected minor cracks and cuts on the skin. Staphylococci of human origin contaminating meat or confectionery constitute the source of most outbreaks, but about 10 per cent of them are milk borne, and the organism is then usually of bovine origin. The conditions needed to cause food poisoning of this type are contamination of a suitable food—most foods will support the growth of staphylococci—and a period of some hours after preparation during which the organisms are able to multiply. This may occur during a period of slow cooling after cooking or if food is held at ambient temperature in a warm climate after preparation. Later reheating or even boiling will not then prevent illness, because this is caused by preformed, heat-stable toxin and not by the ingestion of living staphylococci.

Pathogenesis. Detailed study of staphylococcal enterotoxin has been hindered by many technical difficulties. Strains which form enterotoxin are almost always coagulase positive, but enterotoxin production is otherwise not related to any easily measurable metabolic activities. Moreover, study of the toxin has hitherto been limited by lack of a satisfactory animal model; most workers use intraperitoneal injection of toxin in kittens as the test system. Some progress has been made in recent years, notably the differentiation of four antigenic types: enterotoxins A, B, C, and D. Enterotoxin B has been isolated in relatively pure form by Bergdoll and his colleagues. The types are antigenically specific and do not cross-react, but one staphylococcal strain may produce more than one type. The toxin, like the crude extracts, is relatively heat resistant and resistant to trypsin. Its precise mode of action is still in dispute, but experiments in monkeys suggest that this so-called enterotoxin probably has its primary site of action in the central nervous system, and that vomiting is a centrally induced response.

Clinical Manifestations and Treatment. The period between ingestion and illness is short, one to six hours, occasionally a little longer, and the illness is characterized by abdominal cramping pain with violent and often repeated retching and vomiting. Diarrhea is variable; it may be profuse, mild, or absent entirely. Although often violent, staphylococcal food poisoning is short lived, usually subsiding in six or eight hours and rarely lasting as long as 24 hours. It may occasionally threaten life in patients who are old or suffering from other serious disease. The patient is often recovering when first seen by a doctor, but may require an intramuscular injection of prochlorperazine, 12.5 mg or metoclopramide, 10 mg, to control vomiting. Patients with evidence of serious depletion of extracellular fluid may require intravenous treatment using isotonic sodium chloride with added potassium.

Prevention. Careful training of food handlers in personal hygiene and immediate refrigeration of foods not due for immediate consumption are the most important preventive measures. Enterotoxin is not produced at ordinary domestic refrigerator temperatures. Foods should not be left to cool slowly, especially in large containers, and should be taken from the refrigerator and reheated, if this is required, immediately before serving.

Epidemiologic work on outbreaks of staphylococcal food poisoning involves standard methods of bacteriophage typing in identifying the source of the responsible strain. Since, however, terminal heating may kill the organisms in food without inactivating enterotoxin, staphylococci may not be grown from food under suspicion. Animal assays for the detection of enterotoxin are now being replaced by serologic methods based on gel diffusion after preliminary extraction and concentration.

CLOSTRIDIAL FOOD POISONING

Etiology.   *Clostridium perfringens* type A is responsible for about one third of the reported cases of food poisoning both in the United States and in Great Britain. It occurs in fairly large outbreaks, with an average of 35 affected people in each episode. The organism is ubiquitous. Strains can be isolated from the feces of man and of most domestic and farm animals, and samples of raw meat may often be contaminated with this organism. It has also been found in flies, soil, and dirt from kitchens. The conditions necessary for an outbreak are well defined. A meat or poultry dish, in the form of either a stew or a solid preparation such as a joint, pie, or mince, is cooked at a temperature not higher than 100° C, allowing the spores to survive. During a period of slow cooling the spores germinate, this process being provoked by "heat shock"; rapid multiplication of vegetative forms is encouraged by the rich medium and the low oxidation-reduction potential after cooking. These conditions are especially likely to apply with a large bulk of food, in which slow cooling and anaerobic conditions are likely to occur. Food eaten cold or merely warmed before serving may then cause an outbreak of food poisoning.

Pathogenesis.   Human volunteer experiments indicate that ingestion of living organisms is necessary for the production of this form of food poisoning, and the responsible strain may often be found in large numbers in the feces of affected patients. Strains of *Cl. perfringens* type A which cause food poisoning do not differ from other strains in any way easily identifiable by routine methods, although outbreaks in Britain have most commonly been caused by strains with heat-resistant spores. The pathogenesis of the disease has yet to be defined in detail. It was believed for some time that phosphoryl choline, an end product of the action of alpha toxin (= lecithinase-phospholipase-C) was responsible for the outpouring of fluid into the bowel, but this substance has no effect in experimental systems and is probably inactive in the bowel. Recently, however, partial purification has been achieved of a toxin from strains which cause diarrhea in human volunteers as well as accumulation of fluid in isolated loops of rabbit ileum. The toxin is a heat-labile, nondiffusible protein, antigenic and different from other known toxins produced by *Cl. perfringens.*

Clinical Manifestations.   The incubation period is 8 to 12 hours after ingestion of the infected food, occasionally as little as 6 or as long as 24 hours. The main features are diarrhea and griping abdominal pain. The feces are liquid but do not contain blood or mucus. A small proportion of patients suffer from nausea and vomiting. The illness is usually not severe, lasts less than 24 hours, and

is unaccompanied by systemic disturbance or fever. A few deaths have been recorded in old or infirm patients.

Drug treatment is rarely necessary, but in longer attacks a kaolin mixture may be given, and patients with severe abdominal pain may need an analgesic.

Prevention.   Preferably food should be served immediately after cooking. If it has to be kept, it should be rapidly cooled and held at a safe temperature. Cooked meat should always be kept either cold, below 5° C, or hot, over 60° C. Careful techniques of food hygiene are especially important in institutions in which large amounts of meat or poultry are cooked.

ENTERITIS NECROTICANS
(Pig-Bel)

Outbreaks of severe intestinal disease have been associated with ingestion of *Cl. perfringens* type C. A large outbreak was reported from Germany in 1948, and a similar syndrome known as pig-bel has more recently been described from parts of New Guinea in which pig feasts have an important economic and social function. The syndrome is characterized by severe abdominal pain, bloody diarrhea, and vomiting. Operation or autopsy reveals a severe hemorrhagic jejunitis and ileitis. Some patients die and some recover after resection of strangulated, perforated, and necrotic bowel. Others may pass through the acute phase to develop chronic small bowel obstruction and malabsorption, and some recover completely.

VIBRIO PARAHAEMOLYTICUS FOOD POISONING

V. parahaemolyticus is a halophilic marine vibrio long recognized as an inhabitant of coastal waters of Japan and as a cause of gastroenteritis associated with sea foods. More recently it has been found in American and British coastal sea waters. Techniques for its isolation and differentiation from nonpathogenic marine vibrios are now well established.

In Japan gastroenteritis of this type is confined to the summer months. It is the most common cause of infective food poisoning in Japan, accounting for 59 per cent of 22,000 cases of identifiable cause in 1963. *V. parahaemolyticus* causes an infectious type of gastroenteritis and is associated with ingestion of raw fish or shellfish. Outbreaks in Japan have been associated with semidried young sardines, and especially with sushi, a food composed of cooked rice, raw fish, and shellfish. In 1971 three outbreaks of *V. parahaemolyticus* were identified in the United States, associated with ingestion of indigenous crabs and shrimps.

Incubation periods varying from 2 to 66 hours have been recorded, but the most frequent interval between ingestion and infection is 12 to 24 hours. The chief clinical features are severe diarrhea accompanied by cramping abdominal pain, nausea, and vomiting. Most patients also exhibit systemic symptoms of fever, chills, and headache. Less commonly the organism causes a dysenteric form of illness with fever and bloody diarrhea. The illness lasts for one to five days, and recovery appears to be complete. As with staphylococcal and clostridial food poisoning, the disease is rarely fatal, but old and debilitated patients may be at special risk.

BACILLUS CEREUS FOOD POISONING

Bacillus cereus is an aerobic, spore-bearing, gram-positive bacillus of wide natural distribution, and several outbreaks of food poisoning have been associated with high counts of the organism in the responsible food. Contamination has been traced to corn flour, rice, and other dried foods. In large outbreaks in Norway affecting as many as 600 people, the incubation period was 12 hours, and the main features were watery diarrhea, abdominal pain, and nausea lasting about 12 hours. More recently, fried rice in restaurants has been incriminated. Large quantities of rice are prepared and kept at warm kitchen temperatures for many hours, small portions being refried for a few minutes as orders are placed. In one such episode the rice contained 450×10^6 organisms per gram. The incubation period has been as short as 15 minutes to 3 hours when large inocula such as these are ingested.

OTHER FORMS OF BACTERIAL FOOD POISONING

Many outbreaks cannot be assigned to one of the specific pathogens generally accepted as a cause of food poisoning, but many other bacteria have been implicated at one time or another as possible causes of acute gastrointestinal illness. The evidence is often inconclusive and is frequently based on high counts of the presumptive pathogen in samples of food which may have been kept at room temperature for long periods before reaching the laboratory, or on the isolation from patients' stools of organisms which form part of the normal fecal flora. Volunteer studies have often proved equivocal. With these reservations, it seems likely that diarrhea and vomiting may occasionally be caused by a considerable variety of bacteria, if circumstances have allowed their multiplication to high enough concentrations before ingestion. The genera most often implicated have been the enterococci (group D streptococci) and various members of the Enterobacteriaceae, notably *E. coli,* Proteus, Providencia, Pseudomonas, and Citrobacter.

23. BOTULISM

Etiology. Botulism is a life-threatening illness characterized by muscle paralysis and variable gastrointestinal symptoms. It is caused by absorption from the gastrointestinal tract of ingested toxin produced by *Clostridium botulinum.* Botulism resulting from wound infection by this organism has also been recorded several times.

Incidence. The unexpectedness of outbreaks of botulism, the dramatic and frightening nature of the illness, and its high mortality have attracted much attention from both laymen and doctors, but botulism is in fact an uncommon disease. From 1899 to 1969 there were 659 outbreaks in the United States, with 1696 cases and 959 deaths. Outbreaks have also been recorded in many other countries, especially in Canada, Japan, Western Europe, Scandinavia, and the U.S.S.R.

Epidemiology. The six strains of *Cl. botulinum* cause disease in man and in a variety of animals. Human disease is caused by types A, B, and E and occasionally by type F. Toxins produced by the different types are antigenically distinct. *Cl. botulinum,* a spore-bearing anaerobic bacillus, is widely distributed in nature. The organism has been identified in many parts of the world, in cultivated and virgin soils, in a variety of marine environments, and in many animals and animal products. The distribution of types varies in different areas, so that type A botulism is more common than type B in the United States, especially in the Western states, whereas in Europe this order is reversed. In recent years type E has superseded both types A and B in frequency. Type E organisms are especially but not exclusively associated with the aquatic environment in northern latitudes, being found in the sea bed of coastal and lake waters and in the intestinal tract of fish. However, types A and B may also be associated with a marine source.

Pathogenesis. Contamination of fresh food by spores of *Cl. botulinum* does not cause botulism. The spores must have germinated and toxin must have been produced by the vegetative organisms. Spores are destroyed at a temperature of 121° C or greater, as used in commercial canning processes, but can usually survive a temperature of 100° C. Type E spores are relatively heat sensitive, but smoking and light cooking may not kill them, so that food processed in these ways or preserved in the raw state may act as a vehicle of the disease. Another factor predisposing to type E botulism is the production of toxin by this organism at temperatures as low as 5° C. The cooking or preserving process is conducive to the germination of spores and, by reason of the lowered redox potential, to multiplication of the vegetative forms. Multiplication is inhibited in acid media, and botulism is rarely associated with food of pH below 4.5. All types of botulinum toxin are heat labile, and botulism could be entirely prevented by terminal heating for 20 minutes at 80° C or for 10 minutes at 90° C.

The types of food associated with botulism as a result of these contributory factors vary, with local food customs, from country to country. In the United States home-preserved vegetables constitute the most frequent source, followed by preserved fruit and fish products. Meat and meat products are more commonly responsible in Europe. Preserved fish is the chief source of botulism in Japan, Scandinavia, and the U.S.S.R. Although most outbreaks are associated with domestic methods of preparing and preserving foods, outbreaks from commercially prepared foods also occur. Recent sources have included canned tuna fish, canned vichyssoise, and vacuum-packed smoked fish.

Ingested toxin is rapidly absorbed from the gastrointestinal tract. Toxemia may be demonstrated for periods of up to ten days or even three weeks, and it is possible that toxin continues to be absorbed from the bowel for some days after ingestion. Type E toxin is potentiated by proteolytic enzymes, including trypsin, and this phenomenon has been invoked as a mechanism which contributes to the pathogenicity of this type. Botulinum toxin is active in extremely low doses, nanogram quantities of pure toxin being lethal to mice. It prevents conduction in peripheral nerves by a presynaptic block, thus preventing release of acetylcholine without direct action on the acetylcholine release mechanism. Anticholinesterase drugs do not affect its action.

Clinical Manifestations. Illness usually begins between 12 and 36 hours after ingesting the toxin-containing food. The first manifestations are often gastrointestinal, especially in type E disease, with nausea, vomiting, abdominal pain, and distention. Other common early symptoms are weakness, unsteadiness, and dryness of the mouth and throat. Neurologic symptoms may accompany the early gastrointestinal illness or may follow at an interval of 12 to 72 hours. Early features are blurring of vision, dysphagia, dysarthria, and weakness of a variety of muscles. Weakness spreads as the disease advances, affecting especially the respiratory system, the external ocular muscles, and muscles of the neck and proximal limb groups. The pupils are usually dilated and fixed, and retention of urine is common. Deep tendon reflexes are preserved. The patient remains mentally clear, and fever is not observed except as a terminal event. Paralysis may continue for many days or weeks.

One recent outbreak of type A botulism showed atypical features; the pupillary reactions remained normal, and two of the six patients showed myasthenic features not usually observed in botulism. Defects of cardiac conduction have occasionally been noted.

The chief causes of death are respiratory or bulbar paralysis or both, along with the infective complications resulting from these paralyses.

Diagnosis. The illness is easily recognized if a group of patients, known to have eaten food of a type associated with botulism, present with characteristic symptoms. By contrast, diagnosis of the individual patient, in whom there may be no suspicion that the illness is a form of food poisoning, has often proved extremely difficult. The gastrointestinal features may be so severe as to simulate intestinal obstruction, and the epigastric pain may be mistaken for that of myocardial infarction. The dry and sometimes painful throat may suggest various forms of acute pharyngitis, and the combination of sore throat and neurologic disease can cause confusion with diphtheria. The neurologic illness has been mistaken for acute polyneuritis (Guillain-Barré syndrome), encephalitis, a stroke, or myasthenia gravis. The dry mouth and fixed dilated pupils suggest atropine poisoning, as is produced by *Datura stramonium* (jimson weed). Paralytic poisoning caused by shellfish or by puffer fish (see below) is accompanied by prominent sensory symptoms not found in botulism.

Circulating toxin may sometimes be detected in the patient's blood, even long after onset of the disease. It is detected by intraperitoneal injection in mice, controls simultaneously receiving antiserum of the different types. Suspected food is also tested for toxin in the same way, and the organism is sought by anaerobic culture.

Treatment. Since the greatest risk of botulism is respiratory failure, treatment is dominated by the prevention and management of this complication. Bulbar paralysis is treated by early tracheostomy, employing a cuffed endotracheal tube. Coincident or supervening respiratory muscle paralysis indicates the need for artificial ventilation applied through the tracheostomy. Specific antitoxin is probably effective in reducing the mortality of type E botulism. Although there is no such evidence in other forms of botulism, the high mortality of the disease and the difficulty of obtaining statistically valid data justify the use of antitoxin in all forms of the disease. Antitoxin should be given irrespective of the duration of illness when the diagnosis is made, because toxin may be present in the blood for many days. Unless the type of botulism is definitely known, multivalent antitoxin should be administered, because the type cannot be reliably inferred from the food source. After a prelimi-

nary test for hypersensitivity to horse serum, two vials of trivalent antitoxin (each containing 7500 IU type A, 5500 IU type B, and 8500 IU type E antitoxin) are administered by intravenous injection, and this is repeated in two to four hours. For botulism of known type, preparations containing A and B antitoxin or E antitoxin alone are available, as is a small stock of monovalent F antitoxin.

Until 1968 no method had been proposed by which the effects of botulinum toxin could be counteracted, but recently guanidine has been claimed as a useful adjunct in treatment. Both clinical and electromyographic improvement were observed in a number of patients who received guanidine by nasogastric tube in a dose of 15 to 50 mg per kilogram per day.

Since it is uncertain whether the long duration of toxemia in botulism is attributable to continued absorption from the bowel, gastric aspiration and colonic washouts are also used in treatment. A solution of sodium bicarbonate may be left in the stomach to promote breakdown of toxin.

Prognosis. The over-all mortality of botulism is high, 60 to 70 per cent for type A, 10 to 30 per cent for type B, and 30 to 50 per cent for type E. Patients with type E botulism tend to die more quickly than those affected by other types, usually within three days of onset. Improved management of respiratory failure should lower the death rate, especially because patients who survive the stage of severe paralysis can recover completely.

24. POISONOUS PLANTS AND ANIMALS

PARALYTIC SHELLFISH POISONING

Shellfish may act as the vehicle of transmission of many pathogens, for example, infective hepatitis, *Vibrio parahaemolyticus* gastroenteritis, and diarrhea and vomiting of unknown cause. Ingestion may also give rise to an acute neurologic syndrome caused by the transmission to man of a neurotoxin acquired by shellfish from plankton on which they feed. Outbreaks are especially likely to follow a sudden increase in the population of dinoflagellate protozoa, the "red tide." The main responsible species in the Pacific Ocean is *Gonyaulax catanella*, which produces the paralytic poison *saxitoxin*, first isolated from the Alaskan butterclam *Saxidomus giganteus*. The toxin of *G. tamarensis*, responsible for outbreaks on Atlantic coasts, produces the same pharmacologic effects, although it may not be identical with saxitoxin. The toxins are water-soluble, heat-stable compounds, rapidly absorbed from the gastrointestinal tract and active in vitro at concentrations of 1 to 10 μg per milliliter. They act on vertebrate nerve fibers and on skeletal muscle fibers, abolishing action potentials by preventing depolarization.

Clinical Manifestations. Symptoms may begin as soon as 20 minutes after ingestion, with paresthesias of the hands and mouth, weakness of the limbs, and a floating feeling. Other common features are ataxia, headache, and vomiting, whereas in severe cases bulbar and respiratory paralysis supervene and may cause death. Mortality rates between 5 and 18 per cent have been reported in various outbreaks, but the illness is less likely to be severe if water used in cooking the shellfish has been discarded. Treatment is that of respiratory paralysis. No specific treatment is available, but patients are likely to recover if they survive the first 12 hours of the illness.

A different form of paralytic shellfish poisoning is associated with ingestion of red whelk, *Neptunea antiqua*. This is caused by tetramine (tetramethylammonium hydroxide) which is produced in the salivary glands of this mollusk and causes curare-like effects on muscle.

FISH POISONING

A number of different mechanisms are involved in fish poisoning. Some species are inherently poisonous; the toxins of other species are acquired from organisms on which they feed; yet another form of fish poisoning is caused by breakdown products of bacterial action.

Ciguatera Poisoning. This can be acquired from a large number of species, about 300 in all, whose common characteristic is the narrow range of reef or coastal tropical waters which they inhabit. The toxin is thought to originate in blue-green algae consumed by herbivorous fish which are in turn the prey of carnivorous species. The toxin accumulates in the tissues and is excreted very slowly. Poisoning of this type is difficult to prevent, because the toxin is stable to heat, cold, and drying, and the taste and smell of the fish are unaffected. Symptoms commonly begin several hours after ingestion, but may be almost immediate. Nausea and vomiting are followed by paresthesias of the face, mouth, and limbs, dizziness, ataxia, muscular weakness, and severe muscle pain. The patient may die from respiratory paralysis during the first day, and in nonfatal cases the neuritic symptoms may persist for many weeks. No immunity is gained by an attack; indeed, a second episode of poisoning may be more severe.

Tetraodon Poisoning. Many puffer fish found in the Pacific, Atlantic, and Indian Oceans are inherently toxic. The neurotoxin contained in their viscera *(tetraodontoxin)* is identical with that formerly known as tarichatoxin, found in the Californian newt *Taricha torosa*. Its mode of action is similar to that of saxitoxin, and this is reflected in the syndrome of tetraodon poisoning which bears clear resemblances to paralytic shellfish poisoning (see above). Symptoms begin soon after ingestion and include paresthesias, dizziness, ataxia, and paralysis, often together with diarrhea, vomiting, and abdominal pain. The patient may die of respiratory paralysis.

Scombroid Poisoning. Some species of the mackerel family, such as tuna and bonito, are susceptible to decomposition by *Proteus morganii*. Toxic products result from the breakdown of histidine normally contained in fish flesh. Within a few minutes of ingesting contaminated fish, the patient develops nausea, vomiting, headache, epigastric pain, dysphagia, dryness of the mouth, and severe urticaria. The illness usually lasts less than 24 hours.

Other Fish Poisons. Neurologic symptoms may follow ingestion of several other types of fish. Some of the toxins responsible are probably acquired from dinoflagellates, as in paralytic shellfish poisoning, but the source of other neurotoxins is still uncertain. In addition to these forms of fish poisoning, some species of the Gempylid group such as castor oil fish and snake mackerel contain a purgative oil, whereas the roe of some freshwater fish is toxic during the reproductive period, causing acute gastrointestinal symptoms with headache and fever.

MUSHROOM POISONING

In poisoning by muscarine-containing species such as *Amanita muscaria* (fly agaric) and *Amanita pantherina*, symptoms begin two or three hours after ingestion and consist of abdominal cramp, sweating, salivation, miosis, and bradycardia. Poisoning by these species is rarely fatal. By contrast, death-cup poisoning, by *Amanita phalloides* and *Amanita verna*, carries a mortality of 30 to 50 per cent or more. Two groups of toxins are contained in these mushrooms. Cyclic heptapeptides known as *phallotoxins* cause the violent symptoms of abdominal pain, vomiting, and diarrhea which begin 6 to 15 hours after ingestion. Symptoms then remit for about 48 hours. During this time tests of liver function become abnormal, and signs of hepatic and renal failure then develop, often accompanied by confusion, coma, and paralysis of the extremities. This phase of the illness is probably caused by cyclic octapeptides known as *amatoxins*.

No specific treatment is available, but the stomach should be emptied by induced vomiting or gastric lavage, and atropine administered if muscarinic effects are observed. Otherwise, the general principles of management in acute hepatic and renal failure should be observed. For example, peritoneal dialysis or hemodialysis may be necessary in renal failure, and modern methods of managing acute hepatic failure may help to reduce the high mortality.

In experimental conditions, the mortality rate in mice poisoned by alpha-amanitin (the principal amatoxin of *A. phalloides*) is much reduced by administration of a number of agents—penicillin and sulfamethoxazole, penicillin and phenylbutazone, and chloramphenicol—which are thought to act by displacing toxin from plasma albumin-binding sites and thus promoting its excretion. Whether this approach to treatment would be useful in human mushroom poisoning is unknown.

POISONING BY FLOWERING PLANTS

An immense number of plant species may contain constituents toxic to man, and only a few of the more common and important forms of plant poisoning can be considered here.

The first examples are all members of the family of *solanaceous plants,* in which toxic species are especially well represented.

Atropa belladonna (deadly nightshade) poisoning is caused by ingestion of the prominent black berries, which contain a number of alkaloids of the belladonna group. The symptoms and signs are those of atropine poisoning: dry mouth, dry skin, blurring of vision, dilated pupils, tachycardia and excitement, hallucinations, and delirium followed by coma—"hot as a hare, blind as a bat, dry as a bone, red as a beet, and mad as a hen."

Datura stramonium (thorn apple, jimson weed) also contains stramonium alkaloids, as do other species of this genus, and they may cause poisoning by ingestion of their seeds, of extracts of leaves, and even of nectar.

Clinical manifestations are generally similar to those of atropine poisoning.

Other familiar members of the Solanaceae are *Solanum americanum* and *S. nigrum* (common nightshade, black nightshade), *S. dulcamara* (woody nightshade, bittersweet), *Hyoscyamus niger* (henbane), and the potato plant, of which the green parts and tuber sprouts may be poisonous. Plants of this group contain a mixture of the stramonium alkaloids and of solanine, itself a mixture of alkaloids.

No specific treatment is available for these forms of poisoning. Peripheral effects caused by atropine can be antagonized by pilocarpine, but this does not affect its cerebral actions. Vomiting should be induced or the stomach emptied by gastric lavage.

The family Umbelliferae also includes many toxic species, in addition to familiar food species such as carrot, parsnip, and celery. *Conium maculatum* (hemlock) is a common weed which contains several toxic alkaloids causing nausea and vomiting, progressive weakness, respiratory paralysis, and convulsions. Various species of Cicuta, the water hemlocks, are also toxic, the root containing cicutoxin, an unsaturated alcohol. Ingestion is followed by vomiting, salivation, delirium, convulsions, and paralysis.

25. CHEMICAL FOOD POISONING

Various forms of metallic poisoning are discussed in Ch. 27 to 33 and Ch. 626. Occasionally patients react idiosyncratically to a normal constituent of food, or to a food additive or preservative. The headache and hypertension induced by certain foods in patients receiving monoamine oxidase inhibitors are attributable to their natural tyramine content. The two examples which follow illustrate peculiar reactions to additives in food.

Chinese Restaurant Syndrome. A few people develop dramatic symptoms 10 to 20 minutes after eating some kind of Chinese food. These include tingling and burning in the back of the neck, radiating to the upper back, arms, and front of the chest. Some of them experience throbbing pain in the temples and infraorbital region. The symptoms fluctuate in severity and usually last for 45 minutes to 2 hours. The cause of this syndrome has been much disputed, but is probably the monosodium glutamate used in seasoning certain Chinese foods.

Hot Dog Headache. A patient experienced several hours of bitemporal headache and facial flushing, starting within 30 minutes of eating certain kinds of cured meat. His symptoms were shown to be caused by sodium nitrite used in the curing process.

Cherington, M. and Ryan, D. W.: Botulism and guanidine. N. Engl. J. Med., 282:195, 1970.

Dadisman, T. A., Nelson, R., Molenda, J. R., and Garber, H. J.: *Vibrio parahaemolyticus* in Maryland. 1. Clinical and epidemiological aspects. Am. J. Epidemiol., 96:414, 1972.

Editorial: Death cap poisoning. Lancet, 1:1320, 1972.

Evans, M. H.: Mechanism of saxitoxin and tetrodotoxin poisoning. Br. Med. Bull., 25:263, 1969.

Gangarosa, E. J., Donadio, J. A., Armstrong, R. W., Meyer, K. F., Brachman, P. S., and Dowell, V. R.: Botulism in the United States, 1899–1969. Am. J. Epidemiol., 93:93, 1971.

Koenig, M. D.: Drutz, D. J., Mushlin, A. I., Schaffner, W., and Rogers, D. E.: Type B botulism in man. Am. J. Med., 42:208, 1967.

Koenig, M. G., Spickard, A., Cardella, M. A., and Rogers, D. E.: Clinical and laboratory observations on type E botulism in man. Medicine, 43:517, 1962.

Loewenstein, M.: Epidemiology of *Cl. perfringens* food poisoning. N. Engl. J. Med., 286:1026, 1972.

Murrell, T. G. C., Roth, L., Egerton, J., Samels, J., and Walker, P. D.: Pigbel; enteritis necroticans. Lancet, 1:217, 1966.

Nakamura, M., and Schulze, J. A.: *Clostridium perfringens* food poisoning. Ann. Rev. Microbiol., 23:359, 1970.

Riemann, H. (ed.): Food-borne infections and intoxications. New York, Academic Press, 1969.

Ryan, D. W., and Cherington, M.: Human type A botulism. J.A.M.A., 216:513, 1971.

Zen-Yoji, H., Sakai, S., Terayama, T., Kudo, Y., Ito, T., Benoki, M., and Nagasaki, M.: Epidemiology, enteropathogenicity and classification of *Vibrio parahaemolyticus*. J. Infect. Dis., 115:436, 1965.

26. COMMON ACCIDENTAL POISONING

Robert J. Haggerty

Definition. The term "accidental poisoning" is usually limited to clinical illness that results from the introduction of exogenous chemicals into the body. These chemicals may be medications in excessive dose, other chemicals not intended for human metabolism, or biologic products, both plant and animal. The term, however, generally excludes disease produced by toxic products of microorganisms. An accident is (1) an observable tissue or biochemical injury that is (2) unplanned. This definition is too restrictive for accidental poisoning, for in many instances the physician is called upon to treat patients who have only ingested a poison but do not yet have any observable symptoms or signs of tissue or biochemical injury. Also, although most poisonings are unplanned in children, the same tissue or biochemical damage occurs when a chemical is introduced for homicidal or suicidal intent.

Etiology. Accidental poisoning is best understood as a problem of multiple causes—the interaction of an agent (the poison) with a host (the patient) in a particular environment. The major agents and the number of accidental poisoning deaths caused by each are listed in Table 1. In nonfatal accidental poisoning the agents responsible are quite different from those in fatal cases. The most common agents responsible for nonfatal accidental poisoning are listed in Table 2, together with the number of such accidents in different age groups. Strictly speaking, these are the etiologic agents, but to understand why a particular poisoning occurs requires knowledge of the interaction of the agent, environment, and host; this is discussed under Pathogenesis.

The route of entry of the poison (agent) is most often oral for solids and liquids, but may occasionally be by absorption through skin, rectum, or lung, or by parenteral injection.

Incidence. Nearly 3000 accidental poison fatalities occur each year in the United States. Only 10 per cent of these occur in children, but nearly two thirds of all accidental poisonings occur in preschool children. Not so evident from Table 2 is the second peak in the late teens and early twenties owing to suicide attempts. In children there are from 300 to 1000 nonfatal poison ingestions for each poison fatality. Some estimates place the total number of nonfatal poisonings as high as 300,000 to 500,000 per year in children in the United States. It is

TABLE 1. Mortality: Agents Responsible for Accidental Poison Deaths in the United States, 1969

	Less Than 5 Years of Age	Total
Medications		
Salicylates and analgesics	68	554
Sedatives and hypnotics	8	687
Psychotherapeutic drugs	12	103
Others	49	467
Total drugs	137	1811
Household products		
Alcohol	1	189
Petroleum and solvents	29	67
Pesticides	25	56
Heavy metals	18	39
Other	32	725
Total other than medications	105	1076
Grand total	242	2887

the most common medical, i.e., nonsurgical, emergency seen in preschool children. In one study, 12 per cent of all two-year-old children had experienced an accidental poisoning within the previous year. In addition to differences in the agents responsible for fatal as compared with nonfatal poisoning, the agents responsible for accidental poisoning vary considerably in their frequency between children and adults. Salicylates are the most common agent involved in children, whereas barbiturates and carbon monoxide are more common in adults. A multitude of household products (such as cleansers, solvents, and insecticides) are potentially poisonous and are available in the American home. They are more likely to be the cause of childhood than of adult poisonings.

Epidemiology. There are more epidemiologic data available on the role of the agent in causing accidental poisoning than on the host and environmental factors, and very few data on the complex interrelations of these three factors in causing accidental poisoning (Wehrle et al.). Most of the available information is of the retrospective epidemiologic type for accidental poisoning in children. It documents incidence by age (peak childhood age one to four years), sex (males more than females, except for the poison suicides of the late teens and early twenties), socioeconomic class (no difference), season (no overall significant variation, although there are some special

variations such as medications that are more frequent in the winter and pesticides in the summer), hour of day (peak in midmorning), geographical area (lye and petroleum distillates more common in the South), and place where poisoning occurred (kitchen, bedroom, and bathroom are most common). Unfortunately, this information has not led to effective prevention, for the death *rate* for all age groups from accidental poisoning has remained steady for the past two decades at about 1 per 100,000 for all age groups. There has been a significant decrease in both the *actual number* of deaths in children under five years of age from accidental poisoning (from 422 in 1958 to 242 in 1969) and in the *rate* (from 2.5 per 100,000 in 1958 to 1.5 in 1969). The most dramatic drop has occurred in aspirin poisoning. Over 20,000 total ingestions were reported to the National Clearinghouse in 1965 and only about 8000 in 1972, whereas the number of all ingestions reported actually increased. The reasons are probably multiple, but are likely to be from public and professional education, better therapy, safety enclosures for dispensing medicines (Schertz et al.), and limitation of the number of tablets in children's aspirin (1 1/4 grains) to 36 per bottle.

Since poisonous agents such as aspirin are available in nearly every home, the very real question is why more children are not poisoned when one considers the ubiquity of potentially poisonous agents.

Some children seem peculiarly susceptible to accidental poisoning (Sobel and Margolis). A child with a history of one poisoning episode is nine times as likely to have a second episode in the following year than is a child from a matched control group. Poisoned as compared to non-poisoned control children appear to have different personalities. They are more impulsive and overactive and are likely to strike back when disciplined, to have more disturbed relationships with their parents, and to have other behavior problems. Their social environment is also different, for their parents are more likely to have marital problems, to be suffering acute illness at the time of the ingestion, or to show a more distant and tense family relationship. Whether this knowledge can lead to identification of the high-risk group before poisoning occurs and whether one can change the incidence of poisoning in this high-risk group are not known; prevention by alteration of social and environmental therapy has never been documented. Among adults, suicide and homicide by poisoning obviously present a very different

TABLE 2. Most Common Agents Responsible for Accidental Poisoning Reported to the National Clearinghouse for Poison Information Centers, 1972*

	<5 Yrs.	5–14 Yrs.	15+ Yrs.	Unknown	All Ages
Medicines	47,625	4742	27,044	4721	84,132
Aspirin	8146	734	1871	310	11,061
Other internal	30,919	3570	24,294	3674	62,457
External	8560	438	879	737	10,614
Cleaning and polishing agents	17,369	852	1203	1819	21,243
Petroleum products	4571	429	610	472	6082
Cosmetics	8660	194	191	491	9536
Pesticides	5336	530	745	1043	7654
Turpentine, paints, etc.	6282	370	479	620	7751
Plants	5503	772	449	663	7387
Gases and vapors	157	178	564	379	1278
Miscellaneous	8599	1731	1357	1578	13,265
Unknown	916	248	1182	150	2496
	105,018	10,046	33,824	11,936	160,824

*Data from National Clearinghouse for Poison Information Centers, May–June, 1973.

epidemiologic picture. Unlike immunization for infectious diseases, no one method of control can be expected to be effective for all types of poisoning.

Prevention. Prevention of accidental poisoning, in spite of these negative statements about its effectiveness, should be attempted by many groups, including physicians. Better labeling of household products and prescriptions is of importance, but it should be remembered that children of the age most often poisoned cannot read. Parents should store such medications in safe places, but locked medicine cabinets are of little practical use because they are usually left unlocked when in use. Physicians treating adults should especially warn grandparents that the digitalis, quinidine, or other potent drugs they are receiving are toxic to small children and are often taken by the child from the grandmother's pocketbook. When prescribing analgesics, especially aspirin, for an acute illness in adults, the physician should warn that these are poisonous to children and should prescribe only the minimal amounts needed for an illness. All prescriptions should be dispensed in safety cap enclosures. New laws also require household cleansers to be dispensed in safety cap containers and should be effective. A common scenario of an accidental poisoning starts with a mother with an influenzal syndrome who may have aspirin prescribed; she falls asleep, and her two-year-old child ingests a fatal amount of aspirin left on the bedside table. Other acute family crises, social as well as medical, also seem to be factors in the pathogenesis of childhood poisoning (Meyer et al.). The physician who cares for such adult crises may be the most effective person to prevent childhood accidental poisonings by seeing that adequate supervision of children is arranged when parents are sick or upset.

Most poisonings in adults are the result of suicide attempts, and of course prevention is aimed at recognition of the person at risk.

Community aspects of poison prevention include public education concerning the hazards of poisons. The Federal Hazardous Substances Labeling Act requires special labeling of hazardous substances and the listing of toxic ingredients on the label. This important step is but one of many that have been taken by the community in an effort to reduce the frequency of accidental poisoning.

National Poison Prevention Week during the third week in March serves as a focal point for health education programs. But to have any chance of success, such measures should be carried out throughout the year. The rapid development of poison information centers since the first one was formed in Chicago in 1953 to the now more than 500 in the United States is another important community action. The National Clearinghouse for Poison Information Centers of the Public Health Service coordinates activities of the local centers and is a valuable repository of information, both for treatment of poisoned patients and for preventive programs. The Association of Poison Control Centers, a voluntary national group, has produced educational material designed to prevent poisonings, has established standards for operation of poison control centers, including an approved list of antidotes, their indications, and doses, and has promoted scientific study of poisonings. It seems clear that these multiple approaches to prevention of poisoning need to be continued, but there is a need to critically evaluate their effectiveness and to add imaginative new programs aimed at prevention.

Diagnosis. Diagnosis of accidental poisoning is made from (1) the label on the poison container, (2) the characteristic signs and symptoms in the patient, and (3) chemical analyses, in that order of importance. In most cases of acute poisoning, especially in children, there is no problem in determining that ingestion of a poison has occurred. The patient is often observed to ingest the poison or is found with the empty container. Here the problem is only to determine the chemical ingredients of the compound ingested, how much was taken, and what toxicity is to be expected. On the other hand, unlabeled prescriptions or trade-name household products (of which there are estimated to be over 250,000 potentially poisonous ones available in American homes) may present a serious problem in identification of the precise chemical involved. Poison information centers are especially equipped to deal with this aspect of diagnosis, for they keep on file trade names of potentially poisonous products and their ingredients. Most operate 24 hours a day and are listed in the telephone book. Information on management will also be provided by these centers. Of great use to the physician in diagnosis of poisoning, as well as in therapy, is a book (Gleason et al.) which contains a section with over 17,000 trade-name household products, their ingredients, toxicity, symptoms, and treatment.

When the label is missing, identification of the poison may be aided by knowing that certain ingredients are common to household products used for the same specific purpose; e.g., most solvent cleansers contain ketones or hydrocarbons. Federal labeling legislation, which requires most hazardous household chemicals to bear a label that plainly lists ingredients, has helped in diagnosis. *The label on the container is the single most useful diagnostic bit of information in accidental poisoning.*

When the patient has not been observed to ingest a poison, the problem of diagnosis may be great. Although some poisons produce pathognomonic signs or symptoms, most do not. Almost any acute disease may be simulated, and the range of symptoms and signs that may result is so vast that one can only advise that any symptoms or signs of unknown cause must be suspected of being due to poisoning until proved otherwise. Lists of such symptoms and signs with the various poisons that can produce them are available in standard toxicology texts.

Toxicologic analysis of body fluids or of the ingested substance itself plays a numerically small but important role in the diagnosis of accidental poisoning. Its main usefulness is for certain common medications, e.g., the ferric chloride urine screening test for salicylates and phenothiazines, and barbiturate or salicylate determinations of blood specimens; and for some heavy metal determinations (lead, thallium, mercury). It is usually impossible for a chemist to analyze a specimen of a completely unknown poison. Even when analysis is possible, the results will not be available for several hours or days; and except for certain patients with chronic poisoning, treatment must be begun much sooner than that. In those few instances in which analysis is useful, it is usually much easier to analyze the remains in the container from which the poison came than to analyze body fluids in which great dilution of the poison has occurred. Recent developments suggest that chemical analysis may play a more important role in the future. Such techniques as thin-layer and gas chromatography make possible the identification of the minute amounts of poisons present in body fluids.

Once the poison that was ingested has been identified,

TABLE 3. Toxicity Rating*

Rating	Probable Lethal Dose	
	mg/kg	For 70 kg Man
6 – Super toxic	<5	A taste < 7 drops
5 – Extremely toxic	5–50	7 drops to 1 tsp
4 – Very toxic	50–500	1 tsp to 1 oz
3 – Moderately toxic	500 mg–5 gm	1 oz to 1 pint
2 – Slightly toxic	5–15 gm	1 pint to 1 quart
1 – Practically nontoxic	>15 gm	>1 quart

*From Gleason, M., Gosselin, R., Hodge, H., and Smith, R.: Clinical Toxicology of Commercial Products. 4th ed. Baltimore, Williams & Wilkins Company, 1973.

there remains the problem of determining its potential for harm to the patient. This depends on the amount ingested and the toxicity of the agent. The amount can sometimes be estimated by observers who may have seen the patient ingest the poison and by the amount remaining in the container. The toxicity of a particular poison can be assessed by reference to known data on LD_{50} and minimal lethal dose. A table has been prepared that is most useful in then estimating the degree of risk to the patient (Table 3).

Treatment. A common mistake in the therapy of acute poisoning is to search for a specific antidote, of which there are very few, and to delay general therapy, which may be very effective and which is all that is available for the majority of poisonings.

General principles of therapy are (1) elimination of the poison from the body, (2) inactivation of the poison, and (3) supportive measures.

Elimination of the Poison. INDUCED EMESIS. One of the most common poison problems brought to the physician is that of a child or adult who has just ingested a potential poison but is still asymptomatic. The most important part of therapy is removal of the poison from the stomach before significant absorption can occur. It is now clear that gastric lavage, the time-honored method for removal of gastric contents, is much *less* effective than induced vomiting because the stomach normally traps large quantities of material in several pouches inaccessible to the lavage tube. The most effective way to induce vomiting is to administer a large dose of syrup of ipecac (15 ml for a child one to four years old, 30 to 45 ml for adults), followed by a repeat dose if no vomiting occurs within 20 minutes (Robertson). This dose is considerably larger than is recommended in older texts, but it has been found safe and much more rapidly effective than smaller doses. Many physicians now prescribe a 1-ounce bottle of syrup of ipecac when children reach age one in order that parents will have it on hand in case of need. Vomiting is more complete if the patient drinks several ounces of fluid three to five minutes after administration of the syrup of ipecac. Mechanical induction of vomiting by gagging, although having the merit of speed, is so often not effective that it is not the first choice of methods. Parenteral administration of apomorphine (1 mg for a one- to three-year-old, 6 mg for an adult) has received renewed interest as a very effective emetic, especially if Naloxone (adult dose, 0.4 mg) is then used as an antidote for the depressant effects, once vomiting has occurred. Vomiting should be induced even if several hours have elapsed after ingestion, for many poisons remain for long periods in the stomach when ingested in large quantities. Other methods of inducing vomiting such as

use of a solution of powdered mustard or soap suds are not very effective.

CAUTIONS REGARDING INDUCED EMESIS. The only contraindications to induced emesis in the treatment of accidental poisoning are in patients who have ingested caustics (lyes, acids, etc.), strychnine, and hydrocarbons, and in the comatose patient. With any cause of altered consciousness, gag reflex may be altered sufficiently to increase the risk of aspiration. Ipecac does not work well if antiemetics or some tranquilizers with antiemetic properties have been ingested. Whether one should remove hydrocarbons by careful gastric lavage is still a disputed point. A collaborative study suggests that it may be of slight advantage. At least lavage does not seem to be dangerous, but emesis should not be used to remove hydrocarbons. Saturated salt and sodium bicarbonate solutions should not be used as emetics.

GASTRIC LAVAGE. Even though less effective than emesis, gastric lavage is indicated for comatose poisoned patients to remove the poison from the stomach with less risk of aspiration than with emesis. A large-bore gastric lavage tube should usually be employed, and the stomach should be irrigated with copious amounts of water or physiologic saline. Aspiration can be prevented by having the patient lie on his side with the head slightly lower than the body. Sodium bicarbonate should not be used because it increases absorption of many poisons (salicylates) and causes large amounts of carbon dioxide to be released in the stomach, increasing the risk of aspiration.

OTHER METHODS OF POISON REMOVAL. No data are available on the *effectiveness of catharsis* or *colonic irrigations.* Most do not use cathartics today, for ipecac will cause catharsis and there is often diarrhea produced by the original poison.

Exchange transfusion has proved useful for removal of some poisons when plasma protein binding makes any form of dialysis less effective, i.e., with boric acid and some barbiturates.

Peritoneal dialysis and hemodialysis are effective means of removing many poisons. For preschool children, and even for many adults, peritoneal dialysis (Etteldorf et al.) is preferred because proper equipment and an experienced team for hemodialysis are less available. Use of commercially prepared solutions that contain properly balanced electrolytes and albumin, together with simple multiple-holed polyethylene tubing for insertion into the peritoneal cavity, provides a relatively convenient and simple technique. In certain adult patients in whom renal failure from the poisoning is the major problem, e.g., ethylene glycol poisoning, or for whom prolonged dialysis is needed, hemodialysis has proved very useful.

The kidney is the most effective organ for removal of many poisons. If renal function was normal prior to the poisoning, this route of excretion should be facilitated by adequate fluids, usually intravenously, and in some situations by the use of *osmotic diuretics,* such as mannitol (Cirksens et al.). In salicylate poisoning renal excretion is enhanced as much as twentyfold by making the pH of the urine alkaline with sodium bicarbonate. For patients who are seriously ill, several of these routes of elimination of the poison should be used simultaneously, i.e., gastric lavage, enhancement of urinary excretion, and peritoneal dialysis.

Inactivation of the Poison. A time-honored agent designed to inactivate many poisons has been the "universal antidote" made of two parts charcoal, one part tannic acid, and one part magnesium oxide. This mixture is of no value, but there are new data to support the use of specially prepared activated charcoal to absorb poisons in the intestinal tract. Five to 6 teaspoonfuls of such charcoal (not burnt toast) mixed in a glass of water should be swallowed or administered by gastric tube and then, after absorption has occurred, within 30 minutes, removed from the stomach (Holt and Holz). Neutralization of ingested acids or alkalis is probably of little value, because the tissue necrosis that results from such poisons occurs almost immediately upon contact. The use of demulcents, such as olive oil or milk, makes the patient who has ingested an irritant poison more comfortable but probably does little else and should be avoided if the poison is fat-soluble.

Supportive Measures. More lives are likely to be saved by careful, early, symptomatic treatment of complications such as peripheral vascular collapse, respiratory obstruction, urinary retention, fluid imbalance, and central nervous system excitement or depression than by frantic and usually unsuccessful search for specific antidotes. All these complications are treated by the standard methods that are used when they are due to other causes.

Poisonings for Which Specific Antidotes Exist. *Cyanide poisoning* produces death within minutes. Specific antidotes are available, but unless poisoning occurs in a laboratory there is rarely time to administer them. The antidotes are sodium nitrite injected intravenously (6 to 8 ml per square meter of body surface of a 3 per cent solution at a rate of 2.5 to 5 ml per minute), which produces methemoglobinemia, followed by sodium thiosulfate intravenously (50 ml of a 25 per cent solution). Amyl nitrite inhalation may be of value immediately while the sodium nitrite is being prepared.

Heavy metal poisoning can often be successfully treated by various chelating agents—BAL, EDTA, or penicillamine (see Ch. 27 to 33 and 626).

Iron salts produce acute gastroenteritis, shock, liver necrosis, and, frequently, death. As few as 10 tablets of the usual size (0.3 gram) may be fatal. The specific antidote, desferrioxamine, is useful intravenously to bind absorbed iron (2.0 grams in 5 per cent of levulose solution intravenously, dose 90 mg per kilogram); 140 mg of desferrioxamine can bind about 1 gram of ferrous sulfate—200 mg of iron. It is contraindicated orally, for it probably enhances absorption. Fluid replacement, including blood plasma, should be used for shock.

Morphine and other opium derivatives can be successfully antagonized by Naloxone HCl (adult dose 0.4 mg), repeated up to three times at three-minute intervals. If no improvement occurs, another cause of symptoms should be suspected. Since the action of the antagonist lasts only one to two hours and that of morphine for six or more hours, repeat doses may be needed after two hours (see Ch. 341).

Phosphate ester insecticides such as parathion are powerful anticholinesterases. In addition to peripheral parasympathetic stimulation they produce voluntary muscle paralysis, the most serious being to the muscles of respiration. Red cell cholinesterase is a valuable laboratory test to make the diagnosis and to follow therapy. Atropine in very large doses of 1 mg subcutaneously for a child, 2 to 3 mg for an adult, every 15 to 60 minutes until symptoms subside will antagonize these peripheral parasympathomimetic toxic effects. 2-Pyridine aldoxime methiodide (PAM), a cholinesterase regenerator, is dramatically effective in relieving skeletal muscle paralysis (1 gram intravenously over a five- to ten-minute period and repeated as a slow intravenous drip as needed for respiratory paralysis). Atropine is used first. PAM is not used alone. Airway obstruction must be treated by aspiration, positioning, and occasionally tracheostomy.

Treatment of Specific Common Poisons. A few words should be said about general management of the most common poisonings, but reference to standard texts is necessary for details of treatment of these as well as for the many poisonings that cannot be discussed here.

Amphetamine poisoning is common from an overdose of reducing pills or pep pills. After removal from the stomach, chlorpromazine should be administered in full dose to counteract mania and delirium. Barbiturates should not be used because the late-stage depression that occurs with amphetamines may be compounded.

Atropine poisoning may be produced by overdose or accidental ingestion of the drug or by accidental ingestion of one of several plants, such as the jimson weed. Symptoms include those of parasympathetic blocking, intense erythema, fever, and delirium. Peripheral parasympathetic blockade can be treated with pilocarpine, but this will not counteract the more serious central nervous system symptoms, which must be treated symptomatically with sedatives such as chloral hydrate or paraldehyde.

DDT and other chlorinated hydrocarbon insecticides are relatively uncommon causes of acute poisoning, for fatal doses in man are in the range of 250 mg per kilogram, and this amount is difficult to ingest. Central nervous system stimulation and convulsions are the most serious symptoms. Treatment is entirely symptomatic.

Hydrocarbon ingestion, especially of gasoline and kerosene, produces a severe pneumonia due mainly to direct aspiration into the lung rather than to bloodstream transport to the lungs. Most of the aspiration probably occurs during the initial swallow, but some may also occur during subsequent vomiting. *Emesis is therefore contraindicated.* If large amounts have been ingested, careful lavage is useful. The head should be lower than the chest to prevent aspiration, and the procedure should be performed with a small Levin tube passed through the nose. This is most effective if done before vomiting and consequent aspiration can occur. Varying degrees of central nervous system depression occur, but this rarely needs therapy except with lighter fluid, a common poisoning today with the use of outdoor charcoal cooking. It should be removed by lavage. Probably the only effective therapy for the patient with severe pneumonia is oxygen. Although adrenocortical steroids and prophylactic antimicrobials have been used, there is little evidence that they are the crucial element in successful therapy of this poisoning. Again lighter fluid is the exception, and adrenal steroids do seem useful for pneumonia caused by this agent.

Carbon tetrachloride produces prompt central nervous system depression and abdominal pain. Early death is due to depression of vasomotor and respiratory centers and convulsions. If the patient survives this, he may develop renal and hepatic necrosis. The management at this stage is the same as for other causes of failure of these organs.

Methyl alcohol can cause severe metabolic acidosis and blindness with a fatal dose from as little as 2 ounces. Treatment includes emesis, ethyl alcohol to inhibit the metabolic oxidation of methanol (whiskey, 30 ml every three to four hours for adults), and sodium bicarbonate intravenously for the metabolic acidosis.

Lye and other caustics produce severe, deep burns of the esophagus that may perforate or may later cause esophageal stenosis. Initial pain, airway obstruction, and shock are treated symptomatically. Early esophagoscopy, to determine whether burns have occurred, is followed by cortisone if burns are found. After several days for healing to progress, careful dilatation of the esophagus can be begun. Management should be a team effort with the esophagoscopist.

Salicylate poisoning is the single most common cause of poisoning in children. Emesis should always be carried out if the patient is awake, even though several hours have elapsed after ingestion. Salicylates produce an initial respiratory alkalosis that is transient in children but less so in adults, followed by severe metabolic acidosis, dehydration, and loss of body potassium. With severe poisoning several routes of elimination may have to be used, i.e., by increasing urinary excretion and by peritoneal dialysis. Initial hydration should be vigorous to initiate brisk diuresis, and the fluids should include sodium bicarbonate, 14 to 20 ml of 7.5 per cent solution per 500 ml of fluid. Once diuresis has begun, potassium salts, approximately 35 mEq per liter of fluid, should be added to the solution. Monitoring of serum pH and electrolytes and adjustment of fluid and electrolyte administration appropriately are important for optimal therapy. Milder degrees of poisoning can usually be treated with alkali and intravenous fluids alone. Other symptoms, such as respiratory depression or convulsions, are treated symptomatically.

Cirksens, W. J., Bastian, R. C., Malloy, J. P., and Barry, K. G.: Use of mannitol in exogenous and endogenous intoxications. N. Engl. J. Med., 270:161, 1964.
Etteldorf, J. N., Dobbins, W. T., Summitt, R. L., Rainwater, W. T., and Fischer, R. L.: Intermittent peritoneal dialysis using 5 per cent albumin in the treatment of salicylate intoxication in children. J. Pediatr., 58:226, 1961.
Gleason, M., Gosselin, R., Hodge, H., and Smith, R.: Clinical Toxicology of Commercial Products. 4th ed. Baltimore, Williams & Wilkins Company, 1973.
Holt, L. E., Jr., and Holz, P. H.: Activated Charcoal as an Antidote for Poisons. Nat. Clearinghouse Poison Control Cent. 1963, Jan.-Feb., pp. 1–3.
Meyer, R. J., Roelofs, H. A., Bluestone, J., and Redmond, S.: Accidental injury to the preschool child. J. Pediatr., 63:95, 1963.
Robertson, W. O.: Syrup of ipecac—a slow or fast emetic? Am. J. Dis. Child., 103:136, 1962.
Schertz, R. G., Latham, G. H., and Stracener, D. E.: Child-resistant containers can prevent poisonings. Pediatrics, 43:84, 1969.
Sobel, R., and Margolis, J. A.: Repetitive poisoning in children: A psycho-social study. Pediatrics, 35:641, 1965.
Wehrle, P. F., DeFreest, L., Penhollow, J., and Harris, V. G.: The epidemiology of accidental poisoning in an urban population. III. Pediatrics, 27:614, 1961.

HEAVY METAL POISONING

Edmund B. Flink

27. INTRODUCTION

Many features of poisoning by the heavy metals are similar. The important metals from the standpoint of toxicology are arsenic, lead, mercury, antimony, cadmium, and thallium. The toxic and lethal doses of each metal are small. Antimony, arsenic, lead, mercury, and thallium all have effects on enzymes of the body. Antimony, arsenic, and mercury poison sulfhydryl groups. Mercuric ions even in fairly dilute solutions denature proteins and cause protein precipitation. Thallium and cadmium have recently assumed importance industrially.

Other metals may be toxic also. *Beryllium* intoxication is discussed in Ch. 526, and *bismuth, copper, gold, iron, silver, and uranium* intoxications are discussed in Ch. 626. *Barium* ions cause epigastric pain, nausea, vomiting, diarrhea, chills, cramps, muscle contractions, convulsions, hypertension, tachyarrhythmia, and cardiac arrest. Sodium sulfate or magnesium sulfate should be given immediately to precipitate the barium as sulfate. *Cobalt* was added to beer from 1957 to 1967. Ingestion of large volumes of this beer caused serious and often fatal myocardiopathy. Cobalt has been eliminated as an additive. *Manganese* poisoning occurs in mining and smelting of manganese ores. Damage to the basal ganglia of the brain occurs with attendant Parkinson-like symptoms. When symptoms begin, removal from exposure is mandatory. Proper ventilation of mines and processing plants will prevent intoxication.

Dubois, K. P., and Geiling, E. M. K.: Textbook of Toxicology. New York, Oxford University Press, 1959.
Gleason, M. N., Gosselin, R. E., Hodge, H. C., and Smith, R.: Clinical Toxicology of Commercial Products. 4th ed. Baltimore, Williams & Wilkins Company, 1973.
Goodman, L. S., and Gilman, A.: Pharmacological Basis of Therapeutics. 4th ed. New York, The Macmillan Company, 1970.

28. ARSENIC POISONING

Exposure. Many household and garden pesticides contain arsenous oxide, copper acetoarsenite (Paris green), or calcium or lead arsenate. Drugs that contain arsenic include sodium cacodylate, Fowler's solution, and the arsphenamines (now obsolete). Fowler's solution continues to be used in treatment of asthma in certain regions. Fruits sprayed with insecticides may contain enough arsenic to be toxic. Bootlegged whiskey has occasionally been contaminated with arsenicals. Arsenic trioxide (As_2O_3) or white arsenic has been a favorite for homicidal purposes. Accidental ingestion of arsenic-containing poison continues to be an important source of exposure especially for children.

Although toxic exposure occurs in a variety of industries, only a few cases are reported. Poisoning does occur among agricultural workers using insecticide sprays or dust. Arsine (AsH_3) is a very serious industrial hazard. It is produced accidentally by the exposure of nascent hydrogen to arsenic trioxide.

Arsenic is stored in liver, nervous system, nails, hair, and other viscera and can be detected in them after excretion in urine has ceased. A single dose requires 10 to 70 days for excretion, so accumulation is possible from small daily doses.

The minimal lethal dose of arsenic trioxide (As_2O_3) is 60 to 180 mg, but there is a great variability in susceptibility. The lethal dose of arsine is smaller than this.

Manifestations. *Acute poisoning* may be overwhelming and may produce shock and death within 20 minutes to 48 hours. Ingestion of smaller doses causes vomiting, diarrhea, abdominal pain, and muscle cramps, but does not cause corrosion of mucous membranes. If the victim survives acute poisoning, he may recover without sequelae, or he may develop symptoms of chronic poisoning.

Intravascular hemolysis and renal damage are characteristic of arsenic poisoning, so hemoglobinuria, nausea, vomiting, and abdominal pain develop within six hours after exposure. This initial illness may be quickly fatal, or recovery may begin in a few days. Instances of chronic arsine poisoning have been reported.

Chronic poisoning results from repeated ingestion of small doses. This is the usual method for homicide. Weight loss, diarrhea or constipation, nausea, anorexia, fatigue, drowsiness, peripheral neuropathy, headache, confusion, pigmentation and scaling of the skin, hyperkeratoses of palms and soles, and transverse white lines of all fingernails (Mee's lines) are the important symptoms and signs. Hyperkeratoses may go on to malignant changes in the form of multiple basal cell cancers (Bowen's disease). Perforation of the nasal septum is common. Myocardiopathy induced by arsenic may be fatal.

Hematologic findings of chronic arsenic poisoning include anemia, leukopenia, thrombocytopenia, basophilic stippling, and disturbed erythropoiesis, and myelopoiesis.

Diagnosis. The diagnosis can be established by determining arsenic in the urine. Normal persons excrete an average of 0.015 mg per day, with a range of 0.005 to 0.04 mg. Most patients with manifestations of arsenic poisoning excrete more than 0.1 mg per day.

As in lead poisoning, urine coproporphyrin III excretion is increased markedly, but delta amino levulinic acid is not increased in experimental arsenic poisoning in rabbits and probably not in human intoxication.

Hair and nails store arsenic, so analysis of arsenic content may be of diagnostic value, particularly after removal of the patient from exposure. Hair and nail samples must be very carefully washed to exclude adhering dust and extraneous material. Normal values have ranged from 0.025 to 0.088 mg per 100 grams of hair. Over 0.1 mg per 100 grams is abnormal.

Treatment. When a poison has been ingested, immediate induction of emesis or gastric lavage is of prime importance. Dimercaprol (BAL) should be given immediately. The initial intramuscular dose of BAL is 2.5 to 3.0 mg per kilogram of body weight, followed by the same dose every four hours for six doses. For very severe poisoning, the initial dose should be 5.0 mg per kilogram, followed by 2.5 mg per kilogram, as indicated above, with additional doses at 6- to 12-hour intervals for six doses, depending on the status of the patient. BAL has not proved to be effective in arsine poisoning or in chronic poisoning, probably because the damage has already occurred. Removal from exposure in chronic poisoning is mandatory and usually suffices.

Severe anemia must be treated by transfusion. Treatment of acute renal insufficiency requires the same considerations as that resulting from a variety of causes.

Prevention. Proper storage and labeling of poisons in general should prevent accidental poisoning of children. Avoiding direct contact with insect sprays and wearing appropriate masks when using dusting powders will control this industrial exposure.

Heyman, A., Pfeiffer, J. B., Jr., Willet, R. W., and Taylor, H. M.: Peripheral neuropathy caused by arsenical intoxication: A study of 41 cases with observation of the effects of BAL. N. Engl. J. Med., 254:401, 1956.

Kyle, R. A., and Pease, G. L.: Hematologic aspects of arsenic intoxication. N. Engl. J. Med., 273:18, 1965.

Vallee, B. L., Ulmer, D. D., and Wacker, W. E. C.: Arsenic toxicology and biochemistry. A.M.A. Arch. Industr. Health, 21:132, 1960.

29. LEAD POISONING

Etiology. Exposure to lead in the home is chiefly by ingestion of white lead paint scales by children (pica), from new water systems in which white lead has been used in joints of pipes, by ingestion of soluble lead salts in foods, wines, and distilled liquors, by use of pewter dishes, and by use of tetraethyl lead gasoline for cleaning purposes. Drinking of "moonshine" whiskey distilled by use of an auto radiator as a condenser has resulted in epidemics of acute lead poisoning and constitutes an important cause of lead poisoning of adults.

Ingestion of lead paint scales by young children in areas of poor and old housing constitutes the greatest problem in the United States today. In New York City 4000 cases of lead poisoning were found in 1970 and 1971 because of increased interest and availability of appropriate tests. The incidence in children is greatest in summer months and reaches a peak at the age of one to three years. Black children are at greatest risk. Siblings of children with lead intoxication should be examined also, because about a third of them have been found to have serious exposure.

Lead is dissolved and absorbed from the gastrointestinal tract, deposited in the liver, and then released into the systemic circulation. The respiratory tract epithelium may absorb lead fumes or may propel particles into the pharynx, where they are swallowed. Tetraethyl lead and related compounds may be absorbed through the skin. Soluble lead salts, such as lead acetate or lead carbonate, are readily absorbed and can cause acute poisoning when ingested.

There are many industrial uses of lead and, therefore, many opportunities for exposure. In recent years the industrial consumption of lead in the United States has averaged about 1,110,000 tons a year. The industries using or producing lead are petroleum, mining and smelting, storage battery manufacture, printing, paint and pigment, ceramic and glass, construction (mainly plumbing and insulation), ammunition, wrecking and salvage (acetylene torch and electric arc volatilizing lead paints and alloys), battery reclaiming, and brass polishing. Any procedure that produces lead vapor, mist, or dust exposes workers to inhalation and absorption of lead from respiratory tract epithelium.

The lead-using trades have set up standards and checking procedures that have controlled industrial hazards well. Smoking and eating are restricted to uncontaminated areas. Washing hands and changing clothes before eating and leaving work are the most important personal preventive measures. The gasoline industry has rigid standards for tetraethyl lead workers, but exposure to dangerous amounts still occurs when there is a break in procedure. Cleaning and repairing large storage tanks pose a particular hazard.

Pathology. In chronic poisoning no gross or microscopic lesions are pathognomonic of lead poisoning. Lead is stored in an inert form in bone and is not harmful except when mobilized. Most of the remaining lead is found in the bone marrow, blood, liver, and kidneys. An increased amount of lead in tissues indicates exposure but not necessarily toxicity. Absence of an increased concentration of lead in tissues practically excludes lead poisoning.

In the encephalopathic type, small perivascular hemorrhages, necrosis of cells, and serous exudate around blood vessels may be found anywhere in the brain. In children with acute poisoning, nuclear inclusions are found in liver cells and renal tubular cells. Occasionally inclusions are found in renal tubule cells of lead workers. In Australia chronic lead exposure from the dust of white lead paint has been incriminated as a common cause of chronic renal failure in young adults.

Clinical Manifestations. Lead poisoning is usually divided into acute and chronic forms. Although "chronic poisoning" correctly describes prolonged exposure, manifestations often are acute. It is convenient for descriptive purposes to divide symptomatology into an alimentary form, a neuromuscular form, and an encephalopathic form.

Anemia and attendant pallor and weakness are present in most patients with chronic exposure. *Insomnia, headache, dizziness,* and *irritability* are common symptoms without evidence of more serious encephalopathic disturbances. In a patient with poor oral hygiene, lead sulfide is deposited along the gingival margin of some or all teeth and produces a blue-black *"lead line."* *Stippling of the retina* adjacent to the optic disc has been described as an early sign in lead poisoning. Chronic renal failure results from chronic lead intoxication. *Saturnine gout* is particularly common in lead poisoning from "moonshine" whiskey. The renal clearance of uric acid decreases.

Alimentary Form. *Painter's* or *lead colic* is the cardinal feature and is the result of spasm of the bowel. Constipation is a natural consequence, and nausea, vomiting, and weight loss are common. Colic is intermittent and often severe enough to double the patient up. Between attacks there is merely a sense of pressure. Absence of tenderness differentiates the condition from appendicitis or other causes of peritoneal inflammation. Relief actually may be produced by pressure on the abdomen. Colic is not invariably present.

Neuromuscular Form. Extensor muscles of the upper extremities are more often paralyzed than flexors or lower extremity muscles. *Wrist drop* is a common and characteristic example. Muscle soreness and stiffness or hypertonus precede and accompany paralysis. The absence of sensory disturbance is important in differentiating this from other forms of peripheral neuropathy. Paralysis is confined to a functional muscle group and is not determined by the distribution of an entire motor nerve. Atrophy may occur after longstanding paralysis and may result in incomplete recovery of muscle function after termination of exposure (see Ch. 456 to 474).

Encephalopathic Form. At present this occurs primarily in children. The diagnosis is not suspected until a large amount of lead has been ingested. Because of the good safeguards in industry now, it rarely occurs in adults and then only after massive exposure to lead fumes or tetraethyl lead in a salvage operation, in cleaning large gasoline storage tanks, or in accidental breaks in techniques. Tetraethyl lead is lipid-soluble, so that exposure results almost exclusively in the encephalopathic form.

The presenting manifestations include *convulsions, mania, delirium,* or *coma.* There may be a history of antecedent behavioral changes such as irritability, insomnia, restlessness, loss of memory, hallucinations, and confusion.

Children may suddenly become very ill. Increased intracranial pressure may occur and is manifested by projectile vomiting, lethargy, convulsions, and coma. In very young children fontanelles bulge. The optic discs may not reflect increased pressure when the process is very acute in onset. Scattered neurologic findings indicate cerebral and cerebellar abnormalities. Blindness and deafness may occur and persist.

Laboratory Findings. The hematologic findings depend on the action of lead on hemoglobin synthesis. Lead interferes with enzymes ALA synthetase, ALA dehydrase, and heme synthetase. ALA and coproporphyrin III accumulate and are excreted in the urine in excessive amounts, and protoporphyrin accumulates in erythrocytes as a result of the blocks in synthetic process. Normally 2 mg of ALA or less is excreted per 24 hours. Lead poisoning results in a 20- to 200-fold increase in excretion of ALA. ALA excretion is a sensitive indicator of lead intoxication. Normally 60 to 280 μg of coproporphyrin is excreted per 24 hours.

In lead poisoning free erythrocyte protoporphyrin (FEPP) ranges from 300 to 3000 μg per 100 ml (normal 15 to 60) and free erythrocyte coproporphyrin (FECP) ranges from 1 to 20 μg per 100 ml (normal 0 to 2). It is noteworthy that iron deficiency anemia and thalassemia result in FEPP values that overlap those of lead poisoning, but the range is not quite as great. If a fresh wet film of blood of a patient with lead poisoning is examined under ultraviolet light, 75 to 100 per cent of the erythrocytes have a red fluorescence. This fluorescence is the result of increased FEPP.

Lead poisoning and *hereditary acute intermittent porphyria* have manifestations that are similar. Both are characterized by colicky abdominal pain, mental symptoms, and paralysis. Acute intermittent porphyria regularly has a great increase in porphobilinogen excretion and uroporphyrin excretion, but lead poisoning usually does not result in excessive excretion of either substance.

Normochromic microcytic anemia, decreased red cell life span, decreased osmotic fragility, but increased mechanical fragility are found. Acute hemolytic anemia with hemoglobinemia, hemoglobinuria, and renal damage occur occasionally in acute poisoning. Death from shock may occur in two to three days. *Basophilic stippling* is nonspecific, is rarely found in tetraethyl lead intoxication, is seldom found in acute poisoning of children, and cannot be relied on for screening purposes. Nevertheless, it frequently furnishes the initial clue for clinical recognition of chronic lead poisoning.

Aminoaciduria, renal glycosuria, fructosuria, hyperphosphaturia, and citraturia result from changes in the epithelium of the proximal convoluted tubules. Other toxins also cause these manifestations. The changes are usually reversible.

Diagnosis. In children, particularly, the normal blood level is low. If the higher range is used with the upper limit of some 0.06 mg per 100 grams, children with serious acute poisoning will have normal levels (see accompanying table). In adults the upper limits of normal coincide with the mean of "safe" exposure.

A diagnosis of tetraethyl lead intoxication is made on the basis of history of exposure. Urine lead determination is the most valuable test. Blood values usually are normal.

Because of the medicolegal implications, it is important to be certain that there is evidence of increased lead excretion. Detection of an earlier exposure may be accomplished by the use of 1.0 gram intravenously of calcium disodium edetate (CaEDTA). Striking augmentation of lead excretion to over 1.0 mg per day usually

Normal and Abnormal Values in Exposure to Lead

| | Adults | | |
	Normal Industrial Exposure	"Safe" Industrial Exposure	Dangerous Industrial Exposure
Urine mg per liter	Range: 0.00 to 0.06 Mean: 0.03	0.01 to 0.15 0.08	0.08 to 0.4 0.2
Blood mg per 100 grams	Range: 0.01 to 0.05 Mean: 0.03	0.01 to 0.07 0.06	0.07 to 0.2 0.09
Feces mg per specimen	0.25	0.6 to 1.0	1.1+

| | Children | |
	Normal Range	Poisoning
Blood mg per 100 grams	British series American series	0 to 0.04 0.003 to 0.055	0.04 to 0.4 0.06+

occurs. This proves previous exposure but not intoxication.

Collection of samples for analysis must be done with great care to avoid contamination. Pyrex bottles or polyethylene flasks should be rinsed with nitric acid and distilled water. Urine and stool specimens should be passed directly into acid-cleaned containers. Tissues should be placed directly in acid-cleaned containers.

Blood now can be collected in special vacutainer 20 ml tubes (Becton, Dickinson Company) with pure gum rubber stoppers. These tubes have been chemically cleaned for lead analyses. The needle is a straight stainless steel tube. Duplicate samples are desirable.

Lead determinations on blood and urine can now be performed quickly and accurately, using an atomic absorption spectrophotometer. All state and many large city departments of health have such facilities available.

Treatment. Cessation of exposure is of prime importance. A saline cathartic should be given to rid the gut of any unabsorbed lead before chelation of lead is attempted, especially in the encephalopathic form in children.

Colic may be controlled temporarily by intravenous infusion of 1.0 gram of calcium gluconate. The infusion may be repeated as needed.

Fluid intake should be high unless there is increased intracranial pressure. Electrolyte concentrations should be determined and corrected if abnormal.

Chelation of lead by calcium disodium edetate, U.S.P. (CaEDTA), is now the initial treatment of choice for inorganic lead and tetraethyl lead intoxication and is much more effective than any previous method. The chelated lead is excreted in the urine. CaEDTA in doses of 1 to 2 grams per day for an adult and not more than 75 mg per kilogram for a child is given in six to twelve hours intravenously. This dose is repeated for two to three days with a five- to ten-day rest period between courses. Nephropathy has resulted rarely from therapy, but this usually has occurred with larger doses than those outlined above. If symptoms are severe, treatment should not be delayed to obtain results of lead analyses. Lead excretion should be determined during as well as before treatment.

D-Penicillamine not only chelates lead but also supplies sulfhydryl groups. A dose of 30 mg per kilogram up to a total of 2.0 grams per day in four divided doses given orally is satisfactory. It is particularly useful to follow the initial CaEDTA therapy. It has the additional advantages that it can be given orally continuously, and that it is much less toxic than CaEDTA. For moderate lead intoxication, penicillamine is the agent of choice. Successful treatment with CaEDTA or penicillamine results in a return of ALA and coproporphyrin excretion to normal. Erythrocyte protoporphyrin declines very slowly after successful treatment.

The most serious manifestation is lead encephalopathy, which requires prompt and skillful treatment. Increased intracranial pressure may occur suddenly and must be treated vigorously. Infusion of urea solution in a dose of 100 mg per kilogram to 1000 mg per kilogram as 30 per cent urea in 10 per cent glucose solution or of mannitol solution (20 per cent) in a dose of 7 to 10 ml per kilogram can alleviate increased pressure effectively, but the benefit may last only a day or two, and repetition may be necessary. Dexamethasone sodium phosphate in a dose of 10 mg intravenously initially followed by 4 to 6 mg intramuscularly every four to six hours in adults is an effective alternative. Craniotomy may even be required for relief of pressure. Chelation of lead with CaEDTA must be started immediately for patients who are gravely ill.

Physiotherapy is important for patients with neuropathy. Splinting to support the weak extremity prevents overstretching of muscles; otherwise, permanent disability can follow.

Prognosis. In the gastrointestinal form the outlook is good for complete recovery after adequate treatment and prevention of re-exposure. Recovery from paralysis is usually complete even after many months of paralysis.

Encephalopathy is very serious. It causes a mortality rate of 25 per cent or more, and often leaves mental retardation and various permanent neurologic lesions in those who survive. In adults permanent blindness, extraocular muscle paralysis, or other lesions may result. The acute form caused by tetraethyl lead either is fatal or is followed by complete recovery. There is great urgency in treatment of this form. One cannot wait to get results of lead analysis before starting treatment.

Albahary, C.: Lead and hemopoiesis. Am. J. Med., 52:367, 1972.
Ball, G. V., and Sorensen, L. B.: Pathogenesis of hyperuricemia in saturnine gout. New Eng. J. Med., 280:1199, 1969.
Beattie, A. D., Moore, M. R., and Goldberg, A.: Tetraethyl-lead poisoning. Lancet, 2:12, 1972.
Byers, R. K.: Lead poisoning. Review of literature and report on 45 cases. Pediatrics, 23:585, 1959.
Einarsson, O., and Lindstedt, G.: Nonextraction atomic absorption method for the determination of lead. Scand. J. Clin. Lab. Invest., 23:367, 1969.
Feldman, F., Lichtman, H. C., Oransky, S., Ana, E. S., Reiser, L., and Malemud, C. J.: Serum delta aminolevulinic acid in plumbism. J. Pediatr., 74:917, 1969.
Fleming, A. J.: Industrial hygiene and medical control procedures. Arch. Environ. Health, 8:266, 1964.
Guinee, V. F.: Lead poisoning. Am. J. Med., 52:283, 1972.

30. MERCURY POISONING

Etiology. Acute mercury poisoning results from accidental or intentional ingestion of soluble mercuric salts such as mercuric chloride ($HgCl_2$, corrosive sublimate) and is characterized by very serious corrosive effects on the entire gastrointestinal tract and serious renal tubular cell damage.

Mercury is a liquid and is highly volatile at room temperature. In 1957 over 4 million pounds of mercury were used in the United States. It is used widely in medical research and clinical pathology laboratories, as well as in the manufacture of scientific instruments, electric meters, mercury vapor lamps, amalgams with copper, tin, silver or gold, in solders, and in the production of organic mercurial compounds. Mining cinnabar (HgS), refining mercury from it, and cleaning mercury distilling apparatus involve substantial hazards. Photoengraving, bronzing, and the production of certain paint colors such as vermilion and antifouling agents for hulls of ships all use mercury compounds.

As little as 0.1 gram of $HgCl_2$ may cause poisoning, but fatal doses are usually in excess of 1.0 gram. It is caustic and produces cell destruction by protein precipitation on direct contact. In more dilute solutions, such as concentrations effected by absorption from the intestinal tract after ingestion of a toxic dose, its effect is primarily due to selective affinity for sulfhydryl (-SH) groups of proteins, especially of enzymes. This property is counteracted by dimercaprol.

Chronic mercury poisoning results from inhalation of mercury vapor or ingestion of small amounts of mercuric nitrate or other salts, and is characterized by mental symptoms and stomatitis.

Alkyl mercury compounds (ethyl and methyl mercury) have become an important environmental problem. The compounds are soluble in organic solvents, and the covalent carbon-mercury bond is not degraded by biologic processes. Methyl mercury particularly is found in tuna and swordfish taken from waters heavily contaminated with mercury. Epidemics have occurred in Minamata and Niigata, Japan, and in several countries where seed grain treated with alkyl mercury compounds (as antifungal agents) has been diverted into food. Nearly complete intestinal absorption occurs; the liver excretes most of it into the intestine, resulting in continuous enterohepatic circulation. Methyl mercury passes the placental barrier very well and accumulates in the fetus with resultant cerebral palsy and mental retardation of the child.

ACUTE POISONING

See Ch. 626.

CHRONIC POISONING

Clinical Manifestations. *Stomatitis.* Excessive salivation and a metallic taste are common. A blue line develops along the gingival margin. Gums become hypertrophied, bleed easily, and are sore. The teeth become loose.

Erethism. The term "erethism" is applied to the psychic disturbance characterized by irritability, shyness, and deterioration of family and social activities, suggesting hyperthyroidism. Since felt hat makers formerly used mercury salts in the manufacturing process and often became "mad," these symptoms gave rise to the phrase "mad as a hatter."

Tremors. Tremors of the eyelids, lips, tongue, fingers and extremities are characteristic of chronic poisoning. Coarse jerky movements and gross incoordination interfere with fine movements such as writing and eating. Atrophy of the cerebellar cortex and, to a lesser extent, of the cerebral cortex occurs. Microscopic changes occur in the granular layer of the cerebellum, ganglion cells, and posterior columns.

Nephrotic Syndrome. Contact with ammoniated mercury and other compounds has caused proteinuria and frank nephrotic syndrome. Removal from exposure is mandatory, so a careful history of medicinal or occupational exposure is needed.

Hypersensitivity. Hypersensitivity reactions to mercurial diuretic agents include asthma, urticaria, exfoliative dermatitis, and sudden death. Fatal accidents can be prevented by avoiding intravenous injections. Death is usually due to ventricular fibrillation.

Hypersensitivity to calomel (HgCl) results from long-term ingestion of HgCl. Hypersensitivity to ammoniated mercury or other compounds results from topical application. Fever, morbilliform rash, leukopenia, eosinophilia, and enlargement of the spleen and lymph nodes characterize this condition. Mercury fulminate used in percussion caps and detonators may cause dermatitis of exposed parts, with pruritus, papules, vesicles, and pustules.

Acrodynia or "Pink Disease." This disorder of infants and young children is characterized by irritability, insomnia, stomatitis, loss of teeth, hypertension, erythema of fingers, toes, nose, cheeks, and buttocks, and even acral gangrene. Fever, leukocytosis, and albuminuria occur. In 1948 Warkany and Hubbard suggested that sensitivity to mercury might be the cause, and that hypothesis is now fairly generally accepted. The diagnosis is established by finding excretion of more than 0.1 mg of mercury per day in the urine. An organic mercury compound, phenyl mercuric propionate, has been incorporated into house paint to prevent growth of mold. This paint has been incriminated as a source of toxic exposure.

ORGANIC MERCURY INTOXICATION

Ethyl and methyl mercury compounds have an affinity for the central nervous system and produce fatigue, headache, loss of memory, apathy, emotional instability, paresthesia, generalized ataxia, deafness, dysarthria, progressive visual deterioration, dysphagia, and, occasionally, coma and death. Changes in the central nervous system similar to the lesions of chronic mercury poisoning are found.

Diagnosis. Industrial exposure and characteristic symptoms usually make recognition of chronic mercury poisoning relatively straightforward, but, in the absence of known exposure, the diagnosis may be elusive. Patients with chronic mercury poisoning excrete in excess of 0.3 mg of Hg per liter of urine. Normal values range from 0.0001 to 0.001 mg per liter. An excretion of 0.1 mg per liter is considered evidence of toxic exposure. In instances of exposure to metallic mercury for more than five years, a brown reflex from the anterior lens capsule can be seen by slit lamp. Some observers consider it an early sign of mercury poisoning. Albuminuria and hematuria are common findings in chronic poisoning.

Treatment. Removal of the patient from all possible exposure is of paramount importance. The use of BAL in chronic poisoning has not been established as effective treatment. However, n-acetyl-DO-penicillamine, in a dose of 500 mg four times a day, increases mercury excretion and has been used successfully in therapy of chronic mercury poisoning and acrodynia. This treatment is ineffective in methyl mercury poisoning, but promising results have been obtained here, using ion-absorbing resin to interrupt the enterohepatic circulation of mercury.

Prognosis. Recovery is slow even after removal from exposure. Patients with advanced intoxication fare poorly. Only 15 per cent of the more severely involved patients recovered completely in one series. Signs of cerebellar and cerebral damage persisted and prevented return to normal activities.

Prevention. Removal of $HgCl_2$, calomel, and mercury ointments from the market would eliminate acute poisoning and many instances of chronic poisoning. Good safe substitutes are available for each compound. Elimination of mercuric nitrate from the felt-processing industry has already occurred. Mercury salts for fingerprinting by police departments have been replaced by barium, zinc, or bismuth. Silver has replaced mercury in the manufacture of mirrors.

Mercury-containing paints should have a warning label "For Outside Use Only." Mercury cannot be replaced in many electrical apparatuses and scientific instruments. Proper exhaust ventilation, scrupulous avoidance of any exposed metallic mercury, and good personal hygiene are necessary precautions. The maximal allowable concentration of Hg has been set at 0.1 mg per cubic meter of air. Medical supervision is necessary wherever potential exposure exists. Neurologic signs and especially visual field changes, tremor, ataxia, and dysarthria are serious danger signals.

Battigelli, M. C.: Mercury toxicity from industrial exposure. A critical review of the literature. J. Occup. Med., 2:337, 1960.

Hirschman, S. Z., Feingold, M., and Boylen, G.: Mercury in house paint as a cause of acrodynia. N. Engl. J. Med., 269:889, 1963.

Joselow, M. M., Louria, D. B., and Browder, A.: Mercurialism. Environmental and occupational aspects. Ann. Intern. Med., 76:119, 1972.

31. ANTIMONY POISONING

Antimony and potassium tartrate (tartar emetic) is used for emetic purposes, and other organic antimony compounds are used in treatment of schistosomiasis, filariasis, and certain fungal infections. Antimony is encountered in metallurgic processes, mining and smelting, and in rubber manufacturing, but industrial poisoning is rare. Finely divided antimony is more toxic than compounds of antimony. Trivalent antimony combines with sulfhydryl groups of enzymes. The symptoms of acute poisoning are similar to those of acute arsenic poisoning. Vomiting is a prominent symptom. Dimercaprol (BAL) is an effective agent for treatment of antimony poisoning, and the regimen is like that for arsenic and mercury. Dermatitis and conjunctivitis occur from exposure to dust in the smelting process. Stibine (SbH_3) is more volatile than arsine and is very toxic also. It attacks the central nervous system and causes acute hemolysis. Death occurs when there is a 0.01 per cent concentration in the air. The chemical process of formation and the effects are like those of arsine.

32. CADMIUM POISONING

Cadmium sulfide is associated with zinc minerals and particularly with zinc sulfide. Cadmium exposure can

occur in the manufacture of alloys, vapor lamps, and storage batteries, grinding and polishing alloys, cadmium plating, welding, zinc ore smelting, and glass blowing. Inhalation of cadmium fumes results in pulmonary edema, followed in two to three days by proliferative interstitial pneumonia. Various degrees of permanent lung damage and fibrosis occur. Cadmium can be inhaled in fatal concentrations without enough discomfort to warn the worker. The inhalation of fumes with cadmium produces dryness of throat, cough, headache, vomiting, sensation of constriction in the chest, severe dyspnea, and prostration. There is no effective treatment except symptomatic treatment of pulmonary edema. Foods prepared and stored in cadmium-plated containers may be contaminated sufficiently to cause poisoning. Cadmium ingestion usually does not produce fatal poisoning, but causes rather violent gastrointestinal symptoms, with sudden onset 20 to 30 minutes after eating.

33. THALLIUM POISONING

Thallium sulfate (Tl_2SO_4) is an extremely toxic cumulative poison (lethal dose 0.2 to 1.0 gram). It has a mild metallic taste. Thallium is absorbed from the gut and from the intact skin. It has had wide use as a rodent, ant, and cockroach poison. Because of serious and frequent accidental and deliberate (homicidal) toxicity, the U.S. Department of Agriculture banned thallium formulations for household use in 1965. Unfortunately, some of it can still be found on shelves in homes and stores.

Alopecia is a very important and unique sign. *Accumulation in nervous tissue* accounts for critical symptoms which include ataxia, choreiform movements, vomiting, constipation, restlessness, delirium with hallucinations and delusions, and, finally, coma. Blindness, loss of other special senses, facial paralysis, paresthesias, and peripheral neuropathy occur. Central lobular necrosis of the liver and renal damage also occur. Liver radiopacity increases in some patients. Urinary excretion of 10 mg per day or more indicates serious poisoning.

Various therapeutic trials, including dithiocarb, dithizone, BAL, and KCl, have been used but either have failed to bring improvement or may even be dangerous because of mobilization of thallium and redistribution to the brain. Gastric lavage should be done immediately after diagnosis up to four hours after exposure. Prussian blue (potassium ferric hexacryanoferrate II) is an excellent chelator of thallium by exchange of potassium for thallium. Prussian blue is not absorbed from the gut and is nontoxic. It must be introduced into the duodenum by tube because of gastric dilation produced by thallium. The recommended dose of colloidal solution is 250 mg per kilogram per day in two to four divided doses. A vigorous laxative such as castor oil is necessary for the first day or two. After this an osmotic agent such as 50 ml of 15 per cent mannitol solution will suffice. Therapy should continue until thallium excretion is less than 0.5 mg per 24 hours.

Huff, J. E.: Special communication: Thallium poisoning. Clin. Toxicol., 5:89, 1972.

Kamerbeck, H. H., Rauws, A. G., TenHam, M., and VanHeijst, A. N. P.: Prussian blue therapy of thallotoxicosis. Acta Med. Scand., 189:321, 1971.

34. CARBON MONOXIDE POISONING

Bertram D. Dinman

Definition. Carbon monoxide, a product of incomplete combustion of carbonaceous materials, is an odorless, colorless gas; its density is slightly less than air. The gas is commonly produced by the internal combustion engine, poorly vented heating devices, or gas refrigerators. Certain industrial operations such as those associated with blast furnaces and coke ovens, foundry cupolas, petroleum refineries, and underground mines also present risks of serious carbon monoxide intoxication. Less severe but potential exposures may exist in automobile repair shops, among traffic policemen, or in arc welding. Frank intoxication caused by vehicular exhausts is usually due to impaired integrity of exhaust systems and/or the automobile body. Poisoning associated with engine operation for in-car heating purposes occurs only with such defects or when the motor is run in confined spaces, e.g., deep snowdrifts, garages. Natural gas has replaced manufactured gas in the United States; since the former is free of carbon monoxide, illuminating gas per se no longer presents any risk of injury. However, carbon monoxide may be produced by the incomplete combustion of natural gas in faulty heating or other gas-burning apparatus. Chronic cigarette smokers develop 3 to 8 per cent carboxyhemoglobin (COHb) concentrations. Although the foregoing exogenous sources of carbon monoxide have long been recognized, the phenomenon of endogenous carbon monoxide production is now well established; as a result of cleavage of the α-methylene bridge in the heme portion of hemoglobin, 0.3 to 1.0 ml per hour is normally produced. This leads to a normal blood COHb concentration of 0.5 to 0.8 per cent.

Pathogenesis. Since carbon monoxide usually exists in a gaseous form, the only significant portal of entry is via the respiratory tract. The gas diffuses across the alveolar membrane in amounts proportional to the pressure gradient for carbon monoxide between alveolar air and blood. The rate of uptake is directly proportional to the respiratory rate, duration of exposure, and carbon monoxide concentration in air. The high affinity of carbon monoxide for hemoglobin (218 times greater than that of oxygen) is responsible for its primary pathologic effect, i.e., reduction of erythrocytic oxygen-carrying capacity. As a result, all signs, symptoms, and pathologic alterations are those of tissue hypoxia. In addition to reducing blood oxygen tension, carbon monoxide in association with hemoglobin (i.e., carboxyhemoglobin) impedes that pigment's discharge of oxygen at the capillary bed. Thus capillary oxygen tensions must be decreased lower than normal in order to dissociate oxygen from the erythrocyte to the tissues. This impairment of oxygen dissociation is expressed by a shift in the oxyhemoglobin curve to the left. Such effects are further complicated in that respiratory chemoreceptors respond only to decreased blood oxygen tension; since this is not decreased (i.e., there is simply a decrease in blood oxygen content), physiologic compensatory mechanisms are not brought into play.

Aside from the formation of carboxyhemoglobin and the resultant hypoxia, there is little evidence that carbon monoxide has any significant direct effect upon tissue except at extremely high concentrations.

Pathology. Carboxyhemoglobin is characteristically cherry red in color. Accordingly, the tissues and skin of poisoned individuals always grossly present a characteristic pink color when blood levels of carboxyhemoglobin exceed 30 per cent concentration levels. (Rarely, severely poisoned individuals may not manifest this change at autopsy; this results from reduction of COHb below the 30 per cent level owing to therapeutically induced respiratory clearance prior to death.) The skin may present areas of vesiculation and ulceration at pressure points. Ischemic necrosis of the cardiac papillary muscles and renal tubular degeneration may be noted. Although animal experiments suggest that repeated carbon monoxide exposures may accelerate the development of coronary atherosclerosis, the design of these experiments makes extrapolation of the results to humans difficult. Although the brain of patients dying of acute intoxication (i.e., within the first 24 hours) is congested, pink, and edematous, under these conditions this organ does not usually demonstrate specific, localized degenerative lesions. However, those surviving this acute episode can later develop diffuse degenerative changes prominently involving the cerebral cortex, globus pallidus, cerebellum, and basal ganglia. It is frequently stated that carbon monoxide–induced lesions have a predilection for certain locations in the brain, e.g., basal ganglia, hippocampal region, but in fact a consistent pattern of brain localization is not evident.

Clinical Manifestations. This disease is characteristically an acute poisoning. Although chronic forms of carbon monoxide intoxication have been claimed to exist, they are not adequately documented. Repeated episodes of mild acute poisoning can occur without cumulative effects.

The clinical picture of carbon monoxide poisoning is closely correlated with the blood concentration of carboxyhemoglobin. Although levels of less than 10 per cent COHb are said to produce no clinical effects, subtle changes of central nervous system function have been consistently demonstrated at the 5 to 10 per cent COHb level (e.g., increased visual threshold, impaired higher cognate function). In addition, precipitation of anginal episodes has been noted in patients with coronary artery disease during exercise with COHb levels of 3 to 5 per cent.

Although frontal, bandlike headaches may be experienced in the 10 to 20 per cent COHb range, more commonly these occur at the upper reaches of this range. In the 20 to 30 per cent COHb range the headaches become more severe. Dyspnea on exertion may be the only other manifestation. At the 30 to 40 per cent COHb levels, headaches become very severe, and are associated with nausea and vomiting, weakness, dizziness, dimness of vision, and possibly collapse. At the 40 to 50 per cent COHb level, ataxia, syncope, and collapse may be observed, in addition to tachycardia and tachypnea. As blood levels of 50 to 60 per cent COHb supervene, there may be coma associated with intermittent convulsions, and Cheyne-Stokes respiration may develop. In the 60 to 70 per cent COHb range, coma deepens, intermittent convulsions occur, and there is clinical shock. Death may terminate such exposures, although profound shock, respiratory and cardiovascular failure, and death have been reported to be delayed until 70 to 80 per cent COHb concentrations are attained. In severe cases, leukocytosis, proteinurea, glycosuria, hematuria, and cylindruria are usually demonstrated, in addition to temperature elevation of 39° C or more.

Diagnosis. Diagnosis is established by quantitative determination of blood carboxyhemoglobin concentration; analysis of alveolar air for carbon monoxide correlates well with blood COHb. The method of Coburn, utilizing a nondispersive infrared meter, is highly accurate; the helium-ionization detector equipped gas chromatograph also provides high sensitivity. Although spectrophotometry has long been used, its sensitivity and specificity are less than with more modern techniques.

The cherry-red skin and mucous membrane coloration are highly characteristic of carbon monoxide poisoning. However, it is not readily detected until a 30 to 35 per cent COHb concentration is attained.

Treatment. The patient must be immediately removed from the contaminated environment. In mild cases clearance of carbon monoxide from the blood is spontaneously accomplished if respiration is sustained. Fresh air and absolute rest are sufficient in such cases; attempts at exertion of any type within four to six hours can cause a rapid recrudescence of signs and symptoms. In the event of unconsciousness—no matter how transient—hospital management and emergency treatment are indicated. Respiration must be sustained by whatever method is available—i.e., artificial respiration, intermittent positive pressure breathing apparatus. Regardless of the level of COHb initially found, normal air breathing will result in 50 per cent clearance of blood carbon monoxide in about 250 to 300 minutes; 100 per cent oxygen inhalation will achieve a similar reduction of carbon monoxide loading in 35 to 80 minutes, and oxygen at three atmospheres of pressure results in the same clearance in about 25 minutes. The use of a 95 per cent oxygen–5 per cent carbon dioxide mixture hastens oxygenation, largely owing to the Bohr shift.

Persistence of coma and the presence of shock require the usual supportive treatments. Induction of hypothermia may help prevent irreversible brain damage.

Prognosis. Patients who do not become comatose usually recover without permanent sequelae. Persistence of hyperthermia, shock, or acute hypoxia-induced clinical laboratory signs for two days after intoxication holds a grave prognosis. Among those who survive such severe intoxication, a small proportion will demonstrate residual changes—e.g., major seizures, dysphasia, parkinsonism or varying degrees of hyperkinesia, mental impairment. Such severely affected patients usually manifest such signs within one week of the acute episode. However, in approximately half of these severe cases there may be apparent recovery followed by relapse after a latent period of one to three weeks. In either case, if recovery is to supervene, it should be expected within two years of the acute episode.

Coburn, R. F. (ed.): Biological effects of carbon monoxide. Ann. N.Y. Acad. Sci., 174:430, 1970.

Haldane, J.: The action of carbonic oxide in man. J. Physiol. (London), 18:430, 1895.

Meigs, J. W.: Acute carbon monoxide poisoning. An analysis of one hundred five cases. A.M.A. Arch. Indust. Hyg. Occup. Med., 6:344, 1952.

Peterson, J. E., and Stewart, R. D.: The post-exposure relationship of carbon monoxide in blood and expired air. Arch. Environ. Health, 21:165, 1970.

Richardson, J. C., Chambers, R. A., and Heywood, P. M.: Encephalopathy of anoxia and hypoglycemia. Arch. Neurol., 1:178, 1959.

Shillito, F. H., Drinker, C. K., and Shaughnessey, T. J.: The problem of nervous and mental sequelae in carbon monoxide poisoning. J.A.M.A., 106:669, 1936.

DISORDERS DUE TO HEAT AND COLD

Paul Webb

35. INTRODUCTION

When thermoregulation fails or is overwhelmed, life-threatening disorders develop from severe heat stress or cold stress. Profound hypothermia is the result of serious loss of body heat, whereas a major accumulation of body heat produces heat stroke. Both conditions require prompt and vigorous treatment. There are other, less serious disorders from heat exposure, in which heat is not stored in large quantity; these are the more common and more easily managed heat syncope and heat exhaustion. Cold and heat can cause local tissue injury, of course, as in frostbite, immersion foot, and burns, but this chapter deals only with the general disorders.

36. HEAT STROKE

A medical emergency, heat stroke is easily diagnosed when it is expected. Thus when military men begin training in hot climates or when seamen work in the engine rooms and galleys of ships in tropical waters, heat casualties are common, and some of them may be heat stroke. In young, healthy men who have been working hard in heat, unconsciousness, high body temperature, strong rapid pulse, and hot flushed skin are presumptive evidence of heat stroke in the absence of another obvious diagnosis such as head injury or massive infection. But in older people who have not been exerting themselves in hot work places, the diagnosis of heat stroke is not so obvious. Deaths from "excessive heat and insolation" in the United States range from 1 to 12 per 100,000 in people over 65, and many cases are missed or not reported. Heat deaths in the elderly are presumably similar in mechanism to classic heat stroke.

Prodromal symptoms, which may not be notable, include faintness, dizziness, staggering, headache, and nausea. There is a clear history of heat exposure or of heavy exertion in heat. Classically the patient in heat stroke is unconscious, although any degree of impairment of the central nervous system may present initially, from lethargy, confusion, or irrational agitation, to coma and convulsions. The body temperature is high, 40° C (104° F), or higher measured in the rectum; but if the patient is not seen immediately, and if even simple measures have been started to relieve heat stress and to start cooling, the body temperature may be lower. The pulse is strong, and its rate is usually 140 or higher. Blood pressure measurement will show a normal or elevated systolic pressure and a lowered diastolic pressure. However, in the late and severe stage of the disorder, blood pressure is low as the circulation fails. The skin is flushed, and sweating may be present, or—a bad sign—reduced or absent. Heat stroke is easily distinguishable from heat syncope or heat exhaustion, with their mildly elevated body temperatures, transient disturbances of consciousness, and mild circulatory signs. Heat stroke results from excessive heat storage, with high cardiac output, cutaneous vasodilation, and low peripheral resistance. Cessation of sweating and circulatory failure are late signs. There is evidence that the heart failure is right-sided, with low resistance in the systemic circulation and high resistance in the pulmonary circulation.

One should not always expect to see all the signs of heat stroke in an elderly person whose circulatory function is not what it used to be, and in whom there may be some pre-existing infectious disease. The diagnosis should be thought of if body temperature stays high and circulation is failing. Heat deaths during heat waves typically increase one or two days after the heat wave begins, and continue for one or two days after it is over. Predisposing factors are age, obesity, lack of acclimatization, and preceding infection or gastrointestinal upset.

The greater the heat storage and the longer it has been present, the worse the prognosis. Damage is done by general cellular degeneration and widespread hemorrhages, especially those in the central nervous system, kidneys, and liver. Laboratory findings in severe cases include reduced blood coagulation, low prothrombin, and low platelet count; low urine volume, high specific gravity, albumin, and renal casts; elevated blood urea; hemoconcentration; low serum potassium and normal to high serum chloride; changes in liver function; elevation of serum enzymes; and a hyperdynamic circulatory pattern unless circulatory failure has already developed.

Treatment of heat stroke should begin at once. Its aim is to lower body temperature and to support the circulation. Effective cooling methods, in ascending order of effectiveness, are wet towels and a strong fan in a cool dry room; icebags over much of the body; water-cooled sheets such as are used to induce hypothermia; and a tub bath of cold water. The higher the body temperature, the more aggressive the cooling technique should be. Sedation may be needed to control the patient, who may struggle or who may begin to convulse. A tranquilizing cocktail of pethidine, chlorpromazine, and phenergan may be used to prevent both convulsions and shivering, or simpler means of calming a person may suffice. Cooling should be continued until the rectal temperature goes below 38° C. After the initial lowering of body temperature, continued temperature monitoring is vital, for strong cooling may produce an after-drop of temperature, and somewhat later, patients will often start to store heat again despite being in a thermally comfortable environment.

Shock must be treated with fluid replacement and possibly isoproterenol. Fluid therapy should be started judiciously, with the amount and electrolyte content guided by laboratory findings. Other supportive measures are begun when problems are identified, e.g., platelet transfusions or renal dialysis.

37. HEAT SYNCOPE

A person who becomes dizzy or suddenly tired after exercising in the heat may abruptly faint. As soon as he is recumbent, and especially if he is removed from direct exposure to heat, he recovers. In contrast to the patient with heat stroke, the person with heat syncope has a cool, sweaty, pale skin; his pulse is weak and either mildly elevated — 100 to 120 beats per minute — or slow, as in vasovagal syncope. His blood pressure falls just

before fainting, and recovers quickly when he lies down or sits with head lowered.

Lack of acclimatization and lack of training for the exercise undertaken predispose to heat syncope. Cutaneous vasodilation and blood pooling in the erect position contribute to the hypotension. Treatment is a matter of allowing the person to rest, cool down a little, and drink some extra liquid.

38. HEAT EXHAUSTION

Taking much longer to develop than heat syncope (often several days), heat exhaustion results from loss of fluid or loss of fluid and salt. The symptoms of prolonged water depletion are thirst, fatigue, giddiness, elevated body temperature, oliguria, and finally delirium. The water depletion results from sweating and inadequate replacement by drinking, whether voluntary or involuntary. Voluntary dehydration in heat — the failure to replace water loss even though water is available — is common, but most people catch up at the end of the day when they get out of the heat. In the tropics it is sometimes not possible to cool off at night or keep up with water replenishment. This causes problems for the non-native dweller especially.

When both water and salt become depleted, muscle cramps are added to the picture of fatigue, nausea, and giddiness. The urine chloride will be low to absent, and serum chlorides reduced.

Heat exhaustion is treated by rest in bed away from heat, and restoration of body water, or water and electrolytes. Cool liquids should be given by mouth, up to 6 or 8 liters the first day. If body temperature does not return to normal spontaneously, alcohol sponging or wet towels and a fan may be used. If the patient cannot drink, intravenous therapy should be started. Continuation of fluid and electrolyte replacement should be guided by laboratory analyses.

Prevention of heat exhaustion is a matter of ensuring an adequate fluid intake, which means enough to replace losses from sweating. These losses can be as high as 6 to 8 liters per day in men working hard in hot dry conditions. People who are not yet acclimatized to heat need supplemental salt, because their sweat contains more electrolyte than that of the acclimatized. A daily intake of 15 to 25 grams of NaCl is recommended for newcomers to hot environments; about 10 grams of this can be consumed with a meat-containing diet. The additional 5 to 15 grams is best taken in the form of salted fruit drinks and enteric-coated salt tablets. But if water and fluids are in short supply, salt tablets should not be used. The routine use of salt tablets in hot situations is no longer encouraged except possibly for people who have little experience, and then only during the first days of becoming acclimatized.

39. HYPOTHERMIA

When the rectal temperature is below 35° C (95° F), hypothermia is said to be present. This major loss of body heat occurs in hikers and climbers exposed to cold, in elderly people who live alone in meagerly heated homes, in people who have been drinking heavily and have fallen asleep out of doors, in accident victims, and in people accidentally immersed in cold water. In profound hypothermia people are often assumed to be dead, for their vital signs are so depressed as to be missed even by trained observers. If only a clinical mercury thermometer is available, it will fail to register low enough to point to the diagnosis.

Estimates of the frequency of hypothermia vary widely, but the incidence is possibly higher than anyone suspects. In England it has been shown that elderly people are often forced to tolerate being chronically depleted of body heat, and the same may well be true in the United States for isolated old people. This would seem to be an ideal initial condition from which to develop hypothermia. Added hunger, fatigue, or minor injury could increase the heat depletion by rendering such people helpless. Drugs such as chlorpromazine may also contribute to it.

A person in profound hypothermia is in coma and cold to the touch. The skin is pale, usually grayish in color; the neck and extremities resist bending. No peripheral pulse can be found, breathing appears to be absent, and pupillary reflexes are absent. If a low-reading thermometer can be found, the rectal temperature will show 30° C or lower. Less profound hypothermia differs in degree; there will be some signs of consciousness, reaction to pain, a detectable if slow pulse, and flexible joints.

Additional findings are hypotension; cardiac irregularities on the EKG, typically atrial fibrillation and a J wave associated with the QRS complex; low pH in the blood from metabolic acidosis, especially in patients whose hypothermia was preceded by exhaustion and prolonged shivering; low blood CO_2 content; and high blood glucose.

Rewarming is the first order of business, and a decision must be made about passive or active rewarming and, if active, whether by external or core first means. A person who is still somewhat conscious, who has a reasonable heart rhythm, and whose rectal temperature is between 31 and 35° C is probably best handled by rewarming in a warm room or in a bed with blankets. If a person is acutely hypothermic from cold water immersion, the preferred approach is immersion in a warm tub bath whose temperature is kept at 40 to 42° C. A person with slowly developed hypothermia, in whom fatigue, injury, or old age has produced a poor condition beyond the hypothermia, should probably be warmed actively but less aggressively, e.g., with a heating blanket kept at 37° C. Rewarming the core first may be undertaken for profound hypothermia, for there is grave danger of ventricular fibrillation at heart temperatures from 27 to 30° C. The core-warming method avoids the early return of cold blood from the arms, legs, and skin, which commonly causes an unwanted after-drop in central temperature during external rewarming. But the methods of core-warming first are not simple ones; warm peritoneal dialysis and an extracorporeal blood circuit with a heater are examples.

Other than a determined approach to restoring body heat, the management of hypothermia should be as conservative as circumstances warrant, i.e., trauma or infection must be heeded. Respiratory support, for example, should include intubation or tracheostomy only if absolutely necessary. These procedures affect an already irritable heart. Cardiac irregularities should be watched rather than treated; if arrest occurs, it should be treated by external cardiac massage, and use of a defibrillator for ventricular fibrillation. Fluid therapy should be guided by laboratory findings rather than by some predetermined rule; thus one should combat acidosis or hypokalemia specifically if present.

Anderson, S., Herbring, B. G., and Widman, B.: Accidental profound hypothermia. Br. J. Anaesth., 42:653, 1970.

Ellis, F. P.: Mortality from heat illness and heat-aggravated illness in the United States. Environ. Res., 5:1, 1972.

Fernandez, J. P., O'Rourke, R. A., and Ewy, G. A.: Rapid active external rewarming in accidental hypothermia. J.A.M.A., 212:153, 1970.

Fox, R. H., Woodward, P. M., Exton-Smith, A. N., Green, M. F., Donnison, D. V., and Wicks, M. H.: Body temperatures in the elderly: A national study of physiological, social, and environmental conditions. Br. Med. J., 62:200, 1973.

Leithead, C. S., and Lind, A. R.: Heat Stress and Heat Disorders. Philadelphia, F. A. Davis Company, 1964.

O'Donnell, T. F., Jr., and Clowes, George H. A., Jr.: The circulatory abnormalities of heat stroke. N. Engl. J. Med., 287:734, 1972.

Patton, J. F., and Doolittle, W. H.: Core rewarming by peritoneal dialysis following induced hypothermia in the dog. J. Appl. Physiol., 33:800, 1972.

Shibolet, S., Coll, R., Gilat, T., and Sohar, E.: Heatstroke: Its clinical picture and mechanism in 36 cases. Quart. J. Med., 36:525, 1967.

Zingg, W.: The management of accidental hypothermia. Can. Med. Assoc. J., 96:214, 1967.

40. RADIATION INJURY

Niel Wald

Definition. Radiation energy from sources of ionizing radiation which interacts with human cells, tissues, and organs produces a variety of clinical manifestations, depending on the magnitude and duration of radiation exposure and on the size and function(s) of the body area irradiated. The source of the radiation energy absorbed may be external, such as an x-ray machine, or it may be internal contamination from a radioactive isotope inhaled, ingested, injected, or absorbed through the skin or a wound.

Clinical manifestations of radiation energy absorption may be acute, with or without late sequelae, or they may be delayed and chronic. The acute manifestations include the acute radiation syndrome which typically follows whole body radiation exposure; local tissue or organ injury with little or no systemic manifestations after partial body exposure; and growth and developmental disturbances after exposure of the fetus. The clinical effects of intermittent or constant low level radiation exposure from external or internal sources may present as chronic progressive impairment of certain tissues or organs, or solely as the relatively late appearance of one or another of the long-term sequelae of radiation exposure, such as cancer and leukemia. In addition, any of these forms of exposure which impinge on the gonads may produce germ cell changes or mutations which can cause sequelae in subsequent progeny.

Tissue injury may be produced by cellular interactions with radiations of any part of the electromagnetic spectrum, including the output of the sun, lasers, or microwave equipment. Some of these, such as x-rays, gamma rays, and neutrons, are capable of penetration, and can produce internal tissue damage. Other radiations, such as alpha rays and low energy beta rays, have a very limited range in tissue and are only injurious when given off within the body by incorporated radioactive isotopes. The radiations *emitted* by ionizing radiation sources are quantitated in roentgens (r) of exposure, whereas the radiation energy *absorbed* by the tissues exposed is quantitated in rads. The same absorbed dose delivered at different rates will produce very different effects.

Etiology. Typical radiation injury is caused by exposure to *ionizing radiations*. Since the recognition of man-made radiation by Roentgen in 1895 and of natural radioactivity by Becquerel the following year, occupational and medical exposures have been the most usual sources of radiation injury, the use of nuclear weapons in World War II producing a major addition in human cases of radiation injury. Injury from external sources occurred among the early x-ray workers, the employees of the nuclear weapons project, and the subsequent nuclear energy research and industrial organizations. In addition, unavoidable injury has been produced in some radiation therapy patients through exposure of normal tissues adjacent to the lesion under treatment.

Internal radionuclide exposure resulted in injury to employees of the radium watch dial painting industry in the 1920s. More recently, fallout from nuclear weapons tests has produced some internal radionuclide deposition in the general public. In the medical patient population, the uses of radium as a therapeutic agent and thorium as a diagnostic x-ray contrast medium have resulted in clinical sequelae decades after administration. Also, there have been instances of diagnostic and therapeutic radioisotope misadministration producing acute injury and occasionally causing death.

Incidence and Prevalence. The frequency with which radiation injury occurs is closely related to the availability of sources for radiation exposure and the understanding and care with which they are maintained and used. The largest potential source of radiation casualties is the military use of *nuclear weapons*. The Joint Commission for the Investigation of the Effects of the Atomic Bomb in Japan estimated the incidence of radiation injury in Hiroshima to be about 40 per cent and in Nagasaki about 50 per cent in the injured survivors. In Hiroshima about 30 per cent of the deaths in those who survived longer than one day were ascribed to radiation injury either alone or combined with blast and/or burn damage. In the survivor study population of 113,000, 117 cases of leukemia developed between 1950 and 1966. It is probable that the modern nuclear weapons would exceed these results. In nuclear weapons tests, some 300 people have inadvertently been exposed to local high levels of radioactive fallout, with resultant clinical manifestations in about 25 per cent.

Early peacetime uses of radioactivity led to an initial high incidence of injury. Within seven years of the demonstration of x-irradiation by Roentgen in 1895, some 200 cases of x-ray injury had been reported. After recognition of the hazard, radiation protection standards were developed internationally. There has been a marked reduction in this type of injury, although hand injuries still occur occasionally in industrial radiographers and the users of x-ray diffraction and other analytic equipment in research and development laboratories.

The discovery of natural radioactivity by Becquerel in 1896 led to the purification of radium by the Curies in 1911 and its use in medicine and industry. About 5000 watch dial painters, industrial chemists, and medical patients were involved. A subset of this population, 777 cases, had developed 51 bone sarcomas and 20 carcinomas, mainly paranasal, by 1971. The development of man-made radioactive material during and after World War II led to a nuclear industry population of several hundred thousand workers, but only 97 cases of clinical radiation injury had developed by 1969. Although data collection concerning medical misadministrations of radioactive isotopes designed for diagnostic and therapeutic purposes has not been systematic, several deaths and a number of injuries are known to have occurred in the very large American patient population receiving these materials.

Epidemiology. The manifestations of acute or of late radiation injury are not produced solely by irradiation. It is therefore essential to utilize epidemiologic methodology in order to establish the relationship of the etiologic agent to the clinical symptomatology. Two most helpful features have been the temporal relationship of the exposure to the development of clinical effects and the quantitative dose-response relationship.

The etiologic role of radiation in the clinical syndrome of *acute* radiation injury has been shown in epidemiologic studies of the Japanese atomic bomb survivors, the Marshall Island and Japanese fishermen exposed to fallout from a nuclear weapon test, several groups of radiation therapy patients, and the workers involved in various industrial radiation accidents. Epidemiologic studies relating *late* radiation effects such as neoplastic diseases and life-shortening to radiation exposure have dealt with radiologists and other physicians, the Japanese population under long-term follow-up by the Atomic Bomb Casualty Commission, the radium watch dial painters, therapeutically x-irradiated patients (particularly those receiving thymic irradiation in infancy), and patients receiving radioactive iodine therapy.

Pathogenesis. The basic pathology begins with the interaction of the radiation with tissue within the first second of exposure. The radiation energy in photons or particles penetrating the protoplasm may interact at the atomic level to produce ion pairs. These ions combine radiochemically with cell water, producing free radicals such as H and OH which further react to produce such forms as H_2O_2 and HO_2. These, in turn, may interact with critical molecules of the cell protoplasm such as nucleic acids or enzymes. If the dose is high and interactions are numerous, the cell may be killed directly by the radiation. At lower doses, the ability of the cell to divide may be impaired permanently or temporarily. If the DNA is involved, sublethal damage of this molecule may result in reproduction of the alteration (i.e., mutation) in daughter and descendant cells. Direct cell killing begins with exposures of one or more thousands of rads, in general, although some cells such as lymphocytes and spermatogonia are affected at much lower doses. Those cells which are rapidly dividing and differentiating are most vulnerable. Mitotic arrest occurs after several hundreds of rads and is characterized by continuing function of the existing cells but no new divisions. The continuing synthesis of proteins and enzymes, despite an irreversibly impaired mitotic apparatus, leads to "giant cells" which die after several weeks because their excessive size interferes with nutrition and metabolism. At doses of about 100 rads or more, mitotic delay results from temporary impairment of the mitotic mechanism. At still lower doses transient chromosomal "stickiness" is seen, presumably caused by denaturation of the DNA-histone molecules. Also, beginning at exposures as low as a few rads, are chromosome aberrations, i.e., breaks, deletions, gaps, and abnormal forms such as ring and dicentric chromosomes.

The effects of these cellular abnormalities on the various organs depend on the rate of proliferation of new cells required. In high turnover tissues such as the blood-forming tissue and the gastrointestinal tract, the relatively short life span of the predominant cells leads to rapid depletion before the onset of mitotic recovery and new cell production. In the period of mitotic inhibition of the blood-forming tissue, for example, the consequent depletion of mature cells results in increased probability of infection and hemorrhage. The resultant pathologic manifestations are nonspecific, although the inflammatory changes accompanying infection are deficient in polymorphonuclear cells.

In tissues which have little or no continuous proliferation, such as the liver or brain, this type of radiation injury is not apparent; however, functional impairment may be detected by appropriate means. In very slow turnover tissues, such as the lens of the eye or the thyroid gland, the manifestations of acute radiation effects may require months to years before becoming evident. Also, the small arterioles damaged by local radiation injury may show a compensatory increase in cell production, leading to endothelial thickening, obliterative endarteritis, and extensive fibrosis over a prolonged period of time.

Chromosomal abnormalities produced in injured cells may be reproduced and perpetuated for decades. A long-lived component of the lymphoid cells may even carry the original radiation damage for many years before dividing. Clones of cells with the same specific chromosome abnormality may develop over a period of years as well.

Clinical Manifestations. Clinical manifestations of radiation injury can be subdivided into three major forms: the acute radiation syndrome, acute local radiation injury, and delayed effects. External penetrating irradiation, as well as external and internal radionuclide contamination and local traumatic injury with radionuclide contamination, may produce these manifestations.

Acute Radiation Syndrome. This syndrome is seen typically after exposure of most or all of the body to external sources of penetrating ionizing radiation, although high doses of ^{32}P, ^{131}I, and ^{198}Au have also evoked it. It appears in three major forms, in ascending severity of injury. These are the hematologic, the gastrointestinal, and the central nervous system–cardiovascular forms. Four discernible clinical stages can be recognized, particularly when the severity of injury allows for ultimate survival. These are the initial or prodromal stage which subsides into a latent stage, followed by a stage of manifest or overt illness, and a recovery stage. The duration of each stage is inversely related to the severity of injury.

Typical manifestations of the *hematologic form* are seen after an exposure in the midlethal range (300 rads). Prodromal anorexia, nausea, and possibly vomiting may commence within several hours and generally subside within 48 hours. Transient waves of skin erythema and conjunctivitis may be observed over the same period or longer. The patient may be asymptomatic after the prodromal stage for one to three weeks. Then the increasing inadequacy of the body's defenses against infection and hemorrhage becomes manifest, with development of fever, oropharyngeal lesions, abscesses, petechiae, purpura, and bleeding from body orifices. Other findings include scalp pain and epilation, and recurrent anorexia and nausea accompanied by weakness, fatigue, weight loss, and emaciation. Gradual recovery ensues, beginning about the fifth to sixth week after exposure and requires several months.

The earliest laboratory finding is lymphopenia, reaching absolute lymphocyte levels below 1000 per cubic millimeter within the first 48 postexposure hours. The reticulocytes may disappear in the same time period. A gradual fall in granulocyte counts begins during the first two weeks, reaches a plateau, or even shows an abortive rise, followed by a steep fall to a low point at about 30 days postexposure. The platelet count nadir occurs at the same time, after a more continuous fall. If the individual survives, an abrupt increase in all the cell lines mentioned, except the lymphocytes, will occur within the next week and rapidly reach normal levels. An initial increase in granulocyte count in the first 24 hours may occur on the basis of a nonspecific "alarm reaction," and should not mislead one to exclude radiation injury on this basis. Blood biochemical analyses may show nonspecific indicators of major cell and tissue damage such as creatinuria, increased excretion of DNA breakdown products such as beta-aminoisobutyric acid, deoxycytidine, and various other amino acids. Serum enzyme measurements such as LDG, SGOT, and SGPT may be elevated. Within 24 hours chromosome breakage and abnormal forms can be seen in peripheral blood cytogenetic preparations, with the frequency related to the magnitude of the radiation exposure.

The *gastrointestinal form* is associated with anorexia, nausea, vomiting, and diarrhea within the first few hours after exposure. These may be of sufficient severity to require active treatment but usually subside within 48 hours. A latent period follows which may last only a few days to a week before there is a major recurrence of all the gastrointestinal systems as well as those of infection and hemorrhage as described above. These patients generally die with a fulminating enterocolitis before the full appearance of epilation and other slower developing radiation sequelae.

Laboratory abnormalities in the gastrointestinal form of radiation injury are similar to those of the hematologic form but occur more promptly and with greater magnitude. In addition, the hematocrit may be increased as a result of hemoconcentration caused by fluid loss, which, with hypoglycemia and electrolyte imbalance, results from the loss of a functional intestinal mucosal lining.

In the *central nervous system and cardiovascular form*, immediate nausea, projectile vomiting, and explosive diarrhea are characteristic. These may be accompanied by disorientation, hyperesthesia, ataxia, sweating, prostration, and shock. There may be some improvement after several hours, but alternations develop between evidences of central nervous system hyperexcitability, including convulsions, and CNS depression, such as somnolence and coma. This is accompanied by hypotension which gradually becomes irreversible, as does oliguria, leading to a fatal outcome in 24 to 48 hours.

Laboratory observations in the central nervous system and cardiovascular form of acute radiation injury show marked telescoping of the previously described injury syndromes with abnormalities occurring sooner and with greater severity. Complete lymphopenia and an initial granulocyte level of 30,- to 40,000 may be present within the next few hours. Prompt chromosome examination may show marked increase in chromatid and chromosome aberrations, but as the circulating lymphocytes disappear, it may become difficult to find dividing cells. The biochemical evidences of tissue damage are much more striking in this form of the syndrome. In addition, biochemical evidences of azotemia secondary to hypotension become prominent. Transient hyperbilirubinemia may be observed.

Local Radiation Injury. Localized radiation injury may occur with acute and/or chronic clinical manifestations, depending on the total dose and dose rate with which the exposure takes place.

The early changes result in three major clinical findings: erythema, epilation, and transepidermal injury. *Erythema* comparable to a mild sunburn or a thermal burn of the first degree may appear on exposure to more than 200 to 300 rads. A transient first wave may be present within hours after exposure, associated with hyperesthesia, burning, or itching. The major redness appears two or three weeks later, the interval depending on the dose. In the lower dose range no further changes other than tanning may occur, and medical care is not necessary. A counterpart to this reaction has been described in the conjunctiva and in the anterior chamber of the eye, with inflammatory changes observed promptly after exposure.

Epilation, or loss of hair, may occur after exposure to any form of radiation, beginning with exposures of about 200 to 300 rads. It generally becomes apparent only two or three weeks after exposure. Associated skin or scalp tenderness may occur one or two days preceding the actual hair loss. With doses greater than about 500 rads, epilation may be complete. If the exposure is much greater than 600 rads, hair may not regrow.

Transepidermal injury (dry or wet dermatitis) is comparable to a thermal second-degree burn with erythema, blistering, and pain. Confluent bullae may develop in about one and one-half to three weeks, depending on dose (usually exceeding 1000 rads). These may rupture, leaving open, weeping lesions vulnerable to infection.

With higher doses, probably on the order of 5000 rads, a more serious version of transepidermal injury occurs, in which the lesion resembles a third-degree burn. Pain occurs promptly and is intense. The raw areas may be very slow in healing, or may not heal until surgical resection and skin grafting are performed. Epilation is permanent.

Still higher doses may produce immediate tissue damage to structures below the skin. Such injuries, which have occurred in the abdominal wall, male genitalia, and extremities, are irreversible, requiring surgical excision and further reconstructive management.

Delayed Effects. Delayed effects of radiation exposure are of two varieties: those finally appearing in organs whose cells received the radiation exposure and are relatively slow in responding; and those late effects occurring in organs and tissues in which descendent cells ultimately express the initial radiation injury after a latent period which may be many years in duration. The first type of delayed effect can be seen in the male gonad, for example. Doses as low as 15 rads will produce *impairment in fertility* owing to moderate oligospermia beginning about 50 days after the exposure. Azoospermia will occur with doses of more than 200 to 300 rads for a period of roughly one to one and one half years. Doses of 500 to 600 rads may produce permanent sterility in male or female survivors.

The lens of the eye is another late-responding tissue, with opacities appearing in the posterior subcapsular region in months to several years after exposures of about 200 rads or more. *Cataracts* of the posterior lens may develop in the majority of patients who receive more than 600 rads. The gradual development of *hypothyroidism* several years after exposure of several hundred rads is another example of delayed response. *Skin changes* constitute another late response to either acute injury or repeated low level radiation exposure. There may be loss of the detailed finger-ridge pattern and hair, abnormalities of the fingernails, and dryness of the skin. Localized hyperkeratosis may be seen, as well as breakdown of previously healed but atrophic skin, and, ultimately, neoplastic skin changes may develop in such areas.

In the *fetus* the clinical manifestations will depend largely on its age and the magnitude of exposure. If the exposure takes place in the first one to two weeks, resorption of the conceptus is probable. Between the second and sixth weeks, the effect will be on the particular organs under development at the time. Further along in gestation, there will be more subtle generalized effects ultimately expressed as deficits in growth and development, including microcephaly and mental retardation.

The most common *late effects* of radiation exposure are *neoplastic diseases.* The earliest to appear are the acute leukemias and chronic granulocytic leukemia, with a peak incidence of approximately four to seven years after the radiation exposure. Chronic lymphocytic leukemia is not increased by radiation exposure. Other neoplasms whose induction appears significantly increased by radiation exposure include cancer of the thyroid and salivary glands, lung, bone, and female breast tissues. Internally deposited radionuclides have been associated particularly with malignant neoplasms of bone and reticuloendothelial tissues such as liver, spleen, and lymph nodes. Radium deposition has involved the mastoid bones and those surrounding the paranasal sinuses in particular, whereas internally administered thorium dioxide has produced an increase of hemangiosarcomas of the liver. In addition, a generalized increase in incidence of all forms of cancer has been documented in the Japanese atomic bomb survivors. *Shortening of life expectancy* through somewhat earlier death from all causes has been documented in the radiologist population but not yet in the Japanese A-bomb survivors.

Diagnosis. *Acute Radiation Syndrome.* The manifestations of acute radiation injury are not unique to this causative agent. Therefore the diagnosis rests on the history and the evolving clinical pattern defined by time of onset and duration of the clinical signs, symptoms, and laboratory abnormalities, particularly the hematologic changes.

In the absence of an adequate history of radiation exposure, the diagnosis may be elusive. The various manifestations may suggest a wide range of conditions. Prodromes suggest psychoneurosis, food poisoning, or gastrointestinal viral infection; symptoms in the period of manifest illness may mimic aplastic anemia, leukemia, infectious gastroenteritis, typhoid fever, and even mumps (for radiation parotitis). When a radiation exposure history is elicited, hematologic and cytogenetic examinations may be used as well as physical dosimetry data obtained by personnel monitoring equipment, if any, and by reconstruction of the exposure situation, in order to obtain confirmatory and quantitative information concerning the potential severity of the injury. However, it must be kept clearly in mind that the evolving clinical pattern is the final diagnostic criterion for the recognition and management of this form of injury.

Local Injury.   Local radiation injury, particularly as it appears on the upper extremities, is often confused with thermal and chemical burns. Differentiating features are absence of waves of erythema in the latter as well as the more severe prolonged pain and slower healing associated with radiation. Recurrent tissue breakdown after healing is also suggestive of radiation injury as opposed to the other possibilities.

Delayed Effects.   No clinical characteristics of the late effects of radiation exposure are unique to this etiologic agent.

Radionuclide Contamination.   Radionuclides deposited on the surface of the skin may be absorbed, inhaled, or ingested into the body where they may act to produce delayed effects. In order to prevent such sequelae, the recognition of their presence is essential even though no immediate clinical manifestations are present. Such diagnostic procedures must involve close collaboration between the physician and the health physicist, the professional trained to recognize and quantitate radiation exposure in order to prevent deleterious effects of radiation. Radioactivity surveys of the suspected individual with appropriate radiation detection equipment should be carried out. It is most important to collect all urinary and fecal excretions in separate containers until sufficient data of the nature and magnitude of contamination are obtained. Some radionuclides such as radon may be sought in breath samples. An early postexposure blood sample should also be collected and preserved for radionuclide analysis. Finally, it may be necessary to carry out chest or whole body low-level radiation counting in an appropriate facility, i.e., a so-called "whole body counter."

If a traumatic wound is present, radionuclide contamination may be sought by measuring radioactivity of swabs used in cleaning the wound as well as by surveying over the surface with appropriate detectors. If the wound is the sole contaminated area, excreta samples will show whether the contaminant has been absorbed into the body and therefore is sufficiently soluble for circulation and translocation to remote sites from the wound.

Treatment.   *Acute Radiation Syndrome.*   The treatment of acute radiation syndrome is based on an understanding of its pathophysiology. The prodromal symptoms in the acute radiation syndrome are self-limited, but sedatives and antiemetics may be used if needed. Throughout the syndrome it is important to reduce anxiety by keeping the patient informed about the nature of his injury, the expected transient health impairment, and its anticipated duration and treatment. The prolonged weakness associated with this syndrome even during convalescence may be in some measure secondary to the prolonged anxiety and fear of the unknown often associated with radiation injury.

In the *hematologic form,* the inhibition of mitosis responsible for the overt illness is self-limited. Thus management is directed toward maintenance of the patient through the period in which his defenses against infection and hemorrhage are deficient. This is best achieved by conservative means. The threat of exogenous bacterial and viral infection is reduced by strict reverse isolation of the patient with maintenance of a clean environment by use of a laminar air flow or "life-island" methods. Attendant personnel must be screened

for potential pathogens and treated prophylactically if necessary.

Prophylactic oral antimicrobial drugs to clear pathogenic bacterial and fungal organisms from the gastrointestinal tract have been used when the total granulocyte level falls below 1000 per cubic millimeter. Various blood elements may be given to replace deficiencies when needed. Red cells are needed only if significant bleeding has occurred. Fresh platelets should be available for use if significant hemorrhage develops. Their use has been advocated even in the absence of bleeding when the platelet count falls below 10,000 per cubic millimeter. If available in concentrated form, normal granulocytes may be administered in the face of overt infection during the granulocytopenic phase. If not available, in the presence of a clearly life-threatening infection the use of the much greater numbers of granulocytes of patients with chronic granulocytic leukemia has been suggested, because they are capable of phagocytosis. On recovery, it is assumed that the patient's immune system will rid the body of such donor cells.

In the situation in which both biologic and dosimetric indicators suggest the high probability of a fatal outcome, bone marrow transplantation may be warranted. Because such marrow requires about two weeks to correct the deficit in circulating blood cells, such a decision should not be delayed much beyond the first postexposure week. The hazards of a graft reaction by the host if his radiation-induced immunosuppression is not sufficient and of "graft versus host" reaction if it is too long lasting define the narrow boundaries within which therapeutic benefit may be expected. The availability of an identical twin or a very close matching relative on tissue compatibility testing will also influence the decision.

Management of the *gastrointestinal form* of acute radiation syndrome has not been successful thus far in the few human occurrences. Animal studies by Bond and Cronkite suggest that the vigorous and early utilization of adequate anti-infection agents, blood components, nutrients, electrolytes, and fluid may influence mortality favorably.

In the few human instances of the *central nervous system–cardiovascular form,* the progressive hypotension has not been improved by the administration of pressor agents, and the fluid administration involved has augmented the congestive heart failure which has ensued.

Local Radiation Injury.   The treatment of local radiation injury is generally similar to that of thermal burn of the same severity. This includes the maintenance of asepsis, eventual removal of devitalized tissue to the degree necessary, and the use of skin grafting to cover nonhealing ulcerations. An additional feature in management is very careful and prolonged observation for possible early neoplastic changes of the skin.

Delayed Effects.   Clinical management of the delayed effects of radiation exposure does not differ in any way from the management of similar pathologic conditions not caused by radiation.

Radionuclide Contamination.   In the event of an accident in which radionuclide contamination is likely, only urgent first aid should be given and the patient evacuated from the site. Contaminated skin and wounds should be washed promptly, and all excreta collected.

Useful preparations for skin decontamination include soap and water, surgical and laundry detergents, and oxidizing agents. These should be accompanied by brushing and rinsing, with care taken not to abrade the skin.

Contamination of the eyes, nose, and mouth is treated initially with copious water washing as soon as possible. Isotonic irrigants may be substituted as soon as available.

For definitive wound care, the usual surgical principles apply, with modifications only in the aseptic procedures and debridement in order to avoid introduction of skin contamination into the wound. It may also be desirable to give diethylenetriaminepentaacetic acid (DTPA), a chelating agent available from the U.S. Atomic Energy Commission for investigational use, intravenously prior to surgery to minimize the ultimate deposition of any contaminant which may get into circulation during surgery.

If radioactivity measurements of excreta and of the whole body suggest a residual body burden of a larger quantity than seems acceptable on the basis of medical judgment and regulatory agency guides, various treatments may be used to minimize the absorption and enhance the excretion of the radionuclide.

To minimize respiratory absorption, the use of irritants, expectorants, and pulmonary lavage is under current investigation. Inhalation of DTPA aerosol mist is also currently being tested for transuranic isotope contamination.

To minimize gastrointestinal absorption, the simplest measure is to accelerate excretion with a mild laxative. For strontium-90, sodium alginate and aluminum hydroxide gel have been used orally to prevent uptake from the gut. For cesium-137, Prussian blue (ferric ferrocyanide) does the same. To promote excretion of nuclides already within the body and to reduce deposition in target organs, such as bone, a variety of agents are available. For plutonium, americium, yttrium, lanthanum, and fission products, intravenously administered chelating agents are useful, DTPA being the most effective. For strontium, the combination of high calcium intake and acidification of the blood with ammonium chloride has effectively reduced bone absorption.

Prognosis. *Acute Radiation Syndrome.* The estimated short-term radiation exposure which would be lethal for 50 per cent of an untreated human population in 60 days is about 300 rads mean midline absorbed dose. This exposure would be expected to produce the hematologic form of the acute radiation syndrome, with half the exposed population dying within 60 days. However, an accidentally irradiated worker survived an estimated 600 rads absorbed whole body dose, with postexposure treatment, including isogeneic marrow transplantation, by Wald, Thomas, and co-workers, despite tissue damage severe enough to necessitate subsequent amputation of all four extremities; and Thomas et al. have used pre- and postexposure treatment, including isogeneic marrow, successfully in patients with leukemia receiving up to 1600 rads.

Thus it appears that successful management of the hematologic form of acute radiation injury is possible under optimal therapeutic circumstances with great expenditure of medical resources. Clearly, such prognostic optimism would not apply to the large-scale population exposure situation such as occurred in Hiroshima and Nagasaki. Furthermore, even the best clinical management has not yet succeeded in allowing the survival of those few individuals who accidentally have received exposures resulting in major gastrointestinal or central nervous system–cardiovascular damage.

Local Radiation Injury. The outlook for good recovery from local radiation injury depends in part on the adequacy of management of the acute changes, including the removal of devitalized tissue and the prevention of secondary infection. However, the main determinant of the ultimate outcome will be the severity of injury to the underlying blood vessels.

Delayed Effects. The prognosis for the various delayed effects of radiation exposure is similar to that of the same pathology in the absence of such exposure.

The likelihood of a radiation-exposed individual's developing a late effect of the exposure is increased in relationship to the exposure dose. The statistical probability can be assessed for leukemia only on the basis of its occurrence in the population exposed to the atomic bombs in Hiroshima and Nagasaki. There, the increased likelihood is one to two cases per year per million people observed per rad of exposure for a period at least 15 to 20 years after the exposure. Epidemiologic studies of thyroid cancer in patients who received thymic irradiation in childhood suggest a similar incidence. It is not known whether this dose-response ratio holds for all malignant tumors.

Prevention. Since the foregoing discussion has indicated that there are no specific methods of reversing the course of events initiated by radiation exposure, the best measure against radiation injury is prevention. The largest *potential* source of radiation exposure to the general population is the nuclear weapon. It is therefore essential that all measures be taken to minimize the possibility of any human population receiving such an exposure again. Another potential source of population exposure, the widespread and increasing utilization of nuclear energy as a source of electric power generation, has been controlled successfully thus far.

The largest *actual* source of population exposure consists of users of radiation in the healing arts. It is evident that such usage of ionizing radiation has produced untold benefit to the same population. Nevertheless, it is incumbent on the users of medical radiation sources to minimize the exposures needed to obtain the necessary diagnostic information. This requires not only optimal operation of existing equipment by current techniques but also a continuing research and development effort to improve the efficiency of such exposure to allow reduction of exposure while obtaining the necessary biomedical information. Adequate specialized education of all users of radiation sources in the philosophy and methods of radiation protection is another factor in the preventive approach to radiation injury.

Andrews, G. A., Balish, E., Edwards, C. L., Kniseley, R. M., and Lushbaugh, C. C.: Possibilities for Improved Treatment of Persons Exposed in Radiation Accidents. *In* Handling of Radiation Accidents. Vienna, International Atomic Energy Agency, 1969, p. 119.

Basic Radiation Protection Criteria. NCRP Report No. 39, Washington, D.C., National Council on Radiation Protection and Measurements, 1971.

Bond, V. P., Fliedner, T. M., and Archambeau, J. O.: Mammalian Radiation Lethality. A Disturbance in Cellular Kinetics. New York, Academic Press, 1965.

Brent, R. L., and Gorson, R. O.: Radiation exposure in pregnancy. Current Problems in Radiology, Vol. II, No. 5. Chicago, Year Book Medical Publishers, 1972.

Fabrikant, J. I.: Radiobiology. Chicago, Year Book Medical Publishers, 1972.

Ionizing Radiation: Levels and Effects. A report of the United Nations Scientific Committee on the Effects of Atomic Radiation to the General Assembly, with annexes, Vols. I and II. New York, United Nations, 1972.

Manual on Radiation Haematology, Technical Reports Series No. 123, Vienna, International Atomic Energy Agency, 1971.

Michaelson, S. M.: Human exposure to nonionizing radiant energy. Po-
    tential hazards and safety standards. Proc. I.E.E.E., 60:389, 1972.
Rubin, P., and Casarett, G. W.: Clinical Radiation Pathology. Philadelphia,
    W. B. Saunders Company, 1968.
Stannard, J. N.: Toxicology of radionuclides. Ann. Rev. Pharmacol.,
    13:325, 1973.
The Effects on Populations of Exposure to Low Levels of Ionizing Radia-
    tion. Report of the Advisory Committee on the Biological Effects of
    Ionizing Radiations. Washington, National Academy of Sciences–Na-
    tional Research Council, 1972.
Thoma, G. E., and Wald, N.: The diagnosis and management of accidental
    radiation injury. J. Occup. Med., 1:422, 1959.
Wald, N.: Radiation injury and its management. In Wang, Y. (ed.): Hand-
    book of Radioactive Nuclides. Part IX. Cleveland, The Chemical Rub-
    ber Co., 1969, p. 837.

41. ELECTRIC SHOCK

Charles E. Billings

The effects of electricity on the body are determined by a great variety of physical, anatomic, and physiologic factors, and possibly by demographic factors as well. Before going on to a discussion of the effects, it is well to review briefly the most important of these factors.

Physical factors: Ohm's law reminds us that a certain electromotive force or potential, measured in volts, is necessary to permit the flow of a current, measured in amperes, through a conductor having a certain resistance, expressed in ohms. The rule applies whether the conductor is a wire, a volume conductor containing a salt solution, or an interface such as the skin.

Direct currents (DC) exert effects different in some respects from alternating currents (AC); in the latter case, the frequency is very important. In general, the effects of frequencies in the 50 to 60 Hz range are greater than those of AC at very high frequencies. The duration of current flow must also be considered. The electrical properties of shoes, gloves, and clothing through which the current passes are of importance.

Anatomic and physiologic factors: The interior of the body is an excellent volume conductor of low resistance. The skin, however, through which electrical energy usually enters the body, has much higher resistance to the passage of current. Heavily callused, dry skin may have a resistance of several hundred thousand ohms. Thin skin, moist with perspiration, especially if it is lightly abraded to induce hyperemia, may have resistance as low as 1000 to 2000 ohms. Sweating causes marked decreases in skin resistance, both by wetting it and by providing additional conduction pathways to the interior of the body through the glands themselves.

Within the body, current densities are determined by the resistivities of the tissues in the path of current. Most accidental shocks travel either from hand to hand or from hand to foot.

Incidence. Electric currents are used therapeutically; electroconvulsive treatment, cardioversion, and electrical cardiac pacing are their major present uses. In the past, iontophoresis was a method of introducing certain drugs through the intact skin. All these techniques present the danger of overdosage and injury.

Accidental electric shock, with which this chapter is primarily concerned, is encountered most commonly in four settings: industry, the home, lightning strikes, and, increasingly, in medical diagnostic and treatment settings. Each year more than 1000 persons in the United States are killed by electrical injuries, with industrial accidents accounting for more than half the total.

Pathophysiology. Electric currents of sufficient magnitude can cause gross disruption of tissues, especially the brain. More commonly, however, two types of injuries occur. Burns caused by conversion of electrical to thermal energy at sites of relatively high resistance are common, especially in the skin and underlying fat. Interruption of physiologic function may occur, however, especially in neural and neuromuscular tissue, without any obvious anatomic effects in those tissues. Such functional effects in the central nervous system and heart are the major dangers of accidental electric shock.

Clinical Manifestations. The threshold for perception of a direct current is in the neighborhood of 5 mA (range 2 to 13 mA); the predominant sensation is of warmth at the contact site. Much lower thresholds are observed with alternating currents at 60 Hz; the median in one study was below 1.1 mA (range 0.4 to 1.9 mA). Subjects described a tingling sensation at these levels.

Pain thresholds are more difficult to obtain owing to the subjective nature of this symptom. In various studies, ranges of 3 to 10 mA have been found with 60 Hz AC.

As current flow increases beyond these levels, a point is reached at which involuntary muscle spasm is produced. If the current is entering or leaving the body through the hands, the victim is unable to free himself from the electrode. The maximal level of current at which an electrode can be released has been called the "let-go" current by Dalziel et al. They found that mean direct currents of 74 mA (range 61 to 83) and mean alternating currents of 16 mA (range 10 to 22) were maxima in normal subjects. After extensive studies, they concluded that the following were maximal safe current flows through the hands for 99.5 per cent of persons:

	DC	60 Hz AC
Men	62 mA	9 mA
Women	41 mA	6 mA

Without question, the most dangerous effect of electric current is its ability to induce ventricular fibrillation. In transverse current flow in animals, about 3 per cent of the current flows through the heart. If the current pathway is parallel to the body axis, however, 9 to 10 per cent of the total current flows through the heart.

There is a relatively short period during the repolarization phase of each cardiac cycle when the heart is extremely sensitive to exogenous electrical stimuli. An electric current of 0.75 mA applied to the surface of the heart during its sensitive period can induce fibrillation. It appears, from extensive studies of this phenomenon, that maximal safe currents for the arm-to-leg pathway are below 100 mA. Currents much above this level, applied for periods longer than one to two seconds, may be expected to induce ventricular fibrillation.

There are other manifestations of electrical injury. An alternating current of several hundred milliamperes passing transversely through the brain rarely causes respiratory disturbances except during the grand mal seizure which results, but such a current traversing the brainstem along a longitudinal pathway will cause respiratory arrest, which may persist for a considerable period of time after interruption of current flow. Thrombotic phenomena in the brain or elsewhere are not uncommon after electrical injury. Still other changes, including burns, cerebral edema, and perivascular hemorrhages, appear to be due to thermal injury rather than to the passage of the electric current per se.

Diagnosis and Treatment. Diagnosis of a serious electrical injury must be immediate, and treatment must begin immediately if the patient is to be saved. Since most electric shock deaths are due to hypoxia secondary to ventricular fibrillation, respiratory arrest, or both, treatment must consist of artificial respiration and closed chest cardiac massage, begun as soon as possible after the current path is interrupted and continued until satisfactory respiratory and cardiac function have returned. This may take several hours. Cardiac defibrillation should be employed if indicated; cardiotonic drugs and other supportive measures may be required. It is most important to realize that even severely shocked patients may have suffered only functional impairment; if hypoxia can be prevented until spontaneous function resumes, they may recover completely.

Complications. Aside from problems caused by severe surface or deep burns (which may require surgical treatment), the most ominous early complication of electrical injury is nephrosis with resultant oliguria or anuria. Cataract formation may occur as late as months after the initial injury; in laboratory animals, this has been observed more frequently after direct current shocks.

Subjects may complain of weakness or paralysis of extremities for many hours after a shock; pain, muscular stiffness, and minor personality changes may persist for months.

Prognosis. There are so many variables in each case of electrical injury that no meaningful data on recovery rates are available. As in the case of ventricular fibrillation from other causes, the likelihood and the completeness of recovery are largely functions of the promptness with which cardiopulmonary resuscitation is begun and of its adequacy thereafter.

Prevention. A word should be said here about primary prevention of electrical injuries, especially in medical settings, in which preventive measures can be controlled by medical personnel. *Any* electrical device, a lamp, electric bed, TV control unit, or patient intercom, poses a very real threat to life. Continuous monitoring of patients in surgical and intensive care units has vastly increased the opportunities for electrical injuries owing to passage of stray currents through monitoring leads attached in ways which minimize skin resistance and maximize the likelihood of internal injury should such currents occur. Cardiac catheters containing sensor leads are another and particularly dangerous source of such injuries.

These catastrophes are totally preventable if, and only if, proper fail-safe protective devices are an integral part of *all* electrical circuits which can involve the body. Protective fuses must be incorporated in all such circuits; adequate grounding of all electrical equipment used in patient areas is mandatory.

Fischer, H.: Pathologic effects and sequelae of electrical accidents. Electrical burns (secondary accidents, renal manifestations, sequelae). J. Occup. Med., 7:564, 1965.

Franco, S. C.: Electric shock and cardiopulmonary resuscitation. Arch. Environ. Health, 19:261, 1969.

Jude, J. R., Kouwenhoven, W. B., and Knickerbocker, G. G.: Cardiac arrest. J.A.M.A., 178:1063, 1961.

Morley, R., and Carter, A. O.: First aid treatment of electric shock. Arch. Environ. Health, 25:276, 1972.

MOTION SICKNESS AND PROBLEMS OF AIR TRAVEL

Harold V. Ellingson

42. MOTION SICKNESS

Manifestations and Occurrence. Motion sickness is a syndrome characterized by pallor, sweating, salivation, and nausea that frequently progresses to vomiting. Prostration may be severe if exposure to precipitating factors is prolonged. It may occur in persons riding in airplanes, ships, automobiles, or trains, or sometimes in children after prolonged or vigorous sessions in playground swings. Among air travelers, the incidence has declined with introduction of newer jet transports that fly at altitudes above the layers of most turbulent air. The disorder still remains a problem among passengers in small aircraft and others flying at low altitudes in stormy or hot weather, when turbulence may be severe.

Etiology. Causative factors are not completely understood. Labyrinthine stimulation resulting from repetitive pitching, rolling, rotating, or up-and-down motion is clearly a most important factor, since persons with nonfunctioning labyrinths are often totally insusceptible to motion sickness, and since incidence and severity are commonly proportional to severity and duration of the motion. Psychic factors also appear to be important. Apprehension undoubtedly predisposes to motion sickness; a few unfortunates feel nauseated on stepping aboard a motionless airplane or a ship at a pier. Some people can tolerate motion without distress until they smell an unpleasant odor such as that of cigar smoke or the vomitus of a fellow passenger. Visceral sensations of motion appear to be contributory, since abdominal restraint reduces incidence of reactions. Visual stimuli apparently may play a part; symptoms sometimes occur in an immobile subject who watches moving pictures depicting motion.

Prevention and Treatment. Prophylaxis may often be achieved by the use of any of a number of drugs, given 30 minutes to an hour before the trip begins. Hyoscine, 0.6 mg, with d-amphetamine, 10 mg, meclizine (Bonine), 25 to 50 mg, cyclizine (Marezine), 50 mg, and dimenhydrinate (Dramamine), 50 mg, are among the most effective agents. For prolonged journeys, the same dose of meclizine or hyoscine-d-amphetamine should be given every 24 hours; doses of cyclizine or dimenhydrinate should be repeated every four to six hours as required. A traveler who senses the onset of an attack may often avert nausea and vomiting by reclining as far as possible, by holding his head firmly against a pillow or head rest, by closing his eyes or fixing his gaze on a point, and by increasing his ventilation with cool air. In treatment, the same drugs mentioned above are useful, though retention may be difficult if vomiting has already occurred. Fortunately, symptoms usually disappear soon after the journey is concluded or motion has ceased. Recovery after prolonged vomiting may be hastened by fluid replacement.

43. PROBLEMS OF AIR TRAVEL

For the normal person, and for most ambulatory patients under a physician's care, air travel is no more trying than is travel by any other means. However, a physician should be informed of factors encountered in flight that may have an influence on his patient's welfare. Besides accepting as passengers many ambulatory patients under the care of physicians, most airlines are prepared to carry litter patients; special litters can be accommodated by adjustment or removal of several seats. In remote areas, private flying agencies sometimes provide air ambulance service to large medical centers. Before a patient travels or is moved by air, the physician should consider the hazards mentioned below and should, if necessary, discuss the case with a medical official of the carrier. The patient's condition, the altitude and duration of the flight, the cabin pressure altitude, and the availability of oxygen in flight all have a bearing on suitability of air travel by, or movement of, a patient. With proper precautions, all but a few patients can safely be carried by air.

Factors to be Considered. Aside from the possibility of motion sickness, the two most important factors to be considered in air travel by patients are reduction in air pressure and reduction in oxygen content of air at altitude. Cabin pressurization in larger and newer aircraft minimizes these changes, but hazards may be present for a few persons.

In pressurized airplanes, cabin pressure is normally maintained at a fixed excess over that of the outside air. The amount of excess varies with the type of aircraft, but the differential is commonly in the neighborhood of 8 pounds per square inch. This gives a cabin pressure that does not fall below that of sea level until the aircraft reaches 22,000 feet. Above this, internal pressure falls until at 40,000 feet the cabin has an "altitude" of 7000 feet above sea level. In older aircraft, pressure differentials are smaller, and cabin pressures on some flights may be equivalent to as much as 9000 feet. Only a few light aircraft are pressurized; these are often flown at 10,000 to 12,000 feet, or even more over mountainous terrain.

Hazards of Reduced Pressure. A bubble of gas trapped within the body will expand as air pressure is reduced. At an altitude of 5000 feet, trapped gas expands to 125 per cent of its sea level volume, and at 10,000 feet to 150 per cent of its sea level volume. Expansion causes pressure on surrounding tissues; this may jeopardize blood supply, and may cause rupture of containing walls.

Persons with *unreduced hernia* should not fly, since if gas is trapped it may expand and interfere with circulation. A *perforating wound of the eyeball or the skull* may allow entrance of a bubble of air that might expand at altitude. Patients with these injuries should not travel or be moved by air until absorption is complete. Patients with *pneumothorax* should not fly until all air has been absorbed. The same caution applies after *pneumoencephalography.* Expansion of abdominal gas causes some distention, and patients who have had *abdominal surgery* should not fly for two weeks after surgery. A patient with a *colostomy* may expect filling of the bag on ascent. Patients with *acute upper respiratory tract disease* may have discomfort in the sinuses or middle ear because of closure of the ostia of the sinuses or the eustachian tube and consequent failure of pressure adjust-ment during ascent or descent; use of decongestant nose drops or inhalers before flight may avert difficulty. A similar precaution is useful for the patient with *chronic sinusitis* or *allergic rhinitis.* Patients with *lung cavities, abscesses,* or *bullous emphysema* should not fly because of the danger of rupture.

Hazards of Reduced Oxygen. Oxygen content of alveolar air is reduced at increasing altitudes. Though oxygen saturation of the blood is less markedly reduced, patients whose tissue oxygenation is marginal for any reason (whether from impaired pulmonary function, reduced oxygen-carrying capacity of the blood, or impaired tissue circulation) should not fly unless prior arrangement has been made with the airline for oxygen to be continuously available in flight. Patients should not fly after *myocardial infarction* until they are symptom-free with moderate exertion, usually at least six weeks after an attack. Patients with *angina pectoris* that is symptomatic on climbing a flight of stairs should have supplemental oxygen available during flight. *Anemia,* when the hemoglobin is less than 50 per cent, should preclude flight unless oxygen is available. Patients with *developing gangrene* or *carbon monoxide poisoning* should not be moved without supplemental oxygen in flight. Any *pulmonary disease,* when severe enough to cause cyanosis at ground level, to seriously impair exercise tolerance, or to reduce vital capacity below 50 per cent of normal, is a contraindication to flight unless supplemental oxygen is made available.

Sickle cell trait has been the cause of some concern as a possible risk for air travelers and aircrew members. The concern has been based on earlier reports of splenic infarction at moderate altitude, in unpressurized aircraft, or on the ground in persons with sickle cell trait and most commonly after exertion, vomiting, or anesthesia. It should be noted that in no case was the cause-effect relationship with reduced oxygen tension established. Moreover, no reaction attributable to sickle cell trait has been reported from flight in a pressurized aircraft. For prospective passengers in commercial aircraft, screening for sickle cell trait has not been considered warranted. With respect to aircrew members, some airlines in the past have screened prospective employees and have declined to hire those with the sickle cell trait. This policy has been based on the assumption that, if an aircraft accidentally lost its pressurization, the aircrew members might be called upon for physical exertion, possibly rendering themselves vulnerable to splenic infarction. Fears have been allayed by the small number of depressurization incidents in flight, by the uneventful performance of Olympic athletes with known sickle cell trait in Mexico City at an altitude of 2240 meters (7349 feet), and by the documented normal performance of professional football players with sickle cell trait, often at altitudes over 1524 meters (5000 feet). Most airlines no longer screen for sickle cell trait or exclude from employment as cabin attendants those who have it; some, however, do not accept them as pilots. The National Academy of Sciences–National Research Council has recommended that "except for pilots or copilots, persons with the sickle cell trait should not be restricted from flight duty." This exclusion from pilot duty of persons with the trait may be overcautious and unwarranted. At least one major airline accepts pilots with sickle cell trait without question, and has had no incident attributable to this disorder.

Aerial movement is sometimes considered for a patient who has recently suffered from an attack of *poliomyelitis.* In general, such a patient should not be moved by air until his condition has become stabilized. If respiratory paralysis has occurred, the patient who is able to be out of a respirator for 8 to 12 hours a day can usually be moved safely by air. For those requiring a respirator continuously, portable equipment is available that can be carried in aircraft. Such patients should be observed carefully in flight by an experienced attendant, with special attention to the maintenance of normal ventilatory exchange and the avoidance of dehydration, as this tends to make secretions thicker and more difficult to aspirate. If bulbar involvement has caused difficulty in swallowing, a tracheostomy should be performed prior to flight to ensure adequacy of the airway.

Time Zone Changes. Subjective fatigue and delays in adjustment to time zone changes after east-west or west-east travel are matters of common observation. Not only sleeping habits, but more profound cycles of deep body temperature, water and electrolyte excretion, plasma lactic dehydrogenase, and other physiologic measures are involved. The time required for a traveler to "get on schedule" at the destination depends upon many factors, including individual characteristics, the number of time zones passed, the opportunities for rest before and after flight, and, for some, the direction of flight. A traveler to the west is not likely to have trouble in going to sleep at night in the new time zone, but he may have morning insomnia; one traveling several time zones to the east is likely to experience evening insomnia and retarded awakening. If the traveler has a tendency toward insomnia, travel may cause a troublesome accentuation.

Studies have indicated some actual impairment of psychologic performance in the 24 hours immediately after travel through 7 to 12 time zones. Performance has commonly returned to normal after one good night's sleep. Adjustment of sleeping habits and the overcoming of subjective fatigue may take several days; the deeper physiologic cycles require longer periods—from four to eight days for adjustment to a time differential of 7 to 12 zones.

Travelers can minimize problems by giving special attention to rest before and after long flights. If circumstances permit before the trip, the prospective traveler may benefit from modifying his sleep schedules toward those of the destination. If possible, a flight departing in the morning should be chosen. Overindulgence in food and alcohol en route should be avoided. Trusted somnifacients for a few nights after arrival may speed the adjustment. Some experienced travelers recommend that "million dollar decisions" be avoided in the first 24 hours after a long flight.

Other Hazards. Prolonged sitting and inactivity may be hazardous for persons with a history of *thrombophlebitis* or other circulatory disorder of the lower extremities. These patients should be advised to move about frequently during long flights. A patient with a *fractured jaw* treated by fixation should not fly because of the danger of aspirating vomitus in case of motion sickness. If he must fly, a quick-release fixation should be devised.

Common Questions. Physicians are often asked questions about flying. *Normal infants* tolerate air travel well, but feeding should be given during descent, to facilitate aeration of the middle ear by swallowing. *Old age* in itself is no contraindication to flight, if significant disease is not present. *Pregnancy* is no contraindication to flight, but if the mother is near term, the airline may require a physician's statement that delivery is not likely to occur during the flight. There is no evidence that the mild oxygen deficit in the atmosphere is harmful to the fetus. *Hypertension* is not adversely affected by air travel, though preflight sedation may be appropriate. Patients with *communicable diseases* should, of course, not travel when hazards of transmission to others exist. *Patients whose conditions make them objectionable to others,* such as those with urinary incontinence or malodorous discharges, should not travel in the crowded cabins of commercial aircraft. *Mild asthma* is not ordinarily adversely affected by flight. Patients subject to severe asthmatic attacks should carry their tested medications, and should ensure in advance the availability of oxygen if needed. In *epileptics,* oxygen deficiency and hyperventilation attending excitement in flight may precipitate seizures. Persons subject to frequent seizures should have proper medication, including sedation, prior to travel by air and if possible should be accompanied by an attendant. *Psychiatric disorders* require individual evaluation; the likelihood of disturbance or agitation under the minimal stress of travel and the safety and comfort of fellow passengers should be considered. Questions regarding other conditions should be referred to the airline's nearest medical official. Indeed, it is advisable to discuss with the airline's medical official any prospective passenger whose condition might be unfavorably influenced by flight.

Beighton, P. H., and Richard, P. R.: Cardiovascular disease in air travelers. Br. Heart J., 30:367, 1968.

Bergin, K. G.: Transport of invalids by air. Br. Med. J., 3:539, 1967.

Buley, L. E.: Formula for determining rest periods on long distance air travel. Aerosp. Med., 41:680, 1970.

Committee on Medical Criteria: Medical criteria for passenger flying. Arch. Environ. Health, 2:124, 1961.

McFarland, R. A.: Influence of changing time zones on air crews and passengers. Aerosp. Med., 45:648, 1974.

Money, K. D.: Motion sickness. Physiol. Rev., 50:1, 1970.

Murphy, J. R.: Sickle cell hemoglobin (Hb AS) in black football players. J.A.M.A., 225:981, 1973.

National Academy of Sciences–National Research Council: The S-Hemoglobinopathies: An Evaluation of Their Status in the Armed Forces, 1973.

Wood, C. D., and Graybiel, A.: Theory of anti-motion sickness drug mechanisms. Aerosp. Med., 43:249, 1972.

ALTERATIONS IN ATMOSPHERIC PRESSURE

Robert L. Johnson

44. INTRODUCTION

The physiologic and pathologic effects of alterations in atmospheric pressure are governed by the physical behavior of gases. The individual gaseous molecules of the earth's atmosphere have mass and therefore weight owing to the effect of gravity. Atmospheric pressure represents the weight of the mass of air extending upward from the earth's surface. At sea level this amounts to 760 mm of mercury (1.013×10^5 Newtons per square meter, 1013 millibars, 14.7 pounds per square inch, or 1 atmosphere). Atmospheric air (dry) contains 20.94 per cent oxygen, 0.03 per cent carbon dioxide, and approximately 79 per cent nitrogen at all altitudes. However, the partial pressures of the individual gases of the atmosphere, in accordance with Dalton's law, vary directly as the total atmospheric pressure. At sea level, where atmospheric pressure is 760 mm of mercury, the partial pressures of oxygen, carbon dioxide, and nitrogen are 159 (760 × 0.2094), 2.3 (760 × 0.0003), and 600 (760 × 0.79) mm of mercury, respectively, in dry air.

Water, being much denser than air, exerts a much greater pressure. The weight of a 33-foot column of sea water equals that of a like-sized column of air extending through the entire atmosphere. Since water is incompressible, pressure increases in linear fashion with further descent, each 33 feet adding an additional atmosphere of pressure.

The medical problems created by changes in atmospheric pressure may be grouped into direct and indirect effects. The former result from mechanical forces created when pressure differentials develop across the walls of air-containing spaces within the body or upon its surface. Indirect effects result from alterations in partial pressures of the individual gases of the atmosphere.

45. DIRECT EFFECTS OF CHANGES IN ATMOSPHERIC PRESSURE

Gases respond to pressure changes in accordance with Boyle's law. Their volume varies inversely and their density, or molecular concentration, directly as the absolute pressure. The fluids and solids of the human body, being incompressible, transmit pressure freely and thus assume the pressure exerted upon the body's surface. Any alteration in the latter is reflected almost instantly by an identical pressure change in body fluids and tissues. Pressure within air-containing spaces of the body can be maintained equal to external pressure only by appropriate adjustments either of the number of molecules of gas within the space or of the volume of the space. No medical difficulties arise as long as air can pass freely between such spaces and the environment. If additional air cannot enter such a space to increase its pressure during descent, fluids and tissues of the surrounding walls, whose pressure is increasing with increasing ambient pressure, tend to move in to reduce its volume and eradicate the pressure differential. The lining of the walls becomes hyperemic and swollen. Serum or blood may move into the relative vacuum. Conversely, during ascent, pressure within the tissues surrounding the space declines with declining environmental pressure. Unless air can be vented from the space, an increasing pressure gradient creates a distending force against the walls.

The natural air-containing spaces of the body are the paranasal sinuses, the middle ear, the airways and lungs, and the gastrointestinal tract. Small pockets of air may also exist beneath fillings or in diseased teeth. In addition, pockets of air against various surfaces of the body may be produced by goggles, tight-fitting hoods, ear plugs, or wrinkles in diving suits. The middle ear is very susceptible to barotrauma during descent. The sinuses are much less frequently affected, but may also incur barotrauma during ascent. Respiratory infection greatly increases the likelihood of injury. Descent in water may

damage tissues beneath air-containing structures closely applied to the surface of the body. All these injuries, including barotitis with ruptured tympanic membranes, tend to heal spontaneously.

The most serious mechanical injuries resulting from pressure changes involve the lungs. If the breath is held during diving, the increasing pressure compresses the thoracic cage to the position of maximal expiration. On further descent air within the lungs can no longer be compressed to counter the increasing external pressure. The relatively negative intrapulmonary pressure results eventually in pulmonary congestion, edema, and hemorrhage, a condition known as "thoracic squeeze." Breathing the denser air at depth through equipment with excessive air flow resistance or breathing through a snorkel tube which is too long may also create a relatively negative pressure within the lungs, leading to similar consequences.

After breathing the denser air at depths, air must be released from lungs during ascent to prevent expanding air from building up sufficient pressure to overdistend or rupture lung tissue; if this occurs, pneumothorax, mediastinal emphysema, or air embolism may ensue. Air embolism has been reported during ascents of as little as 9 feet and is said to be exceeded in frequency only by drowning as a cause of accidental death among divers. Lung tissue distal to a poorly communicating diseased bronchial passage may be similarly damaged even if the diver vents his excess air during ascent. The air traveler with such bronchopulmonary disease, or one who happens to be holding his breath, may be similarly injured during a sudden loss of cabin pressure at high altitude.

Knowledge of the character of the dive, including depth, duration, air supply, and patterns of descent and ascent in relation to symptoms, often simplifies the problem of diagnosing lung injury in divers. Frothy, bloody sputum may be produced in either thoracic squeeze or lung rupture. If the victim has been skin-diving or using a snorkel tube, thoracic squeeze is likely. In a scuba diver, however, the first consideration must be lung rupture with potentially fatal aeroembolism. (The term "scuba" is derived from "self-contained underwater breathing apparatus.") The unconscious diver must be presumed to have aeroembolism or decompression sickness. Either aeroembolism or serious decompression sickness requires treatment by recompression at the earliest possible moment. Transport to a recompression chamber should be by the fastest method available. The gain from prompt treatment far outweighs the potential danger of further decompression during air transportation at low altitudes. Meanwhile artificial respiration by the mouth-to-mouth method should be carried out if necessary, and oxygen should be administered. Placing the victim on his left side may be beneficial if aeroembolism is suspected. Thoracic squeeze usually requires no more than supportive measures.

46. INDIRECT EFFECTS OF CHANGES IN ATMOSPHERIC PRESSURE

Gases in contact with liquids dissolve in direct proportion to their partial pressures and their solubility coefficients. Gases enter and leave the body in response to gradients of partial pressure between blood and alveolar gases. Gradients of partial pressure likewise determine the movement of gases within body fluids.

Only brief mention can be made here of the effects of increases in the partial pressures of nitrogen, oxygen, and carbon dioxide. At 4 atmospheres absolute pressure (100 feet in water), divers or occupants of hyperbaric chambers may show the narcotizing effect of nitrogen. Judgment, thought processes, and motor ability may become impaired and deteriorate with further increases in atmospheric pressure. Fortunately, the symptoms clear rapidly and completely on return to lower atmospheric pressure.

Hypercapnia normally produces subjective distress and stimulation of respiration, but may cause unconsciousness without warning. Scuba divers who restrict their breathing in an attempt to conserve their air supply expose themselves to this potential hazard. Loss of consciousness in skin divers resulting from "shallow-water blackout" is attributed to a large rise in partial pressure of carbon dioxide associated with an inadequate subjective or respiratory response to hypercapnia.

Convulsive seizures and coma may occur with little warning during exposure to high partial pressures of oxygen. The minimal partial pressure of oxygen capable of producing convulsions appears to be less than 2 atmospheres ($Po_2 = 1520$ mm Hg). Divers breathing air are at little risk of oxygen convulsions. If they use pure oxygen, however, depths greater than 25 feet become hazardous.

Hyperbaric oxygenation is achieved by increasing atmospheric pressure within sealed chambers to levels varying from 2 to 4 atmospheres absolute ($Po_2 = 320$ to 640 mm Hg). Increased oxygenation of tissues occurs chiefly as a result of increased solution of oxygen in plasma. Hyperbaric oxygenation has been reported to be of value during surgical correction of certain congenital cardiovascular disorders and in the treatment of carbon monoxide poisoning and certain anaerobic infections. Precautions must be taken to protect the patient and medical personnel from all the direct and indirect effects of altered atmospheric pressure.

DECOMPRESSION SICKNESS
(Caisson Disease)

In decompression sickness the manifestations are due to formation of nitrogen bubbles in body tissues and fluids. On exposure to lower atmospheric pressure the partial pressure of nitrogen dissolved in body fluids and tissues exceeds nitrogen partial pressure in the lungs. If this pressure reaches the point where nitrogen evolves from tissues and fluids faster than it can be transported by blood to the alveolar membrane to diffuse into alveolar air, bubbles will form. Bubbles large enough to produce symptoms develop when the partial pressure of nitrogen in tissues rapidly becomes more than twice as great as nitrogen partial pressure in the atmosphere. This situation can arise in a diver whose tissues are saturated with nitrogen at a depth somewhat in excess of 33 feet who surfaces rapidly, or by a flier who rapidly ascends from sea level to higher than 18,000 feet.

The processes of nitrogen diffusion and transport necessary for equilibration between tissues and alveolar air require time. Since nitrogen must be transported by blood, equilibration in highly vascular tissues occurs more rapidly than in those that are poorly vascularized. Fatty tissue is not only poorly vascularized but in addi-

tion takes up larger volumes of nitrogen since nitrogen is far more soluble in lipids than in water.

The complete elimination of excess nitrogen from the body after exposure to a lower partial pressure of nitrogen in the atmosphere requires about 12 hours. About 75 per cent of the total is eliminated within $2\frac{1}{2}$ hours, mainly from aqueous solution in plasma and interstitial tissue. The slower component arises mainly from tissues high in lipid content such as fat deposits, bone marrow, and spinal cord.

The total amount and the rate at which nitrogen is taken into solution during a dive will depend not only upon the depth but the time spent at depth. The magnitude of this depth-time factor and the rate of ascent determine whether decompression sickness occurs. Beyond certain depth-time values, it is necessary to ascend in stages with time to allow an adequate amount of denitrogenation to occur before ascending further. Stage decompression is based on never exceeding the 2:1 ratio of alveolar to tissue partial pressure of nitrogen. These general principles also apply in altitude decompression sickness, in which tissues are saturated at 1 atmosphere when ascent begins.

Manifestations. The symptoms produced depend primarily upon the site of bubble formation. The size of the bubbles and their rate of growth influence the severity of symptoms. Although bizarre clinical pictures may occur, certain patterns occur frequently, suggesting a predilection to bubble formation in some tissues and organs. The most common and familiar manifestation is *"bends."* This consists of deep, boring, and usually constant pain in the vicinity of large joints, the knees and shoulders being most frequently involved. Pain may be so severe as to be incapacitating. Most cases of bends occur within the first 30 minutes after decompression, that is, after reaching a critical altitude or after surfacing following a dive in which the depth-time factor was exceeded. Bends in flight disappear completely during descent.

Subjective skin manifestations, usually prickling or burning sensations, termed the "itches" or "creeps," occur rather commonly in fliers. Although objective skin manifestations occur uncommonly, a characteristic pale, cyanotic mottling of the skin sometimes appears, usually over the upper trunk and typically later than bends.

Chokes, believed to be due to bubbles in the pulmonary vasculature, occurs later than bends, and consists of burning retrosternal distress and cough. Relieved at first by shallow breathing, the symptoms progress in severity until coughing becomes paroxysmal and uncontrollable. Recompression by descent produces partial relief, but symptoms may persist for several days. Often associated with cyanosis and syncope, the syndrome has ominous significance because shock and coma may ensue.

Homonymous scintillating *scotomas* are neurologic manifestations of decompression sickness. Although apparently not observed in divers, they are common manifestations at high altitude. They are transient, and frequently disappear while still at altitude.

One or more of the manifestations already mentioned usually precede more serious stages of decompression sickness, which are characterized by neurologic manifestations and sometimes vasomotor instability that may progress to circulatory collapse with cyanosis, shock, and coma. Almost every possible neurologic sign has been observed, including motor paralysis. In altitude decompression sickness, neurologic findings are usually limited to transient paresis and dysthesias. The lower segments of the spinal cord are most frequently involved in divers, and permanent residuals may occur. In decompression sickness a period of apparent recovery from the earlier manifestations may precede the appearance of circulatory collapse and shock. During this latent period vague symptoms can usually be elicited, and signs of instability of blood pressure and heart rate and at least minor focal neurologic signs can be detected. Hemoconcentration, with hematocrit as high as 60 to 70 per cent, is a characteristic finding that presumably results from widespread vascular injury and loss of plasma into tissues.

Treatment. All the varied manifestations of decompression sickness respond rapidly to early and adequate treatment by recompression. Descent from altitude produces sufficient recompression to abolish the early manifestations, but merely retards the appearance of the more slowly developing serious forms of decompression sickness. In such cases widespread bubble formation has presumably already occurred, and descent is entirely analogous to inadequate recompression therapy during which symptoms subside only temporarily. The clinical picture of decompression sickness in divers and fliers might also be expected to differ because of the greater volumes of nitrogen that must be eliminated in divers on decompression.

Divers can prevent decompression sickness by knowing and following established limits for depth and time at depth. Limitations of air supply unfortunately often prevent ascent in stages after depth-time limits have been exceeded. Adequate denitrogenation by breathing 100 per cent oxygen prior to and during ascent is an effective preventive measure in fliers. Divers should avoid the increased hazard of repeating a dive before adequate time at surface to eliminate excess nitrogen from the previous dive. Similarly, fliers who have experienced decompression symptoms during a flight should delay return to even relatively low altitudes because the expansion of bubbles still present in tissues may cause a rapid recurrence of more serious symptoms. The hazard of exposure to altitudes as low as 7000 feet after even safe depth-time dives should be recognized.

Adequate recompression performed at the earliest possible time is the specific therapy for decompression sickness. All other measures are adjunctive. Those reported to be beneficial include oxygen by mask, low molecular weight dextran and standard replacement fluids to correct hypovolemia, heparin in doses of 50 to 100 mg twice daily, and injectable steroids such as dexamethasone, 8 mg initially with diminishing doses every six hours.

Undersea Medical Society: Modern aspects of treatment of decompression sickness. Aerosp. Med., 39:1055, 1968.

OTHER DIVING HAZARDS

Diving, by its nature, either with or without scuba, involves certain respiratory patterns that are potentially hazardous under water. Hyperventilation and breathholding, for example, may initiate cardioinhibitory and vasodepressor reflexes capable of causing syncope, cardiac arrhythmias, and arrest. Bradycardia, apparently more pronounced than might occur simply from breathholding and the head-down position, and various cardiac arrhythmias have also been reported during breath-hold

diving. Vigorous hyperventilation by skin divers prior to a dive may lead to lowering of arterial P_{CO_2} sufficient to abolish the stimulus to breathe and may allow dangerous levels of hypoxemia to develop. In addition, compression of air within the lungs during descent may maintain adequate alveolar P_{O_2} levels despite a diminishing oxygen supply. Distress from air hunger may not occur because alveolar P_{CO_2} has been reduced by prior hyperventilation. During ascent the expansion of the air remaining within the lungs results in a sharp reduction in P_{O_2}, possibly to levels that result in loss of consciousness before the diver is able to reach the surface, and he may drown unless help is available for prompt rescue and resuscitation. Divers using properly functioning open-circuit scuba are unlikely to experience hypoxia if they restrict their dives to well within the limits of their air supply. The rate of air utilization increases in proportion to the increase in absolute pressure when using open-circuit scuba. Total duration of air supply is, for example, only one third as long at 66 feet as at the surface. Increased utilization from heavy exertion causes a proportionately greater expenditure of air.

The availability of scuba has enabled large numbers of untrained people to enter an unfamiliar and hostile environment previously restricted to trained professional divers. The increasing number of serious diving accidents attests to a general lack of understanding of basic underwater principles. The greatest medical problem is education of those who participate in this sport. Physicians in almost any locality may now be called upon to manage a diving emergency. Excellent publications concerning this subject, such as the United States Navy Diving Manual and others, should be available for this purpose.

Bennett, P. B., and Elliott, D. H.: The Physiology and Medicine of Diving and Compressed Air Work. Baltimore, Williams & Wilkins Company, 1969.

Dewey, A. W., Jr.: Decompression sickness, an emerging recreational hazard. N. Engl. J. Med., 267:759, 812, 1962.

Ferris, E. B., and Engel, G. L.: The clinical nature of high altitude decompression sickness. In Fulton, J. F. (ed.): Decompression Sickness, Diver's and Flier's Bends and Related Syndromes. National Research Council, Committee on Medical Sciences. Philadelphia, W. B. Saunders Company, 1951, p. 4.

Lambertsen, C. J. (ed.): Underwater Physiology. Proceedings of the Fourth Symposium on Underwater Physiology. New York, Academic Press, 1971.

United States Air Force: Flight Surgeon's Guide. No. AFP 161–18. Washington, D.C., Department of the Air Force, 1968.

United States Navy: U.S. Diving Manual. NAVSHIPS 0994–001–9010. Washington, D.C., 1968.

HYPOXIA

Hypoxia refers to the reduced partial pressure of oxygen at altitude. It thus represents an indirect effect of altered atmospheric pressure. The clinical manifestations at a given altitude are influenced primarily by duration of exposure, rate of ascent, and individual tolerance. However, the level of physical activity, the degree of health, physical conditioning, altitude acclimatization, and such factors as temperature, wind, and humidity may all modify the response in varying degrees.

The transfer of gases between lung, blood, and tissues depends upon differences in partial pressures. Alveolar air is saturated with water vapor, which exerts a constant pressure of 47 mm of mercury. Carbon dioxide normally contributes about 40 mm of mercury pressure to total alveolar pressure. Although total alveolar pressure is in equilibrium with atmospheric pressure, the space available for oxygen and other components of inspired air is approximately 87 mm of mercury less than existing atmospheric pressure. Mixing of inspired with residual air further reduces alveolar partial pressure of oxygen from that in the atmosphere. The alveolar pressure constantly contributed by water vapor and CO_2 occupies an increasingly large proportion of alveolar pressure as atmospheric pressure declines. At sea level (alveolar Po_2 = 103 mm of mercury) hemoglobin is normally 95 to 98 per cent saturated. Not until altitudes of 10,000 feet (P_B = 523 mm of mercury and alveolar Po_2 = 61 mm of mercury) does hemoglobin saturation begin to fall below 90 per cent. Thereafter saturation declines rapidly with further increases in altitude and decline in alveolar partial pressure of oxygen.

Manifestations.   The first important physiologic effect of hypoxia occurs at about 5000 feet, when night vision begins to be impaired. Ventilatory and cardiovascular adjustments are minimal until about 10,000 feet, above which respiratory rate and depth and heart rate increase progressively to increase alveolar Po_2 and cardiac output. Exertional dyspnea may appear, and in some people mental concentration becomes difficult. Vagal cardioinhibitory reflexes may lead to bradycardia and sometimes ectopic cardiac rhythms, and may precipitate syncope. Headache, slight giddiness, and restlessness are common.

Above 15,000 feet some persons experience lassitude and indifference whereas others exhibit increased activity, irritability, euphoria, and other disturbances of affect. The impairment of judgment that begins at these altitudes jeopardizes the safety of fliers and mountain climbers. Cyanosis, loss of peripheral vision, dimming of vision, and variable degrees of muscular incoordination appear at altitudes of around 18,000 feet. Somewhere between this level and 25,000 feet, consciousness can no longer be retained for more than a few minutes. Rapid descent or administration of oxygen is essential to prevent death. If corrective action is taken soon enough, recovery is rapid and complete.

High-flying jet aircraft make it possible for many people of various ages and states of health to be exposed to the potential hazard of sudden hypoxia from rapid decompression. Should cabin pressure be abruptly lost at high altitudes, only a short period of consciousness would be possible with the breathing of ambient air. At altitudes between 30,000 and 45,000 feet oxygen transfer across alveolar walls would be reversed, and the duration of consciousness would shorten progressively from about 1 minute to 15 seconds, or the lung-to-brain circulation time of about 9 seconds plus around 6 seconds from oxygen already present in brain tissue. Rapid donning of oxygen masks and descent of the aircraft would shorten the period of severe hypoxia and minimize the possibility of serious injury.

Lamb, L. E.: Aerospace medicine *In* Dock, W., and Snapper, I. (eds.): Advances in Internal Medicine, Vol. XII. Chicago, Year Book Medical Publishers, 1964, p. 175.

ACUTE MOUNTAIN SICKNESS

This is a clinical syndrome observed in unacclimatized persons usually within a few hours after rapid exposure to high altitude. Individual tolerance varies widely. Some experience symptoms at altitudes as low as 7000 to 8000 feet, although others tolerate altitudes of 14,000 feet with minimal symptoms. There appears to be no way to predict unusual susceptibility, but rapid ascent, physical exertion, and poor physical condition increase the likelihood. Initial symptoms are usually mild to incapacitating headache, exertional dyspnea, malaise, and weakness. Insomnia, anorexia, nausea, vomiting, diarrhea, and abdominal pain may occur. Mental capacity and judgment may be impaired. Inability to sleep is a common problem. Cyanosis of the lips and nail beds, Cheyne-Stokes breathing, and tachycardia are usually present. These manifestations usually subside gradually over a period of several days, but may recur at higher altitudes. In some instances the symptoms are severe and unrelieved except by oxygen or descent to a lower altitude. Gradual ascent with periodic halts of several days to allow acclimatization will prevent or reduce the severity of symptoms. Acetazolamide, given in dosages of 250 mg every eight hours prior to and during exposure to altitude, has been reported to reduce the frequency and severity of symptoms. The mechanism of its effect is not clear, but increased ventilation and alveolar oxygen tension, decreased carbon dioxide tension and serum bicarbonate, and absence of alkalosis were observed in treated subjects. Furosemide, 80 mg every 12 hours, has produced relief of symptoms and signs usually within 48 hours, apparently in association with the induced diuresis.

Forward, S. A., Landowne, M., Follansbee, J. N., and Hansen, J. E.: Effect of acetazolamide on acute mountain sickness. N. Engl. J. Med., 279:839, 1968.
Singh, I., Khanna, P. K., Srivastava, M. C., Lal, M., Roy, S. B., and Subramanyam, C. S. V.: Acute mountain sickness. N. Engl. J. Med., 280:175, 1969.

HIGH ALTITUDE PULMONARY EDEMA

Acute pulmonary edema is an uncommon but serious and sometimes fatal complication of rapid exposure to altitudes above 9000 feet. Hypoxia is considered the primary etiologic agent. Many earlier fatal cases were erroneously diagnosed as pneumonia. Young, unacclimatized persons and acclimatized residents who have sojourned at lower altitudes for a few days or weeks appear most susceptible. Recurrences are common in those who have experienced an attack. Rapid ascent and heavy physical exertion increase susceptibility.

Autopsy findings have included wet lungs congested with serosanguineous edema fluid. Bronchiolar and alveolar edema with hyaline membranes, resembling those seen in hyaline membrane disease of the newborn, over the internal walls of alveoli, alveolar sacs, and alveolar ducts have been characteristic findings. Dilatation of preterminal arterioles and thrombosis of septal capillaries and of small and medium-sized pulmonary arteries have also been observed. The exact pathogenic mechanism is conjectural. A comparative increase in capillary pressure is thought to be responsible for the alveolar edema. In a few cases pulmonary artery pressure has been elevated and electrocardiograms have suggested acute right ventricular overloading. The hyaline membrane formation, not a characteristic finding in death caused by simple hypoxia, has not been explained, but a deficient pulmonary fibrinolysis system has been postulated.

Symptoms usually appear 6 to 36 hours after exposure

to altitude and may be preceded by acute mountain sickness. Exertional dyspnea, weakness, malaise, and a persistent, dry, irritating cough are the characteristic initial symptoms. Later, noisy respiration, rales, cyanosis, orthopnea, and hemoptysis develop. Unless continuous oxygen therapy is carried out or the patient descends to a lower altitude, these symptoms progress, and death occurs. Gradual acclimatization and avoidance of undue physical exertion during the early period of exposure to altitude are important preventive measures.

CHRONIC MOUNTAIN SICKNESS
(Monge's Disease)

Chronic mountain sickness is a clinical syndrome that occurs in residents at high altitudes, usually over 14,000 feet, characterized by loss of tolerance to hypoxia in a previously acclimatized person. The cause is not known, but associated are increased polycythemia, decreased pulmonary ventilation, increased Pco_2, lowered arterial saturation, and impaired sensitivity of the respiratory center as compared with asymptomatic residents at high altitude. Hemoglobin and hematocrit may be increased to as much as 25 grams per 100 ml and 80 per cent, as compared with 21 grams and 60 per cent in native residents. Hyperplasia and hyperactivity of marrow erythroid cells and pulmonary hypertension are greater than in the healthy residents.

The clinical manifestations are similar to those of erythremia. They include marked cyanosis, dyspnea, cough, palpitations, headache, giddiness, muscular weakness, pain in the extremities, sensory and motor changes, and episodic stupor. The condition can be cured only by returning to a lower altitude or to sea level.

Monge also described a less severe form of chronic mountain sickness in mountain residents that he called *subacute mountain sickness.* Many of the symptoms resemble those of acute mountain sickness, but they persist unless the patient descends to sea level or receives oxygen. The marked cyanosis and alveolar hypoventilation of chronic mountain sickness does not occur, and the laboratory findings are like those in asymptomatic natives.

Hultgren, H. N., and Grover, R. F.: Circulatory adaptation to high altitude. Ann. Rev. Med., 19:119, 1968.
Lenfant, C., and Sullivan, K.: Adaptation to high altitude. N. Engl. J. Med., 284:1298, 1971.
Weihe, W. H. (ed.): Physiological Effects of High Altitude. New York, The Macmillan Company, 1964.

47. DROWNING

Charles J. Stahl

Definition. Drowning is a pathologic condition, terminating in death, which may result from the complex biochemical, respiratory, and cardiovascular changes that follow the aspiration of fluid during immersion, or—less commonly—from asphyxia associated with obstruction of the airway.

Etiology. Accidents account for most drownings. The victims are often children or other persons who have not learned to swim. Less frequently, it may result from suicide or homicide. The circumstances for accidental

drowning may include the following: (1) disasters such as floods, tidal waves, shipwrecks, and vehicular accidents; (2) hazardous environmental conditions or careless acts while engaged in fishing, aquatic sport, or occupational activities; (3) impaired ability to swim because of pre-existing illness, intoxication, exhaustion, or exposure to cold water; and (4) unintentional falls into water.

Incidence and Prevalence. Nearly 8000 deaths by drowning and approximately the same number of near-drownings occur annually in the United States. This is the third most common type of accidental death. The majority of the victims are young men under 25 years of age. Several million Americans engage in the sport of underwater swimming, using either self-contained underwater breathing apparatus (scuba) or snorkel. When underwater accidents are considered alone, drowning is the most common cause of death. It occurs more frequently than deaths from barotrauma, including air embolism and decompression sickness, discussed in Ch. 44 to 46.

Pathogenesis. Survivors of near-drowning have provided some knowledge of the sequence of events. The victim usually experiences panic at the time of immersion and struggles to reach the surface, unless previously incapacitated by alcohol, drugs, or injury. Breath-holding is common and persists until accumulation of carbon dioxide stimulates the respiratory center. When the victim can no longer restrain the urge to breathe, high pulmonary carbon dioxide and low pulmonary and arterial oxygen tensions are present. Gasping may result in aspiration of water or other liquid. In about 10 per cent of fatal cases, however, it is believed that the victims do not aspirate fluid, but die from asphyxia during reflex laryngospasm or breath-holding. Swallowing of water, vomiting, and coughing may occur. Convulsions precede death in some cases.

The pathophysiologic changes in drowning were poorly understood until the studies with experimental animals reported by Swann and Spafford. They demonstrated that the hemodynamic and biochemical changes during drowning of dogs are affected by the type of fluid encountered. When drowning occurs in *fresh water,* rapid absorption of hypotonic water from the lungs into the circulation results in hypervolemia, hemodilution, and hemolysis. Serum electrolytes are decreased, except for potassium, which increases because of hemolysis. The altered ratio between sodium and potassium, as well as anoxia, may cause ventricular fibrillation in dogs. The mechanism for drowning in *sea water,* however, is probably different. As the result of the aspiration of sea water, salts pass into the circulation and fluids diffuse into alveoli. Serum electrolytes, particularly chloride and magnesium, increase markedly. Hypovolemia, hemoconcentration, and hypoproteinemia, as well as pulmonary edema, occur.

Recent studies of drowning and near-drowning in laboratory animals by Modell indicate that the biochemical and cardiovascular changes are dependent not only upon the tonicity of fluid but also upon the quantity of fluid aspirated. Sea water, volume for volume, is twice as lethal as fresh water, and causes more profound changes in serum electrolytes. The serum electrolytes of animals that survived aspiration of either fresh water or sea water quickly returned to normal concentrations. These studies confirm prior observations by Fuller that life-threatening changes in electrolytes may not occur in human victims of drowning. After near-drowning with aspiration of water by dogs, the most significant changes include hypoxemia, hypercarbia, and acidosis. Pulmonary edema and decreased pulmonary compliance are evident. Fresh water alters or destroys the normal surface-tension properties of *pulmonary surfactant.* Sea water only partially removes surfactant. The pathophysiologic effects are alveolar collapse, uneven ventilation, pulmonary edema, and hypoxemia. At least 20 ml of fresh water per pound of body weight must be aspirated by dogs to cause changes in electrolytes or ventricular fibrillation.

Although the pathophysiologic mechanisms seem less well understood and may differ from experimental findings, clinical evaluations of near-drowning victims indicate that fluid and electrolyte balance are restored rapidly. The majority of human drowning victims aspirate 10 ml of fluid or less per pound of body weight. Hemodilution has not been demonstrated, and hemolysis is uncommon. The changes in serum electrolytes and blood volume are often transient and depend upon the quantity and tonicity of fluid aspirated. Nonspecific electrocardiographic changes occur as the result of hypoxia. Ventricular fibrillation is uncommon in human victims. The initial effect of the aspirated fluid on the alveolar membranes and pulmonary surfactant results in collapse of alveoli, decreased compliance, and shunting of blood through nonventilated alveoli. Subsequently, hypoxia also occurs from the diffusion deficit resulting from pulmonary edema or pneumonia. The hypoxia caused by near-drowning with aspiration in human victims is manifested by arterial hypoxemia and metabolic acidosis.

The pathologic findings of drowning are often nonspecific. White or bloody foam, usually seen in the mouth, nose, and tracheobronchial tree, may not be evident after attempts at resuscitation. The skin of the palms and soles is often wrinkled and pale. These changes are consistent with prolonged immersion, but are not pathognomonic of drowning. Lacerations or incised wounds of skin, without evidence of vital reaction, reflect the effects of tides, collision of the body with underwater obstacles, and postmortem injuries inflicted by sharp objects such as motorboat propellors. Mutilation of a body by aquatic animals is common, particularly about the soft tissues of the face.

The lungs are heavy and edematous. In children, however, the lungs are often pink and distended with entrapped air. Pressure on the cut surfaces of the lungs yields variable degrees of frothy fluid. Foreign material from the aquatic environment, as well as vomitus, is often seen in the mouth, upper airway, and tracheobronchial tree. Depending on the postmortem interval, the pleural cavities contain variable quantities of straw-colored to dark watery fluid, which is a transudate from the edematous lungs. A relatively dry appearance of the lungs, attributed in some cases to death by reflex laryngospasm and closure of the glottis, may also result from agonal absorption and elimination of water from the lungs after cessation of respiration. Water may be found in paranasal sinuses, and hemorrhagic fluid is frequently observed in the middle ear and mastoid air cells. The latter finding is not specific for drowning, as it is also seen in other asphyxial deaths. Diatoms are microscopic unicellular or colonial algae containing silica. The significance of diatoms in the diagnosis of drowning is controversial. They may offer evidence of the aspiration of water when the same types of diatoms are demonstrated not only in the lungs but also in the water in which the body was found. After prolonged immersion in water, the changes of decomposition and the effects of aquatic life obscure the usual anatomic findings, but the pleural spaces may contain unusual amounts of sanguineous, watery fluid. The microscopic findings in the lungs may include pulmonary edema, focal intra-alveolar hemorrhage, disruption of alveoli, and demonstration of diatoms.

In laboratory animals (rats), Reidbord and Spitz observed differences in the ultrastructural changes of lungs in drownings in fresh water from those in sea water. With sea water, cellular swelling and vacuolation, as well as discontinuity of alveolar lining cells, were noted. After drowning in fresh water, the lungs of rats showed endothelial destruction, mitochondrial swelling, and cellular disruption. Histochemical changes were also reported by Spitz. An acute perivasculitis, consisting mainly of neutrophils, was seen in the lungs of rats after drowning in sea water. Similar changes, but to a lesser extent, were seen in fresh-water drowning. The distribution and amount of peroxidase-positive granules in the histologic sections parallel the density of the neutrophilic infiltration around vessels. These experimental studies may serve as the basis for a distinction between drowning in sea water and drowning in fresh water.

Numerous chemical and physical tests have been applied to the diagnosis of drowning. They include tests for concentrations of chloride or magnesium in whole blood, plasma, or serum; specific gravity of plasma; refractive index, electrical conductivity, and osmolarity of blood. None of them is entirely reliable, and all require considerable judgment in interpretation. There is yet no specific laboratory test for the diagnosis of drowning.

Clinical Manifestations. The victim of drowning usually experiences breath-holding and a substernal burning sensation. Loss of consciousness and aspiration of fluid may occur. Most victims have a violent struggle prior to loss of consciousness, but a few people show passive behavior. After rescue, the patient is usually unconscious, flaccid, cold, and cyanotic. Respirations are absent, and the pulse is imperceptible. If the patient is conscious, tinnitus and visual abnormalities are often reported. Frothy fluid may be seen in the nose and mouth, and examination of the chest may disclose signs of pulmonary edema. If a significant amount of water has been swallowed, nausea and vomiting may occur and gastric distention may be evident. Nonspecific electrocardiographic changes are related to the effects of hypoxia. Cardiac arrhythmias such as ventricular fibrillation, as reported for animals, are uncommon in man. Evidence of arterial hypoxemia and metabolic acidosis is provided by studies of gas and pH in blood. Serum electrolyte changes are usually transient and depend on the quantity and tonicity of fluid aspirated. The postimmersion period is sometimes complicated by pneumonia, hemoglobinuria, acute tubular necrosis, or brain damage from prolonged cerebral anoxia.

Diagnosis. When the patient is a victim of near-drowning, other physical causes for disability should be considered, including injury to the cervical cord from a dive into shallow water. In the differential diagnosis of near-drowning, other causes for aquatic accidents, especially air embolism and decompression sickness, must be considered. These untoward effects of barotrauma (see Ch. 45 and 46) are usually associated with underwater swimming, diving, or the use of self-contained underwater breathing apparatus (scuba). Recognition and differentiation from near-drowning are extremely important, as recompression, the appropriate method of treatment, may bring dramatic and lifesaving results.

The diagnosis of near-drowning is usually not difficult after the circumstances are known. Diagnostic studies include chest films, electrocardiograms, electroencephalogram, central venous pressure, serial determinations of arterial gas and pH, and appropriate laboratory tests, including hematocrit, hemoglobin, leukocyte count, serum electrolytes, and serum protein determinations. Respiratory complications, particularly pneumonia, are invariably present when fever, leukocytosis, pulmonary infiltrate on chest x-ray films, and decreased arterial oxygen tension are evident.

When the body of a dead person is found immersed in water, the diagnosis of drowning alone requires exclusion of other possible causes for death. A careful appraisal of the circumstances of death and of findings from pathologic and toxicologic studies and from postmortem chemical and physical tests is required. The role of a preexisting illness, such as heart disease, as a precipitating factor in drowning depends on demonstration of pathologic features of the disease, as well as careful correlation with the circumstances and consideration of the hazards in the environment occupied by the victim immediately before the fatal incident. In some cases of suicide, particularly in bathtubs, if a concentration of a drug sufficient to cause coma is found in the blood, the investigator should suspect that the victim ingested a lethal dose of the drug, then went into coma, and drowned subsequently. Failure to find evidence of injury, intoxication, or pre-existing disease, as well as evidence that the person was alive during the period of immersion, favors the presumption that death was caused by drowning.

Treatment. Prompt rescue, first aid, and resuscitation offer the best chance for survival of drowning victims. The airway is cleared of any obstructions, and dentures are removed. Resuscitation by artificial ventilation is continued until oxygen is available, spontaneous breathing occurs, or signs of death are evident. If a heart beat or carotid pulse is not detectable, closed-chest cardiac massage, as well as artificial ventilation, is required. As soon as it is available, 100 per cent oxygen, with or without intermittent positive pressure, is administered continuously en route to a hospital. Survival depends not only upon the emergency care but also the prior health of the victim, the duration of immersion, and the amount of water aspirated.

Since there are both immediate and delayed effects of near-drowning, admission to a hospital for intensive pulmonary care is indicated. If the patient survives the first 24 hours, he is likely to recover. Reoxygenation should be started, followed by aspiration of the airway and suction of the stomach. Tracheostomy is rarely necessary. After insertion of an endotracheal tube, 100 per cent oxygen is given with either intermittent positive pressure or positive end-expiratory pressure, as well as with periodic hyperinflation of lungs. The administration of sodium bicarbonate solution intravenously in a dose of 0.3 to 0.4 mEq per pound of body weight is recommended upon admission to the hospital, for a significant number of near-drowning victims have metabolic acidosis associated with hypoxia. Based on serial determinations of gases and pH in the arterial blood, arterial hypoxemia

and acid-base concentrations are corrected by effective ventilation, oxygenation, buffers, or bicarbonate. Respiratory stimulants are contraindicated. As indicated, bronchodilators, diuretics, digitalization, or transfusion of whole blood, plasma, or packed red cells are given. The need for antimicrobial drugs is determined by clinical signs and roentgenographic changes, as well as by culture of tracheal secretions. Although the role of steroids in the treatment of near-drowning is uncertain, the intravenous administration of methylprednisolone sodium succinate, 5 mg per kilogram per 24 hours divided into six equal doses, has been proposed. Intensive care is continued as long as necessary to correct hypoxemia and acidosis. As the patient improves, oxygen is given by catheter or mask and reduced in concentration to 40 per cent.

Bucklin, R.: Drowning: A review of the physiological, experimental, and pathological findings. *In* Wecht, C. H. (ed.): Legal Medicine Annual, 1972. New York, Appleton-Century-Crofts, 1972, pp. 93–104.

den Otter, G.: Low-pressure aspiration of fresh water and sea water in the non-anoxic dog. An experimental study on the pathophysiology of drowning. Forensic Sci., 2:305, 1973.

Editorial: Drowning. Lancet, 2:691, 1972.

Edmonds, C.: A salt water aspiration syndrome. Milit. Med., 135:779, 1970.

Edmonds, C., and Thomas, R. L.: Medical aspects of diving. Part 2. Med. J. Aust., 2:1256, 1972.

Fuller, R. H.: The clinical pathology of human near-drowning. Proc. R. Soc. Med., 56:33, 1963.

Modell, J. H.: The Pathophysiology and Treatment of Drowning and Near-Drowning. Springfield, Ill., Charles C Thomas, 1971.

Sladen, A., and Zauder, H. L.: Methylprednisolone therapy for pulmonary edema following near drowning. J.A.M.A., 215:1793, 1971.

48. LEECHES AS AGENTS OF DISEASE (Hirudiniasis)

Philip D. Marsden

The leeches belong to the class Hirudinea of the phylum Annelida. All blood-sucking species of medical importance live in fresh water or are terrestrial. They possess anterior and posterior suckers used for locomotion and attachment; the anterior sucker contains the mouth and cutting plates. When attachment to a host is gained, the skin is quickly perforated, and suction begins until the leech has taken several times its own weight in blood. In sucking blood, leeches secrete an anticoagulant, hirudin, the action of which continues after detachment. Leeches can survive for years without food. They can pass through boot eyelets and the fabric of loosely woven cloth to reach the skin of the host.

Both external and internal forms of hirudiniasis occur. *External hirudiniasis* is due to both land and aquatic leeches. In Southeast Asia particularly, as well as in India, tropical Australia, and parts of South America, land leeches drop in considerable numbers from jungle vegetation onto man. Large numbers may result in considerable blood loss, and even one or two may have a considerable psychologic impact. To remove these leeches, a lighted cigarette, match, or salt applied to the leech will cause it to release its jaws. The wound should be washed in antiseptic and an antibiotic cream or dressing applied; otherwise, secondary infection commonly occurs. The rarer *internal hirudiniasis* is usually due to accidental ingestion of small immature leeches in raw drinking water. They become attached to the buccal mucosa, pharynx, or larynx, and may grow there to produce signs of hemorrhage and obstruction. Manual removal of the leech with forceps may be difficult. An epinephrine nasal spray may induce it to release its hold. In the rare cases of urethral or vaginal involvement, strong salt solution has caused detachment prior to surgical removal.

Protection against aquatic and terrestrial leeches can be in the form of protective clothing or the use of repellents. Some repellents are rather soluble in water and need to be reapplied, but the use of diethyltoluamide in lanolin may overcome this problem.

Chin, T. M.: A further note on leech infestation of man. J. Parasitol., 35:215, 1949.

Mann, K. H.: Leeches (Hirudinea): Their Structure, Physiology, Ecology, and Embryology. Oxford, Pergamon Press, 1962.

Salzberger, M.: Leeches as foreign bodies in the upper passages in Palestine. Laryngoscope, 38:27, 1928.

Walton, B. C., Traub, R., and Newsom, H. D.: Efficacy of clothing impregnants M-2065 and M-2066 against terrestrial leeches in North Borneo. Am. J. Trop. Med. Hyg., 5:190, 1956.

ARTHROPODA OF MEDICAL IMPORTANCE

Philip D. Marsden

49. INTRODUCTION

The phylum Arthropoda is the largest in the Animal Kingdom, containing at least three quarters of a million species. Some classes of arthropods include species of medical importance. These are the Pentastomida (tongue worms), Chilopoda (centipedes), Diplopoda (millipedes), Arachnida (scorpions, spiders, ticks), and Insecta. The latter are especially important. The major characteristic of arthropods is a segmented body that is invested with a rigid or semirigid cuticle of chitin.

The disorders produced by venoms of arthropods are discussed in Ch. 59.

50. PENTASTOMIDA

(Pentastomiasis, Porocephalosis, Porocephaliasis, Linguatulosis, Armilliferosis)

Although the members of the class Pentastomida that occasionally infect man look very much like helminths, in fact they are modified arthropods with rudimentary legs and annulated but not segmented bodies. Two families of medical interest, the Linguatulidae, and the Porocephalidae, contain the genera Linguatula (with flattened adults) and Porocephalus (with cylindrical adults).

Linguatula serrata is found in adult and nymphal stages in the nose and paranasal sinuses of carnivorous animals and as larvae and encapsulated nymphs in herbivorous animals throughout the world. Rarely, human infection with the adult occurs in the lungs. More com-

monly larvae and nymphs encyst in the mesenteric lymph nodes, liver, spleen, kidneys, and intestinal wall. Infection is acquired by ingesting eggs discharged in the nasal secretions of canines. This parasite is found in 4 per cent of necropsies in Chile. The syndrome of parasitic pharyngitis (halzoun) may be caused by the larvae.

The genus Porocephalus contains 20 species, of which two, *P. armillatus* and *P. moniliformis,* have been found in man in Africa and Asia, respectively. The adult is a parasite of the respiratory tract of snakes (pythons and others) and crocodiles, and the nymph is found in a wide variety of mammals. Humans acquire infection by ingesting pond or drinking water contaminated by snakes or by eating snake meat. The ingested eggs hatch in the intestine, and the larvae bore through the wall to lodge in any viscus, where they undergo nine molts in six months to a year to form infective nymphs. In man the infection usually comes to a blind end, as they have to be ingested by the definitive host. Human infection with encysted larvae or nymphs on the surface of the liver or in the intestinal mucosa, peritoneal cavity, or lung is fairly common in Africa, particularly in the Republic of the Congo. Painful inflammatory lesions may result, or the parasites may be asymptomatic and their resultant calcification give a characteristic crescentic opacity between 4 and 7 mm in size (1.4 per cent of abdominal x-rays, in Ibadan, Nigeria, show this sign).

A recent report describes the findings of encysted nymphs in 45 per cent of autopsies on Malaysian aborigines. A range of lesions was observed from the encysted pentosomal nymph still viable with relatively little reaction, to the formation of a necrotic granulomatous reaction, with death followed by fibrosis and calcification. It is worth noting that this parasite must also be considered because a blood eosinophilia can occur, especially after the death of the larvae. Rarely, the parasite has caused intestinal obstruction, pneumonitis, meningitis, pericarditis, nephritis, and obstructive jaundice.

Burns Cox, C. J., Prathap, K., Clark, E., and Gillman, R.: Porocephaliasis in Western Malaysia. Trans. R. Soc. Trop. Med. Hyg., 63:409, 1969.

Prathap, K., Lau, K. S., and Bolton, J. M.: Pentastomiasis: A common finding at autopsy among Malaysian aborigines. Am. J. Trop. Med. Hyg., 18:20, 1969.

Schacher, J. F., Saab, S., Germanos, R., and Boustany, N.: The aetiology of halzoun in Lebanon: Recovery of Linguatula serrata nymphs from two patients. Trans. R. Soc. Trop. Med. Hyg., 63:854, 1969.

Steinbach, H. L., and Johnstone, H. G.: The roentgen diagnosis of Armillifer infection (porocephalosis) in man. Radiology, 68:234, 1957.

51. TICK PARALYSIS

Tick paralysis is a rapidly progressive flaccid paralysis, usually symmetrical, with loss of tendon and superficial reflexes. It follows tick bite and is probably caused by a neurotoxin in tick saliva. Several pathogenic chains have been suggested, including a conduction block in the somatic motor fibers, interference of the monosynaptic pathways, a depolarizing block at neuromuscular junctions, and an actual muscle lesion.

Symptoms may not come on until five to six days after attachment of the tick, when the patient becomes restless and irritable and may have numbness or tingling of the extremities, lips, throat, and face. Difficulty in walking is rapidly followed by inability to stand. Within a day or two there is paralysis of the limbs and trunk muscles, and a bulbar lesion will lead to dysphagia, slurred speech, and impaired vision. Death may result from respiratory failure or aspiration pneumonia. Pain and fever are rare, but there may be local skin change around the site of the bite, and morbilliform rashes have been reported. Providing that the paralysis is not too far advanced, rapid and complete recovery follows removal of the tick, although recovery may take more than a week. The cerebrospinal fluid is normal; bulbar and respiratory failure must be treated symptomatically, and a respirator may be lifesaving. *The paralysis is often confused with poliomyelitis.* In polyneuritis, myelitis, syringomyelia, and spinal cord tumor, sensory loss is usually present. Sensory signs are very rare in tick paralysis. *Like leeches, ticks should not be pulled off* but should be persuaded to detach by the application of a lighted cigarette or carbon dioxide snow to their posterior end.

Children are more frequently affected than adults. In one series of 119 cases, 79 per cent, including all the fatal cases, were in children under 16; two thirds were girls. Late removal of ticks is more probable in children, particularly in girls with long hair, for in these patients 70 per cent of the ticks are attached to the head and neck. There appears to be no correlation between mortality and the proximity of tick attachment to the brain. With rapid overseas travel, this diagnostic problem may confront a physician anywhere in the world. Various tick species are responsible. *Dermacentor andersoni* and *D. variabilis* are the chief offenders in the Rocky Mountains of North America, *Ixodes holocyclus* in Australia, and *Rhipicephalus simus* in Africa. The paralysis occurs in travelers to tick-infested areas who are likely to intrude into tick habitats by camping, picnicking, fishing, or hunting.

Ransmeier, J. C.: Tick paralysis in the eastern United States. J. Pediatr., 34:299, 1949.
Tick paralysis. Br. Med. J., 2:314, 1969.

52. SCABIES

Scabies is the most common skin disease encountered in some parts of the world, and is usually associated with poor living conditions. It is due to infection of the skin by the mite *Sarcoptes scabiei.* Hyperinfections with crusting and pustulation are termed "Norwegian" scabies. Scabies should be considered in every patient who complains of a persistent itch, and this symptom, together with papules, vesicles, and pustules on the extremities and follicular papules on the trunk, should be regarded as being due to scabies until proved otherwise.

The female mite is acquired by sharing a bed with an infected person or by other close personal contact, and in this sense in adults it can be likened to a venereal disease. The mite burrows into cracked and folded regions of the skin, the tunnel being limited to the stratum corneum except at the anterior end. Burrowing is by means of jaws and the sharp cutting edges on the terminal joints of the first two pairs of legs. Both copulation and egg production occur in the burrow, the rarely seen male ranging over the skin in search of the female. About two eggs are produced daily for two months. The hatched six-legged larvae make their own burrows and develop into adulthood in a fortnight. About one month after the establishment of the first burrow the patient begins to itch, probably because he becomes sensitized to

acarine products. The scratching limits the population of mites by depriving them of a roof over their heads and crushing them. In experimentally induced infections Mellanby found that the population reached a maximum within three months and varied from 20 to 400 egg-laying females. Examination of nearly 900 men with scabies showed a mean population of 11.3 adult females per man, and more than half the patients harbored five adult acari or fewer.

The skin eruption has two aspects: the burrows which have to be searched for, and the changes resulting from sensitization and secondary infection which are obvious. The burrow of the ovigerous female appears as a narrow, slightly raised white gray or black line. The white shiny dot sometimes seen at one end, which may be associated with a small vesicle, is the site of the mite.

The *burrows* are commonly found on the sides and webs of the fingers, the ulnar border of the hand, the volar aspect of the wrists, the points of the elbows, the axillary folds, the areolae of the nipples in women, the external genitalia in men, the buttocks, and the margins or soles of the feet. The face and scalp are never affected in adults. Sometimes a typical burrow cannot be found. *There is a widespread rash* of follicular papules usually well marked on the abdomen, buttocks, inner sides of the thighs, and axillary folds. Scratch marks, crusted papules, and pustulation demonstrate the effects of scratching. An infected eczema sometimes develops on the fingers and wrists, nipples, or glans penis. Patients who are unable to scratch do not develop such lesions.

The *diagnosis of scabies* is probable if other members of the household are found infected. The mite can be identified by scraping a burrow along its length with the edge of a scalpel blade held at a right angle to the skin. The resultant material is mounted in 10 per cent potassium hydroxide under a coverslip, and microscopy reveals the mite. It has a body shaped like a tortoise with two pairs of legs in front and two pairs behind. The forelegs end in "suckers" and the hindlegs in long bristles. The female is about 400 μ long and coated in short bristles. Eggs or immature forms may also be present.

The typical clinical picture of scabies is subject to a number of variations. In babies the scalp may be affected, which means that the topical preparation must be carefully applied. Clean people usually have few lesions, and scabies may be overlooked in nurses for this reason. A localized eczema may be the presentation, or persistent sepsis of the skin. The amount of itch is very variable. In Norwegian scabies two million mites may be present, and the stratum corneum may be honeycombed with burrows on biopsy. Clinically, Norwegian scabies resembles exfoliative dermatitis. Often itching is absent, and this has been offered as the explanation of this hyperinfective state. However, some of these patients do itch, and other hypotheses attribute this state to topical or systemic corticosteroids or vitamin A deficiency.

The differential diagnosis includes atopic eczema, neurodermatitis, dermatitis herpetiformis, and two conditions considered in Ch. 54, pediculosis and papular urticaria. Papular urticaria is due to the bites of various insects, often fleas or bedbugs, but may also result from bites of various mites, either cheese straw or grain mites or the Sarcoptes of dogs and cats mentioned at the end of this chapter.

The three essential aspects of treatment are to treat all members of the household simultaneously, to use an application that will kill the parasites, and to apply it to the whole skin area. Since the acaricides mentioned below destroy all adults, larvae, and nymphs, but not the eggs, a further treatment should be given after a week. Suitable topical preparations for total body application are as follows: (1) *Benzyl benzoate, 25 per cent emulsion (60 ml for each application).* It is slightly irritating and may cause secondary eczematization and conjunctivitis if it is carried to the eyes. It has a rather penetrating smell, but is a very effective acaricide. (2) *Gamma benzene hexachloride (Gamma BHC) as a 1 per cent cream (25 grams for each application).* This is odorless, nonirritant, and effective against associated pediculosis as well.

A bath before the first application is desirable, and clean underclothes and sheets should be used after it. The itch may persist for some weeks after treatment, and soothing calamine lotion can be prescribed. Oral antimicrobial drugs may be necessary to combat skin infection and should be given concurrently. Most "failures" of treatment are due to unsatisfactory therapy, but it has recently been suggested that there may be benzyl benzoate-resistant Sarcoptes. As scabies is often transmitted in the course of sexual contact, the possibility of an associated venereal disease should be borne in mind. For effective treatment of scabies in a community where it occurs in high incidence, a treatment center is necessary. During World War II in Britain, scabies clinics brought the disease under control, and a scabies order gave personnel powers to enforce treatment. This species of parasite is comprised of a number of physiologic forms specific to the various vertebrate hosts; the disease in man is produced by *Sarcoptes scabiei var. hominis.* Other forms include *S. scabiei var. canis,* the cause of sarcoptic mange. This parasite and the cat mite *Notoedres cati* can cause severe papular urticaria in man although the classic burrow is not seen as these mites are specific to their normal hosts and incapable of burrowing and breeding in man.

Herridge, C. F.: Norwegian scabies (crusted scabies). Br. Med. J., 1:239, 1963.
Lyell, A.: Diagnosis and treatment of scabies. Br. Med. J., 1:223, 1967.
Mellanby, K.: Scabies. New York, Oxford University Press, 1943.
The scabies epidemic. Br. Med. J., 2:193, 1967.
Thomsett, L. R.: Mite infestations of man contracted from dogs and cats. Br. Med. J., 2:93, 1968.

53. MYIASIS
(Maggots)

Myiasis may be defined as the infection of vertebrates with the larvae (maggots) of Diptera (flies) which feed on the tissues of the host. The maggots are usually identified by the form of their posterior spiracles, but this may be difficult to define in the early molts. Rearing the larvae to adults makes identification easier, especially with immature stages. Myiasis is a far greater problem in sheep, cattle, and deer than in man, and there is no form of myiasis found exclusively in man. For the purposes of a textbook of medicine, it is permissible to abandon the scientific classification of the responsible species and consider the clinical type of myiasis produced. For a description of the genera of flies, a textbook of entomology should be consulted. Primary myiasis occurs in the absence of debility of the host or tissue injury; this is in contrast to secondary myiasis.

PRIMARY MYIASIS
Furuncular Myiasis

Furuncular myiasis is a good descriptive term, because the skin lesion looks like a boil but in fact contains a maggot which breathes through a hole in the tip of the lesion. When mature, the maggot drops to the ground to pupate. There are two distinct types occurring in Africa and the Americas, respectively. (1) The African Tumbu fly *(Cordylobia anthropophaga).* The eggs are sometimes laid on clothing or else the larvae actively seek the host and burrow into the skin to feed. Multiple lesions are common. The normal hosts are wild rodents. (2) The human botfly *(Dermatobia hominis).* The botfly is found in South America, Central America, and Mexico. The eggs are frequently laid on a hematophagous insect (mosquito or stable fly) by the female and thence transported to the host. The secondarily infected "boil"-like lesion also occurs in other mammals in endemic areas.

The application of petroleum jelly to the lesion to block the spiracles often brings the suffocating larvae wriggling out backward, especially when mature. Immature larvae can be excised, but if possible it is better to let them mature and drop out.

Creeping Myiasis

Creeping myiasis is a form of larva migrans caused by flies of the genera Gastrophilus and Hypoderma. The former larvae do not mature and, being restricted to the stratum corneum, leave an obvious trail. Hypoderma penetrates more deeply and can complete its development in some instances and perforate the skin to escape.

The behavior of these two species is easily understood if their lives in their normal hosts are mentioned. *Gastrophilus,* normally a parasite of Equidae, has a period of migration as a young larva in the tongue epithelium but matures in the lumen of the intestine. *Hypoderma* is classically a parasite of bovids. *H. bovis* migrates via nerve trunks to gain the spinal canal and paravertebral muscle mass, and *H. lineatus* penetrates, migrating via the mucosa of the upper gut and gaining the same muscles via the esophagus. Both cause voluminous subcutaneous paravertebral abscesses, ruining the hide. It is not surprising, therefore, that when man is the host, the larvae may wander widely and even gain the eye, causing blindness.

Ophthalmomyiasis

A painful conjunctivitis can be produced by the first-stage maggots of *Oestrus ovis* hatching from eggs laid by the female near the conjunctiva. Hypoderma maggots may penetrate the globe of the eye. Such maggots can be irrigated from the conjunctiva or mechanically removed.

Other Forms of Primary Myiasis

Genitourinary myiasis owing to Fannia or Calliphora maggots has been rarely reported, the eggs being laid in the vicinity of the urethra. Maggots of these genera and the genera Sarcophaga and Musca have been found in freshly passed stools and can develop in the fecal stream. Tetrachloroethylene is effective. Intestinal myiasis is cosmopolitan and relatively common. In North America the drone fly *(Tubifera tenax)* larvae is the most frequently encountered species. The larvae of *Auchmeromyia luteola* (the Congo floor maggot) are temporary blood-sucking parasites of Africa; the larvae emerge from hiding places at night to suck blood, but after a meal retire to rest.

SECONDARY MYIASIS

Invasion of the body by maggots can occur in very debilitated individuals and in those with destructive or ulcerative lesions. Thus wounds may be infected by maggots of various fly genera, including Wohlfahrtia, Callitroga, and Chrysomyia. Similarly, myiasis of the nose, upper respiratory passages, or ear is caused by the screwworm fly maggots invading infected debilitated tissues. They should be picked out with forceps; otherwise they can penetrate the base of the skull and invade the brain.

PREVENTION

Reduction of screwworms, botflies, and warble fly maggots in sheep and cattle reduces the chances of human infection. This can be done with various dips of insecticides. Auchmeromyia larvae can be killed by dusting houses with insecticides. Clothing should be ironed and not hung out of doors for Cordylobia to lay eggs on it. Repellents and bed nets will reduce the incidence of Dermatobia lesions. The proper control of refuse disposal will reduce the number of blue- and greenbottle flies. It is worth noting that the eradication of the screwworm fly from Curaçao by releasing sexually sterile males is one of the few instances of a successful form of biologic control.

Baumhover, A. H.: Eradication of the screwworm fly: An agent of myiasis. J.A.M.A., 196:240, 1966.
Flew, G. P., and Grundy, J. H.: Infection with *Dermatobia hominis* occurring in British Guiana. J. Royal Army Med. Corp., 113:148, 1967.
Günther, S.: Furuncular Tumbu fly myiasis of man in Gabon, Equatorial Africa. J. Trop. Med. Hyg., 70:169, 1967.
James, M. T.: The flies that cause myiasis in man. United States Department of Agriculture Misc. Publ. No. 631, 1947.
Palmer, E. D.: Entomology of the gastrointestinal tract. Milit. Med., 135:165, 1970.
Zumpt, F.: Myiasis in Man and Animals of the Old World. London, Butterworth and Company (Publishers), Ltd., 1965.

54. ECTOPARASITIC INSECTS
(Fleas and Lice)

Both fleas and lice are ectoparasites of man in the sense that they live outside his body on the skin but are dependent on him for food. Lice are more dependent than fleas and cannot survive long if separated from man because they need his body warmth and his tissues for their frequent feedings. Fleas are more exploratory and are capable of fantastic leaps, thus enabling them to transfer easily from host to host. Lice are flattened dorsoventrally, enabling them to hug the surface of the skin, whereas fleas are laterally compressed, enabling them to slip between the upright hairs. Lice have no true metamorphosis in their life cycle, the young resembling the adults, whereas fleas have a conventional true cycle of metamorphosis with larvae and pupae.

Both ectoparasites play important roles in the transmission of human disease. Louse-borne typhus *(R. pro-*

wazeki) and louse-borne relapsing fever *(Borrelia recurrentis)* are mainly transmitted by the body louse, and in conditions of poverty, war, and famine, great epidemics have occurred. Apart from plague, fleas also transmit endemic or murine typhus caused by *Rickettsia typhi (R. mooseri)*.

PEDICULOSIS
(Head, Body, and Pubic Lice)

Man provides food and shelter for two genera of lice. *Pediculus humanis var. capitis* infests the head and *P. humanis var. corporis,* the body and clothing. *Phthirus pubis* (crab lice) usually lives in the pubic area, but on occasion extends its range to the axilla, chest hairs, and even the eyebrows and eyelashes. The eggs or nits are found attached to the hairs of the host, and in the case of the body louse are found in clothing. All three lice suck blood frequently and can exist only a short time away from the host. Their saliva produces an *irritant roseate papular dermatitis.* Scratching leads to secondary bacterial infection of the skin with crusting and induration, and pigmentation may be present in severe infestations (vagabond's disease). Enlargement of local lymph nodes is common, especially the posterior auricular group in severe capitis infections. *Phthirus pubis* infestation of the eyelashes leads to blepharitis. The irritant cutaneous lesions suggest the diagnosis, which is confirmed by finding the eggs or adults. The eggs can be combed out of the hair with a fine-toothed comb.

Treatment. In the treatment of head lice an ointment of 1.0 per cent hexachlorocyclohexane in vanishing cream (Kwell) should be rubbed on the scalp thoroughly. This treatment is also effective for pubic lice when the ointment is massaged into the skin of the infested area. Lice and eggs can be removed individually from the eyelashes or eliminated by the application of 0.25 per cent physostigmine ophthalmic ointment. Body lice are destroyed by sterilizing the clothing by heat, using the ointment on infested areas of the body. A 10 per cent DDT in pyrophyllite dusted onto the head, body, and clothing without undressing is highly effective. Lice in Korea and Egypt have developed resistance to DDT, and 1 per cent hexachlorocyclohexane or pyrethrum powder may be substituted for it. The secondary pyoderma should be treated with appropriate antimicrobial drugs.

Prevention. The prevention of lousiness consists primarily in personal cleanliness and the avoidance of infected persons, bedding, and clothes. *Phthirus pubis* is usually transmitted by sexual intercourse. The rise of the "hippies," with their low standards of personal hygiene and tendency to increasing sexual promiscuity, has resulted in an increase in the incidence of crab lice. Lice are quite host-specific; thus, unlike fleas, the lice of domestic animals are not attracted to man.

Ackerman, A. B.: Crabs—the resurgence of *Phthirus pubis*. N. Engl. J. Med., 278:950, 1968.
Buxton, P. A.: Louse: An Account of the Lice Which Infect Man, Their Medical Importance and Control. London, Edward Arnold (Publishers), Ltd., 1939.

FLEAS

Pulex irritans is primarily a human flea. The fleas of the cat and dog (Ctenocephalides) and of the rat and mouse (Xenopsylla) also frequent man. They usually migrate over the body until a tight garter or belt obstructs their passage, and there they proceed to suck blood. Individuals vary greatly in their reaction to the salivary secretion of fleas. Some are unaffected. On those who are severely irritated, raised red edematous lesions are produced (papular urticaria). Fleas are sensitive to applications of DDT.

The control of fleas requires their destruction in the home. Vacuum cleaning of rugs and removal of debris will eliminate adults as well as eggs, larvae, and pupae. Insecticide sprays such as 5 per cent DDT in oil are effective. The living quarters of dogs and cats and the animals themselves should also be treated. As DDT is rather toxic to young cats, a 4 per cent Malathion powder can be used for them. Bird fleas can also cause papular urticaria; hen runs may require treatment, and birds' nests should be removed from under eaves of affected houses.

TUNGIASIS
(Tunga Penetrans)

The common names jigger or chigoe are to be avoided because they are easily confused with chigger, the name given to trombiculid harvest mites. A highly modified flea, *Tunga penetrans*, parasitizes man, pigs, and dogs, as well as a variety of other mammals. It is common in Africa and South America. The adult female is a permanent parasite of the subcutaneous tissues of warm-blooded animals and is embedded in the skin with just the anal pore having access to the exterior. The male copulates with the embedded female, and several hundred eggs are laid, after which the female dies.

The embedded females are most common on the sole of the foot and the root of the nail, where they cause pain. In debilitated people lying in infested huts many lesions may be present, all on one side of the body including the face. Secondary infection commonly results from the severe irritation. Septicemia, thrombophlebitis, tetanus, and gas gangrene may be complications. The swelling containing the ovigerous female is about the size of a pea and may be mistaken for myiasis. However, the lesion is recognized by the tip of the flea's abdomen appearing as a black dot in the center of the lesion.

Embedded females are best removed individually. After cleansing the skin with antiseptic, the opening hole of the flea pustule is enlarged with a sterile needle, and the intact insect can then be enucleated or expelled by gentle pressure. Antimicrobial therapy may be needed for secondary bacterial infection. Prophylaxis with DDT powder to the feet and socks or benzyl benzoate application is effective.

Bolam, M. R., and Burtt, E. T.: Flea infestation as a cause of papular urticaria. Br. Med. J., 1:1130, 1956.

Jelliffe, D. B.: Tungiasis. *In* Simons, R. D. G. P. (ed.): Handbook of Tropical Dermatology. New York, American Elsevier Publishing Company, Inc., 1953, p. 895.

55. ARTHROPODS AS MECHANICAL CARRIERS OF DISEASE

FLIES

The common house fly and its relatives, the stable fly, greenbottle, bluebottle, blow fly, and flesh fly, breed and feed on human and animal feces and garbage. Typhoid fever, bacillary dysentery, amebiasis, and cholera may be transported on the fly's body from feces to man's food, and are found in the feces and vomitus of flies. Poliomyelitis and infectious hepatitis conceivably could also be transmitted in this way. Small flies called eye gnats may act as carriers of pathogens causing acute purulent conjunctivitis and yaws.

Control of flies by spraying breeding habitats with 10 per cent DDT in kerosene is effective. Garbage should be tightly sealed or destroyed to prevent fly access. Houses and particularly food cabinets should be rendered fly-proof. Outdoor privies and septic tanks should be disinfected.

COCKROACHES
(Blattidae)

These common hospital and home insects may serve as mechanical transmitters of intestinal bacteria, virus, or Protozoa by their contact with filth and food. Cleanliness in the kitchen is essential for their control. The following are effective against roaches: Chlordane, 5 to 10 per cent dust; Chlordane, 2 per cent, and DDT, 5 per cent, in kerosene; or Malathion, 2 per cent in oil.

BEDBUGS
(Cimex)

Bedbugs are reddish brown and wingless, and have a disagreeable odor. As with fleas, the bites of bedbugs may result in papular urticaria. Because they suck human blood, they would seem to be likely disease transmitters, but all attempts to demonstrate this have failed. Although in the laboratory they can be infected with numerous human pathogens, they do not appear to transmit them in nature. In small African babies numerous bites are said to have resulted in iron deficiency anemia. A 5 per cent kerosene solution of DDT or 0.1 per cent lindane oil on infested bed frames, furniture, and wall crevices will control this insect. Infested mattresses should be discarded.

56. ARTHROPODS AS INTERMEDIATE HOSTS OF INFECTIOUS DISEASE

The infectious agents for which arthropods serve as vectors and the hosts in which these pathogens can develop are considered elsewhere in this book. In concluding this discussion of arthropods, it is worth emphasizing that for the medical man with biologic interests the field of medical entomology still holds considerable research possibilities and is worthwhile exploring. To aid in this interest some general references are given below.

Busvine, J. R.: Insects and Hygiene. London, Methuen and Company, Ltd., 1951.

Gordon, R. M., and Lavoipierre, M. M. J.: Entomology for Students of Medicine. London, Blackwell Scientific Publications, Ltd., 1962.

Herms, W. B.: Medical Entomology. 5th ed. Revised by M. T. James. New York, The Macmillan Company, 1961.

Horsfall, W. R.: Medical Entomology, Arthropods, and Human Disease. New York, The Ronald Press Company, 1962.

Leclercq, M.: Entomological Parasitology. Translated by G. Lapage. New York, Pergamon Press, Inc., 1969.

Smart, J.: A Handbook for the Identification of Insects of Medical Importance. London, The British Museum, 1965.

VENOM DISEASES

57. SNAKEBITE

Sherman A. Minton, Jr.

Identification, Distribution, and Classification of Venomous Reptiles.   Recognition of venomous snakes is difficult, for the only character common to all species is the presence of venom-conducting maxillary fangs. Handbooks for identification of snakes of most geographic areas are available from natural history museums or government agencies. Local information about reptiles is often untrustworthy, and erroneous beliefs are widespread even among educated and professional persons. Harmless reptiles are often believed dangerous; dangerous species may sometimes be considered innocuous. The number of species of poisonous snakes is nearly always greater in tropical countries; nevertheless, certain species may be abundant in temperate regions, e.g., the prairie rattlesnake in the northern Great Plains of the United States. Even in the tropics it is unusual for more than three or four species to be important in a given area.

Following is a brief classification of venomous reptiles:

Lizards. FAMILY HELODERMATIDAE. Two species known as Gila monsters are restricted to parts of Mexico and the southwestern United States. There are venom-conducting teeth in the lower jaw; the venom has local irritant and neurotoxic effects.

Snakes. FAMILY COLUBRIDAE. This family includes most of the world's snakes, about 2500 species. A few hundred, mostly tropical and subtropical, have grooved fangs on the posterior maxilla. The fangs frequently are not engaged in defensive biting. Little is known concerning the venoms, but some are powerfully hemorrhagic. Nearly all rear-fanged snakes are harmless for practical purposes, but bites of the African boomslang (*Dispholidus typus*) and bird snakes (*Thelotornis kirtlandii*) have caused deaths.

FAMILY ELAPIDAE.   These snakes have fixed fangs on the anterior ends of the maxillae; the fangs may be followed by solid teeth. The venoms are predominantly neurotoxic and often very potent. Some are also hematotoxic and necrotizing. About 120 species are confined to the Old World, and almost 50 species of coral snakes inhabit tropical and subtropical America.

FAMILY HYDROPHIDAE.   These are marine or brackish water snakes characterized by laterally flattened tails and, in nearly all species, by great reduction or absence of enlarged ventral scales. They have fixed, short fangs followed by solid teeth. Their venoms in man act primarily on skeletal muscle, and are often extremely potent but small in quantity. About 50 species inhabit the coastal waters of south Asia, northern Australia, and islands of the southwest Pacific; one species reaches the western coasts of tropical America.

FAMILY VIPERIDAE.   Single, large fangs on short and otherwise toothless maxillae rotate, permitting the fangs to be erected or folded against the roof of the mouth. Venoms usually cause local necrosis and hemorrhage, but some are predominantly neurotoxic. One subfamily, *Crotalinae* or pit vipers, is characterized by a deep pit lined with sensitive heat receptors situated between the eye and nostril. There are about 100 species of pit vipers, .nostly in the Americas and Southeast Asia.

All dangerous snakes of the Americas except the coral snakes belong in this group. The other subfamily, *Viperinae*, lacks the sensory pit. There are about 50 species confined to Africa, Asia, and Europe.

Epidemiology.   World mortality from snakebite is estimated as 20,000 to 25,000 annually. The greatest number of reported snakebite deaths occur in the Indian subcontinent (10,000 to 12,000 annually); high figures are also reported from Burma, Ceylon, Thailand, and other Southeast Asian countries, Brazil, and other countries in the American tropics. Mortality is believed moderately high in tropical Africa, although reliable figures are not available. Moderate to low incidence is reported from southern Europe, the Middle East, Australia, and New Guinea, the temperate regions of Africa and South America, Japan and associated islands, and the United States (fewer than 20 deaths annually in recent years). Snakebite mortality is very low to nil in northern Europe and Asia, Canada, the West Indies (exclusive of Trinidad), New Zealand, the Malagasy Republic, and Oceania.

High snakebite mortality and morbidity are seen in localities where a dense human population lives in close proximity to dangerous snakes. Some southeast Asian venomous snakes (Indian cobra, kraits, bamboo vipers) are singularly adapted to life in local villages and even in suburbs of large, modern cities. Dangerous pit vipers of the genus Bothrops in Latin America are plentiful in sugar cane and banana plantations; Russell's viper in Southeast Asia often frequents cultivated fields. Local practices in agriculture, irrigation, and construction may provide good refuges for snakes, or may bring about increase in the rodents and lizards that are the food of many venomous snakes.

Snakebite is most common in adult males. The incidence is next highest in children because of their carelessness and curiosity. Adult females are the least frequently bitten. Persons at greatest risk from snakebite are those who deliberately handle or work with venomous snakes, be they scientists, entertainers, or religious zealots. If this small, high-risk group is excluded, snakebite is chiefly a hazard to farmers who till their land by primitive methods, plantation laborers, and those engaged in construction work or brush-clearing by largely manual methods. Practices of fish netting and trapping sometimes expose fishermen to bites by sea snakes and other aquatic species. Recent studies indicate that snakebites in the eastern United States are usually sustained near the victim's home, and involve persons in the 5- to 19-year age group predominantly.

Ethnic factors increasing the incidence of snakebite include types of dress that do not protect the legs and feet, sleeping outdoors on mats on the ground, and religious protection of venomous snakes or their use in rituals.

Control of snakes is best accomplished by indirect means: better construction of dwellings, disposal of rubbish, and control of rodents. Direct control campaigns have not been successful, except in small areas, and may be undesirable as many beneficial snakes are also destroyed.

Properties of Snake Venoms.   Snake venoms are slightly viscid fluids, usually pale yellow to amber, occasionally white or colorless. Most medically important species yield 0.1 to 1.5 ml of fluid venom; yields of 5 ml have been reported for large vipers. Snakes may inject the entire content of their venom glands in biting, but usually do not do so. It has been shown experimentally that the Palestine viper injects about 15 per cent of its venom in an average strike, but in some cases may inject up to half the contents of its glands. Sometimes snakes bite without injecting venom.

Venoms dry as platelets, representing 15 to 45 per cent of the original weight of the sample. In this form they are stable for years if kept in sealed vials at cool to moderate temperature.

Average venom yields from representative species of snakes and the estimated fatal doses for man are given in the accompanying table. It should be emphasized that both the amount of venom and its toxicity are subject to wide variation, according to geographic distribution, age, season, and other factors.

Numerous enzymes have been identified in snake venoms. Hyaluronidases, present in most venoms, account for the rapidity of absorption. Proteases cause local inflammation, necrosis, and damage to vascular epithelium. Phospholipase A alters membrane permeability and releases histamine, thus contributing to hemorrhage and shock. Phosphodiesterase may be responsible for some of the hypotensive effect of venoms. Esterases in many viper venoms liberate bradykinin. Mamba venoms are high in acetylcholine. Many snake venoms inactivate complement.

Many snake venoms interfere with the normal process of blood coagulation and may do this by several mechanisms operating either sequentially or simultaneously. In clinical situations, concomitant intravascular coagulation and fibrinolytic activity frequently produce a defibrination syndrome with nonclotting blood.

About 40 polypeptide toxins have been isolated from elapid and sea snake venoms. The structure of many is known, and synthesis of a peptide with the amino acid sequence of cobrotoxin (from Chinese cobra venom) has been accomplished. Most of these toxins have molecular weights of about 7000 and are composed of a chain of 61 to 74 amino acids linked by disulfide bonds. They produce a nondepolarizing neuromuscular block by acting on the postjunctional membrane of the motor endplate. A few (e.g., β-bungarotoxin) are larger molecules that block the neuromuscular junction by reducing acetylcholine output from presynaptic nerve terminals. Others have cardiotoxic and cytolytic activity. Some additional polypeptide toxins have been isolated from rattlesnake and other viperid venoms. In composition and mode of action, they appear to be more diverse than the elapid toxins.

Snake venoms are antigenically complex, those of vipers generally containing more antigens than those of elapids, whereas sea snake and colubrid venoms contain fewest antigens. With some exceptions, venoms of phylogenetically related snakes have similar antigenic

Snake Species	Geographic Distribution	Venom Yield* (mg)	Lethal Dose for Man† (mg)
Beaked seasnake, *Enhydrina schistosa*	Coastal waters southern Asia and northern Australia	10–15	1.5
ELAPIDAE			
North American coral snake, *Micrurus fulvius*	Southern United States	3–5	5
Indian krait, *Bungarus caeruleus*	Most of India and Pakistan	8–12	2
Tiger snake, *Notechis scutatus*	Australia	35–45	3
Mamba, *Dendroaspis angusticeps*	East Africa	75–100	15
Death adder, *Acanthophis antarcticus*	Australia and New Guinea	70–100	10
Indian cobra, *Naja naja*	Southeast Asia to Indonesia and Formosa	150–200	20
Ringhals, *Hemachatus haemachatus*	South Africa	80–120	60
VIPERINAE			
Puff adder, *Bitis arietans*	Most of Africa; southern Arabia	160–200	100
Saw-scaled viper, *Echis carinatus*	Northern and western Africa to northern India and Ceylon	20–35	5
Russell's viper, *Vipera russelli*	West Pakistan to Formosa	150–250	50
Palestine viper, *Vipera xanthina*	Middle East	90–140	60
CROTALINAE			
Cottonmouth moccasin, *Agkistrodon piscivorus*	Southern United States	100–150	100
Fer-de-lance, *Bothrops atrox*	Mexico to Argentina	100–160	50
Jararaca, *Bothrops jararaca*	Tropical South America	40–70	40
Habu, *Trimeresurus flavoviridis*	Ryukyu Is.; closely related species in Formosa and southeastern part of the People's Republic of China	100–300	100
Western diamondback rattlesnake, *Crotalus atrox*	Southwestern United States and northern Mexico	200–300	70
Neotropical rattlesnake, *Crotalus durissus*	Southern Mexico to Argentina	25–40	10
Western rattlesnake, *Crotalus viridis*‡	Western United States and southwestern Canada	90–130	50

*Venom extractions from adult snakes of average size; maximal yields may be two to four times the upper limit of the average range.

†Estimated for an adult of 70 kg.

‡There are 13 other species of rattlesnakes in the United States. At least one species occurs in every state except Maine, Delaware, Alaska, and Hawaii.

makeup, a matter of practical importance in production and use of therapeutic antisera.

Clinical Manifestations. The clinical picture in snakebite is difficult to summarize briefly. Several syndromes are seen.

In the United States, most snakebites are characterized by severe local pain, edema spreading from the bite, painful lymphadenopathy, and local ecchymosis, often with serum-filled blebs. Systemic manifestations include nausea and vomiting, thirst, sweating, and fever rarely exceeding 38° C. If no additional symptoms develop, the prognosis is excellent, although there may be local necrosis occasionally severe enough to require skin grafting. Danger signs include numbness and tingling of the face, pronounced drop in blood pressure, violent muscle spasms or convulsions, hematuria, hematemesis, cyanosis, and difficulty in breathing. Increased clotting time and a drop in hemoglobin indicate severe envenomation. This syndrome is seen after bites of most rattlesnakes, the copperhead and cottonmouth moccasin, and a number of Old World vipers.

Hemorrhagic manifestations dominate the picture in bites by certain Latin American lancehead vipers (Bothrops), *some African and Asian vipers,* particularly the saw-scales (Echis), a few elapids such as the Australian genus Pseudechis, and the rear-fanged boomslang (Dispholidus). Local symptoms resemble those listed in the previous paragraph, but there is usually less edema. Persistent oozing of blood from fang punctures, bleeding gums, fever, and headache are prominent even in mild cases. Ecchymoses may be seen anywhere, particularly at sites of mild trauma. Gross hematuria, hematemesis, hemoptysis, and blood in the feces are common. Prothrombin time and sometimes clotting time are greatly prolonged; return to normal is a favorable prognostic sign. The usual cause of death is massive cerebral, retroperitoneal, or intestinal hemorrhage that may occur as much as 12 days after the bite. Some patients die of anemia and exhaustion, particularly when there is associated scurvy, malnutrition, hookworm disease, or malaria.

Elapid neurotoxins rapidly involve the bulbar centers, causing ptosis, strabismus, slurred speech, and dysphagia with drooling of saliva. Other early symptoms are vomiting, giddiness, muscular weakness, and drowsiness. Respiration is labored; the patient may complain of a sensation of weight on the chest. The temperature is normal or subnormal. Violent abdominal pain sometimes occurs after krait and coral snake bites. General symptoms usually begin within 30 minutes after the bite; sometimes there is a latent period of several hours. Local symptoms vary. Cobra bites usually cause considerable pain and swelling, occasionally followed by necrosis. Bites by many types of elapids cause little immediate local reaction, but pain radiating from the bite may begin after an hour or more. Hemoglobinuria and albuminuria are common. Death usually occurs within 15 hours after onset of systemic symptoms; patients surviving longer generally recover. Despite severe nervous system involvement, permanent neurologic sequelae do not occur.

A somewhat different neurotoxic syndrome accompanies bites by crotamine-secreting tropical rattlesnakes. Local pain and swelling are slight to moderate. The outstanding symptoms are dizziness, intense headache, impairment of vision that may progress to blindness, paralysis of the neck muscles, and respiratory depression. Albuminuria and hematuria are seen, and suppression of urine flow may supervene. The prognosis is poor.

Seasnake bites show little or no local symptoms. After a latent period of 30 minutes to a few hours, the patient complains of muscular pain, stiffness, and progressive weakness. Trismus, ptosis, and loss of tendon reflexes are seen. In severe cases blurring of vision, thirst, vomiting, and difficulty in breathing occur. The urine contains myoglobin, albumin, and erythrocytes, although gross hematuria is rare. Tubular necrosis may be followed by acute renal failure. When symptoms are severe the prognosis is grave, but many seasnake bites are mild, probably because of the small amount of venom injected.

A singular type of envenomation is ophthalmia, caused by the so-called spitting cobras, of which there are two species in Africa and one in Malaysia. Venom is ejected in a fine spray through an opening on the anterior aspect of the fang. On contact with mucous membranes of the eye, it produces violent pain and sometimes temporary blindness. Permanent ocular damage is rare, and systemic symptoms do not occur. Prompt washing with water or other nonirritant fluids is usually adequate therapy; local use of dilute antivenin has been recommended. Venoms of these snakes have the same effect as other cobra venoms if the snake bites rather than spits.

Diagnosis. The diagnosis of snakebite is materially simplified if the snake has been captured or killed and correctly identified. Differential diagnosis involves distinction between (1) snakebite and other injuries, (2) bites of poisonous and nonpoisonous snakes, and (3) minimal envenomation, in which conservative management is indicated, and severe envenomation, which demands more active therapy.

Injuries by objects such as thorns and spines of plants must occasionally be distinguished from snakebite. Usually these are recognized readily by the nature of the wound and lack of progressive symptoms. Differentiation between snakebite and injuries by other venomous animals may be difficult if the patient did not see the animal that injured him, or is too young to give a reliable history. Wounds inflicted by arthropods such as scorpions, centipedes, spiders, and insects are usually smaller than those caused by fangs of snakes and bleed less. Fish spines and teeth of small mammals usually cause deeper, more ragged wounds.

The pattern of puncture wounds will not reliably differentiate bites of poisonous snakes from those of nonpoisonous species. The writer has been bitten hundreds of times by many species of nonpoisonous snakes and sustained injuries ranging from single punctures to six rows of multiple punctures. Bites by poisonous snakes showing a single fang puncture are not rare, and may terminate fatally. Bites in which the palatine and mandibular teeth cause wounds in addition to those made by the fangs are also seen. Nonpoisonous snakebites show very little local swelling, usually bleed freely, and cause little pain. Unfortunately, bites of some dangerous snakes also show little local reaction.

In North American pit viper (rattlesnake, moccasin) bites, the development of more than 30 cm of edema and erythema in the first 12 hours plus any of the more serious symptoms mentioned in the paragraphs on clinical manifestations calls for administration of antivenin and supportive measures. Cases with less edema and mildness or absence of systemic symptoms need only observation and symptomatic therapy. In bites by snakes with hemorrhagic venom, hemoptysis, hematuria, and increased prothrombin time are early evidences of serious poisoning. Early clinical signs of severe neurotoxic poisoning are impaired vision, ptosis, slurred speech, and drowsiness. The presence of trismus, muscle pain on passive movement, and myoglobinuria differentiates severe seasnake bites from mild ones and from injuries by other venomous marine organisms.

Treatment. Therapy in snakebite has four aims: (1) retarding absorption of venom and removing as much as possible by mechanical means, (2) neutralization of venom by immune serum, (3) counteracting specific pharmacologic activities of the venom, and (4) relief of symptoms and prevention of complications.

Local Treatment. Clinical and experimental evidence indicates that appreciable amounts of rattlesnake and other viperine venoms may be removed by incision and suction. A ligature should be applied immediately and tightly a few centimeters proximal to the fang wounds and released for 90 seconds every 15 minutes. It may be moved proximally as swelling increases. Two to four incisions about 1 cm long are made completely through the skin through or near the fang wounds. Suction is applied intermittently over the incisions for approximately one hour after the bite. A breast pump, modified plastic syringe, or the devices in commercial snakebite kits may be used; oral suction should not be used if other means are available. Bracelet or multiple incisions are not advised. If circulation distal to the bite becomes badly impaired, fasciotomy may be necessary.

Incision and suction increase the danger of infection, and oozing of blood from incisions may be a problem after bites by snakes with powerfully anticoagulant venoms. Absorption of some highly neurotoxic venoms is so rapid that incision and suction are ineffective.

After the first hour, the ligature is released. The bitten part should be immobilized 24 to 96 hours.

After acute symptoms of poisoning have subsided, treatment of vesicles and necrotic areas is similar to that advocated for severe burns.

Serum Therapy. Snake venom antisera or antivenins are prepared by hyperimmunization of animals (usually horses) against one or more snake venoms. The antibody-containing fraction of the serum is concentrated by methods used in preparation of bacterial antitoxins. Sometimes the product is lyophilized for greater stability. Antivenins are prepared by approximately 30 laboratories in various parts of the world. Most are intended for treatment of bites by the important venomous snakes of a particular geographic area. Some success has been achieved in preparation of antivenins against entire phylogenetic groups of venoms; e.g., polyvalent Crotalidae antivenin appears to be effective against venoms of most medically important species of pit vipers. There are no international standards for preparation and assay of antivenins. Products differ widely in potency and stability. The toxin-neutralizing capacity is low in comparison with bacterial antitoxins, and large doses are required. An initial dose of 20 to 50 ml diluted with five times its volume of physiologic saline should be given by intravenous drip over a 30 to 45 minute period. More antivenin should be given as the patient's condition dictates. A total of 100 to 150 ml in the first 24 hours may be required in a severe bite. If intravenous injection is not practicable, undiluted antivenin should be given intra-

muscularly. Infiltration of the bitten area with antivenin gives no advantage, and is contraindicated on fingers and toes. Allergic reactions to antivenin are common, and fatal anaphylaxis has been reported. A skin test for hypersensitivity should be done before administering serum; a positive reaction is contraindication to its use except in very severe cases. In bites by snakes known to be not highly dangerous (the copperhead in the United States, the European viper) or in bites by small snakes of more dangerous species, antivenin should be withheld unless the patient is a small child or there are signs of severe intoxication.

Supportive and Symptomatic Treatment. Except when it is obvious that only a minimal amount of venom has been injected, snakebite victims should be hospitalized at least 12 hours and kept in bed.

Blood transfusion is valuable therapy for bites by snakes with strongly hematotoxic venom. Blood typing should be done at the earliest opportunity, because the action of some venoms may make the procedure difficult. Adjustment of fluid and electrolyte balance is indicated in presence of shock, severe vomiting, hematuria, and albuminuria.

Oxygen is helpful in cases of hypoxia from blood destruction or respiratory impairment from the action of neurotoxins. In the latter, aspiration of secretions from the throat and trachea may be necessary, and the use of a respirator may be advisable. A tracheostomy may be required.

The presence of necrotic tissue, interference with local blood supply, and the toxic action of venoms on leukocytes and other phagocytic cells increase the hazard of infection even in relatively mild snakebites. Antimicrobial therapy should be instituted in most cases. Tetanus prophylaxis with toxoid or antitoxin is advisable; gas gangrene antitoxin is not recommended as a regular measure.

The necrotizing action of some pit viper venoms is reduced by local infiltration of tissue with 20 to 100 ml of 0.1 M ethylenediamine tetraacetic acid (EDTA). This must be done as soon as possible after the bite. Lethal factors of the venom are *not* neutralized by EDTA.

A corticosteroid preparation in doses of 100 to 500 mg of hydrocortisone or its equivalent may have beneficial antihypotensive and anti-inflammatory effects and is also helpful in treatment or prevention of serum reactions. The replacement of antivenin by repeated large doses of corticosteroids is not recommended. Antihistaminics have not proved effective in snakebite therapy.

Pain is often severe in viper bites, and may require codeine or meperidine. Anxiety and fear, sometimes to the point of hysteria, commonly accompany snakebite. Verbal reassurance and a confident attitude on the part of the physician are often more helpful than any medication; nevertheless, light barbiturate sedation is often advisable. An old and much maligned remedy, an ounce or so of whiskey or brandy, may accomplish the same purpose.

Extensive trials of immunization with snake venom toxoid are being undertaken in the Ryukyu Islands, an area of very high snakebite incidence. Preliminary results have been encouraging but not conclusive.

Nonpoisonous snakebites generally require no treatment unless the snake was a python or other large species. Precautions against infection should be taken. The snake's teeth frequently break off in the wound and should be removed. No specific diseases are transmitted by snakes in biting.

Behringwerk Mitteilungen: Die Giftschlangen der Erde, Wirkung und Antigenitat der Gifte. Therapie von Giftschlangenbissen. Marburg-Lahn, N. G. Elwert, 1963.

Minton, S. A.: Venom Diseases. Springfield, Ill., Charles C Thomas, 1974.

Reid, H. A.: Snake-bite in the tropics. Br. Med. J., 3:359, 1968.

Russell, F. E.: Clinical aspects of snake venom poisoning in North America. Toxicon, 7:33, 1969.

U.S. Navy Bureau of Medicine and Surgery: Poisonous Snakes of the World. Washington, D.C., U.S. Government Printing Office, 1968.

Yang, C. C.: Chemistry and evolution of toxins in snake venoms. Toxicon, 12:1, 1974.

58. MARINE VENOMS

Sherman A. Minton, Jr.

Venomous species occur in most phyla of marine animals. Their relative medical importance is increasing with the growing popularity of travel and of aquatic sports and with expanding exploitation of marine resources. Recognition of these animals and knowledge of their habits minimize opportunities for injury.

Most marine animal venoms appear to be proteins; however, quarternary ammonium compounds, epinephrine, 5-hydroxytryptamine, histamine, and other pharmacologically active compounds have been detected. Zootoxicologic properties of these venoms are too diverse for brief summary. Mechanisms of action for most species are poorly understood.

Jellyfish Stings. The pelagic coelenterates known as jellyfish belong to two main groups, the Portuguese men-of-war or bluebottles of the class Hydrozoa and the "true" jellyfish of the class Scyphozoa. Medically important species occur in all oceans; however, more serious stings are reported from Australian and south Asian waters. The venom apparatus consists of tentacles that may be up to 30 meters long and are thickly studded with highly specialized stinging capsules or nematocysts. Their primary function is capture and immobilization of food. Coelenterates never *attack* man; indeed, they are physically incapable of doing so. Injuries usually occur through contact with floating or stranded coelenterates or their detached tentacles. Such contact is followed by intense burning pain and development of linear, erythematous wheals that may progress to vesiculation. Muscular cramps, dyspnea, and nausea may be seen. Local necrosis may follow severe jellyfish stings. A systemic reaction clinically similar to anaphylactic shock may follow stings by sea wasps *(Chiropsalmus* and *Chironex)*; death has occurred three to four minutes after contact. Irukandji sting, caused by the Australian jellyfish *Carukia barnesi,* is characterized by a mild nettling rash followed after 10 to 60 minutes by sweating, cramps, severe myalgia, vomiting, and, sometimes, cough with hemoptysis. Recovery occurs within a day or two.

If tentacles are clinging to the skin, they should not be pulled or rubbed off, as this may discharge additional nematocysts. Prompt application of alcohol to the tentacle will inactivate the nematocysts. If alcohol is not available, the tentacles should be covered with sugar, salt, or dry sand and left alone 15 to 20 minutes before being scraped off. Local application of analgesic cream or spray, preferably one containing an antihistaminic or corticosteroid, may give some relief. Systemic reactions have been successfully counteracted by epinephrine (0.5 to 1 ml subcutaneously) plus 10 ml intravenously of calcium gluconate, antihistaminics, artificial respiration, and oxygen. Antivenin for the sea wasp, *Chironex,* is available from Commonwealth Serum Laboratories, Australia. Morphine or meperidine may be required to control pain.

Cone Shell Stings. Large marine snails of the genus *Conus* inflict injury with a harpoon-like tooth that can be rapidly extruded and is used for capture of prey as well as defense. Nearly all injuries are seen in shell collectors. Mild cases show only local symptoms resembling those of wasp stings. In severe cases, initial pain is followed by numbness, paresthesia, paresis beginning in the region of the injury and occasionally spreading to involve the entire skeletal musculature, sensation of constriction of the chest, dysphagia, visual disturbances, and collapse. Fatalities are on record, nearly all of them ascribed to the large species, *C. geographus,* widely distributed in the warmer parts of the Pacific and Indian Oceans.

The active principle of cone shell venom appears to be a protein-carbohydrate complex. Treatment is symptomatic with support of respiration essential in severe cases.

Miscellaneous Venomous Invertebrates. Spines of sea urchins cause painful injuries; systemic effects are very rare. A species of spiny Australian starfish inflicts a wound followed by bouts of vomiting lasting several days. Various sessile coelenterates such as hydroids, sea anemones, and stinging corals cause nettle-like stinging, sometimes with zosteriform hemorrhagic lesions and necrosis. Abdominal cramps, chills, diarrhea, and leukocytosis with eosinophilia may accompany severe stings. There is no specific treatment for any of these envenomations.

Venomous Fishes. Stonefish (Synanceja), scorpionfish (Scorpaena), lionfish (Pterois), weeverfish (Trachinus), and related species have venom glands associated with spines, especially those of the dorsal fin. Except for the greater weever, these are shallow-water fish particularly common about reefs, where they lie partly buried or concealed in crevices. Here they are apt to be accidentally touched or trodden upon. In open water the fish may adopt a more active defense, swimming so that the venomous spines are presented to an enemy. Skin divers and aquarium keepers have been injured under such circumstances. Fishermen may be injured when removing the fish from nets or traps. Fresh fish in markets may sting the buyer. Similarity of symptoms and of venom activity in laboratory animals suggests common or similar active principles in their venoms. *Synanceja verrucosa,* found from Oceania to the east coast of Africa, appears to be the most dangerous member of this group.

After injury by spines of these fishes, there is local pain that tends to spread and is often followed by hypesthesia or paresthesia at the site of puncture. Victims invariably describe the pain as almost unbearable, and it is regularly accompanied by hyperactivity often manifest by rolling about on the ground. There is severe local swelling, sometimes with formation of blisters and sloughing. Profuse sweating, dyspnea, hypotension, cyanosis, and collapse are seen especially with Synanceja stings; death may occur within an hour. Those who survive a severe sting may complain of weakness, dyspnea, and muscular aches for several weeks.

Immersion of the injured site in water as hot as can be tolerated is the most effective first aid.

Antivenin for Synanceja is available from Commonwealth Serum Laboratories of Australia; it may be expected to have some effect in stings by related species of fishes. The initial intramuscular or intravenous dose of 2 ml may be repeated in severe cases. Infiltration of the wound with emetine hydrochloride solution (65 mg per milliliter) is recommended if antivenin is not available.

Stingrays are widely distributed in warm coastal waters, including mouths of rivers; one family is restricted to fresh water. There are about 30 medically important species; the larger ones are 8 to 10 feet long, and weigh more than 100 pounds. Venom-secreting tissue is in the grooves and sheaths of barbed bony spines on the dorsum of the tail; in large species of rays, the spine may be 35 to 40 cm long. Stingrays typically bury themselves in sand or mud, where they may be stepped upon or grazed by persons diving. The fish lashes with its tail, driving the sting into its victim. Stings of large rays can readily penetrate the abdominal or thoracic wall. The wound is a puncture or laceration often surrounded by a zone of blanching for the first 30 minutes or so; later the area becomes hyperemic and edematous. Pain is severe, and sweating, nausea, weakness, and syncope are common. Muscular twitching, convulsions, irregular respiration, and cardiac arrhythmia indicate severe poisoning. Of 1097 stingray injuries reported in the United States during a five-year period, 62 patients required hospitalization, and two deaths resulted.

First aid for stingray injuries is immediate irrigation with salt water and removal of any fragments of the sting sheath that can be seen. This is followed by soaking in hot water for 30 to 90 minutes, administration of analgesics, and tetanus prophylaxis. Injuries by large rays, particularly when the chest or abdomen has been penetrated, require surgical management. There are no specific pharmacologic antagonists to stingray venom, nor is antivenin available.

Halstead, B. W.: Poisonous and Venomous Marine Animals of the World (3 Vols.). Washington, D.C., U.S. Government Printing Office, 1965–1970.
Keegan, H. L., and Macfarlane, W. V. (eds.): Venomous and Poisonous Animals and Noxious Plants of the Pacific Region, New York, Pergamon Press, 1963.
Nigrelli, R. F. (Ed.): Biochemistry and pharmacology of compounds derived from marine organisms. Ann. N.Y. Acad. Sci., 90:615, 1960.
Russell, F. E.: Marine toxins and venomous and poisonous marine animals. Adv. Marine Biol., 3:255, 1965.

59. VENOMOUS ARTHROPODS

Philip D. Marsden

CHILOPODA
(Centipedes)

Flattened dorsoventrally, centipedes have a single pair of legs to each body segment. They feed on other arthropods, and the appendages of the first segment are modified as poison claws through which venom is injected into the prey. Although not fatal to man, their bite can produce intense fiery pain, and the area at the site of the bite may be inflamed. Regional lymph nodes enlarge, and rarely there are signs of meningism. Treatment consists of analgesics and the use of local anesthetics at the site of the bite. Recurrence of the local edema and arthritis has been noted. Corticosteroids have been helpful.

Haneveld, G. T.: Centipede bites. Br. Med. J., 2:592, 1957.

DIPLOPODA
(Millipedes)

These have a rounded body contour and two pairs of legs per segment. They are vegetarian, but as a defense mechanism they secrete noxious fluids from body pores when attacked. These secretions may produce a vesicular dermatitis in man.

ARACHNIDA
(Scorpions and Spiders)

Scorpionida
(Scorpions, Eight Legs)

Envenomation of man or scorpiasis is common in some tropical areas. About 20,000 cases of scorpion sting occur annually in Mexico, and approximately 5 per cent are fatal, these deaths occurring mainly in small children. There are ten times more deaths from scorpion stings in Mexico than from snakebite. Scorpions are armed with a single curved caudal sting with which they inject their venom and paralyze their prey—usually other arthropods. Scorpions are nocturnal and hide beneath debris during the day.

The effects of envenomation vary with the species. Violent pain may occur at the site of the sting with radiation into the affected limbs. Chills with abundant cold sweats may be associated with severe thirst and vomiting. Venoms may have neurotoxic effects with paralysis and convulsions or cardiovascular effect with myocarditis and tachycardia, or may cause intravascular hemolysis. Death is often due to respiratory paralysis. Pancreatitis and defibrination syndromes have recently been described. Stings by scorpions with neurotoxic venom may not produce much local reaction.

Immediate treatment, as with snakebite, is aimed at delaying absorption of the venom. A tourniquet is applied to the limb and released every 20 to 30 minutes. If available, ice packs should be applied to the site and the patient kept at rest. Specific antiserum is available in some areas and should be given if signs occur in the central nervous system. Phenobarbital may control convulsions. Spraying DDT or benzene hexachloride (BHC) will cut down the scorpion population.

Bartholomew, C.: Acute scorpion pancreatitis in Trinidad. Br. Med. J., 1:666, 1970.
McIntosh, M. E., and Watt, D. D.: Biochemical immunochemical aspects of the venom from the scorpion *Centruroides sculpturatus. In* Russell, F. E., and Sanders, P. R. (eds.): Animal Toxins, London, Pergamon Press, 1967, p. 47.
Poon-King, T.: Myocarditis from scorpion stings. Br. Med. J., 1:374, 1963.
Sita Devi, S., et al.: Defibrination syndrome due to scorpion venom poisoning. Br. Med. J., 1:345, 1970.
Whittlemore, F. W., Jr., Keegan, H. L., and Barowitz, J. L.: Studies of scorpion antivenoms: 1. Paraspecificity. Bull. WHO, 25:185, 1961.

Spiders
(Eight Legs, Abdomen Joined to Cephalothorax by a Narrow Waist)

Most spiders possess venom apparatus in the form of a pair of chelicerae terminating in sharp fangs and associated venom glands. The degree of development of this apparatus varies, and the glands contain only a small amount of venom suitable for paralyzing other arthropods. Of the 200 genera described, only eight contain species reported to be poisonous to man. Human fatalities have occurred after the bite of species of Latrodectus, Loxosceles, Phoneutria, and Atrax.

Latrodectus. It is likely that all species in this genus are poisonous to man, but the black widow (*L. mactans*) and the gray widow (*L. geometricus*) are most important. Males have much less venom than the aggressive females. These spiders are represented in most warm parts of the world and occur in the Americas from Southern Canada to Chile. They spin their webs in dark places, often outhouses. In Texas 90 per cent of spider bites occur on the buttocks and genitals because of the tendency to spin webs under lavatory seats in outside privies. The bite may pass unnoticed; two tiny red spots may be seen at the site, or a severe local reaction occurs. The neurotoxic fraction in the venom is a protein of low molecular weight which affects the cord and nerve endings. Absorption is accompanied by pain and numbness in the affected part. In 15 minutes to a few hours generalized agonizing muscular pains appear, together with symptoms of shock. The blood pressure falls, and there are marked sweating, a feeling of weakness and nausea, and labored respiration. The marked rigidity of the muscles of the abdominal wall may simulate tetanus or an acute abdomen. Paralysis and coma may be followed by cardiac or respiratory failure in severe cases.

An intravenous injection of 10 ml of a 10 per cent solution of calcium gluconate administered slowly will relieve muscular spasm. If this fails, a muscle relaxant such as mephenesin can be given. An antivenin is available in some endemic areas where there is a demand for it. It is effective against most species of Latrodectus. The spiders are sensitive to DDT spraying.

Loxosceles. The hairy brown spiders, *L. reclusa*, of the United States and *L. laeta* of Central and South America, occur in houses among furniture. Pain occurs at the site of their bite, followed by erythema, edema, and local necrosis. A rarer cutaneovisceral form is associated with toxic nephritis and hepatitis, the venom being cytotoxic. Local pain and edema decrease after parenteral antihistamine and corticosteroids have suppressed systemic reactions.

Phoneutria. This is a genus responsible for fatalities in children in some South American countries (Chile, Brazil). The venom acts on both the central and peripheral nervous systems.

Atrax. The Australian funnel web spider also produces neurotoxic symptoms.

Editorial: Spider bites. Lancet, 2:509, 1969.
Horen, W. P.: Arachnidism in the United States. J.A.M.A., 185:839, 1963.
Levi, H. W., and Spielman, A.: The biology and control of the South American brown spider *Loxosceles laeta* (Nicolet) in a North American focus. Am. J. Trop. Med. Hyg., 13:132, 1964.
McCrone, J. D., and Hatala, R. J.: Isolation and characterisation of a lethal component from the venom of *Latrodectus mactans*. *In* Russell, F. E., and Sanders, P. R. (eds.): Animal Toxins. London, Pergamon Press, 1967, p. 29.
Smith, C. W., and Micks, D. W.: Comparative study of the venom and other components of three species of Loxosceles. Am. J. Trop. Med., 17:651, 1968.

ACARINA
(Ticks and Mites)

Families in the order Acarina (ticks and mites) are responsible for carrying some important human infections. The family Ixodoidea contains the hard ticks responsible for transmitting the rickettsia of tick typhus. The Argasidae are the soft ticks, some of which transmit tick-borne relapsing fever (*Borrelia duttoni*). The mites are also of medical importance. The family Trombiculidae contains the important genus of red mites, Trombicula, which transmit scrub typhus caused by *Rickettsia tsutsugamushi (orientalis)*. The larvae of other similar mites cause an unpleasant, irritating skin rash (chiggers, red bugs, or harvest mites). About 24 hours after feeding, small red macules appear, and there may be hundreds if infection is severe. The diagnosis is made by finding the six-legged orange red larvae on the skin. BHC dusting powder destroys mites in their habitats and dibutyl phthalate or benzyl benzoate is quite effective for about a week if dusted over clothing. The house mouse mite Allodermanyssus transmits *Rickettsia akari* of rickettsialpox. One other mite, *Sarcoptes scabiei*, which is responsible for one of the most prevalent skin diseases in the world, is considered in Ch. 52. Tick paralysis, a little-diagnosed entity, is discussed in Ch. 51.

STINGING INSECTS

Hymenoptera
(Bees, Wasps, Hornets, Ants)

All stinging insects are included in this order, which contains 60,000 species. The stinging apparatus consists of a modified ovipositor and paired poison glands that discharge into a reservoir—the poison sac. In bees the venom apparatus is usually torn away from the body when the insect is brushed off. The average bee sting contains 0.3 mg of venom. The venom of bees and wasps contains a number of fatty acids and saponin-like substances.

A direct action (increase in vascular permeability at the site of the sting) is associated with the presence of histamine, serotonin, and a particular kinin. In addition to the effect of these substances there is an indirect effect, depending, among other things, on the properties of histamine liberated from the damaged tissues, probably by an enzymatic mechanism. The position of the sting is of great importance. If it occurs in the buccal or pharyngeal mucosa, a serious edema of the glottis and asphyxia may result. If venom is directly inoculated into a blood vessel, rapid absorption can cause syncope and even death.

In parts of Africa and Asia some varieties of bees are especially aggressive, and a number of deaths have resulted from multiple stings. The total number of simultaneous stings necessary for a fatality is about 500. Apart from deaths owing to multiple stings, many fatalities occur in hypersensitive patients, in whom death may occur in one hour owing to anaphylaxis and laryngeal edema. The allergen occurs in all parts of the insect, and hypersensitive patients can be desensitized by injection of wasp and bee extract. In the United States more deaths were caused by stinging insects than by snakes in the period 1950 to 1954. In such allergic states intense pruritus after sting is followed by severe angioneurotic edema and asthma. Severe abdominal pain and convulsion may occur.

Stings should be removed from the wound, with care taken not to express more venom into the wound by squeezing the poison sac. Acute allergic reactions should be treated with 0.5 ml of 1:1000 epinephrine intramuscularly. This can be repeated as often as necessary, together with an intramuscular injection of an antihistamine. Hydrocortisone, 100 mg, should be injected intravenously in patients with severe laryngeal edema; tracheostomy may be lifesaving. Milder reactions can be relieved by black coffee plus 30 mg of ephedrine. Sensitized persons should carry sublingual tablets of isoproterenol and antihistamines and have epinephrine ampules available (see also Ch. 77).

Barnard, J. M.: Cutaneous responses to insects. Types and mechanism of reactions. J.A.M.A., 196:259, 1966.
Beard, R. L.: Insect toxins and venoms. Ann. Rev. Entom., 8:1, 1963.
Mann, G. T., and Bates, M. R., Jr.: The pathology of insect bites: A brief review and report of eleven fatal cases. South. Med. J., 53:1399, 1960.
Shaffer, J. H.: Stinging insects: A threat to life. J.A.M.A., 177:473, 1961.

Ants

Although most ants possess venom apparatus, only a few are capable of injuring man. The Tucandeira ant of the Central American forests possesses a powerful sting that may result in fever for several hours. Allergic reactions to ants have been reported. The fire ant *(Solenopsis saevissima* richteri) has now established itself in the southern United States, and after multiple stinging produces a pustular, markedly erythematous rash caused by a necrotizing toxin solenamine.

Adrouny, G. A.: The fire ant's fire. Bull. Tulane Univ. Med. Fac., 25:67, 1966.
Cavill, G. W. K., and Robertson, P. L.: Ant venom, attractors and repellents. Science, 149:1337, 1965.
Middleton, E.: In combined staff clinic on poisoning by venomous animals. Am. J. Med., 42:118, 1967.

URTICATING INSECTS

A number of moths and butterflies (Lepidoptera) and beetles (Coleoptera) possess urticating qualities and can cause irritant dermatitis and conjunctivitis.

Lepidoptera

The caterpillars of a large number of moths and some butterflies possess urticating hairs or spines singly or in clusters over the body. If such a caterpillar is handled, these penetrate the skin, and venom passes through an opening at the tip. The hairs frequently break and remain in the skin. When the caterpillar pupates, the urticating hairs are frequently present in the cocoon that surrounds the pupa, and are also carried on the wings and body of the adult insect when it emerges.

Dermatitis produced by caterpillars is very widespread. Outbreaks have occurred in Israel and Japan. In 1956, 250,000 cases of dermatitis were estimated on Honshu Island. In Texas 2130 cases of caterpillar stings were reported in 1968. The hairs can be removed by application of adhesive tape. If cellophane tape is used, the hairs can then be mounted on a slide for microscopic examination. Washing the affected area with mild antiseptic should be followed by the application of calamine. Severe urticaria may require parenteral epinephrine and antihistamines. Adult moths have been recorded as producing similar lesions.

Hellier, F. F., and Warin, R. P.: Caterpillar dermatitis. Br. Med. J., 1:346, 1967.
Zaias, N., Ioannides, G., and Taplin, D.: Dermatitis from contact with moths (Genus Hylesia). J.A.M.A., 207:525, 1969.

Coleoptera
(Beetles)

Two families of beetles that contain urticating substances are the Staphylinidae (rove beetles) and the Meloidae (blister and oil beetles). Eight staphylinids of the genus Paederus cause dermatitis, especially in tropical countries. The irritant is present in the coelomic fluid, and when the beetle is crushed on the skin, erythematous blistering and pigmentary lesions occur. Pederin, a powerful vesicating toxin, constitutes 1 per cent of the tiny beetle's body weight. Staphylinids are so small that they are not usually noted in the skin.

Several genera of Meloidae have urticating properties, including Mylabris, Epicanita, and Lytta. *Lytta (Cantharis) vesicatoria* is familiarly known as Spanish fly. These beetles are night-flying and are frequently attracted to artificial light. The urticating substance occurs in the hemolymph, which is extruded through the integument if the insect is disturbed or escapes when the insect is crushed. Large blisters are produced if the insect contacts the human skin, and blindness may occur if the conjunctiva is affected. The pathogenesis of these lesions is explained in a way similar to that of attacks by gaseous vesicants, namely, by a blocking of enzymes of the SH groups. Like these enzymes, cantharidin inhibits glucide metabolism. *It should be noted that cantharidin has no aphrodisiac effect, and that the fatal dose is less than 60 mg.* Topical treatment of the blisters with magnesium sulfate and methyl alcohol packs has been recommended. Other tropical beetles producing vesicants are in the families Paunidae and Oedemeridae.

Two other conditions associated with beetles can be mentioned here.

Scarabiasis is the term used for the presence of adult dung beetles in the stool of man. Certain beetle larvae survive in the fecal stream, notably the meal worms (Tenebrio) ingested in contaminated cereals.

Carpet beetles can be used as an example of harmless insects which may be associated with delusions of parasitosis and the production of a type of dermatitis artefacta. However, there is at least one report of a patient who became sensitized to the varied carpet beetle *(Anthrenus verbasci)* which can be brought into the house on cut flowers.

Armstrong, R. K., and Winfield, J. L.: *Paederus fuscipes* dermatitis. An epidemic on Okinawa. Am. J. Trop. Med. Hyg., 18:147, 1969.
Ayres, S., and Mihan, R.: Delusions of parasitosis caused by carpet beetles. J.A.M.A., 199:675, 1967.
Browne, S. G.: Cantharidin poisoning due to a blister beetle. Br. Med. J., 2:1290, 1960.
Cormia, F. E.: Carpet beetle dermatitis. J.A.M.A., 200:799, 1967.
Giglioli, M. E. C.: Some observations on blister beetle, family Meloidae, in Gambia, West Africa. Trans. Roy. Soc. Trop. Med. Hyg., 59:657, 1965.
Halprim, K. M.: The art of self mutilation. II. Delusions of parasitosis. J.A.M.A., 198:1207, 1966.
Kerdel Vegas, F., and Gothman Yahr, M.: Paederus dermatitis. Arch. Derm., 94:175, 1966.
Rosin, R. D.: Cantharides intoxication. Br. Med. J., 3:33, 1967.
Scarabiasis. J. Trop. Med. Hyg., 70:49, 1967.

Part IV
IMMUNE DISEASE

60. INTRODUCTION

Henry G. Kunkel

Immunology represents one of the most rapidly expanding areas of biology, and many new techniques for the study of alterations in disease have become available recently. This is particularly true at the cellular level, and much has been learned of the lymphocyte which is clearly the key cell involved in both cellular and humoral immunity. The concept of two major types of lymphocytes, T cells (thymus derived) and B cells (bone marrow derived), is firmly established. Alterations in level and defects in these cells are now recognizable.

Immunologic alterations, both at the cellular level and with respect to immunoglobulins (Igs) and antibodies, have been found in a wide variety of different diseases. However, in many instances it has proved uniquely difficult to pinpoint the abnormality as primary in the disease etiology. It is well recognized that similar changes can occur secondarily, particularly as a result of certain viral infections. In some diseases the significance of the immunologic alterations is clear, as for example in the allergic disorders, in thyroiditis, and in certain types of immune deficiency. In other diseases, such as systemic lupus erythematosus (SLE), Graves' disease, acquired hemolytic anemia, and pemphigus, immunologic alterations are present which appear to be involved in the disease process, but their origin and relative significance remain less clear. Finally, there are diseases such as rheumatoid arthritis, ulcerative colitis, and pernicious anemia in which the evidence for an immunologic disorder remains very tentative. Interest has centered in particular on the challenging question of autoimmunity and its possible pathogenic role in many of these disorders. One difficulty which has hampered investigators stems from the gradual realization that the occurrence of autoantibodies is by no means a rare phenomenon limited to specific diseases. Many normal persons appear to possess such antibodies. Some autoantibodies appear to be without harmful effects, and the possibility exists, at least in certain instances, that they may be of benefit.

Examples of widely prevalent autoantibodies that in most situations appear to be without harmful effects are immunoconglutinin or antibody to complement, the antigamma globulins frequently termed rheumatoid factors, and the antinuclear antibodies of many different types. All of these have been found in the serum of normal persons as well as in those with a wide variety of microbial diseases. Evidence has been obtained, however, that under certain conditions harmful effects can be produced by certain types of antinuclear and anti-gamma globulin antibodies. Characteristics such as concentration in serum, exact specificity (particularly toward antigens encountered in the serum), and physical properties such as solubility appear to govern this question.

One immunologic mechanism of tissue injury that is coming increasingly to the fore is the direct effect of antigen-antibody complexes from the circulation. This is particularly true of renal injury. Such a process appears to be involved in a number of diseases in which renal injury is manifest such as systemic lupus erythematosus and glomerulonephritis. The antigen reacting with antibody to form complexes may come from external sources such as streptococci and administered drugs, or it may come from autologous tissue breakdown products. The injury from such complexes is not limited to the kidney, a particularly sensitive target organ, but may also involve the blood vessels as a potential mechanism of vasculitis. Platelet damage represents a well documented example; complexes of drugs such as quinidine and its antibody in sensitive individuals adhere to platelets and bring about their destruction.

TYPES OF ANTIBODIES AND THEIR PROPERTIES

Five major classes of human antibodies have been characterized: IgG, IgM, IgA, IgD, and IgE. In addition the IgG class has been divided into four subclasses which differ markedly in biologic properties: IgG 1, IgG 2, IgG 3, and IgG 4. The concentration in serum and some of the special properties of these classes and subclasses are shown in the accompanying table. All these proteins migrate in the gamma-beta area by electrophoresis, with IgG 4, IgA, IgD, and IgE showing the most rapid mobility at pH 8.6. They have been determined quantitatively primarily through the use of specific antisera in radial immune diffusion assays. The five major classes are very distinct antigenically, and specific antisera are readily obtained. The four subclasses of IgG show marked cross-reactions, and it is primarily because of this distinction that they have been termed subclasses.

It is now apparent that all Igs and antibodies consist of two major polypeptide chains, the heavy or H chain and the light or L chain. Both the H and L chains have a variable and a constant area. The variable portions are directly involved in the antibody combining site. The constant areas of the heavy chains differ among the classes and subclasses and are responsible for the different biologic properties shown in the table. Figure 1 illustrates the basic Ig chain structure, showing the variable and constant areas as they apply to IgG 1 immunoglobulins. There are two L-H chain pairs which make up the two antigen combining sites of this type of molecule. Enzymatic splitting of the molecule has proved of great utility in the study of the various properties of antibodies. Papain produces an Fab and an Fc fragment, and each of these is readily isolated. Most of the properties of the different classes and subclasses shown in the table are based on structural differences in the Fc part of the molecule.

As shown in Figure 1, the common IgG globulin is made up of a single four-chain unit. In the case of IgM or 19S Ig as it is sometimes called, a similar four-chain monomeric unit is further polymerized into a macroglobulin consisting of five such units linked by disulfide bonds. The IgA globulin is more variable and sometimes consists of a simple four-chain 7S molecule and in other instances is polymerized to various larger sizes. Less is known about the IgD type, but this also appears to be a

Biologic Properties of Human Immunoglobulins

	IgG 1	IgG 2	IgG 3	IgG 4	IgA	IgM	IgD	IgE
Concentration mg/ml*	9.4	3.2	1.0	0.6	1.9	0.5	0.03	0.0003
Placental transfer	+	+	+	+	0	0	0	0
Complement fixation†	+	±	+	0	0	+	0	0
PCA‡ reactivity	+	0	+	+	0	0	0	0
P-K§ reactivity	0	0	0	0	0	0	0	+
Lymphocyte receptors¶	±	±	0	0	+	+	+	0
Macrophage binding	+	0	+	0	0	0	0	—

*Mean values in adult whites.
†Classic complement pathway.
‡Passive cutaneous anaphylaxis.
§Prausnitz-Küstner.
¶Ig receptors for antigen on the membranes of B lymphocytes.

7S protein made of two light and two heavy chains. The proteins of the IgE class also consist of two light and two heavy chains. However, longer heavy chains are present, making the four-chain molecule considerably larger. These classes differ from each other in carbohydrate content, which plays an important role in solubility differences. They also differ in their ability to cross the placenta, an important property with regard to maternal-infant antibody relationships. The IgM and the IgA show little or no placental passage, in marked contrast to IgG globulin, which in cord blood reaches similar levels to those in maternal serum. A very significant special property of IgA antibodies is their occurrence as the dominant antibody in all external secretions. Saliva, tears, intestinal secretions, colostrum, and other body fluids contain primarily IgA antibodies.

Recently it has been demonstrated that IgD is of special significance on the membrane of B type lymphocytes. It appears that IgD and IgM act as the primary receptors for antigen on the lymphocyte surface.

The total amino acid sequence is now available for a number of Igs and it is clear that marked differences occur in the variable areas of the heavy and light chains, particularly in special regions which have been termed the hypervariable areas. These amino acid substitutions account for the specific combining properties of individual antibodies for antigen. The genetic mechanism by which the huge diversity of antibody molecules is produced with amino acid differences in the hypervariable areas remains unknown. The germ line theory proposes that there are sufficient DNA units in the genome to code for all the different antibodies. The somatic theory, on the other hand, considers a variety of different mechanisms arising during cell development and involving somatic mutations from a very limited number of DNA units.

Antibodies with autospecificity have been found that belong in each of the five main classes of Igs, with the exception of IgD and IgE. Most of the diverse antibodies encountered in the sera of SLE patients are of the IgG type, which goes along with the usual marked elevation in the total serum IgG globulin. A few, however, have been described that fall into the IgM and IgA class, particularly among the antinuclear antibodies. The rheumatoid factors as well as the majority of other anti-gamma globulins are primarily IgM macroglobulins. Most of the cryoglobulins are macroglobulins; this is also true of the cold agglutinins. Decreased solubility in the cold is a general characteristic of the antibodies of high molecular weight. It is known that these antibodies are also very sensitive to sulfhydryl compounds such as cysteine and penicillamine, which act on the disulfide bonds responsible for their polymeric structure. Attempts have been made to utilize this effect for therapeutic purposes, particularly for the cold agglutinin disease, but with limited success thus far. The antibodies of high molecular weight usually fix complement very effectively and as a result produce severe cellular injury when cells are involved as antigens. Many such antibodies are involved in hemolytic reactions of erythrocytes. In other instances the specific properties of macroglobulin antibodies make them more benign. The IgG–anti-IgG complexes found in rheumatoid arthritis sera are readily soluble under most conditions, permitting them to circulate at high concentrations with surprisingly few harmful effects. However, some of the IgG–anti-IgG complexes have been shown to have very harmful effects. This is particularly true in the disorder known as mixed cryoglobulin disease in which severe kidney disease is frequently found.

The skin-sensitizing antibodies or reagins that appear to be responsible for most of the harmful effects in the allergic diseases have many unique properties. The most striking of these is the persistence in the skin for periods

Structure of Immunoglobulins

Figure 1. Diagrammatic illustration of the basic structure of the Ig molecule. There are two L chains and two H chains linked by disulfide bonds; the amino terminal ends of the chains are on the left and the carboxy terminal ends at the right. The undulating lines represent the variable portions of both the H and L chains. The sites of cleavage by papain and pepsin to give Fab and Fc fragments are indicated. The Greek letters refer to the kappa and lambda light chains and the heavy chains of the various Ig classes. The position of a carbohydrate side chain (CHO) is shown.

of weeks after transfer to normal persons. The demonstration that these properties are characteristics of antibodies of the IgE class has been a significant recent development in immunology. Quantitatively this is a very minor class, representing only approximately 0.05 per cent of the total immunoglobulins of the serum. However, it has become clear that it is specifically involved in histamine release from leukocytes and other cells. The finding of several myeloma proteins of the IgE type has aided greatly in our understanding of the specific characteristics of proteins of this class. Their molecular weight is somewhat higher than IgG proteins and their sedimentation rate is approximately 8S. They are rich in carbohydrate and do not fix complement. It is of particular interest that IgE forming cells are concentrated in the mucosal system of the nose and respiratory tract as well as the regional lymph nodes, raising the possibility that locally formed IgE may be involved in respiratory allergy. Other types of antibodies to allergens are also found in the sera of sensitive patients that do not have the unique skin-sensitizing properties and rapidly diffuse away from the site of the injection. These antibodies, which have been termed blocking antibodies, appear to be typical IgG globulins, in contrast to the reagins. They also combine with antigen and may prevent a reaction with the skin-sensitizing antibody.

LYMPHOCYTES AND OTHER IMMUNOLOGICALLY SIGNIFICANT CELLS

Two major classes of lymphocytes are now well documented which differ strikingly in their biologic properties. The B cell is distinguished by the presence of immunoglobulin receptors for antigen on its surface, and it becomes a plasma cell after stimulation; it is the primary antibody-producing cell. The T cell, on the other hand, plays a number of very different roles. It too has a receptor for antigen on the membrane surface, but the nature of this receptor remains obscure. After stimulation it enlarges to a blast cell that does not produce antibody but produces a wide variety of mediators that are significant in many immunologic processes. One of these has a significant effect on B cells and is the means by which the T cell cooperates with the B cell, thus aiding in the production of antibodies. Another very important function of T cells is their direct participation in cellular immune reactions such as graft rejection. Figure 2 illustrates diagrammatically the pathways that have been envisioned for the evolution of B and T cells from a progenitor stem cell.

A wide variety of other mediators have been described which are released by activated lymphocytes. None of these have been isolated, and it is not clear that they all represent different substances. The best known of these is "transfer factor," which is a low molecular weight dialyzable constituent that appears to transfer delayed hypersensitivity to specific antigens from a positive individual to a negative one; sensitivity to tuberculin, to diphtheria toxoid, and to coccidioidin represent three examples out of many that have been studied. Special interest has centered on "transfer factor" because of its potential value in therapy. Patients with various fungal infections, those with immune deficiency disorders, and even cancer patients have been injected with concentrated material prepared from donor lymphocytes in an attempt to produce a cellular immunity that may aid the

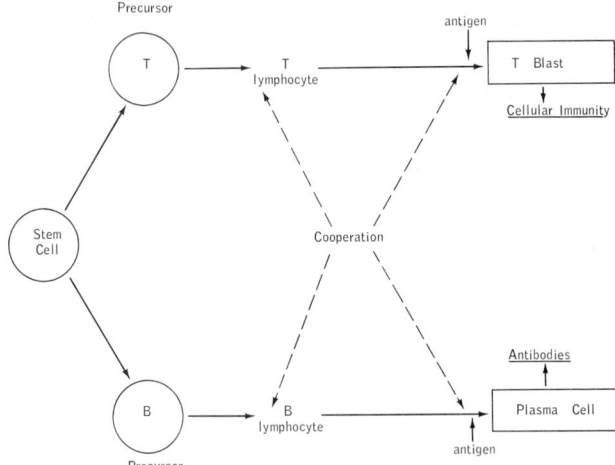

Figure 2. Diagrammatic representation of the development of immunologically active lymphoid cells of the T and B cell types from a common stem cell. Terminal differentiation to plasma cells producing antibodies and to T blasts responsible for cellular immunity follows antigenic stimulation.

immune response of these patients. Evidence has been obtained of therapeutic value for "transfer factor," but the final word on its usefulness is not in.

Migration inhibition factor (MIF) is another mediator released by T cells which has been widely studied. It is released in response to antigen and inhibits the migration of macrophages. This is usually measured by determining the diameter of the ring of macrophages moving out of the end of a capillary tube. It has become a widely used assay for the determination of cellular immunity to specific antigens. Other mediators include interferon, lymphotoxin, chemotactin, and skin reactive factor.

The macrophage clearly plays a key role in cellular immunologic reactions. Many aspects of this role remain poorly understood, but it is evident that a number of the mediators described above affect the macrophage directly and increase its activity against bacterial or other targets. Evidence is available for the release of a variety of enzymes from macrophages after stimulation. In addition, the macrophage has been shown to play an important role in the interaction of antigen with T cells. Some workers view this as a presentation of antigen which otherwise would not activate the T cell.

Another cell type which appears to have broad significance is the K or killer cell. This cell appears to hold a high affinity for antibody and acts in conjunction with antibody to attack target cells, the so-called antibody mediated lympholysis. Little is presently known about this cell and its relation to B cells or macrophages. It is clearly an important cell in tumor rejection in various animal models.

CHARACTERISTICS AND ESTIMATION OF B AND T LYMPHOCYTES

A number of different methods have been developed for differentiating B and T lymphocytes, and some of these provide quantitative results which are of use in assessing these immunologic parameters in diseased individuals. The most characteristic aspect of the B cell is the surface Ig which can be detected readily by a variety of techniques. The most widely used of these is the fluorescent antibody method in which anti-Ig antiserum that is fluorescent is used to stain the Ig on the cell. Figure 3 illustrates the dot-like staining obtained with such an antiserum on the surface of a B cell, whereas a T cell in the same field is entirely negative. This procedure reveals positive staining for Ig on approximately 15 per cent of normal peripheral blood lymphocytes. The Ig is primarily IgM and IgD and has been shown to be synthesized by the B cells. In certain individuals with various disease states, lymphocyte antibodies are found which attach to autologous lymphocytes and give falsely high levels for B cells by the surface Ig staining criterion. Short-term cultures of such lymphocytes aid in distinguishing this type, because the antibody is lost from the surface while the receptor immunoglobulin remains.

Another useful method for determining B cells stems from the presence of a receptor for the third component of complement which is not found on T cells. Red cells that are coated with antibody and complement form rosettes around B cells, and the number of such rosettes is readily quantitated. A third procedure utilizes the B cell characteristic of reacting with the Fc portion of IgG immunoglobulins. This is a weak interaction, and stable binding occurs only when the Ig is aggregated or is in the form of an immune complex. Large aggregates of IgG are readily visualized by a variety of methods attached to B cells specifically. The complement receptor and the Fc receptor procedures give results for B cell levels that are close to those obtained by Ig staining.

The T lymphocyte in the human can be detected by its selective binding of sheep red blood cells to give rosettes. This is a simple and accurate quantitative method that has come into wide use. The explanation for this useful binding procedure remains obscure. Both thymocytes and peripheral blood T cells give the rosettes. Approximately 80 per cent of blood lymphocytes are positive; this figure when added to the B cell population of 15 per cent gives a value close to 100 per cent. Specific antisera that are T cell specific are also available and can be utilized in fluorescent antibody studies or cytotoxic assays to quantitate the T cell population. Results with the antisera usually give a lower percentage figure for blood lymphocytes than is obtained with the rosetting procedure. Specific mitogen stimulation of T cells is also used as an assay of T cell competence. Phytohemagglutinin and concanavallin A are the primary mitogens for this purpose, and the T cell response is measured by determination of the blast cells produced or through the incorporation of tritium labeled thymidine. The advantage of the mitogen procedures is that the functional competence of T cells is determined, rather than just an enumeration of T cells. The disadvantages lie in the difficulty in quantitation and the influence of other cells such as the macrophage in the response.

The *mixed lymphocyte culture* (MLC) reaction is also used as an assay of T cell function. This is usually carried out in a unidirectional system with a known stimulating lymphocyte population that is treated with mitomycin C. The latter reagent prevents these cells from responding but preserves their stimulating potential. The response is measured by the uptake of tritiated thymidine, and cells from different patients can be analyzed in terms of their response. The primary use of the MLC reaction, however, is in histocompatibility testing prior to grafting, in which compatibility is detected through an absence of any response, which is determined primarily by the MLC genes. These appear to differ from the HL-A genes that are separate but closely linked and determine the HL-A antigens that can be determined serologically. Because of the difficulties of the MLC test systems, the different phenotypes are only partially recognized, but their significance for graft survival is clearly recognized.

Alterations in the level and functional capacity of T and B lymphocytes have been found in a wide variety of diseases. The most striking findings are in the immune deficiency disorders (see Ch. 61 to 69), and analyses of the lymphocytes that are present are providing new insight into the basic defects. In Graves' disease and thyroiditis an increase in T cells and a fall in B cells have been demonstrated clearly. Alterations in Hodgkin's disease, leprosy, cancer, and connective tissue disease have been described. However, these studies are only beginning, and their significance remains to be determined. It is of special interest that the leukemic lymphocytes in the vast majority of cases of chronic lymphatic leukemia are of the B cell type; in acute lymphatic leukemia they appear to be of T cell character.

DELAYED TYPE OF HYPERSENSITIVITY

Delayed type of hypersensitivity is clearly a reaction of T cells which have been stimulated by antigen to react against targets such as infectious agents, grafts, and tumors. Antibody is not involved in this phenomenon, and disagreement exists among immunologists concerning the role of macrophages. The term "delayed type of hypersensitivity" arose from the delayed skin response of sensitive subjects to antigen; the reaction does not

Figure 3. Surface Ig staining by the fluorescent antibody technique of a B type lymphocyte (lower frame). The upper frame shows two lymphocytes by phase contrast microscopy. One lymphocyte of the T type fails to show any Ig.

begin for several hours and reaches a maximum after two or three days. The term "cellular immunity" has also been used, although, as mentioned above, some types of cellular immunity also involve antibodies. Two major types of delayed hypersensitivity have been most widely studied: that induced by infection, and the other, termed contact sensitivity, resulting from exposure to a variety of substances ranging from oily resins of plants to simple chemicals employed for domestic, industrial, and medical purposes. Delayed hypersensitivity to autologous antigens has been difficult to demonstrate in humans, although it can be produced in laboratory animals by immunization with autologous antigens.

Delayed-type hypersensitivity is more strikingly evident in certain specific infections such as tuberculosis, brucellosis, lymphogranuloma venereum, mumps, vaccinia, and some fungal infections. Skin tests that depend on this type of cellular immunity have been utilized in these diseases. Tuberculin reactions have been extensively studied in humans and laboratory animals as a model for the delayed type of hypersensitivity. The skin reactivity to tuberculin can be transferred to normal recipients by means of cells from lymphoid tissue, peritoneal exudate, and peripheral blood. In laboratory animals viable cells are required, but in humans the supernatant fluid of disrupted leukocytes can transfer the reactivity. "Transfer factor," mentioned above in the discussion of mediators, represents the active principle involved.

Graft versus Host Reaction.   Another probable manifestation of delayed-type hypersensitivity, or at least cellular immunity, is the graft versus host reaction. This has sometimes been termed "homologous disease." Initially it was largely a disorder of laboratory animals that are able to accept foreign bone marrow or lymphoid cells because they have been irradiated or otherwise treated so that these cells are not rejected. More recently it has been encountered frequently in humans who have received certain grafts, particularly bone marrow. The foreign cells react against various antigens in the host animal, resulting in a variety of clinical manifestations. The skin lesions are most characteristic: edema, erythema, and ulceration, followed by thickening, scaling, and loss of hair. Lesions of the joints and of the heart are also observed and these have aroused considerable interest because of certain similarities to those observed in some of the connective tissue disorders. Hemolytic anemia with a positive Coombs reaction has also been described. The possibility has been raised that in certain human diseases immunologically active cells react against the host in a fashion similar to that of the transferred cells in the laboratory animal experiments. The origin of such cells has been ascribed to some type of failure of tolerance mechanisms or to an alteration of host cells through somatic mutation.

SENSITIVITY TO FOREIGN ANTIGENS

Direct sensitivity to foreign antigens, the most common type of potentially injurious immunologic reaction in man, is usually a result of antigenic stimulation by foreign protein or polysaccharide antigens. These may gain entrance to the body through parenteral, oral, respiratory, or other routes. The classic example is serum sickness, usually resulting from the administration of horse or rabbit immune serum. An Arthus reaction is initiated through the direct union of antigen and antibody in the tissue spaces. Precipitates in and around small blood vessels cause secondary damage to cells, or, when antigen is in excess, soluble complexes are formed that may deposit in certain sensitive organs in the blood vessel walls and cause local inflammatory reactions.

In most of the human allergies such as hay fever and food allergy the exact mode of sensitization to external antigens is not directly apparent. Numerous factors such as heredity, intestinal absorption, respiratory secretion, and even emotional state appear involved. In such sensitive or atopic individuals the reaction to foreign antigens is more commonly of the anaphylactic type. Here the binding of antibody to tissue cells appears to play an important role. Local anaphylaxis results from the association or passive absorption of antibodies to local sites that come in contact with antigen. Not all antibodies have this property, and the IgE class is primarily involved. The antigen in turn reacts with the antibody and alters these cells, which then cause the release of histamine and other pharmacologic mediators into the tissue fluid and circulation. In the skin this gives rise to the wheal and erythema at the site of antigen introduction, as in ordinary prick and scratch diagnostic tests. Hay fever and allergic asthma are local manifestations of such reactions. Extensive urticaria may also represent an expression of local cutaneous anaphylaxis.

The antigens involved in these local allergic reactions are a very diversified group. A number have been isolated and partially characterized. The major allergen of *ragweed pollen* has been found to be a protein of approximately 37,000 molecular weight and represents a very small portion of the extractable solids of the pollen. The biologic activity of the isolated material is very high; as little as 10^{-12} grams cause a positive intracutaneous wheal and erythema reaction in sensitive individuals. A highly active protein has also been isolated from the *timothy hay pollen*. Low molecular weight nonprotein allergens have also been isolated. The best example of these is chloragenic acid, which is the active material from castor beans. Just how this is effective is not clear, but the general hypothesis is that it acts as a hapten and combines with body proteins to become a complete antigen. Similar sensitivity to a wide variety of chemicals, particularly those belonging to the group of nitrogenous aromatic substances, has been observed.

The *drug reactions* represent an analogous type of sensitivity that may become manifest in an extremely variable manner. There is a growing awareness of the possibility that sensitivity to unknown foreign materials may play a role in a variety of diseases that at present remain obscure or have been classified as possibly autoimmune in nature. Particular insight into a variety of mechanisms of immunologic cell injury has been gained from the study of the sensitization caused by drugs, particularly quinidine. In some persons thrombocytopenic purpura is the result of such sensitivity; in others it is a hemolytic anemia. It now appears that this effect is primarily the fortuitous result of the physical characteristics of the antibody produced. If the antibody is of low molecular weight, it forms a type of antigen-antibody complex with quinidine that has a particular predilection for platelets; if it is of high molecular weight, complexes are formed on union with the drug that affect primarily the erythrocytes. Complement is also intimately involved in the different effects. This system illustrates the vagaries involved in the selective action against individual target organs and may be of importance in consideration of disorders of unknown origin such as idiopathic thrombocytopenic purpura and "autoimmune" hemolytic anemia. The possibility of involvement of unknown foreign antigens, particularly haptens, is not excluded.

It has become increasingly evident that many antigens gain entrance into the body via the intestinal tract through the consumption of *food*. This has been demonstrated best for bovine milk proteins, and antibodies to a wide variety of these proteins have been found in the serum of many children and some adults. Clear precipitin reactions between bovine protein fractions and these human sera are readily observed. Usually, apparently, no ill effects result from these antibodies despite the fact that some bovine products that remain antigenic continue to gain entrance into the circulation. However, this is only one example of an antibody response to food products; many others must exist that may have important implications in, for example, certain of the intestinal disorders of unknown origin such as ulcerative colitis.

A somewhat different but very important type of reaction to foreign antigens is that produced by maternal-infant incompatibility in which the foreign antigen is introduced from the fetus. *Hemolytic disease of the newborn* is the outstanding example in which the mother produces antibodies that cause destruction of the erythrocytes in the fetus or newborn. The incompatibility leading to such effects may involve Rh antigens or those of the ABO system. Analogous phenomena have been described for leukocytes and platelets. Cytolytic or cytotoxic reactions occur in which complement is usually but not always necessary to effect the cellular damage. Many other antigens are probably involved in similar maternal-infant incompatibility, but the extent to which they lead to disease is not clear at present. One outstanding example that has become manifest recently is that for genetic types of gamma globulin. A high percentage of infants who lack the genetic gamma globulin character of the mother develop antibodies. These usually appear at approximately the sixth month after delivery and remain throughout the life of the individual. Antibodies to IgA globulins appear to have special significance with regard to transfusion reactions. Most of these appear in individuals who lack all IgA in their serum and probably arise either through maternal immunization or through the administration of blood products.

Another indirect type of reaction to foreign antigens involves antigenic cross-reactions between such antigens and autologous tissues. In this situation an immune response is stimulated by a foreign antigen such as a bacterium, but since a constituent of the organism is antigenically similar to a constituent of the host the immune reaction damages the host tissue. Such cross-reactions have been identified, but the exact role of this mechanism in disease remains to be determined; the possibility exists that presumed autoimmune reactions may be initiated in certain instances by such foreign stimuli. Evidence has been obtained that material from the cell wall of hemolytic streptococci is related antigenically to human cardiac myofibers and the smooth muscle of blood vessel walls. This finding has led to the hypothesis that the cardiac damage of rheumatic fever thus results secondarily from the immune response to the streptococcal infection that preceded it.

SENSITIVITY TO AUTOLOGOUS ANTIGENS

It has become amply clear that many persons develop immunologic reactivity against autologous tissue antigens, but the mechanism by which this sensitivity arises remains obscure. In some instances it may be through the reaction to an unknown foreign organism that contains antigens, particularly polysaccharides, that cross-react with similar polysaccharides in the body tissues. In other instances it may arise through tissue breakdown with release of antigens into the circulation that are ordinarily buried and not subject to the usual tolerance mechanisms. Recent studies in laboratory animals indicate that autologous proteins such as gamma globulin readily become antigenic through slight alteration of the molecule. Antibodies are produced to new determinants not ordinarily exposed but, in addition, as immunization continues, additional antibodies may be produced that involve the native configuration of the protein and will react directly.

One of the best examples of autosensitization in human disease is that found in thyroiditis. There are many features that remain poorly understood, but the evidence is overwhelming that the various degrees of lymphadenoid change in the thyroid gland, particularly in Hashimoto's disease, involve some type of immune reaction against antigens in the thyroid gland. The fact that similar lesions can be produced in laboratory animals by immunization with autologous thyroid antigens lends strong support to such a view. Even in laboratory animals it remains unclear whether some type of cytotoxic antibody or a cellular autoimmunity plays the dominant role in the tissue injury.

In Goodpasture's disease antibodies reactive with autologous antigens of basement membranes have been demonstrated. These react primarily with renal and pulmonary tissues and have been eluted from these diseased organs obtained at autopsy. Clear evidence of a pathogenic role of the basement membrane antibodies in the renal disease of these patients has been obtained. The antibodies eluted from the human kidneys produce glomerulonephritis in monkeys after infusion. The evidence for a role in the pulmonary disease of these patients is more indirect. It has been demonstrated that antibodies eluted from the lung fix to renal glomerular basement membrane, and antibodies eluted from the kidney fix to pulmonary membranes. The origin of these antibodies remains obscure. Similar antibodies also appear to be involved in a few cases of idiopathic glomerulonephritis.

In many blood diseases antibodies occur in the serum that react with autologous cells and in some instances clearly produce disease. The cold agglutinin syndrome is perhaps the clearest from the standpoint of the effect of the abnormal antibody in producing erythrocyte destruction. Anemia, jaundice, and hemoglobinuria can all be traced directly to the action of the cold agglutinin. An "idiopathic" type of the syndrome and one associated with histiocytic lymphoma and lymphocytic lymphoma offer no clues as to the mechanism by which the cold agglutinin was produced. Another type of disease that is usually of shorter duration follows viral or mycoplasmal pneumonia. Paroxysmal cold hemoglobinuria of the Donath-Landsteiner type is closely related and usually is associated with prenatal syphilis, although many non-syphilitic cases have been reported. The much more common idiopathic, acquired hemolytic anemia of the warm antibody type presents a more obscure picture. Here the relationship of the erythrocyte damage to a variety of red blood cell antibodies is much more tentative. Only in a minority of cases can the antibodies be shown to have a definite specificity. In these instances it is directed against an Rh antigen, usually anti-e. Again no clue is available concerning the origin of these gamma globulins that react with autologous erythrocytes.

Idiopathic thrombocytopenic purpura is another disease in which circulating antibodies react with autologous cells—in this case platelets—and cause disease through the resulting cellular injury. These antibodies have proved surprisingly difficult to detect by conventional immunologic methods, but it is now clear that they are present. The role of leukocyte autoagglutinins as a cause of leukopenia has proved even more difficult to assess. Many of the antibodies reported by early workers have been shown to result from transfusions given to these patients, with the production of isoantibodies. However, most workers still believe that autoagglutinins do occur and are responsible for some cases of leukopenia.

Systemic lupus erythematosus (SLE) is probably associated with a greater variety of antibodies with autospecificity than any other condition. The best known of these are the antinuclear antibodies, certain of which are responsible for the LE cell phenomenon. Special interest has centered on the DNA antibodies because of evidence for an association with disease activity. Antibodies to native double-stranded DNA as well as antibodies specific for the single-stranded form are found in the sera of these patients. Recently antibodies to double-stranded RNA have been detected. It has become evident that antibodies to a wide spectrum of polynucleotides are uniquely present in this disease. Numerous additional antibodies to protein and carbohydrate antigens extracted from the cytoplasm as well as the nucleus of human cells have been described. Some of these appear to be responsible for various secondary manifestations of the disease as, for example, hemolytic anemia. This is associated with a positive Coombs test, suggesting the occurrence of antibodies to autologous erythrocytes. Idiopathic thrombocytopenic purpura, probably involving antiplatelet antibodies, also occurs in these patients. Abnormalities involving blood coagulation have been of special interest to investigators; antibodies to specific clotting factors appear to be involved. The origin of these many antibodies as well as others not discussed remains obscure. Some of them appear to represent a marked elevation of antibodies found at low levels in normal persons, which is compatible with the concept that in SLE a general hyperreactivity of the immune system exists. The high prevalence in females and the familial trend of the disease have not as yet been fitted into the immunologic concepts. Recent work with various strains of mice, particularly the New Zealand NZB strain, has shown that manifestations of a disease with many features resembling SLE occur in a high proportion of the animals. Most striking is the renal disease and the hemolytic anemia. This experimental model shows a marked similarity to

the human disease, and the unique antibodies to double-stranded DNA and RNA are present. Studies in these mice have suggested a significant role for secondary viral infections in potentiating various disease manifestations. Whether this also applies to the human disease remains to be proved.

The possibility has been considered that a large number of other diseases in which the cause is unknown may have as their origin some type of autoimmune mechanism. This is particularly true of rheumatoid arthritis, primarily because it is associated with uniquely high incidence and levels of an unusual group of antibodies called rheumatoid factors. These have been clearly demonstrated to be antibodies to gamma globulin and are capable of reacting with autologous gamma globulin. No evidence is available to suggest that the rheumatoid factors play a direct role in the arthritis; however, many workers think they may be indicative of an as yet undefined immunologic reaction. The fact that they are produced at least in part in the synovial tissue of the joints from local accumulation of plasma cells adds some weight to this concept. On the other hand, it has also become clear that the rheumatoid factors could develop as a response to some type of foreign organism. Antibodies to the organism after reaction with the particulate antigen or fragment thereof would form secondary anti-gamma globulins to these antigen-antibody complexes. This possibility has been strengthened by the experimental production of anti-gamma globulins in rabbits after injection of coliform organisms, as well as their appearance in human sera after various types of infection. In bacterial endocarditis, for example, the rheumatoid factors disappear after elimination of the organism with antimicrobial therapy. Similar attempts with such therapy in rheumatoid arthritis patients is without effect on the rheumatoid factors. The accumulated evidence indicates that there must be some profound immunologic stimulus present in the rheumatoid arthritis patient to sustain the rheumatoid factors at the extreme levels often observed and for the prolonged periods in which they are present. The nature of this stimulus remains unknown.

Another disorder showing profound immunologic abnormalities associated with arthritis similar to that in rheumatoid arthritis is Sjögren's syndrome. It also has been considered a possible connecting link between rheumatoid arthritis and SLE. Extreme elevation of gamma globulin similar to that found in SLE patients is observed along with many similar antinuclear and anticytoplasmic antibodies. In addition, the vast majority of these patients have rheumatoid factors, often at extreme levels. Serologically they show the findings of both rheumatoid arthritis and SLE. The lesions observed in the lacrimal, salivary, and other glands of patients with Sjögren's syndrome are highly suggestive of a local immunologic reaction. They closely resemble those observed in the thyroid gland in chronic thyroiditis, in which an immunologic alteration has been more evident.

The immunologic aspects of pernicious anemia are of considerable interest. Antibodies to intrinsic factor have been demonstrated in a large number of cases, and antibodies to the parietal cells of the gastric mucosa are frequently found. These have been revealed by a variety of classic immunologic procedures. In addition, the intrinsic factor antibody inhibits labeled B_{12} absorption in tests in vivo. Many of the antibodies appear to be autoantibodies and are found in untreated cases; others appear to represent antibodies to hog intrinsic factor as a result of therapy. A direct role in the pathogenesis of the disease has not been established, but they at least are important in certain therapeutic considerations.

The serum of patients with myasthenia gravis contains a number of unusual antibodies directed at muscle constituents. These have been demonstrated primarily by fluorescent antibody techniques, a procedure that has proved unusually difficult when dealing with muscle sections. However, precipitating and complement-fixing antibodies have also been found. No direct role for these antibodies in the disease has been demonstrated, but they certainly raise the possibility of an immunologic mechanism. The frequent association of thymic disease with myasthenia gravis is well documented and adds further weight to a possible immune basis for this disease. One of the most important developments in immunology in recent years is the recognition of the profound role of the thymus gland in the development of immunity. It is also known that some infants born of myasthenic mothers have a transient myasthenic syndrome that could be due to placental transfer of antibody.

Antibodies with autospecificity of various types have been found in a variety of other diseases. In ulcerative colitis, antibodies to colon tissue and cellular immunity to colon cells have been described. Patients with liver disease show a wide variety of antibodies to autologous cell constituents. Antibodies reactive with mitochondria are of special interest because of their specific occurrence in primary biliary cirrhosis. They are of diagnostic value, but a pathogenic role remains to be demonstrated. Pancreas antibodies have been described in patients with pancreatitis, and adrenal antibodies in patients with Addison's disease. In all these instances the major possibility that these represent antibodies secondary to tissue breakdown in the disease has not been excluded. As stressed earlier, autoantibodies are far more common than had previously been thought, and any assessment of an injurious role in a specific disease is extremely difficult.

IMMUNE COMPLEX DISEASE

When artificially made antigen-antibody complexes are injected into laboratory animals, they are deposited in a number of organs with resultant tissue injury. By far the most sensitive organ is the kidney, and acute and chronic renal disease has been produced in a number of species by this procedure. The complexes are trapped in the glomeruli and form lumpy deposits along the glomerular basement membrane. These have distinct histologic characteristics by electron microscopy and by fluorescent antibody staining techniques. In human glomerulonephritis similar deposits are frequently observed when these same procedures are utilized. In systemic lupus erythematosus such deposits in the glomeruli are particularly striking, and a large accumulation of additional evidence for antigen-antibody complex mediated renal injury is available.

Extensive studies in a number of different laboratories have demonstrated that DNA-anti-DNA complexes represent one type involved in SLE. Antibodies to DNA aroused considerable interest when they were first described in SLE approximately 17 years ago. However, they were relegated to the position of scientific curiosi-ties, and it has only been recently that their harmful potential has been realized. Antibodies to double-stranded DNA have special significance because double-stranded DNA antigens can appear in the circulation as a result of tissue breakdown; antigen-antibody complexes are formed with fixation of complement and deposition in the most vulnerable organ, the kidney. Elution of antibody from isolated glomeruli of diseased kidneys has proved to be a very effective technique for the detection of antibodies deposited in the kidney. DNA antibody has been found in such eluates at specific concentrations as high as 1000 times those in the serum. DNA antigen has also been demonstrated in the granular deposits observed in the glomeruli. Other, more indirect evidence such as the close clinical relationship among the appearance of DNA antibodies, serum complement depression, and exacerbations of disease has also aided in establishing the significance of the DNA system. Further studies are required to determine the relevance of the many other antibodies in the serum of these patients; some of these, if they can encounter specific antigen, may be involved as well.

Another type of renal disease in which evidence for immune complexes is rapidly accumulating is that associated with various types of drugs. Some of these may present a picture very analogous to that of serum sickness; in others, chronic drug administration may lead to a slowly progressive glomerulonephritis. The latter situation is well illustrated in the case of penicillamine. Numerous instances of nephritis have been reported after long-term administration of this material for the treatment of cystinuria, Wilson's disease, or rheumatoid arthritis. Granular deposits of gamma globulin and complement along the glomerular basement membrane are readily visualized in fluorescent antibody studies which closely resemble those produced in experimental animals by injection of complexes.

The presence of granular and "lumpy" deposits of gamma globulin and complement detected by fluorescent antibody techniques may be well visualized in renal biopsy specimens and have been found in a variety of different conditions such as malaria, bacterial endocarditis, and thyroiditis. Cases of chronic glomerulonephritis of unknown cause frequently show such a pattern. However, supporting evidence for specific antigen-antibody complexes is as yet unavailable for most of these. In poststreptococcal nephritis similar characteristics of complex-induced nephritis are present, and suggestive evidence for streptococcal antigens in the deposits has been obtained.

Eluates obtained from glomeruli isolated at autopsy from kidneys of patients who had subacute and chronic glomerulonephritis have in a number of instances shown high concentrations of gamma globulin. This appears to represent specific antibody, but its nature remains a mystery. The search is on in a number of laboratories for specific antigens that might react with such gamma globulin. Particular attention is being paid to various human viruses, because recent work in laboratory animals has demonstrated complexes of virus and antibody in the kidneys of mice. The task is a difficult one, however, and human tissue antigens, bacterial antigens, and even unknown drugs may be equally reasonable candidates. The possibility also seems likely that multiple antigen-antibody systems are involved in the different cases of idiopathic glomerulonephritis.

Another type of antigen-antibody complex that appears to be involved in some types of renal disease is that composed of IgG globulin and anti-IgG globulin. Such complexes are widely distributed in human sera and reach unusual levels in rheumatoid arthritis. Usually these are quite soluble, but in some patients they precipitate out in the cold as mixed cryoglobulins. Patients with such mixed cryoglobulins show a rather ill-defined clinical syndrome, but renal lesions are common. The components of such complexes along with complement have been identified in the glomeruli of these patients.

Evidence has been obtained that injury to circulating cells, particularly platelets, may be mediated by antigen-antibody complexes. A number of drug-induced thrombocytopenias fall into this category. Particular interest is currently centered on similar mechanisms in the joint inflammation of SLE and rheumatoid arthritis. Gamma globulin complexes are well known in the latter, and high concentrations have been observed in joint fluid, in which they appear to be involved in local complement depletion. Much work remains before a direct cause-and-effect relationship can be established. Lack of an adequate experimental model similar to those available for immunologic renal injury has hampered progress in this field.

Eisen, H. N.: Immunology. *In* Davis, B. D., Dulbecco, R., Eisen, H. N., Ginsberg, H. S., and Wood, W. B., Jr. (eds.): Microbiology. New York, Harper & Row, 1973, pp. 349–595.
Moller, G. (ed.): T and B lymphocytes in humans. Transplant. Rev., 16:3, 1973.
Natvig, J. B., and Kunkel, H. G.: Human immunoglobulins: Classes, subclasses, genetic variants and idiotypes. *In* Dixon, F. J., and Kunkel, H. G. (eds.): Advances in Immunology, Vol. 16. New York, Academic Press, 1973.
Robinson, R. R. (ed.): Immunological aspects of renal disease. Kidney, 3:55, 1973.
Spiegelberg, H. L.: Biological activities of immunoglobulins of different classes and subclasses. *In* Dixon, F. J., and Kunkel, H. G. (eds.): Advances in Immunology, Vol. 19. New York, Academic Press, 1974.

THE PRIMARY IMMUNODEFICIENCY DISEASES

Robert A. Good

61. INTRODUCTION

Knowledge of the lymphoid cells, their functions, and their organization into two separate major immunity systems has advanced rapidly in recent years. Current views are summarized in Table 1. Current understanding of the immunity functions has derived in consider-

able measure from study of the primary immunodeficiencies of man. In turn, new knowledge and understanding of the relation of structure to function in the lymphoid system have made possible better definition of the several primary immunodeficiencies. A continuing interplay between clinical analysis and advancing basic understanding of immunity and the immunologic apparatus represents a fine model of how progress in medicine can proceed most rapidly to the maximal benefit of man. Consequently, study of the primary immunodeficiencies has had importance to medicine in recent years far beyond the numerical frequency of patients who suffer from these relatively infrequent diseases.

In Table 2 is a listing of those diseases currently recognized by a WHO expert panel as the major primary immunodeficiencies of man. Included in Table 2, as well, is an effort to analyze each of the diseases in terms of its genetic basis and in terms of the types of cells primarily involved in the deficiency. Such an analysis must be recognized as ephemeral because of the rapidity of development of our knowledge and because rapid changes in understanding continue. Nevertheless, for the present these several diseases can be usefully viewed in light of this classification.

62. X-LINKED INFANTILE AGAMMAGLOBULINEMIA

Soon after Bruton initially described agammaglobulinemia in an eight-year-old boy, groups of patients, including multiple cases in several families, were studied in Boston, Minneapolis, and New York. From these studies, one form of agammaglobulinemia could be clearly established as being of sex-linked nature. This form has been called the Bruton type of agammaglobulinemia in recognition of the monumental contribution of the pediatrician who discovered the first of the primary immunodeficiencies and associated disease with absence of gamma globulin in the blood. Bruton's discovery launched a period in which immunology has been maximally influenced by the "experiments of nature" represented by the several forms of primary immunodeficiency.

X-linked agammaglobulinemia is a disease in which fully developed B lymphocytes and plasma cells are absent from blood and blood-forming tissues. Production of immunoglobulins and synthesis and secretion of antibodies are grossly deficient or lacking altogether. Figure 1 represents a characteristic immunoelectrophoretic pattern comparing normal with agammaglobulinemic patients. Figure 2 compares an antigen-stimulated lymph

TABLE 1.   The Cellular Basis of Immune Responses

T cell system:	+PHA or Con-A† →	Blast cells	Cell-mediated immunity
Thymus-dependent T lymphocytes*	——————→	Killer cells (e.g., graft rejection)	
	+antigen →	Soluble lymphocyte factors	
B cell system:	+antigen →	Plasma cell line	Humoral antibody synthesis
Thymus-independent, "bursa-equivalent" B lymphocytes			

*There is evidence that T cells plus antigen can cooperate with B cells to produce antibody.
†Phytohemagglutinin or concanavallin.

TABLE 2

Type	Suggested Cellular Defects			Inheritance		
	B Cells		T Cells		Autosomal	
	(a)*	(b)†		X-linked	Recessive	Other§
X-linked agammaglobulinemia	X	(X)‡		X		
Thymic hypoplasia			X			X
Severe combined immunodeficiency	X	(X)	X	X	X	X
With dysostosis	X	?	X		X	
With adenosine deaminase deficiency	X		X		X	
With generalized hematopoietic hypoplasia	X		X		X	
Selective Ig deficiency						
IgA	?	X	(X)			X
Others		?				X
X-linked immunodeficiencies with increased IgM		X		X		
Immunodeficiency with ataxia telangiectasia		X	X		X?	
Immunodeficiency with thrombocytopenia and eczema (Wiskott-Aldrich syndrome)			X	X		
Immunodeficiency with thymoma	X*		X			X
Immunodeficiency with normo- or hypergammaglobulinemia	X	X	(X)			X
Transient hypogammaglobulinemia of infancy		X				X
Varied immunodeficiencies (largely unclassified and common)	X	X	(X)		(X)	X

*Absent or very low.
†Easily detectable or increased.
‡Some cases with circulation B-lymphocytes without detectable surface Ig have been found.
§Implies multifactorial or unknown genetic basis or no genetic basis.

node from a normal person (A) and a stimulated node from an eight-year-old agammaglobulinemic child (B). Absence of germinal centers and absence of plasma cells characterize the node of the agammaglobulinemic patient. Plasma cells are not found anywhere in the body. Even the lamina propria of the intestinal tract and exudates of chronic inflammatory processes such as bronchiectasis are devoid of plasma cells in these patients.

Clinically, children with X-linked agammaglobulinemia are normal at birth, but during the second half of the first year of life they begin to have infections with the encapsulated, virulent pathogens such as pneumococci, *Hemophilus influenzae,* and *Pseudomonas aeruginosa.* Infections in these children usually respond well to appropriate drug therapy; but because of lack of humoral immunity, resistance to these infections is minimal. Untreated, the bacterial infections spread rapidly, and recurrent episodes of pneumonia, otitis, sinusitis, dermatitis, meningitis, and osteomyelitis are characteristic. By contrast, these patients seem able to resist well many other infections such as tuberculosis, histoplasmosis, and fungal and viral infections. Herpes, vaccinia, chickenpox, measles, paralytic poliomyelitis, and hepatitis, however, are unusually frequent in these children. Leukemia also occurs with inordinate frequency in these children.

Even though immunoglobulins are virtually absent in serum and antibody synthesis is minimal or absent altogether, cell-mediated immunities, including delayed and contact allergies, are normal. Skin allograft rejection occurs with nearly normal vigor. Specific delayed allergic reactions can be transferred from the agammaglobulinemic child to an immunologically normal person, using large numbers of peripheral blood lymphocytes. Modern techniques for studying the peripheral blood lymphocytes reveal that X-linked agammaglobulinemia may be heterogeneous. The majority of patients with this disease are completely lacking B lymphocytes, as defined by the presence of readily demonstrable immunoglobulins at the cell surface. In these patients T cells are somewhat increased in number, and one finds in the blood a population of lymphocytes whose exact nature is not absolutely clear. The latter may possess receptors for the third component of complement and also receptors for the Fc portion of the IgG molecule. Whether they are incompletely developed B lymphocytes or a separate lymphoid cell remains to be determined.

Diagnosis is established by analysis of the immunoelectrophoretic pattern of serum and by quantitation of each of the several immunoglobulins, using the Manchini radioimmunodiffusion or other suitable immunochemical analyses. IgM, IgA, IgD, and IgE are regularly

Figure 1. Normal immunoelectrophoretic pattern (above) compared with immunoelectrophoretic pattern from a patient with X-linked infantile agammaglobulinemia. Note absence of demonstrable IgM, IgA, and IgG on the immunoelectrophoretic pattern.

Figure 2. Comparison of normal lymph node *(A)* and lymph node of patient with X-linked infantile agammaglobulinemia *(B)* after antigenic stimulation. Note abundant germinal center formation in the normal node and absence of germinal centers in the stimulated node from the agammaglobulinemic patient.

absent, and IgG is absent or present in extremely low concentrations, 100- to 1000-fold less than that of normal persons.

Treatment involves early detection and intensive and specific treatment of the bacterial infections, as well as prophylaxis using gamma globulin concentrates injected intramuscularly at frequent intervals. We have found 0.3 ml of 16 per cent gamma globulin solution given intramuscularly every two weeks to be a good regimen with which to start prophylactic management. Exudative enteropathy is a common complication and is often due to infestation with *Giardia lamblia.* This infection and the exudative enteropathy can be treated specifically with Flagyl. The usual immunizations may be given, although no antibodies will be formed. Although vaccinia has been tolerated, we recommend that no live virus vaccines be used in any patient with primary or secondary immunodeficiency disease.

63. DiGEORGE'S SYNDROME

Counterpart to patients with X-linked agammaglobulinemia are those born without a thymus who as a consequence lack T lymphocytes in their blood and tissues. Such patients also frequently have no parathyroids. Their ears are often of abnormal appearance, and they have a characteristic facies with prominent forehead and bowed mouth. Frequently they also have abnormalities of the first portions of the great vessels and the outflow tract from the heart. Absence of thymus is not always complete. Absence of thymic shadow on chest roentgenograms and absence of T lymphocytes and T lymphocyte functions on immunologic analysis are characteristic. The stimulated lymph nodes show well developed far cortical areas, and in some cases germinal centers are present. In other cases, germinal centers have been deficient. In all instances, the thymic dependent lymphoid areas are very grossly depleted. Plasma cells are present and may be present in normal numbers in the lymphoid tissues. Absence of thymus and T cells

may be incomplete. Treatment of the endocrinopathy requires appropriate use of vitamin D and sterol therapy to raise serum calcium level. The immunodeficiency has now been repeatedly treated successfully, using transplantation of thymus obtained from allogeneic embryos. This form of treatment has in several instances seemed to correct completely the deficiency of T cells and the defects of immunologic functions. Failure of thymus and T cell development of nude mice represents an autosomal recessive defect that seems to be an experimental counterpart of DiGeorge's syndrome. The cause of the human disease is unclear, and a genetic basis has not yet been established for this rare disease. Selective deficiency of thymic and T lymphocyte development without the associated hypoparathyroid or great vessel anomalies has been called Nezelof's syndrome. This disease has also apparently been treated successfully by allotransplantation of fetal thymus.

64. SEVERE COMBINED IMMUNODEFICIENCIES (SCID, Swiss Type Immunodeficiency)

Several different genetically determined primary immunodeficiency diseases in which both T and B lymphocyte systems fail to develop normally have now been described. Each of these diseases is genetically determined. Forms with either autosomal recessive or X-linked inheritance have been defined. Infants with each of these distinct forms of severe combined immunodeficiency disease have very gross deficiencies of both T and B immunity systems. Lymphocyte numbers, generally under 1000 per cubic millimeter, are low but not absent from blood. Both T and B cells are either missing or very much reduced. Levels of all classes of immunoglobulin are low.

The thymus, lymph nodes, and spleen are small and poorly developed. Indeed, these lymphoid organs are often almost completely devoid of lymphoid cells. Antibody production and development of cell-mediated immunities is extremely deficient or absent, and in vitro lymphocyte responses to lectins such as PHA, concanavallin A, and pokeweed mitogen fail to occur. In some of these children, responses of blood leukocytes to stimulation with allogeneic cells have been noted.

If these patients are not treated, they regularly succumb early in life to any of many different forms of infection, i.e., *Pneumocystis carinii*, cytomegalovirus, other viruses, fungi, or low- or high-grade bacterial pathogens. Live virus immunization often leads to lethal infections. Attempts to help these children, or children with DiGeorge's syndrome, by blood transfusion often leads to death from fulminating graft-versus-host disease, because these patients cannot defend themselves against the immunologically competent lymphocytes invariably present in whole blood. If blood or blood products must be given, they should be given only after irradiation of well oxygenated blood with 3000 R or after freezing and centrifugation.

Since both B and T immunity systems are lacking in these children, attempts to correct the immunodeficiency by transplantation of bone marrow have been made. In more than 30 instances, marrow transplantation from an appropriately matched donor has made possible apparently complete restoration of both T and B immunity systems in these children. Whenever definitive markers have been available, it has been possible to establish that the new immunity systems in such marrow-reconstituted children have been derived from the bone marrow cells of the donor. For successful marrow transplantation, a sibling donor selected by HL-A tissue typing and mixed leukocyte culture matching has generally been necessary.

More recently, however, in absence of a matched sibling, a satisfactory matching of an uncle by mixed leukocyte reaction with an SCID child has permitted reconstitution of immunity function. Recently techniques have been developed which promise sufficient matching, even among unrelated persons, to permit reconstitution of the two missing immunity systems in such patients by marrow transplantation with a donor selected from the general population. Definitive diagnosis and immunologic reconstitution of the rare children with this disease are highly technical undertakings that should be done only by those who specialize in this therapeutic approach.

65. SEVERE COMBINED IMMUNODEFICIENCIES WITH ADENOSINE DEAMINASE DEFICIENCY

An autosomal recessive genetically determined disease similar to the severe combined immunodeficiency disorders described in Ch. 64 has recently been found to be associated with absence of adenosine deaminase (ADA) in red blood cells, lymphoid cells, and other cells of the body. Clinical manifestations, immunodeficiencies, cellular defects, and susceptibility to infection in this disease are all similar to those occurring in the X-linked and autosomal recessive forms of SCID, except that, quantitatively, the functional and cellular defects seem more variable in this disease. In the patients with

SCID and adenosine deaminase deficiency, however, some lymphoid tissue development does occur and the thymus contains Hassall's corpuscles and has characteristics of an involuted rather than an underdeveloped thymus. Two patients with ADA deficiency and SCID have now been reconstituted by marrow transplantation.

The relationship between ADA deficiency and this form of severe combined immunodeficiency is not yet clear, but it is of great interest that at least one primary immunodeficiency disease can now be associated with an inherited inability to produce an enzyme—adenosine deaminase. Whether the immunodeficiency is due to some toxic product consequent to the enzyme deficiency or whether this enzyme is essential in some crucial step in development of the lymphoid cells remains to be determined. When the immunodeficiency associated with ADA deficiency is corrected by marrow transplantation, the lymphoid cells possess normal amounts of adenosine deaminase, but the red cells continue to lack the enzyme completely.

66. THYMOMA WITH IMMUNODEFICIENCY

More than 50 patients have been studied in which broadly based immunodeficiency, thymoma, and hypogammaglobulinemia have been associated. The first such case provoked the extensive laboratory inquiry which established the major role played by the thymus in developmental immunobiology. Both cellular and humoral immunity functions, and both T and B cell numbers are deficient. Patients are susceptible to a broad range of bacterial, viral, and fungal infections. In one such instance encountered by Siegal et al., normal serum possessed a factor that permitted the patient's lymphoid cells to develop in vitro into B lymphocytes with easily demonstrable surface immunoglobulin. This factor was absent from the blood or serum of the patient with the thymoma-agammaglobulinemia syndrome. Anemia caused by insufficient generation of red blood cells may sometimes be associated. Removal of the thymus tumor which is composed primarily of nonlymphoid spindle-shaped stromal epithelial cells does not correct the immunodeficiency.

67. COMMON VARIABLE IMMUNODEFICIENCY

Among the most frequent forms of primary immunodeficiency disease is that presently called the common variable immunodeficiency. This rather cumbersome term is used as temporary nomenclature for what may indeed be several different diseases. However, in this form the immunodeficiency is variable from time to time in the same patient and from patient to patient in the same family. Inheritance may be autosomal recessive or autosomal dominant. In still other patients the disease is sporadic, and because of its onset later in life has been thought to be acquired. The initial agammaglobulinemic patient described by Bruton probably would now be classified with this group.

Immunodeficiency in these patients is associated with decreased concentrations of all or several immunoglobulins. Antibody production is feeble, and even cell-mediated immunity responses may be decreased. Pneumonia, sinusitis, otitis media, gastrointestinal infection and malfunction, and *Giardia lamblia* infestation are common concomitants. A wide variety of autoimmune phenomena and autoimmune diseases have been frequently encountered. Pernicious anemia, histaminefast achlorhydria, and gastric cancer occur with high frequency early in life in patients with this syndrome.

The occurrence in these patients of much autoimmunity, autoimmune disease, e.g., Coombs-positive hemolytic anemia, autoimmune thrombocytopenic purpura, pernicious anemia, and many collagen-vascular or mesenchymal diseases, including rheumatoid arthritis and vasculitis, has represented a set of fascinating but perplexing relationships. Sprue-like syndrome with or without giardiasis is frequent.

Diagnosis is made by history of frequent and persistent infections, immunoelectrophoretic pattern, and quantitation of each of the immunoglobulin classes by radial immunodiffusion. Enumeration of T and B lymphocytes is of interest because, in spite of deficiencies in producing immunoglobulins, most of these patients have normal or only slightly reduced numbers of B lymphocytes in the circulating blood. Plasma cells are deficient in the lymphoid tissue in direct proportion to the deficits of antibody production and immunoglobulin levels. In patients possessing normal or increased amounts of IgM who have low levels of IgG and IgA, lymph nodes, spleen, and intestinal lymphatic tissue may be grossly enlarged. Germinal centers may be extraordinarily hypertrophied, suggesting the erroneous diagnosis of follicular lymphoma.

Treatment, as in other forms of primary immunodeficiency, involves early recognition and specific antimicrobial therapy of the frequent bacterial infections. Careful diagnosis and specific treatment of *Giardia lamblia* and fungus infections are also important. Prophylactic administration of gamma globulin concentrates in very large doses, 0.6 ml per kilogram every three to four weeks, is helpful in reducing the frequency of infections in some patients. However, in these patients even more than in patients with Bruton's X-linked infantile agammaglobulinemia, prophylaxis with currently available preparations of gamma globulin is inadequate. More satisfactory prophylaxis has been achieved, using frequent infusions of plasma from carefully selected donors free of history of hepatitis and free of both Australia antigen and antibody to Au antigen. The latter precaution is extremely important, because chronic progressive hepatitis has been an especially difficult and sometimes lethal consequence of administration of blood products to these patients. What is needed are adequate preparations of gamma globulin concentrates that are suitable for intravenous administration.

In addition to the more specific forms of therapy, prophylactic regimens such as those introduced by Mathews for the ideal pulmonary toilet are helpful. Postural and positional pulmonic drainage, breathing exercises, and inhalation therapy have all been helpful in treating and apparently in preventing pulmonary disease in these patients. The autoimmune diseases should be treated as they are in persons of greater immunologic vigor, but with cognizance of the facts that the patients are immunologically compromised and that large doses of adrenal steroids, immunosuppressive agents, and splenectomy can further debilitate the bodily defense.

68. ISOLATED ABSENCE OF IMMUNOGLOBULINS—SELECTIVE DEFICIENCY OF IgA

Selected absence of any of the immunoglobulin classes or subclasses can occur, and such selective deficiencies have already been described for several, e.g., selective absence of IgG 2. However, none of the other immunoglobulins are so frequently lacking from blood as is IgA. The frequency of selective absence of IgA ranges from 1/700 to 1/3000, according to studies of blood bank donors from several parts of the world. Many patients lacking IgA seem to be quite healthy, but a high proportion have severe atopy, autoimmune phenomena, and autoimmune diseases. Respiratory disease is frequent, especially in those patients who possess IgE. Gastrointestinal disease is also frequent, and severe progressive sprue has been reported. Recently Soothill and his associates have observed that classic atopy caused by production of antibody of IgE class occurs especially when the IgA system is slow to develop. One possible basis for the increased frequency of autoimmune phenomena and disease with deficiency of IgA is that the dimeric form of IgA antibodies is transferred across the epithelial barrier onto the gut surface from the site of production in the lamina propria of the gastrointestinal tract. This antibody system normally provides a barrier to absorption of foreign proteins and other antigens, as has recently been shown by Walker and Isselbacher. Consequently, when the local immunity system is lacking or deficient, antigens that are cross-reactive with host constituents can be absorbed and provide excessive stimulation of the systemic immunity systems. This stimulation leads to production of antibodies and immune cells that in some instances cross-react with host constituents, producing autoimmune phenomena and autoimmune disease. Patients lacking IgA frequently develop antibodies to IgA, serum proteins of the bovidae, and many other antigens in food and flora in amounts far in excess of those produced by normal persons. Most patients who fail to produce IgA antibody have in their circulation at least normal numbers of B lymphocytes that produce and have at their surface IgA molecules. For reasons currently poorly understood, these cells do not differentiate to IgA-secreting plasma cells. If these cells could be induced to develop to B cells capable of secreting IgA, these patients might be much improved. Recently Wu et al., using pokeweed mitogen, and Waldmann et al., using blast forms of putative T lymphocytes obtained from patients with Sézary's syndrome (presumably T-cell leukemia), have induced such differentiation of these IgA-producing to IgA-secreting B cells.

69. IMMUNODEFICIENCY DISEASES WITH ATAXIA TELANGIECTASIA AND WISKOTT-ALDRICH SYNDROME

Immunodeficiency diseases also accompany the Wiskott-Aldrich and ataxia telangiectasia syndromes. The former is a disorder of X-linked inheritance that is featured by a clinical triad, including eczema, thrombocytopenic purpura, and increased susceptibility to infection. The immunodeficiency in this syndrome is accompanied by low levels of IgM. These patients form antibody poorly to certain antigens, especially polysaccharide and small protein antigens, and show a progressive deficiency of T cell numbers and functions. The basic genetic fault is unknown, but the patients frequently succumb to infection with any of several viruses, bacteria, or fungi. Nearly 10 per cent of patients with the Wiskott-Aldrich syndrome die of cancer. Usually, but not always, the cancer takes the form of lymphoreticular sarcoma. Bleeding, especially accompanying infection, and intracranial bleeding are also frequent causes of death in these children. Treatment has thus far been unsatisfactory, but platelet transfusions and plasma infusions from selected donors have been helpful in some instances. Patients with *ataxia telangiectasia* also reflect a familial and probably autosomal recessive genetically determined clinical triad of progressive cerebellar ataxia, cutaneous telangiectases, and immunodeficiency. In this disease the thymus fails to develop normally and retains an embryonic appearance. T lymphocytes and T cell functions are regularly grossly deficient, and some 70 to 80 per cent of the patients lack IgA. IgE also is frequently absent from the circulation both in ataxia patients and in healthy family members. These patients are troubled with frequent sinopulmonary infections which seem to relate to the deficiency of IgA but not clearly to the deficiency of IgE.

More than 10 per cent of the patients with ataxia telangiectasia thus far studied have developed malignancies. The malignancies reported are predominantly reticulum cell sarcomas, lymphosarcomas, leukemias, and gastrointestinal cancers. Waldmann recently found that alpha-fetoprotein is present in inordinately high concentration in a majority of patients with ataxia telangiectasia (see also Ch. 446).

70. OTHER PRIMARY IMMUNODEFICIENCIES

Many other forms of immunodeficiency have been discovered in recent years, and the diseases and syndromes associated with them are only now being clarified. For example, selective deficiencies of the components of the complement system are associated with serious immunodeficiency in very high frequency. These deficiencies render the patients susceptible to infection, collagenvascular diseases, overwhelming pneumonia, or skin and bowel infections, depending on which complement component is lacking. Ongoing studies will define these associations more clearly. It seems fair to predict, however, that deficiencies of each of the specific proteins involved in the defenses of the body will occur and that diseases have been or will be associated with these deficiencies. Such deficiencies will include deficiencies of each immunoglobulin class or subclass, deficiencies of essential lymphokines, complement components, and components of the major effector processes. The latter already include diseases in which malfunction or deficiencies of development of granulocytes occur, as in congenital neutropenia or chronic granulomatous disease. Deficiencies or abnormal function of monocytes or

other cells and molecular elements involved in bodily defense are being defined. Each disease will represent an experiment of nature capable of teaching us a new lesson about how the immunity system functions. Each will require treatment, which will be made possible by the advancing knowledge of immunity functions and their organization and development. It is thus to be anticipated that the constructive interplay between clinic and laboratory will continue to produce new knowledge and to test our advancing understanding of the immunologic systems in the bodily defense.

Bach, F. H., and Good, R. A. (eds.): Clinical Immunobiology, Vol. 1. New York, Academic Press, 1972.

Bach, F. H., and Good, R. A. (eds.): Clinical Immunobiology, Vol. 2. New York, Academic Press, Inc., 1972.

Bergsma, D., Good, R. A., and Finstad, J. (eds.): Immunodeficiency in Man and Animals. Stamford, Conn., Sinauer Press, 1974 (in press).

Boder, E., and Sedgwick, R. P.: Ataxia-telangiectasia. *In* Goldensohn, E., and Appel, S. (eds.): Cellular and Molecular Bases of Neurological Disease. Philadelphia, Lea & Febiger, 1973.

Bruton, O. C.: Pediatrics, 9:722, 1952.

Cooper, M. D., Faulk, W. P., Fudenberg, H. H., Good, R. A., Hitzig, W., Kunkel, H. G., Roitt, I. M., Rosen, F. S., Seligman, M., Soothill, J. F., and Wedgwood, R. H.: Meeting report of the Second International Workshop on Primary Immunodeficiency Diseases in Man. St. Petersburg, Florida, February 1973. Clin. Immunol. Immunopath., 2:416, 1974.

DiGeorge, A. M.: Congenital absence of the thymus and its immunologic consequences. *In* Good, R. A., and Bergsma, D. (eds.): Immunologic Deficiency Diseases in Man. New York, The National Foundation Press, 1968, pp. 116–121.

DiGeorge, A. M.: Discussion of paper by M. D. Cooper et al. J. Pediatr., 67:907, 1965.

Dupont, B., Anderson, V., Ernst, P., Faber, V., Good, R. A., Hansen, G. S., Henriksen, K., Juhl, F., Killmann, S. A., Koch, C., Muller-Berart, N., Park, B. H., Svejgaard, A., Thomsen, M., and Wiik, A.: Immunological reconstitution in severe combined immunodeficiency with HI-A incompatible bone marrow graft. Donor selection by mixed lymphocyte culture. Transplant. Proc., 5:905, 1973.

Fudenberg, H., Good, R. A., Goodman, H. C., Hitzig, W., Kunkel, H. G., Roitt, I. M., Rosen, F. S., Rowe, D. S., Seligman, M., and Soothill, J. R.: Primary immunodeficiencies. Report of a World Health Organization Committee. Pediatrics, 47:927, 1971.

Gitlin, D., Janeway, C. A., Apt, L., and Craig, J. M.: *In* Lawrence, H. S. (ed.): Cellular and Humoral Aspects of the Hypersensitive States. New York, Harper & Row, 1959, p. 375.

Good, R. A.: Studies on agammaglobulinemia II. Failure of plasma cell formation in bone marrow and lymph nodes of patients with agammaglobulinemia. J. Lab. Clin. Med., 46:167, 1955.

Good, R. A.: Morphological basis of the immune response and hypersensitivity. *In* Felton, H., et al.: Host Parasite Relationships in Living Cells. Springfield, Ill., Charles C Thomas, 1957, pp. 68–161.

Good, R. A.: Immunodeficiency in developmental perspective. Harvey Lecture Series, 1972. New York, Academic Press, 1973, Vol. 67, pp. 1–107.

Good, R. A., and Bach, H. F.: Bone marrow and thymus transplants: Cellular engineering to correct primary immunodeficiency. *In* Good, R. A., and Bach, F. H. (eds.): Clinical Immunobiology, Vol. 2. New York, Academic Press, 1974, pp. 63–114.

Good, R. A., and Bergsma, D.: Immunologic Deficiency Diseases in Man. Birth Defects Original Article Series, Vol. 4. New York, The National Foundation Press, 1968.

Good, R. A., and Zak, S. J.: Disturbances in gamma globulin synthesis as experiments of nature. Pediatrics, 18:109, 1956.

Janeway, C. A., and Rosen, F. S.: The gamma globulins. IV. Therapeutic uses of gamma globulin. N. Engl. J. Med., 275:826, 1966.

Lawton, A. R., Wu, L. Y. F., and Cooper, M. D.: The cellular basis of IgA deficiency in humans. Proc. International Symposium on the Immunoglobulin A System. October 23–25, 1973 (in press).

Rosen, F. S., and Janeway, C. A.: The gamma globulins. III. The antibody deficiency syndromes. N. Engl. J. Med., 275:709, 769, 1966.

Soothill, J. F.: Interactions in immunodeficiency. *In* Immunodeficiency in Man and Animals. Stamford, Conn., Sinauer Press, 1974 (in press).

Waldmann, T. A., Broder, S., Suer, M., and Blackman, M.: Regulation of synthesis of immunoglobulins. Proceedings, Sixth Symposium on Plasma Proteins (L. Donato [ed.]). New York, Elsevier Publishing Company, 1974 (in press).

Walker, W. A., Isselbacher, K. J., and Bloch, K. G.: Intestinal uptake of macromolecules: Effect of oral immunization. Science, 177:608, 1972.

71. SERUM SICKNESS

Fred S. Kantor

Definition. Serum sickness is a disease characterized by fever, arthralgia, skin eruptions, and edema which appears after injection of a foreign serum or serum proteins and is dependent upon an immune response of the patient to the injected serum. Hypersensitivity reactions to a variety of drugs may produce an identical illness.

Etiology. With the advent of antimicrobial therapy, the use of serum for the treatment of microbial diseases has declined markedly; the most common cause for "serum sickness" at present is not serum itself but exogenously administered drugs, particularly the antimicrobials. Serum therapy is still used primarily for the neutralization of bacterial toxins such as tetanus and botulinus toxins and also in the form of rabies antiserum.

The incidence and severity of the disease are clearly related to the type of serum preparation as well as to the amount administered. Of patients given prophylactic tetanus antitoxin prepared in horses, approximately 2 to 5 per cent will develop symptoms of serum sickness. The figure is considerably higher for those patients receiving equine rabies antiserum; approximately 16 per cent of these patients develop serum sickness. In general, there is an increasing incidence and severity through childhood, adolescence, and adulthood. Reactions in children are quite mild, lasting from one to four days, whereas in patients over the age of 15, the disease is more frequent and more severe.

Different methods of production of various equine antisera may have a profound effect upon the serum sickness liability of the product. Most tetanus antitoxin preparations involve a peptic digestion which does not impair antitoxic properties while hydrolyzing many of the proteins present in the serum. In contrast, antirabies antiserum is not subjected to peptic digestion because of the great loss of antibody encountered with the enzymatic treatment. The most important factor concerned with the development of serum sickness is the total amount of serum administered. Recommended doses of tetanus antitoxin and rabies antisera vary considerably from time to time; from 5 to 10 ml of tetanus antitoxin may produce serum sickness in 5 to 10 per cent of patients, whereas 80 ml will almost always result in illness. Age and dose relationships in serum sickness resulting from drugs are not as clear cut as with serum or serum proteins. In most cases the drug by itself is not capable of inducing the disease and must combine with a protein of the patient to form a complete antigen or immunogen. In such a situation the genetic potential of the patient of forming complete antigens and producing antibodies to them must be considered in addition to the patient's age and the dose and duration of the drug given.

Mechanism. The essential basis of serum sickness is antigen-antibody interaction. A blood level of circulating foreign protein can be measured in patients shortly after beginning serum treatment. In the early stages the administered protein is catabolized in a manner similar to that seen in the animal from which it came. This is the latent period and usually lasts from four to ten days, during which time the patient develops an immune response that is evidenced by the appearance of antibody directed against the injected protein. As soon as antibody appears, it combines with circulating foreign protein antigen to form soluble complexes. These complexes have a varied fate, depending upon their nature and the ratio of antigen to antibody in the complex. Experimental studies, in the rabbit primarily, have shown a deposition of antigen-antibody complexes beneath the endothelium of blood vessels and within the basement membrane of these vessels. Complexes containing antibodies of the IgM or the IgG classes may initiate fixation and activation of the complement sequence. With localization of complement-containing complexes in the walls of blood vessels, polymorphonuclear leukocytes are attracted to the site and appear to injure the vessel by release of potent enzymes found in their lysosomal granules. The vascular injury mediated by complement and polymorphonuclear leukocytes may lead to thrombosis and hemorrhage, typified by the petechial or ecchymotic rash attendant on serum sickness.

Another manifestation of the interaction of antigen and antibody is the release of potent vasoactive materials such as histamine, serotonin, bradykinin, and slow-reacting substance (SRSA), all of which lead to vasodilatation and leakage of protein and fluid from the vascular space into the tissues, resulting in edema. The disease varies from species to species in laboratory animals. As most of the work has been done in the rabbit, it is pertinent to note that the renal disease, which is a frequent and important aspect of immune complex disease in the rabbit, is often nonexistent or a very mild component in the usual human patient.

Continuation of disease is dependent upon a continual supply of antigen. Removal by the reticuloendothelial system of the immune complexes is signified by a rise in serum antibody directed against the foreign proteins, and reduction of symptoms and signs of illness. Unless the foreign proteins are readministered, the disease is self-limited. During convalescence and for long periods thereafter, antibodies against the foreign proteins are readily demonstrable in the patient's serum. Readministration of foreign antigen promptly leads to formation of immune complexes and clinical manifestations of disease, which continue until antigen is entirely removed from the circulation.

Clinical Manifestations. The onset of disease is often heralded by itching and discomfort, frequently at the site of serum injection. Fully developed serum sickness is a miserable disease. The unfortunate patient lies on his side in bed with a swollen, distorted face, often resulting in closure of both eyes so that he cannot see, with a skin itching all over and often covered with an urticarial or erythematous rash. He is reluctant to scratch his skin because of the pain in all his muscles and joints upon movement, and so he lies quietly in bed suffering from headache, itching, and joint pain. Especially frightening and discomforting is the appearance of neurologic manifestations which may result in weakness of an extremity or a sensory deficit, or occasionally an isolated facial palsy. Compounding the patient's difficulties may be abdominal pain, nausea, and vomiting. Upon examination a generalized lymphadenopathy may be palpated, especially prominent in the regions draining the site of injection of the serum. At that site there may be a local rash with erythema and either urticaria or tenderness, and this may provide a potent clue for the physician as to the nature of the illness. Occasionally, auscultation of the chest reveals a cardiac arrhythmia or a pericardial friction rub. The spleen is usually not palpable. A common manifestation is fever of 38.3 to 39°C (101 to 102°F), and, in addition to the subjective complaints of joint pain, the patient may manifest objective arthritis with swelling, redness, and accumulation of fluid in joints. The skin may show a petechial or purpuric rash in addition to the more common urticarial eruption.

Laboratory Studies. Examination of the blood may reveal a mild leukocytosis, and circulating plasma cells have been observed. The sedimentation rate is usually normal or only slightly elevated. Eosinophilia occurs, but is relatively uncommon. The urine may show slight proteinuria, a few red cells, and occasionally a few casts; but there are rarely significant evidences of renal impairment. Examination of the serum proteins of the patient reveals circulating horse gamma globulins and macroglobulins present early in the disease, and predominantly anti-horse IgA globulin antibodies late in the disease and during convalescence. The development of antibodies to horse alpha-2-macroglobulin in the sera of patients recovering from serum sickness suggests that this component of the equine serum which lacks any antibody value could be deleted in manufacture without impairing the antitoxic benefits of the serum. Serum complement levels are reduced for variable periods during the disease and then return to normal.

Treatment and Prognosis. Very mild symptoms of pruritus and skin rash may be controlled by an antihistamine, such as brompheniramine, 4 mg given every four hours. Epinephrine and sympathomimetic amines have been recommended in the past for the treatment of the urticaria of serum sickness, and salicylates for the treatment of joint pains. However, for all but the mildest symptoms, adrenocortical steroids in the form of prednisone can be given with great safety and efficacy, and the patient need not suffer with less effective medications. As this is a self-limited disease with a natural course of one to three weeks, the usual hazards of steroid therapy are not realized before treatment is stopped. A treatment course of 40 mg per day for four or five days may be sufficient, even for quite severe disease. Symptomatic improvement appears often within hours of the onset of steroid therapy and sometimes is remarkable within 24 hours.

Prevention. Tetanus antitoxin prepared from *human* serum is now commercially available in many parts of the world. When this is available, there is no reason to choose horse serum to obtain antitoxic benefits. When equine sera must be used in treatment, patients should be carefully questioned concerning prior exposure and for allergic symptoms to other horse products, such as horse dander or horsehair, as found in horsehair mattresses. All patients, regardless of history, should be skin tested by production of a minimal wheal (0.01 to 0.02 ml) of a 1:10 dilution of the serum to be tested. After 15 to 20 minutes the skin site is examined for an urticarial wheal, and in its absence treatment may be instituted. If the patient is allergic and the necessity for serum treatment is great, desensitization may be attempted by repeatedly injecting small amounts of serum beginning in dilutions of 1:100 and doubling the tolerated amount about every 15 or 20 minutes until the appropriate dose is achieved. Such treatment is hazardous because of possible anaphylaxis, and the indications for it should be scrutinized carefully.

In patients who have developed serum sickness after tetanus antitoxin, active immunization should be begun during the patient's convalescence from serum sickness.

It is generally advisable to immunize against tetanus all individuals who are seen by the physician in connection with unrelated allergic disease and found to be sensitive to horse dander or horse products. The immunization can be accomplished by use of tetanus toxoid.

Occasionally, in the course of serum therapy *an acute anaphylactic reaction* occurs, consisting of sudden vascular collapse, severe pruritus of the face, hands, and feet, often accompanied by bronchospasm and incontinence of stool and urine. Such events must be treated promptly *with epinephrine and not adrenocortical steroids.* A tourniquet should be placed proximal to the injection site of the drug or serum, and 0.2 ml of epinephrine injected into the site of injection which will slow absorption from the site. An additional 0.3 to 0.5 ml of 1:1000 aqueous solution of epinephrine should be given subcutaneously above the tourniquet if the patient has an effective blood pressure. In the absence of adequate blood pressure, the epinephrine must be given intravenously notwithstanding the hazard of production of cardiac arrhythmia, because the drug will not be absorbed from the periphery. After epinephrine administration, diphenhydramine (Benadryl), 50 mg, should be given orally or subcutaneously. The outcome of anaphylactic reactions is usually decided in the first few minutes; rapid restoration of blood pressure with prompt treatment is an excellent prognostic sign. Fatalities are few but tend to occur when the possibility of anaphylaxis is not considered *prior* to the administration of serum or drug so that effective measures are delayed.

Kojis, F. G.: Serum sickness and anaphylaxis. Am. J. Dis. Child., 64:93, 313, 1942.
Kunkel, H. G. (Chairman): Symposium on immune complexes and disease. J. Exp. Med., 134:1s-330s, 1971.
Vaughan, J. H., Barnett, E. V., and Leadley, P. J.: Serum sickness: Evidence in man of antigen-antibody complexes and free light chains in the circulation during the acute reaction. Ann. Intern. Med., 67:596, 1967.
von Pirquet, C., and Schick, B.: Serum Sickness. Baltimore, Williams & Wilkins Company, 1951.

72. DRUG ALLERGY

Fred S. Kantor

The value of therapeutic agents should constantly be weighed against their potential liability. Hypersensitivity reactions must be distinguished from two other untoward effects of drugs. The first is that of intolerance, in which the usual undesirable toxic effects occur at dosages of the drug well below that expected in a normal population. An example of this type of reaction includes visual disturbances and alterations in cardiac rhythm with very small doses of digitalis. The second form of drug reaction to be distinguished from hypersensitivity is that of idiosyncrasy. Whereas intolerance is a quantitative difference, idiosyncrasy is qualitative and is based upon a biochemical alteration in the way the patient handles the drug. Such a reaction does not depend on prior exposure to the drug, is not dose dependent, and does not resemble the other pharmacologic manifestations of the drug. An example of idiosyncrasy is the hemolytic anemia produced in patients with glucose-6-phosphate dehydrogenase deficiency when treated with primaquine. Altered reactivity (von Pirquet combined these two words to produce the word "allergy") on the part of the patient always follows prior exposure, even though this may not be apparent, and its mechanism is related to the hypersensitive state as reflected by delayed hypersensitivity or antibody production.

Incidence. Any drug may produce a hypersensitivity reaction, but some drugs have a much higher liability in this regard than do others. Digitalis and tetracycline have a low liability in producing allergic drug reactions, even though reports of documented cases have appeared. On the other hand, several of the antimicrobials, notably novobiocin, and certain anti-inflammatory agents, such as phenylbutazone, may have a high incidence of drug reaction. In addition to the variations produced by different drugs, equal liability is not shared by all patients for development of drug reactions to a single drug, such as penicillin. Patients with a history of allergic disease or previous drug reactions, as well as patients with certain inflammatory diseases such as lupus erythematosus, are generally thought to be more prone to the development of new drug allergies.

Pathogenesis. Certain therapeutic agents such as insulin are complex protein molecules which are known to be immunogenic. The majority of drugs represent classes of simple chemicals which require complexing with a tissue or serum protein of the patient in order to form an antigenic or immunogenic molecule. Drugs which are highly reactive chemicals usually are the most frequent sensitizers, and conversely the more inert members of the drug armamentarium are of less allergenic potential. Sensitization by means of a simple chemical involves the formation of covalent bonds with host protein which forms a hapten-carrier conjugate. Antibodies and hypersensitivity are directed against the hapten or the hapten and a closely adjacent portion of the carrier molecule, but never to the carrier protein itself. To form a hapten-protein conjugate, the administered drug may have to undergo considerable chemical rearrangement. This may occur during the metabolism of the drug, producing an antigenic determinant which is different from the administered drug. The necessity of chemical rearrangement of the drug to form the allergenic hapten-protein complex predicts difficulty of testing in vitro for drug allergy, because the laboratory must know what the antigenic determinant is.

Drug allergy has been investigated with respect to the antigenic determinant in only a limited number of cases. One of the most recent and extensive investigations has been in the case of penicillin and a derivative, the penicilloyl determinant. This has been labeled the major determinant, and as many as three—and perhaps many more—as yet undescribed chemical rearrangements may account for minor determinants, all of which can produce sensitization in given individuals and produce allergic symptoms upon administration of the drug. It should be borne in mind that not all drug immunization implies drug allergy. A good example of this is that all patients recently treated with penicillin will have developed antibodies directed against the penicilloyl determinant.

Hypersensitive reactions have been divided into *delayed hypersensitivity* and two varieties of immediate hypersensitivity: *wheal-and-flare* and *Arthus reactivity.* Serum sickness, which was discussed in Ch. 71, is an excellent example of an immediate type of hypersensitivity involving complement-fixing antibody and producing reactions to the so-called "Arthus" type.

The other type of immediate hypersensitivity, i.e., wheal-and-flare, is manifested in two major, clinically recognizable situations, urticaria and anaphylaxis. In these cases, the interaction of the drug-protein conjugate with IgE antibodies leads to release of active mediators resulting in vasodilatation and smooth muscle contraction. In this form of reaction, the hapten-protein conjugate and its respective antibody do not enter into the pathogenesis of the reaction but merely cause the release of the vasoactive material which produces the clinical effects. The last type of well-recognized mechanism is that of cellular or delayed hypersensitivity. In this form of immunity, circulating antibody is not important, and the interaction of the drug-protein conjugate is with sensitized cells, causing a release of a variety of biologically active materials which lead to perivascular accumulation of mononuclear cells and the development of induration. The best example of delayed hypersensitivity induced by drugs is skin sensitization resulting from direct contact with a variety of medications. Paradoxically, antihistamines, which have been incorporated into a variety of topical preparations for treatment of itching, burning, or allergic skin conditions, are themselves skin-sensitizing, and by combining with skin proteins form potent sensitizing agents which lead to delayed hypersensitivity and the development of the typical skin lesions of contact sensitivity. A combination of reaction types is often present in typical drug allergy, but one or another of the reaction types usually predominates and treatment is most efficacious when directed against this reaction type.

Clinical Manifestations. Fever may develop immediately after administration of a drug or, more commonly, may increase in a stepwise fashion after the seventh or eighth day of administration. The fever may show a sustained or remittent course and is usually low-grade in the range of 37.8 to 39° C (100 to 102° F), although hectic fevers are often observed, accompanied by constitutional symptoms. In general, the patient appears less ill than would be anticipated from the height of the fever. A drug reaction may mimic the septic picture entirely, but it usually pursues a more indolent course. Cessation of fever within a day or two of discontinuing the offending drug is to be expected. In some cases of fever alone, and if the drug reaction involves other organ systems, such as the skin and the joints, it may take several days, up to a week, for the symptoms to slowly subside. Penicillin, diphenylhydantoin (Dilantin), and barbiturates are frequent causes of drug fever.

Skin Rash. Skin rash as a manifestation of drug allergy may take several forms. A maculopapular, very fine rash appearing in the softer skin of the axillary line and on the extensor surfaces of the extremities and along the trunk may be unnoticed by the patient. Usually, urticarial rashes are reported because they are accompanied by pruritus. Persistent administration of an offending drug causing maculopapular eruptions may lead to confluent erythroderma and subsequent exfoliative dermatitis. Similarly, a rash may progress to an eczematous eruption with weeping papulovesicular lesions and ill-defined patches of erythema and edema, accompanied by intense pruritus. Erythema multiforme-like eruptions may be produced by a variety of drugs and are characterized by the formation of sharply circumscribed lesions that are usually symmetrical in distribution. The individual lesions seem to spread peripherally and clear centrally to form an annular pattern with secondary and tertiary rings evolving into a "target" or "iris" lesion.

Symmetrical lesions of the lower extremities closely resembling typical erythema nodosum may also be caused by drugs, including sulfones, penicillin, and iodides. The term "fixed eruption" is used to describe an erythematous and sharply defined lesion which recurs at the same site and in the same form upon re-exposure to the same drug. Withdrawal of the drug usually leads to healing, but hyperpigmentation of the area involved may remain. Photosensitivity reactions characterized by erythema, edema, and mild scaling are sharply limited to areas exposed to light, and a clue to the examiner may be provided by the **V**-shaped area at the neckline, usually at the site where the collar leaves the skin exposed to light and it becomes involved. Sulfonamides and thiazide derivatives are examples known to engender photoallergic reactions.

Other Organ Systems. Drug allergy is often manifested by reactions involving the hematopoietic system. Sedormid, a once popular sedative, resulted in thrombocytopenic purpura, which was shown to depend upon the presence of drug, a serum factor demonstrated to be antibody, and the presence of platelets. Several other drugs, such as quinine and quinidine, thiouracil, and the anticonvulsant hydantoin group, have been implicated as causes of thrombocytopenic purpura. Hemolytic anemia and agranulocytosis are also common adverse reactions ascribed to drugs. Sulfonamides and thiouracil have caused both types of reaction, but aminopyrine and phenylbutazone produced mainly agranulocytosis. Care should be taken in the interpretation of allergic causality of pathologic events leading to agranulocytosis or hemolytic anemia. One of the outstanding examples of a purported allergic hemolytic anemia was that induced by the fava bean. It was later shown that the presence of an enzyme defect in the red cells of these patients resulted in their shorter life span when exposed to drug and that sensitization in the immunologic sense was not required. Aplastic anemia, involving all the formed elements of the blood, is occasionally associated with drug administration; in particular it is described with chloramphenicol, gold, and the sulfonamides.

Gastrointestinal symptoms are common adverse reactions to the administration of therapeutic agents, but the mechanism of action is rarely allergic in nature. The kidney is involved in periarteritis nodosa caused by drugs. In this disease, antimicrobial drugs, notably the sulfonamides, have been frequently implicated. Interstitial nephritis has been described with the penicillinase-resistant penicillin preparation methicillin in association with hematuria, rash, and marked eosinophilia.

The lupus erythematosus syndrome has been described following ingestion of certain drugs, particularly hydralazine, procainamide, and the hydantoin derivatives. The severity of the syndrome induced by drug ingestion may vary from only a serologic manifestation, such as a positive lupus test, to the full-blown picture of fever, arthritis, polyserositis, and hematologic manifestations. Pulmonary infiltration and eosinophilia (PIE syndrome), peripheral neuritis, and hemorrhagic encephalitis have all been ascribed to allergic drug reactions, and probably represent varieties of allergic vascular injury resident in the particular organs involved. Liver damage has been attributed to treatment with heavy metals, thorazine, and sulfonamides; the evidence supporting the allergic basis of these reactions is meager. In recent times, the introduction of halothane, a potent, widely used anesthetic agent, has led to a series of symptoms, primarily involving liver dysfunction, which in some patients strongly suggest an allergic basis.

GENERALIZED ANAPHYLAXIS. Generalized anaphylaxis as a manifestation of drug allergy is a clinical catastrophe with which the physician must be prepared to deal promptly. The condition is usually initiated by an injected drug, although an orally administered tablet has been reported to produce a fatal reaction. Frequently the initial symptoms are generalized pruritus, particularly on the soles of the feet and the palms of the hands, and the general development of a hyperemia of the skin, particularly about the ears, so that the individual often looks as though he had acquired a recent sunburn. Angioneurotic edema may cause distortion of the face, swelling of the eyelids, and rapid loss of effective plasma volume, leading to vascular collapse and shock. The risk of developing an anaphylactic reaction, particularly to penicillin, is enhanced by the patient's having had a prior, less serious reaction, such as a maculopapular rash.

Diagnosis. Avoidance and challenge is still the best diagnostic means available to the physician, although it is often inadvisable because of the danger to the patient. Certainly in cases of anaphylactic reactions or urticarial eruptions, the challenge to the patient subsequent to the subsidence of the symptoms is not warranted and is extremely dangerous. However, in drug fever, when that condition appears alone, a fractional dose may be administered after the fever subsides to further identify the cause. Unfortunately, laboratory tests performed in vitro have been very disappointing. The basophil degranulation test, lymphocyte stimulation test, skin window technique, and others have been reported with some success from isolated laboratories, but in general they have been found to be difficult to reproduce and have not come into general usage. The necessary information concerning the intermediary metabolites of each drug and the development of specific antigenic determinants is not available for the majority of drugs which cause allergic reactions. Until this information is known, laboratory tests are not likely to be useful in this area. The leukocyte count may be high or low, and therefore not useful; eosinophilia is not a regular occurrence.

Treatment and Prophylaxis. Subsidence of allergic reactions to drugs usually occurs promptly after discontinuance of the drug, often within one or two days, but in many instances prolongation of symptoms for several days and, indeed, in some instances for several weeks and months, is well recognized. Many of our foodstuffs are contaminated with drugs: Chickens are fattened with estrogenic hormones, hogs are fed antimicrobials, and cows, when suffering from mastitis, may be treated with large doses of penicillin which appears in the milk. When strongly suspecting a drug hypersensitivity which fails to subside after cessation of the drug, inadvertent environmental drug administration should be carefully investigated. In general, treatment of the drug reaction should be directed against the altered physiology. In the reactions involving vasoactive substances, the use of a direct vasoconstrictor such as epinephrine may be lifesaving and should be used first, instead of the more glamorous, but less effective, group of adrenocortical steroids. The latter group of agents are very useful in the treatment of the Arthus type of immediate hypersensitivity as manifested by serum sickness and polyarteritis, as well as in many forms of delayed hypersensitivity. Epinephrine should be given in dosages of 0.5 to 1 ml of 1:1000 dilution of aqueous epinephrine, given subcutaneously. Antihistaminics such as diphenhydramine (Benadryl, 50 mg) or brompheniramine (Dimetane, 4 mg) may be administered orally or parenterally, but the intravenous use of diphenhydramine is to be avoided because serious adverse reactions to this medication have occurred. Drug reactions are self-limited diseases, and the use of steroids in these diseases is most efficacious and generally does not impose the usual liabilities of steroid therapy. Accordingly, therapy may be instituted with full doses of 40 to 60 mg a day, and 40 mg a day may be given for three or four days, dropped to 20 mg a day for an additional several days, and discontinued without a long tapering regimen.

Ackroyd, J. F.: Sedormid purpura: An immunological study of a form of drug hypersensitivity. In Kallos, P.: Progress in Allergy, Vol. 3. New York, Interscience Publishers, 1952, p. 531.

Chase, M. W.: Hypersensitivity to simple chemicals. Harvey Lectures, 62:169, 1966.

Demis, D. J.: Allergy and drug sensitivity of skin. Ann. Rev. Pharmacol., 9:457, 1969.

DeWeck, A. L.: Drug Reactions. In Samter, M. (ed.): Immunological Diseases. 2nd ed. Boston, Little, Brown & Company, 1971, p. 415.

Levine, B. B.: Immunochemical mechanisms of drug allergy. Ann. Rev. Med., 17:23, 1966.

Shulman, N. R.: Mechanism of blood cell destruction in individuals sensitized to foreign antigens. Trans. Assoc. Am. Physicians, 76:72, 1963.

73. ALLERGIC RHINITIS (Hay Fever)

Fred S. Kantor

Definition. Hay fever is the common name applied to allergic rhinitis which recurs each year at a specific season—usually spring or fall. It is characterized by rhinorrhea, sneezing, itching of the eyes, nose, ears, and palate, and edema of the nasal mucous membranes. Nonseasonal allergens, such as feathers and animal danders, may produce year-round disease called perennial allergic rhinitis; vasomotor rhinitis is a "wastebasket" term which designates perennial rhinitis without an identifiable allergic basis.

Etiology and Epidemiology. Susceptible persons exposed each year to airborne pollen of many varieties of plants, particularly trees, grasses, and weeds, develop a "wheal and flare" type of immediate hypersensitivity to protein components of the pollen grains called allergens. The exact hereditable basis of hay fever is still unclear, but clustering of a variety of diseases which involve "wheal and flare" hypersensitivity in certain individuals, and in families, strongly supports the view that such a basis exists. Recent evidence suggests that sensitivity to a particular allergen, such as ragweed, may be dependent upon transmission of a specific immune response gene and therefore might be predictable in an individual before development of the disease.

Drab, colorless plants, unattractive to birds and bees, must depend upon the wind for pollination and release of huge amounts of airborne pollen. In contrast, colorful blossoms and odoriferous plants generally release smaller amounts of heavier, stickier pollen which is not widely disseminated. "Rose fever," a form of allergic rhinitis prevalent in early summer, is a misnomer; while roses are visually in full bloom, it is the pollen from grasses such as timothy, June, and orchard grass which produces the disease.

Ragweed and grass pollen are the most common causes of allergic rhinitis in the United States. Ragweed abounds in the midwestern states, and is prevalent in the eastern and southeastern part of the country. West of the Rocky Mountains and in the dry Southwest, very little ragweed appears. Each area has a distinctive potentially sensitizing flora, and sufferers fleeing from one part of the country to another are often disappointed when symptoms rapidly reappear in their new location. In the northern United States early spring hay fever (April and May) is usually due to tree pollen; the grasses pollinate and produce symptoms in early summer (June and early July) and the ragweed in late summer and early fall. Spores of ubiquitous molds are present throughout the year but increase in numbers at different times because of increased mold growth on decaying vegetation. Spores of Homodendrum peak in number in July, whereas spores of Alternaria increase in the fall, overlapping the ragweed season, and may be the basis of an erroneous diagnosis of ragweed hay fever.

The trees are a varied and an important group; ash, beech, birch, cedar, hickory, maple, oak, sycamore, and poplar all produce important windborne pollen, whereas the less antigenic pollens of the firs and pines are not usual sources of disease. Each species of tree produces an antigenically distinct pollen with a relatively short period of pollination lasting two to four weeks. Hypersensitivity to multiple species of trees with overlapping pollinating periods, and to grasses, molds, and ragweed, may blur the seasonal aspects of the patient's problem and suggest a perennial allergic rhinitis. Unlike the trees, grasses such as timothy, fescue, orchard, redtop, and June (Kentucky bluegrass) share important antigenic determinants and in the extreme South and West may produce year-round symptoms. A careful account of seasonal variations in symptoms coupled with a knowledge of the flora of the patient's locality and the pollinating periods of the indigenous plants is vital to the specific diagnosis and management of this group of diseases. In the British Isles and the European continent, trees and grasses are important causes of pollinosis; allergic travelers would do well to check the season of their proposed trip. Europe has little or no ragweed, so American sufferers may doubly enjoy a late summer European vacation.

Pollen grains are about 20 to 40 μ in diameter, and each species has a distinctive appearance. By collecting grains on a glass slide with a simple timed exposure or with more sophisticated air-sampling devices, pollens may be identified and enumerated. The severity of symptoms of an allergic population will vary with the pollen numbers in an approximate way, but the use of daily radio broadcast pollen numbers as a diagnostic or predictive aid is of little value. The "counts" are derived from samples obtained the previous day, and at different locations and altitudes. Often the patient will ask why he doesn't feel better (or worse) because of the low (or high) pollen count!

Allergic rhinitis may be caused by any inhaled antigen; those often implicated, in addition to plant pollen, are house dust, feathers, fungus spores, and animal danders. Food allergy is often suggested as a basis for inhalant symptoms, but manifestations in the skin such as urticaria or angioneurotic edema (see Ch. 75 and 76) are the rule, and the respiratory tract is an unlikely target organ for this type of hypersensitivity.

Pathogenesis. Sensitization may occur at any time of

life but usually occurs in childhood or adolescence. It is curious that an adult may become sensitized to a pollen to which he has been exposed each previous year of his life; this suggests that factors other than genetic proclivity and exposure are necessary. When pollens impinge upon the nasal mucous membrane, they release a variety of protein antigens called allergens which initiate the immune response. The major allergens of grasses and ragweed have been partially purified and are low molecular weight proteins of relatively low antigenicity. This means that for a given amount of antigen, the immune response in terms of amount and avidity of antibody produced is small. The important point is that this type of antigen in low doses tends to elicit an unusual response characterized by production of reaginic antibody, which is largely or completely of the IgE class. Such antibodies are present in nanogram quantities in serum, and "fix" to the surface of cells so that passive administration will sensitize a particular skin site for weeks. Because of this quality, reaginic antibodies are sometimes called homocytotropic. Contact with the specific allergen will cause "sensitized" cells to release potent vasoactive substances, largely histamine and slow reacting substance of anaphylaxis (SRS-A). These materials cause capillary vasodilatation with leakage of fluid and colloid into the tissues leading to the major symptoms of allergic disease.

Although the symptoms produced by inhalation of pollen are localized to the mucosa with which it comes in contact, the sensitization is systemic. When peripheral leukocytes of sensitive individuals are exposed to allergen in vitro, they release histamine. This reaction affords a rapid measurement of sensitivity, usually expressed in terms of amount of allergen necessary to produce release of 50 per cent of the cellular histamine. It also provides an objective measurement of the efficacy and mechanism of treatment. Production of IgE antibody is not limited to allergic individuals; normal subjects or laboratory animals will develop this class of antibody response after subcutaneous injection of allergens. The presence of extracts of roundworms such as ascaris facilitates production of IgE antibody in an unknown way. Similarly, the nasal route of allergen exposure in an allergic individual facilitates development of IgE antibody. Nonimmunologic factors also play a role in producing what may be called the "inertia" of allergic disease; patients who are well tend to remain well, whereas those who are sick tend to remain sick. Nonspecific irritants of all sorts can cause incapacitating sneezing and rhinorrhea in a patient suffering from allergic rhinitis; these might be tolerated without a sniffle at another time of year. Upper respiratory infections, particularly sinusitis, occur more frequently in the allergic patient owing to edema and obstruction of normal drainage. Similarly, the normal effects of emotional states upon the nasal mucosa are often exaggerated in the allergic patient.

Clinical Manifestations. The abrupt onset of morning sneezing, usually in paroxysms of several sneezes in rapid succession, accompanied by rhinorrhea, itchiness of eyes, palate, and pharynx, are characteristic of allergic rhinitis. Symptoms recur each year at approximately the same time, corresponding to the appearance of the offending pollen in the air. Increased exposure will intensify symptoms: dry, windy days, riding in an open car, and working in a garden are frequently reported to worsen the symptoms. A hay fever sufferer notes that the morning and evening hours are the worst, with a relatively better period during the midday. Mucosal congestion and edema often lead to total blockage of the airway, necessitating mouth breathing. The conjunctivae are red and weepy, and the lids and periorbital tissues may be puffy.

Hay fever is not often accompanied by temperature elevations, and the name is therefore misleading. Fever should alert one to the common complications: sinusitis, otitis, or mastoiditis. Cough, wheezing, and dyspnea are frequent companions of allergic rhinitis. Because pollen grains are too large to affect the terminal bronchioles, it was thought that the allergic reaction in the upper respiratory tract could trigger lower airway obstruction, but recent studies indicate that pollen fragments small enough to reach the bronchioles are present in the inspired air.

Diagnosis. Early in the course, the differentiation of allergic rhinitis from that caused by irritants or infections is difficult, but in retrospect the patient will usually remember similar but milder symptoms at the same time in previous years. The seasonal history is the most important of all clues to correct diagnosis. Allergic rhinitis may be differentiated from viral upper respiratory infections when pruritus of eyes, nose, and pharynx is present, and by the absence of fever, sore throat, and malaise. The nasal mucous membranes appear swollen, pale, and boggy in allergic rhinitis, and red and "angry" in viral infections; but inflammation secondary to sneezing and frequent blowing to clear the nose may blur these differences. Nasal secretions may be obtained by asking the patient to blow his nose into a piece of ordinary wax paper; smears stained with Wright's or Giemsa stains show an abundance of eosinophils in allergic rhinitis, whereas in infectious rhinitis smears reveal polymorphonuclear leukocytes.

Environmental allergens other than pollen are more difficult to diagnose as the basis of allergic rhinitis, but a careful history will often elicit them. Inquiry should be made into the home: How old is it? What is the heating system? What are the floor, wall, and window coverings? What types of pillows, mattresses, quilts, and comforters are used by the patient and by his or her spouse? Frequently the nonallergic marriage partner will sleep on a feather pillow not five inches from the allergic one sleeping on a nonallergenic pillow. The question of what makes symptoms worse or better has a special significance in the allergic history. Often patients can specify a place or activity associated with symptoms which when avoided keeps them symptom-free.

Skin Tests. Since sensitization is systemic, the allergic individual reacts whenever contact with allergen occurs. Injection of minute quantities of allergens into the skin produces a wheal in 10 to 15 minutes in individuals with reaginic antibodies. Unfortunately, the presence of a positive skin test does not prove that the patient's symptoms are related to the allergen provoking the skin response. Often allergic individuals will have multiple positive skin reactions, such as to ragweed and grass allergen, but express symptoms in only one season and not the other. Skin tests are performed as either scratch tests or intradermal injections. Sets of skin test allergens are readily available and are often used indiscriminately. The patient may be tested with 200 to 300 skin tests with confusing results and erroneous diagnosis. A limited number of tests, 10 to 20, including house dust, common animal danders, feathers, common molds, and pollen, should suffice in all but the most difficult cases.

If skin tests are not diagnostic, why do them? They are often helpful in confirming a suspicion based on the history. The degree of skin reactivity in the untreated patient bears an approximate relationship to the degree of sensitivity and the amount of specific IgE antibody. Occasionally a positive skin test will point to a new direction of inquiry; e.g., a positive test to horse dander led to the finding that the patient was sleeping on a mattress with horse hair. Finally, when a decision is made to hyposensitize with allergen injections (see below), the degree of skin test reactivity provides guidance for a starting dosage.

Allergenic materials for testing and treatment are made by extraction of the solid allergen in a neutral buffer; usually a weight-to-volume ratio is employed, such as 1 gram of defatted ragweed pollen extracted with 100 ml of buffer producing 1:100 allergenic extract. In recent years, Kjehldahl analysis has led to standardization of extracts in protein nitrogen units (PNU) per milliliter. One PNU is equal to 10^{-8} gram N.

This "scientific"-sounding quantity may mislead the user, because only a small fraction of the extract contains the allergenic proteins and all the nitrogen is measured. Until the content of specific allergens is assayable, it is likely that the crude weight per volume or PNU per milliliter standard will be used. Extracts prepared in the same manner at different times may have wide variation in the amount of active allergen per milliliter. It is essential to be careful when using a new extract.

Intradermal tests are more sensitive than scratch tests and carry a greater likelihood of causing a constitutional reaction in a highly sensitive individual. Reactions are read after 10 to 15 minutes. A slight but definite wheal is considered 1+; a moderate reaction (wheal 6 to 10 mm) without pseudopods is read as 2+; a wheal of 10 to 15 mm with pseudopod formation is read as 3+; and wheals larger than 15 mm with a wide flare are read as 4+.

The initial intracutaneous tests with pollens should be made with solutions of antigen containing no more than 10 protein nitrogen units per milliliter, and not more than five to ten tests should be done at any one time. A minimal wheal (0.01 to 0.02 ml) is produced in the skin with a 27 needle attached to a tuberculin syringe. If little or no reaction is obtained, subsequent tests may be made with solutions containing 100 units and then 1000 units per milliliter. Reactions less than 2+ at 1000 PNU per milliliter are of doubtful significance in the untreated patient, whereas strongly positive reactions at 10 PNU per milliliter are almost always associated with symptomatic disease. The interpretation of positive reactions must be made in relation to the prevalence of the antigen in the area and the patient's history.

Passive transfer of allergic patient's serum to normal volunteers' skin will sensitize the site to antigenic challenge. Such tests, called P-K reactions (Prausnitz-Küstner), are useful when it is not possible to perform skin tests in young children, or on patients with generalized dermatitis. They are rarely done any more because of the danger of hepatitis and the availability of in vitro tests for histamine release and IgE measurement.

Treatment.   Treatment is directed toward avoiding the allergen, modifying the state of hypersensitivity, and ameliorating the symptoms. By far the most effective means is strict avoidance of the offending allergen. When this is due to an increased sensitivity to an animal dander such as that of horse or cat, merely identifying the cause will help greatly in avoidance. Often patients will "hide" their pets from the physician's inquiry because they have a strong suspicion of the offender but hope that something else will be found. Effective filtration of the air within the patient's house is now possible with a variety of electrostatic and barrier-type filters. Dust control and attention to bedding and furniture filling will be rewarding in selected cases.

Treatment with repeated injections of specific allergens has been in vogue for 70 years, and recent studies have confirmed the efficacy of this mode of therapy and given insight to its mechanism. Preseasonal, coseasonal, and perennial administration of allergens all have their proponents, but perennial administration avoids the necessity of building up the dosage each year and results in the same number of patient visits. Increasing amounts of allergen are injected subcutaneously once or twice weekly, starting with a dose shown to be tolerated by skin tests. The goals of hyposensitization are two: production of a nonreaginic (blocking) antibody which can effectively compete with reaginic antibody for allergen, and reduction of the amount of reaginic antibody produced (tolerance induction), thereby decreasing cellular sensitivity to allergen. Addition of serum from a treated individual to sensitized leukocytes in vitro may increase by 100-fold the amounts of allergen necessary for 50 per cent histamine release from these leukocytes.

The increment of allergen injected at each visit is determined by the patient's skin reaction to the previous injection. If redness and swelling exceed the size of a 50-cent piece, the dose should be repeated or lowered until it is better tolerated. Often an increase in sensitivity occurs early in treatment; this may lead to a worsening in symptoms if it coincides with the patient's season. Usually patients are treated for two or more years after maximal benefit has been achieved, at which time hyposensitization is stopped. A proportion of patients will maintain their improvement whereas, in many, a slow return of symptoms during the following year or 18 months is common. Patients should always be advised to remain in the office for 30 minutes after the injection, because the allergen may provoke a constitutional reaction. This is often heralded by reddening of the conjunctivae, nasal swelling, red ears and nose, and a feeling of faintness. Tourniquets should be applied above the injection sites and 0.2 to 0.5 ml of aqueous epinephrine 1:1000 injected above the tourniquet. Such reactions are uncommon. They are usually easily managed in the office or clinic; but if the patient leaves the office immediately after an allergen injection, the reaction at best will be very frightening and might possibly be fatal.

A variety of repository allergen preparations, including mineral oil emulsions, and alum-precipitated allergens, have generated interest because of a putative ability to administer more allergen in fewer injections with less likelihood of systemic reactions. The efficacy and safety of these preparations are still to be determined.

Symptomatic Treatment.   Antihistamines are often helpful in ameliorating symptoms of allergic rhinitis. In general they are only partially effective, and patients complain of the soporific side effects. Brompheniramine (Dimetane) and chlorpheniramine (Chlor-Trimeton) are both available in 4 mg tablets and in long-acting preparations containing 8 or 12 mg. Both these preparations seem to have less soporific effects than Benadryl, which should be used only at bedtime. Response to these drugs is often quite variable in different patients, and several preparations should be tried if results are poor or side effects great. Dexamethasone (Decadron), administered locally by a special nasal spray inhaler, delivers 0.1 mg per spray, and it is often efficacious. Its use once on each side twice a day is often all that is necessary during a short pollen season. The local effect without systemic liability makes this therapy attractive. Systemic steroids are very effective but are used rarely because of their considerable side effects. A short course of four to five days of 30 mg per day of prednisone will help a new patient over the worst symptoms before other measures become effective or the peak of the season passes.

A variety of sympathomimetic drugs, such as Neo-Synephrine, 0.5 per cent, phenylephrine, 0.25 per cent, or Privine, 0.1 per cent, have been used intranasally to shrink the nasal mucosa, but the effects are short-lived and all cause a "rebound" swelling of the nasal mucosa which may be a self-propagating disease. These drugs are not recommended in allergic rhinitis. For relief of allergic conjunctivitis accompanying pollinosis, eye drops containing epinephrine (0.025 per cent), or dexamethasone (0.1 per cent drops) may be used for a brief period with excellent relief. Prolonged use of steroid eye drops is not recommended because of corneal thinning and cataract formation.

Ishizaka, K., and Ishizaka, I.: Identification of γF antibodies as a carrier of reaginic activity. J. Immunol., 99:1187, 1967.

Lichtenstein, L. M., Ishizaka, K., Norman, P. S., Sobotka, A. K., and Hill, B. M.: IgE antibody measurements in ragweed hay fever: Relationship to clinical severity and results of immunotherapy. J. Clin. Invest., 52:472, 1973.

Lowell, F. C., and Franklin, W.: A double-blind study of the effectiveness and specificity of injection therapy in ragweed hay fever. N. Engl. J. Med., 273:675, 1965.

Samter, M. (ed.): Immunological Diseases. 2nd ed. Boston, Little, Brown & Company, 1971.

74. VASOMOTOR RHINITIS

Fred S. Kantor

Vasomotor rhinitis is a vague term describing chronic rhinitis without an allergic basis. It is indistinguishable from allergic rhinitis except for chronicity, absence of geographic or seasonal influences, and prevalence of coexistent nasal polyps. Frequently the patient has sought the use of sympathomimetic drugs administered as nose drugs such as Neo-Synephrine or Privine. The problem is compounded by the recurrent rebound rhinitis produced by these agents. Often they are the sole propagating cause of rhinitis which was once allergic or viral in origin, but which has become chronic through the use of these drugs.

The causes of vasomotor rhinitis have been ascribed to bacterial and food allergies, but documentation of these agents is meager and the mechanism is really unknown. Occasionally, a patient with allergies to a variety of ubiquitous substances may present without a clear-cut seasonal environmental history because of the overlapping allergens. These patients may recall a time when

their symptoms were seasonal, and skin tests may be helpful in sorting out the problem. In general, however, the bulk of patients with perennial rhinitis at home or away, in summer and winter, will not yield a definite etiologic agent.

Treatment is symptomatic. If nose drops or sprays have been abused, it is useful to discontinue these agents on one side only for a few days and then on the other side so that the patient can breathe through the treated side while the other is recovering from the rebound effects of the drug. Antihistaminics such as brompheniramine (Dimetane), 4 mg every four hours, are sometimes helpful but rarely very successful. Some patients are helped by a nasal dexamethasone spray (Turbinaire) once on each side twice a day. This may produce relief without administering an effective systemic dose and thereby avoid the undesirable side effects.

75. URTICARIA

Fred S. Kantor

Definition. Urticaria, or hives, is an eruption of the skin characterized by elevated, erythematous, sharply demarcated wheals, usually intensively pruritic, lasting hours to days but often recurrent for weeks and sometimes years.

Etiology and Pathogenesis. The characteristic lesion is produced by capillary dilation in the dermis, leading to loss of fluid into the tissues. Swollen collagen bundles, widening of the dermal papillae, and flattening of the rete pegs are seen microscopically. It is useful to divide the causes into immunologic, paraimmunologic, and nonimmunologic categories.

By far the most common *immunologic cause* of acute hives is food allergy. In this circumstance, vasoactive mediators such as histamine, kinins, and slow-reacting substance of anaphylaxis (SRS-A) are released from mast cells, basophils, and other tissues, producing capillary dilation. The release of mediators is typically due to interaction of antigen with circulating, or fixed, reaginic antibody, usually of the IgE variety. This antibody can be passively transferred by the serum of an affected individual to the skin of a volunteer. A wheal is produced at the transfer site upon ingestion of the offending food antigen. This is the classic Prausnitz-Küstner (PK) reaction. Reactions of IgE antibody with antigen are not complement dependent and produce no vascular necrosis. Complement-dependent IgG-antigen interactions may also cause mediator release by cytotoxic action on mediator-containing cells. These reactions may be produced by antibodies directed against cell antigens, such as isohemagglutinins, and may also be due to antibodies directed against foreign antigens in which the antigen or the complex is passively affixed to the cell surface. The urticaria of serum sickness (see Ch. 71) is such an example. The most frequent route of antigen presentation in the production of acute urticaria is oral ingestion. Inhalation uncommonly produces hives, and occasionally contact with allergen on the skin may suffice. People sensitive to animal dander often report that contact with the fur or saliva of the animal may cause hives; patients allergic to bees may develop hives of the lips and mouth upon contact with honey.

The "paraimmunologic" causes are likely to involve similar mechanisms to those of the first category, but the relationship of the antigens and antibodies involved is less apparent. Infection with viruses, bacteria, and fungi may present with hives; hepatitis is a common example. Intestinal parasites, particularly the roundworms, are often associated with hives and eosinophilia. Bites of common insects such as mosquitoes, bedbugs, lice, and other biting insects may produce not only local manifestations but generalized urticaria. Neoplastic diseases, particularly lymphomas of the Hodgkin's variety, and the myeloproliferative diseases are commonly associated with hives. Finally, in the paraimmunologic category are the diseases in which immune complexes have been demonstrated and are thought to play an important etiologic role. In this group, hives are most often associated with systemic lupus erythematosus and dermatomyositis, but the palpable purpura of leukocytoclastic angiitis (Henoch-Schönlein purpura) may first appear as urticaria and then become purpuric.

The nonimmunologic causes of urticaria include physical stimuli such as cold, heat, actinic energy (solar urticaria), and pressure. Cold urticaria may be a familial or sporadic disease in which areas exposed to cold develop urticarial wheals. In about 50 per cent of the sporadic cases, a factor in serum is capable of "sensitizing" normal skin so that a wheal develops when an ice cube is applied to the site. Cold urticaria may be symptomatic of an underlying systemic disease; multiple myeloma, cryoglobulinemia, and syphilis have been reported. The mediators responsible for cold urticaria are presumed to be similar to those released by allergic reactions, but the mechanism of release remains unclear.

Solar urticaria is produced by two spectra of actinic rays of 3100 to 3700Å and 4000 to 5000Å in wavelength. Marked sun exposure in a sensitive individual has led to generalized vascular collapse. Urticaria to sunlight can be passively transferred by serum from individuals who are sensitive to the lower spectrum. The mechanism of mediator release is unknown but, unlike cold urticaria, treatment with drugs and barrier creams is quite effective (see below).

Certain drugs and chemical compounds have the capacity to cause mast cell degranulation directly, resulting in mediator release without an antigen-antibody reaction. Surface-active materials such as saponin, highly negatively charged molecules like polylysines, and many drugs share this property. Common drug examples are morphine, quinine, polymixin B, curare, decholin, hydralazine, and meperidine. Nonimmunologic release of histamine may be the basis of many "drug reactions" which have failed to yield immunologic mechanisms such as the rare reactions to radiographic contrast agents which are iodinated organic compounds. Indeed, the warm "glow" produced by good brandy is probably more a factor of mediator release than alcohol content, as any ethanol sampler can attest.

A special form of urticaria which consists of small, almost papular, wheals surrounded by a large axon flare is called cholinergic urticaria. Affected individuals will produce a similar eruption when injected with small amounts of mecholyl or acetylcholine. The mechanisms are obscure, but clearly emotional stress, exposure to heat, such as a warm bath, or exercise may bring out the eruption.

Urticaria pigmentosa, or systemic mastocytosis, is due to infiltration of the skin by mast cells; it is believed to be a true neoplasm of very slow growth in which the chemical manifestations are much more distressing to the patient than the invasive ones. Areas of infiltration are marked by freckle-like hyperpigmentation which, upon stroking, will produce a typical linear bumpy wheal, because the skin between the accumulation of mast cells does not urticate.

Chronic urticaria implies recurrent lesions for a period of six weeks or more. The clear causal relationship of certain foods to acute urticaria has led to the assumption that the chronic form is due to an extended exposure to an unidentified allergen or urticator. Investigation of such patients yields a single causal factor in very few, and the bulk of these patients defy elucidation of a specific etiologic factor. Many writers have emphasized psychologic factors in chronic urticaria, supporting their arguments with numerous cases of acute urticaria in response to a specific stress—a heavy date, an important examination, or the like. Although these factors must play some role, their magnitude in a particular patient is very difficult to assess.

Clinical Manifestations. Typically, the wheal is 1 to 5 cm in diameter, often irregular, with a blanched center ("target" lesion) and surrounding erythema. The individual lesions are evanescent, often fading within hours. Successive crops appear for the duration of the disease. The lesions tend to appear at pressure points—e.g., the belt line, the brassiere straps, or the garters. Rarely are the soles and palms affected; but when they are, the patient may complain of difficulty in walking. Pruritus is common and sometimes so severe that the patient cannot wait to get home and fling off his or her clothes. When urticaria is due to a single exposure to a food or drug, it usually appears within minutes. An ingestant taken more than 24 to 48 hours before onset is rarely the cause. Occasionally summation of two allergic stimuli may be responsible; e.g., some patients may eat frozen strawberries in winter with impunity, but during the pollen season the same strawberries will cause hives.

Treatment. Acute or sporadic urticaria usually responds well to antihistaminics such as brompheniramine (Dimetane), 4 mg every four hours, or tripelennamine (Pyribenzamine) 50 mg every four hours. If the patient is in acute distress, 0.3 ml of 1:1000 epinephrine subcutaneously will often provide relief until the antihistaminic effect is apparent. In severe or unresponsive cases of sporadic urticaria, four days of prednisone, 40 mg per day may be necessary and very helpful.

In chronic urticaria the cause is rarely evident and therefore hard to remove. Most patients have been treated with antihistaminics without benefit. The use of a rigid elimination diet may not only remove hidden allergens, but more likely may also remove foods such as spices which are direct releasers of histamine. In addition to the elimination diet, liberal doses of brompheniramine (Dimetane), 8 mg every four hours, and hydroxyzine, 10 to 25 mg three times a day, are helpful. After a period of relief, cautious reduction of the drug regimen and addition of selective foods in groups, such as eggs, milk, and milk products, one at a time every three to four days, will often result in cessation of symptoms. The result is frequently a grateful patient on a full diet; the doctor, however, remains perplexed.

Cold urticaria is often refractory to treatment with all the agents mentioned above, and often the patient has to adjust his life style to avoid the cold. In contrast, solar urticaria is readily treated with barrier creams that filter out the actinic energy of the appropriate wave length. Hydroxychloroquine (Plaquenil), 200 mg, once daily or even twice a week, may protect a sensitive person who anticipates sun exposure.

Beall, G. N.: Urticaria: A review of laboratory and clinical observations. Medicine, 43:131, 1964.
Sheffer, A. L., and Austen, K. F.: Urticaria and angioedema. In Fitzpatrick, T., Clark, W., VanScott, E., Eisen, A., and Vaughan, J. (eds.): Dermatology in General Medicine. New York, Grune & Stratton, 1971.
Sheldon, J. M., Lovell, R. G., and Mathews, K. P.: A Manual of Clinical Allergy. 2nd ed. Philadelphia, W. B. Saunders Company, 1967.

76. ANGIONEUROTIC EDEMA

Fred S. Kantor

Definition. Angioneurotic edema (angioedema) is characterized by painless swelling in the subcutaneous tissues or submucosa, usually occurring about the face (eyes, lips, tongue), but any part of the body may be involved. Two types are now well recognized: sporadic, transient angioedema, related to giant urticaria but involving deeper vessels, caused primarily by food allergy; and hereditary angioedema, which is transmitted as an autosomal dominant trait and is marked by severe deficiency in function of an inhibitor to the activated first component of complement—C'1 esterase.

Etiology. The causes of the sporadic type are the same as in urticaria (see Ch. 75) and most frequently involve food allergy, although occasionally an inhalant or contactant may be incriminated. In some, emotional factors can trigger an attack. A definite relationship between aspirin ingestion and angioedema has been documented in some individuals. Often asthma and nasal polyps are also associated. Evidence does not favor an immunologic basis for this syndrome, and the mechanism is unknown; the recently reported effect of aspirin upon prostaglandins may provide an important lead.

The lesion of the familial variety is indistinguishable from the sporadic type but is not related to hypersensitivity. Serum from affected persons who are heterozygotes (the trait is dominant) has very low inhibitor activity between attacks and often none measurable during the attack. In a variant of the disease the inhibitor is present but in an inactive form. Deficiency of the inhibitor is due to impaired synthesis, because catabolic rates in affected patients are normal.

Pathogenesis. Sporadic angioedema may be thought of as a variant of giant urticaria, with dilation of subcutaneous instead of cutaneous vessels and leakage of fluid and colloid into the tissues. It is generally believed that interaction of ingested allergens with reaginic antibody causes release of vasoactive mediators, including histamine, slow-reacting substance of anaphylaxis (SRS-A), and, possibly, bradykinins. Because the affected capillaries are deep, redness and intradermal swelling are not features. Respiratory and gastrointestinal symptoms occur rarely; the latter should raise a strong suspicion of hereditary angioedema, because abdominal pain is a common feature of the familial disease.

The relationship of the deficiency of C'1 esterase inhibitor to the attacks of angioedema is a complicated one. Attacks are associated with the presence of active C'1, depletion of its natural substrates which are C'4 and C'2,

and elevation of bradykinin levels. In addition to inhibiting C'1 esterase activity, the inhibitor is known to inhibit kallikrein and plasmin. Kallikrein converts a serum alpha globulin to bradykinin; plasmin is a broad tryptic-like enzyme which digests fibrin, may cleave C'3 to produce anaphylatoxin (a vasoactive mediator), and may digest Hageman factor into active fragments which can convert prekallikrein to kallikrein. C'1 esterase inhibitor also reduces the capacity of active Hageman factor or its fragments to convert prekallikrein to kallikrein and to convert plasminogen proactivator to the active form. To sum up: the C'1 esterase inhibitor acts at several places, and its deficiency favors the formation of vasoactive mediators from the complement sequence (C'2a, C'3a) and indirectly from the formation of active plasmin and kallikrein.

Clinical Manifestations. The lesion is a tense, rounded, nonpitting swelling several centimeters in diameter which may last two or three days. In addition to the face, the hands, feet, and genitalia are often affected. In the familial form, laryngeal edema accounts for death in 30 per cent of the patients. Severe abdominal pain, vomiting, and the appearance of an acute intra-abdominal condition is common in the familial type and is an important differentiating feature from the sporadic variety. During abdominal attacks a characteristic pattern of bowel wall edema can sometimes be demonstrated in x-rays of the gastrointestinal tract. Attacks may be initiated after minor trauma such as tooth extraction, supporting the relationship to the clotting mechanism and the role of Hageman factor activation.

Diagnosis. The sudden appearance of profound swelling without trauma or underlying infection is strongly suggestive of angioneurotic edema. Accompanying urticaria or a history of food allergy is helpful, but an inapparent insect bite can sometimes cause swelling of the eyelid or lip and must be considered. The familial form often presents with abdominal complaints accompanying the subcutaneous swelling, and laryngeal edema is also frequently noted. Symptoms of hereditary angioedema may rarely first appear in adult life, and the presence of active C'1 esterase inhibitor should be confirmed in any case involving laryngeal edema or abdominal complaints.

Prognosis. The sporadic variety tends to recur either because all the causative factors are not identified, or, more likely, because the patient "cheats" and samples a forbidden food. The hereditary form of the disease is often fatal in early life, although not before reproductive age.

Treatment. Like urticaria, sporadic angioedema is treated with epinephrine, 0.3 to 0.5 ml, 1:1000, or an aqueous solution containing crystalline epinephrine 1:200 (Susphrine), 0.6 to 0.8 ml, given in conjunction with antihistamines. Brompheniramine (Dimetane), 4 mg, tripelennamine (Pyribenzamine), 50 mg, or diphenhydramine (Benadryl), 50 mg, may be given every four hours. Resolution is slow, because resorption of tissue fluid is required. Prednisone, 40 mg per day, may be given for three to four days in severe or prolonged cases. The patient should be carefully questioned about activities within the 12- to 24-hour period preceding the onset, with special reference to items passing the lips such as food, chewing gum, toothpaste, or aspirin. Usually the patient knows the culprit.

In the hereditary form of disease the aforementioned measures are useless. Poor responses to epinephrine, antihistamine, and corticosteroids are well documented. Some salutary effects of methyltestosterone have been claimed, but recent controlled studies revealed that epsilon-aminocaproic acid (EACA), a potent plasmin inhibitor, prevented or ameliorated attacks when given in doses of 7 to 16 grams per day. The mechanism is unknown. Plasmin may activate C'1, producing the clinical attack, and the drug works by inhibiting plasmin. Infusions of plasma have had only limited trials, because, in addition to providing the inhibitor, plasma contains more substrate for the activated enzymes and could theoretically produce adverse effects.

Fink, A. I., and Gay, L. N.: A critical review of 170 cases of urticaria and angioneurotic edema followed for a period of from two to ten years. Bull. Johns Hopkins Hosp., 55:280, 1934.

Ruddy, S., Gigli, I., and Austen, K. F.: The complement system of man. N. Engl. J. Med. 287:489, 1972.

Thompson, J. S.: Urticaria and angioedema. Ann. Intern. Med., 69:361, 1968.

77. INSECT STINGS

Fred S. Kantor

Allergy to antigens contained in the venom of the Hymenoptera insects (bee, wasp, hornet, yellow jacket) may produce a fatal reaction when an otherwise healthy victim is stung. Often a history is obtained of a previous sting which produced local swelling more extensive and longlasting than usual. The patient may rapidly develop shock with or without respiratory difficulty, urticaria, or angioedema, and prompt treatment is vital. If the site of the sting is known, and on an extremity, a tourniquet should be placed above the site to delay further absorption of venom. Epinephrine, 1:1000, 0.3 to 0.5 ml, should be given subcutaneously. If the patient is in shock, the intravenous route must be used, despite the hazard of arrhythmia, to ensure absorption of the drug. Bees have barbed stingers and leave the stinger and venom sac at the site. These should be removed with a forceps or scraped off with the edge of a fingernail so that the venom remaining in the venom sac is not injected through the stinger into the patient. Antihistaminics and steroids are given as adjuncts to epinephrine as described in Ch. 76.

After the acute episode is controlled and before leaving, the patient should be given an emergency kit which contains two tourniquets (stings may be multiple), forceps, or an eyebrow tweezer, a syringe for epinephrine injection (1 ml, 1:1000), and antihistamine tablets. If restung, the patient is instructed to place the tourniquet above the site, take one antihistaminic tablet (diphenhydramine [Benadryl], 50 mg), and prepare the epinephrine syringe while obtaining help from others. Muscular activity enhances the rate of absorption of venom; the patient should be urged to walk, not run, toward help. Since a generalized reaction may lead to temporary skin-test refractoriness, the patient is urged to return in three weeks for testing and hyposensitization treatment. This is clearly effective in preventing fatal reactions upon subsequent exposure in the majority of patients. Results of treatment and a wider discussion of insect stings may be found in the November, 1973, issue of The Journal of Allergy and Clinical Immunology.

Part V

CONNECTIVE TISSUE DISEASES ("COLLAGEN DISEASES") OTHER THAN RHEUMATOID ARTHRITIS

78. INTRODUCTION

K. Frank Austen

The connective tissue ("collagen") diseases or systemic rheumatic diseases are a group of clinicopathologic entities considered together because of common or overlapping clinical and histologic features. The term "collagen diseases" was introduced by Klemperer for such reasons and not because of any conviction about a common etiology. Each of the major entities within this grouping has prominent nonspecific constitutional manifestations coupled with patterns of organ involvement which determine the clinical designation, i.e., rheumatoid arthritis, rheumatic fever, systemic lupus erythematosus, scleroderma, dermatomyositis, and periarteritis nodosa (polyarteritis nodosa). Except for rheumatic fever (see Ch. 191), these entities are considered in this Part and in Part VI. The common histologic features of the group are widespread inflammatory damage to connective tissues and blood vessels, at times associated with deposition of fibrinoid material. Fibrinoid refers to an amorphous material staining deeply eosinophilic with hematoxylin and eosin, which is deposited along connective tissue fibers and within vessel walls, and most probably represents a nonspecific response of connective tissue to injury. Clinical findings which have been invoked to support a common grouping include cardinal features of more than one entity in the same patient; transitions between one entity and another within the same patient; possible familial aggregation; and serologic abnormalities which may predominate in one entity but have an appreciable incidence in others.

Progressive systemic sclerosis (scleroderma), polymyositis alone or with cutaneous manifestations (dermatomyositis), and systemic lupus erythematosus (SLE) have distinct clinicopathologic and/or serologic features. By contrast, periarteritis nodosa has neither a characteristic morphologic, biochemical, or immunochemical abnormality nor a clinical presentation that is easily distinguished from systemic necrotizing angiitis of other types, including those which may be associated with any of the other connective tissue diseases. It seems pertinent, therefore, to review historically the problem of necrotizing angiitis and to include an operational classification based almost entirely upon clinical considerations. Detailed consideration of the structure and function of the structural proteins, collagen and elastin, ground substance, and cellular elements of connective tissue is presented first.

CONNECTIVE TISSUE

Connective tissues are composed of various combinations of collagen, elastin, proteoglycans, and other less well characterized glycoproteins. The unique proportions and distribution of these individual components give different organs of connective tissue their particular qualities. The proteoglycans and the specific arrangement of collagen fibers at various layers give cartilage its smooth, translucent quality and its toughness with elasticity; in contrast, bone has a lesser amount of proteoglycans and a rigid structure related to mineralization within and around collagen fibers. The lens of the eye is transparent because of the precise planes in which collagen fibrils are laid down. Skin and blood vessels are rich in elastin which confers upon these tissues a capacity for distensibility. Basement membrane, a specialized form of collagen and glycoprotein, separates epithelium and endothelium from their environment in multiple tissues. Only in very rare diseases is a primary abnormality of the connective tissue responsible for symptoms or pathology. However, in all forms of arthritis or vasculitis the connective tissues are the site in which inflammation occurs. Although playing a passive, secondary role in pathophysiology, it is damage to connective tissue that results in the signs and symptoms of disease.

Collagen is synthesized by fibroblasts, chondrocytes, and osteoblasts. Different genes code for synthesis of distinct collagen polypeptides in different organs. Thus skin and bone collagens are triple helical structures with two similar α chain polypeptides ($\alpha1$ [I]) and one $\alpha2$ polypeptide chain, whereas cartilage collagen is composed of three $\alpha1$ (II) chains which have a different primary sequence. Collagen α chains are synthesized on polyribosomes as a procollagen. The pro-α chains of collagen undergo hydroxylation of numerous proline residues to give hydroxyproline and certain lysine residues to yield hydroxylysine; several of the hydroxylysine residues are then glycosylated. Procollagen has an additional peptide attached to the amino terminus which is cleaved off when pro-α chains are released from the cell. The hydroxylated glycosylated collagen molecule then precipitates with other similar molecules in precise register to form collagen fibrils. This precise register gives the 640 to 700 Å periodicity on electron microscopy characteristic of collagen fibrils. After fibril formation an additional change in primary structure of the molecule occurs, that of cross-linking within and between different molecules. Cross-links are derived by oxidation and aldol condensation between lysine, hydroxylysine, and histidine residues on adjacent polypeptide chains of the same molecule and on other molecules as well. Cross-linking makes collagen more stable and may retard its susceptibility to specific collagenases.

Recently synthesized collagen has a more rapid turn-over than mature collagen. Since hydroxyproline is present only in collagen and elastin, and since collagen is the most abundant protein in the body, the excretion of urinary hydroxyproline serves as a rough index of collagen turnover. Collagen is degraded by collagenases, present in mesenchymal tissues and in certain epithelial tissues, which cleave through one site on each collagen triple helix. The reaction products uncoil, are thermally denatured at body temperature, and become immediately susceptible to multiple tissue proteases. In rheumatoid arthritis and certain skin and bone diseases, proliferation of cells which synthesize collagenase may result in excessive destruction of collagen.

The so-called "collagen diseases" are not primary diseases of collagen, and there are few examples of true collagen disease. In *dermatosparaxis*, a disease of calves, procollagen is not cleaved to collagen, and the resulting fibrils in the skin lack tensile strength, allowing the animals to become denuded. In humans, a heritable disease with an expression similar to Ehlers-Danlos syndrome occurs in which the enzyme activity which hydroxylates lysine to form hydroxylysine in collagen and other proteins is markedly decreased. In *homocystinuria* an abnormal collagen may be formed because significant quantities of homocysteine inhibit cross-link formation between collagen molecules. Ascorbic acid is one of the cofactors (along with ferrous iron and α-ketoglutarate) essential for hydroxylation of proline and lysine residues in collagen; since poorly hydroxylated collagen forms a less stable helix, this may explain the decrease in tensile strength of healing wounds in ascorbic acid deficiency (scurvy).

Basement membranes provide elastic support and act as a filtration barrier between epithelial and endothelial cells and their environment. The amino acid composition of basement membrane resembles that of collagen except that it has a high concentration of carbohydrate, many sulfur-containing amino acids, and very high concentrations of hydroxylysine relative to other collagens.

Proteoglycans have a role in connective tissue not unlike that of cement in reinforced concrete. The proteoglycans are formed of subunits of disaccharides linked together and joined to a protein core. In articular cartilage this core is a protein with a length of 20,000 to 50,000 Å. The disaccharide chains, many of which are sulfated, have a length of 15,000 to 36,000 Å. Each proteoglycan subunit (core protein plus disaccharide chains) is joined with others to form large aggregates by a link glycoprotein. The physiologic implications of this macromolecular organization are probably related to the excluded volume effect; that is, in connective tissue, they control by virtue of size and domain the passage of other molecules to and from cells. In the polysaccharide component of proteoglycans one of the hexose residues of each disaccharide group is a hexosamine, and the other is a uronic acid or galactose moiety. Proteoglycans are synthesized by mesenchymal tissues by a complicated process involving assembly of the polysaccharide units, sulfation, and covalent linkage to the protein core.

Proteoglycans have a more rapid turnover than collagen and are degraded primarily by acid hydrolases found in lysosomes. Factors such as vitamin A which destabilize lysosomal membranes can result in general-ized depletion of proteoglycans from many connective tissues. Proteoglycan destruction is accentuated by products of the inflammatory cells in the connective tissue, but there is no evidence to suggest that there is a primary abnormality of the proteoglycans in the "collagen" diseases. A possible exception may be *degenerative* or *osteoarthritis* in which increased autolysis of proteoglycans by chondrocytes may be an initial factor.

Elastin has covalent cross-links, desmosine and isodesmosine, which are similar to cross-links in collagen and are formed from condensation of lysine residues on different parts of the same chain or other elastin polypeptides. Unlike collagen, which is a rigid rod, elastin is an amorphous random coil aggregate linked by these cross-links; this structure assures its return to an original configuration after it is distorted and gives rise to its elastic properties.

HISTORICAL REVIEW OF ANGIITIS

The term *periarteritis nodosa* was aptly introduced by Kussmaul and Maier in 1866 to designate a morbid process manifested by numerous nodules along muscular-type arteries. Infiltration of the media with polymorphonuclear leukocytes and to a lesser extent eosinophils, plasma cells, and lymphocytes, disruption of the internal elastic lamina, fibrinoid necrosis, and extension to the adventitia and intima are characteristic. Proliferation of the intima leads to partial or total occlusion, and segmental scarring of the entire wall is responsible for the visible and/or palpable aneurysms. It is characteristic of the lesions to be in all stages of evolution from acute to healed. Additional characteristic features of periarteritis nodosa are the sparing of capillaries and veins except for involvement by spread from contiguous arteries, and the absence of involvement of pulmonary arteries despite the location of nodules in the bronchial arteries.

In 1923 Ophüls reported a patient with a periarteritis nodosa–like illness with the additional features of pulmonary vessel lesions, extensive involvement of small arteries and veins, granulomatous vascular and extravascular reactions, and an intense eosinophilic infiltration of vascular and pulmonary parenchymal lesions. The granulomas often included an eosinophilic core of altered collagen and necrotic eosinophils surrounded by radially arranged macrophages, lymphocytes, plasma cells, and varying numbers of polymorphonuclear leukocytes, both neutrophilic and eosinophilic. A detailed study of similar patients in 1951 by Churg and Strauss emphasized the striking clinical feature of severe progressive asthma with peripheral eosinophilia followed by fever, and prompted these authors to term this entity *allergic angiitis and granulomatosis*. Rose and Spencer (1957) also appreciated these unique clinicopathologic features but preferred the term polyarteritis with pulmonary involvement to distinguish this group from classic polyarteritis.

In 1926 von Glahn and Pappenheimer considered that the *arteritis of rheumatic fever* could be distinguished from periarteritis nodosa by the absence of arterial thrombosis (or eosinophils), involvement of small arteries, and minimal fibrinoid necrosis. In the heart, Aschoff bodies represent a key extravascular histologic finding, although the clinical manifestations are predominantly related to rheumatic carditis.

Still another type of necrotizing vascular lesion, originally believed to be limited to the cranial arteries and characterized by the presence of multinucleated giant cells, was recognized by Horton, Magath, and Brown in 1934 and established as a clinical entity by Kilbourne and Wolff in 1946. The process usually involves the innermost layer of the media with predominantly a lymphocyte infiltration, the presence of multinucleated giant cells, fragmentation of the internal elastic lamina, and associated fibrinoid necrosis. The infiltration may extend to involve the adventitia and the intima, leading to intimal thickening with subsequent thrombosis. This entity, *giant cell arteritis,* can be predominantly local—presenting as cranial, especially temporal, or aortic arch (Takayasu's) arteritis—or it may be systemic. The syndrome of polymyalgia rheumatica seems to be associated with a local or systemic form of giant cell arteritis with or without arterial occlusion.

Necrotizing vascular lesions associated with the administration of horse antiserum and the development of clinical serum sickness were described by Clark and Kaplan in 1937. Rich observed similar lesions (1942) which he considered to be periarteritis nodosa not only in cases of serum sickness but also in circumstances of sulfonamide hypersensitivity. However, the more recent and prevailing view proposed by Zeek in 1952 is that hypersensitivity to drugs and serum, termed *hypersensitivity angiitis,* is distinguishable from periarteritis nodosa. Hypersensitivity angiitis involves small arteries, arterioles, and venules in a process of fibrinoid necrosis, occurring in the subendothelial ground substance and extending from the intima to involve the entire vessel wall; the accompanying cellular reaction is pleomorphic with polymorphonuclear leukocyte predominance frequently including eosinophils. Hypersensitivity angiitis often involves the pulmonary system and is characterized by virtually all lesions being at a similar evolutionary stage.

An unresolved issue is whether or not allergic granulomatosis and angiitis as defined by Churg and Strauss encompasses *Wegener's granulomatosis.* This disease, described by Wegener in 1936, is characterized by necrotizing granulomatous lesions of the upper and lower respiratory tract, generalized focal necrotizing lesions of both arteries and veins, and a glomerulitis typified by fibrin thrombi, focal necrosis of tufts, and on occasion a granulomatous reaction. This complex is somewhat similar to allergic granulomatosis and angiitis, but it is noteworthy that Wegener's granulomatosis is not associated with progressive asthma and prominent peripheral eosinophilia and does not exhibit a prominence of eosinophils in the necrotizing lesions. Thus for the present it seems reasonable to list this entity separately; lethal midline granuloma may be a related condition or a local variant. (See Ch. 105.) More recently, variants of Wegener's granulomatosis have been recognized in which the granulomatous reactions are predominantly lymphoid- and sarcoid-like, respectively.

The final category includes miscellaneous entities. Atrophic malignant papulosis, described by Degos in 1954, refers to a characteristic clinical triad associated with necrotizing vascular lesions of the skin, gastrointestinal tract, and brain. Erythema elevatum diutinum is manifested by a chronic erythematous-papular and often purpuric skin eruption with or without systemic signs such as arthritis; it will probably be shifted to the hypersensitivity angiitis group when more information

is available. A variety of purely cutaneous vasculitis syndromes have been described, and only time will tell whether these are distinct or are merely limited manifestations of a systemic entity.

OPERATIONAL CLASSIFICATION OF NECROTIZING ANGIITIS

Necrotizing angiitis is a convenient generic term for the entire group of syndromes in which vascular lesions, arterial or venous or both, may involve all three layers of the vessel wall with fibrinoid necrosis and various cellular infiltrates (see accompanying table). The clinical manifestations are caused largely by partial or complete vascular occlusion; the lesions are segmental, and the clinical patterns depend on the size and characteristic distribution of the lesions. Zeek recognized five major syndromes in this group: periarteritis nodosa, allergic angiitis and granulomatosis, rheumatic fever, giant cell arteritis, and hypersensitivity angiitis. With some modification this tabulation continues to be operationally useful.

Rheumatic fever can be placed under a category broadened to include those collagen diseases in which necrotizing vascular lesions are present but are not the most prominent aspect of the entity, i.e., rheumatoid arthritis, scleroderma, dermatomyositis, polymyositis, Sjögren's syndrome, and erythema nodosum. The category of hypersensitivity angiitis is particularly diverse and contains a variety of clinical entities distinguishable on the basis of precipitating events, serologic abnormalities, and relative frequency of involvement of various organ systems—drug reactions, Henoch-Schönlein purpura, serum sickness, systemic lupus erythematosus, mixed cryoglobulinemia (IgG-IgM complexes), hypergammaglobulinemic purpura, C2 deficiency with vasculitis, occasional instances of chronic urticaria, and Goodpasture's syndrome. The problems of any effort at

Necrotizing Angiitis

Periarteritis nodosa (polyarteritis nodosa)

Allergic angiitis and granulomatosis of Churg and Strauss ("polyarteritis nodosa with pulmonary involvement")

Connective tissue disease ("collagen disease"), associated with
  Rheumatoid arthritis
  Scleroderma
  Poly- and dermatomyositis
  Rheumatic fever
  Erythema nodosum
  Sjögren's syndrome

Giant cell arteritis

Hypersensitivity angiitis
  Drug reaction
  Henoch-Schönlein purpura
  Systemic lupus erythematosus
  Mixed cryoglobulinemia
  Goodpasture's syndrome
  Hypergammaglobulinemic purpura
  C2 deficiency with vasculitis
  Australian antigenemia with vasculitis

Wegener's granulomatosis and variants

Miscellaneous
  Degos' disease (malignant papulosis)
  Erythema elevatum diutinum

classification are highlighted by the vasculitis associated with Australian antigenemia and designated periarteritis nodosa by some. The clinical manifestations of urticaria, arthralgia, fever, eosinophilia, and azotemia; the pathologic findings of fibrinoid necrotizing lesions of arterioles with deposition of immunoglobulin, viral antigen, and complement; and the serologic presence of circulating immune complexes with hypocomplementemia are entirely consistent with hypersensitivity angiitis. The demonstration of arterial abnormalities by angiography presumably reflects the continuum from periarteritis nodosa to hypersensitivity angiitis under these etiologic circumstances. Separate categories are introduced for Wegener's granulomatosis and for a miscellaneous grouping.

Such an operational classification is a justified interim measure because there are associated implications as to prognosis, treatment, and etiology. A classification based on mechanism is a further goal, and to this end a few cautionary comments about the immunopathologic approach are in order. The fibrinoid in the lesions of systemic lupus erythematosus contains protein residues of nuclear origin, acid mucopolysaccharides derived from altered ground substance, and fibrinogen (or derivatives), immunoglobulins, and complement proteins. These findings are interpreted to mean the presence of immune complexes, consisting of nuclear antigen and antibody, complement fixation, and secondary deposition of fibrinogen and alteration of ground substance. In Goodpasture's syndrome the fibrinoid necrosis of the alveolar wall and in the glomerulus is associated with deposition of complement and immunoglobulins with a specificity against basement membrane. In vasculitis associated with Australian antigenemia, immune complexes with specific antigen have been isolated from the plasma and recognized in tissues along with complement by immunofluorescent studies. Whereas in systemic lupus erythematosus, vasculitis with Australian antigenemia, mixed cryoglobulinemia, and Goodpasture's syndrome the specificity of the antibodies contributing to or responsible for the clinicopathologic manifestations of the disease is known, such is not the case for the other entities shown in the table. Thus, the contribution of immunologic events to their lesions is a matter of speculation. Immunoglobulins and complement have been observed in the glomerular lesions of Henoch-Schönlein purpura, in the vascular lesions of rheumatoid arthritis and of periarteritis nodosa, and in the granulomatous response of allergic angiitis and granulomatosis (often with fibrinogen), but not in Wegener's granulomatosis. Such proteins could deposit nonspecifically owing to trapping, transudation or exudation, or because of aggregation of gamma globulin. Studies should be directed toward determining the specificity of the deposited immunoglobulins. Arguments to favor specific deposition could be based on demonstration of antigen in the lesion, recognition of the antibody specificity following elution, and demonstration that the predominant L chain type or H chain subgroup in the deposit is different from the ratio observed in the circulation. Each of these criteria has been met with regard to the lesions of systemic lupus erythematosus.

Churg, J., and Strauss, L.: Allergic granulomatosis, allergic angiitis, and periarteritis nodosa. Am. J. Pathol., 27:277, 1951.

Frohnert, P. P., and Sheps, S. G.: Long-term follow-up study of periarteritis nodosa. Am. J. Med., 43:8, 1967.

Gocke, D. J., Morgan, C., Lockshin, M., Hsu, K., Bombardieri, S., and Christian, C. L.: Association between polyarteritis and Australian antigen. Lancet, 2:1149, 1970.

Grant, M. E., and Prockop, D. J.: The biosynthesis of collagen. N. Engl. J. Med., 286:194, 242, 291, 1972.

Harris, E. D., Evanson, J. M., Dibona, D. R., and Krane, S. M.: Collagenase and rheumatoid arthritis. Arthritis Rheum., 13:83, 1970.

Kilbourne, E. D., and Wolff, H. G.: Cranial arteritis: Critical evaluation of syndrome of "temporal arteritis," with report of a case. Ann. Intern. Med., 24:1, 1946.

Klemperer, P.: The concept of collagen disease in medicine. Am. Rev. Respir. Dis., 83:331, 1961.

Kussmaul, A., and Maier, R.: Über eine bisher nicht beschreibene eigenthümliche Arterienerkrankung (Periarteritis nodosa), die mit Morbus Brightii und rapid fortschreitender allgemeiner Muskellähmung einhergeht. Deutsch. Arch. Klin. Med., 1:484, 1866.

Liebow, A. A.: Pulmonary angiitis and granulomatosis. Am. Rev. Respir. Dis., 108:1, 1973.

Silbert, J. E.: Biosynthesis of muco-polysaccharides and proteinpolysaccharides. In Perez-Tamayo, R., and Rojkind, M. (eds.): Molecular Pathology of Connective Tissues. New York, Marcel Dekker, Inc., 1973.

Wegener, F.: Über generalisierte, septische Gefässerkrankungen. Verh. Deutsch. Ges. Path., 29:202, 1936.

Zeek, P. M.: Periarteritis nodosa: A critical review. Am. J. Clin. Pathol., 22:777, 1952.

79.   SYSTEMIC SCLEROSIS
(Scleroderma)

Edward D. Harris, Jr.

General Considerations. *Scleroderma* is a disease involving blood vessels and connective tissue. The clinical picture is dominated by symptoms of vascular insufficiency caused by abnormalities in small arterioles and capillaries, and by progressive fibrosis in multiple organs. Most patients have involvement predominantly of the arms and hands with Raynaud's phenomenon and acrosclerosis. The face and upper chest may be affected as well, but it is interesting that the legs and feet are involved less often, and it is rare that diffuse involvement of the entire skin is seen. Associated with the cutaneous manifestations are dysfunctions of certain viscera, particularly the esophagus, lungs, and kidneys.

Localized scleroderma, a term which includes morphea and linear scleroderma, involves the skin exclusively.

The diagnosis of systemic sclerosis is made most often in patients between the ages of 35 and 55. Between three and five new cases per million population appear each year. Only 8 per cent of cases begin in the first two decades of life. The disease is three times more common in females than in males. There is some evidence that black women have a poorer prognosis than white women, and males a poorer prognosis than females.

Pathogenesis and Pathology. *Pathogenesis.* Data are accumulating to indicate that abnormalities in the vascular system are primarily involved in the pathogenesis of this disease. Raynaud's phenomenon with its characteristic blanching and pain followed by suffusion is a very common initial complaint in systemic sclerosis. Patients with Raynaud's phenomenon have been shown to have significantly decreased cutaneous fingertip blood flow compared with that of normal controls when both were cooled to 18°C. In clinically unaffected muscle tissue, patients with scleroderma have been shown to have loss of 80 per cent of the normal amount of capillaries; those remaining capillaries have a diameter increased over normal, swollen endothelial cells, and reduplication of the basement membrane. Surface microvessels of the nail fold in systemic sclerosis are also decreased in number and increased in diameter. Digital arteriograms in patients with Raynaud's syndrome and scleroderma often have shown obstruction of the proper digital arteries, and plethysmography has demonstrated decreased amplitude of reflection of the pulse. There may be a common factor of altered vascular reactivity in the development of Raynaud's phenomenon, depressed sensitivity to cholinergic agonists of the lower esophageal sphincter, pulmonary hypertension, and reduced renal cortical blood flow—all abnormalities associated with systemic sclerosis. Resting venous catecholamine concentrations and urinary catecholamine excretion patterns in scleroderma have been normal.

Studies of the proliferative lesion of scleroderma (the appearance of excessive and inappropriate collagen deposition) have revealed no significant abnormality of physical properties, amino acid analyses, cross-linking, or solubility of collagen. Detailed sequence studies have not been carried out in scleroderma collagen; it is not known whether the thin "beaded" filaments in collagen of scleroderma which resemble "embryonic" fibrils actually do represent $\alpha 1$ (III) collagen—a genetically different type of collagen α chains recently characterized from many soft tissues, including blood vessels and fetal skin.

Numerous studies have indicated that there is an increased rate of collagen synthesis in scleroderma. Increased activity of protocollagen proline hydroxylase has been found in skin biopsies from scleroderma. Medium from cultures in vitro of scleroderma skin fibroblasts has been found to contain significantly more collagen than does medium from control cells. A similar increase in the synthetic rate of sialic acid, a proteoglycan component of connective tissue, has been found. No defect in the collagenolytic system in scleroderma has been reported.

To sum up: A leading yet unproved hypothesis for the development of systemic sclerosis is that a primary abnormality of the small blood vessels causes change in connective tissue sufficient to alter normal patterns of collagen and proteoglycan metabolism.

There is very little evidence that tissue damage in scleroderma is mediated by immune complexes or activation of the complement or kinin systems. Although only rare reports have revealed gamma globulin deposited along renal basement membranes in scleroderma, fibrin as a component of fibrinoid material in walls of small vessels of "scleroderma kidneys" is commonly found.

Pathology. The result of systemic involvement in scleroderma is sclerosis. The *reticular dermis* is usually thickened. It may have a normal collagen-bundle pattern or may show broad, homogeneous, acellular deposits of collagen with indistinct bundle patterns. Other findings include atrophy of the rete pegs of the epidermis, atrophy of the hair follicles and sweat glands, perivascular lymphocytic infiltration, and hyalinization of arterioles. During acute, early phases of the disease, edema may be present in the dermis. The subcutaneous tissue is replaced by thick collagen bundles which bind the dermis to deeper structures. Pathologic changes in the musculoskeletal system include acute and chronic inflammation in the *synovium* with no pannus formation and with more sclerosis than is found in rheumatoid synovium with an equivalent inflammatory response. Fibrin deposits are laid down around *tendons,* and in *muscles* there are a variety of abnormalities, the most common being fibrosis of the perimysium and epimysium, scattered cellular infiltrates, and atrophy and necrosis of muscle fibers similar to that seen in polymyositis.

In the internal organs, microvascular abnormalities (see Pathogenesis), mild inflammation, and edema in connective tissue are followed by increased deposition of fibrous tissue in both appropriate and inappropriate loci. This leads to distortion of the architecture of the tissues affected. In the *lungs,* a relatively low-grade interstitial pneumonitis is followed by interstitial fibrosis, most marked in lower lobes. After this, cyst formation and bronchiectasis may develop. Arteriolar thickening (concentric intimal proliferation or medial hypertrophy) is seen, particularly in those patients with clinical evidence of pulmonary hypertension. In the gastrointestinal tract, the *esophagus* is frequently involved with muscle atrophy and fibrosis. Lesions secondary to reflux of gastric contents are present in 20 per cent. Fibrosis around Brunner's glands in the submucosa of the *duodenum* occurs and can be recognized on specimens obtained by peroral biopsy. Involvement of the *small bowel* begins with patchy subserosal fibrosis and may progress to almost complete replacement of smooth muscle with fibrous tissue and marked thickening of the serosa. The small bowel may develop multiple sacculations, presumably at sites of weakness in the continuity of the wall. Dilation, muscle atrophy, and fibrosis are seen in the *colon;* the fibrosis is irregular, leading to the characteristic sacculations and diverticula. The *heart* is frequently enlarged and may be the only organ weighing more than predicted for the subject's body weight. Small patches of interstitial myocardial fibrosis are commonly found. In very severe cases, as much as 60 per cent of cardiac muscle is replaced by dense, relatively acellular and avascular fibrous tissue. Endocardial or valvular thickening is unusual and is rarely of hemodynamic significance. Fibrinous pericarditis is found quite often, even in the absence of uremia. *Kidneys* in scleroderma are normal in size when renal involvement has not been present clinically. In patients dying with uremia they may be small and frequently have small cortical infarcts. Histologically, intimal proliferation in the interlobular arteries, fibrinoid necrosis of small arteries and arterioles (including the glomerular tufts), and thickening of the basement membrane (the "wire-loop" lesion) may all be present. These changes are similar to those seen in kidneys from patients with malignant hypertension and occasionally may be present in the absence of renal failure or severe hypertension.

Clinical Manifestations and Diagnoses. The disease usually begins insidiously. Raynaud's phenomenon, vague weakness, weight loss, diffuse stiffness and aching, polyarticular arthritis, and diffuse edema of the hands are the most common initial symptoms. If the illness progresses, it generally does so slowly, and is marked by characteristic organ system changes. Rarely, rapid progression to severe cutaneous and visceral involvement may occur in less than six months.

Cutaneous System. The patient with classic, well-developed acrosclerosis presents with taut, thickened, or edematous skin bound tightly to subcutaneous tissues in the hands and fingers. Feet and toes are involved less often than hands, forearms, and neck. Normal skin folds at the knuckles disappear. Chronic recurrent painful ulcerations at the ends of the digits develop, and the fingers themselves may shorten through progressive resorption of the terminal phalanges. Joints become immobilized from tight encasement in thickened skin as well as from contractures of muscles and tendons and palmar fascia. Telangiectasia, increased or decreased pigmentation, and subcutaneous calcification are common. Hair becomes thin, and the skin of the face appears smooth and waxy. The skin around the mouth may constrict, restricting lip movement and preventing adequate dental hygiene. The normal sweating mechanism is often impaired; the involved skin feels leathery and dry and may scale and itch. The CRST syndrome (calcinosis, Raynaud's phenomenon, sclerodactyly, and telangiectasia) and the Thibierge-Weissenbach syndrome (diffuse deposition of insoluble calcium phosphates in subcutaneous tissue in the presence of acrosclerosis) are variants of the cutaneous expression of systemic sclerosis.

Musculoskeletal System. Almost half the patients with systemic sclerosis present with joint pain or develop it during the first year of their illness. Small joints are involved more often than large ones. Joint deformity and immobility in systemic sclerosis do not result from an invasive, erosive synovitis as in rheumatoid arthritis, but are the result of encasement as subcutaneous tissue is replaced by bundles of collagen. Muscle wasting is often severe in areas such as the hands, in which joint mobility is impaired by progressive tightening of the overlying skin.

Gastrointestinal Tract. Of the internal organ systems, the gastrointestinal tract is the one most often involved in systemic sclerosis. *Oral* symptoms include xerostomia and a progressive decrease in the size of the mouth. Sjögren's syndrome is seen often, and the frequency of its association with systemic sclerosis is probably underestimated. Symptoms referable to the *esophagus,* ranging from simple dysphagia to heartburn, nausea, and substernal fullness, are found in 45 to 60 per cent of cases. The dysphagia is related to diminished peristalsis in the lower segments of the esophagus and incompetence of the lower esophageal sphincter. If reflux esophagitis becomes a persistent complication, stricture may develop. There is a very frequent association of Raynaud's phenomenon and decreased esophageal peristalsis, although this association is not limited to patients with scleroderma. Vomiting, abdominal distention, and pain or diarrhea may indicate involvement of the *small intestine.* As in the esophagus, motility of the small bowel is decreased, and there may be malabsorption secondary to intraluminal stagnation with concomitant bacterial overgrowth. Functional bowel complaints secondary to pathologic changes in the *colon* are common. Disease of both large and small bowel may produce a clinical picture identical to paralytic ileus with incomplete obstruction at any level. Pneumatosis cystoides intestinalis (air-filled cysts in the mesentery which may rupture, causing peritonitis) is a rare but striking complication of scleroderma bowel disease.

An association between primary biliary cirrhosis and scleroderma with CRST syndrome is now recognized.

Heart and Lungs. Dyspnea is the most common cardiorespiratory symptom in systemic sclerosis and is present in more than 50 per cent of patients. Fine, dry crackles at the bases of the lung are the first abnormality found on physical examination. In some patients, progression to respiratory insufficiency and death from hypoxemia is related to progressive pulmonary fibrosis. The earliest abnormality of pulmonary function is a decrease in pulmonary diffusion capacity. Those exposed in their occupation to silicate dust have a predilection to develop this form of the disease. Restriction of chest wall expansion by dermal fibrosis around the thorax rarely affects respiratory function. A few patients with severe cystic and fibrotic changes in the lungs have developed multifocal alveolar cell carcinomas.

Signs of elevated pulmonary vascular resistance may develop independent of parenchymal changes in the lungs and lead to cor pulmonale and congestive heart failure.

Replacement of myocardium with fibrous tissue on a primary basis ("scleroderma heart disease") is an occasional cause of heart failure. In addition, impaired cardiac function can be attributed to right ventricular failure secondary to pulmonary hypertension.

Kidneys. The sudden development of malignant hypertension resistant to therapy and uremia progressing rapidly to death is a dreaded complication of systemic sclerosis. Most patients have had skin changes before development of abnormal renal function. Plasma renin is elevated, and renal arteriograms reveal narrowed interlobular arteries and afferent arterioles with focal or generalized loss of the cortical nephrogram. It is rare for patients with this complication to survive longer than four months unless nephrectomy and hemodialysis and/or transplantation are carried out.

Nervous System. Involvement of the nervous system is rare. Facial pain, questionably related to a trigeminal neuropathy, is seen in occasional patients and may be disabling. Significant reduction in mean conduction velocity of peripheral nerves has been reported.

Laboratory Findings. The erythrocyte sedimentation test is elevated in most patients with systemic sclerosis, and a mild anemia of chronic disease may be present. In addition, iron deficiency anemia may result from bleeding from esophagitis, and vitamin B_{12} and/or folic acid deficiency from overgrowth of organisms in an atonic bowel. Hemolysis is unusual, although microangiopathic hemolytic anemia has been described in scleroderma (presumably related to fragmentation of erythrocytes from contact with diseased blood vessels and/or intravascular fibrin). A number of serologic abnormalities link systemic sclerosis to other connective tissue diseases. Mild hypergammaglobulinemia is present in 30 to 50 per cent of patients, rheumatoid factor in 25 to 35 per cent, antinuclear antibodies (often with a speckled or a nucleolar pattern) in sera of 30 to 60 per cent, and LE cells in less than 10 per cent of patients. Urinary hydroxyproline excretion, an index of collagen turnover, has been shown by Rodnan to be greater than normal in some patients, particularly in those with active disease.

The electrocardiogram shows nonspecific abnormalities in almost 50 per cent of patients. The pattern of conduction defects with very low voltage is seen only in those uncommon patients with marked myocardial replacement by fibrous tissue.

Roentgenography. Roentgenograms are important for diagnosis and follow-up evaluation. The findings of soft tissue atrophy, subcutaneous calcinosis, and resorption of the tufts of the terminal phalanges without loss of apparent joint spaces between phalanges are virtually pathognomonic of systemic sclerosis when seen on hand films. The periodontal membrane is occasionally thickened. Upper gastrointestinal films reveal a dilated, atonic esophagus in about 60 per cent of patients. Small bowel studies may demonstrate segmental atony, dilation, and sacculation in the duodenum and jejunum. Linear pneumatosis (air in the wall of the gut) is occasionally seen in flat plates of the abdomen of patients with severe small bowel involvement. Barium studies of the colon reveal wide-mouth, asymmetrical diverticula in 20 to 40 per cent of patients; progression to a dilated, atonic megacolon rarely occurs. In patients with pulmonary involvement, chest roentgenograms reveal a diffuse reticular pattern with a honeycomb appearance in the lower lung fields. Serial films may document progression to a picture of dense interstitial fibrosis amid radiolucent cystic areas.

Differential Diagnosis. When systemic sclerosis presents as persistent symmetrical polyarthritis involving the hands without previous skin changes, it may be impossible to differentiate it from rheumatoid arthritis or systemic lupus erythematosus, or, if the overlying skin becomes edematous or red, dermatomyositis. In fact, "overlap" syndromes combining clinical or serologic manifestations of several of these entities are being described with increasing frequency, and one should avoid hasty classification of any clinical picture that is consistent with more than one of the connective tissue diseases.

Diseases or pathologic findings associated with Raynaud's phenomenon which must be differentiated from scleroderma include occupational trauma; anatomic lesions, e.g., scalenus anticus syndrome and cervical ribs; vasomotor syndromes resulting in disuse atrophy, e.g., Sudek's atrophy or the shoulder-hand syndrome; peripheral vascular arteriosclerosis; heavy metal or ergot poisoning; and hematologic abnormalities, e.g., polycythemia vera, paroxysmal cold hemoglobinuria, and presence of cold agglutinins or cryoproteinemia.

The atrophic changes in the skin in systemic sclerosis must be differentiated from those seen in Werner's syndrome, progeria (Hutchinson-Gilford syndrome), chronic hypostatic edema or myxedema, lichen sclerosus et atrophicus, porphyria cutanea tarda, and/or scleredema. Unlike systemic sclerosis, Werner's syndrome affects the feet more severely than the hands, and has associated with it a high-pitched voice, growth abnormalities, and premature cataracts, arteriosclerosis, and diabetes. Sclerodermatous changes have been reported in skin of patients with progeria, but the dwarf-like stature, characteristic facies, and premature death from coronary insufficiency set this syndrome apart. Porphyria cutanea tarda may have skin changes simulating scleroderma but can be differentiated on the basis of urinary or fecal porphyrin excretion. Scleredema (scleredema adultorum of Buschke) is a brawny edema which appears abruptly, involves skin of the neck and chest initially, and is characterized pathologically by the presence of a material resembling acid mucopolysaccharide diffusely interspersed among collagen bundles in the dermis. This is a self-limited process, perhaps related to a previous bacterial infection, and has a good prognosis. The cutaneous telangiectasia of scleroderma resembles Osler-Weber-Rendu disease (hereditary telangiectasia).

Involvement of viscera in systemic sclerosis can mimic many other illnesses. The abnormalities in pulmonary function and the roentgenographic findings seen are similar to those found in idiopathic pulmonary fibrosis (Hamman-Rich syndrome) and the pulmonary fibrosis of rheumatoid arthritis or advanced sarcoidosis. Scleroderma heart disease must be differentiated from infiltrative cardiomyopathies as well as fibrosis from diffuse coronary artery disease. The dysphagia of scleroderma is completely nonspecific, and disease of the bowel rarely can simulate sprue or any of the malabsorption syndromes, partial intestinal obstruction, or megacolon.

Course Untreated. The course of systemic sclerosis is variable. Those patients with primary acrosclerosis and decreased esophageal motility may have slowly progressive disease with no significant increased probability of early death. Others, particularly patients with pulmonary, cardiac, or renal involvement, may progress rapidly to early death. Renal failure is the cause of death of scleroderma in 20 to 40 per cent of patients. Recent data obtained using life-table methods suggest that there is a 50 to 70 per cent five-year survival. Chances for survival are worse if the patient is a black male, diagnosed over the age of 40 years, with cutaneous lesions of the trunk, pulmonary involvement, and an abnormal electrocardiogram or blood urea nitrogen greater than 40 mg per 100 ml.

Treatment. Patients with acrosclerosis can lead productive and useful lives. The most important goal in therapy is to preserve function in and prevent injury to the hands. Vocational and/or climatic change may be indicated. Hand care must be stressed, including instructions for active and passive exercises that the patient may do himself several times each day in order to prevent further deformity. Early signs of local infection in fingertips must be treated immediately before they progress to large ulcerations. Psychologic support can be of great value in helping a patient adjust to the discomfort and apparently inexorable progression of his disease.

Because so little is known about the underlying defect in scleroderma or its pathogenesis, no specific treatment is available. The one possible exception to this is the use of broad-spectrum antimicrobials in treatment of malabsorption associated with bacterial overgrowth in the upper small intestine. If esophageal motility is decreased, antacid therapy is used liberally to prevent secondary esophagitis and stricture. If stricture develops, bougienage will be needed. Salicylates in pharmacologic doses may decrease clinical signs of inflammation, e.g., elevated sedimentation rates, joint pain, and erythema, which is present in most patients at some time in the course of their disease.

Corticosteroids are ineffective in the treatment of systemic sclerosis; neither the vascular lesions nor the fibrosis are improved by their use. However, there is a subgroup of patients with an overlap syndrome called "mixed connective tissue disease" who present with a variety of symptoms, including Raynaud's phenomenon, arthritis, and skin changes consistent with scleroderma, but with features (including LE cells, leukopenia, inflammatory myositis, and lymphadenopathy) of other connective tissue diseases as well. Many of this group will have high titers of antinuclear antibody in a "speckled" pattern directed against an extractable nuclear antigen (not DNA). In general, this group of patients does not develop renal disease and responds very well to corticosteroid therapy.

Recently, use of intra-arterial reserpine has been advocated to decrease the frequency of Raynaud's phenomenon and potentiate healing of ulcers. Given intra-arterially (0.5 to 1.0 mg), benefit without side effects has been noted up to seven months after a single injection. A decrease in finger vasoconstriction in response to cooling in patients with scleroderma given reserpine in the ipsilateral brachial artery has been documented. The placebo effect of this type of procedure and potential hazards of intra-arterial reserpine must be continually evaluated. Oral reserpine in doses sufficient to relieve symptoms of Raynaud's phenomenon often causes central depression, but when used in small doses (≤ 0.5 mg per day), combined with oral sympathetic or ganglionic blocking agents, may increase capillary blood flow without causing intolerable side effects.

Potassium p-aminobenzoate, ethylenediaminetetra-acetic acid, 6-aminocaproic acid infusions, and dimethyl sulfoxide applications have been employed by a number of investigators. D-penicillamine, capable of inhibiting formation of cross-links in collagen and some mammalian collagenases in vitro, has not been of proved benefit in scleroderma. Pilot studies of immunosuppressive therapy are being evaluated; initial results show no clear-cut role for these drugs in systemic sclerosis.

Initial results in few cases in which "scleroderma kidneys" were removed and hemodialysis and/or renal transplantation carried out have demonstrated that life of good quality can be prolonged by these aggressive approaches. It is not yet known whether the transplanted kidneys will develop vascular changes, but it is now clear that patients with systemic sclerosis who develop renal disease need not die from rapidly progressive renal failure.

D'Angelo, W. A., Fries, J. F., Masi, A. T., and Shulman, L. E.: Pathologic observations in systemic sclerosis (scleroderma). Am. J. Med., 46:428, 1969.
Rodnan, G. P.: Progressive systemic sclerosis (scleroderma) and calcinosis. In Hollander, J. L., and McCarty, D. J. (eds.): Arthritis and Allied Conditions. 8th ed. Philadelphia, Lea & Febiger, 1972.

80. POLYMYOSITIS AND DERMATOMYOSITIS

H. Richard Tyler

General Considerations.   The disorder termed polymyositis refers to an illness first described by Wagner in 1863 in which muscle weakness is the principal clinical feature. Inflammatory, degenerative, and regenerative changes can be seen in the muscles. When skin changes occur and are prominent, the cases are referred to as dermatomyositis. This subgroup was first delineated by Unverricht in 1887. The muscular lesions of dermatomyositis, however, are identical to those seen in polymyositis. Because of the dramatic skin lesions, dermatomyositis was more widely recognized. Appreciation that muscular syndromes are more common than dermatomyositis resulted from the increased use of muscle biopsy and the clinical awareness that an insidious onset and absence of muscle pain are common. If there are changes indicative of nerve damage, the term neuromyositis is occasionally used. Some authors prefer the non-specific and noncommittal term polymyopathy and identify as separate entities only those cases whose specific cause is known. Others reserve the term polymyositis for cases with evidence of inflammatory changes in muscles. Until the cause of the majority of the cases is more clearly identified, one has to accept the need to re-evaluate nomenclature periodically. All these disorders form a large spectrum which ranges from the very acute cases with myoglobinuria to the very chronic localized disorders that mimic muscular dystrophy.

The incidence of the disease has been estimated between 0.1 and 0.6 per 100,000 population, with a prevalence of 6.3 per 100,000. As a cause of acute or subacute muscle weakness in an adult, polymyositis is much more common than muscular dystrophy.

The disease can appear at any age, but it is most common between the ages of 40 and 60. Females are affected about twice as frequently as males. In most instances, no precipitating cause is obvious, but some cases have followed a viral-like illness or the use of antimicrobial drugs. Virus-like particles have been noted in muscle in some cases. Their role in relation to the disease has not been defined. Hypersensitivity has been implicated by some because of the association with malignancy, the frequent relation to a previous infection, and the association with symptoms common to the other collagen diseases.

In most instances, it is not possible to establish a definite etiology. Specific infections (such as toxoplasmosis) may cause a polymyositis, but in most cases there is no evidence of an infectious cause. It has not been possible to demonstrate antimuscle antibodies in these patients. The presence of antimyosin antibody and other antibodies in some patients is nonspecific, as it is also found in patients with muscular dystrophy and neuronal atrophy. It has been possible to produce a myositis in guinea pigs similar to human polymyositis by use of muscle plus Freund's adjuvant. In tissue culture preparations of rat skeletal muscle, "sensitized" lymph node cells from animals previously injected with muscle plus adjuvants destroyed the muscle cells when added to the culture, whereas unsensitized lymph node cells did not. The significance of these experiments for human disease remains uncertain.

Lymphocytes or their products from affected patients have cytotoxic activity toward muscle cells in 79 per cent of cases in one series, suggesting a cell-mediated immune response to muscle antigen. Intramuscular vascular deposits of immunoglobulin and C_3 have been demonstrated, especially in the childhood form of dermatomyositis.

Pathology.   Muscle biopsy may show inflammatory cells around vessels and in the interstitium frequently associated with individual muscle fiber necrosis. These necrotic muscle fibers are frequently in various stages of being phagocytized. Attempts at regeneration characterized by basophilic fibers having prominent sarcolemmal nuclei are usually impressive. It should be emphasized that histologic findings vary greatly in the same muscle and between different muscles so that sampling is important. The muscle tissue from the more chronic cases often shows surprisingly little change under the light microscope. This may consist of smaller muscle fibers, which vary significantly in cross-section diameter, associated with proliferation of sarcolemmal nuclei. In the polymyositis associated with Sjögren's syndrome, the muscle may be heavily infiltrated with plasma cells and lymphocytes. In the few studies utilizing the electron microscope, changes such as thickened basilar membranes, myofibrillary degeneration and, rarely, virus particles were seen. These studies have not contributed any new insight into the disease.

In the childhood form of dermatomyositis, there is intense perivascular inflammation with active arteritis and phlebitis. There is often occlusion of vessels with fibrin thrombi and infarction of muscles, nerves, and viscus (Banker and Victor). Other forms of more limited or less intense polymyositic syndromes in children have pathologic changes similar to those previously described.

The three useful laboratory tests, serum enzymes, electromyography, and muscle biopsy, are not always abnormal. Any one or even two may yield normal findings in a particular case. In one series, electromyography was abnormal in 89 per cent and muscle biopsy was confirmatory in 63 per cent. Serum enzymes are usually elevated except in some slowly progressive or chronic cases.

Clinical Manifestations and Diagnosis. The patient usually first notes the insidious development of *weakness in proximal muscles*. The weakness is more common at the hips than in the shoulders. Some weakness in the flexors of the neck is almost always present. Muscle discomfort or tenderness is common but can be completely absent. When present, it is more common in the shoulders, back, and arms than in the thighs. Muscular wasting is a late sign, and when it occurs it is usually in proximal muscles such as the quadriceps. The weakness is out of proportion to the loss of muscle bulk. Reflexes are depressed in proportion to muscle weakness.

The development and the rate of progression of the weakness may show great variations from patient to patient, and even in the same patient at different stages of the illness. Weakness can progress until the patient becomes bedridden, but this is unusual. Contracture of muscles may develop quickly.

A *skin rash* may or may not be present. It usually takes the form of an erythema over the face, shoulders, and arms. It can mimic erythema nodosum, eczema, or exfoliating dermatitis, or can manifest itself by thickened, brawny, edematous skin. On occasion, the skin lesions appear primarily in areas exposed to sunlight. Erythematous, slightly raised lesions occur over bony prominences, i.e., elbows, knuckles, knees, and medial malleoli. These lesions often become scaly and atrophic. Hyperemia around the nail beds is not uncommon. In childhood forms a violaceous suffusion of the upper eyelids, called a "heliotrope" rash, is diagnostic of this disorder. This may also be seen in adults.

Dysphagia, secondary to weakness of pharyngeal muscle and hypotonicity of the upper part of the esophagus, is frequent. About one third of the patients have arthralgias and/or Raynaud's phenomenon. Other visceral manifestations are rare. Many patients have a tachycardia. Electrocardiograms may show nonspecific T wave changes. Interstitial fibrosis and pericarditis have been noted on histologic examination. A transitory pneumonitis has also been reported. Transitional cases with some features suggesting scleroderma have occasionally demonstrated severe gastrointestinal symptoms with malabsorption, severe myopathy, and only slight skin changes. If the muscle weakness comes on acutely with much muscle necrosis, myoglobinuria will occur. This can result in acute renal failure. Polymyositis may also be seen with Sjögren's syndrome.

The *childhood form of dermatomyositis* may be much more pernicious. It starts out with skin changes, anorexia, and fatigue. Weakness, stiffness, and pain in muscles customarily follow. Low-grade fever, dysphagia, contractures, and calcinosis usually develop. A perforated viscus or mediastinitis is often the immediate cause of death.

Course Untreated. The condition can progress to severe disability and death, but most patients either improve spontaneously or proceed to a chronic phase. In earlier series, including patients primarily recognized as having dermatomyositis, case fatality rates of 50 per cent were common. In a later series of adult patients with polymyositis, it was noted that about two thirds were alive after ten years. About 50 per cent of these had complete recoveries, and the rest had some degree of residual disability. Many of the patients in this series had received some steroid therapy.

In a survey by Sheard in which adult cases were accumulated from the literature, tumors were present in nearly 20 per cent, or five times the expected incidence. When polymyositis develops in an adult male, a greater than 50 per cent chance exists that a tumor will be discovered. In another series described by Shy, it was noted that when polymyositis appeared after the age of 50 a *cancer* was found in 71 per cent of males and 24 per cent of females. The muscular weakness may precede the detection of the tumor by two or three years despite diligent search, and in this series all nine males above 50 who were followed for three years or more had an associated neoplasm. In the male, the usual carcinoma is in the lung, stomach, intestine, or prostate; and in the female, in the ovary, uterus, or breast.

Childhood dermatomyositis appears to be a very specific subgroup of polymyositic disorders. It is severely disabling and is associated with a very high fatality rate.

Laboratory Findings. The sedimentation rate is usually elevated, and there may be mild leukocytosis, especially in the acute cases. A number of enzymes which derive from muscle are usually elevated in serum. Creatine phosphokinase and aldolase are the most specific, but lactic dehydrogenase and transaminase (SGOT) are usually elevated also. Serum protein changes occur in about 50 per cent of the patients. These most commonly consist of elevations of the $\alpha 2$ and γ globulins. Rheumatoid factors are positive in 10 to 50 per cent, depending on the series. About 5 per cent will have a positive LE prep. Myoglobinuria is transient and is found only with acute and severe muscular degeneration.

In patients with dysphagia, the roentgenograms often reveal pooling of barium in the vallecular and pyriform sinuses. Hypomotility of the esophagus is present in about one third of the cases. The roentgenograms frequently reveal no abnormalities except the rare deposition of subcutaneous calcification in the childhood form of the disease. Electrocardiograms often show minor abnormalities.

Electromyography is almost always abnormal in the clinically affected muscles. There is excessive irritability of muscle when the needle is initially inserted. The motor units (which are made up of many muscle fibers supplied by a single nerve) often show a loss of amplitude, indicating a reduction in the number of functioning muscle fibers in each motor unit. The mean duration of the units is often shortened. Polyphasic discharges are common, indicating a loss of individual muscle fibers of the unit. Positive denervation waves of 20 to 50 msec and fibrillary potentials are seen, indicating some denervation or separation of a portion of the muscle from its afferent nerve supply. Repetitive discharges of pseudomyotonic firing are not uncommon. When the changes indicating denervation are prominent, the term "neuromyositis" has been used. The electromyogram is useful in indicating which muscles to biopsy. The site of biopsy should be selected to ensure that a proper sampling of abnormal muscle is being taken. It should not be taken at the site of previous electromyographic needle insertion.

Differential Diagnosis. The major causes of weakness, which must be differentiated from polymyositis, are those due to muscular dystrophy and disorders of the peripheral and central nervous system. Muscular dystrophy is usually a familial disorder which is longstanding and can often be traced to childhood. The involvement of proximal muscles and neck flexor weakness would be unusual in most adult forms of muscular dystrophy. In myotonic dystrophy, the only dystrophy which often demonstrates neck flexor weakness, there is a distal weakness of muscles in the extremities. There are also cataracts and myotonia to percussion. Fascioscapulohumeral muscular dystrophy and other proximal dystrophies usually spare neck flexors. All the dystrophies are characterized by family history, significant muscle wasting, and weakness; the deep tendon reflex loss is usually early and prominent. In polymyositis, reflexes are often relatively spared until severe weakness occurs. In some cases it may be impossible to distinguish a dystrophy from polymyositis. The family history may be difficult to verify, and the biopsy in chronic cases may not be characteristic. A few cases of familial polymyositis have been reported.

The weakness in peripheral neuritis tends to be distal, and careful examination usually enables one to find mild sensory loss, autonomic dysfunction, and distal areflexia. Weakness from spinal cord disease has characteristic reflex changes, such as extensor plantar responses and hyperreflexia. Occasionally, motor neuron disease (the primary muscular atrophy variant) presents as a myopathic disorder. Muscle biopsy and EMG usually distinguish between the two conditions. On occasion a subacute variety of Guillain-Barré disease can cause proximal weakness. Elevation of cerebrospinal fluid protein is helpful in establishing this entity and is not seen in polymyositis.

Of the muscular syndromes, the metabolic myopathies most closely mimic the distribution of muscle weakness and the weakness seen with polymyositis. Chronic thyroid myopathy is characterized by its involvement of proximal muscles with significant loss of muscle bulk. The reflexes are usually quite brisk. Although there are no distinctive features, the clinical signs of thyrotoxicosis and the presence of clinical tests to support hyperthyroidism usually make it easy to distinguish this group. The most common myopathy seen today is probably the one induced by excess or chronic use of corticotrophin or steroids. This is especially true of the fluorinated steroids. It is identical to that seen with hyperadrenocorticism. The weakness is primarily proximal, most often involving the pelvic girdle. Early wasting of the quadriceps muscle is especially prominent. Pain and discomfort are unusual. Reflexes usually persist, and severe disabling syndromes are unusual. Muscle biopsy tends to show surprisingly little change, and then only very scattered and in single muscle fibers. These changes are usually much less than one would anticipate from the clinical status of the patients.

Since steroids are often used in the treatment of a number of clinical syndromes, it may be very difficult to establish whether progressive weakness is due to the underlying disease or the steroid treatment. Often one will have to either decrease the steroid dose sharply or increase it significantly to make such judgments. If pain is a significant problem, one must be cautious about the clinical evaluation of weakness or its disappearance with the use of high doses of steroids.

Hyperparathyroidism and hyperinsulinism have rarely been associated with syndromes of muscular weakness and must be separated from idiopathic polymyositis primarily by the associated laboratory findings. Muscle weakness is often associated with osteomalacia.

There are a number of parasitic diseases such as trichinosis and toxoplasmosis which should be considered in acute or subacute syndromes, especially when generalized symptoms and eosinophilia are noted. These are fully discussed elsewhere in this text.

Polymyalgia rheumatica is characteristically associated with significant muscular discomfort and a high sedimentation rate. Changes in serum enzymes or muscle biopsy are usually not present to any significant degree. There are noticeable short-term and even daily fluctuations of symptoms. Significant objective weakness is not common, although complaints of pain and fatigue and feelings of muscular weakness are often voiced by the patient. Although the findings in some are related to those seen with temporal arteritis, the findings in others are very similar to those of some patients seen with epidemic neuromyasthenia.

Treatment. The physician's obvious goal is to eradicate the active disease process, if possible, and improve the functional capacity of the patient. In almost all cases prolonged management and long-term follow-up will be necessary. Often the chronic nature and the severe disability caused by the illness make it essential for the physician to play an active role as a counselor and friend.

Many of these patients achieve significant symptomatic improvement of muscle function when treated with corticotrophin, steroids, or salicylates. The use of immunosuppressive medication has been promising in a few cases. Methotrexate has been used, especially in dermatomyositis. The disorder is rarely "cured," however, and relapses are common, especially if steroids are abruptly withdrawn. Patients may require medication for many years. The initial dose of corticotrophin or steroids should be high (60 to 80 mg of prednisone) and tapered over months. It is useful to monitor serum enzymes during this period, as they often give an early indication of the patient's likely course. Relapses are common when steroids are withdrawn in the first two years, but less frequent if treatment lasts at least three years. When possible, steroids should be used on an alternate-day basis to decrease side effects. When steroid-treated and presteroid series of patients are compared in terms of long-range follow-up, as by Rose and Walton, the group receiving steroid treatment has fared better. Patients with some of the adult forms usually do well. Those with the childhood forms of dermatomyositis usually do not respond satisfactorily to steroids alone.

Banker, B. Q., and Victor, M.: Dermatomyositis (systemic angiopathy of childhood). Medicine, 45:261, 1966.
Pearson, C. M.: Polymyositis. In Milhorat, A. T. (ed.): Explanatory Concepts in Muscular Dystrophy and Related Disorders. Amsterdam, Excerpta Medica Foundation, 1967.
Rose, A. L., and Walton, J.: Polymyositis: A survey of 89 cases with particular reference to treatment and prognosis. Brain, 89:747, 1966.
Sheard, C.: Dermatomyositis. Arch. Intern. Med., 88:640, 1951.
Shy, G. M.: The late-onset myopathy. World Neurol., 3:149, 1962.
Walton, J. N.: Disorders of Voluntary Muscle. 2nd ed. London, J. A. Churchill, Ltd., 1969.
Walton, J. N., and Adams, R. D.: Polymyositis. Edinburgh, Livingstone, Ltd., 1958.

81. SYSTEMIC LUPUS ERYTHEMATOSUS

Peter H. Schur

General Considerations. Systemic lupus erythematosus (SLE) is a chronic, inflammatory disease of unknown cause affecting skin, joints, kidneys, nervous system, serous membranes, and often other organs of the body. The classic facial "butterfly rash" facilitates diagnosis, although the rash need not be present. The clinical course may be fulminant or indolent, but generally is characterized by periods of remissions and relapses. Patients with SLE develop distinct immunologic abnormalities, especially antinuclear antibodies. A diagnosis of SLE has frequently been established or confirmed by the finding of these antibodies, especially the one causing the LE cell phenomenon.

Lupus, which is Latin for wolf, has been used since about 1230 to describe cutaneous conditions which resemble the malar erythema of a wolf. Numerous publications in the nineteenth century by, among others, Bateman, Biett, Hebra, and Kaposi, described what we know now as lupus of the skin. In 1851, Cazenave first used the term "lupus erythemateux." Kaposi, in 1872, noted the systemic involvement in lupus, and in 1875 noted that the rash resembled a butterfly. Osler described the systemic complications of lupus and noted that they could occur in the absence of skin disease. The clinical recognition of SLE has changed greatly since Hargraves first described the LE cell test in 1948 and since the development of the immunofluorescent antinuclear factor test by Friou in 1957.

Incidence and Etiology. SLE is not a rare disorder. The prevalence rate is approximately 5 per 100,000 population. The disease appears to occur more frequently in blacks than in whites and is rare among Asians. It occurs five to ten times more frequently among females than males and has been diagnosed in patients ranging from 2 to 97 years old. However, the majority of patients are first discovered to have SLE while in their third and fourth decades of life.

The cause of SLE remains unknown. Exposure to sunlight or ultraviolet radiation, viz., sunlamps, often leads to the prompt appearance of the facial butterfly rash or a rash on other exposed skin surfaces. Many other factors, including infections, surgery, and certain drugs, have been shown to be associated with exacerbations of SLE. Recent attention has focused on procainamide, hydralazine, hydantoins, and other drugs which may precipitate a lupus-like illness.

In view of the preponderance of the disease in females, endocrine factors have been thought to influence the development of SLE. The disease tends to remit during the last two trimesters of pregnancy and to relapse post partum. Inhibitors of ovulation can cause an exacerbation of SLE.

Genetic factors may influence the development of SLE in susceptible individuals. Much evidence supports this hypothesis. The high incidence of SLE among females might be considered an X-chromosome-related factor. Connective tissue disorders, dysgammaglobulinemia and autoimmune phenomena are observed frequently among relatives of many patients with SLE. Genetic control of immune responses to certain antigens correlates closely with histocompatibility types in some animals. An association between particular HLA antigens and SLE has been noted, suggesting that SLE patients may hyperreact to some antigens. Additional evidence for a genetic role in SLE comes from studies in certain strains of inbred mice and dogs. NZB and NZW mice develop an illness which includes hemolytic anemia, renal disease, and immunologic abnormalities, and is similar to human SLE. The F_1 hybrid generation, especially the females, develop the illness more frequently, at an earlier age, and with a much higher incidence of autoimmune phenomena.

Lupus erythematosus is characterized particularly by autoimmune phenomena. Patients develop antibodies to many of their own cells, cell constituents, and proteins. The origin of these autoantibodies is as obscure as is the cause of SLE. However, they do appear to represent a loss of tolerance to self antigens. Mice of the NZB strain have been found to lose their tolerance for foreign antigens much more rapidly than do other mice.

A possible viral cause for SLE has also been proposed. Loss of tolerance may be influenced by viral infections. Structures resembling viral nucleocapsids have been found much more frequently in endothelial cells in SLE patients than in normal persons. Antibody titers to certain viruses are elevated in SLE sera, but no one virus has been implicated. The presence, in many SLE patients, of antibodies to double-stranded RNA suggests reaction to an RNA virus (infection). "C" type RNA virus particles have been found in NZB mice; other viruses, including DNA and RNA viruses, can provoke the development of autoantibodies and nephritis in NZB mice. Cell-free filtrates, presumably containing a virus, have been prepared from spleens of dogs with lupus. These filtrates, when injected into normal dogs and mice, induce the formation of antinuclear antibodies; they also activate latent leukemia viruses in mice.

These data suggest that an abnormal immune response in genetically predisposed SLE patients may alter the delicate balance between immunity and tolerance and result in the development of antibodies to intracellular contents released during chronic viral infection or to new antigens in cells which result from viral infection or transformation.

Pathogenesis and Pathology. Many of the manifestations of SLE appear to result from the deposition of antigen-antibody complexes in tissues. Although immune complexes have not been isolated from SLE patients, certain evidence is consistent with their presence. In laboratory animals, when immune complexes are formed in the circulation, serum complement levels fall and nephritis develops. In patients with SLE, especially in those with anti-DNA antibodies, a fall in complement levels is often associated with the development of nephritis. In addition, some patients with serum antibodies to DNA develop fever and nephritis as the antibody disappears and is replaced by free DNA, a sequence which presumably represents immune complex formation and deposition followed by antigen excess. Furthermore, some sera from SLE patients with nephritis, when treated with deoxyribonuclease, have a rise in anti-DNA antibody levels. This fact suggests that DNA has been bound in vivo to the antibody as an immune complex. Using the immunofluorescent technique, immunoglobulins (especially IgG), complement components, and antigens (viz., DNA) have been detected in a granular and lumpy distribution along the renal glomerular basement membrane. After elution of the gamma globulin from the glomeruli, it has been possible to demonstrate that it consists primarily of antinuclear and some anticytoplasmic antibodies. Similar immune complexes have been demonstrated at the dermal-epidermal junction of lupus skin lesions. It is hypothesized that, as the complement system is activated during immune complex formation and deposition, chemotactic factors are released and that damage to normal cells and extracellular tissue is caused both by activated terminal sequences of complement and by lysosomal enzymes released by polymorphonuclear leukocytes.

The pathologic changes of SLE, even in clinically uninvolved organs, are often minor when examined by routine histologic methods. Fibrinoid, an eosinophilic amorphous material, is commonly deposited along tissue fibers and in blood vessels. Fibrin and serum proteins (including immunoglobulins, complement, and DNA) have been detected in fibrinoid and possibly represent deposits of immune complexes. Synovium and serous membranes, including pleura and pericardium, may be edematous and contain deposits of fibrinoid. Vasculitis can involve venules, capillaries, arterioles, and occasionally arteries. Hematoxylin bodies are rounded, hematoxylin-stained masses, roughly the size of nuclei, and are found in areas of inflammation. They are believed to represent in vivo LE bodies analogous to the cytoplasmic inclusions in LE cells.

Skin biopsies may show acute inflammation with liquefaction, degeneration of the basal layer with vacuolization of basal cells, edema of the dermis, and fibrinoid necrosis in the dermis and local blood vessels with cell infiltration. In chronic lesions, hyperkeratosis with follicular plugging is seen.

The spleen is the site of "onion skin lesions," which are characterized by concentric perivascular fibrosis around central and penicilliary arteries.

Libman-Sacks verrucous nonbacterial endocarditis consists of nonbacterial vegetations on the heart valves or chordae tendineae. Fibrinoid is deposited in the superficial connective tissue with infiltration of neutrophils, lymphocytes, and histiocytes. The myocardium may be involved by vasculitis.

Renal lesions are highly variable, from mild to severe. The mildest form of renal lesion consists of deposits of immunoglobulin and complement in the mesangium and along the glomerular basement membrane without any other observable histologic abnormality. The most common renal lesion is focal glomerulitis with minimal increase of cellularity, focal thickening of the capillary basement membrane, and fibrinoid change. In glomerulonephritis, these lesions are more generalized and severe and are usually a mixture of proliferative and membranous changes with hypercellularity of endothelial, mesangial, epithelial, and inflammatory cells, capsular inflammation leading to crescent formation, and focal thickening of the basement membrane. Some kidneys are found to have only a diffuse membranous glomerulonephritis with few cells but considerable thickening of the basement membrane. Basement membrane thickening, when associated with fibrinoid changes, results in the so-called "wire loop" lesions. There may also be hyaline thrombi in glomeruli, focal necrosis, and, occasionally, hematoxylin bodies. Tubular degenerative changes are common.

Clinical Manifestations. The characteristic picture of a patient with well-advanced lupus is one of a young woman with fever, weight loss, arthralgia, a butterfly rash, pleural effusion, and nephritis. With better methods of detection (the antinuclear antibody tests), much larger groups of patients with less obvious and more varied symptoms and signs are being recognized. Most patients complain of some fatigue, arthralgia, rashes, and fever. When specific organs are involved, other symptoms may develop: pleurisy, pericarditis, edema, dyspnea and cough, Raynaud's phenomenon, bleeding, and purpura or seizures. The disease is now considered a chronic illness with periods of remission and activity.

Musculoskeletal System. Most patients complain of pain in their joints (arthralgia) at some time. Commonly the hands, wrists, knees, ankles, and elbows are affected. Arthritis of joints, that is, local redness, swelling, or heat, is observed less frequently than is arthralgia. Although slight deformities at the metacarpophalangeal and proximal interphalangeal joints may occur, major joint swelling with synovial thickening, flexion deformities with subluxations, and deviation are uncommon. It is unusual for joint narrowing or cystic changes such as those seen in rheumatoid arthritis to be found on radiologic examination. The appearance of deforming or destructive joint lesions suggests a diagnosis of an overlap syndrome (rheumatoid arthritis–lupus). Muscle pain is a frequent complaint and is accompanied, occasionally, by proximal muscle atrophy. The bones are rarely affected, but an increased prevalence of aseptic necrosis of the femoral head or condyle has been noted, especially in those patients receiving corticosteroid therapy.

Mucocutaneous Manifestations. The classic "butterfly rash" is seen in less than half the patients with SLE.

TABLE 1. Frequency of Clinical Symptoms in Systemic Lupus Erythematosus*

	Per Cent
Weight loss	62
Fever	83
Arthralgia, arthritis	90
Skin	74
Butterfly rash	42
Photosensitivity	30
Mucous membrane lesions	12
Alopecia	27
Raynaud's phenomenon	17
Purpura	15
Urticaria	8
Renal	53
Nephrosis	18
Gastrointestinal	38
Pulmonary	47
Pleurisy	45
Effusion	24
Pneumonia	29
Cardiac	46
Pericarditis	27
Murmurs	23
EKG changes	39
Lymphadenopathy	46
Splenomegaly	15
Hepatomegaly	25
Central nervous system	32
Psychosis	15
Convulsions	15
Cytoid bodies	11

*Adapted from Dubois, E. L.: Lupus Erythematosus, New York, McGraw-Hill Book Company, 1966; Estes, D., and Christian, C. L.: Medicine, 50:85, 1971; and Fernandez-Herlihy, L.: Lahey Clinic Found. Bull., 21:49, 1972.

There may be only a blush and swelling or a scaly erythematous maculopapular rash on both cheeks and the bridge of the nose after exposure to the sun. This may clear spontaneously, only to recur. Other skin areas, particularly those exposed to the sun, may be involved. The lesions are called "discoid" when they scale, are associated with follicular plugging, and heal with atrophy, scarring (telangiectasia), hyperpigmentation, or hypopigmentation (vitiligo). Discoid lupus per se is not accompanied by systemic complications. Involvement may also occur on the forehead, pinna, and scalp, resulting in alopecia. Patchy hair loss is frequent and usually reversible, but discoid lupus with scarring can lead to permanent partial baldness. In these days of well-fitted hairpieces, alopecia is often undetected on cursory examination. Periungual erythema and telangiectasia are found in about 10 per cent of patients with SLE. Small ulcerations signifying an underlying vasculitis often develop on the fingertips and may progress to gangrene. Raynaud's phenomenon may occur in both hands and feet. Painful ulcers are seen on the buccal mucosa, hard and soft palate, and gums. Purpura and ecchymoses usually reflect an underlying blood platelet and clotting problem, renal insufficiency, or the side effects of corticosteroids. Urticaria and angioedema may be present.

Renal Disease. Kidney involvement is found in about half of SLE patients and usually occurs within two years of the onset of symptoms. Acute nephritis or the nephrotic syndrome may be the presenting manifestation of SLE. The most common abnormality is a mild glomerulitis which is associated with minimal proteinuria or hematuria, or both. This lesion generally responds well to therapy initially, but often recurs in mild form or as even more severe renal involvement. Acute lupus glomerulonephritis occurs less often and is associated with varying degrees of pyuria, hematuria, proteinuria, fluid retention, edema, hypertension, and azotemia. The nephrotic syndrome is associated with variable proteinuria, with fluid retention, and frequently with normal serum cholesterol levels. The finding of pyuria with fever in patients with SLE, especially in young women receiving corticosteroids, may reflect a urinary tract infection rather than lupus nephritis; a renal biopsy may be necessary to make the correct diagnosis.

Most patients recover well from attacks of acute nephritis, with loss of edema and azotemia, but usually some proteinuria and decreased glomerular filtration rate (GFR) persist. Patients have recurrences, and some develop chronic glomerulonephritis with hypertension and proteinuria.

Cardiovascular Manifestations. The endocardium, myocardium, and pericardium are involved in nearly half the patients with SLE. Although electrocardiographic changes, such as nonspecific ST, T wave changes, are not uncommon, clinical myocarditis is seen less frequently. Myocarditis should be suspected when tachycardia is disproportionate to either fever or anemia. Cardiomegaly with congestive failure is rare. Precordial chest pain may be caused by either pleurisy or pericarditis. Careful, frequent auscultation may be rewarded by discovery of a pericardial friction rub. Tamponade or constrictive pericarditis is rare. Libman-Sacks or nonbacterial verrucous endocarditis usually occurs on the mitral valve and is recognized by murmurs which cannot be explained by fever or anemia; but generally this is a postmortem diagnosis. Bacterial endocarditis may de-

velop on a previously damaged valve, especially in patients receiving corticosteroids. Thrombophlebitis may be the first manifestation of SLE. Occlusion of major arteries occurs rarely. Equally rare is pulmonary hypertension.

Pulmonary Involvement. Pleuritic pain is a common complaint and is often the first clue to the diagnosis of SLE. It is generally accompanied by a friction rub and a variable amount of fluid accumulation, but the effusions are often painless. There may be pulmonary infiltrates which are quite difficult to distinguish from those due to infections. The x-ray examination shows bilateral patchy infiltrations which may shift from lobe to lobe. The involvement can progress to atelectasis and to marked pulmonary insufficiency and cyanosis. Most pulmonary symptoms respond well to intensive corticosteroid therapy; but infections must be carefully considered as a cause of the infiltrate.

Neurologic and Psychologic Manifestations. Many patients have read in a dictionary or have heard that SLE is invariably a fatal illness, and this fact understandably leads to great anxiety. Similarly the patient may be told that he or she has arthritis, which leads to ungrounded fears of disabling deformities. These natural fears and anxieties of a chronic illness are complicated frequently by organic neurologic disturbances. The latter manifest themselves as behavioral disturbances, including hyperirritability, confusion, hallucinations, obsessional and paranoid reactions, and frank organic psychosis. The psychosis of SLE may easily be confused with, and in fact is difficult to differentiate from, a steroid-induced psychosis; other symptoms and signs of active SLE usually accompany the organic diease. Organic brain damage most commonly manifests itself as convulsions, which occur in at least 15 per cent of patients. Other less frequent neurologic findings include peripheral neuropathy, hemiparesis, motor aphasia, ptosis, diplopia, and nystagmus.

"Cotton wool spots" are fluffy white exudates (containing cytoid bodies) in the superficial layers of the retina. They are usually associated with some visual disturbance, are present with other signs of active SLE, and are generally reversible.

Gastrointestinal Manifestations. Anorexia, nausea, vomiting, and abdominal pain are common. The cause is obscure, but may be from peritonitis, enteritis, pancreatitis, or a paralytic ileus. Diarrhea and hematochezia have been noted. The liver is often found to be enlarged because of chronic passive congestion, but this is usually transitory. Liver biopsy may be normal or show fatty infiltration and/or fibrosis.

These manifestations in SLE should not be confused with *lupoid hepatitis,* which is a condition primarily of young women with progressive active hepatitis leading to chronic liver disease and failure. Nephritis is said not to occur. Patients have high levels of gamma globulins, positive LE cell preparations, or positive tests for antinuclear factor (ANF); serum complement levels remain normal or elevated.

Lymph Nodes and Spleen. Lymph nodes, characteristically, are enlarged in SLE but are not tender. The enlarged nodes have been mistaken for lymphoma. Splenomegaly, considered very common years ago, is seen now in about 15 per cent of patients.

Menses and Pregnancy. Menses are frequently irregular or heavy, or both. In patients with circulating anticoagulants, bleeding may be profound. Although pregnancy carries some increased risk of miscarriage in the first trimester, most SLE patients without renal disease do well through term. It should be noted, however, that there is a considerable risk of postpartum exacerbation of the disease.

Course Untreated. Until recent years the natural course of untreated SLE was considered to be bleak. The average patient was considered to have but a few months or, at best, a few years to live. Since 1948, this situation has changed for the better. The reason for this improvement lies in the recognition of many cases of mild lupus through the development of very sensitive diagnostic tests (antinuclear antibodies), as well as in the development of improved forms of therapy. The disease in most patients is characterized by periods of remissions and relapses, which may be protracted or brief. The same individuals usually have recurrences of the same symptoms they had previously, such as arthritis, pleurisy, nephritis, or rashes. However, variable symptoms and signs may develop years apart. If nephritis develops, it generally does so early in the course.

The prognosis for patients seems to improve each year, but mortality rates remain high during the first year after diagnosis. Whereas in 1956, patients were given only a 50 per cent chance of surviving four years, today they have a better than 90 per cent chance to survive ten years. Prognosis still remains poor for patients with diffuse proliferative glomerulonephritis or with central nervous system involvement.

Laboratory Findings. *Hematologic.* Anemia occurs in many patients with SLE and is generally mild, normochromic, or normocytic. Anemia may also be due to infection, renal insufficiency, or bleeding. Autoagglutination of red blood cells may be observed. The Coombs test is frequently positive, but severe hemolytic anemia is uncommon. Leukopenia occurs in about one half the patients. The differential cell count is usually normal, although mononuclear cells may be more suppressed than neutrophils. Complicating infections generally result in a rise of the white blood cell count either into the normal or elevated range. Corticosteroid therapy also causes leukocytosis. Thrombocytopenia, with or without purpura, may precede other manifestations of SLE by years or may disappear, leaving other manifestations of the disease. A circulating anticoagulant may be present in as many as 25 per cent of patients with SLE. This anticoagulant, either as antibody to factor VIII or, more commonly, as an inhibitor to the formation of "prothrombinase," results in prolonged clotting and prothrombin times and may be associated with mild or, rarely, severe hemorrhages.

Renal. Renal dysfunction occurs in over half the patients. Most patients have only some impairment of concentrating ability, a few red and/or white blood cells in the urine, and perhaps some proteinuria (< 0.5 gram per day). Active nephritis is defined when there is hematuria (> 5 rc per hpf), pyuria (> 5 wc per hpf), erythrocyte casts, increasing proteinuria, or a decreasing glomerular filtration rate. Hematuria and pyuria are rarely seen in lupus nephritis in remission.

Plasma Proteins. The erythrocyte sedimentation rate is often elevated. Serum albumin levels are low, especially in the nephrotic syndrome. Gamma globulin levels which are elevated in many patients may be low in nephrotics. Cryoglobulins, consisting of immunoglobulins and complement components, have been noted frequently, especially in patients with renal disease.

TABLE 2. Laboratory Abnormalities in SLE*

	Per Cent
Anemia	71
Leukopenia	56
Thrombocytopenia	11
Hemolytic anemia	8
Circulating anticoagulant	2
Rheumatoid factor	19
Biologic false-positive test for syphilis	15
Hypoalbuminemia	50
Hyperglobulinemia	37
LE cell	82
Antinuclear antibodies	96
Anti-double stranded DNA	32
Anti-single-stranded DNA	46
Anti-double-stranded RNA	51
Anti-nucleoprotein	41
Anti-"Sm"	68
Hypocomplementemia	66
CH50	66
C4	64
C3	52

*Adapted from Dubois, E. L.: Lupus Erythematosus, New York, McGraw-Hill Book Company, 1966; Estes, D., and Christian, C. L.: Medicine, 50:85, 1971; and Fernandez-Herlihy, L.: Lahey Clinic Found. Bull., 21:49, 1972.

Abnormal Immunologic Reactions. Biologic false-positive tests (BFP) for syphilis have been noted in about 15 per cent of the patients with SLE, especially in those with circulating anticoagulants. The BFP may be the first laboratory clue to the diagnosis of SLE and may precede symptoms by years. Rheumatoid factors have been found in some patients with SLE, even in the absence of clinical rheumatoid arthritis.

Most characteristic of SLE are the large number of autoantibodies which react with cells and their nuclear and cytoplasmic constituents. Historically of greatest significance is the LE cell phenomenon. The LE cell is formed in vitro as follows: some leukocytes are traumatized and release nucleoprotein (DNA-histone); the nucleoprotein reacts with an IgG antibody, and the complex is phagocytized by the remaining viable leukocytes. The LE cell consists of a leukocyte with a large purple-red homogeneous globulin inclusion body which compresses the nucleus against the cell membrane, leaving only a thin rim of cytoplasm. Because LE cells are not always present in patients with SLE, more sensitive tests have been developed for the detection of various antinuclear antibodies (ANA). An immunofluorescent (IF) technique, employing rodent liver or kidney as the source of nuclei, detects ANA in over 99 per cent of SLE patients. The antibodies may be of IgG, IgA, IgM, IgD, or IgE classes. Circulating DNA and other antigens may rarely block the detection of the ANA. With this immunofluorescent technique, different patterns of nuclear fluorescence reflect antibodies to different nuclear structures. The "homogeneous" or "diffuse" pattern reflects antibodies to nucleoprotein. The "peripheral," "rim," or "shaggy" pattern reflects primarily antibodies to DNA. The speckled pattern reflects antibodies to a group of nuclear proteins, including "Sm" and ribonucleoprotein. A nucleolar pattern has also been observed and appears to represent antibodies to a nuclear RNA.

Antibodies to some antigens, especially to DNA, have also been detected by other methods, including precipitation, diffusion in agar, complement fixation, agglutination, binding (Farr technique), and fluorescent spot test. The titers of antibodies to DNA and, to some extent, to nucleoprotein, double-stranded RNA, and ribosomes, tend to be higher during periods of clinical activity, especially of active nephritis, than during clinical remissions.

Complement levels are depressed in most patients with SLE at some time during their illness, especially when disease activity is present. Markedly depressed complement levels are seen primarily in patients with active lupus nephritis. The low levels reflect in vivo activation and fixation of complement components by circulating immune complexes. Serial determination of whole complement levels (CH5O) or of individual complement components (especially C4 and C3) may be useful in following and managing patients with SLE. "Lupus" has also been seen in some patients with congenital deficiency of C1r or C2.

Diagnosis. The diagnosis of SLE can be made if any four or more of the following manifestations are present, serially or simultaneously, during any interval of observation: butterfly rash, discoid lupus, Raynaud's phenomenon, alopecia, photosensitivity, oral or nasopharyngeal ulceration, arthritis without deformity, LE cells, chronic false-positive STS, profuse proteinuria, cellular casts, pleuritis or pericarditis, psychosis and/or convulsions, or hemolytic anemia, leukopenia, or thrombocytopenia. SLE should also be suspected—especially in young females—with unexplained fever, purpura, easy bruising, diffuse adenopathy, hepatosplenomegaly, peripheral neuropathy, endocarditis, myocarditis, interstitial pneumonitis, peritonitis, or aseptic meningitis.

Patients are frequently first diagnosed as having rheumatoid arthritis, rheumatic fever (especially children), glomerulonephritis, tuberculosis, scleroderma, vasculitis (including periarteritis), idiopathic thrombocytopenic purpura, lymphoma, anemia, or neutropenia. The LE cell is specific for SLE, if rheumatoid arthritis, lupoid hepatitis, or drug reactions can be excluded. Although the LE cell test is quite often negative, the antinuclear factor test is positive in virtually all patients with SLE. The antinuclear antibodies have also been detected in 68 per cent of patients with Sjögren's syndrome, 40 to 75 per

cent of patients with scleroderma, especially the speckled pattern, 22 per cent of patients with juvenile rheumatoid arthritis, and 25 to 50 per cent of patients with rheumatoid arthritis, especially the homogeneous pattern. However, the antinuclear factors are present in higher titers in patients with SLE than in other disorders. Antibodies to double-stranded DNA are highly diagnostic of SLE.

Diagnostic problems always arise in patients with the so-called overlap syndromes, mixtures of signs and symptoms of SLE and other related diseases, such as rheumatoid arthritis, Sjögren's syndrome, scleroderma, and dermatomyositis. These patients are best considered, and treated, for their primary symptoms and complaints.

Drug-Induced Lupus. Drugs that induce lupus can be divided into two categories: drugs that induce lupus in many individuals, and drugs associated with exacerbations of SLE. In the former group are hydrazides (hydralazine, isoniazid), anticonvulsants (Dilantin), and procainamide. Over 50 per cent of subjects taking procainamide develop antinuclear antibodies; about 25 per cent develop symptoms and signs of lupus. Arthralgia, pleurisy with effusion, fever, and weight loss are common features, but renal disease and hypocomplementemia are not seen. Symptoms generally clear in a few weeks after discontinuation of the drug, even though antinuclear antibodies persist for months. Antinuclear antibodies appear less frequently in subjects taking hydralazine. Patients with the hydralazine lupus syndrome may have arthritis, dermatitis, serositis, leukopenia, antinuclear antibodies, and anti-DNA antibodies, but rarely have renal or central nervous system disease. Symptoms usually stop after cessation of the drug. Patients with hydralazine lupus are slow acetylators of the drug. These studies suggest that certain subjects may have a genetic predisposition for developing drug lupus. Other drugs, including penicillin, sulfonamides, and oral contraceptives, are associated with exacerbations of SLE, and rarely cause lupus-like symptoms or antinuclear antibodies in other subjects.

Therapy and Management. As there are no specific remedies for the treatment of the underlying processes of SLE, the main goals of management must be limited to the treatment of acute relapses and prevention of exacerbations. Certain measures are helpful in prevention of relapses. Sunlight, ultraviolet radiation, immunizations, blood transfusions, penicillin, and sulfonamides should be avoided when possible. Surgery or infections may lead to a relapse and may require more aggressive concurrent management of the lupus. In the long-term management of this illness, both patient and physician must learn to recognize those symptoms and signs that herald relapses. Although these symptoms may involve fever and arthralgia in some patients, they may appear as hair loss, mucosal ulcers, pleurisy, weight loss, or simply fatigue in others. Before frank clinical symptoms develop, many patients will develop abnormal laboratory tests such as a reduced level of hemoglobin or serum complement or a reduced white blood cell or platelet count; an abnormal urinalysis or creatinine clearance; or a rising titer of anti-DNA antibodies.

Many of the patients seen in the hospital by physicians or students have severe but not life-threatening disease. By contrast, many of the patients seen in the office have much milder disease. The patient fearing the unknown or having heard the worst must be reassured

TABLE 3. Autoantibodies in SLE

Antinuclear	Nucleoprotein
	DNA
	Histone
	Sm
	RNA
	Ribonucleoprotein
	Residue
Anticytoplasmic	Mitochondria
	Lysosomes
	Microsomes
	Ribosomes
	Cytoplasmic sap glycoprotein ("Ro")
	RNA protein
Anti-RNA	Ribosomal RNA
	Double-stranded RNA (? viral)
	Single-stranded RNA
Anticell	Red cell
	White blood cell
	Platelet
Anticlotting factors	
Antithyroid	
Rheumatoid factor	
Biologic false-positive test for syphilis	

that a majority of patients have mild to moderate disease and that with proper management many of the more serious complications can now be controlled.

Active disease should be treated aggressively to prevent permanent tissue injury. The general measures to be taken include rest when the disease is active, sunscreens, and physical therapy for muscle weakness and deformities. For those patients on moderate to high dosages of corticosteroids, salt restriction and diuretics may be of benefit. Drugs used for the treatment of SLE include topical steroids, salicylates, antimalarials, corticosteroids, and immunosuppressives. The use of corticosteroids is indicated in most patients with SLE and has improved survival. Dosage should be individualized according to the activity of the disease and side effects. *Immunosuppressives* are best used according to the guidelines of Schwartz and Gowans, whose indications are life-threatening or seriously crippling disease; presence of reversible lesions; failure to respond to conventional therapy or intolerable side effects; no active infection; no hematologic contraindication; meticulous follow-up; and objective evaluation.

The acute erythematous maculopapular rash responds well to the avoidance of sunlight, local application of corticosteroid cream, and the systemic introduction of antimalarials such as hydroxychloroquin. Systemic corticosteroids are rarely warranted. The chronic lesion, or discoid lupus, responds to these same measures to a variable degree. Severe, extensive lesions have been treated with large doses of antimalarials when all else has failed. However, the patient should be cautioned about the relative risks of retinal damage when taking large doses of antimalarials. Arthralgia and arthritis respond well to rest, physical therapy, splinting, salicylates, and antimalarials. Steroids should not be needed.

Fever often responds to rest and salicylates. Antimalarials may be beneficial. Persistent fever not responsive to these measures usually coincides with other signs of activity and responds to moderate doses of corticosteroids. Infections must be excluded.

Pericarditis and pleurisy respond well to rest and corticosteroids. Fluid, if present in moderate amounts, is best removed. Myocarditis should be treated with moderate doses of steroids, fluid restriction, and careful administration of digitalis.

Hemolytic anemia and thrombocytopenia need not be treated unless symptomatic. They generally respond well to steroids. If not, immunosuppressives or a splenectomy may be necessary.

Involvement of the central nervous system responds poorly to treatment. Organic psychosis, in addition, may be difficult to differentiate from a steroid-induced psychosis. Because of the risk of permanent brain damage, large doses of steroids (2 to 3 mg of prednisone per kilogram of body weight per day) are recommended until maximal improvement is achieved, at which time the dosage of steroids is gradually tapered. Immunosuppressives may be necessary.

Mild focal glomerulitis with minimal urinary abnormalities may respond on occasion to bed rest; however, these patients and those with acute glomerulonephritis generally require systemic corticosteroid therapy. Prednisone has been given with good results, according to the following schedule, depending on renal function: blood urea nitrogen (BUN) less than 30 mg per 100 ml, 1 mg of prednisone per kilogram of body weight per day; BUN 31 to 100 mg per 100 ml, 2 mg per kilogram; BUN over 100

mg per 100 ml, 3 mg per kilogram. Patients unresponsive to these regimens may benefit from immunosuppressives. Medication is maintained until hematuria clears and serum complement levels return toward normal; this usually occurs within about three weeks. The LE cells, proteinuria, elevated sedimentation rate, and high titers of antinuclear antibodies may persist. The prednisone dosage is then tapered slowly – 10 mg every five days. Complete blood counts, urinalyses, serum creatinine levels, and serum complement levels are checked weekly to detect relapses; relapses usually respond either to maintaining the dosage at that level or increasing it by 5 to 10 mg of prednisone per day. Many patients can be maintained at a dosage of 5 to 10 mg per day; some can tolerate steroids on alternate days; a few can discontinue steroids and remain asymptomatic. Continued careful monitoring and early treatment of slight relapses may avoid more severe exacerbations.

Patients with chronic membranous glomerulonephritis and nephrotic syndrome respond less well to corticosteroids or immunosuppressives. Some, usually those with normal complement levels, may have fixed proteinuria.

Dubois, E. L., and Tuffanelli, D. L.: Clinical manifestations of systemic lupus erythematosus. J.A.M.A., 190:104, 1964.
Estes, D., and Christian, C. L.: The natural history of systemic lupus erythematosus by prospective analysis. Medicine, 50:85, 1971.
Harvey, A. M., Shulman, L. E., Tumulty, A., Conley, C. L., and Schoenrich, E. H.: Systemic lupus erythematosus: Review of the literature and clinical analysis of 138 cases. Medicine, 33:291, 1954.
Rothfield, N. F., and March, C. H.: Lupus erythematosus. In Fitzpatrick, T. B., Arndt, K. A., Clark, W. H., Eisen, A. Z., Van Scott, E. J., and Vaughan, J. H. (eds.): Dermatology in Internal Medicine. New York, McGraw-Hill Book Company, 1971, pp. 1493–1518.
Schur, P. H., and Sandson, J.: Immunological factors and clinical activity in lupus erythematosus. N. Engl. J. Med., 278:533, 1968.

82.   PERIARTERITIS NODOSA
(Polyarteritis Nodosa)

K. Frank Austen

Definition. Kussmaul and Maier introduced the term periarteritis nodosa in 1866 to designate a morbid process manifested by numerous grossly visible or palpable nodules along the course of medium-sized muscular arteries. The lesions are segmental in distribution, have a predilection for the crotch of bifurcations and branchings, and involve all but the pulmonary arteries. The clinical manifestations are disparate and polymorphic, and result from partial or complete arterial occlusion, hemorrhage, and glomerulitis. In view of the necrotizing nature of the process, involving the entire arterial wall, Ferrari in 1903 suggested the alternate name of polyarteritis acuta nodosa.

The incidence, age distribution, and male-to-female ratio of periarteritis nodosa are difficult to determine because a diagnostic serologic procedure is lacking, and the spotty distribution of lesions makes biopsy uncertain. Nonetheless, the condition has been reported to occur from infancy to old age, with a peak incidence in the fifth and sixth decades of life, and the male to female ratio has been estimated at from 2 to 3:1.

Pathology. The lesions of polyarteritis involve arteries of medium and small caliber, especially at bifurcations and branchings. The segmental process involves the media, with edema, fibrinous exudation, fibrinoid necrosis, and infiltration of polymorphonuclear neutrophils and varying numbers of eosinophils, and extends to the adventitia and intima. Thrombosis and infarction or hemorrhage occur at this stage. Subsequently, the regions of fibrinoid necrosis are replaced by cellular granulation tissue, and the intima proliferates. Finally the involved segment is replaced by scar tissue with associated intimal thickening and periarterial fibrosis. These changes produce partial occlusion, thrombosis and infarction, and palpable or visible aneurysms with occasional rupture.

The glomerulitis is characterized by capillary microthrombi, focal fibrinoid necrosis, polymorphonuclear neutrophil infiltration, and capsular proliferation. With progression, the necrotizing feature of the glomerulitis is less apparent, and the process is difficult to distinguish from glomerulonephritis of other causes.

Clinical Manifestations and Diagnosis. The widespread distribution of the arterial lesions produces diverse clinical manifestations, which reflect the particular organ systems in which the arterial supply has been impaired. In addition, no study including a large number of living patients has or even can limit its patient population to those with classic periarteritis as defined by Kussmaul and Maier. The available studies are likely to include an admixture of patients with allergic angiitis and granulomatosis and hypersensitivity angiitis (see Ch. 78). Among the early general symptoms and signs of periarteritis nodosa are tachycardia, fever, weight loss, and pain in viscera and/or the musculoskeletal system so that the differential diagnosis is of fever of unknown origin. Striking and specific presenting signs may relate to abdominal pain, acute glomerulitis, polyneuritis, or myocardial infarction. Pulmonary manifestations, especially intractable bronchial asthma, would indicate allergic angiitis and granulomatosis rather than classic polyarteritis nodosa.

Renal. Renal involvement in two forms, renal polyarteritis and a glomerulitis, may occur separately or together. Renal polyarteritis was the most common lesion in the postmortem studies of Rose and Spencer (see accompanying table), and in the comparable analysis performed at the Armed Forces Institute of Pathology by Mowrey (1954). Manifestations of the renal involvement include intermittent proteinuria and microscopic hematuria with occasional hyaline and granular casts. The glomerulitis is manifested by marked microscopic and even macroscopic hematuria, proteinuria, cellular casts, and progressive renal failure; survival of the acute phase is followed by progressive hypertension. It is no longer the prevailing view that hypertension precedes or occurs in the initial phase of periarteritis nodosa, but rather that it reflects healing renal polyarteritis, progressive glomerulitis, or both. Such renal involvement is the cause of death in about two thirds of patients with classic periarteritis nodosa and about one third of those with allergic angiitis and granulomatosis.

Gastrointestinal. Characteristic arterial lesions are commonly found in one or more abdominal viscera. The principal manifestation is pain, especially in the umbilical region or right upper quadrant; anorexia, nausea, and vomiting are less prominent. Impaired arterial supply to the bowel can produce mucosal ulceration, perforation, or infarction with melena or bloody diarrhea. Involvement of appendix, gallbladder, or pancreas can simulate cholecystitis, appendicitis, or hemorrhagic pancreatitis. Liver involvement can range from hepatomegaly with or without jaundice to the signs of extensive hepatic necrosis. Splenomegaly is uncommon. The vasculitis associated with Australian antigenemia and considered by some to be representative of periarteritis nodosa is, of course, characterized by evidence of parenchymal liver disease.

Central and Peripheral Nervous System. Neurologic manifestations are generally late occurrences in the course of periarteritis nodosa, and their particular presentation reflects the specific brain area compromised. Headache, convulsive seizures, papillitis, and retinal hemorrhages and exudates occur with or without localizing signs referable to the cerebrum, cerebellum, or brainstem; meningeal irritation may occur as a result of subarachnoid hemorrhage. Multineuritis multiplex, that is, involvement of several or even many individual nerves at the same or different times, is a common finding and is attributed to arteritis of the vasa nervorum. The peripheral neuropathy is usually asymmetrical with both sensory and motor distribution. The former can be extremely painful, but the latter, with attendant muscular degeneration, has on occasion been so severe as to dominate the clinical presentation.

Articular and Muscular. Arthralgia and myalgia are frequent in polyarteritis nodosa. Arthralgia is migratory, generally without swelling, and apparently due to small localized arterial lesions rather than extensive synovitis. The interpretation of those rare instances of synovitis with deformity and arterial changes of periarteritis nodosa is difficult, but it seems preferable to consider such cases as rheumatoid arthritis. Muscle pain or weakness reflects either direct involvement of the arterial supply or a peripheral neuropathy from involvement of the vasa nervorum.

Cardiac. Polyarteritis of the coronary arteries and their branches has a frequency approaching that of renal polyarteritis, and heart failure is responsible for or contributes to death in one sixth to one half of the cases. The clinical manifestations of cardiac involvement are those of partial or complete arterial occlusion as modified by

Incidence of Necrotizing Angiitis in Various Organs at Necropsy*

	Polyarteritis Nodosa (Classic)	Allergic Angiitis and Granulomatosis ("Polyarteritis with Pulmonary Involvement")
	Per Cent	Per Cent
Lungs (pulmonary arteries)	0	47
Heart	35	60
Kidneys: Glomerulitis	30	57
Renal polyarteritis	65	60
Stomach and intestines	30	40
Liver	54	37
Pancreas	39	17
Spleen	35	43
Brain	4	3
Periadrenal connective tissue	41	40
Voluntary muscle	20	33

*Reproduced in modified form from Rose and Spencer: Quart. J. Med., 26:43, 1957. There were 54 cases in periarteritis group and 30 with the diagnosis of allergic angiitis and granulomatosis.

the superimposition of renal hypertension and an appreciable incidence of acute pericarditis without effusion. Whereas the combination of infarction and hypertension commonly leads to left-sided failure, an occasional patient with allergic angiitis and granulomatosis will present with predominantly right-sided decompensation.

Genitourinary. Involvement of the ovaries, testes, and epididymis is frequent, though usually asymptomatic. Mucosal ulceration in the bladder can occasionally precipitate gross hematuria with dysuria.

Cutaneous. Cutaneous involvement of some form is believed to occur in over 25 per cent of those affected with periarteritis nodosa. The acute cutaneous manifestations of periarteritis nodosa include polymorphic exanthemata—purpuric, urticarial, and multiform in character—and severe subcutaneous hemorrhage, resulting from necrotizing arteritis, with secondary gangrene. Ulcerations and a persistent livedo reticularis are associated with the more chronic stage of the disease. A most characteristic but uncommon finding is cutaneous and subcutaneous nodules; these occur at any time in the disease course. The nodules tend to group, appear in crops, are usually movable, may regress in days or persist for months, range in size from a pea to a walnut, and may cause the overlying skin to become reddened or to ulcerate.

Allergic Angiitis and Granulomatosis ("Polyarteritis with Pulmonary Involvement"). Pulmonary lesions are absent in classic polyarteritis nodosa but almost always precede the onset of polyarteritic lesions in other organs in the process termed allergic granulomatosis and angiitis by Churg and Strauss. Such patients typically present with bronchitis, bronchial asthma, or the findings of pneumonia. The asthma is intractable and associated with a marked peripheral eosinophilia. The pneumonic episodes are transient or progressive and can include hemoptysis or pleuritic pain. The appearance and superimposition of polyarteritis in other organs is followed by a rapid deterioration, respiratory involvement accounting for half the deaths.

Course Untreated. The course of periarteritis nodosa is progressive with destruction of vital organs. Intermittent acute episodes resulting from thrombosis of vital or nonvital structures are prominent. Death is most frequently attributed to renal involvement in cases of classic periarteritis nodosa and to pulmonary lesions in those cases classified as allergic angiitis with granulomatosis. Cardiac failure caused by a combination of infarction and renal hypertension is an additional frequent cause of death in both groups, and acute vascular accidents in the gastrointestinal tract or central nervous system account for much of the remaining mortality. In the retrospective postmortem study of Rose and Spencer, the five-year survival rate was about 10 per cent in classic periarteritis nodosa, and about 25 per cent in allergic angiitis and granulomatosis if onset was dated from the start of respiratory symptoms. The more recent report of the British Medical Research Council in 1960 placed the 54 months' survival rate in polyarteritis nodosa at nearly 50 per cent. A similar survival rate atributed to early steroid treatment has been noted in a Mayo Clinic series in which pulmonary involvement did not appear to influence the prognosis. Rare patients with polyarteritis limited to nonvital sites have been reported to experience an unusually long course or even a lasting remission. The entire issue of prognosis will be influenced by the criteria for entry into a series until the entity of periarteritis is more definitively separated from the more favorable grouping of hypersensitivity angiitis.

Laboratory Findings. Leukocytosis, predominantly polymorphonuclear, is apparent in over 75 per cent of the cases of periarteritis nodosa or allergic angiitis and granulomatosis, eosinophilia often being marked in the latter group. The erythrocyte sedimentation rate is customarily elevated with or without some increase of the globulins. Abnormalities in the urine sediment, especially hematuria and proteinuria, reflect renal involvement. Abnormalities of the electrocardiogram and electroencephalogram are those expected on the basis of arterial occlusive disease or those secondary to the metabolic disturbances of uremia. Lesions apparent on chest roentgenograms are the rule in patients with allergic angiitis and granulomatosis. The findings range from transient or progressive infiltration to consolidation, cavitation, or scarring; upper and lower lobes are involved with equal frequency. As none of these findings is specific, antemortem diagnosis of polyarteritis depends upon biopsy. Since the arterial involvement is segmental and spotty in distribution, it is advisable to obtain tissue from a symptomatic site, and it is essential to section completely the entire specimen. A deep, open surgical biopsy, including subcutaneous tissue and underlying muscle, should be obtained whenever possible from a skeletal muscle exhibiting pain and tenderness. Involvement of the epididymis and testes is sufficiently common to make this a useful biopsy site, if palpation reveals the typical nodularity of segmental vascular lesions. There are insufficient data on needle and surgical biopsies of internal organs, such as liver or kidney, to permit assessment of their usefulness or complications. As an alternative or additional procedure, arteriography of several organs to detect aneurysms of medium-sized muscular arteries may be helpful. Whether or not arteriography will prove definitive depends upon more experience with patients manifesting periarteritis nodosa and other forms of necrotizing vasculitis.

Differential Diagnosis. The differential diagnosis of classic periarteritis nodosa includes all those conditions associated with necrotizing angiitis (see Ch. 78). The absence of pulmonary lesions distinguishes classic periarteritis nodosa from allergic angiitis and granulomatosis. The other connective tissue diseases are recognized by their clinical characteristics even when necrotizing arteritis becomes prominent. For example, cases of rheumatoid arthritis with ulcerating cutaneous lesions and peripheral neuropathy often exhibit prominent rheumatoid nodules and a high titer of rheumatoid factor. Giant cell arteritis, in its limited form, cranial (especially temporal) or aortic arch (Takayasu's) arteritis, or in its disseminated state lacks the glomerulitis, peripheral neuropathy, and cutaneous manifestations notable in periarteritis nodosa. The drug-induced hypersensitivity angiitis group may be difficult to separate on purely clinical grounds, although the history of antecedent drug administration, the frequency of pulmonary involvement, infrequency of gastrointestinal manifestations, and absence of nodules along arteries are useful points. The clinical presentation in Henoch-Schönlein purpura, mostly in children and with a relatively good prognosis, is distinctive. The combination of progressive nephritis and pulmonary hemorrhage seen in Goodpasture's syndrome is unlike polyarteritis nodosa. The findings in the immunoglobulins which accompany active systemic lupus erythematosus or mixed cryoglobulinemia are distinctive; in addition, in the presence of active renal disease both entities manifest a reduced serum complement level not observed in periarteritis nodosa. Necrotizing vasculitis with or without renal disease in C2 deficiency, Australian antigenemia, and hypergammaglobulinemic purpura are differentiated by the unique features responsible for designating the entity.

The key morphologic differences between periarteritis nodosa and other causes of necrotizing angiitis are noted in Ch. 78 and include the absence of extravascular granulomas, sparing of the pulmonary arteries, failure of venous involvement except by contiguous spread, and predilection for medium-sized arteries. For allergic angiitis and granulomatosis the striking granulomatous response excludes all but Wegener's granulomatosis. The prominence of bronchial asthma, peripheral eosinophilia, and the usual absence of necrotizing lesions in the upper respiratory tract permit a tentative clinical distinction between allergic angiitis and granulomatosis (termed by some polyarteritis nodosa with pulmonary involvement) and Wegener's granulomatosis. Additional entities to be considered in the differential diagnosis are certain microbial and occlusive diseases with diverse manifestations, notably chronic meningococcemia, subacute infective endocarditis, trichinosis, certain rickettsial diseases, leptospirosis, and syphilis. A few vascular occlusive diseases, including Degos' disease and thrombotic thrombocytopenic purpura, must also be considered. Necrotizing papulosis of Degos, with its occlusive arterial lesions of the skin, gastrointestinal tract, and brain, is best characterized by the cutaneous manifestations. These lesions typically involve the trunk and extremities, begin as pink to gray papules, undergo central umbilication, and persist for variable periods with depressed (porcelain-like) centers covered with a removable scale and surrounded by a red elevated margin. The absence of both thrombocytopenia and intravascular hemolysis distinguishes periarteritis nodosa from thrombotic thrombocytopenic purpura. Additional points of help in the differential diagnosis of periarteritis nodosa in general are the rarity of Raynaud's phenomenon, the absence of the nephrotic syndrome, and the lack of lymphadenopathy.

Treatment. The therapy of periarteritis nodosa and allergic angiitis and granulomatosis is clearly unsatisfactory. Nonetheless, such patients can remain ambulatory and professionally active for periods of months to years after the clinical onset of the disease. The commonly employed antiinflammatory agents such as salicylates or phenylbutazone have little or no clear effect, and thus corticosteroids have been employed most widely. Large doses, in the range of 40 to 60 mg of prednisone per day, afford symptomatic relief and apparently do improve the one-year survival statistics. On the other hand, the study by the Medical Research Council of England did not reveal a better 54 months' survival period in a steroid-treated group as compared with a control series, whereas early steroid treatment was considered efficacious in the Mayo Clinic series. Experience with antimetabolites, such as azathioprine or cyclophosphamide, is insufficient to allow a conclusion as to their efficacy in periarteritis nodosa. The effect of these classes of compounds and drugs with related activities has been considered beneficial in diverse cases falling within the general classification of necrotizing vasculitis.

Churg, J., and Strauss, L.: Allergic granulomatosis, allergic angiitis, and periarteritis nodosa. Am. J. Pathol., 27:277, 1951.

Collagen Diseases and Hypersensitivity Panel: Report to Medical Research Council. Br. Med. J., 1:1399, 1960.

Mowrey, F. H., and Lundberg, R. A.: The clinical manifestations of essential polyangiitis (periarteritis nodosa) with emphasis on the hepatic manifestations. Ann. Intern. Med., 40:1145, 1954.

Rose, G. A., and Spencer, H.: Polyarteritis nodosa. Quart. J. Med., 26:43, 1957.

Part VI
DISEASES OF THE JOINTS

Charles L. Christian

83. INTRODUCTION

Although the terms "arthritis" and "rheumatism" have similar connotations, the former is restrictive, denoting inflammatory disease of joints. "Rheumatism" embraces a wide variety of illnesses that affect components of the musculoskeletal system: joints, muscles, ligaments, tendons, and bursae. Rheumatic syndromes can be classified as either inflammatory or degenerative, but the pathologic processes are sometimes less distinct than the nomenclature implies. A joint damaged by inflammatory disease is more vulnerable to degenerative influences, and syndromes that appear to be primarily degenerative in nature may be associated with the cardinal signs of inflammation. Musculoskeletal pain and stiffness, although characteristic of rheumatic syndromes, can be significant manifestations of virtually every disease of man. Errors in diagnosis and management result from uncritical elicitation of the medical history, physical signs, and, probably most frequently, from unbalanced interpretations of laboratory data. Hyperuricemia, rheumatoid factors, and antinuclear factors are not disease specific; and radiographic evidence of degenerative joint disease does not constitute proof that pain in an extremity is due to that process.

The accompanying classification of rheumatic disease (table), condensed and somewhat amended from the American Rheumatism Association's recommended (tentative) nomenclature, indicates the diversity of illnesses that can cause manifestations of rheumatic disease.

ARTHRITIS ASSOCIATED WITH KNOWN INFECTIOUS AGENTS

84. BACTERIAL ARTHRITIS

The great majority of cases of bacterial arthritis result from hematogenous spread of infections. Much less frequently, bacterial infection may result from joint aspiration or injection or by spread from contiguous osteomyelitis. In adults, gram-positive cocci (*Staphylococcus aureus, Streptococcus pyogenes, Diplococcus pneumoniae*) and *Neisseria gonorrhoeae* account for most

Rheumatic Disease — Classification

1. Polyarthritis of unknown etiology:
   a. Rheumatoid arthritis
   b. Juvenile rheumatoid arthritis
   c. Ankylosing spondylitis
   d. Psoriatic arthritis
   e. Reiter's syndrome
   f. Others
2. "Connective tissue" disorders (acquired):
   a. Systemic lupus erythematosus
   b. Progressive systemic sclerosis (scleroderma)
   c. Polymyositis and dermatomyositis
   d. Necrotizing arteritis and other forms of vasculitis
3. Rheumatic fever
4. Degenerative joint disease (osteoarthritis):
   a. Primary
   b. Secondary
5. Nonarticular rheumatism:
   a. Fibrositis
   b. Intervertebral disc and low back syndromes
   c. Myositis and myalgia
   d. Tendinitis and peritendinitis (bursitis)
6. Diseases with which arthritis is frequently associated:
   a. Sarcoidosis
   b. Relapsing polychondritis
   c. Schönlein-Henoch purpura
   d. Ulcerative colitis
   e. Regional enteritis
   f. Whipple's disease
   g. Sjögren's syndrome
   h. Familial Mediterranean fever
   i. Others
7. Arthritis associated with known infectious agents:
   a. Bacterial
   b. Rickettsial
   c. Viral
   d. Fungal
   e. Parasitic
8. Traumatic and/or neurogenic disorders:
   a. Traumatic arthritis (the result of direct trauma)
   b. Neuropathic arthropathy (Charcot joints)
   c. Shoulder-hand syndrome
   d. Mechanical derangement of joints
   e. Others
9. Arthritis associated with known or strongly suspected biochemical or endocrine abnormalities:
   a. Gout
   b. Chondrocalcinosis articularis ("pseudogout")
   c. Alcaptonuria (ochronosis)
   d. Hemophilia
   e. Sickle cell disease and other hemoglobinopathies
   f. Agammaglobulinemia (hypogammaglobulinemia)
   g. Gaucher's disease
   h. Hyperparathyroidism
   i. Acromegaly
   j. Hypothyroidism
   k. Scurvy
   l. Hyperlipoproteinemia type II (xanthoma tuberosum and tendinosum)
   m. Hemochromatosis
   n. Others
10. Neoplasms
11. Allergy and drug reactions
12. Miscellaneous disorders:
    a. Pigmented villonodular synovitis and tenosynovitis
    b. Behçet's syndrome
    c. Erythema nodosum
    d. Avascular necrosis of bone
    e. Juvenile osteochondritis
    f. Erythema multiforme (Stevens-Johnson syndrome)
    g. Hypertrophic osteoarthropathy
    h. Multicentric reticulohistiocytosis

cases. (Other areas of this text contain more detailed accounts of the problems and management of sepsis caused by specific bacterial organisms. The emphasis here is on principles of diagnosis and management that are common to all types of bacterial arthritis.)

Certain organisms appear to exhibit a tropism for joints: *N. gonorrhoeae, N. meningitidis, Hemophilus influenzae,* and *Streptobacillus moniliformis.* Host factors associated with debilitating chronic disease, rheumatoid arthritis, sickle cell anemia, hypogammaglobulinemia, and immunosuppressive therapy increase the risk of bacterial arthritis. A problem of increasing frequency is the development of low-grade infection complicating prosthetic joint placement. The recognition of infection may be delayed many months after joint replacement. Organisms of low virulence, especially *Staphylococcus albus,* predominate.

Clinical Manifestations. Although inflammatory signs in a single joint should heighten one's suspicion of bacterial sepsis, the disease may be polyarticular, a pattern that predominates with gonococcal arthritis. Rigor and high temperature, common manifestations of bacterial arthritis, are rare in rheumatoid arthritis and other types of noninfectious joint disease. Inflammatory signs tend to be marked; but in the presence of debilitating disease or treatment with adrenocorticosteroids or immunosuppressive agents, pain, swelling, and erythema may be masked. In patients with chronic rheumatoid arthritis, a preponderance of inflammatory disease in one or a limited number of joints should arouse suspicion of complicating bacterial arthritis.

Diagnosis. Since accurate diagnosis and effective management depend on isolation and characterization of the microbe, the highest priority is to be given to careful and complete bacteriologic studies. Although synovial fluid leukocyte counts in excess of 50,000 per cubic millimeter and reduced synovial fluid glucose content are common manifestations, no level of either is diagnostic of infection. Stained smears of joint fluid may demonstrate bacterial forms in the absence of a positive culture, especially when there has been chemotherapy. Synovial fluid and blood for microbiologic studies should be delivered without delay to the laboratory, preferably by someone involved in the patient's management. In addition to routine aerobic and anaerobic cultures, special media are needed for the isolation of *N. gonorrhoeae.* Obviously, bacteriologic studies of other materials, such as sputum, urine, and cervical exudate, may help to identify the organism causing arthritis.

Radiographic signs indicating loss of articular cartilage or erosion of bone are uncommon during the first week of disease.

Management. Success in management, as in diagnosis, rests with identification of the pathogen. The selection of appropriate antimicrobial agents and recommendations regarding dose and duration of therapy are covered in other areas of this text (see Ch. 268). It should be remembered that bacterial arthritis is usually a part of systemic sepsis and that the involvement of the synovial bursae behaves like a closed space infection. Since there is adequate transport of the commonly employed antibiotics from blood to joint fluid, there are rarely if ever indications for intra-articular therapy. When response to therapy is inadequate, measurement of bactericidal levels of drugs in synovial fluid may be indicated.

The decision whether to drain the joint bursae is influenced by the character of the exudate. When there is gross suppuration, and fluid cannot be easily aspirated with a large-bore needle, surgical incision and drainage are usually performed. When fluid can be aspirated with a needle and syringe, this is the preferred method for periodic decompression. The frequency of aspiration depends upon the extent and rate of reaccumulation. Gross joint destruction and the presence of contiguous osteomyelitis are indications for surgical drainage.

Physical therapy is inappropriate during the acute phase of bacterial arthritis. Maintenance of rest may be facilitated by removable splints. The rate at which gentle passive exercises can be graded into active motion should be tailored to each patient. Even in the absence of structural damage of weight-bearing joints, activity should not be resumed until signs of acute inflammation have subsided. The prognosis for full recovery is good when effective therapy is initiated within a week of the onset.

Gonococcal Arthritis. Gonococcal infection is discussed in Ch. 199. Because of its frequency and somewhat unique manifestations, this form of bacterial arthritis deserves emphasis. It is most common in females and homosexual males whose primary infections, because they are often asymptomatic, are untreated. The manifestations vary, but the most common pattern is migratory polyarthritis associated with tenosynovitis (especially in the hand and foot), followed by a "settling" in one or two joints. Shaking chills often precede or accompany the synovitis. Erythematous skin lesions, which may be macular, vesicular, or pustular (often with a necrotic center), are common in gonococcemia. The same clinical pattern can be associated with *N. meningitidis* and *H. influenzae* infections, although the latter is rare in adults.

Tuberculous Arthritis. The general decline in the frequency of tuberculosis is reflected in the relative rarity of tuberculous bone and joint disease. During the past few decades tuberculous arthritis has been predominantly an adult disease with evidence of pulmonary or disseminated disease frequently lacking. It is usually manifest in a single joint, most commonly hip, knee, or wrist, but any articulation may be affected, and occasionally two or more may be involved. Tuberculous *spondylitis,* predominantly a disease of children, has dramatically decreased in western countries.

Signs of acute inflammation are usually absent. Tuberculous arthritis is most commonly confused with monarticular rheumatoid arthritis. The ultimate differentiation, in a tuberculin-positive subject, often requires synovial biopsy and subsequent histologic and bacteriologic studies. Modern chemotherapy (see Ch. 242) has made surgical procedures (drainage, synovectomy, or fusion) unnecessary except in a rare patient with severe joint destruction.

85. VIRAL ARTHRITIS

Prevailing theories regarding the pathogenesis of rheumatoid arthritis, systemic lupus erythematosus, and related syndromes implicate atypical microbial infection. Although evidence supporting such speculations is indirect, there are well-defined, common viral infections associated with polyarthritis, notably rubella and viral hepatitis. Other viral syndromes associated with arthritis include mumps, infectious mononucleosis, and several arborvirus infections. Polyarthritis resembling acute rheumatic fever or acute rheumatoid arthritis occurs in approximately one third of women with natural or vaccine *rubella* infection. Lower frequencies of this complication are seen in men and children. Rubella arthritis usually follows the onset, or the fading phase, of the characteristic rash. The virus has been isolated from affected joints. The duration of joint inflammation varies from a few days to two weeks, rarely longer. There has been no documentation of chronic arthritis resulting from rubella infection. The management of pain and stiffness, which may be severe, should require nothing more than salicylate therapy.

Transient polyarthritis—more commonly polyarthralgia—is a significant prodromal manifestation of viral *hepatitis*. As with rubella, the pattern of arthritis resembles that of acute rheumatoid arthritis. It is frequently associated with fever and an urticarial skin eruption. These antedate the signs and symptoms of hepatitis by a few days to a few weeks, and have generally receded by the time icterus is apparent. Persistent polyarthritis has not been observed as a complication of viral hepatitis, although a small percentage of individuals with chronic active hepatitis have mild chronic or recurrent synovitis. The role that hepatitis B (Australia) antigen plays in the pathogenesis of the arthritis is not known, but certain manifestations, i.e., depressed serum complement and urticarial rash, are consistent with the hypothesis that immune complexes may be involved. Treatment is symptomatic.

86. OTHER FORMS OF INFECTIOUS ARTHRITIS

Syphilitic Arthritis. Syphilis is discussed in Ch. 246. Syphilitic arthritis, in its various forms, is now rare. A mild chronic synovitis, usually of the knees, may occur at about the age of puberty in patients with prenatal syphilis (*Clutton's joints*). Earlier skeletal manifestations of prenatal syphilis are related to periostitis and osteochondritis. Rheumatic manifestations have been attributed to secondary syphilis, but these, along with gummatous involvement of bones and joints, must have more historical than current importance. The most common rheumatic expression of syphilis, neuropathic arthropathy or Charcot joint, is reviewed in Ch. 97.

Mycotic Arthritis. Any of the invasive *mycoses* such as histoplasmosis, coccidioidomycosis, blastomycosis, and actinomycosis can affect joints, usually by extension from adjacent bone. Their manifestations generally resemble those of tuberculosis. Coccidioidomycosis can also cause the joint inflammation of erythema nodosum (see Ch. 911).

Alpert, E., Isselbacher, K. J., and Schur, P. H.: The pathogenesis of arthritis associated with viral hepatitis: Complement component studies. N. Engl. J. Med., 285:185, 1971.

Davidson, P. T., and Horowitz, I.: Skeletal tuberculosis: A review with patient presentations and discussion. Am. J. Med., 48:77, 1970.

Keiser, H., et al.: Clinical forms of gonococcal arthritis. N. Engl. J. Med., 279:234, 1968.

Schmid, F. R.: Principles of diagnosis and treatment of infectious arthritis. *In* Hollander, J. L., and McCarty, D. J., Jr. (eds.): Arthritis and Allied Conditions. 8th ed. Philadelphia, Lea & Febiger, 1972.

Sharp, J. T. Gonococcal arthritis. *In* Hollander, J. L., and McCarty, D. J.,

Jr. (eds.): Arthritis and Allied Conditions. 8th ed. Philadelphia, Lea & Febiger, 1972.

Smith, J. W., and Sanford, J. P.: Viral arthritis. Ann. Intern. Med., 67:651, 1967.

87. RHEUMATOID ARTHRITIS

Definition. In 1858 Sir Alfred Garrod introduced the term rheumatoid arthritis for a syndrome which he recognized as distinct from gout and acute rheumatic fever. With only minor exceptions (Garrod included Heberden's nodes as features of rheumatoid arthritis) his description matches the modern definition. The American Rheumatism Association's criteria for "classical, definite, probable and possible rheumatoid arthritis" have led to more consistent reporting in clinical studies, but the diagnosis still rests mainly on exclusion of other causes of synovitis.

Rheumatoid arthritis is a systemic disease of unknown cause. The frequency of extra-articular manifestations justifies the concept of "rheumatoid disease," but in the majority of patients clinical and pathologic findings and disability are the result of chronic inflammation of synovial membranes. There is striking heterogeneity among patients regarding mode of onset, pattern of joint involvement, frequency of extra-articular manifestations, and clinical course. There is a tendency for symmetrical involvement of hands, wrists, and feet. Spontaneous remissions and exacerbations are characteristic. Ten to 20 per cent of patients have complete remissions, whereas the remainder have sustained fluctuating activity. Joint injury results from formation of chronic granulation tissue (pannus), products of proliferative and exudative synovitis; this is capable of altering articular and periarticular structures.

Incidence and Epidemiology. The frequency of rheumatoid arthritis, based on limited population surveys in Europe and North America, is in the range of 1 to 3 per cent. It is two to three times more common in females. The onset is most frequent in the fourth and fifth decades of life, but it may occur at any age. There are no consistent trends relating prevalence to geography, climate, or culture. The apparent relative rarity in tropical climates may reflect the age of indigenous populations and the level of available medical care. Multiple family members in selected kindreds may be affected; but in general, familial patterns (even in monozygotic twins) are not striking.

Pathology. The pathologic elements of chronic synovitis include exudation, cellular infiltration, and the proliferation of granulation tissue. Although polymorphonuclear leukocytes predominate in synovial fluid, the principal infiltrating cells in synovial membranes are lymphocytes. These are often arranged in nodular aggregates, occasionally as true lymphoid follicles with germinal centers. Rarely, the majority of infiltrating cells are plasmacytes. Multinucleated giant cells may be seen. None of the aforementioned histologic features are diagnostic of rheumatoid arthritis.

Pannus, presumably by its content of hydrolytic enzymes, is capable of eroding articular cartilage, subchondral bone, ligaments, and tendons. Products of exudation in synovial fluid may also contribute to cartilage injury. The variable pattern of joint disability (subluxation, loss of motion, or ankylosis) relates to destructive processes in articular and periarticular structures.

Extra-articular manifestations, although clinically evident in a minority of patients, may give rise to widespread pathologic features of rheumatoid arthritis. Many of these appear to result from focal perivascular inflammation. Ten to 20 per cent of patients with rheumatoid arthritis form *subcutaneous or periosteal nodules* over pressure or friction points. The histologic appearance of nodules (central areas of necrosis surrounded by palisading connective tissue cells and an envelope of granulation tissue) is characteristic. In rare instances, the same granulomatous process can occur in multiple organs. More commonly (probably in the range of 50 per cent of cases) there is a mild perivascular infiltration of mononuclear cells in *muscle and peripheral nerves.* An uncommon but significant complication of the disease is the development of diffuse *necrotizing arteritis* with visceral involvement indistinguishable from polyarteritis nodosa. Milder forms of vasculitis, manifested by peripheral neuropathy and *chronic skin ulcers* of the lower extremities, are much more frequent. In such patients chronic inflammation of the sclera is common.

Cardiac pathology is less evident clinically than it is histologically. At necropsy, between one third and one half of rheumatoid patients have evidence of pericarditis (usually healed). Granulomatous lesions resembling rheumatoid nodules rarely may be found in the epicardium, myocardium, valves, and proximal aorta.

Pulmonary lesions, although infrequent, are significant expressions of rheumatoid disease. They include (1) chronic *pleural effusion,* (2) *Caplan's syndrome* (exaggerated pulmonary nodule formation in rheumatoid patients exposed to silica dust), (3) involvement with *granulomatous lesions resembling rheumatoid nodules,* and (4) *interstitial fibrosis.*

The most common patterns of neurologic involvement are peripheral neuropathy and nerve root irritation or myelopathy secondary to vertebral involvement (especially at C1-C2).

Pathogenesis. The role of *inflammation* in the production of articular, periarticular, and extra-articular injury is evident. A variety of lysosomal enzymes, neutral proteases, and synovial collagenase are capable of hydrolyzing constituents of connective tissue, and the role of such enzymes in the induction of tissue injury seems explicit. A more basic question, however, is: What initiates and perpetuates the inflammatory response? In this regard, immunologic theories predominate.

Immunologic Features. Synovial tissue in rheumatoid arthritis often displays histologic features characteristic of lymphoid organs, with prominent collections of lymphocytes and plasma cells (sometimes in the form of germinal centers). Immunoglobulin synthesis has been demonstrated in rheumatoid synovial tissue by immunohistologic and tissue culture studies. There is evidence for a role of immune complexes in the induction of inflammation. Synovial fluid exudate cells and synovial lining cells contain deposits of immunoglobulin and complement. Complement levels in synovial fluid are reduced in a pattern consistent with immune activation, and complexes of immunoglobulins are detectable in joint fluid. Detailed characterization of these has not been accomplished, but in part they consist of rheumatoid factors.

Rheumatoid Factors. Rheumatoid factors are autoantibodies reactive with the Fc portion of IgG. Antigammaglobulin activities are associated with the three major classes of immunoglobulins (IgM, IgG, and IgA), but, because of the enhanced agglutinating property of IgM antibodies, standard tests measure predominantly IgM rheumatoid factors. Rheumatoid factors form soluble complexes with their antigen (IgG). The complexes of IgM rheumatoid factor with IgG have a sedimentation coefficient of approximately 22S, whereas the complexes formed with IgG rheumatoid factors are very heterogeneous, sedimenting in the "intermediate" range between IgG and IgM. These intermediate complexes, which comprise at least part of the complexes measurable in rheumatoid synovial fluid, are capable of reacting with IgM rheumatoid factors to form insoluble aggregates. It is postulated that such complexes in joint fluid, perhaps augmented by their reactivity with IgM rheumatoid factor, activate complement-dependent mediators of inflammation and promote phagocytosis and subsequent release of hydrolytic enzymes. Although this hypothesis is attractive, there are a variety of reasons why one cannot assign an exclusive and primary role to rheumatoid factors in the induction of rheumatoid synovitis. On the basis of current evidence, it is more likely that rheumatoid factors are products of the host response to a more primary event. The nature of this postulated primary event is still unknown, but there is renewed interest in an old concept that microbial disease may underlie the development of rheumatoid arthritis.

Infectious Agents. A number of clinical and pathologic features of rheumatoid arthritis are mimicked by animal models of disease where microbial causes are explicit—in particular, chronic arthritis in swine induced by species of Mycoplasma and by *Erysipelothrix insidiosa.* An interesting aspect of these experimental models is that by the time chronic disease has developed, the inducing microorganism is often not demonstrable. By analogy, if the microbial hypothesis for rheumatoid disease is correct, the generally negative results of efforts to recover microorganisms may thus be explained. Although speculation regarding an infectious cause of rheumatoid disease has been augmented by modern concepts of viral persistence and by studies of animal models, direct evidence in its support is lacking. There have been periodic reports of the isolation of Mycoplasma and bacterial forms and of demonstrations that rheumatoid synovial cells are resistant to infection by exogenous viruses, but these observations still lack confirmation.

Clinical Manifestations. *Mode of Onset.* Usually, rheumatoid arthritis has an insidious onset, often beginning with poorly localized aching and stiffness. These early symptoms may be attributed to "grippe," and the subsequent evolution of frank synovitis may be sufficiently slow that the patient does not seek medical attention for many weeks. A variety of "precipitating" factors have been entertained (trauma, environmental change, infections, and psychologic stress), but none of these is constant in the antecedent history. Most patients manifest symmetrical polyarthritis early in the course of their disease, but a significant number (approximately one third) will have inflammation limited to one or two joints. Occasionally limited expressions of the disease, i.e., monarthritis or even tenosynovitis, may persist for many weeks or months. In contrast to the gradual onset of disease that characterizes the majority, the onset is precipitous in some patients, almost to the hour of a given day.

Symptoms. Pain, the dominant symptom, corresponds to the pattern and intensity of joint involvement, whereas *stiffness* is more generalized and is characteristically maximal after periods of physical inactivity. *Morning stiffness* is an almost invariable feature: its intensity and duration can guide one in assessment of disease activity.

The majority of patients experience *constitutional symptoms* such as weakness, increased fatigability, and diminished appetite. Temperature elevation in excess of 37.8° C is uncommon. Higher temperatures should prompt search for superimposed infection, but occasionally temperatures as high as 40° C have no other explanation than active rheumatoid arthritis. Many patients complain of coldness and hypesthesias and paresthesias in the hands and feet (in the absence of signs of nerve entrapment).

Physical Signs. The physical signs of rheumatoid arthritis vary enormously according to anatomic patterns, severity, and stage of disease. The "classic" articular and extra-articular expressions are features of *chronic* rheumatoid arthritis.

GENERAL EXAMINATION. Observations of gait and performance of simple tasks, such as removal of clothing, may reveal evidence of stiffness or specific anatomic patterns of disease. Many, but not all, patients appear chronically ill and undernourished. Generalized lymphadenopathy and splenomegaly are features in some subjects (approximately 10 per cent); rarely this picture is so striking that it mimics lymphomatous disease. Dependent edema not attributable to other causes is an infrequent but significant feature. Easy bruising and increased fragility of skin are common in patients with chronic disease; both are amplified by corticosteroid therapy. Nodules are most commonly found in subcutaneous tissue, but they can occur within the dermis and periosteum. Nodules are characteristically localized over points of pressure or friction, most commonly the extensor surfaces of the proximal forearms. In a bedridden patient they may be found over the posterior aspects of the head, trunk, and spine.

SKELETAL MANIFESTATIONS. The invariable signs of swelling, tenderness, and pain on motion in early cases may seem poorly localized to joints. A common mode of

Figure 1. Early rheumatoid arthritis manifest as symmetrical swelling and slight flexion deformities of proximal interphalangeal joints of the hands. Roentgenograms were normal except for evidence of soft tissue swelling.

onset, with symmetrical involvement of the distal upper extremities, is diffuse swelling of the hands and wrists. More discrete enlargement of articulations (Fig. 1) may not appear for weeks or months. Warmth is usually evident, especially over the large joints such as the knee, but skin erythema is infrequent. Swelling reflects varying degrees of synovial thickening and proliferation and an increased volume of synovial fluid. From palpation and ballottement, the examiner can usually estimate the relative roles of effusion and synovial proliferation.

The characteristic deformities of joints which are products of sustained chronic disease are attributable to a variety of events: loss of articular cartilage, destruction or weakening of ligaments, tendons, and capsular structures, muscle imbalance, and the physical force associated with use of the affected joints (Fig. 2). In addition, there are biologic variations which in some patients favor joint subluxation and instability and in other patients result in bony or fibrous ankylosis.

Muscle atrophy of the affected extremities may be evident within weeks of onset of rheumatoid arthritis. Whether this relates to primary myopathic change or disuse is moot, but rarely an overt myopathy, indistin-

Figure 2. Hand deformities characteristic of chronic rheumatoid arthritis. *A,* Subluxation of metacarpophalangeal joints with ulnar deviation of digits. *B,* Hyperextension ("swan neck") deformities of proximal interphalangeal joints.

guishable from polymyositis, may be a feature of the disease.

Extensions or rupture of synovial bursae beyond the confines of joint capsules can result in features of special importance to the internist. The most common example of this is the communication of joints of the wrists with the tenosynovium of the finger extensors. Popliteal cysts associated with knee synovitis may rupture into the calf and produce an inflammatory reaction that very closely resembles deep vein thrombophlebitis. The sudden onset of this complication, often associated with forceful flexion of the knee, and the intense inflammation help distinguish it from phlebitis, but this differentiation is best accomplished by arthrography. Rarely, extensions from hip synovitis may result in the formation of pelvic or inguinal masses.

EXTRA-ARTICULAR MANIFESTATIONS. Many of the features of rheumatoid arthritis that are associated with diffuse vasculitis have been discussed previously under Pathology. The clinical expressions of vasculitis (neuropathy, chronic skin ulcers, digital gangrene, and rarely visceral arteritis) and the clinical patterns associated with disseminated granulomata (heart, lung, sclera, and dura mater) are invariably features of chronic "classic" disease and are rarely encountered in patients who lack the rheumatoid factor.

For reasons unknown, pulmonary involvement (pleural effusion, granulomatous pneumonitis, and diffuse interstitial fibrosis) is more common in males. Cavitating pulmonary nodules occasionally result in pneumothorax or chronic bronchopleural fistulas. The glucose content of rheumatoid pleural effusions is frequently less than 10 mg per 100 ml.

There are usually no problems in interpretation of neurologic signs related to peripheral neuropathy, nerve entrapment (median nerve involvement at the wrist is common), and radiculopathy. In contrast, the insidious progression of muscle weakness secondary to myelopathy from C1-C2 subluxation can mistakenly be attributed to "arthritis" and associated constitutional symptoms.

Other extra-articular manifestations of rheumatoid arthritis include amyloidosis, keratoconjunctivitis sicca, and Felty's syndrome.

Clinical Course and Prognosis. Statistics regarding the natural history of rheumatoid arthritis are based on studies in large rheumatic disease units where patients are not representative of the entire population of rheumatoid arthritics, i.e., they tend to be patients with more severe and sustained disease. Patients with more remitting patterns of disease are less apt to be entered into prognostic studies. However, even the published figures allow one to present a reasonably optimistic outlook to the patient. After 10 to 15 years of disease, over 50 per cent of patients remain fully employed and only about 10 per cent are completely incapacitated. Ten to 20 per cent of patients have virtually complete remissions; the course followed by the remainder is extremely varied. The average patient with episodic exacerbations and partial remissions will experience gradual progression of deformity and disability. The minority, with sustained disease activity and only slight remissions, may become completely disabled within a few years of onset. The *features associated with a poor prognosis*, in a statistical sense are (1) classic pattern of disease (symmetrial polyarthritis with subcutaneous nodules and high titers of rheumatoid factor), (2) sustained disease of more than

one year's duration, (3) onset below age 30, and (4) extra-articular manifestations of rheumatoid arthritis.

Roentgenographic Findings. Early in the disease roentgenograms of affected joints are usually negative except for evidence of soft tissue swelling and joint effusion. Osteoporosis, especially in juxta-articular locations, may be evident within weeks of onset of disease. Loss of articular cartilage, shown by reduction in the apparent "joint space," and bone erosions are rarely evident before several months of sustained disease. Subluxations, dislocations, and bony ankylosis, if they occur, are still later phenomena. Diffuse osteoporosis is common with chronic disease and is heightened with adrenocorticosteroid therapy. The frequency of avascular osteonecrosis, especially of the femoral heads, is also increased with such therapy.

Laboratory Findings. Mild *anemia,* similar to that associated with chronic infection, is common in rheumatoid arthritis. Serum levels of both iron and iron-binding protein are frequently depressed. Anemia is usually normocytic and normochromic, but if there is accompanying iron deficiency, the erythrocytes may be slightly hypochromic and microcytic. Leukocytosis, eosinophilia, and thrombocytosis are occasional laboratory features. (See Ch. 88 for discussion of neutropenia associated with Felty's syndrome.)

The *erythrocyte sedimentation rate* (ESR) is increased above the normal range in virtually all patients with active rheumatoid arthritis. There are a variety of other "acute phase reactants" in the serum which reflect inflammatory activity, but none of them match the simplicity of the ESR or exceed its sensitivity.

Rheumatoid *synovial fluid* is usually turbid with reduced viscosity, increased protein content, and slight reduction of glucose levels relative to the blood. Leukocyte counts (predominantly polymorphonuclear cells) vary between a few thousand and more than 50,000 cells per cubic millimeter. Cells containing inclusions are common, but these may be seen in other types of exudative synovitis. Complement in synovial fluid, relative to protein content, is commonly reduced, a finding usually associated with positive tests for rheumatoid factors.

There are no tests that are specific for rheumatoid arthritis, although the term "rheumatoid factors" has been applied to autoantibodies reactive with IgG (see Pathogenesis above). A variety of test systems are available, but most laboratories utilize the *latex fixation test,* in which polystyrene latex particles coated with IgG are agglutinated by rheumatoid factors. Less commonly applied systems include the *bentonite flocculation test* and a variety of *hemagglutination tests* employing erythrocytes coated with immunoglobulins. The latex fixation test is positive (1:80 titer or higher) in approximately 70 per cent of rheumatoid subjects. Although less than 5 per cent of healthy control subjects are positive, the rheumatoid factor is associated with other connective tissue syndromes, liver disease, and a variety of infectious diseases such as bacterial endocarditis, tuberculosis, syphilis, and leprosy. The frequency of positive tests for rheumatoid factor in the general population increases with age.

Differential Diagnosis. *General.* Differential considerations are numerous and vary according to the pattern of disease. There is seldom confusion in identifying "classic" rheumatoid arthritis, but symmetrical involvement of hand and wrist joints can be a feature of other syndromes (see below). Differentiation is more difficult and complex in patients with early acute polyarthritis or in those with arthritis limited to one or a few joints.

Chronic Polyarthritis. The most common form of chronic arthropathy, degenerative joint disease, is usually quite distinct from rheumatoid arthritis. Minimal inflammatory signs, absence of constitutional symptoms, ESR determinations in the range of normal, and the characteristic radiographic findings usually serve to identify degenerative joint disease. A clinical pattern of degenerative joint disease which has been termed "primary generalized osteoarthritis" (see Ch. 98) may be mistaken for rheumatoid arthritis, especially when there is symmetrical enlargement of interphalangeal joints in the hands. *Bouchard's nodes*, the bony enlargement of proximal interphalangeal joints of the hand (see Fig. 4B) are rather frequently misinterpreted as signs of rheumatoid arthritis.

Gout and *chondrocalcinosis* (see Ch. 821 and 97, respectively) may mimic chronic rheumatoid arthritis. The most definitive basis for their identification is polarized light microscopy of synovial fluid.

Other connective tissue syndromes such as *systemic lupus erythematosus* (SLE) and *progressive systemic sclerosis* are infrequently associated with chronic deforming joint change. Their differentiation from rheumatoid arthritis is based on characteristic multisystemic patterns of disease. Certain serologic features of SLE, especially hypocomplementemia and the antibodies to native deoxyribonucleic acid, are rare in rheumatoid arthritis. A few patients, with mixed clinical and laboratory features of two or more syndromes, defy classification.

The majority of patients with arthritis and *psoriasis* are indistinguishable from patients in the spectrum of rheumatoid arthritis. The designation psoriatic arthritis as a separate entity is in part arbitrary, but certain clinical and laboratory features of psoriatic arthritis (see Ch. 92) aid in its differentiation from rheumatoid arthritis.

Rheumatic manifestations of a wide variety of systemic diseases, including sarcoidosis, ulcerative colitis, regional enteritis, Whipple's disease, amyloidosis, acromegaly, chronic infection, and malignancies, can resemble rheumatoid arthritis. This list emphasizes the importance of exclusions in formulating a diagnosis of rheumatoid arthritis.

Acute Polyarthritis. The range of differential considerations for acute polyarthritis includes those listed above plus a variety of disorders that rarely if ever result in chronic joint disease. The most frequent set of diagnostic considerations for acute polyarthritis includes rheumatoid arthritis, acute rheumatic fever, infection, and drug hypersensitivity. Acute arthritis associated with chills and fever should be considered infectious until proved otherwise. The presence of carditis, evidence of recent streptococcal infection, fever, and prompt response to salicylate therapy contribute to the recognition of acute rheumatic fever. Important differentiating features of gonococcal arthritis are prominent tenosynovitis, the cutaneous manifestations, and, most important, isolation of the bacteria from blood or joint fluid. The common viral infections that can resemble acute rheumatoid arthritis are rubella and viral hepatitis. There are other remitting forms of polyarthritis in which viral causes are suspected but not established. A careful clinical history and the recognition of other allergic phenomena will help in the identification of drug hypersensitivity.

Monarthritis or Oligoarthritis. All the conditions listed above under Acute and Chronic Polyarthritis are appropriate to the differential diagnosis of arthritis affecting one or a limited number of joints; but when the pattern of joint involvement is restricted, the most important differential consideration is infection. A complete medical evaluation, including chest x-ray, tuberculin tests, and appropriate microbial studies, is indicated. When there is continued suspicion of bacterial or mycobacterial infection, synovial biopsy may be required.

Management. *Basic Principles.* In the management of rheumatoid arthritis, the physician should keep the following facts in mind: (1) in most patients the disease is chronic; (2) spontaneous remissions occur in almost all patients; (3) the majority of subjects can continue to lead active lives with varying degrees of restrictions; and (4) complications of drug therapy, most notably adrenocorticosteroids, can cause greater morbidity than the underlying disease.

The patient and the doctor must be educated not to expect and seek a short-term solution. The physician can present a reasonably optimistic prognosis, based on knowledge of the natural history of rheumatoid arthritis, and can assure the patient that there are conservative means of ameliorating symptoms and minimizing disability.

There are no specific dietary recommendations; rather, the general nutritional status of the patient and associated medical conditions influence diet selection. Weight reduction, in obese patients, should have high priority. Providing that the diet is well balanced, there are no indications for vitamin supplementation. The anemia of rheumatoid arthritis does not respond to hematinic therapy except to the extent that iron deficiency may be a complicating feature. Rarely the anemia may be so severe as to require transfusion.

Psychologic depression is a common consequence of chronic rheumatoid arthritis. From the physician, the patient needs sympathetic understanding of his problems and a willingness to help solve them. When depression is severe, these efforts may be facilitated by the use of antidepressive medication. If anxiety, restlessness, and insomnia are complicating features, the use of mild sedatives or tranquilizers may be indicated.

A basic program that is applicable to all patients includes (1) rest, (2) employment of salicylates for the relief of pain and suppression of inflammation, and (3) maintenance of joint function by physical measures. Some but not all patients will be candidates for medicinal therapy other than salicylates and/or orthopedic surgical procedures.

REST. Patients and physicians alike tend to be confused by the apparently conflicting goals of rest and exercise. They are not mutually exclusive (see Physical Measures below). It is clear that physical work, applied to an affected extremity, will intensify the synovitis of rheumatoid arthritis. The specific prescription of rest will vary according to the severity and pattern of involvement, but all patients should be directed to respect their symptoms of pain and fatigue and to restrict physical activities to the essentials. Any way that occupational duties can be modified to lighten the work load should be tried, and daytime rest periods are important. Occasionally when symptoms are very severe, hospitalization for attainment of more complete rest is indicated.

EMPLOYMENT OF SALICYLATES. All students of rheumatoid arthritis agree that salicylate therapy is part of the basic management. The majority of patients can tolerate acetylsalicylic acid in doses of 3.6 grams daily or more, if the physician is persistent in his recommendations. When gastrointestinal symptoms complicate therapy, ingestion of the drug with meals or the use of enteric-coated or buffered products may be helpful. When doses of acetylsalicylic acid in the range of 3.6 grams daily are tolerated but rheumatic symptoms are poorly controlled, gradual increase in the dose is warranted. It is too often concluded, on the basis of inadequate trials, that "aspirin was not effective." Measurement of blood salicylate levels is appropriate when there is a question of toxicity or absorption.

PHYSICAL MEASURES. The choice of various heat modalities (warm pool, tank, bath, shower, diathermy, or ultrasound) depends primarily on the areas affected and the availability of services. Diathermy and ultrasound treatments are contraindicated in patients with metal implants. A warm pool permitting exercise under water is optimal for the patient with very severe symptoms, but for most individuals a hot bath or shower will suffice. Morning stiffness and pain will be minimized by ingestion of salicylates followed by a hot bath.

The *goals of an exercise program* are (1) maintenance of motion of affected joints, and (2) prevention of muscle atrophy. Both of these can be achieved without submitting inflamed joints to the task of work. An active exercise program for the lower extremities can maintain motion and strength without heavy weight bearing, allowing the right combination of rest and exercise. The rate of progression from gentle passive exercises, required for the most symptomatic patient, to a more active program will vary according to the pattern of involvement and the response to therapy. In order that the patient avoid assuming a passive dependent role, it is crucial that emphasis be placed on what he or she can do independent of supervision. The average doctor is not sufficiently trained in physical medicine to write detailed prescriptions, but he should be very specific in what his goals are when referring the patient to a physical medicine service. Furthermore, he should review the program periodically with the patient and reinforce its importance in the total management. It is a moot point whether forceful active exercises are appropriate for the distal upper extremities; evidence suggests that heavy work will aggravate hand and wrist deformities. For a patient with acutely inflamed joints, removable splints to achieve rest are helpful, but there are no convincing demonstrations that such devices prevent development of chronic hand deformities.

The role of orthopedic surgery in the management of rheumatoid arthritis is discussed subsequently in this chapter.

Other Antirheumatic Therapy. For the patient whose response to salicylate therapy has not been adequate, several other anti-inflammatory agents can be employed. These include indomethacin, phenylbutazone (and oxyphenbutazone), antimalarial drugs (chloroquine and hydroxychloroquine), and gold compounds. At the time of this writing, several other nonsteroidal anti-inflammatory agents are under evaluation but are not yet licensed for use in the United States. The adrenocorticosteroid drugs are the most potent anti-inflammatory medications available, but their value, for reasons stated below, is limited. Unfortunately all medications employed for the treatment of rheumatoid arthritis, except

gold compounds, have in common the property of promoting peptic ulceration.

Among those who specialize in the management of rheumatic disease, there is no uniformity of habit regarding the employment of agents listed above, although the majority, at some time, will institute gold therapy for the patient with sustained rheumatoid arthritis. Codeine and related analgesics may be required on a temporary basis, but their chronic use should be discouraged.

Phenylbutazone is a reasonably potent anti-inflammatory agent, but there is limited enthusiasm for its use in long-term management of rheumatoid disease. In doses of 200 to 300 mg daily, this drug may be helpful in the treatment of intermittent exacerbations. The incidence of serious toxicity (exfoliative dermatitis and hematologic complications) is infrequent but a source of concern. The occasional patient who is helped by long-term therapy should be under close medical supervision and should have periodic blood counts.

Indomethacin, although chemically unrelated to other analgesic and anti-inflammatory drugs, has a pattern of efficacy similar to that of phenylbutazone. Both are more effective in gout and ankylosing spondylitis than in rheumatoid arthritis. In the dose range of 50 to 200 mg per day, a few patients will experience sufficient benefit to warrant its continuation. Gastrointestinal symptoms and vascular headaches are common side effects, but serious complications are rare. Concomitant aspirin therapy appears to diminish gastrointestinal absorption of indomethacin.

Antimalarial compounds such as chloroquine and hydroxychloroquine have moderate anti-inflammatory activity in the treatment of rheumatoid arthritis. Because of the occasional association of irreversible retinopathy, the use of antimalarials has sharply declined.

Although soluble *gold compounds* have been employed in the treatment of rheumatoid arthritis since the 1930s, their mode of action is not known. There is no evidence that they have anti-inflammatory activity; rather, clinical impressions suggest that, in some unknown way, they increase the likelihood of remission. The level of enthusiasm for chrysotherapy varies considerably among rheumatic disease specialists. Some advocate such treatment within weeks of onset of disease; others reserve it for patients who have had sustained disease for several months or more in spite of more conservative therapy. There is a cumulative effect of gold compound administration. Sensitive assays can detect trace amounts many months after discontinuation of therapy. Gold is excreted primarily in the urine. The most common complications are dermatitis and stomatitis. Renal damage, manifested by proteinuria and microscopic hematuria, and hematological dyscrasias (thrombocytopenia and granulocytopenia) are rare but significant complications of chrysotherapy.

The preparations employed are sodium aurothiomalate (Myochrysine) and aurothioglucose (Solganal). Both are administered by deep intramuscular injection at weekly intervals. It is common practice to use small doses (10 to 25 mg) for the first two or three injections, followed by 50 mg at weekly intervals thereafter. Complete blood count and urinalysis should be obtained prior to each injection for several weeks and every few weeks after that as long as therapy is continued. If there is any sign from these tests or from clinical assessment (pruritic rash or stomatitis) of gold toxicity, therapy should be interrupted. If unequivocal evidence of gold toxicity develops, such as severe stomatitis or exfoliative dermatitis or renal or hematologic complications, treatment should not be resumed. In the case of mild, transient skin reactions, it is common practice to reinstitute the medication at reduced levels after the rash has cleared. Experience indicates that remissions, if they occur on gold therapy, will occur during the course of 20 weekly injections (approximately 1 gram total dose). In the absence of improvement during this course, there is no point in continuing therapy. For the patient experiencing a remission, it is recommended that maintenance therapy be continued (50 mg at three- to four-week intervals). The decision as to maintenance therapy in patients who experience only partial remission is more difficult.

Mild gold-induced dermatitis may persist for several weeks or more, but usually requires no therapy other than topical corticosteroids. The most common presentation consists of several scattered, well-circumscribed pruritic lesions associated with mild scaling. The discomfort associated with severe dermatitis may warrant a course of systemic corticosteroid therapy (10 to 20 mg of prednisone daily) or the use of BAL (dimercaprol). Hematologic complications, most commonly thrombocytopenia, are also indications for dimercaprol therapy. Dimercaprol, 2.5 mg per kilogram of body weight, is given every four hours for two days, followed by the same dose twice daily for approximately a week. An alternative means of promoting gold excretion is the employment of penicillamine, although there is less clinical experience to recommend it.

Adrenocorticosteroid Therapy. SYSTEMIC THERAPY. Since the early therapeutic trials of cortisone in 1949, several related compounds with potent anti-inflammatory activity have been introduced. These include prednisone, prednisolone, triamcinolone, methylprednisolone, dexamethasone, betamethasone, and paramethasone. Electrolyte and water-retaining properties, associated with cortisone and hydroxycortisone therapy, are minimal with the newer drugs, but the more serious side effects are common to *all* adrenocorticosteroid preparations (see below). The approximate milligram equivalent of the various drugs that yield comparable pharmacologic effects are cortisone (25 mg), hydrocortisone (20 mg), prednisone (5 mg), triamcinolone (4 mg), methylprednisolone (4 mg), dexamethasone (0.75 mg), betamethasone (0.6 mg), and paramethasone (2 mg).

Because of frequent and potentially life-threatening complications of adrenocorticosteroid therapy, it should not be employed in the management of rheumatoid arthritis until there has been a sustained trial of more conservative therapy. In general, the more experienced the physician is in the management of rheumatoid disease, the more reluctant he is to begin adrenocorticosteroid therapy. The following facts should be pondered before initiating such treatment: (1) adrenocorticosteroid drugs suppress inflammation, but they do not correct or change the underlying process; (2) small doses, in the range of 5 to 10 mg of prednisone, often provide only partial and temporary gains; (3) over periods of months or years, there is a tendency for the dose to increase; (4) once instituted, it is very difficult to discontinue therapy; and (5) the morbidity and mortality associated with long-term adrenocorticosteroid therapy often exceed those of the underlying disease.

In the light of these facts, it is difficult to summarize indications for adrenocorticosteroid therapy of rheumatoid arthritis. If a conservative effort, employing less toxic drugs and physical measures, fails to check progressive disability and if the alternative to adrenocorticosteroid therapy seems to be chronic invalidism, then the former may be indicated. In such cases the daily dose should not exceed 10 mg of prednisone or its equivalent; as little as 5 to 7.5 mg in divided doses may provide some benefit. Although pituitary-adrenal unresponsiveness and other complications of therapy are minimized by alternate-day or single daily dose regimens, most patients with rheumatoid arthritis do not tolerate such programs. Occasionally, sustained disease may be less severe but may compromise the occupational activity of a wage earner or mother of a household. A small dose (5 or 7.5 mg daily of prednisone or equivalent) may allow continuation of employment, but the physician and patient should make the decision deliberately and with full realization of the toxic potential of such therapy.

COMPLICATIONS OF ADRENOCORTICOSTEROID THERAPY. The frequency and severity of *osteoporosis,* a feature of rheumatoid disease regardless of therapy, are increased by adrenocorticosteroid treatment. Compression fractures of vertebral bodies are common. (Detailed discussions of the management of osteoporosis are presented in Ch. 879 to 884). There are theoretic bases for employment of high calcium intake, vitamin D, fluorides, and anabolic steroids, but their efficacy in preventing or reversing osteoporosis is uncertain. Another frequent skeletal complication of adrenocorticosteroid therapy is *avascular osteonecrosis,* most commonly affecting the femoral head.

Although most antirheumatic drugs are associated with *peptic ulceration,* the frequency of this complication is probably highest in patients treated with adrenocorticosteroids. The problem is sometimes compounded, because the signs and symptoms of perforation and peritonitis may be masked by therapy.

Decreased host resistance to acquired or reactivated *infections* is a well-documented feature of adrenocorticosteroid therapy. It is common practice to institute isoniazid prophylaxis of tuberculin-positive patients receiving steroid therapy.

Aggravation of latent or overt diabetes mellitus and psychic disturbances ranging from mild euphoria to frank psychosis are infrequent with the doses of adrenocorticosteroids used in the treatment of rheumatoid arthritis.

Any patient receiving daily adrenocorticosteroid therapy must be assumed to have an *inadequate pituitary adrenal response* to stress. With intercurrent illnesses, or with surgery, the dose should be increased and the patient observed closely for signs of adrenal insufficiency. The same precautions apply to those whose treatment has been discontinued up to two years prior to the stressful illness. The value of intermittent corticotrophin therapy in the amelioration of pituitary adrenal unresponsiveness is unproved.

INTRA-ARTICULAR ADRENOCORTICOSTEROID THERAPY. Several adrenocorticosteroid preparations suitable for intra-articular therapy will temporarily suppress signs and symptoms of synovitis. This mode of therapy is helpful for a patient whose disability relates primarily to disease in one or two joints. With rigorous antiseptic technique, the risk of infection is low. If there is any question of antecedent infection at the time of arthrocentesis, intra-articular steroids should not be administered. The usefulness of intra-articular therapy is dependent upon the duration of symptomatic benefit. Because of clinical suspicions and experimental evidence that steroid compounds are deleterious to articular cartilage, most physicians will not inject a joint more frequently than every four to six weeks.

Immunosuppressive (Cytotoxic) Therapy. Several drugs initially developed for cancer chemotherapy have been applied in the treatment of rheumatoid arthritis. The categories of compounds include alkylating agents, purine and pyrimidine antagonists, and folic acid analogues. There is no basis for concluding that one compound is superior to another in immunosuppressive and anti-inflammatory properties, but the best data with regard to the treatment of rheumatoid arthritis derive from a controlled study of cyclophosphamide therapy. Patients receiving up to 150 mg daily of cyclophosphamide sustained significantly fewer new bone erosions over the period of study. In spite of these observations, the use of immunosuppressive agents is to be viewed as experimental therapy. Acute toxicity, especially myelosuppression, is potentially fatal and, as well, there is concern that immunosuppressive therapy may foster the emergence of primary malignant tumors.

Other Experimental Drugs. Penicillamine, in a well-controlled study in England, had moderate efficacy in the suppression of severe chronic rheumatoid arthritis and resulted in reductions of rheumatoid factor titers. As an antirheumatic agent, penicillamine remains in the experimental category, primarily because of potentially serious toxicity (agranulocytosis and nephropathy).

Orthopedic Surgery. Orthopedic surgeons are playing an increasingly important role in the management of rheumatoid arthritis. The value of reconstructive surgery in the rehabilitation of selected subjects is well established. Techniques of arthroplasty and prosthetic joint replacement have improved dramatically during the past decade. The rationale for synovectomy is sound, i.e., the removal of chronic pannus and its destructive potential, but proof of its efficacy is lacking. Disease frequently recurs in regenerated synovium, but the intensity of recurrent inflammation tends to be less. On the basis of current experience, synovectomy is probably warranted for patients with sustained (several months or more) proliferative synovitis affecting knee, hand, and wrist joints.

Cooperating Clinics Committee of the American Rheumatism Association: A controlled trial of cyclophosphamide in rheumatoid arthritis. N. Engl. J. Med., 283:883, 1970.

Duthie, J. R. R., et al.: Course and prognosis in rheumatoid arthritis. Ann. Rheum. Dis., 23:193, 1964.

Freyberg, R. H., Ziff, M., and Baum, J.: Gold therapy for rheumatoid arthritis. *In* Hollander, J. L., and McCarty, D. J., Jr. (eds.): Arthritis and Allied Conditions. 8th ed. Philadelphia, Lea & Febiger, 1972.

Hollingworth, J. W.: Local and Systemic Complications of Rheumatoid Arthritis. Philadelphia, W. B. Saunders Company, 1968.

Ruddy, S., and Austen, K. F.: The complement system in rheumatoid synovitis: I. An analysis of complement activities in rheumatoid synovial fluids. Arthritis Rheum., 13:713, 1970.

Short, C. L., Bauer, W., and Reynolds, W. E.: Rheumatoid Arthritis. Cambridge, Harvard University Press, 1957.

Winchester, R. J., Agnello, V., and Kunkel, H. G.: Gammaglobulin complexes in synovial fluids of patients with rheumatoid arthritis: Partial characterization and relationship to lowered complement levels. Clin. Exp. Immunol., 6:689, 1970.

Zvaifler, N. J.: The immunopathology of joint inflammation in rheumatoid arthritis. *In* Dixon, F. J., and Kunkel, H. G. (eds.): Advances in Immunology. vol. 16. New York, Academic Press, 1972.

VARIANTS OF RHEUMATOID DISEASE

88. FELTY'S SYNDROME

Splenomegaly is observed in approximately 5 per cent of patients with rheumatoid arthritis. Felty originally described a syndrome consisting of rheumatoid arthritis, splenomegaly, and neutropenia. Anemia and thrombocytopenia are occasional features. This syndrome is most common in older individuals who have had longstanding chronic rheumatoid disease. Other extra-articular manifestations of rheumatoid disease such as rheumatoid nodules, chronic skin ulcers, and keratoconjunctivitis sicca are common. Rheumatoid factor tests are invariably positive, and antinuclear phenomena are more common than in uncomplicated rheumatoid arthritis. The indications for splenectomy are influenced primarily by the frequency and severity of infectious complications. Most patients experience hematologic remissions after splenectomy, but relapses occur in many of them.

89. SJÖGREN'S SYNDROME

In 1933 Sjögren called attention to the combination of rheumatoid arthritis, keratoconjunctivitis sicca, and xerostomia. The characteristic ocular and oral mucous membrane involvement may occur in the absence of rheumatic disease. In addition to its association with rheumatoid arthritis, it can be a manifestation of other connective tissue syndromes such as systemic lupus erythematosus, progressive systemic sclerosis, and polymyositis. The sicca complex is clinically manifest in approximately 10 to 15 per cent of patients with rheumatoid arthritis, but pathologic expressions, such as lymphoid infiltration of the minor salivary glands in the lip, are much more frequent. More than 90 per cent of affected patients are women, and most have had longstanding chronic arthritis.

The symptoms related to salivary insufficiency include difficulty with chewing and swallowing, dental caries, and ulcerations of the buccal mucous membranes. Dryness may also involve the upper respiratory tract, larynx, and tracheobronchial tree. In common with Felty's syndrome, patients with Sjögren's syndrome frequently manifest extra-articular features attributed to vasculitis. A small but significant number of patients with Sjögren's syndrome have developed reticulum cell sarcoma or a more benign lymphoproliferative disorder termed "pseudolymphoma." Because lymphomatous complications have occurred primarily in patients with a history of irradiation for parotid gland enlargement, this mode of therapy has been discouraged.

Rheumatoid factor tests are positive in the majority of patients, and antinuclear and a variety of other autoimmune reactants are associated with Sjögren's syndrome.

The treatment is symptomatic. Artificial tears of 0.5 per cent methylcellulose are helpful. Adrenocorticosteroid or immunosuppressive drugs are restricted to those patients with severe disability or life-threatening complications.

Barnes, C. G., Turnbull, A. L., and Vernon-Roberts, B.: Felty's syndrome: A clinical and pathological survey of 21 patients and their response to treatment. Ann. Rheum. Dis., 30:359, 1971.

Shearn, M. A.: Sjögren's Syndrome. Philadelphia, W. B. Saunders Company, 1971.

Whaley, K., Williamson, J., Chisholm, D. M., et al.: Sjögren's syndrome. I. Sicca components. Quart. J. Med., 42:279, 1973.

OTHER FORMS OF POLYARTHRITIS OF UNKNOWN ETIOLOGY

90. ANKYLOSING SPONDYLITIS
(Marie-Strümpell Spondylitis, von Bechterew's Syndrome, Rheumatoid Spondylitis)

In this syndrome there is prominent involvement of spinal articulations, sacroiliac joints, and paravertebral soft tissues. Because one third to one half of patients with ankylosing spondylitis manifest synovitis in peripheral joints (especially hips and shoulders), the syndrome was formerly viewed as a variant of rheumatoid arthritis. However, several features of ankylosing spondylitis are distinct from those of rheumatoid arthritis: (1) prominent ligamentous calcification and ossification with a tendency to bony ankylosis; (2) male preponderance; (3) impressive evidence of genetic transmission in selected kindreds; (4) symptomatic benefit with medications, notably phenylbutazone and indomethacin, that are minimally effective in rheumatoid arthritis; (5) absence of rheumatoid factor and rheumatoid nodules; and (6) the association of certain extra-articular manifestations such as iridocyclitis and aortitis.

Etiology. The cause of ankylosing spondylitis is unknown. The disease has been found to be 30 times more prevalent among the relatives of spondylitic patients than among relatives of controls. Recent studies have demonstrated a striking association between ankylosing spondylitis and HL-A 27, but the manner in which this histocompatibility antigen influences pathogenesis is unknown. Infectious causes have long been suspected but never established. Spinal involvement indistinguishable from ankylosing spondylitis is occasionally a feature of Reiter's syndrome, psoriatic arthritis, and inflammatory bowel disease.

Incidence and Prevalence. Ankylosing spondylitis is a common cause of back pain in young men. The male-to-female ratio is approximately 8:1. In an English survey, the incidence of ankylosing spondylitis was 1 in 2000 among the population at large.

Pathology. On the basis of symptoms and early radiographic findings, the disease appears to begin in the sacroiliac joints, with subsequent involvement of zygapophyseal and costovertebral articulations, interspinous ligaments, and paravertebral tissues. The characteristic immobility of the spinal column results from bony ankylosis of zygapophyseal joints and ossification of paravertebral structures. Syndesmophytes, the bony bridges which unite adjacent vertebral bodies, form in the outer lamellae of the anulus fibrosus and adjacent connective tissue fibers. The pathologic character of synovial inflammation is not distinct from that of rheumatoid arthritis. Aortic involvement resembling syphilitic aortitis can result in aortic insufficiency. Iridocyclitis occurs in approximately 25 per cent of patients. The incidence of amyloidosis complicating ankylosing spondylitis is approximately 5 per cent. Rarely, a pattern of pulmonary fibrosis, sometimes associated with cavitation, has been described.

Clinical Manifestations. In the majority of cases the onset of ankylosing spondylitis, usually in the second or third decade of life, is insidious. The initial symptoms are usually low back pain and stiffness; rarely, the first symptoms may relate to involvement of hip, shoulder, or peripheral joints. Symptoms may be sufficiently mild that the patient seeks no medical attention for months. At the other extreme, there may be debilitating pain at the outset, associated with fever, severe fatigue, and weight loss. In most patients, however, constitutional symptoms are not prominent. Pain and stiffness, which are maximal after periods of inactivity, often interrupt sleep in the early morning hours. Radicular and sciatic patterns of pain are common. The pattern and rate of spinal ankylosis are varied. The majority of patients experience gradual cephalad progression of spinal immobility, but the disease may remain confined to the sacroiliac joints and lumbar segments. The development of the poker back type of spinal deformity usually evolves gradually over a period of ten years or more. The majority of patients remain fully employed. Hip involvement, the most common cause of occupational disability, is now amenable to prosthetic surgery.

Physical signs are limited in the early stages of disease. Sacroiliac joint involvement may be evident from palpation of these joints or from orthopedic maneuvers which produce sacroiliac joint movement. Paravertebral muscle spasm and tenderness are common. Physical signs associated with the chronic phase of ankylosing spondylitis relate primarily to spinal immobility. The most accurate estimate of lumbar flexion is accomplished by comparing midline measurements from the sacrum to T-12 in flexion and extension. The normal difference in these two measurements is approximately 3 inches. The presence and progression of costovertebral joint involvement can be documented by measurements of chest expansion.

The most important extra-articular manifestations of ankylosing spondylitis are *iridocyclitis,* occurring in approximately one quarter of patients, and aortitis. The frequency of *aortic insufficiency* has been as high as 4 per cent in some series. *Cardiac conduction disturbances,* most frequently first degree A-V block, occurs in about 10 per cent of cases. *Cauda equina involvement,* a rare but significant complication of longstanding spondylitis, is manifest as urinary or rectal sphincter incompetence and pain and sensory loss in the sacral distribution.

Roentgenographic Findings. Characteristic roentgenographic findings of ankylosing spondylitis involve the following structures: sacroiliac joints, zygapophyseal articulations, vertebral bodies, and paravertebral soft tissues. Changes in the sacroiliac joints are the earliest and most consistent findings. The margins of subchondral bone are blurred, followed by subchondral sclerosis and bony erosions. Progressive narrowing of the interosseous joint space and sacroiliac fusion develop slowly over a period of years. Sclerotic and erosive changes in zygapophyseal and costovertebral articulations are common but less readily demonstrated by x-ray. Alterations in vertebral bodies, loss of anterior concavity, and anterior marginal erosions are features of longstanding disease. Calcification and ossification of the anulus fibrosus and adjacent paravertebral ligaments give rise to the characteristic syndesmophytes that gradually bridge adjacent vertebral bodies. In advanced cases this results in the so-called *bamboo spine*. In addition to sacroiliac joints, other cartilaginous articulations such as the symphysis pubis and sternomanubrial joints may be involved. There is a tendency for ossification of ligaments and tendon insertions. Roentgenographic changes in the hips and shoulders, less commonly in more peripheral joints, are not distinct from those of rheumatoid arthritis, although the incidence of bony ankylosis of the hips is greater in ankylosing spondylitis.

The full set of roentgenographic findings, described above, is a product of many years of progressive disease. In a minority of patients with ankylosing spondylitis, the disease appears to go into remission after involvement of restricted segments of the spine.

Diagnosis. Ankylosing spondylitis should be suspected in anyone, particularly a young male, with persistent or recurrent low back pain and stiffness or recurrent sciatic pain. Although associated phenomena such as elevation of erythrocyte sedimentation rate, thoracic girdle pain, arthritis in the lower limbs, and iridocyclitis will enhance the suspicion, early diagnosis should not be excluded on the basis of normal roentgenograms, because several months or, rarely, a few years may elapse before development of roentgenographic changes. Although degenerative joint disease can result in back pain and loss of spinal motion, this is a problem of later decades of life, and the roentgenographic features are distinct from ankylosing spondylitis. Joint disease identical to ankylosing spondylitis can be a feature of *ulcerative colitis, regional enteritis, Reiter's syndrome,* and *psoriasis.*

Treatment. The highest priority goal in the management of ankylosing spondylitis is the maintenance of a functional posture. It is doubtful that any medication will prevent ankylosis of those spinal segments involved, but the suppression of pain and inflammation is essential before an appropriate physical medicine program can be instituted.

Indomethacin and phenylbutazone are usually more effective than other antirheumatic agents in the control of pain and stiffness, but an initial trial on salicylate therapy (3.6 to 4.5 grams daily) is recommended. For those patients who do not experience sufficient relief of symptoms with salicylates, indomethacin in doses of 100 to 150 mg daily or phenylbutazone (100 to 300 mg daily) is indicated. With control of symptoms, the dose of either indomethacin or phenylbutazone should be gradually reduced to the lowest level that will maintain improvement. With continuous use of phenylbutazone, the risk of hematologic complications should be kept in mind and periodic blood counts obtained. Adrenocorticosteroid therapy is rarely indicated for ankylosing spondylitis. If all other efforts to control progressive disability fail, such therapy may be indicated, as outlined under rheumatoid arthritis (see Ch. 87). Systemic adrenocorticosteroid therapy may be required for the control of iridocyclitis. Although roentgen therapy, directed at areas of involvement, is effective in control of symptoms, this mode of treatment is not recommended because of the

demonstrations of chromosomal injury and an observed incidence of leukemia that is ten times greater in patients so treated than in the general population.

For the management of ankylosing spondylitis, emphasis should be given to the institution and maintenance of an exercise program. In order that flexion deformity of the spine be avoided, the patient should sleep on a very firm mattress, preferably without a pillow. There should be a twice daily performance of exercise directed at the maintenance of erect posture, strengthening of paraspinal muscles, and promotion of chest cage motion. A hot bath or shower will often facilitate exercise activity. If physical medicine measures fail to check the progression of flexion deformity, back splints or braces may be tried. In carefully selected individuals with advanced flexion deformity, spinal osteotomy can improve posture, but this is associated with significant risk of neurologic complications. For the patient with severe hip involvement, the most frequent cause of major disability, prosthetic hip replacement offers dramatic relief.

91. JUVENILE RHEUMATOID ARTHRITIS

Although the definition of juvenile rheumatoid arthritis is somewhat arbitrary (onset of disease under age 16), there are clinical features which tend to distinguish it from rheumatoid arthritis in adults. These include high fever, transient morbilliform rash, leukocytosis, uveitis, local growth disturbances, low frequencies of rheumatoid factor and subcutaneous nodules, and a higher incidence of monarticular disease than is observed in adults.

The discussions of etiology, pathogenesis, and pathology of rheumatoid arthritis (see Ch. 87) are relevant to juvenile rheumatoid arthritis except for speculations regarding a pathogenic role of rheumatoid factors.

In approximately 20 per cent of children with juvenile rheumatoid arthritis, the onset is acute and fulminating and is associated with systemic manifestations such as fever, rash, pericarditis, and splenomegaly *(Still's disease).* Occasionally these features may persist for several weeks before synovitis is evident. (A similar systemic pattern of disease has been observed, rarely, in adults.) In approximately half of patients, the onset is polyarticular, resembling rheumatoid arthritis in adults. In one third of juvenile rheumatoid arthritis patients, the onset is monarticular. Many patients in this group continue to have disease limited to one or a few joints, often in an asymmetrical pattern, and manifest no systemic disease except for iridocyclitis (10 to 15 per cent). The frequency of cervical spine and sacroiliac joint involvement exceeds that of adults. Abnormal skeletal growth adjacent to inflamed joints results from varied degrees of accelerated local growth and premature closure of epiphyseal plates.

Leukocytosis in the range of 15,000 to 25,000 is common. Serologic evidence of recent streptococcal infection is found in a third to a half of subjects, adding to the problem of differentiation from acute rheumatic fever. No more than 10 per cent of sera are positive in the commonly employed tests for rheumatoid factor. The frequency of antinuclear antibody is higher than in adults with rheumatoid arthritis. This is especially so in children with iridocyclitis.

Distinctive roentgenographic findings include local growth disturbances (noted above), abnormal periosteal bone accretion, and prominent involvement of cervical zygapophyseal joints.

Differential considerations vary according to the pattern of juvenile rheumatoid arthritis. The systemic form of disease resembles certain infectious syndromes. Recognition of the characteristic morbilliform rash, if it is present, is important in diagnosis. The polyarticular onset of disease, when accompanied by high fever and signs of carditis, is easily confused with acute rheumatic fever. Features of juvenile rheumatoid arthritis that may aid in this distinction are frequent onset of disease under age 5, nonmigratory pattern of polyarthritis, cervical spine involvement, marked leukocytosis, and rash. The immediate suppressive effect of salicylate therapy is less striking in juvenile rheumatoid arthritis than it is in rheumatic fever.

Fifty per cent or more of patients with juvenile rheumatoid arthritis experience complete remissions. The serious consequences of extra-articular involvement relate to carditis, chronic iridocyclitis, and amyloidosis.

Principles of management outlined for rheumatoid arthritis (see Ch. 87) apply to children with chronic arthritis. Contractures and restricted motion of articulations are more common in children than in adults. The patient's parents must be given important roles in the maintenance of a physical medicine program. Aspirin in the range of 90 to 130 mg per kilogram daily is the treatment of choice. Early in the course of the disease, adrenocorticosteroid therapy should be reserved for patients with severe systemic manifestations, such as carditis, that do not respond to salicylate therapy. Periodic ophthalmologic consultation, at approximately six-month intervals, is recommended, since iridocyclitis may be asymptomatic and missed by casual examination. Because of the threat of blindness from sustained iridocyclitis, systemic adrenocorticosteroid therapy may be indicated if this complication is severe and fails to respond to local treatment. In addition to the usual complications and limitations of adrenocorticosteroid therapy, growth retardation, a natural feature of the disease, is augmented by such treatment. The indications for the employment of gold therapy are similar to those presented for rheumatoid arthritis. The dose of gold thioglucose or gold thiomalate is 1 mg per kilogram per week. A course of therapy consists of approximately 20 weekly injections.

92. PSORIATIC ARTHRITIS

The recognition that psoriatic arthritis is a disease entity, as opposed to the coincidental occurrence of two common diseases, i.e., rheumatoid arthritis and psoriasis, is relatively recent. Based on population surveys, approximately 5 per cent of patients with cutaneous psoriasis have chronic arthritis. One quarter to one third of such patients manifest rheumatoid nodules or positive tests for rheumatoid factor, and probably represent cases of coexistence of two diseases. Patients with psoriasis and chronic arthritis are clinically heterogeneous, but some of them manifest sufficiently unique features to justify the term psoriatic arthritis.

Several clinical subtypes of psoriatic arthritis are recognized. The most common pattern is of a scattered asymmetrical involvement of interphalangeal joints of the hands and feet, frequently manifest as "sausage digits" (Fig. 3). Much less common, but recognized by all as "classic psoriatic arthritis" is the exclusive involvement of distal interphalangeal joints. In approximately one quarter of patients with psoriasis there is a symmetrical pattern of arthritis indistinguishable, apart from negative serology, from rheumatoid arthritis. In this group, there is a tendency for severe osteolytic involvement with resorption of bone and telescoping of digits (arthritis mutilans). Approximately 5 per cent of patients with psoriasis and arthritis manifest features identical to those of ankylosing spondylitis, although the roentgenographic character of syndesmophytes tends to differentiate the two syndromes.

It is important to recognize that there may be asynchronous onset of cutaneous involvement and arthritis and that a patient with typical psoriatic arthritis may have minimal or hidden cutaneous involvement. Psoriatic nail involvement occurs in over 80 per cent of patients with psoriatic arthritis, in contrast to only a 30 per cent incidence in patients with uncomplicated psoriasis. Typical psoriatic arthritis, especially spondylitis, may evolve after recurrent attacks of Reiter's syndrome.

The unique clinical patterns of psoriatic arthritis such as bone resorption, asymmetric involvement of interphalangeal joints, and spondylitis are represented in roentgenographic findings. An increased incidence of

Figure 3. Common patterns of psoriatic arthritis in the hands. *A,* Asymmetrical enlargement of interphalangeal joints of right thumb and left ring finger. *B,* "Classic" involvement of distal interphalangeal joints and nails of digits two, three, and five of left hand.

hyperuricemia in psoriatic patients probably reflects the increased metabolism of skin. Other than the absence of rheumatoid factor in patients with psoriatic arthritis, there are no immunologic, biochemical, or pathologic distinctions from rheumatoid arthritis.

Principles of management of psoriatic arthritis do not differ from those of rheumatoid arthritis. Antimalarial drugs are contraindicated, because they have been observed to provoke exfoliative dermatitis in psoriatic subjects. Reliance should be placed on a basic regimen of salicylates and physical therapy. Adrenocorticosteroid drugs should be employed only as a last resort. For the patient with very severe psoriatic arthritis, immunosuppressive therapy, in spite of its experimental status and considerable toxicity, is probably more appropriate than adrenocorticosteroid therapy.

93. REITER'S SYNDROME

Although the association of arthritis, urethritis, and conjunctivitis was recorded early in the nineteenth century, this triad of clinical manifestations bears the name of the German physician who, in 1916, described a patient with nongonococcal urethritis, conjunctivitis, and arthritis after an episode of diarrhea. Other common manifestations of the syndrome include fever, oral and genital mucous membrane lesions, cutaneous keratosis, and iritis. Most patients are young males; it is rare in women regardless of age.

Etiology. The cause of Reiter's syndrome is unknown, but most attention has focused on infectious causes. Venereal transmission seems apparent in many cases; in others the onset of Reiter's syndrome follows diarrheal illness. In several large epidemics of bacillary dysentery, a small percentage of patients have developed typical Reiter's syndrome, including genitourinary tract involvement. Mycoplasmal and chlamydial species are suspect as etiologic agents. The significance of sporadic isolation of such organisms from synovial fluid or synovial tissue is unknown. In preliminary studies there appeared to be a high association of HL-A 27 with Reiter's syndrome equivalent to that observed with ankylosing spondylitis.

Clinical and Laboratory Manifestations. All the clinical features of Reiter's syndrome may appear simultaneously, but more commonly genitourinary or gastrointestinal symptoms precede the onset of ocular or rheumatic features by several days or a few weeks. Occasionally the classic pattern evolves slowly over weeks or months after the appearance of a single manifestation. Polyarthritis is frequently asymmetrical with predilection for involvement of articulations of the lower extremities, but the pattern of joint involvement can be varied. The majority of patients experience complete remissions within weeks or a few months of onset. A minority (range of 10 per cent) manifest persistence of synovitis in articulations of the extremities or spine and will have disability that parallels that of sustained rheumatoid arthritis or ankylosing spondylitis. Rarely, the clinical picture of chronic or recurrent Reiter's syndrome evolves into typical psoriatic arthritis.

There are no distinctive laboratory features. Peripheral blood leukocytosis is common. Properties of synovial fluid are similar to acute rheumatoid arthritis, although complement levels in joint fluid are invariably high.

Roentgenographic abnormalities, equivalent to those associated with rheumatoid arthritis, are found in those patients with sustained synovitis. Periostitis, adjacent to involved joints, is a common but not distinctive feature of Reiter's syndrome.

The most common diagnostic alternative to Reiter's syndrome is *gonococcal arthritis*. The past literature is confusing because of the failure to distinguish these two syndromes and to recognize that gonococcal infection may be coincident to Reiter's syndrome. In a minority of patients, typical mucocutaneous lesions, particularly balanitis circinata and keratoderma blennorrhagica, leave no question regarding diagnosis, but the failure to isolate *N. gonorrhoeae* and the resistance of the manifestations to antimicrobial therapy are the main bases for differentiating Reiter's syndrome from gonococcal arthritis.

Treatment. The management of Reiter's syndrome is similar to that of rheumatoid arthritis. If salicylate therapy in the range of 3.6 to 4.5 grams daily fails to suppress synovitis or constitutional symptoms, phenylbutazone or indomethacin (both in the range of 100 to 200 mg daily) may be beneficial. There is no experience to recommend gold therapy. There are a few reports describing remissions of very severe disease coincident to treatment with immunosuppressive agents; but in the light of their immediate and long-term toxicity, such therapy is considered experimental.

94. PALINDROMIC RHEUMATISM

This term has been applied to a recurring pattern of polyarthritis which results in no permanent joint deformity. The syndrome resembles gout in its acute onset and marked inflammatory signs. Rapid subsidence of signs and symptoms occurs within hours or a few days of onset. The frequency of episodes and the anatomic areas affected are variable, but for individual subjects the pattern of recurrent disease tends to be constant.

Since recurrent polyarthritis can be a feature of many rheumatic syndromes, the term palindromic rheumatism, if it is used at all, requires rigorous exclusion of other causes of synovitis. A significant number of patients, the majority in some series, with palindromic rheumatism eventually manifest typical features of rheumatoid arthritis. Systemic and constitutional symptoms are generally lacking. Since the brief episodes terminate spontaneously, there is no uniformity of opinion regarding response to therapy.

95. INTERMITTENT HYDRARTHROSIS

This term has been applied to the pattern of recurrent joint effusions, usually the knees, in which other inflammatory signs are minimal. The interval between episodes varies from one to a few weeks. In most reports of intermittent hydrarthrosis, there has been female preponderance. Occasionally recurrences correlate with menstruation. The diagnosis of intermittent hydrarthrosis, like palindromic rheumatism, should be restricted to individuals who have been followed long enough to exclude other causes of recurrent synovitis. A significant number of patients will eventually manifest chronic synovitis consistent with rheumatoid arthritis. When discomfort and restricted motion are attributable to joint space distention, simple arthrocentesis may be beneficial; there is no agreement regarding the efficacy of medicinal therapy in suppressing or preventing attacks.

Ansell, B. M., and Bywaters, E. G. L.: Rheumatoid arthritis (Still's disease). Pediat. Clin. North Am., 10:921, 1963.
Calabro, J. J., and Marchesano, J. M.: The early natural history of juvenile rheumatoid arthritis. A ten year follow-up of 100 cases. Med. Clin. North Am., 52:569, 1968.
Kinsella, T. D., MacDonald, F. R., and Johnson, L. G.: Ankylosing spondylitis: A late re-evaluation of 92 cases. Can. Med. Assoc. J., 95:1, 1966.
Moll, J. M. H., and Wright, V.: Psoriatic arthritis. Semin. Arthritis Rheum., 3:55, 1973.
Ogryzlo, M. A.: Ankylosing spondylitis. In Hollander, J. L., and McCarty, D. J., Jr. (eds.): Arthritis and Allied Conditions. 8th ed. Philadelphia, Lea & Febiger, 1972.
Schlosstein, L., et al.: High association of an HL-A antigen, W27, with ankylosing spondylitis. N. Engl. J. Med., 288:704, 1973.
Sharp, J. T.: Reiter's syndrome. In Hollander, J. L., and McCarty, D. J., Jr. (eds.): Arthritis and Allied Conditions. 8th ed. Philadelphia, Lea & Febiger, 1972.
Williams, M. H., et al.: Palindromic rheumatism: Clinical and immunological studies. Ann. Rheum. Dis., 30:375, 1971.

96. DISEASES WITH WHICH ARTHRITIS IS FREQUENTLY ASSOCIATED

Arthritis may be a significant feature of all of the syndromes listed in this chapter. Discussion here is brief and is limited to rheumatic manifestations of the various disorders. More detailed considerations will be found elsewhere in the chapters devoted to those diseases.

INFLAMMATORY BOWEL DISEASE

The reported incidence of arthritis complicating *ulcerative colitis* and *regional enteritis* (Crohn's disease) has varied, but it is generally in the range of 10 per cent. The most common rheumatic pattern is an asymmetric polyarthritis involving a few joints. In the majority of patients the disease is intermittent and results in minimal joint damage. The frequency and severity of arthritis are generally higher in those subjects with sustained and extensive bowel involvement, but occasionally rheumatic manifestations will antedate the recognition of enteric disease. *Erythema nodosum* and *uveitis* are three to four times more common in patients with enteritis and arthritis than in patients without rheumatic manifestations. In contrast to the generally benign character of rheumatic complications of enteritis, a small number (approximately 10 per cent of those with arthritis) experience a pattern of disease and disability equivalent to rheumatoid arthritis.

The incidence of *spondylitis,* which is indistin-

guishable from ankylosing spondylitis, in patients with ulcerative colitis and regional enteritis has varied between 2 and 6 per cent. This represents at least a twenty-fold increase in the frequency of spondylitis over that in the general population. Clinical, laboratory, or roentgenographic findings do not distinguish spondylitis complicating enteritis from ankylosing spondylitis unassociated with bowel disease, except that male predominance in the former is less striking.

There are no special recommendations regarding the management of arthritis associated with enteritis: the general principles outlined for the treatment of rheumatoid arthritis and ankylosing spondylitis (see Ch. 87 and 90) are appropriate. The main management effort is directed at the intestinal disease. Remissions of arthritis frequently follow surgical resection of diseased bowel, but rheumatic complications rarely affect the decision regarding surgical therapy.

WHIPPLE'S DISEASE

This is a rare syndrome, probably bacterial in cause, characterized by diarrhea, malabsorption, fever, anemia, increased skin pigmentation, and migratory polyarthralgia or polyarthritis. Permanent joint damage is rare.

FAMILIAL MEDITERRANEAN FEVER

Musculoskeletal pain occurs in approximately 7 per cent of patients with this heritable disease. The arthritis is usually monarticular or limited to a few joints; most commonly involved are knees, ankles, hips, or shoulders. Severe pain and tenderness are out of proportion to other modest signs of inflammation. Arthritis, like other manifestations of this syndrome, is usually recurrent, but permanent damage to joints is rare. None of the anti-inflammatory medications have been found to be effective in the treatment of this form of arthritis. Management is limited to analgesics and local physical measures.

SARCOIDOSIS

The most common rheumatic manifestation of sarcoidosis is a transient acute polyarthritis associated with erythema nodosum and hilar adenopathy. Lower extremity joints are primarily involved. At times it is difficult to be certain whether inflammatory symptoms and signs reflect true synovitis or the cellulitis of erythema nodosum. Recovery is uniform. Most patients can be managed with salicylates but, if pain and disability are severe, a course of adrenocorticosteroid therapy may be indicated. Much less common than the acute rheumatic syndrome is chronic granulomatous synovitis that clinically resembles rheumatoid arthritis.

HYPOGAMMAGLOBULINEMIA

A mild polyarthritis, rarely deforming in character, has been observed in as many as one third of patients with congenital and acquired hypogammaglobulinemia. The pattern of joint disease resembles that of rheumatoid arthritis, although other connective tissue syndromes such as systemic lupus erythematosus, systemic sclerosis, and dermatomyositis have been associated with immune deficiency states. A variety of autoimmune phenomena and connective tissue syndromes have been observed in patients lacking IgA, the most common selective deficiency. Regression of arthritis frequently follows institution of gamma globulin therapy.

POLYCHONDRITIS

Relapsing polychondritis is a rare disorder characterized by inflammation and destruction of cartilage. In the majority of patients there is intermittent involvement of cartilage in ears, nose, trachea, pharynx, costochondral junctions, and peripheral joints. With subsidence of inflammation there may be collapse and deforming change of the ears, nose, and laryngotracheal structures. The pattern of joint involvement is usually that of recurrent polyarthritis associated with minimal residual deformity. Other manifestations include fever, iritis, episcleritis, cataracts, deafness, and aortic insufficiency. Aortic involvement, occurring in 14 per cent of reported cases, and involvement of cartilaginous structures of the respiratory tract are the two life-threatening complications of polychondritis. Pathologic studies demonstrate varying degrees of inflammation and loss of cartilage matrix. The cause is unknown. Adrenocorticosteroid therapy has been employed for life-threatening manifestations, but the generally remittent character of the disease makes it uncertain whether any mode of therapy changes its natural history. Aortic involvement has necessitated prosthetic valve replacement in a few reported patients.

BEHCET'S SYNDROME

This syndrome was initially described as a triad (recurrent aphthous stomatitis, genital ulcerations, and iritis), but other manifestations are common: pyoderma, erythema nodosum, erythema multiforme, thrombophlebitis, and polyarthritis. Central nervous system involvement, in a minority of patients, may be fatal. Intermittent or chronic polyarthritis is usually limited to one or a few joints and rarely results in significant deformity. There is a strong suspicion that viral infection underlies the development of Behçet's syndrome, but attempts at microbial isolation have been equivocal or negative. Adrenocorticosteroid therapy is indicated if iritis is severe or if there are neurological manifestations.

HEMOCHROMATOSIS

Joint involvement has been observed in as many as half of patients with idiopathic hemochromatosis. Joint swelling with bony enlargement is particularly common in the small joints of the hands, but other joints may be affected. The clinical and roentgenographic features resemble degenerative joint disease more than rheumatoid arthritis. There is narrowing of the joint space with subchondral erosions and sclerosis. Roentgenographic evidence of chondrocalcinosis is present in a third or more of patients with arthropathy and may account, via crystal-induced synovitis (see Chondrocalcinosis and

Pseudogout in Ch. 97), for occasional acute inflammatory manifestations. The management of arthropathy is similar to that described for degenerative joint disease.

ACROMEGALY

The majority of patients with acromegaly develop an atypical form of degenerative joint disease. Increased levels of growth hormone result in hypertrophy of articular cartilage, subchondral bone, and periarticular tissues. Hypermobility of joints, a common manifestation, may contribute to degenerative change. The fingers and knees are most frequently affected. Radiographic features demonstrating overgrowth of bone are pathognomonic. Median nerve entrapment secondary to wrist synovitis is common.

HYPERPARATHYROIDISM

Patients with hyperparathyroidism are subject to a variety of associated rheumatic disorders which may occur singly or in combination. These include (1) hyperuricemia and gouty arthritis, (2) chondrocalcinosis with episodes of calcium pyrophosphate dihydrate crystal-induced synovitis, and (3) degenerative joint disease resulting from deformation of atrophic subchondral bone. Rheumatic symptoms, particularly those associated with chondrocalcinosis (see Chondrocalcinosis and Pseudogout in Ch. 97) may be the first manifestation of hyperparathyroidism.

SICKLE CELL DISEASE AND RELATED HEMOGLOBINOPATHIES

Severe polyarthralgia is a frequent manifestation of the crises of sickle cell disease. Occasionally pain is accompanied by transient joint effusion or other evidence of inflammation. The most common rheumatic symptoms result from avascular osteonecrosis of the femoral head, less commonly of other bony structures. This complication is also associated with sickle cell trait, hemoglobin C disease, SC disease, and sickle cell–thalassemia. In children, periostitis may result in transient diffuse swelling of the hands and feet. Sickle cell disease is associated with an increased incidence of bacterial arthritis and osteomyelitis, especially those caused by gram-negative organisms.

Bluestone, R., et al.: Acromegalic arthropathy. Ann. Rheum. Dis., 30:243, 1971.

Bywaters, E. G. L., Dixon, A. St. J., and Scott, J. T.: Joint lesions of hyperparathyroidism. Ann. Rheum. Dis., 22:171, 1963.

Ferguson, R. H.: Enteropathic arthritis. *In* Hollander, J. L., and McCarty, D. J., Jr. (eds.): Arthritis and Allied Conditions. 8th ed. Philadelphia, Lea & Febiger, 1972.

Hamilton, E., et al.: The arthropathy of idiopathic haemochromatosis. Quart. J. Med., 37:171, 1968.

Hughes, R. A. C., et al.: Relapsing polychondritis: Three cases with a clinicopathological study and literature review. Quart. J. Med., 41:363, 1972.

McEwen, C.: Arthritis accompanying ulcerative colitis. Clin. Orthop., 59:9, 1968.

McEwen, C., et al.: Ankylosing spondylitis and spondylitis accompanying ulcerative colitis, regional enteritis, psoriasis and Reiter's disease. A comparative study. Arthritis Rheum., 14:29, 1971.

O'Duffy, J. D., Carnery, J. A., and Deodhar, S.: Behçet's disease: A report of ten cases, three with new manifestations. Ann. Intern. Med., 75:561, 1971.

Spilberg, I., Siltzbach, L. E., and McEwen, C.: The arthritis of sarcoidosis. Arthritis Rheum., 12:126, 1969.

97. MISCELLANEOUS FORMS OF ARTHRITIS

NEUROPATHIC JOINT DISEASE (CHARCOT JOINTS)

This chronic progressive degenerative arthropathy is a complication of a variety of neurologic disorders. Impairment of proprioceptive and pain sensation deprives the affected joint of the normal protective reactions when exposed to forces of weight bearing and motion. Although any neuropathic process which impairs sensory innervation may underlie neuropathic joint disease, syphilitic tabes dorsalis, in spite of its declining frequency, and diabetic neuropathy are the most common associated conditions. Syringomyelia, myelomeningocele, and congenital indifference to pain are less frequent neurologic bases for neuropathic arthropathy. The distribution of joints affected correlates with the pattern of neuropathy. In tabes dorsalis, the knees, hips, ankles, and vertebrae are frequently involved. In diabetic neuropathy, destructive changes are limited to the distal lower extremities, and in syringomyelia the shoulder and elbow joints are most commonly affected.

Although pain is generally present, discomfort tends to be disproportionately mild relative to signs of joint destruction. Clinical, pathologic, and roentgenographic features of chronic neuropathic joint disease reflect severe degrees of destruction and disorganization of affected joints. In the early cases, the differentiation from other causes of joint derangement depends upon the demonstration of sensory neuropathy.

Management includes immobilization of affected joints and restriction of weight-bearing activities with crutches, splints, and braces. Surgical arthrodesis, although frequently unsuccessful, is indicated in select subjects. Depending on the anatomic pattern and extent of involvement, the application of prosthetic devices after amputation may improve function.

HEMARTHROSIS

Recurrent or chronic hemarthrosis is the most common manifestation of a group of heritable disorders of blood coagulation (see Ch. 796 to 798). Hemarthrosis can be a complication of anticoagulant therapy or trauma in an otherwise normal subject.

In hemophilia, joint bleeding usually begins before the age of five and tends to recur repeatedly during childhood in response to minor injury. The most commonly affected joints are the knees, elbows, and ankles, but any articulation may be involved.

Acute hemarthrosis usually results in marked local inflammatory signs and symptoms which recede within a few days. Approximately half the patients with hemophilia develop chronic deformities in one or more joints. Some of them suffer a chronic progressive synovitis, restricted to one or a few joints, which clinically and roentgenographically resembles rheumatoid arthritis. There may be marked synovial membrane hyperplasia, destruction of articular cartilage, and erosions of subchondral bone. This chronic progressive pattern probably results from a low level of continuous or intermittent bleeding into affected joints. Joint fluid, in the chronic cases, usually contains blood and very high levels of leukocyte-derived proteases. Other musculoskeletal manifestations of hemophilia result from bleeding into muscle and bone. The resolution of large hematomas may cause formation of chronic cysts.

The first principle in management is to prevent trauma, a goal not easily achieved in children. Acute hemarthrosis should be managed by immobilization, analgesic therapy, and the administration of plasma products which contain the appropriate coagulation factor. In the choice of analgesics, it is probably wise to exclude salicylates and other drugs which alter platelet function. If there is marked distention of the joint bursae, aspiration can be accomplished after the defect in coagulation has been corrected. When pain and acute inflammation have subsided, an exercise program directed at restoration of motion should be instituted. For the patient with chronic deforming joint disease, the availability of potent plasma products has permitted application of certain surgical procedures such as synovectomy and arthroplasty.

SCHÖNLEIN-HENOCH PURPURA

Nondeforming polyarthritis, most frequently affecting knees and ankles, is a common manifestation of this syndrome, other features being nonthrombocytopenic purpura, abdominal pain, and glomerulonephritis. The syndrome is rare in adults.

MULTICENTRIC RETICULOHISTIOCYTOSIS
(Lipoid Dermatoarthritis)

This rare disorder usually begins in the middle decades of life and affects females three times more than males. It is characterized by the development of multiple histiocytic nodules in the skin and mucous membranes and severe polyarthritis which may simulate rheumatoid arthritis. The firm reddish-brown or yellow papular nodules are most commonly found on hands, forearms, head, neck, and chest. Mutilating joint destruction, especially in the distal interphalangeal joints, occurs in approximately half the patients with this syndrome. Diagnosis is by demonstration of histiocytes and multinucleated giant cells, containing PAS-positive material, in skin or synovium. Similar infiltrates have been observed in other organs. A few reports of apparent benefit from adrenocorticosteroid or immunosuppressive therapy are difficult to interpret because of the tendency for spontaneous remissions.

HYPERTROPHIC OSTEOARTHROPATHY

This term refers to a syndrome which includes clubbing of fingers and toes, periostitis with new osseous formation at the ends of long bones, arthritis, and signs of autonomic disorders such as flushing, blanching, and profuse sweating. The syndrome occurs with a wide variety of underlying disease states. Less commonly there are hereditary and idiopathic (pachydermoperiostosis) forms of disease. The fully expressed pattern is usually associated with intrathoracic disease: lung carcinoma, lung abscess, empyema, bronchiectasis, chronic interstitial pneumonitis, or tuberculosis. Clubbing, usually without periostitis, may be seen with cyanotic heart disease, bacterial endocarditis, biliary cirrhosis, ulcerative colitis, regional enteritis, and thyroid disease.

The distal ends of metacarpals, metatarsals, and long bones of the forearms and legs are most frequently affected. There are inflammatory changes of periosteum, synovial membranes, and periarticular structures. The periosteum is "lifted" by the deposition of new bone matrix and subsequent mineralization. Clubbing results from edema, cellular infiltration, and connective tissue proliferation of the nailbeds.

The production of a humoral substance that mediates increased vascularity and/or connective tissue proliferation has long been suspected as the pathogenic factor in hypertrophic osteoarthropathy, but no such factor has been convincingly demonstrated. Evidence that neural factors are involved derives from observations of striking resolution of signs and symptoms after denervation of the hilum or vagotomy on the same side as the thoracic lesion. Regression of osteoarthropathy has also been observed after resection of pulmonary neoplasms.

Pain, tenderness, and enlargement of the distal portions of extremities may be accompanied by acute polyarthritis that resembles rheumatoid arthritis. The differentiation of the acute polyarthritis syndrome is aided by the recognition of clubbing and roentgenographic evidence of periostitis and intrathoracic disease.

Aside from therapy directed at the associated illness, there is no effective treatment of hypertrophic osteoarthropathy. Symptomatic benefit may be obtained from salicylates, other analgesics, or adrenocorticosteroids.

CHONDROCALCINOSIS AND PSEUDOGOUT

Chondrocalcinosis is defined as the presence of calcium-containing salts in cartilaginous structures of one or more joints. These salts include calcium pyrophosphate, calcium hydroxyapatite, and calcium orthophosphate. The term pseudogout refers to the acute and/or chronic synovitis associated with the appearance of calcium pyrophosphate dihydrate crystals in joint fluid.

There is a tendency to chondrocalcinosis in patients with hyperparathyroidism, alcaptonuria, hemochromatosis, Wilson's disease, and acromegaly, and perhaps with gout as well. There appears to be a significant association of diabetes mellitus with pseudogout, and a familial pattern of chondrocalcinosis has been described. Pseudogout, like true gout, appears to be an expression of crystal-induced synovitis.

The incidence of chondrocalcinosis increases with age. Several clinical patterns have been recognized. The most common is of a progressive arthritis of large joints, especially the knee and hip. This is usually indistinguishable from degenerative joint disease, although superimposed acute inflammatory episodes are common. The intermittent acute pattern of synovitis, which resembles gout, is less common. In a small percentage of patients there is a sustained progressive synovitis that resembles rheumatoid arthritis. Since many patients with calcification of articular cartilage manifest no rheumatic signs or symptoms, the terms chondrocalcinosis and pseudogout are not synonymous.

Attacks of *pseudogout* are usually monarticular; less commonly two or more joints may be involved simultaneously. The knee is the most frequently affected joint.

The diagnosis rests on roentgenographic criteria, but proof requires the demonstration of calcium pyrophosphate dihydrate crystals under polarized light microscopy. These crystals usually have rod or rhomboid shapes and show weak positive birefringence.

Roentgenographic evidence of calcification of articular fibrocartilage may be found in many structures, including menisci, intervertebral discs, and symphysis pubis. Since punctate and linear radiodensities may be more evident in asymptomatic joints, suspicion of pseudogout should direct a survey of more than the affected articulation.

The metabolic basis for crystal deposition in chondrocalcinosis is not known. There are speculations regarding inhibition or deficiency of pyrophosphatases in cartilage, synovial tissue, or joint fluid.

Aspiration of an acutely swollen joint is often sufficient therapy in itself. If inflammatory signs are marked, aspiration may be followed by intra-articular adrenocorticosteroid therapy or the oral administration of phenylbutazone.

SYNOVIAL TUMORS

Pigmented villonodular synovitis is the most commonly applied term for a syndrome characterized by villous or nodular growths affecting synovial linings of joints, bursae, or tendons, and a characteristic histopathological picture, i.e., presence of inflammatory granulomas containing hemosiderin and cholesterol crystals and multinucleated giant cells. There is dispute as to whether this condition should be classified as a form of synovitis or as a true neoplasm. Joint involvement is usually monarticular. The knee is most frequently affected, less commonly the hip, elbow, ankle, or foot. Synovial fluid is usually hemorrhagic or xanthochromic. The inflammatory mass frequently invades cartilage, subchondral bone, and periarticular structures. Pigmented villonodular synovitis may affect extra-articular bursae and tendon sheaths or may occur as a localized tumor in only part of a joint. The treatment of choice is synovectomy. Recurrence is uncommon.

Synovial chondromatosis is an uncommon disorder characterized by the presence of multiple foci of cartilage metaplasia in synovial membranes. Bits of metaplastic growths frequently detach and grow as loose bodies in the joint cavity and ultimately become ossified. In the latter state, this condition is referred to as synovial osteochondromatosis. The knee is most commonly affected; the disease is rarely polyarticular. Symptoms include pain, swelling, limitation in motion, and intermittent locking of the affected joint. The treatment is surgical synovectomy.

A variety of benign tumors (lipoma, chondroma, hemangioma, and xanthoma) may affect joints.

Primary malignant tumors are rare. Synovioma is a highly malignant fibroblastic sarcoma which probably originates in periarticular structures. This usually occurs in late childhood or early adult years. The recommended therapy is wide excision (frequently requiring amputation), regional lymph node dissection, and irradiation. With the most aggressive management the five-year "cure" rate is usually less than 50 per cent. Synovial chondrosarcoma is a rare neoplasm that may simulate synovial chondromatosis. Radical excision or amputation is the treatment of choice.

Barrow, M. V., and Holubar, K.: Multicentric reticulohistiocytosis. Medicine, 48:287, 1969.

Eichenholz, S. M.: Charcot Joints. Springfield, Ill., Charles C Thomas, 1966.

Howell, D. S.: Hypertrophic osteoarthropathy. *In* Hollander, J. L., and McCarty, D. J., Jr. (eds.): Arthritis and Allied Conditions. 8th ed. Philadelphia, Lea & Febiger, 1972.

McCarty, D. J., Kohn, N. N., and Fares, J. S.: The significance of calcium phosphate crystals in synovial fluid of arthritic patients: The pseudogout syndrome: Clinical aspect. Ann. Intern. Med., 56:711, 1962.

Moskowitz, R. W., and Katz, D.: Chondrocalcinosis and chondrocalsynovitis (pseudogout syndrome): Analysis of 24 cases. Am. J. Med., 43:322, 1967.

98.   DEGENERATIVE JOINT DISEASE
(Osteoarthritis)

Early degeneration of articular cartilage probably begins in all subjects by the end of the second decade of life. In the pathologic sense, degenerative joint disease is a "normal" response to aging. If the incidence of degenerative joint disease is estimated by minimal roentgenographic criteria, approximately 90 per cent of the population by the age 40 is affected. Although only a small proportion of those with abnormal roentgenograms are symptomatic, degenerative joint disease is the most common cause of chronic disability.

Degenerative joint disease is sometimes classified as primary and secondary. The latter denotes the acceleration or augmentation of wear by abnormal stresses associated with injuries, obesity, and mechanical joint disturbances. Primary degenerative joint disease, in which there is no abnormal wear or forces, is probably influenced by one or more biochemical abnormalities that impair cartilage metabolism.

Pathology. The earliest lesions of degenerative joint disease are microscopic alterations of articular cartilage. These include diminution of metachromatic material, decreased numbers of chondrocytes, fatty degeneration, alteration of collagen fibrils, and surface irregularities. Later morphologic changes include localized softening of the cartilage with surface flaking and fibrillations. Abrasion of fibrillated cartilage results in progressive loss of cartilaginous surfacing and exposure of subchondral bone.

Subsequent to ulcerations of cartilage, new bone formation occurs at the margin of articular cartilage. These marginal osteophytes are represented in roentgenograms as the characteristic "spurs." Other osseous changes include cysts of varying size beneath the joint surface and remodeling of subchondral bone.

Changes in synovial membranes, including fibrosis, hypertrophy, and occasionally synovitis, appear to be secondary to events affecting articular cartilage. Rarely the pathologic features of inflammation mimic those of rheumatoid arthritis.

Etiology and Pathogenesis. Accepting the likely premise that primary changes in articular cartilage underlie the development of degenerative joint disease, etiologic considerations may relate to the reparative processes of cartilage. In response to injury, the metabolic activity of chondrocytes increases, but their capacity to replicate and form new matrix is limited. Secondary degenerative joint disease occurs when the forces of wear and tear exceed the restricted capacity for repair. When degenerative joint disease develops (frequently in familial patterns) in the absence of abnormal stresses, it is presumed that accelerated degeneration results from one or more biochemical abnormalities affecting cartilage metabolism. Chemical studies of degenerative cartilage have revealed several abnormalities: decreased water and chondromucoprotein contents and alterations in the profile of glycosaminoglycans. Some of these changes could be mediated by the action of lysosomal hydrolases, but the nature of the presumed biochemical defect in degenerative cartilage remains unknown.

Conditions which alter mechanical properties of joints or which affect the osseous support of articular cartilage are numerous. They include obesity, trauma, hypermobility of joints, neuropathy, acromegaly, Paget's disease of bone, hyperparathyroidism, and alterations of articular or periarticular structures by inflammatory joint disease.

Clinical Patterns of Degenerative Joint Disease. Pain is the dominant symptom of degenerative joint disease but, as noted earlier, disease which is roentgenographically moderate to severe may be asymptomatic. Pain is aggravated by joint motion or weight bearing. Transient stiffness after periods of inactivity is common. Loss of articular cartilage and osseous hypertrophy result in bony enlargement and malalignment of joints and crepitation on motion. Mild tenderness to palpation and effusions are common, but other inflammatory signs are usually absent.

Figure 4. Hand deformities of degenerative joint disease. *A,* Bony enlargement of distal interphalangeal joints (Heberden's nodes) and similar change in one proximal interphalangeal joint (Bouchard's node). *B,* Symmetrical degenerative changes in proximal interphalangeal joints (Bouchard's nodes), a pattern that is frequently mistaken for rheumatoid arthritis.

The present discussion of clinical manifestations of degenerative joint disease is developed largely on anatomic lines, since signs and symptoms reflect regional patterns of involvement.

The Hand. *Heberden's nodes* are bony protuberances at the dorsal margins of distal interphalangeal joints. Early Heberden's nodes have a soft cystic consistency and may be associated with prominent inflammatory signs. The chronic stage of Heberden's nodes, characterized by bony enlargement and angular deformities (Fig. 4A), is usually minimally symptomatic. Heredity and sex are prominently involved in the development of Heberden's nodes. They are much more common in women. On the basis of family studies, it has been postulated that a single autosomal gene is involved which is dominant in females and recessive in males.

Patients with Heberden's nodes frequently show degenerative changes in other joints of the hands. The misinterpretation of proximal interphalangeal joint involvement (Bouchard's nodes) as rheumatoid arthritis is a common error (Fig. 4B). Metacarpophalangeal joint involvement is rare. Pain on the radial side of the wrist caused by degenerative disease in the first carpometacarpal joint is a frequent manifestation.

Coxarthrosis (Malum Coxae Senilis). Symptoms of *primary degenerative hip disease* usually appear in the later decades of life, but in as many as half the cases there is evidence of antecedent hip disease such as congenital dysplasia, slipped capital femoral epiphysis, or Legg-Calvé-Perthes disease. In addition, a variety of acquired disorders such as rheumatoid arthritis and avascular necrosis of the femoral head may lead to degenerative hip disease. Groin pain on motion or weight bearing is the dominant symptom, and this is often referred to the medial aspect of the thigh or knee. Over a period of months to a few years, the majority of patients become seriously disabled because of pain and restricted motion.

Degenerative Disease of the Knee. Involvement of the knees is the most common source of major disability in degenerative joint disease. Although mild synovitis and effusion may be present, joint enlargement primarily reflects bone proliferation. Crepitation on motion is a consistent finding. Degenerative changes are usually more prominent in the medial compartment of the knee, leading to varus deformity.

An early manifestation of degenerative change in the patellofemoral joint is termed *chondromalacia patellae.* This syndrome of knee pain and mild effusion, usually associated with trauma, is seen predominantly in young adults.

Vertebral Degenerative Joint Disease, Including Herniated Disc Syndromes. Two sets of articulations are present at all levels of the spinal column: the intervertebral discs and the posterior zygapophyseal joints. In addition to these, the cervical spine (between C2 and C7) has articulations between the lateral aspects of adjacent vertebral bodies, usually referred to as *joints of Luschka.* Degenerative changes in joints of Luschka are the most common cause of pain in the cervical area. In lumbar levels degeneration and herniation of the nucleus pulposus of intervertebral discs are usually the bases for symptoms.

CERVICAL SPINE. The close proximity of cervical nerve roots to the joints of Luschka makes them vulnerable to irritation or compression from any derangement in or about the joints. Since the greatest amount of stress in the cervical spine occurs at C4-C5 and C5-C6 levels, degenerative changes in the intervertebral discs and joints of Luschka are most common there. Osteophytic spurs at the margins of joints of Luschka may impinge upon nerve roots as they leave the intervertebral foramina. The pattern of pain and neurologic findings varies according to the level involved: pain is frequently in the supraclavicular and upper trapezius regions but can be referred into the occiput and more distal upper extremity. Discomfort is aggravated by motion of the neck, particularly rotation and lateral bending.

If there is degeneration of the intervertebral discs in the cervical spine, the joints of Luschka provide a barrier against lateral herniation of the nucleus pulposus. The protrusion and subsequent osteophytic reaction may therefore encroach directly on the spinal cord rather than nerve roots. The progression of the resulting cervical myelopathy may be insidious and painless.

LUMBAR SPINE. Symptoms of degenerative disease of the lumbar spine are nearly always attributable to involvement of intervertebral discs. Protrusion or extrusion of degenerated discs is directed posteriolaterally, impinging upon nerve roots or the cauda equina. Although any of the lumbar discs can herniate, this most commonly occurs at L4-L5 and L5-S1. Patients with herniated lumbar discs frequently have a history of mild or recurrent backache prior to development of more acute discomfort. Pain radiates distally into one or the other lower extremity and is aggravated by spinal movement, particularly bending to the side of the pain. There is usually marked paravertebral tenderness and aggravation of pain by straight leg raising. Loss or suppression of the ankle jerk and sensory deficit in the lateral border and sole of the foot and toes suggest L5-S1 root compression. No reflex change, sensory deficit in the lateral leg and mediodorsal aspect of the foot, and weakness of the toe extensors suggest L4-L5 root compression.

Primary Generalized Hypertrophic Osteoarthritis. This is more a concept than a disease: it describes a polyarticular pattern associated with somewhat more inflammatory reaction than is customary with degenerative joint disease. There is usually involvement of the hands, including Heberden's and Bouchard's nodes, along with changes in the first carpometacarpal joints. Women in the middle years of life are most commonly affected, and a familial pattern is prominent. A closely related syndrome of degenerative joint disease has been termed *erosive osteoarthritis.*

Laboratory Findings. There are no specific laboratory abnormalities of degenerative joint disease. The erythrocyte sedimentation rate is usually normal. Synovial fluid is clear and exhibits high viscosity and normal mucin clot test. Leukocyte counts in synovial fluid vary in the range of 200 to 2000 per cubic millimeter. Fragments of cartilage are frequently identified in the fluid.

Roentgenographic Features. Osteophyte formation at the margins of affected joints is the basis for the most striking roentgenographic feature of degenerative joint disease, but earlier and more common findings, resulting from destruction of articular cartilage, are narrowing of the interosseous joint space and subchondral bone sclerosis. Radiolucent cysts, varying in size from a few millimeters to several centimeters, may be seen in periarticular bone.

Degeneration of cervical and lumbar discs results in interspace narrowing. Exostoses at the margins of vertebral bodies may coalesce with adjacent osteophytes, causing fusion at one or more levels. Roentgenographic documentation of intervertebral herniation requires contrast myelography. Disc degeneration is best observed by anteroposterior and lateral roentgenograms. For visualization of osteophytes encroaching on foramina, especially important in the cervical spine, oblique projections are required.

Differential Diagnosis. In their typical expressions, degenerative joint disease and rheumatoid arthritis are easily distinguished. The latter is usually associated with evidence of systemic disease, prominent signs of joint inflammation, and the characteristic symmetrical pattern of disease affecting the hands and wrists. When a patient presents with signs of mild inflammation in one or two weight-bearing joints of the lower extremities, the differentiation between these two syndromes is more difficult. In that setting a normal erythrocyte sedimentation rate, negative rheumatoid factor test, and minimal abnormalities in synovial fluid support the diagnosis of degenerative joint disease. No test singly or in combination can be viewed as diagnostic; even the roentgenographic demonstration of marginal osteophytes may be a secondary change in rheumatoid arthritis. In the most experienced hands, there is a small percentage of patients in whom the diagnosis remains indeterminate.

A common diagnostic error is the interpretation of degenerative changes in proximal interphalangeal joints of the hands as evidence of rheumatoid arthritis (Fig. 4B). The deformities that characterize Heberden's and Bouchard's nodes may be marked, but this pattern of degenerative joint disease is not associated with prominent signs of inflammation, and the metacarpophalangeal joints and wrist joints are rarely if ever affected.

Important aspects of differential diagnosis involve the recognition of syndromes in which secondary development of degenerative joint disease may occur. These include hemochromatosis, neuropathy, chondrocalcinosis, alcaptonuria, hypermobility of joints (including the Ehlers-Danlos syndrome), mechanical derangements of joints, and a variety of metabolic disorders that affect the support of articular cartilage by subchondral bone.

There should never be confusion in the differentiation of degenerative joint disease of the vertebral column from ankylosing spondylitis. Patients with the latter are almost invariably young men, and the roentgenographic features are distinct from those associated with degenerative joint disease.

Treatment. The management of degenerative joint disease is highly varied, depending upon anatomic patterns and the degree of joint deformity. An optimistic forecast is appropriate for most individuals. Patients should understand that disability can be minimized even though there is no specific remedy. The common statement that "nothing can be done for your kind of arthritis" is a false cliché.

Drugs. No medication has been shown to retard the development or progression of degenerative joint disease. The requirement for analgesic drugs is varied; many patients have so little pain that they require no medicinal therapy. Aspirin in moderate dosage (0.6 gram three to five times a day) is usually helpful for the patient with pain. Sustained salicylate therapy is superior to intermittent or erratic dosage. A common problem in degenerative joint disease, regardless of anatomic location, is the occurrence of intermittent episodes of increased pain which tend to subside spontaneously. For these recurrent episodes, phenylbutazone (100 to 300 mg daily) or indomethacin (75 to 150 mg daily) may be beneficial. Continuous use of drugs other than salicylates is rarely indicated in degenerative joint disease. Some patients with disabling hip pain, however, experience sufficient relief of symptoms with phenylbutazone or indomethacin to warrant maintenance therapy. It is common practice to prescribe muscle relaxants, such as diazepam or carisoprodol, for pain and muscle spasm of vertebral disease, but objective assessment of their efficacy is lacking.

Physical Measures. There are two general goals in the design of a physical medicine program for degenerative joint disease: minimizing the forces of work and weight bearing that apply to affected joints, and maintenance of normal joint alignment and motion. The patient with hip or knee disease should be instructed to avoid unnecessary walking or stair climbing. This recommendation is not inconsistent with the performance of an exercise program (in nonweight-bearing attitude) which can maintain muscle power and joint motion. Quadriceps isometric exercise for degenerative joint disease of the knees is particularly important. There is a powerful rationale for weight reduction for the obese patient with involvement of the spine or lower extremities. The use of a cane or a crutch can reduce forces of weight bearing applied to a symptomatic hip or knee by as much as 50 per cent. In selected patients with an unstable knee, fitting of a brace may be beneficial.

Certain physical measures are selectively relevant to degenerative joint disease of the spine. Patients need to learn to live with the altered mechanics of their spine. With cervical involvement, hyperextension and hyperflexion should be avoided. The patient should sleep supine with no more than one pillow. Most, but not all, patients with cervical radicular pain will be helped by intermittent traction. If this is beneficial, there are inexpensive devices for applying intermittent cervical traction at home. When symptoms are acute, wearing a cervical collar will restrict movement and minimize pain.

The patient with symptomatic degenerative disease of the lumbar spine should sleep on a hard mattress and avoid bending and lifting activities. A program of graded postural exercises is important when pain has subsided. External support provided by a lumbosacral corset will frequently minimize mild chronic symptoms. When lumbar disc herniation results in severe pain or nerve deficit, hospitalization is usually indicated. The majority of such patients will experience a remission of symptoms within a two- to three-week period. Consideration of surgical therapy is appropriate for those patients who fail to respond to conservative management.

Surgical Management. The main anatomic areas affected by degenerative joint disease that are amenable to orthopedic surgical therapy are the hip, the knee, and the vertebral column. Several surgical procedures are appropriate for the patient with debilitating hip pain. These include arthrodesis (if the disease is unilateral), mold arthroplasty, osteotomy, and total joint replacement. In most centers, the last is the preferred procedure. Operative procedures for the knee with degenerative joint disease include debridement, osteotomy, and a variety of prosthetic arthroplasties. If there is reasonable preservation of motion and stability of the malaligned knee, tibial or femoral osteotomy is frequently beneficial. When there is a serious disability attributable to malalignment and instability of the knee, one or another prosthetic procedure may be indicated. However, the successes, to date, of knee joint replacement have not been as predictable as have comparable procedures for the hip.

Virtually all orthopedic surgeons agree that surgical procedures for degenerative disease of the spine are appropriate *only* after there has been a systematic and sustained trial of conservative management. If radicular pain is relentless or if there are increasing neurologic deficits from nerve root involvement or myelopathy, surgical correction is warranted.

Armstrong, J. R.: Lumbar disc lesions. 3rd ed. Baltimore, Williams & Wilkins Company, 1965.

Friedenberg, Z. B., and Miller, W. T.: Degenerative disc disease of the cervical spine. J. Bone Joint Surg., 45A:1171, 1963.

Kellgren, J. H., Lawrence, J. S., and Bier, F.: Genetic factors in generalized osteo-arthritis. Ann. Rheum. Dis., 22:237, 1969.

Mankin, H. J.: Biochemical and metabolic aspects of osteoarthritis. Orthop. Clin. North Am., 2:19, 1971.

Sokoloff, L.: The Biology of Degenerative Joint Disease. Chicago, University of Chicago Press, 1969.

99. THE PAINFUL SHOULDER

Because shoulder pain is frequent and due to diverse mechanisms, this subject deserves special attention. Of prime importance is recognition that pain in the shoulder may be referred from disease affecting cervical, intrathoracic, and diaphragmatic areas. Shoulder motion is affected by the action of muscles through a "joint complex" consisting of independent articulations—glenohumeral, acromioclavicular, and sternoclavicular, as well as the scapulothoracic surface relationship. In addition, shoulder function requires movement of gliding surfaces of periarticular structures—the musculotendinous cuff, the subdeltoid bursa, and the long head of the biceps. Any of the syndromes associated with synovitis may be responsible for shoulder pain. The primary concern in this chapter is a group of painful disorders which affect the periarticular soft tissues of the shoulder.

CALCIFIC TENDINITIS AND BURSITIS

The most common cause of shoulder pain results from degeneration of the supraspinatus and infraspinatus tendons. Approximately 3 per cent of people in their middle years have calcific deposits in these rotator tendons. Although the majority of such subjects have few or no symptoms, a significant percentage develop pain because of inflammation of the parietal surface of the overlying subdeltoid bursa. An inflammatory exudate containing calcareous matter may rupture into this bursa. The symptoms may be acute, subacute, or chronic. The acute syndrome is characterized by sudden onset of pain in the shoulder area, often with radiation into the neck and proximal arm. Any motion of the shoulder girdle elicits pain. There is frequently exquisite local tenderness over the anterior and anterolateral aspect of the shoulder joint. Night pain is a prominent feature. Roentgenographic studies usually demonstrate linear calcific deposits in the involved tendon or a more diffuse calcific

pattern in the subdeltoid bursa. In most instances acute symptoms abate after a few days, but in a minority subacute discomfort persists for weeks.

The treatment is influenced by the severity and duration of symptoms. Anti-inflammatory agents, such as phenylbutazone or indomethacin, and analgesics are usually sufficient to control acute symptoms. In most patients there is a spontaneous remission of pain and a disappearance of calcific deposits. When the symptoms are very acute, aspiration of calcified material and injection of adrenocorticosteroid preparation may give prompt relief. The prospects of more chronic disability can be minimized by the institution of an active exercise program as soon as the level of discomfort permits. If the patient is not making progress toward regaining normal shoulder motion with a home exercise program, supervised therapy in a physical medicine department is important. A small percentage of patients with refractory pain and persistent roentgenographic findings may require surgical exploration for removal of calcific deposits.

BICIPITAL TENDINITIS

The long head of the biceps originates from the superior surface of the glenoid. It emerges from the glenohumeral bursa to lie in the bicipital groove of the humerus where it is covered by a synovial sheath. The shoulder pain of bicipital tendinitis frequently radiates along the biceps to the forearm, and is aggravated by abduction and internal rotation. Tenderness over the bicipital groove and accentuation of pain with resisted supination of the forearm, with the elbow flexed at 90 degrees, aid in the recognition of bicipital tendinitis. The management is similar to that described for calcific tendinitis: local injection of adrenocorticosteroid preparations, systemic anti-inflammatory agents, and an exercise program. In refractory cases, surgical exploration with tendon transfer usually yields good results.

ROTATOR CUFF TEARS

The same degenerative changes that underlie the development of shoulder tendinitis can weaken the musculotendinous rotator cuff and predispose it to rupture. In most patients with this problem, there is acute onset of shoulder pain after trauma or performance of strenuous work. If the tear is complete, the patient is unable to abduct the arm, but it can be held in abduction, once elevated to 90 degrees, by the action of the deltoid muscle. With incomplete tears, the patient has only mild pain and moderate weakness. The diagnosis of rotator cuff tears can best be established by contrast arthrography. With complete rupture of the supraspinatus tendon, surgical repair is usually warranted. In patients with partial tears, partial immobilization followed by an exercise program is appropriate.

THE SHOULDER-HAND SYNDROME
(Reflex Neurovascular Dystrophy)

This is a poorly understood disorder characterized by pain and stiffness in the shoulder, together with pain, swelling, and vasomotor phenomena in the hand. Involvement of the distal upper extremity is frequently followed by dystrophic change that resembles *Sudeck's atrophy*. The syndrome is presumed to result from reflex sympathetic stimulation analogous to that proposed for causalgia. It principally affects patients above the age of 50 and is often associated with acute illness such as myocardial infarction, trauma to the distal upper extremity, cerebrovascular accident, or pulmonary disease. The significance of associated degenerative change in the cervical spine is uncertain, because of its high frequency in the population at risk. When the disease is bilateral (approximately 25 per cent of cases), the differentiation from acute rheumatoid arthritis may be difficult. There is marked variability in intensity and duration of acute symptoms and extent of dystrophic change. In a small percentage of patients the end result is "frozen shoulder" and dystrophic changes in the hands that resemble those of systemic sclerosis.

There is probably no condition for which aggressive physical therapy is more important than for the shoulder-hand syndrome. An active exercise program, facilitated by analgesic medication, should be instituted as soon as possible. When refractory pain impedes progress in the physical medicine program, a trial of systemic corticosteroid therapy (10 to 20 mg per day of prednisone or equivalent) or stellate ganglion block is warranted.

FROZEN SHOULDER

A minority of patients with any of the shoulder conditions discussed above develop chronic restriction of motion of the glenohumeral joint. When there is no apparent relationship of frozen shoulder to other shoulder disease, such as tendinitis or rotator cuff injury, the condition is sometimes termed *adhesive capsulitis*. This condition may be clinically indistinct from the shoulder-hand syndrome. Pain is generally less severe and less well localized relative to other conditions causing shoulder pain. The most important aspect of management of frozen shoulder is prevention. Early attention to the underlying cause of shoulder pain and the institution of an effective exercise program is nearly always successful in combating the progression of shoulder immobility. Management of the chronic frozen shoulder is much more difficult. Manipulation under general anesthesia followed by intensive physical therapy may be indicated when patients are not helped by conservative management.

DePalma, A. F., and Kruper, J. S.: Long-term study of shoulder joints afflicted with and treated for calcific tendinitis. Clin. Orthop., 20:61, 1961.
Steinbrocker, O.: The painful shoulder. *In* Hollander, J. L., and McCarty, D. J., Jr. (eds.): Arthritis and Allied Conditions. 8th ed. Philadelphia, Lea & Febiger, 1972.

100. NONARTICULAR RHEUMATISM

This term designates a group of painful disorders resulting from involvement of tendons, bursae, and other periarticular structures. Conditions causing shoulder pain are considered separately in Ch. 99.

BURSITIS

Bursae are closed synovial sacs located at sites of friction between skin, ligaments, tendons, muscles, and bones. Trauma is the most common cause of bursitis, but almost any illness characterized by joint synovitis may be associated with involvement of the lining of bursae. Bursae commonly involved include the following: subdeltoid, trochanteric, olecranon, and prepatellar. Septic or gouty bursitis can be documented by appropriate studies of aspirated fluid. Protection of an inflamed bursa from friction and trauma is the most important aspect of treatment, but moderate doses of salicylates, phenylbutazone, or indomethacin may be helpful. Local injection with an adrenocorticosteroid preparation is indicated if symptoms are severe or refractory to other treatments.

TENOSYNOVITIS

Tendon sheaths, like bursae, have synovial linings and can be involved by any process capable of inducing joint synovitis. Tenosynovitis in the hand or foot is a frequent manifestation of gonococcemia. Calcific tendinitis, a common source of shoulder pain, (see Ch. 99) may be associated with marked inflammatory signs resembling acute gout. Focal thickening of the tendon sheath and adjacent tendon can result in "locking or triggering" phenomena. This problem, termed stenosing tenovaginitis, is common in the flexor tendons of the fingers. Involvement of the abductor pollicis longus and extensor pollicis brevis tendons of the thumb *(de Quervain's syndrome)* results in pain and tenderness at the radial aspect of the wrist. There are no generalizations regarding management, since tenosynovitis may be a manifestation of various disease states, including rheumatoid arthritis and other connective tissue syndromes, infection, gout, and hypercholesterolemia. The common form of tenosynovitis, unassociated with systemic disease, will often subside with rest. If symptoms are severe or recurrent, local injections of adrenocorticosteroid preparations are usually effective. Surgical excision of the affected tendon sheath is indicated for those patients with persistent disability.

TENNIS ELBOW
(Epicondylitis)

This common condition is characterized by pain over the lateral aspect of the elbow. Tenderness is localized in the area of the common extensor insertion in the region of the lateral epicondyle. The problem, most common in middle-aged males, is related to sports or occupations that involve repetitive wrist extension or pronation–supination. Pain is accentuated by resisted wrist extension. If symptoms fail to respond to rest, injection of local adrenocorticosteroid preparations is usually successful. For the rare patient with persistent disability, surgical therapy may be needed.

CARPAL TUNNEL SYNDROME

This problem results from entrapment of the median nerve as it passes deep to the transverse carpal ligament of the wrist. Inflammation of the adjacent flexor tendon sheaths, the most common basis for median nerve entrapment, may be a feature of rheumatoid arthritis; but in most patients the tenosynovitis is localized and unassociated with systemic disease. The majority of patients are middle-aged women. The most consistent symptoms are dysesthesia, paresthesia, and hypesthesia in the middle three digits of the hand. Referred pain in the more proximal upper extremity is common. Symptoms are usually intermittent, occurring most frequently during the night. Forced flexion of the wrist or nerve compression locally may induce the characteristic symptoms. In a minority of patients, there is progressive wasting of the muscles of the thenar eminence. Conservative management consists of fitting a removable dorsal splint to hold the wrist in slight extension and the local injection of an adrenocorticosteroid preparation. Surgical release of the transverse carpal ligament is indicated for patients with persistent disability.

TIETZE'S SYNDROME

This mysterious benign disorder is characterized by painful enlargement of the upper costal cartilages. It is usually unilateral and limited to a single costochondral juncture. Occasionally the manubriosternal and sternoclavicular joints are affected. The disease may be recurrent, but remission is the rule. Some patients are concerned that they have cardiac disease; reassurance alone may be sufficient management. If discomfort is severe or recurrent, analgesics, heat, or local infiltration (adrenocorticosteroid or local anesthetic agents) may be beneficial.

FIBROSITIS

This term has been applied to a poorly defined symptom complex which is characterized by pain and stiffness in varying areas, most commonly in the neck, shoulder girdle, and posterior aspect of the trunk. Physical signs except for questionable nodules or thickening of the deep fasciae are lacking, and laboratory and roentgenographic studies are negative. The term fibrositis is based on vague hypothesis and common usage rather than on anatomic abnormalities. Localized areas of tenderness, commonly in the paravertebral areas medial to the scapula, have been termed "trigger points." The syndrome usually begins in the middle years of life. Because the majority of patients appear tense and anxious and have no recognizable objective basis for symptoms, the syndrome is often considered psychogenic. Since pain and stiffness can be manifestations of a variety of musculoskeletal, neurologic, and systemic disorders, the diagnosis of fibrositis requires the exclusion of more defined illnesses. The patient and his physician tend to share an unhappy experience in efforts to control symptoms. The results of strong reassurance, that serious disease is lacking, are variable, as are the results of therapy with salicylates, sedatives, tranquilizers, and muscle relaxants. Temporary relief is occasionally achieved by injection of local anesthetic into tender points or by chilling the overlying skin with ethyl chloride.

Levey, G. S., and Calabro, J. J.: Tietze's syndrome: Report of two cases and review of the literature. Arthritis Rheum., 5:261, 1962.

Phalen, G. S.: The carpal tunnel syndrome: Seventeen years' experience in diagnosis and treatment of 654 hands. J. Bone Joint Surg., 48A:211, 1966.

Swannell, A. J., Underwood, F. A., and Dixon, A. St. J.: Periarticular calcific deposits mimicking acute arthritis. Ann. Rheum. Dis., 29:380, 1970.

Part VII
GRANULOMATOUS DISEASES OF UNPROVED ETIOLOGY

101. INTRODUCTION

Paul B. Beeson

The chapters to follow include a variety of rather uncommon and difficult-to-classify syndromes. These are characterized by long and fluctuating clinical courses, and the affected tissues show the picture of chronic inflammation, usually with formation of granulomas. Sarcoidosis is the most common and best known. The others are comparatively rare, and their natures and classifications are subject to controversy. For the purpose of textbook exposition the best recognized clinical forms have been described as separate diseases. It should be noted, however, that there are shades of similarity and that each of these is thought by some students to be merely a variant expression of one of the other processes, e.g., Wegener's granulomatosis and lethal midline granuloma. Some of these syndromes could well have been discussed with the diseases of connective tissue, as in fact they used to be in former editions. In the present state of knowledge — ignorance is more accurate — the editors have elected to place the descriptions of these syndromes under a heading with a noncommittal title.

102. SARCOIDOSIS

D. Geraint James

Definition. Sarcoidosis is a multisystemic granulomatous disorder of unknown cause most commonly affecting persons in the middle period of life. It is characterized by widespread epithelioid cell granulomas, depression of delayed-type hypersensitivity, and lymphoproliferation. The Kveim-Siltzbach skin test is frequently positive, and there may be abnormal calcium metabolism.

The diagnosis is most securely established when consistent clinicoradiographic findings are supported by histologic evidence of granulomas with minimal necrosis. The course and prognosis are related to abruptness of clinical onset; an acute onset usually heralds a self-limiting course and spontaneous resolution, whereas an insidious onset is often followed by unrelenting progression.

Etiology, Immunology, and Pathogenesis. Since the cause remains unknown, theories abound. Any hypothesis should endeavor to explain certain cardinal immunologic upsets, so it is currently fashionable to try to intertwine possible causal agents with these immunologic abnormalities and produce a working hypothesis of the pathogenesis. It should be remembered that any such theory, however attractive, remains but a tentative

bridgehead for a final assault on the still unknown cause. We still do not know whether sarcoidosis is one disease resulting from one cause or a collection of similar reactions to multiple causes. At present most authorities favor the unitarian concept of a single disorder rather than a multicausal syndrome. There are, of course, numerous causes of granulomatous disorders, including infections, chemicals, neoplasms, inhaled allergens, immunologic deficiency states, and at least one inherited enzyme defect (chronic granulomatous disease of childhood). When all these have been excluded, there remains a hard core which we term multisystemic sarcoidosis. It presents in all parts of the world with a similar clinical, radiographic, histologic, chemical, and immunologic pattern, and responds predictably and in similar fashion to treatment. It is this condition which we believe to be one disease resulting from one cause.

Causal Agents. Claims of an infective agent have included human and anonymous mycobacteria, the leprosy bacillus, fungi, viruses, and protozoa. Many organisms provoke a nonspecific granulomatous reaction, but this should not be misconstrued as multisystemic sarcoidosis. Epstein-Barr virus antibody titers of 1:640 and over are significantly more frequent in sarcoidosis than in control subjects. This again should not be misconstrued as evidence of yet another etiologic agent but rather as a reflection of widespread lymphoproliferation, for there may also be raised antibody titers to herpes simplex, rubella, measles, and parainfluenza viruses.

Beryllium and zirconium are known to produce sarcoid granulomas in individuals sensitized to these elements, but other tested elements in the periodic table do not seem to be granulomagenic.

Other agents for which etiologic claims have been made include pine pollen, peanut dust, and clay eating in various parts of the world.

Immunology. The cardinal immunologic upsets in sarcoidosis are threefold: (1) thymus-mediated lymphocyte (T cell) misbehavior, as indicated by depression of delayed-type hypersensitivity; (2) vigorous lymphoproliferation with considerable bursa-dependent (B) mononuclear cell activity; and (3) granuloma formation in all organ systems.

T CELL BEHAVIOR. Depression of delayed-type hypersensitivity is revealed by cutaneous anergy using tuberculin or many other antigens such as dinitrochlorobenzene, and also in vitro by various tests of lymphocyte function. There is a good correlation between in vivo and in vitro anergy in sarcoidosis. Sarcoid lymphocytes show a diminished response to phytohemagglutinin (PHA). When patients recover from sarcoidosis, tuberculin sensitivity returns to what it was before the onset of sarcoidosis. If the T cells were sensitized to tuberculin prior to sarcoidosis, they lose their ability to react with tuberculin during the acute disease but sometimes return to normal with cure. The more obvious the depression of delayed-type hypersensitivity during the acute phase of the disease, the more likely it is to remain depressed. This generalization also applies to in vitro PHA-stimulated lymphoblastic transformation, which may remain below par for many years.

VIGOROUS LYMPHOPROLIFERATION. Whereas there is cutaneous anergy and impaired cellular immunity, the very reverse holds for humoral antibodies, serum immunoglobulins, and other circulating factors in sarcoidosis. At the same time as T cell eclipse, there is vigorous lymphoproliferation, with increased immunoglobulin formation. Simultaneously, there may be significantly increased circulating antibodies to the Epstein-Barr virus, herpes simplex, rubella, measles, and parainfluenza viruses, and an increased antibody response to mismatched blood. The precise immunologic impact which causes this galaxy of high-titer serologic antibodies and profuse immunoglobulins is obscure.

GRANULOMA FORMATION. Granulomas develop in all organ systems at the time of T cell eclipse and lymphoproliferation, possibly reflecting a reaction to circulating immune complexes.

Hypothesis of Pathogenesis. An antigenic insult, whether by one of the aforementioned infective or chemical agents or even by vegetable matter, is met by a reticuloendothelial response in which both thymus-derived (T) cells and plasma (B) cells participate. The T cells are transformed, possibly by undergoing antigenic alteration on their cell surface, and become depleted. Depletion may be due not only to T cell transformation but also to T cell interaction with transformed T cells. Depletion results in depression of delayed-type hypersensitivity, which is recognized by cutaneous anergy and by in vitro lymphocyte transformation tests. At the same time there is vigorous lymphoproliferation, and the B cell response is reflected by an increase in circulating immunoglobulins. During this same phase, transformed T cell circulating immune complexes are probably responsible for such clinical phenomena as erythema nodosum and uveitis. The antigenic insult may be airborne, for bilateral hilar lymphadenopathy is such a frequent mode of onset. The more acute the onset and the more active the reticuloendothelial response, the more likely there will be spontaneous remission with full restoration of T cell function. If this does not occur spontaneously, then it may be induced by corticosteroids, which restore normal T cell function.

The antigen responsible for lymphoproliferation, T cell transformation, and granuloma formation almost certainly resides in Kveim-Siltzbach antigen, possibly linked to and altered by transformed T cells into an immune complex.

Pathology. A granulomatous reaction is the wasteland laid bare by the engagements between indigestible antigen and macrophages, thymus-mediated lymphocytes, and humoral antibodies. Phagocytic cells aggregate into epithelioid and giant cells, which are the hallmarks of a sarcoid granuloma. *Epithelioid cells* are large mononuclear cells about 20 μ in diameter with round or oval nuclei showing a loose chromatin pattern with prominent nucleoli; when stained with hematoxylin and eosin, the cytoplasm is pale, granular, and often vacuolated. *Giant cells* are up to 300 μ in diameter, containing as many as 30 nuclei, usually arranged peripherally. Within these epithelioid and giant cells may be found three types of inclusion bodies—Schaumann, asteroid, and residual bodies—all of which are nonspecific (Fig. 1).

Schaumann bodies are concentrically laminated, deeply basophilic conchoidal bodies, 100 μ in diameter, often with brilliant birefringent crystals. They are made up of calcium carbonate, phosphate, and iron. *Asteroid bodies* are star-shaped lipoproteins, 1 to 5 μ in diameter, with a central core and with radiating, slightly curved spines. They occur in only 2 per cent of patients with sarcoidosis. *Residual bodies* are cytoplasmic lipomucoprotein granules, 1 μ in diameter, and are end-products of activated lysosomes. All three inclusion bodies in turn have been confused with tubercle bacilli and other organisms and parasites.

The granuloma may also contain sparse, inconspicuous plasma cells and a fringe of lymphocytes. Necrosis is minimal in the sarcoid granuloma, and the reticulin fiber framework remains intact in this sparse necrosis. As the lesion ages, reticulin fibers ramify between the epithelioid cells which thicken and become converted into collagen. It loses its outline and becomes a solid amorphous eosinophilic mass of hyaline material.

Williams and his colleagues have shown, by enzyme histochemistry, that the epithelioid cells are identical in the granulomas of sarcoidosis, Kveim-Siltzbach test biopsies, regional ileitis, tuberculosis, swimming-pool granuloma, and chronic beryllium disease; all show strong biosynthetic and phagocytic enzyme activity. The epithelioid cells of all these granulomas are metabolically active in synthesizing nucleic acid and attempting to digest extracellular material. Also within this granuloma are the immunoglobulins IgG, IgA, IgM, and IgD,

Figure 1. Features of a granuloma.

LYMPHOCYTE (T)

EPITHELIOID CELL 20 μ

GIANT CELL 300 μ

SCHAUMANN BODY 100 μ

ASTEROID BODY 5 μ

RESIDUAL BODY 1 μ

PLASMA CELL (B)

which can be identified in variable amounts by immuno-fluorescence.

Epidemiology. Sarcoidosis has a worldwide distribution but is more frequently recognized in sophisticated communities. Mass radiography figures show an over-all prevalence of 20 per 100,000 population in Great Britain, rising to a figure of 120 in Irishmen and 200 per 100,000 in Irishwomen examined in London. In the United States, it is ten times more prevalent in blacks than in whites, regardless of birthplace or residence. The black African appears not yet affected to a significant degree, but this may be due to obscuring tuberculosis or to lessened awareness, or both. It is certainly being recognized more frequently in less sophisticated areas, suggesting that the detection of asymptomatic cases depends on advanced screening techniques.

Irishwomen in London and Puerto Ricans in New York are prone to develop erythema nodosum. Likewise, there is an increased prevalence of sarcoidosis in Martinican subjects living in Paris and in West Indians in Britain. Hormonal factors may play some part, for erythema nodosum caused by sarcoidosis is more common in women of the childbearing years of life, during early pregnancy, and also in women taking oral contraceptives.

Familial sarcoidosis has been reported sufficiently often in various parts of the world to give rise to the suggestion that it is due to a recessive mode of inheritance which finds partial expression in affected homozygotes. Various relationships include brother-sister and mother-son, but father-offspring is exceedingly rare.

Clinical Manifestations. The numerous masquerades of sarcoidosis (Table 1) are reminiscent of syphilis in the days before penicillin. It was always important to remain alert to the possibility of syphilis; otherwise it was occasionally overlooked. The same may now be said for sarcoidosis. Many cases of sarcoidosis remain undetected; instead they are merely termed idiopathic pulmonary fibrosis, hilar adenopathy, iridocyclitis, erythema nodosum, or nephrocalcinosis. Sarcoidosis should always be considered when a middle-aged patient attends several different outpatient clinics, particularly respiratory, ophthalmic, and dermatologic clinics. It is sometimes postulated that the manifestations of sarcoidosis differ in various parts of the world. There are certainly minor differences, but the major patterns of disease which emerge from a comparison of sarcoidosis in London, New York, and Paris are surprisingly similar. This is a retrospective survey of patients attending sarcoidosis clinics at the Mount Sinai Hospital, New York City (Dr. Louis Siltzbach), at the Hôpital Bichat, Paris (Professor J. Turiaf), and ours at the Royal Northern Hospital, London (Tables 2 and 3). From these series, certain generalizations emerge as helpful guidelines. Sarcoidosis has an equal sex distribution, being observed in 302 women (56 per cent) of the Royal Northern Hospital series of 537 patients. It is most prevalent in those under age 40, for 358 of the 537 (67 per cent) presented in this age group, compared with one third over 40. It may be detected for the first time in a routine chest x-ray or because troublesome respiratory symptoms lead to a chest film. It may also present as erythema nodosum or other skin lesions, iridocyclitis, peripheral lymphadenopathy, salivary gland enlargement, or nervous system involvement. Asymptomatic or silent sarcoidosis, detected by routine chest x-ray, is so common that sarcoidosis may be regarded as an iceberg syndrome in which the un-

TABLE 1. Modes of Presentation of Sarcoidosis

Chest Physician	Dermatologist	Ophthalmologist
Breathlessness	Erythema nodosum	Iridocyclitis
Bilateral hilar	Lupus pernio	Keratoconjunctivitis
lymphadenopathy	Plaques, scars,	sicca
Pulmonary fibrosis	keloids	Sjögren's syndrome
Cor pulmonale	Maculopapular erup-	Choroidoretinitis
	tions	Glaucoma, cataract

Neurologist	Gastroenterologist	Cardiologist
Cranial nerve palsy	Hepatic granulomas	Cardiac arrhythmias
Myopathy, neuropathy	Splenomegaly	Bundle branch block
Space-occupying	Similarity to Crohn's	Cardiomyopathy
lesions	disease	Complete heart
Meningitis		block

General Physician	Rheumatologist	Urologist
Acute rheumatism	Polyarthralgia	Hypercalciuria
Lymphadenopathy	Bone cysts	Renal calculi
Parotid enlargement	Dactylitis	Nephrocalcinosis
Peripheral		Uremia
lymphadenopathy		

diagnosed silent subclinical variant is far more frequent than is realized.

Physical Examination. General examination of the patient must be thorough (Fig. 2). It is incomplete unless accompanied by a chest radiograph, slit-lamp examination of the eyes, and estimation of the 24-hour urinary calcium. Multisystem involvement is a characteristic feature of sarcoidosis, with intrathoracic involvement in nine tenths of patients, ocular and skin involvement each occurring in about one quarter, and, depending on the series and country, erythema nodosum in up to one third of patients. Involvement of other tissues includes peripheral lymphadenopathy in 29 per cent, the spleen in 12 per cent, neurosarcoidosis in 7 per cent, and salivary gland enlargement or bone cysts in about 6 per cent of patients (Table 3).

Intrathoracic Sarcoidosis. It is convenient to refer to three abnormal chest x-ray appearances:

STAGE 1. Bilateral hilar lymphadenopathy is the earliest and most frequent change, comprising about one half of chest radiographic abnormalities. The right paratracheal chain of lymph nodes is frequently enlarged in this early stage of sarcoidosis and is radiographically visible in at least 25 per cent; hence the popularity of right scalene node biopsy and mediastinoscopy at this stage. Hilar adenopathy is the hallmark of acute early reversible sarcoidosis, and it may be associated with erythema nodosum and acute iritis.

STAGE 2. In one quarter of patients, the chest radiograph shows both bilateral hilar lymphadenopathy and parenchymal mottling of the lungs. The mottling takes the form of localized or disseminated fine miliary or occasionally coarse miliary nodulation, or a fluffy cotton-wool appearance, sometimes with margins sharply circumscribed. Miliary infiltration is a subacute transient stage, usually resolving and certainly changing during one year of observation.

STAGE 3. In one of seven patients, the chest radiograph discloses that the disease has already reached a late stage of diffuse pulmonary mottling on presentation, persisting as coarse or fine reticulation intermixed with nodular densities 1 to 5 mm in diameter. In some in-

TABLE 2. Features of Sarcoidosis Patients in New York, London, and Paris

Features		Mount Sinai Hospital, New York		Royal Northern Hospital, London		Hôpital Bichat, Paris	
		No.	%	No.	%	No.	%
Total		311	100	537	100	329	100
Sex	Women	211	68	302	56	146	45
Race	White	111	36	474	86	277	84
	Negro	146	47	2	<1	3	1
	Caribbean	54	17	33	6	39	12
	Other	–	–	28	5	10	3
Age at presentation (years)	Under 40	221	71	358	67	238	72
	Over 40	90	29	179	33	91	28
Onset	Routine chest x-ray	124	40	119	22	156	47.5
	Respiratory symptoms	59	19	49	9	53	16
	Erythema nodosum	33	11	150	28	22	7
	Other skin lesions	20	6	37	7	14	4
	Ocular symptoms	22	7	53	10	29	8.5
Presenting chest x-ray stage	0	26	8	85	16	20	6
	1	133	43	243	45	123	37.5
	2	108	35	129	24	162	49
	3	44	14	80	15	24	7.5
Skin tests	Positive Kveim-Siltzbach	285	92	384	82	187/243	77
	Negative tuberculin	191	63	246	55	266/329	81
Blood tests	Hyperglobulinemia	158	61	85	34	48/212	22.5
	Hypercalcemia	33	14	57	24	17/249	7
Treatment	Corticosteroids	103	33	185	34	224	68.5
	No steroids	208	67	352	66	89	27
Mortality	Due to sarcoidosis	17	5	25	5	6	1.8
	Due to other causes	9	3	8	1.5	7	2

stances confluence of the mottled areas is noted, pulmonary fibrosis is irreversible, and upward retraction of the lung roots has developed. Bulla formation, gradual enlargement of the right ventricle, and pulmonary hypertension are serious prognostic signs.

Extrathoracic Sarcoidosis. Ocular lesions occur in about one quarter of patients. They include acute and chronic iridocyclitis and choroidoretinitis, papilledema, keratoconjunctivitis, conjunctival follicles, and the late complications of cataract and secondary glaucoma. There are certain well-defined ocular syndromes. Acute iritis, erythema nodosum, and bilateral hilar lymphadenopathy have a benign self-limiting course, whereas chronic iridocyclitis with associated lupus pernio or skin plaques, bone cysts, and pulmonary fibrosis are persistent and troublesome. Keratoconjunctivitis sicca with or without parotid and lacrimal gland enlargement mimics Sjögren's syndrome. Parotid gland enlargement, anterior uveitis, and facial nerve palsy are features of Heerfordt's syndrome.

Skin lesions, other than erythema nodosum, are noted in one quarter of patients. They include lupus pernio, plaques, scars, keloids, and transient maculopapular eruptions.

Erythema nodosum is associated with bilateral hilar lymphadenopathy and polyarthralgia. It occurs predomi-

TABLE 3. Frequency of Involvement of Various Tissues in Sarcoidosis in New York, London, and Paris

Organs Involved	Mount Sinai Hospital, New York (311)		Royal Northern Hospital, London (537)		Hôpital Bichat, Paris (329)	
	No.	%	No.	%	No.	%
Intrathoracic	285	92	452	84	300	90
Hilar nodes	241	77	372	70	227	70
Lung parenchyma	152	49	209	40	186	56.5
Peripheral lymph nodes	116	37	153	29	75	23
Eyes	62	20	147	27	37	11
Skin	59	19	135	25	39	12
Erythema nodosum	33	11	167	31	22	6.5
Spleen	57	18	62	12	20	6
Bone cysts	13/139	9	19/475	4	6/165	3.5
Salivary glands	25	8	33	6	21	6
Nervous system	13	4	38	7	14	4

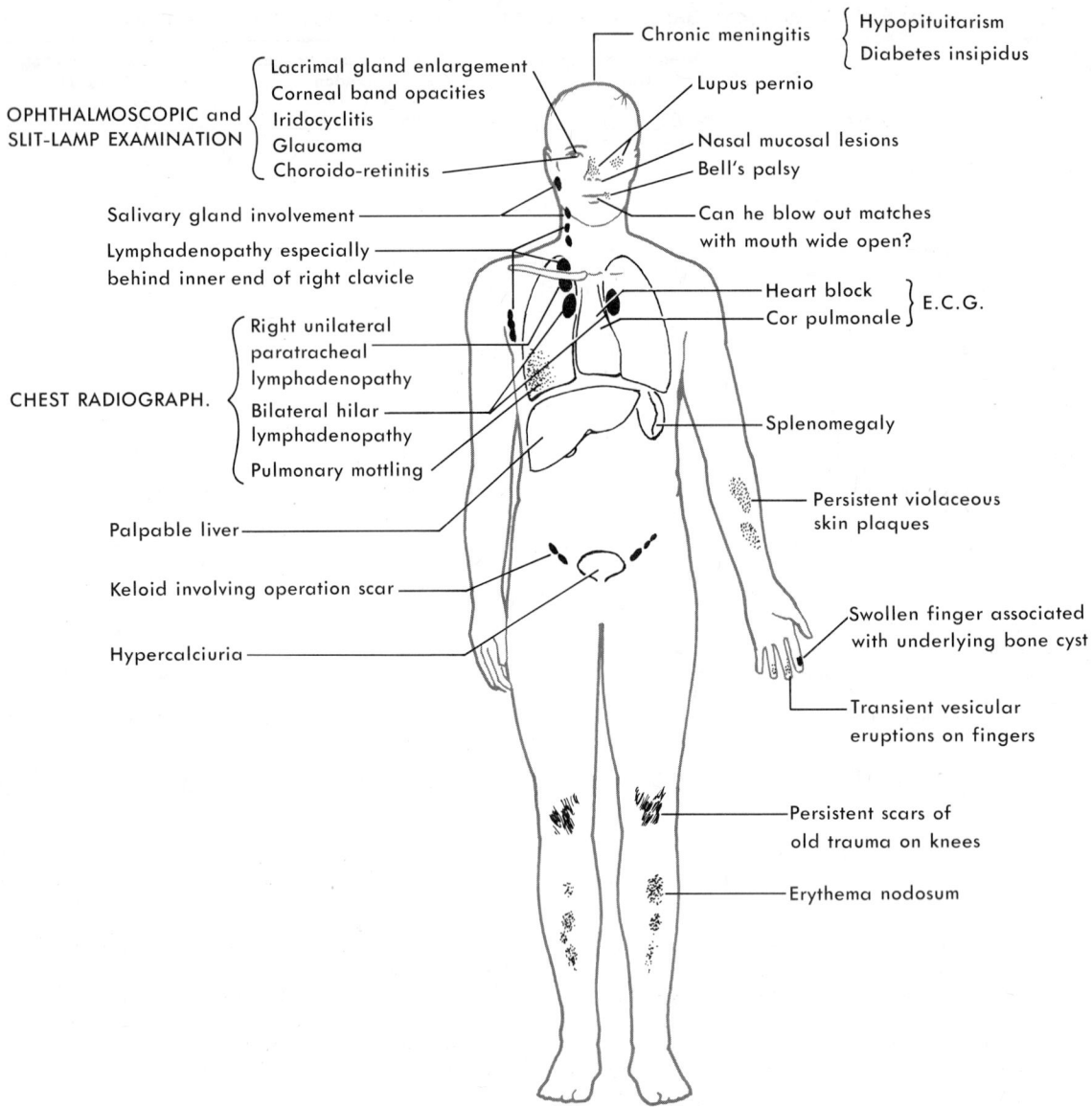

Figure 2.   Clinical examination of a patient with suspected sarcoidosis.

nantly in women of childbearing age, often associated with pregnancy or lactation; such patients should be reassured that it is a benign syndrome which will not affect the fetus or leave complications.

Reticuloendothelial system involvement occurs in 215 of 537 patients (40 per cent), comprising peripheral lymphadenopathy in 153 (28 per cent) and splenomegaly in 62 (12 per cent). Splenic enlargement is usually silent, but rarely it may cause hypersplenism or lead to presinusoidal portal hypertension.

Neurosarcoidosis is far less common, occurring in 38 of 537 patients (7 per cent). Facial palsy is a frequent neurologic presentation either alone or with other cranial palsies or with papilledema. Other presentations include peripheral neuritis, myopathy, meningitis, and space-occupying brain lesions.

Bone cysts occur in about 6 per cent of patients; they are most commonly seen in conjunction with chronic skin lesions, so the dermatologist is far more likely than

the chest physician to detect them. Bone cysts reflect chronic persistent irreversible sarcoidosis in all systems.

Myocardial sarcoidosis is difficult to recognize clinically. It should be considered if a patient with florid multisystem sarcoidosis develops heart block, bundle branch block, arrhythmias, congestive heart failure, or clinical evidence of cardiomyopathy. Sudden death without previous evidence of a heart lesion may occur in sarcoidosis.

Endocrine involvement in sarcoidosis. The pituitary is more frequently involved than any other endocrine gland, the diagnosis being suggested by the development of polydipsia and polyuria in sarcoidosis without evidence of renal disease. Since 1909, about 60 cases of diabetes insipidus caused by sarcoidosis have been reported. Histologic proof is necessary to distinguish this syndrome from histiocytosis X, in which diffuse infiltration of the lungs coincides with diabetes insipidus. Apart from diabetes insipidus, deficiency of one or more anterior pituitary hormones may occur, comprising gonadotropin, thyroid-stimulating hormone, and adrenocorticotropic hormone in that order of frequency. Hypothalmic involvement may be associated with galactorrhea and raised serum prolactin levels. Adrenal, thyroid, or pancreatic involvement by sarcoidosis is extremely rare.

Special Clinical Situations. Pregnancy. Sarcoidosis is not a contraindication to pregnancy. In fact, patients improve and are able to abandon steroid therapy from the second trimester onward. Chest radiography is unnecessary until after delivery; thereafter it should be performed, because relapse, if it does occur, is more likely during the six months after parturition. The only precaution is to check the serum calcium level, as it is liable to rise with excessive vitamin D intake during pregnancy.

CHILDHOOD. Sarcoidosis is rarely a pediatric problem. In the Royal Northern Hospital series, it was observed in one child under ten years of age and occurred in only 25 of 537 patients (5 per cent) under 20 years of age. When multisystemic granulomas are observed in young children, sarcoidosis should not be considered until the several other causes of granulomatous disorders are excluded, particularly helminth infestation, mycobacterial infection, and chronic granulomatous disease of childhood.

Unusual Features. Fever is not a feature of sarcoidosis, except under certain circumstances. It is commonly associated with erythema nodosum, uveoparotitis (Heerfordt's syndrome), acute meningitis, hypersplenism, and secondary infection complicating end-stage pulmonary fibrosis and nephrocalcinosis. If there is persistent fever in the absence of these features, it is important to consider such alternatives as Hodgkin's disease or Wegener's granulomatosis.

Ulceration, even when a biopsy of the ulcer reveals sarcoid tissue, is not a feature of sarcoidosis, and it is sufficient to raise alternative diagnostic possibilities. A granulomatous nasal or laryngeal ulcer raises the possibility of Wegener's granulomatosis; a leg ulcer in a child might be due to swimming-pool granuloma and an ulcer in the neck due to cat scratch disease.

It should be remembered that all that glitters is not sarcoidosis.

Diagnosis. *Kveim-Siltzbach Test.* Kveim-Siltzbach antigen is a saline suspension of human sarcoid tissue prepared from the spleen of a patient suffering from active sarcoidosis. The antigen, 0.15 ml, is injected intradermally very superficially into the flexor surface of the forearm, and the inoculation site is observed for the development of a visible and palpable nodule during the ensuing six weeks. Any palpable nodule is examined by biopsy, usually one month after the injection, using a Hayes-Martin drill. This core of tissue is serially sectioned for evidence of sarcoid tissue or of a foreign body giant-cell reaction; this decision is made blind, i.e., without knowledge of the clinical picture. A Kveim-Siltzbach test is reported as positive if the intradermally injected antigen produces a nodule in the course of three to six weeks and if this nodule shows evidence of sarcoid tissue, as distinct from a foreign body giant-cell reaction. A parallel may be drawn between it and the beryllium patch test in beryllium disease, the zirconium skin reaction in patients with zirconium deodorant granulomas, and the lepromin reaction in leprosy. All tests are individually specific for their own disease states. That these are delayed hypersensitivity phenomena is suggested by

the fact that they occur only in patients who have been in contact with, say, beryllium or zirconium; they are not positive before contact; a positive result can be obtained, using extremely high dilutions of the element; and the reaction is specific.

Several factors influence the Kveim-Siltzbach reaction, which must still be regarded as a crude but most useful biologic test. Potent antigen is essential, and this means that it must be obtained from the spleen of a patient with active sarcoidosis. Another important factor is the histologist's interpretation of the biopsy material, for an inexperienced observer could confuse sarcoid tissue with a nonspecific foreign body giant-cell reaction, particularly if doubly refractile crystals are not sought by polarized light. Finally, the Kveim-Siltzbach test is suppressed by oral corticosteroids, just as any sarcoid tissue is suppressed by these agents. An occasional false-positive result is inevitable with a biologic test of this kind, but a figure of less than 2 per cent is acceptable. The Kveim-Siltzbach test is positive in three quarters of patients with sarcoidosis. It is particularly helpful when histologic confirmation is otherwise lacking or equivocal. It is useful in the differential diagnosis of diffuse pulmonary mottling, uveitis, or erythema nodosum; and it is also worth performing in obscure cases of subacute meningitis or cranial nerve palsies. It is negative in patients with nonspecific local sarcoid-tissue reactions and in all other granulomatous disorders.

It is unfortunate that there is no standardized commercial supply of Kveim-Siltzbach antigen. Various institutes prepare their own antigens from sarcoid spleen or lymph nodes, and it is then necessary to carry out skin tests with these antigens in sarcoidosis and other subjects to assess their specificity. Poor nonspecific antigens are discarded, but a potent specific supply will last for years. Undoubtedly the world's best antigens have been, and continue to be, prepared by Dr. Louis Siltzbach at the Mount Sinai Hospital, New York City. We have a satisfactory one at the Royal Northern Hospital, London, as does Professor J. Turiaf at the Hôpital Bichat, Paris. Dr. Andrew Douglas has recently prepared a promising new specific antigen in Edinburgh, and Dr. Behrend's antigen in Hanover, Germany, is effective and specific. Instead of endeavoring to meet the world's needs, what we are all trying to do is discover the specific granuloma-provoking principle and therefrom produce a standardized synthetic and accurately reproducible agent.

KMIF Test. Efforts are being made to develop in vitro Kveim-Siltzbach tests by investigating the response of peripheral lymphocytes from patients with sarcoidosis and controls to stimulation by Kveim-Siltzbach antigen, using guinea pig macrophages as the indicator cells. The technique is termed the Kveim-induced macrophage inhibition factor (KMIF) test. Sarcoid lymphocytes when stimulated in vitro with sarcoid material produce a macrophage inhibition factor with a migration index of less than 0.8 in three quarters of subjects (positive KMIF test). There is a good correlation with the cutaneous Kveim-Siltzbach test. Also resembling the skin test is the effect of steroid therapy which makes the KMIF test negative.

Tuberculin Reaction. The tuberculin reaction is negative in all conventional strengths in about 60 per cent of patients with sarcoidosis. Those exhibiting some degree of tuberculin hypersensitivity have only weakly positive reactions. Insensitivity to tuberculin and to other antigens such as dinitrochlorobenzene is only relative, and the insensitivity does not appear to be as profound as it is in malignant lymphomatous diseases.

Biochemical Findings. ABNORMAL CALCIUM METABOLISM. Hypercalcemia and hypercalciuria may be short-lived and self-limiting, or they may progress to nephrocalcinosis with excretion of renal calculi and eventual uremia. Hypercalcemia occurred in 10 (13 per cent) and hypercalciuria in 37 (49 per cent) in our series of 75 patients with sarcoidosis in whom simultaneous serum and 24-hour urine calcium levels were determined. Thus hypercalciuria is much more common than hypercalcemia and is the more sensitive index of abnormal calcium metabolism. Fortunately it is usually transient and self-limiting.

HYDROXYPROLINURIA. Hydroxyproline excretion is considerably increased in acute sarcoidosis, returning to normal as the chest x-ray abnormality resolves, whereas excretion is normal in chronic sarcoidosis.

ALKALINE PHOSPHATASE. Elevation of the alkaline phosphatase level is due to hepatic involvement by space-occupying miliary granulomas and not because of bone cysts.

Lung Function Studies. The two most useful practical tests are the single-breath diffusing capacity and the vital capacity. Impairment of the diffusing capacity can be observed even at the early stage of bilateral hilar lymphadenopathy when the lung fields are radiographically clear. The deficit may become more marked because of the natural fall in diffusing capacity with increasing age, and also because of reduction in lung volume and impaired perfusion of ventilated lung. Reduction of vital capacity is also observed with advancing disease.

Immunoglobulins. Serum IgG is elevated in one half, IgA in one quarter, and IgM in one eighth of patients. There is a relative deficiency of IgD associated with the rise in IgM. There is no clear-cut association between clinical patterns of disease and the abnormal immunoglobulin, and certainly none of diagnostic value.

Other Factors. Serum complement activity is increased, haptoglobin is decreased, and cryoglobulins have been identified in serum in erythema nodosum. Serum autoantibodies, including thyroid, gastric, mitochrondrial, and antinuclear factor, are similar in incidence to those found in the normal population.

Monocytes from sarcoidosis patients show an increase in rosette erythrophagocytosis, compared with controls for both IgG and C3 complement receptors, indicating an increase in monocyte phagocytic capacity and membrane receptor function. These observations should help to explain circulating immune complexes in this disease.

Anemia and Eosinophilia. These are not characteristic features of sarcoidosis. When a patient is found to have biopsy evidence of a granuloma and this is associated with anemia and/or eosinophilia, it is necessary to consider disorders other than sarcoidosis in the first instance. If noted in a child, helminthic infestations, such as Toxocara infection, should be considered. If these are the findings in a young male adult, granulomatous Hodgkin's disease should be ruled out before considering sarcoidosis.

Sedimentation Rate. This test is of limited value in the management of sarcoidosis. It is grossly elevated when there is associated erythema nodosum, and its elevation may also reflect raised, abnormal serum immunoglobulin levels. Finally, it is raised when there is

TABLE 4. Differences Between the Multisystemic Disorder Sarcoidosis and a Nonspecific Local Sarcoid Tissue Reaction

	Sarcoidosis	Sarcoid Reaction
Number of systems involved	Several	Usually one
Age group	20–50 years	Any
Chest radiograph	Abnormal in 84%	Normal
Slit-lamp examination of eyes	Abnormal in 25%	Normal
Tuberculin test	Negative in 66%	Variable
Kveim-Siltzbach test	Positive in 84%	Negative
Calcium metabolism	Abnormal in 20%	Normal
Response to corticosteroids	Good	Variable
Other treatments	Oxyphenbutazone, chloroquine, p-aminobenzoate	Depends on cause—anti-infective, immunosuppressive

secondary infection associated with end-stage pulmonary fibrosis or with nephrocalcinosis.

Comment. The diagnosis is most securely established when consistent clinical and radiographic findings are supported by histologic evidence of noncaseating epithelioid cell granulomas by organ biopsy in more than one system and/or a positive Kveim-Siltzbach test.

When confronted with a patient suspected of having sarcoidosis, certain steps in the management are essential. (1) Seek histologic confirmation of the clinical diagnosis as soon as possible. The patients who are troubled in later years by their disease are almost always those in whom the clinical diagnosis was not supported by histologic confirmation initially, and so treatment was delayed until it was too late to be effective. (2) Make sure that granulomas found in one system are part of the multisystemic disorder and not just a nonspecific local sarcoid tissue reaction. There are several points of differentiation (Table 4)—clinical, radiologic, and immunologic—but the simplest and most secure way of distinguishing them is by the Kveim-Siltzbach test, which is positive in sarcoidosis and negative in local sarcoid tissue reactions. (3) Judge whether the disease is acute or chronic (see Course and Prognosis).

Differential Diagnosis. It should be remembered that there are many causes of nonspecific local sarcoid tissue reactions and other unrelated granulomatous disorders. The disorders with which sarcoidosis is confused depend to some extent on the discipline and interests of the clinician concerned. The chest physician must distinguish it from tuberculosis and extrinsic allergic alveolitis; the gastroenterologist must differentiate it from Crohn's regional ileitis or primary biliary cirrhosis; and the general physician may have to distinguish it from Hodgkin's disease. The modes of presentation of sarcoidosis involve most disciplines (Table 1); it cannot be overemphasized that sarcoidosis is a multisystemic disorder, and the diagnosis should be entertained when the patient is seen to attend many different outpatient clinics, particularly respiratory, ophthalmic, and dermatologic.

Tuberculosis. It is more important to recognize tuberculosis than to overlook sarcoidosis. Now that tuberculosis is becoming less common and sarcoidosis more frequently recognized, there remains considerable confusion, particularly between tuberculin-positive sarcoidosis and tuberculin-negative tuberculosis. There are several distinguishing features (Table 5), and the

Kveim-Siltzbach test may be of crucial help. With steroid therapy the negative tuberculin skin test in sarcoidosis may become positive and the strongly positive tuberculin test in tuberculosis may wane.

Hodgkin's Disease. Disseminated Hodgkin's disease is similar to sarcoidosis from clinical, radiographic, and immunologic standpoints (Table 6), but histology is distinctive. Hodgkin's disease has a male preponderance, and the patient is usually ill with weight loss, fever, pruritus, and anemia, whereas sarcoidosis has an equal sex distribution and the patient is usually asymptomatic and well.

Intrathoracic Hodgkin's disease most frequently involves the upper mediastinum; the subcarinal and posterior mediastinal nodes are seldom involved without enlargement of the upper mediastinal nodes. The hilar nodes tend to fuse with the right cardiac border, whereas in sarcoidosis the right hilar nodes stand away from the right border of the heart.

Primary Biliary Cirrhosis (PBC). Sarcoidosis and PBC are both chronic granulomatous disorders, which may provide superficial confusion to the gastroenterologist who has found hepatic granulomas by aspiration liver biopsy or sarcoid tissue in abdominal lymph nodes at laparotomy. However, the clinical presentations and physical signs are quite different (Table 7). The two most helpful distinguishing tests are the Kveim-Siltzbach test, which is always negative in PBC, and the serum antimitochondrial antibody test, which is negative in sarcoidosis.

Crohn's Regional Ileitis. This is a chronic granulo-

TABLE 5. Differences Between Sarcoidosis and Tuberculosis

Features	Sarcoidosis	Tuberculosis
Age incidence (years)	20–50	<20 or >50
Fever	Rare	Common
Erythema nodosum	Common	Uncommon
Uveitis / Skin involvement / Enlarged parotids / Bone cysts	Common	Very rare
Ulceration and sinuses	No	Common
Involvement of: Pleura / Peritoneum / Pericardium / Meninges / Small intestine	Very rare	Common
Caseation	Minimal	Maximal
Acid-fast bacilli	Absent	Present
Tuberculin test	Negative in 55%	Positive in most
Kveim-Siltzbach test	Positive in most	Negative
Hypercalcemia	Yes	No
Hypercalciuria	Yes	No
Calcification	No	Yes
Hilar lymphadenopathy	Bilateral	Unilateral
Pulmonary cavities	Rare, late	Common, early
Ghon focus	No	Yes
Corticosteroids	Helpful	Harmful alone
Antituberculous drugs	Unhelpful	Treatment of choice

TABLE 6. Comparison Between Sarcoidosis and Hodgkin's Disease

Features	Sarcoidosis	Hodgkin's Disease
Age (years)	20 to 50	20 to 40
Sex	Equal	Males, 3:1
Weight loss	Rare	Common
Splenomegaly	Rare	Frequent
Submental lymph nodes	Infrequent	Frequent
Erythema nodosum	Common	Rare
Gut symptoms	Absent	Common
Pruritus	Absent	Common
Bone lesions	"Punched out" phalangeal cysts	Sclerotic lesions of spine and pelvis
Sclerotic lesions	No	Mixed sclerotic/osteolytic in 16%
Leukocytosis / Lymphopenia / Eosinophilia	Absent	May be present
Hilar lymphadenopathy	Bilateral	Bilateral or unilateral
Hilar gland pressure symptoms	No	Yes
Pulmonary infiltration	Common	Uncommon
Pulmonary infiltration followed by hilar adenopathy	Never	Yes
Pleural effusion	Rare	Common
Skin lesions	Distinctive histology	Specific histology with eosinophilia
Secondary infections	Rare	Common
Delayed-type hypersensitivity	Depressed	Depressed
Immunoglobulins	Abnormal	Normal
Kveim-Siltzbach test	Positive	Negative
Histology	Distinctive	Distinctive
Radiotherapy	Unhelpful	Curative
Corticosteroids	Therapy of choice	Helpful
Immunosuppressive regimens	Not indicated	Indicated
Prognosis	Good	Poor

matous disorder of the intestinal tract. In contradistinction to sarcoidosis, it is almost never multisystemic. Distinguishing features are the over-all clinical picture, radiographic changes, calcium metabolism, serum antireticulin antibodies, and Kveim-Siltzbach test (Table 8).

Extrinsic Allergic Alveolitis. There are several different inhaled antigens which provoke an antigen-antibody reaction and a granulomatous histology in the lower reaches of the bronchi. The prototype is farmer's lung; others include suberosis, bird fancier's, thatcher's, maplebark stripper's, and sequoia tree feller's asthma. The keys to the diagnosis are the occupational history, the clinical picture of asthma, the histology of a granuloma encompassing the inhaled foreign body, the presence of serum precipitins against the provoking inhaled antigen, and the negative Kveim-Siltzbach test (Table 9).

Course and Prognosis. There are two forms of sarcoi-

TABLE 7.   Features Distinguishing Sarcoidosis from Primary Biliary Cirrhosis

Features	Sarcoidosis	Primary Biliary Cirrhosis
Sex	Equal	Females, 8:1
Decade of onset	3, 4	5
Onset over 40 years	Rare	Frequent
Erythema nodosum	Yes	No
Uveitis	Yes	No
Respiratory	Yes	No
Pruritus	No	Yes, nearly always
Jaundice	No	Yes
Xanthomas	No	Yes
Clubbing	No	Yes (in 25%)
Hepatomegaly	No	Yes (in 100%)
Splenomegaly	Yes (in 12%)	Yes (in 50%)
Skin pigmentation	No	Yes (in 71%)
Steatorrhea	No	Yes
Bilateral hilar lymphadenopathy	Yes	No
Kveim-Siltzbach test	Positive in 75%	Always negative
Depression of delayed-type hypersensitivity	Yes	Yes
Circulating anti-mitochondrial antibodies	No	Yes (in 99%)
Calcium metabolism	Hypercalcemia Vitamin D sensitivity	Hypocalcemia (Steatorrhea)
Raised alkaline phosphatase	Yes, minority	Yes, majority
Raised serum cholesterol	No	Yes, majority
Liver granulomas	Yes	Yes
Corticosteroids	Helpful	Contraindicated
Vitamin D	Contraindicated	Helpful
Cholestyramine	Not necessary	Helpful
Prognosis	Very good	Poor; dead in five years

TABLE 8.   Differences Between Sarcoidosis and Crohn's Regional Ileitis

Features	Sarcoidosis	Crohn's Regional Ileitis
Histology	Granulomas	Similar
Involvement		
Intestine	Rare	Invariable
Intrathoracic	Yes in 90%	No
Skin	Yes in 25%	Mucocutaneous ulceration extending to involve genitalia
Erythema nodosum	Yes	Yes
Eyes	Yes in 25%	No
Associated ankylosing spondylitis	No	Yes
Complicating		
Malabsorption	No	Yes
Amyloidosis	No	Yes
Peritonitis	No	Yes
Hepatic granulomas	Yes	Yes
Depression of delayed-type hypersensitivity	Yes	Yes
Kveim-Siltzbach test	Positive in 75%	Negative
Abnormal calcium metabolism	Hypercalcemia and hypercalciuria	Hypocalcemia associated with malabsorption
Serum antireticulin antibodies	Negative	Positive in 25%

It is not possible, unfortunately, to define such a clear-cut natural history in other forms of sarcoidosis, except to predict that maculopapular eruptions, conjunctivitis, salivary gland enlargement, Bell's palsy, and peripheral lymphadenopathy usually regress without treatment in the course of one year. On the other hand, chronic iridocyclitis, keratoconjunctivitis sicca, lupus pernio, plaques, and keloids persist unchanged or with minor fluctuations indefinitely.

TABLE 9.   Comparison of 95 Patients with Extrinsic Allergic Alveolitis and 68 Patients with Sarcoidosis by Villar (Lisbon)

Features	Extrinsic Allergic Alveolitis	Sarcoidosis
Age	Older	Younger
Erythema nodosum	Absent	Common
Hilar adenopathy	Rare	Frequent
Multisystem	No	Yes
Depression of delayed-type hypersensitivity	Yes	Yes
Kveim-Siltzbach test	Negative	Positive
Serum precipitins	Yes	No
Histology	Granuloma encompassing foreign body	Granuloma
Prognosis	Good if removed from exposure to antigen	Good

dosis, acute and chronic, with clear-cut differences in onset, natural history, course, prognosis, and response to treatment (Table 10).

Acute sarcoidosis has an abrupt explosive onset, a high spontaneous remission rate, a predictable response to anti-inflammatory drugs, and a good prognosis. From the onset to complete resolution usually occupies less than two years.

Chronic sarcoidosis has an insidious, ill-recognized onset and progresses inexorably; treatment relieves symptoms but rarely leads to resolution of the fibrotic process, and pulmonary fibrosis, cor pulmonale, secondary cataract formation, and nephrocalcinosis are liable to supervene.

It is important to distinguish acute (transient) from chronic (persistent) sarcoidosis, because their natural history and prognosis vary as greatly as in acute and chronic nephritis or acute and chronic hepatitis.

Undoubtedly the most predictable course and the best prognosis accompany erythema nodosum. It usually subsides within a month of its onset, and accompanying hilar adenopathy will regress in the course of one year. Recurrence and sequelae are rare.

TABLE 10. Differences Between Subacute (Transient) and Chronic (Persistent) Sarcoidosis

	Subacute	Chronic
Natural history	Transient	Persistent
Age at onset	Under 30 years	Over 30 years
Onset	Abrupt	Insidious
Skin	Erythema nodosum, maculopapular rash, vesicular eruptions	Lupus pernio, plaques, scars, keloids
Eyes	Conjunctivitis, acute iritis, papilledema, hemorrhages, exudates	Keratoconjunctivitis sicca, chronic uveitis, cataract, glaucoma
Lungs	Hilar adenopathy	Pulmonary mottling
Bone cysts Parotitis Lymphadenopathy Splenomegaly Bell's palsy	Usually transient	Rarely permanent
Histology	Epithelioid and giant cells	Hyaline fibrosis
Calcium metabolism	Hypercalcemia, hypercalciuria	Nephrocalcinosis
Kveim-Siltzbach test	Positive	May be negative
Hydroxyproline excretion	Increased	Normal
Spontaneous remission	Frequent	Rare
Steroid therapy	Abortive effect	Symptomatic relief
Alternative treatments	Oxyphenbutazone	Chloroquine, para-aminobenzoate, phosphate
Recurrence after steroid therapy	Rare	Frequent
Low calcium diet	Unnecessary	May be necessary
Prognosis	Good	Poor

Skin and pulmonary lesions follow a very similar course and likewise parallel each other's response to treatment. Transient skin lesions are usually associated with hilar adenopathy, whereas chronic skin lesions are more likely to be accompanied by pulmonary fibrosis. The former tend to clear without treatment, and the latter fail to do so despite prolonged therapy. Resolution of all types of pulmonary sarcoidosis may be expected in two thirds of patients. It is less likely to be achieved in older patients and in those in whom there is accompanying extrathoracic disease — particularly in bone or skin. The combination of pulmonary and cutaneous sarcoidosis constitutes the hallmark of chronicity, presumably because longstanding fibrosis has supervened. Clearing of the abnormal chest x-ray occurs in only one third of patients with bone cysts, in only one fifth with skin lesions, and in only one sixth in whom bone and skin lesions accompany pulmonary sarcoidosis. The other significant factor influencing the course is treatment by corticosteroids, chloroquine, or oxyphenbutazone (see Treatment).

Complications. Sarcoidosis would remain a relatively benign and unimportant disease but for the development of certain devastating complications, namely, irreversible fibrosis in the lungs and eyes and abnormal calcium metabolism affecting the kidneys. In assessing the prognosis, it is important to assess the degree of functional failure of lungs, heart, eyes, and kidneys. In the practical management of sarcoidosis, it is the physician's duty to diagnose the condition sufficiently early so that effective therapy may prevent these unfortunate sequelae.

The over-all mortality is 8 per cent, comprising a mortality of 5 per cent directly caused by sarcoidosis and the remaining few deaths resulting from unrelated causes. Comparative figures indicate that the patient seems to have the same chance of survival whether he lives in London, New York, or Paris (Table 2).

Two forms of sarcoidosis — acute and chronic, with clear-cut differences in onset, course, and prognosis — have been defined, because this concept is important in the practical management and treatment of the individual patient with sarcoidosis. What we do not know is whether the two forms represent different diseases. The balance of evidence favors two forms of the same disease in which the differences reflect varying interplay between the causative seed and the receptive soil. Acute sarcoidosis is probably triggered by active circulating immune complexes with the development of acute vasculitis and iritis, whereas chronic sarcoidosis is maintained at a slower pace by a fibrotic hyaline reaction on the part of the tissues involved.

Acute and chronic forms of the same disease are well exemplified by beryllium disease, nephritis, and hepatitis.

Treatment. Corticosteroids, the sheet anchor of therapy, are indicated in about one third of patients (Table 2).

Various Preparations of Corticosteroids. The profound influence of corticosteroids on clinical, radiologic, immunologic, and biochemical abnormalities is well established. The range of available preparations for oral administration or topical application is wide; a combination of oral and topical steroid therapy is often the most effective. For instance, iridocyclitis may be brought under control by prednisolone eye drops, particularly if reinforced by one subconjunctival depot injection of hydrocortisone. Likewise, triamcinolone acetonide may be injected directly into the disfiguring skin plaques with great benefit, alone or in conjunction with oral corticosteroids or chloroquine. Oral corticosteroids may contribute several unpleasant side effects, not the least being fluid retention and cushingoid facies. These undesirable sequelae may be overcome by using prednisolone-21-stearoylglycolate (Sintisone) which does not seem to be fluid retaining. When treatment is changed from other steroids to Sintisone, patients appear to lose fluid, the weight drops a little, and mooning of the face lessens. Preliminary evidence would also suggest that it is less likely to cause a rise in intraocular pressure, and thereby less likely to contribute to secondary glaucoma. The potency of one 6.65-mg tablet is approximately equivalent to that of one 5-mg tablet of prednisolone or prednisone. It is particularly indicated for patients who are fluid retainers and for those who have or are likely to develop glaucoma or patients with a family history of glaucoma. Oral steroid therapy in a dose of 30 mg daily for about six months is necessary in one third of patients with sarcoidosis. Indications for treatment are now well established.

Indications for Corticosteroid Therapy. OCULAR INVOLVEMENT. Topical corticosteroids should always be administered for iridocyclitis, in eye drops applied frequently during the day, reinforced with a corticosteroid eye ointment at night. If there is no substantial and continuing improvement during ten days, then the concentration of corticosteroid in the anterior segment of the eye may be increased by a local subconjunctival depot of cortisone. Oral corticosteroids are indicated if local treatment does not lead to a rapid response or if ophthalmoscopy reveals posterior uveitis. In addition, the inflamed iris should be rested by local atropine eye drops to maintain a dilated pupil.

ABNORMAL CHEST RADIOGRAPH WITHOUT SPONTANEOUS IMPROVEMENT IN SIX MONTHS. Bilateral hilar lymphadenopathy is likely to subside without treatment, particularly if it is associated with erythema nodosum. On the contrary, pulmonary infiltration which remains static or worsens during the course of six months is an indication for oral steroids in an effort to prevent irreversible pulmonary fibrosis.

BREATHLESSNESS. If this symptom is present, the disease has already reached a stage of irreversible pulmonary fibrosis or disturbed gas transfer. Steroid treatment provides symptomatic relief but does not influence the grave prognosis at the irreversible stage of breathlessness.

PERSISTENT HYPERCALCIURIA. Steroids will prevent excessive gastrointestinal absorption and excessive urinary excretion of calcium. Calcium metabolism usually reverts to normal within ten days.

DISFIGURING SKIN LESIONS. When lupus pernio or other unsightly lesions distress patients, oral and local corticosteroids may correct the deformity. Unfortunately, small doses of steroids must be continued indefinitely if the cosmetic improvement is to be maintained. In order to minimize the side effects of oral corticosteroids, local intralesional steroids or chloroquine, or both, are helpful alternatives.

NEUROLOGIC INVOLVEMENT. The more acute the presentation, the more likely it is to respond to systemic corticosteroids, which should be administered as soon as the diagnosis has been established. Most patients are aged 20 to 50 years. There is evidence of intrathoracic involvement in 82 per cent, ocular disease in 58 per cent, cutaneous sarcoidosis in 29 per cent, peripheral lymphadenopathy in 26 per cent, parotid enlargement in 16 per cent, and splenomegaly in 10 per cent. This multisystem involvement is a key to the diagnosis of neurosarcoidosis; it is supported by evidence of a positive Kveim-Siltzbach test in 76 per cent and a negative Mantoux status in 60 per cent of patients.

Neurosarcoidosis carries a mortality of 10 per cent, which is twice the over-all mortality of sarcoidosis. Resolution of neurosarcoidosis is more likely to occur in younger patients with an explosive onset such as meningitis. The response to treatment is better (1) with accompanying erythema nodosum than with chronic skin lesions, (2) with acute than with chronic uveitis, and (3) with hilar adenopathy than with old diffuse pulmonary infiltration.

GLANDULAR INVOLVEMENT. Glandular involvement occurs particularly if there is disordered function, e.g., dry eyes caused by lacrimal gland involvement, dry mouth caused by salivary gland enlargement, or hypersplenism resulting from sarcoidosis of the spleen. The indication for treatment is disordered function rather than anatomic enlargement of the gland in question.

MYOCARDIAL INVOLVEMENT. It is easy to include involvement of the heart in a theoretical list of indications for corticosteroid therapy, but much more difficult in practice to recognize myocardial sarcoidosis. It is, of course, suspected and treated when a patient with multisystemic sarcoidosis develops cardiac arrhythmia or bundle branch block.

Other Drugs. Treatment may be necessary when there are contraindications to corticosteroid therapy or when it has proved fruitless. Under these circumstances it is proper to consider treatment with oxyphenbutazone, chloroquine, potassium para-aminobenzoate, or immunosuppressive agents such as azathioprine.

OXYPHENBUTAZONE. In a controlled trial comparing oxyphenbutazone, prednisolone, and a placebo in the management of pulmonary sarcoidosis, both active drugs were significantly better than the placebo. Prednisolone and oxyphenbutazone were equally effective. Although one in six patients showed spontaneous regression of pulmonary sarcoidosis in six months, this trial showed that the number is increased to one in two patients by oxyphenbutazone or prednisolone. Not only does oxyphenbutazone influence the radiologic picture; like corticosteroids, it can also prevent the development of sarcoid tissue, for it may delay the evolution of sarcoid tissue in the Kveim-Siltzbach nodule. Oxyphenbutazone is of value only in acute exudative sarcoidosis and not in the chronic fibrotic form of the disease.

CHLOROQUINE. The way in which chloroquine acts is unknown, but it is helpful in the management of lupus pernio and pulmonary fibrosis. It is of no value in acute sarcoidosis.

POTABA. Potassium para-aminobenzoate is known to have an antifibrotic effect, and it is worth considering in pulmonary fibrosis and lupus pernio caused by sarcoidosis. Three-gram envules should be taken by mouth four times daily for several months. This form of treatment is an effective alternative to corticosteroids and chloroquine, and giving all three in rotation helps to overcome the undesirable long-term complications of steroids and chloroquine.

Immunosuppression. Azathioprine, chlorambucil, and methotrexate have met with mixed success, possibly because patients for such treatment have been incorrectly selected. They have usually been patients with hard-core chronic fibrotic sarcoidosis who have already resisted all other forms of treatment. Azathioprine can be used with advantage in combination with long-term steroids, allowing the dose of the latter to be reduced and thereby minimizing the adverse effects of steroids. Thus far, there have been no trials of the effect of antilymphocytic globulin or of transfer factor in sarcoidosis.

Treatment of Hypercalciuria. Hypercalciuria is swiftly brought under control by oral corticosteroids. If they are contraindicated, then sodium phytate or an oral phosphate preparation is an alternative means of preventing overabsorption of calcium. There is an effective and palatable effervescent phosphate preparation containing 500 mg elemental phosphate and also sodium cellulose phosphate which is recommended as 5-gram doses three times daily with meals. A high chapati diet may also be considered because of its phytate content. Calcitonin has not yet been assessed adequately in sarcoidosis.

Drugs Which Should Not Be Used. Patients with sarcoidosis are peculiarly sensitive to vitamin D, which causes unpleasant symptoms associated with hypercalcemia, hypercalciuria, and elevated blood urea levels. In precorticosteroid days, *calciferol* was often given in sarcoidosis. It is useless, toxic, and obsolete. Vitamin D preparations should be withheld during pregnancy.

Antituberculous drugs have no influence on the course of sarcoidosis and should not be used for the treatment of sarcoidosis. An argument could be made for prophylactic isoniazid along with corticosteroids in countries where there is considerable tuberculosis.

Tuberculin injections had a vogue, especially for sarcoid uveitis, but they are no longer indicated.

Radiotherapy is no longer used even for the lymphoproliferative forms of sarcoidosis.

James, D. G.: The Lettsomian Lectures on "The Granulomatous Disorders." Trans. Med. Soc. Lond., 88:116, 1973.
James, D. G.: Modern concepts of sarcoidosis. Chest, 64:675, 1973.
Jones Williams, W., Pioli, E., Jones, D. J., and Dighero, M.: The Kmif. (Kveim-induced macrophage migration inhibition factor) test in sarcoidosis. J. Clin. Pathol., 25:951, 1972.
Scadding, J. G.: Sarcoidosis. London, Eyre & Spottiswoode, 1967.
Siltzbach, L. E.: Sarcoidosis: Clinical features and management. Med. Clin. North Am., 51:483, 1967.
Siltzbach, L. E.: Proceedings of the Sixth International Conference on Sarcoidosis held in Tokyo, September 1972. In press.
Villar, T. G.: Proceedings of the Sixth International Conference on Sarcoidosis held in Tokyo, September 1972. In press.
Williams, D., Jones Williams, W., and Williams, J. E.: Enzyme histochemistry of epithelioid cells in sarcoidosis and sarcoid-like granulomas. J. Pathol., 97:705, 1969.

103. POLYMYALGIA RHEUMATICA AND CRANIAL ARTERITIS
(Temporal Arteritis, Giant Cell Arteritis, Polymyalgia Arteritica)

Paul B. Beeson

The two clinical syndromes of cranial arteritis and polymyalgia rheumatica are described together, because they are often associated and because of the probability that they represent different expressions of one process. The age distribution of patients is almost unique, and the diseases seem to follow similar courses. Most persons affected are more than 60 years of age; occurrence before age 50 is exceedingly rare. Although symptoms may come on quite abruptly and may cause serious incapacity for a time, the natural tendency is toward gradual improvement, with complete subsidence after a period of several months to a few years. The remarkable age incidence and self-limited course must figure prominently in any attempt to determine the nature of these disorders.

POLYMYALGIA RHEUMATICA

Polymyalgia rheumatica is a distinctive kind of muscular rheumatism in old people, more frequent in women than in men. It is characterized by pain and stiffness in the neck, shoulders, and back, and sometimes of the pelvic girdle. Tenderness and true muscle weakness are usually lacking. The stiffness may be particularly troublesome in the morning so that patients are barely able to get out of bed. There may be headache or painful areas over the cranium. Systemic manifestations aside from occasional low-grade pyrexia are not prominent. The patients have a vague sense of malaise simply described as "feeling rotten." Unfortunately these people are too often dismissed with the assumption that symptoms are caused by degenerative processes about which little or nothing can be done.

The distinctive laboratory finding is marked elevation of the erythrocyte sedimentation rate, i.e., more than 80 mm by the Westergren method. Mild anemia is not uncommon, and some hematologists are reporting cases of unexplained anemia in old people which, like the muscular symptoms, respond promptly to steroid therapy. Other laboratory tests are of little help. Muscle biopsy generally reveals no significant inflammatory change even when the tissue is taken from areas which seem to be the site of much pain and stiffness. Blood enzymes which sometimes become elevated in other disorders of muscle are normal in this disease. There may be slight elevation of the alpha 2 globulin. Electromyographic findings are normal. A possible element of autoimmunity is indicated by the observation that lymphocyte transformation occurs in the presence of muscle tissue, especially during acute phases of the symptoms. The affected muscles do not atrophy.

Because of the frequent association of polymyalgia rheumatica with cranial arteritis, and especially because cranial arteritis may cause sudden blindness, some experienced clinicians believe that biopsy of a temporal artery should be carried out in all patients with polymyalgia rheumatica. When this has been done as a routine procedure, the artery has shown the characteristic changes in more than half the cases, regardless of clinical manifestations of arteritis. Others regard this as unnecessary because a trial of steroid therapy, which would be appropriate for cranial arteritis as well as for polymyalgia, will be carried out in any event.

In the differential diagnosis rheumatoid arthritis and degenerative joint disease may present problems; however, careful questioning and examination will show that polymyalgia is a disease of muscles, not joints. Various neoplastic diseases, including multiple myeloma, have to be considered in the differential diagnosis. Similarly the collagen diseases, especially polymyositis, may resemble polymyalgia rheumatica.

Therapy with adrenal steroids is remarkably effective, usually bringing about prompt amelioration of symptoms. It should be begun with a moderately large dose, e.g., 40 to 60 mg of prednisone daily for the first week, with gradual reduction over the next few weeks to a maintenance dose of 7 to 12 mg daily for several months. Some experienced observers recommend at least two years of this low-dose therapy for all patients. There are cases on record in which the symptoms have persisted for as long as ten years. Usually, by occasional trials of reduced dosage and by following the sedimentation rate, the physician can determine when to terminate steroid therapy.

Esiri, M. M., MacLennan, I. C. M., and Hazleman, B. L.: Lymphocyte sensitivity to skeletal muscle in patients with polymyositis and other disorders. Clin. Exp. Immunol., 14:25, 1973.
Fessel, M. J., and Pearson, C. M.: Polymyalgia rheumatica and blindness. N. Engl. J. Med., 276:1403, 1967.
Hamrin, B.: Polymyalgia arteritica. Acta Med. Scand., Suppl. 533, pp. 1–131, 1972.

CRANIAL ARTERITIS

This entity, like polymyalgia rheumatica, occurs only in people past middle age. In a substantial proportion of cases, symptoms resembling those of polymyalgia rheumatica are present weeks or months before the onset of the severe headache which characterizes cranial arteritis. In contrast with polymyalgia rheumatica there is a distinctive histologic lesion in the large and medium-sized arteries of the upper part of the body, especially the temporal vessels.

Cranial arteritis often has an abrupt onset, with severe pain usually in one temple but sometimes in the occipital area, face, jaw, or side of the neck. This may be associated with exquisite hyperesthesia so that the patient dislikes touching the scalp, combing the hair or washing. The pain may have a throbbing character. Pain in the tongue, blanching of the tongue, and even gangrene of the tongue have been described in this disorder, doubtless ascribable to involvement of lingual arteries. Peripheral neuropathy with both sensory and motor components has also been described. When the temporal artery is affected it may be tender, thickened, and nodular. Conversely the vessel may be pulseless and impalpable. The erythrocyte sedimentation rate is elevated, and there may be a substantial fever and polymorphonuclear leukocytosis.

The most feared complication of cranial arteritis is impairment of vision. This may lead to sudden onset of blindness in one or both eyes. The pattern of involvement may be uniocular, resulting from disease of the ophthalmic artery, or occipital, resulting from disease of the vertebral artery. A precise estimate of the frequency of this complication cannot be made because patients with visual symptoms receive special medical attention. The danger is real, and it is generally agreed that all patients with active cranial arteritis should receive steroid treatment for some months, especially to prevent visual loss. There is also suggestive evidence that patients with cranial arteritis are at special risk of certain other vascular accidents, including brainstem strokes and coronary occlusion.

Although it cannot be doubted that the arteries most often affected are branches of the external carotid (accounting for the use of such names as cranial arteritis and temporal arteritis), it should be recognized that other arteries may also be the site of giant cell arteritis. Autopsy has disclosed arteritis in the aorta and even in the hepatic and renal vessels. Instances of aortic aneurysm thought to be due to giant cell arteritis are on record. These may result from an associated pathologic process described under a variety of names such as medial aortopathy.

Steroid therapy should be given according to the plan outlined for polymyalgia rheumatica.

Fauchald, P., Rygvold, O., and Oystese, B.: Temporal arteritis and polymyalgia rheumatica. Ann. Intern. Med., 77:845, 1972.
Marquis, Y., Richardson, J. B., and Ritchie, A. C.: Idiopathic aortopathy and arteriopathy. Am. J. Med., 44:939, 1968.
Wilkinson, I. M. S., and Russell, R. W. R.: Arteries of the head and neck in giant cell arteritis.,Arch. Neurol., 27:378, 1972.

104. LETHAL MIDLINE GRANULOMA

Paul B. Beeson

Lethal midline granuloma is a horrid, rare, chronic destructive disease affecting the midline structures of the face and nearly always terminating in death. The process most often affects males aged 20 to 50 and usually begins with symptoms of nasal obstruction with purulent, sometimes bloody discharge. Months or years later the skin of the nose and inner eyelid become red, then necrotic, with the formation of fistulas and with progressive loss of facial tissue. Owing to a tendency to thrombosis of blood vessels it progresses by causing necrosis of hard or soft tissues, leading to destruction of the nasal septum, the hard or soft palate, the paranasal sinuses, and the orbital cavities. There is little tendency for regional lymph nodes to become enlarged, and the process does not ordinarily affect the lungs. Pain and fever are variable. Death may result from inanition, hemorrhage, or sepsis (notably when the destructive process has exposed the meninges).

A disease conforming to the aforementioned description can be caused by several specific infections, e.g., syphilis, yaws, leprosy, mucormycosis, by carcinoma arising in the nose or paranasal sinuses, and by lymphomas. Sometimes, despite prolonged and intensive study including repeated biopsy, the specific causes are identified only late in the disease or at autopsy. Some writers have classified lethal midline granuloma and Wegener's granulomatosis together, but that seems unwarranted. Kassel and his colleagues take the view that most cases of lethal midline granuloma are forms of neoplastic disease, some of which eventually are found to resemble accepted types of lymphoma, others a less easily recognized form which has been called "polymorphic reticulosis." Others, who agree with the neoplastic concept, have suggested the designation "midline malignant reticulosis." They feel that the old term lethal midline granuloma should be used only as a clinical designation for a process which can have several causes.

As might be expected from scattered reports of an unusual clinical disorder probably comprising more than one pathogenetic entity, recommendations as to treatment have varied. Radiation therapy to the affected regions seems the procedure most likely to palliate or arrest the process. Occasional benefits from the use of cytotoxic drugs (cyclophosphamide, methotrexate, chlorambucil) are on record. Steroid hormones do not help. Antimicrobial therapy may be called for from time to time to combat secondary infection by bacteria or fungi.

Eichel, B. S., and Mabery, T. E.: The enigma of lethal midline granuloma. Laryngoscope, 78:1367, 1968.
Fechner, R. E., and Lamppin, D. W.: Midline malignant reticulosis. Arch. Otolaryngol., 95:467, 1972.
Kassel, S. H., Echevarria, R. A., and Guzzo, F. P.: Midline malignant reticulosis (so-called lethal midline granuloma). Cancer, 23:920, 1969.

105. WEGENER'S GRANULOMATOSIS

Paul B. Beeson

The central pathologic lesion in this disease is a granuloma which tends to affect blood vessels, with resulting necrosis of tissue. Lesions usually appear first in the upper and lower respiratory tract, but at some stage an associated generalized vasculitis develops and causes severe damage in the kidneys and other organs.

Persons of both sexes and all ages are affected, but the highest incidence appears to be in mid-adult life. In the "classic" picture, i.e., that which was first identified, the initial involvement is usually in the nose and paranasal sinuses. The patient suffers for months with symptoms of nasal stuffiness and discharge and is treated for recurrent sinusitis or chronic otitis. Later there is extension to the lower respiratory tract, with symptoms and signs caused by single or multiple lesions in the lungs. This may lead to an erroneous diagnosis of neoplastic disease. At some time after this the generalized vasculitis becomes evident, and there may then be rapid deterioration, with manifestations of disease in the nervous system, the gut, the joints, the skin, and subcutaneous tissues. At autopsy there may be destructive lesions in spleen and liver. The most sinister aspect of the disease is its tendency to cause severe damage to the kidneys, and renal insufficiency is the most common cause of death. Hypertension rarely develops despite severe renal disease. After onset of manifestations of disseminated disease the course rarely lasts more than a few months without treatment.

Limited Forms of Wegener's Granulomatosis. Carrington and Liebow have called attention to a group of cases in which the major pathologic change is in the lungs, and in which there is little evidence of disease in the nose or paranasal sinuses, or of generalized vasculitis.

Lymphomatoid Granulomatosis. Liebow et al. have now described another subgroup, which they consider to be related to Wegener's granulomatosis; in this the principal sites of involvement are the lungs, skin, and central nervous system. The histologic findings are those of angiitis with extensive necrosis and an infiltrative process resembling some form of lymphoma. The dominant clinical manifestations are cough, fever, and massive hemoptyses. This form of disease, despite the local "lymphomatoid" appearance, generally does not spread to lymphoid tissues, such as hilar nodes or spleen.

Diagnosis. The diagnosis can be suspected on clinical grounds but can only be made by histologic examination of affected tissue. Routine blood studies, including eosinophil counts, are usually normal. Biopsy from the nasal structures or lung will show the characteristic granuloma with special involvement of arteries and resulting tendency to necrosis. Biopsy of the kidney may show focal necrotizing glomerulitis.

Course. As already mentioned, once there is evidence of dissemination, especially with renal involvement, the downhill course may be rapid. On the other hand, in the "limited forms," some patients have lived several years and in some of them the disease has appeared to go into remission. Generally, however, this still must be regarded as a disease which tends to progress and to end fatally.

Treatment. Most patients are treated with antimicrobials; these may be required from time to time to deal with secondary infections, but certainly do not affect the primary disease. Steroid therapy has been generally disappointing; in fact, some writers regard this as a diagnostic feature. Others recommend that steroids should be given, along with cytotoxic drugs. Although comparative clinical trials have not been carried out, there is now a rather convincing volume of individual case reports which seem to show definite benefit from use of cytotoxic drugs with or without steroids. Several seem to have had an effect, including azathioprine, 2 to 3 mg per kilogram, chlorambucil, 0.2 mg per kilogram, cyclophosphamide, 1 to 2 mg per kilogram, or methotrexate. The last can be given in intermittent intravenous courses, 15 to 50 mg once a week, provided that renal function is reasonably good, and may have the advantage of rapid effect. If remission is obtained, these therapies can sometimes be stopped without reappearance of symptoms, but it is impossible to predict how long remission will last.

Carrington, C. B., and Liebow, A. A.: Limited forms of angiitis and granulomatosis of Wegener's type. Am. J. Med., 41:497, 1966.

Fahey, J. L., Leonard, E., Churg, J., and Godman, G.: Wegener's granulomatosis. Am. J. Med., 17:168, 1954.

Fauci, A. S., and Wolff, S. M.: Wegener's granulomatosis: Studies in eighteen patients and a review of the literature. Medicine, 52:535, 1973.

Leading article: Wegener's granulomatosis. Lancet, 2:519, 1972. (References to cytotoxic drugs in therapy.)

Liebow, A. A., Carrington, C. R. B., and Friedman, P. J.: Lymphomatoid granulomatosis. Hum. Pathol., 3:457, 1972.

106. WEBER-CHRISTIAN DISEASE
(Relapsing Febrile Nodular Nonsuppurative Panniculitis, Panniculitis)

Paul B. Beeson

The designation Weber-Christian disease will be used to describe several clinical syndromes which may or may not be variants of the same disease. The feature shared by all is the occurrence of localized inflammatory lesions in adipose tissue. Histologically these show chronic inflammation with mononuclear cell infiltration; sometimes the mononuclear cells are filled with fatty material. Giant cells occur occasionally, and in more acute lesions polymorphonuclear leukocytes may be present. There is a tendency to inflammatory occlusion of small blood vessels, and necrosis is common.

The term *Weber-Christian disease* is usually applied to a clinical syndrome in which the principal involvement is in the panniculus adiposus. Women are affected more frequently than men with this form of the disease. It is characterized by development of multiple tender nodules in the subcutaneous fat, from 5 mm to 10 cm in diameter. The lesions are located principally on the thighs and trunk and in the breasts. They are tender, and there may be some reddening of the skin. Occasionally necrosis of the skin leads to sinus formation with discharge of an oily liquid. The course is usually indolent; crops of lesions develop from time to time over periods of months or years. When the inflammation subsides, there often remains an area of loss of subcutaneous tissue which cause dimpling of skin. Systemic manifestations are usually mild, but may include malaise, low-grade fever, leukocytosis, and eosinophilia. Enlargement of the liver and spleen are reported in some cases. The illness may grumble along for months or several years and then cease.

A more serious expression of this pathologic process has been termed *systemic Weber-Christian disease.* Here there is widespread inflammation affecting not only the panniculus adiposus but similar tissue within the abdominal and thoracic cavities. There may be parenchymatous inflammation, affecting thoracic or abdominal organs, including lungs, pericardium, pleura, bowel, spleen, kidneys, and adrenal glands. At least a dozen cases are recorded in which this form of disease has led to death.

The term *mesenteric panniculitis* has been applied to an obscure disease characterized by inflammation of the mesenteric fat. This has been encountered mainly in males, and reports of the syndrome have appeared principally in surgical journals. Symptoms include recurrent episodes of fever, abdominal pain, nausea, vomiting, and malaise. At operation the mesentery is found to be thickened, with red or yellow patches, and biopsy reveals the characteristic panniculitis, which cannot be differentiated from the lesions of Weber-Christian disease.

Several writers have suggested that these forms of inflammation in the retroperitoneal adipose tissue may represent the initial lesion in at least some cases of retroperitoneal fibrosis.

There is no specific therapy. Considerable relief of symptoms by use of large doses of steroids has been reported, but in other instances this has not proved helpful. Antimicrobial drugs should not be given. The use of immunosuppressive or cytotoxic agents could be considered, especially when there is evidence of systemic extension of the panniculitis.

Milner, R. D. G., and Mitchinson, M. J.: Systemic Weber-Christian disease. J. Clin. Pathol., 18:150, 1965.
Ogden, W. W., II, Bradburn, D. M., and Rives, J. D.: Mesenteric panniculitis. Ann. Surg., 161:864, 1965.

107.   FIBROSING SYNDROMES
(Multifocal Fibrosclerosis)
Paul B. Beeson

In rare instances the delicate fibrous areolar tissue in certain anatomic regions becomes the site of a chronic low-grade inflammatory process, leading to deposition of dense sclerotic plaques, which may obstruct or limit the movement of adjacent viscera. When the process is in the active phase, there are characteristic findings of chronic or granulomatous inflammation, featured by mononuclear cell infiltration and occasional giant cells. In the end stages the pathologic lesion is simply that of scar tissue so that by the time this process causes clinical manifestations there may be little evidence of the initial inflammatory reaction. As a general rule the process tends to originate in the midline, around the great vessels, and then to spread laterally. At the periphery of the lesion there appears to be an inflammation of fatty tissue; this is gradually converted to a dense fibrous mat, with little or no sign of inflammation. In most cases a clue to the inciting mechanism is lacking, hence the frequent use of the term "idiopathic" in describing the various syndromes. Indubitably this pattern of response may follow different kinds of injury. For example, there is an association between therapy with methysergide and some cases of retroperitoneal fibrosis, and the suggestion has been made that fibrosing mediastinitis can occur as a sequel to infection with *Histoplasma capsulatum.* In a number of instances the disease has developed concurrently with a neoplastic process such as reticulum cell sarcoma or carcinoid tumor.

Although most of these syndromes have been described as separate entities, depending on the clinical manifestations and the interests of the writers who have reported them, it should be emphasized that several anatomic areas may become affected in one person. For example, retroperitoneal fibrosis and sclerosing mediastinitis may be present at the same time. Even more interesting is the report by Comings and his associates of two brothers, offspring of a consanguineous marriage, who exhibited varying combinations of retroperitoneal fibrosis, mediastinal fibrosis, sclerosing cholangitis, Riedel's thyroiditis, and pseudotumor of the orbit. This remarkable constellation of syndromes in two siblings brings up the possibility of a genetic predisposition to disease of this character, but of course does not exclude other precipitating factors, e.g., common exposure to some chemical.

RETROPERITONEAL FIBROSIS
(Periureteral Fibrosis)

In retroperitoneal fibrosis the fibrosing process is most commonly located over the promontory of the sacrum with extension laterally to the ureters and up as high as the level of the second or third lumbar vertebra. Less commonly the lesion develops in other extraperitoneal areas, for example, contiguous with the kidneys, duodenum, descending colon, or urinary bladder.

In some cases there has been an associated vasculitis in the skin and subcutaneous tissues, manifested by the formation of nodules, erythematous discolorations, and ulcerations. Similarly, inflammatory changes in small vessels at the sites of the sclerosis have been noted.

The occurrence of retroperitoneal fibrosis in patients taking methysergide for migraine has been reported with greater frequency than could be due to chance, and that drug must be listed as one etiologic factor. It has also been thought that continued use of amphetamine compounds may evoke this process.

The manifestations of retroperitoneal fibrosis are variable, depending on the anatomic location of the process. Pain is the most common symptom; it is vague and tends to be located in the low back and may be accompanied by symptoms referable to the gastrointestinal tract. The patient is likely to lose weight and have low-grade fever. There may be some anemia and elevation of the erythrocyte sedimentation rate. Although the ureter is the structure most often affected, symptoms referable to the urinary tract are uncommon until obstructive uropathy has led to azotemia and other clinical manifestations of renal insufficiency. The fibrosing process may surround the inferior vena cava, but signs of obstruction of that vessel are uncommon; this contrasts with mediastinal fibrosis in which the most common expression is superior caval obstruction.

Diagnosis of retroperitoneal fibrosis is difficult because of the lack of localizing manifestations. It is most often suggested by the findings at intravenous pyelography: displacement of the ureters toward the midline and evidence of obstruction usually at the level of the pelvic brim. One or both ureters may be affected. Less often a mass can be palpated in the pelvis or on the posterior abdominal wall. Once the presence of a mass has been disclosed, by roentgenography, by palpation, or at laparotomy, the main problem in differential diagnosis lies in distinguishing retroperitoneal fibrosis from retroperitoneal tumor.

Surgical treatment, if employed before there has been

severe renal damage, is often highly successful. Inasmuch as the fibrosing process is seldom invasive, the constricted organ can often be freed by blunt dissection so that normal movement or flow is restored. Relief of ureteral obstruction is usually achieved simply by dissecting this structure free of its fibrous encasement and bringing it out on the anterior surface of the sclerotic mass. Occasionally, however, the obstruction recurs months or years after such treatment. The claim has been made that prolonged steroid therapy may be helpful, but the evidence for this is unconvincing, and prompt surgical relief should be attempted whenever the risk is not very great. Nevertheless, many people who have had experience with this disease recommend that steroid treatment should be employed as an adjunct to surgical measures. When the inferior vena cava is obstructed, surgical relief is technically difficult and risky; here it may be preferable to temporize, in the hope that development of collateral pathways may alleviate the circulatory block.

The long-term outlook is fairly good if the disease is recognized and if its obstructive consequences can be treated suitably by surgical means. Prolonged observations of some successfully treated patients indicate that the disease tends to run its course and subside so that the life expectancy may not be shortened. Most deaths have been caused by renal failure.

MEDIASTINAL FIBROSIS

Taut bundles of collagenous tissue form in the superior and anterior mediastinum with impingement on the aorta, trachea, and pericardium, but the predominant manifestations are those caused by obstruction of the superior vena cava: puffy, suffused appearance of the face and conjunctivae, nonpitting edema of the face, neck, and upper extremities, and distended veins in the neck and upper extremities. The main task in differential diagnosis is to distinguish this relatively benign condition from obstruction caused by tumor. Roentgenographic examination of the chest may reveal little or no abnormality, but angiographic studies will show the obstruction of the superior vena cava and its large tributaries. Thoracotomy may be required for histologic diagnosis.

As already mentioned, some evidence suggests that histoplasmosis may be a cause of mediastinal fibrosis; therefore it should be considered, and when tests for this infection are positive a trial of appropriate chemotherapy seems justified.

Some patients with this syndrome have shown gradual improvement over months or years, presumably because of development of collateral circulation. Attempts to remove the fibrosing tissues from the large veins are technically difficult and hazardous.

SCLEROSING CHOLANGITIS

A diffuse fibrous sheath sometimes envelops the common bile duct, the hepatic ducts, and the gallbladder. The clinical manifestations are pain and tenderness in the right upper quadrant and prolonged, gradually deepening jaundice. Liver function tests reveal changes of extrahepatic biliary obstruction. This condition may progress to death, with the picture of biliary cirrhosis.

Treatment is not very satisfactory. Steroid therapy has rarely seemed to help. It is suggested that prolonged T-tube drainage of the bile ducts may ameliorate the situation until the disease regresses.

FIBROSCLEROSIS IN OTHER ORGANS

Riedel's thyroiditis is a rare form of fibrotic disease affecting the structures in the anterior part of the neck. This differs from Hashimoto's thyroiditis in being equally common in males and females and in the tendency of the fibrotic process to involve not only the thyroid but also its neighboring structures.

Peyronie's disease is a sclerotic induration of the corpora cavernosa of the penis. This disease has been encountered in association with sclerosing processes in other parts of the body.

Pseudotumor of the orbit causes unilateral exophthalmos and is likely to be confused with tumor. It has been seen in association with Riedel's thyroiditis, as well as in other fibrosclerosing syndromes.

Dupuytren's contracture has been thought by some to be another expression of the systemic fibrosclerosing syndromes; however, it is so often independent that the case for similar pathogenesis seems weak.

Alpert, L. I., and Jindrak, K.: Idiopathic retroperitoneal fibrosis and sclerosing cholangitis associated with a reticulum cell sarcoma. Gastroenterology, 62:111, 1972.

Carton, R. W., and Wong, R.: Multifocal fibrosclerosis manifested by vena caval obstructions and associated with vasculitis. Ann. Intern. Med., 70:81, 1969.

Catino, D., Torack, R. M., and Hagstrom, J. W. C.: Idiopathic retroperitoneal fibrosis: Histochemical evidence for lateral spread of the process from the midline. J. Urol., 98:191, 1967.

Comings, D. E., Skubi, K. B., Van Eyes, J., and Motulsky, A. G.: Familial multifocal sclerosis. Ann. Intern. Med., 66:884, 1967.

Glenn, F., and Whitsell, J. C., III: Primary sclerosing cholangitis. Surg., Gynecol. Obstet., 123:1037, 1966.

Hewlett, T. H., Steer, A., and Thomas, D. E.: Progressive fibrosing mediastinitis. Ann. Thorac. Surg., 2:345, 1966.

Salmon, H. W.: Combined mediastinal and retroperitoneal fibrosis. Thorax, 23:158, 1968.

Wagenknecht, L. V., and Auvert, J.: Symptoms and diagnosis of retroperitoneal fibrosis. Urol. Int., 26:185, 1971.

108.   EOSINOPHILIC SYNDROMES

Paul B. Beeson

GENERAL CONSIDERATIONS

Many diseases characterized by eosinophilia are dealt with in other areas of this book, for example, parasitic infestations, polyarteritis nodosa, and Hodgkin's disease. In addition there remains a group of poorly understood, uncommon syndromes in which substantial eosinophilia is a striking clinical feature. Some of these will be described in this chapter, and some bibliographic citations are appended. It must be emphasized that these conditions almost certainly comprise a heterogeneous group; doubtless with further study better understanding and more rational classification will be possible.

Despite a considerable amount of investigation there remains a vast ignorance about the role of the eosinophil. In the minds of many people it is merely a granulocyte which stains peculiarly and tends to proliferate when an allergic reaction develops. It resembles the neutrophil in morphology and has similar phagocytic ability, but differs in possessing a peroxidase not found in the neutrophil, in having a crystalline structure (the internum) within its granules, and in its behavior after administration of adrenal cortical steroid. It tends to lodge in tissues that have contact with the environment and to congregate in the neighborhood of antigen-antibody complexes and to ingest them. Although much has been written about the relationship of the eosinophil to histamine, there is no convincing evidence in man that the eosinophil makes histamine, neutralizes histamine, or is subject to a chemotaxis by histamine.

Indubitably the behavior of eosinophils is altered in some allergic states and immune processes. Their number in the circulation increases, and this is almost certainly a reflection of increased production in the marrow. Common factors of many diseases characterized by eosinophilia are constant or repeated exposure to comparatively large quantities of foreign material. Increased production of eosinophils by hematopoietic tissue follows the general pattern of immune responses and is mediated by the lymphocyte.

EOSINOPHILIC PULMONARY SYNDROMES

The term *Löffler's syndrome* is applied to a benign illness usually lasting less than a month, characterized by transient pulmonary infiltrations, low fever, and peripheral eosinophilia. Characteristically the infiltrates are located in peripheral areas of the lungs; when in the apices, the radiologic appearance may simulate that of tuberculosis. Some instances of this are associated with parasitic infestations in which circulating parasites lodge in the lungs, causing inflammatory reactions there. More often, however, the same clinical picture is found in patients who show no sign of parasitic infestation. A somewhat similar clinical picture may develop as a manifestation of sensitivity to nitrofurantoin. In most instances steroid treatment causes prompt amelioration of symptoms and clearing of the infiltrates.

A form of illness which resembles Löffler's syndrome except for longer duration and greater severity has been designated *pulmonary infiltration with eosinophilia* or *PIE syndrome.* This can cause marked disability because of fever, cough, and breathlessness and can persist for some years. Here again there is no clue to the etiology. Steroid therapy should be tried and may bring about improvement, but may have to be maintained for many weeks or months because of the tendency to relapse.

A wide variety of etiologic entities goes by the name *tropical pulmonary eosinophilia.* Doubtless many of these are either parasitic disorders or allergic responses to an inhaled antigen. This term has been used so broadly that it has little more significance than "nephritis" or "dermatitis."

Some patients exhibit pulmonary infiltration and eosinophilia during the course of *bronchial asthma* or *polyarteritis nodosa.* These entities can usually be distinguished from the aforementioned syndromes.

Liebow and Carrington have described a group of patients who had chronic pneumonia characterized by infiltration with eosinophils. They make the point that, although there is usually an increased number of

eosinophils in the blood, this is not always true; but on the basis of the lung lesions they use the diagnostic term *eosinophilic pneumonia.* The consistent anatomic feature is an alveolar exudate made up of a mixture of large mononuclear cells and eosinophils. In most cases of this type the etiology cannot be determined; certainly the clinical picture can be caused, among other things, by parasites, fungi, and drugs or other chemical agents.

EOSINOPHILIC SYNDROMES AFFECTING OTHER ORGAN SYSTEMS

Eosinophilic Endomyocardial Disease (Löffler's Endocarditis). Löffler described cases in which there was a marked and prolonged eosinophilia of the blood, associated with increasing cardiac disability. Autopsy in such cases discloses cellular infiltration of the myocardium and a fibrotic process on the parietal endocardium in which eosinophils are prominent. Frequently there is also an eosinophilic infiltrate in other tissues. Therapy with steroids has little or no beneficial effect. Differentiation between Löffler's myocarditis and diffuse eosinophilic collagen disease (see below) is sometimes impossible.

Eosinophilic Meningitis. From countries bordering on the Pacific come case reports of a subacute meningitis characterized by the presence of more than 10 per cent eosinophils in the cerebrospinal fluid. A striking clinical feature is pain and paresthesia in the extremities. There may be palsy of the sixth and seventh cranial nerves. Epidemiologic investigations point to a nematode, *Angiostrongylus cantonensis,* as the causative agent; the infestation seems to be acquired by eating raw or insufficiently cooked snails. The case fatality rate is only about 1 per cent (see Ch. 315).

Eosinophilic Collagen Disease. Many cases have been reported of a multisystemic illness, resembling dermatomyositis, in which there is marked eosinophilia. Muscle and joint pain are common, and the myocardium may be affected (as in Löffler's myocarditis). The kidneys are seldom injured.

Eosinophilic Gastroenteritis. See Part XIV, Section Three.

Eosinophilic Leukemia and the Hypereosinophilic Syndromes. Whether there is such an entity as *eosinophilic leukemia* continues to provoke controversy. Numerous cases have been described under that title. They have been characterized by prolonged clinical course, marked elevation of the eosinophil count in blood and bone marrow, hepatomegaly, splenomegaly, and fatal termination; at autopsy eosinophilic infiltration of various tissues has been noted. Doubt has been expressed about the designation of leukemia in some of these, principally because the eosinophils in the blood and tissues are mature forms; nevertheless some of those reported seem to satisfy conventional criteria for the diagnosis.

Hardy and Anderson believe that it is possible to depict a broad spectrum of hypereosinophilic syndromes extending from the most benign, Löffler's syndrome, to a clinically malignant form often confused with eosinophilic leukemia. This last group is characterized by manifestations of cardiac and pulmonary infiltration as well as marked enlargement of the liver and spleen, and often terminates fatally.

Steroid Treatment in the Eosinophilic Syndromes. In this heterogeneous group of diseases the efficacy of steroid treatment has been variable. Sometimes there has been a prompt and dramatic response, with apparent clinical cure. In others prolonged therapy has been required to suppress the cardiac and pulmonary manifestations. In a further group steroid therapy has had little or no beneficial effect.

Benvenisti, D. S., and Ultmann, J. E.: Eosinophilic leukemia. Ann. Intern. Med., 71:731, 1969.

Hailey, F. J., Glascock, H. W., Jr., and Hewitt, W. F.: Pleuropneumonic reactions to nitrofurantoin. N. Engl. J. Med., 281:1087, 1969.

Hardy, W. R., and Anderson, R. E.: The hypereosinophilic syndromes. Ann. Intern. Med., 68:1220, 1968.

Klein, N. C., Hargrove, L., Sleisenger, M. H., and Jeffries, G. H.: Eosinophilic gastroenteritis. Medicine, 49:299, 1970.

Liebow, A. A., and Carrington, C. B.: The eosinophilic pneumonias. Medicine, 48:251, 1969.

Pierce, L. E., Hosseinian, A. H., and Constantine, A. B.: Disseminated eosinophilic collagen disease. Blood, 29:540, 1967.

Punyagupta, S., et al.: Eosinophilic meningitis in Thailand. Am. J. Trop. Med. Hyg., 19:950, 1970.

Reeder, W. H., and Goodrich, B. E.: Pulmonary infiltration with eosinophilia (PIE syndrome). Ann. Intern. Med., 36:1217, 1952.

Part VIII
MICROBIAL DISEASES

109. INTRODUCTION TO MICROBIAL DISEASES

Walsh McDermott

Microbial diseases are all those produced by a transmissible agent capable of multiplication in living tissue and sufficiently small in its individual units to be visible only by light or electron microscopy. One might question whether a useful purpose is served by including under the one label such diverse entities as diseases produced by protozoa and those caused by the smallest viruses. Certainly at one level of analysis a grouping of this sort is not particularly useful. For this reason, protozoa have been removed from the present Part and, with the helminths, form one of their own (Part IX); general discussions of the rest of the microbial diseases have been placed with the individual subdivisions, such as viral or bacterial diseases. But there is a larger sense in which all these diseases are usefully regarded as a single group separate from and unlike all other diseases. For the non-microbial diseases, except for those resulting from undernutrition, are essentially individual, private affairs which, if uncontrolled, represent personal tragedies but seldom have wide public impact. By contrast, a society unable to employ contemporary technology to manage its microbial diseases is condemned to misery; infant and childhood deaths are a commonplace, pregnancy is virtually a permanent way of life for all women from their mid-teens to their mid-forties, and back-breaking toil is the lot of most people. To gain understanding of microbial disease in a scientific and technologic sense is thus an essential prerequisite to the building and maintenance of a modern society.

With that understanding of microbial disease is an appreciation of the tremendous adaptive plasticity of microbes—their great capacity for *change* both in themselves and in the conditions of their parasitism. This ability to adapt to change means that the microbial world is an enduring potential source of new diseases. It also means that there is no real prospect for a world free from microbial diseases, either those of man or of the plants and other animals. Thus if we are to continue our long record of successes in meeting microbial challenges to man, there can be no letup in our search for greater knowledge of the subject at the bedside, in the field, and in the laboratory. Our brilliant successes in the prevention and treatment of so many microbial diseases are not founded on the extermination of the microbe. They are all based on making the environment outside or within the human host a place in which the microbe cannot flourish to its full capacity. To exploit some weak link in the pathogenic chain in this way requires exact scientific and clinical knowledge. The incapacitation of the microbe thus affected may or may not jeopardize its survival as a species. Paleontology has taught us that species or genera have disappeared from this planet. Our systematic study of microbes is not yet of sufficient age to document such extinction of a disease-producing microbe, but there is no reason to doubt that it could occur. There is considerable reason to doubt, however, that it can be produced by the purposeful actions of man. A far greater body of knowledge would be necessary than is now available to produce such purposeful extinction of a microbial species. This is so not only because of microbial adaptability, but also because we have so little ability to identify and successfully interrupt *all* significant ecologic relationships involved. The story of the malaria eradication campaign (see Ch. 271) is a case in point. Whether the situation with smallpox will be any different remains to be seen. In the writer's judgment, it seems most unlikely. "Final victories" in the form of microbial extinction are not to be expected, but neither are they necessary or particularly desirable. Our existing conceptual base and pluralism of practical approaches have yielded an array of triumphs that make our current management of microbial disease one of the finest chapters in the whole history of science for man's benefit. To a considerable extent, however, these practical cures and preventives rely upon the change in hygienic habits in and around the home that come with, or are made possible by, improved socioeconomic status. What is needed now is not only a continued effort in the same direction but also a new massive effort of a different sort. This new effort should be devoted to reviewing those major microbial diseases for which we already have effective technologies, with the object of developing new and quite different methods suitable for wide application in economically underdeveloped regions.

Dubos, R. J.: Man Adapting. New Haven, Yale University Press, 1965, pp. 369–399.
Morrison, R. S.: The concept of eradication and public education. The Pharos, 23:3, 1963.

Section One. VIRAL DISEASES

110. INTRODUCTION TO VIRAL DISEASES

Edwin D. Kilbourne

The thread that binds together such differing diseases as influenza, mumps, smallpox, and yellow fever for common consideration in this section is the tenuous one of viral etiology. All are the result of infection with viruses, and all viruses share in common submicroscopic size and complete and intimate dependence on the cells of the host that they infect. Yet these tiny packages of protein-coated nucleic acid are as different as the diseases discussed in these pages. They vary in size from the 30 mμ RNA-containing particle of yellow fever virus to the 250 mμ antigenically complex particle of smallpox virus, with its DNA core. The relation of design and function of viruses is now being appreciated. Certain myxoviruses, including the influenza and parainfluenza viruses, possess a potent neuraminidase that probably abets their attack on the mucin-coated cells of the respiratory tract. The myxoviruses are fragile and unstable in the environment, whereas the enteroviruses, including poliovirus, can pass unscathed through the barrier of gastric acidity in their journey to the target cells of the small intestine.

Neither structural nor chemical similarity of viruses, however, is any sure guide to the diseases that they may cause. Mumps and parainfluenza viruses are indistinguishable by electron microscopy and even share antigens in common, but one invades the salivary glands, pancreas, or meninges, whereas the other produces mild upper respiratory tract infection or infantile croup. Nor does viral dissimilarity predict dissimilar disease. The structurally amorphous, genetically plastic RNA virus of influenza and the geometrically precise DNA-bearing adenovirus, with its potential for latency, both evoke clinical syndromes that may be difficult to differentiate.

With this caution in mind about the great dissimilarities among viruses and their associated diseases, the common features of viral infections can be considered as useful generalizations.

Most viral infections occur in childhood, at which time any of the 200 obligate human viruses ordinarily produce acute but benign disease or no disease at all. However, the unborn child may be peculiarly vulnerable to the effects of rubella, and the newborn – if unprotected by maternal antibody – may be severely damaged by infection with the ordinarily innocuous virus of herpes simplex. With the exception of the neonatal period, the severity of disease associated with primary or initial viral infections increases with the age of the patient. Poliomyelitis is more frequent and more severe in adult infection; varicella pneumonia is essentially limited to adults; the postpuberal complications of mumps are notorious; and jaundice occurs more frequently in older than in younger patients with infectious hepatitis. It is necessary to emphasize the evidence for greater potential susceptibility of the adult because it may *appear* that the adult is less vulnerable to viral disease, protected as he is by a legacy of immunity to many viruses from his childhood experience with them. This fact of age-related susceptibility is increasingly important as the epidemiologic patterns of viral infections change with changes in man's environment and with the introduction of new vaccines. If a vaccine induces impermanent immunity so that infection is merely postponed, the consequences might be disastrous.

Although firm and enduring immunity attended by persisting humoral antibody follows most viral infections, it is unlikely that antibody formation per se is the essential mechanism of recovery. Interferon, a nonspecific and nontoxic product of virus-infected cells, is more closely related temporally to the decline of virus in tissues and to recovery from infection, but its role in the self-termination of viral infections is still conjectural. Experimental evidence that corticosteroid hormones are inhibitory to interferon synthesis may explain the deleterious effect of these hormones or of stress on certain viral infections of man – notably on the extension of recurrent herpes simplex keratitis or on varicella in children already receiving steroid therapy.

The enduring immunity of viral infections has few exceptions. The frequency of common colds is now explicable as the result of multiple infections with multiple antigenically unrelated viruses; the seemingly transient

immunity of influenza reflects the changing nature of the virus itself. For most viral infections there is no indication whether protracted immunity is maintained by recurrent subclinical infection or by persistence of the virus in the host. With a few – varicella-zoster, herpes simplex, and cytomegalic inclusion disease – all associated with herpesviruses which replicate in the cell nucleus, viral genomes undoubtedly persist throughout life in the tissues, and there may be reactivated to produce recurrent disease in the partially immune host. In the growing number of patients who are immunologically crippled with cancer or subjected to chemical immunosuppression for transplantation surgery, such reactivations may occur as new and sometimes terminal diseases.

Evidence is increasing that viruses are involved in a variety of mammalian cancers and also in chronic diseases of the central nervous system. In man, the association of the herpes-like Epstein-Barr virus (EBV) with Burkitt's lymphoma and cancer of the retropharyngeal space is striking, although an etiologic relationship has not been proved. The human papilloma virus (associated with the common wart) is a member of a group of mammalian viruses – the papovaviruses – two of which have recently been proved to be capable of genetic integration with the host cell chromosome in the manner of lysogenic bacteriophages.

The recent direct demonstration of a measles-like virus in patients with subacute sclerosing panencephalitis suggests the awesome potential of common agents of acute infection.

In contrast to the bacterial diseases of man, the viral diseases are relatively insusceptible at present to chemotherapy, but the efficient immunity of natural viral infection can be duplicated with vaccines. The coat proteins of all viruses are antigenic, and it is reasonable to conclude that vaccines could be made for all viruses that can be cultivated in the laboratory. The great number of viral pathogens limits the feasibility of this approach, however, as does our uncertain knowledge of the ultimate potential of these viruses for good or evil. The vaccine itself may be a two-edged sword: if a living virus, it may be contaminated with alien viruses or nucleic acid; if inactivated, it may be poorly antigenic. At its best, however, the vaccine may be the ultimate weapon if eradication of the virus can be effected by substitution in the community of vaccine virus for wild type. A trend in this direction is evident with poliomyelitis.

The intractability of viral infections to chemotherapy is a corollary of the intimacy of virus-host association. To the extent that the viral parasite subverts the host's cellular machinery to its own synthesis, it cannot be interrupted without compromising the host as well. But the recent discovery of new, virus-coded enzymes in infected but not in normal cells suggests the possibility of employing highly selective antimetabolites specifically directed against virus synthesis. Indeed, this effect has already been realized in vitro, and in man limited success in arresting the progression of recurrent herpes simplex keratitis has been achieved even with antimetabolites not specific for virus. Chemoprophylaxis of smallpox and effective therapy of progressive vaccinia have attended the semi-empiric use of isatin β-thiosemicarbazone.

Man may never be free of viruses, but, hopefully, he may gradually replace the plagues of the past with more peaceful coexistence in the future.

VIRAL (AND FILTER-PASSING MICROBIAL) INFECTIONS OF THE RESPIRATORY TRACT

111. THE COMMON COLD (Acute Coryza)

George Gee Jackson

Definition. The common cold is a symptom complex caused by viral infection of the upper respiratory passages. Most precisely, the term applies to afebrile, acute coryza of viral origin. In the broadest sense, the common cold refers to any undifferentiated upper respiratory infection. The terms rhinitis, pharyngitis, laryngitis, and "chest cold" are sometimes used to designate the principal anatomic site of infection. The main difference between the common cold and other viral or bacterial respiratory infections is the absence of fever and the relatively mild constitutional symptoms and signs.

Etiology. Many viruses can cause the common cold. No single strain of virus accounts for more than a small proportion of the illnesses. Among the viruses recently identified, rhinoviruses comprise the largest single etiologic group. Isolates have been made from about 70 per cent of acute coryzal illnesses in young adults and about 35 per cent of common colds in children. The viruses listed in Table 1 comprise six categorical groups that have been etiologically related to the common cold in some investigations. (The coxsackie- and echoviruses listed therein are also considered separately in Ch. 126 to 136.)

The increasing ability to recover viruses and better serologic means for the diagnosis of viral infections have shown that 5 to 10 per cent of common colds are associated with more than one virus, and definite evidence of simultaneous dual infection is not rare. The causative agents of some of the infections have not been revealed by tissue culture methods currently in use. Certain of the more labile or fastidious viruses have been grown only in unusual cultures of human cell strains or in organ cultures of human embryonic trachea. Other viruses can be shown only by the transmission of illness to volunteers. More than 90 antigenically different strains of rhinoviruses are known to cause the common cold syndrome. Well over 100 viruses that can cause mild respiratory illnesses in man may be prevalent in the population at any one time.

TABLE 1.   Viruses Sometimes Associated with the Common Cold

Myxoviruses:
Influenza A, B, C
Paramyxoviruses:
Parainfluenza 1, 2, 3, 4
Respiratory syncytial
Measles
Coronaviruses: > two types
Reovirus 1
Adenoviruses:
Types 1, 2, 5, 6; 3, 4, 7, 14
Picornaviruses:
Coxsackievirus A 21, 24
Coxsackievirus B 3, 4, 5
Echovirus 7, 8, 11, 15, 19, 20 (others rarely)
Rhinovirus > 90 types or subtypes

Incidence and Prevalence. The incidence of common colds is related to age and environment. Preschool children have an average of six to twelve respiratory illnesses per year, most of which are common colds. Parents with young children have approximately six viral respiratory illnesses per year, and other adults have two to three per year. Statistics gathered by the United States Public Health Service show that in the winter quarter of the year at least one half of all persons acquire a common cold; 20 per cent of persons have a similar illness in the summer quarter.

The prevalence of common colds is approximately 15 per cent of persons per week during the winter months. Surveillance of a group of student nurses during one winter revealed that individuals had common cold symptoms on 10 per cent of the days. Among industrial employees in the United States, common colds accounted for nearly one million person-years lost from work among an industrial force of 60 million. This amounts to one half of all absences and one quarter of the total time lost. Similarly, acute respiratory illness is highly prevalent among military forces, especially recruits, and is a major cause of disability.

Epidemiology. The common cold is spread by direct person-to-person contact. Under conditions of household association, 10 per cent of adults acquired the disease from an index case. From studies in volunteers, it was shown that some persons became infected and shed virus without having symptoms.

It is a common observation that an increase in the frequency of colds occurs in the winter. Sometimes this has been correlated with sharp changes in the temperature, humidity, or pollution of the air, but the popular belief that cold weather causes common colds cannot be substantiated from epidemiologic observations in the Arctic or tropics or from studies in volunteers. Exposure of volunteer subjects to cold did not activate latent respiratory viruses. The reason for the apparent relation between the season and common colds remains unclear. In the United States, it is usual to observe three waves of common colds per year. One occurs in the autumn a few weeks after the opening of schools, another in midwinter, and a third wave in the spring. The separate epidemics have usually been shown to be due to different viruses, each of which may have its own seasonal epidemiology.

Pathology. The pathologic changes in the mucous membranes of the respiratory passages are edema, hyperemia, transudation, and exudation. The severity of the cytopathic effect is related to the type and virulence of the infecting virus and the extent of infection. Picornaviruses (rhinoviruses and enteroviruses) have been observed to cause more metaplasia and degeneration in smears of exfoliated cells from the nasal turbinates than the myxoviruses. This generalization does not hold for infections of the lower respiratory tract. During the acute phase of infection, protein components of the respiratory secretions are altered, and serum globulins become more abundant. Abnormal soluble substances of cellular origin also can be found. The secretion is rich in glycoprotein. Repair is relatively rapid and, insofar as is known, occurs without residual pathologic damage. Recently, however, inquiry has been made regarding the role of repeated viral respiratory infections in the pathogenesis of later degenerative diseases, such as bronchitis and emphysema.

Viral infection induces swelling and some exudation, but it causes no significant change in the bacterial flora of the nasopharynx. When the inflammatory changes are of sufficient magnitude, channels connecting the paranasal sinuses and middle ear to the airway become obstructed. Suppuration can develop from secondary bacterial growth under these conditions.

Mechanisms of Infection and Immunity. Viruses from infected persons are airborne in droplet spray that is emitted during respiration, talking, sneezing, and coughing. Particles in the size range of 5 to 50 μ are probably the most infectious. Transmission can also be made by hand contact. The nasopharynx is the portal of infection. The incubation period is short, usually one to four days. Proliferation of virus can often be demonstrated within 24 hours after the infection of volunteers. Virus shedding usually precedes the onset of symptoms by one to two days, and the peak excretion occurs a few days later, during the symptomatic phase of the illness. Virus excretion ceases after several days, and symptoms decrease concomitantly. Later studies from the same person as well as attempts to recover viruses from well persons indicate that the carrier state after infection is transient, and the prevalence of asymptomatic chronic carriers is not great. Rhinoviruses have not been recovered from more than 1 to 2 per cent of well persons in populations where colds are occurring.

Host susceptibility or resistance to infection is determined primarily by the immunologic status resulting from recent previous infection with the same or related viruses. Some physiologic functions, such as menses and fatigue, and constitutional factors, such as an allergic diathesis and vasomotor rhinitis, are secondary determinants of host susceptibility. Emotional distress and overconcern with personal health increase symptoms, whereas stoical and ascetic personality traits decrease overt susceptibility. In controlled studies, chilling did not increase the susceptibility of volunteers to infection nor did ventilation with frigid air.

The nasal secretion is the first barrier against infection of the epithelial cells of the respiratory tract. In addition to the mechanical movement of mucus, the secretion contains glycoprotein inhibitors for some myxoviruses that can compete with cell receptors for the virus. Because virus union with inhibitors is reversible whereas cellular infection is not, these inhibitors probably do no more than delay and decrease the multiplicity of infection. Specific gamma globulins of low molecular weight, principally IgA and IgG, also are contained in nasal secretion. The former is primarily the result of local antibody production and plays an important role in immunity from prior infection. The activity of IgG is related to, but poorly correlated with, the height of specific antibody in the plasma. In one study, the gradient between nasal and serum antibody was 1 to 30. During the early stages of infection, before symptoms have begun, there is an easily demonstrable increase of globulins in nasal washings.

Infection with some respiratory viruses stimulates the local production of a protein or proteins referred to as interferon. Noninfected cells exposed to interferon are protected against viral infection. The mechanism offers an attractive thesis for the termination of infection and repair of the mucosa before specific antibody is formed.

A response in serum-neutralizing antibody against the infecting virus is not always sufficiently prompt or of great enough magnitude to permit diagnosis of the causative role of a virus in the infection. Specific immunity against illness from reinfection with the same strain of virus, however, is readily demonstrable in volunteers. This clinical immunity is apparent for a period of about two years after infection. Asymptomatic infections are not entirely prevented. Reinfection in the presence of serum antibody usually results in a modified illness. The specificity of the antibody and its concentration at the site of infection on the surface of the mucosa appear to be critical factors. Although serum antibody reduces infection and illness, it is possible for infection of the respiratory mucosa to occur. In such cases, the acute inflammatory response can be exaggerated, presumably as a result of the local antigen-antibody reaction or hypersensitivity of the persons resulting from earlier infection.

Clinical Manifestations. The common cold is in large part a subjective symptomatic diagnosis. The major symptoms for any individual tend to be repetitive, but they differ appreciably from person to person. Some persons have only "head colds," whereas others complain regularly of pharyngitis or cough as characteristic principal symptoms of their colds. The occurrence of symptoms that 100 young adults described as characteristic of a naturally acquired common cold is shown in Table 2.

The same symptoms occur in volunteers challenged with an infectious virus, and their time of occurrence and duration have been observed. Sneezing, headache, and malaise are the initial symptoms, followed by chilly sensations, sore throat, rhinorrhea, and nasal congestion. The chilly sensations may be associated with some lowering of oral temperature that is sometimes interpreted as the initiating cause in natural colds. Fever of any significant degree is absent. The constitutional symptoms are transient, lasting only one or two days. There is sometimes a lull for a day between the early symptoms and the development of characteristic nasopharyngeal symptoms of a full-blown cold. The dry or sore throat tends to recede as the cold progresses. Nasal discharge is the hallmark of the common cold. At the onset, the secretion is clear, watery, and often profuse. Later, secretions thicken, become mucopurulent, yellow-green, and tenacious. Nasal obstruction is at first an intermittent symptom associated with an exaggeration of the rhythmic physiologic turgescence of the nasal turbinates. Later, the turbinates become swollen and boggy,

TABLE 2. The Syndrome of the Common Cold

Symptoms	Frequency
Severe:	
Nasal discharge	100
Nasal obstruction	99
Moderate:	
Sore or dry throat	96
Malaise	81
Postnasal discharge	79
Headache	78
Cough	76
Mild:	
Sneezing	97
Feverishness	49
Chilliness	43
Burning eyes and mucous membranes	28
Muscle aching	22

encroaching on the nasal lumen, which contains increased secretions. These symptoms ordinarily run their course within a week. As the illness progresses, cough may appear as an increasingly prominent symptom, and persists for one to two weeks. It may be dry or productive of a variable amount of mucoid sputum.

Physical signs are limited to the nasopharynx, the surrounding sinuses, and middle ears. Usually, mild hyperemia, congestion, or both, are all that can be seen, and the deviation from normal may be insufficient to recognize as pathologic.

Hematologic changes have been observed in volunteers when the initial blood values and the time sequence of infection were known. Mild leukopenia with relative lymphocytosis is the initial response, followed after a day or two by a slight leukocytosis with some increase in polymorphonuclear leukocytes. A fall in the hematocrit and rise in the erythrocyte sedimentation rate can also occur. Although the aforementioned changes can be related to the infection in volunteers, their deviation from normal is not great enough to be useful in isolated cases.

Complications of a cold are usually bacterial in origin. They are infrequent and consist of suppuration in the nasopharynx and its contiguous passages. Serous effusion, however, may appear in the middle ear and perhaps in the sinuses.

Diagnosis. The diagnosis of a common cold is made on the basis of history and symptoms. At the peak of the illness, signs of the infection also are apparent. Examination is important for the recognition or exclusion of illnesses of more severe nature that patients may be prone to designate as a cold. The differential diagnosis includes prodromes of other infections and infectious, vascular, allergic, and neoplastic processes in the nose, pharynx, sinuses, or ears. Other serious diseases, such as bacterial endocarditis, tuberculosis, bronchitis, bronchiectasis, and lung abscess have been called "chest colds" because of lack of characteristic symptoms and incomplete examination of the patient by a physician. The diagnosis of common cold therefore should be avoided as a designation for a broad category of respiratory symptoms of diverse causes.

The clinical symptoms do not permit discrimination with regard to the specific viral cause of a cold. The overlap in the symptoms produced by infection with any one of many viruses that cause the common cold is so great as to preclude more than a judgment regarding the general group of viruses to which the etiologic agent might belong. Under the controlled conditions of studies in volunteers, different viruses cause appreciably different syndromes. For each, the clinical manifestations are also related to the dose, size of particle inhaled, and modifications by host factors. The diagnosis of the specific viral cause of a common cold is based on laboratory procedures.

Treatment and Prevention. In considering treatment and prevention of the common cold, the following factors that have been discussed must be kept in mind: (1) The number of antigenically distinct viruses that cause the common cold is large. (2) Except for the time and economic loss, the infection is benign and the duration of severe symptoms is brief. (3) Viral infection does not significantly change the bacterial flora of the nasopharynx, and bacterial complications are infrequent. (4) Infection initiates production of interferon and antibodies that naturally limit the infection. (5) Specific immunity to illness with the same virus exists for one to two years after infection. (6) Reinfection can occur in the presence of antibody in the plasma.

At present there are no antimicrobial drugs of practical effectiveness in man against the viruses responsible for the common cold; hence the use of such drugs is not recommended. Carefully controlled trials with unlicensed drugs in volunteers indicate that effective chemoprophylaxis against the common cold is possible. The development of such products could initiate a more optimistic position regarding drug treatment. Suppurative complications are caused by obstruction more often than by the virulence of local bacteria. Routine antibacterial chemoprophylaxis selects resistant bacterial strains and does not prevent suppurative complications.

Supportive treatment is desirable and helpful. Additional rest in bed, warm clothing, and prevention of chilling increase the patient's comfort. If ventilatory insufficiency, stridor, and anoxemia that may accompany a cold are present, steam inhalation, a decongestant, a bronchodilator, or an expectorant may be indicated. Postural changes can help in the drainage of secretions and the raising of sputum. Because of the diverse causes and syndromes, there is no one regimen to be recommended. Aspirin in a dose of 0.6 gram for an adult or 10 mg per kilogram of body weight for children can reduce headache and malaise. However, it increases virus shedding and should generally be avoided. Oral phenylpropanolamine hydrochloride (15 to 50 mg), inhalation of hexamine vapor, or nose drops with 0.5 per cent ephedrine or phenylephrine shrink the vascular bed of the mucosa and provide temporary nasal decongestion. Nose drops in any oily vehicle should be avoided, and potent vasoconstrictors with transient action and physiologic rebound, such as epinephrine, are not desirable. Increased fluids or hard candy lozenges may be adequate for control of coughing. Cough syrups, such as elixir of terpin hydrate with codeine (64 mg per 30 ml), are more effective if necessary. Antihistamines have no effect on the common cold, except that a person prone to severe inhalant allergy may experience some reduction in the volume of nasal secretion. Large doses of vitamin C (ascorbic acid) have no significant protective effect against viral infections causing the common cold and no appreciable inhibitory effect on rhinoviral colds. Excessive amounts which have been recommended are rapidly excreted in the urine and can cause urinary symptoms owing to the increased acidity of the urine. The numerous compounded remedies, including those with vitamins, bioflavonoids, quinine, alkalinizers, multiple analgesics, antihistamines, decongestants, and tranquilizers, are developed for sales profit in a large market of uninformed and uncritical people and are not for the benefit of the patient or his physician. Their widespread and repeated use invariably leads to cases of fatal hematologic disorders, eruptive or exfoliative dermatitis, and anaphylaxis or other severe idiosyncratic reaction.

Prevention of common colds by quarantine or isolation of cases is without effect because of the number of infected but asymptomatic persons and because virus excretion usually precedes the symptoms. The hygienic collection and disposal of respiratory secretions to reduce airborne dissemination from coughing and sneezing should be encouraged as common courtesies. Interruption of the airborne phase of transmission by increasing space, higher rates of air ventilation, alterations in temperature and humidity, vaporization of disinfectants, and ultraviolet irradiation of overhead air all have been given trials without clearly significant results.

Vaccines for protection against the common cold are not available. Former "cold vaccines" were bacterial suspensions and have no basis for effectiveness. The large number of antigenically distinct viruses augurs numerous difficulties in the production of an effective vaccine. Nevertheless, promising vaccines are being developed for specific groups of viruses.

Andrewes, C. H.: Rhinoviruses and common cold. Ann. Rev. Med., 17:361, 1966.
Badger, G. F., Dingle, J. H., Feller, A. E., Hodges, R. G., Jordan, W. S., Jr., and Rammelkamp, C. H., Jr.: A study of illness in a group of Cleveland families. II. Incidence of the common respiratory diseases. Am. J. Hyg., 58:31, 1953.
Hendley, J. O., Fishburne, H. B., and Gwaltney, J. M., Jr.: Coronavirus infections in working adults: Eight-year study with 229E and OC43. Am. Rev. Respir. Dis., 105:805, 1972.
Jackson, G. G., Dowling, H. F., Anderson, T. O., Riff, L., Saporta, J., and Turck, M.: Susceptibility and immunity to common upper respiratory viral infections—the common cold. Ann. Intern. Med., 53:719, 1960.
Jackson, G. G., Dowling, H. F., Spiesman, I. G., and Boand, A. V.: Transmission of the common cold to volunteers under controlled conditions. I. The common cold as a clinical entity. Arch. Intern. Med., 101:267, 1958.
Johnson, K. M., et al.: Role of enteroviruses in respiratory diseases. Am. Rev. Respir. Dis., 88:240, 1963.
Paul, J. H., and Freese, H. L.: An epidemiological and bacteriological study of the "common cold" in an isolated arctic community (Spitzbergen). Am. J. Hyg., 17:517, 1933.
Tyrrell, D. A. J.: Common Colds and Related Diseases. Baltimore, Williams & Wilkins Company, 1965.
WHO Technical Report Series, No. 408: Respiratory Viruses. Geneva, 1969.

112. RHINOVIRAL RESPIRATORY DISEASE

George Gee Jackson

Etiology. For many decades, attempts were made to isolate the common cold virus. On some occasions, propagation of infectious material was accomplished for a brief period, but the viruses could not be sustained. In 1954, the virus known as 2060 and the closely related JH strain were isolated from adults with acute coryza. These viruses were believed to be enteroviruses and were designated echovirus 28. Soon thereafter, several different workers isolated similar viruses that were designated in the early literature as Salisbury agents, ERC viruses, entero-like viruses, coryzaviruses, muriviruses, and unclassified common cold viruses. Because of common biologic properties, these are all designated now as rhinoviruses. There are approximately 90 different serotypes of rhinoviruses capable of infecting man. They comprise a subclass in the family of picornaviruses, which also includes the coxsackie-, polio-, entero- and echoviruses. These are all small viruses (10 to 30 mμ) of the ribonucleic acid type that are not inactivated by ether. The acid lability (pH 3) of rhinoviruses is probably the reason for their absence from the intestine, and is the major property that distinguishes them from enteroviruses. Rhinoviruses characteristically grow best in tissue cultures held at a reduced temperature (33° C) similar to that found in the nose of man.

Prevalence and Epidemiology. It is likely that rhinoviruses infect persons in all countries and climates. Nearly all adults have evidence of earlier infection with several different serotypes of rhinoviruses. Similar viruses have been recovered from cattle, but transfer from other animals to man has not been shown. In human infections, some serotypes may occur annually, but the occurrence of different serotypes has been haphazard. About 15 per cent of a young adult population will have neutralizing antibody against any one serotype. Infection with rhinoviruses is more prevalent among adults than among children. In persons with colds, one third of adults and 10 to 15 per cent of children have had rhinovirus recovered from the nasal secretion. Infection with these viruses is relatively more frequent in summer, fall, and spring than in midwinter. Rhinoviruses have been recovered in 1 to 3 per cent of well adults observed during epidemic disease. Infection is believed to occur by the airborne route, but transmission can also occur by hand transfer from contaminated surfaces.

Clinical Manifestations and Diagnosis. Rhinovirus infections begin with headache, malaise, chilliness, a dry, scratchy sore throat, and burning nasal membranes and eyes. Nasal discharge and obstruction of the upper air passages rapidly become the dominant symptoms. Cough is a variable and later symptom. Fever is absent or of slight degree and transient. No pharyngeal exudate is observed, but cervical adenopathy can occur. In children, rhinoviruses sometimes cause croup or lower respiratory tract disease. Adults occasionally develop symptoms of lower respiratory disease, and sensitive tests of bronchial clearance are abnormal even if lower respiratory symptoms are minimal or absent. The incubation period is one to three days, and the course of illness is about one week. Rhinovirus appears in the nasal secretion a day or two before the onset of nasal symptoms, and is shed during the period of illness. The pathologic findings and pathogenesis are described in Ch. 111. A rise in neutralizing antibody in the convalescent serum occurs in only about one half of the infections.

Treatment. There is no specific treatment directed against propagation of the rhinovirus. Supportive measures are those given under treatment of the common cold. Quarantine is not necessary. Interferon produced by rhinovirus infection may be a principal factor in the amelioration of the disease. Recently, pretreatment of volunteers by topical administration of high doses of interferon obtained from human leukocytes was shown to reduce infection and illness. Also, the prior administration of a substituted propanediamine, which induces interferon, was effective in reducing infection, illness, and virus shedding. Although these products are not currently available, both are under development. They are attractive because interferon inhibits rhinoviruses without regard to serotype. In similar studies, vitamin C (ascorbic acid) in doses of 3 grams per day by mouth failed to prevent infection and illness. No polyvalent vaccine is available, but experimental vaccines have been effective against a single type of rhinovirus. The large number of distinct serotypes is discouraging to the prospects of developing an effective vaccine unless strains that cause heterotypic responses are found. Immunity to reinfection is quite specific and probably lasts only several months to two years after most infections, although detectable serum antibody may persist longer.

Beem, M.: Rhinovirus infections in nursery school children. J. Pediat., 74:818, 1969.
Bloom, H. H., Forsyth, B. R., Johnson, K. M., and Chanock, R. M.: Relationship of rhinovirus infection to mild upper respiratory disease. J.A.M.A., 186:38, 1963.

Dick, E. C., Blumer, C. R., and Evans, A. S.: Epidemiology of infections with rhinovirus types 43 and 55 in a group of University of Wisconsin student families. Am. J. Epidemiol., 86:386, 1967.

Douglas, R. G., Jr.: Pathogenesis of rhinovirus common colds in human volunteers. Ann. Otol. Rhinol. Laryngol., 79:563, 1970.

Douglas, R. G., Jr., Lindgren, K. M., and Couch, R. B.: Exposure to cold environment and rhinovirus common cold. Failure to demonstrate effect. N. Engl. J. Med., 279:742, 1968.

George, R. B., and Mogabgab, W. J.: Atypical pneumonia in young men with rhinovirus infections. Ann. Intern. Med., 71:1073, 1969.

Hendley, J. O., Gwaltney, J. M., Jr., and Jordan, W. S., Jr.: Rhinovirus infection in an industrial population. IV. Infection within families of employees during two fall peaks of respiratory illness. Am. J. Epidemiol., 89:184, 1969.

Kawana, R., Yoshida, S., Matsumato, I., Kaneko, M., and Wako, H.: Rhinovirus isolated from Japanese children with common cold. Jap. J. Microbiol., 10:127, 1966.

Monto, A. S., and Johnson, K. M.: A community study of respiratory infections in the tropics. II. The spread of six rhinovirus isolates within the community. Am. J. Epidemiol., 88:55, 1968.

Person, D. A., and Herrmann, E. C.: Experiences in laboratory diagnosis of rhinovirus infections in routine medical practice. Mayo Clinic Proc., 45:517, 1970.

Scott, E. J., Grist, N. R., and Eadie, M. B.: Rhinovirus infections in chronic bronchitis: Isolation of eight possibly new rhinovirus serotypes. J. Med. Microbiol., 1:109, 1968.

113.　VIRAL PHARYNGITIS, LARYNGITIS, CROUP, AND BRONCHITIS

George Gee Jackson

The same viruses that cause the common cold also cause other syndromes of respiratory illness. Pharyngitis, laryngitis, croup, or bronchitis may be even more characteristic of infection with some of the viruses than acute afebrile coryza. This clinical classification of the illnesses according to the anatomic site of predominant symptoms is the principal (although unreliable) way the physician has of differentiating diseases of different etiology. The mildest infections are those limited to the upper respiratory tract. As progressively more caudal sites are involved, the infections become more severe and cause more constitutional symptoms. *Acute rhinitis* (the common cold) and *nonexudative pharyngitis* nearly always occur without fever, whereas *exudative viral pharyngitis*, which is relatively uncommon among civilians, is a febrile illness. When adenovirus is the cause, *conjunctivitis* is very likely to be a prominent part of the syndrome. With viruses that cause pharyngitis the inflammation may extend into the eustachian tubes and cause *primary* or *secondary otitis media* and *sinusitis*. The lymphoid hyperplasia can include cervical adenitis. *Croup* is a distinctive clinical syndrome resulting from involvement of the larynx with resultant edema and stridor. It is a relatively common manifestation of respiratory viral infection in children. The classes of viruses most often causing croup are the myxoviruses and parainfluenza viruses. Bronchitis, bronchiolitis, and bronchopneumonia are severe manifestations of viral respiratory infection. They cause fever, respiratory difficulties, and symptoms that often require hospitalization of the patient. The course may be quite abrupt, including sudden unexpected death. The occurrence of these different clinical syndromes resulting from infection with some of the viruses responsible for the common respiratory infections is indicated in Table 3. Further details about the illnesses and their management are given in the discussions of the specific viruses.

The spectrum of diseases is caused not only by the fact that viruses are relatively nonspecific in the clinical syndrome produced, but also because the age and status

TABLE 3.　Spectrum and Relative Importance of Clinical Syndromes Caused by Different Respiratory Viruses

Virus	Coryza	Pharyngitis (Conjunctivitis) (Otitis)	Croup	Bronchitis	Pneumonia or Systemic Disease
Influenza A, B	++			++	++++
Influenza C	++			+	
Parainfluenza 1, 3	+++	++	+++	+	+++
Parainfluenza 2	+		++++		
Parainfluenza 4	++++	+			
Respiratory syncytial	+++		++	++++	+
Coronavirus	++++	+		+	
Reovirus 1	+				
Adenovirus 1, 2, 5	+	++			+
Adenovirus 3, 4, 7, 14, 21	++	++++		+	+
Coxsackievirus A 2, 3, 4, 6, 8, 10	+	++++	+		++
A 21, 24	++++	+			
Coxsackievirus B 2, 3, 4, 5	+	+	+	+	++++
Echovirus 7, 8, 11, 15, 19, 20 (others rarely)	++	++	+		++
Rhinoviruses	++++	+		+	
Mycoplasma		+			+++

of individuals influence the site and severity of the symptoms. In infants and children, the airway is smaller and the amount of lymphoid tissue is relatively greater than in adults. In the former, croup and bronchitis are more common manifestations of infection with the same viruses that may cause only coryza or pharyngitis in adults. A stronger effect on the amelioration of viral respiratory illness, however, is exerted by the immunologic responses of the host to previous infections.

FACTORS RELATED TO THE MANIFESTATIONS AND PREVALENCE OF VIRAL RESPIRATORY INFECTIONS

The initial infection with a virus may be resolved without establishing solid immunity to reinfection, or if immunity is established, it may be transient. The capacity of many of the respiratory viruses to cause reinfection has now been established. Reinfection in a partially immune host causes different illnesses from the initial infection. Usually the disease is milder on successive reinfections, but the dose of virus, manner of infection, season, presence of dual infection, and other factors may be of more importance. Sometimes, reinfection in the presence of antibody appears to increase the tissue response and exaggerate the symptoms.

In order for a viral infection to maintain a high prevalence of infection, one or more of several conditions is required. Some of these are virologic; others are epidemiologic or immunologic, as exemplified in Table 4. All these mechanisms are found in the case of one or another of the different viruses that cause common respiratory infections. The result is that we experience a continual endemic and cyclic epidemics of viral respiratory disease, with a large number of viruses infecting various sites of the respiratory tree and producing different anatomically designated clinical syndromes. The level of disease is exaggerated by new types of viruses or new exposures of susceptible hosts and is moderated by a progressive buildup of herd immunity developed by aging, naturally acquired infections, and vaccines. Likewise, the clinical syndrome is affected by these viral, epidemiologic, and host conditions. An appreciation of these factors is essential to the understanding of the problem of viral respiratory infections, their treatment, and control.

TABLE 4. Mechanisms That Contribute to the High Prevalence of Viral Respiratory Infection

Mutagenic or recombinant production of new types:
  Influenza A, B
Multiple antigenically distinct types simultaneously present:
  Rhinoviruses
Virus shedding before recognition of disease (or with asymptomatic infections):
  Rhinoviruses, parainfluenza, influenza
Social congregation of infected and uninfected persons:
  Rhinoviruses, adenoviruses
Latent infections:
  Adenovirus 1, 2, 5, 6; herpes simplex
Inadequate antibody response from infection (children):
  Respiratory syncytial, rhinoviruses
Reinfection in the presence of circulating antibody:
  Parainfluenza 3, 1; respiratory syncytial
Transient specific immunity from infection or vaccine:
  Rhinoviruses, influenza
Lasting immunity but recurrent epidemic disease among susceptibles:
  Adenovirus 4, 7; measles

Chanock, R. M., and Parrott, R. H.: Acute respiratory disease in infancy and childhood: Present understanding and prospects for prevention. Pediatrics, 36:21, 1965.
Ferris, J. A. J., Aherne, W. A., Locke, W. S., McQuillin, J., and Gardner, P. S.: Sudden and unexpected deaths in infants: Histology and virology. Br. Med. J., 2:439, 1973.
Foy, H. M., Cooney, M. K., and Maletzky, A. J.: Incidence and etiology of pneumonia, croup, and bronchiolitis in preschool children belonging to a prepaid medical care group over a four-year period. Am. J. Epidemiol., 97:80, 1973.
Glezen, W. P., and Denny, F. W.: Epidemiology of acute lower respiratory disease in children. N. Engl. J. Med., 288:498, 1973.
Hope-Simpson, R. E., and Higgins, P. G.: A respiratory virus study in Great Britain: Review and evaluation. Prog. Med. Virol., 11:354, 1969.
Kevy, S. V.: Current concepts: Croup. N. Engl. J. Med., 270:464, 1964.
Monto, A. S., and Cavallaro, J. J.: The Tecumseh study of respiratory illness. I. Plan of study and observations on syndromes of acute respiratory disease. Am. J. Epidemiol., 94:269, 1971.
Mufson, M. A., Webb, P. A., Kennedy, H., Gill, V., and Chanock, R. M.: Etiology of upper respiratory tract illnesses among civilian adults. J.A.M.A., 195:1, 1966.

114. ADENOVIRAL INFECTIONS

George Gee Jackson

Definition and Etiology. The adenoviruses comprise a distinct group of viruses of the deoxyribose nucleic acid variety. The viral particle has a coat (capsid) consisting of 254 capsomeres arranged in an icosohedron, which is a structure with 20 equilateral triangular faces; it is 60 to 90 nm in size. Most of the capsomeres (240) are six sided, called hexons; the other 12, at the junctions of the triangles are five sided, called pentons. The hexons have a common group-specific antigen characteristic of all adenoviruses. Each type has specific hexon and penton antigens. There are more than 31 specific serotypes among the strains of human origin. Only a few of them cause infections of the respiratory tract. The common types involved are 1, 2, 3, 4, 5, and 7. Types 14 and 21 also have caused acute respiratory illness. Type 8 is the principal cause of epidemic keratoconjunctivitis.

Some early isolates were recovered from surgically removed adenoids grown as tissue culture explants. These were reported as adenoidal degenerative or AD agents. The first strains from respiratory illnesses were designated RI agents. A later name, used briefly, was adenoidal-pharyngeal-conjunctival or APC agents. All the strains are now included under the term adenoviruses.

Incidence and Prevalence. Adenoviruses types 1, 2, and 5 infect virtually all persons early in childhood. They have been associated with febrile pharyngitis, with lower respiratory disease (sometimes fatal), and with gastrointestinal symptoms in infants. In older children and adolescents, adenoviruses, predominantly types 3 and 7 in the United States and 3, 4, 7, 14 and 21 in Europe, cause about 5 per cent of the viral respiratory illnesses. The incidence among college students may be as great as 8 per cent. At military recruit camps, infection with adenovirus types 4 and 7 is highly prevalent. It is often the predominant cause of respiratory illness, and 70 to 80 per cent of all incoming recruits become infected. Among civilian adults, adenoviruses cause only 1 to 3 per cent of respiratory illness.

Epidemiology. Adenoviruses occur in all parts of the

world. Man is the principal reservoir of infection. Many species of animals also are infected with adenoviruses, but these are of different serotypes, and cross-infection between man and animals either does not occur or is rare. Transmission is by person-to-person contact, but spread occurs only when the contact with an infected person is close or prolonged. The incubation period is from three to eight days. Swimming pools have been an effective vehicle for the transmission of adenovirus conjunctivitis. Such epidemics occur in the summer and have been referred to as Greeley disease and pseudomembranous conjunctivitis. As noted above, military inductees often become infected with adenoviruses 4 or 7 in the first few weeks in training and develop the syndrome called acute respiratory disease (ARD) of recruits. Season affects the transmission and symptoms of infection, with incidence of clinical disease being highest in the autumn and winter. Asymptomatic enteric infections are common.

Pathogenic Mechanisms. During the acute infection and for a period of one to three weeks, virus is excreted in the respiratory secretions or in those of the eye, or in both. A high proportion of infected persons have virus in the stool, which may be a source for the spread of infection. Viruria also has been observed during the acute respiratory illness. Adenoviruses replicate in the nucleus of the cell and, when the concentration is high, form crystals of virus. The nuclear chromatin becomes clumped, and the cells may undergo lysis. A most remarkable aspect of adenoviral infections with types 1, 2, 3, and 5 is the capacity of the virus to persist as a latent infection in lymphoid tissue for years after the initial infection. Fifty to 90 per cent of surgically removed adenoids yield adenovirus of one of these types. Whether this provides a source for infection of others or any harm to the host is unknown.

Some of the adenoviruses are capable of producing tumors when injected into newborn hamsters. Among the respiratory strains, some isolates of type 7 and type 3 have been oncogenic in baby hamsters. These studies on the tumorigenicity of adenoviruses also have shown the capacity of adenoviruses to combine within the same envelope (capsid) the oncogenic genome of some other tumor-producing viruses of DNA type, specifically the simian virus, SV-40. Thus under defined experimental conditions, adenoviruses can be oncogenic in their own right or act as a carrier for oncogenic material. There is no evidence that these properties give the virus any oncogenic capacity in man, but the phenomena are of basic biologic importance.

Some adenoviruses have an associated smaller virus (AAV). It is a defective DNA virus which can multiply only in the presence of adenoviruses. The significance of AAV in the pathogenesis of adenoviral infections is not known.

Clinical Manifestations and Differential Diagnosis. Different clinical syndromes produced by adenoviral infections in older children and adults are characteristic. Fever and pharyngitis are the hallmarks; catarrhal otitis occurs frequently, cervical adenopathy is common, conjunctivitis may be present, and a few patients develop pneumonia. The syndromes have been given descriptive names, as follows: (1) acute febrile pharyngitis, (2) nonstreptococcal exudative pharyngitis, (3) acute respiratory disease of recruits, (4) pharyngoconjunctival fever, and (5) adenoviral pneumonia. Any single type of virus

among those that cause natural respiratory infections in man can produce the entire spectrum of these clinical manifestations and also the common cold. The age of the patient and the route of inoculation are important. In newborn infants, giant cell pneumonia, myocarditis, and encephalitis have been described. In young children, mesenteric adenitis and intussusception have been reported. Infection with adenovirus types 1, 2, 5, and 6 may occur in the preschool child without any overt illness, whereas type 7 causes severe illness in this age group, with 5 per cent fatality. The former types infect nearly all children, but type 7 infections are infrequent. The common adenoviruses have been associated in a possible interrelated role with *H. pertussis* in whooping cough. Type 11 has been found as a cause of acute hemorrhagic cystitis in children (girls).

Conjunctivitis, when present, is an acute follicular lesion, often unilateral, with marked erythema, suffusion, and narrowing of the palpebral fissure. Keratoconjunctivitis, caused by adenovirus type 8, is a serious infection of the eye with corneal infiltrates; it rarely occurs in pharyngoconjunctival fever. Pharyngeal exudate, if present, is more likely to appear on the pharyngeal wall than as follicular tonsillitis. Cervical lymph nodes are enlarged and firm but less tender than with streptococcal infections. A macular rash that is difficult to distinguish from rubella has been described in a few cases. The leukocyte count is normal or slightly elevated. A prompt antibody response usually accompanies the infection. It can be measured in the serum by complement fixation or virus neutralization tests.

Treatment and Prevention. Treatment is supportive and with few exceptions recovery occurs without sequelae, excluding those of type 8 keratoconjunctivitis. Immunity to reinfection is demonstrable, but second infections have been observed with types 1, 2, 3, and 5. These types cause latent infections, and it is possible that later episodes represent an activation or recrudescence of the latent infection. Reinfection, if it occurs, usually causes mild illness.

Vaccine administration can elicit protective antibody and effectively prevent specific adenovirus infections. Live, enteric-coated, oral adenovirus vaccines of types 4 and 7 have been extensively evaluated in military recruits at stations where the incidence of infection and disease is high. Given prophylactically, it stimulates antibody, prevents specific adenovirus illness, and reduces pharyngeal infection after natural exposure by about two thirds. In epidemic situations mass immunization with live virus vaccine promptly interrupts the epidemic. Use of the vaccine is not recommended for civilians because of the low incidence and sporadic occurrence of infection with adenovirus types 4 and 7 among them. No adenovirus vaccines are available commercially.

Becroft, D. M.: Bronchiolitis obliterans, bronchiectasis, and other sequelae of adenovirus type 21 infection in young children. J. Clin. Pathol., 24:72, 1971.

Bell, J. A., Rowe, W. T., Engler, J. I., Parrott, R. H., and Huebner, R. J.: Pharyngoconjunctival fever. Epidemiological studies of a recently recognized disease entity. J.A.M.A., 157:1083, 1955.

Brandt, C. D., Kim, H. W., Vargosko, A. J., Jefferies, B. C., Arrobio, J. O., Rindge, B., Parrott, R. H., and Chanock, R. M.: Infections in 18,000 infants and children in a controlled study of respiratory tract disease. I. Adenovirus pathogenicity in relation to serologic type and illness syndrome. Am. J. Epidemiol., 90:484, 1969.

Chou, S. M., Roos, R., Burrell, R., and Gutmann, L.: Subacute focal adenovirus encephalitis. J. Neuropathol. Exp. Neurol., 32:34, 1973.

Dudding, B. A., Top, F. H., Jr., Winter, P. E., Buescher, E. L., Lamson, T. H., and Leibovitz, A.: Acute respiratory disease in military trainees. The adenovirus surveillance program, 1966–1971. Am. J. Epidemiol., 97:187, 1973.

Fox, J. P., Brandt, C. D., Wasserman, F. E., Hall, C. E., Spigland, I., Kogon, A., and Elveback, L. R.: The virus watch program: A continuing surveillance of viral infections in metropolitan New York families. VI. Observations of adenovirus infections: Virus excretion patterns, antibody response, efficiency of surveillance, patterns of infection, and relation to illness. Am. J. Epidemiol., 89:25, 1969.

Hamory, B. H., Couch, R. B., Douglas, R. G., Jr., Black, S. H., and Knight, V.: Characterization of the infectious unit for man of two respiratory viruses. Proc. Soc. Exp. Biol. Med., 139:890, 1972.

Klenk, E. L., Gaultney, J. V., and Bass, J. W.: Bacteriologically proved pertussis and adenovirus infection. Possible association. Am. J. Dis. Child., 124:203, 1972.

Levy, J. L., Jr.: Etiology of "idiopathic" intussusception in infants. South. Med. J., 63:642, 1970.

Manalo, D., Mufson, M. A., Zallar, L. M., and Mankad, V. N.: Adenovirus infection in acute hemorrhagic cystitis. A study in 25 children. Am. J. Dis. Child., 121:281, 1971.

McCormick, D. P., Wenzel, R. P., Davies, J. A., and Beam, W. E., Jr.: Nasal secretion protein responses in patients with wild-type adenovirus disease. Infect. Immun., 6:282, 1972.

115. RESPIRATORY SYNCYTIAL VIRAL DISEASE

George Gee Jackson

Definition and Etiology. Infection with respiratory syncytial virus (RS) causes epidemic acute respiratory disease. The illnesses are rather acute in onset and may be mild or severe. Since its recognition in 1956 as an infection of man, RS has produced regular epidemics of influenza-like respiratory disease.

Respiratory syncytial virus is a paramyxovirus that resembles influenza and parainfluenza viruses in its structure and many biologic characteristics. It is serologically distinct from them, does not agglutinate erythrocytes as they do, and does not cause lesions in eggs or common laboratory animals. The virus was first isolated from chimpanzees and was designated chimpanzee coryza agent (CCA). The name respiratory syncytial virus is descriptive of the cytopathic effect of the virus in infected tissue cultures. Only one type of the virus is known; some isolates have shown minor differences when tested against specific immune serum, but these appear clinically insignificant with regard to man.

Epidemiology. Respiratory syncytial virus has been recovered at several locations in the United States and elsewhere; it is likely that it has worldwide distribution. The epidemiologic pattern of infection lies somewhere between the epidemicity of influenza A and the endemicity of the parainfluenza viruses. Usually there are sharp, well defined limits to each epidemic. In the interepidemic period, the virus is detected much less frequently, but RS virus has been isolated from illnesses in every month of the year. Epidemics recur at intervals of 8 to 16 months. These have appeared simultaneously in geographically widely separated locations. During an epidemic, a large proportion of the population may experience infection, even persons who have had prior infection and have residual serum antibody. The pattern of the epidemic spread is characteristic of airborne or direct contact transmission. The incubation period is three to seven days.

Incidence and Prevalence. The high prevalence of infection is indicated by the fact that 70 per cent of infants at birth have appreciable amounts of maternal antibody against RS virus. During the first few months of life this declines, and between 3 and 12 months about 35 per cent develop antibody as a result of natural infection. By five years of age, 95 per cent of children have been infected. The incidence of infection with RS virus varies because of its epidemicity, but it makes a significant contribution in the production of serious respiratory diseases of children. Among hospitalized pediatric cases, RS infection has been found to be etiologic in approximately 20 per cent. In this respect, it ranks ahead of the parainfluenza viruses or adenoviruses and is also more prevalent than influenza. In the first year of life, RS virus is the single most frequent clinical infection causing lower respiratory illness and is a major cause of death in this age group. Among adults, the incidence is less well documented because of the milder nature of the disease, but an increase in hospital admission of adults with lower respiratory disease occurs during periods of RS virus infection.

Pathogenesis. Infection causes inflammation of the respiratory mucosa with a tendency for necrotizing bronchiolitis, bronchiolar obstruction, focal atelectasis, and patchy pneumonia. Infants and adults with chronic bronchopulmonary disease are especially at risk of fatal or severe illness. Bacterial pneumonia can be a complication. The annual epidemiologic recurrences of disease, the reisolation of virus from the same children in successive years, and investigations in adult volunteers have all emphasized the importance of reinfections with respiratory syncytial virus. The pathogenesis of the reinfections is not antigenic differences among strains. The studies in volunteers show convincingly that the presence in the serum of neutralizing antibody against the challenge strain does not prevent reinfection or illness. The high prevalence and importance of RS virus in the causation of respiratory disease appears to reside in this capacity to produce reinfections with clinical symptoms.

Clinical Manifestations. Fever and bronchiolitis are the characteristics of infection in children. Rhinitis and pharyngitis are usually present. Otitis may occur. In one study, pneumonia was shown roentgenographically in more than two thirds of the cases. Croup may develop, but it is relatively infrequent. The average maximal temperature is 39° C, but in individual patients it may reach 40.5° C. Ordinarily, fever lasts for three days. Dyspnea, cough, and wheezing are obvious symptoms. Tachypnea, rhonchi, and crepitant rales are present on examination. A few of the patients are cyanotic. The leukocyte count is elevated to between 10,000 and 20,000 per cubic millimeter in many cases. This clinical syndrome cannot be distinguished with certainty from epidemic influenza. Ordinarily, there is more rhinitis, and the onset is less abrupt. A fatality rate of 2.5 per cent has been estimated for hospitalized patients. Sudden death of infants and young children in their cribs at home after mild respiratory symptoms has been suspected by epidemiologic association to be of RS etiology.

In about two thirds of the documented cases there is a less severe syndrome, which has been diagnosed in outpatient clinics. These patients have fever, but they have fewer constitutional symptoms than those who are hospitalized. Rhinitis and pharyngitis are relatively more prominent. Cough is frequent, but rales and rhonchi are scarce.

Among adults with prechallenge antibody, the clinical manifestation of infection is acute coryza. At least, this is the conclusion reached from studies in volunteers and by isolation of RS virus from patients with common colds. An analysis of proved cases in adults admitted to a hospital in one study, however, indicated that persons with chronic bronchitis (one half of the cases studied) had an acute exacerbation of bronchitis; in one fourth of them infection caused bronchopneumonia, and in one fourth it produced the influenza syndrome with severe constitutional symptoms. Thus the entire spectrum of viral respiratory illness is produced in adults by RS virus.

Diagnosis.   The suspicion of RS virus infection is based upon clinical and epidemiologic observations. The diagnosis can be made by virus isolation from the respiratory secretions or by serologic tests. Respiratory syncytial virus is recovered by the inoculation of secretions into cultures of a human epithelial cell line or diploid cell strain. The specimens must be fresh or collected and frozen in a stabilizing medium, because of the extreme sensitivity of the virus to freezing and thawing. Several days are required before the virus becomes apparent in the tissue culture and can be identified; hence virus isolation is not of immediate value in the diagnosis of an ill patient. The use of specific immunofluorescent antibody to recognize viral antigens in nasopharyngeal secretions has been recommended for rapid diagnosis.

Serodiagnosis can be made by either complement-fixation (CF) or neutralization tests, using paired sera collected as early as possible after the onset of illness and again after two to three weeks. A fourfold or greater rise in the serum antibody titer is regarded as diagnostic of infection.

Treatment and Prevention.   Careful assessment of respiratory competence, close observation, and supportive care are important, especially in children, in view of the relative severity of the involvement of the lower respiratory tract. Anticipation of the possible need for tracheostomy (to reduce respiratory dead air space and assist in the removal of secretions) and mechanical assistance with ventilation in occasional patients is wise. Antimicrobial drugs have no effect on the RS virus or on the outcome of the usual infection. Isolation of the patient from other susceptible contacts should be done during hospitalization, but the spread of infection in the community is not controlled by isolation procedures.

The annual occurrence of epidemic infection and the clear demonstration of reinfections, often with equally severe second episodes, might suggest that immunoprophylaxis would have little effect on the infection. On the other hand, the mildness and lower frequency of infections in adults are circumstantial support for the development of immunity. The antigens of the RS virus are labile and poorly antigenic. Use of investigational inactivated vaccine that produced nonprotective levels of serum antibody augmented the clinical severity and fatality of subsequent infection. Similarly, the high fatality among infected infants in the first few months of life, when maternal antibody is demonstrable, suggests that passively acquired antibody may have a paradoxical aggravating effect. Attenuated, temperature-sensitive mutants that can be given as live virus vaccines into the

respiratory passages are being developed. Perhaps the larger amount of viral antigen and repeated doses that can be given in this way will induce protection.

Beem, M.: Repeated infections with respiratory syncytial virus. J. Immunol., 98:1115, 1967.
Berglund, B.: Respiratory syncytial virus infections in families. A study of family members of children hospitalized for acute respiratory disease. Acta Paediatr. Scand., 56:395, 1967.
Cradock-Watson, J. E., McQuillin, J., and Gardner, P. S.: Rapid diagnosis of respiratory syncytial virus infection in children by the immunofluorescent technique. J. Clin. Pathol., 24:308, 1971.
Fransen, H., Sterner, G., Forsgren, M., Heigl, Z., Wolontis, S., Svedmyr, A., and Tunevall, G.: Acute lower respiratory illness in elderly patients with respiratory syncytial virus infection. Acta Med. Scand., 182:323, 1967.
Hilleman, M. R.: Respiratory syncytial virus. Am. Rev. Respir. Dis., 88:181, 1963.
Hornsleth, A., and Volkeit, M.: The incidence of complement-fixing antibodies to the respiratory syncytial virus in sera from Danish population groups aged 9-19 years. Acta Pathol. Microbiol. Scand., 62:421, 1964.
Jacobs, J. W., Peacock, D. B., Corner, B. D., Caul, E. D., and Clarke, S. K. R.: Respiratory syncytial and other viruses associated with respiratory disease in infants. Lancet, 1:871, 1971.
Kapikian, A. Z., Mitchell, R. H., Chanock, R. M., Shvedoff, R. A., and Stewart, C. E.: An epidemiologic study of altered clinical reactivity to respiratory syncytial (RS) virus infection in children previously vaccinated with an inactivated RS virus vaccine. Am. J. Epidemiol., 89:405, 1969.
Mufson, M. A., Levine, H. D., Wasil, R. E., Mocega-Gonzalez, H. E., and Krause, H. E.: Epidemiology of respiratory syncytial virus infection among infants and children in Chicago. Am. J. Epidemiol., 98:88, 1973.
Sommerville, R. G.: Respiratory syncytial virus in acute exacerbations of chronic bronchitis. Lancet 2:1247, 1963.
Urquhart, G. E., and Gibson, A. A. M.: RSV infections and infant deaths. Br. Med. J., 3:110, 1970.

116. PARAINFLUENZA VIRAL DISEASES (Croup)

George Gee Jackson

Definition.   Infection with parainfluenza viruses is a common and recurrent cause of respiratory illness. Croup is a prominent syndrome in children, but the spectrum of illness varies from the common cold to pneumonia and systemic illness.

Etiology.   Parainfluenza viruses are members of the myxovirus family. They closely resemble influenza virus but differ from it serologically and in some biologic respects. Four distinct types of parainfluenza viruses are recognized that cause infections in man. They are closely related to one another and have some characteristics in common with mumps, measles, and respiratory syncytial virus. Types 2 and 4 differ somewhat from types 1 and 3 in the clinical illnesses produced and in their epidemiology.

Parainfluenza viruses were first designated as hemadsorption or HA viruses, owing to their property of causing erythrocytes to adsorb and stick to infected cells in tissue cultures. Type 2 was recovered from cases of croup and initially was called the "croup-associated" or CA virus.

A strain of parainfluenza type 1, the Sendai virus, was first isolated in mice and called influenza D. Mice and other rodents were then recognized to have natural infection with parainfluenza viruses. The Sendai and other animal strains of parainfluenza type 1 have slight serologic differences from strains of human origin. A simian myxovirus (SV-5) is commonly found in monkey kidney tissue cultures, occasionally in eggs and other tissues. It resembles parainfluenza type 2; virus isolates from cattle with shipping fever (SF-4) were found to be parainfluenza type 3.

Incidence and Epidemiology. Few, if any, persons escape infection and reinfection with the different types of parainfluenza viruses. Most children develop antibody from infection with parainfluenza type 3 before the age of four years. By the time they enter school, 70 per cent of children have antibody against more than one type. Among older children and adults, nasopharyngeal reinfection with types 1 and 3 is common regardless of the presence of serum antibody. Reinfection with parainfluenza viruses accounts for an appreciable proportion of common colds and upper respiratory illnesses in adults.

Parainfluenza types 1 and 3 are endemic and cause illness in all seasons of the year. A study in Glasgow, Scotland, indicated that infections in the autumn were usually type 1 and those in the summer type 3. The former tended to have a biennial epidemic cycle; the latter had annual endemicity. All types can cause epidemics of respiratory disease in the winter season. Together, the parainfluenza viruses cause about 40 per cent of all cases of croup. A greater proportion of infections with types 1 and 2 cause croup, but because of its greater prevalence and transmissibility, type 3 is a more common cause of the croup syndrome. Type 3 virus spreads easily from person to person. It infects virtually all contacts who have no antibody and reinfects many persons with a demonstrable level of antibody in the serum. Type 1 virus does not spread as efficiently as type 3, but is nevertheless highly transmissible. Type 2 infection has been less prevalent and more episodic in its occurrence than either types 1 or 3. Infections caused by type 4 have been entirely sporadic and infrequently recognized.

Although many animal species have a high incidence of infection with the parainfluenza viruses, spread to man from these sources has not been well established.

Clinical Manifestations. The clinical syndrome of croup in children is the most common characteristic of infection with parainfluenza viruses. Involvement of the trachea and bronchi also increases the amount of mucous secretions which can become inspissated and cause additional respiratory obstruction. Type 3 infections may be symptomatically more severe and cause more lower respiratory tract disease. Although croup is the most distinctive syndrome, parainfluenza virus infections cause rhinitis or pharyngitis more than twice as often as croup, and bronchitis, bronchiolitis, or pneumonia at least as frequently as croup. Over-all, croup is a symptom in fewer than 10 per cent of infections.

The initial infection with parainfluenza viruses produces more severe disease than reinfection and produces fever of 39 to 40° C in about three fourths of the cases. Among adults, parainfluenza viruses cause mostly upper respiratory tract disease, predominantly the common cold or afebrile coryza. About one third of patients with reinfection will have fever. In dual viral infections, a parainfluenza virus has been recognized as a common member of the pair with a resultant increase in the severity of the symptoms.

Diagnosis. Clinical differentiation of the type of parainfluenza viral infection and even the differentiation from other viral infections of the respiratory tract cannot be made with confidence. The virus can be isolated from nasopharyngeal secretions during the illness and for a brief period thereafter. This is the most certain and may be the only way to identify the specific type of parainfluenza virus involved. Serologic responses are often heterotypic owing to the nearly universal infection of persons with type 3 early in life and the common infection with types 1, 2, and mumps viruses. A rise in antibody against one of these viruses does not permit confidence in a strain-specific diagnosis.

Treatment. The treatment is supportive, as described for the common cold. The croup syndrome may be very acute, and cause respiratory insufficiency requiring urgent and decisive management. A comfortably warm, draft-free environment with high humidity (steam) is recommended for reducing laryngeal stridor. Maintenance of an adequate airway is essential. Antimicrobial drugs are usually contraindicated. Vaccines have been produced for types 1, 2, and 3, and their antigenicity has been shown, but their effectiveness in the prevention of natural infection has not been convincing.

Banatvala, J. E., Anderson, T. B., and Hocking, E. D.: Parainfluenza infections in the community. Br. Med. J., 1:537, 1964.
Chanock, R. M., Parrott, R. H., Johnson, K. M., Kapikian, A. Z., and Bell, J. A.: Myxoviruses: Parainfluenza. Am. Rev. Respir. Dis., 88:152, 1963.
Gardner, S. D.: The isolation of parainfluenza 4 subtypes A and B in England and serological studies of their prevalence. J. Hyg. (Camb.), 67:545, 1969.
Herrmann, E. C., Jr., and Hable, K. A.: Experiences in laboratory diagnosis of parainfluenza viruses in routine medical practice. Mayo Clinic Proc., 45:177, 1970.
Kim, H. W., Vargosko, A. J., Chanock, R. M., and Parrott, R. H.: Parainfluenza 2 (CA) virus: Etiologic association with croup. Pediatrics, 28:614, 1961.
LaPlaca, M., and Moscovici, C.: Distribution of parainfluenza antibodies in different groups of population. J. Immunol., 88:72, 1962.
Lennette, E. H., Jensen, F. W., Guenther, R. W., and Magofin, R. L.: Serologic responses to parainfluenza viruses in patients with mumps virus infection. J. Lab. Clin. Med., 61:780, 1963.
McLean, D. M., Bach, R. D., Larke, P. B., and McNaughton, G. A.: Myxoviruses associated with acute laryngotracheobronchitis in Toronto, 1962–63. Can. Med. Assoc. J., 89:1257, 1963.
Miller, W. S., and Artenstein, M. S.: Aerosol stability of three acute respiratory disease viruses. Proc. Soc. Exp. Biol. Med., 125: 222, 1967.
Mogabgab, W. J., Dick, E. C., and Holmes, B.: Parainfluenza 2 (CA) virus in young adults. Am. J. Hyg., 74:304, 1961.
Parrott, R. H., Vargosko, A., Luckey, A., Kim, H. W., Cumming, C., and Chanock, R. M.: Clinical features of infection with hemadsorption viruses. N. Engl. J. Med., 260:731, 1959.
Pierson, M., deLavergne, E., Gelgenkrantz, S., and Worms, A. M.: Aspect clinique et épidémiologique de quelques cas d'infection à myxovirus Parainfluenza III (EA 102). Arch. Gesamte Virusforsch., 13:257, 1963.
Starke, J. E., Heath, R. B., and Curwen, M. P.: Infection with influenza and parainfluenza viruses in chronic bronchitis. Thorax, 20:124, 1965.
Von Euler, L., Kantor, F. S., Hsuing, G. D., Isaacson, P., and Tucker, G.: Studies of parainfluenza viruses: I. Clinical, pathological, and virological observations. Yale J. Biol. Med., 35: 523, 1963.
Wenzel, R. P., McCormick, D. P., and Beam, W. E.: Parainfluenza pneumonia in adults. J.A.M.A., 221:294, 1972.

117. INFLUENZA

Edwin D. Kilbourne

Definition. Influenza is an acute, contagious disease that is usually attended by fever and prostration and is ordinarily benign in outcome. The headache, myalgia, and asthenia that characterize the disease are severe out of proportion to the symptoms originating from involvement of the respiratory tract—the primary and perhaps exclusive site of infection with the causative virus.

History. Epidemics of respiratory disease similar to modern influenza have been recorded through the centuries. Since the year 1510 there have been 31 pandemics described. The calamitous nature of these epidemics may have led to the naming of the disease by the Italians as an "influenza" or influence of the heavenly bodies or perhaps as an "influenza di freddo" (influence of the cold).

In 1933 the isolation of a virus in ferrets by Smith, Andrewes, and Laidlaw established the specific infectious etiology of the disease, and led rapidly to accurate definition of its epidemiology and clinical variations. The virus isolated in 1933 is now known as influenza A virus.

A second type of virus was isolated independently in 1940 by Francis and by Magill (influenza B virus). In 1950 influenza C was isolated from a patient in nonepidemic circumstances by Taylor, and later was shown by Francis and his associates to be the cause of epidemic disease.

The discovery by Burnet (1940) that the influenza viruses could be cultivated readily in the chick embryo led directly to simplified methods of studying influenza and to the development of an inactivated viral vaccine. Hirst's discovery (1941) that the virus could agglutinate erythrocytes in vitro (hemagglutination) (also noted by McClelland and Hare in 1941) provided not only a new technique for basic virology but a practical method for the precise measurement of virus and antibody.

In 1941 Horsfall and associates published the first evidence of protection of man against influenza by a vaccine containing inactivated influenza A virus. The Commission on Influenza of the Armed Forces Epidemiological Board has demonstrated the feasibility of mass immunization, and has developed the vaccines now in standard use.

Etiology. Influenza is a consequence of infection with certain *myxoviruses* that have common physical, chemical, and biologic properties. These viruses comprise three groups (A, B, and C), which are completely unrelated antigenically, do not induce cross-immunity to one another, and have different epidemiologic characteristics. Four major subgroups of influenza A viruses have been identified since discovery of the virus in 1933, one having replaced the other in chronologic succession. Serologic studies defined a virus that first appeared in swine in 1918 (HswN1) as the probable cause of the notorious human pandemic of that year. Influenza A virus subtypes are defined on the basis of antigenic analysis of their two outermost proteins. These biologically active glyoproteins (hemagglutinin [H] and neuraminidase [N]) are the primary determinants of immunity and mutate independently, as was clearly evident in the replacement of H2N2 by H3N2 (Hong Kong) virus in 1968 (see accompanying table). The hemagglutinin (H) is responsible for binding the virus to the cell; antibody to this protein therefore neutralizes the virus and is the major determinant of immunity. The viral neuraminidase (N) is instrumental in release of virus from cells; antineuraminidase antibody is not neutralizing, but limits viral replication and therefore the course of infection. As ex-

ternal spike-like projections from the viral envelope, H and N are in immediate contact with host antibody during infection and therefore are under selective pressure (see Epidemiology). Beneath these "spikes" the virus particle is bounded by a lipid bilayer derived from the host cell (Fig. 1). Just beneath the lipid layer the core of the particle is surrounded by the M or membrane protein. The nucleoprotein (NP) occurs in helical form in association with the viral RNA. The internal M, NP, and P proteins (of undefined location and function) are common to all influenza A viruses and do not differ significantly in antigenic nature from one subtype to the other. Type-specific A, B, or C categorization of virus thus depends on serologic reactions (usually complement-fixation) mediated by these internal antigens.

The viral genome within comprises segments of RNA (totaling 3.9×10^6 daltons) capable of reassortment during infection to provide an unusually high frequency of genetic recombination. Isolated viral RNA(s) is not infectious, because it does not constitute the message. Transcriptase is necessary for viral replication. It is not known which of the viral proteins described above has transcriptase function.

Influenza B and C viruses have been less thoroughly studied, but appear to be structurally similar to influenza A viruses. Little antigenic variation of influenza C virus has been remarked, and antigenic variation of influenza B virus has been of lesser magnitude than that observed with influenza A. However, a new variant that appeared in 1972 (prototype strain B/Hong Kong/5/72) is markedly different from earlier strains and appears to be emerging to predominance.

The influenza viruses are of medium size (approximately 850 Å in diameter), and by conventional electron microscopy they appear spherical or filamentous in form, with spike-like projections.

Epidemiology. The arbitrary designation of the three types of influenza virus as A, B, and C coincides fortuitously with their relative rank as causes of severe epidemic disease. Influenza B and C viruses have been associated chiefly with sporadic epidemics in children and young adults, notably in school or other institutional populations. Most adults carry antibodies to these viruses, probably as the result of recurrent subclinical infection. There is no evidence that pandemics of influenza B or C have occurred.

Major Subtypes of Influenza: Antigenic Variations in Hemagglutinin (H) and Neuraminidase (N) of the Virus in Relation to Pandemic Severity of Influenza*

Year of Appearance	Virus		Former Designation	Change in	Extent of Change	Result
1918	Hsw	N1	(Swine)	?	?	Pandemic (severe)
192?	H0	N1	(A₀)	H	++	No evident pandemic
				N	+	
1947	H1	N1	(A₁)	H	++	Pandemic (mild)
				N	+	
1957	H2	N2	(A₂)	H	+++	Pandemic (severe)
				N	+++	
1968	H3	N2	(HK)	H	+++	Pandemic (moderate)
				N	0	

*Modified from Kilbourne, E. D.: J. Infect., Dis., 127:478, 1973.

Vertical connecting lines indicate antigenic relatedness (i.e., shared antigenic determinants). Double lines indicate close similarity. H0N1 is new subtype designation for A₀, etc. Plus signs indicate grading of extent of antigenic change from immediately preceding viral subtype. The severity of the subsequent pandemics appears to be related to the degree of antigenic change in the virus.

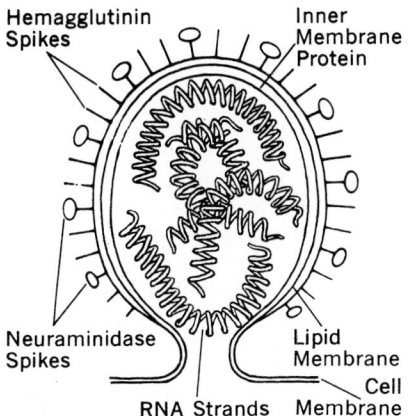

Figure 1. Schematic representation of influenza virus particle as it buds from the plasma membrane of the infected cell, incorporating host lipid and carbohydrate in the process. The surface proteins, hemagglutinin, and neuraminidase are subject to mutations that permit the virus to escape previously established immunity. (Reprinted, by permission, from Kilbourne, E. D.: Man's adaptable predator. Natural History, 82:72, 1973. Copyright © The American Museum of Natural History, 1973.)

Discussions of influenza are usually concerned with the influenza A viruses, for these are the important and apparently more mutable viruses that cause widespread epidemic and pandemic disease. The complicated and still puzzling epidemiology of influenza A is most conveniently considered by separate discussions of the *pandemic, epidemic*, and *endemic* infections — all attributable to the same virus under different conditions.

Pandemic Influenza. The isolation of a virus of the influenza A group from the pandemic of 1957 established that pandemic influenza was etiologically linked with the less extensive epidemic disease from which viruses had been recovered during the 1933–1956 period.

Influenza A virus is an obligate human parasite which is transmitted directly from man to man under conditions of close interhuman contact, presumably via the respiratory tract. With *human* viruses survival of the virus appears to depend on its serial transmission from man to man.

When a major antigenic change in the virus oc-

curs — perhaps as a reciprocal of high immunity in the general population — this mutation may be so extreme that acquired immunity in the population to previously existing influenza A viruses is inadequate to prevent infection or disease initiated by the new virus, which replaces the older virus completely. Under these conditions, people of all ages and in all places are susceptible to influenza, and a worldwide epidemic or pandemic may ensue (Fig. 2). The source of the markedly different strains of virus that suddenly appear to initiate pandemics is unknown. Direct mutation from the antecedent virus seems unlikely in view of the magnitude of change in H and N antigens. Therefore recombination in nature of human and animal influenza A viruses has been proposed to explain the recurrent decennial introduction of apparently novel viruses into the human population.

The incubation period of influenza is only 24 to 48 hours, so that, once progressive spread begins, the impact on the community is sudden and devastating. Both the incidence and the severity of illness are highly variable and are influenced by age, pregnancy, and pre-existing chronic disease and by such environmental factors as crowding and season of the year. Morbidity is usually first noted among schoolchildren, then in young adults, and finally in older, less active, and presumably less exposed members of the community. Infection of the aged is more frequently followed by bacterial pneumonia. As a consequence, a "second wave" of increased community mortality may coincide with the delayed appearance of influenza in this age group — *at a time when influenza is no longer apparent in the community* by the usual criteria of absenteeism from school or industry.

Specific immunity to influenza develops rapidly after infection, but it may decline within one or two years so that recurrence of infection and disease from the same antigenic type of virus may occur *under conditions of heavy exposure* as in military barracks or boarding schools. On the other hand, the steady decline in community morbidity after the initial pandemic wave obviously points to the acquisition of immunity of some durability by most of the population.

Interpandemic "Epidemic" Influenza. Influenza occurs in its characteristic acute epidemics in the early months of the year in the north temperate zone. In a par-

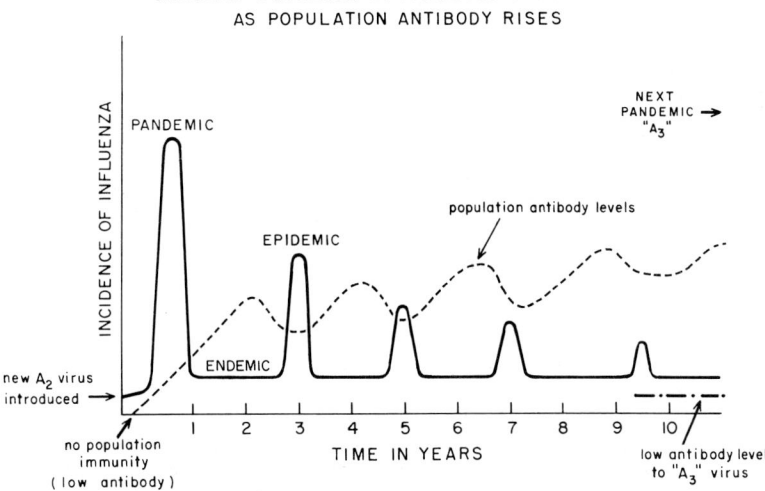

Figure 2. Schematic representation of the correlation of influenza incidence and mean population antibody levels after introduction of a new influenza virus variant. (From Kilbourne, E. D.: Sandoz Panorama, 6:7, 1968.)

ticular community the epidemic usually comes and goes within a month, rising to a peak in 12 to 14 days, and subsiding almost as rapidly. Although the case fatality rate is less than 1 per cent, the presence of influenza may be detected by a sudden increase in unspecified total mortality in the community. This mortality occurs at both extremes of age, and is occasioned principally by the bacterial pneumonias that may complicate influenza in the very young and very old.

Epidemics of influenza A have been demonstrated to occur every year since discovery of the virus, but communities are usually spared recurrence for two or more years after an epidemic.

After a pandemic, the frequency and extent of epidemics gradually abate with the development of population immunity to the new virus. Minor antigenic variations of the virus may be detected during this time, but at least a decade seems to be required for change sufficient to establish a truly "new' subtype (Fig. 2).

Endemic Influenza. The interepidemic survival of influenza virus has long been a puzzle in view of the fragility of the virus and its apparently obligate restriction to human hosts. It has become increasingly clear, however, that influenza virus infections may occur continuously within the population, either as sporadic instances of disease that are not recognized as influenza or as clinically inapparent infections. As more and more members of the population develop immunity, infections without disease become more and more frequent and serve to maintain the virus in the community. Such infections are recognized by serologic studies.

Pathology and Pathogenesis. The primary lesion of influenza is a necrosis of the ciliated epithelium of the respiratory tract. In the uncomplicated infection epithelial damage is probably confined to the upper and middle portion of the respiratory tract, the trachea being the most strikingly involved. Early in infection the necrotic ciliated cells are desquamated, leaving intact the basal cell layer. On about the fifth day of illness regeneration begins in the basal layer with the development of undifferentiated "transitional" epithelium, which may simulate metaplasia. After two weeks ciliated cells may again be seen.

When influenza is complicated by bacterial pneumonia, the pathologic findings are variable and depend on the nature of the secondary invader. However, *primary influenza virus pneumonia* presents a characteristic picture. The lungs are dark red, heavy, and edematous. The trachea and bronchi contain bloody fluid, and the mucosa is hyperemic. Microscopy shows ciliated epithelium to have been lost from the trachea, bronchi, and bronchioles, but evidence of epithelial regeneration may be seen. In the submucosa, focal hemorrhage, edema, and slight leukocytic infiltration may occur. Capillary thrombosis with focal leukocytic exudate has been described. The alveolar spaces contain neutrophilic and mononuclear cells admixed with fibrin and edema fluid. Intra-alveolar hemorrhage is common in the lower lobes. The alveolar septa may be thickened, and acellular hyaline membranes may line alveolar ducts and alveoli.

Pathologic changes attributable to influenza occur only rarely outside the respiratory tract. There are no physiologic or biochemical changes in the patient that are pathognomonic of influenza. Although "leukopenia" is often stated to be characteristic, total leukocytic counts in the uncomplicated disease may vary from 2000 to 14,000 cells per cubic millimeter, and are usually in the normal range. However, *lymphocytopenia* is commonly detectable, especially in the first four days of illness. The erythrocyte sedimentation rate may be moderately elevated or normal. No characteristic changes occur in the bacterial flora of the respiratory tract.

The Complicated Disease. In primary influenza viral pneumonia, *leukocytosis* is the rule, even in the absence of bacterial pathogens, although the erythrocyte sedimentation rate may not be elevated. *Serum glutamic oxaloacetic transaminase concentrations* are elevated in proportion to the severity of pulmonary involvement and may exceed 60 units per milliliter. *Oxyhemoglobin saturation* is reduced to 46 to 85 per cent. *Partial pressure of CO_2* is elevated, and the *pH of arterial blood* is lowered. The *proteinuria* and elevated *blood urea nitrogen* concentrations that may be noted are the results of fever and dehydration and do not reflect primary renal damage. No notable changes in *serum electrolytes* or in *blood clotting* occur.

Clinical Manifestations. Infection with influenza virus may be asymptomatic, may be attended only by slight fever, or may result in the "typical" prostrating disease that identifies epidemics. This disease is remarkably constant in its expression from year to year, and the uncomplicated case of pandemic influenza does not differ from the "three-day fever" of nonpandemic outbreaks. The higher fatality rates associated with the 1918 pandemic were usually attributable to secondary bacterial pneumonia. Significant variations in the disease caused by any of the A or B subtypes of virus have not occurred. Influenza C appears to be a less severe disease, but it has not yet received adequate study.

Patients with influenza almost invariably *cough*, although this symptom may not be bothersome or even noted by the patient. The cough is brief and spasmodic, and usually not productive of sputum. Other symptoms related to the destruction of respiratory epithelium are *substernal burning pain* (from the trachea), *dryness or soreness of the throat*, and *nasal obstruction and discharge*. Neither sore throat nor evidence of rhinitis is particularly prominent in influenza. Slight *pharyngeal injection* may be noted. *Epistaxis* is rare, but is valuable diagnostically when it occurs. *Conjunctival burning and injection* are common.

In 5 to 10 per cent of patients with uncomplicated disease, crepitant or musical *rales, roughened breath sounds,* or *pleural friction rub* may be detected. Such signs rarely persist for more than one or two days. *Chest pain* may accompany the friction rub, or more often is substernal and referable to the trachea.

The prostrating effects of influenza are associated with *fever, chilly sensations* (seldom with rigors), *headache,* and *myalgia. Fever* usually exceeds 38° C and may reach 41° C. It is usually abrupt in its onset and decline and lasts for only two to five days in the absence of complications. *Headache* is often frontal and is of the throbbing sort associated with fever; its severity is proportional to the degree of fever. *Extraocular myalgia* is a characteristic but not universal complaint that may be elicited only by examination. *Myalgia* may be generalized or confined to the back or lower extremities. *Gastrointestinal symptoms* are uncommon, and occur more often in patients with pre-existing gastrointestinal disease.

In sum, the picture of uncomplicated influenza is that of a patient with flushed face and reddened eyes who lies flat in bed and coughs occasionally with a dry spasmodic cough. He moves about fitfully, complaining of headache or backache. By contrast, the rare patient with influenza virus pneumonia (see below) sits erect, is extremely anxious and agitated, gasps for breath, and manifests *cyanosis* of the lips and nailbeds.

Course and Complications. In both pandemic and epidemic influenza the disease, although acute and prostrating, is brief, so that it is uncommon for any symptom to last beyond seven to ten days, and fever usually subsides earlier (Fig. 3). A protracted *postinfluenzal asthenia* has been emphasized in some reports. It is not clear to what extent secondary bacterial infections or psychogenic factors contribute to the state. Nevertheless, the alerting of the patient to the possibility may save some apprehension during the convalescent period. *Encephalitis* and *myocarditis* have been described infrequently as complications of influenza, and have rarely been well documented or associated with virus isolation from the brain or heart.

The important and potentially lethal complications of influenza derive from infection of the lung, either with the influenza virus itself or with bacterial pathogens. The pulmonary complications of influenza may be considered as (1) *primary influenza virus pneumonia*, (2) *combined influenza virus and bacterial pneumonia,* and (3) *influenza complicated by secondary bacterial pneumonia.* All three types of complication are more frequent in patients with pre-existing cardiac or pulmonary disease or in women late in pregnancy. The aged, in whom apparent or inapparent chronic disease is more frequent, are also understandably more vulnerable to pulmonary complications of influenza. Neurologic complications have been temporally associated with influenza, as with other respiratory viral infections. Evidence for a clearcut causative role of the virus in such sequelae is lacking. Recently, Reye's syndrome in children (see Ch. 397) has occurred with increased frequency after influenza epidemics, especially influenza B.

Primary Influenza Virus Pneumonia. Primary influenza virus pneumonia is a severe disease that is usually fatal. Within 24 hours of the onset of typical symptoms of influenza, the patient experiences high fever (39.5 to 40° C), a cough productive of bloody sputum, and profound dyspnea and anxiety. Cyanosis is notable, and poor air exchange is indicated by the generalized pulmonary findings, which include suppression of breath sounds, expiratory wheezing, and diffuse, moist rales. Signs of consolidation are absent. Chest roentgenograms disclose diffuse bilateral nodular infiltrates that radiate outward from the hilum, sparing the lung periphery.

The patient almost always dies within five to ten days of the onset of illness after a course characterized by unremitting fever, progressive pulmonary involvement, and terminal vascular collapse (Fig. 4). Antibacterial drugs, oxygen, bronchodilators, and corticosteroids are usually unavailing.

Pathogenic bacteria are not recoverable from the sputum, blood, or lung during life or post mortem, and influenza virus is demonstrable in high concentrations in the lung.

Primary influenza virus pneumonia is restricted almost invariably to patients with pre-existing cardiac or pulmonary disease or pregnancy. Still more specifically, the victim usually has rheumatic cardiovascular disease and mitral stenosis. The predilection of this complication for the patient with mitral stenosis suggests that hemodynamic factors such as pulmonary hypertension are more important in its pathogenesis than general debility or the absence of specific immune mechanisms.

There appears to be a graded spectrum of severity of the disease caused by influenza virus, so that, intermediate between the uncomplicated case with transient rales and the fatal virus pneumonia, occasional instances of "mild segmental influenza virus pneumonia" have been described.

Combined Influenza Virus and Bacterial Pneumonia. In patients with primary influenza virus pneumonia, infection with bacterial pathogens may supervene. In such patients the characteristic and dramatic onset of the virus pneumonia may be attended or closely followed by such symptoms of bacterial pneumonia as *productive cough, shaking chills,* or *pleuritic pain.* Signs of focal consolidation may be engrafted upon the diffuse pulmonary findings of the viral infection. Pneumococcus, Staphylococcus, *Hemophilus influenzae,* or, more rarely, group A streptococci may be demonstrated by culture of lung, blood, or sputum. In 1957–1958, pneumococcus and Staphylococcus were the most frequent bacterial invaders.

The host setting and course of the combined infection are basically the same as in the pneumonia associated with influenza virus infection alone.

Influenza Complicated by Secondary Bacterial Pneumonia. Bacterial pneumonia, characterized by focal consolidation, may occur after influenza in previously healthy persons as well as in the ill and infirm. This complication is further distinguished from influenza virus pneumonia by (1) the lag between influenzal symptoms and the appearance of pneumonia, sometimes with brief interval of freedom from symptoms; (2) the presence of focal and not diffuse pulmonary involvement; and (3) the absence of influenza virus in throat washings, but the presence of bacterial pathogens in the sputum. This "late" type of pulmonary complication is by far the most common.

Diagnosis. In the context of an epidemic, influenza may easily be distinguished from other acute respiratory diseases, although diagnosis of the isolated case may be difficult. In its typical form influenza is characterized by relatively high fever, which sets it apart from the syn-

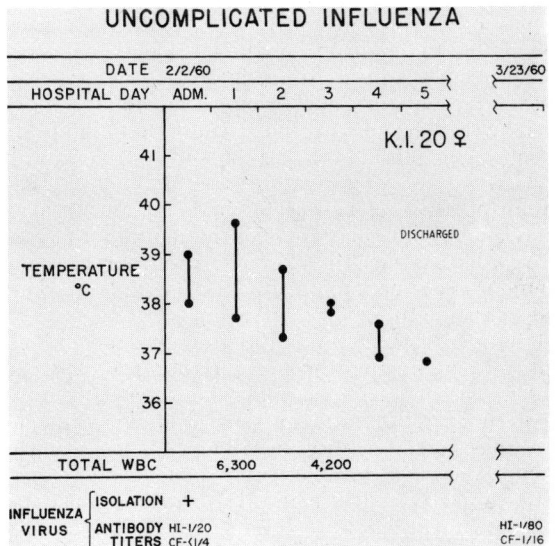

Figure 3. (From Kaye, D., et al.: Am. Rev. Respir. Dis., 85:9, 1962.)

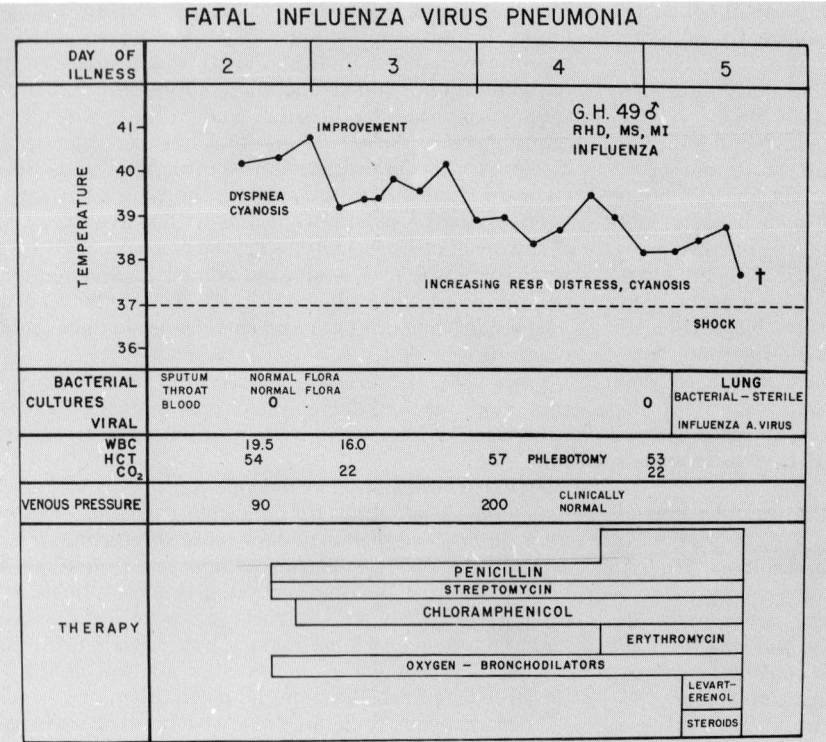

Figure 4. (From Kaye, D., et al.: Am. Rev. Respir. Dis. 85:9, 1962.)

drome of the *common cold.* With the common cold, nasal symptoms predominate, but they are usually minor in influenza. *Adenoviral infections* are the most difficult to distinguish from influenza, but, in general, fever and prostration are less, onset is less sudden, and sore throat and laryngitis are more prominent in adenoviral disease. One of the clinical forms of respiratory syncytial viral disease may closely mimic influenza. The aching, febrile, minor illnesses associated with infection by various arbo- or enteroviruses may also simulate influenza but are notably unattended by cough, although sore throat may occur. In *streptococcal pharyngitis,* the greater frequency of vomiting, the predominance of sore throat, and the occurrence of cervical adenitis and leukocytosis are helpful in differential diagnosis. *Primary atypical pneumonia* is usually distinguishable clinically from influenza virus pneumonia by its more gradual onset, purulent sputum, and indolent, ordinarily benign course.

The *definitive diagnosis* of influenza depends upon isolation of the virus from throat washings or sputum and the demonstration of an increase in specific humoral antibodies. Viral isolation is most successful in the first two to three days of illness and is best accomplished by the intra-amniotic inoculation of chick embryos. Primary cultures of mammalian cells may also be used but are less satisfactory. If virus grows to high enough titer on the first passage, isolation and identification of the agent may be accomplished within 48 to 72 hours of inoculation of the specimen. Recently, fluorescent antibody staining of exfoliated nasal epithelial cells has been applied as a quick and specific diagnostic test.

Antibody may be detected in the patient's serum by neutralization, hemagglutination-inhibition, or complement-fixation tests as early as eight to nine days after the onset of illness, but maximal response is evident only after 14 days. The diagnosis cannot be made with a single serum specimen because of the prevalence of antibody in the population; rather an *increase* in antibody titer of fourfold or more must be demonstrated by the study of two or more serum specimens obtained early in illness and in convalescence.

Prognosis. The prognosis is ordinarily favorable in this brief and self-limited disease. However, the severity of the disease is a reciprocal of host susceptibility, and the outcome may be fatal in those with prior cardiac or pulmonary disease. The prognosis is also influenced by the prevalence of potential respiratory bacterial invaders in the community and the prospects for their control.

Treatment. There is no specific treatment for influenza. The general measures used in the symptomatic treatment of other infections are useful, including especially aspirin (0.3 to 0.6 gram) for the headache, malaise, and myalgia, and codeine sulfate (0.016 to 0.064 gram) for irritability, cough, and substernal pain. Diet may be regulated by the patient with the warning that high fat foods are not well tolerated. Fluids should be given in abundance.

Routine antibacterial prophylaxis is unnecessary and inadvisable, but may be considered for those with chronic disease with the view of forestalling the sequel of pneumococcal pneumonia. In this case, full therapeutic doses of penicillin should be given.

Treatment of primary influenza viral pneumonia is highly unsatisfactory, but oxygen therapy with positive pressure breathing devices has shown some promise.

Prevention. Influenza may be prevented by the parenteral injection of vaccines of influenza viruses that have been produced in the chick embryo and rendered noninfective (inactivated) by formalin or ultraviolet irradiation. The duration of protection usually does not exceed one year under conditions of epidemic exposure. Present vaccines are principally *bivalent* in that they contain the contemporary influenza A virus (Hong Kong) component and also lesser amounts of influenza B antigen. These newer vaccines have been purified by density gradient centrifugation or chromatography and are far less toxic than preparations of the past. A so-called "hemagglutinin" vaccine contains antigens of the disrupted virus. It is of low reactogenicity, but may be less immunogenic than vaccines made from whole virus.

In experimental field trials amantadine hydrochloride has had a chemoprophylactic effect in influenza, as evidenced by lower infection rates and less severe illness in subjects who received the drug shortly before exposure to the infection. After infection, antibody titers were lower in drug-treated subjects, presumably reflecting a decreased antigenic stimulation from reduced viral replication. The drug is presumed to act by inhibiting virus penetration and not intracellularly on virus replication. Some evidence suggests that amantadine may have a slight therapeutic effect if given soon after the initiation of infection. Central nervous system toxicity may limit the usefulness of this compound in older people.

Because protection provided by influenza vaccine is transient, immunization of the general population is not feasible. The vaccine is useful in three special situations: (1) to reduce *morbidity* in groups essential for the community life, such as policemen, physicians, and the military; (2) to reduce *morbidity* in groups particularly subject to the occurrence of epidemics, as in boarding schools, institutions, and military camps; and (3) to prevent disease and hence reduce *mortality* in those peculiarly vulnerable to the effects of infection, especially those with chronic cardiac and pulmonary disease. In these groups, especially the latter, vaccine should be administered annually in the autumn.

Live virus vaccines for influenza are in use in the Soviet Union, but are still under experimental evaluation in the United States.

International Conference on Hong Kong Influenza. Bull. W.H.O., 41:335, 1969.

Kilbourne, E. D.: The molecular epidemiology of influenza. J. Infect. Dis., 127:478, 1973.

Louria, D. B., Blumenfeld, H. L., Ellis, J. T., Kilbourne, E. D., and Rogers, D. E.: Studies on influenza in the pandemic of 1957–1958. II. Pulmonary complications of influenza. J. Clin. Invest., 38:213, 1959.

Smith, W., Andrewes, C. H., and Laidlaw, P. P.: A virus obtained from influenzal patients. Lancet, 2:66, 1933.

VIRAL DISEASES THAT MAY INVOLVE THE CENTRAL NERVOUS SYSTEM

For a detailed description of these diseases, the reader is referred to Ch. 387 to 403.

VIRAL DISEASES CHARACTERIZED BY CUTANEOUS LESIONS

118. MEASLES
(Moribilli, Rubeola)

Edwin D. Kilbourne

Definition. Measles is an extremely contagious, febrile disease of high morbidity characterized by rash and catarrhal inflammation of the eyes and respiratory tract. It is principally a benign disease of children, but may afflict with equal frequency persons of any age not previously immunized by infection or vaccination.

Etiology. Measles is caused by a medium-sized RNA *paramyxovirus* approximately 1400 Å in diameter. The virus is of a single antigenic type and resembles other paramyxoviruses (e.g., parainfluenza and mumps viruses) in structure and biologic activity, except that it lacks a neuraminidase. Thus measles virus is an enveloped, lipid-containing virus that is released from the infected cell by budding evagination. The virus bears external spikes that contain a hemagglutinin capable of agglutinating erythrocytes of certain primates. Hemolytic and fusing activity is dissociable from the virus particle. In contrast to the genome of influenza viruses, the RNA is not segmented and high frequency genetic recombination of the virus does not occur. Antigenic variation of the virus has not been noted. Measles virus is antigenically and biologically related to the viruses of canine distemper and bovine rinderpest.

Measles virus replicates most readily in primary cultures of human embryonic tissue or primate kidney cells. However, adaptation of virus to a variety of primary or continuous mammalian and avian cell cultures has been achieved. (Vaccine viruses are propagated in chick embryo cells.)

Subhuman primates have long been known to be susceptible to measles; recently, propagation of the virus in the brains of mice, hamsters, and ferrets has been achieved, demonstrating its neurotropic potential.

Prevalence and Epidemiology. Measles is a disease of cosmopolitan distribution, endemic in all but isolated populations. It may occur at any time of the year, but most outbreaks are in the late winter and early spring, with a peak at the end of April. The disease recurs in epidemic cycles at two- to three-year intervals in most civilized communities that have been studied. This epidemic periodicity is best explained as a result of the introduction of new susceptibles into the population by birth or ingress from other areas. When the proportion of nonimmunes reaches a certain crucial concentration (45 to 50 per cent), disease and coincident dissemination of virus may occur to produce an epidemic. It is likely that virus is introduced from sources external to the involved population, probably by incoming susceptibles. Isolated communities such as the Faröe Islands (Panum) are infrequently attacked by measles, at which times manifest illness appears in virtually all persons not previously infected. In Greenland, a country not known to have been invaded previously by the disease, an epidemic resulted in overt measles in 99.9 per cent of the indigenous population (Christiansen et al.).

Throughout most of the world, measles is a disease of children; most adults possess acquired immunity. Beyond the age of ten more than 90 per cent of the population have specific antibody. Although the peak attack rate coincides with the beginning of school (age six) in technologically advanced societies, it occurs between the ages of two and three in most developing countries. Morbidity and mortality rates do not appear to be influenced by sex or race. Case fatality rates are highest in children less than five years of age, and are also relatively high in the aged. Congenital infection has occurred.

There is no evidence that the virus may vary in virulence in nature. The oft-cited and notorious virulence of the disease in primitive, isolated, or crowded populations may be explained as a corollary of (1) more prevalent infection of feeble and aged adults, (2) poor environmental conditions, (3) inadequate medical care, and (4) secondary bacterial infections. A strikingly increased mortality rate is observed in areas such as West Africa in which protein-calorie malnutrition is prevalent. Because measles virus per se rarely induces fatal disease, it is evident that fatalities attributable to measles may vary in incidence according to the prevalence of bacterial pathogens and the resistance of the population to their presence.

Communicability.   Measles is one of the most contagious of infections. Demonstration of virus in nasopharyngeal secretions is in accord with epidemiologic evidence that infection is disseminated and acquired by the respiratory tract. Close physical proximity or direct person-to-person contact is the usual requisite for infection.

Immunity.   An unmodified attack of measles is usually followed by lifelong immunity. This observation is in accord with the observed persistence of both complement-fixing and neutralizing antibodies after infection and the relatively high titer of antibodies present even in older persons. The mechanism of persistent immunity after measles is undefined. Although persistence of infective virus after infection seems not to occur, the internal nucleocapsid of measles virus or a closely related variant is demonstrable years after infection in the brain and peripheral lymph nodes of those rare individuals afflicted with subacute sclerosing panencephalitis (SSPE) (see Ch. 401). Thus the potential for viral persistence exists, and in those afflicted with SSPE, antibody levels to measles virus are higher than in those who have experienced uncomplicated measles.

A more likely explanation for the persistent immunity in measles is the maintenance of such immunity by subclinical exogenous reinfection. Careful studies of isolated or closed populations after administration of live virus vaccine have demonstrated a more rapid decline of antibody titer than in populations in which measles virus is circulating. Anamnestic antibody response in the absence of disease has been shown in immune contacts of patients with measles. Thus achievement of eradication of the virus may be compromised as vaccination (see below) is more and more effective in curtailing the circulation of the wild virus; then the booster immunization provided by natural reinfection will become inoperative, and repeated vaccination in the same subject may be required. Passively transferred maternal antibody protects the young infant from measles but also reduces the possibility of effective immunization by live virus vaccines at that age.

Pathology and Physiologic Responses.   Pathologic changes in fatal measles usually represent the compound effect of viral and secondary bacterial infection. Pneumonia is almost invariably present; it is most frequently interstitial, but may produce purulent exudate within the alveoli. More representative are changes of the uncomplicated viral disease within the tonsillar, nasopharyngeal, and appendiceal tissue removed during the prodrome. These changes consist of subepithelial round cell infiltration and the presence of multinucleated giant cells. The latter are so characteristic that skilled pathologists have predicted the development of rash from their presence in surgical specimens. Similar cells are commonly observed in tissue cultures infected with measles virus. Cytoplasmic and nuclear inclusions may be seen in epithelial cells. The lesions clinically apparent as Koplik's spots derive from inflammatory mononuclear cell infiltration of buccal submucous glands and necrosis of focal vesicular lesions of the mucosa. Rash is the result of proliferation of capillary endothelial cells in the corium and the coincident exudation of serum, and occasionally erythrocytes, into the epidermis. Viral microtubular aggregates within nuclei and cytoplasm of syncytial giant cells of skin lesions and Koplik's spots attest to the direct role of the virus in the production of these lesions.

No consistent or characteristic physiologic aberrations are observed with measles. The transient hemoconcentration and albuminuria found with other febrile diseases may occur. A normal total leukocyte count or leukopenia is observed throughout the febrile period. Initially, the leukopenia is occasioned by a decline in lymphocytes on the first day of fever; subsequently, granulocytopenia ensues as well. The incubation period is characterized by neutrophilia, and convalescence by a relative lymphocytosis. Measles virus has been isolated from the leukocytic fraction of blood, and is propagable in suspensions of leukocytes in vitro. A false-positive serologic test for syphilis may be observed.

Hormone-Like Effects of Measles Infection.   Several striking physiologic effects of measles, although poorly understood, mimic the influence of corticotrophin or the adrenal corticosteroids. These are transient suppression of the tuberculin reaction (observed also with measles vaccines), improvement in eczema and allergic asthma, delay in wound healing, and the induction of remissions in leukemia, Hodgkin's disease, Burkitt's lymphoma, and lipoid nephrosis. Whether these effects are directly attributable to the virus or are hormonally mediated is not known. In recent in vitro experiments, addition of measles virus to human lymphocytes depressed the usual proliferative response of such cells to phytohemagglutinin P or antigen.

Clinical Manifestations.   After an incubation period that averages 11 days, measles becomes clinically manifest with symptoms of fever, malaise, myalgia, and headache. Within hours *ocular symptoms* of photophobia and burning pain are evidenced by conjunctival injection, tearing, and exudate in the conjunctival sac. Concomitantly, or soon thereafter, *catarrhal inflammation of the respiratory tract* is manifested by sneezing, coughing, and nasal discharge. Less commonly, hoarseness and aphonia may reflect laryngeal involvement. In this prodromal stage of one to four days' duration, petechial lesions of the palate and pharynx or tiny white spots on the buccal mucosa (*Koplik's spots*) may herald the appearance of skin rash. The white lesions described by Koplik characteristically occur lateral to the molar teeth, and typically are mounted on red areolae of injected mucosa, which may coalesce to form a diffuse red background. Not invariably present, they constitute a valuable, if not pathognomonic, diagnostic sign. The enanthem may involve other mucous membranes such as the vaginal lining. It may "overlap" the subsequent appearance of the cutaneous rash by one to three days. Rarely, a transient, erythematous exanthema may occur in the prodromal period.

Upper: Early measles eruption. (Reproduction from Therapeutic Notes, by Courtesy of Parke, Davis & Company.) *Lower:* Koplik's spots in measles (Hecker, Trumpp, and Abt).

The *rash* of measles follows the prodromal symptoms by two to four days, occasionally as late as seven days. It first appears behind the ears or on the face as a blotchy erythema, spreads downward to cover the trunk, and finally is manifest on the extremities. The hands and feet may escape involvement. Initially, the eruption consists of discrete, reddish-brown macules that blanch with pressure. Subsequently, these lesions become slightly elevated, tend to coalesce, and may develop a hemorrhagic, nonblanching component. Rash is sometimes very extensive in children with protein-calorie malnutrition, and skin lesions associated with kwashiorkor may develop at the site of the exanthem. The rash fades in the order of its appearance; its disappearance about five days after onset is attended by a fine, powdery desquamation that spares the hands and feet. At its maximum the exanthema usually marks the termination of malaise and fever in the uncomplicated illness.

The *fever* of measles is commonly of the typhoidal, progressively rising type, and falls by lysis. It persists for about six days, and frequently reaches 39.5° C. In the adult, fever may follow rather than antedate the catarrhal symptoms. Throughout the febrile period, productive *cough* and auscultatory evidence of bronchiolitis may be evident. These manifestations may persist after defervescence, and cough is often the last symptom to disappear. It is probable that bronchopulmonary symptomatology is an integral part of the primary viral infection; roentgenographic evidence of pulmonary involvement is frequently seen in the uncomplicated disease in the absence of leukocytosis and obvious bacterial infection.

Complications. It is difficult to distinguish between those complications directly attributable to the virus of measles and those resulting from secondary bacterial infections. The persistence or recurrence of fever and the occurrence of leukocytosis are presumptive evidence of the usual bacterial sequelae of *otitis media* or *pneumonia*. The pneumonia resembles other forms of viral pneumonia and is often caused solely by a specific reaction to the measles virus. Superimposed bacterial infection is common, however, and accounts for most of the severe or fatal cases. Pneumococcus, *Streptococcus hemolyticus, Staphylococcus aureus,* and *Hemophilus influenzae* are the usual secondary invaders. The incidence of bacterial complications is increased by crowding, debility, and the prevalence of bacterial pathogens in the population. Bacterially engendered sequelae may be unduly frequent in crowded contagious disease hospitals.

Serious complications directly related to the measles virus are rare. *Laryngitis* of sufficient severity to embarrass respiration has been observed, and may warrant tracheostomy. *Electrocardiographic abnormalities* may be found in as many as 30 per cent of children, but clinical evidence of cardiac disease is meager in such cases. *Abdominal pain* or *diarrhea* may be related to invasion of lymphoid tissue of the appendix or Peyer's patches. These symptoms may lead to unnecessary surgery before the appearance of the typical rash. The frequency of stomatitis and gastrointestinal symptoms is greater in malnourished children in tropical areas and may reflect coincident bacterial and parasitic infection.

Encephalomyelitis. A rare (0.1 per cent) but serious consequence of measles is a demyelinating encephalomyelitis that may appear from 1 to 14 days after the onset of infection. This complication is associated with a recurrence of fever, and headache, vomiting, and stiff neck. Stupor and convulsions occasionally follow. Localizing neurologic symptoms may or may not be present. Death ensues in about 10 per cent of patients; about half of survivors suffer permanent residuals of varying severity. Measles virus has been recovered from the brain of a patient with fatal measles "postinfectious" encephalitis six weeks after onset of measles. Recently, abnormal electroencephalograms were recorded in 51 per cent of children with measles *without evidence of encephalitis.* In some of the children the abnormal encephalographic findings were persistent. As noted above, the presence of virus has been demonstrated in patients with subacute sclerosing panencephalitis.

Other late sequelae of measles are thrombocytopenic purpura and exacerbation or activation of pre-existing pulmonary tuberculosis.

Giant-Cell Pneumonia. In children with severe disease involving the recticuloendothelial system (especially leukemia), measles virus may induce an interstitial pneumonia characterized by giant cells and intracellular inclusion bodies. The disease is usually fatal; if the patient survives, persistence of virus and poor antibody formation are evident in convalescence. The pneumonia may occur in the absence of rash so that its etiologic relation to measles may be unsuspected.

Measles Modified by Vaccine or Antibody Administration. Attenuation of the natural disease by antibody prophylaxis may result in an illness of lessened severity comparable with the milder infection of the maternally immunized newborn. Fever alone may be observed, but some degree of exanthema is usually apparent. Koplik's spots may not appear. In general, the course is truncated and relatively uncomplicated. Similar attenuated disease may occur in children partially immunized with inactivated viral vaccine.

Unfavorably Modified Measles—A New Disease. After administration of inactivated measles vaccine (no longer in general use), infection of vaccinees with either live measles vaccine or wild-type natural measles virus led to the development of a new syndrome characterized by dermal hypersensitivity to measles virus and an atypical (petechial, vesicular, or urticarial) rash atypical in distribution. In some cases pulmonary complications occurred. The exact mechanism of this reaction is unknown, but it is almost certainly a manifestation of delayed hypersensitivity to the viral proteins engendered by alum-precipitated inactivated viral vaccine. No such sequelae have followed use of live virus vaccine (see below).

Diagnosis. The experienced layman can diagnose typical measles. The querulous, bleary-eyed child, his face blotched and his nose crusted with exudate, presents a characteristic, if miserable, picture as he breathes open-mouthed between paroxysms of sneezing and coughing. The severity of the catarrhal symptoms distinguishes the disease from other eruptive fevers. In the prodromal period the diagnosis should be suggested by (1) fever higher than that of the usual common cold, (2) known measles in the community, and (3) Koplik's spots on the buccal mucosa.

Differential diagnosis (see accompanying table) includes consideration of rubella, scarlet fever, exanthema subitum, infectious mononucleosis, secondary syphilis, drug eruptions, and infection with certain coxsackie- and echoviruses. Of value in excluding these possibilities are the milder course and pinker rash of rubella, the sore throat and leukocytosis of scarlet fever, and serologic tests for infectious mononucleosis and syphilis. The rash of exanthema subitum does not appear until the termination of fever. Fever, enanthema, and catarrh are uncommon with the cutaneous manifestations of drug hypersensitivity.

Specific Diagnosis. Specific diagnosis depends on the isolation of measles virus from throat washings, blood, or urine by inoculation of various types of tissue culture with materials obtained during the first five days of illness. Increase in specific antibody may be detected as early as the first or second day of rash by the complement-fixation test. Antibody is also demonstrable by neutralization and hemagglutination-inhibition procedures.

Presumptive diagnosis may be made if giant cells are detected in stained smears of nasal exudate in the pre-eruptive period.

Prognosis. Uncomplicated measles is rarely fatal, and complete recovery from the disease is the rule. Fatalities are almost always the result of secondary streptococcal or pneumococcal pneumonia, occurring principally in children below the age of five who become infected after the dissipation of passive neonatal immunity. Mortality in developing countries may be 250 times that observed in the United States or northern Europe. Case fatality rates are also high in elderly and tuberculous patients. Congestive cardiac failure is a common cause of death in patients over 50 years old.

Antimicrobial drugs effective against the usual secondary invaders have reduced the case fatality rate of measles sharply. The incidence of otitis media and pneumonia may be lowered by the prophylactic use of penicillin or a tetracycline early in illness.

Encephalitis occurs as frequently in mild as in severe measles (i.e., about one in a thousand cases). However, the incidence of neurologic sequelae after administration of attenuated live virus vaccine is only one in a million.

Treatment. There is no specific treatment for measles.

Symptomatic Therapy. In the absence of complica-

A Guide to the Differential Diagnosis of Measles

	Conjunctivitis	Rhinitis	Sore Throat	Enanthem	Leukocytosis	Specific Laboratory Tests Available
Measles	++	+	0	+	0	+
Rubella	±	±	±	±	0	+
Exanthema subitum	±	±	0	0	0	0
Enterovirus infection	0	±	±	0	±	+
Scarlet fever	±	±	++	0	+	+
Infectious mononucleosis	0	0	+	0	±	+
Drug rash	0	0	0	0	0	0

0 Not usually present; no test available.   +   Present; test available.
± Variable in occurrence.   ++ Present and severe.

tions, bed rest is the essence of treatment in this usually benign, self-limited disease. Codeine sulfate (0.015 to 0.06 gram) is useful in the amelioration of headache and myalgia and is effective in the management of cough. Aspirin (0.3 to 0.6 gram) may be employed for its analgesic and antipyretic actions. Diet should be unrestricted. Bright light is not an ocular hazard, but photophobia may require darkening of the patient's room.

Antimicrobial Prophylaxis. The course of uncomplicated measles is not influenced by antimicrobial therapy. In common practice the incidence of serious bacterial infections is not sufficient to justify the routine prophylactic use of antimicrobials. Certain special circumstances may warrant full therapeutic dosage with penicillin or the tetracyclines in anticipation of the potentially fatal sequelae of pneumococcal or beta-hemolytic streptococcal infections. These circumstances include treatment of the chronically ill, the very young, or the aged, and the treatment of patients under crowded conditions that foster the increase and dissemination of pathogenic bacteria, as may occur in contagious disease hospitals. If careful observation of the patient is possible, rational therapy is based on the prompt recognition and etiologic definition of complications, followed by initiation of the appropriate antimicrobial drug in proper dosage.

Prevention. Vaccination. Highly effective vaccines are now available for the prevention of measles. Most are derived from the Edmonston strain of measles virus isolated in the laboratory of Dr. John Enders. This strain, although it proved very effective in early trials as a live virus vaccine, produced febrile and other reactions (attenuated measles) with such high frequency that it has been supplanted by *"further attenuated" (live virus) vaccines* that are almost as effective as the original vaccine in inducing immunity. These live virus vaccines produce immunity by infection, and therefore need be given only as a single injection. They induce antibody response of somewhat lesser magnitude than that following natural infection. In children over one year of age, seroconversion after vaccination is 90 to 97 per cent. Although a gradual fall in antibody titer occurs in the absence of exposure to wild type virus (see Epidemiology; Immunity), serum antibody is demonstrable in most individuals eight to ten years after a single administration of vaccine. Reinfection with disease has occurred in a small fraction of vaccinated subjects under epidemic conditions. The vaccine virus is not contagious.

Live virus vaccine is given as a single parenteral injection to persons more than one year of age. The coincident injection of standardized *measles immune globulin* (0.01 ml per pound of body weight) at a different site will greatly reduce the incidence of fever and other symptoms. If *live "further attenuated" vaccine* is used under the same conditions, gamma globulin is unnecessary.

Contraindications to live virus vaccine include pregnancy, leukemia and other systemic malignant diseases, active tuberculosis, and administration of resistance-depressing drugs such as corticosteroids and antimetabolites.

Inactivated vaccine produces impermanent immunity and unfavorably alters response to later infection. It therefore is no longer recommended (see Complications, above).

Eradication of measles through administration of live virus vaccines is a scientifically reasonable possibility. The introduction of immunization in the United States in 1963 led to a decrease in annual incidence of from 4,000,000 to 250,000 cases in five years. However, a subsequent resurgence of disease was undoubtedly attributable to underutilization of vaccine in susceptible groups, particularly nonwhite populations in impoverished circumstances. The reinstitution of Federal funds for measles vaccine in 1971 reversed the upward trend of disease in the following year.

Christiansen, P. E., et al.: An epidemic of measles in southern Greenland, 1951. Acta Med. Scand., 144:313, 430, 450, 1952–53.

Enders, J. F., Katz, S. L., Milovanovic, M. V., and Holloway, A.: Studies on an attenuated measles-virus vaccine. I. Development and preparation of the vaccine: Technics for assay of effects of vaccination. N. Engl. J. Med., 263:153, 1960.

Koplik, H.: The diagnosis of the invasion of measles from a study of the exanthema as it appears on the buccal mucous membrane. Arch. Pediat., 13:918, 1896.

Linnemann, C. C., Jr.: Measles vaccine: Immunity, reinfection and revaccination. Am. J. Epidemiol., 97:365, 1973.

Panum, P. L.: Observations Made During the Epidemic of Measles on the Faröe Islands. Delta Omega Society, 1940.

Tyler, H. R.: Neurological complications of rubeola (measles). Medicine, 36:147, 1957.

119. RUBELLA
(German Measles)

Edwin D. Kilbourne

Definition. Rubella is an acute, benign, contagious disease of children and young adults. The cardinal manifestations of the illness are a pale pink rash and posterior cervical lymphadenitis. Paradoxically, this mild disease is one of the few viral infections convincingly associated with the genesis of fetal abnormalities. When infection is acquired in utero, it often results in generalized disease of the infant and protracted excretion of virus after birth. Accordingly, recognition and prevention of the disease are matters of far-reaching consequence.

Etiology. Rubella virus is a small, spherical RNA virus with a mean diameter of 550 to 600 Å. The particle is ether sensitive—an attribute of lipid-containing enveloped viruses. The virus develops by budding from marginal and intracytoplasmic membranes. Classification of the virus is uncertain at present, but similarities of structure and development to certain group A togaviruses (including the infectious nature of its isolated RNA) have been noted. (There is no evidence of arthropod transmission.) Thus the virus is clearly unrelated to the virus of measles.

The virus agglutinates the erythrocytes of newly hatched chicks—a characteristic that permits measurement of both virus and antibody. Rubella virus replicates with the production of cytopathic effects in a number of commonly employed cell culture systems, including African green monkey and human diploid cells. Virus replication and production of embryopathic effects similar to those in humans have been experimentally induced in rats.

Incidence and Epidemiology. Accurate information on the incidence of rubella is not available, but approximately 80 per cent of young adults have specific hemagglutination-inhibiting (HI) antibodies against the virus. The mildness and brevity of clinical signs of rubella may confound the diagnosis and reporting of many instances of infection. Studies of the experimental disease lend support to prior clinical evidence that infection may occur without rash, and indicate a further diagnostic pitfall. It can be said, however, that the disease is seen on every continent, may occur in epidemic form, and has its highest incidence in the early spring. The disease is less frequently acquired in childhood than measles, as is attested by serologic studies and by the fact that rubella is more common than measles in young adults. The higher incidence of infection in younger age groups in institutional outbreaks argues against a greater susceptibility of the adult. It is probable that rubella is spread by the respiratory route by close and sustained personal contact. The usual infection is contagious during the period of prodromal symptoms and for as long as seven days after the appearance of rash. However, it is now recognized that the infant with congenitally acquired infection may excrete virus for months after birth and is contagious during this time. The epidemiologic implications of this fact—first established in the large epidemic of 1963–1964—are yet to be determined. There is evidence that the newborn may be unusually contagious, and that although he may have no obvious stigmata of infection, yet he may be shedding virus.

Immunity is lasting. HI antibodies have been demonstrated 30 years after initial infection. Authenticated second attacks are rare, and require serologic documentation because of the nebulous nature of the clinical syndrome. *Subclinical* reinfection demonstrated by increase in IgG serum antibody has been documented with increasing frequency as better serologic methods and increased surveillance have become available. Reinfection occurs most commonly in crowded populations in which the density of infection and probably of spread are high. It is important to note that most such reinfections are not associated with viremia and thus probably pose little threat in pregnant women. As in many other infections, IgM response serves to distinguish primary from reinfection. Presumably, as in measles, inapparent infections may boost immunity throughout life. Immunity that follows artificial immunization with live virus vaccine is of a lesser degree. (See Prevention, below.)

Pathology.   Death from uncomplicated postnatally acquired rubella is unknown. Histologic changes characteristic of the disease have not been demonstrated. The onset of disease is attended by leukopenia resulting from a decrease in both lymphocytes and neutrophils. After five days, absolute lymphocytosis is manifest. The total leukocyte count is normal at the tenth day.

Congenital Rubella.   Necropsies of fetal and infantile victims of maternal infection have shown a variety of embryonal defects related to developmental arrest involving all three germ layers. Those defects most consistently associated with maternal rubella are microcephaly, cataract, patency of the ductus arteriosus, and defects of the interventricular septum. However, recent studies have revealed a wide spectrum of tissue damage in association with virologically proved disease of varying severity. In some infants hepatic and renal degeneration and myocardial necrosis without inflammation have been noted, whereas in others thrombocytopenia and purpura may be the sole abnormality. It has been proposed that the generalized visceral involvement and characteristic residua of the disease may result from a sequence of platelet damage, intravascular coagulation, and thrombosis. Another theory holds that the smaller size of the rubella-infected infant and some abnormali-

ties may reflect inhibition of multiplication of embryonic cells by the virus.

Clinical Manifestations.   *Postnatally Acquired Rubella.*   Fourteen to 21 days after exposure to the infection, the onset of rubella is evidenced by symptoms variable in their occurrence and severity. Cough, sore throat, and coryza may initiate the illness, but are often absent; headache, malaise, and myalgia may precede the eruption, especially in young adults. Commonly, fever and obvious enlargement of posterior cervical nodes antedate the appearance of the rash. Fever, when present, rarely exceeds 38° C and seldom persists beyond 48 hours. Injection of the bulbar conjunctivae may be noted. Palpable, tender, and occasionally visible lymphadenopathy involves postauricular and suboccipital nodes with sufficient frequency to be an important diagnostic sign. Generalized peripheral lymphadenitis, and, more rarely, splenomegaly, may occur.

The exanthema of rubella is usually apparent within 24 hours of the first symptoms as a faint macular erythema that first involves the face and neck. Characterized by its brevity and evanescence, it spreads rapidly to the trunk and extremities, sometimes leaving one site even as it appears at the next. The pink macules that constitute the rash blanch with pressure and rarely stain the skin. Rubella virus has been isolated from the skin lesions. Diffuse erythema on the second day of rash may closely simulate scarlet fever. The eruption has vanished by the third day. Rubella may occur without rash. An enanthema has been described that is inconstant in form and occurrence, and lacks the premonitory significance of the Koplik spots of measles. The lesions consist of red macules that usually involve the soft palate.

Complications.   Recovery is almost always prompt and uneventful, although relapse occurs with greater frequency than in most viral diseases (5 to 8 per cent). Secondary bacterial infections rarely occur. Rare complications are arthralgia, neuritis, gingivitis, thrombocytopenic purpura, and increased capillary fragility. Heart block has been described. A *meningoencephalitis* of short duration may occur one to six days after the appearance of rash. Its incidence is estimated at 1 in 6000 cases, and it is fatal in approximately 20 per cent of those afflicted. Rubella encephalopathy is not associated with demyelinization (in contrast to other postviral encephalitides). Survivors may have electroencephalographic abnormalities, but intellectual function seems to be preserved.

Congenital Rubella.   The fortuitous coincidence of the development of cell culture systems for the isolation of rubella virus and the occurrence of a global epidemic of rubella (in 1963–1964) demonstrated that the classic ocular and cardiac "teratogenic" effects of rubella are but isolated manifestations of a continuing and persisting fetal infection. It is now clear that congenital transplacental infection of the fetus occurs as a consequence of maternal infection (which may or may not be clinically evident), usually in the first trimester of pregnancy. Virus is demonstrable in placental and fetal tissues obtained by therapeutic abortion at that time. If pregnancy is not interrupted (and spontaneous abortion is uncommon), fetal infection persists, and upon delivery of the infant, virus is recoverable from the throat, urine, feces, conjunctivae, bone marrow, and cerebrospinal fluid of the living infant and from most organs at autopsy. About 10 to 15 per cent of infants born to mothers infected in the first trimester of pregnancy have stigmata of infection readily recognizable in the first year of life. These include *cardiac lesions, cataracts, glaucoma, microphthalmia,* and *esophageal atresia.* Most infants in whom virus is detectable do not have evidence of disease at birth or may simply have a lower than normal birth weight. In others, disease of intermediate severity has been recently recognized. Most prominent of the newly observed manifestations is *thrombocytopenic purpura,* which disappears soon after birth. *Hepatosplenomegaly* may persist for months. Other signs include *corneal clouding, fullness of the fontanels, lesions of the long bones,* and *electroencephalographic abnormalities.*

A most striking finding has been the persistence of virus in the pharynx, gastrointestinal tract, and cerebrospinal fluid for as long as one year after birth (9 per cent). Infective virus was present in a congenital cataract after three years, and in the urine of a victim of congenital rubella 29 years after her birth. This evidence of continuing viral synthesis occurs coincidentally with circulating antibody (initially of maternal origin) and originally suggested a form of "immunologic tolerance" to the virus. However, it has been shown that the character of the antibody changes during the first year from IgG (presumably maternal) to IgM, indicating a primary response of the infant to the persisting viral antigen. Studies of older infants and children with stigmata of congenital rubella show them to be free of demonstrable virus and to possess the IgG immunoglobulins that characteristically persist after other viral infections. The defect in host response that is responsible for viral persistence has not yet been defined.

Diagnosis. Rubella may be diagnosed clinically with assurance only during an epidemic. It may be difficult to distinguish from mild or modified measles, infectious mononucleosis, or scarlet fever. Distinction from measles may be made on the basis of pinker, nonstaining rash, the milder course, and the lesser catarrh of rubella. Sore throat is a more prominent complaint in scarlet fever; the course of infectious mononucleosis is often more protracted, and splenomegaly is more frequent than in rubella. Specific diagnosis of rubella is made by isolation of the virus in any of several cell culture systems, or by demonstration of neutralizing, hemagglutination-inhibiting, or complement-fixing antibody response during infection. The high incidence of dermatoglyphic abnormalities (50 per cent) and increased percentage of chromosome breaks described in patients following congenital rubella may prove to have diagnostic value when studied further.

Prognosis. Complete recovery from postnatally acquired rubella is almost invariable. The rare deaths attributable to rubella follow the infrequent complication of meningoencephalitis. Infection in pregnancy constitutes a hazard to the fetus but not to the mother.

Treatment. There is no specific treatment for the disease. Few patients suffer discomfort severe enough to warrant symptomatic medication. Headache and myalgia may be controlled by aspirin; bed rest is advisable for the duration of the fever.

Prevention. *Passive Immunization. Administration of gamma globulin to the pregnant woman may only mask her symptoms of infection yet not protect the fetus from viral invasion.* Its use may thus only obscure the picture and confound decision about the need for therapeutic abortion. Hence the practice seems inadvisable and is now seldom carried out.

Active Immunization. Rubella may be prevented in children and adults by the parenteral administration of attenuated live virus vaccines either produced in duck embryo cell cultures and derived from passage of virus in African green monkey kidney cells or derived from primary rabbit cell kidney passage. Seroconversion rates after immunization are approximately 95 per cent. As with other live virus vaccines, serum antibody titers are lower than those that follow natural infection. However, antibody persists for at least four years after vaccination, but the permanence of vaccine-induced immunity must still be established by further observation. Natural infection of individuals immunized with vaccine is not uncommon, although such infection is usually asymptomatic. In children, vaccination is attended by little, if any, reaction; but in women, rash, malaise, arthralgia, and mild, acute arthritis occur frequently, the incidence being directly related to age. For this reason, and in order to induce "herd immunity" to depress circulation of the virus, it is currently recommended in the United States that immunization be carried out principally in childhood. However, since the epidemic threshold—at least in semiclosed populations—is low (between 4.7 and 8.4 per cent), containment of the disease by mass immunization may prove difficult. A high level of vaccine-induced immunity in elementary school children (83 per cent) failed to prevent the spread of rubella in one community. Despite the higher reaction rates in adults, it seems advisable to immunize adolescent girls or women of childbearing age for whose unborn children rubella may have tragic consequences. Of this population, only seronegative individuals should be immunized, and contraception (when appropriate) should be carried out for at least three months after vaccination. The inadvertent administration of vaccine to pregnant women has demonstrated that attenuated vaccine viruses can infect the fetus and thus have the *potential* for teratogenesis.

Cooper, L. Z.: Rubella: A preventable cause of birth defects. *In* Bergsma, D. (ed.): Birth Defects: Original Article Series, Vol. IV, No. 7, Intrauterine Infections. The National Foundation, December, 1968, pp. 23–35.
Gregg, N. M.: Congenital cataract following German measles in the mother. Trans. Ophthal. Soc. Austral., 3:35, 1941.
Horzinek, M., Maess, J., and Laufs, R.: Studies on the substructure of togaviruses. Arch. Gesamte Virusforsch., 33:306, 1971.
Leedom, J. M., Wilkins, J., Portnoy, B., and Salvatore, M. A.: Important assumptions, extrapolations, and established facts which underlie the use of live rubella virus vaccines. Am. J. Epidemiol., 92:151, 1970.
Proceedings of the International Conference on Rubella Immunization. Am. J. Dis. Child., 118, July 1969.

120. EXANTHEMATA ASSOCIATED WITH ENTEROVIRAL INFECTIONS

Edwin D. Kilbourne

Infection with any of a number of enteroviruses may be associated with erythematous, macular eruptions. In some patients occipital and cervical lymphadenopathy may be noted, so that the infection may closely simulate rubella. However, differential diagnosis is aided by the frequency of a vesicular ulcerative enanthem and aseptic meningitis in patients with enteroviral disease and also by its summertime occurrence. Those enteroviruses most frequently associated with rash are the group A coxsackieviruses 9 and 16, and (quite fortuitously) echoviruses bearing the same numerical designations (i.e., echovirus 9 and echovirus 16). The eruptions associated with the coxsackieviruses may include small vesicles, especially notable with coxsackievirus A16 (hand, foot, and mouth disease). Echovirus 16 and coxsackievirus B5 produce eruptions that mimic roseola infantum. Rash seems to be more common in children than in adults.

Lerner, M. A., Klein, J. O., Cherry, J. D., and Finland, M.: New viral exanthems. N. Engl. J. Med., 269:678, 1963.
Wenner, H. A., and Lou, T. Y.: Virus diseases associated with cutaneous eruptions. Prog. Med. Virol., 5:219, 1963.

121. VARIOLA AND VACCINIA

C. Henry Kempe

INTRODUCTION AND HISTORY

Immunization against the dread disease of smallpox is perhaps the most widely applied immunization procedure currently in use. Over the past 150 years it has demonstrated its effectiveness beyond question. The vaccinia virus (Poxvirus officinale), which is in effect a laboratory strain carried for many generations in a variety of laboratory animals, differs from the newly isolated virus of cowpox (Poxvirus bovis), which was originally employed by Jenner (1798) and his predecessors for the immunization of man against the smallpox virus (Poxvirus variolae).

Smallpox was described in detail by Rhazes in the tenth century, and had been described previously by Galen in the second century. Spread from Asia to Europe and North Africa occurred in the Middle Ages, and the disease was prevalent in the sixteenth century. At approximately the same time the disease was introduced into the West Indies by African slaves and from there into Mexico and South America. The best studied epidemics are those in the eighteenth century in England when over 90 per cent of the cases occurred in children under ten years of age and when smallpox accounted for one third of all deaths in children. Smallpox occurred in epidemic form less frequently in North America until 1752 when over 30 per cent of the inhabitants of Boston, Massachusetts, were affected and the mortality rate was over 30 per cent (Creighton, 1894). In 1721 deliberate inoculation of smallpox as protection against the natural disease was introduced in England. It consisted of the inoculation of pustular material by puncturing the skin. This resulted in a febrile disease after an eight-day incubation and a general eruption on the ninth day. The mortality rate from this procedure was 1 to 2 per cent, and it is stated that 17 of 897 inoculated persons died from the disease (Woodville, 1796). Needless to say, modified infection did give rise to highly virulent natural disease in susceptible contacts. In 1738 variolation was successfully used in Charleston, South Carolina, with material that had been allowed to dry. With better care of the patients, the death rate was somewhat reduced; it was thought to be about one or two out of 500, whereas the mortality from the naturally acquired smallpox was 10 to 20 per cent. Variolation was followed by inoculation of cowpox after widespread acceptance of Jenner's studies published in 1798. In truth, this practice had been current among a number of colleagues of Jenner's at a previous time, and he made no claim to originality. Jenner, however, did play a decisive role in popularizing this method of protection against smallpox, and variolation was outlawed in England in 1840. It is possible that the endemism of smallpox in England during the eighteenth century was due to the practice of variolation rather than to natural epidemic occurrence.

VARIOLA
(Smallpox)

Etiology. Smallpox virus is readily visible with any microscope equipped with darkfield illumination or by phase contrast microscopy. With electron microscopy, the smallpox virus resembles elementary bodies of vaccinia virus. The elementary bodies are small, brick-shaped structures with a diameter of about 200 mμ. They can be demonstrated by direct examination of smears of early skin lesions. The virus is very resistant to drying, and living virus can be demonstrated from scabs kept at room temperature for over three years. Virulent virus has survived on clothing of patients and on bedclothes of hospitalized patients, and has caused the disease in laundry workers who were not protected.

Incidence. In 1967, when an intensified eradication program was begun, there were 42 countries reporting a total of 131,000 cases of smallpox. Since it is likely that only about 5 per cent of cases were actually reported, it is estimated that at least 2,500,000 cases occurred in 1967 in 30 countries that had endemic smallpox and in 12 others that experienced importations. In contrast, in 1972, 19 countries reported 65,000 cases at a time when reporting had been vastly improved.

By 1973 only five countries had endemic smallpox—Ethiopia, Sudan, India, Bangladesh, and Pakistan—whereas 14 others had cases as a result of importations.

In South America, Brazil was the last country to become smallpox free. It seems likely now, after 450 years, that smallpox has been eliminated from the Western Hemisphere. In Asia, on the other hand, the difficulty of eradication is still a serious problem.

Epidemiology. The principal natural reservoir of smallpox is thought to be the patient suffering from the disease. The patient is not infective until the third day of the clinical disease, that is, one day before the maculopapular phase of the skin eruption is noted. Contacts may be allowed at large until they actually become ill, because they are not infective during the early pre-eruptive febrile disease.

Intensive efforts are currently being made to determine a possible nonhuman host, the most likely of which is the nonhuman primate. The surprising and significant animal reservoirs of yellow fever and malaria, which have materially affected the eradication campaign for those two diseases, have, understandably, also been of concern to those working in the field of smallpox.

In 1970, 13 cases of pox infection occurred in humans in areas of Africa which had been free of smallpox for two years or more (Foege, 1973). In ten of these, the illness was typical smallpox; all but one of these patients had not been vaccinated. No human source of infection was discovered, but none of over 100 unvaccinated close contacts subsequently contracted the disease. Virus was isolated and appeared indistinguishable from monkeypox virus isolated among outbreaks in captive monkeys, but there was no illness among monkeys in the area (Ladnyr, 1973). Therefore although it is possible that monkeypox can cause a clinical illness resembling smallpox in man, its infectivity appears to be low.

Pathology and Pathogenesis. It is likely that the site of entry of the smallpox virus is the upper respiratory tract and, possibly, the eye. In the 12-day incubation period the virus probably multiplies in the regional lymphoid tissues. The fact that no patient is infectious during the incubation period suggests that in this interval an open lesion does not exist in the respiratory mucosa. In the unmodified case, a massive viremia occurs at the onset of the fever, and remains during the first two or three days of the pre-eruptive phase. In this way the virus localizes in the mucous membranes and in the skin as well as in the internal tissues. After the virus disappears from the blood and the skin eruption appears, the patient feels better, and the temperature tends to decrease. Antibodies are noted in the blood as early as the fourth day of the disease. The virus multiplies in the epithelial cells of the skin while being relatively protected from the action of circulating antibody so that cell destruction continues for some time. When pustulation occurs, the temperature tends to rise again, probably because of the absorption of the toxic products of cell necrosis. It is of interest that patients become infectious on the third day of the disease, probably because saliva has been contaminated through the early mucosal lesions noted in the pharynx and mouth. Skin lesions become infective after the superficial corneal layer has been severely damaged. Scabs remain infectious throughout the illness and until their separation during the third to fourth week of illness. The pitting is generally confined to the face, even in severe cases, and is due to destruction of sebaceous glands followed by organization and subsequent shrinking of granulation tissue and fibrosis. In cases of hemorrhagic smallpox numerous blood cells are present in the corium. *Cytoplasmic inclusions* are characteristic of infection with the vaccinia-variola group of viruses. Inclusion bodies can be shown best in epithelial cells, particularly of the involved skin and mucous membranes. Skin scrapings stained with hematoxylin and eosin show the inclusion to be round or oval homogeneous masses, either basophilic or acidophilic, located in the cytoplasm fairly close to the nucleus. The appearance of the inclusion bodies varies with the stage of infection but also with the method of fixation and staining, and this suggests that they consist of masses of elementary bodies. Intranuclear inclusions have also been described, but these are not invariably seen. With antimicrobial therapy, pathologic changes from bacterial complications are not found, and bacterial cultures, in this situation, are usually sterile.

Clinical Manifestations. The incubation period of smallpox is generally 12 days. The illness begins with intense malaise and high fever lasting for four to six days. There is intense prostration, and the clinical impression is often that of dengue. Severe headache, photophobia, and, occasionally, vomiting are noted. A small number of patients show a prodromal or "toxemic" rash, most easily noted in the groins, the axillae, and the flanks. On the fourth day the *focal rash* occurs, the fever diminishes slightly, and the patient feels much better, just at a time when the first macular skin lesions begin to form. The focal rash usually occurs first on the mucosa of the mouth and pharynx, the face, or the forearms, and it then spreads to the trunk and legs. A feature of variola is the fact that lesions in any one area are all at the same stage of development, whereas in varicella they are in all stages. The initial rash is macular and quickly becomes papular. Within two days the papules have developed into vesicles and these, within a few hours, become cloudy and pustular. On the eighth or ninth day from the beginning of the rash, drying and crusting begin. From three to four weeks from the onset of the disease, scabs have generally fallen off, leaving pigment-free skin, frequently with some scarring or pitting. The eruption is characteristically more severe on the face and the distal parts of the arms and legs, and less severe over the trunk and abdomen. The groins and axillae may be entirely spared. This centrifugal distribution is distinct

from the characteristic rash of varicella, which tends to be centripetal. Lesions are generally found on the palms of the hands and the soles of the feet, a situation uncommonly seen in varicella of childhood, although these parts are often involved in the adult form. Fever generally recurs during the pustular stage, but the temperature returns to normal as the lesions become crusted. The characteristic pustular lesions of smallpox are round, raised, and tense, with a tendency to central depression as they begin to dry out. Clinical classification of disease from the mildest form (variola sine eruptione) to modified, to confluent, to malignant confluent, to hemorrhagic indicates degrees of severity of smallpox influenced in part by age, state of immunity, and state of hormonal balance. It is of great interest that women within a short time of term, either before or after delivery, tend to have a much more severe disease than those not pregnant.

In cases modified by vaccination or transplacental immunity in the first few months of life, the rash may be scant and the evolution of lesions may be very quick. *Regardless of how mild an index case of smallpox may be, the susceptible infected contacts suffer unmodified disease,* and overlooked early cases are frequently the cause of severe epidemics. Permanent scarring or pitting may result even in the absence of purulent infection of lesions with secondary bacterial pathogens (staphylococci and streptococci) in patients who have deep lesions and serious disease.

In previous years, the bacterial complications were incriminated as the principal cause of death, particularly after the pustular phase had commenced. It is now known that the mortality rate is chiefly related to the amount of virus present in the blood during the viremic phase that occurs in the first two days of the disease before any eruption is noted. It has been shown that if the amount of virus in the blood is so great that the whole blood of the patient in the viremic pre-eruptive phase can be used as the antigen in the complement-fixation test, the patient will almost surely die, although death may be delayed for nine or ten days. Patients who do die in the first week of illness often show evidence of heart failure and terminal pneumonia. Even in the absence of any antimicrobial therapy, the lungs are often sterile, indicating that the pneumonia is caused by the smallpox virus itself. The majority of deaths occur, however, in the pustular stage toward the end of the second week of the disease. Occasionally an encephalitis has been described that is indistinguishable from that associated with measles, varicella, or smallpox vaccination and tends to occur between the eighth and sixteenth days of disease.

Infection in Utero. No congenital anomalies have been described in infants of mothers infected with smallpox, but abortion is common because of the frequent bleeding that occurs during the toxemic phase. Infection of the fetus in utero may occur during the viremic phase in the mother; if this occurs near the end of pregnancy, the child will show clinical disease within a few days after birth. Infection has also been shown to occur at the time of birth if the disease is still active in the mother. There are two reports of smallpox in babies infected in utero a few days before birth, although the mothers showed no signs of the disease (Bancroft, 1904; Lynch, 1932).

Variola Minor. In the twentieth century, a milder clinical form of smallpox became prevalent in this hemisphere. It was recognized in Brazil in 1910, when a widespread outbreak of this mild form of the disease was recorded with a mortality of only 1 per cent. To this mild type of smallpox the name alastrim — variola minor — was given. Similar mild forms of the disease were recognized in South Africa, and it is now accepted that alastrim probably existed in Jenner's day side by side with variola major, the mortality of which has remained steady at about 30 per cent.

The vast majority of epidemics seen in this century in North America and Europe have been due to variola minor. Thus there were 12,000 cases in 1927 in England and Wales and over 48,000 cases in 1930 in the United States. In the 1930's, with the widespread application of smallpox vaccination in infancy, smallpox began to decrease in the United States. An important factor in this decrease was the better preservation of smallpox vaccine with the wider availability of refrigerators. It is likely that more potent vaccines and widespread improvement of health services also contributed to the decline in the number of cases. The two types of disease (variola major and variola minor) appeared to be distinct with a markedly different mortality for the two. At present there would appear to be no evidence that an outbreak of alastrim gives rise to cases of classic variola major, although the two types may produce coexistent separate outbreaks, as they apparently did in Detroit in 1924.

There is complete cross-protection for these two infections as there is from vaccinia. The clinical picture is similar in the prodromal or pre-eruptive phase to that of variola major, but hemorrhagic and toxic cases are almost never seen. The lesions tend to be more superficial and develop more rapidly; the total illness is shorter than in classic variola major. There may be no secondary fever during the pustular stage.

Differential Diagnosis. Smallpox is easily diagnosed, particularly during an epidemic period. More difficult to diagnose is the first and unsuspected case in those countries where smallpox is not endemic. This is particularly true if the first case is hemorrhagic. In this situation meningococcemia, a bleeding diathesis as a part of a blood dyscrasia, or typhus may be the suspected diagnosis. Very mild smallpox, modified by previous vaccination or alastrim, may be thought to be varicella, a drug eruption, or erythema multiforme. Except after known exposure, the clinical diagnosis cannot be made with certainty during the febrile phase, because the picture is indistinguishable from that of dengue, enteroviral infections, and other febrile diseases. In the eruptive phase, the most useful clinical points to remember are (1) the centrifugal distribution of lesions; (2) the fact that in a given area all the lesions are at the same stage of development; (3) the fact that there is a relative progression of eruptions from the face and arms to more recent lesions on the arms or legs; (4) the presence of a severe, febrile, three-day pre-eruptive disease; and, on occasion, (5) a known contact at least 12 days previously.

Laboratory Tests. Laboratory diagnostic procedures are of great value in quickly establishing the diagnosis of smallpox in the first case that appears in a community. These consist of (1) light microscopic or electron microscopic demonstration of viral particles in stained smears of vesicular fluid, (2) serologic or fluorescent demonstration of viral antigen in materials from cutaneous lesions, (3) isolation of virus from such materials, and (4) detection of antibodies in the serum early in the eruptive phase. The results of such tests are particularly helpful in differentiating varioloid from varicella and

the hemorrhagic forms of the disease from other conditions (see Ch. 388). A detailed description of these procedures may be found in the 1969 article by Downie and Kempe.

Treatment. No specific treatment for smallpox is currently available, although a number of promising antiviral drugs are under study. Penicillin and broader-spectrum antimicrobials have been used in the prevention and treatment of bacterial complications. There is suggestive clinical evidence that secondary late bacterial complications, including pneumonia and staphylococcal involvement of skin and bones, are decreased by the use of antimicrobial therapy. But even with such therapy the mortality rates have not been reduced below 25 per cent in most outbreaks of variola major. Good nursing care and maintenance of fluid and electrolyte balance are essential. Convalescent smallpox serum and vaccinia-immune gamma globulin have been used in the treatment of severe cases without any evidence of success.

Prevention of Smallpox. *Management of Recently Exposed Persons.* The use of vaccinia-immune gamma globulin (see below) has been successful in the prophylaxis of smallpox and has reduced the incidence after known contact fourfold in control trials (Kempe et al., 1956, 1961). This compares with approximate six-, four-, 3.5-, and twofold reductions in attack rates in methisazone-treated groups reported in the studies of Bauer (1963, 1969) doValle (1965), Rao (1969), and Heiner (1971), respectively. In Heiner's study only the vaccinated contacts showed significant reduction in attack rates (twofold), and no difference in mortality or morbidity was noted between tested and placebo groups.

Community Control. There is no evidence that we owe our freedom from smallpox in the United States to routine vaccination. Compulsory routine vaccination was discontinued in Great Britain in the late 1950's, and 90 per cent of the population has either never been vaccinated or not vaccinated in the past ten years. Since 1969 there have been 12 smallpox importations into England, but the experience with secondary cases, deaths, and generations of cases until control has been no different in that country than in Germany, which has a far higher level of immunity in its population. Public health policy in the United States long held that high immunity levels are vital, and that an 80 per cent vaccination rate would give "herd protection." This has been thoroughly discredited, because importations have caused repeated outbreaks even though as many as 90 per cent of the population in an area were vaccinated. Only one third of the adults in the United States have been vaccinated in the past ten years, and fewer than 20 per cent of them in the last three years. Individuals who have not had a recent successful vaccination can be infected and may have a difficult-to-diagnose case, but they can, nevertheless, transmit the infection in its most virulent form, as has, in 1973, been shown again in the case of the English laboratory worker who had a greatly modified case of smallpox but still was able to transmit the infection in a fatal form to two contacts. There has been no smallpox in the United States since 1949, because we have been fortunate in not having the virus introduced rather than because our population is adequately protected. If variola major had been introduced, secondary cases would have resulted; but their number would have depended on early versus late diagnosis, prompt versus delayed ring vaccination of contacts, and careful immunologic survey and case finding, as well as the presence of a high level of immunity in our hospital staff personnel. In 1964, because of the persistent concern with the number of serious complications of smallpox vaccination, we recommended the discontinuation of nonselective routine vaccination of American children. *Selective* vaccination as a general policy has been endorsed in 1971 by all major public health and professional groups, except for the American Medical Association. Vaccination is now limited to (1) hospital personnel, (2) travelers to endemic areas, and (3) contacts of those with proved cases of smallpox. If the global eradication programs now underway should not be successful, it will be necessary to remain constantly alert that foreign quarantine procedures and selected traveler surveillance are maintained at a high level, and that adequate measures are taken, from both the clinical and laboratory points of view, in making the proper diagnosis at the earliest possible time.

With currently available techniques, an importation of smallpox and the development of some secondary cases in an unprotected population will, even with failures in early diagnosis, not result in any greater number of deaths than have occurred in the past 40 years from universal infant vaccination itself.

Control of Infected Persons, Contacts, and Environment. All cases should be reported to the local health authority, and patients should be isolated in a hospital until all crusts have disappeared. All oral, nasal, fecal, and urinary discharges and articles associated with patients should be disinfected by burning, high-pressure steam, or boiling. All contacts at home, place of work, or elsewhere should be vaccinated or revaccinated with a potent product and kept under daily surveillance for 16 days from the time of last contact. Any fever during surveillance calls for prompt isolation until smallpox can be excluded. The patient's source case should be sought assiduously. Adults with chickenpox or patients with hemorrhagic or pustular lesions of the skin need careful review for possible errors in diagnosis.

Epidemic Measures. In an epidemic the measures to be taken are as follows: (1) All smallpox patients and suspects should be isolated in hospital until they are no longer infectious. (2) All contacts should be carefully listed, vaccinated, and kept under surveillance for 16 days. (3) A public statement of the situation should be made by all available methods, and all possible contacts should be urged to be vaccinated. Potent vaccine should be provided and arrangements made for early vaccination of inner-ring and outer-ring contacts. (4) The use of vaccine, immune gamma globulin, and chemoprophylaxis with N-methylisatin B-thiosemicarbazone for close household contacts should further decrease the number of secondary cases. (5) Mass immunization of the entire population of a community or larger area is an emergency measure to be used only when an outbreak has given evidence of material spread.

International Measures. The World Health Organization and countries adjacent to the one in which an outbreak occurs should be notified by telegram of the existence of any cases of smallpox. At all times, the measures applicable to ships, aircraft, and land transport arriving from smallpox areas should be enforced, as specified in International Sanitary Regulations. It should be noted that evidence of protection by successful vaccination or revaccination (within a period of three years) is a widely enforced requirement for entry to the United States for *travelers from endemic countries but from no others.*

Vaccination vs. Chemoprophylaxis. Vaccination remains the best method of prevention for any individual likely to be exposed through travel in the smallpox-endemic regions of Asia or Africa. To be fully effective, successful revaccination every three years or, better, each year is recommended.

Upon exposure to a case of smallpox, vaccination and revaccination should be supplemented by chemoprophylaxis with methisazone, 3 grams given twice only 12 hours apart. For children three to ten years old, 1.5 grams twice only should be given, and for infants under three years of age, 0.75 gram twice only. Vaccination after exposure is generally inadequate to prevent disease, but should be done because in an epidemic situation subsequent repeat exposures may occur. The use of vaccinia-immune gamma globulin also markedly reduces clinical incidence and severity when used in full doses of 10 ml intramuscularly once for adults and 5 ml intramuscularly once for children under 12 years. Vaccinia-immune globulin and methisazone can and should both be given, when available, for a limited number of known contacts, such as may occur in aircraft exposures and to family contacts. A common but harmless side effect of methisazone is emesis. If vomiting occurs less than one hour after the dose, the full dose should be repeated with an antiemetic such as dimenhydrinate (Mavezine or Dramamine). Alcohol is strictly contraindicated because of the similar structure of methisazone and of the antialcoholic Antabuse.

WHO and health agencies of member countries in which there is endemic smallpox successfully depend on vaccination alone and concentrate on the elimination of specific smallpox foci, attempting to break the transmission chain rather than to rely on mass vaccination campaigns, which had been the time-honored method of eradication in the attempts at eradication in the past. It is believed that, particularly in Africa and Asia, it is much more efficient and economical to try to interrupt transmission at a time of low seasonal incidence of smallpox. Current strategy consists of an attempt to contain outbreaks of smallpox by the early detection and containment of cases so as to reduce smallpox incidence as quickly as possible, rather than the institution of mass vaccination.

In an outbreak in central Java in 1969, when more than 95 per cent of the 23,000,000 inhabitants in the province bore vaccination scars, almost 1700 cases of smallpox nevertheless occurred, 85 per cent of them developing in persons who had never been successfully vaccinated. In other words, in a population in which only 5 per cent were unimmunized, continued transmission was readily possible—definite evidence that "herd immunity" does not work. The incredible success obtained in West and Central Africa, and parts of Indonesia and Ethiopia, is entirely due to this change of strategy based on early detection of outbreaks and the establishment of trained teams to investigate and contain them. Case-finding requires a reporting network which had to be developed. The use of freeze-dried potent vaccine replaced liquid vaccine in all WHO programs. A very useful tool for case-finding is the WHO photo recognition card often given to schoolchildren, who proved to be one of the most fruitful sources of information in remote villages in

Asia and Africa. The schoolchild through recognition cards, visits to the principal markets which are held every week in different locations, and searching out through walking from village to village are the three bases for case-finding which lead to case identification and subsequent vaccination.

VACCINIA
(Vaccination)

Smallpox vaccine commonly in use is prepared from the vaccinia lesions on the skin of inoculated calves or sheep or from the allantoic membranes of chick embryos. All currently used smallpox vaccine contains infective virus, and all successful vaccinations are deliberately induced mild viral infections. It is thought that within one year after primary vaccination the chance of an attack is reduced to one one thousandth of that in the unvaccinated; within three years, to one two hundredth; within ten years, to one eighth, and within twenty years, to one half; after twenty years there is little if any protection against infection. However, the mortality in smallpox patients successfully vaccinated many years before is less than in the unvaccinated. There is no question that regular revaccination induces a high degree of immunity even with very massive exposure to the disease. Targeted vaccination and surveillance with case-finding in the remaining endemic areas of Asia and Africa will, in time, reduce the susceptible population below that necessary to permit the survival of the pathogenic virus.

Recommended Program for Vaccinations in the United States. We can look forward to the time when the present eradication program will have eliminated smallpox as a threat to man. At that time, vaccination will no longer be necessary, and jennerian vaccinations will then be a matter of only historic importance. Until this is achieved, however, smallpox vaccination will continue to be necessary for those at risk, namely, travelers to endemic areas and those who, by their occupation, are likely to come into contact with such travelers. These include hospital personnel and those involved with transportation services, as well as those in the armed forces.

Contraindications to Vaccination. Primary *routine* vaccination is no longer performed on North American infants, but even *selective* vaccination is generally contraindicated in infant patients who fail to thrive; in persons with dysgammaglobulinemia, blood dyscrasias, eczema, or other dermatitides; in the presence of radiation or other immunosuppressant therapy; in those exposed to infectious diseases; or in unvaccinated siblings of children with eczema. In the eczematous child, vaccination can be performed safely with attenuated vaccine when travel to endemic regions is contemplated. If exposure is likely, elective vaccination of the eczematous child *should* be performed, because the eczema vaccination in this situation is only 1 in 150 and the mortality is zero. Vaccination or revaccination is absolutely contraindicated for adult patients with neoplastic diseases, including Hodgkin's disease, lymphomas, and other conditions involving the prolonged use of corticosteroids, nitrogen mustard, or radiation therapy.

When travel outside the limits of the United States to nonendemic areas is contemplated, vaccination is no longer required for re-entry into the United States. At most, telephonic health surveillance for 14 days after re-entry to the United States may be required. This is much to be preferred to life-threatening disease from vaccination. Vaccination has not been carried out by the Quarantine Service when the patient's physician has presented written evidence that the procedure should not be performed. If such a person must travel to an endemic area, the use of vaccinia-immune gamma globulin should be considered so as to provide temporary protection and to act as a substitute for the use of vaccination with live vaccinia virus.

Recommended Vaccination Techniques. To minimize the risk of unnecessary complications, the following practices are recommended:

Age for Primary Vaccination. In nonendemic areas, primary vaccination is not routinely done or is performed when the child is over two years of age. There are no conclusive data indicating the exact period when complication rates are minimal. The presence of some transplacental maternal immunity, provided that the mother has been vaccinated, may be desirable in modifying the primary vaccination reaction, and vaccination may be carried out in the first months of life. Vaccination of newborn infants has been done without complications (Kempe et al., 1952). However, in such cases in endemic areas, revaccination should be performed after an interval of six months. If primary vaccination is delayed for several months, children who are at increased risk, such as those suffering from the Swiss type of agammaglobulinemia, will have been readily identified by their clinical course and will therefore not become casualties of smallpox vaccination. The 1966 experience in the United States fails to show a higher risk of postvaccinia encephalitis for the two-to-ten age group (Neff et al., 1968), but some European authors have stressed that the first years of life may be a safer period. The case mortality for encephalitis is certainly highest among the youngest children (Berger, 1964; Coneybeare, 1948; Muller, 1946; Neff, 1968).

Site for Vaccination. Primary vaccination and revaccination are best performed on the outer aspects of the upper arm, over the insertion of the deltoid muscle or behind the midline. Reactions are less likely to be severe on the upper arm than on the lower extremity or other parts of the body. With proper technique, resultant scars are small and unobtrusive.

Preparation of the Vaccination Site. With a clean skin, the best preparation is none at all. The use of chemical skin cleaners may leave a residue that contains virus-inactivating material, and vigorous physical cleansing of the site may create minute abrasions that then can become sites of secondary vaccinia eruptions, with resultant involvement of a comparatively large skin area.

Vaccination Technique. Regardless of age, primary vaccination should be performed with no more than two or three pressures with the side of a needle. These pressure points should be as close together as possible, and should be made only at one site. With the highly potent vaccines currently in use, more numerous pressure points are not necessary and certainly should not be utilized for a nonimmune person. When children or adults are to be revaccinated after a lapse of more than five years, the same small number of pressure points should be used. For revaccination within a five-year period of those persons known to have had a major reaction, the full complement of 30 strokes can safely be used (Leake, 1946).

Vaccination Reaction. The description of the reactions after vaccination or revaccination should follow the criteria recommended by the Expert Committee on Smallpox of the World Health Organization. A successful primary vaccination is one that on examination after seven to ten days presents a typical jennerian vesicle. If this is not present, vaccination must be repeated with fresh vaccine and a few more strokes of the needle. The successful revaccination is one that on examination one week (six to ten days) later shows a vesicular or pustular lesion *or* an area of definite palpable induration and congestion surrounding a central lesion; this lesion may be a scab or an ulcer. These reactions are termed *major reactions;* all others should be called *equivocal reactions.*

A major reaction indicates virus multiplication with consequent development of immunity. An equivocal reaction may merely represent an allergic response, which could be elicited by inactive vaccine or poor technique in someone who had been sensitized by earlier vaccination; or the equivocal reaction may result from sufficient immunity to prevent virus multiplication. Since the allergic response cannot be readily differentiated from the one caused by true immunity, another vaccination should be performed, using a different lot of vaccine if there is the possibility that the first was of weak potency, and the procedure should be completed with an additional number of pressures. The site should be examined one week later; if the result is again equivocal, revaccination should be repeated, using a full 30 pressures as recommended by Leake. For the sake of expediency, an equivocal reaction to revaccination with a minimal insertion may be followed by vaccination at two sites, not less than 2 inches apart, using known potent vaccine. This method will make a third return unnecessary in almost all instances.

In summary, successful smallpox vaccination consists of the production of a major reaction. When potent vaccine and good technique are used, repeated inability to produce a major reaction can be assumed to be due to solid immunity from previous immunization.

Frequency of Vaccination. Revaccination is essential to reinforce the immunity conferred by previous vaccination. This not only maintains a high level of immunity against smallpox, but minimizes the risk of complications on revaccination. To maintain adequate immunity against smallpox, revaccination should be carried out at approximately five-year intervals. Those persons at some increased risk, such as hospital and public health personnel, members of the armed forces, and those working at port or airline offices, as well as shipping personnel, should be revaccinated at least once every three years. When exposure to smallpox is probable, by travel or residence in a smallpox-endemic area, annual revaccination is desirable.

Complications of Vaccination. With the abandonment of universal routine vaccination of infants in 1971, complications in the United States have markedly decreased. Life-threatening complications of primary vaccination include eczema vaccinatum, postvaccinial encephalitis, and vaccinia gangrenosa (progressive vaccinia). The principal danger after revaccination is vaccinia gangrenosa, a condition in which the impairment of the patient's immune mechanism permits the continuing multiplication of the vaccinia virus. Vaccinia gan-

grenosa is seen in seemingly normal subjects as well as in those suffering from dysgammaglobulinemia, Hodgkin's disease, leukemia, blood dyscrasias, and other conditions in which corticosteroid therapy or ionized irradiation has been administered therapeutically. The presence of these conditions is an absolute contraindication to vaccination.

Human vaccinia-immune globulin has been shown to be effective in the prevention and treatment of eczema vaccinatum and has also been used extensively in the treatment of other complications, in which it also produces a significant reduction in mortality. Vaccinia-immune globulin reduces the incidence of postvaccinial encephalitis. In the Royal Netherland Army, 53,630 of 106,174 recruits received hyperimmune vaccinia-immune gamma globulin, and the remaining 52,544 recruits received a placebo. In the group treated with gamma globulin, 3 cases of postvaccinial encephalitis occurred in contrast to 13 cases in the control group. There was one fatality in each group. Gamma globulin failed to have an effect on the severity and duration of the encephalitis produced by the vaccination, and it was not effective in treatment. There is evidence that transplacental maternal immunity is also effective in modifying the course of primary vaccination; significant reactions are rarely reported in very young infants whose mothers have been vaccinated in the past. In cases of vaccinia gangrenosa, the simultaneous use of vaccinia-immune globulin and N-methylisatin beta-thiosemicarbazone appears to be of value. The therapeutic dose of the drug is 200 mg per kilogram orally initially, followed by 50 mg per kilogram every six hours for three days. After an interval of three days, another three-day course may be required. Adequate early treatment of the complications of smallpox vaccination can materially reduce the morbidity and mortality. Through the Center for Disease Control in Atlanta, Georgia, a group of experts is available for telephone consultation (day: [404] 633-3311; night: [404] 633-2176). When such consultation is used in conjunction with vaccinia-immune globulin and chemotherapeutic agents, effective diagnostic and therapeutic aids are available for all.

Bauer, D. J., St. Vincent, L., Kempe, C. H., Young, P. A., and Downie, A. W.: Prophylaxis of smallpox with methisazone. Am. J. Epidemiol., 90:130, 1969.

Downie, A. W., and Kempe, C. H.: Variola and vaccinia viruses. *In* Lennette, E. H. (ed.): Diagnostic Procedures for Viral and Rickettsial Diseases. New York, American Public Health Association, 1969, Chap. 25.

DoValle, L. A. R., DeMelo, P. R., De Salles Gomes, L. F., and Proenca, L. M.: Methisazone in prevention of variola minor among contacts. Lancet, 2:976, 1965.

Heiner, G. G., et al.: Field trials of methisazone as a prophylactic agent against smallpox. Am. J. Epidemiol., 94:435, 1971.

Kempe, C. H., et al.: The use of vaccinia hyperimmune gamma globulin in the prophylaxis of smallpox. Bull. WHO, 25:41, 1961.

Kempe, C. H., et al.: Smallpox vaccination of eczema patients with a strain of attenuated live vaccinia (CVI-78). Pediatrics, 42:980, 1968.

Neff, J. M.: Complications of smallpox vaccination. I. National Survey in the United States, 1963. N. Engl. J. Med., 276:125, 1967.

Rao, A. R., et al.: Chemoprophylaxis and chemotherapy in variola major. I. An assessment of CG 662 and Marboran in prophylaxis of contacts of variola major. Indian J. Med. Res., 57:477, 1969.

WHO Expert Committee on Smallpox: Second Report, Publication 393, World Health Organization Technical Report Series. Geneva, World Health Organization, 1968.

For more detailed lists of references see the following:

Dixon, C. W.: Smallpox. London, J. & A. Churchill, Ltd., 1962.

Downie, A. W.: Smallpox. *In* Horsfall, F. L., Jr., and Tamm, I. (eds.): Viral and Rickettsial Infections of Man. 4th ed. Philadelphia, J. B. Lippincott Company, 1965.

122. ORF
(Ecthyma Contagiosum, Contagious Pustular Dermatitis)

Clayton E. Wheeler, Jr.

Orf is a worldwide viral infection of sheep and goats that is occasionally transmitted to the skin of man. The disorder occurs most often in sheepherders and shearers, meat porters, butchers, veterinarians, technicians engaged in vaccine manufacture, and children or adults caring for pet lambs.

The virus is a round-ended, brick-shaped particle that measures 260 by 160 mμ and is classified with the paravaccinia viruses. Inoculation into the glabrous skin of sheep produces erythematous macules in three or four days, followed by pustular, granulomatous, papillomatous, and crusted phases. Healing occurs in four to six weeks. Infected animals show crusted, warty, or granulomatous lesions about the lips, nose, and eyelids that have occasioned the term "scabby mouth." The agent proliferates in primary tissue cultures of human amnion, monkey kidney, and bovine testis, in which a characteristic appearance is produced. Neutralizing and complement-fixing antibodies have been demonstrated in the blood of recovered animals and man.

Human lesions are usually single and appear most often on the hands, fingers, forearms, or face. There is often a history of trauma at the site of the lesion, followed in four to eleven days by the appearance of a red macule or papule. In a week or two this becomes a multiloculated vesicle from which little fluid can be expressed upon incision. In the next two weeks the surface becomes white and sodden, a crust usually forms, and a granulomatous reaction often develops. Healing takes place with little or no scar formation in four to six weeks. Mature lesions are 1 to 4 cm in diameter, elevated, dome-shaped, plateau or tumor-like, and well demarcated from normal skin. Regional lymphangitis or lymphadenopathy may occur as part of the viral infection or as a result of secondary bacterial involvement. Erythema multiforme is an uncommon complication. Persistent, giant orf has been observed in an immunosuppressed individual.

Microscopically, proliferation, ballooning, and reticular degeneration of epidermal cells, multilocular vesiculation, and pseudoepitheliomatous hyperplasia may be found. A granulomatous reaction is present in the dermis.

Treatment is symptomatic and is directed toward prevention or cure of secondary bacterial infection. Vaccination with live virus provides effective control in animals but it is not practicable in man.

Leavell, U. W., Jr., McNamara, M. J., Muelling, R., Talbert, W. M., Rucker, R. C., and Dalton, A. J.: Orf: Report of 19 human cases. J.A.M.A., 204:657, 1968.

Nagington, J., Newton, A. A., and Horne, R. W.: The structure of orf virus. Virology, 23:461, 1964.

Nagington, J., and Whittle, C. H.: Human orf. Isolation of the virus by tissue culture. Br. Med. J., 2:1324, 1961.

Savage, J., and Black, M. M.: Giant orf of finger in a patient with lymphoma. Proc. R. Soc. Med., 65:766, 1972.

123. MOLLUSCUM CONTAGIOSUM

Clayton E. Wheeler, Jr.

Molluscum contagiosum is an infection of the skin, and occasionally of the conjunctiva, with the largest of the true animal viruses. The viral particle is oval or brick shaped and measures approximately 300 by 220 mμ. It does not grow in the skin or cornea of animals or in tissues of the chick embryo, and its growth in tissue culture is questionable, although a cytopathic effect occurs, and interferon production is induced. Experimental inoculation of ground, filtered molluscum material into human skin is followed by a new lesion at the inoculation site in 14 to 50 days. Studies of immunity are fragmentary, although there is suggestive evidence for the development of complement-fixing antibodies and cutaneous sensitivity of the delayed type.

The pathologic change is confined to the epidermis, which grows into the dermis as multiple, closely packed, pear-shaped globules. Epidermal cells undergo characteristic degeneration as they progress from the basal layer to the surface, where they form a cavity at the center of the growth. Cellular degeneration is produced by intracytoplasmic growth of viral particles that form huge inclusions. These enlarge and distort the cell and crowd the nucleus to one side. Inclusions contain large amounts of deoxyribonucleic acid and stain deeply with hematoxylin and eosin.

This common disorder is worldwide and usually affects children. The disease is autoinoculable and mildly contagious, but the source of the infection and method of spread are often unknown.

Lesions are most often seen on the trunk, face, arms, or genital areas, although they occur almost anywhere. Conjunctival infection may result in epiphora, discharge, conjunctivitis, or keratitis. Lesions may be solitary, few and localized, numerous and generalized, or eruptive in association with atopic dermatitis or immunosuppressive therapy. They vary in size from barely visible to 0.5 cm or larger. They are usually discrete, but they may be grouped or form plaques or tumor-like masses. Characteristic papules are skin colored or slightly pink, pearly, circumscribed, elevated, firm, rounded, or semiglobular, and present central umbilication from which a curdlike material can be expressed. Inflammation is usually absent, but it may develop from irritation or secondary infection. Systemic infection with the virus is unknown.

The clinical appearance of the papules and the expression of a gelatinous central core usually suffice for diagnosis. The microscopic picture is diagnostic. Molluscum contagiosum is most often confused with nevi, warts, epithelioma, pyogenic granuloma, folliculitis, and other forms of pyoderma. Cure can usually be accomplished by curettage or light electrodesiccation. Spontaneous involution is not uncommon.

Lynch, P. J.: Molluscum contagiosum venereum. Clin. Obst. Gynecol., 15:966, 1972.

Postlethwaite, R.: Molluscum contagiosum. A review. Arch. Environ. Health, 21:432, 1970.

Sturt, R. J., Muller, H. K., and Francis, G. D.: Molluscum contagiosum in villages of the West Sepik district of New Guinea. Med. J. Aust., 2:751, 1971.

124. FOOT-AND-MOUTH DISEASE
(Aphthous Fever)
Walsh McDermott

Foot-and-mouth disease is a viral infection of animals, chiefly cattle, which occurs in man only with great rarity. Infection, when it does occur in man, presumably results from direct contact with the agent either in the laboratory or from handling the tissues or body fluids of infected animals. The disease in man is characterized by a short incubation period followed by the appearance of a febrile illness with vesicular lesions of palms, soles, and the oropharyngeal mucosa. Neurologic involvement has not been reported, and the disease is self-limited. There is no treatment of established value; the tetracycline drugs have yielded inconclusive results in the treatment of laboratory animals. Prevention of the disease in man has not been extensively studied, for man generally has a high degree of resistance to the infection. Spread among cattle is presumably by the airborne route. An effective vaccine for use in cattle has been developed. As in influenza, however, there are many types and subtypes of foot-and-mouth (FMD) virus, and it is believed that for optimal effectiveness the homologous viral strain, i.e., the "epidemic" strain, should be present in the vaccine.

Annotations: Spread of foot-and-mouth disease. Lancet, 2:580, 1969.
Flaum, A.: Foot-and-mouth disease in man. Acta. Pathol. Microbiol. Scand., 16:197, 1939.
Hyslop, N. St.G., Davie, J., and Carter, S. P.: Antigenic differences between strains of foot-and-mouth disease virus of type SAT 1. J. Hyg. (Camb.), 61:217, 1963.

125. MUMPS
Dorothy M. Horstmann

Definition. Mumps is an acute contagious viral infection, most commonly manifested by nonsuppurative swelling of the parotid glands. Other salivary glands, the testes, pancreas, and central nervous system are among the various organs that may also be involved.

Historical Note. Hippocrates described mumps in the fifth century B.C. Because of its characteristic manifestations, it was one of the earliest diseases to be recognized as a clinical entity. A classic description was written by Hamilton (1790), who was the first to stress the importance of orchitis as a complication. He also noted that central nervous system signs sometimes accompany the parotitis, but it was early in the twentieth century before clinicians recognized meningoencephalitis as a relatively frequent manifestation. In 1940 Wesselhoeft called attention to the occurrence of oophoritis and pancreatitis, and later others reported involvement of many organs and tissues. Not until 1934 did Johnson and Goodpasture prove the viral etiology of mumps by reproducing the disease in monkeys inoculated with filtrates of infective human saliva. The virus was adapted to growth in hens' eggs in 1945 by Habel, and by Levens and Enders, who demonstrated its hemagglutinating properties. Enders and his associates also described the appearance of dermal hypersensitivity and of complement-fixing (CF) antibodies after mumps. The availability of a skin test and of serologic tools allowed the demonstration that infection with mumps virus can occur without parotitis and not infrequently without any signs at all. Immunization with a killed virus vaccine was tried in the 1950's with limited success. In 1966 Bunyak and Hilleman developed a highly effective live attenuated mumps virus vaccine, prepared in chick embryo tissue culture, which is currently widely used.

Etiology. Mumps is an RNA virus, a member of the myxovirus family that includes the influenza and parainfluenza viruses. These agents all have the property of agglutinating chicken, human, and other erythrocytes. In monkeys, mumps virus induces parotitis, and in suckling mice or hamsters it may cause fatal meningoencephalitis. The virus multiplies in embryonated chick embryos and in a variety of tissue culture cells. For primary isolation (usually from saliva), eggs or preferably cell cultures derived from monkeys or humans are used. In tissue cultures the presence of the virus is recognized either by the appearance of cytopathic changes or by means of the hemadsorption test, which depends on the ability of the virus-infected cells to adsorb guinea pig erythrocytes. In infected cultures these are seen firmly attached to the cell sheet, whereas in control tubes the erythrocytes float in the media. The specificity of the reaction is established serologically, using the hemadsorption inhibition test. Mumps virus is associated with soluble (S) and viral (V) complement-fixing (CF) antigens and a skin test antigen. Infection induces CF, hemagglutination-inhibiting, and neutralizing antibodies.

Epidemiology. Mumps is a common disease, endemic all over the world. It occurs throughout the year, but there is a seasonal prevalence, with a regular increase in cases in winter and spring. Epidemics are frequent, large outbreaks tending to have a seven- or eight-year cycle. The disease incidence is the same in both sexes, but males are more prone to develop central nervous system complications. Most cases occur between the ages of 5 and 15 years; young adults are nevertheless sometimes susceptible, as evidenced by epidemics in military camps and schools.

The only known reservoir of infection is man. In experiments in volunteers, Henle et al. showed that the virus may be present in the saliva from two to six days before the occurrence of parotid swelling, and as long as seven to nine days after onset. *Transmission* is thought to be by direct contact, air-suspended droplets, or fomites contaminated with saliva. Rather more solid contact appears to be necessary for transmission of mumps than is the case with measles or chickenpox.

Although it is a common disease, only about 60 per cent of the adult population gives a positive history, in contrast to more than 90 per cent for measles. The difference is due in part to the frequency of inapparent infection with mumps virus. About 50 per cent of those with a negative history give a positive serologic test, indicating previous silent infection. One experience with mumps virus appears to confer lifelong immunity.

Pathogenesis and Pathology. The widespread involvement of glandular and other tissues in the body indicates that mumps is a systemic infection. The virus apparently enters and multiplies first in the upper respiratory tract; it then invades the bloodstream, and localizes in the salivary as well as other glands and in the central nervous system. The parotids are one of many target organs, the greater frequency with which they are involved being simply a reflection of greater sensitivity.

Limited observations on pathologic specimens indicate that the reaction in the parotid gland is a nonspecific inflammatory one, which is not extensive. The testes and pancreas also demonstrate inflammatory and degenerative changes. Lesions induced by the virus in the central nervous system are of two types: those induced by direct viral invasion, resulting in a primary encephalitis; and the demyelination characteristic of postinfectious encephalitis. Mumps virus has been shown to cause hydrocephalus in laboratory animals, and there is some evidence that this lesion may also occur rarely in man.

Clinical Manifestations. The incubation period is 17 to 21 days, usually 18; extremes of 12 and 35 days have been reported. In most cases, pain and swelling in the parotid region are the first signs of the disease, although occasionally in adults pain in the testicle may be the initial symptom. Rarely, meningitis appears first, followed later by parotitis. In more severe cases, there is often a prodromal period, sometimes lasting as long as two or three days, with fever, malaise, headache, chills, sore throat, earache, and tenderness along the region of the parotid ducts.

Parotid swelling is first observed below the ear, usually obliterating the hollow between the mastoid process and the ascending ramus of the lower jaw. The gland increases in size over a two- to three-day period, but there is great variation in the degree of swelling; in mild cases it may be scarcely apparent, but in severe ones the associated edema may eventually spread superiorly to the eyes, posteriorly to the mastoid region, and inferiorly below the chin and over the anterior aspect of the neck. For the first two days, unilateral involvement is the rule, but eventually both glands are affected in about 70 per cent of cases. The skin over the swollen parotids is not usually reddened, but is tense and tender on pressure. Not infrequently the submaxillary and sublingual glands are also affected. Involvement of the sublingual glands can result in swelling of the tongue, with attendant painful swallowing. Presternal pitting edema is also occasionally present, apparently because of obstruction of the lymphatics by the enlarged salivary glands.

The patient seldom suffers severe pain except on movement of the jaws, e.g., in talking or chewing. If Stensen's duct becomes partially occluded as the gland swells, there is sharp pain on taking food or an acid drink, which stimulates the secretory mechanism. Because this occurs only with partial occlusion of the duct, it is not a constant sign. The papillae at the opening of Stensen's or Wharton's duct may be reddened, but this also is inconstant.

Constitutional symptoms vary greatly and may be virtually absent. They are especially mild in children, but tend to be more severe in adults, in whom the incidence of extraparotid lesions is higher. Fever varies with the extent of involvement, ranging between 38 and 39.5 C in full-blown, uncomplicated cases, but going as high as 40.5 and 41° C if orchitis, meningoencephalitis, or both develop.

The duration of parotid swelling and fever is dependent upon the extent and severity of the process. Usually the temperature is normal within five days, and swelling has disappeared by seven to ten days. A peculiar tendency to relapse with recurrence of parotid swelling has been noted in buglers, horn players, and others whose occupations involve similar exertion.

Neurologic Manifestations. The incidence of *aseptic meningitis* varies widely in different epidemics, but can be as high as 25 per cent. Serial examination of the cerebrospinal fluid indicates that the cell count is elevated in approximately one half of all cases of mumps. Clinically evident neurologic involvement may occur preceding, simultaneously with, or after parotitis. It affects males three to five times more commonly than females, and may be the only manifestation of the infection. The clinical picture of headache, fever, stiff neck, and lethargy is similar to that in other forms of viral meningitis, but the cerebrospinal fluid findings may differ in several respects. Thus cell counts tend to be higher; 500 to 1000 cells, predominantly lymphocytes, are common, and occasionally even several thousand are present. The pleocytosis in mumps is also more prolonged, and may persist for several weeks. Glucose levels below 40 mg per 100 ml have recently been reported in 10 to 20 per cent of cases. The protein levels are moderately elevated. *Encephalitis,* whether resulting from direct attack by mumps virus or occurring as postinfectious encephalitis, is rare.

Other rare neurologic complications include permanent nerve deafness, either unilateral or bilateral; labyrinthitis; polyneuritis, sometimes affecting the facial or trigeminal nerves; disturbances in accommodation; optic neuritis, iritis, and iridocyclitis; and possibly hydrocephalus.

Orchitis. Orchitis is rare before puberty. After puberty, its incidence varies, but is usually about 25 per cent; there is considerable variation in different epidemics. Testicular involvement is most often unilateral, but may be bilateral, one following the other by one to nine days. The onset is commonly between the fifth and tenth days of illness, as the parotid swelling is subsiding. In mild cases there may be nothing more than discomfort, with tenderness and slight fever. In others, onset is abrupt, with a chill, fever to 40° C or higher, nausea, vomiting, sweats, backache, prostration, and severe testicular pain. Swelling of the testicle may be moderate, or the gland may rapidly reach three to four times normal size, in which case it is excessively hard, tender, and so painful that even 0.030 gram of morphine is not always effective. In severe cases, the epididymis, spermatic cord, or tunica vaginalis may be involved, and straw-colored hydrocele fluid sometimes collects.

In mild cases the testicle may be normal in four days, although in the most severe, it may require three or four weeks before all evidence of inflammation has disappeared. Some degree of atrophy, apparently caused by pressure necrosis, occurs in about a third to a half of all cases of orchitis, *but in most instances it is unilateral. Even when both testes are involved, the distribution of the inflammatory reaction and loss of functional tissue are apt to be spotty, and seldom result in sterility.*

Oophoritis. Oophoritis occurs occasionally in adult females, but it may be more frequent than suspected, as mild forms are difficult to recognize. High fever, chills, lower quadrant or back pain, and palpable ovarian enlargement have been described. Sterility resulting from mumps oophoritis is virtually unknown.

Pancreatitis. Pancreatitis has been estimated to occur in less than 10 per cent of cases. Severe epigastric pain, vomiting, diarrhea or constipation, and fever are characteristic; abdominal tenderness and muscle spasm may be marked.

Other Organs. More rarely, other glands or organs are involved, particularly in adults. The following have been reported as complications of mumps: prostatitis, bartholinitis, and mastitis (in both males and females); involvement of the thyroid, thymus, and lacrimal glands; splenomegaly; and hepatitis. Transient abnormalities of renal function occur frequently, but persistent nephritis is unusual, although fatal cases have been reported. Polyarthritis, occurring ten days to two weeks after onset, is a rare complication. Myocarditis, accompanied by precordial pain or heart block, has been described. Serial electrocardiograms on patients with mumps have revealed some abnormality in as high as 15 per cent, although very few patients show clinical evidence of myocarditis.

Diagnosis. Sudden onset of parotitis in a previously healthy patient with a negative history of mumps presents no diagnostic problem. Other causes of parotid swelling are suppurative parotitis, an acute bacterial infection in which there is marked tenderness, the skin over the gland is red and hot, and pus can often be expressed from the duct; preauricular and anterior cervical lymphadenopathy; and salivary calculi obstructing the duct and giving rise to recurrent parotitis. Chronic enlargement of the gland occurs with tumors, Mikulicz's disease, and uveoparotid fever of sarcoidosis.

Mumps infection in the absence of parotitis is often difficult to recognize. Orchitis can be due in rare instances to infection with other viruses such as coxsackievirus B, echovirus, and lymphocytic choriomeningitis virus. A variety of viral agents cause aseptic meningitis or meningoencephalitis that cannot be distinguished clinically from central nervous system involvement caused by mumps. In such situations specific laboratory tests are necessary to establish the etiology. Mumps virus can be isolated from saliva, urine, and, in meningitis, from the cerebrospinal fluid. More commonly, confirmation of the diagnosis is based on the demonstration of a significant rise in antibody titer (either complement-fixing or hemagglutination-inhibiting) when acute and convalescent serum samples are tested. If only a single convalescent specimen is available, the presence of a high titer is suggestive of recent infection. The *skin test* is of no value in diagnosis, because dermal hypersensitivity usually does not develop until three to four weeks after onset; it is less reliable than serologic tests in determining immune status.

Routine laboratory tests frequently indicate a relative lymphocytosis in uncomplicated parotitis; with orchitis, pancreatitis, or aseptic meningitis, the total leukocyte count often reaches 15,000 to 20,000, with a high percentage of polymorphonuclear cells. The blood amylase is usually elevated as a result of parotitis and is therefore not a reliable indication of pancreatic involvement.

Prognosis. Complete recovery is the rule, and mortality is virtually nil. A few fatal cases of encephalitis have been reported; bilateral testicular atrophy with resultant sterility (see above) and permanent nerve deafness are rare residua.

Treatment. Bed rest and symptomatic therapy are all that can be offered. For parotid pain, aspirin or codeine is effective. Some patients find an ice bag applied to the parotid region comforting, but others prefer heat. The headache associated with meningitis may be relieved by lumbar puncture. If orchitis is mild, no special treatment is required; if severe, meperidine (Demerol) (0.05 to 0.1 gram) or morphine (0.01 to 0.015 gram) may be necessary to control the pain. Local support and provision of warmth by means of a nest of absorbent cotton are more effective than an ice bag to the scrotum. Corticosteroids relieve the pain but do not appear to alter the duration of illness, nor do they protect against the subsequent development of atrophy. They are not indicated in mild cases, but in severe ones hydrocortisone, 10 mg per kilogram per day, may be given for three to four days.

Prevention. A live attenuated mumps virus vaccine, grown in tissue cultures of chick embryo cells, was licensed in 1968. To date, more than 10 million persons have been immunized in the United States. The vaccine is available as a monovalent preparation or combined with measles and rubella vaccines. It is given subcutaneously, causes virtually no clinical reaction, and induces antibody conversions in more than 95 per cent of susceptibles. The serum titers are lower than those that follow natural infection, but they have persisted satisfactorily for the six-year period over which antibodies have been tested. Vaccinees have been shown to be resistant to mumps when subsequently exposed to siblings with the disease.

The vaccine may be given to persons of any age over 12 months; it is not recommended for infants under one year because of the possible presence of residual maternal antibody which interferes with the development of active immunity. Immunization is recommended particularly for boys approaching puberty who give no history of mumps. If the vaccine is given after exposure, it is unlikely that it will protect. However, it may be given under these circumstances so that if contact infection failed to develop in a susceptible subject who was exposed, he will be protected when he next meets the virus.

Mumps vaccine should not be given to persons with allergy to egg proteins or to neomycin. It is contraindicated for those with any disease that results in compromised immune mechanisms and for patients on immunosuppressive therapy. Since the vaccine contains live virus, it should not be given during pregnancy.

Henle, W., and Enders, J. F.: Mumps virus. *In* Horsfall, F. L., Jr., and Tamm, I. (eds.): Viral and Rickettsial Infections of Man. 4th ed. Philadelphia, J. B. Lippincott Company, 1965, pp. 755–768.

Johnstone, J. A., Ross, C. A. C., and Dunn, M.: Meningitis and encephalitis associated with mumps infection. A 10-year survey. Arch. Dis. Child., 47:647, 1972.

Reed, D., Brown, G., Merrick, R., Sever, J., and Feltz, E.: A mumps epidemic on St. George Island, Alaska. J.A.M.A., 199:113, 1967.

Roseman, R. D.: Mumps orchitis. Clin. Proc. Children's Hospital, Wash. D. C., 14:239, 1958.

Weibel, R. E., Bunyak, E. B., Stokes, J., Jr., and Hilleman, M.: Persistence of immunity following monovalent and combined measles, mumps, and rubella vaccines. Pediatrics, 51:467, 1973.

ENTEROVIRAL DISEASES

Albert Z. Kapikian

126.   COXSACKIEVIRUSES, ECHOVIRUSES, AND NEWLY RECOGNIZED ENTEROVIRUSES: INTRODUCTION

The coxsackieviruses, groups A and B, echoviruses, and polioviruses comprise the enterovirus subgroup of the picornaviruses of humans. It has been proposed recently that newly recognized serotypes of the enterovirus subgroup be designated simply as enteroviruses rather than as members of a specific enterovirus subgroup (i.e., polio-, coxsackie-, or echovirus) on account of overlapping properties among certain enterovirus strains. In this system, the first newly recognized serotype has been designated enterovirus 68 in order to avoid confusion with enterovirus numbers proposed previously, and, in addition, because 67 enteroviruses, comprised of 3 polio-, 30 coxsackie-, and 34 echoviruses, had already been described (1 coxsackievirus and 3 echoviruses have been reclassified [see below]). Previously recognized serotypes of the polio-, coxsackie-, and echoviruses would not be affected by this proposal, for they would retain assigned subgroup and number designations. In addition to the enterovirus subgroup, picornaviruses of humans include two other subgroups: the rhinoviruses (described in Ch. 112), and the unclassified picornaviruses representing those viruses that cannot be classified with certainty into the proper subgroup. The picornaviruses are grouped on the basis of certain common biochemical and biophysical properties, such as small size (15 to 30 nm), ribonucleic acid (RNA) core, and resistance to inactivation by ether. The term picornavirus was chosen to signify two of these properties: "pico" implying small, and "rna" referring to the nucleic acid type.

COXSACKIEVIRUSES

The isolation of the first of the group A coxsackieviruses during a study of a small poliomyelitis outbreak was reported by Dalldorf and Sickles in 1948. Suspensions of fecal specimens from two patients with paralytic poliomyelitis were found to cause paralysis in suckling mice, with widespread degeneration of the skeletal musculature. Since polioviruses were not known to cause illness in suckling mice and since these newly recovered agents (unlike the polioviruses) produced no illness in monkeys, it was assumed that a new agent distinct from the polioviruses had been isolated. As neither the anatomic lesions nor the range of symptoms induced by infection with this agent in man was known, it was suggested that the virus be called "Coxsackie virus," because the first strains were isolated from residents of Coxsackie, New York. The following year, additional types, including the first of the group B coxsackieviruses, were isolated. In the ensuing years, numerous other group A and B coxsackieviruses were isolated; at this writing, there are 23 group A coxsackieviruses (numbered A1 to A22 and A24) and 6 group B coxsackieviruses (numbered B1 to B6). Coxsackievirus A23 is omitted because it has been reclassified as echovirus type 9.

The coxsackieviruses are divided into groups A and B on the basis of differences in lesions induced in suckling mice. In this animal the group A viruses characteristically produce flaccid paralysis with widespread degeneration of skeletal musculature and no other lesions, whereas the group B viruses produce fewer and less severe skeletal muscle lesions, but produce in addition encephalitis, fat necrosis, pancreatitis, hepatitis, and myocarditis; clinically, group B–infected suckling mice develop tremors, spasticity, and spastic paralysis. All group B coxsackieviruses (and polio- and echoviruses [except echovirus 21]) grow readily in monkey kidney cell cultures, but none of the group A coxsackieviruses (with the exception of A9) are capable of consistently growing in these cultures.

ECHOVIRUSES

The first echoviruses were isolated in the early 1950's as a result of the introduction of cell culture techniques as an efficient tool for the isolation and study of polioviruses. During the course of studies attempting to isolate poliovirus from fecal specimens in cell cultures, agents were found that not only were not neutralized by either poliovirus or coxsackievirus antisera, but also were incapable of inducing illness in suckling mice or in monkeys. These new "human enteric" or "orphan" viruses were later termed enteric cytopathogenic human orphan viruses (echo), because they were isolated predominantly from the lower alimentary tract, caused cytopathogenic changes in monkey and human cell cultures, and were recovered from humans. Moreover, they had neither been associated etiologically with disease in humans nor shown to be pathogenic in selected laboratory animals. The term "orphan" was suggested because of this lack of etiologic association with disease.

The echoviruses were numbered from 1 to 34. Currently, 31 serotypes are recognized as types 10, 28, and 34 and have been reclassified. Type 10 was found to be considerably larger in size than other echoviruses and was reclassified as reovirus type 1; type 28 was found to possess certain properties (such as inactivation at pH 3) not shared by other echoviruses and was reclassified as rhinovirus 1A; and type 34, although nonpathogenic in suckling mice, was found to be antigenically related to coxsackievirus A24 and was therefore reclassified as a strain of coxsackievirus A24.

NEWLY RECOGNIZED ENTEROVIRUSES

Enteroviruses 68, 69, and 70 are the most recent additions to the enterovirus subgroup and are classified according to the new system described above because of overlapping properties among certain enterovirus strains. For example, one strain of enterovirus 68 induces characteristic group A coxsackievirus lesions in suckling mice, whereas three other strains of this serotype do not. In addition, among the classified coxsackie- and echoviruses, certain strains of coxsackievirus A24 are not pathogenic in suckling mice, whereas the prototype strain is; and certain strains of echovirus 9 are pathogenic in suckling mice, whereas the prototype strain is not.

DISEASES DUE TO COXSACKIEVIRUSES, ECHOVIRUSES, AND NEWLY RECOGNIZED ENTEROVIRUSES

A definitive presentation of diseases caused by coxsackie- and echoviruses is difficult, because these agents have been isolated from an ever-increasing list of specific diseases and clinical syndromes. The mere isolation of the virus from a patient's throat or anal swab and/or the demonstration of serologic evidence of infection is not sufficient evidence to establish an etiologic relationship between the virus and the patient's illness. Isolation of virus from blood, cerebrospinal fluid (CSF), or diseased tissue is more meaningful evidence for an etiologic association than the above, but even more meaningful evidence may be obtained from controlled epidemiologic studies. The establishment of an etiologic association is especially difficult with the coxsackie- and echoviruses. These viruses not only commonly cause subclinical infections but also are frequently shed in the stools for several weeks after either subclinical or clinically apparent infection. Therefore an isolation could occur by chance during various periods of illness or well-being. Only those specific diseases or clinical syndromes in which either satisfactorily controlled epidemiologic studies have established the etiologic relationship between coxsackievirus, echovirus, or newly recognized enterovirus infections and an illness, or in which virus isolations have been made from blood, CSF, or diseased tissue will be presented in the following discussions (see accompanying table).

Epidemiology. Coxsackie- and echoviruses are widely distributed throughout the world. They are found most commonly in human feces, but may also be found in the oropharynx or in nasopharyngeal washings; in patients with aseptic meningitis these agents may also be recovered from the CSF. They are resistant not only to the common antimicrobial drugs such as penicillin, streptomycin, and the tetracyclines, but also to many of the commonly used antiseptics such as 70 per cent alcohol, 5 per cent Lysol, and 1 per cent quaternary ammonium compounds. The occurrence of these infections is not influenced by sex or race. They have been isolated from all age groups, but it is apparent that in most instances infants and children are most susceptible to infection. The prevalence of these agents in surveys of presumably normal infants and children has ranged from less than 5 per cent to 50 per cent, depending on the location of the survey. Season appears to be an important factor in the epidemiology of coxsackie- and echovirus infections, for the majority of infections occur during the summer and early autumn months. The incubation period may vary widely, but usually ranges from 1 to 15 days. Recently, enterovirus 70 and a strain related to coxsackievirus

Diseases Caused by Coxsackieviruses, Echoviruses, and Newly Recognized Enteroviruses

Coxsackieviruses group A, types 1–22, 24:
  Herpangina (types 2, 3, 4, 5, 6, 8, 10, 22)
  "Hand, foot, and mouth disease" (types 5, 16)
  Acute lymphonodular pharyngitis (type 10)
  Aseptic meningitis (types 1, 2, 4, 5, 7, 9, 10, 14, 16, 22, 24)
  Epidemic exanthemata (type 9)
  "Common-cold like" (type 21)
  Acute undifferentiated respiratory or nonrespiratory illnesses
    (all types listed above with clinical syndromes)
  Acute hemorrhagic conjunctivitis (epidemic conjunctivitis) (type 24)
Coxsackieviruses group B, type 1–6:
  Epidemic pleurodynia or Bornholm disease (types 1–5)
  Aseptic meningitis (types 1–6)
  Myocarditis of newborn infants (types 1–5)
  Myocarditis and pericarditis of infants beyond newborn period,
    children, and adults (types 1–5)
  Orchitis (types 1–5)
  Acute undifferentiated respiratory or nonrespiratory illnesses
    (types 1–6)
Echovirus types 1–9, 10–27, 29–33:
  Aseptic meningitis (types 1–9, 11, 12, 14–19, 21, 22, 25, 30, 31, 33)
  Epidemic exanthemata (types 9, 16)
  Diarrhea (type 18, possibly types 6, 7, 14, 19)
  Acute undifferentiated respiratory or nonrespiratory illnesses
    (all types listed above with clinical syndromes, plus type 20)
Enterovirus types 68–70:
  Acute hemorrhagic conjunctivitis (epidemic conjunctivitis) (type 70)

A24 have been recovered from the conjunctiva during outbreaks of acute conjunctivitis; these outbreaks have had some unusual epidemiologic characteristics (see below).

As shown in the table, these viruses produce a broad spectrum of clinical manifestations, ranging from inapparent infection and mild undifferentiated respiratory or nonrespiratory illnesses to severe illnesses with varying involvement of the central nervous system. Illnesses associated with these agents are described in Ch. 127 to 136.

PREVENTION OF COXSACKIEVIRUS, ECHOVIRUS, AND NEWLY RECOGNIZED ENTEROVIRUS INFECTIONS

The ability to produce effective inactivated and live poliovirus vaccines offers hope that such vaccines can also be produced for the other enteroviruses. However, at present, the need and demand for such vaccines have not been determined.

127. HERPANGINA

Definition. Herpangina is a specific infectious disease characterized by the presence of small papulovesicular lesions on the anterior pillars of the tonsillar fauces and the soft palate; it occurs frequently in outbreaks among infants and children during the summer and early autumn.

History. It was first described in 1920 as a distinct clinical syndrome by Zahorsky in a report of 82 cases of "herpetic sore throat"; he subsequently suggested that this "peculiar throat disease . . . the clinical features of which are sufficiently clear to separate . . . from other diseases of the mouth and throat" be named "herpangina." Two other outbreaks of illness resembling herpangina were reported in 1939 and 1941.

Etiology. Herpangina was not described again until 1950 when Huebner et al. described studies in which certain group A coxsackieviruses were recovered from 32 of 37 herpangina patients, and on the basis of epidemiologic evidence an etiologic association was suggested. Numerous clinical and epidemiologic reports from many parts of the world have confirmed an etiologic relationship between certain group A coxsackieviruses and herpangina (see table). Reports have appeared recently relating certain group B coxsackievirus and echovirus infections temporally with herpangina-like syndromes; further epidemiologic studies are needed to elucidate the role of the group B coxsackieviruses and echoviruses in the pathogenesis of herpangina-like syndromes.

Epidemiology. Herpangina is a common infectious disease occurring frequently in outbreaks, but also sporadically, in most parts of the world predominantly during the summer and early autumn. Although it occasionally occurs in adults, the highest incidence is found in infants and young children. Multiple cases in a family are frequently observed. Spread is from person to person with an incubation period of about four days. Subclinical infections as well as illnesses without the characteristic herpanginal lesions commonly occur in family members infected with the same serotype as that recovered from the herpangina case. Immunity to the infecting type appears permanent, but recurrent attacks occur as a result of infection with a different serotype.

Pathology. The pathologic process of herpangina in man is not known, as no deaths have been reported.

Clinical Manifestations. The illness is characterized by a sudden elevation of temperature (37.8 to 40.5° C) and the development of the characteristic throat lesions in association with variable systemic signs and symptoms. In a study of 69 group A coxsackievirus-positive infants and children with herpangina, 89 per cent developed a fever which lasted an average of two days with a range of one to four days; 5 per cent of patients with temperature elevations developed febrile convulsions. Anorexia, dysphagia, or sore throat was evident in 70 per cent, vomiting in 38 per cent, abdominal pain in 21 per cent, and headache in 16 per cent (Parrott and Cramblett, 1957). The disease is characterized by the presence of discrete 1 to 2-mm grayish papulovesicular pharyngeal lesions on an erythematous base. These lesions, which gradually progress to slightly larger ulcers, may appear on the anterior pillars of the tonsillar fauces, the soft palate, the uvula, and the tonsils, and are usually present for four to six days after the onset of illness. In one herpangina case in a seven-year-old girl, small ulcers were also observed on the labia and skin near the genital region (Mitchell and Dempster, 1955). White blood cell counts usually reveal no characteristic abnormality; cerebrospinal fluid examinations have been normal.

Diagnosis. In a typical case, careful, repeated examination of the oral cavity and pharynx should facilitate the diagnosis. Herpangina can be differentiated from acute infectious gingivostomatitis resulting from infection with herpes simplex virus, because the lesions in the latter disease are located on the gums, lips, tongue, or buccal mucous membrane. In acute infectious gingivostomatitis, lesions may also be found on the anterior pillars of the faucial tonsils or soft palate (as in herpangina), but almost always occur in association with similar lesions in the anterior portions of the mouth. In addition, gingivostomatitis caused by herpes simplex

virus infection occurs sporadically in all seasons of the year. In recurrent aphthosis the lesions do not usually occur in the pharynx and are not generally accompanied by fever. Herpangina should also be differentiated from "hand, foot, and mouth disease" and acute lymphonodular pharyngitis, both of which are described below.

Prognosis and Treatment. Herpangina is a self-limited disease, with complete recovery occurring usually within four to six days. There is no specific therapy for the coxsackievirus infection. Treatment is supportive and symptomatic.

128.   HAND, FOOT, AND MOUTH DISEASE
(Vesicular Stomatitis and Exanthem)

An outbreak in Toronto of a new clinical syndrome caused by coxsackievirus A16 was reported in 1958 (Robinson et al.). Observed mostly in infants and children, and occasionally in young adults, the new syndrome was characterized by vesicular and ulcerative lesions of the mouth and oropharynx or fauces and a vesicular eruption involving the hands, feet, and legs. In 1960 the term "hand, foot, and mouth disease" was first used to describe a similar outbreak in England (Alsop et al.). Coxsackievirus A5 has also been found to be associated with sporadic cases (Flewett et al., 1963).

129.   ACUTE LYMPHONODULAR PHARYNGITIS

An outbreak in Kentucky of a new clinical syndrome caused by coxsackievirus A10 was reported in 1962 (Steigman et al.). Observed chiefly in children, the illness was characterized by lesions on the uvula, anterior pillars, and posterior pharynx. The lesions were raised and discrete, whitish to yellowish in color, solid and not vesicular, and surrounded by a 3 to 6 mm zone of erythema. Patients experienced fever, headache, and sore throat, with symptoms lasting 4 to 14 days. The incubation period was estimated at 5 days.

130.   EPIDEMIC PLEURODYNIA OR BORNHOLM DISEASE
(Epidemic Myalgia, Devil's Grip)

Definition. Epidemic pleurodynia or Bornholm disease is a specific acute infectious disease of viral etiology, characterized by the sudden onset of severe abdominal and/or chest pain, fever, and headache. It occurs most often in the summer or early autumn, frequently in outbreaks, but may also occur sporadically.

History. Numerous outbreaks of this disease were described in early medical literature. Windorfer relates that Hannaeus described an outbreak occurring in Schleswig-Holstein in 1732. In 1872, Daae and Homann each reported an epidemic in Drangedal, Norway. Two years later Finsen, using the term pleurodynia, described outbreaks in 1856 and 1865 in Iceland. In 1888, Dabney provided the first description of such an outbreak in the United States; a patient described the severe chest pain as the "devil's grip"—a term subsequently applied on occasion to designate this disease. Hanger, McCoy, and Frantz reported 16 cases in 1923 and called the syndrome epidemic pleurodynia. Sylvest in 1930 described an outbreak on Bornholm, a Danish island in the Baltic; in 1933 he wrote a classic monograph "Epidemic Myalgia," in which he reviewed the world literature and presented detailed case histories of 93 patients with the disease in Bornholm and Copenhagan; the designation Bornholm disease was frequently applied following Sylvest's descriptions.

Etiology. The group B coxsackieviruses are recognized as the etiologic agents of epidemic pleurodynia or Bornholm disease. In 1949 Curnen, Shaw, and Melnick recovered a group B coxsackievirus from the feces of a 14-year-old boy with acute pleurodynia; in addition, they reported the occurrence of illnesses resembling pleurodynia in several laboratory personnel working with this virus. Subsequently, numerous studies appeared relating temporally epidemic pleurodynia and group B coxsackievirus infections (see table in Ch. 126).

Epidemiology. Outbreaks of Bornholm disease have been reported from most parts of the world. It is noteworthy that they generally occur in the summer and early autumn. Although all age groups can be affected, children and young adults experience the highest incidence. Intrafamilial spread is common, multiple cases in a single family being observed frequently; however, absence of intrafamilial spread should not exclude the diagnosis. In one large study, about one third of the patients developed the illness as single cases in a household (Warin et al., 1953). Although both large outbreaks and sporadic cases have been described, epidemic pleurodynia is not a common disease in that it is not generally prevalent each summer and early fall, but rather occurs in sharp outbreaks confined to geographically limited areas. The mode of transmission is probably by person-to-person contact, with an incubation period of about two to five days.

Pathology. The specific pathologic manifestations in humans are unknown, as no deaths have been reported.

Clinical Manifestations. Epidemic pleurodynia is characterized typically by the sudden onset of abdominal and/or chest pain, fever, and headache. The spasmodic abdominal or chest pain which may range from mild to extremely severe and which is often aggravated by respiration and movement is the most characteristic feature. In a report on 22 patients with epidemic pleurodynia who had a mean age of 25 years, Huebner et al. described the sensation of difficult breathing as particularly striking, and cited some characteristic descriptions of this symptom: "I can't breathe," "pain cut off my breath," "can't get a real long breath," and "it hurts to breathe." In a study of 114 patients hospitalized with epidemic pleurodynia in Boston, Finn et al. reported that the typical severe paroxysmal pleuritic type of pain was often described as "smothering," "stabbing," "knifelike," "catching," and "like a vise around the lower ribs." It is noteworthy that, although the onset of pain is typically

the initial symptom, in the Boston study about one quarter of the patients had prodromal symptoms one to ten days before the onset of pain—symptoms such as "head cold," headache, anorexia, and myalgia.

Review of several outbreaks reveals that the location of the characteristic pain in infants and young children tends to be more abdominal than thoracic, whereas in older children and adults it tends to be more thoracic than abdominal. For example, in the 1949 Boston study in which almost three quarters of the patients were between 10 and 30 years of age, the characteristic pain was located in the chest alone in 48 per cent, in the chest and abdomen in 37 per cent, and in the abdomen alone in 14 per cent. In contrast, in a 1953 Birmingham, England, study of 104 hospitalized children whose average age was $5\frac{1}{2}$ years, the characteristic pain was located in the abdomen alone in 81 per cent, in the abdomen and chest in 11 per cent, and in the chest alone in 9 per cent (Disney et al.). Similar findings were reported in a South African outbreak in which 32 (80 per cent) of 40 children had abdominal pain alone, 4 both abdominal and chest pain, and 4 chest pain alone (Patz et al., 1953).

In the Boston study the chest pain was located "over the lower ribs and for varying distances up the chest, usually on the lateral aspect but not infrequently over the front and back" except in six patients whose thoracic pain was limited to the substernal region only; about one third of patients with chest pain experienced referral of such pain to one or both shoulders, one or both scapulae, the interscapular region, or the neck. Among those with abdominal pain, approximately three quarters experienced epigastric or upper abdominal pain; it was noteworthy that in two patients the site of pain was in the right lower quadrant. Other symptoms among the total group included moderately severe or severe headache (44 per cent), cough (33 per cent), anorexia (26 per cent), nausea (24 per cent), chilly sensations (21 per cent), chills (18 per cent), "head cold" (16 per cent), vomiting (16 per cent), sore throat (12 per cent), and diarrhea (7 per cent). Physical examination revealed that 95 per cent were febrile (37.2 to 40° C) with a mean temperature of 38.3° C; the fever lasted a mean of $3\frac{1}{2}$ days with a range of 1 to 14 days. Recrudescences of fever after the temperature had returned to normal or nearly normal were common. The pulse rate was proportional to the temperature. Visible splinting of the chest was observed commonly, especially during paroxysms of pain. In addition, a pleural friction rub confined to the lower half of the chest was heard in about one quarter of all cases. Localized tenderness to pressure was found in about one quarter of cases and was usually confined to those areas of the chest where pain was present. Tenderness confined to the abdomen (in 29 per cent), or tenderness in both abdomen and chest (in 9 per cent) were the most common abdominal findings, although "splinting and rigidity of the upper abdominal area were not infrequently present, especially when the pain was severe" (Finn et al.). In the Birmingham children's study, generalized abdominal tenderness was present in 34 per cent and right iliac fossa tenderness in 13 per cent (Disney et al., 1953). Roentgenographic examinations of the chest have revealed no characteristic abnormalities. The white blood cell count is usually within normal limits; occasionally a moderate leukopenia, leukocytosis, or eosinophilia may be present. The majority of patients are well within one week of onset, but longer periods of illness are not unusual. It is noteworthy that not infrequently relapses may occur a few days or more than one month after recovery.

Complications. Complications of epidemic pleurodynia occur relatively infrequently and include orchitis, aseptic meningitis, and pericarditis. Cases of group B coxsackievirus myocarditis of newborn infants have occasionally been reported during outbreaks of epidemic pleurodynia. It is noteworthy that myocarditis has only very rarely been reported as a complication in a patient with epidemic pleurodynia; however, the possibility should be borne in mind.

Diagnosis. A clinical diagnosis is usually not difficult once the presence of an epidemic is known. However, during the early stages of an outbreak or when a sporadic case is encountered, it may be quite difficult, if not impossible, to make the correct diagnosis. A vivid illustration of this difficulty is provided by a children's hospital study in which it was found that, until the house staff and other medical personnel in the community became aware that a pleurodynia outbreak was occurring, admission diagnoses on children eventually shown to have epidemic pleurodynia included the following: acute abdomen, possible appendicitis, possible duodenal ulcer, pyelonephritis, pneumonia, pleurisy with pneumonia, rheumatic fever, pain of unknown origin, trauma (fractured rib), myositis (influenzal), collagen disease, tuberculosis, and intussusception (Bain et al., 1961). Symptoms of common duct obstruction, pancreatitis, coronary occlusion, and intestinal infections may also be mimicked by epidemic pleurodynia.

Laboratory Findings. Laboratory diagnosis of group B coxsackievirus infection is made by isolation of the virus from throat washings or stools during the early phase of illness and by demonstrating a rise in neutralizing antibody against one of the group B coxsackie viruses in paired acute and convalescent phase sera. Unfortunately results of such tests become available too late to be of assistance in making a diagnosis in the acute case.

Treatment and Prognosis. There is no specific therapy for the coxsackievirus infection. Treatment is supportive and symptomatic. Recovery is usually complete and follows after variable periods as noted above. However, some patients may experience lingering aftereffects of tiredness and weakness, with a gradual return to normal health.

131. CARDIAC MANIFESTATIONS OF COXSACKIEVIRUS INFECTIONS

MYOCARDITIS NEONATORUM
(Epidemic Myocarditis of Newborn; "Acute Aseptic Myocarditis")

Group B coxsackieviruses were first recognized as a cause of severe, often fatal myocarditis in the newborn infant in the mid-1950's when investigators in South Africa, the Netherlands, and the United States reported 14 fatalities among 20 newborns who developed the disease from 3 to 21 days after birth (Montgomery et al., 1955; Javett et al., 1956; van Creveld and De Jager, 1956; Verlinde et al., 1956; Kibrick and Benirschke, 1956). Isolation of a group B coxsackievirus from the myocardium in six fatal cases provided firm evidence of an etiologic association. In most cases infection undoubtedly occurred soon after birth; however, in several it may have occurred in utero. It was noteworthy that outbreaks of other syndromes etiologically associated with group B coxsackieviruses (such as Bornholm disease, "summer grippe," and aseptic meningitis) were occurring concurrently in the general population.

The onset of the disease is typically acute and is characterized by dyspnea, cyanosis, pallor, and tachycardia. Some patients may have a fever, and in others the temperature may be subnormal. Vomiting and coughing attacks may also be present. Initially the disease may be mistaken for pneumonia, but symptoms of cardiac decompensation with enlargement of the heart and liver soon appear. Significant cardiac murmurs are not usually present. The electrocardiogram shows evidence of severe damage to the myocardium. In fatal cases the infant rapidly develops severe prostration and circulatory collapse. Pathologic examination of the heart reveals both a diffuse and focal infiltration of lymphocytes, polymorphonuclear leukocytes, plasma cells, and reticulum cells. In some areas the striations of the myocardial fibers are distinct but in others degeneration and necrosis may be present. Encephalitis, meningitis, and lesions in the lungs, liver, pancreas, spleen, kidneys, adrenal glands and pituitary glands may also be present in newborns with myocarditis. There is no specific therapy for coxsackievirus infections. Treatment is supportive and symptomatic (see Ch. 580). Individuals suspected of having group B coxsackievirus infections (based on epidemiologic, clinical, or other evidence) should, of course, be denied access to maternity and nursery units; medical personnel suspected of having such infections should also be denied access to such units. In addition, appropriate quarantine measures should be taken if a patient in a maternity or nursery unit develops an illness suggestive of a group B coxsackievirus infection.

MYOCARDITIS AND PERICARDITIS IN INFANTS BEYOND THE NEWBORN PERIOD, IN CHILDREN, AND IN ADULTS

Cases of myocarditis and pericarditis in infants beyond the newborn period, in children, and in adults have also been found to be associated with group B coxsackievirus infections. In addition to occurring as a distinct clinical entity, pericarditis may also occur as a complication of Bornholm disease. Myocarditis has only rarely been reported as a direct complication of Bornholm disease, but the possibility should be borne in mind.

It is not possible at this time to estimate the relative importance of the coxsackieviruses in the over-all etiology of myocarditis or pericarditis; epidemiologic and laboratory studies are needed to answer this important question (see Ch. 571 to 576 and Ch. 580).

132. "ASEPTIC MENINGITIS" DUE TO COXSACKIE- AND ECHOVIRUSES

Coxsackie- and echoviruses are important causes of aseptic meningitis in infants and children, as numerous serotypes have been implicated etiologically with this syndrome (see table). The epidemiology, clinical manifestations, and diagnosis of aseptic meningitis caused by coxsackie- and echoviruses (and other agents as well) are presented in Ch. 389.

It is noteworthy that sporadic cases of paralytic illness resembling paralytic poliomyelitis have been associated temporally with certain coxsackie- and echovirus strains (especially coxsackievirus A7, which also causes neuronal lesions in monkeys); in addition, sporadic cases of encephalitis have been associated with these viruses. Further epidemiologic studies are needed to elucidate the role of these viruses in the pathogenesis of such illnesses.

133. EXANTHEMATA AND "ASEPTIC MENINGITIS WITH RASH" DUE TO COXSACKIE- AND ECHOVIRUSES

In 1954 Neva et al. described the isolation of a new virus, later classified as echovirus 16, from patients with a mild exanthematous illness. The same virus was recovered during a similar outbreak occurring three years later, and it was suggested that the disease be called "Boston exanthem," because the first outbreak had occurred in and around that city. The illness, which affected infants and children, and adults as well, was characterized by several days of fever and a macular or maculopapular rash which usually appeared soon after the fever and other signs and symptoms had subsided; no central nervous system (CNS) manifestations were observed. It is noteworthy, however, that echovirus 16 was also recovered during the Boston outbreak from hospitalized patients with aseptic meningitis without rash (Kibrick et al., 1957).

In the mid and late 1950's numerous outbreaks of aseptic meningitis with rash caused by echovirus type 9 were observed in many parts of the world; in a few of the outbreaks an exanthem was not present. In typical outbreaks the clinical manifestations may vary widely from a very mild illness to the classic aseptic meningitis syndrome with or without rash. The eruption, which is characteristically macular or maculopapular, usually appears during the febrile period and occurs most often in infants and young children.

Coxsackievirus A9 has also been found to be a cause of an illness characterized by fever and a maculopapular or vesicular eruption with or without signs of CNS involvement; CNS involvement without rash may also occur. "Hand, foot, and mouth disease" has been associated etiologically with coxsackievirus A16 and A5 infections and is discussed in Ch. 128. In addition, it is noteworthy that various other coxsackie- and echovirus serotypes have been associated with sporadic cases or small outbreaks of exanthematous illnesses.

134. ACUTE UNDIFFERENTIATED RESPIRATORY AND NONRESPIRATORY ILLNESS DUE TO COXSACKIE- AND ECHOVIRUSES

Most of the coxsackie- and echovirus serotypes that are etiologically related to specific or severe illnesses such as aseptic meningitis, epidemic pleurodynia, herpangina, various exanthemata, myocarditis, and pericarditis have also been shown to be capable of producing mild acute undifferentiated febrile or afebrile respiratory or nonrespiratory illnesses that are indistinguishable from such illnesses caused by other agents (see table in Ch. 126). These mild illnesses are the most common clinical manifestations of coxsackie- and echovirus infections in infants and children, and are frequently described as "summer grippe." It is of interest that these nonspecific illnesses occur with greater frequency than the specific ones and often in the total absence of any concomitant occurrence of the more specific illness usually regarded as characteristic of these viruses.

Coxsackievirus A21 (Coe) virus has been shown to be the etiologic agent of an upper respiratory illness in an outbreak in a military population in which the agent was shed by 32 (26 per cent) of 122 patients with respiratory illness and by only 6 (6 per cent) of 108 of the controls (Bloom et al., 1962). A "common cold syndrome" was the most frequent illness observed, a fever of at least 37.8° C occurring in 14 of the virus-positive patients; fever in 5 of the 14 patients reached 38.9° C. Studies of this agent with volunteer subjects have also shown its ability to induce a characteristic upper respiratory illness (Parsons et al., 1960). It is of interest that coxsackievirus A21 was isolated much more frequently from throat swabs than from anal swabs in both the naturally occurring and artificially induced illnesses. Coxsackievirus A21 does not appear to be a major cause of upper respiratory illnesses in civilian populations. In volunteer studies, echovirus types 11 and 20 have been shown to be capable of inducing mild undifferentiated illnesses in adults (Philipson, 1958; Buckland et al., 1959, 1961).

135. COXSACKIE- AND ECHOVIRUSES IN DIARRHEAL DISEASES OF INFANTS

The relative importance of the coxsackie- and echoviruses in the etiology of gastroenteritis and epidemic diarrhea in infants and young children is difficult to determine at this time and awaits further epidemiologic studies, although it appears that these agents are not major causes of viral gastroenteritis. In 1958 epidemiologic data were presented on the etiologic association of echovirus type 18 in an epidemic of summer diarrhea which was not severe and which occurred in 12 premature and 5 older full-term infants in a hospital in New York City (Eichenwald et al.).

Controlled studies among infants and young children under four years of age conducted in Cincinnati demonstrated that enteroviruses were recovered approximately 2.5 times more frequently from patients with diarrhea than from controls (48 per cent versus 20 per cent) (Ramos-Alvarez and Sabin, 1958). Echoviruses were recovered approximately six times more often from children with diarrhea than from controls (31 per cent versus 5 per cent), whereas the recovery of polioviruses and coxsackieviruses was about the same in the diarrhea and control groups. Echovirus types 6, 7, and 14 were isolated from the majority of echovirus-positive children. In a controlled study of infants and children with diarrhea in the summer and fall in Mexico, it was found that echovirus infections occurred 8.5 times more often in diarrheal patients than in controls (Ramos-Alvarez and Olarte, 1964). Two other controlled studies (one in Texas, the other in Scotland) have failed to demonstrate statistically significant differences in the recovery rate of enteroviruses from infants and children with and without diarrhea (Yow et al., 1963; Sommerville, 1958). The recovery rate of echoviruses was greater in the diarrheal patients than in the controls in both studies, although the differences were not statistically significant. It is noteworthy that recent studies have indicated that "reovirus-like" viruses may be major etiologic agents of diarrhea of infants and children (Bishop et al., 1973, 1974; Flewett et al., 1973; Middleton et al., 1974; Tan et al., 1974; Cruickshank et al., 1974; Sexton et al., 1974; Kapikian et al., 1974; Bruce White et al., 1974). In addition, other recent studies have shown that a 27 nm "parvovirus-like" particle (Norwalk agent) was associated with a community outbreak of viral gastroenteritis (Kapikian et al., 1972, 1973; Dolin et al., 1972). Additional studies should aid in assessing the relative importance of different virus groups as etiologic agents of gastroenteritis.

136. ACUTE HEMORRHAGIC CONJUNCTIVITIS (Epidemic Conjunctivitis)

Acute hemorrhagic conjunctivitis is a recently described clinical entity which occurred in parts of Africa in 1969–1971, and in parts of Asia in the early 1970's, afflicting large numbers of people—predominantly adults—and spreading in pandemic fashion (Lancet, 1973). A small outbreak occurred in England in 1971; no cases have been reported in North and South America, Australia, or New Zealand. Certain epidemics have been associated etiologically with either of two distinct enterovirus serotypes—enterovirus 70, the more prevalent strain, and a strain related to coxsackievirus A24 (Mirkovic et al., 1974; Schmidt et al., 1974). The disease, which is highly contagious, is estimated to have an incubation period of about 24 hours and is characterized by a sudden swelling of the eyelid, and "redness," congestion, and pain in the eye, with excess lacrimation (Kono et al., 1972). Subconjunctival hemorrhage, which may vary from minute petechiae to large hemorrhagic areas, is the most characteristic symptom in most outbreaks. In the Singapore epidemics, however, subconjunctival hemorrhage was not as prevalent as in other outbreaks (Lim and Yin-Murphy, 1971). Complete recovery usually occurs within two weeks of onset. Corneal involvement is rare. It should be noted that during an outbreak of acute hemorrhagic conjunctivitis in India, radiculomyelopathy, predominantly lumbar, was observed infrequently as a complication; viral studies were not reported from this outbreak (Bharucha and Mondkar, 1972; Wadia et al., 1972).

Acute Haemorrhagic Conjunctivitis. Lancet, 1:86, 1973.
Dalldorf, G., and Melnick, J. L.: Coxsackie viruses. In Horsfall, F. L., Jr., and Tamm, I. (eds.): Viral and Rickettsial Infections of Man. 4th ed. Philadelphia, J. B. Lippincott Company, 1965, p. 474.
Finn, J. J., Jr., Weller, T. H., and Morgan, H. R.: Epidemic pleurodynia; Clinical and etiologic studies based on one hundred and fourteen cases. Arch. Intern. Med., 83:305, 1949.
Horstmann, D. H.: Viral exanthems and enanthems. Pediatrics, 41:867, 1968.
Huebner, R. J., Beeman, E. A., Cole, R. M., Beigelman, P. M., and Bell, J. A.: The importance of Coxsackie viruses in human disease, particularly herpangina and epidemic pleurodynia. N. Engl. J. Med., 247:249, 1952.
Kibrick, S.: Current status of Coxsackie and echoviruses in human disease. Progr. Med. Virol., 6:27, 1964.
Melnick, J. L.: Echoviruses. In Horsfall, F. L., Jr., and Tamm, I. (eds.): Viral and Rickettsial Infections of Man. 4th ed. Philadelphia, J. B. Lippincott Company, 1965, p. 513.
Rosen, L., Melnick, J. L., Schmidt, N. J., and Wenner, H. A.: Subclassification of enteroviruses and echo type 34. Arch. Gesamte Virusforsch., 30:89, 1972.
Weller, T. H., Enders, J. F., Buckingham, M., and Finn, J. J., Jr.: The etiology of epidemic pleurodynia: A study of two viruses isolated from a typical outbreak. J. Immun., 65:337, 1950.

POLIOMYELITIS

See Ch. 392.

ARTHROPOD-BORNE VIRAL FEVERS, VIRAL ENCEPHALITIDES, AND VIRAL HEMORRHAGIC FEVERS

(Arboviruses and Arenaviruses)

137. INTRODUCTION

Karl M. Johnson

Arthropod-borne viruses (arboviruses) are defined on an epidemiologic basis. Thus any virus is an arbovirus if it actually multiplies in one or more arthropods and if it is biologically transmitted to vertebrates with sufficient frequency by arthropods to make this an important means of virus survival. More than 300 distinguishable agents have been tentatively so classified. Many have similar physical and chemical properties and could reasonably be placed within families on this basis as well; others have fundamental properties relating them to animal virus groups not generally associated with recognized arthropod transmission.

Immunologic properties are currently used to cluster individual arboviruses. Viruses having such relationships are included in groups that historically began with A, B, and C; thereafter, the name of the first virus to be discovered was used to designate the group. Originally virus names were derived from antecedent diseases, e.g., yellow fever, dengue, and equine encephalitides. Later, geography in combination with disease syndrome was favored, providing names such as St. Louis encephalitis and Colorado tick fever. Finally, there are many geographically named arboviruses for which no clinical syndromes have been defined, either because they rarely infect man or because they have not been associated with morbidity of dramatic proportions.

About 90 arboviruses are known to infect man, and most of these have been shown to produce illness. With rare exceptions, such as dengue and urban yellow fever, these are zoonoses in which man is an accidental host of no apparent importance in the fundamental natural history of the virus.

Clinical syndromes produced by arboviruses share the common properties of fever and myalgia accompanied by viremia. Beyond that, classification is inevitably arbitrary, because the same virus can induce a wide variety of patterns in different patients, and different viruses have been linked to remarkably similar syndromes. Emphasis is given here to the often infrequent but spectacular severe diseases some of the agents evoke. Thus individual descriptions are placed in one of the following groups: (1) *fevers of a relatively undifferentiated type,* with or without rashes, usually benign; (2) *encephalitides,* often severe and with significant case fatality rates; and (3) *hemorrhagic fevers,* also frequently severe and fatal.

The largest number of viruses have been associated exclusively with milder, undifferentiated disease. The majority of these are encountered most commonly in tropical and semitropical countries (see table in Ch. 140). The classic clinical prototype is *dengue.* Those to be described represent but a small sample. Of these, *Chikungunya, Mayaro, O'nyong-nyong,* and *Ross River*

are group A viruses, *dengue* and *West Nile* belong to group B, and the remainder are unclassified or are in the *sandfly fever* group. Although each gained entry to this book because of its proved epidemic disease potential for man, clinical differentiation even during epidemics is generally difficult; epidemiologic and laboratory methods are more important. When more than one such virus is simultaneously endemic, the latter techniques are essential.

All arboviruses conspicuously associated with encephalitis and hemorrhagic fever are included. In the case of the latter syndrome, all but one of the viruses belong to antigenic group B. Yellow fever is listed among the hemorrhagic fevers because many cases do not display the "classic" picture of jaundice, but manifest gastrointestinal hemorrhage (black vomit), epistaxis, and melena with fatal shock and thus fit this description better than either of the other two arbovirus clinical syndromes. Arenavirus-caused hemorrhagic fevers, although not arthropod borne, are described here because of their clinical similarity to those induced by arboviruses and because they are zoonotic infections.

It should be emphasized that all these viruses frequently provoke only mild clinically undifferentiated infections. Thus specific virologic diagnostic tests are of fundamental importance in sporadic infections as well as during epidemics. Specific diagnosis of all arboviral disease depends upon isolation of virus and/or detection of a homologous antiviral immune response. In many parts of the world malaria is first sought in acute febrile disease with or without neurologic manifestations. The findings of such parasites, however, may not solve the problem; it should be remembered that either a simultaneous arbovirus infection or a drug-resistant parasite may account for the lack of response to supposed specific chemotherapy.

Virus isolation, together with an antibody rise to that agent between acute and convalescent phase sera from the patient, provides nearly incontrovertible evidence for an etiologic association between virus and disease. Blood is the best source of virus for all the diseases here described except for Venezuelan equine encephalitis which may be gotten from pharyngeal swabs at least as readily. *Such specimens should be obtained on the very first day the patient is seen,* because viremia rarely persists for long into the encephalitic period. Since antibodies are often present at the end of the first week of symptoms, it is important to obtain the acute phase serum specimen for serologic diagnosis at this time. A convalescent serum obtained 10 to 30 days after onset will usually reveal an increase in specific antibodies when measured by the complement-fixation (CF), hemagglutination-inhibition (HI), or neutralization test. No more than 10 ml of blood need be obtained for any of these specimens unless special studies are contemplated. Materials for virus isolation should be kept chilled, or frozen at temperatures of at least −60° C if shipment for testing involves great distances.

Hammon, W. McD., and Sather, G. E.: Isolation and identification of arthropod-borne-viruses. *In* Lennette, E. H., and Schmidt, J. J. (eds.): Diagnostic Procedures for Virus and Rickettsial Diseases. 4th ed. New York, American Public Health Association, 1969, pp. 227–280.

Horsfall, F. L., Jr., and Tamm, I. (eds.): Viral and Rickettsial Infections of Man. 4th ed. Philadelphia, J. B. Lippincott Company, 1965.

Taylor, R. M. (ed.): Catalogue of Arthropod-Borne Viruses of the World. Washington, U.S. Government Printing Office, 1967.

UNDIFFERENTIATED FEVERS

138. DENGUE

Karl M. Johnson

Definition. Dengue is an acute, febrile, self-limited infectious disease caused by an Aedes mosquito-borne dengue virus. Malaise, prostration, and pain of muscles and joints are characteristic, accompanied by lymphadenopathy, leukopenia, and one or two episodes of exanthem. Typically an illness of about one week is followed by one or more weeks of depression and weakness.

Etiology. Four distinct immunologic subtypes of dengue virus have been recovered from patients. These agents produce partial cross-immunity such that a primary infection will protect against another subtype only for a few months, although homologous immunity is of long duration. Sequential infection with any two subtypes, however, appears to confer long-term clinical protection against infection with any of the remaining two subtypes.

Epidemiology. Man and certain Aedes mosquitoes are the essential links in the recognized natural virus cycle. Size of human populations and ecologic factors affecting the mosquito vector and multiplication of virus in that host are of prime importance. Thus the disease has occurred in all continents and many islands, but only in "summer-like" temperatures where there are large numbers of *Aedes aegypti, Aedes albopictus,* or *Aedes scutellaris* mosquitoes. Since infection is usually clinically apparent in adults and frequently inapparent in children, various combinations of human and Aedes ecology may produce nearly silent continuous endemic infection, repeated seasonal epidemics, or massive outbreaks affecting populations previously free of dengue for many years.

Viremia adequate for mosquito infection is present just prior to and for the first three days of illness. An infected mosquito requires eight to twelve days to become infective at warm temperatures. Such a mosquito is infective for life and may transmit the virus to one or more susceptible persons on whom it feeds or probes. The incubation period in man is five to six days.

Aedes aegypti, by far the most important vector, breeds, rests, and feeds in or near human habitations. It is primarily attracted to man, biting in daylight and twilight. These attributes make it an ideal virus vector and explain why dengue is principally an urban disease. In rural areas other Aedes species such as *A. albopictus* may transmit infection, but their habits and relatively sparse human populations render explosive epidemics uncommon.

No extrahuman virus reservoir has been conclusively documented, but there is suggestive evidence that monkeys and forest mosquitoes may be capable of virus maintenance.

Pathology. Since dengue is rarely if ever fatal, the only information available is that from biopsy of the skin rash. Such lesions consist of endothelial swelling, perivascular edema, and mononuclear infiltration of small vessels. Petechiae are characterized by extravasation of blood without significant inflammatory reaction.

Clinical Manifestations. Dengue in adults is typically sudden in onset with rising temperature and only minor chilliness, headache, and fatigue. By the second day temperature is frequently 40° C, headache with ocular or retrobulbar pain is severe, and the patient complains of back pain, generalized myalgia, and aching joints. During this interval there is a diffuse blushing of the face and upper trunk, sometimes accompanied by a fleeting *erythematous macular* or *pinpoint rash* of the limbs. General lymphadenopathy is usually apparent, but hepato- or splenomegaly is rare. The leukocyte count at this stage is apt to be essentially normal.

At about the third to fifth day a *maculopapular* or *scarlatiniform rash* appears, beginning on the trunk and spreading in centripetal fashion. This generally lasts at least three days, becomes itchy as it fades, but rarely desquamates. The fever is generally of five to seven days' duration, sometimes with a fall at about the fourth day, giving a saddleback curve. The second bout of fever is often more severe, accompanied by relative or absolute bradycardia and by leukopenia. Monocytes, lymphocytes, and segmented leukocytes all decrease in absolute numbers, although there may be an absolute increase in immature polymorphonuclear cells. A few small petechiae may appear, especially on the lower extremities.

Dengue in young children is definitely a milder disease; recent longitudinal population studies in cities of endemic virus activity confirm an impression formed down the years by the paucity of description of pediatric cases during epidemics. Clinical manifestations may also vary with infecting subtype. Halstead retrospectively documented that volunteer studies done nearly 50 years ago in the Philippines employed subtype 1 and 4 viruses, the disease associated with the latter being milder and less "classic" than that caused by the former.

Diagnosis. During sharp epidemics occurring in places where ecologic factors are compatible, clinical diagnosis of many cases of average severity will usually be correct. But several other arboviruses as well as rubella may be the cause. Thus laboratory confirmation of a *few* cases during an epidemic and of *every* case when the pattern is sporadic is important. Travel history during the previous ten days is essential whenever dealing with a suspect case in areas where the disease is rare.

Virus may be isolated from blood or serum of patients early in the course of illness by inoculation of suckling mice, Aedes mosquitoes, or cell cultures. Serologic diagnosis is also possible, using acute and convalescent (two weeks) sera, but is frequently complicated by previous infection with one or more viruses of arbovirus group B. A laboratory competent to execute and interpret tests for a number of different arboviruses is required.

Treatment and Prognosis. There is no specific therapy. Bed rest is indicated, as well as the usual supportive measures to maintain fluid and electrolyte balance and alleviate discomfort. Secondary bacterial infection is uncommon but should be anticipated and appropriately treated. Except in severely debilitated persons, the prognosis is uniformly excellent. Final recovery is complete, although temporary depression and lassitude are common during convalescence, and patients should not be rushed back to normal occupations.

Prevention. Vaccines for dengue viruses are not generally available, although experimental work on the problem continues. Individual protection is difficult, because mosquito attacks occur during daytime, and continuous use of repellent is not practical. Community protection is possible through effective control or eradication of the Aedes vector. Patients should be protected from mosquitoes during the first five days of illness in order to prevent further virus transmission, and space-spraying of buildings frequented by patients should be done to eliminate mosquitoes possibly infected prior to the diagnosis of the disease.

139. WEST NILE FEVER
Karl M. Johnson

Definition. West Nile fever is an acute febrile mosquito-borne illness marked by headache, lymphadenopathy, and a macular skin eruption. It is generally self-limited, although rare cases of mortality caused by encephalitis occur in aged persons. The disease is caused by a group B arbovirus.

Etiology. West Nile virus is a small ribonucleic acid–containing virus belonging to an antigenic complex within the B group of arboviruses, which includes *Japanese B, Murray Valley,* and *St. Louis encephalitis* viruses, as well as *Ilheus* virus. Immunologic relationships are shared to a somewhat lesser degree with *yellow fever* and *dengue* viruses. Immunologic cross-protection is readily demonstrable experimentally among members of this antigenic complex. Despite the fact that such closely related viruses are frequently distributed geographically in a discontinuous manner, reflecting a long process of evolutionary segregation, West Nile and *Japanese B* viruses have been repeatedly recovered from the same mosquitoes in the same localities in southern India.

Epidemiology. Millions of people have been infected with West Nile virus, which is endemic in many parts of Africa, the Middle East, Southwest Asia, and southern Europe. Continuous human migration into Israel over the past 30 years has resulted in repeated epidemics among adults. Elsewhere the disease is mainly an affliction of children. Annual summer epidemics are correlated with seasonal peaks in populations of culicine mosquitoes. In Egypt and Israel, *Culex univittatus* is the principal epidemic vector. Much lower levels of virus transmission occur in winter when the suspected vector is *Culex pipiens.*

In ecologic terms, West Nile virus is one of the least evolved arboviruses. In addition to moquitoes, it multiplies in, and can be experimentally transmitted by, the bite of various species of hard and soft ticks. It has been recovered from Argas and Hyalomma ticks in nature. Although the primary natural virus cycle appears to comprise mosquitoes and wild birds, virus or antibody has been detected in rodents, camels, cattle, horses, and monkeys.

The incubation period in man is about three to six days. Most infections are clinically apparent. A number of documented laboratory infections suggest that the agent also can be transmitted by the respiratory route.

Clinical Manifestations. Sudden onset of fever, lasting three to six days, is accompanied by photophobia, myalgia, and chilling. Nausea and vomiting may occur early in the febrile period. A saddleback fever curve is seen in a minority of patients, and there is usually a definite leukopenia with absolute reduction of polymorphonuclear cells by the third day of illness. At about this time a fine *maculopapular* rash is observed on the trunk and occasionally on the extremities. It is more common in children than in adults, is *nonirritating,* and fades rapidly without desquamation. Lymphadenopathy is often demonstrable at the time the patient is first seen.

Although mild meningismus is demonstrable in a minority of patients and may be accompanied by increased cells and protein in the cerebrospinal fluid, clinical encephalitis is not a feature of West Nile infection except in a handful of very old patients. Pathologic studies were not done in the few fatal cases reported. Convalescence is generally uneventful, although older patients may complain of generalized weakness for several weeks. No permanent sequelae have ever been observed.

Diagnosis. Clinically this disease is so similar to dengue that laboratory diagnosis is essential in all cases. Virus isolation is by far the best hope, and blood specimens obtained as late as the fourth symptomatic day yield a reasonably high percentage of strains when inoculated into suckling mice or the yolk sacs of embryonated eggs. Serologic diagnosis may also be attempted with the usual paired serum samples, but previous infection with related group B arboviruses, including 17D live yellow fever vaccine, may render interpretation of results extremely difficult beyond the confirmation that infection was due to a mosquito-borne member of this large antigenic group.

Treatment and Prevention. Management of patients is completely symptomatic. Complications are unusual, and the only reason to keep patients under observation after the rash has faded is to ensure the collection of appropriate diagnostic specimens in situations in which knowledge of the specific cause of illness may have public health implications.

Although there is an impression that prior infection with related group B viruses may lessen the symptomatology of West Nile fever, this has not been rigorously established. Inactivated or attenuated West Nile virus has been used in combination with other group B agents in experimental attempts to produce broad-spectrum immunity to this virus group. Such vaccines are not ready for general use. Thus mosquito control and individual protective measures against mosquito bite represent the only available means of prevention of this infection. Since the main epidemic mosquito vectors are not concentrated around human dwellings and since infection rarely causes severe human disease, expensive systematic mosquito control systems have not often been mounted.

140. FEVERS CAUSED BY GROUP A ARBOVIRUSES: CHIKUNGUNYA, O'NYONG-NYONG, MAYARO, AND ROSS RIVER
Karl M. Johnson

Definition. Chikungunya, O'nyong-nyong, Mayaro, and Ross River fevers are acute nonfatal diseases caused

Etiologic and Epidemiologic Features of Undifferentiated Arbovirus Fevers

Fever	Virus	Vector(s)	Vertebrate Host(s)	Geographic Distribution	Human Epidemiologic Features
Dengue	Group B (4 types)	*Aedes aegypti*	Man	Tropics and subtropics; Old and New World	Varies from continuous endemic to repeated epidemic pattern based on human-Aedes population cycles
West Nile	Group B	Culex mosquitoes Argas, Hyalomma ticks	Wild birds	Mediterranean basin, Middle East, Soviet Union, Southwest Asia	Continuously endemic (tropics) to annually epidemic in Mediterranean climates
O'nyong-nyong	Group A	*Anopheles funestus, Anopheles gambiae*	Man	East Africa	Singular massive epidemic; malaria control may affect pattern
Chikungunya	Group A	*Aedes aegypti, A. africanus,* Culex mosquitoes	Man, monkeys?	Africa, Southern Asia, Philippines	Basically similar to dengue
Mayaro	Group A	Haemagogus, Psorophora mosquitoes	Monkeys, marsupials	Northern South America and Central America	Endemic, forest-associated infection; localized outbreaks during forest destruction
Ross River	Group A	Culex, Aedes mosquitoes	Wild mouse	Eastern Australia	Endemic infction in subtropical north; summer-fall epidemics farther south
Rift Valley	Ungrouped	Aedes, Culex mosquitoes	Large wild and domestic animals	East and South Africa	Sporadic rainy season transmission to man; mainly contact infections during livestock epizootics
Colorado tick	Bluetongue group	*Dermacentor andersoni* tick	Ground squirrels, chipmunks	Rocky Mountains of North America	Sporadic and focal summer infections during recreational and occupational activity
Sandfly	Phlebotomus fever group (15 types)	Phlebotomus, Lutzomyia sandflies	Man, monkeys, small wild mammals	Mediterranean basin, eastward to southern Asia; forests of tropical America	Annual seasonal transmission to children; epidemic whenever large numbers of susceptible adults introduced; forest-associated infections in American tropics.

by an antigenically related, geographically dispersed complex of group A arboviruses. Maculopapular rashes and arthralgia are common features of these infections, which occur in Africa, Southeast Asia, tropical America, and Australia.

Epidemiology.   Each of these viruses has caused epidemic disease in human populations. Perhaps the most dramatic was that due to O'nyong-nyong in East Africa from 1959 to 1962, when an estimated two million persons of all ages were affected. The important mosquito vectors of each disease are listed in the accompanying table. Chikungunya virus is often transmitted by *Aedes aegypti;* because of the rash and minor hemorrhagic phenomena associated with infection, this agent has at times been considered responsible for cases of hemorrhagic fever during outbreaks basically caused by dengue virus infection. O'nyong-nyong virus is the only known arbovirus transmitted principally by anopheline mosquitoes. Sylvan maintenance cycles involving arboreal mosquitoes and monkeys have been postulated for Mayaro and Chikungunya viruses. Epidemic behavior of these agents is far from understood. Irregularly occurring outbreaks during warm rainy months are the rule. There is strong circumstantial evidence that Chikungunya virus has moved steadily eastward into Asia from Africa during the last 25 years, employing a simple cycle composed of man and *Aedes aegypti* mosquitoes. The incubation periods of these agents in man vary from about two to twelve days. Clinical attack rates are high in relation to those for infection, with the exceptions of Ross River and Mayaro viruses, which induce mild or inapparent infection in children.

Clinical Manifestations.   Onset is typically abrupt, and arthralgias or rashes are more likely to be the chief complaints than are headache and fever. Fever is usually mild, and is virtually absent with Ross River virus. Chikungunya virus frequently induces a saddleback fever curve, but the second episode, in contrast to dengue, is usually less severe. Arthralgias may or may not be symmetrical in distribution and usually involve terminal joints most severely. The maculopapular rashes are generally irritating, distributed over the trunk and extensor surfaces of the extremities, and may appear early or late in the course of the first week of symptoms. Leukopenia is a common feature of these diseases, and cervical lymphadenitis is frequently reported in cases caused by O'nyong-nyong and Ross River viruses.

Diagnosis.   All these viruses except Ross River can be recovered readily from the blood of patients during the initial three days of illness. Standard serologic techniques are highly reliable in making specific diagnosis, provided a second serum specimen is obtained 10 to 14 days after onset of symptoms. Differentiation of O'nyong-nyong and Chikungunya viruses in East Africa may present problems. Malaria, rubella, enterovirus infection, and other nonviral causes of acute arthralgia must be considered in the differential diagnosis of individual cases.

Treatment and Prognosis.   Treatment is symptomatic, and prognosis is uniformly excellent, although polyarthritis may persist or recur over an interval of several weeks to months. Corticosteroid therapy is contraindicated for joint pain in adults, at least until the third week, when hormonal antibodies have appeared. Children possibly infected with Chikungunya virus in areas where *Aedes aegypti* and dengue viruses are endemic should be hospitalized, because it is impossible to differentiate this disease from the prodrome of the dengue shock syndrome.

141. COLORADO TICK FEVER
Gordon Meiklejohn

Definition. Colorado tick fever is an acute, tick-transmitted viral disease which occurs throughout the Rocky Mountain area and is characterized by a biphasic febrile course and leukopenia.

Etiology. Colorado tick fever virus is an arbovirus which has not yet been shown to be related to other members of this group. The virus has been isolated from a wide range of ticks and a number of small mammals in the Rocky Mountain area. Only the wood tick, *Dermacentor andersoni,* is important in transmission. Cases occur throughout the Rocky Mountain area, including western Canada and the eastern parts of California and Oregon.

Epidemiology. The disease occurs in the spring and summer when tick exposure is common. The reservoir of the disease is in small mammalian hosts which infect the larvae or nymphs of ticks. The ticks maintain the virus over the winter months, and the adult tick then transmits the virus to other small mammals or to man.

Pathogenesis. Viremia can be detected at the time of onset of fever and persists throughout the febrile course. The virus may persist in, or in association with, the red blood cells for long periods.

The disease is characterized by a profound leukopenia and occasionally thrombocytopenia which is usually greatest during the second febrile episode. Pathologic data on the disease in man are meager because there have been only two reported fatal cases. In those instances, the pathologic changes were those of an extensive hemorrhagic diathesis associated with encephalitis.

Symptoms and Clinical Course. The onset is usually sudden, with chilly sensations, malaise, and fever. Muscle aching and pain about the joints are common manifestations, along with headache and backache. In children, anorexia, nausea, and vomiting are common. The disease is characteristically biphasic. The first episode of fever usually lasts two or three days, after which the temperature returns to normal. After a day of normal temperature, the fever again rises, and the second cycle usually approximates the first in length. Rashes are uncommon, but a small proportion of patients have petechial or macular rashes. Involvement of the central nervous system with meningitis or, less frequently, encephalitis may occur, especially in children. Patients who develop encephalitis have findings similar to those infected with other arboviruses, such as disorientation, coma, and convulsions. Hemorrhagic manifestations, including epistaxis and gastrointestinal bleeding, occur very infrequently and are most commonly seen in patients with encephalitis.

Diagnosis. The diagnosis is based on a history of tick exposure during the preceding three to seven days, followed by a biphasic febrile course with leukopenia. During the first febrile episode, the disease cannot be differentiated from many other acute febrile illnesses, including Rocky Mountain spotted fever during the first day or two of that illness before a rash becomes obvious. The differentiation between these two diseases is extremely important, because early treatment of Rocky Mountain spotted fever with tetracycline will abort the illness and cure the patient. Laboratory procedures to confirm the diagnosis include viral culture from blood, demonstration of viral antigen on red cells by fluorescent antibody techniques, and serologic tests with paired serum specimens.

Prevention. Protection against ticks by appropriate clothing or repellents is possible but usually impractical. Experimental vaccines have shown promise but are not currently available.

Prognosis. The disease almost invariably runs a benign course and produces a lifelong immunity. The rare exception is the patient who develops either an encephalitis or a hemorrhagic diathesis.

Treatment. Treatment is symptomatic. When the patient is seriously ill and the diagnosis of Rocky Mountain spotted fever is entertained, it is advisable to give tetracycline in doses of 2.0 grams per day. If the patient has Rocky Mountain spotted fever, the temperature usually falls to normal within 48 hours, whereas the course of Colorado tick fever is not altered by this regimen.

142. RIFT VALLEY FEVER
Karl M. Johnson

Definition. Rift Valley fever is a febrile illness of short duration characterized by headache, myalgia, prostration, photophobia, and leukopenia. It is the only such arbovirus infection accompanied by significant complications which are ocular. The virus is mosquito borne, enzootic in wild game animals, epizootic in domestic livestock, and restricted geographically to East and South Africa.

Etiology. Rift Valley virus is a 30 to 50 nm, ribonucleic acid–containing arbovirus antigenically unrelated to any other known agent. Historically it was the second disease-producing, mosquito-borne virus ever described, the first being yellow fever.

Epidemiology. The virus was initially recovered from sheep in East Africa. Subsequent investigations showed that infection was common among large wild mammals of the region, and that virus was naturally present in a variety of mosquito species of the genera Aedes, Culex, and Erethmapodites, many of which are now known to feed primarily on wild game. After seasonal rains which lead to high mosquito populations, the virus spills over from this wild cycle, causing epizootics with high mortality in sheep, cattle, and even fowl. The agent is pantropic in these animals, the most striking lesion being a severe necrotizing hepatitis, reminiscent of yellow fever in man.

Human infection can be acquired in at least two ways: by mosquito bite, which is usually associated with big-game hunting or with ranching activity, and by direct or aerosol contact with the virus through the handling of tissues of affected livestock, or working with the agent in the laboratory. More human disease has been associated with the latter than the former transmission mechanism. This virus is so infectious to man, and of such potential economic hazard to the livestock industry, that it is now prohibited in the United States, even for experimental purposes.

Clinical Manifestations. After an incubation period of three to six days, onset of symptoms is usually abrupt, with fever, photophobia, and severe generalized headache. There may be severe prostration, myalgia, nausea, and vomiting. Epigastric pain is a frequent complaint. Temperature oscillates between 38 and 40° C, is often "saddleback" in evolution, and may persist up to one week. Leukopenia is common, as is a relative bradycardia. Skin eruptions are almost never observed, although minor hemorrhages in skin and from mucous membranes are infrequently present. Convalescence is usually, although not always, uneventful.

Complications. These consist of a *central serous retinopathy* with an associated *central scotoma*. The fundus shows exudates involving the macula that may be secondary to thrombosis of vessels. Whether such lesions represent direct viral damage or result from an immunopathologic reaction to infection is not known. The exudates usually shrink and disappear over the course of several weeks, but in a minority of patients *retinal detachment* has ensued.

Diagnosis. This is above all a disease of place and of particular human activity. A history is more valuable than any other procedure. Blood obtained during the first three days of illness almost always contains virus which is lethal when inoculated into mice. Serologic diagnosis of this infection is also definitive, because interpretation of antibody responses in paired sera is never compromised by heterologous reactions with any other agent.

Treatment and Prevention. Management of patients, as for other arthropod-borne fevers, is symptomatic. Serial examination for retinal complications should be done, and continued rest is indicated for persons in whom such lesions occur. Since the ocular complications appear to have an acute episodic rather than a subacute or chronic allergic pathogenesis, corticosteroids are of no benefit in their management.

Prevention of infection is principally through individual anti-mosquito measures. A live attenuated vaccine has been used in animals and man in South Africa, but this has more recently been replaced for human use among persons at high risk of infection, such as veterinarians, by a formalin-killed preparation which appears to confer complete clinical protection for at least two years.

143. SANDFLY FEVER

Karl M. Johnson

Definition. Sandfly fever is a self-limited viral disease consisting of fever, headache, and myalgia. Leukopenia and conjunctival injection are characteristic. It occurs during the warm season in the littoral of the Mediterranean Sea and eastward through Asia Minor, Pakistan, and northern India. Sporadic cases have been recognized in tropical America.

Etiology. Although the classic syndrome in the Old World is caused by two antigenically related viruses, Sicilian and Neapolitan, recent ecologic studies in various parts of the world have led to the recovery of at least 15 distinct but related agents from phlebotomine sandflies. These are now referred to as members of the Phlebotomus fever group of arboviruses. Many can be isolated in suckling mice or hamsters, but cell cultures, especially an African green monkey continuous cell-line (Vero), appear to be uniformly susceptible to infection with cytopathic effect.

Epidemiology. The vector of classic sandfly fever is *Phlebotomus papatasii*, and the only known vertebrate host is man. The fly has a very short flight range, stays close to ground level, and breeds best during warm dry periods in small collections of organic debris beneath stones, in masonry cracks, and in other protected sites. It has a short life span, probably not more than three weeks, but because of its small size it can readily penetrate the usual barriers of screens or netting which exclude mosquitoes. Serial man-fly transmission probably accounts for much of the virus activity during the season of peak fly populations, but transovarial transmission by the vector appears to be an important mechanism for long-term virus survival in view of the repeated recovery of virus in nature from nonbiting male sandflies.

Although antibodies have been found in forest-dwelling rodents and especially arboreal mammals in tropical America, equivalent isolation rates of some serotypes from male and female flies strongly suggest that the transovarial mechanism is a basic biologic adaptation for maintenance of viruses of this antigenic group.

Human disease patterns are determined by geographic and ecologic distribution of vector and virus. In highly endemic areas most infections occur during childhood and are rarely recognized in epidemic form. Epidemics in such regions are generally the result of introduction of large numbers of susceptible adults, such as during wars and national immigration.

Pathogenesis. Since there are no fatalities, the pathology of this disease in man is unknown. Experimental studies in man, however, disclosed that after intracutaneous inoculation the incubation period is three to six days. Viremia is brief, usually being confined to the day prior to and that of the onset of symptoms. Postinfection immunity is type specific and is clinically complete for at least two years. It may be lifelong.

Clinical Manifestations. Inapparent infection during experimental studies was rare. Onset is sudden, and peak fever is usually attained in the first 24 hours, subsiding after two to four days. It is accompanied by headache, myalgia, photophobia and ocular pain, and definite conjunctival injection. There may be erythema, but not a true eruption, over the face and upper trunk. Constipation and diarrhea sometimes occur. Bradycardia is not a feature of this disease, although the typical viral leukopenia is common. Cerebrospinal fluid remains normal. A few patients experience a second bout of fever and symptoms during the second week of evolution, but convalescence is otherwise uneventful and complete.

Diagnosis, Treatment, and Prevention. Epidemiologic history represents the best clue to diagnosis. Virus isolation and serologic procedures may be carried out but serve principally to exclude other possible causes such as dengue and influenza. Management of patients is purely symptomatic. No vaccine is generally available, but DDT and other insecticides have proved highly effective in control of the classic Phlebotomus vector.

Anderson, C. R., Downs, W. G., Wattley, G. H., Akin, N. W., and Reese, A. A.: Mayaro virus: A new human disease agent. II. Isolation from blood of patients in Trinidad, B.W.I. Am. J. Trop. Med. Hyg., 6:1012, 1957.

Barnett, H. C., and Suyemoto, W.: Field studies on sandfly fever and Kala-azar in Pakistan, in Iran, and in Baltistan (Little Tibet). Trans. N.Y. Acad. Sci., Sec. II, 23:609, 1961.

Clarke, J. A., Marshall, I. D., and Gard, G.: Annually recurrent epidemic polyarthritis and Ross River virus activity in a coastal area of New South Wales. I. Occurrence of the disease. Am. J. Trop. Med. Hyg., 22:543, 1973.

Doherty, R. L., Barrett, E. J., Gorman, B. M., and Whitehead, R. H.: Epidemic polyarthritis in Eastern Australia, 1959–1970. Med. J. Aust., 1:5, 1971.

Eklund, C. M.: Natural history of Colorado tick fever virus. J. Lancet, 82:172, 1962.

Emmons, R. W., and Lennette, E. H.: Immunofluorescent staining in the diagnosis of Colorado tick fever. J. Lab. Clin. Med., 68:923, 1966.

Florio, L., Stewart, M. O., and Mugrage, E. R.: The etiology of Colorado tick fever. J. Exp. Med., 83:1, 1946.

Halstead, S. B., Nimmannitya, S., and Margiotta, M. R.: Dengue and chikungunya virus infection in man in Thailand, 1962–1964: II. Observations on disease in outpatients. Am. J. Trop. Med. Hyg., 18:972, 1969.

Hotta, S.: Twenty years of laboratory experience with dengue virus. I. Epidemiology—past and present. In Sanders, M., and Lennette, E. H. (eds.): Applied Virology. Sheboygan, Wisc., Ellis Corporation, 1965, pp. 228–256.

Robinson, M. C.: An epidemic of virus disease in Southern province, Tanganyika Territory in 1952–1953. I. Clinical features. Trans. R. Soc. Trop. Med. Hyg., 49:28, 1955.

Sabin, A. B., Philip, C. B., and Paul, J. R.: Phlebotomus (pappataci or sandfly) fever. A disease of military importance. Summary of existing knowledge and preliminary report of original investigations. J.A.M.A., 125:603; 693, 1944.

Schrire, L.: Macular changes in Rift Valley fever. S. Afr. Med. J., 25:926, 1951.

Shore, H.: O'nyong-nyong fever: An epidemic disease in East Africa. III. Some clinical and epidemiological observations in the Northern province of Uganda. Trans. R. Soc. Trop. Med. Hyg., 55:361, 1961.

Silver, H. K., Meiklejohn, G., and Kempe, C. H.: Colorado tick fever. Am. J. Dis. Child., 101:30, 1961.

Spigland, I., Jasinska-Klingberg, W., Hofshi, E., and Goldblum, N.: Clinical and laboratory observations in an outbreak of West Nile fever in Israel. Harefuah, 54:275, 1958.

Taylor, R. M., Work, T. H., Hurlbut, H. S., and Rizk, F.: A study of the ecology of West Nile virus in Egypt. Am. J. Trop. Med. Hyg., 5:579, 1956.

Tesh, R. B., Chaniotis, B. N., Peralta, P. H., and Johnson, K. M.: Ecology of viruses isolated from Panamanian phlebotomine sandflies. Am. J. Trop. Med. Hyg., 23:258, 1974.

Weiss, K. E.: Rift Valley fever. A review. Bull. Epizoot. Dis. Afr., 5:431, 1957.

Wisseman, C. L., Jr.: The ecology of dengue. In May, J. M. (ed.): Studies in Disease Ecology. New York, Hafner Publishing Company, 1961, Chap. 2, p. 15.

ARTHROPOD-BORNE VIRAL ENCEPHALITIDES

Karl M. Johnson

144. INTRODUCTION

The arthropod-borne viral encephalitides comprise a group of clinically similar diseases induced by a variety of small viruses containing ribonucleic acid. Although infection usually occurs through the bite of an infectious arthropod, some of the agents are also transmitted by contact through mucous membranes, by aerosol, and by ingestion. In general, arthropods become infectious only after an extrinsic incubation period of one week or longer, which may be modified further by environmental temperature. Once infectious, however, such vectors remain so for long periods, in many cases for life. Encephalitis is usually an infrequent manifestation of human infection, but the agents to be considered all cause this dramatic and life-threatening syndrome with sufficient frequency that the term has been included as an integral part of viral nomenclature. This exposition is designed to provide the physician with the key clues necessary to aid him in sorting the variables involved in diagnosis and prognosis of infection, and to suggest areas where ignorance rather than understanding characterizes the state of knowledge concerning these diseases and their clinical management. Because of the very real public health significance attached to the occurrence of even a single case of some of the encephalitides, the importance of specific diagnosis of arboviral encephalitis cannot be overstressed.

It is possible to subdivide these diseases in a variety of ways. They are distributed nearly worldwide, occurring in both temperate and tropical climates; they are caused by different viruses, some of which are antigenically related; they are transmitted by mosquitoes or ticks; they cause central nervous system (CNS) disease predominantly in adults or in children; and they may or may not clinically affect domestic livestock.

Pathogenesis and Pathology of Arboviral Encephalitis. After deposition in the skin, virus may multiply locally and spread via lymphatics to cells of the reticuloendothelial system localized in lymph nodes, small vessels, and other organs such as spleen. In vitro studies suggest that macrophages are inherently susceptible to virus replication but that lymphocytes are resistant unless "blast transformed." Release of virus from such cells leads to viremia and widespread dissemination to other organs. Clinical symptoms and pathologic changes in many of these organs suggest that vascular endothelial cells are regularly damaged, but no direct or indirect visualization of virus in such cells in man has yet been achieved.

Although myocarditis, focal hepatic necrosis, and damage to lungs and kidneys may occur, the hallmark of these agents is their ability to induce damage to the brain. Despite some variation from virus to virus, a basic similarity exists in the gross and microscopic pathology of arbovirus-induced encephalitis. Brains are minimally edematous grossly with occasional small hemorrhages. Microscopic edema and hyperemia are present in the leptomeninges and cortex. There are small hemorrhages in many parts of the brain, sometimes with small arteriolar thrombi. Most striking of all are conspicuous collections of mononuclear, occasionally polymorphonuclear leukocytes around small vessels, the so-called "perivascular cuffs." Neuronal lesions are often focal and reveal nuclei and cytoplasm in various states of degeneration. Microglial and polymorphonuclear accumulations often present a picture of focal nodules. These lesions are most common in the gray matter, midbrain, basal nuclei, brainstem, and cerebellum, although some of the viruses induce destruction of anterior horn cells of the upper spinal cord.

Leukocytes and modest increases in protein concentration in cerebrospinal fluid are almost always seen. Although polymorphonuclear cells may be slightly more numerous early in the course of disease, there is always an evolution to a pleocytosis. It is of interest also that clinical encephalitis is almost always marked by a moderate leukocytosis rather than the leukopenia so characteristic of undifferentiated and primary hemorrhagic fevers produced by arboviruses.

A central question is how much of the CNS damage produced by these arboviruses is due to direct virus-induced destruction of neurons and how much may be the result of immunologically mediated injury to small vessels and/or neurons. In most instances virus is difficult to recover at autopsy from the brain, and it is not readily obtained from cerebrospinal fluid either. This has been explained in the past on the basis that antiviral antibodies are usually present at death in fatal encephalitis such that in vivo or in vitro neutralization obscures the real sequence of events. Although some neuronal destruction almost certainly occurs, the clinical course in the majority of patients who make rapid and nearly complete recovery and the pathognomonic *mononuclear* perivascular cuffs strongly point to an immune-induced inflammatory lesion as a major contributor to disease. What is wanted are new investigations of general and local immunologic reactions in patients with these diseases. The problem is of more than theoretical interest, because an elucidation of pathogenesis might well lead to a rationale for employment of therapeutic measures which present wisdom must continue to regard as potentially more harmful than helpful.

Clinical Manifestations. The shifting, protean neurologic manifestations seen in arbovirus encephalitis suggest a mixture of permanent neuronal damage and temporary central dysfunction secondary to intermittent anoxia and edema. This pattern accounts also for the observed wide range of convalescent behavior and permanent sequelae.

The temperature course is frequently bizarre, indicating an anoxic effect on central thermoregulatory function. Indeed, persistent high fever is the most ominous clinical sign, and *external artificial control of temperature may be the most important measure available* for the management of the severely ill patient.

Although statistically significant differences in the frequency of specific neurologic symptoms and signs of encephalitis caused by individual arboviruses are slowly emerging, it remains evident that the range provoked by each agent is quite broad. Symptomatology in the individual patient rarely provides assurance as to the specific etiologic agent. Unexplained differences in patterns correlated with human age, however, are sometimes striking. Thus death caused by St. Louis encephalitis virus (SLE) is almost invariably restricted to the elderly, as though the vascular reserves available to cope with an acute inflammatory anoxia were compromised. By contrast, CNS disease and death caused by Venezuelan equine encephalitis virus (VEE) are observed almost exclusively in children. Major upper motor neuron destruction leading to permanent paralysis is largely attributable to Japanese B and Russian spring-summer encephalitis viruses. Sophisticated clinical investigation of all these diseases is nearly nonexistent. More work such as that of the Dallas group who measured cerebral blood flow and certain hormonal functions in patients with St. Louis encephalitis virus is urgently needed.

Differential Diagnosis. The most common disease clinically indistinguishable from arbovirus encephalitis is that caused by *herpes simplex* virus. Previous clinical herpetic infection and the fact that this disease occurs throughout the year may offer clues to its recognition (see Ch. 390).

Enteroviruses and *leptospira* may produce disease which mimics arboviral encephalitis, and the seasonal pattern is often coincident. Indeed mixed arboviral and enteroviral epidemics are not infrequently recognized.

Meningitis and rarely encephalitis caused by *mumps* virus may also be confused with that caused by arboviruses (see Ch. 125).

Postinfectious or *postvaccinal* encephalitis after measles, rubella, or varicella infection or inoculation

with rabies or vaccinia vaccines must always be considered in such cases. History is the key to these diagnoses (see Ch. 118 to 121 and Ch. 396).

Rabies and *lymphocytic choriomeningitis* viruses can also resemble arboviral encephalitis. History of animal bite usually establishes the former diagnosis, but the latter must usually be separated by viral diagnostic procedures.

An assortment of acute febrile encephalopathies marked by hypoglycemia, diarrhea, convulsions, and coma, with or without visceral pathologic changes, has been described. These syndromes of undetermined etiology generally do not induce significant cerebrospinal fluid pleocytosis, nor do they display the marked central inflammatory changes so typical of arbovirus infection.

Bacterial and *fungal meningitides* can usually be distinguished by reduced sugar, high protein, and a mixture of cells, as well as by presence of stainable organisms in cerebrospinal fluid. Not uncommonly, however, incompletely treated bacterial meningitis may present a real diagnostic challenge.

Tumors and *abscesses* are usually separable by strong localization of neurologic signs, by absence of high fever unless septicemia is present, and by suitable tests to document abnormal space-filling lesions. *Toxic encephalopathies* must be thought of. History and chemical determinations are the best aids to establishment of such diagnoses.

It should thus be apparent that competent microbiologic diagnostic facilities are essential to establishing the specific diagnosis, and that such competence must extend beyond the arboviruses per se.

145. WESTERN EQUINE ENCEPHALITIS

Etiology. Western equine encephalitis (WEE) virus was the first such agent to be recovered from equines and humans. Isolated from an encephalitic horse in 1930 by Meyer, this agent represents the prototype for arboviruses immunologically collected into group A by Casals. The agent produces inapparent infection, mild febrile illness, or clinical encephalitis in both equines and humans.

Epidemiology. This virus, as well as its immunologic relatives, eastern equine encephalitis (EEE) and Venezuelan equine encephalitis (VEE), is limited in distribution to the Western Hemisphere. Virologic and serologic studies have disclosed seasonal mosquito-bird activity cycles in many areas of the United States and Canada and in parts of southern and eastern South America as well. It is not present in tropical Middle America. In North America clinical infection of man has been recognized in the Mississippi drainage basin, the Great Plains, and the valleys between the western mountains. In most of these regions the mosquito vector is *Culex tarsalis,* and a variety of small birds appear to provide the principal blood virus source for mosquito infection. Equines and humans are frequently infected, as disclosed by population surveys for specific antibodies, but do not develop viremia of sufficient concentration to serve as hosts for further amplification of the basic cycle. Seasonal temperature fluctuations play a decisive role in disease transmission, exerting effects on mosquito population, on virus incubation period in mosquitoes, and on migratory behavior of birds. Thus WEE is a disease of summer and early fall.

Experimental work has shown that WEE virus may persist during winter in hibernating snakes, and claims for such a mechanism in nature have been made but are as yet not generally accepted as valid. Human attack rates are highest in young adult males and in infants less than one year old. This pattern is due to the strong geographic localization of WEE virus and to the fact that agricultural irrigation projects vastly increase the breeding habitat available for *Culex tarsalis*. Incubation period of infection in man is generally five to ten days. Mortality among patients with encephalitis may reach 10 per cent.

Clinical Manifestations. A two- to four-day prodrome of fever, headache, and myalgia commonly precedes the appearance of CNS signs in children; adults more often experience abrupt onset of stiff neck and drowsiness with fever and muscle aching. Clinically, CNS disease is almost always more severe in children, who, in addition to the hallmark signs of disorientation, somnolence, and coma, often suffer convulsions, abnormal reflexes, and flaccid or spastic paralyses. Fever lasts for a week or more, but rarely for two, and ranges from 39 to 40° C. Higher temperatures are prognostically ominous and should be reduced by external means.

Clinical improvement at the end of the febrile period is often dramatic in adults, most of whom make uneventful recoveries without residual motor or psychologic residua. Children, especially the very young, are not so fortunate; more than half of them are left with permanent damage, producing mental retardation, emotional instability, or spastic paralyses.

Although leukopenia may be present early in the course of illness, a mild leukocytosis with polymorphonuclear cells predominating is more common. Cerebrospinal fluid is clear, contains normal sugar concentration but moderately increased protein, and nearly always shows a mild pleocytosis.

Diagnosis. Encephalitic signs occurring in both children and adults during summer should immediately raise suspicion of an arboviral causation. The major differential is similar disease caused by enteroviruses. Specific laboratory diagnosis is required in both instances.

Although WEE virus has been recovered on occasion from brain tissue of patients dying during the first week of disease, isolation of the agent from blood or cerebrospinal fluid is difficult even during the initial three days of symptoms. Specific diagnosis thus depends on demonstration of increasing anti-WEE antibody titers in sequentially collected sera. A specimen should be obtained and frozen as part of the initial examination of the patient, because such antibodies often appear during the first week of symptoms. The second serum can be taken 10 to 14 days later. Although single convalescent sera are of limited usefulness in areas where WEE infection is common, detection of specific antibodies of the IgM class is good evidence for very recent infection. This test is of proved utility in cases occurring among infants who have residual IgG antibodies from their immune mothers.

Treatment. Control of high fever and maintenance of water and electrolyte balance are the essential measures in management of patients. When necessary, reduction of fever should be by use of external chilling techniques rather than by use of analgesics such as aspirin. Contin-

uous care should be taken to see that a patient's airway and normal respiratory function are maintained.

Convalescence is usually prolonged and should never be forced. Children should be thoroughly examined at intervals up to a year after acute encephalitis in order to detect those who may require psychiatric or special educational and motor therapy.

Prevention. During epizootics or epidemics the prime objective is to prevent mosquitoes from biting babies. Houses should be screened; cribs, bassinets, and carriages should be covered by fine mesh netting. Transmission of WEE virus can also occur in utero; thus *pregnant women* should be specially protected against mosquito attack by restricting outdoor activity, by using repellents, and by use of residual and knockdown insecticides within and near their homes.

Community-wide organized control programs to reduce mosquito populations are important in areas where repeated epidemics have occurred. Based on combinations of insecticide and management of irrigation water, the value of such measures has been documented in California, Colorado, and Texas.

Epizootics of WEE in equines frequently precede human epidemics. An effective formalin-killed chick embryo virus vaccine is now used to protect horses, thus reducing the "sentinel" value of this species as a warning of an impending epidemic. The vaccine is not licensed for use in human medicine.

146. EASTERN EQUINE ENCEPHALITIS

Etiology. Eastern equine encephalitis (EEE) virus is a group A arbovirus which produces severe encephalitis and death in a high proportion of equine and human infections. It was first isolated in 1933 by Ten Broeck and Merrill and has been shown to be the most common cause of summertime epizootic-epidemic arboviral encephalitis in the eastern United States. Most outbreaks have occurred along the seaboard from northern Florida to Canada. Sporadic disease outbreaks also have been documented in some of the Caribbean islands during the fall. An antigenically distinguishable EEE virus variant is present in Middle and parts of South America. To date this variant has been associated with acute neurologic disease in equines but not in man.

Epidemiology. Basic elements in the natural cycle of EEE virus in North America are the mosquito *Culex melanura* and a large number of species of small wild birds. Although reminiscent of WEE epidemiology, that of EEE differs significantly owing to the fact that *Culex melanura* distribution is strongly localized to a series of coastal fresh water hardwood swamps. Virus activity in these swamps occurs each summer, commencing later as one moves from south to north. Two possible mechanisms may account for this seasonal chain; either the virus overwinters in each swamp by infection of vertebrates (hibernating turtles as well as contact infections among rodents have been proposed), or the Culex-bird cycle is maintained through the winter in the most southerly swamps where frost is unusual. In the latter case spring migration of birds could provide the means for reintroduction of virus into northern swamps each year. Southward fall bird migration definitely seems to account for the Caribbean outbreaks because EEE-infected migrants have been detected in the southern United States and on the islands, and virus strains recovered during these autumnal epizootic epidemics were identified antigenically as North American rather than South American in origin.

Epizootics in equines and in exotic gallinaceous birds such as pheasants, chukar partridges, and Pekin ducks usually precede by one to three weeks the appearance of human encephalitis. Evidence has accumulated indicating that accessory mosquito vectors such as the salt-marsh *Aedes sollicitans* and the widely dispersed *Aedes vexans* may be important in transmission of virus to these abnormal hosts. As with WEE virus, equines and humans are of no or very limited significance as hosts for further mosquito infection. Disease patterns observed in game-bird farms strongly suggest, moreover, that direct contact infection is important in the epizootics which at times devastate these exotic species.

Although EEE infection of wild birds is usually not symptomatic, the reverse is true for horses and humans. More than half of equine infections are clinically overt, and mortality among such animals may approach 90 per cent. Serologic surveys among human populations resident very close to the fresh-water swamps have revealed individuals with specific antibodies and no history or stigmata of encephalitis. Nevertheless, it is probable that clinical encephalitis occurs in a high proportion of human North American EEE infections. Mortality among hospitalized patients runs to 50 per cent or higher, and many survivors have residual neurologic dysfunction regardless of age.

Clinical Manifestations. The incubation period is assumed to be about seven to ten days, after which there is sudden onset of high fever, headache, conjunctivitis, nausea, and vomiting. This pattern, particularly common in adults, progresses rapidly from drowsiness to delirium and coma. There is stiff neck and irritability, at times accompanied by positive Kernig's sign, absent or hyperactive reflexes, and muscle spasticity in the extremities, often asymmetrical. Patients, if conscious, may be unable to speak or swallow. Excessive salivation is common. The disease terminates fatally within the first two weeks, usually within seven days, or shifting signs of deep CNS involvement may continue for several weeks, the patient gradually returning to consciousness. Serial neurologic examination usually discloses which centers and nerve supplies have sustained permanent damage.

Polymorphonuclear leukocytosis which can reach 50,000 cells per cubic millimeter is characteristic. During the first days of disease the CSF, usually under considerable pressure, also contains such cells in numbers up to 1000. Protein is elevated; as illness progresses, the cells become predominantly mononuclear.

A diphasic disease pattern is often seen in children. After a day or two of fever, headache, and gastrointestinal upset, followed by two or three days of clinical improvement, there is fulminating onset of high fever, vomiting, delirium, convulsions, and coma. There may be intermittent or persistent opisthotonos, generalized rigidity, and localized paralyses. Circulatory stasis or mechanical obstruction leads to clinical cyanosis, especially in the very young.

Convalescence is slow, and during this time neurologic residua become apparent. There may be permanent damage to cranial nerves, as to those regulating muscle function of one or more extremities. Mental or emotional deterioration, or both, may be so severe as to require permanent institutional care.

Diagnosis. Although EEE virus can be isolated from the brains of persons who die during the first week of illness, little success attends attempts to recover the agent from blood or CSF specimens during the acute illness. Sera taken during the first seven days of disease may contain neutralizing and hemagglutination-inhibiting antibodies for EEE virus. If so, the diagnosis is likely, because such substances are rarely found in the general population. A second serum obtained at about 14 days usually shows rising titers of specific antibodies.

Treatment. There is no specific chemotherapy, and there is no evidence that passively administered anti-EEE antibodies alter the course of clinically apparent disease. Thus management is that of any desperately ill patient: careful control of fluid and electrolyte balance, constant maintenance of a patient's airway, and external treatment of direct life-threatening hyperthermia. Secondary bacterial infections, if they occur, generally appear after the most acute primary phase of disease, and are those attendant to mechanical maintenance of respiratory and urinary function, physical inactivity, and bed sores. Physiotherapy to minimize paralytic contractures should begin after the febrile period.

Prevention. The principles are similar to those for WEE infection. There is a killed virus vaccine for equine, but not human, use. Since the ecology of EEE virus is centered in natural rather than man-modified habitats, organized mosquito-control efforts directed specifically at annual disease prevention are not economically feasible. Insecticides, however, are of some value both near residences and in accessible areas of mosquito-virus activity whenever a human epidemic exists or is threatened by the appearance of an epizootic.

Convalescent human plasma has been used to prevent disease after inadvertent direct exposure to EEE virus in laboratory workers. It is of unproved value and appears to be of no help unless given within 24 hours of the accident.

147. VENEZUELAN EQUINE ENCEPHALITIS

Etiology. Venezuelan equine encephalitis (VEE) virus is a group A arbovirus which causes fatal CNS disease in equines and an acute influenza-like syndrome in humans. During large epidemics cases of encephalitis are seen in young children, but the incidence of neurologic signs in this age group rarely exceeds 1 to 3 per cent of infections.

First isolated from horses by Kubes and Rios during a 1938 epizootic in Venezuela, the virus was not associated with human disease until several years later. Investigation of arbovirus ecology in tropical America during the past three decades has resulted in the recognition of several antigenic subtypes of VEE virus which differ in pathogenicity for equines and possibly humans and which have distinct cycles of maintenance and transmission. Taken together, VEE viruses have killed more equines and produced more human illness in the Western Hemisphere than any other arbovirus.

Epidemiology. Enzootic VEE virus cycles have been carefully studied in Trinidad, Colombia, Panama, Brazil, Mexico, and the United States (Florida Everglades). Virus activity was always focal, localized to shaded fresh-water swamps or to slow-moving bodies of water where floating water lettuce plants, *Pistia*, were common. The vector mosquitoes in each instance were members of the taxonomically complex subgenus *Culex melanoconion*. Small rodents, or in some cases water birds, are the principal vertebrate hosts. These animals develop high levels of virus in blood without significant mortality. Humans resident near or entering such enzootic foci suffer overt clinical infection, because the mosquito vectors are opportunistic rather than highly specialized blood feeders.

For some time it was thought that such enzootic foci were the sources for the periodic equine-human VEE outbreaks that swept large parts of Venezuela, Colombia, Ecuador, and Peru. But antigenic analysis of virus strains from all countries where VEE occurs together with experimental studies in horses has disclosed that enzootic VEE viruses were never involved in epizootics. Such strains, although capable of infecting and inducing cross-immunity, produced no encephalitis or sufficient viremia to infect mosquitoes when inoculated into equines. In contrast, antigenically distinct epizootic virus strains are highly pathogenic for equines, and induce truly dramatic viremias in them. Many genera and species of mosquitoes are thus infected and capable of further transmission of virus to equines, humans, and other vertebrates. Unlike the related WEE and EEE viruses, then, the equine is the single major host responsible for amplification and dissemination of the classic VEE strains. At present no mechanism has been discovered to account for interepizootic maintenance of such viruses in nature. Epizootics of VEE typically take place in rural tropical regions characterized by climates having a pronounced dry season. Cattle raising is the dominant land use, and outbreaks most often occur after the advent of the rainy season. Although human-mosquito transmission chains are possible, the timing of human disease one to two weeks after appearance of equine encephalitis suggests that epidemic VEE in man is mainly a spillover from the fulminant equine-mosquito cycle. At times nearly all equines and large fractions of rural human populations are infected during such outbreaks. Many thousands of human infections, most of them clinically apparent, can thus occur in a few weeks.

A unique outbreak occurred recently in Central America, with the apparently exotic epizootic virus finally reaching into southwestern Texas during the summer of 1971.

All subtypes of VEE virus are highly infectious for humans and other vertebrates when administered via the respiratory route. Thus many laboratory infections have been recorded.

Clinical Manifestations. Onset of illness is typically abrupt, patients frequently reporting the exact time of appearance of severe headache, chills, fever, and explosive vomiting and diarrhea. These symptoms ensue two to four days after infectious mosquito bite but can occur within 24 hours after exposure to highly infectious aerosols. Conjunctival injection and mild sore throat are present early in the clinical course, and myalgia is usually intense. Fever often reaches 40° C. In general the first day of symptoms is the worst, and the fever curve shows daily evening peaks which regress to normal after three to five days. Mild somnolence is common, but severe neurologic signs are seen in only a small percentage of cases, nearly always among children. Individual cases may thus be readily confused with influenza, acute infectious or toxic gastroenteritis, or leptospirosis.

During the first day of illness blood leukocytes are usually normal or slightly increased in numbers, with a strong shift toward polymorphonuclear dominance and a conspicuous eosinopenia. There follows a definite leukopenia, and by the fourth or fifth day a relative lymphocytosis is usual. Normal total and differential values are re-established by about the tenth day.

Nuchal stiffness is unusual, and the CSF generally shows no cells or a very mild pleocytosis with normal protein. Children exhibiting more serious neurologic signs, including abnormal reflexes, spastic paralyses, convulsions, and coma, usually experience a biphasic febrile course with the second fever spike associated with CNS signs. Epilepsy, paralyses, tremors, hallucinations, and emotional instability may persist as permanent sequelae of infection in children, and occasional cases of residual epilepsy and intention tremors have been cited among adults.

Most fatalities occur in children under five years of age. Autopsies revealed gross and histologic changes similar to those seen with other arboviruses causing encephalitis, but in addition were noteworthy for the presence of scattered gross focal hemorrhages in brain, heart, and lungs.

Diagnosis. Since clinical presentation of VEE infection is rarely overtly encephalitic, the diagnosis will be missed unless it is considered in a patient with high fever, respiratory symptoms, and gastrointestinal upset who resides in or has recently visited either an enzootic focus or an epizootic area of tropical America. Virus can be recovered with ease, however, from either blood or throat swab specimens taken during the initial 72 hours of symptoms. Since patients are potentially infectious for humans and mosquitoes during this phase, the importance of establishing the cause is obvious. Paired serum samples obtained early in illness and about 10 days later will reliably reveal rising levels of specific anti-VEE antibodies.

Treatment. There is no specific treatment. Analgesics and external chilling may be required to control hyperthermia. Life-threatening fluid and electrolyte imbalance may result from vomiting and diarrhea in children and must be alertly detected and corrected. Patients frequently complain of lassitude and inability to concentrate mentally for one to four weeks after fever has subsided, but convalescence is otherwise usually uneventful.

Prophylaxis. Formalin-inactivated vaccines have been used to protect equines in South America for 30 years. The potency of these products is borderline at best, and the frequent persistence of live VEE virus in them may well have been the cause of subsequent major epizootics. An experimental live attenuated vaccine, strain TC-83, has been used with success in immunizing laboratory personnel at high risk of aerosol infection. This vaccine, which produces febrile reactions in up to 20 per cent of adult recipients, has not been tested in children or pregnant women. It has been associated with birth defects when inoculated into pregnant rhesus monkeys and seems unlikely ever to be generally safe for human protection.

Nevertheless, this vaccine is the single most important tool available for interdiction of human VEE epidemics. Most mosquitoes acquire virus from equines, and it has been shown that mass vaccination of equines prevents further viremic infection of these animals within three days. Once horse infections cease, transmission to man generally comes to an end within a short interval as infected mosquitoes die. Insecticides are useful in killing infected mosquitoes when temporally combined with equine vaccination.

Since patients are potentially infectious, precautions should be taken to prevent them from mosquito bite. Although medical personnel attending patients are potentially at risk of acquiring the disease by aerosol, the infrequent occurrence of significant coughing during VEE infection may explain the absence of well-documented instances of such transmission.

148. CALIFORNIA ENCEPHALITIS

Definition. California encephalitis is an acute CNS disease which occurs during summer in many areas of the United States and is caused by one or more antigenically related viruses of the California arbovirus complex.

Etiology. The original virus strain of this antigenic complex was recovered from *Aedes dorsalis* and *Culex tarsalis* mosquitoes in the San Joaquin Valley of California in the 1940's. Serologic studies showed this agent to be associated with a few cases of childhood encephalitis previously thought clinically to be caused by WEE or St. Louis encephalitis viruses.

In 1960 the La Crosse strain was recovered from the brain of a six-year-old child who died of encephalitis. Although very few other isolates have been made from man, antigens prepared from the La Crosse agent have been used in recent years to document many cases of acute CNS disease in different regions of the United States.

At least six antigenically related California arboviruses have been recovered from a variety of mosquitoes and wild vertebrates in the United States. Related agents are known from tropical America, Europe, Africa, and Asia. One variant is annually active in the far north of western Canada and Alaska.

Epidemiology. Frequent epidemics of California encephalitis have been documented in Wisconsin, Indiana, and Ohio, and sporadic cases are on record from North Carolina and Florida. It is probable that the disease occurs over a much wider area of the midwestern and southern United States, but is not diagnosed because specific serologic tests are not generally employed and because cases often appear sporadically in a large number of small rural communities.

The La Crosse virus is transmitted principally by tree-hole breeding mosquitoes of the genus Aedes. Small mammals such as rabbits, chipmunks, and squirrels provide sources of virus for new mosquito infection, but the basic mechanism of virus maintenance is probably transovarial transmission of virus through the various life stages of the mosquito. This behavior was recently proved for *Aedes triseriatus*, the first known instance of insect maintenance of a mosquito-borne arbovirus.

More than 90 per cent of human cases of encephalitis occur in persons 15 years old or under. Males are more often affected than females, probably because exposure to the virus is most frequently related to the outdoor recreational pursuits of camping, fishing, or hunting in woodlands where infected day-biting Aedes mosquitoes are present. Although mortality from California encephalitis has not been established, it is low, not exceeding 5 per cent. Serologic studies also show that human infection with these viruses is far more common than clinical encephalitis.

Clinical Manifestations. Although not accurately known, the incubation period is probably between five and ten days. Onset of symptoms is typically insidious, with mild fever and headache for several days. As these symptoms increase, the headache usually becomes frontal, and the complaints are sometimes ascribed by patient or relatives to a minor traumatic incident. Mental confusion may or may not precede the sudden occurrence of convulsions, which may be the only overt sign of CNS disease on admission to hospital. Coma may supervene, and meningeal signs are occasionally seen, but shifting deep neurologic signs such as paralyses and reflex changes are rarely observed.

Mild to severe leukocytosis is characteristic of the acute stage of illness, counts sometimes reaching 30,000 per cubic millimeter. Cerebrospinal fluid is clear under moderate pressure and contains up to several hundred leukocytes, predominantly polymorphonuclear early, becoming mononuclear as illness progresses.

Fever generally subsides by lysis after a course of less than two weeks. Motor and sensory neurologic sequelae have not been observed, but emotional and learning dysfunction has been noted in children several months after physical convalescence is complete.

Diagnosis. The differential diagnosis of importance is that between viral encephalitis and post-traumatic *subdural hematoma*. Favoring the former are season of occurrence, history of forest exposure, the presence of leukocytosis, a clear cerebrospinal fluid, and the absence of localizing neurologic signs.

Specific diagnosis of California encephalitis must be made serologically, no isolate having yet been obtained from blood or excretions of acutely ill patients. Thus a fourfold or greater increase in CF, HI, or neutralizing antibodies between acute and early convalescent serum specimens provides the only confirmation of etiology.

Treatment and Prophylaxis. Management of patients is completely symptomatic. Hyperthermia and respiratory failure, although unusual, are the dangerous signs that must be detected and corrected without delay. No vaccine is available, nor has any experimental work been reported in this direction. Mosquito control is virtually impossible on a large scale because of the specialized breeding habits of the vector species. Protective clothing, nets, and repellents are the only effective measures available to individuals entering the woodlands where infected mosquitoes are present.

149. ST. LOUIS ENCEPHALITIS

Definition. St. Louis encephalitis (SLE) was the first recognized and is the most important arboviral encephalitis in the United States. It occurs sporadically and in major outbreaks during late summer and fall, afflicting rural populations in the West and urban-suburban communities elsewhere in the nation.

Etiology. St. Louis encephalitis virus is a group B arbovirus, most closely related antigenically to Japanese B and Murray Valley encephalitis viruses. It occurs only in the Western Hemisphere.

Epidemiology. The causative virus was first recovered from fatal cases during a major outbreak of encephalitis in St. Louis in 1933. Since that time sporadic cases and outbreaks of varying intensity have occurred in rural Washington and California, and in suburban and urban areas of Florida, Texas, the lower Ohio Valley, Pennsylvania, and New Jersey. Presence of virus is indicated by antibodies and/or isolation of virus strains from wildlife in Mexico, Central America, South America, and several Caribbean islands.

The basic virus cycle leading to human outbreaks involves birds and certain Culex mosquitoes. Although the possible mechanisms for virus survival during winter are not precisely known, they include reintroduction by northward migrating birds, recrudescent infection in nonmigratory birds, persistence of infected adult mosquitoes, and persistent infection in hibernating bats. The principal mosquito vector in the western United States is *Culex tarsalis,* especially abundant in irrigated agricultural areas. The vectors of urban-suburban epidemics elsewhere in the country are *C. pipiens, C. quinquefasciatus,* and *C. nigripalpus.* The virus has been recovered from many different mosquitoes in tropical America, many of them strongly arboreal in activity pattern, but it is not clear which are the most important in ecologic terms.

Although the distribution of SLE virus in the United States overlaps to a considerable degree with that of both EEE and WEE viruses, two important epidemiologic features distinguish the former from the latter group A viruses. First, although all three agents "spill over" from birds to horses, only EEE and WEE cause equine disease. Second, because the extrinsic incubation period in the mosquito is longer for SLE than for the equine viruses, St. Louis encephalitis always occurs later in the summer and is not found as far north (Canada) as the group A encephalitides.

Clinical Manifestations. Acute disease probably occurs in no more than 1 to 2 per cent of St. Louis encephalitis virus infections. Usually the course is benign, comprising a few days of fever and pronounced headache followed by complete recovery. More severe disease is occasionally seen in young children and occurs in a substantial number of adults more than 40 years of age. After an incubation period variously estimated at up to two weeks, there is acute onset of fever and altered sensorium. Convulsions are more common in children than in adults. The most common neurologic signs are stiff neck, tremors of the hands and face, dysdiadochokinesia, and nystagmus. Cranial nerve abnormalities are found in about 20 per cent of cases. Myalgia, photophobia, and conjunctival suffusion are common, and acute urinary symptoms with unexplained mild pyuria and increased blood urea nitrogen concentration occur in nearly one fourth of patients.

White blood cell counts are usually normal to moderately elevated, and increased numbers of immature polymorphonuclear leukocytes may be found early in the course. Although an occasional patient has no cells in the cerebrospinal fluid on admission to hospital, all eventually are found to be positive, the total number of leukocytes rarely exceeding 500. Although some polymorphonuclear cells may be present at the beginning, later examinations reveal only lymphocytes. Cerebrospinal fluid protein is typically increased, but rarely exceeds 100 mg per 100 ml.

Diagnosis. Given appropriate season and place, the differential diagnosis of St. Louis encephalitis virus infection centers on other arboviruses and enteroviral meningitis in children and on *acute cerebrovascular accidents* in the elderly. An infectious cause may not even be considered in the latter group until a cluster of cases demands explanation. The virus itself has never been recovered from blood or cerebrospinal fluid of patients, and only rarely from brains of persons who die during the first week of illness. Specific diagnosis is thus dependent upon serologic testing of paired sera. The most practical technique is that of complement fixation, although the neutralization test provides the most definitive result if the early acute specimen is recovered before significant levels of antibody have been produced.

Treatment and Prognosis. Treatment is purely symptomatic. Persistent fever above 40° C is an ominous sign and should be vigorously controlled. About 10 to 25 per cent of adults with acute encephalitis die, most of them from complications of underlying diseases. Such deaths generally occur after the first 10 days of illness when most of the neurologic manifestations have subsided. Hyponatremia is a frequent problem in management of the acute phase of disease, and in some cases has been ascribed to a partial persistent elaboration of antidiuretic hormone. Convalescence is often quite prolonged, and long-term examination of patients reveals frequent persistence of personality changes and emotional disturbance. Motor deficits are uncommon.

Prevention. There is no specific vaccine. Surveillance of seasonal mosquito-avian activity patterns of the virus in endemic regions is valuable as a guide to the timing of measures designed to reduce populations of vector mosquitoes. Emergency use of insecticides against adult mosquitoes during urban-suburban epidemics is probably of considerable help in reducing morbidity.

150. JAPANESE B ENCEPHALITIS

Definition. Japanese B encephalitis is a severe arbovirus disease which occurs in eastern Asia. Summer-fall outbreaks occur in Siberia, Korea, Japan, Taiwan, and other Pacific islands. Continuous endemic virus transmission has been proved or is suspected in Southeast Asia, the Philippines, and East Indies.

Etiology. The causative agent is a group of B arbovirus closely related antigenically to St. Louis, Murray Valley, and West Nile viruses. Unlike these agents, however, Japanese B virus is pathogenic for certain monkeys and equines, and has been shown to induce abortion or stillbirth in pregnant sows, a fact of major economic significance to the porcine industry of Japan and Taiwan.

Epidemiology. The basic cycle of infection in both temperate and tropical areas is mosquito-vertebrate-mosquito. In temperate areas the primary vector is *Culex tritaeniorhyncus,* and the important vertebrate hosts are herons, egrets, and pigs. Virus is detected in a given locale annually, first in mosquitoes in July, and then in birds and pigs within a few weeks. Epidemics of encephalitis occur later, in August and September, and by November virus has apparently disappeared. Winter survival has not been elucidated. Epidemics tend to be larger in alternate years for reasons not clearly understood.

In tropical areas virus transmission is less strongly seasonal, and although the basic cycle is similar to that of temperate zones, other vectors such as *C. gelidus* in Malaysia, Thailand, and Vietnam and *C. annulirostris* on Guam are important. Regardless of area, the ratio of inapparent to disease-associated infections in man is very high. Annual infection rates in children may reach 10 per cent, but only 1 in 300 to 500 infections results in clinical disease. This ratio apparently declines with increasing age, one case of encephalitis occurring per 25 infections in American troops.

Clinical Manifestations. Japanese B infection is similar to that of St. Louis encephalitis virus in the high frequency of inapparent infection or mild illness, in onset, and in the signs or symptoms of central nervous system disease. But urinary tract symptoms and signs are less common, and the over-all severity of neurologic disease is more severe in Japanese B infections. Children commonly evidence paralysis of the face or extremities. Adults tend toward bilateral paresis without sensory changes. Sensorial changes, spastic rigidity, cerebellar signs, and coma are frequent in adults. The fever usually peaks four or five days after onset, then slowly subsides. Relative bradycardia is often seen, accompanied by a modest transient leukocytosis. Cerebrospinal fluid pressure is often increased moderately, and pleocytosis and increased protein are invariably present.

Diagnosis. Although epidemiologic considerations may strongly suggest it, specific diagnosis requires a variety of virologic procedures. Isolation of virus from blood has been reported but is uncommonly achieved. Virus or, more often, fluorescent antigen can sometimes be demonstrated in brain tissue of fatal cases. Serologic diagnosis offers the best possibility of establishing the cause, but in many areas of Southeast Asia and India this is often confounded by the prior presence of antibodies to other related group B viruses. In Japan, where fewer such problems exist, it has been shown that primary infection induces early IgM antibodies reactive in neutralization and HI tests only, whereas IgG antibodies reactive in CF test are detectable eight or more days after onset of disease. Depending on the timing of serum specimens, diagnosis may thus require use of any or all three procedures. Detection of specific IgM HI antibodies has increased the precision of diagnosis in areas where related group B viruses are endemic.

Treatment and Prognosis. Intensive supportive care is mandatory and is all that is available. Artificial control of hyperthermia is frequently required. Anticonvulsant drugs may be needed, although prognosis in such cases is generally poor. The mortality rate varies from about 30 per cent for those under 20 years of age to nearly 80 per cent in older persons. Severity of clinical disease is directly correlated with quantitative antibody response. It has also been shown that early appearance of IgG antibodies was more common in persons who had received one dose of inactivated vaccine or who were more than 50 years old. Correlation of disease severity with early IgG immune response has not yet been reported.

Permanent sequelae are most common in children under age ten, with severe residual damage generally being reserved for the very young. These changes run the gamut of upper motor paralyses, cerebellar syndromes, personality changes, and mental deterioration frequently requiring permanent institutional care.

Prevention. Formolized vaccine has been widely used in Japan and, providing that two or more doses are given, is credited with significant protection. A live attenuated vaccine has been tried in pigs in an effort to prevent annual amplification of the natural virus cycle; but although individual animals can be thus protected, the suppression of vaccine virus replication by passively acquired antibodies and the rapid turnover of this economically exploited species in Japan effectively preclude large-scale use of this measure. Specific vector control is not practical either, although modernization of rice culture techniques with attendant increased use of insecticides has apparently reduced peak mosquito vector populations in both Japan and South Korea, and is credited with significant reduction in epidemic disease transmission in recent years.

151. MURRAY VALLEY ENCEPHALITIS

Murray Valley encephalitis is similar to Japanese B encephalitis in pathogenesis and clinical features, and is caused by a very closely related virus. Diagnosis requires laboratory studies similar to those for other group B encephalitides.

The disease almost certainly was recognized in 1917–18 when an epidemic of 134 cases, then called *Australian X disease,* occurred in the Murray and Darling River valleys of Victoria and New South Wales. Virus strains isolated at the time were lost. Sporadic cases occurred during the next three decades, but the present designation was established during an outbreak of some 40 cases in 1951, more than a third of them fatal. This time the virus was recovered and completely characterized. Many inapparent human infections were detected. Endemic infection is maintained in a bird-mosquito cycle in Northern Australia and New Guinea, and it has been postulated that the virus is intermittently brought south by migratory birds, where an amplifying cycle involving domestic fowl, waterbirds, and *Culex annulirostris* mosquitoes produces epidemic disease, most commonly among children. An epidemic early in 1974 promises further elucidation of this disease in the Murray Valley.

152. TICK-BORNE GROUP B ARBOVIRUS DISEASES: RUSSIAN SPRING-SUMMER ENCEPHALITIS, LOUPING ILL, KYASANUR FOREST DISEASE, OMSK HEMORRHAGIC FEVER

Definition. The tick-borne complex of group B arboviruses cause mild to severe febrile illness with frequent neurologic abnormalities and in two instances (Kyasanur Forest disease [KFD] and Omsk hemorrhagic fever [OHF]) acute hemorrhagic manifestations. These agents are distributed throughout Eurasia (KFD, OHF, Russian spring-summer encephalitis [RSSE]) and Great Britain (louping ill). Powassan virus occurs in Canada and the western United States but has so far caused only a single recognized case of human disease.

Etiology. The group B tick-borne arboviruses constitute an antigenic complex readily distinguishable from most mosquito-borne group B agents, and separable into several closely related subtypes. With the exception of RSSE and OHF, which overlap geographically, these viruses are found in distinct regions of the world. Suckling mice and a variety of cell cultures have proved most satisfactory for virus isolation, and a complete range of serologic techniques is available for differential classification. Hemorrhagic pneumonia is induced in muskrats by inoculation of OHF virus, encephalitis with occasional hemorrhagic diathesis follows administration of KFD virus to langur and bonnet monkeys, and varying clinical encephalitis occurs upon intracerebral inoculation of monkeys, sheep, and goats with the remaining members of the complex.

Epidemiology. The viruses persist in discrete geographic foci by interchange between wild and domestic vertebrates and ixodid ticks, principally of the genera Ixodes, Dermacentor, and Haemaphysalis.

Many vertebrates, including rodents, birds, bats, sheep, goats, and cattle, experience clinically silent viremic infection. The capacity of the tick vectors to transmit virus transovarially has been experimentally documented, thus providing a fundamental mechanism for winter survival of some of the viruses. Persistent infection of hibernating species such as bats and hedgehogs has also been demonstrated. In the case of OHF and KFD viruses, respectively, viremia and overt fatal infection occur naturally in muskrats and monkeys, and major epizootics among these animals often precede or accompany outbreaks in man.

In addition to tick transmission, RSSE infection in man may be acquired through *drinking raw milk* of infected goats. Tick-transmitted infection may result from factors affecting residence, occupation, or recreation. Residents of rural forested areas, particularly agricultural, veterinary, and forest workers, are at highest risk. Seasonal disease patterns reflect temperature-dependent tick activity, with peaks ranging from late spring to autumn, depending on the tick and the geographic locality. Some of the agents can also apparently infect man by the respiratory route, as evidenced by winter outbreaks among trappers and skinners of muskrats (OHF) and by aerosol-associated laboratory infections (OHF, KFD).

Clinical Manifestations and Pathology. Onset is typically abrupt after an incubation period of three to twelve days. The pattern is frequently diphasic except for OHF, the initial phase consisting of fever, headache, myalgia, gastrointestinal disturbances, and, in KFD, mild to moderate hemorrhages from the nose and intestines. Leukopenia is common during this phase which lasts five to ten days.

The second phase usually begins with high fever and severe headache. Louping ill is usually mild to moderate in over-all severity, but RSSE infection tends to be progressively more severe from Europe to Far Eastern Asia. Although serous meningitis is the most common form over-all, infection in the easternmost part of the Soviet Union is frequently grossly encephalomyelitic, with transient or permanent flaccid paralysis, nystagmus, deafness, and somnolence. Bulbospinal disease is the most serious, resulting in neck and shoulder paralysis or even death. The second phase of KFD also is predominantly neurologic, although severity is usually moderate. Moderate leukocytosis and cerebrospinal fluid pleocytosis and elevated protein are characteristic of this phase. The latter abnormalities have been shown to persist in louping ill for weeks after apparent clinical recovery.

Pathologically the lesions produced by these viruses are generally similar to those observed with other arbovirus encephalitides or hemorrhagic fevers (inflammatory vasculitis in brain or focal capillary hemorrhages without inflammation). But not infrequently RSSE virus produces neuronal damage in the cervical cord reminiscent of poliomyelitis, and the viruses of OHF and KFD induce a focal hemorrhagic bronchopneumonia with occasional necrotic foci in the liver and gastrointestinal tract.

Diagnosis and Treatment. Specific diagnosis, in contrast to disease caused by most mosquito-borne encephalitides, can often be made by isolation of the virus from blood during the initial febrile phase, or from brain in rapidly fatal infection. Serologic diagnosis is even more reliable, although access to all three common techniques is necessary to establish the cause in some instances. With the exception of RSSE-OHF, anamnestic responses to infection with related agents are usually not a problem. Treatment is symptomatic. Blood loss in OHF and KFD is rarely sufficient to warrant transfusion.

Prognosis and Prevention. Louping ill virus infection has not caused fatalities or permanent neurologic sequelae. Far eastern RSSE, in contrast, has a fatality rate of more than 15 per cent and leaves many survivors with permanent paralysis of an arm or the shoulder girdle. Soviet workers also claim that 3 to 5 per cent of paralytic patients follow a chronic progressive course that develops into clonic spasms, epilepsy, and death. Strong indirect evidence for chronic virus persistence in the brain of one patient during a period of 14 years with final deterioration and death has been obtained by Japanese workers. Fatality rates do not exceed 5 per cent for KFD and OHF, and there are no permanent sequelae associated with these diseases.

Soviet workers have administered formolized mouse brain RSSE vaccine to thousands of persons with reported good results. Work proceeds in that country on a live attenuated vaccine. Otherwise, protection is largely individual against tick bite, consisting of adequate clothing and insect repellents. Aerial spraying of insecticides has been tried on a large scale for tick control in parts of Russia but has been abandoned as too expensive.

Anderson, S. G., et al.: Murray Valley encephalitis in the Murray Valley, 1956 and 1957. Med. J. Aust., 2:15, 1958.

Blaskovic, D., and Nosek, J.: The ecological approach to the study of tick-borne encephalitis. *In* Melnick, J. L. (ed.): Progress in Medical Virology. Vol. 14. Basel and New York, S. Karger, 1972, pp. 275–320.

Eklund, C. M.: Human encephalitis of the western type in Minnesota in 1941: Clinical and epidemiological study of serologically positive cases. Am. J. Hyg., 43:171, 1946.

Feemster, R. F.: Equine encephalitis in Massachusetts. N. Engl. J. Med., 257:701, 1957.

Finley, K. H.: Post-encephalitis manifestations of viral encephalitides. *In* Fields, W. S., and Blattner, R. L. (eds.): Viral Encephalitis, Springfield, Ill., Charles C Thomas, 1958, pp. 69–94.

Grabow, J. D., Mathews, C. G., Chun, R. W. M., and Thompson, W. H.: The electroencephalogram and clinical sequelae of California arbovirus encephalitis. Neurology, 19:394, 1969.

Hart, K. L., Keen, D., and Belle, E. A.: An outbreak of eastern equine encephalomyelitis in Jamaica, West Indies. I. Description of human cases. Am. J. Trop. Med. Hyg., 13:331, 1964.

Hilty, M. D., Haynes, R. E., Azimi, P. H., and Cramblett, H. G.: California encephalitis in children. Am. J. Dis. Child., 124:530, 1972.

Johnson, K. M., and Martin, D. H.: Venezuelan equine encephalitis. *In* Brandly, C. A., and Cornelius, C. E. (eds.): Advances in Veterinary

Science and Comparative Medicine. Vol. 18. New York, Academic Press, 1974, pp. 79–115.

Lincoln, A. F., and Sivertson, S. E.: Acute phase of Japanese B encephalitis. Two hundred and one cases in American soldiers, Korea, 1950. J.A.M.A., 150:268, 1952.

Matthews, C. G., Chun, R. W. M., Grabow, J. D., and Thompson, W. H.: Psychological sequelae in children following California arbovirus encephalitis. Neurology, 18:1023, 1968.

Parkin, W. E., Hammon, W. McD., and Sather, G. E.: Review of current epidemiological literature on viruses of the California arbovirus group. Am. J. Trop. Med. Hyg., 21:964, 1972.

Quick, D. T., Thompson, J. M., and Bond, J. O.: The 1962 epidemic of St. Louis encephalitis in Florida. IV. Clinical features of cases occurring in the Tampa Bay area. Am. J. Epidemiol., 81:415, 1965.

Southern, P. M., Jr., Smith, J. W., Luby, J. P., Barnett, J. A., and Sanford, J. P.: Clinical and laboratory features of epidemic St. Louis encephalitis. Ann. Intern. Med., 71:681, 1969.

Venezuelan Encephalitis: Washington, D.C., Pan-American Health Organization Publication Number 243, 1972, pp. 416.

Wallis, R. C.: Recent advances in research on the eastern encephalitis virus. Yale J. Biol. Med., 37:413, 1965.

Weaver, O. M., Haymaker, W., Pieper, S., and Kirland, R.: Sequelae of the arthropod-borne encephalitides. V. Japanese encephalitis. Neurology, 8:887, 1958.

Webb, H. E., and Rao, L.: Kyasanur Forest disease: A general clinical study in which some cases with neurological complications were observed. Trans. R. Soc. Trop. Med. Hyg., 55:284, 1961.

White, M. G., Carter, N. W., et al.: Pathophysiology of epidemic St. Louis encephalitis. Ann. Intern. Med., 71:691, 1969.

VIRAL HEMORRHAGIC FEVERS

153. INTRODUCTION

Karl M. Johnson

The viral hemorrhagic fevers form a group of acute diseases in which bleeding is a prominent clinical manifestation. These diseases occur in distinct parts of the world, are caused by ribonucleic acid–containing viruses, and may be transmitted to man by mosquitoes, by ticks, or by direct contact with excreta of virus-infected rodents (see table on opposite page). Despite its long-standing fame as a cause of acute hepatocellular necrosis, *yellow fever* is included under this heading because of its recognized ability to induce gastrointestinal hemorrhage and a shock syndrome similar to that seen with other viruses of the group.

After a variable period of a few days to one to three weeks, during which virus multiplies in lymphoid cells and produces a viremia, hemorrhagic fever patients experience fever, myalgia, and other nonspecific symptoms. Bleeding ensues, generally near the end of the febrile period, and although usually not sufficient per se to account for it, such hemorrhage is the harbinger of a clinical crisis dominated by hypovolemic shock. In at least two instances, epidemic hemorrhagic fever and dengue hemorrhagic fever, there is evidence that shock is caused by a widespread capillary vascular lesion in which plasma protein escapes the circulation much faster than erythrocytes. Thrombocytopenia and deficits in various circulating hemostatic factors are frequently present, but it is not clear whether they are etiologically related to this condition.

How the hemorrhagic syndrome is produced thus remains a mystery. No evidence for a direct virus-induced lesion of capillary endothelium has been obtained to date. Disseminated intravascular coagulation (DIC) has been shown in a few instances and postulated in others. But even assuming that DIC occurs, we have no clear idea about the vital pathophysiologic triggers for this chain reaction. Certain facts suggest, however, that altered immunologic function may be important in the pathogenesis of hemorrhagic fever. First, the pathology of such viral disease, unlike that associated with arboviral encephalitis, is characterized by the absence of inflammatory tissue reaction. Second, the high evidence of secondary bacterial infections and the delay of specific humoral antibody response observed in arenavirus-caused disease and Crimean hemorrhagic fever implies a direct suppression of B-cell lymphocyte function. Finally, there is the possibility that antigen-antibody complexes may be important in the genesis of some of these conditions. Available data include long incubation period, leukocytosis, and acute, reversible renal insufficiency in epidemic hemorrhagic fever; the temporal association between hemorrhagic disease and secondary dengue virus infection together with reduction of circulating complement components is even more suggestive. As for the arboviral encephalitides, elucidation of the operative variables is important. Clinical management of disease and vaccine development appear to offer more hope of averting fatal infection than does interruption of the nonhuman natural virus cycles.

154. YELLOW FEVER

Wilbur G. Downs

Definition.   Yellow fever is an acute viral disease characterized by sudden onset, prostration, moderately high fever, and a pulse rate slow in relation to temperature. Severe cases are often characterized by vomiting of altered blood, albuminuria (sometimes massive), and jaundice, and may progress to collapse and death. The disease is endemic in tropical rain forest regions of Africa and South America. There are two epidemiologic types of the disease. When the virus is transmitted from man to man by the domestic mosquito, *Aedes aegypti,* it is called *urban yellow fever,* but when it occurs in a forest environment and is transmitted to man by some forest mosquito, usually in the absence of *A. aegypti*, it is called *sylvan* (or *jungle) yellow fever.*

Etiology and Epidemiology.   Yellow fever is a group B arbovirus, is small, $38m\mu \pm 5 \ m\mu$, and readily passes Berkefeld V and N and Seitz filters. Unadapted virus exhibits both viscerotropic and neurotropic characteristics. Viscerotropism is manifested by involvement of liver, kidneys, and heart, and neurotropism by infection of cells of the central nervous system. By successive brain-to-brain passage in mice, the virus becomes adapted and manifests more neurotropism, losing its viscerotropic properties almost entirely. Prolonged passage of the virus in chick embryo tissue culture has produced an attenuated strain, 17D, widely used as a vaccine.

Man is universally susceptible to the virus, and characteristic symptoms and lesions of yellow fever in man are reflections of its viscerotropism. Certain monkey species, including *Macacus rhesus* and Alouatta species, are very susceptible to infection and usually die, whereas other species — for example, Cebus species — may be readily infected but usually recover. Albino mice,

Viral Hemorrhagic Fevers: Etiologic and Epidemiologic Considerations

	Causative Agent	Vector(s)	Vertebrate Host(s)	Geographical Distribution	Epidemiologic Features of Involvement of Man	Control	Remarks
Yellow fever (urban)	YF virus—a group B arbovirus	*Aedes aegypti* in cities	Man	Human populations (usually urban) in tropics of South and Central America and Africa	Person-to-person passage by *Aedes aegypti*	*Aedes aegypti* control; vaccination	Sylvan YF can spread to cities
Yellow fever (sylvan)	YF virus—a group B arbovirus	*Haemagogus* mosquitoes in New World; *Aedes* species in Africa	Monkeys of several genera and species	Forests and jungles of South and Central American and West, Central, and East Africa	Man infected by exposure in jungle (i.e., woodcutters, hunters, etc.)	Vaccination	Human cases sporadic and unpredictable; disease often a "silent" endemic in forests
Dengue hemorrhagic fever	Dengue viruses of four types; group B arboviruses	*Aedes aegypti*	Man (involvement of other primates has been postulated)	Tropical and subtropical cities of Southeast Asia and Philippines	Small children usually involved in cities where *Aedes aegypti* densities are high	*Aedes aegypti* control; mosquito repellent, screens, etc.	Disease may represent an immunologic over-response to a sequential infection with a different dengue strain
Omsk hemorrhagic fever	Two distinguishable subtypes of HF virus	Ticks of genus *Dermacentor*	Small rodents and muskrats	Omsk region of USSR; northern Roumania	People exposed in fields and wooded lands.	Tick repellents and protective clothing	
Kyasanur forest disease	KFD virus—a group B arbovirus	Ticks of several species in genus *Haemaphysalis*	Monkeys (Rhesus and langur) and small rodents and birds	Mysore State, India	People exposed in fields and wooded lands	Tick control; tick repellents and protective clothing	Monkey mortality signals epidemic activity
Argentine hemorrhagic fever	Junin virus, an arenavirus LCM-related	None proved; mites suspected	Small rodents: Akodon; *Calomys laucha, musculinus*	Argentina: NW of Buenos Aires extending west to Province of Cordoba	Field workers at harvest time are particularly at risk	Rodent control in fields	Infected rodents contaminate environment with urine
Bolivian hemorrhagic fever	Machupo virus, an arenavirus LCM-related	None recognized	Small rodent, *Calomys callosus*	Beni Province of Bolivia	Residents of small, rodent-infested villages and homes; 1971 nosocomial outbreak in Cochabamba, Bolivia	Rodent control in villages; full isolation in hospital patient care	High mortality in man
Lassa fever	Lassa virus, an arenavirus LCM-related	None required	Small rodent; *Mastomys natalensis*	West Africa: Nigeria, Liberia, Sierra Leone	Residents of small rodent-infested villages; dramatic nosocomial outbreaks	None known; possibly rodent control	High mortality in man
Crimean hemorrhagic fever	CHF-Congo virus; an ungrouped arbovirus	Ticks of several genera	Larger domestic animals implicated; also African hedgehog	Southern USSR, Bulgaria, East and West Africa	Cowhands and field workers in USSR; nosocomial outbreaks reported	Tick control relating to livestock; full isolation in patient care	Human disease important in USSR; importance to man in Africa not known
Korean hemorrhagic fever (hemor. nephroso-nephritis)	Not known; virus suspected	Not known	Possibly small mammals	Korea; northern Eurasia to and including Scandinavia	Rural or sylvan exposure (military, forest occupations, farmers)	None	A baffling epidemiologic and clinical entity

especially of the Swiss strain, are highly susceptible to the neurotropic element of virus strains recovered from nature, provided they are inoculated intracerebrally.

In urban yellow fever, the *A. aegypti* mosquito transmits the virus by biting a human host during the initial period of viremia and later biting a susceptible person. An extrinsic incubation period of nine to twelve days in the mosquito must elapse before the mosquito can transmit infection by bite.

In sylvan yellow fever, man acquires his infection through the bite of some mosquito other than *A. aegypti*.

Since 1934 no large epidemics of urban yellow fever have been reported from the Western Hemisphere. In Africa, in areas contiguous to the rain forest areas where sylvan yellow fever is endemic, there are still frequent epidemics of urban yellow fever. The announcement of

urban yellow fever, *A. aegypti*-transmitted, in a seaport or airport brings strict international quarantine regulations into effect.

There is no evidence that yellow fever has ever been present in the Orient.

Pathology. Yellow fever produces characteristic lesions in the liver of man. There are necrosis and necrobiosis of the parenchymal cells, most evident in the midzones of the lobules, with normal or much less involved cells around the central and portal veins. The necrosis is scattered and irregular rather than massive and uniform. Scattered among the necrotic cells are Councilman bodies, parenchymal cells that have undergone eosinophilic hyaline necrosis. There are also fatty changes in the parenchymal cells. The liver lobules are not collapsed. Pathologic changes in the kidneys are seen mainly in the tubules, with extensive damage to the epithelium and with lumina containing debris, casts, and basophilic concretions.

Clinical Manifestations. Most attacks of yellow fever are mild and show few if any of the classic symptoms. The only symptoms may be fever and headache, both of short duration. The epidemiologic implications of this disease make diagnosis of great importance, and it is essential to maintain a high index of suspicion with regard to undiagnosed fevers (vernacular terms: "PUO," "FUO," "flu," etc.) in regions where yellow fever is known to be, or can be suspected of being, endemic.

The incubation period is from three to six days. The onset is sudden, often with a chill, and without prodromal symptoms. The first stage of the disease, which lasts about three days, is the *period of infection.* The symptoms are feverish feeling, severe headache, backache, pain in the legs, and prostration. The face is flushed, and the eyes are injected; there is photophobia. The tongue is bright red at the tip and edges. There is no jaundice at the onset of illness. The temperature rises abruptly to about 40° C, sometimes higher. The pulse rate may rise to 90 or 100 initially, only to become increasingly slow in relation to the temperature (Faget's sign). The pulse is strong and full during this stage. Nausea and vomiting are the rule, as are epigastric distress and tenderness. Constipation is to be expected. A progressive leukopenia, sometimes pronounced, has frequently been observed early in the disease. The sudden development of intense albuminuria about the third or fourth day is characteristic.

After a short remission, the *period of intoxication* begins about the fourth day. The remission in fever is often indefinite or absent, and it may be accompanied by a deceptive temporary improvement. In this period, lassitude and depression may replace restlessness and agitation. Headache may diminish, and jaundice gradually develops. Although jaundice is always present in severe cases, it is usually not so intense as the name of the disease would indicate. Various hemorrhagic manifestations are evident. The gums are swollen and bleed easily, either spontaneously or when pressed; the nose may bleed. There may be petechiae in the skin. Hemorrhages from the stomach, intestine, or uterus, or subcutaneously, may be massive. The pulse rate falls progressively and may go below 50 per minute. Even in otherwise mild cases there may be dilatation of the heart and low blood pressure as evidence of myocardial damage. Vomiting may be frequent and distressing, and the vomitus in this stage usually contains altered blood, whence the name "el vomito negro" often applied to the disease in Latin America. The amount of albumin in the urine rises, often to 3 to 5 grams per liter, sometimes much higher. Fatal cases often exhibit hiccup, copious vomiting of altered blood, tarry stools, and anuria. Coma may last two or three days, or death may be immediately preceded by a short period of wild delirium. Death occurs most frequently from the sixth to the ninth day.

When there is recovery from a severe case, the temperature is likely to reach normal by the seventh or eighth day. Convalescence begins then and progresses rapidly to complete recovery with rapid disappearance of the albuminuria. Relapses do not occur, and there are no sequelae. Complications are rare. A lifelong immunity follows the attack, whether it be mild or severe.

A feature of yellow fever is the great variation in the degree to which different organs are affected. With much renal involvement there may be no cardiac symptoms, and vice versa. In mild and moderate cases there is little or no albuminuria, jaundice, or hemorrhage.

Diagnosis. In a severe illness with "black vomit," intense albuminuria, jaundice, and melena, as a group or in combinations, yellow fever must be suspected. Diseases that must be differentiated from severe yellow fever include hepatitis, carbon tetrachloride poisoning, other jaundices, malaria, and typhoid. In mild cases, which have been confused with dengue and influenza, clinical diagnosis is notoriously inaccurate. The necessary laboratory procedures are highly specialized. The isolation of virus in mice, rhesus monkeys, or certain tissue cultures from serum of the acutely ill patient or from serum or liver of a deceased patient, affords convincing diagnosis. Specialized procedures are needed for the identification of the isolate. Serologic tests on paired acute-phase and convalescent serums, using techniques of complement-fixation, hemagglutination-inhibition, and virus neutralization, can also give positive diagnosis. Although the tests must be done in a specialized laboratory, nevertheless under primitive conditions the serum specimens can be collected and submitted to such a laboratory.

For postmortem diagnosis, specimens of liver and other tissues should be preserved in 10 per cent formalin for histologic examination. Virus recovery can be attempted from such tissues if small pieces are placed in 50 per cent glycerol-saline and shipped, under refrigeration if possible, to a laboratory.

Prognosis. Early in the disease the prognosis should be guarded, because sudden changes for the worse may occur. If early symptoms are mild, rapid recovery is probable. Some patients with severe disease will recover, but symptoms of hiccups, copious black vomit, melena, and anuria imply a very grave prognosis.

The over-all average case fatality rate is less than 10 per cent, and rates of less than 5 per cent have been observed in epidemics involving completely susceptible populations. Rates based on hospitalized cases may be higher.

Treatment. There is no specific treatment. A patient should be moved as little as possible and should be kept quiet in bed. Heroic efforts to get a patient from some remote area to a district hospital should be discouraged. The severe headache and body aches may require relief with an analgesic. The heart should be watched carefully throughout the illness and into early convalescence.

Water should be given in adequate amounts, parenterally if necessary. Easily assimilated food should be given to the extent that the patient will tolerate. Milk in moderate quantities can be recommended. When vomiting has ceased and the temperature is down, full diet may be given. Full activity should be resumed only gradually.

Prevention. If a case of yellow fever is treated in a place in which vector mosquitoes exist, the patient must be kept under a bed net or in a mosquito-proof room during the first four days of illness.

Vaccination is essential for persons who intend to visit yellow fever endemic areas and for the people resident in such areas. Yellow fever is notorious for existence in endemic areas with no overt signs of its presence, and despite negative reports of the weekly international epidemiologic bulletins relative to a given area, vaccination for persons going to an endemic area must be stressed.

Two strains of living virus have been used extensively for immunization of man. The 17D vaccine, developed by Rockefeller Foundation workers, is prepared in chick embryos and is inoculated subcutaneously. The French neurotropic vaccine, developed by Institut Pasteur workers, is prepared from mouse brains suspended in gum arabic solution and is given by scarification. With either strain, an effective immunity to yellow fever is readily induced. The 17D vaccine is currently recommended, because it produces fewer undesirable reactions, particularly in small children. Vaccination ordinarily gives protection in a week, and the consequent immunity has been shown to last at least ten years. An urban epidemic can be stopped by mass vaccination of the population combined with vigorous anti-*aegypti* measures.

155. HEMORRHAGIC FEVER CAUSED BY DENGUE VIRUSES

Karl M. Johnson

Definition. These hemorrhagic fevers of Southeast Asia and India are acute, infectious, urban, mosquito-borne diseases caused by dengue viruses. Endoepidemic in pattern, dengue hemorrhagic fever is clinically defined as a dengue disease that worsens two or more days after onset, and is characterized by hypoproteinemia and one or more hemostatic abnormalities such as thrombocytopenia, prolonged bleeding time, or elevated prothrombin time. The dengue shock syndrome consists of hemorrhagic fever plus shock (hypotension or a pulse pressure of 20 mm Hg or less) and hemoconcentration (hematocrit at least 20 per cent greater than convalescent value). Chikungunya virus infections fulfilling these criteria are rarely encountered.

Etiology. All evidence suggests that these diseases are caused by each of the four recognized dengue virus subtypes. How they produce such disease is still not clear. A current hypothesis is that severe dengue disease is produced by an immunologic reaction that occurs in some individuals experiencing a second dengue infection. However, in a 1972 outbreak on Niue Island, Oceania, several hemorrhagic cases were seen in children with no possibility of prior dengue infection.

Epidemiology. These hemorrhagic fevers were first seen in epidemic proportions in Manila and Bangkok (1954) and in Singapore (1960). Other outbreaks have been reported from Malaysia, South Vietnam, India, Indonesia, and Oceania. In Bangkok age-specific rates in children have reached 7 to 8 per 1000. In most outbreaks cases occur only in children, principally below the age of 8 years; otherwise, the epidemiology of infection leading to dengue hemorrhagic fever is basically similar to that associated with ordinary dengue fever; outbreaks occur during the rainy season in large urban centers where *Aedes aegypti* is well established. Halstead has proposed that dengue hemorrhagic fever is an immune disease, brought on usually by a second (but not a third) dengue virus infection in a previously sensitized host. The syndromes have not been observed in many places where dengue is or has been prevalent, including the New World and many parts of Southeast Asia, Australasia, and Oceania.

Pathology. Autopsy data are scant. The chief abnormalities include generalized vascular congestion and dilatation with edema and multiple focal hemorrhages in most organs, mild to moderate pleural effusion and ascites, mononuclear cell infiltration of interstitial tissues and alveolar walls of lungs, focal myocardial congestion, and a decrease in mature lymphocytes with proliferation of mononuclear forms in the germinal centers of lymph follicles.

Necrosis is unusual, and no specific damage of the blood vessels has been observed. Perivascular infiltration by mononuclear cells is common, but there is no evidence for significant vasculitis or for platelet or thrombin thrombosis of vessel walls. About one third of cases show evidence of globulin on endothelial surfaces and the walls of arterioles. The bone marrow often shows maturation arrest of megakaryocytes, and sometimes there is marked generalized cellular hypoplasia with rapid restoration to normal after emergence from shock.

Pathologic change in the liver, although generally inconspicuous, consists of focal lesions and varies greatly in degree of severity. These lesions are of particular interest, because occasionally Councilman bodies and other changes characteristic of yellow fever are observed.

Pathogenesis or Mechanism of Disease. The pathogenesis is as yet poorly understood. The vascular congestion, dilatation, and increased permeability lead to the extensive edema and hemorrhage observed in the gastrointestinal tract, the skin, and other tissues. The cause of these vascular changes is unknown, but they result in loss of plasma volume and associated electrolyte disturbances. Platelet deficiency probably plays a role in the hemorrhages. Bleeding time is usually prolonged, prothrombin times are somewhat prolonged, clot retraction is poor, and the blood fibrinogen is slightly reduced. None of these changes is very profound. The circulatory collapse and shock observed appear to be far in excess of what might be expected from the extent of loss of edema fluid and blood. The adrenal changes suggest exhaustion of steroid reserve. Death in some cases has been accompanied by severe hyperkalemia.

Clinical Manifestations. The onset is that of a dengue infection, usually abrupt, with fever. Nausea and vomiting are common. The throat appears injected, and there may be a dry cough. About the second or third day petechiae appear, usually first on the face or distal portions of the extremities but sparing the axillae and chest. The tourniquet test may be conspicuously positive before petechiae appear. Purpura and large ecchymoses as well as other manifestations of bleeding tendency are occasionally prominent. There may be severe abdominal pain and tenderness. About the third or fourth day, vomiting may produce copious coffee-ground material. Melena also is not uncommon, but gross bleeding from the intestines is rare. Shock is likely to occur in severe cases about the fourth day, and this critical state lasts about 12 to 24 hours. At this time the temperature falls to normal, the blood pressure and pulse pressure are low or unmeasurable, and the limbs are cool and present a purple or brownish mottled appearance. Perspiration is frequently profuse. The face and hands appear edematous. Restlessness and apprehension are conspicuous as the patient enters shock. This state of shock is entirely out of proportion to the apparent loss of blood. Thrombocytopenia is noted during this period, and bleeding time is prolonged. Leukocytes remain at approximately normal levels, but are elevated in number in serious cases more frequently than they are depressed. The total and differential leukocyte counts are not those observed in dengue. Although the numbers of both immature and mature polymorphonuclear cells are decreased, there is an increase in lymphocytes and sometimes in monocytes.

Diagnosis. Hemorrhagic fever begins as an extension of a classic dengue infection, and the early dengue syndrome intergrades into the milder and atypical manifestations of the later hemorrhagic syndrome. The diagnosis in a febrile child acutely ill for only two or three days is rendered highly probable by the presentation of petechiae, purpuric lesions, and unusual ecchymosis of the skin with most prominent distribution on the extremities and face, together with melena, thrombocytopenia, and a relatively normal leukocyte count. In a milder case or at an earlier stage, the tourniquet test may be of great assistance in detecting unusual capillary fragility. The rapid development of circulatory collapse and shock during the fourth to sixth day, associated with the aforementioned findings, differentiates this from most other exanthematous diseases. Meningococcemia and the Waterhouse-Friderichsen syndrome need careful consideration. Thrombocytopenic purpura can be expected to have an entirely different onset and is usually not associated with fever. Laboratory methods available for diagnosis are those described for dengue fever.

Treatment. There is no specific therapy, but case fatality rates can be greatly reduced by skillful management directed toward combating shock. Close monitoring of pulse, respiration, and blood pressure during the course of treatment is essential for at least 48 hours, because shock can occur and recur. Oxygen should be administered if there is cyanosis or labored breathing. Hypovolemia should be treated by administration of lactated Ringer's solution or 5 per cent glucose in normal saline, on the basis of 20 ml per kilogram of body weight, administered rapidly. In profound or unresponsive shock, plasma or a plasma expander (dextran in normal saline) can be given at the rate of 20 ml per kilogram of body weight. When signs improve, 5 per cent glucose in normal saline or in lactated Ringer's solution should be given at the rate of 10 ml per kilogram per hour, and continued until vital signs are normal. Acidosis should be corrected with sodium bicarbonate as necessary.

Whole blood should be given only if blood loss is known to be large. Administration of whole blood to a patient with elevated hematocrit may result in heart failure. Paraldehyde or chloral hydrate may be required for children who are markedly agitated. Salicylates administered during the febrile period may cause bleeding and acidosis, and they should not be given to febrile patients during a hemorrhagic fever outbreak. Pressor amines, alpha-adrenergic blocking agents, and steroids have not been demonstrated to be of value in treatment.

Prognosis. Death is almost always associated with shock, and rarely occurs after the sixth day of illness. Case fatality rates among hospitalized patients have ranged from 5 to 50 per cent, depending to a large extent upon the condition of patients on admission and the facilities available for treatment. Careful management should be able to save all but the 5 or 10 per cent of patients admitted in a moribund state. Residual effects have not been observed, and, in contrast to primary dengue, recovery is usually prompt and complete seven to ten days after onset. Mental depression is seldom observed.

Prevention. The control of this hemorrhagic fever is the same as that for dengue, and consists of mosquito control or protection from mosquito bites and isolation of the patient from mosquitoes. No vaccine is available, and if the immunologic theory of causation is confirmed, vaccines as presently conceived would be specifically contraindicated.

156. CRIMEAN HEMORRHAGIC FEVER

Karl M. Johnson

Definition. Crimean hemorrhagic fever (CHF) is an acute febrile disease, often marked by severe hemorrhage and high mortality, occurring in the Soviet Union and Bulgaria.

Etiology. The CHF agent is an arbovirus first isolated from human blood specimens in 1967. It is pathogenic for suckling mice and grows in several types of cultured cells. This virus is indistinguishable from Congo virus of Africa in CF and neutralization tests. Strains from Eurasia and Africa are thus referred to as CHF-Congo virus.

Epidemiology. CHF-Congo virus is naturally transmitted by several species of hard ticks belonging to the general Hyalomma, Rhipicephalus, Amblyomma, and Boophilus. Active foci of infection with transmission to man exist in the lower Don and Volga river basins and the Central Asian republics of Kazakstan and Uzbekistan of the Soviet Union. A single tick isolate has been reported from Pakistan. Few human cases have been recognized in Africa. The disease occurs most frequently among adults who are heavily exposed to ticks while working among cattle. Cases begin to appear in April and reach a peak during summer months. Proved or presumed vertebrate hosts for the virus include cattle, goats, hares, rooks, and hedgehogs. Transovarial tick transmission is suspected but not yet proved. Nosocomial human infections have occurred repeatedly in Central Asia, suggesting transmission by aerosol. The incubation period is estimated at about one week.

Clinical Manifestations. Onset is typically abrupt with high, unremitting fever, chills, headache, and myalgia. There may be hyperemia of the upper trunk and neck, conjunctival effusion, vomiting, and diarrhea. Hepatomegaly is noted in about half the cases; splenomegaly is uncommon. Pronounced panleukopenia is almost invariably present, as is thrombocytopenia. Bleeding begins on about the fourth day of illness. Petechiae appear in the oral mucosa and skin, at times presenting as frank *purpura hemorrhagica.* Nose, gums, and intestinal tract are the most common sites of bleeding, and in this disease above all other viral hemorrhagic fevers, blood loss per se may be life threatening. Stiff neck, hyperexcitability, or coma occurs in about 10 per cent of cases and these are grave prognostic signs. The cerebrospinal fluid, however, contains no leukocytes or increased protein. There may be proteinuria and microscopic hematuria, but renal function is rarely compromised. The fever and bleeding generally resolve by lysis at about the eighth day. Hypovolemic shock with a paradoxical rising hematocrit may appear just prior to the end of fever and is the most common cause of death.

Diagnosis. Virus can be gotten easily from blood of patients during the first few days of illness. Specific CF and neutralizing antibodies appear in the sera of most patients 30 to 60 days after onset of symptoms.

Treatment and Prognosis. Therapy is symptomatic. Management of fluid, electrolyte, and erythrocyte balance forms the continuous clinical challenge. Shock is a grave problem and should be anticipated and treated as outlined in Ch. 157. Whole blood transfusion may be necessary. Intercurrent bacterial infection is very common, especially pneumonia. Mortality in the Soviet Union ranges from 20 to 50 per cent. Patients surviving the acute illness generally recover completely, albeit quite slowly. Several instances of mono- or polyneuritis persisting for several months have been recorded.

Prevention. There is no vaccine yet available; thus avoidance of the disease in endemic foci depends on personal measures designed to prevent tick bites.

157. HEMORRHAGIC DISEASES CAUSED BY ARENAVIRUSES: ARGENTINE AND BOLIVIAN HEMORRHAGIC FEVERS AND LASSA FEVER*

Karl M. Johnson

Definition. Argentine and Bolivian hemorrhagic fevers and Lassa fever are acute diseases caused respectively by Junin, Machupo, and Lassa viruses. Clinically, the diseases share the common features of fever, severe myalgia, leukopenia, hemorrhagic manifestations, shock, and (excluding Lassa fever) neurologic abnormalities.

Etiology. The three viruses are serologically and morphologically related, and related to lymphocytic choriomeningitis virus, in a grouping designated as arenaviruses.

Geographical Distribution, Incidence, and Prevalence. Argentine hemorrhagic fever is localized to the provinces of Córdoba and Junin in northern Argentina, where several hundred to several thousand cases occur annually, principally in agricultural field hands, in the harvest months. Bolivian hemorrhagic fever has been reported only from Beni province of Bolivia, between the rivers Mamore and Branco, with the exception of a hospital outbreak in Cochabamba, Bolivia, in 1971, traceable to contact with a person from Beni province. Infections are seen in inhabitants of certain of the small towns, as well as in rural populations. Lassa fever has been reported from Nigeria, Liberia, and Sierra Leone, and hospital outbreaks account for most of the cases reported. Case fatality rates are estimates in the usual absence of prompt and specific diagnosis, but may be as high as 50 per cent in hospitalized cases of Lassa, and 10 to 20 per cent for the South American diseases.

Epidemiology and Probable Mode of Transmission. The viruses have been isolated from wild rodents: Junin, most commonly from *Calomys musculinus, Calomys laucha,* and also *Akodon arenicola;* Machupo, from *Calomys callosus;* and Lassa, from *Mastomys natalensis.* An attractive current hypothesis is that infection is acquired by direct human contact (ingestion, inhalation, or entrance through mucous membranes or skin breaks) with virus-containing rodent excreta. For all three agents, persistent infection in rodents has been demonstrated, with viremia readily detectable for months. A similar pattern of chronic virus infection in rodents has been described for lymphocytic choriomeningitis virus.

Pathology. Few cases have received full study. Findings include irregularly focal diapedesis and capillary hemorrhage without much evidence of inflammatory reaction. Gross hemorrhages may be seen in the mucosa of the stomach and intestines and in the brain. Pulmonary infection, probably intercurrent, is frequently seen.

Clinical Manifestations. Although as many as half of all etiologically confirmed cases appear as acute undifferentiated fevers, the findings and clinical cause of "full-blown" Argentine and Bolivian infections are so nearly identical as to justify joint description. The same holds for Lassa fever. Onset is usually gradual, with increasing fever, headache, diffuse myalgia, and anorexia. By the third day the temperature may be 39.5 to 40.5° C, with severe myalgia, particularly in the lumbar regions (or legs in Lassa fever). Conjunctival injection is present, a flush involving the upper trunk and face is frequently observed, and there may be a relative bradycardia. Beginning about the fourth day, scattered fine petechiae may appear on the face and neck, about the pectoral girdle, and/or in the buccal mucosa or palate. Aphthous ulcers of the oral mucosa have been a noteworthy feature of Lassa infections. The Rumpel-Leede test is frequently positive. Frank hemorrhages from one or more sites, including the stomach, intestines, nose, gums, and uterus, accompanied by microscopic hematuria, may occur. Hemorrhagic phenomena are not a common feature of Lassa infections. Although hemorrhage per se is rarely the precipitating cause, a hypotensive crisis frequently develops between the sixth and eighth days, coincident with a rapid return of temperature to normal after five or more days of sustained fever. Patients surviving this stress for 48 hours generally make slow but complete recovery.

Perhaps a fifth of the patients with the Bolivian or Argentinian disease develop neurologic signs. These are quite characteristic, and begin on about the fifth or sixth day with a fine intention tremor of the tongue. This may become so severe as to render speech unintelligible and to preclude oral ingestion of solid or even liquid food. If so, gross intention tremors of the extremities usually appear, occasionally accompanied by an intermittent nystagmus. Such patients often become delirious, and may experience generalized clonic and tonic convulsions. The cerebrospinal fluid appears normal, however, and contains neither leukocytes nor virus. Convalescence is marked by weakness and signs of autonomic nervous system lability such as postural hypotension, spontaneous flushing and blanching of the skin, and episodes of diaphoresis.

Neurologic findings have not been described for Lassa fever, but a state of mild euphoria during the initial several days of fever has been noted, as well as blurring of the sensorium and semicomatose state in later stages of the illness. Some Lassa fever patients have shown electrocardiographic evidence of myocardial involvement.

Transient loss of scalp hair and typical Beau's lines in the nails, particularly those of the fingers, are observed in a majority of cases several weeks after subsidence of

---

*The author wishes to express his thanks to Dr. Wilbur G. Downs for his considerable assistance in the preparation of this chapter, particularly with reference to the material on Lassa fever.

the high, sustained fever. Many patients are not able to resume full activity for at least one month after illness.

Leukopenia is almost invariably present, and cell counts may be as low as 1000 per cubic millimeter by the fourth or fifth day. All elements are reduced nearly equally, and there is often a mild to moderate thrombocytopenia during the first week. Usually the peripheral blood picture returns to normal rapidly after defervescence, although there may be transient relative lymphocytosis and mild anemia. During the latter portion of the febrile period, progressive increase in hematocrit similar to, but usually milder than, that of hemorrhagic nephrosonephritis (q.v.) is frequently observed. At about the same time, moderate proteinuria is common, although renal function is rarely compromised seriously, and frank azotemia and hyperkalemia are almost never present.

Diagnosis. The presence of high fever, severe myalgia, and leukopenia should arouse immediate suspicion of viral hemorrhagic fever within the known endemic areas of its occurrence. Potential intimate contact with wild rodents in a rural or semirural setting serves to strengthen the likelihood of this diagnosis. Since these findings and all others described cannot be relied upon to differentiate the disease clinically from other infections such as yellow fever, typhoid and paratyphoid fevers, typhus, malaria, and leptospirosis, specific identification of cases depends upon laboratory confirmation. Virus can sometimes be isolated from blood, throat washing, and urine during the febrile period. At autopsy splenic tissue almost always yields the agent. Serologic detection of infection is a reliable method if paired acute and convalescent serums are employed. Both group-reacting complement-fixing antibodies and virus type-specific neutralizing antibodies appear in three to four weeks and reach peak values in seven to ten weeks after the onset of illness.

These three agents have been responsible for several fatal laboratory infections, and work with the viruses should be carried out only with strictest precautionary measures, and complete isolation from other laboratory activities, in special high-risk laboratories.

Treatment. In the absence of any specific therapy, successful treatment presents an acute challenge in the science and art of physiologic management. Patients require complete rest and maximal comfort. Mild sedatives and analgesics should be judiciously used. Careful measurement of fluid intake and output is mandatory. The electrolyte balance should be checked regularly; marked underhydration and overhydration are to be avoided, because these conditions appear to compromise the patient's ability to weather the hypotensive crisis. Daily hematocrit determinations and examinations of urine for protein are the most valuable tests for anticipating and managing this problem. Frequent measurement of blood pressure is also important, because many patients enter the shock phase with persistent relative bradycardia and warm, dry skin. Raising the foot of the bed may suffice to stabilize the pressure at levels adequate to preserve vital urinary output. If not, careful administration of human plasma or concentrated albumin (not whole blood) is indicated. In one instance of a Lassa infection, administration of plasma from a recovered patient appeared to be effective. Great care should be exercised in administering plasma or other fluids intravenously during shock, because intractable pulmonary edema is readily induced. Complications, particularly

bacterial infections, should be anticipated and promptly treated. Convalescence should never be hurried.

Prognosis. Although the case mortality may exceed 20 per cent, there is no single finding early in the disease that aids prognosis in the individual case. In general, the very young and the very old, as well as those who do not receive medical attention prior to the sixth day of disease, are subject to the highest risk. The onset of severe shock and neurologic abnormalities are both ominous prognostic signs, and at least half the patients exhibiting these signs succumb. The prognosis in Lassa fever is even poorer in diagnosed cases.

Prevention. Effective elimination of intimate human contact with certain wild rodents represents the only proved method for prevention of disease. This may be achieved by maintaining sound standards of personal and environmental hygiene. Campaigns to eliminate rodents, repair buildings, and clean rubbish near dwellings are highly successful when the disease is acquired mainly from peridomestic animals. There is insufficient evidence at present to warrant recommendation of systematic measures to control attacks by any potential arthropod vector.

Hospital outbreaks involving hospital staff have provided most of the Lassa fever cases to date. There has been a recent hospital outbreak of Machupo virus in Cochabamba, Bolivia. Such outbreaks can be extremely dangerous to personnel and demoralizing to hospital operation.

158. EPIDEMIC HEMORRHAGIC FEVER: HEMORRHAGIC NEPHROSONEPHRITIS

Karl M. Johnson

Definition. Epidemic hemorrhagic fever is an acute disease of unknown cause that occurs in northeastern Asia and, in milder form, in northern European U.S.S.R., Scandinavia, Czechoslovakia, Rumania, and Bulgaria. It is characterized by fever, prostration, vomiting, proteinuria, hemorrhagic manifestations, shock, and renal failure.

History. The disease was first described in the far east of the Soviet Union in the 1930's, with suggestive history as far back as 1913. An epidemic in United Nations troops in Korea, beginning in 1951, attracted much attention.

Etiology. Soviet investigators detected a filtrable virus, by parenteral inoculation of serum or urine of patients prior to the fifth day of illness into human volunteers. Despite repeated claims, no agent has yet been established in any other experimental host system.

Epidemiology. The disease is rural, characterized by isolated cases widely separated in place. Environmental exposure in forests or fields near forests is invariably noted. Person-to-person transmission does not occur. Soviet workers believe that the disease is transmitted directly from asymptomatically infected rodents to man by means of virus-contaminated rodent excreta. Some outbreaks in Europe have coincided with population "explosions" of the redbacked vole *(Clethrionomys glareolus),* involving invasion by rodents of fields, barns, and even houses.

Pathology. Profound, protein-rich retroperitoneal edema is characteristic of early death in shock, but not of later deaths. Changes in various organs apparently have a similar pathogenesis and consist of widespread, often focal, congestion and hemorrhage, sometimes accompanied by necrosis, without significant inflammatory response. The "pathognomonic" lesion is found in the kidneys, which appear swollen and, when incised, exhibit extreme hemorrhagic congestion sharply localized to the medulla. Gross congestion or hemorrhage derived from dilated, congested small blood vessels is also found frequently in the right atrium, the pituitary, and the stomach, and less often in intestines, adrenals, lungs, and central nervous system. Liver and spleen are usually not grossly involved. Petechial hemorrhages may occur in the skin, heart, adrenals, brain, and serous surfaces.

Clinical Manifestations and Pathologic Physiology: The following description is based on the minority of patients (about 20 per cent) who exhibit the more severe form of disease, which can be divided into five clinical phases. All patients, however, have fever, proteinuria, and isohyposthenuria.

The febrile phase lasts three to eight days and is characterized by fever, malaise, a flush over the face and neck, and injection of the eyes and palate. Toward the end of this period, petechiae occur, blood platelets decrease, traces of protein appear in the urine, and the hematocrit begins to rise.

The hypotensive phase develops suddenly during defervescence and lasts one to three days. Shock is insidious with warm dry extremities and initially no increase in pulse rate. The dominant feature is a reduction in effective blood volume owing to a loss of plasma from the vascular system. Hematocrit values may reach 70 per cent, and erythrocytes are sequestered in dilated capillaries. Nausea and vomiting are common, as are back and abdominal pain, the latter having occasioned ill-advised exploratory laparotomy in misdiagnosed cases. Heavy proteinuria and oliguria progressing to acute renal failure occur during this interval. Capillary hemorrhages are most prominent at this time also, and blood leukocytes, earlier normal or reduced, now show a leukemoid reaction.

The oliguric phase begins as the sequestered plasma returns to the vascular system and the hematocrit falls. Deaths during this three- to five-day interval are due to pulmonary edema, hyperkalemia, and shock secondary to dehydration or secondary pulmonary infections. Some patients become hypertensive and display a reactive hypervolemic syndrome that responds to phlebotomy. Biochemical abnormalities associated with renal failure appear at this time.

The diuretic phase, lasting for days or weeks, usually initiates clinical recovery but is fraught with problems in clinical management. Diuresis of 3 to 8 liters daily and isohyposthenuria lead to an extremely brittle situation with respect to hemodynamics and salt balance. Hypokalemia and hypernatremia can be problems. Shock may occur, and bacterial pulmonary infections are common. Nearly a third of all deaths occur during this phase.

Convalescence requires three to twelve weeks and is marked by gradual return of appetite, strength, and urinary concentrating ability.

Diagnosis. In the absence of any specific test, the diagnosis must be made on clinical evidence and should be suspected when an acute febrile illness associated with the characteristic flush and petechiae occurs in a subject who has been in an endemic area. The subsequent developments such as hypotension or shock, increased hematocrit, thrombocytopenia, oliguria, and renal failure assist in establishing the diagnosis, but proteinuria and isohyposthenuria developing near the time of defervescence are the most useful diagnostic signs.

Prognosis and Treatment. Because antimicrobial drugs, convalescent serum, hormones, and other agents are entirely ineffective, the management of hemorrhagic fever must be supportive and based on an understanding of its physiologic and biochemical characteristics and on frequent clinical observations. Adequate sedation with barbiturates or opiates is frequently required for restlessness. Contrary to the practice in other febrile diseases, fluid intake must be limited because any excess will simply leak out of damaged capillaries and increase edema and symptoms. When intravenous fluid is required, it usually should be 10 per cent dextrose in water, and must be given very slowly. If shock fails to respond to simple measures such as shock blocks, then concentrated (salt-poor) human serum albumin to restore plasma volume may be required. Treatment in the oliguric phase is that of acute renal failure, with careful control of electrolytes and particular attention to hyperkalemia. If oliguria persists, hemodialysis or peritoneal dialysis is indicated. Soviet workers have so treated 60 severe cases and report only three deaths. The chief problem of the diuretic phase is one of careful matching of fluid and electrolyte intake against the brisk urinary output, so as to avoid excessive dehydration and shock, on the one hand, and hypervolemia and pulmonary edema, on the other. Electrolyte abnormalities are still a problem, especially potassium deficiency. Over-all mortality under optimal conditions seldom surpasses 5 per cent.

Prevention. Preventive measures are based on the assumption that the disease is transmitted by rodents with or without the aid of an associated arthropod vector. Vigorous rodent control measures, as well as dipping of clothing in acaricidal solutions and the individual use of insect repellents, are recommended in endemic areas during seasonal periods of disease activity.

Barnes, W. J. S., and Rosen, L.: Fatal hemorrhagic disease and shock associated with primary dengue infection on a Pacific island. Am. J. Trop. Med. Hyg., 23:495, 1974.

Bokisch, V. A., Top, F. H., Jr., Russell, P. K., Dixon, F. J., and Muller-Eberhard, H. J.: The potential pathogenic role of complement in dengue hemorrhagic shock syndrome. N. Engl. J. Med., 289:996, 1973.

Casals, J., Henderson, B. E., Hoogstraal, H., Johnson, K. M., and Shelokov, A.: A review of Soviet viral hemorrhagic fevers, 1969. J. Infect. Dis., 122:437, 1970.

Casals, J., Hoogstraal, H., Johnson, K. M., Shelokov, A., Wiebenga, N. H., and Work, T. H.: A current appraisal of hemorrhagic fevers in the U.S.S.R. Am. J. Trop. Med. Hyg., 15:751, 1966.

Frame, J. D., Baldwin, J. M., Jr., Gocke, D. J., and Troup, J. M.: Lassa fever, a new virus disease of man from West Africa. I. Clinical description and pathological findings. Am. J. Trop. Med. Hyg., 19:670, 1970.

Groot, H., and Bahia Ribiero, R.: Neutralizing and hemagglutination-inhibiting antibodies to yellow fever 17 years after vaccination with 17D vaccine. Bull. WHO, 27:699, 1962.

Halstead, S. B., et al.: Observations related to pathogenesis of dengue hemorrhagic fever. Yale J. Biol. Med., 42:261, 1970.

Hammon, W. McD., Rudnick, A., Sather, G., Rogers, K. D., and Morse, L. J.: New hemorrhagic fevers of children in the Philippines and Thailand. Trans. Assoc. Am. Physicians, 73:140, 1960.

Johnson, K. M., Halstead, S. B., and Cohen, S. N.: Hemorrhagic fevers of Southeast Asia and South America: A comparative appraisal. *In* Melnick, J. L. (ed.): Progress in Medical Virology, Vol. 9. Basel/New York, S. Karger, 1967, pp. 105–158.

Mertens, P. E., Patton, R., Baum, J. J., and Monath, T. P.: Clinical presentation of Lassa fever cases during the hospital epidemic at Zorzar, Liberia, March–April 1972. Am. J. Trop. Med. Hyg., 22:780, 1973.

Sabattini, M., and Maiztegui, J. I.: Fiebre hemorrágica argentina. Medicina (Buenos Aires), 30: Supp. 1, 111, 1970.

Simpson, D. I. H., Knight, E. M., et al.: Congo virus: A hitherto undescribed virus occurring in Africa. Part I. Human isolation — clinical notes. East Afr. Med. J., 44:87, 1967.

Smithburn, K. C., et al.: Yellow Fever Vaccination. Geneva, World Health Organization Monograph Series No. 30, 1956.

Smorodintsev, A. A., Kazbintsev, L. I., and Chudakov, V. G.: Virus Hemorrhagic Fevers (Y. Halperin, translator). Washington, D. C., Office of Technical Services, U. S. Department of Commerce, 1964.

Strode, G. K. (ed.): Yellow Fever. New York, McGraw-Hill Book Company, 1951.

Symposium on Epidemic Hemorrhagic Fever. Am. J. Med., 16:617, 1954.

VIRAL DISEASES CHARACTERIZED BY PROTRACTED, RECURRENT, OR LATENT INFECTION

These diseases are discussed in detail in Ch. 398 to 403.

VIRAL DISEASES (PRESUMPTIVE)

Paul B. Beeson

159. CAT SCRATCH DISEASE

The essential feature of cat scratch disease is lymphadenitis, usually limited to one anatomic region, developing as a sequel to accidental injury of the skin. In two thirds of the reported cases there has been a history of scratch or bite by a cat.

Epidemiology. The disease occurs in all parts of the world, most often in winter. Children are affected more frequently than adults. Although injuries by cat claws or teeth are the most common form of skin injury, other puncture wounds, by wood splinters, thorns, and metallic objects have appeared to be responsible at times. Cats thought to have caused human infection show no sign of illness, do not react to the cat scratch antigen, and probably merely convey the causative agent on claws or teeth. "Epidemics" of cat scratch disease, though reported, are difficult to evaluate because they may simply reflect special interest and awareness of certain physicians. There are, however, several reports of more than one case developing in a family over a period of a few months.

Etiology. Although this disease has the features of a specific infection, efforts to demonstrate a causative bacterium, fungus, or filterable virus have met with failure. Perhaps the most impressive evidence for viral etiology is in a report of electron microscopic examination of affected lymphatic tissue, in which herpes-like viral particles were observed. Serologic investigations have failed to yield evidence pointing to Epstein-Barr virus. The hypothesis has been offered that the clinical manifestations result from an immunologic reaction; hence the inciting agent may no longer be demonstrable at the time the patient seeks medical help. Several groups of workers have reported serologic evidence that the causative agent is related to viruses of the psittacosis–ornithosis–lymphogranuloma venereum–trachoma group, but the proportion of patients exhibiting such positive serologic reactions has varied considerably, and, furthermore, patients with cat scratch disease do not react to intradermal injection of antigens prepared from this group of viruses.

Pathogenesis. An indolent or subacute inflammatory lesion develops at the site of primary inoculation in approximately one third of cases. It becomes clinically evident one to several weeks after the injury. Lymphadenitis, the hallmark of the disease, appears a few days later. Initially this takes the form of a granulomatous inflammation, sometimes containing giant cells. In cases of some duration microabscesses can nearly always be found; in about one fourth of cases these coalesce to form a grossly evident abscess.

Clinical Manifestations. The site of inoculation is most likely to be on the hand, forearm, or face. It may exhibit one or more erythematous papules. Less frequently there is vesicle formation going on to rupture and production of a small eschar. The lesion usually heals without scar formation. The lymph nodes most frequently affected are in the epitrochlear, axillary, or cervical groups, but when the injury has been on the legs the inguinal nodes may be the site of the disease. The process varies in clinical severity and acuteness, sometimes smoldering for weeks with enlarged and tender nodes, at other times progressing more quickly to pronounced swelling, with redness and edema of the overlying skin. There may be fluctuation, and in rare instances the skin undergoes necrosis, permitting discharge of exudate. The usual course is for the swelling and tenderness gradually to subside in two to eight weeks. Systemic manifestations are not prominent, although young children sometimes have high fever for a few days. The erythrocyte sedimentation rate may be elevated; there is often a moderate leukocytosis, and sometimes mild eosinophilia. Transient morbilliform rashes may accompany the adenitis; occasionally lesions are developed which have the appearance of erythema nodosum. Pulmonary and arthritic manifestations are extremely rare, perhaps only coincidental. Development of osteolytic lesions near the adenitis has been described.

The most serious complication is *encephalitis*, evidenced by fever, delirium, cranial nerve palsies, and pleocytosis in the cerebrospinal fluid. The encephalitis usually subsides without residual damage. When the primary lesion affects the conjunctiva, the preauricular nodes are affected, giving the clinical picture of *Parinaud's oculoglandular syndrome.*

It has been suggested that cat scratch disease may present as *mesenteric lymphadenitis,* because positive skin tests have been associated with that clinical picture. The presumption is that the portal of entry in such cases is the intestine.

Diagnosis. The diagnosis is based largely on the clinical circumstances, i.e., a subacute lymphadenitis limited to one region with or without suppuration, with or without a primary skin lesion distal to the node, and history of cat scratch or bite or of some comparable trauma to the skin. Several other processes must be considered in the differential diagnosis. Among infections are tuberculosis, infectious mononucleosis, tularemia, lymphogranuloma venereum, and sporotrichosis. Hodgkin's disease may cause difficulty, because the granulomatous picture in the lymph node of cat scratch disease may bear some resemblance to that of Hodgkin's disease; but the presence of microabscesses usually serves to differentiate these.

The Hanger-Rose test appears to be relatively specific for cat scratch disease. This employs an "antigen" prepared from the purulent matter aspirated from nodes of other patients, in a manner comparable with that formerly employed for lymphogranuloma venereum (Frei test). The exudate is diluted 1 to 5 in saline, and sterilized by heating at 60° C for one hour on two occasions. After intradermal injection of this material, the reaction is read at 24 to 48 hours. A positive result consists of induration 5 mm or more and erythema 10 mm or more in diameter. Unfortunately test material is not available commercially.

Treatment. There is no evidence that antimicrobial therapy, including tetracycline, is of value. Bed rest is advisable when fever and general malaise are present. If fluctuation becomes evident in the affected lymph node, it is recommended that the pus be aspirated (and used for the preparation of skin test antigen). Incision of an abscess is inadvisable, because sinus formation with prolonged drainage sometimes results, but biopsy of intact nodes seems safe in the presuppurative stage.

Daniels, W. B., and MacMurray, F. G.: Cat scratch disease. Report of one hundred sixty cases. J.A.M.A., 154:1247, 1954.
Kalter, S. S., Kim, C. S., and Heberling, R. L.: Herpes-like virus particles associated with cat scratch disease. Nature, 224:190, 1969.
Lyon, L. W.: Neurologic manifestations of cat scratch disease. Arch. Neurol., 25:23, 1971.
Warwick, W. J.: The cat scratch syndrome, many diseases or one disease? Prog. Med. Virol., 9:256, 1967. (This useful review lists nearly every publication up to 1966.)

160. NONBACTERIAL GASTROENTERITIS
(Epidemic Nausea, Epidemic Vomiting, Winter Vomiting Disease, Epidemic Diarrhea)

Acute illnesses characterized by nausea, vomiting, and diarrhea are among the most common of human ailments, especially in children of school or preschool age.

This pattern of indisposition has many of the characteristics of infectious disease: occurrence in epidemics, short incubation period, sudden onset, fever, brief course, and complete recovery. Indeed, these features may also be manifestations of gastrointestinal infections by recognized pathogens: Salmonella, *Entamoeba histolytica,* Shigella, and the enteroviruses. Furthermore, especially in young children and in travelers, such illness may be attributed to colonization of the bowel by strains of "normal" gut flora, a mechanism thought by some to be involved in the extremely serious syndrome known as infant (or "weanling") diarrhea. There remains, however, a large residue of gastroenteritis in which no microbial etiologic agent can be indicted, and it is generally assumed that as yet unidentified viruses are responsible. Progress in this connection has been made, both in the United States and in Britain. Competent groups of workers have succeeded in transmitting the illness to volunteers by oral administration of bacteria-free fecal filtrates. It seems likely that the causative virus or viruses will soon be characterized (see Ch. 135).

The presenting symptom may vary in different epidemics; this has given rise to reports of "epidemic nausea," "epidemic vomiting," and "epidemic diarrhea." Nevertheless in nearly all of them the clinical descriptions show that the allied symptoms were also present. In some epidemics, especially those affecting schoolchildren, hysteria appears to have played a role in determining the prominence of various symptoms.

The onset is abrupt, usually with nausea and vomiting, followed within a few hours by diarrhea. In young children there may be rise of body temperature, but fever is less common in older persons. The illness usually begins to subside within 24 hours, and recovery is established by the second to fourth day.

In the majority of cases the illness is easily dealt with at home; indeed, the best management could be characterized as masterful inactivity. Bed rests and sips of water or carbonated drinks are sensible therapy during the acute phase. Neither antimicrobial drugs nor purges should be given. If diarrhea is exceptionally troublesome, diphenoxylate hydrochloride (Lomotil), 5 mg every 4 to 6 hours, or paregoric may be used. In rare instances admission to hospital may be advisable so that fluids and electrolytes can be given parenterally.

Clarke, S. K. R., et al.: A virus from epidemic vomiting disease. Br. Med. J., 3:86, 1972.
Dolin, R., et al.: Transmission of acute infectious nonbacterial gastroenteritis to volunteers by oral adminstration of stool filtrates. J. Infect. Dis., 123:307, 1971.
Jordan, W. S., Jr., Gordon, L., and Dorrance, W. R.: A study of illness in a group of Cleveland families. VII. Transmission of acute nonbacterial gastroenteritis to volunteers: Evidence for two different etiologic agents. J. Exp. Med., 98:461, 1953.
Leading Article: Viruses of vomiting. Br. Med. J., 4:442, 1972. (Useful references.)

161. EPIDEMIC NEUROMYASTHENIA
(Iceland Disease, Benign Myalgic Encephalomyelitis)

Between 1934 and 1960, several epidemics were reported of symptoms resembling those of poliomyelitis.

The acute phase was often followed by a prolonged period of disability, with headache, muscular weakness, fatigue, and mood depression.

Most outbreaks have occurred in summer, and about half of those reported have involved hospital personnel, especially student nurses. In all instances the attack rate has been much higher in women. Sporadic cases have been reported, but the diagnosis is difficult in the absence of an epidemic.

Severe generalized headache is nearly always a prominent complaint at the onset, and frequently there are pain and stiffness of the neck. Generalized tenderness of the muscles is common, and they frequently exhibit a characteristic of rapid fatigue and loss of motor power on repeated contraction. In perhaps 40 per cent of affected persons, areas of muscle weakness or paralysis appear during the first two weeks. These may be in the trunk or the extremities, and the pattern of involvement often changes from day to day. Cranial nerve signs, bladder dysfunction, and paresthesia may also be noted. In most cases complete recovery of neurologic function occurs within four to eight weeks, but relapses and exacerbations are common during the next few months.

Fever is inconspicuous or absent. The cerebrospinal fluid is usually normal, and routine tests of blood and urine reveal nothing of significance.

A striking feature of this illness is the prolonged period of disability after subsidence of the acute phase.

Particularly troublesome are the behavioral manifestations of irritability and mood depression, which together with easy fatigue may interfere with normal living for months and even years after the acute episode. In this stage the subject may present a picture of hysteria or of simple neurasthenia.

Deaths have not been reported; therefore nothing is known of the pathology.

Extensive laboratory investigations failed to yield evidence of participation of any known pathogenic microorganism; nevertheless, the presumption had seemed warranted that it was an infectious disease. However, McEvedy and Beard have cast doubt on the likelihood of an infectious etiology. They carefully reviewed the reports of 15 recorded outbreaks, with special attention to the well-documented epidemic among nurses at the Royal Free Hospital, London. They suggest alternatively that these epidemics represented psychosocial phenomena: either mass hysteria among the subjects or altered medical perception. Their analysis and argument are persuasive, but the question remains unanswered.

Acheson, E. D.: The clinical syndrome variously called benign myalgic encephalomyelitis, Iceland disease and epidemic neuromyasthenia. Am. J. Med., 26:569, 1959.
Dillon, M. J., Marshall, W. C., Dudgeon, J. A., and Steigman, A. J.: Epidemic neuromyasthenia: Outbreak among nurses at a children's hospital. Br. Med. J., 1:301, 1974.
McEvedy, C. P., and Beard, A. W.: Concept of benign myalgic encephalomyelitis. Br. Med. J., 1:11, 1970.

Section Two.   RICKETTSIAL DISEASES

162.   INTRODUCTION

Edward S. Murray

The rickettsial diseases are caused by a family of microorganisms (Rickettsiaceae) that have characteristics common to both bacteria and viruses. They are now considered to be more like bacteria, because among other characteristics they (1) possess metabolic enzymes, (2) have cell walls, (3) utilize oxygen, and (4) are susceptible to broad-spectrum antimicrobial drugs. They resemble viruses by virtue of the fact that they grow only within living cells. These microorganisms were named "rickettsiae" to honor Dr. H. T. Ricketts, who died in 1910 while investigating the etiology of epidemic typhus and Rocky Mountain spotted fever.

The rickettsial diseases are grouped together because they possess a number of common characteristics. (1) The etiologic agents are similar in size and shape and can be seen as pleomorphic coccobacillary forms under the light microscope. (2) All rickettsial organisms occur under natural conditions in either fleas, lice, ticks, or mites, and these arthropods are in all cases except Q fever the primary means by which the diseases are transmitted to man. (3) All rickettsiae take on a characteristic red color with the Gimenez stain. (4) In all rickettsial infections except Q fever and rickettsialpox,

agglutinins are produced to either the OX-19 or OX-K strains of the bacillus *Proteus vulgaris* (Weil-Felix reaction). (5) The characteristic pathologic lesion is a widespread peripheral vasculitis. (6) All are acute infectious diseases characterized clinically by fever, headache, and a rash (except Q fever, which has no rash). Finally, as previously noted, all rickettsial diseases in the early stages are readily susceptible to optimal doses of broad-spectrum antimicrobial drugs, e.g., chloramphenicol and the tetracyclines.

All rickettsial organisms, except the antigenically heterogenic strains of scrub typhus, produce complement-fixing antibodies. Data from these tests when combined with results of Weil-Felix reactions and clinical and epidemiologic features constitute definitive criteria for the diagnosis of each disease.

The immunity produced by any one of the rickettsial diseases is usually of long duration. Although the members of one group confer either partial or complete immunity to diseases caused by other members of the same group, there is, in general, no cross-immunity between groups. A minor degree of cross-immunity does exist, however, between some members of the typhus and spotted fever groups.

Since incubation periods for all the rickettsial diseases vary from 2 to 14 days, any of the rickettsial diseases can appear in air travelers reporting ill in any part of the world.

TABLE 1. Summary of Certain Important Epidemiologic and Clinical Characteristics of Rickettsial Diseases

Disease	Epidemiologic Features		Reservoir	Usual Incubation Period (Days)	Eschar	Rash	
	Geographic Occurrence	Usual Mode of Transmission to Man				Distribution	Type
Typhus group							
Primary louse-borne typhus	Worldwide	Infected louse feces rubbed into broken skin or as aerosol to mucous membranes	Man	12 (8-15)	None	Trunk to extremities	Macular, maculopapular
Brill-Zinsser disease	Worldwide	Recrudescence months or years after a primary attack of louse-borne typhus	–	–	None	Trunk to extremities	Macular, maculopapular
Murine typhus	Scattered pockets, worldwide	Infected flea feces rubbed into broken skin or as aerosol to mucous membranes	Rodents	12 (6-14)	None	Trunk to extremities	Macular, maculopapular
Spotted fever group							
Rocky Mountain spotted fever	Western Hemisphere	Tick bite	Ticks, rodents	6 (2-12)	None	Extremities to trunk; palms and soles	Macular, maculopapular, petechial
Tick typhus	Mediterranean littoral, Africa, Asia	Tick bite	Ticks, rodents	12 (7-18)	Frequent	Trunk, extremities, face, palms, soles	Macular, maculopapular, petechial
Rickettsialpox	USA, USSR, Korea	House mouse, mite bite	Mites, mice	12 (9-24)	Usually present	Trunk, face, extremities	Papular, vesicular
Scrub typhus	Japan, SW Asia, W and SW Pacific	Mite bite	Mites, rodents	11 (6-21)	Frequent	Trunk to extremities	Macular, maculopapular, evanescent
Q fever	Worldwide	Inhalation of dried dusts from environment of infected animals	Ticks, mammals	14 (9-20)	None	None	None

163. THE TYPHUS GROUP

Edward S. Murray

The typhus group is made up of three diseases: *epidemic louse-borne typhus fever, Brill-Zinsser disease* and *murine flea-borne typhus fever.* Clinically and pathologically, these three illnesses are very similar. Differences occur only in the intensity of the symptoms and signs, the severity of the course, and the case fatality rate. Epidemiologically, however, the three members of the typhus group are very different, and hence will be described under separate headings.

EPIDEMIC LOUSE-BORNE TYPHUS FEVER
(Classic, Historic, Human, European Typhus; Jail Fever, War Fever; Camp Fever; Fleckfieber [German]; Typhus Exanthématique [French]; Tifus Exantemático, Tabardillo [Spanish]; Dermotypho [Italian])

History. It is probable that typhus fever has afflicted mankind since ancient times. Although the plague of Athens in 430 B.C. is believed to have been epidemic typhus (MacArthur, 1954), the account of Fracastorius in 1546 is the earliest medical record that describes typhus fever with sufficient accuracy to permit its definite identification. Despite the work of Fracastorius, typhoid and typhus fevers were usually regarded as one entity by physicians until 1837, when Gerhard in Philadelphia clearly differentiated the two disorders on the basis of the important clinical and pathologic differences. Even today, however, confusion in terminology persists in those parts of Europe where *typhoid* fever is called "typhus abdominalis."

Typhus fever has played a major role in the history of the past four centuries. It followed in the wake of wars, famines, and human misfortunes. It often has had a more decisive effect on military campaigns than the actual battles themselves, a subject admirably treated by Zinsser in his book, *Rats, Lice and History.* Typhus epidemics in eastern Europe and Russia between 1918 and 1922 are estimated to have caused 30,000,000 cases and at least 3,000,000 deaths. Millions of cases occurred again during World War II in Nazi prison camps, in the Eastern European combat zone, among Yugoslav partisan forces, and in North Africa.

Etiology. In 1916 da Rocha Lima showed that typhus was caused by the microorganism that he named *Rickettsia prowazekii.* This organism has a protean morphology with coccobacillary forms predominating. However, the most typical form is a diplobacillus which has slightly pointed ends with a transparent band between the two bacilli. The organism takes on a characteristic red color when stained by the Gimenez method (Hoeprich). *R. prowazekii* possesses a soluble antigenic moiety which is shared also by *Rickettsia mooseri,* the other member of the typhus group.

R. prowazekii is readily killed by common antiseptics and dies in a few hours if exposed to room temperature. It remains viable for several days in blood at $+5°$ C. Hence, a specimen of blood from a suspected case of typhus can be held for a day or more in a refrigerator pending isolation procedures. Organisms remain viable for several months in dried louse feces, and have survived for over 20 years when quick frozen in an alcohol bath and stored at $-60°$ C.

Living *R. prowazekii* organisms contain a toxin that is lethal for mice as well as a substance that is hemolytic for the red blood cells of many animals.

Transmission. The role of the human body louse in the transmission of typhus was first demonstrated experimentally by Nicolle, Comte, and Conseil in 1909. A few years later mechanisms of transmission were precisely worked out by Wolbach, Todd, and Palfrey (1922) in their classic experiments in Poland on the etiology of typhus fever.

Man and the louse are the only known natural hosts of *R. prowazekii*. There is no passage of *R. prowazekii* organisms from one louse vector generation to the next via the egg. Furthermore, there is no confirmed evidence of an animal reservoir (Ormsbee). The chain of typhus infection starts when *R. prowazekii* appears in a patient's blood during the febrile period. A louse becomes infected during one of its frequent blood meals. The rickettsiae multiply in the cells lining the gut of the infected louse. First these cells become greatly distended and then burst, discharging myriads of microorganisms into the gut where they invade other lining cells or pass out in the feces. The disease is invariably fatal to the louse owing to the ultimate complete destruction of its intestinal epithelium. Transmission of rickettsiae from an infected louse to a new human host can occur by several mechanisms. When a louse takes a blood meal, it makes a small puncture wound in the skin, defecating at the same time. The louse bite is irritating, causing the patient to scratch and thus rub infected feces into the wound. It is also possible for one to become infected if dried infected louse feces gain access to the mucous membranes of the eye or respiratory tract. In an epidemic the spread of typhus from patient to patient and community to community is clearly related to the temperature preferences of the louse. Lice choose a 29° C environment which they find in the folds of the garments of a healthy man. Here they live and lay their eggs. Lice tend to leave a typhus patient when his temperature rises to 40° C or higher. Also, they quickly abandon a corpse in search of a warm host. Transmission of typhus from man to man occurs only by means of the louse; hence, once deloused and bathed, a typhus patient cannot transmit the disease.

Pathology. The microscopic pathology of typhus is characteristic. Rickettsiae multiply in the endothelial cells lining the small blood vessels. Endothelial proliferation and perivascular infiltration lead to thrombosis and leakage. Such vascular lesions when they occur in the skin produce the rash, whereas lesions in the meninges most probably account for the highly characteristic rickettsial headache. The myocardium is also a frequent focus of vascular lesions. Gangrene is directly related to thrombosis of capillaries, small arteries, and veins in affected areas (McAllister).

Clinical Manifestations and Course. The incubation period is approximately ten days to two weeks. Prodromata of vague malaise and headache are not uncommon, especially in vaccinated individuals. The *onset* is usually abrupt, and the patient can frequently state the exact hour when his illness began. The major clinical signs and symptoms are fever, headache, and rash. The fever may rise to 39 to 40° C the first day, or it may take two or three days to reach this level. However, once the temperature reaches 40° C it tends to remain at this level or higher with only slight fluctuations until altered by treatment or recovery. A remittent (or widely fluctuating) temperature is not characteristic of untreated typhus except very late in the disease or in vaccinated persons.

The headache is characteristic. It is intense, persists night and day, and is intractable to all efforts at alleviation. The rash makes its appearance on the fourth to sev-

Temperature curve in a case of classic louse-borne typhus. (From Horsfall, F. L., Jr., and Tamm, I. [eds.]: Viral and Rickettsial Infections of Man. 4th ed. Philadelphia, J. B. Lippincott Company, 1965.)

enth day of illness and consists at first of pinkish macules that fade on slight pressure. These discrete macules usually appear first on the upper trunk in the axillary area. In the course of one or two days the rash spreads over the entire body, usually sparing the face, palms, and soles which are involved only rarely. The macules soon become darker, fixed, and maculopapular. In severely ill patients the rash may progress to petechial, hemorrhagic, or confluent forms.

Patients often have a slight cough without sputum as in mycoplasmal pneumonia. An accompanying patchy pulmonary consolidation is more often diagnosed roentgenographically than by physical examination. Respirations may be increased out of all proportion to findings in the chest.

At first the pulse rate is slow in relation to the temperature, but by the end of the first week it becomes rapid (110 to 140), weak, and frequently undulating or irregular. The blood pressure is usually low, and there may be brief episodes of severe hypotension. Conjunctivitis and flushing of the face are frequent findings. The spleen is palpable in about half the cases. Renal insufficiency of varying degree is a common occurrence. During the acute phase, deafness and ringing in the ears are common complaints, as is also myalgia of the back and legs.

In fatal cases the terminal period is usually characterized by a profound stupor, peripheral vascular collapse, and severe renal failure. In cases without complications, the temperature begins to drop rapidly by lysis between the thirteenth and sixteenth days of illness. Recovery of normal mental and physical powers is remarkably rapid, although the patient may not regain his full strength for two to three months.

Typhus Fever in Previously Immunized Persons. The symptoms and clinical course of typhus are greatly modified as a consequence of prior active immunization. The illness may consist merely of a mild headache and fever of several days' duration. Most patients, however, go on to develop a transient macular rash and suffer from a relatively severe headache and fever for about a week. Complications are rare; mortality has not been reported, and the diagnosis can be established only by serologic or isolation studies.

Typhus Fever Modified by Specific Treatment. If specific treatment is begun early, the clinical course of typhus is usually arrested at whatever stage is present when treatment begins. The temperature usually drops to normal within 36 to 72 hours, and the major clinical signs and symptoms (including the rash) disappear soon thereafter. However, weakness of a greater or lesser extent almost always persists for days or weeks after recovery. On the other hand, if the disease is allowed to progress untreated beyond the eighth or ninth day, treatment becomes less and less effective. In such cases clinical recovery will depend largely upon the extent of vascular damage produced in the heart, brain, and kidneys before therapy was begun.

Diagnosis. *Clinical Diagnosis.* Before the characteristic rash appears, it is impossible to assert on clinical grounds alone that a patient is suffering from epidemic typhus. The early stages of a number of acute infectious diseases closely resemble the first few days of epidemic typhus—for example, smallpox, relapsing fever, malaria, typhoid fever, meningococcal infection, yellow fever, and several of the other rickettsial diseases. Of major help in the differential diagnosis is the characteristic maculopapular typhus rash that begins on the upper trunk and extends centrifugally to the extremities. The rash may be evanescent in children as well as in mildly ill adults. It is also difficult to recognize in dark-skinned subjects.

Laboratory Diagnosis. SPECIFIC SEROLOGIC TESTS. Complement-fixing antibodies first appear in the serum of patients between the seventh and twelfth days of the disease. Soluble antigens that are commercially available detect group antibodies common to both murine and epidemic typhus. In most instances epidemiologic considerations such as geographic location and type of vector involved (flea or louse) will suffice to distinguish between these two diseases in the typhus group. When confusion in diagnosis arises, specific washed antigens (available in special rickettsial laboratories) can be used to differentiate between murine and epidemic typhus. In performing the complement-fixation test it is important to use 4 to 8 units of either type of antigen employed in order to detect the early IgM type of antibodies. Evidence has accumulated over the years indicating that serologic cross-reactions frequently occur between the typhus and Rocky Mountain spotted fever groups of diseases. Hence clinicians must evaluate any serologic results along with clinical and epidemiologic data before arriving at a final diagnosis.

Other special serologic tests that can be used in laboratory diagnosis include immunofluorescence (Elisberg), mouse toxin neutralization, and rickettsial agglutination. Agglutination can also be carried out using sheep or human group O erythrocytes sensitized with a serologically active fraction derived from rickettsiae treated with ether, heat, and alkali (erythrocyte-sensitizing substance or ESS). These special tests are available in rickettsial research laboratories, but are rarely if ever needed to establish a diagnosis.

Persons recovered from typhus regularly show significant antibody titers in their sera for years after an attack of the disease. Hence for definitive diagnosis it is important to demonstrate a rise or fall in antibody titer related to the acute or convalescent period of the clinical disease.

WEIL-FELIX TEST. The Weil-Felix reaction, although nonspecific, is of great value in indicating the strong probability of a typhus infection. The test is positive in over 90 per cent of bona fide cases of primary epidemic typhus. The basis for the Weil-Felix reaction is related to the fact that a certain antigenic component found in

some rickettsiae is shared by various strains of *Proteus vulgaris*. Thus *R. prowazekii* can stimulate antibodies that will agglutinate the OX-19 strains of Proteus. Since low levels of Proteus OX-19 antibody are present in many healthy individuals, diagnostic significance is only attached to titers of 1 to 160 or greater. Such titers are usually demonstrable between the seventh and eleventh days after onset of typhus. The rapid slide method which can be carried out in only three to five minutes is quite satisfactory when performed with controls. Occasionally agglutinins develop for the OX-2 Proteus strains but none for OX-K. Proteus OX-19 antibody titers also develop in other rickettsial diseases, notably murine typhus and Rocky Mountain spotted fever.

ISOLATION OF RICKETTSIAE FROM THE PATIENT. The laboratory diagnosis of typhus may be made by inoculating blood from a patient into a susceptible species such as the guinea pig or chick embryo if facilities are available for the further manipulation required to establish the identity of the microorganisms thus obtained.

Prognosis. The prognosis in untreated cases is closely correlated with age. In children under ten years the disease is usually mild, and fatalities are uncommon. In adults the mortality ranges from 10 per cent in the second and third decades of life to more than 60 per cent in those over 50. However, active immunization and the use of specific therapy greatly affect mortality figures.

In the absence of specific treatment, the appearance of renal insufficiency is an early sign that a patient's illness will be severe or fatal. The extent and severity of the typhus rash is also roughly indicative of the severity of the disease. Complications such as pneumonia or gangrene of the skin are likewise serious prognostic signs. A fall in systolic blood pressure to values below 80 mm or mercury for a few hours or longer may cause damage from which the patient may not recover, even though the blood pressure rises after the period of severe hypotension.

Treatment. Chloramphenicol or the tetracyclines are highly effective when given early and in adequate dosage. The clinician must decide on the basis of his own preference which drug he will use. Recent reports suggest that doxycycline is an effective drug in the treatment of rickettsial infections.

Prompt and optimal specific therapy is urgent. A maximally effective rickettsiostatic blood level of drug should be obtained at the earliest possible moment. Since large doses of chloramphenicol are well absorbed from the gastrointestinal tract, this drug may be preferred in gravely ill patients. For chloramphenicol the following dosage schedule is considered optimal: Therapy is begun with an initial loading dose of 50 mg per kilogram of body weight, followed by a daily dose of 50 mg per kilogram of body weight divided into three or four equal doses during each 24-hour period. For an adult this schedule would amount to approximately 5 grams of chloramphenicol given over the first 24-hour period (an initial loading dose of 3 grams followed by 0.5 gram every six hours). This dosage of chloramphenicol for the first 24 hours of illness is higher than that recommended in bacterial diseases. However, a large body of experience in using high initial doses of this drug in treating rickettsial diseases fully justifies such a schedule.

Since large single doses of tetracyclines are irregularly absorbed from the gastrointestinal tract, a loading dose of these drugs is not indicated. The daily recommended dose of the tetracyclines is calculated on the basis of 25 mg per kilogram of body weight. Treatment is more effective if the daily dose is divided and administered at intervals of three or four hours rather than on a six- to eight-hour schedule.

As the temperature approaches normal, the daily dosage of the antimicrobial being administered can be cut in half and then continued for two or three more days. Relapses are uncommon even when treatment is begun as early as the first or second day of illness.

Intravenous preparations of chloramphenicol and tetracyclines are available, and should be used in critically ill patients when oral medication is not possible because of vomiting or uncooperativeness. For adults, 1 gram of chloramphenicol sodium succinate in glucose or saline solution can be given intravenously, followed by 500 mg every four to six hours. Intravenous tetracycline can be administered in glucose or saline solution, 1 gram initially, followed by 500 mg every six hours. Intravenous therapy should be discontinued as soon as the patient is able to take the drug by mouth.

Penicillin and streptomycin have very little, if any, effect. Their use should be considered only when secondary bacterial infections develop for which they are specifically indicated. The sulfonamides may have a harmful effect, and are contraindicated. Steroid therapy has been used by some clinicians in severely ill patients. Carefully controlled hormone therapy may be of practical value in patients first seen late in the course of illness at a time when supplemental antitoxemia measures could be lifesaving.

Special nursing care is of utmost importance. Comatose patients should be turned frequently to prevent decubitus ulcers and hypostatic pneumonia. Vomiting necessitates small frequent feedings. Sedatives should be used with care so that the course of the disease is not obscured. Excessively high temperatures should be controlled by alcohol sponging.

It should be kept in mind that because of the widespread endothelial damage in epidemic typhus, as well as in all the other rickettsial diseases, a severely ill patient may be even more desperately ill than he appears. Therefore all laboratory and other manipulative measures that disturb and exhaust him should be reduced to a minimum. The antimicrobial drugs are rickettsiostatic only; hence the patient's own defense and recuperative powers are major factors in his recovery.

Prevention. Two highly effective measures, immunization and louse control, are available for the prevention and control of typhus. Both are applicable to an individual as well as a community. Killed typhus vaccines produced from yolk sacs of infected chick embryos have been widely used. Immunization with killed vaccines does not fully protect against infection. However, when vaccinated individuals do contract typhus, the course of illness is shorter and milder, and fatalities have not been reported. An experimental living attenuated "Strain E" typhus vaccine (Fox) is under trial in the United States, the USSR, and Africa. Moderately severe illness has occurred in a small percentage of those inoculated with minimal immunizing doses of this vaccine. However, the prompt development and prolonged duration of the immunity resulting from a single dose of Strain E vaccine indicates that under certain circumstances this vaccine may be found to play a useful role in typhus control.

Louse control with DDT and the newer developed in-secticides offers a powerful weapon against typhus epidemics. Both infected and noninfected lice can be eliminated almost completely by mass delousing of a population. A major factor in the efficacy of DDT is the persistence of its lethal effect on lice for two to four weeks after being dusted into garments.

Recent reports indicate that in several areas lice have become partially resistant to DDT. Other insecticides such as malathione or lindane may have to be used under these circumstances.

BRILL-ZINSSER DISEASE AND THE CARRIER STATE

History. In 1898 Nathan Brill in New York described sporadic cases of a typhus-like illness with fever, headache, and a maculopapular rash which occurred characteristically in immigrants from Russia and Poland. The disease was clearly distinguishable from typhoid, because the Widal test was negative. However, the illness was not typical of typhus, as all cases were sporadic with no spread to family or other contacts.

Over the next three decades many clinicians in the large cities of the eastern United States reported cases that were referred to as Brill's disease. In 1912 Anderson and Goldberger demonstrated by cross-immunity tests in monkeys that Brill's disease was a form of typhus, and for a period thereafter Brill's disease and murine typhus were confused with each other. However, by 1931 murine typhus was clearly defined as a flea-borne disease and Brill's disease remained an isolated syndrome of unknown etiology.

In 1934 Hans Zinsser carried out extensive epidemiologic studies on 538 cases of Brill's disease occurring in New York and Boston. Almost invariably patients were immigrants from eastern Europe where louse-borne typhus was prevalent. This led Zinsser to postulate that the syndrome represented a relapse of a prior typhus infection. He reasoned that man was a carrier and through the medium of recrudescent "Brill's disease" cases served to maintain the disease between epidemics. Over the next two decades Zinsser's hypothesis was widely accepted. To acknowledge the contributions of the two scientists whose observations revealed the interepidemic reservoir of typhus, the syndrome was renamed Brill-Zinsser disease.

Typhus, the Carrier State, and Recrudescence. Clinical and epidemiologic features of Brill-Zinsser disease are consistent with the view proposed by Zinsser that it represents a relapse or recrudescence of a primary louse-borne typhus infection suffered at some time in the past. This makes Brill-Zinsser disease analogous in many ways to a relapse of malaria occurring years after an original malarial attack. Zinsser's hypothesis has received additional confirmation recently from laboratory studies in which normal lice were fed on patients during the acute phase of Brill-Zinsser disease. From these lice microorganisms were isolated that proved to be identical to *R. prowazekii*—the etiologic agent of primary louse-borne typhus.

Brill-Zinsser disease, however, differs from primary louse-borne typhus in a number of respects. (1) Clinically the disease is shorter, milder, and frequently without a rash. This picture is consistent with the fact that the syndrome represents an *R. prowazekii* infection in an individual already partially immune. (2) No louse vector or exogenous source of the infection is apparent. (3) The majority of patients give a history of having suffered an attack of primary louse-borne typhus in the past. But it is the serologic data that provide the most sharply distinguishing characteristics of these two disease entities caused by the same organism. In primary louse-borne typhus the acute phase antibodies are IgM in type, whereas the antibodies in Brill-Zinsser disease are from their very earliest appearance of the IgG class. These differences are characteristic of the primary and secondary immune response.

An interesting feature of the Brill-Zinsser syndrome is the frequent absence of a significant Weil-Felix reaction.

TABLE 2.   Distinguishing Characteristics of Primary Louse-Borne Typhus and Brill-Zinsser Disease

	Primary Louse-Borne Typhus	Brill-Zinsser Disease
Epidemiologic		
Past history of typhus	No	Yes
Occurrence of cases	Epidemic	Sporadic
Seasonal occurrence	Winter-spring	Year round
Transmission	By infected lice	Occurs in absence of lice
Clinical		
Duration of fever	12-18 days	7-11 days
Rash	Regularly present	Frequently absent or evanescent
Mortality	10-50% depending on age	Rare
Laboratory		
Specific antibody rise	Slow—begins 7th to 10th day, maximum 15th to 20th day	Rapid—begins 4th to 5th day, maximum 9th to 11th day
Type of immunoglobulin response during acute phase	Primary—IgM	Secondary—IgG
Weil-Felix reaction	Regularly present in titers of 1/160 or higher	Frequently absent (see text)
Cross-reacting specific *R. mooseri* antibodies in acute phase	No	Yes

In fact the reaction is almost always negative when a Brill-Zinsser disease relapse occurs within the first few years after the primary attack at a time when immunity from the original illness is presumably still quite high. As the interval between the original attack and the recrudescence lengthens, positive Weil-Felix reactions occur more frequently. The Weil-Felix reaction is usually also negative in those who develop primary louse-borne typhus after prophylactic vaccination, as well as in typhus patients who receive antimicrobial therapy very early in the course of their illness.*

Brill-Zinsser disease has now been reported from many parts of the world. Wherever it has been recognized, it has always occurred in individuals who were born or had lived for some time in an area where louse-borne typhus occurs in epidemic form—particularly the countries of eastern Europe. Brill-Zinsser disease also occurs in eastern Europe itself. In this area, particularly in Bosnia, Yugoslavia, small family epidemics of primary epidemic typhus in children have been described in which a direct relationship could be traced from the children's infection to an adult recrudescent case of Brill-Zinsser disease that occurred several weeks earlier in the same family.

The epidemiologic significance of Brill-Zinsser disease cases is clear. They indicate the existence of carriers with latent infection who constitute the interepidemic reservoirs of typhus. Thus in a community where louse infestation is prevalent, when a latent carrier relapses and becomes an overt Brill-Zinsser disease case, the scene is then set for a possible epidemic of louse-borne typhus.

Pathology.   The findings in Brill-Zinsser disease are the same as those described under Louse-Borne Typhus.

Diagnosis.   The clinical diagnosis of Brill-Zinsser disease should be considered when a fever of unknown origin with an intense persistent headache occurs in a patient who has lived at some previous time in an area where louse-borne typhus occurs in epidemic form. A macular or maculopapular rash, if present, is of additional help in diagnosis.

The diagnosis can be confirmed in the laboratory by employing the complement-fixation test. A negative Weil-Felix test in the presence of rising CF antibodies is highly suggestive of Brill-Zinsser disease rather than primary louse-borne typhus, because more than 95 per cent of cases of the latter disease show a significant rise in Proteus OX-19 agglutinins. However, it should be kept in mind that the Weil-Felix test may be positive in Brill-Zinsser disease if the period elapsed between the original and the recrudescent attack is ten years or longer. The demonstration of only the IgG class of antibodies in the early acute phase of illness is highly diagnostic of Brill-Zinsser disease.

Prognosis and Treatment.   Statements in the paragraphs on Prognosis and Treatment of Louse-Borne Typhus apply to Brill-Zinsser disease as well.

Control of the Interepidemic Typhus Reservoir.   The factors that precipitate an attack of Brill-Zinsser disease are unknown, and methods to prevent recrudescent attacks have not yet been discovered. However, the spread of infection from recrudescent Brill-Zinsser disease cases to nonimmune contacts can be curtailed. When Brill-Zinsser disease occurs in an area such as the United States where louse infestation is extremely rare, no spread of the disease will occur, and no measures are required beyond treatment of the Brill-Zinsser disease itself. However, when Brill-Zinsser disease cases occur in a community where louse infestation is prevalent, one practical method of control is the "fire brigade" technique. This consists of a surveillance network throughout the community organized to report promptly the occurrence of a Brill-Zinsser disease case or the first ensuing cases of primary louse-borne typhus. A centrally based control team should then be available to come in with insecticides to eliminate all lice in the environment, including lice on all contacts near and far.

*Weil-Felix reactions are related to the fact that certain Proteus organisms share a common antigen with certain of the rickettsiae. Because the amount of this common antigen in each individual rickettsia is extremely minute, a relatively large mass of rickettsiae may be required to stimulate the Proteus agglutinins. The partially immune status of a Brill-Zinsser disease patient as well as that of a typhus-vaccinated individual may prevent the rickettsial mass in the blood and tissues from obtaining the necessary level to evoke a Proteus response. Likewise, early antimicrobial treatment may reduce the likelihood of a Proteus response by contributing to an early and rapid elimination of rickettsiae from the infected individual.

TABLE 3. Complement Fixation and Weil-Felix Reactions in Rickettsioses

Group	Disease	Rickettsial Complement Fixation (CF)*			Weil-Felix (WF) Agglutination*		
		Group Antigen Type			Proteus Strain		
		Typhus	RMSF	Q Fever	OX-19	OX-2	OX-K
I	Primary louse-borne typhus	+++	±	0	+++	+	0
	Brill-Zinsser disease	+++	±	0	0 or +++	0	0
	Murine typhus	+++	±	0	+++	+	0
II	RMSF	±	+++	0	+++†	+++†	0
	Tick typhus	0	+++	0	+++†	+++†	0
	Rickettsialpox	0	+++	0	0	0	0
III	Scrub typhus	0	0	0	0	0	+++
IV	Q fever	0	0	+++	0	0	0

*+++ = Strong reactions in CF 1:40 to 1:280.
      Strong reactions in WF 1:160 or greater.
  + = OX-2 reactions relatively weaker than OX-19.
  0 = Negative at 1:5 dilution in CF.
      Negative at 1:40 dilution in WF.
  ± = Recent evidence indicates that frequent cross-reactions occur between the typhus group and Rocky Mountain spotted fever (see text).
†In RMSF or tick typhus, agglutinins to either OX-19 or OX-2 or both can be present in either high or low titer.

MURINE FLEA-BORNE TYPHUS FEVER
(Endemic Typhus, Rat Typhus, Flea Typhus, Urban or Shop Typhus of Malaya)

History. Murine typhus fever probably has occurred for centuries as a sporadic or endemic disease, but only since 1931 has it been clearly distinguished from classic epidemic louse-borne typhus. During the early part of this century in the United States murine typhus was confused with Brill's disease. However, in 1926 Maxey, after extensive investigation, concluded that the typhus occurring in the southeastern United States must have a reservoir other than man, and he mentioned mice and rats specifically. He further suggested that fleas, mites, or ticks could be the vector. Mooser, in 1928, observed a basic difference in behavior of certain strains of typhus rickettsiae in the tissues of guinea pigs. Dyer and colleagues isolated typhus rickettsiae from rat fleas in Baltimore (1931), and Mooser, Zinsser, and Ruiz Castaneda found the agent in rats in Mexico City. Mooser subsequently named the disease "murine typhus" to indicate its presence as a natural infection of rats. Reports showing the worldwide distribution of murine typhus rapidly accumulated. In the United States the incidence of the disease was increasing up to 1946. The rapid decrease in incidence since that time has been attributed, in part, to vigorously applied control measures.

Etiology. The etiologic agent, *Rickettsia mooseri,* is similar to *Rickettsia prowazekii* in metabolic, biochemical, and staining characteristics; however, in size, *R. mooseri* is slightly smaller and more uniform. *R. mooseri* and *R. prowazekii* are classed together in the typhus group by virtue of the fact that they possess a common soluble antigenic moiety.

Epidemiology and Transmission. Rats infected with murine typhus are found scattered throughout the world in circumscribed areas. In the United States reservoirs of the disease are found along the southern Atlantic seaboard and in states bordering on the Gulf of Mexico. Other known areas of infection are Mexico, South America, the Mediterranean littoral, and Manchuria. However, the disease is widespread, occurring elsewhere in such areas as Ethiopia, Malaysia, and Australia.

Murine typhus is maintained in nature as a mild infection of rats, and is transmitted from rat to rat by the rat louse or by the rat flea, *Xenopsylla cheopis.* A flea becomes infected while feeding on a rat during the acute phase of an infection. The rickettsiae multiply in the flea without causing any damage to the host. Once infected the flea continues to discharge rickettsiae in its feces for the remainder of its life; however, infected female fleas do not transmit *R. mooseri* via their eggs to the next generation of fleas. Man usually acquires the disease when bitten by an infected flea. Rat fleas generally prefer to feed on rats, but they will attack man if rats become scarce. At the same time that an infected flea sucks blood it deposits feces that are teeming with rickettsiae. These may be rubbed into the flea bite wound or, as dried aerosol of feces and microorganisms, they may gain access to the body through the mucous membranes of the conjunctivae or respiratory tract. Infection of man is an accidental occurrence and is not related to the maintenance of the disease in nature.

Pathology. Information on the pathology of murine typhus is limited, because death from this form of typhus is rare. It is usually assumed that the lesions are essentially the same as those in louse-borne typhus.

Clinical Manifestation and Course. The incubation period of murine typhus lasts from six to fourteen days. The symptoms are similar to those of louse-borne typhus, the principal differences being that murine typhus is milder and shorter, the rash is less extensive and persists for shorter periods, there are fewer complications, and the case fatality rate is lower.

Diagnosis. *Clinical Diagnosis.* The diagnosis of murine typhus may be suspected when a patient has a sustained fever of several days' duration accompanied by headache, generalized aches and pains, and a macular or maculopapular rash appearing on the fifth or sixth day after onset of fever. The rash is first noted on the trunk and later spreads to the extremities; the face, palms, and soles are rarely involved. Since murine typhus is present in many of the areas where Rocky Mountain spotted fever (RMSF) occurs, it is helpful to remember that the rash of RMSF first appears on the wrists and ankles, rapidly spreads up the extremities to the trunk, and regularly involves the palms and soles. The patient with murine typhus usually gives a history of activities that have brought him into contact with places where rats are numerous. However, there is often no definite recollection of a flea bite.

It is impossible on clinical evidence alone to distinguish an ordinary case of murine typhus from a case of Brill-Zinsser disease or a mild case of louse-borne typhus. Epidemiologic and laboratory data will almost always be required to arrive at a definitive diagnosis.

Laboratory Diagnosis. Both the complement-fixation and Weil-Felix tests are employed in the laboratory to confirm the clinical suspicion of a murine typhus infection. Rising antibodies to the soluble typhus group antigen indicate either a primary louse-borne typhus, Brill-Zinsser disease, or murine typhus infection. From the time of onset Brill-Zinsser disease antibodies are IgG in type. In contrast, the antibodies produced in the acute phase of murine and louse-borne typhus are characteristically IgM. One may have to resort to specific washed rickettsial antigens to distinguish between louse-borne and murine typhus. In murine typhus as in primary louse-borne typhus 4 to 8 units of antigen are required to obtain optimal fixation of complement during the acute phase of illness.

The Weil-Felix test employing Proteus OX-19 strains is regularly positive in murine typhus. Isolation of *R. mooseri* from patients may be accomplished early in the course of the disease by inoculating blood into guinea pigs, mice, or chick embryos. (See Laboratory Diagnosis in Louse-Borne Typhus.)

Prognosis. Even when untreated, murine typhus is usually a mild disease with fatalities occurring only in the elderly. The use of specific therapy further reduces the duration and severity of the disease.

Treatment. Treatment of murine typhus is similar to that for louse-borne typhus. However, the usual mildness of murine typhus permits more leeway in a therapeutic regimen. For example, tetracycline can be used as the preferred drug, thus avoiding the greater potential toxicity of chloramphenicol.

Prevention and Control. Measures to prevent and control murine typhus depend upon limiting the rat population. The first step is to reduce the flea population of rat colonies by dusting rat runs with DDT or its equivalent. After this, rat populations are reduced by poisoning, trapping, eliminating rat harborages, and rat-proofing buildings.

A vaccine has been produced and demonstrated to be effective. However, its use is hardly justified in view of the clinical mildness and sporadic nature of the disease.

Elisberg, B. L., and Bozeman, F. L.: Serologic diagnosis of rickettsial diseases by indirect immunofluorescence. Arch. Inst. Pasteur Tunis, 43:193, 1966.

Fox, J. P., Montoya, J. A., Jordan, M. D., Cornojo Ubillus, J. R., Garcia, J. L., Estrada, M. A., and Gelfand, H. M.: Immunization of man against epidemic typhus by infection with avirulent *Rickettsia prowazeki* (strain E). Arch. Inst. Pasteur Tunis, 36:449, 1959.

Gear, J. H. S.: Rickettsial vaccines. Br. Med. Bull., 25:171, 1969.

Hoeprich, P. D. (ed.): Infectious Diseases. New York, Harper & Row, 1972.

MacArthur, W. P.: The Athenian plague: A medical note. Classical Quarterly, 4:171, 1954.

McAllister, W. B.: The pathology of louse-borne typhus fever from the epidemic of 1943-5 in Egypt. Nav. Med. Res. Inst., Proj. NM 007 017 (X-696), Rep. No. 1, 25 January 1949.

Murray, E. S., O'Connor, J. M., and Gaon, J. A.: Differentiation of 19S and 7S complement-fixing antibodies in primary versus recrudescent typhus by either ethanethiol or heat. Proc. Soc. Exp. Biol. Med., 119:291, 1965.

Murray, E. S., and Snyder, J. C.: Brill-Zinsser disease: The interepidemic reservoir of epidemic louse-borne typhus fever. Proceedings Sixth International Congress of Microbiology, Rome. 4, Section 11, 31-44, 1953.

Ormsbee, R. A., Burgdorfer, W., Peacock, M., and Hildebrandt, F.: Experimental infections of *R. prowazeki* among domestic livestock and ticks. Am. J. Trop. Med. Hyg., 20:117, 1971.

Proceedings of the International Symposium on the Control of Lice and Louse-borne Diseases. Washington, D.C., December 4–6, 1972. Pan American Health Organization Scientific Publication No. 263.

Smadel, J. E.: Status of the rickettsioses in the United States. Ann. Intern. Med., 51:421, 1959.

Snyder, J. C.: The typhus fevers. In Horsfall, F. L., Jr., and Tamm, I. (eds.): Viral and Rickettsial Infections of Man. 4th ed. Philadelphia, J. B. Lippincott Company, 1965, Chapter 50.

Wolbach, S. B., Todd, J. L., and Palfrey, F. W.: The Etiology and Pathology of Typhus. Cambridge, Mass., Harvard University Press, 1922.

Zdrodovskii, P. F., and Golinevich, H. M.: The Rickettsial Diseases. New York, Pergamon Press, 1960 (in English).

Zinsser, H.: Rats, Lice, and History. Boston, Little, Brown and Company, 1935.

164. ROCKY MOUNTAIN SPOTTED FEVER
(Spotted Fever, Tick Fever, Tick Typhus [England], Fiebre Manchada [Mexico], Fiebre Petequial [Colombia], Febere Maculosa [Brazil])

Herbert L. Ley, Jr.

Definition. Rocky Mountain spotted fever is a relatively severe, self-limited rickettsial infection transmitted to man by various species of hard ticks. The disease is characterized by fever, headache, bone and muscle pains, and a generalized rash that frequently may become petechial or hemorrhagic.

Etiology. The disease is caused by *Rickettsia rickettsi (Dermacentroxenus rickettsi)*, the prototype rickettsia of the spotted fever group of organisms. These include, in addition to *R. rickettsi*, the agents of rickettsialpox, north Asian tick-borne rickettsiosis, and African and Queensland tick typhus, all of which are distinctive among rickettsiae in their ability to multiply in the nucleus as well as in the cytoplasm of mammalian and tick cells. All these agents share an antigen common to the group, and each possesses an individual species-specific antigen as well. Serologic differentiation among members of the group has been complicated by the shared antigen; specific antisera, prepared in mice, are useful in laboratory identification of the individual members of the group. All the tick-borne rickettsioses of the Western Hemisphere have proved, to date, to be caused by *R. rickettsi*, regardless of the country of origin or the local name given the disease. The incubation period of the disease may vary from 2 to 14 days; severe illnesses appear to be associated with short incubation periods.

Distribution and Incidence. Rocky Mountain spotted fever is limited in distribution to North and South America. The disease was first described in the United States in Montana at the turn of the century, and for some time was thought to be limited to that area. Beginning in the 1930's, the disease was recognized in the eastern United States, Canada, Mexico, Brazil, and Colombia. Incidence and mortality data are difficult to obtain outside the United States, but in this country an average of 300 cases has been reported annually for the ten-year period from 1950 to 1959, with an average mortality rate of 6 per cent. During the 1960's about 300 cases have been reported annually in the United States, approximately half occurring in the Atlantic seaboard states from Delaware to Florida.*

Epidemiology. Rocky Mountain spotted fever is widely disseminated in nature and is principally a disease of ticks and small mammals. Man is rarely involved except when he intrudes into the "silent" wild cycle of disease. The hard ticks involved in transmission, the Ixodidae, feed on small mammals during their development through the larval and nymphal stages to tick adulthood. Once infected with *R. rickettsi* the tick may transmit the rickettsiae to its progeny transovarially or to man and other animals by feeding upon them. Thus the tick is both a vector and a reservoir of infection. The species of tick involved in the disease cycle varies according to geographic area. In the northern United States, the rabbit tick, *Haemaphysalis lepori-palustris,* rarely bites man, but appears to be responsible for maintaining the disease among rabbits and small mammals. Human infection in the United States is most commonly acquired in the West from *Dermacentor andersoni* (the wood tick), in the East from *Dermacentor variabilis* (the dog tick), and in the South from *Amblyomma americanum* (the Lone Star tick). Many other species of hard ticks have been implicated in transmission of the disease in Central and South America. Under laboratory conditions soft ticks of the genus Ornithodorus are also capable of transmitting the agent, but appear to be unimportant as vectors in nature. Among the animals believed to be involved in the natural cycle of disease are squirrels, rabbits, porcupines, chipmunks, weasels, several species of feral rats and mice, and, perhaps most important from the human viewpoint, dogs. All these animals have been shown to be susceptible to infection with *R. rickettsi;* the disease produced is usually mild and limited in duration but is associated with a rickettsemia sufficient to infect ticks feeding on the animal at the time.

Although it was once considered that the western form of the disease was more serious than the eastern, the higher mortality rates in the western United States appear to be a reflection of a much higher average age among patients. Formerly the disease was one of the adult male in the West and of children of both sexes in the eastern United States. In recent years more than half the patients reported nationally have been less than 15 years of age. As might be expected, the disease has a striking seasonal pattern in which nearly 90 per cent of all cases occur during the period from May through September.

Pathology and Physiologic Responses. Histopathologically, the disease is an endangitis, starting in the endothelial cells and extending into the smooth muscle of the vessel walls. Rickettsiae may be demonstrated in the lesions by appropriate stains. Thrombi are formed at the points of inflammation and lead to areas of focal necrosis and hemorrhage. The major organ systems involved are the skin, subcutaneous tissues, and the central nervous system, although mononuclear cell infiltration may also be found in the lungs, heart, liver, and spleen. Except for the rash, gross findings at autopsy are minimal.

Clinical laboratory findings in the milder cases are usually limited to a moderate leukocytosis. Peripheral

vascular collapse, the most serious consequence of the disease, may result from the pooling of blood in the damaged capillaries and from loss of water, electrolytes, and proteins into the extravascular space. Patients having this complication will show a decrease in hematocrit, blood chloride, and serum protein levels, and an increase in serum nonprotein nitrogen levels. Thrombocytopenia has also been observed in severe illnesses.

Clinical Manifestations. Headache and fever, frequently accompanied by mild chills, appear as initial symptoms of infection 2 to 14 days following contact with ticks. Within the first day of fever the patient usually complains of pains in the bones, joints, and muscles, photophobia, and increasing prostration. Initial physical examination usually reveals only flushing of the skin, conjunctival injection, and minor respiratory signs referable to a dry cough. By the second day the fever usually rises to 40 to 40.5° C and stays at that level until the end of the second week. Between the second and sixth days of fever a generalized macular rash develops that resembles the eruption of measles. Initially the rash blanches with pressure, but after 24 to 48 hours the eruption frequently becomes petechial or, in the more severe cases, hemorrhagic. In mild illnesses, or in previously vaccinated persons, the rash may be minimal. Central nervous system symptoms in the form of agitation, insomnia, delirium, or coma usually appear by the end of the first week of fever. It is during the second week of fever that the most critical circulatory and pulmonary complications of the disease occur. Gangrene of the extremities or other dependent parts and pneumonia are sometimes seen in untreated patients. Fever usually abates by the end of the second week, and full recovery commonly takes several weeks or months in untreated patients.

Diagnosis. Rocky Mountain spotted fever should always be considered in the differential diagnosis of a febrile illness with rash occurring in the months of May through September in the United States. The most common initial diagnosis of illness for patients subsequently found to have Rocky Mountain spotted fever is measles, despite the fact that measles usually does not occur during the period when Rocky Mountain spotted fever is most common. As in all the rickettsial diseases, the initial diagnosis must be made solely on clinical grounds because confirmatory laboratory tests are of no assistance until relatively late in the illness. The symptoms, physical findings, and history of exposure in an area known to harbor ticks must be weighed carefully by the physician, and, if the diagnosis is considered probable, treatment should be initiated. Two other rickettsial diseases, rickettsialpox and murine typhus, may mimic mild cases of Rocky Mountain spotted fever. Fortunately both respond equally well to treatment appropriate for Rocky Mountain spotted fever.

Laboratory confirmation of the clinical diagnosis may be obtained by isolation of *R. rickettsi* from the blood during the first week of illness. *Isolation studies in guinea pigs or embryonated eggs should be attempted only by laboratories equipped for such work because of the danger of infection of laboratory personnel.* More commonly, laboratory diagnosis depends upon serologic tests with paired serum samples, the first obtained as early as possible during illness and the second about the fifteenth to twenty-fifth day of disease. These tests utilize either the Weil-Felix Proteus OX-19 and OX-2 agglutination reactions or the complement-fixation test with yolk sac antigen. In the agglutination test, positive results may be

---

obtained with either or both of the OX-19 or OX-2 antigens; approximately 15 per cent of patients may show no rise in Weil-Felix titers even though complement-fixation tests are positive.* A fourfold or greater rise in titer with the complement-fixation test is considered confirmatory.

Treatment and Prognosis. Until 1945 treatment of Rocky Mountain spotted fever was limited to supportive therapy; mortality rates were 20 per cent or greater. In 1945, para-aminobenzoic acid (PABA) was shown to be effective in treatment, producing defervescence in approximately three days and reducing mortality virtually to zero. By the early 1950's, chloramphenicol and the tetracyclines replaced PABA in the treatment of this disease because the newer antimicrobial drugs were equally effective as PABA and far better tolerated. In the majority of patients, headache and other symptoms abate within 24 to 48 hours, and fever disappears within three to four days after beginning therapy with 25 mg per kilogram per day of the tetracyclines or 50 mg per kilogram per day of chloramphenicol, given in four divided doses by mouth. With either regimen, treatment should be continued for 24 to 48 hours after the patient becomes afebrile. The physician must weigh the disadvantages of gastric irritation or the dangers of use in renal insufficiency associated with the tetracyclines against the risks of blood dyscrasias with chloramphenicol. In general, because of the greater seriousness of the toxicity to chloramphenicol, tetracycline is the preferred therapy. For patients too ill to take oral medication, parenteral preparations must be used; when these are necessary, the patient will also require intravenous fluids to correct electrolyte or fluid abnormalities. Corticosteroids may also be of help for severely ill patients.

The most important step in treatment is early diagnosis; no amount of drug therapy can modify the course of the disease in the patient who is admitted in extremis. Heroic measures such as corticosteroid therapy and parenteral administration of antimicrobials are completely unnecessary if the diagnosis is made and treatment begun early in the course of the disease. Early treatment will also prevent sequelae such as brain or heart damage, which have been observed in patients who have been treated late in their illness.

Prevention. Although protective vaccine is available, its use has descreased markedly in recent years, presumably because effective antimicrobial therapy is now available. Nevertheless, use of the vaccine is appropriate for selected persons who may be exposed to the danger of infection in remote areas in which medical treatment may be difficult or impossible to obtain.

Because ticks cannot transmit infection to man without having been attached for several hours, a degree of protection can be achieved by careful examination of one's person and careful removal of attached ticks on a twice daily schedule. Considerable difference of opinion exists regarding the safest method of removal. The use of a lighted cigarette or the application of kerosene, both highly regarded in some circles, appears to have the disadvantage that agonal responses of the tick may cause actual expression of rickettsiae into the wound. Another method appears to be preferable: the tick is grasped by the head and thorax with a pair of fine forceps and pulled gently but firmly until the mouth parts are extracted from the skin. The third category of control measures is directed against the tick vector of the disease. The use of clothing impregnated with tick repellents provides significant protection to those who must travel through tick-infested areas. When groups of people may be exposed to ticks in summer camps or recreational areas, the selective use of residual insecticides, such as DDT, dieldrin, or lindane, has proved effective in limited areas in reducing tick populations.

Lackman, D. B., Bell, E. J., Stoenner, H. G., and Pickens, E. G.: The Rocky Mountain spotted fever group of rickettsias. Health Lab. Sci., 2:135, 1965.

Ricketts, H. T.: Contributions to Medical Science by Howard Taylor Ricketts, 1870–1910. Chicago, University of Chicago Press, 1911, p. 278.

Wisseman, C. L., Jr. (ed.): Symposium on the Spotted Fever Group of Rickettsiae. Medical Science Publication No. 7, Walter Reed Army Institute of Research. Washington, D.C., U.S. Government Printing Office, 1960.

Woodward, T. E., and Jackson, E. B.: Spotted fever rickettsiae. *In* Horsfall, F. L., Jr., and Tamm, I. (eds.): Viral and Rickettsial Infections of Man. 4th ed. Philadelphia, J. B. Lippincott Company, 1965, p. 1095.

Zdrodovskii, P. F., and Golinevich, H. M.: The Rickettsial Diseases. New York, Pergamon Press, 1960, p. 277.

165. TICK-BORNE RICKETTSIOSES OF THE EASTERN HEMISPHERE

*Herbert L. Ley, Jr.**

Definition. The three diseases that constitute this group, i.e., *African tick typhus, North Asian tick-borne rickettsiosis,* and *Queensland tick typhus,* are caused by rickettsiae that are closely related to one another and to the agent of Rocky Mountain spotted fever. Each is transmitted by the bite of an ixodid tick.

African tick typhus *(Boutonneuse fever)* may be regarded as the prototype of the group. It is the most widely distributed geographically, occurring throughout the African continent, in those parts of Europe and the Middle East adjacent to the Mediterranean, Black and Caspian Seas, and in India. Boutonneuse fever is a mild to moderately severe febrile illness of a few days' to two weeks' duration. It is characterized by a primary lesion that develops at the site of the infected tick bite and a generalized maculopapular erythematous rash that appears about the fourth day. As in Rocky Mountain spotted fever, agglutinins against Proteus OX-19 (Weil-Felix reaction) usually appear during convalescence, as do specific complement-fixing antibodies against the rickettsial organisms.

History, Distribution, Etiology, and Epidemiology. Boutonneuse fever was first recognized in 1910 in Tunisia by Conor and Bruch. During the next several decades the occurrence of similar diseases was noted in Africa, Europe, and the Middle East; these were given various local names. However, it was not until modern serologic methods employing specific rickettsial antigens were applied that *Rickettsia conori* was shown to be the etio-

---

*See Ch. 163 for discussion of the Weil-Felix reaction.

*Ch. 164 to 169 have been written to replace articles on the same subjects prepared for previous editions by the author's former teacher and colleague, the late Dr. Joseph E. Smadel. Thus, Dr. Smadel's many contributions to these subjects understandably permeate the whole section. For this chapter on Tick-Borne Rickettsioses, however, the present author found it inadvisable to do more than make trivial changes and update the references so that, to all intents and purposes, it is as it was originally prepared by Dr. Smadel.

logic agent for a single widely disseminated disease, African tick typhus. Queensland tick typhus caused by *R. australis* was established as an entity during World War II. Although the rickettsial nature of North Asian tick-borne rickettsiosis was demonstrated in 1938, only in recent years has its etiologic agent, *R. siberica,* been clearly differentiated from other members of the spotted fever group of organisms.

The etiologic agents of the three diseases of the Eastern Hemisphere are all members of the spotted fever group of rickettsiae. Together with *R. rickettsi* and *R. akari* they possess common group antigens that are readily demonstrated by agglutination and complement-fixation procedures. In addition, type-specific antigens characterize each member of the spotted fever group; these are demonstrated by similar in vitro serologic procedures employing specially purified antigens. *Rickettsia conori, R. australis,* and *R. siberica* may be differentiated from one another and from *R. rickettsi* and *R. akari* by complement-fixation tests using antisera from mice, by cross-vaccination tests performed in guinea pigs, or by cross-neutralization tests using the mouse lethal toxin obtained from each agent and homologous antisera. Experimental infection of animals with one member of the spotted fever group of rickettsiae induces appreciable resistance to infection with other members.

For the most part, the *epidemiology* of the three tick-borne rickettsioses of the Eastern Hemisphere resembles that of spotted fever in the Western Hemisphere. Thus, the rickettsial agents are maintained in nature by cycles involving ixodid ticks and small wild animals; man, if he intrudes into the cycles, serves as a dead end in the chain of transmission. Boutonneuse fever in the Mediterranean area has a more domesticated and urbanized pattern. Here, another cycle is also involved with the brown dog tick as the vector and the dog as the animal host.

Pathology. In fatal cases, which are few and usually limited to the aged and debilitated, the findings are similar to those in Rocky Mountain spotted fever except for the presence of the *tache noire,* the black button-like necrotic primary lesion that is generally found on the surface areas of the body ordinarily covered by clothing. The basic pathologic changes are found in the small blood vessels (see Ch. 164).

Symptoms, Laboratory Findings, and Diagnosis. The three tick-borne rickettsioses that occur in different parts of the Eastern Hemisphere resemble one another closely. After an incubation period of about five to seven days, the disease begins with fever, headache, malaise, and conjunctival injection. The primary lesion, which is present in most cases at the onset of fever, consists of a small ulcer 2 to 5 mm in diameter with a black center and a red areola; the regional lymph nodes are enlarged. The generalized erythematous maculopapular rash appears about the fourth day and quickly involves most of the body, including the palms and soles and often the face. In severe cases the rash becomes hemorrhagic. Fever abates during the second week. The prognosis is good except in the aged and debilitated. Complications and sequelae are unusual.

The laboratory findings of greatest importance are those derived from the Weil-Felix and rickettsial complement-fixation tests. Agglutinins against Proteus OX-19 develop during the second week and complement-fixing antibodies appear shortly thereafter.

Diagnosis is established by the clinical picture, including the *tache noire,* the geographic location, and positive serologic reactions. In the differential diagnosis the typhus fevers, meningococcal infections, and measles must be considered.

Treatment. Adequate information is available to indicate that treatment with the broad-spectrum antimicrobial drugs is as effective in patients with African tick typhus as in those with other rickettsioses (see Ch. 164 for details of therapy). Presumably, these measures are also applicable to the other two tick-borne rickettsioses of the Eastern Hemisphere.

Prophylaxis. Prevention of human disease is based on avoiding the bites of infected ticks. In Ch. 164 are set forth details regarding personal prophylaxis, including the use of chemical insect repellents, and for reduction of tick population by measures involved in terrain control. Experimental vaccines prepared from formalin-treated yolk sac tissue infected with each of the Eastern Hemisphere rickettsiae under discussion are effective in animals, but commercial vaccines for human use are not available.

Bozeman, F. M., Humphries, J. W., Campbell, J. M., and O'Hara, P. L.: Laboratory studies of the spotted fever group of rickettsiae. *In* Wisseman, C. L., Jr. (ed.): Symposium on the Spotted Fever Group of Rickettsiae. Medical Science Publication No. 7, Walter Reed Army Institute of Research. Washington, D.C., U.S. Government Printing Office, 1960, p. 7.
Freyche, M. J., and Deutschman, Z.: Human rickettsioses in Africa. Epidemiol. Vital Stat. Rep., WHO 3:161, 1950.
Woodward, T. E., and Jackson, E. B.: Spotted fever rickettsiae. *In* Horsfall, F. L., Jr., and Tamm, I. (eds.): Viral and Rickettsial Infections of Man. 4th ed. Philadelphia, J. B. Lippincott Company, 1965, p. 1095.
Zdrodovskii, P. I., and Golinevich, H. M.: The Rickettsial Diseases. New York, Pergamon Press, 1960, p. 292.

166.　RICKETTSIALPOX

Herbert L. Ley, Jr.

Definition. Rickettsialpox is a mite-borne rickettsial disease, mild and self-limited, which is characterized by an initial eschar-like lesion and a fever of a week's duration accompanied by headache, backache, and a generalized papulovesicular rash.

Etiology. The disease is caused by *Rickettsia akari,* a member of the spotted fever group of rickettsia. Although *R. akari* possesses an antigen in common with *Rickettsia rickettsi,* it is most closely related to *Rickettsia australis,* the agent of North Queensland tick typhus. The organism is transmitted to man, with an incubation period of 10 to 24 days, by the bite of the mouse mite, *Allodermanyssus sanguineus.*

Incidence and Distribution. The incidence of the disease is difficult to determine. In the first three years after the disease was described in 1946, 500 cases were reported in the United States, most of them from New York City. Reporting of the disease has decreased markedly since that time. It is likely that small numbers of cases continue to occur without being reported because the disease is one in which national reporting is not required. The disease has been reported from Boston, West Haven, Connecticut, New York, Philadelphia, Pittsburgh, and Cleveland in the United States, and from the U.S.S.R.

Epidemiology. When the disease was first described in 1946–1947, in a New York apartment housing project, the investigators demonstrated the presence of the agent in both the commensal mouse, *Mus musculus,* and its mite ectoparasite, *A. sanguineus,* both of which were present in large numbers. The single piece of information that was missing from the initial study was the manner in which the disease agent, *R. akari,* entered the mouse and mite populations. The subsequent isolation from a field mouse in Korea of a rickettsial agent indistinguishable from *R. akari* suggests that the agent may be widely distributed among feral rodents and their ectoparasites. If this view is correct, the disease may be expected to occur in areas of expanding suburbia where man and commensal populations of domestic mice come into contact with feral mice and their ectoparasites.

Pathology. Because rickettsialpox is a benign infection with no reported deaths, pathologic examination has been limited to biopsy material. The initial lesion or eschar resembles the eschars of scrub typhus and boutonneuse fever. The skin lesion of the early rash is characterized by perivascular infiltration with mononuclear cells. During the later stages of the rash when vesiculation occurs, the histologic changes are highly characteristic and consist of necrosis of the superficial epithelial cells, leading to an intra-epidermal vesicle. Clinical laboratory findings are limited to a minimal leukopenia during the febrile period.

Clinical Manifestations. The first sign of infection is the initial lesion or eschar, which appears approximately a week before onset of fever. Most patients are unaware of the small papule that develops at the site of the infecting mite bite, or if they note it, they interpret it as a "pimple." The lesion begins as a small papule that enlarges slowly to 0.5 to 1.5 cm in diameter, develops a central vesicle, and finally forms a dark crust without pustulation. Except for the lack of itching, tenderness, or pustulation, the lesion resembles that of a primary vaccinia reaction, and usually leaves a small scar. When searched for carefully, the initial lesion will be found in over 90 per cent of cases.

About a week after the appearance of the initial lesion, fever of an intermittent type develops, with chills or chilly sensations and drenching sweats. After approximately a week the fever gradually subsides. The early febrile period is characterized by headache, photophobia, marked lassitude, and muscle pains, including backache. Beginning on the first to fourth days of fever a maculopapular rash appears, which develops into a vesiculopapular rash. The vesicles are firm, sometimes surrounded by erythema, and on drying form a dark crust that falls off without leaving a scar. In contrast to chickenpox, the rash appears on many areas of the body at almost the same time and does not itch; it is absent from the palms and soles.

Physical examination during the febrile period yields little additional information. An enlarged spleen or lymphadenopathy will be found in only a few cases. The differential diagnosis very early in the disease should include measles, chickenpox, and smallpox; with the appearance of the vesicles only the latter two diseases need be considered. The presence of an initial lesion, the more superficial position of the vesicle, and the persistence of the papular base throughout the period of rash argue strongly for rickettsialpox rather than chickenpox. Smallpox lesions resemble those of rickettsialpox, but progress to pustules. In addition, the constitutional symptoms of most patients with smallpox are considerably more severe than those of patients with rickettsialpox.

Diagnosis. The clinical characteristics of the disease are so distinctive that in most patients a presumptive diagnosis may be made on clinical grounds. Chickenpox in adults poses the most difficult diagnostic problem. Laboratory confirmation of the diagnosis is possible by isolation of the agent from blood obtained during the acute phase of illness and also by complement-fixation tests on paired specimens of serum. Because the agent of rickettsialpox is closely related to that of Rocky Mountain spotted fever, complement-fixation tests may be performed with antigen prepared from either organism. A fourfold or greater rise in antibody titer may be expected in patients with rickettsialpox when the acute phase specimen is collected early in the febrile period and the convalescent specimen is collected three to four weeks after onset of disease. The Weil-Felix agglutination reaction is of no diagnostic value in rickettsialpox.

Treatment and Prognosis. The disease may be so mild in some patients that no specific treatment may be indicated. When therapy is desirable, the tetracyclines may be used in oral doses of 25 mg per kilogram per day for three or four days. Response to treatment is rapid; most patients become afebrile in 24 to 36 hours. Relapses of infection have not been reported. The course of the disease is benign and the prognosis is excellent.

Control. The principal target of preventive measures is the mite vector of the disease, *A. sanguineus,* which may be controlled by the use of residual insecticides (DDT or dieldrin) in areas of mouse harborage. Vector control should be achieved prior to initiating mouse control measures to avoid further dispersal of the mites in their search for food. No vaccine is currently available.

Dolgopol, V. B.: Histologic changes in rickettsialpox. Am. J. Path., 24:119, 1948.

Greenberg, M., Pelliteri, O., Klein, I. F., and Huebner, R. J.: Rickettsialpox—a newly recognized rickettsial disease. II. Clinical observations. J.A.M.A., 133:901, 1947.

Lackman, D. B.: A review of information on rickettsialpox in the United States. Clin Pediatr. (Phila.), 2:296, 1963.

Roueché, B.: The alerting of Mr. Pomerantz. *In* Roueché, B.: Eleven Blue Men. Boston, Little, Brown and Company, 1954, p. 48.

167. SCRUB TYPHUS
(Tsutsugamushi Disease, Mite-Borne Typhus, Japanese River Fever, Tropical Typhus, Rural Typhus)

Herbert L. Ley, Jr.

Definition. Scrub typhus is a mite-borne rickettsial disease that occurs in Southeast Asia and adjacent areas and is characterized by fever, headache, lymphadenopathy, conjunctival injection, a maculopapular rash, and, in most patients, a distinctive eschar or skin lesion.

Etiology. The disease is caused by *Rickettsia tsutsugamushi (R. orientalis),* a group of rickettsial agents that produces a single distinctive clinical syndrome in man, but is characterized by extreme variation in antigenic composition of organisms isolated in different geographic areas and even in adjacent foci of the disease within the same country. All strains of *R. tsutsugamushi* can be propagated in mice and embryonated eggs; some strains will also produce disease in the guinea pig. Because of antigenic variation in the organisms, complement-fixing antibodies produced in response to infection in man appear to be specific only for the infecting or closely related strains. Nevertheless, all strains of *R. tsutsugamushi* have the potential of stimulating Weil-Felix Proteus OX-K agglutinins in man.

Distribution and Incidence. The disease occurs in a roughly triangular area of Southeast Asia and adjacent countries approximately 5,000,000 square miles in extent. The western apex of the triangle is located in Pakistan, the northern in north Japan, and the southern in the north coastal areas of Australia. It is impossible to obtain reliable data on the incidence of the disease among the indigenous populations of the area. However, World War II provided numerous examples of explosive outbreaks of the disease in military units in the Asiatic-Pacific area. In one such outbreak among British troops in Ceylon, 756 patients were hospitalized with scrub typhus as a result of a four-day jungle training exercise. American forces operating on the islands of Owi and Biak experienced over 1000 cases of the disease in less than two months. During the period from 1942 to 1945, nearly 16,000 cases of the disease occurred in American, British, and Australian troops alone. At present the disease is reported sporadically among the people of Southeast Asia and becomes a major medical problem only when development projects or recreational activities bring groups of people into contact with foci of the disease in nature.

Epidemiology. Like Rocky Mountain spotted fever, scrub typhus is principally a disease of rodents and their ectoparasites that is propagated in a "silent" cycle in nature, involving man only when he unwittingly comes into contact with the mites that transmit the disease. A variety of rodents, chiefly rats and feral mice, have been shown to be infected in nature. The disease in these animals is relatively mild but is associated with a rickettsemia that provides an opportunity to infect mites feeding on the animals during their illness. In some areas ground birds have also been implicated in the disease cycle in nature. The vector mite in most areas is a species of the genus Leptotrombiculidium highly adapted to the local ecology, although mites of the genus Schongastia have been shown to transmit the agent in the less important jungle cycle of the disease. The mite vectors are free-living, feeding upon vegetation and insect eggs, except in their larval stage, during which they must obtain a meal of tissue fluid from a vertebrate host in order to complete their maturation to the adult stage. The mites are not only capable of transmitting *R. tsutsugamushi* to their vertebrate host during this feeding but are also capable of transmitting the agent to their offspring transovarially. Thus the mite is both a vector and a reservoir for scrub typhus, just as is the tick for Rocky Mountain spotted fever. The highly specific ecologic requirements for propagation of the mite in terms of temperature, humidity, and food sources, coupled with its limited range of locomotion, lead to the formation of "mite islands," highly localized in terms of both geographic and seasonal distributions. In some exceptional areas, such as Malaysia, the mite population is present throughout the year. More commonly, the mites are highly seasonal in appearance, and are most numerous during the warm, moist months of the year, although one focus of infection in southern Japan is characterized by a winter peak of mite population. The seasonal distribu-

tion of scrub typhus understandably parallels the distribution of the mite vector. Man exposes himself to infection by transferring mites from vegetation to his body; most infections have followed contact with grassy "scrub" areas or straw cut from them. The disease may occur elsewhere because infected mites have been found in other habitats.

Pathology. As with the other rickettsioses, the basic lesion is one of inflammation of the walls of the small blood vessels with perivascular infiltration of mononuclear cells. Pneumonitis and a diffuse myocarditis with mononuclear infiltration of the myocardium are frequently observed at autopsy. Gross pathologic findings are usually limited to enlargement of the spleen, lymphadenopathy, and the cutaneous eschar of the disease.

Clinical Manifestations. The initial symptoms of the disease, frontal headache and temperature of 40 to 40.5° C, follow the infecting mite bite by 6 to 21 days. Physical examination at onset reveals only generalized lymphadenopathy, conjunctival injection, and, in most Caucasian patients, the developing eschar. This skin lesion, absent in most Asian patients, appears first as a small papule at the site of the mite bite and enlarges during the first few days of fever to approximately 1 cm in size. On this papular base a multilocular vesicle develops that evolves into the flat, black eschar characteristic of the disease. Regional lymph nodes draining the area of the eschar may become painful, and may enlarge to the size of an acorn. About the end of the first week of fever a generalized macular rash appears, which may last only a few hours or may develop to a livid maculopapular eruption of a week's duration. In untreated patients complications such as pneumonitis, encephalitis, and cardiac failure occur late in the second week of fever; if the patient survives, defervescence begins about the fifteenth day of fever.

Diagnosis. Early diagnosis of the disease must be based on the clinical findings and the history of exposure in an endemic area. Laboratory confirmation of the diagnosis is based on isolation from blood of the agent in mice or on a rise in Weil-Felix OX-K agglutinins in serum during the course of illness. If the acute specimen is obtained before the tenth day of fever and the late specimen is obtained during the third week of illness, fourfold or greater rises in Weil-Felix OX-K titers will be observed in almost all untreated patients and in three fourths of those receiving antimicrobial therapy. Because of strain variation in the etiologic agent, the complement-fixation test is unsatisfactory in the laboratory diagnosis of the disease. Clinical laboratory data are of little assistance in diagnosis; patients usually show only a moderate leukopenia. The differential diagnosis of the disease should include leptospirosis, typhoid fever, dengue, murine typhus, and malaria.

Treatment. The tetracyclines are the therapeutic agents of choice for scrub typhus at oral dosage levels of 25 mg per kilogram per day. Chloramphenicol has also been used at oral dosage levels of 50 mg per kilogram per day. Both drugs carry with them some risk of toxicity, but the nature of the major risk with chloramphenicol (aplastic anemia) is such that its use is distinctly less preferable. Drug therapy may be discontinued 24 hours after defervescence, which usually occurs within 36 hours after beginning therapy. Relapses have been observed in patients treated during the first week of fever; continuation of therapy through the fourteenth day of disease, or the administration of single 3.0 gram oral doses of drug on the seventh and fourteenth days after cessation of the initial course of antimicrobial therapy will prevent recrudescences of infection. The relapses occur because the antimicrobial drugs are not eradicative.

Prognosis and Mortality. Before effective treatment was available, mortality from scrub typhus was appreciable, varying from 5 to 40 per cent. Early antimicrobial therapy has essentially limited deaths from the disease. If the patient is treated in the first week of illness he is usually ready to resume full activity in several weeks.

Prevention. Preventive measures are directed at minimizing contact of man with the mites transmitting the disease. The application of residual miticides such as dieldrin or lindane to large areas of terrain will permit safe continuation of operations in rubber plantations and similar industrial activities that bring workers into contact with areas previously known to be the source of numerous infections. When area miticide application is impracticable, as in military operations, the use of clothing impregnated with mite repellents provides significant protection against infection.

Audy, J. R.: The ecology of scrub typhus. *In* May, J. M. (ed.): Studies in Disease Ecology. New York, Hafner Publishing Company, Inc., 1961, p. 389.

Sheehy, T. W., Hazlett, D., and Turk, R. E.: Scrub typhus: A comparison of chloramphenicol and tetracycline in its treatment. Arch. Intern. Med., 132:77, 1973.

Smadel, J. E.: Influence of antibiotics on immunologic responses in scrub typhus. Am. J. Med., 17:246, 1954.

Smadel, J. E., and Elisberg, B. L.: Scrub typhus rickettsia. *In* Horsfall, F. L., Jr., and Tamm, I. (eds.): Viral and Rickettsial Infections of Man. 4th ed. Philadelphia, J. B. Lippincott Company, 1965, p. 1130.

Tamiya, T. (ed.): Recent Advances in Studies of Tsutsugamushi Disease in Japan. Tokyo, Medical Culture Inc., 1962.

Traub, R., and Wisseman, C. L., Jr.: Ecological considerations in scrub typhus. Bull. WHO, 39:209, 1968.

168. TRENCH FEVER
(Five-Day or Quintana Fever, Shin Bone Fever, Volhynian Fever)

Herbert L. Ley, Jr.

Definition. Trench fever is a self-limited louse-borne rickettsial disease characterized by intermittent fever, generalized aches and pains, negligible mortality, and multiple relapses.

Etiology and Epidemiology. The disease is caused by *Rickettsia quintana,* a rickettsial agent that grows extracellularly in the louse intestine and is excreted in louse feces. Transmission takes place by rubbing louse feces into skin abrasions or into the bite wound left by the louse. The incubation period of the disease may vary from 5 to 38 days, but is usually two to four weeks. The disease was a major military problem during World War I, when an estimated 1,000,000 cases occurred in western Europe. It was not seen in epidemic form again until World War II when 80,000 cases were reported in eastern Europe. Recent studies have demonstrated the disease in endemic form in Mexico. During epidemics man is clearly the principal reservoir. He may also be the major long-term reservoir because the disease agent has been isolated from asymptomatic patients years after their initial infection.

Pathology and Clinical Manifestations. Because the disease has a negligible mortality, information on the histopathologic changes is limited. Biopsy studies reveal only perivascular inflammation, principally in the form of lymphocytic infiltrations. The presenting symptoms of the disease are recurrent fever, severe weakness, headache, dizziness, back and leg pains (particularly in the shins), and photophobia. Physical and laboratory examinations are not remarkable except for slight enlargement of the spleen and liver, areas of cutaneous tenderness distributed over the body, and a moderate leukocytosis. A transient rash of erythematous macules or papules occurs in about 70 per cent of patients. The patient's fever may rise as high as 40.5° C in an irregular fashion with intervals of nearly normal temperature between peaks of fever. The fever may last for only four or five days in the more fortunate patients. In others, the initial pyrexia may be followed after five or six days of normal temperature by one to eight relapses of fever similar to the initial episode. In still other patients, the initial fever may decline, shading into relapses without a true afebrile period, producing a "saddleback" or "typhoidal" fever curve.

Diagnosis. The most important fact supporting the diagnosis of trench fever is a history of contact with lice within the incubation period of the disease. Xenodiagnosis—the feeding of clean uninfected lice on a patient suspected of having the disease—is a useful diagnostic aid. The lice are examined a week after feeding on the patient for the presence of rickettsiae in the lumen of the gut. The technique of cultivation of *R. quintana* on blood agar containing 10 per cent of fresh blood has also been used diagnostically. Recently developed serologic tests appear promising in the diagnosis of the disease. The differential diagnosis of the disease should include leptospirosis, dengue, malaria, relapsing fever, and the typhus fevers.

Treatment and Prognosis. Although the tetracyclines and other antimicrobials may be expected to be as effective in the treatment of trench fever as in the treatment of the other rickettsial diseases, in the absence of epidemics of trench fever no reliable information about their efficacy is available. Because the disease has a negligible mortality, the long-term prognosis is excellent. Even without treatment the majority of patients are able to return to full activity within one to two months after onset, although a few continue to experience recurrences of the symptoms of infection for months or years.

Prevention. The only practicable method of control of trench fever is the elimination of the louse vector of the disease by dusting clothing with residual insecticides. Ten per cent DDT powders proved highly effective for louse control during the World War II period, but the development of DDT resistance in lice in many parts of the world has forced the use of 1 per cent lindane or 1 per cent malathion powders. For additional comments on louse control, see Ch. 163.

Trench Fever: Report of Commission on Trench Fever. American Red Cross Medical Research Committee. London, Oxford University Press, 1918.

Varela, G., Vinson, J. W., and Molina-Pasquel, C.: Trench fever. II. Propagation of *Rickettsia quintana* on cell-free medium from the blood of two patients. Am. J. Trop. Med., 18:708, 1969.

Vinson, J. W., Varela, G., and Molina-Pasquel, C.: Trench fever. III. Induction of clinical disease in volunteers inoculated with *Rickettsia quintana* propagated on blood agar. Am. J. Trop. Med., 18:713, 1969.

Warren, J.: Trench fever rickettsia. *In* Horsfall, F. L., Jr., and Tamm, I. (eds.): Viral and Rickettsial Infections of Man. 4th ed. Philadelphia, J. B. Lippincott Company, 1965, p. 1161.

169. Q FEVER

Herbert L. Ley, Jr.

Definition.   Q fever is a self-limited rickettsial infection characterized by fever, headache, and constitutional symptoms, associated, in approximately half the patients, with a pneumonitis. It is unique among the rickettsial diseases of man in that human infection is most commonly acquired by inhalation of the agent rather than by contact with an arthropod vector.

Etiology.   The disease is caused by *Coxiella burnetii,* a rickettsial agent having the general biologic characteristics of this class of microorganisms but possessing, in addition, a resistance to desiccation and to exposure in dusts and soils that is unique among the rickettsiae. The organism may be propagated in embryonated eggs and in mice, hamsters, and guinea pigs, and has frequently infected laboratory personnel engaged in isolation studies on clinical material. Both patients and animals develop agglutinating and complement-fixing antibodies for the agent. On the other hand, *C. burnetii,* unlike most of the other rickettsiae, does not stimulate the production of Weil-Felix Proteus agglutinins in man.

Incidence and Distribution.   The true incidence of the disease in the human population is impossible to determine because the majority of infections are undiagnosed. Isolated serologic surveys have revealed that many persons exposed to infection in sheep and cattle ranches, abattoirs, meat packing plants, or wool processing plants present serologic evidence of past infection. More detailed investigation of animals and arthropods on a worldwide basis has shown *C. burnetii* to be ubiquitous in distribution except for the countries of Denmark, Finland, Ireland, the Netherlands, Norway, and Sweden. In the United States the disease, first recognized in the states of Montana and California, is now recognized as prevalent in most of the states in which sheep and cattle are produced. Small numbers of cases have been reported for most of the remaining states.

Epidemiology.   The epidemiology of the disease is complex because it involves two major patterns of transmission. The first pattern, described in Australia, is a disease cycle in wild animals with transmission of the agent from animal to animal by a tick vector. Although the species of animal and arthropod vary from country to country, such a cycle has been demonstrated in Australia in two forms, bandicoot-tick-cattle and kangaroo-tick-sheep. In both these cycles the agent can be transmitted indefinitely as an inapparent infection in the wild reservoir (bandicoot or kangaroo) by ticks, but it may also be transmitted laterally by arthropod to a domestic animal in close contact with man. In these and similar cycles recognized in other parts of the world, *C. burnetii,* like the other rickettsial agents of human disease, is vector-transmitted.

However, Q fever patients rarely give a history of tick bite. Human infection with the agent has now been shown to occur almost exclusively by a second transmission pattern capable of sustaining itself independently of the wild animal cycle. The reservoirs of infection in the second pattern are animals domesticated by man, principally cattle, sheep, and goats, in which *C. burnetii* produces only an inapparent or mild infection. In sheep, Q fever organisms are excreted in very large numbers in placental tissue, and to a lesser degree in birth fluids, milk, and feces. In the cow, and probably the goat, excretion occurs mainly through the placenta and milk. *With all infected animals, the period of parturition is associated with the formation of a primary infectious aerosol, easily demonstrated by air-sampling studies.* Such aerosols infect other cattle in the herd and also the human population in direct contact with the animals. Further, because contaminated clothing, wool, hides, bedding, and soil may be the source of secondary aerosols, *the infections may be transmitted via these vehicles at considerable distances from the infected cattle;* in certain circumstances these distances are measurable in miles. The unique resistance of *C. burnetii* to prolonged exposure in nature contributes to the spread of the agent by such infectious microenvironments. Within California, where the local epidemiology of the disease has been studied in great detail, sheep are the major reservoir for human infection in the northern part of the state and cattle in the southern part. In the latter area milk may be a vehicle of infection if consumed raw. Although the pulmonary route is the most important portal of access of the agent to man, the transmission of the rickettsia from man to man by this method is rare, despite the occurrence of an infectious pneumonitis in some patients.

Pathology.   Because the mortality rate is low, postmortem studies have been limited. In those patients having a pneumonitis, the histopathology is similar to that seen in the viral pneumonias and psittacosis. Recent studies in patients have directed attention to hepatic pathology during the acute phase of the disease, demonstrable both in biochemical abnormalities of liver function (elevated cephalin-cholesterol flocculation, alkaline phosphatase, and thymol turbidity tests) and in histologic abnormalities in biopsy specimens (focal inflammation and granulomas). Q fever endocarditis, producing valvular vegetations from which rickettsiae may be isolated, has also been described.

Clinical Manifestations.   After an incubation period of 9 to 20 days after respiratory exposure, most patients complain of an abrupt onset of fever, headache, muscle pains, and severe malaise. The temperature may rise as high as 40° C and remain elevated, with considerable fluctuation, for one to three weeks. Occasionally, patients may suffer a prolonged fever of several months' duration. In contrast to the other rickettsial infections, there is no rash. In approximately half the patients there is roentgenographic evidence of pneumonitis, manifested clinically as a slight, nonproductive cough developing in the second week of fever.

Diagnosis.   Q fever should always be suspected in a patient having a febrile illness for which no obvious cause can be found. If the patient's occupation brings him into contact with sheep, cattle, or goats, or byproducts such as wool or hides, particular care should be exercised to exclude Q fever from consideration. The presence of Q fever should be suspected in any patient in whom the differential diagnosis includes viral pneumonia, psittacosis, primary atypical pneumonia, pulmonary mycotic disease, or comparable infections. Furthermore, recent data would also support consideration of Q fever in the differential diagnoses of endocarditis and of hepatitis with or without jaundice.

Diagnostic laboratory studies usually must be limited to serologic studies because of the extensive history of accidentally acquired laboratory infections resulting from attempts at isolation. Either complement-fixation or agglutination tests may be employed, and with either test a fourfold or greater rise in titer of antibody may be expected to occur between the first and fourth weeks of illness. Recent reports have emphasized the importance of both strain and phase variation in the selection of antigens for diagnostic use.

Treatment and Prognosis. The tetracyclines or chloramphenicol are both effective in treatment of acute infections with *C. burnetii,* but because of the nature of chloramphenicol toxicity, the tetracyclines are definitely to be preferred. The dosage of antimicrobial given should be the same as that for epidemic typhus or Rocky Mountain spotted fever. The mortality is low (1 per cent or less), even in untreated patients, and is lower still in those treated with antimicrobial drugs. Therapy should be continued for approximately one week even though the patient usually becomes afebrile within 48 hours. Patients occasionally may experience relapses after treatment, and when this complication occurs additional drug therapy should be administered. Prognosis is less favorable for the rare patient in whom Q fever endocarditis develops. In some of these patients the disease has been reported to have been unresponsive to antimicrobial therapy, although favorable results have been reported in one patient treated with trimethoprim and sulfamethoxazole.

Prevention. Experimental lots of yolk-sac vaccines have been effective in prevention of clinical disease in volunteers experimentally infected via the respiratory route. Because this vaccine is not commercially available, control measures are limited to minimizing exposure to the agent. In particular, milk from cattle, sheep, and goats in endemic areas should be pasteurized or boiled before use. Because rickettsiae are excreted in the sputum and urine of patients, these materials should be disinfected by autoclaving to prevent secondary infection in hospitals.

Freeman, R., and Hodson, M. E.: Q fever endocarditis treated with trimethoprim and sulphamethoxazole. Br. Med. J., 1:419, 1972.

Grist, N. R.: Q fever endocarditis. Am. Heart J., 75:846, 1968.

Johnson, J. E., and Kadull, P. J.: Laboratory-acquired Q fever: A report of fifty cases. Am. J. Med., 41:391, 1966.

Ormsbee, R. A.: Q fever rickettsia. *In* Horsfall, F. L., Jr., and Tamm, I. (eds.): Viral and Rickettsial Infections of Man. 4th ed. Philadelphia, J. B. Lippincott Company, 1965, p. 1144.

Powell, O. W.: Liver involvement in "Q" fever. Aust. Ann. Med., 10:52, 1961.

Tigertt, W. D., and Benenson, A. S.: Studies on Q fever in man. Trans. Assoc. Am. Physicians, 69:98, 1956.

170. BARTONELLOSIS
(Carrión's Disease, Oroya Fever, Verruga Peruana)

Herbert L. Ley, Jr.

Definition. Bartonellosis is an insect-borne microbial disease limited to South America. It is characterized by two distinctive clinical stages. The first of these (Oroya fever) presents a severe febrile infection associated with a marked anemia, bone and joint pains, bacteremia, and an appreciable mortality. The second stage (verruga peruana) is more benign and is distinguished by the appearance of a generalized eruption of hemangiomatous papules and nodules.

Etiology. The disease is caused by *Bartonella bacilliformis,* a small gram-negative pleomorphic bacillus that may be cultivated readily in enriched bacteriologic media. The disease is transmitted to man by the bite of sandflies of the genus Phlebotomus, with development of the characteristic symptoms of Oroya fever after an incubation period of two weeks to three months.

Prevalence and Distribution. Although a number of epidemics of the disease have been reported, it is more commonly seen as sporadic cases among populations of Peru, Colombia, and Ecuador, and is restricted within these countries to those who live at altitudes of 1500 to 9000 feet on both slopes of the Andes. In general, the distribution of the disease coincides with the ecologic zones supporting populations of Phlebotomus.

Epidemiology. In Peru the disease is transmitted by *Phlebotomus verrugarum,* a night-biting sandfly. The biting habits of the vectors in the other countries are similar, although the species of Phlebotomus involved in transmission in the other areas are not conclusively identified. The principal reservoir of the disease appears to be man; no additional animal reservoirs have as yet been implicated in nature. Reports of cultivation of the agent from apparently healthy persons suggest that as much as 10 per cent of infections may be subclinical. Persons convalescent from the disease are known to have a low-level bacteremia for months or years, providing frequent opportunities for infection of the disease vector.

Pathology and Physiologic Responses. In the Oroya fever stage of illness the causative organism may be found in peripheral blood smears stained with Giemsa or Wright's stain as well as in the reticuloendothelial cells of the viscera and lymphatics. In the blood the parasite is found both free in the plasma and adhering to the erythrocytes. The parasitization of the erythrocytes causes an increased mechanical fragility and also an increased sequestration of the cells in the spleen and the liver. A hypochromic and macrocytic anemia develops rapidly during the febrile period, erythrocyte counts decreasing within a period of only a few days to levels of one million to two million cells per cubic millimeter. The bone marrow is hyperplastic, with an abundance of nucleated erythrocytes. The pathologic findings secondary to the anemia are absent in the verruga stage of infection. The histopathology of the skin lesions is that of dilation of the capillaries and proliferation of the vascular endothelial cells that may be shown to contain the causative agent.

Clinical Manifestations. The presenting symptoms of patients with Oroya fever are intermittent high fever, painful muscles and joints, tender enlarged lymph nodes, and the systemic symptoms and prostration of a severe anemia. These symptoms may persist from several weeks to several months in untreated patients, half of whom may die within the first three weeks of fever. If the patient survives, gradual convalescence is punctuated, after a few days to a month, by the appearance of the cutaneous lesions of the second phase of the disease. The verrugae may persist for a month to a year in untreated persons, but mortality is negligible. Occasional patients may experience only the fever and anemia without the skin manifestations or only the cutaneous lesions without the initial fever. Although these two aspects of the infection were once thought to be different diseases, there is no doubt that both syndromes are manifestations of infection with the same organism. The current interpretation that the skin lesions are an expression of developing immunity in the patient is supported by the observation that second attacks of the disease are exceedingly rare even in highly endemic areas and that the attacks are almost always caused by verruga rather than by Oroya fever.

Diagnosis.   In endemic areas the diagnosis can usually be made on the basis of clinical findings. In the acute stage of Oroya fever both blood smears and blood culture usually reveal the presence of the agent. As the patient progresses toward the verruga stage of infection, or with treatment, the organism becomes more difficult to demonstrate.

Treatment and Prognosis.   The prognosis in the untreated patient depends upon both the nature and the severity of his infection. Mortality in the Oroya fever phase of the disease may exceed 50 per cent, particularly when the infection is complicated by concurrent attacks of malaria, amebiasis, tuberculosis, salmonellosis, or other diseases. The disease responds well to treatment with penicillin, streptomycin, chloramphenicol, and the tetracyclines. Chloramphenicol is favored by many South American clinicians because of the frequency of concurrent salmonella infections, but the risks of its potentially more serious toxicity must be weighed against the fact that the other drugs mentioned are therapeu-

tically effective. In general, as in the rickettsial infections, the tetracyclines are the preferred form of antimicrobial therapy for bartonellosis. When the broad-spectrum antimicrobials have been used, oral doses of 1 to 2 grams per day have been used for a period of a week or more with excellent results. Patients become afebrile in 24 to 48 hours, and, if they receive transfusions, recover strength rapidly. Although the mortality of the verruga stage of infection is less than 5 per cent, antimicrobial therapy is desirable to hasten the disappearance of the skin lesions.

Prevention.   Control measures are directed principally against the Phlebotomus vector. Because the insect is a night feeder and moves by a series of short "hops" between surfaces, the application of a residual insecticide to the exterior and interior of doorways, windows, and other avenues of entry to human habitation is effective. Where insecticide application is impracticable, bed nets or insect repellents provide significant protection. Control of breeding of the vector is difficult, but may be undertaken when it is otherwise impossible to prevent contact of the vector with man. No protective vaccine is available. Patients need not be isolated in hospital wards if the vector is absent because the disease cannot be transmitted by person-to-person contact.

Reynafarje, C., and Ramos, J.: The hemolytic anemia of human bartonellosis. Blood, 17:562, 1961.

Urteaga, B. O., and Payne, E. H.: Treatment of the acute febrile phase of Carrión's disease with chloramphenicol. Am. J. Trop. Med., 4:507, 1955.

Weinman, D.: The Bartonella Group. *In*: Dubos, R. J., and Hirsch, J. G. (eds.): Bacterial and Mycotic Infections of Man. 4th ed. Philadelphia, J. B. Lippincott Company, 1965, p. 775.

DISEASES CAUSED BY CHLAMYDIAE

171. TRACHOMA AND INCLUSION CONJUNCTIVITIS

Ernest Jawetz

Definition.   Trachoma and inclusion conjunctivitis are chronic infectious diseases of the eye and genital tract, caused by closely related microorganisms and exhibiting overlapping spectra of clinical manifestations and epidemiologic patterns. These range from mild and self-limited to severe and blinding eye disease, with or without involvement of the genital tract.

Etiology.   The agents of *trachoma and inclusion conjunctivitis* (TRIC agents) are members of the psittacosis-lymphogranuloma venereum–trachoma group. Formerly these agents were considered viruses; now they are called *chlamydiae*. They are nonmotile, gram-negative, obligate intracellular parasites which multiply in the cytoplasm of their host cells by a distinctive developmental cycle. Chlamydiae differ from viruses in many important respects: they possess both RNA and DNA; they multiply by binary fission; they possess bacterial types of cell walls and ribosomes; they produce a variety of metabolically active enzymes; and their growth can be inhibited by several antibacterial drugs. It is probable that chlamydiae are closely related to gram-negative bacteria,

but lack some significant mechanism for the production of metabolic energy so that they are restricted to an intracellular existence.

TRIC agents can infect epithelial cells of conjunctiva, cornea, urethra, and cervix of man and monkey, but do not replicate in most other tissues of the body. The infective particle ("elementary body") is a sphere with a diameter of 250 nanometers (millimicrons) and stains purple with Giemsa's or red with Macchiavello's stain. The infective particle is taken into the host cell by phagocytosis and, after replication, results in the development of an inclusion body. This is an oval or crescent-shaped mass of "elementary bodies" embedded in a matrix of glycogen, lying in the cytoplasm of an epithelial cell often adjacent to the nucleus. Inclusion bodies can be stained brightly with specific immunofluorescence.

TRIC agents can be grown in the yolk sac of embryonated eggs and in X-irradiated cells in culture. The growth of TRIC agents is markedly inhibited by tetracyclines, sulfonamides, erythromycins, penicillins, and chloramphenicol, but not by aminoglycosides. Therefore aminoglycosides can be used to suppress bacterial contaminants in clinical specimens and to aid in isolation of TRIC agents in the laboratory.

TRIC agents share with other chlamydiae a heat-stable group antigen. These are lipopolysaccharides detectable by complement-fixation tests. In addition, species- or strain-specific antigens have been detected in the cell wall. Infected persons may develop antibodies to both types of antigens in serum and tears. By immunofluorescence tests specific antigens and antibodies can be identified. Thus genital TRIC isolates often fall within certain antigenic groups (D, E, F, etc.), whereas ocular TRIC isolates from endemic trachoma areas often fall within other groups (A, B, C). At least nine specific antigenic groups have been identified to date. There exist cross-reactions between the specific antigens of the chlamydiae of lymphogranuloma venereum and of certain TRIC agents. However, to date there is no specific laboratory characteristic that can always differentiate isolates of trachoma from isolates of inclusion conjunctivitis agents.

TRIC agents can persist in man for years, with or without symptoms and signs of infection. Subclinical infection can be activated by trauma, corticosteroid administration, and perhaps bacterial superinfection. The development of scarring and blindness in some endemic trachoma regions is attributable to a large extent to recurrent bacterial infections of the eye, especially with Hemophilus or Neisseria.

Prevalence and Epidemiology. Since antiquity, trachomatous infection was recognized in the Mediterranean basin and in the Orient. Today, trachomatous eye disease is very prevalent in Africa and Asia. It has been estimated that up to 400 million persons may be infected with TRIC agents, and up to 20 million may be economically blinded as a result. Trachoma flourishes in areas that are hot and dry, and that have a shortage of available water and poor hygienic customs. In such areas endemic levels are high, and initial infection commonly occurs in early childhood. In certain parts of the world, e.g., in North Africa, virtually the entire population is infected with TRIC agents before reaching adulthood. The high prevalence of bacterial superinfection in such populations undoubtedly contributes to the severity of eye disease and to its causing widespread blindness. In parts of the United States, e.g., Indian reservations of the Southwest, endemic TRIC infection is relatively common, but it rarely leads to major visual impairment, perhaps because bacterial superinfection is infrequent. Throughout the world sporadic cases of ocular TRIC infection occur, often with a clinical picture resembling trachoma. It is probable that some of these originate in genital infections rather than in contact with ocular trachoma.

Active cases of ocular TRIC infection shed the infective agent in desquamated conjunctival cells, conjunctival exudate, or tears. The infectious agent may be transmitted by fingers, fomites, and perhaps flies. Patients with early active infection probably shed more infective TRIC agent, and thus are more infectious for contacts than are those with chronic infection. However, even patients with longstanding scarred eye disease, and without signs of current activity, may shed TRIC agent and thus serve as a source of infection.

These comments concern ocular TRIC infection, particularly typical endemic trachoma. *Typical inclusion conjunctivitis* has a radically different epidemiologic pattern. Inclusion conjunctivitis is fundamentally an infection of the adult human genital tract, transmitted as a venereal disease. In the female the TRIC agent grows mainly in the transitional epithelium of the cervix. These cells may contain typical inclusions, and occasionally a mild cervicitis is present. In the male, genital infection may produce ("nonspecific") *urethritis,* as the TRIC agent replicates in urethral epithelium. In both sexes, adult genital tract infection and proctitis are often asymptomatic. Adults may transfer genital secretions to their own or other eyes by fingers, by fomites, and — occasionally — in swimming pools. The infection may pass from the cervix of the infected mother to the eye of her newborn during passage through the birth canal. The newborn infant may then develop eye disease between 5 and 14 days after birth.

The epidemiologic patterns described for typical trachoma and typical inclusion conjunctivitis may be mixed. Thus the genital tract of women in endemic trachoma regions may harbor TRIC agents, and these may produce either inclusion conjunctivitis or clinically typical trachoma in the offspring. Genital isolates from adults in nonendemic areas may, upon inoculation into the eye, give rise to disease resembling either inclusion conjunctivitis or trachoma.

Pathology and Pathogenesis. TRIC agents invade mainly the epithelium of the conjunctiva, cervix, and urethra. The earliest sign of infection is the appearance of inclusion bodies within epithelial cells and neutrophil infiltration of the epithelium of mucous membranes. Subepithelial infiltration with plasma cells and lymphocytes and the development of lymphoid follicles then follow. In the cornea, epithelial keratitis is often accompanied by the formation of subepithelial opacities. Blood vessels from the limbus, accompanied by fibroblasts, may invade the cornea to form a pannus. Progression of the inflammatory process leads to necrosis and scar formation in the conjunctiva. In classic trachoma, these changes occur more markedly in the upper half of the conjunctival sac and cornea; in inclusion conjunctivitis, more markedly in the lower conjunctiva. Inflammatory changes, lymphoid infiltration, necrosis, and scar formation have also been observed in TRIC agent infection of cervix and urethra.

Classic inclusion conjunctivitis of the newborn is an acute purulent conjunctivitis; in the adult it is a follicular conjunctivitis. However, all pathologic changes from limited follicular conjunctivitis to full-blown "trachoma" with scars and pannus may follow inoculation of genital isolates into the adult eye.

Classic, chronic, severe trachoma in hyperendemic areas progresses to marked lid deformation and loss of vision. As a result of cellular infiltration and scarring near the lid margins, the tarsal plate is bowed and the lid margins inverted (entropion), and some eyelashes turn inward (trichiasis), rubbing against the cornea with each lid movement, and aggravating corneal opacification. The scarring may destroy tear function, with resulting keratinization of corneal epithelium.

TRIC agents exhibit a pronounced tendency to persist in infected tissues for years even in the absence of signs of active disease, and this predisposes to relapses and to chronicity.

Clinical Manifestations. In experimental human infection with TRIC agents the incubation period is from two to seven days. *Inclusion conjunctivitis* of the newborn usually begins between the fifth and fourteenth days of life (whereas gonococcal ophthalmia usually begins two days after birth). The incubation period of naturally occurring trachoma is uncertain because the onset is often insidious, particularly in children. Early symptoms of TRIC infection are those of irritation, lacrimation, and mucopurulent discharge. The earliest physical signs are conjunctival hyperemia, mucopurulent discharge, papillary hypertrophy in infants, and follicular hypertrophy in adults.

Typical *trachoma* in children and adults begins as a follicular conjunctivitis, most noticeable in the conjunctiva of the upper lid and the tarsal plate. There are epithelial keratitis and subepithelial corneal infiltration, followed by gradual corneal vascularization from the upper limbus downward. This evolves into a dense fibrovascular pannus extending over part, or all, of the cornea, grossly impairing vision. Linear or stellate scars appear on the conjunctiva. Progressive scarring of the subepithelial tissues leads to deformation of the tarsal plate, resulting in entropion, trichiasis, and further corneal damage. These changes often follow secondary bacterial infection, which may also produce corneal ulceration and accelerate loss of vision. Typically there are no systemic symptoms or signs of infection, and the eye is the sole involved organ.

Typical *inclusion conjunctivitis* of the newborn presents as an acute purulent conjunctivitis with papillary hypertrophy but little involvement of the cornea. Over a period of weeks or months this tends to regress spontaneously and eventually heal without any scars or with only fine linear conjunctival and corneal scars and minimal, if any, pannus. In the adult, inclusion conjunctivitis is an acute mucopurulent conjunctivitis, often accompanied by preauricular adenopathy. Follicular hypertrophy is most noticeable in the conjunctiva of the lower lid, and tends to persist for weeks or months, occasionally accompanied by epithelial keratitis and subepithelial corneal infiltrates. Some adults with chronic inclusion conjunctivitis develop a limited pannus and a few scars of conjunctiva and cornea.

Adult genital TRIC infection usually precedes the eye involvement. Adult *cervicitis* and *urethritis* either are asymptomatic or produce only slight discharge and discomfort. This so-called nongonococcal urethritis forms as much as half of the acute urethritis in the male seen in venereal disease clinics (see Ch. 199).

All intermediate stages between minimal self-limited inclusion conjunctivitis and typical progressive trachoma can occur as a result of infection with TRIC agents of either ocular or genital origin. The typical, severe trachoma that leads to blindness and is seen in hyperendemic areas occurs probably as a result of long-standing infection with many relapses of TRIC agent activity, hypersensitivity reactions, and repeated bacterial superinfections. Conversely, the self-limited inclusion conjunctivitis of the newborn may be characteristic of a first infection, without hypersensitivity reaction, and without bacterial complications in an immunologically immature host. The basis for different clinical patterns of mild or severe disease seen in different areas of the world is not clearly understood.

Diagnosis. The traditional criteria for the diagnosis of trachoma are the triad of follicular hypertrophy, most prominent on the upper tarsal conjunctiva, pannus, and conjunctival scars. The last two signs may be detected only by biomicroscopic examination (slit lamp).

The diagnosis of inclusion conjunctivitis rests on finding typical inclusions in a purulent conjunctivitis of the newborn or in a follicular conjunctivitis of the adult. There should be only minimal vascular invasion of the cornea. Examination of the adult genital tract may reveal cervicitis and urethritis with moderate discharge and inclusions in epithelial cells. Proctitis may be present.

Among laboratory tests for TRIC infections, the demonstration of typical intracytoplasmic inclusions in conjunctival or genital cells is most widely used. Specific immunofluorescent stain is more sensitive than Giemsa stain. Polymorphonuclear leukocytes are often prominent in scrapings that contain TRIC inclusions. Isolation of TRIC agents in embryonated eggs or in irradiated cell cultures remains a specialized laboratory procedure. Serologic tests can support the diagnosis only if a rise in complement-fixing or immunofluorescence antibodies occurs during acute disease. The cytologic appearance of expressed follicular material may be helpful. Among follicular diseases of the conjunctiva, only TRIC infections (especially trachoma) produce the necrotic changes in follicles that are evidenced by the presence of many macrophages engorged with cell fragments.

Differential Diagnosis. In differential diagnosis of ocular TRIC infections, adenovirus infections, herpetic keratoconjunctivitis, folliculosis of children, chronic follicular conjunctivitis (Axenfeld type), reactions to allergens and irritating chemicals, and certain bacterial infections must be considered. Some of these entities may coexist with TRIC infections, and repeated competent ophthalmologic examinations and elaborate laboratory assistance may be required to establish a correct diagnosis. The demonstration of morphologically typical inclusions by immunofluorescent or Giemsa stain is most helpful in the diagnosis of TRIC infections, when combined with efforts to isolate viruses or bacteria of possible etiologic significance.

The single most difficult differential diagnosis may be between ocular trachoma and oculogenital inclusion conjunctivitis, as described above. This differentiation requires epidemiologic considerations, clinical and laboratory examination of the genital tract, and—if a TRIC agent has been grown—a "typing" of the isolate by immunofluorescent tests. At times the eye lesions of trachoma and of oculogenital inclusion conjunctivitis in the adult cannot be distinguished. The most important differential diagnosis of inclusion conjunctivitis of the newborn is chemical or bacterial conjunctivitis.

Treatment and Prognosis. TRIC agents are susceptible to several antibacterial drugs. Tetracyclines and sulfonamides have been most widely used in treatment. Tetracycline suspensions or ointments can cling to the conjunctiva for prolonged effect. Ophthalmic topical tetracycline preparations have been administered in various dosage schedules for several months in chronic endemic trachoma. Sometimes there was clinical improvement, but often active disease recurred, and the over-all efficacy of topical tetracyclines in chronic TRIC infections is being questioned. In inclusion conjunctivitis of the newborn, there is a strong natural tendency toward healing. The administration of topical tetracycline two to four times daily for three weeks further accelerates healing.

Oral tetracycline hydrochloride, 1 to 2 grams in three divided daily doses, or doxycycline, 2.5 to 4.0 mg per kilogram in a single daily dose, or oral trisulfapyrimidines, 4 grams daily in divided doses for five to six weeks, often suppress signs of activity in chronic trachoma of adults. However, these treatment regimens often fail to eradicate the infectious agent. By contrast, in acute TRIC infections these oral drug regimens alone, or combined with topical tetracycline, may result in permanent cure. This is probably true for both eye infections and genital tract infections, providing that they are of short duration.

In areas of hyperendemic trachoma, mass treatment

must be applied to early infection of children and must be repeated at intervals in order to control TRIC infection before scarring occurs. No conclusive evidence exists that mass drug treatment can eradicate trachoma from a population, but repeated courses of drug treatment are probably beneficial by reducing the reservoir of infection, by temporarily suppressing TRIC agent and clinical activity in the patient, and by controlling bacterial superinfection.

Drug therapy has no influence on established scars or pannus. Surgical correction is required in serious entropion or trichiasis. Topical corticosteroids and caustics have no place in therapy.

Prevention. Endemic trachoma is favored by ignorance, poverty, and cultural patterns that oppose hygienic improvement and medical treatment. In addition, the sheer lack of water available for washing seems to be important.

The most potent preventive measures include efforts to increase the total supply of water, simple cleanliness such as frequent hand washing, avoidance of common towel or common eye pencil, and measures to reduce flies. It is also important to detect mild, early infection in young children in endemic areas and to apply effective drug treatment repeatedly. This prevents the blinding progression of the disease, and probably reduces the infective reservoir. Detection and treatment of adults who already suffer visual impairment can probably reduce the source of infection for children.

Prevention of genital TRIC infections requires the control of sexual promiscuity, early diagnosis and effective treatment of cases and sexual contacts, and prolonged follow-up to establish that the genital or ocular infection is not relapsing. Effective treatment of pregnant women with genital TRIC infection can prevent inclusion conjunctivitis in the newborn. The usual instillations into the eye of the newborn (silver nitrate or penicillin) do not prevent inclusion conjunctivitis. A newborn baby with inclusion conjunctivitis should be isolated to prevent spread to others.

Experimental vaccines against TRIC infections have been prepared. In field tests no vaccine has given unequivocal protection against infection, or against progression of disease. Work is continuing in the hope of developing preparations of greater immunogenicity.

However, natural infection engenders only minimal protection against reinfection. The most that could be expected of artificial immunization is an attenuation of the disease resulting from infection. The best current hope for control of TRIC infections rests on a combination of public health measures and drug treatment.

Dunlop, E. M. C., Jones, B. R., Darougar, S., and Treharne, J. D.: Chlamydia and non-specific urethritis. Br. Med. J., 2:575, 1973.

Dunlop, E. M. C., Vaughan-Jackson, J. D., Darougar, S., and Jones, B. R.: Incidence of chlamydiae in nonspecific urethritis. Br. J. Vener. Dis., 48:425, 1972.

Jawetz, E.: Chemotherapy of chlamydial infections. *In* Garattini, S., Goldin, A., Hawking, F., and Kopin, I. J. (eds.): Advances in Pharmacology and Chemotherapy. Vol. 7. New York, Academic Press, 1969, pp. 253–282.

Jawetz, E., Hanna, L., Dawson, C., Wood, R., and Briones, O.: Subclinical infections with TRIC agents. Am. J. Ophthal., 63:1413, 1967.

Jones, B. R.: Ocular syndromes of TRIC virus infection and their possible genital significance. Br. J. Vener. Dis., 40:3, 1964.

Moulder, J. W.: The relation of the psittacosis group (Chlamydiae) to bacteria and viruses. Ann. Rev. Microbiol., 20:107, 1966.

Thygeson, P.: Trachoma Manual and Atlas. U.S. Department of Health, Education and Welfare, U.S. Public Health Service Publication No. 541, Revised 1960.

Wang, S. P., and Grayston, J. T.: Immunologic relationship between genital TRIC, lymphogranuloma venereum, and related organisms in a new indirect immunofluorescence test. Am. J. Ophthalmol., 70:367, 1970.

172. LYMPHOGRANULOMA VENEREUM

Ernest Jawetz

Definition. Lymphogranuloma venereum (LGV) is an acute and chronic venereal disease with prominent systemic manifestations, caused by a chlamydial agent closely related to trachoma and inclusion conjunctivitis (TRIC) agents. LGV produces early genital lesions followed by enlargement and suppuration of regional lymph nodes and a variety of febrile systemic manifestations. Late results are prominent inguinal draining sinuses in men and fibrosing proctitis and rectal strictures in women and homosexual males.

Etiology. The chlamydiae of LGV resemble TRIC agents (see Ch. 171) in many respects, including the formation of compact intracytoplasmic inclusions with a glycogen matrix, inhibition of growth by sulfonamides, and antigenic features. All LGV chlamydiae carry the chlamydial group reactive antigen. Specific antigens have been defined by immunofluorescence, thus permitting classification of LGV isolates into three specific antigenic types. These antigens cross-react with type-specific antigens of certain TRIC agents. LGV chlamydiae differ from TRIC agents in growing more readily in cell cultures and in several animal tissues.

Prevalence and Epidemiology. LGV is transmitted almost exclusively by sexual contact. The genital tract and rectum of chronically infected persons serve as reservoirs of infection. The highest incidence of the disease has been reported from subtropical and tropical areas, but the infection occurs all over the world. Definitive serologic surveys of LGV infection by appropriate specific methods have not been performed.

Pathogenesis and Pathology. A primary vesicular or ulcerative lesion develops at the site of inoculation one to four weeks after infection. The chlamydiae spread rapidly to regional lymph nodes which become enlarged and inflamed. From the penis or vulva the spread is mainly to inguinal and iliac nodes. From the vagina or rectum the spread is mainly to perirectal and pelvic nodes. The involved nodes become matted and suppurate and may discharge pus through multiple sinus tracts.

During the stage of early, active lymphadenitis, the chlamydiae may become widely disseminated by the bloodstream and may reach various organs, including the central nervous system. In the late, chronic stages of infection, fibrosis, obstruction, and strictures develop. Lymphatic obstruction may lead to elephantiasis of external genitalia (penis, scrotum, vulva). Chronic proctitis may lead to progressive rectal strictures, with obstruction of the bowel lumen and fistula formation.

The histologic appearance of involved lymph nodes shows acute and chronic inflammation, suppuration, and fibrosis, but is not specific or diagnostic of LGV.

Clinical Manifestations. Several days to several weeks

after exposure, a small, evanescent papule or vesicle develops on any part of the external genitalia, anus, or rectum. The lesion may ulcerate, but usually — especially in women — it remains unnoticed and heals in a few days. Soon thereafter the regional lymph nodes enlarge and tend to become matted and often painful. In males, inguinal nodes are most commonly involved both above and below Poupart's ligament, and the overlying skin often turns purplish as the nodes suppurate and eventually discharge pus through multiple sinus tracts. In females, the perirectal nodes are prominently involved with proctitis and bloody mucopurulent anal discharge. This is also seen in homosexual males.

During the stage of active lymphadenitis, there are often marked systemic symptoms, including fever, headaches, meningismus, conjunctivitis, skin rashes, nausea and vomiting, and arthralgias. Rarely is there meningitis, arthritis, or pericarditis. Unless effective antimicrobial therapy is instituted at that stage, the chronic inflammatory process progresses to fibrosis, lymphatic obstruction, and rectal strictures. The lymphatic obstruction may lead to elephantiasis of the penis, scrotum, or vulva. The chronic proctitis of women or homosexual males may lead to progressive rectal strictures, rectosigmoid obstruction, and fistula formation.

Diagnosis. LGV must be considered in every case of enlarged, matted, tender inguinal lymph nodes, active proctitis, draining inguinal or perianal fistulas, and rectal strictures. It must be distinguished from inguinal adenopathy of any cause, including pyogenic infection of lower extremities, plague, tularemia, chancroid, granuloma inguinale, syphilis, and inflammatory or neoplastic lesions of the rectum. A clinical impression of LGV can be supported by the demonstration of the chlamydiae, a skin test, or a meaningful serologic response, but histologic appearance of biopsied tissue is not specific.

Material from fluctuant suppurating nodes may be obtained by aspiration or biopsy. When inoculated into x-irradiated cell cultures, into embryonated eggs, or, by intracerebral injection, into mice, LGV chlamydiae can sometimes be isolated. Only rarely can chlamydial inclusions be seen in stained smears of such material.

The skin test (Frei test) consists of the intradermal injection of LGV antigens, prepared in embryonated eggs, and a suitable control of egg material. The test is considered positive if an indurated area or papule — at least 6 mm larger than the control site — develops in 48 hours. Reactivity to chlamydial group antigen develops within 3 to 8 weeks after LGV infection and may remain positive for life. This delayed hypersensitivity reaction may be positive after *any* chlamydial infection. A negative skin test cannot exclude LGV infection. Skin tests with commercial antigens are sometimes negative even when LGV chlamydiae are isolated from pus, or when the serologic response unequivocally proves a chlamydial infection. Thus the Frei test is of only limited value in the diagnosis of suspected LGV infection. Early antimicrobial drug treatment may interfere with the development of a positive skin test and antibody response.

The complement-fixation (CF) test with heat-stable group reactive antigen is at present the most generally available test for LGV and other systemic chlamydial infections. In the presence of inguinal adenopathy or proctitis, a rise of antibody titer in sera taken two to three weeks apart strongly supports the diagnosis of LGV. In untreated LGV patients, the CF titer is often 1:64 or more, and such a high titer in a single serum from a pa-

tient with a compatible clinical picture also supports the diagnosis. With effective treatment the titer declines. Persisting high antibody titers suggest chronic persistent infection. Indirect immunofluorescence tests for antibodies to LGV antigens are as sensitive as and more specific than CF tests but are not generally available.

Other abnormal laboratory findings are less helpful. The white blood cell count is often elevated during lymph node suppuration or proctitis, sometimes with a relative monocytosis. Total serum proteins may be elevated with a reversed albumin-globulin ratio. Gamma globulin, cryoglobulins, rheumatoid factor, and IgM are sometimes significantly increased in serum.

Treatment. The growth of LGV chlamydiae can be inhibited by sulfonamides, tetracyclines, and some other antimicrobials. Full systemic doses of a soluble sulfonamide (e.g., trisulfapyrimidines USP, 6 to 8 grams daily) or of a tetracycline (e.g., tetracycline HCl, 2 to 4 grams daily) are administered for three to four weeks as early in the course of LGV infection as possible. LGV acquired since 1967 in Southeast Asia has responded more regularly to tetracycline than to sulfonamides. In some patients, two or three courses of treatment are required. Supportive therapy consists of bed rest, compresses to inflamed areas, analgesics, and aspiration of fluctuant sites. Treatment is guided by the subsiding of constitutional symptoms and of lymph node swelling, closure of fistulas, and resolution of proctitis. If the infection is eradicated, the serum antibody titer drops markedly over a period of six to eight months.

Prognosis. Although the acute illness in early LGV is usually self-limited, the chronic complications resulting from lymphatic blockade or rectal stricture are debilitating and often require surgical correction. It is important therefore to prevent these late complications by early diagnosis and prolonged or repeated treatment. Death from LGV uncomplicated by bacterial superinfection is very rare. There may be an increased incidence of anorectal carcinoma in persons with anorectal chronic LGV.

Prevention. Since LGV is generally acquired as a venereal disease, all measures applicable to the prevention of venereal diseases are pertinent. No active immunization is available.

Abrams, A. J.: Lymphogranuloma venereum. J.A.M.A., 205:59, 1968.
Jawetz, E.: Chemotherapy of chlamydial infections. Adv. Pharmacol. Chemother., 7:235, 1969.
Management of Chancroid, Granuloma Inguinale, and Lymphogranuloma Venereum in General Practice. U.S. Public Health Service, Publication No. 255. Washington, D.C., U.S. Government Printing Office, 1968.
Schachter, J., Smith, D. E., Dawson, C. R., Anderson, W. R., Deller, J. J., Hoke, A. W., Smart, W. H., and Meyer, K. F.: Lymphogranuloma venereum. Comparison of the Frei test, complement fixation test, and isolation of the agent. J. Infect. Dis., 120:372, 1969.
Sigel, M. M.: Lymphogranuloma Venereum. Coral Gables, University of Miami Press, 1962.

173. PSITTACOSIS
(Ornithosis, Parrot Fever)
David E. Rogers

Definition. Psittacosis is a specific infection of birds produced by the obligate intracellular bacteria, *Chlamydia psittaci*. When transmitted to man, this agent can produce asymptomatic infection, a transient influenza-like illness, or serious pneumonic disease characterized by high fever, headache, cough, myalgia, pulmonary infiltrates, and a significant mortality. Because it is now recognized that many species of birds other than the order Psittaciformes transmit psittacosis, *ornithosis* has been suggested as a more accurate title. Usage has made psittacosis the accepted term for the human disease.

History. In 1879, Ritter, a Swiss physician, described seven cases of an unusual pneumonia that occurred after contact with tropical birds. Morange, in 1894, established the parrot as a vector and termed the disease *psittacosis* after the Greek *psittakos* (the parrot). During 1929–1930 a serious epidemic of pneumonia occurred in Europe and America after shipments of infected South American parrots. This epidemic led to clearer recognition of psittacosis as a human disease. The etiologic agent was demonstrated to be a filterable agent by Bedson, Western, and Simpson in 1930. Subsequent studies have shown that over 90 species of birds can harbor the agent, and its worldwide distribution has been documented. Reported cases in the United States have declined since 1960, probably as a consequence of requiring tetracycline treatment of imported psittacine birds.

Etiology. *C. psittaci* is an obligate intracellular parasite. It is morphologically and serologically related to lymphogranuloma venereum and to a number of mammalian agents producing pneumonitis, meningoencephalitis, and abortion in their native hosts. To date, these agents have not been shown to produce human disease. Because of their large size (250 to 400 mμ), possession of both RNA and DNA, a demonstrable cell wall containing muramic acid, division by binary fission, and their susceptibility to chemotherapeutic agents known to inhibit bacterial enzyme systems, these agents have recently been reclassified as bacteria. Parrots and parakeets are the most common carriers and until recently represented the major source of human infection. With better control of psittacine disease in aviaries, other birds now contribute more human infections, and cases have resulted from contacts with turkeys, pigeons, ducks, chickens, pheasants, finches, and other fowl. Although individuals of both sexes and all ages are susceptible, overt clinical infections in children are uncommon. Persons working with birds are at greatest risk of infection, and there is an increased incidence of psittacosis in pet shop employees, pigeon handlers, and poultry workers.

The agent is present in the blood, tissue, and discharges of infected birds. It is hardy and can withstand drying. Although the avian disease can be fatal, infected birds frequently show only minimal evidence of illness, such as ruffled feathers, lethargy, and failure to eat. Birds having active infections are most likely to transmit the disease, but asymptomatic carriers are common, and birds that recover can shed transmissible agent for many months. In general, human psittacosis acquired from psittacine birds or turkeys has been more severe than that acquired from pigeons, ducks, chickens, or pheasants. Bird ectoparasites can harbor the agent and may serve as a source of reinfection for domestic flocks. Antimicrobials incorporated in bird foodstuffs may not eradicate psittacosis from infected parrots or parakeets but can render them less infectious for man.

Psittacosis is generally acquired by the respiratory route through inhalation of infected dried bird excreta, more rarely by handling the feathers and the tissues of infected birds. On rare occasion the disease may be acquired through an open lesion or the bite of a bird. Mouth-to-beak intimacies have led to infection in man. Small epidemics have been attributed to aerosols of dust laden with dried excreta. Cases have been reported after only brief exposure to birds. There is some evidence that the incubation period may be shortened by a large inoculum. Person-to-person transmission of psittacosis, although rare, has been documented. These cases of "human" strain psittacosis have been severe, with high mortality.

Pathology. In birds, the principal sites of disease are the liver, spleen, and pericardium. In man, the lung is most commonly involved. The psittacosis agent generally gains access to the human body via the respiratory route, and then rapidly enters the blood and produces systemic disease involving the lungs and the reticuloendothelial tissues. The agent can be isolated from the blood and sputum during the first two weeks of illness, and has been found in the spleen in fatal cases. The mature pulmonary lesion is a lobular pneumonitis. The process is initiated by inflammation and progressive edema of the alveolar cells. Exudation is often accompanied by small hemorrhages. Polymorphonuclear leukocytes appear early in the process. Later inflammatory exudates show lymphocytes and large numbers of mononuclear leukocytes within the alveoli and interstitial spaces. The mucosa of the trachea and bronchi generally remains intact but is edematous and invaded with mononuclear cells. Thick, gelatinous plugs of mucus may fill major and minor bronchi and may account for the severe cyanosis and progressive anoxia seen in fatal cases. Foci of necrosis may occur in more severely affected areas of the lung and are sometimes associated with capillary thrombi. The process is generally most severe in dependent bronchopulmonary segments. Vasculitis and thrombosis may account for many findings. Large monocytes and macrophages containing cytoplasmic inclusion bodies, which may represent the agent (LCL bodies), are characteristic of psittacosis infection. Hyperplasia and monocytic infiltration of pulmonary and hilar lymph nodes and splenic enlargement with occasional areas of focal necrosis may occur. Rarely the liver may show intralobular focal necrosis and swollen Kupffer cells containing the psittacosis elementary bodies. Changes in the myocardium, pericardium, meninges, brain, adrenals, and kidneys have been reported.

Clinical Manifestations. Wide variations can occur in the clinical picture. The incubation period ranges from 7 to 15 days but may occasionally be longer. Asymptomatic infection or mild influenza-like infections probably are the rule. Moderate or severe infections, although less frequent, are more commonly diagnosed. The onset of illness may be insidious, but it often starts with chills and a fever that rises slowly from initial levels of 38 or 39 to 39.5 to 40.5° C during the first week of illness. The pulse may be slow relative to the height of the fever. Headache is severe. Malaise, anorexia, severe myalgias, particularly in the neck and back, and arthralgias are common. Cough is generally prominent but may be delayed until late in the first week. Small amounts of mucoid sputum with occasional blood streaking are the rule, and pleuritic pain is rare. Changes in mentation are often seen. Delirium or stupor may occur in severe cases toward the end of the first week, and is usually associated with severe pulmonary involvement, cyanosis, and other evidences of anoxia. Other neurologic manifestations are uncommon. Nausea and vomiting are frequent. Epistaxis may occur early in the course of the illness. A macular rash resembling that seen in typhoid has occasionally been described. Jaundice and progressive nitrogen retention have been reported in severe cases. Severe dyspnea, tachypnea, tachycardia, cyanosis, jaundice, delirium, and stupor are all poor prognostic signs.

The physical findings of pneumonia are often sparse. Chest roentgenograms may reveal evidence of infiltrates not detected at the bedside. Examination may reveal only fever, painful muscle groups, an elevated respiratory rate, and a relative bradycardia. Fine, crepitant rales may be heard in localized areas over the lungs. Frank percussion or auscultatory changes suggestive of true consolidation are less common. Pleurisy with effusion can occur but is unusual. Mild hepatomegaly is frequent. A palpable spleen has been noted in a substantial number of patients. An erythematous pharynx may be noted. In rare instances there may be signs of pericarditis or myocarditis. In prolonged, severe illness, thrombophlebitis and pulmonary infarction have been reported as late complications.

Patients with mild cases may recover in 7 to 8 days. More severe infections may last 12 to 21 days without specific treatment. Fever is ordinarily sustained or remittent, and when accompanied by bradycardia, resembles the fever seen in untreated typhoid infections. Defervescence is generally slow, and a prolonged convalescence is common. Relapses have been reported even after appropriate treatment. Secondary bacterial infections are rare.

Laboratory Findings. Simple laboratory studies are not helpful in establishing a diagnosis. The leukocyte count is usually normal, but leukopenia or low-grade leukocytosis ranging to over 20,000 cells per cubic millimeter may occur. The erythrocyte sedimentation rate is generally elevated. Proteinuria is common during the febrile period. Chest roentgenograms generally show soft patchy infiltrates radiating outward from the hilum, which tend to be more prominent in dependent lobes or segments. Occasionally diffuse miliary, nodular, or frank lobar distribution of infiltrates is seen.

A specific diagnosis can be made only by isolation of the agent or by serologic studies. The agent is present in the blood and sputum during the first two to three weeks, but isolation is hazardous, and should not be attempted except in special laboratories. Diagnosis is generally made by a fourfold rise in complement-fixing antibodies against a heat-stable group antigen prepared from psittacosis agent grown in eggs. Paired acute and convalescent sera should always be tested. A significant change in antibody titers is generally present by the twelfth to fourteenth day of disease; the titers are usually maximal by 30 days, then slowly disappear. Treatment can delay

or suppress antibody response. There is considerable cross-reaction between antigens prepared from psittacosis and lymphogranuloma venereum viruses. False positive complement-fixation tests may occur with Q fever or brucellosis. Cutaneous hypersensitivity to the Frei antigen may develop during psittacosis.

Differential Diagnosis. Specific diagnosis of psittacosis is of extreme importance because of its potential severity (reported fatality rates range from 5 to 40 per cent), its response to antimicrobials, and the public health significance of psittacosis infection. All cases should be reported to the local health department. The syndrome of viral pneumonia accompanied by protracted high fever, unusually severe headache, and relative bradycardia should suggest psittacosis. Often a history of contact with birds is the only clue to diagnosis and may be elicited only by repeated questioning of the patient and family. When pneumonic symptoms are prominent, psittacosis must be differentiated from viral pneumonias, mycoplasmal pneumonia, influenza, Q fever, tuberculosis, histoplasmosis, coccidioidomycosis, bacterial pneumonia, and other processes that produce pulmonary infiltrates. If pneumonic symptoms are not prominent, psittacosis can be confused with other systemic febrile illnesses such as typhoid fever, brucellosis, infectious mononucleosis, infectious hepatitis, miliary tuberculosis, or the viral meningoencephalitides.

Treatment. The tetracyclines are the drugs of choice, and early diagnosis and initiation of treatment may be lifesaving. After institution of therapy with 2 to 3 grams daily, both fever and symptoms are generally controlled within 48 to 72 hours, although the response may be indolent. Although the disease apparently responds to penicillin in doses above 2 million units daily, tetracycline remains the drug of choice. Treatment should be continued for at least 10 days. The high fever and progressive anoxia secondary to extensive pulmonary involvement in severe cases may require appropriate measures directed at these problems.

Favour, C. B.: Ornithosis (psittacosis). Am. J. Med. Sci., 205:162, 1943.
Harding, H. B.: The bacteria-like chlamydiae of ornithosis and the diseases they cause. CRC Crit. Rev. Clin. Lab. Sci., 1:451, 1970.
Meyer, K. F.: The ecology of psittacosis and ornithosis. Medicine, 21:175, 1942.
Schaffner, W., Drutz, D. J., Duncan, G. W., and Koenig, M. G.: The clinical spectrum of endemic psittacosis. Arch. Intern. Med., 119:433, 1967.
Wilson, G. S., and Miles, A. A.: The psittacosis-lymphogranuloma group. *In* Wilson, G. S., and Miles, A. A. (eds): Topley and Wilson's Principles of Bacteriology and Immunity. 5th ed. Baltimore, Williams & Wilkins Co., 1964, vol. 2. pp. 2246–2267.

Section Three.   MYCOPLASMAL DISEASES

Robert B. Couch

174.   INTRODUCTION

The mycoplasmas (formerly called pleuropneumonia-like organisms, PPLO) are the smallest free-living organisms. They share a number of properties with bacteria, e.g., growth outside the host cell, susceptibility to antimicrobial drugs, generation of metabolic energy, reproduction by fission, and possession of both RNA and DNA. In contrast to bacteria, they do not possess a cell wall. The mycoplasmas are commonly confused with L-forms of bacteria, because L-forms also lack a cell wall

The Human Mycoplasmas

Species	Usual Site of Occurrence
M. pneumoniae	Respiratory tract
M. salivarium	Oropharynx
M. orale 1	Oropharynx
M. orale 2	Oropharynx
M. orale 3	Oropharynx
M. fermentans	Oropharynx and genital tract (rarely detected)
M. hominis	Genital tract
T-mycoplasmas	Genital tract

and their colonial morphology resembles that of mycoplasmas. However, L-forms are related to their bacterial parents and are unrelated to the mycoplasmas.

Members of the genus Mycoplasma cause a variety of diseases in animals. These include sinusitis, pneumonia, arteritis, arthritis, and neurologic disease. Because of these varied pathologic states in animals, it has been proposed that many inflammatory diseases of man of unknown etiology are caused by mycoplasmas. In this regard, extensive efforts to incriminate mycoplasmas in the etiology of rheumatoid arthritis have thus far been inconclusive. At present, eight species of human mycoplasmas have been identified. Only one species, Mycoplasma pneumoniae, has been clearly shown to produce disease in man, and the disease is essentially limited to the respiratory tract. Two species have been incriminated as causing disease of the male and female urogenital tract, and the other known species appear to be commensals. Nevertheless, because of the variety of animal diseases described, it would be surprising if some other human diseases are not caused by mycoplasmas.

The eight species of human mycoplasmas and their usual anatomic site of occurrence are shown in the accompanying table. M. pneumoniae is a significant cause of acute respiratory disease, including pneumonia (see Ch. 175). M. salivarium and M. orale 1 are common inhabitants of the oropharynx, particularly if oral hygiene is poor. M. orale 2 and 3 are uncommon inhabitants of the oropharynx, and M. fermentans has on rare occasions been recovered from the oropharynx and genital tract. None of the latter 5 species have been shown to cause human disease. M. hominis and the T-mycoplasmas (so called because of the "tiny" colonies produced on agar medium) have been collectively called the genital mycoplasmas and have been incriminated as etiologic agents in several disease syndromes (see Ch. 176).

175. PNEUMONIA AND OTHER RESPIRATORY DISEASES CAUSED BY M. PNEUMONIAE

Definition. Pneumonia is the most severe manifestation of respiratory infection with Mycoplasma pneumoniae. Bronchitis, pharyngitis, and asymptomatic infections are frequently seen, particularly in young children; pneumonia occurs predominantly among older children and young adults. The disease responds to treatment with the tetracyclines and erythromycins.

History. A pneumonia that was unlike lobar pneumonia of Diplococcus pneumoniae was recognized in the 1930's. Extensive bacteriologic studies failed to reveal a specific etiology in many of these cases, and Dingle and Finland in 1942 applied the term primary atypical pneumonia to this group of nonbacterial pneumonias. In 1943 the discovery that cold hemagglutinins developed in the sera of many of the patients provided a useful diagnostic test. During World War II the Armed Forces Commission on Acute Respiratory Disease described many of the clinical and epidemiologic characteristics of an atypical pneumonia, retrospectively identified by serologic tests as caused by infection with M. pneumoniae.

The causative agent was first isolated by Eaton in cotton rats, and subsequently was shown to infect hamsters and chicken embryos. It is filterable and for this reason was considered to be a virus for many years. In 1957, Liu reported an immunofluorescent test for antibody, using sections of infected chicken embryo bronchi for antigen, and Chanock in 1961 reported that the organism was the cause of most cases of pneumonia associated with the development of cold hemagglutinins. Subsequent to these studies and the demonstration that the organism was a Mycoplasma, it was given the name Mycoplasma pneumoniae.

Etiology. Mycoplasma pneumoniae can readily be distinguished from the seven other known human species of Mycoplasma. The organism is about 200 nm in size. It will grow aerobically or anaerobically on artificial media, but the medium must be enriched with 20 per cent horse serum and yeast extract. The small granular colonies grow embedded in the surface of the agar, and are best detected by microscopic examination. Tentative identification procedures utilize the fact that M. pneumoniae ferments glucose, exhibits hemadsorption, hemolyzes guinea pig and sheep red blood cells, and is resistant to methylene blue. Final identification requires serologic procedures.

Analysis of the lipids of M. pneumoniae has partially explained some of the serologic responses noted in this infection. The protective antigen appears to be a glycolipid contained in the membrane of the organism. A phospholipid which reacts with some Wassermann-positive sera has been identified, and cross-reactions with glycolipids of Streptococcus MG and the I antigen of human erythrocytes probably account for these occasional serologic responses. The anti-tissue antibodies noted in this infection may have a similar explanation.

Epidemiology. M. pneumoniae infection is endemic in large populations, but numerous localized outbreaks have occurred in schools and military populations. There is no periodicity such as occurs with influenza and no seasonal prevalence as with bacterial and viral respiratory illnesses.

The basic epidemiologic unit is the family, where the infection is often introduced by five- to nine-year-old schoolchildren. Infection spreads slowly but will ultimately involve 80 to 90 per cent of family members who are not immune. Though most common in young school-age children, the very young, adolescents, and young adults frequently acquire the infection. It is rare above age 50 when serum antibody is almost universally present.

Roentgenographic evidence of pneumonia occurs in 30 to 50 per cent of infected family members, but studies in the military have suggested that less than 10 per cent of infections result in pneumonia. This disparity may be accounted for by the finding that illness is more likely to occur and to be more severe with advancing age.

Pathogenesis. M. pneumoniae is a primary pathogen of the respiratory tract that is spread by close and frequent contact between infected and susceptible persons. The organism can be recovered from sputum and throat swab specimens two to three days prior to onset of illness. Thereafter, the concentration of organisms in secretions rises to the time of occurrence of illness and remains high for four to six days. After illness subsides, the agent may persist in respiratory secretions for several weeks in a considerable percentage of cases, and positive cultures frequently occur after antimicrobial treatment.

The organism grows on the ciliated border and between respiratory epithelial cells. All evidence indicates that it does not invade lung parenchyma. It has been suggested that the peroxide produced by the organism might produce cell damage; more recently it has been suggested that the illness may be a result of hypersensitivity to the organism or one or more of its products.

Resistance to infection has been shown to correlate with presence and magnitude of serum antibody, and this mechanism may also influence recovery from illness. Antibody is detectable in respiratory secretions, and recent data suggest that resistance more closely correlates with this antibody than with serum antibody. The association between antibody and resistance probably accounts for prevalence of the infection in younger age groups, as most adults have detectable serum antibody. Nevertheless, reinfection with mild illness has been shown to occur.

Pathology. From the limited studies available, it is apparent that a great variety of pathologic findings may occur in pneumonia, including patchy or confluent bronchopneumonia, interstitial pneumonia, and lobar pneumonia. Pleuritis with a small pleural effusion may be present, but significant pleural effusion is rare. Gross pathology usually reveals patchy areas of lung infiltration and inflamed bronchial and bronchiolar lumina containing mucoid and occasionally purulent exudate. Microscopic sections reveal mononuclear peribronchial and peribronchiolar infiltrates with edema and mononuclear cell infiltration of neighboring alveolar septa. Mucosal cell lining of respiratory passages usually remains intact, and polymorphonuclear cell infiltration is prominent only if necrosis and sloughing of the mucosal cell lining occur. No pathologic alterations have been described in other areas of the body.

Clinical Manifestations. Infection may be manifested by pneumonia, tracheobronchitis, pharyngitis, or bullous myringitis. Pneumonia is the most serious and best described syndrome. The incubation period to onset of illness is about three weeks, most cases occurring in 15 to 25 days.

Pneumonia. The onset of pneumonia is usually insidious, with malaise and headache as prominent symptoms. For a period of two to three days these symptoms increase in severity, and feverishness, myalgias, and sore throat may also occur. Cough is usually not prominent until two to three days after onset of illness. It is either nonproductive or productive of small amounts of mucoid sputum that occasionally contain flecks of blood. *Despite the delayed appearance of cough, it becomes the dominant respiratory symptom in mycoplasmal pneumonia, and its absence or the occurrence of only mild cough makes a clinical diagnosis questionable.* In some cases cough occurs early, and patients may exhibit the paroxysms, substernal discomfort, and tracheal tenderness characteristic of acute tracheobronchitis. Headache is commonly reported as the most distressing symptom in an adult. Ear discomfort, owing to myringitis, mild nasal symptoms, and prominent sore throat may also occur, especially in the younger age groups. Substernal or diffuse chest discomfort on inspiration is common, but typical pleuritic pain is rare.

Patients usually do not appear seriously ill. Tachypnea, dyspnea, and cyanosis are rare and are not seen unless pulmonary involvement is extensive or other disease is present. The degree of fever is variable, but fever is present in virtually all cases of pneumonia.

Physical examination usually reveals mild nasal obstruction and discharge and mild to moderate injection of the posterior pharynx. Mild injection of the tympanic membranes is commonly seen, and about 15 per cent of patients will exhibit frank myringitis, some of whom will develop blebs or bullae. Hemorrhage into the blebs or bullae is common, and these patients usually complain of severe ear pain. Tender cervical lymphadenopathy is a common finding, particularly when pharyngitis is also present.

Findings on chest examination may be minimal, and roentgenographic findings that seem out of proportion to physical findings frequently occur. Auscultation of the chest may reveal rhonchi and wheezes over the involved area of the lung owing to mucus in large bronchi and bronchioles, and fine to medium moist rales may also be heard. In the occasional patient with more extensive disease, signs of consolidation may be detected.

Tracheobronchitis. Tracheobronchitis alone may occur from infection with *M. pneumoniae* and is more common than pneumonia. The onset and clinical picture are little different from that described for pneumonia, and a significant proportion of cases clinically diagnosed as tracheobronchitis will exhibit infiltration when x-rays are obtained. The cases in which the chest x-rays are normal tend to be less severe.

Pharyngitis. Pharyngitis frequently accompanies the tracheobronchitis and pneumonia caused by *M. pneumoniae;* however, pharyngitis alone may also occur. The onset and constitutional manifestations are similar to those described for pneumonia, but sore throat appears early and persists as the predominant symptom. Mild nasal symptoms and some cough may also occur. Pharyngeal examination may reveal a diffusely erythematous pharynx with or without pharyngeal and tonsillar exudate, or only mild pharyngeal congestion may be present. Tender cervical lymph nodes frequently accompany pharyngitis.

Ear Disease. Myringitis, occasionally accompanied by blebs or bullae, is most commonly seen in association with disease of the respiratory tract; however, it has also been reported as an isolated disease occurrence. Such patients complain of ear pain which on occasion may be severe.

Roentgenographic Findings. No roentgenographic changes can be considered typical of mycoplasmal pneumonia. Infiltrates are usually unilateral, confined to a lower lobe, and more prominent near the hilum. Frequently a single segment is involved, but on occasion the infiltrate may be extensive and lobar or may involve more than one lobe. Small pleural effusions are not uncommon.

Laboratory Findings. In pneumonia and the other mycoplasmal respiratory diseases, the leukocyte counts are usually within normal limits and rarely exceed 10 to 15,000 per cubic millimeter. Differential counts usually reveal slight neutrophilia with counts of 60 to 85 per cent neutrophils. During the period of acute illness lymphopenia may be seen. The erythrocyte sedimentation rate is usually elevated. Urinalysis is within normal limits except for occasional albuminuria, which may be attributed to fever. Gram stain and culture of sputum usually reveal normal flora.

Course and Complications. The clinical course is variable and is best described for pneumonia. Illness on occasion may be severe, but very few deaths from pneumonia have occurred. Fever is variable in duration, lasting from three days to two weeks. Fever usually subsides by lysis, and when this occurs, slow but progressive improvement in the cough, malaise, and lethargy ensues. However, symptoms may persist for three to six weeks. Roentgenographic abnormalities frequently persist for two to four weeks.

The most common pulmonary *complication* is relapse soon after clinical recovery. This appears to occur in about 10 per cent of cases, and the disease may involve the same or a different lobe of the lung. Cases of residual pleural abnormality have also been reported. Clinically significant intravascular hemolysis in association with demonstrable cold hemagglutinins occurs in a small percentage of cases. Such patients exhibit cold hemagglutinin titers of 1:500 or greater and also have demonstrable hemagglutinins at room temperature. Hemolysis usually occurs when fever subsides or chilling of peripheral tissues occurs.

M. pneumoniae has been associated with central nervous system and cutaneous manifestations. The former patients have had psychosis, meningitis, meningoencephalitis, or radiculopathy. A variable number and type of cell have been noted in the cerebrospinal fluid. Skin manifestations have included urticaria, vesiculopustular eruptions, maculopapular eruptions, erythema multiforme, and erythema nodosum, although many patients were simultaneously receiving drugs, so that causation is not certain. A reported association with Stevens-Johnson syndrome is perhaps of special significance as these cases are frequently preceded by respiratory symptoms and accompanied by pneumonia. Evidence of *M. pneumoniae* infection should be sought in such cases.

Hemorrhagic bullous myringitis (see under Clinical Manifestations), bronchiectasis, pericarditis, myocarditis, Guillain-Barré syndrome, arthritis, and thrombocytopenic purpura have also been reported as complications of *M. pneumoniae* infection.

Diagnosis. Early diagnosis can be made only by clinical means. The presence of marked headache, lassitude, myalgias, definite nasopharyngeal findings, and nonproductive cough suggests nonbacterial pneumonia. Absence of the usual features of bacterial pneumonia, such as sudden onset, shaking chills, pleuritic pain, and purulent or bloody sputum, offers important support for the diagnosis. Other causes of pulmonary infiltration such as tuberculosis, mycotic infection, pulmonary infarction, and malignancy must be considered.

Among the causes of nonbacterial pneumonia that may mimic mycoplasmal pneumonia are psittacosis and Q fever, for which an exposure history should be sought, and adenoviral and influenzal pneumonias, which are usually more acute in onset and occur primarily during recognizable epidemics. If the age of the patient is 5 to 30 years and other similar cases have occurred in a family, diagnosis is more certain, but the only clinical finding that makes mycoplasmal pneumonia almost a certain diagnosis is the additional presence of myringitis with a bleb or bulla on the tympanic membrane.

Isolation of *M. pneumoniae* may be accomplished from sputum or throat swab specimens. Either enriched solid or special liquid medium may be used, although identifiable isolations are not usually detected for at least five days after inoculation, and 14 to 21 days of incubation may be required.

The cold hemagglutinin test is generally available and useful. Sera of about 50 per cent of patients with *M. pneumoniae* pneumonia will develop this autoantibody which agglutinates human red blood cells when reacted in the cold (4°C). It is more likely to occur in more severely ill patients, and usually appears toward the end of the first week or the beginning of the second week of illness. *Serum for this test should be separated from red blood cells before refrigeration.* Positive direct Coombs tests and an occasional false positive serologic test for syphilis may occur.

A variety of serologic procedures have been described for detecting rise in specific serum antibody titer to *M. pneumoniae* between acute and convalescent sera. Complement fixation is the most available procedure and will demonstrate a rise in titer in 75 to 80 per cent of cases. Growth inhibition is a more sensitive and specific method and is preferred, but it requires experience with cultivation techniques which is not widely available.

Treatment. Tetracycline and its derivatives and erythromycin have been shown to hasten the disappearance of fever, rales, and cough in treated cases of pneumonia. Since definitive diagnosis is not possible within the first few days after onset of illness, decisions regarding administration of antimicrobials must be made on clinical grounds. Patients presumed to have mycoplasmal pneumonia should receive tetracycline or its equivalent in doses of 0.25 gram every six hours. Erythromycin in doses of 0.5 gram every eight hours appears to be an acceptable alternative. Incomplete relief of cough, occasional relapse, and continued shedding of the organism frequently follow six- to eight-day courses of treatment with these antimicrobials. It is possible that continuing treatment for two to three weeks will provide more complete recovery, and therefore this duration of treatment is recommended. The additional use of antipyretics, antitussives, intermittent positive pressure breathing, oxygen, and the like is determined by individual needs.

It is recommended that all patients with bullous myringitis be treated with erythromycin or tetracycline for 10 to 14 days. Treatment of patients with pharyngitis and tracheobronchitis on a routine basis is not recommended unless the organism has been isolated, because these illnesses are indistinguishable by clinical techniques from the great majority of acute respiratory illnesses caused by viruses. However, if protracted illness occurs and *M. pneumoniae* has been isolated, the antimicrobials listed above may be used.

Prevention. No established method is presently available to prevent *M. pneumoniae* infection. Patients in the acute stage of pneumonia should probably be isolated and attempts made in the home to prevent close contact with ill individuals. There is no vaccine currently available.

Chanock, R.: Mycoplasma infections of man. N. Engl. J. Med., 272:1257, 1965.

Couch, R.: *Mycoplasma pneumoniae. In* Knight, V. (ed.): Viral and Mycoplasmal Infections of the Respiratory Tract. Philadelphia, Lea & Febiger, 1973, pp. 217–235.

Dingle, J. H., and Langmuir, A. D.: Epidemiology of acute respiratory disease in military recruits. Am. Rev. Respir. Dis., 97 (Supplement):1, 1968.

Hayflick, L. (ed.): The Mycoplasmatales and the L-phase of Bacteria. New York, Appleton-Century-Crofts, 1969.

Mufson, M., Manko, M., Kingston, J., and Chanock R.: Eaton agent pneumonia: Clinical features. J.A.M.A., 178:369, 1961.

176. GENITOURINARY DISEASE CAUSED BY MYCOPLASMAS

Etiology. *Mycoplasma hominis* and T-mycoplasmas may cause genitourinary disease. *M. hominis* typically produces colonies on agar with the often-described "fried-egg" appearance. Colonies are usually 200 to 300 μ in diameter and are best visualized by microscopy. This colony size contrasts to that of the T-mycoplasmas, which is 10 to 30 μ in diameter. On agar medium *M. hominis* grows well under aerobic conditions, whereas T-mycoplasmas grow best anaerobically. Both grow well in broth, and tentative identification procedures employ the preferential metabolism of arginine by *M. hominis* and the fact that T-mycoplasmas possess a urease system and grow best in an acidic medium. The T-mycoplasmas are antigenically heterogeneous, and the number and significance of types and subtypes has not yet been delineated. A recent report suggests that *M. hominis* is also antigenically heterogeneous.

Epidemiology. The genital mycoplasmas may be recovered from the distal urethra of both the male and female and the vulva, vagina, and cervix of the latter. Presumably because of intimate association with mucosal surfaces, specimens that contain epithelial cells are superior to urine or secretion specimens for isolation tests.

Infants may become colonized with genital mycoplasmas at birth, presumably acquiring them from the birth canal. The frequency of recovery of organisms decreases for the first year or two of life, and most individuals then remain free of genital mycoplasmas until puberty. Mycoplasmas then reappear, and frequencies are directly proportional to extent of sexual activity and promiscuity, suggesting the possibility of the disease being acquired venereally.

Despite the fact that genital mycoplasmas are commonly recovered from the urogenital tract, disease is uncommon. This suggests a low order of pathogenicity for these organisms.

Clinical Manifestations. *Nonspecific Urethritis.* The syndrome of dysuria, urgency, and frequency of urination with urethral discharge and without evidence of gonococcal infection has been called nonspecific or nongonococcal urethritis. A negative urine culture for bacteria and absence of prostatitis if the patient is a male are essential supportive findings. Patients with postgonococcal urethritis in which the gonococcus disappears but symptoms of urethritis remain are also included in this category of patients. The urethritis may be caused by a T-mycoplasma but apparently not by *M. hominis.*

Pelvic Inflammatory Disease. Patients with lower abdominal pain and fever who exhibit tenderness on movement of the cervix and in the adnexal areas are usually designated as having pelvic inflammatory disease. In most instances acute or subacute salpingitis is present, although tubo-ovarian abscesses or pelvic abscesses elsewhere may present similar findings. *M. hominis* may cause the disease in many of these cases.

Cervicitis and vaginitis as separate disease entities may occasionally be caused by *M. hominis,* although the data are inconclusive in this regard.

Mycoplasmal Disease in Pregnancy. Both *M. hominis* and the T-mycoplasmas have been recovered from the uterus, amnion, and fetus. Infection is more likely to occur with *M. hominis* than with T-mycoplasmas and to occur during therapeutic or spontaneous abortion, or when premature rupture of the membranes has occurred. Blood cultures are occasionally positive, and such patients exhibit fever and serum antibody responses. The frequency and significance of *M. hominis* infection of the uterus and products of conception are uncertain, but it seems probable that *M. hominis* is responsible for some cases of septic abortion and puerperal infection.

Postpartum fever in patients with normal pregnancy and delivery may occasionally be caused by invasion of the bloodstream with *M. hominis* or T-mycoplasma. The frequency of such cases attributable to mycoplasmas is probably low.

Treatment. All mycoplasmas are susceptible to the tetracyclines. *M. hominis* is susceptible to lincomycin and resistant to erythromycin, whereas the converse is true for the T-mycoplasmas. Patients with nonspecific urethritis should receive tetracycline or its equivalent in doses of 0.25 gram every six hours for five to seven days. Although T-mycoplasmas are also susceptible to erythromycin, results of treatment have been somewhat better with tetracycline. When erythromycin is used for therapy of nonspecific urethritis, patients should receive 0.5 gram every eight hours for five to seven days. Relapse and/or reinfection occurs in about 20 per cent of patients within three months. Second courses of the drug are frequently beneficial, but the sexual contacts of such patients should be examined for T-mycoplasmas. Recurrent nonspecific urethritis is an indication for urologic evaluation for structural abnormality of the urethra.

Since pelvic inflammatory disease may be caused by gonococci, *M. hominis,* and perhaps other bacteria, and since the site of disease is not accessible for obtaining culture specimens, antimicrobial therapy directed toward the specific cause is often not possible. In nonhospitalized patients tetracycline has been reported to be effective treatment. In most instances of postpartum fever caused by mycoplasmas, spontaneous cure without specific antimycoplasmal therapy occurs. Patients considered as candidates for treatment should receive tetracycline in doses noted above.

McCormack, W. M., Braun, P., Lee, Y. H., Klein, J. O., and Kass, E. H.: The genital mycoplasmas. N. Engl. J. Med., 288:78, 1973.

Section Four. BACTERIAL DISEASES

177. INTRODUCTION

Walsh McDermott

For the past few decades the problems presented by bacterial and mycotic diseases have presented themselves in two different forms depending upon the nature of the society. In the economically underdeveloped parts of the world, the individual diseases have presented in classic form, each occupying its traditional niche in the over-all pattern. By contrast, in nations with highly developed health services, the familiar bacterial diseases have by no means disappeared, but their menace has been largely nullified by vaccines and by prompt and appropriate antimicrobial therapy. For example, one hears that lobar pneumonia "has largely disappeared." In actuality is *has* become much less prominent, not because its major cause, pneumococcal infection, is any less frequent, but because with prompt chemotherapy the early pneumonic lesion is halted in its progress well short of the confines of the lobe. It is the same old pneumonia, but it is no longer "lobar." Expressed differently, without any change in the annual incidence of pneumococcal infection or disease, the annual incidence of *serious problems* from this cause has substantially diminished. In place of such clinical problems there are now essentially new menaces in the serious systemic disease produced by *E. coli,* Proteus, Pseudomonas, Candida, and other microbes that were formerly regarded as essentially harmless inhabitants of man. The disease caused by staphylococci and tubercle bacilli can likewise be regarded as being partially of this sort, in that the microbes can subsist harmlessly in the tissues for considerable periods between eruptions as destructive disease. In effect these new clinical patterns represent *endogenous microbial disease*—clinical entities that appear almost exclusively in people with some temporary or sustained lowering of local or general defenses. Because of the resulting changes in the tissue environment, disease-producing microbes are evoked from the dormant or latent state. Generally speaking, these changes in the internal milieu represent a direct or indirect consequence of our modern therapies. They are the unsought-for effects of practical therapeutic gains that in themselves represent great scientific achievements. The practices involved include the use of corticosteroids and immunosuppressants; the suppression of customary microbial flora by drugs, thus compromising the protection to the host afforded by *bacterial interference;* surgical procedures, e.g., subtotal gastrectomy or splenectomy that can reduce previously acquired host resistance; and the longer survival of many patients despite protracted, severe, and ultimately fatal illness.

This increasing ability to alter man's internal environment has had the effect that virtually no microbial species today can be considered nonpathogenic, for in appropriate circumstances virtually any can give rise to disease. All these mechanisms unleash what are, in effect, "new" microbial diseases. There are other "new" diseases that may have been similarly unleashed or may have merely become easier to recognize by virtue of the selectivity of drug action. The separation of "atypical" pneumonia from bacterial pneumonia by the introduc-tion of sulfonamide back in the 1930's and the growing importance of "atypical" mycobacteria as disease agents are cases in point. What is happening was biologically predictable, and the changing nature of the situation may be expected to continue.

To be capable of staying with this change the physician must know considerably more about the behavior of microbes, as they cause disease and are exposed to drugs within an otherwise normal or a compromised host, than he had to master only one or two decades ago. This knowledge is of two sorts: certain concepts and principles related to the microbe-drug-host interactions, and a body of knowledge sufficient to permit him to make microbiologically relevant diagnosis on clinical grounds. Knowledge of the latter sort is presented in the individual chapters that follow. For discussion of host defenses and their behavior during administration of immunosuppressive drugs, the reader is referred to Ch. 60 to 70 and Ch. 771 to 775. Endogenous microbial disease itself is discussed in Ch. 178, whereas the concepts and principles related to microbe-drug-host interactions are considered in Ch. 267 and 268.

McDermott, W.: Inapparent infection. The Dyer Lecture. Public Health Rep., 74:485, 1959.

Rogers, D., et al.: Infections in the altered host. *In* Year Book of Medicine, 1972, 1973, 1974. Chicago, Year Book Medical Publishers.

178. HOSPITAL-ASSOCIATED INFECTIONS: ENDOGENOUS MICROBIAL DISEASE

Jay P. Sanford

A startling metamorphosis has occurred in the disease pattern presented by microbes in the highly industrialized countries as contrasted with the classic pattern in most of the economically underdeveloped world. The nature of this pattern is illustrated by the data of Rogers, based upon a comparison of life-threatening infections demonstrated at necropsy in a group of patients who were hospitalized in 1938–1940 and a group who were hospitalized in 1957–1958 (see accompanying table). It

Changing Pattern of Life-Threatening Microbial Diseases at Necropsy (%)

Etiology	Year of Study	
	1938–1940	*1957–1958*
Pneumococci, streptococci, tubercle bacilli	20	2
Staphylococci	8	8
Gram-negative bacilli (aerobic)	4	11
Mycotic	1	4
"Hospital-associated infections"	7	54

should be noted that, although infections caused by *D. pneumoniae*, *Strep. pyogenes*, and *M. tuberculosis* had dropped significantly, there had been a concomitant two and a half–fold increase in infections caused by aerobic gram-negative bacilli, especially Enterobacteriaceae and Pseudomonadaceae, and a fourfold increase in those caused by fungi. Over-all, infections were either the major or a significant contributory cause of death in 28 per cent of patients hospitalized in 1938, but remained the major or a significant contributory cause of death in 14 per cent of patients hospitalized in 1958, at a time when antimicrobial drugs, corticosteroid agents, and other therapeutic modalities were available. The problem is essentially summarized by the observation that in 1938 most patients were admitted to hospitals with infection, less than 10 per cent being hospital associated, whereas by 1958 over 50 per cent of the life-threatening infections were acquired while the patient was hospitalized originally for a noninfectious problem. *Current studies in community hospitals suggest that about 5 per cent of patients who are admitted to general hospitals will acquire an infection while hospitalized.*

This metamorphosis in the pattern of infectious diseases reflects the impact of control and better management of infections caused by more virulent or invasive microorganisms and the introduction of medical practices which compromise the antimicrobial defense mechanisms of the patient. The organisms currently responsible for hospital-associated infections often were considered as "saprophytes" which were present in the environment or the "normal flora" of the patient. The antimicrobial defense systems include local mechanisms which depend upon the integrity of skin and mucosal barriers, the occurrence of bacterial interference, the inflammatory defense mechanisms which are evoked when the local defenses have been breached, and immune mechanisms, both humoral antibody (B lymphocyte-mediated) and cellular (T lymphocyte- and macrophage-mediated).

This change in the pattern of hospital-associated infections is well illustrated by the sequence of infections which have occurred in patients with extensive thermal burns with the progressive application of control measures and therapy. Before the introduction of penicillin G, group A streptococci were a leading cause of infection in the burned patient; subsequently, staphylococci became the leading cause of death. With better control of contact transmission of staphylococci and the development of more effective antistaphylococcal drugs, the staphylococci were superseded by aerobic gram-negative bacilli, such as *Pseudomonas aeruginosa*, *Serratia marcescens*, and *Providencia stuartii*. These organisms are the major problem in most burn centers today, but where control has been achieved, burn wounds have become infected with fungi such as members of the genus Mucor and viruses such as *Herpesvirus hominis* (simplex). This susceptibility of the burned patient is not only the consequence of the loss of the integumentary barriers; these patients also have a defect in granulocyte responsiveness and depression of cellular immunity.

The common hospital-associated infections include *urinary tract infections,* these usually being associated with the use of indwelling urethral catheters; *pneumonia,* which often may be attributed to the use of contaminated ventilatory therapy equipment; *cellulitis, phlebitis, and bacteremia* associated with the use of indwelling venous and arterial cannulas or improperly sterilized intravenous fluids; and *postsurgical wound infections.* These four categories of infection account for about 85 per cent of hospital-associated infections. The causative microorganisms include both bacteria and fungi such as *Candida spp.* Most of these causative organisms are present in the external environment of the patient and are delivered by contact transmission or through contaminated materials such as contaminated "disinfectants." Control of many of these infections can be accomplished by meticulous attention to good nursing practices. However, knowledge is lacking in many basic areas, such as the question as to why "sick" patients lose their ability to resist colonization of the skin and oropharynx with aerobic gram-negative bacilli, even if they have not received antimicrobial drugs.

In addition to these hospital-associated infections, there is a broad category of infections which are increasing in frequency both in hospitalized and in nonhospitalized patients. These infections occur in patients whose antimicrobial defenses are severely impaired and in whom the causative microorganisms not only include the usual "pathogens" such as staphylococci and hospital-associated microorganisms such as Pseudomonas, but also include the patient's endogenous microorganisms such as *Clostridium perfringens;* organisms in the environment which are of very low virulence such as *Aspergillus spp.;* and viral and parasitic agents whose epidemiology still is poorly defined — for example, infections caused by cytomegaloviruses and *Pneumocystis carinii* in the renal transplant patient on immunosuppressive therapy. These infections are termed "opportunistic" infections and are often caused by microorganisms considered as "saprophytes" or "commensals."

Advances in biomedical engineering and in the chemotherapy of malignant disease have blurred the traditional boundaries between pathogens and nonpathogens. Today physicians must consider virtually all microorganisms as capable of producing human disease in the patient whose antimicrobial defenses are compromised and who is placed in an environment which often is contaminated; hence we learn of infections caused by *Serratia marcescens,* a nonpathogen used as a marker organism 20 years ago, *Bacillus subtilis,* and even *Erwinia spp.,* a "coliform" of tulips.

Curry, C. R., and Quie, P. G.: Fungal septicemia in patients receiving parenteral hyperalimentation. N. Engl. J. Med., 285:1221, 1971.
Eickhoff, T. C., Brachman, P. S., Bennett, J. V., and Brown, J. F.: Surveillance of nosocomial infections in community hospitals. I. Surveillance methods, effectiveness, and initial results. J. Infect. Dis., 120:305, 1969.
Kunin, C. M., and McCormack, R. C.: Prevention of catheter-induced urinary-tract infections by sterile closed drainage. N. Engl. J. Med., 274:1155, 1966.
Pierce, A. K., and Sanford, J. P.: Bacterial contamination of aerosols. Arch. Intern. Med., 131:156, 1973.
Rogers, D. E.: The changing pattern of life threatening microbial disease. N. Engl. J. Med., 261:677, 1959.

PNEUMONIA

179. INTRODUCTION

Walsh McDermott

To discover that a pneumonia, i.e., an intrapulmonary process of some sort, is present in an adult patient is no very difficult feat; neither is that knowledge particularly helpful unless two further steps can be taken. These are detection of evidence that the disease is indeed microbial in origin and not an infarct or neoplasm, and identification of the specific microbe or kind or microbe that is involved. Every aspect of management—the choice of treatment, the complications to be watched for, and the hour-by-hour prognosis—depends on the nature of this information. To obtain it accurately *and in proper time* requires that the physician be wholly familiar with the various ways in which each one of the microbial pneumonias expresses itself. Some of these—for example, plague pneumonia—he may never see. Yet he must know at least enough about plague pneumonia so that he could avert its terrible consequences for others should he ever encounter a case. Other forms of pneumonia encountered relatively rarely arise as complications of some familiar microbial disease such as measles or tuberculosis or streptococcal disease. Occasionally, well-known viruses such as influenza or chickenpox cause pneumonia, or the physician may be asked to see a patient with psittacosis. In the compromised host, necrotizing pneumonias caused by Pseudomonas and other gram-negative bacilli are being recognized increasingly as one form of the endogenous microbial disease mentioned in the preceding two chapters. Most of the time, in an adult patient the physician is dealing with *mycoplasmal pneumonia* or with *one of three bacterial pneumonias,* pneumococcal, staphylococcal, or some other form of necrotizing pneumonia in an obviously altered host. This narrowing of the probabilities does not really lighten the seriousness of making the correct choice. The most effective treatment for pneumococcal pneumonia is utterly without value in Klebsiella pneumonia; a choice of therapy based on a diagnosis of mycoplasmal pneumonia when the patient actually has staphylococcal pneumonia could result in a fatality.

As *staphylococcal pneumonia* is so closely related to viral influenza, it is discussed both under staphylococcal disease (Ch. 195) and under influenza (Ch. 117). *Mycoplasmal pneumonia* is discussed in Ch. 175; the other major bacterial pneumonias, *pneumococcal, Klebsiella,* and the other *necrotizing pneumonias,* are presented in Ch. 180 to 183. Klebsiella pneumonia, although infrequent, is of great importance because of its potential severity and the ease with which it can be misdiagnosed. The pneumonias caused by the individual viruses and by rickettsial (and chlamydial) agents are considered in earlier chapters of Part VIII. Pneumococcal pneumonia is the most important of all pneumonias, not only in numerical terms, but because in large measure, and especially in its complications, it is the prototype of all the bacterial pneumonias.

180. PNEUMOCOCCAL PNEUMONIA

*Edward W. Hook**

Definition. Pneumococcal pneumonia is an acute bacterial infection of the lungs caused by *Streptococcus pneumoniae* (the pneumococcus) and characterized clinically by an abrupt onset, rigor, fever, chest pain, cough, and bloody sputum. Bacterial pneumonia occurring in otherwise healthy persons is usually caused by the pneumococcus.

Bacteriology and Immunology. The somatic portion of the lancet-shaped pneumococcal cell is gram positive. In its virulent form (smooth, S), the pneumococcus has an outer capsule consisting of a high molecular polysaccharide polymer that is specific for each serologic type. In addition to the type-specific capsular antigen, there is a species-specific carbohydrate in the cell wall, known as the "C" substance. The capsule of pneumococcus acts as an armor against phagocytic cells and thus contributes significantly to the pathogenicity of the organism. Pneumococcal variants having no capsules (rough, R strains) are essentially avirulent. Antibody to the type-specific carbohydrate promotes phagocytosis by combining with the highly polymerized polysaccharide of the capsular gel. The pneumococcus also produces hyaluronidase, a hemolysin that causes greenish discoloration around colonies on blood agar, and autolytic enzymes that, when activated, render the organism gram negative and eventually cause its dissolution.

Pneumococci grow rapidly on a variety of bacteriologic media. Blood agar and beef infusion broth containing 0.5 per cent dextrose and 5 to 10 per cent blood or serum are the media most commonly used. On blood agar virulent strains form circular, glistening, dome-shaped colonies that are alpha hemolytic. Because of the great quantity of capsular polysaccharide formed by type 3 pneumococcus, its colonies are more mucoid and usually much larger than those of other types. Unlike the alpha-hemolytic Streptococcus, pneumococcus is soluble in bile, sodium deoxycholate, and other surface-active agents, is highly sensitive to ethyl hydrocuprein chloride (optochin), and is mouse virulent.

The extraordinary virulence of pneumococci for mice may be made use of in isolating the organisms from sputum. The technique usually used consists in injecting intraperitoneally 0.5 ml of sputum previously emulsified by having been drawn repeatedly into a tuberculin syringe. When virulent pneumococci are present, the mouse usually dies within 48 hours, and a pure culture of the organism can be isolated from the heart's blood. Since other bacteria in the sputum do not ordinarily produce fatal infections in mice, the animal serves as a convenient and highly sensitive differential "culture medium" for the isolation of pneumococci.

More than 82 different serologic types of pneumococci have been identified by agglutination tests with specific antiserums or by the quellung test. The latter is based upon the fact that when pneumococci come in contact with homologous anticapsular serum, a capsular precipitin reaction and swelling occur, rendering the capsule easily visible under the microscope.

Anticapsular antibody usually appears in the blood of patients with pneumococcal pneumonia between the fifth and tenth days of the disease. In some untreated patients, its appearance coincides with recovery; in others no such relation is demonstrable. Specific polysaccharide, which has diffused away from the bacteria, can often be identified in the urine and blood. Using counterimmunoelectrophoresis, circulating polysaccharide

---

*Dr. W. Barry Wood, the author of this chapter for many years, died on March 9, 1971. Dr. Hook has revised the chapter but has retained much of the original material.

can be detected in the blood of one third to one half of patients with pneumococcal bacteremia but much less often in the absence of demonstrable bacteremia. The technique may have diagnostic usefulness because it can give specific diagnostic information in about one hour. Patients frequently continue to excrete the capsular carbohydrate in the urine for days and even weeks after recovery.

Epidemiology. Pneumococcal pneumonia may occur at any season, but it is most common during the winter and early spring, when viral respiratory infections are most prevalent.

The types of pneumococci that most commonly cause pneumonia in adults are types 1, 3, 4, 5, 7, 8, 12, 14, and 19. Together, these nine types account for about three quarters of all cases. The most common types encountered in childhood pneumonias are 1, 6, 14, and 19.

Pneumococci, particularly of the higher types, are frequently present in the respiratory tracts of normal subjects. Ordinarily the prevalence of carriers of highly pathogenic types is relatively low, except for type 3, which is a common inhabitant of the normal pharynx. Nevertheless, there is evidence that normal carriers play a more important role in the dissemination of infective types than do patients ill with pneumonia. Occasionally, in relatively closed communities, high carrier rates of pathogenic types are encountered. In such circumstances the occurrence of widespread viral disease of the respiratory tract may result in an epidemic of pneumococcal pneumonia. Except for these rare epidemics, most of which occur in hospitals or custodial institutions, the disease is sporadic. Pneumococcal pneumonia occurs frequently in patients with multiple myeloma or hypogammaglobulinemia.

Pathogenesis and Pathology. The lung is the only major viscus of the body exposed to air. As the atmosphere, particularly in congested places, contains many pathogenic bacteria, it is remarkable that pneumonia is not more common. The failure of normal subjects to acquire acute bacterial pneumonia as an airborne infection is due to efficient defense barriers of the lower respiratory tract. These include (1) the epiglottal reflex, which prevents aspiration of infected secretions; (2) the sticky mucus that lines the bronchial tree and to which airborne organisms adhere; (3) the cilia of the respiratory epithelium, which keep the mucus moving constantly toward the pharynx at the rate of 1 to 3 cm per hour; (4) the cough reflex, which serves to propel mucus or foreign bodies out of the lower tract; (5) the lymphatics that drain the terminal bronchi and bronchioles; (6) phagocytic cells, especially alveolar macrophages that are ever present in the normal alveoli; and (7) opsonins and specific antibody. In addition, the alveoli themselves are relatively dry and thus offer a poor medium for growth of bacteria that succeed in reaching them. Acute bacterial pneumonia results only when the defense barriers of the normal respiratory tract fail.

The thesis that bacterial pneumonia usually results from aspiration of infected secretions from the upper respiratory tract is strongly supported by both experimental and clinical observations. Rats infected with pneumococci in the nasopharynx regularly exhibit pulmonary lesions only when subjected to experimental procedures involving chilling of the body, anesthesia, administration of morphine, or alcoholic intoxication, all of which are predisposing factors in human pneumonia and have been shown in laboratory animals to slow the epiglottal reflex and thus to facilitate aspiration. Experimental pneumonia can best be produced by intrabronchial inoculation of organisms suspended in mixtures of gastric mucin or starch having viscosities similar to that of mucus. Viral infection of the upper respiratory tract in man usually precedes the onset of acute bacterial pneumonia by several days. Not only is the volume of secretion from the nasopharynx greater than normal during viral infections such as the common cold, but also the number of pathogenic microorganisms in the secretions is significantly increased. Thus the stage is set for aspiration of infected mucus. That such aspiration often occurs at the onset of pneumonia in man is suggested by the usual sites of initial involvement of the lung. The earliest lesions of bacterial pneumonia usually appear in those parts of the lungs into which aspirated fluid is most likely to drain. Whereas most airborne bacteria are caught on the sticky surfaces of the bronchial tree and never reach the alveoli, organisms contained in thin nasopharyngeal secretions are readily carried into the alveoli by the liquid mucus. The latter, like Lipiodol, cannot all be ejected by ciliary action, and much of it penetrates to the farthest reaches of the bronchial tree, where it establishes the initial focus of infection.

Other factors known to predispose patients to acute bacterial pneumonia include exposure to noxious gases and anesthetics, cardiac failure, influenza viral infection of the lungs, and trauma to the thorax. A feature common to all these conditions is the accumulation of fluid in the alveoli. Harford (1950) has shown that the dry lungs of normal mice are able to rid themselves of large numbers of inspired bacteria, whereas lungs containing fluid are readily infected. This observation suggests that pulmonary edema, by providing a suitable culture medium for the bacteria, may facilitate the establishment of active infection within the alveoli. Influenza also causes destruction of the ciliated columnar epithelial cells lining the tracheobronchial tree, thus interfering with function of cilia. In addition, influenza virus also apparently inhibits phagocytosis.

Pneumococcal pneumonia may also occur as a complication of bronchogenic carcinoma, chronic pulmonary disease, such as bronchiectasis or lung abscess, or any process that produces obstruction of a bronchus.

Splenectomy carries an increased risk of severe bacteremic infections which are predominantly although not exclusively pneumococcal in etiology. The clinical course is often fulminant, frequently associated with evidence of diffuse intravascular coagulation and a high mortality rate. Although it appears that even healthy adults with post-traumatic splenectomies show increased susceptibility, the risk is greatest in infants and young children, in patients with underlying diseases which compromise reticuloendothelial function, and during the first postsplenectomy years. The mechanism of this relationship is unknown, but it appears that the spleen is important in removing encapsulated bacteria in the absence of antibody.

Children with sickle cell anemia and other sickle cell hemoglobinopathies also seem especially vulnerable to severe pneumococcal infections, especially meningitis. The pneumococcus, not *Hemophilus influenzae,* is the most common cause of bacteremia and meningitis in patients with sickle cell anemia. The causes of this relationship are probably multiple and include deficient pneumococcal opsonizing activity, functional asplenia in some instances and actual splenic atrophy in others, and impaired phagocytic and killing capacity of reticuloendothelial cells.

In patients with severe pneumococcal disease with bacteremia and pneumonia or extrapulmonary sites of infection in cerebrospinal, pleural, or peritoneal fluids, the frequency of underlying disease exceeds 50 per cent.

Early Lesion. Once the infection has gained a foothold within the alveoli, the lesion evolves in a characteristic manner. The first response of the lung to bacterial invasion is an outpouring of edema fluid into the alveoli which serves to "float" organisms into new alveoli through the pores of Kohn and terminal bronchioles.

a, Pneumococci in edema-filled alveoli at margin of spreading pneumonic lesion (×800).

b, Beginning stage of polymorphonuclear exudation in zone of early consolidation. Note leukocytes in alveolar capillaries, some in process of diapedesis (×800).

c, Leukocytic exudate (still predominantly polymorphonuclear) in inner zone of advanced consolidation. Pneumococci have been phagocytized and destroyed (×800).

d, Alveolar macrophage reaction characteristic of late stage of resolution (×800).

e, Pneumococci in edema fluid contained within lumen of a large bronchus. Such infected bronchial fluid causes spread of pneumonia to other lobes of the lungs (×1250).

f–i, Surface phagocytosis of encapsulated microorganisms in formalin-fixed rat lung (×1250). Bacteria shown in these photomicrographs are klebsiella, but same results have been obtained with pneumococci.

f, Polymorphonuclear leukocyte is seen approaching bacteria near alveolar wall. Time 12:30.

g, Leukocyte has reached alveolar wall and is about to trap organisms against the tissue surface. Time 12:31.

h, Cell has trapped some of the encapsulated bacteria against the wall and is in the process of phagocytizing them. Time 12:32.

i, Having ingested several of the organisms, the leukocyte is moving up the alveolar wall. Time 12:35.

(Photomicrographs from studies on experimental pneumonia. W. B. Wood et al.: J. Exp. Med., Vol. 73; and Smith and Wood: *ibid.,* Vol. 86.)

Centrifugal spread of infection occurs. After the outpouring of edema fluid, polymorphonuclear leukocytes and some erythrocytes accumulate in the infected alveoli, first in small numbers but later in such quantities as to fill each alveolus and thus render the area completely consolidated. Once the infected alveoli become crowded with leukocytes, phagocytosis of bacteria takes place, and the invading organisms are destroyed. Macrophages appear in the exudate, and resolution begins only after most of the organisms have been ingested.

Spreading Lesion. Three stages in the inflammatory reaction account for the distinguishing histologic features of the spreading pneumonic lesion. In the outermost portion there appears an "edema zone" in which the alveoli are filled with acellular serous fluid containing bacteria. Inside the edema zone a second zone may be identified in which there are signs of early consolidation with leukocytes in most of the alveoli. Here phagocytosis is often noted. Still more centrally a third transition to a "zone of advanced consolidation" is noted where the alveoli are packed with cells and where beginning resolution may be evident.

All stages of inflammation can be found in a spreading lesion. In the most recently invaded areas at the periphery, edema and hemorrhage predominate, causing "red hepatization," whereas in the older, more central parts of the lesion, dense consolidation with leukocytes accounts for the characteristic color of "gray hepatization."

Not all pneumococcal pneumonia causes lobar consolidation. Lesions may be patchy in distribution and concentrated particularly about the bronchi. Because a clear-cut distinction between pneumococcal bronchopneumonia and lobar pneumonia cannot always be made even by the pathologist, and because management of the two conditions is the same, it is rarely important for the clinician to differentiate them. The etiology rather than the anatomy of the lesion determines therapy.

Interlobar Spread. The spread of the pneumonic process may be stopped by the pleural boundaries of the lobe. Often, however, the infection spreads to other lobes of the lungs by flow of infected edema fluid from bronchi of the involved lung into the bronchial tree of a new lobe.

Bacteremia. Bacteremia is common during the course of pneumococcal pneumonia, particularly when the infection is fulminating. The fact that organisms appear in the thoracic duct in experimental pneumonia before they appear in the systemic circulation suggests that the bacteria reach the bloodstream via the lymphatics. Blood cultures are positive in 20 to 30 per cent of patients with pneumococcal pneumonia. The prevalence of bacteremia increases with age, and is more common with type 2 pneumonia and less common with type 3 pneumonia than with other pneumococcal types.

Invasion of Pleura and Pericardium. The exact mechanism whereby pneumococci invade the pleura or pericardium is not known. As the lymphatics at the periphery of the lung drain outward toward the pleura, it is possible that pleural invasion results from lymphangitic spread. When infection of a pleural or pericardial cavity occurs, there results an outpouring of serous fluid followed by the deposit of fibrin. Leukocytes accumulate in the infected cavity, and, if infection persists, a purulent focus results. The pus in such cavities is at first thin but later becomes thick and stringy as a result not only of fibrin formation but also of the precipitation of deoxyribonucleic acid derived from the nuclei of disintegrating leukocytes. Finally, the thick fibrinous pus becomes walled off, forming loculated foci of chronic suppuration.

Similar purulent foci may occur in the meninges, peritoneum, or joints, as a result of hematogenous spread. Acute vegetations on the endocardium of the heart valves are sometimes encountered. Children with nephrotic syndrome are more prone to pneumococcal peritonitis than normal children. Pneumococcal peritonitis also occurs as a complication of hepatic cirrhosis with ascites.

Mechanism of Recovery. SURFACE PHAGOCYTOSIS. Owing to the antiphagocytic properties of their capsules, fully encapsulated, virulent pneumococci are resistant to phagocytosis when suspended in a fluid medium devoid of opsonins. In the presence of relatively immovable cellular surfaces, however, as in the alveoli, leukocytes are able to trap the encapsulated organisms and ingest them without the aid of opsonizing antibody.

HEAT-LABILE OPSONINS. Leukocytes in vivo are also assisted, right from the start of infection, by heat-labile opsonins that are present in normal plasma. These opsonins, which gain access to acute inflammatory exudates, are immunologically polyspecific, i.e., they act on all sorts of bacteria, in contrast to the monospecific anticapsular antibody that is eventually generated. Their opsonizing action on pneumococci has been shown to involve multiple components of the complement system, including C3. Its cleavage product, C3b, appears to act as a ligand between the organism on which it is deposited and the surface of the phagocyte.

ANTICAPSULAR OPSONINS. Most patients with pneumococcal pneumonia who survive long enough eventually generate an excess of monospecific anticapsular antibody. The process usually takes five to ten days. These newly formed immunoglobulins not only agglutinate the pneumococci in the edema zone of the lesion and thereby inhibit their spread, but also act as potent accessory opsonins and further increase the efficiency of phagocytosis.

MACROPHAGE REACTION. The exact role of the "macrophage reaction" in the recovery process is not entirely clear. Because the appearance of macrophages in the alveolar exudate coincides in general with the disappearance of organisms from the lesion, it has long been assumed that these large mononuclear phagocytes take an active part in destroying the bacteria, and in the final analysis tip the scales in favor of the cellular defenses of the host. Studies relating to experimental lymphadenitis cast some doubt upon this assumption. The "macrophage reaction" in a regional lymph node draining an area of active infection can be artificially initiated at any stage of the nodal inflammation by merely cutting the afferent lymph vessels bringing bacteria to the node. Thus it appears that macrophages accumulate in the exudate only when the active stimulus of direct bacterial invasion has been eliminated. If this interpretation is correct, the polymorphonuclear leukocytes may be looked upon as the "shock troops" that play the major role in controlling the infection, whereas the macrophages serve primarily to remove the particulate debris from the resolving exudate and thus promote clearing of the lesion.

RESOLUTION. One of the most remarkable features of pneumococcal pneumonia is the completeness with which it resolves. Even when several lobes are completely consolidated, recovery usually results in restoration of the entire pulmonary parenchyma to its normal state within a few weeks. Not all the processes that take part in this dramatic resolution have been identified, but they include (1) the action of cytolytic enzymes upon disintegrating leukocytes; (2) transport of cells from the lesion via lymphatics; and (3) phagocytosis and digestion of cellular debris by macrophages. The rarity with which tissue necrosis occurs in pneumococcal pneumonia, despite the violence of the inflammatory response, appears to account for the completeness of the healing. Occasionally recovery proceeds more slowly than usual and leads to "delayed resolution." The factors responsible for delaying the removal of exudate from the lesion in such cases are not known. In rare instances, as the result of irreversible damage to the pulmonary parenchyma, resolution fails to take place altogether, and the lesion becomes the site of intense fibroblastic activity that leads to permanent scarring or "organized pneumonia."

Infection with type 3 pneumococcus may occasionally lead to pulmonary necrosis and abscess formation. This pneumococcus has a large capsule that interferes with phagocytosis and accounts, at least in part, for its extraordinary pathogenicity.

SUPPURATIVE EXTRAPULMONARY FOCI. Suppurative pneumococcal lesions, which usually occur in such extrapulmonary sites as the pleura, pericardium, meninges, joints, mastoids, or accessory sinuses, resolve much less readily, even with intensive chemotherapy, than does uncomplicated pneumococcal pneumonia. In such areas of suppuration, phagocytosis appears to be relatively inefficient, because trapping of bacteria by leukocytes in the exudate is inefficient and many of the leukocytes in the exudate are not viable. Although a drug like penicillin may reach the organisms in a purulent focus, it may not destroy them, because pneumococci do not multiply rapidly in pus of long standing, and "resting" bacteria are not susceptible to the bactericidal action of penicillin. In fact, suppurative pneumococcal lesions may respond satisfactorily only when chemotherapy is combined with some form of drainage that removes the bulk of the necrotic exudate.

Clinical Manifestations. *Symptoms.* Victims of pneumococcal pneumonia are often seriously ill when first seen. The degree of prostration may be such that an adequate history can be obtained only from the family. The story of a mild nasopharyngitis preceding by several days the onset of major symptoms is frequently elicited. The first distressing symptom is usually a shaking chill, lasting for several minutes to a half hour. More than 80 per cent of patients with pneumococcal pneumonia experience one or more chills during the earliest stages of the disease. The initial rigor is often so violent as to cause the bed to shake and the patient's teeth to chatter. It is followed in about one case in three by vomiting. The initial chill usually coincides with bacterial invasion of the lung and marks the onset of fever. Several chills may occur at the start of pneumococcal pneumonia, but repeated attacks of rigor late in the disease suggest an extrapulmonary complication such as empyema, pneumonia caused by some other bacterium, or administration of antipyretics.

CHEST PAIN. In approximately 70 per cent of cases, severe chest pain occurs at the onset and may even precede the rigor. The pain, which is "stabbing" in character and exaggerated by cough and respiration, is caused by inflammation of the pleura resulting from the characteristically peripheral location of the initial lesion. There may be local tenderness in the chest wall at the site of the pleurisy. When the diaphragmatic surfaces of the pleura are affected, the pain may be referred either to the corresponding side of the lower chest wall and upper abdomen or to the shoulder. The patient may gain some relief from the knifelike pain by lying on the affected side, thereby splinting that half of the thorax.

COUGH. A cough may be absent at the onset, but usually is a prominent symptom during the course of the disease. Stimulation of the cough reflex results from irritation of the lower respiratory tract and from accumulation of mucus and exudate within the bronchial tree. Approximately 75 per cent of patients raise diffusely bloody or "rusty" sputum in contrast to "blood-streaked" sputum. The thorough mixing of the blood appears to be due to the fact that bleeding occurs directly into the alveolar exudate and thus constitutes an integral part of the inflammatory response to the infection. When the sputum is particularly sticky or jelly-like, type 3 pneumococcus or Klebsiella should be suspected, because both these organisms produce an inordinate amount of capsular polysaccharide that causes the exudate to be highly viscous.

FEVER AND TOXEMIA. Constant features of the disease are fever and toxemia, with the temperature usually ranging between 39.5 and 41°C. During the febrile period complaints of malaise, anorexia, weakness, myalgia, and general prostration are extremely common. Pneumococcal pneumonia may occasionally progress with great rapidity, and the general condition of the patient may deteriorate alarmingly within a few hours.

Physical Signs. Patients with well-established pneumococcal pneumonia appear acutely ill. There is moderate to severe respiratory distress. The nostrils dilate with each inspiration. Paroxysms of hacking cough, often productive of bloody or rusty sputum, occur during the examination. The chest pain, which is usually unilateral, may be so severe as to interfere with the patient's breathing and coughing; in these circumstances grunting expiration results. The location of the pain indicates immediately the approximate site of at least part of the lesion. The patient occasionally appears apprehensive and may even be delirious.

The temperature, pulse rate, and respiratory rate are usually elevated by the time the patient seeks the aid of a physician. The temperature should be taken by rectum, because oral measurement with the subject breathing rapidly through the mouth is likely to be inaccurate. The pulse pressure is characteristically widened, as in any high fever.

The skin is usually hot and moist, with beads of perspiration visible on the face and forehead. Cold extremities may indicate impending shock. Herpetic blisters are frequently noted about the mouth. The lips, mucous membranes, and nail beds are often cyanotic as a result of blood passing through poorly aerated lung. The cyanosis may be exaggerated by lowered respiratory exchange associated with rapid shallow breathing, often resulting from pleural pain. Icterus of the sclerae should be carefully looked for because of the prognostic significance of overt jaundice in pneumonia.

The ears should always be examined with an otoscope to exclude the presence of active otitis. Tenderness over a mastoid process or over an accessory nasal sinus should also be noted. The presence of exudate in the pharynx or over the tonsils suggests the possibility of streptococcal or adenoviral pneumonia. Definite nuchal rigidity may indicate pneumococcal meningitis, a serious complication of pneumonia. The neck veins must be carefully examined to detect the presence of increased venous pressure caused by complicating congestive heart failure. Deviation of the trachea constitutes an important sign of either atelectasis (toward the involved side) or pleural effusion (away from the involved side).

EXAMINATION OF THE CHEST.   Diminished respiratory excursion or a slight inspiratory lag of one side of the chest often reveals the site of the principal lesion. A localized area of tenderness in the chest wall, noted during percussion, may be one of the earliest signs of pleural invasion. Careful percussion and auscultation do not always reveal signs of consolidation. In early cases, particularly, there may be no conclusive physical signs. Lesions at a distance from the chest wall are difficult to outline by percussion. When consolidation is extensive, the typical findings of dullness to percussion, bronchial or tubular breath sounds, and fine crackling rales are easily elicited, except in the presence of complicating bronchial obstruction or extensive pleural effusion. A coarse "leathery" friction rub is frequently audible in the region of consolidation.

Examination of the heart may be difficult because of loud respiratory sounds. An apical systolic murmur is frequently heard during high fever and is often of no significance. Diastolic murmurs, on the other hand, arising from either the mitral or aortic valve, are usually indicative of underlying organic heart disease or complicating pneumococcal endocarditis. A pericardial friction rub often constitutes the first sign of spread of the pneumococcal infection to the pericardial cavity. Ventricular premature contractions are not uncommon in the presence of any moderate or severe infection.

ABDOMINAL DISTENTION.   Distention of the abdomen is frequently encountered. When tympany is noted in the left axilla and left upper quadrant, acute gastrectasia should be suspected. Occasionally, the examiner will note rigidity and even tenderness in one or both upper quadrants of the abdomen, suggesting a subdiaphragmatic lesion. This sign is usually due to referred pain resulting from involvement of the parietal pleura over the outer part of the diaphragm.

The neurologic examination is rarely abnormal in pneumococcal pneumonia except in the presence of meningitis or brain abscess. Digital examination of the rectum may be postponed if the patient is acutely ill, but in women a sufficiently complete pelvic examination should be performed to exclude the possibility of an infected abortion, which may lead to metastatic bacterial pneumonia.

Laboratory Findings.   As in most acute bacterial infections, the total leukocyte count in pneumococcal pneumonia is elevated, and there is a "shift to the left" in the differential count. The number of leukocytes in the peripheral blood during the active infection usually ranges from 15,000 to 40,000 per cubic millimeter; counts above 40,000 are occasionally encountered. Leukopenia (with a "shift to the left") is observed in fulminating pneumococcal infections, particularly in the presence of bacteremia and in alcoholics.

Although the presence and location of the pulmonary lesion can usually be determined by physical examination, confirmatory roentgenographic evidence is often helpful. Both posteroanterior and lateral views of the chest should be taken. Pneumococcal infection of the lungs usually begins in the right middle lobe or in one of the lower lobes. The pulmonary process is limited to a single lobe in the majority of patients. In fact, it is not unusual for the process to be limited to a single pulmonary segment. In the series of Austrian and Gold, collected since the introduction of antimicrobial drugs, fewer than one third of the patients with pneumococcal pneumonia and bacteremia had more than a single lobe involved. Bulging interlobar fissure may be observed occasionally in pneumococcal pneumonia, although it is much more characteristic of Friedländer's pneumonia.

Whenever the diagnosis of pneumococcal pneumonia is suspected, the patient's blood should be cultured. Anaerobic as well as aerobic cultures are recommended to ensure detection of pneumonia caused by a microbe other than pneumococcus. A blood culture positive for pneumococci provides important information regarding both etiology and prognosis.

Pneumococci are usually present in sputum, nasopharynx, and material aspirated from the trachea. Sputum for smear and culture may be difficult to obtain, but this usually can be accomplished by urging the patient to cough, or a paroxysm of cough can be induced by passing a nasal catheter into the trachea. If a sputum specimen cannot be obtained, a nasopharyngeal culture should be collected, because there is a high positive correlation between specific pneumococci isolated from cultures of the nasopharynx and from the sputum of patients with pneumococcal pneumonia. Transtracheal aspiration or lung puncture is not indicated for the diagnosis of bacterial pneumonia in the usual patient.

The sputum in pneumococcal pneumonia shows large numbers of gram-positive, lancet-shaped diplococci in association with polymorphonuclear leukocytes. Gram-positive cocci which are not pneumococci are frequently observed in sputum smears and account for the poor correlation of results of studies to identify pneumococci on Gram-stained sputum smears and on sputum cultures. Omniserum, a pool of antibody against 82 pneumococcal types, can be used for definitive identification of pneumococci in sputum. The results of the quellung reaction using omniserum correlate with the results of cultures in about 90 per cent of cases. Because the carrier rate of pneumococci in the general population may be quite high, positive identification of pneumococci in sputum or nasopharynx does not establish a definitive diagnosis of pneumococcal pneumonia.

Other laboratory examinations that may be of value in the management of the patient include blood electrolyte and urea determinations.

Clinical Course.   During the course of the disease the patient should be examined carefully once a day. More frequent physical examinations may unduly exhaust an acutely ill subject. The common complications of pneumococcal pneumonia should be specifically looked for during each examination, particularly when fever persists.

Defervescence.   The fever of untreated pneumococcal pneumonia either may terminate abruptly by "crisis" five to ten days after onset or may gradually subside by lysis. When effective antibacterial therapy is used, a dramatic crisis may occur within 24 hours, or the fever may persist for several days. Physical signs in the chest may also change, coarse sticky rales of resolution replacing the fine crepitant rales and tubular breath sounds of consolidation. Complete clearing of the pulmonary lesion may occur within a few days, but usually the auscultatory signs of resolution persist for a week or more after defervescence. If resolution is not complete within 21 days, it is arbitrarily classified as delayed. The promptness of defervescence and the speed of resolution are in general inversely proportional to the age and extent of the lesion at the time treatment is begun.

Crisis marking the start of recovery must be differentiated from the "pseudocrisis" occasionally noted at the onset of shock or at the time of interlobar spread of the infection. Although the temperature may fall precipitously during a pseudocrisis, the pulse rate remains elevated, and the patient's general condition fails to improve.

Relapse. Relapse may occur in pneumococcal pneumonia when chemotherapy is discontinued too soon. If fever, tachycardia, and other signs of active infection recur while the patient is still receiving penicillin therapy, it may usually be assumed that a previously unrecognized purulent complication of the pneumococcal infection (such as empyema) exists, that a drug-resistant secondary invader has gained a foothold in the lung, or that hypersensitivity of the patient to penicillin has caused the development of drug fever.

Complications. *Pleural Effusion.* The most common specific complication of pneumococcal pneumonia is pleurisy with effusion. In somewhat less than 10 per cent of cases, fluid can be demonstrated in the pleural cavity by either physical or roentgenographic examination. Such effusions are usually small, and, when sterile, are rarely of significance. They result from inflammation of the pleura overlying the lesion in the lung. Occasionally they may be of sufficient volume to cause respiratory embarrassment and necessitate thoracentesis. Whenever pleural effusion is detected in a patient who has failed to respond promptly to treatment, a thoracentesis should be performed in order to determine whether the fluid is infected and thus represents an early empyema.

Empyema. Empyema, though less common than sterile pleural effusion, is far more serious. Before the advent of chemotherapy, the incidence of this complication was approximately 5 per cent. With the use of penicillin, empyema is much less common (less than 2 per cent). Its presence is indicated by continued fever (often irregular), persistent leukocytosis, and signs of pleural effusion. Localized tenderness is frequently noted in the chest wall overlying the site of the lesion. The exudate in the pleural cavity may become loculated by thick, fibrinous adhesions. When the lesion is confined to an interlobar fissure or is located in the thoracic "gutter" adjacent to the spine, it may be detectable only by roentgenographic methods. Repeated exploratory thoracenteses, done preferably with the help of fluoroscopy, may be required to prove the presence of empyema. Its detection is of the greatest importance, because, once discovered, it is amenable to proper therapy, whereas, if left untreated, it may eventually drain exteriorly through the chest wall *(empyema necessitatis)* or rupture into a bronchus and cause a bronchopleural fistula. Rarely, empyema heals spontaneously, causing calcification of the pleura.

Meningitis and Endocarditis. Two serious complications of pneumococcal pneumonia that are often associated with one another are endocarditis and meningitis. Pneumococci usually localize on the aortic valve, producing aortic insufficiency. The development of pneumococcal endocarditis is rare at present. Equally serious is *pneumococcal meningitis* resulting from blood-borne metastasis to the meninges. About 20 per cent of cases of pneumococcal meningitis develop secondary to pneumo-

coccal infection of the lung. The meningitis is characterized by the presence in the pia-arachnoid of a heavily infected exudate, which may cause subarachnoid block or may lead to localized subarachnoid abscesses. Unless vigorous therapy is instituted promptly, the prognosis is hopeless. Even when treatment is intensive, the patient may fail to recover, or may sustain permanent damage to the brain.

Pericarditis. Like the other complications of pneumococcal pneumonia, pericarditis has also become relatively rare since the introduction of potent antimicrobial drugs. When the pericardium is invaded, the patient usually experiences precordial pain, and a leathery friction rub may be heard over the heart. Pericardial effusion usually results, causing a "dampening" of the heart sounds. If the fluid is sterile, the condition is benign, unless so large a volume accumulates as to cause cardiac tamponade. Empyema of the pericardium, on the other hand, is a serious complication requiring prompt and vigorous treatment. Pericardiocentesis is mandatory to establish the diagnosis of purulent pericarditis.

Other Specific Complications. Still rarer specific complications include peritonitis and pyogenic arthritis. Occasionally the pulmonary lesion of pneumococcal pneumonia fails to resolve even after many weeks, and finally is replaced by fibrous tissue.

Nonspecific Complications. Acute dilatation of the stomach (gastrectasia) and *paralytic ileus* occur particularly in patients suffering from anoxia and severe toxemia and give rise to gaseous distention of the abdomen (tympanites) that causes discomfort and often increases respiratory embarrassment. *Shock*, likewise, is a complication of severe toxemia and indicates a serious prognosis. *Congestive heart failure* occurs frequently as a complication of severe pneumonia in patients with underlying heart disease. As congestive heart failure is an important predisposing factor in bacterial pneumonia, it is not surprising that they are often associated, and obviously both must be treated. The diagnosis of congestive heart failure in the presence of pneumonia may at times be difficult, but should be considered in any patient with abnormal distention of neck veins, peripheral edema, an enlarged tender liver, and elevated venous pressure. Pulmonary signs of congestion may be unreliable, particularly if the pneumonia is bilateral.

Jaundice, the pathogenesis of which is controversial, may be related to lysis of erythrocytes in pneumonic lesions, depressed liver function resulting from anoxia, or focal hepatic necrosis consequent to the pneumococcal infection. Pneumococcal pneumonia may also precipitate hemolysis and jaundice in persons with glucose-6-phosphate dehydrogenase deficiency. The presence of prominent icterus usually indicates a poor prognosis, and may be associated with chronic liver disease, e.g., cirrhosis. As in any bedridden patient, *phlebothrombosis* may occur during pneumonia. Its early presence should suggest the possibility that the pulmonary lesion is due to infarction of the lung rather than to primary pneumonia. *Herpes labialis* occurs in at least 10 per cent of patients with pneumococcal pneumonia.

Differential Diagnosis. Pneumonia resulting from organisms other than pneumococcus may at times be difficult to differentiate from pneumococcal pneumonia. Only by bacteriologic study of the sputum can pneumonia caused by *Klebsiella pneumoniae* (Friedländer's bacillus), *Staphylococcus aureus,* or *group A Streptococcus* be identified. *Tuberculous pneumonia* rarely causes the acute prostration characteristic of coccal infection. *Mycoplasmal pneumonia* and other infections of the lungs, such as psittacosis and Q fever, do not often cause shaking chills, diffusely bloody sputum, severe pleural pain, or a marked leukocytosis, although they may at times be confused with acute bacterial pneumonia. *Tularemic pneumonia* and pneumonia caused by *H. influenzae,* especially common in young children, must also be considered. When the diagnosis is in doubt, repeated examinations of the sputum should be made, using both the Gram and "acid-fast" stains.

The most important noninfectious processes that must be differentiated from pneumococcal pneumonia are *pulmonary infarction* and *atelectasis.* Pulmonary infarction may be exceedingly difficult to differentiate from pneumonia. The dyspnea, pleural pain, hemoptysis, fever, physical signs of pulmonary consolidation, roentgenographic findings, and leukocytosis are all in keeping with an acute infection of the lungs. Frequently, however, the initial symptom is intense pleural pain of sudden onset; shaking chills rarely occur; there is no preceding history of respiratory infection; the fever is usually not high; frank hemoptysis is common; pulmonary signs, when present, appear early; and the total leukocyte count rarely reaches 20,000 per cubic millimeter. Moreover, although the chest signs develop rapidly in pneumococcal pneumonia, they appear right away with a pulmonary infarct. A combination of perfusion and ventilation scans may serve to differentiate infarction from pneumonia.

When a pulmonary infarct becomes infected, as sometimes happens, differentiation from primary bacterial pneumonia may be extremely difficult. Although in such cases the patients should receive antimicrobial treatment as in pneumonia, recognition of the infarction is of importance because of the need for anticoagulant therapy.

Pulmonary atelectasis, resulting from bronchial obstruction, not only may simulate pneumonia but often leads to serious infection of the lung if the bronchial obstruction is not relieved. Aspiration of mucus during or after surgical anesthesia is a common cause of atelectasis. Dyspnea, cough, chest pain, splinting of one side of the thorax, dullness to percussion, and suppressed breath sounds may all suggest primary pneumonia. Fever and leukocytosis also are noted when infection is present. As pulmonary atelectasis may be relieved by forced coughing and postural drainage or, if necessary, by bronchoscopy, it is important to differentiate it from primary pneumonia. Occasionally, sufficient shift of the mediastinum occurs to make the diagnosis obvious. Collapse of a segment of the lung may also result from chronic bronchial obstruction caused by bronchogenic carcinoma or aortic aneurysm.

Subdiaphragmatic infection may be confused with pneumonia. Subdiaphragmatic abscess, liver abscess, or other infections in the upper abdomen may extend to the diaphragm and produce local inflammation, small collections of pleural fluid, chest pain, and atelectasis secondary to decreased respiratory excursions. Conversely, pneumococcal pneumonia may simulate intra-abdominal disease. Pleurisy may result in pain referred to the abdomen so as to suggest acute appendicitis or cholecystitis.

Even when the diagnosis of pneumococcal pneumonia is established beyond doubt, the possibility of a second underlying lesion of the lung must be borne in mind. Chronic obstructive pulmonary disease or lung abscess may lead to repeated attacks of bacterial pneumonia and often becomes evident only after the pneumonic consolidation has resolved. Bronchogenic carcinoma, as well as pulmonary tuberculosis, must also be looked for in the follow-up examination.

Treatment. The treatment of pneumococcal pneumonia may best be discussed under three headings: (1) antibacterial therapy, (2) supportive measures, and (3) the treatment of complications. Before the advent of effective antibacterial therapy, supportive treatment was of the greatest importance. The introduction, first, of antipneumococcal serum and, later, of sulfonamides, penicillin, and the other antimicrobial drugs has so altered the management of pneumococcal pneumonia that today supportive treatment is rarely crucial, and serious complications are only occasionally encountered.

Antibacterial Therapy. PENICILLIN. Penicillin is at present the drug of choice in the treatment of pneumococcal pneumonia. All strains of the organism isolated in the United States and most other areas of the world are extremely susceptible to penicillin, and most are inhibited in broth by concentrations of less than 0.02 μg per ml. However, pneumococci relatively resistant to penicillin have been isolated frequently in New Guinea and rarely in Australia. The minimal inhibitory concentration of benzylpenicillin for these strains is 0.1 to 2.0 μg per ml. These strains are also relatively resistant to the penicillinase-resistant penicillins and cephalosporins, but are fully sensitive or only slightly resistant to ampicillin.

The effectiveness of antimicrobial treatment is due in part to the natural resistance of the host, which accounts for the destruction of a large proportion of the invading bacteria. Host resistance, which results primarily from the activity of phagocytic cells in the lung, when combined with the bacteriostatic and bactericidal effects of drug therapy, controls promptly all but the most malignant pneumonia. Even with no treatment at all, approximately seven of every ten patients with pneumococcal pneumonia eventually recover, but some will have experienced a very severe illness before recovery has occurred.

Antipneumococcal therapy should be initiated promptly, therefore, in order to halt the spread of the infection both locally and through the bloodstream. An effective method is to give aqueous procaine penicillin G intramuscularly in a dose of 300,000 units at 12-hour intervals. Some authorities recommend the administration of aqueous penicillin G by the intramuscular route in doses of 300,000 units several times during the first 24-hour period of observation in addition to the procaine penicillin. In the presence of shock, penicillin should be given intravenously. Treatment should be maintained for at least one week or until the temperature has been normal for 72 hours; if treatment is discontinued too soon, relapse of the infection occurs.

Penicillin may also be given by mouth. However, in a serious infection such as pneumococcal pneumonia, it is inadvisable to rely on oral penicillin therapy in acutely ill patients. In fact, parenteral therapy throughout probably provides the greatest margin of safety. If parenteral therapy is not feasible or advisable throughout the period of therapy, procaine penicillin G can be given parenterally initially and penicillin V can then be given orally after defervescence. When oral penicillin V is used, it should be given in a dosage of at least 250 mg every six hours.

Response to penicillin therapy is often dramatic. Bacteremia, when present at the start of treatment, clears within a few hours. A crisis, characterized by rapid defervescence and a striking subsidence of symptoms, occurs in less than 48 hours in approximately half the patients. The others experience a more gradual recovery, the temperature falling by lysis over a period of four to seven days. Frequently a secondary rise in temperature occurs after the crisis. This elevation is usually low-grade and subsides spontaneously within a few hours, or at most a few days.

When a patient's pneumonia fails to respond satisfactorily to penicillin therapy, three possible explanations should be considered: (1) that the patient is suffering from a serious complication such as empyema, endocarditis, meningitis, or pulmonary suppuration (possibly secondary to bronchogenic carcinoma); (2) that the primary infection is of nonpneumococcal origin and is due to an agent that is resistant to the action of penicillin, e.g., a penicillin-resistant strain of Staphylococcus or Klebsiella; or (3) that drug fever has developed as a result of penicillin hypersensitivity. Occasionally, patients will respond initially to treatment only to have unmistakable signs of persistent pneumonia subsequently develop, in spite of continued therapy. This sequence of events is usually due to the presence of a mixed infection, the initial response to treatment resulting from control of penicillin-susceptible organisms, and the relapse occurring as a result of persistence of a penicillin-resistant species. Re-examination of the sputum and modification of the antimicrobial therapy are immediately indicated. Patients with underlying chronic pulmonary disease are particularly prone to such mixed infections.

Persons giving a history of having had a penicillin reaction in the past should, of course, not be treated with penicillin.

OTHER ANTIMICROBIAL DRUGS. Cephalothin or cefazolin can be used as effective alternatives to penicillin for parenteral therapy in patients hypersensitive to penicillin. Patients hypersensitive to penicillin sometimes show cross-sensitivity to cephalosporins; a cutaneous scratch test with the cephalosporin to be used should probably be performed in these patients to determine whether the drug can be used as an alternative to penicillin. Cephalothin should be administered in doses of 1 gram every four hours by the intramuscular or intravenous route, and cefazolin should be given in doses of 0.5 gram every six hours. Erythromycin in doses of 250 mg every six hours by the oral route is also adequate for treatment of patients with a history of penicillin allergy, provided they are not severely ill. Methicillin, cloxacillin, and nafcillin are also effective in the treatment of pneumococcal pneumonia. Tetracyclines should not be used in treating pneumococcal infections unless the organism is known to be susceptible. The prevalence of tetracycline-resistant pneumococci has increased greatly in recent years, now exceeding 5 per cent in many areas of the world. Pneumococci are relatively resistant to gentamicin, and pneumococcal pneumonia has been shown to progress during the administration of this drug.

Supportive Treatment. Patients suffering from pneumococcal pneumonia should be kept at bed rest, and visitors to the sick room should be limited to the immediate family. Pleural pain, if mild, may be treated with codeine sulfate (30 to 60 mg) orally. A tight chest binder may relieve pain but is inadvisable because it inhibits effectiveness of cough. Hypoxemia should be treated with oxygen administered by nasal catheter or by mask. Acetylsalicylic acid should not be used, because it interferes with the utilization of the fever curve to evaluate response to therapy.

FLUID AND ELECTROLYTES. During the acute state of pneumococcal pneumonia, considerable fluid is lost from the body, chiefly through the skin as the result of high fever. Dehydration may develop rapidly and, if severe, may become a contributing factor in the development of shock. Intravenous fluids and electrolytes may be required to control dehydration. When hydration is adequate, the specific gravity of the urine should remain below 1.020. Pneumonia may occasionally lead to the syndrome of inappropriate secretion of antidiuretic hormone.

DIET. Many patients with pneumococcal pneumonia are too ill to tolerate a full diet and should receive only liquids during the height of the fever. Fruit juices, ginger ale, and soups are well tolerated. After the crisis a regular diet may be prescribed.

The patient should be kept in bed until the temperature is approximately normal and should be observed closely until the pneumonic lesion has resolved. As already emphasized, all patients should be subjected to a follow-up roentgenographic examination three to four weeks after recovery.

Treatment of Complications. SHOCK. Patients with peripheral vascular collapse (shock) resulting from severe pneumococcal pneumonia usually respond poorly to the accepted forms of antishock therapy. The prognosis is almost invariably grave when this complication develops. Oxygen therapy should be begun immediately, even if cyanosis is absent. The central venous pressure should be used as a guide for fluid replacement. The use of corticosteroids has not been demonstrated to be of value.

ABDOMINAL DISTENTION. Decompression is indicated if distention is severe. Acute gastric and ileal dilatation is best managed with the use of gastric suction; a rectal tube may be indicated if colonic distention is a problem.

DELIRIUM TREMENS. Delirium tremens may sometimes be difficult to control in patients with a history of chronic alcoholism. Restraints may be required. The safest sedative to control hyperactivity in these patients is diazepam (Valium) in a dose of 0.066 mg per kilogram every four to six hours.

EMPYEMA AND PERICARDITIS. The treatment of choice for empyema and purulent pericarditis is systemic antimicrobial therapy and surgical drainage. Injection of penicillin into the pleural or pericardial cavity is not required. Repeated needle aspirations are occasionally effective but do not provide effective drainage in most patients.

The treatment of the remaining two major complications of pneumococcal pneumonia, namely endocarditis and meningitis, is discussed in Ch. 192 and 201.

Prognosis. The case fatality rate in untreated pneumococcal pneumonia ranges from 20 to 40 per cent. The widespread use of sulfonamide drugs in the late 1930's resulted in a lowering of the fatality rate among treated patients to approximately 10 per cent. Penicillin therapy has lowered the rate still further. At present approximately 95 per cent of patients with pneumococcal pneumonia recover when properly treated with penicillin.

The prognosis in pneumococcal pneumonia is influenced adversely by each of the following: (1) old age (and also infancy), (2) late treatment, (3) infection with certain types of pneumococci (particularly types 2 and 3), (4) involvement of more than one lobe of the lung, (5) leukopenia, (6) occurrence of bacteremia, (7) jaundice, (8) the presence of complications (notably shock and meningitis), (9) pregnancy (particularly in the third trimester), (10) the presence of other disease such as heart disease or cirrhosis of the liver, and (11) alcoholic intoxication and delirium tremens. Through a consideration of these factors a rough estimate may be made of the severity of the infection in each case, and therapy may be modified accordingly.

Even with the most intensive penicillin treatment, a significant number of patients will die of pneumococcal pneumonia. A recent study, for example, has revealed that in patients destined, at the onset of illness, to die within five days (because of complicating disease, old age, etc.), penicillin therapy has little if any effect. Similarly, the case fatality rate in type 3 pneumococcal pneumonia with bacteremia still exceeds 50 per cent regardless of treatment.

Prevention. Because pneumococcal pneumonia is not highly contagious and usually responds promptly to early therapy, prophylaxis constitutes less of a problem than in many other infectious diseases. It is estimated that only one in every 500 persons of all ages in the United States may be expected to contract the disease in any one year.

Although pneumococcal pneumonia can undoubtedly be prevented (or at least aborted) in many patients by the intensive treatment of every upper respiratory tract infection with antimicrobial drugs, their use for this purpose should be avoided. The possible inconvenience to the patient of hypersensitivity reactions and the danger of favoring drug-resistant strains of bacteria outweigh the advantages to be gained in preventing such a relatively uncommon and readily treatable disease as pneumococcal pneumonia. Some authorities do recommend penicillin prophylaxis for children with sickle cell anemia less than three or four years of age whose circulating erythrocytes contain Howell-Jolly bodies as an indicator of splenic hypofunction.

During recent years Austrian has redirected attention to the possibility of specific immunization as a means of preventing pneumococcal infection. During World War II, MacLeod and colleagues showed in controlled experiments in man that pneumococcal polysaccharides are effective antigens, evoking the formation of antibody that persists for years and that confers type-specific immunity to pneumococcal infection. Austrian has proposed immunization of that portion of the population at greatest risk with the types of pneumococci that are most often responsible for disease. Austrian's recent data, reported in 1972, show that 62 per cent of 2000 cases of pneumococcal bacteremia in adults were caused by six types (1, 3, 4, 7, 8, 12), that 70 per cent of 100 bacteremias in the pediatric age group were caused by six types (1, 6, 14, 18, 19, 23), and that 70 per cent of 300 isolates from otitis media in children were caused by seven types (1, 3, 6, 14, 18, 19, 23). Since high risk groups can be identified and a large proportion of infections are caused by a few pneumococcal types, studies on the value

of immunization are indicated and are in progress. Whether effective immunization of certain groups by polysaccharide vaccines will be followed by an increasing occurrence of infections with other pneumococcal types is unknown but is a definite possibility.

Patient Isolation. The cross-infection rate in pneumococcal pneumonia is low, and patients receiving chemotherapy are probably not highly infectious. Isolation is not indicated in the usual patient.

Austrian, R.: Current status of bacterial pneumonia with especial reference to pneumococcal infection. J. Clin. Path. [suppl.] 21:93, 1968.
Austrian, R.: Pneumococcal infections in sickle cell anemia. Am. J. Dis. Child., 123:614, 1972.
Austrian, C. R., and Austrian, R.: Pneumococcal pneumonia (lobar pneumonia). In Tice's Practice of Medicine. Hagerstown, Md., W. F. Prior Company, 1959, Vol. 1, p. 1.
Austrian, R., and Gold, J.: Pneumococcal bacteremia with especial reference to bacteremic pneumococcal pneumonia. Ann. Intern. Med., 60:759, 1964.
Bisno, A. L.: Hyposplenism and overwhelming pneumococcal infection—a reappraisal. Am. J. Med. Sci., 262:101, 1971.
Coonrod, J. D., and Rytel, M. W.: Detection of type-specific pneumococcal antigens by counterimmunoelectrophoresis. II. Etiologic diagnosis of pneumonia. J. Lab. Clin. Med., 81:778, 1973.
Heffron, R.: Pneumonia with Special Reference to Pneumococcus Lobar Pneumonia. New York, Commonwealth Fund, 1939.
Kauffman, C. A., Watanakunakorn, C., and Phair, J. P.: Purulent pneumococcal pericarditis. A continuing problem in the antibiotic era. Am. J. Med., 54:743, 1973.
Lukems, J. N.: Hemoglobin S, the pneumococcus and the spleen. Am. J. Dis. Child., 123:6, 1972.
Wood, W. B.: Studies on the Cellular Immunology of Acute Bacterial Infections. The Harvey Lectures, Series 47, 1951–52.
Wood, W. B., and Smith, M. R.: An experimental analysis of the curative action of penicillin. J. Exp. Med., 103:487, 1956.

KLEBSIELLA AND OTHER GRAM-NEGATIVE BACTERIAL PNEUMONIAS

Jay P. Sanford

181. INTRODUCTION

The combination of improved identification of gram-negative bacilli by diagnostic laboratories and the increased frequency of their isolation from clinical specimens has resulted in a striking increase in recognition of various gram-negative bacilli as serious human pathogens. Previously, procedures for the identification of gram-negative bacilli were primarily designed to enable rapid detection of Salmonella and Shigella from fecal specimens and Klebsiella from sputum specimens, with a lumping of the remaining organisms as "coliforms." Today, members of three families of aerobic gram-negative bacteria (Enterobacteriaceae, Pseudomonaceae, and Achromobacteraceae) have been recognized as potential pulmonary pathogens. The family Enterobacteriaceae is composed of numerous interrelated bacilli, all of which are gram-negative, are nonsporing, grow on ordinary media, and rapidly ferment glucose. The following genera are included in the family: Shigella, Escherichia, Salmonella, Arizona, Citrobacter, Edwardsiella, Klebsiella, Enterobacter (formerly Aerobacter), Hafnia, Serratia, Proteus, and Providence. Whereas the Enterobacteriaceae have received considerable attention, the nonfermenting aerobic gram-negative bacilli are being recognized with increased frequency. Organisms that fall into this category include *Pseudomonas aeruginosa, P. maltophilia, P. pseudomallei, P. cepacia, P. stutzeri, Acinetobacter lwoffi* (previously *Mima polymorpha*), *Acinetobacter anitratus* (previously *Herellea vaginicola* and *Achromobacter anitratus*), *Moraxella spp., Alcaligenes spp., Flavobacterium spp.,* and *Aeromonas hydrophilia.*

Pulmonary infections associated with the small aerobic gram-negative bacilli belonging to the genera Bordetella, Brucella, Hemophilus, Pasteurella and Yersinia and nonsporulating anaerobic gram-negative bacilli, e.g., Bacteroides, Fusobacterium, Dialister, will be discussed elsewhere. Infections caused by *Pseudomonas pseudomallei* (melioidosis) are presented in Ch. 220.

182. PNEUMONIA DUE TO KLEBSIELLA PNEUMONIAE
(Friedländer's Pneumonia)

In 1882, Friedländer first cultivated the organism now designated as *Klebsiella pneumoniae* from the lungs of patients who had died of pneumonia. Although he considered it to be the etiologic agent in most cases of pneumonia, four years later the pneumococcus was described and established as the predominant etiologic agent in lobar pneumonia. Consequently for many years *Klebsiella pneumoniae* (Friedländer's bacillus) was thought to be only a secondary invader. It is now recognized that a small but definite percentage, 0.5 to 5.0 per cent, of primary pneumonias are due to *Klebsiella pneumoniae.* This historical background is of interest because it reflects the current disagreements regarding the role of other gram-negative bacilli as primary pulmonary pathogens.

Pathogenicity. Klebsiella may persist in the oropharynx of normal persons, although the prevalence is low, 1 to 6 per cent. There is no tendency for contacts to acquire the organism from a carrier, and Bloomfield was unable to implant organisms in the pharynx of healthy volunteers. Yet the prevalence in pharyngeal cultures increases to 8 to 23 per cent in hospitalized subjects. Pulmonary infections arise most likely from the inhalation or aspiration of organisms from the oropharynx during circumstances when the major pulmonary antibacterial defense mechanisms, the mucociliary blanket, or alveolar macrophages are compromised.

The pathogenesis of experimental Klebsiella pneumonia is similar to that of encapsulated type 1 pneumococcal pneumonia. The outer margin of the spreading lesion is characterized by an edema zone in which the alveoli are filled with fluid containing many bacteria (see illustration in Ch. 180). The organisms multiply freely in the fluid, and are carried mechanically into adjacent alveoli through the pores of Kohn. Phagocytosis is noticeable only in the central zone of consolidation where alveoli are packed with leukocytes, thus allowing "surface phagocytosis." Three differences in experimental Klebsiella pneumonia in comparison with type 1 pneumococcal pneumonia are (1) greater numbers of Klebsiella in the areas of consolidation, (2) destruction of alveolar walls, and (3) organization with fibroblastic activity.

Klebsiella pulmonary infections are usually classified as primary, i.e., infection developing in a patient without underlying disease, or secondary. The demarcation between primary and secondary is often indistinct, as classic primary Klebsiella pneumonia usually occurs in patients with underlying conditions such as alcoholism, chronic obstructive airways disease (emphysema-fibrosis), or diabetes mellitus. Operationally, infections may be considered as primary if Klebsiella organisms are isolated from specimens obtained when the patient first seeks medical aid. The designation "secondary" is then applied to those infections that either represent superinfection of an underlying infection or are opportunistic in origin.

Predisposing Factors. In patients with primary pneumonia, males heavily predominate (80 to 90 per cent), most infections occurring in middle-aged and older patients (average age being the mid-50's). The most common co-existing disease is alcoholism (66 per cent). The few series in which alcoholism is not frequent are drawn from predominantly black populations. Both chronic bronchopulmonary disease and to a lesser extent diabetes mellitus appear to predispose patients to Klebsiella pneumonia.

Pathology. The involvement in fatal primary Klebsiella pneumonia is most often lobar, but may be lobular or a combination of the two. An upper lobe is most commonly involved. The pleural surface is covered by a fibrinous exudate and adhesions form early. Empyema is appreciably more frequent than in pneumococcal pneumonia, probably occurring in one fifth to one quarter of cases. Microscopically in the acute stage, the alveolar walls are congested. Usually the alveoli are filled with an exudate composed of a mixture of polymorphonuclear and mononuclear cells, with a predominance of the former. In rare cases, mononuclear cells may predominate. There is often necrosis of alveolar walls, with abscess formation. Other findings at autopsy may include extrapulmonary sites of dissemination, e.g., pericarditis or meningitis. Evidence of alcoholic hepatosis and alcoholic cirrhosis is common.

Clinical Manifestations and Course. Based upon clinicobacteriologic findings, Klebsiella infections can be classified as primary or secondary (as defined under Pathogenicity, above); pure or mixed, depending upon whether klebsiellae are isolated as the predominant organism or associated with other organisms, especially other gram-negative bacilli; and acute or chronic.

Primary Klebsiella Pneumonia. The "classic" clinical pattern is that of acute primary Klebsiella pneumonia. As with pneumococcal pneumonia, the onset is usually sudden (90 per cent), associated with cough productive of sputum (90 per cent), pleuritic chest pain (80 per cent), and true rigors (60 per cent). Early prostration is a usual feature. Occasionally the acute onset is preceded by an undifferentiated upper respiratory infection and cough. Rarely epigastric pain and vomiting are the initial symptoms. The characteristic sputum has been described as a nonputrid homogeneous thick mixture of blood and mucus, often brick red in color, which is sufficiently thick to be expectorated with difficulty. This typical sputum is seen in one quarter to three quarters of patients. In some patients the sputum is thin, resembling currant jelly, although in most it is either blood tinged or rusty. Frank hemoptysis may occur. On examination, patients appear acutely ill, febrile, dyspneic, and often cyanotic. Although temperatures are often said to be less than those observed with pneumococcal pneumonia, two thirds are between 39 and 40° C. Tachycardia coincides with the fever. Chest examination typically reveals signs of pulmonary consolidation; there may be loss of lung volume as manifested by decreased size and expansion of the involved hemithorax and diaphragmatic elevation. Auscultation may reveal suppressed breath sounds with few rales, even with advanced consolidation. Involvement of more than one lobe is frequent (in two thirds of patients) with a predilection for upper lobes.

Laboratory and Roentgenographic Findings. Peripheral leukocyte counts range from marked leukopenia to leukocytosis, leukopenia and neutropenia being poor prognostic signs. In one quarter of patients the total leukocyte count may be in the normal range. On sputum culture, either gram-negative bacilli other than Klebsiella or pneumococci often may be isolated. A mixed sputum flora containing other gram-negative bacilli such as *Pseudomonas spp.* is especially common in secondary infections. In the prechemotherapeutic era, blood cultures were positive in about 15 per cent of cases during the course of the illness. At present, a pulmonary source is still often incriminated in patients with Klebsiella bacteremia. This is unusual in other types of gram-negative bacillary bacteremia, in which the urinary tract usually represents the major primary source.

The roentgenographic features are variable, and include massive lobar consolidation, lobular involvement, lung abscess formation with either multiple small thin-walled or large abscess cavities, and residual parenchymal fibrosis. Bulging of a fissure, sharp advancing borders of the infiltrates, and abscess formation occur with greater frequency than in other types of pneumonia. The pneumonic infiltrate is relatively dense, but shadows of similar density are seen with other types of pneumonia. Bronchopneumonic distribution is less usual but can occur, and even bilateral perihilar infiltrates are reported. The diagnostic usefulness for any given roentgenographic configuration has been questioned; however, in many instances a correct diagnosis can be suggested from the roentgenogram.

Complications. Rapid destruction of pulmonary tissue with suppuration or residual fibrosis occurs in as many as half of the surviving patients. Necrosis may occur within 24 to 48 hours, and abscess formation may be recognized within four days. Other less common pulmonary complications include pleural effusion and pneumothorax. In the past, activation of quiescent pulmonary tuberculosis has been reported.

The course of illness is not marked by an unusual propensity for extrapulmonary manifestations, but they can occur, and include pericarditis, meningitis, gastroenteritis, erythematous skin rashes, and nonsuppurative polyarthritis.

Prognosis and Treatment. In the pre-antimicrobial era, the case mortality of Klebsiella pneumonia ranged from 51 to 97 per cent. With the advent of drug therapy, the various tetracycline derivatives, streptomycin, and chloramphenicol were found to have an excellent in vitro effect, and clinical use resulted in a marked decrease in mortality in most series. In some series, the mortality remains nearly 50 per cent; in these there has been a predominance of severely ill alcoholic patients, although good results have been reported even in this group. Analysis of the mode of death frequently reveals inadequate removal of tenacious pulmonary secretions to be a signif-

icant factor. The correlation of bloodstream invasion and fatality is frequently close.

In vitro studies reveal the majority of strains of Klebsiella to be susceptible to cephalothin, cefazolin, chloramphenicol, colistimethate, gentamicin, kanamycin, polymyxin B, and tobramycin. The antimicrobial regimen of choice is often varied according to the gravity of the acute clinical situation and the extent of underlying problems. In less seriously ill patients, cephalothin or gentamicin is preferable, but in patients with life-threatening infections combination therapy, e.g., cephalothin or cefazolin and kanamycin, gentamicin, or tobramycin, is usually employed. Meticulous measures directed at supportive care, maintenance of clear airways, adequate but not excessive ventilation and oxygenation, adequate fluid and electrolyte replacement, and often control of delirium tremens are essential.

183. PNEUMONIA DUE TO AEROBIC GRAM-NEGATIVE BACILLI OTHER THAN KLEBSIELLA PNEUMONIAE

The large number of bacterial species other than *Klebsiella pneumoniae* that belong to the families Enterobacteriaceae, Pseudomonaceae, and Achromobacteraceae are considered together because of the similarities in their abilities to produce pulmonary infection.

Until recently the over-all frequency of pneumonia caused by gram-negative bacilli other than Klebsiella received relatively little attention. Between 1963 and 1965, 4.3 per cent of all pneumonias of patients admitted to the Detroit General Hospital were caused by gram-negative bacilli (82 episodes, 78 of which were classified as primary). In 1967–1968, of 292 patients admitted to Grady Memorial Hospital (Atlanta) with pneumonia, the disease in 167 could be attributed to specific bacterial pathogens; of these, 33 (20 per cent) were due to gram-negative bacilli. Among these gram-negative bacillary pneumonias, the following organisms were encountered: *Klebsiella pneumoniae, Enterobacter aerogenes, Escherichia coli, Pseudomonas spp.*, Bacteroides, Proteus, *H. influenzae*, and Achromobacter. In addition, in many hospitals other gram-negative organisms such as nonpigmented *Serratia marcescens* are being encountered, especially in hospital-associated secondary pneumonias. It appears that collectively gram-negative bacilli other than Klebsiella may be more prevalent than Klebsiella in causing both primary pneumonia and secondary hospital-acquired pneumonias.

Predisposing Factors. As with primary Klebsiella pneumonia, in primary pneumonias caused by these other agents, older males are more often affected. Underlying disease conditions occur in almost all patients; these include heart disease, alcoholism, renal disease, diabetes mellitus, and chronic bronchopulmonary disease, especially cystic fibrosis. Primary gram-negative bacillary pneumonia may be more common during the summer.

Infections most frequently occur in patients who are receiving inhalation therapy that incorporates reservoir nebulization and who are also receiving antimicrobial therapy. Adrenocortical steroids, immunosuppressive agents, cytotoxic chemotherapy, and tracheostomy may also be predisposing factors. However, such infections may occur in patients who are not receiving inhalation therapy, as these organisms are ubiquitous and appear with increased frequency in seriously ill patients.

Pathology. On microscopic section, bronchopneumonia with confluent microabscesses is seen. The intraalveolar inflammatory exudate is mixed polymorphonuclear leukocytic and mononuclear. With infection caused by E. coli and Pseudomonas, however, the cellular infiltrates may consist predominantly of mononuclear cells admixed with fragmented pyknotic nuclei of necrotic neutrophils. At a later stage, alveolar spaces are filled with a deeply basophilic granular material containing large macrophage-like cells and dense colonies of gram-negative bacilli.

When caused by Pseudomonas, in the areas of an abscess there is often focal hemorrhage. The dominant microscopic lesion is that of alveolar septal necrosis. In association with these necrotizing lesions, necrosis of arterial walls and secondary thrombosis of vessels have been encountered when the Pseudomonas pneumonia was of bacteremic origin or associated with nebulization therapy equipment. With the primary Pseudomonas pneumonia reported by Tillotson and Lerner, the vascular involvement was not a feature. *Pseudomonas cepacia* was also associated with a necrotizing granulomatous pneumonia. With the other non-Klebsiella gram-negative bacilli, alveolar septal necrosis is not a usual feature.

Clinical Features and Course. The clinical features are generally similar to those observed in patients with primary Klebsiella pneumonia, except that hemoptysis is unusual.

In patients with Pseudomonas pneumonia, apprehension, toxicity, confusion, and progressive cyanosis are characteristic. Relative bradycardia may occur. Alteration in diurnal temperature patterns with the peak temperature in early morning was noted by Tillotson and Lerner. The physical signs over the thorax are not characteristic. The development of empyema is common (22 to 80 per cent). Roentgenograms reveal bilateral bronchopneumonic infiltrates, usually lower lobe, that often are nodular and may undergo necrosis with abscesses which may be small but are often greater than 1 cm in diameter. A pattern of interstitial infiltration may be seen.

Primary E. coli pneumonia tends to present as a bronchopneumonic process in the lower lobes. The pulse is proportional to the temperature. Early findings include rales without consolidation. Empyema formation is less common than with Klebsiella or Pseudomonas.

Proteus species also produce a clinical picture similar to Klebsiella, with fever, chills, dyspnea, pleuritic chest pain, and cough productive of purulent sputum. Signs of consolidation are usual. Roentgenograms reveal dense infiltrates in the posterior segment of an upper lobe or superior segment of the right lower lobe. Progression to lung abscess or empyema is common.

Serratia infections, which are almost always secondary, have been associated with the clinical oddity "pseudohemoptysis" owing to the red pigment prodigiosin produced by some strains of *Serratia marcescens*. Other features may include abscess formation or empyema, or both.

Clinical experience with the other bacterial genera such as Hafnia, Flavobacterium, Mima, and Herellea, is limited, but other characteristics suggest that their clinical features are similar to secondary Klebsiella infections.

Laboratory Findings. The usual laboratory findings such as leukocyte counts are of little help, being either normal or moderately increased. Cultures of sputum are only of moderate help, because these organisms are frequently present as commensals in patients who are receiving antimicrobial therapy or in those who are critically ill. Specimens collected by the transtracheal technique in which neutrophils are present and gram-negative bacilli are stained and cultured are most helpful in making a diagnosis. With empyema, thoracentesis with staining and culture of the fluid will confirm the diagnosis and facilitate the selection of optimal therapy.

Prognosis and Treatment. Prognosis varies with the type of organism as well as with the underlying condition of the patient. Mortality rates in the range of 80 per cent are not uncommon with Pseudomonas pneumonia, whereas they may be lower with the other organisms.

The antimicrobial regimen of choice may be selected according to antimicrobial susceptibilities anticipated in a given community but must be confirmed by tests on an individual patient's organism. In general, *Pseudomonas aeruginosa* and *Enterobacter aerogenes* are most susceptible to carbenicillin, colistimethate, gentamicin, polymyxin B, and tobramycin. In contrast, *Pseudomonas cepacia* may be susceptible only to chloramphenicol. E. coli is susceptible to the same agents as *Ps. aeruginosa*, and in addition most strains are susceptible to cephalothin or cefazolin. *Serratia marcescens* and the indole-positive *Proteus spp.* are most susceptible to gentamicin and tobramycin. As with Klebsiella pneumonia, in pneumonias caused by these other gram-negative bacilli, meticulous attention to supportive care is as important as the antimicrobial therapy.

Bloomfield, A. L.: The fate of bacteria introduced into the upper air passages. V. The Friedländer bacilli. Bull. Hopkins Hosp., 31:203, 1920.
Hyde, L., and Hyde, B.: Primary Friedländer pneumonia. Am. J. Med. Sci., 205:660, 1943.
Jervey, L. P., Jr., and Hamburger, M.: The treatment of acute Friedlaender's bacillus pneumonia. Arch. Intern. Med., 99:1, 1957.
Johanson, W. G., Pierce, A. K., Sanford, J. P., and Thomas, G. D.: Nosocomial respiratory infections with gram-negative bacilli. Ann. Intern. Med., 77:701, 1972.
Manfredi, F., Daly, W. J., and Behnke, R. H.: Clinical observations of acute Friedländer pneumonia. Ann. Intern. Med., 58:642, 1963.
Pennington, J. E., Reynolds, H. Y., and Carbone, P. P.: Pseudomonas pneumonia. Am. J. Med., 55:155, 1973.
Pierce, A. K., Edmondson, E. B., McGee, G., Ketchersid, J., Loudon, R. G., and Sanford, J. P.: An analysis of factors predisposing to gram-negative bacillary necrotizing pneumonia. Am. Rev. Respir. Dis., 94:309, 1966.
Pierce, A. K., Sanford, J. P., Thomas, G. D., and Leonard, J. S.: Long-term evaluation of decontamination of inhalation-therapy equipment and the occurrence of necrotizing pneumonia. N. Engl. J. Med., 282:528, 1970.
Rose, H. D., Heckman, M. G., and Unger, J. D.: *Pseudomonas aeruginosa* pneumonia in adults. Am. Rev. Respir. Dis., 107:416, 1973.
Sullivan, R. J., Dowdle, W. R., Marine, W. M., and Hierholzer, J. C.: Adult pneumonia in a general hospital. Arch. Intern. Med., 129:935, 1972.
Tillotson, J. R., and Lerner, A. M.: Characteristics of pneumonia caused by *Escherichia coli*. N. Engl. J. Med., 277:115, 1967.
Tillotson, J. R., and Lerner, A. M.: Characteristics of nonbacteremic pseudomonas pneumonia. Ann. Intern. Med., 68:295, 1968.

STREPTOCOCCAL DISEASES

184. INTRODUCTION

Gene H. Stollerman

Streptococci constitute a large heterogeneous group of gram-positive bacteria that are very common parasites of man. Their name derives from their growth in liquid media as chains of globular bacteria. Classification of streptococci has been confusing, because a single species may cause a variety of diseases and because several kinds of streptococci can often be cultured from the same site of infection.

CLASSIFICATION

The modern classification of streptococci is based upon Lancefield's identification of the group-specific cell wall "C" carbohydrate antigens which are present in beta-hemolytic streptococci and in some nonhemolytic species as well.

Group A Infections. The most important human streptococcal pathogen, *Streptococcus pyogenes*, can be identified as containing group A carbohydrate with specific rabbit antiserum to the carbohydrate cell wall antigens, and thus can be distinguished from other beta-hemolytic streptococci which are also frequently isolated from the respiratory tract of man. Diseases caused by group A streptococci will be considered in detail in Ch. 185 to 191 and in Ch. 610. Streptococci belonging to other serogroups that are of importance to man will be mentioned briefly here.

The traditional classification of streptococci by their properties of hemolysis on the surface of blood agar plates is clinically useful. It helps to distinguish hemolytic streptococci, to which the more virulent species belong, from the alpha-hemolytic *Streptococcus viridans* ("green" streptococci), the predominant normal flora of the upper respiratory tract, and the nonhemolytic streptococci which include the *enterococci,* a common inhabitant of the gastrointestinal tract.

Beta-hemolytic streptococci are those that produce a completely clear zone around the colony as a result of the formation of either extracellular hemolysin, streptolysin O and streptolysin S, or both. Classification of streptococci based on the type of hemolysis they produce, however, is unsatisfactory for many reasons. Many species belonging to specific serologic groups may be nonhemolytic, such as group D. On the other hand, some enterococci belonging to the usually nonhemolytic group D may produce beta hemolysis, or some apparently nonhemolytic colonies may become alpha hemolytic upon prolonged incubation. Beta hemolysis is therefore primarily useful in the first step of the identification of group A organisms which are, with only rare exceptions, consistently hemolytic.

Group B Infections. The group B organisms are classically represented by the species *Streptococcus agalactiae.* They were well known for many years as the cause of bovine mastitis but produced human disease rarely. Until recently, little attention was paid to group B organisms in man, although it was known that they could colonize the vagina and genitourinary tract and were occasionally found in the upper respiratory tract as well. In fact, between 5 and 10 per cent of hemolytic streptococci isolated from man were identified in many studies as group B. In the past decade, however, group B streptococci have been reported with increasing frequency as a cause of perinatal infections. In the preantibiotic era, group A streptococci were the common agent of puerperal fever. Since the early 1960's, however, group B streptococci have emerged as a major cause of puerperal infection and as a cause of neonatal sepsis, with or without meningitis.

The frequency with which group B streptococci are recovered from the female genital tract (and the male genitourinary tract as well) appears to be increasing, and cervicovaginal carrier rates in normal pregnant women vary from 3 to 6 per cent. In some studies, approximately one third of infants born to such carriers have contracted serious group B infections. Group B organisms also seem to be causing bacteremic complications of pyelonephritis in both men and women more often than heretofore, especially in diabetics and other compromised hosts. These infections have remained susceptible to penicillin so far.

Group D Infections. This group includes *Streptococcus faecalis,* often referred to as *enterococcus* because of the frequency with which it is found in the human gastrointestinal tract. Enterococci may also be cultured from the oropharynx and, although usually nonhemolytic, some strains can produce beta or alpha hemolysis. *S. faecalis* is an exceptionally hardy organism which can resist heat (62° C for 30 minutes), grow well at room temperature, multiply in hypertonic media (6.5 per cent sodium chloride), and grow in the presence of 0.05 per cent sodium azide.

Enterococci are often isolated from the blood in bacterial endocarditis and from the urine in urinary tract obstruction. The precise role of these organisms in the pathogenesis of pyelonephritis has not been fully evaluated. They can be associated with suppurative abdominal lesions, especially after bowel surgery.

The failure of some laboratories to distinguish the enterococci from other streptococci often leads to inappropriate therapy in serious infections. These organisms may also be recovered from the respiratory tract and may be regarded mistakenly as penicillin-resistant group A streptococci. This error occurs most often during the post-treatment follow-up study of cases of group A streptococcal sore throat and may lead to needless overtreatment in an attempt to eradicate the organisms from the pharynx. It cannot be emphasized too strongly that enterococci do *not* cause pharyngitis and tonsillitis.

Streptococci of Other Groups. Strains of groups C, E, G, H, K, and O are isolated from the respiratory tract of man but are of little clinical significance. "Human" group C strains may occasionally cause illnesses that resemble those of group A, but such infections are relatively rare. Moreover, as far as is known, only group A organisms cause rheumatic fever. Group G may occasionally cause mild infections, but these are relatively infrequent and are uncomplicated. Groups A, C, and G all elaborate in vivo antigenically similar streptolysin O, streptokinase, hyaluronidase, and erythrogenic toxin.

Alpha-Hemolytic Streptococci ("Green" Streptococci). The alpha-hemolytic streptococci are often referred to found to be noninfective when inoculated into the throats of human volunteers. Children, among whom infection is commonplace and healthy carriers are abundant, are primarily responsible for the spread of streptococcal disease. The introduction of an untreated, infected five-year-old into a family will be followed by pharyngeal infection of more than half of his siblings and a significant number of adults in the household. The spread of an M-typable, virulent strain of group A Streptococcus through a family occurs much more readily than that of non-M-typable organisms. The problem of control of hemolytic streptococcal disease is complicated by the fact that a very large proportion of infections by these organisms is either exceedingly mild or completely inapparent. Persons with this type of "subclinical" infection are fully capable of disseminating the streptococci, but will not necessarily come under the care of a physician who could apply modern chemotherapy, eradicate streptococci from the pharyngeal tissues, and eliminate the possibility of transmission of the disease.

Epidemiologic factors such as climate, season, and geography are important primarily as they affect close contact of individuals. For example, military recruit populations, particularly when mobilized in large camps in cold climates and crowded housing conditions, provide the most ideal circumstances for the rapid passage of the organism from individual to individual, and such populations give rise to some of the most severe epidemics on record. Streptococcal disease is most severe in civilian populations when poverty and poor housing promote the most crowded living conditions.

In the temperate zones of the United States pharyngeal streptococcal infections vary strikingly with the season of the year. The peak incidence occurs between December and May, and only rare sporadic infections appear during the hot summer months. In recent family studies of a large metropolitan area in the northern part of the United States, it was estimated that a streptococcal infection occurs approximately once every three to four years during childhood and adolescence, and that in a middle class population in this metropolis only about 2 per cent of all respiratory illnesses that occurred were due to group A streptococcal infection.

The epidemiology of *scarlet fever* is the same as that of other group A streptococcal infections except that the strains producing the infection seem to be lysogenized by a bacteriophage that induces the production of erythrogenic toxin in a manner entirely analogous to diphtheria organisms that produce diphtheria toxin. Thus the epidemiology of scarlet fever is essentially that of any other strain of group A Streptococcus that does not produce the erythrogenic toxin. This explains the mild sporadic cases of scarlet fever, the severe epidemics of streptococcal pharyngitis *without* any scarlet fever cases, and the localized outburst of scarlet fever in a single concentrated population such as a school or institution.

The epidemiology of streptococcal pyoderma is strikingly different from that of streptococcal pharyngitis in several respects. Seasonal occurrence of the two is quite disparate in temperate climates: pharyngitis is more common and intense in cold weather, whereas streptococcal pyoderma occurs often in the late summer and early fall. The close indoor contact during the colder months may facilitate respiratory spread, whereas increased exposure of the uncovered skin to minor trauma and insect bites may favor skin infection during the warmer months. Although, geographically, epidemic

streptococcal pharyngitis is more common in temperate or cold climates and streptococcal pyoderma in hot or tropical climates, exceptions are not uncommon in both diseases.

Streptococcal pyoderma affects an even younger age group than pharyngitis, occurring most often in children of preschool age and in infants. Transmission of streptococcal pyoderma may be aided mechanically by insects, particularly flies, that are attracted to skin lesions. Poverty and filth, as well as crowding, are major predisposing factors. Patients with streptococcal pyoderma often harbor the same organisms in the throat that colonize the skin.

The Contrasting Epidemiology of Acute Rheumatic Fever and Acute Glomerulonephritis (see accompanying figure). Students of the nonsuppurative sequels of group A streptococcal infection have long been impressed with the extreme rarity with which ARF and AGN occur in the same patient at the same time, and the antecedent infection is considered, therefore, to be due to a strain that is *either* "rheumatogenic" *or* "nephritogenic," but not both! Simultaneous appearance of both sequelae has not been a feature of the reported experience of large numbers of patients with either disease in severe epidemics in which a single streptococcal strain could be identified as the cause (Rammelkamp, 1953). The route of infection also seems to differentiate rheumatogenic from nephritogenic strains. Acute rheumatic fever seems to be almost always, if not exclusively, a complication of a pharyngeal infection. Acute glomerulonephritis occurs after *either* skin or pharyngeal infection. Although skin strains often parasitize the throat, the best known rheumatogenic pharyngeal strains do not seem to parasitize the skin.

The strains which belong to the M serotypes that have clearly caused pharyngitis followed by rheumatic fever are those commonly encountered in the throats of children in the cities of the temperate zones of the United States and western Europe and include, among others, 1, 3, 5, 6, 14, 18, 19, and 24. *All* strains containing these M

Seasonal distribution of acute rheumatic fever (ARF) and acute glomerulonephritis (AGN) admissions at City of Memphis Hospitals, September 1965–August 1968. (After Bisno, A. L., Pearce, I. A., Wall, H. P., Moody, M. D., and Stollerman, G. H.: N. Engl. J. Med., 283: 561, 1970.)

antigens are not necessarily non-nephritogenic, and from time to time sporadic cases of AGN have appeared which seemed to be due to strains representing some of these serotypes (types 1, 3, and 6).

The identification of M type 12 organisms as the major pharyngeal serotype that has been associated with AGN (Rammelkamp et al., 1952) is of interest because this M serotype is perhaps the most common one encountered in the throats of schoolchildren, and yet AGN does not appear consistently in populations harboring this strain. Thus not all members of a given M serotype are necessarily nephritogenic.

The recent attention to the bacteriology of skin strains of streptococci has revealed them to contain M and T proteins of types hitherto unrecognized (types 49 and 52 to 60). Although AGN has occurred in association with most of the strains in these categories, no specific M or T antigen per se has been related to this complication.

The factors of infection determining the attack rate of rheumatic fever are also quantitative. The attack rate may vary from as low as 0.3 per cent after very mild, sporadic streptococcal infections associated with strains of low virulence to as high as 3 per cent or greater after infections with highly virulent strains of group A streptococci. The two factors that appear to have most influence on the frequency with which rheumatic fever follows a streptococcal infection are (1) the duration of convalescent carriage of the strain after the infection, and (2) the magnitude of the immunologic response associated with the infection. Thus patients with relatively feeble antistreptolysin O responses may show an attack rate of rheumatic fever of considerably less than 1 per cent, whereas those with the most vigorous streptococcal antistreptolysin O responses may suffer attack rates of rheumatic fever as high as 5 to 10 per cent. The acquisition of streptococci in the throat and their subsequent carriage *without* immunologic response has not been associated with reactivation of rheumatic fever in rheumatic subjects, nor do primary attacks of rheumatic fever occur very often without a well defined immune response. The epidemiology of rheumatic fever is therefore a reflection of the prevalence and severity of group A streptococcal pharyngitis.

CLINICAL SYNDROMES OF GROUP A STREPTOCOCCAL INFECTION

Gene H. Stollerman

186. STREPTOCOCCAL SORE THROAT

The classic syndrome described as most typical of group A streptococcal infection in older children and adults is as follows:

Symptoms. Sudden onset of sore throat, sometimes associated with abdominal pain and nausea, especially in children, and accompanied by constitutional symptoms of malaise, headache, and feverishness.

Signs. Redness and edema of the throat, and particularly the presence of an *exudate* on the tonsils or tonsillar fossae; enlargement and particularly *tenderness* of the anterior cervical nodes, and fever of 38.2° C or greater. Helpful laboratory data, other than results of throat culture, include leukocytosis greater than 12,000 leukocytes per cubic millimeter.

Although this classic syndrome is, indeed, associated with group A streptococcal infection, the full clinical picture develops in a minority of patients with pharyngitis, except during epidemics. Much more common in clinical practice is the patient with some, but not all, of the aforementioned signs and symptoms. It is not unusual for mild streptococcal disease to be associated with *nonexudative* pharyngitis, and, conversely, for viral infections, particularly adenovirus, to produce purulent tonsillar exudate and a syndrome indistinguishable from streptococcal tonsillitis. Hemolytic streptococci are the only significant *bacterial* cause of nonexudative pharyngitis. Many viral infections may mimic this clinical state, making the study of upper respiratory infection without bacteriologic control most difficult.

Streptococcal respiratory infection is not accompanied by significant cough or by coryza. The presence of either of these manifestations should suggest a different cause. Rhinorrhea does occur, especially in young children, who frequently develop suppurative sinusitis.

Scarlet Fever. The disease is clinically similar in almost all respects to tonsillitis and pharyngitis caused by nonscarlatinal strains of group A streptococci. Its name, however, comes from the presence of a skin rash caused by the erythrogenic toxin produced by scarlatinal strains. The erythrogenic effect of the toxin on the skin can be neutralized by antitoxin. This is the basis of the diagnostic *Schultz-Charlton reaction*. The injection of 0.1 ml of scarlet fever antitoxin, or of 0.2 to 0.3 ml of convalescent human serum, into an area where the rash is florid will be followed by blanching around the site of injection in 8 to 12 hours. Streptococcal antitoxin is no longer readily available, and usually clinical and bacteriologic studies suffice for diagnosis.

The enanthem of scarlet fever includes a tongue that may be bright red with large papillae (raspberry tongue) or coated with the red papillae protruding (strawberry tongue). These manifestations of the disease are rarely seen in adults. The rash usually appears on the second day of the disease. It consists of a diffuse, bright scarlet erythema with many points of deeper red. The distribution is variable, but the trunk and inner aspects of the arms and thighs are most often affected. In many cases the rash is clearly seen only in the axillae and groins. The face is flushed and red, but a pale area, the *circumoral pallor,* is often seen around the mouth. The palms and soles are not erythematous. Petechiae and occasionally ecchymoses are observed, especially in severely ill patients. The application of a tourniquet to the arm for five minutes will be associated with the appearance of large numbers of petechiae distal to the obstruction in nearly all cases. This is the *Rumpel-Leede* sign; it is not specific for scarlet fever. The erythema disappears usually by the sixth to the ninth day of infection in association with the return of the temperature and the throat to normal. Desquamation of the skin is characteristic of scarlet fever, and it begins as a fine scaling of the face and body that is usually completed during the second week. About this time the extensive and characteristic desquamation of the palms and soles starts and continues for one to two weeks. Often the diagnosis is made retrospectively in patients who show this desquamation after a sore throat and in whom the scarlatinal rash may have been overlooked. Eosinophilia may be a feature of scarlet fever, especially during desquamation, and is sometimes striking (up to 20 per cent).

The course and clinical features of scarlet fever vary greatly with the severity of the disease. Many mild cases are observed in which constitutional symptoms and sore throat are minimal, fever is low grade and of short duration, and the rash is evanescent. A florid eruption is sometimes seen in persons in whom all other evidences of the disease are slight, indicating that the reaction to the erythrogenic toxin per se is not primarily responsible for the systemic manifestations of scarlet fever. Again, the situation is comparable to that in diphtheria. A mild sore throat with a strain that is a potent toxin-producer may result in a clinical picture dominated by the effects of the exotoxin. Conversely, severe pharyngeal infection may be present with a strain that is a relatively mild toxin-producer, and the clinical manifestations resulting from the toxin may be slight.

Course of Steptococcal Pharyngitis. The course of untreated hemolytic streptococcal pharyngitis in older children and adults is benign. Seventy-five per cent of patients are afebrile within 72 hours after onset, but sore throat, abnormal signs in the pharynx, and tender adenitis may persist for two or three days after the return of the temperature to normal. Although the whole process is shortened by appropriate antimicrobial therapy by 24 to 48 hours, it is not always easy to distinguish the treated from the untreated patient. An acute pharyngitis that *fails to respond* to adequate penicillin therapy is virtually never due to group A streptococcal infection. On the other hand, the course of viral pharyngitis is often also very brief, and a spontaneous defervescence in 24 to 48 hours may mislead the clinician who has treated the patient into believing the patient has had a therapeutic response to penicillin therapy. In severe streptococcal infections, leukocytosis, when present in the acute stage, may persist in more than one half of untreated patients for a week or more, but this disappears more quickly after the institution of antimicrobial therapy. The erythrocyte sedimentation rate returns to normal in 80 per cent of patients by the third week.

Group A streptococci tend to persist in the pharynx for long periods after recovery if antimicrobial therapy has not been employed. In general, the more virulent the strain, the longer and more consistent is the duration of convalescent throat carriage. Under epidemic conditions, 80 per cent of untreated patients may carry the infecting strain for as long as four weeks. On the other hand, sporadic and mild streptococcal infections among schoolchildren studied in recent years are not as frequently associated with such prolonged throat carriage.

Streptococcal pharyngitis in infants and small children lacks an acute and well defined onset, has rhinorrhea as a dominant manifestation, is rarely associated with high fever, and runs a protracted and indeterminate course. The physical signs in the throat are nondescript, and usually do not permit an accurate clinical diagnosis. Suppurative complications such as otitis media and cervical lymphadenitis occur frequently.

The change of the pharyngeal response after the first few years of life to an explosive onset with fever, sore throat, and exudative pharyngitis may be a reflection of the sharp increase in delayed hypersensitivity (cellular immunity) that appears after the first or second year of life as a result of repeated infection with different types of group A streptococci. It is noteworthy that rheumatic fever is very rare before heightened cellular and humoral immunity to the Steptococcus occurs, whereas acute glomerulonephritis is common.

Diagnosis of Steptococcal Pharyngitis. Streptococcal tonsillitis and pharyngitis in its typical form needs to be differentiated from diphtheria, nonstreptococcal exudative pharyngitis (usually adenovirus), and infectious mononucleosis. When streptoccal infection is nonexudative, however, it cannot be differentiated (in the absence of scarlet fever) from a variety of viral agents producing an identical clinical picture. Cough, coryza, and rhinorrhea (in adults) make a nonbacterial disorder more likely. Unfortunately therefore the clinical diagnosis of the kind of streptococcal pharyngitis that now occurs most commonly as a sporadic infection in civilian communities is usually a crude guess. It is possible, however, to *exclude* the diagnosis of streptococcal disease in considerably more than half the patients studied for sporadic pharyngitis by the use of throat cultures. The incidence of throat cultures positive for beta-hemolytic streptococci decreases progressively with age in patients with sporadic acute respiratory diseases in civilian communities. In several large cities in the northern sections of the United States, surveys have shown that less than 5 per cent of adults who had routine cultures for upper respiratory infections harbored group A streptococci in their throats. It is obvious therefore that without bacteriologic confirmation, the clinical diagnosis of viral versus streptococcal pharyngitis is quite unsatisfactory.

Before any antimicrobial therapy is administered, swabs should be passed through the mouth under direct vision, using a good light, and rubbed over the tonsils and posterior pharynx. The swab should be streaked directly, with a minimum of delay, on sheep blood agar plates of low dextrose content. After incubation overnight, the number of hemolytic streptococci present should be recorded in a roughly quantitative manner. These organisms will be very numerous in nearly all cases if they are the cause of the infection. The presence of a few does not provide convincing evidence that they are responsible for the illness, because 5 to 10 per cent of the general population are nasopharyngeal carriers of these organisms. Serologic grouping and typing of the isolated organisms are usually not necessary for routine clinical diagnosis. Because all group A streptococci are susceptible in vitro to discs containing less than 0.02 unit of bacitracin, some laboratories determine the bacitracin susceptibility of hemolytic streptococci routinely. A hemolytic Streptococcus resistant to such low concentrations of bacitracin is virtually never a group A Streptococcus. On the other hand, approximately 5 per cent of non-group A hemolytic streptococci are also susceptible to this low concentration.

Immunologic Diagnosis of Streptococcal Pharyngitis. The immunologic diagnosis of group A streptococcal infection is of no value in the treatment of the acute illness, because an antibody response will not usually be detected until 10 to 20 days after the onset of the disease. Measurement of antistreptolysin O, antihyaluronidase, antistreptokinase, anti-NADase, or anti-DNAse B is of great value in determining whether or not there has been preceding streptococcal pharyngitis in patients with possible rheumatic fever or glomerulonephritis. The presence of low titers of such antibodies during convalescence virtually excludes recent streptococcal disease except in patients who have been intensively treated early in the illness. Helpful in excluding the diagnosis of recent streptococcal infection is a hemagglutination test which employs red blood cells sensitized with all the streptococcal extracellular antigens contained in a crude filtrate of a group A culture (Streptozyme). When human sera are reacted with such cells, an increase in antibody to any of these numerous antigens can be detected readily, and low titers therefore denote freedom from recent streptococcal infection. It should be noted that streptococcal pyoderma does not produce an equally strong immune response to all streptococcal antigens. In particular, antistreptolysin O and anti-NADase are increased relatively infrequently, whereas anti-DNAse B and antihyaluronidase, particularly the former, are better indicators of recent streptococcal pyoderma. The clinician should be aware that elevated serum levels of streptococcal antibodies may persist for long periods of time after an immune response has occurred. Such elevated serum levels do not necessarily imply an unfavorable prognosis, and are not an indication for additional prolonged antimicrobial therapy.

The Value of Throat Cultures in Deciding When to Treat. There may be some difficulty in interpreting the significance of a throat culture weakly positive for hemolytic streptococci when streptococcal disease is mild and sporadic. Such a positive culture may represent the acquisition of a strain temporarily in the pharynx that does not actually invade the deeper tissues of the host, does not produce a significant immune response, and does not lead to acute rheumatic fever. Such a positive culture may also represent the convalescent carriage of an infection that occurred several weeks previously and may bear no relation to subsequent acute symptoms of viral pharyngitis from which the patient may now be suffering. The physician's problem in deciding which patient with pharyngitis to treat with antimicrobial drugs will be clarified if he obtains throat cultures routinely in all such patients whom he examines. By doing this he becomes alert to the epidemiology of the infections he encounters. A throat culture negative for beta-hemolytic streptococci will exclude a great many patients from unnecessary and promiscuous use of expensive antimicrobial drugs. In outbreaks of exudative pharyngitis, negative throat cultures in a succession of patients will immediately reveal the nonstreptococcal nature of the disease encountered. Conversely, a succession of strongly positive cultures leaves little doubt that a local outbreak of streptococcal pharyngitis is in progress.

When exudative pharyngitis is associated with a throat culture heavily seeded with beta-hemolytic streptococci, there is little argument with the general recommendation for prompt and adequate antimicrobial therapy. Moreover, when a succession of such cases is observed, the practitioner is immediately alerted to the need to culture material from the throats of asymptomatic contacts to prevent the spread of an epidemic. It is with the sporadic cases of nonexudative pharyngitis that are associated with positive throat cultures that some argument has been raised as to the need to employ intensive penicillin therapy in the regimens recommended for the prevention of rheumatic fever (see below). In some populations and under some conditions, such intensive

treatment may not be necessary. At present, however, these conditions have not yet been sufficiently defined to justify broad generalizations. Until further studies define more precisely the risk of withholding or modifying chemotherapy of such infections, it is safer to err on the side of overtreatment and thus to ensure the prevention of passage of streptococcal strains through a population. Indeed, with the assistance of the throat culture, all contacts of patients with well diagnosed exudative streptococcal pharyngitis may be studied for acquisition of potentially dangerous strains, and those identified as carriers may be treated. The consequence of such practice would undoubtedly have a profound influence on the epidemiology of streptococcal infection and therefore upon the incidence of rheumatic fever and glomerulonephritis.

Complications of Pharyngitis. Suppurative and nonsuppurative complications may follow untreated streptococcal tonsillitis and pharyngitis.

Suppurative Complications. *Peritonsillar abscess* or *quinsy sore throat* is an interesting and infrequent complication of streptococcal tonsillitis. Its exact pathogenesis is unknown. Suppuration extends through the capsule of the palatine tonsil into the loose connective tissue of the neck. This is associated with formation of brawny edema of the affected side with movement of the tonsil toward the midline of the throat. An abscess eventually forms and drains in untreated cases, *but the pus does not regularly contain streptococci.* It is probable that the initial streptococcal infection does not cause this lesion directly, but may permit other organisms such as anaerobic gram-negative bacilli of the Bacteroides group and anaerobic nonhemolytic streptococci to gain a foothold in the affected tissues. The onset of this complication is marked by an abrupt increase in soreness and swelling of the neck, and often by increased fever and malaise. The involved tonsil and anterior pillar are greatly swollen, the cervical nodes are large and tender, and eventually a fluctuant mass may be felt in the affected area with the gloved finger. Complications of peritonsillar abscess arise when the infection extends further into the neck or leads to the development of suppurative thrombophlebitis. Peritonsillar abscess is only rarely seen today, because severe hemolytic streptococcal tonsillitis is often treated early in its course with effective antimicrobial agents.

Direct extension of hemolytic streptococci from the locus in the throat to the surrounding tissues may result in certain suppurative complications. Paranasal sinusitis, otitis media, mastoiditis, suppurative cervical adenitis, and impetigo are the most common, and will occur most frequently in untreated children less than four years old. It has been demonstrated that otitis media occurring early in the course of streptococcal respiratory infection is caused by the same serologic type that was present in the throat at the onset. A similar complication that develops after the first week is likely to be the result of a reinfection, and a different type will be recovered from the purulent exudate. Bacteremia was once observed rather frequently during the course of streptococcal respiratory infection and was often associated with metastatic lesions in the joints, bones, and elsewhere. Such cases are now almost unknown, even if antimicrobial therapy is withheld. Similarly, there has been a nearly complete disappearance of group A streptococcal meningitis. Pneumonia has always been a surprisingly uncommon complication of streptococcal upper respiratory infections. Tender cervical adenitis is regularly present and is not to be regarded as a complication unless the lymph nodes become very large and fluctuant. All the various suppurative streptococcal complications may be prevented by early and adequate antimicrobial therapy. Response to similar management is excellent if any such complications should develop in an untreated patient.

Nonsuppurative Complications. The principal nonsuppurative complications of streptococcal disease, acute rheumatic fever (ARF), and acute glomerulonephritis (AGN), are discussed in Ch. 189 (ARF) and in Ch. 610 (AGN).

187. STREPTOCOCCAL SKIN INFECTIONS

STREPTOCOCCAL PYODERMA

Clinical Features. Aside from secondary infections of wounds or burns, group A streptococci can cause at least two kinds of skin infection, *pyoderma* and *erysipelas.* These differ markedly in clinical appearance, in epidemiology, in pathogenesis, and perhaps in the strains of streptococci causing infection. The term streptococcal pyoderma includes all kinds of streptococcal skin infections, other than erysipelas, many of which are secondary infections. The term *impetigo,* or *impetigo contagiosa,* describes what often appears to be a *primary* infection, is initially and transiently vesicular, and presents as crusted, nonscarring lesions in its later stages.

The initial lesion of streptococcal impetigo is a papule that develops rapidly into a vesicle with a small surrounding area of erythema. The vesicles are often missed clinically because of their evanescence and rapid transformation into pustules with thick, amber-colored crusts that appear to be "stuck on" the skin. Aside from occasional itching and burning, the lesions are not painful unless they become deep seated. Regional lymph nodes are commonly involved even without extensive local cellulitis. Often an apparently innocuous lesion may yield large numbers of group A streptococci in cultures taken beneath dried crusts, and such indolent-appearing lesions can produce full-blown acute glomerulonephritis. Bacteremia, which is rare in streptococcal pharyngitis, occurs more frequently with skin and wound infections, and occasionally scarlet fever has been reported. Superficial streptococcal skin infections often pursue a chronic course of weeks or months, and their onset is often difficult to establish. A deeply ulcerated form is known as *ecthyma.*

Contagiousness of streptococcal skin infections is evident from the tendency of multiple cases to occur in a family and from their tendency to occur in epidemics. The importance of antecedent skin trauma is apparent in the epidemiology of streptococcal pyoderma (see above). Its preponderance in the summer when insect bites and trauma to exposed parts of children are most common, especially in populations in which poverty results in poor hygiene, neglect, flies, and crowding, suggests the conditions for maximal opportunity of invasion of the skin by virulent strains. Because of the frequency, especially in children, of such minor skin trauma as mosquito bites, abrasions, burns, eczema, scabies, and pediculosis, it is often difficult to determine whether or not group A streptococci invade the unbroken skin. In epidemic conditions owing to particularly virulent strains, the clinical appearance of the lesions often suggests direct invasion, but it is virtually impossible to exclude minute and transient antecedent trauma.

Diagnosis. The frequency with which staphylococci colonize the skin makes contamination of skin lesions with these organisms almost the rule. Cultures of lesions more clearly considered streptococcal pyoderma are frequently also associated with staphylococci, and the relative role of each organism in the etiology of impetigo has caused much confusion and controversy. Although the issue is not entirely settled, current evidence suggests that impetigo can be divided on clinical, bacteriologic, and epidemiologic grounds into two basic forms: a bullous type, in infants, which forms thin, varnish-like crusts and is primarily staphylococcal in origin, and a vesicular type, which develops thick "stuck-on" crusts and is primarily streptococcal in etiology. Whereas the classic bullous impetigo caused by staphylococci yields a pure culture of phage Type 71 organisms, the early vesicular stage of streptococcal impetigo may yield pure cultures of group A streptococci, but in the purulent and crusted stages large numbers of staphylococci may be present also. The latter are of a variety of phage types suggesting secondary colonization.

Skin cultures of pyodermas should be made after careful cleansing of the surface of the lesions with gauze soaked in sterile warm water, avoiding antiseptics, soaps, and detergents that kill or suppress the more fastidious streptococci and favor the survival of the more adaptable Staphylococcus. Often the removal of crusts and careful culture of the serous exudate beneath will yield large numbers of hemolytic streptococci in almost pure culture. Sheep blood agar plates incubated anaerobically or in 10 per cent CO_2 favor the growth of streptococci.

The higher numbered M and T serotypes associated with pyoderma strains of group A streptococci set them apart from the primarily pharyngeal strains, although it should be noted that throat carriage of the "skin strains" may be high in populations in which much pyoderma is present, especially during the summer months.

The weak antistreptolysin O response to pyoderma strains should be borne in mind, and anti-DNAse B or antihyaluronidase titers should be measured when studies of the immune response to these streptococcal infections are indicated (see above), as in the diagnosis of poststreptococcal AGN.

ERYSIPELAS

This form of group A streptococcal skin infection has special characteristics and may be considered in greater detail. Erysipelas usually involves the face and head, but may affect any area of the body. Other than an occasional case of a group C strain that has been recognized, erysipelas is caused by group A streptococci. The precise way in which the bacteria are introduced into the skin in primary facial erysipelas has not been determined. Large numbers of group A streptococci are fairly constantly present among the nasopharyngeal flora of patients with early erysipelas. It may be that the primary infection is a nasopharyngitis from which the organism is transferred to the skin.

After reaching the face, the streptococci may enter the skin through minute abrasions that are not recognizable after the disease is well established. In surgical and wound erysipelas, it is probable that streptococci are introduced into the traumatized areas from external sources, usually the nose and throat of attendants and other patients. The epidemiology of facial erysipelas differs somewhat from that of group A streptococcal infection in the affected age groups. This disease, when large numbers of cases were observed in the past, was rather common in infancy, rare between the ages of six and thirty, and predominantly a disorder of middle age. There has been no explanation for this discrepancy in age distribution.

Erysipelas usually begins as an abrupt onset of fever with a shaking chill. A history of preceding acute or subacute upper respiratory infection is obtained in about one third of adult cases and more frequently in infants. Very early in the disease a definite zone of redness and edema of the skin appears, most frequently around the bridge of the nose or around a surgical incision, traumatic wound, area of dermatitis, or the newly severed umbilical cord. Facial erysipelas is usually self-limited if no antibacterial therapy is administered. Under these circumstances, the temperature remains at a high level for four to ten days and then falls by lysis or crisis. During this interval a local process involves a large part of the face. As the lesion develops and spreads from the central focus, the skin is red, hot, edematous, and glistening. Blebs are frequently formed. The advancing edge of the lesion is sharply defined and slightly elevated. Great swelling occurs when the infection involves the eyelids.

The disease may involve one or both sides of the face, and usually remains active and spreading until the cheeks and eyelids are affected. Very often the inflammatory process does not extend over the bony prominences, and is limited to the area between the mandible, the malar eminence, and the hairline. In certain cases the ear is included, but spread to the scalp and trunk is rare except in infants.

Untreated *erysipelas of the trunk or extremities,* which usually occurs in infants or persons who have undergone surgery or have been injured, is a more malignant disease. Large areas of skin are often involved rapidly, prostration frequently occurs, and death is a common event. In this form of the disorder it is often possible to observe the characteristic recovery of the skin first affected while the process advances elsewhere. Healing of the skin requires one to two weeks after the temperature has returned to normal.

188. HEMOLYTIC STREPTOCOCCAL PNEUMONIA

Group A hemolytic streptococci were once responsible for 3 to 5 per cent of cases of bacterial pneumonia, but this form of the disease is now rarely seen. It usually appears as a complication of influenza or other viral respiratory infection or in persons with underlying pulmonary disease. It is almost never observed as a sequel to streptococcal tonsillitis and pharyngitis or scarlet fever.

The pneumonic process is lobular in distribution in the lung. Empyema develops in 30 to 40 per cent of untreated cases. It is present early in the illness and is characterized by the formation of large amounts of thin fluid. Bacteremia is demonstrable in 10 to 15 per cent of the cases of streptococcal pneumonia. The demonstration of large numbers of hemolytic streptococci in the sputum by cultural methods, or the isolation of these organisms from the blood or pleural fluid, is required for diagnosis.

189. TREATMENT OF GROUP A STREPTOCOCCAL INFECTION AND CHEMOPROPHYLAXIS OF NONSUPPURATIVE COMPLICATIONS

Gene H. Stollerman

The management of the various group A streptococcal illnesses should include those general measures that are applied in all acute infections. Bed rest, light or liquid diet if pharyngeal discomfort is present and severe, and adequate but not excessive fluid intake are indicated.

Most important is the prompt institution of appropriate antimicrobial therapy, which has four goals: (1) the prompt control of the acute suppurative process in the respiratory tract or elsewhere, (2) the prevention of suppurative complications, (3) the prevention of nonsuppurative complications, and (4) the elimination of the carrier state and the prevention of transmission of the organism to others. The third and fourth goals will be fully attained only if the organism is permanently eradicated from the tissues. This can best be accomplished by the administration of penicillin. Sulfonamides are not effective either in eradicating the carrier state or in preventing an immunologic response, and thus do not prevent nonsuppurative complications. Erythromycin is an acceptable second choice to penicillin in the presence of allergy to penicillin. Tetracycline-resistant group A streptococci have been described with increasing frequency, and this drug is therefore an unreliable choice. It is essential that treatment in full doses be given over a period of at least ten days, regardless of which of the effective drugs is used.

Group A streptococci are among the most susceptible of all bacteria to the action of penicillin. The range of susceptibility for all strains of this serologic group is extremely narrow, between 0.01 and 0.04 unit per milliliter of culture. Moreover, no penicillin-resistant strains of group A streptococci have been demonstrated.

Duration of exposure to penicillin is the most important factor in therapy. Prolonged exposure to small concentrations of penicillin therefore is just as effective as a more intensive form of treatment of group A streptococcal pharyngitis. A single intramuscular injection of 600,000 units of benzathine penicillin provides blood levels that are barely detectable but that persist for about ten days; 1.2 million units results in levels that persist for at least two to four weeks or more. Such doses cure streptococcal pharyngitis, terminate carriage in the throat, and prevent rheumatic fever with optimal efficiency. Shorter-acting penicillin salts, such as aqueous procaine penicillin, must be administered still more often (usually daily for ten days) in a dose of 300,000 or 600,000 units intramuscularly to accomplish the same results. In the treatment of streptococcal pharyngitis, combinations of aqueous, procaine, and benzathine penicillin have no advantage over a single injection of benzathine penicillin G alone if a dose of at least 600,000 units or, preferably, 1.2 million units of the latter is employed.

If given orally, penicillin G must be administered in doses of 200,000 to 250,000 units four times daily for ten days. Thus, penicillinemia of about ten days' duration, regardless of the choice of preparation, is necessary to ensure bacteriologic cure. Sulfonamides are ineffective in preventing rheumatic fever when used to treat streptococcal pharyngitis. They do not suppress the immune response, do not terminate pharyngeal carriage of streptococci, and thus do not reduce the attack rate of subsequent rheumatic fever. They may be used, however, as continuous prophylaxis to *prevent* new infections (see below).

PREVENTION OF RHEUMATIC FEVER

Although the more promptly penicillin therapy is instituted, the more effective is prevention of subsequent rheumatic fever, there is no harm in delaying therapy for 24 hours to await report of a throat culture. It has been shown that the incidence of acute rheumatic fever can be partially reduced by treatment instituted as long as nine days after the onset of pharyngitis. When the patient has been seen within the first day or two of his infection, withholding treatment for one day more has not proved to constitute a risk. One exception to this statement involves the patient with a history of rheumatic fever. In such a patient, the prevention of rheumatic recurrence is not always possible unless treatment is instituted at the first clinical sign of streptococcal infection. In such a patient, any delay of therapy entails the risk of reactivation of the disease. Certain features of the chemoprophylaxis of rheumatic fever are also presented in Ch. 191.

Patients with more serious streptococcal infections, such as streptococcal pneumonia, severe wound infections with sepsis, or suppurative complications of ordinary respiratory infection, should receive 600,000 units of procaine penicillin G per day intramuscularly for several days until the illness is well controlled, when a shift to a single dose of benzathine penicillin or to oral penicillin may be made. The response of extrapharyngeal suppurative complications of streptococcal infection to penicillin is good, and recovery without surgical intervention is the rule, with one exception. Sterilization of abscesses in well-established suppurative cervical adenitis is most difficult. Incision and drainage is usually required in such cases unless spontaneous rupture occurs. As in all situations of antimicrobial therapy in the presence of pus and necrosis, prolonged therapy for as long as several weeks may be required when adequate debridement is not possible. For patients allergic to penicillin, erythromycin is recommended in doses of 1 gram per day, which may be given in four divided doses for a period of ten days. Severely ill patients may receive 500 mg of erythromycin twice daily intravenously for a short time until they are able to accept the drug by mouth.

PREVENTION OF GLOMERULONEPHRITIS

As in rheumatic fever, initial attacks of glomerulonephritis can be prevented by prompt and adequate penicillin treatment of streptococcal pharyngitis. However, the latent period between streptococcal infection and glomerulonephritis is generally shorter than for rheumatic fever. Therefore glomerulonephritis is not as efficiently prevented by treatment of the antecedent streptococcal infection with penicillin as is rheumatic fever. When the clinician is aware of the appearance of other cases of acute glomerulonephritis or rheumatic fever in the population he attends, he should treat sore throat promptly and vigorously and should be more energetic than ever in obtaining throat cultures from the contacts of his patient.

The treatment of streptococcal pyoderma has been studied far less methodically than pharyngitis and has varied widely in practice. The principles guiding the treatment of pyoderma may be somewhat different from those of pharyngitis in which prevention of rheumatic fever requires thorough eradication of group A streptococci. Unlike pharyngeal infections, topical treatment of skin infections may be adequate for mild cases of impetigo. Whether or not parenteral antimicrobial drugs are used, the removal of crusts and cleansing of the affected skin surfaces with soap seems to be an important part of the treatment of streptococcal pyoderma. In patients with extensive, persistent, or recurring impetigo, intramuscular benzathine penicillin is the treatment of choice.

190. PROPHYLAXIS OF STREPTOCOCCAL INFECTION

Gene H. Stollerman

Mass Prophylaxis. Mass prophylaxis is the term applied to the treatment of an entire population, both healthy and affected persons, to interrupt or prevent an epidemic, impending or in progress. This has been done frequently in military populations when epidemic streptococcal pharyngitis and its aftermath of rheumatic fever or glomerulonephritis have appeared. Occasionally, similar measures have been taken against local epidemics in schools or institutions. A single injection of 1.2 million units of benzathine penicillin G intramuscularly has proved extremely effective for this purpose because it (1) is therapeutic in those actually infected, (2) terminates pharyngeal carriage, and (3) protects against the acquisition of new infections for four to five weeks.

Unfortunately, no form of immunization is of avail. However, alert medical practitioners who will promptly detect and adequately treat streptococcal infections, a good system of public health reporting of rheumatic fever and acute glomerulonephritis, and good facilities for routine use of throat cultures should reduce extensive epidemics of streptococcal disease to a rarity. This should so alter the spread of streptococcal infections as to diminish the virulence and epidemicity of the Streptococcus and thereby continue the present trend in the decline of nonsuppurative complications of streptococcal disease.

Tonsillectomy has been employed prophylactically in the past, but is now known to be useless for this purpose, as it does not prevent infection by hemolytic streptococci. Subsequently acquired streptococcal respiratory illnesses may be less severe, but the frequency of occurrence of nonsuppurative complications is not reduced.

Continuous Chemoprophylaxis. Continuous chemoprophylaxis against group A streptococci has proved to be highly effective in preventing recurrences of rheumatic fever (see below) and may be attained by one of three regimens listed here in order of their apparent efficacy and practicability:

1. Benzathine penicillin G in a single injection of 1.2 million units will provide protection for about 30 days. The disadvantages and discomfort of this regimen have to be weighed against the susceptibility to rheumatic recurrences of the individual patient. Those with rheumatic heart disease, those who have had a recent attack of rheumatic fever, and those exposed to an environment in which the incidence of streptococcal infection is frequent deserve the most effective protection. For such patients, benzathine penicillin by injection monthly is recommended.

2. Sulfonamide in daily administration by mouth of 1.0 gram of sulfadiazine or one of the other sulfapyrimidines provides satisfactory prophylaxis, but failures will occur. Toxic reactions may be observed during the first 60 days of continuous treatment. These have been rare, however, with the small doses of sulfadiazine that have been employed extensively.

3. Oral penicillin in doses of 200,000 (125 mg) units of penicillin G has been employed widely for prevention of streptococcal infections. This regimen has not been any more effective, however, than the daily dose of 1.0 gram of sulfadiazine. Indeed, 200,000 units of penicillin *twice* daily has not proved as yet to be clearly superior to the single dose. It is possible that the oral dose of penicillin may have to be increased to nearly therapeutic proportions to be more effective than sulfonamides, and this would increase further its expense and impracticability.

Franciosi, R. A., Knostman, J. D., and Zimmerman, R. A.: Group B streptococcal neonatal and infant infections. J. Pediatr., 82:707, 1973.

Lancefield, R. C.: Current knowledge of type-specific M antigens of group A streptococci. J. Immunol., 89:307, 1962.

Parker, M. T., Bassett, D. C. J., Maxted, W. R., and Arneaud, J. D.: Acute glomerulonephritis in Trinidad: Serologic typing of group A streptococci. J. Hyg. (Camb.), 66:657, 1968.

Rammelkamp, C. H., Jr.: Epidemiology of Streptococcal Infections. Harvey Lectures, Series 51, 1955–56. New York, Academic Press, 1957, p. 113.

Rheumatic Fever Committee, American Heart Association: Prevention of rheumatic fever. Circulation, 43:983, 1971.

Seegal, D., and Seegal, B. C.: Facial erysipelas: A study of 281 cases treated at the Massachusetts General Hospital from 1870–1927. J.A.M.A., 93:430, 1929.

Siegel, A. C., Johnson, E. E., and Stollerman, G. H.: Controlled studies of streptococcal pharyngitis in a pediatric population. I. Factors related to the attack rate of rheumatic fever. N. Engl. J. Med., 265:559, 1961.

Stetson, C. A., Rammelkamp, C. H., Jr., Krause, R. M., Kohen, R. J., and Perry, W. D.: Epidemic acute nephritis: Studies on etiology, natural history, and prevention. Medicine, 34:431, 1955.

Stollerman, G. H.: Factors determining the attack rate of rheumatic fever. J.A.M.A., 177:823, 1961.

Stollerman, G. H.: Rheumatogenic and nephritogenic streptococci. Circulation, 43:915, 1971.

Stollerman, G. H., and Pearce, I. A.: The changing epidemiology of rheumatic fever and acute glomerulonephritis. Adv. Intern. Med., 14:201, 1968.

Uhr. J. W. (ed.): The Streptococcus, Rheumatic Fever and Glomerulonephritis. Baltimore, Williams & Wilkins Company, 1964.

Wannamaker, L. W.: Infections of the throat and skin. N. Engl. J. Med., 282:23, 78, 1970.

Wannamaker, L. W., and Matsen, J. M. (eds.): Streptococci and Streptococcal Diseases. New York, Academic Press, 1972.

Wood, H. F., Feinstein, A. R., Taranta, A., Epstein, J. A., and Simpson, R.: Rheumatic fever in children and adolescents. III. Comparative effectiveness of three prophylaxis regimens in preventing streptococcal infections and rheumatic occurrences. Ann. Intern. Med., 60 (Suppl. 5):31, 1964.

191. RHEUMATIC FEVER

Richard M. Krause

Definition. Rheumatic fever is an uncommon, but by no means rare, delayed sequel of an upper respiratory tract infection caused by group A hemolytic streptococci. The pathogenesis remains obscure. Multiple focal aseptic inflammatory lesions are the basis for the acute manifestations, which may include migratory arthritis, carditis, chorea, erythema marginatum, and subcutaneous nodules, as well as a number of less prominent signs and symptoms. Recurrences of rheumatic fever are common after an untreated streptococcal infection in patients with a previous history of this disease. The acute disease is of limited duration, but the carditis may lead to permanent valvular damage. It is for this reason that extensive studies have been concerned with methods to prevent first attacks as well as recurrences of rheumatic fever. Prevention can be achieved only by the prompt detection, diagnosis, and treatment of streptococcal pharyngitis.

Etiology and Pathogenesis. Despite the decline in recent years in the incidence of rheumatic fever, interest in the disease is unabated because of its unique relationship to streptococcal infections. All the available evidence indicates that only group A streptococcal infections of the upper respiratory tract lead to rheumatic fever. Further, the two episodes are separated by a latent period during which the signs and symptoms of either illness are commonly absent. Although streptococci may be present in the throat from the onset of pharyngitis to the onset of rheumatic fever, there is no satisfactory evidence that foci of living streptococci contribute to the occurrence of rheumatic inflammatory lesions. Thus rheumatic fever appears to be a reaction to the streptococcal infection, and not a continuation of the infectious process.

The epidemiologic, clinical, and laboratory evidence for the association between streptococcal infections and rheumatic fever deserves special comment. Numerous epidemiologic studies have described a temporal relationship between these two diseases. Prior to the days of penicillin, an epidemic of scarlet fever in a closed population, such as a boarding school, was followed in two to four weeks by an uncommonly high incidence of rheumatic fever. But the certain relationship between the two diseases was only established once there had been major advances in the bacteriology of streptococci. The advent of methods to delineate the antigenic structure of the group A Streptococcus and the immune response to the various streptococcal antigens permitted the identification of the group A Streptococcus as the only pathogen that causes the pharyngitis leading to rheumatic fever. The serologic methods to detect antibodies to streptococcal antigens played an especially important role in establishing this relationship. With such methods, it was possible to determine for the first time that nearly every patient with rheumatic fever had a preceding streptococcal sore throat. This was not always evident from the results of throat cultures taken at the onset of rheumatic fever. Although group A streptococci may persist in the throat during the interval between streptococcal pharyngitis and rheumatic fever, it is not uncommon for repeated cultures of the pharynx to be negative for these organisms.

The most persuasive argument in favor of a relationship between streptococcal pharyngitis and acute rheumatic fever stems from the treatment schedules that have been devised to prevent primary as well as recurrent attacks of rheumatic fever. In brief, it is clear that adequate antimicrobial therapy of streptococcal pharyngitis will prevent a subsequent attack of rheumatic fever.

Once the bacteriology of streptococcal pharyngitis was clarified, the recurrent nature of rheumatic fever was no longer a mystery. Almost all serologic types of group A hemolytic streptococci are apparently capable of causing a pharyngitis that can lead to rheumatic fever (the possible exceptions to this rule are some of the recent new types of streptococci that have been most prominently isolated from skin lesions, some of which are associated primarily with the occurrence of acute nephritis). Because immunity to streptococcal infections is M-type specific, infection with one type results in no significant protection against the many other types. Thus, it is common for a child to experience several different streptococcal infections during the school years, and this, in turn, makes possible repeated attacks of rheumatic fever. A child who has had an attack of rheumatic fever retains a special susceptibility to repeated attacks in subsequent years. However, the reason for this special susceptibility remains to be explained.

Although most, if not all, serologic M types of group A streptococcal infections of the pharynx can lead to rheumatic fever, it should be stressed that only 3 per cent or less of all patients who do not receive adequate antimicrobial therapy for a streptococcal infection will develop subsequent rheumatic fever. Epidemiologic evidence indicates that rheumatic fever occurs only after streptococcal pharyngitis, but not in association with streptococcal skin infections, e.g., impetigo. It is conceivable that the response to the pharyngeal infection is qualitatively and quantitatively different from the response to skin infections. It is known, for example, that the antibody response to streptolysin O is more likely to be elevated after pharyngeal infections than after skin infections, whereas the antibody response to DNAse B occurs with high frequency after infection at either site. Thus it is conceivable that the special consequences of a pharyngeal infection set the stage for the occurrence of rheumatic fever.

The selective occurrence of rheumatic fever in only a few people with pharyngitis argues for the importance of host factors in addition to the infectious process in the pathogenesis of rheumatic fever. It is possible that the accumulative effects of repetitive streptococcal infections in any one individual are a factor that increases the risk. Young children under the age of three have streptococcal pharyngitis, but rheumatic fever is uncommon in this age group. Throughout the remainder of childhood repetitive streptococcal infections lead to delayed hypersensitivity to streptococcal products, but such hyper-

tivity is not commonly present in children less than three years of age. It is after the age of four that rheumatic fever is most common in children. The possible importance of genetic factors in predisposition has been suggested. Although it has been observed that rheumatic fever may occur in families, no clear-cut genetic pattern has been found. In a study of monozygotic twins, less than one fifth were concordant for rheumatic fever. Unsatisfactory and inconclusive though these studies are, the selective occurrence of rheumatic fever in only a few of all those infected with streptococci suggests that predisposing factors work in conjunction with the infectious process to produce rheumatic fever, but the nature of such contributory causes has remained obscure.

Although the central role of streptococcal infections in the etiology of rheumatic fever is now established beyond question, the mechanism by which the hemolytic streptococci initiate the disease process is unknown. For convenience, evidence can be marshaled for the support of three different theories of pathogenesis. Each of these theories is less than satisfactory.

The most currently attractive hypothesis is that rheumatic fever is a consequence of an immunologic response or hypersensitivity reaction, or both, to streptococcal antigens. An immunologic mechanism is suggested by the intriguing parallel between the latent period of serum sickness and rheumatic fever. Patients who develop rheumatic fever appear to have an exaggerated antibody response to streptococcal antigens. Such patients commonly, but not always, have a higher antistreptolysin O response than those who do not develop this complication after streptococcal pharyngitis.

The arguments suggesting that autoimmunity may be of importance in pathogenesis cannot be recorded in detail here. The occurrence of autoantibodies that react with mammalian muscle in the sera of patients with rheumatic fever in concentrations greater than in the sera of patients who do not develop this complication has been emphasized. What remains to be determined is the source of antigenic stimulus for this autoantibody a the pathologic significance of such autoantibody cause this autoantibody cross-reacts with a strep antigen, it has been argued that these anti only another manifestation of the immune the preceding streptococcal infection. It i however, that the host's own tissues w the toxic processes at the time of th tered tissue antigens became the tibody production. In addition to source of the stimulus that g tibodies, there is the addit pathologic significance. It in the genesis of the ir similar to the autoa pear to be intimat lesions of lupus

Another p rheumatic conseque toxins mar st

little bacteriologic evidence for a direct infection of the heart valves, the myocardium, or other organs involved in rheumatic fever. Nevertheless, because the prevention of rheumatic fever requires the successful and complete eradication of the infecting Streptococcus from the pharynx by drug therapy, the view lingers that persistence of the infecting Streptococcus in some form may be a factor in the disease process.

Epidemiology. It is obvious from what has been said that the epidemiology of acute rheumatic fever and the epidemiology of streptococcal pharyngitis are clearly interrelated. The incidence of the two diseases is related. Any environmental or host factor that enhances the occurrence of streptococcal pharyngitis will enhance the occurrence of rheumatic fever. Streptococcal disease is most common between the ages of five and fifteen years, with a peak incidence between six and eight years, and this is the age group with the highest attack rate of rheumatic fever. Although adults have fewer streptococcal infections than children because of acquired immunity and less exposure to streptococci, the special circumstances of military service or close association with children enhance the risk of higher attack rates for adults.

As is the case for most other respiratory diseases, the occurrence of streptococcal pharyngitis fluctuates widely with the seasons. The occurrence of acute rheumatic fever parallels such fluctuations. The peak occurrence falls in the late winter and early spring months, although not uncommonly the number of cases increases sharply for a brief period shortly after the onset of school in the early fall.

Classic epidemiologic studies indicate that rheumatic fever occurs most commonly in the temperate zones. But recent scattered reports from Africa, India, and countries of Southeast Asia suggest that rheumatic heart disease

in the large cities of the United States, and suggest that the over-all decline in cases stems primarily from the prevention of recurrences and less from the prevention of first attacks. Recently it has been estimated, for example, that no less than 200 cases of acute rheumatic fever occurred in the city of Cleveland during one year.

For the United States at large, the yearly incidence of first attacks of rheumatic fever has been estimated at about 50,000 to 100,000 children, but for a variety of reasons such estimates are unsatisfactory. The disease is not reportable in all states and, in addition, without unequivocal pathognomonic signs and symptoms that clearly establish diagnosis, the disease is both over- and underreported. Some idea of the continued occurrence of rheumatic fever in the population can be obtained by the examination of schoolchildren, college students, and military recruits for the prevalence of rheumatic heart disease. Among schoolchildren, the prevalence is between 0.7 and 1.6 per 1000. The prevalence for freshmen college students and servicemen is between 6 and 9 per 1000.

Clinical Manifestations. The most striking clinical manifestations are due to arthritis, carditis, and chorea. Each sign and symptom of rheumatic fever may be either mild or severe, and the severity of each may vary independently. Thus severe carditis may be associated with minimal or no evidence of arthritis, and vice versa. Because the manifestations of rheumatic fever at first glance appear so variable, and because no single set of manifestations is typical for rheumatic fever, the Jones criteria have been devised as a guide to aid in the differential diagnosis. The signs and symptoms that comprise the Jones criteria are listed in the accompanying table. Use of these criteria for guidance in differential diagnosis will be discussed later.

Although a history of a preceding streptococcal pharyngitis is common, this infection may have been so mild as to have escaped medical attention. Indeed, a number of patients can recall no recent sore throat. The

Clinical and Laboratory Manifestations of Acute Rheumatic Fever

Major Manifestations	Minor Manifestations

1. Carditis
2. Polyarthritis
3. Chorea
4. Erythema marginatum
5. Subcutaneous nodules
	1. Clinical
	  a. Previous rheumatic fever or
	    rheumatic heart disease
	  b. Arthralgia
	  c. Fever
	2. Laboratory
	  a. Acute phase reactions, erythrocyte
	    sedimentation rate, C-reactive
	    protein, leukocytosis
	  b. Prolonged P-R interval

plus

...nce of preceding streptococcal infection (increased ASO ...occal antibodies, positive throat culture for group A ...ent scarlet fever)

...ria (revised) have been employed as a guide in the diag...ic fever, but this scheme has not received universal ...presence of two major manifestations, or of one major ...anifestations, indicates a high probability of the pres...c fever *if supported by evidence of a preceding strepto*...The absence of the latter should make the diagnosis ...in situations in which rheumatic fever is first dis...ong, latent period from the antecedent infection, e.g., ...ea or low-grade carditis.

...he recommendations of the Committee of The American ...n (Circulation, 32:664, 1965.)

interval between the pharyngitis and the onset of rheumatic fever has been termed the latent period. This is a period of one to four weeks, and during this time the patient usually appears entirely well. On some occasions, however, laboratory examination will reveal evidence of disease activity.

The onset of rheumatic fever, with characteristic signs and symptoms, is usually sudden, but it may be insidious. In the latter case, diagnosis depends on observation of the clinical course and the interpretation of laboratory data. Usually the first symptoms are fever and joint pain. Fever may be high and sustained in severe cases, but more frequently it is moderate and often low grade. Sore throat is not uncommon, even though examination reveals minimal evidence of acute inflammation. Epistaxis occurs commonly both at the onset and throughout the acute stage of the disease, and in some cases results in serious loss of blood. In children, severe abdominal pain is not uncommon, and vomiting may occur. Localization of such pain in the right lower quadrant with fleeting signs of peritoneal inflammation may suggest the diagnosis of appendicitis.

Arthritis. The arthritis in rheumatic fever may involve multiple joints, but a characteristic feature is that the inflammation occurs and subsides in the joints first affected, only to occur in others that were initially spared. This phenomenon has been termed migratory polyarthritis. The large joints of the extremities are most frequently affected, but all are potentially susceptible. Arthritis can occur in the hands, feet, or spine, or in such joints as the sternoclavicular and the temporomandibular.

The manifestations of arthritis may be either mild with vague discomfort in the joints of the extremities, or severe. Acutely inflamed and swollen joints are commonly very painful. In mild cases there may be no objective evidence of arthritis. When arthritis is severe, the skin over the joint shows local redness and heat, the joint is swollen, and fluid is obviously present within the joint cavity. Passive or active movement of the joint is extremely painful. The fluid in such cases is turbid and contains inflammatory leukocytes, but is sterile on bacteriologic culture.

Although uncommon, the arthritis may not affect multiple joints. Experienced clinicians have observed the occasional case in which arthritis may persist for prolonged periods in only one joint, with minimal evidence of arthritis in the others.

There is usually a difference between the pattern of arthritis in children and that in adults. Frank arthritis is less common in children between four and six years of age. Only mild joint pains may be noted, or merely vague localized aching in the extremities. It is this type of complaint that has been referred to in the past as "growing pains." Such symptoms and low-grade fever suggest a mild illness, but examination of the heart may reveal severe carditis. It bears repetition that rheumatic fever can occur without any evidence of joint involvement whatever.

Carditis. Palpitation and precordial chest pain or discomfort are common symptoms. If the carditis is severe, symptoms of cardiac failure may occur in addition to those of rheumatic fever. The final and definitive diagnosis of carditis depends upon the physical, roentgenographic, and electrocardiographic examinations.

The carditis may be mild or severe. In mild cases,

tachycardia, persistent during sleep, may be the only sign suggesting carditis. Persistent bradycardia has been well documented in rheumatic fever, but it is far less common than tachycardia. In the more severe cases, generalized cardiac enlargement frequently occurs, often associated with a diffuse precordial impulse.

On auscultation, the heart sounds in the apical area may be muffled, indistinct, and of poor quality. The second sound in the pulmonic area is usually greatly accentuated in comparison with the second aortic sound. Gallop rhythm may occur, and is usually an indication of serious myocardial disease. The sounds may seem distant if precordial effusion is present, and the pericarditis may produce a to-and-fro friction rub (see Ch. 571 to 576).

The most common cardiac murmur during the acute phase of the initial attack of rheumatic fever is a blowing systolic murmur best heard in the apical area. Such murmurs are caused by dilatation of the valve rings as a result of general dilatation of the heart. Less commonly, soft diastolic murmurs are heard along the left sternal border in the third and fourth interspaces. It is difficult to determine whether inflammation of the valve leaflets contributes significantly to these murmurs in all cases. As the murmurs may disappear permanently on recovery, their final significance cannot be determined except by repeated examinations during and after convalescence. Mitral stenosis and aortic stenosis are late manifestations of cardiac damage that do not develop until months or years after the initial or repeated attacks.

Disturbances of the conduction system are a common feature of rheumatic carditis. Although certain irregularities, such as second-degree heart block, can be recognized clinically, the electrocardiogram is the best method to detect all potential conduction system disturbances. One of the most commonly observed electrocardiographic changes is the prolongation of the P-R interval. In some cases, the Wenckebach phenomenon is observed. Further delay in conduction may lead to drop beats, with the occurrence of couplets and triplets. Finally, complete dissociation is indicated by an independent rhythm for both the ventricles and the atria. Atrial fibrillation is uncommon during the acute attack.

In addition to these conduction abnormalities, the electrocardiogram may show T wave changes, such as inversion of the T wave in one or more leads. When pericarditis is present, elevation of the S-T segment is observed initially. Late in the course, the configuration of the T wave simulates that seen in coronary disease.

Although cardiac enlargement, when present, is usually detectable on physical examination, the dilatation of the various chambers of the heart is more accurately determined by roentgenography of the chest. It is not uncommon for dilatation to arise rapidly when severe myocarditis is present.

The recurrence of active rheumatic fever should be suspected in patients with chronic rheumatic heart disease when the character of the murmurs changes over a short period of time. Cardiac failure may occur, but the carditis associated with recurrent rheumatic fever in such cases poses several diagnostic problems, because the manifestations of acute rheumatic carditis are superimposed on those of chronic valvular disease. Furthermore, the status of the pre-existing heart disease is often unknown. When there is evidence of advanced valvular deformity, any final assessment of the extent of cardiac damage must await convalescence from the acute attack.

Erythema Marginatum. *Erythema marginatum* or *circinatum* of the skin is one of the characteristic manifestations of acute rheumatic fever and occurs in 10 to 20 per cent of the childhood cases. It is a multiform type of erythema, and consists of roughly circular lesions that may be distributed over the extremities, the trunk, and sometimes the face, and that spread centrifugally, leaving a clear center. The lesions tend to coalesce so that, although individual areas are iris-like, the larger areas are serpiginous in outline. The erythema blanches on pressure and may be evanescent, disappearing and later reappearing at the same sites. The lesions are usually not elevated, although in some cases a slight papular quality may be detected. Most commonly, no discomfort is associated with the lesions. Erythema marginatum is uncommon in other diseases.

Subcutaneous Rheumatic Nodules. These lesions are one of the physical findings that lend strong support to the diagnosis of rheumatic fever, but in recent years they have occurred less commonly than was the case in the past. They are firm, insensitive nodules that occur over the bony prominences of the various joints and tendons of the extremities, the spine, and the back of the head. They are loosely attached to the underlying tissue, and the skin is freely movable over them. If the joint can be flexed without undue pain, the nodules are more readily apparent because of the tension of the skin. If nodules are numerous, they may occur in a symmetrical distribution. The nodules are more frequently encountered in the more severe cases of rheumatic fever with serious cardiac involvement.

Sydenham's Chorea. Chorea may occur in combination with other symptoms of rheumatic fever, but it is commonly seen as the sole manifestation of the disease. This phenomenon is explained by the fact that chorea tends to make its appearance late in the course of rheumatic fever. The onset may be delayed for as long as six months after the initiating streptococcal infection, although the delay is usually less than this. Patients with chorea may have had an easily recognizable preceding attack of arthritis and carditis, and, indeed, may have been hospitalized with it, only to have the chorea occur as a late manifestation at a time when all other evidence of any inflammatory process had disappeared. When the onset of chorea is delayed and the other manifestations of rheumatic fever have abated, the laboratory findings are often normal. It is not uncommon for chorea to occur in patients who can recall no earlier illness. It seems likely that such individuals had an attack of acute rheumatic fever in the recent past which was so mild that it escaped clinical detection. It is for this reason that patients with so-called "pure chorea" may develop rheumatic heart disease.

The onset of chorea is usually insidious, and the parents of the child with chorea may first note increased awkwardness and a tendency to spill food or drop objects that is attributed to carelessness. Even the appearance of involuntary purposeless movements of the extremities may be discounted as nervousness. However, with further progression of the disease, the irregular and uncontrollable movements become obvious. They may become extensive, and may involve not only the hands, feet, arms, and legs, but the tongue and facial muscles. The severity may range from no more than minimal involuntary movements observed only by close inspection, to violent, continual activity, totally incapacitating the patient and requiring protection from self-injury. In moderate cases, interference with all coordinated activity, such as writing and eating, is common. On occasion, chorea may be limited to one side of the body. The disease appears to affect females somewhat more frequently than males.

Miscellaneous Clinical Manifestations. Rheumatic pneumonitis may occur, but this is difficult to detect clinically, particularly if there is superimposed heart failure. Rheumatic pneumonia has seldom been seen in recent years, probably because the disease process itself appears to be much more mild than in former times. Such few cases as do occur are in patients with severe rheumatic fever.

Erythema nodosum is less common than erythema marginatum. The dull, red nodular lesions occur most frequently on the extensor surfaces of the extremities in various sizes from less than 1 cm to several centimeters in diameter. They are extremely tender on pressure, and the pain is aggravated by movements of the extremities. These lesions occur in patients in whom there is little or no other clinical evidence to suggest acute rheumatic fever. They have been seen in association with a number of infections, including tuberculosis, as well as streptococcal pharyngitis. For these reasons, the presence of erythema nodosum is not considered a major sign for the diagnosis of rheumatic fever.

Laboratory Findings. *Hematology.* There are no characteristic abnormalities of the leukocyte differential count that are indicative of rheumatic fever. Leukocytosis is common, but not always present, with a total count from 12,000 to 24,000 per cubic millimeter. This is associated with an increase in the percentage of polymorphonuclear cells.

A moderate degree of anemia is generally seen, which is normochromic with proportional decreases in the hemoglobin concentration and the erythrocyte count. The anemia usually persists for as long as the rheumatic process is active. The most severe anemias are obviously encountered in patients who have an associated blood loss owing to epistaxis.

Urinary Findings. Some proteinuria and an increase in the number of red and white cells in the urine are common during the acute phase of the disease. However, it is seldom that these abnormalities are as great as those characteristically encountered in acute glomerulonephritis. When this is the case, simultaneous acute nephritis and rheumatic fever must be considered, but such a combination is a most uncommon event.

Evidence for a Prior Streptococcal Infection. The most important laboratory information for establishing the diagnosis of rheumatic fever is data that substantiate the prior occurrence of streptococcal pharyngitis. The detection of group A beta-hemolytic streptococci by a throat culture is helpful in this regard, but of greater usefulness is the serologic detection of antibodies that are indicative of a previous streptococcal infection.

Because the streptococci that caused the initial infection may persist for many weeks in the pharynx in those instances in which antimicrobial therapy was not given or was inadequate, a throat culture may detect the infecting group A streptococci at the time of the onset of rheumatic fever. But such a finding is only suggestive of a preceding streptococcal pharyngitis and is not an unambiguous indication of it. This stems from the fact that 5 to 30 per cent of the healthy population may carry group A streptococci in the pharynx during the respiratory disease season. Thus the recovery of this organism from a patient may be an inadvertent finding and not indicative of a preceding streptococcal sore throat. Nevertheless, the throat culture is helpful, and should be obtained in all cases. When the patient has a negative throat culture, it is frequently possible to isolate the group A streptococci from other members of the family. Such a finding is indicative of a recent intrafamilial spread of streptococci.

The most helpful information that is indicative of a recent streptococcal infection is obtained with tests that detect serum antibodies to streptococcal antigens. The most widely employed test is the antistreptolysin O determination. As with all antibody tests, the detection of an antibody rise over a one- to three-week interval is the only unequivocal evidence for the recent occurrence of a streptococcal infection. If a patient is seen in the first few days after the onset of rheumatic fever, the antistreptolysin O titer at that time may be less than the titer seen several weeks after onset of rheumatic fever. Not uncommonly, however, the titer has reached a maximal plateau so that it is not possible to detect a progressive increase in titer. When this is the case, the antistreptolysin O titer should be at least 250 units in adults and at least 333 units in children over five years of age to be acceptable as an indication of a previous streptococcal infection. Obviously, a certain proportion of the individuals in the normal population have had a recent streptococcal infection at any one time, and they will have antistreptolysin O titers similar to these.

Approximately 15 to 20 per cent of the patients with rheumatic fever and nearly all patients who exhibit only chorea have a low or borderline low antistreptolysin O titer. In such instances, it is helpful to employ another antibody test. The anti-DNAse B test is becoming widely accepted as a second antibody test, and it is a useful means to obtain additional evidence for the occurrence of a previous streptococcal infection. When both these antibody tests are used, it is possible to obtain antibody evidence for a preceding streptococcal infection in almost all cases of rheumatic fever.

One other serologic test should be mentioned because it may be used more widely in the future. It has been noted that nearly all patients with rheumatic fever have readily detectable serum autoantibodies that react with muscle tissue, including heart, whereas the concentration of these antibodies is very much less or absent in sera of patients with other rheumatic diseases. Such findings suggest that this antibody test may have clinical usefulness for the differential diagnosis of rheumatic fever.

Other Laboratory Tests. An elevated sedimentation rate and a positive C-reactive protein are present in rheumatic fever, but these findings are nonspecific indicators of inflammation, and they cannot be used to differentiate rheumatic fever from other diseases. However, a normal C-reactive protein and a normal sedimentation rate are helpful in excluding active rheumatic fever. In patients with mild symptoms, such as vague arthralgia and lassitude, if the sedimentation rate and the C-reactive protein are normal, active rheumatic fever is unlikely.

Diagnosis and Differential Diagnosis. A history of severe sore throat in the recent past, migrating polyarthritis, carditis, fever, and an elevated antistreptolysin O titer is such a classic combination of signs and symptoms that the diagnosis can seldom be questioned. But the problem is often not as straightforward as this.

The various major manifestations of rheumatic fever that have been described above are considered to be part of the same disease because they occur together with a frequency that far exceeds chance. Because they may occur singly or in various combinations in any individual patient, the diagnostic criteria originally proposed by Jones have been suggested as a guide to diagnosis. These criteria are listed in the table. Any combination of these criteria can occur in patients with other disorders. It is for this reason that stress is placed on supporting evidence for a preceding streptococcal infection. When this is the case, the diagnosis is weighed in favor of rheumatic fever and against the other connective tissue disorders that may mimic it.

The designations major and minor for the various criteria are based on the diagnostic importance of the particular findings. The major ones are more indicative of rheumatic fever than the minor. The occurrence of two major manifestations is strong presumptive evidence for rheumatic fever. Only one major manifestation and any combination of the minor suggest possible rheumatic fever. In any case, if evidence is lacking for a preceding streptococcal pharyngitis, the possibility of other diseases must be kept in mind.

In many ways the most useful purpose of the criteria is their value in reducing overdiagnosis. For example, not uncommonly, patients, after streptococcal infections, may have vague pains in the extremities, an increased sedimentation rate, and a borderline temperature elevation. Careful follow-up of such patients has not revealed the delayed occurrence of rheumatic heart disease. Therefore the diagnosis of rheumatic fever should be made with caution and only with clear evidence of one or more of the major manifestations. When the diagnosis is in doubt, because the symptoms are of such a mild nature, treatment with aspirin and steroids should be withheld until the signs and symptoms are unmistakable. Early treatment of a questionable case may so depress the disease activity that clear-cut clinical signs and symptoms do not develop.

In the early stages, during the acute onset, *rheumatoid arthritis* and *systemic lupus erythematosus* may mimic rheumatic fever. Indeed, if the streptococcal antibody tests are elevated, the diagnosis may be in question unless the special diagnostic tests for the other diseases are clearly positive. Usually as time progresses, the special distinctive clinical features of rheumatoid arthritis and lupus serve to exclude the diagnosis of rheumatic fever. On occasion, at the onset, Still's disease may be confused with rheumatic fever, but again the clinical course will aid in differentiating the two.

Subacute bacterial endocarditis can occur in persons with valves previously damaged by rheumatic fever, and it often presents a clinical picture that is not readily distinguishable from a rheumatic recurrence. Vague pains in the extremities are more common than overt arthritis, but these symptoms together with fever and debility in a known rheumatic patient are sufficient to suggest a rheumatic recurrence. The difficulties are increased by the fact that in some cases it is not possible to recover the offending organism in a blood culture. The characteristic petechiae and painful septic emboli of endocarditis are helpful in differential diagnosis (see Ch. 192).

The so-called *benign idiopathic pericarditis*, which is apparently not rheumatic in origin, is indistinguishable in the acute phase from those cases of rheumatic fever in which pericarditis is the major detectable manifestation.

The diagnosis of idiopathic pericarditis is dependent primarily on elimination of other possibilities and on the subsequent course of the disease, which is characterized by complete recovery without residual damage. Thus the final conclusion is often reached only in retrospect, and must remain somewhat uncertain because rheumatic pericarditis with minimal involvement of the myocardium and endocardium could conceivably behave in a similar fashion.

Fever, arthritis, and positive acute phase reactants may also occur in bacterial arthritis, serum sickness, subacute bacterial endocarditis, sickle cell anemia, and acute aleukemic leukemia. In such cases in which confusion exists, only a careful assessment of the clinical course, physical examination, and laboratory findings will exclude rheumatic fever.

Persistent monarticular arthritis, without other major manifestations of rheumatic fever, is usually not due to rheumatic fever, and osteomyelitis or local injury must be considered.

Therapy. There is no specific treatment for rheumatic fever. Therapeutic measures are devised to promote, or at least hopefully not to hinder, the natural healing processes. Bed rest is always prescribed, and most students agree that it should continue for as long as there is unequivocal evidence of disease activity. It is not at all clear that absolute bed rest without bath privileges is essential. Nevertheless, hospitalization has an advantage over home care because the degree of activity is more readily supervised. This is particularly true because aspirin and steroids will generally eliminate all painful manifestations, and the patient sees no necessity for remaining at rest and in bed. A program for a progressive increase in recreational and occupational therapy has important psychologic value and should be an integral part of the long-term bed rest management. Schooling should not be neglected during this time. Hospital or home visit teaching programs, or both, are available in many cities, and instruction should be begun as soon as the acute manifestations of the disease are brought under control by anti-inflammatory therapy.

After the first few weeks of bed rest in patients without carditis, gradual ambulation can be started. In patients with carditis, this is usually delayed until six to ten weeks after onset of the disease. As long as the presence of carditis is suspected, even though masked by treatment, ambulation should not be started. During the period of bed rest, the patient is permitted a number of activities in increasing amounts, such as sitting up in a chair, occupational therapy, and schoolwork.

The period of bed rest is a good time for patients of all ages to be informed about the nature of the illness and the optimistic prospects for an active, long life. The need for a continuous program to prevent streptococcal pharyngitis should be discussed in detail. It is at this time, also, that patients with more severe forms of heart disease should be advised that some curtailment of normal physical activity may be necessary during convalescence. But pessimism is not warranted. All too often, patients are left with the impression that their useful, active life is at an end. This is almost invariably not the case.

It is recommended that all patients with acute rheumatic fever be treated with a course of penicillin to eliminate the hemolytic Streptococcus from the pharynx. This is recommended even if the throat culture does not reveal group A beta-hemolytic streptococci, because these organisms may persist in areas where they remain undetected, such as the interior of the tonsils. Parenteral penicillin is the drug of choice unless there is a history of allergy to it. Three hundred thousand units of penicillin G once a day in children and twice a day in adults for ten days is an effective dose. A single dose of 1.2 million units of long-acting benzathine penicillin is preferred by many, as the one injection facilitates administration. Oral penicillin, 200,000 units four times a day, also for ten days, is acceptable therapy, but requires careful supervision in order to be sure that all doses are taken without fail. If there is a history of penicillin allergy, the drug of choice is erythromycin. The dose is 250 mg four times a day for ten days. Sulfonamide in any form should never be used. After completion of the ten-day course of penicillin or erythromycin, a continuous prophylaxis regimen should be started to prevent reinfection with group A streptococci and to reduce the risk of recurrent attacks of acute rheumatic fever (see Ch. 189).

Aspirin and Steroid Therapy. Most patients respond rapidly to either steroid or aspirin therapy. After one or two weeks, arthritis and fever have disappeared, and the acute phase reactants frequently have returned to normal, or nearly so. On occasion, neither fever nor arthritis responds to full aspirin dosage, and steroids are required to control the disease. Most clinicians favor use of steroids in nearly all patients with carditis. It is certainly indicated in patients with severe carditis and pancarditis. Some prefer to withdraw the steroid treatment after several weeks and continue treatment by substituting aspirin. Others continue steroid therapy for the full course. The arthritis in nearly all patients responds readily to aspirin alone. The evidence remains equivocal for the beneficial effect of steroid therapy in preventing the development of permanent rheumatic heart disease, even though there is apparent clinical improvement in the acute carditis when steroids are used.

It should be stressed again that when full and adequate treatment eliminates all the clinical manifestations of the disease, including laboratory abnormalities, the underlying disease process is still continuing unabated for its natural course. If the drugs are withdrawn before the process is at an end, the disease with all its clinical manifestations will recur. Duration of therapy is discussed below.

The daily dose of aspirin is 60 mg per pound of body weight. The actual total dose per day varies from 3 grams in young children to 10 grams in adults. It is preferable to give this total amount in at least six divided doses. Aspirin should be given throughout the 24-hour day, at least during the early stages of the disease. Individual variation in the efficacy of absorption or excretion of the drug and in its therapeutic effectiveness requires readjustment of the dose in many cases. The aim is to give the minimal dose that results in full control of symptoms and to avoid serious toxic side reactions because of overdosage. Studies on the concentration of salicylates in the blood have shown that optimal therapeutic effect usually requires at least 25 mg per 100 ml of serum. The optimal therapeutic range is between 25 and 35 mg per 100 ml of serum. Levels greater than the upper limit are associated with toxicity. When aspirin is given in conjunction with the prednisone, it is frequently necessary to give a daily dose of aspirin larger than that recommended above in order to achieve the therapeutic salicylate level. Furthermore, as aspirin is continued upon the withdrawal of prednisone, less aspirin is frequently required to maintain an adequate serum salicylate level.

The most common toxic manifestations of aspirin therapy are nausea, vomiting, and gastric distress. Tinnitus and partial but temporary impairment of hearing usually occur only at full therapeutic dosage. Hyperpnea frequently results from central stimulatory action in respiration and can lead to alkalosis. It is uncommon to see the more severe metabolic disturbances of acute salicylate toxicity.

In practice, nausea and vomiting are the most frequent complications that result from starting aspirin. This can be minimized if the initial daily dosage is below the optimum and is then gradually increased over a period of a few days. Attempts to achieve full and optimal salicylate levels within 24 hours often result in severe nausea and vomiting. In such cases it may be difficult to reach an effective therapeutic level of salicylate, and in such instances steroids afford an alternative therapeutic approach. The use of sodium bicarbonate to reduce gastric irritation is not recommended, as it increases the excretion of salicylate and interferes with the maintenance of an anti-inflammatory concentration of the drug in the blood. If a portion of the aspirin is given as enteric-coated pills, some degree of gastric irritation can be eliminated.

Prednisone is the recommended steroid because a low salt diet and added potassium are usually not required. There is no firm agreement on the dosage of this drug. The usual procedure is to begin with a relatively large daily dose until activity of the disease appears to be under control, and then to reduce the dosage to the minimal amount that will maintain the full effect. In the experience of many, the total daily dosage of 0.5 mg per pound given in divided doses is adequate to bring the signs of inflammation, including fever, rapidly under control. Almost all signs and symptoms are suppressed in two or three days. It is at this point that the daily dose may be reduced. After two or three weeks of steroid therapy, some prefer to shift to aspirin, particularly for those patients without carditis. The advantage of this is that most side effects of prolonged steroid therapy, such as the mild manifestations of Cushing's disease, are avoided. Prolonged use of steroid therapy may lead to complications, such as infections, growth retardation, gastric ulcers, and toxic psychoses.

The treatment of chorea is symptomatic. There is no evidence that either steroids or aspirin have any influence on the symptoms of chorea. The usual case lasts from two weeks to several months, but in rare instances it may persist longer. Many patients show improvement when bright light, noise, and undue activity are eliminated from their bedroom. In some cases, measures must be taken to prevent self-injury from violent chorea movements, including tongue-biting. Phenobarbital and other sedatives may be helpful.

Duration of Therapy. The duration of therapy bears some relationship to the severity of the acute manifestations. The disease process in the typical mild case without carditis subsides in three to four weeks. When severe arthritis and carditis are present, the natural course lasts two to three months. Such estimates for the duration of the disease can be used to determine the termination of therapy, recognizing, however, that disease activity in the occasional case may persist for many months.

Laboratory tests such as determination of the sedimentation rate and the C-reactive protein assume normal values during the course of adequate therapy. For this reason, they cannot be used to determine the duration of therapy.

Many clinicians prefer to withdraw either aspirin or steroid therapy gradually over a period of one or two weeks. After withdrawal, a clinical "rebound" is commonly seen. This may be so mild that only the acute phase reactants indicate its occurrence, but not uncommonly clinical manifestations are present. These may be mild or severe, and include fever, arthritis, and tachycardia. Usually the rebound subsides in five to ten days without use of anti-inflammatory drugs. The occurrence of positive C-reactive protein, an elevated sedimentation rate, and an elevated white count, without significant clinical manifestations, is not sufficient grounds for reinstituting therapy. But progressive clinical severity and particularly the emergence of severe carditis may require reinstitution of therapy. In such instances, it is assumed that the natural duration of the disease has yet to run its course. In practice, if therapy must be reinstated because of the emergence of carditis, the drugs are continued for another three to four weeks.

If no significant rebound occurs, ambulation should begin, and usually full activity, except vigorous exercise, may be permitted three to four weeks after the termination of therapy. If persistent rheumatic heart disease is present, the permissible level of physical activity is determined by an assessment of its severity.

Prevention. Prior to the days of antimicrobial drugs, measures were not available to prevent recurrences of rheumatic fever. Now properly supervised continuous chemoprophylaxis is effective in preventing these recurrences, and it should be employed for all patients with a well-documented history of rheumatic fever or unequivocal evidence of rheumatic heart disease. Prophylaxis prevents streptococcal pharyngitis and therefore the recurrences of rheumatic fever.

A detailed consideration of drug regimens for prophylaxis has been presented in Ch. 189. Intramuscular benzathine penicillin, 1.2 million units each month, is the preferred drug and route of administration. Such a route of administration does not leave open to question the degree of patient compliance, as is the case with orally administered penicillin.

The duration of antimicrobial prophylaxis should be extended through childhood. In the case of adolescents and adults, it should not be terminated as long as the patient is associated with population groups that have high attack rates of streptococcal infections, such as military recruits, schoolchildren, medical personnel, and school teachers. Because of the risk of additional valvular damage during a recurrence, prophylaxis should be continued for life for all patients with definite rheumatic heart disease. Contrary to popular belief, people in late middle age can have a recurrence of rheumatic fever after streptococcal pharyngitis.

Epidemiologic studies clearly indicate that streptococcal disease spreads in the home and in the school. The physician must be alert to the occurrence of streptococcal pharyngitis in the family and the school of the patient on prophylaxis. This is a potential risk to the patient, and strict compliance with the prophylaxis must be urged. If streptococcal disease occurs in the family, it should be treated with adequate antimicrobial drugs.

For a number of reasons, the prevention of first attacks

of rheumatic fever is difficult to achieve. Prompt recognition and treatment of streptococcal pharyngitis is hampered in a number of cases by the fact that the symptoms are so mild that the patient does not see a physician. Not uncommonly, when the patient is seen by a doctor, the disease is misdiagnosed or the antimicrobial therapy prescribed is inadequate. For example, the tetracyclines should never be used to treat streptococcal pharyngitis, because 25 to 40 per cent of all group A streptococci are now resistant to this family of drugs.

The occasion arises when special measures are needed to control epidemics of streptococcal pharyngitis in a school or a community or in an army recruit camp. Several unexpected cases of rheumatic fever in a short period of time in a small population group should alert the physician to the possibility that there is a serious streptococcal epidemic in the community in question. Methods to curtail such epidemics have been described in Ch. 190.

Prognosis.   Recovery from the acute attack is the rule. Death at this stage is very rare, even in cases of severe carditis, because of the anti-inflammatory effects of steroid therapy. The disease process in mild cases of rheumatic fever without carditis usually subsides in two to four weeks, and the patient usually makes a complete recovery. When carditis is present, the disease usually persists for six weeks to three months. Patients with carditis during the acute attack may progress to valvular rheumatic heart disease. This is less common in patients without carditis, but absence of carditis during an acute attack is unfortunately not an absolute guarantee against the development of subsequent valvular deformity.

Chronic disability and death owing to rheumatic heart disease are related to recurrent attacks. In former years, before antimicrobial therapy, patients who had had rheumatic fever usually suffered recurrences. Additional valvular deformity was the frequent outcome of each recurrence. As a result, a progressive severity of rheumatic heart disease was common. In current times the prognosis is more optimistic. Progressively severe valvular deformity after an initial attack, if recurrences are prevented, appears to be much less common than in former times, but this point requires further epidemiologic study. The efficacy of adequate chemoprophylaxis in the prevention of recurrences is clearly documented. In one study more than two thirds of the patients with a history of rheumatic fever who were not on prophylaxis had one or more recurrences over an eight-year follow-up period. If prophylaxis is adequately supervised and the drug is taken without fail, a recurrence is an extremely uncommon event.

Kuttner, A. G., and Mayer, F. E.: Carditis during second attacks of rheumatic fever: Its incidence in patients without clinical evidence of cardiac involvement in their initial rheumatic episode. N. Engl. J. Med., 268:1259, 1963.

Lendrum, B. L., Simon, A. J., and Mack, I.: Relation of duration of bed rest in acute rheumatic fever to heart disease present 2 to 14 years later. Pediatrics, 24:389, 1959.

Markowitz, M., and Gordis, L.: Rheumatic Fever. 2nd ed. Philadelphia, W. B. Saunders Company, 1972.

McCarty, M.: Missing links in the streptococcal chain leading to rheumatic fever: The T. Duckett Jones Memorial Lecture. Circulation, 24:488, 1964.

United Kingdom and United States Joint Report: The natural history of rheumatic fever and rheumatic heart disease: Ten-year report of a cooperative clinical trial of ACTH, cortisone, and aspirin. Circulation, 32:457, 1965.

Wood, H. F., and McCarty, M.: Laboratory aids in the diagnosis of rheu-

matic fever and in evaluation of disease activity. Am. J. Med., 17:768, 1954.

Zabriskie, J. B., Hsu, K. C., and Seegal, B. C.: Heart-reactive antibody associated with rheumatic fever: Characterization and diagnostic significance. Clin. Exp. Immunol., 7:147, 1970.

192.   INFECTIVE ENDOCARDITIS
(Bacterial Endocarditis, Prosthetic Valve Endocarditis)

Paul B. Beeson

GENERAL CONSIDERATIONS

In the group of diseases to be considered here, an infective agent colonizes a focus in the heart (or much less commonly in a large vascular channel elsewhere), producing a disease characterized by fever, heart murmur, splenomegaly, embolic manifestations, and bacteremia. This clinical state is of special importance because it almost invariably leads to death unless recognized and treated properly.

In common clinical parlance the term *bacterial endocarditis* is usually employed. The adjective "bacterial" is inadequate inasmuch as the same clinical disease can be caused by fungi, rickettsiae, or spirillar organisms; hence "infective" appears more nearly correct and is gaining in popular usage. The word "endocarditis" is itself misleading, because most of the endocardial surface remains unaffected, and the lesion is more or less restricted to a focus on a cardiac valve leaflet. In rare instances the same form of infection develops at the site of coarctation of the aorta or in a large arteriovenous fistula.

It is customary, and indeed helpful, to speak of either "acute" or "subacute" infective endocarditis. There are major differences between these two forms, and the practice of lumping them together has been responsible for inexactness and confusion. The important differences between acute and subacute endocarditis are shown in the accompanying table.

Having emphasized the difference between the two groups, a qualification must now be entered, because there are borderline cases with both acute and subacute features. Thus infections caused by such organisms as enterococcus or one of the fungi may be difficult to classify. Nevertheless it seems preferable to emphasize,

Differences Between Subacute and Acute Infective Endocarditis

	Subacute	Acute
Causative agent	Normally noninvasive, usually *Strep. viridans*	Capable of primary invasion, e.g., *Staph. aureus*
Pre-existing valve damage	Usually present	May not be present
Other foci of infection by same organism	None	Nearly always
Duration if untreated	Months to 1 to 2 years	Days to weeks
Response of infection to appropriate chemotherapy	Majority cured	Less than half cured

rather than to blur, the division between subacute and acute infective endocarditis.

A special new category of infective endocarditis has been created by cardiac surgery, namely, that engrafted on prosthetic devices.

SUBACUTE INFECTIVE ENDOCARDITIS

Definition. As a rule this form of illness begins insidiously and pursues a long clinical course lasting several months. The causative agent survives only in the endocardial vegetations, and consequently there are no other foci of infection either prior to or after the establishment of the focus. Deaths are due to heart failure, renal failure, embolism, or hemorrhage.

Age and Sex Incidence. The disease is comparatively uncommon before puberty, but may be encountered at any later period of life. It is by no means a rarity in advanced age, when recognition may be especially difficult. The incidence is higher in males.

Microbiology. Literally hundreds of different microbes have been reported as the causative agents in this illness. Most of them are commensals that seem incapable of invading other parts of the body and are pathogenic only when growing in the privileged sanctuary of an intravascular vegetation. Despite the long list of possibilities, the *viridans streptococci* are by far the most common causes of this infection, accounting for 50 to 80 per cent of the reported cases. These organisms are normally present in the mouth and intestine. Classification of the viridans group is unsatisfactory, but the variety called *Streptococcus sanguis,* characterized by the production of dextran, is the one most commonly encountered in infective endocarditis. Other streptococci which may cause the disease include group D or enterococcus and some microaerophilic organisms. Second to the streptococci are *Staphylococcus epidermidis* or *albus;* other well known causes include *diphtheroids* and *Hemophilus spp.* The list of possible etiologic agents is not confined to bacteria, but also includes the *rickettsiae of Q fever,* some spirillar organisms resembling *Spirillum minus,* and a number of *fungi.* Viruses have not been implicated as yet, although the coxsackievirus agents have been shown capable of producing endocardial lesions in laboratory animals. There has been much interest in the possibility that *L forms* of bacteria can be the etiologic agents, and indeed some have been recovered from valve leaflets in patients who had received penicillin therapy, but there is no clear evidence yet that these can be the primary causes of the disease.

It is accepted that organisms become established in some sort of pre-existing nidus on a heart valve, having been carried there in the circulating blood. The frequency with which various microbes are encountered in this disease does not seem to parallel the frequency with which various species enter the bloodstream. For example, *Streptococcus sanguis* is not the predominant organism among the streptococci found in the mouth, although it is the most common single cause of endocarditis. In those cases that arise after instrumentation of the urinary tract, enterococcus is far more important than the coliform bacteria which are the most common organisms in bacteremia associated with urinary tract infection. As a matter of fact, one of the striking features of this disease is the comparative rarity of infections caused by coliform bacteria. Conceivably this may be

related to their susceptibility to lysis by the combined action of complement and antibody without requiring assistance from phagocytes. Another possible factor may be the surface properties of different organisms, whereby some are more likely than others to adhere to a small mass of platelets.

Pathogenesis. In infective endocarditis the organisms find shelter in a structure which develops on a heart valve (or elsewhere in the circulatory system), which provides them with optimal growth conditions as well as protection from phagocytic cells. In a sense one should look on this infection as comparable to that which sometimes develops in the presence of a foreign body or mass of necrotic tissue, in that phagocytes cannot reach the parasite.

It is known that bacteria gain access to the bloodstream fairly commonly: for example, during dental treatment or even vigorous chewing, cleansing of the teeth, parturition, or at the time of urethral instrumentation. In the vast majority of instances such bacteremias are asymptomatic and harmless, but when a suitable nidus is available within the cardiovascular system, circulating microorganisms may stick to it and find conditions there which permit their survival. The original nidus for such growth could be a tiny platelet thrombus on a roughened surface. Angrist, who has studied this question extensively, has offered evidence that the pre-existing lesion is probably so-called *nonbacterial thrombotic endocarditis.* He feels that lesions of this type may, when colonized during an episode of bacteremia, be converted into the vegetation of bacterial endocarditis. Studies of experimental endocarditis in rabbits have shown that such lesions are indeed very susceptible to infection; bacteria lodging there multiply in a manner comparable to that observed under optimal conditions in vitro. Sequential studies of such lesions appear to show that, when the population of bacteria on the surface of a small lesion reaches a certain point, it stimulates the laying down of a covering blanket of platelets and fibrin. Beneath such "blankets" bacterial colonies develop, safe from phagocytes.

Subacute infective endocarditis usually affects valves which have already been damaged. In the past, rheumatic valvulitis was the factor in about 70 per cent, and congenital defects were responsible for another 10 per cent. Syphilitic valvulitis is only rarely complicated by bacterial endocarditis, and perhaps the cases in which this has been reported simply represent the coincidence of syphilis and infective endocarditis. With the present diminishing prevalence of rheumatic heart disease, a higher proportion of cases of infective endocarditis seems to occur in middle-aged and elderly people who have not previously been known to have a valvular defect. In them one presumes that changes associated with aging may render the valve susceptible. The disease is much more common on the left side than on the right. The approximate percentages in autopsied cases are as follows: mitral, 85; aortic, 55; tricuspid, 15; and pulmonic, 1. More than one valve may be affected.

The tendency of subacute bacterial endocarditis to develop in some valve areas and to spare others has excited much speculation. Vegetations are usually found on the downstream side of a leaflet where there is a regurgitant stream. Rodbard points out that the dynamics of flow in such areas during the regurgitant phase would provide little or no lateral pressure; this could either interfere with nutrition of surface tissues or create a situation in which platelets and fibrin could collect, thus offering protection to circulating bacteria. Factors identified by Rodbard are (1) a high pressure source (left ventricle, aorta); (2) a narrow orifice (insufficient valve, ductus arteriosus); and (3) a low pressure chamber beyond the orifice (atrium, ventricle during diastole, and pulmonary vein). This fits with the frequent development of endocarditis on the mitral and aortic valves or in small ventricular septal defects, coarctation of the aorta, ductus arteriosus, or peripheral arteriovenous fistula, and with the rarity of endocarditis on the roughened aorta or in association with atrial septal defect or a large ventricular septal defect. Also in line with this concept is the tendency of subacute bacterial endocarditis to occur in patients with comparatively mild heart disease without failure and without atrial fibrillation. In the presence of the latter complications, decreased pressure gradients and flow rates would perhaps be less favorable to the initiation of a lesion. The concepts of Rodbard and Angrist are thus compatible, and they comprise the most acceptable explanations currently available for development of this unique infection.

After infection has been established on a heart valve or other intravascular focus, steady and continuous *bacteremia* usually ensues. Study of the dynamics of this bacteremia, whereby samples of blood were withdrawn simultaneously from different parts of the circulatory system, has shown that the apparent constancy of the bacteremia is due to an equilibrium between steady replenishment of the arterial blood with fresh organisms and their removal from blood passing through organs containing reticuloendothelial tissue. The notable characteristic of this constant bacteremia is absence of metastatic foci of infection. Most of the organisms must be filtered from the blood and destroyed in reticuloendothelial tissue; those that lodge elsewhere are prey to phagocytes and do not seem capable of establishing infection.

The distinguishing feature of subacute bacterial endocarditis is its chronicity and durability. This lesion, caused by microorganisms incapable of persisting in or infecting other tissues, becomes responsible for a progressive disease, nearly always fatal unless treated with antimicrobial drugs. The host responds with formation of antibodies which react with the infecting organism. Capillaries do not extend into all areas of the vegetation; consequently, comparatively few phagocytic cells can reach the nests of bacteria. It appears therefore that bacteria can colonize superficial portions of the vegetations, safe from phagocytosis, yet capable of drifting out into the circulating blood at a comparatively even rate. Their presence in the vegetation doubtless provides a stimulus to further deposition of fibrin and platelets, causing a gradual enlargement. The lesion may at the same time lead to erosion of the underlying structures, with destruction or perforation of the valve leaflet and worsening of a pre-existing insufficiency.

Pathology. The *vegetation* is composed of masses of platelets, fibrin, and bacteria. In the deeper areas next to the endocardium there may be beginning organization and some capillary blood supply. Attempts at healing may be seen—endothelialization of the surface and organization of the deeper parts. Bacteria are never found in the deeper parts of the vegetation; they tend to be distributed in discrete colonies lying just beneath the surface of the vegetation, adjacent to the moving blood.

Other features of the disease may be attributed either to the bacteremia or to embolization of fragments of vegetation. Enlargement of the *spleen* with follicular hyperplasia is doubtless an example of acute splenic tumor developing in response to continued bacteremia or to antigen administration. The spleen may also be the site of infarction by emboli from the vegetations. The *kidney* may be infarcted grossly or may show evidence of multiple small emboli ("flea-bitten kidney"); there may also be glomerulitis. The last-named lesion has received much study lately. It appears to be an example of immune complex disease, and is probably the factor responsible for renal failure in some longstanding cases, as it is doubtful that embolic injury is ever sufficient to result in renal insufficiency. Major embolization may affect the *brain* and *mesentery.* Myocardial infarction caused by emboli in the coronary vessels is an occasional event, especially in patients with endocarditis on the aortic valve; more commonly the heart shows focal myocarditis, which is probably caused by multiple small emboli. *Mycotic aneurysms* may develop in the walls of large or medium-sized arteries, usually at sites of bifurcations, also occasionally at the base of the aorta. They are thought to result from embolization in vasa vasorum. They are especially dangerous when in the cranial cavity, where rupture may produce manifestations of subarachnoid or intracerebral hemorrhage. Rupture elsewhere can cause severe localized pain and swelling.

Manifestations. In well over half of all cases the disease begins without an identifiable predisposing factor. Some patients give a history of a respiratory infection at about the time the cardiac infection seems to have begun, but this may represent only the coincidental occurrence of a common ailment or erroneous interpretation of early nonspecific symptoms. In 5 to 10 per cent of cases there is a history of dental extraction or other manipulation within three weeks of the onset. In an even smaller proportion of cases the illness has been preceded by urologic instrumentation or by parturition. Opinions differ about the role of dental sepsis, but probably gingival or peridental infection adds to the hazard.

The *onset* in most cases is subtle, with malaise and low-grade fever; patients usually think they have "the flu." Occasionally there is a more dramatic beginning, with greater initial prostration or with an embolic accident. *Fever,* although present in nearly every case, is variable in extent, sometimes not more than $0.5°$ C above normal; in other cases there may be hectic variations accompanied by chilliness and sweating. In addition to malaise, other accompaniments of fever such as fatigue, weight loss, and anorexia may be noted.

Heart murmur is present in nearly all cases of subacute endocarditis. Percentages as high as 98 or 99 have been reported, but this is too high. There is no cardiac murmur if the vegetations are outside the heart, as in coarctation or infected arteriovenous fistula. Occasionally, even when the infection is on a valve leaflet, auscultation may reveal nothing early in the illness, but a murmur may be detected later. This seems especially common in middle-aged men with aortic valve endocarditis. Right-sided endocarditis, too, is especially noted for the absence of heart murmur. Changing murmurs are often said to be characteristic of subacute bacterial endocarditis; actually the day-to-day changes are often simply caused by fluctuations of body temperature and heart rate. However, the abrupt appearance of an aortic diastolic murmur is of great significance. Infected patent ductus arteriosus may be accompanied by significant changes in character of the murmur from time to time. *Pericardial friction rubs* are notably rare in this disease. *Splenomegaly* is present in about 80 per cent of cases, but the organ seldom becomes greatly enlarged. It may be tender after infarction. *Clubbing of the fingers and toes* develops in at least half the longstanding cases, but nowadays, with early recognition and effective therapy, this physical sign should not have time to develop.

Findings in the *skin* and *mucous membranes* may be helpful in diagnosis, especially late in the course. *Petechiae* appear on any part of the body. These are small, are red or purple, and do not blanch on pressure. It may help to mark the locations of red spots and to inspect them again after a day or two, an interval in which petechiae should fade. Petechiae in the conjunctiva or oral mucosa are especially easy to recognize and not likely to be confused with any other lesion. Sometimes they have white centers. Small areas of hemorrhage may be seen in the ocular fundi. Hemorrhages in the nail beds usually have a linear distribution near the distal end, hence the name "splinter hemorrhages." These can be helpful diagnostic signs, but it must be emphasized that *they are by no means pathognomonic of bacterial endocarditis.* They often occur in patients with other chronic diseases of the heart and lungs, apparently caused by dissemination of tiny thrombi, and they can frequently be found in people who do manual work. *Osler's nodes* are acute, tender, barely palpable nodular lesions in the pulps of the fingers and toes. There may be reddening of the overlying skin. They tend to appear abruptly and then to subside within a few days. *Pallor* caused by anemia is present when the disease has existed for a few weeks or longer. Older descriptions of the disease mention a *café-au-lait color of the skin.* This is rarely seen today; it may have been related to longstanding untreated infection with renal decompensation. *Neurologic manifestations* are common, and may constitute the chief complaint, especially in older patients. Cerebral embolism may simulate an ordinary stroke. Less commonly there may be encephalopathy, meningitis, or convulsions. Peripheral neuropathy has been reported.

The *blood picture* is not distinctive in bacterial endocarditis. Mild normochromic anemia, without reticulocytosis, develops in patients untreated for more than a few weeks. The leukocyte count is moderately elevated or in the high normal range because of increase in granulocytes. *Abnormal histiocytes* may be found in the peripheral blood in this disease, especially when the specimen examined is the first drop of blood obtained by puncture of an ear lobe. The characteristic cells are bizarre in appearance and may contain erythrocytes or other leukocytes. Their demonstration has occasionally been helpful in diagnosis.

Dramatic clinical events may follow lodgment of large emboli in arteries throughout the body, and these can occur some days after institution of appropriate treatment. *Cerebral* or *coronary* embolism may cause *cerebral* or *myocardial infarction. Splenic infarction* is manifested by tenderness and sometimes by pain on respiration. *Renal infarction* is usually asymptomatic but may reveal itself by the sudden appearance of hematuria. Embolism of the *mesenteric arteries* can cause severe abdominal pain, ileus, distention, and melena. Occlusion of a distal artery may result in *gangrene* of a digit, the tip of the nose, or the ear.

Heart failure is a frequent and important complication that merits discussion under manifestations of bacterial endocarditis. The mechanism of failure may be either further impairment of valvular efficiency or injury to the myocardium. The former may be due to perforation of a valve cusp or leaflet or from rupture of a papillary muscle or chorda tendinea. It is especially likely when the aortic valve is affected; here there may be sudden intensification or alteration in character of the regurgitant murmur, accompanied within hours by evidence of worsening circulatory status. The myocardium may be injured by multiple small emboli or by larger ones affecting whole segments of the coronary circulation. In any event the development of signs of heart failure during the acute or convalescent stage of bacterial endocarditis has grave prognostic significance. Deciding when to resort to cardiac surgery because of this complication is an important aspect of modern management.

Rheumatic Manifestations. Pains in muscles and joints are fairly common in bacterial endocarditis. Occasionally there are swelling and heat in one or more joints that may be difficult to differentiate from an exacerbation of rheumatic fever; indeed the conditions can probably coexist.

Mild or moderate *proteinuria* is common, and microscopic *hematuria* is a useful diagnostic finding; needle biopsy of the kidney has revealed active lesions of glomerulitis even when urinalysis showed nothing. In untreated cases, death may result from *renal failure;* this is rare now except when the true nature of the underlying disease is unrecognized. As already mentioned, the serious form of kidney damage is that which resembles glomerulonephritis morphologically. Interestingly, renal function may improve after institution of effective antimicrobial therapy.

ACUTE INFECTIVE ENDOCARDITIS

In this kind of endocarditis the course is generally more fulminating than in the subacute form. The determining factor is the kind of etiologic agent. Here we are dealing with microorganisms that are recognized pathogens. The most common is *Staphylococcus aureus,* but many others may produce the same clinical disease: *β-hemolytic streptococcus, pneumococcus, gonococcus, Pseudomonas, Proteus, Brucella, Bacteroides, Candida,* and *Histoplasma.*

This type of infection of a heart valve often develops secondary to infection elsewhere, e.g., meningitis, pneumonia, or septic thrombophlebitis such as that which may arise at the site of an indwelling catheter. As a consequence, the existence of bacterial endocarditis must be recognized in the setting of an acute microbial disease. On the other hand, it may come on without evidence of a pre-existing focus. Whatever the beginning, metastatic infections are frequent elsewhere, especially in the lungs, kidneys, meninges, and joints.

This disease can exhibit all the clinical manifestations already described in the subacute form. Although more frequent on the left side of the heart, the proportion of tricuspid valve infections is greater: 25 to 50 per cent in different reported series. Two physical findings seen only in acute endocarditis are the *Janeway lesion* and the *Roth spot.* The first is a painless red-blue lesion a few millimeters in diameter, found on the palm or sole. The second is in the optic fundus: an oval pale area near the disc, perhaps a quarter the area of the disc, surrounded by hemorrhage. Acute endocarditis frequently develops in patients with no pre-existing valvular disease; consequently there may be no murmur at the onset. However, damage to the valve and adjoining structures is likely to occur, and perforation of an aortic cusp or rupture of a chorda tendinea may cause sudden appearance of signs of aortic or mitral insufficiency. Another frequent lesion is *myocardial abscess in the valve ring area*—a complication with grave prognostic significance.

Since a heart murmur may not be present at the onset, and since significant foci of infection may be evident elsewhere, the existence of endocarditis may not be obvious. Its possibility must always be kept in mind, especially when appropriate antimicrobial therapy fails to bring about clinical improvement within a few days. Patients must be examined frequently for the appearance of a murmur or signs of heart failure.

The treatment and prognosis of all forms of infective endocarditis will be dealt with in one section. Nevertheless, it is worth emphasis here that antimicrobial therapy in acute endocarditis is substantially less effective than in the subacute forms. Furthermore the need for cardiac surgery is more likely to arise in acute than in subacute bacterial endocarditis.

PROSTHETIC VALVE ENDOCARDITIS

As the number of operations to implant prosthetic valves in human hearts has increased, a new, third category of infective endocarditis has been created. This can take either the acute or the subacute form. The vegetations are most often found along the line of suturing of the device; they may spread on to adjacent endothelium or on to the device itself.

The reported incidence of endocarditis as a complication of prosthetic valve surgery has varied from as low as 1 per cent to as high as 6 per cent. The variation is doubtless related to differences in the length of follow-up after the operative procedure, in operative techniques, in materials employed, and in the kind of prophylactic antimicrobial therapy. The risk of infection appears far higher with aortic than with mitral valve replacement; in one series 17 per cent of aortic valves became infected, in contrast to only 1.5 per cent of mitral valves.

There are probably at least three modes of infection in prosthetic valve endocarditis. In some cases microbes may be implanted during the operative procedure, from air, circulatory pumps, and the like. Prophylactic therapy at the time of surgery doubtless diminishes the frequency of such infections but cannot be expected to bar all possible invaders. Second, during the postoperative period, infection can establish itself on the prosthesis secondary to a suppurative process elsewhere, e.g., sternal infection, empyema, or infection around a venous catheter. Finally, endocarditis may originate "spontaneously" at any time after surgery as a chance event in a transient bacteremia, as has been described in discussing the genesis of subacute infective endocarditis. It is reasonable to assume that the risk of endocarditis in persons with prostheses is at least as great as in patients with rheumatic or congenital heart disease. If that is correct, we can expect this form of endocarditis to become increasingly common as patients live longer after cardiac surgery.

The bacteriology of prosthetic valve infections is variable, and may include pathogens as well as commensals.

In those instances which appear to have had their onset at the time of surgery, the organisms have been mainly *Staphylococcus epidermidis* and diphtheroids. Those developing secondary to sepsis elsewhere have most commonly been due to *Staphylococcus aureus,* but other pathogens such as Pseudomonas and Proteus and Candida also constitute a threat. Among late cases, i.e., those becoming evident more than two months after surgery, *Staphylococcus epidermidis* and *Streptococcus sanguis* are particularly important.

SPECIAL SITUATIONS

Infected Arteriovenous Fistula. Perhaps 20 such cases have been reported. The infecting organism in most of them has been a viridans streptococcus. In about a third of reported cases, bacterial endocarditis has later developed on the aortic valve. Presumably the fistula, by causing circulatory strain, has rendered the valve liable to infection. This seems analogous to the observations of Lillehei on susceptibility to endocarditis in dogs with surgically induced arteriovenous fistulas.

Chronic Hemodialysis. Numerous reports have appeared of infective endocarditis as a complication of chronic hemodialysis for renal insufficiency. In some there has been an obvious pre-existing septic process, such as the site of the shunt. The infecting organisms in such cases have been *Staphylococcus aureus,* Candida, or Pseudomonas. In several others the causative organism has been a viridans streptococcus; this suggests an analogy with the cases developing in association with arteriovenous fistula, just described.

Heroin Addiction. Acute bacterial endocarditis is one of the hazards of heroin addiction, for the drug is usually self-administered intravenously with little or no aseptic technique. There appears to be a special likelihood of tricuspid endocarditis. Because of the resulting embolization, the principal clinical manifestations may be pulmonary (pleuritic pain, cough, hemoptysis, and multiple shadows in radiogram). Heart murmur may not be detected. The clinical impression is thus likely to be that of pneumonia with septicemia. The most common infecting organism is *Staphylococcus aureus,* and other possibilities include enterococcus, Candida, and such gram-negative bacilli as Pseudomonas or Proteus. The bacteriology of the endocarditis of heroin addiction must vary according to local mores: in Detroit there are many Pseudomonas infections, whereas in New York City *Staph. aureus* is by far the most frequent cause.

Pneumococcal Endocarditis. In some instances pneumococcal endocarditis has appeared to be associated with chronic alcoholism and malnutrition. The possible coexistence of endocarditis should always be considered in pneumococcal meningitis, and Austrian has estimated that endocarditis will be found in a quarter to a third of patients with pneumococcal meningitis. Rupture of the aortic valve cusp is likely to occur in this disease, and it is almost invariably followed by severe heart failure.

Enterococcal Endocarditis. Middle-aged or elderly men with urologic disease and women in the child-bearing period are at special risk of enterococcal infection; hence, there is little question that instrumentation of the urogenital tract is an important pathogenetic event. The clinical features are intermediate between the subacute and acute forms, because there is a tendency to metastatic suppurative foci, especially splenic abscess.

Gonococcal Endocarditis. Two distinctive features have been reported. About half the patients show an unusual kind of fever; a double rise and fall during each 24-hour period. This has not been characteristic of any other form of endocarditis, and an explanation is lacking. The second noteworthy feature is evidence of hepatic dysfunction. The liver is conspicuously spared in most kinds of endocarditis, but jaundice is relatively common when gonococcus is the infecting organism.

Bacteroides Endocarditis. Portals of entry include the respiratory, gastrointestinal, and genitourinary tracts. The clinical picture is one of acute bacterial endocarditis, and septic thrombophlebitis may be a feature. Some strains are penicillin sensitive, and in them the prognosis is better.

Fungal Endocarditis. The clinical features in fungal endocarditis may be those of either acute or subacute bacterial endocarditis. In some the valvular involvement has been only one aspect of an overwhelming septicemic process, but in the majority the endocarditis has been the central lesion. One notable characteristic is embolic occlusion of large arteries; this may be related to the bulkiness of vegetations induced by fungi. The most frequent fungal infections are by Candida or Histoplasma, but a few cases of infection with Aspergillus, Blastomyces, Coccidioides, Cryptococcus, and Mucor have also been reported.

Q Fever Endocarditis. This kind of infection should be thought of, and tested for, in patients with the clinical manifestations of subacute infective endocarditis, in whom blood cultures yield no growth, and in whom a trial of penicillin therapy fails to cause clinical improvement. The majority of reported cases have been in males with aortic insufficiency, and the progress has been slow. Serologic tests for *Rickettsia burnetii* should reveal antibodies in high titer. Some apparent cures have been reported by use of tetracycline, chloramphenicol, or cotrimoxazole, plus valve replacement.

Diagnosis. The possibility of bacterial endocarditis must always be kept in mind, because it is a curable disease, yet fatal if unrecognized. Unexplained fever lasting more than a week in a patient with a heart murmur imposes on the physician an obligation to consider the likelihood of bacterial endocarditis *and to draw blood cultures.* Delay until the appearance of such "cardinal" manifestations as clubbing of the fingers, splenic enlargement, anemia, changing murmurs, and petechiae is inexcusable.

Firm diagnosis can be achieved only by demonstration of bacteremia, which is possible in about 95 per cent of cases. As already discussed, bacteremia, if present at all, is usually a fairly steady, continuous process. Cultures are not more likely to be positive at a particular time of day or when the patient's body temperature is high or low. The best practice therefore is to draw four to six samples of blood for culture during the first day or two. Blood from the antecubital vein is as likely to yield positive cultures as arterial blood or bone marrow. If the patient had been receiving antimicrobial therapy, it may be necessary to stop treatment and wait a few days before obtaining the cultures. If an organism with unusual growth requirements is suspected, special culture media may have to be employed.

Diagnosis is considerably more difficult in abacteremic cases. It is impossible to say why, in a small proportion of cases, bacteria rarely gain access to the bloodstream, in contrast to the more common state of affairs when they are demonstrable almost continuously. Some agents cannot be demonstrated by the usual blood culture techniques; for example, cases caused by the Rickettsia of Q fever will be identified only by testing specifically for serologic evidence of this infection. Likewise in some cases of fungal endocarditis the organisms may not show up in blood cultures; in such situations help may be obtained from serologic tests or by demonstrating the organism in biopsy of another tissue. At any rate, the clinician must recognize the existence of this type of case and must weigh the indications for proceeding with a "blind" trial of antimicrobial therapy, as described later under Treatment.

Differential Diagnosis. Subacute infective endocarditis is one of the most familiar causes of prolonged fever of obscure origin. When bacteremia can be demonstrated, the diagnosis is relatively easy; it is the abacteremic cases that present the main difficulty. A treatise on the differential diagnosis of this disease could be of great length; here it is possible only to mention some of the most common diseases with which infective endocarditis can be confused.

Systemic lupus erythematosus may present many of the findings of bacterial endocarditis, e.g., fever, heart murmur, anemia, hematuria, arthralgia, and petechiae. A positive LE test or demonstration of antinuclear factor and negative blood cultures are the usual criteria for differentiation. Therapeutic trials of antimicrobial drugs and of steroids may give assistance.

It may be extremely difficult to distinguish between *acute rheumatic fever* and infective endocarditis. Erythema marginatum, pericarditis, and severe disabling arthritis would point toward acute rheumatic fever. Changing titers of antibody to beta-hemolytic streptococcal antigens would also favor that disease.

Sickle cell disease can cause fever, anemia, heart murmur, arthralgia, and abnormal kidney function. Demonstration of sickling or of abnormal hemoglobin should clarify the issue.

Atrial myxoma can mimic infective endocarditis. There may be fever, arthralgia, changing heart murmur, petechiae, splinter hemorrhage, and embolic manifestations. Several patients with this rare disease have been treated for infective endocarditis—a fatal clinical error in view of possible surgical cure.

Nonbacterial thrombic endocarditis is a common finding at autopsy in people who have suffered long wasting illnesses, especially lung cancer. It is now well accepted that embolization by pieces of these structures can occur, with manifestations of infarction, in spleen, kidney, and brain. Thus these patients may have heart murmur, fever, and embolic manifestations.

Drug reactions resulting in fever and anemia can resemble infective endocarditis. The finding of eosinophilia would help to differentiate such reactions from endocarditis, and the results of discontinuing drug therapy will resolve the issue.

Other well-known causes of obscure febrile illness such as *miliary tuberculosis* and *lymphoma* or *other neoplasms* may cause confusion if the patient happens to have a heart murmur.

The differential diagnosis in *acute bacterial endocarditis* includes various major acute infectious processes such as pneumonia, meningitis, pyelonephritis, and biliary tract infection. In these, the existence of endocarditis may be overlooked because of the prominence of local manifestations.

Prosthetic valve endocarditis developing soon after the surgery may be exceedingly difficult to identify. The differential diagnosis includes various kinds of postoperative sepsis and postcardiotomy and postpump syndromes as well as drug fever. When it develops two or more months after operation, the picture is likely to be that of subacute infective endocarditis, and here the correct diagnosis should be reached more easily.

Treatment. *General Considerations.* Bacterial endocarditis stands out among infectious diseases as the one in which cure depends on use of drugs capable of killing bacteria without assistance of phagocytes. The difficulty doubtless stems from the protection that is offered when microbes grow in a mass of platelets and fibrin that cannot be penetrated by phagocytes. Ample clinical experience has shown that the bacteriostatic antimicrobial drugs, such as sulfonamides, tetracycline, and chloramphenicol, seldom cure this infection. Although their administration may result in clinical improvement and sterile blood cultures, relapse occurs each time treatment is terminated. *The penicillins are by far the most valuable agents,* and it should be said that when the infecting organism is not killed by a member of this family, or when the patient is so allergic that one dare not give penicillin, the chances of successful result are reduced. Nevertheless, cures have resulted from treatment with several other bactericidal drugs, including the cephalosporins, neomycin, kanamycin, vancomycin, gentamicin, carbenicillin, and colistin. In a few cases fungal infection has been cured with amphotericin B or 5-fluorocytosine.

The place of streptomycin as an adjunct to penicillin therapy deserves special consideration. There can be no question of its value in combination with penicillin in the treatment of enterococcal infections, and there are also reports which show a similar enhancement of the efficacy of vancomycin. Authorities disagree on the need for streptomycin when dealing with infections caused by microorganisms highly sensitive to penicillin. Certainly, literally thousands of these have been cured by treatment with penicillin alone. There is reason to argue, however, on the basis of in vitro tests as well as studies of experimental endocarditis in rabbits that bacterial killing proceeds more rapidly and more completely with combined treatment than with penicillin alone. Because of this, and in view of the minimal risk of toxicity from streptomycin in the dose recommended, it seems reasonable to combine streptomycin therapy with penicillin as a general rule.

A second requirement for success is prolonged therapy. Unlike most infections, in which an antibacterial effect sufficient to tip the balance in favor of the host will suffice, the cure of bacterial endocarditis seems to depend on the ability of the drug to sterilize the vegetation unaided by host defenses. Therefore opportunity must be provided for every germ present to enter a phase of growth in which it is susceptible to killing by the agent or agents being used. Perhaps also some time is required for erosion of the surface of the vegetation, exposing the nests of bacteria that lie embedded there so that they can be carried off to other tissues for destruction. A few cures have been reported in cases treated for only ten days, and hundreds of patients have been successfully treated in 14-day courses. On the other hand, there is ample experience to demonstrate that treatment should extend for far longer periods in certain kinds of cases, as will be described subsequently.

The question of combining antimicrobial therapy with anticoagulant or fibrinolytic agents to inhibit further deposition of fibrin and platelets on the vegetations has often been raised. There is little evidence to show that this is beneficial; and indeed it adds a serious hazard of fatal hemorrhage, usually intracranial, from mycotic aneurysms. Therefore *this form of treatment is to be avoided* if possible. The risk is great enough to call for cessation of anticoagulant treatment for such indications as atrial fibrillation or deep vein thrombosis, but perhaps it must be accepted in patients with prosthetic valves.

Certain considerations influence the decision on how soon to begin therapy once the diagnosis seems probable and blood cultures have been obtained. Because excessive delay in instituting treatment undoubtedly permits further damage to heart valves and opportunity for serious embolic accidents, there is a tendency to commence antimicrobial therapy immediately. Indeed, when the clinical course is acute and the causative microorganism is probably a pathogen, or when the aortic valve is affected, it is advisable to begin treatment without delay, using the best guess as to appropriate drugs and doses, and making changes later when laboratory results are available. On the other hand, waiting until the diagnosis has been confirmed by blood culture, so that chemotherapy can be based on secure knowledge of the etiology, also has advantages. When the clinical manifestations are mild, and viridans streptococcus infection seems likely, there is comparatively little danger in waiting until the diagnosis can be confirmed by blood culture. Sensitivity tests can then provide information on the best drug to use and the proper dosage.

When bacteremia has been demonstrated, the organism should be kept viable in the laboratory until conclusion of treatment, because further tests to confirm or improve the efficacy of the treatment regimen may be desired. It is useful to test the patient's serum during treatment for bactericidal effect on the causative organism. For probability of favorable clinical result, bacterial killing by a dilution of 1 to 8 or greater is desirable.

It is generally believed that antimicrobials should be administered parenterally in this disease, although some successes have been obtained by giving penicillin orally. It would be essential in this situation to ascertain that suitable levels in body fluids are being attained, by testing the antibacterial activity of the patient's serum from time to time during the course of therapy.

Penicillins. Even when penicillin appears to be the drug of choice, the necessary dosage may vary considerably. When the etiologic agent is a viridans streptococcus, sensitive to 0.05 μg per milliliter or less, therapy consisting of 2 million units of penicillin daily, given parenterally at six-hour intervals, is sufficient. For strains less sensitive to penicillin, e.g., 0.05 to 1.0 μg per milliliter, considerably larger amounts of penicillin, up to 10 or 20 million per day, may be required, and it is common practice to add probenecid, 0.5 gram four times a day, to retard penicillin loss via the kidneys. In cases of enterococcal infection, one is dealing with an organism generally exhibiting a considerable resistance to penicillin, i.e., 5 or more μg per milliliter. Here the requirement is for large daily doses of penicillin, and the need for streptomycin as an adjunct is unquestioned. The amount of penicillin required may be 20 million to 100 million units daily, together with 1.0 gram of streptomycin per day, in four doses. Quantities of penicillin of this magnitude must be given by continuous intravenous infusion because of the pain caused by intramuscular injection. Ampicillin may be better than penicillin G in some enterococcal infections; streptomycin should be given here, too.

When the causative organism is a penicillinase-producing organism, especially *Staphylococcus aureus,* cure may be effected by use of a semisynthetic penicillin such as oxacillin. The dose is 4 to 18 grams daily intramuscularly or, with less pain, intravenously.

Occasionally the patient is so allergic to penicillins that their administration would threaten his life. Attempts may be made to suppress the allergic manifestations by steroid therapy, but this can lead to most serious difficulty. Here it may be preferable to try another bactericidal drug.

Other Antimicrobials. When the causative organism is not sensitive to one of the penicillins, or in the rare event that the patient is impossibly allergic to drugs of this family, it becomes necessary to treat with other agents.

The *cephalosporins* are valuable assets in this situation, and a substantial number of patients have been successfully treated with them. In view of the need for prolonged treatment with large doses, the best-tolerated method of administration is cephaloridine or another analogue by continuous intravenous drip, in a dose of 1 to 3 grams every six hours.

Vancomycin treatment has also succeeded against a number of gram-positive organisms, including the enterococcus; it must be given intravenously, 0.25 to 0.5 gram every six hours.

In *gram-negative bacterial endocarditis* the drugs mentioned so far may all be ineffective, but cure may be achieved with other agents. The choice must be made with the aid of detailed laboratory tests, but the following are among the most likely possibilities: *kanamycin,* 10 to 20 mg per kilogram of body weight per day divided into three equal doses, intramuscularly or intravenously; *gentamicin,* 3 to 5 mg per kilogram of body weight per day divided into three equal doses, intramuscularly or intravenously; *carbenicillin,* 10 to 30 grams per day, by continuous intravenous infusion. The last-named agent can be given with either of the first two, though not in the same vehicle. It is necessary to be on the alert for signs of toxicity with gentamicin or kanamycin, especially to kidney or eighth nerve; nevertheless, their use even to the point of serious injury may be justified when nothing else seems able to cure the infection.

Treatment of *prosthetic valve endocarditis* by chemotherapy alone is rarely successful, and there is a growing tendency to combine it with surgery, as discussed subsequently. There may be some advantage to be gained by a preliminary course of chemotherapy for a few weeks, on the assumption that surgery will be technically easier if inflammation of surrounding tissues has been lessened by control of active infection. However, worsening of the circulatory status is an overriding indication to proceed with surgery immediately.

In rare instances, resistant cases of bacterial endocarditis have been handled successfully by use of unusual combinations of antimicrobials, e.g., rifampicin and erythromycin; or tetracycline, chloramphenicol, and streptomycin. Laboratory guidance concerning combinations of drugs is difficult, and the results are somewhat unreliable because of the changing concentrations that take place in the patient's body fluids. Perhaps the best guide is to test the bactericidal effect of the patient's serum while he is under treatment.

The chemotherapy of the various mycotic infections is discussed in Ch. 255 to 266.

Treatment of abacteremic cases is difficult because there is no guide to the selection of drugs and dosages. In view of the probability of gram-positive infection, a reasonable program of treatment is the following: Begin with 10 million units of penicillin and 1 gram of streptomycin daily. If the patient's condition improves and his temperature level falls during the next 72 hours, continue with this program. If there is no evidence of clinical effect in three days, raise the dose of penicillin to 100 million units daily, and continue treatment for three days. If there is still no sign of benefit, discontinue penicillin and streptomycin and try oxacillin, 12 grams daily for four days. If this does not appear to be effective, change to vancomycin, 2 grams daily, by continuous intravenous drip, for another four days. If the causative agent is a gram-positive bacterium, one of the foregoing plans of treatment should have produced some sign of improvement. Because the possibility of gram-negative bacterial infection must also be considered, one could then try the effects of kanamycin, gentamicin, or carbenicillin, in the doses already described. If all these fail, the possibility of infection by something like *R. burnetii,* Candida, or Aspergillus must be given special consideration.

In the decision on *duration of antimicrobial drug treatment,* some variation is permissible and proper. There is no convincing clinical evidence that all cases must be treated for several weeks; on the other hand, it seems prudent in some instances to continue therapy for three or more months. As stated earlier, therapy must be maintained for many days, no matter how prompt the clinical response. At present the minimal time for any treatment is thought to be two weeks. This would be reasonable in a case in which all the auguries are favorable, e.g., *Streptococcus sanguis* sensitive to less than 0.05 μg of penicillin per milliliter, short duration of illness before therapy is begun, prompt defervescence after institution of treatment, and patient under 50 in good general health. Contrarily, in dealing with infection of a prosthetic valve by *Staphylococcus aureus,* one would be ill advised to think of discontinuing treatment in less than two months, regardless of apparent clinical response. In some instances, with indolent but stubborn infections of prostheses by, say, *Staphylococcus epidermidis,* oral treatment with a semisynthetic penicillin has had to be maintained for two or more years and even then has succeeded only in suppressing bacterial growth.

At the conclusion of a planned course of therapy, if the infection has been eradicated, the patient's temperature should be normal, the spleen should have diminished in size, and he should be free of complaints. After cessation of therapy he should be watched for signs of recurring infection. Blood cultures should be obtained during the first week, and at two weeks and six weeks. If there has been no return of symptoms by the end of six weeks and if blood cultures have remained negative, it is safe to assume that cure has been accomplished. Second attacks of bacterial endocarditis are by no means rare, whereas relapse of the original infection after a free interval of six weeks would be unlikely. Prophylactic chemotherapy to prevent development of a second infection is not advisable, because it may cause the next infection to be associated with a more resistant organism.

Surgical Measures. Even before the advent of modern chemotherapy, a few cures of this disease were achieved by closure of an infected arteriovenous fistula or patent ductus arteriosus. Simply by obliterating the vascular channel in which the vegetation was placed, the infection has been caused to burn itself out. This point is worth bearing in mind even in the "chemotherapy era," as it may encourage the undertaking of radical surgical treatment in emergency situations.

Prosthetic valve implantation during the active phase of infective endocarditis has now become fairly common practice, and the indications for it are becoming better defined. Review of recent experience at the Henry Ford Hospital showed that surgery had been employed in 15 per cent of cases of infective endocarditis. There are two main indications for surgery: (1) *Insufficiency of the valve resulting from damage caused by infection.* This may result from injury to a natural leaflet, or a paraprosthetic leak caused by infection at the suture line. Aortic valve infection is especially dangerous from this standpoint. The delicate leaflets are subject to erosion or perforation, and such damage may throw the patient into very severe pump failure which cannot be controlled by digitalis and diuretics. Sometimes it becomes necessary to operate within hours because of a shocklike state. This is a desperate situation, but nothing is gained by delaying surgery in the hope that the patient's condition can be improved by medical measures. The likelihood that viable microorganisms may still be present should not argue against operation. The surgeon may be able to remove some infected tissue when implanting the new valve, and if circulatory efficiency is improved, there may then be time for chemotherapy to cure the infection: (2) *Inability to cure the infection with drugs alone.* In some cases the removal of an infected prosthesis and its vegetations, with the placement of a new one, together with intensive chemotherapy, has served to eradicate a previously intractable infection. In acute tricuspid endocarditis caused by Pseudomonas the entire valve has been excised, with subsequent cure by chemotherapy, and the patients have been described as hemodynamically stable one or two years later even without their tricuspid valves.

Prophylaxis. *Care of the Teeth.* It is a general impression that the incidence of *Streptococcus viridans* endocarditis is lower in edentulous persons than in subjects with teeth. This has led to an extreme view in some clinics that teeth should be removed as a prophylactic measure in all patients with valvular heart disease. The majority opinion, however, is that otherwise healthy teeth should not be sacrificed. Nevertheless, it is reasonable to recommend that special attention be given to oral hygiene in patients with valvular heart disease, and that indications for extraction be interpreted liberally.

Chemoprophylaxis When Bacteremia Is Anticipated. In view of the indubitable role of manipulations likely to produce transient bacteremia in the origin of some cases of bacterial endocarditis, it has become accepted practice to "protect" persons with valvular or congenital heart disease by giving a short course of antimicrobial drug therapy at the time of such procedures. This is recommended in all textbooks and is the subject of special educational programs by national heart associations in many countries. The specific recommendations have been based on the probable infecting organisms and their in vitro sensitivities. It must be pointed out, however, that these are based only on what seems to be a good idea, for the efficacy of such prophylaxis has never been proved. There are, in fact, a number of reports of endocarditis caused by penicillin-sensitive organisms after tooth extraction despite the fact that penicillin had been given according to one of the "approved" regimens. Actual proof of value of such therapy would be almost impossible to achieve by clinical experiment, because the risk of endocarditis, even in patients with valvular heart disease who must have tooth extraction, is very small — perhaps one in several hundreds.

Recently a suitable experimental model for producing endocarditis in rabbits after a single intravenous injection of bacteria has permitted for the first time an evaluation of current recommendations for chemoprophylaxis. This has revealed that dosage schedules comparable with those recommended for clinical use are rarely successful in preventing development of endocarditis in the test animals. Giving the antimicrobial drug just before or just after the bacterial inoculum does not affect the result. Tetracycline, commonly recommended for use after genitourinary manipulations, is worthless even though the therapy is maintained for seven days. Penicillin, to be effective, must be given in large dosage, and a bactericidal level maintained for some hours. The effectiveness of penicillin is enhanced when streptomycin is given with it. Vancomycin appears to be excellent, even with a single injection, but has the drawback of intravenous administration.

On the basis of present information derived from the animal work, the following is here recommended: (1) *For dental extraction:* in order of probable efficacy, (a) penicillin G, 1,000,000 units intramuscularly, plus 0.5 gram of streptomycin intramuscularly; (b) vancomycin, 1.0 gram intravenously; (c) penicillin G, 2,000,000 units, plus procaine penicillin, 600,000 units intramuscularly. All can be given immediately before or immediately after the procedure. (2) *For urethral or gynecologic procedures:* ampicillin, 1 gram, plus streptomycin, 0.5 gram, intramuscularly, just before and six hours after the procedure.

Chemoprophylaxis at Time of Cardiac Surgery. Cardiac surgeons are likely to have their own views about this, but at present a reasonable scheme would be 1 gram each of ampicillin and oxacillin intramuscularly or intravenously every 6 hours for 10 to 14 days, beginning just before surgery.

Prognosis. Most reports of series of cases of infective endocarditis treated with modern chemotherapy indicate that the infection can be eradicated in 60 or 70 per cent of cases; a few have claimed success in as high as 80 per cent. Both figures are far too high for acute bacterial endocarditis, in which a 25 to 30 per cent recovery rate would be felt to be a considerable achievement. It must also be emphasized that eradication of infection is not the whole story, because a significant proportion of patients have nevertheless suffered additional cardiac injury, either by valve damage or by coronary artery embolization. In some of these the valvular defect can now be alleviated surgically. Aside from circulatory insufficiency, a few patients are permanently disabled by cerebral embolism. As an over-all figure, including both acute and subacute cases, it may be said that somewhat less than 50 per cent of treated patients will be well and free of cardiac failure five years later. Such results are remarkably good, however, when viewed in the light of the almost certain fatal outcome without chemotherapy and surgery.

The following factors indicate a poor outlook: (1) *Insusceptibility of the causative organism* to penicillin and other bactericidal drugs. Results are likely to be less favorable in infections caused by staphylococci, gram-negative bacteria, enterococci or fungi. (2) *Heart failure,* appearing during treatment. This is likely to resist supportive therapy and may lead to death within a few weeks or months. It carries with it the added risk of surgery if the failure is due to valvular insufficiency. (3) *Aortic valve involvement.* The likelihood of serious valvular damage and intractable failure seems much greater when the aortic valve is one of those infected. (4) *Old age.* The death rate is high in all forms of endocarditis after the age of 60. (5) *Abacteremic disease.* In most reports the survival rate for abacteremic patients is about half that for bacteremic patients. Diagnosis is likely to be delayed and treatment begun later. Without laboratory aid the treatment must be by guesswork and evidence of clinical response; this means further delay before an effective program is hit upon. (6) *Infection of a prosthetic device.* Chemotherapy seldom eradicates infection established on a prosthesis. (7) *Delay in institution of therapy.* Failure to think of the possibility of this diagnosis may lead to loss of precious days or weeks. The common practice of prescribing a broad-spectrum antimicrobial such as tetracycline for any patient with fever may lead to serious delay.

Angrist, A. A.: Pathogenesis of bacterial endocarditis. J.A.M.A., 183:249, 1963.

Arbulu, A., Thoms, N. W., and Wilson, R. F.: Valvulectomy without prosthetic replacement. J. Thorac. Cardiovasc. Surg., 64:103, 1972.

Black, S., O'Rourke, R. A., and Karliner, J. S.: Role of surgery in the treatment of primary infective endocarditis. Am. J. Med., 56:357, 1974.

Dreyer, N. P., and Fields, B. N.: Heroin-associated infective endocarditis. Ann. Intern. Med., 78:699, 1973.

Durack, D. T., and Beeson, P. B.: Experimental bacterial endocarditis: I. Colonization of a sterile vegetation. Br. J. Exp. Pathol., 53:44, 1972.

Durack, D. T., and Petersdorf, R. G.: Chemotherapy of experimental streptococcal endocarditis. I. Comparison of commonly recommended prophylactic regimens. J. Clin. Invest., 52:592, 1973.

Griffin, F. M., Jr., Jones, G., and Cobbs, C. G.: Aortic insufficiency in bacterial endocarditis. Ann. Intern. Med., 76:23, 1972.

Gutman, R. A., Striker, G. E., Gilliland, B. C., and Cutler, R. E.: The immune complex glomerulonephritis of bacterial endocarditis. Medicine (Baltimore), 51:1, 1972.

Kerr, A., Jr.: Subacute Bacterial Endocarditis. Springfield, Ill., Charles C Thomas, 1955.

King, L. H., Jr., Bradley, K. P., Shires, D. L., Jr., Donohue, J. P., and Glover, J. L.: Bacterial endocarditis in chronic hemodialysis patients. Surgery, 69:554, 1971.

Kristinsson, A., and Benthall, H. H.: Medical and surgical treatment of Q-fever endocarditis. Lancet, 2:693, 1967.

Lerner, P. I., and Weinstein, L.: Infective endocarditis in the antibiotic era. N. Engl. J. Med., 274: 323, 388, 1966.

Nastro, L. J., and Finegold, S. M.: Endocarditis due to anaerobic gram-negative bacilli. Am. J. Med., 54:482, 1973.

Quinn, E. L., Madhavan, T., Salahuddin, N., Cox, F., and Fisher, E.: The increasing role of surgical therapy in bacterial endocarditis. Surg. Clin. North Am., 52:1467, 1972.

Reyes, M. P., Palutke, W. A., Wylin, R. F., and Lerner, A. M.: Pseudomonas endocarditis in the Detroit Medical Center, 1969–1972. Medicine, 52:173, 1973.

Rodbard, S.: Blood velocity and endocarditis. Circulation, 27:18, 1963.

Rosen, P., and Armstrong, D.: Nonbacterial thrombotic endocarditis in patients with malignant neoplastic disease. Am. J. Med., 54:23, 1973.

Slaughter, L., and Morris, J. E.: Prosthetic valve endocarditis. Circulation, 47:1319, 1973.

Westenfelder, G. O., Paterson, P. Y., Reisberg, B. E., and Carlson, G. M.: Vancomycin-streptomycin synergism in enterococcal endocarditis. J.A.M.A., 223:37, 1973.

STAPHYLOCOCCAL INFECTIONS

F. Robert Fekety

193. INTRODUCTION

Staphylococci are the most common cause of suppurative skin infections of man. They also cause bacteremia and serious infections of lungs, pleura, endocardium, meninges, muscles, bones, joints, and other viscera. Troublesome staphylococcal infections have been recognized with increasing frequency since antimicrobial drugs were introduced. Pathogenic staphylococci are ubiquitous in our environment and are constituents of our normal flora. Some strains are resistant to many of our most useful antimicrobial drugs and increase in prevalence when they are used. Hospitalized patients are frequently exposed as well as being highly susceptible to this organism. They are particularly likely to develop these infections and to have great difficulty in handling them.

Bacteriology. Staphylococci are spherical gram-positive cocci that grow well on simple laboratory media, both aerobically and anaerobically. Grapelike clusters of organisms are seen in stained smears from cultures; small irregular clusters, pairs, and short chains are seen in smears of pus. When gram-positive cocci are seen *within* leukocytes in smears, it is very likely that they are staphylococci, since other cocci are usually killed and digested soon after phagocytosis, but staphylococci are not.

Staphylococci are the most important pathogens in the genus Micrococcus, which also includes many saprophytes. Pathogenic staphylococci *(Micrococcus pyogenes, Staphylococcus pyogenes)* are noteworthy for their metabolic and biochemical versatility. Two species can be tentatively identified by lipochrome pigment production on agar: *S. aureus* is characteristically golden yellow, and *S. epidermidis* (formerly *S. albus*) is white. Differentiation according to pigment production is unreliable, because *S. aureus* often grows as white colonies on primary isolation. Cream-colored, orange, golden, or lemon-yellow colonies of *S. aureus* are also seen. *S. aureus* is the most important pathogenic Staphylococcus.

Pathogenic staphylococci usually produce a variety of toxins with hemolytic, necrotizing, leukocidal, vasospastic, or lethal properties. They are also capable of fermenting mannitol and other sugars. They produce a number of other potentially important extracellular substances, including lysozyme, catalase, enterotoxin, exfoliatoxin, fibrinolysin, hyaluronidase, lipase, nuclease, beta lactamase, phosphatase, deoxyribonuclease, protease, and coagulase (a plasma-clotting substance). The pathogenetic role of these toxins and enzymes is still uncertain, but coagulase production and mannitol fermentation correlate best with pathogenicity for man. By convention, coagulase-positive mannitol-fermenting staphylococci are called *S. aureus.* The tube coagulase test is more reliable than the slide test, which measures bound coagulase (clumping factor).

Coagulase-negative and mannitol-negative isolates are called *S. epidermidis. S. epidermidis* does not often cause infection of man unless susceptibility is increased or there is a nidus of infected foreign material, such as an intracardiac prosthesis or an intravascular plastic catheter or shunt. However, such appropriately susceptible hosts are now commonplace in hospitals. Consequently, these opportunistic organisms are being recognized more and more frequently as the etiologic agents in serious infections, and *they can no longer be dismissed automatically as contaminants whenever they are isolated from cultures of blood or other specimens.*

Pathogenesis.   Abscess formation is the characteristic feature of staphylococcal infection. When staphylococci lodge in susceptible tissues and begin to multiply, an acute inflammatory reaction rapidly ensues. Thrombosis of small blood vessels occurs, and fibrin is deposited in the lesion, which becomes avascular, necrotic, and surrounded by a fibroblastic wall. The tissues become hypertonic, edematous, congested, tense, and painful. The center of the lesion gradually liquefies, forming the characteristic thick, creamy yellow pus which is slightly acidic and comprised mostly of dead organisms, leukocyte debris, and proteinaceous substances. Further evolution of the lesion is slow, even under drug therapy, until it drains, after which it usually begins to heal. Thus antimicrobial drugs do not affect undrained abscesses very much.

Granulomatous reactions are occasionally seen at sites of chronic staphylococcal infections. These may contain masses of staphylococci resembling "sulfur granules," and can be confused with actinomycosis (staphylococcal botryomycosis). Granulomas are also characteristic of staphylococcal lesions in association with the leukocytic deficiency syndromes, such as the chronic granulomatous disease of childhood.

Very little that is conclusive has been established about the mechanisms of the pathogenicity of staphylococci. There are obvious but unproved clinical implications for the dermonecrotic, lethal, and leukocidal toxins. Fibrin products of coagulase activity may help to wall off the lesion and protect the organism from granulocytes, but the resultant fibrin network may also enhance surface phagocytosis. The pathogenetic role of hyaluronidase, fibrinolysin, hemolysins, and the other extracellular products is entirely speculative. The factors important in promoting phagocytosis and intracellular killing of the organism are incompletely understood.

Some of these substances that may be involved in pathogenesis have been used as antigens in experimental vaccines, but immunization as a means of enhancing resistance to staphylococci has met with little success. Most adults possess serum antibodies to a number of staphylococcal antigens, but high titers of these antibodies have not correlated well with protection from disease. Protein A, a component of staphylococcal cell walls, nonspecifically binds antistaphylococcal antibodies at the Fc fragment instead of appropriately at the Fab fragment. This reversed attachment of immune globulins appears to render them functionally ineffective, and may be the explanation for the observation that neither vaccination nor the disease seems to result in immunity despite the production of large amounts of antibody. In addition, there is some evidence that hypersensitivity reactions to antigenic products of the microorganism may deleteriously influence local susceptibility to infection. Additional studies are required if safe and effective vaccination against staphylococci is to become possible.

Epidemiology.   Pathogenic staphylococci are normally acquired by a high percentage of healthy infants within a few days or weeks of birth. Most healthy humans harbor virulent staphylococci in the anterior nares or on the skin, either occasionally or consistently. Clinical disease occurs in exposed persons or asymptomatic carriers when local or general resistance is decreased or when the exposure is heavy. Staphylococci are abundant in our environment and can survive in dust for long periods, but implantation of large numbers of staphylococci derived from air and other exogenous sources seems an uncommon explanation for disease. To produce skin infections experimentally in healthy persons, more than a million pathogenic staphylococci must be inoculated, and no significant differences have been demonstrated between strains derived from lesions or from healthy mucous membranes. The experimental evidence that certain strains of pathogenic staphylococci are especially virulent is inconclusive, but the epidemiologic evidence suggests that this factor may be important in nursery outbreaks and in recurrent furunculosis. Factors that increase host susceptibility to relatively small numbers of ordinary staphylococci thus seem of great importance in explaining the high frequency of staphylococcal disease.

Although numerous conditions are known to predispose to staphylococcal disease, the mechanisms causing the organism to become invasive in these patients are not well understood. Skin infections usually begin about hair follicles, sebaceous glands, or at sites of wounds, abrasions, or foreign body penetration. Greasy substances, oils, sunburn, and other conditions causing blockage of the ducts of cutaneous glands predispose to infection. In some cases infection results because of massive multiplication of the organism within exudates or devitalized tissues. Burns, surgical wounds, and dermatitic lesions frequently become secondarily infected with staphylococci. Sutures enhance local susceptibility to staphylococcal infection, possibly because bacteria can multiply within their interstices as in a protected sanctuary or because a tight suture may reduce local blood flow and thus impair cellular or humoral defense mechanisms. Furthermore, the inflammatory response to sutures may lower local resistance. Similar mechanisms may explain infection at the site of other foreign bodies, such as prosthetic devices and intravenous catheters. Diabetics seem to have an increased frequency of cutaneous staphylococcal infections, possibly because their acute defensive inflammatory responses may be delayed and deficient (especially during ketoacidosis), because of vascular disease and gangrene, and because of the frequent exposure that diabetics have to hospitals and medical procedures that increase the risk of infection. The chronic granulomatous disease of childhood is characterized by serious infections with catalase-positive organisms such as staphylococci, because the granulocytes of the affected individuals are unable to generate sufficient hydrogen peroxide to permit intracellular bactericidal mechanisms to operate normally. Other congenital or acquired conditions characterized by defective leukocyte formation and frequent staphylococcal infections have recently been described. Malnutrition and a wide variety of serious chronic debilitating diseases predispose to serious staphylococcal infection. In some cases this may be attributable to treatment with antimicrobial drugs that encourage overgrowth of pathogenic staphylococci. In others it may be the consequence of therapeutic efforts or disease processes adversely affecting cellular or humoral defense mechanisms. Neoplasms, uremia, extensive operations, and treatment with adrenal steroids and cytotoxic or immunosuppressive agents predispose to serious staphylococcal infection. Influenza, measles, diabetes mellitus, and cystic fibrosis predispose to staphylococcal pneumonia. Newborn infants are hypersusceptible to this organism, and are subject to severe spreading skin infections and primary staphylococcal pneumonia with pneumatocele formation.

Because of their ubiquity, versatility, and resistance to antimicrobial drugs, staphylococci have become a major cause of serious infections in highly susceptible persons who tend to congregate in hospitals. Bacteriophage typing of staphylococci has contributed to understanding the modes of transmission of these infections. Man is the major source of the organism. Patients and personnel in hospitals are more commonly asymptomatic carriers of the organism than are those without hospital contact. The organism is most often found in the anterior nares, in intertriginous areas of hair, and on the hands. Carriers and infected patients readily contaminate their environment, and staphylococci can be isolated from air, dust, floors, mops, blankets, clothing, dressing carts, and other fomites. The usual habitat of S. epidermidis is the skin and mucous membranes of man and animals.

Studies in nurseries for the newborn have shown that transmission of the organism occurs primarily via the hands of personnel who either are carriers or have recently handled infected or colonized newborns. The spread of organisms from heavily colonized infants via the airborne route ("cloud babies") may occur, but this seems much less frequent than transmission via hands. Postoperative wound infections are more frequent in nasal carriers and often appear to be attributable to strains carried by the patient prior to operation (endogenous infection). Infected patients or personnel are also important sources of strains causing wound infections (exogenous infections); the usual mechanism is contact spread via hands. Transmission via air, environment, or fomites is a less common route of wound infection. All these mechanisms contribute to the perpetuation of the reservoir of staphylococci in the hospital and to the spread of organisms to personnel and highly susceptible patients.

Most authorities believe that special attention in hospitals to measures such as isolation and frequent handwashing with antiseptics in order to prevent the spread of staphylococci is worthwhile. Infected patients can shed large numbers of bacteria into the environment and should be isolated unless the infection is at a closed site (e.g., blood, meninges). Personnel with clinical infections should not have contact with susceptible patients. The indiscriminate use of antimicrobial drugs favors the transmission and survival of drug-resistant strains. Few surgical patients deserve chemoprophylaxis, for there is little evidence that prophylaxis is capable of preventing staphylococcal infection. Because so many persons are asymptomatic carriers of pathogenic staphylococci, it is not practical to exclude all of them from contact with susceptible persons in hospitals. Actually, healthy carriers of ordinary strains seem unlikely to acquire new and potentially more dangerous strains, which is probably an example of *bacterial interference*. However, it may be necessary during outbreaks to exclude carriers of *especially dangerous* staphylococcal strains (as demonstrated by *both* bacteriophage typing and clinical experience) from nurseries, delivery rooms, and operating rooms.

Treatment. Although antimicrobial therapy has markedly improved the prognosis in serious staphylococcal infection, it must be emphasized that surgical drainage of abscesses and removal of infected foreign bodies are not only equally important, but may be the only way to achieve a cure. Patients with staphylococcal infections usually respond relatively slowly to drug therapy, and despite optimal treatment the mortality rate is high in persons with compromised defense mechanisms. Although antimicrobial therapy is considered elsewhere in detail (Ch. 267 and 268), there are certain points that should be stressed here.

Appropriate cultures and drug-susceptibility tests should always be obtained to confirm the diagnosis of serious staphylococcal disease and to guide therapy. Although many antimicrobial drugs are now available for treating these infections, the often unpredictable susceptibility of the organism narrows the initial choice to only a few. Bactericidal penicillin analogues are preferred unless the patient is allergic to them. Because most strains causing infection in the hospital and also in the community are resistant to penicillin G and ampicillin, the choice should be limited to drugs that are not significantly inactivated by staphylococcal penicillinase. Toxic-appearing patients with serious infections are best treated parenterally. Methicillin, oxacillin, nafcillin, cephalothin, and cefazolin are recommended for serious infection. Used properly, they seem to produce equally good therapeutic results. Many if not most experts still prefer methicillin, but nafcillin has become increasingly popular because it is the most active derivative and rarely causes nephritis or other serious side effects. The cephalosporins are especially useful with mixed infections because of their relatively broad spectrum. Cephaloridine should rarely be used because of its nephrotoxic potential in doses greater than 4.0 grams per day. Cefazolin is a well-tolerated new cephalosporin preparation providing good serum antistaphylococcal activity, and is preferred over the other cephalosporins for intramuscular use. Cephalothin should be avoided in treating central nervous system staphylococcal infections, because its less active desacetyl metabolite tends to accumulate in the cerebrospinal fluid.

For oral therapy of less serious infections, cloxacillin, dicloxacillin, and the more expensive cephalexin are suitable and equally efficacious when given orally in proper amounts. Oxacillin and nafcillin are not recommended, because their oral absorption is too erratic.

The penicillinase-resistant penicillin analogues are also adequate for the treatment of infections caused by more sensitive organisms such as penicillin-susceptible staphylococci, pneumococci, and group A beta streptococci when the dosages commonly recommended for staphylococcal disease are used. It is *not* necessary to add penicillin G to the regimen when these organisms are suspected of playing a role in the illness. However, many persons prefer to use both penicillin G and methicillin or nafcillin initially and switch to the more active drug when the nature of the etiologic agent becomes clear. If the organism is susceptible to it, penicillin is preferred, because it is usually the most active drug as well as the most convenient and inexpensive one to administer. Penicillin V is better than penicillin G for oral therapy of staphylococcal infections because of its better absorption.

If the patient is allergic to penicillin, all the semisynthetic penicillins should be avoided. Vancomycin, clindamycin, gentamicin, cephalothin, cefazolin, or cephalexin are suitable substitutes. Allergic cross-reactions between penicillin and the cephalosporins have been observed. Kanamycin, erythromycin, and bacitracin are occasionally useful. Tetracyclines, including minocycline, and chloramphenicol are less frequently employed because of frequent drug resistance, fear of toxicity, or lack of bactericidal action.

Because of the numerous suitable antimicrobial agents and variable clinical situations, only general guidelines for dosage and duration of treatment of staphylococcal infections can be given here. A delay in initiating appropriate therapy is often deleterious. Severe infections respond slowly and require large doses given for long periods. Relapses are common if therapy is terminated too early, especially if the lesion has not drained or foreign bodies are not removed. It is unusual for the organism to become resistant to the penicillin derivative during therapy. Endocarditis and other serious infections are usually treated for at least four to six weeks. In serious infections, parenteral therapy is preferred because of the desirability of ensuring the maintenance of high concentrations of the antimicrobial in blood and tissues. In order to maintain adequate serum antistaphylococcal activity, the interval between intravenous doses of penicillins and cephalosporins should not exceed four hours in critically ill patients, and the drugs should not be given rapidly as an "intravenous bolus."

Although methicillin-resistant strains of *S. aureus* have been encountered frequently in Europe, they are not common in the United States. Faulty drug-susceptibility discs occasionally result in their spurious detection. Methicillin-resistant organisms usually show multiple resistance to other semisynthetic penicillins and cephalosporins. Resistant strains grow better at 30 than at 37° C and in high salt media. They may be recognizable only after prolonged incubation (48 hours) in the presence of methicillin or oxacillin, presumably because the isolates contain only a small proportion of resistant clones. Most laboratories do not employ these special conditions routinely. These organisms seem less virulent than methicillin-susceptible staphylococci, but they have occasionally been of clinical importance. Wide misuse of the new penicillins will probably result eventually in an increase in the prevalence of these strains. Vancomycin, gentamicin, clindamycin, or a combination of kanamycin or gentamicin with cephalothin or methicillin has been recommended for treatment of infections with these organisms.

Cephalosporins, vancomycin, gentamicin, and the macrolides are the most active drugs against *S. epidermidis.* These coagulase-negative organisms are often surprisingly resistant to methicillin and the other semisynthetic penicillins.

194. CUTANEOUS STAPHYLOCOCCAL INFECTIONS

FURUNCLES

A furuncle (boil) is an acute circumscribed staphylococcal abscess of the skin and subcutaneous tissues. The term folliculitis refers to pustular furuncles involving hair follicles. Folliculitis is common in persons with oily skin, poor hygiene, or occupational exposure to cutting oils. Deep folliculitis of the beard area is known as *sycosis barbae.* Patients with multiple or recurrent furuncles are said to have *furunculosis,* but otherwise normal adults commonly experience an average of five or six furuncles per year.

Furuncles are most common on the face, neck, buttocks, thighs, perineum, breasts, and axillary skin. Most furuncles begin at the base of a hair follicle and take three to five days to evolve. Itching or pain may be the earliest symptom. As the center of the lesion becomes necrotic and hypertonic, fluid is drawn into the furuncle and it swells, thinning the overlying erythematous skin. Spontaneous drainage usually occurs soon thereafter. A hard core of necrotic debris is sometimes extruded from the center of the abscess. Relief of pain and onset of healing are usually rapid after drainage occurs, although erythema and swelling may persist for several weeks. A furuncle may regress without draining and form a "blind boil" that is indolent and prone to exacerbation after minor local trauma.

When the sebaceous glands of the face and upper back are extensively involved with furuncles, the condition is referred to as *pustular acne vulgaris. Juvenile acne* is not caused by staphylococci, but these organisms may secondarily infect acne lesions.

Furuncles involving blocked apocrine sweat glands *(hidradenitis suppurativa)* frequently become chronic. This troublesome infection tends to spread to other local sweat glands and hair follicles and leads to interconnecting draining sinuses and extensive scarring. Lesions occur in the axillary, perianal, and genital areas. Hydradenitis is difficult to cure with antimicrobial drugs and drainage alone. Excision of the involved tissues and skin grafting are frequently necessary and usually successful.

Although systemic symptoms and bacteremia are unusual with an ordinary furuncle unless the lesion is squeezed or manipulated, asymptomatic bacteremia related to a furuncle is probably fairly common. Furuncles are believed to be important in the pathogenesis of endocarditis, osteomyelitis, pyarthrosis, and other metastatic infections developing after hematogenous dissemination of the organism. Septic thrombophlebitis caused by local extension of infection is another serious complication of furuncles. Lesions in the middle third of the face are especially dangerous, because they may spread intracranially via emissary veins and cause cavernous sinus thrombophlebitis.

CARBUNCLES

A carbuncle is a large furuncle or an aggregate of interconnected furuncles. Carbuncles often drain through multiple skin openings. They represent an acute suppurative inflammation of subcutaneous tissues extending between hair follicles in clefts along fibrous and adipose tissues. They occur where the skin is thick (such as the back of the neck), possibly because thick skin promotes internal and lateral extension rather than external drainage. Carbuncles may attain the size of lemons, and are often associated with extreme pain, chills, fever, leukocytosis, malaise, prostration, bacteremia, and sometimes death.

IMPETIGO

Impetigo is a superficial primary pyoderma caused by group A beta streptococci, *S. aureus*, or both. It is most common in infants and children. It begins as macules and progresses to vesicles and bullae, which rupture, releasing a cloudy yellow fluid which forms crusts, and reveal a weeping denuded area. Central healing occurs, and the lesions may become chronic and resemble fungal infections. The lesions are superficial, rarely larger than 2 cm, and they spread by autoinoculation. Streptococci are usually responsible for these lesions, but there is good evidence that staphylococci of bacteriophage type 71 may be involved in some cases.

THE SCALDED SKIN SYNDROME

An association of bacteriophage group II staphylococci with exfoliative dermatitis has been recognized in three distinct but related clinical entities. (1) *Generalized exfoliative dermatitis (scalded skin syndrome, pemphigus neonatorum, Ritter's disease, staphylococcal toxic epidermal necrolysis)* is severe and characterized by generalized painful erythema, formation of bullae, and shedding of the upper epidermis in large sheets. The focus of infection may be at a distant site. The disease is usually seen in newborns but has been recognized in adults, and is often confused with pemphigus. (2)*Bullous impetigo* is a localized form of the scalded skin syndrome in which the infection occurs at the site of the lesion. (3) *Staphylococcal scarlet fever* is a mild variant of the generalized scalded skin syndrome and is clinically similar to streptococcal scarlet fever. A localized infection is the usual focus of toxin production. Antibodies to the streptococcal erythrogenic toxin do not seem to be cross-reactive.

These three clinical variants appear to represent the spectrum of a disease process with a common etiology—the exfoliative exotoxin produced by group II staphylococci (especially types 3A, 3C, 55, and 71). The disease has been duplicated in a laboratory model. The characteristic lesion consists of intraepidermal cleavage through desmosomes of the stratum granulosum. Other forms of toxic epidermal necrolysis can be distinguished because they show necrosis of the entire epidermis with cleavage near the dermoepidermal junction.

TREATMENT OF CUTANEOUS INFECTIONS

Some authorities believe that furuncles and pustules can be aborted at early stages by the administration of an antimicrobial drug or by the local application of an antiseptic such as alcohol. Once drained, small lesions require no further therapy, but they should be kept covered with a dressing or zinc oxide ointment to help prevent contamination of other sites. More severe lesions require local and systemic therapy. Rest, heat, and elevation of the affected site tend to relieve pain and minimize spread of the infection. Warm compresses hasten maturation of the lesion, but care should be taken to ensure that they do not cause maceration of the skin. Incision should be delayed until frank suppuration and fluctuance are detectable, because early incision is ineffective and may promote local extension and bacteremia.

Antimicrobial drugs should be given if the furuncle is large, on the face or neck, or accompanied by lymphaden-itis, fever, or other systemic reaction. They should also be given if the patient has diabetes or another underlying disease predisposing to complications, or if surgical incision is to be performed. Oral therapy with a penicillin analogue, erythromycin, or clindamycin is usually satisfactory. Therapy should be continued until signs of active inflammation have disappeared; a week is usually sufficient. Gamma globulin, adrenal steroids, and vaccines are of no proved value.

Impetigo responds rapidly to treatment with appropriate systemic antimicrobial therapy, but topical bacitracin ointment may be adequate in mild cases.

PREVENTION OF CUTANEOUS INFECTIONS

Furuncles are difficult to prevent, because the patient usually continues to be susceptible and the organism is ubiquitous. However, measures that protect the skin and minimize contact with the organism may be worth the trouble they entail. Predisposing conditions should be treated or eliminated. Skin irritants and abrasive tight clothing should be avoided. The fingernails should be kept short, and frequent handwashing should be stressed. Draining lesions should be considered highly contaminated and kept covered. Daily bathing and shampooing with antiseptic soap may be useful. Very rarely it may be possible to treat carriers with antimicrobial drugs for several weeks or months and eliminate the organism and thus prevent recurrences. Antimicrobial ointments or 2 per cent hexachlorophene cream may be applied several times daily to susceptible areas or to the anterior nares to suppress the organism. It is sometimes possible to get rid of a troublesome organism by intentionally inducing nasal carriage with a relatively nonpathogenic species after the more virulent Staphylococcus strain has been suppressed by drug therapy (bacterial interference). The 502A strain of *S. aureus* has been employed for this purpose in patients with recurrent furunculosis. Small numbers of organisms of the 502A strain have been used to intentionally colonize the umbilicus and nares of newborn infants in order to prevent acquisition of more dangerous strains. Outbreaks in nurseries have been terminated in this way. Minor but definite infections have been caused in infants and adults by strain 502A, and its use is still experimental. Staphylococcus vaccines, toxoids, and bacteriophage lysates are of no proved value in prevention, and irradiation to produce atrophy of sebaceous glands is not recommended.

195. STAPHYLOCOCCAL PNEUMONIA

Staphylococci cause less than 5 per cent of all bacterial pneumonias, except during influenza epidemics, but the disease is especially important because of its high mortality rate (up to 50 per cent) (see Ch. 179).

In so-called primary staphylococcal pneumonia, the organisms gain access to the lung via the tracheobronchial tree. Primary staphylococcal pneumonia is most often seen in infants; in children with cystic fibrosis or measles; in adults with influenza; or in debilitated, hospitalized persons being treated with antimicrobials, steroids, cancer chemotherapy, or immunosuppressants.

The diagnosis of primary staphylococcal pneumonia in adults with serious underlying diseases is often difficult. High spiking fever, multiple chills, cyanosis, rapidly progressive dyspnea, chest pain, and the production of thick, creamy yellow, salmon-colored, or reddish-yellow sputum should lead to the suspicion of staphylococcal pneumonia. Peripheral vascular collapse and marked signs of toxicity should also cause one to suspect the diagnosis in patients with pulmonary filtrates. Staphylococcal pneumonia developing in association with influenza or an underlying debilitating illness characteristically begins with a sudden and marked worsening of the illness, accompanied by prostration, cyanosis, tachypnea, bloody or purulent sputum, and high fever. Fever, cough, sputum production, dyspnea, and chest pain may be minimal during early stages of staphylococcal pneumonia. In infants the sudden development of pneumothorax, pneumatoceles, or empyema is a characteristic feature. Necrosis of lung tissue and formation of multiple abscesses is characteristic in adults.

Hematogenous or *secondary staphylococcal pneumonia* is seen most frequently in narcotic addicts with endocarditis and in others with bacteremia from a primary focus elsewhere. Secondary staphylococcal pneumonia is characterized by multiple peripheral infiltrates resembling embolic lesions which progress to necrosis and abscess formation, with a high frequency of pleuritic pain, empyema, and pneumothorax, and infrequent signs of consolidation. The signs of septicemia frequently overshadow the pulmonary disease in these patients.

The physical signs in patients with staphylococcal pneumonia are highly variable. A toxic appearance and low-grade fever may be the only detectable manifestations, particularly when the pneumonia is in a central location or interstitial, which is common. Patchy bronchopneumonia with multiple small abscesses is another common presentation, and can be detected by the presence of either coarse or fine rales. Dullness to percussion is not an early sign, and signs of frank consolidation are rarely found. Pleural effusion and empyema are frequent, but the fluid is commonly loculated in intralobar fissures and may not be readily detected or aspirated.

The leukocyte count is usually elevated to between 15,000 and 25,000 per cubic millimeter. A leukocyte count greater than 15,000 in an adult with influenza should raise the question of a secondary bacterial pneumonia. Chest roentgenograms show patchy infiltrates, most often near the hilum, multiple cavities, and pleural effusions. The Gram-stained smear of the sputum usually shows polymorphonuclear leukocytes and large numbers of clustered gram-positive cocci. When cocci are seen within leukocytes in sputum, staphylococcal pneumonia is the presumptive diagnosis. The blood culture is *not* often positive unless the pneumonia is secondary to staphylococcal bacteremia originating at some other site.

Differential Diagnosis. All other forms of pneumonia must be considered. The distinction from pneumonia caused by gram-negative organisms is especially important in patients developing pneumonia in the hospital. A carefully performed Gram stain of a good sample of sputum is the keystone of choosing initial therapy, and may be helpful in interpreting subsequent culture reports. Abscess formation, salmon-colored sputum, and an ap-

propriate setting for the development of staphylococcal pneumonia are helpful clues.

Since drug-resistant staphylococci frequently colonize the respiratory tract soon after the administration of antimicrobial drugs, one should not diagnose staphylococcal pneumonia solely on the basis of a sputum culture revealing rare or moderate numbers of the organism in someone under treatment for other pulmonary infections.

Prognosis. Even under the best of circumstances, the case fatality rate for pneumonia is 15 to 20 per cent. Higher fatality rates are seen in very young infants and in elderly debilitated patients. As this pneumonia is characterized by necrosis of lung parenchyma, recovery is usually slow. Improvement after the initiation of therapy is often not evident for 48 to 72 hours, and the illness usually lasts three to four weeks. Convalescence may be markedly prolonged when empyema is present. Bronchiectasis is frequently a consequence of staphylococcal pneumonia.

Treatment. Once the diagnosis is tentatively established, vigorous antimicrobial therapy by the parenteral route should be initiated promptly. Methicillin, oxacillin, nafcillin, cephalothin, or cefazolin, in doses of at least 1 gram every four to six hours, are preferred and equally good. The organism should be considered resistant to penicillin and ampicillin until it is demonstrated to be susceptible. If the organism is susceptible, penicillin G (20 million units intravenously per day) is the drug of choice. If the patient is allergic to penicillin, vancomycin (0.5 gram intravenously every six to eight hours), gentamicin, or clindamycin (600 mg four times per day) may be used. Therapy should be continued for 10 to 14 days or more after the patient shows a definite clinical response. The clinical response is usually very gradual. When empyema is present, it may be helpful to administer antimicrobial drugs directly into the pleural cavity, and proteolytic enzymes may be instilled to help thin the exudate. Surgical drainage of empyema with a chest tube is usually required, because the pus is often loculated or too thick for needle aspiration. Oxygen, bronchodilators, expectorants, fluids, and other supportive measures are important.

196. STAPHYLOCOCCAL OSTEOMYELITIS

Staphylococcus aureus is the etiologic agent in the majority of instances of primary or hematogenous osteomyelitis. The disease is becoming uncommon and is readily cured if treated early with appropriate antimicrobial drugs. Bacteremia occurring from a skin infection which may be no more serious than a furuncle is the usual inciting event. Secondary staphylococcal osteomyelitis is related to penetrating trauma, surgery, or a contiguous focus of infection. It is also seen in patients with diabetes mellitus or peripheral vascular disease after local cutaneous infections.

Hematogenous staphylococcal osteomyelitis is primarily a disease of children, adolescents, and intravenous drug abusers. It is more frequent in boys. It usually begins in the metaphyseal area of the diaphysis near the epiphyseal plate, and is uncommon after epiphyseal closure. The metaphysis is a weak spot in growing bones. It has a terminal blood supply subject to bacterial embolization and thrombosis. The capillary and venous networks in this area are extensive, and strains and other minor injuries readily result in hematomas which afford a nidus for bacteria. Furthermore, the capillaries in this area are deficient in phagocytic lining cells. The most common sites of involvement are the lower femur, upper tibia, ankle, wrist, or hip, but any metaphyseal area can be involved. The vertebrae are more commonly involved in adults, particularly narcotic addicts. As the infectious process develops in the metaphysis, the arterial blood supply is usually compromised because it is terminal and encased in rigid bony canals. Thromboses and vascular insufficiency develop and lead to necrosis of bone. An early radiologic sign of the inflammatory process is decalcification or rarefaction of bone caused by hyperemia and injury to osteoclasts. If the infection is untreated, a sequestrum of necrotic bone will separate in six to eight weeks. Treatment with antimicrobial drugs has practically eliminated this result. In pyogenic osteomyelitis it is characteristic for the periosteum to react to the infection by forming a layer of reparative bone (osteosclerosis) called the involucrum. Reactive bone formation is much less common in tuberculous osteomyelitis, unless the process has been going on for more than six months.

The infection tends to spread along the diaphysis or outward to the subperiosteal space where an abscess often forms, particularly in children. From there the infection may extend and involve nearby joints. This is seen in about 10 per cent of cases, and is more frequent when the hip or shoulder bones are infected. It is uncommon for the infection to enter the joint by crossing the epiphyseal plate barrier in children, but this is not unusual in adults. In addition, sterile joint effusions are not uncommon when there is an osteomyelitic focus nearby.

If not treated early or adequately, the infection tends to become chronic, with recurrent exacerbations, metastatic lesions, the formation of draining sinuses, and extensive scarring, eventually requiring surgical debridement and saucerization of bone. Amyloidosis occasionally develops after longstanding osteomyelitis.

Staphylococcal infections of vertebrae and intravertebral discs are especially frequent in intravenous drug addicts. They are also seen after pelvic and urinary tract infections. The patients usually complain of back pain accentuated by straining or coughing, pain radiating down the leg, or abdominal pain. *Paravertebral abscesses* are a frequent complication. Narrowing of the disc space, erosion of the vertebral end plates, and bridging of the disc space by new bone formation are important radiologic findings. The condition may be mistaken for tuberculous spondylitis, but osteophytic bridging or isolated involvement of the vertebral arches or processes is unusual in tuberculosis. Acute endocarditis is an occasional complication of staphylococcal vertebral osteomyelitis.

High fever, chills, and throbbing pain in the bone are the early signs of osteomyelitis. Local muscle spasm, splinting, or limping are the early local signs. Redness, swelling, and warmth are seen later. Bacteremia is frequent in osteomyelitis, and the patient may appear delirious and critically ill. The systemic signs and symptoms may overshadow the local manifestations. Leukocytosis and anemia are common. Rarefaction of bone is the earliest radiologic sign, but may not appear until 10 to 14 days after onset. Periosteal reaction with new bone formation is seen after the disease has been present for at least a month. Bone scans, using radioactive strontium or fluorine, can localize the lesion prior to x-ray changes. They are particularly useful in drug addicts who present with fever and vague somatic complaints referable to the lower back.

Rheumatic fever, traumatic lesions, leukemia, scurvy, pyogenic arthritis, hemoglobinopathies, Ewing's tumor, and other neoplasms should be considered in the differential diagnosis of osteomyelitis.

Treatment. With appropriate treatment, death from acute osteomyelitis is rare, and progression to chronic osteomyelitis is not likely. Mixed infection with other organisms, such as Pseudomonas, is seen fairly often. Empirical treatment without the aid of exudate or operative specimens of bone for culture and histologic study is hazardous and should be avoided. Since early treatment is important, therapy directed against the Staphylococcus should be started as soon as cultures have been obtained when this organism appears likely. Intensive parenteral therapy should be given initially. One of the penicillins, cephalosporins, or clindamycin is recommended. Gentamicin is useful in addicts when Pseudomonas as well as Staphylococcus is suspected. Immobilization is important. Some evidence of a clinical response should be noted within four days. It may be necessary to aspirate the subperiosteal abscess, or to drain it surgically. Vigorous treatment should be continued for at least three or four weeks. Ideally, oral therapy should then be continued for two or three months. Radiologic signs of the infection may never become apparent if treatment is given early. Although small sequestra usually absorb spontaneously, larger pieces of dead bone require surgical removal, especially if there is a slow or incomplete clinical response. Operative removal of foreign bodies is frequently necessary to achieve a cure in secondary osteomyelitis.

With chronic osteomyelitis, antimicrobial therapy should be given, and sequestrectomy, saucerization of infected bone, and removal of sinus tracts should be performed. Only rarely will such patients respond to drug therapy alone. Closed irrigation with antimicrobial agents is occasionally a useful adjunct to surgery.

197. STAPHYLOCOCCAL BACTEREMIA AND ENDOCARDITIS

Bacteremia may occur with any localized staphylococcal infection, but is relatively uncommon with minor postoperative wound infections and pneumonia, unless of hematogenous origin. Carbuncles and other serious skin infections; infected intravascular shunts, catheters, and other foreign bodies; endocarditis; and osteomyelitis are the most common foci causing bacteremia. Staphylococci bacteremia is frequent in patients with marked granulocytopenia or serious chronic debilitating diseases. It is usually associated with hectic fever, temperatures to 40° C or more, repeated shaking chills, and marked systemic toxicity. Widespread metastatic abscesses may develop in kidneys, lungs, bone, skin, brain, meninges, myocardium, and other viscera. The case fatality rate with staphylococcal bacteremia is 50 per cent when there is predisposing underlying disease, and about 20 per cent when there is not.

Bacteremia with coagulase-negative staphylococci sometimes pursues an indolent course for many weeks with remarkably few clinical manifestations. Bloodstream infections with these organisms are usually seen after ventriculoatriostomy shunting or cardiac surgery with insertion of prostheses. A proliferative and membranous glomerulonephritis and the nephrotic syndrome may be seen as a result of chronic S. epidermidis bacteremia in patients with infected shunts, and prompt improvement in the renal disease may follow removal of the shunt.

Endocarditis frequently complicates staphylococcal bacteremia from another site. The disease is usually of the acute, malignant, or ulcerative type with S. aureus, but a form indistinguishable from that caused by S. viridans is occasionally seen, especially when S. epidermidis is responsible. The illness usually has an acute onset, with shaking chills, high fever, changing cardiac murmurs, cutaneous pustules and petechiae, splinter hemorrhages, metastatic abscesses, hematuria, progressive anemia, and marked leukocytosis. Thrombocytopenia and disseminated intravascular coagulation may be seen. Normal heart valves may be infected and destroyed in just a few days. Abscess of the myocardial valve ring occurs frequently and should be suspected when serious arrhythmias develop.

The distinction between endocarditis and bacteremia originating from another focus may be difficult. Continuous bacteremia suggests endocarditis or other intravascular focus; intermittent bacteremia suggests an extravascular focus.

Acute staphylococcal endocarditis in heroin addicts is characterized by frequent involvement of the tricuspid valve. Multiple septic pulmonary emboli and infarcts with abscess formation and empyema are the usual presenting manifestations. The classic peripheral cutaneous manifestations of endocarditis such as splenomegaly, Osler's nodes, and splinter hemorrhages may be lacking in right-sided endocarditis, but blood cultures are usually positive. Cerebral manifestations relative to abscess formation, embolization, meningitis, and subarachnoid hemorrhage are frequent. Panophthalmitis is occasionally a complication. A murmur from the tricuspid lesion is usually present but often overlooked initially until pulmonary emboli call attention to its presence. Other clues to tricuspid involvement are atrial or ventricular diastolic gallops along the lower left sternal border and the external jugular vein, or a short soft murmur along the lower left sternal border which is increased with inspiration (Carvallo's sign) and with the patient standing.

Acute proliferative glomerulonephritis of the immune complex type may develop during the course of staphylococcal endocarditis and is sometimes confused with an allergic reaction to drugs used in treatment.

Treatment. Even with appropriate therapy, staphylococcal bacteremia still has a mortality rate of almost 50 per cent. Patients over the age of 50 have a particularly poor prognosis. Parenteral therapy is necessary, and the regimen must be bactericidal. Therapy for bacteremia should be continued for no less than four weeks, and preferably for six to eight weeks if it is believed that the patient has endocarditis as well as bacteremia. In doubt-

ful cases, therapy should be given for six to eight weeks. Surgical treatment of the focus of infection is important to consider, and early replacement of damaged valves may be necessary if there is severe or intractable heart failure. When the site of infection is an intravascular foreign body, the infection is rarely cured until the foreign material is removed. However, infected cardiac prostheses are not usually replaced until at least one course of intensive treatment has proved unsuccessful, because 5 to 10 per cent of these infections may be cured with medical therapy alone.

MISCELLANEOUS INFECTIONS

Staphylococci are commonly found in *nose* or *throat* cultures, but they do not cause pharyngitis or tonsillitis, except rarely in patients with agranulocytosis or leukemia. Their presence usually represents nothing more than colonization, and does not by itself justify treatment with antimicrobial drugs.

Staphylococcal pyarthrosis represents a diagnostic and therapeutic challenge in adults. It may occur after orthopedic surgery or in association with osteomyelitis. Skin ulcers and contaminated intra-articular injections or aspirations are often important in pathogenesis. Rheumatoid factor may bind antistaphylococcal antibodies, and may contribute to lowered resistance. Joint infection should be suspected in all patients with rheumatoid arthritis who show an apparent exacerbation of joint disease with fever, pain, effusion, and leukocytosis. Chills favor the diagnosis of septic arthritis over rheumatoid disease. Joint fluid aspiration is essential for early diagnosis. Immobilization, repeated aspiration, surgical drainage when indicated, and appropriate antimicrobial drugs are the treatment.

Staphylococcal meningitis is uncommon. It is usually the result of penetrating trauma, local surgery, or bacterial endocarditis. Therapy must be vigorous. If the organism is known to be susceptible to penicillin G, 24 to 30 million units should be given daily by the intravenous route. If it is resistant to penicillin G or of unknown susceptibility, methicillin (12 to 24 grams per day), oxacillin (12 grams per day), or nafcillin (12 grams per day) may be used. Cephalosporins are not recommended. If gentamicin is used, it should be given intrathecally (5 mg) as well as by the usual routes. Bacitracin (5000 to 10,000 units in 5 to 10 ml of sterile saline) has also been used successfully intrathecally as supplemental therapy.

Primary spinal epidural abscess is a neurosurgical emergency in which prompt recognition and treatment are indicated to prevent permanent spinal cord damage. It is sometimes seen in narcotic addicts in association with vertebral osteomyelitis. The process is usually acute, is located dorsally in the lower thoracic or lumbar regions, and is most often caused by staphylococci. Fever, localized spinal tenderness, and rigidity of the spine are followed by root pain, localized weakness, progressive paresthesias, sphincter changes, and evidence of spinal cord compression. The lumbar spinal fluid usually is under reduced pressure and shows pleocytosis, but may be normal. Myelography localizes the lesion, but is seldom necessary. Antimicrobials are merely adjuncts to treatment, for total recovery depends on early diagnosis followed by prompt surgery, usually laminectomy, and drainage (see Ch. 384).

Staphylococcal pericarditis usually occurs after bacteremia, often in association with osteomyelitis or endocarditis, with formation of focal myocardial abscesses and spread to the pericardium. The Staphylococcus is the most frequent cause of purulent pericarditis. Treatment consists of antimicrobial therapy and pericardiocentesis, but if rapid improvement is not noted, open surgical drainage should be instituted.

Staphylococcal parotitis is seen in debilitated adults who become dehydrated and receive inadequate mouth care. Extensive edema, erythema, and tenderness are seen in the parotid area, and pus may be seen oozing from Stensen's duct. The patient usually has a high fever and disorientation. Shock and death are common. Irradiation of the gland may be a useful adjunct, but appropriate antimicrobial therapy and supportive care are more important.

Staphylococcal (tropical) pyomyositis is a relatively common disease of indigenous residents of hot, humid tropical areas. It is occasionally seen in temperate climates, where it is usually misdiagnosed. Bacteremia resulting from minor superficial lesions is followed by abscess formation beneath the deep fascia of skeletal muscles, especially in the leg. Local trauma may be important in determining the site of the infection. There is diffuse swelling of the limb, but usually no fluctuance or regional adenopathy. The skin may become tense and cellulitic, but is often normal. Fever may be minimal during the first week of illness. The diagnosis is frequently made at operation, at which time multiple abscesses are found to have coalesced and extended between muscle fasciculi and within fascial compartments. It is uncommon for osteomyelitis to coexist. Staphylococci of bacteriophage group II are usually implicated. Surgical drainage and antimicrobial therapy are efficacious.

198. STAPHYLOCOCCAL GASTROENTERITIS AND ENTEROCOLITIS

The enterotoxins produced by staphylococci are an important cause of acute epidemic gastroenteritis or food poisoning. The toxin is formed prior to ingestion of contaminated and usually improperly refrigerated or stored food (see Ch. 22).

Staphylococci are normal inhabitants of the intestines, although their presence is not usually recognized unless selective media are used. They may increase during antimicrobial therapy, and patients may concomitantly experience mild diarrhea. Much more rarely the organisms cause acute necrotizing pseudomembranous enterocolitis. Most common after abdominal surgery, shock, or antimicrobial therapy or in leukemia, this syndrome has a high mortality rate. Locally produced enterotoxin is thought to be responsible for the manifestations of the disease. Symptoms include abdominal pain, distention, ileus, fever, diarrhea, bloody stools, electrolyte depletion, dehydration, and shock. Gram stain of the stool reveals leukocytes and large numbers of cocci in sheets and clumps, and establishes the diagnosis. Vancomycin given by *mouth* is useful in treatment; a dose of 1.0 gram hourly for four doses and then every four hours has been used. Parenteral therapy with another appropriate drug may also be given. Oral neomycin is no longer recommended, because many staphylococci in hospitals are resistant to it. Shock and electrolyte imbalance should be treated vigorously with appropriate fluids.

Andriole, V. T., and Lyons, R. W.: Coagulase-negative Staphylococcus. Ann. N.Y. Acad. Sci., 174:533, 1970.

Banks, T., Fletcher, R., and Ali, N.: Infective endocarditis in heroin addicts. Am. J. Med., 55:444, 1973.

Boyle, J. D., Pearce, M. L., and Guze, L. B.: Purulent pericarditis: Review of literature and report of eleven cases. Medicine, 40:119, 1961.

Cohen, J. O. (ed.): The Staphylococci. New York, Wiley-Interscience, 1972.

Elek, S. D.: Staphylococcus Pyogenes. Edinburgh, E. & S. Livingstone, Ltd., 1959.

Fekety, F. R.: The epidemiology and prevention of staphylococcal infection. Medicine, 43:593, 1964.

Keys, T. F., and Hewitt, W. L.: Endocarditis due to micrococci and *Staphylococcus epidermidis*. Arch. Intern. Med., 132:216, 1973.

Levin, M. J., Gardner, P., and Waldvogel, F. A.: "Tropical" pyomyositis. N. Engl. J. Med., 284:196, 1971.

Lillibridge, C. B., Melish, M. E., and Glasgow, L. A.: Site of action of exfoliative toxin in the staphylococcal scalded skin syndrome. Pediatrics, 50:728, 1972.

Mailbach, H. I., Strauss, W. G., and Shinefield, H. R.: Bacterial interference: Relating to chronic furunculosis in man. Br. J. Dermatol., 81: Suppl. 1, 69, 1969.

McCloskey, R. V.: Scarlet fever and necrotizing fasciitis caused by coagulase-positive hemolytic *Staphylococcus aureus*, phage type 85. Ann. Intern. Med., 78:85, 1973.

Shinefield, H. R., Ribble, J. C., Boris, M., and Eichenwald, H.: Bacterial interference: Its effect on nursery acquired infection with *Staphylococcus aureus*. Am. J. Dis. Child., 105:646, 1963.

Van Prohaska, J., Mock, F., Baker, W., and Collins, R.: Pseudomembranous (staphylococcal) enterocolitis. Surg. Gynecol. Obstet., 112:103, 1961.

Waldvogel, F. A., Medoff, G., and Swartz, M. N.: Osteomyelitis: A review of clinical features, therapeutic considerations and unusual aspects. N. Engl. J. Med., 282:198, 260, 316, 1970.

Watanakunakorn, C., Tan, J. S., and Phair, J. P.: Some salient features of *Staphylococcus aureus* endocarditis. Am. J. Med., 54:473, 1973.

Waxman, A. D., Bryan, D., and Siemsen, J. K.: Bone scanning in the drug abuse patient: Early detection of hematogenous osteomyelitis. J. Nucl. Med., 14:647, 1973.

DISEASES CAUSED BY NEISSERIA

199. GONOCOCCAL DISEASE

Donald Kaye

Definition. Gonorrhea is an infection of the mucous membrane of the urethra and genital tract caused by *Neisseria gonorrhoeae*. Involvement of the pharynx and rectal mucosa is common. Infection is almost always the result of sexual contact. After invasion of mucosal sites, gonococci may spread and cause infections such as arthritis, tenosynovitis, perihepatitis, endocarditis, and meningitis.

Etiology. *N. gonorrhoeae* is a gram-negative coccus that was first described by Neisser in 1879 in exudates from patients with gonorrhea. In stained smears of exudates the organisms appear as diplococci with flattened or slightly concave adjacent sides and resemble a pair of kidney beans. A considerable portion of the organisms in exudates are within polymorphonuclear leukocytes.

Gonococci grown in laboratory media assume an oval or spherical form, and single cocci and clumps of cocci may be found in addition to diplococci. *N. gonorrhoeae* can be distinguished from other Neisseria by its ability to ferment glucose but not maltose or sucrose.

Primary isolation of the gonococcus is difficult. The organism is fastidious in its growth requirements, and is susceptible to toxic substances that are present in many media. Blood, serum, ascitic fluid, or other agents must be added for enrichment, as growth will usually not occur on plain agar. Blood is commonly used, and the medium is heated (chocolate agar) to reduce the deleterious effect exerted by certain amino acids toxic to the gonococcus. Commercial media are available that satisfy the various growth requirements of *N. gonorrhoeae*. Most strains require an atmosphere of 2 to 10 per cent carbon dioxide. Colonies of *N. gonorrhoeae* are round, gray-white, and translucent. Overgrowth with other bacteria occasionally occurs in cultures of exudate from the urethra, vagina, and cervix and is frequent in cultures from the pharynx and rectum if nonselective media are used.

All Neisseria produce an oxidase that can be used for tentative identification of colonies of *N. gonorrhoeae* (colonies turn purple on exposure to 1 per cent para-aminodimethylaniline monohydrochloride). With cultures from the genital tract, the combination of colonies of typical morphology composed of gram-negative diplococci and a positive oxidase test is strong presumptive evidence of the presence of *N. gonorrhoeae*. However, other Neisseria and members of the tribe Mimeae resemble *N. gonorrhoeae* both in colonial morphology and microscopic appearance and give a positive oxidase reaction (*Mima polymorpha* var. *oxidans* is the only Mimeae that is oxidase positive). Therefore cultures that are presumptively positive for *N. gonorrhoeae* should be confirmed by fermentation reactions or by fluorescent antibody techniques.

Thayer-Martin selective medium, containing vancomycin, sodium colistimethate, and nystatin, permits growth of *N. meningitidis* and *N. gonorrhoeae* but inhibits growth of many other bacteria frequently found in specimens from urethra, cervix, vagina, rectum, and pharynx. Growth of other Neisseria and of *Mima polymorpha* var. *oxidans* is inhibited.

Incidence and Prevalence.   There has been an increase in the reported incidence of gonococcal infections in recent years. However, the true incidence and prevalence of gonorrhea are unknown because of problems in diagnosis, antimicrobial therapy by nonmedical persons, incomplete reporting by physicians, and the presence of many undetected asymptomatic female carriers. It has been estimated that over 2 million new cases of gonorrhea occur annually in the United States. The magnitude of the problem of asymptomatic gonorrhea in females may be demonstrated by the fact that there is about a 5 per cent prevalence of asymptomatic gonorrhea in pregnant women.

Gonorrhea is a disease of the sexually active, and most cases occur in patients 15 to 24 years of age. Gonorrhea rates are higher among military personnel, migrant groups (such as itinerant laborers and seafarers), homosexuals, and prostitutes. In surveys 10 to 33 per cent of prostitutes have gonorrhea.

Epidemiology.   *N. gonorrhoeae* is a parasite of man; it does not cause disease in animals. Gonorrhea is almost always acquired from sexual con-

tact, exceptions are gonococcal conjunctivitis (which occurs primarily in infants) and vulvovaginitis. Conjunctivitis results either from passage of the infant through an infected genital tract (ophthalmia neonatorum) or from contamination after birth. Vulvovaginitis is an infection of the genital tract of infants and preadolescent girls that results from direct contact with infected adults or, rarely, can be spread by contact with towels or linens contaminated with gonococci.

Repeated attacks of gonorrhea are common; therefore individual attacks seem to confer little or no immunity. However, individual variation in susceptibility to infection has been demonstrated after inoculation of *N. gonorrhoeae* into the urethras of male volunteers. Trauma to the urethra probably increases susceptibility to gonorrhea. After an episode of acute gonorrhea, *N. gonorrhoeae* may remain in the genital tract for months. Chronic asymptomatic carriers of the gonococcus are important in the epidemiology of gonorrhea because they are difficult to detect and therefore are rarely treated. It has been common knowledge that most women with gonorrhea are relatively asymptomatic, but only recently has it been appreciated that as many as 10 per cent of males with gonorrhea seen in a venereal disease clinic may be asymptomatic (Pariser).

Pathogenesis and Pathology.   *N. gonorrhoeae* are unable to penetrate stratified squamous epithelium, but penetration and infection of columnar and transitional epithelium readily occur. In males the urethra is attacked first, resulting in purulent urethritis and involvement of the urethral glands. Direct spread of infection may result in prostatitis, epididymitis, or seminal vesiculitis. During stages of healing, stricture formation may occur. Gonococcal proctitis in the male is almost always the result of rectal intercourse.

In the female, urethritis is mild and transient. Bartholin's and Skene's glands and glands of the cervix may become infected with or without involvement of the urethra. Contiguous spread of infection can cause salpingitis. Proctitis may result from contiguous spread or rectal intercourse. Gonococcal salpingitis is usually bilateral and may cause pyosalpinx and formation of a tubo-ovarian abscess. The inflammation tends to heal with fibrosis and adhesions that may produce obstruction of the fallopian tubes and sterility. Ascent of infection to the fallopian tubes often occurs during or just after menstruation. Although endometrial infection is usual when *N. gonorrhoeae* invades the fallopian tubes, it is not serious and tends to subside promptly. The vagina does not become infected in adults, probably because of the presence of squamous epithelium with many layers of cells and the lack of glands.

Conjunctivitis is the most common manifestation of gonococcal disease in infants. It is a destructive inflammation of the eye and before the use of antimicrobial agents frequently caused blindness. Between one year of age and pubescence, gonococcal infection is rare in males but causes vulvovaginitis in females. The increased susceptibility to gonococcal infection of the immature vaginal mucous membrane in contrast to the resistance of the mucosa of adults is probably explained by the thin mucous membrane present prior to adolescence.

Gonococcal infection of the pharynx is common and results from oral-genital contact. Gonococcal pharyngeal infection has been demonstrated in up to 20 per cent of homosexual men and 20 per cent of women practicing fellatio who had gonococcal infection at any site. In 3 to 4 per cent of these patients, only pharyngeal cultures were positive for gonococci (Pariser; Wiesner et al.).

Occasionally invasion of the blood occurs and *N. gonorrhoeae* may disseminate and produce infection at distant foci. Joints are the most frequent extragenital sites of localization, but tenosynovitis, endocarditis, meningitis, skin lesions, and infection at other foci may also occur.

Dissemination of gonococcal infection is more common in women than in men and is probably more common in homosexual males than in heterosexual males. This is probably explained by the fact that men with gonococcal urethritis are usually symptomatic and therefore are treated promptly, greatly decreasing the chances of dissemination of infection. In contrast, women with gonorrhea and males with gonococcal proctitis or pharyngitis (almost always homosexuals) are usually asymptomatic and are therefore unlikely to be treated. Although asymptomatic urethritis is relatively uncommon in men with gonorrhea, there seems to be a disproportionately high incidence of these men among males with disseminated gonococcal infection. The source for dissemination may be the genital tract, rectum, or pharynx. It has been estimated that dissemination of gonococcal infection occurs in up to 3 per cent of women with gonorrhea and is most prone to occur during pregnancy or during or just after menstruation.

Clinical Manifestations. *Gonorrhea in the Male.* The incubation period of gonococcal urethritis in the male is usually two to eight days. There is sudden onset of dysuria, urgency, and frequency associated with mucoid urethral discharge that rapidly becomes purulent and profuse. Gonococcal urethritis usually does not cause fever, but prostatitis, seminal vesiculitis, or epididymitis is frequently associated with fever. Acute urinary retention may result from involvement of the prostate. Rectal examination reveals tenderness of the affected organ in the presence of prostatitis or seminal vesiculitis. Epididymitis causes severe pain and tenderness of the epididymis.

Untreated gonorrhea subsides over a period of weeks, but a small amount of mucoid discharge from the urethra may continue to be found each morning for months. Gonococci may persist, usually in the prostate. Urethral stricture is a common sequela of untreated urethritis, especially after recurrent attacks of gonorrhea. Epididymitis can result in sterility.

Gonorrhea in the Female. In females the disease may begin with dysuria, urgency, and frequency after an incubation period of two to eight days. However, the urethritis is frequently of short duration and often is mild or completely asymptomatic. Cervicitis gives rise to a mucopurulent discharge that varies from scant to profuse. Involvement of Skene's ducts or Bartholin's glands is common, and abscess formation may occur. Gonococci can be isolated from the rectum in 20 to 50 per cent of women with gonorrhea, and occasionally can produce symptomatic proctitis. In 5 per cent of women with gonococcal infection only the anorectal culture contains gonococci. The duration of symptoms from an untreated infection that remains localized in the lower genital tract is usually no longer than a month or two. However, the patient may remain a carrier of the disease for many months.

Salpingitis is manifested by acute onset of fever and lower abdominal pain. Physical examination usually reveals lower abdominal tenderness, pain on movement of the cervix, and tenderness of the adnexa (with or without palpable masses). Acute pelvic inflammatory disease tends to recur, and pelvic pain and fever are present intermittently. Sterility is common.

Extragenital Gonococcal Infection. PROCTITIS. Gonococcal proctitis is usually asymptomatic but may be manifested by anal discharge, burning rectal pain, blood and pus in the stools, and pain on defecation.

PHARYNGITIS. Gonococcal infection in the oropharynx can probably cause symptomatic pharyngitis, tonsillitis, and gingivitis but is usually asymptomatic.

ARTHRITIS. Arthritis is the most common form of clinically recognized disseminated gonococcal infection; it usually occurs within one to three weeks after initial infection in the genital tract or may follow pharyngeal or rectal infection. Onset may be gradual with migratory polyarthalgias leading to frank arthritis in one or more joints, or it may be sudden with hot, swollen, and extremely painful joints. Fever and leukocytosis are usually present. Over 75 per cent of patients have polyarthritis. The joints that are most commonly involved are the knees, ankles, and wrists, but any joint may be involved, including the spine and sternoclavicular and temporomandibular joints. *Tenosynovitis,* which is rarely observed in other types of pyogenic arthritis, is common in gonococcal arthritis and most often occurs about the wrists and ankles. The skin lesions associated with gonococcal bacteremia are also frequently present.

N. gonorrhoeae can be isolated from joint fluid in only 25 to 50 per cent of cases. The fluid ranges from serous to frankly purulent, has the protein content of an exudate and usually contains increased numbers of leukocytes that are mainly polymorphonuclear. Muscle wasting about the joint and permanent deformity may result. Some authorities have described two types of arthritis produced by the gonococcus: (1) polyarticular arthritis, usually with no or small effusions that tend to be sterile, often associated with bacteremia and skin lesions, and (2) frank pyogenic arthritis (often involving one joint from which gonococci can frequently be isolated) without bacteremia or skin lesions. The first type has been attributed by some to hypersensitivity, but it seems more likely that it represents the initial or bacteremic phase during which organisms localize in joints. Frank pyogenic arthritis may occur after a clinically apparent or inapparent bacteremic phase. Sterility of the joint fluid in patients during the bacteremic phase may be due to taking cultures early in the disease, before microorganisms in the joint have sufficient time to proliferate.

GONOCOCCAL BACTEREMIA. Gonococcal bacteremia can produce a syndrome with recurrent episodes of fever, skin lesions, arthralgia or arthritis, mild to severe constitutional symptoms, and intermittently positive blood cultures. This syndrome occurs with infection in the genital tract, rectum, or pharynx, and, if untreated, can recur over a period of months or even years. The rash usually appears during the first day of symptoms and may recur with each episode of fever. The rash is found on the distal part of the extremities and consists of scanty pin-point erythematous macules that rapidly become maculopapular, vesiculopustular, and frequently hemorrhagic. Bullae can form. The mature lesion is elevated, has a dirty gray necrotic center, and is surrounded by erythema. It heals in three to four days. Gram-negative cocci can often be seen in stains of fluid from the lesions, but cultures for *N. gonorrhoeae* are usually negative. Immunofluorescent studies on the exudate from the pustules demonstrate *N. gonorrhoeae* in a high percentage of patients. Identical skin lesions may be seen in patients with meningococcemia, which can present an indistinguishable clinical sydrome.

GONOCOCCAL ENDOCARDITIS. Gonococcal endocarditis is extremely rare at present. In most patients, previously normal valves are attacked. The valves on the left side of the heart are involved most often, but valves on the right side are affected with a higher frequency than with endocarditis caused by other bacteria. A double daily temperature elevation (double quotidian) is common in patients with gonococcal endocarditis.

PERIHEPATITIS [FITZ-HUGH–CURTIS SYNDROME]. Perihepatitis is a rare complication in women with gonococcal pelvic inflammatory disease and results from direct spread of gonococci from the pelvis to the upper abdomen. It is manifestated by fever, upper quadrant pain (usually right upper quadrant), tenderness and spasm of the abdominal wall, and occasionally a friction rub over the liver. During the acute stage the gallbladder temporarily may not be visualized on cholecystography; this can lead to an erroneous diagnosis of cholecystitis. The patient often has a recent history of pelvic pain or vaginal discharge, and physical examination may reveal evidence of pelvic inflammatory disease. *N. gonorrhoeae* can frequently be demonstrated in the cervical or vaginal discharge.

The symptoms respond to antimicrobial therapy. The untreated disease subsides after one to four weeks of fever and abdominal pain, leaving "violin-string" adhesions between the anterior surface of the liver and the anterior abdominal wall. Recently this syndrome was reported in a male, probably caused by lymphatic or hematogenous dissemination.

Diagnosis. In the male the combination of urethritis and the presence of intracellular gram-negative diplococci in smears of exudate from the urethra is strong presumptive evidence of gonorrhea. Confirmation is obtained by culture or, if available, fluorescent antibody studies. Anorectal cultures should be obtained in homosexual males.

For routine screening, cervical cultures will detect the vast majority of females with asymptomatic gonorrhea. Gonorrhea should be suspected in any female contact of an infected male. Similarly the asymptomatic carrier state should be suspected in asymptomatic male contacts of symptomatic females or asymptomatic females detected by routine cultures. In the female with suspected gonorrhea, cultures of exudate from the cervix and anorectal area should be obtained in addition to urethral cultures.

Pharyngeal cultures for *N. gonorrhoeae* should be obtained from homosexual males and females practicing fellatio. In all patients with suspected disseminated gonococcal infections, cultures of the pharynx and anorectal area should be obtained in addition to genital tract cultures.

Gonococci die within hours if allowed to dry. Therefore exudates should be inoculated as soon as possible on Thayer-Martin medium or on a suitable transport medium for *N. gonorrhoeae*. Transgrow, a commercially available antibiotic-containing medium, is packaged in a bottle with an increased carbon dioxide tension, and is preferred for transporting specimens containing gonococci or meningococci to central laboratories.

With use of fluorescent antibody it is frequently possible to make a definite identification of *N. gonorrhoeae* in exudate within one hour of obtaining a specimen.

Genital tract infection with the chlamydiae of inclusion conjunctivitis may occur in both sexes, and in the male can present as urethritis. Strictly speaking, it is the genital infection that is primary, with the conjunctivitis representing a secondary involvement. This disease is a common finding in venereal disease clinics where its incidence may approach that of gonococcal urethritis in the male. Since the discharge in the chlamydial infection is not grossly purulent, it is seldom confused with acute gonorrhea, but it can resemble gonococcal urethritis at the time of onset of post-treatment relapse. The chlamydial form of urethritis is discussed in Ch. 171. It is not established whether this infection is responsible for any cases of *Reiter's syndrome,* or whether the latter represents a separate entity (see Ch. 93.)

Salpingitis. Acute salpingitis must be differentiated from appendicitis and tubal pregnancy. The presence of bilateral tenderness in the adnexa with or without masses, a history of recent sexual intercourse followed by urethritis or vaginal discharge, and demonstration of gonococci on cervical smear are strongly suggestive of gonococcal salpingitis. When it is impossible to differentiate acute salpingitis from appendicitis or tubal pregnancy, the diagnosis must be established at laparoscopy or laparotomy.

Arthritis; Blood-Borne Lesions. The diagnosis of gonococcal arthritis or bacteremia with skin lesions should be suspected in a patient with the appropriate clinical syndrome, especially if there is a recent history of urethritis or vaginal discharge. Tenosynovitis is suggestive of disseminated gonococcal infection. Isolation of *N. gonorrhoeae* from the genital tract, rectum, or pharynx is supportive evidence, and demonstration of gonococci in skin lesions, blood, or joint fluid is confirmatory. The serum complement-fixation test for gonococci may be of aid in suggesting gonococcal arthritis, especially if titers are rising. However, this test is not well standarized. Other serologic tests which look promising are currently under investigation.

When stains and cultures of joint fluid are negative for gonococci (50 to 75 per cent of cases), it is frequently difficult to differentiate gonococcal arthritis from Reiter's syndrome (nonbacterial urethritis, conjunctivitis, and arthritis). The problem in differential diagnosis is compounded by the fact that patients with Reiter's syndrome may have concomitant gonococcal urethritis. Urethritis and arthritis in a female suggest gonococcal arthritis, because this disease is more common in females, whereas Reiter's syndrome is rare in females. The presence of tenosynovitis and response to antimicrobial therapy strongly imply gonococcal arthritis. Patients with Reiter's syndrome frequently have prolonged courses with recurrences and do not respond to antimicrobial therapy. Keratodermia blennorrhagica (a symmetrical eruption with a predilection for the soles, palms, and genitals) occurs in Reiter's syndrome and is probably not associated with gonococcal arthritis. After an initial polyarthritis in Reiter's syndrome, ankylosing spondylitis may develop.

Gonococcal arthritis can often be differentiated from acute rheumatic fever, rheumatoid arthritis, and gout by the absence of carditis, lack of rheumatoid factor in serum, and failure to respond to colchicine, respectively.

When *N. gonorrhoeae* cannot be isolated from the joint, the response to penicillin therapy is often the strongest confirmatory evidence of gonococcal arthritis.

Treatment and Prognosis. Penicillin is the drug of choice for all gonococcal infections. Prior to 1954 a single injection of 300,000 units of penicillin cured almost all cases of gonorrhea. In recent years gonococcal strains of increased resistance to penicillin (requiring up to 2.0 μg per milliliter for inhibition) have constituted as much as 50 per cent or more of all isolates. Concomitantly there has been a striking increase in the incidence of failure of therapy with 600,000 to 2,400,000 units of penicillin. It must be stressed that penicillin remains the drug of choice for gonorrhea but that much larger doses are required than in previous years. If the trend in increasing resistance to penicillin continues, the point will soon be reached at which the doses of penicillin required will preclude the use of parenteral penicillin for routine therapy of uncomplicated gonorrhea.

N. gonorrhoeae organisms have also been becoming more resistant to tetracycline. Although the level of resistance to tetracycline is not yet of clinical importance in the United States, more resistant strains are being isolated in certain areas of the Far East. The same strains of N. gonorrhoeae that are relatively resistant to penicillin also tend to have increased resistance to tetracycline and ampicillin but not to spectinomycin.

The current recommendations of the Venereal Diseases Branch of the Center for Disease Control for treatment of uncomplicated gonorrhea (urethral, cervical, pharyngeal, or rectal) in men or women or in patients with known exposure to gonorrhea are as follows:

Aqueous procaine penicillin (4.8 million units) should be administered intramuscularly at one visit (two sites of injection) together with 1 gram of oral probenecid preferably 30 to 60 minutes before the penicillin; or 3.5 grams of oral ampicillin simultaneously with 1 gram of probenecid. When penicillin or ampicillin is contraindicated, alternate regimens are: spectinomycin, 2 grams in one intramuscular injection; or tetracycline hydrochloride orally, 1.5 grams initially, followed by 0.5 gram four times a day for four days (9 grams) for both men and women.

Spectinomycin (Wiesner et al.) and ampicillin do not seem to be effective in eliminating N. gonorrhoeae from the pharynx. With this exception, the cure rates with these regimens are over 90 per cent in the United States. Aqueous procaine penicillin and spectinomycin have the important advantage of one-visit parenteral therapy which guarantees absorption of the total course of treatment. A major advantage of the procaine penicillin regimen (although clearly more painful) is that it will cure incubating syphilis (Schroeter et al.). The advantage of the tetracycline regimen is that it will usually prevent postgonococcal urethritis in males (see below).

Urethritis should subside within two to three days after therapy. A watery urethral discharge may persist in males for weeks despite elimination of gonococci and usually requires no treatment (postgonococcal urethritis or nongonococcal urethritis). Several studies have demonstrated that postgonococcal urethritis can usually be prevented by use of tetracycline for therapy of gonorrhea and that postgonococcal urethritis will usually respond to tetracycline treatment.

Relapse of gonorrhea occurs most commonly during the first week after treatment. Therefore to evaluate cure, a culture should be obtained one week after therapy and, if possible, at two more weekly intervals. In homosexual males and in females, anorectal cultures should be obtained as well as cervical cultures to evaluate cure of genital tract gonorrhea. If relapse occurs (and relapse is often difficult to differentiate from reinfection), the patient may be retreated with one of the alternative regimens, preferably spectinomycin.

Causes of failure of therapy, other than infection with gonococci relatively resistant to penicillin, are failure to distinguish between relapse and reinfection; failure to identify nongonococcal urethritis, e.g., Reiter's syndrome or infection with chlamydiae; and possibly the presence of penicillinase-producing bacteria at the site of infection.

Patients with gonococcal prostatitis, seminal vesiculitis, epididymitis, salpingitis, arthritis, perihepatitis, or the syndrome of gonococcal bacteremia with skin lesions should be treated with bed rest and 10 to 20 million units of aqueous penicillin G intravenously each day. Patients who are allergic to penicillin may be treated with tetracycline, 0.5 gram orally four times a day; cephalothin in doses of 6 to 12 grams intravenously each day may be used in pregnancy. The duration of therapy should be seven to ten days (two weeks for arthritis) or longer until signs of infection have subsided and cultures become negative. Response to therapy usually occurs within two to three days. However, arthritis frequently responds more slowly, and it may take seven to ten days for the patient to become afebrile. Recent evidence suggests that gonococci that are relatively resistant to penicillin are less likely to cause disseminated infection (i.e., are less virulent), and that after several days of intravenous penicillin therapy the course can be completed with oral ampicillin in treatment of disseminated infection.

In acute gonococcal disease in the genital tract, surgery is indicated only for drainage of abscesses. However, in the chronic stage in some female patients it may become necessary to remove involved pelvic organs. In gonococcal arthritis, pus should be aspirated by needle when possible, but occasionally surgical drainage of the joint becomes necessary. Injection of penicillin into the joint is not indicated. Physiotherapy should be started during the period of convalescence to promote return of function of the joint.

For gonococcal endocarditis or meningitis, 20 million units of aqueous penicillin G should be administered parenterally each day (four to six weeks for endocarditis and two weeks for meningitis).

About 3 per cent of patients with gonorrhea may be in the incubation period of syphilis. The doses of procaine penicillin recommended for therapy of uncomplicated gonorrhea will cure incubating syphilis but will not cure established syphilis. Therefore serologic tests for syphilis should be performed prior to initiation of therapy in all patients treated for gonococcal infections. If the serologic test is positive, therapy for syphilis must be initiated. If the serologic test is negative, no follow-up tests are required if procaine penicillin is used to treat the gonorrhea. Ampicillin, spectinomycin, and tetracycline in the doses recommended for gonorrhea have not been shown to abort incubating syphilis. Therefore serologic tests for syphilis should be obtained monthly for four months after therapy for gonorrhea with these regimens.

Prevention. Use of a condom provides a high degree of protection for the uninfected partner. Past experience has indicated that prophylactic use of oral penicillin in a dose of 250,000 units within two to three hours after exposure markedly decreases the incidence of infection. Sexual partners of patients with gonorrhea should be identified and treated as quickly as possible to prevent further spread of disease.

The instillation of 1 per cent silver nitrate (Credé method) or an antimicrobial drug into the eyes of the newborn has largely eradicated gonococcal ophthalmia neonatorum.

Barr, J., and Danielsson, D.: Septic gonococcal dermatitis. Br. Med. J., 1:482, 1971.
Brown, W. J.: Trends and status of gonorrhea in the United States. J. Infect. Dis., 123:682, 1971.
Holmes, K. K., Counts, G. W., and Beaty, H. N.: Disseminated gonococcal infection. Ann. Intern. Med., 74:979, 1971.

Martin, J. E., Jr., and Lester, A.: Transgrow, a medium for transport and growth of *Neisseria gonorrhoeae* and *Neisseria meningitidis.* HSMHA Health Rep., 86:30, 1971.

Owen, R. L., and Hill, J. L.: Rectal and pharyngeal gonorrhea in homosexual men. J.A.M.A., 220:1315, 1972.

Pariser, H.: Asymptomatic gonorrhea. Med. Clin. North Am., 56:1127, 1972.

Schroeter, A. L., Turner, R. H., Lucas, J. B., and Brown, W. J.: Therapy for incubating syphilis. Effectiveness of gonorrhea treatment. J.A.M.A., 218:711, 1971.

Sparling, P. F.: Antibiotic resistance in *Neisseria gonorrhoeae.* Med. Clin. North Am., 56:1133, 1972.

Venereal Diseases Branch, State and Community Services Division, Center for Disease Control: Recommended treatment schedules for gonorrhea. Ann. Intern. Med., 76:991, 1972.

Vickers, F. N., and Maloney, P. J.: Gonococcal perihepatitis. Report of three cases with comments on diagnosis and treatment. Arch. Intern. Med., 114:120, 1964.

Wiesner, P. J., Tronca, E., Bonin, P., Pederson, H. B., and Holmes, K. K.: Clinical spectrum of pharyngeal gonococcal infection. N. Engl. J. Med., 288:181, 1973.

200. MENINGOCOCCAL DISEASE

Harry A. Feldman

Definition. Meningococcal infections may affect the upper and lower respiratory tracts, blood (meningococcemia), central nervous system (meningococcal meningitis, cerebrospinal fever, spotted fever, or epidemic cerebrospinal meningitis), joints (arthritis), heart, pericardium, eyes, skin, urethra, and other organs, singly or in any combination in a given patient. First recognized in 1805 by Vieusseux in Geneva and in 1806 by Danielson and Mann in Massachusetts, meningococcal meningitis, the best known form, occurs sporadically and as localized or widespread epidemics.

Etiology. *Neisseria meningitidis,* a gram-negative coccus, variable in size and occurring singly or as biscuit-shaped diplococci, was established as the causative agent by Weichselbaum in 1887. Metabolically fastidious, the organism grows best on enriched culture media at 37° C in an atmosphere of increased CO_2. Mueller-Hinton or meat infusion broths, or agar containing 10 per cent of blood (rabbit, sheep, or horse), or human ascitic fluid are excellent. Chocolate agar is especially good for initial isolation. Incorporating the vancomycin and colistin with or without nystatin (Thayer-Martin agar) makes this especially useful for isolation from throats or other areas of marked contamination. Cultures incubated in an atmosphere of 5 to 10 per cent carbon dioxide grow more luxuriantly, improving the isolation rate. Meningococci are very susceptible to chilling or drying, so all cultures should be inoculated and incubated promptly. Some meningococcal strains are exquisitely susceptible to sulfonamides so that media inoculated with specimens from such patients should have para-aminobenzoic acid (5 mg per 100 ml) added to them.

Identification of meningococci is based on morphology, Gram staining, fermentation of glucose and maltose but not sucrose, and immunologic reactions. The four classic immunologic groups, A, B, C, and D, have been expanded to include X, Y, Z, 29-E, and W-135. The most common are A, B, C, and Y. Group D is so rare that such identification is almost suspect. The groups are usually identified by their agglutination with specific antisera. A and C organisms are encapsulated so young cultures quell (capsular swelling) with specific antisera. This reaction is especially useful for the rapid, precise identification of such meningococci in cerebrospinal fluid, but requires potent antisera. Subgroups of B and C have been described, but the techniques are complex and the results are mainly of epidemiologic significance.

Lipopolysaccharides or "endotoxins" in purified form have been prepared from meningococci. Although these are toxic for animals and probably play significant roles in the pathogenesis of human disease, this remains to be defined. A true, group-specific exotoxin has not been demonstrated.

Epidemiology. Any discussion of the epidemiology of meningococcal infections is complicated by the multiplicity of serogroups. Sporadic infections may be seen almost constantly in all areas. Major epidemics are generally caused by Group A organisms and seem to occur in 20- to 30-year cycles. For example, during World Wars I and II there were massive civilian and military outbreaks which persisted for several years. Groups B and C produce lesser outbreaks, usually in the intervening years. The remaining groups are usually detected in carriers or sporadic cases, with Group Y the most frequent. Thus the over-all picture is that of high waves about every 20 to 30 years and lower ones in the interims. There are localized exceptions to this generalization. Detroit had a major Group A epidemic in 1929, with 724 cases reported in an eight-month period and a general mortality rate of 50 per cent. In infants, however, the mortality rate was 84 per cent, and in those over 40 years, 72 per cent. Santiago, Chile, had a severe Group A epidemic in 1941 to 1942 with 5885 cases; of these, 15.9 per cent were fatal. The contrasting mortality rates probably reflect the effectiveness of sulfonamide treatment.

In recent years the most devastated area has been that portion of Africa which lies below the Sahara and north of the Equator. This "meningitis belt" now averages about 10,000 cases per year with about 1200 deaths, but from 1939 to 1962 it reported 593,738 cases with 102,956 (17 per cent) deaths! In earlier outbreaks in the same area, as many as 85 per cent of cases were fatal. Here, as in South Africa, Group A organisms continue to predominate. The latter has also produced major outbreaks recently in Morocco, Finland, and Canada, but has been detected only rarely in the United States.

Infants and children are most frequently affected, about 60 per cent of cases occurring in those under 15 years. Military recruits for some unknown reason are especially vulnerable. About 80 per cent of their cases occur within the first 90 days of service, most often in the first month. The incidence of both cases and carriers is usually higher in males. Race and color do not seem to influence either incidence or susceptibility, but socioeconomic level does. The higher rates reported among blacks in certain urban areas probably reflect increased poverty with its concomitant crowding. The exact incubation period is often nondeterminable, but the range is probably one to ten days. There are a few instances in which this seems to have been longer—about three weeks.

The portal of entry of meningococci is the upper respiratory tract, and transmission from person to person occurs by direct or intimate contact, by airborne droplets, or by articles contaminated with fresh secretions from the respiratory tract. Mouth-to-mouth resuscitation has resulted in several cases in physicians, and in one instance nasopharyngeal carriage followed a kidney transplant from a donor who had died of meningococcemia. Yet even during severe epidemics, the majority of clinical infections seem to be unrelated to others, so that case-to-case spread is usually impossible to trace. Posterior nasopharyngeal culture surveys during outbreaks may demonstrate as much as 90 per cent of the population to be carriers of meningococci, constantly or intermittently, without clinical evidence of disease. Although the carrier rate often is less than 5 per cent during interepidemic periods, much of the population may harbor meningococci at some time, because the respiratory tract flora is constantly undergoing change.

Group A meningococci and, to a lesser extent, Group B and C strains have been the usual causes of epidemics in the past. Organisms of these groups were highly susceptible to sulfonamides so that such drugs were exceedingly effective for both the treatment of cases and mass prophylaxis. This changed in 1963 when sulfonamide-resistant Group B meningococci were noted to be prevalent. Subsequently, markedly resistant Group C strains were detected, and more recently, and perhaps even more disturbing, sulfonamide-resistant Group A strains first were isolated during an epidemic in North Africa, and subsequently in the "belt" below the Sahara, South Africa, Greece, Finland, Norway, Canada, Australia, and Southeast Asia. This phenomenon is now so widespread that all cases must be considered to be due to sulfonamide-resistant strains unless specifically proved to be otherwise. The same holds for carrier strains and for those of the other, less frequent, serogroups.

The physician is often concerned with the question of whether family members or other contacts of meningococcal patients are at excessive risk from this disease. Fortunately, secondary cases are unusual, but they do occur. In the Detroit epidemic of 1929, 4 per cent of cases were in affected households. In the Santiago epidemic of 1941–1942, the over-all secondary attack rate was 2.5 per cent. Because most of these follow within ten days (many four days) of the index case, they are often considered to be co-primaries. Acceptance of this concept leads to another control approach which will be dealt with subsequently (see Prevention). Household *carrier* rates, on the other hand, are high. In several studies of families of meningococcal patients, 45 to 50 per cent were found to be carrying organisms of the same group as the patient. These figures provide some justification for the anxieties of both families and physicians when cases occur which, unfortunately, cannot be resolved by the relatively simple procedure which was possible when sulfonamide-susceptible strains were the rule.

Pathogenesis and Pathology. In meningococcemia the essential lesion is vascular, with endothelial damage, inflammation of vessel walls with necrosis and thrombosis, and focal hemorrhages into cutaneous, subcutaneous, submucosal, and synovial tissues. In rapidly extending meningococcemia the Waterhouse-Friderichsen syndrome is often present. This is usually but not necessarily accompanied by bilateral adrenal hemorrhages.

Involvement of the central nervous system is characterized by acute purulent meningitis, although, if suspected early, there may be only hyperemia. Some degree of encephalitis usually accompanies the meningitis. When treatment is delayed or ineffective, permanent damage to some cranial nerves is to be expected.

The pathogenesis of meningococcal infections is usually initiated by the colonization of the posterior nasopharynx and adjoining structures by bacteria entering through the upper respiratory passages. Symptoms and signs of an acute upper respiratory infection may result, although this is not accepted by all observers. Invasion of the bloodstream follows, but this may be relatively asymptomatic. The resulting dissemination of the meningococci leads to metastatic lesions in skin, meninges, joints, eyes, ears, lungs, pericardium, urethra, and in other organs and tissues. The sites of these localizations determine the symptoms and signs that follow.

We are totally at a loss to explain why meningococcal infections are so limited and innocuous in some individuals and so extensive and overwhelming in others. No microbe can kill more quickly; deaths have been observed within several hours after the first symptom.

Chemical alterations reflecting the severity of the meningococcal infection may be profound. Their cause is not known, but it is assumed that to some degree they are endotoxic in origin. They may be furthered by the release of various substances from damaged tissue cells. Hemorrhagic manifestations may be owing to direct vascular damage because of a Shwartzman-like reaction, to thrombocytopenia, or to both. Other changes are those found in acute sepsis: fever, dehydration, reduction in blood volume, altered acid-base balance, and negative nitrogen balance. In severely ill patients, cyanosis, circulatory collapse, and other signs of shock appear, probably the result of the combined actions of bacterial endotoxins and tissue anoxia. Alterations suggestive of acute adrenal insufficiency, low serum sodium, elevated potassium, low chloride, and hypoglycemia may be present and are consistent with absent or diminished cortical secretion by damaged adrenal glands. There is no evidence that adrenal insufficiency as judged by the degree of excretion of corticosteroids in fulminating infections per se occurs independently of glandular destruction.

Clinical Manifestations. A sequential development of clinical manifestations of meningococcal infections can be discerned from a number of cases, but any one patient may present with symptoms and signs of advanced diffuse illness. The usual sequence consists of infection of the upper respiratory tract, bacteremia, septicemia, meningitis, and/or other metastatic localization. One stage will appear to dominate, giving the appearance of mild illness, grave illness, or none.

Infection of the Upper Respiratory Tract. The upper respiratory tract is the most frequent site of meningococcal infection. Most patients have no or inconsequential symptoms so that the organism is detectable only by culture of the posterior nasopharynx. Whether symptoms result from such colonization is contested by many observers, because descriptions of this stage usually have been derived from military recruits who also are subject to many viral and mycoplasmal respiratory infections. On the other hand, many but not all patients with meningococcal illnesses give histories of preceding or concurrent nasopharyngitis.

Meningococcemia. Bacteremic meningococcal infections may vary from acute fulminating illnesses of a few hours' duration to indolent, chronic infections lasting days, weeks, or, rarely, months. Symptoms may be relentlessly progressive or intermittent, with relapses and recrudescences at different times.

MILD OR SUBACUTE MENINGOCOCCEMIA. The most common form of meningococcemia is that of a relatively mild, acute, or subacute infection. Prodromal symptoms are frequently absent except for those of a mild upper respiratory infection in some. Onset is usually sudden, with fever, chilliness or frank chills that may be recurrent, malaise, myalgia, and apathy. The presenting symptoms may be any combination of these, but frequently the initial complaints are those of recurrent fever, rash, arthralgia, acute mono- or polyarthritis, nausea and vomiting, and conjunctivitis. The symptoms may regress or persist if the disease progresses. Fever may be remittent and irregular with spikes to 39 or 39.5° C. The pulse rate is proportionate to the fever. Respirations are usually normal or only slightly increased except when pneumonia or pleurisy is present.

The most striking feature on physical examination is the rash, which occurs often. It appears soon after onset, is variable (the severest is petechial or purpuric), measuring from 1 or 2 mm to 1 cm or more in diameter, and is pink to reddish blue (see accompanying figure). Early in the disease there may be a generalized, mottled erythema which appears dusky in slightly cyanotic patients. Light pink macules resembling the "rose spots" of typhoid, wheals, or nodules like erythema nodosum may appear before petechiae and ecchymoses. *Careful search in good daylight may be necessary to detect early lesions.* Occasionally, vesicular, pustular, or bullous lesions are present. Superficial or deep ulcerations may result from petechiae, especially when coalescent. These are sometimes very extensive and ultimately may require grafting. *The rash often appears first on the wrists and ankles,* but any area may be involved, including the conjunctivae and the mucous membranes. Hemorrhagic lesions fade to a brown, rusty color three or four days after their appearance; if new crops appear, often after chills, multiple skin lesions may be present at the same time. This is more likely when treatment is delayed or unsuccessful.

Other physical findings, including splenomegaly, are inconstant. Herpetic lesions of the lip are found in about 10 per cent of the cases. Unless meningismus develops, symptoms referable to the central nervous system are absent, although those resulting from metastatic localizations are usually self-evident, depending upon their site.

The firm diagnosis is established with laboratory aids. Leukocytosis up to 40,000 cells per cubic millimeter with 80 to 90 per cent neutrophils is almost always present. In overwhelming cases, gram-negative intracellular diplococci may be seen within leukocytes in stained smears from capillary blood, buffy coat, or directly from skin lesions. A blood culture positive for meningococci furnishes final etiologic proof. It should be emphasized that several cultures of the blood may be necessary to detect meningococci and that growth of the organism in liquid medium may be slow. Other laboratory examinations are either normal or compatible with any febrile illness.

The subsequent course is dependent on therapy, although some patients with very mild disease recover spontaneously after several weeks or months. Any of the complications and sequelae of meningococcal infections may develop.

ACUTE FULMINATING MENINGOCOCCEMIA. This differs from the milder form in the rapidity with which it progresses and in its overwhelming character. The onset is usually abrupt and quite dramatic, with a shaking chill, severe headache, dizziness or vertigo, collapse, or unconsciousness. Patients with massive purpura, low blood pressure, rapid, quiet respiration, and overwhelming bacteremia are said to have the Waterhouse-Friderichsen syndrome. They are often clear mentally. Their extensive rash (see figure) involves skin and mucous membranes as well as internal organs such as skeletal muscle and, classically, the adrenal glands. Leukopenia is another indicator of the gravity of the patient's condition. Body temperature may be subnormal, normal, or slightly elevated. Within a few hours there may be circulatory collapse with intravascular coagulation. Often there is a consumptive coagulopathy (see Ch. 201).

Others may have the encephalitic form, which is characterized by rapidly developing coma, rapid stertorous

Skin lesions in fulminating meningococcemia. (Courtesy of Dr. Worth B. Daniels.)

breathing, a petechial but not massive purpuric rash, and normal blood pressure. Some may present with a combination of encephalitis and adrenal involvement with early deep coma, purpura, and low blood pressure. Occasionally, the pituitary gland, like the adrenals, is damaged by hemorrhage. These severe illnesses are often rapidly fatal. It is in the attempt to prevent or to reverse this rapid course that so much emphasis is placed upon early, intensive treatment.

CHRONIC MENINGOCOCCEMIA. Chronic meningococcemia is an uncommon form of meningococcal disease in which episodes of fever of a few days' duration recur at intervals of days, weeks, or more rarely, months. Chills and arthralgic symptoms are frequent, but rash may be absent or evanescent. Repeated cultures of the blood may be necessary before meningococci are recovered. Failure to suspect, recognize, and treat chronic meningococcemia may result in meningitis or endocarditis.

Meningitis. Although it constitutes only a relatively small percentage of the total number of meningococcal infections, meningitis is the most characteristic and important manifestation. The onset and symptoms are often indistinguishable from those of a generalized infection; in some, meningeal involvement seems to predominate. In others, both groups of symptoms appear almost simultaneously, but there may be great variations in their intensity and severity. In addition to the signs of sepsis and the rash, patients with meningitis have evidence of inflammation of the meninges: pain in the neck and back on forward flexion of the head, stiff neck, retraction of the head or severe opisthotonos, Kernig's and Brudzinski's signs, hyperesthesia, hyperirritability, and exaggerated reflexes. Unequal reflexes are unusual, but may be present. Involvement of the cranial nerves, when present, may result in strabismus and deafness. The increased intracranial pressure may lead to severe headache, nausea, vomiting, dilated or irregular pupils, engorgement of the fundal veins, choking of the discs, irregular slow pulse, and moderately elevated blood pressure. Cheyne-Stokes or Biot's respiration may appear. As the disease progresses, restlessness and irritability may be followed by delirium or by generalized or jacksonian type convulsions; the patient may become greatly depressed, somnolent, and finally stuporous and comatose. In infants the signs of meningitis may be no more than refusal of feedings, vomiting or regurgitation, diarrhea, irritability, and fever. Convulsions and bulging of the fontanelles, when present, are extremely useful signs.

LABORATORY FINDINGS IN MENINGITIS. The cerebrospinal fluid is under increased pressure and varies from clear to frankly purulent. The cell count is elevated, often to thousands per cubic millimeter, mostly neutrophils. Gram-negative intra- and extracellular diplococci can be seen in variable numbers in stained smears of the sediment. The total protein in the cerebrospinal fluid is increased, and its sugar content is usually reduced. Meningococci may be grown from the fluid by proper cultural methods. Fluid obtained early in meningitis may have few or no cells and no reduction of its glucose content, but cultures nonetheless will often be positive.

COURSE OF MENINGITIS. Extremely variable, the course is greatly influenced by therapy. In untreated cases the temperature is erratic, and symptoms progress to early death or to chronic meningitis with severe sequelae or delayed death.

Complications of Meningococcal Infections. The complications of the different forms of meningococcal infections include intercurrent infections, metastatic localizations, and permanent damage to the central nervous system. These may appear during the acute stage or subsequently. Intercurrent infections of the respiratory tract with other agents may occur. Bacteremic or metastatic complications include conjunctivitis, panophthalmitis, otitis, purulent mono- or polyarthritis, pneumonia, pleurisy, pericarditis, myocarditis, endocarditis, orchitis, epididymitis, jaundice, hepatorenal failure, transient albuminuria and hematuria, and adrenal hemorrhage with necrosis. Infection of the central nervous system may produce transient or permanent paralyses, hemiplegia, neuroradiculitis, encephalitis, encephalomyelitis, altered cerebration, convulsions, cranial nerve damage, cerebral thrombosis, and brain abscess. Organization of exudate in the ventricular channels and the subarachnoid space may mechanically obstruct the flow of cerebrospinal fluid, producing hydrocephalus. The accumulation of subdural fluid of high protein content, which when encapsulated resembles a subdural hematoma, is fairly frequent in infants and young children. Recurrent meningitis caused by meningococci or other bacteria is usually due to structural defects of bone resulting from trauma or other causes which sometimes require surgical repair. Complications resulting from therapy can be avoided or minimized, if anticipated.

Permanent sequelae may result from almost any complication; the most frequent are deafness, ocular palsies, blindness, changes in intellectual ability, psychoses, and hydrocephalus.

Diagnosis. The specific diagnosis of meningococcal disease depends primarily upon differentiation from other acute systemic and meningococcal infections. Final confirmation of the diagnosis requires bacteriologic identification of the causative organism as a meningococcus. During an epidemic, especially in a recruit military camp or a closed population, all cases of fever with abrupt onset, of prostration with or without fever, of petechial or purpuric rash, of drowsiness or coma, and of meningitis should be treated vigorously as meningococcal infections whether or not organisms are found in initial smears and cultures.

Meningococcal infections in their early stages may resemble any acute systemic infection. In sepsis caused by pyogenic organisms such as staphylococci, streptococci, or pneumococci, there may be a preceding upper respiratory infection, recurrent fever, malaise, arthralgia, and leukocytosis. A rash similar to that of severe meningococcemia and even signs of the Waterhouse-Friderichsen syndrome occasionally may be present in such cases. Final proof is accomplished by isolation of the offending organisms from the blood, joint fluid, sputum, and so forth. Meningococcal infections must also be differentiated from the acute exanthemata, typhus (both endemic and epidemic), typhoid and other enteric fevers, subacute bacterial endocarditis, rheumatic fever, brucellosis, and others.

Diagnosis of Meningitis. The diagnosis of meningococcal meningitis requires differentiation from meningismus, other bacterial meningitides, viral meningoencephalitis, myeloencephalitis resulting from bacterial toxins (tetanus, botulinus) or chemicals, and noninfectious problems such as subarachnoid or cerebral hemorrhages or thrombosis, diabetic coma, and uremia. In most cases of meningococcal meningitis, the diagnosis is readily established by the specific identification of the organism; in others the etiology may not be determinable when the patient is first seen, but a number of helpful procedures can be carried out. The usual medical history should be obtained, but a careful inquiry should be made into recent localized infections, especially of the ear, and trauma to the head, because these predispose to secondary bacterial meningitides, more likely to be caused by *H. influenzae* or pneumococci.

Physical examination should include a thorough search for diseases of the eyes and upper respiratory passages, sinuses, and ears and for evidence of injury to the head, in addition to careful general and neurologic examinations. A complete blood count should be made and cultures of the blood and posterior nasopharynx obtained. Any suspected localized areas of infection likewise should be cultured. Urinalysis and determinations of serum electrolytes and the blood nonprotein nitrogen may aid in the differential diagnosis and help to indicate precautions to be observed in therapy. In seriously ill, if not in all patients, blood coagulation analyses should be performed to determine the presence of a consumptive coagulopathy. Bleeding from the upper gastrointestinal tract ("stress ulcers") should be suspected in the very sick, especially those in shock.

Lumbar puncture should be performed as soon as possible and before specific treatment is instituted. After determining the initial pressure, fluid should be removed slowly until the pressure is reduced to an approximately normal level. The dynamics of the cerebrospinal fluid can then be estimated by jugular compression for evidence of block or sinus thrombosis. Examination of the cerebrospinal fluid should include the following: gross appearance, total and differential cell counts, determination of sugar (compare with blood level) and protein, and cultures and examination of Gram-stained smears. If organisms are seen, they can often be identified tentatively from their appearance and precisely with proper and *potent* antisera by a positive direct quellung test if of Group A or C.

A presumptive diagnosis can usually be made from the Gram-stained smear, the differential cell count, and the sugar content of the cerebrospinal fluid. Caution should be exercised in the interpretation of smears, because even experienced personnel may be misled by overdecolorized or dead gram-positive diplococci or other bacteria. Final identification depends on serogrouping organisms from culture. The leukocytes are almost entirely neutrophils in purulent meningitides, except syphilitic or tuberculous. In the latter, as in viral infections (mumps, herpes, coxsackieviruses, echoviruses, and others), mononucleated cells predominate except in their early stages. The sugar content is usually low in bacterial meningitis and normal in viral infections. In meningismus the fluid is usually normal. The proportion of erythrocytes to leukocytes is similar to that in whole blood in cases of subarachnoid hemorrhage. The history, other physical findings, and special laboratory tests should help to differentiate myeloencephalitides resulting from toxins or chemicals.

Treatment. During the past 30 years, Groups A, B, and C meningococci have been responsible for almost all meningococcal infections regardless of their clinical forms. Until about 1963 practically all meningococcal strains were exquisitely susceptible to the sulfonamide drugs, whether in carriers or cases. For these reasons, the sulfonamides were the agents of choice for both treatment and prophylaxis. They are still excellent, providing

that one is certain that the patient or carrier has a sulfonamide-susceptible organism. Without suitable tests of the homologous strain, this assumption is no longer permissible.

Since sulfonamide-resistant Group A, B, C, and Y strains are now commonplace, the treatment of patients requires penicillin G in massive dosage. For adults, this means 20,000,000 units per day intravenously or 1,000,000 units every two hours intramuscularly. The latter should not be used for patients in, or on the verge of, shock. When the 20,000,000 unit dose is used intravenously, it is best to divide it into four or more doses per day rather than to administer it by continuous drip. Doses in children should be reduced in accordance with pediatric therapeutic principles.

Ampicillin may be used as an alternative, although an occasional patient does not seem to respond adequately to this drug. Close observation of the patient's course will alert the physician to this problem, should it arise. The dose should be at least 150 mg per kilogram per day for children and 10 to 12 grams per day for adults, parenterally, divided into six to eight doses.

In patients known to be truly allergic to penicillin, chloramphenicol is the alternative drug of choice. The use of this drug imposes precautions of its own. These can be managed, but close watch should be kept on the hematopoietic system and the drug withdrawn immediately if a complication appears. Thus far, no meningococci resistant to penicillin or chloramphenicol have been identified. If the patient's organism is found to be susceptible to sulfonamide, treatment can be altered accordingly. *Cephalothins and lincomycin should not be used, because therapeutic failures have followed their administration.*

Patients with meningococcal disease are usually more dehydrated than they appear. Care should be taken to ensure a daily urine output of more than 1000 ml. Treatment should be continued at least until all signs and symptoms have been normal for a minimum of two days and preferably for five. It may be stopped abruptly. Relapse occurs occasionally and requires prompt treatment.

Patients with fulminating meningococcemia or meningitis, or both, should be started on therapy as soon as the diagnosis is suspected and specimens obtained, without waiting for bacteriologic confirmation. Penicillin should be given by vein. (Patients allergic to penicillin are best treated with chloramphenicol.) The central venous pressure should be monitored and corrected as necessary. Disseminated intravascular coagulation when diagnosed should be managed as in any other disease state (see Ch. 201). Norepinephrine, intravenously, may be required to maintain blood pressure. Steroids are clearly required if there is evidence of adrenal collapse; such patients are managed as are those with acute adrenal insufficiency. Otherwise, there is no good evidence that steroids are of any positive value. These severely ill patients are the most likely ones to bleed from gastric lesions ("stress ulcers") which require special handling, contraindicating steroids. Intravenous infusions will be required to correct dehydration, but an excess should be avoided. Oxygen therapy should be instituted and maintained as long as cyanosis or dyspnea is present. Blood transfusions have not been shown to be of significant value in this type of circulatory failure.

Certain laboratory tests such as hematologic examinations should be repeated as aids in monitoring the patient's course. This is especially true for patients admitted with severe leukopenia or thrombocytopenia. Their reversal is of considerable prognostic importance. Blood cultures should be repeated if the fever persists or returns, for continued bacteremia suggests the presence of endocarditis or other metastatic localization. Repeat lumbar punctures are indicated if there is persistent increased intracranial pressure, failure to respond to adequate therapy, or relapse of meningitis.

Symptomatic and supportive treatment is essential for patients with meningococcal infections. Sedation should be minimal, yet sufficient to assure adequate rest but not to interfere with the assessment of the patient's course. Approximately one month of convalescence is required for complete recovery in most cases and even more for those with severe illnesses.

The treatment of complications of meningococcal infections is primarily that of the underlying disease. Should fever or signs of meningeal irritation reappear, then the most probable causes are recurrence of infection with the meningococcus because of inadequate treatment, drug fever, or superinfection with another organism. In such circumstances, the cerebrospinal fluid and blood should be re-examined and cultured. If the meningococcal infection has relapsed, intensive treatment should be reinstituted and maintained until the patient has fully recovered.

Prognosis. The prognosis in meningococcal infections has improved enormously because of the efficacy of the sulfonamides and penicillin. In untreated cases of meningococcemia and meningitis the mortality formerly varied from 20 to 90 per cent, averaging about 70 per cent. The introduction of serum therapy reduced this to about 50 per cent. With the sulfonamides the case fatality rate has been reduced to 5 to 10 per cent, depending upon age and complicating conditions. The recent recognition of sulfonamide-resistant meningococci has not altered this significantly, because cases can be treated as successfully with penicillin. Age is perhaps the most important factor in prognosis, for the greatest mortality, despite adequate therapy, occurs in those less than two or more than 40 years old. In the U. S. Army during World War II, the over-all mortality was slightly less than 5 per cent and, in some series, even below 1 per cent. More than 90 per cent of these cases were caused by sulfonamide-susceptible Group A strains. In addition to a most favorable age distribution in the Army, the excellent physical condition of patients, early diagnosis, and the prompt institution of effective therapy were probably responsible for this remarkable recovery rate. The prognosis is still poor in fulminating cases with abrupt onset, extensive cutaneous lesions, and circulatory collapse. In spite of rapid, intensive therapy, such cases frequently terminate fatally. Relapses, recurrences, and complications have been greatly reduced by specific treatment so that the prognosis for total recovery is generally good. *The most frequent permanent sequelae despite adequate treatment* are deafness, cranial nerve paralyses, mental deficiency, and, less often, blindness and hydrocephalus. These are all relatively uncommon and usually result from treatment delays for whatever cause.

Prevention. Prophylaxis as applied to meningococcal infections during the past 30 years represented an outgrowth of the World War II experience which demonstrated not only that sulfadiazine rapidly cured meningococcal disease but also that the nasopharyngeal carrier state was reversed soon after such treatment was begun. After several successful trials in military recruits, a policy was adopted whereby small amounts of sulfadiazine were administered simultaneously to all members of recruit training centers, schools, ships, and similar groups upon the recognition of a predetermined number of cases. This resulted in an immediate reduction in carriers, accompanied by a sharp decrease in cases. Thus was reflected the interaction of a susceptible organism with an effective drug when administered to a total population at risk.

Because of the fears often generated by the diagnosis of meningitis, the same sulfadiazine regimen was adopted for general use by physicians and health departments to treat family and hospital (staff) contacts of sporadic cases. But the "secondary" cases which occasionally occur in households usually begin within 96 hours or less of that of the index patient, suggesting that they are co-primary rather than secondary. Sometimes this interval is as long as 7 to 10 days. It would seem then that if *disease* is to be prevented under such circumstances, therapeutic rather than "prophylactic" medication is needed. Unless the causative strain is known to be sulfonamide susceptible, it must be assumed to be resistant, requiring penicillin for treatment with dosage in the therapeutic range. If taken orally, this will require 8 million or more units per day in young or older adults. Suitably reduced doses should be prescribed for children. Either oral or parenteral regimens for streptococcal prophylaxis provide *no* protection for meningococcal infections.

The recommendation for meningococcal disease is really for *intervention* rather than *prevention*. Alternatively, one can observe closely (including nasopharyngeal cultures) and treat immediately upon the appearance of any symptoms. But over-all, the risk is very low and should not induce the hysteria which so often accompanies the hospital admission or diagnosis of a case of meningococcal meningitis. The isolation of patients after 24 to 48 hours of adequate therapy is not indicated.

Although the foregoing is suitable for the immediate contact or family, it is not applicable to a population group such as in a camp, school, or mental institution. In such instances the objective is to rapidly reduce the over-all carrier level to a point where transfer is impeded, decreasing the case rate. Again, sulfonamides are the most effective drugs for this purpose, but only when the causative organisms are susceptible. Penicillin, in contrast to sulfonamides, often fails to eliminate the carrier state, even in therapeutic doses. Both rifampin (600 mg daily for five days) and minocycline (200 mg, then 100 mg twice daily for five days), singly, sequentially, and together, have been used for this purpose in military units and in modified dosage in an elementary school population. Meningococcal carrier rates are reduced quite effectively, but resistance to rifampin does occur and increases with reuse. Some toxic effects have been noted, especially in children, so that additional experience will be required for further definition. Caution with regard to the widespread use of rifampin in populations with high tuberculosis rates is probably well advised because of possible increased resistance among tubercle bacilli. At no time should either rifampin or minocycline be used for the treatment of actual cases of meningococcal disease.

There is considerable reason for optimism regarding meningococcal vaccines. Potent group-specific polysaccharides have been prepared from meningococci of

Groups A and C, but not yet from B. After very careful graduated trials, Group C meningococcal polysaccharide vaccine was made a routine for all American military recruits in single subcutaneous doses of 50 μg. Disease caused by this serogroup has all but been eliminated from that population. Currently, field trials with Group A polysaccharide vaccine are under way, and the early results are encouraging. The duration of protection has not yet been established, nor has either effectiveness or usefulness been defined in children. Measurable responses to polysaccharide vaccines are quite different and less in children (especially under two years) than adults. No polysaccharide vaccine has been licensed, and thus such vaccines are not yet available for general use.

Artenstein, M. S., Gold, R., Zimmerly, J. G., Wyle, F. A., Schneider, H., and Harkins, C.: Prevention of meningococcal disease by Group C polysaccharide vaccine. N. Engl. J. Med., 282:417, 1970.

Evans, R. W., Glick, B., Kimball, F., and Lobell, M.: Fatal intravascular consumption coagulopathy in meningococcal sepsis. Am. J. Med., 46:910, 1969.

Feldman, H. A.: Neisseria infections other than gonococcal. In Bodily, H. L., Updyke, E. L., and Mason, J. O. (eds.): Diagnostic Procedures for Bacterial, Mycotic and Parasitic Infections. 5th ed. New York, American Public Health Association, Inc., 1970.

Feldman, H. A.: Meningococcal Infections. In Stollerman, G. H. (ed.): Advances in Internal Medicine. Vol. 18. Chicago, Year Book Medical Publishers, 1972, pp. 117–140.

Gotschlich, E. E., Goldschneider, I., and Artenstein, M. S.: Human immunity to the meningococcus. V. The effect of immunization with meningococcal Group C polysaccharide on the carrier state. J. Exp. Med., 129:1385, 1969.

201. BACTERIAL MENINGITIS

Robert G. Petersdorf

Definition. Meningitis is an inflammatory process involving the coverings of the central nervous system. Bacteria, viruses, spirochetes, parasites, and fungi may be the offending pathogens. This chapter is concerned with meningitis caused by bacteria other than meningococci and mycobacteria; these are discussed in Ch. 200 and 236, respectively.

Etiology. With the exception of *Mycobacterium tuberculosis,* the three most common microorganisms causing meningitis are *Diplococcus pneumoniae, Neisseria meningitidis,* and *Hemophilus influenzae.* The meningitis caused by *H. influenzae* is usually of type B and occurs uncommonly after the age of 6 and rarely after 12. When it occurs in adults, a deficiency in immune globulins, a parameningeal focus, or head trauma should be suspected. Meningococcal disease is found in both children and adults, but is rare after the age of 50. Pneumococcal meningitis is most common in infancy and old age. Other, less common pathogens are *Staphylococcus aureus,* which is usually found in association with epidural or brain abscess, in thrombosis of the cavernous sinus, or after cranial trauma and neurosurgical procedures; *Escherichia coli,* a common offender in meningitis in newborns; and other enteric organisms, including Proteus species, Klebsiella-Enterobacter, Paracolon, Salmonella, and Pseudomonas. Infection with Pseudomonas has followed lumbar puncture, spinal anesthesia, and the establishment of shunting procedures to relieve hydrocephalus. Gonococcal meningitis, which is quite indistinguishable from meningococcal infections, is being

reported with increasing frequency. The group A Streptococcus, formerly a common offender, is now a relatively rare cause of meningitis, although enterococci and anaerobic streptococci continue to be isolated, primarily from patients with brain abscess and meningitis. Rarer organisms include *Listeria monocytogenes,* a small gram-positive rod resembling nonpathogenic diphtheroids; *Mima polymorpha,* a pleomorphic gram-negative organism that is difficult to differentiate on Gram stain (but not culture) from *H. influenzae* and *N. meningitidis;* and *Cl. perfringens* and *Past. multocida.*

Incidence. The precise incidence of bacterial meningitis is difficult to determine, because, except for meningococcal infections, meningitis is not reportable. There appears to be a decrease in incidence of all forms of meningitis except perhaps for *H. influenzae.* However, the mortality rate has remained relatively constant. This may reflect the susceptibility of aged or "poor risk" patients to meningeal infections. Like many infections, most forms of bacterial meningitis are more prevalent among individuals of low socioeconomic status.

Pathology. There is considerable variation in the pathologic picture, depending in part on the duration of the disease, the infecting organism, the resistance of the host, and the type and duration of therapy. Although bacterial meningitis is usually localized to the subarachnoid space, infections caused by viruses, spirochetes, parasites, and fungi are commonly complicated by cerebritis or encephalitis. In bacterial meningitis, grossly purulent exudate is present over the cortical and basal surfaces of the brain, and may invest the spinal cord as well. The pus is often localized to the cerebellopontine angles. Cortical phlebitis with its consequences of vascular congestion, thrombosis, and infarction may be prominent findings. Microscopically, exudate consisting of several hundred layers of polymorphonuclear leukocytes is present over the surface of the brain and in the ventricular system, where the pus may produce noncommunicating hydrocephalus. Occasionally, the exudate penetrates the arachnoid, forming a subdural empyema. Although migration of inflammatory cells into subjacent neuronal tissue and necrosis of nerve cells may occur, in general, the meninges provide remarkable protection to the neurons, which are usually spared from the inflammatory process and invasion by bacteria.

Pathogenesis. The routes by which microorganisms penetrate the blood–cerebrospinal fluid barrier and establish infection in the subarachnoid space have not been clearly defined. In a number of instances, bacterial meningitis follows infection of the middle ear, mastoid, paranasal sinuses, and trauma or surgery to the face and head. In these instances, it seems likely that bacteria enter through a rent in the leptomeninges or that infection in a neighboring focus may render the meninges more permeable to microorganisms. Pneumococci, streptococci, staphylococci, and (more rarely) *H. influenzae* and gram-negative enteric bacilli have been implicated in this type of meningitis. Meningococci, which are usually carried in the nasopharynx, have been assumed to ascend to the meninges via the small venules and via arachnoid sheaths investing the olfactory nerves and accompanying them through the lamina cribrosa. However, there is no direct evidence for this route of infection in man. It has been postulated that infection emanating from distant foci, such as pneumococcal meningitis that follows pneumonia, or infection without a primary focus, is blood borne. In laboratory animals, bacteremia is not associated with meningitis unless the meninges are subjected to microtrauma (in the form of needle puncture) at the height of bacteremia. It is conceivable that this situation exists in man and that a microscopic defect in the meninges is a prerequisite for entry of bacteria from the blood. Occasionally, meningitis follows the rupture of a brain abscess. Anaerobic streptococci, enterococci, staphylococci, mixtures of bacteria, and actinomycetes may be isolated under these circumstances.

Clinical Manifestations. *History.* Most patients with meningitis report fever, lethargy, confusion, headache, vomiting, or stiff neck. The mode of onset may vary. Some patients rapidly develop headache, confusion, and loss of consciousness within 24 hours; they usually do not have antecedent respiratory symptoms. Others complain of headache, fever, and stiff neck associated with otitis, rhinorrhea, sore throat, or cough for one to seven days prior to the appearance of the full clinical picture. Still others have symptoms referable to the respiratory tract for several weeks before meningitis sets in. *Cough* is a common symptom in pneumococcal meningitis which is often accompanied by pneumonia; *earache* often antedates infection with *H. influenzae,* and a *sore throat* may precede neisserial meningitis. Other symptoms of bacterial meningitis include backache, weakness, dizziness, ataxia, photophobia, and generalized myalgias. Additional clues are a history of sickle cell disease, a common accompaniment of pneumococcal meningitis in children; previous or recent infection or surgery involving the nose, throat, or sinuses; head trauma; recent lumbar puncture or spinal anesthesia; and close and intimate contact with a patient who has a meningococcal infection.

Physical Findings. Most patients demonstrate the signs of meningeal irritation, i.e., stiff neck and positive Kernig or Brudzinski signs. Patients without these signs are often very young, very old, or severely obtunded. A *petechial eruption* is relatively rare in meningitis caused by bacteria other than meningococci unless bacterial endocarditis is present. There may be physical signs of pneumonia, particularly in patients with pneumococcal meningitis, and evidence of aural infection may also be found. Often, however, a primary focus (otitis, mastoiditis, sinusitis, pneumonia, or empyema) is not apparent on physical examination and should be carefully sought by other means, because failure to eradicate the primary focus may result in failure of therapy or post-treatment relapse. Although intracranial pressure is characteristically elevated, papilledema is rare. When it is encountered in the course of acute bacterial meningitis, it should call to mind the possibility of subdural empyema, brain abscess, or venous sinus thrombosis. The level of consciousness in most patients with meningitis may vary from confusion and mild lethargy to deep coma. About 10 to 15 per cent are remarkably alert. In approximately 50 per cent, however, other signs of neurologic damage develop during the course of infection. These include major motor seizures, hemipareses, which are often transient and probably postictal, signs of diffuse central nervous system damage (bilateral Babinski signs and fixed, mid-stage pupils), or paresis of the second, third, sixth, seventh, and eighth cranial nerves.

Associated Disease. With the exception of epidemics of meningococcal meningitis, which are usually confined to closed environments such as army camps or schools, bacterial meningitis occurs sporadically, usually in a setting of some associated disease. Pharyngitis antedates meningitis in many patients with meningococcal and Hemophilus infection. Otitis with or without mastoiditis, although much rarer nowadays than 20 years ago, remains an important precursor of Hemophilus and pneumococcal meningitis, which is also frequently associated with pneumonia. Pneumonitis is also often present in meningitis caused by gram-negative pathogens. A number of patients with pneumococcal meningitis have multiple myeloma; patients with this neoplasm are generally prone to recurrent pneumococcal infections. A similar propensity has been described for children with sickle cell disease. In addition to the common meningeal pathogens, meningitis in patients with diabetes mellitus is likely to be caused by uncommon organisms such as Klebsiella-Enterobacter, and *Staphylococcus aureus.* Enteric bacteria not uncommonly are seen in meningeal infections among patients with leukemias or lymphomas. Cranial trauma may precede meningitis by several days and occasionally months or years; in such instances *D. pneumoniae,* hemolytic *Staph. aureus,* or coliform bacteria are usually the offending organisms. Cranial osteomyelitis may intervene between head trauma and the development of meningitis. Patients undergoing shunt procedures for relief of hydrocephalus tend to have infections with bacteria that are ordinarily not pathogenic such as *Staphylococcus epidermidis* or micrococci; gram-negative enteric bacterial and Pseudomonas meningitis also complicate shunting procedures. Occasionally, subcutaneous or mucosal infections such as furunculosis, decubitus ulcers, omphalitis in neonates, and endometritis precede leptomeningitis.

Rare Types of Meningitis. MIMA POLYMORPHA MENINGITIS. *Mima polymorpha* is a gram-negative pleomorphic bacillus that is easily confused on Gram stain with members of the Neisseria group and *H. influenzae.* It can be separated from these organisms, however, by cultural and serologic techniques. Meningitis caused by *Mima polymorpha* closely resembles meningitis caused by the more common pathogens and cannot be differentiated from them on clinical grounds. Separation of mimae from Neisseria is of more than academic importance because mimae may be resistant to penicillin and sulfonamides and respond only to the tetracyclines.

LISTERIA MENINGITIS. The most common clinical illness caused by Listeria is meningitis, and any patient with clinical and laboratory evidence of meningeal infection said to be caused by a diphtheroid should be assumed to harbor Listeria in the cerebrospinal fluid. Clinically, the illness cannot be distinguished from meningitis caused by other bacteria (see Ch. 222).

OTHER ORGANISMS. Bacteria that have caused infections usually in patients with antecedent head trauma or neurosurgical procedures include *Cl. perfringens* and *Past. multocida,* although any organism can occasionally produce infection in this setting.

Recurrent Meningitis. Recurrent bouts of meningitis are most frequently related to remote as well as to recent head trauma. The individual episodes are usually caused by the same bacterial species that are associated with meningitis occurring in the absence of trauma, except that pneumococci of higher serologic types are isolated most commonly, and may account for 80 per cent of these infections. Bouts of meningitis may be separated by an interval of several years. Cerebrospinal fluid rhinorrhea owing to a defect in the cribriform plate is often associated with recurrent meningeal infection. These patients also usually have evidence of a recent or remote skull fracture involving the frontal bone. All patients with repeated bouts of meningitis should be subjected to vigorous search for a communication between the subarachnoid space and the nasopharynx. This should include laminagrams of the frontal and ethmoid bones, and instillation of radioiodinated albumin or a dye such as indigo carmine intrathecally, followed by testing for these substances in nasal secretions. Testing these secretions with glucose oxidase (Dextrostix) may give a positive test, connoting CSF rhinorrhea.

Rarer situations predisposing to recurrent meningeal infections include chronic mastoiditis or petrositis, congenital abnormalities of the cranial vault, and congenital dermoid sinus tracts. Ventriculomastoid shunts aimed at relief of hydrocephalus are also complicated by recurrent infections, which are often heralded by otitis media. Recurrent bouts of meningitis have been reported in children who have undergone splenectomy; this does not appear to be true of adults. Nor is there evidence that the incidence of meningitis is increased in children with hypo- or dysgammaglobulinemia.

Infections with Multiple Organisms. Meningitis caused by two or more organisms occasionally occurs in infants, young children and neonates, who may develop brain abscesses after surgery or birth trauma. *H. influenzae* is usually one of the organisms, and has been found in conjunction with *N. meningitidis, D. pneumoniae,* group A Streptococcus, and *E. coli.* In adults infections with multiple organisms most commonly follow rupture of a brain abscess into the subarachnoid space, and streptococci, staphylococci, and gram-negative enteric pathogens may all be isolated from the same specimen of cerebrospinal fluid.

Complications of Bacterial Meningitis. *Disseminated Intravascular Coagulation.* This syndrome, which is also called consumptive coagulopathy, is manifested by multiple petechiae, ecchymoses, purpura, bleeding from other surfaces, hypotension progressing to shock, and gangrene of distal extremities (see Ch. 200).

Although fulminant meningococcemia (with or without meningitis) is an important cause of disseminated intravascular coagulation (DIC), other gram-negative infections (particularly when accompanied by endotoxin shock), pneumococcal bacteremia in asplenic patients, Rocky Mountain spotted fever, disseminated herpes and congenital rubella, and falciparum malaria are among the other infectious causes of this syndrome. (See also Ch. 801.)

Clinical manifestations of DIC are due to the consumption of platelets and clotting factors and the anticoagulant effects of fibrin degradation products, leading to actual or potential bleeding; the deposition of fibrin, resulting in capillary thrombosis and ischemic infarction; and the distribution of red cells, leading to microangiopathic hemolytic anemia. Treatment should be directed at the underlying meningococcal infection.

Temporal and Cerebellar Herniation. These complications are commonly found in fatal meningitis, and may be recognized by distinct respiratory, ocular, and motor signs that indicate loss of diencephalic, midbrain, pontine, and medullary function in an orderly rostral-caudal sequence. In the presence of these signs, repeated lumbar punctures should be avoided.

Endocarditis. Endocarditis, most often involving the aortic valve, is found in 10 to 15 per cent of fatal cases of pneumococcal meningitis. Pneumonia is also frequent in this setting. Rheumatic or congenital valvular disease may antedate development of endocarditis, but frequently normal valves are involved. Staphylococci and coliform organisms and gonococci may also be the cause of the endocarditis-meningitis syndrome. Endocarditis may be difficult to detect clinically but should be seriously considered in patients with meningitis, pneumococcal, staphylococcal, gonococcal, and coliform bacteremia, and heart murmurs. The appearance of an aortic diastolic murmur when none was present previously is diagnostic of endocarditis in this setting.

Purulent Arthritis. Purulent arthritis may complicate pneumococcal, meningococcal, and staphylococcal meningitis. In general, it responds to antimicrobials, although aspiration of synovial fluid may be necessary.

Subdural Effusions. Subdural effusions have been a frequently reported complication of Hemophilus meningitis, but may also follow other types of meningitis in children. Prolonged unexplained fever, confusion despite adequate antimicrobial therapy, and convulsions after the apparent subsidence of infection are classic manifestations of accumulating subdural fluid that is usually sterile. Aspiration of this fluid, which may need to be repeated, results in relief of symptoms.

Neurologic Residua. Residual damage to the nervous system occurs in 10 to 20 per cent of patients, and is most common after pneumococcal meningitis in adults and *H. influenzae* meningitis in children. *Deafness* remains the most common sequel of pyogenic meningitis; hemiparesis, convulsive disorders, and dementia are seen occasionally.

Diagnosis. *General Considerations.* The diagnosis of bacterial meningitis is not difficult, provided a high index of suspicion is maintained. Meningeal infection should be considered in every patient with a history of upper respiratory illness interrupted by vomiting, headache, lethargy, confusion, or stiff neck. When first seen, some of these patients present only with low-grade fever, mild headache, or occasional emesis. Nevertheless, the possibility of meningeal infection must be carefully considered. In patients with pneumonia it is particularly dangerous to ascribe confusion to age or "toxemic" depression. Meningitis may be present in addition to pulmonary infection, and the dosage of antimicrobial drug used to to treat pneumonia is often inadequate to control meningeal infection. The susceptibility of alcoholics to pneumococcal meningitis cannot be emphasized too strongly, and may be related to the high prevalence of pneumonia in this group. Fever and confusion in these patients should not be attributed to alcoholic intoxication, delirium tremens, or hepatic encephalopathy unless the cerebrospinal fluid has been examined.

Two unusual types of recurrent meningitis may mimic bacterial infection, at least initially. *Mollaret's meningitis* consists of recurrent febrile attacks, malaise, headache, and meningeal signs accompanied by a marked polymorphonuclear inflammatory reaction in the CSF. Attacks last two to three days and subside spontaneously. *Behçet's syndrome* is characterized by recurrent oral and genital ulcerations and relapsing ocular lesions along with meningitis. Other neurologic abnormalities may include cranial nerve palsies, seizures, hemiparesis, extrapyramidal signs, and chronic brain syndromes.

Cerebrospinal Fluid. The cerebrospinal fluid should be examined in any patient with evidence of meningeal irritation. In patients with papilledema or other evidence of elevated cerebrospinal fluid pressure, lumbar puncture should be performed with care, employing a small-gauge needle. Papilledema does not constitute a contraindication to lumbar puncture in patients in whom the diagnosis of meningitis is suspected. The cerebrospinal fluid pressure is usually elevated, and the gross appearance of the fluid may vary from slight turbidity to gross pus. The fluid should be centrifuged immediately, and the sediment stained by Gram's method and cultured on blood and chocolate agar under increased CO_2 tension and anaerobically in thioglycollate. Some common pitfalls encountered in Gram staining include washing the organisms off the slide, decolorizing gram-positive bacteria, and interpreting particles of stain as bacteria. Nevertheless, carefully performed Gram stains are accurate in 90 per cent of cases in which organisms are seen. Pneumococci are more easily identified than meningococci. Although immunofluorescent techniques have been used to expedite the diagnosis in a variety of bacterial meningitides, they appear to be no more accurate than a well-performed Gram stain. The cause of pneumococcal, meningococcal, and *H. influenzae* meningitis may be determined by counterimmunoelectrophoresis. However, this technique requires potent antisera for accurate results.

The number of cells in the cerebrospinal fluid is always elevated and varies between 100 and 100,000 per cubic millimeter. Initially, polymorphonuclear leukocytes predominate; these are replaced by lymphocytes as the inflammatory process progresses. Early in the infection one may find a plethora of bacteria with only a few cells. This is particularly true in pneumococcal and staphylococcal infections.

A low cerebrospinal fluid sugar is the hallmark of bacterial meningitis, and distinguishes it from the viral meningitides. Usually the value is below 40 mg per 100 ml and may be close to 0. Patients who have diabetes mellitus or who are receiving intravenous infusions of glucose may have falsely high glucose values. However, the ratio of blood to cerebrospinal fluid sugar in these patients is always higher than the normal value of 1.5 to 1. For example, a cerebrospinal fluid sugar of 150 mg per 100 ml in the presence of a blood sugar of 500 mg per 100 ml is highly significant. The information obtained from blood sugar, which should be obtained routinely at the time of initial lumbar puncture, is frequently critical.

The protein content of the cerebrospinal fluid is generally elevated and may be as high as 800 mg per 100 ml. Higher values are usually obtained in pneumococcal meningitis than in infections with other pathogens. The development of subarachnoid block is usually heralded by very high CSF protein values (800 to 1500 mg per 100 ml).

Other Cultures. Blood cultures should be obtained routinely in patients suspected of having meningitis; they are positive in approximately 50 per cent of cases. Occasionally, when the cerebrospinal fluid cultures are negative, the blood cultures may provide the only clue to the etiologic agent. Nose, throat, and ear cultures may not reflect the meningeal pathogen and are misleading too often to be of more than ancillary value in diagnosis.

Roentgenographic Studies. All patients with meningitis should have roentgenograms of the chest, skull, mastoid, and paranasal sinuses as soon as their condition permits. Frequently these provide the clue to the portal of entry of the pathogen. Eradication of these foci with antimicrobial therapy or surgical drainage may be essential for control of the meningeal infection. When a mass lesion is suspected, brain scan and arteriography should be performed.

Other Laboratory Tests. Most patients with meningitis are sufficiently ill to warrant determination of blood urea nitrogen and serum electrolytes, particularly because water intoxication and severe hyponatremia are not uncommon. Blood sugar should be determined routinely (best in conjunction with determination of the cerebrospinal fluid sugar). Lactic dehydrogenase and its isozymes are elevated in bacterial meningitis. Most of this increase is due to a rise in fractions representing leukocytes, but a rise in LDH isozyme fractions emanating from brain occurs only in patients who die or who are destined to develop neurologic sequelae.

Prognosis. Untreated meningitis is almost always fatal. Antimicrobial therapy has dramatically improved the outlook for patients with meningeal infections. However, except for recurrent pneumococcal meningitis in which the prognosis is remarkably good, the mortality in adequately treated pneumococcal meningitis remains between 10 and 70 per cent, and 50 per cent of infections with staphylococci and gram-negative enteric bacilli are lethal. On the other hand, the mortality rate associated with meningococcal and *H. influenzae* meningitis is less than 10 per cent. In addition to the difference in prognosis engendered by different microorganisms, factors that adversely influence outcome include (1) improper or delayed diagnosis, usually a consequence of falsely attributing confusion or delirium to "toxemic" depression of the central nervous system or hepatic encephalopathy; (2) fulminating infection with rapid loss of consciousness; (3) bacteremia; (4) old age or the neonatal period; (5) certain underlying and complicating illnesses, including bacterial endocarditis, brain abscess, diabetes mellitus, and pneumonia; and (6) development of coma, localizing neurologic signs, and convulsions.

Treatment. *Choice of Therapy.* Antimicrobials are the mainstay of therapy in bacterial meningitis and should be administered parenterally at the earliest possible moment. If the Gram stain of the cerebrospinal fluid reveals the causative microorganism, specific treatment may be instituted from the beginning. However, if microscopy of the stained smear has been inconclusive, the initial therapy must be sufficiently broad to be fully effective against the most reasonable possibilities. For example, purulent meningitis in an adult without evidence of an overt portal of entry is most apt to be pneumococcal or meningococcal; in a young child, *H. influenzae* must also be considered. Primary staphylococcal meningitis would be rare in a previously healthy adult, but should be considered in a long-hospitalized patient, particularly if neurosurgery has been performed.

Penicillin is the drug of choice for pneumococcal and meningococcal meningitis, and should be administered parenterally in a dosage of 10 to 20 million units a day. For patients who are sensitive to penicillin, chloramphenicol in dosage of 4.0 to 6.0 grams per day should be used. The cephalosporins enter even the inflamed meninges poorly and should not be used for the treatment of meningitis.

There is still considerable debate whether *H. influenzae* meningitis should be treated with chloramphenicol (4.0 to 6.0 grams a day) or ampicillin (6.0 to 12.0 grams a day). Both drugs are probably equally effective, but ampicillin has the additional advantage of being bactericidal for pneumococci and meningococci. Use of this agent should, for all practical purposes, eliminate multiple drug therapy in "undiagnosed meningitis." A few "ampicillin failures" have been reported in children with *H. influenzae* meningitis. These were probably related to inadequate dosage or poor absorption of the drug, although a few resistant strains of *H. influenzae* have been reported. Staphylococcal meningitis should always be treated with one of the penicillinase-resistant penicillins, e.g., methicillin, oxacillin, or nafcillin in dosage of 6.0 to 12.0 grams parenterally. For the rare cases of meningitis caused by the Enterobacteriaceae or Pseudomonas, gentamicin in dosage of 5 mg per kilogram parenterally plus 4 to 8 mg intrathecally is the regimen of choice.

In patients with mastoiditis, an infected ventriculomastoid shunt, or cranial osteomyelitis, surgical attack on these primary foci while the patient is receiving appropriate antimicrobial therapy is indicated, but may be postponed until the acute meningeal episode is over.

Duration of Therapy. The duration of antimicrobial therapy in meningitis cannot be prescribed categorically. The cerebrospinal fluid should be examined every 24 to 48 hours during the early days of therapy, but once the patient is recovering, the intervals between lumbar puncture may be as long as a week, and numerous examinations of the CSF are rarely necessary. In the absence of extrameningeal foci, a seven- to ten-day course of antimicrobial therapy should suffice.

Other Measures. If there is evidence of increased intracranial pressure, and supratentorial or cerebellar herniation, therapy with mannitol, urea, or dexamethasone should be instituted. Adrenal cortical hormones also have been used as an adjunct to antimicrobial therapy, but have not resulted in noteworthy improvement. They should never be used unless the etiologic organism has been clearly identified and the appropriate drug is being administered. There have been some enthusiastic reports about proteolytic enzymes in the treatment of pneumococcal meningitis, but these agents have not been evaluated in sufficient detail to recommend their general use.

Other supportive therapy includes administration of adequate but not excessive parenteral fluids and anticonvulsants when indicated. Sedation should be employed with caution, even for delirious patients; of the many agents available, paraldehyde continues to be safe and effective.

Barrett, F. F., Taber, L. H., Morris, C. R., Stephenson, W. B., Clark, D. J., and Yow, M. D.: A 12 year review of the antibiotic management of *Hemophilus influenzae* meningitis. J. Pediatr., 81:370, 1972.

Beaty, H. N., and Oppenheimer, S.: CSF lactic dehydrogenase and its isoenzymes in infections of the central nervous sytem. N. Engl. J. Med., 279:1197, 1968.

Carpenter, R. R., and Petersdorf, R. G.: The clinical spectrum of bacterial meningitis. Am. J. Med., 23:262, 1962.

Coonrod, D. J., and Rytel, M. W.: Determination of aetiology of bacterial meningitis by counterimmunoelectrophoresis. Lancet, 1:1154, 1972.

Hand, W. L., and Sanford, J. P.: Post-traumatic bacterial meningitis. Ann. Intern. Med., 72:869, 1970.

Harter, D. H., and Petersdorf, R. G.: A consideration of the pathogenesis of bacterial meningitis: Review of experimental and clinical studies. Yale J. Biol. Med., 32:280, 1960.

Mangi, R. J., Kundargi, R. S., Quintiliani, R., and Andriole, V. T.: Development of meningitis during cephalothin therapy. Ann. Intern. Med., 78:347, 1973.

Oppenheimer, S. J., O'Toole, R. D., and Petersdorf, R. G.: Bacterial meningitis: *In* Shy, G. M., Goldensohn, E. S., and Appel, S. H. (eds.): The Cellular and Molecular Basis of Neurological Disease. Philadelphia, Lea & Febiger (in press).

Rahal, J. J.: Treatment of gram-negative bacillary meningitis in adults. Ann. Intern. Med., 77:295, 1972.

Rapaport, S. I.: Defibrination syndromes. *In* Williams, W. E., Beutler, E.,

Erslev, A. J., and Rundles, R. W. (eds.): Hematology. New York, McGraw-Hill Book Company, 1972.

Snyder, S. N., and Brunjes, S.: *H. influenzae* meningitis in adults. Am. J. Med. Sci., 250:658, 1965.

Swartz, M. N., and Dodge, P. R.: Bacterial meningitis—a review of selected aspects. N. Engl. J. Med., 272:725, 779, 842, 898, 954, 1003, 1965.

202. HEMOPHILUS INFLUENZAE INFECTIONS

Walsh McDermott

Although principally a pathogen for young children, *H. influenzae* may occasionally cause serious disease in the adult. In addition, the microbe is frequently present as a secondary "invader" in chronic obstructive lung disease and has played a similar role in the past in epidemics of presumed viral influenza. Virtually all severe primary infections are caused by serotype b, although other types may be present in the secondary "invader" role. The microbe is recognized as the most frequent cause of purulent meningitis in children; it is also the cause of a form of croup known as *obstructive laryngitis with epiglottitis*. Both conditions are quite serious. The *meningitis* is described in Ch. 201. The *laryngitis/epiglottitis* presents quite a characteristic picture. The onset is sudden and the course fulminating. Mild fever and dysphagia develop during an apparently innocuous respiratory infection. Dyspnea starts abruptly, and laryngeal obstruction requiring tracheotomy develops. High fever develops along with laryngeal redness and edema, and when the tongue is pressed downward, the enlarged, distorted, red, and edematous epiglottis is easily seen.

The diagnosis of an *H. influenzae* infection can be made rapidly by microscopy of Gram-stained smear or the demonstration of capsular swelling (quellung) of bacterial cells found in the appropriate biologic fluid. For initial culture, chocolate agar incubated in a candle jar may be used. Further cultural studies may be necessary of autoclaved blood agar, or yeast agar extract.

Therapy of the laryngitis/epiglottitis in children should be prompt and should include tracheostomy and appropriate antimicrobial therapy. Treatment of the meningitis is discussed in Ch. 201. Ampicillin, tetracycline, and chloramphenicol are all effective agents. As it has not been possible to demonstrate the superiority of any one drug in clinical trials (Nelson et al., 1972; Barrett et al., 1972), it seems advisable to use ampicillin.

Another disease caused by Hemophilus is *chancroid*, which is a localized venereal disease caused by *H. ducreyi*. It is characterized by painful, nonindurated ulceration involving the genitalia, accompanied by enlargement and suppuration of regional lymph nodes. Early syphilis often occurs simultaneously with chancroid. Tetracycline and erythromycin are both quite active against *H. ducreyi;* they have the disadvantage that conceivably they could mask a concurrent initial syphilis. Careful attention must be paid to the possibility of syphilis; otherwise, sulfadiazine should be used in the treatment of chancroid.

H. parainfluenzae, another member of the Hemophilus species, is an occasional cause of bacterial endocarditis.

Nelson, K. E., Levin, S., Spies, H. W., and Lepper, M. H.: Treatment of *Hemophilus influenzae* meningitis: A comparison of chloramphenicol and tetracycline. J. Infect. Dis., 125:459, 1972.

203. WHOOPING COUGH (Pertussis)

Stephen I. Morse

Definition. Whooping cough is an acute respiratory illness that classically affects infants and young children. The etiologic agent is usually *Bordetella pertussis;* occasionally *B. parapertussis* and rarely *B. bronchiseptica* produce a similar syndrome. The descriptive name derives from a distressing, prolonged inspiratory effort that follows paroxysmal coughing. Whooping cough is still responsible for a significant number of deaths in infants in areas where pertussis immunization is not practiced.

History. The disease was first recorded in the middle of the sixteenth century by Moulton and by DeBaillou. Whether whooping cough was indigenous to Europe or had been transported there in the preceding century is uncertain. Sydenham applied the name "pertussis" to any illness accompanied by violent coughing, but the term became restricted to the epidemic disease that was a well-recognized clinical entity by the middle of the eighteenth century. In 1900 Bordet and Gengou observed coccobacilli in the sputum of a child with whooping cough, but it was not until 1906 that they were able to culture the organism. Many years passed before the Bordet-Gengou bacillus was universally accepted as the etiologic agent of whooping cough. *B. pertussis* undergoes marked biologic and morphologic changes on prolonged cultivation, thereby accounting for the difficulties in establishing the etiologic role of the agent and the inconstant protective effect of immunizing preparations. Although the mortality rate of whooping cough in the United States began to decline in the early part of this century, the incidence in young children did not significantly decrease until after the use of prophylactic vaccines became widespread.

Etiology. When first isolated, *Bordetella pertussis* is a minute, nonmotile, weakly staining, gram-negative coccobacillus, 0.5 to 1.0 μ in length. Capsules can be demonstrated by special procedures, and bipolar metachromatic granules are present. The complex medium containing blood originally employed by Bordet and Gengou is still often used for cultivation. Primary isolates, phase I organisms, will not grow on conventional laboratory media, but will do so after prolonged passage. At the same time colonial morphology changes, marked pleomorphism of individual cells is evident, and there is an alteration in antigenic composition. The change from phase I to phase IV has been likened to the smooth to rough transition of other microbes. Only phase I organisms are virulent, and only phase I organisms provide effective immunizing material.

Members of the Bordetella genus were formerly regarded as species of Hemophilus. However, the Bordetella group does not have the strict requirement for X and V growth factors, and they are antigenically distinct. The addition of blood to Bordet-Gengou medium is required for the growth of phase I organisms, but the blood acts to neutralize bactericidal substances, probably fatty acids, rather than to provide nutrients. Charcoal, starch, or ion exchange resins can be substituted for blood.

B. pertussis produces a heat-stable toxin (endotoxin) and a heat-labile toxin. A role of toxins in the development of disease has not been demonstrated. A hemagglutinin has also been isolated. The capsular material does not swell in the presence of antiserum. A species agglutinogen has been recognized as well as agglutinating factors that differ between strains. Serotyping is therefore a useful epidemiologic tool. The role of the interaction between the organism and phagocytes has not been defined, although the presence of antisera appears to increase uptake of *B. pertussis* by leukocytes.

Remarkable biologic effects are induced in laboratory animals by the injection of killed phase I organisms. These include development of heightened sensitivity to histamine and serotonin; increased susceptibility to anaphylaxis and to experimental allergic encephalomyelitis; increased antibody production, including reaginic antibody, in response to heterologous antigens; and hyperleukocytosis and hyperlymphocytosis. The factors responsible for these reactions have not been characterized fully.

It should be emphasized that none of the cellular components or products of *B. pertussis* has been shown to be of central importance in the pathogenesis of whooping cough.

Approximately 5 to 10 per cent of clinical whooping cough is caused by *B. parapertussis*. The animal pathogen *B. bronchiseptica* is responsible for a very minor percentage of cases. These organisms can be differentiated from *B. pertussis* by appropriate further bacteriologic or serologic procedures. It has recently been suggested that adenoviruses, alone or in concert with *B. pertussis,* may play an etiologic role in some cases of whooping cough.

Incidence and Epidemiology. In communities of susceptibles the family attack rate is 80 to 90 per cent, which is extremely high for a bacterial disease, approaching that seen in varicella or measles. Transmission is by droplet infection. Carriers of *B. pertussis* are found infrequently, and the reservoir is therefore unknown. Disease usually occurs in late winter in the northern climates and in late spring in southern zones, but there is great variation.

The mortality rate from whooping cough has fallen since the turn of this century owing to improved supportive therapy. The incidence of whooping cough, however, did not change until after the 1940's, when immunization of young children became standard practice. In the five-year periods 1926–1930, 1936–1940, 1956–1960, and 1965–1969, the fatality rate per thousand cases in the United States was 39.1, 19.4, 6.8, and 5.9, respectively. In the same time frames, the number of reported cases was 909,705; 956,262; 146,989; and 32,329, respectively. The majority of deaths, over 70 per cent, occur in children under one year of age, with the preponderance in infants under the age of six months.

Neither immunization against pertussis nor natural disease provides lifelong protection. In the case of artificial immunization, an attack rate greater than 50 per cent has been reported when the interval after immunization exceeds 12 years, a rate no different from that in unimmunized individuals of the same age. Thus in the face of routine immunization, it is possible that pertussis will become primarily a disease of older children and adults.

Pathology. Interpretation of pathologic material obtained at autopsy is difficult because of the common presence of complicating respiratory infections. Lesions caused by *B. pertussis* are found principally in the bronchi and bronchioles, but changes are also seen in the nasopharynx, larynx, and trachea. Masses of bacteria are intertwined with the cilia of the columnar epithelium together with mucopurulent exudate. There is also necrosis of the midzonal and basilar epithelium with infiltration of polymorphonuclear leukocytes and macrophages. Peribronchial accumulation of lymphocytes and granulocytes produces the picture of interstitial pneumonitis. Secondary atelectasis and localized emphysema are common. The alveoli in uncomplicated whooping cough do not contain exudate.

Clinical Manifestations. After an incubation period of 7 to 16 days, symptoms appear. It is customary to divide the clinical course into three stages, each of two weeks' duration, but variation is frequent, particularly in the immunized community.

Catarrhal Stage. Whooping cough begins with symptoms indistinguishable from those of a mild viral upper respiratory infection or common cold. Sneezing is frequent, the conjunctivae are injected, and a nocturnal cough appears. The temperature may be slightly elevated at this time. Infectivity is greatest during the catarrhal stage.

Paroxysmal Stage. Seven to 14 days after onset, the cough becomes more frequent, diurnal, and then paroxysmal. In a typical paroxysm there is a series of 15 to 20 short coughs of increasing intensity, and then with a deep inspiration the air is drawn into the lungs, making the "whoop." A tenacious mucus plug is usually expelled, and vomiting frequently follows the spasmodic episode. Paroxysms may occur as often as every half hour, and are accompanied by signs of increased venous pressure. The conjunctivae are deeply engorged; there is periorbital edema; and petechial hemorrhages, particularly about the forehead, as well as epistaxis are common. During the attack the infant may be cyanotic until the crowing whoop occurs. In between paroxysms the child usually feels well though justifiably apprehensive.

Physical examination of the chest is usually unremarkable, although scattered rhonchi may be heard. The chest roentgenogram sometimes reveals hilar and mediastinal nodal enlargement. The presence of fever immediately suggests the development of a secondary infectious process.

Convalescent Stage. Gradually the paroxysms become less frequent and less intense, vomiting ceases, and slow recovery ensues. Often for many months even a mild, unrelated respiratory infection will be manifested by a return of paroxysmal cough and whoop.

It is important to recognize those patients with whooping cough in whom variation from the pattern frequently occurs. In young infants the paroxysms and the whoop are often absent; instead, choking spells and apneic periods may be the major manifestations. Second attacks of whooping cough as well as disease occurring in previously immunized individuals often present simply as an upper respiratory illness or bronchitis.

Complications. Complications may be related to the primary disease or to secondary events. Alterations in acid-base balance occur as a result of metabolic alkalosis when vomiting is severe. Recurrent vomiting can also lead to malnutrition. Anoxemic manifestations are seen when ventilation is markedly impaired. Central nervous system changes can result from cerebral anoxia or hemorrhages consequent to the elevated venous pressure. Rarely, cortical degeneration occurs, but the exact pathogenesis of the encephalopathy is unknown. A serous meningitis with lymphocytosis of the cerebrospinal fluid has been described. Localized areas of emphysema and atelectasis generally return to normal after the disease has run its course, and pneumothorax and interstitial emphysema are infrequently seen.

The major cause of death in whooping cough is complicating pneumonia or bronchopneumonia caused by other bacteria or viruses. In addition, secondary bacterial otitis media occurs frequently.

Diagnosis. There is little difficulty in making the clinical diagnosis of whooping cough in a patient who, after a variable period of coryzal symptoms, develops paroxysmal coughing with a terminal inspiratory whoop. Toward the end of the catarrhal stage, or early in the spasmodic phase, leukocytosis often occurs. In contrast to the leukocytosis found in most bacterial diseases, the predominating cell type is the mature small lymphocyte. Characteristically the leukocyte count ranges from 15,000 to 30,000 per cubic millimeter, and 80 per cent of the cells are small lymphocytes. However, the leukocyte count either may be normal or may reach a level greater than 100,000 per cubic millimeter. Polymorphonuclear leukocytosis suggests a secondary bacterial complication.

Difficulty in recognizing whooping cough occurs in the catarrhal stage, in abortive or mild cases, and in young infants. Epidemiologic awareness may suggest the possibility, but microbiologic identification of the organisms is required. During the early stages of whooping cough *B. pertussis* can be isolated from approximately 90 per cent of patients. By the third or fourth week of illness the organism can be recovered in only 50 per cent of cases, and in the convalescent stage it is unusual to obtain a positive culture.

Adequate specimens and appropriate media are essential if bacteriologic diagnosis is to be efficient. *Specimens are best obtained by pernasal swab rather than by the cough plate method.* A sterile cotton swab wrapped about a flexible copper wire is passed through the nares, and mucus is obtained from the posterior pharynx. The swab must not be allowed to dry out because *B. pertussis* is readily killed by desiccation. As quickly as possible the specimen is plated onto fresh Bordet-Gengou medium, to which penicillin has been added to prevent overgrowth of adventitious organisms. Incubation is at 35° C, and although the trained observer can recognize the small, bisected pearl colonies of *B. pertussis* within 48 hours, at least 72 hours of growth is usually required. Presumptive identification can be made by agglutination tests with appropriate antisera. It is virtually impossible to distinguish between Bordetella species on primary isolation except by serologic means.

A fluorescent antibody staining procedure that can be applied directly to clinical specimens as well as to organisms grown in culture is now in more general use.

Serologic procedures are of little help in the diagnosis of whooping cough because a rise in titer of most antibodies does not occur until at least the third week of illness.

It is difficult to distinguish abortive or mild cases of pertussis from tracheobronchitis caused by other agents except by bacteriologic means. On the other hand, paroxysmal coughing may be associated with pulmonary lesions such as allergic bronchitis, atypical pneumonia, or cystic fibrosis.

Treatment. Mild cases of pertussis require only supportive treatment. Specific therapy of severe whooping cough has been disappointing despite the in vitro susceptibility of *B. pertussis* to various antimicrobial agents and the protective effect of passively administered antibody in experimental disease.

Antimicrobials. A number of antimicrobial drugs have significant in vitro activity against *B. pertussis*. Agents that readily eradicate the organisms in human disease may shorten the course of the illness if given in the catarrhal or early paroxysmal stages. In the established paroxysmal stage the organisms can also be readily eliminated by antimicrobials, but the course of the illness is unaltered. Even in the paroxysmal stage the use of drugs is justified in order to render the patient noninfectious.

Erythromycin, oxytetracycline, and chloramphenicol are more effective in eliminating organisms than ampicillin. On the basis of drug safety and efficacy either erythromycin or tetracycline is the drug of choice. The daily dose for each is 50 mg per kilogram of body weight given in four divided doses. The organism is eliminated after a few days of therapy, but because bacteriologic relapse may occur, treatment should be continued for ten to fourteen days.

Immunotherapy. Hyperimmune human gamma globulin is often used in therapy of unimmunized patients, particularly small infants. The usual dose is 1.25 or 2.5 ml intramuscularly for three successive days.

Supportive Therapy. Particularly in the young infant, supportive measures combined with careful nursing care are of paramount importance. Specific attention must be devoted to the maintenance of proper water and electrolyte balance, adequate nutrition, and sufficient oxygenation. Constant alertness for the presence of secondary infectious complications such as pneumonia is required, and appropriate therapy should be promptly instituted upon discovery.

Prevention. The great communicability of whooping cough, particularly during the first few weeks of illness, makes it desirable to isolate the patient for four to six weeks, or, ideally, until cultures are negative. Unfortunately, the diagnosis is usually not made until the end of the catarrhal stage, and by then spread of the disease has already occurred. Exposed susceptibles should be isolated from social groups until it is determined whether disease is present. Unimmunized contacts, especially infants, should receive 2 to 4 ml of hyperimmune gamma globulin intramuscularly, the dose to be repeated in five days. Those young children who have not received a booster dose of vaccine in more than a year should receive an injection upon exposure.

Recent studies have suggested that erythromycin may be effective in prophylaxis against pertussis in exposed, susceptible persons.

Active Immunization. The fall in incidence of whooping cough in the very young is directly related to widespread immunization with suitable, killed suspensions of *B. pertussis*. The highest risk of serious morbidity and mortality is in the young infant. Women of childbearing age generally do not have significant levels of protective antibody in their sera, and consequently the newborn are not protected by maternal antibodies. Therefore active immunization is begun as early as is commensurate with the production of a satisfactory immune response. At present, it is recommended that the infant receive three injections of pertussis vaccine at one-month intervals beginning at 6 to 12 weeks of age. Each injection provides four NIH* units. The NIH unitage is based upon the ability of a vaccine to protect mice against a standard intracerebral infection. The pertussis suspension is usually incorporated into a triple vaccine with alum-precipitated diphtheria and tetanus toxoids (DPT). Booster injections are given one, three, and five years after completion of the initial course. Administration of pertussis vaccine to those over six years of age is not generally recommended because of an apparent in-

creased incidence of untoward reactions. However, low doses have been administered to adults without incident. There is no protection against parapertussis.

As previously noted, immunization does not confer lifelong protection. Approximately 80 per cent of those vaccinated within four years of exposure will be protected, whereas 80 to 90 per cent of a matched unimmunized group with similar exposure will contract pertussis. However, as the time after immunization increases, the attack rate in both groups approaches 50 per cent.

Instances of "vaccine failure" have usually been shown to be due to the use of preparations of low potency. However, it has recently been suggested that a change in the dominant serotype causing disease, unrepresented in certain vaccine preparations, may be of importance. This controversial point is under study.

Local reactions as well as fever may occur after injection of pertussis vaccine. The exact incidence of the more severe complication of encephalopathy is uncertain, but both fatalities and residua have been reported. The occurrence of neurotoxicity appears to be decreasing as more refined immunizing suspensions are used, and certain soluble extracts of *B. pertussis* may prove to be effective without engendering serious side effects. Despite the small, but real, incidence of neurologic complications of pertussis immunization, the risk still seems far less than the hazards of whooping cough in the young child. Nevertheless, in infants with a personal or family history of convulsions or other neurologic disorders, pertussis immunization should be deferred, or very small doses should be cautiously administered. Care should also be exercised in the immunization of children with a family history of an allergic diathesis.

Klenk, E. L., Gaultney, J. V., and Bass, J. W.: Bacteriologically proved pertussis and adenovirus infection. Am. J. Dis. Child., 124:203, 1972.
Kurt, T. L., Yeager, A. S., Guenette, S., and Dunlop, S.: Spread of pertussis by hospital staff. J.A.M.A., 221:264, 1972.
Morse, S. I.: The Hemophilus-Bordetella group. *In* Davis, B. D., Dulbecco, R., Eisen, H. N., Ginsberg, H. S., and Wood, W. B., Jr. (eds.): Microbiology. 2nd ed. Hagerstown, Md., Harper & Row, 1973.
Pittman, M.: *Bordetella pertussis*—bacterial and host factors in the pathogenesis and prevention of whooping cough. *In* Mudd, S. (ed.): Infectious Agents and Host Reactions. Philadelphia, W. B. Saunders Company, 1970.
Preston, N. W., and Stanbridge, T. N.: Efficacy of pertussis vaccines: A brighter horizon. Br. Med. J., 3:448, 1972.

204. GRANULOMA INGUINALE

Walsh McDermott

Granuloma inguinale is an indolent granulomatous and ulcerative disease usually localized to the genitalia and caused by a pleomorphic coccobacillus, *Donovania granulomatis*, the so-called "Donovan body." When grown on artificial medium, the organism develops a large capsule that reacts immunologically with klebsiella capsular material. *Donovania granulomatis* also resembles *K. pneumoniae* in morphology. Presumably, the infection is customarily transmitted during coitus or other close bodily contact, and the degree of communicability appears to be relatively low. The lesion tends to be

*National Institutes of Health.

single, and may rarely appear on surfaces of the body other than the genitalia. Systemic infection, notably with the production of arthritis or osteomyelitis, has been reported. Usually, the lesion appears on the genitalia or in the perianal area as a relatively painless nodular infiltration that soon breaks down, leaving a sharply demarcated ulcer with friable granulation tissue at the base. On histologic examination, the lesion appears well vascularized and is the site of considerable cellular infiltration, especially with polymorphonuclear leukocytes and monocytes. In appropriately stained tissue scrapings, the causative microbe, *Donovania granulomatis*, may be seen situated principally within the monocytes, although smaller numbers of extracellular microorganisms can usually be identified. The lesion spreads by direct extension, it is highly destructive to the skin and subcutaneous tissue, and secondary infection with other microorganisms is common. Rarely, if sufficiently extensive, the process may cause elephantiasis of the genitalia.

There is nothing particularly characteristic about the lesions of granuloma inguinale, and the early lesion is indistinguishable from those produced by *T. pallidum, H. ducreyi*, or other processes that involve the genitalia. The diagnosis can be established only by appropriate microbiologic techniques, and these should be employed whenever the physician encounters a genital lesion (or an indolent ulceration elsewhere) that is not clearly caused by some other process. Microscopy of deep scrapings or impression smears from the lesion of granuloma inguinale stained by the Wright method usually reveals *Donovania granulomatis* within the monocytes. The ease with which the microorganisms can be detected varies to some extent with the age of the lesion. In a relatively old lesion, the scrapings should be made from the depth of the lesion, and an extensive search of the smears may be necessary. The microorganisms can also be cultured in medium containing chick embryo yolk by methods originally developed by Anderson and her associates. Antigen prepared from capsular material of *D. granulomatis* has been employed in a complement-fixation reaction and in a cutaneous reaction, but these have not yet been developed to the point of general application.

Granuloma inguinale has been successfully treated with streptomycin and the tetracyclines. As initial therapy, tetracycline should be employed in a total daily dosage of 2.0 grams administered by mouth in divided doses for a two-week period. In unusually extensive lesions it may be necessary to continue the treatment for a longer period in order to attain complete healing. If relapse occurs or the lesions appear refractory to tetracycline treatment, streptomycin should be administered intramuscularly in a total daily dosage of 2.0 grams in divided doses for a two-week period.

No detailed studies are available concerning the prevention of granuloma inguinale. It seems likely, however, that thorough washing of the genitals with soap and water immediately after sexual intercourse has a significant influence in reducing the probability of infection.

Anderson, K., Goodpasture, E. W., and DeMonbreun, W. A.: Immunologic relationship of *Donovania granulomatis* to granuloma inguinale. J. Exp. Med., 81:41, 1945.
Davis, B. D., Dulbecco, R., Eisen, H. N., Ginsberg, H. S., and Wood, W. B., Jr.: Microbiology. New York, Hoeber Medical Division, Harper & Row, 1970, Chap. 36.
Sheldon, W. H., Thebaut, B. R., Heyman, A., and Wall, M. J.: Osteomyelitis caused by granuloma inguinale. Am. J. Med. Sci., 210:237, 1945.

205. DIPHTHERIA

Heonir Rocha

Diphtheria is an acute infectious disease caused by a bacillus, *Corynebacterium diphtheriae*. The infection usually localizes in the pharynx, larynx, and nostrils and occasionally in the skin, and gives rise to both local and systemic signs. The latter are related to the production of a potent soluble exotoxin elaborated by the microorganisms multiplying at the site of infection.

Etiology. *Corynebacterium diphtheriae* is a gram-positive, nonsporulating, nonmotile pleomorphic bacillus, which grows best aerobically and does not form gas. In stained smears diphtheria bacilli are frequently club shaped in appearance and are arranged in palisade form. The most common media used to isolate the bacilli are Löffler's and potassium tellurite agar. By the appearance on tellurite agar and the ability to ferment starch and glycogen, three distinct types of colonies can be identified: *gravis, mitis,* and *intermedius*. All three types can produce the same powerful toxin, which is a complex protein, with a molecular weight of 64,000, produced by bacterial cells infected with a lysogenic bacteriophage. In so-called avirulent diphtheria strains no parasitism with bacteriophages can be demonstrated, and the bacilli fail to produce toxin. The amount of toxin produced depends on genetic and nutritional factors. The ability to produce toxin under laboratory conditions is not entirely related to potential for causing severe disease, because several virulent strains are poor toxin formers.

It is usually said that the *gravis* strain is more frequently associated with epidemic diphtheria; also, that the case fatality rate associated with any epidemic is determined by the proportion of cases infected with the *gravis* or *mitis* types. However, these views are not generally accepted. Although there seems to be a trend toward more severe infection with the *gravis* and *mitis* types, without question the same clinical picture can be produced by all three types.

Epidemiology and Immunity. Diphtheria has a worldwide distribution, its natural incidence being greatest in temperate climates. The disease occurs predominantly in poor socioeconomic conditions where inadequately immunized hosts and crowding are common. It exhibits a tendency to be most prevalent in autumn and winter but can give rise to epidemics at any time of year.

The human host is the only significant reservoir of *Corynebacterium diphtheriae,* which is transmitted directly or indirectly from one person to another. The usual habitat of *Corynebacterium diphtheriae* is the respiratory tract. The organism can multiply in the mucous membranes of the respiratory tract (pharynx or nares) of immunized hosts without giving rise to clinical disease. The transmission of diphtheria is mainly via droplets, although fomites and dust may have a minor role. Milk has been shown to be a vehicle of infection in rare instances. Duration and closeness of contact are the important factors in transmission. In some tropical areas the skin has been implicated as a major reservoir of *Corynebacterium diphtheriae* infection.

Immunity against the disease depends basically upon the existence of antitoxin in the blood of the host, which is formed in response to direct stimulation of diphtheria toxin either by artificial immunization or by clinical or subclinical infection. Infants under the age of six months are normally protected by passive immunity received through the placenta from immune mothers. Adults are usually protected by artificial immunization or subclinical infection. It has been suggested that cutaneous diphtheria may be the main method whereby natural immunization is acquired in tropical countries.

A relatively simple way to gain valuable information concerning a patient's immune status is obtained by observing the reaction after the intradermal injection of 0.1 ml of diluted, highly purified diphtheria toxin (Schick test). A positive reaction is interpreted to mean that the patient is susceptible to the disease; a negative reaction indicates that the levels of antitoxin exceed 0.03 unit per milliliter and that the host is not likely to acquire the clinical disease.

The maximal age incidence of diphtheria lies in the period of two to six years. The disease is an unusual occurrence in adults in endemic areas. However, recently in the United States, approximately 25 per cent of the cases occurred in persons 15 years of age or older.

Pathogenesis. The most serious consequences of *Corynebacterium diphtheriae* infection are the result of production and absorption of an extremely active and damaging exotoxin. The organisms multiply on epithelial cells at the infected site (usually pharynx), secreting the specific toxin which produces local signs and is absorbed, producing a systemic illness. The initial cytotoxic effect of the toxin is in tissues immediately adjacent to the bacterial growth, resulting in necrotic changes. As a consequence, an exudate which tends to coalesce is formed during the initial 24 to 48 hours. This fibrinous exudate contains leukocytes, necrotic epithelial cells, red blood cells, and the growing diphtheria bacillus. The exudate forms a tough membrane (so-called pseudomembrane) which is firmly attached, with a white shiny center and a gray or brownish periphery. If this membrane is forcibly removed, bleeding occurs. Occasionally it extends throughout the tracheobronchial tree, forming a cast. Edema of soft tissues subjacent to the membrane may be intense. These local lesions when present in the larynx can result in encroachment of the airway with varying degrees of respiratory obstruction.

From the local site of production the soluble toxin is disseminated by the blood and lymphatics and can produce degenerative changes in the heart, nervous system, and kidneys. The diphtheria toxin is regularly lethal to the affected cells. It becomes adsorbed to the cell membrane, penetrates into the cell, and alters the protein synthesis by interfering with the transfer of amino acids from RNA to the growing polypeptide chain. As a result, the cell degenerates and dies. Specific antitoxin may neutralize even adsorbed toxin, but does not prevent the chain of events once the toxin penetrates the cell.

Diphtheria infection may be localized infrequently in wounds, buccal mucosa, vagina, and conjunctiva. These extrarespiratory locations usually give rise to milder disease with much less systemic illness.

Clinical Manifestations. The incubation period of diphtheria varies from one to seven days, but is most commonly two to four days. *The clinical picture* depends upon the anatomic location of the lesions and the severity of the toxic process. The most common localization of infection is the oropharynx.

Faucial diphtheria is the most common clinical form and includes the most toxic forms. In a typical case the onset is usually sudden, with low-grade fever (37 to 38° C), malaise, and mild sore throat. The pharynx is only moderately injected, and a thick tonsillar exudate is frequently seen. This exudate usually spreads from one tonsil to the other and may invade the pillars, uvula, and soft palate. Moderate tonsillar as well as cervical lymph node enlargement is usually present.

In some cases the membrane or exudate is limited to the tonsils *(tonsillar diphtheria),* and toxic manifestations are inconspicuous. In other cases, there is spread of the original process to the uvula, posterior pharyngeal wall, and posterior nasal mucosa *(nasopharyngeal diphtheria),* sometimes with massive cervical lymphadenopathy (bullneck appearance) and signs of toxemia. In this clinical form the child is pale, lethargic, prostrated, restless at times, and extremely weak. The pulse is rapid and thin; heart beats become muffled; respiration is labored and frequently noisy. This state of toxemia may result in death within a few days if the condition remains untreated. Finally, in some patients the infection spreads downward to the larynx, producing a clinical picture of progressive laryngeal obstruction *(laryngeal diphtheria).* When the larynx is involved, the first symptoms are hoarseness, dyspnea, a brassy cough, and an increasing expiratory and inspiratory stridor. In a few instances laryngeal involvement may be the first sign of infection.

As the obstruction progresses, dyspnea becomes more severe, bronchial secretions accumulate, the accessory muscles of respiration come into full play, and there are supra- and infrasternal retraction at each stridulous breath. If obstruction is not relieved, the patient becomes extremely restless, anxious, and cyanotic, and the condition then merges into severe exhaustion and a comatose stage.

In some cases the infection is basically localized in the anterior nasal area *(anterior nasal diphtheria).* Clinically it is manifested by bilateral serous or serosanguineous discharge which causes crusted lesions on the upper lip. Small rounded ulcers, some of them covered with a whitish exudate, are usually seen in the anterior part of the nasal septum. Constitutional symptoms are lacking, and this process is chiefly important because of its epidemiologic implications. It is frequently undiagnosed in an endemic area, and may be an important source of spreading the disease.

Other parts of the body may be the site of primary or secondary diphtheric lesions, the most commonly described being the skin. *Cutaneous diphtheria* takes the form of chronic nonhealing ulcers, sometimes covered with a grayish membranous exudate. It seems probable that these ulcers, mainly described in the tropics, have a complex etiology. Treatment with antitoxin alone usually gives disappointing results. Involvement of the conjunctiva, vagina, or ear by *Corynebacterium diphtheriae* has been rarely reported.

Diagnosis. In most instances of diphtheric oropharyngeal infection, a presumptive diagnosis must be made on clinical grounds, without awaiting laboratory confirmation, because therapy should be started at once.

The clinical manifestations which should arouse suspicion of *nasopharyngeal diphtheria* are (1) insidious onset of a painless pharyngitis associated with an exudate (usually localized or predominantly in one tonsillar area); (2) association of a faucial exudate with insidious and progressive signs of laryngeal obstruction, or with a serous or serosanguineous nasal discharge; and (3) the presence of faucial exudate with marked cervical adenopathy and signs of toxicity (prostration, tachycardia, marked pallor).

For laboratory diagnosis, a swab from the suspected site should be promptly inoculated on a Löffler slant, a tellurite plate, and a blood agar plate. Identification of the etiologic agent can be made after overnight incubation on the basis of colony formation, cellular morphology, and sometimes fermentation reactions. Immunofluorescence techniques have been tried for the rapid diagnosis of diphtheria. For reliable results the specimen has to be incubated four hours before applying the fluorescent antibody technique. Slides prepared directly from throat swabs are unsatisfactory. The fluorescent antibody technique is not of value for the identification of toxigenic strains.

Several conditions may be confused with diphtheria, especially during an epidemic bout. This is the case, for instance, with streptococcal pharyngitis. In this condition there is usually high fever (39 to 40°C) with frequent chills, the throat is fiery red, the exudate is thin and easily removable, and swallowing is painful. Other pharyngeal infections which may be accompanied by an exudate are adenoviral exudative pharyngitis, infectious mononucleosis, Vincent's angina, and angina of agranulocytosis. Rhinitis associated with diphtheria must be differentiated from rhinitis of simple colds and from foreign bodies in the nostrils. The distressful laryngeal manifestations of diphtheria should be differentiated from acute laryngotracheobronchitis.

Complications. The most important complications of diphtheria are related to the cardiovascular and nervous systems. They are most frequently associated with the severe forms of the disease.

Although electrocardiographic changes have been described in a high percentage (25 per cent) of cases of diphtheria, clinically manifest myocarditis is less common. The onset of myocarditis is often insidious, appearing in the second or third week of the infection. Characteristically, the patient exhibits a weak rising pulse with distant heart sounds and a profound weakness and lethargy. When heart failure ensues, the patient becomes dyspneic, with marked pallor and epigastric pain, and he develops cardiac enlargement and an apical diastolic gallop. The most common electrocardiographic changes are T wave flattening or inversion, bundle branch block or intraventricular block, and several types of disorders of rhythm (premature contraction and atrial fibrillation).

Diphtheria myocarditis, particularly when associated with heart block, carries an extremely poor prognosis. Despite vigorous treatment, including steroids and digitalis, the mortality rate is very high. Glucagon has also been tried but is ineffective.

Nervous system involvement is manifested by cranial nerve or peripheral nerve paralysis. The most common form of cranial nerve palsy is paralysis of the soft palate, which is suspected by the development of nasal regurgitation of fluid upon attempted swallowing. Nasal speech may be present but is frequently slight. This condition is mild, and recovery usually occurs within two weeks. Ciliary paresis and oculomotor paralysis (affecting both sides) make up the next most common form. Rarely, facial, pharyngeal, or laryngeal paralysis is observed.

Peripheral neuritis, usually affecting the limbs, may appear from about the fourth to the eighth week. It varies greatly in extent but is frequently manifested by weakness in the dorsiflexors of the feet, accompanied by decreased or absent tendon reflexes in the lower extremities. Less commonly, the upper limbs, the neck, and the trunk may be involved. The prognosis is good. Diphtheric polyneuritis has been described after cutaneous diphtheria.

It must be emphasized that recovery from the complications of diphtheria is nearly always complete insofar as can be determined by clinical examination. It has been suggested that a lowering of cardiac reserve can persist in some cases, but this assumption needs further documentation.

Treatment. The most important act in the treatment of diphtheria is to administer antitoxin as soon as the diphtheria is suspected on clinical grounds without awaiting laboratory confirmation. Admittedly this practice will result in the unnecessary use of antitoxin in some cases. But this is of little consequence in view of the considerable improvement in prognosis in severe forms of the disease when antitoxin is administered early and in adequate amounts.

Opinions vary as to what constitutes an efficient dose. It is usually accepted that in mild or moderate cases a dose of 20,000 to 40,000 units, injected intramuscularly, is enough. In severe cases, 50,000 to 100,000 units is the recommended dose, half of it being given by slow intravenous infusion. As the antitoxin is a horse protein, precautions should be observed to avoid severe hypersensitivity reactions (anaphylaxis). It is mandatory to inquire if allergy to horse serum is known, and to perform a conjunctival or intracutaneous skin test with a 1:10 saline dilution of the antitoxin. If a positive reaction is obtained by either method, desensitization with increasing doses of antiserum is recommended. Epinephrine must be at hand before antitoxin is administered by any route.

As the *Corynebacterium diphtheriae* is susceptible to several antimicrobials, these drugs have been used routinely, in addition to antitoxin, in cases of diphtheria. Penicillin G is still the drug of choice, and is usually given as procaine penicillin, 400,000 units intramuscularly every 12 hours, for a period of 10 to 12 days. Erythromycin, also very active against the diphtheria bacillus, is an alternative drug and is recommended in a dosage of 30 to 40 mg per kilogram of body weight for a similar period. In suspected cases, these drugs must not be administered without the antitoxin, because they may mask the infection and thus may make it impossible to establish a laboratory diagnosis.

Bed rest is essential in all patients during the acute phase of the disease; this can vary in completeness and duration, depending on the degree of toxicity and the presence of cardiac involvement. In any event, the patient's return to activity should be carefully guided by the physician. Complications such as dehydration, shock, and congestive heart failure should be promptly diagnosed and properly treated.

In cases exhibiting marked toxicity and in patients with severe laryngeal involvement and/or shock, corticosteroids (prednisolone, 3 to 5 mg per kilogram of body weight per day) have been advocated along with the antitoxin and antimicrobials. Cases of laryngeal obstruction may require emergency tracheostomy and careful postoperative aspiration to avoid complications. Such patients need special nursing for safety.

Patients with diphtheria should be isolated, preferably in hospital. Before their discharge from isolation, cultures from throat and nose (or local lesion) should be taken, and at least two consecutive negative cultures should be obtained.

Prevention. Diphtheria may be effectively prevented by *active immunization.* The primary course of immunization should be administered within the first year of life, preferably between the third and sixth months. Of the preparations available, *fluid toxoid* and *alum-precipitated toxoid* are the most commonly used. The primary course of fluid toxoid consists of three intramuscular injections (0.5 ml, 1.0 ml, and 1.0 ml) at weekly intervals (one to three weeks). For immunization with the alum-precipitated toxoid, two 1-ml intramuscular injections administered at intervals of one to two months are enough. Despite its greater antigenic potency, the alum-precipitated toxoid also has a greater sensitizing ability, and may induce sterile local abscesses at the injection site owing to the irritating effect of the alum upon tissues. Both fluid and alum-precipitated toxoid are excellent immunizing agents, conferring immunity to at least 90 per cent of those receiving a primary course. After this immunization in infancy, one stimulating dose should be given one or two years later, and another given at the time the child enters school.

Diphtheria toxoid has been combined with immunizations against tetanus and pertussis and should be given within the first year of life. All children under eight years of age who are not immunized are susceptible to diphtheria and should be actively immunized without preliminary Schick testing. In older children and adults, before immunization with toxoid, a sensitivity test should be done. The development of a local reaction within 48 hours of the intracutaneous injection of 0.1 ml of 1:10 dilution of toxoid in normal saline *(Moloney test)* is a warning that toxoid should be administered cautiously in multiple small diluted doses.

Passive immunization against diphtheria may be rapidly conferred by subcutaneous inoculation of 1500 units of diphtheria antitoxin. This procedure should be limited to persons peculiarly at risk of infection, such as nonimmunized children heavily exposed to an infected case. The protection is limited to a period of two to three weeks, and active immunization with a toxoid preparation should be started at the same time. Human diphtheria antitoxin is not yet available.

Treatment of Diphtheria Carriers. Whenever diphtheria is common, carrier rates are high. In approximately 15 to 20 per cent of cases, the cultures will remain positive for as long as one month after the disease, but they will subsequently become negative in most instances. Erythromycin in a dosage of 30 to 40 mg per kilogram of body weight has been found effective for treatment of carriers. Tonsillectomy and adenoidectomy have also been advocated to eliminate the carrier state.

Belsey, M. A., Sinclair, M., Roder, M. R., and LeBlanc, D. R.: *Corynebacterium diphtheriae* skin infections in Alabama and Louisiana. N. Engl. J. Med., 135:135, 1969.

Bray, J. P., Burt, E. G., Potter, E. V., Poon-King, T., and Earle, D.: Epidemic diphtheria and skin infections in Trinidad. J. Infect. Dis., 126:34, 1972.

McCloskey, R. V., Eller, J. J., Green, M., Mauney, C. V., and Richards, S. E. M.: The 1970 epidemic of diphtheria in San Antonio. Ann. Intern. Med., 75:495, 1971.

McCracken, A. W., and Mauney, C. V.: Identification of *Corynebacterium diphtheriae* by immunofluorescence during a diphtheria epidemic. J. Clin. Pathol., 24:641, 1971.

Naiditch, M. J., and Bower, A. A.: Diphtheria: Study of 1433 cases observed during 10-year period at Los Angeles County Hospital. Am. J. Med., 17:229, 1954.

Scheid, W.: Diphtherial paralysis. An analysis of 2292 cases of diphtheria in adults, which included 174 cases of polyneuritis. J. Nerv. Ment. Dis., 116:1095, 1952.

Tasman, A., and Lansberg, H. P.: Problems concerning the prophylaxis, pathogenesis and therapy of diphtheria. Bull. WHO, 16:939, 1957.

CLOSTRIDIAL DISEASES

206. INTRODUCTION

Emanuel Wolinsky

The clostridia are spore-forming anaerobic gram-positive bacilli that for the most part lead a saprophytic existence in nature. The may be found in large numbers in the intestinal tracts of humans and animals, and in the soil. They are capable of producing disease by virtue of their elaboration of powerful exotoxins, but special conditions must be present in the tissues to allow the organisms to germinate, proliferate, and elaborate toxins. The mere presence of clostridia in the wound or on the surface of the body is not significant. Most clostridial disease is caused by *C. perfringens,* although occasionally *C. novyi (oedematiens), septicum, sordellii (bifermentans), histolyticum,* and *fallax* may be human pathogens.

The pathologic states attributable to clostridial infection cover a wide range of severity and localization, from the relatively benign wound infection to the highly fatal gas gangrene; from transient bacteremia to life-threatening septicemia; from relatively mild food poisoning to necrotic enteritis; and from pleural empyema to purulent meningitis. The neurotoxic disease caused by *C. tetani* is discussed below, and that caused by *C. botulinum* is discussed in Ch. 23.

BACTERIOLOGY

All the clostridia owe their pathogenicity to the elaboration of exotoxins that have enzymatic activity. Four major toxins and eight minor ones have been described and given Greek letters. The most important of them is the alpha toxin, which is a lecithinase capable of splitting lecithin in the red cell envelope and causing severe hemolysis. Many of the species of clostridia have been separated into types according to their ability to elaborate specific exotoxins. *C. perfringens* may be divided into five or six toxigenic types; Type A elaborates more alpha toxin than any other type or species and is by far the most important variety of Clostridium in human disease, particularly gas gangrene.

207. CLOSTRIDIAL MYONECROSIS (Gas Gangrene)

Emanuel Wolinsky

The clostridial gas gangrene is best called *clostridial myonecrosis* because the outstanding feature is rapidly progressive muscle necrosis with relatively little inflammatory reaction, and because other organisms can produce skin and subcutaneous gangrene with gas formation. The disease most often arises from traumatic or surgical wounds in which anoxic conditions prevail as a result of ischemia or crushed muscle. Battle wounds of World Wars I and II supplied plentiful case material for study; gas gangrene occurred in approximately 10 per cent of World War I wounds and in 1 per cent of those that occurred in World War II. In civilian practice the rate of gas gangrene among 188,000 major open wounds has been estimated to be 1.8 per cent. The rate of contamination or local infection of open wounds, on the other hand, amounts to 30 to 80 per cent. The soil is the usual source of the clostridia in exogenous infection, the intestine or biliary tract in autogenous infection.

Pathogenesis. The factors that predispose to the invasion of muscle by the bacilli with the subsequent elaboration of exotoxins are related to lack of oxygen and lowering of the oxidation-reduction potential of the tissues. These factors are (1) impaired local vascular supply owing to vessel trauma or pressure from foreign bodies, casts, or tourniquets; (2) presence of metallic bodies, clothing, or dirt in the wound; (3) presence of necrotic tissue or hemorrhage; and (4) growth of aerobic microorganisms in the wound.

Under these circumstances the bacilli can multiply anaerobically and elaborate toxins, which diffuse out and damage surrounding muscle, which in turn becomes colonized with the bacilli. Thus the disease spreads rapidly to surrounding muscles and gains momentum. The severe generalized toxemia remains poorly explained. Alpha toxin is not found in the blood, and it is postulated that a toxic factor that acts on certain vital centers or enzymes is produced by the interaction of clostridial toxin with infected muscle.

Clinical Manifestations. The clinical picture of gas gangrene is dominated by rapidly progressive toxemia and shock. After a relatively short incubation period of one to four days the patient suddenly exhibits restlessness and anxiety; the temperature and pulse rate begin to rise and the blood pressure to fall. He is noted to be pale and sweating. The wound becomes painful and markedly swollen. Some hours later, after progression of the signs and symptoms, a thin brownish exudate begins to ooze from the wound, and a small amount of crepitus may be noted in the surrounding tissues. A bronze discoloration starts at the edge of the wound and progresses outward. Blebs filled with purplish fluid may appear. An odor characterized as "mousy" or "sickly sweet" is described by many observers. By this time the patient may be anuric and in irreversible vascular collapse. When the muscle is exposed by incision, it appears to be "cooked" or dead—it does not bleed when cut or retract when pinched. Smears from *involved muscle* show many large gram-positive rods and no other organisms, but very few pus cells. Smears and cultures from the *wound exudate* at the surface may reveal other organisms in addition to the clostridia, especially in grossly contaminated wounds. Roentgenograms reveal the presence of gas in and around muscle bundles in the form of fernlike, lacy patterns. Untreated, fully developed clostridial myonecrosis is almost always fatal.

Myonecrosis must be differentiated from clostridial and nonclostridial *crepitant cellulitis,* from *anaerobic streptococcal myonecrosis,* and from *physical* and *chemical* causes of gas in the tissues. *Clostridial cellulitis*

(anaerobic cellulitis, local gas gangrene, epifascial gas gangrene, or gas-forming fasciitis) is a gas-forming infection of connective tissue mainly localized to subcutaneous areas with spread in fascial planes, but healthy muscle is not involved. It arises as a result of clostridial infection of tissue already necrotic from ischemia or trauma. The onset is gradual, and toxemia, pain, and swelling are less than in gas gangrene. A large amount of gas is distributed in the form of large bubbles along the fascial planes, but not in the muscle. Incision will show that the muscle is viable, and smears from muscle tissue away from the open wound will not reveal organisms.

Nonclostridial crepitant cellulitis is similar to clostridial cellulitis, except that the infection is associated with other organisms usually in a mixed flora consisting of two or more of the following: aerogenic coliforms (*E. coli,* Klebsiella, Enterobacter), anaerobic streptococci, Bacteroides, and gamma streptococci. In many cases this mixed bacterial flora in gas-forming cellulitis includes clostridia; these cases do not appear to differ in prognosis from those in which clostridia are absent.

Anaerobic streptococcal myonecrosis was described by MacLennan in infected war wounds from the Middle East in 1948, but there have been few reports since then. Other organisms, especially group A streptococci and *Staph. aureus,* were always found with the primary agent, and 3 of 19 patients had anaerobic streptococcal bacteremia.

Simple contamination of wounds with clostridia is not uncommon. The organisms, usually in association with a mixed flora, exist as saprophytes on necrotic tissue and debris and do not invade further. Clostridia may also be found in localized collections of purulent material in wounds, or in a collection of foul-smelling brownish fluid known as a "gas abscess" or a "Welch abscess." Drainage will usually suffice to bring these conditions under control. There is not always a clean-cut distinction among the various pathologic states described above, nor is it clear how often one can recognize an orderly progression in the severity of clostridial invasion from simple contamination to full-blown myonecrosis.

Diagnosis. The diagnosis of gas gangrene is essentially a clinical one. Upon first suspicion of the disease, dressings and casts must be removed and the wound or suspected area thoroughly inspected. Roentgenograms may help to show the fine bubbles of gas distributed in and around muscle bundles. Incision should be made into

TABLE 1.   Classification of Histotoxic
Clostridial Disease

Traumatic
  A. Wound infection (war and civilian)
    1. Simple contamination
    2. Localized (purulent or "gas abscess")
    3. Gas-forming cellulitis
    4. Myonecrosis
  B. Uterine infection (postabortion and postpartum)
  C. Burns, panophthalmitis, brain abscess, etc.

Nontraumatic
  A. Postoperative (abdominal, amputation)
  B. Postinjection
  C. Spontaneous
    1. Localized (pneumonia, empyema, cholecystitis, myonecrosis)
    2. Septicemic (malignant disease, intestinal lesion)
  D. Bacteremia without hemolysis or sepsis (from decubitus ulcer, gangrenous extremity, uterus)

TABLE 2. Gas-Forming Soft Tissue Infections

	Clostridial Myonecrosis	"Anaerobic" Cellulitis	Streptococcal Myonecrosis
Onset	Sudden	Gradual	Gradual
Toxemia	Extreme	Slight	Slight
Pain	May be severe	Slight	Gradually increasing
Swelling	Marked	Slight	Marked
Skin color	Bronze	No change	Erythematous
Exudate	Thin, brown	Thin, bloody; later purulent	Profuse, thin seropurulent
Gas	Little, in muscle	Profuse, large bubbles in fascial planes	Little, in muscle
Muscle	Dead, "cooked," healthy muscle invaded	Not involved	Initially edematous, then hemorrhagic
Bacteriology	Mixed flora from exudate or open wound; from muscle aspirate pure gram-positive rods	May be pure clostridia or mixed flora from exudate or subcutaneous tissue; no organisms in muscle aspirate	Anaerobic streptococci, along with Group A Streptococcus, *Staph. aureus, etc.,* from exudate and muscle
Prognosis	Serious	Good	Good
Treatment	Radical surgery, penicillin, antitoxin, hyperbaric oxygen	Surgical drainage and debridement, appropriate antimicrobials	Surgical drainage and debridement, penicillin

the muscle so that the characteristic appearance may be appreciated. At the same time a specimen of muscle may be examined by Gram stain and by anaerobic cultural techniques. Slides may also be made for staining by the fluorescent antibody technique (Clark et al., 1969). Smears and cultures from the exudate around the wound surface may be misleading. Tables 1 and 2 summarize the most important findings for the differential diagnosis.

Treatment. Treatment must be prompt and vigorous. Most important is thorough *debridement* and *excision* of all devitalized tissue and dead muscle. Hopelessly involved extremities usually need to be amputated except perhaps under the influence of hyperbaric oxygen. It is said that if any infected muscle is left behind, it will prevent cure. General *supportive measures* should include intravenous fluids and blood, other measures to combat vascular collapse and shock, and peritoneal dialysis when necessary. *Antimicrobial* treatment is given to prevent bloodstream invasion and to suppress further spread of infection. Penicillin is the drug of choice given in large doses of 10 to 20 million units per day intravenously. Erythromycin may be substituted in patients allergic to penicillin. In a recent study it was found that 11 per cent of clostridial strains were resistant to tetracycline. *Antitoxin* is recommended, especially during the first few hours of the disease, in the hope of neutralizing any free toxin in the body fluids, although its usefulness is doubtful because the exotoxins are very rapidly bound to cells. The recommended dose is 40 thousand units of trivalent or pentavalent antitoxin intravenously at once and 20 to 40 thousand units repeated at four- to six-hour intervals. The usual precautions for horse serum must be observed. *Hyperbaric oxygen* at 3 atmospheres has been recommended by some as a dramatically successful mode of therapy that should take precedence over immediate surgical treatment and antitoxin. It is said that debridement may be deferred until systemic toxicity has been relieved and demarcation between necrotic and viable tissue is clear. In this way loss of tissue may be minimized and amputation sometimes avoided. If a suitable chamber is not available locally, it is probably unwise to delay surgical extirpation in favor of a long journey.

Treatment of "anaerobic" cellulitis and streptococcal myonecrosis need not be so radical. Usually wide excision and debridement along with supportive measures and appropriate antimicrobials will suffice. A Gram-

stained smear of wound exudate and muscle aspirate will help one to decide whether penicillin alone should be given (for pure Clostridium or Streptococcus) or whether antistaphylococcal or anticoliform agents should be added or substituted. For the former, one should use a semisynthetic penicillinase-resistant penicillin (methicillin, nafcillin, or cephalothin) to initiate treatment; for the gram-negative bacilli one can add tetracycline, gentamicin, or kanamycin.

Prevention. The prophylactic use of antitoxin and antimicrobials at the time of injury does not prevent gas gangrene. Careful attention to good surgical technique is most important. All devitalized tissue must be excised and vascular supply left intact. Care must be taken with tourniquets and casts to prevent undue ischemia. Plaster of Paris itself may be contaminated with clostridia.

UTERINE INFECTION

Postabortion and postpartum clostridial infections of the uterus are still important causes of serious disease in obstetrics. At least 5 per cent of women harbor clostridia in the vagina as simple contaminants. Fulminant infection usually follows criminal abortion or prolonged and difficult labor, and presents a clinical picture similar to that seen in traumatic gas gangrene. Unlike wound gas gangrene, however, uterine infection is frequently accompanied by clostridial sepsis leading to jaundice, hemolysis, hemoglobinemia, hemoglobinuria, and renal shutdown. As in wound infection, there may be various grades of clostridial involvement, from simple contamination to secondary invasion of necrotic matter in the uterus or a dead fetus to true invasion of intact uterine muscle producing myonecrosis or "physometra." Clostridial infection must be differentiated from the more slowly progressive uterine infection produced by anaerobic streptococci and Bacteroides which commonly leads to pelvic thrombophlebitis and septic pulmonary infarcts.

Treatment is essentially the same as that outlined above, except that a decision must be made quickly on whether to do a hysterectomy or merely to empty the uterus. Evidence for uterine perforation or necrosis will call for the more radical procedure. Antimicrobial therapy should probably include clindamycin or chloramphenicol in addition to penicillin to control Bacteroides.

POSTOPERATIVE GAS GANGRENE

Nontraumatic gas gangrene that follows surgical operations is probably the most common variety of the disease in civilian hospitals today. Of 42 cases of *C. perfringens* infection reported from a single hospital, 18 followed operations and 10 were secondary to trauma (Pyrtek and Bartus, 1962). Most of these infections involve the abdominal wall after biliary or intestinal surgery, or the leg or hip after amputation or correction of hip fractures, although the complication has been described after many other kinds of surgical procedures. Recent investigation in England indicated that most of these infections were sporadic and autogenous in origin, probably as a result of fecal contamination of the skin. Parker called attention to the importance of adequate preoperative sterilization of the skin with sporicidal agents and the advisability of giving prophylactic penicillin from a few hours before operation to one week after to those patients at greatest risk from postoperative clostridial infections—elderly patients who will have hip surgery or thigh amputations.

208. OTHER CLOSTRIDIAL DISEASES

Emanuel Wolinsky

SEPTICEMIA

Clostridial septicemia occurs rarely from traumatic wound gangrene, occasionally from postoperative gas gangrene, and commonly from uterine infection. In addition, nontraumatic or spontaneous clostridial septicemia has been described from such conditions as acute cholecystitis, perforated peptic ulcer, ulcerating carcinoma of the colon, acute pancreatitis, diverticulitis, appendiceal abscess, decubitus ulcer, and gangrenous limbs. Septicemia may occur in terminal cancer patients from portals of entry such as ulcerations of the respiratory or alimentary tracts. A study of 21 patients suffering from various malignant diseases who had septicemia caused by *C. septicum* has been reported (Alpern and Dowell, 1969). As a result of septicemia, infection may localize in the pleura, myocardium, endocardium, and meninges. Benign clostridial bacteremia without hemolysis was observed in a series of 20 patients, all of whom survived (Rathbun, 1968).

MISCELLANEOUS FORMS

Pneumonia and empyema may be associated with clostridial infection, usually as a result of aspiration of contaminated material from the mouth or the stomach, but occasionally by way of the bloodstream. Penetrating injuries may lead to serious clostridial infections of the eye, brain, and meninges. Severe gas gangrene may result from injections into the buttock or thigh, presumably from inadequately sterilized skin. In at least one instance the organism was also isolated from cotton sponges soaked in alcohol.

209. CLOSTRIDIAL GASTROENTERITIS

Emanuel Wolinsky

Clostridial food poisoning has been the second most common variety reported to the Communicable Disease Center, representing 16 per cent of the total outbreaks and 34 per cent of the cases. There is no seasonal preference, and the most common vehicles have been beef and turkey products. *C. perfringens* type A may be recovered from the stools of patients and from the suspected food product. The disease is characterized by a short incubation period, acute onset, absence of fever, and a relatively benign course. The outbreaks are self-limiting, and the disease is not spread to other people directly. Evidence points to an infection rather than an intoxication as the primary mechanism of the disease. *Enteritis necroticans* ("Darmbrand") was first described shortly after World War II in Germany. Other outbreaks occurred in North Germany and the Rhineland; then the disease apparently vanished. The disease was characterized by severe diarrhea, collapse, high mortality, and patchy hemorrhagic necrosis of the small bowel. It was originally attributed to a new type of *C. perfringens* called type F, but these organisms are now considered to be members of type C. It corresponds in many ways to certain clostridial enterotoxemias of animals.

Altemeier, W. A., and Culbertson, W. R.: Acute non-clostridial crepitant cellulitis. Surg. Gynecol. Obstet., 87:206, 1948.
Ayliffe, G. A. J., and Lowbury, E. J. L.: Sources of gas gangrene in hospital. Br. Med. J., 2:333, 1969.
Bornstein, D. L., Weinberg, A. N., Swartz, M. N., and Kunz, L. J.: Anaerobic infections—Review of current experience. Medicine, 43:207, 1964.
Cabrera, A., Tsukada, Y., and Pickren, J. W.: Clostridial gas gangrene and septicemia in malignant disease. Cancer, 18:800, 1965.
MacLennan, J. D.: The histotoxic clostridial infections of man. Bact. Rev., 26:177, 1962.
Parker, M. T.: Postoperative clostridial infections in Britain. Br. Med. J., 3:671, 1969.
Roding, B., Groenveld, P. H., and Boerema, I.: Ten years' experience in the treatment of gas gangrene in hyperbaric oxygen. Surg. Gynecol. Obstet., 134:579, 1972.
Unsworth, I. P.: Gas gangrene in New South Wales. Med. J. Aust., 1:1077, 1973.

210. TETANUS

Alexander Crampton Smith

Tetanus, often called "lockjaw," is a disease of the nervous system characterized by intense activity of motor neurons resulting in severe muscle spasms. It is caused by an exotoxin of *Clostridium tetani*.

History. Tetanus has caught the imagination of physicians since Hippocrates, and this is probably in part due to the horrifying nature of the clinical picture in the established untreated case. The presence of the causative organism in soil was demonstrated by Nicolaier, who produced tetanus in animals by soil injections. The Clostridium was isolated in pure culture in 1899 by Kitasato, and in 1892, Nocard immunized horses by injections of antitoxic horse serum. Passive immunization after wounding saved many lives in World War I, and active immunization with toxoid almost eliminated tetanus in the allied armies in World War II. Curare was first suggested as having an application in the treatment of tetanus in 1811, but as curare in sufficient dosage to abolish the spasms of severe tetanus will certainly paralyze the muscles of ventilation, the large-scale use of curare had to wait almost 150 years until intermittent positive pressure ventilation (IPPV) through a cuffed tracheotomy tube was introduced into the treatment of tetanus in Denmark in 1953 (Bjørnboe et al.).

ETIOLOGY AND PATHOGENESIS

Clostridium tetani is a gram-positive actively motile bacillus, which in its spore-bearing form has a characteristic "drumstick" appearance. Spores may develop at either end of the bacillus, giving a "dumbbell" appearance. It is a strict anaerobe, and spores will not germinate in the presence of even the smallest amount of oxygen. An oxidation-reduction potential of + 0.01 volt or less at pH 7 is required if germination is to take place. The Clostridium grows well on laboratory media at 37° C, and growth occurs slowly at 22° C. Vegetative bacilli are readily killed by antiseptics and by heat, but spores are highly resistant to antiseptics and, to a certain extent, are resistant to heat. To kill most spores, boiling for one hour is necessary, but the most resistant may require boiling for four hours. Autoclaving for ten minutes at 120° C may, however, be relied on to sterilize contaminated objects. *Clostridium tetani* is commonly found in soil and in the feces of domestic animals and humans. Presumably by contamination with soil and feces, spores can be recovered from dust and clothing; in suitable surroundings like dried earth, spores will survive for many years.

Clostridium tetani produces two exotoxins, *tetanospasmin* and *tetanolysin,* and of these tetanospasmin is the neurotoxin which produces the typical muscle spasms of tetanus. It is extremely potent, each milligram of crystallized toxin containing 50 to 75 million mouse lethal doses. This extreme toxicity may be the reason why an attack of tetanus does not confer immunity, as it is postulated that the fatal dose of tetanus toxin is less than the amount required to provoke an immune response. Tetanolysin can cause hemolysis on blood agar plates, but does not seem to play any significant part in the pathologic process caused by the Clostridium.

There have been differences of opinion about the site of action of tetanospasmin and about the route by which it spreads, but it now seems firmly established that the toxin acts in the spinal cord and the brainstem and that it spreads centrally along motor nerve trunks and up the spinal cord. Tetanus will follow the intravenous injection into animals, but the route by which toxin in the blood enters the nervous system is not clear. Toxin injected intramuscularly apparently spreads not only by passing up motor nerves but also by absorption into the blood, and it has been suggested that vascular spread is the more important route in generalized tetanus. Payling Wright surveyed the evidence for neural and vascular spread, but research, notably with radioactive isotopes (Fedenec, 1967), is continuing.

EPIDEMIOLOGY

The incidence of tetanus is difficult to establish because it is not a notifiable disease in many countries. The total world deaths each year, however, probably exceed 160,000, and if the average crude fatality rate is about 45 per cent (and it may be much higher), there must be more than 350,000 cases in the world every year. Tetanus is thus still a major public health problem in devel-oping countries. The organism is found in soil and human and animal feces, and tetanus is common in warm climates and in rural areas that are highly cultivated and consequently have a large population of men and animals. Agricultural workers, in whom injuries may easily be contaminated with the Clostridium, are particularly at risk. *Clostridium tetani* can also be found in urban areas, but the degree of contamination is not high, and it is likely that the increased standards of living and hygiene which urbanization implies also contribute to a lower incidence of tetanus in cities. Further evidence of the importance of education and hygiene is the absence of neonatal tetanus in countries where obstetric hygiene is good, compared with the high incidence in countries where dung is sometimes used as a dressing for the umbilical stump.

PREVENTION OF TETANUS

Before Injury

Active Immunization. The U.S. Public Health Service Advisory Committee has stated that the need for active immunization against tetanus is universal and that such immunization is the only way by which tetanus may be eliminated as an important health problem. There is little doubt that active immunization with adsorbed tetanus toxoid will convey a remarkably high degree of immunity. LaForce et al. (1969) have calculated that the incidence of tetanus in the under-ten age group in the United States of America was about 3.8 per 100 million. This underscores the excellent results obtained by active immunization of American and British military personnel in World War II.

In the United Kingdom, the recommended course of injections is three doses of adsorbed toxoid in a mixed vaccine, one injection at six months of age, and two others, with six to eight weeks between first and second and six months between second and third. A "booster" is advised at school entry and another at 15 to 19. Thereafter, "booster" doses should be given at ten-year intervals. The American Academy of Pediatrics suggests three injections of toxoid no less than one month apart in infancy, a reinforcing dose about twelve months later, and a fifth or "booster" injection on entering school. Subsequent routine toxoid "boosters" should be administered at intervals of approximately ten years.

After Injury

Prevention of Contamination. Simple measures that prevent contamination can contribute significantly to the prevention of tetanus, and the effect of attention to treatment of the umbilical stump on the incidence of neonatal tetanus is a good example of the effectiveness of simple hygiene. The aim of surgery in prophylaxis is to remove all dead tissue and foreign bodies from a wound. This will not only remove spore-bearing material, but will also deny the spores the anaerobic conditions necessary for their growth. As Adams et al. suggest, it is probably realistic to recognize a "tetanus-prone" wound. Such wounds include deep penetrating puncture wounds in which anaerobic conditions are likely to exist and surgical exposure is difficult or impossible. Tetanus-prone wounds also include wounds heavily contaminated with soil or manure, wounds with dead or devitalized tissue or retained foreign bodies, and wounds seen more than six to eight hours after infliction.

Active Immunization. In the United Kingdom a "booster" dose of toxoid is recommended if an injury occurs more than three years after the completion of the last course or more than three years after a "booster." If the wound is judged to be "tetanus prone," a "booster" should be given. The American Academy of Pediatrics recommends that an emergency injection of toxoid should be given if injury occurs more than one year after the last "booster." In spite of this, it has been suggested (Peebles et al., 1969) that if there is a valid history of an accepted immunization program, special tetanus boosters on admission to camps, schools, and colleges and emergency injections at times of injury are unnecessary and should be abandoned to minimize toxoid reactions. If a wounded patient's immune status is in doubt, he should be regarded as unimmunized, and other means of preventing tetanus should be used. If passive immunization with antitoxin is chosen, active immunization should be commenced at the same time with an injection of toxoid in another limb. Antitoxin will not influence active immunization conferred by a full course of adsorbed toxoid.

Passive Immunization. The use of passive immunization by means of antitoxin has probably resulted in the saving of many lives. The absence of a controlled trial precludes certainty, but circumstantial evidence is very strong. Animal experiments show that antitoxin given soon after inoculation with tetanus will protect against the disease, and Bruce (1920), reviewing 1458 cases of tetanus occurring in World War I, showed that the incidence of tetanus, after prophylactic antitoxin was available in large quantities, fell from 9 per 1000 wounded to 1.4 per 1000 wounded. Other improvements in surgical care could have been contributory, but it seems likely that antitoxin was an important factor in the decrease in incidence.

Antitoxin has two disadvantages, both relative. The antitoxin commonly used is produced by the active immunization of horses, first with toxoid and then with tetanus toxin. If a patient has had a previous injection of horse serum, he may develop antibodies against horse serum proteins very soon after an injection of prophylactic equine antitoxin. This will result in immune elimination of the subsequently injected equine antitoxin so that protection is absent or incomplete. This elimination may be accompanied by sensitivity reactions, either local redness and swelling of the injected limb or generalized serum sickness. If circulating antibodies are present, immune elimination may be very rapid and may be accompanied by fatal anaphylaxis. The dose of equine antitoxin for prophylaxis is 1500 units, but prophylactic antitoxin should not be given if either local or general reactions follow the subcutaneous injection of a test dose of 75 units. Epinephrine, 1 per 1000, should always be available whenever equine antitoxin is given; in cases in which antitoxin is indicated and either a history of previous injections of horse serum or a reaction to a test dose has been elicited, prophylaxis with human antitetanus immunoglobulin, 250 units, will be more effective and much safer.

Chemoprophylaxis. Antimicrobial drugs can inhibit the multiplication of *Clostridium tetani* and kill the vegetative form of the organism. By killing aerobic organisms coexisting with the Clostridium, antimicrobial drugs can prevent multiplication by denying the Clostridium the conditions favorable to its growth; they have no effect, however, on tetanus toxin. Because of the dangers of passive immunization, some centers in the United Kingdom have largely abandoned the use of antitoxin in favor of chemoprophylaxis, and at least one of these has provided data showing no increase in the incidence of the disease. Although the efficacy of chemoprophylaxis is not yet certain, it seems clear that in certain circumstances it may provide an alternative to prophylaxis by antitoxin.

For effective chemoprophylaxis certain criteria must be fulfilled: the organism must be susceptible to the drug chosen, and the patient must not be sensitive to the drug. *Clostridium tetani* is susceptible to a variety of drugs, including penicillin, tetracycline, and erythromycin, so that it is probably not difficult to make a suitable choice for a particular patient. Chemoprophylaxis must be started early. Smith (1964) has shown that in mice inoculated with tetanus spores, chemoprophylaxis was effective if it was started four hours after inoculation but not if started eight hours after inoculation. The time interval in humans is not established, but it is suggested that in injuries seen later than six hours after infliction, some other form of prophylaxis should be chosen. Antimicrobial therapy must be continued for a sufficient time to ensure that tetanus spores cannot survive, and this means for at least five days.

PATHOGENESIS

If tetanus is to supervene, the Clostridium must be introduced into human tissue, and the disease may follow a trivial or a serious injury. In countries with good medical services, serious wounds receive effective treatment, and tetanus is usually avoided. Apparently minor wounds then become a common cause of the disease, but in quite a high proportion of cases no responsible injury can be identified. The site of action and method of spread of the exotoxin have been mentioned, but it is rather surprising that no unequivocal evidence of recognizable pathologic lesions caused by tetanus has yet been forthcoming even after careful postmortem studies.

CLINICAL FEATURES AND CRITERIA OF SEVERITY IN TETANUS

The criteria of severity may be established in two ways: from the history and from the symptoms and signs.

From the History. The severity of an attack of tetanus is related to the incubation period (the period from injury to the first sign of tetanus) and the onset period, described by Cole (1940) as the period from the first sign to the first generalized spasm. If the former is less than 9 days and the latter less than 48 hours, the attack of tetanus may be expected to be severe. The length of the onset period is, in general, the more reliable guide to the expected severity of the attack.

From the Symptoms and Signs. *The Mild Case.* Tetanus usually presents with rigidity of muscles, and this rigidity may be severe enough to cause pain. The patient with mild tetanus may have "local tetanus" in which rigidity affects only one limb, or the patient may have mild generalized rigidity. Stiffness of the jaw muscles causes trismus, and stiffness of the facial muscles may cause a change of expression. Stiffness of the muscles of the neck and back may cause discomfort or even pain on attempted flexion of the spine.

The Moderate Case. The patient has more severe generalized rigidity. Trismus is pronounced, the mouth can hardly be opened, and rigidity of the muscles of the face may cause the sneering "risus sardonicus." Opisthotonos may be pronounced, but more typically the stiffness of the antagonist muscles makes the patient lie "at attention" in bed, and the muscles of back and abdomen are hard to the touch. Patients with moderate tetanus may show mild exacerbations of this generalized rigidity as "reflex spasms." These spasms may arise spontaneously or more commonly as a result of stimuli. The important difference, however, between the patient with mild and the patient with moderate tetanus is the presence or absence of dysphagia. Spasm of the pharyngeal muscles makes swallowing difficult, and the patient coughs or splutters while drinking. This will predispose to the inhalation of pharyngeal contents and is the diagnostic characteristic of the moderate case.

The Severe Case. The patient who represents a severe case is distinguished from the patient with a moderate case by the presence of reflex spasms that may be of appalling intensity. If the spasms are untreated opisthotonos becomes extreme, and the intense muscle spasm may fracture vertebrae. Spasm of the laryngeal muscles, the diaphragm, and the intercostals prevents ventilation, and cyanosis occurs. The occurrence of reflex spasms that cause cyanosis and cannot be controlled except by powerful relaxants such as curare is the characteristic feature of the severe case of tetanus.

Patients with severe tetanus may also show a group of signs that have often been described but have been attributed by workers in Oxford to overactivity of the sympathetic nervous system (Kerr et al.). Many patients sweat profusely and, in some, oxygen uptake and carbon dioxide output are increased. In some patients most severely affected, extreme peripheral vasoconstriction develops with a glove-and-stocking distribution and a sharp line of demarcation between warm skin and cold skin. Hyperpyrexia may also develop, and probably reflects the inability of the vasoconstricted patient to lose heat. The most striking features of this syndrome, however, involve the cardiovascular system. Sinus tachycardia occurs and may progress to multifocal ventricular ectopic beats. The blood pressure is generally elevated, and superimposed on this elevation are peaks, often associated with spasms or stimuli, in which the systolic pressure may reach 300 mm Hg, and the diastolic 150 mm Hg. The syndrome may progress to hypotension that does not respond to pressor agents.

Perhaps fortunately, patients with severe tetanus often remember little of their illness and have failed to remember such bizarre incidents as a Union Jack being waved in the ward during the playing of "Rule Britannia." Electroencephalography shows a sleep pattern, with arousal during stimulation such as tracheal aspiration.

DIAGNOSIS

The diagnosis of the established case of tetanus is all too easy, and strychnine poisoning is the only condition which is truly similar to established tetanus. Trismus may occur from dental infections, and the author has seen one case of hysterical tetanus. More recently, overdose with the phenothiazine group of drugs has been confused with tetanus, but the movements in this condition usually include grimacing and jaw movements in which the jaw is opened widely.

CAUSES OF DEATH IN TETANUS

One of the most remarkable features of tetanus is that when patients recover, even from the most severe forms of the disease, they recover completely. It would therefore seem reasonable to study the causes of death carefully in tetanus so that by avoiding them the natural tendency of the disease toward recovery may be exploited. In a survey in Oxford, the causes of death in 18 of 82 patients were bronchopneumonia, 4; pulmonary embolus, 3; technical failure, 2; coincidental causes, 5; and no identifiable cause of death, 4.

Bronchopulmonary complications of tetanus are becoming less common now that the management of patients receiving IPPV through a tracheostomy tube is better understood, and it is likely that chest complications will become still less common in the future. In general on the writer's service, pulmonary embolus is not a common cause of death in patients with other diseases treated by tracheostomy and IPPV. However, the difference in the incidence of pulmonary embolus between *patients with tetanus* requiring treatment with curare and IPPV and patients *with other diseases similarly treated* is so striking that anticoagulants are now used in patients with tetanus severe enough to merit treatment in this way. The incidence of technical failure underlines the complexity of treating the fully paralyzed patient; the coincidental causes of death apparently had nothing to do with the main disease. No identifiable cause of death could be found in four patients who had all displayed a syndrome suggestive of sympathetic overactivity. Careful study of patients with similar symptoms and signs admitted subsequently has reinforced our belief that in some patients with severe tetanus the sympathetic nervous system is as grossly uninhibited as is the motor nervous system (Prys-Roberts et al.).

TREATMENT

There are certain forms of treatment required by all patients with tetanus.

Control of Rigidity and Reflex Spasms. Drugs to control rigidity vary with the severity of the case. *Barbiturates* have been used for many years, and in mild or even moderate cases are useful, but the amount of barbiturate necessary to obtund severe reflex spasms would cause coma. *Chlorpromazine* has proved antispasmodic properties in tetanus and is a sedative. It also is useful in mild and moderate cases, but has been shown by a clinical trial (Adams, 1958) to be no more effective than barbiturates, and like the barbiturates is inadequate to obtund the spasms in the severest cases. It may be used in doses of up to 50 mg intramuscularly every four to six hours. *Mephenesin* is a centrally acting muscle relaxant that has been used extensively in the treatment of tetanus with good results, especially in moderate cases, but it must be given frequently and in large doses. The effect of a dose as large as 1 gram can be observed to have diminished significantly in one hour, and this dose, continued at hourly intervals, is close to that which will paralyze ventilation. If it becomes necessary to give paralyzing doses of mephenesin to control rigidity or reflex spasms, it is clearly not the drug of choice. Mephenesin is a local anesthetic and must be given by nasogastric tube. If given intravenously, except in extremely dilute solutions, it will cause hemolysis and hemoglobinuria. *Diazepam* is currently popular and has been used in mild and moderate cases in doses from 10 mg every four hours intramuscularly, to 600 mg intravenously per day. Like the other drugs mentioned above, it will not control the spasms of the severest case, and it is probably unwise to use very large doses. The severity of the case should be admitted and treatment changed to curare and IPPV. *Curare* and similar powerful relaxants will completely abolish the reflex spasms of the severest case of tetanus, but will also paralyze the muscles of ventilation. It is therefore necessary in addition to apply IPPV through a cuffed tracheostomy tube. Curare can be given intramuscularly in doses from 15 to 30 mg.

Wound Excision.   Wound excision has been discussed under Prevention and seems a logical course of action if the causal injury can be identified. It has been suggested that excision of the wound is ineffectual in established tetanus because all the exotoxin produced by the organism has been fixed by the nervous system before symptoms and signs develop. Francis (1914) inoculated animals with tetanus and killed them when symptoms and signs began. He was able to recover many thousands of mouse lethal doses of toxin from the site of the inoculation, and this would seem to make the case for wound excision unassailable. A careful search should be made for foreign bodies in any wound excised, and excision should probably be conducted under cover of antitoxin.

Chemotherapy.   Antimicrobial therapy has also been discussed under Prevention. As a therapeutic measure all patients with tetanus should have large doses of penicillin or another active antimicrobial for a sufficient time to ensure that the Clostridium cannot survive. This should be for at least five days.

Antitoxin.   The advisability of using equine antitoxin as a therapeutic measure has been a controversial matter for many years. There is some, but not clear-cut, evidence that the use of equine antitoxin reduces mortality in established tetanus. On general grounds, however, the work of Francis cited above suggests that toxin is still being produced at the time when symptoms and signs begin, and hence it would seem reasonable to neutralize any accessible toxin. Therapeutic antitoxin is subject to the same objections and hazards as prophylactic antitoxin, and its dangers must be balanced against the possible gain by its use. A suitable dosage regimen, including subcutaneous, intramuscular, and intravenous injections, should be designed to uncover sensitivity if present, and to avoid anaphylaxis. Ten thousand units intravenously is a suitable dose, but up to 100,000 units has been used. If a history of previous injections of horse serum can be obtained, or if a sensitivity reaction occurs, equine antitoxin should not be used. If available, human antitoxin in the same dose is more effective and much safer.

Mild Tetanus

The patient with mild tetanus needs only these general measures, including a relaxant and sedative such as diazepam. The patient should be encouraged to drink water under supervision every two hours in the early stage of the disease when it may be progressing. If a patient coughs or splutters while drinking, dysphagia is present, and the patient moves into the moderate group.

Moderate Tetanus

The patient with moderate tetanus differs from the mild case by the presence of dysphagia. He needs the general measures applicable to all patients with tetanus, but in addition he must have a tracheostomy and have a cuffed tracheostomy tube inserted into the trachea to make inhalation of pharyngeal contents impossible. The operation is performed under general anesthesia with a cuffed endotracheal tube in situ so that the operation may be careful and unhurried. A cuffed tracheostomy tube should be inserted through a high U-shaped incision into the trachea so that the tube lies easily in the trachea where it is approximately parallel to the skin. If the tracheostomy is high, there is sufficient distance between the tracheostome and the carina to make it unlikely that the tube will enter the right main bronchus. The wound should not be covered and should be cleaned frequently with a mild antiseptic. It is necessary to aspirate secretions from the trachea, and disposable gloves should be worn during this procedure, not only to prevent contamination of the trachea with organisms carried on the aspirating catheter, but also to avoid contamination of the tracheostomy wound. The patient with moderate tetanus must be fed by nasogastric tube, and may require large amounts of fluid to offset excessive sweating. A high calorie diet of about 3000 calories a day is necessary, but too much protein should not be given. Patients with moderate tetanus may have a considerable degree of muscle rigidity and may even have occasional mild reflex spasms. Diazepam in divided doses of up to 400 mg intravenously per day has a considerable effect on the rigidity of tetanus without interfering with ventilation. In spite of treatment, muscular rigidity is painful and uncomfortable, and the patient should be turned every two hours to lessen this discomfort and avoid pressure sores.

Severe Tetanus

The patient with severe tetanus differs from the patient with moderate tetanus in that he has frequent reflex spasms that cannot be controlled by muscle relaxants other than curare, and needs to be paralyzed with curare or another powerful relaxant. Curare may be given by intramuscular injection of 15 to 30 mg; if the patient must be paralyzed, there seems little to be gained by withholding the drug. At Oxford the nurses are instructed to give a further dose of curare when reflex spasms become obvious, and 400 mg of curare per day has been necessary. The high incidence of pulmonary embolus in patients with severe tetanus has led to the use of anticoagulants in patients severely enough affected to require treatment with curare and IPPV. Anticoagulants are not, however, used within 24 hours of tracheostomy. The treatment of a paralyzed patient with IPPV is complex, and appropriate monographs should be consulted (Adams et al., 1969; Spalding and Crampton Smith, 1963). The patient cannot breathe, and IPPV must be applied through the cuffed tracheostomy tube. It has become common practice in recent years to ventilate with a large tidal volume at a slow rate, for example, with a tidal volume of 1 liter and a rate of 12 to 14 per minute. An artificial dead space is introduced between ventilator and patient so that rebreathing of expired air may bring the tension of carbon dioxide in the arterial blood to about 30 mm Hg. Large tidal volumes seem to contribute to the health of the lungs, but the patient must also be turned every two hours to promote lung drainage, the inspired air must be fully humidified and at body temperature, and chest physiotherapy three times a day is indicated. Frequent chest films are necessary, and tracheal aspiration must be carried out with aseptic precautions. The patient cannot drink and must be fed by nasogastric tube or by vein if absorption fails. Patients with severe tetanus sweat profusely and may need large quantities of fluid, but the urine specific gravity is not always a good guide to hydration, and the patient should be weighed daily. It is not uncommon to observe a patient seriously ill with tetanus who is having a large fluid intake and gaining weight, but who still produces a high specific gravity urine. Later in the disease a diuresis may occur, and the patient may lose weight abruptly. A patient with severe tetanus needs 3000 calories per day, but too much protein is not advised, even though the patient, being functionally denervated by curare, may show muscle wasting. Urine is voided normally, but manual extraction of feces may be necessary. The patient cannot communicate, and sedation is probably indicated for patients paralyzed with curare. Withdrawal of sedation in severely ill patients may, however, disclose that the patient is unconscious.

Some patients most severely affected by tetanus develop a syndrome suggesting sympathetic overactivity. The cardiovascular component of this syndrome, tachycardia, arrhythmias, and hypertension, should be treated with beta- and alpha-adrenergic blockers (Prys-Roberts et al.). If it is thought necessary to administer a beta blocker intravenously, this should be done with great caution. Propranolol in 0.2 mg aliquots to a total of 2 mg has been successfully used to control arrhythmias and severe tachycardia. Control can sometimes be maintained by intragastric propranolol, 10 mg every eight hours, but larger doses may be required. In some cases, when hypertension is not severe, control of the heart rate may be all that is necessary, but if the blood pressure is elevated, alpha-adrenergic blockade is also indicated. Bethanidine, 5 mg by nasogastric tube every two hours, has been used successfully, and as this drug acts at postganglionic nerve endings, an overdose could be counteracted by pressor agents. The receptors, however, remain susceptible or perhaps hypersensitive to circulating catecholamines, and other combinations of antihypertensive drugs may be more effective. The author is aware of a patient successfully treated with propranolol, reserpine, and bethanidine. It is important not to reduce the heart rate to a point at which the cardiac output fails, because the depressed heart is working against an increased peripheral resistance. Moderate control of heart rate should be effected with a beta blocker, but hypertension when the heart rate is 100 or less must be controlled by alpha blockade.

In summary, in *a mild case* the patient needs (1) wound excision, (2) human or equine antitoxin, (3) penicillin or another appropriate antimicrobial drug, and (4) a centrally acting relaxant and sedative drug, such as diazepam.

In *the moderate case* the patient needs in addition (5) tracheostomy and the insertion of a cuffed rubber tracheostomy tube to separate the pharynx from the trachea and to make inhalation of foreign material impossible, and (6) nasogastric tube feeding.

In *the severe case* the patient needs in addition (7) virtually complete paralysis with curare or another powerful relaxant and IPPV, (8) anticoagulant drugs, and (9) if sympathetic overactivity is present, treatment with alpha- and beta-adrenergic blockers.

PROGNOSIS

The patient with mild tetanus will almost certainly survive whether treated or not. The patient with moderate tetanus, if untreated, is at risk from inhalation of foreign material. Repeated episodes of this kind may lead to fatal pneumonia. The patient with moderate tetanus, if treated, should not die except from causes unrelated to the primary disease. The patient with severe tetanus who is having reflex spasms severe enough to cause cyanosis will certainly die if untreated. Even with treatment, the severity of the illness and the complexity of the therapeutic regimen make the outlook uncertain. In the United Kingdom in 1967, even in the best centers the mortality in patients with tetanus severe enough to indicate treatment with curare and IPPV varied between 10 and 40 per cent. Over-all mortality in the best hands is often still as high as 20 per cent, and at the extremes of age the mortality may be higher. It is paradoxical that in advanced countries where the immunization programs are efficient, mortality in the cases that do occur is high, not only because unimmunized patients are generally at the extremes of age, but also because patients who escape the immunization programs tend to have a poor physical status. Tetanus is becoming increasingly common among drug addicts.

Adams, E. B., Laurence, D. R., and Smith, J. W. G.: Tetanus. Oxford, Blackwell Scientific Publications, 1969.

Bjørnboe, M., Ibsen, B., and Johnson, S.: Et tilfaelde af tetanus behandlet med curarisering, tracheostomi of overtryksventilation med kvaelstofforilte og ilt. Ugeskr. Laeger., 115:1535, 1953.

Kerr, J. H., Corbett, J. L., Prys-Roberts, C., Smith, A. C., and Spalding, J. M. K.: Involvement of the sympathetic nervous system in tetanus. Br. Med. J., 2:236, 1968.

Prys-Roberts, C., Corbett, J. L., Kerr, J. H., Smith, A. C., and Spalding, J. M. K.: Treatment of sympathetic overactivity in tetanus. Lancet, 1:542, 1969.

Wright, G. P.: Neurotoxins of *Clostridium botulinum* and *Clostridium tetani*. Pharmacol. Rev., 7:413, 1955.

ANAEROBIC BACTERIA

211. DISEASE DUE TO NONSPOREFORMING ANAEROBIC BACTERIA

Sydney M. Finegold

Definition. Essentially every type of infection may be caused by nonsporeforming anaerobes. No organ or tissue of the body is immune to infection with these organisms. The majority of anaerobic infections involve two or more anaerobes, but infection with a single species of anaerobe does occur. Aerobic or facultatively anaerobic organisms may also be present in mixed infections. In mixed anaerobic infections, clostridia may be found together with nonsporeforming anaerobic bacilli and cocci. There are a number of unique features associated with certain clostridial infections, however, and it is convenient to consider these infections separately (see Ch. 206 to 210). Actinomycosis may also show distinctive clinical features; this disease (also often a mixed infection) is discussed in Ch. 224.

Etiology. The nonsporulating anaerobic bacteria are distributed widely throughout the body as indigenous flora. Numerically, they are the dominant flora on the various mucosal surfaces.

The anaerobic gram-negative bacilli and the anaerobic cocci are the major etiologic agents in anaerobic infections. They are encountered at least 15 times as frequently as clostridia. Gram-positive nonsporeforming anaerobic bacilli are encountered less commonly.

Anaerobic Gram-Negative Bacilli. The anaerobic gram-negative bacilli found in human infections belong to the genera Bacteroides and Fusobacterium, the former being encountered with much greater frequency. *Bacteroides fragilis* is the most commonly seen of all anaerobes. It is of added importance because it is the most resistant of the anaerobes to antimicrobial compounds. The subspecies of *B. fragilis* recovered most often from infections are, in order, *ss. fragilis, ss. thetaiotaomicron,* and *ss. vulgatus. B. fragilis,* like other gram-negative anaerobic rods, stains poorly. The staining is usually irregular, with bipolar staining (and a central clear or light area) especially common. There is a variable amount of pleomorphism. Two other Bacteroides species seen relatively often, though rarely as single infecting agents, are *B. melaninogenicus* (coccobacilli) and *B. oralis* (morphologically similar to *B. fragilis*). *Fusobacterium nucleatum,* the fusiform bacillus, is the most frequently found of the fusobacteria. This organism is long and thin, with tapered ends; they are often in pairs end to end. Long filaments may also be noted. Granules (sometimes gram-positive) may be seen. *F. necrophorum,* formerly commonly encountered, is now seen much less. Other species of Fusobacterium seen include *F. mortiferum* and *F. varium,* the latter being relatively resistant to antimicrobials. Medically important fusobacteria other than *F. nucleatum* tend to be highly pleomorphic, with long filaments containing central swellings, large, free round bodies, and considerable irregularity of staining.

The spirochetes of the genus Treponema, also gram-negative anaerobes, which are part of the indigenous flora, are very likely not pathogenic, judging from experimental studies. The old terms "fusospirochetal infection" and "Vincent's infection" are therefore no longer appropriate.

Anaerobic Cocci. The anaerobic cocci include gram-positive streptococci (Peptostreptococcus), gram-positive cocci in pairs or masses (Peptococcus), and gram-negative cocci (Veillonella, Megasphaera, Acidaminococcus). The anaerobic cocci are not usually pleomorphic, but many are smaller than facultative streptococci. Veillonella are tiny cocci in masses. As a group, anaerobic cocci are found in human disease almost as often as are the gram-negative anaerobic bacilli. The most commonly encountered species include *Peptostreptococcus anaerobius, intermedius,* and *micros* and *Peptococcus magnus, asaccharolyticus, prevotii,* and *variabilis.*

The microaerophilic cocci and streptococci are a very poorly characterized heterogeneous group. They are best defined as organisms which tolerate reduced oxygen tension (18 per cent oxygen) – with or without added carbon dioxide. Most of these are probably actually facultative streptococci. These organisms are encountered in serious infections with some frequency, not uncommonly in pure culture. They are considered with the obligate anaerobes, because they will often be overlooked unless good anaerobic techniques are used for transporting and culturing clinical specimens.

Gram-Positive Nonsporeforming Anaerobic Bacilli. The most commonly encountered gram-positive anaerobic nonsporeforming bacilli belong to the genus Eubacterium, particularly *E. lentum, E. alactolyticum,* and *E. limosum.* Gram-positive anaerobic bacilli in general destain readily and may appear gram-negative. Eubacterium strains may be filamentous. Propionibacterium strains, chiefly *P. acnes,* are seldom involved in infections of significance other than endocarditis (in patients with pre-existing valvular disease or artificial heart valves) or other infections related to implanted artificial prostheses. *Bifidobacterium eriksonii* is another well-established pathogen. Actinomyces may also be involved in infections without the distinctive clinical features of actinomycosis.

Features of Infections Due to Various Organisms. There are differences in the types of infection involving various anaerobes related to differences in their distribution in the body as normal flora. Thus the anaerobic cocci are encountered more often in oral and pulmonary infections and in female genital infections than in intra-abdominal disease. *Bacteroides fragilis,* which is the dominant member of the colonic flora, is involved in intra-abdominal infection commonly but is less frequently involved in dental infections or lung abscess. Aside from these differences, all the nonsporeforming anaerobes may be involved in any of the infections to be discussed in this chapter. Furthermore, the clinical picture is basically the same in these conditions regardless of the specific flora involved. Minor exceptions include distinctive odors related to end-products of metabolism (e.g., butyric acid produced in large amounts by Fusobacterium strains), the occasional formation of soft granules resembling sulfur granules by Fusobacterium, and the production of black color in blood-containing exudates by *B. melaninogenicus.*

Relative Importance of Various Organisms in Mixed Infections. It is difficult to determine the role of each species recovered from a mixed anaerobic infection and to assess the relative importance of the anaerobes and aerobic or facultative bacteria in mixed infections. Quantitative culture techniques may help. A small number of patients with pulmonary and intra-abdominal mixed infections of mild to moderate severity have been treated with agents active only against the anaerobes and have done well. This suggests that the anaerobes may have been the key pathogens.

Incidence and Prevalence. Anaerobic infections are the most frequently overlooked or misdiagnosed of all bacterial infections. Fortunately, the introduction of simplified anaerobic cultural procedures and an increased awareness of anaerobes and their importance on the part of bacteriologists and clinicians are beginning to overcome the problem.

Good data on the incidence of anaerobes in various infections are not always available. One big problem has been a tendency to overlook anaerobes in mixed cultures when one or more aerobic or facultative forms are present. Problems in specific identification have interfered with accurate determination of the involvement of particular organisms in various anaerobic infections.

A major reason for the lack of good information is the fact that most published studies focus on only clinical aspects or bacteriologic features, but not both. Nevertheless, there are studies supporting the view that anaerobes are common causes of infection. Some years ago Stokes (1958) found anaerobes in over 10 per cent of 4737 positive cultures of clinical specimens. Lodenkämper and Stienen (1955) detected 690 anaerobic infections in an eight-year period. Mattman et al. (1958) found anaerobic cocci in 45 per cent of 437 positive cultures from hospitalized patients. Recently, Martin et al. (1972) isolated 601 anaerobes from clinical specimens in an eight-month period.

Several recent studies have combined good clinical and bacteriologic analysis to yield reliable information on the incidence of anaerobes in certain infections. Thus Heineman and Braude (1962) have shown that anaerobes are the dominant cause of brain abscess. Bartlett and coworkers (1972, 1973) have established that lung abscess and aspiration pneumonia are most often due to anaerobes and that these organisms are important causes of necrotizing pneumonia and of empyema. Several groups have data to indicate that at least half to two thirds of cases of intra-abdominal abscess and of peritonitis involve anaerobes. Very likely over half of all cases of pyogenic liver abscess also involve these organisms. Rotheram and Schick have demonstrated that anaerobes are the most prevalent pathogens in postabortal sepsis. Other types of infections in which anaerobes play an important role include chronic otitis media and sinusitis, gingivitis and other oral infections, dental infections, bronchiectasis, other pulmonary infections, breast abscess, appendicitis, diverticulitis, abdominal wound infections, puerperal sepsis, various other obstetrical and gynecologic infections, ischiorectal and perirectal abscess, infected pilonidal sinuses, gas-forming cellulitis, necrotizing fasciitis, and septic thrombophlebitis.

Pathogenesis or Mechanisms. Anaerobic bacteria basically are saprophytic members of the indigenous flora. Under certain conditions, however, they may invade and produce disease.

A simplistic definition of anaerobic bacteria would be bacteria which cannot survive in the presence of air. However, it is well known that a number of anaerobes generally regarded as fairly fastidious will tolerate 2 to 8 per cent oxygen in the atmosphere, and a number of these organisms will tolerate considerably more. A more important factor determining whether or not the environment is suitable for growth of anaerobic bacteria is the oxidation-reduction potential of the medium. This is a measure of the tendency of the system to give up electrons and is usually expressed as the Eh value in millivolts. The Eh of a system is a function not only of its inherent reducing tendency but also of its hydrogen ion concentration, the Eh becoming more negative as the hydrogen ion concentration decreases.

One of the major defenses of the body against infection by anaerobes is the normal Eh (+120 mv). Lowering of the redox potential permits anaerobic growth in tissues, even those exposed to air. Lowered oxidation-reduction potential results from impaired blood supply, tissue necrosis, and growth of facultative bacteria in a wound. Thus vascular disease, epinephrine injection, cold, shock, edema, trauma, surgery, presence of a foreign body, malignancy, gas production by microorganisms, and aerobic infection all may predispose to anaerobic infection. The predisposition of diabetics to anaerobic infection is undoubtedly related at least partially to impaired blood supply and lowering of Eh. The association of malignancy (particularly of the colon, the bronchus, and the uterus) and anaerobic infection is well established; at times, anaerobic infection may be the first clue to the malignant process.

Certain toxins such as collagenase, hyaluronidase, deoxyribonuclease, and proteinases account for the virulence of some anaerobic infections.

The septic thrombophlebitis seen commonly in anaerobic infections may relate to production of heparinase by anaerobic bacteria. This lesion may lead to metastatic infection and helps account for the difficulty in eradicating anaerobic infections. Tissue destruction and abscess formation are also common manifestations of anaerobic infection.

Previous antimicrobial therapy is a not uncommon background for anaerobic infection. Preoperative "bowel preparation" with oral neomycin often results in a residual anaerobic flora, as many anaerobes tolerate even the very high concentrations achieved in the bowel lumen with such therapy. The popular combination of gentamicin plus cephalothin (given parenterally) may lead to anaerobic superinfection, particularly with *Bacteroides fragilis.*

Conditions which predispose to infection in general (malnutrition, severe debilitating disease, corticosteroid and other immunosuppressive therapy, granulocytopenia) also facilitate anaerobic infection.

Aspiration and poor dental hygiene are common background factors in anaerobic pulmonary infection.

The unique involvement of only certain subspecies of *B. fragilis* in infection is probably related to resistance to normal serum bactericidal factors (Casciato et al., 1973). Under anaerobic conditions the granulocyte phagocytic bactericidal system may not function efficiently.

Clinical Manifestations.   For the most part the manifestations of anaerobic infection are those of the basic process (e.g., peritonsillar abscess, cholangitis, endometritis). Tissue necrosis, abscess formation, and septic thrombophlebitis are common with anaerobic infection, as are a foul odor and gas in tissues or in discharges.

Tonsillitis, Ludwig's Angina.   Exudative tonsillitis (Vincent's angina) used to be a common anaerobic infection, usually caused by *Fusobacterium necrophorum*. The local tonsillar infection undoubtedly still occurs but is rarely recognized as an anaerobic process. The dreaded Ludwig's angina (cellulitis of the submandibular space), probably an anaerobic infection in most cases, is also uncommon now.

Bacteremia, Endocarditis.   In recent years, bacteremia caused by anaerobes has dominated clinical reports on anaerobic infections. Most likely this is because anaerobes are much more likely to be present in pure culture in bacteremia than in other sources of anaerobic infection, and consequently it is much easier to isolate the offending organism. On the other hand, it is clear that anaerobic bacteremia is relatively common. At both the Mayo Clinic and the Oschsner Clinic, bacteroides are the second most common isolates from blood cultures. The primary sources of anaerobic bacteremia at present are gastrointestinal and gynecologic infections. Less common sites include infected decubitus ulcers and other wounds. Gram-negative anaerobic bacilli possess endotoxin, and septic shock and disseminated intravascular coagulation have been described in the course of anaerobic bacteremia.

In large series of endocarditis, only 1 to 2 per cent of positive blood cultures have yielded anaerobes as a rule. As high as 15 per cent, however, were sterile in the presence of strong clinical or pathologic evidence of endocarditis. Our experience is that approximately 10 per cent of cases of endocarditis are caused by anaerobic or microaerophilic cocci. The main portals of entry for anaerobes in bacterial endocarditis are the mouth, the gastrointestinal tract, and, to a lesser extent, the genitourinary tract. The incidence of pre-existing heart disease is lower in the case of anaerobic endocarditis, and there is evidence to indicate that embolization may be more common in the case of the disease involving anaerobes.

Pleuropulmonary Infection.   Anaerobic pulmonary infection is commonly overlooked. Unfortunately, even when suspected, it has often not been confirmed by proper culture of appropriate specimens. Coughed sputum culture is unsatisfactory because of the presence of anaerobes as normal upper respiratory tract flora. The clinical course of anaerobic pulmonary infection ranges from incidentally discovered infection to fulminant infection. Most patients present with a smoldering illness. The most common underlying condition is a predisposition to aspirate caused by altered consciousness or dysphagia. Important clues to anaerobic etiology are aspiration, pulmonary necrosis, indolent course, and foul-smelling sputum or pus. The principal types of anaerobic pulmonary infection are lung abscess, necrotizing pneumonia, and pneumonia without necrosis; many patients have an associated empyema.

Anaerobes are probably second only to the pneumococcus as causes of pneumonia in hospitalized patients, because aspiration pneumonia is a common event.

Intra-abdominal Infection.   Anaerobes are a prime cause of peritonitis and intra-abdominal abscess and are involved in virtually all cases of complicated appendicitis or diverticulitis.

Anaerobes (especially nonsporeformers) play a relatively minor role in gallbladder infection.

Genitourinary Tract Infection.   Various urinary tract infections may involve anaerobes, but these organisms are not common causes of such infection. Factors predisposing to anaerobic urinary tract infection are stones, malignancy, obstruction, and previous renal tuberculosis.

A large variety of female genital tract infections involve anaerobic bacteria. Clostridia cause the most serious female genital tract infections, but infections in this system are much more commonly produced by nonsporeforming anaerobic bacteria. Predisposing conditions include pregnancy, the puerperium (particularly with premature rupture of the membranes, prolonged labor, or postpartum hemorrhage), abortion (spontaneous or induced), malignancy, radiation, surgery, cauterization, stenosis, uterine fibroids, and old gonococcal salpingitis.

Skin, Soft Tissue, and Muscle Infection.   These infections include such entities as cellulitis, pyoderma, infected cysts, infection of decubitus and other ulcers, abscesses, bacterial synergistic gangrene, chronic undermining ulcer of Meleney, necrotizing fasciitis, bite infection, noma, and tropical ulcer. Anaerobes are common infecting agents in hidradenitis suppurativa. Subcutaneous abscesses involving anaerobes are seen in narcotic addicts who are "skin-poppers."

Anaerobic (gas-forming) cellulitis is an acute soft tissue infection, seen particularly in diabetics and commonly ascribed to coliforms. Although gas-producing nonanaerobes may be involved, it is our experience that anaerobes predominate. Muscle is not involved, but it is essential that clostridial myositis be ruled out. This differentiation may require surgery which, in any case, is important therapeutically.

Anaerobic streptococci may produce a myositis simulating "gas gangrene," but the infection is much less severe. Rarely, Bacteroides may be involved in a mild form of myositis.

Bone and Joint Infection.   Osteomyelitis caused by anaerobes is probably overlooked often. Anaerobes are relatively common in infected diabetic ulcers of the foot with bony involvement.

There are a number of well-documented cases of purulent arthritis caused by anaerobes, chiefly gram-negative bacilli. Predisposing factors include underlying joint disease and local or systemic corticosteroid therapy. Any joint may be affected, but there is a peculiar susceptibility of the sternoclavicular and sacroiliac joints.

Diagnosis.   *Clues Suggesting Anaerobic Infection.* Features indicating the likelihood of anaerobic infection include foul or putrid odor, infection located near mucosal surfaces (particularly with manipulation of the associated organs), tissue necrosis, gas in tissues or discharges, infection associated with malignancy or other tissue-destructive process, endocarditis with negative routine blood cultures, infection related to the use of aminoglycoside antimicrobials (by any route) and/or broad-spectrum penicillins or cephalosporins, septic thrombophlebitis, infection after bites, black coloration or red fluorescence under ultraviolet light of discharges or lesions (*B. melaninogenicus* infection), unique morphology on Gram stain of exudate, and failure to obtain growth on routine culture (particularly when organisms are seen on Gram stain of exudate).

Specimen Collection. The major consideration is to avoid "contaminating" a specimen with normal flora, because anaerobes are prevalent as indigenous flora.

Expectorated sputum is not suitable for anaerobic culture. Bronchoscopically obtained specimens are also not suitable, because the instrument becomes "contaminated" during insertion; however, fiberoptic bronchoscopy through a nasotracheal tube may prove to be satisfactory. Transtracheal needle aspiration or direct lung puncture is the optimal method of obtaining specimens.

In the case of uterine infection, the patient must be positioned to provide maximal exposure. The cervical os is decontaminated. Then material is obtained from the uterine cavity by syringe or swab technique, using great care to avoid normal vaginal flora. Rough quantitation of growth may help to distinguish between infecting organisms and normal flora, because a certain degree of contamination may be inevitable in this situation.

In the case of abscesses, unbroken skin or mucosal surface is decontaminated, and pus is removed with a syringe. This is preferable to using a swab on a portion of an exposed lesion.

Voided midstream urine may contain anaerobes from the urethral flora; therefore percutaneous suprapubic bladder aspiration is necessary.

Specimen Transport. Proper transport of specimens to the laboratory is crucial for recovery of anaerobes which may be present. Since some anaerobes are tolerant to oxygen contact, a laboratory which isolates such organisms as *B. fragilis* and *C. perfringens* may not realize that it is overlooking more demanding anaerobes. Many anaerobes responsible for clinical infections do not tolerate oxygen exposure well, so that special transport methods are needed to ensure their survival. Various means for proper anaerobic transport include the following:

1. Syringe technique—eliminate all air from specimen in syringe and needle and then stick needle into a sterile rubber stopper.
2. Gassed-out tubes—inject specimen into butyl rubber-stoppered tube which has been gassed out with oxygen-free CO_2. Commercial vials of this type are available.

Treatment. *General Aspects.* Surgical aspects of therapy are extremely important. Drainage of collections of pus and excision of necrotic tissue are commonly necessary, and in minor infections they may be all that is required. Obstructions must be relieved.

Anticoagulant therapy or venous ligation may be indicated in patients with septic phlebitis. Treatment of shock and disseminated intravascular coagulation, when they occur, and general supportive measures are important aspects of therapy.

Local use of hydrogen peroxide or zinc peroxide is useful. Hyperbaric oxygen therapy is not indicated in infection with nonsporeforming anaerobes.

Antimicrobial Therapy. In vitro susceptibility tests, properly performed, serve as a good guide to drug therapy of anaerobic infections. Standardized disc susceptibility tests are available for most anaerobic bacteria but are most satisfactory with organisms which have been identified. Use of a disc test without measurement of zones of inhibition, or application of standards which were developed for aerobic and facultative organisms, yields completely undependable results. Conventional tube or plate dilution tests with incubation in an anaerobic jar are reliable. Patterns of susceptibility to selected drugs are noted in the accompanying table.

Penicillin is active against most anaerobes other than *Bacteroides fragilis;* however, this organism is the anaerobe most commonly isolated from infection. Certain strains of anaerobic cocci require as much as 8.0 μg per milliliter for inhibition, and occasional strains of *Fusobacterium varium* are resistant to penicillin. Dosage of penicillin G should be at least 6 to 8 million units daily in the case of seriously ill patients or infection with relatively resistant strains. Ampicillin and cephaloridine are usually comparable to penicillin G, but several other penicillins and cephalosporins are less active. Some agents in these classes may be useful because very high blood levels are achieved safely or because of their resistance to beta lactamases.

Tetracycline is no longer valuable in many geographic areas, because many strains of anaerobes of all types are now resistant. Two new tetracycline derivatives, doxycycline and minocycline, are more active in vitro but have not yet been studied extensively clinically.

Lincomycin, erythromycin, and vancomycin are active against certain anaerobes; more information is needed, however, on the validity of in vitro tests with these drugs, and they are not approved by the Food and Drug Administration for use in anaerobic infections.

Chloramphenicol is active against all anaerobes, with only rare strains resistant, and is very effective clinically. It penetrates the central nervous system well. However, because of its serious and unpredictable toxicity, it should be reserved for seriously ill patients and used only until bacteriologic data indicate that a less toxic drug would be suitable. Nevertheless, chloramphenicol is the drug of choice for serious anaerobic infection of uncertain cause. Initial dosage of chloram-

Susceptibility of Anaerobes to Selected Antimicrobial Agents

	Microaerophilic and Anaerobic Cocci	Bacteroides fragilis	Bacteroides melanino-genicus	Fuso-bacterium varium	Other Fusobacterium Species	Eubacterium
Penicillin G	++++	+	++++	+++*	++++	++++
Clindamycin	+++	+++	+++	++	+++	+++*
Metronidazole†	++	+++	+++	+++	+++	?
Chloramphenicol	+++	+++	+++	+++	+++	+++

++++ Drug of choice.   ++ Moderate activity.
+++ Good activity.   + Poor or inconsistent activity.

*A few strains are resistant.
†Experimental for anaerobic infections.

phenicol in such a patient should be 40 to 50 mg per kilogram of body weight daily; once the patient has shown a good response, 30 mg per kilogram per day should be adequate.

Clindamycin (7-chlorolincomycin) has broad activity against anaerobes, with only *Fusobacterium varium,* among the nonsporeformers, commonly resistant. However, a number of strains of Clostridium other than *C. perfringens* are not uncommonly resistant. At the time of this writing it would be regarded as one of the drugs of choice for nonsporeforming anaerobic infections, except in very serious infections in which the nature of the infecting organism and its susceptibility to clindamycin are not yet known. Oral dosage for adults is 150 to 450 mg every six hours, and parenteral dosage is 600 to 2700 mg per day (in two to four equal doses), depending on the severity of the infection. Daily doses as high as 4.8 grams have been given intravenously to critically ill patients.

Metronidazole has broad activity against anaerobic microorganisms and is consistently bactericidal versus *Bacteroides fragilis* and other anaerobes. Its use for anaerobic infections is still on an experimental basis.

Although it is true that *Bacteroides fragilis* infections are more common below the diaphragm and that most anaerobes recovered from infections above the diaphragm are penicillin susceptible, there is too much overlap for practical application of this knowledge in the individual case — particularly if the patient has a serious infection. For example, *B. fragilis* is part of the infecting flora of 20 to 25 per cent of anaerobic pulmonary infections. It has also been recovered from such infections as sinusitis, mastoiditis, and brain abscess.

Therapy with antimicrobial agents in anaerobic infections must be intensive and prolonged. These infections have a considerable tendency to relapse.

Prognosis. In general, infection with nonsporeforming anaerobes carries a relatively good prognosis, provided the diagnosis is suspected and confirmed early and appropriate therapy instituted promptly. To some extent, of course, the prognosis varies with the site and extent of the lesion. Brain abscess is still a very serious infection with a significant mortality (50 per cent). The over-all

mortality in anaerobic pulmonary infections is 15 to 20 per cent, with a distinctly higher mortality in the case of necrotizing pneumonia (greater than 30 per cent). The mortality in liver abscess varies greatly from series to series, depending primarily on whether or not cases were discovered ante mortem and on how early they were picked up. On the whole, the mortality is in the range of 25 to 50 per cent. The mortality in sepsis caused by nonsporeforming anaerobes is 30 per cent. In patients with endocarditis caused by gram-negative anaerobic bacilli, mortality is also 30 per cent, but it is higher in cases caused by *Bacteroides fragilis* than in those caused by other, more sensitive gram-negative anaerobic bacilli. The mortality in endocarditis caused by anaerobic cocci is not significantly different from that caused by facultative streptococci. The availability of a number of effective drugs has permitted a reduction in mortality and morbidity resulting from anaerobic infection.

Prevention. The major principles in prophylaxis are avoidance of conditions which reduce the redox potential of the tissues and avoidance of the introduction of anaerobes from the indigenous flora into sites where they may set up infection. Discriminate use of antimicrobial drugs will minimize anaerobic superinfection.

Early appropriate therapy of anaerobic infections will prevent metastatic infection.

Precautions to minimize the possibility of aspiration will be helpful in preventing anaerobic pulmonary infection. Good surgical technique (e.g., minimal devitalization of tissue, use of closed methods of resection) will prevent postoperative anaerobic infections.

Bartlett, J., and Finegold, S. M.: Anaerobic pleuropulmonary infections. Medicine, 51:413, 1972.
Finegold, S. M., and Rosenblatt, J. E.: Practical aspects of anaerobic sepsis. Medicine, 52:311, 1973.
Goldsand, G., and Braude, A. I.: Anaerobic infections. D. M., November 1966.
Marcoux, J. A., Zabransky, R. J., Washington, J. A., II, Wellman, W. E., and Martin, W. J.: Bacteroides bacteremia: A review of 123 cases. Minn. Med., 53:1169, 1970.
Rotheram, E. B., Jr., and Schick, S. F.: Nonclostridial anaerobic bacteria in septic abortion. Am. J. Med., 46:80, 1969.
Saksena, D. S., Block, M. A., McHenry, M. C., and Truant, J. P.: Bacteroidaceae: Anaerobic organisms encountered in surgical infections. Surgery, 63:261, 1968.

TYPHOID FEVER AND SALMONELLOSIS

212. TYPHOID FEVER*

Abram S. Benenson

Definition. Typhoid fever is an acute, often severe illness caused by *Salmonella typhi* and characterized by fever, headache, apathy, cough, prostration, splenomegaly, maculopapular rash, and leukopenia. Typhoid fever is the classic example of enteric fever caused by salmonellae.

Incidence and Prevalence. Typhoid fever is a disease of major importance in areas of the world that have not at-

tained high standards of public health. A progressive decrease in incidence of typhoid fever has occurred in the United States since 1900, but sporadic cases and limited outbreaks continue to occur. About 400 cases per year have been reported in recent years; over a third of these were in persons under 15 years of age, and in about 10 per cent the patients were under 5 years. About 40 per cent of these infections were acquired in other areas of the world, but most were acquired in the United States from food contaminated by chronic typhoid carriers. In the United States more than 3000 chronic typhoid carriers are under supervision by health departments, but the actual number of chronic carriers is probably considerably higher. Typhoid fever will continue to occur on a limited scale in countries with high standards of public health because of the frequency of typhoid in other areas of the world, the magnitude of intercontinental travel, and the existence of reservoirs of chronic carriers.

---

*In the two previous editions the chapter on Typhoid Fever was written by Dr. Edward W. Hook. Significant portions of that chapter are included in the present version prepared by Dr. Benenson, who joins with the Editors in expressing indebtedness to Dr. Hook.

Epidemiology. The ultimate source of infection with *S. typhi* is man, either a patient with typhoid fever or a typhoid carrier. The patient with typhoid excretes large numbers of *S. typhi* in feces or urine, and viable bacilli may also be present in vomitus, respiratory secretions, or pus. Chronic enteric carriers, the most important source of infection, often excrete 10^6 or more viable bacilli per gram of feces. The typhoid bacillus can survive for weeks in water, ice, dust, and dried sewage. Water containing typhoid bacilli has been responsible for many outbreaks in the past; it may be contaminated directly by excreta containing *S. typhi* or by excreta washed down from remote sites by rain or introduced by faulty sanitation or plumbing. Foods may be contaminated by dirty hands or water contaminated by *S. typhi* and occasionally by contaminated dust. Flies are excellent mechanical vectors for the transmission of infection. Oysters and other shellfish may be infected in polluted tidal waters. In areas where typhoid fever is common, the incidence usually increases during the summer.

Pathogenesis. The portal of entry of *S. typhi* is almost always the gastrointestinal tract. In studies with human volunteers, bacilli were recovered from the stools within 24 hours after the organisms were swallowed; within a few days the stool usually became negative. The bacilli penetrate the intestinal epithelial lining without causing appreciable inflammation, and apparently enter the small lymphatics, reaching the mesenteric lymph nodes where they enter mononuclear cells within which they multiply. Although transient bacteremia may occur, the involvement of the reticuloepithelial cells in a proliferative process in liver, spleen, bone marrow, and other lymph nodes may be the response to circulating endotoxin. The incubation period represents the period for significant intracellular multiplication; its length is inversely proportional to the number of organisms ingested. When the symptoms do appear, there is a bacteremia; this has been considered to cause the clinical manifestations, although asymptomatic bacteremias have been observed not infrequently. Incidental to the systemic dissemination of bacilli, hepatomegaly occurs frequently, and infection of the biliary tract occurs regularly. Typhoid bacilli multiply in bile, with subsequent seeding of the intestinal tract with millions of bacilli. Infection of the gallbladder is usually asymptomatic, although symptoms of cholecystitis occasionally do develop.

The similarity of many manifestations of typhoid fever to the events observed after the intravenous injection of purified endotoxin of *S. typhi* suggests that the clinical picture is produced by these endotoxins. Both typhoid fever and injected endotoxin produce headache, chills, fever, anorexia, abdominal discomfort, myalgia, thrombocytopenia, and leukopenia. The specific pathologic findings of typhoid fever can be produced in the rabbit by intravenous administration of the purified endotoxin. Tolerance to the pyrogenic action of endotoxin is present during the convalescent phase of typhoid fever, and vascular hyper-reactivity to epinephrine or norepinephrine (exaggerated blood pressure rise after intravenous injection and local hemorrhagic lesions after intradermal injection) appears during the febrile phase of the disease and persists into convalescence. Both the development of tolerance and the vascular hyper-reactivity can be produced by endotoxin and strongly suggest that endotoxin does play an important role in human typhoid fever. However, volunteers made tolerant to endotoxin prior to challenge with *S. typhi* develop a clinical disease indistinguishable in severity and incubation period from that of controls, an observation apparently in conflict with the hypothesis that endotoxin released during infection is responsible for the early fever and other manifestations.

The infective dose of *S. typhi* is influenced by many factors. Epidemiologic data suggest that a few organisms, possibly 10 or 100, could initiate infection. Among human volunteers, 50 per cent developed overt disease after the oral ingestion of 10^7 viable *S. typhi* organisms of a strain containing the Vi antigen. When the same dose of non-Vi strains was administered, only 26 per cent developed disease, indicating the potential influence of different bacterial strains. Animal studies with *S. enteritis* have indicated that alteration in intestinal flora may increase susceptibility; pretreatment of human volunteers with streptomycin was followed by clinical disease in one of four volunteers given 1000 typhoid bacilli, a dose which produced no clinical disease in 14 untreated volunteers.

Pathology. A granulomatous proliferation of mononuclear cells with the formation of ill-defined nodular masses of reticulohistiocytic elements, principally in the mesenteric lymph nodes and spleen, together with a marked reactive follicular hyperplasia of lymphoid tissue, characterizes the pathology of typhoid fever. Hypertrophy of the lymphoid tissue of the small intestine, especially of the Peyer's patches in the terminal ileum, is followed by superficial coagulation necrosis; this sloughs to form an ulcer usually confined to the mucosa and submucosa. Erosion of blood vessels results in hemorrhage; extension of the ulcer into the muscularis and serosa leads to intestinal perforation. The liver is enlarged, and areas of focal granulomatous lesions form by the third week. Focal necrosis is also found in spleen, cardiac muscle, and lymph follicles. Bronchitis is common, and pneumonia caused by *S. typhi* or *Diplococcus pneumoniae* is not unusual.

Clinical Manifestations. The incubation period usually is eight to 14 days but varies from five days to five weeks. The duration of illness in an untreated case of average severity is about four weeks. The onset is usually gradual and associated with anorexia, lethargy, malaise, headache, general aches and pains, and fever. During the first week there is a gradually increasing remittent fever. Dull, continuous headache is a prominent symptom in almost all cases. About two thirds of the patients have a nonproductive cough, and epistaxis occurs in about 10 per cent. The majority of patients have vague abdominal pain or discomfort. Constipation is frequent and more common than diarrhea, which occurs in only about 20 per cent of the patients. During the second week of illness the fever shows less of a tendency to remit and is often sustained at around 40° C. During this phase patients are often severely ill with marked weakness, abdominal discomfort, and distention. Mental dullness is prominent, and delirium may occur. Diarrhea is more common during the second week than during the first, and stools may contain blood. As the illness extends into the third week, the patient continues to be febrile and becomes increasingly exhausted and weak. Patients without complications usually begin to improve during the third and fourth weeks. The fever gradually begins to decline, and the temperature may be normal by the end of the fourth week.

The physical signs vary with the stage of the disease.

During the first week fever and slight abdominal tenderness may be the only findings. However, during the second and third weeks findings characteristic of typhoid fever may develop. The patient appears acutely ill with a dull, expressionless, lethargic face. The mental state varies within wide limits from normal to frank mental confusion and delirium. The pulse is often not as fast as might be expected to accompany the degree of temperature present. Rhonchi or scattered moist rales may be present as a manifestation of bronchitis. The majority of patients have slight abdominal tenderness, most pronounced on the right side and in the upper abdomen. Abdominal distention may be severe. A soft spleen can be palpated in about three fourths of the patients. Maculopapular skin lesions appear during the second or third week of illness in about 80 to 90 per cent of patients with typhoid fever. These "rose spots" are 2 to 5 mm in diameter, blanch on pressure, are located predominantly on the upper abdomen or anterior chest, and are sparse, usually not exceeding 20 in number. The skin lesions last for two to four days and then disappear, but may be followed by fresh crops. The signs of illness subside as fever diminishes. Convalescence is slow; a month or more is often required to regain normal status.

Variation in the typical course described in preceding paragraphs is common. The illness may be mild and last only a week or may be prolonged, with a febrile course as long as eight weeks.

Laboratory Findings. Normochromic anemia develops during the course of the disease. Anemia may be aggravated by blood loss in stools. Leukopenia is frequent, and is characterized by a relative decrease in the number of polymorphonuclear leukocytes and an absence of eosinophils. Thrombocytopenia is common. Albuminuria is common during the febrile period of the disease. Feces often give a positive reaction for occult blood during the third and fourth weeks of illness.

S. typhi can be isolated from the blood in about 90 per cent of patients during the first week of disease and in about 50 per cent at the end of the third week; positive blood cultures are infrequent after the fourth week. The bacilli may persist in the bone marrow after blood cultures are negative. *S. typhi* can be isolated from feces at any stage of illness, but the greatest incidence of positive results is obtained during the third to fifth week when 85 per cent of the patients have positive cultures. Many reports indicate that typhoid bacilli can be cultured from the urine in about 25 per cent of those with typhoid fever during the third and fourth weeks of illness. Care should be taken in collection of urine to avoid contamination with feces containing typhoid bacilli.

The frequency of positive stool cultures begins to decrease rapidly about six weeks after onset of illness; two or three months after onset only 5 to 10 per cent of patients continue to excrete bacilli. Other patients become negative for typhoid bacilli during subsequent months, but approximately 3 per cent continue to excrete organisms for periods in excess of one year, becoming chronic enteric carriers. This occurs approximately three times more frequently when the disease occurs in an adult than in a child, and approximately two to three times as often among women than men. Many carriers give no past history of typhoid fever. Chloramphenicol therapy has not reduced the frequency of the chronic carrier state; among chloramphenicol-treated women in Chile a chronic carrier state existed in 2.3 per cent of

those who had been under 15 years old at time of disease versus 25 per cent among those who had been 35 years old or older. There was increased likelihood of the carrier state when the disease was more severe, when there was a relapse, when therapy was delayed, and when there were symptoms of gallbladder disease. Organisms persist in the gallbladder or biliary tract and enter the intestinal tract in large numbers in bile, resulting in as many as 10^6 or more virulent organisms per gram of feces. Chronic carriers will continue to excrete organisms for many years, usually for life, unless measures are taken to terminate the carrier state.

An increase in titer of agglutinins against the somatic (O) antigens and flagellar (H) antigens of *S. typhi* (Widal reaction) usually occurs during the course of typhoid fever, reaching a peak during the third week of illness. A fourfold or greater increase in titer in the absence of typhoid immunization during the previous four to six weeks should be considered highly suggestive of infection. In occasional cases there is no increase in agglutinins during the course of typhoid fever. The use of the agglutination reaction as a diagnostic test should always be subordinated to direct cultural demonstration of the causative organism.

Complications. *Intestinal hemorrhage* and *perforation* may occur during the second or third week of illness. Severe hemorrhage occurs in about 2 per cent of patients, although gross blood in feces is present in 10 to 20 per cent of cases, and a positive test for occult blood is even more common. Intestinal perforation, usually in the lower ileum, develops in about 1 per cent of cases and is the most serious of all complications of typhoid fever. The first signs of hemorrhage or perforation may be a sudden drop in temperature and an increase in pulse rate. Often, however, one or more episodes of bleeding will precede a perforation. The perforation is usually associated with acute abdominal pain, tenderness, and rigidity, which are most marked in the right lower quadrant of the abdomen. Signs of peritonitis develop rapidly after perforation, and temperature returns to febrile levels. Thrombophlebitis, particularly of the femoral vein, pneumonia, and cholecystitis occur in a small proportion of patients. Other complications include osteomyelitis, meningitis, and localized infection of almost any organ. Alopecia was a well known sequel of typhoid fever in the preantimicrobial era. The incidence of abortion is increased when typhoid fever occurs during pregnancy, especially during the first trimester.

Relapse. One or two weeks after defervescence illness may recur with signs and symptoms similar to those during the initial illness, including bacteremia. Relapse occurs in 8 to 10 per cent of patients with typhoid fever who do not receive antimicrobial therapy and in 10 to 20 per cent of patients treated with chloramphenicol. The relapse is usually milder than the initial episode but may be severe, even fatal. Manifestations may last as long as three weeks during a relapse. Second and third relapses have been described.

Diagnosis. The diagnosis of typhoid fever can often be suspected on the basis of the clinical picture. Definitive diagnosis is established by isolation of the organism from blood or feces, or, occasionally, from sputum or purulent exudates. A fourfold or greater increase in agglutinin titers, in the absence of recent immunization, provides confirmatory evidence of infection. However, when the rise in antibodies is only against the O antigen, infection with other salmonellae in Group D, which share common somatic antigens (IX, XII), must be considered.

Since in the early stages the patient frequently appears ill, is highly febrile, and has a leukopenia and no localizing signs, the differential diagnostic possibilities include many diseases. Prominent among these are systemic infections with other salmonellae, disseminated tuberculosis, malaria, leptospirosis, brucellosis, shigellosis, murine typhus fever, tularemia, Rocky Mountain spotted fever, acute bronchitis, influenza, and pneumonia caused by viruses or *Mycoplasma pneumoniae*. Central nervous system manifestations may suggest meningitis or encephalitis. Certain nonmicrobial diseases associated with fever and abdominal complaints, such as Hodgkin's disease, may also be confused with typhoid fever. Herpes labialis is rare in typhoid fever, and its presence should lead to a consideration of other diagnoses.

Prognosis. The fatality rate prior to effective antimicrobial therapy varied among different socioeconomic and age groups but was around 10 per cent. Death was usually associated with profound toxemia, intestinal perforation, intestinal hemorrhage, or intercurrent pneumonia. The fatality rate since the introduction of chloramphenicol is 1 or 2 per cent when facilities are available for appropriate supportive care.

Treatment. Chloramphenicol has been employed successfully in the management of typhoid fever since 1948 and is still the antimicrobial agent of choice. However, in 1972 and 1973, typhoid bacilli isolated in Mexico, Kerala (India), Saigon, and Bangkok were resistant to chloramphenicol, tetracycline, streptomycin, and sulfonamides; all but a few were susceptible to ampicillin. Thus isolates should be tested for drug susceptibility, especially if infection may have been acquired in these areas or if the response to therapy is disappointing. Chloramphenicol is given orally in doses of approximately 50 mg per kilogram per day in four divided doses until the temperature is normal; thereafter, the dose may be reduced to 30 mg per kilogram per day. Chloramphenicol therapy should be continued for a total of two weeks. Response to treatment is not rapid. Patients usually show subjective improvement after one or two days, but the temperature does not return to normal until three to five days after the beginning of therapy. Hemorrhage and perforation may develop during chloramphenicol therapy, even in afebrile patients. Treatment of relapse is the same as for the initial episode. Chloramphenicol may result in suppression of agglutinin response in patients treated during the early phase of typhoid fever.

Ampicillin is also effective in the treatment of typhoid fever. As mentioned above, ampicillin is particularly valuable for treatment of infections with chloramphenicol-resistant strains, but the response appears to be slower with ampicillin than with chloramphenicol. If ampicillin is used in the treatment of typhoid fever, a total daily dose of 150 to 200 mg per kilogram of body weight should be administered intravenously in four divided doses until the patient is afebrile, and should then be continued orally for a total of two weeks of therapy. With highly susceptible strains, 40 mg per kilogram per day intramuscularly may suffice.

Typhoid organisms whose multiple-drug resistance is due to the prevalent R factor, a plasmid transferable to other enterobacteria, retain their susceptibility to a variety of other antimicrobial drugs, none of which have yet been evaluated for effectiveness in treatment of typhoid fever. Several studies have suggested that trimethoprim-sulfamethoxazole is comparable to chloramphenicol in treatment of typhoid, and that it was effective in the management of chloramphenicol-resistant infections. The use of prednisone or drugs with similar activity should be considered for patients with severe toxemia and pyrexia. Prednisone should be given in a dose of 60 mg per day in four divided doses for the first day, 40 mg during the second day, and 20 mg on the third day; corticosteroid therapy should be discontinued after the third day. In patients treated with prednisone, temperature returns to normal or occasionally decreases to hypothermic levels within hours, and the toxic state rapidly ameliorates. Prednisone should be administered only in conjunction with appropriate antimicrobial therapy, and under these conditions it does not increase the risk of complications.

Perforation, although previously managed by surgical means, is now usually treated conservatively without surgical intervention. When perforation occurs, the antityphoid drug therapy should be continued, and additional antimicrobial drugs administered to control multiplication of intestinal flora in the peritoneal space. Transfusion is required for large hemorrhages.

Patients with typhoid fever are unusually sensitive to the antipyretic effect of salicylates and may develop profound hypothermia after small doses. Tepid sponge baths are effective in lowering temperature and should be used instead of salicylates. Laxatives and enemas should not be used because of the danger of inciting intestinal perforation or hemorrhage.

Treatment of Carriers. Cholecystectomy results in termination of the chronic enteric carrier state in about 85 per cent of cases. When the organism has been shown to be susceptible to it, ampicillin, in a total dose of 6 grams per day given orally in four equal doses for a period of six weeks, combined with probenecid, will apparently terminate the carrier state in most patients without gallstones and with normal gallbladder function as indicated by cholecystogram. Ampicillin occasionally terminates the carrier state in persons with evidence of gallbladder disease or gallstones, but the proportion of apparent cures is less than 25 per cent. Penicillin G in doses of 12 million units or more daily combined with probenecid for 14 days has also been successful in terminating the carrier state in some persons. Chloramphenicol has not been shown to be effective in the treatment of the chronic carrier state and should not be used in this situation.

Prophylaxis. Controlled field trials have shown that typhoid vaccine is effective in reducing the incidence of disease, and that acetone-killed and dried vaccine was more effective than the heat phenol product. Protection has not been correlated with any specific antibody response. The immunity is relative and can be overcome by exposure to a large number of organisms; no protection could be demonstrated in healthy volunteers against an oral dose of 10^7 organisms, a dose known to produce disease in 50 per cent of normal subjects. Immunization should be considered for inhabitants of areas where the incidence of the disease is high, for travelers to these areas, and for persons working with *S. typhi*. A course of immunization consists of two subcutaneous injections of 0.5 ml of vaccine separated by four or more weeks. Booster doses should be given at three-year intervals if exposure continues. Local discomfort and fever frequently follow administration of the vaccine; these can be alleviated by an antipyretic. Booster doses of the heat phenol vaccine can be inoculated intradermally in doses of 0.1 ml with less systemic reaction. The acetone-killed and dried product, however, should *not* be injected intradermally, because it produces local pain and tenderness more marked than after subcutaneous injection.

Patients with typhoid fever should remain in isolation during hospitalization. Persons known to be carriers should not be permitted to work as food handlers; members of their households should be immunized against the disease.

Second attacks of typhoid fever have been observed, but as a general rule one attack confers lifelong immunity comparable to that elicited by the inactivated vaccine.

Armijo, R., Pizzi, A., and Lobos, H.: Prevalence of typhoid carriers after treatment with chloramphenicol. Bol. Of. Sanit. Panam., 62:295, 1967.

Ashcroft, M. T., Singh, B., Nicholson, C. C., Ritchie, J. M., Sobryan, E., and Williams, F.: A seven-year field trial of two typhoid vaccines in Guyana. Lancet, 2:1056, 1967.

Cvjetanovic, B., and Uemura, K.: The present status of field and laboratory studies of typhoid and paratyphoid vaccines. Bull. WHO, 32:29, 1965.

Dinbar, A., Altman, G., and Tulcinsky, D. B.: The treatment of chronic biliary Salmonella carriers. Am. J. Med., 47:236, 1969.

Hornick, R. B., Greisman, S. E., Woodward, T. E., DuPont, H. L., Dawkins, A. T., and Snyder, M. J.: Typhoid fever: Pathogenesis and immunologic control. N. Engl. J. Med., 283:686, 739, 1970.

Huckstep, R. L.: Typhoid Fever and Other Salmonella Infections. Edinburgh, E. and S. Livingstone, Ltd., 1962.

Lawrence, R. M., Goldstein, E., and Hoeprich, P. D.: Typhoid fever caused by chloramphenicol-resistant organisms. J.A.M.A., 224:861, 1973.

Marselis, J. G., Jr., Kaye, D., Connolly, C. S., and Hook, E. W.: Quantitative bacteriology of the typhoid carrier state. Am. J. Trop. Med. Hyg., 13:425, 1964.

Overturf, G., Marton, K. I., and Mathies, A. W., Jr.: Antibiotic resistance in typhoid fever. N. Engl. J. Med., 289:463, 1972.

Robertson, R. P., Wahab, M. F. A., and Raasch, F. O.: Evaluation of chloramphenicol and ampicillin in Salmonella enteric fever. N. Engl. J. Med., 278:171, 1968.

Stuart, B. M., and Pullen, R. L.: Typhoid: Clinical analysis of three hundred and sixty cases. Arch. Intern. Med., 78:629, 1946.

Woodward, T. E., and Smadel, J. E.: Management of typhoid fever and its complications. Ann. Intern. Med., 60:144, 1964.

213. SALMONELLA INFECTIONS OTHER THAN TYPHOID FEVER

Edward W. Hook

Definition. The genus Salmonella consists of more than 1700 serotypes and variants. These organisms with a few exceptions are primary pathogens for animals that are readily transmitted to man. The outstanding exception is *S. typhi,* which is a parasite only of man and does not cause disease in lower animals in nature.

Human infection with Salmonella may be expressed as *acute gastroenteritis, enteric fever* (paratyphoid fever), *bacteremia,* or *localized metastatic infection* at almost any site. The clinical syndromes resulting from Salmonella infection cannot always be sharply differentiated and sometimes overlap.

Transient *asymptomatic infection* of the intestinal tract is also common with most serotypes. A *chronic carrier state* may occur occasionally after infection with Salmonella other than *S. typhi,* and is characterized by prolonged excretion of the organism in feces or urine.

Typhoid fever is considered in a separate chapter (see Ch. 212) because of its historical identity, the host specificity of the pathogen, and the wealth of data on basic and clinical aspects of the disease. This separation is unrealistic to the extent that an illness closely resembling typhoid fever can result from infection with other salmonellae, and *S. typhi* can on occasion produce all the clinical syndromes described for the other Salmonella serotypes.

Etiology. Salmonellae are gram-negative, aerobic, nonsporing rods that grow readily on simple culture media. Presumptive identification of salmonellae involves relatively simple biochemical and agglutination reactions, but definitive identification of serotype depends on precise analysis of the somatic (O) and flagellar (H) antigens of the organism. Subdivision of certain serotypes, for example *S. typhimurium,* can be achieved by bacteriophage typing. Specific identification of all isolates is desirable, especially for epidemiologic reasons, and can be obtained through local, state, or federal health agencies.

Salmonella serotypes most frequently isolated from human infections in the United States during 1972 were, in descending order of frequency, *S. typhimurium, S. newport, S. enteritidis, S. infantis, S. heidelberg, S. saintpaul, S. thompson, S. derby, S. oranienburg,* and *S. javiana.* These ten serotypes accounted for about 66 per cent of the total Salmonella isolates from man during 1972. *S. typhimurium* is the serotype most frequently isolated year after year, usually accounting for 20 to 30 per cent of the total.

Incidence and Prevalence. Salmonellae are widespread among members of the Animal Kingdom in all parts of the world. Virtually all domestic and wild animal species have been shown to harbor these organisms, and infection rates range from 1 per cent to more than 40 per cent. For example, in certain studies salmonellae have been isolated from 41 per cent of turkeys, 7 to 50 per cent of swine, and 24 per cent of apparently healthy cattle.

In 1972, 26,110 isolations of Salmonella from humans were reported in the United States. The annual incidence of reported isolations has remained approximately constant since 1963, the first full year of operation of the Salmonella Surveillance System in the United States. The true incidence of human salmonellosis is probably much higher than the number of reported cases.

The prevalence of asymptomatic human carriers of salmonellae in the general population has been estimated to be about 0.2 per cent. The carrier state in the vast majority of these people is transient and probably represents persistence of organisms in the stools after asymptomatic or mild intestinal infection. The transient carrier state is more frequent in persons whose occupations provide opportunity for contact with Salmonella in foods, such as professional food processors or abattoir workers, than in the general population.

Epidemiology. Man almost always acquires Salmonella infection by the oral route. Any item of food or drink can be contaminated directly or indirectly with viable bacilli from infected animals or man and can serve as a source of infection. Although the role of human carriers in the spread of salmonellosis must not be minimized, the majority of infections of man in the United States are related to the enormous reservoirs of salmonellae in lower animals.

The greatest single source of human disease is poultry products, including chickens, turkeys, ducks, and eggs. Other animal meats, especially pork, beef, and lamb, also serve as sources of infection. Salmonellae on meats or other foods contaminate utensils, tables, and other items in the processing plant, market, or kitchen, and may be transferred from these items to previously uninfected foods. A significant proportion (1 to 58 per cent) of raw meat purchased in retail markets is contaminated with salmonellae.

Eggs or egg products are common sources of Salmonella infection. The bacilli may be found on the external surface of the eggshell, between the shell and the shell membranes, or in yolks of eggs from hens with ovarian infection. The incidence of infection of eggs is low, but pooling of large numbers for freezing or drying increases the possibility of contamination of large quantities of materials. Prepared food mixtures containing dried eggs have been implicated many times in outbreaks of Salmonella infection.

Sterilization of contaminated foods is not always achieved by cooking. Viable salmonellae contaminating large birds such as turkeys, especially if the fowl is stuffed, may persist despite the baking process, and organisms in eggs occasionally survive frying, scrambling, or boiling in the shell.

The numerous byproducts of the meat-packing industry, such as bone meal, fertilizer, domestic animal food, and fish meal, often contain salmonellae and may serve as sources of infection, especially among lower animals. Finally, in considering potential sources of infection, household pets, including dogs, cats, birds, and turtles, should not be overlooked; all have been shown to harbor salmonellae.

Direct transmission from man to man without food as the intermediate source does occur. Person-to-person transmission appears to be a relatively common mode of spread in hospital outbreaks, especially those occurring in nurseries or pediatric wards. For example, salmonellae may be introduced into a nursery by a newborn infected at birth from an infected mother and then spread to other babies by nursery attendants. Several nursery and hospital outbreaks have also been described in which infection appeared to be perpetuated by airborne spread of salmonellae.

S. choleraesuis bacteremia has been reported in immunologically compromised patients who received platelet transfusions from a donor with chronic intermittent bacteremia secondary to minimally symptomatic osteomyelitis.

Pathology. Death from Salmonella gastroenteritis occurs primarily in infants, the aged, and persons with underlying diseases. The intestinal mucosa is red and swollen and often shows petechial hemorrhages. The pathologic findings in paratyphoid fever are qualitatively similar to those of typhoid fever, although the involvement of Peyer's patches is less prominent and ulcerations are much less frequent. Intestinal lesions are usually absent in patients with Salmonella bacteremia, and the findings are similar to those of any acute generalized infection. Blood-borne salmonellae may localize in almost any organ, producing single or multiple suppurative lesions.

Pathogenesis. Multiplication of salmonellae in the intestinal tract is associated with invasion of mucosal cells of the small intestine, inflammation of the intestinal mucosa, and symptoms of gastroenteritis. Gastroenteritis is a true infection of the mucosa; ingestion of a large number of dead bacilli will not produce the disease. An enterotoxin analogous to that produced by *Vibrio*

cholerae and certain other enteric pathogens has not been demonstrated.

Salmonellae multiplying in the intestinal tract occasionally gain access to the blood, producing transient bacteremia or localized infections that can serve as sources of persistent bacteremia. The pathogenesis of enteric or paratyphoid fever is similar to that of typhoid fever.

The prevalence of salmonellae in foods for human consumption makes it almost inevitable that man come in contact with these organisms relatively frequently. The outcome of such exposures depends on many factors, especially the characteristics of the Salmonella serotype, the number of bacteria ingested, and the status of the host.

Every serotype of Salmonella has the capacity to produce asymptomatic infection, acute gastroenteritis, bacteremia with or without localized infection, or paratyphoid fever. However, some serotypes are much more likely to produce certain of these clinical syndromes than others. For example, *S. anatum* usually produces inapparent infection or gastroenteritis and only rarely invades the blood. In contrast, *S. choleraesuis* only occasionally produces gastroenteritis or inapparent infection but is a common cause of bacteremia or metastatic infection. Differences in pathogenicity are observed not only between serotypes, but also between strains of the same serotype.

Limited information is available on the number of organisms required to produce salmonellosis in man. Experiments in volunteers suggest that a large number (approximately 10^5 to 10^6) of viable salmonellae are usually required to produce gastroenteritis in normal adults. A transient carrier state may follow ingestion of inocula 10 or 100 times smaller than those required to produce disease.

The resistance of the host also plays a major role in determining the wide range of responses from no disease to rapidly fatal illness observed in human salmonellosis. Local factors in the stomach and intestine may be the first lines of defense. It is known that salmonellae are rapidly killed at pH of 2, a level readily attained in the stomach, and that concomitant administration of certain antacids reduces the challenge dose of organisms required to initiate infection under experimental conditions. It has been established that major gastric surgery, including subtotal gastrectomy, gastroenterostomy, and/or vagotomy, predisposes to Salmonella gastroenteritis. The mechanism of this effect is unknown, but may be related to reduced bactericidal acitivity of gastric juice or altered intestinal flora. It has been shown in experimental Salmonella infections of mice that the microbial flora of the normal intestine exerts a protective action by suppressing multiplication of salmonellae. In these studies alteration of intestinal flora by antimicrobial drugs increased susceptibility to infection with *S. typhimurium* 100,000 times, and resistance was restored by re-establishing the normal enteric flora. Prior antimicrobial therapy also enhances susceptibility of man to symptomatic intestinal infection with salmonellae.

The incidence of severe Salmonella infections is increased in patients with certain underlying diseases. Another process, such as hepatic cirrhosis, lupus erythematosus, leukemia, lymphoma, or neoplasm, is present in one third to one half of patients with Salmonella bacteremia. These conditions are associated with a general depression of resistance to microbial invasion, and secondary infection is not unexpected. However, in a few diseases – acute bartonellosis, sickle cell anemia, and, perhaps, malaria – there appears to be a predisposition to infection with salmonellae that exceeds any general susceptibility to other bacterial species. The acute hemolytic phase of bartonellosis is complicated by the development of Salmonella bacteremia in as many as 40 per cent of cases. Patients with sickle cell anemia and other sickle hemoglobinopathies are unusually susceptible to invasion of the blood by Salmonella, and there is a strong tendency for localization of infection in bone. In fact, Salmonella species, not staphylococci, account for the vast majority of instances of osteomyelitis in patients with sickle cell anemia. Osteomyelitis is probably related to the localization of organisms in the areas of ischemia and necrosis of bone so common in sickle cell anemia; this is but one example of the striking tendency of salmonellae to localize at sites of pre-existing disease. Localization of salmonellae has been reported in vascular aneurysms, bone compressed by aortic aneurysms, hematomas, areas of infarction, and a variety of cysts and neoplasms.

Clinical Manifestations. *Salmonella Gastroenteritis.* Symptoms of gastroenteritis develop 8 to 48 hours after ingestion of contaminated food. The relatively long incubation period represents the time required for multiplication and invasion by the organism. Nausea and vomiting are common initial manifestations and are rapidly followed by colicky abdominal pain and persistent diarrhea, occasionally with mucus or blood. Nausea and vomiting are rarely severe or protracted. An initial chill is not unusual, and fever of 38 to 39° C is common. Symptoms usually subside in two to five days, and recovery is uneventful.

Considerable variation in the severity of Salmonella gastroenteritis is observed, even among patients infected at the same meal. Some patients have a mild afebrile disease with a few loose stools, whereas others have high fever and 30 to 40 liquid stools per day. Severe diarrhea occasionally occurs in an afebrile patient. Abdominal pain may be intense, localized, and associated with rebound tenderness, suggesting appendicitis or some other acute intra-abdominal process. Symptoms of gastroenteritis persist in some patients for as long as two weeks.

The leukocyte count is usually normal, and blood cultures are sterile in almost all cases. The causative organism can be isolated from the feces of almost all patients during the acute illness. About 50 per cent of the patients continue to have stool cultures positive for salmonellae at two weeks after onset of gastroenteritis, but only 15 per cent remain positive at the end of the fourth week. A small proportion of patients continue to excrete organisms after two months, but in most of these the cultures become negative in the next six months. The period of excretion of organisms in stool tends to be longer in infants than in older children or adults. The term "chronic enteric carrier" should be reserved for the patient shown to have persistently positive stools with the same Salmonella species for one or more years.

Enteric or Paratyphoid Fever. Salmonellae other than *S. typhosa* may produce an illness with all the features of typhoid fever, including prolonged sustained fever, respiratory and gastrointestinal symptoms, rose spots, leukopenia, and positive blood, stool, and urine cultures. Although paratyphoid fever may be clinically indistinguishable from typhoid fever, it is usually milder with a shorter course and a lower mortality rate. The or-

ganisms most likely to produce this syndrome are *S. paratyphi A*, *S. paratyphi B*, and *S. choleraesuis.* Paratyphoid fever is occasionally preceded by manifestations of Salmonella gastroenteritis.

Bacteremia. Salmonellae also produce a clinical syndrome that is characterized by chills, prolonged intermittent fever, anorexia, and weight loss. The characteristic features of typhoid or paratyphoid fever, such as rose spots, sustained fever, and leukopenia, are absent. Patients with this form of illness usually have no gastrointestinal complaints, and, indeed, stool cultures are usually negative for the causative organism despite its presence in blood. The leukocyte count is normal in most cases.

A prolonged febrile illness lasting weeks or months and characterized by weight loss, anemia, hepatosplenomegaly, and bacteremia with salmonellae, including *S. typhosa,* has been described in South America and the Middle East in patients with schistosomiasis. The organisms apparently find a protected environment for multiplication within the gut of the worm. Eradication of the worms may also result in cure of the bacterial infection (see Ch. 296).

Localized Disease. Signs of localized infection appear in many cases of Salmonella bacteremia. Abscess formation may occur at almost any site, or bronchopneumonia, empyema, endocarditis, pericarditis, pyelonephritis, osteomyelitis, or arthritis may develop. Meningitis is a focal manifestation more common in newborns and infants than in adults. Patients with localized infections usually have striking polymorphonuclear leukocytosis as high as 20,000 to 30,000 cells per cubic millimeter of blood.

Diagnosis. Salmonella gastroenteritis must be differentiated from other acute diarrheal diseases, especially shigellosis, invasive and enterotoxigenic *Escherichia coli* infection, staphylococcal food poisoning, and enteritis produced by viral agents. A short incubation period, absence of fever, and prominence of nausea and vomiting are characteristic of staphylococcal food poisoning, whereas tenesmus, dysentery, and numerous fecal leukocytes suggest a diagnosis of shigellosis. However, differentiation on the basis of clinical information alone is difficult, especially in sporadic cases, and definitive diagnosis depends on isolation of the causative organism from the stool.

In patients with enteric fever, blood cultures are usually positive early in the course of the disease, and feces and urine become positive somewhat later. In patients with Salmonella bacteremia, the organisms can be isolated from blood, or in some cases from pus or exudate from localized infection.

Patients with salmonellosis may show during the course of illness a fourfold or greater increase in titer of agglutinins against the causative organism or closely related species. However, agglutination tests performed in the ordinary clinical laboratory are usually not helpful in diagnosis, because only a limited number of Salmonella antigens are used.

Treatment. The most important aspect of the management of patients with Salmonella gastroenteritis is prompt correction of dehydration and electrolyte disturbances. Diphenoxylate hydrochloride with atropine (Lomotil), paregoric, or small doses of morphine may be used to relieve abdominal cramps and diarrhea if contraindications do not exist. There is no convincing evidence that antimicrobial drugs, including chloramphenicol, ampicillin, or trimethoprim combined with sulfonamide, reduce the duration of illness or the period of excretion of organisms in the stool. In fact, recent studies indicate that the period of excretion of salmonellae in the stool during convalescence after symptomatic intestinal infection is actually longer in patients who have been treated with antimicrobial drugs during the acute illness than in patients who have received no antimicrobial therapy.

In Salmonella bacteremia, paratyphoid fever, or localized infections of bones, joints, meninges, and other sites, chloramphenicol is the drug of choice and should be administered in divided doses of about 50 mg per kilogram per day for at least two weeks. Four to six days may be required for defervescence in favorable cases and even longer in patients with localized infection. In patients with localized infections, it may be necessary to continue antimicrobial therapy for four to six weeks, and surgical drainage of collections of pus may be required. Salmonellae persisting in tissues during chloramphenicol therapy may be responsible for relapse after the antimicrobial is discontinued. Relapse is not related to the emergence of chloramphenicol-resistant strains during therapy, and clinical response to a second or third course of therapy usually differs in no way from the first.

Ampicillin has also been shown to be effective in treating paratyphoid fever, but the response to ampicillin is slower than the response to chloramphenicol. Ampicillin is also often effective in the treatment of other systemic Salmonella infections if the causative organism is susceptible to this drug. Ampicillin is preferred over chloramphenicol for patients requiring prolonged therapy. Approximately 10 to 20 per cent of the *S. typhimurium* strains isolated in the United States and a somewhat higher proportion in England are resistant to ampicillin. Ampicillin resistance is mediated by transferable resistance determinants or R factors, and is uncommon among serologic types other than *S. typhimurium*. Strains of Salmonella resistant to chloramphenicol do occur but are not common, with the exception of *S. typhi* in Mexico, Vietnam, and certain areas of India. Nevertheless, the physician must remain alert to the possibility of chloramphenicol resistance among nontyphoidal strains.

Excretion of salmonellae in stool after clinical or subclinical infection ceases spontaneously in almost all patients; the convalescent carrier state is not an indication for antimicrobial therapy. Chronic enteric carriers of salmonellae other than *S. typhi* are managed as are typhoid carriers.

Prognosis. The case fatality rate in Salmonella gastroenteritis rarely exceeds 1 or 2 per cent, and probably averages about 0.3 per cent. Fatalities occur almost entirely in infants, the aged, and persons with major underlying disease. The case fatality rate in the more serious systemic infections is high; it approaches 20 per cent in *S. choleraesuis* bacteremia.

Prevention. Every effort should be made to prevent the spread of salmonellae among the population by the excreta of patients with acute illness and convalescent or chronic carriers. Patients with acute illness should be isolated, and convalescent or chronic carriers should not be employed as food handlers and should practice strict personal hygiene.

The control of salmonellosis among animals and prevention of spread of infection to man present many problems. Progress is being made in developing methods of detection and control of salmonellosis in domestic animals and in improving hygienic conditions in food-processing and food-dispensing establishments.

Aserkoff, B., and Bennett, J. V.: Effect of therapy in acute salmonellosis on salmonellae in feces. N. Engl. J. Med., 281:636, 1969.
Bauer, H.: Growing problem of salmonellosis in modern society. Medicine, 52:323, 1973.
Bennett, I. L., Jr., and Hook, E. W.: Infectious diseases (some aspects of salmonellosis). Ann. Rev. Med., 10:1, 1959.
Center for Disease Control: Salmonella Surveillance Annual Summary, 1972. Issued November 1973. Atlanta, Georgia.
Musher, D. M., and Rubenstein, A. D.: Permanent carriers of nontyphosa salmonellae. Arch. Intern. Med., 132:869, 1973.
Rhame, F. S., Root, R. K., MacLowry, J. D., Dadisman, T. A., and Bennett, J. V.: Salmonella septicemia from platelet transfusions. Study of an outbreak traced to a hematogenous carrier of *Salmonella choleraesuis*. Ann. Intern. Med., 78:633, 1973.
Wahab, M. F. A., Robertson, R. P., and Raasch, F. O.: Paratyphoid A fever. Ann. Intern. Med., 70:913, 1969.

OTHER BACTERIAL INFECTIONS

214. ENTERIC BACTERIAL INFECTIONS

Calvin M. Kunin

Definition. The wide variety of microorganisms commonly found in the gastrointestinal tract, particularly the gram-negative, nonsporulating bacilli, have become increasingly important in clinical medicine. They are the principal organisms found in infections of the abdominal viscera, peritoneum, and urinary tract, as well as being frequent secondary invaders of the respiratory tract, burned or traumatized skin, and sites of decreased host resistance and instrumentation. Currently, they are the most frequent cause of life-threatening bacteremia. Infections with these organisms will be considered together because of their common habitat in the gut and on mucous surfaces, the similarity of epidemiologic and pathogenic characteristics, and the common approach used in diagnosis, treatment, and prevention.

Bacteriology. The gastrointestinal flora is exceedingly complex. The large intestine contains about 10^{10} to 10^{11} organisms per gram of contents. Of these, 90 to 95 per cent are obligate anaerobes. Most common are the gram-negative bacilli, Bacteroides and Fusobacterium, gram-positive bacilli, including Bifidobacterium, Eubacterium, and Corynebacterium species, and a wide variety of anaerobic streptococci. Other anaerobes include the gram-positive spore-forming rods of the clostridia species and gram-negative cocci, Veillonella. Enterococci are also present. The well-known aerobic gram-negative rods, which are members of the family Enterobacteriaceae, account for only 5 to 10 per cent of the total flora. These include the most common, *E. coli*, as well as the Klebsiella-Enterobacter group, Proteus, Providencia, Edwardsiella, Serratia, and, under pathologic conditions, Salmonella and Shigella. Pseudomonas is an entirely unrelated species, and is usually found in only small numbers in the bowel. Various yeasts are also found in lesser numbers in the normal large intestine.

Although the human gastrointestinal tract is usually considered to be colonized in the anatomic regions proximal to the cardia of the stomach and distal to the ileocecal valve, recent studies have demonstrated organisms in the jejunum and almost always in the ileum. Moderate changes in the diet do not affect the ratio of predominant bacteria in the feces, but antimicrobial therapy has a strong selective effect and is the single most important reason for the increasing emergence in human infection of these heretofore unusual organisms.

All the microorganisms of the gastrointestinal tract are potentially pathogenic under conditions of altered host resistance. The major diagnostic problem is to differentiate superficial colonization from actual tissue invasion.

Endotoxin. The gram-negative bacteria of the gastrointestinal tract produce disease by invasion of tissue and by release of a pharmacologically active lipopolysaccharide from the cell wall, known as endotoxin. Endotoxins from a wide variety of unrelated species behave quite similarly, regardless of the inherent pathogenicity of the microorganism from which they are derived or their antigenic structure.

In the intact microorganism they exist as complexes of lipid, polysaccharide, and protein. The biologic activity seems to be a property of a lipid and carbohydrate portion. The cell wall of gram-negative bacteria may be roughly divided into three regions. The outermost region contains the chains of specific sugars which characterize the O-specific antigens and determine individual serotypes within a species. This is linked to a core polysaccharide which is of similar structure among related groups of bacteria. This is in turn linked through 2-keto-3-deoxy-octonate trisaccharides to the major lipid component termed lipid A. Evidence has now accumulated to indicate that all the properties of endotoxin may be accounted for by this complex lipid substance. Lipid A is a polymer containing glucosamine disaccharide units linked through pyrophosphate bridges and esterified with lauric, palmitic, and myristic acids. Perhaps the most important finding in recent years is that lipid A is immunogenic and will induce antibodies which cross-react among the gram-negative bacteria. Animal studies reveal that antibody prepared against the active component of endotoxin will protect against challenge from heterologous gram-negative bacteria. The frequency of shock and death in patients with gram-negative bacteria appears to be lower in individuals with initially high titers of cross-reacting antibody to the Re or core lipopolysaccharide (lipid A) component. These findings hold promise for development of immunoprophylaxis and therapy.

When inoculated intravenously, the endotoxins cause fever, leukopenia, circulatory collapse, capillary hemorrhages, necrosis of tumors, and the Shwartzman phenomenon. Noteworthy is the remarkable tolerance that develops after repeated injections of endotoxin. For example, the first intravenous injection in man of as little as 0.01 ml of typhoid vaccine will give rise to a violent response, with chill and high fever; yet after 10 to 14 daily injections of increasing quantities, the subject can accept 25 ml or more without symptoms and with only a slight rise in temperature. This state of tolerance is not obviously dependent on specific antibodies; it extends to endotoxins of unrelated bacterial strains. The clinical features of gram-negative bacteremia resemble the reaction of laboratory animals or man to intravenous injection of purified endotoxic preparations, and may well represent a direct "pharmacologic" response to bacterial endotoxin. In other types of infectious process there is reason to doubt that such phenomena as fever, leukocytosis, and leukopenia are direct effects of endotoxin liberation.

The phenomenon of endotoxin tolerance may explain the remarkable tendency of the symptoms of pyelonephritis to subside spontaneously. By contrast, endotoxin tolerance is not a feature of experimental typhoid fever, but, rather, volunteers infected with this organism have been shown to be hypersensitive to its effects. Endotoxin tolerance is currently under intensive study because of the presumed important pathologic effect of this substance. The often conflicting observations on tolerance to the fever-producing property of endotoxin now appear to be due to the fact that multiple phenomena are operating simultaneously. Endotoxin is believed to be pyrogenic by inducing macrophages (monocytes, Kupffer and related cells) to release a protein, termed endogenous pyrogen. This protein is carried in the circulation to the temperature-regulating nuclei in the hypothalamus, producing an alteration in thermoregulation. Frequent, repeated doses of endotoxin are thought to exhaust the cells' capability of releasing this substance. More prolonged exposure is believed to induce antibodies which block the action of endotoxin.

Antibodies. Antibodies reacting with most Enterobacteriaceae can be demonstrated in sera of normal animals and man, probably because of the continual production of antigen in the gastrointestinal tract. Gram-negative bacteria contain a wide variety of antigenic determinants. The best studied include the H or flagellar antigens which are heat-labile proteins present in motile strains. They have not been shown to be of pathogenetic significance. Some of the enteric bacteria contain K or capsular polysaccharides (they are particularly prominent among Klebsiella, but are not confined to this group). These surface slime layers interfere with phagocytosis and may be important in imparting virulence to encapsulated strains. They appear to account for invasiveness but not toxicity. The *Enterobacteriaceae* share a common antigen (CA). Antibody to core lipopolysaccharide, described above, is currently thought to be the key determinant of resistance to endotoxin damage. Antibodies to the O or somatic antigens of *E. coli* have been most extensively studied. Very low titers are present in human newborns, presumably because they are mostly of the high molecular weight IgM variety, and do not readily pass the placenta. Human colostrum is rich in O antibody, but this is not absorbed during breast feeding. Colonization of the digestive tract, however, is soon accompanied by appearance of a wide variety of antibodies in serum, which contains virtually all the *E. coli* O antibodies by one year of age. It is likely that the great susceptibility of the newborn to overwhelming gram-negative bacterial sepsis is related to lack of maternal antibodies.

As a rule, most strains are susceptible to opsonization and lysis by the combined effects of antibody and complement. Some strains, however, seem insusceptible to lysis in vitro. Nonetheless, this system may be of great importance in preventing strains from invading and persisting in the blood.

Tests for Endotoxemia. A remarkably sensitive test for endotoxemia has been developed, based on the finding that small amounts will cause gelation of lysates of amebocytes of the horseshoe crab. The test must be currently considered primarily as a research test, because, although it is commonly positive in gram-negative bacteremia, this is not always true, and a positive test does not correlate well with the outcome of infection. Since endotoxemia does not require living organisms, the test may be positive in the absence of detectable bacteremia. A less sensitive test is based on the enhanced cutaneous vasoconstriction that follows intradermal injection of the patient's serum into rabbits given endotoxin intravenously. This test must also be considered as investigational. Perhaps the most important aspect of these tests is that they offer strong evidence that endotoxin is indeed often present in the blood of patients with gram-negative sepsis.

THE ROLE OF ENTERIC BACTERIA IN PYOGENIC INFECTIONS OF THE ABDOMINAL CAVITY

The mixed flora of the intestinal tract participate in infections that originate from lesions of the bowel, such as appendicitis, cholangitis, diverticulitis, and perforation (from ulcerative colitis, ileitis, or carcinoma). These may lead to subdiaphragmatic, hepatic, and pelvic abscesses, which are frequent causes of fever of unknown origin in the patient recovering from abdominal surgery or trauma to this region. Because enteric bacteria grow luxuriantly in both aerobic and anaerobic media and therefore are likely to predominate in cultures, their relative importance tends to be exaggerated. There is good reason to believe that anaerobic bacteria — bacteroides, clostridia, and anaerobic streptococci — play more important roles in this kind of process. It should be pointed out here that a "fecal" odor of pus, though often ascribed to coliforms, is doubtless caused by associated anaerobic bacteria. Anaerobic bacteria are usually present as mixtures of two or more species. They should be suspected when there is foul pus and when organisms can be visualized microscopically but fail to grow under routine conditions.

OTHER INFECTIONS CAUSED BY THE ENTERIC BACTERIA

Gastroenteritis. A significant proportion of cases of gastroenteritis occurring in the neonatal period of life appear to be caused by enteric bacteria. About ten serologic strains of *E. coli* have been identified with this capability; they are spoken of as enteropathogenic strains. Outbreaks of diarrhea among adults, particularly travelers abroad, have been associated with enterotoxigenic strains of *E. coli*. Sporadic epidemics with invasive strains have been reported after ingestion of imported cheese. Certain strains of Proteus and Pseudomonas have at times also been held responsible for similar illness.

Meningitis and Brain Abscess. During the first four weeks of life, purulent meningitis is frequently caused by members of the enteric group of bacteria. Such cases occur sporadically in nurseries, and may be associated with infection of any other tissue of the body. Infants with meningoceles are especially liable to enteric bacterial meningitis. In adults, such infections are rare, but

may occasionally be seen as complications of gram-negative bacteremia or in association with other diseases affecting host resistance, e.g., diabetes mellitus or lymphoma (see Ch. 201). Nontraumatic brain abscess is frequently due to infection by multiple species of anaerobic organisms similar to those found in the gastrointestinal tract. The sites of origin include chronically infected ears, sinuses, lung, abdomen, and pelvis.

Bacteremia in Hepatic Cirrhosis. Occasionally persons with cirrhosis of the liver develop an acute febrile illness and are found to have bacteremia caused by one of the enteric organisms, usually *E. coli*. Occasionally these patients have signs of peritonitis, but in most of them the event comes "out of the blue" without evidence of localized sepsis anywhere. The illness is short and self-limited or responds to appropriate chemotherapy. Speculation as to its pathogenesis has included the possibility of shunting bacteria away from the filtering action of the liver, impairment of humoral or cellular defense mechanisms, or complement inactivation owing to high blood ammonia. In actuality a satisfactory explanation is lacking at present.

Surface Infection. Enteric bacteria, particularly Proteus and Pseudomonas, are commonly recovered from the surfaces of burns, varicose ulcers, decubitus ulcers, tracheostomy sites, and the like. Generally, these organisms appear to play no pathogenic role, and satisfactory healing may proceed regardless of their presence. They can at times result in fulminant gram-negative sepsis, particularly in the patient with severe burns. The exudate from the sinus of a chronic osteomyelitis or chronic otitis media often contains Proteus as the dominant organism. Otitis of the external auditory canal owing to Pseudomonas may give troublesome local symptoms, especially in swimmers.

Perirectal Abscess. This is an important complication in patients with marked granulocytopenia. Rectal examination should be carefully performed in such patients, particularly when they develop fever and perianal pain.

Abscesses at Sites of Subcutaneous Injections. Rarely, enteric bacilli cause abscesses in subcutaneous tissue at sites of hypodermic injections, notably in diabetic subjects who inject their own insulin. These are sometimes characterized by gas formation, and they thus arouse fear of more serious clostridial infection, whereas, in fact, they are usually of minor clinical importance.

Metastatic Infections. Despite the frequency with which enteric bacteria succeed in invading the blood, metastatic localization of infection is rare. There are, however, occasional instances of such suppurative lesions as arthritis and panophthalmitis in patients with bacteremia originating in acute pyelonephritis. Of special interest in this regard is osteomyelitis of the spine. This is usually seen in men with prostatic disease, chronic cystitis, and posterior urethritis. Possibly the method of spread here is by way of septic emboli to the spine through the vertebral venous plexus.

Superinfection. Enteric bacteria frequently predominate in the bronchial secretions of patients under treatment with large doses of penicillin or broad-spectrum antimicrobial agents. In most instances, this is not of significance and simply represents emergence of unaffected bacterial strains after the suppression of the primary pathogens. Transtracheal aspiration, followed by gram stain and culture of the secretions, is a useful method to distinguish between colonization of the pharynx versus true infection of the lower respiratory tract. It is not an indication for cessation or change in antimicrobial therapy unless there is clinical evidence of tissue invasion by the newly emergent organism. Primary gram-negative bacterial pneumonia often superimposed on viral influenza, however, does occur and may be exceedingly difficult to manage.

GRAM-NEGATIVE BACTEREMIA

Bacteremia caused by gram-negative bacilli has become a problem of greater relative importance since the advent of penicillin and better control of gram-positive coccal infections. Urinary tract infection accounts for about two thirds of all cases of blood invasion by the enteric bacteria. Other causes include surgical disease of the gastrointestinal tract, infections developing at the site of "cut-downs" and intravenous catheters, postpartum or postabortal sepsis (including the so-called "placental bacteremia"), and infection of wounds, ulcers, burns, and internal prosthetic devices such as heart valves. Sometimes there is a clearly apparent precipitating factor such as cystoscopy, surgical or obstetrical procedure, or manipulation of an infected wound.

These bacteremias have clinical characteristics closely resembling the recognized biologic effects of gram-negative bacterial endotoxins. Onset of symptoms may occur with a shaking chill and rise in temperature of 38 to 40.5° C. There is an initial leukopenia, but after 6 to 12 hours usually there is leukocytosis. An *important and highly significant accompaniment is circulatory embarrassment with lowering of the blood pressure.* This may be manifested only by some alteration in the patient's state of consciousness, and the skin may continue to feel warm, although sometimes the skin is cold and clammy. Occasionally patients slip into a shocklike state without much elevation of temperature; hence infection of this kind must always be taken into consideration in evaluation of peripheral circulatory failure. Petechial hemorrhages and purpura are not common. Some patients, however, do develop the syndrome of disseminated intravascular coagulation (DIC). This phenomenon is not unique to gram-negative bacteremia and may be due to such diverse causes as rickettsial and gram-positive bacterial infections. The most common findings are reduced platelet count, low factor V levels in plasma, and fibrin split products in serum. Serum complement is low only in the most seriously ill patients. There are diminution in urine output, increase in proteinuria, and often a rise in nonprotein nitrogen of the blood. The cardiac output may be unpredictably low, normal, or elevated. Some patients show shifts in acid-base balance in the direction of metabolic acidosis, whereas others have compensatory hyperventilation. The pH of the blood, however, often remains normal. Lactic acidosis is common in severely ill patients. It is characterized by a marked anion gap with low levels of both serum bicarbonate and P_{CO_2}. These findings are often confusing, particularly if they occur in patients with complicating problems such as pulmonary or renal insufficiency or congestive heart failure. Serum lactate levels are helpful in sorting out these factors. Much depends on the nature of the underlying disease and the renal reserve. The outlook is grave, being influenced by age, associated disease, and evidence of shock. When obvious signs of circulatory collapse are present, the fatality rate may be as high as 75 per cent.

UNIQUE FEATURES OF PSEUDOMONAS INFECTIONS

Pseudomonas infections, although often similar to those caused by other gram-negative bacteria, sometimes have unique characteristics. As already mentioned, this organism frequently appears in necrotic tissue, as in ulcers, burns, or draining sinuses. Usually such colonization is of little clinical significance, and mere removal of necrotic tissue may cause it to disappear. Nevertheless, under certain circumstances, especially in chronically debilitated persons or in patients with agranulocytosis or acute leukemia, severe sepsis may be produced by this class of bacteria.

Pseudomonas is notoriously resistant to antimicrobial therapy; hence it tends to emerge as the dominant microorganism after eradication of other bacteria by drugs, and it may then be responsible for the phenomenon of superinfection, as in the bronchopulmonary infections that may complicate prophylactic chemotherapy of chronic lung disease.

Because Pseudomonas commonly occurs in tap water, and because it may be resistant to antiseptics used in sterilizing instruments, it is likely to be carried into the body by such procedures as cystoscopy. Furthermore, most of the reported instances of meningitis after lumbar puncture have been associated with this organism.

Tissue invasion, most often seen in patients with leukopenia or relapse in leukemia, is characterized by necrotizing vasculitis with bacterial invasion of the walls of arteries and veins. This leads to a distinctive necrotic skin lesion (called ecthyma gangrenosum) that is found most commonly along the axillary folds or in the anogenital area, but may also develop on any part of the body. It may begin as a vesicle that later becomes necrotic. The typical lesion of ecthyma gangrenosa is a round, indurated ulcer with a black center that varies from a few millimeters to several centimeters in diameter.

TREATMENT OF ENTERIC BACTERIAL INFECTIONS

General Principles. The major clinical problems in management of enteric bacterial infections are (1) differentiation of superficial contamination that often requires no treatment from true or potential tissue invasion, (2) early recognition and drainage of abscesses, (3) anticipation of the role of anaerobic bacteria that cannot be readily cultured, and (4) early recognition of bacteremic shock. *Many of these infections are preventable,* particularly those arising from instrumentation of the urinary tract, intravenous catheters and contaminated fluids, suction, and ventilation equipment. *Every physician must consider elimination of such sources of contamination as one of his prime responsibilities.*

Gram-Negative Bacteremia. The presence of gram-negative organisms in the blood should alert the physician to search for a site of origin such as intravenous or urinary catheters and abdominal or perirectal abscesses. Removal of devices and drainage of abscesses should be done as soon as possible. Antimicrobial therapy should be guided as often as possible by in vitro drug-susceptibility tests because of the remarkable ability of enteric bacteria to develop resistant strains. Among the aminoglycoside antimicrobials, gentamicin and kanamycin are most reliable, followed by streptomycin. Rapid emergence of resistant strains is a major problem with streptomycin. It should rarely be used alone. The so-called broad-spectrum drugs such as tetracycline and chloramphenicol are also useful against the Enterobacteriaceae, as are ampicillin and cephalothin. They are most often effective when not previously used in the patient, because emergence of resistant strains is common. Drug susceptibility tests are essential to guide the choice of drugs. Large doses of penicillin G are effective against many of the gram-positive and some gram-negative anaerobes. Chloramphenicol, clindamycin, and occasionally tetracycline are useful for Bacteroides, whereas Pseudomonas will generally respond only to drugs such as polymyxin B or colistin methane sulfonate (polymyxin E) and gentamicin. Carbenicillin is a new semisynthetic penicillin that may be of considerable value in treatment of Pseudomonas, Enterobacter, and Proteus infections. The problems are the large doses required, development of resistance, tendency for sodium overload (4.7 mEq per gram), and high cost. It should be reserved for clearly established infection caused by a susceptible organism. It is generally advisable to use two and sometimes more agents, including gentamicin, in severe gram-negative sepsis, particularly when bacteriologic identification is delayed.

Antimicrobial therapy in severe gram-negative sepsis is often a guessing game, but it can be approached with a reasonable rationale rather than, as is often the practice, merely by giving large doses of the most currently popular antimicrobial drugs. It should be remembered that gram-negative bacteremia is more common than is usually suspected and is often transient and without complication. For example, bacteremia may occur after gastrointestinal endoscopy, urinary instrumentation, and manipulation of the bowel during surgery. These events often go undetected, or there is a single temperature rise and no further complications. Antimicrobial therapy probably plays little role in management of these transient episodes. The main problem is caused by the release of endotoxin. Endotoxin is not affected by antimicrobial drugs. Judgment will therefore have to be made to determine whether there is an infected site which requires treatment.

The site of origin of the infection, the underlying illness of the patient, and prior receipt of antimicrobial agents are key determinants in planning therapy. For infection arising in the urinary tract in a patient not previously on chemotherapy, relatively safe drugs such as ampicillin, tetracycline, or a cephalosporin should be effective. For patients previously receiving multiple antimicrobials, gentamicin is preferred. Mixed anaerobic infections in patients with a perforated abdominal organ or a brain abscess should receive large doses of aqueous penicillin G plus chloramphenicol. Clindamycin also shows great promise as an effective agent for the anaerobic intestinal flora. A cephalosporin may be substituted for penicillin G in the allergic patient, although cross-sensitization has been described. Acute cholecystitis is often associated with E. coli in the gallbladder. Ampicillin or tetracyclines or chloramphenicol are recommended as the first drug, provided they have not been used previously. Gentamicin should be added if the course is complicated. Pneumonia caused by gram-negative bacteria is usually overdiagnosed. It is best established by transtracheal aspiration or culture of the blood, pleural fluid, and, occasionally, percutaneous lung aspiration.

The clinician must distinguish this from the superficial gram-negative bacterial colonization of the oropharynx which commonly accompanies debility or antimicrobial therapy. It almost uniformly occurs in patients with tracheostomies and usually should not be treated. In addition, patients with debility or difficulty in clearing secretions will often aspirate the oral contents and develop a mixed anaerobic infection of the lung. This problem is best treated with large doses of penicillin or clindamycin rather than with drugs used for aerobic gram-negative infections. True gram-negative pneumonia (as defined above) should be treated with the most potent agents, depending in part on drug susceptibility tests. Gentamicin is probably the single most effective agent. Cephalosporins are useful for Klebsiella; ampicillin tends to be more effective for Enterobacter, whereas gentamicin alone or with carbenicillin is useful for Pseudomonas. Gram-negative sepsis in patients with burns or leukemia is often due to Pseudomonas and should be treated with gentamicin and carbenicillin. The subject of antimicrobial therapy is considered in greater detail in Ch. 267 and 268.

Management of bacteremic shock is complex, requiring corrective measures designed to improve cardiac function, tissue perfusion, and electrolyte imbalance, particularly acidosis. This requires monitoring of the central venous pressure by a well-placed catheter in the superior vena cava or right atrium in an attempt to achieve a pressure of about 8 to 12 cm of water, and following the dynamics of pressure changes as fluid replacement is given. Replacement fluids include blood, dextran, and saline solutions. Drugs such as isoproterenol may be used to increase cardiac output and improve tissue perfusion; vasopressors such as metaraminol should be used sparingly except in severe shock. High doses of corticosteroids are widely used, but their efficacy has not been established by controlled studies. Heparin may be useful in the syndrome of disseminated intravascular coagulation.

Blair, E., Wise, A., and MacKay, A. G.: Gram-negative bacteremic shock. J.A.M.A., 207:333, 1968.
Editorial: Consumption coagulopathy in septicemic shock. N. Engl. J. Med., 279:884, 1968.
Moore, W. E. C., Cato, E. P., and Holdeman, L. V.: Anaerobic bacteria of the gastrointestinal flora and their occurrence in clinical infections. J. Infect. Dis., 119:641, 1969.
Steinhauer, B. W., Eickhoff, T. C., Kislak, J. W., and Finland, M.: The Klebsiella-Enterobacter-Serratia division. Clinical and epidemiologic characteristics. Ann. Intern. Med., 65:1180, 1966.

215. SHIGELLOSIS

Leighton E. Cluff

Definition. Shigellosis is an enteric infection with one of the species of Shigella bacilli, which may be asymptomatic or may cause dysentery.

Bacillary dysentery is usually a self-limited, acute illness characterized by diarrhea with mucous-bloody feces, tenesmus, fever, and abdominal colic and tenderness. Symptomless infected persons and those convalescing from dysentery may harbor Shigella in the stool for several days, serving as a source of infection for others. The infection is worldwide and is most common among persons living in crowded unhygienic circumstances. Man is the principal host to the microorganism, and the infection is usually transmitted from person to person, directly or indirectly.

History. Dysentery has been recognized for centuries. Delineation of dysentery attributable to Shigella, however, was not possible until 1896, when epidemic diarrhea in Japan was shown by Shiga to be caused by a specific microorganism.

Association of the bacillus isolated from feces of patients with the disease was possible by demonstration of rising titers of specific serum agglutinins in a significant proportion of patients. Subsequently, Flexner, Boyd, and Lentz identified other species of Shigella bacilli responsible for dysentery in man. From the beginning, dysentery has been a nemesis to encamped military troops, persons living in unhygienic conditions, and patients in mental institutions. It has occasionally caused epidemic disease in hospitals, nurseries, and schools. Currently, Shigella infection is responsible for a significant proportion of diarrheal disease particularly among children and older persons living in crowded urban areas. There was a progressive increase in the number of infections identified in England and Wales after 1940. Over 40,000 cases were noted in 1960.

Etiology. Strains of Shigella can be characterized antigenically, and there are four serologic groups responsible for disease in man. These are usually identified as serotypes of *Shigella dysenteriae* (shiga), *Shigella flexneri, Shigella boydii,* and *Shigella sonnei.* Another group, formerly referred to as *Shigella alkalescens,* may also produce enteric infection in man, but biochemically and antigenically it is more closely related to coliform bacilli.

The shigellae are gram-negative, slender, nonmotile, nonsporulating bacilli, which on primary isolation resemble coccobacilli. They are aerobic and facultative anaerobic, growing readily on relatively simple media at 37° C. They can be selectively grown in the presence of various bile salts (SS and desoxycholate media), thereby being distinguished from most coliform bacilli. Species and strains of Shigella can be identified by carbohydrate fermentation and antigenic analysis with specific antiserum. As with other enteric pathogens, Shigella bacilli do not ordinarily ferment lactose.

Epidemiology. Shigellosis is most common in tropical countries under unhygienic, crowded conditions, but is endemic throughout the world.

Young children appear to be more susceptible than adults to bacillary dysentery, but the disease is less common in the first six months of life than in older infants and children. Eighty per cent of children under nine years of age infected with Shigella will develop dysentery, whereas only about 50 per cent of infected older persons develop illness. Under the age of 20 years the frequency of shigellosis in males is greater than in females, but over the age of 20 years the reverse is true. Nevertheless, the case fatality rate is higher in men at all ages. In some countries bacillary dysentery has its peak incidence in summer months, often after heavy rains, whereas in other areas, such as the United States, the highest incidence may be in winter, spring, or autumn. The months when shigellosis is particularly prevalent in tropical and semitropical countries correspond with the time of year when flies are prevalent. Shigella may be found in the intestinal tracts of flies having contact with infected human feces, but carriage of the bacilli on the insect's feet is probably the means by which it may spread infection. In countries with a high standard of sanitation flies play an inconsequential role in transfer of infection.

Infection is usually transmitted by patients with dysentery, ambulatory persons convalescing from the disease, or asymptomatic carriers. Inadequately washed hands or contaminated inanimate articles are the principal means of transmission. The seats of toilets may become contaminated during flushing and serve as a source of infection. Epidemics of shigellosis have been related to milk, ice cream, and other foods and water contaminated by the hands or feces of infected persons. Shigella in dust has also been incriminated in outbreaks of bacillary dysentery. These sources of infection are also important in perpetuation of endemic infection. Outbreaks of shigellosis in winter usually spread from an infected person in a school or institution to other persons. Secondary cases may result in extension of the disease to other schools or institutions such as hospitals or nurseries. Relapsing disease, reinfection, and chronic infection may enable perpetuation of infection among patients in nursing homes and inmates of mental hospitals. In this setting, outbreaks are often not explosive.

Endemic and epidemic shigellosis is commonly characterized by isolation of several different serologic types of Shigella. Major outbreaks caused by a single serotype are rare, but small outbreaks may be attributable to a single serologic type.

Shigella dysenteriae (shiga) is an uncommon cause of infection in Britain, Europe, and North America, but is responsible for a significant proportion of cases in Asia. *Shigella sonnei* is the prominent cause of bacillary dysentery in countries where personal contact and endemic infection, rather than poor sanitation and unhygienic conditions, are responsible for spread of the disease.

After infection, the bacilli may be isolated from feces or rectum for only a week or slightly longer. Rarely does carriage of the bacilli persist as long as three months. Carriage of *Shigella dysenteriae* (shiga), however, persists longer than with other species, and carriage of *Shigella flexneri* may be intermittent during convalescence from infection. Generally, however, persistent carriers of *Shigella dysenteriae* remain ill, whereas carriers of *Shigella flexneri* are well. Convalescence from infection caused by *Shigella sonnei* is not associated with prolonged excretion of the bacilli in feces except in the very young and very old.

Although Shigella infection is largely confined to human beings, primates have been shown occasionally to be a source of infection in man. Shigella survive in eggs, oysters, clams, and shrimp for many days, but these serve as sources of infection only when contaminated by infected persons and their excreta.

Pathogenesis and Pathology. Shigella species possess an endotoxin similar to that of other gram-negative bacteria, but it seems unlikely that it plays a significant role in the pathogenesis of bacillary dysentery. *Shigella dysenteriae* (shiga) produces an exotoxin that can exert a deleterious effect upon the nervous system and may affect the intestinal epithelium like cholera enterotoxin and cause diarrhea. The occurrence of paralytic manifestations in dysentery produced by this species may be attributable to the exotoxin.

Bacillary dysentery is infrequently associated with bacteremia, and the infection is confined to the intestinal mucosa, occasionally invading mesenteric lymph nodes. Morphologic lesions are most frequently observed in the colon, occasionally involving the terminal ileum. Ulceration of the mucosa develops, with intervening inflamed membrane but no undermining of the ulcer edges as in amebic dysentery. The bowel wall is infiltrated with granulocytes, there is edema of the submucosa, and occasionally the involvement may extend to the serosa. If ulceration is not extensive, healing occurs without scarring, but when it is severe, fibrosis and even stenosis of the bowel may develop.

Clinical Manifestations. Patients with shigellosis may have simple self-limited diarrhea, acute gastroenteritis, true dysentery, or no symptoms of illness. It has been proposed that bacillary dysentery may occasionally be responsible for chronic colitis, but it has been difficult to establish this relationship with certainty.

The incubation period of dysentery is usually about 48 hours, but it may be shorter. The illness begins abruptly with abdominal cramps, pain relieved by defecation, and watery diarrhea. This is followed promptly by the development of tenesmus, feverishness, and passage of mucous stool, occasionally containing blood. Abdominal tenderness, most pronounced in the lower quadrants, is found, and the bowel is hyperactive on auscultation. The temperature rarely rises very high, except in children, in whom it may become 40° C or more. Without treatment the illness persists for a few days and then subsides.

Acute gastroenteritis, associated with nausea, some vomiting, and diarrhea, is seen particularly in outbreaks of infection by *Shigella sonnei*.

Shigella dysenteriae (shiga) infection is often more severe than that caused by the other species. The fever may be higher, hypotension develops more frequently, and the intestinal symptoms are more intense. Recovery may be delayed, and debility may persist for several weeks. Peripheral neuritis more commonly complicates infection by *Shigella dysenteriae*.

Conjunctivitis, iritis, and nystagmus are occasional complications of bacillary dysentery, appearing between the first and second weeks of disease. Nonsuppurative arthritis may also develop. Fluid and electrolyte depletion may be considerable, particularly in infants and children, producing severe dehydration and acidosis. Potassium deficit may be recognized, particularly as the patient's fluids are replenished. Convulsions develop occasionally in children, but appear to be correlated to the degree of fever.

At times, bacillary dysentery seems to have been precipitated by onset of measles, and almost half the cases may be accompanied by infection with enteropathic viruses, including adenovirus, echovirus, poliovirus, and coxsackievirus. The association of a virus with the disease, however, does not influence its clinical manifestations. The frequency of serious underlying disease in persons with shigellosis is not as common as in salmonellosis. Massive intestinal bleeding occurs in severe bacillary dysentery when there is extensive intestinal necrosis and ulceration.

Diagnosis. Isolation and identification of Shigella in the stool or from swab culture of the rectal mucosa are the only means of establishing the diagnosis of shigellosis. The serum agglutinin titer will rise in about half the patients with bacillary dysentery, but it is not ordinarily useful for diagnostic purposes. Shigella survive in feces for only a short while. Therefore feces should be promptly cultured, or the specimen should be collected in a 30 per cent glycerol-saline solution for preservation. Examination of the feces microscopically in bacillary dysentery will usually reveal a large number of granulocytes, comprising about 90 per cent of all cells, apart from erythrocytes. As convalescence begins, mononuclear cells become predominant. Specific immunofluorescence techniques have been developed for the rapid detection of Shigella in feces. This test agrees with cultural results in over 90 per cent of instances.

Viral enteritis caused by echovirus, coxsackievirus, and poliomyelitis virus may be epidemic and may be confused with shigellosis. Fever is uncommon, however, in viral enteritis unless there is severe dehydration, and the feces contain no blood or pus. *Staphylococcal enterocolitis* develops usually in hospitalized patients undergoing abdominal surgery who have received antimicrobial therapy. *Amebic dysentery* usually has a gradual onset, the diarrhea is ordinarily not severe, there is often little or no fever, and microscopic examination of the feces will reveal a predominance of mononuclear cells. Sigmoidoscopy reveals undermined ulcers with normal intervening mucosa. *Salmonellosis* is more often accompanied by nausea and vomiting at onset and occasionally by a chill and very high fever. Blood cultures are often positive. *Staphylococcal food poisoning* and many forms of viral gastroenteritis are more prominently associated with nausea and vomiting than with diarrhea.

Treatment. Sulfonamides were effective in treatment of shigellosis when they were first used. Resistant bacilli emerged, however, and sulfonamides are not now considered to be the most effective drugs for the infection. Resistance of Shigella to multiple antimicrobials has been induced by episomal transfer from other enteric bacilli. Conceivably, therefore, drug-susceptible Shigella may become drug resistant from other drug-resistant bacilli in the intestinal tract.

Tetracycline has been an effective drug against Shigella, but resistant strains have been identified. A few strains of Shigella are resistant to chloramphenicol. Colimycin and neomycin are almost always effective in vitro, but a few strains resistant to ampicillin have been found. Streptomycin given orally has been used to treat shigellosis, but strains resistant to this drug have also been identified. Cephalothin and massive doses of penicillin G may be effective.

At present, ampicillin in a dosage of 2 or more grams orally each day in divided doses for five days is the preferred agent in treatment of shigellosis in adults. Tetracycline or (in very serious circumstances) chloramphenicol may be effective alternatives if either the microorganism is resistant to ampicillin or the patient is allergic to the penicillins. Oral streptomycin, 0.5 gram twice daily, is also recommended in Great Britain.

Fluid and electrolyte replacement should be given to the patient who is in collapse or who is dehydrated. Diphenoxalate hydrochloride and atropine (Lomotil) and opiates such as paregoric or morphine may alleviate the abdominal discomfort and tenesmus but should be used cautiously.

Prognosis. The mortality rate in untreated bacillary dysentery is about 0.1 per cent or less, but it may be higher during famine or starvation. In addition, the fatality rate with dysentery caused by *Shigella dysenteriae* (shiga) is higher than with that attributed to other Shigella. Death rarely occurs when appropriate treatment is prescribed.

Dammin, G. J.: The pathogenesis of acute diarrheal disease in early life. Bull. WHO, 31:29, 1964.
Gordon, J. E., Behar, M., and Scrimshaw, N. S.: Acute diarrheal disease in less developed countries: I. An epidemiological basis for control. Bull. WHO, 31:1, 1964.
Levine, M. M., et al.: Pathogenesis of *Shigella dysenteriae* (Shiga) dysentery. J. Infect. Dis., 127:261, 1973.
Ramos-Alvarez, M., et al.: Diarrheal disease of children. The occurrence of enteropathogenic viruses and bacteria. Am. J. Dis. Child., 107:218, 1964.
Reller, L. B., et al.: Shigellosis in the United States, 1964–1968. J. Infect. Dis., 120:393, 1969.
Watanabe, T.: Infective heredity of multiple drug resistance in bacteria. Bact. Rev., 27:87, 1963.

216. CHOLERA
(Asiatic Cholera)

Leighton E. Cluff

Definition.   Cholera is a specific infectious disease of man caused by *Vibrio cholerae*. It is characterized by diarrhea with fluid and electrolyte depletion, occurring endemically and epidemically in Asia and occasionally pandemically.

Etiology.   In a classic study in 1857, Snow described an outbreak of cholera in London and incriminated contaminated water as the source of disease. In 1883, Koch identified *Vibrio cholerae* in the feces of a large number of patients with cholera. The cholera vibrio is a comma-shaped, gram-negative, flagellated, and motile microorganism that grows aerobically on nutrient media at 37° C, preferentially at an alkaline pH. There are two biotypes of *Vibrio cholerae*, the "classic" and the El Tor. The El Tor strain is hardier than the classic strain, persists longer in nature and in man, is more resistant to chemical agents, is hemolytic, and is antigenically separable from the classic strain. *V. cholerae* can be differentiated from noncholera vibrios by its fermentative, hemolytic, pathogenic, and antigenic reactions.

Incidence and Prevalence.   Cholera is endemic in India, Burma, Pakistan, Thailand, and a few other areas in Asia. It has occurred in epidemics throughout the world. Prior to the nineteenth century, cholera was unknown outside India, but during that century it was observed sporadically and as an epidemic in Europe, England, Russia, and North America. In the twentieth century, cholera has largely disappeared from the Western Hemisphere and Europe but continues to occur endemically and epidemically in Asia, primarily along the Ganges River in India and in Pakistan. The pandemic of cholera extending from 1898 to 1907 was responsible for at least 370,000 deaths in India. A current pandemic, attributable to the El Tor strain, began in 1961 in Indonesia and has spread through most of Asia, the Middle East, Africa, and recently (1972–1973) into Western and Eastern Europe.

Epidemiology.   Only man is naturally infected with *V. cholerae*. The infection is transmitted most commonly by contaminated water, but it can be transmitted by contamination of fresh leafy or root vegetables and fruit fertilized with human feces or with water containing the microorganism. *V. cholerae* has been isolated from flies, roaches, and other insects, but these may be an unimportant source of contagion. Doctors and nurses caring for patients with cholera rarely contract the disease, suggesting that direct contact under hygienic conditions is an uncommon mode of transmission of the infection. Cholera is primarily a disease of persons who live in poverty or who have poor standards of living and sanitation. The case-infection ratio in classic cholera is about 1:7, but in El Tor cholera this ratio can be 1:25 or 1:100. Asymptomatic infected persons who travel may establish new foci of cholera. *V. cholerae* does not survive long in fresh water, but can survive for long periods in sea water, particularly along beaches contaminated with human sewage.

Outbreaks of cholera usually appear during dry, hot weather preceding a rainy season. The reason for this seasonal occurrence of cholera is unexplained. Although sporadic cases may occur throughout the year, there are rare chronic carriers of *V. cholerae*, as there are of typhoid bacilli, and the principal reservoir of the organism in interepidemic periods is unclear. In endemic areas around river basins, *V. cholerae* can be isolated from the water throughout the year, although most cases of cholera occur seasonally.

Pathology and Pathogenesis.   Recent studies of cholera indicate that the small intestine is most severely involved. The gastrointestinal epithelium remains intact, even in the acute phase of the disease, but there are mononuclear cell inflammation of the mucosa, vascular congestion, and goblet cell hyperplasia. This acute stage may be followed by increased "turnover" of the epithelial cells. These morphologic changes are similar to those seen in nonspecific diarrhea but do not explain the clinical features of the disease. Chronic atrophic gastritis may precede and persist after the infection. It is likely that nutritional and other chronic affections of the intestine and stomach are predisposing causes of cholera. Occurrence of the disease in impoverished and malnourished persons further suggests this possibility. A cholera-like disease has been produced in dogs by feeding them vibrio with bicarbonate.

The cholera vibrio produces an enterotoxin which is responsible for the disease manifestations. The enterotoxin is a heat-labile protein with a molecular weight of 10,000 to 90,000 which binds to intestinal epithelium, initiating intense secretion of isotonic fluid, but does not interfere with absorption of glucose and electrolyte. One step in this sequence is activation of adenyl cyclase–producing cyclic AMP and providing the energy for ion secretion and water transport into the gut lumen.

The primary difficulty in cholera is severe fluid and electrolyte depletion. The feces contain mucus, epithelial debris, large quantities of water, sodium, potassium, and bicarbonate, but little plasma protein. There is no significant loss of albumin into the intestines, as illustrated by the failure of intravenously injected Evans blue dye to appear in the feces.

Clinical Manifestations.   Cholera begins as an acute diarrhea with abdominal pain. Vomiting may appear early, but is not prominent. Fever and chills are usually absent. The oral and axillary temperature may be depressed, whereas the rectal temperature may be elevated slightly above normal. Over a few hours the diarrhea increases in severity, and the volume of feces may be as great as 15 to 20 liters in 24 hours. Initially, the feces are bile stained, but as the diarrhea worsens, the feces become watery, mucoid, and odorless, and occasionally may contain blood. The feces of patients with cholera may resemble rice water or starch water and may contain cellular debris and masses of cholera vibrios. The patient becomes rapidly dehydrated, the skin is cold and withered, and the face becomes drawn. As dehydration increases, the patient becomes stuporous, comatose, hypotensive, and cyanotic, and may die in shock. Urine output decreases, mouth and eyes become dry, but lacteal and sweat secretion may persist. Muscular cramps may be severe. Thirst is intense, and the ingestion of fluid rarely induces vomiting. Recovery ordinarily is prompt after replacement of fluid and electrolytes, but the patient may continue to have anuria or oliguria and may die in renal failure. The renal insufficiency may be attributable to hypokalemia, shock, or reduced renal blood flow owing to dehydration.

With severe dehydration the hematocrit, leukocyte

count, and specific gravity of the plasma rise. The plasma sodium chloride and total serum protein are increased above normal. The plasma potassium may be slightly elevated or normal, although potassium depletion is severe. Metabolic acidosis is usually severe.

In cholera the fecal sodium and chloride concentrations are increased above normal, as is fecal osmolarity, but these are consistently lower than the plasma values. Fecal potassium and carbonate concentrations, however, are higher than those of the plasma. These electrolyte changes in cholera resemble those in other diarrheal disease, but are more severe.

Many patients with cholera are anemic before onset of the disease; therefore the rise in hematocrit with dehydration may not be demonstrable. Infection by El Tor vibrio often causes no symptoms or mild diarrhea difficult to distinguish from other acute enteric illnesses.

Diagnosis. In endemic areas and during epidemics, cholera is easily recognized clinically. Sporadic cases must be differentiated from other diarrheal diseases such as typhoid fever, bacillary dysentery, amebiasis, other forms of intestinal parasitism, viral enteritis, staphylococcal food poisoning, and chemical poisoning. The epidemiologic and fulminant characteristics of cholera, however, are helpful diagnostically. Bacteriologic and immunologic identification of *V. cholerae* from the feces is usually possible. Microscopic examination of the feces may reveal masses of the microorganism. *V. cholerae* may be cultured from the feces of patients convalescing from cholera, but ordinarily disappears within a few days or a few weeks.

Strains of *Escherichia coli* and other enteric organisms may elaborate an enterotoxin similar to that of cholera vibrio and cause a cholera-like illness. Cholera-like diarrhea also can be caused by *Clostridium perfringens*, Salmonella, and Shigella.

Many patients with cholera will have a positive serologic test for *V. cholerae* antibodies on the day of onset of disease. Serum antibody titers, measured by hemagglutination or vibriocidal assay, however, rise to maximal levels in about seven days after onset of cholera. Vibriocidal titers fall rapidly after illness.

Other Vibrio Infections. Noncholera vibrios are widespread in surface water throughout the world and have been associated with diarrheal disease. *Vibrio fetus* produces disease in human beings but is primarily an infection of cattle causing septic abortion, and can be differentiated serologically from *V. cholerae*. Man is infected after occupational exposure to diseased animals or animal products. *V. fetus* infection of man does not produce diarrhea, but is responsible for bacteremia, abortion, pneumonia, endocarditis, thrombophlebitis, and an illness resembling acute brucellosis.

Treatment. The treatment of cholera is correction of the fluid and electrolyte depletion attributable to the severe diarrhea. Urine output and the patient's clinical appearance are indices of hydration if the patient does not have renal failure. The degree of hydration can be estimated clinically. The hemoglobin or hematocrit determination may be misleading because of pre-existing anemia. When the patient is first seen, the blood electrolyte determinations also may be unreliable as indices of the degree of electrolyte depletion and dehydration. Plasma protein concentration, and particularly plasma specific gravity, can serve as an index for administration of fluids and electrolyte.

A good replacement solution for intravenous administration to adults contains 133 mEq sodium, 98 mEq chloride, 13 mEq potassium and 48 mEq bicarbonate, prepared by addition of 5 grams sodium chloride, 4 grams sodium bicarbonate, and 1 gram potassium chloride to 1 liter sterile, pyrogen-free distilled water. In hypotensive adults the initial infusion should be given rapidly (50 to 100 ml per minute) until a strong radial pulse is restored. Subsequently, fluids are infused in quantities equal to fecal losses, measured preferably by having the patient on a "cholera cot" (a cot with a centrally placed hole to collect feces). If fluid loss cannot be accurately determined, fluid should be given to maintain radial pulse, blood pressure, and skin turgor. Overhydration can be avoided by observation of neck veins and auscultation of lungs. In children, sodium loss is less, and potassium loss is greater than in adults. Therefore the intravenous fluid used for replacement should be different (94 mEq sodium, 15 mEq potassium).

Many liters of fluid will be needed (25 or more) until the administration of fluid is no longer required. The cholera patient, even if in shock and comatose when first seen, will often be able to take oral feeding after four hours. At that time potassium, as juices or in other form, may be fed. Otherwise, if the diarrhea continues for more than 24 hours, the intravenous fluids should contain 10 mEq of potassium per liter. Oral fluid therapy of cholera patients is effective in adults and children. The fluid may contain 100 mEq sodium, 10 mEq potassium, 70 mEq chloride, 40 mEq bicarbonate, and 120 mM per liter glucose, with an osmolarity of 327 mOsm per liter.

Tetracycline given orally (40 mg per kilogram per day) or in a dosage of 100 mg per liter of intravenous fluid and administered in a total dosage of 250 to 500 mg during the first day of treatment shortens the period of diarrhea and decreases the requirement for fluid replacement. This is associated with a hastening of the disappearance of *V. cholerae* from the feces. Advances in understanding the action of cholera enterotoxin indicate the possibility that an antagonist of adenyl cyclase or an agent lowering intracellular levels of cyclic $3'5'$ adenosine monophosphate may reverse the disease.

Prognosis. The case mortality rate from untreated cholera in persons 10 to 20 years of age is 50 per cent; in persons over 50 it is 70 per cent. Death is more common among those less than 10 years of age than among patients between 10 and 20 years of age. Almost invariably, death can be prevented if the fluid, electrolyte, and alkali therapy is begun early in the illness and if there is no serious associated disease or renal failure.

Prevention. Cholera can be eliminated by improved standards of living, public health, and sanitation. In those parts of the world where water supply and sewage disposal are controlled effectively, cholera no longer occurs.

There is a killed bacterial vaccine for immunization against cholera that provides some temporary protection. It may be useful in reducing the incidence of the disease in endemic areas. A toxoid of cholera enterotoxin is being evaluated and may add to the effectiveness of cholera vaccine in protection against the disease. Administration of cholera vaccine is no longer a requirement for entrance into the United States from cholera endemic areas.

Barua, D., and Burrows, W.: Cholera. Philadelphia, W. B. Saunders Company, 1974.
Carpenter, C. C. J.: Cholera: Diagnosis and treatment. Bull. N.Y. Acad. Med., 47:1192, 1971.

Gangarosa, E. J.: The epidemiology of cholera, past and present. Bull. N.Y. Acad. Med., 47:1140, 1971.

Hendrix, T. R.: The pathophysiology of cholera. Bull. N.Y. Acad. Med., 47:1169, 1971.

Holmgren, J., et al.: Experimental studies on cholera immunization. Infect. Immun., 5:662, 1972.

Mahalanabis, D., et al.: Oral fluid therapy of cholera. Johns Hopkins Med. J., 132:197, 1973.

Phillips, R. A.: Asiatic cholera. Ann. Rev. Med., 19:69, 1968.

Snow, J.: Snow on Cholera. The Commonwealth Fund. London, Oxford University Press, 1936.

217. PLAGUE*

Fred R. McCrumb, Jr.

Definition. Plague is an acute or chronic disease of wild and commensal rodents transmissible among these lower animal hosts and to man through the bite of infected ectoparasites. The infection in man is acute and frequently fulminant and usually is characterized by abrupt onset of high fever, lymphadenopathy near the site of exposure, bacteremia, and prostration. Secondary or embolic pneumonia may result in direct respiratory spread of the disease from man to man. Thus two clinical types of human infection are recognized: *bubonic plague,* characterized by either regional lymphadenopathy or bacteremia wherein organisms invade the blood by way of the lymphatics and produce overwhelming sepsis, and *primary plague pneumonia.*

Etiology. *Yersinia pestis* (formerly *Pasteurella pestis*) is a nonmotile, aerobic gram-negative bacillus that grows readily but slowly on artificial media. Small, convex dewdrop colonies become grayish and present a surface appearance like that of beaten copper after 48 hours' incubation at 37° C on blood agar. Virulent organisms are sticky because of the presence of a protein capsule. In liquid media, a surface pellicle and stalactites are characteristic. *Y. pestis* is highly virulent for a variety of laboratory animals. The microorganisms may be seen on microscopy of suitably stained node impressions, peritoneal exudate, and peripheral blood of these hosts as coccoid or large ovoid "safety-pin" bacilli. This bipolar staining is best demonstrated with Giemsa or Wayson's stain, and may be conspicuous in lymph node aspirates and sputum of infected human beings. The organism is destroyed quickly by sunlight and common chemical disinfectants and is noninfectious after 15 minutes at 55° C. *Y. pestis* may survive for several weeks in dry flea feces and human sputum, and may be kept viable and virulent in the frozen state for months. Although streptomycin-resistant mutants have been encountered in experimental plague infections, all naturally occurring human strains of *Y. pestis* studied to date are inhibited in vitro by low concentrations of streptomycin, chloramphenicol, and the tetracyclines.

Incidence and Prevalence. The first adequate description of widespread disease deals with an outbreak of plague in the Egyptian port of Pelusium in 542 A.D. During the next 50 years, plague spread widely into Asia and Europe and it has been estimated that 100 million people perished at that time. Plague assumed catastrophic proportions again during the fourteenth century when it appeared not only in Europe and the Middle East but also in China and India. Pneumonic plague was prominent in this pandemic, which, for unclear reasons, became known as the "Black Death." In Europe alone, 25 million, or one fourth of the population, succumbed. The spread of plague resulted in the establishment of numerous widely distributed permanent natural foci among wild rodent populations.

During recent years, human plague has occurred in Vietnam, Burma, Indonesia, India, Iran, the Malagasy Republic, Central and South Africa, the United States, and several countries of South America. There has been a continuing decline in the incidence of human plague, however, and, in many instances, this decrease in incidence is unquestionably spontaneous. Certain endemic areas are characterized by a constant low human case rate resulting from sporadic infections that occur as a result of man's accidental contact with wild rodent foci. In the United States between 1908 and 1974, some 145 human plague infections associated with wild rodents were distributed over 15 western states. Under certain circumstances, however, such as those now prevailing in Vietnam, plague continues to reach epidemic proportions.

Epidemiology. The ecology of plague varies from one region to another, and the extent to which man is affected by enzootic infections is determined in part by the proximity of human and rodent habitations and the bionomics of rodent ectoparasites. Although ticks and lice are capable of transmitting *Y. pestis* to susceptible animals, practically speaking, the important vectors are fleas. Occasionally man contracts plague by handling the carcass of an infected animal. Epidemics of plague usually arise from infected commensal rats such as *Rattus rattus* and *Rattus norvegicus,* the causative organism being transmitted to man by *Xenopsylla cheopis,* the common rat flea. There is general agreement that natural foci of plague infection among so-called wild rodents (mice, field rats, gerbils, ground squirrels) account for the persistence of this disease in endemic areas. In some instances, man's intrusions into natural foci may result in outbreaks of human plague, and there is ample evidence of an interchange of fleas between commensal and wild rodent species. Flea-borne plague in man is usually of the bubonic variety, and as such does not represent a serious risk to other human beings. By contrast, plague pneumonia secondary to bacteremia may initiate a series of direct transmissions to susceptible contacts in whom the disease is manifest by a fulminant primary pneumonia. Primary pneumonic plague may spread among a susceptible human population with alarming rapidity.

Age and sex distribution of plague is dependent upon the nature of rodent foci and the habits of the human population at risk. Thus domestic rat plague will be distributed evenly among both sexes of all ages when the home is infested with rat fleas. When field rodents constitute the source of infection, the disease will occur predominantly among field workers.

Pathology. Evidence of infection is usually not present at the portal of entry into the skin, although a small pustule is observed in a few patients with bubonic plague. Similarly, lymphatics leading to regional nodes are grossly normal. The primary bubo is usually enlarged, exquisitely tender, and surrounded by a broad zone of subcutaneous edema. There is an intense hemorrhagic inflammatory reaction with infiltration of polynuclear cells. As the inflammation progresses, necrosis and suppuration of the bubo occur. There is a characteristic gelatinous edema of contiguous connective tissue along with dilatation of small blood vessels. Occasionally, infection of the oropharyngeal mucous membrane will lead to tonsillar or mediastinal reaction of the type seen in lymph nodes. Pathologic changes noted in other organ systems can be ascribed to small blood vessel disease, as evidenced by hemorrhages in serous membranes and gastrointestinal mucosa. In addition, degenerative

---

*The assistance of Colonel Dan C. Cavanaugh, MSC, in the revision of this chapter is gratefully acknowledged.

changes of renal tubular epithelium and parenchymal cells of the liver are frequent. There may be slight enlargement of the liver and spleen. Vascular congestion of the meninges is accompanied by cerebral edema.

Secondary or embolic plague pneumonia is characterized by perivascular foci of inflammatory cells and colonies of *Y. pestis*. As the disease progresses, distinction from primary plague infection of the lung is less obvious, and both may show gradation from lobular pneumonia to lobar consolidation. It is not unusual for several lobes to become involved within a period of 24 to 48 hours. In all instances, reaction in the lung is intense, there being cellular infiltration, gross hemorrhage, and copious exudation of watery sputum. There is overwhelming growth of plague bacilli in the lung that can be readily demonstrated in impression smears of cut lung surface. Bronchial lymph nodes are usually enlarged and hyperemic.

Pathogenesis. After the ingestion of plague bacilli, the proximal digestive tract of the flea becomes obstructed as organisms multiply in the proventriculus. Refeeding results in regurgitation of the freshly ingested human blood as well as *Y. pestis* into the feeding site. Organisms are then carried to regional lymph nodes, where a local inflammatory reaction leads to the formation of a bubo. In most instances, bacteremia occurs early in the disease and may assume enormous proportions in fulminant infections. Plague pneumonia is associated with the production of infectious droplets and respiratory spread of *Y. pestis*. Epidemiologic studies suggest that intimate contact is a prerequisite to successful respiratory transmission of this organism, and the nature of the primary lung lesion favors spread by particles of small size.

Although much has been said about intoxication in human plague infection, evidence of specific toxin activity in human beings is wanting. Extraction of virulent and attenuated strains of *Y. pestis* has revealed the presence of a water-soluble toxic substance that is highly lethal for Swiss mice. Although this material is antigenic in laboratory animals and antibodies may be demonstrated in the sera of patients recovered from plague, its role in the pathogenesis of plague has not been established. However, a classic gram-negative endotoxin has been identified in the plague bacillus, and Shwartzman-like reactions have been described in severe cases.

Clinical Manifestations. Most plague infections make their appearance abruptly with high fever, tachycardia, malaise, and aching of the extremities and back. Temperature usually rises to 39.5 to 40° C within a few hours of onset, and the patient has the general appearance of profound illness, with flushed face and anxious expression. As the disease progresses, delirium may become a prominent feature of the clinical syndrome, and anxiety gives way to depression.

Bubonic Plague. The incubation period in bubonic plague varies from one to six days in most instances and progresses to fulminant bacteremia, death ensuing within three to five days of the onset of symptoms. The case fatality in untreated bubonic plague is variously estimated at 60 to 90 per cent. Regional lymphadenopathy or buboes of flea-borne plague are found in the groin in more than 50 per cent of patients with this form of the disease. Femoral and inguinal buboes are followed in frequency by axillary and cervical node involvement.

The site of infection is influenced by the nature of exposure to vectors, there being a high frequency of lower extremity exposure among working adults and axillary and cervical buboes among children exposed as they sleep in a flea-infested dwelling. The involved node may not be greatly enlarged but is invariably painful and exquisitely tender. Within a few hours, there is periadenitis with edema of surrounding tissue. Buboes may involute slowly or suppurate with discharge of necrotic material in patients who survive the acute phase of infection. When bacteremia progresses relentlessly, the clinical picture is one of overwhelming sepsis, and death is associated with peripheral vascular collapse.

Plague Pneumonia. Plague pneumonia acquired as a result of respiratory spread of *Y. pestis* is even more fulminant, untreated patients rarely surviving for more than three days. The disease is characterized by an explosive onset of high fever, tachycardia, tachypnea, and restlessness. Flushing of the skin, conjunctival suffusion, and anxious expression are common. Headache and myalgia may be severe, but are inconstant. During the early phase of illness, the paucity of signs is disproportionate to the obvious severity of the infection. Cough may be absent until six or more hours have passed. Subjective symptoms referable to the chest may be absent, or the patient may complain of pleural pain or dull substernal oppression. Physical signs of pneumonitis may be lacking at this time; however, as the disease progresses, rales, suppressed breathing, and impaired percussion appear. Signs of consolidation are not encountered frequently until after therapy has been instituted. The general clinical state rapidly deteriorates, and patients with this disease are gravely ill after 10 to 15 hours of fever. The patient may find it difficult to produce more than small amounts of sputum in the early hours of illness; however, blood-tinged sputum usually appears within the first 12 hours. Bloody, frothy, liquid sputum typical of plague pneumonia is produced in large quantities late in the disease at a time when the prognosis is uniformly poor.

Laboratory Findings. Peripheral blood leukocytosis with total counts of 12,000 to 15,000 and neutrophilia usually occur in both types of human plague. There is elevation of the erythrocyte sedimentation rate, but other hematologic abnormalities have not been observed. Proteinuria and mild hematuria may accompany the acute febrile phase of plague.

Diagnosis. The clinical diagnosis of plague is confirmed by conventional bacteriologic techniques and inoculation of susceptible laboratory animals. *Y. pestis* may be isolated in pure culture after 48 to 96 hours from bubo aspirates, blood, and sputum, using blood agar and infusion broth. Inoculation of these materials into mice or guinea pigs produces bacteremia and death of the animal in two to five days. A smear of heart's blood of these animals will reveal numerous bipolar staining rods.

In all instances, however, a tentative diagnosis of plague must be made on clinical and epidemiologic grounds, there being dire consequences of a missed diagnosis, especially of plague pneumonia. Careful examination of stained smears of bubo aspirates or sputum will usually reveal the presence of small gram-negative bacilli, and proper isolation precautions and specific therapy must be based on the judgment of this examination. Stained smears from organs of cadavers in cases of sudden death in plague endemic areas should be examined with great diligence to avoid catastrophic spread of this disease.

Patients recovering from plague develop specific antibodies that may be demonstrated in convalescent-phase serum by bacterial agglutination, agglutination of erythrocytes sensitized with capsular antigen, complement-fixation, and mouse protection tests. Antibodies make their appearance early in the second week of disease and continue to rise up to the fourth or fifth week. In all cases, serodiagnosis is retrospective but of value in establishing the presence of infection with *Y. pestis* as well as the immune status of a vaccinated population.

Plague infections in man must be differentiated from tularemia, lymphogranuloma venereum, and other causes of localized lymphadenopathy. The disease is frequently confused with malaria, influenza, enteric fevers, and various causes of acute pneumonia, among them Klebsiella, staphylococcal, tularemic, and viral infections of the lung. In the absence of buboes or pneumonia, bacteremia caused by a variety of gram-negative organisms may resemble acute septicemic plague.

Treatment. *Y. pestis* is readily inhibited in vitro by relatively small concentrations of streptomycin, chloramphenicol, and the tetracyclines. The disease responds readily when antimicrobial therapy is started during the early phase of illness, but it rapidly becomes refractory to specific treatment as it progresses. In view of the ease and uniform success of early therapy, delay in diagnosis and administration of chemotherapy is a grave error in clinical judgment. Pneumonic plague is uniformly fatal, and becomes difficult to treat after the twelfth to fifteenth hour of fever. Bubonic plague is generally less severe, but may progress to death with equal swiftness.

Early studies with sulfonamides revealed that mortality from bubonic plague could be reduced to 5 to 20 per cent by the administration of sulfadiazine or sulfamerazine at the rate of 12 grams daily for four to seven days. These drugs were found to be ineffective in plague pneumonia.

Streptomycin or the broad-spectrum antimicrobials represent the therapy of choice in all plague infections. Streptomycin should be administered parenterally at the rate of 4 grams daily for two days followed by 8 to 10 grams given over a period of five additional days. Chloramphenicol should be administered at the rate of 6 to 8 grams daily for the first 48 hours followed by 3 grams (50 to 75 mg per kilogram) daily for a total dosage of 20 to 25 grams. Chloramphenicol should be given intravenously and orally during the first 48 hours of therapy if the latter route of administration is feasible. Tetracyclines should be administered in a similar manner, large doses (4 to 6 grams daily) being given during the first 48 hours of therapy. Intravenous therapy during the first 24 hours is mandatory in severely ill patients but should be supplemented by oral administration of the drug if this is tolerated by the patient.

When specific therapy is not instituted within the first 15 hours of overt illness in plague pneumonia, antimicrobial therapy usually will not favorably alter the outcome of the disease.

Supportive care includes the use of intravenous fluid therapy, pressor drugs to support failing peripheral circulation, and oxygen therapy when respiratory function has been compromised by widespread pneumonitis. Tracheostomy frequently results in improved pulmonary function and facilitates care of patients severely ill with primary respiratory disease.

Prevention. Prevention of plague is best accomplished by control programs to reduce rodent infections in endemic foci. Improvement in living standards is usually associated with spontaneous disappearance of this disease or at least its confinement to natural foci. However, there are many areas where such an evolution is not likely to occur and natural foci will probably always exist. Under such circumstances, three general approaches to plague control are available. In practice, rodent control has proved to be the least effective method in most endemic regions, primarily because human living standards cannot be sufficiently improved. Rodenticides in common use include sodium fluoroacetate (1080), arsenic trioxide, red squill, alpha-naphthylthiourea (ANTU), and anticoagulants such as warfarin. In economically underdeveloped areas, vector control with insecticides is probably the most effective single control method. The residual effect of 10 per cent DDT dust or 5 per cent spray dispersed around rat habitations and human dwellings is sufficient to reduce sharply the flea populations and thus eliminate large numbers of vectors. However, resistance to DDT has been observed in the most important vector, *X. cheopis,* and local vectors should be tested for susceptibility to various insecticides. In practice, the application of insecticides should always precede any employment of rodenticides. Finally, although millions of human beings have been inoculated with living, attenuated or formalin-killed plague vaccines, the protective effect of these immunoprophylactics has not been assessed adequately. However, there is evidence to support the concept that the production of specific antibodies in man is associated with a significant degree of resistance to plague infection. Protection of human populations against plague is best assured in endemic areas when all available control measures are employed.

Baltazard, M.: Déclin et destin d'une maladie infectieuse: La peste. Bull. W.H.O., 23:247, 1960.
Burkle, F. M.: Plague as seen in South Vietnamese children. Clin. Pediatr., 12:291, 1973.
Butler, T.: A clinical study of bubonic plague. Am. J. Med., 53:268, 1972.
Cavanaugh, D. C., and Steele, J. H.: Trends in research in plague immunization. J. Infect. Dis., 129:S1, 1974 (Supplement, May).
McCrumb, F. R., Jr., Mercier, S., Robic, J., Bouillat, M., Smadel, J. E., Woodward, T. E., and Goodner, K.: Chloramphenicol and Terramycin in the treatment of pneumonic plague. Am. J. Med., 15:284, 1953.
Meyer, K. F.: Effectiveness of live or killed plague vaccines in man. Bull. W.H.O., 42:653, 1970.
Poland, J. D.: In Hoeprich, P. D. (ed.): Infectious Diseases. New York, Harper & Row, 1972, p. 1141.
Pollitzer, R.: Plague. W.H.O. Monograph 22, Geneva, 1954.
W.H.O. Expert Committee on Plague. W.H.O. Tech. Rep. Ser. No. 447, 1970.

218. TULAREMIA

Theodore E. Woodward

Definition. Most cases of tularemia are characterized by the formation of a focal ulcer at the site of entry of the causative bacillus, enlargement of regional lymph nodes, and a constitutional reaction of fever, prostration, myalgia, and headache. There may be pneumonia, which is occasionally accompanied by pleurisy or a typhoid-like illness.

Franciscella tularensis, the microbial agent, is

transmitted to humans by insect vectors such as ticks or deer flies, by the handling or ingestion of infected animal tissues, or by inhalation of infected aerosols. The clinical diagnosis is confirmed by demonstration of bacteremia, by isolation of the bacillus from the sputum, tissue exudates, or gastric washings, and by demonstration of serum agglutinins in early convalescence.

Historical Features. The knowledge of the ecology and clinical features of tularemia has been developed in the United States through the pioneering work of Francis and other Public Health Service investigators. McCoy described the disease in 1911 while studying a plaguelike illness in ground squirrels in Tulare County, California. The first clinical description and bacteriologic proof of illness is attributed to Wherry and Lamb in 1914. In a series of studies conducted in Utah and elsewhere, Francis (1928) incriminated rabbits as important animal hosts and established the transmissibility of disease by deer flies.

Etiology, Specific Laboratory Diagnosis, and Epidemiology.
Tularemia is of considerable interest because the causative microorganism is a member of the important gram-negative group characterized by intracellular parasitism about which basic information on immunity mechanisms is incomplete. The bacillus is pleomorphic and nonmotile, and propagates best on such artificial media as blood-glucose-cysteine agar or after inoculation of animals with suspensions of infected tissues.

Culture. During the early stages of illness, *F. tularensis* is isolated readily by direct culture in appropriate media or by the subcutaneous or intraperitoneal inoculation of exudate into mice or guinea pigs. Positive cultures are obtained from the local ulcer or regional lymph nodes during the first several weeks in patients with ulceroglandulary type of illness. Regardless of the clinical type of tularemia, viable organisms may be isolated from nasopharyngeal or gastric washings during the active systemic phases of illness. Pleural fluid and bronchial secretions are suitable for cultural purposes. Bacteremia may be demonstrated in all forms, although isolation from the blood by culture on an artificial medium is difficult because of the paucity of organisms present. Organisms have been isolated from cerebrospinal fluid or bone marrow, although such cultural procedures are rarely indicated. Under ideal conditions, if suitable media are inoculated with appropriate material, the organism may be identified within two to four days. Impression smears of splenic tissues often reveal the characteristic coccal or bacillary forms intracellularly after preparation with Giemsa or Wayson's plague stain.

Serologic Diagnosis. The conventional serum agglutination reaction is a very useful diagnostic test, because specific agglutinins appear within eight to ten days from the onset of illness. Maximal titers are reached in about four weeks. Demonstration of a rise in titer through examination of serial specimens is confirmatory evidence of infection, although single titers of 1:160 or more are usually significant. Sera from patients with brucellosis or tularemia may show cross-agglutination, although the titer is usually higher with the homologous antigen.

Cutaneous Test. Foshay described a diagnostic skin test that consists of the intradermal inoculation of a purified antigen consisting of a killed suspension of *F. tularensis.* The reaction is of the delayed tuberculin type, becoming positive in 48 hours. The test is highly specific and becomes positive during the first week of tularemia either prior to or coincident with the development of agglutinins. The test remains positive for years.

Epidemiology. Tularemia has been detected in many countries of the Northern Hemisphere, including Japan, Central Europe, Asiatic and European Russia, and Scandinavia. *F. tularensis* has been found in practically all animal species. In much of North America cottontail rabbits are the most important animal host and were formerly a very common source of the ulceroglandular and typhoidal forms of tularemia. Restricted sale of wild rabbits in metropolitan areas resulted in a sharp decline of the disease.

The clinical infection develops after puncture wounds by bony spicules of infected rabbits or by the ingestion of improperly cooked food. Foxes, squirrels, rats, mice—indeed, all rodents—have been incriminated as sources of infection. Streams are contaminated for variable periods by infected animal carcasses (or by other less well understood routes), so that drinking the water or handling aquatic mammals such as muskrats may be hazardous.

Many cases have their origin from infected arthropods such as ticks, deer flies, or mosquitoes. In North America the ticks *Dermacentor andersoni, Dermacentor variabilis,* and the Lone Star tick are important reservoirs and vectors. Infected female ticks transmit *F. tularensis* transovarially. A primary ulcer often forms at the site of tick attachment.

Tularemia occurs in all seasons: among hunters and trappers in the fall and winter, and during the spring and summer when ticks and deer flies are active. All ages and both sexes are susceptible. Since 1967, fewer than 200 cases have been reported annually in the United States. During a four-week period in the spring of 1968, 47 patients acquired the disease in Vermont after the handling of muskrats.

Mechanism of Infection and Pathology. The disease may present in a variety of forms with two major subdivisions, depending on whether or not the initial site of entry can be visualized. In all forms there is lymph node involvement. In most instances there is a primary ulcer, variable in size, which may be located on the skin (ulceroglandular), in the eye (oculoglandular), or in the nasopharynx with necrotizing lesions. Sometimes the cutaneous lesion may be insignificant, so that the picture is that of "glandular tularemia" without an overt primary lesion. The entry also may be through the intestinal tract (enteric or typhoidal) or via the lungs (pulmonary).

After infection, *F. tularensis* reaches the blood via the lymphatics and nodes; the microbe, although phagocytized, resides intracellularly without loss of viability. Granulomatous lesions develop within the reticuloendothelial system, particularly in lymph nodes, liver, and spleen. These lesions, usually hyperplastic, bear some resemblance to tuberculosis and may caseate or form small local abscesses. The macrophage is the predominant cell type that surrounds an area of caseous necrosis. Langhans' cells are observed occasionally, and the larger lesions are liable to central abscess formation.

Bronchopneumonia is a common development in tularemia, occurring in approximately 30 per cent of patients who acquire the disease, regardless of the type of infection. Histologically, the early lesion is edematous, and consists of fibrin and leukocytes associated with necrosis of alveolar walls. In non-necrotic areas the exudate consists of the large mononuclear type. The gross lesions resemble the bronchopneumonia of tuberculosis, although histologically there is less epithelioid cell transformation. Tubercle-like nodules are more common in lymph nodes than in the lungs. Mediastinal nodes are involved frequently.

Clinical Manifestations. The incubation period of tularemia ranges from two to ten days. Headache, fever, and toxic signs characterize all forms of the illness and are in no way dissimilar to those in other infectious illnesses. The pertinent historic and epidemiologic features are often helpful clues, and in approximately three fourths of all patients there is a primary lesion associated with adenopathy.

Ulceroglandular Tularemia. The initial lesion begins as a reddish papule, which is often undermined and more extensive than the small area of superficial induration indicates. Neighboring and draining lymph nodes are enlarged, tender, and discrete. Fluctuation of these nodes occurs later in the illness, after two or more weeks, when other acute signs may have partially abated. Such diseased nodes may subsequently require incision and drainage. The lymph nodes during the early stages are laden with *F. tularensis* and, if incised, may provoke bacteremia and toxemia. Fluctuant buboes four or more weeks old are usually sterile. Generalized lymphadenopathy occurs. Systemic signs of toxemia may be severe in ulceroglandular tularemia, although most cases are mild or moderate in severity. Pneumonia of all gradations may accompany this type of infection.

Occasionally, tularemia referred to as the glandular type may occur as generalized adenopathy and toxemia but without cutaneous lesions.

Enteric Form of Tularemia (Typhoidal or Cryptogenic). After ingestion of infected animal tissues or water, ulcerative lesions of the buccal mucosa, pharynx, and intestine, and subsequent involvement of cervical, pharyngeal, and mesenteric lymph nodes may occur. The course of illness may be fulminant and fatal unless the disease is recognized and treated properly. Certain of these patients manifest illness that is similar to various forms of gastroenteritis and typhoid fever. These patients may be severely ill with sustained high fever, profound toxicity, stupor, and delirium or coma. This typhoidal systemic reaction may typify any of the clinical varieties of tularemia regardless of the presence of a cutaneous lesion. The term "cryptogenic" has often been used to connote the absence of an obvious portal of entry.

Pulmonary Tularemia. Lung involvement occurs in all forms of tularemia, subsequent to the bacteremia. Available evidence suggests that primary tularemic pneumonia is an entity, particularly in those persons such as laboratory workers who are exposed to infected aerosols. The incubation period varies from two to five days, depending upon the number of viable bacteria inhaled. In addition to headache, fever, malaise, and prostration, there is a nonproductive harassing cough and a sensation of substernal discomfort. Later the sputum may be mucoid or bloody and, in severely ill patients, pleural pain, dyspnea, tachycardia, and cyanosis occur.

In spite of extensive pulmonary involvement, there may be a paucity of physical signs. The early roentgenographic signs, seldom evident before the second to the fourth day of fever, consist of small irregular oval lesions with hilar adenopathy. Later in the illness, the infiltrate may be annular. True abscess formation is rare, although during resolution and convalescence, which in untreated patients or in those treated late may be prolonged, shadows suggesting abscess formation may be noted. Pleuritis with effusion is not uncommon.

Oculoglandular Tularemia. After ocular contamination there may be pain, photophobia, intense congestion, itching, lacrimation, chemosis, and a mucopurulent discharge. Small yellowish granulomatous lesions may appear on the palpebral conjunctivae or cornea and may eventually ulcerate. The preauricular and other regional lymph nodes may enlarge and ultimately suppurate. In untreated patients, serious ocular complications, including corneal perforation or optic atrophy, may ensue.

Other General Manifestations. Initially, in severely ill patients, there is a rigor followed by pyrexia that persists for a month or more. The fever may be continuously high or remittent, and defervescence is usually gradual. Hepatomegaly and splenomegaly with tenderness over the respective organs are relatively common. Toxic signs in all cases include fever, headache, myalgia, and nausea. Rashes are very uncommon; when present, they consist of localized papular lesions along the peripheral lymphatics or maculopapular body eruptions. In untreated patients or in those first given antimicrobial therapy late in the course of illness, convalescence may be prolonged with sporadic episodes of fever, weakness, muscular pains, and chronic respiratory signs.

Nonspecific Laboratory Findings. The erythrocyte sedimentation rate and C-reactive protein are elevated during the active stages. In contrast, the total blood leukocyte count is usually normal or low. Occasionally there may be moderate leukocytosis. Mild albuminuria may occur at the height of illness.

Differential Diagnosis. Ulceroglandular tularemia is recognized readily in endemic areas. Punctate lesions with surrounding erythema at the site of prior arthropod attachment suggest *Rocky Mountain spotted fever,* particularly when associated with fever, headache, and toxic signs. The absence of a rash would favor tularemia, because patients with rickettsial disease develop a characteristic exanthem. *Meningococcemia* is recognized by its fulminant character, the typical exanthem, leukocytosis, and the bacteriologic findings. Fever, toxic signs, pharyngitis, adenitis, hepatomegaly, and splenomegaly are common to tularemia and *infectious mononucleosis.* The hematologic and serologic findings are usually distinctive. *Cat scratch disease* is characterized by peripheral ulceration and regional adenopathy; a history of contact with cats, the cutaneous reaction to specific antigens, and the absence of agglutinins for *F. tularensis* are distinguishing features. *Ecthyma* and *furunculi* are similar in some respects to this form of tularemia, although lymphadenitis and systemic signs are less likely to develop.

The lesions of *sporotrichosis* are multiple, occur along the course of lymphatics, attach themselves firmly to the skin, and are freely movable.

Certain forms of tularemia may present with clinical features similar to those of psittacosis, Q fever, and mycoplasmal pneumonia. Broad-spectrum antimicrobial drugs are effective in each of these conditions. Appropriate serologic tests or viral isolation may be required to define the precise cause. Influenza with associated pneumonia is similar but does not respond to specific drugs, and its clinical course is short. Fungal diseases, such as *histoplasmosis* and *coccidioidomycosis,* may be acute and may simulate pulmonary tularemia. Consideration of the history, the epidemiologic data, and the cutaneous manifestations, as well as the bacteriologic and serologic findings, usually will permit proper identification.

The presence of unexplained pleural effusion, similar to tuberculous fibrinous pleurisy, requires differentiation. The results of cultural and serologic tests will aid in differentiation.

Complications. Pericarditis and meningitis are distinctive but unusual complications of tularemia. Pericardial involvement may develop by direct extension from the pulmonary lesions or lymph nodes, and is characterized by a fibrinous or fibrocaseous exudate. In untreated patients constrictive pericarditis may ensue. Tularemic meningitis is characterized by a lymphocytic pleocytosis in the cerebrospinal fluid, and was usually fatal prior to the availability of specific antimicrobial drugs. Rare instances of tularemic peritonitis, perisplenitis, osteomyelitis, and endocarditis have been reported.

Treatment. *Specific Therapy.* Tularemia is very amenable to treatment with antimicrobial drugs. Streptomycin is preferable, but the broad-spectrum antimicrobials are equally beneficial in ameliorating the active manifestations. They are less effective, however, in eradicating the organism, primarily because of their bacteriostatic mode of action. With the latter drugs, relapses are liable to occur if treatment is initiated within the first week of illness.

STREPTOMYCIN. Streptomycin, when given in doses of 1.0 gram daily to adults for about one week, results in prompt recovery. Most patients are improved within 24 hours, and are afebrile within 48 hours. Relapses are uncommon with streptomycin except when insufficient drug is given during the very early stages of illness. Strains resistant to streptomycin do appear, a fact which is of no clinical significance when infection is acquired naturally.

TETRACYCLINE AND CHLORAMPHENICOL TREATMENT. Broad-spectrum antimicrobials are very effective in rendering the patient afebrile and free from toxicity within 48 to 72 hours. Relapses are uncommon when therapy is initiated 10 to 12 days after the onset of illness, but are frequent if it is given during the first week. *F. tularensis* does not develop resistance to chloramphenicol or tetracycline; hence, retreatment leads to prompt response.

The following dosage schedule is considered optimal: for tetracycline, an initial oral dose of 25 mg per kilogram of body weight; and for chloramphenicol, 50 mg per kilogram of body weight. Subsequent daily doses are calculated on the same basis as the initial loading dose, dividing the requirement equally and giving it at six- to eight-hour intervals. Antimicrobial therapy is continued until the patient is improved and has been afebrile for about five to seven days.

No supplementary chemotherapy is necessary with any of the aforementioned regimens. Tetracycline is preferred solely because reactions to it are potentially less serious.

General Management. An adequate diet with appropriate protein intake is advisable. Oxygen treatment is indicated for all severely ill patients with pneumonia whether or not cyanosis is present. Other supportive measures useful for treating patients with pneumonia, such as frequent turning and the performing of a tracheostomy to provide a proper airway, are indicated. Thoracentesis for removal of fluid will allay respiratory embarrassment. The presence of any superimposed infection is detected by appropriate examination of the sputum, blood, or tissues.

The local ulcer requires no special measures. During the early several weeks of illness, lymph nodes should not be manipulated unduly or incised. Later, fluctuant buboes, which are usually sterile, may require incision and drainage. Recovery ensues rapidly.

Prognosis and Postinfection Immunity. In untreated patients, the case fatality rate in ulceroglandular tularemia was formerly approximately 5 per cent. However, of those patients with typhoidal tularemia or with pulmonary manifestations, about 30 per cent succumbed. With the advent of streptomycin and later the broad-spectrum antimicrobials, death from tularemia has been virtually eliminated and the morbidity shortened drastically to several days after institution of treatment, even among severely ill patients.

Second attacks of tularemia with systemic complications are uncommon, because recovery from the initial episode usually confers immunity. However, it is not unusual for patients to develop primary lesions when reinfected long after the initial systemic infection. Viable *F. tularensis* may be isolated from such recurrent primary ulcers, which resemble a Koch reaction. Under these conditions, systemic manifestations are unusual.

Under test conditions in volunteers, when streptomycin is given soon after intradermal infection (before the onset of clinical illness), an attack may be aborted fully. Immunity does not develop, agglutinins fail to appear, and such subjects are prone to further infection. This phenomenon is of little practical significance, as patients are usually encountered after a week or more of active clinical illness. Partial to complete resistance to infection follows such antigenic stimulation.

Control Measures. *General.* In infected areas those measures designed to repel ticks, mosquitoes, or deer flies should be employed. Gloves should be used for handling all potentially infected animals, particularly rabbits, and animals to be consumed should be cooked thoroughly. Laboratory workers exposed to infected aerosols should exercise care by wearing suitable masks and utilizing other protective devices.

Vaccination. The available killed vaccines afford only partial protection to man against tularemia. Viable attenuated preparations have been used with considerable success in the Soviet Union. The vaccine is administered intradermally and provokes a reaction similar in severity to that which follows smallpox immunization. Significant protection has been demonstrated in volunteers in the United States vaccinated with a similar viable product and who subsequently were exposed to virulent strains of *F. tularensis* by the respiratory or cutaneous routes. In those subjects who have developed clinical illness after immunization, the disease has been mild.

Foshay, L.: Tularemia. Ann. Rev. Microbiol., 4:313, 1950.
McCrumb, F. R.: Aerosol infection of man with *Pasteurella tularensis*. Bact. Rev., 25:262, 1961.
Meyer, K. F.: Pasteurella and franciscella. *In* Dubos, R., and Hirsch, J. G. (eds.): Bacterial and Mycotic Infections of Man. 4th ed. Philadelphia, J. B. Lippincott Company, 1965, Chap. 27, p. 659.
Young, L. S.: Tularemia epidemic, Vermont, 1968. Forty-seven cases linked to contact with muskrats. N. Engl. J. Med., 280:1253, 1969.

DISEASES CAUSED BY MALLEOMYCES

Leighton E. Cluff

219. GLANDERS
(Farcy)

Definition. Glanders, or farcy, is an infectious disease of horses, mules, and donkeys caused by *Malleomyces* *mallei.* The infection is occasionally transmitted to man, and is characterized by an acute fulminant febrile illness or a chronic indolent disease with abscesses of the respiratory tract or skin. Farcy refers to the nodular abscesses observed in skin, lymphatics, and subcutaneous tissues.

Etiology. Glanders was described by Aristotle about 330 B.C., and the occurrence of the disease in horses was observed by Apeyrtos about 375 A.D. Royer's (1837) monograph on glanders in man remains the classic description of the disease. The microorganism responsible for glanders was isolated in 1882. It is a gram-negative bacillus culturable aerobically on ordinary nutrient media. It is variously called *Malleomyces mallei, Bacillus mallei,* or *Pfeiferella mallei.* *M. mallei* is nonmotile. It elaborates a specific antigen (mallein) upon lysis that is used as a skin test material for diagnostic purposes. The bacillus is antigenically separable from *M. pseudomallei,* which causes melioidosis. When grown on potato slices or potato infusion agar, *M. mallei* produces a brown pigment resembling that of *Pseudomonas aeruginosa.* The bacillus produces fatal infection experimentally in guinea pigs and hamsters but will not cause disease in rats, cattle, hogs, or fowl.

Incidence and Prevalence. Glanders has probably never been a common disease in man. It occurs almost exclusively in persons handling horses, and therefore is an occupational disease. It has been reported from all parts of the world. It has been eradicated in the United States and the United Kingdom, but may still occur in Asia and South America.

Epidemiology. Glanders is a communicable disease among horses, and it may occur sporadically in other animal species in contact with horses. In horses, glanders is manifested by nasal symptoms and abscesses and by cutaneous nodules or abscesses (farcy). Glanders is transmitted to man by direct contact with infected horses, the bacillus preferentially invading areas of abraded or injured skin. Experimental infection can be induced in animals by inhalation of the bacillus, and certain laboratory-acquired infections indicate that infection may develop in man after inhalation of the microorganism. *Unlike melioidosis, glanders can be transmitted from person to person.*

Pathology and Pathogenesis. Characteristically glanders is associated with cellulitis, necrosis, abscess, and thromboses with septic embolization. Healing occurs by fibrosis, and, rarely, by calcification.

Clinical Manifestations. Glanders may occur as a fulminant acute febrile disease, as a chronic indolent and relapsing disease, or as a subclinical occult infection detectable incidentally at postmortem examination or by serologic test. The two principal features of glanders are (1) nasal cellulitis and necrosis-producing septal perforation, palatal and pharyngeal ulceration; or (2) cutaneous cellulitis, vesiculation, and ulceration at the site of inoculation of the bacillus into the skin, followed by lymphangitis with nodular abscesses along the lymphatics and lymphadenopathy (farcy).

Pulmonary involvement is common in glanders, producing pneumonia, abscesses, pleural effusion, and empyema. Occasionally, in chronic indolent glanders, small nodular granulomatous lesions may be found in the lungs. Hilar lymph node enlargement is common in pulmonary glanders.

When glanders becomes disseminated, destructive polyarthritis, subcutaneous and muscular abscesses, osteomyelitis, meningitis, and pustular skin lesions, particularly over the joints and face, are seen. Prostration and stupor may develop, and are followed by death in two to three weeks.

Chronic glanders may be punctuated by recurrent acute relapses with bacteremia, often resulting in a fulminant course and death. Amyloidosis may be a complication of chronic glanders.

Fever and chills, headache, and backache are common in acute glanders. Leukopenia or a normal leukocyte count is the rule, but leukocytosis has been observed.

Diagnosis. There are no pathognomonic clinical features of glanders. The nodules along lymphatics resemble those seen in sporotrichosis. The respiratory lesions may be difficult to distinguish from other ulcerative infections of the nose and mouth. The cutaneous lesion often resembles streptococcal cellulitis. The multiple abscesses mimic many mycotic and staphylococcal infections and are difficult to distinguish from those of melioidosis. The acute fulminant illness may resemble typhoid fever or disseminated tuberculosis. The diagnosis of glanders can be established by combination of a history of exposure to horses, isolation of M. mallei, serologic tests (agglutination, complement-fixation), and skin test with sterile culture filtrate (mallein). Inoculation of infected material into guinea pigs may facilitate identification of the microorganism.

Treatment. There are reports of successful treatment of glanders with sulfonamides. Tetracycline, chloramphenicol, and streptomycin may be useful, but there is little clinical experience with these drugs in glanders. Because of the serious prognosis and the lack of documented experience with drug therapy, it is advisable to administer daily streptomycin (1.0 gram) in association with a sulfonamide or a tetracycline until all evidences of disease have disappeared. Incision, drainage, and excision of abscesses must be done with caution, for the infection may be disseminated by such manipulation.

Prognosis. Although a few patients have been cured with chemotherapy, the effect of treatment on the mortality rate is not known. *More than 90 per cent of patients with glanders will die from the disease if untreated.* However, the frequency of occurrence of occult or subclinical glanders is not known.

Prevention. Infected horses have been identified by skin tests with mallein and by serologic tests. Destruction of infected animals has eliminated glanders as a public health problem in the United States and most other countries.

Eghbal, M., Rafyi, A., Chamey, H. M., and Farvar, B.: Development of bacterial resistance to sulfonamides during therapy of glanders in man. Presse Méd., 61:1535, 1953.

Howe, C., and Miller, W. R.: Human glanders. Report of six cases. Ann. Intern. Med., 26:115, 1947.

Mendelson, R. W.: Glanders. U.S. Armed Forces Med. J., 1:781, 1950.

220. MELIOIDOSIS

Definition. Melioidosis is a rare disease of man caused by *Malleomyces pseudomallei.* It has been observed most frequently in Malaysia, the People's Republic of China, Burma, India, and other parts of the Far East and Southeast Asia, but has only rarely been observed in North and South America. It is a disease of wild rodents and some domesticated animals, and probably is transmitted to man by contact with diseased animals or animal excreta and possibly by contact with contaminated soil. The disease in man appears in a subclinical (only positive serologic tests), pulmonary, septicemic, or extrapulmonary form. The septicemic and pulmonary disease may be acute and fatal. The pulmonary and extrapulmonary infection with abscesses may be chronic and debilitating.

Etiology. Melioidosis was first identified by Whitmore and Krishnaswami (1912) in Rangoon. The disease was recognized as similar to glanders and attributable to a gram-negative bacillus resembling but differing from *Malleomyces mallei.* The microorganism causing melioidosis has been variously called *Malleomyces pseudomallei, Bacillus whitmori,* and *Pfeiferella whitmori.* It is a motile bacillus that grows aerobically on nutrient agar. Culturally it may resemble Klebsiella and *Pseudomonas aeruginosa. M. pseudomallei* is antigenically distinguishable from *M. mallei.* It produces fatal infection in guinea pigs, rabbits, and other laboratory animals.

Epidemiology. *M. pseudomallei* has been found to cause disease sporadically, endemically, and epidemically among a wide variety of animal species, including rats, rabbits, goats, hogs, dogs, cats, and horses. In addition, the bacillus has been found to be harbored by mosquitoes and fleas. Frequently, the initial manifestations of melioidosis in man are cutaneous abscesses, diarrhea, and pneumonia; therefore it is probable that the disease is transmitted by direct contact with infected animals or by ingestion or inhalation of contaminated material. All these routes of inoculation can produce the disease experimentally in animals. It is unlikely that melioidosis is ever transmitted from man to man. Infection has been observed in narcotic addicts, and in infants, or in patients with diabetes mellitus, renal or liver disease, and pregnancy as predisposing factors.

Clinical Manifestations. Melioidosis may appear acutely or insidiously, and most often follows a fulminant course with septicemia or a chronic indolent course with multiple abscess formation. The incubation period of the disease is not known. The acute illness is often associated with fever, chills, cough, production of bloody and purulent sputum, diarrhea, or abdominal pain. Physical examination may reveal signs of pneumonia, empyema, lung abscess, hepatomegaly, jaundice, and splenomegaly. *A subacute or chronic illness may follow the acute disease or may develop in the absence of an acute illness.* In this situation the patient often has osteomyelitis, suppurating lymphadenopathy, subcutaneous abscesses, psoas abscess, lung abscess, pyelonephritis, or liver or spleen abscess. Bronchocutaneous and other types of fistulas may appear. Patients with this chronic illness may survive for many months, and occasionally may recover.

Diagnosis. Melioidosis may resemble typhoid fever, malaria, mycotic infection, and occasionally acute staphylococcal septicemia or staphylococcal pneumonia. The chronic pulmonary disease most resembles tuberculosis. Melioidosis can be differentiated from these diseases only by bacteriologic identification of the bacillus from blood, sputum, urine, or pus. Hemagglutination and complement fixation tests may be useful when acute and convalescent serologic titers are compared. A single positive test may only indicate previous clinical and subclinical infection.

The leukocyte count of the peripheral blood often is normal in melioidosis, but may rise to levels of 20,000 per cubic millimeter. Urinalysis may show pyuria and hematuria.

Treatment and Prevention. There is no available antigen for active immunization against melioidosis. Prevention of the disease is possible by controlled sanitation and improved standards of living. Patients have been successfully treated with chloramphenicol, sulfonamides, or tetracycline, given over long periods of time. The drug susceptibility of *M. pseudomallei,* however, is variable. In adults, 3 grams of tetracycline a day orally for 90 days, or, alternatively, in septicemia, large doses of chloramphenicol are preferred. Surgical drainage of abscesses is essential for proper management.

Buchman, R. J., Kmiecik, J. E., and LaNove, A. M.: Extrapulmonary melioidosis. Am. J. Surg., 125:324, 1973.
Khaira, B. S., Young, W. B., and Hart, P. DeV.: Melioidosis. Br. Med. J., 1:949, 1959.
Prevatt, A. L., and Hunt, J. S.: Chronic systemic melioidosis. Review of literature. Am. J. Med., 23:810, 1957.
Spotnitz, M., Rudnitsky, A., and Rambaud, J. J.: Melioidosis pneumonitis. J.A.M.A., 202:950, 1967.

221. ANTHRAX

Leighton E. Cluff

Definition. Anthrax is an infectious disease of wild and domesticated animals caused by *Bacillus anthracis.* Occasionally it is transmitted to man. A necrotic ulcer of the skin or mucous membranes is the most common feature of the disease, but hemorrhagic mediastinitis and disseminated infection with hemorrhagic meningitis may also develop. Depending upon the most prominent feature of the disease, anthrax has been variously referred to as *malignant pustule, splenic fever, woolsorters' disease, milzbrand,* and *charbon.*

Etiology. *Bacillus anthracis* was identified in 1849 by Davaine, and was further characterized by Koch in 1877. It is a gram-positive, spore-forming, encapsulated, hemolytic, aerobic microorganism. It resembles *B. subtilis* and *B. cereus* but can be differentiated from these organisms by its virulence for laboratory animals such as the mouse and rabbit, by its lack of hemolytic activity on blood agar, and by lysis of *B. anthracis* with specific bacteriophage. In broth, the bacillus elaborates an antigen that can be used for specific immunization ("protective antigen"). The spores of *B. anthracis* are killed by boiling for ten minutes but survive for long periods of time in soil, in animal carcasses, and after aerosolization.

Epidemiology. Anthrax has occurred sporadically and in epidemics throughout the world. Cattle, sheep, goats, horses, and swine are most commonly found to have anthrax; outbreaks of the disease in these animals rarely occur in the United States. Although the disease has been acquired by butchering, skinning, or dissecting infected carcasses, human infection in the United States is observed almost exclusively in persons handling imported contaminated hides, wool, goat hair, or other animal products. There has been a progressive decrease in anthrax in the United States in the past several years (17 cases from 1956 to 1964). The infection may be transmitted to man by direct contact, inhalation, and ingestion of infected material.

Pathology and Pathogenesis. Anthrax is characterized by edema, hemorrhage, necrosis, and various degrees of inflammation. *B. anthracis* possesses a glutamyl polypeptide capsule that interferes with phagocytosis, and this contributes to its pathogenicity. The gelatinous edema of anthrax infection contains large amounts of bacterial capsular material. The serum of many animals has lytic activity against the bacillus, but this anthracidal substance seems to bear little, if any, relationship to natural resistance. It is probable that *B. anthracis* initiates infection in the skin only through abrasions, cuts, or other types of injury. During the course of lethal anthrax infection in laboratory animals a bacterial toxin is produced that is responsible for death. This lethal toxin can be neutralized by specific antitoxin.

Clinical Manifestations. The skin lesion of anthrax usually begins as a small erythematous papule that becomes vesicular, necrotic, and covered with a dark crust or eschar. Intense nonpitting edema, which may not be erythematous, often surrounds and may extend a considerable distance from the eschar. Characteristically the lesion is pruritic but not very tender or hot. The skin lesion is commonly on exposed areas of hands, arms, neck, or face; and there may be mild regional lymph node enlargement. Lymphangitis is not usually observed. Constitutional symptoms and fever are frequently absent unless the skin disease is severe or the infection becomes disseminated, when high fever, prostration, and death may occur.

Infrequently anthrax may develop without a lesion, possibly after inoculation into the skin, but probably more commonly after inhalation of spores of the bacillus in contaminated air. Characteristically, this form of anthrax is severe and is associated with disseminated infection. *Hemorrhagic mediastinitis*, often without pneumonia, and *hemorrhagic meningitis* may occur. Death is common in this form of anthrax; the illness may begin abruptly, be of short duration, and terminate rapidly. Dyspnea and cyanosis are indicative of respiratory or ventilatory insufficiency. Roentgenographic examination of the chest in inhalation anthrax reveals widening of the mediastinum. Leukocytosis is ordinarily not pronounced. Pleural effusion may complicate pulmonary anthrax. Anthrax in man from ingestion of bacilli is rare.

Diagnosis. Anthrax is most readily diagnosed in persons known to have been exposed to animals or animal products potentially contaminated with *B. anthracis*. Cutaneous anthrax can be differentiated from many other bacterial infections of the skin by the insignificance of regional adenopathy, lymphangitis, and cellulitis in relation to the severity of the eschar and edema. Furthermore, pruritus, lack of tenderness, and intense nonpitting edema are characteristic of anthrax. Small skin lesions, however, may be more difficult to recognize. Pulmonary anthrax can be identified by a history of occupational exposure and acute widening of the mediastinum shown by roentgenographic examination. Anthrax meningitis is confused with subarachnoid hemorrhage or cerebrovascular accident, but is usually associated with prominent signs of infection, and gram-positive bacilli can be seen in the cerebrospinal fluid.

In disseminated anthrax infection, blood cultures are often positive. Occasionally, the bacilli may be identified in the centrifugal sediment of blood treated with 3 per cent acetic acid solution and stained with Wright's stain.

In cutaneous anthrax, the bacilli can usually be cultured from the lesions, or typical encapsulated bacilli will be seen when stained with a polychrome eosinmethylene blue stain (Wright or Giemsa). Their direct cultivation on peptone agar should always be attempted.

If the specimen has to be shipped, the specimen should be dried on silk threads or on a sterile glass slide. In view of the occurrence of anthrax-like bacilli on the skin, it is imperative that diagnoses be confirmed by animal inoculations, preferably in guinea pigs or mice or by specific bacteriophage lysis. In pulmonary anthrax, the bacillus has been found microscopically in the sputum and in the pleural exudate.

Prognosis. Cutaneous anthrax is often a self-limited disease, but dissemination of the infection and death may occur in 20 per cent of patients. A fatal outcome in cutaneous anthrax can be averted by appropriate treatment, but treatment of disseminated infection is often unsuccessful in preventing death.

Treatment. *B. anthracis* is susceptible to the action of penicillin and the tetracyclines. Penicillin G should be given in total daily doses of at least 1.2 million units, starting as soon as anthrax is diagnosed or seriously suspected. The effectiveness of the tetracyclines is probably not quite so great as that of penicillin; nevertheless, they are effective in cutaneous anthrax and may be administered in a total daily dose of 2.0 grams. Therapy with penicillin or the tetracyclines should be continued for seven days. It should be emphasized that in patients with disseminated anthrax, the progressive course may be so rapid that antimicrobial drugs may not save the patient's life.

Prevention. Anthrax can be prevented in man by control of infected animals or animal products. Sterilization of wool during manufacture is often impracticable, although this is the means employed to prevent infection from clothing and other products, such as shaving brushes, made of potentially infected materials. Vaccination with "protective antigen" is effective in preventing infection in persons likely to be occupationally exposed.

Brachman, P. S.: Human anthrax in the United States. *In* Hobby, G. L. (ed.): Antimicrobial Agents and Chemotherapy. Baltimore, Williams & Wilkins Company, 1965.

Brachman, P. S., Plotkin, S. A., Bumford, F. H., and Atchison, M. M.: An epidemic of inhalation anthrax. II. Epidemiologic investigation. Am. J. Hyg., 72:6, 1960.

Gold, H.: Anthrax: Report of 117 cases. Arch. Intern. Med., 96:387, 1955.

Hughes, M. H.: Anthrax. Br. Med. J., 1:488, 1973.

Plotkin, S. A., Brachman, P. S., Utell, M., Bumford, F. H., and Atchison, M. M.: Epidemic of inhalation anthrax, first in twentieth century. I. Clinical features. Am. J. Med., 29:992, 1960.

Smith, H., and Keppie, J.: Studies on the chemical basis of pathogenicity of *Bacillus anthracis* using organisms grown in vivo. *In* Howie, J. W., and O'Hea, A. J. (eds.): Mechanisms of Microbial Pathogenicity. London, Cambridge University Press, 1955.

222. LISTERIOSIS

Leighton E. Cluff

Definition. Listeriosis is an infectious disease of animals and man with exceptionally protean manifestations, including meningitis, disseminated granulomas, lymphadenopathy, respiratory symptoms, and ill-defined acute febrile illness. It can produce abortion and fetal or neonatal death. The infection is caused by a gram-positive bacillus called *Listeria monocytogenes* and is worldwide in distribution.

Etiology. Infection of the human being with *Listeria monocytogenes* was identified in 1929 by Nyfeldt. The microorganism was first characterized, however, by

Murray, Webb, and Swann in 1926, during an epizootic among rabbits and guinea pigs. Subsequently the microorganism has been identified as a cause of disease in fox, raccoon, goat, lemming, mouse, rat, hamster, pig, horse, cow, dog, domestic fowl and wild birds, and other animals. *L. monocytogenes* is a gram-positive, nonspore-forming, aerobic or microaerophilic, motile bacillus. It ferments a number of sugars, with formation of acid but no gas. It can be grown on nutrient agar or broth, preferably containing 1 per cent glucose, and produces beta hemolysis on blood agar. *L. monocytogenes* resembles *Erysipelothrix rhuziopathiae* and diphtheroids, but can be differentiated from these bacteria by its motility (best at 20 to 30° C), its specific antigenicity, and its animal pathogenicity. Listeria regularly — and Erysipelothrix occasionally — produces purulent keratoconjunctivitis in rabbits after inoculation into the conjunctival space, whereas diphtheroids do not.

Incidence and Prevalence. Listeriosis in man and animals has been observed throughout the world. It has been recognized more frequently in humans in recent years, but its true incidence is not known. Confusion in bacteriologic differentiation accounts largely for inadequate recognition of listeriosis. In addition, the diverse manifestations of the disease render it difficult to identify clinically.

Epidemiology. Listeriosis may develop after inhalation, ingestion, or direct contact with contaminated food or animal products. The disease is most common in persons living in rural areas. Although infection with Listeria occurs in many domesticated and wild animals, there are only rare instances of epizootics or outbreaks in animals other than man. Transmission of infection from person to person probably occurs under some circumstances, notably in nursery outbreaks. Women can carry Listeria in the vagina, and infection may be transmitted venereally. Whether or not man can be an asymptomatic carrier of Listeria under other conditions is not known.

Pathology and Pathogenesis. Human listeriosis is characterized by disseminated granulomas and focal necrosis or suppuration in involved tissues. Lesions may develop in liver, intestinal tract, gallbladder, skin, mucous membranes of the respiratory tract, lung, heart, spleen, lymph nodes, placenta, and brain. The fetus may be infected transplacentally through the umbilical vein, with production of septicemia. Debilitating diseases such as chronic infection and cancer predispose to the occurrence of listeriosis. Pregnancy may increase susceptibility to infection, but the disease in pregnant women may be less severe than in other persons. Administration of adrenal cortical steroids may also increase susceptibility to listeriosis. Infection also occurs in persons with no underlying disease.

Clinical Manifestations. *Meningitis* is the most commonly recognized form of listeriosis in the United States. It is characterized at onset by symptoms of headache, myalgia, fever, chills, nausea, vomiting, and photophobia, followed by the development of stiff neck, stupor, convulsions, somnolence, and, finally, death. The onset may be abrupt or gradual, and the initial symptoms may be those of gastrointestinal or respiratory illness. Examination reveals manifestations of meningitis or encephalitis in varying degrees of severity. There may be pharyngitis, rhinitis, otitis media, neck rigidity, ocular palsy, and signs of depressed cerebral function. Leukocytosis is common, with granulocytosis and, occasionally, monocytosis, in the early phase of the disease. The cerebrospinal fluid, with decreased sugar, elevated protein, and cell counts of 150 to 3000 per cubic millimeter, is indistinguishable from that in many purulent meningitides. Early, the cells in the fluid may be principally granulocytes, but later there may be a predominance of mononuclear cells.

Febrile pharyngitis with cervical and generalized lymphadenopathy can be caused by Listeria, and may be difficult to differentiate from *infectious mononucleosis*. Patients with this type of illness, however, may have an abrupt onset of fever, chills, headache, myalgia, conjunctivitis, macular rash, and sore throat. Lymph nodes in the neck and elsewhere may enlarge, and there may be hepatosplenomegaly. Blood leukocytes occasionally increase in number with a more or less pronounced monocytosis. The absorbed heterophil serologic test for infectious mononucleosis is negative, Listeria can be isolated from blood and pharynx, and there will be a rising serum agglutinin titer for Listeria.

Lymph node enlargement in the neck and elsewhere without respiratory symptoms may also be attributed to listeriosis. In addition, lymph node enlargement associated only with conjunctivitis may occur. Isolated acute upper respiratory illness may be attributable to listeriosis, although for obvious reasons this diagnosis is seldom established. Chronic urethritis in men has been described, and possibly may be responsible for subclinical or occult infection, demonstrable by culture of the bacillus from bone marrow.

Papular skin lesions associated with disseminated listeriosis have been seen in infants, but adults may acquire primary cutaneous infection after direct contact with infected animal tissues.

Disseminated listeriosis in infants has been reported frequently in Europe, but infrequently in the United States. The disease may arise by transplacental infection of the fetus, causing abortion, fetal death, or serious illness within several days after birth. Outbreaks of infection may develop in newborn nurseries, probably by person-to-person transmission. The disease is characterized by disseminated visceral granulomas and abscesses. When it manifests itself in infants a few weeks old, it often begins as a mild febrile illness with cough, coryza, gastrointestinal symptoms, and pneumonia. Granulomas may be formed on the posterior pharyngeal wall. Granulocytosis and occasionally mononucleosis are present. Pleural and pericardial effusions may develop. Listeriosis has been reported as a common cause of neonatal death and fetal damage in Europe.

Listeriosis in pregnancy may be subclinical or may be associated with an acute febrile illness resembling influenza and occasionally pyelonephritis; it is rarely severe. Its occurrence after the fifth month of pregnancy, however, is likely to affect the fetus seriously. A woman may become a vaginal carrier of Listeria and may possibly infect her infant at birth.

Disseminated listeriosis in adults has an abrupt onset with chill and fever. Meningitis can occur, as well as bacterial endocarditis. Blood cultures are usually positive, and there may be a consumptive coagulopathy. This type of listeriosis is observed most often in patients with carcinoma or debilitating disease, and its development may have been facilitated by adrenal steroid therapy.

Diagnosis. There are no pathognomonic clinical features of human listeriosis. The diagnosis rests on isolation of the microorganism or rising agglutinin titers in the serum. It is likely that the recognition of listeriosis has been difficult because of the failure to differentiate Listeria from diphtheroid bacilli in culture. The isolation of microorganisms resembling diphtheroids from infectious material or blood should alert one to the necessity for further bacteriologic characterization.

Listeriosis may resemble influenza, miliary tuberculosis, typhoid fever, mycotic infections, and several bacterial infections with septicemia. *Infectious mononucleosis* is most often confused with listeriosis in adults, for the two diseases may be clinically alike. However, listeriosis is infrequently associated with monocytosis, does not produce a positive absorbed heterophil serologic test, and in systemic disease the bacillus can be isolated from blood, bone marrow, urine, or upper respiratory tract.

Treatment. *Listeria monocytogenes* is susceptible in vitro to sulfonamides, penicillin, tetracycline, chloramphenicol, erythromycin, novobiocin, and occasionally streptomycin. Penicillin is the drug of choice, but the tetracyclines and erythromycin are also effective. Some have recommended use of the aminoglycosides, but most strains of Listeria are susceptible to less toxic antimicrobial drugs, and these are preferred unless in vitro resistance is demonstrated. Treatment should be continued for a period of several days, depending upon the characteristics of the disease.

Prognosis. Listeria meningitis has a fatality rate of 70 per cent in untreated patients. The fatality rate in treated patients has not been defined, but is considerably lower. The prognosis in adults with pharyngitis and lymph node enlargement is good, whether treated or not, but meningitis may supervene. Recovery from meningitis may leave residual symptoms of central nervous system damage. Infection of the newborn is very serious; the fatality rate and the incidence of congenital defects are high. Untreated, disseminated listeriosis is usually a fatal disease.

Prevention. Listeriosis must be regarded as primarily a contagious disease of animals; prevention of human infection would require elimination of animal reservoirs, but this would not prevent person-to-person transmission. Pasteurization prevents transmission of the disease by contaminated milk. Animal products, including meat, should be declared unfit for consumption if the disease is found in slaughtered animals. Better recognition of the disease should clarify its epidemiology and indirectly facilitate control measures. There are no effective agents for immunization.

Gray, M. L., and Killinger, A. H.: *Listeria monocytogenes* and listeric infections. Bact. Rev., 30:309, 1966.

Hoeprich, P. D.: Infections due to *Listeria monocytogenes*. Medicine, 37:143, 1958.

Lowenstein, M. S., Fox, M. D., and Martin, S. M.: Human listeriosis in the U.S. J. Infect. Dis., 123:328, 1971.

Medoff, G., Kunz, L. J., and Weinberg, A. N.: Listeriosis in humans: An evaluation. J. Infect. Dis., 123:247, 1971.

Moore, R. M., and Zehmer, R. B.: Listeriosis in the U.S., 1971. J. Infect. Dis., 127:610, 1973.

223. ERYSIPELOID OF ROSENBACH

Leighton E. Cluff

Erysipeloid of Rosenbach is a specific infectious disease attributable to *Erysipelothrix rhuziopathia*. It occurs in man after contact with infected animals or animal products, particularly swine, cattle, sheep, fish, birds, dogs, horses, reindeer, rabbits, mink, rats, and mice. The disease in man therefore usually arises in abattoir employees, butchers, kitchen workers, those handling fish, those handling animal hides and pelts, and those working with bone or bone meal. Most infections in human beings can be related to skin injury. The causative microorganism is a gram-positive bacillus, nonspore-forming, that can be grown aerobically or anaerobically on nutrient broth containing 1 per cent glucose or upon blood agar. It produces death in laboratory animals, particularly mice, causing focal abscesses in the liver or cutaneous cellulitis. The bacillus is susceptible in vitro to tetracycline, penicillin, and chloramphenicol.

Erysipeloid in man occurs seasonally, usually in summer and early fall, and is worldwide in distribution. Most commonly it is characterized by a nonsuppurative violaceous lesion of the hand or fingers that is swollen, very slightly tender, and has a sharply defined margin rarely extending above the wrist. In contrast to streptococcal cellulitis there are usually burning, tingling, and itching, but little pain in the involved area; rarely does the patient have systemic symptoms of fever, chills, malaise, or headache. Lymphangitis is infrequent, and when it develops it is often attributable to secondary infection with staphylococci or streptococci. The localized disease is self-limited, lasting a few days, and resolution is rapid, associated with brownish discoloration of the involved skin and rarely desquamation. A bacteriologic diagnosis can be made by culture of material aspirated or biopsied from the margin of the lesion, but isolation of the bacillus is not invariable. Ordinarily, the lesion is sufficiently distinctive to permit a clinical diagnosis when the microorganism is not cultured.

Infrequently Erysipelothrix infections may become disseminated, causing a diffuse involvement of skin. Rarely, bacteremia may develop, and bacterial endocarditis can occur.

Erysipeloid continues to occur frequently in exposed persons. The ubiquitousness of the bacillus has made it difficult to eradicate the disease. The ordinarily benign character of the infection, however, has made it an insignificant public health problem. Treatment of erysipeloid with penicillin has been shown to shorten the illness, but relapses of the disease have occurred in persons who are untreated or who receive inadequate treatment.

Ewing, M.: Erysipeloid. Med. J. Aust., 1:449, 1957.

Klauden, J. V.: Erysipeloid as an occupational disease. J.A.M.A., 111:1345, 1938.

Price, J. E. L., and Bennett, W. E. J.: The erysipeloid of Rosenbach. Br. Med. J., 2:1060, 1951.

Sneath, P. H. A., Abbott, J. D., and Cunliffe, A. C.: The bacteriology of erysipeloid. Br. Med. J., 2:1063, 1951.

224. ACTINOMYCOSIS

John P. Utz

Definition. Actinomycosis is a chronic, systemic disease characterized by multiple indurated abscesses and sinus tracts characteristically in the face, neck, chest, and abdomen.

History. Lebert is credited with the first report, in 1857, of actinomycosis in man. Bollinger described the disease in cattle in 1876. In 1877 Harz named the causative organism *Actinomyces bovis.* In 1878 Israel clearly defined the disease in man by a summary of the clinical and pathologic characteristics observed in 38 patients. The same author in collaboration with Wolff in 1891 succeeded in growing the microorganism in anaerobic culture. In 1910 Lord observed *A. bovis* in and about carious teeth and tonsillar crypts in the mouths of otherwise normal persons.

Etiology. Actinomycosis in man is caused by *A. israelii* and in cattle by *A. bovis,* but species characteristics overlap. In the normal mouth *A. israelii* grows as a pleomorphic rod-shaped bacterium and in tissues as a granule. In draining pus, mycelial clumps measuring 1 to 2 mm in diameter and colored white to yellow have been termed "sulfur" granules. Microscopically these are composed of 0.5 to $1.0\,\mu$ filaments which stain gram-positive. On agar media under strictly anaerobic conditions, *A. israelii* grows as a white spherical or lobulated colony. Laboratory animals are generally not susceptible to experimental infection. Although long considered to be a fungus, the microbe is now classified under the bacteria, a designation that more closely fits certain of its major characteristics, including susceptibility to penicillin.

Epidemiology. The disease is worldwide in distribution. During the first part of the twentieth century it was viewed as being the most common of the "systemic mycoses," but the incidence has been decreasing of late. Males are affected almost twice as frequently as females, and the illness seems most common among farmers and in rural areas. Disease is produced by direct invasion of contiguous tissues by *A. israelii* commonly present in the mouth or bowel. There is virtually always concurrent infection with other anaerobic bacteria. Disease in the brain, heart valves, or extremities may be exceptional instances of hematogenous dissemination. Disease in cows, dogs, or swine has no contagious relation to that in man.

Pathology. In tissues the characteristic and classic findings are the actinomycotic granules. These are usually found in abscesses and are surrounded by polymorphonuclear leukocytes. Chronic granulomatous reactions are also seen with giant cells, especially about granules.

Clinical Manifestations. *Cervicofacial Form.* The cervicofacial form occurs in less than half of all cases. Infection probably spreads secondarily to trauma or to carious teeth or infected tonsils. The subcutaneous tissues at the angle of the mandible and of the neck have a characteristic "woody" or indurated feeling, and the skin over these areas is reddened and may have single or multiple draining sinus tracts. Pain is seldom prominent even with osteomyelitic or periosteal lesions of bone.

Thoracic Form. This form of disease arises from aspiration into the bronchi of *A. israelii* or in a few instances from extension of disease from the esophagus to mediastinal tissues and secondarily to pleura and lung. Fever and cough are minimal early in the illness. As disease progresses to consolidation, pleurisy, and draining sinuses, prominent symptoms are weight loss, night sweats, and high fever. Rib involvement occurs occasionally, pleural effusion rarely.

Abdominal Form. Actinomycosis of the abdomen generally follows appendicitis, appendiceal abscess, a perforating lesion of the stomach, or a diverticulum of the large bowel. An abdominal mass is usually palpable, and may be extensive; and there may be burrowing sinus tracts, some of which may open to the skin in the inguinal or other regions. Retroperitoneal and thoracic spread through the diaphragm are common.

Other Forms. Approximately 10 per cent of patients have lesions in the brain, heart valves, anorectal area, or subcutaneous tissue of the extremities. Rare instances of actinomycosis of the finger have been attributed to injury to the hand by an adversary's tooth.

Diagnosis. The diagnosis of actinomycosis is supported by the finding in pus of granules that microscopically are composed of gram-positive, branching, often beaded filaments. It should be emphasized that granules may be expressed from otherwise normal tonsils and may not be found in cerebrospinal fluid in cases of central nervous system disease. The diagnosis is confirmed by the isolation of the microorganism in anaerobic culture from a lesion.

Skin test and serologic methods of confirmation are unreliable and unavailable.

Cervicofacial forms of actinomycosis must be distinguished from Ludwig's angina, tuberculosis, osteomyelitis, and malignancy. The thoracic form of disease is suggestive of tuberculosis, other fungal infections, and malignancy. Abdominal actinomycosis is often suspected of being tuberculosis, malignant disease, and, occasionally, amebiasis.

Treatment. Penicillin, first used for actinomycosis in 1944, continues to be the best drug in treating all forms of the disease. Although most strains are inhibited in vitro by levels of 0.1 unit per milliliter, the nature of the pathologic process leads often to treatment failures and necessitates prolonged therapy. Doses of 10 to 20 million units parenterally daily for at least six weeks or until lesions have healed are recommended. In penicillin-allergic patients, alternative agents are tetracycline, clindamycin, or chloramphenicol.

Surgical resection and incision and drainage of chronically infected tissues are important adjunctive therapeutic measures.

Prognosis. Prior to antimicrobial therapy, prognosis for life was poor in all forms. With penicillin therapy, the approximate recovery rates are as follows: cervicofacial, 90 per cent; abdominal, 80 per cent; and thoracic, 40 per cent.

Cope, V. Z.: Actinomycosis. London, Oxford University Press, 1938.
Lerner, P. I.: Susceptibility of pathogenic actinomycetes to antimicrobial compounds. Antimicrob. Agents Chemother., 5:302, 1974.
Peabody, J. W., Jr., and Seabury, J. H.: Actinomycosis and nocardiosis. J. Chronic. Dis., 5:374, 1957.

225. NOCARDIOSIS

John E. Bennett

Definition. Nocardiosis is an uncommon acute or chronic suppurative infection, most often originating in the lung, with a marked tendency to spread to brain and other organs.

History. Eppinger described the first case in 1890 and isolated the etiologic agent.

Etiology. *Nocardia asteroides* is the etiologic agent in most cases of nocardiosis. *Nocardia brasiliensis* causes an occasional case of nocardiosis, but this organism more typically is responsible for mycetoma or, rarely, a lymphocutaneous disease resembling sporotrichosis. Both Nocardia species are aerobic, higher bacteria with branching hyphae 0.5 to $1.0\,\mu$ wide. Hyphae are gram-positive and weakly acid fast. Nocardia grow readily at

25 or 37° C on many antibiotic-free culture media. Colonies are initially smooth and white or cream colored, later becoming chalky with an orange or yellow hue. Growth is often apparent in the first week of incubation. Identification of an isolate as *N. asteroides* or *N. brasiliensis* is a complex task, best assigned to a reference laboratory.

Epidemiology. Nocardia organisms are soil saprophytes. Portal of entry is the lung or, rarely, through trauma to the skin or gastrointestinal tract. Man-to-man transmission is unknown. Nocardiosis is infrequent but worldwide. Infection in males is two to three times as common as in females. Disease occurs at any age but is more frequent in older adults. No occupational predisposition is known. Many patients have pre-existing debilitating conditions, such as neoplasia, immunosuppressive therapy, or alveolar proteinosis.

Pathology. The lung lesion is a bronchopneumonia, with a tendency to suppuration, empyema, and abscess formation. Brain lesions are poorly encapsulated abscesses, often multiple. Purulent meningitis may result from rupture of a brain abscess into the cerebrospinal fluid. Neutrophils are the most prominent inflammatory cell in all sites, but lymphocytes and plasma cells also occur. Giant cells or epithelioid cells are unusual. Branching filaments of Nocardia are scattered in the lesion, with no granule formation. Hyphae are best demonstrated histologically by a tissue Gram stain, such as Brown and Brenn. An overstained Gomori methenamine silver procedure can also be used.

Clinical Manifestations. Presenting symptoms usually refer to the lung, brain, or subcutaneous tissue, in that decreasing order of frequency. Pulmonary infection may be acute or of many months' duration. Symptoms include fever, cough, purulent sputum, weight loss, anorexia, fatigue, dyspnea, and chest pain. Radiologic appearance of the lung lesion is variable, but typically there are one or more areas of dense pneumonia. Lesions tend to cavitate with time. Empyema is frequent. Infection sometimes extends from the lung into the chest wall, forming a subcutaneous abscess. The central nervous system is infected in 30 per cent of cases. This may be the initial or sole manifestation of the disease or may be a late complication of pulmonary nocardiosis. Clinically the neurologic disease presents as a brain abscess or purulent meningitis. Skin or subcutaneous abscesses also occur in about 30 per cent of cases, usually in the presence of pulmonary nocardiosis. Dissemination to many other organs may occur, particularly heart, kidney, spleen, and liver.

Diagnosis. A refractory, suppurative pneumonitis should suggest the possibility of nocardiosis, particularly in the presence of chest wall extension, brain abscess, or skin abscesses. Sputum, bronchoscopic washings, pleural fluid, percutaneous lung aspirates, and pus aspirated from other sites should be Gram stained and cultured for Nocardia. Cultures of blood, bone marrow, urine, or cerebrospinal fluid are rarely positive. Branching, gram-positive filaments on smear raise the possibility of actinomycosis or nocardiosis. Nocardia can usually, but not always, be distinguished from Actinomyces on smear by the absence of granules and weak acid-fastness of the former. Acid-fastness is best demonstrated by a modified Ziehl-Neelsen stain or in tissue by a modified Fite-Faraco stain. Use of 1 per cent sulfuric acid during destaining is critical. Diagnosis of nocardiosis by culture alone is fraught with problems. Nocardia organisms are

difficult to isolate from heavily contaminated specimens, such as sputum, and accurate culture identification of Nocardia requires both time and expertise.

Nocardia is sometimes isolated from a specimen, usually sputum, but the patient's condition is best explained by other diagnoses. Either the Nocardia is a laboratory contaminant or it is causing a mild, self-limiting disease. Although this situation does occur, it is much more common for subsequent developments to indicate that nocardiosis had been the cause of symptoms incorrectly ascribed to tuberculosis, neoplasm, or another disorder.

Treatment. Treatment of choice is enough sulfadiazine to give serum concentrations of 10 to 15 mg per 100 ml. Six to nine grams per day is usually required for an adult. Copious fluid intake and urine alkalinization with oral sodium bicarbonate are necessary to prevent crystalluria. After about a month, if the patient is improving, sulfadiazine dosage may be reduced to 4 to 6 grams per day, or an equivalent amount of sulfisoxazole or trisulfapyrimidines may be used instead. Therapy is usually continued at this dose for 12 to 18 months. Pus in the brain, pleura, or soft tissues should be drained. Whether or not drugs other than sulfonamides are useful is an open question. Only a few patients not receiving sulfonamides have survived. It is common practice for patients responding poorly to sulfonamides to be given an additional drug, particularly ampicillin, 150 mg per kilogram per day. Cycloserine, erythromycin, and minocycline also have their advocates.

Prognosis. Clinically apparent nocardiosis is usually fatal without treatment. With appropriate therapy, nocardiosis confined to the lung has the best prognosis (50 to 60 per cent survival) and central nervous system infection the worst (13 per cent survival). The occurrence of nocardiosis in the presence of immunosuppressive therapy portends a poor prognosis.

Grossman, C. B., Bragg, D. G., and Armstrong, D.: Roentgen manifestations of pulmonary nocardiosis. Am. J. Roentgenol., 96:325, 1970.
Kurup, P. V., Randhawa, H. S., and Gupta, N. P.: Nocardiosis: A review. Mycopathologia, 40:193, 1970.
Murray, J. F., Finegold, S. M., Froman, S., and Will, D. W.: The changing spectrum of nocardiosis. Am. Rev. Respir. Dis., 83:315, 1961.
Orfanakis, M. G., Wilcox, H. G., and Smith, C. B.: In vitro studies of the combined effect of ampicillin and sulfonamides on *Nocardia asteroides* and results of therapy in four patients. Antimicrob. Agents Chemother., 1:215, 1972.

226. BRUCELLOSIS
(Undulant Fever, Malta Fever)
Vernon Knight

Definition. Brucellosis is an infectious disease caused by microorganisms of the genus Brucella, transmitted to man from lower animals. The disease may be acute, subacute, subclinical, chronic, or relapsing, and infection may localize in various viscera and tissues.

Etiology. Brucellae are small, gram-negative, aerobic, nonmotile, and nonspore-forming coccobacilli. Three species, characterized by their affinity for a particular animal host, account for most human infections: *Brucella abortus* (cattle), *Brucella melitensis* (sheep and goats), and *Brucella suis* (pigs). A newly described species,

Brucella canis, causes abortion in beagles and has, on infrequent occasions, been transmitted to humans in contact with infected dogs.

History. Brucellae were first isolated by Bruce in 1887 from the spleens of British soldiers dying on the island of Malta. This disease, now known to have been caused by infection with *B. melitensis,* was contracted by drinking raw goat's milk. Bang, in 1897 in Denmark, isolated a strain of the species now designated *B. abortus* from cattle with infectious abortion. Traum in 1914 isolated the third species, *B. suis,* from an infected sow.

Epidemiology. In the United States, reported cases of brucellosis in man now number slightly less than 200 per year, representing a low plateau after a steady decrease since 1947, when 6300 cases were reported. The cases occur principally in persons associated with swine- and cattle-slaughtering operations and to a lesser extent among workers involved in producing and marketing livestock. Two thirds of infections result from exposure to swine, and a smaller proportion results from exposure to cattle. In keeping with this, the majority of isolations of Brucella from human cases have been *B. suis,* and less frequently *B. abortus* or *B. melitensis. B. canis,* the cause of disease in dogs, has been isolated from a few human patients. A small number of patients reported exposure to milk or cheese as a possible source of infection. Of interest is the fact that in recent years about two thirds of American cases have occurred in Iowa, California, Virginia, Texas, and Minnesota.

The decrease in human brucellosis in this country is a result of almost uniform pasteurization of milk and milk products and reduction of the infection in cattle. The latter has been accomplished by a State-Federal eradication program whereby movement of infected or exposed animals is restricted and infected animals are slaughtered. In addition, a program of vaccination of calves with live strain 19 Brucella vaccine has contributed to control of the disease. Recently a program to eradicate porcine brucellosis was started.

In Great Britain about 300 cases of brucellosis in man are reported annually. These arise from ingestion of milk and milk products and contact with infected cattle. It is estimated that 300,000 cattle, involving one third of the dairy herds in Britain, are infected. In Britain, brucellosis occurs chiefly in cattle, and infections caused by *B. melitensis* and *B. suis* do not occur except for a small number of cases whose infection was acquired from sources outside Britain. In other countries that use sheep and goats more extensively, these animals may be the principal sources of infection.

Pathogenesis and Pathology. In the case of ingested dairy products, the organism penetrates the gastrointestinal mucosa; with direct contact the organism enters through breaks in the skin or the conjunctiva. It presumably may also be inhaled, because brucellae have been isolated from the air of a slaughterhouse where infected animals were killed, and infection is readily transmitted to laboratory animals by aerosol. Many persons have become infected with the organism in the laboratory, and one laboratory accident involving apparent airborne spread has been described. Brucellae are destroyed in milk and milk products by pasteurization; otherwise, they may remain viable in refrigerated milk for 10 days and in cheese up to 90 days. They may persist in meat for several weeks.

After penetration of skin or mucous membranes, the organisms spread via lymphatics to regional nodes and thence to thoracic duct and the bloodstream. Hematogenous dissemination leads to localization in spleen, bone marrow, liver, kidneys, endocardium, and elsewhere. In cattle, swine, sheep, and goats, organisms also localize in mammary glands, male and female genital organs, and in the pregnant uterus, fetal fluids, and membranes, causing abortion. Correlated with genital, uterine, and fetal infection is the finding in these tissues of a 4-carbon, polyhydric alcohol, erythritol, which promotes the growth of brucellae. Although erythritol is apparently not present in the human testicle, orchitis is paradoxically a complication of human Brucella infection. Erythritol is not present in human placentas, and brucellosis is rarely associated with abortions in humans.

Characteristically, Brucella infections are granulomas consisting of foci of lymphocytes, epithelioid cells, plasma cells, and multinucleated giant cells. In severe cases, necrosis and abscess formation may occur, a finding most characteristic of infection with *B. suis.* Brucella infection causes the development of the usual array of humoral antibodies which can be measured as agglutinins, opsonins, bacteriocidins, and precipitins, and by complement fixation. These apparently participate in the control of acute infection, aided by macrophages which ingest and destroy large numbers of organisms. Despite increased capacity of macrophages from infected animals to destroy brucellae, infection may persist in intracellular foci in macrophages or in other cells at local sites of infection, to become the source of chronic or relapsing infections.

Clinical Manifestations. The incubation period varies from a few days to a few weeks or even months. Onset may be insidious, with nonspecific findings such as low-grade fever, headache, weakness, joint pains, insomnia, sweats, and low back pain. Less commonly, onset may be abrupt, with high fever, chills, and prostration, but with few localizing signs. It is probable that fever and some of the other acute manifestations of infection are an effect, at least in part, of Brucella endotoxin, which resembles endotoxin from other gram-negative bacteria. Some lymphadenopathy occurs in about one half of cases, and splenomegaly occurs in about one third, usually in the more severely ill.

The initial illness, when untreated, may persist a few days to several weeks, and improvement may be followed by one or more relapses. Disability may persist for a year or more. Treatment is usually followed by prompt recovery, but relapse may occur in a small percentage of patients. The accompanying figure illustrates the prompt response to treatment with tetracycline of a patient with acute *B. melitensis* infection. Her disease relapsed a few weeks later but was successfully retreated with the same drug.

Infrequent but severe complications of brucellosis include *meningoencephalitis, spondylitis, endocarditis, orchitis, pancytopenia, nephritis, hepatic and splenic suppuration, cholecystitis, arthritis,* and *uveitis.* When the complication is the presenting complaint, as is sometimes the case, the diagnosis of brucellosis may not be suggested. For that reason the varied involvement possible with this disease should be kept in mind. Suppurative lesions of the liver and spleen often calcify with the passage of time, and calcific densities in roentgenograms of liver or spleen may be a clue to diagnosis. Such cases usually respond to treatment, although recovery is slow, and relapses may occur.

Brucellosis has been diagnosed occasionally in patients with Hodgkin's disease and other forms of reticu-

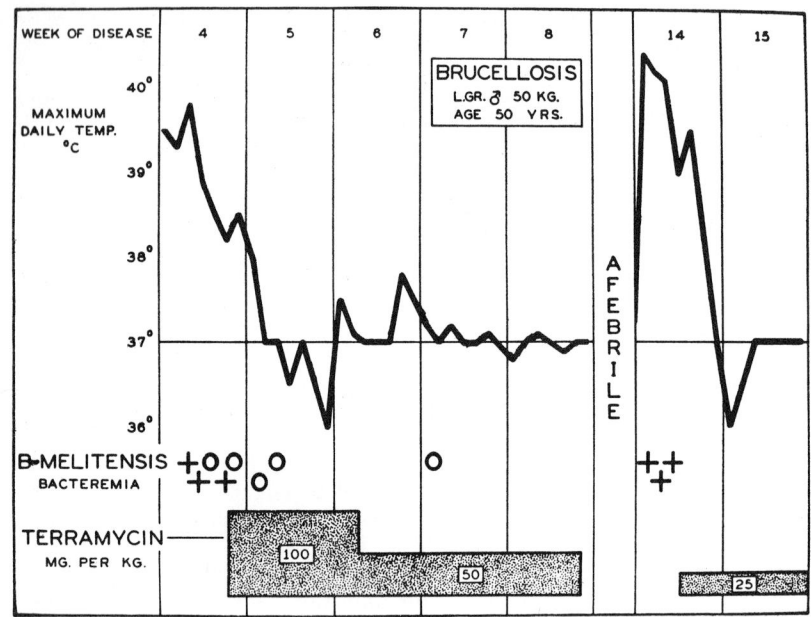

Bacteremic relapse in *B. melitensis* infection and successful retreatment with oxytetracycline. (Case of Dr. F. Ruiz Sanchez, Guadalajara, Mexico; from Knight, V.: Ann. N.Y. Acad. Sci., 53:332, 1950.)

loendothelial neoplasia. Apparently, when such neoplastic processes affect patients with Brucella infection, the neoplasia may interfere with cellular immunity and lead to dissemination of the organism from localized foci of infection.

Subclinical Disease. "CHRONIC BRUCELLOSIS." Occasionally the physician will be consulted by a patient who is chronically ill with something called "chronic brucellosis." Usually such patients have chronic arthralgias, intermittent low fever, lassitude, and a considerable overlying anxiety. Serologic tests for anti-Brucella antibodies may be present, but are of low titer (less than 1:100); the skin reaction to Brucella antigen is positive; but multiple blood cultures are negative for Brucella. Such patients seldom give a history of a well-documented attack of acute brucellosis, although they may well have received anti-Brucella chemotherapy. As a general proposition, it is extremely difficult to establish with certainty that any particular infection is *not* present. With due recognition of this fact, it can be stated that as a practical matter (1) almost certainly these patients do not have brucellosis; (2) the possibility of a Brucella infection should not be accepted as a satisfactory explanation for whatever symptoms they do have; and (3) they should not receive anti-Brucella chemotherapy. There are two sorts of experience in support of these assertions. First, a high proportion of persons occupationally exposed to infection show clean-cut bacteriologic evidence of infection, yet such subclinical infections are an asymptomatic affair. Second, the clinical syndrome of the alleged "chronic brucellosis" does not progress to detectable Brucella disease, nor is it suppressed by anti-Brucella chemotherapy.

SUBCLINICAL INFECTION. Among those occupationally exposed, unless stimulated by further exposure, the titer of antibody declines to normal in a few months to a few years. In the absence of symptoms, in this form of undoubted Brucella infection, antimicrobial treatment is probably not indicated. However, disseminated infection and bacteremia may occur with mild illness. Persons repeatedly exposed maintain high titers of antibody, and may display hypersensitivity to the Brucella organism as evidenced by excessive reaction to accidental exposure to live strain 19 Brucella vaccine or the occurrence of skin rash after handling of Brucella-infected animal tissues. As discussed previously, however, illness in people with Brucella antibody should not be assumed to be brucellosis without other diagnostic studies, in order not to miss infectious mononucleosis and other diseases which mimic brucellosis.

Diagnosis. Definitive diagnosis is best made by isolation of the organism from blood, bone marrow, or local sites of involvement. Cultures should be examined for growth every four to five days, and not be discarded before six weeks of incubation.

The organisms may be isolated in trypticase soy or tryptose phosphate broth; the primary isolation of *B. abortus* requires the presence of 10 per cent carbon dioxide. Virulent organisms possess a capsule and grow as small, glistening translucent colonies on agar. This property is gradually lost by cultivation on artificial media (smooth → rough mutation). *B. abortus* is inhibited by thionine, whereas *B. suis* and *B. melitensis* are inhibited by basic fuchsin and crystal violet. *B. suis* may be distinguished from the other species by production of H_2S. Within species, patterns of metabolic activity and other characteristics permit the definition of several "biotypes," which may be of value in epidemiologic work.

Cross-reacting agglutinating antibodies are formed in response to two principal antigenic determinants common to virulent strains of the three major species. Studies suggest that the antigens are specific, surface polysaccharides. They are designated M and A (M for *melitensis,* which predominates in this species, and A for *abortus,* which predominates in *B. abortus* and *B. suis*). These characteristics permit serologic differentiation of *B. melitensis* from the other two species.

Agglutinating antibody is usually present by the time the patients are first seen. In primary infections a large fraction of the antibody may be IgM, but IgG later becomes the predominant antibody moiety. Titers of 1:80 or greater are indicative of past or present infection. There is considerable variation in the titer of agglutinating antibody in both acute and chronic brucellosis, but a rising titer of antibody suggests the presence of active infection. In some cases, lower dilutions of serologic tests will not show agglutination when higher dilutions are positive (prozone reaction). This reaction is caused by incomplete or blocking antibodies, and can be avoided by using 5 per cent sodium chloride or albumin solution as a diluent instead of physiologic saline. A Coombs-type antiglobulin test will also reveal Brucella antibody obscured in the prozone reaction. A complement-fixing antibody test is also available.

An *intradermal skin test* is available, utilizing several preparations of Brucella antigen. It is of the delayed hypersensitivity type, and has about the same significance as the tuberculin test. As positive skin tests are frequent in endemic areas, the test is of little value in diagnosis of individual cases; moreover, the test may elicit a low titer of circulating Brucella agglutinins.

Differential Diagnosis. Acute febrile brucellosis must be differentiated from diseases whose onset is associated with fever but without localizing signs. These include influenza, other viral respiratory infections, infectious mononucleosis, early stages of infectious hepatitis, malaria, typhoid, primary histoplasmosis, disseminated tuberculosis, and lymphoma. The possibility of other illness in patients with subclinical brucellosis should be kept in mind. *The skin test should not be depended upon for diagnosis of brucellosis.*

Treatment. Tetracycline and its derivatives are usually effective in relieving the acute manifestations of the infection. Tetracycline, 0.5 gram four times daily for a period of 21 days, is recommended for uncomplicated Brucella infection in adults. Some patients in the first few hours of treatment will have a Herxheimer-like reaction characterized by increased fever, weakness, hypotension, and generalized discomfort. These manifestations clear spontaneously and, in the writer's experience, have not been a serious problem. In more severe cases streptomycin, 0.5 gram twice daily, may be given during the first two weeks of tetracycline treatment. Relapses can be retreated by the same regimen used initially.

Trimethoprim and sulfamethoxazole in combination have produced remission in acute brucellosis. Treatment prolonged to six weeks may prevent the occasional relapses seen with shorter periods of treatment. The dose used was 10 mg of trimethoprim and 50 mg of sulfamethoxazole per kilogram per day, equivalent in an average adult to 4 tablets, each containing 80 mg of trimethoprim and 400 mg of sulfamethoxazole.

In patients with the rare but serious complication of pancytopenia, steroids, such as prednisone, 40 to 60 mg per day, should be given for the first seven to ten days of antimicrobial treatment. Steroids may also be beneficial in relieving the prostration of more severely ill patients.

Prognosis. Most acute cases of brucellosis respond to a course of antimicrobial therapy with a prompt and lasting recovery. Relapse may occur one or more times in about 5 per cent of cases treated 21 days or longer, but responds to retreatment. There is some evidence that there may be residual damage in patients with Brucella nephritis. In untreated brucellosis, the mortality is less than 2 per cent, and the majority of the patients make a complete recovery within three to six months. When symptoms are prolonged in brucellosis, it may be due to hypersensitivity to Brucella antigen. The exact mechanism of such reactions is not known, but both cellular and humoral immune responses may be involved.

Prevention. Present programs in the United States to control the disease in cattle and pigs are succeeding, and the disease in man is expected to disappear here in the next few years. Elsewhere control measures are less advanced. The major preventive measure for the general population is to consume only pasteurized dairy products. There is no way to prevent spread of infection to workers from infected animals or animal tissues.

Busch, L. A., and Parker, R. L.: Brucellosis in the United States. J. Infect. Dis., 125:289, 1972.
Hassan, A., Erian, M. M., Farid, Z., Hathout, S. D., and Sorensen, K.: Trimethoprim-sulphamethoxazole in acute brucellosis. Br. Med. J., 3:159, 1971.
Henderson, R. J., and Hill, D. M.: Subclinical Brucella infection in man. Br. Med. J., 3:154, 1972.
Morgan, W. J. B.: Brucellosis in animals: Diagnosis and control. Proc. R. Soc. Med., 62:1050, 1969.
National Brucellosis Committee (subcommittee of Office of Veterinary Public Health Services): Brucellosis in the United States, 1970. Arch. Environ. Health, 25:66, 1972.
Swenson, R. M., Carmichael, L. E., and Cundy, K. R.: Human infection with *Brucella canis*. Ann. Intern. Med., 76:435, 1972.

DISEASES DUE TO MYCOBACTERIA

227. TUBERCULOSIS

Roger Des Prez

GENERAL CONSIDERATIONS

Tuberculosis is a chronic infection, potentially of lifelong duration, caused by two species of mycobacteria, *M. tuberculosis* and, rarely, *M. bovis*. It is almost always initiated by inhalation of infectious material, rarely by ingestion, and more rarely still by cutaneous inoculation (prosector's wart). Early in infection a silent bloodstream spread seeds the lymphatic system and other organs throughout the body, leaving foci which may cause clinical illness after long periods of latency. Tuberculosis must be differentiated on bacteriologic grounds from chronic infections caused by other species of mycobacteria.

Although paleopathologic evidence indicates that humans were infected with tuberculosis in neolithic times, the infection became epidemic with the Industrial Revolution, which produced the crowded living conditions most favorable to its spread. In the mid-nineteenth century, it is said to have accounted for one quarter of adult deaths in Europe. During that century three great strides led to an accurate conception of the disease and its cause. In 1804 Laennec published the opinion that the many different forms of tuberculosis in the lungs and elsewhere, previously regarded as different diseases, were actually different manifestations of one disease. By 1839 the term *tuberculosis* came into use, reflecting the unifying anatomic feature of tubercle formation. In 1865, Villemin established the contagious nature of the process by infecting laboratory animals with diseased tissue. In 1882 Koch reported isolation and culture of the tubercle bacillus and successful production of disease in animals by these isolates.

The sanatorium movement, which began because of emphasis on climate in treatment, received further impetus from the demonstration of the infectious nature of the process. As a result, phthisiology became a distinct and sophisticated medical specialty but one which was separated from the mainstream of medicine. The development of diagnostic radiology led to an appreciation of the pivotal importance of cavity formation. Treatment, other than general supportive measures and bed rest, became directed almost entirely at the goal of cavity closure, utilizing methods such as pneumoperitoneum, therapeutic pneumothorax, and collapse of the chest wall by surgical measures (thoracoplasty).

By 1947 it had become established that streptomycin (SM) was a truly effective antituberculous drug, initiating the chemotherapy era. Soon after, it was shown that combination of SM with para-aminosalicylic acid (PAS) tended to prevent treatment failures associated with development of bacterial resistance to SM, establishing the principle of combined drug therapy. The availability of effective drug treatment also made it possible for the first time to resect diseased tissue, a procedure which had previously frequently resulted in spread of infection. Some form of pulmonary resection became a part of treatment of many if not most cases. This attitude persisted for some 15 years until it became clear that resection added very little to the long-term results of effective and extended drug therapy.

In 1953 isoniazid (INH) was established as an antituberculous drug of a different and higher order than SM, and tuberculosis became a medically curable illness in most cases. Since patients on treatment became rapidly noninfectious and required little bed rest or specialized therapeutic methods aimed at cavity collapse, the need for sanatoriums disappeared, and tuberculosis became, perhaps for the first time, the legitimate province of the general physician and general hospital. Treatment began to be applied not only to patients with demonstrably active cases but also to individuals in whom active disease seemed only reasonably likely to develop (chemoprophylaxis). Finally, the more meticulous bacteriologic techniques required to determine drug susceptibility of infecting strains was, more than anything else, responsible for the recognition and eventual definition of many other pathogenic mycobacteria, all of which are less susceptible to isoniazid.

BACTERIOLOGY

Mycobacteria are acid-fast, nonmotile, nonsporulating, weakly gram-positive rods classified in the order Actinomycetales. Until recently, only *M. tuberculosis,* the human tubercle bacillus, and *M. bovis* were regarded as pathogenic for man. *M. avium,* which causes tuberculosis in poultry and swine, is thought to produce human disease only rarely. Recently other mycobacteria, previously either unrecognized or regarded as saprophytes, have become recognized as human pathogens. The clinical importance of these "atypical" mycobacteria is discussed in Ch. 244.

Such distinguishing characteristics as slow growth rate, resistance to chemical disinfectants, and the ability to survive within phagocytic cells are attributed to the hydrophobic, lipid-rich (60 per cent of dry weight) mycobacterial cell wall. Its relative impermeability accounts for the typical diagnostic staining characteristics. In the Ziehl-Neelsen method, staining with carbolfuchsin is facilitated by steaming the smear. Subsequent treatment with acid-alcohol elutes carbolfuchsin from other bacteria and organic material, but "acid-fast" mycobacteria resist decoloration.

When pulmonary tuberculosis is sufficiently advanced to cause symptoms, most cases will demonstrate a positive sputum smear. Sputum for culture is usually collected over a 24-hour period, but some authorities prefer the first sputum raised in the morning. When sputum is not produced, the respiratory secretions can be obtained by gastric aspiration or by inhalation of heated, hypertonic aerosols (10 per cent saline). The aerosol is inhaled for 15 minutes, and all sputum raised then and for a 15-minute period thereafter is collected.

Differentiation of Clinically Important Mycobacterial Species

Definitive identification of mycobacteria is usually accomplished by reference laboratories, but good species identification can be achieved by a few simple observations. Rate of growth and production of pigment were used by Runyon to classify the so-called "atypical" mycobacteria into four groups; Group I is characterized by formation of yellow colonies after brief exposure to light (photochromogens), Group II by production of yellow or orange colonies without light stimulation (scotochromogens), Group III by nonpigmented colonies, and Group IV by growth within seven days. These characteristics, together with nonsusceptibility to isoniazid, lack of production of niacin, and production of the enzyme catalase, suffice for tentative identification of those mycobacteria known to be of pathogenic importance in man. *M. tuberculosis* usually requires two or three weeks for visible growth. Colonies are rough, and no pigment is produced. It is the only species which produces a positive niacin test. Isoniazid-susceptible strains of *M. tuberculosis* produce catalase, whereas isoniazid-resistant strains are usually catalase negative. *M. bovis* resembles *M. tuberculosis* but does not produce niacin. The *photochromogenic* property of *M. kansasii* (Runyon Group I) is its most distinguishing characteristic. Growth is slow, colonies are either rough or smooth, moderate isoniazid resistance is usual, catalase production is marked, and niacin is not produced. *M. marinum* (Runyon Group I) resembles *M. kansasii* except that growth is poor at 37° C and good at room temperature. *M. avium* and *M. intracellulare* (the Battey bacillus) grow slowly, produce smooth, thin, nonpigmented colonies, are highly resistant to isoniazid, produce catalase, and do not produce niacin. They are serologically closely related and differ only in that *M. avium* grows well at 45° C and *M. intracellulare* does not. They are classified in Runyon's Group III. *Scotochromogenic mycobacteria* (Runyon Group II) produce yellow to orange pigment in the dark, grow slowly, have smooth colonies, are highly resistant to isoniazid, produce catalase, and do not produce niacin. *Rapid growers* (Runyon Group IV) produce colonies within seven days, are catalase positive, niacin negative, and very resistant to isoniazid.

EPIDEMIOLOGY

In much of the world, bovine tuberculosis remains a significant problem and infection by mouth is frequent. In Western nations, however, infection is almost always by inhalation. Most importance is attached to the dried residues of droplets aerosolized by cough, called *droplet nuclei,* which may remain suspended in air for prolonged periods and are sufficiently small to reach terminal air passages where removal is difficult and bacterial multiplication can begin. Well-studied epidemics in certain closed environments such as naval vessels and boarding schools indicate that one person with cavitary disease may "poison" the environment with droplet nuclei and infect virtually all susceptibles in the same environment, even in the temporary absence of the infectious person himself. A tuberculosis ward is probably not a place of great risk when care is taken, because persons receiving chemotherapy become rapidly noninfectious. Infected urine may be contagious, especially for young children using the same toilet facilities, owing to droplet nuclei formed from urine aerosolization. Transmission of tuberculosis by the genital route is rare. Inoculation of abraded skin by contaminated tissues at autopsy examination may produce a primary skin infection in tuberculin-negative individuals (prosector's wart). Fomites are not important in the spread of infection.

Incidence and Prevalence. The decline in tuberculosis mortality which began in the middle of the last century was probably due to improved living conditions and heightened social awareness. In the past 20 years of drug treatment, mortality has declined somewhat more rapidly, but the incidence of new cases has fallen less, suggesting a residue of older individuals infected in earlier years. In the young, it is clear that the new case rate has drastically fallen in urban United States. In 1928, 53 per cent of 16-year-old schoolchildren in Philadelphia were tuberculin positive. By 1968, this had decreased to 1.4 per cent. The incidence of new disease in older groups will eventually also surely decline, but active tuberculosis in the United States is at present most frequently seen in nonwhite older males, presumably infected while young and succumbing to age- and race-dependent factors favoring evolution of infection into disease.

IMMUNOLOGIC RESPONSE AND PATHOLOGIC FEATURES

Tuberculosis is the prototype of infections which require cellular immune responses for control. Infection induces a rich antibody response, but what role, if any, these antibodies play in control of infection is not clear. In the first few weeks after infection, the previously unexposed host has virtually no defense against multiplication of the infectious inoculum either at the initial site or at various metastatic foci established by lymphohematogenous dissemination. During this silent period, lymphocytes genetically coded to react with antigens of the tubercle bacillus proliferate and circulate throughout the lymphatic system. At some interval, usually three to six weeks after infection, the population of specifically reactive lymphocytes usually reaches sufficient size and dissemination to bring the infection under control. The mechanism by which this is accomplished is the elaboration, by reactive lymphocytes in contact with antigen, of a series of lymphocyte products which attract or entrap macrophages at the site of the lymphocyte-antigen interaction, stimulate them to a metabolically more active state in which their mycobactericidal activity is greatly enhanced, and cause some macrophages to differentiate into epithelioid cells and fibroblasts. This sequence of events results in a quite efficient control of infection. However, activated lymphocytes may also elaborate cytotoxic materials which in some instances, particularly when large concentrations of antigen interact with large populations of reactive lymphocytes, may cause cellular necrosis, an event of central importance in the progression of the infection. Although the details of these antigen-lymphocyte-macrophage interactions are by no means clear, *in a general sense tissue hypersensitivity, as manifested by the tuberculin reaction and by cellular necrosis, and cellular immunity, as manifested by successful containment of the infection, are parallel consequences of the appearance of a population of specifically reactive lymphocytes.*

The pathologic response to tuberculous infection is determined in large part by interaction of these two factors, the population of specifically reactive lymphocytes present in the host and the mass of antigen present in the lesion, as modified by structural characteristics of the tissue involved. Small numbers of bacilli in a host with well established lymphocyte reactivity to tuberculosis antigens induce *tubercle formation*, characterized by central multinucleated giant cells surrounded by a cluster of epithelioid cells. More peripherally, lymphocytes are seen admixed with fibroblasts and, in older lesions, fibrosis. Visible bacilli are few or absent. Lesions of this histologic character are termed *productive* and represent successful local containment of infection. When large bacterial concentrations coexist with high levels of lymphocyte reactivity, an exudate rich in fibrin and a nonspecific inflammatory reaction containing polymorphonuclear leukocytes, monocytes, and small numbers of epithelioid and giant cell results; such lesions, termed *exudative*, may progress to *caseous necrosis*. In contrast to many other infections, tissue autolysis in tuberculosis is initially incomplete. The term caseous depicts its cheesy, semisolid, or solid consistency, which appears microscopically as amorphous, homogeneous, eosinophilic material. When specific lymphocyte reactivity has waned because of age or intercurrent illness, and breakdown of a previously quiescent chronic focus leads to extensive bacteremia, the cellular response may be minimal or lacking entirely in the presence of large concentrations of multiplying bacteria in the miliary foci. This histologic picture has been termed *nonreactive tuberculosis*.

Since the histopathologic response is determined in part by local factors, quite different patterns may occur simultaneously in the same individual and even in different parts of the same lesion, some representing progression and some successful containment. In pulmonary caseous foci, for instance, the histologic response at increasing distances from the caseous center (where antigen concentration is greatest) comes more and more to resemble that associated with successful containment of infection, with tubercle formation and fibrosis predominating. It is important to emphasize that these histologic features are not diagnostic of tuberculosis and may be seen in some combination in a wide variety of other conditions.

PATHOGENESIS

The tubercle bacillus requires ready access to oxygen for growth, and even under the most favorable circumstances cell division occurs no more frequently than every day or two, explaining the chronic character of tuberculous disease. In unfavorable circumstances it may become metabolically dormant and persist in necrotic tissue for years. Infection by inhalation requires very few infectious units under favorable circumstances. The initial focus is usually in the mid or lower lung fields where there is greater ventilation. Bacterial multiplication proceeds with little or no reaction, spreads to regional nodes in the hilum of the lung, and thence gains access to the bloodstream. *It is important to emphasize that asymptomatic lymphohematogenous dissemination of the primary infection before the acquisition of tuberculin hypersensitivity probably occurs in all instances; it is this event which sets the stage for the development of chronic pulmonary and extrapulmonary tuberculosis at a later time.* The metastatic bacterial colonies throughout the body also multiply in unimpeded fashion prior to development of tuberculin reactivity. Circulating bacilli are most efficiently cleared from the bloodstream by reticuloendothelial organs, but bacterial multiplication is favored in those areas known to be associated with clinical tuberculosis, notably the apices of the lungs, lymph nodes, kidneys, richly vascularized skeletal areas, and the central nervous system.

As mentioned, the subsequent development of *tuberculin hypersensitivity* and *cellular immunity* greatly alters the balance in favor of the host. Activated macrophages reduce the bacterial population at both initial and metastatic foci, and further bacterial growth is inhibited. It is likely, however, that slowly metabolizing viable bacilli persist at most foci. When antigen concentration at the site of initial infection and in the regional lymph nodes is sufficiently large, cellular necrosis may develop and eventually calcify, producing the so-called *Ghon complex*. This roentgenographic finding, for years considered pathognomonic of tuberculosis, is now known to be also caused by certain fungi, notably histoplasmosis and coccidioidomycosis, and other mycobacteria.

Fate of the Primary Infection. In possibly 99 per cent, the infection remains quiescent after the development of tuberculin hypersensitivity and is of no further clinical significance. In very few, infection may evolve into clinical tuberculosis in a number of ways. In some, particularly the very young, the preallergic bacteremia (early hematogenous dissemination) may progress directly into generalized acute hematogenous tuberculosis. The resemblance of the resulting disseminated tubercles to millet seeds led to the designation, *miliary tuberculosis*. At times it is the strategic location of miliary tubercles rather than progression of the bacteremia which is critical, particularly with respect to development of *tuberculous meningitis*, because subependymal foci in brain or spinal cord may rupture into the subarachnoid space and produce spread of the infection via the subarachnoid fluid. Meningitis may occur in the setting of obvious, progressive bloodstream infection but also may be due to a nonprogressive and otherwise asymptomatic bacteremia.

Local rather than hematogenous events will also determine the outcome. The initial focus may directly evolve into progressive pneumonia (*progressive primary*); rarely cavitation may result. Large hilar nodes may become necrotic, liquefy, discharge into the bronchial tree, and produce tuberculous pneumonia in this fashion, or, particularly in the young, often partially compress the major bronchi, producing bronchial obstruction and collapse of a pulmonary segment or lobe. When the site of the initial infection is subpleural in location, rupture into the pleural space may occur, producing the clinical picture of *serofibrinous pleurisy with effusion*. A hematogenous focus located near the pleural surface can also produce this syndrome.

Numerically, the most frequent serious sequel of the preallergic bacteremia is chronic pulmonary tuberculosis. Pulmonary sequestration of blood-borne bacteria occurs in a distribution proportional to blood flow, but conditions in the superior and posterior aspects of the lungs greatly favor bacterial multiplication. Over the years it has been a matter of controversy whether chronic apical pulmonary tuberculosis of the so-called *reinfection type* results from breakdown of latent residua seeded at the time of the initial infection (*endogenous reinfection*) or from acquisition of new infection from the environment (*exogenous reinfection*). Many authorities assume that both can occur. However, it now seems likely that exogenous reinfection is considerably less important, and that apical pulmonary tuberculosis is almost always a direct consequence of the primary infection, with progression (then or later) in that area caused by local factors favoring bacterial growth, whereas the initial focus in the mid or lower lung fields almost always regresses.

The time at which apical pulmonary tuberculosis appears depends on three factors: first, the period of life in which infection occurs; second, normal, age-dependent factors favoring or inhibiting growth of the apical lesion; and third, non-age-related factors altering resistance to progression of the infection. All mortality curves from urban populations in the early part of this century, in which infection in childhood was the rule, demonstrate a peak in the first three years of life owing to the relative deficiency in cellular immunity which characterizes this period of life. In very young children, progressive hematogenous tuberculosis, particularly miliary and meningeal disease, constituted a large part of the over-all mortality. Older prepubertal children (roughly between 5 and 15), although in no way resistant to *infection,* very seldom manifested progressive *disease.* After puberty a second mortality peak was seen which continued through the second and into the third decade and was more pronounced in females than in males. Thereafter, the death rate continued at a lower level until old age, when a third, less dramatic mortality peak was seen. At present, in countries with low prevalence, clinical tuberculosis is becoming more a disease of the elderly, particularly the older male, presumably caused in part by waning immunologic competence in old age.

As mentioned, persons infected during the disease-resistant period of childhood (roughly 5 to 15) are prone to develop clinical tuberculosis in the postpubertal and early adult period of life, presumably owing to age-dependent host factors favoring evolution of the infection. In contrast, apical pulmonary tuberculosis caused by infection after childhood most often becomes manifest within two years of initial infection. Beyond this period of maximal jeopardy, quiescent foci in the lungs and elsewhere may evolve to produce clinical disease at any time when a combination of local and systemic factors favor reactivation.

The importance of local factors in reactivation of previously quiescent foci is illustrated by development of tuberculous arthritis after injury, activation of pulmonary tuberculosis by destructive lung disease such as lung abscess, and the appearance of late hematogenous dissemination after trauma. Thus any tuberculin-positive individual is at risk to develop any form of tuberculosis, often as a result of a remote and clinically undetectable primary infection. The role of immunologic senescence or other processes altering cellular immunity needs to be emphasized; reactivation of tuberculosis becomes progressively likely as individuals become more aged.

Endobronchial Spread of Chronic Pulmonary Tuberculosis: The Importance of Cavity Formation. In contrast to the earliest stages of tuberculous infection in which lymphohematogenous dissemination is the rule, once chronic pulmonary tuberculosis has become established, further spread occurs for the most part via the bronchial tree. The cavity, which is responsible both for progression of pulmonary disease in the individual and for infection of others, has provided the environment which has nurtured the tubercle bacillus through so many centuries of coexistence with the human species. *Especially in the era prior to the availability of effective drugs, cavity formation was the pivotal event in the course of pulmonary tuberculosis, to the prevention or treatment of which most forms of therapy were directed.*

Late Hematogenous Dissemination. Foci seeded at the time of the preallergic bacteremia may, after prolonged quiescent periods, break down and liberate bacteria into the bloodstream. Chronic pulmonary foci may cause late bacteremia in this manner, but extrapulmonary and often clinically inapparent foci, particularly in lymph nodes, bones, and the urogenital system, cause most instances of miliary and meningeal tuberculosis in older individuals.

THE TUBERCULIN TEST

The tuberculin test is best performed by intracutaneous injection of 0.1 ml of purified protein derivative (PPD of Seibert). Proper introduction will be indicated by a raised white area that persists for some minutes after injection. PPD in solution rapidly adsorbs to glass or plastic with loss of potency. Accordingly, injection should be made promptly after mixing the tablet with the provided diluent; preferably a solution containing an agent preventing adsorption of antigen (Tween-stabilized tuberculin) should be employed. Dosage is expressed in terms of tuberculin units (1 TU is 0.00002 mg, bioequivalent to 1:10,000 Old Tuberculin or OT; 5 TU is 0.0001 mg; 250 TU is 0.001 mg, bioequivalent to 1:100 OT). In children or in persons with coincidence of ocular involvement, the 1 TU dose is used. In adults a 5 TU dose is employed first. *Production of visible and palpable induration over 10 mm in diameter after 48 to 72 hours is considered virtually diagnostic of infection with M. tuberculosis.* A smaller reaction is of uncertain significance, because it may be due to other mycobacterial infections. If this is negative, retesting with 250 TU is carried out. A positive reaction to this larger (second-strength) dosage is also of uncertain significance, because it may reflect cross-reactivity. A negative reaction in a *nonfebrile, relatively well individual* is strong evidence against tuberculosis. However, as many as 15 per cent or more of persons constitutionally ill with proved tuberculosis may fail to react to 250 TU when first tested, becoming reactive again as health returns. Associated illnesses such as Hodgkin's disease, sarcoidosis, less commonly other neoplasias, and acute infections, notably the viral exanthemata, may also cause false negatives. False positives are almost always due to infections with other mycobacterial species.

FACTORS MODIFYING THE COURSE OF TUBERCULOSIS

Nutritional status, mental and physical stress, and exhaustion modify the course of tuberculosis, as is well illustrated by the peak in mortality statistics observed during the major wars in both belligerent and nonbelligerent nations. *Pregnancy, delivery, and the puerperium,* long regarded as risk periods, have probably been overemphasized. Although statistical evidence is lacking, there is little doubt that *prolonged therapy with corticosteroids* predisposes to exacerbation of tuberculosis, as does *therapy with oncolytic or immunosuppressive agents. Diabetes* predisposes to clinical tuberculosis and the disease tends to be more fulminant, particularly in young, poorly controlled diabetics. *Silicosis* or *anthracosilicosis* alters host repsonse to tuberculosis in important ways. Instances of infection with the usually nonpathogenic *M. avium* is observed in silicotics. Once established, silicotuberculosis may produce massive conglomerate fibrosis with little potential for resolution and little response to antituberculous drugs. Moreover, conglomerate fibrosis often contains quite small bacterial populations, making bacteriologic diagnosis difficult. In times past, *sarcoidosis* was thought to predispose to the progression of tuberculosis, but this no longer appears to be the case. *Hodgkin's disease, leukemia, and other lymphatic neoplasms* are often confused with tuberculosis and may also be complicated by active tuberculosis caused presumably by the detrimental effects of these diseases on cellular immune mechanisms. *Carcinoma* and *destructive infections* such as histoplasmosis, other mycobacterial infections, and lung abscess may erode an old tuberculous focus, releasing tubercle bacilli which may or may not produce disease. Severe viral illness, notably rubella and influenza, may have detrimental effects on the course of tuberculosis. *Gastric resection,* for unknown reasons, favors the development of pulmonary tuberculosis. *Pulmonary surgery* may also cause progression of quiescent pulmonary foci. The role of various types of trauma in activating latent foci has been mentioned previously.

PREVENTION OF TUBERCULOSIS

Vaccination

BCG (bacille Calmette Guérin) is a strain of *M. bovis* with attenuated virulence for man. Several large studies have produced convincing evidence that vaccination with an effective strain of BCG will result in a significant decrease in the incidence of clinical disease. Also of benefit is the fact that vaccinated persons who do become ill develop less progressive forms of tuberculosis. Miliary and meningeal disease in young children, for instance, is rare after BCG vaccination, a major advantage, considering the gravity of these conditions in the very young. (Disseminated infection with BCG itself is so rare as to be of no importance.) The difficulty with BCG stems from the lack of a satisfactory animal model for testing its immunizing potency, and by no means could all "vaccines" be called effective. This problem with BCG is not unlike that with antityphoid vaccine and, in the case of BCG, has been largely solved by the use of dry frozen vaccine from a batch known to have shown full effectiveness in large-scale field trials.

BCG vaccination programs have been carried out with substantial success in some European countries and the United Kingdom. In the United States the irregular performance of the early vaccines acted against its general use. By the time a generally effective dry frozen vaccine was developed, the falling rates of infection and disease in the United States made employment of the vaccine a procedure of value in only specialized circumstances (see below). One source of reluctance has been the fact that tuberculin positivity is induced by BCG, thus destroying the major indicator of early infection, an important consideration in areas of low prevalence. The success of isoniazid prophylaxis (see below) was another factor that weighed against widespread vaccination. Almost all authorities advise the use of BCG in tuberculin-negative children in areas in which 20 per cent or more of secondary schoolchildren are tuberculin-positive. (Vaccination is, of course, of no use in tuberculin-positive persons.) Vaccination may also be appropriate for missionary or government personnel prior to assignment to areas of known high prevalence, in groups of health professionals with high (over 20 per cent) incidence of infection, and even in some military personnel. Vaccination of infants born to tuberculous mothers or who must live in known high-risk environments is the procedure of choice, but is compromised somewhat by the problem of keeping the infant isolated for the four- to ten-week period required for development of tuberculin hypersensitivity in response to BCG vaccination. A strain of *M. microti* (the vole bacillus), naturally attenuated for man, is of the same order of effectiveness as BCG, but this has not been widely used.

Chemoprophylaxis

The term chemoprophylaxis has been applied to two distinct situations: first, the treatment of tuberculin-negative individuals in the hope of preventing infection in high-risk situations; and second, treatment of tuberculin-positive persons in the hope of preventing evolution of infection into disease. In a practical sense, it means treatment with isoniazid, because of its effectiveness, convenience, low cost, and relatively low toxicity.

Circumstances in which *infection prophylaxis* (primary prophylaxis) is indicated are few. When an infant cannot be isolated from a mother with active tuberculosis long enough to establish tuberculin hypersensitivity with BCG, isoniazid may be administered to the child until and for a few months after the mother achieves a negative sputum under treatment. When the period of risk cannot be defined, such as in households with recalcitrant infectious patients or in geographic pockets of known high risk, it may be useful to continue therapy for two years or more, because the morbidity associated with meningitis is less in older children. Alternatively, it may be reasonable to stop chemoprophylaxis at some point for a period long enough to achieve vaccination and tuberculin conversion and then to resume therapy for another year, assuming that the conversion might be due to either vaccination or infection, and that in either case protection would result. Prophylactic treatment of tuberculin-negative household contacts of newly discovered active cases is advised by many. The decision to do so should take into consideration the hepatotoxicity of isoniazid, particularly as related to the age of the individual and the practical aspects of monitoring for this toxic manifestation (see below).

Certain exposure to highly contaminated material, as in laboratory accidents or in mouth-to-mouth resuscitation of positive patients, may be covered with prophylactic isoniazid for a period of several months. In the latter situation, attention should be given to the possibility of isoniazid resistance if these data are available, and therapy adjusted accordingly. The status of the tuberculin test during and after treatment should be monitored.

In certain conditions, notably sarcoidosis and Hodgkin's disease, cutaneous anergy may make it impossible to determine whether or not infection has occurred. Moreover, both roentgenographic and histologic abnormalities in sarcoidosis and to a lesser degree in Hodgkin's disease may resemble those produced by tuberculosis. Further, both these conditions may require corticosteroid therapy (see below). For these reasons, many persons with sarcoidosis, Hodgkin's disease, and related lymphomas are treated with isoniazid without certain knowledge as to whether or not infection has in fact occurred. Similarly, prolonged corticosteroid therapy in gravely ill individuals is ordinarily accompanied by isoniazid, because all debilitating conditions may produce cutaneous anergy, making it impossible to exclude either old or active tuberculosis.

In contrast, *disease prophylaxis* (secondary prophylaxis) is a frequently employed and well established procedure. Its greatest use is in the recent tuberculin converter, which in point of fact represents treatment of an early and active infection. Treatment of children under five years with a positive reaction to a 5 TU dose of tuberculin is recommended without exception. This may also be the case in older persons in whom tuberculin conversion is known to be a relatively recent (within two years) event. The degree of tuberculin reactivity is important in reaching the decision to treat; most weak tuberculin reactions (requiring large tuberculin doses to be elicited) have entirely different implications and do not require treatment. It seems likely, although not yet established, that the incidence of tuberculosis in later life will be substantially reduced by early treatment of the tuberculin converter.

In addition to treatment of the preclinical infection, as defined above, a number of situations known to be prejudicial to the course of tuberculous infection constitute sufficient reason for chemoprophylaxis in tuberculin-positive individuals. These include silicosis, severe and poorly controlled diabetes, the postgastrectomy state, progressive neoplastic disease of the lung or of the myeloid or lymphatic systems (particularly when treatment with oncolytic agents is employed), and prolonged treatment with corticosteroids. The occurrence of severe viral illness in a tuberculin-positive individual is regarded by some as an indication for chemoprophylaxis. Persons with an undiagnosed pulmonary infiltrate and a positive tuberculin reaction, in whom for one reason or another definitive diagnosis is not indicated, may be given prophylaxis. It is essential in such circumstances, however, to ensure that the period of prophylaxis does not serve to postpone appropriate diagnostic approaches for more serious diseases. Finally, persons with known, presumably arrested tuberculosis never treated with chemotherapy should receive isoniazid. Often, previously stable infiltrates will regress under this therapy, demonstrating that the presumed inactivity was illusory.

Chemoprophylaxis in adults consists of isoniazid in dosage of 300 mg once daily for a period of a year or two, depending on the circumstances. In children, the dose is 6 to 8 mg per kilogram. The indications for the use of isoniazid in these uncertain situations should be balanced against the real risk of hepatotoxicity, particularly in older persons. It must be recalled that transient liver function test abnormalities are observed in 10 per cent of persons receiving isoniazid and clinical jaundice in 1 per cent; in one large study at least, death from severe hepatitis occurred in approximately 0.1 per cent. These figures undoubtedly overestimate the extent of the problem because of the difficulty of sorting out hepatic diseases of other causes. Nevertheless, everyone receiving isoniazid should be told of the symptom complex which might represent drug-induced hepatitis, and ideally should be seen monthly by a knowledgeable medical worker. If careful surveillance of symptoms is maintained, periodic liver function testing is probably not necessary. As mentioned above, the presence of established unrelated liver disease complicates the picture. There is no clear evidence that liver disease predisposes to an increased incidence of isoniazid hepatotoxicity. However, the detection of isoniazid-induced hepatotoxicity is rendered more difficult by the presence of unrelated liver disease. Finally, it is reasonable to assume that the consequences of hepatotoxicity might be more serious in the presence of an already damaged liver. Age appears to be an important factor; toxic reactions are rare in childhood and seem to be particularly severe in postmenopausal women. The histologic picture of isoniazid-induced hepatitis resembles viral hepatitis, including chronic active hepatitis, and prolonged reactions may lead to cirrhosis. These severe and at times fatal reactions have always been associated with continual ingestion of the drug for a week or more, usually for a much longer period, after the appearance of symptoms, emphasizing the need for patient education and continued supervision.

228. PULMONARY TUBERCULOSIS

Robert Goodwin

SYMPTOMATIC PRIMARY INFECTION

The primary infection is most often symptomatic in infants and young children because of an age-related tendency to extensive lymphadenitis and lymphohematogenous spread, and accordingly has traditionally been termed childhood tuberculosis. At the time of tuberculin conversion, fever and lassitude may be briefly present; rarely *erythema nodosum* or symptomatic inflammation of the eye *(phlyctenular keratoconjunctivitis)* will develop. Hilar lymphadenitis may partially compress the major bronchi, producing a brassy cough and occasionally sputum and localized bronchial obstruction. The chest roentgenogram will often reveal hilar adenopathy, usually unilateral, and at times a small parenchymal infiltrate. Diagnosis is based on a positive and usually vigorous tuberculin test. Microscopy of the sputum smear is occasionally positive, and positive cultures can probably be demonstrated in most patients if obtained repeatedly. Symptoms are most often either lacking or evanescent, but syndromes based on hilar adenopathy, pleural effusion, and, rarely, direct progression of the initial pulmonary infiltrate may be seen.

Hilar adenopathy may compress the small and relatively flaccid bronchi in the very young, thus producing partial or complete bronchial obstruction and obstructive pneumonitis. Involvement of the bronchial wall and mucosa by direct extension from contiguous tuberculous lymphadenitis can seed tuberculous foci distally. Prolonged obstruction and endobronchial scarring may result in distal bronchiectasis. Occasionally a node will rupture into a bronchus, producing intense bronchitis and pneumonitis which may go into caseation. (This may also occur in the adult [see below].) *Tuberculous pleurisy and effusion* (see Part XI, Section Nine) is an important and not uncommon complication occurring soon after infection in both children and young adults. Although this syndrome is itself usually self-limited, three fourths of the patients will subsequently develop progressive pulmonary or extrapulmonary tuberculosis; accordingly tuberculin-positive patients should be treated as having active tuberculosis unless another cause of the effusion can be definitely established. The term *progressive primary* connotes direct evolution of the initial infiltrate into a pneumonic, caseous process. It differs from apical chronic pulmonary tuberculosis in that hilar adenopathy is prominent and the process involves the middle or lower lung fields.

Features characteristic of childhood tuberculosis may also be seen in isolated populations into which tuberculous infection has only recently been introduced. In such circumstances, instead of being infected in childhood, the major portion of the population acquires infection in young adulthood.

Treatment. Children are usually given a larger dosage of isoniazid (10 to 15 mg per kilogram) than adults, because the risks of isoniazid toxicity are negligible in the young. An uncomplicated infection is usually treated with isoniazid alone except when drug resistance seems likely on epidemiologic grounds (contact with a patient with a known drug-resistant strain). Symptoms caused by bronchial compression may be benefited by brief corticosteroid treatment (prednisone, 20 to 40 mg daily). Treatment of progressive, caseous pulmonary parenchymal disease requires more than one drug (see below).

CHRONIC PULMONARY TUBERCULOSIS

Pulmonary tuberculosis in adults is predominantly an apical parenchymal process almost always caused by evolution of hematogenous foci seeded during the preallergic phase of the initial infection. This may occur fairly promptly or after long periods of quiescence. Whether or not a latent period intervenes, these metastatic foci gain largest size and are therefore most unstable in the superior areas of the lung in which local factors favor bacterial growth.

Chronic pulmonary tuberculosis begins as a small patch of bronchopneumonia surrounding a growing bacterial colony, most commonly in the posterior or apical segment of an upper lobe or the apical segment of a lower lobe. The inflammatory response in the sensitized host produces fibrin-rich alveolar fluid containing a mixture of inflammatory cells. Intense inflammation may progress to caseous necrosis which, while intact, is an effective mechanism of host defense, causing the death of most organisms. (Invariably, however, a few metabolically dormant organisms persist.) The critical factors which may reverse this favorable trend are the tendency of caseous foci in upper lung zones to liquefy and discharge into the bronchial tree, producing a cavity in open communication with inspired air, from which infectious secretions spread via the bronchi to other areas of the lung and to the outside environment. *Once reactivation occurs, the progressive nature of tuberculosis in the sensitized host is largely due to the combination of these three factors: the tendency of apical caseous foci to liquefy; the access of liquefied infectious material to the bronchial tree; and the aerobic nature of the organisms, resulting in extremely large bacterial populations within open cavities.*

Bronchogenic spread of infectious material is enhanced by coughing, which aerosolizes infectious material and then on inhalation distributes it widely throughout the lung. Sooner or later new foci of disease develop, which then may undergo caseous necrosis and then heal, or liquefy, slough, and produce another cavity. New lesions usually appear first in the segment or lobe initially involved, producing scattered, patchy disease. The apical posterior areas of the contralateral lung are quite apt to become involved. In addition to the exudative response, some associated productive tissue reaction is usually found, characterized by giant cells and epithelioid cells forming tubercles and leading eventually to fibrosis and healing. This is particularly true in the anterior and basal portions of the lung and in areas which respond to continual bronchogenic seeding from apical cavities with granuloma formation, fibrosis, and scarring but very rarely become necrotic or cavitary. Almost all lesions will contain some mixture of exudative and productive tissue responses, with progression in one area and regression in another. Moreover, the pace and tempo of progressive disease is highly variable from one patient to the next and in the same individual at different times. Intercurrent or genetic factors, vigorous hypersensitivity reactions, and large numbers of organisms favor acute and rapidly progressive reactions which may produce confluent pneumonia *(tuberculous pneumonia or phthisis florida)*. At the other end of the spectrum, relatively effective immunity and low bacterial populations favor predominantly productive lesions with a greater tendency to spontaneous healing. Large thick-walled cavities in a shrunken, extensively carnified lobe *(chronic fibroid tuberculosis)* may persist for years without causing symptoms but will nevertheless be highly contagious.

Mechanisms of healing are basically the same whether they occur spontaneously or after drug treatment. Theoretically, the exudative component of the early infiltrate could resolve with preservation of normal lung architecture. More often it is replaced with fibrous tissue. Solid caseous foci may become encapsulated by fibrosis. An open cavity may occasionally become obstructed by granulation tissue at the bronchocavitary junction, and become inspissated and encapsulated, producing a tenuous form of healing. An open cavity probably always remains infectious except after prolonged antimicrobial therapy, which may eliminate all necrotic and infectious tissue and result in a clean fibrotic cavity wall. Regardless of the type and extent of healing, however, it is probable that dormant organisms capable of renewed growth and reactivation of disease persist in all cases.

Symptoms. Small apical infiltrates may persist for months or even years in tenuous balance, undergoing minor extensions and regressions and producing no symptoms. Discovery of such cases by chest roentgenogram is a fortunate event. When the infection reaches a certain size, however, absorption of antigenic substances results in entirely nonspecific *constitutional symptoms* such as anorexia, fatigue, fever, chilliness, night sweats, and wasting. Constitutional symptoms usually begin insidiously and progress slowly. Weight loss and fatigue are more likely to lead to medical attention than is fever, which usually occurs in the afternoon and is often unrecognized. Often the magnitude of the illness becomes apparent to the patient only when viewed in retrospect after drug treatment.

Symptoms caused by local pulmonary inflammation are also variable in degree and in time of onset. *Cough* and *sputum* are the most consistent, both because of bronchial involvement and because of secretions from a cavity. Accordingly, their presence indicates advanced disease. Material from cavities mechanically irritates draining bronchi and, since it is highly infectious, eventually causes superficial mucosal and submucosal tuberculous disease. Depending upon the degree of bronchial reaction, the size of cavities, and the quantity of drainage, cough may vary from mild to severe, and sputum may be scant and mucoid or copious and purulent.

Hemoptysis and *chest pain* are unpredictable symptoms which cause the patient great concern. Hemoptysis may be due to slough of a caseous lesion or bronchial ulceration. It is usually minor in degree but is most often associated with advanced disease. Particularly in late chronic disease, bleeding may be copious and sudden, owing to rupture of an artery within the fibrous wall of a cavity (Rasmussen aneurysm). Exsanguination is unusual, but, particularly in extensive disease, there may be a real threat of drowning, requiring prompt positioning for draining (prone or Trendelenburg) and avoidance of drugs which suppress cough. *Pleural pain* is usually due to extension of inflammation to the pleural surface with involvement of the parietal pleura without production of pleural fluid *(dry pleurisy)*. Much less commonly, pleural pain will be associated with serofibrinous pleurisy with effusion (which usually occurs prior to established apical pulmonary tuberculosis), and rarely tuberculous empyema will be discovered. Hemoptysis and chest pain are the symptoms most likely to lead to a diagnosis of tuberculosis. Rarely, medical attention is not sought until disease occurs in other tissues bathed in highly infectious pulmonary secretions, such as in painful pharyngeal ulcers; hoarseness and dysphagia caused by laryngeal involvement; tuberculous otitis media; or anal pain caused by a tuberculous perirectal abscess. Shortness of breath is common in pneumonic or extensive destructive disease.

Lower and Middle Lobe Tuberculosis in Older Persons. As tuberculosis in young adults becomes less frequent, certain atypical presentations in older persons are being recognized. A progressive infiltrate in the lower or midlung field may rarely be due to a progressive primary infection, presumably because of deficient immune mechanisms in the elderly. Also, tuberculous hilar lymph nodes from a remote infection may rupture into a bronchus, causing tuberculous pneumonia in the associated lobe or segment.

Physical Examination. Although there are no physical findings diagnostic of tuberculosis, examination does provide valuable information regarding the degree of illness, the presence of associated disease, and anatomic and functional pulmonary changes. In patient assessment, information derived from the physical findings must be correlated with the chest roentgenogram. *Neither is adequate without the other.* Physical findings usually underestimate the extent of involvement and may be entirely normal, even with advanced disease. In spite of these inadequacies, physical examination provides some information not obtainable in any other way, such as asymmetry in respiratory excursion, contraction of the hemithorax, and deviation of the trachea. Dullness associated with decreased fremitus may detect pleural thickening or pleural fluid. Auscultation may reveal rales, but very frequently these can be detected only during quick inspiration after a short cough (post-tussic rales). (Interestingly, rales may persist for years after disease has become inactive, presumably owing to permanent distortion of small bronchi.) With large or fortuitously located lesions, tubular breath sounds and whispered pectoriloquy may be heard. Distant, hollow tubular breath sounds heard over cavities are termed amphoric, because they resemble sounds made by blowing across the mouth of a jar (amphora). Forced hyperventilation may detect local stenosis and obstruction of a bronchus. Careful funduscopic examination may reveal choroidal tubercles. In a particular situation any one of these observations from a careful physical examination may be of considerable help in arriving at a correct diag-

nosis. It can hardly be too strongly emphasized, however, that in the usual course of events, the physical examination of the chest of a patient with tuberculosis can be completely normal. Consequently, the diagnosis of pulmonary tuberculosis must not be excluded on the basis of a normal chest examination.

Roentgenologic Findings. The chest roentgenogram is central to diagnosis, determination of extent, and character of disease, and evaluation of response to treatment. Although not diagnostic, the finding of a patchy infiltrate located in the apical posterior area is highly suggestive of tuberculosis. Cavities can usually be seen on the standard posteroanterior chest roentgenogram, but may be overlooked, and are much more clearly seen with planigrams. Certain histopathologic characteristics of the infiltrates can be estimated from the chest roentgenogram. Exudative lesions tend to have soft indistinct margins. Increased density suggests caseation. Productive lesions tend to be small and nodular with sharply defined margins. Scar tissue produces quite sharp margins and tends to contract. Healing exudative lesions first become smaller and less dense and then, as scarring develops, become more sharply defined. When the roentgenographic changes have stabilized except for slow further contraction, one criterion indicating achievement of quiescent or inactive status is met.

Other Laboratory Findings. A normocytic, normochromic anemia is usual and may be severe. The white blood count is usually normal; a monocytosis of 8 to 15 per cent may be seen. Prolonged and severe infections may cause hyperglobulinemia and hypoalbuminemia. Hematuria or pyuria may disclose coexisting renal tuberculosis; marked albuminuria may indicate amyloidosis. A low serum sodium is sometimes found in extensive chronic pulmonary tuberculosis, more often caused by abnormal retention of water (inappropriate secretion of antidiuretic hormone) than by coexistent Addison's disease. It is important to exclude the presence of diabetes.

Diagnosis. A strong presumptive diagnosis may often be made on the basis of roentgenographic characteristics alone. A sputum smear positive for acid-fast bacteria on microscopy, a usual finding in extensive disease, will, in the proper setting, provide nearly conclusive evidence of pulmonary tuberculosis. It must be remembered, however, that any destructive process in the lung, particularly in the apical posterior area, may erode an inactive focus and cause appearance of acid-fast bacilli in the sputum without development of new, active tuberculosis. This should seldom be a cause of confusion, however, because such excretion of tubercle bacilli is apt to be short lived and, above all, because such a necrotizing pneumonia should be recognizable in other ways (see Ch. 181 to 183 and 195). A positive tuberculin test, although of great use in children, has limited diagnostic significance in older age groups. A negative reaction to 250 TU is strong but not conclusive evidence against active tuberculosis. *Histologic demonstration of granulomatous disease* provides only presumptive evidence of tuberculosis, and even demonstration of acid-fast bacteria is not definitive in that they may represent mycobacteria other than *M. tuberculosis*. Definitive diagnosis requires culture and speciation of the organism.

Differential Diagnosis. Although tuberculosis may be confused with virtually any intrathoracic condition, certain diseases are frequently considered in differential diagnosis. *Fungal disease,* particularly histoplasmosis, and disease caused by other mycobacteria can be indistinguishable from chronic cavitary or fibroid tuberculosis. (Coexistence of histoplasmosis and tuberculosis in the same individual is not rare.) *Bronchiectasis* may present with symptoms suggesting tuberculosis, and bronchiectatic areas surrounded by infiltrate may mimic cavitation roentgenographically. *Cavitary lung abscess* often involves the dorsal segments of the lower lobes and posterior segments of the upper lobes owing to patterns of aspiration during unconsciousness. Typically, lung abscess causes little in the way of physical findings, may have a fluid level, and is not associated with patchy bronchogenic infiltrates. *Acute bacterial pneumonias* may resemble florid tuberculosis in all particulars except for the sputum examination and response to antimicrobial drugs. *Neoplasm* may resemble tuberculosis, as in an isolated coin lesion, an obstructing and inconspicuous endobronchial tumor causing distal chronic inflammation, or a cavitating neoplastic mass. (An irregular cavity wall suggests necrotic neoplasm.) The association between neoplasm and tuberculosis is complex: first, in that cancer may erode into and reactivate a latent tuberculous focus; second, in that saprophytic mycobacteria may be found in association with a destructive neoplasm; and third, in that chronic scarring in a tuberculous focus may induce neoplastic degeneration. New roentgenographic progression of a previously stable, fibrotic tuberculous focus may be due to "scar cancer" rather than to progressive infection.

Classification of Pulmonary Tuberculosis. Previous classifications included the following description of the extent of disease. *Minimal:* The total area of disease, taken in the aggregate, is less than the area from the second chondrocostal junction and the fifth vertebral body to the apex of the lung on one side, and no cavity is demonstrable (planigrams usually required). *Moderately advanced:* The aggregate total area of scattered, small lesions is less than one lung field, or of dense, confluent lesions less than the equivalent of one third of one lung field. The total diameter of cavitation, if present, is less than 4 cm. *Far advanced:* Disease greater in extent than moderately advanced.

The present classification (American Thoracic Society, 1974) is as follows:

Basic Classification

0. *No tuberculosis exposure, not infected* (no history of exposure, negative tuberculin skin test)
I. *Tuberculosis exposure, no evidence of infection* (history of exposure, negative tuberculin skin test)
II. *Tuberculous infection, without disease* (positive tuberculin skin test, negative bacteriologic studies [if done], no roentgenographic findings compatible with tuberculosis, no symptoms due to tuberculosis)
   Chemotherapy status (preventive therapy):
   A. None
   B. On chemotherapy since (date)
   C. Chemotherapy terminated (date)
      1. Complete (prescribed course of therapy)
      2. Incomplete
III. *Tuberculosis: infected, with disease*
   The current status of the patient's tuberculosis shall be described by the following characteristics:
   A. *Location of disease*
      1. Pulmonary
      2. Pleural
      3. Lymphatic
      4. Bone or joint
      5. Genitourinary
      6. Miliary
      7. Meningeal
      8. Peritoneal
      9. Other
      The predominant site shall be listed for each patient. Other sites may also be listed if significant. More precise anatomic sites may be specified.
   B. *Bacteriological status*
      1. Positive by
         a. Microscopy only (date)
         b. Culture only (date)
         c. Microscopy and culture (date)
      2. Negative (date)
      3. Pending
      4. Not done
   C. *Chemotherapy status*
      1. None
      2. On chemotherapy since (date)
      3. Chemotherapy terminated (date)
         a. Complete (prescribed course of therapy)
         b. Incomplete
   The following data are necessary in certain circumstances:
   D. *Roentgenogram findings*
      1. Normal
      2. Abnormal
         a. Cavitary or noncavitary
         b. Stable or worsening or improving
   E. *Tuberculin skin test*
      1. Positive reaction
      2. Doubtful reaction
      3. Negative reaction
      4. Not done

Tuberculosis suspect: Patients may be so classified until diagnostic procedures are complete. This classification should not be used for more than three months.

TREATMENT OF PULMONARY TUBERCULOSIS

The capacity of the tubercle bacillus to retreat into a metabolically dormant state allows some viable cells to survive all drugs presently available. Therefore, although effective drug therapy may control the active phase of pulmonary tuberculosis, slow drug-independent healing processes are required for permanent control and the disease is chronic, its course measured in many months or years.

Principles of Drug Therapy

Controlled clinical trials have established certain basic principles, but new concepts gradually emerge, many of which have not been fully evaluated and are in some cases controversial (see also Ch. 267 and 268). A textbook presentation must offer a definite and simple plan of approach which in the author's judgment is the most reasonable at the time; it cannot present both sides of all controversial points.

Effective use of drugs now available should provide cure in 95 to 100 per cent of previously untreated cases. In actual practice, results are less satisfactory. In part this may reflect poor medical direction, but much more important is the often carefully obscured failure of the patient to follow his drug regimen.

The Antituberculous Drugs. *Isoniazid* (INH) remains the keystone of original treatment of pulmonary tuberculosis. It is highly effective (bactericidal against actively metabolizing cells, bacteriostatic against metabolically dormant cells), well absorbed, distributed throughout all tissues in effective concentrations, of low toxicity, and inexpensive. Drug resistance may emerge in the presence of very large bacterial populations such as are associated with pulmonary or renal cavities, and one or more companion drugs must be added to prevent this. However, isoniazid, in contrast to all other antituberculosis drugs, may retain some in vivo effectiveness even when in vitro studies indicate resistance, probably caused in part by a slightly decreased pathogenicity of isoniazid-resistant strains. Accordingly, it is advisable to continue administration of isoniazid in spite of development of in vitro resistance, while adding other effective drugs. The incidence of isoniazid-resistant isolates from previously untreated patients has remained for some years at approximately 2 per cent in the United States and England, although in other areas this figure may be higher. Allergic reactions to isoniazid are uncommon. Transient elevations of SGOT occur in 10 per cent of patients, and isoniazid-related hepatitis, reversible in its early stages, occurs in less than 1 per cent below age 35 but up to 2.5 per cent in higher age groups, particularly in subjects using alcohol excessively. Isoniazid depletes body pyridoxine stores and may induce peripheral neuritis, particularly in nutritionally compromised patients such as alcoholics. Pyridoxine (50 mg a day) is often given with isoniazid and is mandatory with doses greater than 300 mg daily and in severe alcoholics. Isoniazid dosage is 5 mg per kilogram of body weight, which in most adults is usually rounded off to 300 mg in a single daily dose. Larger doses (10 to 15 mg per kilogram) may be given at the cost of greater toxicity (pyridoxine always added) in extensive caseous disease and in isoniazid-resistant infections, particularly when supporting drug therapy is weak.

Rifampin (RMP) is a new antituberculous agent of the same order of effectiveness, low incidence of toxicity, and high degree of patient acceptance as INH. Its cost is almost prohibitively high. Its effectiveness (with companion drugs) in INH-resistant treatment failures has radically changed the prognosis in such cases from uncertain at best to favorable in the majority. Its role in initial treatment has yet to be established. Clinical and experimental evidence indicates that RMP plus INH is more effective than any other regimen. However, to date the evidence for increased clinical effectiveness is confined to patients treated for only six months. In these it is clear that INH plus RMP leads to fewer relapses after discontinuation of therapy than is the case with any other regimen administered for this period of time. However, when therapy is continued for 18 months, which is routinely recommended although at times hard to achieve, the advantage of the combined use of these two most potent agents disappears. Further, it seems likely that hepatotoxicity is increased by the use of INH and RMP together in comparison to regimens containing only one or the other. Finally, in contrast to INH, RMP loses all effectiveness when resistant strains emerge. At present it seems justifiable to employ both agents in treatment of cases of extraordinary gravity such as extensive miliary or caseous pulmonary tuberculosis associated with marked debility. At the time of this writing, however, it is the author's practice to reserve RMP for retreatment in the usual case of pulmonary tuberculosis.

Rifampin is excreted by the liver and rarely if ever should be used in the presence of liver disease. Rarely it may cause bilirubinemia, usually with larger than ordinary dosage. Its use combined with INH increases the incidence of liver function abnormalities. Thrombocytopenic purpura and a serum sickness type of reaction have been observed. These allergic phenomena are rare at conventional daily dosage but are not uncommon when larger than usual dosage and intervals greater than 24 hours are employed. The recommended dosage is 450 to 600 mg administered by mouth in a single daily dose given at least an hour before or after meals, because food makes absorption unreliable.

Streptomycin (SM) is the second major commonly used antituberculosis drug. It is often administered for a few months as the third drug in three-drug therapy (INH plus EMB plus SM) of severe disease. In conjunction with INH, it offers a strong two-drug regimen for hospitalized patients. SM is excreted by the kidneys, and toxic levels may develop when renal function is compromised. Eighth nerve toxicity (especially the vestibular branch) is a troublesome complication, more serious in those over 50, in whom the ability to compensate for loss of vestibular function is less effective. Streptomycin is administered intramuscularly in a dose of 1 gram daily in active treatment circumstances but may be reduced to 1 gram two or three times weekly in suppressive usage.

Ethambutol (EMB) is the most useful oral companion drug for INH (replacing para-aminosalicylic acid) in original treatment cases, and, if not previously used, for RMP in retreatment (INH-resistant) cases. A tendency to induce optic neuritis (loss of visual acuity, field constriction, and loss of green color discrimination) limits dosage. An acceptable incidence of 2 per cent allows the use of 25 mg per kilogram of body weight in hospitalized patients, but 15 to 20 mg per kilogram is recommended for outpatient treatment, at which dosage the incidence of optic neuritis is negligible.

Para-aminosalicylic acid (PAS), the principal companion drug to INH for years, has now been replaced by the much less toxic EMB. PAS is difficult to take and is poorly tolerated because of gastric irritation. In addition, it causes serious hypersensitivity reactions more frequently than any other antituberculous drug. PAS is now used mainly as a companion drug in retreatment cases with limited drug options. It is usually administered as the sodium salt in a dose of 5 grams three times daily with meals or 10 grams in a single daily dose given on a full stomach.

Pyrizinamide (PZA) follows SM in antimicrobial effectiveness, but its value is limited by early development of drug resistance (as early as six weeks in an active infection). This may be offset by its use with multiple drugs, with a strong drug, or in an already fairly well controlled infection. SM plus PZA is a good combination. Hepatotoxicity is a limiting factor, with 15 per cent showing altered liver function tests and 3 per cent frank jaundice, and with reported fatal hepatitis in as high as 1 per cent. The usual oral dosage is a total of 2 to 3 grams daily given in two to three divided doses.

Ethionamide (ETH) is moderately effective in retreatment cases as a companion drug with a strong agent or as one of three or more weak drugs. Patient intolerance is moderately high owing to central nervous system mediated nausea. It is administered by mouth in a dose of 500 to 1000 mg daily, most often 250 mg three times daily.

Cycloserine (CS) is a toxic and rather ineffective drug used in retreatment with a strong drug or as a member of a combination of three or more drugs. Its tendency to induce a variety of central nervous system symptoms, including convulsions, limits the dosage to 0.5 to 1.0 gram daily, the lower being of questionable effectiveness and the higher a dose that few tolerate. A regimen of 250 mg three times daily is a reasonable compromise.

Capreomycin (CM) is an aminoglycoside that approaches SM in effectiveness, with similar dosage requirements and toxicity. There is no cross-resistance with SM, and in general it can be substituted for that drug, but it is best to include it in a three-drug regimen.

Viomycin (VM) and *kanamycin* (KM), aminoglycosides that are less effective and more toxic than SM or CM, are used only in retreatment when

the drug options have become quite limited. The aminoglycosides have additive toxicities, and only one can be used at a time.

Combined Drug Therapy. Drug resistance may be *primary* (in previously untreated patients) or may emerge during treatment. Although a matter of continuing concern, primary resistance is not yet a major problem in most areas. Continuing surveys in the United States, Great Britain, and elsewhere indicate a rather stable level of 2 to 3 per cent of previously untreated infections primarily resistant to either INH or SM, and less than 1 per cent to both drugs. However, some careful studies have demonstrated a higher incidence of primary drug resistance in children in urban areas of known high prevalence.

Drug resistance emerging during treatment is a major problem recognized ever since earliest drug trials. Canetti's detailed studies provide insight into the mechanisms of this phenomenon. Naturally occurring mutants resistant to INH appear at a predictable rate of 1 per 10^5 or 10^6 bacterial cells. This is true with respect to SM and probably other antituberculous drugs. When INH is administered alone and the bacterial population is large, drug-susceptible cells are killed or suppressed and resistant mutants may in time repopulate the site of infection. This is of little practical importance in closed lesions with a low bacterial population (10^3 to 10^5 cells per gram of tissue), but is extremely important in open lesions associated with very large bacterial populations. Pulmonary cavities usually contain 10^7 to 10^9 but occasionally 10^{10} or more organisms; therefore as many as 10^3 or more INH-resistant bacteria might be present from the outset, providing an ample nidus for establishment of a drug-resistant infection once the larger susceptible population is suppressed. Under these circumstances, significant numbers of resistant organisms may appear in the sputum in a few weeks, and after three to four months the major portion of the bacterial population may be INH resistant. If two effective drugs are used at the same time, and organisms resistant to each are present in a ratio of 1 to 10^5 bacterial cells, then the population of organisms resistant to both would be approximately 1 in 10^{10} bacteria, making emergence of resistance unlikely. This is the basis of the principle of combined therapy in which two or more effective drugs are used, each active against organisms resistant to the other.

Although combined therapy is primarily intended to prevent development of drug resistance, it may also increase drug effectiveness. It is important to accomplish either or both of these aims with minimal drug toxicity. The character and severity of the disease should determine the drug combinations used. Cavities with thick necrotic walls and large areas of caseation provide both the greatest hazard of drug resistance and the severest test of drug therapy. Consequently, two or three drugs, including two of the most potent (INH, SM, RMP), are recommended for severe disease.

Prolonged Therapy. The principle of prolonged therapy was also established early by the occurrence of relapse when treatment was terminated too soon, ordinarily caused by organisms still susceptible to the agents administered. Since the antituberculosis drugs are bacteriostatic for dormant organisms, suppressive therapy must be continued until the slow processes of host healing mechanisms secure control of residual infection. Strangely, there have been few studies designed to determine how long is "prolonged" and what circumstances should modify the duration of suppressive therapy. General experience indicates that for disease without residual cavity or large areas of caseation, two years of overall drug treatment usually secures permanent healing. For years, persistent cavities were resected to diminish risk of relapse. As more prolonged periods of drug therapy came into use, it became clear that the persistent "open negative" thin-walled cavity was not a serious threat and eventually became sterilized. Two to three years of drug therapy is usually indicated when thin-walled cavities persist. Caseous "open negative" thick-walled cavities require longer suppressive therapy, and surgical excision may occasionally be advisable. Some patients with extensive, necrotic disease are treated with indefinite administration of INH.

Stages of Therapy. Drug treatment consists of an *active treatment phase* during which a combination of drugs is administered in the presence of large numbers of organisms, and a *suppressive phase* during which isoniazid, usually as a single agent, is continued when the infection is reduced to a few dormant organisms.

Patient Participation. Drug regimens are always dependent on patient cooperation. Patient failure to take drugs is the most frequent and important cause of treatment failure. There are many reasons such as simple forgetfulness, the illusion of health associated with disappearance of symptoms, and the always underestimated reluctance of almost all individuals to subject themselves to any discipline for prolonged periods. Some discontinue drugs when they feel well. Alcoholics frequently forget or don't care. There are many less obvious reasons, including imagined drug reactions, queer health ideas, and rumors passed on by other patients. There is a strong tendency to cover up lapses. Every physician who treats tuberculosis has often observed relapse in a patient who indignantly maintains that he has taken his drugs faithfully, only to find that the infection is still drug susceptible and that the disease promptly responds to the same drugs given under supervision. It is important that the physician remain constantly aware of this human element.

A Plan of Drug Therapy

Initial Treatment. *Active Phase of Therapy.* Usually treatment is best initiated in a hospital where the patient can be isolated, observed, and kept at reduced activity, and where appropriate roentgenologic laboratory facilities are available. In ideal circumstances, treatment can be initiated in the home. But even under the worst circumstances, reasonably good results may be obtained if only the patient will take the drugs. The first consideration in any event is institution and maintenance of effective drug therapy.

In selecting initial drugs, it is reasonable to assume that the organism is susceptible to all agents (see above, Combined Drug Therapy). The first choice is always INH. The decision concerning companion drugs must be based on the character and severity of the disease, assessed primarily by roentgenologic findings. In *severe cavitary disease,* INH, plus daily SM and EMB, provides maximal drug effectiveness and protection against development of resistance. In *moderate cavitary* or *noncavitary disease,* two drugs are sufficient, usually INH and EMB. The antimicrobial activity of INH suffices, and ethambutol is adequate to prevent emergence of resistant strains. Since this clinical category includes the

major portion of pulmonary tuberculosis, INH-EMB is the most frequently employed regimen.

In *minimal, noncavitary disease* with at most a very few organisms in the sputum, it is permissible to use INH alone, but in most cases it is preferable to begin with INH and EMB, continuing the EMB for only two or three months if the sputum becomes promptly noninfectious.

Ordinarily a bacteriologic diagnosis is established at least by smear before institution of drugs. If smears are negative on microscopy, five or six adequate sputum specimens should be cultured before initiating drugs. In severely ill patients, drugs should be started immediately, because a few days of antituberculous drugs will not interfere with demonstration of tubercle bacilli in a sputum smear or culture. Complete roentgenographic studies, including, if possible, planigrams, should be obtained at the outset and during progress on treatment. During the early course of treatment, it is best that the hemogram and urinalysis be repeated at weekly intervals and that liver and renal function be monitored frequently. Throughout the active treatment phase, chest roentgenograms and sputum specimens should be obtained at least monthly. During the early period, it is best to obtain sputum specimens at weekly intervals or clusters of three at fortnightly intervals in order to establish convincingly that tubercle bacilli either have disappeared from the sputum or are now drug resistant. Drug susceptibility studies for the commonly used drugs should be obtained before treatment, again in three or four months if the sputum still contains tubercle bacilli, or at any time of bacteriologic relapse.

The most significant event in the course of the active treatment phase is the disappearance of tubercle bacilli from the sputum. In noncavitary disease or in patients with small thin-walled cavities, this frequently occurs within one or two months. In some patients with extensive cavitary disease, reversal of infectiousness occurs rapidly, i.e., in about two months. This has important prognostic significance, because such patients demonstrate lower relapse rates than those in whom reversal of infectiousness requires four months or longer. The persistence of tubercle bacilli in the sputum after four months is associated with a rapidly rising incidence of drug resistance, and after six months the finding of drug resistance is likely. Between the four- and six-month period, therefore, there is need to consider strengthening the drug regimen in patients who continue to discharge bacilli in the sputum. A more potent companion drug, such as SM, may suffice, particularly if there are few organisms in the sputum. If there are many organisms still present in the sputum, two new drugs are needed. If the original regimen was INH and SM, it is best to continue these drugs and add RMP or EMB, or EMB and ETH, pending drug susceptibility studies. Significant resistance to any of these drugs requires a regimen containing at least two drugs (one major) to which the organisms are susceptible, and three if the new regimen does not contain a major drug. INH is always continued, even with high degrees of in vitro resistance; other drugs to which resistance is demonstrated are usually discontinued.

When discharge of tubercle bacilli in the sputum has been shown to have ceased for three consecutive months, when appropriate roentgenologic improvement has occurred (much less important), and when no cavities or large areas of caseation persist, the active treatment phase may be superseded by the suppressive phase (usually INH alone). If cavities persist ("open negative"), combined therapy should be continued for a longer time. For thin-walled cavities, the total period of combined drug therapy should be at least nine months. Persisting thick-walled cavities require combined drug therapy for at least a year and perhaps a good deal longer. Expert judgment is required in these cases.

The persistence of tubercle bacilli in the sputum after six months of drug therapy ordinarily means either drug resistance or patient noncompliance. Drug susceptibility studies will determine which possibility is present. If the patient's cooperation cannot be relied on, surgical excision may be advisable before all effective drugs are dissipated.

Decisions as to length of hospitalization, isolation, and return to work must be individualized, taking into consideration young children in the patient's environment, his social responsibility (covering cough), reliability in drug taking, history of alcoholism, and similar factors. Under ideal circumstances, in limited infections shedding relatively few organisms, work may be resumed or even continued without interruption after two or three weeks of effective drugs. Individuals with more severe infections may leave the hospital and return to work when control of the infection seems imminent or is accomplished.

Suppressive Phase of Therapy. Once control has been stabilized during the active phase, combined therapy is supplanted by a prolonged period of suppressive treatment. In all but the most severe cases, the patient will have returned to work by this time. Ordinarily, INH alone in a single daily dose of 300 mg is used. In disease without significant residual cavitation (none or thin-walled cavities), therapy is continued until 18 to 24 months after tubercle bacilli have disappeared from the sputum. The presence of thick-walled residual cavitation, persistence of large areas of unsloughed caseation, and slow bacteriologic conversion require longer periods of suppressive therapy. Decisions must be individualized under these circumstances, but total treatment periods of three or even four years may be reasonable, and occasionally therapy is continued indefinitely.

Retreatment. In most retreatment circumstances it is very important that the patient be managed in a hospital experienced with tuberculosis. Expert judgment is particularly important in drug-resistant tuberculosis in order to attain maximal effectiveness from limited drug resources. Even though resistance to INH is demonstrated or suspected, it is important to continue the use of this drug, usually in higher (up to 10 to 15 mg per kilogram) than normal doses (see above).

There is an infinite variety of circumstances attending each retreatment case. The determination of the susceptibility of the organism to all available drugs is critical to proper management. Some circumstances and principles of retreatment are tabulated here: (1) A relapse after prompt reversal of infectiousness almost always indicates that drugs have been stopped too soon, usually by the patient. If drugs were stopped completely, most will harbor drug-susceptible strains and respond again to the initial drug regimen. (2) If lapse in treatment and relapse is followed by irregular drug ingestion, resistant organisms will probably be present. (3) A patient who continues to shed tubercle bacilli in the sputum for more than six months is probably excreting drug-resistant organisms. (4) Under circumstances of suspected or presumed drug resistance, a two- or three-drug combination, including an unused strong drug (INH, RMP, SM) and an unused companion type drug (EMB, PZA, ETH, PAS, CS), may be added to INH while awaiting drug susceptibility studies. (5) CM can replace SM in the aforementioned regimens. VM and KM are less effective and more toxic, and their use is limited to last resort situations. (6) SM, CM, VM, and KM have similar and additive toxicities, and no more than one should be used at the same time.

Other Forms of Treatment. The effectiveness of drug therapy in untreated disease has made most other forms of treatment largely unnecessary. Bed rest and surgery may still have a place in retreatment cases and treatment failures.

Bed Rest. Strict bed rest, long the mainstay of treatment, is insignificant compared to effective antimicro-

bial drug therapy, and is no longer generally used in any circumstance. Modified bed rest is beneficial during the symptomatic stage of the early treatment period. In treatment failures, with infections resistant to all drugs, modified bed rest and continued use of INH may together in time salvage many apparently hopeless cases. In retreatment cases with tubercle bacilli resistant to all but the weakest drugs, modified bed rest will improve chances of success.

Surgery. Surgery is now rarely used, because effective use of combined and prolonged drug therapy has demonstrated the relative innocuousness of the "open negative" status. Surgery is no longer recommended for the thin-walled cavity when the sputum becomes promptly noninfectious. Surgical resection remains important and is advisable (1) in cases of drug treatment failure, provided there is sufficient pulmonary reserve and sufficient drug coverage available to avoid complications, and (2) in cases with any persistent cavity in which lack of patient cooperation compromises the prospects of prolonged drug therapy. When a drug-resistant strain is present, lobectomy is less apt to lead to complications than is segmental resection.

Adjunctive Therapy with Corticosteroids. Corticosteroids will suppress the hypersensitivity state in tuberculosis, and relatively low doses (30 mg daily of prednisone) will abolish constitutional symptoms. High dosage (60 to 80 mg of prednisone) is required to block the local inflammatory reaction, and the cost in terms of side effects is usually greater than the benefit. Steroid therapy may, however, be of great benefit in extensive disease in which hypersensitivity-induced debility may be fatal before the stores of absorbable antigen are significantly reduced (several weeks after control of bacterial growth by antimicrobial agents); the use of corticosteroids will abolish these constitutional symptoms and may tide the patient over this critical period. Also, in less serious disease in which fever, anorexia, and anemia of infection lead to weeks of serious morbidity, corticosteroids will produce prompt symptomatic recovery and repair of the anemia. In these two circumstances a moderate dose of corticosteroids (approximately 10 mg of prednisone three times daily) will suffice; it is usually possible to taper the dose by 2.5 mg decrements every four or five days. In the rare instance of hypoxia caused by a diffusion defect, usually in severe miliary tuberculosis, a large anti-inflammatory dose of corticosteroids (60 to 80 mg of prednisone daily) may be necessary for a few days before quickly decreasing to 30 mg of prednisone daily and then tapering. The unusual coexistence of Addison's disease and active pulmonary tuberculosis should be borne in mind. The adverse effect of steroids on tuberculous infection can be disregarded in the presence of effective antituberculous therapy.

Hospitalization. The classic reasons for hospitalization (bed rest and isolation) are no longer pertinent. Bed rest is not necessary in initial drug treatment, and effective drug therapy reduces the period of significant infectiousness to a few weeks. However, proper management of pulmonary tuberculosis requires a variety of services, including roentgenographic facilities, a bacteriologic laboratory competent to culture tubercle bacilli and to determine drug resistance, availability of a variety of laboratory studies for evaluation of possible drug susceptibility reactions, diagnostic facilities for evaluation of associated disease, opportunity for frequent patient observation during the early stages of treatment, and, above all, the availability of expert judgment in severe or difficult cases. Home care is entirely adequate if these services are available, but in most circumstances they are best provided through the specialty service of the hospital, either on an ambulatory basis or as an inpatient. Hospitalization is actually more important in retreatment cases, because frequent drug susceptibility studies, the advice and skills of an experienced thoracic surgical service, and expert judgment are critically important when drug resources are limited.

Desensitization. In most instances there will be sufficient alternative therapies to make it unnecessary to resort to desensitizing patients to any of the antituberculous drugs. In the rare incidence in which this might become necessary, the reader is referred to Simpson and Hubaytar (Am. Rev. Respir. Dis., 84:738, 1962), for a simple and effective method of desensitization to SM and INH.

EXTRAPULMONARY TUBERCULOSIS

Roger Des Prez

229. INTRODUCTION

Extrapulmonary tuberculosis falls into two groups on the basis of pathogenesis. The first comprises conditions resulting from *lymphohematogenous dissemination (miliary tuberculosis, tuberculosis of bones and joints, renal tuberculosis,* most cases of *tuberculous lymphadenitis, female genital tuberculosis, peritonitis, pericarditis, meningitis,* and some instances of *pleural effusion).* These illnesses may coexist with tuberculosis elsewhere or *may be isolated clinical manifestations.* The second comprises conditions which complicate pulmonary tuberculosis, caused either by bronchial or gastrointestinal spread of infectious secretions (*intracanalicular spread*) or by direct contiguous invasion (pleura, pericardium, esophagus). Urogenital tuberculosis may represent a combination when a hematogenous renal focus cavitates and seeds the lower urinary tract via the ureters.

230. PRINCIPLES OF DRUG THERAPY

Most extrapulmonary tuberculosis responds more readily to drugs than does advanced pulmonary tuberculosis, because the bacterial populations are small. The exception is cavitary renal tuberculosis which may contain large bacterial populations, requiring combined drug therapy. In the remainder, the likelihood of drug resistance developing on therapy is negligible, and the choice of a drug regimen depends on how life-threatening the illness is judged to be. Those conditions carrying a threat of early mortality (miliary and meningeal tuberculosis, and probably spondylitis and pericarditis) are treated with maximal drug therapy (isoniazid and daily streptomycin, or isoniazid and rifampin) at least until response is established, thus increasing antimicrobial potency and eliminating the small possibility of a primarily isoniazid-resistant infection. Less threatening

conditions such as involvement of serous membranes, lymph nodes, the skeletal system (excluding the spine), and genital tuberculosis may be treated with isoniazid alone. Usually response is good, and only prolonged isoniazid therapy is required. When it is not, other drugs may be added without significant loss.

231. TUBERCULOSIS OF THE PLEURA

Substantial subpleural foci established prior to tuberculin hypersensitivity may, when this develops, rupture into the pleural space, evoking a brisk allergic reaction and the clinical syndrome of *primary serofibrinous pleurisy with effusion.* This occurrence, of itself usually self-limiting, is important in identifying rather extensive initial infections which are very likely to result in progressive tuberculosis elsewhere at a later time (see Part XI, Section Nine). Pleural effusion may also result from subpleural hematogenous foci and, uncommonly, as a complication of established chronic pulmonary tuberculosis, which more frequently causes local inflammation and adhesions (dry pleurisy), precluding sudden delivery of large amounts of antigenic material into the pleural cavity. Rarely, rupture of a necrotic chronic focus into the pleural space may produce tuberculous empyema and secondary bronchopleural fistula.

232. ENDOBRONCHIAL TUBERCULOSIS

Cavitary tuberculosis inevitably produces bronchial mucosal infection in the immediate vicinity of the cavity and usually in spotty distribution elsewhere. In the days before drug therapy, such involvement at times obstructed the bronchocavitary junction or even a whole segment or lobe, with subsequent inspissation, fibrosis, and contraction, an important although tenuous healing mechanism. Superficial bronchial lesions respond promptly to chemotherapy, and now usually require little attention. However, partial degrees of bronchial cicatrization may cause nontuberculous complications such as atelectasis and obstructive pneumonitis. Some degree of permanent bronchial distortion probably occurs in all moderately extensive pulmonary tuberculosis. Tuberculosis of the trachea, now rare, is an extension of florid endobronchial tuberculosis. The consequences of bronchial involvement in childhood are discussed in Ch. 228.

233. TUBERCULOSIS OF THE LARYNX

Prior to drug therapy, tuberculosis of the larynx was a dread late complication of extensive pulmonary tuberculosis. The onset of hoarseness, dysphagia, and perhaps pain referred to the ear often initiated downhill course, with extensive bronchogenic spread throughout both lung fields from copious, thin, laryngeal secretions. This is now almost never seen, even in patients with a drug-resistant strain and highly infectious sputum. Rarely, isolated ulcers or nodules with intact mucosa, resembling carcinoma, are diagnosed as tuberculosis either by biopsy or by association with active pulmonary tuberculosis. Hematogenous laryngeal tuberculosis is usually accompanied by hematogenous involvement of the lung as well. Response to drug therapy is excellent, and surgery is usually unnecessary.

234. GASTROINTESTINAL TUBERCULOSIS

Gastrointestinal tuberculosis frequently complicated extensive pulmonary tuberculosis in years past, and was also caused by ingestion of milk containing tubercle bacilli. It is now rare, but occasionally complaints related to a gastrointestinal focus may lead to recognition of pulmonary tuberculosis; even more rarely, gastrointestinal tuberculosis presents without recognizable active pulmonary disease.

Tuberculosis of the tongue and mouth may present as painful ulcers or as a nonhealing tooth socket after dental extraction. Untreated, the process is indolently progressive, but response to chemotherapy is rapid. Extension of oropharyngeal disease via the eustachian tube may produce *tuberculosis of the middle ear and mastoid bone. Tuberculosis of the tonsil and pharyngeal lymphatic tissue* was common when bovine tuberculosis was epidemic; draining regional nodes were termed *scrofula. Tuberculosis of the esophagus* may very rarely result from penetration of an adjacent node, leading to bronchoesophageal fistula or to ulcerative or hyperplastic disease of the esophageal wall. *Tuberculosis of the stomach* may resemble diffuse neoplastic involvement (linitis plastica type) or a nonhealing ulcer, and may, if caused by extension from an adjacent lymph node focus, present as an isolated clinical manifestation. Hyperplastic or ulcerative *duodenal tuberculosis* may resemble peptic or neoplastic obstructive disease. Tuberculosis of the intestine may produce ulceration with bleeding and a tendency to perforation and fistula formation, hyperplasia with obstructive symptoms, or a combination of the two. *Tuberculosis of the small intestine* is more liable to produce perforation than disease elsewhere. *Ileocecal tuberculosis* is the most frequently observed form of bowel involvement, presumably because of cecal pooling of infectious fecal material producing mucosal disease, occult bleeding, obstruction, or fistula formation. *Tuberculosis of the ascending and transverse colon* is much less common, and may present as a concentric, hyperplastic lesion producing obstruction. *Tuberculosis of the sigmoid colon* may resemble carcinoma, atypical ulcerative colitis, or diverticulitis. All these lesions may perforate and produce *tuberculous perirectal and pelvic abscesses* and fistula in ano. Diagnosis is now almost always an unexpected finding at surgery; but if it is established by nonsurgical means, the effects of chemotherapy should be determined, because even advanced lesions may respond satisfactorily.

235. MILIARY TUBERCULOSIS

The term *miliary tuberculosis* was coined to describe the appearance of lungs and other organs from fatal cases of progressive tuberculous bacteremia in which the disseminated small tubercles suggested millet seeds. It is at present applied to any form of persistent or recurrent hematogenous dissemination. The hematogenous phase of the primary infection is especially liable to evolve into miliary tuberculosis in very young children, and, together with the associated meningitis, accounts for most tuberculosis deaths in this age group. In adults miliary tuberculosis may be due to old residua of remote infections which reactivate, undergo necrosis, and seed the circulation. A pulmonary focus may be responsible, but more frequently a previously undetected extrapulmonary focus in the lymphatic, genitourinary, or skeletal system is the cause. Such foci may cause multiple bacteremic episodes, and the process may be protracted, intermittent, and low grade. Host factors such as debility, advanced age, intercurrent therapy with oncolytic agents, immunosuppressives, or corticosteroid hormones, malignant disease, particularly of the lymphatic and hematopoietic systems, and occasionally local injury are frequently associated with activation of latent foci.

Clinical Features and Diagnosis.   In the very young, the illness is acute and severe, with high intermittent fevers, night sweats, and occasionally rigors. Complications such as pleurisy, peritonitis, or meningitis occur in as many as two thirds, usually developing several weeks after the onset of constitutional symptoms. A similar acute illness is usual in adults as well. The presenting syndrome is similar to that seen in an acute viral or rickettsial infection or in typhoid fever or brucellosis. The onset, although perhaps not actually abrupt, can nevertheless be dated. The patient is prostrated, frequently has a moderately severe headache, and, although conscious and oriented, usually seems to wish to be left alone. A leukopenia is present, sometimes as low as 3500 to 4000 cells per cubic millimeter, and there is a considerable increase of immature forms. Although meningeal signs may be absent, eventually meningitis appears in about two thirds of patients. In some patients, however, miliary tuberculosis may be covert and subtle, with weeks or months of nonspecific, slowly progressive, constitutional symptoms such as weight loss, weakness, and low-grade or absent fever. This clinical picture, ascribed to small, intermittent bacteremic episodes, has been designated *chronic hematogenous tuberculosis.* As in the more acute form, the presenting complaint may be due to serous membrane involvement, meningitis, or, less commonly, disseminated lymphatic involvement. Choroidal tubercles are often absent. Splenomegaly is uncommon.

Diagnostic studies are usually initiated because of the appearance of a typical miliary infiltration on chest roentgenogram. However, *individuals may succumb to miliary tuberculosis before the miliary pulmonary infiltrate has become roentgenographically detectable.* The tuberculin test is of little help, because as *many as one fourth of proved cases may be initially tuberculin negative,* reactivity returning when treatment results in improvement. Anemia is usual. The white blood count is usually normal or depressed initially (see below). Gastric and urine cultures, although frequently positive for *M. tuberculosis,* are of little immediate diagnostic help. Culture of the cerebrospinal fluid may be positive for tubercle bacilli despite the absence of pleocytosis, protein elevation, or meningeal signs. Evidence of associated tuberculosis is helpful but often lacking. In many, a tentative diagnosis is made when granulomatous lesions are discovered on bone marrow aspiration or liver biopsy. Culture of these tissues may be positive without histologic evidence of disease, and negative findings do not exclude the diagnosis.

Primary Hepatic Tuberculosis. In rare cases the sole clinical manifestations of miliary tuberculosis may be hepatic dysfunction and fever. The hepatic findings may resemble those of neoplastic or nontuberculous granulomatous origin (elevation of serum alkaline phosphatase, less elevation of serum bilirubin, and little indication of hepatocellular damage). At times the presenting findings will resemble those of extrahepatic obstruction with ascending cholangitis. Diagnosis is made by liver biopsy.

Miliary Tuberculosis of the Aged. Miliary tuberculosis in older persons may present simply as a wasting illness with intermittent, low-grade fever or no fever at all, commonly misdiagnosed as neoplasm, and frequently discovered only at autopsy. In such cases, a therapeutic trial of isoniazid will often be diagnostic and may be a conservative alternative to diagnostic laparotomy.

Miliary Tuberculosis and Hematologic Disease. Many hematologic illnesses may be mimicked by miliary tuberculosis (leukemoid reaction, leukopenia, thrombocytopenia, aregenerative anemia, hemolytic anemia, leukemia, myelofibrosis, and even polycythemia). The often associated histologic picture of foci containing myriads of acid-fast organisms but little specific cellular reaction has been termed *nonreactive tuberculosis.* Many such cases are misdiagnosed as leukemia, a confusion compounded by the fact that miliary tuberculosis may complicate true leukemia. Further, the steroid therapy administered for a hematologic illness may reactivate a latent tuberculous focus, leading to secondary miliary tuberculosis. Since steroid therapy is often indicated for serious hematologic disease, awareness of the possibility that the underlying cause may be cryptic miliary tuberculosis is very important.

Electrolyte Abnormalities. A surprising number of patients with miliary tuberculosis, especially but not exclusively those complicated by meningitis, will demonstrate hyponatremia. Although coexistent adrenal insufficiency is always a concern, the syndrome of inappropriate secretion of antidiuretic hormone is a much more frequent cause.

Treatment and Prognosis. Treatment of miliary tuberculosis with regimens including isoniazid should be successful in virtually all patients except those dying within the first few weeks or those with serious underlying disease. The prognosis with concurrent meningitis is less favorable. Maximal drug therapy with isoniazid and rifampin is recommended. When a good response has been established and the infecting strain is known to be isoniazid susceptible, rifampin may be discontinued. Isoniazid should be continued for a total of at least two years. (A good response to isoniazid in a therapeutic trial of unproved disease makes it unnecessary to add another drug.) Response to treatment may be dramatic or require some weeks. Adjunctive therapy with corticosteroids is advisable in severe cases with extensive pulmonary involvement and serious hypoxemia, and also in cases with poor response owing to severe debility. It is, of course, mandatory in the rare instance of coexistent adrenal insufficiency. Other causes for poor response to treatment, such as miliary disease caused by mycobacteria other than *M. tuberculosis* or by isoniazid-resistant *M. tuberculosis,* are rare, presumably owing to the decreased virulence of these organisms.

236. TUBERCULOUS MENINGITIS

Tuberculous meningitis is invariably fatal when untreated and is often associated with incapacitating neurologic damage, particularly in the very young, even with prompt therapy. It was long regarded as primarily a children's disease, but at present one half or more of cases are observed in adults. Meningitis complicates the majority of untreated cases of miliary tuberculosis. The infection reaches the subarachnoid space by direct extension from a subjacent focus, most frequently a small, subependymal tubercle, less frequently a tuberculoma or parameningeal focus in the spine, middle ear, or elsewhere. Since the critical factor is location, extensive bacteremia merely enhances the probability of meningeal involvement, which may also follow a small, transient, otherwise inapparent hematogenous phase. Once infectious material ruptures into the subarachnoid space, an allergic inflammatory response spreads infection via the cerebrospinal fluid, implanting bacilli elsewhere on the meningeal surfaces. Involvement is usually most marked at the base of the brain and may produce a grossly thickened space-occupying exudate, causing pressure injury to adjacent cranial nerves and long tracts. Obstructed basilar foramina may cause hydrocephalus. Vascular thrombosis and ischemic brain damage may also occur.

Clinical Features and Diagnosis. The illness may be abrupt and severe, or subtle and chronic. In some instances defects in mentation or affect may develop, with little to suggest infection. Extrameningeal tuberculosis is clinically apparent in half the patients and the tuberculin test is positive in three fourths, *but the absence of both does not exclude the diagnosis.* A variety of neurologic abnormalities may develop, including cranial nerve palsies, blindness, deafness, long tract signs, subarachnoid block, disorders of consciousness ranging from mild confusion to dementia or coma, and, as mentioned, the syndrome of inappropriate secretion of antidiuretic hormone.

An increase of cells in the cerebrospinal fluid, more than half mononuclear cells, is the rule. Cell counts are rarely over 1000 per cubic millimeter, more frequently in the 50 to 200 range, and may be as low as only a few lymphocytes. In acute severe disease, the cerebrospinal fluid may contain predominantly polymorphonuclear leukocytes, thus resembling pyogenic meningitis. The cerebrospinal fluid protein is almost always elevated and glucose is usually depressed in comparison with simultaneously determined blood glucose. Smears of the cerebrospinal fluid sediment will be positive for acid-fast bacilli in less than 25 per cent; this return may be improved if the pellicle on the top of the fluid specimen is stained and examined. Culture will eventually be positive for *M. tuberculosis* in at least 75 per cent of cases. Of the cerebrospinal fluid abnormalities, only the degree of pressure elevation has prognostic import, higher pressures being associated with a tendency to herniation at the base of the brain. Accordingly, the cerebrospinal fluid should be removed cautiously and slowly.

Treatment and Prognosis. Therapy should always include isoniazid and either rifampin or streptomycin, probably the former. Early in the course, isoniazid should be administered in larger than conventional dosage (8 to 12 mg per kilogram in the adult, and 15 to 20 mg per kilogram in children) with pyridoxine (100 mg per day). If response is favorable, these dosages may be reduced after four weeks or so. Isoniazid may be given by mouth or by intramuscular administration if oral therapy is not possible (equal total dose). Rifampin is administered as described for pulmonary tuberculosis. Intrathecal therapy is not indicated.

Bacteriologic cure should be achieved in three fourths or more of the patients, but permanent neurologic residua (weakness, paralysis, blindness or deafness, other cranial nerve palsies, hydrocephalus, compromised intelligence, and, rarely, symptoms and signs of pituitary or hypothalamic dysfunction such as precocious puberty, obesity, diabetes insipidus, and panhypopituitarism) may result in as many as 25 per cent. These are local complications of the inflammatory response, and accordingly adjunctive anti-inflammatory therapy might be advantageous. Use of *corticosteroid hormones or corticotrophin* has received wide acceptance. Although evidence is conflicting, most studies reveal a slight but definite survival advantage in groups receiving adjunctive corticosteroid therapy, particularly in prevention of brainstem herniation. The response to corticosteroid therapy may be dramatic, with rapid clearing of sensorium, regression of abnormalities in the cerebrospinal fluid, defervescence, and loss of headache. Even if long-term benefits are slight, this symptomatic improvement justifies corticosteroid therapy. Prednisone (60 to 80 mg per day) is recommended in all cases of tuberculous meningitis complicated by altered consciousness, neurologic abnormality, subarachnoid block, or cerebrospinal fluid pressures in excess of 300 mg of water. This will include most cases. The corticosteroid therapy may be tapered rapidly in the second or third week to a level of 30 mg, and then decreased at a slower rate every third or fourth day, using the signs and symptoms of meningeal inflammation as a guide to reduction of dosage. The hormone can usually be discontinued entirely after six to eight weeks.

237. TUBERCULOMAS

Tuberculomas, once the most frequent cause of intracranial mass lesions in children, are now rare. Except in cases in which meningitis develops owing to extension to the subarachnoid space, the symptoms are those of an expanding cerebral or cerebellar mass. Diagnosis is usually made at surgery. Antimicrobial therapy should be administered when the diagnosis is made, both in hope of some resolution and to prevent development of meningitis.

238. TUBERCULOUS PERICARDITIS

The subject of pericarditis is covered in Ch. 571 to 576, and this discussion concerns only aspects unique to tuberculous pericarditis. The pericardium is most often contaminated by an adjacent mediastinal node, less frequently by a pulmonary focus, and rarely via the bloodstream, evoking an allergic effusion which disseminates the infection over the entire pericardial surface.

Associated pleural effusion is present in approximately one half of the patients, and peritoneal involvement may also occur, a syndrome termed *tuberculous polyserositis.* Although always associated with other tuberculosis foci, frequently pericarditis is the only clinically apparent manifestation. Prior to the era of chemotherapy, tuberculous pericarditis was fatal in 90 per cent or more of the cases, with deaths caused both by progressive infection and by acute and chronic cardiovascular complications such as tamponade, constriction, restriction, and myocardial and coronary artery involvement.

Features tending to differentiate tuberculosis from other causes of pericarditis are the somewhat chronic course, less prominent pain and rub, and symptoms of chronic systemic infection, although frequently a symptom complex resembling progressive right heart failure leads to diagnosis. Etiologic diagnosis of tuberculous pericarditis, once the anatomic process has been established, is always difficult. The tuberculin test is usually positive (over 90 per cent), but may be negative. *Pericardiocentesis* is often employed for both diagnosis and relief of tamponade. *This procedure is associated with significant morbidity and mortality, and, if done, should always be preceded by unequivocal evidence of pericardial fluid.* It is not only risky; it also provides meager diagnostic information. The character of the fluid will not differentiate tuberculous disease from other causes of pericardial exudate (with the possible exception of pyogenic pericarditis). The fluid is rarely positive for acid-fast bacilli on microscopy, and culture (positive in approximately 40 per cent) requires too much time to be of immediate therapeutic assistance. It is the writer's preference to advise pericardiocentesis only for temporary relief of tamponade or to exclude the possibility of a pyogenic process when associated clinical manifestations (high spiking fever, marked leukocytosis, associated nontuberculous infection) make this uncommon process a serious consideration. Pericardiocentesis is best carried out in association with right heart catheterization and only after arrangements for prompt thoracotomy have been made, should this become necessary. When the presence of documented tuberculous disease elsewhere makes tuberculous pericarditis likely and little hemodynamic compromise is present, therapy may be initiated with isoniazid and rifampin and the course carefully followed. If, because of uncertain diagnosis, unfavorable hemodynamic conditions, or less than prompt improvement, this approach becomes unsatisfactory, and if the general condition of the patient is otherwise fairly good, we advise thoracotomy and anterior pericardial stripping. The advantages of this approach are (1) accurate diagnosis; (2) relief of tamponade and very probably prevention of some instances which would otherwise progress to constrictive or restrictive disease; (3) a favorable surgical technical situation prior to the development of chronic inflammation, scarring, and fibrosis; and (4) relief of right atrial hypertension which favors fluid retention, venous thrombosis, and pulmonary embolization. Our personal experience with patients succumbing to pulmonary embolic disease has led us to this rather prompt and decisive diagnostic and therapeutic approach.

Some authorities advise the use of corticosteroids to favor resolution of the inflammatory process. Although this is acceptable in the presence of a certain diagnosis and the absence of substantial right atrial hypertension, such circumstances rarely obtain in the individual case.

Further, the risk of an infectious process not susceptible to antituberculous drugs, although minor, is always present.

239. TUBERCULOUS PERITONITIS

Tuberculous peritonitis usually results from rupture of an adjacent caseous lymph node, fallopian tube, or subserosal tubercle into the peritoneal cavity, and is often the only clinical manifestation of infection. Peritoneal involvement from a bowel focus is rare. The process may become loculated or may involve the entire peritoneal surface, and the response may vary from copious, thin ascitic fluid with a few inflammatory cells to a hyperplastic reaction with gelatinous exudate tending to fibrosis or caseation. The onset may resemble pyogenic peritonitis, or may be quite subtle, suggesting occult malignancy, fever of unknown origin, bowel obstruction, or unexplained ascites. Fever may be absent and the tuberculin test negative. Recognition of tuberculous peritonitis in cirrhotics may be difficult, because the symptoms may resemble those of uncomplicated cirrhosis with ascites, requiring paracentesis for detection (ascitic fluid in uncomplicated cirrhosis usually contains less than 200 cells).

Diagnosis is usually made at laparotomy or on the basis of response to specific antituberculous chemotherapy. The peritoneal fluid resembles that found in tuberculous pleurisy with effusion, but is indistinguishable from that which may occur in peritoneal carcinomatosis. In acute cases the leukocytosis may be predominantly polymorphonuclear, suggesting a pyogenic process. Acid-fast stain of the fluid sediment is rarely positive and tubercle bacilli can be cultured in less than 20 per cent of cases. Needle biopsy of the parietal peritoneum (Cope or Abrams needle) will be diagnostic in most patients, but has resulted in death from occult intraperitoneal bleeding. Accordingly, if tissue is required, a limited exploratory laparotomy is preferable. When the therapeutic implications of tissue diagnosis are limited to the question of whether or not to treat for tuberculosis, a trial of isoniazid is often an acceptable alternative. Multiple drug therapy is advised by some authorities, but single drug therapy with isoniazid for a period of 24 months has produced completely satisfactory responses in all cases known to the writer.

240. TUBERCULOUS LYMPHADENITIS

Prior to the control of bovine tuberculosis, cervical tuberculous lymphadenitis or *scrofula* was commonplace, owing to local infection of the oropharynx and draining cervical lymphatics. This mode of acquisition of tuberculous cervical lymphadenitis is now extremely rare in areas with no bovine tuberculosis problem. In contrast, cervical granulomatous lymphadenitis in children caused by mycobacteria other than *M. tuberculosis* and *M. bovis* is almost certainly acquired by the oral route (see Ch. 244).

The term tuberculous lymphadenitis is now used to describe superficial lymph node involvement either caused by extensive lymphatic spread from a primary pulmonary focus or as a part of a generalized lymphohematogenous dissemination. The cervical and mediastinal nodes are most frequently involved. Clinical evidence of associated tuberculosis is lacking in more than half of the cases. Painless or, less frequently, painful node enlargement is the usual presenting complaint, but many patients have symptoms of systemic infection. The nodes may become fluctuant and drain.

Drugs should be administered before surgery is resorted to, because often even large, necrotic, chronically draining nodes will resolve completely and resection is rarely needed. Drug therapy should be given for at least a year and probably two. Most recommend use of isoniazid and a companion drug, but isoniazid given as a single agent is adequate therapy in almost all instances. Prolonged rest or hospitalization is not necessary once a favorable response has been established. Careful bacteriologic investigation is particularly important in view of the frequency of granulomatous lymphadenitis caused by other mycobacterial species, which are quite drug resistant and require a different therapeutic approach emphasizing surgical removal.

241. GENITOURINARY TUBERCULOSIS

RENAL TUBERCULOSIS

Renal tuberculosis develops from foci in the cortex seeded via the bloodstream. Although usually unilateral when detected, 50 per cent of the cases will become bilateral in the absence of treatment, presumably because of progression of contralateral hematogenous foci. The bacilli lodge in the cortex, but infection does not become progressive until it reaches the medulla (via the renal tubules) where the environment is much more favorable to progression. Foci in the renal papillae may cause obstruction and retrograde involvement of the obstructed segment, or may undergo necrosis, excavate, and seed the ureteral and vesical mucosa. Papillary obstruction with infection may cause segmental renal destruction; scarring in the renal pelvis and ureters may cause obstructive hydronephrosis; and the contaminated urine may cause bladder irritability, contracture, and scarring, as well as infection of the male genitalia.

Symptoms are usually subtle and are often lacking even with advanced cavitary renal tuberculosis. Sterile pyuria should suggest tuberculosis, especially with frequency and dysuria. Pyuria may be intermittent and low grade (10 white blood cells per high power field). Intermittent hematuria may also be seen. Fever and backache are uncommon and probably late symptoms. Male genital tuberculosis may be the first clue to renal involvement. History of prior tuberculous infection or coexistent extrarenal foci other than in the bladder and genitalia are the exceptions.

Diagnosis is based on the isolation of tubercle bacilli from early morning specimens of urine. Demonstration of acid-fast bacilli by microscopy of concentrated sediment should be regarded with suspicion, but could be caused by smegma bacilli. Intravenous or retrograde pyelography may provide the first evidence of disease and is necessary to assess the degree of involvement. However, unless calcification is present, the findings are nonspecific.

Treatment with a two-drug regimen, including isoniazid, for a period of at least two years will arrest the disease in most instances. Relapse is usually associated with emergence of drug resistance, and retreatment with two drugs to which the infection is susceptible is advised. Intravenous pyelograms should be obtained at three-month intervals to detect and treat ureteral strictures complicating the healing process. Very rarely obstruction with complicating pyogenic infection or pain may require removal of renal tissue, but this is to be avoided if possible.

MALE GENITAL TUBERCULOSIS

Male genital tuberculosis affects the *prostate,* the *seminal vesicles,* the *epididymides,* and more rarely the *testes;* it may be secondary to recent or remote renal tuberculosis or to lymphohematogenous spread. Most instances present as an epididymal lesion, varying from a firm, painless, small nodule to an inflamed and draining mass. Diagnosis is usually made by prostatic or epididymal biopsy. Some instances may be detected because of poor healing and fistula formation complicating prostatic or scrotal surgery; in these, diagnosis may require a therapeutic trial of isoniazid, because culture of the draining material is often unrevealing. Response to drug therapy is excellent in most patients, and surgery is usually not required except for diagnosis. Combined drug therapy is usually recommended; but in the absence of active renal disease, isoniazid is adequate therapy.

FEMALE GENITAL TUBERCULOSIS

Female pelvic tuberculosis begins as a hematogenous endosalpingeal focus. Infection may spread to the ovary, the endometrium, and rarely the cervix, producing an ulcerating granuloma that resembles carcinoma. Local or generalized peritonitis may also develop. The most common symptoms are menstrual disorders and abdominal pain. Most patients are sterile. In a smaller number, pregnancy and delivery appear to activate a previously latent focus. When conception does occur, tubal disease favors ectopic pregnancy. Pelvic inflammatory disease unresponsive to antimicrobial therapy may lead to the recognition of tuberculosis. In the majority, however, local and constitutional symptoms are mild or absent. Diagnosis is made by histologic study and culture of endometrial scraping, by culture of menstrual blood, and often by exploratory laparotomy. Response to a drug regimen containing isoniazid or to isoniazid alone is usually excellent, and surgery is only rarely necessary to remove large tubo-ovarian abscesses.

242. TUBERCULOSIS OF BONES AND JOINTS

Blood-borne tubercle bacilli tend to lodge in the anterior aspects of vertebral bodies and in the metaphyseal areas of long bones. Evolution of foci in bone may produce cystic areas of osteomyelitis without joint involvement but often erode the end plate and involve the nearby joint space. At present, bone and joint tuberculosis is not common in the United States, but several cases are seen each year on most medical services. It remains a major problem in other areas of the world.

TUBERCULOUS SPONDYLITIS

The most grave form of skeletal tuberculosis is *tuberculous spondylitis* or *Pott's disease.* The originating focus is usually in the anterior aspect of the vertebral body near an intervertebral disc. The developing infection may erode the cortex, destroy the intervertebral disc, and involve the adjacent vertebral body. The roentgenographic picture of rarefaction and destruction of adjacent areas of two vertebral bodies, loss of the intervening disc space, and a tendency to anterior wedging or collapse is typical of tuberculous spondylitis, but is also caused by other infectious processes. The anterior foreshortening and angulation of the spine may result in a visible and tender posterior bony prominence or gibbus. Less frequently, the infection may begin in the center or posterior aspect of the vertebral body. The thoracic, thoracolumbar, cervical, and lumbosacral areas are involved in order of decreasing frequency. More than one area may be involved with intervening normal vertebrae. Characteristically, the infection dissects anterolaterally from the vertebral body, producing a paraspinal abscess. In the thoracolumbar area, this may be seen as mediastinal widening or a pear-shaped retrocardiac density on the chest roentgenogram. In the lumbar area, the psoas shadow may be lost. In the cervical area, the abscess may displace anteriorly and obstruct the esophagus and trachea. The firm paraspinal ligamentous structures may result in high pressure in the abscess and produce ischemic paralysis in the subjacent spinal cord. The abscess pressure also may cause it to dissect along ligamentous planes and present as a fluctuant or firm mass in the groin, the gluteal area, or the supraclavicular space.

Clinical Features and Diagnosis. Symptoms are usually insidious and prolonged and may not include fever, although weight loss is common. Local back pain is frequent, and referred pain imitating renal colic or abdominal disorders occurs. Walking may be painful, and the gait may become stilted. Miliary, meningeal, or pulmonary tuberculosis may develop and dominate the picture in the untreated case. Severe anterior angulation of the spine may eventually produce a hunchback deformity. Frequently, however, it is the development of *weakness or paralysis* which leads to medical attention. Paralysis, now the most serious consequence of Pott's disease, may develop owing to pressure from abscess fluid, to generalized inflammatory edema, or to intrusion of a bony sequestrum or granulation tissue on the anterior aspect of the cord. Paralysis caused by angulation and displacement is unusual, because the anatomic abnormality develops slowly, but violent movement may produce cord transection when spine instability is marked.

In prior years most infectious spondylitis was tuberculous. However, it is now clear that entirely similar roentgenographic and clinical pictures can be produced by several other organisms, notably staphylococci, gram-negative enterobacteria, fungi, and rarely mycobacteria other than *M. tuberculosis.* Accordingly, in the absence of strong ancillary evidence for tuberculosis, aspiration or open biopsy of the vertebral body is indicated.

Treatment. Treatment of Pott's disease is based on antimicrobial therapy and immobilization. Usually isoniazid and streptomycin or rifampin for a period of two years or more is recommended. Most orthopedists advise some form of prompt surgical intervention such as debridement of the abscess cavity and spinal fusion, followed by a prolonged period of body casting. Others, particularly in areas in which surgical facilities are limited, have reported comparable results using just drug therapy and a brief period (two or three months) of bed rest without casting. When paralysis develops or fails to improve on therapy, surgery is required, and the procedure, whether abscess evacuation, debridement of granulation tissue, or removal of sequestra, is dictated by the findings at operation. Usually some form of spinal fusion will also be carried out. Although the course of therapy is usually decided by the responsible orthopedist, it is the writer's preference to assess the effects of drug therapy and bed rest while maintaining close surveillance of the neurologic status, because many individuals will achieve stable spines and remission of neurologic symptoms without operative intervention or casting.

TUBERCULOUS ARTHRITIS

Clinical Findings and Diagnosis. Tuberculous arthritis involves the hips, knees, elbows, shoulders, and small joints of the hands and feet in roughly that order. The initial symptoms are pain on motion or weight bearing, usually with some swelling. The process is usually monarticular, chronic, and associated eventually with considerable muscle wasting, pain, and stiffness. A history of trauma to the involved joint can frequently be obtained. In the absence of proved associated tuberculosis, diagnosis requires biopsy, histologic study, and culture. The need for verification by culture has been emphasized by reports of cases of granulomatous arthritis caused by mycobacteria other than *M. tuberculosis* (see Ch. 244).

Treatment. Most authorities recommend isoniazid and daily streptomycin. It is the writer's practice to utilize isoniazid alone. Intra-articular injection of drugs is not recommended. Many and perhaps most instances of tuberculous arthritis will heal with preservation of joint function when treated with mild immobilization, bed rest in the case of weight-bearing joints, and chemotherapy. When progress is not entirely satisfactory, joint exploration and removal of hypertrophied and fragmented synovial granulation tissue may be required. Casting and procedures to effect joint fusion are rarely necessary and are often detrimental.

OTHER FORMS OF SKELETAL TUBERCULOSIS

Cystic tuberculosis of bone (tuberculous caries or *tuberculosa multiplex cystica*) is a rare condition in which osteolytic cystic areas of long and flat bones and occasionally of the tubular bones of the hands or feet are caused by tuberculosis. *Tuberculosis of the costochondral junction* may present as a cold abscess overlying the area of involvement. *Tuberculosis of the tendon sheaths*

and bursae is usually secondary to involvement of the adjacent joint. These are responsive to antimycobacterial drug therapy with isoniazid alone or combined with streptomycin.

243. RARE FORMS OF TUBERCULOSIS

Ocular tuberculosis is one of the causes of *granulomatous intraocular infection. Phlyctenular keratoconjunctivitis* is a rare allergic external ocular inflammation observed in children at the time of the primary infection and characterized by small blisters (phlyctenules) at the junction of conjunctiva and cornea. *Choroidal tubercles* often provide a clue to the presence of disseminated tuberculosis. They produce no symptoms and are difficult to differentiate from other retinal exudates.

Cutaneous tuberculosis, once important but now only rarely seen, is usually grouped into two categories. The first, in which organisms are present, includes *lupus vulgaris, tuberculosis verrucosa cutis* (anatomic or prosector's wart), *scrofuloderma* (the skin changes surrounding a draining tuberculous sinus or overlying a tuberculous node), and *tuberculosis orificialis* (nodular and ulcerated lesions around the mouth or other orifice through which highly infectious material passes). These are all very responsive to isoniazid. The second group comprises the *tuberculids* (including *erythema induratum* or Bazin's disease). These reactions are thought to be allergic and comprise a variety of erythematous, papular, and ulcerative forms. Their relationship to tuberculosis is poorly understood. *Tuberculosis cutis miliaris acuta disseminata* is a rare complication of overwhelming miliary tuberculosis, usually in children.

Tuberculosis of the adrenals is important only as a now uncommon cause of adrenal insufficiency. Tuberculosis of the *spleen, thyroid, pancreas,* and *breast* may all occur and mimic other infections or neoplastic change in these organs.

Bentley, G., and Webster, J. H. H.: Gastrointestinal tuberculosis. A 10-year review. Br. J. Surg., 54:90, 1967.

Bobrowitz, I. D.: Ethambutol compared to streptomycin in original treatment of advanced pulmonary tuberculosis. Chest, 60:14, 1971.

Brown, A. B., Gilbert, R. A., and TeLinde, R. W.: Pelvic tuberculosis. Obstet. Gynecol., 2:476, 1953.

Canetti, G.: Present aspects of bacterial resistance in tuberculosis. Am. Rev. Respir. Dis., 92:687, 1965.

Diagnostic Standards and Classification of Tuberculosis. New York, National Tuberculosis and Respiratory Disease Association, 1969.

East African/British Medical Research Councils: Controlled clinical trial of short-course (6-month) regimens of chemotherapy for treatment of pulmonary tuberculosis. Lancet, 1:1079, 1972.

Garibaldi, R. A., Drusin, R. E., Ferebee, S. H., and Gregg, M. B.: Isoniazid-associated hepatitis. Report of an outbreak. Am. Rev. Respir. Dis., 106:357, 1972.

Goyette, E. M.: Treatment of tuberculous pericarditis. Prog. Cardiovasc. Dis., 3:141, 1960.

Kent, D. C.: Tuberculous lymphadenitis: Not a localized disease process. Am. J. Med. Sci., 254:866, 1967.

Konstam, P. G., and Blesovsky, A.: The ambulant treatment of spinal tuberculosis. Br. J. Surg., 50:26, 1962.

Mackaness, G. B.: The immunology of antituberculous immunity. Am. Rev. Respir. Dis., 97:337, 1968.

Moulding, T.: Chemoprophylaxis of tuberculosis: When is the benefit worth the risk and cost? Ann. Intern. Med., 76:761, 1971.

Munt, P. W.: Miliary tuberculosis in the chemotherapy era: With a clinical review in 69 American adults. Medicine, 51:139, 1971.

Newman, R., Doster, B., Murray, F. J., and Ferebee, S.: Rifampin in initial treatment of pulmonary tuberculosis. A U.S. Public Health Service tuberculosis therapy trial. Am. Rev. Respir. Dis., 103:461, 1971.

Proudfoot, A. T., Akhtar, A. J., Douglas, A. C., and Horne, N. W.: Miliary tuberculosis in adults. Br. Med. J., 2:273, 1969.

Rich, A.: The Pathogenesis of Tuberculosis. 2nd ed. Springfield, Ill., Charles C Thomas, 1952.

Smith, D. T.: Diagnostic and prognostic significance of the quantitative tuberculin tests. Ann. Int. Med., 67:919, 1967.

Smith, D. T.: Isoniazid prophylaxis and BCG vaccination in the control of tuberculosis. Arch. Environ. Health, 23:235, 1971.

Sochocky, S.: Tuberculous peritonitis. A review of 100 cases. Amer. Rev. Resp. Dis., 95:398, 1967.

Stead, W. W.: Pathogenesis of a first episode of chronic pulmonary tuberculosis in man: Recrudescence of residuals of the primary infection or exogenous reinfection? Am. Rev. Respir. Dis., 95:729, 1967.

Twomey, J. J., and Leavell, B. S.: Leukemoid reactions to tuberculosis. Arch. Intern. Med., 116:21, 1965.

Vall-Spinosa, A., Lester, W., Moulding, T., Davidson, P. T., and McClatchy, J. K.: Rifampin in the treatment of drug-resistant *Mycobacterium tuberculosis* infections. N. Engl. J. Med., 283:616, 1970.

Youmans, G. P., and Youmans, A. S.: Recent studies on acquired immunity in tuberculosis. Curr. Top. Microbiol. Immunol., 48:129, 1969.

244. DISEASES DUE TO MYCOBACTERIA OTHER THAN M. TUBERCULOSIS AND M. LEPRAE

Robert Goodwin

The term tuberculosis traditionally refers to infection associated with *M. tuberculosis (var. hominis* and *var. bovis).* It has long been known that other mycobacterial species exist in nature, some of which cause disease in animals. For years their role in human disease was unappreciated, owing largely to the overwhelming prevalence of *M. tuberculosis.* When found, their significance was denied because of the notion that mycobacteria were human pathogens only if they produced disease in the guinea pig (these did not). In recent years modern culture methods and drug susceptibility studies stimulated by the chemotherapy era have identified many mycobacterial species other than *M. tuberculosis* in human disease tissue.

Much of the most important bacteriologic work on these "atypical" mycobacteria has been carried out by Runyon, who classified them into four groups primarily on the basis of the presence and type of pigment production and growth rate. (See Bacteriology in Ch. 227). Most recently most of the known human pathogens have received tentative species designations, which will be employed herein. The relationship of these to the Runyon classification is as follows: *M. kansasii* and *M. marinum*—Runyon Group I (photochromogens); *M. scrofulaceum*—Runyon Group II (scotochromogens); *M. intracellulare* (Battey bacillus), *M. avium,* and *M. xenopi*—Runyon Group III (nonpigmented species); *M. fortuitum*—Runyon Group IV (rapid growers).

Human infection with many of these organisms is widespread throughout tropical and subtropical areas of the world. Their epidemiology is obscure. Many of the organisms involved are widespread in nature, being found particularly in the soil and in water. *M. kansasii* has been recovered from milk in Dallas and tapwater in California, but its source in nature is not clear. *M. intracellulare* is readily found in soil and in house dust, and has been demonstrated in throat swabs of normal individuals. *M. avium,* also of widespread distribution, is found in chickens and other birds as well as in household mammals. *M. scrofulaceum* has been isolated from soil and water, and is frequently found in oropharyngeal secretions of healthy men. *There is no evidence of man-to-man transmission of any of these, and no source case has ever been identified in human disease.*

The diseases produced by these organisms have roentgenologic, pathologic, and, to some extent, clinical similarities to tuberculosis, but there are distinct differences in virulence, treatment, and prognosis. The term *mycobacteriosis* has been suggested to differentiate them from tuberculosis. However, species orientation is preferable, because there are differences in organ susceptibility, treatment, and prognosis. It is convenient from a clinical standpoint to group these infections according to organ involvement. Pulmonary disease, mainly in older white men, is the most common clinical manifestation. Lymphadenitis in children and granulomatous skin lesions in all age groups are next in frequency. Injection abscesses are not uncommon. Rarely, disseminated disease, meningitis, renal or skeletal involvement, and penetrating wound infection are reported.

PULMONARY DISEASE

M. kansasii and *M. intracellulare* (Battey bacilli), and less frequently *M. avium,* may produce a tuberculosis-like pulmonary disease in susceptible individuals, as may rarely the less virulent *M. fortuitum, M. xenopi,* and *M. chelonei* (subsp. chelonei) and even more rarely *M. aquae, M. szulgai,* and *M. scrofulaceum.*

Prevalence. In the United States and Europe, 1 to 2 per cent of hospital admissions for tuberculosis are due to infection with either *M. kansasii* or *M. intracellulare.* There are geographical variations, particularly in the United States. The prevalence of *M. intracellulare* infections is relatively high in Georgia and northern Florida, and *M. kansasii* infection is much more frequent in the Dallas and Chicago areas. In some localities the incidence is as high as 7 to 10 per cent of annual hospital admissions for tuberculosis.

Clinical Manifestations. Pulmonary disease caused by *M. kansasii, M. intracellulare,* and *M. avium* primarily affects white males over the age of 45, less frequently, females and blacks. Chronic bronchitis and emphysema are present in some series in 40 per cent of patients with disease caused by *M. kansasii* and in 60 per cent of those with disease caused by *M. intracellulare.* Although virulence is less, disease, once established, tends to become cavitary and progressive. The clinical picture at any given time is indistinguishable from that of chronic pulmonary tuberculosis. Although in general slower in tempo than untreated tuberculosis, these infections may produce relentless destruction of pulmonary tissue and lead to death from respiratory insufficiency. Constitutional symptoms are much less prominent, local symptoms of cough and sputum are similar, and hemoptysis may occur somewhat more frequently than in tuberculosis. Roentgenographic studies usually reveal far-advanced disease at the time of discovery. Cavities are more frequently thin walled and pneumonic lesions less prominent than in tuberculosis, but there is much overlap, and roentgenographic differentiation is not possible in the individual case. Lesions have the apical posterior localization characteristic of tuberculosis. Pleural effusions are uncommon, and pleural changes of any sort are inconspicuous. Pathologic changes cannot be distinguished from those of tuberculosis, although in general the process appears more chronic with more fibrosis and less caseation.

Diagnosis is dependent upon bacteriologic identification of the specific organisms. With the exception of *M.*

kansasii, mycobacteria other than *M. tuberculosis* may be found in oropharyngeal secretions of normal persons, and therefore diagnosis of disease requires repeated demonstration of the organism in significant numbers in the presence of compatible pulmonary disease. A tuberculosis-like disease that does not respond to antimicrobial therapy or the demonstration of a high order of primary drug resistance should suggest the possibility of another mycobacterial species.

Treatment. Mycobacteriosis, excepting to some extent *M. kansasii* infection, differs most strikingly from tuberculosis in conspicuous lack of susceptibility to the antituberculous drugs. Pulmonary disease caused by these less virulent agents is therefore much more difficult to treat than drug-susceptible tuberculosis. *M. kansasii* is partially responsive to antituberculous drugs, and their use is usually recommended. Isoniazid-streptomycin-ethambutol is an effective starting regimen, which should be modified when drug susceptibility reports are available. In vitro and animal studies suggest that rifampin may be highly effective. The addition of this drug to the aforementioned regimen or its substitution for ethambutol in serious infection is reasonable, but a final statement awaits further clinical trials. Surgical excision may be necessary in treatment failures. The use of drugs is generally disappointing in disease caused by *M. intracellulare,* and probably entirely ineffective against *M. avium, M. fortuitum,* and other rare atypical pulmonary mycobacterial infections. There is no established plan for drug management of disease caused by *M. intracellulare* or the other drug-resistant mycobacterial infections. Although some strains are occasionally partially susceptible to some of the drugs, this is quite unpredictable. The most commonly useful drugs are isoniazid, ethambutol, ethionamide, pyrazinamide, and cycloserine. Rifampin should be tried. Multiple drugs increase the chance of success but at greater risk of toxicity. When effective, drugs are usually continued for one year after the sputum is free from bacilli. To the degree that drug therapy is less useful, other methods of treatment become more so. Hospitalization and a fairly confining type of rest therapy are recommended. Most agree that residual cavities should be resected, if possible, whether or not the sputum has been rendered noninfectious. The incidence of surgical complications is remarkably low even without effective drug coverage.

A statement of *prognosis* must be quite broad. The persistence of the bacilli in the sputum despite drug treatment is an unfavorable sign. Sputum free from bacilli for a year with no residual cavity (with or without surgery) indicates a good prognosis with a relapse rate perhaps no greater than 5 to 10 per cent. With vigorous treatment, including the use of surgery when indicated, the best success rates in pulmonary disease caused by *M. kansasii* are in the range of 85 per cent, and in disease caused by *M. intracellulare,* 75 per cent.

LYMPHADENITIS

Infants and young children may respond to a primary infection with certain atypical mycobacteria with the clinical manifestations of scrofula. Reports from the United States, Europe, and Australia in recent years indicate that 75 per cent of granulomatous cervical adenitis suggestive of tuberculosis is actually caused by mycobacteria other than *M. tuberculosis. M. scrofulaceum,* a scotochromogen, *M. avium, M. intracellulare,* and, less commonly, *M. kansasii* are the responsible agents. Each of these may be the predominant cause of adenitis in certain geographical areas and not found at all in others. In the vast majority the adenitis is cervical, occasionally preauricular, and rarely inguinal, axillary, or epitrochlear. Cervical adenitis most commonly occurs in the submaxillary and submandibular areas and is almost always unilateral, in most instances representing a regional component of a primary infection. Submaxillary and submandibular involvement suggests that the buccal mucosa is the portal of entry; involvement of the preauricular node implies conjunctival infection. In the extremities the infection usually follows a puncture wound. The pathology of the lesion is similar to that of tuberculosis, as are the clinical manifestations. Enlarged, firm, and nontender single nodes or groups of nodes may appear and persist unchanged or progress to fluctuation, drainage, and sinus formation, sometimes quite rapidly. Surgical excision is usually employed for both diagnosis and treatment. Infections with *M. kansasii* may be an exception, and a trial of drug treatment is indicated (see Pulmonary Disease, above). Isoniazid treatment of granulomatous cervical adenitis is recommended prior to cultural identification, because the infection may be due to *M. tuberculosis.* If antigens are available, the demonstration of skin hypersensitivity to some other mycobacterial species and a negative or smaller reaction to PPD-S *(M. tuberculosis)* is regarded as diagnostic. PPD-B (Battey) may be used for this purpose. Although recurrence may develop in an adjacent lymph node, surgical excision of grossly involved nodes is usually curative.

SUPERFICIAL SKIN DISEASE

In addition to *M. leprae* (leprosy) and *M. tuberculosis,* two other mycobacteria, *M. marinum* and *M. ulcerans,* occasionally produce skin infections. Both have temperature requirements below 37° C, accounting for limitation of infection to superficial areas of the skin. *M. marinum,* previously referred to as *M. balnei,* is a photochromogenic saprophyte first described in marine fish. It is widely distributed in nature, occurring in soil, water and freshwater fish as well. The temperature for optimal growth is 30 to 32° C. It has been implicated in epidemics of granulomatous skin disease traced to infected swimming pools, beaches of several of the Hawaiian Islands, and more rarely tropical fish aquariums. The granulomas occur at the site of minor abrasions, most commonly on the elbows, but also on the knees, toes, fingers, dorsum of the feet, and bridge of the nose, appearing two to three weeks after exposure as papules or nodules which increase slowly in size and may ulcerate. Spontaneous healing is to be expected after several months. Diagnosis may be established by culturing a biopsy of the lesion at 30° C. Histologically, the tissue usually suggests a tuberculosis-like granuloma, but may appear to be a nonspecific chronic inflammatory reaction. Rifampin may speed spontaneous healing.

Disease caused by *M. ulcerans* is relatively rare in most areas of the world but strangely is quite common in the Buruli district of the upper Nile in Africa. This organism has a limited temperature requirement in the range of 32 to 33° C. Disease begins as a painless nodule, usually on the extremities, which may grow rapidly and ulcerate. The ulcers (Buruli ulcers), seldom less than 5 cm in diameter and often much larger, have characteristic undermined margins. They tend to be persistent and progressively destructive. Surgical excision is curative and is much simpler when the lesion is recognized in the preulcerative stage.

OTHER INFECTIONS

More than 100 cases of *injection abscesses* have been reported, mostly caused by the common saprophyte, *M. fortuitum*, but also by *M. chelonei* (subsp. abscessus). These have occurred mostly in adults and respond to incision and drainage. The same organisms, and more rarely *M. kansasii*, have occasionally caused penetrating wound infections. *M. fortuitum* infection may result in corneal ulceration after trauma.

A dozen or so usually fatal cases of *disseminated* infection have been reported in young children and more rarely in immunologically deficient adults. Many different mycobacteria have been implicated, including *M. kansasii, M. avium, M. intracellulare, M. scrofulaceum,* and *M. fortuitum*. Multiple and single *bone and joint* lesions have been reported, mostly in children. Rare cases of *meningitis* in children and adults are reported with *M. avium* and *M. kansasii*. One case of renal infection caused by *M. kansasii* has been found.

Bates, J. H.: A study of pulmonary disease associated with mycobacteria other than *Mycobacterium tuberculosis:* Clinical characteristics. Am. Rev. Respir. Dis., 96:1151, 1967.
Lincoln, E. M., and Gilbert, L. A.: Disease in children due to mycobacteria other than *Mycobacterium tuberculosis*. Am. Rev. Respir. Dis., 105:683, 1972.
Pfuetze, K. H., and Hubble, R.: Nontuberculous mycobacterial diseases. Disease-a-Month, September 1968.
Schaefer, W. B., and Davis, C. L.: A bacteriologic and histopathologic study of skin granuloma due to *Mycobacterium balnei*. Am. Rev. Respir. Dis., 84:837, 1961.
Selkon, J. B.: 'Atypical' mycobacteria: A review. Tubercle (Suppl.), 50:70, 1969.

245. LEPROSY
(Hansen's Disease)

M. F. R. Waters

Definition. Leprosy is a chronic inflammatory disease of man caused by *Mycobacterium leprae*, which displays a wide clinical "spectrum" related to host ability to develop specific cell-mediated immunity (CMI). In high resistant "tuberculoid" leprosy, the localized signs are restricted to skin and nerve. Low resistant "lepromatous" leprosy is a generalized disease involving many systems, with widespread lesions of skin, peripheral nerves, upper respiratory tract, eyes, testes, and the reticuloendothelial system. Common complications include more acute, immunologically mediated, inflammatory episodes ("reactions"), secondary inflammation in the anesthetic areas which result from nerve damage, and deformity of hands, feet, and face.

Etiology and Microbiology. Although Hansen recognized the leprosy bacillus in 1873, as yet *M. leprae* has not been cultured in vitro. There is no known animal res-

ervoir. Past attempts to infect human volunteers were unsatisfactory, and successful experimental transmission was not achieved until 1960, when Shepard reported limited infection in mouse footpads. Since that date, leprosy has been one of the fastest growing points in medical research. In 1967, Rees and his colleagues obtained lepromatous leprosy in thymectomized-irradiated mice. More recently, Kirchheimer and Storrs (1971) have described lepromatous leprosy developing in a proportion of immunologically normal nine-banded armadillos inoculated with leprosy bacilli.

M. leprae is an intracellular, rod-shaped, acid-fast organism, 1 to 7 μ long and 0.25 μ in width; morphologically it resembles *M. tuberculosis*. However, in suspensions prepared from lepromatous tissues, bacilli are frequently arranged in characteristic "cigar-bundle" groups and in larger aggregates or "globi" derived from multinucleate Virchow giant cells. The cytoplasm of many bacilli is fragmented; such bacilli are dead. The percentage of solid-staining, presumed viable bacilli is known as the morphologic index (MI). Dead organisms are only slowly broken down, and may remain in tissues for many months or years.

In normal mice, a footpad inoculum of 5000 or 10,000 bacilli yields 10^6 after about six months, but no subsequent increase occurs. During the log phase of multiplication, the generation time is 12 to 13 days, the longest of any known bacterium. In thymectomized-irradiated mice, yields of 10^9 bacilli per footpad are not uncommon and systemic spread occurs, but the generation time remains unchanged. The footpad technique has been applied to studying the effect of drugs in leprosy, the detection of drug resistance, and the immunology and pathogenesis of the disease.

M. leprae is most easily detected in patients by Wade's "scraped incision" method. After cleansing, the skin is pinched to exclude blood, and a small cut made in the skinfold some 2 to 3 mm deep. One side of the cut is then scraped with the back of the scalpel point. The tissue pulp collected on the blade is spread on a glass slide, dried, fixed, and stained by the Ziehl-Neelsen method, care being taken never to overheat the carbolfuchsin. Leprosy bacilli are very scanty in tuberculoid lesions, and are often not detected by routine methods. They become more numerous as the spectrum is crossed and are present in huge numbers in lepromatous lesions. A lepromatous patient may have more than 10^{12} bacilli in the body. The density of bacilli in smears or tissues is termed the bacterial index (BI).

A standardized, autoclaved suspension of *M. leprae* is used as a prognostic intradermal skin test, the "lepromin test," which gives an accurate assessment of specific CMI in leprosy patients; it is negative in lepromatous and positive in tuberculoid leprosy. However, the test is often positive in nonleprosy patients, including those who have never visited leprosy endemic areas, and shows some cross-reactivity with tuberculin. Therefore it is of no diagnostic or epidemiologic value.

Incidence and Prevalence. Although governmental returns indicate a world total of 11 million leprosy patients, many consider that 15 million is a more accurate estimate, and that 1 million new patients will arise over the next 5 years. The importance of leprosy lies not only in numbers but also in the chronicity of the disease, which frequently disables but now seldom kills. Therefore it makes disproportionate demands on the health services and economies of developing countries.

Leprosy occurs in almost all tropical and warm temperate regions, including Japan and Korea, and is endemic in several states of the United States. It has only recently died out in certain northern European countries and Canada. It seems to be related particularly to overcrowding, so that as living standards rise, the disease becomes less common.

Epidemiology. Because *M. leprae* cannot be cultured, and because there is no simple, specific immunologic test of past or present infection, epidemiologic studies have hitherto been restricted to clinical cases. These have been further hampered by the long incubation period of three or more years. Close (household) contacts of lepromatous patients may show a tenfold higher incidence of leprosy and those of tuberculoid patients a twofold higher incidence than the general population. Lepromatous patients are thought to form the main source of infection in the community.

The lepromatous dermis is full of bacilli, but these are not shed in significant numbers through the intact epidermis. However, leprosy bacilli are excreted freely in lepromatous nasal secretions, so that 24-hour yields are comparable in numbers to those of *M. tuberculosis* coughed up in cavitary pulmonary tuberculosis. Bacilli from dried nasal secretions remain viable after being kept in the dark for at least 24 hours, and thus could be largely responsible for the spread of leprosy. The possibility of insect spread is also being reinvestigated. It has been assumed, without proof, that *M. leprae* gains entry through the skin or the respiratory tract.

Studies in twins and other subjects suggest that lepromatous disease is a host-determined characteristic possessed by a fixed proportion of all people. Godal (1971) has recently developed a specific lymphocyte transformation test (LTT) which may help to clarify the epidemiology of leprosy.

Pathology and Clinical Manifestations. Leprosy has two special features. One is the invasion by *M. leprae* of certain superficial nerves, which may become thickened and firm. The other is the wide range of clinical and histologic manifestations, reflecting the intricacies of the host-parasite relationship. Skin lesions, which are best seen in good oblique light, may occur anywhere, save on the hairy scalp and perineum. Nerves of predilection, which should always be palpated, include the ulnars at and above the medial humeral epicondyle, the superficial radials and medians at the wrist, the great auriculars at the edge of the sternocleidomastoid muscle, and the lateral popliteals (common peroneal) at the neck of the fibula. Appropriate muscle weakness and wasting may occur, resulting in claw hand (ulnar and/or median), foot drop, claw toes, and facial nerve paralysis, the last-named usually incomplete but including lagophthalmos. Wrist drop is comparatively rare.

The spectrum of leprosy has been particularly well defined by Ridley and Jopling, who proposed a five-group system of classification according to certain immunologic features, principally *the cytology* of the host cells of the macrophage-histiocyte series (whether histiocytic or epithelioid), *the bacterial density,* and *the degree of infiltration by lymphocytes.* Their classification enables the majority of patients to be diagnosed accurately from the clinical features, although the intermediate "borderline" (dimorphous) groups are relatively unstable, and tend to move toward lepromatous in the absence of treatment and toward tuberculoid after institution of effective chemotherapy. The five groups are, in order across the spectrum, *tuberculoid* (TT), *borderline-tuberculoid* (BT), *borderline* (BB), *borderline-lepromatous* (BL), and *lepromatous* (LL). Their distinctive clinical manifestations are now described, and these, with their corresponding pathologic, bacteriologic, and immunologic features, are summarized in the accompanying table.

Tuberculoid (TT). The typical tuberculoid lesion is large and annular, with a sharply raised outer edge and a thin erythematous rim which slopes gradually to a hypopigmented, flattened center. In profile, it resembles a saucer the right way up. The surface is dry, hairless, and sometimes scaly, with loss of sweating and marked anesthesia. Sometimes the lesion is a plaque with a dry, pebbly surface, or a macule. The lesion is usually single—at most two or three may be present—and, frequently, running to it may be palpated a thickened cutaneous sensory nerve in which caseation may occur. Sometimes, one of the nerves of predilection in the region of the skin lesion may be enlarged; rarely the only sign is a thickened nerve. Tuberculoid leprosy appears to be related to delay in the development of adequate cell-mediated immunity, and it forms a stable group.

Borderline-Tuberculoid (BT). The skin lesions resemble those of TT leprosy, but are usually multiple, though asymmetrical, and smaller in size, or else small "satellite" lesions may be present near the periphery of larger lesions. Sharp-edged papules may also occur. Enlarged cutaneous sensory nerves are less commonly found, but frequently one or more nerves of predilection are thickened. Therefore BT leprosy is often associated with deformity of one or both hands and/or feet; a patient may present with, or later develop, a plantar ulcer in an anesthetic foot or burns or infection of anesthetic fingers. Lagophthalmos may result in exposure keratitis.

Borderline (BB). The rather numerous, though asymmetrical, skin lesions are erythematous or hyperpigmented, and vary markedly in size. They occur as papules, plaques, and most characteristically as annular lesions with broad rims. The outer edge is often flattish and irregular; it rises to a thick inner edge, and the anesthetic, hypopigmented center is always sharply "punched out." The profile resembles a saucer the wrong way up, except that where the cup should sit is a deep central depression. Satellite lesions are common. Moderate and widespread, though asymmetrical, enlargement of the nerves of predilection may occur with or without associated muscle weakness and wasting.

Borderline-Lepromatous (BL). The skin lesions are numerous, but are not usually bilaterally symmetrical. They consist of erythematous or hyperpigmented papules, nodules, or plaques which appear moist and succulent, and which possess normal sensation or show only mild hypoesthesia. Small, indefinite-edged, hypopigmented macules may also be present. Some nodules may be dimpled, and often one or two lesions, usually the first to appear, have punched-out, hypopigmented, anesthetic centers, indicating progression from BB leprosy. Nerves of predilection close to the latter are often markedly thickened; elsewhere they may be only slightly enlarged. Ear lobes may appear normal, or be asymmetrically (more rarely symmetrically) enlarged. The eyebrows, nasal cartilage, and eyes are unaffected. Although bacilli are very numerous in the lesions, they are often undetected in normal-looking skin.

Lepromatous (LL). Lesions show marked bilateral symmetry. Skin lesions are very numerous, with erythematous, smooth, shiny surfaces, and are neither anes-

Summary of the Clinical, Histological, Bacteriological and Immunological Findings of the
Five Groups of the Leprosy Spectrum

	TT	BT	BB	BL	LL
Skin lesions					
Numbers	1 to 3	Very few to moderate	Moderate	Moderate to many	Very many
Symmetry	Very asymmetrical	Asymmetrical	Asymmetrical	Slightly asymmetrical	Symmetrical
Anesthesia	Very marked	Marked	Marked to moderate	Slight to nil	Nil
Nerve enlargement					
Cutaneous sensory	Common	May occur	0	0	0
Peripheral nerves*	0 or one	Common; asymmetrical	Common; asymmetrical	Moderately asymmetrical	Symmetrical
Skin histology					
Granuloma cell	Epithelioid	Epithelioid	Epithelioid	Histiocyte	Foamy histiocyte
Lymphocytes	+++	+++	+	± or ++	±†
Dermal nerves	Destroyed	Mostly destroyed	Some visible	Visible	Easily visible
Bacilli numbers (routine examination)	0	0, + or ++	+, ++ or +++	++++	+++++
Lymph nodes					
Paracortical infiltrate	Nil; immunoblasts	Sarcoid-like	Diffuse epithelioid	Diffuse histiocytes	Massive infiltrate with foamy histiocytes and Virchow cells
Germinal centers	Normal	Normal	Normal	Some hypertrophy	Gross hypertrophy
Lepromin test	+++	++	± or 0	0	0
Reactions					
ENL	0	0	0	Rare	Very common
Lepra	?	Common	Very common	Very common	(Rare)‡

*Nerves of predilection, i.e. ulnar, median, lateral popliteal, facial, great auricular, and posterior tibial.
†In LL leprosy, the peripheral blood shows an absolute decrease in T and an absolute increase in B lymphocytes.
‡Lepra reactions are occasionally seen in treated LL patients who have developed from borderline (BT, BB, or BL) in the absence of treatment.

thetic nor anhidrotic. Early cases may have numerous, small, hypopigmented macules with vague edges and small papules with indefinite edges; nerves may be but slightly thickened at this stage, although significant involvement of the nasal mucosa is frequently detected. With time, plaques and nodules develop, and the skin progressively thickens as lepromatous infiltrate increases; rarely, but especially in Central America, infiltrate alone occurs. The ear lobes enlarge, and the lines of the face coarsen and deepen (leonine facies). The lips often swell, and the eyebrows and eyelashes become scanty and are lost. Iritis and keratitis are common. Nasal blockage occurs, with ulceration and blood-streaked discharge, and in time the nasal cartilage and bones may be gradually destroyed, resulting in saddle-nose deformity. Lepromatous laryngitis may cause hoarseness. Edema of the extremities may occur, lymph nodes often enlarge, and testicular involvement frequently leads to atrophy and occasionally to gynecomastia. Dermal nerve damage leads to a progressive pseudo-"glove-and-stocking" anesthesia; light touch, pain, and temperature sensation are eventually lost over most of the body except scalp and flexures, but position sense is well preserved. Very numerous bacilli are present not only in the skin, in the draining lymph nodes, and in nerves of predilection, but also in the liver, spleen, bone marrow, and blood; there are relatively few in the kidney, and the lungs, heart, and central nervous system are not clinically involved in the infection.

In some peoples, such as the Chinese, many of the lepromatous cases originate as borderline, and a small number of residual BB-type lesions may be found; otherwise the signs are consistent with LL. In treated LL patients whose disease relapses, the new lesions are usually asymmetrical initially, but otherwise retain lepromatous characteristics.

Indeterminate Leprosy. Some child contacts of adult cases develop a single (occasionally two or three) hypopigmented macule, 2 to 5 cm in diameter, which shows hypoesthesia and decreased sweating. Histologically, there is lymphocytic infiltrate around the dermal appendages and neurovascular bundles. If left untreated, about one quarter later develop leprosy which may be of any type on the spectrum.

Reactions. *Erythema Nodosum Leprosum (ENL)— Lepromatous Lepra Reaction.* More than 50 per cent of treated LL patients, and the occasional untreated LL or treated BL patient, suffer from episodes of erythema nodosum leprosum. Over the course of a few hours, a crop of painful erythematous papules develops, typically on the exterior surfaces of the limbs and the face, but in severe attacks over much of the body except the scalp. The papules last for two to three days, becoming more purple, and then gradually subside, leaving dark staining of the skin. The episodes are usually associated with fever and general malaise. They may be isolated or may occur continuously over months or years, leading, if untreated, to gross prostration, weakness, and occasionally death. In severe ENL, the papules may form sterile pustules and ulcers. A frequent complication is painful neuritis, usually of the ulnar, median, or lateral popliteal nerves, and muscle weakness may increase. Lymphadenitis, iritis, and orchitis may also occur, and more rarely nephritis and large-joint arthritis. The ENL is due to immune complex formation, resulting in vasculitis and polymorphonuclear infiltrate. The antigen is probably derived from the cytoplasm of dead leprosy bacilli, and serum immunoglobulin levels are markedly elevated in LL leprosy.

Nonlepromatous Lepra Reactions. These occur very frequently in BT, BB, and BL leprosy. The leprous lesions themselves become markedly swollen, erythematous, and often scaly, and new lesions may appear. The reaction lasts for many weeks or months. Systemic upset and fever are uncommon, but neuritis may occur, and ulceration of the friable skin may lead to unsightly scarring. The reaction is often associated with change in specific CMI and therefore of a patient's leprosy classification, so that untreated patients become more lepromatous and treated patients more tuberculoid.

Diagnosis and Differential Diagnosis. It is essential to consider leprosy in all patients with skin or peripheral nerve lesions who have resided in endemic areas. The three most helpful findings are (1) thickening of one or more nerves, either of predilection or cutaneous sensory; nerve enlargement is found in some TT, many BT, and the great majority of BB, BL, and LL patients; (2) anesthetic skin lesions, which are found in almost all TT, BT, and BB patients, in many BL patients, and in those LL patients who have evolved from borderline; and (3) acid-fast bacilli (AFB) in skin smears, which are positive in many BT and in all untreated BB, BL, and LL patients. Smears are usually taken from both ear lobes and up to six typical skin lesions. Leprosy should be suspected when skin or nasal symptoms persist despite routine treatment; in chronic, painless, plantar ulceration; in foot drop unassociated with trauma; or in unusual presentations of arthritis and erythema nodosum. Confirmation should be obtained by skin biopsy or, in neural leprosy without skin lesions, by biopsy of a thickened sensory nerve.

Lack of anesthesia differentiates vitiligo, mycotic infections, lupus erythematosus, and psoriasis from TT and BT leprosy. Nerves are not enlarged in neurologic conditions such as syringomyelia, motor neuron disease, and Friedreich's ataxia; they are enlarged in hereditary sensory neuropathy of Déjérine and Sotta, which can be differentiated by the absence of skin lesions and of AFB and by the familial history. Dermal leishmaniasis, yaws, secondary syphilis, and neurofibromatosis may resemble LL leprosy, but there is no nerve thickening, and smears for AFB are negative.

Treatment. Treatment is made difficult by the excessive prejudice and outdated fear of leprosy persisting in many cultures, and by the extreme chronicity of the infection and slowness of response to treatment which is related in part to the unique generation time of *M. leprae.*

Treatment of the Infection. The drug of choice remains DDS (dapsone, 4-4'diaminodiphenyl sulfone), which is as cheap as aspirin and may be administered by mouth or parenterally. In LL and BL patients, clinical improvement is detected from about three months after starting DDS (often earlier in TT, BT, and BB leprosy), and around this time bacilli from nose and skin will no longer infect mice. The MI reaches zero by six months, but the BI takes many years to become negative. Small numbers of viable bacilli have been shown to persist, possibly in Schwann cells and other special sites, in LL patients treated continuously for at least ten years; such patients may relapse if treatment is stopped. Therefore it is recommended that DDS be given for the following minimum periods:

Intermediate and TT	3 years
BT	5 years
BB	7 years
BL	10 years
LL	20 years or for life

Although the minimal effective dose of DDS is less than 1 mg, the recommended standard adult dose in LL and BL leprosy is 100 mg daily by mouth or 300 to 400 mg twice weekly by injection. This results in an incidence of drug resistance of only 2.5 per cent, whereas the incidence may be many times higher on lower dosage, especially if irregularly taken. DDS resistance has not yet been reported from the other types of leprosy (TT, BT, BB, and indeterminate), in which bacillary loads are so much lower. In these, a dosage of 25 to 50 mg DDS daily is acceptable.

Sulfone resistance has been detected 5 to 25 years after the start of treatment, sometimes long after the patient has become smear negative. New active lesions, usually asymmetrical papules and small plaques with high BI and MI, are found on a background of old, resolving, or resolved lepromatous leprosy. Bacilli from these lesions will grow in the footpads of mice treated with DDS mixed in their diet (Pettit and Rees, 1964). Clinically, resistance must be distinguished from relapse off treatment by a therapeutic trial of DDS, 400 mg given regularly twice weekly by injection. In drug-susceptible relapse, uninterrupted improvement occurs. In resistant patients, some initial improvement may occur if there is a mixed bacterial population of partially and highly resistant organisms, but the MI is unlikely to fall to 0, and further new lesions, with raised MI, will sooner or later appear.

Toxic effects of DDS include dose-related sulfhemoglobinemia and hemolytic anemia, the latter especially in glucose-6-phosphate dehydrogenase–deficient patients. Drug allergy, which occurs in one in several hundred cases, may be serious and even fatal; three to seven weeks after starting DDS the patient develops fever, pruritus, and dermatitis, which may become exfoliative, and jaundice and psychosis sometimes occur. DDS must be stopped immediately and prednisolone given for several weeks.

Alternative treatment is required in sulfone allergy and in proved cases of sulfone resistance. *Clofazimine* (B663, Lamprene), a rimino-phenazine dye, is both antimycobacterial and, in high dosage, anti-inflammatory. It is relatively nontoxic, its chief disadvantage being that it causes a reddish-brown pigmentation of the skin which is objectionable to most light-skinned patients. In a dose of 100 mg daily, it appears clinically and bacteriologically approximately as effective as DDS. Clofazimine resistance has not yet been reported, although the drug has been given for over ten years to sulfone-resistant patients. It is used widely in dark-skinned races, in a dose of 100 mg three or four times a day, to control ENL and lepra reactions, although several weeks elapse before its full anti-inflammatory effect is produced.

Rifampin is bactericidal. It kills leprosy bacilli faster than any other drug tried hitherto, so that patients may be rendered minimal public health risks within a few days; clinical improvement is seen in about three weeks, and the MI falls to zero within six weeks. It has been used for over six years in the treatment of DDS-resistant leprosy, usually in combination with the second-line drug thiambutosine, with excellent results, although the

BI falls no faster than with clofazimine. Dosage is 600 mg daily, and intermittent therapy is under trial. Rifampin combined with DDS may also be of value in the initial therapy of sulfone-sensitive LL leprosy, when a rapid therapeutic effect is especially desirable.

Treatment of Reactions. In mild erythema nodosum leprosum, paracetamol or aspirin may suffice. Somewhat more severe episodes often respond to two or three courses of stibophen, 2 ml daily parenterally for five days. In severe continuous ENL, or in all episodes complicated by significant neuritis or iritis, there are three alternative regimens. Prednisolone, given in addition to DDS, rapidly suppresses ENL, but in the long term severe steroid toxicity is common. Therefore steroids are best reserved for short-term cover for operations, childbirth, and similar situations. The drug thalidomide is equally effective in controlling reactions, but its use is contraindicated in women because of its teratogenic potential. The dosage is initially 200 mg twice daily; subsequently it is progressively lowered to a maintenance dose, usually of 50 to 100 mg nightly, which may be continued for years. DDS must not be discontinued. The third alternative is clofazimine in high dosage. In light-skinned males and postmenopausal females thalidomide is probably the drug of choice; in dark-skinned patients and premenopausal women clofazimine is the safest drug, provided that a rapid action is not required. *Lepra reactions* can often be controlled with paracetamol, with or without stibophen. But whenever neuritis occurs or when there is risk of skin ulceration, the signs of inflammation should be suppressed with prednisolone. Although steroids may be required for some months, toxicity is rare, because the dosage is usually less than for ENL and the total duration of the reaction is shorter. In dark-skinned patients, clofazimine can be commenced with the prednisolone, and the latter drug slowly withdrawn. Thalidomide is useless in this type of reaction.

Other Treatment. Patients must be educated to protect their anesthetic limbs. The healing of plantar ulcers is aided by rest and plaster splints. Reconstructive surgery and physiotherapy are valuable in the rehabilitation of deformed patients. The use of transfer factor in LL and BL leprosy is being assessed.

Prognosis. Even without treatment, patients with TT leprosy and three quarters of those with "indeterminate" disease eventually cure themselves; however, the patients with BL, most BB, and many BT forms of disease tend to lose cell-mediated immunity, and their disease becomes more lepromatous. Widespread nerve damage may develop in the BT and BB groups. Patients with the LL form used to die from uncontrolled leprosy, intercurrent infection, or amyloid nephritis, and blindness was common. With correct treatment, the prognosis now is good. Death from leprosy is rare, although amyloidosis is still seen occasionally, especially in inadequately treated ENL. Patients who fail to care for anesthetic extremities may suffer from repeated trauma or infection, resulting in gradual absorption of digits, or amputation may become necessary for chronic osteomyelitis. Even with careful management, reactional neuritis may sometimes cause increased deformity, and ENL may also, if rarely, result in blindness or significant renal damage.

Prevention. Because *M. leprae* cannot be grown in vitro, there is no specific vaccine. The precise value of BCG in protecting against early leprosy is being further assessed. Prophylactic DDS or acedapsone (diacetyl DDS) may be justified in special local situations. Otherwise prevention rests on early diagnosis of cases, and annual examination of known contacts may be rewarding.

Rees, R. J. W., and Waters, M. F. R.: Recent trends in leprosy research. Br. Med. Bull., 28:16, 1972.
Ridley, D. S., and Jopling, W. H.: Classification of leprosy according to immunity. A five-group system. Int. J. Lepr., 34:255, 1966.

TREPONEMAL DISEASES

Thorstein Guthe

246. SYPHILIS

Definition. Syphilis is a chronic infectious disease caused by *Treponema pallidum.* From the portal of entry—usually the genitals—there is lymphatic invasion and blood-borne spread (treponemia), and the infection is generalized from the beginning. Subsequently the disease becomes localized and dispersed. The early lesions are benign and the late manifestations destructive in character. Several organs of the body may be involved, but late treponemia and establishment of further lesions occur rarely in the acquired disease; this reflects the relative stability of the immunity that develops during the course of the disease. The host response includes specific humoral and cell-mediated immunity. Immune responses can be detected by serologic and other tests. Despite its slow evolution and remarkable immunologic

features, syphilis will, if untreated, eventually incapacitate one of five and kill one of ten infected persons.

Treponema Pallidum. *T. pallidum,* discovered by Schaudinn and Hoffman in 1905, is a helical cell about 0.15 μ wide and 6 to 15 μ long. Around its central protoplasmic core is wound a bundle of three to four axial fibrils that provide the "muscle," giving *T. pallidum* a characteristic motility pattern. Treponemes undergo transverse fission. Multiplication time is 30 to 35 hours. *T. pallidum* has not been cultivated in vitro. It can remain viable for many hours on special media, or indefinitely if preserved at extremely low temperatures (carbon dioxide ice, liquid nitrogen).

Transmission. A few treponemes suffice to implant infection (Magnuson et al., 1956). Transmission is facilitated by moist conditions and congenial temperature, and occurs almost exclusively by direct contact with infectious lesions. Injured or inflamed areas will favor implantation. Sexual transmission is the rule. Not infrequently genito-oral, genito-rectal or mouth-to-mouth transmission takes place. The chain of infection sometimes involves both heterosexual and homosexual prac-

---

The author wishes to acknowledge the valuable advice of his colleague Dr. O. Idsøe, Consultant on Treponematoses, World Health Organization, Geneva, concerning this chapter.

tices. As many as 30 to 40 infected persons have been brought to treatment on the basis of a single index case. "Innocent" transmission by adults or children occasionally occurs. Contact between an infector, the moist object, and the susceptible must be rapid to achieve indirect transmission. Inoculation into the skin or a vein has resulted from an accidental needle prick. An initial lesion does not arise in blood-borne transmission when it occurs in utero of pregnant syphilitic women (prenatal syphilis) or more rarely by blood transfusion from an infected blood donor (syphilis d'emblée). A macerated fetus and the mucocutaneous lesions of early prenatal syphilis are highly contagious. Some infected individuals can pass asymptomatically through the early stages of syphilis, as distinct from those whose early trivial symptoms were misinterpreted or "masked" by treatment of other conditions, e.g., gonorrhea. Physiologic secretions (salivary, vaginal, seminal) may contain treponemes from contagious lesions. Direct intrauterine infection of the egg or the fetus from semen of a syphilitic male cannot arise.

Epidemiology. The health of the public is affected when syphilis spreads within and between countries. Propagation is facilitated by the properties of the agent, by its mode of transmission, and by behavioral, social, and several environmental factors. In recent years the climate of opinion concerning sexual behavior has become overtly permissive among the young. The pattern of promiscuity and of heterosexual and homosexual relations has altered. Industrialization, urbanization, migration, and unprecedented tourism have facilitated human contact and sexual encounters with concomitant risk of acquiring sexually transmitted disease. Paradoxically, medical advancements have contributed in the same direction. Thus fear of infection has been removed by easy and effective antimicrobial therapy and fear of pregnancy by oral contraceptives and intrauterine devices. Generally it has become clear that medical advances have been to some extent outweighed by the complex ecologic forces in a rapidly changing environment. It has been recognized that new ways are needed to promote the mental and physical health of individuals and communities, e.g., health education, recreation, city planning.

The long-term trend of syphilis in the last 100 years has been downward. However, the epidemic outbreak of syphilis (and gonorrhea) during World War II was first followed by a rapidly declining incidence until 1958, since which time there has been a noticeable recrudescence of these conditions. Examples of reported incidence of *early syphilis* per 100,000 population are United States, 3.9 in 1958 and 10.1 in 1971; Poland, 18.6 in 1958 and 51.9 in 1971; and France, 3.3 in 1958 and 8.3 in 1971. It has been shown (United States) that for each reported case of early infectious syphilis three additional cases are diagnosed and treated by private physicians but not reported to the health authorities. A decline in *late* cardiovascular and neurosyphilis and in *congenital syphilis* has been observed since the mid-1940's. This decline has occurred despite the experience that late syphilis can be expected to increase after periods of high incidence of early syphilis. *The prevention of the late forms of syphilis by the penicillin treatment of early syphilis is one of the great achievements of the chemotherapy era.*

Host-Treponeme Relationship. Man is the only natural host of *T. pallidum.* Hormonal and genetic factors may affect susceptibility to infection. The host-treponeme interaction is best portrayed by the rhythm and features in the development of lesions during the course of untreated syphilis.

Natural Course of Syphilis. After implantation and local multiplication of *T. pallidum* and extension of the infection to lymph nodes, treponemes spread rapidly to all body tissues via venous blood, the pulmonary circulation, and the arterial system. Human syphilis therefore ceases rapidly to be a local disease (even incubating infection can cause blood-transfusion syphilis). The agent does not grow in the bloodstream, but on passage through the small vessels, numerous metastatic foci are set up in the body, e.g., in the skin, mucous membranes, and nervous system. After the appearance of the initial lesion, some three weeks after infection, multiplication continues for several weeks in these metastatic foci. Some eight to nine weeks after the original implantation the first generalized mucocutaneous outbreak occurs. The primary lesion heals spontaneously within a few weeks, and the secondary eruption within a few weeks or months. The treponemes in the metastatic foci of internal organs are presumably killed in most instances, but sometimes they become only temporarily inactivated (latent), giving rise to further manifestations. In the untreated disease further secondary episodes occur in 25 per cent of patients within the first four years, mostly within two years. With increasing duration of infection the hematogenous "showers" of treponemes generating these contagious episodes become less frequent and less rich in treponemes. The cutaneous lesions tend to group and localize, or may occur solitarily until the mucocutaneous system no longer responds to treponemes with pathologic changes. The further course of the untreated infection is illustrated by data from the University Clinic, Oslo, where by the turn of the century some 1100 patients with diagnosed early syphilis remained untreated under hospitalized conditions and were subjected to follow-up studies. In the last representative follow-up investigation 50 to 60 years after the original infection (Gjestland), late "benign" syphilis had occurred in 15 per cent, cardiovascular syphilis in 10 per cent, and neurosyphilis in 6.5 per cent of these patients. Ten per cent died as a direct consequence of their disease. In about two thirds, latency continued indefinitely after subsidence of the secondary attacks. They went through life without major physical or mental consequences of their disease.

These features of the host-treponeme relationship in syphilis raise the question of the mechanisms concerned in the pathogenesis of lesions and their nature in both early and late disease, and point to the remarkable role of the defense forces of the host against the invading pathogen during the natural course of the infection.

Immunology. The immune response of the host directed against the pathogen is reflected in the natural course of syphilis as outlined above. The underlying waning treponemia, the decrease in demonstrable treponemes in late lesions, and the presence of presumed resistance to superinfection after the initial phase of the disease are among the signals. Moreover, a varying degree of cross-resistance to syphilis in persons infected with yaws and pinta suggests the broader role of immunity in treponematoses. Knowledge is limited, however, concerning the effector mechanisms in the protective host responses. It is possible to demonstrate humoral immunity by passive transfer of immune serum in laboratory animals (Turner et al.,

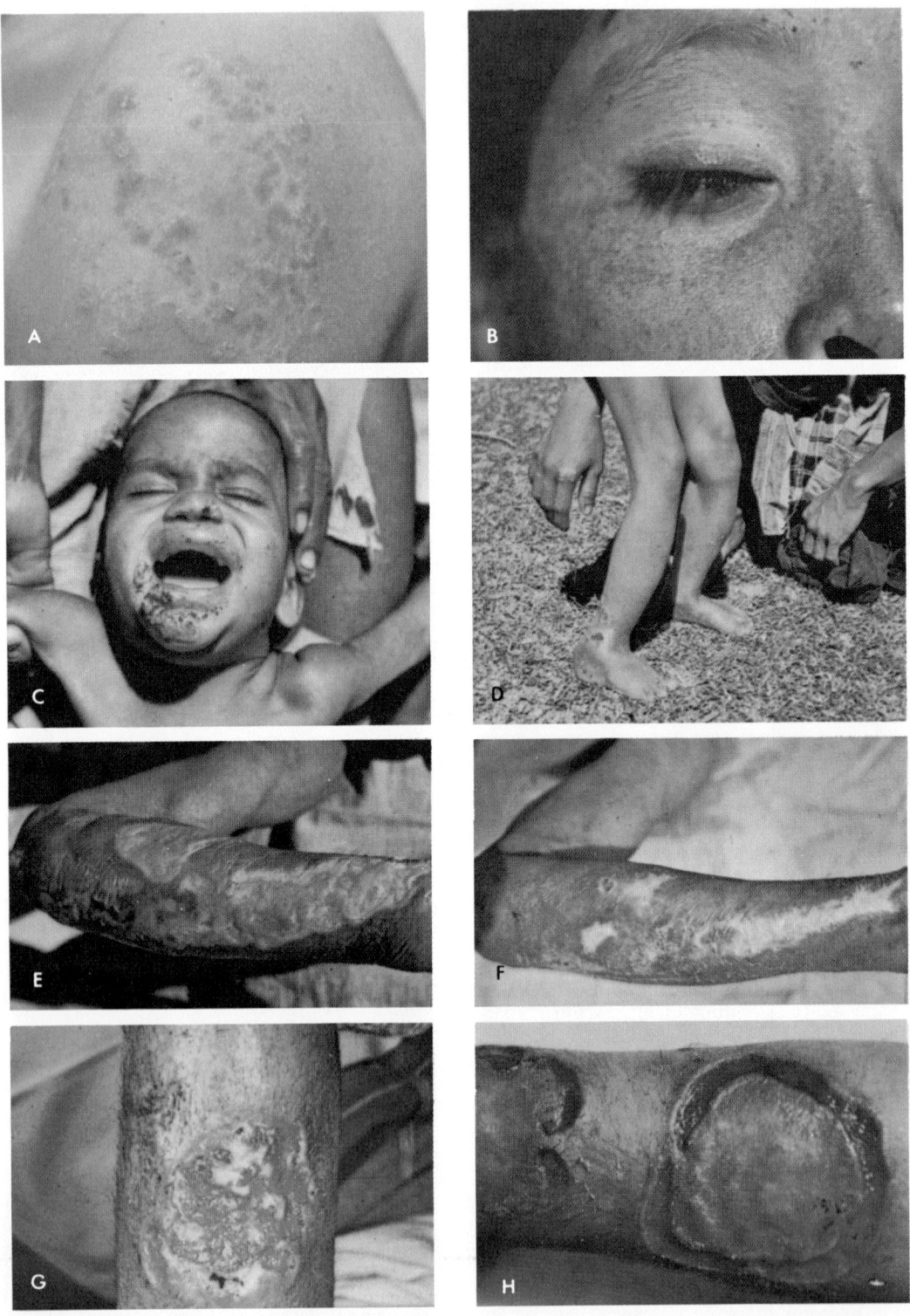

A, Initial lesions in early pinta. *B*, Late pigmented blue variety pinta. *C*, Early papillomatous yaws. *D*, Osteoperiostitis of yaws. *E*, Deep ulcerated late yaws of arm before therapy with long-acting penicillin. *F*, Same patient after treatment. *G* and *H*, Syphilitic tertiarisms.

1973). A cellular immunity response also occurs, but its significance has not been determined (Levene et al., 1971). In animal experimentation successful immunization can reportedly be achieved by the use of gamma-irradiated *T. pallidum* vaccine (Miller, 1973).

The humoral response involves formation of two main antibody types, reagin* and treponemal antibody.

Reagin develops early, four to five weeks after infection, and forms more rapidly than treponemal antibody described below. It declines when the disease moves toward latency, and may fall below detectable levels in late disease. It is affected considerably by therapy in the early phase of syphilis. A rising titer is a precursor of clinical outbreak, and reagin is therefore a useful gauge of disease activity, but of limited value as indicator of immunity. All evidence contradicts a protective role of reagin which is directed against cardiolipin present in the tissues of the antibody-producing host. Reagin is presumably an autoantibody formed in response to tissue destruction during the pathologic process (WHO, 1970; Wright and Doniach, 1971). It is not known if reagin has a pathogenic significance.

Of the *treponemal antibodies* the immobilizin appears to be the more important. Fluorescent and agglutinating treponemal antibodies also appear. Immobilizin is operative in the treponemal antibody immobilization test (TPI). It appears late—two to three months after the infection. It is formed slowly but can persist for life as an indicator of infection. Immobilizin reflects roughly the development of host resistance, although the evidence is equivocal that it has a direct protective role.

In syphilis antibody-producing plasmocytes are characteristically present in early lesions and in lymph nodes. Antibody demonstrated by reagin tests may belong to both IgM and IgG immunoglobulins. IgM is produced early in the infection. IgG exclusively forms the immobilizing antibody when it appears later in the infection. In immunofluorescent tests both IgM and IgG antibodies react with *T. pallidum*. Whether or not formation of antibody continues after treponemes have been eradicated by treatment—as well as the circumstances under which such eradication may take place—is not known (see Persistence of Treponemal Forms, below). IgG antibodies can pass the placenta, in contrast to IgM. The presence of IgM in the serum of newborns suggests local formation of antibodies and therefore prenatal active infection. IgG also passes the blood-brain barrier when the meninges are inflamed. This explains why serodiagnostic tests that mainly identify IgG antibody are preferred in examining the cerebrospinal fluid for syphilis of the nervous system.

Cell-mediated immunity manifests itself as delayed hypersensitivity demonstrable by the response to intradermally injected antigen after 12 to 48 hours. Interaction of antigen with specifically sensitized lymphocytes and cell structures is believed to be the underlying mechanism. Although knowledge is very limited, cell-mediated immunity apparently does not play a major

role during the secondary eruptions of syphilis (Levene, 1969). However, it is believed to be operative in gummatous lesions. Moreover, the striking clinical and histopathologic similarity of late destructive skin and bone lesions in venereal syphilis, bejel, and yaws suggests a common cell-mediated or other mechanism of the host response at this stage.

Immunopathologic mechanisms involving tissue damage are very little known in syphilis. Multiple humoral antibodies circulate in all phases of the disease, antigen is present, and antigen-antibody complexes may have pathogenic significance. Nevertheless a direct cytotoxic effect on host cells has not been established. Immunopathologic mechanisms have been suggested in a few and rare manifestations engendered by syphilitic infection, notably biphasic paroxysmatic cold hemaglobinuria and membranous glomerulonephritis (syphilitic "nephrosis"). The occurrence of cryoglobulins in syphilis has also been reported.

In recent years there have been several important scientific developments in basic immunology concerning humoral and cellular immunity and immunopathology (WHO, 1964 and 1969), which may be expected to be applied also in syphilis and other treponematoses. *At present the clinical and laboratory findings can only illustrate the capacity of immunocompetent cell systems to react to antigenic stimuli in the early phase of syphilis, and to generate protection against further metastatic spread and superinfection with the pathogen. The human host can contain the infection at the time of latency by establishing a notable equilibrium between the pathogenic potential of treponemes and the immune forces, as evidenced by a relatively infrequent disturbance of this equilibrium resulting in occurrence of late injurious manifestations.*

Persistence of Treponemal Forms. Adequate penicillin therapy of early syphilis will usually heal lesions and prevent late manifestations in most instances. Symptomatic manifestations after penicillin therapy of latent syphilis are rare. When occurring, they signal survival of pathogenic treponemes notwithstanding the immune forces and therapy. When not occurring, e.g., late latency, and persistently positive serologic tests have sometimes in the past been considered to be due to persistent antibodies produced by "immunologic memory" rather than to treponemes persisting in the host. However, persistence of treponemal forms (treponeme-like structures) in host tissues has been reported in recent years. Thus in some instances of treated late syphilis treponemal forms were described in lymph nodes and cerebrospinal fluid (Collart et al.), in aqueous humor of the eye (Smith and Israel), and in treated congenital syphilis, as well as in pathologic and nonpathologic ophthalmic situations apparently unrelated to syphilis. Rarely treponemal forms have also been found (lymph nodes) after treatment of early syphilis (Yobs et al.). The treponemal forms that have been demonstrated after treatment of early and late syphilis have only rarely been shown by animal infectivity tests to be viable (Turner). Others may be modified or "dormant" *T. pallidum*, acting as antigenic stimulus for continued treponemal antibody production, whereas others may be saprophytic organisms indigenous to the human host. In some instances these situations may coexist. Persistence of abated forms of microorganisms in the face of normally

---

*The term *reagin* is used throughout this chapter. It is widely accepted by physicians, clinicians, and epidemiologists to denote antibodies to cardiolipin-type antigens formed in syphilis and other treponematoses. Reagin is often referred to by immunologists and allergists to describe antibodies concerned in the immediate types of skin hypersensitivity and anaphylactic reactions.

effective drugs has already been studied in mycobacteria and corynebacteria, and is a phenomenon apart from true drug resistance (McDermott). There is no evidence that penicillinase-producing, resistant pathogenic treponeme strains have developed. Knowledge concerning immunologic tissue and humoral aspects of persistent treponemal forms is extremely limited, but regardless of the extent to which such forms are viable or modified pathogenic treponemes—or related indigenous organisms—their role may be significant in the immunologic life of the host. *For the physician it is important to realize that studies in this area are very few, that accepted treatment practices need not be reconsidered in early syphilis, and that in late syphilis special considerations continue to pertain.*

Pathology. The early treponemia and the resulting metastatic foci are reflected in the diversity of the body organs involved in the pathology of this chronic inflammation. The macroscopic characteristics of skin manifestations are described later. The histopathology of lesions is basically characterized by endarteritis and periarteritis of the small vessels and capillaries, which show infiltration of lymphocytes and plasmocytes and multiplication of histiocytes. Granulomatous inflammation is typical of the late stages of syphilis as of other chronic infections, e.g., tuberculosis.

In the *early skin lesions* in which many treponemes are present, lymphocytosis and plasmacytosis are particularly marked, although varying in intensity. Acanthosis usually occurs. Many treponemes are present. *Lymph nodes* in the early disease show adenitis with prominent follicles, plasmacytosis, sometimes focal necrosis, fine fibrosis, and presence of treponemes. The histologic picture in lesions and lymph nodes is compatible with antibody production by stimulated cells (WHO, 1970). *Late nodular and gummatous lesions* (usually treponeme-free) are the results of delayed hypersensitivity and show chronic granulomatous tissue with lymphocytes, epithelioid cells, and eventually giant cells in addition to the endovascular changes of early lesions. In *cardiovascular syphilis* there is endarteritis of the vasa vasorum, particularly in the ascending aorta and arch. All layers of the large vessel are involved with destruction of elastic and muscle tissue, weakening the entire structure and predisposing to aneurysm. The aortic ring may also be weakened with shortening and thickening of valve leaflets leading to regurgitation. Coronary ostia may become narrowed, resulting in rare ischemic heart disease. *Central nervous system* syphilis is either meningovascular with inflammation of the pia-arachnoid and its vessels or parenchymatous with the nervous tissue attacked. The leptomeningitis may be acute or chronic. Infiltration of small meningeal vessels may cause thrombosis and local brain damage. The parenchymatous process may engender paresis if the brain is predominantly involved, or tabes dorsalis if the spinal cord is predominantly involved. Tabes begins as extradural leptomeningitis around the dorsal nerve roots, followed by degeneration of axis cylinders and demyelinization of posterior columns of the spinal cord. Optic atrophy may occur from basal meningitis or interstitial neuritis in the nerve or chiasma, or central gummatous lesions may affect the optic nerve directly. Involvement of afferent vessels to the spinal cord may lead to degeneration of pyramidal tracts and a rare condition known as Erb's spastic paraplegia. *Ophthalmic lesions* include uveitis with serofibrinous exudate and synechiae in acquired syphilis, and interstitial keratitis with substantial lymphocytic infiltration in congenital syphilis. Rare membranous *glomerulonephritis* ("nephrosis") in early syphilis shows peculiar vascular or granulomatous tissue changes. Other forms of visceral syphilis, e.g., interstitial nephritis, may occur. In *prenatal syphilis* the placenta is often voluminous, thickened, and pale with enlarged cotyledons and perivascular fibrosis throughout the villi, such as can also be seen in erythroblastosis (Rh-negative mother). Fibrous proliferation and monocellular infiltrates characterize fetal tissues in congenital syphilis; but in addition to the placenta changes, the most characteristic findings are in the lungs (pneumonia alba) and the bones (osteochondritis and periostitis), the latter changes being diagnosable roentgenologically.

Notwithstanding the diversity of the organs affected and the multiformity of the lesions underlying the clinical picture, the elementary pathologic changes in all syphilitic processes are of vascular and inflammatory nature.

Clinical Manifestations and Diagnosis. Untreated acquired syphilis shows a great variety of clinical manifestations, depending inter alia on the duration of the infection and the immunologic state of the host. The accepted classification of syphilis into *early syphilis* of less than four years' duration and *late syphilis* of more than four years' duration is based on these immunologic grounds, as well as on clinical and epidemiologic considerations rather than on definite "stages" of disease that may sometimes merge or overlap. In congenital syphilis, in which there is prenatal hematogenous transmission of *T. pallidum* to the fetus from the syphilitic mother, the disease is usually divided into *early congenital syphilis* in children less than two years old and *late congenital syphilis* in those who are older.

Early Syphilis. The incubation period, initial lesions, secondary manifestations, and early latent period are included in this designation.

THE INITIAL LESION (PRIMARY CHANCRE). Following an incubation of two to six weeks after the original infection, the initial lesion appears at the site of implantation of *T. pallidum*: in males usually on the penile shaft, coronal sulcus, glans, or prepuce, and occasionally intraurethrally; and in females on the external genitalia and cervix. In 5 to 10 per cent of patients the initial lesions are extragenital (lips, tonsils, fingers, within the anus, but also anywhere else). The initial lesion is usually a painless lenticular papule, rapidly eroding and becoming a flat indurated infiltrate, usually with elastic consistency, 3 to 20 mm in diameter, and of round or oval shape. However, lesions are frequently "atypical," modified by size, location, and the nature of underlying tissue, if not by treatment. Solitary chancres are usual. Multiple chancres may appear after manifold simultaneous implantation of *T. pallidum,* especially in women. Regardless of site, initial lesions are accompanied by moderate enlargement of regional lymph nodes, usually recognizable clinically within a week of their appearance. The nodes are firm, freely movable, and painless. The initial lesion heals slowly (two to six weeks), and may or may not leave an atrophic scar. Lymphadenopathy may last for several months. With approaching secondary manifestations metastatic lesions of skin and mucous membrane sometimes go unrecognized while the primary sore is still present. On the other hand, the initial lesion is occasionally absent from the beginning, the secondary lesions nevertheless developing in due course (syphilis d'emblée).

In *diagnosis* of a suspected solitary genital or other lesion, careful general clinical examination of the patient should be undertaken in addition to mandatory dark-field examination for *T. pallidum* in material from the sore and the repeated performance of serologic tests, e.g., VDRL. These may be reactive as early as four weeks after the infection and one week after the appearance of the lesion. If treponemes are not found but seroreactivity has been established, the diagnosis is made in conjunction with clinical and anamnestic data. The most common lesions to suggest, erroneously, syphilitic sores are *chancroid* (which may coexist with chancre) and *granuloma inguinale. Balanoposthitis, erosion and carcinoma of the cervix uteri, and lymphogranuloma venereum* should also be considered. Other conditions include *traumatic sore, herpes progenitalis, condylomata acuminata, lichen planus, scabies, fissura in ano,* and *Vincent's angina.* Differential diagnostic considerations may vary from one country to another, according to the prevalence of the various conditions.

From its earliest phases the incubation period of syphilis is one of considerable biologic activity. When the patient with an initial lesion is first seen by the physician, generalized infection has already occurred as a result of the early treponemia, although generalized symptoms may not as yet have appeared. Unless initial lesions give rise to suspicion of disease, the patient may not seek medical care during the early period of infectiousness. Local genital lesions should therefore always be considered suspect of syphilis until proved otherwise.

SECONDARY MANIFESTATIONS AND EARLY LATENCY. About the sixth week of the infection there is *generalized lymphadenitis* with palpable superficial lymph nodes. Lymph nodes, otherwise seldom swollen, are involved, e.g., the pre- and postauricular, occipital, and supratrochlear lymph nodes. All nodes are firm, freely movable, and painless. *Cutaneous rashes,* notably the macular rash, appear six to eight weeks after the initial lesion, the vestiges of which remain in some patients. The macules are pale red, roundish patches 5 to 10 mm in diameter, neither infiltrated nor scaling, and do not itch. They are usually bilateral, and are distributed to the trunk and proximal parts of extremities. On black skin, macules appear as darker patches. Macular rashes last one to two months. *Papular lesions* often develop before disappearance of macules. The papules are coppery-red, round infiltrates 3 to 10 mm in diameter, sometimes leaving pigmented patches on healing, e.g., "necklace of Venus." The papules are distributed anywhere, and include scalp, soles, and palms. The latter show up as flat, slightly scaly lesions or as a characteristic bluish-red rash covered by normal keratin. The papular rash may last two to four weeks.

In its further development and notably during relapses many varieties of papules may appear in syphilis. Large hypertrophic papules ("condylomata lata") are localized to skin folds, e.g., genitals, anus, axillae, under pendulous breasts, and elsewhere, and are often humid and eroded. Split papules at the oral angles resemble perlèche. On black skin circinate and arciform papules are common around the mouth and on the chin. Seborrheic, psoriasiform, and acneiform papules may occur. Varioliform papules are sometimes encountered in the tropics. They may give the impression of smallpox, but the base of the latter is less infiltrated beneath the pustule which shows umbilical depression and later also characteristic crusts. Follicular and corymbiform grouped papules are late manifestations in secondary syphilis. Patchy loss of hair occurs three to eight months after infection and gives a moth-eaten appearance. It is evident from the above that polymorphism characterizes the early and particularly the subsequent relapsing lesions in secondary syphilis, even in the same person. *Mucous membranes,* notably in the mouth, vulva, and anus, may be involved separately or conjointly with skin manifestations. Erosive superficial mucosal patches are often covered by a thin gray membrane with a red halo. Ulceromembranous tonsillitis and pharyngitis may cause moderate symptoms (hoarseness). Mucous membrane lesions are very contagious. At least 20 per cent of patients with early syphilis will have transient *subacute meningitis* ("meningeal rash"), causing headache and increase of cells and protein in the cerebrospinal fluid. *Ophthalmic conditions* may occur, notably iritis with demonstrable synechiae, but seldom before six months after the infection. *Interstitial nephritis* may give minor or no symptoms. *Periostitis,* particularly of the long bones, is common and shows up as swelling, tenderness, and ostealgia (nocturnal pains).

RELAPSING SYPHILIS. Condylomata lata are likely to recur. The skin manifestations tend to be unilateral, the eruptions more dense, marked, with fewer lesions, and sometimes solitary. They are also more infiltrated and of somewhat longer standing, and have some characteristics that resemble the skin lesions in late syphilis. This reflects the increasing immunity with the duration of the early disease. Neurorecurrences, as well as ophthalmic and other relapsing manifestations, may occur. If the patient has been inadequately treated, relapses may be delayed.

DIAGNOSIS OF SECONDARY SYPHILIS. The diagnosis of secondary syphilis is made on the basis of lymphadenopathy, mucocutaneous lesions, demonstration of *T. pallidum* by dark-field examination of lesion fluid or lymph node aspirate, and seroreactivity in reagin tests. The history may or may not be helpful. In the presence of mucocutaneous manifestations, the necessary serologic tests are usually obtained by the physician. Errors arise from a syphilitic lesion that is misinterpreted as representing some localized body lesion of nonmicrobial origin, e.g., an anal fissure, or from solitary lesions that may be considered "trivial." Close search for clinical manifestations other than the presenting symptom may well reveal lesions on other parts of the skin or simultaneously occurring mucosal eruption, e.g., oral or genital mucous patches, loss of hair, palmar or volar lesions, pointing to the serious systemic nature of the condition.

The most common eruptions that should be considered in differential diagnoses of early generalized secondary syphilitic rashes are *acute microbial disease, exanthemata,* and *drug eruptions.* In the later phase of secondary syphilis when lesions become more localized, the following conditions are of differential diagnostic importance: *pityriasis rosea, perleche, psoriasis,* and *superficial fungus infections.* Also *lichen planus* and sometimes certain forms of *tuberculids, scabies, venereal warts,* and *Reiter's disease* may come into purview. *Aphthous stomatitis* and *Stevens-Johnson* syndrome are among oral cavity manifestations to be considered.

As a whole it is noted that manifestations of secondary syphilis have a very wide range; they involve the skin and other body systems, often extensively, but sometimes in a more limited way and discretely, with corresponding variation of clinical symptomatology in patients who are usually not feeling subjectively ill. *Hardly in any other disease is it of such importance as in suspected syphilis to make a careful and complete examination of the entire skin, mucous membranes, and body systems. Laboratory examination should always be undertaken in suspected cases.*

EARLY ASYMPTOMATIC (LATENT) SYPHILIS. This designation serves to identify seroreactive persons who have no signs and nonreactive cerebrospinal fluid within the first four years of infection. *In view of the tendency of early syphilis to contagious secondary relapses and the potential seriousness of neurosyphilis, which sometimes may develop after two years' duration of the infection, patients in whom a diagnosis of early latent syphilis is established should be treated and kept under surveillance by the physician in the same way as is done for symptomatic secondary syphilis.*

Late Syphilis. In the natural course of syphilis, further infectious mucocutaneous relapses seldom occur after the second, and hardly ever after the fourth year. "Refractory" or premunitory immunity has then been established, and persists for life in two thirds of patients who remain asymptomatic. In the remainder, slow chronic destructive inflammation and fibrosis continue in various affected tissues, giving rise to late manifestations.

LATE ASYMPTOMATIC (LATENT) SYPHILIS. Latent syphilis has reactive serologic tests as its sole evidence. The cerebrospinal fluid is nonreactive, and there is absence of all manifestations at the time of diagnosis four years or more after the original infection. The history, antecedent treatment, and previous serologic tests are important in establishing the diagnosis. Confirmatory treponemal antibody tests (FTA/TPI) are essential to exclude biologically "false" seroreactivity. In addition to careful clinical examination of skin, mucous membranes, and eyes, examination of the cerebrospinal fluid and roentgenologic studies of the heart and aorta are mandatory.

LATE SYMPTOMATIC SYPHILIS. Late symptomatic syphilis may cause inapparent to severe damage of body systems. *Late "benign" syphilis* may show mainly nodular or squamous skin lesions of destructive character, containing few or no treponemes, with tendency to peripheral extension, central healing, and scar formation, a pattern usually not encountered in other skin lesions except lupus vulgaris. Certain forms of *skin tuberculosis, deep mycosis,* and occasionally *cancer* are the main differential diagnostic problems. Serologic examination is obviously important. The typical lesion of late syphilis is the *gumma,* which can involve the skin, mucous membranes, skeletal system, and viscera. Nodular ulcerative lesions spread peripherally, the subcutaneous gumma infiltrating and later perforating the skin, creating a roundish ulcer with cut-out, not undermined, borders in contrast to tuberculous ulcerations. The hard and soft palate can be perforated. In rare instances the total anterior or central part of the palate and nose may be mutilated by gummatous and other involvement of skin and bones, a condition known as rhinopharyngitis mutilans ("gangosa"), which is also encountered in late yaws

and bejel. *Skeletal lesions* involve mostly periosteum, more rarely cortex and medulla, and are of a diffuse or localized gummatous nature, particularly affecting the long bones, e.g., tibia, clavicle. Pain, swelling, and roentgenologic findings are diagnostic characteristics. Syphilitic joint lesions are less frequent. Charcot's joints, frequently associated with tabes dorsalis, are considered as a neuroarthropathy. *Nervous system syphilis* includes affliction of cranial nerves from basal syphilitic meningitis, giving symptoms according to the nerve involved, e.g., eighth-nerve deafness, diplopia. Damage to the central nervous system can otherwise give rise to a very wide range of neurologic and other signs and symptoms which characterize meningovascular and parenchymatous neurosyphilis, e.g., general paresis, tabes dorsalis. The latter is frequently associated with primary optic atrophy. *Cardiovascular syphilis* manifests itself primarily as aortitis of the ascending aorta and may lead to aortic insufficiency and aneurysm. Roentgenography is as essential as cerebrospinal fluid examination for the diagnosis of late syphilis. (See Ch. 386 and 587.)

A relatively frequent coexistence of cardiovascular syphilis with neurosyphilis (10 to 15 per cent), neurosyphilis with "benign" late syphilis (13 per cent), and the latter with cardiovascular syphilis (10 per cent) should be kept in mind by the physician. Almost all fatalities in syphilis result from neurosyphilis or syphilis of the heart or aorta. These most serious forms of the disease are discussed elsewhere in Ch. 386 and 587 and in a monograph on venereology (Willcox).

Maternal and Prenatal ("Congenital") Syphilis. The manifestations of maternal syphilis depend on the stage of disease; diagnosis is established on usual anamnestic, clinical, and serologic criteria. Serologic screening may detect pregnant women with no past history of disease. These should be investigated and treated as early latent syphilis. During the first years of infection most pregnancies will terminate in fetal death if the mother is left without treatment. Later in the course of the infection the risk decreases, and untreated syphilitic women may give birth to healthy children. Presumably this is related to the lessening likelihood of the occurrence of treponemia with time. Nevertheless, occasionally an untreated syphilitic woman may deliver a congenitally syphilitic child many years after infection.

EARLY PRENATAL SYPHILIS. Early congenital syphilis is prenatally acquired infection diagnosed in children less than two years old. The fetus is infected after the fourth month of pregnancy. The lesions on delivery depend on the time of infection, and may vary from marasmic to apparently healthy infants. Fibrotic visceral lesions are characteristic. Osteochondritis is diagnosed by roentgenographic examination. The child may be born with "snuffles" from affliction of the nasopharynx with mucous and sometimes hemorrhagic discharge. The cutaneous rash after birth can be impressive papular and bullous eruptions in the palms and soles (exceptional in acquired syphilis), and tend characteristically to affect facial, circumoral, anogenital, and diaper areas, and palms and soles. Such lesions are highly contagious, and *T. pallidum* can easily be demonstrated. Infants without signs of disease, who are suspected of being infected by a seroreactive mother, should be clinically and serologically kept under surveillance for at least six months to establish active infection or passive reaginemia.

LATE PRENATAL SYPHILIS. Late congenital syphilis is a prenatally acquired infection that has persisted and developed in children over two years of age. On discovery the condition is often latent and should be confirmed by FTA/TPI tests. Residual manifestations of early lesions may be present, notably rhagades radiating from the prolabium and frontal bosses and saber tibia from periostitis of the shaft. There may be osseous destruction (saddle nose) and dental deformities, with wedge-shaped, widely spaced, often notched permanent upper central incisors (Hutchinson's teeth). Other "signs" include eighth nerve deafness and syphilitic synovitis in both knee joints (Clutton's joints). The most common affliction is *interstitial keratitis,* usually appearing in late childhood and eventually becoming bilateral. There is photophobia, ground glass appearance of the cornea, and vascularization of adjacent sclera. Other late manifestations resemble those of acquired late adult syphilis of similar duration. Meningovascular syphilis, paresis, and tabes occur, but cardiovascular syphilis is rare.

The profound pathologic processes of prenatal syphilis and the personal and social limitations that they impose are preventable through routine serologic testing of all pregnant women and adequate treatment of those found infected.

Interpretation of Laboratory Findings. In addition to clinical and anamnestic examination, the diagnosis of syphilis depends on laboratory findings. In early syphilis dark-field examination of lesions and serologic tests are indispensable; in late syphilis in addition to serologic tests examination of the cerebrospinal fluid is the most important laboratory procedure.

Dark-Field Examination. T. pallidum cannot be readily identified in dried, fixed fluid, or tissue specimens by silver, chromatic, or fluorescent staining. Its presence can best be ascertained in the living state by microscopic dark-field examination which can be done by the trained physician. Material for examination includes tissue fluid from initial and secondary lesions after saline washing and gentle squeezing or an aspirate from an enlarged lymph node. Preferably, specimens should be examined on the spot. They can, however, be collected in a capillary tube, sealed with wax, and mailed to a competent laboratory. Care must be taken in interpreting the findings. T. pallidum may resemble spirochetes normally inhabiting genitalia and the oral cavity. The regular corkscrew-like coils, the slow, rotating, forward-backward motions, and graceful sideways bendings help in identification of T. pallidum. *Repeated failures to demonstrate T. pallidum with adequate technique in a suspected lesion may mean that the lesion is healing, that the patient has received topical or systemic treatment, or that the lesion is nonsyphilitic. Before the lesion is diagnosed as nonsyphilitic, an examination of lymph node aspirate should be made.*

Serologic Tests. Serologic tests are indispensable for individual diagnosis of syphilis, for following the effect of therapy, for routine screening of pregnant women, blood donors, and other "risk groups," and for case and contact finding in community, national, and international health programs. It is essential for the physician to utilize laboratories that employ standard reagents and methods and that partake in a proficiency testing program of sensitivity, specificity, and reproducibility in cooperation with a regional or national reference center. Serologic tests detect antibodies formed during the course of the syphilitic infection.

Reagin tests use cardiolipin antigen according to different methods. These may vary from one country to another, but are based on either complement fixation or flocculation techniques, e.g., VDRL.*

The pattern of antibody production has been outlined under Immunology, indicating that treponemal antibody, notably the immobilizin, is specific and reflects roughly the immunity status of the patient, whereas reagin is rather an indicator of disease activity. *The use of quantitative reagin methods† is essential to permit the physician to assess the effect of treatment and compare antibody titers of periodically examined serum specimens in the post-treatment surveillance of the patient.*

Three types of *treponemal antibody tests* are in use: (1) The treponema immobilization test (TPI) uses live T. pallidum as antigen, immobilized by antibody in the presence of complement. It is the only test in which the biologic action of serum antibody can be determined directly under the microscope. (2) The fluorescent treponemal antibody test (FTA) uses killed treponemes as antigen. Syphilitic serum is bound to the surface of treponemes fixed onto a slide, and the antibody is made visible by use of fluorescein-tagged antiserum against human globulin. Nonspecific antibodies are removed either by dilution of serum (FTA$_{200}$ test) or "absorbed" (FTA/ABS test). (3) The passive treponemal hemagglutination test (TPHA) uses disrupted T. pallidum as antigen, coated onto tannin-treated sheep erythrocytes which are agglutinated in the presence of specific antibody.

"False" reaginemia occurs in certain pathologic conditions not caused by syphilis. Transient low-titer seroreactivity may, for example, arise from acute bacterial and viral infections, or after vaccinations, e.g., for smallpox. "False" seroreactivity occurs also from disease of connective tissue, e.g., disseminated lupus erythematosus, leprosy, and malaria; from the continued use of heroin; or from conditions affecting serum globulins, e.g., malnutrition. Moreover, both reagin and treponemal serologic tests for syphilis are also reactive by definition in other treponematoses (yaws, pinta, and bejel). *It should be realized, however, that syphilis remains the most common cause of reagin seroreactivity and that in screening examinations only one of ten VDRL seroreactive persons may be a problem case requiring confirmation with a specific treponemal test.* If TPI or FTA tests, or both, are needed and such tests are not undertaken by a local recognized laboratory, serum specimens can be mailed for examination to a laboratory of repute. If there is doubt about the interpretation of serologic tests, consultation should be arranged with a syphilologist.

Reagin tests may generally confirm a diagnosis of syphilis when a suspected initial lesion is present, although they are usually subordinate to dark-field findings of T. pallidum in the early stage. Reagin tests are reactive in all instances of secondary syphilis; they are im-

---

*Among the reagin tests, flocculation reactions, e.g., VDRL, Kline, Eagle, and complement fixation reactions, e.g., Kolmer, are used. In the present chapter the Venereal Disease Research Laboratory (VDRL) test is referred to as the prototype of reagin tests. It is subjected to national proficiency testing within and between laboratories in several countries and is based on the use of antigens referable to International Standard Preparations for the components used.

†In quantitative serologic tests a series of a progressively higher dilution of serum is made and each dilution is tested separately. The highest dilution that is reactive represents the titer.

portant in the diagnosis of congenital syphilis, offer a clue in latent syphilis, and have supplementary value in late syphilis. Treponemal antibody tests are essential for diagnosis in patients with repeated low or fluctuating reagin titers, in patients without anamnestic and/or clinical evidence, and in acquired and congenital disease, as well as in suspected late manifestations.

Cerebrospinal Fluid Examination. Lumbar puncture* can be undertaken at the physician's office or at a clinic. Examination of the cerebrospinal fluid serves to establish a diagnosis of latent syphilis by exclusion of asymptomatic neurosyphilis, aids in following the effect of therapy once such diagnosis has been made, and generally assures surveillance of patients in different phases of the disease. In syphilitic meningitis there occurs an increase of lymphocytes, proteins, and in some instances antibody. The first sign of asymptomatic neurosyphilis or meningitis arising from latency is pleocytosis of more than four cells per cubic milliliter, closely followed by an increase in protein to 40 mg or more (depending on laboratory method) and reactive antibody tests. When progressing to parenchymatous neurosyphilis, 150 cells or more, marked protein increase (globulin) and strongly reactive antibody tests are encountered. Complement-fixation tests for reagin (Kolmer) and treponemal antibody tests (TPI/FTA) are most suitable in cerebrospinal fluid examinations. When reactive they are pathognomonic of neurosyphilis; flocculation tests are sometimes nonreactive when antibody is present. Successful treatment leads to rapid regression of the cell count. Normalization of protein requires more time. Reversal of serologic tests may take several years.

---

*In some countries suboccipital puncture is preferred.

Therapy. Mahoney and co-workers (1943) introduced penicillin therapy in syphilis, and this drug has replaced previous metal therapy. Benzyl penicillin G is a more effective antitreponemal agent than the newer penicillins, e.g., ampicillin, methicillin. Injection therapy is preferred, and oral therapy is not recommended. The reproduction time of treponemes is of long duration (30 to 35 hours), and they may lodge in places where they do not multiply. Sustained, uninterrupted treponemicidal blood and tissue levels are therefore held to be more effective than intermittent penicillinemia and also minimize the arising of resistant mutants. Long-acting penicillin preparations such as procaine pencillin G in oil and monostearate (PAM) and benzathine penicillin G (DBED) as well as short-acting aqueous penicillin G preparations are all effective when used in treatment schedules providing adequate time:dose relationships. Aqueous preparations require frequent injections, higher dosages, and more involved patient management. The characteristics of the penicillin preparation used are more important than number, frequency, and total dosages of treatment schedules of undefined preparations. The accompanying table shows generally accepted treatment schedules.

Early Syphilis. Usually *T. pallidum* disappears from initial lesions within 24 hours, somewhat more slowly from secondary lesions. There is rapid involution of the lesion after adequate penicillin therapy, and the long-term outcome is highly satisfactory. A cooperative international study of 688 seronnreactive and 494 seroreactive patients with primary syphilis, adequately treated and followed up to 11 years, showed no clinical relapses. Among 499 adequately treated patients with secondary syphilis, also followed up to 11 years, fewer than 5 per cent were retreated for clinical relapse, seroresistance, and—in most cases—reinfection. In 2485 patients with

---

Penicillin Treatment Practices in Syphilis

Indications for Syphilis Therapy[†]	Dosage and Administration*		
	N,N-Dibenzylethylenediamine Dipenicillin G (DBED) or Benzathine Penicillin G	Procaine Penicillin G in Aluminium Stereate Suspension (PAM)	Aqueous Benzyl Penicillin G or Procaine Penicillin G
Primary, secondary, and early latent syphilis with nonreactive cerebrospinal fluid and adequate opportunity for follow-up; epidemiological treatment	Total of 2.4 megaunits; single dose of two injections of 1.2 megaunits in one session	Total of 4.8–6.0 megaunits; first dose of 2.4 megaunits, and 1.2 megaunits at each of subsequent injections 3 days apart (over 9 days)	Total of 6.0 megaunits in doses of 600,000 units daily for 10 consecutive days
Late latent or when cerebrospinal fluid not examined in "latency": asymptomatic neurosyphilis, symptomatic neurosyphilis, cardiovascular syphilis, late benign (cutaneous, osseous, visceral gumma)	Total of 6 to 9 megaunits in doses of 3 megaunits at 7-day intervals, over 14–21 days	Total of 6 to 9 megaunits given in doses of 1.2 megaunits at 3-day intervals, over 15–21 days	Total of 6–9 megaunits in doses of 600,000 units daily, over 15 days
Congenital Early Up to 2 years of age	Total of 50,000 units per kg in a single or divided dose at one session	Total of 100,000 units per kg given in three divided doses at 2- to 3-day intervals	Total of 100,000 units per kg as 10,000 units per kg per day for 10 consecutive days[‡]
Late 2 to 12 years, weight 32 kg (71 lb) or less	Same as early congenital syphilis	Same as early congenital syphilis	Same as early congenital syphilis
Over 12 years, or over 32 kg	Same as adult latent syphilis	Same as adult latent syphilis	Same as adult latent syphilis

*Individual doses can be divided for injection in each buttock to minimize discomfort.
[†]In *pregnancy,* treatment is dependent on the stage of syphilis.
[‡]Preferable in very small children.

nonspecified "early syphilis" followed up to 12 years, re-treatment in different subseries of patients varied from 1 to 9 per cent with an average of 1.5 per cent retreated for serorelapse, seroresistance, and clinical relapse, the remainder being reinfections (Idsøe et al., 1972). *For the physician it is therefore unnecessary to subject all patients with early syphilis to the intensive treatment required by the few patients who experience seroresistance or relapses after currently accepted therapy schedules. But the need for proper post-treatment observation and surveillance of the patient is obvious. For community health reasons it is essential that a large "epidemiologic dose" of penicillin be administered immediately on diagnosis of infectious syphilis (see table), rendering the patient rapidly noninfectious and providing protection against spread of infection should the patient default from further treatment.*

After adequate penicillin treatment of *early syphilis,* the VDRL titers begin to descend, usually after two months, and a subsequent rapid fall is to be expected in most cases. As a whole, the time to reach seronegativity depends on the duration of infection when treatment was started, although in the majority of cases it is achieved within six months. At the ninth month 5 to 10 per cent may still be seroreactive at a low titer.

A few patients will retain seroreactivity at the end of the second year, mostly those treated in the late secondary and early latent phases. Fluctuations of titers during post-treatment surveillance examinations may occur. Only a persistent rise from nonreactivity or a fourfold titer increase from previous titer level should be considered as *serologic relapse.* Failures occur within one to two years, most of these within three to nine months. Serologic relapse usually precedes or accompanies infectious clinical relapse in which the mucocutaneous lesions are often localized. Cerebrospinal fluid examination is then essential, and retreatment should be provided at once. Occasionally, titers fail to decrease the first six to nine months after therapy. Retreatment is also then indicated. Retreatment should be intensive, usually effected by doubling the previous dosage scheme. The few patients who retain a residual low reagin titer after the second year and who after CSF examination have no evidence of syphilis may safely be followed without further treatment. Both these as well as the reagin nonreactive patients can be considered as "cured" of syphilis when the surveillance scheme has been completed. Whether or not the last treponeme has been eliminated—or will eventually be eliminated by the immunity forces—is another matter. *Long-term practical experience shows no convincing evidence that late clinical manifestations occur after penicillin therapy of early syphilis, providing that it was adequate and that the exceptional early failures were retreated; the assurance that can be given to the patient is thus of a high order.* Distinction between infectious relapse and reinfection is sometimes not possible except on epidemiologic grounds. If the patient is cured of his infection before his immunity defenses have been mobilized, reinfection may occur on renewed exposure to *T. pallidum.*

Late Syphilis. During the course of untreated late syphilis, regression or reaginemia as a rule takes place very slowly and may occasionally reach nondetectable levels by usual reagin tests. Such reagin nonreactivity may be encountered in parenchymatous or cardiovascular syphilis. Treatment does not substantially affect reagin reactivity, or serologic nonreactivity is reached only after many years. Treponemal antibody tests (TPI/FTA) are normally reactive in late syphilis, and despite treatment may remain so throughout life.

The considerable capacity of the immunity in untreated syphilis to prevent progression of late latent infection to symptomatic disease has already been emphasized. This function cannot, however, be accurately measured by serologic tests as distinct from the clinical effect of therapy, although the latter is convincing. It has been estimated by McDermott (1967) that probably less than 2 per cent of diagnosed late latent syphilitics may develop serious manifestations after proper penicillin therapy. Principally, these are older patients with pre-established unrecognizable manifestations, e.g., aortitis, at the time they are treated for their presumed late latent infection. In the treatment of actual late manifestations, the character, location, and extent of the latter dictate the amount of specific therapy; the indications given in the table—mainly based on the generally accepted schedules applied in the United States Public Health Service VD control program—should be considered only as norms in this respect. Functional and other damage caused by the syphilitic processes require supporting therapy and collateral medical care.

As gummatous lesions may coexist with or precede cardiovascular and/or neurosyphilis, routine physical examination, including roentgenologic examination of the cardiovascular system and examination of the crebrospinal fluid, should be made before treatment, which should be adjusted to the findings. Gummas resolve rapidly, but require several months to heal, depending on size and location.

Maternal and Prenatal ("Congenital") Syphilis. The provision of treatment in diagnosed maternal syphilis is often urgent. Even with diagnosis late in pregnancy, a normal infant can be expected after adequate penicillin therapy. Treatment of maternal syphilis depends on the stage of disease as in other infected persons. With solely anamnestic or serologic evidence of syphilis, the need for treatment should be evaluated at each pregnancy. Confirmation of past adequate therapy and subsequent absence of evidence of active syphilis justify withholding treatment unless reinfection occurs. *If doubt exists concerning diagnosis or previous therapy, pregnant women should be retreated adequately, regardless of reagin titer.*

Infants with manifest early congenital syphilis are often seriously ill and require treatment and medical care in hospital. Penicillin is provided by body weight of children and preadolescents. Patients with interstitial keratitis should be hospitalized for intensive treatment (0.3 megaunit of benzyl penicillin G daily for three weeks) and local hydrocortisone application. Treatment of ocular, aural, osseous, and late systemic manifestations requires consultation with specialists.

Prophylactic Treatment. In persons with suspected or known exposure to infectious syphilis lesions, it is fallacious to await development of clinical or serologic symptoms before treatment. If the chain of infection involves a pregnant woman, it is generally accepted that prophylactic treatment should be given immediately. However, prophylactic treatment is increasingly being accepted in other circumstances also, because considerations applicable in previous arsenical therapy (long-treatment courses and toxicity) do not apply to present-day antimicrobial drugs. Syphilis is often acquired from promiscuous heterosexual or homosexual practices. Physicians cannot influence behavioral patterns of contacts. In individual cases, however, the physician can endeavor to elicit contact information comprising the three previous months in primary, six months in secondary, and twelve months in latent syphilis as a basis for epidemiologic action and treatment by a local clinic or health authorities.

When prophylactic treatment is given by the physician, it should be adequate, meaning curative for early syphilis, so as to prevent any hidden or asymptomatic infection from developing, and appropriate clinical and laboratory post-treatment surveillance should be arranged.

Patients Previously Treated. Older patients sometimes confront the physician with information concerning previous injections of arsenicals and/or bismuth or penicillin. Such patients may show low titer reagin tests and TPI/FTA seroreactivity. The physician is justified in treating these patients as newly discovered cases of late latent syphilis after exclusion of systemic involvement when adequate history of disease or therapy cannot be obtained.

Penicillin Side Reactions. An acute systemic febrile reaction—the Herxheimer reaction—with intensification of lesions occurs in about half the patients with early syphilis when treated with antitreponemal drugs, e.g., penicillin. It occurs within 12 to 24 hours, and lasts for 6, seldom for 24 hours after the first injection. Corticosteroid preparations appear to attenuate Herxheimer symptoms. Reaction to subsequent penicillin injections signals intolerance to the antimicrobial drug in late syphilis, e.g, aortitis or paresis. The Herxheimer reaction can be severe, but does not—according to modern authorities—indicate interruption of therapy, gumma of larynx being among particular exceptions.

Penicillin may give rise to drug-induced hypersensitivity based on antigen-antibody reactions. The *immediate* or accelerated type shows urticaria, angioneurotic edema, and anaphylactic shock. It is common practice therefore for the patients to be observed for 20 to 30 minutes after penicillin administration, which should not be used in those with known or suspected penicillin hypersensitivity. Syphilis in allergic, e.g., asthmatic, or atopic patients should be managed with caution during treatment sessions. The physician should always have resuscitation remedies readily available, notably epinephrine (Adrenalin), 0.5 ml subcutaneously, which may be lifesaving, aminophylline, and corticosteroids. The *late* or delayed penicillin hypersensitivity reaction causes dermatitis, various skin eruptions, and exfoliation, and occurs within days or weeks after challenge. The condition is successfully treated with corticosteroids and antihistamines (see Ch. 72).

The true extent of penicillin hypersensitivity is unknown, but reactions appear to be relatively rare. The frequency varies from 0.07 to 10 per cent, depending on degree of selection in patient material studies in different countries. Fatality from anaphylactic shock is 15 to 20 per million treated patients (Idsøe et al.). Most deaths are preventable if resuscitation remedies are used immediately. Objective prediction of adverse reactions is not possible. Immunodiagnosis (skin testing, serohemagglutination) is not yet suitable for general practical use.

Alternatives to Penicillin. In persons with suspected or known penicillin hypersensitivity, other antimicrobial drugs must be used. None are as effective as penicillin in the treatment of syphilis. The experience with cephaloridines, for example, must be regarded as experimental; others have marked side effects. The usefulness of orally administered erythromycin and tetracycline, on the other hand, has been demonstrated. A total dose of 30 to 40 grams over 10 to 15 days (750 mg four times daily) of either erythromycin or tetracycline is given. In pregnant women erythromycin and not tetracycline should be used. The latter in large dosages may cause serious conditions in the mother (pancreatitis, azotemia, fatty liver), and teratogenic effects, e.g., dental deformities, in the offspring. In indicated retreatment of early syphilis and in late manifestations, the total dosage should be doubled or another drug used.

Surveillance. The short period of actual penicillin treatment is in contrast to the relatively long post-treatment surveillance required. The demonstrated persistence in host tissues of treponemal forms after presumably adequate therapy and the continued TPI reactivity that may signal presence of *T. pallidum* in host tissues suggests a prudent attitude to be justified in post-treatment surveillance of syphilis patients.

Early Syphilis. Quantitative reagin tests should be undertaken at 1, 2, 3, 4, 5, 6, 9, 12, 18, and 24 months after treatment, with FTA/TPI tests at 18 and 24 months; in addition to periodic clinical examinations, the cerebrospinal fluid should be examined at 24 months. (1) If all serologic tests are nonreactive and the cerebrospinal fluid normal at 24 months, the patient can be discharged. (2) If reagin titers are persistently low or nonreactive, the cerebrospinal fluid normal, and FTA/TPI tests reactive at 24 months, further six-monthly serologic follow-up examinations are indicated, with renewed cerebrospinal fluid examination four years after original treatment. (3) If the cerebrospinal fluid is reactive in (1) or (2), it is necessary to proceed as in neurosyphilis.

Late Latent Syphilis. Quantitative reagin tests should be undertaken at 3, 6, 9, 12, 18, and 24 months and FTA/TPI tests at 1, 12, and 24 months, with examination of the cerebrospinal fluid and radiologic examination of the heart and aorta *before* treatment. Unless there is roentgenographic or other evidence of cardiovascular syphilis, the patient can be discharged from observation.

Neurosyphilis. In asymptomatic neurosyphilis, clinical examination, quantitative reagin tests, FTA/TPI tests, and cerebrospinal fluid examination should be undertaken every six months for four years. If the cerebrospinal fluid becomes reactive, the patient should be retreated, the cerebrospinal fluid examination repeated six months later, and the subsequent follow-up observations conducted as above. In symptomatic neurosyphilis, quantitative reagin tests, FTA/TPI tests, and cerebrospinal fluid examination should be obtained at six-month intervals for four years. If there is no improvement at six months, the patient should be retreated and the surveillance continued. If two nonreactive cerebrospinal fluid tests are obtained a year apart, no further tests are necessary (see Ch. 386).

Cardiovascular Syphilis. In addition to clinical and roentgenographic surveillance, quantitative reagin tests and FTA/TPI tests should be undertaken every six months for four years, cerebrospinal fluid examination having been made before treatment. In cases of reactive fluid, the patient should be treated as in neurosyphilis (see Ch. 587).

Late "Benign" Syphilis. The follow-up observations for late "benign" syphilis are the same as for late syphilis when cardiovascular and/or neurosyphilis are present.

Maternal and Prenatal ("Congenital") Syphilis. In the first pregnancy, clinical examination and quantitative reagin tests should be undertaken preferably at monthly intervals after treatment until term, and thereafter as appropriate for the stage of disease. In subsequent pregnancies in women with previously adequately treated syphilis, quantitative reagin tests should be undertaken at least on the initial visit and during the last month before delivery. Thereafter they should be obtained whenever appropriate in terms of the stage of disease. In *early prenatal syphilis* when lesions are present, the patient should be treated as in "early syphilis." If no lesions are apparent, quantitative reagin testing of child and mother should be carried out at one, two, three, four, five, and six months to ascertain possible differential titers. If reaginemia of the child is passive and no diagnosis of syphilis appears justified, this decision should be reconfirmed at 12 and 24 months. If disease is "active," the patient should be treated as appropriate for early latent syphilis. In *late prenatal syphilis* (over two years) quantitative reagin tests should be obtained at three-month intervals in the first year, at six-month intervals in the second year, and thereafter at yearly intervals for four years. If the cerebrospinal fluid is reactive or if other late involvement is present, the patient should be treated accordingly.

Aspects of Prevention. Efforts at containment of syphilis and other sexually transmitted diseases through broad social and educational prevention have apparently been outweighed by behavioral and environmental changes in a permissive society. Moreover, sex education—when undertaken in schools—does not always include sufficient information on venereal diseases. Even in enlightened community programs concerning sex and family-life education, the sexually transmitted diseases are often ignored. Although the physician can provide a measure of health education, prevention of disease ultimately depends on individual decisions influenced by knowledge, motivation, and convenience. These decisions concern protection from risk of infection by some (chemoprophylaxis, condoms, postexposure measures), while causing others to report for early treatment should symptoms occur.

The physician should take into account the *psychologic effect* of a diagnosis of syphilis and give the patient sufficient time to alleviate his anxiety, distress, and ignorance; on the other hand, the indispensability for the patient to provide contact information, to complete treatment, and to accept post-treatment surveillance should be emphasized. The physician should put forward a balanced view concerning the communicability of the disease to others, risk of late manifestations, anticipated course of serologic tests, and similar matters. To patients contemplating marriage, interpartner transmission of infection and the chances of having nonsyphilitic children are particularly important. The physician should advise against marriage until the danger of infectious relapse is minimal. Such advice has less meaning if the couple are already living together. Advice concerning pregnancy prevention may then be required, and the physician should specifically inquire as to the need. Late manifestations, e.g., neurosyphilis, should receive consideration similar to other physical handicaps. General paresis is a contraindication for marriage. A dilemma arises when syphilis has been acquired from an extramarital source. The patient must then be urged to arrange for examination of the spouse. Careful surveillance is obviously needed.

The early stages of syphilis and other sexually transmitted diseases are health problems for large numbers of people. The late stages are also chronic social and economic burdens of the individual and the community. To those not seeking the services of the private physician, the community should in its prevention program make available *treatment facilities free of charge* in addition to laboratory, case finding, and social services. In several countries these are provided by state or national public health services. Internationally, the Brussels Agreement administered by the World Health Organization provides these facilities to seafarers in major ports regardless of nationality. *It is important that the private practitioner and specialist diagnosing syphilis in any community take advantage of the epidemiologic facilities of the health authorities so as to have contacts of infectious cases and their associates brought for examination and treatment by him, by a colleague, or at a clinic.*

Collart, P., Borel, L. J., and Durel, E.: Étude de l'action de la pénicilline dans la syphilis tardive: persistance due tréponème pâle après traitement. Première partie: La syphilis tardive expérimentale. Seconde partie: La syphilis tardive humaine. Ann. Inst. Pasteur, 102:596, 692, 1962.

Gjestland, T.: The Oslo Study of untreated syphilis: An epidemiologic investigation of the natural course of the syphilitic infection based upon a re-study of the Boeck-Bruusgaard material. Acta Derm. Venereol. (Stockh.), 35, Suppl. 34, 1955.

Idsøe, O., Guthe, T., and Willcox, R. R.: Penicillin in the treatment of syphilis. The experience of three decades. Bull. WHO (Suppl.), 47:1, 1972.

Levene, G. M., Wright, D. J. M., and Turk, J. L.: Cell-mediated immunity and lymphocyte transformation in syphilis. Proc. R. Soc. Med., 64:426, 1971.

McDermott, W.: Microbial persistence. Yale J. Biol. Med., 30:257, 1957/58.

McDermott, W.: Microbial Persistence. The Harvey Lectures, Series 63. New York, Academic Press, 1969.

Miller, J.: Immunity in experimental syphilis. Successful vaccination of rabbits with *Treponema pallidum*, Nichols strain, attenuated by irradiation. J. Immunol., 110:1206, 1973.

Smith, J. L., and Israel, C. W.: The presence of spirochetes in late seronegative syphilis. J.A.M.A., 199:980, 1967.

Syphilis and other venereal diseases. Med. Clin. North Am., 48:613, 1964.

Turner, T. B., Hardy, P., Newman, B., and Nell, E.: Effect of passive immunization on experimental syphilis in the rabbit. Johns Hopkins Med. J., 133:241, 1972.

United States Department of Health, Education and Welfare: Syphilis: A Synopsis. Public Health Service publication No. 1660. Washington, D.C., U.S. Government Printing Office, 1968.

Willcox, R. R.: A Textbook of Venereal Diseases and Treponematoses. 2nd ed. Springfield, Ill., Charles C Thomas, 1964.

World Health Organization: Cell-mediated immunity responses. Report of a Scientific Group. WHO, Tech. Rep. Ser. 423, 1969.

World Health Organization: Report of a Scientific Group on Treponematoses Research. WHO, Tech. Rep. Ser., 455, 1970.

Wright, D. J. M., and Doniach, R.: Recent advances in the immunology of syphilis. Proc. R. Soc. Med., 64:419, 1971.

Yobs, A., Clark, J. W., Jr., Mothershed, S. E., Bullard, J. C., and Artley, C. W.: Further observations on the persistence of *Treponema pallidum* after treatment in rabbits and humans. Br. J. Vener. Dis., 44:116, 1968.

NONSYPHILITIC TREPONEMATOSES: YAWS, BEJEL, PINTA

247. INTRODUCTION

The course and manifestations of venereal syphilis include many of the features of other nonsyphilitic treponematoses endemic among children and adults in tropical, subtropical, or adjoining regions, where rural populations reside in unhygienic and poor socioeconomic conditions. Clinical features have given distinct names to each of these conditions: yaws, bejel, and pinta. Each is caused by treponemes morphologically indistinguishable from *T. pallidum,* and a scale of pathogenicity can be established based on the degree and type of tissue damage. *T. carateum (pinta)* is the least invasive, affecting only human skin. *T. pertenue (yaws)* affects both the cutaneous and osseous systems. The *treponeme of bejel* affects, in addition, mucous membranes. In contrast to venereal syphilis, there is as a rule no cardiovascular and nervous system involvement or congenital disease in the nonsyphilitic treponematoses.

In addition to the treponemes causing the human infections, the related *T. cuniculi* is responsible for a naturally occurring sexually transmitted spirochetosis of rabbits. The organism is morphologically indistinguishable from pathogenic human treponemes and gives rise to the formation of reagin and treponemal antibodies; the condition responds to antisyphilitic drugs and shows some degree of reciprocal immunity to syphilis and yaws. Finally, cynomolgous monkeys in Africa sometimes have a naturally occurring, apparently asymptomatic treponematosis with significant treponemal serum antibody levels. When isolated and "reactivated" by experimental hamster passages, the treponemes found in lymph nodes are apparently closely related to *T. pertenue* of yaws (Fribourg-Blanc et al.; Sepetjian et al.).

In controlled laboratory experiments, each disease condition usually reproduces itself. However, long-term exposure of infected animals to different environmental conditions may, in some circumstances, modify the biologic characteristics of the particular treponemes. The extent to which this phenomenon occurs in nature has given rise to several speculations concerning the origin and phylogenesis of treponematoses through the ages (Hudson; Willcox; Hackett).

All persons with nonsyphilitic treponematoses develop reagin and treponemal antibodies just as in venereal syphilis; there is a varying degree of cross-immunity between these conditions, and all respond to penicillin and other antisyphilitic drugs. This group of infections—including venereal syphilis—is therefore referred to as treponematoses, notwithstanding individual clinical, biologic, and epidemiologic differences within the group, reflected in problems of diagnosis, treatment, prevention, and community control.

In the past two decades yaws, pinta, and bejel have been subjected to mass penicillin campaigns in the areas of the world where they prevail. Millions of persons with clinical or latent infections or contacts have been treated with long-acting penicillin preparations under the aegis of the World Health Organization, resulting in a remarkable regression of disease and infection, as evidenced in long-term seroepidemiologic postcampaign studies. The application of such methods has become of interest also in the study of "disappearing disease" in relation to the dynamics and theory of epidemic diseases in general (Guthe et al., 1972).

Fribourg-Blanc, A., Niel, G., and Mollaret, H. H.: Note sur quelques aspects immunologiques du cynocéphale Africaine. Bull. Soc. Pathol. Exot., 59:54, 1966.
Guthe, T., Ridet, J., Vorst, J., D'Costa, J., and Grab, B.: Methods of sur-

veillance of endemic treponematoses and sero-immunological investigations of "disappearing" disease. Bull. WHO, 46:1, 1972.
Hackett, C. J.: On the origin of the human treponematoses. Bull. WHO, 29:7, 1963.
Sepetjian, M., Tissot-Guerraz, F., Salussola, D., Thivolet, J. Z., and Mournier, C.: Contribution à l'étude du tréponème isolé du singe par A. Fribourg-Blanc. Bull. WHO, 40:141, 1969.
Willcox, R. R.: Evolutionary cycle of treponematoses. Br. J. Vener. Dis., 36:78, 1960.

248. YAWS
(Frambesia Tropica, Pian, Bouba, Parangi, Patek)

Definition.   Yaws is produced by a spirochetal microorganism, *T. pertenue,* which causes a chronic human infection, most often with onset in childhood. An initial cutaneous lesion usually appears, followed by relapsing infectious secondary nondestructive lesions of the skin, periosteum, and bones, frequently interspersed with symptom-free periods. Late manifestations include destructive and deforming lesions of skin, bones, and joints. Hyperkeratosis, notably of the soles, may develop in secondary and late yaws. There is no evidence of cardiac or nervous system involvement or of prenatal manifestations. Infected persons slowly develop relative immunity, and humoral antibodies can be detected by serologic tests reactive also in other treponematoses (syphilis, pinta).

History.   Yaws probably existed in Africa from remote times. Early accounts suggest that it was brought to the West Indies with the slave trade in the sixteenth century. By the eighteenth century it had become a serious health problem of the Antilles, Central America, and South America, as well as in areas of Oceania and Southeast Asia. Sauvages (1778) proposed the name frambesia for the disease because of the raspberry-like appearance of its papillomatous secondary lesions. Moseley (1800) observed its clinical course, notably that yaws ends in enlarged nodes and destructive lesions. Maxwell (1839) determined its incubation period to be three to four weeks after inoculation of lesion material into humans. Castellani (1905) identified *T. pertenue* as the causative microorganism of yaws. Lambert (1923) first attempted community-wide treatment with arsenicals in the Pacific Isles. The advent of long-acting penicillin preparations and single injection therapy revolutionized case treatment and made possible important reduction of yaws by mass penicillin campaigns (World Health Organization, 1950–1970) in the tropics.

Etiology.   The causative agent, *T. pertenue,* is a helical cell 8 to 12 μ in length and about 0.2 μ in diameter, with several closely set spirals. It resembles *T. pallidum* (syphilis) and *T. carateum* (pinta) morphologically in dark-field illumination and structurally in electron microphotographs. *T. pertenue* has not been grown in vitro, but will survive in special media for several days without multiplication. Strains stored in glycerin remain virulent for many years at $-70°$ C (CO_2 ice) or lower temperatures, e.g., liquid nitrogen or helium. *T. pertenue* is pathogenic for the same animal species as *T. pallidum.* The latter causes subclinical "silent" infection in the hamster, whereas *T. pertenue* causes a specific dermatitis—a procedure sometimes used to differentiate between treponemes in the laboratory (Vaisman, 1969). Pathogenic treponemes closely resembling or identical with *T. pertenue* have been isolated from wild cyno-

The author wishes to acknowledge the valuable advice of his colleague Dr. J. Ridet, Medical Officer, Communicable Diseases Division, World Health Organization, Geneva, concerning this chapter.

molgous African monkeys (Fribourg-Blanc et al.; Sepet-jian et al., 1968).

Epidemiology and Pathogenesis. Despite mass penicillin campaigns in recent years, yaws has remained a disease of many rural communities in the intertropical zone in Africa, the Americas, Southeast Asia, and Oceania. Areas of high prevalence of active yaws sometimes lie within a few miles of communities where the disease is rarely observed, depending on the ecologic situation, the evolutionary stage of endemicity, and the number of susceptibles at any given time. There is also a higher frequency of early yaws lesions in the rainy than in the dry season (Harding, 1947). Moreover, skin lesions are less frequent in cooler climates in mountainous tropical communities where they also become less moist and where papillomas tend to erupt in sweaty, mucocutaneous junctions and skin folds rather than involving the flat body surfaces (Ramsey, 1925). Furthermore, the occasional yaws lesions encountered after mass penicillin campaigns appear to be less extensive and less moist. In areas where no further lesions are encountered after such campaigns, continued specific seroreactivity (TPI) in a small proportion of children born after the campaigns could suggest the possibility of asymptomatic infection taking place in the new circumstances.

T. pertenue is incapable of penetrating unbroken skin. It is also unable to pass the placenta and cause congenital yaws. Transmission usually occurs through contact of skin abrasions, cuts, or lesions, e.g., trauma, injury, dermatoses, with infectious yaws lesions of another person. Indirect transmission via contaminated hands is believed to occur among children. Nursing mothers are sometimes infected directly by their infants. In addition to early infectious lesions, untreated latent yaws cases—which are liable to relapse with active lesions—form an important part of the reservoir maintaining the disease in rural communities. Humidity, moisture-holding soil, and mean annual temperatures of 27° C or more are also necessary for the spread of yaws. Moreover, transmission is favored by scant clothing, bare feet, crowded dwellings, and deficient personal hygiene. The gradual improvement of environmental and socioeconomic conditions will reduce the attack rate of yaws (Saxena and Prasad, 1963).

No true vector has been found in which *T. pertenue* actually multiplies, but it has been shown that disease can be transmitted by experimentally infected gnats. In some areas *Hippelates pallipes* may serve as mechanical carriers (Kumm and Turner, 1936). Geographic coexistence of foci of human yaws and natural treponematoses of wild cynomolgous monkeys have been observed in Africa (Baylet et al., 1970).

The age distribution of yaws depends on the rate of transmission and level of endemicity. In hyperendemic communities, e.g., the former Netherlands New Guinea (Kranendonk), the highest incidence of infectious lesions was in the two- to five-year-olds, with a seroprevalence of more than 90 per cent, pointing to an early, almost complete epidemic "saturation" of the community with yaws. In areas of moderate or low endemicity the highest seroprevalence is in older age groups. After mass penicillin campaigns, maximal seroprevalence was in the 45- to 59-year-olds, e.g., Nigeria, signaling regression of a hyperendemic situation many years ago. In the latter instance many more young individuals are susceptible to yaws in the new generation, but there are also more barriers to impede renewed

spread of the infection, e.g., education, health consciousness, chemotherapy, and health services. On the other hand, the greater number of serologically nonreactive young people in the new generation have, when reaching puberty, less protective cross-immunity to infection with venereal syphilis. This, in turn, has been reported to be among the reasons for the increased incidence of syphilis noted in tropical countries in the last decade.

Pathology. A main pathologic feature of yaws is the involvement of the skin. In early lesions the epidermis is thickened. There are cell infiltration ("plasmocytoma") of the dermis, hyperplasia, edema, and the presence of many treponemes. The papillae are elongated, often with thickening of the interpapillary pegs. Proliferation of vascular endothelium and obstruction of vessels are less characteristic of yaws than of syphilis. The epithelium may show hyperkeratosis, become superficially eroded, and be covered by dried exudate. The acanthotic epidermis and the papillary proliferation give rise to a fungating, frambesiform, crust-covered lesion. Diffuse periostitis and cortical rarefaction of the long bones are common in early yaws and are more marked than in venereal syphilis. The late lesions of yaws are due to a different tissue response, and endarteritis is observed histopathologically. Late lesions include ulcerating granulomatous nodules and gumma of the skin and bones. The gumma is built of elements similar to syphilitic lesions. Late skeletal affliction is mostly characterized by periosteal proliferation, rarefaction, or destruction of multiple areas of the long bones which can lead to extensive deformities.

Clinical Characteristics. At the site of entry of *T. pertenue* an initial lesion usually develops after an incubation period of three to four weeks. The implantation is facilitated by previous breaks in the skin (abrasion, injury, vaccination). The lesion is a papule situated on the legs in more than half the cases. In babies and toddlers it often appears on the buttocks or in the perineum. The papule grows into a round, broad-based granulomatous lesion ("mother yaw") covered by a serous crust from which *T. pertenue* can be recovered. The regional lymph nodes are frequently enlarged, not "shotty," and do not suppurate. An initial lesion will heal spontaneously within three to six months; ulcerating initial lesions require more time to heal.

As a result of early treponemia a generalized secondary eruption appears before or after the healing of the initial lesion. The most frequent and characteristic eruptions are roundish, raised, rough, granulomatous papules ("yaws" or frambesides), often covered by a brownish crust. These lesions appear anywhere on the skin, but rarely on the scalp. They sometimes show arciform arrangements. Secondary lesions may last for more than six months. A new crop may appear before the preceding lesions heal. Relapsing crops tend increasingly to become localized, e.g., to periaxillary, perianal, or circumoral areas. Sometimes the papilloma may be solitary. Plantar papules appear late, often after the generalized eruption, and are modified by a thick keratotic layer characteristic of barefoot people: a cherry-like granuloma appears in a well of cracked horny layer, frequently giving rise to painful disability ("crab yaws"). On the body, micropapular as well as various forms of macular or desquamative macular ("pian dartre") lesions may also appear. Lesions of mucous membranes are rare, but occur. Desquamatous macules can develop in the palms and notably on the soles, which are sometimes covered by a thick hyperkeratotic layer. In addition to skin eruptions in early yaws, there is superficial lymph node enlargement. In many cases there are pain and tenderness of the tibial shaft and other long bones owing to early periostitis. Such periostitis sometimes leads to saber tibia and polydactylitis. In many cases the general health of the patient appears little affected; in others there are systemic manifestations, with irregular fever, loss of appetite, and weight loss.

The secondary lesions begin to regress after several months, but relapses may occur on and off for four to five years before true latency is reached. The latter can be interrupted by late lesions of several types. (1) *Superficial ulcerations* of the skin with central healing tendency are observed, and *cutaneous and subcutaneous nodules* with ulceration and marginal healing may leave markedly dyspigmented atrophic scars, sometimes with deforming contractures. (2) *Diffuse or more localized hyperkeratosis* of the soles — less frequently of the palms — with fissuring and pitting can result in a characteristic mottled pattern, occasionally complicated by ulceration and sometimes developing more than 15 years after the infection. (3) *Osteal or periosteal gummatous lesions* of the tibia and other long bones may penetrate subcutaneous and cutaneous tissues, resulting in chronic ulcerations. These may also affect tarsal and carpal bones, the scapula, the sternum, and the skull. Affliction of palatonasal structures may lead to gangosa (rhinopharyngitis mutilans), a spectacular condition similar to that in syphilis. The osteitis and periostitis can occur both in association with generalized skin lesions and after these have receded.

Other yaws lesions are less common and include painless subcutaneous fibromatous juxta-articular nodes, paranasal egg-shaped swelling of the superior maxillary bone (goundou), chronic late macular or hyperkeratotic lesions of palmar surfaces, and volar aspects of wrists and insteps of soles, frequently followed by depigmentation.

Diagnosis. Typical early yaws lesions are generally not confused clinically with other conditions. Ulcerated initial leg lesions may sometimes be mistaken for other ulcerations, e.g., tropical ulcer. Also, spirochetes found in tropical ulcers resembling *Borrelia vincentii* may be mistaken for *T. pertenue*. Facial yaws papules may look like crusted impetigo. Individual lesions may resemble those of secondary syphilis or cutaneous leishmaniasis. Demonstration of treponemes by microscopic dark-field examination of exudate from the lesion and seroreactivity in reagin and treponemal antibody tests (VDRL, FTA, TPI, TPHA) serve to distinguish yaws from other conditions except those of the treponematosis group. Reagin tests become positive in serum about a month after the initial lesion (Li and Soebekti, 1955), and TPI titers can be very high (1:2560) in early yaws (WHO, Eastern Nigeria, 1968). Ulcerating contractures and mutilating lesions may present differential diagnostic problems in relation notably to leprosy and tuberculosis. Hyperkeratosis of the soles is often confused with other plantar conditions, mainly keratoma plantare sulcatum, plantar pitting, and tropical hyperkeratotic conditions of unknown origin (Hackett and Lowenthal).

Prognosis. In infected persons the prognosis is favorable when early treatment is provided. Otherwise, periodic infectious recurrences over many years give rise to months of incapacity. An undetermined number of infected persons develop late lesions. Others go on to spontaneous clinical cure; some also become serologically nonreactive ("burnt-out yaws"). Among those developing late chronic lesions, extensive invalidism and deformities often result.

Treatment and Control. The aim of treatment of individual patients is cure of the early disease and prevention of late manifestations. Intramuscular injection of 1.2 megaunits of benzathine penicillin (DBED) or 2.4 megaunits of PAM (procaine penicillin G in oil and 2 per cent monostearate) in adults and half doses for children suffices to cause disappearance of early lesions and prevent relapses. The response is dramatic. The early lesions usually become dark-field-negative within 48 hours, and healing takes place within 1 to 2 weeks. Serologic titers decline, but many retain low-titer reagin seroreactivity, depending on the duration of the infection (D'Mello and Krag, 1955). Penicillin sometimes causes a Herxheimer reaction. The usual safeguards against hypersensitivity reactions to penicillin should be taken (see Ch. 246). Persons with late yaws lesions may require repeated therapy. Oxytetracycline and chlortetracycline are reported to be useful in cases of deforming osteoperiostitis, indolent gummas, or ulcerations. Two grams daily for five to ten days in adults and proportionately less for children are given. Ulcerations of late yaws may also require application of local antiseptic dressings. Deformities caused by chronic osteitis and contractures may necessitate local surgery in addition to drug therapy.

In the efforts to achieve community-wide control of yaws, the previous work of the Jamaica Yaws Commission (1936) was in recent years extended under the auspices of the World Health Organization. Since 1950 some 200 million people in 45 countries were examined, and some 50 million treated with long-acting penicillin in large-scale control programs. The aim was (1) to survey entire area populations so as to control the reservoir of infection, (2) to interrupt the spread of yaws through mass treatment, rendering early cases noncontagious, preventing infectious recurrences, and aborting incubating disease, and (3) to undertake postcampaign yaws surveillance by periodic resurveys to detect and promptly treat overlooked cases or new infections that might arise. Untreated early cases free of clinical symptoms between outbreaks form an important part of the reservoir of infection and contribute to maintain the disease in rural communities. Accordingly, mass treatment criteria in these campaigns were based on a certain association in the population between the occurrence of clinically active lesions and of seroprevalence owing both to such lesions and to clinically symptom-free infections (Hackett and Guthe, 1956). The criteria for mass treatment are as follows: (1) When the prevalence of active yaws cases is 10 per cent or higher (hyperendemic areas), more than 50 per cent of the population is seroreactive, and all members of the community are to be treated. (2) When there are 5 to 10 per cent of active cases (mesoendemic area), all children and their obvious contacts are treated, because most contagious cases occur in the lower age groups. (3) When there are less than 5 per cent active cases (hypoendemic areas), solely case and contact treatment is provided. This wide use of penicillin results in rapid regression of active lesions. The prevalence thus has declined within a few years from more than 20 per cent to less than 1 per cent after mass campaigns in many areas. Examples of reduction in *infectious* yaws are: in N. Nigeria from 4.2 (1954) to 0.1 per cent (1964); in W. Samoa 3 per cent (1955) to nil (1965).

Indifference must be anticipated in rural populations toward long-term surveillance after mass campaigns that resulted in "disappearance" of community-wide diseases. In the case of yaws, seroepidemiologic studies have shown continued low-level transmission with tendency to focal outbreaks ten to fifteen years after mass campaigns (Guthe). Using cardiolipin serology, 40 per cent of children in areas of Indonesia remained seroreactive four to eight years after treatment, and 13 per cent of the seroreactive children still had high seroreactivity titers. A potential for clinical relapses therefore remains. It is really not possible to drive a community disease out of existence by the use of a drug alone even if the population coverage in mass campaigns is nearly complete. Broader measures are needed, notably development of basic health services, into the functions of which the continued surveillance of communicable diseases can be integrated following mass campaigns, e.g., against yaws. (World Health Organization, 1970).

Prophylaxis. Prevention of yaws depends on avoidance of minor injuries to the skin, and of shielding of open wounds and abrasions from contamination by flies. Open infectious lesions should be protected. Health education should aim at improvement of personal hygiene (soap) and community hygiene (water). Children with infectious lesions should be treated and excluded from school until noninfectious. Mass therapy represents an important control measure. No method of artificial immunization is available.

Fluker, J. L., and Hewitt, A. B.: Late yaws. Br. J. Vener. Dis., 46:264, 1970.

Guthe, T.: Clinical, serological and epidemiological features of framboesia tropica (yaws) and its control in rural communities. Acta Dermatovener. (Stockholm) 49:343, 1969.

Hackett, C. J., and Guthe, T.: Some important aspects of yaws eradication. Bull. WHO, 15:869, 1956.

Hackett, C. J., and Lowenthal, L. J. A.: Differential Diagnosis of Yaws. WHO Org. Monograph Series No. 45, Geneva, 1960.

Kantor, I., et al.: Test patterns of yaws antibodies in New Zealand. Arch. Dermatol., 103:226, 1971.

Turner, L. H.: Notes on the Treponematoses with an Illustrated Account of Yaws. Kuala Lumpur, Government Press (Institute for Medical Research, Federation of Malaya, Bulletin No. 9), 1959.

Turner, T. B., and Saunders, G. M.: Yaws in Jamaica: 1. An epidemiological study of two rural communities. Am. J. Hyg., 21:483, 1935.

World Health Organization: Bibliography on yaws 1905–1962. Geneva, 1963.

World Health Organization: Scientific Group of Treponematoses Research. WHO Techn. Rep. Ser., No. 455, 1970.

249. BEJEL
(Endemic Syphilis, Nonvenereal Childhood Syphilis, Belesh, Dichuchwa, Njovera, Skerljevo)

Definition. Bejel is a chronic, inflammatory childhood disease of the treponematosis group. The early disease is characterized by infectious mucocutaneous lesions and osseous manifestations resembling those of secondary syphilis. After disappearance of early lesions and an undetermined latency period, late manifestations may develop. There are skin and bone lesions similar to those of late "benign" venereal syphilis. If they occur at all, cardiovascular, nervous system, and prenatally acquired manifestations are extremely rare.

Etiology. The bejel treponeme is morphologically indistinguishable from *T. pallidum, T. pertenue,* and *T. carateum.* It is present in early lesions or lymph node aspirate. The organism has not been cultivated in vitro. In laboratory animals Turner and Hollander showed consistent differences in clinical reaction as compared with that of yaws and venereal syphilis treponemes. The bejel treponeme is apparently an intermediate between the two (Paris-Hamelin et al., 1968). Like other treponematoses, bejel is accompanied by antibody formation with seroreactivity in reagin, e.g., VDRL, and treponemal antibody (TPI/FTA) tests. Childhood infection with bejel protects against later infection with syphilis.

Epidemiology. Humans are the reservoir of bejel. Treponemes are most likely transmitted directly among children by skin-to-skin contact, or by hands moistened with treponeme-containing saliva, or indirectly via drinking flasks, the spouts of which have been demonstrated to contain treponemes (Grin). Treponeme implantation is generally facilitated by labial and oral fissures, occurring in dry climates, or by small mucosal lesions. Bejel is a household disease. In some instances 60 to 70 per cent of rural community populations have been reported to be infected. Narrow huts, crowded dwellings, unhygienic living conditions, and low socioeconomic standards favor transmission.

There are many scattered endemic centers of bejel in backward rural areas north and south of the tropics. Bejel occurs along the Kalahari and Sahara deserts in Africa, in the countries of the Balkans and the Eastern Mediterranean region, on the Arabian peninsula, in central Asian countries, and in Australia. It prevails in arid areas in contrast to yaws, which is encountered in moist, tropical jungle regions. Bejel was first described as a disease of nomadic people, subsequently to occur in settled rural populations, e.g., among the Dogons of Mali, the Islamic descendants of Bosnia, and the Bakwenas of Botswana. Previously it was widespread in the Middle East and Europe. Bejel has not been observed in the Western Hemisphere, where pinta and yaws are the prevailing childhood treponematoses. Bejel is in regression from its higher prevalence of two to three decades ago as a result of extensive mass penicillin campaigns and some improvement of health services. In certain areas the prevalence of bejel has remained higher than that of yaws because of occurrence in nomadic tribes, on account of geographic inaccessibility of endemic foci, and inadequacy of health services (Basset, 1963). It is likely to recur when mass treatment has been incomplete. Thus in Niger infectious lesions (5 per cent) and seroreactivity (30 to 40 per cent) were found some years after a mass treatment campaign.

Clinical Manifestations and Diagnosis. The experimental incubation period is approximately three weeks. Initial lesions are rarely encountered. The earliest lesions are "mucous patches" of the secondary type localized to the oral and faucial mucosa. "Split papules" occur at the oral angles. Local papular condylomata lata or anal, genital, or other intertriginous skin areas were observed in 25 per cent of infected children in Iraq (Guthe and Luger). Generalized secondary rashes and alopecia are relatively rare. Regional lymphadenopathy is common. Polyadenitis is rare. The early disease is followed by a latency period of undetermined duration, with seroreactivity as the sole sign of infection. Late "benign" manifestations of the skin develop in some patients. They do not differ in character from those in late venereal syphilis. Superficial tuberoulcerative skin lesions and characteristic serpiginous nodular ulcers occur. Nasopharyngeal ulcerations may occur and range from palate perforation to rhinopharyngitis mutilans as in yaws and syphilis (gangosa). Gummatous ulceration of the breast may occur in women previously infected with bejel who are suckling a child with oral lesions, a phenomenon which supports the concept that gumma may be delayed hypersensitivity reactions from repeated exposure (see Ch. 246). Juxta-articular nodes have been described in some geographic areas.

Bone lesions are the most frequent manifestations of late bejel, affecting the clavicle, other long bones, and the frontal bones, giving rise to swelling, tenderness, and pain. There is periosteal and endosteal proliferation, and deformities may result. Isolated cases of cardiovascular and neurologic system involvement have been described in Bosnia (Grin) and Botswana (Murray et al.). Incidental cases of prenatally acquired disease have also been reported. No case of prenatal or systemic disease was observed in several thousand examinations in a WHO project in Syria which included radiologic and cerebrospinal fluid examinations. When observed, the systemic manifestations may be due to the occurrence also of venereal syphilis in the geographic area concerned.

Diagnosis. The diagnosis of early bejel is established on epidemiologic and clinical grounds. It may be confirmed by dark-field demonstration of treponemes in the lesions or in node aspirate and by serologic tests (VDRL), reactive in nearly 100 per cent of cases. Serodiagnostic tests cannot differentiate latent bejel from latent yaws or syphilis. Because late clinical lesions are similar to those of yaws and syphilis, the local epidemiologic situation is an important diagnostic consideration. As distinct from the manifestations of late prenatal syphilis, dental deformities and interstitial keratitis are not observed in bejel.

Treatment and Prevention. Penicillin is as effective against bejel as it is against yaws, syphilis, and pinta. In the control campaigns initiated by the World Health Organization in several countries, one dose of 1.2 mega-units of long-acting penicillin PAM or benzathine penicillin G (DBED) was given intramuscularly in early cases, with two further doses at three- to seven-day intervals to patients with late manifestations. Half doses are used for contacts. The longer acting benzathine penicillin is preferred in contact treatment among nomadic tribes. Rapid healing of early lesions was followed by seroreversal in a large proportion of cases. Late destructive lesions required more time. Healing with scars progressed slowly but definitely and with some reduction in reaginemia, but with little or no effect on treponemal antibody tests (TPI/FTA), as in syphilis.

Seroepidemiologic studies undertaken in Bosnia, Yugoslavia, 20 years after the penicillin mass campaign—which was followed by systematic periodic surveillance over ten years—showed that childhood infection had been reduced to nil, the community seroimmunologic profiles indicating complete interruption of transmission. During this period adequate basic health services were provided, health education promoted, and general socioeconomic development took place. Bosnia remains the only example of eradication of endemic treponematoses. However, eradication of childhood infection has resulted in a population susceptible to venereal syphilis in later life. The absence of protective cross-immunity has thus created a new epidemiologic situation in which sporadic cases of the sexually transmitted treponematosis occurs.

Grin, E. I., and Guthe, T.: Evaluation of previous mass campaigns against endemic syphilis in Bosnia and Herzegovina. Br. J. Vener. Dis., 49:1, 1973.
Guthe, T., and Luger, A.: Epidemiological aspects of non-venereal "endemic" syphilis. Dermatologica, 115:248, 1957.
Hudson, E. H.: Non-venereal Syphilis. Edinburgh and London, E. & S. Livingstone, Ltd., 1958.
Turner, T. B.: Syphilis and the treponematoses. In Mudd, S. (ed.): Infectious Agents and Host Reactions. Philadelphia, W. B. Saunders Company, 1969.
Turner, T. B., and Hollander, D. H.: Biology of the Treponematoses. WHO Monograph series no. 35, Geneva, 1957.

250. PINTA
(Mal del Pinto, Carate)

Definition.   Pinta is a chronic skin infection caused by *Treponema carateum*, giving rise to an initial lesion and a generalized secondary rash, both containing treponemes. Late skin manifestations comprise extensive dyschromic (treponeme-containing) and achromic (treponeme-free) conspicuous splotches. Antibodies are produced, detectable by serologic tests reactive also in syphilis and yaws. Organ systems are not involved, physical health is not impaired, and prenatal disease is not known.

History. Manifestations of pinta were described in Berochea and by Corona (1811). Frequent seroreactivity (Wassermann complement fixation test) in pinta patients led Menck (1926) to imply association with syphilis and made Herrejon (1927) assume a treponeme to be the causative microorganism. Armenteros and Triana (1938) identified *T. carateum* in Cuban pinta. Leon Blanco (1939) obtained early generalized eruptions by self-inoculation of dark-field-controlled material from lesions. In therapy Corona (1811) showed the usefulness of mercury, Maria Graz (1913) of arsenobenzoles, and Varela (1944) of penicillin.

Etiology.   The etiologic agent, *T. carateum,* is a slender helical cell, 8 to 35 μ long and 0.2 to 0.3 μ wide. It has regular spirals, performs characteristic movements in microscopic dark-field examination, and is morphologically indistinguishable from the treponemes causing syphilis and yaws. *T. carateum* has not been cultivated in vitro.

Epidemiology.   Pinta is an endemic treponematosis of large rural populations in tropical forest and valley regions of Central and South America. For example, in rural areas of Mexico the prevalence of pinta varied from 1.3 to 9 per cent (1964) of the census population. Pinta cases occasionally reported from Pacific islands, India, Indonesia, and West Africa have not been verified and may have been "pintide" yaws. Unlike yaws, pinta is not a disease of earliest childhood. Community data (Mexico) indicate age-specific prevalences of early pinta lesions to be 2.5 per cent below five years of age, 8.8 per cent between five and ten years, and 12.2 per cent between ten and fifteen years. In late life some early lesions occur also after 40 years of age.

Transmission presumably takes place by person-to-person contact and is facilitated by poor hygiene, low economic standards, and limited health services. Treponemes are present in early lesions as well as in

The author wishes to acknowledge the valuable advice of his colleague Dr. S. Christiansen, Scientific Adviser, WHO Reference Centre for Treponematoses, State Serum Institute, Copenhagen, Denmark, concerning this chapter.

extensive late dyschromic lesions, where they can be found up to 40 years after the infection. Pinta does not appear to be very contagious, because an infected spouse with treponeme-containing lesions may sometimes not infect a serologically nonreactive partner or other family members. Scratches and insect bites may provide portals of entry for the agent. Blanco found 63 per cent of 257 initial lesions located on the legs and dorsum of feet. Arthropods (Simuliidae, Hippelates, or Ornithodorus) have not been convincingly demonstrated to be reservoirs of treponemes or biologic vectors, although mechanical transmission cannot be excluded.

Host-Treponeme Relationship. Experimental animal infection has been achieved in the chimpanzee (Kuhn et al., 1968). Man is the only known natural host of *T. carateum.*

As in syphilis, two types of antibody are formed during the human infection: (1) *Reagin,* detectable by cardiolipin antigen tests (VDRL), appears two to six months after the infection. (2) *Treponemal antibody,* identified in treponemal tests (fluorescent [FTA], hemagglutinating [TPHA], and immobilizing [TPI] antibody tests), is produced notably during dyschromic late manifestations but possibly before this stage. In untreated pinta the antibodies persist for many years. Asymptomatic seroreactors in communities affected by pinta are rare or absent. Superinfection can be achieved experimentally during the early generalized erythrosquamous stage of disease, but not after establishment of dyschromic late lesions. Varying degrees of cross-immunity between pinta, syphilis, yaws, and bejel have been reported (Medina, 1965). However, knowledge of humoral and cell-mediated immunity mechanisms is lacking. The same applies to immunologic (immunopathologic) processes possibly concerned in the genesis of lesions. Related aspects are discussed in Ch. 246.

The histopathology of pinta is characterized by a perivascular infiltrate of inflammatory cells composed of lymphocytes, some plasma cells, histiocytes, and macrophages. Swollen endothelial cells show no proliferation, arterioles and capillaries are not obliterated (as is the case in syphilis), and granulomatous tuberculoid structure is not observed. In dyschromic lesions accumulation of melanin-filled chromatophores in the upper corium is characteristic, and is caused by pigment "fallout" from the epidermis. This might be a consequence of the primary process. In achromic lesions the picture is quite different—epidermis is atrophic with flattened rete pegs, melanocytes and melanin are lacking, elastic fibers are destroyed, and there is collagenic sclerosis, which explains the porcelain whiteness of achromic lesions. The pigment changes may result from direct action of *T. carateum* on the epidermal "melanin unit" (a melanocyte with a pool of associated malpighian cells [Duchon et al., 1968]). Pinta lesions are localized to skin areas exposed to sunlight. This is unrelated to the number and distribution of melanocytes. A photosensitization process is therefore unlikely.

Clinical Manifestations and Diagnosis. The incubation period in experimental pinta is 7 to 21 days. In man, the initial manifestation is a small papule developing by extension or by coalescence with satellite lesions into a scaly maculopapular lesion. There is regional lymphadenopathy. A generalized erythrosquamous rash develops three to nine months after infection, and can be of the "wandering" type. Palpable polyadenitis is not a feature of secondary pinta in contrast to secondary syphilis.

One to three years after the initial lesion, sizable dyschromic macules develop. These late lesions develop from secondary pintides or independently, and pass from slate blue through violet to brown and white—the final achromic phase of the pathogenic process. The time required to pass through these stages varies for different patches in the same individual, and the coexisting colored and white skin areas present a mottled appearance. Dyschromic lesions are usually located on frontal skin, cheeks, ears, forearms, back of hands, and dorsum of feet, but never the scalp. Blue lesions may be punctate, but most often appear as smudges on the brow, cheeks, and side of nose, and may last for one to two years. Brown lesions last much longer, and white elements are of lifelong duration. The achromic lesions are porcelain white and exhibit a "geographic coast" appearance; the skin is not supple and has no skin lines or lanugo. A different clinical course of pinta has been described in Cuba (Pardo-Castello, 1942), where the early phase is limited to palms and soles, with hyperpigmented spots turning into keratotic elements. The hyperpigmentation extends to the backs of hands and forearms. In Cuba implication of the cardiovascular and nervous systems has also been suggested. Such systemic involvement has not been verified in other pinta-affected areas of Central and South America. For instance Mazotti (1966) found nonreactive treponemal antibody tests (TPI) in the cerebrospinal fluid of a series of advanced pinta patients in Mexico. Neither were abnormalities found in the cerebrospinal fluid of pinta patients in Venezuela (Lawton-Smith and Medina, 1971).

Early pinta may be difficult to differentiate from *neurodermatitis* (dark-field examination is decisive even if there is seroreactivity); *trichophytosis of the glabrous skin* (pinta does not have vesicles or pustules); *pityriasis alba* (early pinta is more infiltrated); *tinea versicolor* (secondary pintides are more sharply delineated and infiltrated); or *psoriasis* (on removal of scales in pinta no bleeding points appear on a smooth surface). In *late pinta* the leukoderma may closely resemble similar lesions in *syphilis* and *yaws* (scarring); *vitiligo* (supple skin in scalp and perianal areas); *chloasma* (pregnancy and disorders of female genitals); *melanosis* (telangiectasis and poikiloderma are not features of pinta); or *incontinentia pigmenti* (urticaria prior to spots in infancy, pattern of splotches different, concomitant retinal and organ disease).

Laboratory Methods. A diagnosis of pinta depends on microscopic dark-field demonstration of *T. carateum* in fluid from early initial and secondary generalized lesions and late dyschromic lesions, as well as on serologic reagin and treponemal antibody tests. Methodologic considerations and interpretations concerning these are related to those in syphilis.

Treatment. The treatment of choice is repository, long-acting penicillin, notably procaine penicillin G in oil with aluminium monostearate (PAM) and benzathine penicillin G (DBED). The considerations regarding time-dose relationship, oral therapy, and alternative antimicrobial drugs in persons hypersensitive to penicillin are the same as are discussed in Ch. 246. Rein et al. (1952) obtained highly satisfactory treatment results with 2.4 to 4.8 megaunits of PAM in early and late pinta. Injections of 2.4 megaunits of the longer-acting benzathine penicillin G can be effectively applied in a single dose or two injections of 1.2 megaunits in each buttock in one session.

Prognosis. Pinta neither endangers life nor gives rise to prenatal disease. It has little appreciable effect on general health of patients. Treatment causes treponemes to disappear rapidly from the lesions, which sometimes regress very slowly, depending on their extent. Achromic patches in which atrophy of the epidermis has occurred do not change. However, the disfigurement from pinta, notably of younger persons, is sometimes associated with psychologic misery and social ostracism. Freedom of choice of habitat, mate, and employment is curtailed.

Prevention. Pinta prevention consists in examination and treatment with long-acting penicillin, of all patients and their contacts, along with improvement of rural health services, hygiene, and economic standards. In the frame of the international treponematoses program of the World Health Organization (WHO) and the Pan-American Health Organization (PAHO) extensive peni-cillin treatment campaigns have been undertaken in rural endemic pinta areas by several national health administrations in Central and South America during the last two decades. For instance, in Mexico more than 350,000 pinta patients and contacts have been treated since 1959. Prevalence was reduced from 5.9 to 0.4 per cent in five main states.

Chandler, F. W., Kaufmann, A. F., and Kuhn, U. S., III: The histopathology of experimental pinta in the chimpanzee. J. Invest. Dermatol., 58:103, 1972.

Mazotti, L.: Negatividad de la prueba de inmovilizaciom de treponemas (TPI) en el liquido cefalorraquideo de 10 enfermos de pinto (carate). Rev. Inst. Salubr. Enferm. Trop., 22: Nos. 1 and 2, 1962.

Rein, C. R., Kitchen, D. K., Marquez, F. and Varela, G.: Repository penicillin therapy of pinta in the Mexican peasant. J. Invest. Dermatol., 18:137, 1952.

Smith, J. L., et al.: Neuro-ophthalmological study of late yaws and pinta. II. The Caracas project. Br. J. Vener. Dis., 47:226, 1971.

SPIRILLARY AND LEPTOSPIRAL DISEASES

251. RELAPSING FEVERS
(Recurrent Fever, Famine Fever, Tick Fever, Mianeh Fever, Carapate Disease, Kimputu)

Thorstein Guthe

Definition. Human relapsing fevers are acute arthropod-borne infections characterized by toxemia and febrile episodes that subside and recur over a period of weeks. They are caused by spirochetes of the genus Borrelia and occur in an epidemic form usually transmitted through the louse *Pediculus humanis,* and an endemic form transmitted through tick species of the genus Ornithodoros. The ecology and epidemiologic features are not alike. The clinical course and manifestations tend to be similar, although some characteristics are different.

History. Rutty (1739) first described the disease clinically. Henderson (1843) reported an epidemic in Edinburgh, differentiating the disease from typhus. Obermeier (1868) discovered spirochetes in the blood of relapsing fever patients. Munch (1874) and Motchoukoffski (1876) confirmed the etiology of the disease by self-inoculation of blood from relapsing fever patients. Flugge (1891) suggested the body louse to be a vector. Ross and Milne (1904) showed that "tick fever" mentioned by Livingstone in 1857 was caused by spirochetes in the peripheral blood. Dutton and Todd (1905) described the mechanism of infection in *Ornithodoros moubata* and the passing of the infection to its progeny. Koch (1906) confirmed the mechanism of ovarian transmission.

Etiology. Relapsing fever spirochetes are classified in the genus Borrelia. They are delicate helical organisms with length varying from 8 to 30 μ and width from 0.3 to 0.5 μ, with five to ten loosely wound irregular coils. These vary in different strains or in the same strain in varied conditions. The organism divides by transverse fission, is actively motile, and colors readily with usual blood stains.

Among numerous species of relapsing fever spirochetes, *B. recurrentis (B. obermeierei)* is generally accepted as the louse-borne species pathogenic for man. *B. carteri, B. berbera,* and *B. aegypti* — also louse-borne — may be subspecies or possibly only synonyms. Among tick-borne spirochetes *B. persica, B. hispanica, B. duttoni, B. turicatae,* and *B. venezuelensis* are strains with affiliation to natural transmitters of related tick species in different parts of the world. Morphologically the organisms do not differ significantly. They induce essentially the same clinical syndromes in humans. Based on animal experimentation and epidemiologic features, a distinction between louse-borne and tick-borne fevers is generally maintained. Staining methods, antigenic characteristics, serologic, and other methods have not shown consistent differences between strains as a basis for classification. Distinction of the tick-borne strains according to their Ornithodoros species vector has been attempted.

Borreliae cannot withstand desiccation and are susceptible to many chemical agents. They survive in citrated blood for three months at 0 to 2° C. When frozen at −72° C, strains are viable for long periods of time. Present culture methods on artificial media have maintained the organism alive for several months without multiplication. Borreliae multiply abundantly in developing chick embryos. Rodents can also be used for maintenance of strains (rats, hamsters). The long life of ticks (O. tholozani can live for 25 years) makes these insects suitable for preservation of tick-borne strains.

Transmission. Under natural conditions relapsing fevers are transmitted by body lice and ticks, although head lice, bedbugs, and fleas have sometimes also been implicated as vectors. (1) When *lice* feed on patients during attacks of relapsing fever, borreliae enter the midgut. Within five to six days the organisms penetrate into the celomic cavity outside the gut, and feces do not contain Borrelia. These do not reach the salivary glands, ovaries, or eggs. Thus borreliae are not injected into humans who are bitten by infected lice. Mutilation or crushing is necessary to transfer infection through abraded skin or by the hand to the conjunctiva, or to the gastrointestinal tract by ingestion. The louse remains infected during its short lifetime (27 to 50 days). Since transovarian transmission is not generally accepted, it is assumed that man is the only host. (2) The many *tick vectors* of relapsing fever — mainly belonging to genus Ornithodoros — attach themselves to the host for a short time, taking up blood. Several methods of infection have been reported, including infected saliva reaching capillaries opened by the bite, gut content being evacuated by the end of the meal and excreta being passed from the malpighian tubules, and infected coxal gland fluid being passed while feeding. Continued transovarian passage of Borrelia to the progeny takes place, and Ornithodoros are invertebrate hosts acting as chronic vectors in the transmission of relapsing fever to man.

Epidemiology. The epidemicity or endemicity of relapsing fevers is dependent on the biology of the vectors.

Louse-Borne Relapsing Fever. Louse-borne relapsing fever is typically epidemic under conditions in which overcrowded poor populations live under unhygienic conditions that facilitate wide dissemination of body lice. Louse-borne fever has been the scourge of armies campaigning in the field, as with typhus, with which it is sometimes confused. Cold spells or climates and heavy clothing favor lousiness and transmission of infection. Louse-borne disease has occurred in sporadic outbreaks, spreading with great rapidity across whole continents, thereafter dying down and disappearing, often for long periods. Epidemics with extensive mortality include those in Russia and Central Europe (1919 to 1923), and in West Africa and French Equatorial Africa (1920 to 1930). More recently a serious epidemic in North Africa (1942 to 1944) spread to the Eastern Mediterranean region and Europe. An estimated one million persons became ill, and some 50,000 died. Since then louse-borne relapsing fever has mainly been reported to occur in the cooler highlands of West, East, and Central Africa, representing possibly a transition from louse- to tick-borne disease. Cases of louse-borne disease have also been reported in the Far East and in several countries in the Americas (Felsenfeld, 1973).

Tick-Borne Relapsing Fever. Tick-borne relapsing fever is endemic with many circumscribed centers in the Eastern and Western Hemispheres, and has been reported from the Far East, Africa, Central America, tropical and temperate South America, the United States (western and central western states), and Canada (British Columbia). Wild rodents and other small animals constitute the vertebrate reservoir for many Borrelia species (rats, foxes, weasels, jackals, chipmunks, squirrels, owls, marmosets, and bats). A variety of tick species of genus Ornithodoros are of ecologic importance. They feed on these animals as well as on man. The frequency of relapsing fever transmission by ticks to man depends on the contact opportunities with humans. Many small animals which are common hosts of ticks bring these into houses and dwellings.

Pathology. Borreliae circulate in the peripheral blood during the pyrexial attacks, disappear prior to the crisis, and are probably present in the internal organs during remissions. In autopsy material their presence can be demonstrated notably in the spleen and brain. The pyrexial attack, the intercalate period, and subsequent relapses probably reflect an immunity pattern in which antibody is first produced against the original Borrelia strain with subsequent formation, persistence, and multiplication of antigenic variants. These in turn give rise to further specific antibody varieties in a cyclical manner. Eventually lysins and immobilizins seem to be the most important antibodies in modifying and eliminating Borrelia from the body of animals and man (Felsenfeld). Knowledge of immunologic aspects is inadequate.

Clinical Characteristics. Variations occur in symptoms of toxemia, severity of clinical manifestations, and recurrence of febrile periods, not only between louse-borne and tick-borne fevers, but also within outbreaks of each of these varieties. Generally, louse-borne fever has a longer incubation (up to 15 days), fewer relapses (usually one or two), longer pyrexial episodes (four to seven days), and longer intercalate periods (seven to ten days) than tick-borne fever. The incubation of the latter has been reported as short as one day (*B. hispanica*). As many as 14 waning relapses with pyrexial periods of two days' duration have been described (*B. persica*).

In both types of fever the initial attack is ushered in with chills, nausea, vomiting, joint and muscle pain, photophobia, and fever. The temperature rises rapidly to 40 to 40.5° C, remains elevated during the attack, except for slight morning remissions, and usually falls by crisis. Cough and bronchitis are frequent. An erythematous, evanescent macular or petechial rash develops in some patients, notably in louse-borne fever. The rash involves the neck, shoulders, chest, and abdomen. There are abdominal pain, splenomegaly, hepatomegaly, and sometimes jaundice of varying intensity. Epistaxis, hemoptysis, hematuria, or hematemesis occurs. Uterine hemorrhages and abortion are not infrequent. Headache, delirium, and symptoms of meningeal irritation may occur; pleocytosis and Borrelia in the cerebrospinal fluid have been described. The initial attack ends with crisis. There are profuse sweating, sometimes prostration, and occasionally cardiac weakness or collapse. In the intercalate period there is usually noticeable clinical improvement. The relapse sets in acutely with remanifestation of previous symptoms, although milder with each subsequent attack. The pyrexial attacks become shorter and the intercalate period longer.

In tick-borne fever ophthalmic and neurologic manifestations are special features. Iritis, iridocyclitis, retinitis, choroiditis, and temporary blindness may occur. Cerebral involvement may generate coma, focal hemiplegia, meningitis, aphasia, and cranial nerve palsies. These may appear late and remain as sequelae.

Convalescence in both fevers is protracted. The mortality is reported at from 2 to 8 per cent. It can be much higher in epidemic outbreaks of louse-borne fever.

Diagnosis. Except in epidemic periods, definitive diagnosis of relapsing fever depends on demonstration of borreliae present in the peripheral blood, mostly in the early pyrexial period. Borrelia can sometimes also be found in the lesions of the rash. In wet blood films borreliae can be seen under the light microscope, but preferably by dark-field illumination. The organisms are diagnosed in Wright- or Giemsa-stained films. When these methods fail, intraperitoneal inoculation of infected whole or citrated blood (0.2 to 0.5 ml) into young white mice or rats gives rise to detectable borrelemia within 24 to 48 hours.

From the onset there is a marked polymorphonuclear leukocytosis, 15,000 to 25,000 per cubic millimeter, with increase in immature forms. Blood sedimentation is accelerated. There are secondary anemia and urobilinuria, and sometimes also albuminuria and hematuria.

Agglutinating, complement-fixing, immobilizing and borrelicidal antibodies can readily be demonstrated in the serum of infected persons. IgG hyperglobulinemia occurs initially after infection, followed by a rise in IgM immunoglobulin (Felsenfeld, 1969). Inconstant variations between species and strains and variability of antigen and antibodies, even during the fever attack in the same person, limit the usefulness of serodiagnostic procedures. Reagin tests, e.g., VDRL for syphilis are reactive in 10 to 20 per cent of cases. The Weil-Felix test is reactive in titers of 1:80 or higher. Lice removed from patients can be shown to contain borreliae after grinding, suspension, and inoculation of mice. Demonstration of borreliae in ticks in this way is only presumptive evidence, because some ticks carry the organism but are unable to transmit it to the human host. Chick embryos can be infected, and this is the basis for a method of detecting positive ticks collected in nature (Bairamova).

In the differential diagnosis of relapsing fever, confusion may arise with other acute infectious fevers, notably *malaria, typhus,* and *dengue,* but also *influenza* and *early smallpox.* When jaundice is present, *yellow fever* and *leptospirosis* should be considered. The differences emerge as the attack develops. However, definitive diagnosis depends on detection of Borrelia.

Treatment. The patient with relapsing fever is extremely ill. Bed rest, careful nursing, ample fluid, and careful diet are necessary. Antimicrobial drugs are therapeutically effective. One of the tetracyclines (tetracycline, oxytetracycline, or chlortetracycline) is the treatment of choice (Bryceson et al., 1970). When proper medical and nursing care of individual sporadic cases is possible, intravenous injection is preferred during the later phase of febrile attacks. Oral administration is indicated during afebrile intervals or in older patients, e.g., 0.5 gram every four to six hours for three to five days, and then 1 gram twice daily for another three to five days. In children under ten years of age, half doses are used. Chloramphenicol, streptomycin, and novobiocin are also effective, but for various reasons are not the preferred treatment. In epidemic situations with many cases and when individual nursing care is not possible, repository or other penicillin preparations should be given in large doses to prevent failures. All borrelicidal drugs may give rise to initial exacerbation of symptoms in a Herxheimer type of reaction similar to that observed in treponematoses. A more cautious therapeutic approach and subsidiary treatment of the general and particular symptoms of the patient may then be required (e.g., hydrocortisone prior to drug administration).

Prevention. No effective vaccine has been developed. Antimicrobial drugs, e.g., repository penicillin used prophylactically, have been described to be effective under epidemic conditions. Prevention of louse-borne relapsing fever is through avoiding exposure to body or head lice, notably by personal hygiene, cleanliness, and disinfestation of louse-infested clothing and persons. DDT-resistant louse strains have developed since World War II, and control may depend on the use of other insecticidal powders or residual sprays, e.g., the dimethyldithiophosphate group (Malathion).

Tick-borne relapsing fever is much more difficult to control, because the vectors do not live on the victim. The ticks inhabit cracks of walls and floors of houses, caves, burrows of small animals, and so forth. Some ticks are night feeders and require intensive search to be discovered. Newer insecticides have a high, but not complete, degree of success against ticks, e.g., benzene hexachloride (Lindane), dimethyl dithiophosphate (Malathion), naphthylmethylcarbamate (Carbaryl). In rural endemic relapsing fever areas, avoidance of ticks might mean a change in the domestic environment and habits of residents. Exclusion of animals, maintenance of smooth walls and floors, installation of windows, and upgrading of housing are generally necessary for long-term prevention.

Bairamova, R. A.: Experience in infecting chick embryos with tick spirochetes by means of infected Ornithodoros. Journal Microbial (Moscow), 40:83, 1963 (English summary).
Bryceson, A. D. M., Parry, E. H. O., Perrine, P. L., Warrell, D. A., Virkotich, D., and Leithead, C. S.: Louse-borne relapsing fever. Quart. J. Med., 39:130, 1970.
Coffey, E., and Eveland, W. C.: Experimental relapsing fever initiated by *B. hermsi.* J. Infect. Dis., 117:23, 28, 29, 1967.
Correa, P.· Baylet, R. J., and Brougein, P.: À propos d'un cas de fièvre recurrent chez un nouveau-né ou l'infection par voie transplacentaire parait peu contestable. Bull. Soc. Med. Afr. Noire Lang. Fr., 9:215, 1964.
Felsenfeld, O.: Borrelia. Strains, Vectors, Human and Animal Borreliosis. St. Louis, W. H. Green, 1971.
Felsenfeld, O.: Borrelia. *In* Burrows, W. (ed.): Textbook of Microbiology. 20th ed. Philadelphia, W. B. Saunders Company, 1973.
Gefel, A., Anzarut, A., and Pruzanski, P.: Clinical picture and therapy of tickborne relapsing fever. Israel Med. J., 23:211, 1964.
World Health Organization: Louseborne relapsing fever. Wkl. Epid. Rec., 44:425, 1969.

252. PHAGEDENIC TROPICAL ULCER

Thorstein Guthe

Ulcerative skin processes are often encountered in outpatient clinics and hospital practice in the intertropical zone. In addition to clinical types recognizable etiologically, as in treponematoses, leprosy, blastomycosis, and leishmaniasis, the phagedenic ulcer is sufficiently common and characteristic to be considered as a distinct entity. It prevails in tropical Africa, the West Indies, Central and South America, Asia, and Oceania.

Repeated experimental ulcer production in human volunteers (Panja, 1951) supports attributing an *etiologic role* to spirochetes resembling *Borrelia vincentii* and/or fusiform bacilli which are present in sloughs and deep tissues of phagedenic tropical ulcers. Proteus, staphylococci, and hemolytic streptococci are invaders of ulcers of one week's duration. Hot, humid climate furthers the occurrence—sometimes epidemic—of phagedenic ulcers in the intertropical zone, notably in jungle-forest regions. Trauma is a precipitating factor, whether by excoriation, insect bite, or wound. They provide portals of entry for the infective agents on unprotected skin, usually of young males with an active occupation, rarely in females. Forest and plantation workers, labor gangs, campaigning soldiers, and similar workers, as well as individuals of all races, are attacked. Some 90 to 95 per cent of lesions occur on the lower third of the limbs. Deficiency of protein, vitamin A, and other nutrients may favor the occurrence of ulcers, if not their chronicity. The latter is also ascribed to impaired local circulation, anoxemia, and formation of arteriovenous shunts, as in varicose ulcers.

The *course* of phagedenic ulcers is characterized by an acute phase of one to ten days' duration. A papule rapidly develops into an angry hemorrhagic bulla with surrounding inflammation and necrotization, which leads to a round, cup-shaped, fetid, painful ulcer, 3 to 6 cm in diameter, with ragged edges and a sloughing debris-covered base. The ulcer is usually single. In serious cases it may extend and affect deeper tissues, exposing muscle tendons and periosteum. Regional lymphadenopathy is usually absent; fever is moderate and inconsistent. In the later indolent phase the pain subsides and the ulcer base becomes cleaner, with hypertrophic edges owing to epithelial hyperplasia and dermal sclerosis. Ulcers may recur in the same or other areas in 8 to 10 per cent of the cases, suggesting absence of immunity. Prior to penicillin therapy, ulcers sometimes required hospitalization and local treatment for many months. Acute complications are rare (septicemia, gangrene). Chronic complications include carcinomatous changes in ulcers of long duration (Serafino and Menye).

Diagnosis is established on the basis of anamnestic information and the characteristics of the lesion. Demonstration of fusospirochetal organisms is of relative value. Histopathologic characteristics are nonspecific unless malignant changes occur. Among early differential diagnostic considerations are ecthyma, boils, and gangrene, and later the ulcerations of leprosy and treponematoses (notably yaws), leishmaniasis ("oriental sore"), and septic sore ("desert sore"). Phagedenic ulcers may become papillomatous when *T. pertenue* of yaws is implanted. Varicose ulcers are rare in indigenous populations in the intertropical zones. Sickle cell anemia is a not uncommon cause of ulceration, and the presence of sickling should be excluded by appropriate hematologic examinations.

Treatment in the acute stage includes bed rest and local application of mild antiseptic dressings. Intramuscular injections of long-acting benzathine penicillin G (DBED), 1.2 megaunits a week apart with half doses for children (Basset), usually control infection within a few days. Reinforcement of dietary proteins and vitamins has been recommended. In old chronic cases skin grafting is required.

Prevention of phagedenic ulcers is aided by improvement of rural sanitation, development of local health services, and health education. The latter is directed toward bodily cleanliness, protective clothing and footwear, prompt disinfection when injuries occur, and correction of dietary deficiencies.

Basset, A.: Tropical phagedenic ulcer. *In* Simons, P., and Marshall, J. (eds.): Essays on Tropical Dermatology. Amsterdam, Excerpta Medica Foundation, 1969, pp. 25–33.
Castellani, A.: The common ulcers of the leg, cosmopolitan and tropical. J. Trop. Med. Hyg., 60:55, 91, 1957.
Panja, G.: Tropical phagedenic ulcer (Vincent's ulcer.). *In* Gradwohl, R. B. H., Soto, L. B., and Felsenfeld, O. (eds.): Clinical Tropical Medicine. St. Louis, C. V. Mosby Company, 1951, pp. 641–646.
Serafino, X., and Menye, P. A.: Les ulcères phagédéniques cancérisés de jambe. Bull. Cancer (Paris), 55:353, 1968.

253. THE RAT-BITE FEVERS
(Sodoku, Haverhill Fever)
Thorstein Guthe

Definition. Rats are sometimes infected with two independent agents, *Spirillum minus* and *Streptobacillus moniliformis*, also called *Actinobacillus muris*. Rat-bite fever in humans is a clinical syndrome characterized by local lesion, irregular septicemia, metastatic rash, and febrile episodes that commonly follow bites by infected rats, infrequently bites by some other rodents, and rarely bites by carnivores or other animal sources of in-

fection. In humans both the spirillary fever (Sodoku) and streptobacillary fever (Haverhill fever) have similar clinical courses with certain differential characteristics. An etiologic diagnosis can best be established by laboratory means.

Etiology. *S. minus* is a short, thick spirillum 2 to 5 μ long and 0.2 μ wide with three to four regular coils and pointed extremities with tufts of flagella. It exhibits rapid, darting motions in the dark-field microscope. Cultivation in vitro has not been achieved. *Str. moniliformis* is a pleomorphic, nonmotile, gram-negative bacillus 2 to 15 μ long and 0.1 to 0.4 μ wide. It grows in liquid media showing single rods, chains, or long filamentous forms. On solid media symbiont microscopic colonies appear adjacent to or beneath other colonies, and are made up of pleuropneumonia-like stable L-form organisms. Serologic evidence suggests that *Str. moniliformis* may be an intermediate between Corynebacterium and its own L-form (Peace).

Epidemiology. The distribution of both rat-bite fevers is worldwide and coincidental with reservoirs of infected rats where these live in close association with man. Although the rat is the principal natural host, both agents may also inhabit other rodents, e.g., mice, squirrels, ferrets, weasels, and some higher species such as cats, dogs, and pigs. By bites or ingestion of infected cadavers animals infect each other and in turn infect humans. Infection with *S. minus* is usually inapparent in its natural hosts. The agent is mainly in the blood and lacrimal secretion in rodents transmitting infection. Traumatic bleeding of gums and mucosal lesions of the oral cavity may explain nasopharyngeal presence of the agent. Reported prevalence of *S. minus* in rats varies greatly, i.e., 25 per cent in London, 2 to 22 per cent in India, 6 to 14 per cent in Japan, and nil in Atlanta (Brown and Nunemaker). *Str. moniliformis* is found in the saliva and nasopharynx of rodents with inapparent infection. The agent has also been reported to be associated etiologically with epizootics of septicemic infections of wild and laboratory rodents. Apart from bites, streptobacillary fever in humans can also occur by ingestion of food containing infected excreta. Epidemics caused by contaminated raw milk were reported in Haverhill, Massachusetts, and "Haverhill fever" became synonymous with streptobacillary rat-bite fever in the literature (Place and Sutton). Sporadic cases, sometimes in the late stages, continue to be reported (Osimani et al., 1962; McCormack et al., 1967).

Pathology. In spirillary rat-bite fever at the bite site there are intense cellular infiltration, edema, and degeneration leading to necrosis. Degenerative changes occur in the liver and kidneys. Hyperemia of cerebral cortex has been noted. *S. minus* is present at the bite site, in regional lymph nodes, and sometimes in the blood, whereas *Str. moniliformis* can invariably be recovered from the blood as well as from local tissues. The morbid anatomy and histopathology of the rat-bite fevers have not been thoroughly studied. This also applies to the possible role of humoral or cell-mediated immunity in the pathogenesis of the disease. Spirillolytic substances appear in the serum. Cardiolipin antigen tests for treponematoses can be reactive in spirillary infection. In the streptobacillary infection serum agglutinates antigens of the bacillus.

Clinical Manifestations. The clinical features are similar but not identical in both fevers. The incubation periods described vary with averages of two to three weeks in spirillary fever and three days to a week in streptobacillary fever. The modes of presentation of septicemias are diverse, although the onset of symptoms is usually ushered in by chills, nausea, and fever. There is activation of the quiescent bite lesion in spirillary fever, with pain, swelling, edema, and sometimes ulceration of the site of the infecting bite. Regional lymph nodes are also swollen, firm, and nonadherent (Gilbert et al., 1971). This is not a prominent feature in streptobacillary fever. General symptoms include muscle pain, tenderness, and prostration. With each of several episodes of spirillary fever, pain returns with exacerbation of local symptoms. In the streptobacillary variety there may be few fever episodes, even a single one. Migrating arthralgias are encountered in *S. minus* infections, whereas polyarthritis with fibrinous synovial fluid characterizes streptobacillary fever. In spirillary fever the temperature may rise to 40° C and last for two to three days with abrupt fall. All symptoms fade and temperature returns to normal between pyrexial periods. There can be six to eight attacks separated by three to seven days. The attacks then get less frequent, shorter, and milder. The rash may develop with the first or a subsequent fever attack. It is macular or maculopapular in both fevers, and in the spirillary variety sometimes petechial. In spirillary fever the color is notably of a deep purplish shade. The rash is distributed to the trunk and extremities and is not associated with itch. It fades and disappears with the fall of the temperature. It reappears in periods of remission. Endocarditis is reported as a late complication in both fevers; pericarditis has also been described in streptobacillary fever (Carbeck et al., 1967). Sometimes motor and sensory disturbances occur. Urticaria is occasionally observed. The fatality rate in the spirillary fever previously reported at 2 to 10 per cent is greatly reduced by antimicrobial therapy. Most untreated cases subside spontaneously, but others may go on indefinitely.

Diagnosis. A history of rat or other animal bite, infiltration at the bite site, the pattern of the fever, and the rash will in many instances justify a presumptive diagnosis by the physician. Differentiation from other relapsing or trench fevers may be difficult. Malaria may coexist. Weil's disease is rarely transmitted by actual rat bite. The rash may be confused with secondary syphilis or yaws.

Dark-field examination of exudate from the bite site, serous fluid from rash, or aspirate from lymph nodes may confirm a diagnosis of suspected spirillary fever. It is difficult to demonstrate *S. minus* in thick blood drop preparations even at the height of fever attacks. The serum agglutinates spirillum in low dilutions. Reagin tests for treponematoses may be reactive in individuals known not to have had syphilis, yaws, pinta, or bejel. Diagnosis is best confirmed by inoculation of blood, lymph, or excised bite site into the scrotal skin of guinea pigs or intraperitoneally in mice. In streptobacillary fever the microorganism can readily be recovered by culture from the blood, wound serum, or synovial fluid. High serum agglutination titers after three to four weeks are considered of diagnostic value. Reagin tests for treponematoses are usually nonreactive.

Treatment. Lourie and Collier (1943) demonstrated the *spirillocidal* effect of penicillin. This drug is also effective against *Str. moniliformis,* although possibly less so. Time-dose relationship studies in rat-bite fevers concerning choice of short-acting or long-acting penicillin

have not been published. Benzyl penicillin G structured preparations are preferable. The extensive appraisal of therapy in rat-bite fevers by Roughgarden emphasizes that intramuscular dosages of penicillin should (in both fevers) be no less than 0.4 to 0.6 megaunit daily for seven days in the early disease, and that the dosages should be doubled if little or no effect is observed. In endocarditis the dosages should be as in similar conditions of streptococcal origin: 10 to 15 megaunits daily for three to four weeks. Streptomycin, 0.5 gram twice daily for three to four days and half dose for children, and oxytetracycline 0.5 gram initially and half-maintenance doses for several days, have been shown to be effective. These drugs are in reserve for use in penicillin-hypersensitive persons and in patients with streptobacillary infection attributed to persistence of penicillin-resistant L-forms of the organism.

Prevention. Prevention rests on rat destruction. Antiplague measures to extinguish rats also affect the distribution of rat-bite fever, as shown in Manila. Rat-bite wound in children and adults should be treated promptly with antiseptic dressing and a prophylactic dose of penicillin or other effective antimicrobial drug.

Brown, T. M., and Nunemaker, J. C.: Rat-bite fever: A review of the American cases with re-evaluation of etiology; report of cases. Bull. Hopkins Hosp., 70:201, 1942.

Gilbert, G. L., Cassidy, J. F., and Bennet, N. M.: Rat-bite fever. Med. J. Aust., 2:1131, 1971.

McCormack, R. C., Kaye, D., and Hook, E. W.: Endocarditis due to streptobacillus moniliformis. J.A.M.A., 200:77, 1967.

Mollaret, P.: Infektionen nach Katzen- oder Rattenbisse. Münch. Med. Wschr., 111:13, 1969.

Peace, P.: Evidence that *Streptobacillus moniliformis* is an intermediate stage between a corynebacterium and its L-form or derived PPLO. J. Gen. Microbiol., 29:91, 1962.

Roughgarden, J. W.: Antimicrobial therapy of rat-bite fever. Arch. Intern. Med., 116:39, 1965.

Tiriba, A. da C.: Rat bites: Clinical and epidemiological considerations on subsequent infections. Med. Bras., 17:127, 1971.

254.   LEPTOSPIROSIS

Jay P. Sanford

Definition. Leptospirosis is an inclusive term applied to disease caused by all leptospires regardless of specific serotype. Correlation of clinical syndromes with infection by differing serotypes indicates that a single serotype of Leptospira may be responsible for a variety of clinical features; likewise, a single syndrome, e.g., aseptic meningitis, may be caused by multiple serotypes of leptospires. Hence, the general term leptospirosis is preferred rather than the synonyms such as Weil's disease, Canicola fever, etc.

Etiology. The genus Leptospira contains only one species, *L. interrogans,* which may be subdivided into two complexes, interrogans and biflexa. The interrogans complex includes most of the pathogenic strains, whereas the biflexa complex includes mainly saprophytic strains with no recognized hosts. Within each complex the organisms show antigenic heterogeneity which is stable and allows classification into serotypes. Certain serotypes with common antigens are arranged into serogroups. Despite contrary common usage, an example of the correct designation of leptospira is as follows: pomona serogroup of *L. interrogans,* not *L. pomona.* The interrogans complex now contains about 130 serotypes arranged in 16 serogroups (the number in parentheses refers to number of serotypes within the serogroup): Icterohemorrhagiae (13), Hebdomadis (28), Autumnalis (13), Canicola (11), Australis (10), Tarassovi or Hyos (10), Pyrogenes (9), Bataviae (8), Javanica (6), Pomona (6), Ballum (3), Cynopteri (3), Celledoni (2), Grippotyphosa (2), Panama (2), and Shermani (1). At least 22 serotypes of Leptospira occur naturally in the United States.

Prevalence. Leptospirosis, although not a common disease, has been reported from all regions of the United States. Between 1960 and 1973, about 75 cases have been reported annually. Occasional upswings in the number of cases have been the result of common source outbreaks.

Epidemiology. Infection in man is incidental and is not essential to the maintenance of leptospirosis. The infection occurs in a wide range of domestic and wild animal hosts. In many species, such as opossums, skunks, raccoons, and foxes, infectivity ratios in the range of 10 to 50 per cent are not unusual. Interspecies spread of specific serotypes of leptospires between animal hosts is frequent, e.g., *pomona*, a serotype principally associated with livestock, has been demonstrated in dogs. The infection in animals may vary from inapparent illness to severe fatal disease. The carrier state may develop in many animals wherein the host may shed leptospires in its urine for months to years.

It has not been established that pathogenic leptospires are capable of multiplication outside a host. Survival in nature is governed by factors including pH of the urine, soil, or water into which they are shed and ambient temperature. Acid urine permits only limited survival; however, if the urine is neutral or alkaline and is shed into a similar moist environment which has low salinity and is not badly polluted with microorganisms or detergents, and with a temperature above 22° C, leptospires may survive for several weeks. Human infections can occur either directly by contact with urine or tissue of an infected animal or indirectly through contaminated water, soil, or vegetation. The usual portals of entry are abraded skin, particularly about the feet, and exposed mucous membranes, conjunctival, nasal, and oral. The concept that organisms can penetrate intact skin has been questioned. Although leptospires have been isolated from ticks, they appear to be unimportant in transmission.

With the ubiquitous infection of animals, leptospirosis in man can occur in all age groups, at all seasons, and in both sexes. However, it is primarily a disease of teenage children and young adults (at least 50 per cent of patients are between ages 10 and 39 years), occurs predominantly in males (75 per cent), and develops most frequently in hot weather (in the United States two thirds of infections occur from June to October). The wide spectrum of animal hosts results in both urban and rural human disease. Leptospirosis has been considered an occupational disease; however, improved methods of rat control and better standards of hygiene have reduced the incidence among occupational groups such as coal miners and sewermen. Currently less than 20 per cent of patients in the United States have direct contact with animals, i.e., farmers, abattoir workers, or veterinarians. The majority of patients have incidental exposure, two thirds being children, students, or housewives. Swimming or partial immersion in contaminated water has been implicated in one fifth of patients and has ac-

counted for most of the recognized common source outbreaks.

Pathology. In patients who have died with hepatic involvement (Weil's syndrome), renal involvement, or both, the significant gross changes include hemorrhages and bile-staining of tissues. The hemorrhages, which vary from petechial to ecchymotic, are widespread but are most prominent in skeletal muscle, kidneys, adrenals, liver, stomach, spleen, and lungs.

In skeletal muscle, focal necrotic and necrobiotic changes thought to be rather typical of leptospirosis occur. Biopsies early in the illness demonstrate swelling, vacuolation, and subsequently hyalinization. Leptospiral antigen has been demonstrated in these lesions by the fluorescent antibody technique. Healing ensues by the formation of new myofibrils with minimal fibrosis.

The renal lesion in the acute phase involves the tubules predominantly and varies from simple dilatation of distal convoluted tubules to degeneration, necrosis, and basement membrane rupture. Interstitial edema and cellular infiltrates, consisting of lymphocytes, neutrophilic leukocytes, histiocytes, and plasma cells, are uniformly present. Glomerular lesions either are absent or consist of mesangial hyperplasia and focal foot process fusion, which are interpreted as representing nonspecific changes associated with acute inflammation and protein filtration. Microscopic alterations in the liver are not diagnostic, and correlate poorly with the degree of function impairment. The changes include frequent double nuclei and cloudy swelling of hepatocytes, disruption of liver cords, enlargement of Kupffer cells, and bile stasis in biliary canaliculi. The changes in the brain and meninges are also minimal and are not diagnostic. Thickening of the meninges with a polymorphonuclear leukocytic infiltration has been observed. Microscopic evidence of myocarditis, including focal hemorrhages, interstitial edema, and focal infiltration with lymphocytes and plasma cells, has been recorded. Pulmonary findings consist of a patchy, localized hemorrhagic pneumonitis. Special staining techniques utilizing silver impregnation methods have demonstrated organisms in the lumina of renal tubules but rarely in other organs.

Clinical Manifestations. *General Features.* The incubation period after immersion or accidental laboratory exposure has shown extremes of 2 to 26 days, the usual range being 7 to 13 days and the average, 10 days.

Leptospirosis is typically a biphasic illness. *The leptospiremic or first phase* is characterized by the presence of leptospires in the blood and cerebrospinal fluid. The onset is typically abrupt (75 to 100 per cent of patients). Initial symptoms include headache, which is usually frontal, less often retro-orbital, but occasionally may be bitemporal or occipital. Severe muscle aching occurs in most patients, the muscles of the thighs and lumbar areas being most prominently involved and often accompanied by pain on palpation. The myalgia may be accompanied by extreme cutaneous hyperesthesia. Chills followed by high fever are prominent. The leptospiremic phase typically lasts four to nine days. Features during this interval include recurrent chills, high spiking temperatures (usually 39° C or greater), headache, and continued severe myalgia. Anorexia, nausea, vomiting, and abdominal pain are encountered in about one half of patients. Occasional patients have diarrhea (7 to 29 per cent). Pulmonary manifestations, usually either cough or chest pain, have varied in frequency of occurrence from less than 25 to 86 per cent. Hemoptysis occurs but is rare. Examination during this phase reveals an acutely ill febrile patient. A relative bradycardia may be noted. The blood pressure is usually normal, although European authors comment on early hypotension. Disturbances in sensorium may be encountered in up to 25 per cent of patients. The most characteristic sign is conjunctival suffusion which usually appears on the third or fourth day. It may be lacking in some patients, but more often it is overlooked because of its benign nature. This may be associated with photophobia, but serous or purulent secretion is unusual. Less common findings (in 10 to 50 per cent of patients) may include pharyngeal injection, nuchal rigidity, lymphadenopathy, cutaneous hemorrhages, and skin rashes that are usually macular, maculopapular, or urticarial, and usually occur on the trunk. Uncommon findings (usually less than 10 per cent) are splenomegaly, hepatomegaly, or jaundice. Defervescence and improvement in symptoms coincide with the disappearance of leptospires from the blood and cerebrospinal fluid.

The second phase has been characterized as the "immune" phase and correlates with the appearance of circulating antibodies which have been characterized as predominantly IgM class antibodies. The clinical manifestations of this phase exhibit greater variability than those during the first phase. After a relatively asymptomatic period of one to three days, the fever and earlier symptoms recur and meningismus may develop. The fever rarely exceeds 39°C and is usually of one to three days' duration. It is not uncommon for fever to be absent or quite transient. Even when symptoms or signs of meningeal irritation are absent, routine examination of cerebrospinal fluid after the seventh day has revealed pleocytosis in 50 to 90 per cent of patients. Less common features include iridocyclitis, optic neuritis, and other nervous system manifestations, including encephalitis, myelitis, and peripheral neuropathy.

Some clinicians recognize a third or convalescent phase, usually between the second and fourth weeks, when fever and aching may recur. The pathogenesis of this stage is poorly understood.

Leptospirosis during pregnancy may be associated with an increased risk of fetal loss.

Specific Features. WEIL'S SYNDROME. Weil's syndrome, which may be due to serotypes other than *icterohemorrhagiae,* is defined as severe leptospirosis with jaundice, usually accompanied by azotemia, hemorrhages, anemia, disturbances in consciousness, and continued fever. There is uncertainty as to the pathogenesis of the syndrome, i.e., whether it represents direct toxic damage caused by leptospires or whether it is the consequence of immune response to leptospiral antigens. The consensus favors toxic damage.

The onset and first stage are identical with the less severe forms. The distinctive features of Weil's syndrome appear from the third to the sixth day but may not reach their peak until well into the second stage. As in the other forms of leptospirosis, there is a tendency for the fever to lyse about the seventh day; however, with its recurrence it is marked and may persist for several weeks. Either renal or hepatic manifestations may predominate. Hepatic disturbances include tenderness in the right upper quadrant and hepatic enlargement, both of which are common when jaundice is present. SGOT values are rarely increased more than two- to threefold regardless of the degree of hyperbilirubinemia, which is predominantly conjugated (direct); e.g., serum bilirubin

39 mg per 100 ml, SGOT 105 Sigma Frenkel units. The mechanism of hyperbilirubinemia appears to be an intracellular block to bilirubin excretion.

Renal manifestations consist primarily of proteinuria, pyuria, hematuria, and azotemia. Dysuria is rare. The maximal level of blood urea nitrogen is usually reached on the fifth to seventh day. Serious renal damage usually occurs in the form of acute tubular necrosis associated with oliguria. Hemorrhagic manifestations include epistaxis, hemoptysis, gastrointestinal bleeding, hemorrhage into the adrenal glands, hemorrhagic pneumonitis, and subarachnoid hemorrhage. These have been explained on the basis of capillary injury. In addition, in some patients hypoprothrombinemia and thrombocytopenia have been observed.

ASEPTIC MENINGITIS. A leptospiral cause has been incriminated in 5 to 13 per cent of patients with aseptic meningitis. The pleocytosis is not present before the immune phase, when it develops rapidly. There are usually tens to hundreds of cells, occasionally 1000 per cubic millimeter, which may be neutrophils or mononuclear cells. The cerebrospinal fluid glucose level is almost always normal, i.e., greater than 60 per cent of the concomitant blood glucose, but occasional instances of lowered glucose levels have been recorded. In contrast to the observations with many viral causes of aseptic meningitis, with leptospirosis the cerebrospinal fluid protein may exceed 100 mg per 100 ml early in the course. Xanthochromic cerebrospinal fluid has been observed in the presence of jaundice. Each of the serotypes of leptospires that are pathogenic for man is probably capable of association with this syndrome. The most prevalent serotypes have been *Canicola, Icterohemorrhagiae,* and *Pomona.*

PRETIBIAL (FORT BRAGG) FEVER. An illness was observed in the summer of 1942 that had an onset identical with that of the first phase of leptospirosis. The most distinctive feature was the development of a rash on about the fourth day, characterized by 2 to 5 cm slightly raised erythematous lesions that were usually symmetrically distributed over the pretibial areas. In contrast to other leptospiral syndromes, splenomegaly occurred in 95 per cent of these patients. This outbreak, which related to exposure while swimming, was caused by the Autumnalis serogroup. Subsequently Pomona has been observed in association with rashes, which are usually truncal in distribution but have also been pretibial in location.

MYOCARDITIS. Cardiac arrhythmias, including paroxysmal atrial fibrillation, atrial flutter, ventricular tachycardia, and premature ventricular contractions, have been described, but are usually of little clinical significance. However, on rare occasions definite cardiac dilatation with acute left ventricular failure has been observed. Associated manifestations have included jaundice, pulmonary infiltrates, arthritis, and skin rashes. The serogroups thus far incriminated have included Icterohemorrhagiae and Pomona.

Laboratory Features. Leukocyte counts vary from leukopenic levels to mild elevations in the anicteric patients. In patients with jaundice, leukocytosis as high as 70,000 per cubic millimeter may be present. However, regardless of the total leukocyte count, neutrophilia of greater than 70 per cent is very frequently encountered during the first stage.

Hemolytic substances have been demonstrated in cultures of pathogenic leptospires. In contrast to many hemolysins of bacterial origin, which are not hemolytic in vivo, the leptospiral hemolysins appear active in vivo. In patients with jaundice, anemia may be severe and is most characteristically due to intravascular hemolysis. Anemia owing to leptospirosis is unusual in anicteric patients.

Rarely thrombocytopenia sufficient in magnitude to be associated with bleeding is encountered. The erythrocyte sedimentation rate is elevated in more than one half of patients but is usually less than 50 mm per hour.

Urinalyses during the leptospiremic phase reveal a high frequency of abnormalities, including mild proteinuria, casts, and an increase in cellular elements. In anicteric infections, these abnormalities rapidly disappear after the beginning of illness. Proteinuria and abnormalities in urine sediment are usually not associated with elevations in blood urea nitrogen values. Since the anicteric form of the disease has often gone undiagnosed, estimates of the frequency of azotemia and jaundice are probably high. Azotemia has been reported in approximately one fourth of patients. In three fourths of these patients the blood urea nitrogen is less than 100 mg per 100 ml. Azotemia is usually associated with the occurrence of jaundice. The serum bilirubin levels may reach 65 mg per 100 ml; however, in two thirds of patients the levels are less than 20 mg per 100 ml.

Diagnosis. Diagnosis is based upon either cultural or serologic studies. The most common initial diagnostic impressions in patients with leptospirosis are meningitis, hepatitis, nephritis, "FUO," and influenza. Leptospires may be isolated quite readily during the first phase from blood and cerebrospinal fluid or during the second phase from the urine. Leptospires may be excreted in the urine for up to 11 months after the onset of illness. Whole blood should be inoculated immediately into tubes containing semisolid medium, such as Fletcher's. If culture medium is not available, leptospires reportedly will remain viable up to 11 days in blood anticoagulated with sodium oxalate. Animal inoculation (preferably of either suckling hamsters or guinea pigs) may also be used and is of particular value if specimens, e.g., urine, are contaminated. Direct examination of blood or urine by dark-field methods so frequently results in failure or misdiagnosis that it should not be employed as the only diagnostic test. Antibodies appear from the sixth to the twelfth day of illness. Four serologic tests are available: the macroscopic plate agglutination test (the easiest to perform but a relatively insensitive technique), hemolytic test (complex in performance but requiring only a single antigen), microscopic agglutination test (complex in performance but most specific), and complement-fixation test. Serologic criteria for diagnosis include a fourfold or greater rise in titer during the course. Cross-agglutination reactions between various serotypes commonly occur so that the infecting serotype often cannot be determined with certainty without isolation of leptospires.

Prognosis and Sequelae. Between 1965 and 1968, there were 10 deaths (4 per cent) in 277 patients reported in the United States. Age is the most significant host factor related to increased mortality. In a representative series, the mortality rose from 10 per cent in men less than 50 years of age to 56 per cent in those over 51 years of age. The virulence of the infecting leptospires correlates best with the development of jaundice. In anicteric patients, mortality is essentially unknown. With the occurrence of jaundice, mortality in various series has ranged from 15 to 40 per cent. The long-term prognosis after the acute renal lesion of leptospirosis is good. However, a few patients exhibit residual tubular dysfunction, e.g., a defect in renal concentrating ability, and a patient with permanent renal damage has been recorded.

Therapy and Management. A variety of antimicrobial drugs, including penicillin, streptomycin, the tetracycline congeners, erythromycin, and oleandomycin, have been effective in vitro and against experimental leptospiral infections. The data obtained from controlled observations in man are conflicting as to over-all efficacy. If antimicrobial drugs have any beneficial effect, they must be administered within four days, and preferably within two days, of the onset of illness. The agents most studied have been penicillin G and the various tetracycline congeners. Turner states that large doses of penicillin G or tetracycline are indeed advantageous. Within four to six hours after initiation of penicillin G therapy, a Jarisch-Herxheimer type reaction may occur, which suggests antileptospiral activity. There is general agreement that antimicrobials administered after the fifth day have no beneficial effect. Since diagnosis within the first five days requires a very high index of suspicion, management is primarily supportive. The clinical impression exists that early bed rest may minimize the subsequent morbidity. The presence of azotemia and jaundice requires meticulous attention to fluid and electrolyte therapy.

Alston, J. M., and Broom, J. C.: Leptospirosis in man and animals. Edinburgh and London, E. S. Livingstone, Ltd., 1958.
Berman, S. J., Tsia, C. C., Holmes, K., Fresh, J. W., and Watten, R. H.: Sporadic anicteric leptospirosis in South Vietnam. Ann. Intern. Med., 79:167, 1973.
Edwards, G. A., and Domm, B. M.: Human leptospirosis. Medicine, 39:117, 1960.
Heath, C. W., Jr., Alexander, A. D., and Galton, M. M.: Leptospirosis in the United States. Analysis of 483 cases in man, 1949–1961. N. Engl. J. Med., 273:857, 915, 1965.
Nelson, K. E., Ager, E. A., Galton, M. M., Gillespie, R. W. H., and Sulzer, C. R.: An outbreak of leptospirosis in Washington State. Am. J. Epidemiol., 98:336, 1973.
Ooi, B. S., Chen, B. T. M., Tan, K. K., and Khoo, O. T.: Human renal leptospirosis. Am. J. Trop. Med. Hyg., 21:336, 1972.
Turner, L. H.: Leptospirosis. Br. Med. J., 1:537, 1973.

Section Five.   THE MYCOSES

255.   INTRODUCTION

John P. Utz

Recent developments in epidemiology and histopathologic techniques and the development of amphotericin B as an effective antifungal drug have led to a great increase in awareness of the medical problem of systemic fungal disease. The fact that infection occurs with fungi that are free-living forms in soil, decaying vegetation, and bird excreta poses a difficult problem of control. The deliberate impairment of immune response, e.g., to decrease host versus graft reactions in patients with organ transplants, has created still another setting for infection by "opportunistic" fungi. It is a safe speculation that systemic mycotic infection will continue to be an increasing cause of human disease.

Although the chapters that follow are devoted to the mycoses per se, it should be pointed out that fungi have other pathways through which they can produce disease. P. K. C. Austwick has well summarized these phenomena:

Fungi cause three main types of animal and human disease:

Mycoses: diseases resulting from the invasion of living tissues by the fungus.

Allergies: diseases resulting from the development of hypersensitivity to fungal antigens.

Toxicoses: consisting of the *mycotoxicoses* resulting from the ingestion of toxic fungal metabolites formed in food, and the *mycetisms* resulting from the ingestion of toxic fungal fruiting bodies.

There are also two indirect ways in which fungi can be involved in pathogenic processes in animals, viz., by inducing the formation of toxic substances (including estrogens) by a host plant which is then eaten by an animal; by so degrading a foodstuff that macro-nutrient deficiencies appear in animals feeding on it; and by forming substances such as enzymes, which, although not acting directly on metabolic processes themselves, affect the availability of growth substances to the animal, e.g., vitamins, which may lead to micro-nutrient deficiency.

Fungal pathogenicity thus covers a much wider range of activity than that seen in other pathogenic microorganisms, and its height of complexity may be realized when it is possible for all three types of disease to be present in one individual animal, each caused by the same species of fungus playing three different roles at one and the same time. After all, infection and allergy together due to *Aspergillus fumigatus* are not uncommon in man.

Further complications arise in the existence of two types of fungal thallus morphology in vivo. Firstly, apical hyphal growth leads to spherical or disc-like colonies whose spread is by peripheral extension and by fragmentation, a process compensating for its slowness of dissemination by the provision of relatively large inocula for its extension, and so of more certainty of success. Secondly, the self-replication of single cells either as yeast cells or endosporulating spherules can more readily play a leading role in the dissemination of infection in the body, but for this the fungus is generally dependent upon phagocytosis. It may be said that, in the first instance, the fungus is essentially active, making its own way through the tissues and, in the second, passive and dependent on the bloodstream or blood cells for transport. The latter type of growth is also directly comparable to that in many bacterial and viral infections, being frequently accompanied by acute pyrexial symptoms, while the former is generally associated with a chronic inflammatory process extending sometimes over many years.

Failure to understand this fundamental difference in the behavior in vivo of fungi has led to much confusion in the classification of fungal disease, and it still remains a major problem when trying to generalize on the pathogenesis of the mycoses. The ability of fungi to adopt a wide range of vegetative morphology according to their environment is being increasingly observed, and a number of filamentous saprophytic fungi are now known to be capable of budding as yeast cells under defined experimental conditions, e.g., *Mucor rouxii* and *Aspergillus parasiticus* (Bartnicki-Garcia and Nickerson, 1962; Detroy and Ciegler, 1971). The possession of hyphae or of a unicellular state therefore bears no relationship to the classification or to the potential pathogenicity of the species.*

The systemic mycoses have important properties in common in addition to this point of origin in nature. With few exceptions, they are not contagious from animal to man or man to man, and epidemics or outbreaks arise from a common source. Infection is acquired by inhalation or, in a few instances, by traumatic implantation. The primary focus is usually the lung, and infection spreads hematogenously or, less commonly, by direct extension. The gross and microscopic appearance of infected tissue is that of a granulomatous process. The immunologic response is generally effective (reinfection is rare), and cellular and serologically mediated immune mechanisms have been demonstrated (see Ch. 60 to 70).

256.   HISTOPLASMOSIS

John P. Utz

Definition.   Histoplasmosis is a systemic fungal disease, respiratory in origin, that spreads to the pulmonary lymphatics and by the blood to the mediastinal lymph nodes, spleen, liver, adrenals, gastrointestinal tract, kidneys, skin, central nervous system, heart, and other organs. It may be asymptomatic, acute, and benign, or progressive and eventually fatal.

History.   Darling in Panama in 1905 reported three fatal cases of disseminated disease, which he considered to be due to a *"plasmodium"* with a rigid wall or *"capsule,"* in *histiocytes* which he termed *Histoplasma capsulatum.* In a study of tissue section, da Rocha Lima concluded in 1913 that the agent was a fungus. In 1934 De Monbreun correctly identified the fungus in cultural and laboratory animal studies. Ten years later Christie and Peterson recognized the benign form of human disease with pulmonary calcification and associated skin hypersensitivity to histoplasmin. Subsequently, Palmer

---

*From Austwick, P. K. C.: The pathogenicity of fungi. *In* Microbial Pathogenicity in Man and Animals. Twenty-second Symposium of the Society for General Microbiology, Imperial College, London. Cambridge, England, Cambridge University Press, 1972.

showed widely varying rates of hypersensitivity according to geographic areas in this country.

Etiology. *H. capsulatum* has two morphologic forms, *yeast* and *hyphal*, dependent upon a variety of environmental factors. The yeast form seen in tissues measures 2 to 3 by 3 to 4 μ and has a clear area resulting from shrinkage of cytoplasm from the rigid cell wall. In artificial media or natural substrate the yeast form is converted readily at room temperatures to the hyphal form with the production on Sabouraud's glucose medium of a white to brown cottony mold. On microscopic examination this is composed of branched hyphae, characteristic spherical forms with spiny projections (tuberculate macroconidia) 8 to 14 μ in diameter, and smaller forms (microconidia) measuring 2 to 5 μ. Conversion of the hyphal to the yeast form occurs characteristically after inoculation into animals or less readily on enriched media at 37° C. Skin hypersensitivity, complement-fixing, and other antigens have been demonstrated. Mice and guinea pigs are susceptible to experimental infection.

Epidemiology. Histoplasmosis occurs with highest frequency in infancy and old age and equally in the sexes except more often in the male in old age. It has been reported in more than 30 countries in both temperate and tropical zones. Skin hypersensitivity rates are as high as 80 to 90 per cent in some parts of the eastern and midwestern United States. Rates of skin reactivity increase rapidly with age to young adulthood and then more slowly thereafter. Man and animals are infected by inhalation of the fungus in dust. Soil from chicken houses or from areas contaminated or composted by bat or bird dung is especially rich in organisms. Massive exposure through such activities as destruction of chicken houses, exploration of caves, or community "clean-up" activities has resulted in outbreaks. Fifty per cent of dogs and cats in some areas and many species of wild animals are known to be infected. *Histoplasma duboisii*, a closely related fungus, produces in African patients a disease marked by lymphadenopathy and bone, joint, and skin involvement.

Pathology. The tissue reaction is characteristically engulfment of yeast forms by histiocytes or macrophages derived from organs of the reticuloendothelial system. Epithelioid or histiocytic granulomas are formed, with tubercle-like nodules, caseation necrosis, and calcification in the lung, lymph nodes, liver, spleen, adrenals, and other organs. The organism can best be identified in tissues by culture or by use of special stains (periodic acid–Schiff, Gridley, or Gomori methenamine silver methods). However, fungal cells may be few, crowded, and not differentiated with certainty from those of *H. duboisii, Blastomyces dermatitidis, Torulopsis glabrata,* or *Candida albicans.*

Clinical Manifestations. On the basis of delayed cutaneous hypersensitivity studies, it appears that primary infection with *H. capsulatum* is usually asymptomatic or produces a respiratory illness that is not distinctive.

Primary Acute Form. The primary acute form is characterized by respiratory symptoms of cough, shortness of breath, pleuritic chest pain, hoarseness, hemoptysis, and cyanosis in that order. Associated generalized symptoms are commonly fever, chills, myalgia, malaise, and weight loss. In focal outbreaks where there is exposure to large numbers of spores, sudden onset and pleuritic pain are common. Pleural effusion, however, is rare. The chest film may show bilateral disease with the characteristic diffuse miliary type of lesion, or, more commonly, localized infiltrations, especially in the lower lobes. There may be hilar and peritracheal lymphadenopathy unaccompanied by other lesions. That infection is not localized to lungs alone is attested to by the frequent splenic calcification seen later and the occasional isolation of *H. capsulatum* from urine during the acute illness. In many patients lesions resolve completely, but in others calcification or fibrotic scarring persists. Calcified peribronchial nodes may compress the bronchus leading to bronchiectasis or may erode and result in broncholithiasis. A distinctive residue of primary infection is the solitary nodule of the lung, located just beneath the pleura, appearing roentgenographically as a "coin lesion."

Progressive Disseminated Form. Rarely the disease progresses and resembles that form originally described by Darling. Pulmonary findings are often not prominent; illness is characterized instead by fever, enlargement of the liver and spleen, generalized lymphadenopathy, weight loss, anemia, and leukopenia. One particular feature may predominate, and illness then appears as endocarditis, pericarditis, meningitis, adrenal insufficiency, or multiple ulcerations of mouth, pharynx, larynx, stomach, or small or large bowel. Granulomatous uveitis has been considered, but not yet proved, to be due to *H. capsulatum.*

Chronic Cavitary Form. In older adult males especially, a chronic, cavitary pulmonary disease occurs that closely simulates and is often labeled tuberculosis. This form is characterized by cough, weight loss, dyspnea, low-grade fever, chest pain, and hemoptysis. This form is most likely a reactivation of a previously quiescent primary infection.

Diagnosis. The isolation in culture and microscopic identification of the fungus establish the diagnosis. In suspected cases of acute primary disease both sputum and urine should be cultured. In the widely disseminated forms, blood, bone marrow, cerebrospinal fluid, ulcer swabs, urine, sputum, lymph nodes, and material from liver biopsy may yield the fungus on culture. Conversion of a skin test from negative to positive and a titer of the complement-fixing antibodies that rises and falls or is in excess of 1:32 only support the clinical impression. A single positive histoplasmin skin test indicates only recent or remote exposure to this or related antigen. Frequently, both skin and complement-fixation tests will be negative in a patient with severe or early disease. Careful microscopic study of properly stained tissue sections may reveal characteristic fungal forms, providing additional supporting evidence for the clinical diagnosis (see Pathology).

Acute primary histoplasmosis should be considered in the differential diagnosis of any persistent febrile respiratory disease, especially those occurring after exposure to chicken or other bird excreta and in any pneumonia without appropriate bacteria in sputum. Hepatosplenomegaly, lymphadenopathy, anemia, and leukopenia of the severe disseminated form may closely simulate Hodgkin's disease and leukemia. Mucosal alterations so closely resemble cancer that repeated biopsies for tissue study have been performed, all with negative results, before cultures were done. As a general rule, histoplasmosis should be suspected in any patient with findings suggestive of tuberculosis but without supporting laboratory data.

Treatment. Amphotericin B is the most active of the

presently available antifungal drugs for the treatment of the disease in man. The drug is customarily given intravenously; a dose of 1.0 mg dissolved in 500 ml of a 5 per cent glucose solution is recommended as the first dose. Dosage should be increased daily by increments of 5 to 10 mg. At present there are many recommendations and no consensus as to optimal daily dosage (from 0.5 to 1.0 mg per kilogram), duration of therapy (from 6 to 14 weeks), or total dosage (from irrelevant to at least 2 grams). Each infusion should be administered over at least a two-hour period. Such undesired side effects as local thrombophlebitis, fever, chills, nausea, vomiting, anorexia, rise in serum urea nitrogen, hypokalemia, and anemia may occur in approximately 80 per cent of patients but should not require abandonment of the therapy. After treatment is stopped, most indices of renal function return toward normal, but in about 80 per cent of patients on higher drug doses values are never again the same as before treatment. Salicylates, antihistamines, and corticoids reduce the severity or frequency of such side effects of treatment as nausea, chills, and fever.

A few patients with localized disease in the lungs have been helped by surgical excision of lesions.

Sulfonamides have a measurable benefit in infections in laboratory animals and a reported activity in disease in children.

Prognosis. Except in localized outbreaks with inhalation of large numbers of fungi, acute primary histoplasmosis is almost always a benign illness from which the patient recovers rapidly. Therapy usually has not been administered.

Since progressive disseminated disease is fatal in 80 to 90 per cent, and the chronic cavitary form in 30 per cent of cases, chemotherapy is indicated. Approximately 80 to 90 per cent of patients with severe disease have recovered with amphotericin B treatment.

Corticoid treatment has been associated with deleterious effects in experimental infections of animals and with relapse after amphotericin B therapy in man.

Austwick, P. K. C.: The pathogenicity of fungi. In Microbial Pathogenicity in Man and Animals. Twenty-second Symposium of the Society for General Microbiology, Imperial College, London, April 1972. Cambridge, England, Cambridge University Press, 1972.
Butler, W. T.: Pharmacology, toxicity and therapeutic usefulness of amphotericin B. J.A.M.A., 195:371, 1966.
Drutz, D. J., Spickard, A., Rodgers, D. E., and Koenig, M. G.: Treatment of disseminated mycotic infections: A new approach to amphotericin B treatment. Am. J. Med., 45:406, 1968.
Furcolow, M. L., Doto, I. L., Tosh, F. E., and Lynch, H. J., Jr.: Course and prognosis of untreated histoplasmosis. J.A.M.A., 177:292, 1961.
Vanek, J., and Schwarz, J.: The gamut of histoplasmosis. Am. J. Med., 50:89, 1971.

257. COCCIDIOIDOMYCOSIS (Valley Fever)

Demosthenes Pappagianis

Definition. Coccidioidomycosis is a fungal infection usually acquired by the respiratory route. In most cases it is arrested in the lungs, but it may spread to virtually all organs or tissues. Chronic persistent infection may ensue. Infrequently the infection is fatal.

History. The disease we recognize as coccidioidomycosis was first described in 1892 by Alejandro Posadas in an Argentinian man in Buenos Aires. In the infected tissues a cystlike organism thought to be a protozoan

was observed. The second case was reported in 1894 by Rixford in California, the place of origin of the succeeding several hundred recognized cases, and resemblance of the organism to the protozoan Coccidia led to the name Coccidioides. Ophuls and Moffitt in 1900 recognized the causative organism to be a cultivable mold in vitro. Most early recognized cases of coccidioidal infection were severe, often with widespread cutaneous and visceral lesions, and frequently fatal, but Gifford and Dickson in the early 1930's established that San Joaquin or valley fever was a mild infection caused by *Coccidioides immitis*. Introduction of amphotericin B in 1956 led to successful therapy in coccidioidal infections with an otherwise dismal outlook.

Etiology. In the infected host, *C. immitis* exists as a spherule (sporangium), 20 to 100 μ in diameter, and reproduces by formation of few to several hundred endospores. These endospores are released and in turn enlarge to mature spherules. The filamentous septate *mycelial* form usually found in cultures and in nature produces chains of *arthrospores*. These arthrospores (about $2 \times 5 \mu$) are readily airborne and constitute the inhaled infectious form of the organism. Confirmation of the identity of *C. immitis* requires demonstration of the spherule form of the organism in the patient or by animal inoculation, and constitutes the single best diagnostic procedure.

Epidemiology. Coccidioidomycosis is usually encountered in the southwestern United States (California, Arizona, New Mexico, Texas, southern portions of Nevada and Utah), Mexico, Central America, Argentina, Paraguay, Venezuela, and Colombia. These areas correspond to location of *C. immitis* in the soil. Travelers may acquire the infection during brief visits to these areas. Rarely exportation of the fungus on some product of the endemic region can lead to infection elsewhere. The true *incidence* is likely greater than the 300 to 400 cases reported per year in California, or the more than 500 per year in Arizona. Some 50 deaths per year caused by coccidioidomycosis are reported in the United States. It has been estimated that 25,000 to 35,000 new infections occur per year in California. About a fifth of those so affected will have symptomatic infections that bring them to a physician. The *prevalence* of coccidioidomycosis increases during the dry, dusty summer and fall. An occupational risk of infection exists in agricultural or other disturbers of the soil. In some endemic areas the proportion of the population which has been infected increases with time of residence and may exceed 85 per cent. *C. immitis* survives for months at −20 to 42° C and a pH of 4 to 9. It can be found in rodent burrows and elsewhere, persisting for years in the soil. Rodents, dogs, cattle, sheep, and other animals are also infected by inhalation of arthrospores. The infection is not spread from animals to man or from man to man (although one case of in utero infection has been reported).

Humans from a few weeks to 85 years of age have been infected. In general, infection may be milder in children. In adults, about 60 per cent of infections are asymptomatic. Of the 40 per cent with symptomatic infections, most will recover. Approximately 1 in 100 adult white males with symptoms will develop disseminated coccidioidomycosis. Filipinos and blacks have higher rates of dissemination. Adult white females less frequently develop disseminated coccidioidomycosis, perhaps because of their greater tendency to develop the prognostically favorable erythema nodosum.

Pathogenesis and Pathology. The nature of the response to infection with *C. immitis* appears related to the morphologic states of the organism and to the development of delayed hypersensitivity. Endospores appear to induce a granulocytic response, spherules a macrophagic response. Lesions may resemble closely the granulomatous lesion of tuberculosis or sarcoid, but frequently there is juxtaposed suppuration. The mixed inflammatory reaction may yield amorphous necrosis, hyalinization, fibrosis, and calcification. The contribution of delayed hypersensitivity to pathogenesis is not clear, but anergy to coccidioidin is prognostically unfavorable.

Primary infection usually presents as a pneumonitis. (Fewer than 20 cases of primary cutaneous coccidioidomycosis have been reported.) The infection is usually arrested in the pulmonary parenchyma and regional nodes. Occasionally the organisms spread lymphogenously and hematogenously to virtually any tissue (the gastrointestinal mucosa has not been involved, and the brain and the endocardium only rarely). Such dissemination usually ensues early after the primary infection, but occasionally the pulmonary lesion has cleared by the time dissemination is apparent. In about 5 to 10 per cent of patients with primary pulmonary coccidioidomycosis, a chronic cavity or granuloma will develop. Viable *C. immitis* may persist for years in such lesions, although the patient's clinical status remains favorable. Pulmonary cavities occur and recur more frequently in patients with diabetes mellitus.

Clinical Manifestations. Clinically apparent primary pulmonary coccidioidomycosis will develop in 7 to 28 days (average, 10 to 16 days) after inhalation of the spores, presenting with fever, malaise, pleuritic pain, dry cough, night sweats, anorexia, headache, and weight loss. Chest pain is common and may be severe. Early after onset of symptoms, a macular, urticarial, scarlatiniform or morbilliform rash may develop transiently. It may be seen particularly in the inguinal areas and on the palms and soles, and often before coccidioidin sensitivity develops. Such a rash is seen more frequently in children.

Along with the respiratory component, "valley fever" classically includes erythema nodosum of the anterior tibia or erythema multiforme of the extensor aspects of the upper extremities, palms, and upper thorax and neck. This may be seen in about 40 per cent of adult white females and 5 per cent of adult white males who have symptomatic infections, and is accompanied by arthralgia and swelling of ankles and knees. Erythema nodosum indicates marked sensitivity to coccidioidin and is not likely to be coccidioidal in cause if the skin test is negative. Initially primary coccidioidomycosis may be bronchial or peribronchial. The chest x-ray may reveal pneumonitis resembling acute bacterial, mycoplasmal, viral, or other fungal pneumonias with lobar, lobular, or scattered patches of infiltrate. Hilar densities (parenchymal and adenopathy) and pleural effusion are common. Infrequently there is pericardial effusion. A transient cavity occasionally develops during the acute phase. Primary infection of the skin yields an ulcerative lesion and regional adenopathy. Resolution of primary pulmonary coccidioidomycosis usually occurs within several weeks, although asthenia and easy fatigability may last for several months. There may be persistent and unexplained chest pain despite recovery from the acute infection.

Dissemination of the infection to metapulmonary tissues usually occurs during the early weeks or months of infection. However, meningitis or other forms of dissemination may also be recognized only after the primary pulmonary lesion has faded. The progression is sometimes difficult to discern clinically until an overt lesion of bone, skin, lymph node, or meninges is detected. It may be suspected from deterioration of the patient with persistent fever, weight loss, marked bronchomediastinal adenopathy, or mental deterioration (in meningitis), or from labratory parameters to be discussed below.

Chronic cavities, coccidioidomas, or *bronchiectasis* may remain after apparent clearing of the primary pneumonitis, or they may be detected on routine roentgenograms years after the primary infection. Hemoptysis may be the first indication of a pulmonary cavity.

Diagnosis. Awareness of the extreme variability of clinical patterns offered by coccidioidomycosis is essential. It may resemble influenza; bacterial, mycoplasmal, or other mycotic pneumonia; acute or chronic tuberculosis or histoplasmosis; or neoplasms. The hilar or bronchomediastinal adenopathy may resemble that of sarcoid or lymphomas. The chronic pulmonary cavity is characteristically thin-walled on x-ray, but may resemble a pulmonary abscess or be partially filled with fluid. Coccidioidal fibrosis or bronchiectasis may resemble that of other causes. Lesions of bones or soft tissues may resemble those of blastomycosis, tuberculosis, or other bacterial infections. The erythrocyte sedimentation rate is elevated, and there is often a moderate leukocytosis, sometimes with eosinophilia. Sustained eosinophilia is unfavorable.

Coccidioidal meningitis may resemble tuberculosis or other mycotic meningitis. Decrease in the cerebrospinal fluid (CSF) glucose is often an early significant change. Occasionally in the early stages there may be a polymorphonuclear pleocytosis, but the onset is usually more insidious and the CSF changes in cell and protein are suggestive of chronic or "aseptic" meningitis. A "paretic" colloidal gold curve often accompanies these changes.

Coccidioidomycosis is confirmed by direct demonstration of endosporulating spherules in biopsied tissue or exudates utilizing special fungal stains. *Cultures* from lesions or sputum also yield a diagnosis, provided that animal inoculation is used to confirm the production of spherules. The CSF should be cultured but often fails to yield *C. immitis*.

The time involved and hazard of working with *C. immitis* cultures require that appropriate skin test and serologic studies be carried out. The coccidioidin (mycelial phase antigen) skin test may become positive in three days to three weeks after onset of symptoms. A positive coccidioidin skin test means past or present infection. A negative test does not exclude a coccidioidal cause, for the test is often negative in disseminated infections or with old pulmonary lesions (cavities or coccidioidomas). The skin test should be repeated in following the course of the illness, for anergy is unfavorable. The skin test does not interfere with coccidioidal serologic studies. A newly developed skin test antigen derived from spherules may be more sensitive in detecting sensitivity. Precipitins (IgM) are produced early and assist in diagnosis of primary infections. These are detected by a tube test and by a latex particle agglutination test. They fade within the first few weeks but may persist in severe infections and may reappear, e.g., with a bronchopleural fistula or in reinfection via ventriculoperitoneal or ventriculoatrial shunt. Complement-fixing (CF) antibodies (IgG) appear later and may persist for many months or years after recovery. They are readily detected by immunodiffusion. The CF antibody titer rises proportional to severity (extent of involvement). Thus metapulmonary dissemination is usually reflected in an elevated titer (usually above 1:16, but this level may vary between laboratories), and declining titer indicates improvement. Pleural, joint, and cerebrospinal fluids may contain CF antibody, although usually at lower titer than in the serum. Indeed in coccidioidal meningitis the CSF is occasionally seronegative but the serum positive. The basilar meningitis may yield CF-positive cisternal and lumbar fluids even though the ventricular fluid is negative. Complement fixing by the CSF is usually diagnostic of coccidioidal meningitis, although an extradural (paravertebral) abscess can yield CF antibody in the CSF. In this instance the CSF protein is up, with glucose and cells normal.

The CF test is positive in about 60 per cent of cases with chronic coccidioidal cavities, but is often negative in patients with asymptomatic coccidioidomas. Thus diagnosis of the latter is often not assisted by serologic tests. Cross-reactions occur between *C. immitis, Histoplasma capsulatum,* and *Blastomyces dermatitidis* in serologic and skin tests. Primary coccidioidal infections are sometimes accompanied by higher CF titers with Histoplasma and Blastomyces antigens. Sequential sera should yield higher homologous titers.

Treatment.   Symptomatic therapy is indicated for primary coccidioidomycosis. Amphotericin B is the only useful antifungal agent in coccidioidomycosis and should be applied in most cases of disseminated disease. Occasionally, as with a small single cutaneous lesion, excision may be curative. In the absence of overt evidence of dissemination, systemic amphotericin may be administered for severe primary coccidioidal infection or when the clinical or laboratory picture indicates likelihood of dissemination. Amphotericin may be administered intravenously on alternate days, with the dose gradually raised to 1.0 mg per kilogram of body weight or according to the sensitivity of the strain of *C. immitis.* Prolonged therapy is often needed in coccidioidomycosis, increasing the risk of nephropathy, hypokalemia, anemia, phlebitis, and other side effects. Meningitis can be treated preferably by intracisternal administration of up to 1.0 mg, usually three times a week. Arachnoiditis has frequently complicated lumbar administration; however, recent experience with amphotericin given with 10 per cent (hyperbaric) glucose had less of this complication. Under some circumstances amphotericin may be given by the intraventricular route via the Ommaya reservoir and catheter. The total dose required must be determined by the progress of the patient. Therapy of meningitis should be continued for at least three months after the CSF becomes normal, but continued vigilance for years is required because of the possibility of relapse.

Excisional therapy may also be needed for osseous, articular, or soft tissue lesions. Pulmonary cavities, although generally benign, may be resected if complicated by progressive enlargement, rupture into the pleural space, hemorrhage, or secondary infection. Pre- and postoperative therapy with amphotericin is advisable, although some thoracic surgeons have had few complications without such coverage. The usually benign solitary pulmonary nodule may have to be resected for differentiation from other lesions.

Immunotherapy with Lawrence's leukocyte transfer factor from coccidioidin-sensitive donors has had limited trials. This may provide an important additional therapeutic modality, particularly in anergic patients who have not responded to amphotericin or who may be at risk of recurrence of cavities, e.g., diabetics.

Prognosis.   Prior to amphotericin therapy, more than half the patients with disseminated infections and all with coccidioidal meningitis died. With amphotericin therapy, patients with coccidioidal meningitis have survived for 10 to 15 years, some apparently cured. Nonmeningeal disseminated infections have also been successfully treated, although infections involving joints may be recurrent despite treatment with amphotericin B. Recovery from infection leads to resistance to reinfection (exogenous reinfection has occurred only in a very few laboratory workers). Immunosuppressive therapy of intercurrent disease such as Hodgkin's disease with accompanying cytotoxic therapy may reactivate old arrested coccidioidomycosis.

Prevention.   A vaccine prepared from killed spherules has provided good protection of laboratory animals and has appeared safe in humans. However, it has not had a field trial in humans exposed to infection. Avoidance of exposure to the arthrospores would prevent infection, but the widespread distribution of the organism and impracticality of eradicating if from the soil make avoidance difficult in those who are occupationally tied to the soil. The use of lightweight masks or other measures to reduce inhalation of spores during overt dusty exposures is justified.

Ajello, L. (ed.): Coccidioidomycosis. Tucson, University of Arizona Press, 1967.

Einstein, H.: Coccidioidomycosis, *In* Buechner, H. A. (ed.): Management of Fungus Diseases of the Lungs. Springfield, Ill., Charles C Thomas, 1971, Chap. 4.

Fiese, M. J.: Coccidioidomycosis. Springfield, Ill., Charles C Thomas, 1958.

Huntington, R. W., Jr.: Coccidioidomycosis. *In* Baker, R. D. (ed.): Human Infection with Fungi, Actinomycetes and Algae. New York, Springer-Verlag, 1971, Chap. 6.

Smith, C. W., Saito, M. T., and Simons, S. A.: Pattern of 39,500 serologic tests in coccidioidomycosis. J.A.M.A., 160:546, 1956.

258.   BLASTOMYCOSIS (North American)

John P. Utz

Definition.   Blastomycosis is a chronic systemic fungal disease, respiratory in origin, which, classically, disseminates to the skin and occasionally to subcutaneous tissue, bone, and other organs.

History.   In 1894 Gilchrist and in 1898 Gilchrist and Stokes reported the first two cases and named the responsible fungus *Blastomyces dermatitidis.*

Etiology.   *B. dermatitidis* is a dimorphic fungus existing in tissue as a yeastlike form (8 to 15 μ, rarely 30 μ), with a characteristic thick wall (0.5 to 0.75 μ). The yeast form reproduces by budding, and the typical bud is characterized by its large size and attachment to the parent cell by a persistent wall and a wide pore. On Sabouraud's glucose medium *B. dermatitidis* grows as a white mycelium composed of slender hyphae to which are attached, either directly or by lateral slender stalks (conidiophores), smooth spherical 2 to 10 μ forms (conidia). Skin hypersensitivity, complement-fixing, and other antigens have been demonstrated. Mice and other laboratory animals are susceptible to experimental infection.

Epidemiology.   Blastomycosis was at first exclusively American in distribution: Canada, Mexico, Central

America, northern Latin America, and, in 98 per cent of reported cases, the United States. Recently, however, cases have been reported from widely separated sites in Africa. The disease affects all ages, but there is a slightly higher frequency in the third and fourth decades. Males are affected six to nine times more frequently than females. Man is usually infected by inhalation of conidia, but the saprophytic source of the fungus in nature is not known. In one reported instance genital infection was acquired conjugally. Benign, subclinical cases have been reported, but skin test studies do not support a high incidence of infection in certain areas similar to that of histoplasmosis and coccidioidomycosis. Multiple cases in one small town have been reported.

Pathology. The characteristic tissue response to *B. dermatitidis* is a combination of suppuration and epithelioid and giant cell granulomas. In the lung the disease may be localized or may spread as a bronchopneumonia. Cavitation and circumscribed, calcific nodules are rarely encountered. The skin lesions reveal characteristically pseudoepitheliomatous hyperplasia and microabscesses in which *B. dermatitidis* may be seen. In bone, subcutaneous tissue, meninges, prostate, epididymis, and other organs the histologic appearance is again a combination of suppuration and granulomas.

Clinical Manifestations. *Primary Pulmonary Form.* Primary pulmonary blastomycosis begins usually as a mild respiratory infection (rarely as a fulminant pneumonia) with cough, pleuritic chest pain, and, occasionally, hemoptysis. As the disease progresses, generalized symptoms of fever, night sweats, anorexia, and weight loss appear. Physical signs may not be prominent. However, there may be dullness, bronchial breath sounds, and rales characteristic of consolidation. Roentgenographically, manifestations vary from those of a consolidated lobar pneumonia to multiple infiltrations. Hilar adenopathy is common, localized nodules are less so, and cavitation is rare. Although pleural disease is common, effusion is characteristically extremely rare.

Cutaneous Form. Although cutaneous blastomycosis represents spread from a primary pulmonary infection, the presenting complaint of many patients is a cutaneous lesion, either solitary or multiple. The initial papule or pustule progresses within weeks or months into an ulcerated or warty lesion. The advancing border of this lesion is serpiginous, dusky red, or violaceous, elevated 1 to 3 mm, and has an outer edge that slopes abruptly. The base of the lesion contains small abscesses, from which characteristic budding yeast cells can be demonstrated. The central area may become crusted or, in older lesions, may be healing with a thin atrophic scar. In contrast to the skin lesion that follows accidental laboratory implantation, regional lymphadenopathy does not occur.

Other Systemic Forms. A subcutaneous form of the disease consists of single or more often multiple soft to firm nodules, palpable deep beneath the skin. These may enlarge to become bulging abscesses, but in various stages contain pus. The skin over the nodules may have a slightly reddish hue.

Osteomyelitis or periostitis of long bones or spine occurs frequently. The first manifestation of disease may be a psoas abscess. A septic arthritis may occur either alone or by extension from bone.

Genitourinary blastomycosis is frequently seen in men and is manifested by pain and swelling of the epididymis, prostate, or seminal vesicles.

There may also be involvement of the central nervous system, eye, adrenals, thyroid, and larynx. In contrast to paracoccidioidomycosis, the gastrointestinal tract is almost never involved.

Diagnosis. Although skin lesions may be strongly suggestive, the diagnosis of blastomycosis is confirmed by the finding of typical budding yeast cells in direct preparations or by the culture and identification of *B. dermatitidis* from pus or lesions. When appropriate, sputum, urine, cerebrospinal fluid, bone marrow, or other biopsy and autopsy tissue should also be cultured. Skin tests are almost always negative and, especially in earlier stages of the disease, serologic procedures may show a higher titer or a positive reaction only to *Histoplasma capsulatum.*

The pulmonary form of the disease is rarely diagnosed clinically or roentgenographically and is usually thought to be tuberculosis or, less frequently, sarcoidosis, acute bacterial pneumonia, malignancy, or other fungal infections more common in the geographic area. Skin lesions are suggestive of basal cell carcinoma, tuberculosis, nodulo-ulcerative syphilid, pyoderma, or other fungal infections. Other systemic manifestations mimic those of tuberculosis or other chronic bacterial infection.

Treatment. Amphotericin B has been used extensively for all forms of blastomycosis. Details of administration are given in Ch. 256. Rather less drug is necessary, however, and for involvement of organs and tissues other than bones, 1 to 2 grams is usually sufficient.

2-Hydroxystilbamidine, administered intravenously, is probably less toxic than amphotericin B. It is a satisfactory alternative only in nonprogressive cutaneous disease. The usual dosage has been 225 mg per day and 8.0 grams per course of therapy.

Surgical drainage of abscesses is frequently indicated. Chemotherapy before and after surgery is advisable.

Prognosis. Pulmonary infection of an inapparent or benign form occurs only rarely. Blastomycosis is, if untreated, a chronic and usually progressive disease. Cutaneous and other disseminated disease is eventually fatal in 10 to 30 per cent of cases.

Except with moribund patients chemotherapy usually effects a prompt recovery. Relapse requiring additional therapy has occurred, however, in at least 10 to 15 per cent of patients.

Lockwood, W. R., Allison, F. L., Batson, B. E., and Busey, J. F.: The treatment of North American blastomycosis: Ten years' experience. Am. Rev. Respir. Dis., 100:314, 1969.

Witorsch, P., and Utz, J. P.: North American blastomycosis. A study of 40 patients. Medicine, 47:169, 1969.

259. PARACOCCIDIOIDO-MYCOSIS
(South American Blastomycosis)
John P. Utz

Definition. Paracoccidioidomycosis is a chronic systemic fungal disease, probably respiratory or gastrointestinal in origin, with dissemination to the lymph nodes, skin, lung, and other organs.

History. Lutz in 1908 first described the disease and the organism observed in tissues of a Brazilian patient. In 1909 and 1912, Splendore described more fully the characteristics of the disease and the fungus.

Etiology. The disease is caused by a dimorphic fungus, *Paracoccidioides brasiliensis,* which appears in tissues and exudates as a multiple-budding yeast 2 to 60 μ in diameter. The bud is characterized by a thin wall (0.2 to 1.0 μ) and narrow pore. At temperatures less than 30° C on Sabouraud's glucose medium, a white (later brown) membranous or wrinkled mycelium appears that microscopically is composed of branching hyphae and oval forms (conidia). Delayed cutaneous hypersensitivity and complement-fixing antigens have been demonstrated. Guinea pigs and mice can be experimentally infected.

Epidemiology. Except for reports of occasional patients in North America, the disease occurs exclusively in residents of Central and South America and is especially prevalent in Brazil. It is approximately ten times more frequent in males, and is slightly more frequent in persons 40 to 50 years of age. Manual laborers and farmers seem especially susceptible. Infection is probably acquired by the respiratory route, but a saprophytic, environmental source of fungi is not known. Disease in animals and animal-to-man or man-to-man spread are unknown. Widespread infection of a benign form has been suggested by skin test surveys.

Pathology. The histopathologic reaction to *P. brasiliensis* may be suppurative with abscess formation; in other sites it may be granulomatous with fibroblasts, macrophages, lymphocytes, caseation, and giant cells containing organisms. Lesions are seen in the mucosa of the gastrointestinal tract, lymph nodes, spleen, lungs, and liver.

Clinical Forms. *Primary.* The primary lesion is commonly on the oral or nasal mucosa. Rarely, the conjunctival or anorectal mucosa may be involved. The earliest lesion is a papule that ulcerates and spreads to adjacent tissue.

Cutaneous Form. A variety of skin lesions may be seen, most of which progress to an ulcerative, crusted form suggestive of blastomycosis. In contrast, however, regional lymphadenopathy frequently accompanies skin lesions only in paracoccidioidomycosis. A keloidal form (Lobo's disease) of milder nature, without lymphadenopathy and caused by a different species (*P. loboi*), may be another type of paracoccidioidomycosis.

Lymphangitic Form. In this form there are lymphangitis and enlargement of regional lymph nodes, which suppurate and drain. Cervical and submandibular nodes are most commonly affected.

Visceral Form. The gastrointestinal tract is frequently involved as a primary site of infection. The spleen, adrenals, lungs, and liver may be affected by hematogenous spread. Bone, myocardium, and central nervous system involvement are less frequently seen.

Diagnosis. The diagnosis is established by the culture and identification of *P. brasiliensis* and is only supported by positive skin and complement-fixation tests.

The disease must be differentiated from syphilis, tuberculous adenitis and skin disease, yaws, leishmaniasis, and other fungal infections.

Treatment. Amphotericin B (see Ch. 256) is the drug of choice. In the past, continuous sulfonamide therapy resulted in remission but not cure.

Prognosis. All forms of the disease are fatal if un-treated. Over 90 per cent of cases are cured by amphotericin B.

Furtado, T. A., Wilson, J. W., and Plunkett, O. A.: South American blastomycosis or paracoccidioidomycosis. Arch. Dermatol., 70:166, 1954.
Hildick-Smith, G., Blank, H., and Sarkany, I.: Fungus Diseases and Their Treatment. Boston, Little, Brown & Company, 1964.
Kroll, J. J., and Walzer, R. A.: Paracoccidioidomycosis in the United States. Arch. Dermatol., 106:543, 1972.

260.   MADUROMYCOSIS
(Mycetoma, Madura Foot)

John P. Utz

Definition. Maduromycosis is a chronic systemic fungal disease that follows traumatic or imperceptible implantation of the skin. It is characterized by swelling, induration, suppuration, and draining sinuses of the skin, subcutaneous tissue, and bone, typically of the foot.

History. The disease was first recognized and described in 1712 by Kaempfer in India, and was called Madura foot, after the city of that name. It has been suggested, however, that Madura foot was described by Sophocles in the hero of *Philoctetes.*

Etiology. Many species of ten genera have been reported as etiologic agents; the most common of these have been *Madurella mycetomi, Nocardia brasiliensis,* and, in the United States, *Allescheria boydii.* In tissues or pus these fungi, except for Nocardia (see Ch. 225), are characterized by the appearance of "grains" of oval or irregular shape measuring 0.5 to 2.0 mm, and of white, red, black, or yellow color. Microscopically they are composed of 2 to 4 μ segmented, branched hyphae or round encysted forms (chlamydospores).

A. boydii grows rapidly on Sabouraud's glucose medium, forming a white (later gray or brown) cottony, aerial mycelium, which microscopically consists of thin hyphae to which are attached short or long stalks (conidiophores) bearing a single 8 to 10 by 5 to 7 μ pyriform or ovoid form (conidium). Large (50 to 200 μ) flask-shaped vessels containing asci and spores (4 to 7 μ) can be seen when material from the surface of agar is crushed and examined.

When inoculated intraperitoneally into mice, *A. boydii* is pathogenic, but progressive disease similar to that in humans has not been produced.

Epidemiology. Although occasionally reported from temperate areas, the disease is seen most often in those tropical zones where few people wear shoes. The disease occurs chiefly in adults and more often in males. Most causative organisms are saprophytes of soil or plants. The disease has been reported in the dog, cow, and horse, but animal-to-man or man-to-man spread has not been reported.

Pathology. The typical swollen foot has numerous draining sinuses communicating with abscesses of the skin, subcutaneous tissue, or bone. Drainage sites have characteristic collars of fibrous or epithelial tissues. Suppuration with epithelioid, plasma, and giant cells is intermingled with areas of fibrosis, and one or the other reaction may predominate. With Gram, hematoxylin or eosin, or periodic acid–Schiff stains, fungal cells may be seen either in pus or within macrophages or giant cells.

Clinical Forms. Although lesions have been reported on the leg, torso, hand, and face, the characteristic site of disease is the foot. The first manifestation consists of a papule, small nodule, indurated area with a vesicle, or an abscess that ruptures with sinus tract formation. Infection spreads and new nodules appear, leading to generalized swelling and distortion of the toes. Pain is infrequent, and there are few generalized symptoms. Roentgenographic examination may show lytic lesions with reaction and proliferation of the bone.

Diagnosis. Diagnosis is confirmed by the demonstration of granules in draining material, but the specific cause is dependent on isolation of the fungus in culture. Serologic and skin tests have not been developed for most of the responsible fungi. Maduromycosis must be distinguished from other fungal infections and from tuberculosis, yaws, neoplasms, and elephantiasis.

Treatment. With the variety of antimicrobial agents available, each with specific activity, it is essential that definitive mycologic studies be done prior to treatment to determine the identity and, if feasible, the drug susceptibility of the causative fungus. The failure to do so in many past reports is undoubtedly a factor in the generally pessimistic attitude toward treatment and the early resort to amputation.

The drug of choice for infections caused by *Nocardia brasiliensis* is a sulfonamide (see Ch. 225), whereas for those caused by Aspergillus, amphotericin B is indicated (see Ch. 265). Tetracycline and diaminodiphenylsulfone have been reported to be successful in a few cases of *M. mycetomi* infections. Amphotericin B has been reported ineffective in two cases of *A. boydii* infection. Recently, there have been intriguing reports of benefit in this latter infection related to experimental or clinical use of estrogens.

Prognosis. The disease is usually progressive and rarely self-limited.

Butz, W. C., and Ajello, L.: Black grain mycetoma. Arch. Dermatol., 104:197, 1971.
Carrion, A. L., Hutner, M. S., Nadal, H. M., and Belaval, M. F.: Maduromycosis: An unusual case with a description of the causative fungus. Arch. Dermatol., 82:371, 1960.
Mohr, J. A., and Muchmore, H. G.: Maduromycosis due to *Allescheria boydii*. J.A.M.A., 204:335, 1968.
Zeisler, E. B.: A case from Sophocles. Arch. Dermatol., 84:136, 1961.

261. CHROMOMYCOSIS

John P. Utz

Definition. Chromomycosis is a chronic systemic fungal disease, acquired in the cutaneous form by traumatic or imperceptible implantation, and characterized by wartlike, ulcerated, crusted lesions of the skin and subcutaneous tissues.

History. Although rare in this country, chromomycosis was first reported from Boston in 1915, separately by Lane and Medlar, and the organism responsible was named *Phialophora verrucosa* by Thaxter. Subsequently, cases caused by other genera of fungi were described by Brumpt and Carrion.

Etiology. A number of fungi have been incriminated, but chiefly *Phialophora verrucosa, P. pedrosoi, P. compactum,* and *Cladosporium carrioni.* In tissues these fungi resemble each other and appear as single or clustered, round, thick-walled, 6 to 12 μ budding cells of a striking brown color, from which the disease draws its name. On culture, mycelia are produced that vary according to genus and species. Skin hypersensitivity and complement-fixing antigens have been demonstrated in some fungal species. Laboratory animals are susceptible to experimental infection, but the equivalent of natural disease in man is not produced.

Epidemiology. The disease is seen more often in adult males in the rural areas of the tropics, especially in Brazil, Puerto Rico, and Cuba. The responsible fungi are saprophytes of soil, but are found more often in decaying wood and vegetation. Infection in animals has not been reported, and animal-to-man or man-to-man spread is unknown.

Pathology. Varying degrees of hyperkeratoses, acanthosis, and pseudoepitheliomatous hyperplasia are seen. In the cutis the reaction may be granulomatous with mononuclear, epithelioid, and Langhans' giant cells. Fungal cells are seen readily with hematoxylin and eosin stains.

Clinical Forms. Chromomycosis is a disease of the skin and subcutaneous tissue.

The first patient reported had lesions of the buttock. The most common site is the lower extremity. The disease appears also, in descending order of frequency, on the hand, forearm, arm, neck, and shoulders. The earliest lesion is a nodule or pustule that, over a period of weeks to months, ulcerates, drains, enlarges, dries, and becomes violaceous and wartlike. There is rarely pain, but itching is common. Lesions do not spread generally, but scratching results in autoinoculation and satellite or secondary distal lesions.

Diagnosis. Although older typical skin lesions may be clinically and histologically suggestive, the diagnosis is confirmed by the culture and identification of the causative fungus.

Early lesions may be confused with blastomycosis, tuberculosis, leprosy, yaws, and syphilis.

Treatment. Surgical resection of early skin lesions has been the most common and efficacious therapy. Amputation has been required in a small number of cases. Most of the fungi causing chromomycosis are resistant to amphotericin B, but successful treatment has been reported in two cases when the drug was injected locally into the skin. This drug needs further trial in this disease.

Prognosis. The cutaneous form of chromomycosis is chronic and compatible with long life (in one case, 40 years).

Costello, M. J., De Feo, C. P., Jr., and Littman, M. L.: Chromoblastomycosis treated with local infiltration of amphotericin B solution. Arch. Dermatol., 79:184, 1959.
Vanbreuseghem, R.: Mycoses of Man and Animals. London, Sir Isaac Pitman & Sons, 1958.

262. CRYPTOCOCCOSIS (European Blastomycosis, Torulosis)

John E. Bennett

Definition. Cryptococcosis is a systemic fungal infection, its most common and most lethal manifestation being meningoencephalitis.

History. Busse, who reported the first case in 1894, observed the fungus in tissue and isolated the causative agent. That same year Sanfelice isolated from peach juice the same fungus, naming it *Saccharomyces hominis*. The fungus received no less than 37 additional names until 1952, when Lodder and Kreger-Van Rij's monumental taxonomic study of yeast gave the fungus its current name, *Cryptococcus neoformans*. The fungus was rarely isolated from natural sources until 1955, when Emmons demonstrated that *C. neoformans* was a frequent saprophyte in weathered pigeon droppings. This lent support to the emerging concept that the disease was acquired by inhalation of fungus-laden dust. The discovery of amphotericin B, reported by Gold and co-workers in 1956, was to provide the first successful chemotherapy of cryptococcosis.

Etiology. Cryptococcosis is caused by *Cryptococcus neoformans,* a round or oval yeastlike fungus measuring 4 to 7 μ in diameter. It reproduces by budding. This fungus is unique among systemic mycoses of man in that it is highly encapsulated in tissue. The polysaccharide capsule releases into the host the soluble antigen which provides a means of serologic diagnosis. The fungus can be isolated as a smooth, creamy white colony on a variety of common laboratory media. Culture identification is by gross and microscopic appearance, biochemical reactions, and growth at 37° C.

Epidemiology. The disease is sporadic throughout the world, with no clear focal outbreaks in man or sharply defined areas of high endemicity. Disease occurs occasionally in warm-blooded feral and domestic animals, excluding birds. Cryptococcal mastitis may spread through dairy herds, probably by way of milking machines, and contaminate unpasteurized milk. No spread of infection from animal to man or man to man has been reported. Reservoir of infection is probably saprophytic sources in nature, such as weathered pigeon droppings. Presumed portal of entry is the lung, although this site is often clinically inapparent. The fungus is not a part of the normal flora of man or animals, although occasionally it appears to colonize a patient's damaged bronchial tree. No occupational group is known to be predisposed to cryptococcosis. Infection is uncommon before puberty and is more frequent in males. Predisposing factors include Hodgkin's disease, lymphoma, leukemia, sarcoidosis, and supraphysiologic doses of adrenal corticosteroids.

Pathology. The most frequent and characteristic abnormality on gross examination occurs in the brain, which shows basilar arachnoiditis and focal collections of small, glistening, gelatinous cysts, particularly in the cortical gray matter and basal ganglia. Microscopic examination reveals the cysts to be clumps of cryptococci, with little surrounding inflammation. A dense inflammatory response to the fungus may be noted in meninges or brain but is more characteristic of extraneural lesions. Cellular response consists of macrophages, giant cells, and lymphocytes. Necrosis is seen occasionally at the center of a dense inflammatory response, particularly in the lung. Features notable for their infrequency include polymorphonuclear leukocytes, calcification, extensive scarring, and hemorrhage.

Clinical Manifestations. *Meningoencephalitis.* Symptoms begin with the insidious onset of headache, followed by nausea, vomiting, blurred vision, or decreased mental acuity. Less frequent symptoms include photophobia, diplopia, and gait ataxia. Gradually the patient becomes lethargic and prefers to remain undisturbed. Somnolence or irritability may appear. Fever is low grade or absent. Although no one physical finding is highly frequent or characteristic, examination may disclose papilledema, mild to moderate nuchal rigidity, cranial nerve palsies, or extensor plantar response.

Extraneural Cryptococcosis. Pulmonary cryptococcosis is the second most common clinical manifestation. Even patients with no clinically apparent pneumonitis but with cryptococcosis elsewhere in the body are often found to have a pulmonary focus on careful postmortem examination or sometimes on sputum culture. Chest symptoms and radiologic findings, when present, commonly mimic primary or metastatic carcinoma in the lung. Pleural effusions, cavitation, and hilar adenopathy are not common. Skin lesions occur in 10 per cent of patients with cryptococcosis, and bone lesions occur in about 5 per cent. Either may be the sole clinical manifestation of the infection or may be associated with disease in other organs. Skin lesions begin as asymptomatic papules, pustules, or soft subcutaneous nodules. They tend to become painful as they slowly enlarge, ulcerate, and drain glary pus. Osteolytic lesions may appear in almost any bone and present as a cold abscess. Rare clinical manifestations include prostatitis, hepatitis, endocarditis, pericarditis, renal abscess, and endophthalmitis.

Diagnosis. Lumbar puncture in patients with symptomatic cryptococcal meningoencephalitis usually reveals one or more of the following abnormalities: elevated opening pressure, pleocytosis predominantly composed of mononuclear cells, increased protein concentration, and hypoglycorrhachia. A smear of cerebrospinal fluid sediment, mixed with India ink, reveals encapsulated yeast in about half the cases. The smear may be difficult to interpret and provides only a tentative, albeit useful, diagnosis. Another rapid diagnostic aid is serologic detection of cryptococcal antigen in serum and cerebrospinal fluid. With current techniques, about 70 to 80 per cent of patients with cryptococcal meningitis have detectable antigen if both sites are tested. Extraneural cryptococcosis may result in serum antigen if infection is extensive. A falling antigen titer during recovery is a favorable prognostic sign.

Final diagnosis depends upon culture or biopsy. Several milliliters of cerebrospinal fluid should be cultured for cryptococci in cases of indolent meningoencephalitis and also in every case of documented extraneural cryptococcosis, in order to detect subclinical extension to the central nervous system. The frequency of subclinical renal infection in disseminated cryptococcosis makes urine culture useful. Sputum, blood, prostatic fluid, and pus from cutaneous lesions may also yield the fungus. Biopsy may be required to diagnose cryptococcosis in the lung, skin, or bone. Histologic diagnosis can usually be made with accuracy by those experienced in this area.

Therapy. Intravenous amphotericin B is the treatment of choice for cryptococcosis of the central nervous system. Treatment should be continued for at least four weeks after all weekly cultures become negative. 5-Fluorocytosine should rarely if ever be used alone, but studies currently in progress with combinations of 5-fluorocytosine and amphotericin B appear promising. Intrathecal amphotericin B may be a useful adjunct in patients failing an adequate trial of intravenous therapy or with such poor renal function that reduced doses of intravenous amphotericin B are obligatory. Development of communicating or noncommunicating hydrocephalus may require neurosurgical intervention.

Intravenous amphotericin B is the usual treatment of choice for extraneural cryptococcosis. A probable exception is the patient without either hematologic malignancy or immunosuppressive therapy who, on thorough study, has infection confined to one focus in lung, skin, or bone. Surgical excision of skin or lung lesions, curettage of bone lesions, or simply prolonged observation may be warranted if the lesion is not extensive and is stable or regressing.

Prognosis. Cryptococcal meningoencephalitis is invariably fatal unless treated. With currently available therapy, the case fatality rate is about 25 per cent. Patients with Hodgkin's disease, lymphoma, or leukemia or who require continued immunosuppressive therapy fare less well. Death usually results from the sequelae of coma or from brainstem compression. Despite successful therapy, patients may be left with optic atrophy, hydrocephalus, personality changes, or decreased mental acuity.

Fetter, B. F., Klintworth, G. K., and Hendry, W. S.: Mycoses of the Central Nervous System. Baltimore, Williams & Wilkins Company, 1967.

Littman, M. L., and Zimmerman, L. E.: Cryptococcosis. New York, Grune & Stratton, 1956.

Salfelder, K.: Cryptococcosis. In Baker, R. D. (ed.): Human Infections with Fungi, Actinomycetes and Algae. New York, Springer-Verlag, 1971, pp. 383–464.

263. SPOROTRICHOSIS

John P. Utz

Definition. Sporotrichosis is a chronic systemic fungal disease, acquired usually by traumatic implantation and localized to cutaneous lymphatic tissues, or rarely by the respiratory route with dissemination throughout the body.

History. From a patient at Johns Hopkins Hospital, in 1896 Schenck isolated a fungus that was identified by E. F. Smith as Sporotrichum; it was called *Sporotrichum schenckii* by Hektoen and Perkins in 1900. A great number of cases were seen subsequently in France, and more than 2800 cases in a single epidemic in the gold mines of South Africa.

Etiology. *Sporothrix schenckii,* a dimorphic fungus, is occasionally observed in tissues as round to cigar-shaped yeast- or bacteria-like forms. On Sabouraud's glucose medium at room temperature, a white, cottony, aerial mycelium appears that in three to seven days becomes wrinkled and changes in color from cream to black. Microscopically, branching, septate hyphae are seen, 2 μ in width, bearing directly or on lateral branches ovoid to spherical bodies (conidia) measuring 2 to 4 by 2 to 6 μ in diameter. Mice are susceptible to experimental infection. Delayed cutaneous hypersensitivity and agglutinogen antigens have been demonstrated.

Epidemiology. The disease is worldwide in distribution; it has appeared epidemically in South Africa and in localized outbreaks in Mexico and Florida. It is more common in the male. It frequently affects laborers, farmers, and florists and is considered a true occupational disease. The fungus exists in its saprophytic form in soil, peat moss, and decaying vegetation and on thorns. In the cutaneous lymphatic forms, infection results from accidental implantation into the skin. In disseminated forms, the mode of entry is probably respiratory. Spontaneous sporotrichosis has been reported in dogs, horses, mules, cats, and other animals, and human disease has resulted from animal contact. Direct transfer from man to man is not known to occur.

Pathology. The histopathologic reaction to *S. schenckii* is varied, frequently acute and suppurative, but also subacute or chronic. In some instances granulomas are seen with epithelioid and giant cells either diffusely distributed or localized in a typical tubercle. Fungi may be seen more readily after staining with a modified Schiff-MacManus technique.

Clinical Forms. *Cutaneous Lymphatic Form.* The earliest lesion is a pustule, papule, or nodule of the skin appearing characteristically on a finger and at a site where the patient may recall an earlier, seemingly insignificant scratch or prick. The nodule enlarges, becomes red to violaceous, and is followed by a chain of subcutaneous nodules along regional lymphatics. These at first freely movable nodules may become attached to the skin, and may ulcerate and drain a thin gray to yellow pus. Streaking and pain characteristic of acute lymphangitis are not present. Generalized symptoms are rare.

Other Forms. Other forms may appear secondary to the cutaneous lymphatic lesion either by direct extension to contiguous, subcutaneous tissue, bone, and joint or by hematogenous spread to distant sites. Sometimes the original site of infection is inapparent, and the disease presents as a septic arthritis or osteomyelitis. Less frequently, there may be involvement of the eye, lungs, gastrointestinal tract, central nervous system, or skin. In disseminated disease, systemic symptoms of fever, weight loss, inanition, malaise, pain at sites of lesion, anemia, and leukocytosis are commonly present. Disease limited to the lungs or localized there suggests that there is a respiratory form acquired by inhalation of the fungus. Too few cases have thus far been reported to characterize this form at present.

Diagnosis. Although the diagnosis may seem readily apparent in the cutaneous lymphatic form of disease, the clinical impression is confirmed by the culture and identification of the fungus. Agglutination or complement-fixation serologic and skin tests may be helpful, but are not generally available.

Cutaneous lymphatic sporotrichosis must be distinguished from tularemia, pyoderma of bacterial origin, and other fungal infections. Disseminated disease resembles tuberculosis, staphylococcal osteomyelitis, or neoplastic disease.

Treatment. The cutaneous lymphatic form of disease responds slowly but progressively to the oral administration of iodides in the form of a saturated solution (1 gram per milliliter) of potassium iodide given in dosage of 2 ml four times daily. Treatment should be prolonged one to two months beyond the time of apparent healing.

Disseminated disease, especially of bone and joints, is frequently resistant to iodide therapy. Dramatic improvement has been seen in a few patients treated with amphotericin B, and for this form of disease this drug is recommended.

Prognosis. Untreated cutaneous lymphatic sporotrichosis may persist for many months to years. Treated lesions respond slowly but completely. Disseminated disease is progressive and usually fatal unless treated.

Baum, G. L., Donnerberg, R. L., Stewart, D., Mulligan, W. J., and Putnam, L. R.: Pulmonary sporotrichosis. N. Engl. J. Med., 280:410, 1969.

Gladstone, J. L., and Littman, M. L.: Osseous sporotrichosis. Am. J. Med., 51:121, 1971.

Wilson, D. E., Mann, J. J., Bennett, J. E., and Utz, J. P.: Clinical features of extracutaneous sporotrichosis. Medicine, 46:265, 1967.

264. MUCORMYCOSIS

John E. Bennett

Definition. Mucormycosis is an acute, often fatal infection caused by fungi of the order Mucorales. Phycomycosis is a term which encompasses mucormycosis and several other mycoses.

History. Two cases of pulmonary mucormycosis reported by Fürbringer in 1876 were probably the first cases described with enough clarity to permit any confidence in the diagnosis. It was not until 1943 that Gregory described mucormycosis originating in nose and paranasal sinuses.

Etiology. Rhizopus and Mucor species are the principal pathogens of mucormycosis. These fungi appear in tissue as hyphae 6 to 50 μ wide, rarely septate, irregular in contour, and tending to branch at nearly right angles. Hyphae may be demonstrated histologically by staining with hematoxylin and eosin, Gomori methenamine silver, or periodic acid–Schiff. Growth at 25 or 37° C is profuse and rapidly spreading on most media. Identification of the culture is based largely on microscopic appearance. Only very specialized laboratories are competent to pursue identification beyond a tentative designation of genus.

Epidemiology. Mucormycosis is uncommon and sporadic around the world, usually afflicting patients with serious pre-existing disease. *Cranial mucormycosis occurs predominantly in patients with poorly controlled diabetes mellitus.* Pulmonary and disseminated mucormycosis occurs occasionally in diabetics but is most prevalent in immunosuppressed patients, particularly treated leukemics. Among the varied underlying disorders present in patients with gastrointestinal mucormycosis, uremia, severe malnutrition, and diarrheal diseases seem prominent. Mucormycosis occurs at any age, with no strong predilection for race or sex. It does not spread from man to man. Disease is probably acquired by inhalation of fungal spores. Mucorales are ubiquitous in the environment, growing on decaying vegetation, dung, and foods of high sugar content.

Pathology. Necrosis is the predominant gross and microscopic finding. This is accounted for in part by the propensity of hyphae to proliferate within small and medium-sized arteries, producing thrombosis. Infarcted areas may be ischemic or hemorrhagic. Neutrophils predominate in the inflammatory response.

Clinical Manifestations. Mucormycosis originating in the nose and paranasal sinuses produces a characteristic clinical entity. Initial symptoms mimic bacterial sinusitis, with low-grade fever and sinus pain. However, nasal discharge is not purulent but is thin and sometimes blood streaked. Over the next few days, infection spreads to contiguous structures. Invasion of the orbit may lead to reduced range of ocular motion, proptosis, chemosis, or blurred vision. Direct invasion of the globe or thrombosis of the ophthalmic artery may occur. Nasal turbinates or hard palate develop areas which are black, friable, and bloodless. Frontal or temporal lobes of the brain may be infected by direct extension, producing headache and deepening stupor. Invasion of the carotid artery within the cavernous sinus may cause embolization, mycotic aneurysm, or thrombosis. Without treatment, the patient usually dies in coma a few days to a few weeks from onset.

Pulmonary mucormycosis presents as a rapidly progressive dense bronchopneumonia, accompanied by high fever, toxicity, and tachypnea, but with little cough or sputum. The necrotic central portion of a lesion is sometimes expectorated, producing hyphae in sputum and a cavity on chest x-ray. Gastrointestinal lesions of mucormycosis begin as one or more shallow ulcerations in esophagus, stomach, or intestine. The ulcer tends to enlarge, deepen, and perforate the viscus. Disseminated mucormycosis may originate in nasal area, lung, or gastrointestinal tract. Sometimes no portal is evident. Hematogenous spread may involve brain or other organs. Pulmonary and disseminated mucormycosis are clinically indistinguishable from invasive aspergillosis.

Diagnosis. *Cranial mucormycosis* is easily mistaken for bacterial sinusitis with cavernous sinus thrombosis. The diagnosis requires biopsy of infected mucosa in the nose or sinus. Hyphae are often abundant on histologic section or wet smear of crushed tissue. Hyphae seen in cross-section may be mistaken for yeast. Occasionally hyphae are confused with capillaries, or vice versa.

Pulmonary and disseminated infections caused by Mucorales, Aspergillus, and *Pseudomonas aeruginosa* have many similarities. Diagnosis of mucormycosis, like aspergillosis, requires biopsy. In the proper clinical setting, demonstration of broad, nonseptate hyphae in bronchial brush specimens or sputum would be strongly suggestive. Culture of biopsy specimens is certainly of interest, but isolation of a ubiquitous organism like Mucorales must be interpreted with caution. Blood cultures are very rarely positive for the fungus.

Treatment. Mucormycosis originating in the nose and paranasal areas should be treated by optimal regulation of diabetes mellitus, extensive surgical debridement, and intravenous amphotericin B. After debridement, sinus cavities can be irrigated daily with amphotericin B, 1 mg per milliliter. Although good guidelines for dose and duration of intravenous amphotericin B are not available, it has been customary to treat vigorously at least until disease progression halts. Treatment should probably continue for another month beyond that. Tomograms of the orbit and sinuses can be very helpful in evaluating disease progression. Carotid arteriogram may demonstrate extension to the ophthalmic artery or carotid siphon. Electroencephalogram and lumbar puncture provide late evidence of intracranial extension.

Intravenous amphotericin B is probably useful in other forms of mucormycosis, but too few patients have been treated for this question to be answered.

Prognosis. A substantial number of cures have been reported recently in mucormycosis of the nose, sinus, and orbit. Prognosis is poor once central nervous system signs appear. Other forms of mucormycosis have largely been diagnosed post mortem.

Baker, R. D.: Mucormycosis. *In* Human Infection with Fungi, Actinomycetes and Algae, New York, Springer-Verlag, 1971, pp. 832–918.

Bartrum, R. J., Watnick, M., and Herman, P. G.: Roentgenographic findings in pulmonary mucormycosis. Am. J. Roentgenol., 117:810, 1973.

Battock, D. J., Grausz, H., Bobrowsky, M., and Littman, M. L.: Alternateday amphotericin B therapy in the treatment of rhinocerebral phycomycosis (mucormycosis). Ann. Intern. Med., 68:122, 1968.

Meyer, R. D., Rosen, P., and Armstrong, D.: Phycomycosis complicating leukemia and lymphoma. Ann. Intern. Med., 77:871, 1972.

Price, D. L., Wolpow, E. R., and Richardson, E. P.: Intracranial phycomycosis: A clinicopathological and radiologic study. J. Neurol. Sci., 14:359, 1971.

265. ASPERGILLOSIS

John E. Bennett

Definition. The term aspergillosis embraces a variety of diseases which have in common growth of the fungus Aspergillus in tissue or within air-containing spaces of the body, such as bronchus or pulmonary cavity.

History. Micheli first described the genus Aspergillus in 1729. The first case of aspergillosis in man was probably observed by Sluyter in 1847, although disease in birds had been reported before then. In 1856 Virchow reviewed the literature and reported four autopsied cases. Renon's classic paper of 1897 attracted attention to the disease.

Etiology. The etiologic agent Aspergillus is a fungus largely composed of septate hyphae about 4 μ in diameter. Sporulating structures, called conidial heads, may be seen when the fungus is growing in nature, on artificial medium, or within air-containing spaces of the body. The most frequent pathogen for man is *Aspergillus fumigatus*. However, many other species can clearly cause either invasive or noninvasive disease in man, particularly *Aspergillus flavus*. Aspergilli grow rapidly on many routine laboratory media and, because of their ubiquity, are encountered in the laboratory as airborne contaminants. Identification is by gross and microscopic appearance.

Epidemiology. Aspergilli are often found growing on decaying vegetation. Under proper conditions millions of spores, about 2 to 4 μ in diameter, may be released into the air. Inhalation of these spores must be a common event, but disease is infrequent. Both insects and animals may acquire aspergillosis. The disease is an economically important cause of mycotic abortion in cattle and horses. In man the disease is sporadic and worldwide, with no clear occupational predisposition. Transmission from animal to man or man to man has not been encountered.

Pathology. The fungus is capable of eliciting a wide variety of tissue responses, depending upon site and host. A ball of hyphae may be situated within an ectatic bronchus or epithelialized lung cavity and provoke little or no histologic response. During invasion of tissue in a markedly immunosuppressed host, blood vessel invasion by hyphae, thrombosis, necrosis, and hemorrhagic infarction are prominent features. In invasion of more normal tissue, a pyogenic necrotic reaction is common, but epithelioid granulomas with giant cells may be observed instead. Chronic, fibrosing, non-necrotizing granulomatous inflammation has typically been seen in the paranasal sinus and orbit.

Inhalation of Aspergillus spores may provoke an allergic response without invasion of the body, but this condition will not be considered here. Certain aspergilli, given proper growth conditions, produce proteolytic enzymes or toxins. As far as is known, these substances play no important role in aspergillosis.

Clinical Manifestations. *Pulmonary Aspergillosis.* Aspergillus can colonize ectatic bronchi, cysts, or cavities in the lung. Colonization is usually a sequel of a chronic inflammatory process, such as tuberculosis, bronchiectasis, histoplasmosis, or sarcoidosis. A ball of hyphae may form within an air-containing space, particularly in the upper lobes, and is termed an aspergilloma. The fungus rarely invades the wall of the cavity, cyst, or bronchus in such patients. During bacterial pneumonia, lung abscess, or empyema in a colonized patient,

Aspergillus may appear in the inflammatory process, although its role is uncertain. In most patients it is difficult to determine clinically whether specific symptoms or signs of disease progression are due to the underlying condition or to some allergic, inflammatory, or obstructive process caused by Aspergillus. The most common symptoms are chronic productive cough and hemoptysis. Uncommonly, Aspergillus appears to be the sole cause of chronic pulmonary inflammation. In a few instances, acute bilateral bronchopneumonia has occurred in normal persons, usually after a presumed massive inhalation of spores. However, the majority of patients with invasive aspergillosis now being encountered are markedly neutropenic or are receiving corticosteroid therapy, or both. A patch of bronchopneumonia appears and steadily becomes larger and denser. The lesion may remain focal or, at any time, may spread hematogenously to one or more sites in the lung, brain, or other organs. The lung lesion may also erode directly through the diaphragm or pericardium.

Lesions of Extrapulmonary Origin. Necrotizing lesions originating in the palate, paranasal sinuses, epiglottis, or gastrointestinal tract may occur in the immunosuppressed patient. Aspergillus may infect intracardiac or intravascular prostheses. Chronic granulomatous inflammation may originate in the paranasal sinuses and spread to orbit or brain. Progressive mycotic keratitis caused by Aspergillus may follow corneal trauma. Growth of Aspergillus on cerumen and detritus within the external auditory canal is termed otomycosis.

Diagnosis. Culture of Aspergillus from sputum usually has no clinical significance. Repeated isolation of Aspergillus from sputum or demonstration of hyphae on sputum smear suggests endobronchial colonization. Precipitins to Aspergillus antigens are often demonstrable in the sera of such colonized patients. Radiologic appearance of an aspergilloma is distinctive. In the severely immunosuppressed patient, isolation of Aspergillus from even a single sputum should raise suspicion of possible invasive infection. Biopsy is usually required to diagnose invasive aspergillosis in lung, paranasal sinus, orbit, or brain. Histology may provide evidence of tissue invasion and permit a presumptive diagnosis of aspergillosis. For absolute confirmation and determination of species, the biopsy should be cultured. Neither serologic tests nor cultures of blood, cerebrospinal fluid, or urine are helpful in most forms of invasive aspergillosis.

Treatment. Surgical excision may be helpful in fungus ball of the lung or in aspergillosis of the paranasal sinus and orbit. Measures to improve bronchopulmonary drainage may assist the patient with endobronchial colonization. Intravenous amphotericin B is not helpful in endobronchial or endocavitary aspergillosis, but in invasive pulmonary aspergillosis a prolonged course of treatment will occasionally arrest progression. Ultimate cure of invasive pulmonary aspergillosis requires not only intravenous amphotericin B but also significant restoration of the host's defense mechanisms.

Prognosis. Endobronchial or endocavitary aspergillosis rarely becomes invasive or disseminated. Although the condition is not usually the sole cause of death, it may contribute problems to an already damaged lung. Cure is infrequent in invasive aspergillosis of the lung, heart, paranasal sinus, orbit, or brain.

Green, W. R., Font, R. L., and Zimmerman, L. E.: Aspergillosis of the orbit. Arch. Ophthalmol., 82:302, 1969.

Kilman, J. W., Ahn, C., Andrews, N. C., and Klassen, K.: Surgery for pulmonary aspergillosis. J. Thorac. Cardiovasc. Surg., 57:642, 1969.
Young, R. C., Bennett, J. E., Vogel, C., Carbone, P. P., and DeVita, V. T.: Aspergillosis. Spectrum of the disease in 98 patients. Medicine, 49:147, 1970.

266. CANDIDIASIS
(Candidosis, Moniliasis, Thrush)

John E. Bennett

Definition. Candidiasis is an infection of the skin, mucous membranes, or viscera caused by species of Candida, a yeastlike fungus. Thrush refers to candidiasis of mucous membranes, as in the mouth or vagina.

History. Thrush as a clinical entity has been appreciated for centuries, but its relationship to fungi was unknown until Langenbeck isolated the pathogen from a patient's throat in 1839. Among the many names applied to this fungus, the most significant have been *Oidium albicans* (given by Robin in 1853), *Monilia albicans* (Zopf, 1890) and *Candida albicans* (Berkhout, 1923).

Etiology. *Candida albicans* is the usual cause of candidiasis. A substantial number of cases of disseminated candidiasis have been caused by other species of Candida, particularly *C. tropicalis* and *C. parapsilosis*. The size and shape of Candida cells are variable, but most commonly the cells are oval and 4 to 6 μ in their longest axis. Growth usually appears within a few days of incubation at 25 or 37° C. Deep inoculation into certain media, such as corn meal Tween 80 agar, causes Candida to grow as long tubules called pseudohyphae. Individual species of Candida are distinguished by their ability to utilize or ferment certain sugars. For routine laboratory purposes, *C. albicans* can be identified by its ability to form chlamydospores or, in the presence of serum, to form germ tubes. Candida species look very similar in infected tissue, but usually can be distinguished from other fungi. Candida generally, but not always, grows in tissue as both budding yeast and pseudohyphae. Both tissue forms are well demonstrated by Gomori methenamine silver, periodic acid–Schiff, or tissue Gram stains.

Epidemiology. *C. albicans* is a frequent commensal in the human mouth, gastrointestinal tract, and vagina. Candida is also commonly isolated from the gut of animals. Isolation of this fungus from the environment is unusual, and most of the exceptions could have represented contamination by animals or man. This leads to the presumption that the fungus is spread from man to man and animal to animal. It is usually impossible to trace this spread, because colonization is asymptomatic. A probable exception is the newborn infant, in whom colonization usually leads to oral thrush. Later in life, disease seems to occur when a previously colonized patient becomes more vulnerable to tissue invasion. A wide variety of conditions predispose to candidiasis, particularly diabetes mellitus and therapy with either broad-spectrum antimicrobials or adrenal corticosteroids. Chronic maceration predisposes to cutaneous candidiasis, as in paronychia of bartenders and housewives, intertrigo of obese patients, or diaper rash. Women in the later months of pregnancy are particularly susceptible to vulvovaginal candidiasis. Patients with acute leukemia are prone to gastrointestinal and systemic candidiasis. An important route for acquiring systemic candidiasis is through unsterile intravenous injections of narcotics or through use of plastic intravenous catheters.

When the infusion through the catheter is designed to meet the patient's total caloric requirement, the risk of systemic candidiasis goes even higher.

Pathology. In mucocutaneous candidiasis, pseudohyphae and yeast tend to be confined to the epithelium. Leukocytes infiltrate the epithelium as well as the submucosa or corium. Parakeratosis is usual. Ulceration and hyphal invasion of the submucosa is a more frequent characteristic of gastrointestinal candidiasis. In systemic candidiasis, abscesses may be found in almost any organ, but kidney, lung, spleen, heart, and liver are frequent sites. Such abscesses on gross inspection may appear as small, white, firm, cheesy nodules. Histologically these foci show necrosis, leukocytes, pseudohyphae, and yeast. Giant cells are seen occasionally. In the immunosuppressed patient, inflammatory cells may be scanty or absent. Patients with plastic intravenous catheters may develop at the catheter tip an endovenous fibrin sleeve containing Candida. Presumably, this can continue to seed the bloodstream for several days after withdrawal of the catheter.

Clinical Manifestations. The mouth is the most common site of candidiasis. *Oral thrush* is usually an acute, self-limiting disease which presents as discrete and confluent white plaques on the oral and pharyngeal mucosa. The plaque is a pseudomembrane which can be scraped off with difficulty, exposing a red base. *Candida denture stomatitis* is characterized by well-circumscribed areas of erythema and edema in the mucosa under the upper dentures. Candida also appears to cause chronic hyperplastic oral lesions resembling leukoplakia. All the aforementioned oral lesions tend to be asymptomatic. *Cutaneous candidiasis* can present as diaper rash, red macerated areas in large skin folds, fissuring and desquamation in interdigital areas, angular cheilitis, paronychia, balanitis, or pruritus ani. *Chronic mucocutaneous candidiasis,* also called *Candida granuloma,* is an uncommon disease, usually beginning in early childhood, in which hyperkeratotic lesions wax and wane in the skin and mucous membranes for many years. The most severe skin lesions occur on the face, scalp, and hands. Involvement of mouth, vagina, and nails is usual. Children with this disorder frequently seem to have defective function of thymus-derived lymphocytes and tend to develop hypofunction of the parathyroid, thyroid, or adrenal glands.

The most common symptom of *Candida vaginitis* is pruritus. Other frequent symptoms include discharge and burning pain, the latter being worse on urination or intercourse. Speculum examination reveals an inflamed vaginal mucosa and a thin exudate, sometimes with white curds. Within the gastrointestinal tract, the *esophagus* is the most common site of candidiasis and the only site likely to be symptomatic. Substernal burning and either pain or a sense of obstruction on swallowing may occur. Blood-borne *Candida abscesses* are usually manifest only as fever and toxicity. Hematogenous dissemination to the choroid is detected on funduscopic examination as fluffy white retinal exudates. The abscesses gradually enlarge and extend into the vitreous humor, which becomes increasingly hazy. Cells and flare may also appear in the anterior chamber. The most common symptoms are orbital or retro-orbital pain, blurring, scotoma, and opacities floating across the visual field. *Candidiasis of the endocardium* or around the edges of an intracardiac prosthesis resembles bacterial infections in these sites. *Candida meningitis* clinically mimics cryptococcosis. *Pulmonary and renal candidiasis* are usually hematogenous in origin and cause no focal symptoms. Extensive renal cortical abscesses may cause azotemia. *Candidiasis in the lining of the bladder or renal pelvis* usually appears in a diabetic patient with chronic or recurrent bacterial urinary tract infections or after instrumentation or surgery on the urinary tract. Dysuria, pyuria, and passage of pseudohyphae in the urine are frequent findings. Rarely, pseudohyphae will be found packed in a necrotic renal papilla. A sloughed papilla, largely then a ball of fungus, may obstruct a ureter.

Diagnosis. Demonstration of pseudohyphae on smear with confirmation by culture is the procedure of choice for diagnosing candidiasis of epithelial surfaces. Scrapings for this purpose may be made of skin, oral mucosa, vagina, or nails. Cerebrospinal fluid and joint fluid cultures are helpful in diagnosing Candida meningitis or arthritis. Progression of funduscopic findings usually permits an operational diagnosis of Candida endophthalmitis. Esophagram and esophagoscopy can aid the diagnosis of Candida esophagitis. Biopsy is required to diagnose candidiasis of lung or liver. Blood cultures are very useful in diagnosing Candida endocarditis but are less commonly positive in other forms of systemic candidiasis. The fungus can be isolated from blood, using the same routine media employed for bacteria, but one to three weeks of incubation are often required. Rarely, Candida is seen on blood smear. Skin tests with Candida antigens are so commonly positive in normal people that they are not useful in diagnosing candidiasis. Diagnostic interpretation of serologic tests for candidiasis remains controversial.

Treatment. Oral thrush is best treated by rinsing the mouth with and then swallowing nystatin suspension, 100,000 units four times daily. Painting the lesions with 1 per cent aqueous gentian violet is a messy but effective alternative. Vaginal thrush usually responds to deep insertion of a nystatin vaginal suppository once or twice daily for two weeks. Cutaneous candidiasis of macerated areas requires measures to keep the skin dry plus topical nystatin or amphotericin B. Mild symptoms of Candida esophagitis may respond to the patient's sucking on a nystatin suppository three or four times daily. With pronounced esophageal symptoms, a short course of intravenous amphotericin B is more beneficial. Bladder thrush may be eradicated by bladder irrigation with amphotericin B, 50 μg per milliliter. If a Foley catheter is not in place, oral 5-fluorocytosine is an alternative. Isolation of Candida from blood may or may not indicate the need for intravenous amphotericin B. If the patient is febrile and severely immunosuppressed, a single positive blood culture for Candida is generally an indication for prompt chemotherapy. All too often the patient dies before additional blood cultures are reported positive. In the patient who is not immunosuppressed, significance of candidemia depends upon the number of positive cultures and the presence or absence of a plastic intravenous catheter. Multiple positive blood cultures in the absence of such a catheter indicate the need for chemotherapy. In the presence of such a catheter, discovery of candidemia should prompt removal of the catheter and culturing of its tip. If the patient is not seriously ill and is improving, treatment may be postponed to await clinical progress and the results of subsequent blood cultures. The species of Candida isolated is irrelevant to the decision about therapy. Temporization is inappropriate when endocarditis, endophthalmitis, arthritis, or other hematogenous lesions are detected. Systemic candidiasis is treated with the same daily doses of intravenous amphotericin B as are used with other systemic mycoses. Adequate guidelines for judging duration of therapy are not known. There is also inadequate information to judge whether 5-fluorocytosine has a role in the treatment of systemic candidiasis.

Prognosis. Most forms of mucocutaneous candidiasis are benign and respond to local treatment, although relapse is not rare. Chronic mucocutaneous candidiasis of children responds to intravenous amphotericin B, but relapse is virtually inevitable. For some reason these children rarely develop systemic candidiasis. The ability of treatment to prevent death from most forms of systemic candidiasis and to eradicate candidiasis of the urinary and gastrointestinal mucosa depends largely on the severity of the underlying condition. Candidiasis of the endocardium or around an intracardiac prosthesis is usually fatal despite treatment.

Eras, P., Goldstein, M. J., and Sherlock, P.: Candida infection of the gastrointestinal tract. Medicine, 51:367, 1972.

Fishman, L. S., Griffin, J. R., Sapico, F. L., and Hecht, R.: Hematogenous Candida endophthalmitis—a complication of candidemia. N. Engl. J. Med., 286:675, 1972.

Kirkpatrick, C. H., Rich, R. R., and Bennett, J. E.: Chronic mucocutaneous candidiasis. Ann. Intern. Med., 74:955, 1971.

Winner, H. I., and Hurley, R.: Candida Albicans. Boston, Little, Brown & Company, 1964.

Section Six.   CHEMOTHERAPY OF MICROBIAL DISEASE

267.   DRUGS AND MICROBES

Walsh McDermott

In choosing the initial therapy for a patient with a presumed microbial disease, the physician is confronted with a formidable dilemma. On the one hand, if therapy is to be maximally effective, the correct drug or drug-pairing must be chosen quickly so that it may be administered before significant tissue damage or irreversible physiologic changes have occurred. On the other hand, if the choice is to be made quickly, it is difficult to make it exactly; for there are still only a few techniques by which the cause of an infection can be positively identified during the early hours of acute illness. Thus the physician is in the uncomfortable position of knowing that if he is to obtain the greatest advantages of antimicrobial therapy for his patient, he must make the correct choice of drugs one to five days before solid evidence of the identity of the infection will be forthcoming.

An obvious way out of the dilemma would be by the introduction of rapid diagnostic methods illustrated by techniques such as the use of fluorescent-tagged antibody to swiftly identify organisms. However, surprisingly little effort has been devoted to developing a better, more rapid diagnostic technology. Given this situation, the physician has to rely on his *clinical* acumen and a full knowledge of all the microbial diseases that might reasonably be expected to institute threats to his patients. In actuality, to make this choice of the initial drug regimen from evidence obtained at the bedside is not as difficult as it sounds once the physician realizes what it is that he should be trying to do. While doing it, he can also be comforted by the thought that the expert consultant must go through exactly the same exercise; for he, too, seldom has any secret diagnostic weapons, and is equally hampered by the slowness of the available diagnostic tests. Attempts should be made to differentiate, on clinical grounds, those situations or syndromes that require immediate and intensive action from those that properly may be left to unfold until precise identification becomes possible. Moreover, when a choice of therapy is made, it should be made on the basis of careful consideration of the most serious threats to the patient that are likely. The drug or drugs chosen should be the ones that do most to protect the patient overnight or for a somewhat longer interval against the reasonably likely threats, while at the same time do the least to mask the identity of other infections that might conceivably be present. Above all, once the identity of the infecting microbe *is* established, the physician should be quick to discontinue all but the scientifically relevant therapy.

An example of the exercise involved is as follows:

A young man was first seen with a high fever, a cough, and obviously excruciating pleural pain. His systolic blood pressure was 90 mm of mercury; his leukocyte count was 4000 per cubic millimeter, with a marked increase in immature neutrophils. Less than four hours previously, he had been enjoying himself at the theater, although he had had a mild respiratory infection for the preceding five or six days.

It was apparent that he had an infection, that it was progressing rapidly, and that it involved lung and pleura. What reasonable inferences could be drawn concerning the identity of the infection and hence both its relative threat to him and the appropriate choice of therapy?

At least four microbial species, Pneumococcus, Streptococcus, *S. aureus*, and Klebsiella (Friedländer's bacillus), are capable of producing this particular syndrome, and faced with the individual case there is absolutely no way of differentiating one from another at the bedside. Nevertheless, the clinician knows that this syndrome occurs in such a severe fulminating form in less than 5 per cent of pneumococcal pneumonias, whereas such severity is the characteristic picture of the rapidly necrotizing pneumonias caused by staphylococci, streptococci, or klebsiellae. He also knows that primary staphylococcal pneumonia is extremely rare in the absence of viral influenza, but that as a complication of viral influenza it is by no means uncommon. Here his day-to-day "community epidemiologic knowledge" can stand him in good stead, for he should know whether viral influenza "is around" or has not been seen for some time; in this case, it has been "around." He likewise is aware that staphylococci acquired from hospitalized patients are more apt to be penicillinase-producers than staphylococci acquired in the world at large, so to speak, and he knows that his patient is a medical student. He knows that primary streptococcal pneumonia of this severe type is a rarer phenomenon than primary staphylococcal pneumonia except in the middle of an outbreak of viral influenza. By contrast, Klebsiella pneumonia, although a not unlikely possibility in such a severe pneumonia syndrome, characteristically occurs in middle-aged weakened hosts and would be a most unlikely happening in an otherwise healthy young man.

In this situation as described, the amount of immediately useful knowledge that was produced is considerable. Armed with this knowledge, the physician who knows that he must start drug therapy right away actually has a pretty good idea of the nature of the problem. Indeed, the assembled information made it seem most likely that the patient had a primary staphylococcal pneumonia. Be that as it may, the physician knows the drug regimen he chooses must provide maximal protection against pneumococcus and Streptococcus (penicillin); maximal protection against Klebsiella (streptomycin or gentamicin); and maximal protection against Staphylococcus, including penicillinase producers (oxacillin or a similar drug, along with streptomycin

or gentamicin). Eighteen to 24 hours later when the identity of the infection presumably would become known, the therapy could be modified appropriately. It so happened that the cause of the illness was discovered to be a penicillinase-producing strain of *S. aureus* which was well controlled by the therapy. It should be stressed that once the microbe is identified, the physician's responsibility to modify the therapy is great. Almost invariably the patient has been receiving one or more drugs that are now known to be unnecessary, and the risks of their toxicities should be terminated promptly.

The body of knowledge from which selectivity of the sort described can be obtained is presented in the various chapters on bacterial and mycotic diseases. There are other sorts of knowledge also necessary to the clinician—knowledge about antimicrobial therapy and the drugs themselves (see Ch. 268) and information about some of the microbial mechanisms whereby the impact of drug therapy could be withstood and the microbe survive. One form of survival, viewing the microbial world as a whole, is the "new diseases" that emerge as *endogenous microbial diseases* (see Ch. 178). These "new diseases" are a form of microbial survival of drug challenge, because they ensure that *some* microbes will endure. To ensure the survival of a particular microbial species and hence a particular disease, however, there are two other and quite different survival patterns, *microbial persistence* and *microbial drug resistance*. The latter phenomenon, under the name "drug-fastness," had been recognized since the early days of this century. Microbial persistence, on the other hand, was not recognized—indeed could not be recognized—until the development of penicillin, because it was only then that a powerful antimicrobial drug could be given in virtually any dosage and thus permit exclusion of the obvious possibility that the microbial survival was only a consequence of underdosage.

Microbial Persistence. Microbial persistence can be defined as the phenomenon whereby a microbial strain that is susceptible to a drug in the test tube is nevertheless capable of surviving long-term exposure to that drug in the body. Persistence is thus sharply distinguished from drug resistance, which is a heritable property of a microbial strain and is demonstrable in the test tube as well as in the body. In numerical terms, microbial persistence is of the greater importance, because it is the phenomenon that is responsible for most instances of post-treatment relapse, that interferes with the effectiveness of chemoprophylaxis, and that balks attempts to use drugs for the "eradication" of microbes (see Ch. 268). Once recognized and studied, it became clear that microbial persistence—the drug-related phenomenon—was only one aspect of the larger phenomenon of latent microbial infection with its potentiality for evocation as endogenous microbial disease. As our knowledge accumulates, it is likewise beginning to appear as if microbial persistence and genotypic drug resistance are veering toward each other, and may eventually come to overlap. Persistence thus serves as a link between the other two phenomena, and indeed all three may ultimately be seen to shade into each other. However, we are not yet at that point. Recognition of the present clearly visible difference among the three has been most valuable in that it has made it possible for each to be recognized, reasonably well defined, and isolated for study. For more detailed consideration of these phenomena, the reader is referred to the references at the end of this chapter. Certain aspects of microbial persistence and heritable drug resistance deserve mention at this point.

Until microbial persistence was recognized in the 1940's, the conceptual base of antimicrobial therapy was *therapia sterilisans magna* as originally conceived by Ehrlich; namely, the goal was to effect a total eradication of the infecting microbes from the host. With penicillin and the subsequently introduced drugs, it was discovered that such total eradication did not occur uniformly and predictably. In a significant number of cases of virtually any bacterial disease, drug-susceptible cells of the infecting strain could be isolated well after completion of drug therapy. At times these persisters would increase and produce clinical relapse, which was then easily treatable by the appropriate drug. At other times they would persist in the carrier state or might ultimately disappear either into latency or presumably by leaving the host altogether. Evidence was obtained that this microbial survival could not be explained by failure of drug delivery, namely, that the microbes were located in some sanctuary such as a body compartment or the center of a necrotic area where they could not be reached by the molecules of drug in the extracellular fluid; nor could the phenomenon be explained on the basis that the drug molecules were deviated from making contact with the microbes because the inflammatory-necrotic lesion either chemically degraded the drug or wholly bound it in some way. On the contrary, convincing evidence exists that the capacity to persist is a nonheritable property of a minority of the microbial population, and it is mediated by the ability to assume a metabolic state that has been termed "drug indifference" or "physiologic" spore formation. To what extent bacterial pleomorphism, including such forms as protoplasts, plays a role in persistence is not known. Whatever may be the mechanism or mechanisms, it is also clear that even though an infecting microbial population may be wholly drug susceptible in the conventional sense, actual therapy with that drug will not be uniformly or predictably *eradicative*. This is the case irrespective of whether the drug is classified as "bacteriostatic" or "bactericidal." It is this capacity of drug-susceptible bacteria to survive and outlast periods of drug administration that is responsible for most clinical relapse, failures to eliminate the carrier state, and certain failures of chemoprophylaxis. It is not generally known that Ehrlich in his late years came to perceive that *magna sterilisans* conceived as eradication was untenable. He then subtly changed the *concept* of the "sterilisans" without changing the *word*, and offered the idea that the bacteria in the tissues were in effect rendered sterile, i.e., incapable of having progeny. In the last analysis all that is added to this "latter-day Ehrlich" by the present concept of microbial persistence is the point that the sterile state is reversible.

Drug Resistance. Strictly speaking, any microbial strain that is unaffected by appropriate concentrations of a drug in vitro could be called drug resistant. In actual practice, however, the designation is reserved for the drug-resistant representatives of bacterial species that are customarily susceptible to the drug in question. *Primary resistance* refers to situations in which the infecting bacterial strain is already drug resistant at the time it initiates the infection. *Emergent resistance* refers to the emergence to predominance of a drug-resistant population during the treatment of a microbial disease that was drug susceptible when treatment was started.

All drug-susceptible bacterial species possess the capability to show emergent resistance — that is to say, to escape during therapy — to *some* drug or drugs. But *all* drugs are not associated with emergent resistance. Specifically, no instance of emergent resistance to penicillin has been observed,* and all penicillin resistance is primary. Whether drug resistance can emerge or not thus *depends not on the bacterial species but on the drug*. This clearly indicates that there exists a type of drug action on a microbe wherein the emergence to predominance of drug-resistant forms is not to be feared. The existence of this type of drug action is of obvious importance in considerations of the possible mechanisms involved in multiple drug regimens, as discussed below.

Four Different Forms of Drug Resistance. The pluralistic nature of the broad phenomenon called "drug resistance" can readily be seen by examining different drugs or drug-microbe pairings. At least four distinct forms are identifiable. There is the *sulfonamide-streptomycin form,* in which the resistant bacteria maintain full pathogenic potential and are otherwise altered little, if at all, except for their loss of susceptibility to the drug. There is the *major isoniazid form,* in which certain enzymes have been lost (catalase and peroxidase), and the pathogenicity for laboratory animals, including primates, has been significantly reduced. (There is another, much less frequently encountered form of isoniazid resistance in which full pathogenicity is maintained.) There is a form characterized by *episomal or plasmid transfer,* exemplified by enteric bacteria but also by staphylococci. There is also a form seen most clearly with penicillin and staphylococci in which the critical element in producing the resistance is the *presence of a beta-lactamase,* so-called penicillinase. In some strains of staphylococci the enzyme is inducible; in other strains and species it can be constitutive. Combinations of these various forms of phenomena occur. For example, some strains of isoniazid-resistant tubercle bacilli are of the sulfonamide-streptomycin form, although these are rare; the genetic capability of staphylococci to elaborate penicillinase can be passed from one cell to another by episomal transfer, and the actual enzymatic process of synthesizing penicillinase is induced by exposure to the substrate penicillin.

Episomal transfer is an example of nonchromosomal inheritance, for bacteria not only have chromosomal genes, they also have what are in effect free-floating genes that can pass from one cell to another as if they were a virus. The particles are of two sorts: *the episomes* and *the plasmid.* The difference between them is that the plasmid does not attach itself to the chromosome at any time, whereas the episome can either exist freely in the cytoplasm or at times attach itself to the chromosome. Synergism between an episomal gene and a chromosomal gene can occur. In one such experiment, two genes, one present in the episomal factor and the other in the chromosomal, each of which singly conferred resistance to streptomycin concentrations of 25 mg per milliliter, *co-operated* to yield organisms to 1000 mg per milliliter. It is believed that the synergism was acquired as a direct result of genetic recombination between the chromosome and the episomal factor. The "infection" of the strain of *E. coli* in the form of the episomal factor could be removed by treatment with an acridine dye — in effect, a form of drug therapy in vitro. The last-named observation is of considerable theoretic significance when one attempts to analyze the ways in which two-drug therapy

---

*The penicillin-resistant pneumococci reported from Australia (Hausman et al., 1971) were not isolated in a situation of *emergent* resistance. This also appears to have been the case with the strains isolated by Tempest et al. (1974) at the Navajo Medical Center.

can be more effective than the more powerful drug used alone.

Aid to the Clinician.   In what way is the clinician benefited by acquaintance with this expanding body of knowledge on the multiple forms of what can only loosely be called "drug resistance"? The principal gain—and it is by no means a minor one—is that he is able to perceive that *the results of testing a microbial strain for drug susceptibility in vitro represent only one bit of information, and one that is not always relevant to the therapeutic problem presented by his patient.* The identity of the microbial species, its probable source, e.g., whether acquired in hospital or acquired from a drug-treated household contact, and the *history* of drugs received earlier in the illness and their observed effects usually represent a body of evidence of greater reliability and predictive value than drug-susceptibility tests as they are frequently performed. For example, the highly successful streptomycin-penicillin treatment of enterococcal endocarditis would never have been instituted had the results of the streptomycin-susceptibility tests been the controlling factor. Likewise, a patient's pulmonary tuberculosis may respond well to isoniazid despite isoniazid resistance of the patient's strain when subjected to conventional drug-susceptibility tests. But this is not always the case, which merely reflects that there is obviously more than one form of isoniazid resistance. What is clear is that the clinician should be very wary of abandoning a particular drug therapy that appears to be working satisfactorily and introducing a substitute *solely* on the basis of drug-susceptibility tests. Like many ancillary laboratory procedures, drug-susceptibility tests have a role, but it is usually more a confirming one than a determining one.

Drug Pairings.   Consideration of the mechanisms of drug resistance leads to scrutiny of the use of two antimicrobial drugs together. One of the avowed goals of such multidrug therapy is to postpone or prevent drug resistance of the emergent type; the other is to obtain greater antimicrobial effectiveness per unit of time. Conceivably the same process could be responsible for both effects, although this is not the customary way of looking at the matter. With respect to drug resistance, the orthodox explanation dates from Ehrlich's day and is based on the notion that emergent resistance is prevented or postponed because drug A is effective against those bacterial mutants that are resistant to drug B, and vice versa. By this concept it would be possible for a two-drug regimen to affect emergent resistance without exerting an enhanced antimicrobial effectiveness per unit of time. The enhanced effectiveness phenomenon, which is seen, for example, in the penicillin-streptomycin treatment of enterococcal endocarditis, presumably would have to be explained on some other basis. The issue here is not whether, in appropriate circumstances, two-drug therapy can affect emergent resistance or increase total antimicrobial effectiveness. The question is *how* these phenomena are brought about. If the combined drug action is exerted independently, with drug A acting on cells resistant to drug B, virtually any two-drug regimen would be expected to be effective. Contrariwise, if the respective drug actions are dependent, it would presumably represent a highly specialized phenomenon. To settle this issue would thus be a matter of considerable practical importance. Unfortunately, a reasonably com-

plete and authoritative answer cannot be given at this time.

It can be said from the relatively few sets of observations available that enhancement of antimicrobial effectiveness by concurrent administration of two drugs appears to be a *dependent* phenomenon, *with both drugs generally acting on the same microbial cell.* The phenomenon seems to have considerable specificity in terms of drugs and microbial species involved; hence superior drug pairings are relatively rare, and are not to be expected with just any pairing and any drug-susceptible parasite. Whether the "dependent" mechanism is also the major way by which two-drug regimens influence emergent resistance is less clear. In the writer's judgment, there is considerable reason to believe that this is indeed the case and that *when a drug pairing does exert an influence on emergent resistance, it does so by the action of both drugs on the microbes susceptible to both drugs.* Hence in large measure the action would consist of both drugs acting on the same microbial cell. As in the situation with enhancement, such effective drug pairings would represent highly specialized sets of circumstances.

The indication that drug pairings superior to the more powerful drug alone are special affairs is in agreement with the rarity with which multiple drug regimens are of demonstrated value in clinical medicine. Indeed to all intents and purposes, the examples are largely limited to infections with enterococci, tubercle bacilli, and viridans streptococci. Conceivably with further experience it might be possible to add to the list the gentamicin/carbenicillin treatment of Pseudomonas infections. It is important for the physician to keep reminding himself that, except for these few microbial diseases, the justification for the use of more than one antimicrobial drug at a time is largely limited to situations in which an etiologic diagnosis has not yet (or never) been established. Usually, as discussed above, this occurs only during the early hours of treatment, and the physician should be quick to change to single drug therapy as the situation is clarified.

Need for Selectivity.   The day has gone by when the physician could prescribe all two or three of the available antimicrobial drugs to an acutely febrile patient and relax with the comforting thought that all that modern science could do was being done. With today's multiplicity of drugs, the emergence of "new" microbial diseases, and our considerably expanded knowledge about mechanisms of microbial survival, the physician must be highly selective in his drug choices, and hence must have mastery of a considerably greater body of clinical and laboratory-derived knowledge than was needed even a few decades ago. The physician's "comforting thought" today is of quite a different sort. It consists of the knowledge that, however difficult modern science is making things for *him* in the management of infections, it is making things ever so much better for his patients.

Davis, B. D., Dulbecco, R., Eisen, H. N., Ginsberg, H. S., Wood, W. B., Jr., and McCarty, M. (eds.): Microbiology. 2nd ed. New York, Harper & Row, 1973.
Dubos, R. J.: Man Adapting. New Haven, Yale University Press, 1965.
McDermott, W.: Microbial Persistence. Harvey Lecture Series No. 63, 1969, pp. 1–31.
McDermott, W.: Microbial drug resistance. Barnwell Lecture. Am. Rev. Respir. Dis., 102:855, 1970.

268. ANTIMICROBIAL THERAPY

Richard B. Roberts

The announcement of the first sulfonamide in 1935 ushered in the modern era of antimicrobial therapy, an era characterized by the dramatic reduction in incidence, morbidity, and mortality of many infectious diseases. The most outstanding examples include the reduction in disease incidence or death caused by pneumococcal pneumonia, microbial endocarditis, and tuberculosis. The impact by this class of agents on medical, public health, and economic factors related to disease states has been unparalleled in the history of drug therapy.

The abuse of these therapeutic agents, however, is alarming. In the United States, production of antimicrobial agents and the use of these drugs by physicians has steadily increased in the past decade, i.e., a 60 per cent increase in use over this period of time. Antimicrobial agents are a commonly prescribed medication in office practice (about 15 per cent of all drugs), and approximately one third of hospitalized patients receive such drugs. Surveys have suggested that two thirds of these patients receive the incorrect agent or an inappropriate dose. Indiscriminate use of these drugs may be accompanied by such complications as adverse reactions (allergic or dose related), superinfection, emergence of resistant organisms, and delay in identifying the causative organism.

Since many clinical situations dictate that antimicrobial therapy be instituted prior to identification of the specific etiologic microbe, intelligent use of these drugs requires a thorough knowledge of the suspected infectious process as well as of the changing patterns of microbial resistance. In addition, an understanding of the physical and chemical properties of antimicrobial agents is important, because these properties determine adequate drug levels and toxicity, depending on absorption, distribution, and excretion of these drugs.

SELECTION OF ANTIMICROBIAL AGENTS

Host Determinants

Age and Weight. The dose of an antimicrobial drug is usually calculated on the basis of body weight and, less commonly, body surface (Table 1). The route of administration, dosage, and the incidence of adverse reactions may also vary, depending on the age of the patient. For example, in the neonate and aged patient, renal function may be compromised, and the dosage of drugs excreted by the kidney should be adjusted accordingly. *Tetracycline* should not be used in pregnant women, infants, or young children, because this drug may cause enamel hypoplasia, tooth discoloration, and disturbance in bone growth. *Sulfonamides* should not be given to newborns because of possible elevated serum levels owing to abnormalities in acetylation or kernicterus owing to displacement of bilirubin from serum albumin. Similarly, the liver of premature and newborn babies produces only small amounts of glucuronyl transferase, the enzyme necessary to inactivate *chloramphenicol.* High levels of the biologically active drug may cause the "gray baby syndrome," characterized by abdominal distention, pro-

gressive pallor and cyanosis, vasomotor collapse, and death.

Site of Infection. The anatomic location of an infectious process often determines the choice of the antimicrobial and the route of its administration. Clinical studies have shown that adequate levels of most antimicrobial agents except the polymyxins are achieved in inflamed joints, making intra-articular instillation unnecessary. Antimicrobial drugs also penetrate inflamed pleura. Aminoglycosides should not be instilled into a body cavity (i.e., pleural or peritoneal), because neuromuscular blockade and respiratory paralysis may occur. Adequate drainage in addition to effective drug levels in the blood are necessary in infections associated with obstruction in the respiratory, biliary, or urinary tracts. Adequate levels of an antimicrobial agent in the cerebrospinal fluid are determined in part by the pharmacologic properties of the drug and meningeal inflammation. The penicillins, because of their low toxicity, can be given in sufficient dosage parenterally to achieve adequate levels in the cerebrospinal fluid. Chloramphenicol and sulfonamides cross the blood-brain barrier and are effective in bacterial meningitis. However, therapeutic levels of cephalothin and clindamycin in the cerebrospinal fluid are not achieved in the presence of normal or inflamed meninges, and these drugs should not be used in bacterial meningitis. Gentamicin and polymyxin B cross the blood-brain barrier poorly and should be given intrathecally as well as parenterally to patients with gram-negative bacillary meningitis.

Underlying Disease. Serious and life-threatening infections in the compromised host present as one of the most difficult diagnostic and therapeutic challenges in medicine. A variety of microbes, including bacteria, viruses, fungi, and protozoa, infect patients who have malignant disorders or who receive immunosuppressive and cytotoxic therapy for cancer, rheumatic diseases, and renal transplantation. These patients often require antimicrobial therapy before the etiologic agent or agents are identified. Since infections in the compromised host are usually severe and are caused by a number of diverse microorganisms, an aggressive diagnostic approach, often culminating in invasive biopsy procedures, may be necessary. Initial antibacterial therapy should include a penicillinase-resistant penicillin or a cephalosporin and gentamicin. Carbenicillin is added if the clinical or laboratory findings are consistent with Pseudomonas bacteremia. Clindamycin should be given if anaerobic organisms, especially *Bacteroides fragilis,* are suspected. These drugs should be given in maximal doses parenterally. If the initial bacterial cultures are negative after three to five days, the patient should be re-evaluated. If diagnostic studies are negative, the drug therapy should be discontinued, because superinfection with resistant gram-negative bacilli and fungi may occur. Even with appropriate therapy, clinical response may be delayed and may ultimately depend on remission of the underlying disease or reduction of immunosuppressive therapy.

Function of the liver and kidneys may be affected by many underlying diseases. Since these are the major excretory organs for antimicrobial drugs, either many antimicrobial drugs should not be used or their dosage should be modified in the face of compromised hepatic or renal function. These precautions are discussed subsequently under the heading Excretion.

Genetic Factors. The genetic background of patients

TABLE 1. Antimicrobial Agents for Bacterial, Fungal, and Viral Infections

	Adult Daily Dosage (Time Interval of Divided Doses)	Route	Mechanism of Action
Amantadine hydrochloride	200 mg/day	PO	Unknown
Aminosalicylic acid	12 grams/day (t.i.d.)	PO	Replacement of para-aminobenzoic acid
Amphotericin B	1.0 mg/kg/day or every other day (total dose: 2–3 grams) or 15–50 mg/day × 10 weeks	IV	Interaction with sterols of cell membrane
Bacitracin	t.i.d.	Local	Inhibition of cell wall synthesis
Capreomycin	1 gram/day	IM	Unknown
Cephalosporins			Inhibition of cell wall synthesis
Cephalothin	4–12 grams/day (q. 4–6 hours)	IV	
Cephapirin	4–12 grams/day (q. 4–6 hours)	IM, IV	
Cephaloridine	2–4 grams/day (q. 6 hours)	IM	
Cefazolin	2–6 grams/day (q. 6–8 hours)	IM, IV	
Cephaloglycin	1–2 grams/day (q.i.d.)	PO	
Cephalexin	1–4 grams/day (q.i.d.)	PO	
Chloramphenicol	1–4 grams/day (q. 6 hours)	IV	Inhibition of protein synthesis (50S ribosomal binding)
	1–4 grams/day (q.i.d.)	PO	
Clindamycin	0.6–4.5 grams/day (q. 6–8 hours)	IM, IV	Inhibition of protein synthesis
	0.4–1.2 grams/day (q.i.d.)	PO	
Cycloserine	500–750 mg/day (q. 12 hours)	PO	Inhibition of cell wall synthesis
Cytarabine	10–100 mg/square meter/day	IV	Inhibition of nucleoprotein synthesis
Erythromycins			Inhibition of protein synthesis (50S ribosomal binding)
Erythromycin ethylsuccinate	1–4 grams/day (q. 6 hours)	PO	
	400 mg/day (q. 6 hours)	IM	
Erythromycin stearate	1–4 grams/day (q. 6 hours)	PO	
Erythromycin gluceptate	1–4 grams/day (q. 6 hours)	IV	
Erythromycin lactobionate	1–4 grams/day (q. 6 hours)	IV	
Ethambutol	25 mg/kg/day × 6 weeks, then 15 mg/kg/day	PO	Unknown
Ethionamide	500–750 mg/day (q. 12 hours)	PO	Unknown
Flucytosine	150 mg/kg/day × 6 weeks (q. 6 hours)	PO	Inhibition of nucleoprotein synthesis (competition with cytosine)
Gentamicin	3–5 mg/kg/day (q. 8 hours)	IV, IM	Inhibition of protein synthesis (30S ribosomal binding)
	4–5 mg/day	IT	
Idoxuridine	100 mg/kg/day	IV, Local	Inhibition of nucleoprotein synthesis (competition with thymidylic acid)
Isoniazid	300 mg/day	PO	Inhibition of enzymes requiring pyridoxal as cofactor
Kanamycin	15 mg/kg/day (q. 8–12 hours)	IV, IM	Inhibition of protein synthesis (30S ribosomal binding)
	4–8 grams/day (q. 4–6 hours)	PO	
Lincomycin	2–8 grams/day (q. 6 hours)	IV, IM	Inhibition of protein synthesis (50S ribosomal binding)
	2 grams/day (q.i.d.)	PO	
Methenamine mandelate	4–12 grams/day (q.i.d.)	PO	Unknown
Methisazone	1.5 grams/day × 8 days	PO	Inhibition of nucleoprotein synthesis
Nalidixic acid	2–4 grams/day (q.i.d.)	PO	Unknown
Neomycin	4–8 grams/day (q. 6 hours)	PO	Inhibition of protein synthesis (30S ribosomal binding)
	t.i.d.	Local	
Nitrofurans			Unknown
Nitrofurantoin	5–10 mg/kg/day (q.i.d.)	PO	
Novobiocin	2–4 grams/day (q. 6 hours)	PO	Unknown
	1–2 grams/day (q. 6 hours)	IV	

may play a determinant part in the use of some antimicrobial agents. Although there may be other examples as yet unrecognized, the following known phenomena are important in determining, in part, the response to therapy as well as the risk of adverse reactions.

The rate at which isoniazid and sulfapyridine are conjugated and biologically inactivated in the liver is genetically determined. These drugs are inactivated in the liver by acetylation. Studies have shown that certain groups of patients receiving a sulfonamide or isoniazid acetylate the drug rapidly and others slowly. The rate of acetylation determines the concentration and duration of biologically active drug in the serum. Although sulfapyridine is not commonly used, salicylazosulfapyridine, which is often administered to patients with mild ulcerative colitis, is metabolized by the microbial flora of the colon to sulfapyridine and 5-aminosalicylic acid. The former metabolite is rapidly absorbed into the systemic circulation and is responsible for the adverse reactions that accompany the use of salicylazosulfapyridine.

Acute hemolytic anemia is associated with the administration of certain antimicrobial agents in patients with glucose-6-phosphate dehydrogenase deficiency. This enzyme abnormality is transmitted as a sex-linked partially dominant characteristic with full expression in homozygous males. Affected females are usually heterozygous. The antimicrobial agents that may precipitate acute hemolysis in these patients are chloramphenicol, niridazole, nitrofurantoin, primaquine, and sulfonamides. Sulfonamides may also be responsible for acute hemolysis in patients with certain hemoglobinopathies.

Drug Susceptibility. One of the most important determinants in the selection of an antimicrobial agent is the susceptibility of the causative organism. It is imperative that appropriate stains and cultures of blood, secretions, cavity fluids, and the like be obtained prior to the institution of antimicrobial therapy. Once the organism has been isolated, drug-susceptibility determinations may be performed by either one of two methods: the disc (agar) *diffusion* technique, or the tube (broth) or plate (agar)

TABLE 1. Antimicrobial Agents for Bacterial, Fungal, and Viral Infections (*Continued*)

	Adult Daily Dosage (Time Interval of Divided Doses)	Route	Mechanism of Action
Nystatin	1.5–3 million units (t.i.d.)	PO	Interaction with sterols of cell membrane
Penicillins, penicillinase-sensitive			Inhibition of cell wall synthesis
Aqueous crystalline penicillin G	0.6–20 million units/day (q. 2–6 hours)	IV, IM	
Procaine penicillin G	600,000–4.8 million units/day (q. 6–12 hours)	IM	
Benzathine penicillin G	600,000–2.4 million units (q. 4 weeks)	IM	
Phenoxymethyl penicillin	1–4 grams/day (q.i.d.)	PO	
Penicillins with gram-negative bacillary activity			Inhibition of cell wall synthesis
Amoxicillin	0.75–1.5 grams/day (q. 8 hours)	PO	
Ampicillin	4–12 grams/day (q. 4–6 hours)	IV, IM	
	1–4 grams/day (q. 6 hours)	PO	
Carbenicillin	2–40 grams/day (q. 4 hours)	IV, IM	
	2–4 grams/day (q.i.d.)	PO	
Penicillins, penicillinase-resistant			Inhibition of cell wall synthesis
Cloxacillin	2–4 grams/day (q. 6 hours)	PO	
Dicloxacillin	1–2 grams/day (q. 6 hours)	PO	
Methicillin	6–12 grams/day (q. 4–6 hours)	IV, IM	
Nafcillin	4–8 grams/day (q. 4–6 hours)	IV, IM	
Oxacillin	4–8 grams/day (q. 6 hours)	IV, IM	
	2–4 grams/day (q. 4–6 hours)	PO	
Polymyxins			Disruption of cell wall–membrane complex
Polymyxin B	2.5 mg/kg/day (q. 8 hours)	IV, IM	
	5.0 mg/day	IT	
Polymyxin E			
Colistimethate sodium	5.0 mg/kg/day (q. 6 hours)	IV, IM	
Colistin sulfate	5.0 mg/kg/day (q. 6 hours)	PO	
Pyrazinamide	40–50 mg/kg/day (q. 8–12 hours)	PO	Unknown
Rifampin	600 mg/day	PO	Inhibition of DNA-dependent RNA polymerase
Spectinomycin	2.0 or 4.0 grams/day	IM	Inhibition of protein synthesis (30S ribosomal binding)
Streptomycin	1–2 grams/day (q. 12–24 hours)	IM	Inhibition of protein synthesis (30S ribosomal binding)
Sulfonamides			Competition with para-aminobenzoic acid
Sulfisoxazole	4–6 grams/day (q. 6 hours)	PO, IV	
Salicylazosulfapyridine	4–8 grams/day (q. 3–6 hours)	PO	
Tetracyclines			Inhibition of protein synthesis
Tetracycline HCl	IV: 0.5–1.0 gram/day (q. 12 hours)	IV, PO	
Chlortetracycline		IV, PO	
Oxytetracycline	PO: 1–2 grams/day (q. 6 hours)	IV, PO	
Demethylchlortetracycline	0.6–1.2 grams/day (q. 6 hours)	PO	
Methacycline	0.6–0.9 gram/day (q. 6–12 hours)	PO	
Doxycycline	0.1–0.2 gram/day (q. 12 hours)	IV, PO	
Minocycline	0.1–0.4 gram/day (q. 12 hours)	PO	
Trimethoprim/sulfamethoxazole	4 tablets/day (q. 12 hours) (1 tablet = T80 mg/S400 mg)	PO	Sequential inhibition of folic acid reduction
Vancomycin	2 grams/day (q. 6 hours)	IV	Inhibition of cell wall synthesis
Viomycin	1 gram twice weekly	IM	Inhibition of protein synthesis

dilution technique. The former method is routinely used in most clinical laboratories. Because of the many factors which may influence drug-susceptibility determinations, standardization of this method must take into account the growth of the organism, the inoculum size, the type and quantity of media employed, the size and concentration of drug-impregnated discs, and the duration and environmental conditions of incubation. If these conditions are adhered to, the diameter of the area of growth inhibition about the impregnated disc distinguishes resistant from susceptible strains. In addition, precautions concerning specific bacteria or drugs must also be taken into consideration. Resistance of *Staphylococcus aureus* to methicillin is reliable only if the zones are measured within 20 hours of incubation, because methicillin deteriorates rapidly at incubating temperatures. Fastidious and slow-growing organisms such as Bacteroides and certain streptococci may not produce visible colonies within 24 hours, and reports of susceptibility may not be reliable. Disc susceptibility tests performed in anaerobic jars may give misleading results. Colistin and polymyxin B diffuse poorly in agar, and the drug-susceptibility results may be inaccurate. The standardized disc test is not recommended for gonococci or for *Mycobacterium tuberculosis*.

In certain clinical settings, namely patients with endocarditis and osteomyelitis, a more precise method for determining the susceptibility of an organism may be indicated. The *dilution method* — that is, twofold dilutions of the drug in broth or agar containing a standardized inoculum of the infecting organism — is the technique commonly employed in many laboratories. Results are expressed as the minimal inhibitory concentration or MIC, which is the smallest amount of drug that will inhibit growth after 18 to 24 hours of incubation.

The serum antibacterial activity may also be determined. At a specified time after the drug is given (usually one hour after parenteral administration), serum is collected and serially diluted in a medium inoculated with the organism. A serum dilution of 1:8 or greater that inhibits the growth of the test organism is indicative of an adequate blood level for serious and life-threatening infections. Accurate serum concentrations can be determined by impregnating discs with known concentrations of a drug and other discs with serum dilutions from the patient. These discs are placed on agar previously inoculated with the organism, and zones of growth inhibition are compared after incubation.

Knowledge of the drug-susceptibility patterns of bacteria is important for the intelligent use of antimicrobial agents. For example, despite the common use of penicillin G, group A streptococci, pneumococci, and meningococci have remained susceptible to it. Methicillin-resistant *Staphylococcus aureus* strains, however, have been reported especially from Denmark and less commonly from England and the United States. These strains are also resistant to the cephalosporins. Patterns of susceptibility and resistance of gram-negative bacilli vary from hospital to hospital as well as temporally within the same institution. This phenomenon is principally due to the widespread use of antimicrobial agents active against gram-negative bacilli and the development of emergent resistance. Because of the changing patterns of susceptibility and resistance of bacteria, continuous laboratory surveillance of the incidence and susceptibility of isolates by hospital epidemiologists and clinical laboratories is extremely important. The antimicrobial susceptibilities of various microbes are discussed later in this chapter.

Bactericidal and Bacteriostatic Drugs. Bactericidal agents are drugs that kill organisms at or near the minimal inhibitory concentration. Examples of bactericidal agents include the penicillins, cephalosporins, vancomycin, aminoglycosides, and polymyxins. In general, patients with severe infections should receive bactericidal drugs. This is especially true in patients with abnormal host defense mechanisms involving antibody function, phagocyte function, or cellular immunity. Bacteriostatic drugs inhibit the growth of organisms and include erythromycin, lincomycin, clindamycin, chloramphenicol, tetracycline, and the sulfonamides. Erythromycin, lincomycin, and clindamycin may have bactericidal activity at high concentrations against certain organisms. An intact immunologic system is an important determinant in the response of patients receiving bacteriostatic drugs. In many clinical situations, such as upper respiratory tract infections, anaerobic infections, and uncomplicated urinary tract infections, bacteriostatic drugs are as effective clinically as bactericidal agents.

Combination Therapy. The administration of more than one antimicrobial agent at the same time is indicated for (1) initial therapy in a critically ill patient when the causative organism is not known, (2) polymicrobial infection in which the organisms are not susceptible to one antimicrobial agent, (3) reducing or postponing the emergence of resistance to one or both agents, such as in the therapy for tuberculosis, and (4) synergism. Synergism is best exemplified by the penicillins, the cephalosporins, vancomycin, and the aminoglycosides. In vitro studies suggest that this enhanced antimicrobial effect by bactericidal agents may be due to the inhibition of cell wall synthesis by the penicillins or vancomycin resulting in increased permeability and penetration of the aminoglycosides. The combination of penicillin or vancomycin with streptomycin or gentamicin should be used in patients with enterococcal endocarditis. Limited clinical studies suggest that carbenicillin and gentamicin may be more effective than either drug alone in severe *Pseudomonas aeruginosa* infections. (For additional discussion of multiple drug therapy, see Ch. 267.)

Antagonism between two antimicrobial agents can be demonstrated in vitro. Since bactericidal drugs such as penicillin inhibit cell wall synthesis of rapidly multiplying bacteria, the simultaneous use of a bacteriostatic drug may interfere with bactericidal activity. It is uncommon, however, to detect adverse effects clinically with combined bactericidal and bacteriostatic therapy.

Absorption and Distribution

Pharmacologic properties differ markedly between classes of antimicrobial agents and between agents within the same class. Knowledge of these properties is important for the intelligent use of these drugs. Antimicrobial drugs may be administered by various routes, including topical, oral, and parenteral (intramuscular and intravenous). *Topical administration* should be restricted to special circumstances whenever possible because of possible absorption into the systemic circulation, allergic reactions, and the development of microbial resistance. Examples of appropriate local administration include severe burns, intravenous catheter sites, and purulent conjunctivitis. The *oral route* is used chiefly in initial therapy for mild to moderately severe infections and for the completion of therapy in patients with severe infections. Because of the variable absorption of antimicrobial agents in the presence of gastric acidity, oral medications should be given in the fasting state, i.e., 1 to 2 hours before or after meals. *Parenteral administration* of antimicrobial drugs is indicated for severe infections that require high and sustained blood levels. Many drugs cannot be administered intramuscularly because of severe pain. These include cephalothin, vancomycin, erythromycin, chloramphenicol, and tetracycline. *Intravenous administration* is indicated in patients with severe infections or hypotension, or when appropriate levels cannot be achieved by the intramuscular route. Intravenous appliances must be changed every 24 to 48 hours to avoid thrombophlebitis and local infection with or without bacteremia. In general, medications should be diluted in 50 to 100 ml of solution and allowed to run in over a period of 15 to 30 minutes. Adverse reactions, especially associated with the aminoglycosides and polymyxins, may occur with rapid intravenous administration. Intrathecal and intra-articular therapy may be necessary in gram-negative infections. Complications associated with intrathecal administration include arachnoiditis with severe pain, paresthesias, and transient to permanent paralysis. The intrapleural or intraperitoneal administration of antimicrobial drugs is not recommended.

The distribution of a drug is a complex phenomenon and depends on many factors, including (1) molecular size, (2) electrical charge at pH 7.4, (3) lipid solubility, (4) plasma protein binding, and (5) presence of inflammation. If adequate blood levels are present, most antimicrobial agents will enter infected synovial and serous fluids. However, even in the presence of inflamed meninges, therapeutic levels of cephalothin, clindamycin, polymyxin, or gentamicin may not be achieved.

Excretion

The liver and the kidneys are the two principal excretory organs for antimicrobial agents. Renal clearance, by either glomerular filtration or tubular secretion, or both, is a major determinant of serum levels. Probenecid increases and prolongs the serum level of those antimicrobials excreted by tubular secretion (i.e., the penicillins and cephalosporins). Repeated evaluation of hepatic and renal function must be performed when antimicrobial agents are given in high doses for a prolonged period of time. Ampicillin, nafcillin, erythromycin, tetracycline, chloramphenicol, lincomycin, clindamycin, and novobiocin should be used with caution in patients with liver disease. In the face of impaired renal function, the following agents should be administered with caution, and the dosage reduced accordingly: amphotericin B, cephaloridine, colistimethate, flucytosine, gentamicin, kanamycin, methenamine mandelate, neomycin, nitrofurantoin, penicillins, polymyxin B, streptomycin, sulfonamides, tetracycline, and vancomycin. Many of these agents not only are excreted largely by the kidney but also are nephrotoxic. Although the initial loading dose is the same, subsequent doses are reduced or the duration between doses is prolonged. Formulas for drug dose and interval between doses have been derived based on renal function, i.e., serum creatinine or creatinine clearance. These guidelines are useful but cannot be relied upon alone. Adjustments are best guided by repeated determinations of the serum concentration of the drug. In addition, knowledge of the dialyzability of antimicrobial agents with hemodialysis and peritoneal dialysis is necessary for the management of patients with acute and chronic renal failure.

Adverse Reactions

The administration of antimicrobial agents may be associated with toxic or allergic reactions. Adverse reactions are widely variable, as shown by the following examples: (1) local irritation at the site of administration; (2) hypersensitivity reactions; (3) dose-related hepatic, renal, and bone marrow toxicity; and (4) adverse reactions caused by the composition of the drug preparation (i.e., hyperkalemia with potassium penicillin G, fluid retention with disodium carbenicillin). The adverse reactions associated with specific antimicrobial agents are discussed below.

SPECIFIC ANTIMICROBIAL AGENTS

Antimicrobial agents may be classified as to their chemical structure, mechanism of action, antimicrobial spectrum of activity, and bactericidal versus bacteriostatic properties. Table 1 lists the common antibacterial agents with their route of administration, dosage, and mechanism of action. More detailed descriptions of the indications for each drug are included in the chapters dealing with specific organisms or infectious diseases. The antituberculous drugs (isoniazid, rifampin, streptomycin, para-aminosalicylic acid, pyrazinamide, capreomycin, cycloserine, ethambutol, ethionamide, and viomycin), the antiviral drugs (amantadine hydrochloride, cytarabine, idoxuridine, and methisazone), and the antifungal agents (amphotericin B, flucytosine, and nysta-

tin) are included in Table 1 and are discussed in detail in the chapters dealing with the respective diseases for which they are used. Table 2 lists the antiprotozoan and antimetazoan drugs with their clinical indications, dose, route of administration, and toxicity. The following antiparasitic drugs are not approved by the Food and Drug Administration for general use in the United States: antimony sodium gluconate, bithional, melarsoprol, niclosamide, niridazole, pentamidine, and suramin. These agents, however, may be easily obtained for therapy of the indicated diseases by calling the Parasitic Diseases Branch of the Center for Disease Control at 404–633–3311.

Penicillins. *Penicillinase-Sensitive Penicillins.* The penicillins that are susceptible to penicillinase are penicillin G (benzyl penicillin), phenoxymethyl penicillin, ampicillin, and carbenicillin. Penicillin G has three intramuscular forms which differ in the rate of absorption, thus affecting the concentration and duration of drug in serum. *Aqueous crystalline penicillin G* is well absorbed but is painful and is therefore usually given intravenously. *Procaine penicillin G* is well tolerated intramuscularly and is slowly absorbed so that injections are only necessary every six to twelve hours. *Benzathine penicillin G* is also given intramuscularly and is slowly released from the site of injection over three to four weeks. Procaine penicillin G and benzathine penicillin should not be administered intravenously. Penicillin G is unstable in the presence of gastric acid. *Phenoxymethyl penicillin,* although ten times less active than benzyl penicillin, is acid stable and is preferred for oral therapy. Renal clearance of the penicillins is by glomerular filtration and tubular secretion, and the simultaneous administration of probenecid will increase and prolong serum levels. However, probenecid may cause such adverse reactions as nausea, vomiting, hypersensitivity reactions (rash and fever), and rarely the nephrotic syndrome, hepatocellular injury, and aplastic anemia. Acute gout as well as the development of uric acid stones may be precipitated by probenecid. Penicillin G is active against streptococci of groups A, B, C and G, viridans streptococci, pneumococci, nonpenicillinase-producing staphylococci, *Corynebacterium diphtheriae, Listeria monocytogenes,* anaerobic streptococci, Fusobacterium, Clostridia, treponemes, Leptospira species, Neisseria, Pasteurella multocida, and Actinomyces.

Penicillins with gram-negative bacillary activity include ampicillin and carbenicillin. *Ampicillin* differs from penicillin G only in the presence of an amino group on the side chain. This minor alteration is responsible for the difference in antimicrobial activity. Ampicillin is active against enterococci, *Hemophilus influenzae,* Shigella, Salmonella, *Escherichia coli,* and *Proteus mirabilis.* Indole-positive Proteus species (i.e., *P. rettgeri, P. morgani, P. vulgaris*) and Pseudomonas species are resistant. Ampicillin may be given either parenterally or orally, and the serum half-life is twice as long as that of penicillin G. *Amoxicillin,* an analogue of ampicillin, is available for general use and has several pharmacologic advantages over ampicillin. It is more stable in the presence of gastric acid and thus better absorbed. Serum levels are higher and more prolonged than those of ampicillin. Both drugs have the same spectrum of antibacterial activity.

Carbenicillin is also similar in structure to penicillin G except for a carboxyl group on the side chain. It is active in vitro against *E. coli,* Pseudomonas species, Pro-

TABLE 2. Antimicrobial Agents for Protozoan and Metazoan Infections

Protozoan Infections	Infecting Organism	Antimicrobial Agent	Adult Dose	Route	Adverse Reactions (Most Frequent Are *Italicized*)
Amebiasis Asymptomatic cyst	*Entamoeba histolytica*	Diiodohydroxyquin	650 mg t.i.d. × 3 weeks	PO	*Iodine toxicoderma,* rash, slight thyroid enlargement, nausea
Intestinal disease		Metronidazole	750 mg t.i.d. × 5–10 days	PO	*Nausea,* vomiting, diarrhea; *headache,* vertigo, insomnia, ataxia
Hepatic disease		Metronidazole	750 mg t.i.d. × 10 days	PO	See above
Giardiasis	*G. lamblia*	Metronidazole or	250 mg t.i.d. × 10 days	PO	See above
		Quinacrine	100 mg t.i.d. × 5 days	PO	*Vomiting, vertigo, headache;* psychosis, blood dyscrasia, ocular damage, rash, hepatic necrosis
Leishmaniasis Visceral	*L. donovani*	Antimony Na gluconate	600 mg q.d. × 10 days	IM	Similar to antimony potassium tartrate but less severe
Cutaneous	*L. tropica*	Antimony Na gluconate	600 mg q.d. × 10 days	IM	See above
Mucocutaneous	*L. brasiliensis*	Antimony Na gluconate	600 mg q.d. × 10 days	IM	See above
Toxoplasmosis	*T. gondii*				
Moderate – severe illness		Pyrimethamine and	75 mg first day, then 25 mg q.d. × 4 weeks	PO	*Folic acid deficiency,* blood dyscrasia, rash, vomiting, convulsions, shock
Immunosuppressed host		Sulfadiazine plus	1 gram q.i.d. × 4 weeks	PO	*Rash,* photosensitivity, hepatic and renal toxicity, blood dyscrasia, vasculitis
		Folinic acid	6 mg q. 2 days	IM	
Malaria	*Plasmodium vivax, malariae, ovale*	Chloroquine followed by	1 gram, then 500 mg in 6 hours, then 500 mg q.d. × 2 days	PO	*Vomiting, headache, pruritus,* ocular damage, convulsions, psychosis, rash; hair, nail, and mucous membrane discoloration
		Primaquine	26.3 mg q.d. × 14 days	PO	*Hemolytic anemia* in G-6-PD deficient patients, neutropenia, nausea, hypertension
	P. falciparum Chloroquine-susceptible	Chloroquine	1 gram, then 500 mg in 6 hours, then 500 mg q.d. × 2 days	PO	See above
	Chloroquine-resistant	Quinine and	650 mg t.i.d. × 14 days	PO	*Cinchonism, hypotension, arrhythmias,* blood dyscrasias, photosensitivity, blindness
		Pyrimethamine plus	25 mg b.i.d. × 3 days	PO	See above
		Sulfadiazine	500 mg q.i.d. × 5 days		See above
	Comatose patient	Quinine	600 mg/300 ml saline q. 8 hours until PO tolerated	IV	See above
Trichomoniasis	*T. vaginalis*	Metronidazole	250 mg t.i.d. × 10 days	PO	See above
Trypanosomiasis	*T. gambiense*	Pentamidine	4 mg/kg/day × 10 days	IM	*Nausea, vomiting,* hypoglycemia, hypotension, blood dyscrasias, renal and hepatic toxicity
	T. rhodesiense	Suramin followed by	1 gram on days, 1, 3, 7, 14, and 21 after 100 mg test dose	IV	*Rash, pruritus, paresthesias, vomiting,* peripheral neuropathy, shock
		Melarsoprol	2.0–3.6 mg/kg q.d. for 3 days; repeat after 1 week and, if necessary, after an additional 10–21 days	IV	*Encephalopathy,* vomiting, neuropathy, rash, myocarditis, hypertension
Pneumocystosis	*P. carinii*	Pentamidine	4 mg/kg/day q.d. × 12–14 days	IM	See above

Metazoan Infections	Infecting Organism	Antimicrobial Agent	Adult Dose	Route	Adverse Reactions (Most Frequent Are *Italicized*)
Intestinal nematodes	*Ascaris lumbricoides* (roundworm)	Pyrantel pamoate	11 mg/kg (maximum 1 gram), single dose	PO	*GI disturbance,* headache, dizziness, rash, fever
	Enterobius vermicularis (pinworm)	Pyrantel pamoate	11 mg/kg, single dose; repeat after 2 weeks	PO	
	Necator americanus (hookworm)	Pyrantel pamoate	11 mg/kg, single dose	PO	
	Ancylostoma duodenale (hookworm)	Pyrantel pamoate	11 mg/kg, single dose	PO	
	Trichuris trichiura (whipworm)	Thiabendazole	25 mg/kg b.i.d. × 2 days	PO	*Nausea, vomiting, vertigo, rash,* leukopenia, color vision disturbance, tinnitus, shock
	Strongyloides stercoralis	Thiabendazole	25 mg/kg b.i.d. × 2 days	PO	
Tissue nematodes Filariasis	*Wuchereria bancrofti*	Diethylcarbamazine	2 mg/kg t.i.d. × 14 days	PO	*Allergic and febrile reactions* due to worm disintegration; encephalopathy
	Loa loa	Diethylcarbamazine	2 mg/kg t.i.d. × 14 days	PO	See above
River blindness	*Onchocerca volvulus*	Diethylcarbamazine plus	2 mg/kg t.i.d. × 14 days	PO	See above
		Suramin	1 gram per week × 5 weeks	IV	See above
Trichinosis	*Trichinella spiralis*	Thiabendazole and/or	25 mg/kg q.d. until symptoms subside	PO	
		Corticosteroids	40 mg q.d. for 3–5 days	PO	
Cestodes (tapeworms)	*Taenia saginata* (beef tapeworm)	Niclosamide	2 grams in a single dose	PO	Nausea, abdominal pain
	Diphyllobothrium latum (fish tapeworm)	Niclosamide	2 grams in a single dose	PO	
	Taenia solium (pork tapeworm)	Niclosamide	2 grams in a single dose	PO	
Trematodes (flukes) Schistosomiasis	*S. mansoni*	Stibophen	4 ml q.o.d. to 100 ml	IM	Similar to antimony potassium tartrate but less severe
	S. haematobium	Niridazole	25 mg/kg q.d. × 5–7 days	PO	*Vomiting, diarrhea, dizziness, headache,* EKG changes, rash, insomnia, paresthesias, convulsions, psychosis, hemolysis
	S. japonicum	Antimony potassium tartrate	q.o.d. 8, 12, 16, 20, 24 ml, then 28 ml q.o.d. × 10 doses	IV	*Bradycardia, vomiting, cough,* myalgias with rapid administration, rash, pruritus, colic, diarrhea, hemolytic anemia, hepatic and renal toxicity, shock
Paragonimiasis	*P. westermani*	Bithionol	50 mg/kg q.o.d. × 15 doses	PO	*Photosensitivity, urticaria, abdominal pain, vomiting,* and *diarrhea*

teus species, and some strains of Enterobacter. The minimal inhibitory concentrations for Pseudomonas are very high when compared to other drug susceptibilities (i.e., 75 to 100 μg per milliliter). However, carbenicillin is a relatively nontoxic agent which can be given in doses of 30 to 40 grams per day intravenously with serum levels of 200 to 400 μg per milliliter. One half this dose is usually adequate for *E. coli*, Proteus, and Enterobacter infections. Carbenicillin is principally excreted by the kidneys, and very high urine levels are present after 0.5 or 1.0 gram is given parenterally (1000 μg per milliliter of urine or more). Thus a dose of 4 to 6 grams per day is adequate for uncomplicated urinary tract infections. Since *Pseudomonas aeruginosa* may develop resistance during therapy, especially if the drug is given in suboptimal doses, carbenicillin should not be used alone in patients with severe infections, cystic fibrosis, or chronic urinary tract obstruction when prolonged therapy may be indicated. In addition, superinfection, especially with Klebsiella species and Serratia species, is not uncommon. An oral form of carbenicillin, the indanyl salt of the sodium ester, is indicated only in uncomplicated urinary tract infections caused by susceptible organisms. Whereas serum levels are low after 0.5 to 1.0 gram orally, urine levels are in excess of the minimal inhibitory concentration of susceptible gram-negative bacilli.

Penicillinase-Resistant Penicillins. The semisynthetic penicillins that resist penicillinase are methicillin, nafcillin, oxacillin, cloxacillin, and dicloxacillin. The principal indication for using these penicillins are infections caused by *Staphylococcus aureus* which produce penicillinase. These drugs are also active against group A streptococci and pneumococci. Cloxacillin and dicloxacillin are acid stable and are the preferred agents for oral therapy. Nafcillin is the only penicillinase-resistant penicillin excreted primarily by the liver, and the dose need not be significantly altered in patients with renal failure.

Adverse Reactions to the Penicillins. In general, severe adverse reactions to the penicillins are uncommon, and a wide range exists between therapeutic and toxic serum levels. Hypersensitivity reactions occur in 2 to 5 per cent of patients. These reactions may take two clinical forms: (1) immediate reactions, including anaphylaxis, accelerated urticaria, and angioneurotic edema; and (2) delayed reactions, which are more common and include delayed urticaria, morbilliform eruption, and serum sickness. Hypersensitivity reactions have been reported with all the penicillin derivatives. Patients allergic to one penicillin are allergic to all congeners. Drug fever is not uncommon. Coombs-positive hemolytic anemia may result from the formation of antibody to penicillin-coated red cells. This is most likely to occur when large parenteral doses are given over a long period of time. Central nervous system toxicity, characterized by myoclonus and generalized seizures, may be seen when high doses of parenteral penicillins are administered to patients especially with renal insufficiency. Hyperkalemia may be seen in patients with renal insufficiency, because the potassium salt of penicillin G has 1.6 mEq of K^+ per million units. Diarrhea is common in patients receiving oral ampicillin. Skin rashes have been reported to be more common in patients with infectious mononucleosis who receive oral ampicillin. Carbenicillin must be used with caution in patients in whom sodium restriction is important, because 1 gram of carbenicillin contains 4.7 mEq of sodium. Carbenicillin

may cause elevated hepatic enzymes, neutropenia, and increased clotting and prothrombin times with bleeding in patients with renal insufficiency. Methicillin and, less commonly, penicillin G have been reported to cause interstitial nephritis and reversible azotemia. Bone marrow depression with anemia and leukopenia has also been associated with methicillin therapy.

Cephalosporins. Six cephalosporins are currently marketed in the United States: cephalothin, cephapirin, cefazolin, cephaloridine, cephaloglycin, and cephalexin. The cephalosporins are active against most organisms susceptible to the penicillins, i.e., group A streptococci, viridans streptococci, pneumococci, *Staphylococcus aureus,* and *C. diphtheriae.* Susceptible gram-negative bacilli include *Escherichia coli,* Klebsiella, and *Proteus mirabilis.* Enterobacter species, indole-positive Proteus strains and Pseudomonas species are resistant to the cephalosporins. Cephalothin, cephapirin, cefazolin, and cephaloridine are used parenterally, cephaloglycin and cephalexin, orally. *Cephalothin* is usually given intravenously, because intramuscular injections of greater than 0.5 gram are painful. Renal clearance is rapid, and the drug should be given every four hours. *Cephapirin* has antibacterial spectra and pharmacologic properties similar to cephalothin. *Cefazolin* has several pharmacologic advantages over cephalothin. Because of its low renal clearance and longer half-life, serum levels are two to three times higher and more sustained. Cefazolin may produce less thrombophlebitis than cephalothin and may be given intramuscularly. *Cephaloridine* should be given only by the parenteral route and must be avoided in patients with renal insufficiency. *Cephaloglycin,* the first available oral cephalosporin, is poorly absorbed and is indicated only for urinary tract infections when cephalexin is not available. *Cephalexin* is acid stable and well absorbed. Urine levels are within the therapeutic range after a 0.5 to 1.0 gram oral dose. Since the excretion of the cephalosporins is by tubular secretion, serum levels may be increased and prolonged with the simultaneous administration of probenecid. Since the cephalosporins do not achieve therapeutic levels in the cerebrospinal fluid, these agents should not be used in patients with bacterial meningitis.

Adverse reactions to the cephalosporins are relatively uncommon. The question of cross-allergenicity between the penicillins and the cephalosporins remains controversial. The incidence of cross-sensitization must be low, because cephalosporin compounds have been given successfully to many patients with prior penicillin reactions. However, the cephalosporins should probably not be administered to patients with a documented history of an immediate hypersensitivity reaction to penicillin. Thrombophlebitis is commonly seen with the intravenous use of large doses of cephalothin and cephapirin, and frequent changes of the intravenous site are necessary if these drugs have to be given over an extended period of time. A positive Coombs test without hemolysis may occur with large doses of cephalothin; leukopenia is rare and usually responds to discontinuing the drug. Cephaloridine is nephrotoxic, especially if the dose is greater than 4 grams per day or if patients are receiving ethacrynic acid or furosemide. Acute tubular necrosis has also been reported in patients receiving cephalothin and gentamicin. The specific role of either drug or the combination in this complication is unknown. Nausea and vomiting may accompany the administration of the oral cephalosporins. The presence of cephalexin in the urine may give a false positive test for glucose with Benedict's solution or Clinitest tablets.

Vancomycin. Vancomycin is active against penicillinase-producing *Staphylococcus aureus* and *S. epidermidis,* viridans streptococci, and enterococci. It is an important alternative drug in patients allergic to the penicillins and the cephalosporins who have severe staphylococcal infections or endocarditis caused by penicillin-resistant viridans streptococci and enterococci. Methicillin-resistant *Staphylococcus aureus* strains are usually resistant to the cephalosporins but sensitive to vancomycin. All gram-negative bacilli are resistant to this antimicrobial. Vancomycin can only be administered intravenously. Pain at the site of injection is frequent and thrombophlebitis common. Chills, fever, and urticaria may also accompany its administration. The more severe adverse reactions include reversible nephrotoxicity with albuminuria, casts, and azotemia, and ototoxicity with deafness when very high blood levels are achieved.

Erythromycin, Lincomycin, and Clindamycin. *Erythromycin* is one of two macrolide antimicrobials. It should be classified with lincomycin and clindamycin, because all three drugs have the same mechanism of action (inhibition of protein synthesis by binding the 50S ribosomal unit). The spectrum of activity of these drugs, with a few exceptions, is similar. Erythromycin is active against group A streptococci, pneumococci, and *Staphylococcus aureus. Mycoplasma pneumoniae* and *T. pallidum* are also susceptible to it. Erythromycin may be used in patients allergic to penicillin who have respiratory tract or soft tissue infections caused by pneumococci and group A streptococci, respectively. It may be used as the primary drug in *M. pneumoniae* infections. Erythromycin should not be used for serious *Staphylococcus aureus* infections. Local irritation at the site of parenteral administration is common, and gastrointestinal disturbance may be associated with oral therapy. Erythromycin estolate may produce reversible cholestatic hepatitis, and other preparations of erythromycin should be used. Hypersensitivity reactions, such as rash and eosinophilia, and drug fever are uncommon.

Triacetyloleandomycin is also a macrolide antimicrobial, but it is used infrequently because of adverse reactions.

Lincomycin and clindamycin (a chloro-derivative of lincomycin) are also active against group A streptococci, pneumococci, and penicillinase-producing staphylococci. Enterococci, gram-negative bacilli, and *Mycoplasma pneumoniae* are resistant. Many strains of *Staphylococcus aureus* resistant to erythromycin are also resistant to lincomycin and clindamycin. Staphylococci resistant to erythromycin but susceptible to lincomycin or clindamycin may rapidly develop resistance to the latter drugs during lincomycin-clindamycin therapy (dissociated cross-resistance). Clindamycin is well absorbed from the gastrointestinal tract and produces higher serum levels than oral lincomycin. Clindamycin is also more active against many anaerobes, especially *Bacteroides fragilis,* and has become the drug of choice in the initial therapy of severe anaerobic infections. Erythromycin crosses the blood-brain barrier, but lincomycin and clindamycin do not, and therefore the latter agents should not be used in bacterial meningitis. Gastrointestinal disturbances such as nausea, vomiting, abdominal cramps, and diarrhea occur with clindamycin and lincomycin. Pseudomembranous colitis has been observed

with both drugs. Rapid intravenous administration may be associated with cardiopulmonary arrest. Reversible hepatocellular toxicity and bone marrow depression (leukopenia) have been reported after clindamycin therapy. Hypersensitivity reactions such as rash and generalized pruritus are rare.

Novobiocin. The antibacterial spectrum of novobiocin is similar to that of penicillin G and erythromycin; *Staphylococcus aureus* and pneumococci are susceptible to this antimicrobial. It is well absorbed from the gastrointestinal tract and may also be given intravenously. However, the high incidence of adverse reactions precludes the routine use of this drug, and it is rarely prescribed at present. Toxic reactions include gastrointestinal disturbances (nausea, vomiting, diarrhea, and bleeding), bone marrow depression (pancytopenia), hypersensitivity reactions (eosinophilia, rash, fever, angioedema, exudative erythema multiforme), alopecia, and yellow discoloration of the skin and sclera caused by a degradation product of the drug.

Bacitracin. Bacitracin is a polypeptide antimicrobial agent for topical use only. *Staphylococcus aureus, Staphylococcus epidermidis,* enterococci, viridans streptococci, and group A streptococci are susceptible to it. Gram-negative bacilli are resistant to bacitracin. The antibiotic is stable in ointments only when it is incorporated in petrolatum. Bacitracin is indicated in open superficial skin infections such as eczema, dermal ulcers, and minor wounds infected with drug-susceptible bacteria. Purulent conjunctivitis and infected corneal ulcers may also respond to topical bacitracin when caused by similar organisms. Furunculosis, impetigo, pyoderma, and subcutaneous abscesses should not be treated with topical bacitracin alone. Adverse reactions are rarely seen with this topical antibiotic.

Aminoglycosides. The four drugs that belong to this class of antimicrobial agents are streptomycin, neomycin, kanamycin, and gentamicin. *Streptomycin,* one of the first aminoglycosides available for parenteral administration, was widely used in the 1940's and 1950's, because *Mycobacterium tuberculosis* and gram-negative bacilli, especially *Escherichia coli,* Klebsiella-Enterobacter species, and Proteus strains were susceptible. However, with the development of other drugs for these infections and because adverse reactions, notably vestibular toxicity, are a risk, the use of intramuscular streptomycin is now limited to a few specific diseases. Most strains of enterococci are resistant to streptomycin in vitro. Nevertheless, streptomycin in combination with penicillin or vancomycin is the therapy of choice in patients with penicillin-resistant viridans streptococcal and enterococcal endocarditis. These drug combinations should also be used for prophylaxis against enterococcal bacteremia in patients with underlying congenital or valvular heart disease who have urogenital or gastrointestinal manipulation. Streptomycin has substantial activity against *M. tuberculosis,* and the indications for its use in this disease are discussed in Ch. 228. Streptomycin may also be used in the therapy of plague, tularemia, and brucellosis. *Neomycin,* also discovered in the 1940's, has limited clinical application because of nephrotoxicity and neurotoxicity. The drug is poorly absorbed from the gastrointestinal tract and is therefore useful in patients with severe hepatic disease with impending or frank coma, inhibiting bacterial growth in the intestinal tract and reducing absorption of nitrogenous compounds. Unfortunately, neomycin is widely used in topical antimicrobial preparations, many of which are available without a prescription. There is no evidence from controlled studies that neomycin is effective in healing or preventing skin infections. Indeed, topical neomycin frequently causes contact dermatitis. Injudicious use of neomycin in patients with extensive wounds or burns or instillation into body cavities may result in absorption of the drug and life-threatening adverse reactions.

Kanamycin is closely related to neomycin but is less toxic. It is active against most gram-negative bacilli, including *E. coli,* Klebsiella-Enterobacter species, and Proteus species. The antibiotic is also active in vitro against Shigella, *Staphylococcus aureus,* and *M. tuberculosis,* but is not indicated for clinical use in these infections, because less toxic agents are available. *Pseudomonas aeruginosa* strains are universally resistant to kanamycin. Ampicillin plus kanamycin has been the initial therapy of choice in suspected neonatal sepsis. However, if it is known that kanamycin-resistant gram-negative organisms have been isolated from the nursery, ampicillin plus gentamicin is recommended.

Gentamicin is widely used for serious gram-negative bacillary infections. It is active against Pseudomonas species as well as *E. coli,* Klebsiella-Enterobacter species, and Proteus species. *Staphylococcus aureus* strains are also susceptible to gentamicin; however, less toxic antistaphylococcal agents are available, and gentamicin should not be used for this purpose. Gentamicin may be given by either the intramuscular or the intravenous route. Therapeutic levels in the cerebrospinal fluid are usually not achieved with parenteral administration, and intrathecal injections are indicated in patients with gram-negative bacillary meningitis. In patients with urinary tract infections, the urine should be alkaline for maximal antimicrobial activity. Carbenicillin when mixed with gentamicin in the same solution will inactivate the latter drug over a prolonged period of time.

Adverse reactions are commonly seen with administration of the aminoglycosides. These agents are excreted principally by the kidneys and should be avoided or the dose adjusted in patients with compromised renal function. Furthermore, the therapeutic serum level often approximates the toxic level, and adverse reactions may be unavoidable in patients with life-threatening infections. Since gentamicin has such a wide spectrum of activity against aerobic gram-negative bacilli, it is often used in conjunction with a penicillinase-resistant penicillin or a cephalosporin for the initial therapy in patients with malignancies or who are on immunosuppressive or cytotoxic agents. If the infecting organism proves to be susceptible to a less toxic drug, gentamicin should be discontinued and that agent instituted for the remainder of the patient's therapy. The aminoglycosides should never be injected into body cavities or given rapidly by vein, because neuromuscular blockade with respiratory arrest may ensue. This curare-like effect may be reversed with neostigmine or calcium gluconate. All the aminoglycosides are nephrotoxic and neurotoxic. Neomycin and kanamycin cause auditory toxicity with deafness. Deafness is more commonly seen in patients with renal insufficiency or in patients receiving ethacrynic acid or furosemide. Streptomycin and gentamicin usually cause vestibular damage which may be irreversible. Occasionally deafness may also occur. During long-term therapy, patients must be closely followed with daily tandem-walking and weekly caloric reactions and

audiograms. Paresthesias, peripheral neuropathy, and optic neuritis are rarely observed. Hypersensitivity reactions have been reported with each of the aminoglycosides.

Polymyxins. Polymyxin B and polymyxin E are polypeptide antimicrobials that are active against *E. coli,* Klebsiella-Enterobacter species, and Pseudomonas species. Proteus species are resistant to these drugs. Polymyxin B is given parenterally and may also be administered intrathecally. The polymyxins do not cross the blood-brain barrier and must be given both parenterally and intrathecally in patients with gram-negative bacillary meningitis. Polymyxin E has two forms, parenteral colistimethate sodium and oral colistin sulfate, a nonabsorbable antimicrobial. Although active in vitro against many species of gram-negative bacilli, polymyxin is most useful in the therapy of *Pseudomonas aeruginosa* infections. Since the polymyxins are excreted by the kidneys, caution must be used when these agents are given to patients with renal insufficiency. Serious adverse reactions are dose related. Neurotoxic reactions include circumoral or fingertip paresthesias that are usually reversible. Ataxia, slurred speech, and blurred vision are uncommon. Respiratory paralysis may occur with rapid intravenous administration or in patients receiving succinylcholine and may be reversed by intravenous calcium gluconate but not neostigmine. Azotemia and impaired renal function are seen with high doses. Hypersensitivity reactions have been reported and include eosinophilia and rash.

Spectinomycin. Spectinomycin is active against *Neisseria gonorrhoeae* and has been approved only for use in uncomplicated gonorrhea. The drug does not have treponemicidal activity. It should be considered for use in patients with gonococcal urethritis and cervicitis who are allergic to penicillin, because it can be given as a single dose intramuscularly. There is no cross-resistance between spectinomycin and penicillin. Although spectinomycin inhibits protein synthesis by binding 30S ribosomal subunits (similar to the aminoglycosides), adverse reactions, except for fever and urticaria, have been uncommon to date.

Chloramphenicol. Chloramphenicol has a broad spectrum of activity against the rickettsiae, gram-positive bacteria, gram-negative bacteria, including Salmonella and Shigella, and anaerobic bacteria. The drug is well absorbed from the gastrointestinal tract. It is metabolized by the liver and can therefore be used in patients with renal insufficiency. Adequate levels in the cerebrospinal fluid are present after intravenous injection. Chloramphenicol causes bone marrow aplasia and fatal pancytopenia in 1 of every 40,000 or more courses of therapy or 1 of 25,000 to 50,000 people exposed. This severe toxic reaction is a form of hypersensitivity or idiosyncratic reaction which cannot be predicted before therapy. For this reason, chloramphenicol should be used only for certain specific, severe infections. These indications include (1) typhoid fever or other Salmonella infections, (2) as an alternative drug for ampicillin in *Hemophilus influenzae,* pneumococcal, and meningococcal meningitis, (3) severe anaerobic infections for which clindamycin is not effective, (4) gram-negative bacillary infections that do not respond to other antimicrobial agents, and (5) severe rickettsial infections when tetracycline is not effective.

Anemia which is dose related and not a hypersensitivity reaction may occur with prolonged use. This form of bone marrow depression is reversible and is characterized by interference with iron metabolism, with increased serum iron and saturation of iron-binding globulin, decreased reticulocyte count, and vacuolization of red cell precursors. Patients receiving chloramphenicol must have repeated complete blood counts and serum iron and saturation determinations. This type of anemia is most commonly seen in patients with liver disease or renal insufficiency and in those receiving high doses. Fatal toxicity may develop in neonates ("gray baby syndrome"). Optic neuritis and peripheral neuropathy are rarely seen with prolonged therapy. Hypersensitivity reactions have been reported.

Tetracyclines. The tetracyclines have a broad spectrum of activity. Rickettsia, Chlamydia, *Mycoplasma pneumoniae,* gram-positive and gram-negative bacteria, certain anaerobic organisms, and *T. pallidum* are susceptible to the tetracyclines. At present, 25 to 50 per cent of group A streptococci, 5 to 10 per cent of pneumococci, and most *Staphylococcus aureus* isolates are resistant. In addition, many aerobic gram-negative bacilli and Bacteroides species are also resistant. These changing susceptibility patterns since the introduction of tetracycline in the 1940s have made it necessary to restrict the use of these drugs to the following indications: (1) Rickettsia infections; (2) *M. pneumoniae* infections; (3) Chlamydia infections, including psittacosis, trachoma, lymphogranuloma venereum, and nongonococcal urethritis; (4) granuloma inguinale and chancroid; (5) alternative therapy for gonorrhea and syphilis; and (6) urinary tract infections caused by susceptible gram-negative bacilli.

Tetracycline has replaced *chlortetracycline* and *oxytetracycline* as the agent of choice. It may be given orally or intravenously, although thrombophlebitis often accompanies the latter route of administration. Tetracycline should be avoided in patients with renal insufficiency. Four long-acting tetracyclines are available: *demethylchlortetracycline, methacycline, doxycycline,* and *minocycline.* The rate of renal excretion of these agents is less and oral absorption greater than those of tetracycline, resulting in prolonged serum levels. Minor variations in the degree of antibacterial activity exist among the four preparations which are reflected in the amount of drug recommended per dose. Doxycycline does not accumulate in the serum of patients with renal insufficiency and may be advantageous when the status of renal function is unknown. However, because of the low renal clearance of both doxycycline and minocycline, their usefulness in urinary tract infections may be limited by low urinary concentrations. Unlike the other tetracyclines, minocycline decreases nasopharyngeal carriage of meningococci and may therefore be indicated in prophylaxis of infection caused by sulfadiazine-resistant meningococci. With few exceptions all the tetracycline compounds produce the same adverse reactions. These include gastrointestinal disturbances such as nausea, vomiting, and diarrhea, thrombophlebitis with intravenous administration, staining and hypoplasia of dental enamel and disturbed bone growth in neonates and young children, pseudotumor cerebri with bulging fontanelles and increased cerebrospinal fluid pressure in infants, and acute fatty degeneration of the liver in pregnant women and patients with renal insufficiency. Photosensitivity reactions are not infrequently seen with the long-acting tetracyclines. A variant of the Fanconi syndrome caused by toxic products may occur with administration of outdated tetracycline preparations. Superinfections with resistant gram-negative bacilli, *Staphylococcus aureus,* and Candida may occur with prolonged therapy.

Sulfonamides. For four decades, sulfonamides have been widely prescribed for a variety of clinical infections. However, their present use is limited because of resistance of gram-positive and gram-negative organisms, the availability of more active antimicrobial agents, and adverse reactions. The major indications are (1) nocardiosis; (2) suppressive therapy for paracoccidioidomycosis; (3) prophylaxis in sulfadiazine-sensitive meningococcal infections; (4) alternative prophylaxis for acute rheumatic fever in patients allergic to penicillin; (5) uncomplicated urinary tract infections caused by susceptible organisms, especially *E. coli;* (6) salicylazosulfapyridine therapy in patients with mild ulcerative colitis; (7) certain protozoal infections (toxoplasmosis, *Pneumocystis carinii,* and chloroquine-resistant P. falciparum malaria); and (8) when administered in combination with antifolate compounds, chronic urinary tract infections and possibly also typhoid fever.

Sulfisoxazole is well absorbed from the gastrointestinal tract and may also be administered parenterally if necessary. The drug is chiefly excreted by glomerular filtration and thus is not affected by probenecid. *Sulfamethoxazole* is a congener of sulfisoxazole, but is absorbed less and the renal excretion is delayed. The more potent *sulfadiazine,* once widely used, is less soluble and tends to cause crystalluria. The incidence of crystalluria is decreased by increasing fluid intake and maintaining an alkaline urine. Long-acting sulfonamides, such as *sulfamethoxypyridazine* and *sulfadimethoxine,* although widely used in the past, have no place in clinical antimicrobial therapy because of their toxic effects. The poorly absorbed sulfonamides, *succinylsulfathiazole* and *phthalylsulfathiazole,* are principally used to decrease bacterial counts in the intestine prior to surgery. These agents are of doubtful value. *Salicylazosulfapyridine* may decrease the severity of disease in patients with mild ulcerative colitis. This effect may be due to the antibacterial action of sulfapyridine or the anti-inflammatory effect of 5-aminosalicylic acid.

Adverse reactions caused by the sulfonamides include the following: hypersensitivity reactions with fever, rash, photosensitivity, and rarely vasculitis; nephrotoxicity with crystalluria and renal tubular necrosis; kernicterus in the newborn; hepatitis (occasionally with noncaseating granuloma); agranulocytosis and aplastic anemia; and acute hemolytic anemia in patients with G-6-PD deficiency. Long-acting sulfonamides may cause Stevens-Johnson syndrome and myocarditis.

Trimethoprim-Sulfamethoxazole. This drug combination sequentially inhibits the utilization of para-aminobenzoic acid by bacteria in the synthesis of folic acid. A double sequential blockage is thus produced, and relatively low concentrations of each drug are required for antimicrobial activity. At present, the drug combination (trimethoprim, 80 mg; sulfamethoxazole, 400 mg), has been approved in the United States only for chronic urinary tract infections. Clinical trials suggest that it may be useful in patients with bronchitis, gonorrhea, and possibly typhoid fever resistant to both chloramphenicol and ampicillin. Adverse reactions are the same as those described for the sulfonamides, including the Stevens-Johnson syndrome, and trimethoprim, including nausea, vomiting, skin rashes, and macrocytic anemia caused by folic acid deficiency. Serious nephrotoxicity has been reported in patients with diminished renal function.

Nitrofurantoin. Nitrofurantoin is an oral antibacterial agent that is excreted in the urine by both glomerular filtration and tubular secretion. The drug is most active against *E. coli,* Klebsiella-Enterobacter species, and some strains of enterococci. The susceptibility of Proteus strains is variable, and Pseudomonas species are resistant. Nitrofurantoin should be used only for uncomplicated urinary tract infections or suppressive therapy in patients with chronic urinary tract infections. The drug is most active in the presence of an acid urine, and emergent resistance has not been noted. It should not be prescribed in pregnant women, because it crosses the placenta, or in patients with renal insufficiency. Adverse reactions include nausea and vomiting, hypersensitivity reactions (fever, rash, allergic pneumonitis), paresthesias which may progress to severe polyneuropathy if the drug is not discontinued, acute hemolytic anemia in patients with G-6-PD deficiency, and cholestatic hepatitis.

Nalidixic Acid. Nalidixic acid is also an oral antimicrobial agent used in the therapy of uncomplicated urinary tract infections. The drug is active against strains of *E. coli,* Klebsiella-Enterobacter species, and Proteus species; Pseudomonas species are resistant. Gram-negative bacilli may rapidly develop resistance to this agent, and repeated urine cultures with drug-susceptibility determinations should be performed during therapy. Adverse reactions include nausea, vomiting, hypersensitivity reactions (rash, eosinophilia, photosensitivity), and rarely cholestatic jaundice, blood dyscrasias, visual disturbances, toxic psychosis, and convulsive seizures. Severe headache associated with papilledema has been observed in children.

Methenamine Mandelate and Hippurate. These antimicrobial compounds are the salts of methenamine and mandelic acid and hippuric acid, respectively. They are well absorbed from the gastrointestinal tract and rapidly excreted in the urine. They are bactericidal in acidic urine (pH less than 5.5). An acidifying agent is necessary if the infecting organism forms ammonia. Methenamine mandelate or hippurate may be used for chronic suppression of urinary tract infections. *Escherichia coli* is susceptible to these drugs. Proteus species and Pseudomonas species are usually resistant. Adverse reactions are uncommon and include epigastric pain, dysuria, crystalluria, and metabolic acidosis, especially in patients with renal insufficiency.

FAILURE OF ANTIMICROBIAL THERAPY

The failure of a patient to respond to antimicrobial therapy may be due to factors related to the host and the nature of the disease or to an error in the choice, dosage, or route of administration of the drug. The following causes are most common: (1) incorrect diagnosis; (2) impaired host defense mechanisms; (3) inadequate dose, route of administration, or distribution of drug; (4) closed space infection; (5) presence of a foreign body; (6) superinfection; and (7) microbial drug resistance.

Resistance of microorganisms to antimicrobial agents may be classified as primary (natural) or emergent (acquired) (see Ch. 267). Microorganisms acquire resistance by either mutation or episomal transfer. Mutation patterns may be multi-step, involving a number of genes, or large-step, involving one gene. The efficiency of mutation is increased in the presence of low-dose antimicrobial drug administration. Both gram-positive and gram-negative bacteria develop resistance by mutation. Recognition of episomal transfer of resistance is presently restricted to gram-negative bacilli and *Staphylococcus aureus*. The transfer of cytoplasmic DNA (R factor) requires cell-to-cell contact and is termed conjugation. The transfer of resistance may be single or multiple, and occurs most commonly in the gastrointestinal tract. It is often designated infectious drug resistance.

CHEMOPROPHYLAXIS

Antimicrobial agents are often administered to individuals who are believed to be at some increased risk of acquiring a bacterial infection.

Prophylaxis is usually successful only when a single drug is given for a specific organism. The antimicrobial drugs and their clinical indications which are considered to be of value are summarized in Table 3. Antimicrobial prophylaxis is not effective in viral respiratory diseases, viral exanthems, clean abdominal surgery, and congestive heart failure. Unlike the therapeutic situation in which the identity of the offending microbe might be in doubt and there is urgency in selecting therapy, with chemoprophylaxis there is usually no urgency, and the microbe in question is known. Consequently, the use of antimicrobial drugs in chemoprophylaxis should be more rational than in therapy. Unfortunately, this is not always the case, and in many instances the prophylactic use of antimicrobial agents is unwarranted, ineffective, and often dangerous because of toxic reactions, superinfection, and emergent resistance. The matter of drug toxicity requires comment. Selection of a drug is a matter of

TABLE 3. Recommendations for Antimicrobial Prophylaxis

Disease or Clinical Setting	Etiologic Agent	Antimicrobial Drug
Acute rheumatic fever (recurrent)	Group A streptococcus	Penicillin, erythromycin, sulfonamide
Meningococcal infections	*Neisseria meningitidis*	
	Sulfonamide-susceptible	Sulfisoxazole
	Sulfonamide-resistant	Minocycline
Microbial endocarditis		
Oral cavity instrumentation	Viridans streptococcus	Penicillin, cephalosporin
Urogenital and gastrointestinal instrumentation	Enterococcus	Penicillin or vancomycin plus streptomycin
Open heart surgery	*Staphylococcus aureus* and *epidermidis*	Penicillinase-resistant penicillin, cephalosporin
Newborn nursery epidemics	Enteropathic *E. coli*	Neomycin, Colistin
	Staphylococcus aureus	Penicillinase-resistant penicillin
	Group A streptococci	Penicillin
Tuberculin reactors of certain sorts	*Mycobacterium tuberculosis*	Isoniazid
Malaria	Plasmodia	
	Chloroquine-susceptible	Chloroquine followed by primaquine
	Chloroquine-resistant (*P. falciparum*)	Chloroguanide and sulfone
Ophthalmia neonatorum	*Neisseria gonorrhoeae*	Silver nitrate, penicillin
Burns		Silver sulfadiazine, silver nitrate
Bronchitis (chronic)	Pneumococcus or *Hemophilus influenzae*	Ampicillin, tetracycline

weighing offsetting risks. It is easy to forget that a degree of drug toxicity that is acceptable when weighed against an instance of a particular disease may be unacceptable when weighed against the chance that someone *might* acquire that disease. Finally, although one must emphasize the need for caution in chemoprophylaxis, it is fitting to remember that in terms of the number of people benefited, the use of the drugs in this way represents one of the greatest achievements of modern biomedical science and technology.

Gavin, T. L., et al.: Antimicrobial Susceptibility Testing. American Society of Clinical Pathologists, 1971.

Goodman, L. S., and Gilman, A.: The Pharmacological Basis of Therapeutics. 4th ed. New York, Macmillan, 1970.

Handbook of Antimicrobial Therapy. The Medical Letter on Drugs and Therapeutics (revised ed.), 1974.

Kunin, C. M., et al.: Use of antibiotics. A brief exposition of the problem and some tentative solutions. Ann. Intern. Med., 79:555, 1973.

Pratt, W. B.: Fundamentals of Chemotherapy. New York, Oxford University Press, 1973.

Weinstein, L., and Dalton, A. C.: Host determinants of response to antimicrobial agents. N. Engl. J. Med., 279:467, 1968.

Part IX

PROTOZOAN AND HELMINTHIC DISEASES

269. INTRODUCTION

Philip D. Marsden

With rapid air travel, so-called parasitic infections are becoming more important in temperate climes. They have always been important in the tropics.

Parasitic disease is usually taken to imply infections caused by protozoa and helminths, although, in their relationship to the host, bacteria, viruses, and rickettsiae equally fulfill the general criteria used to describe an organism as parasitic. The reason for this nomenclature is historic; because they are bigger organisms, helminths and protozoa were discovered relatively early by medical investigators. Ascaris and tapeworms are dramatic enough to have been recognized in ancient times, and protozoa were seen with the first crude microscopes.

For the correct diagnosis of parasitic disease the physician must be as competent at the microscope and in using the laboratory procedures to find parasites as he is at defining the clinical presentation at the bedside and interpreting it. As with other infectious diseases, a firm diagnosis rests on finding the infectious agent. Recently serologic tests have been used much more to aid diagnosis, and, interpreted wisely, they are valuable. Broadly speaking, they mean that a patient has developed antibodies of a certain type to a parasitic antigen. Rarely do they give any confirmation about the status of the parasite in the body of man in terms of numbers present or whether they are multiplying. Positive serologic findings should often be an indication for redoubling one's efforts to find the parasite.

Whether a complement fixation test, hemagglutination test, fluorescent antibody test, or gel diffusion test is positive at a significant titer must be decided in the light of known facts about the specificity of the tests.

Many of the drugs used are toxic to man but more toxic to the parasites. We know little of the mechanism of drug action in many cases, e.g., Pentostam in leishmaniasis. With some drugs such as heavy metal containing compounds and emetine the toxic dose for man is near the therapeutic dose. Physicians should be especially careful to check their prescriptions of these drugs, especially if they are not used to prescribing them often.

The National Communicable Disease Center, Atlanta, Georgia, offers unique services to the physician in the United States for the management of parasitic disease. Not only is there a laboratory for diagnostic serology, but recently a number of rare drugs previously not available in the United States and mentioned in this book have become available through the Parasitic Disease Drug Service in the Epidemiology Program. These include drugs for the treatment of both types of human trypanosomiasis, leishmaniasis, amebiasis, pneumocystis infection, and schistosomiasis.

With regard to diagnostic serology, Dr. Irving G. Kagan has kindly provided the accompanying table of serologic tests available for parasitic diseases in the United States.

Immunodiagnostic Tests for Parasitic Infections

	Complement Fixation	Precipitin	Particle Agglutination Tests				Fluorescent Antibody	Methylene Blue Dye
			Bentonite Flocculation	Hemagglutination	Latex Agglutination	Cholesterol Flocculation		
Trichinosis	+	+	+*	±*	+*	+*	+*	
Echinococcosis	+	+	+*	+*	+*		+	
Schistosomiasis	+*		±*	±*		+*	+*	
Ascariasis/toxocariasis			+*	+*			0	
Filariasis	±		+*	+*	0		0	
Cysticercosis	+	0		+*			0	
Chagas' disease	+*	±	0	+*	0		0*	
Leishmaniasis	+			+*			0	
Toxoplasmosis	+*			+*	0		+*	+*
Amebiasis	+*	+	±*	+*	±		±*	
Malaria				±*			+*	

* = Tests available in the U.S.
0 = Under experimental investigation.
± = Used for diagnosis, but requires further evaluation for routine use.
+ = Generally accepted useful routine diagnostic test.
Adapted from data supplied by Dr. Irving Kagan, Center for Disease Control.

Section One. PROTOZOAN DISEASES

270. INTRODUCTION

Philip D. Marsden

Malaria remains the greatest challenge in parasitic disease both in terms of prevalence (over 500 million people still live in malarious areas) and in the amount of morbidity and mortality it causes. In many tropical countries, notably Africa, malaria has a profound influence on the pattern of clinical medicine.

Trypanosomiasis is a good example of geographically restricted disease. *Trypanosoma brucei* infections are restricted to Africa because tsetse flies (Glossina species) are not found elsewhere. African sleeping sickness demands attention because human infections once established are so frequently fatal. Also, this same group of trypanosomes are responsible for widespread fatal disease in cattle, profoundly influencing animal husbandry. South American trypanosomiasis (Chagas' disease) is restricted to the Americas because again the great majority of reduviid bugs occur in this location. The significance of this infection as a public health problem is a matter of current concern. One estimate suggests that 7 million people are infected and 30 million exposed to the risk of infection. Permanent cardiac damage often ensues, and at the time of writing there is no cure.

Also in the family Trypanosomatidae, the genus *Leishmania* is responsible for considerable human suffering. Visceral leishmaniasis is a debilitating infection, and without treatment the terminal event is usually a secondary bacterial infection, often a pneumonia. Cutaneous and mucocutaneous leishmaniasis can be disfiguring infections. Therapy is far from satisfactory.

Amebiasis ranks fourth in this consideration, because, although bowel infections are widely prevalent, invasive disease is less common. Then come a miscellany of rarer protozoal disease entities.

The reader will appreciate that the first three groups of diseases caused by protozoa all have arthropod vectors: Anopheles for malaria, Glossina and Reduviidae for trypanosomiasis, and Phlebotomus for leishmaniasis. It is relevant and important for medical men to have some knowledge of these vectors. A few examples of why this is so will suffice. At the time of writing there have been a few cases of indigenous vivax malaria recognized in the United States. Epidemiologic work has revealed vector Anopheles in the area. Xenodiagnosis using clean Reduviidae is the best way of finding *Trypanosoma cruzi* parasites in a patient with a chronic infection, and because of this these insects are most important, as they are used in diagnostic medicine. Phlebotomus remains very susceptible to DDT, and spraying of this insect's habitats will result in the control of human leishmaniasis.

Another medical consideration worth emphasizing is that blood protozoa can be transmitted by blood transfusion. Particularly important in this respect are malaria and *Trypanosoma cruzi* infections. Suitable selection of donors in temperate countries is necessary to avoid this complication in nonimmune persons exposed to the risk of malaria parasites in transfused blood. *Trypanosoma cruzi* infections transmitted by blood transfusion are said to be particularly acute. It is of interest that recent advances in immunology enable us to screen blood donors for malaria with the indirect fluorescent antibody test, whereas for *Trypanosoma cruzi* the valuable complement-fixation test or an indirect fluorescent antibody test is available.

Belding, D. L.: Textbook of Parasitology. 3rd ed. New York, Appleton-Century-Crofts, Inc., 1965.
Faust, E. C., and Russell, P. F.: Clinical Parasitology. 8th ed. Philadelphia, Lea & Febiger, 1970.
Hunter, G. W., Frye, W. W., and Swartzwelder, J. C.: A Manual of Tropical Medicine. 4th ed. Philadelphia, W. B. Saunders Company, 1966.
Wilcocks, C., and Manson-Bahr, P. E. C.: Manson's Tropical Diseases. 17th ed. Baltimore, Williams & Wilkins Company, 1972.

271. MALARIA

Thomas C. Jones

General Considerations. Malaria is characterized by shaking chills, relapsing fever, prostration, splenomegaly, and anemia. After the initial illness, the disease may follow a chronic or relapsing course. It is caused by four species of the genus Plasmodium (*P. vivax, P. falciparum, P. malariae,* and *P. ovale*). The infection is maintained in nature by the feeding habits of female mosquitoes of the genus Anopheles, in which sporogony occurs, feeding on blood of humans, in which schizogony and gametocytogony occur. Malaria remains a common cause of morbidity and mortality in the world. Delay in diagnosis or inappropriate therapy may lead to severe complications which include coma, acute renal failure, severe anemia, pulmonary edema, or shock. Recognition of the association between malaria and hemoglobinopathies, persistent hypergammaglobulinemia, Burkitt's lymphoma, and the tropical splenomegaly syndrome has emphasized the often subtle but significant influence of malaria on populations living in endemic areas.

History. The term malaria originated in the seventeenth century in Italy where the death of patients after intermittent or so-called Roman fevers was attributed to the bad air (mal'aria) of the marsh and swamp lands. These fevers were recognized in ancient times in China, India, and Mesopotamia, but the earliest record of quotidian, tertian, and quartan fevers was that of Hippocrates in the fifth century B.C. The Greeks and Romans were aware of the association of these fevers with marsh lands and conducted one of the earliest public health campaigns by draining the stagnant water. Cinchona bark was recognized as being effective against fevers in 1600 in Peru, after which it was widely used in Europe. Torti, in 1712, clearly distinguished the fevers that responded to cinchona from those that did not.

The protozoan was first described in the blood of a patient by Charles Laveran in 1880, who observed the parasite in an unstained smear of fresh blood. In 1891 Romanowsky developed a technique for staining blood smears for accurate study of the erythrocytic stage of malaria. In 1897, William MacCallum observed penetration and fertilization of the female gamete, documenting that a sexual cycle occurred in malaria. The role of the mosquito as a vector in malaria was postulated by Sir Patrick Manson after he documented that filaria could develop in the mosquito. Theobald Smith showed a few years later that an insect vector (the tick) could actually transmit disease among cattle. The careful studies of Sir Ronald Ross in 1898 documented that in avian malaria the protozoan developed in the stomach of infected mosquitoes and migrated to the salivary glands, from which it could infect healthy birds. Several months later Bignami, Bastianelli, and Grassi documented the transmission of malaria to man by Anopheles mosquitoes. Our present knowledge of the malaria cycle was completed in 1948 when Shortt, Garnham, Bray, and others confirmed the presence of the pre-erythrocytic stage in man.

A decrease in the prevalence of malaria during this century has resulted from campaigns to control mosquitoes and the widespread use of drug therapy directed against malaria. The systematic approach to mosquito control organized by Col. William Gorgas in the Canal Zone in 1906 was one of the outstanding achievements in preventive medical sciences. Effective insecticides were first introduced in 1939, and a number of synthetic antimalarial drugs were developed. The global program of malaria eradication was instituted during the 1950's with impressive results. It has become clear recently that various technical and socioeconomic problems in some countries have required that careful methods of malaria control be substituted for attempts at eradication of the disease.

Epidemiology. Malaria is an endemic disease in parts of Africa, Asia, and Central and South America, where environmental factors, including temperature, humidity, and standing water, support the breeding of mosquitoes and where there is close contact between the mosquitoes and man. The disease in these areas contributes to a high infant mortality and syndromes of chronic malaria. The prevalence of malaria in endemic areas is usually determined by documenting the proportion of people with large spleens (spleen rate) or the proportion of people with blood smears positive for malaria parasites (parasite rate). It has been estimated that 100 million cases of malaria occur each year. Approximately 1 per cent of these patients die of the disease, although this figure can vary from less than 1 per cent to over 10 per cent, depending on the species of Plasmodium most prevalent, the level of immunity of the host, and the availability of prompt medical care.

Acute disease caused by malaria often occurs when nonimmune persons enter endemic areas. Through the centuries the most impressive effects of malaria have been recorded during time of war when large numbers of nonimmunes are placed in malarious areas. This has certainly been the major factor contributing to the incidence of malaria in American citizens in the past 35 years. The number of cases of malaria in the United States rose from less than 100 in 1960 to 4000 in 1970 as a direct result of the exposure of nonimmune military personnel to the disease in Vietnam.

Epidemics of malaria may occur when the parasite is introduced into a region with a large nonimmune population. This occurred in the Soviet Union after World War I when more than 5 million cases were reported in 1923; and in Ethiopia in 1958 when 3 million cases and 150,000 deaths caused by malaria were reported. Such epidemics are reminders of the potential threat to localities where effective malaria eradication has created a large nonimmune population but where mosquito vectors persist in large numbers. Vectors for transmission of plasmodia, primarily *A. quadrimaculatus* and *A. freeborni*, persist in parts of the United States. Since 1963, 14 cases of malaria have been documented in which infection occurred within the United States.

Falciparum and vivax malaria are widely spread throughout the tropics and subtropics, particularly in hot, humid regions. Malariae malaria is also widespread, but it is of lower prevalence, and it tends to be less evenly distributed. Ovale malaria is primarily seen in West Africa.

During the past decade malaria has been found to be associated geographically with several other conditions, including various erythrocyte abnormalities and Burkitt's lymphoma. Patients with sickle hemoglobin have been shown to acquire falciparum malaria as frequently as those with normal hemoglobin, but their disease is less severe. The malaria parasite appears less able to divide in these abnormal erythrocytes. Other hemoglobinopathies and inherited enzyme defects, including hemoglobin C, D, E, K, O, b-thalassemia, and glucose-6-phosphate dehydrogenase deficiency, have also been shown to occur more commonly in areas endemic for malaria. These defects appear to provide some selective advantage for survival in malarious areas, and their high frequency is a good example of the concept in population genetics of balanced polymorphism. Correlation of the prevalence of Burkitt's lymphoma with prevalence of malaria has led to suggestions that chronic malaria suppresses mechanisms for immunologic surveillance, leading to expression of this tumor. Some work in laboratory animals chronically infected with malaria supports this view, but the relationship needs further clarification.

The epidemiology of malaria is inseparable from the epidemiology of its mosquito vectors. Entomologists must document different and changing characteristics of the numerous species of anopheline mosquitoes, including their flying and resting habits, feeding habits, and degree of resistance to insecticides. For example, a recent change in mosquito living habits from domestic to sylvatic in Central America has rendered the usual technique of household DDT residual spraying less effective. Several instances have been recorded in which mosquito feeding habits changed from cattle to man, resulting in epidemic malaria.

Although the mosquito is the primary vector for malaria, direct transfer of infected erythrocytes from one individual to another by blood transfusion or syringe usage in common by addicts will cause malaria. In these cases the sexual cycle in the mosquito and the pre-erythrocytic stages of malaria in man are bypassed. In the past 15 years 45 cases of malaria transmitted by transfusions were reported in the United States. The American Association of Blood Banks has recommended that blood not be taken from anyone who has emigrated from an endemic area or had malaria during the preceding three years, or who has visited a malarious area during which antimalarial prophylaxis was taken in the preceding two years. Travelers to malarial areas who remained symptom free and who did not take antimalarials may donate blood after six months. An epidemic of vivax malaria (which affected 47 persons) was reported from California after the sharing of heroin injection equipment by drug addicts. One of the members of the group had just returned from Vietnam. In the past, malaria was transmitted intentionally by physicians as a method of causing fever in patients for treatment of neurosyphilis and other diseases. Congenitally acquired malaria has rarely been reported. Transmission of malaria of monkeys, *P. knowlesi* and *P. cynomolgi*, from monkey to man has been demonstrated in the laboratory and rarely documented in nature.

The major thrust against malaria has been the worldwide cooperative program of malaria eradication begun approximately 20 years ago. The program was a unified approach divided into four carefully defined phases: preparatory, attack, consolidation, and maintenance. The techniques included concentrated spraying with residual insecticides, use of antimalarial drugs, and case-detection surveys. Recently, a number of problems have challenged the completion of malaria eradication using these techniques: inadequate finances in some regions; social disorganization during war and natural disaster; resistance of mosquitoes to insecticides; resistance of plasmodia to antimalarial drugs; and the demonstration that the malaria of monkeys can be transmitted to man.

Realization of these limitations has led to programs concentrating on malaria control rather than eradication. Perhaps related to this, there has been an increased interest in malaria immunity, both to define mechanisms of natural or acquired resistance and to develop potentially useful vaccines.

The Protozoan. Over 100 different species of Plasmodium are capable of infecting the red blood cells of mammals, birds, and reptiles. There are several hundred species of Anopheles mosquitoes which can be infected by the protozoan and therefore transmit the disease. Male anopheline mosquitoes feed on nectar and therefore do not transmit the infection. The female requires products of a blood meal for egg production. Female mosquitoes vary in their feeding habits so that only 50 species participate in transmission of human malaria. During the process of feeding, the mosquito injects fluid from the salivary glands. Sporozoites may be released with the salivary fluid if the mosquito ate a blood meal two to four weeks previously which contained male and female malaria gametocytes (Fig. 1).

The sporozoites enter the circulation immediately, and a transient parasitemia occurs which lasts less than one hour. During this period the sporozoites enter hepatic parenchymal cells, initiating the *pre-erythrocytic* stage of plasmodium infection by forming a primary hepatic schizont. The duration of this pre-erythrocytic stage is usually short in *P. falciparum* (5.5 to 7 days) and *P. vivax* (6 to 8 days) but somewhat longer in *P. ovale* (9 days) and *P. malariae* (13 to 16 days). Merozoites are then released from the hepatic cells and enter circulating erythrocytes. Occasionally, when the number of sporozoites inoculated is very low, the period from infection to onset of erythrocyte infection lasts for months or even years. In falci-

---

*The exoerythrocytic state is described in this chapter as "persistent" rather than cyclic, based on the arguments presented by Coatney et al. in the first cited reference. It is recognized that not all malariologists agree with this recent change in terms or the implied change in the nature of tissue schizogony and the mechanism of relapse.

parum malaria the tissue phase terminates at the beginning of the *erythrocyte cycle;* in other Plasmodium species, the hepatic forms persist.* This species variation necessitates different therapeutic approaches in treating malaria. The species also differ in the number of merozoites released after primary hepatic schizogony: *P. falciparum* – about 40,000 from each infected cell; *P. ovale* – 15,000; *P. vivax* – 10,000; and *P. malariae* – 2000. The large number of merozoites released into the circulation in *P. falciparum* may contribute to the high levels of parasitemia seen in this infection and perhaps to the increased frequency with which erythrocytes are observed to contain multiple organisms.

The merozoite enters the red blood cell by inducing erythrocyte endocytosis, and the organism begins to develop within a vacuole in the erythrocyte. Using Giemsa or Wright stains, the parasite is first identified with light microscopy as a characteristic "ring-form," an early *trophozoite* (Figs. 2A and 2B). The organism increases in size, partially filling the red blood cell; this is termed the late *trophozoite*. Later the nuclear material is segregated by schizogony, and the red cell becomes partially filled with the cytoplasm and the multiple nuclei of the *schizont* (Fig. 2C). The erythrocyte cycle is completed when the red blood cells rupture, releasing the merozoites formed from the schizont, which then invade other erythrocytes. This cycle takes 48 hours in *P. falciparum*, *P. vivax*, and *P. ovale* malaria, and 72 hours in *P. malariae* infection. Symptoms of fever and chills coincide with the release of merozoites; hence the clinical descriptions of tertian malaria (fevers on days one and three) and quartan malaria (fevers on days one and four). The number of merozoites formed during erythrocyte schizogony is helpful in species diagnosis. Examination of a mature schizont of *P. malariae* will reveal 6 to 12 developing merozoites, *P. ovale* 6 to 16, and *P. vivax* 12 to 24.

By mechanisms which remain completely unknown, some merozoites do not continue the cycle of schizogony but develop into female and male gametocytes (Fig. 1). These first appear in the peripheral blood several days after the onset of the erythrocytic cycle, and they may

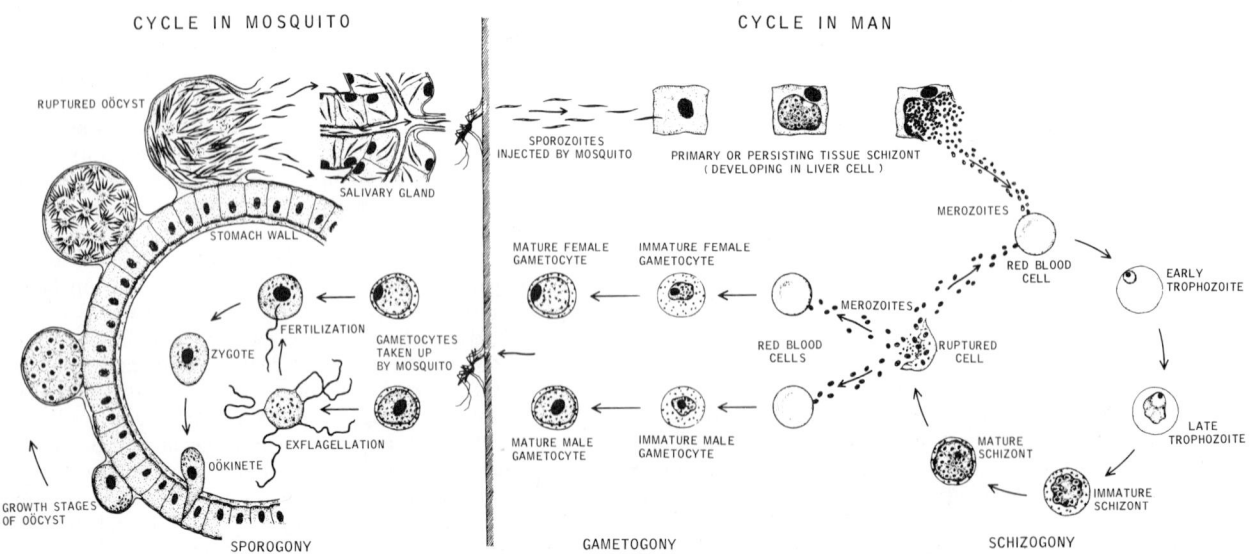

Figure 1. Life cycle of Plasmodium in mosquito and man. (Adapted from Alvarado, C. A., and Bruce-Chwatt, L. J.: Scientific American, Vol. 206, May, 1962. Copyright © 1962, by Scientific American, Inc. All rights reserved.)

persist for weeks after schizogony has been suppressed. During the blood meal of an Anopheles mosquito, the gametocytes are ingested. Conditions exist in the stomach of the mosquito for the male gametocyte to form motile male gametes (exflagellation) which then fertilize the female gamete. After fertilization, the *zygote* becomes a motile *öokinete*, penetrates the stomach wall, and multiplies in an enlarging *oocyst*. Rupture of this cyst allows release of sporozoites which are distributed throughout the mosquito and accumulate in the salivary gland. The formation of sporozoites completes the process of *sporogony*, the sexual or mosquito cycle of malaria.

Pathogenesis and Immunity. There has been no documentation of generalized or significant host injury or response during the periods of sporozoitemia or hepatic schizogony, although antisporozoite antibodies have been demonstrated. After release of merozoites from the hepatic cells into the circulation, however, marked changes occur. Parasitized and nonparasitized red blood cells undergo alterations. In *P. falciparum* infection the erythrocytes develop electron-dense knoblike projections, take unusual shapes, and become less deformable. They also become more adhesive to vascular endothelium and more permeable to sodium, and demonstrate increased osmotic fragility. During the erythrocyte cycle, red blood cells are damaged at the time merozoites are released, leading to intravascular hemolysis and progressive anemia. Damage to vascular endothelium also occurs. B lymphocytes begin to produce IgM and IgG antibodies directed against the merozoites, and excess antibody is seen in the plasma in several days. These antibodies coat merozoites, after which they do not enter uninfected red cells, and they are removed from the circulation by phagocytic cells in the bone marrow, spleen, and liver. T lymphocytes release materials which stimulate increased metabolic and phagocytic activity of macrophages. This series of events produces the clinical and pathologic changes observed in acute and chronic malaria.

In acute falciparum malaria a number of complications result from alteration of the red blood cells and the vascular endothelium. The severe anemia and the adherence of red cells to capillary endothelium decrease oxygen supply to the tissues. The anoxia causes serious functional impairment of the brain and kidneys, less commonly of the liver, myocardium, and bone marrow. In fatal cases of falciparum malaria the brain is edematous, and blood vessels are occluded by parasitized erythrocytes, and surrounded by areas of hemorrhage and necrosis. The kidney may show ischemia of the renal cortex and diffuse glomerulitis, as well as tubular necrosis. The liver may show centrilobular degeneration and necrosis. These changes in the kidney and liver are believed related more to ischemia secondary to severe anemia and hypovolemia than to vascular obstruction by erythrocytes. In patients who die in pulmonary edema unrelated to fluid overload, the cardiac and pulmonary vessels are filled with parasitized red cells. Impaired bone marrow function in man is manifested by thrombocytopenia, absence of reticulocytes, and varying degrees of leukopenia.

Accelerated intravascular coagulation is occasionally documented in patients with malaria; that is, factors V, VII, VIII, X, fibrinogen, and platelets are decreased, prothrombin and partial thromboplastin times are prolonged, and fibrin degradation products are increased.

However, disseminated intravascular coagulation is not a prominent feature at autopsy of patients who die of malaria.

During the acute attack of falciparum malaria, most patients develop vasodilation, just as in some other acute febrile diseases. This results in decreased effective circulating blood volume and orthostatic hypotension. Changes secondary to this include increased aldosterone levels, increased plasma volume, hyponatremia, and reversal of the urinary sodium to potassium ratio.

Some of the clinical and pathologic features of malaria are related to the host immune response. Patients occasionally have a Coombs-positive hemolytic anemia. This may partially explain the rapid intravascular hemolysis which exceeds that attributable to the level of parasitemia alone. "Blackwater fever," the complication of falciparum malaria characterized by rapid hemolysis and acute renal failure, occurs both in patients who have received quinine and in patients who have a history of previous exposure to the Plasmodium who have not received quinine. Antibody damage to red cells has been postulated in both situations. The pathologic changes seen in blackwater fever include renal ischemia and tubular necrosis. Recent evidence has suggested that the glomerulitis seen in some patients with falciparum malaria may be induced by immune complexes.

The pathologic picture in malaria of long duration is in large part that due to the immune response. Marked elevation of the serum immunoglobulins (IgG and IgM) is seen, and the liver and spleen are enlarged consistent with continued stimulation to the reticuloendothelial system. Anemia is common. A number of patients in an area hyperendemic for malaria develop marked splenomegaly (tropical splenomegaly syndrome). Parasites may not be demonstrable in peripheral blood smears, but elevated fluorescent antimalarial antibody titers are present, and the patients respond to prolonged therapy with antimalarials. Liver biopsy frequently shows hepatic sinusoidal lymphocytosis. In *P. malariae* infection of long duration, nephrotic syndrome is not uncommon. There is good evidence that this is related to immune complex injury to the glomerulus. Preliminary evidence has suggested that patients with chronic malaria have depressed cellular immune responses.

Host Resistance. Resistance to malaria involves numerous complex metabolic and immunologic factors. As mentioned previously, certain hemoglobinopathies and enzyme defects of the erythrocytes render patients less vulnerable to the severe complications of malaria. For unknown reasons, blacks appear less susceptible to *P. vivax* infection than whites. *Acquired immunity* to malaria requires both humoral and cellular defense mechanisms. Circulating antibodies are of primary importance in control of the acute infection, documented by studies in which antimalaria IgG was transferred to infected hosts and found to be protective. This protection was species specific. The role of antibody has been shown by the transfer of immunity from mother to fetus, with protection of the neonate during the period in which maternal IgG persists. Whether decreases in immunoglobulin levels contribute to relapse of malaria has not been clearly shown. The importance of cellular defense mechanisms has been assumed because of the intense phagocytic activity of cells of the reticuloendothelial system during malaria infection.

Clinical Manifestations. The patient with malaria experiences chills and fever, often associated with frontal

Figure 2.   *See opposite page for legend.*

headache and myalgias. In the early period of the illness the fever may be persistent for several days before developing into a synchronous periodicity, the hallmark of tertian or quartan malaria. When the typical pattern has been established, the patient has a chill, a rise in temperature to 40 to 41° C, headache, and myalgias. This is followed in several hours by diffuse sweating and a fall in temperature. In vivax and ovale malaria these paroxysms occur every 48 hours (benign tertian malaria) and in malariae malaria every 72 hours (quartan malaria). In falciparum malaria the temperature is usually persistently elevated, but it may occasionally progress to a 48-hour cycle (malignant tertian malaria). Between the paroxysms of chills and fever, the patient often feels well except for some weakness or fatigue.

The illness may begin with nonspecific symptoms such as *sore throat, dry cough,* and *abdominal pain.* Most patients have *nausea* and *anorexia; vomiting* is less common. These symptoms may mislead the physician into making a diagnosis of pharyngitis, influenza, or gastroenteritis. Occasionally, the only sign of malaria is fever. In the postoperative surgical patient, fever caused by malaria is frequently confused with that caused by drug allergy. Rarely fever may be absent.

Physical examination reveals a tachycardia, and the skin is warm and flushed. *Jaundice* is not common, but occasionally it can be a prominent feature of the illness. *Hepatomegaly* is commonly found, and the liver may be moderately tender. The spleen is often palpable in acute malaria and is usually quite soft and occasionally tender. Attempts to palpate the spleen should be made carefully in view of the relative ease with which splenic rupture can occur. *Splenomegaly* is more commonly found in the early stage of vivax and ovale malaria than in falciparum malaria. Orthostatic hypotension can be documented in falciparum malaria. Lesions of herpes simplex virus may be seen.

Examination of peripheral blood after several days of illness reveals a normochromic, normocytic anemia which is usually mild, but it may be severe in prolonged infections or in those presenting with high parasitemia or acute hemolysis. The number of reticulocytes is usually normal until several days after therapy is begun; then reticulocytosis is seen. The white blood cell count is normal or low. Monocytosis may be present, but eosino-philia is not a feature of malaria. Thrombocytopenia of a moderate degree is usually present. Serum $\alpha 1$ glycoproteins are increased, whereas $\alpha 2$ glycoproteins (containing haptoglobin) are decreased. A false positive VDRL may occur. The serum transaminases are almost always elevated to moderate degrees and total bilirubin is often elevated. This is predominantly indirect bilirubin, but occasionally increased conjugated bilirubin is seen. Severe cases of malaria may be associated with sufficient liver dysfunction to be misdiagnosed as infectious hepatitis. Tests for determining intestinal absorption have been shown to be abnormal in some malaria patients. Urinalysis reveals trace amounts of albumin and bilirubin in uncomplicated cases, and rarely marked proteinuria has been documented. In falciparum malaria hyponatremia, reversal of the urinary sodium/potassium ratio, and transient increases in serum creatinine and blood urea nitrogen can frequently be recorded.

Fever and related symptoms gradually subside over several weeks in untreated vivax, ovale, and malariae malaria. However, relapse of vivax or ovale infection may occur months or even years later. The illness at the time of relapse is usually milder and of shorter duration than the initial illness. Death caused by infection with these organisms is very uncommon.

Complications. In falciparum malaria high levels of parasitemia and serious complications may develop rapidly. The most important of these complications are *coma, severe hemolytic anemia, acute renal failure,* and *acute pulmonary edema.* The patient may first demonstrate confusion with increasing lethargy, and within a few hours be unconscious. Focal neurologic signs are uncommon, but hyperreflexia and Babinski signs may be seen. Examination of the cerebrospinal fluid will reveal increased pressure and increased protein, without pleocytosis. *Massive intravascular hemolysis* may result from high levels of parasitemia, quinine therapy, drug administration to patients with glucose-6-phosphate dehydrogenase deficiency, or hypersensitivity after previous malaria infections. Hemoglobinuria, acute tubular necrosis, and renal failure may result. *Hemolysis, hemoglobinuria,* and *renal failure* make up the striking clinical picture of severe malaria known as "blackwater fever." Acute renal failure may occur in the absence of signs of intravascular hemolysis and can be detected early only

---

Figure 2. *A* to *D* show various erythrocyte forms of falciparum or vivax malaria (× 1500).

A, "Ring forms" of *Plasmodium falciparum.* Note the delicate rings and an erythrocyte containing two organisms.

B, Trophozoite of *Plasmodium vivax.* The red cell is enlarged, Schüffner's dots are seen, and the parasite is large and ameboid.

C, Schizont of *Plasmodium vivax* with at least 18 merozoite nuclei.

D, Gametocyte of *Plasmodium falciparum.* The crescent or banana shape is characteristic.

E, *Trypanosoma rhodesiense* in the peripheral blood. It has a nucleus, posterior kinetoplast, an undulating membrane, and flagellum (× 1500).

F, Spleen smear showing a cell filled with *Leishmania donovani.* The rod-shaped kinetoplast and large round nucleus appear as two adjacent red dots.

G, Methenamine silver nitrate stain of clump of Pneumocystis cysts. They appear as black circles against the blue background (× 800).

H, Stool sample observed by light microscopy, showing a motile *Entamoeba histolytica* moving in a straight line across the field. The ameba contains lucent vacuoles and shows a pseudopod directed to the upper right (× 500).

(*A, C, D,* and *F* are photographs taken by T. C. Jones from the Cornell Parasitology teaching slides; *B* is from the collection of H. Zaiman, originally photographed by M. Wittner; *E* and *G* were provided by R. B. Roberts; *H* is a photograph of fresh material provided by T. C. Jones.)

by careful monitoring of the urine volume and serum creatinine or urea nitrogen levels. Acute pulmonary edema is an uncommon complication, but it may develop rapidly and be particularly refractile to therapy. Pulmonary edema may be due to excessive fluid administration, but a number of cases have been reported in which intravascular volume was normal. Patients may present with signs and symptoms of vascular collapse—so-called algid malaria. A rare complication of malaria is splenic rupture, the only complication which is probably more common in vivax than falciparum malaria. Patients who survive untreated falciparum malaria may have recurrences of symptoms for a number of months, but thereafter they remain asymptomatic.

Syndromes Associated with Chronic Malaria. Syndromes associated with chronic malaria are most likely the result of repeated exposure of immune patients to Plasmodium and occur predominantly in hyperendemic areas of malaria. The patients may be asymptomatic, but they have intermittently detectable parasitemia, hypergammaglobulinemia, elevated antimalaria antibody titers, anemia, and splenic enlargement. Some patients develop marked splenomegaly—the tropical splenomegaly syndrome. Patients infected with *P. malariae* may develop nephrotic syndrome (quartan nephrosis). This is most common in children. It is associated with a poor prognosis and does not respond well to corticosteroid administration.

Diagnosis. The diagnosis of malaria must be suspected in every patient with fever, coma, or shock who has lived or traveled in a malarious area, has received a blood transfusion, or may be a drug addict. The only technique for confirming the clinical suspicion of malaria is the identification of plasmodia in fixed, stained blood smears. The diagnosis may be made by an alert technician during examination of a differential white count. However, it is usually only when a high suspicion of the possibility of malaria exists that the proper smears will be done and the necessary time taken to make the diagnosis.

Thin blood smears are made by placing a drop of blood on the end of a glass slide, touching the drop with another slide, and rapidly moving the edge of the second slide along the surface of the first. A thick blood smear is made by placing a drop of blood on a slide, then spreading it to fill a diameter of about 1 cm. The slides are allowed to dry. The thin blood smear is fixed in methanol and stained with Giemsa, or fixed and stained with Wright's. The thick blood smear is first dipped in water to lyse the red blood cells, then fixed and similarly stained. For the inexperienced observer the thin smear is easiest to examine and most likely to yield the diagnosis in the nonimmune patient with malaria. Careful examination of several thousand red blood cells on a properly stained smear will usually reveal the protozoan. When malaria is suspected but smears do not reveal the orgainism, smears should be repeated several times a day. The highest level of parasitemia is said to be demonstrable several hours *after* a chill. A thick smear can be particularly helpful for finding the characteristic gametocyte of falciparum malaria (Fig. 2D), but it may also reveal organisms when they are too infrequent to be easily identified on a thin smear.

The correct diagnosis of the species of plasmodium is critical in determining therapy and prognosis in malaria. The following brief description and the photomicrographs in Figure 2 were selected to aid in differentiating *P. vivax* and *P. falciparum* in peripheral blood.

Differentiation of P. vivax and P. falciparum in Blood Smears. The following characteristics can be used to identify *P. falciparum*. Only the ring forms are usually seen in the peripheral blood; they are small and delicate, often with two chromatin dots (Fig. 2A). The erythrocytes containing these protozoa are not conspicuously enlarged, and red dots (Schüffner's dots) are not present. The level of parasitemia may be high (more than 5 to 10

per cent of the erythrocytes infected), and some erythrocytes may contain several parasites. Organisms may appear to be on the surface of the erythrocyte (appliqué forms). *P. vivax* ring forms are often larger than falciparum rings and in later stages appear quite pleomorphic (Fig. 2B). The infected erythrocytes are usually larger than normal, and if properly stained, Schüffner's dots can be identified. By examining blood films at various times, the maturation of *P. vivax* in the peripheral blood can be documented. The mature schizont (Fig. 2C) contains 12 to 24 chromatin dots, and the parasite cytoplasm almost fills the red blood cell. The gametocyte of *P. falciparum* is very characteristic (Fig. 2D) and should be looked for carefully since it substantiates the diagnosis. It has a crescent or banana shape, whereas the shape of *P. vivax* gametocytes is globular.

Mixed Infection. Even after one species of malaria is identified, it must be kept in mind that the patient could have a mixed infection (1 to 2 per cent of cases). Mixed infection can best be diagnosed by careful review of several thin blood films. Repeated blood films for one to two days after the start of treatment should show decreasing levels of parasitemia. If a *P. vivax* infection is diagnosed and treated with chloroquine but parasitemia is seen to be increasing, a mixed infection with chloroquine-resistant *P. falciparum* should be suspected. At present, *P. falciparum* infection acquired in Southeast Asia and some parts of South America is resistant to chloroquine (see below). All patients diagnosed as having *P. falciparum* should have repeated smears during therapy to ensure that the parasitemia is decreasing.

Chloroquine Susceptibility Test. A technique for documenting whether *P. falciparum* is susceptible or resistant has been developed. At the time of initial diagnosis and before therapy is instituted, a sample of the patient's blood is defibrinated and added to vials (1 ml each) containing varying concentrations of chloroquine and 5 mg of glucose per 100 ml. During 24 hours of incubation, *P. falciparum* will mature to the schizont stage in the vials containing insufficient levels of chloroquine. Chloroquine susceptibility can be calculated from these data.

Antibody Tests. Antibody tests for malaria are not useful in the diagnosis of the acute illness. The indirect fluorescent antibody and hemagglutination tests are of value in testing populations to determine the prevalence of malaria and in screening blood donors when tracing cases of transfusion-induced malaria.

Differential Diagnosis. The differential diagnosis of malaria is lengthy and varies, depending upon the area of the world, the dominant malaria species, and whether the disease is acute or chronic. The fever of malaria must be separated from fever caused by dengue and other arboviruses, typhus, amebiasis, typhoid, relapsing fever, heat stroke, drug allergy, influenza, bacterial pneumonias, and wound infections. Intermittent chills secondary to antipyretics may simulate the chills and fever of malaria in all these conditions. Cerebral malaria must be distinguished from viral encephalitides, drug overdose, and other causes of coma. The jaundice of malaria must be distinguished from viral hepatitis and leptospirosis. In more chronic malaria infection in which splenomegaly and anemia are prominent, one must also consider bacterial endocarditis, schistosomiasis, visceral leishmaniasis, and lymphoma.

Therapy. *Elimination of Parasitemia.* The initial therapeutic goal in the treatment of malaria is to eliminate the erythrocytic stage of the infection, because all the acute symptoms are due to this hematogenous process. Chloroquine, a 4-aminoquinoline, is the drug of choice to accomplish this purpose. It can be given orally, or parenterally if the patient is vomiting. Chloroquine diphosphate is given orally as follows: 1 gram initially (600 mg of base), followed by 500 mg (300 mg of base) at 6 hours, 24 hours, and 48 hours after the initial dose (total dose 2.5 grams; 1.5 grams of base). Children should receive a loading dose of 17 mg per kilogram, followed by 8.5 mg per kilogram at 6, 24, and 48 hours. Chloroquine hydrochloride is available for intramuscular or intravenous injection. It is important to note that the hydrochloride salt contains a different quantity of chloroquine base than the diphosphate salt. Chloroquine base, 300 mg, is given intramuscularly every six hours for three doses (total of 900 mg base). On the second and third days therapy may be changed to oral medication, or single intramuscular injections can be continued until a total dose of 1.5 grams chloroquine base is reached. Intravenous medication with chloroquine is seldom indicated, because the patient in shock or coma will usually be given quinine realizing the possibility of a drug-resistant infection (see below). If intravenous chloroquine is considered necessary, 300 mg of base is diluted in 300 ml of saline and given over 30 to 60 minutes. It can be given every six to eight hours, but not in excess of a total daily dose of 1000 mg of base.

The exact mechanism of action of chloroquine remains unknown. It interrupts the vacuolar digestive mechanisms of protozoa, and it binds strongly to nucleic acids. Higher concentrations of the drug are found in infected erythrocytes than in uninfected cells or plasma. This enhanced uptake of chloroquine by parasitized cells may be very important, as suggested by the observation that chloroquine-resistant strains do not enhance the concentration of chloroquine by erythrocytes. In spite of the fact that chloroquine is also concentrated in the liver, it is ineffective in inhibiting tissue schizogony. Chloroquine is absorbed rapidly from the gastrointestinal tract. Fifty per cent becomes bound to plasma proteins, and only about 10 per cent of the active compound is excreted in the urine. Most of the drug is concentrated in tissue, and degradation probably occurs in the liver. It disappears from tissue over a period of several weeks after the drug is stopped. Chloroquine is usually well tolerated, but it can cause transient headache, visual disturbances, nausea, and vomiting. At toxic levels it can cause delirium, psychotic reactions, and convulsions. Its use is not contraindicated during pregnancy for treatment of malaria. When given for prolonged periods in doses higher than that used in malaria chemoprophylaxis, punctate keratitis and retinitis have been recorded. Amodiaquine is as effective as chloroquine for treating malaria.

Drug-Resistant Plasmodia. When falciparum malaria is diagnosed, a careful history must include the country where the infection was acquired. If the illness was acquired in South America, Central America, or the Philippines and the level of parasitemia is greater than 2 per cent of erythrocytes, or if it was acquired in Vietnam, Laos, Thailand, Malaysia, Cambodia, or Burma, regardless of the level of parasitemia, or if the source of the infection is unknown (such as in transfusion malaria) and parasitemia is high, then quinine sulfate should be used instead of chloroquine. *P. falciparum* acquired in the areas cited has been documented to show varying degrees of resistance to chloroquine.

Resistance of plasmodia to antimalarial drugs has been recognized for many years. Shortly after pyrimethamine and proguanil were introduced, strains resistant to these drugs were identified. This was not unexpected, because protozoa have been known to rapidly develop resistance to inhibitors of folate metabolism. Strains of *P. falciparum* which required higher than standard doses of quinine to be eradicated were recorded many years ago. Only in the past decade, however, has the problem of drug resistance been brought to particular attention by appearance of resistance of *P. falciparum* to previously accepted therapeutic levels of chloroquine. Resistant strains appeared in several parts of the world at about the same time, unrelated to whether chloroquine had been commonly used in the area or not.

Resistance of *P. falciparum* to chloroquine has been divided, based on response in level of parasitemia after initiation of therapy: no reduction (termed RIII level of resistance), and partial reduction (termed RII). The first level of chloroquine resistance (RI), to be considered in more detail below, is one in which *patent* parasitemia is eradicated, but parasitemia and clinical symptoms recur in a few days to several weeks; i.e., recrudescent malaria. At present, quinine is effective in removing patent parasitemia in these cases; however, a number of other drugs are necessary to prevent recrudescence. Careful attention to the diagnosis of chloroquine-resistant malaria is now an integral part of the management of patients with malaria (see Diagnosis).

To eradicate parasitemia in cases suspected to be caused by chloroquine-resistant strains, quinine is given orally, 650 mg every eight hours for seven to ten days. Quinine dihydrochloride is used intravenously in patients unable to take the drug orally. Quinine, 600 mg, is dissolved in 100 to 200 ml of 5 per cent glucose and water and administered over 30 minutes. This is repeated every eight hours. The mechanism of action of quinine against the malaria parasite is unknown. It has been shown to block protein synthetic and glycolytic pathways. It is absorbed readily from the gastrointestinal tract, and over 70 per cent is bound to plasma proteins. Like chloroquine, it is concentrated in tissues, including erythrocytes. Only 5 per cent of administered quinine is excreted unchanged in the urine. The most common side effects of quinine are tinnitus, vertigo, nausea, and vomiting. Although these symptoms are annoying, they are not indications to discontinue medication. A Coombs-positive hemolytic anemia is a rare complication of quinine therapy.

Prevention of Recrudescent Falciparum Malaria. Recrudescence of falciparum malaria occurs frequently in patients whose infection was acquired in Southeast Asia, Central America, or South America. Recrudescence is due to persistence during an asymptomatic period of erythrocytic stages of *P. falciparum* at undetectable levels, followed by increased parasitemia and symptoms several days to six weeks after apparently successful control of the illness by chloroquine or quinine. This is the first level of chloroquine resistance (RI). To prevent this, several drugs have been added to the initial therapeutic program for treatment of falciparum malaria acquired in the areas previously mentioned. Most commonly, pyrimethamine is given, 50 mg orally per day for three days in combination with dapsone, 25 mg orally per day for one month. If dapsone is unavailable, sulfadiazine, 1 gram every six hours for three days, is given concomitant with pyrimethamine. These drugs act by blocking folate metabolism at the paraminobenzoic acid and the dehydrofolate reductase steps. They can cause bone marrow suppression and allergic reactions. Difference of opinion exists over whether these drugs should be started on the first day of chloroquine or quinine therapy or several days later. We recommend that the drugs be started at the end of chloroquine treatment or on the fourth day of quinine therapy. This reduces the possibility of complicating the clinical picture by potential side effects of the drugs. Recently clindamycin or tetracycline has been found effective in combination with quinine against recrudescence of falciparum malaria. In cases in which recrudescence has occurred repeatedly, intravenous quinine has been used in place of oral quinine in combination with these drugs.

Gametocytes usually disappear from the peripheral blood within a few days after schizogony is interrupted, and no specific therapy is needed. Primaquine is an effective gametocidal drug and can be used in the rare patient with prolonged asymptomatic gametocytemia.

Prevention of Relapse Due to Persistent Hepatic Schizonts. Relapse of *P. vivax* and *P. ovale* malaria is caused by the persistence of hepatic schizogony.* Primaquine, an 8-aminoquinoline, is usually effective in preventing relapse (approximately 90 per cent of patients are cured). Since relapse is common in these infections, chloroquine therapy should always be followed by a course of primaquine. The adult dose is 15 mg of base daily for 14 days. Children should be given 0.25 mg per kilogram of body weight per day for 14 days. If relapse occurs after a full course of primaquine, the dose of primaquine should be doubled during a second 14-day period of therapy. The mechanism of action of primaquine is unknown, but it does appear to block glycolysis.

Primaquine can induce hemolysis in patients whose erythrocytes are deficient in glucose-6-phosphate dehydrogenase. Therefore patients should be tested for this deficiency before therapy is started, and if glucose-6-phosphate dehydrogenase deficiency is documented, red blood cell counts should be monitored carefully during treatment.

Supportive Therapy. Treatment of malaria is often accomplished with ease even in cases of falciparum malaria. However, since the course of falciparum malaria is unpredictable and complications may develop rapidly, all cases should be approached as medical emergencies. The management of a patient with malaria includes complete bed rest during the period of orthostatic hypotension. In the occasional patient with very high fever, this should be controlled by continuous antipyretic administration, sponging, and cooling. Frequent determinations of hematocrit, electrolytes, creatinine, urine volume, bilirubin, and transaminases are necessary. The level of consciousness should be carefully monitored.

The patient with falciparum malaria should receive transfusions with packed erythrocytes if severe anemia develops. The vascular volume and cardiac function should be monitored carefully by following the blood pressure, and in severe cases monitoring the central venous pressure may be necessary. Intravenous fluids should be given judiciously with full knowledge of the vascular volume, renal function, and serum electrolytes.

If cerebral malaria develops, the patient should be managed according to procedures used in the care of any comatose patient (see Ch. 319). Corticosteroids have been advocated in these cases to reduce cerebral edema. Heparin therapy should be used in the rare cases documented to have disseminated intravascular coagulation.

If the patient develops oliguria, a trial of furosemide or mannitol may be given. However, when acute renal failure is present, judicious administration of fluids associated with hemodialysis or peritoneal dialysis is indicated (see Ch. 604). The dose of quinine should be reduced to half in patients with renal failure, but maintained at therapeutic levels once hemo- or peritoneal dialysis is instituted.

If signs of pulmonary edema develop, standard therapeutic approaches are indicated, including digitalis preparations and methods to reduce the central venous pressure (see Ch. 520). This complication, however, has been quite refractory to treatment.

Prevention. An individual entering an area where malaria remains endemic must avoid contact with mosquitoes and systematically take drug prophylaxis. Use of mosquito netting, screens, insecticides, and mosquito repellents are the main mechanisms for avoiding contact with mosquitoes. The best repellent available at present is N,N-diethyltoluamide. It remains effective for up to 18 hours, a considerable advance over the odor repellents which are of value for only two or four hours.

The best means of malaria prevention is chemoprophylaxis. This is a cumbersome method, requiring intelligence, compulsiveness, and often willingness to tolerate the mild side effects of the medication. Travelers should check with medical officials in the area they visit for up-to-date advice on malaria chemoprophylaxis. The primary drug recommended for prophylaxis for travelers from the United States is chloroquine diphosphate or sulfate. Five hundred milligrams (300 mg of chloroquine base) is taken once a week. Children of ages 8 to 12 should receive 250 mg; ages 4 to 7, 200 mg; and ages 1 to 3, 125 mg; infants should receive 75 mg weekly. Where malaria is hyperendemic, 500 mg twice weekly has been recommended. Chloroquine should be started one to two weeks before entering the malarious area and continued for six weeks after departure from the area. Chloroquine does not prevent the hepatic infection, but simply suppresses the erythrocytic stage; *therefore the period of prophylaxis after leaving the malarious area is very important.* It is this period which travelers most often ignore and which leads to their illness several weeks after leaving the endemic area. After chloroquine prophylaxis, primaquine (15 mg of base per day) should be given for 14 days to eradicate the hepatic stages of plasmodia infections.

A single tablet containing 300 mg of chloroquine base and 45 mg of primaquine base was used for chemoprophylaxis by the U.S. military during the Vietnam war. This tablet is not recommended for use in preference to chloroquine alone. However, if primaquine is unavailable, this drug combination may be used after the traveler leaves the endemic area; it will prevent chloroquine-sensitive falciparum malaria and relapsing malaria. One table is taken per week for eight weeks. It is important that this combination *not* be used in the *treatment* of malaria, because the dose of primaquine base is at toxic levels when 1.5 grams of chloroquine base is given.

Prophylaxis When Cloroquine Resistance Is Present. Chloroquine prophylaxis may be ineffective in areas

*See footnote, page 474.

such as Southeast Asia and parts of Central and South America where chloroquine-resistant falciparum malaria is encountered. Travelers to these areas must balance their likely level of exposure to infected mosquitoes with the dangers of more vigorous chemoprophylaxis. The Communicable Disease Center has recommended that travelers to these countries take chloroquine in the dose usually recommended for other areas of the world (500 mg once weekly). Chloroguanide hydrochloride (100 to 200 mg per day) is probably an effective alternative to chloroquine chemoprophylaxis. The traveler must be told that these drugs may not be effective, and they should seek medical care promptly if fever occurs. A drug combination which at present is completely effective in preventing chloroquine-resistant falciparum malaria is pyrimethamine, 25 mg, plus sulfadoxine, 500 mg, taken once a week. This combination is not available in the United States, but it can be obtained in many other countries. Another effective drug combination is chloroguanide hydrochloride, 100 mg per day, plus dapsone, 25 mg daily. However, an increased risk of agranulocytosis caused by dapsone makes it less desirable as chemoprophylaxis for civilian travelers unless heavy exposure to infected mosquitoes is anticipated. Further testing will be needed to determine if tetracycline, long-acting sulfonamides, or repository drugs have a place in the chemoprophylaxis of malaria.

Prevention in a Community. Prevention of malaria in communities in endemic areas requires a coordinated effort directed at reducing the number of Anopheles mosquitoes and identifying and treating human cases of malaria. Anopheles are reduced in the environment by draining or filling breeding areas and by the use of larvicides. Effective campaigns against adult mosquitoes usually include spraying of all buildings with residual insecticides twice a year. DDT has been particularly effective for this purpose in the past; however, because of mosquito resistance and potential unacceptable side effects of DDT, other drugs such as hexachlorocyclohexane, dieldrin, malathion, and carbamates are now being used.

In areas endemic for malaria, use of chemoprophylactic drugs is usually reserved for children or pregnant women (to prevent congenital transmission of malaria). In some areas entire populations are treated by including the drug in the salt distribution for daily use. These approaches are used to reduce morbidity and mortality before adequate immunity is acquired. Hopefully, some form of active immunization could replace this method in the future.

Coatney, G. R., Collins, W. E., Warren, M., and Contacos, P. G.: The Primate Malarias. U.S. Department of Health, Education, and Welfare, National Institutes of Health. Washington, D.C., U.S. Government Printing Office, 1971.

Inter-American Malaria Research Symposium. Am. J. Trop. Med. Hyg., 21:613, 1972.

Maegraith, B., and Fletcher, A.: The pathogenesis of mammalian malaria. Adv. Parasitol., 10:49, 1972.

Miller, L. H.: Malaria. *In* Hoeprich, P. D. (ed.): Infectious Diseases. Hagerstown, Md., Harper & Row, 1972, p. 1113.

Neva, F. A., Sheagren, J. N., Shulman, N. R., and Canfield, C. J.: Malaria: Host-defense mechanisms and complications. Ann. Intern. Med., 73:295, 1970.

Powell, R. D., and McNamara, J. V.: Infection with chloroquine-resistant *Plasmodium falciparum* in man. Ann. N.Y. Acad. Sci., 174:1027, 1970.

Russell, P. F., West, L. S., Manwell, R. D., and MacDonald, G.: Practical Malariology. 2nd ed. London, Oxford University Press, 1963.

World Health Organization: Chemotherapy of Malaria and Resistance to Antimalarials. WHO Tech. Rep. Series No. 529, 1973.

TRYPANOSOMIASES

272. AFRICAN TRYPANOSOMIASIS
(African Sleeping Sickness, Maladie du Sommeil, Schlafkrankheit)
W. E. Ormerod

Definition and Etiology. African trypanosomiasis (sleeping sickness) is a meningoencephalitis caused by the protozoan *Trypanosoma brucei* (Plimmer and Bradford, 1899), discovered by Sir David Bruce to be the cause of nagana of cattle in Zululand. The disease occurs in several clinicoepidemiologic patterns. The two principal patterns of disease in man are Gambian sleeping sickness, which is chronic, and Rhodesian sleeping sickness, which is relatively acute. Another form, Zambezi sleeping sickness, although chronic, is more like the acute (Rhodesian) form in its epidemiologic behavior. The terms "Rhodesian" and "Gambian" are used today without geographic implication.

There is no clear-cut difference between the strains of organisms causing Gambian and Rhodesian forms of the disease, but there are strains previously regarded as *T. brucei (sensu stricto)* which, although identical in every other respect, will not infect man. This has given rise to difficulty, because they could not be identified with even moderate precision without experimental infection of man, a procedure which was seldom justifiable. A new test devised by Rickman and Robson and improved by Hawking, which subjects the trypanosome to trypanocidal substances in human serum, is now helping to classify isolates in terms of whether they are likely or not to be infective for man.

Other African species of trypanosomes, *T. congolense* and *T. vivax,* are important causes of disease in domestic livestock, but as they do not infect man they are of no medical interest. Trypanosomiasis can cause serious losses in domestic cattle and, where good husbandry is practiced, can reduce the food supply. By contrast, in Africa where husbandry is usually bad, and the yields are negligible, the existence of cattle trypanosomiasis acts as an important restraint on overgrazing and consequent soil erosion.

T. brucei gives a cyclical infection in the mammalian host but, unlike malaria, the cycles usually overlap, giving a variety of different stages in the blood at any one time. Ormerod and Venkatesan ascribe this cycle to the liberation of "long-thin" blood forms from a visceral stage in the leptomeninges. The blood forms divide until their division is inhibited by the uptake of lipids from the serum with consequent activation of trypanosomal lysosomes. Lysosomal action inhibits some forms completely; they contract into the "short-stumpy" forms which are removed by lysis and phagocytosis. A few, however, partially inhibited, develop multiple nuclei and flagella and, as giant forms, are filtered out of the circulation by mesodermal capillaries to renew the visceral phase.

Epidemiology. *Prevalence.* Although animal strains of *T. brucei* occur throughout the tsetse belt of Africa, that is to say, south of the Sahara and north of the Limpopo River and the Kalahari, human strains are not so widespread. The chronic (Gambian) form is to be found in West Africa from the Gambia to the Congo, penetrating inland to Lakes Chad, Victoria, and Tanganyika. The chronic (Zambezi) form with similar pathology is also to be found in Botswana, Rhodesia, Zambia, and Portuguese East Africa, but, as mentioned above, in its epidemiology it resembles the more acute (Rhodesian) form now found in Tanzania, Uganda, Kenya, and (most recently) Ethiopia. Distinction among these forms is not always useful to the clinician, because today the treatment of all forms is the same. Nevertheless, there is some difference in the prognosis of the different forms, and to the epidemiologist the differences are of great importance.

Transmission. *T. brucei* is transmitted by several species of the tsetse fly Glossina. When the fly bites an infected host, if its feeding is interrupted it can pass the infection to a second host by regurgitating part of the first feed. This mode of infection may occur at the height of an epidemic when other biting flies such as Stomoxys or tabanid (horse) flies may also be involved. Usually, however, the trypanosomes develop in the tsetse into noninfective forms, and this process continues for about 20 days until infective trypanosomes are formed; these remain in the salivary gland of the fly until it dies from other causes. The duration of the developmental cycle in the fly varies with temperature and does not continue below 18° C.

Rhodesian Sleeping Sickness. The Rhodesian strains of *T. brucei* are transmitted mainly by *G. morsitans*. This fly is associated with the edge of Brachistegia woodland (the miombo of Tanzania) and with the woodland that fringes watercourses in which, during the dry season, its habitat resembles that of *G. pallidipes,* also a transmitting agent. Although these flies feed on the blood of a wide range of species of game animals, there is evidence that the only important wild animal reservoir of Rhodesian sleeping sickness is the bushbuck *Tragelaphus scriptus*. This small antelope differs from other game in that it can live in close proximity to man, runs only a short distance when disturbed, and returns to its original "stand" in a thicket where it shares the same population of Glossina with man if he happens to be present. Sporadic Rhodesian disease is spread by this means, but epidemic Rhodesian strains are spread by *G. morsitans,* ranging widely in or between scattered thickets at the edge of the miombo, and under these conditions direct "man-fly-man" transmission occurs. Domestic cattle may also act as a reservoir.

Epidemic Rhodesian sleeping sickness occurred in Tanzania in the 1930's and large areas remain depopulated, because the disease has become "enzootic" and is still liable to break out again and cause acute disease in man. To the north of Lake Victoria, where epidemics have occurred more recently, the disease is spread mainly by *G. pallidipes* which ranges widely in the lakeside thickets. In Kenya a recent epidemic has been attributed to *G. fuscipes,* a fly related to *G. palpalis,* which has otherwise always been associated with Gambian sleeping sickness. This serves to emphasize the unstable and fluctuating epidemiology of the disease in this area, in contrast to the more stable epidemiology of the disease in the more southerly part of its range.

Zambezi Sleeping Sickness. Zambezi sleeping sickness is similar to Rhodesian sleeping sickness in its epidemiology. It is also transmitted by *G. pallidipes* and *G. morsitans,* especially when the fly is concentrated into "fringing forest" during the dry season: the bushbuck is also the most important, if not the only, reservoir. The disease is very sporadic and few of the indigenous population at risk contract it: some present as "healthy carriers"; others develop chronic wasting disease, but outsiders may suffer a very acute infection. Blair et al. point out that the epidemiologic pattern in Rhodesia has remained unchanged for the past 60 years.

Gambian Sleeping Sickness. Gambian sleeping sickness is transmitted mainly by *G. palpalis*. This fly obtains its blood meal from reptiles, birds, and man; it is a shade- and moisture-loving fly, and consequently transmission occurs most readily when a population of flies becomes isolated by unfavorable climate around a small woodland area. Frequently in West African savannah country such woodlands contain the water supply of a village. Here interchange of trypanosomes between fly and man takes place, and a focus of infection is built up. *G. tachinoides,* a fly associated with river thickets of West Africa, also transmits Gambian strains. This fly feeds on the blood of mammals other than man; consequently, it cannot be stated with confidence that there are not other animal reservoirs of Gambian sleeping sickness. Indeed, the dog and the domestic pig have been shown to harbor strains, but there is no evidence that these are of more than occasional epidemiologic importance.

Pathology. The extent of pathologic lesions depends on the duration of the disease. The most acute cases, those in which death occurs within two months, show little effect other than that associated with infectious disease generally. There are general wasting, hemorrhages into lung and bone marrow, and cellular proliferation in lymph nodes and in the malpighian bodies of the spleen. Acute myocarditis is believed to be the cause of death in some cases, but is rarely observed post mortem. Most cases of acute disease show some small round-cell infiltration of the meninges, but the brain appears normal. After about six months, the lymph nodes and malpighian bodies lose much of their cellularity, and fibrosis occurs in lymph nodes and vessels. At this stage the red bone marrow decreases, and a normocytic anemia and a leukopenia with a relative increase in lymphocytes occur. There is slight infiltration of the brain substance with small round cells, but heavy infiltration of the leptomeninges. Where the leptomeninges extend into the Aschoff-Robin space that surrounds meningeal vessels as they penetrate into the brain substance, the lesion known as *perivascular cuffing* is produced; this may vary from a single layer of infiltrating cells surrounding the vessel, in cases lasting for about six months, to a depth of about 20 cells when the disease has continued for two or more years. The nature of the cellular reaction has not been studied in detail, but there is one type of cell, the large

morular cell (Mott's cells) with loculated eosinophilic cytoplasm, that is present in the leptomeninges or the cuffing (rarely in the brain substance). The presence of this cell is considered pathognomonic of advanced sleeping sickness. Thrombosis is liable to occur in the cuffed vessels and gives rise to the cerebral degeneration that causes the progressive mental deterioration and coma from which the disease is named.

Pathogenesis. The tsetse fly feeds by rupturing small vessels and sucking from the subcutaneous pool that is formed. It may inject trypanosomes either into the bloodstream or into the pool where they lodge and grow to form a *chancre,* a hard painful nodule that contains trypanosomes. Initial growth of the trypanosomes is in the blood and, in man, seldom reaches a level greater than one organism per cubic millimeter. With each wave of the infection the organism appears with a different surface antigen, and over 20 have been observed with a single strain. The host responds by production of immunoglobulins in amounts sufficient to produce very high erythrocyte sedimentation rates; these globulins are in the IgM (19S) rather than in the IgG (7S) range, which is normally associated with infectious disease. It is doubtful whether much of the globulins are "protective" or even "specific," and it is likely that the main immunologic action lies in a cell-mediated response against the visceral phase of the organism.

Clinical Manifestations. The clinical diagnosis of sleeping sickness is usually difficult, for there are few reliable physical signs of the disease. A history of exposure to tsetse bite is essential. A chancre may develop at the site of the bite of the infected tsetse fly, although more frequently this passes unobserved or may be confused with the reaction to a normal tsetse bite, which can occasionally be severe. The occurrence, site, and appearance of the chancre vary greatly between different areas and individual patients.

With typical *Rhodesian disease* the bite will have occurred about two weeks before the first symptoms. With *Gambian* and *Zambezi disease,* however, the symptoms may be delayed for several years; the history of, or the scar from, a chancre may be useful in diagnosing the disease in a European.

Irrespective of the demonstration of a previous bite, the most important early symptom of sleeping sickness is the *severe headache*. This is associated with loss of nocturnal sleep and a *feeling of oppression* that African patients will often recognize, causing them to trek many miles to a sleeping sickness clinic. Wasting, mental disturbance, and drowsiness occur only when the disease is established in the central nervous system.

Physical signs in the early stages include fever, which may be high and fluctuating, especially in the Rhodesian and Zambezi disease. A fleeting circinate erythematous rash occurs on the chest and shoulders of some European patients, but is not seen in Africans. Enlarged lymph nodes are associated with Gambian disease and are found characteristically in the posterior triangle of the neck. Periosteal tenderness is described as a diagnostic sign but is neither frequent nor specific; similarly, swelling of the dorsum of the foot is easily confused with famine edema, which may coexist in the type of population at greatest risk of acquiring trypanosomiasis.

Diagnosis. Because there is nothing conclusive about the clinical manifestations of trypanosomiasis, the diagnosis depends entirely on demonstration of the presence of the organism. In the *Rhodesian disease* it is usually made by microscopic examination of a thick (unfixed) blood film stained with Giemsa, a tedious but fairly reliable procedure in the hands of a well-trained microscopist. Injection of blood into rats or mice is of value in doubtful cases. Zambezi strains are more difficult to diagnose by microscopy but are very easily isolated in rats and mice.

Gambian disease cannot with certainty be diagnosed by microscopic examination of the blood or by injection of laboratory animals. Microscopic examination of the fluid obtained by puncture of swollen lymph nodes is the best method in early cases. In later cases microscopy of cerebrospinal fluid is preferable, although concentration of the trypanosomes by centrifugation is often necessary. Culture of the organism as a method of diagnosis is difficult and uncertain as compared with culture of *T. cruzi*. Immunologic methods are not usually successful in the diagnosis of sleeping sickness, except for the fluorescent antibody test which shows promise as a specific diagnostic method. A method of selecting cases for further study is based on the formation of precipitin bands by the patient's serum or cerebrospinal fluid in a gel containing antiserum against IgM, β_2 macroglobulins. Immunodiffusion plates prepared for this purpose can be obtained commercially.

It is impossible at present to distinguish sleeping sickness from other febrile and wasting diseases without demonstrating trypanosomes. These organisms must be sought with care in any patient who has been exposed to tsetse bites in an area in which sleeping sickness has ever been known to occur.

Treatment. The two essential drugs for treatment of sleeping sickness are *suramin* (Bayer 205) and *melarsoprol* (Mel B). Suramin can be used in the early febrile stage of the disease; but because it is a large molecule unable to pass the blood-brain barrier, it becomes ineffective once the central nervous system has been invaded; consequently examination of the cerebrospinal fluid is of importance in deciding which drug to use. If the cerebrospinal fluid is normal, suramin alone may be used, but if trypanosomes, lymphocytes, or a raised protein is found, melarsoprol becomes the drug of choice, preferably after a preliminary course of suramin. Suramin is given intravenously in a course of five doses of 1.0 gram every second day, and this may be repeated after a week. Suramin produces some toxicity to the kidney, with the appearance of casts and albumin in the urine. It causes fetal abnormality in rats, but this has not been noted in man. In Nigeria, 1 in 2000 patients has a dangerous sensitivity to suramin; this can be detected by giving a preliminary dose of 0.2 gram.

Melarsoprol is very dangerous and is contraindicated if suramin can be used, but it is effective in all stages of the disease and is active against most strains of *T. brucei*, including some that are tryparsamide resistant. Doses are given intravenously as the 3.6 per cent solution; three doses of 0.5, 1.0 and 1.5 ml are given at daily intervals, and after a week three more doses of 1.5, 2.0 and 2.5 are given, and so on until a total of 35 ml has been given. Thomson gives slightly higher dosage together with promethazine hydrochloride, 25 mg twice daily throughout the course, and he treats patients showing signs of encephalopathy with BAL, 2 ml every four hours. It must be emphasized, however, that this very high dosage should be reached only if the patient shows no signs of toxicity, notably of arsenic encephalopathy. Sudden death with encephalopathy may occur in the early stages of melarsoprol therapy; this may be due to sensitivity to arsenic or to the rapid liberation of trypanosomal antigen. It is therefore wise to begin therapy of the Rhodesian form with suramin to reduce the number of parasites before continuing with melarsoprol. The effect of melarsoprol therapy can be assessed by following the reduction of protein levels in the cerebrospinal fluid, but it can only be a rough guide because melarsoprol will of itself raise the level of protein for periods up to six months after injection. Melarsonyl potassium (Mel W) may be given intramuscularly, but less experience has been acquired concerning its curative effect. Nitrofurazone, which can be given by mouth (0.5 gram three times a day for 15 days) is even more toxic, but it may be the drug of choice in cases in which the patient is known to be sensitive—or his trypanosomes resistant—to arsenic. It is likely to cause polyneuritis and cardiac arrhythmia, and in patients with hereditary glucose-6-phosphate dehydrogenase deficiency it can cause severe hemolytic anemia (a property which it shares with melarsoprol). Tryparsamide is also used in combination with suramin for mass therapy of Gambian disease; it is not suitable for patients treated individually and is ineffective in the Rhodesian disease. It can produce toxic ambylopia leading to optic atrophy in some patients. The treatment of the trypanosomiasis should always be accompanied by an antimicrobial drug, because sleeping sickness leads to an increased susceptibility to bacterial infection.

Prognosis. Relapse may follow treatment, especially after suramin, when the central nervous system had been already involved at the time chemotherapy was started. Relapse may also occur because of drug resistance. Recovery after treatment is usually complete when the disease is treated at an early stage. If treatment is first given late in the disease, the survivors are often mentally sluggish and sometimes obese. A patient from whom trypanosomes have been isolated will sooner or later be killed by the disease unless it is treated. With Rhodesian disease the patient dies fairly soon, but with both Zambezi and Gambian disease the patient may survive for several years. It is suggested that some patients may be able to overcome the infection by natural means. If this in fact occurs, it is so exceptional that adequate treatment of diagnosed cases should always be performed. The neglect of an outbreak of sleeping sickness may result in extermination of the human population of the locality.

Prevention. African sleeping sickness can be prevented by measures aimed at destroying the habitat of the vector, the shade trees, and the other vegetation upon which the tsetse flies rest. As individual communities become larger, and especially when water sources are provided inside the villages, the risk to the inhabitants is reduced. The use of insecticides may also supplement this process. Elimination of the blood meal of the fly by game destruction programs has no effect on human sleeping sickness; neither has the liberation of sterile male tsetse met with much success.

Probably the most effective measures against the Rhodesian disease involve the isolation of human populations from areas known to harbor infective game and systematic search for and treatment of all infected humans. Search for and treatment of cases are even more important in Gambian disease, because man himself is the reservoir of infection.

Pentamidine, administered intramuscularly, is the

only suitable drug for *chemoprophylaxis,* and is of established effectiveness only against the Gambian disease. Its use is limited to the protection of a controlled population, such as a labor force, exposed to the Gambian disease. Pentamidine should not be used for therapy of individual cases of the disease, because, like suramin, it is not active within the nervous system. A single injection of 4 mg per kilogram is believed to provide a preventive effect in the Gambian disease for at least six months.

Blair, D. M., Burnett Smith, E., and Gelfand, M.: Human trypanosomiasis in Rhodesia. Cent. Afr. J. Med., 14 (Suppl.):1–12, 1968.

Hawking, F.: The differentiation of *Trypanosoma rhodesiense* from *T. brucei* by means of human serum. Trans. R. Soc. Trop. Med. Hyg., 67:517, 1973.

Mulligan, H. W., and Potts, W. H. (eds.): The African Trypanosomiases. London, Allen and Unwin, 1970.

Ormerod, W. E., and Venkatesan, S.: The occult visceral phase of mammalian trypanosomes with special reference to the life cycle of *Trypanosoma (Trypanozoon) brucei.* Trans. R. Soc. Trop. Med. Hyg., 65:722, 1971.

Robertson, D. H. H.: Chemotherapy of African trypanosomiasis. Practitioner, 188:80, 1962.

Thomson, K. D. B.: Melarsoprol tolerance in sleeping sickness patients of the Benue endemic zone. *In* Proceedings of 1st Medical Research Seminar, Yaba, Lagos, 1972, p. 242.

273. CHAGAS' DISEASE

Heonir Rocha

Definition. Chagas' disease is caused by an infection with a protozoan, *Trypanosoma cruzi.* It has a self-limited acute phase, detected only in a minority of infected persons. The disease usually presents as a chronic process, characterized by cardiac and digestive manifestations. In most cases there is no clinical evidence of the infection. In an endemic area, however, Chagas' disease is an important cause of morbidity and mortality.

Etiology. In the blood, *T. cruzi* is a spindle-shaped trypanosome showing a scanty undulating membrane and a large kinetoplast. Following penetration of tissue cells the parasite changes into Leishmania forms, which are round or ovoid bodies containing a large nucleus and a rodlike kinetoplast. Multiplication is cyclical and takes place intracellularly by binary fission. Within tissues there is production of intermediate forms, from which the circulating trypanosomes are derived. There are strains of *T. cruzi* with widely different virulence for mice; also, great differences in tissue tropism and antigenic structure have been documented. These variations have been considered of possible significance in clinical infections, and they could explain some of the diversity of the clinical picture of this disease in different geographic areas.

Epidemiology. Men and probably domestic animals (chiefly dogs and cats) infected with *T. cruzi* are the main reservoirs for contamination of the insect vectors. These vectors are winged but capable of only short flights, and are strictly hematophagous. They belong to the family Reduviidae, subfamily Triatominae, of which several dozen species have been found to be infected. However, only three species, *Triatoma infestans, Panstrongylus megistus,* and *Rhodnius prolixus,* well adapted to human dwellings, are major transmitters of the infection in large areas of South and Central America.

The insect vectors live in cracks and holes in walls and roofs, behind objects hanging on the walls, and in the thatch of primitive adobe houses. Their habits are very much like those of bedbugs; they feed at night or in the dark and seek shelter by day. The flagellate forms of *T. cruzi* are ingested with the blood meal by the insect, and after a series of changes and multiplications in the digestive tract of the vector, the metacyclic trypanosome forms are produced in large numbers and are discharged in the feces. The transmission of the disease usually results from contamination of mucous membranes or broken skin with feces containing the infective trypanosomes (so-called posterior-station transmission).

Occasionally man can be infected by blood transfusion or accidental laboratory contamination. Infection of the newborn via the placenta has also been documented. Transmission via breast milk and by eating infected meat has been reported.

Chagas' disease has been detected in a large area in the Western Hemisphere extending from the southern United States (Texas) to Argentina.

In the United States several species of wild rats, opossums, armadillos, and house mice have been found to be infected; also, several species of triatomid bugs have been found to have *T. cruzi.* However, the disease in humans is practically nonexistent in the United States. The major feature of the epidemiology of Chagas' disease is the association of infection in man and domestic animals with the presence of species of the insect vector in the domestic habitat. This intimate contact of man and vector is apparently lacking in the United States.

The incidence of Chagas' disease has been shown to be greatly variable, depending on the existence of favorable conditions for endemicity. Well-conducted epidemiologic studies are certainly needed to give a better picture of its geographic distribution. So far the disease has been reported only in the Americas, where it has been estimated that at least 7 million people are infected and 30 million are exposed to the risk of infection.

Pathogenesis and Pathology. The invading organism, after penetration through mucous membranes or skin, multiplies within cells of surrounding tissues or regional lymph nodes as Leishmania forms. These forms produce pseudocysts that eventually rupture, causing an inflammatory and lymphatic reaction. The liberated bodies either again penetrate adjacent tissue cells or invade the blood.

The lesions and clinical manifestations of the *acute stage* of the disease are mainly related to the destruction of cells by growth and multiplication of the parasite and the resulting inflammatory reaction. Practically every organ of the body may be invaded, but the reticuloendothelial system, muscle fibers (especially cardiac), and neuroglial cells of the central nervous system are more likely to be involved.

Inflammation is seen mainly around ruptured pseudocysts containing Leishmania, particularly in muscles. In the cardiac muscle there is diffuse interstitial mononuclear cell infiltration and interfibrillar edema, with many pseudocysts of Leishmania in the cardiac fibers; various degrees of muscle degeneration are also seen, waxy and fatty degeneration predominating. In the brain and meninges there is frequently a mild mononuclear infiltration.

Parasitemia may persist for 4 to 12 weeks, after which the parasite remains quiescent in tissues as Leishmania forms with occasional transient blood invasion.

In the *chronic stage,* the main pathologic lesions are observed in the heart and digestive tract. The heart is dilated and hypertrophied, with no valvular or specific vascular lesions. There are frequent mural thrombi, particularly in the right atrium and at the apex of the left ventricle with thinning of this region. Although this thinning may be extreme, leading to aneurysm of the apex, it does not seem to lead to rupture of the ventricle. The myocardium shows a variable degree of mononuclear inflammatory reaction, degenerative changes, and a predominant diffuse interstitial fibrosis. Quantitative studies of the intrinsic nervous system of the heart have shown a pronounced reduction in the number of parasympathetic ganglion cells. The presence of Leishmania within muscle fibers is detected in only about 30 per cent of chronic cases (Fig. 1). Embolic infarcts resulting from intramural thrombi are frequently found in the lungs, spleen, kidneys, and, occasionally, in the brain of patients dying from this disease.

Frequently the patients with digestive tract involvement have megaesophagus and/or megacolon with only minor inflammatory reaction in the myocardium; occasionally there also is severe diffuse myocarditis. In the esophagus and colon there is a marked decrease in the number of cells of the autonomic nervous system, and there are focal inflammatory lesions in the muscular layer. It is thought that megaesophagus and megacolon are the result of destruction of the intramural nervous system, probably related to the parasitic infection and to the secondary inflammatory and vascular lesions.

The detection of widespread inflammation in the myocardium, not associated with the presence of the parasite, the production of similar tissue lesions in mice injected with just an extract of *T. cruzi,* the continuous destruction of muscle fibers, and the necrotizing arteriolar lesions described in muscular layers of the esophagus

Figure 2. Romaña's sign in acute Chagas' disease. Note unilateral periorbital edema. (Courtesy of Professor Aluizio Prata, Salvador, Bahia, Brazil.)

have suggested an immune allergic mechanism for lesions of the acute phase and particularly of the chronic phase of this disease. Furthermore, the reduction of the intrinsic nervous control of the heart and digestive tract has been taken as an important pathogenic mechanism in this parasitic infection.

Clinical Manifestations. In the course of Chagas' disease there are distinct phases with peculiar clinical features.

Acute Form. In an endemic area, the acute manifestations of Chagas' disease usually occur in the first decade of life, and are recognized in only a small minority of infected cases. The local signs at the portal of entry frequently call the attention of the physician to the condition. Characteristically there is *unilateral* painless periorbital edema with mild conjunctival reaction, a bluish or darkish discoloration of the skin, and satellite lymphadenopathy usually with enlarged preauricular lymph nodes. These physical findings are referred to as Romaña's sign (Fig. 2). The subsidence of the palpebral edema usually takes four to eight weeks.

In a minority of cases, the initial lesion occurs in other exposed areas of the skin. It is usually a lesion resembling a furuncle that increases to become a purplish indurated papule, 4 to 6 cm in diameter, with regional adenopathy, leaving a pigmented scar when it subsides.

Concomitantly with the local signs the patient develops a variable clinical picture usually characterized by malaise, anorexia, remittent or continuous fever, mild generalized nontender lymphadenopathy, moderate hepatosplenomegaly, and, in some instances, peripheral edema or a generalized edema of varying degrees which supervenes later on in the course. In a few cases a morbilliform or maculopapular erythematous skin rash is present. The pulse is usually fast (even when fever is absent) and regular. In severe cases there may be marked

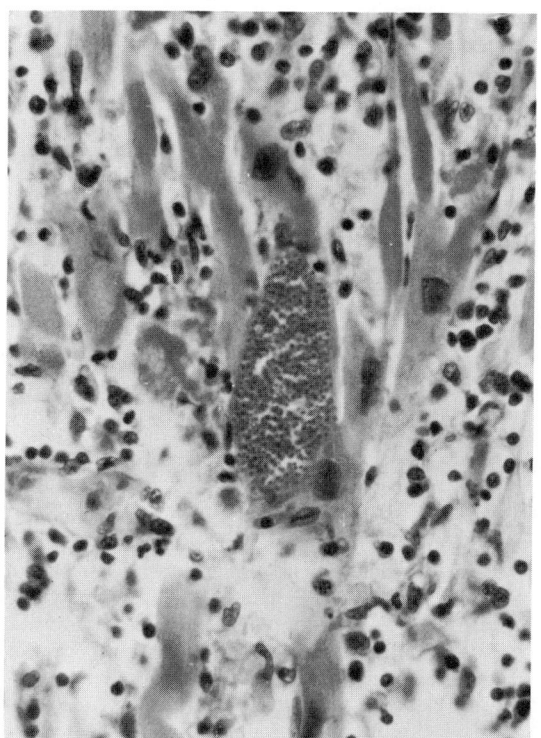

Figure 1. Leishmania bodies within myocardial fiber of a patient with chronic Chagas' heart disease. Note also the mononuclear inflammatory reaction and edema.

cardiac dilatation, gallop rhythm, and signs of heart failure. Myocarditis of variable degree probably occurs in all cases, but it is severe only in a very small percentage. Laboratory findings include a moderate leukocytosis with lymphocytosis, increased sedimentation rate, increase in alpha-2 and gamma globulins, and decrease in serum albumin. The serum glutamic oxaloacetic transaminase (SGOT) has been found elevated in severe cases. Electrocardiographic (EKG) abnormalities are present in about 50 per cent of patients, commonly showing prolongation of P-R interval, low voltage of QRS, and primary T wave changes. These are more pronounced in the most severe cases. The presence of intraventricular block is a very ominous sign.

The disease subsides within two or three months in 90 to 95 per cent of cases. The 5 to 10 per cent fatality rate is usually related to severe myocarditis, acute meningoencephalitis (occurring in the newborn or in the very young), or complicating bronchopneumonia. *In the great majority of patients with the chronic form of Chagas' disease there is no history of an acute phase.* It is thought that probably only 1 per cent of infected subjects have noticeable clinical signs following the initial contamination.

Indeterminate or Latent Phase. Patients who had acute manifestations of the disease, as well as those with inapparent infection, may remain asymptomatic for periods of 10 to 30 years, or for their whole lives. Those patients show only serologic evidence of the disease by complement-fixation (positive Machado-Guerreiro reaction), and occasionally the parasite can be recovered from their blood. This is actually the most common situation in an endemic area. Yet, there are few clinical and anatomic data available concerning this particular stage of the disease.

Chronic Form. The chronic manifestations of *T. cruzi* infection are primarily due to cardiac and digestive involvement.

CARDIAC MANIFESTATIONS. Approximately 20 to 40 per cent of patients with chronic *T. cruzi* infection in an endemic area exhibit evidence of heart damage. This is the most important finding in the chronic phase of this disease. Symptoms and signs are the result of a progressive diffuse chronic myocarditis.

In the early stages the patient may have no symptoms, and the diagnosis of heart disease rests on the electrocardiographic changes.

With the advanced disease the patient may present a clinical picture of heart failure of gradual onset, with serious systemic congestion. Signs of right-sided heart failure usually predominate over those of left ventricular failure. The pulse is weak and irregular because of ventricular premature contractions. The heart is greatly enlarged, the heart sounds are muffled, and there is a systolic murmur of functional mitral insufficiency and sometimes one of tricuspid regurgitation. A widely split second pulmonic sound and an apical third heart sound are commonly heard. The heart shadow roentgenographically shows marked global enlargement, with clear pulmonary fields (Fig. 3). The course of these patients is usually complicated by pulmonary or systemic embolism arising from the frequently occurring mural thrombi. Occasionally, the episode of heart failure begins abruptly, without apparent precipitating cause, usually running a short fatal course; on other occasions it is brought on by pregnancy or delivery, severe pulmonary infection, or an associated severe chronic anemia.

Figure 3. Chest film in a case of chronic Chagas' heart disease. Marked global enlargement of cardiac shadow, with clear pulmonary fields.

In some instances the patient may complain only of palpitation or syncopal attacks resulting from disturbances in cardiac rhythm (ventricular premature contractions or atrioventricular block, Adams-Stokes attacks). In cases of complete atrioventricular block the patient may present with Adams-Stokes syndrome. Rarely, the first manifestation of chronic Chagas' disease is a cerebral embolism owing to dislodgement of a thrombus located in the left ventricle.

A great variety of EKG abnormalities are detected in chronic Chagas' heart disease. Complete right bundle branch block is the most frequent conduction disturbance, occurring in about 50 per cent of cases; similarly, ventricular premature contractions (usually multifocal) are present in half the patients; also frequent are negative symmetric T waves. Atrioventricular block of variable degree occurs in one third of cases, but complete A-V block is detected in only about 10 per cent. Atrial fibrillation or flutter is relatively uncommon (about 10 per cent), and left bundle branch block is rare.

DIGESTIVE MANIFESTATIONS. Megaesophagus and megacolon are important manifestations of chronic *T. cruzi* infection. The evidence for the etiologic role of the parasite in these conditions is (1) the high incidence of these abnormalities in endemic areas of Chagas' disease; (2) the finding of a positive Machado-Guerreiro reaction in 85 per cent of patients with megacolon or megaesophagus in endemic areas. When xenodiagnosis is also performed in these cases, the incidence of *T. cruzi* infection rises to 95 per cent, which is significantly higher than that in the general population of the same area; (3) the frequent detection of EKG changes (about 50 per cent), similar to those described in chronic Chagas' myocarditis, in patients with megacolon or megaesophagus; and (4) the capability of reproducing these lesions in animals chronically infected with *T. cruzi*. This infection in animals and humans produces a marked decrease in the number of cells of the autonomic nervous system in esophagus and colon with disturbance in motility, even in the absence of anatomic changes of these organs. Conversely, fibrosis and degeneration of autonomic ganglia have been demonstrated in the heart of individuals with megaesophagus.

Patients with megaesophagus complain of longstanding progressive dysphagia, regurgitation, retrosternal discomfort, and sometimes paroxysmal attacks of night cough. They may get repeated respiratory infections as a result of aspirations of esophageal contents. The esophagus becomes enormously dilated, and in some cases it can be seen in a plain chest film as a right paramediastinal shadow.

Megacolon is characterized by persistent severe constipation of many years' duration. The incidence of fecal impaction and volvulus with intestinal obstruction is high in endemic areas of Chagas' disease.

The concomitance of megaesophagus, megacolon, and heart failure is not common. Most frequently, patients with digestive involvement present only EKG abnormalities or a moderate enlargement of the heart.

Prenatal Chagas' Disease. Prenatal transmission of *T. cruzi* infection has been verified by clinical and experimental observations. The mother may be in the latent or indeterminate phase of the disease.

The infected newborn may present generalized edema, enlargement of liver and spleen, petechiae or purpuric manifestations, sometimes jaundice, and a picture of meningoencephalitis. The pathologic findings are those of acute Chagas' disease. A microscopic picture of placentitis occurs in those instances. The characteristic feature is the finding of Leishmania within histiocytes of the inflammatory reaction. It has been shown that this infection may be responsible for premature birth or fetal death. The possibility exists of evolution to chronicity of a prenatally transmitted *T. cruzi* infection, but conclusive demonstration in humans is needed.

Diagnosis. In the acute stage, the diagnosis lies mainly in the demonstration of the parasite in the blood of the patient. *T. cruzi* may be seen in a fresh blood smear, in a thick-drop preparation of blood, or in a buffy coat smear up to three months after the onset of the disease. As the parasitemia decreases, or if blood preparations are negative, xenodiagnosis or animal inoculation of freshly drawn blood or blood culture can be used. Xenodiagnosis is a method of having laboratory-bred triatomid bugs feed on patients and examining the insects 40 days later for the presence of *T. cruzi* in the intestinal tract. The method is practical and is very sensitive in the detection of this stage of Chagas' disease. Blood culture in NNN media and inoculation of blood in young mice or guinea pigs require special laboratory facilities, but can be helpful particularly when xenodiagnosis is not available. A precipitin reaction using antigen obtained from *T. cruzi* culture gives positive results in almost every acute case.

The clinical diagnosis of chronic Chagas' heart disease is based on the following: (1) epidemiologic evidence (patient from endemic area, usually of poor socioeconomic group); (2) clinical picture of primary myocardial disease (enlarged heart, with no signs of valvular, coronary artery, or any other cause of heart disease); (3) EKG changes of the types (previously mentioned) usually seen in Chagas' disease; and (4) serologic evidence of infection or isolation of *T. cruzi*.

The most valuable procedure in diagnosing chronic Chagas' disease is the complement-fixation test (Machado-Guerreiro reaction), which is positive in about 95 per cent of cases. Xenodiagnosis is positive in only about 20 per cent of chronic cases.

Differential diagnosis may include rheumatic heart disease, particularly when there is a loud systolic murmur simulating organic valvular disease, in patients under 30 years of age. Coronary heart disease may be another difficult problem in patients over 40. It is often impossible on clinical grounds to dissociate chronic myocarditis owing to Chagas' disease from certain cardiomyopathies of unknown cause. Besides the great help derived from careful evaluation of clinical and epidemiologic data, the Machado-Guerreiro reaction and xenodiagnosis are of major importance in making a definite diagnosis of Chagas' disease.

Clinical Course and Prognosis. Acute Chagas' disease is relatively benign, with subsidence of symptoms in 90 to 95 per cent of cases. The chronic form usually has a slowly progressive course. It is clear that by no means all of those infected ultimately develop the serious forms of the disease, but the exact proportion that do so is not known. This important question could be settled only by a large-scale, long-term prospective epidemiologic study; the need for such a study is great.

Sudden and unexpected death is common in Chagas' disease. Complete A-V block, multifocal premature ventricular contractions, ventricular tachycardia, and marked enlargement of the heart with signs of heart failure are severe prognostic signs. Pulmonary embolism is a frequent terminal complication in patients with heart failure.

Treatment. There is no satisfactory treatment for *T. cruzi* infection. Several chemotherapeutic agents have been tried without success, including primaquine, pyrimethamine, nitrofurans (levofuraltadone), aminopterin, intravenous gentian violet, amphotericin B, and puromycin, among others. These agents may cause transient disappearance of parasitemia, but follow-up studies usually show a relapse. This is probably related to the ineffectiveness of all those agents against the tissue forms of the parasite. Some of them (nitrofurans) may demonstrate great potency against *T. cruzi* in tissue cultures, and also in experimental infection in mice. However, despite extensive killing of intracellular parasites, some intact leishmanial bodies can always be found in the tissues of the laboratory animal. None of the drugs commonly employed in the treatment of African trypanosomiasis have shown value in Chagas' disease (see Ch. 272). Several new drugs are under trial, Bayer 2502 ("Lampit") being one of them. Unfortunately the results have not been uniformly promising.

After a certain degree of tissue damage has occurred, even the eradication of the parasite may not prevent the progression of the disease. In chronic cases, therapy is only symptomatic, comprising the usual measures for heart failure, Adams-Stokes syndrome, megaesophagus, megacolon, or one of its complications. Digitalis preparations should be managed with great care because of the unusual degree of sensitivity to toxic effects.

Prevention. Controlling the transmission of the disease is the most important preventive measure. This requires housing of satisfactory quality; moreover, it requires the repeated systematic application of residual insecticides (benzene hexachloride) effective against the triatomid bugs. For individual short-term protection, fine-mesh bed nets are useful.

Blood transfusion is a potential hazard in endemic

areas. The incidence of positive Machado-Guerreiro reactions among blood donors may be as high as 15 per cent. To prevent infection from transfusions, the addition of gentian or crystal violet to the blood has been used. Persons having a positive complement-fixation test should not be accepted as potential blood donors.

The production of a vaccine to prevent human infection is, certainly, another possible approach. Mice can be protected against a fatal *T. cruzi* challenge by prior inoculation with a strain of mild pathogenicity. However, as it is impossible to predict the potential virulence to man of a *T. cruzi* strain of low pathogenicity to lower animals, only vaccines of killed parasites should be tried at present, and so far they have failed to be protective.

Anselmi, A., and Moleiro, F.: Physiopathology of Chagas' heart disease: Correlations between clinical and experimental findings. Bull. WHO, 44:659, 1971.

Köberle, F.: Chagas' heart disease (pathology). Cardiologia (Basel), 52:82, 1969.

Laranja, F. S., Dias, E., Nobrega, G., and Miranda, A.: Chagas' disease. A clinical, epidemiologic and pathologic study. Circulation, 14:1035, 1956.

Prata, A., Köberle, F., and Puigbo, J. J.: Chagas' heart disease. Cardiologia, 52:79, 1968.

Resenbaum, M. B.: Chagasic myocardiopathy. Prog. Cardiovasc. Dis., 7:199, 1964.

Woody, N. C., and Woody, H. B.: American trypanosomiasis. I. Clinical and epidemiological background of Chagas' disease in the United States. J. Pediatr., 58:568, 1961.

World Health Organization: Chagas' Disease, Report of a Study Group. Technical Report Series No. 202, 1960.

274. PNEUMOCYSTOSIS

Thomas C. Jones

Pneumocystosis is an acute pulmonary disease characterized by fever, tachypnea, dyspnea, and cyanosis which occurs in immunodeficient patients and malnourished or premature infants. It is caused by species of the genus Pneumocystis, organisms of uncertain classification, but probably protozoa. The organisms cause asymptomatic infection in healthy mammalian hosts and are seen extracellularly in cysts in the pulmonary alveoli.

History. In 1909 Carlos Chagas described what he thought was a stage of sporogony of *Trypanosoma cruzi* occurring in the lungs of experimentally infected guinea pigs. The next year Carini observed the same forms in rats infected with *T. lewisi*. In 1912 Delanoe and Delanoe recognized that the "cyst of Carini" was not part of the life cycle of trypanosomes, but was a different organism. The first reports of such an organism in humans appeared in 1938 when Ammich and Beneke independently described them in the lungs of infants dying during the first year of life. Epidemics of the disease in institutionalized children were subsequently described throughout Europe. In 1953 Vanek, Jirovec, and Lukes recognized the relationship between Pneumocystis and the pathologic entity interstitial plasma cell pneumonia. Reports of pneumocystosis have increased since that time, associated with the increased use of corticosteroids and antimetabolites as therapy in malignant disease or in patients undergoing organ transplantation, and with the increased life span of patients with congenital immunodeficient syndromes.

Organism. The life cycle of Pneumocystis is unknown. At present, one can only postulate that the life cycle in lungs of infected mammals includes an extracystic body or trophozoite which changes to a cyst followed by the development of oval bodies within the cyst. These are then released to initiate another cycle. A trophozoite-to-trophozoite cycle may also occur. The cyst stage of the organism is found in exudate within the alveoli. It is 5 to 6 μ in diameter, and its outer wall stains well with meth-

enamine silver nitrate (see Fig. 2*G*, Ch. 271), Gram-Weigert stains or periodic acid–Schiff reagents. Using Giemsa stain, the oval bodies (1 to 2 μ in diameter) can be recognized within the cyst and are usually eight in number. Under the electron microscope these oval bodies are seen to have a nuclear mass, endoplasmic reticulum, ribosomes, and mitochondria. The oval bodies are released from the cyst, after which they are termed trophozoites or extracystic bodies; they move freely about the alveoli, and become the nidus for new cysts to form.

Epidemiology. Pneumocystis species are widely distributed, affecting rodents, rabbits, sheep, dogs, and other mammals, in addition to humans. It is unlikely that animals serve as a reservoir for infection of humans, since organisms of different mammals appear to be host specific. For the same reason, the species name *P. carinii* should not be used to name the organism seen in humans, but should be reserved for the organism identified in rodents. Evidence at present best supports the thesis that infection is transmitted by the respiratory route by droplet spray. In a few cases congenital infection has been considered the most likely route of infection.

Epidemiologic data suggest that the organism is highly infectious, that infection is usually asymptomatic, and that apparently healthy, infected individuals can transmit the disease to immunodeficient patients. This is supported by observations in animals that healthy rats and rabbits when caged communally acquire the infection, and when the animals are rendered immunodeficient by corticosteroid administration, disease may be manifest. It is supported in humans by the high prevalence (4 per cent) of the organism in routine autopsy studies, the increased prevalence of antibodies to Pneumocystis in personnel working in medical institutions (7 to 15 per cent), the epidemics of disease in the institutionalized patients, and the sporadic clusters of cases in hospitalized immunodeficient patients.

Disease that follows recent infection or is associated with latent infection has been seen most commonly in patients with hypogammaglobulinemia of immunoglobulins G or M, in patients in the second to fourth months of life (when passively transferred maternal antibodies first reach low levels), or in patients receiving corticosteroids or antimetabolites. A few patients not on immunosuppressive drugs and with normal immunoglobulin levels and a few patients with isolated defects in cellular immunity have acquired the disease. Organisms reach high numbers in the lungs of infected persons showing clinical disease, and it is likely that these patients can more readily spread the disease than asymptomatic carriers.

Pathology and Pathogenesis. When conditions exist in the alveoli for the multiplication of Pneumocystis, an inflammatory response is elicited which includes transudation of fluid into the alveoli and thickening of alveolar interstitial spaces. The alveoli become filled with foamy, proteinaceous material in which trophozoite nuclei are found along with clumps of the Pneumocystis cysts. The interstitial spaces have been noted to contain predominantly plasma cells and alveolar epithelial cells when pathologic material was studied in malnourished or premature infants; hence the origin of the pathologic description, interstitial plasma cell pneumonia. However, in the immunodeficient child or adult, this pattern is not seen. The inflammatory response in these patients has been described as primarily lymphocytes, macrophages, and occasionally eosinophils. Polymorphonuclear leukocytes are not seen. The lung is usually diffusely involved with this process, although localized disease has occasionally been described. The lung is firm and rubbery in consistency. Other organisms, such as cytomegalovirus or bacteria, are frequently found in association with Pneumocystis. Less commonly, Pneumocystis is found in lungs which also contain mycobacteria, fungi, or toxoplasma. Rarely, pneumocystis may become generalized, involving lymph nodes, spleen, and bone marrow.

Clinical Manifestations. The major symptoms of pneumocystosis are tachypnea and a nonproductive cough. These symptoms often develop insidiously over a period of several weeks and may be associated with fever, dyspnea, and cyanosis. It has been noted that these symptoms may first appear during the period when corticosteroids are being withdrawn. The disease may also present with an abrupt onset (over two to three days) of high, spiking fever, cough, dyspnea, and cyanosis, with the patient reaching a moribund state within a few days. Most of the patients presenting with this rapid course have been on continuous high doses of corticosteroids. In the United States at present the disease which presents with an abrupt onset may be more common than the more insidious onset characteristic of the illness seen in institutionalized infants in Europe. After renal transplantation, pneumocystosis has been recorded as responsible for 10 per cent of pulmonary infections and usually occurs three to four months after transplantation.

On physical examination the patient shows signs of respiratory distress (tachypnea and dyspnea) associated with fever and cyanosis. Auscultation of the lungs may reveal no abnormalities, although scattered rales and rhonchi may be heard.

There are no diagnostic laboratory tests. *The white blood cell count* may reflect the underlying disease of the patient or other complications, but leukocytosis may be seen. Significant eosinophilia has occasionally been reported, particularly in children with humoral immune deficiency. *The blood gases* will usually indicate hyperventilation and decreased oxygen saturation even while the patient is on continuous oxygen, consistent with an alveolar capillary block syndrome. Some have reported associated mild respiratory acidosis. *The chest radiograph* usually shows diffuse mixed alveolar and interstitial pneumonitis. This appears as a granular haziness beginning in the hilar region. A few cases of more localized disease have been seen, giving a segmental distribution. An air bronchogram is often seen. Pleural effusion does not occur.

Course. In immunodeficient patients the course of pneumocystosis will usually be one of progressive deterioration unless improvement occurs in the underlying immune defect. Increasing pulmonary consolidation, cyanosis, and death are the natural history of the disease. After institution of specific therapy against pneumocystis, improvement begins in five to ten days. The roentgenographic findings may become transiently worse after institution of therapy, but will then show gradual improvement over one to three weeks. Some have suggested that pneumocystosis of long duration may lead to interstitial fibrosis or emphysema. This has been difficult to document in view of the many factors leading to pulmonary changes in these patients.

Diagnosis. Once the suspicion of pneumocystis is raised by the clinical setting of immune deficiency and progressive pulmonary symptoms, the patient should be considered for lung biopsy or "brush" biopsy. Most centers now recommend open lung biopsy rather than needle biopsy because the latter provides no visualization of the lung, a smaller sample, and a greater risk of lung collapse or bleeding. Biopsy is required to distinguish pneumocystosis from drug-induced interstitial fibrosis, cytomegalovirus infection, aspergillus or other fungi, unusual forms of bacterial bronchopneumonia, toxoplasmosis, or leukemic infiltration. Impression smears of the biopsy specimen at the time of surgery can be fixed in methanol and stained with Giemsa, methenamine silver, or Gram-Weigert stains and carefully examined for the presence of Pneumocystis cysts. Specimens are also preserved for bacterial and fungal cultures. If the biopsy must be delayed, or if surgery is believed to be contraindicated for other reasons, then a therapeutic trial with specific drugs against Pneumocystis should be instituted. Recently, use of bronchoscopy with a "brush" biopsy has been considered. This may show Pneumocystis; however, the sampling error and absence of tissue for histologic examination make it less valuable than open lung biopsy. Examination of sputum for cysts should be attempted, although in the immunodeficient patient this has usually not been revealing. Increased use of appropriate fixing and staining techniques on sputum and more careful sputum examination may improve the value of this simple test. Immunofluorescent antibody tests are now being evaluated. However, they show significantly elevated titers in only about 30 per cent of cases of pneumocystosis. Although measurement of antibody response using fluorescent antibody techniques is relatively insensitive, it appears to be specific. Thus a change in titer from negative to positive adds support to the diagnosis, whereas the absence of such a change does not exclude it.

Treatment. Therapy for pneumocystosis if started early in the disease has proved to be quite successful. During the past decade pentamidine isethionate has been used. This has reduced mortality from Pneumocystis infection from near 100 per cent to 10 to 50 per cent. The drug is made rapidly available by calling the Parasitic Disease Drug Service, U.S. Public Health Service (404–633–3311). The patient is given 4 mg per kilogram per day intramuscularly for 12 to 14 days. The mechanism of action of the drug remains unknown, but it does cause megaloblastic cell changes, inhibits incorporation of nucleotides into DNA and RNA, and inhibits oxidative phosphorylation. Folinic acid therapy can be used in patients who develop signs of folate deficiency without interfering with action of the drug against the organism. Pentamidine may also cause hypoglycemia, hyperglycemia, and nephrotoxicity. When given intravenously, hypotension can occur. The possibility that pentamidine causes pulmonary interstitial fibrosis has been raised by studies in animals. Because of these observed and potential toxic effects, another drug combination, pyrimethamine and sulfadiazine, has been tested for treatment of pneumocystis. Although there have been fewer patients treated with this combination than with pentamidine, it appears to be effective. These drugs interfere with the synthesis of folinic acid. For treatment of adults, pyrimethamine is given, 25 mg per day, and sulfadiazine, 1 gram four times daily. Folinic acid, 6 mg daily intramuscularly, will prevent significant bone marrow toxicity.

Because of the relationship between the occurrence of

pneumocystis and hypogammaglobulinemia, gamma globulin administration has been recommended. However, commercially available gamma globulin has proved to be of little value when given alone for treatment of pneumocystis. In general, attempts should be made to reduce the dose of corticosteroids when signs of pneumocystosis appear; however, in some patients whose respiratory symptoms developed during tapering of corticosteroids, a transient *increase* in the dose of these drugs while pneumocystosis therapy is started should be considered. Supportive measures such as oxygen therapy, assisted ventilation, and careful fluid and electrolyte balance are important parts of the management.

Prevention. In order to interrupt spread of pneumocystis infection, a great deal must be learned about its life cycle. Since the diseased patient may be able to spread the organism to other patients, healthy personnel, and relatives, appropriate respiratory precautions should be considered when the diagnosis is suspected. Attention to preventing contact between susceptible patients and diseased patients in open wards and in clinics may reduce the spread of the disease. The disease will be controlled only when the relationships between certain types of immune deficiency or corticosteroids and rapid proliferation of the organism are better understood.

Burke, B. A., and Good, R. A.: *Pneumocystis carinii* infection. Medicine, 52:23, 1973.

Norman, L., and Kagan, I. G.: Some observations on the serology of *Pneumocystis carinii* infections in the United States. Infect. Immun., 8:317, 1973.

Robbins, J. B.: *Pneumocystis carinii* pneumonitis. A review. Pediatr. Res., 1:131, 1967.

Rosen, P., Armstrong, D., and Ramos, C.: *Pneumocystis carinii* pneumonia. A clinicopathologic study of twenty patients with neoplastic diseases. Am. J. Med., 53:428, 1972.

Vogel, C. L., Cohen, M. H., Powell, R. D., Jr., and DeVita, V. T.: *Pneumocystis carinii* pneumonia. Ann. Intern. Med., 68:97, 1968.

LEISHMANIASIS

Anthony D. M. Bryceson

275. INTRODUCTION

Definition. Leishmaniasis is an infection with parasites of the genus Leishmania. It is usually a zoonosis transmitted by phlebotomine sandflies between wild or peridomestic animals, especially rodents or canines. Man is infected when he interrupts the natural cycle.

In man the infection is either visceral or cutaneous. Visceral leishmaniasis is a severe chronic infection of the reticuloendothelial system, characterized by fever, chills, weight loss, splenomegaly, leukopenia, anemia, and a high natural mortality. It is caused by *L. donovani*. Cutaneous leishmaniasis is characterized by single or several chronic sores which usually heal spontaneously. In parts of South and Central America, severely mutilating metastatic lesions of the mouth and nose are seen. Cutaneous leishmaniasis is caused by *L. tropica* in the Old World, and by members of the *L. mexicana* and *L. braziliensis* groups in the New World.

Etiology. Leishmania exist in two forms, one in the vertebrate host, including man, and the other in the sandfly and in artificial culture. In the vertebrate host the parasite is in the amastigote (Leishman-Donovan body) stage, so called because it has no flagellum. It is a round or oval body 2 to 3 μ across, containing a nucleus and a smaller kinetoplast which stain respectively red and purple with Geimsa, Wright's, or Leishman's stain, and stand out against the pale blue cytoplasm. Leishmania are strict intracellular parasites and are found in macrophages in which they multiply by binary fission. Heavily parasitized host cells rupture, and fresh cells are invaded. Sandflies become infected when they feed on an infected person or animal and take up parasites from blood or skin. In the sandfly the parasite is in the promastigote (leptomonad) stage, so called because of the anterior origin of its flagellum. Promastigotes are supple, highly motile, spindle-shaped organisms, 15 to 25 μ long and 1.5 to 3.5 μ broad. Promastigotes are found in the midgut of the sandfly, where they divide and whence they migrate forward into the pharynx and buccal cavity, rendering the sandfly infective. The cycle of development in the sandfly takes about seven days. Once inoculated into man, the promastigote rapidly penetrates macrophages, flagellum first, and transforms into an amastigote.

Immunology. The patterns of disease in man are partly determined by the species of parasite (trophism for skin or viscera, differences in immunogenicity and allergenicity) and partly by man's response to the parasite. Resistance to Leishmania depends upon the development of specific cell-mediated immunity. The capacity of individuals to mount such a response varies, and consequently leishmaniasis presents a spectrum of disease in the same way that leprosy does. At one end of the spectrum lie visceral leishmaniasis and diffuse cutaneous leishmaniasis, characterized by abundance of parasites, absence of lymphocytes in lesions, insensitivity to leishmanin, and poor prognosis. At the other end lie the self-healing sores, with relatively scanty parasites, marked lymphocytic infiltration, and leishmanin sensitivity. Accompanying cell-mediated immunity is delayed hypersensitivity to numerous parasite antigens, which causes the destructive pathology of leishmanial ulcers, especially in the chronic conditions of espundia (see below) and leishmaniasis recidiva (see below) in which the normal balance between immunity and hypersensitivity has been lost. The mechanisms underlying these abnormal immune responses are not understood.

Antibody, which is produced in large quantities in visceral leishmaniasis, is not protective, and it has been suggested that it may even contribute to the pathogenesis of hemolytic anemia, nephritis, and amyloidosis. Healing is usually accompanied by long-lasting immunity to the particular species of Leishmania involved, but not to other species.

Leishmanin (Montenegro) Test. Leishmanin is a suspension of 10^6 promastigotes in 1 ml of 0.5 per cent phenol saline. The test is performed by injecting 0.1 ml intradermally into the volar surface of the forearm. A palpable nodule, 5 mm or more in diameter after 48 to 72 hours, is considered positive. The test is an index of delayed hypersensitivity, but not necessarily of immunity to Leishmania. It is not species specific. It is used to map out the extent of past infection in a community and may be of help in diagnosis in individual patients.

276. VISCERAL LEISHMANIASIS (Kala-Azar, Ponos)

Epidemiology. It has been suggested that the zoonotic origin of *L. donovani* was among jackals in the steppes of Central Asia, where sporadic cases of visceral leishmaniasis are still sometimes seen among nomads and in settlers in the outskirts of rapidly expanding towns. From here the disease spread and developed three distinct epidemiologic patterns.

Visceral Leishmaniasis with a Canine Reservoir. This is the pattern in a belt which stretches from Portugal to Peking between latitudes 30 and 48 degrees North, the most important areas being the Mediterranean littoral, including North Africa, the shores of the Caspian Sea, central Soviet Asia, and northeast China. The main vectors are *Phlebotomus perniciosus* in Western Europe, *P. major* in Eastern Europe, *P. papatasii* in the Middle East, and *P. chinensis* in China. In the Mediterranean and Chinese foci, the host-parasite relationship is relatively stable, and the disease is most common among children between one and four years of age. For this reason the parasite is sometimes called *L. infantum,* although adults in areas into which the disease has newly been introduced or visitors of any age are highly susceptible. Domestic dogs and foxes are the reservoir.

Portuguese and Spanish settlers probably introduced *L. donovani,* also called *L. chagasi,* into the New World and initiated a zoonosis among foxes and dogs, although man may still be important as a reservoir. The likely vector is *P. longipalpis.* Visceral leishmaniasis is epidemic in northeast Brazil and sporadic in Amazonia, northern Argentina, and Paraguay and extends up through Venezuela and Colombia as far as Guatemala and Mexico. In Brazil male children are most commonly affected.

Visceral Leishmaniasis with a Rodent Vector. This is the pattern in Africa south of the Sahara from Lake Chad in the west to Somalia in the east, sparing the highlands of Ethiopia. The apparent absence of the disease in West Africa and south of the equator is unexplained. In the Sudan the zoonosis is between the Nile rat (*Arvicanthus niloticus*) and *P. orientalis* on the flood plains of the Nile and its tributaries. Visceral leishmaniasis is found among nomads who occupy temporary villages in riverine acacia woodland and migrant workers from adjoining countries.

In Kenya the disease is associated with termite hills where the vector *P. martini* rests and around which village men gather in the evenings. The reservoir is probably the gerbil *Tatara vicina.* The disease is usually sporadic, but epidemics have occurred. Males are affected four times as often as females, and the disease is most common in teenagers.

Visceral Leishmaniasis with a Human Reservoir. This is true epidemic kala-azar and is the pattern of the disease in northeast India, Bangladesh, Assam, and Burma. Classically the disease spreads along the Brahmaputra valley every 20 years or so. Transmission is by the highly anthroposophilic, domestic sandfly *P. argentipes.* Often, many cases are found to have originated from one house. The age and sex pattern is the same as in Africa. Man is the only reservoir, and *P. argentipes* is readily infected from blood or from the lesions of post-kala-azar dermal leishmaniasis. The disease virtually disappeared over large areas as a result of DDT spraying for malaria control, but could spread again now that spraying has stopped.

Factors Affecting Transmission. Opportunities for contact with infected sandflies largely determine the pattern of disease in a given area. This is modified by the level of immunity of the population or individual. An attack of visceral leishmaniasis confers lifelong immunity, which determines the periodicity of epidemics. Subclinical infections with *L. donovani* or possibly even lizard and rodent species of Leishmania affect the pattern of spread in Africa.

Pathology. The organs most severely affected are the spleen, liver, bone marrow, lymph nodes, intestines, and skin. The patient suffers from hyperplasia within and damage to these organs and from effects secondary to splenomegaly, reticuloendothelial blockage, and chronic parasitemia. Histologically the disease is characterized by massive proliferation of parasitized macrophages with little or no lymphocytic response. In Africa and Central Asia a cutaneous nodule or leishmanioma commonly develops at the site of parasite inoculation. Parasites multiply within histiocytes which may become the focus of a tuberculoid granuloma that heals spontaneously, and the infection proceeds no further. In the majority of cases, however, after a period of months, the infection disseminates.

The spleen is grossly enlarged, smooth, and firm and the capsule thick. The pulp is friable and infarcts are usual. There is massive hyperplasia of reticuloendothelial cells which are heavily parasitized. In the liver, Kupffer cells are hyperplastic and contain parasites. Occasionally parenchymal cells are parasitized. In chronic

untreated cases there is parenchymal cell degeneration which may be followed after several years by fibrosis and even cirrhosis with clinical and biochemical evidence of hepatic dysfunction.

The bone marrow is heavily infiltrated with parasitized macrophages. Erythropoiesis and granulopoiesis are normal in the early stages of the disease, but may be depressed later. The peripheral blood shows anemia and leukopenia. The anemia is probably due to increased plasma volume, sequestration of erythrocytes in the spleen, and hemolysis. Leukopenia is said to predispose the patient to secondary infections. Lymph nodes and lymphoid tissue of the nasopharynx and gut are enlarged and contain many parasitized cells.

Kidneys may show cloudy swelling of tubular cells. In fatal cases hyaline thickening of the glomerular mesangium has been found, and in chronic cases amyloidosis can develop. The skin, although normal in appearance, contains many intracellular parasites. In *post-kala-azar dermal leishmaniasis* there is variable infiltration with lymphocytes, histiocytes, and parasites.

In visceral leishmaniasis there is an enormous overproduction of IgG, only a small fraction of which is specific antibody. Some of it is autoantibody.

Clinical Features. The incubation period is normally two to six months, but may be as short as ten days or as long as nine years. The onset is usually insidious, especially in indigenous peoples who may feel well and have a good appetite despite daily bouts of fever; however, in those who are poorly nourished and have several underlying parasitic infections, the disease may then progress rapidly. In Africa a primary cutaneous nodule may be noticed for a few months before there are any systemic symptoms. The earliest symptom is fever. This is usually gradual in onset and accompanied by sweats, often without preceding chills. Alternatively, the onset is sudden with high fever and chills. This is common in Americans and Europeans who have contracted the disease while visiting an endemic area. Associated with fever there may be dizziness, weakness, and weight loss. Other common early symptoms include cough, diarrhea, pain, or discomfort in the left hypochondrium and symptoms of complicating secondary infections.

The important physical findings are fever, splenomegaly, lymphadenopathy, and skin changes. Fever at first is often inconstant, with apyrexial periods of several days or weeks. In over 80 per cent of cases, however, the fever eventually develops a characteristic pattern with twice daily elevations reaching 38 to 40° C (100 to 104° F), and may then undulate as in brucellosis. In the most acute cases fever and toxemia may be the only signs. Splenic enlargement is not necessarily rapidly progressive, nor does the size of the spleen correlate with the duration of the disease. In many instances, however, it reaches the right iliac fossa. It is firm and not tender unless there has been a recent subcapsular infarct. The liver enlarges more slowly and becomes palpable in about 20 per cent of cases and is likewise firm and not tender. Generalized lymphadenopathy is common in patients from Mediterranean countries, Africa, or China. Various changes have been reported in the skin. Classically there is hyperpigmentation of hands, feet, and abdomen. This may be missed in black Africans; in lighter-skinned Indians it looks gray or black (kala-azar means black sickness). In Africans warty eruptions or ulcers of the skin and oronasal lesions are occasionally seen.

Course and Complications. As the disease progresses,

anemia becomes clinically apparent. There may be bleeding from the nose or gums. In longstanding cases jaundice and signs of hypoalbuminemia may develop, namely, brittle hair, opaque nails, subcutaneous edema and ascites. Finally, after a course which may run for a few months or for five years, the patient becomes emaciated and exhausted. Intercurrent infections are the cause of death in 90 per cent of fatal cases. The most common are cancrum oris, pneumonia, pulmonary tuberculosis, bacillary dysentery, amebic dysentery, and, in Africa, brucellosis. Massive gastrointestinal hemorrhage accounts for another 1 to 2 per cent.

Post-Kala-Azar Dermal Leishmaniasis. About 20 per cent of Indian patients develop a rash one to two years after treatment or spontaneous recovery. The lesions develop slowly and may last for several, even 20, years. In Africa the rash develops in 2 per cent of cases, usually during treatment, and does not persist. It commonly starts as hypopigmented or erythematous macules on the face and sometimes on the arms, legs, and trunk. On the face the rash gradually becomes papular or nodular, especially on the forehead, cheeks, and earlobes, and closely resembles lepromatous leprosy. In 25 per cent of cases the lesions resolve spontaneously.

Diagnosis and Laboratory Findings. The diagnosis must be suspected in any person living in, or having visited, an endemic area who has a prolonged fever. The diagnosis is likely in the presence of splenomegaly, granulocytopenia, anemia, and hyperglobulinemia and is made by isolation of the parasite or by characteristic immunologic changes.

Isolation of Parasite. This is best done by needle aspiration of bone marrow, spleen, liver, or lymph nodes. Material obtained is:

1. Used to make a thin film on a glass microscope slide, stained, and examined under oil immersion for amastigotes, which must be distinguished from platelets. Parasitized macrophages usually rupture on smearing and free parasites must be looked for (see Fig. 2F, Ch. 271). Bone marrow aspiration is the procedure of choice. However, splenic puncture is safe so long as the tip of the spleen is well below the costal margin and the prothrombin and bleeding times are normal. A hypodermic needle on a syringe is inserted into the spleen, allowed to rest a moment, and withdrawn without suction. Organisms are seen in about 90 per cent of splenic aspirates and rather less often from other tissues. Buffy coat preparations show parasites in over 90 per cent of cases in India, but in only about 1 per cent in Africa.

2. Inoculated onto NNN (Novy-MacNeal-Nicolle) medium overlaid with balanced salt solution, containing streptomycin and penicillin (but not amphotericin). Cultures are kept in the dark at 22 to 25° C (not at 37° C), and every three to four days a drop of fluid is taken and examined wet for promastigotes. If after four weeks no parasites are seen, the fluid overlay is reinoculated onto a fresh NNN slope. Culture greatly improves the chances of making a diagnosis.

3. Inoculated intraperitoneally into hamsters, which are susceptible to a single amastigote. Though sensitive, this method is slow and seldom valuable.

Immunologic Tests. Antileishmanial antibodies can be demonstrated by indirect immunofluorescence of promastigotes in 100 per cent of cases and by precipitation in gel in 95 per cent. Cross reactions with *Trypanosoma cruzi* antibodies can be absorbed out. Complement fixation is positive in 65 per cent, but if the older antigen made from Kedrowsky's bacillins is used, reactions may be expected in some patients with mycobacterial disease. Serum obtained by eluting blood dried onto filter paper in the field can be used satisfactorily in all these techniques. The leishmanin test is *negative* in cases of active visceral leishmaniasis, but becomes positive after recovery, being most intense after one to two years, after which it fades slowly.

Total serum proteins are raised up to and over 10 grams per 100 ml. This increase is due almost entirely to the IgG fraction of gamma globulin. On immunoelectrophoresis the IgG pattern is characteristically skewed. In some cases IgM is also slightly increased, but this is said to be transient and to revert rapidly to normal on treatment. In advanced cases serum albumin levels fall. This disturbed globulin pattern underlies the older diagnostic aldehyde test which is also positive in other diseases with a grossly disturbed globulin pattern.

Laboratory Findings. The principal laboratory findings have to do with the blood and with the plasma proteins.

Blood Changes. Leukopenia is the most characteristic finding. The total count is below 2000 cells per cubic millimeter in 75 per cent of cases. There are an absolute neutropenia and eosinopenia and a relative lymphocytosis and monocytosis. Agranulocytosis occasionally develops. Anemia is slower in onset but becomes severe. It is normocytic and normochromic unless complicated by bleeding or deficiency states. There is often a mild reticulocytosis, and erythrocyte half-life is reduced. Thrombocytopenia is usual and progresses with the disease. Early on, tests of clotting are normal but later the prothrombin, partial thromboplastin, bleeding, and clotting times are prolonged. There are no characteristic findings in the urine.

Differential Diagnosis. In Europeans, Americans, and others who are not immune, malaria must be exluded by examination of thick and thin blood films. In immunes, malarial parasites in the blood film are of no diagnostic significance. In many parts of the tropics where malaria and schistosomiasis are endemic, a palpable spleen is commonplace and is usually unrelated to a recent febrile illness. Diseases which can be confused with visceral leishmaniasis include aleukemic leukemia and lymphomas, tropical splenomegaly syndrome (serum IgM, liver biopsy), cirrhosis of the liver with portal hypertension and hypersplenism, miliary tuberculosis, histoplasmosis, acute schistosomiasis, brucellosis, typhoid, and other septicemias, including bacterial endocarditis.

Prognosis. Untreated, 75 to 90 per cent of patients die. Treated, in all early cases, patients should recover. The mortality of late or severe disease in malnourished patients treated under difficult conditions can be over 25 per cent. Bad prognostic signs include extreme emaciation and toxemia, agranulocytosis, and the absence of the lymphocytosis which usually appears during treatment.

Treatment. *Chemotherapy.* Pentavalent antimony is the drug of choice, and, of the available preparations, sodium stibogluconate (Pentostam, Solustibostam) is probably the best. This is marketed as a solution containing 100 mg per milliliter. The dose is 0.2 ml per kilogram of body weight daily by intravenous or intramuscular injection, not exceeding 10 ml per dose. In India six injections are usually adequate, but elsewhere 30 are considered necessary. Alternative preparations include the following: (1) Meglumine antimoniate (Glucantime, 30 mg per ml), 0.4 ml per kilogram of body weight daily for 14 days. (2) Ethyl stibamine (Neostibosan) which must be freshly prepared as a 5 per cent solution. The adult dose is 0.1 ml the first day, 0.2 ml the second day, and 0.3 ml daily thereafter for 8 to 16 doses by intravenous injection. (3) Urea stibamine, 100 to 200 mg intravenously on alternate days for 15 doses. Side effects of pentavalent antimony are cumulative but rare. They are nausea, vomiting, urticaria, bradycardia, and electrocardiographic changes. In 5 to 10 per cent of patients, less in India, more in Africa, the response to antimony is unsatisfactory. The choice then lies between two toxic drugs, pentamidine isethionate (Lomidine, 40 mg per milliliter) and amphotericin B (Fungizone). The dose of pentamidine is 0.1 ml per kilogram of body weight by intramuscular injection every three to four days for ten doses, or less frequently if side effects develop. If the drug is accidentally injected intravenously, the patient will collapse, but recovers quickly if the feet are raised. Cumulative side effects include fatigue, anorexia, nausea, abdominal pain and, in 2 per cent of cases, prolonged hypoglycemia. Ten per cent of patients develop diabetes whose onset is not related to the duration of treatment. If this drug has to be used, a glucose tolerance test should be performed weekly. Amphotericin B is given by slow intravenous infusion in 5 per cent dextrose in a dose of 1 mg per kilogram of body weight on alternate days to a total of 2 grams for an adult. Side effects include rigors, thrombophlebitis, nausea, vomiting, fatigue, anemia, and uremia. This drug is more difficult to administer than pentamidine but is preferable.

Supportive Treatment. Bed rest, good nursing care, oral hygiene, an adequate fluid intake and sufficient food are all desirable. Complicating infections must be sought and treated. Anemia responds as the patient recovers, but if severe, and especially if there is bleeding, blood transfusion should be given. Deficiencies of iron, folate, and other vitamins need treating.

Response to Treatment. Little improvement may be seen until the course of treatment is nearly over. The patient then continues to improve steadily. There are lymphocytosis and reticulocytosis. No criterion of cure has been established. The patient should be seen monthly for six months and at a year. At each visit blood is cultured for Leishmania, spleen size is measured, and hemoglobin and serum IgG estimated. Complement-fixing antibody should not be detectable after six months. The spleen does not always become impalpable, and may indicate cirrhosis.

Relapses and Post-Kala-Azar Dermal Leishmaniasis. These usually respond to a further course or courses of antimony. If not, one of the other drugs may be used. One month should elapse before repeating a course. Rarely, if repeated courses of drugs fail to eliminate the parasite, the spleen remains huge, and the patient suffers from hypersplenism, splenectomy may be indicated. It must be followed by a course of chemotherapy, and in malarial areas by antimalarial prophylaxis for life.

Prevention. On a mass scale the detailed epidemiology of the local disease must be known. This will enable reservoir control (destruction of stray dogs, early detection, and treatment of cases) and vector control (insecticide spraying in the right places) to be carried out, and people may be able to avoid contact with infected flies, e.g., Kenyan termite hills. Personal prophylaxis depends on wearing protective clothing in the evenings, the use of insect repellants, and sleeping under fine mesh netting.

277. CUTANEOUS LEISHMANIASIS OF THE OLD WORLD
(Oriental Sore)

Epidemiology. The innumerable names of this disease (Delhi or Bagdad boil, Biskra button, Aleppo evil, bouton de Crete, little sister) testify to its extent and familiarity throughout the Mediterranean basin, the Near and

Middle East, and parts of India. Four epidemiologic situations are recognized.

"Rural" leishmaniasis throughout these areas is caused by the subspecies *L. tropica major.* The disease is a zoonosis among the desert gerbils (*Rhomobomys opimus*) and is transmitted to man by *Phlebotomus papatasii.* Where village settlements are close to gerbil colonies, up to 100 per cent of the population become infected, usually in early childhood. Travelers, hunters, and soldiers also get the disease. In "urban" leishmaniasis, the parasite *L. tropica minor* is adapted to dogs and to man, either of whom can act as reservoirs. *P. sergenti* is the main vector. This disease was the scourge of Middle Eastern cities; every adult inhabitant bore the scar, and few visitors were spared.

In Africa two distinct zoonoses exist. In West Africa the situation is "rural." Human cases are uncommon and sporadic. The vector and reservoir are not definitely established, but rodents and dogs are probably involved. In Ethiopia the disease is confined to the highlands, where the reservoir is the rock Hyrax (Procavia). The vector is *P. longipes*, which bites villagers at night in their houses.

Pathology. At the site of inoculation there is a massive infiltration with monocytes and histiocytes which take up the parasites and support their growth. The lesion then becomes surrounded by or mixed with lymphocytes and a few plasma cells. Macrophages develop into epithelioid cells, and parasites diminish. In later cases loose tubercles composed of loosely packed cells may develop. The overlying dermis ulcerates. The epidermis shows hyperkeratosis, acanthosis, pseudoepitheliomatous hyperplasia, intraepidermal necrosis, and ulceration. Healing is accompanied by fibrosis and is followed by lifelong immunity. Second infections are seen in only about 2 per 1000 cases, and then often in association with a generalized depression of immunity.

If cell-mediated immunity fails to develop, the patient gets diffuse cutaneous leishmaniasis, the disease spreading to other parts of the skin. Histologic study shows masses of heavily parasitized macrophages with little or no lymphocytic infiltration or epidermal change. The leishmanin test is negative.

In leishmaniasis recidiva, failure to heal is associated with exquisite delayed hypersensitivity, extreme chronicity, a tuberculoid histology with epithelioid giant cells but without caseation, and scanty or undetectable parasites.

Clinical Manifestations. The earliest lesion is a small erythematous papule, appearing two to eight weeks after the sandfly bite. It may itch slightly. The typical "urban" sore grows slowly into a nodule 1 to 2 cm across, and after a period of weeks or months forms a central crust under which is a shallow ulcer. The edge of the lesion is characteristically studded with small satellite papules. The sore usually remains in this state for a few more months and then heals gradually, leaving a depressed mottled scar. The whole process takes from three months to two years. The most common site is the face, followed by the arms and legs. There may be one or several sores. About 1 per cent of urban sores develop *leishmaniasis recidiva (lupoid leishmaniasis).* The ulcer fails to heal completely, scarring centrally but spreading peripherally, or heals and recrudesces at the edge of the scar. The lesion lasts for many years and resembles cutaneous tuberculosis.

There are many variants of the typical pattern of Oriental sore. "Rural" sores are commonly multiple, rapid in evolution, more florid, and produce more scarring. Ethiopian lesions are solitary, facial, milder, and slower in evolution, although lesions affecting the mucocutaneous border of the nose are extremely chronic and disfiguring.

Ethiopia is the only Old World country where *diffuse cutaneous leishmaniasis* is found. It is a rare condition,

Figure 1. Cutaneous leishmaniasis – "Oriental sore."

the extensor surfaces of the limbs, producing infiltrative and nodular lesions which may resemble lepromatous leprosy and do not heal spontaneously. The viscera are not involved, and the patient feels well.

Diagnosis. Leishmaniasis must be suspected as the cause of any chronic nodule or ulcer in a person living in or having recently visited an endemic area. Typical sores are diagnosable on sight. Diagnosis is confirmed by finding parasites in stained slit skin smears taken from a nonulcerated part of the lesion. The slit must reach the dermis, and the smears must contain tissue juice, not blood or pus. If unsuccessful, the crust is removed, the ulcer cleaned of all debris, and smears made of tissue scraped from the base of the ulcer. These methods are simpler and more likely to show parasites than is histology. In healing lesions and lupoid leishmaniasis, parasites are scanty and culture of juice or biopsy tissue may be necessary.

The leishmanin test becomes positive as the lesion ulcerates and is of diagnostic value in patients who do not live in endemic areas; it also may help to distinguish lupoid leishmaniasis from cutaneous tuberculosis, late syphilis, and fungal granulomas, which may be histologically similar.

There are no characteristic blood changes, and antibodies are difficult to demonstrate by usual techniques.

Treatment. Treatment remains unsatisfactory, but, as almost all cases heal spontaneously, the systemic use of toxic drugs is seldom justified. Fortunately most cases respond to a course of pentavalent antimony or to local infiltration with 0.5 ml 2 per cent berberine sulfate or 15 per cent mepacrine. Indolent sores may respond to heating to 50° C by coned infrared rays, to curettage and skin grafting, or to intralesional injections of corticosteroids combined with a course of antimony. Secondary infection is treated with the customary antimicrobial drugs.

Prevention. Detailed epidemiologic knowledge has permitted attacks on the reservoir in Central Asia and in Middle Eastern cities, where demolition of mud buildings and antimalarial spraying have reduced the number of sandflies. Immunization with live, virulent organisms is practiced on a mass scale in Russia and traditionally in the Middle East (see R. A. Neal, 1968).

occurring in perhaps 1 in 100,000 cases. The primary nodule does not ulcerate, but after a period of months or years starts to spread locally, and the disease disseminates to other parts of the skin, notably on the face and

278. CUTANEOUS LEISHMANIASIS OF THE NEW WORLD
(Including American Mucocutaneous Leishmaniasis or Espundia)

Epidemiology and Parasitology. Cutaneous leishmaniasis is endemic in Central and South America as far south as the Parana Estuary in the east and the Peruvian Andes in the west. In this extensive and varied terrain many different zoonoses exist, each associated with its own reservoirs and vectors and a particular pattern of human disease. Two main groups of parasites are now distinguished, those of *L. mexicana* and of *L. braziliensis*. The former, which grows easily in NNN medium and in the hamster, is responsible for most of the cutaneous leishmaniasis in Central America and a little in Brazil. The latter, which grows poorly in NNN medium and in the hamster, is responsible for most of the disease in

Figure 2. Early diffuse cutaneous leishmaniasis in an Ethiopian. Post-kala-azar dermal leishmaniasis may also look like this.

Cutaneous Leishmaniasis of the New World: Epidemiology

Parasite	Vector to Man	Reservoir	Geography	Human Disease
L. mexicana mexicana	*Lutzomyia olmeca*	Numerous rodents	Yucatan, Central America	"Chicle ulcer, bay sore" in forest workers; single skin lesions, healing in six months; diffuse cutaneous leishmaniasis
L. mexicana amazonensis	*Lutzomyia flaviscutellata*	Numerous rodents	Brazil, Trinidad; ? = *L. pifanoi*, Venezuela	Rare, single skin lesions; diffuse cutaneous leishmaniasis
L. braziliensis braziliensis	*Lutzomyia ssp, Psychodopygus ssp.*	Uncertain	All Amazon forests, esp. Brazil	"Espundia"; single or few large persistent destructive skin ulcers; oronasal metastases common
L. braziliensis guyanensis	*? Lutzomyia anduzei*	Unknown	Guyanas, into Brazil, Venezuela	"Forest yaws, pian bois"; multiple, widespread, deep skin ulcers, with nodular lymphatic metastases; ? oronasal metastases
L. braziliensis panamensis	*? Lutzomyia trapidoi*	Rodents, ? sloths	Panama	Single or few deep skin ulcers with nodular lymphatic metastases; ? oronasal metastases
L. peruviana	*? Lutzomyia peruensis*	Dogs	Peru, west slopes of Andes to 3000 meters	"Uta"; single or few skin lesions, healing in one year

South America, including espundia. Epidemiologic details are summarized in the accompanying table.

Cutaneous leishmaniasis presents a formidable obstacle to the development of the Central and South American forests, in large areas of which transmission of the infection is extremely high. This is particularly true in Brazil, where almost all workers on the trans-Amazonian highway become infected and run the risk of developing mutilating oronasal metastatic lesions. Amerindians, on the other hand, very rarely get leishmaniasis, although by the age of 40 years up to 100 per cent are sensitive to leishmanin.

Pathology. The pathology of cutaneous lesions is similar to that of Oriental sore. Metastatic lesions of espundia arise in the mucosa of the nose and mouth and show at first a typical leishmanial granuloma with numerous parasites, which later become scanty, and can be seen also in cells in cartilage, which is rapidly invaded and destroyed. There is vasculitis with edema, necrosis, and fibrosis.

Clinical Manifestations. Cutaneous lesions develop and heal in the same way as Oriental sores, but tend to be less nodular and more ulcerative and destructive. Lesions of the pinna are very chronic. Regional variations are given in the table.

In espundia, from 2 per cent (Panama) to 80 per cent (Paraguay) of primary cutaneous sores are followed after a period ranging from a few days to five years by metastatic lesions of the nose or mouth, most commonly on the mucocutaneous borders, but sometimes on the palate or larynx. These lesions may arise long after the primary lesion has healed. At first there is crusting or polyp formation, and then ulceration and perforation of the septum. Alternatively, large protruding granulomas of the nose and lips develop. The lesion heals slowly, if at all, after many years. Scarring may constrict the nose or mouth, producing gross deformity and making eating difficult. Secondary sepsis is common and increases the patient's debility.

Diffuse cutaneous leishmaniasis is a rare disease found mainly in Venezuela. Its clinical features are the same as in Ethiopia.

Diagnosis. The approach to diagnosis is set forth in Ch. 276 and 277. In late cases of espundia it may be im-

possible to isolate the parasite, but geographic history, clinical pattern, and leishmanin sensitivity make the diagnosis likely. Antibodies are detectable by immunofluorescence in over 90 per cent of patients with cutaneous or oronasal lesions, and disappear when the disease has been successfully treated. Blastomycosis is added to the list of differential diagnoses.

Treatment. The milder varieties of solitary sores seldom need treatment, unless they are disfiguring. Cycloguanil pamoate, 5 mg per kilogram of body weight as a single (painful) repository injection, is said to speed the healing of lesions of *L. mexicana*. If there is any suspicion that a sore has been caused by *L. braziliensis*, it must be treated by a course of pentavalent antimony (see Ch. 276). Established oronasal lesions frequently do not respond to antimony, or are liable to relapse. Amphotericin B (see Ch. 276) is then the drug of choice. Diffuse cutaneous leishmaniasis responds initially to antimony, but becomes resistant in relapse. Amphotericin B should then be tried.

Prevention. Prevention in South America is difficult. Intensity of transmission in the forest and lack of detailed epidemiologic information make mass prophylaxis a hopeless approach at the moment. People who are obliged to enter the forest could attempt to follow a regimen of the application of insect repellents every few hours and of sleeping under a fine mesh netting, but admittedly both of these procedures can produce considerable discomfort.

Lainson, R., and Shaw, J. J.: Leishmaniasis of the New World: Taxonomic problems. Br. Med. Bull, 28:44, 1972.

Manson-Bahr, P. E. C., and Winslow, D. J.: Cutaneous leishmaniasis. *In* Marcial-Rojas, R. A. (ed.): Pathology of Rickettsial and Helminthic Diseases. Baltimore, Williams & Wilkins Company, 1971, p. 97.

Most, H., and Lavietes, R. H.: Kala-azar in American military personnel. Medicine, 26:221, 1947.

Symposium on leishmaniasis. Bull. W.H.O., 44:477, 1971.

Turk, J. L., and Bryceson, A. D. M.: Immunological phenomena in leprosy and related diseases. Adv. Immunol., 13:209, 1971.

Walton, B. C., Brooks, W. H., and Arjona, I.: Serodiagnosis of American leishmaniasis by indirect fluorescent antibody test. Am. J. Trop. Med. Hyg., 21:296, 1972.

Wilcocks, C., and Manson-Bahr, P. E. C. (eds.): Manson's Tropical Diseases. 17th ed. Baltimore, Williams and Wilkins Company, 1972.

Winslow, D. J.: Visceral leishmaniasis. *In* Marcial-Rojas, R. A. (ed.): Pathology of Rickettsial and Helminthic Diseases. Baltimore, Williams & Wilkins Company, 1971, p. 86.

279. AMEBIASIS

Richard Knight

Definition.   Amebiasis is caused by infection with *Entamoeba histolytica.* This species normally lives as a commensal within the large bowel lumen, where it may persist for several years. Symptoms of the disease may be produced by bowel invasion which may lead to submucosal ulcerations or which may allow spread of the organisms to the liver and other organs.

Etiology.   Four species of Entamoeba infect man, but only *E. histolytica* has pathogenic potential. Noninvasive trophozoites of *E. histolytica* within the bowel of an infected host may round up and eliminate their cytoplasmic inclusions to form a precystic ameba. These organisms each secrete a substance which envelops them to become uninucleate spherical cysts (10 to 16 μ in diameter); immature cysts contain a large glycogen vacuole. The cysts mature either within the bowel lumen or outside the body. Most mature cysts have four nuclei resulting from two nuclear divisions; they contain a number of cigar-shaped chromatoid bars that constitute a ribosome store. When these mature cysts are ingested, they undergo one additional nuclear division. The cyst wall is destroyed in the small intestine, releasing eight motile uninucleate amebae or trophozoites. A population of trophozoites can thus become established in the proximal colon and cecum where they live adjacent to the mucosa and multiply by binary fission about every eight hours. These noninvasive forms measure 10 to 20 μ in diameter and feed upon bacteria and exfoliated epithelial cells.

Invasive *E. histolytica* are larger than noninvasive forms, up to 50 μ, and move much more actively by unidirectional pseudopodial movement. They contain ingested erythrocytes—hence the term hematophagous—and few or no bacteria.

Freshly isolated strains of *E. histolytica* behave differently when inoculated intracecally into weanling rats, those from patients with dysentery often being the most pathogenic. In culture, this virulence tends to decrease, although it may usually be restored by animal passage. A few strains have been isolated that differ from *E. histolytica* antigenically and by their ability to grow at room temperature and in hypotonic media. These *E. histolytica*—like amebae are probably never pathogenic; all other strains of *E. histolytica* are potentially virulent.

E. hartmanni is closely related to *E. histolytica* but is smaller, the peripheral nuclear chromatin is more clumped, and the quadrinucleate cysts are less than 10 μ in diameter (mean, 8 μ). *E. hartmanni,* formerly called "small race" *E. histolytica,* is not pathogenic. *E. coli* is another common commensal, whose sluggish trophozoites (20 to 30 μ) have coarse granular endoplasm. The karyosome is eccentric and the peripheral chromatin coarser than that of *E. histolytica.* Mature cysts (12 to 20 μ) have eight nuclei and thin pointed chromatoids. *E. polecki* is primarily a pig parasite and is rare in man except in parts of New Guinea where pigs and man live in close association. The mature cyst has only one nucleus and resembles an immature *E. histolytica* cyst.

Epidemiology.   About 10 per cent of the world's population harbor *E. histolytica.* In the United States the prevalence is 2 to 5 per cent, in some tropical countries over 40 per cent. Poverty and poor sanitation encourage infection. Cysts may survive a month in water but are killed by drying. Rats, dogs, and certain monkeys are sometimes infected, but almost all human infections are from cysts passed by human carriers. *Encystment does not occur outside the body,* so patients passing only trophozoites in their stools are not infectious. Food is the most common vehicle of transmission; it may be contaminated by infected food handlers or flies. Direct contamination with human feces used as fertilizer is most common with uncooked fruit and salad vegetables. Direct fecal spread is important among children or the mentally handicapped in institutions, where infection rates may be very high.

Water-borne infection occurs, sometimes in epidemic form, as in the famous Chicago epidemic in which there were 1400 known cases and more than 100 deaths. Epidemics are probably not often recognized because the incubation period is so variable and many infections asymptomatic. Cysts may appear in the stool as early as four days after infection. The rate of spontaneous loss of infection is perhaps 15 per cent per year, so returning Americans infected in the tropics may remain infected for five years or more. In countries where there is continuous transmission, prevalence rates remain stable from year to year. In certain parts of the world, such as Mexico, parts of South America, the West Coast of Africa, Natal, and Southeast Asia, invasive disease is especially common. The incidence of disease does not necessarily correlate with the prevalence of infection.

Pathogenesis and Pathology.   Commensal trophozoites thrive adjacent to the colonic mucosa where the oxygen tension is moderately low and the pH between 6.0 and 6.5. Host tissues appear to be damaged only by direct contact with amebae; lysosomal enzymes are released, possibly by activating a contact-sensitive surface organelle. The relatively anoxic and acid conditions of cell necrosis favor further penetration of amebae into the tissues. Although some amebic bowel lesions are secondarily infected, the role of intestinal bacteria in pathogenesis is still uncertain. They may act mainly by creating a milieu suitable for amebic growth.

Amebic ulceration is most common in the cecum and rectosigmoid, but may affect any part of the large bowel, appendix, and terminal ileum. The initial lesions are small, discrete superficial mucosal erosions which may then extend more deeply through the muscularis mucosae and spread laterally, producing ulcers that are flask-shaped in cross section. Lesions may coalesce, causing extensive mucosal loss. Blood vessel involvement usually results in local thrombosis. Penetration may extend through the muscle coats, causing *peritonitis,* the most dangerous complication of intestinal amebiasis. Microscopically, tissue necrosis is the main change; amebae occur throughout the lesion, but particularly at the advancing edge, and even beyond into healthy tissue. In tissue sections, amebae may appear shrunken and be surrounded by a clear space. They stain rather indistinctly with ordinary hematoxylin and eosin but stand out clearly as bright red bodies with periodic acid–Schiff stain; iron hematoxylin staining is necessary to show the nuclear structure clearly. The lymphocytic inflammatory response is slight or moderate; some neutrophils are also present, especially if there is secondary bacterial infection.

Ulcers heal rapidly after treatment, and persistent scarring is uncommon. Sometimes localized bowel lesions show a more vigorous host response, with edema and a marked inflammatory reaction producing an amebic granuloma or ameboma. These are most common in the cecum and rectosigmoid and may be multiple.

Although strain virulence may influence the probability of tissue invasion, host factors are also important.

Women in late pregnancy and the puerperium are especially susceptible, as are patients on cytotoxic or corticosteroid therapy. Colonic cancers may be secondarily invaded by *E. histolytica. Trichuris trichiura* infections and intestinal schistosomiasis may also encourage invasion. The high carbohydrate low-protein diets of developing countries perhaps enhance host susceptibility.

Hepatic Involvement. In many patients with invasive intestinal disease, amebae probably reach the liver via the portal vein, but most are destroyed. Hepatomegaly is not unusual in acute amebic dysentery because of products of colonic tissue destruction or bacteria reaching the liver. Established amebic infection of the liver usually causes progressive cytolytic lesions that extend in all directions, with trophozoites proliferating near the advancing edge. Perhaps these lesions begin at the sites of venous embolism or thrombosis. Secondary bacterial infection is rare, and the content of such a "liver abscess" is necrotic liquefied liver tissue. The abscess is sharply demarcated from surrounding liver, which shows edema, hyperemia, and a narrow zone of lymphocytic and polymorphonuclear infiltration; a fibroblastic reaction occurs in longstanding lesions. Most liver abscesses are solitary and occur long after any clinically evident bowel ulceration; but both solitary and the rarer multiple abscesses may develop during or shortly after a bout of dysentery. The term *amebic hepatitis* has been used by clinicians, but there is no pathologic basis for a diffuse lesion of this kind. In adults, 80 to 90 per cent of amebic liver abscesses occur in men, but before puberty both sexes are similarly affected. No other host factors have been definitely identified, although pre-existing liver disease and alcoholism may be relevant. Most complications of liver abscess are due to direct spread to adjacent structures.

Antibody Response. Tissue invasion provokes a humoral antibody response, mainly IgG, and a skin sensitivity to injected amebic antigen. It is not known whether this response has any protective function. Using sensitive techniques, antibodies can be detected in 25 per cent or more of apparently healthy carriers, suggesting that mild self-limiting bowel invasion is more common than has been supposed.

Clinical Manifestations. *Intestinal Amebiasis.* Most persons with *E. histolytica* in the stool have no symptoms, and many will remain symptomless carriers for the whole duration of their infection. Invasive bowel disease begins most commonly between one and six months after infection but sometimes much later, especially in an immunologically compromised host.

Involvement of the colon without diarrhea is the most common form of bowel disease; the ulceration is localized and not severe enough to produce dysentery. The patient complains of colicky pains in the right or left iliac fossa, flatulence, and an altered bowel habit, often with some diarrhea. A little blood or mucus may be noted in the stool; there is little constitutional upset. The cecum or sigmoid colon may be tender or feel abnormal on palpation. Symptoms may persist intermittently for months thereafter, and spontaneous cure is not uncommon.

Widespread colonic or rectosigmoid ulceration produces amebic dysentery with frequent bloody stools. Dysentery may begin abruptly, but often follows a varied period of the milder colonic symptoms noted above. Initially, many patients remain ambulant, but later, fever, colicky abdominal pains, and tenesmus appear. The illness is usually less acute than bacillary dysentery and

dehydration less evident. There may be colonic tenderness and some hepatomegaly. The stool is often offensive and contains some fecal matter; much of the blood present is altered unless there is rectal ulceration. In the rare fulminating form of the disease, toxic megacolon occurs with progressive abdominal distention, vomiting, dehydration, and electrolyte loss; some very ill patients have relatively few bowel actions. Sigmoidoscopy and barium enema examination should not be carried out in patients with severe dysentery; when the diagnosis is in doubt, a limited endoscopy may be justified.

Amebomas may present as a tender abdominal mass, sometimes with fever and constitutional upset. Partial bowel obstruction may occur, especially when the lesion is annular. The appendix may be affected primarily, or secondarily by a cecal lesion. This may resemble simple appendicitis, except that pain begins in the right iliac fossa, and guarding and rigidity are slight unless perforation has occurred.

COMPLICATIONS. A grossly diseased and atonic large bowel may perforate at several points. Absent bowel sounds with relatively little pain, rigidity, or tenderness should suggest this very dangerous possibility. Free gas in the peritoneum confirms it. Less commonly, when perforation is localized, classic signs of peritonitis are produced. Local perforation can also lead to pericolic abscess or retroperitoneal fecal cellulitis. *Fibrous strictures* of the colon rarely follow amebic dysentery or amebomas, but may require surgical relief. Serious hemorrhage is uncommon, but can be life threatening. Amebic ulceration or an ameboma may rarely initiate a cecocolic intussusception. Irritable bowel syndrome may follow amebic colitis and persist for several months. Much rarer is the syndrome of postdysenteric colitis which can continue for several years despite eradication of the amebic infection. It is distinct from simple ulcerative colitis and is associated with very high amebic antibody titers; endoscopy shows reddened edematous mucosa, sometimes with superficial erosions. Barium enema examination will exclude the rare possibility of internal fistulas.

Cutaneous amebiasis takes the form of deep, painful, and rapidly spreading ulceration. The most common sites are the perianal area, perineum, laparotomy incisions, and colostomy stomas. Rarely, the uterine cervix is affected, giving lesions that may resemble carcinoma. Penile lesions may follow anal coitus.

Hepatic Amebiasis. About half of all patients with liver abscess have a history suggestive of amebic dysentery between a week and many years previously. Solitary lesions are most common in the upper part of the right lobe; multiple lesions are often associated with coexistent dysentery. The illness begins insidiously with fever, sweating, and pain in the liver region. If the diaphragm is involved, there may be right pleuritic or shoulder pain. Most patients present within a few weeks of onset; as the disease progresses, there are weight loss and anemia. *Those developing the condition in temperate countries after returning from the tropics rarely have bowel symptoms.* Hepatomegaly is always present, but if enlargement is mainly upward, it may not be very evident on abdominal palpation. Left lobe lesions are palpable as an epigastric mass. Liver tenderness is mainly localized to the site of the lesion, and, in suspected cases, all the lower right intercostal spaces should be carefully palpated. Pain on heavy percussion or compression of the liver is not a very specific sign, because many types of liver and chest disease will be painful with these procedures. Crepitations and signs of lung consolidation or pleural fluid in the lower right chest are quite common. Jaundice occurs only when lesions are very large or numerous. The blood sedimentation rate is raised, and normally there are a polymorphonuclear leukocytosis and some normocytic normochromic anemia. Levels of serum transaminase and alkaline phosphatase are variable and of little diagnostic value. *The most suggestive roentgenographic finding* is an immobile, raised, or bulging right hemidiaphragm; lung or pleural involvement may also be visible. Radioisotope liver scans help considerably to show the site, size, and number of lesions present. *Diagnostic needle aspiration* with the finding of relatively odorless brownish or pink material with no bacteria on Gram staining is almost pathognomonic. An 8 cm pleural aspiration needle 1.5 to 2.0 mm in diameter connected to a large syringe via a three-way tap is normally used. When there is no definite clinical evidence as to the site of the lesion, the eighth or ninth right intercostal space should be explored in the midaxillary line.

COMPLICATIONS. Rupture through the diaphragm can produce amebic lung abscess or empyema and sometimes a bronchohepatic fistula so that the patient coughs up amebic pus. Extension to the body surface may lead to sinus formation and cutaneous lesions. Amebic peritonitis follows rupture into the peritoneum, and the primary source may be evident only at laparotomy. The gut, stomach, vena cava, spleen, and right kidney can also be involved by direct spread. A dangerous complication of left lobe lesions is *amebic pericarditis;* urgent aspiration may be necessary to relieve tamponade, and fibrous constrictive pericarditis is a rare late sequel. More than 100 cases of *amebic brain abscess* have been reported. All have been associated with liver abscess and, so far, all patients have died. This condition should not be confused with primary amebic meningoencephalitis caused by free-living amebae (Naegleria and Hartmanella). Hematogenous lesions also occasionally occur in the lung and perhaps elsewhere.

Differential Diagnosis. *Intestinal Amebiasis.* Amebic dysentery may resemble bacillary dysentery, nonspecific ulcerative colitis, intestinal salmonellosis, and, more rarely, heavy infection with intestinal schistosomiasis or *Trichuris trichiura.* Patients with nondysenteric colitis are often suspected of having irritable bowel syndrome, and blood in the stool may be attributed to hemorrhoids. Diverticulitis, carcinoma, and Crohn's disease of the colon may require exclusion by barium enema and sigmoidoscopy. *The finding of* E. histolytica *should not delay the search for another disease, especially because amebic ulceration may be superimposed upon a carcinoma.* Amebomas may mimic neoplastic, infective, and granulomatous conditions of the large bowel, including lymphogranuloma venereum when the rectum is involved. The interpretation of therapeutic trials with tissue amebicides may be difficult, and the delay can make a tumor inoperable.

Hepatic Amebiasis. In the differential diagnosis of hepatic amebiasis, it is necessary to exclude primary and secondary neoplasms of the liver, abscesses caused by migrating Ascaris worms, and purulent subphrenic or intrahepatic disease. Other conditions to be considered are hydatid cyst, the painful or tender hepatomegaly of viral or alcoholic hepatitis, and various pleural or lung lesions of the right lower chest. Radioisotope hepatoscans are particularly useful in the detection and localization of space-occupying lesions.

Laboratory Diagnosis. *Microscopy and Culture.* Diagnosis is based upon the finding of hematophagous trophozoites in stool specimens or fresh material obtained during endoscopy. Although sigmoidoscopic appearances are not pathognomonic, this procedure is valuable for initial assessment and follow-up. The disease spectrum is wide, and the clinical picture depends upon the severity and extent of bowel involvement.

Hematophagous trophozoites should be sought in temporary wet mounts of dysenteric stools, bowel wall scrapings, material from suspected skin lesions, and in the last portion of pus obtained at liver aspiration. If necessary, the material should be diluted with buffered saline (ideally, pH 6.8). In nondysenteric stools, flecks of mucus or pus should be looked for and examined. Trophozoites remain active and recognizable for about 30 minutes above 18° C (see Fig. 2, Ch. 271). If delay will inevitably be longer than this, the specimen should be kept cool as activity is restored, even after several hours at 4° C. If necessary, amebae may be preserved in polyvinyl alcohol and identified after staining with Heidenhain's iron hematoxylin or Gomori's trichrome stain; alternatively, a smear may be fixed in Schaudinn's fixative and stained later. In wet mounts, the definitive identification of nonhematophagous *E. histolytica* is not possible, and even in stained preparations, it is not easy; for this reason, purged stool specimens are of no help unless hematophagous amebae are obtained. On the other hand, *E. histolytica* cysts can be readily recognized in wet mounts, using dilute Lugol's iodine to define nuclear and chromatoid morphology. Cyst concentration techniques using formol ether sedimentation or zinc sulfate flotation give a diagnostic sensitivity of about 70 per cent per specimen compared with 30 per cent without concentration. Examination of concentrates from stools obtained on three separate days is normally sufficient to exclude an intraluminal amebic infection. Cysts in stool may be preserved in 10 per cent formalin, but this reduces the effectiveness of concentration procedures.

Cultivation of *E. histolytica* from fresh stool is not difficult with appropriate media, and is sometimes helpful in confirming the diagnosis. Stained preparations of isolates must be made for accurate identification. If amebic liver pus is to be cultured, the medium should be preconditioned with *Escherichia coli.*

Serologic Tests. Amebic antibodies may be detected by several techniques; in order of decreasing sensitivity, the most used are indirect hemagglutination, indirect fluorescent antibody, complement fixation, and gel diffusion precipitation. Over 90 per cent of patients with liver abscess normally have positive serologic tests, compared with 60 to 80 per cent of those with invasive intestinal disease. Results must be interpreted with caution; as antibody may persist for several years and in endemic areas, some asymptomatic carriers and noninfected persons will have positive reactions. However, negative serologic tests are quite strong evidence against a diagnosis of liver abscess. Serologic tests are also valuable in suspected amebomas and other localized colonic lesions beyond the reach of sigmoidoscopy.

Treatment. *Clinical Pharmacology.* TISSUE AMEBICIDES. Intramuscular emetine hydrochloride and the synthetic compound, dehydroemetine dihydrochloride, are the most rapidly acting tissue amebicides, but both are toxic and cumulative. Emetine is given in a dose of 1 mg per kilogram of body weight daily (maximum, 65 mg daily) for up to ten days. *Serious cardiotoxicity* is suggested by hypotension, dyspnea, precordial pain, tachycardia, and palpitations, but is unusual until at least six doses have been given. Electrocardiographic changes include T wave inversion, prolongation of PR interval, widening of the QRS complex, and arrhythmias. Less serious side effects are weakness, nausea and vomiting, local myositis at the site of injection, and, rarely, a more generalized myositis. A course of treatment should not exceed ten days and should not be repeated without an interval of at least two weeks. Complete bed rest is essential. The drug should not be given to patients with cardiovascular disease, and is not generally recommended for pregnant women or children. Dehydroemetine is excreted more rapidly in the urine than emetine, and a daily dose of 1.25 mg per kilogram of body weight (maximum, 90 mg daily) is necessary; it is probably less cardiotoxic.

Metronidazole (Flagyl) is a potent and safe amebicide that can only be given by mouth; it is rapidly absorbed from the small bowel to reach all tissues. This compound is also useful in the treatment of intraluminal infections, because some is excreted in the bile in modified form and some directly into the colon. A five- or eight-day course of 750 or 800 mg thrice daily is effective in all forms of invasive amebiasis. Paradoxically, higher doses are required to eliminate a bowel infection than to destroy all tissue-invading amebae. Side effects very rarely necessitate stopping treatment; they include dizziness, nausea, abdominal pain, a metallic taste in the mouth, brownish discoloration of the urine, and a confusional state if alcohol is taken. The effectiveness of metronidazole has greatly simplified the chemotherapy of amebiasis, but its action is slightly less rapid than that of emetine, and there is no parenteral preparation.

The main indication for chloroquine is hepatic amebiasis, because the drug is concentrated by, and accumulates within, the liver. The usual regimen consists of 150 mg base twice daily for three weeks. Some toxicity may occur with this regimen, including T wave changes on the electrocardiogram. *Patients being treated for invasive intestinal amebiasis with drugs other than emetine or metronidazole should be given a two-week course of chloroquine to prevent the development of hepatic lesions.*

LUMINAL AMEBICIDES. Tetracycline can be very useful in some patients with invasive intestinal disease; it acts mainly upon bacteria within the lesions, but also alters the bacterial flora of the gut, and has some direct amebicidal activity. Tetracycline is used especially in children, in situations when a parenteral drug is needed, and when metronidazole or emetine is contraindicated or not available. If the drug is used alone, parasitic cure is uncommon, and there may be clinical relapse. For adults, the dosage is 250 or 500 mg every six hours for five to ten days.

Numerous substances have been used to eliminate the bowel infection in symptomless carriers and in patients with invasive disease who are not given metronidazole. The most effective are diiodohydroxyquin (Diodoquin), diloxanide furoate (Furamide), and paromomycin (Humatin). The only adverse effects of Diodoquin are mild diarrhea, pruritus ani, rashes, and rarely iodism. The related compound clioquinol (iodochlorohydroxyquin) has been incriminated as a rare cause of myelo-optic neuropathy.

Management. INTESTINAL AMEBIASIS. Amebic dysentery and nondysenteric colitis should be treated with emetine, metronidazole, or tetracycline, depending upon drug availability and contraindications. If emetine is given, only a three- to six-day course is normally required to control the acute phase of the disease. It should be combined with or followed by metronidazole or tetracycline with chloroquine. Tetracycline should probably be given to all patients with severe dysentery. Amebic peritonitis should be treated medically with gastric suction and intravenous fluid and electrolytes, together with emetine and parenteral tetracycline. If the diagnosis is made at laparotomy, surgical repair is usually not possible because the bowel wall is so friable. Amebomas may be successfully treated with a full course of metronidazole or a ten-day course of emetine. In all forms of intestinal disease, if metronidazole is not used, a luminally active drug must also be given to eradicate the infection.

In countries where transmission rates are low, such as the United States and Western Europe, it is generally recommended that all detected symptomless infections should be treated to prevent later invasive disease or transmission to others. Suitable regimens for adults are Diodoquin, 650 mg thrice daily for 21 days; entamide furoate, 500 mg thrice daily for 10 days; or paromomycin, 500 mg thrice daily for seven days. Alternatively, a full course of metronidazole can be given, particularly if there is suspicion of tissue invasion or concurrent infection with *Giardia intestinalis.*

HEPATIC AMEBIASIS. Liver abscess may be successfully treated with a ten-day course of emetine plus chloroquine for three weeks and a luminal amebicide. Alternatively, a five- or eight-day course of metronidazole may be used; 400 or 500 mg thrice daily will cure the liver lesion, but 750 or 800 mg should be given to eliminate the coexistent gut infection which must be assumed to be present.

Aspiration of the liver is sometimes necessary for therapeutic purposes as well as for diagnosis. The principal indications are as follows: (1) very large lesions and those in the left lobe, especially when there is clinical or radiologic evidence that rupture is imminent; (2) after rupture, if this has occurred into the pleural cavity or pericardium (these also must be aspirated); and (3) poor clinical response after five days of medical treatment. Sometimes the procedure may have to be repeated two or three times. The principal complications are hemorrhage and introduction of bacterial infection; the latter is suggested if the aspirate changes color, becomes very liquid or offensive, or contains gas. Bleeding is less common than might be expected because in liver abscess the right hemidiaphragm rarely moves with respiration.

Occasionally therapeutic drainage by an elective laparotomy is necessary. The indications are as follows: (1) when aspiration is strongly indicated on clinical grounds, but attempts by percutaneous route have failed to locate or adequately drain the lesion; (2) when the lesion continues to refill despite chemotherapy and several percutaneous aspirations; and (3) in the presence of left lobe lesions when not superficial or when the diagnosis is uncertain. An indwelling soft rubber drain is rarely required after surgical drainage, but if used it must be connected to a sterile underwater seal and removed early.

Amebic lung lesions will respond to treatment given for the associated liver lesion. Cutaneous lesions respond to either emetine or metronidazole.

Prognosis. Despite a normally rapid response to treatment, invasive intestinal disease may relapse if the infection is not eliminated. Host factors may be relevant in some persons, including perhaps those with mild nonspecific colitis. If symptoms recur, care must be taken to exclude other colonic disease. There is so far no evidence of drug resistance by any strain of *E. histolytica.* Amebic peritonitis, especially when there are multiple gut perforations, carries a grave prognosis; but permanent sequelae after any form of amebic colitis are rare. Hepatic scanning suggests that filling defects normally disappear within two or four months after treatment of liver abscess. Failure to aspirate large lesions adequately may lead to clinical relapse or much slower resolution. Healing occurs with little scar formation, but if the lesion was secondarily infected, bizarre hepatic calcification may be seen years afterward. Published reports of unselected patients suggest that a 10 per cent mortality is not unusual in liver abscess, but the prognosis can be much better with early diagnosis and adequate treatment.

After successful treatment for amebiasis, there is no reason why a person from a temperate country should not return to the tropics.

Prevention. Chlorination of water supplies does not destroy *E. histolytica* cysts, but proper filtration is effective. A weak solution of iodine is a more potent cysticide than chlorine. Salads and vegetables may be soaked in vinegar or potassium permanganate solution; these are procedures of doubtful benefit, and for some they render the food inedible. A solution of sodium hypochlorite has been found useful. Visitors to the tropics should avoid purchasing food from street vendors and from premises where flies are evident. Fruit that can be skinned should be safe. Boiling water for five minutes kills cysts. Members of domestic staffs involved in food handling should have their stools examined.

Intermittent mass chemotherapy with entamide furoate and metronidazole has been successfully attempted in Mexico and elsewhere where invasive disease is common; it may also be useful in mental institutions in temperate countries. *Personal chemoprophylaxis* by visitors to the tropics is not recommended, and it is better for such persons to avoid eating uncooked foods and to have their stools examined on return.

Amoebiasis: Report of a WHO Expert Committee. WHO Technical Report Series No. 421, 1–52, 1969.

Biagi, F. F., and Beltran, H. F.: The challenge of amoebiasis: Understanding pathogenic mechanisms. Int. Rev. Trop. Med., 3:219, 1969.

Elsdon-Dew, R.: The epidemiology of amoebiasis. Adv. Parasitol., 6:1, 1968.

Powell, S. J.: New developments in the therapy of amoebiasis. Gut, 11:967, 1970.

Wilmot, A. J. Clinical Amoebiasis. Oxford, Blackwell, 1962.

OTHER PROTOZOAN DISEASES

280. INTRODUCTION

Philip D. Marsden

Apart from *Entamoeba histolytica,* at least four genera and seven species of amebae have been established as living in man. Common stool amebae are *Entamoeba coli, Endolimax nana,* and *Iodamoeba buetschlii.* They are nonpathogenic, but such protozoa have a double importance. First, they must be distinguished from the pathogenic *E. histolytica* by the available clear morphologic criteria. Second, they provide an index of fecal contamination. If any stool protozoan is encountered, it is wise to examine a further specimen, for, because of the variable appearance of protozoa in the stool, the second specimen may reveal a pathogen. *Dientamoeba fragilis* is a delicate ameba without a cystic stage. Some clinicians believe it is a cause of mild diarrhea, but the evidence is not convincing.

Several flagellates are also found in the stool, among them the nonpathogenic *Trichomonas hominis* and *Chilomastix mesnili.* Information on the differential diagnosis of these intestinal protozoa can be found in texts of parasitology. Here we will consider briefly the clinical significance of five pathogenic protozoa: *Giardia lamblia* and *Trichomonas vaginalis* (both flagellates), *Balantidium coli* (a ciliate), *Isospora belli* (a coccidium), and *Naegleria gruberi* (an ameba).

Knight, R., Schultz, M. G., Hoskins, D. W., and Marsden, P. D.: Intestinal Parasites. Gut, 14:145, 1973.

281. GIARDIASIS

Philip D. Marsden

Abdominal pain, distention and flatulence, and recurrent diarrhea may be associated with *Giardia lamblia* infection, especially in children. Inhabiting the duodenum and upper jejunum, the parasite is a pear-shaped flagellate, anteriorly broad and rounded and tapering to a point not unlike a tennis racket. It is convex dorsally with a ventral attachment disc. There are sets of identical structures on either side of the median line. When stained, there are two nuclei, four pairs of flagella, and a parabasal body. In fresh stool this trophozoite is actively motile with an irregular characteristic progression. It reproduces by longitudinal binary fission.

The thick-walled cysts are 10 to 14 μ by 6 to 10 μ and have two to four nuclei with curved rods or axostyles. In some infections several million cysts per gram of feces may be passed. Only in patients with very rapid bowel transit times do trophozoites appear in the stool, although they may be found in duodenal aspirate. Cultivation of Giardia in vitro has recently been achieved.

The infective cysts are transmitted in food and drink, and the infection is cosmopolitan. The great majority of patients are asymptomatic, but there is no doubt that heavy infections are associated with symptoms. Diarrhea is the most common symptom, and the stools are pale and contain mucus. Giardia is in fact a cause of steatorrhea, and patients may have abnormal fat balances and D-xylose tests which return to normal after successful treatment. The hypothesis that this malabsorption is the result of a mechanical barrier produced by large numbers of parasites attached to the microvillar surface is attractive, but effects on digestive enzyme activity and microvillar function are possible. Villous flattening with inflammatory infiltration has been demonstrated in one study.

Diarrhea may alternate with constipation, and apart from these symptoms epigastric pain resembling a peptic ulcer may be a disabling symptom. Anorexia, meat intolerance, and loss of weight may occur. Although Giardia may be found in the gallbladder, the evidence that it is responsible for cholecystitis is unsatisfactory. Giardiasis must be distinguished from other causes of malabsorption and peptic ulcer.

Giardiasis, symptomatic or not, should always be treated. Two drugs are equally effective. Quinacrine hydrochloride (Atabrine), in a dose of 100 mg three times a day after food for seven days, is an established therapy, but the drug has a bitter taste, and nausea and vomiting may result. It may also stain the skin yellow, but psychosis does not occur at this dosage level. Metronidazole (Flagyl), 200 mg three times a day after food for ten days, is equally effective with few side effects. Both drugs have about an 80 per cent cure rate, and in the event of failure of one drug the other can be tried. The follow-up procedures are similar to those in amebiasis.

Hoskins, L. C., Winawer, S. J., Broitman, S. A., Gottlieb, L. S., and Zamchek, N.: Clinical giardiasis and intestinal malabsorption. Gastroenterology, 53:265, 1967.

Yardley, J. H., Takano, J., and Hendrix, T. B.: Epithelial and other mucosal lesions of the jejunum in giardiasis: Jejunal biopsy studies. Bull. Hopkins Hosp., 115:389, 1964.

282.   TRICHOMONIASIS

Thomas C. Jones

Another group of lumen-dwelling protozoa with flagella are the trichomonads. Three species of the genus Trichomonas frequently inhabit man: *Trichomonas hominis, Trichomonas tenax,* and *Trichomonas vaginalis.* Only the last-named is considered pathogenic and is a common cause of infection and disease in the genital tract.

T. vaginalis is a pear-shaped, colorless, single-celled organism 10 to 20 μ in size with two pairs of anterior flagella, an eccentrically located nucleus, an undulating membrane, and a structure termed an axostyle leading to a posterior flagellum. The flagella and undulating membrane move the organisms rapidly through exudative material in a jerky, rotating manner. Vaginal pH may determine its survival since it loses activity at a pH below 5.

The organism can persist in endocervical or urethral glands without causing symptoms, or under appropriate conditions it can induce inflammation on the mucosal surfaces of the vagina, urethra, urinary bladder, or prostate. The inflamed area takes on a characteristic "strawberry-like" appearance owing to vasodilation. Exudate filled with polymorphonuclear leukocytes and mononuclear cells covers the surface. Phagocytosis of the protozoan has been recorded. Trichomonas infection can make interpretation of cervical Papanicolaou smears more difficult for the cytologist. There is no evidence that chronic *T. vaginalis* infection contributes to carcinoma of the cervix.

Patients usually present with symptoms of vaginal itching or burning, and a yellow blood-tinged discharge. These symptoms are more commonly associated with menstruation. If the urethra is involved, symptoms of dysuria and a mild urethral discharge are seen. Approximately 20 per cent of females with documented Trichomonas infection are asymptomatic.

Diagnosis is made by observing the motile organisms in fresh specimens of vaginal discharge. A drop of warm saline is mixed with the exudate and examined immediately, using low-power microscopy. *T. vaginalis* can also be cultured. Metronidazole is effective therapy when given in doses of 250 mg three times daily for ten days. Females should also receive 500 mg vaginal suppositories for ten days. Both male and female partners should be treated at the same time. Failure to do this results in reinfection, so-called "Ping-Pong" vaginitis. The infection is usually acquired by sexual intercourse. It can be transmitted to infants at the time of birth, and may survive on nonmucosal surfaces for a sufficient time to be spread in places such as mental institutions where personal hygiene is poor.

283.   BALANTIDIASIS

Philip D. Marsden

Balantidium coli is the largest protozoan of man, measuring 50 to 70 μ in length by 30 to 60 μ in width. It infects the colon of man and may produce diarrhea and dysentery. When viewed under the low power of the microscope in a saline smear of stool, the grayish-green trophozoite can be seen gliding across the field powered by spiral longitudinal rows of cilia. There is a large oral macronucleus and a smaller micronucleus. A cytostome or mouth ingests organic matter that circulates as food vacuoles. Erythrophagocytosis has been observed. Reproduction is by binary fission or conjugation. A resistant cyst form is passed in formed stools, and this is the infective form. *Cosmopolitan in distribution, it is a rare infection of man although common in pigs.* When man and pig share shelter, human infections are common, and this accounts for the high incidence of human infection in parts of New Guinea (20 per cent) and Peru. *B. coli* of man can be transmitted to monkeys, cats, guinea pigs, and rats, but the importance of these animals as reservoirs is minor. Handling pigs in slaughterhouses may be an occupational risk.

This ciliate can be a tissue invader, and similar factors to those mentioned for *E. histolytica* may well determine this behavior. Proteolytic secretions produce necrosis and ulceration of the mucosa. Columns of balantidia may be seen lying in the submucosa. Secondary infection with bacteria results in an accompanying inflammatory reaction. The ulcers are often quite large and deep, with a broad, indurated base. A liver abscess with *B. coli* in situ has been described, and balantidia have been found in the lung and heart in isolated cases.

Less than one fifth of infected persons have symptoms. Severe infections are associated with diarrhea and the passage of blood and mucus in the stools. Constitutional symptoms of fever, nausea, vomiting, and asthenia are described. Examination of fresh stools reveals the trophozoite or cyst. Culture of the stools on media similar to those used for amebiasis may reveal an infection when conventional microscopy has failed; in symptomatic patients this is usually not necessary. Balantidiasis must be differentiated from amebic dysentery and ulcerative colitis. Although arsenical preparations have been used in the past, oxytetracycline is probably the drug of choice in an adult dose of 500 mg three times a day for ten days. Paromomycin (Humatin) is also effective. Spontaneous recovery has been noted. The infection may be fatal if bowel perforation occurs.

Arean, V. M., and Koppisch, E.: Balantidiasis: A review and report of cases. Am. J. Path., 32:1089, 1956.
Van der Hoeven, J. A., and Rijpstra, A. C.: Intestinal parasites in the central mountain district of Netherlands, New Guinea. An important focus of *Balantidium coli.* Docum. Med. Geog. Trop., 9:225, 1957.

284. COCCIDIOSIS
Philip D. Marsden

Coccidia have alternate asexual and sexual generation in the same host, and the nature of the cycle is not dissimilar to plasmodia in the forms produced. There is probably only one human species, *Isospora belli,* which parasitizes the small intestinal epithelium. The cycles of schizogony and gametogony have now been described in small bowel mucosal biopsies from symptomatic patients, and it has been suggested that this organism causes a malabsorption syndrome. Until recently the case for the pathogenicity of Isospora rested mainly on laboratory infections that resulted in diarrhea lasting about three weeks, accompanied by the passage of the diagnostic form of the parasite in the stool. This is a thick-walled oocyst 25 to 35 μ × 12 to 16 μ in size. Both ends are rounded, and one is contracted to form a neck. This stage is the zygote. Further development in two to four days results in the formation of two sporoblasts, which mature into oval sporocysts. Each sporocyst ultimately contains four sporozoites. These oocysts are very resistant to physical and chemical insult and will readily sporulate in potassium dichromate. Many instances of spurious parasitemia have been reported in man when oocysts of various animals and fish coccidia have passed unchanged through the bowel to appear in the stool and pose a diagnostic problem. The mild persistent diarrhea during the active phase of the infection is usually accompanied only by nausea and abdominal discomfort. In the recent report cited below, the patients had severe diarrhea and steatorrhea unresponsive to therapy, and three died.

Brandborg, L. L., Goldberg, S. B., and Breidenbach, W. C.: Human coccidiosis—a possible cause of malabsorption. The life cycle in small bowel mucosal biopsies as a diagnostic feature. N. Engl. J. Med., 283:1306, 1970.
Smitskamp, H., and Oey-Muller, E.: Geographical distribution and clinical significance of human coccidiosis. Trop. Geogr. Med., 18:133, 1966.

285. PRIMARY AMEBIC MENINGOENCEPHALITIS
Philip D. Marsden

Recently it has been realized that *free-living amebae* are capable of producing severe brain lesions in man. Several species are implicated, but *Naegleria gruberi* has been the species usually identified when cultures are made. They can be cultured on plain agar plates with *Aerobacter aerogenes* as a nutrient source, but we need to know more about their cultural requirements. The Naegleria amebae possess the capacity to transform in culture from ameboid trophozoites to highly mobile flagellates. Another organism, *Acanthamoeba castellani,* was among the first to be recognized. An ameba 6 to 8 μ long, with foamy cytoplasm, a nucleus of 2 μ, and a 1 μ darkly staining central karyosome, it is present as a commensal in human mouths and throats and was

shown to be pathogenic for mice and monkeys before the first cases were reported in man. An initial report from Australia in 1965 described a rapidly progressive meningitis that proved fatal. Early symptoms in the first two days or so are fever, severe frontal headache, defects of olfactory sense, lethargy, sore throat, and obstructed nostrils. By the third day vomiting and impaired consciousness may be present, progressing to deepening coma and death on the fourth day. At postmortem, destruction of the inferior surface of the frontal lobes and olfactory bulbs was seen, associated with a purulent exudate. Histologic examination revealed columns of amebae extending into the brain substance, especially via the perivascular spaces.

This clinical entity has now been reported from several parts of the United States (Florida, Virginia, Texas), Great Britain, and Czechoslovakia. It is usually found in children and young people, and is invariably fatal. It appears to be acquired by swimming, diving, or water skiing in lakes known to contain large numbers of free-living amebae. Pressure changes under water probably force the amebae through the cribriform plate. Naegleria has repeatedly been found in the cerebrospinal fluid of man. The CSF also shows an increased protein level, decreased sugar, neutrophils, and red cells, but is bacteriologically sterile. Most of the patients to date have died, usually because the diagnosis has been missed.

Emetine, arsenicals, sulfonamides, tetracyclines, and metronidazole have been used without success. Amphotericin B therapy has resulted in recovery of a patient in whom Naegleria organisms were recovered from the CSF, and in vitro studies show that therapeutic concentrations are amebicidal. In one recent fatal case *Naegleria gruberi* was recovered from the lungs, liver, spleen, and heart blood, as well as from the central nervous system. Since such free-living amebae are ubiquitous, doubtless reports from other countries will appear in the future.

Culbertson, C. G.: Pathogenic acanthamoeba (Hartmannella). Am. J. Clin. Path., 35:195, 1961.
Duma, R. J., Rosenblum, W. I., McGehee, R. F., Jones, M. M., and Clifford, N. E.: Primary amoebic meningoencephalitis caused by Naegleria. Ann. Intern. Med., 74:923, 1971.
Fowler, M., and Carter, R. F.: Acute pyogenic meningitis probably due to Acanthamoeba sp.: A preliminary report. Br. Med. J., 2:740, 1965.

286. TOXOPLASMOSIS
Thomas C. Jones

General Considerations. Toxoplasmosis is a common infection of mammals and birds which occasionally results in protean disease. It is caused by the protozoan *Toxoplasma gondii.* In man, tissue parasitism during the proliferative phase may occur without signs or symptoms; it may lead to a transient illness characterized by lymphadenopathy, fever, and fatigue; or it may cause extensive damage to the brain, eyes, muscle, heart, liver, or lungs. Severe manifestations of the disease most commonly occur when a fetus is infected (congenital toxoplasmosis) or when infection occurs in patients with impaired immunity. Chronic infection may lead to a recurrent inflammatory process usually recognized by progressive ocular damage. When members of the cat family ingest Toxoplasma organisms, infection of epithelial cells in the intestinal tract results in production of oocysts which, when excreted, provide an important means by which the infection is transmitted in nature. Viable organisms within cysts in muscles and brain of infected animals provide a continued source of infection to carnivores.

History. In 1907 *Toxoplasma gondii* was recognized as a distinct protozoan and named by Nicolle and Manceaux. The first human case of congenital infection was recorded in 1923 by Janku in Prague, and in 1938 Wolf, Cowen, and Paige described the first cases from which the parasite was isolated. Toxoplasmosis in adults was first described by Pinkerton and Henderson in 1941. Eye damage caused by Toxoplasma in adults was first suggested by Frenkel and confirmed after observations made by Wilder in 1952. The present realization that 500 million humans are infected with the protozoan evolved from the extensive epidemiologic studies of Feldman, Desmonts, Thalhammer, and Jacobs, and from the recognition by Siim and others of the varied, often mild clinical patterns of acquired infection. In 1967, Hutchison first suggested that the cat played a role in the life cycle of *Toxoplasma gondii*, a cycle which was subsequently delineated in 1970.

The Protozoan. When mammals or birds ingest either infective oocysts or cysts in muscle or brain of other animals, an *intermediate* or asexual cycle of Toxoplasma infection is initiated. This consists of an obligate intracellular *proliferative* stage and a *cyst* stage. In the proliferative stage, *trophozoites,* which are ovoid or arc shaped, 3 to 4 μ in diameter, 6 to 7 μ in length, enter host cells by endocytosis and then divide by endodyogeny; two daughter cells are formed within each parent. Division continues until the host cell ruptures, releasing organisms which in turn infect adjacent cells. As the host develops immunity, parasite proliferation gradually slows, and a firm wall (cyst) forms around the organism allowing the Toxoplasma to persist for years in this cyst stage.

When *cats* ingest cysts or oocysts of *Toxoplasma gondii*, however, an addition process can occur, i.e., the *definitive* or sexual cycle initiated within the cat's intestinal epithelial cells. Parasites released from cysts or oocysts penetrate the epithelial cells where they first enter a proliferative stage and then mature by gametogony into *macro-* or *microgametocytes*. A *zygote*, formed by union of the gametocytes, matures in one to four days into an infective *oocyst*. The mature infective oocyst is oblong, 9 μ by 13 μ, and it contains two *sporocysts*, each of which contains four *sporozoites*. Oocysts are excreted by the cat for one to three weeks, beginning three to five days after ingestion of the Toxoplasma-containing tissue. Cats generally also acquire a systemic infection (intermediate cycle) at the time of first exposure to Toxoplasma, just as other mammals do. They occasionally repeat the sexual cycle after reinfection, although the period of oocyst shedding may be shorter.

Epidemiology. *Toxoplasma gondii* infects almost all mammals and birds. The usual life cycle in nature is among cats, small mammals, and birds, but man has intruded on this cycle with his taste for uncooked meats and his close association with cats. In some areas, such as Tahiti and the Easter Islands, the prevalence of Toxoplasma infection is near 100 per cent. In most parts of the world the prevalence ranges between 20 and 60 per cent of the population. Only in very dry areas, such as Arizona, and in very cold areas, such as northern Alaska, are low prevalence rates found. A few small islands in the Pacific, where cats have never been introduced, have remained free of toxoplasmosis.

The means by which the parasite is transmitted varies from one area to another: in one, oocyst ingestion seems more likely; in another, cyst ingestion. For instance, the very high rates in certain parts of the tropics are believed to be due to close contact with cat feces. In these areas infection is often acquired in childhood. The oocysts are resistant to drying and to a wide range of temperatures, and may remain infectious in moist soil for a year. Ingestion of oocysts is made more likely by the demonstration that cockroaches and flies can disseminate them to various exposed foods. In the United States the population appears to acquire the infection more commonly by ingesting uncooked infected meat. The infection is acquired at a rate of 1 per cent of the population per year of life from age 15 to age 50. Mutton and pork have been found to be more frequently infected than beef. Rarely, transmission of infection has followed accidental inoculation of trophozoites by laboratory workers, organ transplantation, and leukocyte transfusion from immunosuppressed donors. Blood transfusions from healthy donors have not been shown to be a means of transmitting toxoplasmosis.

Transplacental Transmission. Transplacental transmission in humans occurs only at the time of parasitemia, during the acute infection. The frequency of this secondary form of transmission therefore follows the frequency of acquisition of infection during child-bearing years. In the United States and Europe 0.5 to 1.0 per cent of women have been demonstrated to have rising or very high antibody titers to Toxoplasma during pregnancy. Forty per cent of these adult infections are transmitted to the fetus. This may result in abortion or stillbirth, or an infant with clinical signs of toxoplasmosis (one third to one half of infected infants). Alternatively, infected infants may be completely asymptomatic but may show an antibody response to Toxoplasma antigens as evidence of transplacental infection. These infected asymptomatic infants are believed to make up a population which later in life may show signs of recurrent retinochoroiditis. There is no significant relationship in humans between chronic Toxoplasma infection and either recurrent abortion or prematurity.

Pathogenesis and Immunity. Multiplication of Toxoplasma organisms within cells causes little obvious disturbance to host cell function until the dividing parasites cause the cell to rupture. Adjacent cells are then infected, resulting in progressive tissue necrosis and an acute inflammatory response (edema and infiltration with mononuclear cells and a few polymorphonuclear leukocytes). Organisms are disseminated hematogenously throughout the body. New sites of necrosis and inflammation are initiated, particularly in myocardium and skeletal muscle. In those patients who develop severe generalized toxoplasmosis significant encephalitis, myocarditis, myositis, pneumonitis, hepatitis, and skin rash have been documented.

Generalized lymph node enlargement, along with other signs of systemic infection such as fever and malaise, develops one to two weeks after ingestion of infectious tissue. These lymph nodes show histocytic hyperplasia rather than follicular hyperplasia, giving the hematoxylin-eosin stained section a rather typical appearance of containing predominantly eosin reactive cells. The architecture of the lymph node is preserved. Necrosis and giant cells are not seen, and only rarely can groups of Toxoplasma organisms be identified. Occasionally, even in relatively mild infections, myositis or myocarditis can be demonstrated.

Associated with the development of marked lymphoreticular activity, both humoral and cellular immunity can be demonstrated. Antibodies against various Toxoplasma antigens can be demonstrated in the peripheral blood. Later Toxoplasma antigen induces lymphocyte proliferation and lymphokine production, and mononuclear cells no longer support division of intracellular Toxoplasma. The acute infection resolves, but Toxoplasma organisms remain viable within cysts in the infected tissue for the lifetime of the host.

Congenital Infection; Immunologic Deficiency. Although the healthy adult usually deals effectively with the Toxoplasma infection, the immunologically deficient patient does not. The best example of this is the pathologic changes of congenital toxoplasmosis. The infected placenta may show areas of necrosis, inflammatory cells, and parasites, more frequently on the fetal than on the maternal side of the placenta. The fetal brain shows necrosis, glial cell proliferation, and perivascular lymphocytic infiltration. Toxoplasma can be identified in these lesions. High ventricular fluid protein, aqueductal obstruction, and hydrocephalus are often seen. If the infant survives several months, calcification of these areas occurs. Necrotic lesions in the retina are also seen. Organisms can be isolated from numerous organs of the body, but extensive inflammation is most often identified as pneumonitis, myocarditis, hepatitis, and splenitis.

About half the infections which occur in utero are caused by a sufficiently low number of organisms or are of low enough virulence that infection is manifest only by the appearance of humoral and cellular immune responses. Cysts develop and persist in brain, retina, and cardiac and skeletal muscle. Rupture of these cysts, many years later, can lead to transient episodes of inflammatory response and scarring. These inflammatory lesions are usually well localized, but in the retina they lead to significant organ impairment. The enucleated eye may show areas of necrosis in the retina often associated with proliferating Toxoplasma organisms, as well as a granulomatous inflammation of the choroid and sclera. The eye damage is the result of proliferation of organisms released at the time of cyst rupture which invade other cells, combined with damage caused by the vigorous hypersensitivity reaction.

In the patients with abnormal or suppressed immune responses, primary infection or cyst rupture may lead to symptomatic myositis, myocarditis, retinochoroiditis, or encephalitis.

Clinical Manifestations. Manifestations of toxoplasmosis can be divided into four clinical patterns: acquired disease in otherwise healthy individuals, congenital infection, retinochoroiditis, and disease in the altered host.

Acquired Toxoplasmosis. Patients with acquired toxoplasmosis usually present with lymphadenopathy (90 per cent), fever (40 per cent), or malaise (40 per cent). Lymph node enlargement may be the only sign, and since cervical lymph node enlargement is particularly common, the patient may seek medical attention only because of concern about a neck mass. The nodes are usually nontender and rubbery in consistency. Generalized lymphadenopathy occurs in over half the cases, and transient splenomegaly has been recorded in approximately one third. The fever is usually low grade, but occasionally it may be high and of prolonged duration. Fatigue is often rather marked and may be associated with generalized muscle discomfort. Less commonly recorded signs or symptoms have included sore throat, headache, and a maculopapular rash. The pharynx is usually hyperemic; exudative pharyngitis is not seen. Specific organ involvement in this form of the disease includes

myocardium (rarely pericardium), skeletal muscle, rarely liver, skin, and brain. When such organ involvement occurs, the abnormalities in organ function may dominate the clinical picture. Retinochoroiditis in association with the acute acquired disease is very unusual.

The course of the illness is quite variable. Occasionally fever, malaise, and specific organ involvement are marked and the illness prolonged. More commonly, fever lasts only a few days or weeks, although fatigue and lymphadenopathy may persist for several months. Lymph nodes will occasionally fluctuate in size during the recovery period.

Laboratory tests usually reveal a normal total leukocyte count with a slight monocytosis or lymphocytosis. Atypical lymphocytes may be described, but they are usually not present in large numbers. Hematocrit and hemoglobin are usually normal; however, a Coombs-negative hemolytic anemia has occasionally been reported. Serum transaminases are usually normal, but early in the illness they may be slightly elevated (less than 100 U). The Paul-Bunnell test for heterophil antibodies is negative. The electrocardiogram may show ST and T wave abnormalities in cases in which myocarditis is prominent. The chest film is usually normal; hilar adenopathy is very rare. Lymph node biopsy shows histocytic hyperplasia. Antibodies against Toxoplasma antigens are present in high or rising titers.

Congenital Toxoplasmosis. Cases of congenital toxoplasmosis may be manifested as microophthalmia, microcephaly, seizures, retardation, hepatosplenomegaly, pneumonitis, rash, and fever. If aqueduct of Sylvius obstruction has occurred, hydrocephalus will be prominent. Occasionally, signs may not be obvious at birth, but they may progress during the first months of life. Cerebral calcification may be seen after several months. The infant will show progressive signs of failure to thrive, followed by death. Cases of congenital toxoplasmosis may be mild, demonstrating only mental retardation, a seizure disorder, or retinochoroiditis. Laboratory tests reflect the severity of the specific organ involved. Toxoplasma antibody titers are elevated and will show a persistent or rising titer as maternal antibody disappears.

Toxoplasmic Retinochoroiditis. This form of toxoplasmosis is almost always a late sequela of otherwise asymptomatic congenital infection. Symptoms are usually first noted in the second or third decade of life. Patients have recurrent episodes of ocular pain and decreased vision associated with progressive loss of vision. The lesion is retinal, with an associated posterior uveitis. Toxoplasma infection probably does not cause an isolated anterior uveitis. Systemic signs of Toxoplasma infection are not usually present. Toxoplasma antibody titers are frequently low and tend not to change.

Toxoplasmosis in the Altered Host. Toxoplasmosis may present as a disseminated disease in patients with neoplasms of the lymphatic system, particularly Hodgkin's disease, or in patients being treated with immunosuppressive drugs. The clinical manifestations of the systemic disease are variable. Fever, encephalitis, myositis, hepatosplenomegaly, or myocarditis may occur. Pneumonitis has been described rarely in this setting. Lymphadenopathy may or may not be present. The primary difficulty is in separating the numerous other causes of these signs or symptoms from those caused by toxoplasmosis. At present one clinical pattern seems dominant, that is, progressive signs of encephalitis (confusion, headache, coma). In a patient with altered cellular immunity, these signs should lead to a consideration of and probably treatment for toxoplasmosis. If untreated, this illness is almost always progressive and fatal. Toxoplasma antibody titers are usually elevated.

Diagnosis. The diagnosis of toxoplasmosis rests on the presence of changing or elevated titers of antitoxoplasma antibodies and on isolation of the parasite from infected tissue. The antibody tests available include the indirect fluorescent antibody test (IFA), the Sabin-Feldman dye test, and a complement fixation test. The IFA and dye test show high antitoxoplasma antibody titers usually from the time of earliest symptoms (one to two weeks after infection). A titer of 1:1024 or higher, or evidence of a rising titer, is suggestive of active infection. The high titers will decrease during the subsequent months and after two to four years reach low levels (1:16 to 1:256) for the lifetime of the individual. There has been no cross-reactivity between dye test antibodies and other antigens; thus the test is very specific. An indirect hemagglutination test is also available. However, many feel that the rise in antibody titer is too slow to be as helpful clinically as the Sabin-Feldman dye test.

The complement fixation test becomes positive later than the dye test, three to six weeks after infection, when symptoms are often present. Thus one is often able to see a changing titer over several weeks by using this test in a patient whose dye test is elevated. A significant complement fixation test is a titer of 1:8 or greater or a fourfold increase in titer. This test usually becomes negative within a few years after infection. In conjunction with the dye test it can help separate those patients with persistently high dye test antibody titers from those with recent infection. This may help in deciding if symptoms which began weeks or a few months previously are due to recent Toxoplasma infection or, in an asymptomatic pregnant female, whether the infection was recently acquired. Treatment may transiently decrease complement fixing antibody titers.

In congenital toxoplasmosis the contribution of transferred maternal IgG antitoxoplasma antibody must be excluded. This is done by performing several tests over the first few months; if positive titers are due to maternal antibody, the titer will fall about 50 per cent per month over four to six months. If the infant had been infected, the titer would remain stable, dip transiently, or increase. One may also test for IgM antitoxoplasma antibodies by using an IFA test to determine if the observed antibodies are fetal or maternal in origin. Since IgM antibodies do not cross the placenta, their presence indicates fetal antibody synthesis. In some infected infants this test may be falsely negative.

The diagnosis of Toxoplasma retinochoroiditis by serologic means is difficult. Since the infection is chronic, dye test and IFA titers are usually positive in low titer, and complement fixing antibodies are absent. The diagnosis of toxoplasmic retinochoroiditis may be suggested by finding higher antibody titers in the anterior chamber fluid than in the serum, or by isolating the organism at the time of enucleation. A negative dye test or IFA excludes Toxoplasma as the cause of retinochoroiditis.

The use of serologic tests in the immunodeficient patient to determine "activity" of the infection has also been difficult. Some patients with repeatedly low antibody titers have demonstrated a sudden rise in titer associated with a moribund state and death; however, at autopsy, disseminated toxoplasmosis could not be implicated as a factor contributing to death. Investigators are now examining whether changes in lymphocyte response to Toxoplasma antigen may be of more predictive value. At present, elevated antibody titers, plus progressive encephalitis, should be sufficient to warrant antitoxoplasma therapy in an immunodeficient patient. Evidence of the organism on biopsy of organs such as muscle, kidney, lung, and liver should also be an indication for therapy in these patients.

The diagnosis of toxoplasmosis can be substantiated by isolation of the organism. Biopsy material (particularly lymph node or muscle), tissue at the time of autopsy, or blood, sputum, or cerebrospinal fluid can be inoculated intraperitoneally into Toxoplasma-free laboratory animals. Smears of peritoneal fluid can be made at seven to ten days, stained by Giemsa technique, and examined for the protozoa. If the smear is negative, the peritoneal fluid should be injected intraperitoneally into another animal. If the infected animals survive for three weeks, they are sacrificed and their brains examined for Toxoplasma cysts and their serum for Toxoplasma antibody. Isolation of Toxoplasma organisms from human tissue should be correlated with histopathology of the tissue and antibody titers.

The differential diagnosis in a patient with lymphadenopathy and fever usually rests between lymphoma and infectious mononucleosis, although numerous infections, such as tuberculosis, brucellosis, tularemia, cat scratch disease, and certain systemic viral and rickettsial illnesses, must be considered. Toxoplasmosis can be distinguished from infectious mononucleosis by absence of marked atypical lymphocytosis and heterophil antibodies and normal or nearly normal hepatic transaminases; and from lymphoma by absence of anemia, hilar adenopathy, and a lymph node biopsy which shows histocytic hyperplasia rather than neoplastic cells. The other numerous causes of lymphadenopathy and fever must be excluded by appropriate serologic and skin tests, biopsy, and cultures.

Congenital toxoplasmosis must be distinguished from cytomegalovirus infection. Microcephaly is more common in cytomegalovirus infection than in toxoplasmosis. Ventricular fluid protein content is often higher in toxoplasmosis than in cytomegalovirus infection. Bacterial and fungal meningoencephalitis must be excluded by appropriate cultures. Viral encephalitis, particularly the rubella syndrome, must be considered. Congenital malformations are unusual in toxoplasmosis.

Toxoplasmic retinochoroiditis must be distinguished from cytomegalovirus, herpes, tuberculosis, histoplasmosis, and sarcoidosis by appearance of the retinal lesion and appropriate serologic and skin tests.

Treatment. A combination of pyrimethamine (Daraprim) and sulfadiazine has been shown to be effective in controlling Toxoplasma during the proliferative stage. There is no known therapy for eradicating organisms in the cyst stage. Pyrimethamine is given orally, 75 mg the first day, followed by 25 mg per day for one month. Infants are given 1 mg per kilogram per day for the first three days, and then 0.5 mg per kilogram per day thereafter. An intramuscular preparation is not commercially available. Sulfadiazine is given orally, 4 grams daily in divided doses for one month. Infants can be given 100 mg per kilogram per day. Recently, sulfalene and trimethoprim, a similar drug combination, has been found effective. Other sulfonamides such as the triple sulfonamides can be substituted for sulfadiazine; however, sulfisoxazole (Gantrisin) has been found ineffective. Other drugs such as spiramycin, tetracyclines, and sulfones are less effective than the aforementioned drugs. Since pyrimethamine and sulfonamide inhibit folate synthesis, folinic acid (leucovorin), 6 mg per day, should be used in conjunction with the aforementioned therapy to prevent potential bone marrow toxicity. Platelet counts and white blood cell counts should be performed twice weekly during therapy.

Study of the effectiveness of these drugs in acquired human toxoplasmosis has been limited by the marked variability and spontaneous improvement without therapy. However, in some cases there has been evidence that this treatment shortens the period of fever and malaise, although lymphadenopathy may persist. It has therefore been recommended that only patients with fever, myalgias, or malaise be considered for therapy. Asymptomatic adults should be considered for treatment (1) after accidental laboratory infection and (2) when a pregnant female demonstrates serologic evidence of recent infection, only after appropriate consultations and considerations have led to a rejection of therapeutic abortion and have weighed potential fetal damage from the drugs. There is no adequate evidence to recommend treating dye-test-positive women who wish to become pregnant or who abort habitually, or in treating asymptomatic women after delivery of a congenitally damaged infant.

Congenital toxoplasmosis should be treated whether asymptomatic or symptomatic, because the proliferative stage may continue for several months before adequate cellular immunity has developed to control the infection. Treatment will not be effective when given late in the course of the disease or when severe central nervous system damage has already occurred.

In toxoplasmic retinochoroiditis, the primary therapy should be directed at controlling the hypersensitivity response with corticosteroids. Pyrimethamine and sulfadiazine should be used in conjunction with this therapy to prevent dissemination of infection and to limit local damage caused by proliferating organisms.

In patients with altered immunity and toxoplasmosis, good therapeutic response to this drug combination has been recorded. Fever has been controlled, and evidence of progressive encephalitis has been reversed. In these patients long-term therapy has to be considered because appropriate immunologic responses do not occur, making relapse of the disease likely.

Prevention. Toxoplasmosis is commonly transmitted by consumption of undercooked meat or Toxoplasma oocysts. Thus, dye-test-negative pregnant women or patients with depressed cellular immunity should avoid both these sources of infection. Meat should be cooked at a temperature in excess of 60° C (140° F) for at least 15 minutes. Susceptible individuals should avoid soil or sand boxes where cats may defecate, because oocysts may survive in these places for months. If cats are kept in the house, they should not be fed raw meat or allowed access to wild rodents or birds.

Since infection-immunity in human adults prevents congenital toxoplasmosis, it is reasonable that an appropriate vaccine might be developed in the future. Laboratory workers should take precautions to avoid accidental needle puncture. Baseline antibody testing should be done in patients who are to receive immunosuppressive drugs, who have lymphatic malignancies, or who are to act as organ or leukocyte donors.

Beverley, J. K. A.: Toxoplasmosis. Br. Med. J., 2:475, 1973.
Carey, R. M., Kimball, A. C., Armstrong, D., and Lieberman, P. H.: Toxoplasmosis: Clinical experiences in a cancer hospital. Am. J. Med., 54:30, 1973.
Feldman, H. A.: Toxoplasmosis. N. Engl. J. Med., 279:1370, 1431, 1968.
Frenkel, J. K.: Toxoplasma in and around us. Bio. Science, 26:343, 1973.
Frenkel, J. K.: Toxoplasmosis. In Marcial-Rojas, R. D. (ed.): Pathology of Protozoal and Helminthic Diseases. Baltimore, Williams & Wilkins Company, 1971, p. 254.
Kean, B. H.: Clinical toxoplasmosis—50 years. Trans. R. Soc. Trop. Med. Hyg., 66:549, 1972.
Remington, J. S.: Toxoplasmosis—recent developments. Ann. Rev. Med., 21:201, 1970.
Wallace, G. D.: The role of the cat in the natural history of *Toxoplasma gondii*. Am. J. Trop. Med. Hyg., 22:313, 1973.

Section Two.   HELMINTHIC DISEASES

287.   INTRODUCTION

Philip D. Marsden

Compared to protozoans, helminths are very large organisms with a complex cellular structure. As they feed on host tissue, their metabolism results in various protein secretions and excretions; and because they themselves largely consist of complex protein, it is not surprising that invasion of the body by worms is frequently associated with an eosinophilic response. Thus, in the invasive stage of schistosomes, hookworm, ascaris, and similar parasites, an eosinophilia is usual. Yet when these worms have matured and settled at their site of election, eosinophilia often is not found. It might be argued in the case of intestinal nematodes that this is because they are in the gut and in a strict sense outside the body, but because the phenomenon also occurs with schistosomiasis and tissue filariae this is too facile an explanation. At present the mechanisms and course of

eosinophilia produced in a host in response to a foreign protein are not clearly understood.

With regard to immunology, understandably, complex helminths produce complex crude antigens of low specificity. At the moment, with a few exceptions, group-specific reactions with antigens for schistosomes, hermaphroditic flukes, nematodes, and cestodes are all that are available using tests such as complement fixation or indirect hemagglutination. Skin tests on the whole are much less satisfactory than those based on serology. Many of these helminths are recognized by the presence of characteristic progeny in the form of either eggs in the stools, sputum, or urine, or larvae in the tissues.

The concept of the over-all population or load of worms is important in human disease, as *the parasitic load* is one of the factors determining the extent of pathology (another would be the host response). Today many helminthic infections can be quantitated, and these methods will be mentioned under diagnosis. Another important aspect of worm infections is their relatively long life. Many flukes live for decades after the infection has

TABLE 1.   Prevalence of Common Helminth Infections in Man*

Parasite	Source of Infection	Approximate Locality	Estimated Incidence in U.S. and Canada	Estimated World Incidence
Trematodes (flukes):				
Schistosoma japonicum	Water through skin	Far East	−	46,000,000
Schistosoma haematobium	Water through skin	Africa, Middle East	−	39,200,000
Schistosoma mansoni	Water through skin	Africa, South America, Caribbean	−	29,200,000
Clonorchis sinensis	Fish	Far East	In Chinese immigrants	19,000,000
Opisthorchis felineus	Fish	Far East	−	1,100,000
Paragonimus westermani	Crabs, crayfish	Africa, South America	−	3,200,000
Fasciolopsis buski	Water nuts	Far East	−	10,000,000
Cestodes (tapeworms):				
Diphyllobothrium latum	Fish	Around Arctic Circle, N. Europe, Russia, America	†	10,400,000
Taenia saginata	Beef	Cosmopolitan	10,000	38,900,000
Taenia solium	Pork	Cosmopolitan	†	2,500,000
Echinococcus granulosus	Dog feces	Cosmopolitan	†	†
Nematodes (roundworms):				
Intestinal nematodes				
Strongyloides stercoralis	Human feces	Cosmopolitan	400,000	34,900,000
Hookworm	Human feces	Cosmopolitan	1,800,000	456,800,000
Ascaris lumbricoides	Human feces	Cosmopolitan	3,000,000	644,400,000
Trichuris trichuria	Human feces	Cosmopolitan	400,000	355,100,000
Enterobius vermicularis	Human feces	Cosmopolitan	18,000,000	208,800,000
Tissue nematodes				
Trichinella spiralis	Pork	Cosmopolitan	21,100,000	27,800,000
Wuchereria bancrofti and *Brugia malayi*	Mosquitoes	Africa, South America, South Asia	−	189,000,000
Loa loa	Chrysops	Equatorial Africa	−	13,000,000
Dipetalonema perstans	Culicoides	Africa, South America	−	27,000,000
Mansonella ozzardi	Culicoides	South America	−	7,000,000
Onchocerca volvulus	Simulium	Equatorial Africa, Central America	−	19,800,000
Dracunculus medinensis	Cyclops	Middle East, India, Africa	−	48,300,000

*Based on data calculated by N. R. Stoll (J. Parasit., 33:1, 1947). Since the world population has increased by more than 50 per cent, all the figures given can be regarded as extremely conservative. For instance, it is said that 180 million people in the world are infected with one of the three species of schistosome that infect humans.

†Represents less than 100,000 infections.

been acquired, and similarly many filarial species are long lived. This illustrates the importance of obtaining a very detailed history of the patient's movements around the world because a visit to an endemic area 20 years ago may be connected with a current clinical problem.

It must be remembered that there are a large number of helminths that rarely infect man, and many cannot be included in this book. For information on these a standard textbook on parasitology (see references in Ch. 270) should be consulted. An important topical point is that we are now beginning to realize that for every worm adapted to man there are many others which gain access to man's tissues but fail to mature because they are natural parasites of other mammals or birds. These may cause very puzzling clinical problems. An increasing proportion of unexplained eosinophilia encountered in clinical practice is being explained on a basis of invasion of the body by a worm that will not mature in man because he is not the definitive host.

By a simple classification, worms may be separated into trematodes or flukes, cestodes or tapeworms, and nematodes or roundworms. A check list adapted from H. W. Brown's table in the twelfth edition of this text is given here in Table 1, together with information on the source of infection and the main areas of occurrence in the world. The most important helminthic infections in terms of disease in man and incidence are schistosomiasis, hookworm, and filariasis.

THE CESTODES
(Tapeworms)

Philip D. Marsden

288.   INTRODUCTION

The cestodes are endoparasitic flatworms, the hermaphroditic adults of which are flat and ribbonlike and inhabit the intestinal tract of vertebrates. The larval forms may require more than one intermediate host and develop in the tissues of vertebrates, and in some instances invertebrates. Most adult tapeworms consist of a scolex or head equipped for attachment with suckers, hooks, or grooves and a strobila or tapelike chain of progressively developing segments or proglottides. The neck is the site of segment generation, and mature segments are complete hermaphroditic units with both sets of sex organs. There is no digestive system, food being absorbed directly through the cuticle. There are

TABLE 2. Common Important Tapeworms

Official Name	Intermediate Host(s)	Stage in Man
Diphyllobothrium latum	Water fleas, freshwater fish	Adult worm
Taenia saginata	Cattle (beef)	Adult worm
Taenia solium	Pigs (pork)	Adult worm and larval stage
Hymenolepis nana	Man	Adult worm and larval stage
Echinococcus granulosus	Man, sheep, cattle	Larval stage
Echinococcus multilocularis	Man, sheep, cattle	Larval stage

longitudinal primitive excretory systems and a nervous system. In gravid segments the uterus is loaded with eggs, and these pass out of the bowel either in the segment or free in the stool. The delicate outer membrane of the eggs is often lost, but the thick-walled inner membrane contains a form infective for the intermediate host.

When eggs are ingested by the appropriate intermediate host, larvae (termed onchospheres) are released which are capable of penetrating the intestinal mucosa. The method by which the larvae develop into encysted forms differs among the cestodes and leads to different clinical patterns. Onchospheres in *Taenia solium* each develop into a small (0.5 to 1.0 cm) fluid-filled structure containing a single inverted "head." These are called *cysticerci*, or bladder worms, and many such larvae distributed in various organs cause the disease cysticercosis. The oncospheres in *Hymenolepis nana* penetrate only into the intestinal mucosa. They develop similarly to those just described; however, fluid is usually not present in the larva, and hence it is termed a *cysticercoid*. In the case of *Echinococcus granulosus,* usually only one onchosphere is able to develop (unilocular) within the intermediate host. However, this larva develops an internal germinating membrane capable of producing an entire population of daughter and granddaughter cysts within the primary cyst. This cyst is called an *echinococcal* or *hydatid* cyst. It continues to enlarge as the population of scolices within increases and will commonly reach a diameter of 20 to 30 cm after many years.

The clinical pattern of disease reflects these various methods of development; the cysticercoid of *H. nana* presents as intestinal irritation; the cysticercus of *T. solium* leads to multiple small lesions, often in the brain, causing seizure disorders; the Echinococcus produces a single large space-occupying lesion which often because of its size interferes with liver, lung, or cardiac function.

In the following chapters, we will deal with only the six most common of the 30 or more species of tapeworm which have been found in man. These are listed in Table 2. They will be discussed in the order cited in the table: first those in which man is the definitive host, then those in which he serves as both definitive and intermediate host, and finally those in which only the larval stage can develop in man.

289. DIPHYLLOBOTHRIUM LATUM
(The Fish Tapeworm)

Infection with the fish tapeworm is most common in temperate areas such as Scandinavia and around the Baltic Sea. It also occurs in Canada and in the northern United States, notably Alaska. Central Europe is an endemic focus. In the tropics relatively few reports have appeared from the Philippines, Madagascar, Botswana, Uganda, and Chile. A human parasite, *Diphyllobothrium pacificum,* has been described from Peru. The adult is the largest tapeworm of man, reaching 10 meters and having 4000 segments. (The spatulate head has two deep sucking grooves for attachment to the wall of the ileum.) The gravid segment disintegrates, and operculated ova are passed in the feces.

From the egg a ciliated embryo is eaten by a freshwater flea (Cyclops or Diaptomus species) in which it develops to a *procercoid*. When the infected flea is swallowed by freshwater fish, e.g., salmon, pike, further development takes place in the muscles of the fish to the *plerocercoid,* the form infective to man. The plerocercoid on being liberated into the small intestine grows to an adult in three to six weeks. Although the adult worm causes no pathologic lesion, there is a very important complication to this infection, namely a megaloblastic anemia. This appears to be due to the avidity of the worm for vitamin B_{12}, as 44 per cent of a single dose of Co^{60} labeled vitamin B_{12} was absorbed by the worm, the radioactivity being concentrated in the proximal growing part. Also the nearer the worm is to the jejunum, the greater the chance of developing megaloblastic anemia. It is not clear why the worm needs so much vitamin B_{12}. The worm also appears to require folic acid in the same way. The full range of neurologic symptoms of subacute combined degeneration of the cord may appear, particularly in severe cases of multiple parasitism. Peripheral neuritis appears very early in the parasitism, and recently optic atrophy has been reported.

The *diagnosis* is made by direct examination of the stools, because the eggs are present in very large numbers. Yellowish-brown and operculated, they have to be distinguished from fluke eggs such as Paragonimus, but the large number in the stool favors the diagnosis of fish tapeworm even to the uninitiated. The operculum is actually less conspicuous in Diphyllobothrium, and there is a small knob at the anopercular end (mean size 70 by 45 μ). Because the treatment for the tapeworms of this group and of the Taenia genus is the same, they are considered together later.

Prophylaxis is readily accomplished by thoroughly cooking fish before consumption. Freezing of fish for 48 hours at $-10°$ C will also prevent infection. The infection is not uncommon in New York among Jewish housewives who make their own gefilte fish and sample it in the process.

SPARGANOSIS

This condition requires mention here, because it is the name of an infection caused by the migrating larvae or spargana of several species of tapeworm related to *D. latum* but requiring final hosts other than man. It presents as a migrating subcutaneous painful swelling suggesting a cellulitis. Marked eosinophilia is usually present. The eye may be involved with orbital swelling or even actual penetration of the globe. In China this results from applying infected frogs on poultices to the eye. Biopsy reveals inflammatory tissue reactions and an immature cestode, many of which are quite impossible to identify. *Diphyllobothrium mansonoides (Spirometra mansonoides)* is a common offender. So-called *Sparganum proliferum* is unknown in the adult stage, but may distribute thousands of larvae throughout the body, and in contrast to other forms carries a poorer prognosis. This type of infection is rare, but occurs in many tropical countries, diagnosis being made by finding the plerocercoid larvae in tissues.

290. TAENIA SAGINATA
(The Beef Tapeworm)

The beef tapeworm has a cosmopolitan distribution, being particularly common in the Middle East, Kenya, and Ethiopia. In the last-named country people habitually take a monthly purge of herbs to get rid of an impressive length of worm, but rarely get rid of the head. Beef tapeworm is also common in parts of South America, Mexico, and Russia. In all these countries it is acquired by eating undercooked or raw beef—a delicacy in Ethiopia. In one series in the United Kingdom, fashion models seemed commonly infected because rare steaks were fashionable at the time. In spite of the harmless nature of the parasitism, a fastidious fashion model with a beef tapeworm can be a real problem in medical management. It is doubtful whether *T. saginata* causes any symptoms, although epigastric pain, appetite disturbances, and general malaise have been ascribed to the presence of the worm. It is possible that multiple worms may be associated with symptoms. Very rarely the worm may block the pancreatic or cystic duct or appendix, producing acute inflammation (16 such cases have been reported). The 5- to 10-meter adult worm has four suckers on the head to attach it to the wall of the small intestine. The gravid segments are usually recognized in the stool, but, being muscular, they can traverse the anal sphincter and appear in the underclothing. They contain more than 12 uterine branches, which distinguish them from *T. solium,* although recently some doubt has been cast on the reliability of this criterion. Characteristic Taenia eggs may be found in the stool or on the anal margin. When the eggs are swallowed by cattle, llamas, or buffaloes, the hatched embryos gain the skeletal muscles by the bloodstream after bowel penetration and develop into the encysted bladder-like larval forms or cysticerci which are infective for man.

Man is the only definitive host in which the adult worm can develop. The larval cysticercus form has been reported only three times in man, so host specificity seems to be strict. Treatment will be discussed later; prevention consists in not ingesting beef containing cysticerci.

291. TAENIA SOLIUM
(The Pork Tapeworm Causing Human Cysticercosis Due to Cysticercus Cellulosae)

In contrast to *T. saginata,* both larval and adult forms of this species can develop in man. Again this worm is cosmopolitan in distribution although relatively rare in North America and western Europe; cysticercosis is the most common identifiable cause of epilepsy in the Durban African population and is a serious disease because of the frequency of brain involvement. Man, again the only definitive host of importance, acquires the infection by eating undercooked measly pork containing cysticerci. Pigs and wild boars are the usual intermediate hosts.

The adult worm usually causes no symptoms in the small intestine. For attachment the head has four suckers and two rows of hooklets on a prominent rostellum. It is smaller than *T. saginata* (2 to 4 meters). Its segments are more delicate than *T. saginata* and there are usually less than twelve branches to the uterus in the gravid segment. The eggs are indistinguishable from *T. saginata,* both being approximately 35 μ, thick-walled, brown, and containing an embryonic oncosphere with six hooklets. In *T. solium* infection, however, these eggs are infective to man, but must pass through the stomach and undergo tryptic digestion before hatching occurs. The usual way in which man is infected with eggs is by external autoinfection, transferring eggs from the anus to the mouth or to food fecally contaminated by a carrier of the worm. Internal autoinfection by regurgitating segments of the worm into the stomach is a theoretic possibility, but has not been recorded.

Once free from the egg in the intestine, the oncosphere penetrates the intestinal wall with its hooklets and, as in the pig, settles in the body tissues. The invaded organs in order of frequency are subcutaneous tissue, brain, eye, muscles, heart, liver, lung, and peritoneum. The cysticercus matures in four months to an ellipsoidal translucent cyst, 10 to 20 by 5 to 10 mm, with an opaque invaginated scolex with suckers and hooks. It is gradually surrounded by a thick fibrous capsule and may live for years. Death is frequently associated with calcification.

The invasive phase may be associated with fever, headache, muscle pains, and high eosinophilia. Usually years after this stage more serious symptoms occur owing to brain involvement, with the onset of epilepsy, personality changes, signs of raised intercranial pressure, or long tract signs. In every patient with epilepsy of late onset coming from an endemic area this possibility should be excluded by (1) taking a detailed history, especially in relation to a past history of tapeworm infection; the stool should be examined for Taenia eggs and segments, because rarely the worm may still be in situ; (2) having a full physical examination, especially for subcutaneous nodules containing cysticerci; biopsy will establish the diagnosis; (3) taking roentgenograms of the skull, buttocks, and thighs for calcified cysticerci which have a characteristic size and shape; and (4) performing either a complement-fixation test or an indirect hemagglutination test, using antigen from lyophilized pig cysticerci.

More rarely the globe of the eye is involved, as well as the heart and skeletal muscle. A cysticercus may be visible on the tongue. Sometimes the cysticerci become secondarily infected. In the brain, inflammation around them may produce internal hydrocephalus. Although the adult worm can be eradicated easily, there is no medical treatment for *Cysticercus cellulosae* save palliative anticonvulsants. Rarely surgical intervention may be necessary in cases of raised intracranial pressure. Again prophylaxis rests on avoiding opportunities of eating infected meat and the inspection and thorough cooking of pork.

292. TREATMENT OF INFECTIONS WITH ADULTS OF THE FISH, BEEF, AND PORK TAPEWORM

Quinacrine hydrochloride (Atabrine, Mepacrine) is an effective drug for treatment of all three species of adult worm. The rationale is that a single comparatively large dose of this drug causes the worm to release its hold and it can then be voided. The most successful technique for adults is as follows: Admit the patient to hospital and give only fluids for 36 to 48 hours. Then pass a tube into the duodenum and, with the patient resting quietly, inject 1 gram of quinacrine hydrochloride down the tube in 40 ml of water, using a 20-ml syringe. Half an hour later a saline purge is injected down the tube, and all feces saved for the next 24 hours. Long lengths of the worm stained yellow with the drug are passed, and the head should be identified. If the head is not dislodged, the worm will regenerate in two to three months, and segments will reappear in the stools. The duodenal tube reduces the chances of vomiting the drug, which is a particular hazard with *T. solium* infections. (Obviously, in many endemic areas it will not be possible to get every patient into hospital.) If the head of the worm is found, one can usually reassure the patient that the worm is eliminated unless it is a rare case of multiple infection.

Niclosamide (hydroxychlorobenzamide) is a relatively new drug that may well replace Atabrine, as it is said to be safe, effective, and easy to administer. When the patient wakes in the morning, two tablets of 0.5 gram each are chewed thoroughly and swallowed with a little water. The same procedure is repeated one hour later. No fasting or purgation is necessary, and children receive a proportionately smaller dose. The worm disintegrates so that unfortunately the head cannot be sought as proof of cure. For this reason follow-up at six months is desirable. Although no report has appeared, some authorities believe that this drug should not be used in *T. solium* infection because worm disintegration may be followed by cysticercosis. It must be remembered that feces from patients harboring *T. solium* are an infectious risk. The patient should scrub his hands after defecation and pass his feces into disinfectant.

293. HYMENOLEPIS NANA
(Dwarf Tapeworm)

H. nana is less important as a cause of symptomatic disease than the other tapeworms described here. However, since it is spread directly by contact with contaminated stool, the infection can reach epidemic proportions in institutions where fecal-oral exposure is difficult to control, such as in mental hospitals or schools for young children. In a recent study, almost 8 per cent of the children at Willowbrook State School were found to be infected.

Clinical manifestations of this infection include anorexia, diarrhea, and abdominal pain secondary to irritation of the intestinal mucosa. In addition, systemic signs and symptoms such as headache, dizziness, and occasionally seizures are not infrequent. The treatment of choice is hydroxychlorobenzamide (niclosamide), 2 grams daily for three days, followed a week later by a second course of therapy. This treatment schedule has been developed because relapse occurred when shorter courses of therapy were used. Relapse is thought to occur for two reasons: first, the chlorobenzamide is only effective against the adult; and second, the cysticercoid stage may persist in the mucosa for several weeks before developing into an adult.

294. ECHINOCOCCOSIS
(Hydatid Disease)

There are two species of the genus Echinococcus which infect man, *Echinococcus granulosus* and *Echinococcus multilocularis*. They are the most important cestodes producing serious disease in man because of the size and location of their larval form, the hydatid cyst. Man is only one of a number of intermediate hosts, other important ones being sheep, cattle, and deer. The definitive hosts for these very small adult tapeworms are canines such as dogs, wolves, jackals, and foxes.

Hydatid disease is cosmopolitan because infected stock have been distributed all over the world for breeding purposes. The incidence of human infection is low in many countries, but where the triad of man, dog, and sheep or cattle is common, hydatid disease is relatively frequent. Examples are countries such as Australia, Argentina, Chile, Kenya, New Zealand, and Wales. It has been reported from 15 states in the United States. Canada and Alaska seem to enjoy a distinct variant, *E. granulosus var. canadensis*.

Human infection follows ingestion of the eggs excreted by infected dogs. The adult tapeworm measures only 2.5 to 9.2 mm and has a head with hooklets and suckers, a growing neck, and only three segments: immature, sexually mature, and gravid. Heavy infections of dogs are common, but the worm lives for only about six months in the upper jejunum. The eggs produced are indistinguishable from Taenia eggs and like them produce an oncosphere with six hooklets. On reaching the intestine of the intermediate host such as man, they pass through the intestinal wall and circulate in the blood and can develop in any body tissue. It may take 20 to 30 years before the slowly growing hydatid cyst causes symptoms. Often they remain small (less than 10 cm), but they may grow as large as the human head. The host parasite factors determining growth are not clearly understood, but growth is variable from 0.25 to 1 cm a year. The structure of a developed hydatid cyst is complex. Briefly, it really consists of a whole colony of infective larval forms, for inside the laminated, defined cyst wall is a germinal layer that is constantly budding off new infective individuals. The cyst is filled with fluid, and second and third generation cysts containing thousands of infective forms or scolices are suspended in this fluid. There is little wonder that when a dog eats an infected sheep's liver he acquires many adult Echinococcus organisms.

When the infective embryo or oncosphere passes into the portal circulation of man, it is first held up in the liver where more than half (59 per cent) of those that survive develop. Many are destroyed by phagocytic cells. The next tissue filter is the lungs, where 27 per cent lodge. Finally, 15 per cent escape into the general circulation to involve the abdominal cavity, muscle, kidney, spleen, bone, heart, and brain.

ECHINOCOCCUS GRANULOSUS

Echinococcus granulosus is the common species; there are several types of cysts, as follows: (1) The classic unilocular cyst is usually fertile and surrounded by a false capsule of host tissue fibrosis. Rupture of such a cyst will cause dissemination of daughter cysts with secondary hydatids. (2) Alveolar hydatids have a reticulated irregular outline and resemble those of *E. multilocularis*, but there is no metastatic growth. Owing to irregular growth of the germinal membrane, this cyst usually occurs in the liver and is difficult to remove. It is often sterile, and its contents degenerate. (3) Osseous hydatid. The nature of bone does not permit a host or parasite capsule to form. Daughter cysts form in the bone medulla, erode the cortex, and produce a pathologic fracture. If they escape from the bone, the cysts grow in their normal spherical shape with the usual capsules in the extraosseous tissues.

Clinically, the hydatid cysts may produce signs of a space-occupying lesion in relation to the organ in which it occurs. In the liver abdominal pain and vomiting may be presenting symptoms, a mass being visible or palpable. Usually the cysts are too tense to show fluctuation. In the lung they are usually detected on routine chest films as spherical, well-defined shadows. They are more common in the right lung, and rarely are associated with cough and hemoptysis. Those of the brain are indistinguishable from a cerebral tumor. In the kidney, hematuria or loin pain may be the first sign, whereas hydatid cyst of bone may present as a pathologic fracture.

The *complications* of hydatid disease are important. The most serious is rupture and dissemination of further infective larvae. Patients with suspected hydatid disease should always be gently palpated — a leaking cyst may present as anaphylactic shock with an urticarial rash and high eosinophilia. The cyst may become secondarily infected with bacteria and present similarly to a liver or lung abscess.

A suggestive tumor in a patient from an endemic area demands the following investigations. An eosinophilia may be present. Plain roentgenograms may show calcification in the cyst wall, although this does not mean that the cyst is not infective. An isotope scan of the liver reveals the extent of the tumor, but gives no clue as to its nature. In the chest film the round, uniformly dense shadow is suggestive. A fluid level with air in the cyst means communication with a bronchus and possibly secondary infection. A skin test using cyst fluid is positive in the majority of patients, but it has been shown that the reaction depends on the concentration (nitrogen content) of protein in the fluid injected. A cross-reaction occurs in patients with schistosomiasis. Until there is universal acceptance of a standard skin test antigen, a negative result is meaningless. Hydatid complement-fixation tests, hemagglutination tests, and bentonite flocculation tests are all practicable and are helpful. A scolex antigen is probably the best (Bull. WHO). Rarely cyst fragments, such as scolices, may be found in the sputum or urine. It must be recalled that one in five patients has multiple cysts, so that if a cyst is located in one site, especially if it is not the liver, there may be others. A liver scan should be done in every patient with an extrahepatic cyst. *Diagnostic aspiration is never indicated because of the risk of rupture.* In the liver and lung, carcinoma and abscess are often difficult differential diagnoses.

It should be emphasized that many hydatid cysts never get very large (5 to 10 cm) and never cause symptoms. There is no medical treatment. Surgery is only indicated in cysts that are enlarging, producing pressure symptoms, or developing complications. The physician should consult a surgeon who has experience with this problem. If possible the cyst should be removed entirely. To prevent spillage and dissemination, the cyst is usually aspirated at operation after packing off the site; 20 ml of fluid is withdrawn, and an equal quantity of 2 per cent formalin, 1 per cent iodine, or 30 per cent sodium chloride is introduced to kill the scolices. Injection of a 1 per cent aqueous solution of iodine in a volume amounting to one twentieth of the whole cyst volume is lethal to scolices within one minute. It is said to produce fewer complications than formalin. Anaphylactic reactions owing to spillage during operation may require corticosteroids.

E. granulosus var. canadensis is common in Alaska and Canada where it has a sylvatic cycle in deer and wolves. It produces smaller and more delicate cysts in man than the classic *E. granulosus;* the latter are more frequent in the lung, usually asymptomatic, and almost never cause serious complications so that the distinction is important.

ECHINOCOCCUS MULTILOCULARIS

The medical importance of distinguishing between these two species is that *Echinococcus multilocularis* does not produce large single cysts with endogenous growth and well-defined fibrous tissue encapsulation but rather an aggregate of innumerable small cysts that multiply by exogenous budding to produce the so-called alveolar or malignant hydatid. More than 90 per cent occur in liver, which is progressively honeycombed by a multitude of small cysts. They may become confluent and even metastasize like a malignancy. Intrahepatic or portal hypertension develops with splenomegaly, and biliary obstruction may produce icterus. The hepatic infection may be difficult to differentiate from a malignancy. This species of cestode occurs in south central Europe, Russia, and Alaska. Rarely cases have occurred in Australasia, England, and Argentina.

Prevention of infection with both these species entails elimination of the infection from dogs by worming with arecoline hydrobromide regularly and preventing their eating infected offal. Contamination of the hands, food, and drink with dog feces should be avoided.

295.   OTHER TAPEWORMS

Two other species of adult tapeworms that parasitize the human intestine are usually mentioned, but in comparison with those discussed above they are of little importance in human disease. The rat tapeworm *Hymenolepis diminuta* is acquired by swallowing infected insects carrying the Taenia eggs from rats. *Dipylidium caninum* is the common tapeworm of cats and dogs throughout the world, and is transmitted by their fleas to children handling their pets. The gravid proglottids are shaped like melon seeds and may be seen in the stool. For these parasites niclosamide is usually used, although recently paromomycin has given high cure rates in most of the human intestinal cestodes.

Coenurus infections of man, like hydatid, take the form of cystlike larvae in the tissue; 64 cases have been recorded to date. Infection in temperate regions is proba-

bly due to the larval cyst *Multiceps multiceps* (a dog tapeworm) and usually occurs in the central nervous system. Similar cysts are found in the brain of sheep, producing a fatal disease known as gid, which is characterized by somnolence, loss of weight, visual disturbance, and ataxia. In Africa *Taenia brauni* seems to be responsible for similar "hydatid-like" cysts in the subcutaneous tissues of man.

Araña Iniguez, R.: Hydatid echinococcosis of the nervous system. *In* Spillane, J. D. (ed.): Tropical Neurology. New York, Oxford University Press, 1973, p. 408.

Bjorkenheim, G.: Neurological changes in pernicious tapeworm anaemia. Acta Med. Scand., 140 (Supplement):260, 1961.

Dew, H. R.: Hydatid Disease. Sydney, Australian Publishing Co., Ltd., 1928.

Echinococcosis. Bull. WHO, 39, No. 1, 1968.

Jalayer, T., and Askavi, I.: A study of the effect of aqueous iodine on hydatid cysts in vitro and in vivo. Ann. Trop. Med. Parasitol. 60:169, 1966.

Katz, A. M., and Pan, C.: Echinococcus disease in the United States. Am. J. Med., 25:759, 1958.

Keeling, J. E. D.: The chemotherapy of cestode infections. *In* Goldin, A., Hawking, F., and Schnitzer, R. J. (eds.) Advances in Chemotherapy. London and New York, Academic Press, 1968, Vol. 3, pp. 109–152.

Pawlowski, Z., and Schultz, M. G.: Taeniasis and cysticercosis (*Taenia Saginata*). Adv. Parasitol., 10:269, 1972.

Powell, S. J., Procter, E. M., Wilmot, A. J., and McLeod, I. N.: Cysticercosis and epilepsy in Africans: A clinical and serological study. Ann. Trop. Med. Parasitol., 60:152, 1966.

Swartzwelder, J. C., Beaver, P. C., and Hood, M. W.: Sparganosis in the southern United States. Amer. J. Trop. Med. Hyg., 13:43, 1964.

Templeton, A. C.: Anatomical and geographical location of human Coenurus infection. Trop. Geogr. Med., 23:105, 1971.

Vik, R.: The genus Diphyllobothrium. Exp. Parasitol., 15:361, 1964.

Wilson, J. F., Diddams, A. C., and Rausch, R. L.: Cystic hydatid disease in Alaska: A review of 101 cases of *Echinococcus granulosus* infection. Am. Rev. Respir. Dis., 98:1, 1967.

Yoeli, M., Most, H., Hammond, J., and Scheinesson, G. P.: Parasitic infections in a closed community. Results of a 10-year survey in Willowbrook State School. Trans. R. Soc. Trop. Med. Hyg., 66:764, 1972.

DISEASES CAUSED BY TREMATODES
(Flukes)

296.   SCHISTOSOMIASIS (Bilharziasis)

Kenneth S. Warren

Definition. Schistosomiasis, a chronic infection of more than 200,000,000 people in Asia, Africa, the Caribbean, and South America, is caused by three different worm species, *Schistosoma mansoni, S. japonicum*, and *S. haematobium*. Infection occurs during immersion in fresh water containing schistosome cercariae. These larval forms penetrate the skin and migrate via the lungs and liver to the final habitat of the half-inch-long adult worms: the veins of the intestines and urinary bladder. The worms themselves do not multiply within man, but produce large numbers of eggs, many of which remain in the body, damaging primarily the intestines, liver, and urinary tract. Eggs that are excreted in the urine and feces and that reach fresh water hatch into ciliated miracidia. These organisms penetrate into snails, multiply, and develop into cercariae, the infective form for man.

Etiology. Although the cercariae of many different schistosome species penetrate human skin, there are

three major species that complete their life cycles in man and are thus capable of causing systemic disease: *Schistosoma mansoni, japonicum*, and *haematobium*. The life cycles of these schistosomes are essentially similar, all being digenetic trematodes alternating a sexual phase of reproduction in man (definitive host) with an asexual reproductive phase in snails (intermediate host). Nevertheless, at each phase of the life cycle there are differences among the species that play crucial roles in the epidemiology, pathogenesis, and clinical picture of the disease.

The adult worms or schistosomes are members of the class Trematoda of the phylum Platyhelminthes or flatworms. The male worms (10 to 20 × 0.5 to 1 mm) have cleft bodies within which the longer and thinner females reside, *S. japonicum* being the largest of the three species. The worms may live in man for as long as 30 years, but recent evidence suggests that their mean life span is five to ten years. The habitats of the adult *S. mansoni, japonicum*, and *haematobium* worms are, respectively, the veins of the large intestine, small intestine, and urinary bladder.

The worms absorb metabolites through both their intestines and integument. Their energy processes depend on anaerobic catabolism of carbohydrates; the schistosomes utilize an amount of glucose equivalent to one fifth of their dry body weight each hour and convert 80 per cent of it to lactic acid. In addition, the ingestion of red blood cells appears to be of nutritional significance, as the worms contain a proteolytic enzyme that breaks down globin; the remaining insoluble hematin-like pigment is regurgitated, because the schistosome intestine terminates blindly. The rapid metabolic rate of these worms may in part be related to their continual output of large numbers of eggs, estimated at 1400 to 3000 per day for *S. japonicum* and one tenth that number for *S. mansoni*. The eggs of the last-named species are released singly, whereas those of the other two species are deposited in clutches of as many as ten. They embryonate over a period of six days and increase in size, reaching a mean of $66 \times 155 \mu$ for *S. mansoni*, $60 \times 143 \mu$ for *S. haematobium*, and $67 \times 89 \mu$ for *S. japonicum*. The shape of the eggs is distinctive, *S. mansoni* being ellipsoidal and having a lateral spine; *S. haematobium*, also ellipsoidal but with a terminal spine; and *S. japonicum*, spheroidal with a tiny knob. The eggs remain viable for approximately 21 days after laying, during which time they must pass out of the body if their life cycle is to be completed. Passage from the blood vessels through the tissues and into the lumen of the excretory organs is apparently facilitated by enzymatic secretions of the eggs plus muscular movements of the gut or bladder. A large proportion of the eggs, however, either remain in the intestinal and vesical tissues or break free in the bloodstream and are carried into the liver and lungs.

The eggs that pass out of the body in feces or urine and reach fresh water hatch rapidly into free-swimming ciliated miracidia. The miracidia of *S. mansoni* are negatively geotropic and positively phototropic, although those of *S. haematobium* appear to be the opposite. Their average life span is about six hours. If during this time a snail is encountered, the organisms may penetrate it, and if it is of the genus Biomphalaria for *S. mansoni*, Bulinus for *S. haematobium*, or Oncomelania for *S. japonicum*, the organism can complete its life cycle. The former two snail genera are aquatic, the latter amphibious. The miracidium remains close to the site of penetration, developing into a mother sporocyst. After about ten days daughter sporocysts begin to migrate into the digestive gland of the snail, and at about five weeks from the inception of the process cercariae produced from the daughter sporocysts begin to be shed by the snail. Maximal stimulus for shedding of *S. mansoni* and *haematobium* cercariae is provided by light, but darkness seems to favor the output of *S. japonicum* cercariae. The average daily output of *S. mansoni* and *S. haematobium* cercariae is about 700, but that of *S. japonicum* cercariae is only about two. These organisms may live for two to three days under ideal conditions, but their infectivity begins to decrease by 24 hours. The fork-tailed schistosome cercariae are about 125 to 200 μ in length by 50 to 75 μ in width. *S. mansoni* and *haematobium* cercariae alternate periods of rest, during which they sink slowly, with periods of movement, during which they rise toward the surface of the water. In contrast, *S. japonicum* cercariae attach themselves to the surface film where they tend to remain at rest. When cercariae encounter mammalian skin, they attach themselves with suckers, and by mechanical means, aided by enzymatic secretions, the head penetrates, leaving the tail behind. This process occurs during immersion in water or while the skin remains moist (drying kills the organism), and takes four to ten minutes for *S. mansoni*, but only a few seconds to three minutes for *S. japonicum*.

As the worms do not multiply in the mammalian host, each cercaria that penetrates the skin can develop into only one worm. Many cercariae die in the skin, however, and in the best of experimental hosts only about 60 per cent of the *S. mansoni* organisms reach maturity. Within a few hours to days the schistosomula (the cercariae are completely changed both biochemically and physiologically immediately after penetration) migrate to the lungs by either the blood stream or lymphatics. After a few days in the pulmonary vessels the schistosomula migrate to the liver, either directly through the lungs and diaphragm or by the bloodstream. This phase takes ten to twelve days for *S. mansoni*, a somewhat shorter period for *S. japonicum*, and a longer one for *S. haematobium*. Once in the intrahepatic portal venules the worms rapidly reach maturity, mate, and move against the blood flow to their final habitats. Egg output is detectable at five to six weeks for *S. japonicum*, seven to eight weeks for *S. mansoni*, and ten to twelve weeks for *S. haematobium*.

Epidemiology. *Incidence and Prevalence.* Initial infection in schistosomiasis usually occurs in childhood, and reinfection may continue as long as there is contact with fresh water. It must be remembered that the worms do not multiply in the human body, that complete immunity apparently does not occur, and that the worms may live for decades. Under these circumstances the incidence of schistosomiasis in endemic areas is low and occurs principally in children, but the prevalence of the disease may build up to massive proportions.

The worldwide prevalence of schistosomiasis is now estimated at over 200,000,000 cases. It is known to be endemic in 71 countries that have a total population of 1,362,635,000.

In Africa, *S. haematobium* and *S. mansoni* are widespread. Only the former species occurs in Tunisia, Algeria, Morocco, Mauritania, Portuguese Guinea, Niger, the Congo Republic (Brazzaville), Somalia, and the island of Mauritius. Both species are found in all other countries, including the Malagasy Republic. Sixty per cent of Africans live in areas where exposure to schistosomes is possible, and 40 per cent of these (about 75,000,000 people) are infected.

In Southwest Asia, *S. haematobium* is endemic in Aden, Saudi Arabia, Yemen, Israel, Iraq, Iran, Syria, Turkey, and Lebanon. *S. mansoni* occurs in the first four of these countries, and is particularly prevalent in Yemen, where half the 3,500,000 population are thought to be infected. The highest prevalence rate for *S. haematobium* occurs in Iraq, where 20 per cent of the exposed population of 5,000,000 are infected. Of the 87,003,000 population of Southwest Asia an estimated 10,745,000 are exposed to infection.

In the Orient, *S. japonicum* occurs in China, Japan, the Philippines, and the Celebes. The prevalence in China was estimated at 32,000,000, but it is reported that this number has been substantially reduced by a recent massive control campaign. Schistosomiasis is under control in Japan, but seems to be spreading in the Philippines. Small foci of schistosomiasis japonica have recently been discovered in Thailand and Laos. Of the 868,531,000 population of Southeast Asia, 337,051,500 are estimated to be exposed. A small focus of *S. haema-*

tobium infection was found in India, in Maharashtra State, but it is now believed that transmission there has ceased.

In endemic areas of the New World (population 98,339,000) where only *S. mansoni* is found, 18,199,750 people are estimated to be exposed. Brazil has the largest number of cases, estimated at 8,000,000, and the infection seems to be spreading. Schistosomiasis also occurs in Venezuela, where it is apparently on the wane, and in Surinam. It is endemic in the following Caribbean islands: Puerto Rico, Vieques, Dominican Republic, Antigua, Guadeloupe, Martinique, and St. Lucia. The parasite has not been found in any of the Central American countries.

The one tiny focus of schistosomiasis in Europe, *S. haematobium* in southern Portugal, has now been eliminated.

The life cycle of schistosomiasis will become established only in areas where there is a susceptible snail species. Thus the infection is prevalent on the West Indian island of St. Lucia, although St. Vincent, 30 miles away, is completely free of the parasite. There are 1,450,000 Puerto Ricans now living on the mainland of the United States, and 100,000 immigrants from other areas endemic for schistosomiasis entering this country each year, but the presence of susceptible snails in the continental United States has not been established. Prevalence rates within endemic areas may be exceedingly variable, ranging from close to 100 per cent in some localities to almost none in others. This is governed by the interaction of multiple local ecologic factors relating to both the snail and human populations. Another important factor in the epidemiology of schistosomiasis is the variation in geographic strains of the species; for example, *S. japonicum* on Formosa is highly infective to domestic and wild animals but not to man, and *S. mansoni* in Africa south of the Sahara appears to be relatively avirulent.

Animal reservoirs are undoubtedly of significance in maintaining the life cycle of *S. japonicum* – in particular, cows and dogs. Natural *S. mansoni* infections have been found in rodents, baboons, insectivores, and dogs in Africa, but it is generally believed that animal reservoirs do not play a significant role in the life cycle of this species. *S. haematobium* is rarely encountered in animals.

Although *transmission patterns* differ among the three species of schistosomes, *there is little question that for each species agricultural development, particularly irrigation, may lead to a marked increase in the prevalence of schistosomiasis.* A major epidemic occurred in Egypt after the construction of the low Aswan dam, and in Rhodesia after development of large scale irrigation schemes.

In regard to morbidity and mortality, precise demographic figures are not available, particularly because schistosomiasis is such an insidious disease. The few investigations of morbidity now available show little or no effect of schistosomiasis on educational attainment or work capacity. Most studies suggest, however, that disease and death in schistosomiasis are correlated with intensity of infection. As the worms do not multiply in man, the number of parasites in a given individual is related to the degree of water contact and perhaps the occurrence of partial immunity. Under these conditions, schistosomes have an overdispersed distribution in which most members of the host population bear low worm burdens. As far as has been determined, little or no morbidity occurs in the large majority of the population carrying infections of low intensity. Though the proportion of heavily infected individuals is small, when this figure is multiplied against the vast number of people with schistosomiasis, it becomes obvious that this helminthic infection constitutes a major medical problem. In addition, there is no question that in all its forms schistosomiasis is potentially lethal – Katayama fever in *S. japonicum* infections, portal hypertension with hematemesis in both schistosomiasis japonica and mansoni, uremia in *S. haematobium* infection, and cor pulmonale in all three. Schistosomiasis may also potentiate the development of other diseases such as hepatitis, hepatoma, cirrhosis, and cancer of the urinary bladder.

Pathogenesis and Clinical Manifestations. Basic to an understanding of the disease processes in schistosomiasis are these facts: the schistosomes do not multiply in man; complete immunity does not follow initial infection; repeated infections usually occur; the worms are relatively long lived; most individuals have low worm burdens, but large numbers of worms may accumulate; and a large proportion of schistosome eggs are not excreted but remain within the body. Disease is correlated with the intensity of infection and is related not only to the presence of the various stages of the schistosomes in the body tissues and their secretions and excretions, but to the inflammatory responses of the host as well.

Clinically, three distinct syndromes occur at different stages of schistosome infection. Within one day of cercarial penetration, swimmer's itch, a pruritic papular rash, may appear. Several weeks later Katayama fever, a self-limited but possibly fatal illness resembling serum sickness, may develop. Finally, after many years, during which the infection may be either asymptomatic or associated with relatively mild intestinal or urinary tract symptoms, fibrosis of the liver may result in the signs and symptoms of portal hypertension in schistosomiasis mansoni and japonica; fibrosis of the ureters and bladder in schistosomiasis haematobia may result in changes associated with urinary tract obstruction.

Schistosome Dermatitis. Schistosomiasis begins with penetration of the skin by cercariae. These organisms are not discriminating and will penetrate the skin of most animals whether they are susceptible or insusceptible, living or dead. When nonhuman schistosomes, those that complete their life cycle in animals or birds, enter the skin of man, they die. Even in highly susceptible experimental hosts many *S. mansoni* cercariae die in the skin and perhaps in the lung; in the hamster almost 40 per cent are lost in this manner. In the highest primate thus far studied, the chimpanzee, 4 to 8 per cent of *S. mansoni* cercariae, 14 to 40 per cent of *S. haematobium* cercariae, and 1 to 48 per cent of *S. japonicum* cercariae were recovered as adult schistosomes. In most laboratory animals the recovery rate for *S. japonicum* is higher than that for the other two species.

The death of cercariae in the skin leads to the development of a pruritic papular rash known as *swimmer's itch*. This syndrome occurs in its most severe form after exposure to animal schistosomes, and has been shown to be a sensitization phenomenon, rarely occurring on primary exposure. Papules appear in sensitized persons at 5 to 15 hours, and there is massive round cell invasion of the dermis and epidermis, suggesting a delayed hypersensitivity response. Swimmer's itch has been demonstrated in infected patients experimentally re-exposed to

S. mansoni and *S. haematobium* cercariae. A mild form of swimmer's itch appears to occur in patients exposed to *S. japonicum* cercariae, but the rice paddy dermatitis of the Far East is caused mainly by avian schistosomes.

Katayama Fever. The next clinical phase of schistosomiasis begins 20 to 60 days after exposure and has been known in Japan as Katayama fever since the mid-nineteenth century. This syndrome occurs most frequently and is most severe in *S. japonicum* infections; in schistosomiasis mansoni it is usually found only in patients with very heavy initial infection; it is rarely if ever seen in schistosomiasis haematobia. In addition to fever, the patient suffers from chills, sweating, anorexia, headache, diarrhea, and cough. Hepatosplenomegaly is frequent, and generalized lymphadenopathy and urticaria are often seen. Eosinophilia occurs in most cases, averaging about 40 per cent. The fever may last for several weeks; when it subsides the other signs and symptoms also disappear. Death may occur in the Katayama fever stage of schistosomiasis japonica, but rarely does so in *S. mansoni* infection. At autopsy, massive infection is almost invariably found, with large numbers of eggs in the liver and intestines; 1608 worm pairs were demonstrated at autopsy in a Brazilian child. Katayama fever, which usually appears on initial infection, begins at about the time of onset of egg-laying by the worms; thus large amounts of antigen are suddenly added to moderate levels of cross-reacting antibody formed in response to the developing worms. It is possible, therefore, that this serum sickness–like syndrome may be a form of immune-complex disease.

Chronic Schistosomiasis. A correlation between the number of worms and the development and extent of chronic disease (except for patients with advanced liver fibrosis) was recently demonstrated by techniques quantitating human worm burdens at surgery and at autopsy. Heavy worm burdens were apparently a prerequisite for the development of severe disease, whereas light infections appeared to be of little consequence pathologically. *Thus, patients with few worms may never show any signs or symptoms related to schistosome infection.*

It is said that patients with chronic schistosomiasis mansoni or japonica may complain of fatigue, abdominal pain, and intermittent diarrhea or dysentery. Although this may be true in selected hospital populations, recent controlled field studies have revealed few such signs and symptoms, even in heavily infected individuals. On sigmoidoscopy, particularly in Egypt, granulomatous nodules or polyps may be observed. In *S. haematobium* infection, terminal hematuria, and, occasionally, dysuria and frequency are found. Mild chronic blood loss has been measured by radioisotope labeling in both *S. mansoni* and *S. haematobium* infections, but anemia is not usually seen in areas where there is normal iron intake. All the aforementioned signs and symptoms are related to the passage of eggs through the mucosa of the intestine and the urinary bladder.

Many eggs do not, however, leave the body; in laboratory animals less than half of them are excreted. Over a period of 20 years, for each *S. mansoni* worm pair producing eggs at a rate of 300 per day, at least 1,000,000 eggs will remain in the body. This figure can be multiplied by 10 for each *S. japonicum* worm pair.

In *S. mansoni* and *S. japonicum* infections, some of the eggs remain in the intestinal walls, but many of them enter the circulation and are carried into the liver. In schistosomiasis haematobia many eggs remain in the tissues of the bladder and adjacent organs, but some (usually too few to cause significant disease) enter the lungs via the inferior vena cava as well as the liver via the portal system. Granulomatous inflammation develops around the eggs trapped in the tissues; in the case of *S. mansoni* this has been demonstrated to be an immunologic response of the delayed hypersensitivity type. Both the eggs and the reactions to them are being constantly resorbed, but if large numbers of eggs gather together, the fibrosis subsequent to inflammation may remain. In schistosomiasis mansoni and japonica this leads to hepatic portal fibrosis, and in schistosomiasis haematobia, to fibrosis of the ureters and bladder.

Hepatosplenic Schistosomiasis. As the liver parenchyma is relatively unharmed by the pathologic processes involved in hepatic schistosomiasis japonica and mansoni, the clinical consequences of the disease relate primarily to granulomatous inflammation and portal fibrosis. Pathophysiologically this results in an intrahepatic block to portal blood flow and the development of portal hypertension and portal-systemic collateral circulation. The lesion is presinusoidal; thus intrasplenic and portal pressures are markedly elevated, whereas wedged hepatic vein pressure is normal. Total liver blood flow tends to remain within normal limits owing to a compensatory increase in arterial flow.

Clinically, the earliest sign of significant liver involvement is hepatomegaly. With progression, the spleen enlarges and becomes firm in consistency. Eventually it may extend to well below the umbilicus. At this point the patient tends to be in good general health, but may consult a physician because of a dragging feeling in the left upper abdominal quadrant.

The other major factor bringing the patient to the physician is a sudden hematemesis because of bleeding esophageal varices. Such an episode may not reappear for many years or may recur at fairly frequent intervals. The consequences of hematemesis in schistosomiasis are very different from those in cirrhosis of the liver: the blood ammonia concentration tends to remain normal, hepatic coma rarely occurs, and mortality is very low, being primarily due to exsanguination. This is consistent with relatively normal liver function. Jaundice is almost never seen in uncomplicated schistosomiasis, and the levels of both conjugated and unconjugated bilirubin are usually normal. Serum albumin concentration is normal or only slightly decreased, and globulin is somewhat elevated. As a consequence, ascites and edema are rarely encountered. Even sulfobromophthalein retention is often normal in these patients. Stigmata of chronic liver disease such as palmar erythema, spider angiomas, altered hair distribution, and gynecomastia are rare. Patients may suffer multiple severe hematemeses, but aside from temporary changes, liver function tends to remain relatively normal.

In spite of moderate chronic and occasional severe acute intestinal blood loss, a significant degree of anemia rarely occurs in uncomplicated schistosomiasis. The white blood count is usually within normal limits, but there is a moderate eosinophilia. Splenomegaly, however, may result in hypersplenism, the patient developing leukopenia, thrombocytopenia, and anemia with decreased red blood cell life span.

Patients with decompensated hepatic disease characterized by liver parenchymal malfunction and all the physical stigmata of this state, including jaundice and ascites, are seen in localities in which schistosomiasis is endemic. This is particularly common in the case of schistosomiasis japonica, and may, perhaps, be related to overwhelming embolization of the liver with the large numbers of eggs produced by this parasite. Pathologists have stated, however, that *it has not been possible to prove the transformation of advanced schistosomal fibrosis into true cirrhosis.* In Egypt it has been suggested that patients with schistosomiasis might concomitantly have other forms of liver disease. Finally, it must be recognized that all those infected with *S. mansoni* and *S. japonicum* perforce have some degree of liver involvement, and that the effect of malnutrition, hepatotoxins, and hepatitis may be potentiated; such interrelationships have been demonstrated in laboratory animals.

Pulmonary Schistosomiasis. Pulmonary schistosomiasis, which in its most severe state is characterized by signs and symptoms of cor pulmonale, is a complication of hepatosplenic schistosomiasis. Portal-systemic collateral circulation enables the eggs to bypass the liver, and they are trapped in the pulmonary capillary bed. Arteritis with angiomatoid formation occurs, and there is obstruction to pulmonary blood flow. Pulmonary hypertension is found in every case, but cardiac output usually remains within the normal range. Arterial oxygen saturation is usually normal, and cyanosis is rare. The lungs are often involved in schistosomiasis haematobia because of the passage of eggs from the vesical plexuses into the inferior vena cava, but egg embolization appears to be relatively light, and significant disease is uncommon.

Urinary Tract Schistosomiasis. Severe urinary tract disease may occur in both the early and late phases of *S. haematobium* infection. Initially there may be ureteral obstruction owing to florid granulomatous inflammatory reactions to the eggs in both the ureters and the bladder; these lesions appear to be highly reversible after antischistosomal therapy. Later in the course of the disease irreversible fibrosis may supervene. Bladder fibrosis and calcification lead to frequency and dysuria. On cystoscopy, so-called sandy patches may be seen on the bladder walls; these are made up of large numbers of schistosome eggs. The disease may progress through hydronephrosis, secondary infection, and finally uremia. An association between cancer of the bladder and urinary schistosomiasis has been demonstrated.

In the past decade there has been a growing impression among Brazilian clinicians and pathologists that there is an increased frequency of renal disease in patients with schistosomiasis mansoni. Initially proteinuria was noted in patients with hepatosplenic schistosomiasis, and then, at autopsy, the renal glomeruli of similar patients were found to have pathologic changes. This was followed by ultrastructural and immunocytochemical studies which revealed electron-dense deposits in the glomerular basement membranes which contained immunoglobulins. Similar deposits have been observed in laboratory animals. It should be pointed out, however, that specific schistosomal antigen has not been demonstrated as yet, and comparable lesions have been found in the kidneys of patients with cirrhosis of the liver.

Central Nervous System Schistosomiasis. Schistosomiasis of the central nervous system, although relatively rare, is an important complication of the infection. *S. japonicum* usually involves the brain, whereas *S. mansoni* and *S. haematobium* tend to affect the spinal cord. Schistosomiasis japonica is reputed to be one of the im-

portant causes of focal epilepsy in the Far East. The disease may also present as a space-occupying lesion or occasionally as a generalized encephalitis. Cerebral schistosomiasis japonica may appear at any time in the course of infection from the first three weeks on. At autopsy the lesions almost always consist of large collections of eggs in the venous circulatory system, suggesting the presence of adult worms, although they have never been found. *S. mansoni* and *S. haematobium* in the spinal cord may be associated with a transverse myelitis-like syndrome; at surgery or autopsy large granulomas made up of eggs are usually found.

The development of chronic salmonellosis has been described in schistosomiasis in both man and laboratory animals. In the latter, schistosomiasis has also been associated with increased severity of viral hepatitis and intestinal amebiasis.

Diagnosis. When schistosomiasis is considered as a diagnosis in nonendemic areas, the first question that should be asked is: "Where have you been?" It must then be determined whether there was contact with fresh water, whether transient pruritus was observed soon thereafter, and if there was a febrile episode several weeks later. For schistosomiasis mansoni and japonica, abdominal symptoms and signs might be considered, and for *S. haematobium* infection, terminal hematuria, dysuria, and frequency are important. The presence of eosinophilia is a useful sign of schistosome infection. A wide variety of serologic tests (e.g., complement-fixation, flocculation, fluorescent antibody, and circumoval precipitin) and a skin test of the immediate type are available. *These immunologic methods, which are all based on detection of circulating antibody, essentially have no place in the diagnosis of the individual case,* as cross-reactions with other parasitic infections providing false positive results are relatively common; false negative reactions also occur.

Definitive diagnosis can be made only by finding schistosome eggs in the excreta (feces or urine) or in a biopsy specimen—usually rectal. Eggs may not be present in the early stages of acute schistosomiasis. Schistosome eggs are relatively large, and are easy to identify because of their distinctive shape. Direct fecal smear is too insensitive, but techniques which provide both concentration and quantitation of eggs in the feces have been developed. This is important, because correlations between egg output and intensity of infection have been made. The Kato thick smear technique is a simple and highly effective method for fecal egg counting. A small portion of stool (schistosome eggs are distributed randomly in feces) is passed through 105-mesh stainless steel bolting cloth (W. S. Tyler Co., Cleveland, Ohio) and 50 mg is added to a tared glass slide and covered with a cellophane cover slip (no. 124PD, E.I. DuPont de Nemours, Inc., Film Department, Wilmington, Delaware) impregnated with 50 per cent glycerin. The slides are inverted and pressed onto a bed of filter paper, turned face up, and left for a period of at least 48 hours during which the fecal matter clears. Although the embryo within the egg also clears, the characteristic shape of the egg shell can be easily seen. After counting all the eggs in the sample, multiplication by 20 provides the number of eggs per gram of feces.

Rectal biopsy is a highly efficient method for the diagnosis of *S. mansoni* and *japonicum* infection, and will often help detect *S. haematobium* eggs. Through a proctoscope, snips are taken from the valves of Houston (8 to 10 cm from the anus), pressed between glass slides, and examined immediately under a microscope. Sometimes only opaque dead eggs are observed, suggesting a burnt-out or successfully treated infection. Liver biopsy has been suggested as a means of diagnosis, but will only rarely detect an infection not revealed by the aforementioned methods.

For the diagnosis of schistosomiasis haematobia, urine is collected at midday, because a diurnal variation in egg output has been demonstrated. The urine specimen is centrifuged and the sediment examined. For quantitative data the Bell technique is effective; this involves sieving a 10 ml aliquot of urine collected between 1100 and 1300 hours onto filter paper, staining with ninhydrin and counting the eggs. *S. mansoni* eggs are occasionally found in urine.

For determining the severity of intestinal disease, sigmoidoscopy and barium enema are of value. The extent of liver disease may be estimated by liver biopsy, barium swallow, esophagoscopy, and especially splenoportography with measurement of intrasplenic pressure. In schistosomiasis haematobia, cystoscopy and intravenous pyelography are useful techniques.

Treatment. Antischistosomal treatment should never be instituted without proof of infection by the demonstration of living eggs in excreta or biopsy specimens, except in the rare case of suspected schistosomiasis of the central nervous system. A positive serologic or skin test does not provide a definitive diagnosis. Complete cure is not necessary and indeed is not always desirable in schistosomiasis (particularly in endemic areas where reinfection may occur), because disease is related to intensity of infection, surviving worms do not multiply, and immunity may be premunitive, i.e., dependent on the presence of living organisms. The recent use of quantitative egg counts has shown that in cases in which cure is not achieved by the full course of treatment with an established drug, egg output is usually reduced by over 90 per cent. Thus striving for cure by increasing the drug dosage or repeating the course of treatment is rarely necessary and, because of the toxicity of the antischistosomal drugs, may actually be harmful.

None of the drugs now available for human use have any effect on the schistosomes during their early migratory phases in the body (the first three to six weeks), thus rendering it difficult to treat Katayama fever; steroids have been used to suppress the clinical manifestations during this stage of the infection. The three schistosome species vary considerably in their response to drugs, *S. haematobium* being the most susceptible and *S. japonicum* the most resistant. Under these circumstances it is generally stated that it is still necessary to treat schistosomiasis japonica with the highly toxic antimony potassium tartrate (tartar emetic). In a recent report (1972) of a World Health Organization consultant group, however, it was noted that the cure rates in *S. japonicum* infections with tartar emetic, stibocaptate (Astiban), and niridazole (Ambilhar), respectively, ranged between 40 to 75, 40 to 75, and 40 to 70 per cent. Thus it can be recommended that those infected with any of the three species of human schistosomes be treated with niridazole or stibocaptate, the latter when there are signs or symptoms of liver or cerebral disease. Both these drugs may be obtained from the Parasitic Disease Drug Service of the Center for Disease Control, Atlanta, Georgia 30333.

Particularly in the case of *S. mansoni* infections, it would not be unreasonable to withhold treatment with these drugs in asymptomatic individuals with very low egg counts.

Niridazole is administered orally in two divided daily doses totaling 25 mg per kilogram of body weight for a period of five to seven days. Vomiting, diarrhea, cramps, and dizziness may occur. Side effects are greatly exacerbated in patients with signs and symptoms of liver or cerebral disease. Under these circumstances stibocaptate can be substituted; this antimony compound is administered intramuscularly in a dose of 8 mg per kilogram once per week for five weeks. Antimony compounds are cardiotoxic; stibocaptate is also associated with anorexia, vomiting, abdominal pain, headache, and pain at the site of injection.

Utilizing a combination of surgery and a single dose of an antischistosomal drug, many of the worms can be sieved out of the bloodstream. Although such extracorporeal hemofiltration is a valuable research tool, it should be used as a form of treatment only under special circumstances.

In general, the surgical treatment of schistosomiasis should be approached with caution. Many of the apparently irreversible lesions of urinary tract schistosomiasis will resolve completely after antischistosomal treatment, particularly in young patients. Cerebral schistosomiasis japonica is frequently cured or markedly ameliorated by drug therapy. Finally, prophylactic portacaval shunts should never be performed in hepatosplenic schistosomiasis, because hematemesis is not invariable and is unpredictable in onset, and, when it occurs, mortality is low. If the creation of shunt by surgery is necessitated by repeated bleeding episodes, splenorenal anastomosis is preferable to portacaval shunt because of a much lower incidence of chronic portal systemic encephalopathy. Prior to shunting, however, antischistosomal therapy is necessary to prevent prolonged passage of eggs into the lungs which may lead to the development of cor pulmonale.

Prognosis. The prognosis is usually good. Many patients with schistosomiasis never have symptoms or signs of disease, or have only relatively mild ones. Epidemiologically, both the infection and the disease reach their peak in early adult life and decline with age. Disregarding the factor of death among heavily infected patients, this may be due to decreased exposure to infection, gradual death of the worms, slow development of immunity, and diminution in the inflammatory response to the parasite and its products.

The early stages of hepatic or urinary tract disease appear to be reversible after antischistosomal therapy. Although late disease seems relatively irreversible, progression may be halted and gradual improvement may follow drug therapy. In hepatosplenic schistosomiasis the prognosis in patients suffering a hematemesis is far better than in those with cirrhosis, because the former do not tend to go into hepatic coma. Patients with cerebral schistosomiasis japonica may show remarkable improvement after antischistosome therapy.

Prevention. On the individual level, schistosomiasis may be prevented by avoidance of contaminated waters. If this is not possible, boots should be worn; if contaminated water reaches the skin, rapid drying or rubbing with alcohol will prevent infection. Storage of water for several days will ensure the death of cercariae, as will the boiling of drinking water. Sea water is safe for swimming, although the mouths of rivers and streams should be avoided; chlorination of swimming pools will prevent infection. Repellents are of no great value, and vaccines or prophylactic drugs are not available.

There are three approaches to the control of schistosomiasis on a mass basis: (1) destruction of the snail intermediate host, (2) prevention of snail infection by the treatment of human infection and the construction of privies, and (3) elimination of contact with contaminated water by the provision of safe water supplies. Destruction of the snail is primarily based on the use of molluscicides such as the various copper salts, sodium pentachlorophenate, Bayluscide, and n-trityl-morpholone. Molluscicides, however, are quickly inactivated by sunlight and adsorption to mud and organic matter; they pass rapidly through running water or are diluted in vast bodies of still water, and they often destroy other aquatic fauna and flora. Also, although molluscicides may appear to be highly effective, only a few surviving snails can rapidly repopulate an area. Many biologic control measures have been advocated, including the use of nonsusceptible snail species which may compete for miracidia, food, and space; snail-eating fish and ducks; and snail pathogens. None of these measures has shown outstanding promise. The snails that transmit *S. japonicum* are amphibious and are frequently found along the banks of water courses; their eradication can necessitate the use of earth-moving equipment and flame throwers. When the snails are "buried" in this way, as in the campaigns in the People's Republic of China, it appears to reduce the infectivity of the environment.

An attempt to break the life cycle at the stage of transmission from man to the snail has been hampered by the lack of practical mass therapy. The recent development of effective oral drugs and of a single-dose intramuscular drug offers great promise for the future. An important adjunct to this approach is the construction of privies. Breaking the cycle at the stage of transmission from the snail to man can be accomplished by the provision of safe water supplies for washing and recreational purposes.

Control measures based on the destruction of snails are an end in themselves, and in addition may be inimical to the environment. In contrast, mass antischistosomal treatment coupled with the construction of privies or the provision of safe water supplies should contribute greatly to the general health of the population.

Cheever, A. W.: A quantitative postmortem study of schistosomiasis mansoni in man. Am. J. Trop. Med. Hyg., 17:38, 1968.

Clark, W. D., Cox, P. M., Jr., Ratner, L. H., and Correa-Coronas, R.: Acute schistosomiasis mansoni in 10 boys. An outbreak in Caguas, Puerto Rico. Ann. Intern. Med., 73:379, 1970.

Lehman, J. S., Jr., Farid, Z., Smith, J. H., Bassily, S., and El-Masry, N. A.: Urinary schistosomiasis in Egypt: Clinical, radiological, bacteriological and parasitological correlations. Trans. R. Soc. Trop. Med. Hyg., 67:384, 1973.

von Lichtenberg, F., Edington, G. M., Nwabuebo, I., Taylor, J. R., and Smith, J. H.: Pathologic effects of schistosomiasis in Ibadan, western State of Nigeria. II. Pathogenesis of lesions of the bladder and ureters. Am. J. Trop. Med. Hyg., 20:244, 1971.

Warren, K. S.: The immunopathogenesis of schistosomiasis: A multidisciplinary approach. Trans. R. Soc. Trop. Med. Hyg., 66:417, 1972.

Warren, K. S.: Regulation of the prevalence and intensity of schistosomiasis in man: Immunology or ecology? J. Infect. Dis., 127:595, 1973.

Warren, K. S., Reboucas, G., and Baptista, A. G.: Ammonia metabolism and hepatic coma in hepatosplenic schistosomiasis. Patients studied before and after portacaval shunt. Ann. Intern. Med., 62:1113, 1965.

WHO Reports on Schistosomicidal Drugs. II. Report of a WHO consultant group on the comparative evaluation of new schistosomicidal drugs for use in treatment campaigns. Bol. Of. Sanit. Panam. (English), 6:89, 1972.

HERMAPHRODITIC FLUKES

Philip D. Marsden

297. INTRODUCTION

The hermaphroditic flukes, unlike Schistosoma flukes, have both sets of sex organs in the same worm, and frequently self-fertilization occurs. These flukes are flat leaflike worms with oral and ventral suckers. They have a complex life cycle. The egg hatches to produce a motile ciliated *miracidium,* which penetrates the soft tissue of a snail and undergoes a cycle of development similar to that in schistosomiasis. *Cercariae* are produced by the snail after a few weeks, but unlike schistosomes these cercariae encyst in a second intermediate host, either fish, crab, or plant. These encysted cercariae or *metacercariae* are a relatively resistant form which can survive adverse conditions. If the metacercaria is then ingested by man, it hatches to produce an immature fluke which migrates through the body tissues to gain its site of final development. This varies with the species concerned, being the liver for Clonorchis and Fasciola, the lung for Paragonimus, and the intestine for *Fasciolopsis buski.*

Initial invasion is often accompanied by eosinophilia, but it takes a month or longer before the characteristic eggs are produced. All the eggs have an operculum or lid through which the miracidia escape, unlike Schistosoma eggs. Some of these flukes live for a long time, producing progressive damage in the tissues of the host. When searching for the ova of trematodes in the biliary tree, duodenal aspiration may be more rewarding than stool examination. Therapy, especially in the hepatic hermaphroditic trematodes, is unsatisfactory.

298. HEPATIC HERMAPHRODITIC FLUKES

Clonorchiasis (Clonorchis sinensis). Man is infected by eating the flesh of undercooked or raw freshwater fish in which the metacercariae are encysted. More than 40 species of fish, mainly of the carp and salmon (cyprinoid) group, have been found to harbor metacercariae. The natural definitive hosts other than man are fish-eating mammals, including cats, dogs, mink, and rats. Widespread in the Far East, the main endemic areas of human infection are Japan, Korea, China, and Vietnam. As the flukes live for decades (20 to 30 years) in the biliary tree, immigrants from Asia have been found infected in many countries. A proportion of the Chinese in New York and San Francisco are infected. Infections recorded in Hawaiians are attributed to imports of infected frozen, dried, or pickled fish from Japan.

It appears that most of the larval flukes ascend the biliary tree directly from the duodenum, but some may pass via the portal circulation to the liver. They mature in the bile ducts, and the grayish-brown adults, measuring 10 to 20 mm by 2 to 4 mm, move sluggishly around by means of their suckers in the distal biliary passages. They feed on secretions from the mucosa of the bile duct and possibly also on cellular elements. Occasionally they gain access to the gallbladder and pancreatic ducts. In effect they cause a chronic cholangitis with inflammation of the biliary tree, proliferation of the biliary epithelium, and progressive portal fibrosis. The severity of these changes depends upon the load of flukes.

After ingesting the metacercariae, the patient may present with epigastric pain, malaise, and tender hepatomegaly. An eosinophilia is usually present in the early stages, but no eggs can be found until about one month has passed and the flukes have matured. Light infections are often asymptomatic, but a firm liver edge is often discovered within the costal margin on routine examination. In an Asian, this finding should prompt a careful search for ova in the stool. In heavy infections (10,000 to 20,000 flukes), more serious sequelae occur. The marked portal fibrosis may be associated with signs of portal hypertension. Extension of the fibrosis into the liver parenchyma may be associated with liver cell death and fatty change. Jaundice is more likely to be associated with biliary obstruction owing to a mass of flukes or stone formation. Cholangiocarcinoma is a late complication of severe clonorchiasis, a metaplastic change occurring in the irritated biliary epithelium. In Hong Kong there is a high incidence in males after the fourth decade, the adenocarcinomas showing varying degrees of differentiation. Suppurative cholangitis caused by superimposed bacterial infection may present as hypoglycemic coma. Chronic pancreatitis is a rare complication.

The diagnosis is made by finding the eggs in the stool. Unfortunately they are not characteristic and can be easily confused with a number of other trematodes producing small, similar eggs (Heterophyes, Opisthorcis, Metagonimus). The eggs average 29 by 16 μ; they are light brown and ovoid. There is a definite shoulder in a shell wall near the operculum and a boss at the anopercular end.

The invasive stage must be distinguished from that of other fluke infections, *visceral larval migrans,* and *hepatic amebiasis.* The last-named condition is not associated with eosinophilia. The late stages may resemble cirrhosis and uncomplicated cholecystitis. Hypoglycemic coma can also be a manifestation of a hepatocellular carcinoma. In the elderly, repeated nonparasitic cholangitis is sometimes a difficult diagnosis to establish in patients with pyrexia of unknown origin.

Treatment and Prevention. Most investigators agree that the drugs available for treating this infection are often ineffective and disappointing. Prolonged chloroquine therapy is chiefly suppressive; however, it is still the drug of choice. Chloroquine diphosphate in a dose of 300 mg base (two 250 mg tablets) three times a day for three to six weeks is a standard course. Some workers have increased this dose or used it for periods of up to a year. Various percentages of cures are claimed, but it depends on the criteria used and especially on what stool concentration technique is employed and how frequently. At the higher dosage levels the more severe side effects of chloroquine toxicity may be seen, namely, corneal deposits and retinopathy, central nervous system changes (a parkinsonian-like syndrome), dyspigmentation, cardiac arrhythmias, and peripheral myopathy and neuropathy. A new compound, hexachloroparaxylol, proved effective, but alarming toxicity tests in recent animal studies have resulted in its withdrawal. Biliary obstruction may require surgical relief, and at surgery

as many flukes as possible should be removed from the biliary tree. Prevention of this infection relates to the competent cooking of freshwater fish.

Opisthorchiasis (Opisthorchis viverrini and felineus). *Opisthorchis felineus* is prevalent in the Philippines, India, Japan, and Vietnam, as well as in the USSR and parts of Eastern Europe, whereas *Opisthorchis viverrini* is common in north Thailand and Laos. The life cycles of these flukes are similar to that of *Clonorchis sinensis* and are completed in about four months under favorable conditions. Snails are infected by fecal contaminants of water from infected persons or animal reservoirs, e.g., cats. In northeast Thailand 90 per cent of people more than ten years of age are infected with *O. viverrini,* and 3.5 million in the whole country. With all infections of this type, as might be expected, the incidence rises with age. The source of infection is a popular dish of raw fish, rice, vegetables, and spices.

The pathologic findings are similar to those in *Clonorchis sinensis,* although stone formation is said to be unusual. Cholangiocarcinoma has also been reported to be associated with this infection. The eggs are indistinguishable from Clonorchis. This emphasizes the importance of a geographic history, for the only other way of distinguishing the parasite would be by examination of the adult flukes. Percutaneous transhepatic cholangiography may reveal radiologic changes such as a single cystic cavity or mulberry-like dilatation of the intrahepatic bile ducts.

Dicrocoeliasis. *Dicrocoelium dendriticum* is acquired by eating ants in which the metacercariae have developed following ingestion by the ant of slime balls containing cercariae secreted by the snail. Infections are generally uncommon, but occur in Europe and Asia and around the Mediterranean basin. Being light infections, their main importance is for the physician to recognize the small, fully embryonated thick-shelled eggs (40 μ × 25 μ) for what they are. Spurious parasitism, in which nonhuman species ingested in liver pass through the bowel unchanged, is well documented.

Fascioliasis (Fasciola hepatica). This is also a biliary fluke, but it is less well adapted to man than is *Clonorchis sinensis.* It is a common parasite of sheep, producing marked liver damage. Worldwide in distribution in sheep, it is prevalent in low wet pastures where suitable species of snails are indigenous. The metacercariae encyst on plants, and man is infected mainly as a result of eating wild watercress and other plants gathered in these pastures. Human infections are more common where such salad is favored, e.g., Europe, Cuba, and Chile. In England outbreaks are associated with particularly wet summers.

The adult fluke is large, 2 to 3 cm in length by 0.8 to 1.3 cm in breadth, and may occlude the *common bile duct.* Indeed, many human infections have been first recognized at surgery for biliary obstruction. Again an invasive stage of fever, eosinophilia, and hepatomegaly is associated with larval flukes moving through the liver substance to gain the biliary tract, for the larval flukes produced from the metacercariae in the jejunum pass across the peritoneal cavity to pierce Glisson's capsule and move through the liver substance. Far fewer flukes than Clonorchis are found in man, but again hyperplasia, necrosis, and cystic dilation of the biliary tract, accompanied by leukocytic infiltration and eventually periportal fibrosis, can ensue if the load of flukes is heavy enough. The differential diagnosis is similar to that of clonorchiasis.

The *diagnosis* depends on finding large yellowish operculate eggs 130 to 150 μ in length in the feces or aspirated bile. Liver should be excluded from the patient's diet in areas where raw liver is eaten, because eggs in such livers will pass through the intestinal tract unchanged. A complement-fixation test using an extract of the adult fluke as antigen is a useful diagnostic aid, especially in infections in which the flukes are ectopic. A hemagglutination test has also been developed.

Unlike the other hepatic hermaphroditic flukes, *Fasciola hepatica* and the closely allied *Fasciola gigantica* are occasionally found in sites other than the liver. This could be related to man's being a relatively poor host species. Thus a migrating subcutaneous swelling associated with intense eosinophilia may contain such an immature fluke, and there are records of occurrences in many sites, including the brain.

A further oddity associated with *Fasciola hepatica* infection is the parasitization of the pharynx by young post-metacercarial flukes which are acquired by eating raw liver in which the young flukes are actively migrating. This occurs in Lebanon, where such raw sheep and goat livers are eaten; the patient complains of intense inflammation of the back of the throat. This syndrome of parasitic pharyngitis, known as halzoun, can also be produced by a leech or a pentosomid (a wormlike arthropod).

Emetine hydrochloride is still considered by many the most effective therapy in a dose of 65 mg intramuscularly daily for ten days, but cure is rarely achieved. (For side effects see Ch. 279. It may be replaced by the less toxic dehydroemetine.) Some physicians give chloroquine concurrently, 300 mg of base three times a day for a longer period, although chloroquine alone fails to cure. Bithionol has been shown to be effective in a dose of 50 mg per kilogram on alternate days for 10 to 15 doses, and, being less toxic, may be used as an alternative. Ectopic flukes are removed surgically.

Clonorchiasis

Hou, P. C.: The relationship between primary carcinoma of the liver and infestation with *Clonorchis sinensis*. J. Pathol., 72:239, 1956.
Komiya, L.: Clonorchis and clonorchiasis. *In* Dawes, B. (ed.): Advances in Parasitology. London, Academic Press, 1966, Vol. 4, pp. 53–106.
Viranuvatti, V., and Stitnimankam, T.: Liver fluke infection and infestation in South East Asia. *In* Popper, H., and Schaffner, F. (eds.): Progress in Liver Disease, Vol. 4. New York, Grune & Stratton, 1972, pp. 537–547.
Weng, H. C., Chung, H. L., Ho, L. Y., and Hou, T. C.: Studies in *Clonorchis sinensis* in the past 10 years. Chin. Med. J. (Peking), 80:441, 1960.

Opisthorchiasis

Harinasuta, C.: Opisthorchiasis in Thailand: A review. *In* Harmasuta, C. (ed.): Proceedings of the Fourth Southeast Asian Seminar on Parasitology and Tropical Medicine: Schistosomiasis and Other Snail-Transmitted Helminthiases. Manila, 1969, pp. 177–199.

Fascioliasis

Hardman, E. W., Jones, R. L. H., and Davies, A. H.: Fascioliasis — a large outbreak. Br. Med. J., 3:502, 1970.
Khalil, G. M., and Schacher, J. F.: *Linguatula serrata* in relation to halzoun and the Marrara syndrome. Am. J. Trop. Med., 14:736, 1965.
Neghume, A., and Ossandan, M.: Ectopic and hepatic fascioliasis. Am. J. Trop. Med., 23:545, 1943.
Pantelouris, E. M.: The Common Liver Fluke. Oxford, Pergamon Press, 1964.

299. LUNG HERMAPHRODITIC FLUKES
(Paragonimiasis)

Although *Paragonimus westermani* is the most common species of this group infecting man, recently a number of other human pathogens have been recognized in the genus Paragonimus, which to date numbers more than 31 species. These include *P. africanus* found in Nigeria, the Cameroons, and the Congo, and two new Chinese flukes, *P. skrjabini* and *P. heterotremus*. *P. westermani* is widely distributed in the Far East, occurring as an important human infection in China, Japan, Vietnam, Korea, Formosa, the Philippines, and Thailand. Species also occur in South America in Peru, Colombia, Ecuador, and Venezuela.

Paragonimiasis is a chronic lung infection of man caused by this group of flukes, the adults living in cystic spaces in the lung. Reddish-brown plump oval flukes, they resemble in size a coffee bean (0.8 to 1.6 cm long by 0.4 to 0.8 cm wide). They are covered with little spines and live singly or in pairs in the lung parenchyma, feeding on host exudates. They live five to six years usually. Oval yellowish-brown operculated ova (85 μ by 35 μ) are coughed up in thick, blood-stained sputum. These hatch to produce a miracidium which invades specific snails. The cercariae subsequently produced by these snails encyst as metacercariae in the muscles and viscera of freshwater crabs. Man acquires the infection by eating the crabs raw or partly cooked. The larval flukes released from the metacercariae usually migrate to the lung via the peritoneal cavity, penetrating the diaphragm, but may mature in the abdomen or brain.

For many species man is not the definitive host, felines being preferred. For instance, other hosts apart from man for *P. westermani* are cats, tigers, leopards, mink, badgers, dogs, lions, and rats. *P. westermani* was discovered by Westerman in 1877 in a tiger in the Amsterdam zoo.

Pathogenesis and Pathology. The larval fluke tunnels into the lung at the periphery. There is an inflammatory reaction around it with many eosinophils. Later it forms a cystic space with a fibrous tissue wall. These cysts usually communicate with a bronchus and often become secondarily infected with abscess formation. Death of the fluke is often followed by calcification. Ova may be reaspirated, with an eosinophilic inflammatory response and the formation of small lung granulomas.

Although the target organ for Paragonimus is the lung, it must be realized that often adults go astray, and if the invading species is one less adapted to man, this is more liable to happen. Thus a characteristic feature of *P. skrjabini* infection is migrating subcutaneous nodules that contain active flukes. Such granulomas in the subcutaneous tissue may require excision as in fascioliasis.

In the brain the temporal and occipital lobes are occasionally the site of an eosinophilic granuloma containing flukes and, in a few cases, ova. A transverse myelitis is known. Flukes in the peritoneal cavity produce adhesions and abscesses, and ulceration of the intestine occurs with ova in the stool. Adult and mature flukes have been found in many other organs, including intestine, spermatic cord, testis and scrotum, vagina, and muscles.

Clinical Manifestations. Lung infections are encountered with symptoms of persistent hemoptysis, breath-lessness on exertion, pleural pain, and recurrent pulmonary infections. The condition is known as endemic hemoptysis. Clubbing of the fingers is common, and persistent rales may be heard over the affected lung segments as in nonparasitic bronchiectasis. A lung abscess may be present. Pneumothorax, pleural effusion, and empyema are rarer complications. Chest films early in the disease show infiltrations, but later dense nodular opacities or ring shadows indicate the site of the cysts. Pleural adhesions and calcification are late signs. Coexistent pulmonary tuberculosis occurs in some patients. There are rarely more than 20 parasites in the lungs.

It has been estimated that there were 5000 cases of cerebral paragonimiasis in South Korea in January 1968. Cerebral paragonimiasis may present signs of a space-occupying lesion with epilepsy and paresis of varying degrees. Ophthalmic signs are optic atrophy associated with papilledema or direct involvement with the inflammatory process. The cerebrospinal fluid shows a raised protein, and eosinophils are present. There may be calcifications present on skull roentgenograms; pneumoencephalography may show the site of a pseudotumor. Abdominal paragonimiasis is a difficult condition to diagnose, but an abdominal mass in a patient with lung disease should raise this suspicion.

Diagnosis. This rests mainly on finding ova in the sputum. One third of patients also have ova in the stools because of swallowed sputum or a coincidental intestinal lesion. Complement-fixation tests are useful, and positive results correlate closely with an active infection. Yokogawa has treated patients on this basis alone. The intradermal test remains positive for a long while after active infection and is not a reliable guide. Work goes on defining the antigenic structure of the parasite. The extent to which the Paragonimus antigen cross-reacts with other flukes is not clear.

Pulmonary paragonimiasis may resemble bronchiectasis, lung abscess, bronchial carcinoma, or—most important of all—pulmonary tuberculosis. Cerebral paragonimiasis mimics other space-occupying lesions but especially other helminths in the brain. These include Fasciola, *Schistosoma japonicum, Angiostrongylus cantonensis,* and hydatid.

Prognosis. Fatalities are rare, and lung lesions resolve spontaneously in five to ten years. Cerebral involvement may be associated with persistent epilepsy. Two per cent of lung paragonimiasis is complicated by pulmonary tuberculosis.

Treatment. Bithionol (Actamer, Biton) is 2,2′-thiobis(4,6-dichlorophenol) and is given orally in a dose of 30 mg per kilogram of body weight on alternate days for 20 days. Skin reactions and gastrointestinal irritation are rarely severe enough to interrupt treatment. Results are far superior to those obtained with chloroquine or emetine drugs used in the past. Granulomas containing Paragonimus adults and ova may require surgical removal from the skin, testis, abdominal organs, or brain.

Prevention. It might be thought that it would be a simple matter to dissuade people from eating raw, fresh salted, pickled, or imperfectly cooked crabs and crayfish, but such local delicacies are not easily relinquished. Drunken crab, a favorite dish, involves immersing live crabs in alcohol prior to consumption. In Korea and West Africa, fresh crab juice is used as a home remedy in the treatment of measles.

Chang, H. T., Wang, C. W., Yü, C. F., Hsü, C. F., and Fang, J. C.: Paragonimiasis, a clinical study of 200 adult cases. Chin. Med. J., 77:3, 1958.

Grados, O. B., Cuba, C. C., Morales, F. N., and Mazabel, T. C.: Epidemiologia de la paragonimiasis en el Peru. Arch. Peruanos Pat. Clin., 26:33, 1972.

Miyazaki, I.: Lung Flukes in the Western Hemisphere. Tokyo, Overseas Technical Cooperation Agency, 1972.

Nwokolo, C.: Endemic paragonimiasis in Eastern Nigeria. Clinical features and epidemiology of the recent outbreak following the Nigerian Civil War. Trop. Geogr. Med., 24:138, 1972.

Yokogawa, M.: Paragonimus and paragonimiasis. *In* Dawes, B. (ed.): Advances in Parasitology. London, Academic Press, 1969, Vol. 7, pp. 375–387.

Yokogawa, S., Cort, W. W., and Yokogawa, M.: Paragonimus and paragonimiasis. Exp. Parasitol., 10:81, 139, 1960.

Yokogawa, M., Okawa, T., Tsuji, M., Iwasaki, M., and Shigeyasu, M.: Chemotherapy of paragonimiasis with bithionol. III. The follow-up studies for 1 year after treatment with bithionol. Jap. J. Parasit., 11:103, 1962.

300. INTESTINAL HERMAPHRODITIC FLUKES

FASCIOLOPSIASIS
(Fasciolopsis buski)

Fasciolopsis buski is a large fleshy fluke, 3 cm long and 1.2 cm wide. It is found mainly in China but also in India, Indonesia, Thailand, Malaya, and Taiwan, normally as an intestinal parasite of pigs. The eggs are passed in the feces, and miracidium is released to penetrate a snail. The cercariae subsequently produced encyst as metacercariae on edible water plants called water caltrop or water chestnuts. The tubers and fruits of these plants are eaten fresh and raw from July to September and as they are peeled with the teeth, people are easily infected. The ponds are often fertilized with night soil or contaminated by pigs.

Most infections are asymptomatic, but foci of inflammation may occur at the site of attachment of the worms in the small intestine. In heavy infections abdominal pain may simulate a peptic ulcer, and there may be alternating diarrhea and constipation. A recent investigation does not suggest that malabsorption occurs. Intestinal stasis, ulceration, and even obstruction have occurred. Several thousand worms may be harbored by the patient, and in severe cases, especially in children, edema of the face and trunk has been described. The mechanism of this edema may be complex, as anemia and hypoproteinemia from blood loss in the bowel are possible. Definite allergic edemas do not appear to be reported in the literature, but there is a variable eosinophilia with heavy loads. Brown, in a previous edition of this textbook, suggested that an absorption of toxic metabolites may be responsible for this edema. Ascites and death from exhaustion are rare.

Diagnosis. Diagnosis depends on finding the characteristic eggs in the stool. These are large, 130 to 140 μ by 80 to 85 μ, yellowish, and rather similar to Fasciola but with a smaller operculum. Occasionally an adult fluke may be vomited or passed in the stool. Facial edema may raise the question of differentiating fasciolopsiasis from trichinosis or the nephrotic syndrome.

Therapy. Tetrachloroethylene is effective (see Treatment in Ch. 304). Some advocate hexylresorcinol in an adult dose of 1 gram. Either drug should be given on an empty stomach. Not all the flukes may be eradicated, but the therapy can be repeated after a few days. Prevention entails cooking the offending plants, eradicating snails with molluscocides, and preventing fecal contamination of ponds.

OTHER INTESTINAL HERMAPHRODITIC FLUKES

Two very small intestinal flukes—*Heterophyes heterophyes* and *Metagonimus yokogawai*—deserve mention. The former is found in Egypt, Tunisia, South China, India, and the Philippines, and the latter occurs in the Far East and Indonesia. Both are acquired by eating raw or inadequately cooked fish that contain the respective metacercariae. The adult flukes, 2 to 3 mm long, are attached to the mucosa of the small intestine and are alleged to produce superficial inflammation and ulceration. Usually they are not present in sufficient numbers to produce symptoms. Very rarely eggs may gain access to the circulation and be found in internal organs.

Usually they are passed in the stool and closely resemble Clonorchis eggs, which is perhaps their main importance. Both species can be treated with tetrachloroethylene as used for hookworm. Many species of the genus Echinostoma can also infect man in the Far East, but again rarely produce symptoms. Their eggs resemble those of Fasciola but are smaller. *Gastrodiscoides hominis* is a fascinating fluke with a large ventral sucker. Like the others, it can produce diarrhea. It occurs in Assam, Indochina, India, and Malaysia. In Canada the eggs of *Metorchis conjunctus* are occasionally found in the stools of man.

Barlow, C. H.: The life cycle of the human intestinal fluke *Fasciolopsis buski* (Lankester). Amer. J. Hyg., Monograph 4, 1925.
Cross, J. H.: Fasciolopsiasis in South East Asia and the Far East: A review. *In* Harmasuta, C. (ed.): Proceedings of the Fourth Southeast Asian Seminar on Parasitology and Tropical Medicine: Schistosomiasis and Other Snail-Transmitted Helminthiases. Manila, 1969, pp. 177–199.
Plaut, A. G., Kampanort-Sanyakorn, C., and Manning, G. S.: A clinical study of *Fasciolopsis buski* in Thailand. Trans. Roy. Soc. Trop. Med. Hyg., 63:470, 1969.

THE NEMATODES
(ROUNDWORMS)
Philip D. Marsden

301. INTRODUCTION

Roundworms have an intestinal tract and a large body cavity bordered by a complex cuticle and containing the reproductive, nervous, and excretory systems. They have elongated, cylindrical, bilaterally symmetrical, smooth, nonsegmented, translucent, flesh-colored bodies, often filiform, with a pointed posterior and rounded anterior end. The Nematoda constitute the second largest class in the Animal Kingdom, with 500,000 species. Many are free living. They are unisexual, and the female is usually bigger than the male. There is a great variation in size among the common human species. For example, in the intestinal nematodes a female Ascaris may reach 18 cm whereas a female Strongyloides is smaller than 1 mm. Their bodies are muscular and require high carbohydrate reserves.

The common human nematodes can be roughly divided into the *intestinal nematodes*, of which the common ones in order of importance are hookworms, Ascaris, Strongyloides, Trichuris, and Oxyuris, and the *tissue nematodes*. The latter group includes Trichinella and the various filarial worms. Heyneman has suggested that the life cycles of the intestinal nematodes of man can be shown to demonstrate an increasing dependence upon the host and a decrease in the proportion of metabolically active time in the free-living stages if they are arranged in a certain sequence. This sequence reflects different degrees of adaption by the parasite to the host and is presented in Table 1.

Rhabditis, a free-living nematode which rarely infects man, is but one step away from the relatively common *Strongyloides stercoralis*. Strongyloides represent the first stage in parasitic adaption. Hookworms are obligate parasites with no free-living stage. Both these nematodes and Ascaris have a phase of lung migration by immature larvae in the host, the explanation of which is

not known. Ascaris, Trichuris, and Enterobius have progressively shorter oval maturation times. *Trichinella spiralis* is viviparous; the intestinal phase is transient, and the larvae persist in the host muscle.

Although the adult Trichinella organisms are intestinal nematodes, from a clinical viewpoint trichinosis can be considered as a tissue parasitic infection, as it is the larvae that produce the disease syndrome. The final break from the free-living state is illustrated by the filariae, in which the adult worms live in the host tissue, specific arthropods serving as the intermediate hosts. Whether filariae evolved from insect parasites or arose by adaption of intestinal parasites to insects after ingestion of eggs by coprophagic insects is a matter for speculation.

As in schistosomiasis, the number of worms present in the host determines the clinical manifestations, and many mild infections are asymptomatic. Quantitative

TABLE 1. Sequence for Common Human Intestinal Nematodes (Heyneman)

Species	Details of Life Cycle
Strongyloides stercoralis	Most primitive since parasitism is irregular and exists in free-living adult stage in soil
Necator americanus *Ancylostoma duodenale*	Regular parasitism; no free-living adults, only larvae in soil
Ascaris lumbricoides	All hatched larval stages as well as adults in host; only eggs in soil
Trichuris trichiura	Similar to Ascaris, but newly hatched larvae do not migrate through host's body; all development confined to the intestine
Enterobius vermicularis	Eggs infective shortly after being laid; soil phase for eggs rarely involved
Trichinella spiralis	No eggs laid; larvae hatch within female, are deposited in mucosa, which they penetrate, and migrate via blood stream to encyst in tissues

techniques to determine adult worm load are commonly used in some nematode infections. Among the intestinal nematodes, Strongyloides and Oxyuris infections cannot be quantitated owing to the variability in excretion of progeny. Ascaris produces so many eggs that quantitative techniques are usually not worthwhile, but hookworms and Trichuris eggs can be quantitated by a stool-dilution technique. For example, in Stoll's method 3 grams of stool is emulsified in 42 ml of water in a special flask. Tenth normal sodium hydroxide may be used to soften hard feces. Glass beads and shaking after standing produces a uniform fine emulsion; 0.15 ml volume of this is pipetted onto a glass slide, and all the eggs counted in this volume are equivalent to 0.01 gram of feces. Knowing the number of eggs per gram of stool, the total volume of stool, the egg output per female worm, and the usual sex ratio of the species population, it is possible to calculate the approximate worm load. Tissue helminths can also be quantitated in terms of larval output by expressing results in *Trichinella spiralis* infections as the number of larvae per gram of skeletal muscle or the number of microfilariae per milliliter of blood at a certain time of day. Onchocerca infections are likewise expressed as number of microfilariae per milligram of skin.

Another important feature of nematode infections is the frequency with which infections with nonhuman parasites are encountered as abortive infections, with larvae only rarely maturing to adults, thus suggesting helminths in a process of adaption into man. A number of such parasites will be mentioned in the text that follows, including the genera Oesophagostomum, Toxocara, Anasakis, Angiostrongylus, Dirofilaria, and others of clinical importance.

Heyneman's sequence is followed in the present discussion of the nematodes, although it is important to point out that, in terms of human suffering, hookworm and Bancroftian filariasis are by far the most serious infections.

Beaver, P. C.: Wandering nematodes as a cause of disability and disease. Am. J. Trop. Med., 6:433, 1957.
Beaver, P. C.: The nature of visceral larva migrans. J. Parasitol., 55:3, 1969.
Heyneman, D.: The life cycle of the nematodes parasitic in man: An evolutionary sequence. Med. J. Malaya, 20:249, 1966.
Knight, R., Schultz, M. G., Hoskins, D. W., and Marsden, P. D.: Intestinal parasites, a progress report. Gut, 14:145, 1973.
Marsden, P. D., and Schultz, M. G.: Intestinal parasites, a progress report. Gastroenterology, 57:724, 1969.

INTESTINAL NEMATODES

302. STRONGYLOIDIASIS
(Cochin-China Diarrhea)

Definition. Strongyloidiasis is an infection of the small intestine with the invasive small nematode *Strongyloides stercoralis*. Most infections are asymptomatic, but a few can be life threatening; because of this, treatment is always necessary.

Etiology and Transmission. The parasitic female worm is small (2.2 mm long) and lives in the mucosa of the intestinal villi. The parasitic male has rarely been observed, and experimental work suggests that parthenogenesis is the rule. The eggs produced by the female

hatch rapidly, producing larvae in the small intestine, and these may reinvade the bowel mucosa before being voided in the feces (internal autoinfection). On the other hand, they may invade immediately after voiding via the perianal skin (external autoinfection). Other larvae become infective within hours of contact with the soil, and invasion of a fresh host occurs via the skin. Alternatively, voided larvae may develop into *free-living adults in the soil*. These adults produce further generations of infective larvae in the soil. These alternative cycles make the life history of Strongyloides the most difficult one to grasp.

After skin penetration, the infective larvae undergo the same curious migration as hookworms via the venous system to the lungs (in 24 to 48 hours). Autoinfective forms may take a peritoneal or lymphatic route to the same site. From the lungs the developing larvae ascend the trachea, drop down into the stomach, and mature in the small intestine. Because of the frequency of autoinfection this nematode is self-perpetuating, and infections can last for 30 to 40 years. Man is the only common host, although primates and dogs can be experimentally infected.

Distribution. The parasite is cosmopolitan, but it is more frequent in the tropics. Local habitats where warmth, moisture, and lack of sanitation favor the free-living existence are endemic sites. Curiously enough, in nearly all populations, however, the infection seems to be sporadic and an incidence comparable with that seen in hookworm infection is not encountered. Conceivably, however, this may be due to diagnostic difficulties, as mentioned below. This infection, like all intestinal parasitic infections, has been reported in high incidence from some mental institutions. Resistance to reinfection has been suggested by animal studies.

Pathology and Pathogenesis. The adult female worms burrow through the intestinal submucosa above the muscularis mucosae, depositing eggs as they go. They cause a chronic inflammatory cell infiltrate with many eosinophils. The rapidly hatching larvae are responsible for most of the pathologic findings, and their powers of penetration are such they can be distributed widely throughout the body. For reasons not clearly understood, the whole process may be accelerated (the so-called hyperinfective syndrome). Debility on the part of the host, malnutrition, or corticoid administration favors the development of this syndrome. Obviously prolonged bowel transit time would increase the possibility of internal autoinfection. Inflammation of the small bowel may be so intense as to cause malabsorption, thickening, and edema visible roentgenographically. The mesenteric lymph nodes enlarge, and ulceration and necrosis of the mucosa may occur. The lungs and liver may also show abscess formation, and fatty changes in the liver may indicate primary or secondary malnutrition. In recent years several series of fatal cases have been described from the West Indies, Brazil, and Africa. Acute small bowel obstruction has been described, as well as *E. coli* bacteremia with meningitis, the latter perhaps arising from bacteria being introduced from the bowel on migrating larvae. The gut may be invaded at any level by larvae, and gastric and colonic involvement are well documented. Rarely larvae are found in other abdominal organs. Involvement of the kidney, heart, and endocrine glands is described.

Clinical Manifestations. Dermal invasion, either as a result of primary exposure or by external autoinfection, may be characterized by linear, erythematous, urticarial wheals, which are the sites of migrating larvae. Particularly common around the buttocks, they may occur anywhere, and are often recognized for what they are, as they are relatively fast moving. It is a form of cutaneous larva migrans (see Ch. 305). Lung invasion may be associated with signs of bronchospasm or bronchopneumonia. These may be short-lived or recurrent if several waves of larvae arrive in the lung. Hemoptysis is not uncommon as the larvae burst through the pulmonary alveoli. They may be found in the sputum, and there is usually a marked eosinophilia. Bowel involvement may give rise to a variety of clinical manifestations, but again it must be stressed that many light infections are asymptomatic. The most common gastrointestinal symptom is epigastric pain, which is often to the right of the midline, constant, and of a dull, aching character, mimicking peptic ulcer. Tenderness may be present on abdominal palpation over the duodenum. In heavy infections diarrhea is common; it may not be just the result of inflammation but may also reflect the coexistent malabsorption. Upper abdominal pain and vomiting from the involved upper gut are frequent, but intestinal obstruction is rare. Marked large bowel involvement may resemble ulcerative colitis. In the hyperinfective syndrome death may result from disseminated inflammatory lesions, often with superimposed bacterial infection.

Diagnosis. Strongyloidiasis must always be thought of in patients with unexplained eosinophilia. The high eosinophilia is probably associated with recurrent larval invasion. The diagnosis is made by finding the larvae in the stool, preferably by using a concentration technique. Unfortunately there are a number of difficulties. In warm climates fresh stool should be examined, as hookworm larvae hatch quickly from the eggs; they can be differentiated, but only by an expert. The excretion of larvae in strongyloidiasis is intermittent, and multiple stool specimens should be examined. The Baermann funnel technique and filter paper culture technique have facilitated diagnosis. Sometimes larvae are demonstrated in the duodenal aspirate or sputum when other techniques have failed. Jejunal biopsy may show larvae and adult parasites in section in the mucosa. The filarial complement-fixation test is invariably positive and of diagnostic help in difficult cases. Barium studies may show thickening and deformities of the small bowel owing to inflammatory edema.

Treatment. As so little is known about the conditions governing development of serious infections, all patients should be treated with thiabendazole, 25 mg per kilogram twice daily for two days. Given orally, this drug is effective, with few side effects. The tablets should be chewed; they have an orange taste. Assessment of parasitologic cure requires repeated stool examinations using special techniques. The eosinophilia should fall within eight weeks. The prognosis is good in otherwise healthy subjects, but may be poor in the exceptional circumstances described above. Prophylaxis involves avoiding unsanitary conditions when infection is likely. Strongyloides of nutria and raccoons have caused transient creeping eruptions (cutaneous larva migrans) in Louisiana trappers.

Bras, G., Richards, R. C., Irvine, R. A., Milner, P. F. A., and Ragbeer, M. M. S.: Infection with *Strongyloides stercoralis* in Jamaica. Lancet, 2:1257, 1964.

Kanani, S. R., and Rees, P. H.: The diagnosis of strongyloidiasis with special reference to the value of the filarial complement fixation test as a screening test. Trans. R. Soc. Trop. Med. Hyg., 64:246, 1970.

Stemmerman, G. N.: Strongyloidiasis in migrants. Pathological and clinical considerations. Gastroenterology, 53:59, 1967.

Tanaka, H.: Experimental and epidemiological strongyloidiasis of Amaini Oshima Island. Jap. J. Exp. Med., 28:159, 1958.

303. CAPILLARIASIS

Until recently the genus Capillaria appeared to infect man so rarely that it would not have merited inclusion in a general work of this kind. The most common form, *Capillaria hepatica* (less than 20 cases reported), was recognized by finding Trichuris-like eggs encapsulated in the liver. Species of the genus had also been reported in the lungs and skin of man.

Recently, however, a new parasite of man *Capillaria philippinensis,* has been described from the northern Philippines, where more than 1000 cases and 100 deaths have been confirmed to date. Patients with intestinal capillariasis have colicky abdominal pain, chronic diarrhea, muscle wasting, and edema, which may lead to debility and death in four months. Clinical studies have shown the presence of a severe protein-losing enteropathy in these patients with malabsorption of fats and sugars.

A tiny nematode (3 to 4 mm by 0.03 to 0.04 mm), *C. philippinensis* is confined to the small intestine, particularly the jejunum. The eggs detected in the stool are similar to *Trichuris trichiura* (to which the Capillaria are closely related) but are smaller, are more oval, and have less prominent bipolar plugs. There is evidence that hatching may occur in the small intestine, and tissue invasion of the bowel similar to strongyloidiasis has been noted at postmortem examination. The mode of transmission of the disease is not fully worked out, but three species of fish have been found to contain infective larvae. It is still uncertain whether interhuman transmission occurs.

Apart from intravenous feeding in severe cases, success in eliminating this parasite has been reported by using high doses of thiabendazole.

Cross, J. H., Banzon, T., Clarke, M. D., Basaca Servilla, V., Watten, R. H., and Dizon, J. J.: Studies on the experimental transmission of *Capillaria philippinensis* in monkeys. Trans. R. Soc. Trop. Med. Hyg., 66:819, 1972.

Detels, R., Gutman, L., Jaramillo, J., Zerrudo, E., Banzon, T., Valera, J., Murrell, K. D., Cross, J., and Dizon, J. J.: An epidemic of intestinal capillariasis in man. Am. J. Trop. Med., 18:676, 1969.

Whalen, G. E., Rosenberg, E. B., Strickland, G. T., Gutman, R. A., Cross, J. H., Watten, R. H., Uylangco, C., Dizon, J. J.: Intestinal capillariasis, a new disease in man. Lancet, 1:13, 1969.

304. HOOKWORM DISEASE
(Ancylostomiasis, Miner's Anemia)

Definition. The two common hookworms of man, *Ancylostoma duodenale* and *Necator americanus,* attach themselves to the small bowel by their buccal capsules and suck blood, thereby causing chronic blood loss. Depending on their number and the iron stores of the host, a variable degree of anemia often results. A distinction is made between hookworm infection when the load is too light to produce symptoms and hookworm disease.

Pathogenic Chain. *Etiology.* The human hookworms measure about 1 cm in length, the female being slightly longer than the male, which is recognizable by an expanded posterior end, the copulating bursa. *A. duodenale* is larger than *Necator americanus,* and the two species are differentiated most easily by the fact that *A. duoden-ale* has two pairs of teeth in its buccal capsule, whereas *N. americanus* has a pair of cutting plates only. The eggs of the two species are indistinguishable and are passed in the feces. In warm moist soil the larva hatches within 48 hours. The rhabditiform larva has a free-living cycle in the soil, feeding on bacteria, during which time it molts twice. The filariform larvae resulting from the second molt are the infective stage for man and can survive several months in favorable conditions. They tend to migrate up grass stems or gain any elevation up to 3 feet, and on coming into contact with the skin of man, quickly penetrate it, enter the bloodstream, and are transported to the lungs. Like Strongyloides, there they leave the vascular system and emerge into the alveoli, migrate up the bronchi and trachea, and down the esophagus to reach the small intestine where maturity is attained. Eggs appear in the stool five or more weeks after invasion, and the adults live one to nine years.

Epidemiology. Over 400 million people have hookworm infections, but in the majority the worm load is small. *Ancylostoma duodenale* is the Old World hookworm, being prevalent in Europe, North Africa, and the Middle and Far East. *Necator americanus* is found more in the New World and tropical Africa. During the past 30 years both parasites have become widely distributed, and rigid geographic demarcations are not possible.

The survival of larvae is favored by a damp sandy soil, high in humus content at a temperature of 24 to 32° C. Promiscuous defecation and the absence of shoes are the chief factors responsible for infections. Such conditions occur in mines as well as on the surface of the ground. Urban people tend to have less hookworm than agricultural rural workers at locations where night soil is often used as fertilizer. Infection can be acquired by ingesting or handling contaminated vegetables. Coffee, banana, sugar cane, rice, and sweet potato fields are ideal for the growth and development of larvae. Often one locality is used as a communal latrine in the area, and people reinfect themselves by visiting these sites again and again. *The distinction between hookworm infection and hookworm disease is important.* Methods of estimating the intensity of the infection show that in endemic areas most patients have few worms and no significant anemia. Those who have hookworm anemia have more worms, and these heavy infections could be the result of repeated exposure or a failure of immunity on the part of the host. With canine hookworm, small repeated infections give almost complete immunity. Antibodies have been demonstrated in sera of infected patients.

Pathology and Pathogenesis. Inflammatory cell infiltration is seen at the site of penetration of the hookworm larvae, and in the lungs small hemorrhages occur with eosinophilic and leukocytic infiltration. An eosinophilia is present during the invasive phase. The main feature of the established disease is the active sucking of blood by the worms. They create a negative pressure in the buccal capsule and suck in a piece of mucosa which acts as both an anchorage and a source of blood. It is still not clear what hookworms abstract from the blood. Vital preparations in vitro show red cells being vigorously expelled from the posterior end. Ancylostoma sucks between 0.16 and 0.34 ml of blood per day and Necator, 0.03 to 0.05. The development of anemia depends upon three factors: the iron content of the diet, the state of the iron reserves, and the intensity and duration of infection.

When iron intake is high, a heavy worm load is needed to produce a significant anemia. Up to 60 per cent of the iron from the hemoglobin extracted by the hookworm is reabsorbed in the intestine. At open operation small punctate hemorrhagic spots are encountered at the site of attachment. In addition to anemia, hypoalbuminemia occurs owing to a combination of blood loss and a low rate of albumin synthesis, possibly associated with anoxia affecting liver cell function. Malabsorption is said to occur in a few cases with partial villous atrophy and chronic inflammatory cell infiltration of the lamina propria.

Clinical Manifestations. The site of skin penetration by the larvae is associated with pruritus and the development of an erythematous papular eruption (ground itch) which may last several days or even longer, depending on the host's immune response. Within a week after penetration the patient may have a transient asthmatic attack, but this is not as commonly seen as in invasive ascariasis.

Established hookworm disease is associated with general symptoms of anemia, weakness, fatigue, dyspnea, palpitation, and mental and physical retardation. Pica may be noted. On examination the skin and mucus membrane are pale. Peripheral edema is due possibly to a variety of factors, namely, hypoalbuminemia, a rise of capillary venous pressure, and tissue anoxia. In severe cases there is evidence of congestive cardiac failure. The pulse is rapid with a high pulse pressure. On auscultation of the enlarged heart, a third heart sound and an ejection type of systolic murmur are commonly heard; regurgitant systolic and even diastolic murmurs may occur and disappear when the anemia is corrected. For this reason it is very unwise to diagnose a valvular lesion clinically in such anemic patients until that anemia has been corrected. The hemoglobin may be very low (2 grams per 100 ml) and the patient still ambulant. The patient may complain of upper abdominal pain, and radiologic changes suggestive of a duodenitis have been reported.

Diagnosis and Differential Diagnosis. Stool microscopy, either by a direct smear or by a concentration technique, reveals hookworm ova. Quantitation of the egg excretion enables the physician to decide whether the patient has a significant worm load. This is done by diluting a known volume of stool and counting a sample (Stoll technique). Hookworm ova are 60 to 70 μ long by 35 to 40 μ wide and have a characteristic morphology with a clear shell and developing embryo inside. They must be distinguished, however, from both Trichostrongylus and *Ternidens deminutus,* both of which have larger eggs. Test tube cultivation of ova and differentiation of the resultant larvae are of value in doubtful cases. A skin test using an extract of *Necator americanus* larvae of standard nitrogen content has proved useful in screening a hookworm-infected population. Fluorescent antibody, complement-fixation, and hemagglutination tests have been developed but have little clinical application.

The anemia of hookworm disease is a classic iron deficiency anemia with a low hemoglobin, mean corpuscular hemoglobin concentration and serum iron, and a high iron-binding capacity. On the film the red cells are microcytic and hypochromic. Folic acid deficiency may sometimes be superimposed on macrocytosis. The serum albumin is low, and liver function tests may be abnormal. In the edematous patient there may be confusion with kwashiorkor, wet beriberi, or the nephrotic syndrome. The anemia has to be differentiated from other iron deficiency anemias.

Treatment. Tetrachloroethylene in a dose of 0.1 mg per kilogram of body weight is effective (maximum of 5 ml in a single dose). It is usually dispensed in 1-ml gelatin capsules or in a liquid that should be kept in the refrigerator in a dark bottle. It is given in the morning on an empty stomach; all food should be withheld for six hours and any fatty foods withheld for the rest of the day. Repeated treatments may be necessary. Vertigo, vomiting, and dizziness may follow therapy. Bephenium hydroxynaphthoate (Alcopar) is more expensive but is being increasingly used. The standard dose for an adult is 5 grams containing 2.5 grams of bephenium base; it is taken as granules in a glass of water on an empty stomach. Three daily doses may achieve total eradication. Loose stools, nausea, and vomiting have followed treatment. Both drugs will remove a large number of worms at the first dose, but to get rid of the last 5 to 10 per cent is often very difficult. In many areas total eradication may not be desirable or necessary. In general, tetrachloroethylene is said to be more effective in *Necator americanus* infections. If Ascaris are also present, Alcopar is preferred, or both Ascaris and hookworm will respond to thiabendazole. Tetrachloroethylene irritates Ascaris and may cause migration.

The anemia responds well to ferrous sulfate, 200 or 400 mg three times daily. Occasionally the hemoglobin is so low, or there is an associated acute infection, that the patient presents in extremis owing to heart failure. Pregnancy may also precipitate acute heart failure. Intraperitoneal blood transfusion or exchange transfusions have been life-saving. The prognosis is good in most cases. It is wise to delay treating the hookworm infection until the hemoglobin is above 50 per cent after oral iron. Without treatment of the worm infection, the anemia will relapse when iron therapy is discontinued. *Prevention* involves the sanitary disposal of human excreta and the prevention of soil pollution. The wearing of shoes cuts down the opportunities for infection.

Gilles, H. M., Williams, E. J. W., and Ball, P. A. J.: Hookworm infection and anemia. Quart. J. Med., 33:1, 1964.
Roche, M., and Layrisse, M.: Nature and causes of hookworm anemia. Am. J. Trop. Med., 15:1031, 1966.
Stoll, N. R.: On endemic hookworm, where do we stand to-day? Exp. Parasitol., 12:241, 1962.
Stoll, N. R.: For hookworm diagnosis is finding one egg enough? Ann. N.Y. Acad. Sci., 98:712, 1962.

305. CUTANEOUS LARVA MIGRANS
(Creeping Eruption)

Cutaneous larva migrans is considered at this point because its most common cause is *Ancylostoma braziliense,* although it may be produced by a variety of other helminths. It is characterized by an erythematous, serpiginous, intracutaneous track or burrow, the anterior end of which is observed to migrate at the rate of 1 to 2 cm per day. There is often intense irritation, and secondary infection may result from scratching. This migration is due to the infective larva of *A. braziliense* (the cat and dog hookworm), which does not visceralize in man but wanders around in the skin. This migration may last for

2 to 50 weeks before the larva dies. Rarely some larvae reach the lungs, causing high eosinophilia and patchy pulmonary infiltration.

Patients are often infected by lying on beaches contaminated by dog or cat feces. The feet, legs, and hands are the most common sites, and the appearance of the lesion is usually diagnostic. It is virtually impossible to remove the larva from the skin.

Anyclostoma braziliense is found in the southern United States, Central America, and tropical South America, as well as in tropical Africa and parts of the Far East, especially the Malay peninsula. There have been several reports of the worm maturing in the gut of man and eggs appearing in the feces, so there is not an absolute host specificity. Two other dog hookworms, *Uncinaria stenocephala* and *Ancylostoma caninum,* can produce similar lesions. Occasionally the ground itch of the two common human hookworms may persist and resemble creeping eruption in immune subjects.

The larva migrans track of *Strongyloides stercoralis* tends to be a short line, erythematous and rapidly moving (larva currens). Rodent Strongyloides may produce similar lesions but no mature worms. A form of myiasis with the horse bot fly maggot (Gasterophilus) can produce a larger deeper migrating form of cutaneous larva migrans.

Treatment. Thiabendazole by mouth, 25 mg per kilogram per day for two days, is usually effective. If not, the dose can be doubled and repeated. Alternatively, the advancing end of the burrow can be treated with topical thiabendazole sprinkled on elastoplast or in a cream containing 15 per cent thiabendazole powder in a hydrosoluble base. This drug has completely superseded the other, more unsatisfactory treatments such as ethyl chloride spray and Hetrazan.

Battistini, F.: Treatment of creeping eruption with topical thiabendazole. Tex. Rep. Biol. Med., 27 (Supplement 2):645, 1969.
Beaver, P. C.: Larva migrans. Exp. Parasitol., 5:587, 1956.
Stone, O. J.: Systemic and topical thiabendazole for creeping eruption. Tex. Rep. Biol. Med., 27 (Supplement 2):659, 1969.

306. TRICHOSTRONGYLIASIS

The adult worms of the genus Trichostrongylus are much smaller than hookworms, being under 100 mm long. They lie embedded in the mucosa of the duodenum and jejunum, where they suck a small quantity of blood. Eight species have been reported in man. Infections are most frequent in the Far East, especially in Japan, Korea, and Indonesia. High infection rates have been reported in Iran. South and Western Asia, Chile, and Brazil are areas where human infections also occur. Worm loads in man are usually light and asymptomatic. Infection is acquired by ingesting salad contaminated with infective third-stage larvae. The importance of Trichostrongylus lies in the fact that the egg is frequently mistaken for hookworm, and this group is not very susceptible to antihelminthics used in the treatment of hookworm (e.g., Tetrachlorethylene). These "hookworm eggs" appear to persist after therapy and are termed drug resistant. Frequently, these so-called drug-resistant hookworms turn out to be Trichostrongylus. The eggs of Trichostrongylus are larger and more sharply pointed at one end and have more advanced embryonation than hookworm ova. They are from 73 to

94 μ in length and 40 to 50 μ in width. Larvae recovered from fecal culture of the ova can also be distinguished from hookworm. Treatment is seldom needed, but thiabendazole is probably effective in the majority of cases.

Ghadirian, E., and Arfaa, F.: Trichostrongyliasis, a prevalent zoonotic infection in Iran. In Abstracts of Invited Papers, Ninth International Congress on Tropical Medicine and Malaria, Athens, 1973, p. 156.

Marcial Rojas, R. A.: Trichostrongyliasis. In Marcial Rojas, R. A. (ed.): Pathology of Protozoal and Helminthic Disease with Clinical Correlation. Baltimore, Williams & Wilkins Company, 1971, p. 753.

307. GNATHOSTOMIASIS

Although Gnathostoma species are more closely related to Ascaris, this group is mentioned at this point because it also presents as *creeping eruptions* or, more commonly, as *migratory swelling in the subcutaneous tissues*. More than 100 human infections with the immature stages of *Gnathostoma spinigerum* have been reported from the Far East, particularly Thailand. Normally a parasite of wild felines, dogs, and foxes, Gnathostoma infects man when he eats the larvae in undercooked fish (fermented fish is a Thai delicacy). The larva causes a migratory swelling, often in the subcutaneous tissues, associated with an intense eosinophilia. Occasionally the larva comes to the skin surface and resembles cutaneous larva migrans, but the area of involvement is larger. Sometimes the larva burrows deep into the internal tissues and may lodge in the gut wall or elsewhere and produce an abscess. Indeed, secondary infection frequently occurs. Brain involvement in fatal cases with eosinophilic meningitis has been reported. Eye involvement with iritis and orbital cellulitis is also described. If the worm does not reach the body surface, the symptoms can persist for months. Some recommend extraction of the worm, but Hetrazan has been said to be useful. There is insufficient experience with thiabendazole thus far to permit a definite statement of its value, but its trial seems reasonable.

Miyazaki, I.: On the genus Gnathostoma and human gnathostomiasis with special reference to Japan. Exp. Parasitol., 9:338, 1960.

308. OESOPHAGOSTOMIASIS

Oesophagostomiasis is more closely related to hookworm and Strongyloides than to Gnathostoma, but like Gnathostoma it may rarely form a tumor in the human gut wall. Again, man is not the definitive host. The infection is often carried by pet monkeys, and the clinical picture is usually one of intestinal obstruction. Bacterial infection of the tumor nodule is common. Surgical excision of the tumor shows it to contain worms of Oesophagostomum species.

Anthony, P. P., and McAdam, I. W. J.: Helminthic pseudotumours of the bowel: Thirty-four cases of helminthoma. Gut, 13:8, 1972.

309. ASCARIASIS

Definition. Ascariasis is infection with *Ascaris lumbricoides,* the large roundworm of man. The adults mature in the small intestine and can produce disease by intestinal obstruction or migration. The passage of larvae through the lungs may result in pneumonitis.

Etiology. Ascariasis is a large whitish nematode; the female (20 to 35 cm) is larger than the male (15 to 30 cm), which often has a curly tail. The vulva of the female is situated ventrally at the junction of the anterior and middle thirds of the worm. Frequent copulation is necessary to ensure the continuous production of fertile eggs. A female worm has a reproductive capacity of 26 to 27 million eggs and a daily output of 200,000. The life span of the adult worms is relatively short (12 to 24 months). They are not attached to the wall of the jejunum, but bridge themselves across the lumen and by their muscle tone maintain themselves against the fecal stream. In a largely anaerobic environment they obtain nourishment from the semidigested food of the host and possibly from epithelial cells of the intestinal mucosa. The high protein and vitamin content of the parasite suggests that they deprive the host of nutrients.

The brownish eggs with a thick shell and albuminous coat become infective ten days after being passed in the stool. Fertile and infertile eggs have a different morphology. On ingestion of infective eggs by man, the larvae hatch in the small intestine, and, penetrating its wall, are carried by the blood and lymphatic system to the lungs. It has been suggested that this migration is necessitated by the need for oxygen, which is not available in the intestine, at this stage of the life cycle. Here, like hookworm and Strongyloides, the larvae migrate up the respiratory passages to the epiglottis and down to the esophagus. A new generation of eggs appears in the feces approximately two months after the ingestion of embryonated eggs.

Epidemiology. Although cosmopolitan, this worm is most abundant in the tropics, where sanitation is poor. One in every four people in the world is infected with *Ascaris lumbricoides*. The eggs are killed by direct sunlight and temperatures above 45° C; nevertheless, under optimal conditions they may remain viable for ten years. The eggs pass unchanged through the intestine of animals with the possible exception of the pig. The pig Ascaris, *Ascaris suum*, is morphologically identical to the human Ascaris, and there is some evidence that cross-infections can occur. The susceptibility to infection is greatest in childhood, reaching a peak at puberty, and transmission is by fecal contamination of food and drink. Circulating antibodies appear to play some role in host immunity.

Pathology and Clinical Manifestations. Light infections of a dozen or so worms often pass unnoticed, especially in adults. During the phase of larval migration, especially if many eggs have been ingested, respiratory symptoms may appear 4 to 16 days after infection. The pulmonary migration of larvae is associated with fever, cough, occasionally hemoptysis, and either crepitations or more rarely the signs of consolidation on auscultation of the chest. The sputum contains larvae and eosinophils, and there is a high blood eosinophilia. Sections of the lungs at this stage would show larvae in the bronchioles with patchy infiltration of alveoli with polymorphs and eosinophil leukocytes. Aberrant larvae may lodge in the liver, producing granulomatous lesions and hepatomegaly. More rarely such larvae, which fail to re-enter the circulation, are found in other abdominal organs.

When adult worms are present in the intestine, the established infection is often associated with occasional colicky abdominal pain and some abdominal distention.

These adults may produce complications by mechanical effects within the gastrointestinal tract, or by wandering outside it, or more rarely by producing allergic manifestations in a sensitized host.

Heavy loads of worms may particularly be associated with intestinal obstruction, intussusception, volvulus, appendicitis, and hernial strangulation. A bolus of Ascaris may be a common cause of intestinal obstruction in childhood in an endemic area. Before undertaking bowel surgery, an Ascaris infection should always be excluded, because these worms are difficult to control once the bowel is opened, and considerable peritoneal soiling may result. Migration of adult worms may occur spontaneously or as a result of some stimulus such as fever or tetrachloroethylene. The Ascaris adults may perforate a suture line or cause a bile or pancreatic duct obstruction. Occasionally they migrate into the stomach and are vomited up, or pass down into the large bowel and out with the stool. Adult worms have been described issuing from umbilical fistulas, and even from the nose or ear. Obstruction of the bile duct is associated with cholangitis, and eggs may be deposited in the liver. *A. lumbricoides* has been said by some to be second only to *E. histolytica* in producing liver abscesses. Blockage of the pancreatic duct results in acute pancreatitis. Once the adult worm has left the bowel, it often dies, releasing foreign protein that may produce a reaction in a sensitized host. These reactions range from facial edema and giant urticaria to acute local necrosis and anaphylaxis. Laboratory personnel who work with Ascaris invariably become sensitized to the worms. Young pigs infected with Ascaris do not gain weight normally, and it is possible that heavy loads of human Ascaris may affect children similarly, as the worms will consume much food in the actively growing phase.

Diagnosis. Examination of the feces reveals the characteristic ova. Usually in view of the number of ova produced, they can be found in ordinary direct smear. Although fertilized eggs are easy to recognize, unfertilized eggs assume bizarre shapes and may be mistaken for debris. Rarely one encounters infections of immature worms or only male worms. Sometimes an infection is diagnosed in barium meal examination, as the barium can be seen in the Ascaris gut. Although many serologic tests have been developed for Ascaris, including complement-fixation, hemagglutination, and gel diffusion, they are seldom used for diagnostic purposes.

Treatment. Piperazine citrate is the drug of choice in the treatment of Ascaris infestations. The piperazine salts are simple, safe, and efficient. They act by blocking the neuromuscular junctions of the worm. The paralyzed worm can no longer bridge itself across the intestinal lumen and is carried along in the fecal stream and passed in the stool. Piperazine citrate is given in a dose of 75 mg per kilogram to a maximal single dose of 4 grams. This will clear 75 per cent of patients of their worms, but the dose can be repeated the following day with safety. No special preparation or purgation is necessary. Neurotoxic effects from piperazine have been reported in patients with renal failure who cannot excrete the drug.

Thiabendazole in the same dose as for strongyloidiasis and Alcopar in the same dose as for hookworm are both effective in ascariasis as well. In the presence of Ascaris plus one or another of these intestinal parasites, single drug therapy may be preferred. However, neither of these drugs is as effective in ascariasis as piperazine. In

multiple intestinal helminthic infections, Ascaris should always be treated first.

When examining stools for ova after therapy, it must be remembered that eggs may be passed in the stool for up to a week after the worms have been eradicated owing to the delay in the colonic circulation of feces.

The following regimen is suggested to deal with *intestinal obstruction* owing to Ascaris. Initially conservative treatment with nasogastric suction, intravenous fluids, and piperazine therapy should be tried for 48 hours. If no improvement follows, at laparotomy it is often possible to manipulate the bolus of worms into the large bowel through the terminal ileum. Only if this is not possible should enterotomy and worm extraction be performed.

Prevention. This consists of disposal of human excreta in sanitary privies and toilets. Children must be taught to use these facilities and avoid contamination of food with ova.

Chang, C. C., and Han, C. T.: Biliary ascariasis in childhood. A clinical analysis of 788 cases. Chin. Med. J. (Peking), 85:167, 1966.
Gelpi, A. P., and Mustafa, A.: Seasonal pneumonitis with eosinophilia: A study of larval ascariasis in Saudi Arabia. Am. J. Trop. Med. Hyg., 16:646, 1967.
Lejkina, E. S.: Research in Ascaris immunity and immunodiagnosis. Bull. WHO, 32:699, 1965.
Otto, G. F., and Cort, W. W.: The distribution and epidemiology of human ascariasis in the United States. Am. J. Hyg., 16:657, 1934.
Piggott, J., Hansbarger, E. A., and Neafie, R. G.: Human ascariasis. Am. J. Clin. Path., 53:223, 1970.
The Control of Ascariasis. World Health Organization Technical Report, Series No. 379, 1967.

310. TOXOCARIASIS
(Visceral Larva Migrans)

Toxocariasis is an accidental human infection with the cat and dog Ascaris (*Toxocara cati* and *Toxocara canis*). The eggs of these species are infective two to three weeks after being passed, and if ingested by man the second stage larvae emerge. These penetrate the intestinal wall and reach the liver. The majority remain in the liver but others migrate to other organs, particularly the brain and the eye. Rarely they complete their cycle of development in man and produce adult worms in the bowel. Children are particularly susceptible because of more frequent soiling of the fingers and habits of playing with puppies, in which the incidence of infection is very high. Initially reported from the southern United States, these parasites are common in dogs and cats in many parts of the world. Although many reports have come from North America and Europe, it is likely that this syndrome also occurs in other parts of the world.

The migrating larvae produce "eosinophilic trails" and tissue inflammation in the affected organ. Usually a granuloma forms with epithelial cells, fibroblasts, lymphocytes, plasma cells, and occasional giant cells. A fibrous capsule eventually encloses the larva, which may remain alive for months. The granulomas can be seen macroscopically as small grayish-white spots. Such granulomas have been found in the lungs, eyes, brain, heart, kidney, and striated muscle.

The most common clinical form is that of a patient with a mild fever and tender hepatomegaly. Routine investigation reveals a marked eosinophilia (50 to 60 per cent), and further questioning often brings to light a history of contact with dogs. These signs and symptoms may persist for 18 months. The serum globulins may be elevated and anti-τ globulins are found. Another clinical form is as an *endophthalmitis* with a space-occupying granuloma visibly distorting the contour of the retina on funduscopy. In the past such granulomas were often mistaken for retinoblastomas, and the eye was removed. Several such series of "retinoblastomas" have been examined, and many of the tumors were found to consist of granulomas containing Toxocara larvae. Many mild infections are asymptomatic.

The syndrome of tender hepatomegaly and eosinophilia must be distinguished from invasive schistosomiasis or fascioliasis. A variety of nematodes can produce visceral larva migrans in special circumstances, among them *Ascaris lumbricoides, Necator americanus,* and *Strongyloides stercoralis.* Other nonhuman nematodes such as Gnathostoma, Capillaria, Hepaticola, and Dirofilaria may be involved in granuloma formation in the liver. Sarcoidosis and periarteritis nodosa may mimic this disease. Blind liver biopsy is seldom helpful, but where facilities exist, direct visualization of surface granulomas of the liver with a peritoneoscope may enable biopsy of a granuloma to be made. A definitive diagnosis can often be made by examination of this granuloma. A diagnosis of second-stage rhabdoid Toxocara larva can be made on a section at mid-gut level, showing a maximal width of 12 to 20 μ and lateral alae. A variety of serologic tests are available but lack specificity, as they cross-react with other helminthic infections. However, in areas where such infections are rarely encountered, a fluorescent antibody test or an indirect hemagglutination test may be helpful.

Treatment. Diethylcarbamazine (see Bancroftian Filariasis in Ch. 316) has been used and does kill some larvae in the tissues of infected mice. A resolution of symptoms has followed the use of thiabendazole in one case in a dose of 25 mg per kilogram twice daily for seven days. The prognosis is good if the source of infection is removed by treating the dog with piperazine. Care must be taken to worm pets regularly, especially puppies, if they are in contact with children.

Huntley, C. C., Costas, M. C., Williams, R. C., Lyerly, A. D., and Watson, R. G.: Anti-γ-globulin factors in visceral larva migrans. J.A.M.A., 197:552, 1966.
Kagan, I G.: The serological diagnosis of visceral larva migrans. Clin. Pediatr. (Phila.), 7:508, 1968.
Mok, C. H.: Visceral larva migrans: A discussion based on a review of the literature. Clin. Pediatr. (Phila.), 7:565, 1968.
Nelson, J. D., McConnell, T. H., and Moore, D. V.: Thiabendazole therapy of visceral larva migrans: A case report. Am. J. Trop. Med. Hyg., 15:903, 1966.
Woodruff, A. W.: Toxocariasis. Br. Med. J., 3:663, 1970.

311. ANISAKIASIS

Although the full life cycle is still unknown, it appears that man is occasionally infected by the ascarid *Anisakis marina,* which has its larval stages in herrings. The adult worms develop in marine mammals such as seals, dolphins, porpoises, and whales. Man is infected by eating raw or undercooked herrings, and infection has occurred where such food is considered a delicacy, namely, northeastern Europe (Denmark particularly) and Japan. The larvae appear to burrow into the wall of the stomach or small bowel to produce an eosinophilic granulomatous mass that may be mistaken for a malignancy. Perforation of the bowel wall has been reported, as has stenosis following granuloma formation. Usually the correct diagnosis is not made until the specimen is examined after surgical resection.

Van Thiel, P. H.: The final hosts of the herring worm *Anisakis marina.* Trop. Geogr. Med., 18:310, 1966.
Yokogawa, M., and Yoshimura, H.: Clinicopathologic studies on larval anisakiasis in Japan. Am. J. Trop. Med. Hyg., 16:723, 1967.

312. TRICHURIASIS
(Whipworm Infection, Trichocephaliasis)

In trichuriasis, the adult worms are shaped like a whip. The long anterior threadlike portion of the worm consists of a cellular esophagus buried deep into the submucosa of the colon, making it difficult to dislodge. These adults are pinkish-gray and are 30 to 50 mm long. The male is distinguished from the female by its coiled caudal extremity. The female produces 5000 to 10,000 eggs per day. The eggs are 50 to 55 μ long, golden brown with prominent characteristic bipolar plugs. Under favorable conditions they become infective in three to five weeks, and when ingested by man the first stage larva hatches in the small intestine and spends three to ten days in the intestinal villi. Then it passes down to the large bowel where it matures in 30 to 90 days. The adult worms live for years.

Of worldwide distribution, trichuriasis is most frequently encountered in the tropics. Often in a particular endemic locality, the infestation has a patchy distribution because of dense shade, heavy rainfall, and the clay soils that hold water as well as fecal pollution, thus facilitating transmission. In the United States, whipworm infection is found in the southern Appalachians and southwestern Louisiana; it is not infrequent in Puerto Rico.

The great majority of infections are asymptomatic; only heavy loads of worms cause clinical illness. The worms are distributed throughout the colon and rectum, and heavy infections may be associated with colic and diarrhea with blood. *Trichuris trichiura* abstracts 0.005 ml of blood per worm from the host each day. In children in precarious iron balance a load of over 800 worms may be associated with an iron deficiency anemia. Up to 5000 worms have been recovered from heavily infected children. In such infections rectal prolapse may complicate the diarrhea, and the appearance of the congested mucosa associated with the whitish bodies of the worms has been described as the "coconut cake" rectum. Early infections may be associated with a mild blood eosinophilia. Trichuris has been implicated as a predisposing factor to acute amebic dysentery by causing an initial breach of the mucosa, this suggestion being based on finding a higher incidence of Trichuris in patients with acute bowel amebiasis than is normal for the area. Trichuris is often associated with other helminthic and protozoal infections. Appendicitis and peritonitis with the presence of worms in the peritoneal cavity have been described.

Diagnosis is made by finding the eggs in the feces, either on direct smear or by concentration methods. In the rare Trichuris dysentery the eggs may appear in aggregates in the mucoid stools, together with eosinophils and Charcot-Leyden crystals. Egg counts below 10,000 per gram are unlikely to be associated with symptoms.

Treatment is not very satisfactory. Dithiazanine iodide was formerly used, but it has caused nine deaths, and has been withdrawn from the market. Treatment should be confined to heavily infected individuals presenting with symptoms and to those employed as food handlers, nurses, and so forth. Thiabendazole in a similar dose to that used in Strongyloides (25 mg per kilogram of body weight twice daily for two days) eradicates the infection in one third of cases, and the course can be repeated after one week. Mebendazole, a new broad-spectrum anthelmintic, appears to be effective. An oral dose of 100 mg twice a day for three days gave a cure rate of 64.3 per cent in one trial. It is well tolerated and has a direct ovicidal effect.

Boon, W. H., and Hoh, K. K.: Severe whipworm infection in children. Singapore Med. J., 2:34, 1966.
Franz, K. H., Schneider, W. J., and Pohlman, M. H.: Clinical trials with triabendazole against intestinal nematodes infecting humans. Am. J. Trop. Med. Hyg., 14:383, 1965.
Jung, R. C., and Jelliffe, D. B.: The clinical picture and treatment of whipworm infection. West Afr. Med. J., 1:11, 1952.
Layrisse, M., Apariedo, L., Martinez Torres, C., and Roche, M.: Blood loss due to infection with Trichuris trichiura. Am. J. Trop. Med. Hyg., 16:613, 1967.
Sargent, R. G., Savoury, A. M., Mina, A., and Lee, P. R.: A clinical evaluation of mebendazole in the treatment of trichuriasis. Am. J. Trop. Med. Hyg., 23:375, 1974.
Wagner, E. D., and Chavarria, A. P.: In vivo effects of a new anthelmintic, mebendazole (R 17,635), on the eggs of Trichuris trichiura and hookworm. Am. J. Trop. Med. Hyg., 23:151, 1974.

313. ENTEROBIASIS
(Oxyuriasis, Pinworm or Seatworm Infection)

Infestation with the pinworm, Enterobius vermicularis, is not limited to rural communities and the poor as with many intestinal nematodes, but occurs also in urban communities. Reportedly worldwide in distribution, it appears to be much rarer in the tropics. Children are more commonly infected than adults.

The adult female worm is 8 to 13 mm long, and the male, which is rarely seen, 2 to 5 mm. Both live in the cecum and adjacent large and small bowel. The females migrate at night to the anal orifice, where they deposit their eggs. Within a few hours larvae develop in the eggs, which are then infectious and on ingestion hatch in the duodenum and migrate to the large bowel where they mature in 15 to 28 days. The ova can be transferred from the anal margin to the mouth by contamination of the hands, and ova lodge under the nails after scratching of the anal margin. The eggs also become widely disseminated in the environment, notable in bedclothes and dust samples. It has been suggested that hatching of larvae on the anal margin may result in the colon's being colonized from below as a form of autoinfection. Fortunately the eggs are relatively susceptible to drying, and in a warm dry environment survive only a few days.

Usually pinworm infestation is harmless and is often asymptomatic. Pruritus ani is the chief complaint caused by the migrating female worms. Numerous other symptoms have been described, including enuresis, irritability, and insomnia, which may result from the pruritus. Less convincing reported manifestations are abdominal pain, teeth grinding, nausea, and weight loss.

Rarely the female worm may penetrate into the mucosa of the bowel, where it has been a primary cause of appendicitis. Occasionally female worms migrate into the vagina, causing an intense vulvitis. Prostatitis is a rare complication in the male, and secondary ischiorec-

tal abscesses may follow perianal eczema. Granulomas may form around worms that enter tissues, and such granulomas have been described in the uterus, fallopian tubes, and peritoneum, presumably associated with migration of worms up the female genital tract. A rare case not reported in the literature occurred in a mentally deficient child who developed pulmonary eosinophilic granulomas owing to massive inhalation of Enterobius eggs present in the dust of the mental institution.

The best method for finding Enterobius eggs is by means of the sealing tape (Scotch tape) swab. A piece of Scotch tape 2 inches long is folded, sticky side out, over the end of a wooden tongue depressor and pressed firmly against the perianal region. The tape is then stuck to the slide, acting as a coverslip, and the specimen is scanned for the typical eggs, which are 50 to 60 μ in length, are flattened on one side, and contain a developing embryo. The patient can be given six such swabs, and he does the examination every morning for six mornings on rising and before taking a bath. All can then be examined at the laboratory. Adult worms are rarely observed in feces or on the perianal skin, or seen with the sigmoidoscope. All members of the family should be examined in view of the frequency with which whole families are infected. The eosinophil count is rarely elevated in this infection.

Treatment with piperazine citrate, 65 mg per kilogram (maximal daily dose 2.5 grams) daily for eight days, is usually effective. Single-dose treatment is becoming more fashionable with either pyrvinium pamoate, 5 mg per kilogram (maximum, 250 mg), which can be repeated after two weeks, or thiabendazole, 25 mg per kilogram twice daily for one day, repeated seven days later. Pyrvinium pamoate (Povan) turns the stool red, and may occasionally be associated with vomiting, diarrhea, and skin rashes. The methods of transmission should be explained to the patient, and care of personal hygiene (short nails, frequent baths, and clean underclothes) instituted before treatment. Follow-up tape swabs are necessary. There is a tendency for some patients to become overanxious about this infection, occasionally with the development of a "worm neurosis." They should be strongly reassured.

Cram, E. B.: Studies on oxyuriasis, xxviii. Summary and conclusions. Am. J. Dis. Child., 65:46, 1943.
Deruiter, H., Rijpstra, A. C., and Swellengrebel, N. H.: Ectopic Enterobius vermicularis; variations on its pattern. Trop. Geogr. Med., 14:375, 1962.
Most, H., Gellin, G. A., Yager, R., Aron, B., Friedlander, M., and Quarfordt, S.: Enterobius (pinworm infection): A study of 951 Puerto Rican and 315 non-Puerto Rican children in New York City. Am. J. Trop. Med. Hyg., 12:65, 1963.

TISSUE NEMATODES

314. TRICHINOSIS*
(Trichiniasis, Trichinellosis)

Definition and Etiology.   Trichinosis is a self-limited infection of the intestine (by the adult parasite) and of the striated muscle (by the larvae) produced by a small nematode, Trichinella spiralis. The same animal host

---

*The present chapter is based on the article on trichinosis prepared by Dr. Harold W. Brown for the twelfth edition of this book. Little new clinical information has developed in the interval; what has appeared has been incorporated in the basic article. P.D.M.

thus acts as both the final and the intermediate host, harboring the adults temporarily and the encysted larvae for long periods. When infected meat containing larvae is ingested, these larvae are released into the upper small intestine by the action of digestive juices. They become adult in five to seven days, the males and females mate, and the fertile female begins to deposit larvae into the mucosa. These larvae pass into the circulation through the hepatic and pulmonary filters, and are carried to all parts of the body. They burrow into the muscles and encyst and complete their development in striated muscle. In other tissues such as the myocardium, brain, and eye, the larvae disintegrate and are absorbed. Among the muscles heavily parasitized are the diaphragmatic, masseteric, intercostal, laryngeal, extraocular, nuchal, pectoral, deltoid, gluteus, biceps, and gastrocnemius. A total of 1500 larvae are liberated by each female worm, usually in four to eight weeks but up to 16 weeks, after which the females die.

Larvae attain a size of 0.4 by 0.025 mm in a cyst in the muscle by the thirty-fifth day. The capsule is complete in three months, and calcification occurs within six months to two years. Recent evidence suggests that there may be strain differences in relation to host susceptibility. The parasite is chiefly found in man, hogs, rats, bears, foxes, walruses, dogs, and cats, but any carnivorous or omnivorous animal may be infected.

Epidemiology. Generally of worldwide distribution, the parasite has not been reported from the islands of the Pacific or Australia. It occurs more frequently in the Northern Hemisphere than in the tropics. It is common in Europe and the United States. Fatal cases have recently been described from Kenya and Chile. It is rare east of the Suez Canal. In the United States there has been a marked reduction in the incidence of the infection, owing to laws requiring the cooking of garbage fed to hogs, storage of meat at low temperature, and education of the public resulting in thorough cooking of pork.

Until quite recently, trichinosis was relatively common in New York City, as pork was being obtained from garbage-fed hogs in New Jersey. However, hog-rearing in this way has substantially declined. Pigs become infected by eating infected meat and occasionally infected rats. Rats are infected in the same way. One of the main methods of transmission is in sausages, wursts, or hamburgers in which the beef is diluted (or actually contaminated in mechanical grinders) with a little pork. Infections from bear and walrus meat have been reported. The low incidence in the tropics is probably due to the fact that meat of any kind is a luxury to many people. Hindus, Jews, and Moslems eschew pork, and the Chinese cook it very well.

Pathology and Pathogenesis. Three to four days after invasion of the muscle, the fiber becomes edematous, loses its cross striations, and undergoes basophilic degeneration. The nuclei increase in number and size, and there is interstitial inflammation around the muscle with a chronic inflammatory cell infiltrate. The severity of the disease depends on the adult worm load, the age of the patient, and the degree of host resistance as well as the numbers of organs involved.

In the heart a focal interstitial myocarditis may occur. Acute nonsuppurative meningitis may be associated with larvae in the cerebrospinal fluid. Larvae may cause lesions in the choroid and retina. Catarrhal enteritis, pulmonary edema, and bronchopneumonia may occur in the early stages of the disease.

Clinical Manifestations. The cardinal features of trichinosis are fever, orbital edema, myalgia, and eosinophilia. Only a small percentage of infected patients have sufficient parasites, however, to produce such clinically recognizable disease. The clinical picture can be divided into distinct stages in a symptomatic infection. First, there is the stage of adult maturation during the first weeks after infection associated with transient gastrointestinal symptoms. From the seventh to the fourteenth day larviposition begins, and muscle penetration commences. This is usually associated with an irregular persistent fever (37.8 to 40.5° C), urticarial rash, and occasionally respiratory symptoms in the form of cough and bronchospasm. Muscle pains become prominent and unusual, but the characteristic physical signs are bilateral orbital edema and subungual and subconjunctival hemorrhages. A severe infection may result in death four to eight weeks after infection from toxemia, secondary pneumonia, myocardial failure, or trichinous encephalitis. Severe muscle involvement may render breathing, masticating, swallowing, or locomotion painful. An eosinophilia beginning seven days after the infection may rise to very high levels (70 per cent) and persist for months. Serum transaminases are also elevated in the invasive stage.

Diagnosis and Differential Diagnosis. Although the rising eosinophilia together with a suggestive clinical picture leads one to suspect this diagnosis, it is proved by finding the larvae in a muscle biopsy. This should be done in the fourth week of infection when a small piece of muscle is removed from the deltoid or gastrocnemius. Crushed between two microscope slides and examined under the low-power objective of the microscope, the living coiled larvae can be seen. In light infections when the direct examination is negative, the biopsy specimen can be incubated overnight in an acid-pepsin mixture and the centrifuged deposit examined for larvae.

Calcified cyst and calcified larvae represent older infections, as calcification usually takes 18 months, but the larva may live inside the calcified cyst for many years. Calcified cysts appear as tiny white spots in fresh muscle, but are too small to be detected radiologically.

A variety of serologic tests are available. The bentonite flocculation test is as sensitive as the complement-fixation test and much easier to perform. It is usually positive four weeks after infection, but may be present earlier. A change from a negative to a positive test during the illness is significant. The indirect fluorescent antibody test detects some infections at an earlier stage. Few other parasitic infections are associated with such persistent fever or generalized muscular aches and tender muscles. Polymyositis of nonparasitic cause may present like this and be associated with eosinophilia. Periarteritis nodosa may also mimic trichinosis.

Treatment. Patients with symptomatic trichinosis should be confined to bed and given a smooth high-calorie, high-protein diet. Congestive cardiac failure should be searched for and, if present, should be treated. Mild analgesics can be given for the muscle pain. Anti-inflammatory steroids (prednisolone, 5 mg three times daily) relieve fever, edema, and muscle pain in severe acute cases but are said not to affect the adult worms' fecundity or the number of larvae settling in the muscle. In patients with central nervous system involvement this effect of steroids is dramatic.

Thiabendazole, in a dose of 25 mg per kilogram of body weight for five to seven days, has also produced a marked resolution of the symptoms of fever and muscle pain, but living larvae have still been recovered on muscle biopsy after much larger courses of the drug. In severe infections the use of corticosteroids and thiabendazole may be lifesaving, but when the parasite load is not considerable, the prognosis is good even without treatment.

Prevention. The ultimate prevention of trichinosis is dependent on its elimination in hogs, and the incidence in these animals can be greatly reduced by heat-sterilizing garbage. Freezing meat at −32° C for a few hours (or at 15 to 30° C for several weeks) kills larvae, as does gamma radiation of the meat. Pigs fed on a diet containing 0.1 per cent thiabendazole fail to incubate *T. spiralis* on challenge. Routine meat inspection does not detect the infection, and serologic and skin tests on pigs have not been helpful in detecting infected animals. The chief safeguard at present is the thorough cooking of pork at 60° C for 30 minutes for each pound of meat.

Gould, S. E.: Trichinosis. Springfield, Ill., Charles C Thomas, 1945.
Hennekeuser, M. H., Pabst, K., Poeplau, W., and Gerok, W.: Thiabendazole for the treatment of trichinosis in humans. Tex. Rep. Biol. Med., 27 (Supplement 2):581, 1969.
Maynard, J. E., and Kagan, I. G.: Trichinosis (serology). Practitioner, 191:622, 1963.
Moser, R. H.: Trichinosis from Bismarck to polar bears. J.A.M.A., 228:735, 1974.
Proceedings of the International Commission in Trichinellosis: No. VI. Wiad. Parazyt., 14:127, 1968.
Zimmerman, W. J., Steele, J. H., and Kagan, I. G.: The changing status of trichiniasis in the U.S. population. Public Health Rep., 83:957, 1968.

315. ANGIOSTRONGYLIASIS

Angiostrongylus Cantonensis. Eosinophilic meningoencephalitis, a syndrome caused by *Angiostrongylus cantonensis* (the rat lung worm), was first recognized in New Caledonia in 1950, and has since been reported from Hawaii, Tahiti, other Pacific Islands, Indonesia, and Thailand. The human disease has only been reported from the Far East and the Pacific to date, although infected rats have been found in Madagascar, Mauritius, Ceylon, and Sarawak.

The life cycle was described by workers in Australia in 1955 before the importance of the worm as a human pathogen was known. A delicate filiform nematode, 17 to 25 mm in length, the adult lives in the lungs of rats, and the eggs are coughed up, swallowed, and pass out in the feces as first-stage larvae. Further development occurs in slugs and snails to the third-stage infective larvae. These larvae are ingested by man either while in this intermediate host or after they have been shed by it onto some other article of food, e.g., lettuce. Crabs and freshwater prawns have also been found to be infected with these metastrongyloid larvae, but probably act as paratenic hosts. The dispersal of the giant African land snail *Achatina fulica* may have assisted the spread of the infection. When infective larvae are ingested by the rat, they migrate to the brain and reach young adulthood in four weeks. They then migrate to the pulmonary arteries and after two more weeks start laying eggs. Unfortunately if man accidentally ingests these infective larvae, they migrate to the brain (as in the rat), and there produce the clinical picture of a meningoencephalitis associated with fever, signs of cerebral irritation, mental deficit, and varying degrees of loss of consciousness. Mild blood eosinophilia is present, and lumbar puncture reveals a fluid under increased pressure with increased protein and many eosinophils (from 100 to 3000 per cubic millimeter). Occasionally patients present with a facial nerve lesion or complaints of diplopia and parasthesia. A complement-fixation test using an extract of adult worms as antigen has been developed. The illness usually persists for some weeks or months and then the patient recovers spontaneously.

Young adult worms have been found in the brain and cerebrospinal fluid of man, and experimental infection of monkeys produces a similar syndrome. The pathology of the brain in fatal cases is one of focal areas of softening, the meninges and subarachnoid space being infiltrated with plasma cells, lymphocytes, eosinophils, and neutrophils. There is perivascular cuffing with chronic inflammatory cells in the brain substance. Careful sectioning of the brain is necessary to find the 0.16 to 8 mm nematodes.

This condition must be differentiated from a variety of other parasitic infections involving the central nervous system. In Thailand cerebral gnathostomiasis and Angiostrongylus infections occur. Cerebral paragonimiasis could be an important differential diagnosis in parts of the Far East. In other situations the syndrome of eosinophilic meningitis could be produced by cysticercosis, hydatid, schistosomiasis, fascioliasis, trichinosis, and possibly strongyloidiasis. Refinements of serologic diagnostic techniques will help in this sometimes difficult clinical problem.

The author has been able to trace no references to treatment with thiabendazole, although this would seem to be the drug to try. Prevention entails education regarding dangerous foods such as raw crabs and prawns and undercooked snails, and making sure that lettuce is free of slugs and snails. Freezing of crustaceans and molluscs at −15° C for 12 hours has been found to be effective in destroying the infective larvae of *A. cantonensis*.

Angiostrongylus Costaricensis. Human disease caused by this parasite has recently been described from Costa Rica where 130 cases have been studied. The worm also occurs in Honduras and Panama. Patients, usually children, present with right iliac fossa pain, fever, and blood eosinophilia, and often an abdominal mass is palpable. At operation an eosinophilic granulomatous cecal pseudotumor is found to contain adult worms and eggs.

The intermediate host is a slug, *Vaginulus (Sarasinula) plebius,* and the definitive hosts are at least five species of rodents, including *Rattus rattus.* Infected slugs contaminate lettuce leaves with infective third-stage larvae, and man acquires the disease by ingesting the slug itself on contaminated salad. In the rodent host — and probably in man — the cycle occurs in the abdominal cavity. The third and fourth larval molts occur in lymph vessels. After three months the young adults move to radicles of the mesenteric arteries, mate, mature, and oviposit. Arteritis and thrombosis may be followed by macro- or microinfarcts of the gut, with ulceration and necrosis of the gut wall. Fistulization or generalized peritonitis may ensue. Neither larvae nor eggs are usually detected in the stools of man.

In *Angiostrongylus costaricensis* infection of man, sexually mature adult worms develop, and as such this species is better adapted to man than *Angiostrongylus cantonensis.*

Alicata, J. E.: Present status of *Angiostrongylus cantonensis* infection in man and animals in the tropics. J. Trop. Med. Hyg., 72:53, 1969.
Mackerras, M. T., and Sanders, D. F.: The life history of the rat lungworm *Angiostrongylus cantonensis* (Chen) (Nematoda; Metastrongylidae). Aust. J. Zool., 3:1, 1955.

Morera, P.: Life cycle and redescription of *Angiostrongylus costaricensis* (Morera and Cespedes 1971). Am. J. Trop. Med. Hyg., 22:613, 1973.

Schollhaminer, G., Aubry, P., and Rigaud, J. L.: Quelques réflexions sur la méningite à éosinophiles a Tahiti. Étude clinique et biologique de 165 observations, à propos d'un cas atypique. Bull. Soc. Pathol. Exot., 59:341, 1966.

316. FILARIASIS

GENERAL CONSIDERATIONS

To talk of filariasis as such is to use a general term like anemia, for there are seven types of nematodes found in man belonging to the superfamily Filarioidea, as well as one member of the superfamily Dracunculoidea (the guinea worm), which is usually included in a consideration of this group. Of these Filarioidea, the embryos or microfilariae are found in the blood in five and in the subcutaneous tissues in two species. The adults are viviparous, and the blood microfilariae demonstrate a periodicity in the peripheral blood, depending on the species. They may remain ensheathed in their elongated egg shell or have no sheath. These microfilariae are distinguished on their criteria as well on as the pattern of distribution of nuclei seen in stained specimens in their tails. Giemsa stain can be used, but better results of sheath staining are obtained with Delafield's hematoxylin or Mayer's acid hemalum.

In Table 2 the various species are listed and the characteristics of their microfilariae are shown. The adult worms live for many years, whereas blood microfilariae have a life of three to six months. After being bitten by an infected arthropod it may take 1 year to 18 months before microfilariae are present in the peripheral blood, a long prepatent period. The controlling mechanism for periodicity has never been satisfactorily explained for many of these human species. However, Hawking's recent work suggests that at least two circadian rhythms are involved, one mechanism within the microfilariae themselves, and the other some physiological tide in the host (body temperature for certain animal species). This periodicity fits the habits of the insect vector; for instance, the Loa insect vector flies by day, but most bancrofti infections are transmitted nocturnally. The geographic distribution of these species is of particular importance, because in some it is markedly restricted. For instance *Loa loa* is a filarid of Equatorial Africa, and *Mansonella ozzardi* is only found in South America.

Not all the species listed are significantly pathogenic.

Few symptoms have been ascribed to *Mansonella ozzardi* infections, and the case for the pathogenicity of *D. perstans* is very shaky. Two of these filarial infections are notable in terms of their importance in man. These are the *Wuchereria-Brugia complex*, which produces bancroftian filariasis with lymphatic obstruction and elephantiasis, and *onchocerciasis*, which is a common cause of blindness in endemic areas. Multiple infections occur, in endemic areas, for instance, in parts of West Africa a patient may be seen infected with *Loa loa*, bancrofti, perstans, and onchocerciasis.

This final group of the most modified nematodes will be considered in the order in which they are listed in Table 2, except that the guinea worm will be considered first. Dirofilariasis and pulmonary tropical eosinophilia will then be reviewed.

Hawking, F.: Advances in filariasis. Trans. R. Soc. Trop. Med. Hyg., 59:9, 1965.

Hawking, F., Moore, P., Gammage, K., and Worms, M. J.: Periodicity of microfiliae. XII. The effect of variations in host body temperature on the cycle of *Loa loa, Monnigofilaria setariosa. Durofilaria immitis,* and other filariae. Trans. R. Soc. Trop. Med. Hyg., 61:674, 1967.

DRACONTIASIS
(Guinea Worm)

Infection with the guinea worm (*Dracunculus medinensis*) usually presents as a skin ulceration at the site of emergence of the female adult worm. Man is probably the only reservoir, although monkeys and dogs can be experimentally infected. Human infections are widespread in the tropics, occurring in local distribution in West Africa and the Nile Valley, the Middle East, India and Pakistan, the Caribbean Islands, Guyana, and Brazil. Infection occurs on ingesting infected water fleas (Cyclops) present in drinking water from shallow wells or ponds. The infective larvae in the Cyclops penetrate the intestinal walls and mature in the loose connective tissue under the skin, especially that of legs and feet. The male worm is small and dies after copulation. The female requires a year to become gravid, and then measures up to a meter long and is 2 mm in diameter. When ready to discharge larvae, she approaches the skin surface, and a blister is produced by secretion of a toxic substance from the anterior end of the worm. The blister breaks down to form an ulcer a few centimeters across, and the anterior end of the worm protrudes into this ulcer. On contact with water the head of the worm ruptures, and the uterus periodically discharges the tightly coiled larvae infective to the water flea. Secondary infec-

TABLE 2. Common Filarioidea of Man as Distinguished by Characteristics of Microfilariae

	Periodicity of Microfilariae	Sheathed or Unsheathed	Tail Morphology
Microfilariae in blood:			
Wuchereria bancrofti	Majority nocturnal	Sheathed	Nuclei not to tip of tail
Brugia malayi	Majority nocturnal	Sheathed	Two distinct nuclei in tail tip
Loa loa	Diurnal	Sheathed	Nuclei to tip of tail
Mansonella ozzardi	Nonperiodic	Not sheathed	Nuclei not to tip of tail
Dipetalonema perstans	Nocturnally subperiodic	Not sheathed	Nuclei to tip of tail
Microfilariae in subcutaneous tissues:			
Onchocerca volvulus	Nonperiodic	Not sheathed	Nuclei not to tip of tail
Dipetalonema streptocerca	Nonperiodic	Not sheathed	Nuclei to tip of tail, which is crooked

tion of the ulcer with resultant cellulitis is common. Generalized allergic symptoms may occur prior to the blister formation or when surgical removal of the worm is attempted. Multiple infections are common. The lesion is usually on the lower leg, but may occur on the genitalia, buttocks, or upper limbs. In water carriers lesions have been observed on the back, suggesting that the worm is positively hydrotropic. Alternatively, the mature female may never reach the surface of the body and may be absorbed or calcify in the tissue. The radiologic appearance is pathognomonic because the worm is so large. If a gravid worm dies in situ or is broken during extraction, cellulitis and secondary infection often occur. This may give rise to contractures. Also *Clostridium tetani* may contaminate the wound and tetanus may result. Rarely the adult worm involves serous cavities, the extradural space, or joints. Guinea worm arthritis appears to be due to the presence of the adult worm or larvae in the joint. A microscopic diagnosis can be made by finding embryos in the exudate from the guinea worm ulcer after exposure to a few drops of water.

Gradually winding the worm out of the ulcer by turning it on a stick a few centimeters a day is still common practice. Surgical extraction is also practiced. Recently niridazole (Ambilhar) has been reported to be lethal to the adult worm, which can readily be withdrawn after a course of 25 mg per kilogram of body weight for seven days. Thiabendazole is also effective. Prevention involves contructing water sources that cannot be contaminated and killing cyclops by chlorination or boiling water to be used for drinking.

Muller, R.: Dracunculus and dracunculiasis. *In* Dawes, B. (ed.): Advances in Parasitology, Vol. 9, New York, Academic Press, 1973, p. 73.
Raffier, G.: Efficacy of thiabendazole in the treatment of dracunculiasis. Texas Rep. Biol. Med., 27(Supplement 2):601, 1969.

BANCROFTIAN FILARIASIS

Etiology. Bancroftian filariasis is caused by the filarial worm *Wuchereria bancrofti*. The adult worms reside in the lymphatic system and produce recurrent lymphangitis with fibrosis and obstruction. The infection is transmitted by culicine and anopheline mosquitoes.

The threadlike adult worms are 4 to 10 cm long and live for decades. The female worm is viviparous, producing microfilariae 130 to 320 μ long which are found in the peripheral blood; in some forms this occurs only at night, whereas during the day the microfilariae are in the lungs. If ingested by a suitable mosquito, these microfilariae develop in the thoracic muscles of the insect and are present in the mouth parts after two weeks. They enter the skin through the puncture wound when the mosquito next feeds and, finding their way to the lymphatics of the host, the males and females mate and mature. More than a year after infection microfilariae appear in the peripheral blood.

Epidemiology. Man is the only definitive host of this common type of filariasis. Periodic bancroftian filariasis is found throughout tropical Africa and North Africa, as well as in the tropical coastal borders of Asia and Queensland. It is endemic in the West Indies and the northern countries of South America. In the northern Pacific bancroftian filariasis exhibits nocturnal periodicity, but in the Pacific Islands east of 160 degrees of longitude (including New Caledonia, Fiji, Samoa, the Ellis and Cook Islands, Society Islands, and the Marquesas) the microfilariae are nonperiodic, being present in the peripheral blood throughout the 24-hour period. The term *W. bancrofti var. pacifica* has been applied to this strain.

Pathology. The severity of the lesions probably depends on the adult worm load and their site of development and the susceptibility of the host. Light infections are often asymptomatic, and microfilariae are detected on incidental blood examinations. Maturing adults in the lymphatics are associated with endothelial thickening, fibrin deposition, and infiltration with eosinophils, histiocytes, and lymphocytes. Giant cells occur. Fibrotic and inflammatory changes tend to obstruct the lymphatics, and this process is exacerbated by death of the worms, which may calcify. There is reactive hyperplasia in the lymph nodes, and small granulomas are seen. An eosinophilic endophlebitis of the small veins is present in the lymph nodes. The testicles and epididymis often show similar changes with evidence of chronic inflammation. Worms may not be present at the site of inflammation. Secretions of the worm, especially after molting, are thought to be responsible for some of these changes. As lymphatic obstruction becomes more extensive, chronic edema develops in the infected areas. Recently lymphedema has been produced in laboratory animals with longstanding bancrofti infections.

Clinical Manifestations. Attacks of fever, headache, and lymphadenopathy sometimes associated with urticarial rashes are known as filarial fever and occur in the acute phase of the disease. Often, however, no history of this early phase can be obtained. Epididymitis may occur as a lone lesion. Lymphatics most affected are those of the inguinal region, upper arms, and spermatic cord. Chronic lymphadenopathy is often the only sign of infection for years. Retrograde lymphangitis may be noted. In a small proportion of infected individuals, with increasing lymphatic obstruction over the years, all degrees of chronic edema occur, affecting especially the lower limbs and scrotum. Initially the edema is pitting, but as organization of collagen occurs in the edematous subcutaneous tissues, it becomes nonpitting. Eventually the giant limbs of elephantiasis are produced. The skin over the affected part, at first smooth, later becomes scaly and is fissured at the points where the fascia is attached to the skin. Hyperkeratosis produces warts and nodules. Varicose nodes in the groin are the result of lymphatic dilatation and may lead to scrotal lymphedema. Infection may supervene in any of these lesions with formation of a chronic discharging sinus. Chronic inflammatory disease of the testicle and epididymis with or without hydrocele occurs.

Chyluria may be renal or vesical in origin, depending on the level at which the lymph varix communicates with the urinary tract. Cystoscopy and intravenous or retrograde pyelography help to establish the site of communication.

Diagnosis. In the early stages and when lymphadenopathy only is present, microfilariae are usually present in night blood films. Although the motile microfilariae are easily seen in fresh films, staining is necessary for identification. Microfilariae may be absent in the late stage; thus only 4 per cent of patients with elephantiasis and 30 per cent of patients with hydrocele had microfilariae in one series. Concentration techniques are available for microfilariae, and they may be found in the chylous urine or hydrocele fluid. Eosinophilia is not a constant finding. The filarial complement-fixation test and skin test, although only group specific, are useful in suggesting a filarial cause for a lymphedema. Lymphangiograms reveal the extent of the lymphatic obstruction and may be a useful preoperative measure. It is rarely justified to remove an enlarged lymph node to find the adults because this still further prejudices the lymphatic circulation. In an endemic area surgeons frequently encounter adult worms when operating on the groin.

The differential diagnosis depends on the type of clinical syndrome. Lymphadenopathy caused by other infections and neoplasms must be considered. Elephantiasis may be associated with congenital defects of the lymphatic drainage as well as tuberculous inguinal lymphadenitis. Tuberculosis, *Schistosoma haematobium,* and gonorrhea produce epididymitis, and relatively few hydroceles are filarial. Lymphatic obstruction caused by many other agents may produce lymphedema and chyluria.

Treatment. Diethylcarbamazine (Banocide, Hetrazan) is believed to kill a large proportion of adults as well as microfilariae. A dose of 3 mg per kilogram of body weight is given, rising to a maximum of 12 mg per kilogram over four days. This dose is then given daily for 14 days. Reactions are mild in comparison with those seen in onchocerciasis, but fever, nausea and vomiting, and skin rashes may occur as with any drug. The arsenical Mel W and the antimonial Astiban (sodium dimercaptosuccinate) kill adult filariae, but are too toxic for general use. All patients with microfilaremia should receive an adequate course of treatment.

The management of lymphedema depends on its severity. Mild degrees are best treated with elevation of the foot of the bed and an elastic stocking. Careful instructions regarding foot care should be given, as ascending streptocccal cellulitis is common in the edematous tissues and further prejudices the lymphatic circulation. Some workers believe the Streptococcus to be more important in producing lymphangitis than the worms themselves. Any foot sepsis requires early and vigorous treatment with antimicrobial drugs. Tinea infections should be eradicated. Banocide therapy is often given in elephantiasis on the ground that it may prevent further lymphatic damage, but clinical improvement is seldom observed.

A variety of surgical operations have been devised to remove the edematous subcutaneous tissue from the leg, scrotum, and breasts. Success depends on the type of operation and the skill of the surgeon. In scrotal elephantiasis care must be taken to preserve the testicles. Hydroceles can be treated by the injection of sclerosing agents. Chyluria of bladder origin can be terminated by fulgurating the leaking bladder lymphatics. Renal chyluria is best left alone, although in the past kidneys have been wrapped in cellophane with the subsequent production of renal hypertension.

Prevention. Diethylcarbamazine, 3 mg per kilogram per month for 12 to 18 months, has been effective in mass treatment for preventive purposes. Residual DDT or dieldrin is effective against many of the mosquito vectors, and systematic destruction of mosquito-breeding sites has also met with success. Biologic control of mosquito vectors is receiving intensive field trials, but thus far they have not resulted in methods for mass application.

MALAYAN FILARIASIS

A disease similar to bancroftian filariasis is produced by a closely related filarial worm, *Brugia malayi.* The sheathed microfilariae of this species have two distinct caudal nuclei. Transmitted by mansonoides mosquitoes, it is the only filarial infection of man in Malaya and Borneo, whereas in India, Ceylon, and tropical China it coexists with *W. bancrofti. Brugia malayi* is responsible for only mild lymphedema in man, usually below the knee, with enlargement of the popliteal and femoral nodes. In contrast to bancroftian filariasis, the microfilaremia rates in the Malayan form are quite high in children younger than five years. In this infection, also, there are two types of organisms, one with nocturnal periodicity, and another subperiodic form. The latter is found in many animals (primates, carnivores, and rodents) and is a true zoonosis.

Galindo, L., Von Lichtenberg, F., and Baldison, C.: Bancroftian filariasis in Puerto Rico: Infection pattern and tissue lesions. Am. J. Trop. Med., 11:739, 1962.

Nelson, G. S.: The pathology of filarial infections. Helminth. Abst., 35:Pt. 4, 311, 1966.

Schacher, J. F., and Sahyoun, P. F.: A chronological study of the histopathology of filarial disease in cats and dogs caused by *Brugia phangi* (Buckley and Edeson, 1956). Trans. R. Soc. Trop. Med. Hyg., 61:234, 1967.

Turner, L. H.: Studies on filariasis in Malaya: the clinical features of filariasis due to *Wuchereria malayi.* Trans. R. Soc. Trop. Med. Hyg., 53:154, 1959.

Wilson, T.: Filariasis in Malaya—A general review. Trans. R. Soc. Trop. Med. Hyg., 55:107, 1961.

LOIASIS

Loa loa infection is characterized by the appearance of transient swellings mainly on the limbs; these are thought to be the site of the migrating adult worms in the subcutaneous tissue. Occasionally a worm will traverse the conjunctiva of the eye.

The male adult worm is 30 mm long and the female 70 mm. They live for many years, and gain access to the body through the proboscis of biting flies (deer flies of the genus Chrysops). These worms appear to be in a state of continuous migration in the subcutaneous tissues of the body. It is not clearly understood how the sexes locate each other, but they meet and mate, and the female produces microfilariae that appear in the blood during the day and are infective to the insect vector.

Man is the only reservoir host, with the possible exception of monkeys. Human loiasis is restricted to Africa, mainly the West Coast. It occurs from Sierra Leone to the Cameroons and extends into the heart of Africa in the region of the Congo basin.

Clinical Manifestations. The main clinical manifestation is the repeated occurrence of hot erythematous swellings (5 to 10 cm or more) called Calabar swellings after the endemic area of Calabar. These occur in the upper limbs particularly, are painful, and subside in a few days. They are associated with the presence of an adult worm. A similar swelling occurs around the eye when the adult worm crosses the eye beneath the conjunctivae. The patient notices the worm in his line of vision ("like a submarine, doctor") and it is worth inquiring for such a history. Calabar swellings seem to occur more frequently in the extremities. Why this is so is not known. Routine roentgenography in endemic areas often reveals calcified dead worms lying between the metacarpals. Rarely, neurologic symptoms may be associated with the infection if the Calabar swelling involves a peripheral nerve. Also the parasite has been found in the cerebrospinal fluid associated with a meningoencephalitis.

Diagnosis. The initial diagnosis is usually based on a history of Calabar swellings in a patient coming from an endemic area. Examination of the daytime blood reveals sheathed microfilariae with a characteristic distribution of caudal nuclei. In early loiasis, microfilariae may not be detected even by concentration techniques. Very high eosinophil counts are encountered at this stage (50 to 70 per cent). A positive filarial complement-fixation test is usually present. Occasionally the adult worm can be extracted as it crosses the eye. It has been suggested that another human filarid, *Acanthocheilonema perstans*, may cause Calabar swellings.

Treatment. Diethylcarbamazine (Hetrazan) kills both adults and microfilariae. One course of 12 mg per kilogram of body weight for 14 days is all that is necessary. Reactions are rare.

Woodruff, A. W.: Loiasis. *In* Fairley, N. H., Woodruff, A. W., and Walters, J. H. (eds.): Recent Advances in Tropical Medicine. London, J. & A. Churchill, Ltd., 1961, pp. 178–194.

MANSONELLA OZZARDI

Mansonella ozzardi is found only in the New World, occurring in South America and certain foci in the Caribbean. The adult worms are embedded in visceral adipose tissue. Although they are usually regarded as nonpathogenic, fever, headache, lymphadenitis, and erythematous irritant skin rashes have been reported in association with their presence. Cold extremities, the result of peripheral vasoconstriction caused by a postulated filarial toxin, have been reported. The microfilariae show no particular periodicity and are about twice the size of perstans and have a different caudal morphology. *Simulium amazonicum* has been implicated as the vector, and midges of the genus Culicoides have also been suggested. A recent survey, cited below, showed that of 810 Colombian Indians, 96.2 per cent harbored microfilariae of *Mansonella ozzardi*.

Marinkelle, C. J., and German, E.: Mansonelliasis in the Comisaría del Vaupes of Colombia. Trop. Geog. Med., 22:101, 1970.

Undiano, C.: Importance and present-day concepts of the pathogenicity of Mansonella infections. Fev. Fac. Cienc. Med. Univ. Cordoba, 24:183, 1966.

DIPETALONEMA PERSTANS

Filariasis caused by *Dipetalonema perstans* has an extensive distribution in Equatorial Africa, the Caribbean, and South America, where it sometimes overlaps with *Mansonella ozzardi*. The adult worms are found in association with the serous cavities of the body, usually behind the limiting membrane. They may be seen at postmortem examination moving behind the peritoneum or pleura. The small (100 μ) unsheathed microfilariae are found in the blood throughout the 24 hours, but there is a peak in the peripheral blood population at night. A Culicoides species, a small black midge, is responsible for transmission.

The vast majority of patients exhibiting microfilaremia have no symptoms, but there have been recent reports of clinical symptoms associated with this infection. These reports include fever, Calabar swellings, arthritis, and upper abdominal pain associated with hepatomegaly. A high eosinophilia is often present in cases with scanty embryos, and such a finding in a patient from an endemic area should prompt a careful search for these. Diethylcarbamazine (Hetrazan) has little effect on the adults or on the microfilariae.

Wiseman, R. A.: *Acanthocheilonema perstans:* A cause of significant eosinophilia in the tropics. Comments on its pathogenicity. Trans. R. Soc. Trop. Med. Hyg., 61:667, 1967.

ONCHOCERCIASIS
(River Blindness)

River blindness is a form of cutaneous filariasis caused by infection with *Onchocerca volvulus* and is characterized by skin irritation, corneal opacities, and skin nodules.

Etiology. The threadlike adult worms lie tangled together in fibrous nodules in the subcutaneous tissues or fascial planes. Microfilariae produced by the females become widely distributed in the surrounding skin. Female black flies (buffalo gnats) of the genus Simulium ingest these larvae while taking a blood meal. After development in the fly for one week, the larvae are infective for man and are deposited when the fly next bites. They take more than a year to mature, mate, and produce microfilariae. Adult worms live 7 to 15 years.

Epidemiology. Human onchocerciasis is found on the West Coast of Africa from Sierra Leone to the Congo and in the east from the Sudan to Nyasaland. It also occurs in Guatemala, Mexico, Eastern Venezuela, Northern Brazil, and Surinam. Simulium larvae and pupae are usually found in rapidly running highly oxygenated water. Small insects (3 mm long), the flies bite low on the legs in Africa, but more around the head in Central America, which may account for the high incidence of nodules on the head in the latter locality. In East Africa *Simulium naevi* larvae and pupae evaded detection for many years until they were found on the shells of freshwater crabs.

Pathogenesis and Pathology. An initial inflammatory reaction around the adult worm is followed by a foreign body granulomatous reaction and fibrous capsule formation. The nodules are literally the graveyards of the adult worms, for these eventually die and degenerate, sometimes with secondary abscess formation. The microfilariae in the surrounding subcutaneous tissues produce a low-grade inflammatory reaction with lymphocytes, plasma cells, and eosinophils. Thickening of the epidermis and dermis owing to fibrosis eventually occurs, with destruction of elastic fibers and sometimes reduction in pigmentation.

Microfilariae migrate into the tissues of the eye to produce important inflammatory lesions which may result in blindness. Punctate keratitis is associated with death of microfilariae in the cornea, and such multiple corneal opacities may result in permanent corneal scarring. A low-grade iritis and iridocyclitis result in pupillary distortion and even occlusion. Choroidoretinitis also occurs.

Clinical Manifestations. Any patient who has a persistent irritating skin rash or visual disturbances and has been in one of the endemic areas may have onchocerciasis. More rarely, the presenting complaint takes the form of deep-seated muscular pains. The early skin lesions consist of an erythematous papular irritant rash. In heavy infections definite thickening and hyperkeratosis of the skin occurs (craw-craw or crocodile skin). Rarer late complications are depigmentation and pendulous bags in the groins containing sclerosed lymph nodes.

Nodules vary much in size from a few centimeters to as big as a tennis ball. They are frequently detected over bony prominences such as the greater trochanter, the iliac crest, the olecranons, ribs, and occiput. Often the adult worms are located deep in the fascial planes, and no nodules are palpable. To detect the small milky dots of punctate keratitis near the limbus the eyes should be examined with a strong pencil torch, the beam directed obliquely across the cornea. Signs of iritis may be present. With a slit lamp, microfilariae may be visible in the aqueous humor. Funduscopic examination may reveal the much rarer posterior segment lesion.

Diagnosis. Skin shavings are used to demonstrate microfilariae. Thin sections of the superficial skin are removed with a razor blade, mounted in saline, teased out, and examined. Many motile microfilariae emerge from those snips within an hour after they have been made. Blood contamination can be avoided if the shavings are superficial, and this is important if there is a coexistent blood microfilaremia. If there is a definite site of skin irritation, shavings should be taken from this area. In lightly infected patients multiple shavings may be necessary to detect microfilariae, and quite often they are not found. The reaction to a test dose of 50 mg of diethylcarbamazine (Mazzotti's test) in the form of an exacerbation of the itching rash is suggestive, as are an eosinophilia and a positive filarial complement-fixation test. In up to 35 per cent of cases microfilariae can be found in the urine.

Scabies and superficial mycoses are the most common irritant skin rashes of the tropics and are important differential diagnoses. Streptocerciasis caused by infection with the rare, closely related filarid *Acanthocheilonema streptocerca* also presents as an irritating rash and requires only mention. Although an infection with no mortality, the recurrent irritation of onchocerciasis can be most distressing. Severe ocular lesions may induce total blindness, and this is the blinding filarid.

Treatment. When practicable, all nodules should be excised; this simple measure will reduce the load of adult worms. Suramin is effective in killing adult worms. The side effects and method of administration of this drug are mentioned under African Trypanosomiasis (Ch. 272). A suitable course for onchocerciasis is 1 gram weekly for six weeks. As the drug is nephrotoxic, treatment should be stopped if more than 30 mg per 100 ml of protein appears in the urine.

Diethylcarbamazine is effective in killing microfilariae but does not kill the adult worms. In sensitized individuals, reactions occur when the microfilariae die in the tissues. Skin irritation becomes more intense, and there may be edema of the skin with fever, headache, and malaise. More serious is acute inflammation of the eye which may prejudice sight. As these reactions are dose related, it is usual to start therapy with a small dose of the drug (0.5 mg per kilogram) and increase gradually to the doses recommended in the previous article. Eye reactions can be controlled with 1 per cent cortisone acetate eye drops and the general reactions controlled with antihistamines and, in severe cases, with systemic steroids.

Prevention. Simulium larvae and pupae are very sensitive to small concentrations of DDT in the river water (less than 1 part per million), and this has been the most effective form of control of the insect vector. Personal prophylaxis is possible to a limited extent by avoiding places where biting Simulium are numerous.

Buck, A. A. (ed.): Onchocerciasis. Symptomatology, Pathology, and Diagnosis. Geneva, World Health Organization, 1974.

Duke, B. O. L.: Onchocerciasis. Br. Med. J., 4:301, 1968.

Nelson, D. S.: Onchocerciasis. *In* Dawes, B. (ed.): Advances in Parasitology. Volume 8. New York, Academic Press, 1970, p. 173.

WHO Expert Committee on Onchocerciasis. World Health Organization Technical Report Series No. 335, 1–92, 1966.

Woodruff, A. W., Choyce, D. P., Muci-Mendoza, F., Hills, M., and Pettitt, L. E.: Onchocerciasis in Guatemala: a clinical parasitological study with comparison between the disease there and in East Africa. Trans. R. Soc. Trop. Med. Hyg., 60:695, 1966.

STREPTOCERCIASIS

Dipetalonema streptocerca is carried by midges of the genus Culicoides. It occurs in Central Africa, particularly in the Congo and neighboring countries. The adult worms are found in the region of the shoulder girdle, and the microfilariae produced in the skin cause a reddish brown irritant rash which may be associated with some degree of edema. Skin shavings reveal the unsheathed microfilariae with the crooked tails and the nuclei going down to the tip. Treatment with diethylcarbamazine is effective.

Meyers, W. M., Connor, D. H., Harman, L. E., Fleshman, K., Moris, R. and Neafie, R. G.: Human streptocerciasis: A clinicopathologic study of 40 Africans (Zairans), including identification of the adult filaria. Am. J. Trop. Med. Hyg., 21:528, 1972.

DIROFILARIASIS

Several Dirofilariae have been reported to occasionally cause symptoms in man, particularly in the United States. Such infections have also been reported from the Mediterranean basin, South America, and Africa. In Louisiana and Texas a subcutaneous filarid of raccoons *(Dirofilaria tenuis)* occasionally invades man, but does not mature. It produces a painful subcutaneous nodule, consisting of an eosinophilic inflammatory reaction around the worm; this may be a granuloma or may be located in a lymph node. The diagnosis is usually made after biopsy. Mosquitoes transmit the infection.

Other species found in man include *D. conjunctivae, D. repens,* and *D. immitis.* Adult worms have been detected in the heart and great vessels and in the eye. They have also caused infarcts in the lung and "coin" lesions at the hila which may be mistaken for a bronchial carcinoma and excised before the nature is known. In sections the worm is seen in cross section in the center of an infarcted area infiltrated with eosinophils.

Beaver, P. C., and Orihel, T. C.: Human infection with filariae of animals in the United States. Am. J. Trop. Med. Hyg., 14:1010, 1965.

Beskin, C. A., Colvin, S. H., Jr., and Beaver, P. C.: Pulmonary dirofilariasis, cause of a pulmonary nodular disease. J.A.M.A., 198:665, 1966.

POSSIBLE HUMAN MENINGONEMIASIS

Recently Orihel has pointed out that microfilariae recovered from patients with neurologic disorders in

Rhodesia and thought to be *Dipetalonema perstans* more closely resemble *Meningonema peruzzii*. The adults of this species inhabit the leptomeninges of the brainstem in African monkeys.

Orihel, T. C.: Cerebral filariasis in Rhodesia—a zoonotic infection. Am. J. Trop. Med. Hyg., 22:596, 1973.

PULMONARY TROPICAL EOSINOPHILIA
(Eosinophilic Lung, Weingarten's Syndrome)

Since the early part of this century Indian physicians have recognized a syndrome of paroxysmal cough and nocturnal bronchospasm associated with high eosinophilia, and have called it pulmonary tropical eosinophilia. Low fever, dyspnea, and malaise may be accompanying symptoms. The absolute eosinophil count is above 3000 per cubic millimeter, and may reach very high levels. Chest films may show increased reticulation, prominence of bronchovascular markings, or diffuse miliary mottling of the lung fields. In Ball's series of 1000 cases the great majority were Indian; the condition is much more common among Indians in Singapore. It is now generally accepted that this syndrome is caused by occult filarial infections. The evidence that this is so can be listed as follows: (1) Patients have a consistently high titer of filarial complement-fixing antibodies in the absence of evidence of microfilariae in the blood. (2) There is a clinical, hematologic, and serologic response to therapy with the antifilarial drug diethylcarbamazine. (3) The syndrome has been produced in a volunteer by inoculation of *Brugia malayi* infective larvae and *Brugia pahangi* (a feline filaria). (4) Microfilariae have been demonstrated in lung granulomas in such cases by several groups of workers.

It is possible that eosinophilic lung results from an alteration in host immunity to the filarial parasite, giving rise to allergic phenomena manifested by persistent hypereosinophilia and pulmonary symptoms. What is not yet settled is the precise identification of the parasite. It is likely that several species of filaria of the genera Wuchereria and Brugia, some human, some animal, may be involved, depending on the locality in which the syndrome occurs. The high incidence in Indians is noteworthy and may suggest a genetic predisposition in certain racial groups. The course of diethylcarbamazide recommended is similar to that for bancroftian filariasis. Often the symptoms get temporarily worse after starting the drug, but invariably they resolve, and a second course of the drug or the use of carbarsone as an alternative is seldom necessary.

The question of occult filariasis has recently been reviewed, and it has been pointed out that in many instances it has not been possible to identify the helminth responsible because of the difficulty of interpreting the microfilariae in tissue sections even if they are found. Quite apart from the well defined clinical entity of pulmonary tropical eosinophilia there are patients presenting with signs of reticuloendothelial activation (enlarged lymph nodes, hepatosplenomegaly) and eosinophilia for which it is difficult to find a cause.

Ball, J. D.: Tropical pulmonary eosinophilia. Trans. R. Soc. Trop. Med. Hyg., 44:237, 1950.

Donohugh, D. L.: Tropical eosinophilia, an etiologic enquiry. N. Engl. J. Med., 269:1357, 1963.

Danaraj, T. J., Pacheco, G., Shanmugaratnam, K., and Beaver, P. C.: The etiology and pathology of eosinophilic lung (tropical eosinophilia). Am. J. Trop. Med. Hyg., 15:183, 1966.

Islam, N.: Tropical eosinophilia. East Pakistan, Islam A. Chittagong, 1964.

Lie Kian, J., and Shandosham, A. A.: The pathology of clinical filariasis due to *Wuchereria bancroft* and *Brugia malayi* and a discussion of occult filariasis. *In* Sandosham, A. A., and Zaman, V. (eds.): Proceedings of Seminar on Filariasis and Immunology of Parasitic Infections, and Laboratory Meeting. Kuala Lumpur, Malaysia, Rajiv Printers, 1969, p. 125.

TROPICAL PYOMYOSITIS
Philip D. Marsden

This is a condition of a large deep-seated abscess, single or multiple, occurring in any voluntary muscle. Strange lumps for diagnosis in the tropics sometimes turn out to be deep-seated abscesses. By far the most frequent organism isolated is *Staphylococcus aureus*, and in Uganda 60 per cent of such organisms are phage gpII. Histologically there are areas of focal muscle necrosis with inflammatory cell infiltration. The regional lymph nodes are rarely affected, and there may be no fever or leukocytosis in the peripheral blood. The cause is unknown. Subcutaneous helminthic infection, particularly filaria, and sickle cell disease have been suggested as predisposing conditions, but as yet there is no convincing evidence to this effect. Treatment consists of antimicrobial therapy (initially with penicillin) and surgical drainage.

Elebute, E. A.: Pyomyositis. *In* Schwartz, S. I., Adesola, A. O., Elebute, E. A., and Rob, C. G. (eds.): Tropical Surgery, New York, McGraw-Hill Book Company, 1971.

Marcus, R. T., and Foster, W. D.: Observations on the clinical features, aetiology and geographical distribution of pyomyositis in East Africa. East Afr. Med. J., 45:167, 1968.

EOSINOPHILIA IN RELATION TO HELMINTHIC INFECTIONS
Philip D. Marsden

Hypereosinophilic states are considered elsewhere in this book, and conditions such as periarteritis nodosa, eosinophilic leukemia, and allergic diseases are discussed in the appropriate chapters. However, the author believes that a number of the cases of unexplained eosinophilia seen today in diagnostic units will in time be explained on the basis of helminthic infections, and it is worthwhile making one or two general points in relation to such infections.

As can be seen from the preceding chapters, almost all

helminthic infections in contrast to protozoal infections are at some time or other associated with eosinophilia. In terms of the parasites for which man is the definitive host, the eosinophilia often coincides with the invasive phase of a trematode, cestode, or nematode infection, and the diagnosis may not be apparent until several weeks or months later when the adults begin to produce progeny. For this reason obscure eosinophilia should always be kept under observation, and stool or tissue specimens re-examined. Some parasites are notorious in presenting a problem of eosinophilia for diagnosis, notably Strongyloides and Trichinella infections. After effective treatment of helminthic infections, particularly those in close contact with body tissues, there is often a pronounced rise in circulating eosinophils.

Perhaps more interesting is the clinical situation in which a patient has a significant human helminth load and yet little or no expected eosinophilia in the absence of cortisone therapy. Recent work suggesting that sensitized lymphocytes play an important role in the genesis of eosinophilia may throw some light on this problem.

Eosinophilia is a prominent feature of infections with nonhuman helminths, e.g., Angiostrongylus, and situations in which there is an abnormal host response, e.g., pulmonary tropical eosinophilia. It appears that a small number of nonhuman helminths passing through man's tissues may engender marked eosinophilia and even hypergammaglobulinemia, e.g., toxocariasis, gnathostomiasis. To find the helminths responsible is impossible in many patients, and when found they may be very difficult to identify. Our elucidation of this clinical problem appears to rest on the elaboration of more specific and sensitive serologic tests, and the techniques of indirect hemagglutination, gel diffusion, fluorescent antibody tests, and similar procedures are useful here to detect host response to helminthic antigens. However, much difficult work will be needed to characterize these complex antigens.

Finally, in a clinical consideration of this problem, common things occur commonly. A survey of a series of patients with occult eosinophilia in a large teaching hospital in New York City revealed a few cases of strongyloidiasis, but eosinophilia was most frequently one of the signs of a reaction to drug therapy.

Part X

DISORDERS OF THE NERVOUS SYSTEM AND BEHAVIOR

317.   INTRODUCTION

Fred Plum

Almost all diseases use the nervous system to express themselves and it is this fact that often makes neurology seem complex and difficult to the physician. Pain, sensory loss, weakness, disturbed thinking, and impaired mood or alertness are not specific indicators of specific diseases. To be sure, in many instances, they are symptoms of primary disease of the nervous system. Even more often, however, they reflect disease in some other system or organ of the body. Finally, and perhaps most frequently, these symptoms derive from man's faulty adjustment to his environment. Symptoms are error signals, and the nervous system is as sensitive to symbolic threats as it is to physical ones.

Based on the aforementioned concepts, the goals of the chapters that follow are to present neurologic disease as a problem to be approached logically and for which certain principles repeatedly provide the key for diagnosis and treatment. These principles are based on our current knowledge of how the brain functions as an adaptive organ, adjusting man to his external as well as to his internal environment.

Part X is organized in two main categories. In the first, the more general functions of the nervous system are considered: how it is organized, how it handles certain normal activities, and how it expresses psychologic and somatic symptoms in response to both real and symbolic threat or injury. In the second, the more traditional approach is taken, and neurologic diseases are discussed according to anatomic and causative categories. Heavy emphasis is placed on the biochemistry of disease and the specific physiology of signs and symptoms. It must be recognized, however, that this century's revolution in biologic science is just beginning to attack effectively the problems involved in understanding brain function, behavior, and neurologic disease. Thus these pages often expose our ignorance as much as they do our knowledge.

A word about treatment. Man's brain is his uniquely human organ. Damage it and life loses its meaning in direct proportion, no matter what other physiologic benefits may accrue in the process. The brain cannot be regenerated, repaired, or homotransplanted. It accumulates no metabolic debts and, unless supplied continuously by an effective circulation carrying large amounts of oxygen and glucose, it digests itself irreparably. This means that one cannot "let the brain go" while solving other medical problems. For example, if an elderly man with severe anemia suffers an ischemic stroke while awaiting accurate blood studies, there is no satisfaction later in a correct hematologic diagnosis. If an adolescent girl suffers permanent dementia from hypoglycemia while having her diabetes regulated, the perfect control of glycosuria seems hardly worth it. The integrity of the nervous system must be the first goal in therapeutics.

Section One.   CONSCIOUSNESS AND ITS DISTURBANCES

318.   INTRODUCTION

Fred Plum

William James remarked that everyone knows what consciousness is until he tries to define it. Full consciousness is generally taken to imply not only wakefulness but the total complement of human mental faculties: complete awareness of self and environment. In clinical medicine, when one speaks of consciousness as opposed to unconsciousness or coma, a less encompassing state is usually meant, consisting of behavioral wakefulness plus the capacity to respond appropriately to at least a limited number of external stimuli. *Dementia, apathy, amnesia,* or *aphasia* may impair the content of consciousness, but as long as enough appropriate responses remain in other behavioral functions, consciousness is considered to be preserved. *Obtundation* and *drowsiness* describe states of dull behavior with blunted alertness in which part of the content of consciousness is lost, often with an excessive tendency to sleep. *Stupor* is a state wherein subjects respond when vigorously stimulated, but immediately sink back again as soon as external stimuli are withdrawn. *Coma* is complete unresponsiveness. In light coma, semi-appropriate movements occur in response to noxious stimuli, but in deep coma, subjects retain only primitive reflexes or no response at all.

The present physiologic concept of consciousness is that it depends upon close interaction between the intact cerebral hemispheres and the central gray matter of the upper brainstem. The hemispheres contribute most of the specific components of consciousness, including language, memory, intellect, and learned responses to sensory stimuli. But in order for the cerebrum to function, the organism must be aroused or activated by more caudally placed mechanisms that reside in the thalamus, hypothalamus, midbrain, and upper pons. An important component of this arousal mechanism is located within what Magoun and his colleagues called the ascending reticular activating system; other brainstem systems also influence cerebral cortical activity and the state of consciousness.

The relation of the cerebral cortex to consciousness is more quantitative than qualitative: All hemispheric lesions undoubtedly reduce, at least to some degree, the content of man's consciousness, and the total loss of the cortex causes at least several weeks of coma even if the brainstem is intact. Between the extremes of an injury so small that it is clinically almost undetectable and so large that it causes coma lies a continuum along which the size of the lesion and the impairment of mind, memory, wit, and personality are roughly proportional.

319. THE PATHOGENESIS OF STUPOR AND COMA

Fred Plum

The preceding paragraphs have described how stupor or coma results when a disease process either diffusely and bilaterally blots out the function of the cerebral hemispheres or blocks brainstem-activating structures so that the cortex cannot be aroused. A potentially bewildering series of individual maladies can have one or both of these effects, as may be seen in the accompanying table. However, if one examines the mechanisms by which neurologic diseases cause coma, all these maladies fall into three categories that can be distinguished by their signs and symptoms: (1) supratentorial mass lesions, (2) subtentorial compressive or destructive lesions, and (3) metabolic brain diseases.

SUPRATENTORIAL MASS LESIONS

Supratentorial masses are rarely so large that they produce coma by directly destroying or replacing the ce-

The Common Causes of Stupor and Coma

Supratentorial lesions (causing upper brainstem dysfunction)
  Cerebral hemorrhage
  Large cerebral infarction
  Subdural hematoma
  Epidural hematoma
  Brain tumor
  Brain abscess (rare)

Subtentorial lesions (compressing or destroying the reticular formation)
  Pontine or cerebellar hemorrhage
  Infarction
  Tumor
  Cerebellar abscess

Metabolic and diffuse lesions (see also Table 1 in Ch. 320)
  Anoxia or ischemia
  Hypoglycemia
  Nutritional deficiency
  Endogenous organ failure or deficiency
  Ionic and electrolyte disorders
  Exogenous poison
  Infections
    Meningitis
    Encephalitis
  Concussion and postictal states

rebral hemispheres. Rather, they interfere with consciousness because they shift and squeeze the contents of the supratentorial compartment and, in so doing, compress the diencephalon. The expanding process can originate anywhere in the hemisphere and ultimately produce this reaction because the fibrous tentorium and the bones of the base of the skull resist movement except toward the tentorial opening. As a result, when supratentorial masses demand room for expansion, the diencephalic tectum and adjacent midbrain are particularly likely to be compressed, and sometimes the diencephalon is even displaced downward through the tentorial notch (transtentorial herniation).

How do supratentorial masses progress so that these reactions occur? The brain has certain common responses to injury, including edema, vascular dilatation, and the invasion of leukocytes and proliferation of glial cells. The intensity, tempo, and exact contribution of each of these responses varies according to the nature of the original lesion and the rate at which it appears, but each shares in the brain's defenses against neoplasms, infections, infarcts, and irritants. Thus the original lesion gradually enlarges and tends to impair structures ever more remote from itself in the inexpansible intracranial cavity. The remote effects are due partly to edema spreading away from the edges of the primary lesion and partly to an actual shift of the brain within the skull, compressing normal tissues and blood vessels against rigid structures such as the falx cerebri and the tentorium. At this stage, clinical signs of increased intracranial pressure are common and imply that an intracranial lesion is already exerting generalized deleterious effects.

The clinical picture of supratentorial mass lesions producing stupor or coma has several distinctive features. If a history is available, localizing symptoms such as frontal headache, focal seizures, or other changes consistent with hemispheric disease will usually be found to have preceded unconsciousness. Physically, most patients demonstrate a combination of *focal* hemispheral signs, e.g., sensorimotor defect, aphasia, and visual field defect, reflecting the site of the original pathologic process, plus *diffuse* signs of supratentorial dysfunction, indicating that the lesion is exerting remote effects on the opposite hemisphere and the deep diencephalon. An important negative finding is that, unless the patient is in the terminal stages of illness, no evidence of direct subtentorial brainstem dysfunction can be found: pupillary and oculovestibular reflexes remain intact. If a patient with a supratentorial lesion progresses in his illness, the neurologic signs and symptoms evolve in a characteristic, orderly, rostral-caudal pattern. The more rostrally located neurologic functions first disappear, followed by more caudal impairment, first in the diencephalon and then down the brainstem almost as if the structures were being progressively transected from above downward, each plane of function being removed almost completely before the next is impaired.

The aforementioned description needs amplification to be complete. Some supratentorial masses begin and enlarge in neurologically silent areas such as the frontal lobes or the subdural space and lack a focal signature. Lesions of this type may be revealed only when the patient develops signs of diffuse forebrain dysfunction plus, perhaps, headache and evidence of increased intracranial pressure.

Stupor or coma with supratentorial lesions is ominous

because it implies that the deeply located upper brainstem is already compressed or distorted and that the much more serious complication of herniation of the forebrain downward into the tentorial notch is about to occur. Such herniation begins either with direct downward displacement of the diencephalon (central herniation) or with the uncus of the temporal lobe squeezing into the tentorial notch and against the midbrain (uncal herniation). Either way, if the hernia develops fully, it usually impacts the midbrain and nearly always results in permanent brain damage or death. A characteristic constellation of symptoms heralds each of these patterns of transtentorial herniation. With impending *central* herniation, stupor becomes gradually deeper, and the subjects sigh, yawn, or develop periodic respirations. The pupils shrink to as little as 1 to 2 mm in diameter, but retain their light reflexes. Oculovestibular reflexes are brisk, and the extremities stiffen into bilateral rigidity or spasticity, combined with extensor plantar responses. With *uncal* herniation, signs are in many ways similar to the above except that as the uncus slides over the tentorial edge, it often compresses the third nerve ahead of it, even before the diencephalon is squeezed. The result is that the pupil on the side of the herniation begins to dilate more than its fellow. Eventually, the pupil dilates widely and becomes light-fixed, and the patient becomes stuporous. Shortly afterward, oculomotor functions of the third nerve are usually impaired, and the involved eye turns outward. If the herniating process continues, the opposite third nerve becomes involved as well, and then the brainstem. To initiate effective treatment one must recognize the process before this advanced stage and halt it with osmotic decompressing agents or surgical treatment. Otherwise, when conditions progress this far, few subjects recover without substantial, permanent neurologic injury.

SUBTENTORIAL MASS OR DESTRUCTIVE LESIONS

These conditions cause stupor or coma if they destroy or compress the centrally located activating systems in the brainstem anywhere above approximately the midpons. Expanding lesions of the posterior fossa have the same effect if they compress the midbrain upward. Compression against the medulla oblongata with an ensuing cerebellar pressure cone produces stiff neck, along with respiratory and cardiac irregularities, but does not directly cause loss of consciousness.

The characteristic clinical feature of subtentorial destruction or compression causing coma is the presence of restricted and usually asymmetrical signs of focal brainstem dysfunction, which frequently can be anatomically pinpointed to a single locus by the clinical findings. Seldom do the signs indicate complete brainstem transection. This restricted, discrete localization is unlike metabolic lesions causing coma in which the signs commonly indicate incomplete dysfunction at several different levels of the brain, and also is unlike the secondary brainstem dysfunction and coma that follow supratentorial herniation, in which *all* function at any given level tends to be lost as the process progresses from rostral to caudal along the neuraxis.

Purely compressive lesions of the posterior fossa rarely cause coma until late in their course when the patient is near death. The pathologic process is usually a hemor-

rhage, abscess, or tumor of the cerebellum or fourth ventricle, and occipital headache, nystagmus, diplopia, nausea, vomiting, cranial nerve signs, and ataxia usually precede unconsciousness. Important points in distinguishing both destructive and compressive posterior fossa lesions from metabolic depression of the brainstem are that in metabolic depression oculovestibular responses are generally preserved until the advanced stages, and pupillary light reflexes are nearly always preserved. By contrast, structural brainstem lesions causing coma always disrupt the oculovestibular responses, and those involving the midbrain also interrupt the pupillary reflexes.

METABOLIC DEPRESSION OF THE BRAIN CAUSING COMA

Primary metabolic encephalopathies are intrinsic to the neuron, the glial cell, or the white matter, respectively. They often produce dementia, but rarely cause coma except terminally. *Secondary* metabolic encephalopathies are those in which brain function is disrupted either because the brain is not supplied with a required substance, e.g., thiamine, oxygen, or glucose, or because it is poisoned by an ingested or endogenous toxin, e.g., depressant drugs or the products of uremia. The secondary metabolic encephalopathies are frequent causes of delirium as well as of stupor and coma; their relationship to the normal metabolism of the brain is discussed in detail in Ch. 320.

Experimental evidence conflicts as to whether most metabolic agents causing coma depress mainly the brainstem reticular formation or the cerebral cortex. Clinically, most patients with metabolic encephalopathy appear to suffer depression of the forebrain more than of the brainstem. However, the striking finding with most metabolic agents is that they selectively depress certain susceptible functions at several different brain levels, but at the same time spare other functions that emanate from identical levels. For example, most metabolic poisons depress the reticular and motor functions of the midbrain, yet nearly all of them spare the pupillary light reflex so that reactive pupils persist into the deepest stages· of metabolic coma until asphyxia intervenes. (Poisoning with glutethimide or parasympathomimetics provides the only exception to this rule, both drugs blocking the light reflex in large, coma-causing doses.) Most of the metabolic encephalopathies cause delirium before stupor or coma, and many of them are accompanied in their early stages by asterixis, a flapping irregular tremor of the outstretched hands, or by random myoclonic muscle twitches. Although the metabolic encephalopathies occasionally produce asymmetrical motor signs, they more characteristically impair body movement symmetrically, and they never impair central sensory pathways except as an accompaniment to the over-all depression of the sensorium.

To epitomize, diseases causing stupor or coma fall into three categories:

1. Supratentorial mass lesions, which present with asymmetrical neurologic signs of hemispheral dysfunction combined with evidence of intact subtentorial brainstem function. As supratentorial lesions evolve, the signs indicate progressive rostral-caudal neurologic deterioration, almost as if the brain were being serially sectioned from top to bottom.

2. Subtentorial compressive and destructive lesions, which present from the outset with either cranial nerve abnormalities or other focal brainstem signs, including pupillary and oculovestibular reflex abnormalities. Long tract motor signs are usually present and asymmetrical.

3. Metabolic brain diseases, which present a picture of either diffuse cortical depression or, more often, of impaired function in both the hemispheres and the brainstem accompanied by retained pupillary light reflexes. The multifocal distribution of metabolic encephalopathy is usually symmetrical and not accompanied by sensory impairments.

APPROACH TO THE PATIENT IN STUPOR OR COMA

The physician must ensure that the brain and other vital organs receive no further injury while he obtains whatever history, examinations, and laboratory data are required. Before anything else he must provide a free and open airway and determine that the subject is breathing deeply enough to oxygenate his lungs and eliminate carbon dioxide. Next, the heart and blood pressure should be examined, and possible sources of bleeding checked to be certain that cardiac output and blood volume are sufficient to supply the metabolic needs of the brain and kidney. In all patients in coma an intravenous infusion should be started, using a large-bore needle. Blood samples for typing and cross-matching, as well as for other appropriate laboratory determinations, can be obtained at this time. Whenever the cause of coma is doubtful, and particularly when the clinical signs suggest a metabolic disorder, blood should be taken for sugar determination, and then 50 ml of 50 per cent glucose given intravenously. Hypoglycemic encephalopathy can take many forms, some of which mimic other diseases. If glucose is given promptly, no further cerebral damage occurs while the doctor awaits definitive laboratory diagnosis. Intravenous sugar harms nothing if the coma has another cause.

Beyond these immediate, lifesaving measures, it requires considerable restraint to approach a patient in a coma methodically, for the urge to act without delay is understandably strong, but potentially dangerous. Inquiry into both the past medical history and the circumstances under which the patient lost consciousness generally discloses more of diagnostic value than any other maneuver. Is there any suggestion that head trauma could have occurred recently? Has there been renal, hepatic, or myocardial disease? Could a seizure have preceded the present unconsciousness? Has the subject been taking insulin? Have there been recent changes in mood, behavior, or neurologic function to suggest an evolving intracranial process? Was the subject "blue," depressed, or moody, and did he have access to depressant drugs? Is he a "spree" drinker? These and other questions must be covered comprehensively with relatives, past physicians, friends, police, or ambulance personnel.

One must perform both a meticulous neurologic examination and a thoughtful physical review of every body system, because disease in remote organs often causes or accentuates dysfunction in the brain.

Fever implies infection, or, less often, lymphomatous neoplasm. On the other hand, hypothermia (30 to 36° C

[86 to 96.8° F]) in a patient not severely exposed to cold suggests depressant drug poisoning, hypoglycemia, or severe lower brainstem injury, as by infarction. Hypertension may be the cause of hypertensive encephalopathy or the underlying cause of cerebral hemorrhage. Conversely, an elevated blood pressure can be a symptom of subarachnoid hemorrhage in a subject not previously hypertensive. Hypotension in a supine patient implies low blood volume (hemorrhagic or traumatic shock; severe nutritional and fluid depletion), low cardiac output (myocardial infarction), or low peripheral resistance (depressant drug poisoning). Tachycardia (over 160 per minute) can mean that unconsciousness is the result of lowered cardiac output from a supraventricular cardiac arrhythmia. Bradycardia suggests heart block and the Adams-Stokes syndrome or a myocardial infarct.

The pattern and depth of respiration are often informative in evaluating both neurologic function and acid-base balance, so much so that the evaluation of breathing is discussed more fully in Ch. 320.

The skin should be searched for petechiae (thrombocytopenic or nonthrombocytopenic purpura, meningococcemia, and bacterial endocarditis), bruises, evidence of nutritional deficiency, icterus, angiomatous spiders, and the bright pinkness of carbon monoxide poisoning. Fleshy or clubbed fingertips suggest carcinoma of the lung, or, less often, lung abscess or congenital heart disease (with brain embolism or abscess). A meticulous examination of the optic fundi is imperative but should be completed without cycloplegics, the use of which destroys the potential diagnostic value of pupillary reactions in coma. In the fundus oculi, the pathologic changes of many diseases causing coma can be viewed directly: increased intracranial pressure, hypertensive vascular disease, diabetes, blood dyscrasia, tuberculosis, sarcoidosis, bacterial endocarditis, cryptococcosis, collagen vascular disease, and even subarachnoid hemorrhage producing subhyaloid bleeding.

Chest examination has two potentially rewarding findings: cardiac murmurs suggest bacterial endocarditis with consequent focal, embolic encephalitis; the wheezes and obstructive sounds of the pulmonary cripple suggest CO_2 retention causing narcosis. In the abdominal examination, the presence of masses suggesting polycystic kidneys increases the chances that subarachnoid hemorrhage has occurred, whereas liver enlargement (hepatic coma is common with hepatomas) or splenic enlargement (both blood dyscrasias and infectious mononucleosis can cause encephalitis-like illnesses) can provide valuable leads.

During the neurologic examination, certain potentially informative steps are sometimes overlooked. The skull should always be palpated and inspected meticulously. Edema of the scalp commonly overlies fresh fracture lines, and basal skull fractures predispose to blood pigment stains behind the ear (Battle's sign) and about the orbit (raccoon eyes). Blood also may escape from basal fractures into the ear canals, the middle ears, or the nostrils. The skull should be percussed, because focal or unilateral skull tenderness, manifested by grimacing or withdrawal in a stuporous subject, often overlies an intracranial mass lesion. The neck should be tested carefully: stiff neck can reflect meningitis, cerebellar tonsillar herniation, or, occasionally, simply skeletal muscle spasticity. The stiff neck of acute bacterial meningitis is rarely equivocal; that of impending herniation is commonly less severe and lacks accompanying signs of infection or a prominent Kernig sign. It usually requires several hours or a day or more for stiff neck to develop after subarachnoid bleeding.

It is useful to watch the unconscious patient for a time, observing whether or not the extremities move equally and whether tremor, myoclonus, or single or repetitive seizures involve any part of the body. Status epilepticus with focal continuous epilepsy is not uncommon, but is often overlooked.

Laboratory Examination of the Patient in Coma

Patients should be subjected to a skull roentgenogram (looking for fracture lines, densities, and pineal shifts), a blood count and smear, and a urinalysis. When the clinical findings are consistent with metabolic encephalopathy but the cause is uncertain, the blood glucose and serum sodium, potassium, and bicarbonate should be obtained promptly. Knowledge of the arterial pH often can be almost diagnostic of the cause of metabolic coma (see Table 3 in Ch. 320).

When to do a lumbar puncture is always a serious question. All physicians are aware that in patients with increased intracranial pressure the procedure sometimes induces fatal herniation of the brain through the tentorium or foramen magnum. For this reason, lumbar puncture is best avoided if the physician strongly suspects his patient of having an expanding intracranial mass, particularly in the posterior fossa. However, there are certain treatable diseases such as meningitis that can be diagnosed only by lumbar puncture, and many others in which the procedure yields valuable preliminary diagnostic information. When the advice of neurologic specialists is unavailable, the doctor has no choice but to proceed with lumbar puncture if the diagnosis is in doubt and he believes the procedure has a reasonable chance of offering valuable information. Certain steps minimize the risk. One is to use a small (No. 20), sharp needle. Another is to fill the manometer with saline and attach it to the needle before releasing fluid, a technique that prevents sudden subarachnoid pressure shifts. Finally, jugular manometrics should *never* be performed, for they offer little useful data and increase the risk of impacting potential intracranial herniations.

Magoun, H. W.: The Waking Brain. 2nd ed. Springfield, Ill., Charles C Thomas, 1963.
Petito, F., and Plum, F.: The lumbar puncture (editorial). N. Engl. J. Med., 200:225, 1974.
Plum, F., and Posner, J. B.: The Diagnosis of Stupor and Coma. 2nd ed. Philadelphia, F. A. Davis Company, 1972.

320. DELIRIUM AND EXOGENOUS METABOLIC BRAIN DISEASE

Jerome B. Posner

INTRODUCTION

There are few situations in clinical medicine that confuse and upset the physician so much as when he confronts a patient whose state of consciousness is rapidly changing. The physician's task in such a situation is both enormous and exacting. First he must decide which of three major categories of disease is responsible for the patient's condition: (1) structural brain disease (e.g., brain tumors, subdural hematomas, cerebral infarctions); (2) "functional" brain disease (e.g., schizophrenia, manic-depressive psychosis); or (3) metabolic brain disease or delirium (see definitions below). If the patient's disorder falls into one of the first two categories (discussed elsewhere in this book), the physician can obtain help from highly skilled specialists in those areas (neurologists, neurosurgeons, or psychiatrists). If the patient's behavioral change is due to metabolic encephalopathy, the general physician must then determine himself which of a bewildering variety of metabolic defects is responsible (Table 1) and must rapidly begin treatment to assure that the metabolic defect does not produce irreversible brain damage. While he is carrying out these exacting tasks, he is often impeded by the fact that the patient is noisy, obstreperous, and uncooperative, and by his own knowledge that appropriate treatment is essential and inappropriate treatment (e.g., injudicious use of sedative drugs) potentially deleterious or even fatal. To deal with metabolic brain disease, the physician must understand some pathophysiologic aspects of cerebral metabolism and must undertake a systematic and thorough physical and laboratory examination of the patient.

DEFINITIONS

Metabolic encephalopathy is a term applied to the behavioral changes which result from diffuse or widespread multifocal failure of cerebral metabolism. When the cerebral disorder arises from an intrinsic failure of neuronal or glial metabolism, it is referred to as *primary or endogenous metabolic encephalopathy.* The primary disorders usually begin insidiously, progress inexorably, and produce a clinical picture of dementia, as discussed in Ch. 326 to 331. When the encephalopathy results from interference with brain metabolism by extracerebral disease, it is called *secondary or exogenous metabolic encephalopathy.* The secondary encephalopathies usually begin acutely or subacutely and often subside with time and treatment. They produce a clinical picture in which confusion, thinking errors, behavioral abnormalities, disorders of consciousness, and abnormal motor activity predominate. The causes of secondary metabolic encephalopathy are as many and varied as the illnesses that disturb body chemistry. Some examples of metabolic encephalopathy are listed in Table 1.

Metabolic brain disease is common and often misdiagnosed. When mild, it produces intellectual dullness, social indifference, and vague perplexity easily mistaken by observers for psychogenic depression or simply low intelligence. More severe encephalopathy elicits either a florid picture of tremulous agitation, rich and frightening hallucinations, and periods of seemingly complete loss of contact with the environment, or a more quiet, withdrawn, akinetic state which may fade into stupor or coma. The former, often called *delirium* or *toxic psychosis,* may be confused with a functional psychosis, and the latter, often called *acute* or *subacute confusional state,* is likely to be mistaken for structural brain disease. Although certain specific systemic disorders characteristically cause one or another of the aforementioned

TABLE 1. Causes of Metabolic Brain Disease

I. Deprivation of oxygen, substrate, or metabolic cofactors
  *A. Hypoxia (interference with oxygen supply to the entire brain—cerebral blood flow normal)
    1. Decreased oxygen tension and content of blood
      Pulmonary disease
      Alveolar hypoventilation
      Decreased atmospheric oxygen tension
    2. Decreased oxygen content of blood—normal tension
      Anemia
      Carbon monoxide poisoning
      Methemoglobinemia
  *B. Ischemia (diffuse or widespread multifocal interference with blood supply to brain)
    1. Decreased cerebral blood flow resulting from decreased cardiac output
      Stokes-Adams syndrome, cardiac arrest, cardiac arrhythmias
      Myocardial infarction
      Congestive heart failure
      Aortic stenosis
      Pulmonary embolus
    2. Decreased cerebral blood flow resulting from decreased peripheral resistance in systemic circulation
      Syncope: orthostatic, vasovagal
      Carotid sinus hypersensitivity
      Low blood volume
    3. Decreased cerebral blood flow due to generalized increase in cerebrovascular resistance
      Hypertensive encephalopathy
      Hyperventilation syndrome
      Increased blood viscosity (polycythemia), cryo- and macroglobinemia
    4. Decreased local cerebral blood flow due to widespread small vessel occlusion
      Disseminated intravascular coagulation
      Systemic lupus erythematosus
      Subacute bacterial endocarditis
      Cardiopulmonary bypass
  *C. Hypoglycemia
      Resulting from exogenous insulin
      Spontaneous (endogenous insulin, liver disease, etc.)
  D. Cofactor deficiency
      Thiamin (Wernicke's encephalopathy)
      Niacin
      Pyridoxine
      B_{12}
      Folate

II. Diseases of organs other than brain
  *A. Diseases of nonendocrine organs
      Liver (hepatic coma)
      Kidney (uremic coma)
      Lung (CO_2 narcosis)
  *B. Hyper- and/or hypofunction of endocrine organs
      Pituitary

      Thyroid (myxedema-thyrotoxicosis)
      Parathyroid (hyper- and hypoparathyroidism)
      Adrenal (Addison's disease, Cushing's disease, pheochromocytoma)
      Pancreas (diabetes, hypoglycemia)
  C. Other systemic diseases
      Diabetes
      Cancer
      Porphyria
      Sepsis
      Fever

III. Exogenous poisons
  *A. Sedative drugs
  B. Acid poisons or poisons with acidic breakdown products
      Paraldehyde
      Methyl alcohol
      Ethylene glycol
  C. Other enzyme inhibitors
      Heavy metals
      Organic phosphates
      Cyanide
      Salicylates
  D. Psychotropic drugs
      Tricyclic antidepressants and anticholinergic drugs
      Amphetamines
      Lithium
      Phenothiazines
      LSD-mescaline
      Monoamine oxidase inhibitors
  E. Others
      Penicillin
      Anticonvulsants
      Steroids
      Cardiac glycosides

IV. Diseases producing toxins or enzyme inhibition in CNS
  A. Meningitis
  B. Encephalitis
  C. Subarachnoid hemorrhage

V. Abnormalities of fluid, ionic or acid-base environment of CNS
  A. Water and sodium (hyper- and hyponatremia) (hypo- and hyperosmolality)
  B. Acidosis (metabolic and respiratory)
  C. Alkalosis (metabolic and respiratory)
  D. Potassium (hypokalemia)
  E. Magnesium (hyper- and hypomagnesemia)
  F. Calcium (hyper- and hypocalcemia)

VI. Miscellaneous diseases of unknown cause
  A. Seizures and postictal states
  *B. "Postoperative" delirium
  C. Concussion
  *D. "Sensory deprivation"

*Alone or in combination, the most common causes of delirium seen on medical or surgical wards.

syndromes, each can occur with any of the metabolic brain diseases; thus the terms "delirium," "toxic psychosis," and "confusional state" are used interchangeably in this chapter to describe the wakeful stage of metabolic encephalopathy. A patient who is drowsy but can be coaxed to respond to verbal stimuli is *obtunded*. When he no longer responds to verbal stimuli but responds appropriately to noxious cutaneous stimuli, he is *stuporous*. If he does not respond appropriately to noxious stimuli, he is *comatose*. The term *dementia* is used operationally to describe an irreversible loss of memory and cognitive functions, usually insidious in onset and due to intrinsic disease of the brain. It is the irreversibility of dementia which clearly distinguishes it from delirium. An insidiously developing, quiet delirium may be clinically indistinguishable from the early stages of dementia.

SOME PATHOPHYSIOLOGIC ASPECTS OF METABOLIC BRAIN DISEASE

Pathologic changes in metabolic brain disease depend upon the nature and severity of the illness. The brains of some patients delirious during life are entirely normal at postmortem examination. In most cases, however, at least microscopic pathologic changes can be identified if the process causing delirium has lasted for some hours or days prior to death. The pathologic changes are bilateral, symmetrical, and usually diffusely distributed in the cerebral hemispheres. Lesions may be present in the neurons, the glial cells, or the white matter, depending on the nature of the primary illness.

Perhaps the most common pathologic cerebral changes are observed after anoxia, ischemia, or hypoglycemia.

The mildest abnormalities are visible only microscopically and consist of "microvacuoles" in neuronal cytoplasm of neocortex and hippocampus. The microvacuoles are swollen mitochondria, and this change is probably reversible. With more severe insults there is dissolution of the Nissl granules (particles of ribonucleic acid) and generalized pallor of staining. Finally, the nuclei shrink and become hyperchromatic, and irregular basophilic rings and granules appear in the swollen cytoplasm. These changes are not reversible. After severe and prolonged insults, all neurons in the cerebral cortex may disappear, and the third layer of the cortex may completely degenerate so that the naked eye detects a thin line of spongy necrosis (laminar necrosis). Anoxic changes also affect the basal ganglia to cause grossly visible focal necrosis of the globus pallidus. Occasionally, there may be diffuse demyelination of the subcortical white matter. Characteristically, the brainstem and spinal cord are spared unless the process has been overwhelmingly severe.

A nonspecific but common pathologic change in patients who have died with uremia, hyponatremia, diabetic coma, or CO_2 narcosis is cerebral swelling, recognized grossly by flattened gyri, obliterated sulci, and small ventricles. The cut brain may appear either "wet" or "dry," but, microscopically, large perivascular and perineuronal spaces attest to the presence of edema. Unusual glial cells with ballooned, lobulated nuclei are found in the cortex and basal ganglia of patients who die in hepatic coma, and are relatively specific for this disorder. Widespread perivascular "cuffs" of lymphocytes or polymorphonuclear leukocytes indicate an inflammatory lesion of the brain and meninges from viral or bacterial invasion.

In all cases of metabolic brain disease, the cerebral oxygen uptake declines in rough proportion to the degree of brain dysfunction observed clinically. So far, we understand in only a few instances how systemic illnesses interfere with cerebral metabolism, but these few serve as models to suggest the possible mechanisms for the others. The following material outlines some of our knowledge of normal and abnormal cerebral metabolism.

Glucose. Glucose is the brain's only substrate under physiologic conditions, and is transferred across the blood-brain barrier by facilitated transport. Other substances can serve as substrates of brain in extraordinary circumstances (e.g., ketone bodies during starvation). Under normal circumstances, each 100 grams of brain utilizes about 5.5 mg of glucose per minute, which represents almost the body's entire basal glucose consumption. Eighty-five per cent of brain glucose uptake reacts with oxygen to form CO_2, water, and energy; the remainder is probably accounted for by lactic acid production even in the presence of ample oxygen supplies. Under anaerobic conditions, lactic acid is the end product of glucose metabolism, but the energy so produced is insufficient to maintain neuronal function. There are about 2 grams of reserve glucose (as such and as glycogen) in the brain, an amount that allows the brain of a hypoglycemic patient to survive (although not to function at a normal metabolic rate) for about 90 minutes without suffering irreversible damage. The blood glucose concentration at which cerebral metabolism fails and clinical symptoms develop is variable from patient to patient, but, in general, levels below 30 mg per 100 ml cause confusion, and below 10 to 15 mg per 100 ml, coma.

Oxygen. Oxygen, the other substance vital for normal cerebral function, is not stored by the brain, and a few seconds of anoxia is sufficient to cause coma. After a variable period of time, usually minutes, both hypoxia and ischemia cause irreversible neuronal damage. The normal brain consumes about 3.5 ml of oxygen per 100 grams per minute and produces an equal amount of carbon dioxide (R.Q. = 1). Cerebral oxygen consumption represents 15 to 20 per cent of the total body oxygen consumption at rest and is remarkably constant in normal man, whether awake or sleeping. However, significant deviations in oxygen consumption occur with brain dysfunction. Clinically, delirium usually accompanies oxygen uptakes below 2.5 ml and when the uptake falls below 2.0 ml per 100 grams per minute, most patients are unconscious. The degree of hypoxia necessary to cause clinical symptoms depends not only on the blood oxygen tension but also on hemoglobin concentration, cerebral blood flow, and serum pH. In general, Pa_{O_2} values below 50 mm Hg cause delirium, and below 25 mm Hg, coma.

Blood brings both glucose and oxygen to the brain. Under resting conditions, the brain receives 55 ml of blood each minute, about 15 per cent of the cardiac output. If the flow falls, the brain compensates by extracting more oxygen and more glucose from the blood it receives. Increased extraction of oxygen maintains normal metabolism in the face of a decreased cerebral blood flow up to the point where so much oxygen has been extracted that the oxygen tension of the brain's venous blood falls to about 20 mm of mercury (a level at which hemoglobin is about 35 per cent saturated). At this point, which is reached when cerebral blood flow falls to about half of normal, the oxygen tension is too low to maintain normal metabolism, and the patient loses consciousness. With hemoglobin concentrations below about 8 grams per 100 ml, cerebral blood flow must increase to assure an adequate oxygen supply. Profound anemia thus becomes a potential contributor to cerebral hypoxia.

Other Substances. In addition to glucose and oxygen, the brain requires other substances (e.g., enzymes, vitamins, amino acids, electrolytes) to maintain metabolism, synthesize transmitter substances, preserve cellular structure, and maintain membrane potentials. Abnormalities of any of these essential substances lead to metabolic brain disease. The unique function of nervous tissue is to transmit electrical impulses, both within cells and by synaptic transmission across cells. The integrity of intracellular transmission depends not only on energy from oxidative metabolism (to maintain the sodium pump) but also on finely controlled intra- and extracellular electrolyte balance. Thus, for example, alterations of extracellular sodium, an ion necessary for propagation of the action potential, produce behavioral changes and delirium. Lithium, a cation with properties similar to both sodium and potassium, changes behavior in manic patients and, in overdose, can lead to severe delirium and coma, perhaps by interfering with normal electrolyte function. The integrity of intercellular transmission is regulated by the synthesis, release, re-uptake, and breakdown of transmitter substances and by maintenance of postsynaptic transmitter receptor sites. Several substances have been identified as putative transmitters in the nervous system, including norepinephrine, dopamine, serotonin, acetylcholine, and amino acids, especially glycine, gamma-aminobutyric acid, and glutamic acid. Most psychotropic drugs are believed to exert their behavioral effects by altering the activity of biogenic amines in the central nervous system, and in overdose most of these drugs produce delirium and sometimes coma. By the same token, severe alterations in amino acid metabolism lead to delirium. Interference with transmitter function may occur when the synthesis, breakdown, or release of the transmitter is inhibited, or when a foreign substance having a structure similar to the transmitter competes for sites on the postsynaptic receptor. Such a "false transmitter" may be the mechanism by which hallucinogenic drugs act, and may also be responsible for the production of "hepatic coma." However, despite these considerations, in no instance is the exact mechanism of delirium in either electrolyte or putative transmitter abnormalities clearly understood.

The biochemical common denominator of metabolic brain disease is decreased oxygen uptake: Is there an anatomic common denominator? Two concepts have arisen delineating a principal locus of metabolic brain disease. One is that the neurons of the cerebral cortex are affected first and, as the process becomes more severe, subcortical structures are affected from the rostral end downward, the phylogenetically oldest and most caudal structures resisting most strongly. This view is supported by the pathologic distribution of cerebral anoxic and hypoglycemic changes and by physiologic studies of hypoglycemic animals in which abnormal electrical activity was recorded from the cortex before it appeared in the hypothalamus.

The second concept is that the neurons of the brainstem reticular formation are the most susceptible to metabolic change and, at least at first, the cortical neurons cease to function only because they lose their reticular stimulation. This concept is supported by physiologic experiments on animals, demonstrating that moderate degrees of hypoxia, hypoglycemia, anesthesia, and cyanide poisoning all block electrical conduction through the reticular formation before they block the ability of cortical neurons to receive messages via other afferent pathways (the lemniscal system).

Neither of these experimental concepts fully explains the several human disease states in which metabolic lesions clinically affect several different levels of the neuraxis simultaneously, with the major locus of early dysfunction differing not only from patient to patient but sometimes from one attack to the next in the same patient. This phenomenon is exemplified by the varied picture of hypoglycemia: Some patients first suffer loss of consciousness and have bilaterally synchronous slow waves in the EEG, suggesting an initial reticular involvement. Others first experience restricted cerebral motor or sensory signs unaccompanied by either EEG abnormalities or impaired consciousness. Still other patients convulse with one attack of hypoglycemia but suffer only quiet coma in the next. It appears that in the clinical situation, regional cerebral factors such as blood flow and energy requirements must vary from moment to moment to predispose first one part of the brain and then another to metabolic insult.

CLINICAL FEATURES OF METABOLIC BRAIN DISEASE

The purpose of the physical and laboratory examination in a patient with suspected metabolic brain disease

TABLE 2. Physical Examination of Patients with Suspected Metabolic Brain Disease

History (from relatives or friends)
    Previous medical illnesses (diabetes, uremia, heart disease)
    Previous psychiatric history
    Access to drugs (sedative, psychotropic drugs)
    Recent complaints (headache, depression)

General physical examination
    Evidence of trauma
    Evidence of chronic or acute systemic illness
    Ventilation (see Table 3)

Neurologic examination
    Mental status
        Affect (agitated, depressed, apathetic)
        Alertness (delirium, obtundation, stupor, coma)
        Orientation (time, place, person)
        Perceptual abnormalities (illusions, delusions, hallucinations)
        Psychomotor activity
    Motor examination
        Focal weakness
        Tremor
        Asterixis
        Myoclonus
        Seizures
    Autonomic examination
        Pupillary size and responses
        Temperature
        Heart rate and rhythm
        Diaphoresis

is twofold: first, to establish if the patient is delirious as opposed to suffering behavioral changes from structural brain or psychiatric disease; and second, to determine exactly the type of metabolic defect causing the delirium. In general, examination of the state of consciousness, motor activity, and autonomic activity, as detailed below, helps to answer the first question, whereas the general physical examination, examination of ventilation, and laboratory examination (the latter two detailed below) help to answer the second question. It cannot, however, be overemphasized that, despite the difficulties of examining a delirious patient, a thorough and systematic general physical, neurologic, and laboratory examination *must* be undertaken if a definitive diagnosis is to be established and definitive treatment to be applied. Some principles of the examination are outlined in Table 2.

State of Consciousness and Mental Content. Mental changes are the earliest and most subtle sign of metabolic brain disease. Restlessness or lethargy, emotional lability, insomnia or drowsiness, and vivid nightmares may appear before other mental changes. Patients often appear fearful and anxious, or depressed. They may express the fear that they are "going crazy." Patients may lie quietly or sleep when left alone, and they rarely read or tend to the world around them. Alternately, they may be restless, irritable, and easily distracted. With more severe metabolic disturbances, patients become drowsy and finally stuporous or comatose. The particular affect that prevails in patients with metabolic encephalopathy depends partly on the nature of the illness and partly on the rapidity of its development; previous personality often has surprisingly little influence. Thus, barbiturate- or alcohol-withdrawal syndromes, acute liver necrosis, and porphyria often cause an agitated delirium, whereas uremia, pulmonary encephalopathy, and anoxia usually produce a more quiet illness. Rapidly occurring metabolic processes are more likely to produce agitated delirium than those that develop slowly.

Disturbances in cognition appear along with altered alertness and awareness and are characterized by difficulties with immediate recall and the ability to abstract. Normal subjects readily recall and repeat 6 or 7 digits forward and 5 or 6 backward and can identify the common denominator between such pairs as an apple and an orange or a fly and a tree, but delirious patients cannot. However, innate intelligence and education also determine cognitive abilities and, unless the physician has examined the patient previously, it is difficult to attribute mild disturbances to a metabolic defect. An early sign of delirium, although usually not as early a sign as altered alertness and cognition, is impairment of memory and orientation. Loss of memory for recent events with relative preservation of remote memory is a hallmark of metabolic and other organic brain disease and is tested by asking the patient about the names of his doctors, some important current events, and his recent activities. Orientation to place and time should be specifically tested by asking the date and year, the day of the week, and the present location. Orientation for time, particularly the year, is lost early in patients with delirium and orientation for place a little later.

Perceptual errors, e.g., mistaking the physician for an old friend or family member, illusions, and hallucinations are common accompaniments of delirium. They frighten and agitate some patients, but are quietly tolerated by others. The nature of the illusions and hallucinations seems to be a property of the individual's personality, and often the same hallucinations accompany separate episodes of delirium. A quiet, withdrawn patient must be specifically asked about hallucinations, because he often fails either to volunteer the information or to behave as if he were hallucinating. Hallucinations of metabolic origin are usually visual by contrast with those of schizophrenia, which are usually auditory.

Fluctuations of the mental status are a hallmark of metabolic encephalopathy. Patients may be totally out of contact one moment and lucid the next. Lucid intervals appear unpredictably and last for minutes or hours. Some of the fluctuation is environmentally related. Thus delirious patients characteristically become more disoriented at night, in unfamiliar surroundings, and in situations in which restraints and background noise and unfamiliar activity decrease familiar sensory stimuli. One study demonstrated a significantly higher incidence of postoperative delirium in patients treated in a windowless intensive care unit than in those treated in a similar one with windows.

Motor Activity. Tremor, asterixis, and multifocal myoclonus are characteristic of metabolic brain disease, and the specificity of the latter two makes them the most important physical signs that distinguish metabolic encephalopathy from psychiatric illness or from structural brain disease.

The *tremor* of delirious patients is coarse and irregular at a rate of about eight to ten per second. It is usually absent at complete rest. It is best seen in the fingers of the outstretched hands. It is less specific than asterixis and multifocal myoclonus, and may be seen in patients with psychiatric disease as well as systemic illness not associated with delirium.

Asterixis is an abnormal, involuntary jerking movement elicited in the hands by asking patients to dorsiflex the wrist and spread the extended fingers. In its mildest form there are irregular random lateral jerking movements of the fingers at the metacarpal phalangeal joints. With fully developed asterixis there is sudden palmar flexion of the fingers at the metacarpal phalangeal joint and of the wrist. The movements are asynchronous in the two hands, occur every 2 to 30 seconds, recover quickly, and cannot be controlled by the patient, even when he is aware of their presence. Asterixis may also involve the feet and tongue. In the lightly unconscious patient the same movement can sometimes be evoked by passively dorsiflexing the wrist or the ankles. Bilateral asterixis almost universally accompanies metabolic encephalopathy at some stage of the illness. It is absent in patients with psychiatric disorders unless they are taking large amounts of drugs, and is encountered extremely rarely, and then unilaterally, in patients with gross structural brain disease such as decompensating subdural hematomas or deep hemispheral infarcts encroaching on the diencephalon.

Multifocal myoclonus consists of sudden nonrhythmic, nonpatterned gross muscle contractions in a resting person. The movements are most common in the face and shoulders but occur anywhere in the body. Multifocal myoclonus can often be elicited, if not present at rest, by passive movements of the shoulder and upper arm. It occurs in a later and more severe stage of metabolic illness than does asterixis, and may physiologically represent a more intense and widespread manifestation of that abnormal movement. Multifocal myoclonus makes its most frequent appearance in uremia, hypercarbic-anoxic encephalopathy, and penicillin overdose, but can occur in virtually all metabolic encephalopathies.

Psychomotor activity ranges from extreme hyperactivity to total immobility. Delirious patients may be unwilling or unable to stay in bed, pacing the halls, in constant movement, with outbursts of aggressiveness which may culminate in attacks on others. With more severe delirium, there may be groping movements, picking at the bedclothes, and constant tossing and turning. Such patients may fall out of bed and injure themselves. Increased psychomotor activity is typically observed in acute deliria such as delirium tremens and drug withdrawal states. More commonly, delirium is manifested by reduced activity, with the patient lethargic, drowsy, and generally bradykinetic. The same patient may run the gamut from psychomotor overactivity to reduced activity during the course of the same delirium. *Speech* is often abnormal. Patients with increased psychomotor behavior often speak rapidly, with a muttering or slurred speech which, because of its speed, is incomprehensible. Patients with reduced psychomotor activity may speak slowly, monotonously, and so softly as not to be clearly heard.

Seizures, weakness, and *hyperactive stretch reflexes* frequently accompany severe metabolic brain disease. The seizures are usually generalized, and the motor abnormalities are usually symmetrical. Focal paresis and focal seizures are by no means rare, however, especially with anoxia or hypoglycemia. Signs of focal disturbance make it more difficult to distinguish between metabolic and structural brain disease. However, in metabolic brain disease the focal signs are usually less severe and more fleeting, and they are accompanied by more widespread neurologic dysfunction than in gross structural disease.

Autonomic Activity. Pupillary light reactions are always preserved in metabolic coma with the few exceptions to be mentioned, and absence of the pupillary light reaction strongly suggests a structural lesion. The exceptions are glutethimide intoxication, which may produce mid-position or slightly dilated fixed pupils; anticholinergic drug administration, which produces fixed, dilated pupils; and exposure to severe anoxia, or asphyxia, which produces fixed dilated pupils and, if sustained, probably implies irreversible brain damage.

Hypothermia is common in delirious patients with myxedema, hypoglycemia, and barbiturate intoxication. Hyperthermia with profuse perspiration and tachycardia accompanies most agitated deliria and is especially common with delirium tremens. Hyperthermia without perspiration suggests anticholinergic drug ingestion or infection. Hyperthermia also marks salicylate and occasionally phenothiazine overdosage.

Ventilation. The clinical features of delirium that have been described are common to many metabolic disorders and aid little in the differential diagnosis of specific types of metabolic coma. Ventilation is an exception. A rapid evaluation of the patient's ventilatory status, coupled with an estimate of blood acid-base balance, frequently narrows the range of possible causes of metabolic coma. Some causes of metabolic brain disease associated with ventilatory abnormalities are listed in Table 3. A careful clinical examination of the respiratory rate and depth usually allows the physician to estimate whether his patient is hyperventilating, eupneic, or hypoventilating. Caution must be exercised in evaluating patients with severe emphysema whose respiratory effort is increased and who may be tachypneic but nevertheless hypoventilating because of ineffective lungs. Caution must also be used in evaluating patients poisoned with depressant drugs who appear to be hypoventilating but are actually eupneic because their metabolic needs are so low. Unexplained abnormalities in the respiratory pattern demand rapid determination of blood gas and acid-base status. As may be seen in Table 3, a delirious and clinically *hyperventilating* adult with a low serum pH probably has diabetic ketosis, uremia, lactic

TABLE 3. A Differential Analysis of Hyperventilation and Hypoventilation in Delirious Patients

Clinical and Laboratory Findings	Probable Diagnosis
I. Hyperventilation:	
A. Metabolic acidosis	
(arterial pH <7.30, Pco_2 <35, HCO_3^- <10 mEq per liter)	
1. BUN > 60 mg per 100 ml	Uremic encephalopathy
2. Hyperglycemia (blood sugar > 250 mg per 100 ml)	Diabetic coma
a. 4+ Serum acetone	Diabetic ketoacidosis
b. No acetonemia	Diabetic lactic acidosis
3. Cyanosis (Po_2 <50 mm Hg) − shock	Anoxic lactic acidosis
4. History: diarrhea; hyperchloremia, ±hypokalemia	Diarrheal acidosis
5. Hyponatremia, hyperkalemia, ±hypoglycemia	Addison's disease
6. BUN, sugar, oxygen, blood pressure − normal	Exogenous poisoning
a. Paraldehyde odor on breath	Acidosis secondary to paraldehyde ingestion
b. Hyperemic optic discs, dilated sluggish pupils	Methyl alcohol poisoning
c. Oxalate crystals in urine	Ethylene glycol poisoning
7. None of the abnormal findings above	Spontaneous lactic acidosis
B. Respiratory alkalosis	
(arterial pH >7.45, Pco_2 <35, HCO_3^- >15 mEq per liter)	
1. Po_2 >50, hepatomegaly, serum NH_3 elevated	Hepatic encephalopathy
2. Po_2 <50, cyanosis	Cardiopulmonary disease
a. Rales, elevated venous pressure, cardiomegaly	Pulmonary edema
b. No heart disease	Pneumonia, alveolar-capillary block, pulmonary emboli
3. Absent pupillary and oculovestibular responses, decerebrate rigidity	Central neurogenic hyperventilation
4. Nystagmus on caloric testing, normal examination	Psychogenic hyperventilation
C. Mixed respiratory alkalosis and metabolic acidosis	
(arterial pH >7.35, Pco_2 <35, HCO_3^- <15 mEq per liter)	
1. Fever, tachycardia, hypotension	Gram-negative sepsis
2. Hyperthermia, positive urine $FeCl_3$ test	Salicylate poisoning
3. Abnormal liver function tests	Hepatic encephalopathy
II. Hypoventilation:	
A. Respiratory acidosis	
(arterial pH <7.30, Pco_2 >45, HCO_3^- >20 mEq per liter)	
1. Serum HCO_3^- >20 mEq per liter but <30 mEq per liter	
a. Normal lungs	Depressant drug poisoning
b. Rales, emphysema, Po_2 <40 mm Hg	Chronic pulmonary disease with acute CO_2 retention
2. Serum HCO_3^- >35 mEq per liter	
a. Normal lungs	
(1) Obesity	Pickwickian syndrome
(2) Not obese	"Central alveolar hypoventilation"
b. Rales, emphysema, Po_2 <40 mm Hg	Chronic pulmonary disease with slowly developing CO_2 retention
B. Metabolic alkalosis	
(arterial pH >7.45, Pco_2 <55, HCO_3^- >35 mEq per liter)	
a. Alkali ingestion	
History of peptic ulcer	$NaHCO_3$ ingestion alkalosis
b. Gastric acid losses	
Vomiting, hypotension, hypovolemia	Gastric HCl depletion
c. Renal acid losses	
(1) Edema, heart disease	Diuretic therapy
(2) Hypokalemia, moon face, truncal obesity	Cushing's syndrome secondary to adrenal hyperfunction, steroid therapy, hormone-secreting lung neoplasms
(3) Hypertension, hypokalemia	Primary hyperaldosteronism

acidosis, or poisoning with an acidic product. Severe metabolic acidosis, if not treated, is rapidly lethal. Uremia, diabetes, and Addison's disease can be treated specifically (see Ch. 603, 806, and 846), and the others often respond to prompt and urgent treatment of the acidosis by infusion of bicarbonate. If, however, the serum pH is elevated in the delirious and hyperventilating adult, pulmonary disease, cardiac disease, hepatic coma, or neurogenic hyperventilation are the possible causes. Pneumonia is probably the most common cause of mild respiratory alkalosis in unconscious patients; the others can be evaluated by appropriate laboratory tests. When the serum pH is elevated and the bicarbonate is between 10 and 15 mEq per liter (mixed respiratory alkalosis and metabolic acidosis), sepsis, especially with gram-negative organisms, salicylism (which causes acidosis in children, alkalosis in adults), and severe hepatic coma are the probable causes.

A similar analysis can be applied to *hypoventilating* patients. In these, the severe problems are depressant drug poisoning, which produces a low serum pH with a normal bicarbonate, and chronic pulmonary failure, which produces a low serum pH and usually a high serum bicarbonate. (The serum bicarbonate level indicates the duration of hypoventilation.) Both situations demand ventilatory support.

Electroencephalogram (EEG). The EEG is useful in evaluating patients with metabolic brain disease because it is slower than in normal subjects and because it is symmetrical. The slowing indicates that there is neural dysfunction, and the bilateral symmetry suggests a diffuse process. The degree of slowing roughly parallels the severity of the encephalopathy. The normal EEG has a basic frequency of 8 to 13 per second. In metabolic disease, bilateral, synchronous, paroxysmal bursts of 1 to 3 per second activity are frequently superimposed upon a background of mildly slow 5 to 7 cps activity. A normal EEG is incompatible with severe delirium, and an EEG with focal or unilateral slow activity strongly suggests a structural and not a metabolic brain disorder.

Other Laboratory Tests. The causes of metabolic coma are legion, and a final diagnosis usually depends on extensive laboratory tests. The tests which should be performed immediately to establish the presence of life-threatening metabolic defects are listed in Table 4, along with those whose results are not available immediately but should be done as soon as possible if the diagnosis is unclear.

TABLE 4.   Laboratory Evaluation of Metabolic
Brain Disease

Test	Reason for Test
Immediate:	
Glucose	Hypoglycemia, hyperosmolar coma
Na$^+$	Osmolar abnormalities
Ca^{++}	Hyper- or hypocalcemia
BUN	Uremia
pH, Pco$_2$	Acidosis, alkalosis
Po$_2$	Hypoxia
Lumbar puncture	Infection, hemorrhage
Later:	
Liver function tests	Hepatic coma
Sedative drug levels	Overdose
Blood and CSF culture	Sepsis, encephalitis, meningitis
Full electrolytes, including Mg^{++}	Electrolyte imbalance
EEG	

DIAGNOSIS OF METABOLIC ENCEPHALOPATHY

The physician should consider metabolic encephalopathy as the possible diagnosis for every patient whose thinking, behavior, or state of consciousness has recently become disordered. The diagnosis requires, first, that one establish that metabolic encephalopathy rather than psychiatric disease or a structural brain lesion is causing the abnormal behavior and, second, that one identify the specific metabolic illness responsible.

Psychiatric disease is distinguished in the awake patient by examination of the mental status and the motor function. Patients with psychogenic amnesia who are disoriented claim to be confused about who they are as well as to the place and time; patients with metabolic brain disorders always know who they are. Hallucinations in psychiatric illness are usually auditory; in metabolic illness they are usually visual. Recent memory and cognitive abilities are generally preserved in psychiatric patients but are lost early in patients with metabolic illness. Tremor plagues anxious patients, and occasionally generalized seizures wrack those with catatonic schizophrenia, but asterixis and multifocal myoclonus are never present in psychiatric disease. Asterixis, if carefully searched for, is present in most patients with metabolic brain disease. Rarely, a patient with "hysterical coma" will present a diagnostic problem. Such patients are quietly unresponsive, and all their limbs are flaccid, but they often strongly resist passive eye opening. If the diagnosis is doubtful, irrigating the tympanum with 50 ml of cold water is informative; this procedure produces physiologic nystagmus in the patient with "hysterical coma," but only tonic eye deviation in the comatose patient with metabolic disease. The EEG in "hysterical coma" shows a normal awake record; it is always abnormal in metabolic coma.

Supratentorial mass lesions that encroach on the diencephalon produce diffuse brain dysfunction (see Ch. 319). However, supratentorial lesions produce focal motor and/or sensory signs early in the illness, often before mental changes, and these focal signs either persist or grow worse. Hemiparesis or hemisensory defects, although occasionally present in metabolic disease, are usually mild, often fleeting, and generally appear only after consciousness is lost. Late in the course of mass lesions, when transtentorial herniation has impaired midbrain function, bilateral decorticate or decerebrate rigidity usually replaces unilateral motor signs. These motor signs of midbrain dysfunction may also be present in metabolic coma, but in metabolic coma the pupillary light reflexes are retained, thereby ruling out a structural lesion. The EEG of a patient with a supratentorial mass lesion is usually slow either focally in one area or laterally over one hemisphere; that of a patient with metabolic brain disease, even when focal neurologic abnormalities are present, is symmetrically slow. Skull roentgenograms of patients with structural lesions reveal shift of the pineal gland (if calcified) away from the side of the mass, but the pineal is midline in metabolic disease. If doubt still persists, brain scanning or angiography outlines structural lesions causing coma but is unremarkable in metabolic disorders.

Subtentorial structural lesions are distinguished from metabolic brain disease by the presence in the former of signs of cranial nerve and focal brainstem dysfunction. In patients with subtentorial lesions causing changes in consciousness, the pupils are almost always abnormal, either because pontine and medullary sympathetic pathways are involved or because the third nerve nuclei or fibers are destroyed. Both pupillary light reflexes and the ciliospinal reflex (pupillary dilatation to noxious cutaneous stimuli) are preserved in metabolic disease. Dysconjugate eye movements are common with subtentorial lesions, rare with metabolic disease. Unilateral facial weakness involving both the brow and lower face, unilateral facial anesthesia, absent caloric responses to one side, or eye deviation toward a paralyzed arm and leg all suggest a subtentorial lesion and are against the diagnosis of metabolic disease.

Dementia is the expression of irreversible metabolic brain disease in which the primary metabolic error usually resides in the brain rather than affects the brain secondarily. For this reason, the incipient signs of dementia can resemble delirium, and distinction may sometimes be difficult. In general, dementia begins gradually, whereas delirium begins either acutely or subacutely. Recent memory loss, cognitive difficulties, and disorientation to place occur early in dementia and precede any change in consciousness, whereas lethargy, apathy, decreased awareness, and disorientation in time are early marks of delirium. Tremor, asterixis, and myoclonus are rare in dementia (except myoclonus in Creutzfeldt-Jakob disease). Mild or moderate dementia reduces the brain's defenses against metabolic insults, and thus it is common for a fully reversible delirium to complicate mild systemic illnesses in demented patients. In these cases only treatment of the systemic disorders will separate the delirious component from the dementia (see Ch. 326 to 331).

Differential Diagnosis. Delirium means that a metabolic illness is so advanced that it not only threatens brain function but may threaten life itself unless promptly diagnosed and reversed by treatment. Since the neurologic manifestations of the various metabolic encephalopathies are often similar, specific diagnosis by physical examination is often impossible, so some systematic approach to the problem is needed.

In Table 1 are listed all of the common and many of the less frequent causes of metabolic brain disease. Those marked with an asterisk either alone or in combination account for most of the delirium encountered on general medical wards. The table is designed as a checklist; the specific symptoms, signs, and management of each of the systemic disorders causing delirium can be found elsewhere in this book.

When the cause of delirium is unclear, the first conditions to consider are *hypoxia, hypoglycemia,* and *metabolic acidosis.* Unless promptly treated, all three are potentially rapidly lethal, and the first two very quickly damage the brain irreversibly.

Certain physical signs, such as respiratory abnormalities, convulsions, and fever, suggest specific diagnoses. The examination of respiration aids in the diagnosis of pulmonary encephalopathy, sedative drug poisoning, gram-negative sepsis, and hepatic coma (Table 3). Often an early clue to the diagnosis of hepatic coma is the presence of respiratory alkalosis, which then prompts liver function tests or a blood ammonia determination to support the diagnosis. *Generalized convulsions* occur in many metabolic brain disorders, especially with hypoxia and hypoglycemia. Repeated seizures are dangerous since they create the risk of brain damage and should be treated even before their cause is clear. If hypoxia and hypoglycemia are not the cause, repeated seizures suggest sedative drug withdrawal, uremia, hyponatremia, hypocalcemia, or penicillin encephalopathy.

Agitated delirium accompanied by fever prompts immediate consideration of intracranial infection. Often the patient with meningitis is so combative that nuchal rigidity cannot be adequately assessed, and only lumbar puncture confirms the diagnosis. A lumbar puncture should be performed on any patient who is delirious without obvious cause and who lacks evidence of sustained increased intracranial pressure. Encephalitis and subarachnoid hemorrhage often present initially with delirium accompanied by little or no fever and no nuchal rigidity, and may not be diagnosed unless the cerebrospinal fluid is examined. In any delirious patient with nystagmus or ocular palsies, thiamin deficiency encephalopathy (see Ch. 404 to 406) should be immediately considered, because if this condition is untreated, cardiovascular collapse and death may follow.

Once the dangerous and potentially lethal illnesses detailed above are excluded, there is time to consider the many other causes of metabolic brain disease and to make the tests appropriate to their diagnosis. In most cases, a single cause for delirium is not found. Instead, the patient has multiple metabolic defects, no one of which is sufficient to produce delirium, but the sum total of which in a susceptible patient is responsible. A common example is an *elderly* patient with mild *congestive heart failure, anemia,* and *hypoxia* being given *sedative drugs* for agitation and diuretics which have caused an electrolyte imbalance. The dismay caused by the multiplicity of diagnostic possibilities is partially offset when the physician makes the happy therapeutic discovery that treatment of any one of the metabolic disorders may substantially improve his patient's delirium.

PROGNOSIS AND TREATMENT OF METABOLIC BRAIN DISEASE

Metabolic brain disease can be definitively treated only by correcting the systemic disorder responsible for the delirium, and the effectiveness of this correction, in turn, determines the prognosis of the delirium. With the exception of severe hypoxia, hypoglycemia, or thiamin deficiency, all of which can cause neuronal death, delirium clears as the systemic disorder causing it improves. Often, however, the encephalopathy improves much more slowly than the systemic illness so that severe encephalopathy may persist four to five days or more after the systemic disorder has been fully reversed. Such a delay need not portend an unfavorable outcome, and vigorous efforts to prevent infections and other complications of delirium and coma are indicated during this period, for full recovery of cerebral function still is possible.

Certain general therapeutic measures apply to all delirious patients (Table 5). An adequate *airway* and *oxygenation* of the blood must be assured. For stuporous or comatose patients, this may require an endotracheal tube or tracheostomy. *Blood volume, cardiac output,* and *blood pressure* must be maintained at near normal levels to assure adequate cerebral blood flow. If the cause of coma is not known, a blood glucose should be obtained; but even before the results are reported, intravenous glucose (50 ml of 50 per cent solution) should be given to assure that hypoglycemia will not cause irreversible brain damage. Abnormalities of *acid-base balance* and of

TABLE 5.   Immediate Treatment of Metabolic
Brain Disease

1. Assure oxygenation
2. Maintain circulation
3. Give glucose
4. Restore acid-base balance
5. Treat infection
6. Control body temperature
7. Stop seizures

electrolyte balance should be corrected. Correction should be carried out over several hours, because too rapid correction often leads to other metabolic abnormalities. Infection should be treated and fever lowered.

The awake, delirious patient should be kept in a quiet room, away from the unfamiliar noises and bustle of the general ward. The room should be well lighted, and a light kept burning at night, because darkness accentuates disorientation and hallucinations. Physicians and nurses can reassure the patient by introducing themselves at each contact and quietly apprising him of his whereabouts. All procedures must be carefully and often repetitively explained before they are done. Drugs not essential for treatment of the patient's systemic illness should be withdrawn. This applies particularly to sedatives, narcotics, and tranquilizers, all of which commonly cause or accentuate delirium; it also applies to extensive use of diuretics, antihypertensive drugs, anticonvulsants, and even digitalis, medications that are less widely recognized to cause or accentuate delirium. If the patient is agitated and hyperactive, small doses of diazepam, starting with 5 mg orally or intramuscularly, and increasing as necessary, can be given to quiet him but not to render him unresponsive.

Careful attention is required to other systemic disorders that, although not of themselves sufficiently severe to cause delirium, may increase an already present encephalopathy. Oxygen should be given to mildly hypoxic patients, and transfusions should be administered to those with significant anemia. Mild electrolyte disorders such as hypokalemia and hyponatremia are diagnosed by periodic serum electrolyte determinations and are corrected by appropriate fluid control. Such measures often improve a patient's delirium considerably, even if the primary cause cannot be treated. Fluid losses should be routinely measured and replaced parenterally if the patient is not eating. Vital signs and the state of consciousness must be checked frequently to ensure that sudden worsening does not go undetected.

Lipowski, Z. J.: Delirium, clouding of consciousness and confusion. J. Nerv. Ment. Dis., 145:227, 1967.
Plum, F., and Posner, J. B.: The Diagnosis of Stupor and Coma. 2nd ed. Philadelphia, F. A. Davis Company, 1972.
Sokoloff, L.: Circulation and energy metabolism of the brain. *In* Albers, R. W., Siegel, G. J., Katzman, R., and Agranoff, B. W. (eds.): Basic Neurochemistry. Boston, Little, Brown & Company, 1972, Chap. 15, pp. 299–326.

321.   SLEEP AND ITS DISORDERS

Fred Plum

DEFINITION

Adult man spends one third of each day asleep. Yet why he sleeps and what "rest" does for his tissues are questions which thus far defy satisfactory answers.

Sleep is a recurrent state of relative inactivity of mind and body movement, readily interrupted by external stimuli but largely preventing any awareness of self or environment while it exists. The mere physiologic ability to cycle between sleep and wakefulness requires relatively little brain, although the amount of brain present modifies the cyclic pattern. Newborn babies, in whom the cerebral hemispheres are still little developed, sleep two thirds of each 24 hours in a series of relatively short sleep-wake cycles; anencephalic infants, whose brain stops at the midbrain, tend to do the same, as do adults who have suffered extensive injury to the cerebral hemispheres. Paralleling the evolving functional development of the hemispheres in older children, periods of continuous wakefulness become longer and longer until at about the age of six the adult diurnal pattern of sleep is established. Children up to about the age of 13 sleep more than adults, and women sleep more than men. Data reviewed by Kleitman indicate a mean duration of sleep in healthy adults of about eight hours, with little difference among subjects of different ethnic groups, occupations, or intelligence.

THE PHYSIOLOGY OF SLEEP

Knowledge about the fundamental physiology of underlying states of sleep and wakefulness has accumulated rapidly during the past two decades. These have disclosed that sleep is an active state composed of several identifiable stages regulated by the relations between distinct nuclear areas in the lower brainstem reticular formation and their connections with both more rostral and more caudal neural structures. Sleep is thus a very primitive vegetative function in the organization of the mammalian nervous system. Furthermore, different stages of sleep and wakefulness appear to depend on activity in anatomic pathways employing distinct neurotransmitter agents, lending hope that pharmacologic approaches may lead to better future methods of treating disordered sleep in patients.

The anatomy of sleep, like that of its antithesis, wakefulness, depends upon projections from centers located mainly in the caudal pontine reticular nucleus, the locus caeruleus, the vestibular nuclei, and the oculomotor control centers. Very little brain above the level of the midbrain is required for sleeping and waking to occur, because sleep-wake cycles exist in the most primitive vertebrates as well as in humans born with little or no brain tissue above the midbrain level. Sleep has at least two different forms, one characterized by low voltage fast activity on the EEG and accompanied by skeletal muscle atonia and rapid eye movements (thus the term REM sleep), and the other by increasingly slower waves on the EEG (SW sleep) as sleep becomes deeper. Most dreaming occurs during REM sleep. All evidence indicates that in the healthy state a balance occurs between REM and SW sleep in which REM occupies about one-quarter of the total time and recurs in episodes about every 100 minutes. Drugs which alter sleep affect these different stages in different ways, and there is evidence that human beings have a specific biologic need for a certain minimum of REM sleep as well as of total sleep.

Although few symptoms are more distressing than insomnia, it is not clear just why one needs sleep or what function the state serves. Over-all cerebral metabolism does not change during sleep. However, both Pappenheimer and Monnier have extracted from the cerebrospinal fluid or cerebral blood of sleep-deprived animals a factor that induces sleep when infused into wakeful recipients. Recent studies suggest that the induction and maintenance of the stages of sleep and waking are controlled at least in part by local concentrations in the brainstem of the biogenic amines serotonin and norepinephrine. Furthermore, these amines may serve as transmitters in specific brainstem pathways involved in sleep functions. However, the experimental evidence in the field still has inconsistencies, and it is not yet possible to describe a pharmacologic-physiologic model which fits all the observed requirements. The following references supply the most recent information in this fast-developing field.

Koella, W. P., and Levin, P. (eds.): Sleep. Proc. 1st European Congress of Sleep Research. Basel, Karger, 1973.

Pappenheimer, J. R., Fencl, V., Karnovsky, M. K., and Koski, G.: Peptides in cerebrospinal fluid and their relation to sleep and activity. *In* Plum, F. (ed.): Brain Dysfunction in Metabolic Disorders. Res. Publ. Assoc. Res. Nerv. Ment. Dis., 53:201, 1974.

Williams, H. L.: The new biology of sleep. J. Psychiatr. Res., 8:445, 1971.

DISORDERS OF THE QUALITY OF SLEEP

Too little sleep is known as *insomnia* and too much as *hypersomnia*. Insomnia most frequently results from functional disorders, whereas hypersomnia is often, but not invariably, a sign of organic neurologic disease.

Insomnia. Insomnia has three patterns: difficulty in falling asleep after retiring, intermittent waking throughout the period of attempted sleep, and early awakening. Direct observations on patients suffering from insomnia almost always reveal that they are less wakeful than they think, and there is little evidence that chronic insomnia takes any physical toll. Nevertheless, even brief difficulties in falling or staying asleep cause great subjective distress and lead to a large annual consumption of sedatives.

Physical causes of insomnia are comparatively few. Patients with chronic pain often suffer more at night, which keeps them awake. Those with unrecognized orthopnea resulting from heart disease sometimes translate their difficulties into a primary complaint of sleeplessness; the same is true of patients with marginal pulmonary insufficiency, in whom inability to sleep may be the first sign of respiratory decompensation. Insomnia can be an early symptom of acute infectious illness and is common in Sydenham's chorea and in bulbar poliomyelitis. Aside from these occasional associations with physical illness, difficulty in sleeping reflects mainly anxiety, worry, or depression. Whether insomnia occurs on going to bed or with early awakening helps relatively little in estimating its seriousness as a symptom.

To treat insomnia requires understanding, patience, a close attention to its accompaniments, and a willingness to discuss psychologic issues. Patients with difficulty in sleeping should be advised to eat light evening meals and to avoid stimulants such as coffee or tea after midday. Early morning awakening in the elderly most frequently reflects a declining need for sleep, and is best met by having the subject plan his day better and avoid afternoon naps. All patients are reassured by knowing that sleeplessness will not harm their bodies, and many regain the ability to sleep after a sympathetic physician has taken the time to discuss with them the issues that keep them awake. Patients with insomnia should always be asked sympathetically but directly if they are depressed and particularly if they have considered suicide. Drugs to treat insomnia should be used sparingly. All sedatives are potentially addicting, and most subjects with severe insomnia rapidly develop tolerance to sedation. Alcoholic nightcaps are inadvisable; the sedative effect is moderate and the temptation to "drown" anxiety is great. The most widely used sedatives and their recommended starting dose in grams are chloral hydrate, 1.0; secobarbital sodium, 0.1; pentobarbital sodium, 0.1; and glutethimide, 0.5. Any of these agents are also satisfactory for sedating patients in hospital, and the dosage can be repeated safely at least once or even twice in that setting. When insomnia is associated with depression, amitriptyline, 25 to 100 mg, is useful; the entire dose should be given at bedtime, starting at the lower dose and increasing. Insomnia coupled with more severe symptoms of depression demands close supervision and skilled psychologic management.

Hypersomnia. Hypersomnia occasionally signifies nothing more serious than boredom and mild depression, particularly among adolescents and young adults. Young women sometimes develop transient hypersomnia during menstruation. Occasionally one encounters hysterical hypersomnia, with which patients may claim to sleep for days at a time, then awaken fully. More often, however, excessive sleepiness signifies either narcolepsy or structural nervous system disease; among patients with the latter, the dividing line between prolonged hypersomnia and coma may be difficult to establish. Many neurologic conditions prolong or excessively deepen sleep. These include increased intracranial pressure, neoplasms around the third ventricle or in the posterior fossa, head trauma, encephalitis, and many metabolic disorders, including carbon dioxide retention, hepatic encephalopathy, uremia, pituitary insufficiency, and the surreptitious taking of drugs. With so many potential causes, the approach to hypersomnia of unknown cause resembles that employed to evaluate undiagnosed coma.

A rare condition of recurrent hypersomnia combined with excessive eating is sometimes observed in adolescent males, and is known as the *Kleine-Levin syndrome.* The cause is unknown, but the attacks last several days to a week or more, during which the patient eats voraciously and often develops disturbed behavior. Intervals of months to years of normal behavior separate the attacks. There is no treatment, and the attacks tend to disappear as the patient reaches adulthood.

Narcolepsy. *Definition and Etiology.* Narcolepsy is a chronic disorder characterized by recurrent and excessive drowsiness or sleepiness from which subjects are readily awakened. It is frequently accompanied by cataplexy, sleep paralysis, and, less often, hypnagogic hallucinations. As with most illnesses of unknown origin, many causes have been suggested. Some observers postulate a defect in the reticular formation of the brainstem, particularly since the REM stage tends to appear at the onset of narcoleptic sleep rather than approximately 90 minutes later, as with normal sleep. Other workers have been struck with the high incidence of psychologic disturbances (about 10 per cent of narcoleptics develop schizophrenic reactions), and have tended to regard this as the cause rather than an associated symptom of the illness. A high familial incidence of narcolepsy has been invoked as indirect evidence that the syndrome has a constitutional basis.

Clinical Findings.   Narcolepsy is uncommon but not rare. Both men and women are affected, and there appears to be no ethnic predilection. The onset is usually insidious during adolescence or young adulthood. Once the predisposition to excessive sleepiness starts, it is likely to last a lifetime if not treated. The symptoms range from mild drowsiness, which intrudes upon lecture hours, social events, or after-dinner conversations, to severe sleepiness in which subjects spend nearly the entire day drifting in and out of sleep, unable to work, play, or supervise the home. The sensation is reported as ordinary, uncontrollable drowsiness, perhaps with diplopia, but indistinguishable from that which normally follows severe fatigue. As witnessed by others, the sleep looks natural and is readily interrupted by stimuli. The naps refresh, but only briefly, and somnolence quickly recurs.

Cataplexy is a phenomenon of acute, brief, episodic, generalized muscular weakness, precipitated by feelings of emotion. It affects about three quarters of narcoleptic patients. In general, the stronger the emotion, the greater the muscular paresis, and patients relate that laughter, anger, or surprise "turns them to jelly" and induces brief collapse or aphonia without impaired consciousness. *Sleep paralysis* is a sensation of being unable to move while drifting into sleep or, less often, just upon awakening. Usually, brief contact with another person or strong effort interrupts the sensation, which lasts only a few seconds anyway. *Hypnagogic hallucinations* principally coincide with the early drifting phase of sleep when sleep paralysis occurs. Their intensity, the completeness of the visual or auditory recollections, and the time of onset distinguish them from dreams.

Physical abnormalities are lacking in primary narcolepsy. Laboratory studies are similarly normal. Neither hypothyroidism, hypoglycemia, nor any other endocrine abnormality has been substantiated in these patients, although the basal metabolic rate is low in many, reflecting their tendency to sleep through the test. The blood gases, and particularly the arterial carbon dioxide tension, are normal if obtained while the subject is awake, and no higher than in sleeping normal persons if drawn during drowsiness. The EEG contains normal patterns but a high percentage of sleep frequencies.

Differential Diagnosis.   Narcolepsy must be distinguished from psychogenic hypersomnia on the one hand, and occult central nervous system lesions on the other. Narcoleptic-cataplectic symptoms are intensifications of experiences known in a minor way to nearly everybody, and the exact point where excessive drowsiness, weakness during emotion, and sleep paralysis become a syndrome rather than a psychologic reaction to the environment can be difficult to decide in mild cases. Narcolepsy is favored if the symptoms date back to adolescence or have been present for several years, or if the drowsiness appears as a primary complaint interfering with other activities. Hypersomnia caused by toxins or central nervous system lesions usually resembles narcolepsy very little. Its onset is generally recent and fairly sharply identified in time. Also, the sleep is commonly deep, arousal is difficult, and the patients are slow and apathetic when awake in contrast to narcoleptic patients, who are alert as long as stimulated into wakefulness. Brain lesions causing hypersomnia often produce dementia and headache, neither of which complicates primary narcolepsy. Finally, structural brain lesions causing hypersomnia usually either are large or are situated near the deep midline structures of the third ventricle, and in both cases almost always result in physical signs of oculomotor, skeletal motor, or sensory dysfunction on the neurologic examination. In doubtful cases, lumbar puncture should be obtained as well as an electroencephalogram, which is almost always abnormal when a structural lesion produces hypersomnia.

Treatment.   The treatment of narcolepsy is largely symptomatic. General measures include drinking coffee or tea with meals and otherwise increasing everyday stimuli to a maximum. Most patients can continue to drive automobiles, for enough warning is experienced for them to pull off the road to sleep. Narcolepsy has no relation to epilepsy, and anticonvulsants have no place in treatment. Many individual stimulants have been tried, dextroamphetamine (Dexedrine) and methylphenidate (Ritalin) being most successful. Dextroamphetamine is usually initiated with doses of 10 mg three times daily. If patients require much larger doses, slow-release capsules yield sustained effects. Methylphenidate is the present stimulant of choice and is initiated in doses of 5 to 10 mg three times daily, then gradually increased until it either relieves drowsiness or produces unwanted nervousness and irritability. In addition, the tricyclic antidepressant imipramine in doses of 25 mg three times daily is quite effective in relieving cataplexy and should be combined with methylphenidate. Monoamine oxidase inhibitors have also been used to treat narcolepsy, but produce so many undesirable side effects that their use is not recommended. All stimulant drugs cause anorexia, and subjects must prevent weight loss by making conscious efforts to eat. Serious blood dyscrasias have not been reported. Occasionally the drugs produce excessive excitement or disturbed behavior, and must be discontinued.

Critchley, M.: Periodic hypersomnia and megaphagia in adolescent males. Brain, 62:627, 1962.

Guilleminault, C., Carskadon, M., and Dement, W.: On the treatment of rapid eye movement narcolepsy. Arch. Neurol., 30:90, 1974.

Kety, S. S., Evarts, E. V., and Williams, H. L. (eds.): Sleep and Altered States of Consciousness. Res. Publ. Ass. Res. Nerv. Ment. Dis., Vol. 45, 1967.

Kleitman, N.: Sleep and Wakefulness (revised and enlarged edition). Chicago, University of Chicago Press, 1963.

Zarcone, V.: Narcolepsy. N. Engl. J. Med., 288:1156, 1973.

Section Two. FOCAL DISTURBANCES OF HIGHER NERVOUS FUNCTION

Norman Geschwind

322. LANGUAGE, APHASIA, AND RELATED DISORDERS

Language is one of the most striking biologic attributes of man. Recent evidence suggesting that some potential for language exists in chimpanzees may open up new possibilities for investigation of the neurologic foundations of linguistic behavior. At present, however, nearly all our knowledge of the neural substrate of language is based on man. Detailed postmortem studies of well-described patients have provided the majority of the information, but useful data have been accumulated from patients with other types of disorders and from studies of the effects of stimulation of the brain during operations.

A striking feature of the human brain is dominance, i.e., the superiority of one hemisphere in the performance of certain functions. Dominance is not known to exist in any mammal other than man. About 93 per cent of people are right-handed, and at least 99 per cent of right handers have left hemisphere dominance for speech.

The situation is more complex and less well defined in the non-right-handed, i.e., the left handers and those with varying degrees of ambidexterity. Such a patient becomes aphasic as a result of lesion in *either* hemisphere, although left hemisphere lesions generally produce more lasting disability. A third group, *pathologic left handers*, who have suffered early childhood injury to the left hemisphere, are usually right-brained for speech.

The cause of dominance was in dispute for many years. We now know that the temporal speech region on the left is generally larger than the corresponding area on the right. The nondominant side is, however, endowed genetically with the capacity to develop language. Thus if the dominant hemisphere is damaged before age 10 or 12, there is nearly always excellent recovery of language, although the over-all degree of mental development is slowed. Spontaneous recovery from aphasia can also occur in later life, but much less frequently. Dominance in the intact human can be studied by two recently developed techniques. The Wada test consists of the injection of sodium amytal into the internal carotid artery. This causes a hemiplegia on the side opposite the injection, but aphasia results only from injection on the dominant side. This test is especially useful to neurosurgeons to ascertain the dominant side, especially in non-right-handed patients. Another technique, the *Kimura test,* is that of dichotic listening, in which different words are simultaneously presented to the two ears. Normal individuals tend to report the words presented to the ear opposite the dominant hemisphere.

323. APHASIA

The aphasias may be defined as disorders of language secondary to lesions of the brain. In most cases there is disorder of the output of speech. In the experience of the author, aphasia in spoken speech is invariably accompanied by similar abnormalities in writing. Aphasia in spoken language is of two major types: (1) Nonfluent aphasia, in which few words are produced slowly and with great effort, and sounds are incorrectly articulated. Production of grammatical words is relatively more affected so that sentences tend to be ungrammatical, e.g., "Weather sunny." (2) Fluent aphasia, in the more extreme forms of which the patient produces runs of well-articulated speech, which has the rhythm and melody of normal language and a basically normal grammatical structure, but which tends to convey little information, e.g., "I was at the other one and then I was at this one," a fluent aphasic's circumlocutory manner of explaining that he was in another hospital previously. The speech of these patients usually contains many incorrect words, called *paraphasias. Literal* (or phonemic) *paraphasias* are substitutions of well-articulated but incorrect sounds, e.g., "spoot" for "spoon," and *verbal paraphasias* are incorrect usages of words, e.g., "knife" for "fork," or "department" for "hospital."

In differential diagnosis, one must be wary of describing *mutism* as aphasia, because even severe aphasics are usually not mute. Causes of mutism are (1) uncooperativeness, (2) psychiatric disorders, e.g., severe depression or schizophrenia, (3) widespread disorders of brain, such as trauma, subarachnoid hemorrhage, or metabolic disorders, (4) lesions of mesencephalic and pontine tegmentum, and (5) bilateral lesions of the cranial nerves serving the speech organs, their nuclei, or their supranuclear pathways.

Dysarthria should not be confused with aphasia. Dysarthric speech is incorrectly articulated, but, if transcribed, shows correct grammar and word usage. A helpful clue is that if a patient who is mute or has completely unintelligible speech can produce fully normal language (not just his own name) in writing or on a typewriter, he is almost certainly not aphasic.

A common error is to misdiagnose a fluent aphasia as schizophrenic word-salad. Several clues help to make the differential diagnosis. Fluent aphasia is much more common than schizophrenic word-salad. The schizophrenic speech disorder usually develops in chronic "back ward" schizophrenics. By contrast fluent aphasia may come on abruptly as the result of a stroke in a previously well person. Finally, fluent aphasia from vascular disease usually occurs in older people, whereas schizophrenia almost always is manifest before the age of 30.

Aphasic Syndromes and Their Localizations. *Broca's aphasia* is the result of a lesion of Broca's area, i.e., the portion of the frontal lobe just anterior to the face, lip, tongue, and mouth area of the motor cortex. This produces a nonfluent aphasia, and writing is also involved. Comprehension of language is intact. There is nearly always a right hemiplegia. *Wernicke's aphasia* results from a lesion of Wernicke's area, the posterior portion of the superior temporal gyrus. The aphasia is typically fluent. Written language is equally impaired. Comprehension of spoken and written language is severely impaired. Repetition of spoken language is poor. There is usually no hemiplegia, and other elementary neurologic signs are usually lacking. *Conduction aphasia* results from a lesion of the parietal operculum, i.e., the region lying above the sylvian fissure. There is fluent aphasia involving speech and writing, with severely impaired repetition but intact comprehension. Elementary neurologic signs are usually absent, with the occasional exception of cortical sensory loss on the opposite side. *Anomic aphasia* is characterized by fluent aphasia in speech and impairment of written language, but with intact comprehension and repetition. The components of the Gerstmann syndrome (discussed subsequently) are often present. In this syndrome the lesion, if focal, is at the region of the parietotemporal junction, but a similar syndrome is produced in nonfocal widespread disease of the brain, such as is caused by metabolic disease or by large tumors with raised intracranial pressure.

These four syndromes are the most common, and although overlapping forms are common, relatively pure forms are not rare. Certain other syndromes are much less common.

In *isolation of the speech area* there is a large lesion involving the cortex and underlying white matter in a C-shaped configuration that spares Broca's area, Wernicke's area, and their interconnections, but destroys the cortex and underlying white matter that surround the speech region. These patients either may show little spontaneous speech or may have fluent abnormal speech. The most striking characteristic of this disorder is that despite an almost total lack of comprehension, the patient can repeat well without dysarthria. This lesion is usually the result of anoxia or of carotid insufficiency. *Alexia without agraphia* is a syndrome in which the patient speaks and writes normally but cannot comprehend written language. The lesion, almost always the result of infarction in the distribution of the left posterior cerebral artery, consists of destruction of the left visual cortex and the splenium, i.e., the posterior portion, of the corpus callosum. In *alexia with agraphia* the patient can neither write nor comprehend written language, but other language functions are normal. Other components of the Gerstmann syndrome (see below) may be present. The lesion involves a portion of the left angular gyrus. A right visual field defect may occur if the lesion extends deeply into the white matter but is often absent. *Pure word-deafness* describes a syndrome in which there is dense incomprehension of language in the presence of intact hearing, although other language functions are intact. Two types of lesion produce this: either a single lesion lying subcortically in the posterior temporal lobe or bilateral lesions of the middle portion of the first temporal gyrus. *Pure agraphia* is extremely rare as the result of any focal lesion, but is common in patients with confusional states of toxic, metabolic, or traumatic origin.

324. OTHER DISORDERS OF THE HIGHER FUNCTIONS

Apraxia.   Apraxia is the inability to perform a learned act in response to a stimulus which would normally elicit it, and which cannot be accounted for by weakness, in-

coordination, reflex change, sensory loss, incomprehension, inattention, or uncooperativeness. Three lesions may produce apraxia. With lesions of the corpus callosum there will be apraxia of the left side of the body, but not of the right or of the face. Patients with Broca's aphasia (who usually have a right hemiplegia) will show apraxia that is usually most marked in the face and is also often present in the left limbs. With lesions in the left parietal operculum, producing a conduction aphasia, there is usually apraxia in the face (where it is most marked) and in the limbs of both sides of the body. In all forms of apraxia whole-body movements, e.g., "stand up," "sit down," "turn around," and movements of eye-closing and eye-opening are best preserved. In all forms of apraxia the defect is most marked to verbal command (although the patient comprehends), usually somewhat less marked on imitation of the examiner, and least marked in the handling of objects, although in some patients even this latter category is impaired.

Agnosia.   Agnosia is a failure of recognition of complex stimuli in the face of preserved elementary perception. The most common form is visual agnosia, in which there are usually bilateral posterior occipital lobe lesions. The agnosias are less well understood than the aphasias or apraxias.

Callosal Syndromes.   These were first brilliantly described by Hugo Liepmann in the early 1900's, but have been rediscovered only in recent years. In some cases of anterior cerebral artery occlusion there is infarction of the anterior four fifths of the corpus callosum. The patient will carry out verbal commands with the right hand but not the left. He will name objects held (concealed from vision) in the right hand but not the left. He can, however, with the left hand draw or select from a group of objects the one previously held in the left hand. He manifests, in brief, inability to transfer information between the two hemispheres. Involvement of the splenium of the corpus callosum plays a role in alexia without agraphia (see Ch. 323).

Gerstmann's Syndrome.   This consists of agraphia, right-left disorientation, acalculia (difficulty in carrying out calculations), and finger agnosia (inability to name fingers or to identify them). The patient almost invariably also shows constructional disorder, i.e., a difficulty in drawing or copying designs, especially three-dimensional ones. When all the components of this syndrome are present, the lesion almost invariably lies in the left posterior parietal region. It should, however, be kept in mind that a single component has little localizing value. Thus constructional difficulty without the other components may result from lesions in many locations.

Right Hemisphere Syndrome.   Lesions of the right parietal region produce constructional difficulty that is more severe on the average than that produced from any other site. Patients with lesions in this location may also show a dressing disorder manifested by great difficulty in putting on clothes. Milder degrees of the difficulty may be brought out by such maneuvers as putting one sleeve of the bathrobe inside out; the patient may be unable to get the bathrobe on properly.

A striking feature of acute lesions of the right hemisphere is *anosognosia,* i.e., a tendency to deny or neglect disability, or when admitting its presence, to be unconcerned with it. It is a common experience that the patient with an acute left hemiplegia will show this type of behavior, although by contrast the patient with an acute right hemiplegia will, even if aphasic, show appropriate awareness of disability and will be depressed. These disorders in right hemisphere lesions are always accompanied by a curious mental state, in which the patient shows apathy, poor attention, and often jocularity. These states (and the accompanying unconcern with illness) are usually transient, but are sometimes permanent in cases of large right parietal lesions. Patients with transient cases, however, do not necessarily have parietal lesions.

It should be noted that not all patients who deny illness suffer from right hemisphere disease. Weinstein has shown that a patient with any disability may deny illness if he is sufficiently obtunded. Thus a patient may deny blindness resulting even from disease of the eyes if he develops a confusional state from metabolic disorder or drugs.

325. MEMORY

Memory describes the processes by which past experience is stored and retrieved. Disorders of memory include *anterograde amnesia,* i.e., the failure to store new memories, or *retrograde amnesia,* i.e., disorders of storage or retrieval of memories laid down in the past.

Certain separable stages in memory storage have become clear from clinical observation. There is a stage of *immediate* memory, which is the ability to retain material presented as long as attention is not distracted. This is examined by such tests as digit span, i.e., the ability to repeat a series of digits spoken by the examiner. Most normal persons can immediately repeat a series of seven such digits. The next step is *transfer* to the long-term memory store. The first step in this is *intermediate memory* storage, and the later step is called *remote memory.* The reasons for separating these steps will become clear when we discuss the clinical syndromes.

ANATOMY OF MEMORY

Memories are probably held in short-term store simply by continuation of nervous activity. The transfer to the long-term store probably involves some molecular change either in nerve membrane or in intracellular organelles. The neural structures most involved appear to lie in the limbic system, especially the hippocampal region, mammillary bodies, and, according to some authors, the dorsomedial nuclei of the thalamus (Victor et al.). The intactness of these structures appears to be important, in some as yet undefined way, in the transfer of memories from the intermediate to the long-term stores. The memories are probably not laid down in these limbic structures, because their destruction does not lead to loss of remote memories. They must therefore act on the structures which are the sites of storage. The limbic structures are also important, as will be seen below, in retrieval from the intermediate store.

CLINICAL DISORDERS OF MEMORY

Memory disorder may be evident in widespread disorder of the brain such as may be produced by drugs or metabolic disorders. On the other hand, memory may be relatively or dramatically spared in many of the dementias. Thus memory is much less impaired than such functions as calculation and abstraction in general paresis. By contrast, in Alzheimer's disease, in which involvement of hippocampus is prominent, memory disorder is a salient feature of the initial stages.

Disease processes predominantly affecting the hippocampal-mammillary system will produce significant memory disorder with little or no effect on other intellectual functions. This clinical state is called *Korsakoff's syndrome.* When caused by thiamin deficiency, the most striking lesions are in the mammillary bodies. The hippocampus may be involved in Alzheimer's disease, head injury, or tumors. Disease of the posterior cerebral artery may cause infarction of the hippocampus. Herpes simplex encephalitis has a predilection for all the structures of the limbic system. Occasional cases of severe memory loss have been reported after bilateral removal of the medial temporal structures surgically.

In order to produce a permanent memory deficit, bilateral lesions of the mammillo-hippocampal system are required. However, a unilateral lesion of the *left* hippocampus will produce a transient memory disorder, which may last as long as three months (Geschwind and Fusillo).

The memory disorder that sometimes follows head injury illustrates well the different states of the memory process outlined above. A patient who shows this disorder, let us say a week after the episode, may exhibit the following picture. He will be alert, awake, and cooperative and may, on a standard IQ test, score in a normal or even superior range. In addition his immediate memory, as shown, for example, by digit span, will be normal. By contrast he shows an anterograde amnesia, i.e., an inability to learn new material. He also shows a retrograde amnesia extending back from 3 to 20 years. More remote memories, in particular most of what was learned before the age of 12, are much better preserved. Over the next two or three months the condition improves. The ability to learn new material reappears (but the patient will have a permanent gap in his memory for the period in which he lacked this ability). The retrograde amnesia gradually shrinks until it reaches its permanent form, with a duration of seconds to minutes. The long retrograde amnesia must therefore have been a disorder of retrieval, rather than storage. It thus appears that the integrity of the limbic structures is necessary for the retrieval from intermediate, but not remote memory. In cases of persistent Korsakoff's syndrome, such as occur frequently with other forms of disorders that produce permanent bilateral limbic system damage, the retrograde amnesia does not improve significantly.

A prominent feature of many but not all cases of Korsakoff's syndrome, especially in the early stages, is confabulation, i.e., the tendency of the patient to invent fanciful replies to questions whose answers he doesn't know.

Functional amnesia occurs in hysteria (usually young women) or in older patients who are depressed. A similar clinical picture seen in malingerers is usually easy to recognize. The patient may show either a highly selective memory disorder, e.g., denying that he is married, although all other recent and remote facts are preserved, or a global disorder, e.g., professing total amnesia for all events of his life. Failure of a patient without aphasia to state his own name is invariably not organic in origin.

Another common syndrome is the fugue state in which the patient denies any memory of his activities for a period of time ranging from hours to weeks, during which his external activities appeared normal or during which he disappeared and traveled extensively. Although some short-lasting fugue states may occasionally be the result of temporal lobe epilepsy, the author's experience has been that these are nearly all functional in origin.

Benign memory disorder, a common complaint with onset in the forties or even the late thirties, is the appearance of difficulty in recalling proper names or other specific features which are, however, usually recognized promptly. This problem often arouses great anxiety, but studies indicate that although this delimited difficulty may continue to progress over many years, it is usually not a forerunner of serious intellectual deterioration, and is often compatible with the highest levels of professional activity. It is called "benign" memory disorder to distinguish it from the rapidly progressive and disabling malignant forms in which even in the early stages the memory difficulty involves recollection of the over-all significance of many situations, rather than just isolated facts.

Geschwind, N.: Disconnexion syndromes in animals and man. Brain, 88:237, 585, 1965.
Geschwind, N.: The organization of language and the brain. Science, 170:940, 1970.
Geschwind, N., and Fusillo, M.: Color-naming defects in association with alexia. Arch. Neurol., 15:137, 1966.
Victor, M., Adams, R. D., and Collins, G. H.: The Wernicke-Korsakoff Syndrome. Philadelphia, F. A. Davis, 1971.
Zangwill, O. L.: Cerebral Dominance and Its Relation to Psychological Function. Springfield, Ill., Charles C Thomas, 1960.

Section Three.   DEMENTIA

Paul R. McHugh

326.   INTRODUCTION

General Considerations. Dementia means deterioration in intellectual capacity. The condition is distinguished from mental retardation, in which subnormal intellectual ability has been lifelong and may or may not be caused by brain injury; and from aphasia and Korsakoff's psychosis, in which specific intellectual skills (language and memory, respectively) have deteriorated without a proportional disturbance in other cognitive functions.

Dementia is a clinical entity. Any pathologic process affecting the cerebral hemispheres can lead to an impairment in intellectual capacity. The extent of the brain injury and not the location of injury or the nature of the neuropathology determines its severity. The diagnostic task is twofold: first, the physician must recognize the symptoms of dementia; then, he must identify the cerebral pathology producing it. The first aspect of diagnosis requires skill in testing mental function; the second, knowledge of the mode of onset of different pathologic conditions and of their particular neurologic features and diagnostic laboratory data.

Clinical Manifestations.   The earliest symptoms of dementia can pass almost unrecognized. They appear as disturbances in the patient's capacities for problem solving, grasp of situation, and agility of thought. He may carry out his daily routines at home and at work adequately, but he becomes inefficient in them and may fail in the tasks that are demanding or require his special skills. Thus a physician with dementia manages his familiar patients but is less able to diagnose or prescribe for new ones. A lawyer maintains his office but misses opportunities that depend on judgment and brisk decisions. A teacher spends unusual effort for a routine lesson and is puzzled by questions from his students that go beyond the prepared material. These changes are hard to distinguish from fatigue or boredom. The appreciation of their importance will depend on how well the examiner knows the patient and on how much the patient's liveli-hood depends upon mental capacity. Thus relatives and fellow workers usually notice a change before doctors can be sure of it; and professional, managerial, or skilled workers are more quickly brought for help than are individuals with unskilled occupations.

As a dementia progresses, however, the disability will be obvious to all because its symptoms are defects in basic mental functions. Memory failure is often the first definite symptom. The patient becomes forgetful particularly of the events of the day, overlooks appointments, fails to remember conversations, or forgets the purpose of his errands.

Other symptoms reflect the patient's bewilderment in the face of complexity. He becomes lost in attempting to find his way in the city. He fails to understand a conversation, particularly if several people are involved, as at a meeting. He cannot follow directions that involve a series of steps.

Language presents special difficulties. He is unable to use words with facility and pertinence, but depends on clichés and habitual forms of expression. His conversation becomes rambling and repetitious, his letters long and vague, his directions to others involved and obscure. Defining a word or a proverb for his examining physician is very difficult because he is unable to call up the meaning of abstract words and concepts.

At this stage in a dementing illness, habit sustains the patient's social behavior. Yet this façade of customary manners and speech cannot hide his deficits in mental capacity if examination is carried beyond casual interchange to test his memory, his orientation, or his grasp of situations and concepts.

The dementing patient often suffers from emotional disturbances. Sudden outbursts of emotion, taking the form of anger, tears, or aggressiveness may occur when the patient is attempting a task that is beyond his present mental skill. These *catastrophic reactions* are usually of short duration, but their repeated appearance may be a prominent feature of the illness almost from its onset. They can appear under circumstances in daily life such as during a difficult decision at work or during the mental status examination if a challenging problem is presented. Any such outburst will usually last until the extra demands on the patient are relieved, and during such an outburst the patient will be unable to solve problems that are within his capacity when he is in emotional control.

More sustained and chronic emotional disorders, such as depression and anxiety, are also seen in dementing illness for reasons that are not immediately obvious. They may represent a response of the patient comprehending his growing difficulties but may also represent an injury to central nervous system mechanisms mediating emotional expression.

A symptom seen in some patients and easily confused with depression is a progressive apathy or mental inertia. This may at first be just a loss of sparkle or liveliness of character, but progresses to involve initiative and the physical energy of the patient. Such apathy can result in much poorer performance in daily affairs than can be explained at first by the cognitive disabilities, but worsens as the dementia progresses and can reach such a state of unresponsiveness that the patient is inaccessible to examination.

Finally, if the dementing disorder is relentlessly progressive, the patient will lose all his mental powers. He will be unable to care for himself or appreciate any of his surroundings. He loses his remote memories, now failing to recognize his closest relatives. He cannot care for any of his physical needs and becomes bedridden and totally unaware of his situation. At this point his life is dependent on nursing care and usually is lost to intercurrent infection or malnutrition.

Dementia is thus a decline in all intellectual functions, reflected in every aspect of behavior.

Diagnosis. It is not difficult to recognize intellectual impairment in individuals late in the course of a cerebral disease. The more taxing problem is the recognition of the intellectual impairment when it is slight and potentially reversible. The tests of cognitive function that are part of the neurologic examination of every patient are intended to accomplish this. But they must be interpreted with care.

It is customary to test (1) orientation to time, place, and person; (2) language skills, by naming common objects and comprehending commands; (3) fund of knowledge, such as the names of some capital cities and of presidents; (4) recent memory, by setting three objects to be remembered for 5, 10, and 30 minutes; (5) attention span, by asking for a serial subtraction of 7 from 100 or any other arithmetic task that requires "carrying over"; (6) abstract reasoning power, by asking for definitions of proverbs or the similarity of words such as apple-orange, ear-eye, poem-statue; and (7) constructional capacity, by asking the patient to draw simple objects such as a clock or to copy an abstract design.

The results of these tests must be interpreted in the light of other knowledge about the patient. If the patient was a gifted professional person whose family has noted a decline in his judgment and an increasing forgetfulness, the discovery that he cannot hold three words in mind for five minutes and that he interprets proverbs clumsily provides some evidence that he is suffering from a disturbance to his intellectual power. On the other hand, if the patient was not a person with intellectual achievements in the past and has received a poor education, difficulties in proverb interpretation or fund of knowledge are less likely to represent brain disease. Al-

though it is possible to find all the intellectual functions disturbed in dementia, the tests for recent memory, for attention, and for constructional capacity are most useful. Deficiencies here are easy to document; these functions are affected early in the course of many brain diseases and they are little dependent on education. Also, tests for recent memory are useful in differentiating a patient with mental retardation from an individual of limited intelligence who is developing a brain disease, since memory function is intact in the mildly retarded individual.

It is important to differentiate Korsakoff's syndrome and aphasia. The patient with Korsakoff's syndrome will fail the tests of recent memory. He will be disoriented to time and place, but he will be able to name objects, obey commands, and accomplish tasks of abstract reasoning and drawing if he can hold the question in mind. His disorder is in memory. The rest of his intellectual function is relatively spared. The aphasic patient will have severe problems in naming objects and comprehending words. But if this difficulty can be surmounted, it will be evident that it is language specifically that is disturbed, and other mental functions such as memory, orientation, and the capacity to draw are relatively intact.

It is often useful to supplement the bedside tests of mental function with standardized examination of intellectual skills. The Wechsler Adult Intelligence Scale (WAIS) is most often employed. Nothing about this psychologic examination is different in concept from the bedside tests. It measures the intellectual performance of a patient by asking him to attempt problems in several different areas. Since a mathematical score is given, an objective comparison of his performance with that of others is possible. Although the WAIS includes problems similar to those given at the bedside, it adds several "performance" tests which are actually unfamiliar tasks, such as recognition of errors in pictures, design of patterns from colored blocks, and assembly of parts of puzzles. These tests most specifically examine the ability of a patient to put his mind to an unfamiliar situation and solve it. They are less dependent on learning and decline early in a dementia, producing a discrepancy between these "performance scores" and the "verbal scores" which tend to remain intact for a longer period.

Diagnostic Issues in Dementia. As mentioned previously, the symptoms of dementia appear with an injury to the cerebral hemispheres, and are not specific for a particular pathology. It is the course of their development, the associated neurologic signs, and the laboratory findings that permit diagnosis of the pathologic entities producing the dementia.

Since the same symptoms can be produced by curable, reversible pathology as by incurable and progressive disorders, the first diagnostic consideration should reflect a search for the treatable pathologic entities. Each of the following conditions should be considered in every patient with the symptoms of dementia: general paresis, myxedema, neoplasms and other chronic intracerebral lesions, hepatolenticular degeneration (Wilson's disease), avitaminosis B_{12}, and occult hydrocephalus. Many of these conditions can be diagnosed by evidence derived from the clinical examination; others demand clinical laboratory studies. Thus the Argyll Robertson pupil of cerebral syphilis, lateralized motor-sensory signs of neoplasm, the Kayser-Fleischer ring of Wilson's disease, and a gait disorder caused by a spastic weakness of legs in hydrocephalus should all be sought in the physical examination of the demented patient. A group of laboratory tests are required in the diagnostic evaluation. As a routine, all patients should have a lumbar puncture to measure intracerebral pressure and to obtain a sample of cerebrospinal fluid for analysis. Cell count, protein content, and a test for the syphilitic precipitants will be needed in cerebrospinal fluid. Blood serologic examination, analysis for protein-bound iodine and serum B$_{12}$ analysis are also indicated. An electroencephalogram is useful, as it may reveal a local lesion or a severe generalized slowing of the rhythms characteristic of delirium. Skull roentgenograms can also reveal a local lesion. In many patients it is necessary to proceed to a pneumoencephalogram in order to exclude some of the rarer but curable forms of dementia such as occult hydrocephalus.

The onset and course of a dementing disorder must be carefully analyzed when considering the likely pathologic entities. Was the onset abrupt or insidious, was the subsequent course a gradual and relentless loss of mental faculties, or was it a series of sudden losses producing a steplike decline in the mental faculties? Did it require months or only a few weeks to develop? Different pathologic entities produce different clinical histories in these respects. Thus the dementia associated with vascular disease of the brain will have a sudden onset and increase in an intermittent and variable fashion. The dementia of general paresis tends to be subacute and steadily progressive; that of degenerative disease is more insidious in onset and slow in development.

The characteristics of four known cerebral degenerations will be reviewed as they exemplify some of these general statements about dementia. These conditions are Alzheimer's disease, Pick's disease, Creutzfeldt-Jakob disease, and Huntington's chorea.

327. ALZHEIMER'S DISEASE

Alzheimer's disease is a progressive degenerative process of the brain that produces a dementia in middle to late life.

The brain in Alzheimer's disease gradually atrophies, nerve cells disappearing from the cortex. The major brunt of the atrophic process appears to be in the frontal and occipital regions of the brain, but microscopic examinations will demonstrate pathologic changes throughout the cortex. Many of the neurons that remain show a peculiar alteration of their neurofibrils, which are thickened and twisted into distinctive "neurofibrillary tangles." Within the atrophic cortex there are many "senile plaques." These are microscopic collections of granular argyrophilic particles which tend to form in a halo around an indefinite center containing sudanophilic fat or an amyloid-like substance. Exactly what these plaques are is uncertain, but they appear to represent collections of degenerating brain substance.

The dementia that accompanies Alzheimer's disease has few distinctive characteristics. All the symptoms of dementia enumerated above eventually appear. Onset is insidious and progress slow. A disturbance in recent memory is usually the first symptom. Affective disturbances such as depression or anxiety and disorientation in time and place appear soon after. Often there is a considerable emotional unrest in these patients, prompted

in some 30 to 40 per cent by delusionary false beliefs. A sizable fraction of patients also have auditory and visual hallucinations during illness. Focal neurologic signs are rare early in the course of the disease, but with progression of the illness, focal cortical symptoms of aphasia, apraxia, and agnosia often become prominent. Seizures, both focal and generalized, are common only in far-advanced instances. With these intellectual and emotional disturbances there is the development of a disorder of gait. This takes the form of difficulty in starting the rhythmical movements of walking. A synchronous activation of agonist and antagonist muscles results in a locking of the legs and a hesitant shuffle.

The progress of all these symptoms is much the same in all patients. It is slow, but usually within five to eight years of the onset of symptoms the patient reaches a terminal stage. Here there is a profound dementia and a decerebrate physical state with flexion contractures of all limbs. Death comes from an intercurrent infection or some other complication of the bedfast condition.

The age of onset varies. Because this disorder was first recognized among relatively young people, the term "presenile dementia" has been applied to Alzheimer's disease. This implies a distinction in kind between this condition and "senile dementia" that appears when many other changes of aging are evident. But the cerebral pathology and the clinical course of patients who develop symptoms before or after age 65 are the same. Alzheimer's disease, defined as it is by the cerebral pathology of atrophy with senile plaques and neurofibrillary tangles, is a disorder appearing with increasing frequency as people age.

Alzheimer's disease is not an uncommon disorder, but it is more common in females than in males. Autopsy diagnoses vary from 1 to 10 per cent in mental hospitals, the particular figure depending on whether the observers make a distinction between Alzheimer's disease and senile dementia.

The cause of Alzheimer's disease is unknown. Most examples occur sporadically, but a few patients have a family history of dementia. It is not even certain whether Alzheimer's disease is a specific response to one noxious biologic process or whether it is a more general response of the brain to injurious processes. The latter possibility is suggested by the occasional appearance of Alzheimer pathology in such different situations as the punchdrunk syndrome of boxers, Down's syndrome (trisomy 21), and postencephalitic parkinsonism.

The diagnosis of Alzheimer's disease is made most often by exclusion. An individual who has a slowly progressive dementia without prominent neurologic signs and without any of the clinical and laboratory findings of the treatable conditions mentioned, as well as a pneumoencephalogram demonstrating a moderate dilation of the cerebral ventricles with some atrophy of cortex, is most likely to be suffering from Alzheimer's disease. Only by cerebral biopsy can more conclusive evidence for diagnosis be found, and this cannot be recommended in the usual clinical situation.

328. PICK'S DISEASE

Pick's disease is also a degenerative disorder of the cerebral cortex that produces dementia in middle and late life. It is distinguished from Alzheimer's disease by its morbid anatomy.

In contrast to Alzheimer's disease, in which the cerebral atrophy is diffuse, in Pick's disease the atrophy is relatively circumscribed and confined to the frontal and temporal lobes, where the atrophy is severe. The microscopic pathology is also distinctive in Pick's disease; a particularly degenerating neuron characterized by the accumulation close to the nucleus of a globular argyrophilic mass that distends the neuron into a swollen ballooned form is seen in the disorder. This is the *Pick cell* and it is usually found widespread in the atrophying areas of cortex. There are usually neurofibrillary tangles and senile plaques as well in the atrophic parts of brain.

It is difficult to distinguish an example of Pick's disease from Alzheimer's disease on clinical grounds. Patients with Pick's disease may have less difficulty in gait than patients with Alzheimer's disease. Otherwise, the conditions seem clinically identical. Pick's disease is considerably less common than Alzheimer's disease, but, as in that condition, no definite cause has been identified. Some examples of Pick's disease appear to be transmitted by a dominant gene in a family, but many examples are without a family history.

329. CREUTZFELDT-JAKOB DISEASE

The dementia in Creutzfeldt-Jakob disease is rapidly progressive, advancing noticeably day by day from its onset to a fatal termination, usually within a year. The dementia is accompanied by a variety of neurologic symptoms such as ataxia, aphasia, paralysis, and visual disturbances and by prominent myoclonic jerking of the limbs and body at some stage in the disorder. The EEG is abnormal early in the disturbance, its normal rhythms lost and replaced with a distinctive mixture of slow and sharp waves useful for diagnosis. The condition is the result of a degeneration of cerebral cortex thought to be caused by a transmissible agent of the latent or slow virus variety. It is more thoroughly discussed in Ch. 400.

330. HUNTINGTON'S CHOREA

Huntington's chorea is a distinctive disease entity in which a dementia associated with chorea appears usually in the fourth or fifth decade of life. Its neuropathology is characteristic, and the disease is transmitted as an autosomal dominant.

The dementia of Huntington's chorea appears insidiously but is relentlessly progressive over the 12 to 15 years from onset to fatal termination of the illness. Although most of the cognitive disabilities of these patients are similar to those with other brain diseases, patients with Huntington's chorea can suffer from a profound mental apathy as the illness advances. This apathy can lead to unresponsiveness and mutism late in the course. The absence of aphasia at any stage of the disorder is a noteworthy distinction of this dementia from that in Alzheimer's disease.

Mood changes resembling manic-depressive illness are common in Huntington's chorea. Patients can have discrete periods of severe depression accompanied by psychomotor retardation and delusions of guilt that may prompt suicide attempts. The high incidence of suicide in Huntington's chorea (7 to 10 per cent is reported) is due in most part to these periods of delusional depression. Electroconvulsive treatment combined with antidepressant medication (imipramine, 150 to 250 mg per day) has proved efficacious in the treatment of these depressions. Periods of manic excitement with overactivity and delusions of wealth, strength, and worldly importance can alternate with the depressive periods. The manic symptoms respond to phenothiazine treatment (chlorpromazine, 300 to 500 mg per day).

In some patients symptoms of dementia or mood disorder may appear prior to the onset of choreic movements, and therefore these patients can present diagnostic difficulties. The correct diagnosis is made when the family history is discovered or chorea appears. Of particular interest is the possibility that the degenerative changes in Huntington's chorea may be affecting a particular neurochemical system that might provide a model for the appreciation of biologic mechanisms in both manic-depressive disorder and dementia.

Other characteristics of this disorder are given in Ch. 370.

331. TREATMENT OF THE DEMENTED PATIENT

With the obvious exception of the specific treatments for curable diseases, the issue of treatment for the demented patient is most often that of management of particular symptoms rather than reversal of a pathologic process. Often, a treatment based on some research finding is proposed for the degenerative disorders only to prove of little value when employed in a clinical trial. Thus the discovery that cerebral oxygen consumption is reduced in Alzheimer's disease led to treatments with both oxygen inhalation and hyperbaric chambers. But these treatments failed to produce significant improvement, almost certainly because the observed reduction in oxygen consumption is due to a reduction in the number of viable neurons rather than to an inadequate oxygen supply. Any treatment that is proposed for these distressing conditions is liable to be uncritically acclaimed, with eventual disappointment. The importance of the clinical trial with double-blind technique in assessing these treatments cannot be exaggerated.

Some general principles of management of the demented patient can be emphasized. First, complicating medical conditions such as congestive heart failure, dehydration, iron deficiency anemia, infections, and electrolyte imbalance can, even if not severe in themselves, make the mental condition of a patient with degenerative brain disease much worse. A meticulous correction of all medical complications will do much to aid the patient. Second, much of the emotional unrest in demented patients is due to fear produced by their disorientation, misidentifications, and misinterpretations and to *catastrophic reactions.* Great relief of these symptoms can come from a willingness of nurses and doctors to explain repeatedly to the patient his situation and the proper interpretation of what is happening. Changes in surroundings and in nursing personnel should be minimized; well lighted rooms, preferably with familiar possessions, serve best, and an attitude toward the patient that is accepting and supportive will do much to assist him. Any obligations that require effort beyond his capacity and so produce *catastrophic* reactions must be eliminated. Third, considerable help for individual symptoms can be gained by the use of pharmacologic measures. Sleep disturbances in demented patients are best treated with chloral hydrate, up to 1.0 to 1.5 grams at night. Acute confusional aggression or agitation can be relieved by phenothiazine medication, and thioridazine in doses of 50 to 100 mg three or four times daily has been effective. Depressive symptoms can respond to antidepressant medication (imipramine, 50 mg three times to four times per day).

All these drugs should be used sparingly, as the patient with cerebral degeneration may demonstrate toxic signs at much lower doses than normal patients. Drug toxicity can worsen the condition severely.

In general, the management of the demented patient rests on an appreciation of the nature of his psychologic disabilities and the application of psychosocial medical and nursing principles. The response to this management is often gratifying.

Corsellis, J. A. N.: Mental Illness and the Ageing Brain. London, Oxford University Press, 1962.

McHugh, P. R., and Folstein, M. F.: Psychiatric syndromes of Huntington's chorea. Semin. Psychiat., 1974.

Post, F.: Clinical Psychiatry of Late Life. New York, Pergamon Press, 1965.

Sjogren, T., Sjogren, H., and Lindgren, A. G. H.: Morbus Alzheimer and morbus Pick: A genetic, clinical and pathological study. Acta Psychiat. Scand. (Suppl. 82), 1952.

Strachan, R. W., and Henderson, J. G.: Psychiatric syndromes due to avitaminosis B_{12} with normal blood and marrow. Quart. J. Med., 34:303, 1965.

Wolstenholme, G. E. W., and O'Connor, M. (eds.): Alzheimer's Disease and Related Conditions. Ciba Foundation Symposium. London, Churchill, 1970.

Section Four. PSYCHOLOGIC ILLNESS IN MEDICAL PRACTICE

Paul R. McHugh

332. THE CONCEPT OF DISEASE IN PSYCHIATRY

Any general hospital can provide an experience in psychiatry, because an example of every psychologic disorder will eventually appear among patients admitted to its services. However, many skilled physicians feel unsure of their ability to manage these disorders. They are apt to contrast their knowledge of somatic illness founded firmly in morbid anatomy and pathophysiology with their understanding of psychologic medicine in which classifications seem based on confusing mixtures of symptomatology and speculative theories, and the most effective treatments are empirical. Such physicians will continue uncertain until they grasp how the basic concept of disease can bring order to psychiatry as it does in all of medicine. This they must accomplish before they can profit from a review of the clinical facts of particular psychiatric conditions; hence this chapter.

The term "disease" is difficult to define, because it is a concept and not something concrete or given in nature. It is intended to convey the idea that among all the morbid changes in physical and mental health it is possible to recognize groups of abnormalities as distinct entities or syndromes separable from one another and from the normal and that these separations will prove to have some biologic explanation when the entities have been thoroughly investigated.

All abnormalities can logically be viewed as quantitative changes merging imperceptibly into one another and into the normal, and can then be explained as consequences of disturbed interactions of a few vital processes. The Galenic concept of "humors" is just such a view. In fact the concept of disease based on qualitatively

distinct syndromes is a convention proposed first by Sydenham, and remains but a convention today. However, this has been the most useful convention in the natural sciences. It has become so indispensable in medical thinking that it is taken for granted in most discussions. Neglect of this convention explains much of the difficulty faced by students in psychiatry. Its logic thus needs review here.

The concept of any given disease passes through several stages as knowledge increases. At each stage attention focuses on certain features of the condition which are the "defining characteristics." At the first stage a "clinical disease entity" is recognized and defined as a constellation of symptoms and physical signs running a more or less predictable course or natural history. Dropsy, hemophilia, and epilepsy are typical clinical disease entities. But these entities are not pure species. Each can be the expression of any one of several different pathologic conditions. Dropsy, for example, is found with different pathologic conditions: glomerulonephritis, congestive heart failure, constrictive pericarditis. Thus the second stage is the division of the clinical disease entity into several "pathologic disease entities." When a disease can be conceived as a pathologic entity, the defining characteristics on which concept and diagnosis rest are results of laboratory tests that reveal pathologic function or morbid anatomy. Again, by way of example, the demonstration of an elevated blood urea nitrogen and albumin and casts in the urine of a patient with dropsy leads to a presumptive opinion that the pathologic disease entity responsible for his condition is glomerulonephritis. This presumptive diagnosis is confirmed by studying the histopathology of the kidney. The third and final stage in the concept of a disease is the recognition of a particular etiologic agency. This recognition can derive from any aspect of biologic knowledge:

Genetics, microbiology, and biochemistry have all made their contributions. For glomerulonephritis the etiologic agency is the phenomenon of autoimmunity, and it will be from investigations of this phenomenon that physicians can expect to gain a complete understanding of glomerulonephritis as well as a treatment that can prevent and cure it.

For many medical diseases the mark of the twentieth century has been the discovery of etiologic agencies and their action. Not so for psychiatry. For most psychiatric disorders knowledge has not passed the first stage on the traditional path, and for many even the hold on this stage is insecure. This insecurity arises in part from the difficulty of the subject matter, but also from a neglect of the standards of observation and history-taking that are required in defining a clinical disease entity.

This neglect has been defended by a common opinion in psychiatry that all psychologic disturbances are to be viewed as emotional reactions to some form of environmental distress, and thus are quantitative abnormalities differing from normal in a continuous and smooth fashion rather than grouping into qualitatively distinct entities with separable pathologies and etiologies.

One objection to this view has to be the practical one that it discards for no obvious advantage a convention that has ordered other abnormalities successfully. Another is that it oversimplifies mental disturbances to make them all expressions of a few psychologic mechanisms. A consideration of the forms of disorder for which psychiatry assumes responsibility will demonstrate the utility found in the concept of disease for some of them.

Three groups of disturbances fall into manageable psychiatric categories. *The first holds all those disturbances in mind and behavior that are a result of observable brain pathology.* Represented here are the clinical disease entities of delirium, dementia, and mental retardation. The conceptual and investigative approach to these conditions is indistinguishable from that for other somatic diseases. Such pathologic disease entities as Alzheimer's disease and such etiologic agencies as perinatal hypoxia, infections, and metabolic changes have been discerned.

The second group holds the two functional psychoses in which no obvious brain pathology is evident; schizophrenia and manic-depressive disorder. That these conditions are not unlike somatic disorders and should be conceived as clinical disease entities defined by symptoms and course is impossible to prove at this time. But this view was first prompted by the alien character of the symptoms that seemed unaccountable from an empathic understanding of the patient's temperament and his recent life experiences. It has been strengthened by the discovery of pharmacologic treatments specific to each entity and by the recognition of a few morbid conditions of the central nervous system leading to identical clinical conditions—temporal lobe epilepsy, amphetamine toxicity leading to a schizophrenia-like disorder, and the reserpine reaction that mimics a depressive disorder. It is now more conceivable that we are on the threshold of discoveries that will provide pathologic disease entities and etiologic agencies for these conditions than that they will be explained as quantitative exaggerations of emotional reactions.

The third group of disturbances in mind and behavior are the personality disorders and neurotic symptoms. The concept of disease does not fit these conditions. They seem to be quantitative rather than qualitative abnormalities in psychologic functions. It is difficult to say for these where normal leaves off and abnormal begins since they do seem to be extremes of normal variation. Personality disorders seem no more diseases than are shortness of stature, plainness of face, and dullness of wit. Neurotic symptoms such as anxiety or depression, like any symptoms of disturbance, can be evoked by many causes, including somatic or psychiatric diseases, but they most commonly appear as understandable reactions of an individual with a disordered personality faced with an environment that strikes at his special vulnerability.

Thus the concept of disease does provide in psychiatry a means for organizing clinical material that is similar to that used in general medicine. In the following chapters its application in the detailed consideration of the separate conditions will be attempted.

Jaspers, K.: General Psychopathology. Translated by J. Hoenig and M. Hamilton. Manchester, Manchester University Press, 1963.

Scadding, J. G.: Diagnosis: The clinician and the computer. Lancet, 2:877, 1967.

Taylor, F. K.: Psychopathology. Its Causes and Symptoms. London, Butterworth and Co., Ltd., 1966.

Wightman, W. P. D.: The Emergence of Scientific Medicine. Edinburgh, Oliver and Boyd, 1971.

FUNCTIONAL PSYCHOSES

333. INTRODUCTION

The psychoses form a loose category that gathers together several different clinical entities. To be placed within the category an entity must produce disturbances in thinking and perception that are inexplicable solely as responses to experience and are severe enough to distort the patient's appreciation of the real world and the relationship of events within it. The category psychosis has no uniform foundation as in somatic pathology nor any more objective aspects of psychopathology to mark its distinction from other collections of psychiatric symptoms. It is thus a term difficult to use with precision. Sometimes psychosis is used as a euphemism for insanity, sometimes as a synonym for schizophrenia, one of the entities within the category, and sometimes to draw an elusive and dubious distinction as between neurotic and psychotic depression.

The unmodified term can be qualified by a differentiation into organic psychoses and functional psychoses. Here the term psychosis means only severe mental illness. The organic psychoses, delirium, dementia, and Korsakoff's syndrome, are produced by a variety of cerebral pathologies. The functional psychoses, schizophrenia and manic-depressive disorder, lack a recognizable neuropathology.

This differentiation is practical. It draws a distinction in kind that affects treatment and prognosis, and it indicates the character of the clinical problem. For the organic psychoses the central problem is the cause of the pathologic changes. For the functional psychoses the central problem is consistent diagnosis.

Schizophrenia and manic-depressive disorder are clinical disease entities. The criteria for their diagnosis are their symptoms alone. There are no objective tests verifying a diagnosis. Only the natural history or response to empirically discovered treatments can confirm a diagnostic opinion. Since they lack a recognized neuropathology and are by definition inexplicable as responses to experience, there are no comprehensive etiologic explanations for these disorders. Treatment therefore is symptomatic rather than fundamental. Both prevention and radical cure await a chance discovery or a major scientific advance in understanding the biologic foundations of human behavior.

334. SCHIZOPHRENIA

Schizophrenia is a most devastating mental illness. It is a disturbance of mind and personality appearing in clear consciousness and characterized by several distinctive alterations in mental experiences, modes of thinking, and mood that are seldom completely resolved. The most characteristic features occur during the active phases of the disturbance, and take the form of hallucinations, delusions, and altered behavior toward others. Specific intellectual and affective disabilities varying from minimal to severe can develop insidiously or remain after an attack. A crucial element of the definition is that all these symptoms occur in a patient free of any relevant and discernible pathologic change in his nervous system.

Clinical Manifestations. The symptoms of schizophrenia can begin at almost any stage in life, but most commonly occur during adolescence and early adulthood and then either insidiously or as an acute attack followed by a series of attacks, each leaving behind personality defects of increasing severity.

In some patients it is possible to recognize a particular premorbid personality. They may have seemed more timid or seclusive than others. They may have been bookish, unsociable, and preoccupied with philosophic and religious ideas to the exclusion of friendships and community experiences. But this so-called *schizoid personality* is not found in most patients who develop schizophrenia. At least half of schizophrenic patients had premorbid personalities indistinguishable from normal.

Among the mental changes that mark the onset of a schizophrenic illness, only some are specific to this disorder. Emotional unrest, uncertainty, perplexity, and confusion can be found in many disorders other than schizophrenia, and therefore a diagnosis of schizophrenia cannot rest on them. There are, however, a number of mental changes that are more or less diagnostic. These can be usefully divided into abnormal mental experiences and disturbed modes of expression. The abnormal mental experiences are somewhat more reliable evidence of the illness simply because they are easier to elicit with confidence and less dependent upon interpretation than disturbances in expression.

Hallucinations and delusions are the outstanding schizophrenic mental experiences. Although hallucinations can occur in many disorders such as delirium, dementia, and occasionally manic-depressive disorder, certain forms of hallucinations are more specific for schizophrenia. Thus auditory hallucinations are the most common hallucinations in schizophrenia, and certain kinds of auditory hallucinations are almost diagnostic. Thus hearing one's thoughts aloud or hearing voices commenting about one's every action or several voices engaged in a conversation in which derogatory and praising remarks are passed with the patient discussed in the third person are the most typical schizophrenic hallucinations.

Although delusions, i.e., false beliefs that are incorrigible, idiosyncratic, and preoccupying, can be found in many disorders other than schizophrenia, in this illness delusional experiences are dramatic and well developed. They can begin as vague, fearful interpretations and "half-beliefs" and develop into firm incorrigible convictions. A delusion coming on suddenly, not prompted by any hallucination or previous delusion, nor related in any obvious way to the patient's mood, is called a "primary delusion" and is highly suggestive of schizophrenia. Many other schizophrenic experiences are of delusional form, but have such individual characteristics that they have been named for themselves.

Commonly schizophrenics have delusions about bodily control, the so-called passivity experiences. The patient feels as though he were under the control of some outside force or power making him behave as an automaton without a will of his own. He may feel hypnotized and feel forced to make particular movements, speak with a special voice, or walk to certain areas. The patient may believe these feelings come to him as penetrating waves from electronic or telephonic equipment.

The schizophrenic patient may experience changes in his thinking. Particularly he may feel that his thoughts are disrupted by some outside agency, that his thoughts are withdrawn from his mind, or that other thoughts are inserted into it. He may believe that people can hear his thoughts, which are leaving his mind as waves broadcast to others.

In contrast to these abnormalities of experience are the disturbances in the patient's mode of expression. Particularly noticeable is his abnormal language. Characteristically, he is difficult to understand. His thinking is expressed in a vague and awkward fashion with words poorly chosen and ideas poorly related to one another. Strikingly, the patient makes no effort to correct the vagueness of his thinking or to improve the clarity of his talk. Often, asking a question of the patient, the examiner receives a reply that is off the point and that goes into unnecessary details. Although the questions of the interview seem to start the patient toward a particular answer, it is never reached, but the patient takes up abstract and unnecessary ideas and must be redirected toward his goal. The examiner, laying the responsibility for the confusion on himself, may work to express himself more clearly, and only after considerable effort recognize that the difficulty in communication rests with the odd replies from the patient.

Another prominent disturbance is emotional expression of these patients. They seem distant, unresponsive, and cold. On some occasions the patient's emotional attitude seems incongruous, particularly for the thoughts he is expressing. Thus he may laugh while saying that he is in mortal danger. This cold or incongruous attitude and manner give the schizophrenic patient his most striking features, and even when at their mildest can be baffling and distressing symptoms to his family.

Other abnormal modes of expression of the schizophrenic patient are disturbances in stance and mobility called catatonic symptoms. Gestures may seem stiff, slow, and mannered. Some schizophrenic patients make repetitive movements or facial grimaces. Others may become totally immobile and mute. Still others may assume unnatural postures and hold them for long periods.

During the active phases of the schizophrenic illness the flamboyant subjective experiences are most prominent. During the chronic phase of schizophrenic illness expressive disturbances in thought and emotion are more evident, varying from mild to severe. Although at times some patients seem free of residual symptoms, usually a careful examination will reveal mild disturbances in thinking and emotional responsiveness.

Diagnosis. The diagnosis of schizophrenia rests on recognition of the distinctive clinical symptoms of this disorder and the exclusion of other conditions which may produce similar symptoms.

Many disorders of brain function can imitate schizophrenic symptoms; but with the exception of the three schizophrenia-like disorders to be discussed, patients with the other brain disturbances also manifest disturbed consciousness, disorientation, and disruption of cognitive abilities, particularly recent memory function, that are not found in schizophrenia.

Mania or depression can be confused with schizophrenia (to the considerable embarrassment of the diagnostician when the patient recovers completely on receiving treatment appropriate for these conditions). A source of difficulty is the occurrence of delusions, which are common enough in mania and depression but usually spring directly from the attitudes of self-confidence or self-blame that are so prominent in those disorders.

In schizophrenia disturbances in experience, including the auditory hallucinations and delusions just described, form the most secure basis for diagnosis. Thus, in a person free of brain disease or drug intoxication, recognition of formed auditory hallucinations, primary delusional experiences, passivity experiences, or disturbances in "thought control" permit the diagnosis of schizophrenia to be made with some confidence.

If these symptoms cannot be found, then diagnosis must rest upon recognition of manifest disturbances in thought and emotional expression. It should be pointed out, however, that opinion holding a person's thought to be illogical and vague, or his affective responses to be inadequate or incongruous, is an evaluative judgment and must be held with somewhat less confidence, if the difficulties are minimal or inconstant, than opinion resting on recognition of delusions and hallucinations.

Catatonic symptoms of immobility, posturing, and grimacing, along with the disturbances in behavior described as negativism or reluctance to cooperate, must be carefully interpreted. Only in those patients in whom no evidence of a prominent mood change can be found should a diagnosis of schizophrenia be made. Motility changes in the direction of psychomotor retardation are prominent features of depressive disorder, a condition as common as schizophrenia and more common than the catatonic variety of schizophrenia, and excitement with hyperactivity can appear in mania.

Symptoms of emotional unrest, anxiety, withdrawal, and hostility can be found in schizophrenic patients, but these are common to many other psychiatric disorders, and therefore can never form the basis for a secure diagnosis of schizophrenia. However, that diagnosis is rendered more likely if it can be established that the patient was developing normally without an apparently vulnerable personality, and if these symptoms appeared without a change in the patient's mood or the pattern of his life. Since these more general symptoms can be found in both schizophrenia and many other psychiatric disturbances, it is important to search carefully for the more basic symptoms of hallucinations and delusions from which emotional unrest and unpredictable behavior may stem. Often repeated efforts are required to gain coopera-

tion of the patient so that he will divulge the existence of those basic symptoms that make a diagnosis of schizophrenia certain.

Etiology. There is no neuropathology or consistent pathophysiology that can be observed to develop with progression of the disorder and that might give some hint of causation. An approach to a consideration of etiology has to be more circuitous and the opinions derived held with somewhat less assurance than is true of other clinical entities. Two aspects of etiology can be conveniently separated for the purpose of organizing the information we have. One aspect is "cause," that is, any prerequisite element needed to set in motion a train of events leading to the entity. The other is "mechanism," that is, the particular nature of the train of events, be they psychologic, neurologic, or biochemical, that produce the symptoms. For schizophrenia there is some information relating to "cause" and also to "mechanism," but it is far from conclusive.

"Cause" or Prerequisite Elements in Schizophrenia. The genetic constitution has been decisively demonstrated to be one of the "causes" of schizophrenia. The risk of schizophrenia increases with the closeness of blood relationship to a schizophrenic patient. Thus only 1 per cent of very distant relatives of a schizophrenic patient will themselves suffer from the disorder. This is no higher than the risk in the general population. But 5 to 6 per cent of siblings and 40 to 50 per cent of monozygotic twins of schizophrenic patients will have schizophrenia.

The possible objection that these data merely reflect the increasingly common environment of progressively closer relatives has been refuted by observations on monozygotic twins brought up apart who continue to show an identical high risk. Heston made the same point in a different fashion by studying a group of offspring of schizophrenic mothers. These particular children were raised from earliest infancy in foster homes by normal, nonschizophrenic mothers and fathers. The incidence of schizophrenia in these children was exactly the same as that reported for children raised by a schizophrenic parent. They thus resembled their biologic mother although reared apart from her.

It has nevertheless been impossible to fit schizophrenia into a clear mendelian pattern of dominant or recessive inheritance. Some students of the disease would describe the hereditary contribution to schizophrenia as polygenic, i.e., the sum of a number of contributions from the genes no one of which is solely responsible. The polygenic concept might permit environmental factors to play a larger role in causation. Thus a mild genetic vulnerability might express itself in a schizophrenic phenotype only in those who face stressful environments, whereas those carrying a more severe genetic vulnerability might show the disorder in any environment. It is difficult at the moment to propose a test that would exclude the polygenic hypothesis as a possibility.

Some studies that have established a genetic contribution to the etiology of schizophrenia have also given evidence of the inadequacy of genetics as a sufficient cause for the disorder. That 50 per cent of monozygotic twins of schizophrenic patients are free of this illness means one of the following: (1) Although the genetic constitution is necessary and sufficient to produce schizophrenia, the symptoms employed to define a case fail to provide an adequate means of recognizing all examples of the disorder, and 50 per cent are mistakenly called normal. (2) The defining symptoms encompass a mixed group of disorders, and in only 50 per cent of these disorders are genetic features necessary and sufficient causes for the symptoms. (3) A genetic vulnerability for schizophrenia is necessary but not sufficient. It must be combined with certain life experiences that need not be common for genetically identical individuals.

The present inadequacy of the genetic hypothesis to provide a complete description of the "cause" for schizophrenia reinforces a search for environmental and experiential causes. It has proved just as difficult to determine an environmental contribution as to define the genetic contribution. Thus the experiences of being raised by a cold and distant mother, or of receiving insistent, simultaneous, but incompatible directions from the parents, or of simply living in a disharmonious family incapable of providing a healthy environment for psychologic growth have all been considered causes of schizophrenia.

Such disturbed experiences have been found in the lives of some schizophrenic patients when viewed retrospectively after the onset of the illness. But none has proved to be a common experience in all schizophrenic people. Nor has it been possible to predict an increased incidence of schizophrenia among individuals living in comparably disturbed situations. Presently the most economical view of the role of life experiences in the "cause" of schizophrenia holds that *any* adversity, be it a psychologic shock, abnormality in critical relationships, or physical injury (particularly brain injury) may provide a partial contribution in causing schizophrenia, but that most of these adversities are exerting their causal effects upon a genetically vulnerable individual.

"Mechanism" of the Schizophrenic Syndrome. This is the other aspect of etiology. Given that some combination of genetic and environmental attributes is probably prerequisite for the illness, by what derangements are the symptoms produced? Are they produced by some change in a psychologic function that might have been learned or developed through experience, or are they produced by some morbid change in the nervous system that alters the normal capacity to perceive, integrate, and respond? There have been proposals for each of these "mechanisms."

Many distinguished psychiatric studies have proposed that the mechanism of the disturbance has been through the production of a particular psychologic change fundamental to the whole syndrome and from which all the symptoms can be explained. Thus Federn has proposed a "loosening of ego boundaries" as the essential feature mediating this illness, whereas Bleuler proposed a basic disturbance in associational thinking. A crisis of identity has been proposed by exponents of existential psychiatry. These views have a ring of plausibility perhaps derived from their resemblance to experiences common to all men, part of which can seem to be reflected in the behavior of schizophrenic patients. But they depend on concepts that are difficult to define except in terms of what they purport to explain.

Other studies have attempted to demonstrate the possibility that the mechanism is a change in the central nervous system. No such change has been demonstrated in schizophrenia as yet, so supporters of this possibility have had to reason by analogy.

Three well documented conditions affecting the brain can give rise to a mental disturbance resembling schizophrenia. The most familiar is the syndrome found with *amphetamine intoxication.* In this condition the patient is alert and oriented but preoccupied by auditory hallucinations and delusional ideas indistinguishable from those seen in schizophrenia. The disturbance may last from several days to a few weeks, but disappears eventually after the withdrawal of the stimulant.

Slater, Beard, and Glithero have demonstrated that among patients suffering from *psychomotor epilepsy,* caused by an irritative lesion in the limbic portions of the temporal lobe, a certain number develop a paranoid schizophrenia-like syndrome after 10 to 15 years of epilepsy. This condition displays all the classic delusional and hallucinatory symptoms of schizophrenia, but there is less tendency toward deterioration of thinking and personality.

Finally, certain patients, *withdrawing from excessive alcohol ingestion,* suffer from a period of auditory hallucinations. Although in most of these patients the hallucinatory experience clears within 24 to 48 hours, in a small proportion a chronic condition of persisting auditory hallucinations associated with delusional beliefs, incongruous affect, and disturbed thought develops. This chronic condition may be indistinguishable from the schizophrenic syndrome, and may persist for many years.

For all these schizophrenia-like conditions the possibility exists that the pertinent features might be the expression of a latent predisposition for schizophrenia in the affected individuals. But there is no evidence of a predisposition. The relatives of these patients do not have an increased incidence of schizophrenia, and the patients themselves do not have schizoid traits in their premorbid personalities.

The existence of these conditions demonstrates that the symptoms of schizophrenia are capacities of the damaged human brain. Yet we are ignorant of any common pathologic feature of these brain disorders that could by implication be the fundamental mechanism for schizophrenia. One possibility is that each of these disorders represents an extraexcitatory arousal of the brain, particularly of the reticular formation and limbic system, either directly via amphetamine or epileptic discharge or in rebound from long-continuing action of the depressant ethanol. It may be that the condition of schizophrenia itself is thus produced by some stimulatory action on these same regions evoked by the genetic-environmental "causes" discussed above.

Another proposed mechanism for producing schizophrenia is through some change in body metabolism or chemistry that could itself alter cerebral and psychologic functions. Many students have been prompted to consider this alternative because of the remarkable growth in biochemical methodology. In fact the difficulties in establishing a role for biochemistry in the etiology of schizophrenia rest not with the chemical methodology but with such issues as defining the group being studied, avoiding chemical artifacts related to dietary habits or medications given chronically hospitalized people, and deciding what biochemical change to look for with little knowledge of what kinds of change might produce symptoms. The papers of Kety should be consulted for a more thorough discussion of these difficulties. A rare condition, periodic catatonia, has been documented by Gjessing to be associated with a phasic change in nitrogen balance, but no relationship between this disorder and schizophrenia in general has been found.

Thus our knowledge of "mechanism," as much as our knowledge of "cause," is still fragmentary and provisional. But on the bits of evidence at hand, the view that most examples of schizophrenia will prove to be due to some deranged neural mechanism that itself is produced by an anomaly of the genetic constitution seems easiest to defend.

Treatment. The treatment for any schizophrenic patient is complex and should not be attempted by the inexperienced. A period of hospitalization will usually be required. There a program to include drug therapy, psychologic treatment, and social evaluation can be planned.

The sheet anchor of treatment now for schizophrenia is the *phenothiazine* drugs, discovered in the 1950's almost by accident. To date there is no good explanation for their effectiveness. Clearly they are not simply acting by virtue of their sedative effect, since their remarkable action is not mimicked by other sedatives. They can remove the symptoms of schizophrenia, including the delusions, hallucinations, and disordered thought, and are not restricted to relieving excitement or anxiety as the term tranquilizer might imply.

The most versatile phenothiazine preparation is the original: chlorpromazine. The dose required to treat acute symptoms varies widely from patient to patient, and amounts from 200 to 2000 mg per day may be necessary. Maintenance dosage is similarly an individual matter, but 200 to 300 mg per day is usually an effective range. Since cessation of treatment results in the reappearance of symptoms in 60 to 70 per cent of patients within six months, drug therapy is often given over years. This practice, however, is being re-evaluated in light of a movement disorder (tardive dyskinesia) that may appear with prolonged use of phenothiazines.

The *psychotherapy* suitable for the schizophrenic patient has been a subject of intense controversy. The more radical approaches based on psychologic and particularly psychoanalytic views of the genesis of schizophrenia have not achieved their optimistic goals of curing the patient by relieving some basic psychologic conflict. More modest psychotherapy is indispensable when it is intended to help the patient in his everyday affairs, taking advantage of those personal assets that persist despite his illness, and establishing a relationship of friendly rapport in order to guide him in his management of personal and social issues, which, if mishandled, can lead to distress and further illness. A particularly pressing issue for the schizophrenic patient is the social situation into which he is placed after hospitalization. His psychiatrist, usually at first with the help of a psychiatric social worker, must strive to find a job that is regular and well within the patient's power but not excessively challenging, a domestic arrangement that is calm and supportive but not too emotionally demanding, and a daily routine that combats the tendency to withdraw from all social contacts into an isolated and perhaps fantasy-ridden existence. To accomplish these goals is one of the most challenging exercises in medical treatment. The growth of "halfway houses" as residences for previously hospitalized schizophrenic patients has been prompted by recognition of the need for stable and structured social environments for schizophrenic patients once they have improved enough to leave the hospital.

Prognosis. Prognosis for any patient diagnosed as schizophrenic is always guarded. Certain features carry a good prognosis: high intelligence, a normal premorbid personality, an acute onset, catatonic features in the illness, and a family history of affective disorder. Other features carry a poor prognosis: low intelligence, schizoid premorbid personality, insidious onset of the illness, symptoms of thought disorder, affective blunting in the illness, and a family history of schizophrenia.

The use of phenothiazines has considerably improved the prognosis of schizophrenia, 30 to 50 per cent of patients having complete remissions on follow-up over five years. Another 30 to 40 per cent show some residual symptoms but are able to live in the community, and only 10 to 20 per cent require further hospitalization if phenothiazine treatment is begun and maintained after their first attack of the illness.

Connell, P. H.: Amphetamine Psychosis. Maudsley Monographs, No. 5. London, Chapman and Hall, Ltd., 1958.

Fish, F. J.: Schizophrenia, Bristol, John Wright & Sons, 1962.

Heston, L. L.: Psychiatric disorders in foster home reared children of schizophrenic mothers. Br. J. Psychiatry, 112:819, 1966.

Kety, S. S.: Biochemical theories of schizophrenia, I and II. Science, 129:1528, 1590, 1959, 1969.

Klein, D. F., and Davis, J. M.: Diagnosis and Drug Treatment of Psychiatric Disorders. Baltimore, Williams and Wilkins Company, 1969.

Schneider, K.: Clinical Psychopathology. Translated by M. W. Hamilton. New York, Grune & Stratton, Inc., 1959.

Shields, J.: The Genetics of schizophrenia in historical context. *In* Coppen, A. J., and Walk, A. (eds.): Recent Developments in Schizophrenia. Brit. J. Psychiat., Special Publication No. 1, pp. 25–41, Ashford Kent, 1968.

Slater, E., Beard, A. W., and Glithero, E.: The schizophrenia-like psychoses of epilepsy. Br. J. Psychiatry, 109:95, 1963.

Victor, M., and Hope, J. M.: The phenomenon of auditory hallucinations in chronic alcoholism. J. Nerv. Ment. Dis., 126:451, 1958.

335. MANIC-DEPRESSIVE PSYCHOSIS

The essential feature of this psychosis is an excessive disturbance of mood and self-appraisal from which its other mental symptoms seem to arise. This disturbance can be in the direction of elation and self-confidence or sadness and self-blame. The course tends to be episodic, even periodic, with attacks of elation (mania) or sadness (depression) interspersed with periods of apparent mental health varying in length from weeks to years. Individual patients may suffer attacks of only one kind throughout their lifetime. Single or repetitive attacks of depression seem to be the most common manifestation, but attacks alternately manic and then depressive or even repetitively manic are not unusual.

Clinical Manifestations. *Depression.* During an attack of depression the patient complains of feeling miserable and uncertain of himself. He may give evidence of his sadness by a dejected appearance and by restlessness and distractibility. Some patients are slowed in their activity, and this can progress to a psychomotor retardation of such severity that the patient seems totally unresponsive.

Mental examination of the depressed patient usually brings to light not only his feelings of sadness or misery but also a lowered self-esteem that can vary in intensity from feelings of inadequacy and incompetence to convictions of personal worthlessness, blameworthiness, and evil. This combination of depressed mood with self-blame is the diagnostic sign of this condition. It will also explain most of the other symptoms, modes of behavior, and dangers faced by the depressed patient.

Other symptoms include delusional extrapolations of the attitudes of self-blame. These can increase to a belief that the patient's guilt is notorious, that he is to be arrested, and that he will be condemned to die or to suffer some extraordinary punishment either in this world or the next. Suspiciousness and fear of mistreatment based on these delusional beliefs may be difficult to distinguish from similar attitudes in the paranoid schizophrenic patient. A useful if not cast-iron distinction is the depressive's belief that the suspected ill treatment comes as a justified punishment and not, as with the schizophrenic, as an undeserved persecution.

In some severely depressed patients delusional ideas can become bizarre and even grandiose in concept. Thus they come to believe that they have been the cause of cosmic disasters, that the sun is darkened by them, that whole cities have been deserted because of their presence, or that they and their progeny are accursed in the sight of the Divinity. Delusions of bodily change may take the form that their brains are rotting, their bowels totally blocked, or their bones fractured and dislocated.

Delusional ideas may concern the relationship of the patient to the world and to others. He may believe that he has lost all his money, that he has become a burden to others, that he is universally despised, or even that he gives off such a bad odor that people cannot stand his presence. Again, these beliefs are usually reflective of the patient's inner attitude of self-blame, self-contempt, and hopelessness.

The point about these opinions is that they are delusional and not just false. They are unshakable opinions held in the face of all contrary evidence. Only treatment of the depressive disorder will remove them.

The most worrisome symptom of the depressed patient is *inclination to suicide.* It is easily appreciated that attitudes of such hopelessness and despair as have been described could prompt self-destruction. But it is not necessary to have such exaggerated delusions for suicide to be a distinct risk. Vigilance for suicidal intentions must be maintained throughout the course of the depressive disturbance. There is nothing to prevent a physician's asking any depressed patient about thoughts of self-injury. Often this simple action will reveal both the severity of the mood disturbance and the need to bring the patient into hospital for his own protection.

Homicide is also a possibility for the depressed patient, and is particularly likely in those who harbor beliefs that their family shares in their guilt and accursed characteristics. Any suggestions by the patient that he might prefer death should be most seriously believed.

Along with these psychologic symptoms the depressed patient will often suffer from disturbances in his sleep, particularly waking early in the morning and being unable to return to sleep. Other physical disturbances include bodily aches and pains, loss of appetite, constipation, and weight loss. These features may combine with the retardation to give the appearance of chronic physical ill health. In fact, many depressed patients will first consult internists complaining of such physical symptoms. Helpful to the differentiation of the patient whose somatic symptoms are part of a depressive illness is a discovery of the features of depressed mood, and attitudes of self-blame or hopelessness when these features are combined with complaints of poorly localized pains, with loss of appetite or weight loss, or even with preoccupations about the state of the inner organs.

Mania. Symptoms that are almost the exact opposite of those seen during an attack of depression appear during an attack of mania. Now the patient says that he is in excellent spirits, that he feels well, and in fact has never felt better. He is active and restless, and appears energetic, confident, and quick-witted. These characteristics tend to worsen, and it is in their more extreme form that they become recognized as symptoms. The restlessness and energy become overactivity, with the patient moving constantly and planning progressively less plausible projects. His speech becomes incessant, rapid, and disjointed, one idea following another with little connection between them. His attitude of confidence is that of grandiose self-satisfaction. He may be overbearing and pompous. He often will be irritated by his surroundings, easy to anger, and perhaps suspicious that the efforts being made to control him are unjust.

Although a manic patient can usually be recognized by his overactivity, ebullience, and great self-confidence, he can develop as well ideas of resentment and feelings that he is being in some way unfairly noticed or persecuted. These ideas, on investigation, are found to derive from his own delusional opinion that he is so important that he must be under scrutiny by forces such as foreign powers. Occasionally, these persecutory ideas are so prominent that a diagnosis of schizophrenia is entertained. It is, however, the direct connection of these ideas to the attitude of self-confidence that allows a diagnosis of mania to be made.

With the mental changes manic patients exhibit disturbed social behavior. They may have increased sexual interest and may become promiscuous. They tend to overspend and be reckless with money. They may insult their employers and so be fired from their jobs. In the first attack of mania and before the severe restlessness and disorganization of thought appear, these activities may not be recognized as the products of mental illness, but may be construed as actions for which the patient can be held accountable. Thus the patient can be subjected to severe losses, to legal actions, or to moral criticism that can hamper his life long after his manic attack is over. To protect him from these consequences hospitalization of the manic patient may be required.

Etiology. *"Cause" or Prerequisite Elements in Manic-Depressive Disorder.* As with schizophrenia, an important genetic contribution to the etiology of the manic-depressive disorder seems certain. There is a progressive frequency of incidence with increasing blood relatedness so that with monozygotic twins the concordance rate is over 50 per cent. It is likely that genetic constitution is a necessary but not sufficient cause for this disorder. Certain other features of the illness require consideration. First, the illness does appear in attacks interspersed with periods in which the person appears to be normal. Second, the attacks are somewhat seasonal, appearing more frequently in the spring and fall than in summer and winter. Third, although many attacks occur spontaneously, many seem to be precipitated by some disturbing event. Presumably some other elements must combine with the genetic vulnerability to explain these features. Again, the most easily defended position would hold that a necessary cause for manic-depressive disorder is the genetic constitution of the patient, but that any of a large number of environmental disturbances can bring out the disorder.

Mechanism in Manic-Depressive Disorder. As with schizophrenia, a pharmacologically induced disorder has enhanced confidence that, whatever the "cause," the mechanism for affective disorder is a neural one. Treatment with reserpine for hypertension produced depression in up to one of four patients, and this depression was accompanied by the typical delusional attitudes of the manic-depressive psychosis. The discovery that reserpine depleted brain neurons of biogenic amines, particularly norepinephrine and serotonin, has prompted a variety of hypotheses that propose some lack of norepinephrine, serotonin, or other biogenic amines at synaptic sites in the brain for emotional control. That many effective antidepressant agents also influence these same amines has been a further support to these hypotheses.

Treatment. The first rule in managing either manic or depressed patients is that most of them should be in hospital. Their conditions can bring catastrophe to themselves and their families in the form of financial mismanagement in mania and suicide in depression. If these diagnoses are strongly suspected, then psychiatric opinion should be immediately sought so as to determine whether hospitalization should be imposed. It is critical to have expert help, because the patient can often hide the severity of the disorder in a mass of explanations which may appear quite plausible.

It is crucial to diagnose these patients and separate them from those with other conditions, because new drug treatments have proved effective for them and are specific to the affective disorders. Two classes of pharmacologic agents are effective in *depression.* Seemingly more effective are the so-called *tricyclic antidepressants,* the prototype of which is imipramine. This drug, given in doses of from 75 to 300 mg per day, will relieve a depressive attack in 50 per cent of patients. Maintenance therapy of 100 to 150 mg per day should be continued in such patients for six to eight months after their recovery. If it is ineffective, the logical practice should be to switch to the other class, which includes the drugs that have as their primary action the capacity to inhibit the enzyme monoamine oxidase. These drugs, in doses of 45 to 75 mg per day, have also proved useful in depression.

If *monoamine oxidase inhibitors* are used, the patient must be warned to avoid foodstuffs such as cheese, broad beans, and some yeast extracts, which have pressor amines of the phenyl-ethyl-amine group that includes tyramine. If absorbed by patients whose monoamine oxidase enzyme is depleted, they can cause sudden elevation of blood pressure with headache, blurred vision, and even cerebrovascular hemorrhage.

The mainstay of treatment for severe depression is *electroconvulsive treatment* (ECT). In contrast to the drugs which relieve the symptoms of depression, ECT will terminate an attack of depression usually in four to eight treatments. This treatment can produce the most dramatic and quick recovery from the depths of a life-threatening depression, and should not be withheld from a delusional patient or any seriously depressed patient who has failed to respond to drug treatment after three to four weeks. Maintenance with imipramine, 100 to 150 mg per day for six months, is recommended after ECT for the avoidance of relapse shortly after successful treatment.

The *treatment of mania* is often very difficult, particularly if the patient is suspicious about medicines. Haloperidol in doses of 2 to 10 mg thrice daily taken orally has proved effective. This compound is liable to produce severe extrapyramidal side effects which can be combated with antiparkinsonian drugs and with Benadryl. Chlorpromazine in doses of 300 to 1000 mg per day can also be tried.

A recent and effective measure for controlling mania has been the use of lithium ion in the form of lithium carbonate. This compound is available in 300 mg tablets, and daily intake of 900 to 2400 mg per day can relieve manic excitement. It is, however, essential to follow plasma lithium concentration in these patients, because toxic signs of disorientation, tremor, anorexia, and diarrhea can appear if plasma lithium concentration rises above 2 mEq per liter. The therapeutic level and the toxic level of lithium are close, and therefore the medication must be started when the patient can be carefully supervised in a hospital. Maintenance lithium treatment can be recommended, because there is fair clinical evidence that in this fashion some further attacks of mania may be avoided.

Prognosis. The prognosis for a single attack of mania or depression is excellent. Even without treatment patients tend to recover completely within six months. With antidepressant treatment the medication can be withdrawn after six to eight months with fair assurance that symptoms will not recur at this time.

The longer-range prognosis is not so favorable. Eighty per cent of people who have suffered one attack of affective disturbance will have another at some time in their lives, but this may not be for many years. Some patients, however, will have recurrent attacks of mania or depression interrupted by only brief intervals of normal behavior. A role for lithium in improving their prognosis is presently under study but cannot as yet be considered established.

The best advice to give patients who have suffered from their first affective attack is that they will very likely be quite well for years, but that they and their family should be aware that their mood changes are to be considered seriously, and they should seek psychiatric attention promptly if such a mood change tends to persist or worsen.

Astrup, C., Fossum, A., and Holmboe, R.: A follow-up study of 270 patients with acute affective psychoses. Acta Psychiatr. Scand. (Suppl. 135), 1959.

Lewis, A.: Melancholia. J. Ment. Sci., 80:277, 1934.

Schildkraut, J. J.: The catecholamine hypothesis of affective disorders: A review of supporting evidence. Am. J. Psychiatry, 122:509, 1965.

336. PERSONALITY DISORDERS AND NEUROTIC SYMPTOMS

General Considerations. The concept of disease entities that supports our understanding of the functional psychoses does not suit all psychologic disturbances and particularly those that are described as personality disorders or neurotic symptoms. There is uncertainty both in terms and in concept here. For example, the designation neurosis is ambiguous in that it seems a name for a clinical entity with some sharp distinction from normal, but a cardinal symptom of one neurosis, *anxiety,* is an experience of all people at some time and is an appropriate mood in certain circumstances. What then is abnormal in *anxiety neurosis?* Is this abnormality of a quantative or a qualitative nature? To what kind of patient can the term anxiety neurosis be applied? Should we use it only for patients in the emotional "state" of anxiety, or is it suitable regardless of the present state if a patient has "traits" that make him prone to this emotion?

The term *personality* and particularly its extension, *personality disorder,* can be just as troublesome. Personality seems a word similar to such terms as character or temperament, words intended to describe aspects of human psychologic variation distributed in a smoothly graded fashion in the population. But if that is true, then the distinction personality disorder can seem an arbitrary, socially contrived, or judgmental decision, since no sharp dividing line is to be expected in smoothly graded characteristics. In this chapter an attempt is made to dispel some of these ambiguities while considering several emotional disturbances often called neurotic that occur in a general medical setting.

Although many mental changes and emotional disturbances in patients can be ascribed to known or presumed pathologic changes in brain function, certain varieties of human psychologic constitution and certain life experiences can themselves provoke emotional disturbance and disrupted behavior. The terms personality disorder and neurotic symptoms are intended to describe the disturbances that result from variation in human constitution and experience by invoking the concepts of potential and response. Personality always means *potential.* It encompasses and describes the abiding and distinctive traits or tendencies of an individual to react to circumstances in a particular fashion. Thus by "optimistic personality" is meant an individual who can be expected to respond with cheerfulness and optimism in situations in which others are less likely to do so. An individual's personality is the sum of numerous traits, and a comparison with others is implicit in the description of each trait. Thus every trait can be conceived as a dimension of variation along which people can be dispersed in a fashion similar to their dispersal along the dimensions of height, weight, or intelligence. Any definition of an individual's personality is an attempt to place him in relationship to others in respect to one or more traits. An individual can be said to have a disorder of personality if he deviates to such an extreme along the range of variation for some trait that either he or others complain of its effects.

Whereas personality and personality disorder indicate potential, the neurotic symptoms are emotional *responses* displayed when the individual is troubled by circumstances. For anyone certain environments and life events are conducive to anxiety, others to depression, and still others to suspiciousness. People with a disorder of personality have an increased potential for these responses and are provoked to them by less extreme circumstances and less specific stimuli. Thus paranoid personality disorder is a term used to describe an individual who tends to show attitudes of suspiciousness and feelings of persecution (the neurotic symptoms) in settings so minimally threatening that they will seldom provoke such attitudes in others. If, however, his life is relatively free of threatening features, these feelings will be diminished and, despite his personality traits, symptoms may be avoided.

Before such concepts can be used in the evaluation and management of a particular patient, that patient must be well known to the doctor, and the possibility of other conditions that could produce similar symptoms must be excluded. For this a detailed psychiatric history, mental status, and physical examination are needed. The latter two can be obtained during the first interview, but historical information about the patient's family background, developmental milestones, sexual adjustment, scholastic and occupational achievement, habits, and medical problems may require several hours of examination. Observations from his relatives improve the accuracy of such information, and their descriptions of his personality are indispensable. All these data, combined with the knowledge of the patient's present condition, form the basis for diagnosis, treatment, and prognosis, and to embark on such matters without this information is to commit a capital error. The result is often failure of treatment, because the patient has been misunderstood and emphasis given to minor rather than major features of his problem.

As it becomes clear that a given patient's disturbance is the outcome of the kind of person he is and the situations that he faces, the data of the psychiatric history and the mental status examination can usually be divided into three categories which, although closely related, are usefully distinguished: (1) the predisposing factors for the disturbance, including personality traits and formative life experiences; (2) the precipitating factors; and (3) the symptoms themselves and their effect on the patient.

Predisposing Factors. Predisposing factors are those features special to an individual that make him vulnerable to emotional disturbance. The most critical factor is personality, the traits of which are distinguished in the patient's temperament, attitudes, and predictable responses. But personality is the outcome of genetic constitution, intellectual endowment, and lifetime experiences, and each of these is a predisposing factor in itself. As intriguing examples of studies in these issues, the work of O'Connor on the role of intellectual subnormality in emotional instability and the study of Granville-Grossman on the relationship of parental loss to depression in adulthood can be recommended. Predisposing factors often overlooked are the patient's social status and cultural situation. The scholarly study of Dr. Beatrice Berle, *80 Puerto Rican Families in New York City,* and the recent work of the Dohrenwends in social psychiatry are excellent examples of empirical work in these areas.

Finally, the state of health is an important predisposing feature, because physical illness, through the distress it produces or by direct effects on the central nervous system, interferes with a person's capacity to cope with circumstances and thus leads to psychologic symptoms.

Precipitating Factors. The precipitating factors are events or experiences that have disrupted emotional equilibrium and bear a close temporal relationship to the disturbance for which the patient seeks help. The common-sense expectations that personal illness, or conflict produced by changes in family or occupational circumstances, could precipitate psychologic distress have been confirmed in studies such as those of Brown and Birley. Holmes has attempted to grade life events in a hierarchy of emotional stressfulness, and many workers have found his scale useful for estimating the relative distress different patients have endured. Some psychologic precipitants are more recondite, because they depend on a special meaning an individual gives events, perhaps a symbolic meaning derived from the particular patient's early life experiences. Before emphasizing these more abstruse precipitants of a unique character, it is usually wise to consider the more immediate and obvious ones that may be present.

Symptoms. In this chapter, the symptoms of anxiety,

depression, and hysterical reaction are discussed, because they are common in the general practice of medicine.

All these neurotic symptoms emerge as complaints either of the patient himself or of others who must deal with him. They are symptoms in the sense that they disturb the patient's sense of well-being or they interfere with his behavior and his adaptability to circumstances. They can vary from mild to severe, and they can be acute or chronic.

In the assessment of these symptoms the patient should be encouraged to describe how he feels, how the symptoms developed, what seems to make them worse or better, what they are like when compared to previous emotional reactions, and how they disturb him now. *The aim is to come to appreciate these symptoms as understandable responses of this particular person to his particular circumstances.* The over-all principle is that we are considering here not classes of patients suffering from distinct disease entities, but individuals troubled by their special life circumstances and needing assistance tailored to their particular personal nature and situation. The specific symptoms, their characteristic predisposing and precipitating factors, their effects on behavior, and modes of treatment will be considered in the balance of this chapter.

ANXIETY

Definition. Anxiety is an unpleasant mood of tension and apprehension. It is fear's first cousin and, like fear, has prominent autonomic effects when severe. But fear is an emotion sharply focused on immediate dangers, whereas anxiety is usually imposed by the anticipation of future danger, distress, or difficulties. As an emotional response common to all men, anxiety is useful. Activities that arouse it are avoided and those that diminish it are sustained. Although anxiety may spur people to perform difficult tasks skillfully and admirably, when excessive it is a hindrance, as some well prepared students demonstrate when facing a critical examination. *Anxiety is a medical problem when it is excessive, inappropriate, or without obvious cause.*

Predisposing and Precipitating Factors. Anxiety is the psychologic response to anticipated troubles, real or imagined, dimly or accurately perceived. But men and troubles vary. Some persons, the timid, the inexperienced, the excessively conscientious, are frequently anxious in situations that seem not to affect others. Most people are at least mildly anxious whenever they seek medical advice, and when threatening dangers are intense or prolonged, as in chronic painful illness or in battle, even the most resistant individuals can develop incapacitating anxiety.

Resistance to anxiety varies with physical condition, and when tired, sick, or injured, people are more easily threatened. Also, they are more vulnerable to anxiety when their powers of analysis and discrimination are failing or underdeveloped. Thus, because of inadequate comprehension or imprecise perception, the immature, the elderly, or the person with brain damage may become anxious in situations in which a person with a healthy, mature brain is comfortable. In fact, one of the first indications of a dementia can be an attack of severe anxiety without obvious provocation.

Common precipitants of anxiety in daily life are cir-

cumstances of conflict in which an action is demanded but the correct action may be difficult to discern. Thus a person may be anxious over difficult decisions on which rest his economic and social success or because the decisions produce an unpredictable response in an inconsistent superior. Laboratory models for this kind of situation and its effects on the emotional state have been easy to produce. Pavlov trained dogs to respond to the picture of a circle by rewarding such responses with food. He did not reward responses to an ellipse. Then, by simply compressing the ellipse so that it gradually approached a circle in shape, he made the discrimination progressively more difficult. The emotional response of these dogs was remarkable. They became ferocious and violent when put into harness for the experiment. They tore at their restraints, barked uncontrollably, and refused to attempt the discrimination. In this state, not only did they make many mistakes, but they became unable to make discriminations that had previously been easy. It is not difficult to see analogies in both situation and behavior between Pavlov's dogs and men with emotional conflicts.

An emotional state of anxiety can be produced in other ways than as an understandable response to anticipated difficulties. An intractable anxiety state can follow a head injury as one of the symptoms of the so-called *postconcussional syndrome*. Similarly, a mood of tension and agitation with tremulousness can occur in the delirious states, such as those that follow withdrawal of alcohol or barbiturates and are sometimes produced by the hallucinogenic drugs such as LSD-25. In these situations, it may be disturbed perceptions and misinterpretations that arouse anxiety, but often the anxiety is independent of anything that the patient definitely experiences or understands. Roth describes a peculiar and chronic anxiety state that can follow a calamitous emotional experience. This condition, referred to as the *phobic anxiety syndrome,* occurs in mildly obsessional persons after a severe fright. The disturbance can last for many months. These patients are in a state of considerable anxiety, mostly unformulated, and, associated with this, they have an unwillingness to leave their homes because of vague fears. The peculiar psychologic response of *depersonalization,* which is a change in the awareness of self such that the person feels unreal, is present in many of these patients. In the phobic anxiety syndrome the mood of anxiety follows rather than precedes difficulty, demonstrating that anxiety, normally an anticipatory psychologic response, may take on a self-sustained activity after certain experiences such as severe frights or sudden disasters.

The role of learning and of conditioning has too often been neglected in considerations of anxiety. This probably derived from attempts to explain all anxiety in terms of basic instinctive drives. That a fear-provoking situation could train an individual to experience symptoms of anxiety in circumstances that resembled these situations is very likely, and is indicated by research on emotion in animals. The capacity to develop anxiety via conditioning mechanisms seems the probable explanation for certain cases of phobic anxiety focused on specific objects.

Manifestations of Anxiety. The manifestations of anxiety are divisible into three groups. *First* are the inner feelings of tension, apprehension, and dread that form the anxious mood itself. *Second* are disturbances of the intellectual power of the anxious patient. He is unable to think clearly, to use proper judgment, to learn efficiently, or to remember accurately. *Third* are the autonomic, visceral, and endocrine changes that have been analyzed by Walter B. Cannon and his followers as the companions of emotional excitement and particularly of anxiety or fear. These include tremor, tachycardia, hypertension, increased perspiration, dilated pupils, and reduced salivation and gastric secretion. Increased activity of the sympathetic nervous system and of the adrenal medulla mediates the majority of these visceral responses to anxiety.

A model anxiety state is to be seen among front-line soldiers. The infantryman is a prepared subject for anxiety. He is always threatened with death or mutilation. He must go without sleep, remain exposed to the weather, and often be hungry. He is usually unable to understand what is happening around him. He is repeatedly frightened by gun fire and distressed by the death of comrades. If he is exposed long enough, he develops a severe and persisting anxiety state sometimes called "battle fatigue." He becomes tense and easily startled. His judgment is poor, and he cannot efficiently sustain a complex offensive action. Among other physical complaints, he suffers from headache, anorexia, and diarrhea. He is usually convinced that death is imminent. Almost all men develop this condition if exposed to battle long enough. Wolff reports that the average man in the army of the United States reached this point after 85 days of combat; 75 per cent could be expected to break down by combat day 140, and 90 per cent by combat day 210. These figures vary little among nations, although few are willing to publish them. They make the point that, in his resistance to crippling anxiety, even the bravest man has a "breaking point." On reaching it, he does not betray his group or run from the enemy, but rather he becomes less efficient in protecting himself and runs a high risk of death.

The symptoms of anxiety that physicians see in patients are not different. The patients all have the same three groups of symptoms, but, depending in part on the cause, these symptoms can appear as a relatively brief attack or as a more prolonged, chronic disturbance of mood.

Anxiety attacks may be single episodes or may be periods of exacerbation in a chronic state of tension. They are short periods of tension, varying in severity from mild apprehension to severe panic. An anxiety attack can occur at any time. A favored time is when the patient is traveling in a plane, bus, or train. Most commonly, though, an attack develops at night when, with the disappearance of daytime distractions, a patient begins to ruminate on his troubles. The apprehensions grow to preoccupy his thoughts, and he develops visceral responses of fear. Clear thinking becomes impossible, as does sleep. The heart pounds. A common complaint in an anxiety attack is the sensation of tightness in the chest as though the lungs could not be adequately filled. The patient responds to this sensation by deep and sighing respirations. Sometimes he may produce in this way a respiratory alkalosis with feelings of giddiness and vertigo, tingling of his fingertips, and even tetany with carpopedal spasm. This is the *hyperventilation syndrome,* and the resulting symptoms may add to anxiety.

Full-blown anxiety attacks have an hysterical flavor and may, in part, depend on personal tendencies to self-dramatization and suggestibility. But they also can be the results of a psychic chain reaction, the initial apprehensions and anxiety stirring up cardiac and respiratory changes that are themselves frightening. Granville-Grossman and Turner have provided more evidence that visceral responses to anxiety can increase the subjective symptoms of anxiety by demonstrating that these latter symptoms are improved when an anxious patient is treated with propranolol, a drug that blocks the adrenergic beta-receptors of the sympathetic nervous system and slows the heart rate.

Chronic anxiety may be punctuated by or may begin with an acute attack, but it may be just a steady and distressingly prolonged disturbance of mood. The symptoms are less intense although not different in quality from those of acute anxiety. The patient is tense and "on edge." He may also report some feelings of sadness or hopelessness along with his anxiety. It can be difficult to differentiate his condition from an agitated depression. His intellectual powers are diminished, and he has considerable difficulty in concentration and in thinking. He will score poorly on intelligence tests, particularly on the performance subtests, just as does a patient with dementia. He will have a number of somatic complaints: frontal or occipital headache, anorexia, diarrhea, and weight loss, among other things. On examination, he may have the physical signs of tension, a fine tremor of the extended arms and brisk tendon reflexes, rapid heart beat, increased blood pressure, and pupillary dilatation. More extensive laboratory studies may reveal other visceral and endocrine disturbances, such as reduced gastric acid secretion or increased adrenocortical activity.

Diagnosis. Usually diagnosis is not difficult. In both acute and chronic anxiety, the patient's major complaint is the distressing emotional state. Associated disturbances in thinking and autonomic function serve to confirm the diagnostic impression. For these patients, the major issue is not the diagnosis of anxiety, but rather the question of why they have become anxious now. This question must be answered from knowledge of the circumstances and personality of the patient.

An occasional patient focuses his complaints on his physical symptoms, such as irregularities in the beat of his heart, the change in bowel habits, weight loss, anorexia, or easy fatigability. From these symptoms a more severe illness such as a hidden malignancy, a chronic infection, or some endocrine disorder like hyperthyroidism or Addison's disease may be suspected. Although these conditions are usually seen to be only remote possibilities, laboratory studies may be required to exclude them. As with all psychologically disturbed patients, laboratory studies should not be delayed or protracted but should be decided upon, and this phase of the examination should be finished as promptly as possible.

Treatment. Treatment will vary with the cause and severity of anxiety. Many mildly anxious patients can be helped by a physician who is willing to listen carefully to their difficulties and offer some support and occasional advice. Most patients with anxiety have this mild type. Their disturbances are transient and are based on some particular problem or self-doubt that has developed acutely and is eventually resolved.

Those with more severe anxiety can be aided by a combination of pharmacologic treatment and repeated compassionate discussions of their troubles. Barbiturates have been the preferred agents for relief of anxiety in the past. However, barbiturates can be addictive, and there is the ever-present danger that they may be used in a suicide attempt by an anxious patient who is also depressed. In several double-blind clinical trials, chlordiazepoxide (Librium) has been found as effective as barbiturates for treating anxiety, and can be recommended. Dosage of 10 mg three to four times a day is usually effective. Up to 20 to 25 mg three times daily can be given to severely disturbed patients.

Patients with persisting anxiety can be referred with some confidence to specialists in psychotherapy. The effectiveness of psychotherapy seems to depend on the comfort provided by frequent sympathetic discussions and an increased recognition by the patient of the irrational aspects of his anxiety. The particular school of psychotherapeutic theory subscribed to by the therapist seems less important.

Only the most severely anxious patients need hospitalization and then usually only for an acute attack of anxiety. They are treated best with sedation; chlordiazepoxide in doses of 25 to 30 mg three times daily can be used. The somatic symptoms from the respiratory alkalosis of the hyperventilation syndrome can be treated by placing a bag over the nose and mouth that will retain the expired CO_2 for rebreathing.

Careful consideration should be given to any evidence that the anxious patient may be depressed. Agitated depression can be easily confused with simple anxiety. If depression is thought to be the diagnosis, then antidepressant medication, such as imipramine, 25 to 50 mg three to four times a day, should be given rather than sedatives.

For those individuals with restricted anxieties prompted by particular stimuli, i.e., phobias, there is growing evidence that deconditioning techniques based on learning theory may have an important place in therapy. Certainly some impressive controlled trials have been published indicating a faster response to this mode of management than to interpretive therapy for individuals suffering from a single phobia. This treatment, like any other, should not be attempted without experience and guidance.

DEPRESSION

Definition. Depression is a term for a mood of sadness and gloom. It can be a symptom of manic-depressive psychosis, and Ch. 335 should be consulted for a complete consideration of the subject. Here we are dealing with depression that occurs as a response to troubled life circumstances. Such depression can usually be given a more specific name, such as discouragement, demoralization, or grief—terms that carry specifically the connotation of an emotional reaction.

The troubled mood is usually not hard to recognize. The patient appears miserable, his face expressive of sadness and perhaps tension. He may move without confidence or purpose and report that his energy is decreased and his thinking slow and difficult. Appetite is usually lessened, often with weight loss, and sleep is restless and diminished. Sexual interest will be greatly reduced. The patient may also say that he is irritable and fearful. Depending on the severity of his depression, the patient will seem socially disorganized, proving inefficient in work, failing in duties, and neglectful of appearance. His acknowledged inadequacies in these respects may add to his sense of misery and may prompt thoughts of resigning from work, leaving his family, or even committing suicide.

Although various troubles can provoke depression, there is a specific response that illustrates features common to many depressive reactions. That response is *grief,* well studied recently by Dr. C. M. Parkes.

Grief is an experience in almost every lifetime and is the response that follows the loss, usually by death, of some relative or friend. The severity of the reaction and its duration depend upon many factors, but the most important is the closeness of the relationship and degree of dependence of the mourner on the lost individual.

Grief is a state that follows a pattern of development in which certain stages can be recognized even though the transition from one to the next is not possible to define exactly and features from one can persist in the others. *The first stage,* which lasts several days, begins upon learning of the death. The mourner feels stunned and appears bewildered, does not seem to grasp his loss fully or to relate its implications to his feelings coherently. He may appear irritable, tearful, or anxious, but can also seem calm and capable. Although his emotions and behavior may be unpredictable, they are often culturally modified as he carries out such customs as funeral rituals. He himself will usually report afterward that his emotions were blunted and his thinking uncertain, and that his depressed mood was not fully experienced. Parkes refers to this period as the stage of numbness, blunting, or shock.

This stage ends gradually but usually within one week of the bereavement, when there is an increase in the emotion of sadness and the appearance of an intense sense of loss that comes in waves, called pangs of yearning or pining by Parkes. In this *second stage,* between these surges of distressing feelings, which are so frequent at first as to be almost continuous, the patient is usually irritable and sad, with sleep and appetite diminished. Activity, which often takes the form of aimless moving about rather than productive work, may be increased, particularly so during a depressive surge, a point Parkes uses to support his analogy of this stage of grief to the searching behavior of animals separated from their mates. It is the phenomenon of *surges of misery,* however, that is most characteristic of grief and usually aids in its recognition. With time these occur less often, but it is common experience to have such a wave of depressive feelings sweep over a person following a reminder of the loss years after the bereavement.

The third period of grief appears with a diminution in the attacks of yearning and the anxious restlessness. This phase, usually entered into within several weeks of bereavement, customarily lasts the longest. It is a stage of depressed feelings with apathy and a disinclination to find purpose or interest in work. The patient is no longer restless, sleepless, or without appetite, but his emotional state is one of gloom and discouragement and his capacity for enjoyment or for physical or intellectual work is greatly reduced. Parkes refers to this as the stage of *disorganization,* when the patient seems withdrawn, may complain of ill health, and fails to plan ahead. This state may last over a year and only gradually be replaced with more customary feelings. Recovery may be brought about in part by the natural but chance occurrence of new integrative activities and friendships, and can be facilitated by efforts of the mourner to expose himself to the opportunities for these restorative experiences.

Depressions that are responses to difficulties in life other than bereavement are very similar to this third stage. Symptoms like those in the first two stages of grief can appear briefly in distressing situations that have a sudden onset, such as being informed of an unexpected personal misfortune. But these are usually transient features and are soon replaced by a mood of sadness and discouragement very like that of the third stage.

Precipitating Factors. In this form of depression it is usually not difficult to recognize the change as a response to some difficulty, for the patient is often preoccupied with the trouble itself and is ready to draw the link between it and his present mood. Precipitating situations can be of many kinds. They can be sudden and specific events in which something is lost, such as a relationship or a job. Other provocations are situations chronically thwarting to the sense of achievement and self-esteem, as in an education program in which students are confronted with their errors but given little effective teaching to overcome them. Moving away from home can provoke the very unpleasant depressive reaction, homesickness, especially in persons who depend a great deal on the support of friends and family. In general, circumstances that disturb a person's sense of stability, security, effectiveness, or worth provoke depressive responses.

The more such a precipitant is prolonged or accompanied by a growing realization of his difficulties, the more likely the person is to show a depressive response. A paradigm of these features for a precipitant is found in debilitating physical illnesses such as cancer. Here the protracted and continually worsening clinical situation provides constant reminders of losses suffered and brings more each day. That depression is a universal occurrence in such circumstances has been demonstrated by Hinton in his study of the dying.

For reasons not fully understood, there are some physiologic states and physical illnesses that commonly provoke depressive moods. Patients with hepatitis or influenza are particularly prone to report a depressive mood and to find reasons for it in trifles that did not trouble them when they were well. Endocrine alterations such as the postpartum state, Cushing's disease, or Addison's disease are also precipitants of depressive feelings that can be very distressing to the patient and of such profound degree as to occasionally promote a suicidal action. Certain brain diseases, particularly stroke, may also precipitate a prolonged and distressing depressive state. In all these circumstances the mood of depression may rest on some disturbed physiologic mechanism in the central nervous system as yet unknown. Their possible relationship to manic-depressive disorder is discussed in Ch. 335.

Predisposing Factors. Given that situations of difficulty can lead to depression, there are features of personality that can make an individual more vulnerable to this response, perhaps by making him assess losses and difficulties more acutely and by inhibiting his power to resolve them. Especially vulnerable are those insecure and sensitive individuals who perceive criticism when none is intended and find a source of depressive feelings in their self-doubting.

Another depressive predisposition is that of the self-dramatizing and emotionally unstable and immature individual who tends to amplify emotional reactions of all sorts. When such an individual finds himself in situations of discomfort in which his feelings may be neglected, he seems more prone than others to develop a sense of dissatisfaction, distress, and depression. Slavney and McHugh present empirical evidence of this predisposition in their report of depressive symptoms in 80 per cent of patients hospitalized with the diagnosis of hysterical personality.

Finally, individuals limited in their capacity to cope with difficulties are predisposed to depressive responses. Particularly vulnerable for this reason are the mentally retarded. Even modest impairment in intellectual endowment will interfere with the person's ability to find solutions to situations that present him problems, and his failure and uncertainty tend to provoke a depressive mood. Borderline mental retardation is often overlooked in the search for predisposing factors, and a history of poor occupational and scholastic performance in a depressed patient warrants formal intelligence testing.

Differential Diagnosis. The differential diagnosis of depressive states can be difficult, particularly if it is not carried out methodically. The most important distinction to draw is that between depression as a response to troubled circumstances and depression as a symptom of manic-depressive disorder. This important discrimination rests on clinical grounds and cannot be made with certainty in all situations. Thus, although the depressions of the widow, the homesick, and the patient with a fatal illness can all be recognized as responses, the trap is in making this understandable connection with every depression and explaining it always as being due to some recent difficulty. If the family of the patient says he is more depressed than they would expect him to be under the circumstances, the diagnosis of a depressive response might be questioned. Also, the presence in the patient of remarkable changes in self-attitude such as the appearance of beliefs that he is a criminal or deserves punishment for minor transgressions, or that he is infectious and filled with physical corruption, are not seen in the usual depressive response and should lead to the consideration of manic-depressive psychosis. Finally, a previous history of mania or of depression, or a family history of affective disorder should influence the interpretation of depression and sway the diagnosis away from the depressive response (see Ch. 335).

Treatment. Although the depressive response is characteristic enough to be recognized easily again and again, the particular predispositions, precipitants, and interactions are never the same from one patient to another. Treatment is based on these particulars and is thus unique to some extent on each occasion. It is therefore hard to describe the treatment of depression without some sense of dissatisfaction because, although the principles are simple, no list of them applies to every patient.

An important early decision in treatment is the need for hospitalization. This is usually determined by how severely the mood disturbance interferes with self-care, by the availability of a supportive and protective environment at home, and particularly by the presence of suicidal features. To assess the last, the patient must be asked if he has been considering self-injury. Although judgment is required in evaluating his answers, a sequence of questions probing for suicidal thoughts should be routine for every patient with depression. A proportion of the patients will deny all thought of self-injury and can be assumed to be of lesser suicidal risk. Those who admit to such thoughts should be asked if they have any means in mind. To that question still more patients will reassure the doctor that their thoughts on suicide have not reached so severe an intensity. Those patients, however, who admit to having considered a means (pills, gas, shooting) must be considered of higher risk, and thought must be given to protecting them, perhaps by hospitalization or by guaranteeing that they are under the supervision of friends or relatives. Finally, the patients should be asked if they have acquired any means or done anything to try them out. Again a proportion of patients will say that they have not been that despondent, but those who say that they have done such things are at very high risk and should in most cases be hospitalized.

Once a decision is made about the site of treatment, in a hospital or on an outpatient basis, the act of reaching a secure diagnosis of a depressive reaction in a patient is the first step in its treatment, because this judgment requires that the doctor has come to understand the patient and his predicament. To gain this understanding the doctor's first meetings should be devoted to listening to the patient's description of his circumstances, of his emotional changes, and of the connections he draws between his experiences and his depressive mood. If appropriate, other informants such as relatives can amplify on the patient's statements and give details of his past modes of coping with trouble. All these efforts are intended to bring the doctor an appreciation of this particular individual and the circumstances that he faces.

Such knowledge, combined with the relationships of trust, respect, and empathy that develop naturally in its acquisition, provides the resources for treatment.

The therapeutic efforts from this foundation are directed toward re-engaging the patient in life experiences in which success can be found, replacements for losses enjoyed, and a sense of integrity and control regained. Usually the first need of the patient is some help in simple tactics for the management of his current troubles and for the avoidance of their repetition in the future.

At this stage a sense of helplessness often prompts the patient to abandon many of his activities and efforts, but if at all possible he must be encouraged not to give in to these promptings, because doing so tends to perpetuate the disturbed mood by holding him from opportunities to reassess his situation and to try out solutions. His daily work, even when less efficiently performed, is often helpful in directing his attention to matters other than his troubles.

With assistance in simple matters of personal management, the patient can be helped to some success in his circumstances, bringing him encouragement and promoting a willingness to maintain his efforts and to plan for the future. Educating the patient in how certain circumstances strike his particular vulnerabilities and so provoke depressive responses can be helpful.

The most useful ingredient of the treatment is the support and interest of the doctor. This encourages the patient to express his feelings and discuss his circumstances. In this way not only is the physician provided with more information about assets and vulnerabilities of the patient, but often there is spontaneous recognition by the patient of causal features for his difficulties that brings both relief to his mood and self-perceived tactics for their resolution. If this supportive relationship can be maintained and developed, improvement of depression can be expected. For the occasional patient with whom such a relationship fails or who succumbs frequently to depressive reactions because of some intractable predisposition, more prolonged treatment by specialists in psychotherapy can be recommended.

Finally, treatment with pharmaceutical agents may help. Chlordiazepoxide, 10 mg three times daily, may relieve agitation somewhat in the bereaved or otherwise relatively depressed. A sleeping medication, flurazepam hydrochloride (Dalmane), is helpful for the sleeplessness. *The antidepressant medications,* although most useful in the manic-depressive psychoses, can be tried in some patients with a prolonged depressive response. Imipramine in a dose of 150 to 250 mg a day or the monoamine oxidase inhibitor phenelzine, 15 mg three times daily, has helped individual patients, but this symptomatic relief should be considered a minor part of the treatment plan in patients with this form of depression.

HYSTERIA

Definition. Hysteria is a disturbance of behavior in which symptoms and signs of physical ill health are imitated more or less unconsciously for some personal advantage. As the phrase "more or less unconsciously" implies, hysteria may be hard to distinguish from "malingering," in which the imitation of illness is a well-appreciated fraud. Frank malingering is rare, though, because the power of human self-deception is usually ad-equate to persuade a person of the validity of his own symptoms. The only ones who can be called malingerers with any confidence are some self-mutilating patients and the remarkable pathologic liars, picturesquely called examples of the *Munchausen syndrome,* who travel from hospital to hospital gaining admission by means of dramatic acts of illness.

Predisposing and Precipitating Factors. Hysterical symptoms are to be seen as responses to distressing experiences. They can occur in almost any person facing danger or difficulty, especially if, as with soldiers in battle or prisoners, the distress is intense and prolonged and physical symptoms can provide a viable escape. Dull-witted or immature persons with inadequate powers of introspection and self-control may produce transparently hysterical symptoms in response to milder distress, such as school difficulties or family problems. Some of the exaggerations and elaborations of medical symptoms common in hospitalized patients may be similarly interpreted as responses to the distress of illness by persons whose capacity for self-control has been weakened by somatic illness. Hysterical symptoms can be the first manifestations of a dementing illness or of a depressive or schizophrenic psychosis, and these disorders must be considered when a previously well balanced adult develops a suspiciously hysterical symptom.

Commonly, though, hysteria is a disturbance in the behavior of a person predisposed by an attention-seeking, emotionally unstable, and egocentric personality. In fact, these characteristics form what has become known as the "hysterical personality" even though hysteria can occur in other types of people, and these characteristics do not invariably produce hysterical symptoms. Most easily recognized in such people is their flair for the dramatic. They show this tendency in flamboyant dress and in exaggerated, even melodramatic, responses to questions about their symptoms. They are never so happy as when they are the center of attention. Karl Jaspers characterized the hysterical personalities as those who "crave to appear, both to themselves and others, as more than they are and to experience more than they are ever capable of." The zeal of these patients for exaggeration and drama renders them more liable to hysterical symptoms. But other kinds of people can have these symptoms. In all of them usually a discouraged, depressive mood has been prompted by difficulties in life, and the hysterical symptoms then emerge from this mood state.

Symptoms and Signs. Many of the phenomena of somatic illness can be imitated by hysteria. The accuracy of the imitation depends on the medical sophistication of the patient. A doctor or nurse is more likely to produce a convincing imitation than is an unqualified person.

Common hysterical symptoms are vague subjective disorders, such as generalized weakness, dizziness, indigestion, or pain. Hysterical pain can occur in any part of the body, but the head and neck, the region over the heart, and the low back are particularly favored. Hysterical pain can be of any character, from dull aching to sharp and stabbing pain, but it is often described by the patient in vivid similes such as "like a bullet," "like a bolt of lightning," "aches like an abscessed tooth," or "sore as a hot boil." Usually, hysterical pain is not confined to a local area as around a pathologic lesion, nor is it referred into the distribution of a particular nerve or dermatome. Rather, hysterical pain is felt in a general region of the body and spreads, sometimes in bizarre ways, into contiguous areas without regard to neuroanatomic boundaries. Thus pain beginning in the face may spread along the side of the head and into the back, crossing from the region of the trigeminal nerve into the upper cervical nerve regions. Hysterical pain often varies in its character, intensity, and distribution, changing considerably with attention or suggestion. Occasionally it can be remarkably improved by a small amount of intravenous amobarbital sodium when analgesics do not help.

Although vague symptoms of a subjective kind such as pain or dizziness are the present vogue in hysteria, crude and gross symptoms are still seen. These may be psychologic, such as the amnesia or fugue states, in which memory is partially lost, often in situations in which the patient is depressed or anxious. Other psychologic symptoms shown occasionally include auditory and visual hallucinations and even flamboyant delusions. These must be carefully judged, but appear most commonly in young people who have read popular books on psychology and psychiatry and are apparently suggested into these symptoms by their reading at a time when they are distressed over other matters.

Motor disturbances in the form of abnormal movement, disturbed gaits, seizures, or paralyses are occasionally hysterical symptoms. Hysterical seizures can usually be distinguished from epileptic ones. The patients only rarely injure themselves, bite their tongues, or lose their urine. They do not have the typical tonic and then clonic phases of a seizure, but tend to show a dramatic flailing of the limbs. Consciousness is partially retained, and seizures hardly ever occur when the patient is alone. The EEG is normal.

Sensory disturbances are particularly favored hysterical symptoms. Thus, *blindness* or *deafness* is common, often developing dramatically at a time of emotional distress. Loss of sensation over one side of the body to pin prick or light touch is frequently found after a susceptible patient has been examined by a neurologist.

Diagnosis. Diagnosis of hysteria is seldom easy and never popular. Ideally, it should rest on three supports: first, the *form* of the hysterical manifestation; second, the *personality* of the patient; and third, the *setting* in which the symptoms developed. Often it is not possible to find all three supports to a diagnosis, but all should be sought.

Commonly, hysterical symptoms are vague and variable. In fact, the more definite and consistent a patient's description of the onset, location, nature, and duration of his symptoms, the less likely the symptoms are to be hysterical. Hysterical symptoms and signs are also usually incompatible with what is known of anatomy and physiology. Thus sensory losses do not conform to patterns of nerve distribution; reflexes remain intact and unchanged in the palsies of arm and leg; seizures of the entire body do not disturb consciousness; total blindness appears without a disturbance of pupillary reflex or of opticokinetic nystagmus. The hysterically mute person can phonate on coughing. The hysterically deaf person speaks louder to be heard over increased ambient noises. Many other hysterical symptoms have been analyzed for such inconsistencies by Head.

Knowledge of the personality and past history of the patient is helpful to a diagnosis of hysteria. The recognition that the symptoms are occurring in an hysterical personality should prompt an observer to look very closely at the symptoms before embarking on extensive laboratory tests or upon surgery. Similarly, knowledge

of a previous vague and poorly understood medical disturbance can lend weight to an opinion that a new symptom that has eluded diagnosis is occurring in an individual prone to hysteria. Conversely, hysteria can usually be eliminated as an explanation for symptoms in an emotionally stable, middle-aged person. People who have passed through adolescence and young adulthood without resorting to hysterical behavior are unlikely to employ it when older.

The setting in which the symptoms develop should be carefully scrutinized, and a search made for a distressing event that may have provoked an hysterical reaction or for any purpose that the hysterical symptoms may serve. Occasionally, a clear association between the symptoms chosen and a particular recent disturbance in the life of the subject can be found, such as an amnesia developing in a person who has done something shameful or criminal, or weakness and pain persisting in a person who is seeking financial compensation for an injury. Often, though, motivations behind hysterical symptoms are vague and uncertain. It is usual to find that the patient is unhappy or anxious about some aspect of his life circumstances and that the hysterical symptoms serve to call attention to his distress. Also, it may be possible to demonstrate that the development of particular symptoms has been prompted by suggestion: weakness of legs, for example, developing in a nurse caring for a paraplegic patient, or peculiar falling attacks after the patient has witnessed an epileptic seizure.

A careful study of the symptoms, the personality, and the life setting of a patient usually allows a reasonably certain differentiation of hysterical symptoms from those of a medical illness. There are, however, certain medical problems that are notoriously easily confused with hysteria. These are the diseases that produce vague and changing symptoms that seem to vary with the patient's motivation and, at least in their early phases, lack convincing physical signs. If such an illness occurs in a patient who has features of the hysterical personality and who will therefore describe the symptoms in a dramatic and flamboyant fashion, physicians may be even more persuaded to believe that the illness is only deceptively physical. Examples of diseases frequently confused with hysteria because of their subtle clinical features are the first attack of multiple sclerosis, particularly if sensory changes alone are produced; the weakness of arms and legs seen early in acute idiopathic polyneuritis of the Guillain-Barré type; the difficulty in swallowing of bulbar myasthenia gravis; the attacks of muscular weakness in periodic paralysis; the tonic posturings and oculogyric crises of postencephalitic parkinsonism; the pain of a cauda equina tumor; and the abdominal pain of acute intermittent porphyria.

Management of Hysteria. The management of hysterical patients is difficult. No one method can be recommended unqualifiedly. But there are certain principles that can be followed. To help hysterical patients it is essential to have sympathy for them. Many doctors find these patients irritating. It is just as possible to see them as individuals displaying an intriguing aspect of human behavior that has profound implications in their lives. It is pointless to argue with these patients about the validity of their symptoms. A useful approach is to agree that they have had an illness producing their symptoms, but that they are now improving even though total recovery has not arrived.

It is important to diagnose hysteria promptly. Hesitation in diagnosis leading to several hospital admissions for extensive laboratory investigations is a good way to solidify hysterical symptoms in a patient. Among other things, the uncertainty of doctors helps persuade a patient that the symptoms are real. Repeated examinations increase the consistency with which symptoms are reported. Long hospitalization, mounting bills, and the inconvenience caused to others make it difficult for a patient to abandon symptoms without embarrassment. The gratifying attention given to the patient in the hospital, perhaps as an example of an intriguing diagnostic problem, can feed the self-dramatizing tendencies and so encourage the behavior.

There is always risk of error in any diagnosis, because diagnosis is only a weighing of probabilities. The diagnosis of hysteria, though, depends purely on a physician's judgment and, before relief of symptoms is accomplished, can be confirmed in the laboratory only by evidence of health. Physicians, for obvious reasons, fear more the error of calling a physically sick patient hysterical than the error of mishandling hysteria. They often prefer to exclude, by laboratory examination, progressively more unlikely diseases than to study carefully the symptoms and the individual who has produced them, even though this would lead more directly to a definite diagnosis as well as an understanding of the response. It may be unwise to counsel too strongly against this behavior because medical diagnosis is never easy. A compromise can be found in the admonition to perform immediately the laboratory tests that seem necessary for a patient, but when hysteria is suspected, to bring the period of investigation as quickly as possible to a close so that management of the specific symptom can be begun.

Treatment of the specific symptoms rests basically upon persuasion. The doctor is persuading the patient to perform the functions that the patient claims are disabled. Intravenous amobarbital sodium given to the point where the patient is mildly intoxicated and his speech slurred is particularly helpful in making and establishing a persuasion. Usually, some ingenuity is required for success. The hysterically blind person can, for example, be persuaded first that he can distinguish light from dark and then gradually to distinguish forms, to read large print, and, finally, small newsprint. The person who claims he cannot walk can be encouraged first to move his legs in bed, and then to stand, to make a few tentative shuffles, and finally to stride out. The hysterically deaf person can be persuaded to hear through a stethoscope and then gradually that he can hear without it. A dramatic show of some kind is often helpful in removing these symptoms. If a physician has success in partially removing hysterical symptoms, he should persist in his treatment without interruption in order to bring about as much improvement as possible and even to restore full function. When there is recovery of function, the patient should perform his recovered skills in public – before his family, other patients and several doctors – to prevent his relapsing immediately into his former state.

The fear that sudden removal of hysterical symptoms will result in a disastrous psychologic collapse is exaggerated. Rarely, a depressed patient with hysterical symptoms has an increase in depression, but it is clear that in those situations a depression was overlooked and the more secondary hysterical symptoms were emphasized.

Some hysterical disorders are refractory to treatment.

Among these are the disorders assumed for some material gain, such as compensation. They usually are not improved until some settlement is made. Episodic disorders such as hysterical seizures can be hard to control. Sometimes, however, a statement to the patient that they will not recur, given with full authority by a physician whom the patient trusts and respects, may eliminate these symptoms. The longer the patient has hysterical symptoms, the harder they are to remove. This is a corollary to the aforementioned observation that hysterical symptoms produced for transparent reasons and bordering on malingering are more difficult to eliminate than are the ones produced by an attention-seeking personality in some emotional distress. Symptoms held for a long time cannot be easily abandoned without embarrassing the patient.

Simultaneously with treatment of the specific symptoms, the emotional state and present life of the patient should be studied to discover any distress that may have precipitated the hysterical symptoms. Then advice, social assistance, or guidance can be offered to aid the patient in resolving these difficulties. This aspect of their psychologic treatment depends on developing a relationship of friendship and mutual respect identical to that found necessary in treating an anxious or depressed person.

Long-term management of hysterical patients is much more difficult than treatment of individual symptoms. It is not wise to have the average hysterical patient embark on depth psychotherapy, because he tends to produce more symptoms and to recount involved sexual and other fantasies in order to maintain the interest of his doctor. If possible, these patients should be followed by one physician who understands them and the behavior that they are liable to produce and is also competent to recognize physical illness should it arise. This physician can save these patients from needless surgery and long hospitalization. He can remove hysterical symptoms promptly by being alert to the diagnosis and providing help for the difficulties that precipitate them.

Berle, B. B.: 80 Puerto Rican Families in New York City. New York, Columbia University Press, 1958.

Brown, G. W., and Birley, J. L. T.: Social precipitants of severe psychiatric disorders. In Hare, E. H., and Wing, J. K. (eds.): Psychiatric Epidemiology. New York, Oxford University Press, 1970.

Dohrenwend, B. P., and Dohrenwend, B. S.: Social Status and Psychological Disorder. A Causal Inquiry. New York, John Wiley & Sons, Inc., 1969.

Granville-Grossman, K. L.: The early environment in affective disorder. In Coppen, A., and Walk, A. (eds.): Recent Developments in Affective Disorder. Br. J. Psychiatry, Special Publication No. 2, 1968.

Granville-Grossman, K. L., and Turner, P.: The effect of propranolol on anxiety. Lancet, 1:788, 1966.

Head, H.: The diagnosis of hysteria. Br. Med. J., 1:827, 1922.

Hinton, J. M.: Physical and mental distress of the dying. Quart. J. Med., 32:1, 1963.

Homes, T. H., and Rahe, R. H.: The social readjustment score. J. Psychosom. Res., 11:213, 1967.

Jaspers, K.: General Psychopathology. Manchester, Manchester University Press, 1962.

O'Connor, N.: Psychology and intelligence. In Shepherd, M., and Davies, D. L. (eds.): Studies in Psychiatry. New York, Oxford University Press, 1968.

Parkes, C. M.: The first year of bereavement. Psychiatry, 33:444, 1970.

Roth, M.: The phobic anxiety-depersonalization syndrome and some general aetological problems in psychiatry. J. Neuropsychiatry, 1:293, 1960.

Slavney, P. R., and McHugh, P. R.: The hysterical personality: A controlled study. Arch. Gen. Psychiatry, 30:325, 1974.

Walters, A.: Psychogenic regional pain, alias hysterical pain. Brain, 84:1, 1961.

Wolff, H. G.: Every man has his "breaking point." Milit. Med., 125:85, 1960.

Section Five. PSYCHOLOGIC TESTING IN CLINICAL MEDICINE

Paul R. McHugh

337. INTRODUCTION

The intent of this section is to describe some methods of psychologic testing that have proved helpful in clinical settings. The goal is to provide some capacity to evaluate critically any psychologic test instrument, whether presently in use or likely to be devised in the foreseeable future.

Psychologic tests are intended to assist clinical evaluation of behavioral disorders by bringing accurate measurement to the mental examination. Physicians are familiar with instruments that bring accurate measurement to observations in the physical examination; the clinical thermometer and sphygmomanometer give information in numerical form about body temperature and blood pressure that cannot be collected with such accuracy without their assistance. They are so easy to employ that knowledge of the normal readings in the human population and implications of deviations from normal have been established. Although psychologic tests are aimed at more abstract phenomena such as intelligence or personality, they similarly attempt to bring precision through numerical or graphic measurements and provide a means by which an individual can be compared in these features with others.

The mere provision of a numerical expression does not prove a test useful, as the numbers may not be meaningful. Often in our fascination with a new test and its intriguingly plausible scales for measurement, we overlook its failure to satisfy the criteria of *reliability* and *validity*.

The reliability of a measuring instrument, whether it be for a physical or a psychologic function, is an expression of the accuracy and reproducibility of its findings. No instrument is perfectly reliable, but the range within which it is unreliable must be a small fraction of the potential range of measurement if it is to be capable of detecting a genuine deviation in the variable under study.

The validity of a measuring instrument is an expression of its capacity to measure what it claims to measure. The clinical thermometer does measure body temperature. How can we be sure that psychologic tests are actually measuring the psychologic variables that they claim to measure? How can we be sure that intelligence tests, for example, measure intelligence? The only proof that a psychologic test is valid is the demonstration that scores on it predict behavior in life thought to be the expression of the trait it claims to measure. For example, results on a valid intelligence test should correlate to some extent with scholastic performance.

The issues of reliability and validity can perhaps be made clearer with a homely example. The common ruler is an instrument designed to measure distances. It is a reliable instrument in that repeated measurements of the same object, say a cube one foot to a side, will give the same results. It is also a valid instrument for the measurement of the cube's dimensions. It is not, however, a valid instrument for measuring the cube's weight. This is determined by the material of the cube, and no number of repeated measurements with the reliable ruler will make it give a valid measure of weight.

338. INTELLIGENCE

The quantitative measurement of the mental attribute, intelligence, was first attempted by Binet at the turn of the century. His success and the Stanford-Binet battery of tests developed from his work brought such predictive power to the study of intelligence that they provide an impetus to the development of tests to examine other mental functions. But the tests of intelligence have through their revisions, particularly the *Wechsler Bellevue Intelligence Scale* published in 1939 and the *Wechsler Adult Intelligence Scale (WAIS)* of 1955, remained the most secure and useful tests of mental function.

Intelligence is difficult to define. It is the abstract concept used to explain the observation that individuals vary in their mental capacities and in the effectiveness with which they employ them. Intelligence is more easily defined in practice by pointing to instances of its action. This way is in fact used in our daily life. We judge a man's intelligence by observing his bearing, his speech, his apparent grasp of situations, his judgments, and his emotional control. Then in the light of our past experience of watching other men, we call an individual bright or dull. We are doing nothing conceptually different when we estimate intelligence at the bedside or by means of psychologic tests. We organize the testing so that a series of observations can be made within a reasonable period of time. We add scope to our examination by asking for performance in several different kinds of mental activity. We bring accuracy to the observations by scoring the performance.

The questions on orientation, memory, attention and concentration, fund of knowledge, and capacity to reason abstractly that constitute the tests of cognition routinely carried out at the bedside in the course of the physical and mental examination provide a doctor an estimate of his patient's intellectual functioning. In the light of knowledge of the patient's past life and demonstrated abilities, the doctor makes a judgment whether there has been damage to intellectual functioning. Psychologic tests are able to give a more accurate estimate of the intelligence of a patient at the moment of testing than do these bedside examinations, because these tests have proved both reliable and valid.

All these approaches, from the casual observations to the most refined test, are applications of a fundamentally identical method: an assessment of a performance thought on practical grounds to be a reflection of intelligence. However, any performance will be influenced by other factors, particularly the factors of education and experience. *Since these factors derive from opportunities and social heritage of the subject, every one of these assessments must be qualified and interpreted in the light of the subject's cultural and educational background.*

Subcultural differences that are obvious on bedside examination, being recognized as modifications in expression and in experience, *are allowed for almost automatically in that assessment but are sometimes forgotten when formal intelligence test scores are displayed.* Just as there is no culture-pure bedside examination, there is no culture-pure intelligence test. Test scores must be interpreted in relationship to all that is known about the patient. Particular care in the interpretation is demanded if he is a member of a subculture different from the standard criterion group employed in the development of the formal tests: urban, school-educated whites. The greater his divergence in this respect, the greater the allowance needed in interpreting the scores of his tests. Emotional disturbances or other preoccupations that interfere with the patient's concentration or cooperation will also obviously affect these performances. Allowances must be made for any of these features in assessing test scores, just as allowance is made for these features on bedside examination.

The *Wechsler Adult Intelligence Scale* is the most reliable and valid instrument we have for measuring the intellectual function of the adult. Its reliability has been demonstrated by the close correlation of test scores given on separate occasions to the same individuals and by the similarity of scores when one half of a test is compared with another half (split-half method). Its validity has been demonstrated by its correlation with life performances of individuals it scores as intelligent or dull.

In its present form the WAIS consists of 11 subtests of mental skill. Six of these subtests are "verbal tests." In these the patient is requested to define words, to recognize similarities between words, to do arithmetic, to remember numbers forward and backward, to answer questions on his fund of knowledge, and to judge and interpret proverbs. These tests are followed by five "performance tests," in which a patient is asked to work with rather unfamiliar material and solve problems set to him by that material. Tests here include the putting together of puzzles, work with symbols, the setting out of logical stories from pictures disorganized for the test, construction of patterns from multicolored blocks, and the recognition of things missing from drawings. The performance tests seem somewhat less related to the education of a person than are the verbal tests. All the subtests that have been chosen for the WAIS have a long history of investigation. They are combined together to produce a thorough and accurate instrument.

The scoring of the WAIS is in the form of the *Intelligence Quotient (I.Q.).* In fact, the WAIS derives a verbal I.Q. from the verbal tests and a performance I.Q. from the performance tests. A full-scale I.Q. is derived from the combination of all 11 subtests.

The I.Q. compares an individual with others. Historically it was developed for children. I.Q. then was the ratio of mental age over chronologic age times 100 when mental age was defined in terms of a child's ability to succeed on tests which the average child of a given age could do. Thus a child solving problems which the average nine-year-old could solve had a mental age of nine. If he, himself, was nine years old at the time of the test, he had an average ability and an I.Q. of $9/9 \times 100$, or 100; if his chronologic age was six, he would be an ad-

vanced child with an I.Q. of $9/6 \times 100$, or 150. Terman demonstrated the constancy of I.Q. in the growing child.

But a ratio of mental to chronologic age is unlikely to be useful in adults because tested intelligence does not increase after the late teens. The WAIS and many other tests for adult intelligence continue to use the term I.Q. This is possible because of the fact that tests of intelligence appear to distribute individuals in a "normal" or gaussian fashion. This curve has a mean at I.Q. 100 and a standard deviation of ±15 I.Q. points. It is possible to divide the curve into percentiles of the population. The WAIS score of any person places him in the percentile of the population with similar scores, and his I.Q. can be extrapolated from percentile by means of the distribution curve. Thus an individual whose performance on the WAIS is equal to 50 per cent of the population is said to have an I.Q. of 100, whereas individuals whose test performances exceeded 98 per cent of the population will be said to have an I.Q. of 135 or above.

The WAIS has found its greatest clinical utility in the study of patients with brain disease. Any damage to the cerebral hemispheres will injure intellectual ability and disturb the scores on the WAIS. An intriguing observation is that early in the course of brain disease performance tests are disturbed before the verbal test scores change. This may indicate that verbal tests measure more what an individual has learned and practiced, whereas performance tests measure his capacity to meet new problems. The verbal and performance scores of normal individuals are usually comparable. The verbal I.Q. can be considered a fair estimate of the original intellectual endowment of an individual suffering from a brain injury. The decline of the performance I.Q. is a useful measure of the degree of injury to the cerebral tissue the patient has endured. With an advancing brain disease verbal I.Q. will fall eventually, but a patient will usually continue to demonstrate higher verbal than performance scores.

Emotional unrest such as anxiety or depression will also interfere with WAIS scores. Here, as with cerebral disease, the performance I.Q. will fall below the verbal I.Q., demonstrating that the capacity to work with unfamiliar material is disturbed more than tests of what has been well learned. But because these findings are identical to those in persons with brain disease, the differentiation of an emotional disturbance from dementia cannot come from WAIS results. It must rest on other information such as is derived from the history, physical examination, and mental status.

The WAIS is useful not only in demonstrating deterioration of intellectual function but also when done serially can document recovery of function with treatment. Since it is so simple to employ, its increasing utility in clinical research is assured.

339. PERSONALITY

By personality is meant all the abiding traits of character that constitute an individual's potential to respond in particular ways to circumstances. All physicians are aware of how much information they must acquire through several interviews with the patient and from independent sources before they can have much confidence in their diagnostic opinion on personality. Tests that could elucidate personality more accurately and more rapidly would be useful. Two alternative approaches have been developed, "projective" tests and questionnaires, and each approach has raised particular problems.

In the so-called projective tests of personality ambiguous situations are set before the patient, and his responses are recorded. Thus he is presented with sentences to complete, a picture to interpret, or, in the most well known projective test, the Rorschach test, he is presented with a standardized set of ink blots and asked to describe the forms that he can recognize within them. Since there is nothing in the situations themselves that force any particular response, the responses of the patient are thought to derive from his personal predilections and inner needs, drives, and conflicts. This seems logical. But logic is not the essential criterion for a test intended to aid the clinical examination. It must be demonstrated that the responses on projective tests provide measurements that are reliable and valid. This remains to be done.

Certain features of a patient can be expected to be seen in any set of his responses. For instance, overly conscientious persons will tend to be fixed on details, the schizophrenic patient with his disordered thought will demonstrate this feature in distorted expression, and the depressed patient will speak of unhappy themes as he discusses any matter. These features will appear whether the patient is being examined by his doctor or doing a projective test. Until the reliability and validity of projective tests can be demonstrated, it cannot be known whether they are superior to the clinical examination, and if they are not superior to the clinical examination, they are of doubtful utility to the physician. The question of their value is shrouded in controversy.

The other approach to personality measurement is the questionnaire. This was developed from the clinical examination. Since questions are used there to gain information from the patient, it seemed logical that a questionnaire including these and many other questions would improve on the clinical examination. It came as a surprise when tests developed in this fashion proved to be unreliable and invalid. This was demonstrated when different questionnaires intended to probe similar features of personality, such as introversion, did not correlate well with one another, and in fact could give quite opposite impressions of the same person. Questionnaires developed in this fashion proved so misleading that the method fell into disrepute. It was, however, eventually recognized that these early tests gratuitously assumed that questions would be accurately answered by patients. Consider the question, Do you lack self-confidence, yes or no? To presume that a person will understand this question exactly the same way as the examiner intends and that his criterion for a yes or no answer is the same as that of all other people is to presume too much. Also these early tests failed to consider that many individuals might attempt to show themselves in some more favorable light and therefore not answer questions truthfully.

The most intriguing conceptual advance in the study of personality was the recognition that an objectively truthful answer to questions was not needed for a valid, useful test. In fact, more information can be obtained from observing the patient's replies to questions than from any belief that the statements they agree to or reject are in themselves accurate descriptions of their personality. The task of building questionnaires changed from finding questions that would display the inner feelings of people to finding questions that would be answered differently by different personality types.

To build such a questionnaire the first step was to gather together specific groups of people for study: normal people, anxious patients, hysterical patients, depressed patients, for as many groups as could be differentiated. These patients, the criterion groups, were asked a large number of questions, and the replies were compared from group to group. The questions which differentiated the groups best were then collected for the questionnaire. This questionnaire then given to an individual was interpreted not from the content of questions rejected or affirmed but from the number of questions replied to in the same fashion as in one or more of the criterion groups.

The most useful questionnaire that has been developed is the *Minnesota Multiphasic Personality Inventory (MMPI)*. The questions in that test have been carefully studied and chosen so that they differentiate the groups to the greatest degree possible with it. Because of the complexity of issues of personality, the numbers of questions needed to derive a profile with this test is 550. It was possible in the MMPI to fit in many questions that give an indication of the tendency of the patient to lie, exaggerate, or misunderstand questions.

The results of the MMPI are expressed as a series of ten scales or dimensions along each of which an individual is placed by means of his responses that correspond to responses of nine criterion groups. These scales were originally derived from clinical groups and given clinical names, i.e., hypochondriasis, depression, hysteria, psychopathic, masculine-feminine dimension, paranoid, psychaesthenic, schizophrenic, manic, and social introversion. Three so-called reliability scales are also scored for each test.

The MMPI is a reliable instrument, the accuracy and reproducibility of its readings having been demonstrated in repeated testing of individuals over many years. The validity of its scales varies. Some of the scales measure the personality characteristics for which they are titled. Scores on the psychopathic and manic scales do correlate with the clinical features intended by these terms. Scores on the schizophrenic and hysterical scales do not correlate well with these clinical disorders but with aspects of bizarreness and self-dramatization, respectively, features not specific to schizophrenia or hysteria. In an effort to avoid these invalid implications, the MMPI scales are no longer referred to by clinical titles, but by numbers or letters derived from the original names.

The tendency to look at specific scales for diagnostic impressions has been replaced by consideration of the "profile," or pattern of the several scales together, hoping to derive in this way a more global view of personality structure. This approach emphasizes the multidimensional character of personality. It takes advantage of the features of reliability found in this test. But, once again, the establishment of validity for these profiles must be accomplished. This is being attempted by matching the life course of individuals with predictions from the profiles, but work is still in progress.

Current practice is to find the MMPI useful as a screening and probing instrument that often suggests aspects of personality difficulty that might well be more carefully studied. However, its validity for the differentiation of clinical psychiatric entities or specific personality types is uncertain, and thus it must not be regarded as the arbiter in differential diagnosis.

Butcher, H. J.: Human Intelligence, Its Nature and Assessment. London, Methuen & Co., Ltd., 1968.

Penrose, L. S.: The Biology of Mental Defect. London, Sidgwick and Jackson, Ltd., 1963.

Terman, L. M., and Oden, M.: The Gifted Group at Mid-Life. Genetic Studies of Genius, Vol. V. Stanford, California, Stanford University Press, 1959.

Welsh, G. S., and Dahlstrom, W. G.: Basic Readings on the MMPI. Minneapolis, University of Minnesota Press, 1956.

Williams, M.: Mental Testing in Clinical Practice. London, Pergamon Press, 1965.

Section Six. MEDICAL ASPECTS OF SEXUALITY

Harold I. Lief

THE PHYSICIAN'S ROLE

Once almost completely neglected in medical education, sex counseling is now included in the curriculum of approximately 90 medical schools in the United States. Physicians now recognize the frequency and importance of sexual problems in medical practice. About 40 per cent of the emotional problems for which patients ask their doctors for help are related to marriage, and the most frequent marital difficulties, as perceived by a representative sample of physicians surveyed by Herndon and Nash, are problems of sexual adjustment. In the Marriage Council of Philadelphia clinic, about 75 per cent of couples report some sexual maladjustment, including 15 per cent for whom a sexual problem is a major problem and a primary cause of marital difficulty.

The frequency with which sexual problems arise in practice varies with three factors: the specialty, whether the physician routinely asks about sex problems, and the comfort of the physician in discussing sex with the patient. The highest frequencies, according to Burnap and Golden, are found in the practice of psychiatry, obstetrics-gynecology, urology, and in general practice. If the physician routinely asks about sex problems, the average frequency of patients with sexual problems is 14 per cent, whereas it drops to 7.9 per cent among the physicians who inquire about sexual matters "only when indicated." Among the group of physicians who might be thought to display discomfort with sexuality, the frequency of sexual problems reported in their practices was only 2.7 per cent, as compared with an average of 15 per cent among those physicians who were reasonably comfortable.

The importance of taking a sexual history is emphasized by the results of a study by Pauley and Goldstein, who found that most physicians who routinely take a sexual history from their patients identify significant sexual problems in at least half of them. On the other hand, the great majority of physicians who do not actively inquire about sex activity estimate that less than 10 per cent of their patients have sexual problems.

Most sexual problems presented to physicians are in the context of a marital relationship, as either primary causes of marital dysfunction or as consequences of other areas of marital discord, but which, nevertheless, augment and maintain marital unhappiness. It seems reasonable, then, to make sex and marriage counseling a "package" in the training of the physician and in the delivery of medical care. Even in the case of the pediatrician, it is still logical, for he soon comes to recognize the direct connection between the marital relationship of the parents and the sexual problems of the child.

The busy physician or the physician who shies away from marital therapy may have to treat the couple by dealing with one patient only. And many situations can be handled adequately in this fashion, e.g., the urologist who cures male dyspareunia by clearing up the patient's prostatitis, the internist who helps restore his patient's potency by reassuring him that sexual activity will not give him another coronary occlusion, the gynecologist who reassures his patient that she will suffer no loss of sexual drive after hysterectomy. Yet, sexual behavior involves a relationship, and hence, in most instances, therapy should also be directed toward the relationship.

Not only are marital and sexual problems in medical practice frequent, but they are often overlooked or avoided—either because of the physician's lack of training and his feeling of incompetence in this area or because these problems impinge on his own marital and sexual conflicts or values and make him uncomfortable. Even if he consciously or unconsciously ducks the issue by failing to follow cues, changing the subject by responding with a trite and stereotyped form of reassurance, e.g., "this is just a phase—your problem will disappear in time," he is carrying out counseling of sorts. Vincent has stated it well:

> The theoretical position that the physician cannot or should not engage in any marriage or sexual counseling becomes meaningless when the patients expect this role of their physician and when their illnesses have sexual and marital implications—if not origins. The majority of physicians literally have no choice; even to do and say nothing in response to the patient's questions and/or presentation of symptoms in the sexual and marital areas is, by default, one form of counseling.

In dealing with sexual and marital problems, the physician has an unequaled opportunity to practice preventive as well as therapeutic medicine. By aiding patients to obtain greater sexual satisfaction, he may prevent the escalation of marital discord and consequent family disorganization through emotional conflict with or without divorce. Anything that seems to strengthen family life has positive repercussions on the next generation as well. Early intervention can occur in a number of clinical situations, e.g., premarital counseling, family planning services, during pregnancy, postpartum care, early marriage, as well as through family life education for teenagers and young adults. The pediatrician and obstetrician have especially significant points of entrance into the system of health care, enabling these specialists to practice effective prevention.

To be competent in handling the therapeutic and preventive aspects of the sexual, marital, and family problems he sees almost daily in his practice, the physician must not only have a store of *information,* but must also develop a set of *skills* and *attitudes* that facilitate his making optimal use of his information. Surely the key factor in competent sex and marital counseling is the degree of comfort of the counselor. His skill in interviewing, in eliciting salient data about the most intimate, personal dimension of patients' lives, will depend directly on his capacity to react, not with anxiety, anger, or self-righteousness, but with openness, ease, and a clear desire to achieve an atmosphere of genuine communication—of feelings as well as thoughts. In the absence of these skills and attitudes, his quantity of information, even if vast, is of little use.

SEXUALITY

Sexuality refers to the totality of one's sexual being, of which physical sex is only a part. In this sense, our sexuality is what we "are" rather than what we "do." One's sense of being male and masculine, female and feminine, and the various roles these self-perceptions engender or affect are important ingredients of sexuality. Cognitive, emotional, and physical sex all contribute to the totality.

Sexuality may be described in terms of a system analogous to the circulatory or respiratory system. The components of the sexual system are set forth in the accompanying table.

Abnormalities in biologic sex may be minor or major. Major abnormalities create problems of intersexuality, which may, if not corrected early in life, lead to conflicts in sexual or gender identity. The sex assigned is, with rare exceptions, more important in determining gender identity than is biologic sex, and sex change procedures are usually unwise after the age of 18 months. Some of these patients and some without evident biologic defect have grave difficulties in developing a core gender identity of the same biologic sex. These are transsexuals, mostly biologic males who think of themselves as "a female trapped in a male body."

With these relatively rare exceptions, development of sexuality leads to a secure sense of maleness or femaleness, which is generally complete by the age of three. However, in our culture, doubts and conflicts about masculinity and femininity are ubiquitous. Serious disturbances lead to such sex deviations as transvestitism, fetishism, voyeurism, and exhibitionism.

Homosexuality.   Homosexuality is a special variant of gender identity. Although homosexuals do not question their maleness or femaleness (sexual identity), many, if not most, of them question their masculinity or femininity, at least in cultures which promote heterosexuality

Sexual System (Sexuality)

1. Biological sex—chromosomes, hormones, primary and secondary sex characteristics
2. Sexual identity (sometimes called core gender identity)—sense of maleness and femaleness
3. Gender identity—sense of masculinity and femininity
4. Sexual role behavior: (1) sex behavior—behavior motivated by desire for sexual pleasure, ultimately orgasm (physical sex); (2) gender behavior—behavior with masculine and feminine connotations.

and marriage as much as does ours in the United States. (By the time they are ten years old, 90 per cent of girls and 80 per cent of boys already are fantasizing about marriage.)

The physician should not automatically come to the conclusion that every homosexual who consults him for any medical problem wants to "go straight," i.e., to become heterosexual. In fact, most homosexuals prefer their sexual adaptation, and only those who are in great distress about their homosexual behavior should be considered for psychotherapeutic intervention, and then only after a thorough evaluation of their motivation for change. Family pressure for change is insufficient reason to undertake intervention.

Sexual System and Personality.   Far more commonly, the physician is called upon to deal with less overt conflicts about gender identity that create significant marital problems with sexual connotations, examples of which are the Don Juan who has to prove his masculinity by sexual conquests; the promiscuous housewife who tries to prove to herself her femininity by finding the elusive orgasm, or by demonstrating her attractiveness; the woman who cannot respond sexually because she is afraid of being completely dominated or possessed by a male; and the husband who cannot have sexual intercourse with his wife on top, because it seems unmanly. The "battle of the sexes" is carried out not only in bed, but in every area of marital interaction, generally by people who are uncertain of their masculinity or femininity and who fight to gain self-respect by derogating the partner. Several generations ago, these sexually related social roles were handed down or "assigned" by tradition; today, roles are negotiable, and problems become serious when negotiation is impossible to attain because of faulty communication, or when it breaks down because of disturbed perception or the fear of compromise.

The sexual system develops as such an integral part of personality development that sexuality and personality are inseparably interwoven. The physician who wishes to be an effective sex counselor, therefore, must deal with sexual relations in the context of human, especially marital, relations.

PROBLEM AREAS

Sexual disturbances in marriage may be the result of (1) sufficient psychopathology on the part of one or both spouses, (2) a poor relationship or "fit" between the spouses, or (3) relative ignorance of one or both partners. An example of the first category is the wife whose life experience taught her that sex is nasty and sinful and who cannot experience sexual pleasure, for the pleasure would increase her guilt inordinately. Patients in this category with longstanding sexual dysfunction are generally referred to psychiatrists. Patients whose difficulties stem largely from a poor marital relationship may be seen by the nonpsychiatric physician, who, unless he has had special training in sex and marriage counseling, must be mindful of his own capacities and limitations.

The physician who is comfortable in dealing with sexual problems and whose values do not push him to impose his own standards on his patients can clear up many sexual concerns by giving appropriate information. Sexual misunderstanding and misinformation are extensive; only a few examples are given here: the adolescent boy who thinks his penis is too small, or the teenage girl who thinks she is abnormal because of her sexual urges; the idea that the person who desires sex frequently is a "sex maniac"; the notion that oral-genital sex is a perverse activity; the frequent concept that coital orgasm is the only form of orgasm that is normal; that masturbation leads to mental illness (1650 out of 11,000 medical students who took the Sex Knowledge and Attitude Test, or SKAT, expressed this belief!); that direct clitoral stimulation must be continued until penetration occurs; that waxing and waning of sexual excitement is abnormal; that sexual activity during pregnancy or weeks after recovery from a coronary occlusion is dangerous; or that after the age of 50 or 60 or 70 a person is sexually "over the hill."

In evaluating any sexual problem it is necessary to determine how much weight to attach to the three factors contributing to the problem. Often, all three are represented. The woman who has the concept of sex as a sinful activity and who inhibits her responsivity may have only a hazy idea of what pattern of stimulation (called by Masters and Johnson "sensate focus") is best suited to increase her sexual excitement, and may make all sorts of excuses to her husband ("I'm tired"; "I have a headache"; "It's my period") to avoid sex, or she may grant or withhold sex as a weapon to punish her husband or in bargaining for something she wants.

Although the sexual problems that arise in marriage constitute the most frequent and most important need for professional intervention, additional characteristic sexual problems arise during the life cycle. Including marital sexual problems, some of the more frequent problem areas are the following:

1. Helping children and their parents deal with problems of sexual development. This includes concern about masturbation, sex play among children, menstruation, wet dreams, sexual fantasies, and possible coital activity among teenagers. "How do I, as a parent, talk to my children about sex?" is a question often asked of physicians.

2. Concerns of teenagers about masturbation, penis size, "how far to go during petting," the relation of sex to the relationships between sexes (how does sex relate to love?), erotic arousal for members of the same sex, contraception, and sexual performance. Unwanted pregnancy creates a need for abortion or "problem pregnancy" counseling. Venereal disease may occur at any age level, but it is increasing rapidly among teenagers.

3. Among young adults contemplating marriage, concerns about sexual performance and compatibility, as well as about family planning.

4. During marriage (or other intimate relationships), concerns about sexual interest, frequency, responsivity, coital positions, aspects of noncoital sex such as oral-genital sex, extramarital sex, contraception, abortion, and infertility. Of increasing concern to young people are conflicts about sex-role behavior (what is appropriate for men and women in their relations with each other). Life cycle events such as pregnancy, childbirth, moving to another locality, change of jobs, death, or chronic illness often have important effects on sexual feelings and behavior. Bodily complaints and physical symptoms may mask sexual and marital problems.

5. Other illnesses—psychic, such as depression, or physical, such as heart, lung, metabolic, or neurologic disease—may create special sexual concerns and inhibitions of function, as does ablative surgery.

6. Separation such as occurs with divorce or death in the middle-aged or elderly creates very special sexual problems. The loss of companionship and affection may be even more important than the decrease in sexual opportunities, although the interest in sex itself among the elderly is characteristically unrecognized or minimized by the physician.

Although childhood sex play and masturbation are now recognized as part of normal psychosexual development, parents are frequently concerned enough to ask their physicians about these behaviors. In most instances reassurance is all that is needed. If the sexual activity is "excessive" (and this is often subject to varying interpretation), it indicates a narrowing of the range of healthy social activities of the child, rather than the abnormality of the sexual behavior per se. Parents who ask how to talk about sex with their children can be referred to a number of books on this topic. A list of recommended reading can be obtained from the Sex Information and Education Council of the United States (SIECUS), 1855 Broadway, New York, N.Y. 10023. Similarly, a list of excellent books for teenagers to read can be obtained from the same source. The physician should read any recommended text so that he can answer questions in a more informed manner. The basic points in talking to children or teenagers is to be as comfortable as possible, and to be brief, concise, and factual once the real concerns are elicited by gently encouraging the child to talk, and above all, to avoid lecturing in a pontifical fashion. The physician is more apt to be "heard" if he discusses the pros and cons of sexual decision-making, rather than expressing his own value-position in a forceful manner.

The problem of premarital coitus is characteristically presented by the unmarried girl who asks her physician for the "pill." If freedom of the physician is not restricted by his own set of values, this provides him with an opportunity to discuss with the young patient her feelings and expectations about her relationship with her actual or intended partner. Physicians are often concerned that prescribing contraception for the unmarried girl will be a license for sexual activity. Actually, the young girl asks *after,* rather than before, the initial coital experience. A study of over 500 unwed never-pregnant teenagers aged 13 to 17, who for the first time sought professional help to obtain contraception, shows that 96 per cent of those teenagers who asked for contraception were previously sexually active; most of them had been having intercourse for more than a year; few were using any contraceptives, and still fewer were using one of the most effective methods. It should be clear that if a minor requests contraception, she needs it. This study and others suggest that contraceptive information and educational programs directed at minors will not be a significant factor in their decision to become sexually active.

A special area of increasing concern to physicians is called *"problem pregnancy" counseling.* This is not restricted to teenagers, as the majority of abortions are performed on married women. The unmarried pregnant teenager, however, is in a highly vulnerable position, because pregnancy and childbearing may seriously interfere with her educational and economic status, let alone the negative social sanctions that still persist despite the Supreme Court's decision legalizing abortion. The various options, i.e., continuing with the pregnancy and giving up the baby for adoption, or bringing the baby home, whether to marry or not, or whether to terminate pregnancy, have to be discussed thoroughly, and outside pressures for decision-making separated from internal conflict. The availability of legal abortion has eased the situation greatly, but the decision for abortion should never be made lightly, because the physician should be fairly certain that the patient will not be in the small minority who suffer from depression or remorse after the abortion. This applies to married women as well as to the unmarried. Most patients (who are not harmed by the abortion procedure per se) would derive special benefits by more intensive contraceptive, sex, and family counseling than is ordinarily provided to women seeking abortion.

Family-planning counseling gives the physician an unparalleled opportunity for exploring the connections between sexual attitudes and behavior and contraceptive concerns. The choice of the appropriate method of contraception is influenced by the frequency of coitus, attitudes toward responsibility and decision-making, fears of bodily damage, and desires for greater sexual spontaneity, as well as religious and moral values. Contraceptive failures are related to risk-taking, to the failure to learn how or under what conditions conception occurs, or to the individual's being under stress so that "contraceptive vigilance" is reduced. Adequate communication with the partner about contraceptive planning is an important consequence of appropriate counseling.

Family planning is much more than the prescription of a contraceptive method. It includes the timing of marriage, timing of the first child, child-spacing, the total number of children desired, and sex and marriage counseling, as well as contraception, problem-pregnancy, and sterilization counseling. Genetic counseling may also be a significant dimension of family planning. In this sense, family-planning counseling is an essential feature of premarital counseling, but is of course applicable throughout the child-bearing years.

Patients frequently misperceive the spouse's desired frequency of intercourse; most often the wife overestimates her husband's desired frequency. In one sixth of the cases studied, there was a gross underestimation of the wife's desires. The *perception* of the problem is usually more significant than the *reality*. The physician can often help by asking each spouse separately how often he wants intercourse and his perception of his spouse's desires. Better communication is the first step toward relieving this problem, and in many instances may be all that is required. The physician also has to bear in mind that the sex drive in the male is at a peak between the ages of 15 and 25, whereas in the female it peaks a decade later.

Inadequate responsivity in the female is due either to faulty preparation or to the inhibiting influence of emergency emotions—fear, anger, and guilt. Faulty preparation may be due to ignorance or unconcern of the husband or the inability of the wife to communicate her needs and preferences to her husband. The physician should try to clear away areas of ignorance before tackling the more difficult problems of inhibition caused by emotions designed for emergency "survival" rather than for pleasure. The long-range goal of therapy is to substitute the welfare emotions—love, pride, hope, and joy—for the emergency emotions. Newer techniques of sexual education and re-education, increasing the couple's awareness of the "sensate focus" and increasing each spouse's positive regard for his own body, have been developed by Masters and Johnson.

Premature ejaculation is again due either to a faulty perception of the bodily cues signaling impending ejaculation or to the influence of emergency emotions. Unless the patient is diabetic, impotence is generally related to a fear of failing in penetration, superimposed on emergency emotions related to his feelings about his partner. The vast majority of men with this disorder can be helped by removing the fear of performance, as John Hunter discovered two hundred years ago. He counseled his patients to avoid coitus "in six consecutive amatory experiences" and reported signal success.

Extramarital intercourse is sometimes dealt with more easily by marital partners than one might think. If, however, it threatens to have a destructive effect on the marriage, referral to an experienced marriage counselor is appropriate.

The astute physician has to be on the lookout for the presence of sexual or marital problems that lie behind a host of physical symptoms—headache, backache, fatigue, menstrual irregularities, or dysmenorrhea. Osler said of syphilis that it was "the great imitator" of other disease states. It may be said more accurately that sexual dissatisfaction plays that role today.

Chronic illness often has sexual connotations. Most physicians do not even discuss sex with their postcoronary patients, and when they do they may offer vague and uncertain advice, such as "take it easy." Patients who have chronic illness, or who have had organ ablation such as hysterectomy *are* concerned about their sexual function: How often? Under what circumstances? Am I still virile or attractive? are questions many patients are too embarrassed to ask.

DOCTOR-PATIENT RELATIONSHIP

Many patients are in doubt about what constitutes normal sexual behavior. These include questions about masturbation, oral-genital sex, sexual positions, coital frequency, sex during menstruation, pregnancy, or in the postpartum period, and sex in mid-life or later. The well-informed physician will be able to deal effectively with these concerns if he takes the trouble to inquire about the patient's sex life or is alert to cues that the patient wishes to discuss this area. History taking should utilize open-ended questions that preclude a yes or no answer and that go from less sensitive areas to ones of greater potential discomfort to the patient, e.g., from a discussion of marital relations to sex, or from menarche to petting to coitus, or from frequency to foreplay to coital positions.

If the physician is interested in this area, if he is reasonably comfortable and tactful, and has an appreciation of the role his own feelings and attitudes play in his interviewing and management of his patients' sexual problems, he will be able to establish a feeling of confidence and hope in his patient. This emphatic relationship coupled with the physician's growing fund of information and skills in interviewing makes possible the competent management of marital and sexual problems that heretofore have been either neglected or mishandled. In no other area of his practice can the physician derive greater reward and satisfaction from his efforts.

American Medical Association, Committee on Human Sexuality: Human Sexuality. Chicago, A.M.A., 1973.
Burnap, D. N., and Golden, J. S.: Sexual problems in medical practice. J. Med. Educ., 42:673, 1967.

Calderone, M. S.: Manual of Family Planning and Contraceptive Practice. 2nd ed. Baltimore, Williams & Wilkins Company, 1970.

Group for the Advancement of Psychiatry, Committee on Medical Education: Assessment of Sexual Function: A Guide to Interviewing. Vol. 8, Report No. 88, November 1973.

Herndon, C. N., and Nash, E. M.: Premarriage and marriage counseling: A study of North Carolina physicians. J.A.M.A., 180:395, 1962.

Katchadourian, H. A., and Lunde, D. T.: Fundamentals of Human Sexuality. New York, Holt, Rinehart & Winston, 1972.

Kinsey, A. C., Pomeroy, W. B., and Martin, C. E.: Sexual Behavior in the Human Male. Philadelphia, W. B. Saunders Company, 1948.

Kinsey, A. C., Pomeroy, W. B., Martin, C. E., and Gebhard, P. H.: Sexual Behavior in the Human Female. Philadelphia, W. B. Saunders Company, 1953.

Klemer, R. H.: Counseling in Marital and Sexual Problems: A Physician's Handbook. Baltimore, Williams & Wilkins Company, 1965.

Lief, H. I.: Preparing the physician to become a sex counselor and educator. Pediatr. Clin. North Am., 16:44, 1969.

Lief, H. I.: New developments in the sex education of the physician. J.A.M.A., 212:1864, 1970.

Masters, W. H., and Johnson, V. E.: Human Sexual Response. Boston, Little, Brown & Co., 1966.

Masters, W. H., and Johnson, V. E.: Human Sexual Inadequacy. Boston, Little, Brown & Co., 1970.

McCary, J. L.: Human Sexuality. New York, Van Nostrand, 1973.

Money, J., and Ehrhardt, A. A.: Man and Woman, Boy and Girl. Baltimore, Johns Hopkins University Press, 1972.

Nash, E. M., Jessner, I., and Abse, D. W.: Marriage Counseling in Medical Practice. Chapel Hill, University of North Carolina Press, 1964.

Pauley, I. B., and Goldstein, S. F.: Physicians' perception of their education in human sexuality. J. Med. Educ., 45:745, 1970.

Settlage, D. S. F., Baroff, S., and Cooper, D.: Sexual experience of younger teenage girls seeking contraceptive assistance for the first time. Fam. Plann. Perspect., 5:223, 1973.

Sex Information and Education Council of the United States (SIECUS): Sexuality and Man. New York, Charles Scribner's Sons, 1970.

Sorenson, R. C.: Adolescent Sexuality in Contemporary America. New York, World, 1973.

Trainer, J. B.: Physiologic Foundation for Marriage Counseling. St. Louis, C. V. Mosby Company, 1965.

Vincent, C. E.: Human Sexuality in Medical Education and Practice. Springfield, Ill., Charles C Thomas, 1968.

Vincent, C. E.: Sexual and Marital Health: The Physician as Consultant. New York, McGraw-Hill Book Company, 1973.

Zubin, J., and Money, J. (eds.): Contemporary Sexual Behavior: Critical Issues in the 1970's. Baltimore, Johns Hopkins University Press, 1973.

Section Seven. DRUG ABUSE, ADDICTION, AND INTOXICATION

340. INTRODUCTION

Robert B. Millman

Drug abuse is behavior that results from the complex interaction of an individual, his social and cultural environment, and the pharmacology and availability of particular drugs. There is frequently no sharp line that distinguishes appropriate use from misuse of any drug. Drug abuse may therefore be defined as the use of any substance in a manner that deviates from the accepted medical, social, or legal patterns within a given society. This section will consider the abuse of drugs that are primarily used to induce alterations in mood, perception, and behavior. These may be grouped into six major classes: (1) opiates; (2) central nervous system depressants, including alcohol, hypnotics, and tranquilizers; (3) central nervous system stimulants, including the amphetamine group and cocaine; (4) cannabis; (5) psychedelics; and (6) miscellaneous inhalants.

Abuse of some drugs may be intermittent and lead to little physical, psychologic, or social deterioration. In other cases, the user may become dependent on the drug in order to function at what he perceives to be a satisfactory level. This *psychologic dependence,* or habituation, varies in intensity and may culminate in *compulsive drug abuse,* in which the supply and use of particular drugs become primary concerns of living. In addition, certain drugs have the capacity to produce *physical dependence.* This is an altered physiologic state induced by the repeated administration of a drug that requires the continued administration of the drug to prevent the appearance of a syndrome characteristic for each drug, the *withdrawal,* or *abstinence, syndrome.* The term *"addiction"* has been used in the literature to refer to either behavioral or pharmacologic events. As used herein, it refers to a pattern of compulsive drug use that includes both physical dependence and an overwhelming involvement with the supply and use of a drug. Neither a diabetic who is on insulin nor a well-adjusted patient in methadone maintenance treatment is an addict in this sense of the term, although both are physically dependent on their medication.

Etiology. No single factor is the basis of all drug-taking experience, and no person's drug taking has a single cause. Drugs are taken to reduce pain, to influence mood, to change activity levels, to reduce tension and anxiety, to decrease fatigue and boredom, to facilitate social interaction, to heighten sensation and awareness, to satisfy curiosity, and for many other reasons. If caffeine, nicotine, alcohol, and prescription and over-the-counter depressants and stimulants are included, few people in the United States would be found who take no psychoactive drugs. Some people experiment with drugs that are considered dangerous from a medical or legal point of view and do not repeat the experience. Others persist in drug-abuse behavior patterns for a variety of reasons.

Sociologic Factors. Social and cultural factors determine which drug-abuse patterns are acceptable for a given group; and in some cases, groups derive their identity from particular drug-using behavior. The use of alcohol is condoned and even encouraged in many segments of society. Cannabis and psychedelic use are an integral part of membership in some white middle-class groups. Heroin use, until recently, was an involving, exciting pursuit in inner-city ghetto areas. Given the limited opportunities to experience pleasure, satisfaction, or pride in certain underprivileged groups, moreover, the aggressive, goal-oriented life of a heroin addict may appear attractive to a young boy or girl. Social factors also determine the availability of particular drugs. Heroin is easily available in the inner city, whereas the suburban dweller may have to travel long distances to obtain the drug. Patterns of abuse change rapidly in response to a variety of social and cultural factors. Currently (1974), the incidence of heroin addiction may be decreasing in New York City and some other urban areas, whereas the extent of multiple-drug use, including alcohol and hypnotics, may be increasing.

Psychobiologic Factors. Personality characteristics, in part, determine the psychoactive effects that drugs elicit in individual users and influence the choice of drugs and patterns of abuse. Amphetamines may produce tranquility in some people. Alcohol and barbiturates impair behavior control in others and may permit more aggressive personality types to "act out" in a hostile and violent manner.

Controversy exists whether drug abuse implies a personality disturbance that antedates drug use and that can be classified in distinct groups according to the drug and pattern of abuse. Most authorities agree that the experimental or intermittent abuse of drugs is not necessarily an indication of psychopathology. Compulsive drug use is frequently associated with serious psychopathology. Some workers describe addictive or alcoholic personality types, characterized by a mixture of neurotic traits and character disorders. Narcotic addicts have been described as passive individuals who experience intolerable anxiety related to physical pain, sexuality, hunger, and aggression. Opiates relieve this anxiety and permit the addict to withdraw from these inner tensions.

Evidence is accumulating to suggest that personality characteristics in drug-abusing populations vary considerably and that psychologic factors play a markedly variable role in the etiology of drug abuse. It is well known that some seriously disturbed people have experimented with alcohol, opiates, and other drugs and have not become compulsive users. *Moreover, no predictive test or system has been developed that will determine whether or not a person will become a compulsive user, nor which people will use which drugs.* Although premorbid personality disturbances are crucial in the etiology of some cases of compulsive drug use, the psychopathology noted in other cases may be a reaction to the behavioral patterns of compulsive abuse in a society that condemns the drug-dependent life.

Learning influences the nature of the drug experience and patterns of abuse. Conditioned factors have been implicated in the drug-craving and abstinence symptoms that occur when an abstinent ex-addict returns to a site of former drug use.

Various disease states are treated with psychoactive drugs for prolonged periods. The drug use of a small percentage of patients may come to exceed medically recommended dosages or indications and eventuate in addiction in some cases. Psychologic and sociologic factors should be considered in the etiology of these behavior patterns in addition to the physical and pharmacologic determinants. Genetic and physical factors may also influence the response to drugs in some individuals.

Pharmacologic Factors.   The nature of the psychic and physical effects of particular drugs is a determinant of their initial abuse potential. Considerations of physical dependence and tolerance influence the pattern of abuse. *Tolerance* refers to the decreased effect obtained from repeated administration of a given dose of a drug or to the need for increased amounts to obtain the effects that occurred from the first dose. Tolerance may be either *drug disposition* (metabolic) in type, in which there is more rapid inactivation or excretion of a drug, or *pharmacodynamic* (cellular), in which cells in the nervous system adapt to drug concentrations. Both may occur with the same drug. The physical dependence that develops concurrently with tolerance to opiates, barbiturates, and alcohol is poorly understood and may be related to pharmacodynamic tolerance mechanisms. *Cross-dependence* refers to the ability of one drug to suppress abstinence symptoms produced by withdrawal of another. Cross-dependence may be complete or partial, as with alcohol and the barbiturates.

Diagnosis.   Diagnosis of specific patterns of drug abuse and dependence requires careful history taking, when possible, and a complete physical examination. Drug abusers are often poor historians and may minimize or exaggerate the extent of their drug use, depending on their perception of the situation, their needs, and the attitudes of the examiner. The nature and degree of drug-induced psychoactive effects and any abstinence symptoms and signs should be assessed. Adverse effects of particular drugs should be sought.

Evaluation of the mode of administration of the drugs of abuse is important in establishing a diagnosis. Signs of repeated intravenous injections ("tracks") suggest heroin, amphetamine, or cocaine abuse. These drugs are also "sniffed," whereby the material is inhaled and absorbed through the mucous membranes of the nasopharynx and respiratory tract. Chronic sinusitis or perforation of the nasal septum may suggest this mode of administration. Personal hygiene and patterns of behavior and dress may further define the clinical picture.

Routine qualitative procedures for the detection in urine of morphine (the major metabolite of heroin), methadone, amphetamines, cocaine, and the most frequently abused general depressants are currently available in many laboratories. Results will generally be positive if a dose sufficient to produce pharmacologic effects has been taken within 24 hours prior to the urine sample. Since results are not immediately available or-

dinarily, and since false positives occur, these tests should be used to confirm the clinical impression. They are most useful as an adjunct to the long-term evaluation of patients already in treatment. In emergency situations, blood levels of suspected drugs may usually be obtained immediately.

Treatment and Prevention.   Treatment procedures should vary according to the individual and his social set, the pattern and extent of abuse, and the pharmacology of the abused drugs, as well as the goals of treatment. As distinct from most other patients, drug abusers frequently know more about the behavior and disability incident to drug taking than do their physicians. Serving to further complicate therapeutic efforts, drug abusers are often faced with prejudice and hostility on the part of treatment personnel, e.g., "they did it to themselves." Since many of their personality characteristics and behavior patterns occur in response to the attitudes of society, an inquiring, compassionate attitude is crucial in the treatment of this group of patients.

Drug-abuse prevention programs have focused on educational efforts in which the risks of drug abuse are publicized, and on increased legal stringency. Both approaches have serious deficiencies. Perhaps more important than either of these would be the provision of reasonable, attractive vocational, recreational, and educational alternatives to drug abuse in those most at risk, namely, the young and socially disadvantaged. Finally, physicians must be extremely prudent in their prescribing practices with respect to potentially abusable drugs.

341.   THE OPIATES
Robert B. Millman

Opiates or narcotic analgesics refer to natural or synthetic drugs that have pharmacologic actions similar to the derivatives of opium. Opium is obtained from the poppy plant *Papaver somniferum* and contains more than 20 alkaloids, of which morphine and codeine are relevant to this discussion. Heroin, the principal opiate of abuse in the United States, is converted from morphine by the addition of two acetyl groups (diacetyl-morphine). Demerol and methadone are synthetic narcotic analgesics. Pentazocine is a synthetic analgesic compound that has actions similar to both the opiates and the narcotic antagonists.

Incidence.   People have used opium for medical, religious, or recreational purposes since ancient times. Marked changes have occurred in the characteristics of the opiate-abusing population in the United States during the past 100 years. The use of patent medicines containing opiates was widespread in the middle class during the period from 1850 to 1906, when the labeling requirements of the Pure-Food and Drugs Act caused many preparations to be withdrawn. The Harrison Narcotics Act of 1914 and Supreme Court decisions in the 1920's made possession of narcotics without a prescription a crime and created a climate in which addicts were considered to be criminals and in which physicians could not prescribe narcotics to addicts. The number of oral opiate users declined, and the primary remaining group were those who injected heroin or morphine. Illegal dealers became the only source of opiates. Prices rose precipitously, and addicts frequently resorted to criminal activity to finance their addiction. The addict population from the 1930's to the second world war included predominantly white individuals involved in criminal activity or the entertainment professions who used intravenous heroin as well as morphine, cocaine, and other drugs. The growth of urban black ghettos and the development of efficient production and delivery systems ushered in the present era of extensive heroin use associated with a pervasive street culture that supports the heroin-dependent life. Surveys completed in 1971, estimated between 200,000 and 300,000 heroin addicts in the United States. The majority of these were members of ethnic minority groups and lived in urban areas. Males predominated over females, and the population was quite young. In New York City in 1971, heroin addiction was the major cause of death in males aged 15 to 35. Large numbers of affluent white suburban youths were also becoming addicted. At present, evidence suggests that the incidence of heroin addiction may be decreasing in many urban areas owing to a multiplicity of factors, including changing social and cultural styles, the proliferation of effective treatment programs, and decreased availability of heroin. A recent phenomenon is the oral methadone abuse that is occurring as a result of its increased availability.

Patterns of Abuse. People initially experiment with heroin for many reasons, including a search for pleasure, curiosity, anxiety, immaturity, sexual problems, psychopathology, and peer pressure. In some urban ghetto areas, given the lack of attractive alternatives, using and selling heroin appears to be a rewarding, involving "career" that carries with it the illusion of wealth and significance. Users are generally introduced to the drug by a friend or acquaintance already using the drug. The role of the nonaddicted drug dealer ("profiteer") is minimal in exposing new users to the drug. Street heroin ("smack," "scag," "junk," "dope") is adulterated ("cut") with quinine, lactose, maltose, and other sugars as it passes from the importer to the street user. The final amount of heroin in a street package costing from two to ten dollars may vary from 3 to 30 mg.

Initial street use is generally by "sniffing," in which the material is absorbed through the mucous membranes of the nasopharynx and respiratory tract. A user's first experience with the drug is often characterized as somewhat unpleasant because of nausea, vomiting, and anxiety; these symptoms abate with subsequent use. Effects may then be perceived as a sense of relaxation and peace with relief of worry and tension, a euphoric state in which all things are as they should be. At the outset, use may be intermittent and separated by weeks or months. It is not known how many people experiment with the drug and do not continue its use. Those who do continue to use heroin develop tolerance to its euphoric effects. In an attempt to maximize the euphoric effects of a given street amount, users will begin to inject the drug subcutaneously ("skin-popping") and eventually intravenously ("mainlining"). Intravenous injection produces a warm flushing of the skin and pleasurable sensations in the entire body, described as similar to sexual orgasm and called a "rush" or "kick." Many years of intravenous use of opiates and other drugs may result in obliteration of patent, available veins, necessitating a return to the subcutaneous mode of injection.

As tolerance increases and the awareness of physical dependence becomes manifest, more drug must be used more often. The urban street addict, with little access to legitimate sources of money or drug, must devote all of his time and energy to the acquisition of heroin to support his addiction ("habit"). Involvement in the "junkie" subculture, with its own language and behavioral systems, ensures his supply of drug and provides for the transmission of skills, information, and ideology that makes it possible to live as an addict. Any source of money is acceptable; males frequently engage in theft and forgery, whereas females will be prostitutes and shoplifters. Every user is a potential "dealer" of drugs, since this is the most efficient way of making money.

Food, clothing, sexual desires, and dignity may become subordinate to the ever-present need for opiates. An unknown number of heroin addicts, particularly those in the entertainment professions, are able to maintain their employment and their families and do not become immersed in the behavior patterns of the street "junkie."

If heroin is not available or is in poor supply, addicts will use other opiates, particularly methadone because of its long duration of action, to allay their withdrawal symptoms. Few cases of primary methadone addiction have been noted, since it is usually available in oral form only and the intensity of its euphoric properties is less than that of heroin. Barbiturates, other hypnotics, and alcohol may also be used in this regard. Mixed addictions in this group are frequently seen. An integral part of the natural history of this disease consists of repeated arrests, hospitalizations for the complications of addiction, attempts at self-imposed abstinence, periods when drug is not available ("panic"), and failures in treatment programs. These abstinent episodes may serve to lower an addict's tolerance and so decrease the expense and hardship of his "habit."

The patterns of abuse noted in addicted medical personnel or in those few "medical" addicts, who obtain their drugs through licit channels, are quite different from those of the street "junkie." Meperidine, morphine, and pentazocine are generally the drugs of choice in this group. There is little of the social and physical degradation seen in the general addict population. They are frequently able to maintain their employment and the other elements of their lives.

Opiate addicts are a heterogeneous group. The incidence of premorbid psychopathology is probably quite low in the street addict population. This may be due to the high degree of personality integration and resourcefulness required for survival. There may be a higher incidence of pre-existing personality disturbances in the middle-class addict, whose behavior is more deviant for his social situation. Personality characteristics and behavior patterns frequently result from the interaction of the addict and the drug in the sociocultural environment of addiction.

A small number of people are able to function effectively as street addicts but decompensate acutely when the heroin is withdrawn or when methadone is substituted. The relief of anxiety afforded by the opiates may be important in ensuring continued function in these patients with borderline psychologic adjustments. The very structured existence of street heroin addiction may also be useful.

Pharmacology. Opiates are absorbed from the gastrointestinal tract or the nasal mucosa, and after subcutaneous, intramuscular, or intravenous injection. Morphine and heroin lose much of their analgesic potency when taken orally, whereas codeine and meperidine remain quite active and methadone retains most of its analgesic efficacy after oral administration. Heroin is hydrolyzed to morphine in the body, and except for its greater potency and more rapid onset of action, has pharmacologic properties similar to those of morphine. Morphine is concentrated in parenchymatous tissues, skeletal muscle, and, to a lesser extent, brain. It is conjugated with glucuronic acid and excreted primarily in the urine and secondarily in the feces. Traces of morphine can be found in urine for 48 hours, although 90 per cent or more is excreted within the first 24 hours.

Administered subcutaneously, methadone and morphine exert approximately equal analgesic effects; heroin is three times stronger, whereas meperidine and codeine are approximately one tenth as potent. Morphine or heroin taken intravenously is effective almost immediately; duration of action varies from three to six hours. Oral administration prolongs the action of all the opiates, particularly that of methadone, in which the onset of effect occurs within 30 minutes and the duration of action in nontolerant individuals is four to ten hours.

Morphine or heroin administered to a nontolerant individual induces analgesia through a reduction in the anxiety and tension that result from the perception of pain. Somnolence characterized by an inability to concentrate, sleepiness, or "nodding," also occurs. Opiates cause pupillary constriction, depression of respiration by decreasing the responsiveness of the brainstem to carbon dioxide, depression of body temperature, and stimulation of central nervous system centers to produce nausea and vomiting. Other acute effects include decreased motility of the stomach, diminished pancreatic and biliary secretions, decreased propulsive contractions of the small and large intestine, and increased tone of the anal sphincter, leading to constipation. Increased tone of the detrusor muscle leads to a sensation of urgency accompanied by increased tone of the vesical sphincter, resulting in urinary retention. An acute release of antidiuretic hormone is effected, as well as inhibition of release of ACTH, corticotrophin-releasing factor, and gonadotrophin. Peripheral vasodilatation occurs, resulting in pruritus and possibly causing the observed increase in perspiration. Histamine release occurs, frequently resulting in a wheal-and-flare reaction, or "hive," at the site of injection and in a "pins-and-needles" sensation.

Addiction and Withdrawal Processes. Repeated use of narcotic analgesics produces tolerance to most of the acute narcotic effects, and the lethal dose is markedly increased. Whereas a 10-mg dose of morphine may produce euphoria in a nontolerant individual, the daily use of 5 grams has been reported in addicts. The rate at which this tolerance develops depends on the frequency and magnitude of use. Street addicts may spend from $20 to $200 or more daily on heroin and may inject themselves every three to six hours. Tolerance to all the opiate effects does not occur equally, since highly tolerant users will continue to demonstrate pupillary constriction and constipation. Cross-tolerance occurs with all narcotic analgesics. Tolerance to narcotics is primarily due to some form of cellular adaptation to the drug's action, with increased metabolism of lesser importance.

Physical dependence develops concurrently with tolerance and has been demonstrated after only a few exposures on succeeding days. It is marked by the development of an acute abstinence syndrome upon withdrawal of opiates, the "cold-turkey" process. This syndrome is quite variable in severity and characteristics and depends upon the particular drug, the dose, the interval between doses, and the duration of narcotic use, as well as on the personality and immediate environment of the narcotic addict. With heroin, the first withdrawal signs are generally seen shortly before the next scheduled dose. They are purposive in nature and include feelings of anxiety, restlessness, irritability, and drug craving. Lacrimation, rhinorrhea, yawning, and perspiration become apparent 8 to 12 hours after the last dose of narcotic. A restless sleep may intervene, the so-called "yen

sleep," from which the addict awakens with more severe withdrawal symptoms and signs, including dilated pupils, sneezing, coryza, anorexia, nausea, vomiting, diarrhea, abdominal cramps, bone pains, myalgias, tremors, weakness, insomnia, goose flesh, and, very rarely, convulsions or cardiovascular collapse. With morphine and heroin, withdrawal symptoms peak at 48 to 72 hours, and most observable symptoms disappear in seven to ten days. With methadone, the onset of withdrawal symptoms is more gradual, the peak is less pronounced and later, and the duration may be more than two or three weeks. The abstinence syndrome may be precipitated within minutes in opiate-dependent persons by administration of a narcotic antagonist such as nalorphine, levallorphan, or naloxone, although there are no medical indications for this diagnostic procedure.

Pentazocine (Talwin), a drug with weak opiate-antagonist effects and moderate opiate-agonist effects, elicits morphine-like subjective effects in nontolerant individuals. Higher doses produce dysphoric effects, including nervousness, anxiety, and, infrequently, bizarre alterations in perception and behavior. Tolerance and physical dependence occur, and cases of addiction to this drug are reported. Abrupt withdrawal of the drug from persons taking 200 to 700 mg daily results in an abstinence syndrome marked by irritability, abdominal cramps, nausea, vomiting, hyperthermia, lacrimation, and drug-seeking behavior. When pentazocine is administered to opiate-dependent patients, its antagonistic actions may precipitate withdrawal symptoms.

Subsequent to the termination of abstinence symptoms or after a course of detoxification with decreasing doses of opiates, most addicts experience recurrent urges for narcotics and generally resume their use of these drugs. The traditional psychologic theory of relapse presumes that, after withdrawal, the physiologic causes of drug taking have been removed, but that addicts have an "addictive personality" disorder that causes them to return to opiate addiction to escape reality. Psychologic factors play a role, although no predictive test has been developed to distinguish future addicts from future nonaddicts, nor are addicts able to be distinguished from nonaddicts by psychologic evaluation when they are observed under the same abstinent conditions. Evidence is accumulating that metabolic and neurophysiologic changes persist long after the detoxification process is completed, as does some tolerance. Protracted abstinence signs, as indicated by alterations in blood pressure, pulse rate, body temperature, respiratory rate, and pupillary size, have been documented and may relate to the chronic drug craving reported and the high incidence of relapse. The conditioned associations abstinent ex-addicts experience when they are exposed to their old neighborhoods and friends are also involved in the persistence of drug craving. Narcotic addiction with its implicit relapses after periods of abstinence should be viewed as a disease of complex etiology in which a persistent neurochemical disturbance as well as profound psychologic and social factors contributes to the dominance of drug-seeking behavior.

Medical Complications. When a known dose of an opiate is administered under aseptic conditions, either occasionally or chronically, medical complications are almost unknown. There are well-documented cases of long-term opiate addiction in physicians and others in whom no adverse physical effects were found. The patterns of use, including life style, unknown and markedly variable opiate dose, lack of hygienic administration techniques, and the variety of adulterants used to dilute the opiate, are responsible for the extensive morbidity and mortality (estimated to be about 1 to 2 per cent per year) associated with opiate abuse and dependence.

Acute heroin reactions secondary to intravenous use of street drug are responsible for more than three quarters of all fatalities from narcotics. Formerly thought of as true pharmacologic overdoses with respiratory depression, these reactions may be due to opiate-induced cardiac arrhythmias or hypoxia by unexplained mechanisms. Acute reactions to adulterants, including quinine, allergic reactions, and synergistic effects from multiple-drug use, may also be implicated. The syndrome is marked clinically by the rapid development of cyanosis, pulmonary edema, respiratory distress, and coma. Increased intracranial pressure and occasionally convulsive seizures are seen. The pathologic picture includes pulmonary congestion and edema and frequently cerebral edema.

Skin abscesses, cellulitis, and *thrombophlebitis* are the most frequent complications of heroin addiction. Skin manifestations are particularly noted after the subcutaneous injection of heroin and its adulterants. Septicemia and acute and subacute bacterial endocarditis with involvement of either or both sides of the heart are seen. *Staphylococcus aureus* is frequently the causative organism in right-sided lesions. Peripheral and pulmonary embolic phenomena occur. Osteomyelitis occurs infrequently. Malaria was a frequent complication in the 1930's. The introduction of quinine as an adulterant and the eradication of malaria in this country have decreased the incidence of this complication. Syringe-transmitted syphilis occurs infrequently.

Viral hepatitis transmitted by the communal use of contaminated needles is a frequent complication of intravenous drug use. Abnormal liver function tests, hypergammaglobulinemia, and increased serum immunoglobulins that persist for long periods of time after the acute episodes and that occur in addicts with no history of hepatitis are due in some cases to variants of chronic hepatitis, but may also be due to effects produced by alcohol, malnutrition, allergic phenomena, adulterants, and recurrent or chronic infections. False positive serologic tests are due to these factors. The nephrotic syndrome has been seen in association with street heroin use as well.

Pulmonary complications include pneumonia, abscess, infarction, and tuberculosis. Disseminated extrapulmonary tuberculosis has been reported. Angiothrombotic pulmonary hypertension and granulomatosis result from the intravenous injection of foreign bodies, including talc or cotton. Vascular lesions include local arterial occlusion, phlebitis, mycotic aneurysm, and necrotizing angiitis.

Neurologic complications of street heroin use include transverse myelitis, peripheral nerve lesions, and muscle disorders, including acute rhabdomyolysis with myoglobinuria and a fibrosing chronic myopathy. Septic states may lead to bacterial meningitis and brain, subdural, and epidural abscesses. In this country, intravenous narcotism is a leading cause of tetanus.

Menstrual irregularities in addicted women have been described, although it is unknown whether these can be ascribed to narcotic-induced suppression of adrenocorticotrophic hormone and gonadotrophic release or to malnutrition, frequent infections, and the general life style of female addicts. There is a high incidence of toxemia and of prematurity in infants born to addicted mothers, probably because of these life-style factors and the lack of prenatal care. Withdrawal symptoms are noted in a variable percentage of these newborn.

Treatment. Methods of treatment of narcotic dependence vary considerably, depending on the treatment goals, the factors that are thought to be most significant in the etiology of a patient's addiction, and the characteristics of individual patients. The magnitude of the addict's desire to stop using opiates is an important factor in the selection of the appropriate treatment modality as well as in the outcome. These motivational factors are difficult to assess, since most addicts want to terminate their addiction within one or two years after its onset. Nevertheless, many continue the compulsive use of heroin for many years and suffer repeated treatment failures. Approaches are primarily psychosocial, pharmacologic, or combinations of these. Since addiction has physical, psychologic, and social determinants, treatment is best provided by a well-organized team approach rather than by individual practitioners.

Withdrawal Techniques. Withdrawal of narcotics is most effectively accomplished by inpatient or outpatient substitution of oral methadone for any of the natural or synthetic narcotic analgesics (detoxification). Doses ranging from 20 to 40 mg daily are instituted, followed by a gradual reduction of dosage over the course of 10 to 14 days or more. Optimally, psychologic, legal, and vocational supportive services should be provided the patient throughout the process and continuing into the drug-free period. In some cases, patients are withdrawn in a drug-free environment without opiate substitution, although this has proved less justifiable on medical and moral grounds. The chronic nature of this disease necessitates continuing treatment after the withdrawal process is completed.

METHADONE MAINTENANCE

In this country, methadone maintenance has been the most successful and most widely used approach in the treatment of opiate dependence. This mode of therapy emphasizes social and emotional rehabilitation rather than abstinence. The treatment is based on the two major properties that distinguish methadone from other narcotics: good oral efficacy and long duration of action. After oral ingestion in tolerant individuals, the duration of action of methadone is extended to 24 to 36 hours owing to a reservoir of drug in tissues. Initially, oral methadone is administered daily in doses that will allay symptoms of abstinence. The dose is gradually increased until a stabilization level is reached at which patients will be tolerant to the euphoric effects of the drug and will experience no persistent craving for opiates. If the stabilization level is high enough (80 to 120 mg), there is a good degree of cross-tolerance to the effects of other narcotics, such that the effects of even large doses of intravenous opiates will not be felt (narcotic blockade). Approximately 75 per cent of patients in well-run programs remain in treatment. Improvement has been noted in the work and school records of patients retained in the program, and the incidence of their criminal activity has declined markedly. Long-term methadone maintenance has been shown to be medically safe, with minimal side effects and no toxicity when properly administered. Performance and learning are normal in methadone-maintained subjects. Medication should be dispensed in a clinic situation that provides medical care and extensive rehabilitative services so as to facilitate satisfactory reentry into nondrug-dominated ("straight") society. Since methadone is subject to abuse and is potentially lethal in nontolerant individuals, adequate provisions must be made to prevent its illicit dispersal.

Programs utilizing methadone maintenance for varying periods of time followed by a slow-detoxification process have shown promise. Research is presently under way with levomethadyl acetate hydrochloride, a synthetic congener of methadone that extends opiate effects for 72 hours. Various programs that would provide heroin under supervision are also being considered (heroin maintenance). The short-acting nature of the drug, coupled with the necessity for injecting it, renders this form of treatment less potentially useful.

NARCOTIC ANTAGONISTS

Narcotic antagonists such as cyclazocine and naltrexane are being evaluated for the treatment of detoxified addicts. These agents block or attenuate the euphoriant effects of narcotics and prevent the development of physical dependence in patients who continue to use narcotics. Drug-seeking behavior might be extinguished insofar as it depends on conditioned associations to euphoric drug effects or abstinence symptoms. Prevention of the development of physical dependence might also minimize the continuation of narcotic use after a spree, and increase periods of abstinence. These drugs do not relieve the chronic opiate-drug hunger, and patients are prone to omit their dose of antagonist and relapse to heroin. A major advance would be the discovery of a medicine that relieves all symptoms of physical dependence, blocks the opiate-induced euphoria, does not itself produce physical dependence, and is not subject to abuse.

PSYCHOSOCIAL APPROACHES—ABSTINENCE PROGRAMS

A diverse array of programs exist that emphasize abstinence from opiates and other drugs as a primary component of treatment. These take the form of either voluntary groups or supervised institutionalization.

Voluntary groups are generally communities that are self-regulatory in nature and staffed predominantly by former drug users. The individual remains in the closed, drug-free environment for variable periods of time, frequently one to two years, and is encouraged to develop a new set of social and living skills that will enable him to remain drug free upon completion of the program. Outpatient programs are also under way. Intensive therapeutic techniques are utilized to eliminate the social and personality deficiencies of residents that led them to drug use. These facilities serve to reduce the sense of isolation felt by many drug users, and attempt to provide role models for responsible behavior. Some of the well-known groups are Synanon, Daytop Village, Phoenix House, and Sera. Although sharing many common methods and doctrines, these communities vary considerably in the nature of the therapeutic milieu created and in the complex system of rewards and punishments provided residents. Therapeutic communities are valuable for many people, although only a small percentage

of heroin addicts are motivated to enter a community, and follow-up studies of individuals who have returned to society are not presently available.

An alternative approach is programs which involve the nonpunitive incarceration of an addict for the purposes of rehabilitation (civil commitment). These programs generally include a period of enforced abstinence in a prison, hospital, or other locked facility, followed by careful supervision of the individual in the community. If renewed drug abuse or other antisocial behavior is noted, the addict is reinstitutionalized. To date, these programs have met with meager success. If adequate rehabilitative services and facilities are made available in the future, the efficacy of these programs might be increased.

Results of traditional psychotherapeutic techniques have been disappointing for the majority of compulsive opiate abusers. Specialized forms of group psychotherapy may be useful for some patients. After variable and sometimes prolonged periods of addiction, an unknown number of addicts spontaneously cease opiate use. This "maturing-out" process may be related to advanced age and the difficulty of obtaining drugs, a decline of internal psychologic conflicts, and the cumulative effect of various treatment programs.

342. CENTRAL NERVOUS SYSTEM DEPRESSANTS

Robert B. Millman

All central nervous system depressants are subject to abuse. The most frequently abused drugs in this category are the short-acting barbiturates, particularly pentobarbital (Nembutal) and secobarbital (Seconal), and assorted other hypnotics such as glutethimide (Doriden), methyprylon (Noludar), and methaqualone (Quaalude). Tranquilizers, including meprobamate (Miltown), chlordiazepoxide (Librium), and diazepam (Valium), are implicated in abuse patterns less often. Bromide abuse has become rare. Since many of the characteristics of these drugs are similar, this discussion will center on the barbiturates, with other agents considered when relevant.

Incidence and Patterns of Abuse. There is a continuum of depressant use that extends from appropriate use to compulsive abuse and addiction. Massive quantities of depressants are produced yearly in the United States (over 1 million pounds of barbituric acid derivatives alone). These are prescribed by physicians for hypnosis or sedation in a variety of conditions, including insomnia, depressive and anxiety states, and convulsive disorders. The source of drug for one major category of abuser is physicians' prescriptions. The pattern of use may begin as intermittent use at night to decrease anxiety and ensure sleep, progress to nightly use with increased doses, and culminate in prolonged daily use to maintain an adequate level of functioning. An individual may obtain drugs from several physicians at one time, none of whom are aware of the magnitude of their patient's depressant use. In this group there may be no illicit drug use, although alcohol is frequently used in association with the depressants.

Barbiturate and other hypnotic use is also prevalent in urban drug subcultures. Heroin addicts use hypnotics ("downs") to supplement the poor quality of heroin available. Alcoholics will also use hypnotics when they are available, since the quality of the intoxications are similar. Although some people abuse barbiturates preferentially, concurrent physical dependence on alcohol or opiates is more common than pure barbiturate dependence in these groups. Illicit sources of drugs are most often employed, and a wealth of street names have evolved for the most popular hypnotics, including "reds" (secobarbital), "yellows" (pentobarbital), and "double trouble" (amobarbital and secobarbital). Most use is oral, although some individuals inject the drugs intravenously or intramuscularly. The amounts taken vary markedly, but some individuals have ingested as much as 30 hypnotic doses of the short-acting barbiturates daily over many months.

Recently, a marked increase in the use of illicitly obtained hypnotics has been noted in some adolescent and preadolescent populations. Patterns and extent of use vary markedly, but generally multiple-drug use occurs and is considered appropriate behavior within these groups. Intermittent users may take several times the therapeutic dose, possibly in addition to marijuana, alcohol, and amphetamines if they are available, to get "high" enough to enjoy a concert or party.

The "high" that obtains from abuse of depressant drugs has been characterized as the sense of tranquility or peace that occurs just prior to sleep in normal individuals. The world is seen as limited to the immediate. Inhibitions and anxiety are blunted, and there may be a feeling of aggressiveness, freedom, and pleasant numbness. Sexual pleasure and ability are said to be enhanced at low doses of these drugs; higher doses lead to a decreased ability to perform sexually. Violent and antisocial behavior occurs, frequently serving to isolate depressant abusers ("down heads") from other groups of drug abusers.

There appears to be a high incidence of serious psychopathology in compulsive abusers of the depressant drugs. Users may be seeking obtundation in attempts to cope with anxiety arising from a variety of sources.

Pharmacology. Barbiturates and related hypnotics are rapidly absorbed after oral administration and are distributed throughout the body. They are general depressants of nerves and of skeletal, smooth, and cardiac muscles, although at low doses the central nervous system is primarily affected. Central nervous system effects vary from mild sedation to coma, depending on the particular drug, the dose, the route of administration, the degree of excitability of the nervous system, and tolerance. In some individuals under certain circumstances, small doses produce an initial stimulation not unlike that produced by alcohol. Barbiturate-induced sleep is similar to physiologic sleep except for a reduction in the proportion of rapid eye movement (REM) sleeping time. Duration of action varies with the particular barbiturate. After effects, including drowsiness, depression, impairment of judgment and performance, and occasionally hyperexcitability, may persist for many hours.

Both drug-disposition and pharmacodynamic tolerance to the barbiturates and related hypnotics develop rapidly with repeated administration. Drug-disposition tolerance in the short-acting barbiturates and some other depressants results from the activation of drug-metabolizing liver-enzyme systems and is characterized by the more rapid degradation of the drug and a decrease in sleeping time. The range of tolerance is narrow, and individuals tolerant to the sedating and intoxicating effects of 1 gram of pentobarbital may become intoxicated for prolonged periods upon the addition of 0.1 gram. Although the lethal dose of barbiturates varies in individuals, in distinction to the opiates, tolerance does not increase this dose significantly from that of nontolerant individuals. Severe poisoning is likely to occur when more than ten times the hypnotic dose is ingested at one time. Acute barbiturate poisoning may thus be superimposed on chronic intoxication at any time. The combination of sublethal doses of depressants with opiates or alcohol may also result in acute poisoning. Cross-tolerance develops to all barbiturates as well as to paraldehyde, meprobamate, and chlordiazepoxide. Partial cross-tolerance between alcohol and the depressants occurs.

Clinical Manifestations. Acute depressant poisoning may occur either accidentally or incident to a suicide attempt. Accidental overdoses may be due in some cases to "drug automation"; an individual may fail to fall asleep after several hypnotic doses, become confused, and ingest an overdose. Upon recovery, there may be no memory of the excessive drug ingestion. The clinical manifestations and treatment of poisoning are discussed

in Ch. 348. The acute and chronic signs and symptoms of mild hypnotic intoxication resemble those of intoxication with alcohol. The individual shows general sluggishness, difficulty in thinking, slowness of speech and comprehension, poor memory, faulty judgment, emotional lability, and narrowed attention span. Neurologic signs of barbiturate intoxication include thick, slurred speech, nystagmus, diplopia, strabismus, vertigo, ataxic gait, positive Romberg sign, hypotonia, dysmetria, and decreased superficial reflexes. Sensation, deep tendon reflexes, and pupillary responses are unaltered. Skin rashes have been reported. Unexplained seizures in adults should always prompt one to consider chronic depressant drug abuse.

With compulsive users, clothing may be unkempt and nutrition poor; needle marks and abscesses from intramuscular or intravenous use may be present. Adverse effects of chronic barbiturate use are poorly documented, but may be similar to those of alcohol on organ systems and the brain.

Abstinence Syndrome. Physical dependence, as indicated by abstinence signs and symptoms, develops to all the central nervous system general depressants. A characteristic *general depressant withdrawal syndrome* occurs and is similar to the symptoms of withdrawal from alcohol. It varies in severity, depending on the drug, dose, and frequency of use. *In contrast to the opiate withdrawal syndrome, that from depressants may be life-threatening.* The first manifestation of this syndrome might be considered the rebound increase in nightly rapid eye movement sleep, associated with nightmares and a sense of having slept badly, that occurs after discontinuation of use of only therapeutic doses of barbiturates for several nights. After a daily dose of 0.4 gram of pentobarbital for three months, abrupt withdrawal produces paroxysmal EEG changes without other significant symptoms. After 0.6 gram per day for one to two months, 50 per cent of patients experience insomnia, tremors, anorexia, and irritability, and 10 per cent may have a seizure. After continuous intoxication with doses of 0.9 to 2.2 grams per day for one month or less, 75 per cent may have seizures, and 66 per cent delirium; all experience insomnia, tremors, and anorexia. In general, the time required to produce physical dependence is shorter with the short-acting barbiturates and the withdrawal symptoms are more abrupt in onset and more severe than with the longer-acting sedatives.

When short-acting hypnotics are abruptly withdrawn, signs and symptoms of the intoxication clear over the initial 12 to 16 hours, and the patient appears to improve. Increases in restlessness, anxiety, tremulousness, and weakness then occur, which may be accompanied by cramps, nausea, vomiting, and orthostatic hypotension. These symptoms progress, and coarse hand tremors, muscle twitching, hyperactive deep reflexes, and increased blink reflex appear within 24 hours. Symptoms generally attain their peak during the second and third days, and convulsions may occur then or before. Some patients who have seizures may begin to show improvement, but 50 per cent develop a delirium that is marked by sensorial clouding, visual and auditory hallucinations, and disorientation to time and place. During the delirium, which usually occurs between the fourth and seventh days, hyperthermia, tachycardia, and agitation can lead to exhaustion and sometimes to fatal cardiovascular collapse. The abstinence syndrome generally clears by about the eighth day, and there is usually no residual physical damage. Clearing is frequently preceded by a period of prolonged sleep. With longer-acting barbiturates and chlordiazepoxide, seizures may not occur until the seventh or eighth day. Hallucinations sometimes persist for many months, but these may be a manifestation of an underlying psychosis.

Treatment. Treatment procedures include withdrawal and rehabilitative phases. Compulsive abusers of depressants are often considered more difficult to treat than any other class of drug abusers. Outreach and educational programs aimed at intermittent abusers of depressants before they become addicted may be important in this regard. The pattern of use and extent of physical dependence should be evaluated by means of a careful history and physical examination. Depressant abusers frequently distort or are unaware of the magnitude of their use, particularly those with a concurrent addiction to heroin.

If physical dependence is suspected, close observation or hospitalization is indicated. When the diagnosis is established, a suitable general depressant should be administered after the intoxication clears but before major withdrawal symptoms have begun. Pentobarbital orally is a suitable substitute for most of the general depressants, although phenobarbital and secobarbital may also be used. If the patient will not tolerate the oral administration of pentobarbital, intramuscular injections of the same doses may be used. Patients may usually be switched to oral drugs after a few intramuscular injections. Sufficient pentobarbital should be given to produce a mild but manageable level of intoxication, marked by inconstant slow nystagmus on lateral gaze, slight dysarthria, and ataxia. Most patients require from 0.2 to 0.4 gram every six hours, but some may need up to 2.5 grams over a 24-hour period. This "stabilization dose" should be carefully controlled to prevent signs of increased intoxication, such as dysarthria, emotional lability, constant nystagmus, or gross ataxia. Patients should be maintained on this dose for 24 to 48 hours, after which the dose of pentobarbital should be reduced by 0.1 gram or less daily. The patient should be observed carefully for signs of insomnia, tremulousness, and orthostatic hypotension, at which time the withdrawal of pentobarbital should be suspended for one to two days. If symptoms are severe, the patient should be given 0.2 gram intramuscularly immediately, which will usually suppress them. Delirium, convulsions, or fever should be treated as emergencies, with hourly doses until the patient is able to sleep for 8 to 12 hours, after which the stabilization dose is determined, as described above. Once a withdrawal delirium develops, increased doses of pentobarbital may fail to restore equilibrium; agitation and disorientation may persist for several days.

Fluid and electrolyte losses must be replaced, and complicating medical and surgical conditions treated. Increasing fever without evidence of infection necessitates additional sedation, antipyretics, sponging, or cooling blankets. Phenothiazines, butyrophenones, and diphenylhydantoin are not indicated.

In general, the use of the pentobarbital substitution technique may take from ten days to three weeks. It should not be hurried. Patients who are taking large amounts of lesser-known sedatives should probably be withdrawn from the original drug of abuse, if it is known, without substitution therapy. This withdrawal regimen may be carried out concurrently with that for opiates.

After withdrawal is completed, provisions must be made for high-frequency supportive counseling. Patients are frequently withdrawn and depressed, and the danger of relapse or suicide is great. The inclusion of patients in a therapeutic program, either as an inpatient or on an ambulatory basis, should be assured.

Physicians must be cautious when prescribing depressants for the relief of anxiety and insomnia. Attempts should be made to diagnose and treat the source of these symptoms. Whenever possible, tranquilizers such as chlordiazepoxide and diazepam, with a lower abuse potential, should be used in lieu of the short-acting hypnotics to induce sleep.

Bromides. Chronic bromide intoxication (bromism) has become rare, because bromide has been supplanted in modern medicine with more effective and less toxic sedative and analgesic compounds. The bromide ion is very slowly excreted by the kidney, with a half-life in the blood of about 12 days. Consequently, the daily ingestion of small doses will result in an accumulation of the drug to toxic levels over a period of weeks. Central nervous system symptoms and signs are the most common features and include drowsiness, impaired thought and memory, dizziness, and irritability, leading in more severe cases to delirium, hallucinations, lethargy, and coma. High plasma levels are associated with an EEG pattern of diffuse slow waves. Neurologic disturbances include tremors, thick speech, motor incoordination, and decreased superficial reflexes. A characteristic acneiform rash and other skin lesions occur in 20 per cent of cases. Gastrointestinal disturbances include anorexia, foul breath, and constipation. The diagnosis of chronic bromide intoxication is established by serum bromide levels above 9 mEq per liter in association with the aforementioned clinical picture.

Treatment consists of the daily administration of 200 mEq of either sodium or ammonium chloride, together with sufficient fluids to ensure a large urine output. This reduces the half-life of bromide to three or four days. Diuresis with chloruretic drugs may be useful if more rapid displacement of bromide is indicated. Hemodialysis rapidly clears bromides and may be indicated in treating comatose patients.

343. CENTRAL NERVOUS SYSTEM STIMULANTS

Robert B. Millman

Central nervous system stimulants or sympathomimetics that are subject to abuse include the *amphetamines*, *cocaine*, *methylphenidate* (Ritalin), *phenmetrazine* (Preludin), and *diethylpropion* (Tepanil). This discussion will consider the amphetamine group primarily, including amphetamine, dextroamphetamine, and methamphetamine, which are synthetic derivatives of ephedrine, and cocaine, an alkaloid of the coca plant which grows in the Andes in South America.

Incidence and Patterns of Abuse. Amphetamine abuse is widespread in industrial societies, particularly in Japan, Sweden, Great Britain, and North America. Patterns of use vary markedly. Until the recent federal and state regulations severely limiting physicians' prescribing practices with respect to the amphetamines and related drugs, enormous quantities were prescribed for the treatment of a variety of conditions, including obesity, depressive syndromes, behavior disorders, narcolepsy, and the reduction of fatigue. Many patients, frequently middle-class women, became dependent on these drugs when they found that they had to continue to ingest the drug to prevent depression and to perform optimally. The advent of tolerance necessitated increased doses, occasionally five to ten times the original 5- or 10-mg amount prescribed. Amphetamine abuse by students, athletes, truck drivers, and others who want to increase their efficiency or productivity is common. In both these patterns, oral preparations are used. Hypnotics are often used by this group to ensure sleep, and concurrent dependence on both classes of drugs is not unusual.

Another category of amphetamine abuser is composed of multidrug users, primarily young, who use these drugs for their mood-elevating properties. Any amphetamine may be used, although methamphetamine ("speed," "crystal," or "meth") is preferred, because it has more pronounced central effects and less peripheral ones. The drugs are taken orally on occasion, although "sniffing" or intravenous use is common in drug-dominated groups. Most methamphetamine is manufactured in illegal laboratories, but commercially available oral preparations are also dissolved for intravenous use.

Upon "sniffing," or particularly after intravenous use, the user experiences a "flash" or "rush" that is described as a sense of increased mental capacity and physical strength, with little need for food or sleep, and a feeling of power and intensity that is quite distinct from the feeling of satiation induced by the opiates. Increased activity, planning, and talking occur. Dissipation of the drug effects after three to six hours is experienced as an unpleasant sense of fatigue and depression ("crashing"). Use may be intermittent and limited to special occasions such as a party or journey, or may be more regular. Rarely, chronic amphetamine abusers report that the daily, controlled use of these drugs decreases the anxiety and tension they experience normally, and enhances their ability to eat, sleep, and generally function.

Some individuals use the drug continuously, to maintain the "high" or stave off the "crash" for several days or even longer (a "run"). As tolerance develops, the dose is increased and the drug taken more frequently, such that 1 gram may be injected every two to four hours. As this stage, the compulsive user, or "speed freak," is usually nervous, irritable, and suspicious. There may be intense involvement in complicated and often unnecessary tasks such as disassembling a television set or reorganizing a room. When the supply of drug is depleted or the user becomes too disorganized or debilitated to continue, the "run" ends. Cessation of amphetamine use is usually followed by a prolonged deep sleep. Hypnotics or alcohol are often used to minimize the duration of the "crashing" phase and facilitate the induction of sleep. Upon awakening, although much of the paranoid ideation may be gone, a feeling of lassitude, apathy, and depression may be present. Intravenous users frequently inject other drugs alone or in combination with amphetamines. The combination of amphetamines or cocaine and heroin is known as a "speed ball."

Most of the psychoactive effects of cocaine are similar to those of the amphetamines with regard to elevation of mood, decreased need for food or sleep, and hyperactivity. Supply is always through illicit channels; it is more expensive than the amphetamines or heroin, and it is much shorter acting. After intravenous administration, the primary mode in this country until recently, effects last 5 to 15 minutes. Intravenous use is generally seen in the same population that abuses heroin. It is often used in "runs" of varying duration, such that 1 to 10 grams may be used during the course of a day via frequent injections. Psychologic dependence and compulsive use occur, but less frequently than with the amphetamine group. Recently there has been a marked increase in abuse of this drug by affluent and middle-class people in urban areas. Use in this group, by sniffing the much-adulterated white powder, is generally intermittent; and marijuana, alcohol, and hypnotics may be used concomitantly.

Pharmacology. Peripheral sympathomimetic effects of amphetamines and cocaine are minor compared with their potent central nervous system activity. Peripheral effects include increased cardiac contraction, increased blood pressure with reflex slowing of the heart rate, relaxation of the bronchial musculature, increased contractility of the urinary bladder sphincter, increased venous pressure, pulmonary arterial pressure, and renal blood flow. Central effects include stimulation of the cerebrospinal axis and the medullary respiratory center. In low doses these drugs increase alertness and physical and cognitive ability, particularly when performance has been compromised by lack of sleep. The significant appetite depression seen is probably due to a combination of factors, including an inhibitory effect on the feeding center in the lateral hypothalamus as well as the improvement in mood that occurs.

Tolerance develops to both the peripheral and central effects of the amphetamines. Tolerance to cocaine is not thought to occur; there may be some degree of psychologic tolerance to the euphoric effects of this drug, although it apparently dissipates rapidly. Cross-tolerance exists between the amphetamines, but no cross-tolerance has been demonstrated between the amphetamines and cocaine.

Cessation of amphetamine or cocaine use does not produce major physiologic symptoms. The depression, increased appetite, lassitude, and prolonged sleep that ensue might be considered an abstinence syndrome and evidence of some physical dependence. Moreover, during this sleep, a characteristic electroencephalographic pattern is produced that shows a marked increase in the percentage of REM sleep, and nightmares may occur.

Adverse Effects. Adverse physical effects in intermittent users of amphetamines or cocaine by the sniffing route may be limited to irritation of the nasal mucosa or perforation of the nasal septum. Chronic users may be markedly debilitated and subject to numerous infections as a result of lack of sleep and poor nutrition. A sensation of something crawling under the skin is described ("cocaine bugs"), such that chronic users will frequently have excoriations and open sores from constant scratching and pinching. The intravenous use of these drugs is fraught with the numerous complications that result from nonsterile conditions, which are detailed in Ch. 341. Reports of necrotizing angiitis and hepatitis resulting from the direct toxic effect of methamphetamine require further clarification. Severe overdose reactions or death from either amphetamines or cocaine are quite rare. Amphetamine toxicity is marked by extensions of the sympathomimetic effects, culminating in cerebrovascular accidents, convulsions, and coma. Cocaine toxicity is characterized by initial sympathomimetic effects followed by cortical depression and anesthetization of the midbrain and medulla, leading to respiratory failure and cardiovascular collapse. Large intravenous dosages of cocaine may cause cardiac arrhythmias by direct action of the drug on cardiac tissue. The lethal dosage of amphetamines is variable, depending on the extent of tolerance; that of cocaine is estimated to be about 1.2 grams.

There is a high incidence of psychopathology in compulsive amphetamine and cocaine abusers. The most frequent complications of amphetamine and cocaine abuse are paranoid ideation and stereotyped compulsive behavior. Chronic users are frequently aware of these characteristics of the drugs and will not act on ideas of persecution. Antisocial or violent behavior may occur when this insight is lacking. Continued use frequently leads to a well-described *amphetamine or cocaine psychosis* that is often indistinguishable from acute paranoid schizophrenia. These reactions appear to be inevitable if the dose and frequency of use of amphetamines and cocaine are continually increased or high doses maintained. Psychotic episodes have also been precipitated in some individuals after only one small dose. The syndrome is marked by paranoid ideation; stereotyped compulsive behavior; visual, auditory, and tactile hallucinations; and loosening of associations occurring in a setting of clear consciousness and correct orientation. The etiology of these disorders may be related to actions of amphetamines and cocaine in inhibiting the re-uptake inactivation of the catecholamines, dopamine, and norepinephrine, thus potentiating their synaptic effects. The psychotic episodes invariably appear while the patients are under the influence of the drug, and generally abate within a few days to several weeks after cessation of drug use. Prolonged psychotic episodes occur and may relate to the premorbid personality of the user.

Treatment. Amphetamine and cocaine abusers are a heterogeneous group who demonstrate markedly diverse patterns of drug use. Accordingly treatment must be flexible. Treatment of the physical complications of abuse are considered in the appropriate chapters of this textbook. Treatment of paranoid ideation or the overt psychotic episodes must ensure cessation of amphetamine or cocaine use and may necessitate short-term hospitalization or, if possible, confinement in a safe, supportive atmosphere. Phenothiazine drugs or other tranquilizers are frequently benefical in the acute situation.

After recovery, depressive symptoms should be sought and the possibility of suicide must be considered. The compulsive abuser may require long-term supportive care under close supervision, with provision for psychiatric and social rehabilitation.

Physicians would do well to prescribe this class of drugs with great caution. Some authorities suggest that the childhood hyperkinetic disorders and narcolepsy are the only indications for their use.

344. CANNABIS
(Marijuana and Hashish)

Robert B. Millman

Marijuana and hashish are derived from *Cannabis sativa,* the hemp plant, an herbaceous annual which grows readily in many parts of the world and reaches maturation in four to five months. All parts of both the male and female plants contain varying amounts of the major psychoactive principle, delta-9-tetrahydrocannibinol; its active isomer, delta-8-THC; and numerous other cannabinoids. The concentration of delta-9-THC in the flowering tops of these plants is a function of genetic and environmental factors and varies from less than 0.2 per cent in the fiber-type plants to more than 4 per cent in those plants grown for drug content. In the United States, marijuana refers to the dried mixture of crushed leaves and flowering tops with or without the inclusion of stems and seeds. The flowering tops of the plants secrete a clear, varnish-like resin, which when collected and compressed is called hashish and is thought to be four to eight times more potent than marijuana. Cannabis or its products are also called *kif, bhang, ganja, charas,* and *dagga* in various parts of the world.

Incidence and Patterns of Abuse. Cannabis has been used extensively in many societies since antiquity as a form of folk medicine, as a work adjunct, in association with religious practices, and for recreational purposes. The prevalence of cannabis use has increased explosively in the United States and Western Europe during the past 15 years in association with the changing styles of youth culture. Several recent surveys suggest that the number of people in the United States who have ever used cannabis is 15 to 25 million. Users fall heavily into the teenage and young adult group, although increased use is being noted in older age groups as well. Whereas geographic, social, and cultural considerations are determinants of whether a person will use cannabis, personality characteristics are important in determining the frequency and pattern of use. Many people experiment with the drug and do not continue its use; over half are estimated to use the drug one or more times per month; about one in four who use it that often do so three times or more a week.

The drug is peripheral to the life of the occasional user, and frequently there is no other drug use. Others demonstrate a compulsive abuse pattern, in which their lives are dominated by the acquisition and use of cannabis and other drugs. Occasional users generally smoke in groups, where the ritual of preparation and sharing of the cigarette is an integral part of social interaction. Chronic smokers will also frequently smoke alone.

Marijuana is usually smoked in homemade cigarettes ("joints"). Hashish is smoked in a wide variety of small pipes. Both preparations may be ingested in combination with food or drink, although this is less common. The weight of a marijuana cigarette on the street may vary from 0.5 to 1 gram. In imported material, the delta-9-THC content, although generally less than 1 per cent, may be much more potent.

Pharmacology. Cannabis preparations are three to four times more potent when smoked than when taken orally. After inhalation, effects begin within minutes, peak within one hour, and are dissipated within three hours. After ingestion, effects begin in 30 minutes to two hours, peak at three hours, and persist for four to six hours. The effects of cannabis correlate with the appearance in plasma of active polar metabolites of delta-9-THC, principally the 11-hydroxy-delta-9-THC compounds. Nonpsychoactive polar metabolites are slowly eliminated from the body over a period of more than 1 week.

The acute physiologic effects of cannabis are dose related and include an increase in heart rate, conjunctival vascular congestion, decreased intraocular pressure, bronchodilatation, increased airway conductance, and peripheral vasodilatation. Dryness of mouth and throat, fine tremors of fingers, ataxia, nystagmus, nausea, and vomiting have been noted. Orthostatic hypotension and loss of consciousness occur infrequently. Sleep patterns may be altered.

Psychoactive effects are highly variable and depend on the dose, the route of administration, the personality of the user, his prior experience with the drug, his personal expectations, and the environmental and social setting in which the drug is used. Enhanced perception of colors, sounds, patterns, textures, and taste is common. Mood changes are complex; a sense of increased wellbeing is frequently experienced, although anxiety and depression may be increased by the drug, as well. Drowsiness or hyperactivity and hilarity may occur. Ideas may seem disconnected, rapid-flowing, and associated with altered importance. Time seems to pass slowly, and short-term memory may be impaired. Motor performance is variably impaired, as is reaction time. Although attention can be maintained in certain situations, it is probable that alterations in attention are responsible for some of the reported decrements in performance and cognitive function.

Inexperienced users of cannabis report fewer subjective effects, but demonstrate more decrement in perceptual and psychomotor performance than experienced users. A learning process may be involved in the initial perception of psychoactive effects, although enzymatic induction with more rapid conversion of delta-9-THC to active metabolites is also possible. A varying degree of tolerance develops to some of the psychologic and physiologic effects of the drug. Physical dependence on cannabis does not occur in man.

Adverse Effects. There are no documented reports of human fatalities caused by an overdose of cannabis in any form. Decreased pulmonary function has been reported in chronic users, with an increased incidence of bronchitis, sinusitis, and nose and throat inflammations. Chromosome breakage, in vitro inhibition of cell-mediated immunity, and cerebral atrophy have been reported but not confirmed.

Adverse reactions are generally psychologic in nature, infrequent, and dependent on dose, the personality of the user, and the setting. The most common adverse effects are simple depression, acute panic reactions, and paranoid ideation. These symptoms usually abate in several hours. An acute toxic psychosis, transient in nature, with confusion, auditory and visual hallucinations, and depersonalization, has been reported as occurring infrequently though unpredictably. There is disagreement as to whether cannabis may precipitate a psychotic episode in a stable, well-structured personality. It is agreed that the drug may trigger a prolonged psychotic episode in people with borderline psychologic adjustments. Larger doses are associated with an increase in these reactions, though in a nonlinear way. "Flashback" phenomena similar to those seen with psychedelic use occur rarely.

An amotivational syndrome has been described, in which chronic, heavy users who are psychologically dependent on cannabis demonstrate apathy, diminished goal-directed activity, inability to master new problems, poor social and work adjustment, poor judgment, magical thinking, and multiple drug use. In addition to possible drug effects, sociologic and psychologic characteristics of users may be implicated in this syndrome.

There is no evidence that cannabis use leads to criminal activity. Socially or psychologically predisposed individuals may experiment with other drugs as a result of positive experiences with cannabis.

Treatment. Treatment of the frequently seen depressive and panic reactions should be personal, supportive, and reassuring. The patient must be continually reminded of the drug-induced nature of his difficulty. Tranquilizers are sometimes indicated in violent or aggressive states. Psychotherapy and hospitalization may be indicated in more severe or chronic disorders. The chronic use of marijuana is frequently associated with a subculture that rejects conventional mores and orientation. To be effective, treatment efforts should be sensitive to these value systems.

345. PSYCHEDELICS

Robert B. Millman

The distinguishing characteristics of this class of substances is their ability to reliably produce characteristic alterations in perception, thought, feeling, and behavior. They are among the oldest known psychoactive drugs, often having been used as an adjunct to religious practices in some societies. They are sometimes classified as hallucinogens, psychotogens, or psychotomimetics. In this country, the most frequently abused drugs in this category are related either to the indolealkylamines such as the synthetic *lysergic acid diethylamide (LSD, "acid")*, *psilocybin* ("magic mushrooms"), *psilocin, dimethyltryptamine (DMT)*, and *diethyltryptamine (DET)*, or to the phenylethylamines such as *mescaline*, which is derived from the peyote cactus, and the substituted amphetamines such as 2,5-dimethoxy-4-methylamphetamine *(DOM, "STP")*. *Phencyclidine ("angel dust")*, a drug with anesthetic properties, has been abused for its psychedelic effects. Since the pattern of physiologic and psychologic effects produced by other agents is similar to

that seen with LSD, this discussion will center on LSD. By virtue of their ability to produce bizarre alterations in behavior, some anticholinergic compounds will be considered in this chapter. Their psychoactive effects are distinct from the other psychedelics, and they might better be classified as deliriants.

Incidence and Patterns of Abuse. LSD became available through illicit channels in 1960, and use apparently peaked in the 1967–1968 period, when the new styles of youth culture and its leaders were being popularized by the mass media. Estimates vary from 500,000 to one million users at that time, and have been lower since then. The incidence of other psychedelic drug use parallels that of LSD. The decline may be due to the real and potential dangers of the drug, increasingly severe legal penalties, and changing social patterns.

Use has been primarily among middle-class, white, educated youth in this country who are seeking an enriching, ecstatic, mystical, or transcendental experience. A complex set of metaphysical and religious beliefs and social styles further distinguish the user.

Use is generally intermittent, frequently less than one "trip" monthly, separated by periods in which marijuana is used. Rarely, individuals may take the drug more often ("acid heads"), and some remain in intoxicated states for prolonged periods. Opiate and excessive alcohol use are not often seen in this population, although intermittent amphetamine and hypnotic use are not unusual in the intervening periods. The drug is generally taken in groups so that support is available in the event of a "bad trip." A naive user will frequently be attended by a guide who has previously had the psychedelic experience. As in the case of cannabis, a supportive, safe environment is sought for the experience to minimize the effects of unpleasant reactions.

LSD is generally synthesized in illegal laboratories and made available in a variety of forms, including impregnated paper or sugar cubes, capsules, and tablets. Users are often unaware of the dose they ingest or of whether the preparation is actually LSD or another of the psychedelics.

Pharmacology. LSD is the most potent psychedelic known. It is more than 100 times more potent than psilocybin and 4000 times more potent than mescaline in producing psychologic effects. The usual illicit street dose is probably around 200 μg, but doses as low as 20 μg produce psychologic effects in susceptible individuals. It is generally taken orally, although it has been injected on occasion. Central sympathomimetic stimulation occurs within 20 minutes after ingestion, characterized by mydriasis, hyperthermia, tachycardia, elevated blood pressure, piloerection, increased alertness, and facilitation of monosynaptic reflexes. Nausea and occasionally vomiting occur.

Psychoactive effects are fully evident within one to two hours; these are quite variable from subject to subject and in the same subject under different conditions of dose, mood, expectation, setting, and time. Perceptions are heightened and may become overwhelming. After-images are prolonged and overlap with ongoing perceptions. Objects may seem to move in a wavelike fashion or melt. Illusions and synesthesias, the overflow of one sense modality to another, are common. There may be a sense of unusual clarity, and one's thoughts may assume extraordinary importance. Time may seem to pass very slowly, and body distortions are commonly perceived. True hallucinations with loss of insight may occur in susceptible individuals. Mood is highly variable and labile, and may range from expansive reactions characterized by euphoria and self-confidence to a constricted reaction marked by depression and panic.

The syndrome begins to clear after 10 to 12 hours, and fatigue and tension may persist for an additional 24 hours. The biologic half-life of LSD in man is three hours.

The duration of action of mescaline is about 12 hours, that of psilocybin is four to six hours, that of DOM is six to eight hours, and that of phencyclidine is two to four hours. DMT must be injected or sniffed, and effects last less than two hours.

Tolerance to LSD develops rapidly, repeated daily doses becoming ineffective in three to four days. Recovery is equally rapid, so weekly use of the same dose is possible. Cross-tolerance has been demonstrated between LSD, mescaline, psilocybin, and the amphetamine-based psychedelics, but not between LSD and amphetamine. Physical dependence does not occur with LSD or any of the psychedelic drugs.

Mechanisms of action of LSD are unknown, but may depend on a complex interaction of serotonin and norepinephrine systems in the central nervous system. LSD lowers the threshold for reticular arousal via sensory input and may influence the processes concerned with the filtration and integration of sensory information.

Adverse Effects. Acute physiologic toxicity of the psychedelic drugs is low at doses that produce marked psychologic effects. In man, no deaths directly attributable to the use of these drugs have been reported. Controversy exists as to whether the illicit use of LSD increases the rate of chromosome breakage in users and leads to an increased incidence of congenital defects in children born to parents who had taken this drug. Evidence suggests that pregnant women exposed to illicit LSD had an elevated rate of spontaneous abortions. LSD may inhibit antibody formation and disrupt the body's immune system. Additional study of these adverse effects are necessary, because illicit users of LSD frequently take other drugs and may be malnourished and debilitated.

The acute panic reaction ("bad trip," "freak-out") is the most frequent complication of psychedelic use. These vary in intensity and have led to suicide attempts and accidents on rare occasions. Fear of death or insanity and sensations of breathlessness or paralysis are commonly reported. In most cases, this acute reaction subsides as drug effects are dissipated. Other complications include prolonged psychotic disorders, acute and chronic paranoid reactions, and depressive states. "Flashback" phenomena, the recurrence of some aspect of the drug experience when the individual is not under the influence of the drug, have been reported. The intensity, frequency, and duration of these episodes are quite variable. Adverse psychologic reactions are most frequent in emotionally disturbed individuals in crisis situations or insecure environments, who take the drug in unsupervised settings. High doses of psychedelic drugs lead to an increased incidence of these complications. Whether the psychedelics cause prolonged adverse reactions in emotionally stable people is not clear.

Anticholinergic Compounds. Ingestion of the alkaloids *atropine, hyoscyamine,* and *scopolamine* as they occur in their natural plant forms is reported in other parts of the world, but does not occur in the United States. Use in this country is rare and generally incident to the ac-

cidental or voluntary ingestion of these compounds when they are available in pharmaceutical preparations. Excessive use of *antihistaminic* compounds with anticholinergic effects also occurs. Symptoms of the potent peripheral effects of intoxication with these drugs include dilated, fixed pupils, dry skin and mouth, flushing, hyperthermia, and tachycardia. Psychoactive effects are those of an acute toxic psychosis, with clouding of consciousness, delirium, and loss of memory for the period of intoxication. Vivid sensory phenomena are not prominent, although hallucinations may occur.

Treatment. Treatment of the acute panic reaction may usually be accomplished by ensuring a warm, supportive environment with someone in constant attendance and with a minimum of other external stimuli. The user should be reminded continually that the effects he is experiencing are due to the drug and will pass in time. In particularly agitated patients, phenothiazines or diazepam orally or intramuscularly may be used. In the event of precipitation of prolonged psychosis, hospitalization with supportive care may be required. Flashbacks are treated with reassurance and/or psychotherapy when these are severe. In general, the duration and severity of these decrease with time if psychedelic drug use ceases.

Treatment of anticholinergic poisoning is symptomatic and consists of protecting the patient from self-injury, providing fluids, and reducing the fever. Administration of cholinesterase inhibitors is not indicated.

346. MISCELLANEOUS INHALANTS

Robert B. Millman

Nitrous Oxide. Recreational inhalation of nitrous oxide alone or in combination with oxygen is a rarely reported phenomenon that occurs in some youthful populations. Psychoactive effects occur in 15 to 30 seconds and persist for less than five minutes. The experience is described as one of intoxication, euphoria, and hilarity. Adverse effects have not been reported.

Organic Solvents. The inhalation of a wide range of organic solvents, particularly the toluene in glue, has received a good deal of attention from the mass media and law-enforcement agencies. It is likely that this publicity has contributed significantly to the incidence of this practice in the adolescent and preadolescent population. The material is usually squeezed into a plastic bag and the vapors inhaled. Prolonged exposure, as in the case of industrial workers, may have serious adverse effects on a variety of organ systems. As used recreationally, these solvents produce intoxication and dizziness not unlike that experienced with alcohol. Few side effects have been reported, although suffocation caused by the plastic bag has apparently occurred. The inhalation of aerosol sprays containing fluorocarbon propellants has recently been reported. Acute toxicity has not yet been adequately evaluated, although cardiac arrhythmias are considered to be a potentially serious complication.

Amyl Nitrite. Amyl nitrite ("amies," "poppers") inhalation has been reported in the youthful drug-abusing population. Use is intermittent and characterized by an instantaneous feeling ("rush") of dizziness, hilarity, and activity. Effects persist for minutes. Adverse effects include palpitations, postural hypotension occasionally proceeding to loss of consciousness, and headache. Chronic use is extremely rare, and more severe adverse effects have not been reported.

Brecher, E. M., and the Editors of Consumer Reports: Licit and Illicit Drugs. The Consumers Union Report on Narcotics, Stimulants, Depressants, Inhalants, Hallucinogens, and Marijuana, Including Caffeine, Nicotine and Alcohol. Mount Vernon, New York, Consumers Union, 1972.

Cherubin, C. E.: A review of the medical complications of narcotic addiction. Int. J. Addict, 3:167, 1968.

Dishotsky, N. I., Loughman, W. D., Mogar, R. E., and Lipscomb, W. R.: LSD and genetic damage. Science, 172:431, 1971.

Dole, V. P.: Narcotic addiction, physical dependence and relapse. N. Engl. J. Med., 206:988, 1972.

Dole, V. P., and Nyswander, M.: A medical treatment for diacetylmorphine (heroin) addiction. J.A.M.A., 193:646, 1965.

Isbell, H., Altschul, S., Kornetsky, C. H., et al.: Chronic barbiturate intoxication. An experimental study. Arch. Neurol. Psychiat., 64:1, 1950.

Jaffe, J.: Narcotic analgesics and drug addiction and drug abuse. In Goodman, L. S., and Gilman, A. (eds.): The Pharmacological Basis of Therapeutics, Fourth Edition. New York, The Macmillan Company, 1970, p. 237.

Kalant, H., LeBlanc, A. E., and Gibbins, R. J.: Tolerance to, and dependence on, some nonopiate psychotropic drugs. Pharmacol. Rev., 23:135, 1971.

Kreek, M. J.: Medical safety and side effects of methadone in tolerant individuals. J.A.M.A., 223:665, 1973.

Oakley, S. R.: Drugs, Society and Human Behavior. St. Louis, Mo., C. V. Mosby Company, 1972.

Snyder, S. H.: Catecholamines in the brain as mediators of amphetamine psychosis. Arch. Gen. Psychiatry, 27:169, 1972.

347. ALCOHOL ABUSE AND ALCOHOL-RELATED ILLNESS

Jack H. Mendelson

Definition. The most widely accepted operational definition of alcohol abuse is excessive drinking which adversely affects an individual's health, impairs social function, or both. Although it is not difficult to assess the impact of alcohol abuse on biologic function, it is often impossible to quantify alcohol-related social impairment. Experts disagree about both the type and the severity of problem drinking which cause social dysfunction because of wide variations in societal norms for characterizing deviant drinking behavior. Attempts to establish criteria for normative drinking behavior based upon volume and consumption frequency indices have not been satisfactory because of conflicting social, cultural, religious, and even political perceptions of how individuals in various societies may consume alcohol.

The frequently used term "alcoholism" is ambiguous. "Alcoholism" is often not synonymous with alcohol abuse, but denotes a series of problems ranging from deviant drinking behavior (as defined by the society in which it occurs) to alcohol addiction. Some of the phenomena which are reported to occur during the progression of *alcohol abuse* to *alcohol addiction* include excessive drinking in normal social situations; drinking in isolation; drinking to reduce anxiety, apprehension, or anger; drinking to facilitate the induction of sleep during conditions of insomnia; early morning drinking; and alterations in memory function (blackout) during heavy

episodic alcohol intake. All or none of these phenomena may be reported by individuals who demonstrate evidence of addiction to alcohol, and no specific pattern of events is pathognomonic of behavior attributes for transition of alcohol abuse to alcohol addiction.

Addiction to alcohol is characterized by both tolerance and physical dependence. Tolerance occurs when an individual consumes progressively larger quantities of alcohol over a period of time in order to induce changes in feeling states or behavior which previously were induced by smaller doses of alcohol. Physical dependence occurs when an individual develops subjective discomfort and/or overt withdrawal signs after partial or complete cessation of drinking. It is important to emphasize that withdrawal signs and symptoms may occur in alcohol addicts when they reduce drinking but do not completely cease all alcohol intake. Relatively small decrements in sustained high blood alcohol levels may be associated with precipitation of the withdrawal syndrome.

As with most behavior disorders, it is often impossible to establish a precise definition of clinical status, e.g., alcohol abuse versus alcohol addiction. The physician must make a judgment about the presence and severity of an alcohol-related problem on the basis of careful determination of physical and mental status, occupational performance, social interaction, and—not least important—the patient's own perception of how alcohol consumption enhances or compromises his or her health and well-being.

Etiology. No specific biologic, psychologic, or social variable has been shown to have high predictive value for determining which individuals are at high risk to develop and sustain problem drinking behavior. There are no known psychologic tests which can reliably differentiate alcohol abusers from normal drinkers. Many theories have purported to explain the causation of alcoholism in terms of psychodynamic factors, personality profiles, psychosocial developmental and growth characteristics, nutritional idiosyncrasies, allergic disorders, and specific and nonspecific metabolic derangements. To date, none of these theories of the causation of alcohol abuse or alcohol addiction have significant support from well-controlled laboratory and clinical investigations.

The contribution of specific genetic and environmental factors which may enhance the risk for development of alcohol-related problems has not been clarified. Many patients who develop alcohol-related problems have no family history of alcohol abuse or alcohol addiction. But it is also known that individuals with a family history of alcohol abuse, particularly those who report that both parents had alcohol problems, may be at very great risk for developing alcohol abuse themselves. It is likely that this enhanced risk occurs, in part, as a function of growing up in an environment where excessive drinking is employed for coping with or modifying social stress. Moreover, there are recent data which indicate that a genetic component may be associated with the causation of alcohol problems. Studies of adoptees in Denmark have demonstrated that these individuals are more likely to develop alcohol problems if their biologic parents were alcohol abusers than if the adopted parent had abused alcohol. Thus at present it appears reasonable to conclude that both genetic and developmental factors may contribute to the genesis of alcohol-related illness.

Incidence and Prevalence. Surveys of American drinking practices reveal that approximately two thirds of the adult population of the United States use alcohol at least occasionally. It is estimated that about 12 per cent of the American population are heavy drinkers, i.e., individuals who drink almost daily or who once a week consume five or more drinks per occasion. It is obvious that this definition of heavy drinking may be associated with a number of ambiguities, and it is difficult to rate relative degree of drinking (heavy versus light) from self-written reports about the volume and frequency of alcohol consumed. Thus, individuals may consume the same quantity of alcohol during a given interval of time, but variations in the spacing or the concentrating of the drinking may indicate vastly different drinking patterns. For example, alcohol addicts who are spree drinkers may consume enormous amounts of alcohol in a two or three day interval during a month and remain relatively abstinent the remainder of the time.

A recent survey of American drinking practices and problems revealed that the largest population of problem drinkers were city-dwellers of low socioeconomic status. The highest rates of alcohol-related problems were found in young (under 25) urban men; the number of heavy drinkers among white and black males was similar (22 and 19 per cent, respectively). However, black women reported a significantly higher rate of drinking (11 per cent) than white women (4 per cent). American Indians and Eskimos have high reported rates of alcohol abuse and addiction.

Repeated surveys have shown that alcohol problems can be found in anyone who drinks alcohol to excess and that individual variations obliterate the significance of any group, ethnic, or cultural qualities. Case finding in alcoholism is difficult because of the stigma associated with the disorder. However, most agree that alcoholism represents the major drug problem in America today. It has been estimated that about 5 million adults in the United States have significant alcohol-related problems. It is also estimated that an additional 4 million abuse alcohol to the extent that they are at high risk for the development of alcohol addiction. These figures imply that 7 per cent of the adult population have a significant alcohol-related problem.

Pharmacologic Aspects. After the consumption of alcohol, absorption occurs primarily from the small intestine, but gastric emptying and the rate of absorption from the intestine are influenced by a number of factors. The rate of absorption is accelerated with increasing concentrations of alcohol up to a maximum of 40 per cent. Concentrations of ingested alcohol above 40 per cent may be absorbed more slowly as a consequence of delayed gastric emptying. Similarly, high concentrations of congeners in beverage alcohol delay absorption because they impede gastric emptying by inducing pyloric spasm. The ingestion of food along with beverage alcohol also reduces the speed of absorption by delaying the emptying time of the stomach.

After absorption, ethanol is distributed to all portions of the body and achieves equilibrium with body water compartments. Since ethanol is more soluble in lipid fractions, ethanol concentration in body tissues is greatest in those organs and cells containing high concentrations of lipids. No impermeable or semipermeable membranes impede the diffusion of alcohol into any body organ or tissue.

Alcohol is removed from the body primarily by metabolism in the liver, and only 2 to 10 per cent is excreted directly by the kidneys and the lungs. Alcohol is catabolized in the liver by well-known enzymatic mechanisms involving the enzyme alcohol dehydrogenase and the cofactor NAD. The rate of alcohol metabolism in normal drinkers and in abstinent alcohol addicts is not significantly different. However, the rate of ethanol metabolism may increase in alcohol addicts during the course of spree drinking, and it is believed that this increase is due to an ethanol-induced increase in rate of hepatic metabolism.

There are no known pharmacologic agents which may be utilized in clinical practice to enhance the rate of ethanol catabolism in man. Although it has been shown that high dosage administration of fructose may accelerate rates of ethanol metabolism, the clinical use of this is impractical.

Blood alcohol levels depend upon the amount of alcohol ingested and the weight of the individual. For the average man, it has been estimated that the consumption of 180 ml of distilled spirits on an empty stomach will produce a blood alcohol level of approximately 100 mg per 100 ml. Values around 180 mg per 100 ml have been established by most jurisdictions as the legal limit of sobriety for operating a motor vehicle. Blood alcohol levels achieved in usual social drinking situations average about 50 to 75 mg per 100 ml. At this blood level a subjective state of pleasant tranquility and a mild degree of sedation may occur. Overt signs of intoxication usually occur in social (nontolerant) drinkers between 100 and 200 mg per 100 ml. Severe intoxication is observed in social drinkers at levels above 200 mg per 100 ml, but alcohol addicts who are tolerant to the effects of ethanol may appear relatively intact and nonintoxicated with such blood alcohol levels. Regardless of the degree of tolerance, blood alcohol levels above 400 mg per 100 ml produce stupor and/or coma, and concentrations above 500 mg per 100 ml are frequently fatal.

Alcohol and Behavior. *Acute Intoxication.* Although the concomitants of acute intoxication are well known and easily recognized (dysarthria, ataxia, and emotional lability), there is no simple correlation between the volume of alcohol consumed and an individual's ability to carry out cognitive and motor tasks successfully. Indeed, some individuals actually show improved performance on perceptual and psychomotor tasks with low to moderate doses of alcohol. This paradox obtains because small to moderate doses of ethanol may act in a manner similar to a minor tranquilizer, i.e., to reduce anxiety which may affect skill and performance. Individuals who demonstrate little impairment in performance of cognitive and motor tasks with high blood ethanol concentrations (150 to 200 mg per 100 ml) have probably developed tolerance for alcohol as a consequence of recurrent heavy drinking.

Moderate dosage of alcohol usually impairs visual-motor coordination in most social drinkers. In particular, brightness discrimination and visual adaptation after exposure to bright lights is often markedly reduced. Auditory and tactile sensation are usually unchanged. The integration and evaluation of sensory information, rather than the impairment of sensory input itself, are most severely compromised during acute intoxication. An individual's ability to initiate or maintain sustained attention to stimuli and to judge the qualities of stimuli is usually significantly diminished after moderate alcohol intake. Individuals under such conditions tend to underestimate the speed and distance of objects as well as to show impairment in making judgments regarding the passage of time.

Impairments of behavior associated with acute intoxication are also determined by factors related to the setting. If a person consumes alcohol in a situation in which drunkenness is both expected and tolerated, this anticipation may influence his behavior more than the dosage of alcohol ingested. Similarly, individuals who fear the consequences of intoxicated behavior may successfully mask the manifestations of acute inebriation even though they consume relatively large amounts of alcohol.

Alcohol, Aggression, and Accidents. Although it is well known that alcohol ingestion and acute intoxication are significant factors in accidents, the causal significance of alcohol ingestion per se is not a simple one. Alcohol intoxication may effect a number of patterns of behavior which combine to produce enhanced risk for an accident. These include compromised judgment, enhanced emotional lability, and inability to suppress expression of aggression. Acute alcohol intoxication also contributes to situations which result in death and injury as a function of violence and aggressive behavior. Homicide, armed robbery with aggravated assault, and other crimes of violence are frequent in perpetrators or victims who are acutely intoxicated.

Acute alcohol intoxication has been frequently implicated in fatal accidents. For example, over half of the nonhighway accident fatalities involve alcohol addicts or abusers. A recent survey carried out in a general hospital emergency room in which blood alcohol values were determined in accident victims showed that 30 per cent of the individuals involved in highway accidents, 22 per cent involved in home accidents, and 16 per cent involved in occupational accidents had elevated blood ethanol levels.

Alcohol abuse is a significant contributing factor to over 50 per cent of motor vehicle fatalities, and it has been estimated that 28,000 highway deaths during a recent 12-month period were associated with alcohol intoxication. There is increasing evidence, however, that alcohol-related automobile fatalities may not be simply associated with episodic acute intoxication in social drinkers, but rather are phenomena related to chronic intoxication and alcohol addiction. Statistics obtained from studies of blood alcohol levels in individuals involved in single vehicle fatalities indicate that a majority had blood ethanol values above 150 mg per 100 ml. Such high blood levels suggest that the accident victims were not social drinkers but alcohol addicts. Thus it is possible that the preponderance of motor vehicle accidents and deaths in which alcohol is implicated is associated with addiction to alcohol, as defined in pharmacologic terms, and is not a consequence of occasional intemperate drinking.

Alcohol and Sexual Function. The effect of acute intoxication on sexual behavior and function is poorly understood. The classic reference is Shakespeare's perception that intoxication increases desire but impairs sexual performance. Although the effects of acute alcohol intoxication on sexual behavior in moderate drinkers may be quite idiosyncratic, by contrast, sexual function and behavior are often markedly impaired in alcohol addicts. Male alcohol addicts often report sexual impotence and diminished heterosexual desire. A tendency to initiate or increase alcohol intake has been reported by female alcoholics during premenstrual periods. Gynecomastia and testicular atrophy have been reported in male alcohol addicts, particularly those who also show evidence of alcohol-related liver disease. Recent studies have demonstrated that alcohol administration to alcohol addicts is associated with suppression of plasma testosterone levels.

The "Hangover." A well-known consequence of acute alcohol intoxication is a syndrome of generalized somatic discomfort, headache, nausea, agitation, and mild tremulousness which has been termed the "hangover." The physiologic mechanisms related to the hangover have not been determined. Current evidence indicates that the hangover may be the equivalent of a mild withdrawal syndrome. There is no evidence that any specific characteristic of beverage alcohol, such as its congener content, or any unique pattern of drinking, such as mixing different beverages, is the causal basis for the hangover. No specific form of pharmacotherapy is available for treatment of the problem, and there is little evidence that the plethora of popular remedies have any efficacy.

Addiction to Alcohol. Addiction to alcohol is characterized by the presence of both tolerance and physical dependence. Although many individuals may frequently abuse alcohol, not all become physically dependent. Moreover, it is difficult to predict addiction liability on the basis of dosage of alcohol and frequency of consumption alone. There is no question, however, that physical dependence on alcohol is analogous to physical dependence induced by a number of other centrally acting drugs and is not caused by intercurrent illness, vitamin, or nutritional disorders. Withdrawal signs and symptoms have been observed in otherwise healthy alcohol addicts exclusively as a concomitant of cessation of drinking. Physical dependence has also been induced in a number of species of laboratory animals without producing derangements in nutritional or metabolic function.

Tolerance appears to develop more rapidly than physical dependence for alcohol and other drugs which affect the central nervous system (i.e., narcotics, barbiturates, and psychotropic drugs). Three forms of tolerance may be observed in the alcohol addict: behavioral tolerance, pharmacologic tolerance, and cross-tolerance to certain other drugs which have their primary effect on central nervous function.

Behavioral tolerance is manifest when the alcohol addict can consume relatively large amounts of ethanol without impairment in social behavior or psychomotor coordination. It has been observed clinically and demonstrated in research ward studies that some alcohol addicts can consume as much as 1 quart of beverage alcohol per day without evidence of gross intoxication. It has also been shown that many alcohol addicts can perform relatively complex tasks without error when their blood alcohol levels are twice the legal limit of intoxication for many state jurisdictions.

Pharmacologic tolerance reflects a metabolic adaptive change in the alcohol addict as a consequence of long-term drinking. Evidence of pharmacologic tolerance was originally inferred from the finding of low blood alcohol levels in alcohol addicts who had consumed large amounts of alcohol (up to 1 quart of bourbon per day for 20 consecutive days). Subsequent studies demonstrated an enhanced rate of ethanol metabolism in alcohol addicts during protracted episodes of drinking. The pharmacokinetics of alcohol-induced enhancement of ethanol metabolism have not been clarified, but they appear not to persist after long periods of sobriety. Pharmacologic tolerance may contribute to some small aspect of behavioral tolerance, but adaptive processes in the central nervous system are probably far more important for behavioral tolerance than alcohol-induced enhancement in rates of ethanol metabolism.

Clinical reports have stressed that alcohol addicts may show reduced sensitivity and responsivity to a number of other drugs: *cross-tolerance*. There are reports that alcohol addicts require significantly higher doses of both the barbiturate and volatile anesthetics for induction and maintenance of appropriate levels of surgical anesthesia. Alcohol addicts frequently show cross-tolerance for barbiturates, hypnotics, and psychotropic agents such as the minor tranquilizers. However, cross-tolerance and cross-dependence have not been demonstrated between alcohol and the opiates. It is important to point out that cross-tolerance occurs in alcohol addicts when they are temporarily abstaining from drinking. When alcohol addicts are intoxicated, both synergism and potentiation with narcotics, opiates and analgesics, barbiturates, and a variety of other psychotropic agents may occur. In fact, there is some evidence which indicates that the consumption of drugs such as barbiturates during heavy alcohol intake is associated with a decreased catabolic degradation of both agents.

Although tolerance for ethanol may appear to be very great for some alcohol addicts, the degree of tolerance which can be developed for ethanol is much smaller than that which can potentially occur in opiate or barbiturate addiction. Barbiturate addicts may ingest as much as 2 grams of secobarbital or pentobarbital daily without gross impairments of behavior. Heroin addicts may eventually employ a dosage 50 times larger than their initial intake. On the other hand, blood alcohol levels exceeding 450 mg per 100 ml for any drinker, social or addicted, are rarely observed, because this level is almost invariably associated with a comatose state. Moreover, the lethal level of 500 to 600 mg per 100 ml is no different for alcohol addicts as opposed to normal drinkers, because such blood alcohol levels cause severe and often irreversible respiratory depression.

Physical dependence upon alcohol is characterized by the appearance of withdrawal signs and symptoms after cessation of drinking. Tremulousness, delirium, and seizure disorders were first reported by Hippocrates to accompany alcohol abuse, and detailed descriptions of the abstinence syndrome are reported in the medical literature of the late eighteenth century. Systematic studies by Victor and Adams in 1953 are the basis for the classification of the withdrawal syndromes currently identified in clinical practice. Three types of withdrawal states have been differentiated: tremulous states, seizure disorders, and delirium tremens.

Tremulousness is the most frequent and benign type of abstinence syndrome. Although the onset of tremulousness usually occurs 12 to 48 hours after reduction of alcohol intake or initiation of abstinence, this sign may be observed as early as six hours after cessation of drinking. Tremor is usually mild with involvement of the hands, but in some instances it may be generalized with involvement of all extremities as well as the tongue and trunk. Tremor may be increased when the patient extends the arms with the palms upright and the fingers separated. Tremulousness usually remits or is significantly diminished by 72 hours after cessation of drinking, but in rare instances it may persist for five days.

Hallucinosis may be associated with a tremulous state or may occur independent of tremor. Hallucinations also may occur in alcohol addicts during conditions of severe intoxication as well as during conditions of complete or partial cessation of drinking.

Seizure disorders usually occur 12 to 24 hours after cessation of drinking. Seizures may be associated with tremulousness, but may be present without any other evidence of withdrawal signs. The seizure disorder is of the grand mal type, usually not preceded by auras but almost always followed by a postictal state. Seizures may be observed in patients who have no overt evidence of a neurologic disorder and who have no abnormalities of the electroencephalogram. Victor and Adams have emphasized that approximately one third of all patients who have seizure disorders after cessation of drinking progress to develop delirium tremens.

Delirium tremens is the rarest form of the alcohol withdrawal syndrome. Delirium tremens is characterized by confusion, disorientation, delusions, hallucinations, psychomotor agitation, and autonomic dysfunction. The peak incidence of this syndrome is 72 to 96 hours after cessation of drinking. The severe confusional states and delirium which are the hallmark of delirium tremens are rarely observed in the more frequent instances of tremulousness after cessation of drinking. Patients who develop delirium tremens also often have profuse sweating, tachycardia, hypertension, and fever. Delirium tremens is a potentially lethal illness which requires hospitalization and intensive medical care.

Although the basic mechanisms underlying the alcohol withdrawal syndrome remain to be determined, a number of associated disorders affect the severity of the disorder. Significant disturbances in acid-base, water, and electrolyte homeostasis may be associated with the abstinence syndrome. After cessation of alcohol intake, many alcohol addicts develop episodic hyperventilation which may produce respiratory alkalosis and elevations in blood pH. This condition is usually associated with hypomagnesemia. The low serum magnesium levels observed in alcohol addicts during the withdrawal syndrome are probably caused both by poor dietary intake of magnesium during heavy drinking and by magnesium shifts from the intravascular to the intracellular fluid compartments associated with the pH shift of respiratory alkalosis. It is also important to remember that alcohol addicts who develop withdrawal syndromes may be not dehydrated, but in fact, overhydrated.

Intercurrent Illness and Associated Disorders. Alcohol addicts are at high risk for developing a number of disorders which are observed frequently in general medical practice. These are discussed individually in other chapters of this text, but a few merit mention here.

Alcohol-related hepatic disease is a leading cause of morbidity and mortality in adult males. It has been demonstrated that alcohol intake alone without concomitant nutritional deficiency may induce hepatic disorders such as fatty metamorphosis, alcoholic hepatitis, and Laennec's cirrhosis (see Ch. 709). However, since many people consume large quantities of alcohol without developing these disorders, the crucial determinants of the interrelationships between heavy alcohol consumption and hepatic disease remain to be determined. Gastritis and pancreatitis (see Ch. 640 and Ch. 645 and 646) are also frequently in those who abuse alcohol. A variety of malabsorption syndromes may be associated with heavy alcohol intake (see Part XIV, Section Three).

The most severe neurologic disorders seen in alcohol

addicts are peripheral neuropathies (see Ch. 456 to 474) which are characterized by motor and sensory impairments in the upper and lower extremities. Pain, paresthesia, motor weakness, and paralysis may occur as a consequence of poor dietary intake in conjunction with heavy ethanol intake.

Diseases of the central nervous system may also be associated with chronic alcohol abuse. Wernicke's disease and Korsakoff's psychosis (see Ch. 406) are characterized by derangements of memory function and disorders of thought processes. The genesis of many "organic brain diseases," which at present constitute the majority of first admissions to state mental hospitals, may be related to nutritional and metabolic derangements associated with alcohol abuse.

There is accumulating evidence that alcohol abuse may be a factor in the development of coronary artery disease. Individuals who have a familial Type IV hyperlipidemia (see Ch. 817) are at high risk for developing elevations in blood triglyceride levels with even moderate alcohol intake. A number of cardiomyopathies have been found in alcohol addicts. Finally, it has been shown that chronic alcohol abuse may cause derangements in hematopoiesis, produce muscle wasting, and suppress immune mechanisms with consequence of higher risk for infection.

Affective Disorders and Psychosis. Some individuals with neurotic and psychotic affective disorders drink excessively, but many others with severe depression never abuse alcohol. In manic-depressive illness patients are more prone to drink excessively during the manic phase of their disorder than when they are depressed. There is also evidence to indicate that chronic alcohol abuse enhances rather than reduces feelings of depression.

Approximately 25 per cent of all suicide victims have detectable amounts of alcohol in body fluids on necropsy examination. It is estimated that one third of all suicides are associated with chronic alcohol abuse, but these findings may relate mainly to white middle-aged males. Suicide rates for black males over 35 are low, even though drinking problems may be high.

Treatment and Prevention. Although there are occasional reports of children who die of respiratory failure associated with ethanol overdosage, death from *acute ethanol poisoning* is rare. Rapid ingestion of large amounts of ethanol ususally induces vomiting. Those who consume large amounts of ethanol slowly usually become stuporous before they can ingest a dose necessary to produce significant respiratory depression. The rate of ethanol catabolism in man ranges from 15 to 22 mg per 100 ml per hour, and there are no clinically useful or efficacious methods for rapidly decreasing blood alcohol levels.

Acute ethanol intoxication may be complicated by concurrent intoxication with other centrally acting drugs. There appears to be an increasing degree of polydrug abuse in the United States, particularly drugs which act synergistically with or potentiate the actions of ethanol. Alcohol abusers also frequently abuse barbiturates and minor tranquilizers. The most commonly reported form of drug abuse in narcotic addicts maintained on methadone is with alcohol. In hospital practice it is advisable to obtain blood determinations for other possible central nervous system depressants when a severe depression of consciousness is noted in patients who appear only to be intoxicated with ethanol.

Many persons who seek a physician's aid during conditions of acute ethanol intoxication have other medical disorders. These patients should receive the most careful physical examination and diagnostic workup. Most states have adopted legislation requiring that patients with alcohol-related illness, including acute intoxication, should not be denied admission to hospitals and medical facilities. In addition, the American Medical Association and the American Hospital Association have endorsed resolutions against discriminatory policies for patients with alcohol-related problems who seek admission to general medical facilities. Some patients may request hospital treatment for detoxification after chronic alcohol intake when there is no evidence of any significant intercurrent illness. If the patient's motivation for receiving medical assistance appears good, the physician should attempt to provide the best available hospital care. However, involuntary commitment of patients with alcohol problems is not legal in most jurisdictions if hospitalization is initiated only on the basis of a diagnosis of alcoholism without evidence of a serious psychotic disorder.

Treatment of the *alcohol withdrawal syndrome* has improved significantly during the past decade. Less than 15 years ago many hospitals reported a 15 per cent mortality in patients with delirium tremens. The current mortality rate associated with delirium tremens is less than 1 per cent. The major factor affecting reduction in both mortality and morbidity is the application of good general medical care. Patients requiring treatment for the withdrawal syndrome should have the following procedures carried out on a systematic basis: (1) a careful physical and roentgenologic examination to identify any traumatic injuries (especially trauma to the skull); (2) a search for infection of the pulmonary and genitourinary systems; (3) a search for hepatic, gastrointestinal, and cardiac disorders; and (4) an evaluation of the state of hydration, electrolyte, and acid-base status, with appropriate measures instituted to correct any derangements. It should not be assumed that patients exhibiting the withdrawal syndrome are dehydrated or have any particular derangement in electrolyte or acid-base balance status unless demonstrated by appropriate clinical and laboratory examinations.

Chlordiazepoxide is the best drug for reducing psychomotor agitation in patients who have withdrawal syndromes, provided the agent is used judiciously. In general, the dosage employed should permit reduction of tremor and anxiety without compromising the patient's ability to tolerate fluid and foods orally. Patients exhibiting the withdrawal syndrome should not be sedated deeply simply to produce long periods of sleep. Whenever possible, medication should be given orally, although at the initial stages of the withdrawal syndrome it may be necessary to use the intramuscular route. The routine use of corticosteroids is contraindicated, and the efficacy of diphenylhydantoin (Dilantin) in controlling seizure disorders is questionable. Administration of multivitamins orally or intravenously should be based upon judgment of the patient's nutritional status.

The *treatment of chronic alcohol abuse* is often difficult because most patients with alcohol-related problems tend to deny the severity of their illness and to avoid or reject assistance by physicians and other health care professionals. It has been postulated that the patient's acceptance of treatment can be greatly improved if initial contacts with the physician and the hospital are sympathetic and positive. The point has often been made that treatment for the alcohol abuser and alcohol addict should have limited goals and that alcohol-related illness should be considered as a chronic disease analogous, in some ways, to chronic pulmonary and cardiac conditions. For the most part, physicians treating such illnesses strive to alleviate suffering and to induce compensation rather than achieve absolute cure. A reasonable treatment goal is to restore physical and behavioral status after decompensation in alcohol abusers, even if recidivism is expected. Multimodality therapy suited to the needs of the individual and his resources should be offered. However, the question of which treatment will maximally benefit the patient with alcohol problems remains unanswered.

At present there is no uniformly effective, specific treatment for alcohol abuse. A number of treatment techniques have been employed singly or in combinations which have proved effective for some patients. These include individual and group psychotherapy, Antabuse therapy, referral to self-help groups such as Alcoholics Anonymous, and a number of behavioral modification techniques. It is discouraging that the few relatively well controlled therapy evaluation studies have demonstrated a low rate of alcohol abstinence after therapy. But since these evaluations were carried out in specialized clinic treatment settings, it remains likely that the individual counseling and relationship offered by the family physician will offer a greater degree of success.

The spontaneous recovery rate for alcohol abusers has been estimated to be about 20 per cent over a three-year period. Thus physicians should not assume that alcohol-related disorders are intractable. Since all variants of alcohol abuse are multiply determined, alcohol problems present the treatment challenge of any complex behavioral disorder. Although there is no evidence to indicate that alcohol abuse is invariably associated with a predisposing psychiatric illness, the development of problem drinking rarely occurs in isolation from emotional, interpersonal, and job-related problems.

The physician should employ a multifaceted program of treatment which can be best determined from assessing the patient's motivation, resources, and ability to sustain treatment relationships. For some individuals, self-help groups such as Alcoholics Anonymous may be useful, but one must first explore whether any given patient can effectively utilize this form of assistance. The physician should familiarize himself with all available resources which exist in the patient's community for assistance with alcohol-related problems. It is often essential that the physician involve other members of the family in cooperating with some form of treatment program.

Adequate techniques for *prevention of alcohol-related disorders* have yet to be devised. Although significant emphasis has been placed upon public education and information concerning the responsible use of alcohol, the impact of such programs is difficult to evaluate. Since there are relatively poor incidence and prevalence data for alcohol abuse, it is impossible to argue that public education programs or attempts to shape attitudes have had any impact on alcohol abuse and alcohol addiction. Increased programs of public education and information may appear logical, but it should be remembered that problem drinking usually occurs in situations in which behavior is not determined by logical thinking but rather by internal and external stresses which are not highly amenable to rational persuasion.

Cahalan, D.: Problem Drinkers. San Francisco, Jossey-Bass, Inc., 1970.
Kalant, H.: Absorption, diffusion, distribution and elimination of ethanol: Effects on biological membranes. *In* Kissin, B., and Begleiter, H. (eds.): The Biology of Alcoholism, Vol. 1. New York, Plenum Press, 1971.
Mello, N. K.: Behavioral studies of alcoholism. *In* Kissin, B., and Begleiter, H. (eds.): The Biology of Alcoholism, Vol. 2. New York, Plenum Press, 1972.
Mendelson, J. H., and Mello, N. K.: Alcohol, aggression and androgens. Proc. Assn. Res. Nerv. Ment. Dis., 1974, in press.
Wolfe, S., and Victor, M.: The physiological basis of the alcohol withdrawal syndrome. *In* Mello, N. K., and Mendelson, J. H. (eds.): Recent Advances in Studies of Alcoholism. Washington, D. C., U. S. Government Printing Office, Publ. No. (HSM) 71–9045, 1971.

348.   ACUTE DRUG POISONING

Fred Plum

Accidental or intentional drug overdose has become a common medical problem which almost any physician may be called upon to treat. Suicide ranks high as a cause of death among all age groups beyond early adolescence, and its incidence climbs steadily with age in single white males. Furthermore, psychologically engendered drug abuse plagues many countries, with fatal or near-fatal "accidents" often affecting youngsters of secondary school age as well as adults. No social stratum enjoys immunity. The physician's job is made harder by the fact that the mentally unbalanced or those just seeking new sensations have an ever-expanding roster of pharmaceutical or industrial chemicals to draw from. Nevertheless, changing fashions affect the minority, and the most frequent agents causing drug poisonings will undoubtedly continue to resemble those listed in Table 1.

Table 2 lists the most common drug poisonings presently encountered in the United States, gives their principal signs of toxicity, and outlines their treatment. Clinical appraisal still must be used to diagnose the agent causing several of these reaction patterns, specific chemical tests being either unavailable or impractical. Blood levels or size of the dose are generally unreliable guides to the potential danger with almost any of the drugs listed because tolerance develops to their chronic ingestion, making individuals react differently to similar doses. Also, the mixing of drugs with each other and with alcohol adds to the unreliability of blood levels as a guide to treatment or prognosis of the drugs listed in Table 2. Only the opiates and the sedatives create any appreciable risk of death. Opiate poisoning is discussed in more detail in Ch. 348. The rest of this chapter gives details of the management of sedative drug overdose. For the diagnosis and treatment of suspected drug or chemical poisonings not covered in these pages, physicians should consult the *Physicians' Desk Reference* or the Poison Control Center of a large city.

TABLE 1.   Drugs Used, in Order of Frequency, Among Severe Overdose Subjects, New York Hospital, 1969–1973

Alcohol	Lithium
Barbiturates, glutethimide	Salicylates
Heroin or methadone	Phenothiazines
Methaqualone	Diphenylhydantoin
Meprobamate	Bishydroxycoumarin, Coumadin
Scopolamine	Tolbutamide, phenformin
Amphetamine	Insulin
Imipramine	

TABLE 2.   Common Drug Poisonings, Signs of Toxicity, and Treatment

Drug	Mild Toxic Signs	Tissue for Diagnosis	Treatment	Severe Overdose Signs	Treatment
Opiates: Heroin Morphine Demerol Methadone	"Nodding" drowsiness, small pupils, urinary retention, slow and shallow breathing; skin scars and subcutaneous abscesses; duration 4–6 hrs; with methadone, duration to 24 hrs	Urine	Levallorphan 1 mg iv, nalorphine 10 mg iv, naloxine 0.4 mg iv or im; repeat at 15-min intervals not more than twice; repeat in 3 hrs if necessary	Coma; pinpoint pupils, slow irregular respiration or apnea, hypotension, hypothermia, pulmonary edema	Levallorphan, nalorphine, naloxine; if no response by second dose, suspect another cause; treat shock; find and detect infection
Depressants: Alcohol Barbiturates Glutethimide (Doriden) Meprobamate (Equanil) Methaqualone (Quaalude, Sopor, Mandrax) Chlordiazepoxide (Librium) Diazepam (Valium)	Confusion, rousable drowsiness, delirium, ataxia, nystagmus, dysarthria, analgesia to stimuli Hallucinations, agitation, motor hyperactivity, myoclonus, tonic spasms Usually taken with another sedative if poisoning the attempt	Blood, urine, breath Blood Blood Blood Blood Blood	Alcohol excitement: diazepam or chlorpromazine None needed for acute toxicity; withdraw drug under supervision if patient is a chronic user	Stupor to coma; pupils reactive, usually constricted; oculovestibular response absent; motor tonus initially briefly hyperactive, then flaccid; respiration and blood pressure depressed; hypothermia; with glutethimide, pupils moderately dilated, can be fixed; with meprobamate, withdrawal seizures common; with methaqualone, coma, occasional convulsions, tachycardia, cardiac failure, bleeding tendency	Intubate, ventilate, gavage; drainage position; antimicrobials; keep mean blood pressure above 90 mm Hg and urine output 300 ml/hr; avoid analeptics; hemodialyze severe phenobarbital poisoning As above; diuresis of little help
Stimulants: Amphetamines Methylphenidate	Hyperactive, aggressive, sometimes paranoid, repetitive behavior; dilated pupils, tremor, hyperactive reflexes; hyperthermia, tachycardia, arrhythmia Acute torsion dystonia	Blood	Reassurance if mild Chlorpromazine if intense	Agitated, assaultive and paranoid excitement; ocsionally convulsions; hypothermia; circulatory collapse	Chlorpromazine
Cocaine	Similar but less prominent than above; less paranoid, often euphoric	None: clinical appraisal only	Chlorpromazine Reassure	Twitching, irregular breathing, tachycardia	Sedation
Psychedelics (LSD, mescaline, psilocybin, STP)	Confused, disoriented, perceptual distortions, distractable, withdrawn or eruptive, leading to accidents or violence; wide-eyed, dilated pupils; restless, hyperreflexic; less often, hypertension or tachycardia		Reassure; "talk down"; do not leave alone	Panic	Reassure; diazepam satisfactory; avoid phenothiazines
Atropine-scopolamine (Sominex)	Agitated or confused, visual hallucinations, dilated pupils, flushed and dry skin		Reassure	Toxic disoriented delirium, visual hallucination; later, amnesia, fever, dilated fixed pupils, hot flushed dry skin, urinary retention	Reassure; sedate lightly; (1) avoid phenothiazines; (2) do not leave alone
Antidepressants: Imipramine (Tofranil), amitriptyline (Elavil)	Restlessness, drowsiness, tachycardia, ataxia, sweating	Clinical		Agitation, vomiting, hyperpyrexia, sweating, muscle dystonia, convulsions, tachycardia or arrhythmia	Symptomatic; gastric lavage
MAO inhibitors: tranylcypromine (Parnate), phenelzine (Nardil), pargyline (Eutonyl)	Hypertensive crises, agitation, drowsiness, ataxia	Clinical	Withdrawal	Hypotension; headache; chest pain; agitation; coma, seizures and shock	Symptomatic; gastric lavage
Phenothiazines	Acute dystonia, somnolence, hypotension	Clinical	Benadryl 0.50; withdrawal	Coma; convulsions (rare); arrhythmias; hypotension	Symptomatic; gastric lavage

SEDATIVE OVERDOSE

Pathogenesis.   All the sedative drugs depress the central nervous system, although not equally on a gram-molecular weight basis, and not to the same degree so far as different central structures are concerned. The duration of action varies widely and depends largely on how the particular drug is detoxified or eliminated. The short-acting barbiturates, pentobarbital, secobarbital, and amobarbital, are detoxified by the liver, as is methaqualone. They exert their maximal effects promptly after being absorbed and, even in huge doses, seldom cause neurologic depression lasting longer than three to five days. Barbital and phenobarbital are partially detoxified by the liver and partially excreted in the urine. Severe poisoning with the latter agent can cause coma lasting 10 to 14 days. Glutethimide has a short duration of action comparable to that of secobarbital, but it is poorly absorbed from the gut. This can prolong the effect of an ingested dose. Meprobamate has an intermediate duration of effect lasting for days. Bromide rarely causes full coma, but, once it reaches high levels, it displaces chloride in the blood and tissues, and persists for weeks to cause symptoms without further ingestion.

Although the sedatives have few important effects outside the nervous system, glutethimide and meprobamate in toxic doses tend to produce hypotension. Also, glutethimide possesses unique anticholinergic properties and is the only sedative that predictably produces light-fixed pupils in toxic doses.

A withdrawal syndrome consisting of tremulousness, agitation, and sometimes delirium and convulsions can develop when any of the hypnotic sedatives are stopped after prolonged use. Quantitative information is lacking, but convulsions seem to be a particular problem after withdrawal from meprobamate and methaqualone.

Clinical Manifestations.   Stupor or coma caused by depressant drug poisoning presents the characteristic picture of severe metabolic brain disease. The depression of the central nervous system tends to be bilateral and symmetrical, and the drug affects simultaneously many levels, including the spinal cord. Respiratory and circulatory controlling mechanisms in the lower brainstem are affected only with very high doses or not at all, and, except with glutethimide, the pupillary light reflexes are preserved. Early in the course of poisoning, patients can demonstrate muscular hypertonus or even spasticity as the result of uneven depression of different neurologic levels. Within a short time, usually an hour or less, flaccidity supervenes, and the stretch reflexes tend to disappear. Even moderate degrees of drug depression depress or block the oculovestibular reflexes.

Four grades of coma have been described in order to aid in estimating the severity of poisoning and the effects of treatment. *Grade I* is light coma in which vigorous noxious stimulation evokes withdrawal or groaning. *Grade II* is deep coma in which only minimal grimacing or reflex responsiveness can be evoked by a noxious stimulus. In *grade III* subjects fail to respond in any way to a noxious stimulus. In *grade IV* unresponsive patients remain in deep coma for over 36 hours and, in addition, have serious respiratory or circulatory depression. As mentioned above, a relationship between the blood level of a sedative drug and the depth of coma is only approximate. Generally speaking, however, blood levels of short-acting barbiturates of more than 2.5 mg per 100 ml

and phenobarbital blood levels of more than 12 mg per 100 ml are associated with grades III and IV coma.

Diagnosis.   The combination of unresponsiveness, preserved or sluggish pupillary reactions, absent oculovestibular reactions, motor areflexia, hypothermia, and depression of respiration and circulation is clinically diagnostic of sedative-anesthetic drug poisoning. Only pontine infarction resembles this clinical state, and with lesions of the pons the pupils are usually small or pinpoint, the stretch reflexes are generally preserved or hyperactive, and the plantar responses are extensor. Specific chemical tests will detect barbiturates, glutethimide, meprobamate, methaqualone, and bromides in blood or urine, and are readily done as emergency measures.

Management of Coma.   There are no specific antidotes for the sedative drugs. Treatment consists of physiologic support and preventing complications until the drug is detoxified and is excreted. Proper management saves all but a very few patients if they survive to reach the hospital. Among the writer's series of 356 consecutive patients in coma, 11 or 3.1 per cent died, all but three of whom were older than 45 years. To achieve this low rate required meticulous attention to the airway and ventilation, to the circulation, and to the potential complications of the comatose state. In laboratory animals, the fatal dose of barbiturates is seven times that required to produce apnea and almost twice that which first produces circulatory shock. Similar actions by the drugs in man guide the treatment of poisoning.

Airway and Ventilation.   Several mechanisms threaten to obstruct the airway of patients in coma from sedative drugs. If the subject lies on his back, the tongue and pooled secretions occlude the hypopharynx, with the result that secretions are aspirated into the lungs. The cough reflex and the ciliary action of the tracheobronchial mucosa are depressed. Many subjects aspirate stomach contents into the lungs, particularly if gastric lavage is attempted before tracheal intubation.

Because of these potentially fatal complications, the first step is to secure the airway. An oropharyngeal airway is sufficient to manage patients in light coma who cough when the larynx is stimulated. A cuffed endotracheal tube should be placed in more deeply anesthetized patients who lack a cough reflex. It is wise to precede intubation with atropine, 0.0008 gram intravenously, to reduce the danger of cardiac arrest. How long to leave the endotracheal tube in place in an unresponsive subject is often a difficult question. One practice is to deflate the cuff hourly for 5 minutes, to replace the tube at 24 hours, and to perform a tracheostomy at somewhere between 36 and 48 hours if the cough reflex has not returned or if no other signs indicate a lessening of coma.

To drain the lungs, patients should be placed in the prone position, as illustrated in the accompanying figure, and suctioned gently through the endotracheal tube every half hour, or more often if pulmonary secretions accumulate. It is desirable to administer low concentrations (25 per cent) of moistened oxygen, but not to occlude the tube with a large catheter. Tubes are removed when active coughing or bucking returns.

Hypoventilation should be treated with artificial respiration. Shallow breathing in a deeply comatose patient frequently reflects no more than the subject's depressed metabolism, but if the rate falls below 12 per minute or if the physician entertains serious doubts as to the adequacy of ventilation, artificial respiration is indicated. Ideally, arterial blood gases should be measured in deeply comatose patients and artificial respiration initiated if the arterial Pco_2 climbs above 45 mm of mercury. High concentration (>30 per cent) oxygen therapy should be avoided for patients not receiving artificial respiration, for its use increases the risk of hypoventilation and CO_2 retention.

Circulation. Severe shock is rare with depressant drug poisoning unless the patient has been asphyxiated. However, moderate hypotension is common and significantly reduces glomerular filtration and renal clearance of the barbiturates. Fluids should be given liberally to restore blood volume and promote urine flow, and pressor agents, such as metaraminol or levarterenol, are indicated to keep the diastolic blood pressure above 60 mm of mercury and the systolic above 90 mm of mercury. Digitalis or similar compounds are useful only in patients with heart disease. Corticosteroids are unnecessary.

Prevention of Complications. As long as he remains unconscious, the patient should be kept semiprone in the drainage position and changed from side to side in the semiprone position, but never placed on his back. Since the duration of unconsciousness is to be measured in days, the emergence of drug-resistant bacteria is of less concern than is pneumonia caused by already aspirated material. Thus it is useful to administer penicillin or tetracycline.

The blood pressure, pulse, and respiration should be recorded each half hour, and any abnormalities should be met appropriately. Body temperature elevations imply an infection if stimulants have not been given. Hypothermia above 32° C requires no special treatment. To evaluate the rate of urine flow, most physicians prefer to insert an indwelling catheter.

Other Measures. Gastric lavage is desirable for any patient who has ingested depressant drugs within the preceding few hours. The procedure carries the risk of producing pulmonary aspiration, and is best preceded by tracheal intubation with a cuffed tube in deeply comatose subjects. Subjects too lightly anesthetized to tolerate intubation should be turned prone before being lavaged. Care is required to avoid misplacing the tube and irrigating the lungs.

Forced diuresis and alkalinization of the urine have been recommended as adjuncts in treating barbiturate poisoning. Forced diuresis increases the renal clearance

of both short- and long-acting barbiturates, and the quantity cleared increases proportionately to the volume of urine. Phenobarbital has a relatively high pK value, and raising the urine pH appears to increase its dissociation and excretion. Several programs have been employed to achieve diuresis. The first step is to assure an adequate blood pressure; the second, to infuse a hypotonic electrolyte solution. The infusions are given at hourly rates up to 600 ml, depending upon urine flow. Close attention must be given to hour-by-hour fluid balance and 12-hour electrolyte balance. If urine flow does not match the infusion rate by the second or third hour, infusions should be slowed and more attention given to raising the blood pressure. Chemical and osmotic diuretics are contraindicated. Hypokalemia is a greater risk than hyperkalemia.

For treating bromide intoxication, diuresis should be combined with a high intake of sodium chloride to displace bromide from blood and tissues.

Hemodialysis is not necessary to treat poisoning with the short-acting hypnotics. However, hemodialysis is indicated for patients who have ingested large amounts of long-acting barbiturates such as barbital or phenobarbital as well as for patients who have severe bromide poisoning. In these instances, dialysis can shorten into a day or less a period of coma or stupor that otherwise would last a week or more.

Analeptics and pharmacologic stimulants are contraindicated for coma caused by depressant drug poisoning. Most carry the risk of overstimulating or producing convulsions in lightly poisoned patients.

Recovery and Prognosis. Patients recovering from coma require close medical supervision. Severe pneumonitis can develop as late as three to four days after recovery. If antimicrobial drugs were started during coma, they are best continued for at least 48 hours thereafter. Permanent physical sequelae to coma are extremely rare. Among 356 cases, residual brain injury was observed only once (in a patient who suffered an acute cardiac arrest). Peripheral nerve injuries from pressure developed in 6 subjects, and 14 subjects had pressure skin lesions leaving scars. There were no other residua.

Later management varies according to the patient's underlying psychiatric disorder and his attitudes upon recovery. Serious suicide attempts are never accidents, and reports of near-fatal ingestion caused by misunderstanding the dose or forgetting previous doses carry little validity. The expert opinion of a psychiatrist should be sought before deciding whether to release a patient or to institutionalize him. The immediate prognosis is good, but long-term results are less encouraging, and there is a high incidence of recurrent attempts at self-destruction over the years.

Driesbach, R. H.: Handbook of Poisoning. Diagnosis and Treatment. Los Angeles, Lange Medical Publications, 1971.
Physicians' Desk Reference to Pharmaceutical Specialties and Biologicals. Published annually by Medical Economics Co., Oradell, N.J.

Section Eight.   PROMINENT NEUROLOGIC SYMPTOMS AND THEIR MANAGEMENT

349.   PAIN

Jerome B. Posner

INTRODUCTION

Pain is the symptom for which most patients seek medical assistance. Since only the sufferer and not the observer perceives pain, it can have no precise definition. Sir Thomas Lewis described the situation exactly when he said that pain is "known to us by experience and described by illustration." Webster defines pain as the "sensation one feels when hurt mentally or physically; especially distress, suffering great anxiety, anguish, grief, etc., as opposed to pleasure—or, a sensation of hurting or strong discomfort in some part of the body caused by an injury, disease, or functional disorder and transmitted through the nervous system." Webster's definition suggests that there are two aspects to the perception of pain: the first is an emotionally neutral perception of a stimulus which is usually sufficiently strong to produce tissue damage; the second is an affective response to the perception of that stimulus. Pain implies damage to the organism, either physical or psychologic, and chronic pain, if untreated, will itself damage the organism. It is the physician's twofold therapeutic task to discover and treat the *cause* of pain and also to treat the pain itself, whether or not the underlying cause is treatable. To meet this task, the physician must know something of the anatomy and physiology of pain pathways.

ANATOMY AND PHYSIOLOGY OF PAIN

Three theories have been advanced to explain the physiology of pain. The first, the Doctrine of Specific Nerve Energies, by Müller in 1838, envisioned a specific system of receptors and fibers which respond to pain and to pain only, and are different from other receptors and fibers which respond to other specific sensory modalities. A second theory, the Pattern Theory, by Naff in 1927, suggested that any given fiber and pathway could subserve any modality and that perception of pain depends on the temporal and spatial pattern of the impulses which the stimulus produced. A third concept, the Duplex Theory, by Henry Head in 1920, suggested two interacting sensory systems, one composed of slowly conducting small fibers which subserve pain and the extremes of temperature, and another of large, more rapidly conducting fibers which subserve light touch, localization, and temperature discrimination. Head called these two systems protopathic and epicritic. Clinical and experimental evidence has been presented to support and to refute all three theories, and it is likely that some combination of the three explains the physiology of pain. Whatever the correct hypothesis, certain underlying anatomic and physiologic concepts seem incontrovertible. It is generally accepted that so-called "free" nerve endings are the primary receptors for the pain stimulus. Pain receptors are either nociceptors stimulated by tissue injury or chemoreceptors stimulated by chemical substances. There may be several classes of both types of pain receptors. Several chemicals produce pain when appropriately presented to nerve endings. These include acetylcholine, 5-hydroxytryptophan, hypertonic solutions, strong acids or bases, histamine, and potassium ions. Plasma kinins (e.g., bradykinin and kallidin) are potent producers of pain when injected intradermally or applied to the base of a blister. In the clinical situation, pain probably results when tissue injury, not necessarily structural, releases a substance (probably a proteolytic enzyme) which breaks down cellular proteins into pain-producing polypeptides such as kinins, which in turn stimulate pain receptors.

In the peripheral nerves, the stimulus that leads to pain is carried by two types of small fibers. Fast pain, a sensation of short latency and short duration, usually perceived as pricking or sharp, is mediated by delta fibers (the smallest myelinated fibers) which are 1 to 6 μ in diameter. Slow pain, with a longer latency and duration, is perceived as a poorly localized, burning, exceedingly unpleasant sensation and is mediated by small unmyelinated C fibers which are 0.4 to 1.2 μ in diameter. Both sets of fibers have their cell bodies in the dorsal root ganglia and enter the spinal cord through the dorsal roots into Lissauer's tract. They synapse in the substantia gelatinosa or in the posterior horn of the spinal cord. After synapsing, the delta fibers pass through the anterior white commissure to reach the lateral spinothalamic (neospinothalamic) tract contralaterally and ascend to the thalamus. Postsynaptic C fibers also cross the spinal cord in the anterior white commissure to reach the anterior spinothalamic (paleospinothalamic) tract. These neurons also ascend to the thalamus, but along the way give rise to a large number of collaterals to the reticular formation of the brainstem and hypothalamus. The neospinothalamic tract terminates in the ventrobasal complex of the thalamus, and the paleospinothalamic tract in the intralaminar and perifascicular nuclei of the thalamus. The ventrobasal thalamus also receives fibers from the dorsal column–medial lemniscal system (subserving the modalities of touch, position, and vibratory sensation) and projects to two areas of the cerebral cortex: somatosensory area 1 (which in man is part of the sensorimotor cortex surrounding the Rolandic fissure), and somatosensory area 2 in the parietal operculum. The thalamic intralaminar and parafascicular nuclei (paleospinothalamic tract) project diffusely to the cortex and are considered to be part of the reticular activating system of the brainstem. These anatomic facts, combined with clinical and physiologic observations, have led to the hypothesis that the discretely localized neospinothalamic tract carries rather neutral information about pain localization and intensity, whereas the more diffusely projecting paleospinothalamic tract is responsible for the affective component of pain.

The fast conducting dorsal column–medial lemniscal pathway and the slower conducting spinothalamic pathway interact at several levels of the neuraxis, and it is this interaction which has led to the "gate control theory of pain." According to this speculation, sensory fibers have two functions: to carry patterned information, depending on the specialized properties of each unit, and to modulate the effectiveness of synaptic transmission between peripheral nerve and ascending spinal fibers. The first site of the putative modulating action is in the substantia gelatinosa of the spinal cord where large fibers are presumed to activate an inhibitory system and small fibers stimulate an activating system. If large fiber stimulation is sufficient, synaptic transmission is inhibited, and small pain fiber activity which arrives later is less effective in exciting ascending spinal pathways. If the large fiber stimulus is insufficient or absent, small fibers excite the action system and carry pain messages to higher centers. This hypothesis lacks proof, and some recent contrary evidence has been presented. Similar "gates" in the brainstem reticular formation and in the thalamus which add to the modulation of incoming pain impulses have been proposed to circumvent the objections.

Much of the evidence supporting the aforementioned anatomic concepts has come from clinical and experimental studies in man: There are no known primary diseases of the pain receptors, but pain can be produced either by stimuli which damage tissues (e.g., heat greater than 45°C) or intradermal, intra-arterial, or iontophoretic application of the several chemical substances noted above. In man, the same C fiber ending responds to light needle pressure, pinching, radiant heat, and histamine application. Low concentrations of procaine injected into the peripheral nerve selectively anesthetize small fibers; pain is abolished when light touch, position, and vibration sense—modalities conducted by larger fibers—remain intact. Conversely, ischemia produced by a blood pressure cuff over the nerve blocks conduction in larger fibers so that pain remains after the perception of other modalities is abolished; bright, pricking, or fast pain disappears before the slower, burning, unlocalized pain. Peripheral neuropathies (e.g., diabetic neuropathy, postherpetic neuralgia) which selectively involve large, myelinated fibers often lead to a chronic, burning, spontaneous pain exacerbated by touching the denervated area.

The pathogenesis of pain produced by nerve compression is less well understood. Both herniated intervertebral discs and tumors which compress nerves or nerve roots can produce chronic and severe pain, but when normal nerve roots are compressed or manipulated at surgery, pain is not experienced. It is likely that the compressive lesions cause edema and inflammation which make the nerve susceptible to pain. Evidence adduced at surgical operation suggests that nerve roots which had previously been compressed are painful when manipulated, whereas those not previously compressed are not. Central nervous system lesions are sometimes the cause of chronic pain; direct electrical stimulation of the anterolateral columns in man has shown that approximately 50 per cent of the fibers carry nociceptive information, whereas the remainder are divided between warmth and cold. Although lesions made in these tracts usually relieve chronic pain, stimulation or occasionally even lesions of this area produce chronic, burning, dysesthetic sensations. Spontaneous lesions of the spinothalamic pathways in the spinal cord or midbrain generally produce loss of pain and temperature sensation but occasionally are associated with pain. In the thalamus, a lesion of the ventral-basal complex characteristically produces sensory loss, followed in four to six weeks by a spontaneous burning sensation in that part of the body subserved by the damaged area of the thalamus (thalamic syndrome). Lesions rostral to the thalamus are rarely responsible for the production of pain.

DIAGNOSIS OF PAINFUL DISORDERS

A thorough history, general physical examination, and careful neurologic examination are imperative in any patient complaining of pain. Often the description of the nature and distribution of the pain is so characteristic (e.g., trigeminal neuralgia or tabetic lightning pains) (see below) that it allows no other diagnosis. At times the history is so vague and bizarre and the distribution of pain so unanatomic as to suggest that the pain is a somatic delusion and not due to structural or even physiologic abnormality. Inquiry should be made concerning (1) the temporal pattern of pain, (2) its distribution, (3) exacerbating factors, and (4) relieving factors.

For example, headache beginning early in the morning before arising suggests increased intracranial pressure, whereas headache occurring late in the day is more suggestive of tension. Back pain and sciatica made worse by sitting or walking suggest disc disease, whereas back pain and sciatica which are worse while in bed suggest intraspinal tumor. Pain limited to a specific area is usually due to organ disease, whereas pain distributed in the distribution of a peripheral nerve or nerve root suggests that the nerve itself is diseased. Back pain and sciatica exacerbated by cough or sneeze suggest intraspinal disease, whereas similar pain not exacerbated by cough or sneeze suggests disease in the pelvis. Pain in the back or legs exacerbated by straight leg raising suggests disease of the nervous system, whereas a similar pain exacerbated by rotating the hips suggests pelvic or hip disease. Most pain caused by structural disease is relieved at least to some degree by analgesic drugs, whereas psychogenic pain often is not. Skeletal muscle relaxants or local heat may relieve pain of musculoskeletal origin. Both psychogenic and organic pain are relieved to some extent by distraction and a pleasurable environment. Both are exacerbated by anxiety or stress.

A careful general physical examination must be performed. Both the physical and laboratory examination should begin with the assumption that the site of pathologic change is at the site of pain. The painful areas should be examined for swelling and redness as well as for any obvious deformity. (The pain of herpes zoster usually precedes the rash, and occasionally on examination one may note only the faintest reddening of the skin in a dermatomal distribution.) The areas reported as painful should be palpated, the temperature estimated, and points of tenderness sought. (If the site of pain is in a soft tissue, bone, or joint, it should be tender to palpation as well as spontaneously painful.) Joints should be taken through a full range of motion and the effect of movement on the pain assessed. Nerve trunks going to the extremities should be palpated and stretched by movement of that extremity (e.g., straight leg raising, abduction, and extension of the arm). Inflamed and compressed nerve roots and nerve plexuses are more painful when stretched. A careful neurologic examination must also be performed. If there are neurologic abnormalities (e.g., weakness, sensory loss, reflex changes) in the painful part, one can infer that nervous system disease is responsible for the pain. The absence of specific neurologic abnormalities on first examination does not guarantee, however, that the nervous system is free of disease, because the process may simply not have advanced beyond the stage of selectively involving pain pathways.

Finally, laboratory examinations are performed. If the site of disease appears to be in bones or joints, x-rays of those structures or radioisotope scans may localize it. First attention should be paid to the local site of pain, but the physician should acquaint himself with the common referred patterns of pain (e.g., hip disease commonly causes knee pain, cardiac pain is frequently referred to the ulnar aspect of the arm and forearm, the pain of renal colic may be felt primarily in the groin and testicle, and pain resulting from disease of the throat may be referred to the ear).

Referred pain is pain perceived at a site remote from the source of the disturbance. Usually, referred pain is cutaneous and evoked by disease of deep structures innervated by the same dermatome. Referred pain may be associated with cutaneous hyperalgesia and even relieved by procaine injection into the area of referral. When pain is referred to the same dermatome or myotome as innervates the diseased structure (e.g., pain down the medial aspect of the arm [T1-T2] produced by myocardial infarction or angina pectoris), it is often helpful in diagnosis. However, pain is sometimes referred at a great distance from the primary site to segments not similarly innervated, and there the mechanism is perplexing (e.g., anginal pain referred to the jaw). Various theories have been suggested to account for referred pain. Such theories as division of the same nerve into deep and superficial branches, release of chemical mediators in the nervous system, and convergence of cutaneous and visceral nerves into common synaptic pools at the spinal cord all explain the dermatomal referral of pain but fail to explain pain at remote sites. Knowledge of common sites of referred pain often helps in establishing diagnosis of diseased internal organs.

MANAGEMENT OF CHRONIC PAIN

In some patients, pain is best managed by treating the underlying disorder (e.g., steroids for giant cell arteritis relieve headache and muscle pain promptly; radiation therapy for bone pain caused by cancer is often helpful). In others, a particular kind of pain has a particular treatment (see Specific Pain Syndromes, below), but in many patients the pain is chronic and the physician is able neither to treat the underlying disturbances nor to offer specific therapy for that type of pain. In treating this type of chronic and severe pain, certain general principles should be followed:

1. The pain should be treated by the simplest means which will relieve it, but all efforts should be made to relieve it. Chronic pain is both physically debilitating and psychologically demoralizing. It should be treated by the physician as a serious symptom and all efforts made to relieve it to the extent that the patient is comfortable.

2. Pain should be treated early. There is both clinical and experimental evidence that if chronic pain goes untreated for an extended period of time, abnormal self-excitatory states arise in the central nervous system so that treatment directed toward peripheral structures which initially would have relieved the pain are no longer effective. In general, the earlier one undertakes to treat chronic pain, the more successful one is.

3. Pain should be treated promptly. Clinical evidence suggests that if analgesic drug doses are spaced so far apart that severe pain recurs, the analgesic becomes less effective. Thus patients should be encouraged to take analgesic agents when the pain first reappears rather than wait until it becomes unbearable.

4. Various treatments of pain are additive and should be used together rather than separately.

5. Narcotic drugs should be used sparingly but should not be withheld if there is no alternative effective therapy. Experiments in laboratory animals indicate that enough narcotic given long enough produces physical dependence in every individual. However, the percentage of patients who become addicted to narcotics given for pain is unclear. Many physicians are impressed that narcotic addiction is unusual in patients treated for pain if the pain is later relieved by other means. If a patient has severe pain caused by organic disease and does not respond to non-narcotic drugs or to treatment directed at the underlying disease, narcotics should be used to the degree necessary to relieve pain. In patients with terminal cancer, one need not worry about addicting the patient, and in patients with more chronic disease, judicious use of narcotics, although running the risk of addiction, may restore a debilitated and bedridden individual into a comfortable, working, and useful citizen. Methadone maintenance programs have proved that patients can take narcotics in large doses over long times and continue to function usefully in society.

6. Psychogenic factors always play a role in chronic pain—the pain is more severe when the patient is anxious and stressed and less severe when he is relaxed. The physician must assess the psychologic factors in any patient with pain. If these factors are overwhelming, the chemical and physical methods described below are not likely to be very useful and psychotherapy should be undertaken. However, no patient should be diagnosed as having psychogenic pain until an exhaustive examination has ruled out structural disease.

7. Placebo effects are important. In most clinical studies, about one third of patients report relief of pain when given a placebo, although the extent of relief is rarely equal to that achieved by analgesic drugs. The physician can utilize a patient's desire to be free of pain by approaching the therapy in an enthusiastic and reassuring manner. It is less important whether it is the placebo or the drug which was effective than that the patient be relieved of his pain.

8. Multidisciplinary pain clinics which diagnose and treat intractable pain exist in many centers and should be utilized for severe problems.

Analgesic Agents

Analgesics (or analgetics) are drugs which decrease pain without causing loss of consciousness. Analgesics (Table 1) can be divided for clinical purposes into those which are suitable for mild pain, generally non-narcotic agents; those suitable for moderate pain, usually narcotics or narcotic antagonists with low addiction potential; and those which are suitable for severe pain, generally narcotic agents except for methotrimeprazine. The mild analgesics appear to act peripherally by blocking the pain chemoreceptors and perhaps by relieving inflammation. There is also evidence for a central effect of some of these drugs as well. Aspirin has been shown to be a potent inhibitor of prostaglandin formation, and this may be its mechanism of action peripherally.

The physician's strategy in treating chronic pain should begin with the mildest agents possible and add stronger agents or analgesic adjuvants only when mild agents fail to work. Drugs should always be given in sufficient amounts and at sufficiently short intervals to achieve relief of pain. Treatment should begin with aspirin or acetaminophen, 600 mg every three to four hours. If the pain is due to musculoskeletal spasm or if anxiety is prominent, one of the mild tranquilizers (diazepam or meprobamate) can be added. If the pain fails to respond to this mild regimen, one adds drugs used for the treatment of moderate pain (e.g., codeine or pentazocine). If the pain is still unrelieved and the physician satisfies himself that psychogenic factors are not responsible, the agents used for moderate pain should be discontinued, and agents used for severe pain should be added to the mild analgesic. Levorphanol, 2 mg, or methadone, 10 mg, every three to four hours is probably the agent of choice if oral drugs are to be used, and morphine, 10 mg every three to four hours, if a subcutaneous or intramuscular agent is necessary. Other narcotic drugs may be substituted for these, and often several must be tried to find that which relieves the patient's pain but causes fewest side effects. If the pain continues as a chronic and unremitting problem not relieved by these drugs, or if anxiety and depression appear to be a major contributor to the pain, a major tranquilizer (phenothiazine) or antidepressant agent, or both, may be added to the mild analgesics and narcotic agents. At times a satisfactory resolution of an intractable problem may be achieved by the combined use of a narcotic and non-narcotic analgesic and a tranquilizer or an antidepressant. The physician must be careful to adjust the doses of each so as to produce maximal pain relief with minimal sedation and unpleasant side effects. The physician should be prepared to increase the dose of those particular drugs to which tolerance develops as is necessary to control pain. No tolerance develops to non-narcotic analgesics. The more potent analgesics, including codeine but excepting the phenothiazines, are potentially addicting drugs to which tolerance develops and thus no fixed dose can be defined. These drugs act centrally, probably at synapses.

Non-narcotic Mild Analgesics. Aspirin and acetaminophen (Tylenol, Tempra) are the most useful of the mild analgesics. Either aspirin or acetaminophen may be given in doses of 600 mg every three to four hours, either alone for relief of mild pain or in conjunction with more potent drugs for relief of severe pain. The degree of pain relief is linearly related to the logarithm of the dose of the drug, higher doses being not significantly more effective until doses are reached which produce unpleasant side effects. The side effects of aspirin (clotting disorders, dyspepsia, and gastrointestinal bleeding) make acetaminophen, which has almost no such side effects, a safer drug and probably the drug of choice. There is no evidence that aspirin and acetaminophen together are more effective than either one alone, but either aspirin or acetaminophen plus codeine is more effective than codeine alone. There is no evidence that the other mild, non-narcotic analgesics are superior in any way to the two most commonly used drugs.

Narcotic Analgesics. All these drugs are potentially addicting, and tolerance develops to all. Thus there is no set dose of the drug, and with long, continued usage the dose must increase. *The physician is wise to learn to handle two or three of these drugs and use those consistently rather than using all the drugs occasionally.* He must be prepared to use more than one, because some patients find that side effects of the drugs make one preferable to another. Morphine, 10 mg intramuscularly, is the standard by which other narcotic analgesics are judged.

TABLE 1. Analgesic Agents

Type	Generic Name (Proprietary)	Usual Dose*		Comment
		Oral (mg)	Subcutaneous or Intramuscular	
Some agents used for mild to moderate pain	Aspirin	600 q 3–4 h		Side effects of dyspepsia and GI bleeding
	Acetaminophen (Tylenol)	650 q 3–4 h		Equal to aspirin but without GI side effects; less anti-inflammatory effect
	Phenacetin (aceto-phenetidin)	600 q 3–4 h		Probable renal toxicity with chronic use
	Dextropropoxyphene (Darvon)	65 q 3–4 h		Weak narcotic related to methadone, probably not superior to aspirin
	Phenylbutazone (Butazolidin)	100 qid		Anti-inflammatory agents, probably useful only for pain associated with inflammation (e.g., arthritis)—may cause agranulocytosis
	Indomethicin (Indocin)	25 qid		Useful only for pain associated with inflammation, probably not superior to aspirin
Some agents used for moderate to severe pain	Codeine	30–60 q 4–6 h	120 q 4–6 h	Narcotic with low addiction potential; additive effect if used with mild analgesics
	Oxycodone (with aspirin, phenacetin and caffeine = Percodan)	5 q 4–6 h		No advantages over codeine
	Pentazocine (Talwin)	30–50 q 4–6 h	60 q 4 h	Narcotic antagonist (produces withdrawal in patients physically dependent on narcotics); low addiction potential; hallucinations and dysphoria in doses >80 mg IM or 200 mg po
Some agents used for severe pain: narcotics and antagonists	Levorphanol (Levo-Dromoran)	2 q 3–4 h	2 q 3–4 h	Superior to morphine for postoperative patients in some studies
	Morphine		10 q 3–4 h	The standard narcotic agent for treatment of pain
	Meperidine (Demerol)	50–100 q 3–4 h	75–100 q 2–4 h	More rapid onset and shorter duration of action than morphine; possibly less spasmogenic and better for pain of biliary tree
	Methadone (Dolophine)	10–20 q 4 h	10–15 q 3–4 h	Possibly less sedative effect than morphine
	Fentanyl (Sublimaze)		0.1–0.2	Rapid onset, short duration, used in anesthesia
Non-narcotic	Methotrimeprazine (Levoprome)		20 q 4–6 h	Phenothiazine; no addiction; produces sedation and postural hypotension
Some agents used as analgesic adjuvants (probably little or no analgesic properties per se but used to relieve anxiety and/or depression)	Minor tranquilizers—muscle relaxants: Diazepam (Valium) Meprobamate (Miltown)		5 qid 200–400 qid	Useful with mild analgesics for acute or subacute pain associated with muscle spasm and/or anxiety
	Antidepressants: Amitriptyline (Elavil) Phenelzine (Nardil) Imipramine (Tofranil)		75–100 hs 15 tid 25 qid	Reported useful in pain associated with depressive symptoms (esp. atypical facial pain); may be useful when combined with analgesic agents for chronic pain of many kinds; may cause oversedation or anticholinergic symptoms
	Phenothiazines: Chlorpromazine (Thorazine) Promazine (Sparine) Promethazine (Phenergan) Fluphenazine (Prolixin)		25–50 qid 50–100 qid 25–50 hs 1–3 qd	Reported useful in pain associated with anxiety or depression and in some specific pain syndromes (e.g., thalamic pain, postherpetic pain); these drugs may have analgesic properties or potentiate analgesics; fluphenazine and amitriptyline have been reported to relieve postherpetic pain; may cause oversedation, depression, Parkinson-like syndrome, hypotension, or urinary retention

*Intramuscular dose of narcotics is equivalent to 10 mg of morphine. Since tolerance develops to these drugs, doses must be increased with continued use. Oral doses are not equivalent to intramuscular doses but represent usual starting doses.

Intramuscular morphine has its maximal effect in 60 to 90 minutes and lasts somewhere between three and six hours. It requires 60 mg or more of morphine orally to give the same analgesic effect as 10 mg intramuscularly. Levorphanol has a relatively high oral/parenteral ratio for analgesia; 2 mg given intramuscularly is equal to 10 mg of morphine intrasmuscularly, and 4 mg given orally is equal in total effect to 10 mg of morphine given intramuscularly. Methadone also has a relatively high oral/intramuscular potency ratio; 10 mg intramuscularly or 20 mg orally equals 10 mg of morphine intramuscularly. Codeine and dihydrocodeine are also effective orally and are generally used in doses of 50 to 60 mg as a mild analgesic. They often cannot be used to relieve severe pain, because side effects preclude high doses, but by the same token they are rarely addicting. Pentazocine can be used as a mild analgesic when given in doses of 30 mg and is equal to morphine if given in intramuscular doses of 60 mg. It is a weak narcotic antagonist with a high analgesic potential and has a dependence potential substantially less than that of morphine or meperidine (Demerol). Pentazocine is not included in the Federal Controlled Substances Act. However, hallucinatory effects and toxic psychoses have been noted in its users, and like the other narcotics it can produce respiratory depression. Dextropropoxyphene (Darvon) is structurally related to methadone and is a prescription drug not subject to the Controlled Substances Act of 1970. It is a weak narcotic with low addiction liability and a low analgesic potential.

Other Agents. The phenothiazine methotrimeprazine (Levoprome) is a potent analgesic agent. Given intramuscularly in doses of 15 to 20 mg, it is equivalent to 10 mg of morphine intramuscularly. The drug is not addicting, is an effective antiemetic, and does not suppress cough or respiration but does produce sedation and postural hypotension, making it useful only for hospitalized patients.

Sedative and anticonvulsant drugs as well as other phenothiazines have been utilized by some physicians in the treatment of chronic pain, particularly that associated with depression or other psychologic symptoms. The antidepressant amitriptyline (Elavil), given orally in a single dose of 75 mg at night (when it helps counter insomnia) or orally in divided doses of 25 mg three to four times a day, has been effective in relieving some chronic pain or in decreasing the narcotic dose required. In conjunction with the phenothiazine, fluphenazine, the drug has been reported useful in the treatment of postherpetic neuralgia (see below).

Physical Methods of Pain Relief

There are a bewildering array of physical methods designed to relieve pain (Table 2). These vary from simply rubbing a partially denervated area with a soft towel to placing radiofrequency lesions stereotactically in the thalamic and hypothalamic reticular formations. The simpler procedures can be carried out by the general physician or even by the patient; the more complicated ones, depending on their nature, demand the services of a skilled anesthesiologist or neurosurgeon.

The physician's approach to the use of physical methods for intractable pain should embody certain general principles:

1. Nondestructive procedures should be tried first. Cutaneous stimulation, either by hand or by battery-driven electrodes, or local anesthetic blocks in conjunction with analgesic drugs may be effective in relieving pain. If these simple procedures fail, the services of an anesthesiologist or neurosurgeon should be procured and a treatment plan embodying the use of analgesics and physical procedures outlined.

2. The least destructive procedure which will relieve pain should be tried first. In general, the procedure should be directed first at the peripheral nervous system, and, only if this fails, at the spinal cord, brainstem, or cerebrum. Quantitative data on the incidence of pain relief and its duration are sketchy for most of these procedures and seem to vary from center to center, depending on the skill and enthusiasm of the investigator reporting.

3. Thus the choice of a particular procedure often depends not only on the nature of the patient's disease but on the particular skills, experience, and bias of the physician.

4. If and only if a full trial of analgesic drugs has failed should destructive procedures for relieving pain be tried. These destructive procedures can and should be used in conjunction with analgesic drugs, because, even if the drugs have failed to relieve pain on their own, they may act synergistically with physical methods. Nerve blocks and surgical procedures often yield only temporary relief in patients with chronic pain. Thus many of the enthusiastic reports in the literature refer to patients followed for only a short period of time. When the patients are followed over months or years, the pain which was relieved shortly after the procedure often returns and is as bad as or worse than it was prior to the operation. For this reason, patients with cancer who are not expected to live a long time are often better candidates for surgical destructive procedures than are patients with pain originating from more benign conditions.

5. Patients with chronic pain being considered for destructive procedures must be thoroughly evaluated psychiatrically. If psychogenic factors play a major role in the genesis of pain, surgical procedures will not help, and often the pain will be exacerbated after surgical intervention.

Cutaneous Stimulation. Cutaneous stimulation of a painful area, particularly one which has been partly denervated, is often effective in relieving pain. This procedure, which probably has its greatest use in the treatment of postherpetic neuralgia, consists of rubbing the painful area with a soft cloth or terrycloth towel, almost constantly while awake at first but then with gradually lengthening intervals of rest between rubbing periods. Often a period of rubbing will yield relief which long outlasts the stimulus, and continued intermittent rubbings may totally relieve the pain. The "gate theory" offers an explanation of the rubbing phenomenon, i.e., rubbing stimulates large fiber afferents which may close the gate against incoming pain fibers. Whatever the explanation, the procedure is often useful in the treatment of painful phantom limbs and in chronic cutaneous or extremity pain after surgery. Recently, battery-powered electrical stimulators which give one control over the frequency and intensity of the cutaneous stimulation have become available. The electrodes of the stimulator may be placed over the painful area or over the peripheral nerve supplying the painful area, and stimulation using an intensity and frequency which produces a vibratory sensation is applied.

Acupuncture Analgesia. Acupuncture analgesia has become increasingly popular in the past few years, but no carefully controlled studies have reported on its usefulness. A needle is placed under the skin, often in a place remote from the painful site but at times into the painful site, and the area is stimulated either by twirling the needle or by electrically vibrating it. Several investigators have proposed a "multigate" theory as an explanation for the purported effectiveness of acupuncture, but its mechanism and usefulness in Western medicine for analgesia are still not clear.

Nerve Blocks. Direct block of peripheral nerves, using either anesthetic agents (lidocaine) or neurolytic agents (4 per cent phenol), has been popular in the treatment of thoracic and abdominal pain, particularly that pain which follows surgery. Blocks may be dangerous if used in the extremities, because they may paralyze as well as anesthetize, but in areas where they can be used relief of pain sometimes long outlasts the period of anesthesia. The procedure is a simple one when performed by a skilled anesthesiologist.

Subarachnoid injection of anesthetics or neurolytics directed at nerve roots has been utilized in patients with widespread and intractable pain. Barbotage of nerve roots via lumbar puncture, using either cerebrospinal

TABLE 2. Physical Methods of Pain Relief

1. Directed at end-organs or receptors
   A. Local anesthesia
      Ethyl chloride spray
      Lidocaine injection of painful area — Often useful for pain due to acute muscle spasm or musculoskeletal tension
   B. Local stimulation
      Rubbing painful area (with soft towel)
      Cutaneous electrical or mechanical stimulation (vibrator or battery-powered electrode)
      Acupuncture? — Local stimulation often relieves pain due to partial denervation (e.g., postherpetic neuralgia, postamputation pain, post-thoracotomy pain, causalgia)
   C. Local destruction
      Surgical undercutting of skin — Rarely successful for intractable postherpetic pain

II. Directed at peripheral nerves and roots
   A. Pharmacologic blockade
      Anesthetic block to nerves, plexus, roots
      Subarachnoid block of sensory roots
         Anesthetics
         Neurolytic drugs (phenol, alcohol)
         Mechanical blocks (CSF barbotage)
      Sympathetic block — Repeated anesthetic block to nerves which do not have major motor function may relieve pain for prolonged periods; block should always be tried before surgery is considered; subarachnoid drugs or barbotage often give temporary relief of pain, but motor or autonomic dysfunction may complicate the procedure. For causalgia-like syndromes
   B. Peripheral nerve stimulation — Electrical stimulator placed cutaneously over peripheral nerves is reported to successfully relieve some intractable pain
   C. Surgical procedures
      Peripheral nerve section
      Dorsal rhizotomy
      Dorsal root ganglionectomy — Most useful for thoracic and lumbar pain; good initial results, but long-term results poor; trigeminal rhizotomy effective for tic douloureaux
      Sympathectomy — For causalgia

III. Directed at spinal cord and brainstem
   A. Destructive procedures
      Spinothalamic tractotomy (percutaneous or open) — Most reliable surgical method for pain relief, best for thoracic or lower pain
      Myelotomy — For intractable facial pain, high incidence of paralytic complications
      Trigeminal tractotomy
      Mesencephalic tractotomy — Lesions in spinothalamic tract above cord for head and neck pain
   B. Stimulators
      Dorsal column stimulator — Electrodes placed surgically in dorsal columns and stimulated through the skin reported successful in several kinds of severe pain

IV. Directed at the diencephalon
   A. Destructive lesions (stereotaxic surgery)
      Ventral-basal complex — Not effective for chronic pain; lesions may produce "thalamic" pain
      Centre-médian — Appears effective for pain due to malignancy but not phantom pain; probably best for head and neck tumors
      Pulvinar — Often a delay of two to three weeks before pain is relieved
      Hypothalamus — Only sketchy data available on usefulness or complications

V. Directed at cerebral hemisphere
   A. Destructive lesions
      Cingulomotomy — Designed to relieve "suffering"; only rarely effective; better results if combined with thalamic lesions
      Sensorimotor cortex gyrectomy — Occasional relief of phantom pain or facial pain reported
      Hippocampus — Not fully evaluated; bilateral lesions required; marked personality change
      Frontal lobotomy — Rarely used because of behavioral changes
   B. Other
      Hypnotism
      Acupuncture?
      Psychotherapy
      Psychotropic drugs — All designed to relieve anxiety about pain and perhaps to promote cortical inhibition of pain pathways

fluid, hypertonic saline, or iced saline, appears to destroy enough nerve fibers to relieve chronic pain in the lower extremities, at least for a time. The procedure is sufficiently painful that it must be done under anesthesia. Bladder and bowel dysfunction are occasional complications, and the relief of pain is often transient. Phenol, 4 per cent, can likewise be injected into the subarachnoid space and directed at particular nerve roots by positioning the patient. The mechanism of action is destruction of nerve fibers; if material spills into the cauda equina, bladder and bowel dysfunction are common. The relief of pain is usually longer than that achieved with barbotage but may also be transient.

Each nonsurgical procedure directed at the *peripheral nervous system* has its surgical counterpart. In patients with chronic pain such as that which follows herpes zos-

ter, the skin has been undercut in an attempt to totally denervate it. Postoperative infection is a complication at times and the pain relief is only transient, thus contraindicating this procedure. Peripheral nerves can be cut, particularly in the thorax and abdomen, but this should not be done unless prior nerve blocks have indicated that it will be effective and sustained. The peripheral nerves regenerate after a time, and often the pain returns. Dorsal root ganglia in the thorax and abdomen can be removed for chronic pain or the dorsal roots themselves cut. This procedure also should not be done unless nerve blocks have indicated that it will be effective. Several roots must be cut on either side of the painful area if one is to achieve long-term pain relief.

Surgery of the Central Nervous System. There are three kinds of surgical procedures directed at the central nervous system for the relief of pain. The first, a direct outgrowth of the gate theory, involves the placement of electrodes on the dorsal columns with the power source being led under the skin. The patient then uses a transmitter to deliver a stimulus of known frequency and intensity to the dorsal columns. This increases large fiber input to the spinal cord, causes a mild tingling sensation, and often relieves pain for a prolonged period of time. Enthusiastic reports of this nondestructive surgical procedure have come from several centers, but it has not been performed long enough to fully evaluate its usefulness.

The second kind of procedure involves destruction of pain pathways in the spinal cord, brainstem, or brain. Spinothalamic tracts can be destroyed either surgically, after a laminectomy (open cordotomy), or by the placement of a radiofrequency lesion through a needle (percutaneous cordotomy). These procedures are particularly effective in relieving pain in the lower extremities and have the advantage that, although pain and temperature sensations are lost, cutaneous sensation and motor power remain intact. At times the level of anesthesia approaches within one or two cord segments of the level at which the destructive lesion is placed, but often there is a drop to about five segments below the placement of the lesion. Thus the lesion must be placed considerably higher than the site of pain. If the lesion is placed unilaterally, pain often appears in the other side of the body, necessitating another lesion. Bilateral lesions considerably enhance the risk of motor weakness and bladder and bowel dysfunction, but in skilled hands these risks are low. Occasional patients with bilateral percutaneous lesions in cervical cord suffer loss of automatic respiratory function (Ondine's curse). Percutaneous spinothalamic tract cordotomy, when done by a skilled technician, produces satisfactory pain relief in 70 to 90 per cent of patients, with a small mortality (1 to 5 per cent) and morbidity. The procedure is particularly useful in patients with terminal cancer, because the pain relief is usually sustained until death and the procedure does not require a major operation. An analogous lesion in the low brainstem placed in the descending tract of the trigeminal nerve has been reported useful in relieving facial pain. Pain and temperature sensation are lost, but cutaneous sensation remains intact. Lesions have been placed in the spinothalamic tract of the midbrain, so-called mesencephalic tractotomies. The dangers of this lesion are considerably greater than those of spinal cord lesions, and most centers have abandoned the procedure. Several neurosurgeons have placed lesions in the thalamus, both in the ventral-basal complex and in the interlaminar nuclei. Although good results are occasionally reported for both, the ventral-basal lesions appear only to produce transient relief of pain, whereas those placed in the interlaminar nuclei at the end-point of the paleospinothalamic tract appear to be more successful. There are rare reports of removal of sensory portions of the parietal lobe in relieving chronic pain, but the rarity of the reports implies the ineffectiveness of the treatment.

The third surgical method directed at pain relief is to place lesions in the frontal lobe, particularly the limbic projection to the frontal areas, in an attempt to alter the patient's psychologic response to pain rather than alter the pain pathways themselves. Several different surgical procedures, including frontal lobotomy, frontal leuko-

tomy, and cingulotomy, have been tried with varied success. These procedures, which alter the patient's personality as well as his suffering, probably deserve trial only when all other procedures have failed.

Good statistical data comparing the various surgical procedures for pain are difficult to come by. The best extant data indicate that initial relief of pain occurs with almost all procedures in 50 to 80 per cent of patients, with spinothalamic tract cordotomies yielding the best results. Longer-term follow-up suggests that considerably less than 50 per cent of patients achieve lasting relief, in many series the figure being as low as 20 per cent. Patients with malignant disease seem to have greater pain relief even initially than those with more benign conditions, probably because selection of patients with benign conditions often includes many with psychogenic pain.

SOME SPECIFIC PAIN SYNDROMES

Trigeminal Neuralgia. Trigeminal neuralgia (tic douloureux) is a disease characterized by sudden, lightning-like paroxysms of pain in the distribution of one or more divisions of the trigeminal nerve. The pain is usually unassociated with identifiable structural disease of the nervous system (idiopathic trigeminal neuralgia) but occasionally may be a symptom of a gasserian ganglion tumor, of multiple sclerosis, or of a brainstem infarct involving the descending root of the trigeminal nerve (symptomatic trigeminal neuralgia).

The history is diagnostic. The pain occurs as brief, lightning-like stabs, frequently precipitated by touching a trigger zone around the lips or the buccal cavity. At times, talking, eating, or brushing the teeth serves as a trigger. The pains rarely last longer than seconds, and each burst is followed by a refractory period of several seconds to a minute in which no further pain can be precipitated. The pains, however, often occur in clusters so that the patient first may report each pain as lasting for hours. The pain is limited to the distribution of the trigeminal nerve, usually affecting the second and third division or both, and only occasionally affecting the first division. Spontaneous remissions and exacerbations are common, the exacerbations tending to occur in spring and fall seasons. Between paroxysms of pain, the patient is asymptomatic. Tic pain rarely occurs at night. In idiopathic trigeminal neuralgia, the neurologic examination is entirely normal. In symptomatic trigeminal neuralgia, there may be sensory changes in the distribution of the trigeminal nerve, and such a finding should prompt a careful search for structural disease of the nervous system.

Carbamazepine is the drug of choice for the treatment of trigeminal neuralgia. This anticonvulsant drug is given in doses varying from 400 to 800 mg a day, but because of its sedative properties the initial dose is 100 mg twice daily, gradually increased to the required maintenance dose. No more than 1200 mg should be taken daily. The drug is not an analgesic and is only effective for specific kinds of pain such as trigeminal neuralgia, glossopharyngeal neuralgia, and the lightning pains of tabes dorsalis. Occasional cases of aplastic anemia have been reported, and complete blood counts are procured prior to the initiation of therapy and at frequent intervals thereafter. Other side effects include dizziness and sedation. Diphenylhydantoin in doses of 400 mg a day is also effective in trigeminal neuralgia but less so than carbamazepine. There is no evidence that the two drugs are synergistic. If medical treatment fails, section of the nerve root proximal to the ganglion affords permanent relief. Local anesthesia of the ganglion or the peripheral branches of the nerve at some time prior to surgery is desirable, because some patients find the anesthesia produced by nerve section less tolerable than the pain itself.

Glossopharyngeal Neuralgia. Glossopharyngeal neuralgia is characterized by pain similar to that of trigeminal neuralgia but in the distribution of the glossopharyngeal and vagus nerves. The trigger zone is usually in the tonsil or posterior pharynx, and the pain spreads toward the angle of the jaw and the ear. Occasional patients suffer cardiac slowing or arrest during these attacks as a result of the intense afferent discharge over the glossopharyngeal nerve. Carbamazepine is often effective, but if it fails, glossopharyngeal nerve roots are sectioned in the posterior fossa. Symptomatic glossopharyngeal neuralgia is occasionally the presenting complaint in a patient with a tonsillar tumor, and careful examination of the pharynx and tonsillar fossa for mass lesions must be carried out.

Lightning Pains of Tabes. The lightning pains of tabes are acute, short-lived pains in the trunk or lower extremities which occur with structural lesions of the dorsal roots and particularly with tabes dorsalis. Lightning pains are analogous to trigeminal and glossopharyngeal neuralgia. Like those two disorders, the pain usually responds to carbamazepine. There is no surgical therapy.

"Reflex Sympathetic Dystrophies." This is a term which applies to pain, hyperalgesia, hyperesthesia, and autonomic changes, usually after injury to an extremity. If the injury has involved a peripheral nerve, particularly the sciatic or median nerve, the syndrome is called *causalgia* (hot pain). If the injury has not involved a peripheral nerve, such terms as post-traumatic painful osteoporosis, Sudeck's atrophy, post-traumatic spreading neuralgia, minor causalgia, shoulder-hand syndrome, and reflex dystrophy have been applied, the particular term depending on the outstanding symptom. Whatever the term, the pathophysiology of all these disorders appears to be the same, as do their clinical manifestations and response to therapy.

The disorder may follow either a major or minor injury to an extremity, after which severe pain, usually of a burning quality, develops in the extremity. The pain is continuous but exacerbated by emotional stress and is associated with severe hyperpathia, so that moving or touching the limb is often intolerable. At first the pain is localized to the site of the injury or the distribution of the nerve injured, but with time it spreads, often to involve the entire extremity. Along with the pain there are vasomotor changes, first of vasodilatation (warm and dry skin) but later a change to vasoconstriction (edema, cyanosis, cool skin). Other autonomic disturbances include either hyperhidrosis or hypohidrosis; trophic changes in the skin, subcutaneous tissue, and muscles; and osteoporosis. The entire symptom complex is rarely present in any one patient, and one sign or symptom usually predominates. Untreated, severe reflex sympathetic dystrophy leads to muscle atrophy, fixation of joints, osteoporosis, and a useless extremity. The exact mechanism of the pain and sympathetic changes is not

understood. The various hypotheses include a reverberating "central excitatory state," "artificial synapses" between partially demyelinated nerves, and a central biasing of the spinal cord "gate."

Treatment should be undertaken as early as possible, because there is evidence that the earlier the treatment, the more effective it will be. Treatment begins with local anesthetic infiltration of the painful site, using 2 to 5 ml of 0.5 per cent lidocaine, repeated frequently enough to maintain relief of pain. When local measures fail, most patients are relieved by sympathetic block with lidocaine. This procedure often gives permanent relief, but if repeated local anesthetics produce only transient benefit, surgical sympathectomy should be performed.

Postherpetic Neuralgia. Postherpetic neuralgia refers to severe and prolonged burning pain with occasional lightning-like stabs in the involved dermatome after an attack of herpes zoster. Severe postherpetic neuralgia is usually a disease of elderly patients and, like most chronic pain, is exacerbated by emotional upset and relieved to some degree by distraction. Touching the involved area usually exacerbates the pain. Treatment of postherpetic neuralgia is not entirely satisfactory, but the initial treatment should be directed toward stimulating the painful area. Brisk rubbing for many hours a day with a terrycloth towel or stimulation of the dermatome with a cutaneous electrical stimulator often brings relief which long outlasts the stimulus. Initially, when therapy is undertaken, the hyperpathia may be so severe that the patient is unwilling to have the area stimulated. One can then spray the area with a local anesthetic (e.g., ethyl chloride) before stimulation is undertaken. During the first 48 to 72 hours, stimulation should be done as often as possible while the patient is awake and then decreased gradually. Care must be taken to keep the rubbing light so as not to excoriate friable skin. Relief of pain may take several weeks. Analgesic drugs are sometimes beneficial, and psychotropic drugs (amitriptyline, 75 mg daily, and fluphenazine, 1 to 3 mg daily) have been reported to be useful. If the pain does not respond to conservative treatment, surgical therapy may be considered as a last resort, but the results are usually poor. In many patients the disease runs its course, and after a year or two the pain disappears spontaneously. Thus mutilating surgical procedures are probably not indicated.

Phantom Limb Pain. Phantom limb pain is a chronic and severe pain appearing to be localized in an amputated or totally denervated limb. All patients suffer phantom sensations after amputation, but in only about 10 per cent is it painful, usually when there has been severe pain prior to operation. The pain is frequently similar to that suffered before amputation, or at times it may resemble muscle pain with the phantom seeming to be in a cramped or uncomfortable position. In most instances, the pain lessens and disappears with time, but in occasional patients it is a chronic and severe problem. Therapy is difficult. A search should be made for painful neuromas, but these are an uncommon cause of phantom pain, and even if small neuromas are found and removed, the pain is not usually relieved. Surgical procedures directed at the central nervous system are often not helpful. The pain may be triggered by touching the amputation stump, but over the passage of time healthy areas of the body when touched may also trigger pain in the phantom. Phantom pain is sometimes permanently abolished by cutaneous stimulation, either rubbing or electrical stimulation, or by repeated anesthetic blocks of peripheral nerves proximal to the stump. Narcotic analgesics may be helpful; other analgesic agents are usually not helpful. Sympathetic blocks have been reported to relieve pain in some patients for prolonged periods, but sympathectomy rarely produces relief as lasting as with causalgia. The mechanism of phantom pain is unknown.

Myofascial Pain Syndromes. Pain arising from skeletal muscle is common. Unaccustomed exercise causes soreness and tenderness in the involved muscles but is rarely a source of patient complaint. Prolonged tonic contraction of skeletal muscles, however, has an underlying pathogenesis of psychologic tension, resentment, and anxiety, and may produce pain in which the cause is not immediately apparent to the patient. Examples are tension headache arising from chronic contraction of paraspinous muscles at the base of the skull, anterior chest pain from contraction of pectoralis major, posterior thoracic or lumbar pain from paraspinous muscle contraction, and abdominal pain from rectus muscle retraction. The pain is initially localized over the area of muscle contraction but may spread widely into a distribution characteristic for the muscles involved. The muscles are usually tender to palpation, and there is often a particular tender area somewhere in the muscle, called a trigger area, which, when palpated, reproduces the entire distribution of the spontaneous pain. When the pain is acute, it may be treated with rest, local heat, and mild analgesic drugs, along with muscle relaxant drugs such as diazepam or meprobamate. When the pain is chronic or severe, particularly when a trigger area is found, local anesthesia with ethyl chloride spray or local injection of 0.5 per cent lidocaine sometimes affords relief. At times, a single injection breaks the pain–muscle tension–pain cycle and permanent relief is achieved. At other times, repetitive injections with the addition of analgesic agents and muscle relaxants are required.

Bonica, J. J.: Management of Pain. 2nd ed. Philadelphia, Lea & Febiger, 1974.
Bonica, J. J. (ed.): Symposium Issue: Management of pain. Postgrad. Med., 53:56, 1973.
Jannetta, P. J., et al.: The neurosurgical approach to the relief of pain. In Current Problems in Surgery. Chicago, Year Book Medical Publishers, 1973.
Payne, J. P., and Burt, R. A. P. (eds.): Pain: Basic Principles—Pharmacology—Therapy. Baltimore, Williams & Wilkins Company, 1972.

350. HEADACHE

Fred Plum

INTRODUCTION

Headache is man's most common pain, and in one form or another it affects some 90 per cent of the population. In any consideration of headache, two major points stand out: one is that *most* headaches come from structures *outside* the skull, and the other is that increased intracranial pressure, as such, does not necessarily cause headache. The following is an outline of the principal types:

A. Extracranial headache:
  1. Vascular headaches of the migraine type are recurrent and vary widely in intensity, duration, and frequency. The following subtypes are recognized:

  a. *Classic migraine,* with sharply defined, transient visual, other sensory and/or motor prodromes.
  b. *Hemiplegic or ophthalmoplegic migraine,* featured by sensory and motor phenomena that persist during and after the headache.
  c. *Common migraine,* without striking prodromes and less often unilateral than (a) and (d). Synonyms are "atypical migraine" and "sick headache."
  d. *Cluster headache,* predominantly unilateral, associated with flushing, sweating, rhinorrhea, increased lacrimation and, often, Horner's syndrome. The headaches are usually brief in duration and occur in close-packed groups separated by long remissions.
  e. *Lower half headache,* of possible vascular mechanism, centered primarily in the lower face. In this group are some instances of atypical facial neuralgia, sphenopalatine ganglion neuralgia (Sluder), and vidian neuralgia (Vail).
  2. Muscle contraction headaches are occipitofrontal pains or sensations of tightness, pressure, or constriction associated with sustained skeletal muscle contraction and no permanent structural change. The ambiguous and unsatisfactory terms "tension," "psychogenic," and "nervous" headache refer largely to this group.
  3. Combination of vascular headache of the migraine type and muscle contraction headache.
  4. Anterior headache and nasal discomfort (nasal obstruction, rhinorrhea, tightness, or burning) can result from congestion, edema, and inflammation of nasal and paranasal mucous membranes. This is "sinus" headache.
  5. Nonmigrainous vascular headaches associated with generally nonrecurrent dilatation of intracranial arteries.
  6. Ocular headache due to spread of effects of noxious stimulation, as by increased intraocular pressure, excessive contraction of ocular muscles, trauma, new growth, or inflammation.
  7. Aural headache due to spread of effects of noxious stimulation, as by trauma, new growth, or inflammation.
  8. Dental headache.
  9. Headache due to spread of pain from noxious stimulation of other structures of the cranium and neck (periosteum, joints, ligaments, and muscles or cervical nerve roots).
  10. Cranial neuritides (caused by trauma, new growth, or infection).
  11. Extracranial arteritis.
B. Intracranial headache:
  1. Traction headache. Headache resulting from traction on intracranial structures, mainly vascular, by masses:
  a. Primary or metastatic tumors of meninges, vessels, or brain.
  b. Hematomas (epidural, subdural, or parenchymal).
  c. Abscesses (epidural, subdural, or parenchymal).
  d. Headache following puncture ("leakage" headache).
  e. Pseudotumor cerebri and various causes of brain swelling.
  2. Headache due to overt inflammation of cranial structures resulting from usually nonrecurrent inflammation, sterile or infectious.
  Intracranial disorders: infectious, chemical, or allergic meningitis, subarachnoid hemorrhage, postpneumoencephalographic reaction, arteritis, and phlebitis.
C. Cranial neuralgias: trigeminal (tic douloureux) and glossopharyngeal (see Ch. 349). Trigeminal neuralgia must be distinguished in particular from the brief vascular headache of A 1 c, with which it is often confused.
D. Headaches of a delusional or conversion reaction are those in which a somatic pain mechanism is nonexistent. The diagnosis is rare and must be made cautiously. Closely allied are hypochondriacal and depressive reactions in which tissue abnormalities relevant to headache are minimal.

Pathogenesis of Headache. Wolff and his colleagues identified the principal pain-sensitive structures of the head as (1) *extracranial:* all the tissues, especially the arteries; and (2) *intracranial:* a very limited group of tissues, including the great venous sinuses and their venous tributaries from the surface of the brain, parts of the dura at the base, the dural arteries and the cerebral arteries at the base of the brain, the fifth, seventh, ninth, and tenth cranial nerves, and the upper three cervical nerves.

The cranium (including the diploic and emissary veins), the parenchyma of the brain, most of the dura, most of the pia-arachnoid, and the ependymal lining of the ventricles and the choroid plexuses are not sensitive to pain.

The fifth cranial nerve contains the pathways for pain from sensitive intracranial structures located on or above the superior surface of the tentorium cerebelli.

Pain from these structures is experienced in various regions in front of a line drawn coronally joining the ears across the top of the head.

The ninth and tenth cranial nerves and the upper two or possibly three cervical nerves contain the pathways for pain from pain-sensitive structures on or below the inferior surface of the tentorium cerebelli. Pain from these structures is experienced in various parieto-occipital and upper cervical regions behind the line just described.

HEADACHE FROM INTRACRANIAL SOURCES

Six basic mechanisms of headache from intracranial sources have been formulated: (1) traction on and displacement of the great venous sinuses or of the veins that pass to them from the surface of the brain; (2) traction on and displacement of the middle meningeal arteries; (3) traction on and displacement of the large arteries at the base of the brain and their main branches; (4) dilatation and distention of intracranial arteries; (5) inflammation in or about any of the pain-sensitive structures of the head and portions of the pia and dura at the base of the skull; and (6) direct pressure by tumors on pain-sensitive cranial and cervical nerves. Intracranial diseases commonly cause headaches through more than one mechanism and may also cause secondary extracranial muscle-contraction headache, usually at the occiput, but not elsewhere.

The head pain associated with fever, bacteremia, sepsis, nitrite and foreign protein administration, carbon monoxide inhalation, hypoxia, and asphyxia is due principally to dilatation and distention of intracranial arterial structures. A similar vascular mechanism is the probable basis for the headaches that follow epileptic seizures (with or without convulsions) and certain "hangover headaches," and is a component of many migraine headaches and those associated with arterial hypertension and Meniere's disease. Painful distention of intracranial arteries is likewise responsible for the headaches that accompany sudden brisk rises in the arterial blood pressure, such as occurs with distention of the rectum or urinary bladder in paraplegics, rapid intravenous infusion of epinephrine, and the hypertensive crises occurring with pheochromocytoma.

The headache of meningitis is primarily related to the lowered pain threshold of inflamed tissues. The inflammatory changes are usually most noticeable in the basal dura and pia and in adjacent blood vessels and nerves at the base of the brain. Under these circumstances, even the slight, usually painless arterial dilatation and distention during each cardiac systole become painful; hence, the characteristic throbbing headache.

Lumbar Puncture Headache

Dull, usually pulsating occipital headache develops in about one fifth of patients having lumbar puncture, particularly for the first time. The headache usually begins 12 to 24 hours after the puncture, comes on in the erect position, and subsides if the subject lies flat. The headache usually disappears spontaneously in a day or so, and in most patients is made tolerable by routine analgesics. Occasionally, patients develop more prostrating symptoms that sometimes last as long as 10 to 14 days, accompanied by secondary muscle-contraction headache

as well as nausea and vomiting. Vigorous reassurance and sedatives added to the analgesics may help shorten the course.

The cause of postlumbar puncture headache is probably leakage of cerebrospinal fluid through the torn dural sac. The consequent loss of buoyance results in downward traction on unsupported, pain-sensitive posterior fossa tissues, particularly the veins. The headaches can often be avoided by accurate punctures, using No. 20 caliber sharp spinal needles, which minimize drainage through the dural needle wound.

Headache With Brain Tumor: With or Without Increased Intracranial Pressure

The headache with space-occupying lesions is deep, aching, steady, dull, and seldom rhythmic or throbbing. The pain is continuous in one tenth of the patients and is generally more intense in the morning. Aspirin, 0.3 gram, and local application of cold packs usually diminish the pain, and coughing or straining at stool may aggravate it. Some patients prefer the recumbent to the erect position. The headache is rarely as intense as that associated with migraine, ruptured cerebral aneurysm, or meningitis, and seldom interferes with sleep. Even when the tumor directly compresses and displaces pain-sensitive cranial nerves, headache may be absent or slight, and rarely is it as intense as the pain of tic douloureux, unless the tumor intermittently obstructs the cerebral ventricular system. In this instance, pain is excruciating and generalized, and may last 30 seconds to a half hour and then disappear as quickly as it commenced. During such an attack the sudden increases of intracranial pressure can be fatal.

Severe brain tumor headache is associated with nausea and vomiting. However, vomiting caused by new growth may occur with neither nausea nor headache, and is then usually the result of medullary compression. Being unexpected, such vomiting may be projectile.

When the headache is occipital or suboccipital, it is often associated with "stiffness" or aching of the muscles of the neck and tilting of the head toward the side of the lesion.

Pathogenesis. Increased intracranial pressure, per se, is not necessarily associated with headache. The headache with brain tumor results from traction-displacement of intracranial pain-sensitive structures, chiefly the large arteries, veins, venous sinuses, and the cranial and somatic nerves mentioned.

Local traction and direct pressure may be exerted by the tumor upon adjacent pain-sensitive structures. Extensive displacement of the brain evokes pain from structures remote from, as well as adjacent to, the tumor.

Localizing Value. When the site of the headache is interpreted in terms of the following principles of intracranial pain production and pain reference, it may aid significantly in localization of a brain tumor:

(1) About one third of all headaches approximately overlie the tumor. (2) In the absence of increased intracranial pressure, two thirds of headaches are near or immediately over the tumor, and when unilateral are on the same side. (3) Occipital headache is almost always present and is the first symptom of posterior fossa tumors, except cerebellopontine angle tumors. When headache occurs with cerebellopontine angle tumors, it is frequently and sometimes solely postauricular. (4) Frontal headache is a first symptom in about one third of supratentorial tumors. Occipital headache rarely occurs with such growths unless associated with increased intracranial pressure or early tonsillar herniation. (5) A generalized headache with brain tumor signifies extensive displacement of the brain, usually with increased intracranial pressure, and has little localizing value.

Management. The headache itself rarely determines the management. Nevertheless, the most effective treatment for brain tumor headache is surgical removal of the mass. Transient decompression can be achieved by the intravenous infusion of either 500 ml of a 20 per cent sodium mannitol solution or 250 ml of a solution containing 30 per cent urea in 10 per cent invert sugar. Adrenal corticosteroids in high doses can also be employed to reduce brain edema and transiently decompress the mass. Lumbar drainage is contraindicated, nor does it predictably reduce headache of meningitis or subarachnoid hemorrhage.

If an inoperable tumor causes headache, ventricular drainage or shunting is sometimes employed.

Sometimes x-radiation or surgical procedures are justified in attempts to reduce headache caused by clearly defined metastatic disease. Headache resulting from craniopharyngioma or pituitary tumors does not in itself constitute an indication for surgical procedures, because removal provides no assurance that headache will be diminished or eliminated.

HEADACHES FROM EXTRACRANIAL STRUCTURES

Six main categories of head and face pain from extracranial tissues and related structures can be distinguished: (1) headaches due to painful dilatation and distention of cranial arteries; (2) headaches due to sustained contraction of skeletal muscle about the face, scalp, and neck; (3) headache from disease of the nose, paranasal spaces, eyes, ears, and teeth; (4) craniofacial pain of the major neuralgias and the postinfectious neuralgias and postinfectious neuritides; (5) headache due to nonspecific inflammation of cranial arteries ("cranial arteritis," "temporal arteritis"); and (6) head pain due to trauma, infection, or new growth involving extracranial tissues.

More than 90 per cent of all headaches are in the first two of these categories and occur in a life setting that engenders frustration, resentment, anxiety, emotional tension, and fatigue.

Vascular Headaches

Vascular headaches are principally due to painful dilatation and distention of one or more of the extracranial and, probably, intracranial, i.e., dural, branches of the external carotid artery, with associated edema of adjacent tissues. The most common site of vascular headaches of the migraine type is the temple or the forehead, and one or both frontal, supraorbital, and superficial temporal arteries are most frequently involved. Many headaches at the back of the head and neck are associated with painful dilatation and distention of the postauricular and/or occipital arteries, and comprise one type of "occipital neuralgia."

Finally, the lower half of the head and face and the upper jaw in the vicinity of the back teeth may all be the site of pain of vascular origin, with spread to the neck and even the shoulder. Such headaches may be accompanied by the awareness of unusually forceful throbbing in the neck. "Atypical facial neuralgia" is but one of the many designations applied to such headaches, which very probably result in good part from dilatation and distention of the extracranial portion of the middle meningeal artery, of the internal maxillary artery, and of the other branches and the trunks of the external and the common carotid arteries.

Migraine Syndrome

Clinical Features. The migraine syndrome is a pattern of dysfunction integrated within the central nervous system and manifested as widespread bodily disturbances, both nonpainful and painful. The outstanding feature is periodic headache, usually unilateral in onset but at times becoming bilateral or generalized. The attacks may vary in duration from a few minutes to several days and, in severity, from trifling symptoms to prolonged disabling illness. The headaches are associated with "irritability," nausea, and often photophobia, vomiting, constipation, or diarrhea. Although most common in the temple, headaches may be experienced anywhere in the head, face, and neck. The syndrome runs in families.

For a period of several hours to several days preceding the headache, the cranial arteries undergo a variable contractile state indicated by a facial flushing or pallor and by other transient cranial vasomotor phenomena such as vertigo. In the hour preceding the headache, a variety of visual and other neurologic abnormalities caused by transient local constriction of cerebral or retinal arteries occur in about 10 to 15 per cent of the instances. These prodromes may take the form of scintillating scotomas, visual field defects such as unilateral or homonymous hemianopsia, and, occasionally, hemiplegia. More sustained neurologic defects and even cerebral infarction have rarely occurred. As the vasoconstrictor phenomena recede, vasodilator headache commences, sometimes overlapping, sometimes beginning after a short symptom-free interval. The pain is throbbing and aching, is appreciably reduced by pressure on the common carotid and the affected superficial artery, and is characteristically eliminated or reduced by vasoconstrictor agents, particularly ergotamine tartrate. The walls of the dilated cranial arteries and the adjacent tissues become edematous and tender. With sustained vasodilatation for several hours, the easily compressible arteries become rigid and relatively noncompressible, and the pulsatile pain becomes a steady ache. Redness and swelling of the eye with excessive tearing, and redness and swelling of the nasal mucosa with or without epistaxis, may occur along with the headache. A secondary muscle contraction component of the headache may outlast the vascular pain and will not be modified by vasoconstrictor agents.

One variety of headache closely related to migraine syndrome is the *cluster headache,* sometimes called histamine headache. This head pain is almost always unilateral, affects men much more than women, and usually begins between the third and sixth decades. Attacks come on abruptly with intense throbbing pain arising high in the nostril and spreading to involve the region behind the homolateral eye and sometimes the forehead as well. During the attacks, which last up to two hours, seldom more, the nose and eye water. The skin reddens and a homolateral Horner's syndrome with pupillary constriction and ptosis may develop. The attacks tend to occur from once to several times daily, in clusters lasting weeks or, less often, months. Without apparent reason, the cluster subsides as suddenly as it began, and the patient commonly remains free of headache for weeks or months until another cluster begins. During a cluster period, but not between, alcohol is likely to induce attacks. When headaches recur in close succession, the Horner's syndrome may outlast the headache.

Pathogenesis. Before the onset of migraine headache a generalized accumulation of fluid may occur as part of a nonspecific disturbance in fluid and electrolytes that is found in many persons with and without the migraine syndrome during periods of stress. There is evidence of a general abnormality of vascular behavior in many migraine subjects, and the extracranial vessels of such subjects show more variability in their contractile patterns than those of normal subjects even during headache-free periods. Sympathetic nerve stimulation or section has little effect on these vessels or on the migraine attack, and humoral agents have long been sought as the basis of the migraine syndrome. Local fluid collected from sites of swelling at the point of maximal headache and tenderness during an attack contains a vasodilator polypeptide of the bradykinin type that lowers pain thresholds and may be a factor in a local sterile inflammation. However, neither kinins, histamine, nor substances such as acetylcholine satisfactorily explain the generalized manifestations of the disorder. Several lines of evidence suggest that abnormalities in the metabolism of serotonin may play a role in the migraine syndrome. Reserpine, which induces a drop in serum serotonin levels, will often induce a migraine attack, and serum levels of serotonin have been found to drop spontaneously just before migraine attacks. During migraine attacks, an increased quantity of serotonin metabolites has been found in the urine. Methysergide, a powerful serotonin antagonist, prevents or reduces the frequency of migraine attacks in most subjects.

Management. Headaches of low intensity are usually eliminated by 0.3 to 0.6 gram of aspirin, but sometimes require 60 mg of codeine phosphate as well.

For severe vascular headache, the restoration of the painfully dilated vessels to a nonpainful constricted state and the restoration of pain threshold to normal are accomplished best by the prompt intramuscular administration of 0.25 to 0.5 mg of ergotamine tartrate, not to exceed 0.5 mg in any one week. If the agent is administered in amounts of 1.0 to 2.0 mg by suppository, the side effects of nausea, vomiting, and elevated blood pressure are diminished. Ergotamine tartrate may also be given by mouth in 3.0 mg amounts, to be swallowed or absorbed sublingually. This first dose may be repeated in 30 minutes, and a third given in another 30 minutes if the headache persists. Ergotamine tartrate, 1 mg, can also be given in tablets in combination with caffeine, 100 mg, up to 8 tablets for any single headache attack. The amount of ergotamine so administered should not exceed 10 mg in any one week. Administration by mouth or by suppository is less predictably effective than intramuscular administration

Propranolol, 20 mg four times daily, occasionally adds to the benefit received from ergotamine tartrate or ergotamine-caffeine combinations. Short courses of corticosteroids interrupt periods of cluster headache in about half the affected patients. Methysergide is similarly effective in cluster headache.

Prevention. Of utmost importance is a consideration of the personal problems of the patients. Patients with migraine headaches are generally striving, orderloving persons who, during periods of threat or conflict, become progressively more tense, resentful, and fatigued. Although the disease undoubtedly depends on a con-

stitutional background, feelings of anger, depression, or emotional fatigue often form the backdrop for a recurrence of headache. Treatment is best if it allows the patient free and repeated expression of his conflicts, resentments, and dissatisfactions; enables him to recognize the nature of his dilemma and its relationship to the physiologic basis of his pain; and guides him toward a more flexible attitude and personal adjustment. About two of three patients can be appreciably helped by such aid.

For patients in whom attention to psychologic attitudes and adjustment of life situations fail to bring significant relief, two forms of long-term pharmacotherapy have been useful. One is the monoamine oxidase inhibitor phenelzine sulfate, 45 mg daily, which induces a significant reduction in headache frequency in most patients with migraine, and can be given indefinitely. The other is the serotonin antagonist methysergide, which in doses of 2 mg three to four times daily is effective in about two of three cases in preventing headache of the migraine type. However, methysergide must be used with great caution. Both ergotamine tartrate and methysergide possess the ability to induce profound vasoconstriction and are contraindicated in pregnancy, peripheral vascular disturbance, severe hypertension, coronary artery disease, thrombophlebitis, and renal disease. Serious and unexpected vasospastic and psychic reactions have occasionally occurred with methysergide. Retroperitoneal fibrosis producing back pain and ureteral obstruction has been reported. Any of these serious complications necessitate prompt discontinuance of methysergide, and any single course of the drug should not outlast three to six months.

Muscle-Contraction Headaches

The pain of a muscle-contracting headache is a steady, nonpulsatile ache, unilateral or bilateral, in the temporal, occipital, parietal, or frontal regions. Additional descriptive terms include tightness bitemporally or at the occiput, bandlike sensations about the head, which may become caplike in distribution, viselike ache, weight, pressure, drawing, or soreness. Cramplike head pains and "feeling as if the neck and upper back were in a cast" are described by some patients. Pain may be fleeting, with frequent changes in the site and intensity of recurrences, or localized in one region. The headache may last for weeks, months, or even years.

Pathogenesis. Muscle contraction headaches are due to long-sustained contraction of skeletal muscle about the face, scalp, and neck. Concurrent vasodilatation of the associated cranial arteries frequently contributes to the irritability of the involved muscles and to the headaches.

With prolonged sustained contraction, the muscles of the head, jaws, neck, and upper back become tender, causing the patient to limit their motion. Palpation may reveal sharply localized painful areas or nodules. Commonly, it hurts to comb or brush the hair or to don a hat. Exposure to cold, with shivering, may precipitate or aggravate the headache. Pressure on the contracted, tender muscles may augment the intensity and may elicit tinnitus, dizziness, and lacrimation—features that also occur spontaneously.

Sustained muscle contraction giving rise to headache is often secondary to noxious stimuli from other cranial tissues and structures, e.g., from distended arteries in vascular headache, inflammation or other disease in the eye, ear, nose, paranasal spaces, teeth, or scalp, and from brain tumor. Painful, sustained muscle contraction is also the primary source of many headaches associated with emotional tension states, especially in the adverse life situation of tense, aggressive, frustrated, anxious, or depressed persons.

Management. Reassurance, massage, manipulation, and manual stretching of the nuchal and occipital muscles, aspirin, and phenobarbital (30 mg three times a day) reduce or eliminate most such headaches. Bed rest, local heat, warm baths, and the passage of time are important adjuvants. Removal of the primary source of noxious stimuli may eliminate the headaches secondary to disease of the eye, ear, nose, and sinuses or teeth.

Headaches caused by sustained muscle contraction associated with life stress and emotional tension are only temporarily modified by sedatives or analgesics. Treatment should be directed at improving the patient's adjustment, as outlined under the management and prevention of migraine headache. Particularly among patients susceptible to recurrent headache of this type, the antidepressant amitriptyline in doses of 25 to 75 mg daily may bring considerable relief.

Other Types of Extracranial Headache

Recurrent ("Chronic") Post-traumatic Headache. Head injury may rarely be followed by headaches that stem from intracranial sources such as subdural hematomas or subarachnoid hemorrhages. However, post-traumatic headaches more frequently stem from nonintracranial sources, four types being most common: (1) pain or tenderness resulting from local tissue damage in a scar or at a site of impact, (2) muscle-contraction headache, (3) attacks of throbbing and aching vascular headache, and (4) infrequently, delusional headaches for which no tissue abnormality exists. The first two varieties are most common and are sometimes accompanied by fleeting vertigo with sudden movement or rotation of the head, nausea, irritability, and insomnia.

Many injured patients harbor resentment related to the circumstances of their accident or fear that they have sustained permanent brain injury. These reactions and attitudes are intimately related to the pathophysiology and "chronicity" of post-traumatic headaches, and the headache often fails to subside completely as long as compensation claims remain unsettled.

Headaches Associated with Arterial Hypertension. When otherwise symptom-free and in the absence of hypertensive encephalopathy or pheochromocytoma, about 10 per cent of persons with arterial hypertension may experience severe, even disabling, headaches, particularly during the morning hours. Recent studies show that these are principally vascular and muscle-contraction headaches. Fluctuations in blood pressure correlate only poorly with the headaches, nor is the extent of the elevation directly related to the severity of the attacks. However, headache attacks tend to be less frequent when the blood pressure is least elevated.

The headache associated with arterial hypertension resembles the vascular headaches of migraine and muscle tension and often regresses spontaneously with reassurance, bed rest, sedative medication, and the passage of time, especially when the patient is hospitalized. Ergotamine tartrate and methysergide are contraindicated.

Nasal and Paranasal Structures as Sources of Headache. Sinus headache is predominantly a short-lived problem, always associated with objective evidence of acute sinusitis. Most of the discomfort comes from the ostia, which are many times more sensitive than the relatively insensitive walls of the sinuses. Typically, "sinus" headache commences in the morning (frontal) or early afternoon (maxillary) and subsides in the early or late evening. The pain is dull and aching, is made worse by changing head position, and is seldom associated with nausea and vomiting. It is due to mucosal inflammation, and engorged turbinates, ostia, nasofrontal ducts and superior nasal spaces should be visible. Most patients have sinus tenderness. Headache not associated with turbinate engorgement and inflammation is probably not due to sinus or nose disease. Sinus headache is best treated with decongestants and analgesics. Persistent purulent discharges should be cultured and appropriate antimicrobial drugs employed. Chronic suppurative disease in the frontal, ethmoid, and sphenoid sinuses, or in the mastoid air cells, may result in osteomyelitis and inflammation of adjacent cranial tissues. Headache persisting after surgical drainage of the diseased sinus is evidence for extradural and possibly subdural infection.

Head Pain and Disease of the Teeth. Noxious stimuli in a tooth usually evoke local toothache, but pain can be referred to tissues remote from a diseased tooth. Afferent fibers for sensation in the teeth are contained in the second and third divisions of the fifth cranial nerve. Headache in the areas supplied by the latter is, in rare instances, associated with prolonged, intense toothache, or follows a tooth extraction. More commonly, in association with toothache, tooth extraction or a tender, diseased tooth, distant tissues exhibit surface hyperalgesia, tenderness, and vasomotor reactions, such as tender eyeballs, reddening of the conjunctivae, and tenderness of the auricular and temporal tissues. Because of secondary muscle contraction, other sites of tenderness and pain may be noted behind the ears, behind the lower border of the mastoid process, and in the muscles of the occiput, neck, and shoulders.

The teeth in the upper jaws are frequently the site of tenderness and pain in association with disease of the nasal and paranasal structures. Occasionally, in coronary insufficiency, pain is experienced in the lower jaw because of the close approximation of the fifth cranial and upper cervical neural segments in the cord. The teeth rarely cause craniofacial pains or "neuralgias" in the absence of toothache. Headache may not be attributed to a diseased tooth unless the injection of procaine into the tissues about the suspected tooth greatly reduces the intensity of, or eliminates, such headache.

Head Pain and Disease of the Ear. The fifth, seventh, ninth, and tenth cranial nerves contribute to the sensory innervation of the ear, and branches from the upper cervical roots supply the immediately adjacent scalp and muscles. Severe pain in the vicinity of the ear can be caused by disease of the teeth, acute tonsillitis, inflammatory and neoplastic disease of the larynx and nasopharynx, temporomandibular joint disorders, tumors, and inflammation in the posterior fossa and disease of the cervical spine and its soft tissues. Pain in the ear is also associated with vascular headaches and atypical facial neuralgias as well as herpes zoster of the fifth and seventh cranial nerves and, rarely, the glossopharyngeal nerve. True glossopharyngeal neuralgia causes severe pain radiating from the tonsil into the ear. It has the usual timing feature of "tic."

Primary ear disease is relatively infrequent—but important—as a source of headache, because it almost always indicates inflammation or destructive disease. Acute otitis media (purulent or nonpurulent), furunculosis of the ear canal, traumatic rupture of the tympanum, and fracture of the anterior wall of the bony canal all cause pain in the ear associated with sustained tender contraction of adjacent skeletal muscles. Osteomyelitis of the mastoid bone may be associated with inflammation of the nearby periosteum as well as dura and adjacent tissues (epidural abscess)—both sources of pain in or behind the ear. Pain in this region also accompanies tumors of the acoustic nerve and inflammation and thrombosis of the lateral sinus.

The Eye as a Source of Headache. Errors of refraction (hypermetropia, astigmatism, anomalies of accommodation), disturbances of ocular muscle equilibrium, and glaucoma are universally described as causing headache. Refractive errors are also said to give origin to such other symptoms as aching of the eyes, "sandy" feeling in the eyes, pulling sensations in and about the orbit, and conjunctival congestion. Headache usually starts around and over the eyes and subsequently radiates to the occiput and back of the head.

The pain of increased intraocular pressure at first remains localized in the eyeball, then extends along the rim of the orbit and, finally, throughout most of the area supplied by the ophthalmic division of the trigeminal nerve. Nausea and vomiting sometimes accompany such headaches.

Headache accompanying various ocular disturbances is regarded as secondary to (1) sustained contraction of the intraocular muscles, which is associated with excessive accommodation effort, or (2) sustained contraction of the extraocular muscles, resulting from the effort to produce distinct retinal images, and single binocular vision with fusion. Simple myopia, per se, in contrast to the aforementioned ocular defects, does not evoke headache because the myope, in attempting to improve his vision by the contraction of his eye muscles, actually makes his vision worse and soon abandons the attempt.

With inflammation of the iris and ciliary body, light may cause intense pain in the eye and adjacent areas when the light stimulus is accompanied by movement of the inflamed iris. When the iris is immobilized, pain is allayed.

Anthony, M., Hinterberger, H., and Lance, J. W.: The possible relationship of serotonin to the migraine syndrome. Res. Clin. Stud. Headache, 2:29, 1968.
Anthony, M., and Lance, J. W.: Monoamine oxidase inhibition in the treatment of migraine. Arch. Neurol., 21:263, 1969.
Dalessio, D. J.: Wolff's Headache and Other Head Pain. 3rd ed. New York, Oxford University Press, 1972.
Vinken, P. J., and Bruyn, G. W. (eds.): Headaches and Cranial Neuralgias. Vol. 5. Handbook of Clinical Neurology. Amsterdam, North-Holland, 1968.

351. HEARING LOSS

J. R. Nelson

Approximately 3 per cent of the population suffer from hearing loss sufficiently severe to impair the understanding of speech. A new era of treatment of conductive hearing losses has recently begun with excellent surgical results from use of the operating microscope and new microsurgical techniques. Considerable help is available even to those with hereditary or congenital sensorineural losses through improved audiometric detection methods and rehabilitation programs.

Definition. The two major types of hearing loss are *conductive* losses, usually resulting from involvement of the mechanical sound transmission apparatus in the middle ear, and *sensorineural* losses, in which the cochlea, the cochlear nerve, or more central pathways are affected.

Conductive losses gradually narrow the loudness between air-conducted sounds and those produced by direct vibration of the skull (bone conduction). Discrimination of test words presented above threshold is not disturbed. The proper timing and phase relationships of various sound wave frequencies are maintained even though the mechanical oscillations from ear drum to oval window are dampened by disease processes. Simple tests for conductive hearing loss include the *Rinne test,* in which a 512 cps fork is first held against the mastoid process until the sound fades and then is placed 1 inch from the ear. With 20 to 25 db or more of conductive loss, bone conduction is superior to air conduction. A more sensitive test is the *Bing test,* in which a finger is placed in the ear just as the sound from a fork on the mastoid bone fades away. If the sound then reappears, a normal conductive mechanism is likely. The Bing phenomenon may be absent with as little as 5 db of conductive impairment. The *Weber test* involves the lateralization of sound to the diseased ear when a fork is held at midforehead or on a central incisor.

Sensorineural deafness can be due to either cochlear or retrocochlear pathology. With cochlear pathology there is a paradoxically increased response to successive increments of sound intensity. One test of this is the *recruitment* phenomenon, in which the poorest hearing ear is first determined with a low intensity tone. If a second, higher intensity sound is presented to each ear quickly and the previously poorer ear now appreciates sound best, an abnormal loudness-to-intensity gradient has been demonstrated. A similar phenomenon underlies the short increment sensitivity index test (SISI), in which, in normal hearing, small 1 db pips of sound added to a steady tone 20 db above threshold are not heard; but with cochlear damage a near-perfect reception score of such small increments is found. The illusion that a sound is of a different frequency (diplacusis) is also common. With auditory nerve (retrocochlear) lesions, nerve fatigue occurs whereby a steady tone gradually seems to fade in loudness. More than 20 to 30 db of such "tone decay" is suggestive of a retrocochlear type of sensorineural loss. The *Békésy test* involves presentation of continuous tones and interrupted tones at various frequencies. Because of tone decay, with nerve lesions the audiometric graph for continuous tones will show a greater loss than with interrupted tones when the nerve recovers between stimuli. Such recordings are rated type III or IV in contrast to the normal type I or type II response that occurs in cochlear lesions and in some normal ears. The Rinne test is normal with sensorineural loss, and the Weber test lateralizes toward the normal ear, contrasting with conductive losses.

A battery of simple audiometric tests now can differentiate the various types of deafness. Sensorineural losses can be subcategorized into cochlear and retrocochlear types with about 70 per cent or more accuracy. The

Types of Hearing Loss

	Conductive	Cochlear	Nerve	Pontine
Air > bone conduction	Reversed*	Normal	Normal	Normal
Recruitment	Absent	Present	Absent	Often present
SISI Score†	0–20%	80–100%	0–20%	0–20%
Tone decay	None	None	Present	Present
Bekesy (type)	I	I, II	III, IV	III, IV
Speech discrimination	Normal	Fair to good	Poor	Fair

*Except early, then use Bing test.
†SISI—short increment sensitivity index test (% of pips heard).

idealized findings with various sites of pathology are shown in the accompanying table.

The impedance of the middle ear can also be measured now with a relatively simple device to define abnormal patterns with drum, middle ear, and eustachian tube disfunction. Another exciting new form of testing involves direct recording of cochlear nerve action potentials from the ear drum to evaluate the integrity of the cochlea and nerve directly.

Etiology and Clinical Manifestations. *Hereditary deafness* accounts for up to half of childhood cases and up to a third of adult cases. It is usually of a sensorineural type with either dominant (10 per cent) or recessive inheritance (90 per cent). Onset is usually in childhood with bilateral involvement, but families with adult onset, mostly unilateral findings, or frequency-specific bands of loss are described. Such entities suggest selective abiotrophy ("early aging") of the cochlear neurons. In many cases there are other metabolic defects or malformations of the ear, eye, integument, skeleton, or nervous system (Konigsmark).

Nonfamilial *congenital deafness* syndromes with varying degrees of hypoplasia of the inner ear include complete failure of development of the inner ear (Michel), cochleosaccular dysgenesis (Scheibe), the most common type, and subtotal development of either the membranous labyrinth (Alexander) or the entire osseous and membranous labyrinth (Mondini), both of which may show incomplete hearing loss. These deformities may show characteristic changes on temporal bone laminagrams.

Neurotropic Infections. Both viral and bacterial infections may seriously threaten hearing from embryonic life to adulthood. Maternal German measles (rubella) accounts for at least 20 per cent of congenital deafness and produces a severe bilateral sensorineural impairment in addition to its other teratogenic effects. Reduction of this cause should follow the wide use of the vaccine now available. Only slightly less prevalent are cases of severe postmeningitic hearing loss. The incidence has decreased since the antimicrobial era, but unfortunately it is still all too common in infants and young children. Prematurity probably predisposes to this cause and is an important, poorly understood cause of deafness itself.

Certain cases of sudden, unilateral sensorineural hearing loss are associated with viral upper respiratory infections and produce "cochleitis" with a profound loss, which may be due to direct inflammation or vascular involvement. Some otologists advocate emergency treatment with intravenous histamine for vasodilatation and low molecular weight dextran to reduce blood viscosity.

The rate of recovery may be enhanced, but controlled studies are still needed to clarify this point. Mumps is a well recognized cause of unilateral sensorineural deafness, and vestibular involvement may also occur. Other common childhood viral illnesses may occasionally produce hearing loss. Herpes zoster may simultaneously affect the eighth nerve and geniculate ganglion to produce deafness, vertigo, and facial palsy (Ramsay Hunt syndrome) in addition to ear or throat pain and vesicles. The syndrome of sudden unilateral deafness may also be caused by rupture of the round or oval window membranes with coughing, straining, or other unusual pressure gradients between inner and middle ear. Such perilymph fistulas also cause dizziness, and explorations of the ear may reveal a surgically repairable leak (Goodhill).

Otologic syphilis deserves special mention, because a young adult who may have been sucessfully treated for congenital syphilis may still develop late inflammatory changes of recurrent interstitial keratitis, joint effusion (Clutton's joints), and fluctuating progressive sensorineural hearing loss and vertigo. Eventual total deafness is the rule. A low-tone hearing loss is common early, as with Meniere's disease, but explosive total deafness in one ear suggestive of internal auditory artery occlusion may occur. Such inner ear manifestations may appear even in the absence of a positive VDRL in the blood or serum, and more sensitive tests such as the FTA-ABS test may be required. Some authorities believe that all cases of "bilateral Meniere's" should be considered syphilitic until proved otherwise. Softening of the capsular bone about the oval window occurs so that the stapes moves excessively, but only in an outward direction. This provides the basis for *Hennebert's sign,* which is a positive fistula test (vertigo with middle-ear pressure changes) that occurs only with negative suction applied with a pneumatic otoscope. These cases raise the possibility that treatment failure rather than autoimmune responses or late fibrotic reactions accounts for the late-life damage to the ear. Recent evidence suggests that long-term cortisone treatment may partially reverse or halt the progression of deafness and vertigo. Some authorities also recommend intensive retreatment with oral ampicillin, 1.5 grams, and probenecid, 0.5 gram, four times per day for up to four to five weeks.

Otosclerosis. Otosclerosis is a very common cause of hearing loss in Caucasian adults, and is usually inherited as a dominant trait with up to 40 per cent penetrance. Pathologically, the process consists of an overgrowth of labyrinthine capsular bone around the oval window which leads to progressive fixation of the stapes. Hearing loss begins insidiously in early adult life, with slow progression. Pregnancy may accelerate the condition in females. The audiometric findings in far-advanced cases may be misleading with poor reliability about the amount of sensorineural loss. Careful correlation with tuning fork results is essential. Some patients with no measurable hearing loss by audiometry may still have partial recovery after surgery to the point that use of an aid allows serviceable hearing. The surgical treatment of otosclerosis has developed rapidly in the past 25 years with successive adoption of horizontal canal fenestration, stapes mobilization by fracture, and finally stapedectomy with replacement by Teflon plugs, steel pistons, or wire prostheses that bridge the gap between the incus and a new membrane on the oval window that forms over a fascia or Gelfoam graft. Good to excellent long-lasting results occur in over 90 per cent of cases. Some evidence suggests that administration of 25 to 60 mg of sodium fluoride per day for a year may halt the progression of otosclerosis.

A poorly understood sensorineural component often is seen in longstanding cases, probably owing to involvement of the otic capsule of the cochlea.

Middle Ear Infections. Antimicrobial drugs have not entirely eliminated suppurative otitis media, particularly chronic forms, although acute attacks usually respond to the drugs and to myringotomy. Once chronic drainage and infection have been arrested, several reconstructive surgical procedures are possible even though extensive destruction of middle ear structures has occurred. Modified radical mastoidectomy with tympanoplasty may improve function of the middle ear conductive mechanism. Numerous grafting and artificial prosthetic replacement techniques are available. Recurrent cholesteatoma formation represents a special challenge, as these imbedded epithelial fragments may grow to cause extensive destruction of the middle ear and temporal bone.

Chronic serous otitis media is the most common cause of chronic conductive hearing loss in children. A predisposing factor may be poor eustachian tube function from edema secondary to allergy, inflammation, large lymphoid follicles, large adenoids, or a congenitally small lumen. Insertion of a polyethylene tube in the tympanic membrane for several weeks may allow external drainage, equalize the middle ear pressure, and restore hearing while the eustachian tube hopefully regains its patency.

Traumatic Hearing Loss. There are two major types of temporal bone fractures that may be associated with hearing loss. With a longitudinal fracture along the axis of the petrous pyramid, damage to the inner ear is usually slight, but bleeding from the ear and disruption of the middle ear bones are common and may require surgical repair at a later date. In contrast, transverse fractures perpendicular to the petrous pyramid may cause severe inner ear damage and facial palsy. If facial paralysis is immediate, surgical exploration is mandatory.

Noise-induced acoustic trauma is an important cause of hearing loss in industrial settings, but exposure to gun blasts, airplane engines, and even rock and roll music may cause progressive high tone sensorineural hearing loss. Certain individuals are much more sensitive to acoustic trauma and must be protected with ear molds or protective ear covers if it is necessary to work in high noise levels. The magnitude of this problem is great, and

has been often neglected in spite of advances in prevention.

Meniere's Disease. Although the episodic attacks of vertigo are more disabling, a fluctuating low-tone "cochlear" hearing loss with eventual involvement of other frequencies is common. This condition and acoustic neuroma, which also produces unilateral tinnitus, deafness, and vertigo, are more fully discussed in Ch. 352.

Ototoxic Drugs. Many antimicrobials, mostly when administered by injection, may cause severe cochlear damage. Dihydrostreptomycin fortunately has been removed from use; streptomycin causes semicircular canal and utricular damage with relative sparing of the cochlea and saccule. Other drugs which may cause deafness when blood concentration is high because of large dosage or renal failure are neomycin, kanamycin, vancomycin, gentamicin, ristocetin, ethacrynic acid, furosemide, and quinine. Use of such drugs should be carefully considered, particularly in patients with renal failure.

Central Causes of Deafness. In order to markedly raise the threshold for hearing with central involvement, bilateral damage of the pontine projections or higher centers is required. Other signs of cranial nerve involvement and sensory and motor pathway damage should be sought. Lesions at the cortical level produce complex aphasic impairments, and are beyond the scope of this chapter.

Rehabilitation of the Hard of Hearing. The education of the deaf child and the assistance needed by all hard of hearing persons is a task requiring skilled efforts by the physician, audiologist, and teacher. Selection of hearing aids must not be made before a full professional evaluation reveals the exact cause of the hearing problem.

Davis, H., and Silverman, S. R. (eds.): Hearing and Deafness. 3rd ed. New York, Holt, Rinehart and Winston, 1970.

Goodhill, V., et al.: Sudden deafness and labyrinthine window ruptures. Ann. Otol., 82:2, 1973.

Hardy, D. B.: Fetal consequences of maternal viral infections in pregnancy. Arch. Otolaryngol., 98:218, 1973.

Jerger, J.: Review of diagnostic audiometry. Ann. Otol., 77:1042, 1968.

Jerger, J.: Clinical experience with impedance audiometry. Arch. Otolaryngol., 92:34, 1970.

Konigsmark, B. W.: Hereditary deafness in man. N. Engl. J. Med., 281:713, 1969.

Patterson, M. E.: Congenital luetic hearing impairment. Arch. Otolaryngol., 87:70, 1968.

Pulec, J. L. (ed.): Meniere's Disease. Philadelphia, W. B. Saunders Company, 1968.

Saunders, W. H.: Sudden deafness and its several treatments. Laryngoscope, 72:1206, 1972.

Shambaugh, G. E., Jr.: The diagnosis and treatment of active cochlear otosclerosis. J. Laryngol. Otol., 85:301, 1971.

Sheehy, J. L., Gardner, G., Jr., and Hambley, W. M.: Tuning fork tests in modern otology. Arch. Otolaryngol., 94:132, 1971.

352. DIZZINESS AND VERTIGO

David A. Drachman

THE COMPLAINT OF DIZZINESS

As a *complaint* rather than a *disease*, the term "dizziness" appropriately includes almost any sensation that a patient chooses to call by that name. By usage the term is applied to a number of uncommon sensations that are *not* part of daily experience. It is the thread of unfamiliar spatial disorientation that appears to bind these complaints together. When one listens carefully to a large number of "dizzy" patients, it is possible to sort their complaints into four types: a *rotational sensation, impending faint, dysequilibrium,* and *vague lightheadedness.*

Type I dizziness is a *definite rotational sensation* (vertigo) in which the patient feels that either he or the environment is spinning. Violent vertigo is often accompanied by nausea, vomiting, and a staggering gait. Oscillopsia—a visual hallucination of to-and-fro movement of the environment—may occur. The onset of vertigo is often instantaneous, and patients sometimes describe a sensation of being hurled to the ground. Although full-blown vertigo is unmistakable, with milder forms the patient may describe only a rocking sensation or vague lightheadedness. Recognition of mild vertiginous episodes is often aided by testing with the dizziness simulation battery described below.

Whenever the patient's dizziness is exclusively rotational, it is due to a disorder of the vestibular system: either the peripheral labyrinth or its central connections. Because of this close relationship, it is important to separate definite rotational vertigo accurately from other types of dizziness.

Type II dizziness is a *sensation of impending faint or loss of consciousness.* Pallor, dimness of vision, roaring in the ears, and diaphoresis, with recovery upon assuming the recumbent position, are common. Type II dizziness of cardiovascular origin is of abrupt onset and short duration. When faintness is gradual in onset or of longer duration, the relationship of the episodes to hypoglycemia should be sought.

The complaint of impending faint usually implies an inadequate supply of blood or nutrients to the entire brain, such as occurs in postural hypotension. It is not a feature of *focal* cerebral ischemia, although this mistaken impression is widely subscribed to by physicians.

Type III dizziness is *dysequilibrium:* the loss of balance *without* an abnormal sensation in the head. This experience occurs only when the patient is walking; it disappears as soon as he sits down. It is due to a disorder of motor system control.

Type IV dizziness is *vague lightheadedness* other than vertigo, faintness, or dysequilibrium. This designation includes dizziness that cannot be identified with certainty as any of the other types. When patients complain of lightheadedness, *fractional* or *poorly described* symptoms of vertigo, faintness, or dysequilibrium must first be looked for, e.g., a rocking sensation instead of spinning. Evidence of *hyperventilation* symptoms should next be sought, as well as symptoms pointing to a *psychiatric disorder,* particularly depression or anxiety. Finally, the evidence for *multiple sensory impairment* should be examined, especially a history of peripheral neuropathy, cervical spondylosis, or cataract surgery in an elderly or diabetic patient.

EVALUATING THE DIZZY PATIENT

The *history* must explore four major questions that critically distinguish the disorders producing dizziness: (1) the type of dizziness (I to IV) experienced by the patient; (2) the *abruptness* of attacks or *continuity* of symptoms; (3) the relation or independence of dizziness to

position or motion (standing/sitting/lying; sudden change in position; walking); and (4) the *age* of the patient. The relation of these data to differential diagnosis will be discussed with specific entities.

A neurologic examination allows the distinction between central and peripheral causes of dizziness, and may reveal certain *patterns* of involvement that point to the diagnosis: e.g., brainstem syndrome (hemiplegia alternans), cerebellopontine angle syndrome, multiple sensory impairment.

The dizziness simulation battery is a series of eight bedside maneuvers that have proved valuable in distinguishing the various types of dizziness. Some produce dizziness in all patients, whereas others induce it only in patients with underlying disorders. After each maneuver the patient is questioned as to the similarity of the test-evoked sensation to his own dizziness. Identification of a provoked sensation as identical to the patient's dizziness is often more reliable than a verbal description, particularly if a single maneuver exclusively reproduces his symptoms.

1. *Orthostatic hypotension:* Blood pressure is measured supine, immediately on standing, and after three minutes.
2. *Potentiated Valsalva maneuver:* The patient squats for 30 seconds, then stands and blows into a mercury sphygmomanometer, raising the column to 40 mm Hg for 15 seconds.
3. *Carotid sinus stimulation:* The carotid sinus is unilaterally massaged for 15 seconds without continuous compression of the artery. ECG monitoring is required in the elderly, and the test should be omitted in patients with known cardiac disease.
4. *Neck-twist:* The patient rotates his head in each direction for 15 seconds as if watching an airplane fly past. Dizziness may result from "kinking" of a vertebral artery, cervicogenic dizziness, or a vestibular disorder.
5. *Walking and turning:* The patient walks in one direction and then quickly turns, reversing direction. This test reproduces dizziness occurring with multisensory deficits, gait apraxia, and disorders of balance.
6. *Hyperventilation:* The patient breathes deeply for three minutes.
7. *Nylen-Bárány maneuver:* The examiner carries the patient's head backward from a seated position, so that it is hanging 45 degrees below the horizontal and turned 45 degrees to one side. Vertigo *accompanied by nystagmus* indicates positional vertigo. The characteristics distinguishing a "benign" from a "malignant" form of this condition are listed in Table 1.
8. *Bárány rotation:* The patient is seated in a rotating chair, head tilted 30 degrees forward from the vertical. The examiner spins the patient in one direction ten times within 20 seconds, then abruptly stops the rotation.

Laboratory Tests (Table 2). *Caloric testing* can identify disorders of the labyrinth, vestibular nerve, and central vestibular connections. The patient is positioned so that the horizontal semicircular canals are exactly vertical, and each ear is irrigated with cool (30° C) and warm (44° C) water to produce convection flow of endolymph, which mimics rotational stimulation of each canal. Observations of the amplitude, speed, and duration of the ocular deviation and nystagmus generated by this test provide information on the function of the vestibular apparatus.

Audiometric studies are used to evaluate lesions of the middle ear, labyrinth, and cochlear nerve, particularly in Meniere's disorder and cerebellopontine angle tumors. Routine pure tone audiometry indicates the presence or absence of a hearing loss and may also distinguish banal causes (acoustic trauma, aging, otosclerosis) from specific cochlear and nerve disorders. More elaborate testing, including the short increment sensitivity index

TABLE 1. Positional Vertigo

Benign	Central or Malignant
1. Latency of onset of vertigo and nystagmus	1. Immediate onset of vertigo and nystagmus
2. Adaptation and fatigue of vertigo and nystagmus	2. Persistence of nystagmus
3. Direction-fixed nystagmus	3. Direction-changing nystagmus
4. Severe vertigo and systemic symptoms	4. Mild vertigo; few systemic symptoms

TABLE 2. Laboratory Tests in Dizziness

1. Caloric testing with electro-nystagmography (ENG)	6. Electrocardiogram with rhythm strip
2. Audiometry	7. Serum protein electrophoresis
3. Psychometric testing (MMPI)	8. Thyroid function studies
4. Skull x-rays with Stenvers' views	9. Electroencephalography
5. Cervical spine x-rays	10. Five-hour glucose tolerance test
	Optional: Petrous polytomography 24-hour cardiac monitoring

(SISI), speech discrimination, Békésy, and threshold tone decay tests, improves the accuracy of diagnosis.

SPECIFIC CONDITIONS PRODUCING DIZZINESS

It is not always simple to assemble the clinical and laboratory findings obtained from a dizzy patient into a specific diagnostic entity. A classification is provided here of the causes of dizziness, designed to parallel the four major complaints described earlier.

Vertigo and Other Vestibular Disorders

Vertigo accounts for only about a third of complaints of dizzy patients. When patients present with vestibular disorders, it is most important to distinguish between *peripheral* (labyrinthine) abnormalities and those involving *central* vestibular connections. The key to this distinction is the evidence for or against involvement of neighboring brainstem structures.

Peripheral Causes of Vertigo. *Benign Positional Vertigo.* Benign positional vertigo is probably the most frequent cause of vertigo, accounting for about 25 per cent of patients with this complaint. The patient experiences a sensation of spinning when he rolls over in bed or makes other sudden head movements. Symptoms are greatest when he lies on his side with the affected ear underneath. The vertigo, sometimes accompanied by nausea and vomiting, lasts for less than five minutes, and between episodes the patient is free of symptoms. This condition, brought about *only* on change of position, differs from other vestibular disorders in which vertigo is increased by head motion but is present at other times as well. Benign positional vertigo occurs at any time during adult years; the cause is usually obscure, although it occasionally follows head trauma. The diagnosis is based on the typical history and on finding the "benign" type of vertigo and nystagmus on performing the Nylen-Bárány maneuver (Table 1). Caloric testing reveals depressed labyrinthine function in one ear in about half the patients. In the majority of cases symptoms persist for several weeks, although bouts may recur over a span of years with prolonged symptom-free intervals. This condition must be distinguished from "malignant positional vertigo" (Table 1), which occurs with lesions (tumors, infarcts) involving posterior fossa structures; benign positional vertigo is only rarely associated with such conditions.

Acute Peripheral Vestibulopathy ("Acute Labyrinthitis"; "Vestibular Neuronitis"). This condition is defined as a single bout of spontaneous vertigo, lasting for hours or days. Attacks occasionally follow a trivial respiratory or other infection, but the relation is not clear. Symptoms of vertigo, nausea, and vomiting usually im-

prove within 48 hours, but may persist for 7 to 14 days. On examination the patient appears acutely ill, often pale and diaphoretic, resisting motion of the head. Nystagmus invariably accompanies the vertigo. As the patient recovers, he may feel "off balance" for weeks or months owing to unilateral impairment of vestibular function, present in about 50 per cent of patients. Hearing is not impaired in this condition.

Acute and Recurrent Peripheral Vestibulopathy. Acute and recurrent peripheral vestibulopathy is clinically similar to the entity described above, but consists of *repeated* bouts of vertigo occurring over a period of months or years. This condition occurs in an older age group than acute peripheral vestibulopathy, and is associated with *less* severe vestibular impairment on caloric testing. Approximately half the patients presenting with a single attack of peripheral vestibulopathy experience a recurrence, linking this with the previous condition. The absence of auditory impairment distinguishes this condition from Meniere's disorder.

Meniere's Disorder. Meniere's disorder is widely considered to be one of the most frequent causes of dizziness, but it actually accounts for only about 5 per cent of all dizziness and 10 to 15 per cent of vertigo. It usually occurs in adults and consists of recurring bouts of vertigo associated with *hearing loss* and *tinnitus* which may precede or follow the first bout of vertigo. Patients often complain of "fullness" in the ears, and are sometimes aware of *recruitment* as a sensation of auditory discomfort produced by loud noises. Bouts of vertigo last from hours to days, recurring as often as every week or as infrequently as every ten years. Hearing loss is unilateral in 80 to 90 per cent of patients, with a severe deficit in half the patients. Most patients develop chronic impairment of vestibular function, resulting in the syndrome of vestibular imbalance. In many patients the recurrent episodes of vertigo may "burn out" over the years.

Diagnosis depends on the characteristic history and the audiometric findings (low frequency pure tone impairment, poor speech discrimination comparable to the pure tone hearing loss, and recruitment). Caloric testing demonstrates abnormal vestibular function in 80 per cent of patients.

Pathologic studies have identified distention of the membranous labyrinth with endolymph as the immediate cause of this condition, but the explanation for the excess of endolymph remains obscure.

Toxic Damage to the Labyrinths. Drugs of the aminoglycoside group (e.g., streptomycin) may produce toxic damage to the labyrinths and possibly the eighth nerve. Although toxicity is generally dose related, some patients develop labyrinthine damage after brief treatment with ordinary doses of these drugs, particularly if renal function is impaired. Tinnitus, hearing loss, or vertigo may be the presenting symptom, along with severe impairment of balance, nausea, and vomiting. Vertigo continues for days or weeks. If the ototoxic drug is immediately discontinued, damage to the labyrinth is usually arrested. A characteristic loss of balance follows the acute stage of vertigo and may include blurring of vision on motion owing to loss of the vestibulo-ocular reflexes. With the loss of vestibular sensation, these patients are dependent on visual cues and are unable to walk in the dark. After several months, adaptation to the loss of vestibular sensation develops, and many can lead fairly normal lives.

Diagnosis is based on the history of treatment with one of the ototoxic drugs, followed by the sequence described above. On examination the Romberg test is abnormal. Caloric tests demonstrate bilateral severe hypoactivity of the labyrinths. Bárány rotation may fail to elicit vertigo or nystagmus.

Other Peripheral Causes of Vertigo. Head trauma may be followed by persistent or positional vertigo. Dislocation of the otoliths from the macula of the utricle has been proposed as a cause of this condition. When vertigo immediately follows trauma, the etiologic relationship is clear, but in cases with medicolegal implications vertigo (and other forms of dizziness) may follow head trauma after a lengthy delay. It is often stated that the termination of pending litigation resolves such cases. *Cervicogenic vertigo,* although not vestibular in origin, may present with similar manifestations. Since the articulations and musculature of the cervical region provide extensive input to the brainstem vestibular system, cervical spondylosis or even painful muscular contraction may result in vertigo, nausea, and vomiting. *Dysproteinemias, hypothyroidism,* and *otitis media* are other occasional causes of vertigo.

Treatment. Management of vertigo resulting from most peripheral vestibular disorders is similar. When vertigo is severely disabling, the patient should be placed at bed rest or, in persistent cases, hospitalized. Meclizine, 25 mg four times daily, is of value in suppressing labyrinthine hyperactivity. Atropine tablets, 0.4 mg sublingually at the onset of attacks of vertigo, may abort the development of symptoms. Nausea and vomiting are controlled by trimethobenzamide hydrochloride (Tigan) suppositories, 200 mg every six hours, or in resistant cases by parenteral phenothiazines such as chlorpromazine (Thorazine), 25 mg every six hours. Mild tranquilizers such as diazepam (Valium), 5 mg orally, help control the anxiety that often accompanies vertigo.

Patients with benign positional vertigo may benefit from a soft foam rubber collar that limits cervical motion, thus preventing the stimulus for attacks.

Many patients with peripheral vestibular disorders have residual labyrinthine deficits after the acute vertiginous phase, and benefit from measures to improve their balance. A foam rubber collar is useful to limit neck motion, and methylphenidate (Ritalin) may enable them to react more quickly to the remaining sensory modalities. Balancing exercises help patients to adapt to ambulation in the absence of normal vestibular function.

The treatment of acute attacks of Meniere's disorder is similar to that for other vestibular disorders. A variety of medical and surgical treatments to prevent recurrences of vertigo and/or deterioration of hearing have been proposed; a discussion of their application and merits is beyond the scope of this chapter.

Central Causes of Vertigo. *Cerebrovascular Disease.* Cerebrovascular disease produces vertigo when basilar-vertebral artery ischemia damages the vestibular nuclei or their connections. In virtually all cases injury to adjacent brainstem structures occurs, and vertigo is unlikely to be due to a stroke when other neurologic symptoms or signs are absent. As with other patterns of cerebrovascular disease, elderly hypertensive patients with diabetes, heart disease, or hyperlipidemia are the most likely candidates. Caloric testing may help in the diagnosis by providing evidence of central vestibular involvement.

Transient ischemic attacks may be particularly difficult to diagnose, because at the time of examination the patient may have recovered completely. A reliable history of additional brainstem symptoms is necessary to establish the diagnosis.

The treatment of cerebrovascular disease is discussed in detail elsewhere. Transient ischemia in the basilar-vertebral distribution is a recognized indication for anticoagulation. The role of aspirin, dipyridamole (Persantine) and other agents that affect platelet function is not yet firmly established, but a trial of these relatively safe agents may be justified in those patients in whom differentiation of brainstem ischemia from peripheral vestibulopathy is uncertain.

Multiple Sclerosis. Multiple sclerosis may produce vertigo in young patients, although this condition accounts for no more than 5 to 10 per cent of acute vertigo in those below age 40. Further, although multiple sclerosis may begin with vertigo, this is far less common than onset with optic neuritis or paresthesias. The diagnosis is discussed elsewhere; one must be aware that vertigo associated with ocular motor disorders that cannot be caused by purely peripheral vestibular disease (e.g., persistent diplopia, median longitudinal fasciculus syndrome, ophthalmoplegia) is strongly suggestive of this condition.

Treatment of the vertigo is similar to that for peripheral vestibulopathies; meclizine, atropine, and Tigan are of value in controlling the vertigo and its associated nausea and vomiting.

Cerebellopontine Angle Tumors. Cerebellopontine angle tumors are a *rare* cause of vertigo, but must not be overlooked early in their growth when they are readily removable. The large majority are benign acoustic neuromas arising in the internal auditory meatus. These tumors develop in middle-aged patients who experience vague unsteadiness that progresses over a period of years. Vertigo when present may be of the "malignant" positional type (Table 1), and only rarely does acute spontaneous vertigo occur. Hearing loss, tinnitus, facial numbness or weakness, cerebellar ataxia, and occasional dementia complete the picture. Unilateral or bilateral acoustic neuromas are especially common in von Recklinghausen's disease (neurofibromatosis).

On caloric testing there is a markedly diminished response on the affected side. Audiometry demonstrates the findings of a "retrocochlear" lesion, including rapid tone decay and a Type III or IV curve on Békésy audiometry. Roentgenograms of the petrous bones are diagnostic and show erosion of the affected internal auditory meatus, a finding that is seen even earlier on polycyclic tomography.

Vertiginous Migraine. Vertiginous migraine may occur preceding the headache, during the headache phase, or as a "migraine equivalent" in place of the headache. Since both migraine and vertigo are common conditions, the occurrence of vertigo without a constant time relation to headache may represent only a coincidence in some unfortunate patients. Treatment is directed at prevention of the migraine attacks and control of the symptoms of vertigo, nausea, and vomiting as outlined above.

Viral Infections. Viral infections rarely cause vertigo except when herpes zoster affects the eighth nerve, often in conjunction with the Ramsay Hunt syndrome or geniculate herpes. Facial paralysis, vertigo, and hearing loss occur with herpetic vesicular lesions in the external auditory canal. Lymphocytes and polymorphonuclear leukocytes may be found in the cerebrospinal fluid. The diagnosis is established by demonstrating a rise of antibody titers to herpes zoster. Pathologically, lymphocytic infiltration of the sensory ganglia and nerve roots is seen. Treatment consists of the use of prednisone during the acute phase of the illness and the management of the vertigo, nausea, and vomiting as outlined above.

Vestibular Disorders Not Producing Vertigo. In some patients *hypoactivity* of the labyrinths may occur without antecedent episodes of vertigo. These patients describe lightheadedness on walking, turning, or changing position. The exact cause of the conditions producing these disorders is obscure. With *hyperactive* labyrinths, most often seen in anxious patients, instantaneous vertigo or loss of balance occurs on rapid turning. Caloric testing confirms the abnormal responsiveness of the labyrinths in either case. Patients with hypoactive or asymmetrical labyrinthine function benefit from methylphenidate (Ritalin), head restraint with a foam rubber collar, and a course of balancing exercises. Patients with hyperactive labyrinths are treated with meclizine, 25 mg three times daily.

Faintness: Syncopal and Seizure Disorders

Syncopal Disorders (see also Ch. 353). *Orthostatic Hypotension.* In orthostatic hypotension the patient experiences faintness upon standing, resulting from a fall in blood pressure (at least 25/15 mm Hg). Acquired and idiopathic varieties are described. In the closely related Shy-Drager syndrome (see Ch. 377), manifestations of parkinsonism, peripheral neuropathy, dementia, and cerebellar abnormalities contribute to a multifactorial problem of dizziness.

Cardiac Arrhythmias. Patients with brief dizziness caused by episodic cardiac arrhythmias are often unaware of palpitations and complain only of faintness. When the arrhythmia is constantly present, it is easily recognized by auscultation or electrocardiography. With infrequent runs of abnormal heart rhythm, the use of 12- or 24-hour ambulatory electrocardiographic monitoring is necessary.

Carotid Sinus Hypersensitivity. Carotid sinus hypersensitivity resulting in bradycardia or temporary asystole may also present with Type II dizziness. The dizziness occurs abruptly and disappears rapidly, lasting no more than 15 seconds. The diagnosis is established by reproduction of symptoms with cautious carotid massage.

Vasovagal Syncope. Vasovagal syncope causes confusion with other forms of dizziness when the patient experiences faintness rather than actual loss of consciousness. The tendency to occur in young adults, the relation to precipitating emotional factors, the appearance of pallor at the onset, and the short duration are characteristic.

Cough, Micturition Syncope. Some patients experience faintness upon coughing or, with males, upon micturating while standing. The exact temporal relationship of faintness (or loss of consciousness) to these acts is diagnostic; the reproduction of symptoms by a potentiated Valsalva maneuver confirms the mechanism.

Seizure Disorders. Patients with temporal lobe seizures may describe feelings of "remoteness," "unreality," or, rarely, vertigo. When these events precede a typical psychomotor or generalized seizure, the cause is clearly *epileptic dizziness*. When the dizziness occurs as an iso-lated seizure phenomenon, it presents a diagnostic problem. Such patients *rarely* complain primarily of dizziness, however, because the epileptic phenomena dominate the picture.

Very rarely labyrinthine-induced vertigo may trigger "vestibulogenic epilepsy," a form of reflex seizure akin to reading epilepsy. If caloric testing is carried out while an electroencephalogram is taken, the observation of induced seizure activity establishes the diagnosis.

The reader is cautioned against diagnosing seizure disorders in patients whose dizziness is accompanied by mild abnormalities on electroencephalography without the other criteria mentioned.

Dysequilibrium: Impaired Balance

Bruns' Apraxia of Gait. This is a little-recognized but common disorder of the elderly. The patient walks with a broad-based gait, taking short steps and placing his feet flat on the ground, suggesting a person walking on ice. A tendency to retropulsion increases the danger of falling. On examination, motor power, coordination, and sensation are normal in the legs, although the gait is impaired and hopping on one foot is impossible. The finding of "frontal lobe" deficits, including dementia, grasp and suck reflexes is confirmatory. Most cases of Bruns' apraxia result from a degenerative process similar to Alzheimer's disease. Other causes include such conditions as subdural hematomas, tumors, normal pressure hydrocephalus, or a lacunar state.

When a specific disorder (e.g., a subdural hematoma) is found, treatment is directed toward that condition. In the more common degenerative conditions treatment must be symptomatic. In some patients surprisingly good improvement may result from small doses of L-dopa (1.5 to 3.0 grams per day in divided doses). Mild stimulants (methylphenidate), balancing exercises, and a cane are of benefit, and patients should be encouraged to walk some distance *every day* to avoid lapsing into total dependence.

Parkinsonism. It is not uncommon for patients with parkinsonism and a balance disturbance to complain of dysequilibrium. When tremor is minimal and impaired balance is prominent, it is difficult to distinguish between parkinsonism and gait apraxia. These patients often have a pronounced increase in axial tone, as well as frontal lobe signs and dementia. Treatment is described in Ch. 365.

Cerebellar Lesions. Impairment of balance without other cerebellar signs may be seen in certain cerebellar lesions such as alcoholic cerebellar degeneration or tumors of the vermis. In addition some patients may develop "malignant" positional vertigo. Since a staggering gait and nystagmus are seen in peripheral vestibular disorders, the clinical distinction presents difficulties. Neurodiagnostic studies (radioisotope scan, computerized axial tomography, angiography) may be required to establish the diagnosis.

Astasia-Abasia. Astasia-abasia is impairment of stance and gait on a purely psychiatric basis. In some patients the gait is quite bizarre, but in others it may resemble Bruns' apraxia. The distinction depends on the absence of other frontal lobe signs and on the ability of the patient to walk *normally* under some circumstances, such as only indoors. Other evidence of a phobic or conversion reaction is often present.

Lightheadedness

Vague "lightheadedness" accounts for over 50 per cent of patients' complaints, and includes the largest spectrum of disorders.

Inevitably, some patients provide a *poor description of other types of dizziness* which more introspective or articulate patients would recognize as vertigo, faintness, or dysequilibrium. In addition, *fractional forms of other types of dizziness* are often described as "lightheadedness" even by observant patients. Almost half the patients who initially experience vertigo later complain of lightheadedness as their symptoms subside. The dizziness simulation battery helps to *identify* a sensation which the patient cannot easily *describe* verbally.

Hyperventilation. This is the second most common cause of dizziness after vestibular disorders, and the most common under the age of 40. The disorder is discussed in detail in Ch. 354. In the acute form, young, anxious patients present with brief episodes of shortness of breath, lightheadedness, paresthesias in the fingers and around the mouth, and feelings of panic. More difficult to identify is chronic hyperventilation, seen in patients who periodically sigh deeply. Both forms are recognized by the precise reproduction of symptoms during intentional hyperventilation, but no other maneuver in the dizziness simulation battery reproduces the complaint.

The mechanism of hyperventilation-induced dizziness is presumed to be hypocapnia with secondary cerebral arterial constriction and diminished cerebral blood flow. Treatment of acute attacks with diazepam (Valium), 5 to 10 mg intramuscularly, is often effective.

Multisensory Dizziness. When several sensory modalities are impaired, perception of the environment becomes inadequate to maintain orientation, and the patient experiences dizziness when attempting to walk. The most common combinations of sensory impairment are peripheral neuropathy (with diminished touch, pressure, and proprioceptive sensation), visual loss from cataracts, and cervical spondylosis (with distortion of proprioception from cervical joints). Impaired vestibular and auditory function often add to the sensory disorientation. The aged and diabetic are especially prone to this condition. Patients with multisensory dizziness adopt a broad-based tentative gait, which may superficially resemble Bruns' apraxia of gait, but the "frontal lobe" features are absent. Examination reveals the underlying neurosensory deficit — peripheral neuropathy, visual impairment, cervical arthritis, and hearing loss. Caloric testing may provide evidence of additional sensory impairment. When all five sensory modalities are severely impaired, patients may be unable to walk without assistance.

An important example of this condition is seen in the post-cataract-extraction patient who complains of disabling dizziness despite perfect restoration of visual acuity. Dizziness results from the distortion produced by the corrective lenses used after surgery. Patients who have no other sensory deficits are able to compensate for the visual distortions, but those with peripheral neuropathy cannot. Contact lenses eliminate these distortions, but unfortunately many elderly patients cannot manage them.

Treatment of multisensory dizziness includes balancing exercises and use of a foam rubber collar to eliminate extraneous head motion. A light cane should be used for balance. Methylphenidate (Ritalin) improves the speed of the patient's response to his perceived environment.

Psychiatric Disorders. In addition to patients with astasia-abasia or hyperventilation, some patients experience subjective dizziness on the basis of purely psychiatric disease. Some indicate that their dizziness consists of "difficulty concentrating"; others experience panic states when in crowded places; whereas some frankly psychotic patients describe the bizarre confusion of their perceived environments as "dizziness" for lack of a more explicit term.

In these patients, the diagnosis hinges on elimination of other causes of dizziness combined with evidence of significant psychiatric disease on interview or psychometric testing. It is often useful to demonstrate to such patients the negative findings on extensive tests for organic causes of dizziness, and to assure them that no cause has been overlooked.

Drachman, D. A.: Episodic vertigo. *In* Conn, H. (ed.): Current Therapy 1974. Philadelphia, W. B. Saunders Company, 1974, p. 684.

Drachman, D. A., and Hart, C. W.: An approach to the dizzy patient. Neurology, 22:323, 1972.

Fisher, C. M.: Vertigo in cerebrovascular disease. Arch. Otolaryngol., 85:529, 1967.

Harrison, M. S., and Ozsahinoglu, C.: Positional vertigo: Aetiology and clinical significance. Brain, 95:369, 1972.

Hart, C. W.: The evaluation of vestibular function in health and disease. *In* Otolaryngology. Vol. 1, Chap. 10. Hagerstown, Md., Harper & Row, 1972.

Pulec, J. (ed.): Meniere's Disease. Philadelphia, W. B. Saunders Company, 1968.

353. SYNCOPE

Albert Heyman

Definition. Syncope is the cutting off or transient loss of consciousness. Although the term is usually applied to unconsciousness caused by a temporary decrease in cerebral blood flow, in this discussion a broader definition is employed that includes the brief disturbances in consciousness caused by changes in the chemical composition of the blood as in hyperventilation or hypoglycemia. Syncope is extremely common; in fact, it has been found to occur in as many as 25 to 30 per cent of young, healthy adult males. It should be carefully differentiated from such disorders as epilepsy, vertigo, cataplexy, and strokes, all of which may produce transient disturbances in consciousness, generalized weakness, or inability to stand erect. The loss of consciousness in syncope may not be complete, but may consist of varying degrees of impaired sensorium with transient blurring of vision, weakness, and loss of postural tone. Such attacks may be described by the patient as dizziness, faintness, lightheadedness, or a "drunk feeling." These partial manifestations have the rapid onset, brief duration, and complete recovery characteristic of the fully developed faint.

Pathogenesis. Syncope is most frequently caused by a reduction in cerebral blood flow below a critical level and is usually associated with a sharp fall in blood pressure. This, in turn, is the result of either a loss of peripheral resistance, as seen in vasodepressor faint and in orthostatic hypotension, or a decrease in cardiac output, as in Adams-Stokes attacks. In many patients, however, loss of consciousness is not caused by reduction of blood pressure but by a decrease in such essential blood components as glucose, carbon dioxide, or oxygen. In other instances, as in micturition syncope and cough syncope, the faint seems to result from cerebral ischemia caused by extracardiac disturbances.

There are several features common to almost all types of syncope. Electroencephalographic changes usually appear, and consist of high voltage, 2- to 4-cycle per second slow waves that promptly return to normal after consciousness is regained. Convulsive movements, such as tonic or clonic contractions of the arms or turning of the head, can occur in all types of fainting, depending on the degree and duration of the cerebral ischemia. Fully developed seizures with tongue biting and urinary incontinence, however, are unusual. Recovery is usually hastened in the recumbent posture, which helps restore the normal cerebral circulation. The critical level of cerebral blood flow necessary to maintain consciousness has been estimated to be about 30 ml per 100 grams of brain per minute (normal value is 50 to 55 ml). The duration of asystole or the degree of hypotension necessary to produce critical levels of cerebral ischemia varies, depending upon the posture of the patient, the ability of the cerebral vessels to dilate, and other factors. In normal subjects in the erect posture, a mean arterial blood pressure as low as 20 to 30 mm of mercury or an asystole of four or five seconds' duration is necessary to produce syncope. In the recumbent position, longer periods of asystole may occur before loss of consciousness develops.

Clinical Manifestations. *Orthostatic Hypotension.* Chronic orthostatic hypotension is a disorder of the autonomic nervous system in which syncope occurs when the patient assumes the upright posture. The condition is sometimes seen in diabetic neuropathy and in tabes dorsalis, but in many patients the site of the neurologic lesion is unknown. These people have an abnormality in the baroreceptor reflexes that ordinarily compensates for the pooling of blood in the lower extremities and viscera. When an attempt is made to stand upright, there is an inadequate degree of reflex arteriolar constriction, with a subsequent reduction in venous return. This is associated with an immediate and sharp fall in arterial blood pressure, followed by syncope. The pulse rate remains unchanged during the episode, and there are none of the usual prodromal symptoms of pallor, sweating, and nausea seen in vasodepressor faint. These patients have subnormal values for urinary catecholamines and may have other evidence of autonomic insufficiency such as impotence, bladder disturbances, and loss of sweating in the lower trunk. Orthostatic hypotension has also been associated with a Parkinson-like disorder sometimes referred to as the Shy-Drager syndrome (see Ch. 377).

A new syndrome of orthostatic hypotension known as hyperbradykininism has been reported, in which standing produces a fall in systolic blood pressure, an increase in diastolic pressure and heart rate, and purplish discoloration and ecchymoses over the legs. The disorder is characterized by high plasma levels of bradykinin, which may account for dilatation of the cutaneous venules and capillaries in the legs and reduction in venous return.

Failure of postural adaptation may appear after surgical sympathectomy for hypertension or the administration of vasodilating agents and antihypertensive drugs, especially the sodium-depleting diuretics and ganglionic blocking agents. Syncope has also been noted in patients treated with L-dopa for Parkinson's disease. Patients recovering from chronic wasting illnesses associated

with prolonged bed rest may experience syncope when they attempt to assume the upright position. Shorter periods of bed rest, particularly when associated with dehydration or electrolyte deficits, may also be associated with orthostatic hypotension.

Vasodepressor Syncope (the Common Faint). Vasodepressor syncope is by far the most frequent cause of transient loss of consciousness. The condition is characterized by a fall in blood pressure associated with the development of a variety of autonomic manifestations. In the early presyncopal period, there may be pallor, nausea, and sweating; in later stages pupillary dilatation, yawning, hyperpnea, and bradycardia appear. When the mean arterial pressure falls below critical levels, loss of consciousness and characteristic electroencephalographic changes occur. Bradycardia is often severe at the onset of unconsciousness, and pulse rates of 50 to 60 per minute may be observed even after recovery. The duration of syncope is brief, ranging from a few seconds to several minutes. In the postsyncopal period the patient may complain of headaches, weakness, nervousness, and slight confusion. Vasodepressor faint is most often evoked by sudden emotional stress associated with fear, anxiety, or pain. Hypodermic injections, trauma, minor surgery, and the sight of or withdrawal of blood are common precipitating events. Attacks usually occur in the standing or upright posture, and consciousness returns quickly once the patient is recumbent.

The initial event in this complex vascular and neurogenic reaction is dilatation of the vascular bed throughout the body, particularly in peripheral muscles. Vasodilatation in the limb muscles is a normal response to emotional stimuli, and is thought to represent preparation for "fight or flight." The absence of immediate muscle activity, however, and the fall in peripheral resistance are not compensated for by an increase in cardiac output, and as a result there is a reduction in cerebral blood flow.

Adams-Stokes Syndrome. In the early nineteenth century Morgagni, Adams, and Stokes separately observed and described fainting associated with a persistently slow pulse in the range of 40 per minute. Patients with this syndrome usually have a disordered atrioventricular conduction system, secondary to coronary atherosclerosis. In most instances, the loss of consciousness occurs during the changes in rhythm when there may be asystole, ventricular fibrillation, or tachycardia, or a combination of these arrhythmias. Occasionally sudden death results from cardiac standstill. A rare form of syncope caused by ventricular fibrillation has been reported in children with hereditary prolongation of QT interval in the electrocardiogram, sometimes associated with congenital deafness. The clinical picture of syncope caused by cardiac arrhythmias is often characteristic. Loss of consciousness is abrupt; prodromal signs are not usually present. On regaining consciousness, the patient usually shows little confusion or postsyncopal residua. The attacks may occur several times a day and have no relation to posture or activity. Only a brief period of asystole of four or five seconds' duration will produce loss of consciousness in the erect position, but longer periods of asystole are not uncommon. In such instances, neurologic manifestations such as convulsive movements, pupillary dilatation, and prolonged confusion may be observed. The use of radiotelemetered electrocardiographic tape systems has led to more accurate diagnosis of syncope caused by Adams-Stokes attacks. Such monitoring systems, recorded over periods of 10 to 20 hours, give the frequency and nature of the cardiac arrhythmia during the patient's full activity and provide a firm basis for definitive treatment such as implantation of an intracardiac pacemaker.

Reflex Cardiac Standstill. Syncopal attacks may result from cessation of cardiac action in persons without heart disease. In such individuals, the mechanism for cardiac standstill arises from vagal reflex activity. In a few authenticated cases, swallowing or experimental distention of the esophagus with a balloon has induced complete atrioventricular block and syncope. The alterations in consciousness and electrocardiographic changes disappear when the pressure within the esophagus is relieved or after administration of atropine. The syncopal episode occasionally seen during digital prostatic examination, thoracentesis, or bronchoscopic examination may also be due to such a reflex mechanism. Syncope caused by cardiac arrest has been observed in patients with paroxysmal pain in the throat caused by glossopharyngeal neuralgia.

Carotid Sinus Syncope. In relatively few patients this is the mechanism of syncope. Many persons, particularly those more than 60 years of age, show reflex slowing of the heart and fall of blood pressure during massage of one or both carotid sinuses. Such responses are also seen frequently in patients with cardiac disorders, hypertension, or diseases of the carotid vessels such as atherosclerotic thrombosis or stenosis. The most common response to carotid sinus massage is either sinus bradycardia or sinoatrial block, both of which may be abolished by administration of atropine. Much less frequently, there may be a pure vasodepressor response without slowing of the heart. In a third but rare type of carotid response, fainting may appear in a few seconds without significant changes in either blood pressure or pulse; such instances probably occur only with vigorous pressure and when the opposite carotid is already thrombosed. Carotid sinus syncope is not accompanied by the prodromal symptoms seen in the common faint (nausea, sweating, pallor). It is more frequent in men, and usually occurs in the erect posture. It sometimes follows sudden head turning or pressure of a tight collar.

Only very few of the patients who exhibit bradycardia or a reduction in blood pressure on carotid massage experience loss of consciousness caused by these factors. In eliciting carotid sinus responses, care should be taken to avoid obstructing blood flow to the brain by compression of the carotid vessels. Cerebral infarction and even death have been reported after carotid compression and massage. Massage of both carotid sinuses simultaneously may be hazardous.

Organic Heart Disease. Patients with myocardial infarction or valvular lesions may also have transient periods of unconsciousness. The mechanism of syncope in these disorders is not altogether clear, but may be related to a reduction in cardiac output with inadequate cerebral blood flow. In acute myocardial infarction, fainting probably results from decrease in stroke volume owing to a weakened myocardium. Transient arrhythmias, such as ventricular tachycardia, fibrillation, or heart block, may contribute to the syncopal reaction. Transient loss of consciousness may occur during attacks of angina pectoris, and is probably caused by ventricular fibrillation or various types of heart block associated with temporary periods of myocardial ischemia. Syncope also appears during paroxysmal tachycardia even in the absence of structural heart disease. In such cases the loss of consciousness usually occurs at the onset or at the end of the attack, at which time there may be a brief period of cardiac standstill.

Patients with aortic valvular or subvalvular stenosis often have syncope associated with physical exertion (effort syncope). The loss of consciousness in the early phases of such syncopal episodes may be due to shunting of blood to the peripheral muscles, but the later phases have been shown to be associated with transient ventricular asystole, tachycardia, or fibrillation, presumably caused by diminished coronary arterial blood flow. Sudden death may occur during these attacks. Effort syncope is also seen in patients with congenital heart disease such as patent ductus arteriosus or tetralogy of Fallot, as well as in those with pulmonary hypertension or atrial myxoma.

Cough Syncope. Cough syncope usually follows a paroxysm of explosive and vigorous coughing. It is commonly observed in men but rarely in women. In adults, the condition is often associated with chronic lung disease or bronchitis; in children, it may occur during severe pertussis. The syncope is brief, and there are no postsyncopal residua. The condition has also been described following hearty laughter. The loss of consciousness has been attributed to an increase in the intrathoracic and intra-abdominal pressure caused by vigorous coughing. This, in turn, is thought to produce a sudden sharp elevation in cerebrospinal fluid pressure, thereby "squeezing" blood from the intracranial and cerebral vessels. Other theories maintain that the condition is due to a Valsalva effect with reduction in cardiac output or to cerebral "concussive effect" caused by rapid rise in the cerebrospinal fluid pressure. There is clinical evidence to suggest that the presence of an intracerebral lesion such as brain tumor or stenosis of a major cerebral artery may produce increased susceptibility to syncope after paroxysms of cough. Such cases may have focal neurologic symptoms such as paresthesias or clonic movements of one limb prior to loss of consciousness.

Micturition Syncope. This form of syncope is most often seen during or immediately after micturition in men who rise in the middle of the night to urinate. The loss of consciousness is brief and there is no postsyncopal confusion or weakness. Many such people give a history of drinking large quantities of beer before retiring, and considerable bladder deflation may take place during micturition. A similar fainting may be observed after drainage of a distended bladder in urinary retention or after removal of a large quantity of ascitic fluid by abdominal paracentesis. It has been suggested that the loss of consciousness may be due to a reflex vasodilatation of the peripheral vascular system, a situation thought to be the converse of the paroxysmal hypertension seen in paraplegics during bladder distention. It is not likely to be due to a Valsalva maneuver during micturition but may be related to peripheral vasodilation associated with a warm bed and perhaps the recent consumption of alcohol.

Hysterical Fainting. Hysterical fainting is seen almost entirely in young women with emotional illness. It differs from the vasodepressor faint and the hyperventilation syndrome in that the patient is relatively free of anxiety and shows little concern regarding the fainting episodes. The attack usually occurs in the presence of others. The patient generally slumps to the floor gracefully, sometimes dramatically, without injury or awkwardness. It thus resembles the mid-Victorian drawing-room swoon. In earlier decades, hysterical fainting often occurred in groups of young women during mass excitement, particularly that caused by the presence of screen or television idols. Although unusual behavior is now often observed among young women attending "rock" concerts, swooning is seldom seen.

During the attack the patient may be motionless or may show bizarre resisting movements. The attack may last from several minutes to as long as an hour or more, with fluctuations of responsiveness. There are no abnormalities in pulse, blood pressure, or skin color. The electroencephalogram is normal during the attack, indicating that there may be no actual loss of consciousness. The diagnosis can usually be made without difficulty on the basis of the setting of the episode, the patient's underlying emotional disturbance, and the absence of physical abnormalities.

Cerebral Arterial Occlusive Disease. Patients with generalized atherosclerosis may have frequent episodes of loss of consciousness over a period of days or weeks. In most instances the attack is accompanied by signs of focal neurologic deficits such as motor weakness, sensory loss, or cranial nerve disorders. In such cases the diagnosis can be made without difficulty. Occasionally, however, the patient has no localizing symptoms, and complains of vague dizziness, weakness, and visual disturbances. Many such patients are in the older age group and have evidence of hypertensive disease with coronary or cerebrovascular involvement. These cases of "blind staggers" are difficult to categorize, and a definite diagnosis often cannot be made. The symptoms are probably related to postural disturbance associated with vascular or labyrinthine disease.

Hypoglycemia. Low levels of blood sugar often produce symptoms of weakness, trembling, sweating, tachycardia, hunger sensation, and confused behavior. Syncope is not a common occurrence, but prolonged hypoglycemia may result in seizures, coma, and serious brain damage. The majority of patients with these symptoms have anxiety reaction rather than hypoglycemia. The diagnosis of hypoglycemia must therefore be based on documented low levels of blood sugar at the time of the clinical manifestations which, in turn, can be relieved by ingestion of food or sugar. It is also important that the type of hypoglycemia be established. Reactive hypoglycemia is the most common type and may appear in thin, emotionally tense persons a few hours after ingestion of a high carbohydrate meal. It sometimes follows extensive gastric resection in association with the dumping syndrome and occurs in some people with mild diabetes. Hypoglycemia may also be due to islet cell adenoma of the pancreas. In this condition, nervousness, weakness, trembling, and sometimes convulsions occur after fasting and exercise. The fasting morning blood sugar level may be low, in contrast to that of patients with reactive hypoglycemia, in whom this determination is usually normal. Other conditions such as pituitary insufficiency, Addison's disease, hepatic failure, and large sarcomas may also produce hypoglycemia.

Diagnosis. The diagnosis of syncope depends almost entirely upon a careful history of the attack and the setting in which it occurs. Differentiation of syncope from an akinetic epileptic seizure, such as a petit mal or psychomotor attack, may be difficult. Careful evaluation of the electroencephalographic findings, the onset and duration of the attack, and the postsyncopal manifesta-

tions can usually distinguish these conditions. These factors are also helpful in differentiating the various types of syncope. In vasodepressor faint, the patient usually has prodromal signs of autonomic hyperactivity such as pallor, sweating, salivation, and bradycardia. In cardiac arrest, orthostatic hypotension, and carotid sinus syncope, loss of consciousness occurs abruptly, and prodromal symptoms are not usually present. Postsyncopal confusion, headache, and weakness often follow vasodepressor faint and the hyperventilation syndrome. In chronic orthostatic hypotension and Adams-Stokes attacks, recovery of consciousness is rapid and complete without postsyncopal symptoms. Most types of fainting occur in the erect or upright position, but in cardiac arrest, syncope may appear while the patient is recumbent. The duration of syncope is brief in postural hypotension but prolonged in hyperventilation and hypoglycemia. Most of these differentiating manifestations can be determined by careful history, but special methods of examination may be necessary. These consist of voluntary hyperventilation for approximately two minutes, massage of the carotid sinuses, and observations of pulse and blood pressure during change in posture from recumbency to erect position. An electroencephalogram is indicated whenever convulsive movements develop during the syncopal episode or when focal neurologic symptoms are noted before or after loss of consciousness. An electrocardiogram and blood sugar levels may also be necessary to arrive at a correct diagnosis.

Treatment. Therapy in syncope consists primarily of treatment of the underlying disorder. In all types of fainting, recovery is usually aided by maintaining the patient in a recumbent position with elevation of the lower extremities. Application of cold water to the face and head and inhalation of spirits of ammonia or other pungent aromatics are time-honored and certainly do no harm.

Ad Hoc Committee on Hypoglycemia: Statement on hypoglycemia. Arch. Intern. Med., 131:591, 1973.
Ebert, R. V.: Syncope. Circulation, 27:1148, 1963.
Engel, G. L.: Fainting. 2nd ed. Springfield, Ill., Charles C Thomas, 1962.
Hedeland, H., Dymling, J.-F., and Hokfelt, B.: Catecholamines, renin and aldosterone in postural hypotension. Acta Endocrinol. (Kbh.), 62:399, 1969.
Pedersen, A., Sandoe, E., Hvidberg, E., and Schwartz, M.: Studies on the mechanism of tussive syncope. Acta Med. Scand., 179:653, 1966.
Thomas, J. E.: Hyperactive carotid sinus reflex and carotid sinus syncope. Mayo Clin. Proc., 44:127, 1969.
Weissler, A. M., and Warren, J. V.: Vasodepressor syncope. Am. Heart J., 57:786, 1959.

354. HYPERVENTILATION

Albert Heyman

Hyperventilation Syndrome. The hyperventilation syndrome is one of the most frequent causes of impaired consciousness, usually producing "faintness" and "lightheadedness" without actual syncope. It is almost always a manifestation of acute anxiety. At the onset of an attack, the patient may complain of tightness of the chest and a feeling of suffocation. He may not be aware of overbreathing but usually recalls excessive deep sighing. Later, a sense of unreality develops, accompanied by feelings of apprehension and sometimes panic. Symptoms related to the heart and gastrointestinal tract often appear. These consist of palpitations or pounding of the heart, precordial oppression, fullness in the throat, and epigastric discomfort. The syndrome may last for as long as a half hour or more and may recur several times a day. Sensations of "numbness" and "coldness" of the hands, feet, and perioral areas often develop, and in prolonged attacks tetany with carpopedal spasm may be noted.

The pathogenesis of the individual symptoms of this disorder is not altogether clear. With normal subjects, hyperventilation in the recumbent posture for as long as an hour will not produce loss of consciousness. They may, however, have sensations of decreased awareness, lightheadedness, and blurring of vision, but do not have the trembling, sweating, palpitations, or precordial distress frequently seen in patients with spontaneous overventilation. The high voltage slow wave activity in the electroencephalogram produced by hyperventilation can be prevented by hyperbaric oxygenation, suggesting that these EEG changes, and probably the alterations in consciousness as well, are due to cerebral hypoxia. The serum calcium level remains normal, but there is often a decrease in serum phosphate within 15 minutes after hyperventilation begins. The hypocapnia caused by overventilation results in cerebral vasoconstriction and sometimes a fall in blood pressure owing to muscle vasodilatation. These factors alone are usually insufficient to produce syncope, and the occasional loss of consciousness with this syndrome is probably due to vasodepressor mechanisms as in the common faint.

The hyperventilation syndrome is often precipitated by acute emotional stress and is most common in nervous, anxious women who have other functional disturbances related to tension. The syndrome can often be reproduced by having the patient hyperventilate voluntarily for two or three minutes. Although the patient is often reassured by the fact that he can control the attack somewhat by breath-holding or breathing in a paper bag, therapy directed at the underlying emotional disturbance is usually necessary.

Hyperventilation Combined with Valsalva Maneuver. The physiologic alterations produced by a combination of hyperventilation and increased intrathoracic pressure (secondary to variants of the Valsalva maneuver) account for several unique types of syncope. The "mess trick," a prank often indulged in by schoolboys, consists of sudden manual compression of the chest of the victim after he has been hyperventilating for about a minute. Loss of consciousness may also occur in the "fainting lark," in which the victim is instructed to hyperventilate in the squatting position, stand quickly, and immediately perform the Valsalva maneuver. The loss of consciousness observed in athletes lifting weights ("weightlifter's blackout") is due to similar mechanisms. During competition, these individuals often hyperventilate vigorously and then squat before grasping the weight. Lifting of the weight produces high levels of intrathoracic pressure which reduces venous return and causes decrease in cardiac output, stroke volume, and pulse pressure. These alterations, combined with the peripheral vasodilation caused by squatting and cerebral vasoconstriction caused by hyperventilation, result in a reduction in cerebral blood flow and loss of consciousness. Voluntary syncope has also been observed in muscular teenage boys who can maintain a prolonged Valsalva maneuver by vigorous stretching of the trunk and back muscles. Such instances of "stretch syncope" are often self-induced to provide a curiously satisfying experience.

Brown, E. B.: Physiological effects of hyperventilation. Physiol. Rev., 33:445, 1953.
Klein, L. J., Saltzman, H., and Heyman, A.: Syncope induced by the Valsalva maneuver: A study of the effects of arterial blood gas tensions, glucose concentration and blood pressure. Am. J. Med., 37:263, 1964.
Saltzman, H. A., Heyman, A., and Sieker, H. O.: Correlations of clinical and physiologic manifestations of sustained hyperventilation. N. Engl. J. Med., 268:1431, 1963.

Section Nine.   NEUROLOGIC DIAGNOSTIC PROCEDURES

Richard P. Schmidt

355.   INTRODUCTION

Many special tests and procedures are used to supplement the clinical examination in the establishment of a neurologic diagnosis. These may add precision to the localization and characterization of a disease process, or may record functional alterations as reflected in electrical activity of brain, nerve, or muscle. Their value is related directly to the judgment with which they are used and to the skill with which they are performed and interpreted. Some of the tests outlined below are relatively simple procedures which cause little discomfort, whereas others may be dangerous and must be used only by physicians skilled in the techniques and with full knowledge of potential complications and their treatment. The number of available tests is expanding rapidly, and it has become increasingly important for these to be selectively used and individualized. Those least dangerous and causing the least discomfort are to be used first. Careful clinical examinations may obviate the need for a battery of expensive and time-consuming procedures.

In this section brief descriptions of the useful diagnostic procedures are given. Details of techniques and of interpretations may be found in definitive and specialized monographs.

356.   ROENTGENOLOGIC EXAMINATIONS

Roentgenograms of the skull or spine may demonstrate evidence of disease by deformation or involvement of bony structures, by displacement of normal radiopaque structures such as the pineal body, or by abnormal calcification such as may be seen in tumors, vascular malformations, infectious granulomas, or hematomas. Maximal information should always be obtained from plain roentgenograms prior to the institution of more complex studies. Such studies not only may permit a more satisfactory choice, but may also obviate the need for contrast studies such as arteriography or pneumoencephalography. Brain shift may be evident by displacement of a normally calcified pineal body. Increased intracranial pressure over a long period of time characteristically causes demineralization of the dorsum sellae by pressure from an expanded third ventricle or a beaten silver appearance to the inner table of the skull from pressure of the gyri of the cerebral cortex. Diagnosis of some diseases can be confirmed without further examination. For example, pituitary tumors usually cause enlargement of the sella turcica. Meningiomas are often associated with thickening of bone at the site from which they arise. Abnormalities are observed in plain skull films of about half the patients with brain tumor.

Patterns of calcification as seen roentgenographically may be highly specific in diagnosis of disease. Examples include arcuate densities in the wall of an aneurysm or the veins of an arteriovenous malformation, calcification in the pattern of the cerebral cortex in Sturge-Weber syndrome, and diffuse nodular calcification in congenital toxoplasmosis. Amorphous calcification with or without erosion of the pituitary fossa is typical in craniopharyngioma, and the basal ganglia may be calcified symmetrically in hypoparathyroidism.

Lesions of the skull or spine occur frequently in neoplastic diseases. In some instances the appearance is quite characteristic, as in the "punched-out" rarefactions of multiple myeloma. Special attention may be directed to the foramina at the base of the skull through which nasopharyngeal cancer may invade and cause cranial nerve paralysis. Axial projections of the base of the skull may reveal enlargement of these foramina with special advantage. Acoustic neurinoma characteristically enlarges the internal auditory meatus as shown in special projection.

Diagnosis of congenital malformations of the skull and spine can usually be made without contrast material. In basilar impression there is flattening of the basal angle, frequently associated with malformation of the foramen magnum and cervical spine and with hydrocephalus. Injury to the brain in early life may be associated with asymmetric skull growth. Premature closure of the sutures results in microcephaly or in asymmetric growth in the direction of those sutures which remain open.

In examination of the spine special attention should be given to alignment, integrity of the intervertebral disc space, bony excrescences, and evidences of bone destruction. Intraspinal neoplasms commonly erode and cause separation of the vertebral pedicles. Characteristic patterns are seen in such diseases as tuberculosis of the spine, osteoporosis, metastatic carcinoma, and vertebral hemangioma. Oblique views are especially useful for demonstrating intervertebral foramina, which may be enlarged in tumors such as neurofibromas or compromised by osteophytic spurs causing radicular syndromes.

Body section roentgenography may be used for visualization of abnormalities of skull or spine which are otherwise obscure. This procedure has special value in demonstrating changes near the midline or base of the skull, and may also be used to advantage in intraspinal lesions.

Further stages of neuroradiologic diagnosis depend

upon making visible structures not seen in plain films by use of radiopaque substances injected into arteries or the subarachnoid space, or by gas (usually air or oxygen) to provide radiolucency in cerebrospinal fluid–containing compartments. With increasing sophistication of instrumentation, the techniques of performing such studies are evolving rapidly, demanding high degrees of skill for their performance and interpretation.

Myelography is used when mass impingement upon spinal or posterior fossa neural structures or nerve roots is suspected, and usually when surgical treatment appears to be required. It is usually done using iodized oil, which is heavier than the cerebrospinal fluid, injected into the subarachnoid space at a reasonable distance from the suspected lesion in the lumbar region or, for special purposes, into the cisterna magna. Oil is manipulated up and down by tilting the patient on a table under fluoroscopic control. Introduction of oil into the cranial cavity is usually avoided, and the oil is removed after completion of the procedure. Adequate myelography with fluoroscopy and spot films at various angles is usually satisfactory for demonstrating mass lesions within or impinging upon the spinal subarachnoid space. It has its greatest usefulness in outlining neoplasms, herniations of the nucleus pulposus, or impingements by spondylotic lesions. At times manipulation of fluid pressure may cause acute exacerbation of the patient's symptoms; if a tumor is present, this may call for urgent surgical intervention. *The test is to be avoided unless there is strong and sufficient reason to suspect a mass lesion.* There may, for example, be exacerbation of multiple sclerosis by the procedure. Iodized oil is a foreign substance to the subarachnoid space, and may initiate a sterile meningeal reaction or, rarely, a progressive adhesive arachnoiditis. For these reasons, in some countries myelography is performed using air-contrast or, less commonly, absorbable water-soluble radiopaque material. When more satisfactory, less irritating agents are found, they will probably replace oil.

In *pneumoencephalography,* oxygen or air is introduced in increments into the lumbar subarachnoid space, from which it ascends into the basal cisterns and enters the ventricular cavities. By proper positioning, the entire ventricular system can be visualized, as can the basal cisterns and subarachnoid spaces over the cerebral cortex. Ventriculography may be used in the presence of increased intracranial pressure or when a tumor is suspected, because of lessened danger of initiating herniation as compared with pneumoencephalography. It is performed by introducing gas directly into the lateral ventricle by a needle introduced through a trephine opening in the skull. Pantopaque may be used for special purposes. It has the disadvantage of limiting the examination to the ventricular system because of failure to fill the subarachnoid spaces. In these tests, atrophic processes or obstructions of fluid paths are reflected by enlargement of the ventricles. In the former, there may be concomitant enlargement of the basal cisterns and of the sulci over the convexity of the brain. Space-taking lesions such as neoplasms may obstruct with "upstream" dilatation appropriate to the site or, as is characteristic, may deform and shift the ventricles.

When appropriately used, pneumoencephalography is a safe procedure; however, it is usually distressing to the patient, and may cause severe headache.

The uses of *angiography* are increasing rapidly. By the injection of appropriate root arteries, positioning of the patient, and timing of serial films, it is now possible to demonstrate practically all the intracranial arterial and venous systems and also to study parent vessels from the aorta upward. Techniques for performance vary, but increasing proportions of these examinations are being done by selective catheterization through the femoral arteries, and fewer by direct puncture of carotid or vertebral arteries in the neck. Special radiologic techniques of magnification, subtraction, and stereoscopic visualization are used to increase diagnostic and localizing capabilities. Special angiographic procedures may be used for lesions of the orbit or spinal cord or for visualizing lesions supplied by the external carotid system such as meningiomas.

Cerebral angiography has certain advantages over gas contrast studies. Pathologic processes of blood vessels such as aneurysms or malformations may be demonstrated. Complete or partial occlusions at any site from the level of the aortic arch to the intracranial vascular tree may be visualized. If surgery for occlusive disease is contemplated, all major vessels must be studied. Angiography is the procedure of choice in delineating neoplasms or other space-occupying lesions. Masses may be localized by displacement of arteries or veins from normal positions and by the filling of abnormal vessels within a neoplasm (tumor stain). It is sometimes possible to predict the histologic type of a tumor from its blood supply and vascular pattern. Subdural hematoma is demonstrated to particular advantage by displacement of superficial blood vessels away from the inner surface of the skull, and is seen best on anteroposterior and oblique projections. Angiography may have an added advantage for patients with increased intracranial pressure in that it is less likely to cause herniation and brain shift than is pneumoencephalography. Patients tolerate the procedure well, and do not have the headache, nausea, and vomiting associated with gas insufflation. Complications may occur, however, especially in children, older patients, and those with vascular and systemic diseases. The complications range from transient dysfunction such as hemiparesis or confusion to more unusual permanent neurologic injuries or even death. Puncture of an artery can cause intraluminal rupture of an intimal atherosclerotic plaque or subintimal dissection. Embolization or thrombosis may occur from the site of puncture.

357. RADIOISOTOPE PROCEDURES

Isotope brain scanning depends upon the ability of certain radioactive substances to localize selectively in neoplasms or in injured tissues (such as infarctions) which damage the normally impermeable blood-brain barrier. Isotopes of short half-life, such as technetium[99m] pertechnetate are now preferred because they permit a higher level of radioactivity and a much shorter elapsed time to the completion of the procedure. The scan may be recorded with multiple crystals in a scintillation camera or by more conventional scintillation scanners moving across the head and recording the scanning image instrumentally on paper or film. Several projections are used to "view" the head from different directions. With the scintillation camera, dynamic scans may be obtained, giving some evidence of blood circulation or demonstrating large vascular anomalies. Scans are of special worth for locating lesions relatively near the surface, and may be confusing or "negative" with deep or midline lesions. Artifacts may be produced by bruises of the scalp or by such simple processes as contamination by saliva in which the isotope has been secreted. Scans are excellent as screening procedures because of safety and lack of discomfort or serious inconvenience.

358. ELECTRODIAGNOSTIC EXAMINATIONS

Functions of the brain, nerves and neuromuscular apparatus may be examined by appropriate measurements of electrical activity.

The *electroencephalogram* (EEG) is the recording of amplified potentials generated by the brain by means of electrodes applied to the scalp. Recordings directly from the surface or from the depths of the brain may have application in selected instances such as the surgical treatment of foci generating epileptic partial seizures. An adequate routine examination includes the application of 18 or more electrodes on the scalp and observation of the EEG under conditions of nonattentive wakefulness, in response to overbreathing, and during the course of natural sleep. The instruments now used consist of eight or more matched channels for simultaneous recordings, and by convention the record is written in ink on paper moving beneath galvanometer pens. Variation in rhythm occurs with respect to normal processes such as sleep, and there are marked differences between the EEG of the child and the adult. Although the processes that generate the brain waves are largely unknown, normal or usual patterns and deviation from normal are well recognized and may be highly useful in clinical diagnosis. Deviation from normal may be termed a dysrhythmia, and the type of dysrhythmia and its distribution or localization may correlate with the type of the underlying disease. Highly typical patterns are observed in some of the epilepsies, especially the spike-wave pattern associated with petit mal and localized spikes over the temporal lobe in patients with complex partial seizures (psychomotor). A normal EEG does not preclude the presence of serious disease. Mild deviations from normal may be observed in persons with no evidence of cerebral disease. Intelligence cannot be measured and psychologic diagnoses cannot be made by the EEG. The EEG can be properly interpreted only in concert with the clinical data, and it cannot provide precise diagnosis in and of itself.

The EEG may provide evidence for diagnosis and localization of structural lesions such as neoplasms, infarcts, hematomas, and infections. The tool has the great advantage of relative simplicity of application and harmlessness to the patient. If the brain is infarcted, compressed, or disrupted by neoplasms or hemorrhage, slower than normal (delta) waves are observed and may be localized to areas overlying the pathologic processes. Serial or sequential examinations reflect changes of improvement or worsening in the pathologic process, and thus help to delineate the nature of the underlying disorder. Metabolic abnormalities affecting the brain may be followed by the EEG to ascertain the direction of improvement or worsening.

The *electromyogram* (EMG) records the electrical activity in muscle. Detailed diagnostic examination requires use of needle electrodes inserted into the muscles under study. Instrumentation is analogous to that used for the EEG, except that a cathode ray oscilloscope is necessary because of more rapid potential change. Permanent records may be made on photographic film or magnetic tape. Records are obtained during rest, needle insertion, and voluntary contraction, and in response to physical or electrical stimulation. Auditory monitoring with a loudspeaker is customary in many laboratories. The EMG is most helpful in the diagnosis of disease of the motor unit, which includes the ventral horn cell, ventral nerve root, motor nerve, myoneural junction, and muscle. Neuropathic disorders, such as amyotrophic lateral sclerosis or poliomyelitis, produce signs of muscle denervation, including increased insertion activity, fibrillation potentials at rest, and reduced, altered, or absent normal muscle action potentials. Primary muscle disease (myopathy) frequently reduces the amplitude and duration of the muscle action potentials and increases the complexity of their wave form, although the number of potentials is little changed. Myotonia produces a highly characteristic repetitive pattern. Segmental investigation of muscle innervation may be of use in localization and diagnosis of spinal root compression, such as that caused by intervertebral disc protrusion.

Estimates of motor nerve conduction velocity are made by electrically stimulating the nerve, recording electromyographically from the muscle that it innervates, and measuring the latency. Slowing of conduction is observed in a wide variety of peripheral neuropathies and in many instances of neurologically asymptomatic diabetes mellitus. The site of local nerve compression or conduction block can be demonstrated, an example being the local block of median nerve conduction that is found in the carpal tunnel syndrome. Sensory nerve conduction velocity may be measured by recording nerve action potentials after digital nerve stimulation. Sensory neuropathy may produce slowing of conduction or inability to record the nerve potential.

359. ECHOENCEPHAL-OGRAPHY

High frequency (ultrasonic) sound pulses produced by an electrically activated crystal and conducted in a fluid or solid medium reflect or echo at physical interfaces, and their reflection can, in turn, be detected and recorded. This phenomenon may detect shifts or alterations of structures within the cranial cavity. Present application makes it possible to obtain a rapid, painless, and harmless estimate of the position of midline structures (third ventricle) in the intact cranium. Pulses of ultrasound are delivered to the head through a probe held firmly to the scalp and with liquid or jelly at the interface. A detector may be physically located in the same probe. Proper amplification and display with a cathode ray oscilloscope permit recognition of reflected pulse from skin, ventricle, skull, and other structures. By calibrating the sweep speed of the oscilloscope beam, the distance from the probe to the reflecting surface can be measured in millimeters. Measurement of the position of the midline third ventricle is particularly reliable. This is useful as a screening test for hemispheric mass lesions causing brain shift, and is well adapted to use in emergency hospital services for appraising patients with suspected subdural or epidural hemorrhage. Echoencephalography may also be used to estimate ventricular size and at times to demonstrate abnormal structures such as tumors.

360. NEW AND DEVELOPING TECHNOLOGIES

Improvements in instrument technology and manufacture have greatly expanded the ability to identify and delineate lesions of the central nervous system. Of the recently devised instruments, the EMI-Scanner, developed by EMI Limited in England is achieving acceptance rapidly and is being installed in major centers for neurology and neurosurgery. This instrument uses the principle of differential density absorption of x-rays by lesions and normal structures within the cranial vault. It is composed, in essence, of a rotating x-ray tube and recording device, a small computer, a digital read-out system, and an oscilloscope with its accompanying Polaroid camera. The patient is given no medication before the examination so that it represents a truly noninvasive study. The patient's head is placed in the device, and multiple x-ray pictures are taken by the moving x-ray tube as it courses over the head. These electronic pictures are analyzed by the computer and recorded. Over-all accuracy with the EMI-Scanner appears to be great, and it has the great advantage of being safe and rapid.

Toole, J. F. (ed.): Contemporary Neurology Series, Vol. 3. Special Techniques in Neurologic Diagnosis. Philadelphia, F. A. Davis Company, 1969.

# Section Ten.	THE EXTRAPYRAMIDAL DISORDERS

361. INTRODUCTION

Melvin D. Yahr

The basal ganglia or extrapyramidal diseases comprise a complex group of clinical disorders characterized by abnormal involuntary movements (dyskinesias), alterations in muscle tone, and disturbances in bodily posture. The major clinical states included under this title are parkinsonism, chorea, athetosis, dystonia, and hemiballism. These terms not only are used to denote particular disease entities, but in a descriptive sense refer to a constellation of symptoms that may occur in a variety of central nervous system disorders involving the basal ganglia and/or their connections. They are recognizable, one from the other, by the degree, form, and combination of the triad of symptoms noted above and are distinguishable as disease entities by the age and mode of onset, the identification of particular etiologic and genetic factors, and the rate and manner of progression of symptoms. Although much is known about the clinical aspects of extrapyramidal disorders, our information is deficient in regard to their fundamental anatomic, physiologic, and pathogenic bases.

The conventional anatomic concept of the basal ganglia as a group of nuclear masses in the forebrain has not proved adequate in explaining the clinical manifestations or what is known about the physiologic or pathologic aspects of these conditions. In consequence, neurologists have devised a functional anatomic approach that includes not only the basal ganglia nuclei, but also related structures in the brainstem as well as a neural network of connections with other parts of the nervous system. The structures of importance in this system are the caudate nucleus and putamen, which, because of their similarities in appearance, cellular structure, and phylogenetic development, are collectively known as the striatum; the globus pallidus or pallidum, an older structure but one in which many nonpyramidal pathways converge; the thalamus, another important way station and integrative region; and the subthalamic nucleus, red nucleus and substantia nigra, all brainstem centers with important connections to the basal ganglia. These nuclear masses, along with their connections with each other and with certain parts of the reticular formation, cerebellum, and cerebrum, make up an anatomic-physiologic unit that collectively has been termed "the extrapyramidal system." The role of this system in maintaining normal motor activity in man is not definitely known, and has only been inferred from studies of animals, in which it is more highly developed and not dominated by the cerebral cortex. In submammalian forms in which motor activities are sterotyped and resemble patterned reflexes, this system appears essential for maintaining normal locomotion, feeding, etc. In higher animals, except man, its integrity is necessary for the production of automatic movements and postural adjustments. Some believe that this same function is carried over to man and that coarse, gross automatic movements are mediated by the extrapyramidal system. Others have implied a more secondary role in which this system is incapable of initiating movements but provides a reinforcing and modulating influence on movements of cortical origin. The latter thesis seems more in keeping with our present knowledge of the integrative function of the nervous system; hence it is best to view the pyramidal and extrapyramidal systems as operating in unison and constant balance. Movements having their origin in the cerebral cortex are mediated through the pyramidal tract but are influenced by reflex regulating mechanisms from various components of the extrapyramidal system. In this context, the prime role of the extrapyramidal system is automatic sensorimotor integration, which can be explained in terms of inhibition and facilitation of motor responses to appropriate stimuli. Hence dysfunction within this system results in motor responses that are delayed, slow, and incomplete and especially affect automatic or involuntary movements.

The manifestations of basal ganglia disorders previously noted fall into two general categories: those of a *positive* nature, such as abnormal movements, tremor, and chorea, and those of a *negative* nature, such as postural changes and loss of associated movements. The positive disturbances arise from an excess of neural activity, and as such cannot derive from destruction of neural elements but must represent the function of surviving structures. They are often termed release phenomena, in that a lesion in one structure removes the controlling or regulating influence on another, with the result that the latter becomes overactive. The negative symptoms, on the other hand, are considered to result from the direct loss or destruction of neural elements. Unfortunately, because of the nature of the disease processes affecting this region it has not been possible to correlate intimately the clinical symptoms with structural changes. Further, there are no naturally occurring animal counterparts to the disturbances of upright posture and of movements that occur in human diseases of the extrapyramidal system. Pathologic studies of most of these diseases show widespread neuropathologic changes throughout the cerebrum, although the basal ganglia and brainstem nuclei suffer the brunt of the damage. In some instances, however, the functional impairment is far more than that expected from the changes found on routine autopsy examination. There is a growing body of information that suggests that the abnormalities in such cases may be chemical rather than morphologic. The content of monoamines, such as dopamine and serotonin, is particularly high in structures such as the caudate nucleus, putamen, and substantia nigra. In at least one disease affecting this system, parkinsonism, the level of dopamine has been shown to be markedly decreased. Experimental lesions in the region of the substantia nigra and the pallidum produce similar effects. Since in many instances the chemical abnormalities do not follow the presumed anatomic connections, a neurochemical network is postulated for this system. In such a neural system chemical transmitter substances, such as dopamine, may be stored in nerve endings of axons whose somata or cell bodies are located in distant areas. The observed chemical changes may reflect injury or damage to a specific chemical system in these instances (a dopaminergic neuronal system) and may be similar regardless of the pathologic process. Extrapyramidal structures have other unique biochemical characteristics as indicated by high levels of acetylcholine as well as the enzymes responsible for its synthesis and degradation. All these findings suggest that better understanding of the extra-pyramidal system and its diseases may be derived from intensive study of its chemical topography.

In the clinical evaluation of extrapyramidal disorders it is essential to have a clear understanding of the many and varied symptoms encountered. Those of major significance are abnormal involuntary movements, alterations in muscle tone, and disturbances in bodily posture.

Abnormal Involuntary Movements. *Tremor* is a rhythmic involuntary alternating contraction of opposing muscle groups, fairly uniform in frequency and amplitude. It may involve a limited segment such as fingers or lips, or may be widespread. Characteristically, tremor of extrapyramidal origin is augmented when the part is at rest and diminished or abolished during voluntary movements and sleep. It differs from that of anxiety, thyrotoxicosis, and those due to intoxications by being slower, of greater amplitude, and more rhythmic. Its occurrence at rest and suppression during voluntary movements and sleep distinguishes it from the so-called "action" tremor of cerebellar involvement. The anatomic and physiologic substrate of this type of tremor has not been defined with certainty. In Parkinson's disease in which such tremor is prominent, the substantia nigra invariably undergoes degeneration. However, not all such patients have tremor, and it remains a controversial issue whether the pathologic changes are entirely limited to this structure. Certain thalamic nuclei, particularly the nucleus lateralis posterior, have been implicated, because discharges synchronous with the tremor have been recorded. These findings suggest derangement of a rather complex sensorimotor mechanism with possible multiple pathologic sites.

Athetosis denotes an involuntary movement that results from instability of posture combined with voluntary movement. The result is a slow, writhing, wormlike movement usually most prominent in the fingers and hand, but the face, neck, and feet may also be involved. Multiple areas of the extrapyramidal system, particularly the globus pallidus and striatum as well as the cerebral cortex, have shown pathologic changes when this type of dyskinesia is encountered.

Chorea refers to brief, distal, rapid, explosive movements which at first glance appear to be purposeful and coordinated but on closer inspection are aimless and uncoordinated. They involve upper and lower limbs, face, trunk, and head, and may occur with such rapidity that the individual appears in constant motion. Choreiform movements are accentuated by movement and environmental stimulation, and interfere with normal voluntary function. They are differentiated from tics by being unpatterned, unpredictable, and nonreproducible. Athetosis and chorea may coexist in such a pattern that they are indistinguishable from one another. Pathologic changes accompanying chorea have been found in many areas of the nervous system but especially in the striatum.

Dystonia is a term applied to an abnormally maintained posture resulting from a twisting, turning movement that usually involves the limbs, neck, or trunk. Although there is no specific pattern or posture that describes this disorder, the usual appearance is one of marked distortion of the affected part. The movements appear readily induced by ordinary stimuli, such as walking, talking, or light touch to the skin. The involved muscles appear to be alternately in a state of increased and decreased tone and, usually as the movement starts, the muscles involved appear to gradually build up tone. Patients with this type of movement cannot inhibit, modify, or terminate the posture, and voluntary movements become seriously impaired. In some instances the movements clear, but the abnormal postures become fixed with resultant torticollis, tortipelvis, and deformities of the limbs. Neither the pathologic nor physiologic substrate for this movement disorder has been fully defined. Some have considered it akin to athetosis but different because of the inherent peculiarities of the axial and appendicular musculature that is primarily affected.

Ballism is a violent dyskinesia consisting of forceful, flinging movements of the limbs. The muscles involved are in the shoulder and pelvic girdle, and usually only one side of the body or even one limb is affected. Of all the abnormal movements ballism is the one that appears to be due to a discrete lesion, usually in the subthalamic nucleus of Luys or its immediate connections.

Alterations in Muscle Tone. A wide range of degrees of tension in muscles is to be found in these disorders. Although it is common to associate heightened muscle tonus (rigidity) with extrapyramidal disorders, some, such as chorea and athetosis, may show normal tone or hypotonus of the musculature. Rigidity, which is most commonly encountered in parkinsonism, must be differentiated from spasticity. The former is identifiable by passively flexing and extending the muscles of an extremity or rotating the hand on the wrist. The movement obtained is one of a series of interrupted jerks at regular intervals, the so called cog-wheel effect. Terms such as "plastic" or "lead pipe" are utilized to describe the homogeneous degree of rigidity. Rigidity may be limited to groups of muscles and may be evident only at some joints, or it may be generalized, affecting the entire musculature. The mechanism underlying the rigidity appears to be impairment of reciprocal inhibition of agonist and antagonistic muscle groups. Electromyographic analysis of these muscles shows continuing activity in both groups throughout a movement such as flexion of the forearm. Rigidity reduces muscle power and velocity of movement to some degree, and also contributes to the production of deformities.

Disturbances in Bodily Posture. Patients with extrapyramidal disease in general, and those with parkinsonism in particular, have difficulty in preserving their equilibrium in the erect as well as the sitting position. They also have difficulty in changing from the horizontal to the upright position or in rolling over from back to front. The most profound difficulties are noted in walking, when tendencies to propulsive or retropulsive gait are evident as well as shuffling and festination. Careful analysis of these defects has indicated that the subjects have loss of control of their center of gravity in both sagittal and coronal planes. There are also tendencies to assume abnormal posture such as a flexion of the trunk on standing. There is a notable lack of normal and appropriate use of defense mechanisms, such as putting out the arms when falling. These abnormalities are thought to be due to disturbances in righting reflexes, impairment of vestibular reflexes, and release of proprioceptor mechanisms subsequent to degeneration in the pallidum. They form a distressing and disabling group of symptoms that to date have not been thoroughly investigated.

Denny-Brown, D.: The Cerebral Control of Movement. Springfield, Ill., Charles C Thomas, 1966.

Duvoisin, R.: Clinical diagnosis of the dyskinesias. Med. Clin. North Am., 56:1321, 1972.

Watkins, E. S.: The basal ganglia. In Scientific Foundations of Neurology. London, Heinemann, 1972, pp. 75–83.

Yahr, M. D.: Involuntary movements. In Scientific Foundations of Neurology. London, Heinemann, 1972, pp. 83–88.

Yahr, M. D., and Purpura, D. P. (eds.): Neurophysiological Basis of Normal and Abnormal Motor Activities. Hewlett, N.Y., Raven Press, 1967.

THE PARKINSONIAN SYNDROME
(Paralysis Agitans, Shaking Palsy)

Melvin D. Yahr

362. INTRODUCTION

James Parkinson first described the major manifestations of this syndrome, which is characterized by tremor, muscular rigidity, and loss of postural reflexes. Not only is it one of the most frequently encountered of all the basal ganglia disorders, but parkinsonism is a prominent cause of disability resulting from diseases of all types. Its prevalence has been placed at close to one million patients in the United States, with the addition of 50,000 new cases each year. As a symptom complex its occurrence has been noted in a number of disease processes either as the sole manifestation or in association with other symptoms. However, in the vast majority of cases no definable cause has as yet been found; since the latter seem to have many features in common, particularly in regard to evolution, they have been designated as Parkinson's disease, paralysis agitans, or primary parkinsonism. The cases in which definable processes are found are best classified as secondary or symptomatic parkinsonism. This separation into clinical groups cannot be construed as indicative of a difference in pathophysiology or even pathogenic mechanisms for the production of symptoms, for all parkinsonism may well have a common origin. Indeed, from the standpoint of what is presently known about its chemical pathology, a deficiency of striatal dopamine is common to all types of parkinsonism. In some instances of parkinsonism, regardless of cause, cell loss is consistently found in the substantia nigra in association with other changes diffusely distributed in the corpus striatum and cortex.

363. PARALYSIS AGITANS
(Parkinson's Disease)

The largest number of cases of parkinsonism fall into this category. The disease most frequently makes its onset between the ages of 50 and 65 years. A rarely encountered juvenile form has been described. The disease affects both sexes and all races, and there is no evidence to indicate a hereditary factor, although a familial incidence is claimed by some authorities.

The disease begins insidiously with any of its three cardinal manifestations either alone or in combination. Tremor usually in one or sometimes in both hands, involving the fingers in a pill-rolling motion, is the most common initial symptom. This is often followed by stiffness in the limbs, general slowing of movements and inability to carry out normal and routine daily functions with ease. As the disease progresses the face becomes "masklike," with a loss of eye blinking and failure to express emotional feeling; the body becomes stooped, and the gait becomes shuffling with loss of arm swing; and the patient is unable to readily gain and maintain an erect posture. Speech becomes slow and monotonous. There is a tendency to drool. The skin takes on an oily quality, and there is a tendency to seborrheic dermatitis. Although paralysis agitans is invariably progressive, the rate at which symptoms develop and disability ensues is extremely variable. On only rare occasions is the disease so rapidly progressive that the patient becomes disabled within five years of onset. In the majority, intervals of 10 to 20 years elapse before symptoms cause incapacity.

The major neurologic findings are as follows: (1) *Lack of facial expression,* with diminished eye blinking but ready induction of blepharospasm when the frontalis muscle is tapped (Myerson's sign). (2) *Tremor* of the distal segments of the limbs at rest, accentuated by suspension but decreased during active movements and eliminated in sleep. The tremor is rhythmical, alternately affecting flexor and extensor muscles, and may involve upper or lower limbs, mouth, or head. (3) *Muscular rigidity* is readily evident on passive movement of a joint, and is manifested by a series of interrupted jerks (cog-wheel phenomenon) rather than a smooth flowing, easy motion. (4) *Akinesia* is the tendency to slowness in the initiation of movement and sudden unexpected arrests of volitional movements while carrying out purposeful acts. The parkinsonian patient appears disinclined to move, and in the midst of performing a routine function suddenly finds himself "frozen" and unable to move through the sequence of motion necessary to complete the action. This is especially evident in writing or feeding and can be striking when, in attempting to walk, the patient finds that his feet are suddenly "frozen to the ground." (5) *Postural abnormalities* are most evident in the erect and sitting positions. The patient has a tendency to let his head fall forward on the trunk, and his body tends to fall forward or backward when seated on a stool unless supported; when pushed either from in front or behind in the erect position he falls, making no effort to catch himself with either a step or by movement of his arms. There is a tendency to deformities of the trunk, hands, and feet. Kyphotic deformity of the spine, causing a stooped posture, is a hallmark. There are ulnar deviation of the hand, flexion contractures of the fingers, and an equinovarus posture of the foot.

364. SECONDARY OR SYMPTOMATIC PARKINSONISM

In a long list of diseases and conditions of the nervous system parkinsonism has occurred as the predominant manifestation. These include poisoning with carbon monoxide, manganese, or other metals; brain tumors in the region of the basal ganglia; cerebral trauma; degenerative diseases; intoxication with neuroleptic agents, particularly the phenothiazine group of drugs; and infectious processes, such as encephalitis. Cerebral arteriosclerosis has been implicated by some authorities who have even designated a special form of arteriosclerotic parkinsonism. However, it is exceedingly doubtful that such a disorder exists, and pathologic studies to date have not confirmed a vascular basis for the Parkinson syndrome. In most instances of secondary parkinsonism, neurologic abnormalities involving other areas of the nervous system are found, and the parkinsonism itself may show variations from the usual picture. Of all the conditions noted, only two are frequently encountered: postencephalitic and drug-induced parkinsonism.

POSTENCEPHALITIC PARKINSONISM

One of the most prominent sequelae of the epidemic of encephalitis lethargica (von Economo's disease) that occurred between 1919 and 1926 was the parkinsonian syndrome. The syndrome developed after mild as well as severe encephalitis lethargica, and, although in most instances they immediately followed the acute infectious process, in some patients prominent symptoms were not evident for intervals of up to ten years. The causative agent of encephalitis lethargica was never established. However, recent studies suggest that it was produced by a virus of the influenza A variety. Parkinsonism appears to have been a unique sequela of this form of encephalitis because it has rarely followed any other known viral encephalitides. There are still a significant number of survivors of encephalitis lethargica, and the evolution and consequences of this form of parkinsonism differ from others, so its clinical recognition is of importance.

Postencephalitic parkinsonism has a number of distinctive or unique features, including the following: (1) A history of encephalitis lethargica during the epidemic period 1918–1919. Since the pandemic of influenza occurred concurrently with encephalitis, it is essential that careful documentation be undertaken in differentiating these two infectious processes. (2) In addition to any or all of the parkinsonian symptoms indicated above, one or more of the following neurologic deficits may be found: hemiplegia, bulbar or ocular palsies, dystonic phenomena, tics, or behavioral disorders. (3) The parkinsonism itself is as a rule incompletely developed and has been static or slowly progressive over a period of years. (4) Episodes that have been termed oculogyric crises. These consist of attacks in which spasms of conjugate eye muscles occur so that the eyes are deviated upward, downward, or to one side for minutes or hours at a time.

DRUG-INDUCED PARKINSONISM

The use of neuroleptics as psychotherapeutic or antiemetic agents has resulted in the occurrence of a number of extrapyramidal syndromes. Parkinsonism indistinguishable from that previously described, dystonic movements involving the tongue and face, and akathisia, a restless fidgety state with a desire to be in constant motion, are those frequently encountered. Adults are more likely to develop parkinsonism and akathisia,

whereas dystonic movements predominate in children. In some instances these reactions are dose-dependent; in others they are related to individual susceptibility. The symptoms usually disappear within a few days when the drugs are withdrawn, but occasionally persist for months. In some subjects permanent remnants of parkinsonian symptoms have been found years after elimination of the drugs. Paradoxically, involuntary movements may make their initial appearance after withdrawal of neuroleptic agents. This condition, termed *tardive dyskinesia,* tends to occur in older patients who have been on phenothiazine drugs for extended periods of time, during which they have shown signs of parkinsonism. Stereotyped, repetitive movements of lips, tongue, and mouth and choreiform movements of limbs and trunk characterize this disorder. It may diminish in intensity or disappear spontaneously after weeks or months, but in some patients it has persisted indefinitely. In most instances the occurrence of basal ganglia symptoms, particularly parkinsonism, can be minimized by the simultaneous administration of one of the centrally active anticholinergic agents, such as Cogentin or Artane. Cautious use of neuroleptics, employing restricted doses and drug holidays in those requiring long-term treatment, may be the best preventive measure.

365. MANAGEMENT OF THE PARKINSONIAN SYNDROME

General Principles. Until the etiology and pathogenesis of parkinsonism are defined, its treatment must be considered as symptomatic, supportive, and palliative. It is only in the exceptional case of symptomatic parkinsonism resulting from the use of drugs or occurring in association with specific disease processes that treatment of the causative factor may result in eradication of symptoms. The more frequently encountered patient will require lifelong treatment, consisting of the administration of specific medications, supportive psychotherapeutic measures, physical therapy, and, in rare instances, surgical intervention. Judiciously employed treatment may control the symptoms of parkinsonism in a large proportion of patients for extended periods of time. In most it allows relatively normal activities of living during most phases of this disorder. The introduction of new therapeutic approaches holds promise of forestalling or preventing the progressive disabling nature of this disorder.

Supportive Psychotherapy. The major symptoms of parkinsonism are markedly influenced by psychic factors, and a patient's outlook and motivation will affect the extent to which he can overcome disability. It is important for the physician to provide reassurance, encouragement, and sympathetic understanding to the patient and family so that they may meet the numerous difficulties to be encountered at various stages of the illness. To allay anxieties both should be counseled regarding the meaning of various symptoms, the nature of the disease in terms of its long and variable course, and the potential that most patients can lead active and productive lives for long periods after symptoms begin.

Physical Therapy. Simple measures such as heat and massage will alleviate painful muscle cramps and the muscle contraction headache that often accompanies pronounced rigidity of the cervical musculature. Exercises help in preventing flexion contractures. Gait training, walking exercises, and minor rehabilitative measures may enable the patient to maintain his independence with regard to personal hygiene and daily living activities for many more years than his disabilities might otherwise allow. Physical therapy in parkinsonism need not be elaborate, but when indicated should be done frequently and for an indefinite period. The patient should be instructed in simple home exercises and encouraged to develop a program of physical activity. Most patients in the earlier stages like to take long walks and should be encouraged to continue this habit as long as reasonably possible. Every effort should be made to keep them gainfully employed and to adjust their occupations as indicated by their symptoms.

Drug Therapy.   The drugs now employed in the treatment of parkinsonism are those theoretically capable of restoring normal activity to the striatum. Thus any agent that crosses the blood-brain barrier and enhances the brain's dopaminergic function or that reduces cholinergic activity may be expected to influence parkinsonism favorably. As a general rule a combination of agents with such properties works best.

The dopaminergic system may be functionally enhanced by agents that increase the synthesis of dopamine (this is presumably the modus operandi of levodopa), delay the catabolism of dopamine (monoamine oxidase inhibitors), stimulate its release or its action at receptor sites (amphetamine and its analogues), and block the reuptake of monoamines at the synaptic cleft (anticholinergics). Of the numerous means for improving dopaminergic function that have been tried to date, the most effective thus far has been the administration of levodopa (3,4-dihydroxyphenyl-L-alanine). Given alone or in combination with a peripheral dopa decarboxylase inhibitor (benserazide, carbidopa), it is appreciably more effective and less toxic than any therapeutic agent previously available for the treatment of Parkinson's disease.

In the selection of patients for treatment with levodopa, the over-all severity of parkinsonism and the degree of functional impairment, as well as the existence of concomitant diseases of other organs, must be carefully considered. As previously stated, patients with minimal signs and symptoms who are able to meet the demands of daily living need not involve themselves in a treatment program that may be rigorous and demanding and carries an implicit risk. The presence of occlusive vascular disease involving the heart or brain warrants careful assessment. Severe angina pectoris or transient cerebral ischemic attacks contraindicate the use of levodopa. A history of episodic cardiac arrhythmia presents an additional hazard. When the arrhythmia is associated with myocardial disease, the use of levodopa must be undertaken with extreme caution. Evidence of prior mental illness, particularly affective disorders or major "psychotic breaks," contravenes the use of levodopa. Although requiring careful monitoring, levodopa has been administered without adverse effects to patients with hepatic, renal, gastrointestinal, and hematopoietic disorders. However, the presence of hemolytic anemia and glucose-6-phosphate dehydrogenase (G-6-PD) deficiency contraindicates its use.

Clinical experience with levodopa suggests two phases of treatment with which the physician and patient must be familiar. The first or "introduction phase" extends over a period of weeks or months in which the dosage is slowly built up to the therapeutic range. During this phase, tolerance develops to many of the side effects of levodopa; and although improvement of symptoms occurs in most patients, the optimal therapeutic response may not be evident. A "maintenance phase" follows, in which the full benefits of treatment most often occur, and careful patient monitoring with readjustment of dosage and ancillary therapeutic measures may be required to maintain a stable therapeutic response. Each of these phases requires cooperation on the part of the patient and careful management by the physician to achieve the best therapeutic response.

Levodopa is an aromatic amino acid that is a relatively inert compound by itself, but several of its metabolites have profound pharmacologic effects. These vary, depending on the route of administration, the dosage, and the interval. At present, levodopa has only been validated for oral use in parkinsonism and is available in tablets or capsules of 100, 250, and 500 mg. Treatment may conveniently be initiated with 250 mg given three or four times daily by mouth after meals. If the initial doses are well tolerated, each dose may be increased to 500 mg. Subsequent increments of 125 to 250 mg may be made every two to three days in hospitalized patients or at intervals of one to two weeks in outpatients. It is preferable that no single dose exceed 1.5 to 2.0 grams; hence many patients will be required to take multiple doses throughout a 24-hour period. The dose is gradually increased until either a satisfactory response or a dose-limiting side effect is encountered. The average optimal dose in patients with Parkinson's disease is 5 to 6 grams daily. As a general rule it is often best to settle for a total daily dose that, although failing to control all the symptoms, gives an acceptable degree of improvement and a tolerable level of side reactions. Attempts to eradicate every vestige of the disorder may require doses at which an undue frequency and severity of reactions occur.

It is unusual for patients to enjoy the benefits of levodopa without experiencing some side effects. In most, these effects can be modified to tolerable levels by the judicious use of the drug as well as by ancillary measures. Early on in treatment, the major side effects encountered are nausea, vomiting, and anorexia, requiring reduction of dosage and deferral of further increments until such effects subside. Heightened nervous tension and feelings of anxiety necessitate reduction of dosage and a slower build-up to optimal levels. Acute psychotic episodes with delusions, hallucinations, hypomania, or depression are reactions that make it necessary to withdraw the drug. Cardiac dysrhythmia and/or hypotension with syncope is a combination that rarely permits continued use of levodopa. However, patients with orthostatic hypotension may continue treatment, employing commonly used means for its control. Adventitious involuntary movements develop in most patients on long-term levodopa therapy. When they are mild, treatment may be continued at full dosage. In instances in which the movements are excessive or interfere with function, a reduction in dosage is indicated with an attempt to find a level which compromises between a tolerable level of such movements and some degree of parkinsonian symptoms. Variability in therapeutic response develops in some patients after extended periods of levodopa administration. This apparent loss of "dopa effect" may last for hours or days. Its cause is unknown, and few effective means for relieving it have been found. Occasional transitory alterations in blood chemistry, including elevations of serum glutamic oxaloacetic transaminase (SGOT), alkaline phosphatase, and blood urea nitrogen (BUN), as well as depression of white blood cell count and development of a positive Coombs test, have occurred. To date, these have not been associated with symptoms of dysfunction in organ systems, nor has autopsy material shown structural alterations.

The large daily dose of levodopa required, the delayed onset of therapeutic benefits, and some of its side effects can be avoided by the simultaneous administration of a dopa decarboxylase inhibitor. The use of such a combination prevents the peripheral utilization of levodopa, making it more readily and rapidly available for brain metabolism to dopamine. Hence the beneficial effects make their appearance within a matter of days, and side effects such as nausea, vomiting, and anorexia are virtually eliminated. Those side effects originating in the central nervous system, however, are unaffected. A number of such agents have been developed, but at the time of this writing not all have been validated for general use in all countries. In the United States and some European and South American countries, Sinemet, as tablets containing carbidopa, 10 or 25 mg, plus levodopa, 100 or 250 mg, is marketed. In general, patients will require carbidopa, 100 mg, and levodopa, 1000 mg a day, divided into four equal doses. Available only in some European countries as Madopar is a combination of benserazide, 25 or 50 mg, and levodopa, 100 or 200 mg. The average required daily dose of this combination is benserazide, 200 mg, and levodopa, 800 mg, in four equally divided doses. Aldomet (methyl dopa) in doses of 500 mg (125 mg four times a day) has been used in combination with levodopa, 2 to 4 grams, with some effectiveness, but not to the extent of the previously mentioned compounds. A number of other antiparkinsonian agents are useful as adjunctive drugs with levodopa; they are also indicated for those in whom levodopa is contraindicated and are preferred for patients with very mild symptoms in the very early stages of the disorder. Some are also the drug of choice in drug-induced parkinsonism. Most of these compounds possess central nervous system anticholinergic properties or augment striatal dopaminergic activity. Those most frequently used are trihexyphenidyl (Artane), available in 2 and 5 mg tablets; benztropine (Cogentin), as 1 and 2 mg tablets; cycrimine (Pagitane), as 1.25 and 2.5 mg tablets; and procyclidine (Kemadrin), 2 and 5 mg tablets. All are virtually identical in their therapeutic effectiveness, with little reason except personal preference for choosing one over the other. Treatment should be initiated with small doses such as trihexyphenidyl, 2 mg three times daily, gradually increased until further increases yield no additional benefit or side effects reach an unacceptable degree of severity.

To obtain optimal results with anticholinergic drugs, careful titration of dosage against side effects is required. The goal is to find the dose that yields an optimal compromise between the limited symptomatic improvement of the parkinsonism and the disagreeable symptoms of cholinergic blockade of the central and peripheral nervous systems. Among the latter are blurring of vision, dryness of mouth and throat, anhidrosis, constipation, and urinary urgency or, sometimes, retention. The major symptoms of central anticholinergic intoxication are ataxia, dysarthria, hyperthermia, and a characteristic pattern of mental disturbances, including impairment of recent memory, confusion, delusional thinking, hallucinations, somnolence, and rarely coma.

A number of other agents, not primarily anticholinergics but with mild central anticholinergic properties, are useful. Diphenhydramine (Benadryl), orphenadrine (Disipal), and chlorphenoxamine (Phenoxene) are all similar in pharmacologic action, and there is no reason except personal preference or individual tolerance in choosing one over the other. In general, diphenhydramine has enjoyed the widest use and can be given in divided dosage up to 150 mg a day. It is particularly useful as an adjunct to levodopa, for in addition to benefiting symptoms of parkinsonism, it allays anxiety and tempers insomnia.

The antidepressants imipramine (Tofranil) and amitriptyline (Elavil) are minimally effective when used alone, but in combination with anticholinergic agents or levodopa they may be beneficial. With administration in limited dosage, one may avoid their adverse effects, which may resemble parkinsonism. Not only are they helpful in improving akinesia and rigidity, but depressive symptoms when present are relieved. Imipramine or amitriptyline, 10 to 25 mg given four times a day, can be safely administered for extended periods.

Introduced as an antiviral agent, amantadine HCl (Symmetrel) was accidentally found to have activity against parkinsonism. Its mechanism of action in this regard is unknown, but it has been postulated that it may augment striatal dopaminergic activity or block cholinergic action. When used alone in doses of 100 mg twice a day, its therapeutic effects are evident within 48 to 72 hours, consisting of a mild reversal of symptoms of parkinsonism. More effective action can be achieved when it is added to an existing regimen of treatment consisting of anticholinergic agents or levodopa (or both). On occasion amantadine has proved useful during the induction phase of levodopa therapy. Its effects are short lived, tending to diminish after a month and rarely lasting for more than three months. Many of its side effects are similar to those of the anticholinergic agents, particularly the induction of confusional and delusional states. In some patients after long-term use, edema and a form of livedo reticularis develop over the limbs.

Surgical Measures. Surgical attempts to alleviate parkinsonism are primarily directed to the interruption of one or more neural pathways, the integrity of which appears essential for the production of symptoms, and at a site where normal sensory and motor functions will not be affected. Lesions produced by electrocoagulation or freezing in the ventrolateral nucleus of the thalamus have relieved contralateral tremor and rigidity in the limbs. However, akinesia and disturbances in gait, posture, and voice are not appreciably improved, and multiple lesions are necessary to relieve cervical, truncal, and bilateral limb symptoms. Since in most cases tremor and rigidity are bilateral, a good result on one side often encourages an attempt to do the same for the other. Most surgeons prefer to wait six months to one year before operating on the second side to minimize the complications that are apt to occur with bilateral procedures. Even so, the bilateral procedure frequently produces adverse effects on speech and, though recovery usually occurs, the patient may retain some degree of dysarthria and hypophonia. Since in most cases the manifestations become bilateral within a year or two of the onset, and disability is eventually due not so much to tremor or rigidity but to akinesia and postural abnormalities, stereotactic surgery benefits only a limited number of patients. The best candidate for surgery is the patient whose chief manifestation is unilateral tremor and rigidity, preferably in the upper extremity, and whose disease seems to progress slowly. These characteristics represent an early stage of the disease, and usually the patient is not yet seriously disabled. Thus, proponents of stereotactic surgery urge that thalamotomy be considered early in the course of Parkinson's disease, although its critics have pointed out that surgery does not benefit the more advanced patients who most need help, nor does it prevent progression of the disease. The introduction of more effective pharmacologic therapy with its potential of completely controlling parkinsonian symptoms has diminished the enthusiasm for surgical intervention. A balanced judgment would be that thalamotomy be reversed for cases resistant to other forms of therapy and in which relief of upper limb tremor is desired.

Costa, E., Cote, L., and Yahr, M. D. (eds): Biochemistry and Pharmacology of the Basal Ganglia. Hewlett, N.Y., Raven Press, 1966.
Cotzias, G. C., Papavasiliou, P. S., and Gellene, R.: Modification of parkinsonisim: Chronic treatment with L-dopa. N. Engl. J. Med., 280:337, 1969.
Crane, G. E.: Persistence of neurological symptoms due to neuroleptic drugs. Am. J. Psychiatry, 127:1407, 1971.
Crane, G. E.: Tardive dyskinesia in patients treated with major neuroleptics: A review of the literature. Am. J. Psychiatry, 124:40, 1968.
Duvoisin, R. C., and Yahr, M. D.: Encephalitis and parkinsonism. Arch. Neurol. 12:227, 1965.
Hoehn, M. M., and Yahr, M. D.: Parkinsonism: Onset, progression and mortality. Neurology, 17:427, 1967.
Markham, C. H., Brown, W. J., and Rand, R. W.: Stereotaxic lesions in Parkinson's disease. Arch. Neurol., 15:480, 1966.
Yahr, M. D.: The treatment of parkinsonism: Current concepts. Med. Clin. North Am., 56:1377, 1972.

366. ESSENTIAL TREMOR (Familial Tremor)

Melvin D. Yahr

This is a monosymptomatic condition in which tremor involves the hands and/or head and face. The tremor is usually more rapid than that encountered in parkinsonism, is accentuated by emotional factors, may be worsened by volitional movement, and is usually suppressed by the use of alcohol. The age of onset is variable, but in most cases the disorder begins prior to the age of 25 years and tends to persist throughout life. Some progression of the intensity of tremor and spread to other bodily parts usually occur over the years, which may result in significant physical and social disability. There is a strong familial incidence, with occurrence in several successive generations and members of the same family, but the genetic pattern of inheritance has not been determined. Some have suggested its transmission as an autosomal dominant trait. To date no specific pathologic lesion has been reported in the nervous system of people with this condition. It has been suggested that the condition is an abortive form of parkinsonism, but this concept does not appear justifiable at present. There is no specific effective therapy for controlling the tremor, although beta-adrenergic blocking agents such as propranolol in dosage of 120 to 140 mg a day divided equally into three or four doses are occasionally effective. Sedatives such as phenobarbital, in dosage of 15 mg three times a day, may reduce the intensity of the tremor. It is of utmost importance to differentiate essential tremor from parkinsonism. By and large, the distinguishing characteristics are earlier age of onset; lack of severe progression, akinesia, rigidity, or postural abnormalities; and the strong family history of tremor.

Baughman, F. A., Jr., Higgins, J. V., and Mann, J. D.: Sex chromosome anomalies and essential tremor. Neurology, 23:623, 1973.
Critchley, M.: Observations on essential (heredofamilial) tremor. Brain, 22:113, 1949.
Marshal, J.: Observations on essential tremor. J. Neurol. Neurosurg. Psychiatry, 25:122, 1962.
Scopa, J., Longley, B. P., and Foster, J. B.: Beta-adrenergic blockers in benign essential tremor. Curr. Ther. Res., 15:48, 1973.

367. SENILE TREMOR

Melvin D. Yahr

Tremor is a frequent finding in the elderly, most often involving the upper limbs and head. It differs from parkinsonian tremor in that it is finer and more rapid and at first occurs only with voluntary movements. As time goes on it becomes more constant and is also present while the limbs are at rest. There is no associated weakness or alteration in muscle tone. These features differentiate this form of tremor from parkinsonism. The cause is unknown. Since senile tremor has both cerebellar and extrapyramidal features, in that it occurs at rest and with movement, the assumption is that some critical pathway linking these systems has undergone degeneration. There is no effective treatment, although mild benefit may be derived from sedatives or the use of diphenhydramine (Benadryl) given in 25 mg doses three times a day. Most patients accept it as another of the many changes that come with advancing years. Occasional patients have to be reassured that they do not have parkinsonism or some other progressive neurologic disorder.

THE CHOREAS

Melvin D. Yahr

368. INTRODUCTION

There are a number of disease entities that, though wholly unrelated etiologically, have choreiform movements as their major manifestation. In some, intimate relationships with infectious processes have been found, whereas in others familial tendencies have pointed to a strong genetic component. In the light of newer concepts of inheritance, a common pathogenesis for all may be found. Although controversy exists as to the exact anatomic site from which movements of this type may derive, pathologic changes are commonly found in the striatum, particularly in the small cell components of the caudate nucleus and putamen. The classification of chorea into separate entities is at present somewhat arbitrary and is based on age of onset, association with identifiable disease processes or familial tendency, and occurrence of other neurologic abnormalities.

369. ACUTE CHOREA
(Sydenham's or Infectious Chorea, St. Vitus' Dance)

Acute chorea is a movement disorder encountered primarily during childhood and having its greatest incidence between the ages of 5 and 15 years. Occurrence beyond this age is uncommon, and then is usually in association with pregnancy or in persons who have had symptoms earlier in life. Females manifest these symptoms at least twice as often as males. Acute chorea has been reported in people of all races.

Considered as a symptom complex rather than as a specific disease entity, acute choreiform movements have been encountered as initial manifestations of a variety of conditions. They have been reported in epidemic encephalitis, in the encephalopathies occurring with exanthema, with pertussis and diphtheria, in idiopathic hypocalcemia, hyperthyroidism, systemic lupus erythematosus, carbon monoxide poisoning, vascular disease, tumors, and degenerative processes of the basal ganglia. These instances, however, account for only a small percentage of cases. The closest relationship appears to be with rheumatic fever. In more than half of the cases, rheumatic manifestations consisting of carditis, valvular heart disease, or arthritis occur prior to, coincident with, or following an attack of chorea.

There are no specific pathologic changes or anatomic sites of involvement that can be correlated with acute chorea. In fact, because acute uncomplicated chorea is rarely fatal, there has been a paucity of detailed pathologic studies. Cases that have come to autopsy have shown scattered changes in the cortex, basal ganglia, cerebellum, and brainstem. These have consisted of varying degrees of arteritis combined with cellular degeneration.

The outstanding clinical features of chorea are involuntary movements, incoordination, muscle weakness, and emotional lability. Although the onset of symptoms may be abrupt and obvious, it is more often insidious and subtle. The most frequent initial complaints include clumsiness of the limbs, evidenced by dropping objects from the hands or an awkward gait, particularly during emotionally tense situations. When these are coupled with irritability, poor performance in school, and generally fidgety behavior, frequently a hasty conclusion is reached, blaming the child or implying a psychiatric disorder. The typical choreatic movements may be noted in any part of the body, limbs, face, hands, tongue, or trunk. They may at first appear to be a part of the natural pattern of coordinated movements but are soon noted to be completely random, jerking, aimless, and purposeless. They occur at rest, are accentuated by any attempt at volitional movement, and disappear in sleep. They may be very mild and may minimally affect normal function or may be so forceful and frequent as to be totally disabling. Facial grimacing and difficulty in speech, chewing, and swallowing occur when the muscles subserving these functions are involved. Interruption of voluntary movements by involuntary ones leads to incoordination so that the person drops objects, walks in an awkward, ungainly fashion and, in general, appears uncoordinated. Attempts to maintain forceful muscular contraction are similarly interrupted, and the resultant "waxing and waning" of motor power results in a relative degree of motor weakness. Although actual paralysis is rare, there is a disinclination to use a part of the body that is severely affected by involuntary movements of this type. Generalized reduction of muscle tone is an invariable feature of chorea and is readily demonstrable by hyperextensibility at finger, wrist, and ankle joints. In almost all choreatic children some degree of emotional lability is evident. It varies from total apathy to irritability, restlessness, and, infrequently, wild, inappropriate behavior.

Certain cardinal features can be found in almost all patients. These include (1) pronation of the forearm when the upper limbs are raised and extended; (2) inability to sustain muscle contraction when the examiner grasps the patient's hand or when the patient protrudes his tongue so that it darts rapidly in and out of the mouth; and (3) abnormal posturing of hands in which the wrist is noted to be sharply flexed and the fingers hyperextended at the metacarpal pharyngeal joints.

There are no specific laboratory tests for chorea. The cerebrospinal fluid is normal. The electroencephalogram may or may not show diffuse abnormalities correlated with the severity of the disease. Unless there are associated disease processes that manifest themselves in abnormalities of blood count, chemistry, or sedimentation rate, these studies are normal.

The age of onset and the distinctive involuntary movements readily differentiate acute chorea from other disorders of the basal ganglia. Tics and habit spasms may be confused with mild cases, but their movements are quite different, being stereotyped repetitive patterns localized to a single group of muscles. Huntington's chorea rarely begins in childhood and, in addition, there is a strong familial tendency with associated dementia. Movement disorders associated with cerebral palsy occur in infancy but have an athetoid element. The use of phenothiazines may induce abnormal movements, but the history of drug ingestion will differentiate these.

Acute chorea is a self-limited disease, recovery occurring in two to six months. Recurrence, with as many as two or three attacks over a period of years, appears in almost one third of the cases. There is no specific therapy. Bed rest and reduction of external stimuli to a minimum, combined with sedative drugs such as phenobarbital or chloral hydrate, are beneficial in controlling the severity of the movements. Paradoxically, the phenothiazines, such as thorazine and chlorpromazine, as well as reserpine in doses commensurate with individual tolerance, although capable of inducing chorea, have also been shown to be effective in its control. Because of the high incidence of rheumatic valvular heart disease complicating acute chorea, prophylaxis with antimicrobial drugs over a long interval of time similar to that utilized in acute rheumatic fever is now recommended. If emotional symptoms are intense, psychotherapy may be in order. When specific abnormalities of calcium metabolism or thyroid dysfunction are found, their correction may completely ameliorate the symptoms. With recovery most patients show few, if any, neurologic sequelae.

Aron, A., Freeman, J., and Carter, S.: The natural history of Sydenham's chorea. Am. J. Med., 38:83, 1965.
Schwartzman, J.: Chorea minor. Review of 175 cases with reference to etiology, treatment and sequelae. Rheumatism, 6:89, 1950.

370. HEREDITARY CHOREA
(Chronic Progressive Chorea, Huntington's Chorea)

Hereditary chorea is a progressive degenerative disease of the basal ganglia and cerebral cortex, beginning in adult life and characterized by choreiform movements and mental deterioration. The inheritance of the disease is based on a single dominant autosomal gene. It may be transmitted by either sex, and both sexes are affected in equal numbers. The trait is transmitted from affected individual to affected individual so that those who escape rarely transmit the disease. Only about 50 per cent of the offspring are affected. The disease is relatively rare, although its incidence may be high in geographic regions where affected families have resided for many generations.

Pathologically, widespread degenerative changes with cell loss and reactive gliosis are found, primarily in the cerebral cortex and caudate nucleus. Recently it has been demonstrated that glutamic acid decarboxylase and choline acetylase activity are reduced in the basal ganglia of patients with Huntington's chorea. This results in a deficiency of γ-aminobutyric acid, an inhibitory transmitter substance in brain, as well as depressed function of the excitatory transmitter acetylcholine. Disruption of the homeostatic relationship of these agents may underlie the choreatic manifestations of this disorder.

The clinical manifestations consist of choreatic movements, emotional disturbance, and intellectual deterioration in varying degrees, rate of appearance, and progression. The disease usually makes its appearance between the ages of 35 and 50 years, rather insidiously with any of the aforementioned symptoms, but as a rule with abnormal movements. The movements, though similar to acute chorea, are usually more jerky though less lightning-like and primarily involve the trunk and shoulder girdle and more often the lower limbs than the upper. This pattern of involvement tends to produce a dancing sort of gait, which is a prominent feature of the disease. In rare instances a Parkinson-like rigidity is encountered as the major manifestation rather than involuntary movements. The mental deterioration is similar to that of any organic dementia, with progressive impairment of memory and of intellectual capacity, and inattention to personal hygiene. Emotional disturbances include heightened irritability, bouts of depression, and fits of violent behavior.

With the typical triad of choreiform movements, dementia in adult life, and documentation of similar symptoms in family members, the diagnosis is readily evident. However, there is a tendency for families to deny the existence of mental disease, and it is sometimes difficult to obtain corroborative data even when the diagnosis is strongly suspected. Little difficulty occurs in differentiating hereditary chorea from acute chorea, but senile chorea may raise a problem. The latter, which comes on late in life, involves few mental changes, if any, lacks a familial history, and is usually benign in comparison. Other diseases such as the presenile psychoses, Alzheimer's and Pick's, because of their dementia and similarity in age of onset, may offer some difficulty, especially in instances in which choreiform movements are inconspicuous. Pneumoencephalography demonstrating selective atrophy of the caudate nucleus may help to establish the correct diagnosis in such instances.

There is a tendency to overdiagnose hereditary chorea, applying it to diverse neurologic disorders such as cerebellar degenerations and familial tremors. The dire implications of this form of chorea require strict adherence to the diagnostic criteria.

There is no effective therapy. Theoretically, drugs which are capable of elevating brain γ-aminobutyric acid or enhancing its cholinergic activity should be helpful. Although some, such as phenelzine and dimethyl aminoethanol, are undergoing trial, inadequate reports are available at present to comment on their use. Huntington's chorea is relentlessly progressive, leading to total incapacity and inevitably death, usually within 15 years of onset. In the early stages the patient can be managed at home with supervision and the use of phenothiazines or reserpine to reduce the intensity of the movements and to control the behavior to some extent. As the disease advances, confinement to a psychiatric facility becomes necessary.

Chandler, J. H., Reed, T. E., and DeJong, R. N.: Huntington's chorea in Michigan. Neurology, 10:148, 1960.
Lyon, R. L.: Huntington's chorea. Br. Med. J., 1:1306, 1962.
Perry, T. L., Hansen, S., and Kloster, M.: Huntington's chorea: Deficiency of γ-aminobutyric acid in brain. N. Engl. J. Med., 288:337, 1973.

371. SENILE CHOREA

Infrequently, choreiform movements are encountered as an isolated symptom in persons above 60 years of age. As a rule, the movements are mild and may involve the limbs on one side of the body or bilaterally. Involuntary complex movements of the face, mouth, and tongue may occur, in association with limb movements or as the only manifestation of this disorder. No associated mental disturbance occurs in such patients, and no family history indicative of Huntington's chorea can be obtained. In many instances the symptoms come on abruptly, are unilateral, and show little, if any, progression. This has suggested an underlying vascular lesion, which may be found in an exceptional case. More often than not the pathologic findings are similar to those of Huntington's chorea insofar as involvement of the caudate nucleus is concerned, but the cerebral cortex is spared. This has led to the contrary consideration that these cases are a variant of Huntington's chorea occurring sporadically. Probably this form of chorea has several causes. As a rule, the symptoms are mild and the course benign so that therapeutic considerations are unimportant.

Martin, J. P.: Hemichorea resulting from local lesions of the brain. Brain, 50:637, 1927.
Weiner, W. J., and Klawans, H. L., Jr.: Lingual-facial-buccal movements in the elderly. II. Pathogenesis and relationship to senile chorea. J. Am. Geriat. Soc., 21:318, 1973.

372. TICS
(Habit Spasms)
Melvin D. Yahr

A tic is a sudden, abrupt, rapid, purposeless, involuntary contraction of a muscle or group of functionally related muscles. Usually an irregular sequence of such contractions occurs that may result in eye blinking, head shaking, shrugging of the shoulder, or any sudden gesture of limbs or face. Tics may be voluntarily controlled for brief intervals, but such a conscious effort is usually followed by more intense and frequent contractions. Many persons experience minor transitory tic phenomena under periods of stress that are of no consequence. More persistent, sustained, and gross movements may be related to particular personality disturbances, and may be amenable to psychotherapy. In some instances tics have occurred during the acute phase of encephalitis; these are thought to be an expression of extrapyramidal dysfunction. Tics in younger patients must be differentiated from chorea. Their patterned, predictable, and stereotyped character makes this distinction.

An unusual form of generalized tic (*maladie des tics, Gilles de la Tourette's disease*) involving facial twitching, continuous gestures associated with echolalia, foul language, and obsessional ideas is occasionally encountered in childhood. The disorder is progressive, and sometimes associated with marked personality changes. Recently, however, a number of reports have appeared suggesting that haloperidol (Haldol) in divided dosage of 6 to 20 mg a day may be effective both in reducing the movement disorder and in overcoming the unfortunate verbal outbursts.

Hansen, M., and Eisler, R. M.: Behavioral approaches to study and treatment of psychogenic tics. Genet. Psychol. Monogr., 87:289, 1973.
Shapiro, A. K., Shapiro, E., and Wayne, H.: Treatment of Tourette's syndrome with haloperidol, review of 34 cases. Arch. Gen. Psychiatry, 28:92, 1973.

373. ATHETOSIS
(Mobile Spasms)

Melvin D. Yahr

This involuntary movement disorder is most frequently encountered in early infancy. Although in some respects it resembles chorea and although there are, in fact, transitional forms (so-called choreo-athetosis), the athetotic movements are distinguishable by being slower, coarser, and more writhing. They occur when pathologic conditions involve the basal ganglia, primarily the pallidum, as well as additional motor pathways such as the corticospinal tract. Athetosis is most often found in the heterogeneous group of conditions now lumped together under the term "cerebral palsy" (CP). More often than not, patients with cerebral palsy have marked alteration in muscle tone consisting of a combination of spasticity and rigidity. Their extrapyramidal movements may be widespread or limited and encompass a wide variety of dyskinetic phenomena. Congenital defects, anoxia or trauma at birth, and other degenerative conditions have all been implicated. Some attempt has been made to identify specific entities based on clinicopathologic correlations. One such is athetosis simplex or status marmoratus. Cases of this disorder, which exemplifies all of the features of athetosis, show at autopsy a distinctive marbled appearance of the basal ganglia, the result of an abnormal overgrowth of myelin sheaths and increased numbers of glial cells. The cause of this morphologic abnormality is unknown. Other cases have been grouped together in which the prime pathologic change is cell loss and failure of myelin sheath formation in the region of the basal ganglia—so-called status dysmyelination. Still other cases have been encountered in which abnormal deposits of pigments occur or one of the the lipoidoses or other storage diseases is found with the predominant clinical picture of

athetotic movements. Athetosis is infrequently encountered in adult life, but when it is, tumors, vascular insufficiency, or malformations and the effects of toxic agents have been found in the region of the basal ganglia.

Typical athetosis possesses the following features in varying degrees. One or both sides of the body are involved. The movements involve the upper limbs to a greater extent than the lower and primarily in their distal segments. The muscles innervated by the cranial nerves are invariably involved so that facial grimacing, writhing movements of the tongue, and disturbances in articulation and swallowing are encountered. Abnormal postures of the limbs are assumed. In the upper extremities, these consist of adduction and internal rotation at the shoulder, semiflexion at the elbow, flexion of wrist and metacarpal phalangeal joints, and extension at interphalangeal joints. In the lower limbs the foot is maintained in internal rotation and plantar flexion with dorsiflexion of the toes. Superimposed on these abnormal postures are the athetotic movements described above. Muscle tone is increased during movement but is hypotonic during relaxation, and some degree of weakness is usually found. The reflexes may be hyperactive, with abnormal toe responses. In many instances some degree of intellectual impairment may be found.

The abnormal movements and postural abnormalities are distinctive enough to make this condition readily recognizable. The age at onset, the admixture of other neurologic abnormalities, and the manner in which the symptoms progress identify the disease. Since most instances of athetosis appear in early infancy, before one year of age, diseases of the perinatal period are considered primarily. Athetosis occurring in later childhood or adult life may be a part of other extrapyramidal disorders, such as dystonia, chorea, or hepatolenticular degeneration. Less frequently athetosis is a manifestation of a wide spectrum of neurologic disorders already mentioned in which the pallidum is coincidentally involved.

There is no specific therapy for the relief of athetosis. The use of anticholinergic agents as previously indicated under the treatment of parkinsonism may decrease the intensity of the movements. Thalamotomy has on occasion afforded some degree of relief, but one is hesitant to advocate this surgical procedure on a nervous system already extensively damaged by a variety of pathologic processes.

Courville, C. B.: Structural basis of athetosis in cerebral palsied children. Arch. Pediat., 78:461, 1961.
Mettler, F. A., and Stern, G.: On the patho-physiology of athetosis. J. Nerv. Ment. Dis., 135:138, 1962.
Narabayashi, H., and Nakamura, R.,: Clinical picture of cerebral palsy in neurological understanding. Confin. Neurol., 34:7, 1972.

374. DYSTONIA MUSCULORUM DEFORMANS
(Torsion Dystonia)

Melvin D. Yahr

The torsion dystonias comprise a group of movement disorders characterized by intense, irregular, sustained torsion spasms of the musculature, with resultant marked abnormalities of bodily posture. The dystonic movements may involve any or all of the musculature, but have a predilection for the trunk and shoulder and pelvic girdles. The cause and morbid anatomy of this condition are unknown.

Three forms can be recognized, based on genetic, clinical, and presumed causative factors. These consist of autosomal recessive, autosomal dominant, and acquired or symptomatic types. Symptomatic dystonic movements occur with hepatolenticular degeneration, postencephalitic parkinsonism, and tumors or other diseases involving the basal ganglia; dystonia musculorum deformans is a distinct clinical entity. Glial scarring in the basal ganglia, thalamus, and cortex has been described in some cases, and some have been associated with status marmoratus and dysmyelination, as indicated in Ch. 373.

The autosomal recessive form is found most often in Ashkenazic Jews, beginning between the ages of 5 and 15 years. Its onset is variable but most frequently begins with intermittent spasmodic inversion of the foot, so that on walking the child finds difficulty in placing the heel on the ground. Bizarre stepping or a bowing gait may be noted when the dystonic movements affect the more proximal muscles of the leg or the spine. As the movements become more intense and the proximal musculature is more prominently involved, lordosis and tortipelvis appear. If the muscles of the neck and shoulder girdle are involved, torticollis is an early finding. Facial grimacing and difficulties in speech become evident as the muscles subserving these functions become involved. The continuous spasms over a period of time result in marked distortions of the body of a degree rarely seen in any other disease process. Although muscle tone and power appear to be normal, the involuntary movements interfere with function to such a degree as to make them useless. No changes in the deep tendon reflexes occur, and mentation remains normal.

The autosomal dominant form has its onset in early adult life and generally involves the axial musculature, with torticollis a frequent presenting symptom. In contrast to the recessive form, it remains more restricted in the regions of the body involved and is more slowly progressive. Recently it has been demonstrated that plasma dopamine beta hydroxylase activity is markedly elevated in the dominant form. This finding is strictly empiric, and although it is helpful in classification of the disease, neither the physiologic nor the biochemical significance of this finding has been elucidated.

In its early stages dystonia musculorum deformans must be differentiated from other movement disorders in which dystonic phenomena may occur. The history and physical findings exclude hepatolenticular degeneration and epidemic encephalitis. The age at onset and the involvement of proximal musculature in the movements are enough to differentiate it from athetosis. Chorea is characterized by movements more rapid and of shorter duration than those of dystonia. Hysteria is often a consideration; if it is not positively established by the personality characteristics of the patient, the course of the disease will soon suggest the correct diagnosis.

There is extreme variability in the rate of progression and eventual disability of both forms of the genetically determined disorder. In their early phases there may be complete remission of symptoms or lack of progression of initial symptoms for intervals of up to five years. Because the natural history is subject to wide variations, evaluation of the effects of treatment is difficult. Dys-

tonic movements have been effectively controlled for varying periods of time by both drugs and surgical intervention. The medicines effective are anticholinergic agents such as those indicated for the treatment of parkinsonism, combined with sedative agents such as phenobarbital. In mild cases a combination of these drugs with some general supportive psychotherapy may be enough to control the patient's symptoms for years. On occasion, carbamazepine (Tegretol) in daily dosage of 800 to 1200 mg a day divided equally in four or five doses has proved effective. Levodopa has been reported as being effective in selected cases. In general a lower daily dose (3 grams per day) than that used in parkinsonism has been required. In more serious cases thalamotomy has produced encouraging results. However, because rather extensive lesions must be placed in the thalamic nuclei, multiple operative procedures are required to produce the desired effect. Although the operations are well tolerated by most patients, they do carry an element of risk and are indicated only in selected cases.

Denny-Brown, D. E.: The nature of dystonia. Bull. N.Y. Acad. Med., 41:858, 1965.
Eldridge, R.: The torsion dystonias: Literature review and genetic and clinical studies. Neurology, 20:1, 1970.

375.   SPASMODIC TORTICOLLIS

Melvin D. Yahr

The restriction of dyskinetic movements to neck muscles so that abnormal postures of the head result is the distinguishing characteristic of this symptom complex. Involuntary activity involves the sternocleidomastoids, trapezius, and scalenus muscles in sustained contractions that result in slow, twisting, turning movements of the head (torticollis) or less often forward flexion (anterocollis) or forceful extension (retrocollis). In most instances there is bilateral involvement, and the resultant postural deformity is maintained for varying lengths of time. The muscles of the neck appear under tension, and the continual muscular activity may lead to some degree of hypertrophy, especially evident in the sternocleidomastoid. Similar activity may spread to facial and brachial musculature. The amount of active motion or static postural deformity is extremely variable.

Spasmodic torticollis has variably been described as a psychogenic disorder, a fragment of dystonia musculorum deformans, or a compensatory postural defect in persons with congenital ocular muscle imbalance or defects of the cervical spine or musculature. In some instances it has occurred as part of a wide spectrum of extrapyramidal disorders that follow encephalitis lethargica. There is no information at present regarding either its pathophysiology or pathology.

The disorder has been encountered at all ages, but most frequently makes its appearance during the third to sixth decades of life. The course is extremely variable, being transitory and remitting after a few months in some patients and relentlessly progressive and leading to incapacity in others. Some cases reach a static phase in which movements cease or are minimal, and a minor postural deformity of the head persists.

The evaluation of this condition includes a search for ocular and vertebral signs, major psychiatric disturbances, and other neurologic conditions with which it may be associated. Definable conditions account for only a small percentage of cases. In most, no known cause is uncovered.

There is no specific therapy for torticollis except when an underlying correctible disease process is found. Many measures have been recommended to ameliorate the symptoms. In mild cases or in the initial stages, a combination of drugs previously discussed under the treatment of parkinsonism has proved useful. Symptoms may be reduced to a tolerable degree, and it can be hoped that spontaneous remission will intervene. In those more severely affected a variety of surgical measures have been attempted with inconsistent results. Denervation of the affected muscles by section of the anterior cervical roots and/or the spinal accessory nerve has been utilized. Although the movements decrease on the operated side, they frequently recur in the contralateral group of muscles. Bilateral procedures may result in extensive disability. Recently thalamotomy has been performed with encouraging results. One is hesitant, however, to recommend a procedure of this magnitude except in extreme situations.

Herz, E., and Glaser, G. H.: Spasmodic torticollis. Clinical evaluation. Arch. Neurol. Psychiatry, 61:227, 1949.

376. HEMIBALLISM
Melvin D. Yahr

This rather violent involuntary movement occurs when lesions involve the contralateral subthalamic nucleus, the corpus Luysii. Although a variety of pathologic processes such as tumor and infectious diseases have been found as underlying causes, most are a result of vascular lesions, either hemorrhagic or occlusive. In consequence, they are encountered in older patients, sometimes after a transitory hemiparesis. The event leading to the onset of this movement disorder often is an acute cerebrovascular accident with weakness and/or sensory deficit. As the neurologic signs clear or at a variable interval afterward, the ballistic movements begin. The movements do not occur during sleep, are localized to one side of the body, and involve the limbs in a forceful throwing movement, a result of almost continuous activity of the proximal musculature. Initially, their violence may exhaust and incapacitate the patient to such an extent that death may ensue. However, in most instances, the initial intensity decreases gradually so that they become tolerable, and in approximately six to eight weeks the movements stop spontaneously. Surgical measures, such as thalamotomy, are rarely needed for control. In this regard, it is interesting to note that hemiballism has followed attempted thalamotomy for other extrapyramidal disorders when poor localization for lesion placement has occurred. In such instances, the surgeon has inadvertently placed a lesion in the region of the corpus Luysii.

Carpenter, M. B.: Ballism associated with partial destruction of the subthalamic nucleus of Luys. Neurology, 5:479, 1955.
Hyland, H. H., and Forman, D. M.: Progress in hemiballismus. Neurology. 7:381, 1957.
Martin, P. J., and McCaul, I. R.: Acute hemiballism treated by ventrolateral thalamolysis. Brain, 82:104, 1959.

377. IDIOPATHIC AUTONOMIC INSUFFICIENCY
(Idiopathic Orthostatic Hypotension, Shy-Drager Syndrome)

Fred Plum

Definition. This is an uncommon disorder first clearly described by Bradbury and Eggleston in 1925 as idiopathic orthostatic hypotension; it has been more recently emphasized as including more generalized autonomic and nervous system defects. The cause is unknown and the course progressive; severe disability or death usually occurs within five to ten years after onset.

Pathology and Pathogenesis. Detailed examination of the central and peripheral nervous system at autopsy discloses degenerative changes in the intermediolateral column of the spinal cord, the dorsal motor nuclei, and the pigmented nuclei of the brainstem. In addition, some patients have abnormalities which resemble olivopontocerebellar degeneration, whereas others show striatalnigral degeneration. Peripheral autonomic structures are morphologically normal in most patients. The cause is unknown.

Several observations indicate that the disease begins as a defect in preganglionic autonomic transmitter function. Most of the patients demonstrate a blood pressure hypersensitivity to injected levarterenol, implying the absence of the humoral agent in the sympathetic ganglia. Also, patients with neurogenic orthostatic hypotension have been found not to synthesize norepinephrine and its metabolic products in normal amounts and to have below normal urinary catecholamine levels. Since the drug tyramine, which acts to release norepinephrine from peripheral autonomic nerve terminals, is effective in elevating the blood pressure, at least some epinephrine synthesis must be going on in postganglionic peripheral nerve terminals, but whether this is of a normal or reduced amount is unknown.

Clinical Manifestations. Symptoms of autonomic insufficiency predominate initially. These include impotence in males, constipation, heat intolerance with anhidrosis, and, above all, weakness or faintness or rising to an erect position or during quiet standing. Urinary urgency or retention is common. As the disease progresses, symptoms of more generalized neurologic dysfunction appear. Some patients develop a Parkinson-like illness with hypokinesia, rhythmic postural tremor, and mild to moderate rigidity. Others develop a cerebellar type of incoordination plus a gross rhythmic tremor in the lower extremities. The mind remains clear.

Physical signs include prominent evidence of autonomic insufficiency. Pupillary abnormalities with Horner's syndrome can alternate from side to side. Even with a high environmental temperature there is diffuse anhidrosis of the trunk and extremities. The blood pressure is normal when the subject is supine, but when he stands, systolic and diastolic pressures drop 20 to 40 mm Hg or more but the pulse fails to accelerate. In the early stage of illness the blood pressure can gradually climb during continued standing, but as the disease advances, autonomic compensation decreases and then fails altogether, and syncope with unobtainable blood pressure tends to interrupt any sustained effort to be erect. By this time, many patients have associated signs of generalized neurologic dysfunction, including the Parkinson-like signs mentioned above as well as a cerebellar type of incoordination, muscle wasting and fasciculations, coarse tremors, and extensor plantar responses. Signs of peripheral neuropathy are notably lacking in the idiopathic disease.

Laboratory tests of the usual type are valueless except to exclude other disorders, but confirmation of the autonomic insufficiency makes the diagnosis.

Briefly, the evaluation of autonomic insufficiency investigates the blood pressure response to tilting and quiet standing, the patient's ability to sweat when heated, a cold pressor test (the response is absent), the blood pressure response to injected levarterenol and sublingual nitroglycerin (the responses are hyperactive), and the response to the Valsalva maneuver (the normal blood pressure overshoot with its accompanying tachycardia fails to occur).

Differential Diagnosis.   Orthostatic hypotension can accompany acute cardiac failure (as with myocardial infarction or severe aortic stenosis), blood volume depletion (as with gastrointestinal or other massive hemorrhage), or vasodepressor syncope, but in all these conditions other signs of autonomic activity such as tachycardia and sweating are present and signs of diffuse neurologic illness are absent. Autonomic insufficiency also accompanies some clearly identifiable neurologic diseases, including central thiamin deficiency (Wernicke's encephalopathy), tabes dorsalis, syringomyelia, surgical sympathectomy, the neuropathies of diabetes, amyloidosis, and the Guillain-Barré syndrome, and a small fraction of patients who have vascular occlusive disease producing infarction or ischemia of brainstem autonomic centers. The differentiation from most of these illnesses is readily made by the typical signs, symptoms, and laboratory findings of each, and particularly by the fact that most of them produce sensory impairments in the extremities and other peripheral nerve abnormalities which are altogether lacking in idiopathic autonomic insufficiency.

Course and Treatment.   Although treatment is rarely completely satisfactory and does not affect the disease itself, much can be done to help these patients symptomatically during the early phase of the illness. Nine-α-fluorohydrocortisone given regularly by mouth is often effective in counteracting the orthostatic hypotension; it presumably operates partly by increasing the blood volume. Elastic bandages on the legs may help by reducing venous pooling. Placing the head of the bed on six-inch blocks for sleeping has been found to lessen the next day's degree of orthostatic hypotension. Pressor agents have generally been useless because of their short, intense action and undesirable side effects. However, a combination of monoamine oxidase inhibitors (which reduce the deamination of catecholamines in sympathetic nerve storage pools) and amphetamines (which stimulate norepinephrine release) has been found effective in maintaining the erect blood pressure of some patients previously bedridden from their illness.

Bannister, R., and Oppenheimer, D. R.: Degenerative diseases of the nervous system associated with autonomic failure. Brain, 95:457, 1972.

Bradbury, S., and Eggleston, C.: Postural hypotension: Report of 3 cases. Am. Heart J., 1:73, 1925.

Lewis, R. K., Hazelrig, C. G., Fricke, F. J., and Russell, R. O.: Therapy of idiopathic postural hypotension. Arch. Intern. Med., 129:943, 1972.

Shy, R. M., and Drager, G. A.: A neurological syndrome associated with orthostatic hypotension. Arch. Neurol., 2:511, 1960.

Stead, E. A., Jr., and Ebert, R. V.: Postural hypotension: Disease of sympathetic nervous system. Arch. Intern. Med., 67:546, 1941.

Section Eleven.   CEREBROVASCULAR DISEASES

Fletcher H. McDowell

378.   INTRODUCTION

It is estimated that there are 2 million persons alive today who have neurologic manifestations of cerebrovascular disease and that cerebrovascular disease of all varieties is annually responsible for approximately 200,000 deaths in the United States. Fully a half million Americans each year suffer a new, acute cerebrovascular attack. The over-all problem is even more imposing than the annual incidence and mortality figures. Recurrent vascular accidents are common in nearly all forms of cerebrovascular disease, each recurrence carrying a high risk of mortality. For the survivors, disability and dependency are the usual result. The need for medical care and hospital facilities for these patients is enormous and is an imposing challenge to medical and social service agencies alike.

In the following chapters, the cerebral vascular diseases are divided into two general groups, those producing ischemic *cerebral infarction* and those producing *intracranial hemorrhage.* Much of the material is derived from observations on 966 patients with clinically diagnosed cerebral vascular disease undergoing long-term study at the Cornell Division of Bellevue Hospital in New York City. As a rough index of the frequency of the different types of cerebral vascular accident or "stroke," 88 per cent of these patients had acute infarction or less severe cerebral ischemic attacks, and 12 per cent had intracranial hemorrhage. Of the infarctions, about one in eight was attributed to cerebral embolism.

379. CEREBRAL ISCHEMIA AND INFARCTION

DEFINITION AND ETIOLOGY

Cerebral thrombosis and cerebral emboli produce clinical symptoms by causing cerebral infarction, which means neural death from ischemia. Cerebral ischemia is the result of either a generalized or a localized prolonged reduction of blood flow to the brain. If ischemia is transient, less than 10 to 15 minutes, usually no discernible neurologic deficit remains. If it lasts longer than that, neural damage results, producing neurologic dysfunction, disability, and death.

The causes of cerebral infarction are numerous. The following are the most common ones:

1. Atherosclerotic disease of the intra- and extracranial arteries
2. Cerebral emboli with: (a) rheumatic heart disease, (b) myocardial infarction, (c) cardiac disease and atrial fibrillation, (d) subacute bacterial endocarditis, (e) nonbacterial thrombotic endocarditis
3. Reduced cerebral blood flow from severe hypotension or dysrhythmia of cardiac disease
4. Cerebral arterial spasm following subarachnoid hemorrhage
5. Generalized cerebral hypoxia from (a) cardiopulmonary insufficiency, (b) pulmonary emboli, (c) carbon monoxide poisoning
6. Cerebral thrombosis due to arteritis: (a) collagen vascular disease, (b) giant cell arteritis, (c) bacterial arteritis, including syphilis
7. Cerebral thrombosis due to polycythemia or ischemia caused by severe anemia
8. Cerebral thrombosis adjacent to intracerebral hemorrhage
9. Cerebral arterial vasoconstriction associated with migraine
10. Dissecting aneurysm of the aorta or great vessels in the neck

INCIDENCE AND EPIDEMIOLOGY

Cerebral infarction is most commonly the result of cerebral atherosclerosis and cerebral emboli. In the Cornell-Bellevue series of 873 cases with nonhemorrhagic stroke, 92 per cent were clinically related to cerebral atherosclerosis and 8 per cent to cerebral emboli. In the group with cerebral emboli 20 per cent occurred in association with myocardial infarction, 26 per cent with rheumatic heart disease, most commonly with mitral stenosis, and atrial fibrillation, and the remainder in patients with atrial fibrillation associated with other varieties of heart disease.

Cerebral infarction is almost twice as frequent in males as in females. The peak age period is 60 to 69 years, but the incidence of stroke rises linearly with increasing age. In the Cornell-Bellevue study, stroke occurred earlier than the age of 50 in only 8 per cent of the patients.

NEUROPATHOLOGY

The brain is exquisitely dependent on its oxygen supply. There is no reserve of oxygen in cerebral tissue to sustain cerebral metabolism during periods of reduced or absent cerebral blood flow. When the brain is acutely and completely deprived of oxygen generally or locally, the electroencephalogram changes within 10 to 20 seconds, and irreversible and extensive neural damage occurs in the cerebral hemispheres after three to ten minutes. The determinants of brain ischemia are hypoxia and reduced general or local cerebral perfusion. The more important of the two is a decrease in perfusion. When ischemia is prolonged, the ischemic tissue softens, and the usually distinct margins between gray and white matter become unclear and occasionally hemorrhagic. Under the microscope, neurons are seen to be necrotic and shrunken, i.e., infarcted.

Cerebral infarctions that follow ischemia may be "pale" (nonhemorrhagic) or hemorrhagic. The extravasation of blood into tissues more commonly follows an embolic arterial obstruction, and pale infarcts more frequently follow atherosclerotic or thrombotic arterial obstruction. Often the two varieties of infarction blend together, and there is little advantage in extensively weighing the difference of causation.

A variable amount of *cerebral edema* accompanies cerebral infarction. With large infarctions the edema may be so extensive that portions of the swollen hemisphere shift under the falx or down through the tentorium cerebelli. This change in intracranial space relationships further impairs the flow of blood and cerebrospinal fluid, thus increasing the ischemia and neurologic deficit. This is often followed by secondary congestion and ischemia of the upper brainstem, which is almost invariably fatal.

It is common to find numerous old, small cerebral infarctions in patients dying from other causes, indicating that cerebral infarctions need not always give rise to symptoms. Old infarctions that have been hemorrhagic are identified at postmortem examination by the presence of hemosiderin in the wall of the infarct. As the infarct ages, the necrotic area breaks down, is absorbed, and eventually may be replaced by a fluid-filled cavity lined with glial and fibrovascular tissue.

MECHANISMS

Cerebral infarction is usually accompanied by abnormalities in the state of the arterial conducting system from the heart to the brain or the venous system draining the brain; the efficiency of the heart as a pump in producing a constant blood flow at a sufficient arterial pressure; and the character of the circulating medium (blood), its viscosity, its oxygen-carrying capacity, and its capacity to change from a colloidal suspension to a gel. Most cerebral infarctions are due to simultaneous changes in several of these factors.

The arterial conducting system is most often altered by atherosclerotic disease. In the third decade of life atherosclerosis is usually evident in the arteries leading to the brain, particularly in the larger cerebral arteries. Sites of predilection for plaques (Fig. 1) are the origins of the common carotid artery; just above the common carotid bifurcation; the internal carotid in its siphonous portion; the origin of the middle cerebral artery; and the vertebral arteries just after they enter the skull and the basilar artery. The atheromatous process in cerebral arteries is the same as that found elsewhere in the body, with lipid deposition in the intima, fibrous tissue overgrowth, hemorrhage into the plaques, ulceration of the plaques, and vessel obstruction.

Although atheromatous vascular disease begins early, it is a silent process for most of the life of the patient, and rarely produces symptoms until the middle years, when myocardial infarction, cerebral infarction, and lower extremity infarction occur. Most postmortem studies show

Figure 1. The darkened areas on the arterial diagram show the common sites of atherosclerosis and obstruction in the cerebral vessels.

Labels on figure:
- Anterior cerebral artery
- Middle cerebral artery
- Posterior communicating artery
- Posterior cerebral artery
- Basilar artery
- Internal carotid artery
- Vertebral artery
- Anterior spinal artery
- External carotid artery
- Common carotid artery
- Subclavian artery
- Arch of the aorta

that 80 to 90 per cent of all adult patients examined at autopsy have significant atheromatous disease. Since by no means all of these had experienced adverse clinical effects, the factors determining symptomatic complications assume major importance.

The first factor of importance is the degree and extent of atheromatous vascular disease, both in the arteries in the neck leading to the head and in the intracranial cerebral arteries. In general, persons who have cerebral infarctions have the most extensive cerebrovascular disease in the arteries in the neck and in the head. However, the pathogenesis of infarction depends on several mechanisms, and patients with only small or moderate amounts of vascular disease sometimes suffer serious cerebral infarcts. Conversely, extensive atheromatous disease can be found in large and small intracranial and extracranial cerebral arteries in patients without cerebral infarction.

Diabetes or *hypertension* can be detected in over two thirds of patients who have had cerebrovascular accidents. Patients with either diabetes or hypertension develop atherosclerosis at an earlier age, and the process develops more rapidly than in patients without these complicating illnesses. The atherosclerotic disease is extensive and is found in the smaller intracranial arteries.

The condition of the *cerebral collateral circulation* influences the development of cerebral infarction in persons with atherosclerosis. Most collateral circulation from one major intracerebral arterial system to another is through the circle of Willis via the posterior communicating arteries or the anterior communicating artery. Other sites of collateral circulation include the interconnections of the pial arteries on the cerebral surface between the anterior, middle, and posterior cerebral arteries. Sites of collateral circulation that become func-

tional only when circulation through other routes is impaired are also found between the external and the internal carotid artery system, via the ophthalmic artery, and through muscular branches between the vertebral arteries and the external carotid artery in the neck.

Anomalies of the circle of Willis occur in nearly half the population. The most common is atresia of the posterior communicating artery, which tends to isolate the anterior (carotid system) circulation from the posterior (vertebral basilar) circulation. Anomalies in the circle of Willis are even more common in patients with cerebral infarction, and thus are believed to increase the chances of stroke in patients with cerebral atherosclerosis.

Inflammatory states involving the cerebral arteries are another cause of cerebral infarction. Inflammation produces edema and fibrosis of the vascular wall, which reduces the carrying capacity of the vessel and causes a decrease in cerebral blood flow distally. Collagen-vascular disease is the most common vascular inflammation causing cerebral infarction. Syphilis was formerly the most common inflammation of the cerebral arteries and a frequent cause of cerebral infarction, especially in young persons. Rarely, acute bacterial infections of the pharynx have been followed by vasculitis of the carotid arteries and cerebral infarction. Another uncommon illness is Takayasu's disease, which affects the origin of the cerebral arteries from the aortic arch and its branches, and often results in cerebral infarction, especially in young to middle-aged women.

CEREBRAL EMBOLI

Cerebral infarction can occur without intrinsic arterial disease when emboli block arteries and impair blood flow. The most common cause of cerebral emboli in patients under 50 is rheumatic heart disease with mitral stenosis and atrial fibrillation. Other conditions associated with embolus formation are myocardial infarction with mural thrombi, atrial fibrillation of unknown cause, subacute bacterial endocarditis, thyrotoxicosis with atrial fibrillation, and nonbacterial thrombotic endocarditis. Fat emboli are rare. Paradoxical emboli have been reported as a cause of cerebral infarction. These arise in distal veins, and are shunted through the heart to the brain through a patent foramen ovale.

The neuropathologic changes in the brain that follow embolic infarction are not different from those found with infarction from other causes except that hemorrhage into the infarct is found more often with emboli than with vascular occlusion from atherosclerotic disease. The actual embolic material is often not retrieved from the cerebral vessels at autopsy unless the embolus is large, presumably because most small emboli are lysed. This evanescence means that many instances of embolic cerebral infarction must be inferred by finding a source of emboli in other sites. Multiple small areas of cerebral infarction are commonly found at autopsy in patients with embolic disease.

Cerebral emboli that originate from infected material with bacterial endocarditis or pulmonary infections may cause local inflammation as well as infarction. Infected emboli may produce cerebral abscess, local encephalitis, or mycotic aneurysm.

Recurrent emboli have been postulated as a cause for the transient attacks of neurologic dysfunction often seen in patients with cerebrovascular disease (see below). The surface of atheromatous plaques in the internal carotid artery is frequently ulcerated. A granular lipid debris is present on the ulcer, and the surface of some plaques has been noted to be covered with collections of platelets or organizing blood clot. It is believed that some of the granular or thrombotic material on the surface breaks off, is carried into and obstructs small cerebral vessels, and produces small areas of ischemia. Because only minute vessels are occluded, infarction usually does not occur. In support of this concept is the observation in the optic fundi of some patients having transient ischemic attacks of small white or yellow refractile bodies moving through or blocking the retinal arteries. These emboli have been identified as platelet collections or cholesterol crystals; it is believed that they represent atherosclerotic debris from plaques in proximal vessels and that similar emboli go to brain vessels causing transient occlusion without necrosis. Embolic material from ulcerated atherosclerotic plaques can cause transient ischemic attacks in the absence of significant vascular obstruction.

Cerebral Venous Inflammation and Thrombosis

Cerebral infarction can result from thrombosis of one of the major venous sinuses, i.e., the superior sagittal sinus, the lateral sinus, or the cavernous sinus, or it can follow extensive thrombotic occlusion of cortical veins. The causes of cerebral venous thrombosis include dehydration, head injury, intracerebral hemorrhage, polycythemia vera, leukemia, infection, and the puerperal state. The most common cause is infection of the mastoid, the frontal sinus, or the subdural space. If the superior sagittal sinus is thrombosed anteriorly, both cerebral hemispheres become markedly congested, swollen, and hemorrhagic. The cerebral white matter may be involved, with small hemorrhages and edema. The surface veins become distended and filled with clot.

Thrombosis of surface veins is usually associated with cerebral or subdural abscess. The histologic picture is that of an acute inflammatory reaction with vascular congestion, edema, and neuronal loss.

Cavernous sinus thrombosis usually follows infection of the eye, face, or nose, and in many instances the thrombus extends through the perihypophyseal veins to involve the opposite cavernous sinus as well. Meningitis may follow spread of the infectious process through the sinus to the subarachnoid space.

Cardiac Disease

Hypotension and Hypertension

Cardiac disease contributes to infarction in patients with cerebral atherosclerosis as the result of periods of hypotension after myocardial infarction, congestive failure, and cardiac arrhythmia. In the Cornell-Bellevue series, clinical heart disease not only preceded cerebral infarction in half the patients, but was the actual cause of at least half the deaths after cerebral infarction.

Hypotension. Both hypotension and hypertension have been implicated in the production of cerebral ischemia and infarction. Although cerebral blood flow in the normal person is relatively independent of the systemic blood pressure down to levels of 50 to 60 mm of mercury, it has been suggested that a lesser drop in blood pressure may produce cerebral ischemia when a significant obstruction is present in a vessel leading to the brain. A localized obstruction must reduce the vessel lumen by nearly 80 per cent to produce a significant distal drop in pressure, but luminal encroachment that extends over long distances theoretically could significantly decrease the distal arterial pressure with less severe grades of obstruction. However, the contribution to cerebral infarction of obstruction and distal decreases in blood pressure and flow is still an unsettled matter. Thus Marshall has reported that when patients with transient ischemic attacks were made briefly hypotensive with hexamethonium and tilting, nearly one half showed evidence of generalized cerebral ischemia only, and another one fourth developed evidence of generalized cerebral ischemia before any focal ischemia.

Failure to maintain the blood pressure may occur with cardiac arrhythmias and after myocardial infarction. The asystole that occurs in Stokes-Adams attacks, if prolonged, can reduce the cerebral blood flow so markedly that cerebral ischemia or infarction results.

Hypertension. Longstanding hypertensive cardiovascular disease is probably the single biggest risk factor in stroke; the place of hypertension in the production of acute cerebral ischemia and infarction is less clear. Rapid elevations of blood pressure evoke an increase in cerebrovascular resistance, and model experiments have demonstrated that stenosis coupled with this increased resistance significantly reduces blood flow. In animal experiments, marked hypertension causes constriction in small cerebral vessels leading, in turn, to areas of cerebral infarction. Transient marked increases in blood pressure may contribute to cerebral infarction.

Other physiologic changes in cerebral hemodynamics may contribute to cerebral ischemia. Osteoarthritis in the cervical spine may compress the vertebral arteries so that extension, flexion, or rotation of the head can reduce vertebral artery blood flow to the point that ischemic symptoms occur. Cerebral ischemia will be augmented in these instances if anomalies or extensive atherosclerotic deposits compromise the circle of Willis.

Changes in Blood: Clotting, Viscosity, and Anemia

A variety of blood changes have been linked to cerebral infarction. The most frequent is *thrombus formation,* although in many instances it is unclear whether this is primary or secondary to the ischemic process. Thus infarction is not invariably associated with clot-filled vessels, and when thrombi do occur, they arise most commonly in association with ulcerated atherosclerotic lesions or atherosclerotic plaques, which by themselves produce a marked degree of vessel obstruction. In vessels with greatly reduced or absent flow, clots form readily, and long, wormlike clots have been removed from the distal segment of a partially or completely obstructed internal carotid artery shortly after the development of symptoms and signs of cerebral ischemia. A plausible reconstruction of this sequence suggests that marked stenosis was present first and was suddenly increased by hemorrhage into the atherosclerotic plaque, after which clotting occurred distally to the occlusion.

Alterations in blood clotting suggesting hypercoagulability have been described in patients with cerebral infarctions. However, a state of altered clotting has not been observed before an infarction, and some evidence suggests that hypercoagulability is an epiphenomenon that follows, rather than precedes, infarction.

Other potentially deleterious changes in blood include *increased viscosity* with polycythemia and *decreased oxygen-carrying capacity* with anemia. About 15 per cent of patients with polycythemia die from thromboembolism in the brain. Transient ischemic attacks that occur in patients with polycythemia are believed to result from the increase in blood viscosity that occurs when the hematocrit rises above 55.

Severe *anemia* sometimes precipitates cerebral ischemia, particularly if the hematocrit falls below 20, i.e., if the oxygen-carrying capacity drops more than half. Any degree of anemia may supplement severe atherosclerosis, cardiac disease, or hypotension in causing cerebral ischemia.

Cerebral Infarction and Medication

Stroke in young women of child-bearing age has been related to the use of oral contraceptive agents. The risk of developing stroke in women of this age group is small, but with oral contraceptive agents it is increased an estimated fivefold. Evidence has accumulated relating the increased risk to the estrogen content of the medication which is known to alter blood clotting. Particularly susceptible women are those with migraine and hypertension. In this group, when contraception is needed other means should be used.

THE PATHOGENESIS OF SYMPTOMS AND SIGNS IN CEREBROVASCULAR DISEASE

To make accurate clinical diagnoses in patients suspected of having cerebrovascular disease, the clinician requires an effective working knowledge of the structural and vascular anatomy of the brain. This is presented in the following paragraphs and diagrams, reference to which will explain why patterns of neurologic dysfunction after infarction or ischemia are related more to arterial territories than to specific neuroanatomic systems.

The brain is supplied by four large arteries, the two common carotids and the two vertebrals. One common carotid artery arises from the aortic arch and the other from the innominate artery in the upper thorax. The two vertebral arteries originate from the right and left subclavian artery. The common carotid artery bifurcates in the neck, forming the internal and external carotid arteries. Each internal carotid artery enters the skull through the homolateral foramen lacerum, passes through the cavernous sinus, and gives off branches in the following order: ophthalmic, anterior choroidal, and posterior communicating. It then bifurcates into the anterior and middle cerebral arteries.

The Anterior Cerebral Artery

As may be seen in Figures 2 and 3, the anterior cerebral artery supplies the medial and superior surfaces of the cerebral hemisphere and the whole of the most anterior portion of the frontal lobes. This area contains the motor and sensory cortex for the foot and leg and the supplementary motor cortex. The anterior cerebral artery also supplies several deep structures of importance, including the anterior nucleus of the thalamus and a portion of the anterior limb of the internal capsule.

The Middle Cerebral Artery

The middle cerebral artery (Figs. 3 and 4) supplies the lateral surface of the cerebral hemisphere with the exception of the occipital and frontal poles. The cortex supplied includes the primary motor and sensory area for the face, hand, and arm, the optic radiations, and, in the dominant hemisphere, the cortical areas for speech. The perforating branches of the middle cerebral artery reach the center of the cerebral hemisphere supplying the internal capsule and basal ganglia.

The Posterior Cerebral Artery

As shown in Figures 2 and 3, the posterior cerebral artery supplies the posterior pole of the lateral surface of the cerebral hemisphere and the posterior portion of the medial and inferior surfaces of the hemispheres. This area contains the calcarine cortex or the primary visual receptive area. The short perforating branches of the posterior cerebral artery supply the thalamus, part of

Figure 2. The medial surface of the cerebral hemisphere, showing the course of the anterior and posterior cerebral arteries and the area of brain supplied by each.

Figure 3. The cerebral hemispheres and the vascular supply, in coronal section.

the optic pathways, and other diencephalic structures including the midbrain.

The Vertebral and Basilar Arteries

The vertebral arteries reach the head via a bony canal in the transverse processes of the sixth through the second cervical vertebrae and enter the skull through the foramen magnum. Immediately after entering the skull each vertebral artery gives off a medial branch (these unite to form the anterior spinal artery) and, just distal to this, the posterior inferior cerebellar artery. At all levels along the brainstem, the ventral medial portion is supplied by short paramedian vessels. The ventrolateral portion of the brainstem is supplied by short circumferential branches from the vertebrals or basilar artery. The dorsal lateral portion and cerebellum are supplied by long circumferential branches: the posterior inferior, the anterior inferior, and the superior cerebellar arteries.

The vertebral artery lies on the ventral lateral surface of the medulla oblongata, and from it and the anterior spinal artery short paramedian branches supply the pyramids, the inferior olives and medial lemniscus, the medial longitudinal fasciculus, and the emerging fibers of the hypoglossal nerve as shown in Figure 5.

The more dorsal portion of the medulla includes the spinothalamic tract, the vestibular nuclei, the sensory nucleus of the fifth cranial nerve, the restiform body, and the emerging fibers of the vagus and glossopharyngeal nerves, and is supplied by longer branches from the vertebral artery and branches from the posterior inferior cerebellar artery. The most cephalad and dorsal segment of the medulla includes the vestibular and cochlear nuclei, and it and the posterior portion of the cerebellum are supplied by the posterior inferior cerebellar artery.

At the lower border of the pons, the two vertebral arteries unite to form the basilar artery. From this artery in the pons, short perpendicular branches enter the brainstem to supply paramedian structures including the corticospinal tracts, the pontine nuclei, the medial lemniscus, the medial longitudinal fasciculus, and the pontine reticular nuclei (Fig. 6). Circumferential branches supply the lateral portion of the pons, which includes the

Figure 4. The lateral surface of the cerebral hemisphere and the course of the middle cerebral artery. The sylvian fissure has been opened to better illustrate the course of the vessel.

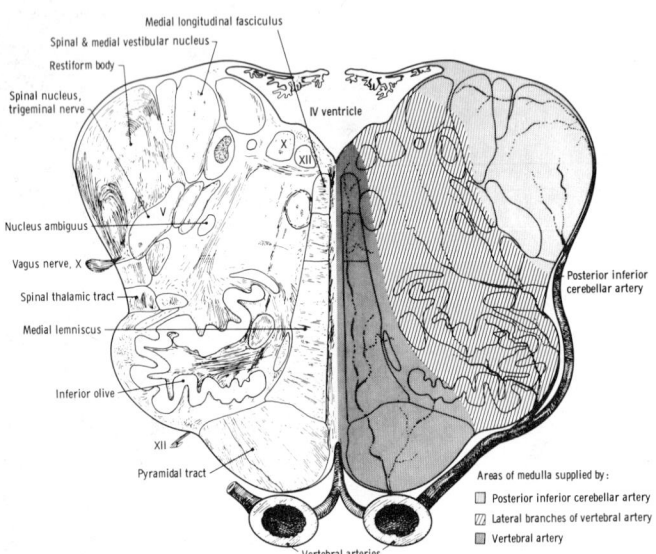

Figure 5. Cross section of the medulla oblongata seen from above at the level of the hypoglossal nuclei. The medial structures are supplied by short branches arising from the vertebral arteries and anterior spinal arteries. The lateral portions are supplied by longer branches and the dorsal and lateral areas by long circumferential branches, at this level called the posterior inferior cerebellar artery.

emerging seventh and eighth cranial nerves, the trigeminal nerve root, the vestibular and cochlear nuclei, and the spinothalamic tracts. The anterior inferior cerebellar artery, the long circumferential branch at this level, also gives branches to the most dorsal and lateral of these structures as it runs dorsally to the cerebellum.

At the level of the midbrain the basilar artery lies in the interpeduncular fossa (Fig. 7). Short branches pass laterally and dorsally to both sides to supply the cerebral peduncles, the emerging third nerve roots, the medial portions of the red nuclei, the medial longitudinal fasciculus, oculomotor nuclei, and the midbrain reticulum. Branches of the posterior cerebral artery supply the lateral portions of the peduncles, the red nuclei, and the medial lemnisci. The superior cerebellar arteries supply some of the dorsal portions of the midbrain, including the colliculi and the anterior portion of the cerebellum on each side.

It will be clear from this review of neurologic and vascular anatomy that infarction can produce a large va-

riety of clinical pictures, depending on the vessels involved. The pattern of most syndromes is helpful in localizing the area of the nervous system damaged by infarction, but only a few reliably indicate exactly which portion of the vascular tree is involved. As an example, diagnoses are often made of middle cerebral artery occlusion, but a review of the vascular anatomy of the brain quickly reveals why, with both anterior cerebral arteries filling from either side, an identical clinical picture can be associated with occlusion of the internal carotid artery at any point along its course.

SIGNS AND SYMPTOMS IN CEREBRO-VASCULAR DISEASE: STROKE SYNDROMES

An adequate exposition of the symptoms and signs of cerebrovascular disease requires a classification of the various clinical entities that make up the stroke syndrome.

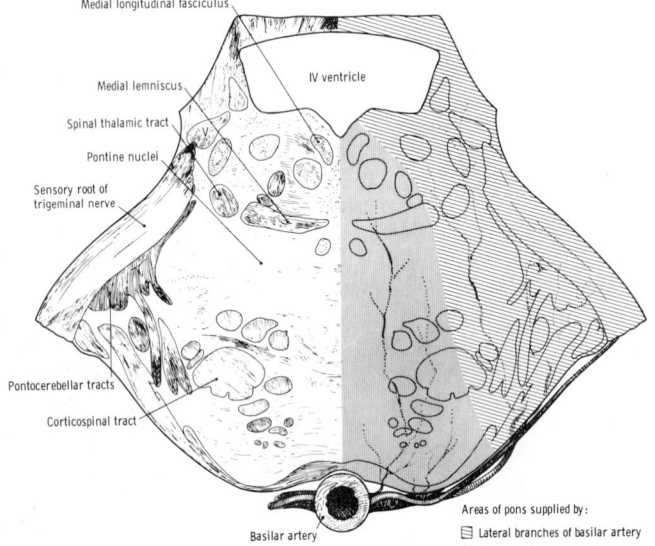

Figure 6. Cross section of the midpons. The most medial regions are supplied by short perforating branches from the basilar artery. The more lateral regions are supplied by lateral branches of the basilar artery. At this level, the more dorsal structures are supplied by the long circumferential branch, the anterior inferior cerebellar artery.

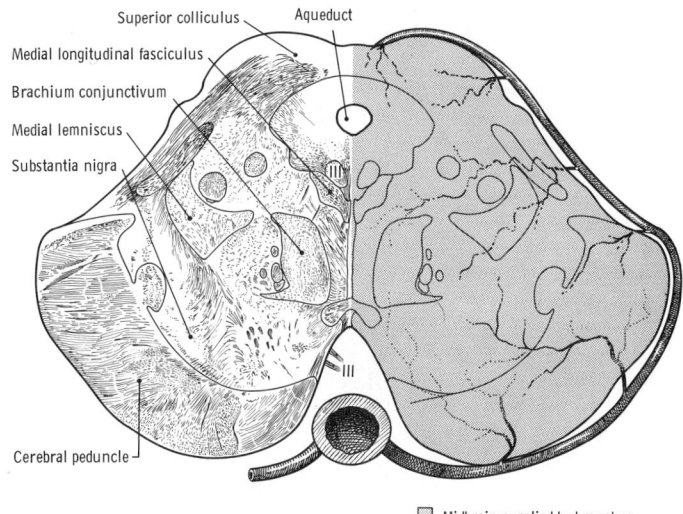

Superior colliculus
Aqueduct
Medial longitudinal fasciculus
Brachium conjunctivum
Medial lemniscus
Substantia nigra
III
III
Cerebral peduncle

Figure 7. Cross section of the midbrain seen from below. The medial, lateral, and dorsal regions are supplied by short branches from the posterior cerebral artery as it passes around the midbrain.

☐ Midbrain supplied by branches of the posterior cerebral artery

Cerebrovascular accidents are classified on the basis of the anatomic site of ischemia or infarction, the cerebral vessels occluded or obstructed, and the temporal character of the entire clinical episode. The latter is clinically the most valuable in that the indicated therapy is often different for the three kinds of temporal profiles found. The three profiles have been defined as *transient ischemic attack, stroke-in-evolution* or *progressive stroke,* and *completed stroke.*

The term *transient ischemic attack* or incipient stroke refers to transient episodes of neurologic dysfunction caused by cerebrovascular disease. The attacks are believed to be caused by cerebral ischemia, and consist of fleeting, 5- to 30-minute disturbances in neurologic function that leave no permanent residue.

Stroke-in-evolution or progressive stroke refers to increasing neurologic dysfunction caused by cerebral ischemia over a period of minutes, hours, or, rarely, days.

Completed stroke refers to the clinical picture seen in patients who have ceased to show further progression in neurologic deficit or in those who have developed a neurologic deficit earlier that is now stable or improving. *Cerebral embolism* is one cause of completed stroke in which the onset is an abrupt monophasic event, and there is clinically a demonstrable source of emboli.

Cerebral Transient Ischemic Attacks

The symptoms vary, depending upon which area of the brain is ischemic, but there are two main types: those associated with ischemia of parts or the whole of a cerebral hemisphere and those associated with ischemia of the brainstem. The symptoms most often include transient contralateral weakness of the lower face, fingers, hand, arm, or leg, but such patients may also experience fleeting sensory symptoms such as tingling, "pins and needles," or numbness in parts of the body contralateral to the ischemia. Ischemia in the dominant hemisphere may cause dysphasia, with impairment in the context of speech and, at times, a transient lack of understanding.

Patients with ischemia in the portion of the brain supplied by the posterior cerebral artery may suffer blurred vision, or may notice transient hemianopic or altitudinal visual field defects or impairment of visual acuity.

Ischemia or insufficiency caused by internal carotid artery stenosis often produces transient retinal ischemia, resulting in monocular blindness or reduced acuity on the side of the stenosis, combined with contralateral weakness of the face, arm, or leg.

Ischemic attacks which result from involvement of the brain supplied by the vertebral and basilar arteries have an extremely wide range of symptoms. Common symptoms include vertigo, tinnitus, diplopia, dysarthria, dysphagia, and dysphonia. Patients may complain of unilateral or bilateral face, arm, and leg weakness and unilateral or bilateral sensations of numbness and tingling in the face, arms, or leg. There may be tinnitus, hearing loss, and ataxia. In addition, patients with brainstem ischemia may experience "drop attacks," in which they suddenly lose postural tone and fall to the ground without losing consciousness, then immediately regain postural control and rise quickly. The most common complaint with transient ischemic attacks from vertebrobasilar insufficiency is dizziness. However, dizziness is commonly associated with other physiologic disturbances and is rarely the only symptom of brainstem ischemia. When patients describe intermittent neurologic episodes with symptoms suggesting a generalized decrease in cerebral blood flow such as dizziness, lightheadedness, and generalized weakness, they should be carefully examined for cardiac dysrhythmia before being studied for the presence of extracranial arterial disease. Cardiac dysrhythmia, with a drop in cardiac output and subsequently in general cerebral blood flow, is a common cause of nonfocal transient ischemic attacks.

Symptoms of vertebral basilar artery ischemia, although variable, tend to occur in combinations that aid in their diagnosis. Vertigo, ataxia, dysarthria, paresthesia, diplopia, tinnitus, dysphagia, and focal weakness in the face, jaw, or pharynx tend to coexist, although not always in the same sequence or combination. Another grouping of symptoms is that of unilateral or bilateral weakness of the extremities with drop attacks and diplopia. The reason for these differences in symptom combinations can be found by referring to the diagrams of the blood supply to the brainstem. Ischemia of the dorsal and lateral portions of the brainstem supplied by the circumferential arteries produces the first group of symptoms. Ischemia of the more ventral portions supplied by the medial perforating arteries causes the second group.

Symptomatic vertebral basilar artery ischemia may occur with stenosis of the subclavian artery proximal to the origin of the vertebral artery. The arm on the side of the stenosis may be supplied by retrograde flow in the ipsilateral vertebral, and, during exercise, enough blood can be diverted from the vertebral system to the arm to cause symptoms of brainstem ischemia. This mechanism of producing brainstem ischemia has been called the *subclavian steal syndrome*. However, most instances of reversed vertebral artery flow with subclavian artery stenosis or occlusion are asymptomatic.

Ischemic attacks may occur many times a day or at weekly or monthly intervals. They may be intermittently present over several months or several years. Some patients with internal carotid artery occlusion have transient ischemic attacks for as long as two years before cerebral infarction occurs. Others have clusters of attacks lasting only a few hours or days before carotid occlusion becomes complete and causes infarction. *The major importance of transient ischemic attacks is that they signal the existence of significant cerebrovascular disease and clearly indicate the potential danger of cerebral infarction.* Studies of the natural history of transient ischemic attacks indicate that about one fourth to one third of patients afflicted will suffer a cerebral infarction within two to five years of onset of the attacks. It cannot always be predicted which patients with cerebral ischemia will develop cerebral infarction or even when it will occur. Transient ischemic attacks become more significant predictors of cerebral infarction if accompanied by extensive atherosclerosis as evidenced by abnormalities in the neurovascular examination, such as arterial bruit in the neck, absent temporal pulse, retinal embolization, and reduction of retinal artery pressure on the appropriate side. Some varieties of cerebral ischemic attacks carry a better prognosis than others. Thus symptoms suggesting involvement of the dorsal and lateral portion to the brainstem, the lateral medullary area, imply the best prognosis. Attacks suggesting ventral brainstem involvement, such as bilateral paresis or unilateral transient paresis or drop attacks, connote a considerably poorer prognosis. Carotid ischemic attacks that occur close together in clusters carry a poor prognosis, for in a large percentage of such patients cerebral infarction rapidly follows.

In the interval between transient ischemic attacks, the neurologic examination is usually entirely normal. During a transient ischemic attack, patients commonly have neurologic deficits corresponding to their symptoms. Thus with ischemia of a cerebral hemisphere, there may be a hemiparesis with reflex asymmetry and an extensor plantar response, or a mild hemisensory or visual field deficit. If the dominant hemisphere is affected, dysphasia may be noted: the patient has difficulty in naming and recognizing objects. Patients examined during a brainstem ischemic attack often exhibit nystagmus, complete facial weakness, palate and tongue weakness, and deviation, dysconjugate eye movements, sensory defects, and weakness on one side or on both sides of the body. The evaluation of patients with transient ischemic attacks must always include careful examination of the optic fundus through a dilated pupil, searching for cholesterol (bronze debris) or platelet emboli (white or invisible plugs) in the arterial tree. The presence of such emboli in one eye is important evidence of an embolic source in the carotid artery. Patients with such emboli should have cerebral angiography, and the presence of ulcerated atherosclerotic plaques should be determined.

Consciousness is usually unimpaired during transient ischemic attacks, although thinking is sometimes slowed. This lack of alteration of consciousness coupled with the absence of either aura or convulsive movements helps to distinguish these attacks from convulsive seizures. Other conditions that must be considered in the differential diagnosis are Meniere's syndrome (which is rare in the elderly), migraine headache, cerebral emboli, or the progressive neurologic deficits caused by cerebral neoplasm.

Stroke-in-Evolution
(Progressive Stroke)

The evolving stroke is characterized by the gradual development of paralysis and sensory impairment over a period of several hours and, at times, one to two days. The symptoms and signs may develop as a series of steplike changes or as an unbroken continuum of worsening. When first examined, a patient may have mild weakness which, as the hours pass, is found to be more and more marked and to involve more and more of the body. The symptoms and signs found are identical to those of completed stroke; only the time course of onset is different. This course also occurs with subdural hematoma and brain tumor, but, for these disorders, the duration usually extends over several days or weeks.

Cerebral Infarction
(Completed Stroke)

Cerebral infarctions resulting from cerebral emboli or from cerebral atherosclerosis and thrombosis, respectively, cannot be distinguished by the neurologic disorders they produce. Differences between these two causes of infarction do exist, however, in the mode of onset of symptoms and in the general physical evaluation.

The pattern of onset of neurologic symptoms and signs in cerebral infarction often suggests the cause. Cerebral embolism causes an abrupt onset of symptoms, and headache often precedes other neurologic symptoms by several hours. Cerebral infarction caused by atherosclerotic vascular obstruction or occlusion often has a less sudden onset. There may be a distinct series of steplike increases in neurologic symptoms and signs, or infarction may be preceded by a series of transient ischemic attacks. A gradual onset with increasing neurologic deficit over several (one to five) hours is characteristic of the progressing stroke. A gradual onset of symptoms and signs over two days or, occasionally, one week, does occur but is uncommon. The frequency of these different patterns can be inferred from the experience of one large series of patients with ischemic infarction; about one third had a sudden onset of symptoms, about one fifth had symptoms that progressively increased over one to 12 hours, and only about one in 20 had symptoms that progressed for as long as 12 to 24 hours. One fifth of the patients with occlusive vascular disease and cerebral embolism had the onset of neurologic signs during sleep.

Headache is present in many patients with embolic or atherosclerotic infarction. The headache is usually mild and localized to the side of the infarction. Headache is believed to be caused by vasodilation of unoccluded vessels near the infarcted area, and is most common when vessels near the base of the brain are occluded.

Consciousness is usually not lost at the onset of infarction of the cerebral hemispheres, but may be reduced, particularly when large infarcts strike the dominant hemisphere. When unconsciousness is present from the onset or is the initial symptom, brainstem infarction is the most likely cause. When large hemispheric infarctions are complicated by rapidly developing and severe brain edema, loss of consciousness caused by diencephalic and upper brainstem compression may occur shortly after the onset of symptoms. This may give the false impression of loss of consciousness from the onset unless a careful history documents a lucid period at the very beginning of symptoms. Convulsive seizures are rare at the onset of cerebral infarction, but they occur in about 8 per cent of patients sometime in the course of the acute or convalescent phase of the illness. They are usually focal, but may be generalized.

When infarction is limited to the cerebral hemisphere, there is weakness or paralysis in the extremities contralateral to the infarction. Patients may also be aware that sensory perception on the side of weakness is impaired and may complain of heaviness or numbness in the arm or leg. They rarely have other sensory symptoms such as pain or paresthesias. Defects in visual fields are common but often escape the patient's notice. The defect is suspected when patients pay little attention to visual stimuli on one side of the body. At times, the eyes may be constantly deviated to the side away from the neurologic deficits.

The most serious consequence of infarction in the dominant hemisphere is dysphasia, which can range from a mild deficit of expression to aphonic mutism. The dysphasia is almost invariably a mixture of difficulty with expression (expressive dysphasia) and difficulty in understanding what is said, written, or indicated by gesture (receptive dysphasia); one or the other may predominate. In patients who have infarction in the nondominant hemisphere, lack of awareness or concern about paralysis of the contralateral side is often evident. Such subjects may, at times, be so completely unaware of their neurologic disabilities that they are hospitalized only after family or friends notice their disabilities. This phenomenon, *anosognosia,* is most common when a patient is obtunded and when there is a significant sensory deficit on the paretic side as a result of infarction of the parietal lobe. It accompanies nearly one fourth of all large strokes, but usually persists only if the patient remains obtunded or confused or has little return of sensation.

Infarctions in the brainstem produce a wide variety of symptoms. Among the most conspicuous are vertigo, diplopia, dysarthria, dysphagia, and ataxia. In addition, the patient may note unilateral or bilateral sensory impairment or weakness. Often patients note clumsiness and difficulty in performing skilled acts without paresis.

Specific Vascular Syndromes

Internal Carotid Artery Occlusion

Occlusion of the internal carotid artery at its origin from the common carotid or intracranially is the site of the major vascular lesion in nearly 20 per cent of strokes. The usual lesion is atherosclerotic with, at first, partial obstruction and, finally, occlusion with a thrombus. Occasionally the internal carotid artery is obstructed by a large embolus.

Symptoms and signs specific for internal carotid artery occlusion in the neck are intermittent visual impairment or blindness in the eye on the side of the occlusion (retinal artery insufficiency) combined with a contralateral hemiparesis and sensory loss (middle cerebral artery insufficiency). This clinical picture often begins with a series of transient ischemic attacks and only later causes permanent weakness and sensory loss. Unless the history of intermittent blindness can be obtained, it is difficult, on clinical grounds alone, to distinguish occlusion of the internal carotid artery from middle cerebral artery occlusion.

On neurologic examination, patients with cerebral infarction caused by internal carotid artery occlusion have paresis of voluntary movement, with weakness most noticeable in the contralateral face and upper extremity. Infarcts produce motility defects as their main manifestations, but there is usually some impairment of sensory perception and, at times, visual field impairment as well.

In the paretic extremities, deep tendon reflexes are hyperactive, and pathologic reflexes such as the Babinski sign (extensor plantar response) are found. Muscle tone becomes increased on the weakened side, and spasticity may be so marked that early contracture is evident. Sensory impairment is most evident in modalities such as position sense, vibration sense, two-point discrimination, and tactile perception of shape and texture. Touch and pain perception may be moderately impaired, and extinction of stimuli on the involved side may be evident on double simultaneous stimulation. The size of the cerebral infarction produced by internal carotid occlusion is extremely variable. When there is no collateral circulation through the anterior communicating, posterior communicating, ophthalmic, or surface collateral arteries, the infarct can involve nearly the whole cerebral hemisphere, both lateral and medial surfaces. With a richer collateral circulation, smaller infarcts and proportionately fewer neurologic defects result. Occasionally occlusion of the internal carotid is asymptomatic, and is discovered only as an incidental finding at autopsy or when cerebral angiograms are done.

Internal carotid artery occlusion or stenosis sometimes causes a partial Horner's syndrome (slight ptosis and miosis) on the side opposite the paresis. The eye changes have been attributed to ischemia of the sympathetic fibers that lie in the adventitia of the arterial wall adjacent to the occlusion, but are more probably due to direct hypothalamic damage, for they can also be observed in patients with similar infarcts who do not have occlusion of the carotid arteries. An audible bruit in the neck at the angle of the mandible is a helpful indicator of stenosis of the internal carotid artery at that site. Occlusion of the internal carotid artery is also suggested when the retinal artery pressure on the affected side, as measured with an ophthalmodynamometer, decreases 25 per cent or more below the arterial pressure in the other eye. Some physicians find that palpation of the internal carotid artery in the pharynx behind the posterior tonsillar pillar is helpful in the diagnosis of carotid artery disease, as the pulse is absent when the artery is occluded. However, patients are often unable to cooperate for the examination, so that the usefulness of the test is limited.

Middle Cerebral Artery Occlusion

The cerebral tissue supplied by the middle cerebral artery is the most common area for infarction from emboli or vascular insufficiency, and the neurologic picture produced by either is the same.

When a middle cerebral artery is occluded, infarction occurs in the lateral portion of the hemisphere and produces varying degrees of contralateral paresis and sensory loss, mainly in the face, the upper extremities, and the hand, and often blindness in the contralateral, homonymous visual field. Occlusions at the origin of the middle cerebral artery produce extensive neurologic disturbance with profound contralateral hemiplegia and sensory loss. Occlusions in branches of the middle cerebral artery may produce a variable clinical picture. At times, only paresis is evident in the arm and face. In some patients, sensory impairment is the dominant and occasionally the only neurologic abnormality, and some patients have only dysphasia.

Anterior Cerebral Artery Occlusion

Anterior cerebral artery occlusion causes infarction in the cortical areas that control motor and sensory functions of the contralateral lower extremity, and impairs voluntary movement and sensory perception of that leg. The upper extremity and face are spared. Cerebral infarction caused by occlusion of the proximal portion of the anterior cerebral artery is uncommon because collateral circulation through the anterior communicating artery is usually adequate to supply both hemispheres.

Posterior Cerebral Artery Occlusion

Posterior cerebral artery occlusion causes infarction of the posterior lateral and posterior medial surfaces of the cerebral hemisphere, including the calcarine cortex. Proximal occlusions of the artery result in infarction of the thalamus and upper brainstem as well. Extensive infarctions in the occipital cortex cause homonymous hemianopic field defects, and those involving the dominant hemisphere may produce disturbances in reading, visual learning, visual recognition, and visual spatial orientation.

Infarction of both occipital poles can follow basilar artery stenosis or occlusion. The result is a double hemianopia and cortical blindness, a striking feature of which is that the patient is usually unaware that he is blind and may vigorously deny it (Anton's syndrome).

Brainstem Infarction

Brainstem infarction, although not as common as hemisphere infarction, produces several distinct clinical syndromes, best categorized by noting whether the clinical picture suggests involvement of ventral paramedian, ventrolateral, or dorsal brainstem structures. As noted in the discussion of neurovascular anatomy, these three areas receive blood supply through different groups of arteries.

Many of the particular groupings of symptoms and signs associated with various brainstem infarctions that have been given eponyms are believed to be common occurrences with brainstem infarction. However, in an analysis of 50 patients with brainstem infarction from the Cornell-Bellevue series, only two clearly fitted into these syndromes as originally described. The remaining 48 had an extensive mixture of symptoms and signs indicating an overlap in the areas believed to be infarcted with occlusions in specific arteries.

Midbrain Infarctions

Occlusion of the paramedian branches from the apex of the basilar artery or of the proximal posterior cerebral arteries causes infarction of portions of one or both cerebral peduncles, the oculomotor nerves, the oculomotor nuclei, the brachia conjunctivae, the red nuclei, and the midbrain reticular formation. The resulting symptoms and signs may be unilateral or bilateral, depending on the extent of the infarction. Unilateral signs include (1) ipsilateral oculomotor palsy and contralateral hemiparesis (Weber's syndrome), (2) ipsilateral oculomotor palsy, ipsilateral ataxia of gait, and poorly coordinated arm and hand movements (Nothnagel's syndrome). Bilateral signs include impaired consciousness, quadriparesis, divergent gaze, impaired vertical eye movements and midposition, or dilated pupils unresponsive to light. Purposeless, flail-like, involuntary movements (hemiballismus) may occur, and usually involve the upper extremity more than the lower. Patients in coma caused by infarction of the midbrain often have an unusual appearance, seeming to be almost awake although unable to communicate in any manner. This state has been called *coma vigil* or *akinetic mutism*. Such patients, although unresponsive, may exhibit a sleep-walking cycle.

When the dorsal area, supplied by the posterior cerebral artery, is ischemic or infarcted, the spinothalamic tract, the red nucleus, the descending sympathetic tracts, and the medial lemniscus are involved. The clinical picture consists of slight ptosis and miosis (Horner's syndrome), ipsilateral ataxia, and choreiform adventitious movements and contralateral impairment of all modalities of sensory perception of the entire body, including the face. This clinical picture is often called the superior cerebellar artery syndrome.

Pontine Infarction

Infarction in the pons is usually associated with basilar artery obstruction. Occlusion of the paramedian branches of the basilar artery causes necrosis of the corticospinal tracts, the pontine nuclei, the medial lemniscus, the medial longitudinal fasciculus, the abducens nucleus, the pontocerebellar tracts, and the pontine reticulum. Ipsilateral abducens palsy, facial weakness, and contralateral corticospinal tract dysfunction (Millard-Gubler syndrome) and the same findings with lateral conjugate gaze palsy (Foville's syndrome) are two unilateral syndromes that occur with occlusion in the paramedian arteries to the pons. Bilateral signs include quadriparesis, reduced reaction to noxious stimuli, and abducens paresis. Other signs include coma, hyperventilation, apneustic or ataxic breathing, small pupils, and internuclear ophthalmoplegia. If only the most ventral portion of the pons is damaged, awareness may be maintained even though the patient is quadriparetic.

With occlusion of arteries to the lateral pons, the signs and symptoms are unilateral and include tinnitus, deafness, nausea, vertigo, impairment of facial sensation, complete ipsilateral facial paralysis, nystagmus, miosis and ptosis (partial Horner's syndrome), and impaired conjugate gaze toward the side of the lesion. Impaired pain and temperature perception of one half the contralateral body below the face is usually found. This clinical picture is often referred to as the syndrome of anterior inferior cerebellar artery occlusion.

Medullary Infarction

Occlusion of the paramedian branches of the vertebral artery in the medulla causes contralateral paresis of the arm and leg, contralateral impaired sensory perception to touch, position sense and vibration sense in the arm, trunk, and leg, and ipsilateral tongue paralysis. With occlusion of arterial branches to the lateral medulla, the clinical picture includes vertigo, nausea, vomiting, dysarthria, dysphagia, nystagmus, ipsilateral Horner's syndrome, ipsilateral vocal cord paralysis, and impaired ipsilateral facial sensory perception to pain with impairment of pain sensation on the contralateral half of the body below the face. This clinical picture is referred to as the syndrome of posterior inferior cerebellar artery occlusion or Wallenberg's syndrome. It results from occlusion of the vertebral artery itself as frequently as or more frequently than it does from occlusion of its branches.

Basilar Artery Occlusion

When the basilar artery is completely occluded, infarction is found mainly in the ventral pons, midbrain, and occipital lobes. The clinical picture is like that seen with occlusion of the paramedian midbrain or pontine branches, but may include various defects in the visual fields and, at times, cortical blindness in addition. The brainstem tegmentum is almost invariably involved, causing major disturbances in consciousness.

Cerebral Embolism

The diagnosis of cerebral embolization is usually not difficult when it is remembered that the onset of neurologic symptoms and signs is abrupt, that they are often preceded by headache for a few hours before paresis is evident, and that a potential source for emboli is usually found on physical examination. Convulsive seizures occur at the onset, but they are uncommon. They are at first focal and later generalized in most patients. Loss of consciousness occurs in nearly one fourth of patients and is usually present for only a few minutes, but, after onset, patients may be confused. The neurologic signs depend upon which artery is occluded; the most common clinical picture is that of middle cerebral artery occlusion. Cerebral emboli can lodge in any major cerebral artery, and emboli commonly recur, often to the same artery. The cerebrospinal fluid is usually clear and without cells. When protein elevation and cells are found, subacute bacterial endocarditis should be suspected. Mitral stenosis with atrial fibrillation, myocardial infarction with mural thrombus, and subacute bacterial endocarditis are the cardiac disorders most commonly found. Normal sinus rhythm does not exclude the diagnosis of cerebral emboli, for it may be found in more than one third of such patients, particularly with a "tight" mitral stenosis or with past myocardial infarcts, respectively. Evidence of embolization to other sites strengthens the supposition that the cause of cerebral infarction is embolic.

Cerebral Venous Thrombosis

The symptoms of local cerebral venous thrombosis are headache, delirium, drowsiness, diplopia, and convulsions. The signs are usually those of increased intracranial pressure with papilledema and focal neurologic abnormalities. Focal fits are common, as are paresis and hemisensory loss. Such patients are restless, confused, and obtunded.

Superior sagittal sinus occlusion produces a somewhat similar clinical picture. At the New York Hospital, 21 patients with noninfective sagittal sinus thrombosis have been studied. Nine had terminal disease and marasmus, six had cyanotic congenital heart disease, and four had other, unexplained episodes of venous or arterial thromboses. Eleven of the 21 patients were children. Below the age of ten, cerebral infarction is more often due to venous than to arterial occlusion. Nearly all patients had fever, and their cerebrospinal fluids were under increased pressure, averaging 260 mm of fluid, and contained more than ten red blood cells. Neurologic symptoms appeared abruptly or progressed rapidly to a maximum, usually within 36 hours. Most patients were obtunded or confused and had headache. The white blood count was elevated in ten patients; in seven it was over 20,000. Nuchal rigidity was common, and papilledema, hemiparesis, and focal epileptic seizures occurred in about half the cases. Two patients presented later with signs of pseudotumor cerebri. The occurrence of hemiparesis or focal epilepsy was usually associated with cortical venous thromboses in addition to the sinus occlusion.

Cavernous sinus occlusion, usually a complication of sinus or paranasal skin infection, is characterized by proptosis, orbital chemosis, and edema, pain around the eye, papilledema, retinal hemorrhages, and fever. Extraocular palsy may be present. The disease carries a high risk of spread to the opposite cavernous sinus. Complications include meningitis and brain abscess.

Transverse or lateral sinus thrombosis, usually secondary to mastoiditis, is now uncommon with the decline in the incidence of that disease. When it does occur, it is usually manifested by headache, tenderness over the mastoid process, and, occasionally, paresis of the structures supplied by the glossopharyngeal and accessory nerve, with dysphagia, dysphonia, and weakness of the ipsilateral sternomastoid and trapezius muscle.

In all varieties of cerebral venous thrombosis, there is usually some evidence of sepsis with fever, malaise, headache, and leukocytosis.

Although the condition is uncommon, a diagnosis of cerebral venous thrombosis should be kept in mind for patients with evidence of cerebral infarction who have focal seizures, increased intracranial pressure, or evidence of infection. Cerebral venous thrombosis is particularly likely as a cause of postpartum cerebral infarction.

PHYSICAL AND LABORATORY FINDINGS

The general evaluation of the patient with cerebral infarction usually reveals evidence of vascular disease at other sites as well as a variety of associated diseases. About one fifth of patients with atherosclerotic cerebral infarction in the Cornell-Bellevue series had had previous strokes, half of which had occurred in the preceding year. Another fifth had had myocardial infarction, usually within the previous year. Over one half of the patients were hypertensive, but the diastolic pressure was above 100 mm of mercury in only one third of the patients. Nearly one fifth of the patients had diabetes mellitus, and one in ten gave a history of peripheral vascular occlusive disease.

Physical Examination. The physical examination of most patients with cerebral infarction discloses a normal or slightly elevated body temperature. Careful examination of the heart should never be overlooked because the presence of cardiac enlargement, atrial fibrillation, and cardiac murmurs, suggesting rheumatic heart disease with mitral stenosis, aids in detecting the presence of cerebral emboli. Patients with cerebral infarction often have atherosclerotic coronary heart disease, and perhaps one fifth have had recent or associated myocardial infarcts.

Palpation may reveal absence of pulsation in easily felt peripheral arteries. In the lower extremities, this is indicative of atherosclerotic vascular disease in the aorta, iliac, femoral or popliteal arteries. In the upper extremities, it may indicate occlusions in the major branches of the aorta, such as the innominate or subclavian arteries. Absence of pulses in one or both upper extremities should alert the physician to such diagnoses as "pulseless disease" (Takayasu's syndrome) or the "subclavian steal syndrome."

Auscultation for bruit over the neck is helpful in identifying sites of extracranial stenosis. A bruit heard in the neck under the angle of the mandible suggests atherosclerotic disease of the carotid artery, and bruit heard just above the clavicles is associated with vertebral or subclavian artery stenosis. Bruit, when loud and localized, is associated with atherosclerotic obstruction at that site in more than three fourths of patients.

Laboratory Examinations. Laboratory tests are aimed at both confirming the diagnosis and identifying complications. Every patient suspected of stroke should have a lumbar puncture and skull roentgenograms, and, if there are any unusual features at all about the illness, an electroencephalogram (EEG) should be obtained.

The cerebrospinal fluid should be examined promptly, for there is no other way to determine the presence of intracranial bleeding or an unsuspected infection. The lumbar puncture must be approached cautiously, however, when patients are in stupor or coma or when it is uncertain whether the illness is caused by stroke or by brain tumor, with increased intracranial pressure. In such instances, it is preferable to proceed with roentgenograms, electroencephalogram, radioactive brain scan, or an arteriogram, because lumbar puncture can inadvertently precipitate tentorial or foraminal herniation when there is an expanding intracranial mass.

The cerebrospinal fluid pressure is rarely over 200 mm of CSF in cerebral infarction. The fluid is usually clear and colorless, but bleeding and xanthochromia from hemorrhagic infarction may be found. The CSF protein level is usually normal, although slight elevations to 60 to 75 mg per 100 ml are found in perhaps one fifth of the patients. Elevations to 80 mg per 100 ml or above are found in less than 10 per cent, but particularly in those with basilar artery disease. With massive cerebral infarction, the protein may be raised to values of nearly 100 mg per 100 ml. Diabetes occasionally accounts for pronounced CSF protein elevations with stroke, probably by a leak of protein through damaged small vessels.

Patients with high values should always be carefully reviewed for the possibility of brain tumor.

Skull roentgenograms should be examined for evidence of fracture, erosion of the posterior clinoids (suggesting chronically increased intracranial pressure), abnormal calcification, and pineal shift.

The *electroencephalogram* (EEG) offers potential help both in differential diagnosis and in distinguishing infarction of the brainstem from that of the hemispheres. The EEG is usually abnormal in patients with cerebral infarction, and the degree of abnormality generally parallels the size of the lesion and the severity of the neurologic deficit. With hemispheric lesions, the abnormality is focal and the normal frequency of brain waves is slowed, so that, acutely at least, the records may resemble those found with brain tumor. In infarction, however, a decrease in the EEG abnormality is expected in serial recordings as the patient improves. With brainstem infarction, the EEG may be entirely normal, paroxysmally abnormal, or generally and diffusely abnormal.

The general evaluation of patients with cerebral infarction should include an electrocardiogram (EKG) and a chest roentgenogram. The EKG may confirm the presence of an arrhythmia or may disclose a silent myocardial infarction. (A potentially confusing point is that the EKG may show minor T wave and S-T segment changes caused by cerebral infarction and not by primary cardiac disease.)

Special Investigations

Arteriography

The technical quality and safety of arteriography has improved to the point that complications develop only in about 1 to 2 per cent of patients with cerebrovascular disease, and permanent worsening and death follow arteriography in less than 1 per cent of patients.

Cerebral angiography is indicated only for certain patients with cerebrovascular disease and has two main values. The first is in differential diagnosis for the patient with an atypical history and findings, or who is unable to give an accurate history because of dysphasia or depressed consciousness.

The second and more important value of cerebral angiograms is the accurate demonstration of the site, extent, and incidence of arterial obstructions and ulcerated atherosclerotic plaques that might be susceptible to surgical correction. Patients with such lesions include predominantly those who suffer transient ischemic attacks or incomplete strokes from which recovery has been substantial. In such cases, it is necessary to outline both the neck vessels and the nature and extent of the intracranial collateral circulation and the collateral channels from extracranial to intracranial vessels.

Rapid roentgenographic exposures have clarified some aspects of the physiology of cerebral blood flow in patients with cerebrovascular disease. Cerebral angiography may identify unusual patterns of blood flow in cerebral vessels, such as retrograde flow down one vertebral artery with proximal subclavian artery stenosis (subclavian steal). Ulceration of plaques can be demonstrated in about 41 per cent of patients with transient ischemic attacks coming to operation. The accuracy of the angiographic diagnosis when compared to findings at surgery is 90 per cent.

Brain scanning, using radiomercury-chlormerodrin or

Tc[99m] Pertechnetate, shows a high uptake of radioactive material in the area of a cerebral infarction. This technique may aid in accurate localization of the infarcted area, but an identical picture can result from brain tumor, thereby limiting its usefulness in differential diagnosis. A normal brain scan during the first few days after the onset of symptoms suggesting a stroke, followed by a positive brain scan, is highly suggestive of cerebral infarction.

Echoencephalography is often helpful in the diagnosis of cerebral infarction. Reflected ultrasound waves are recorded to demonstrate whether midline structures are shifted. Shift of midline structures is uncommon immediately after cerebral infarction, although cerebral edema occurring 24 to 48 hours later can be responsible for a considerable shift. Acutely, at least, a midline shift of more than 2 mm should make one suspect brain tumor or subdural hematoma.

DIFFERENTIAL DIAGNOSIS

The most common sources of error in the diagnosis of cerebral infarction are brain tumors, subdural hematomas, intracerebral hemorrhages, cerebral traumatic lesions, and cerebral infections.

When a clear history of the onset is available, cerebral infarction is seldom confused with other disorders. Stroke caused by cerebral emboli or cerebral thrombosis characteristically produces a maximal neurologic deficit initially, with gradual improvement in function over days, weeks, or months. The first symptoms of brain tumor and subdural hematoma occasionally are mistaken for stroke, but the general tendency is for these two disorders to cause gradually progressive worsening, even though the first symptoms may seem to begin suddenly. In addition, both brain tumor and hematoma tend to produce disturbances in consciousness that are as prominent as or more prominent than focal neurologic defects, which helps in their differentiation from cerebrovascular disease. Often the problem in differential diagnosis is reversed in that the onset of stroke may include a gradual steady progression of symptoms and signs of focal neurologic defects, making the physician think first of tumor and only later of cerebral infarction. When doubt occurs about the diagnoses of infarction, subdural hematoma, and neoplasm, cerebral angiograms and other tests should be done.

Clinically, it is easier to confuse cerebral infarction with intracranial hemorrhage, for the onset is often similar. The cerebrospinal fluid examination usually helps, but blood can be found in both states—although considerably less often in cerebral infarction. Large amounts of blood in a CSF under increased pressure is always caused by intracranial hemorrhage. Angiography helps to settle the problem by demonstrating aneurysm, A-V anomaly, or intracerebral hematoma.

When it is not known whether the patient could have suffered head trauma, it is often impossible to eliminate this as a cause of clinical states resembling cerebral infarction. Careful inspection for scalp lacerations and localized scalp edema and good quality skull roentgenograms identify most instances of trauma if it has been severe enough to cause neurologic injury. If trauma cannot be eliminated and the patient becomes progressively worse, angiography must be done to eliminate consideration of subdural or epidural hematomas. Angiography is preferable to exploratory burr holes, for it will not only indicate a hematoma but will also define other causes of illness such as tumor, intracerebral hemorrhage, or vascular occlusion.

Among the forms of intracranial sepsis only brain abscess is likely to be confused with cerebral infarction. The points that should alert the physician to the possibility of an abscess are a source of infection elsewhere in the body such as an ear, sinus, or chest infection; persistent headache; persistent low-grade fever; white cells, especially polymorphonuclear leukocytes, that persist more than 24 hours in the cerebrospinal fluid; a focal, highly abnormal EEG; and worsening of the clinical state. If abscess is suspected, angiograms performed on the side opposite to the paresis will demonstrate the presence or absence of an intracerebral mass, which, if present, then must be surgically explored and drained to prove the diagnosis.

COURSE

Some improvement in function after the initial neurologic deficit can be expected after almost every cerebral infarction. During the first 72 hours, however, gradual worsening of neurologic deficits and increasing or beginning impairment of consciousness are frequent. This change may indicate extension of the cerebral infarction, but usually is associated with cerebral edema in and around the necrotic area. *Some degree of cerebral edema complicates every infarct.* It appears almost immediately, and with large infarctions may be so extensive as to shift the brain laterally and downward to produce herniation through the tentorium cerebelli and subsequent brainstem compression. This course of events, with its associated impairment of consciousness and other vital functions, is a common cause of death in patients with extensive infarction. The diagnosis of cerebral edema is especially likely when a patient shows a decline in awareness without a significant increase in focal neurologic deficits. Other causes of lethargy and stupor in patients with cerebral infarction are fever, electrolyte imbalance, the injudicious use of sedatives, tranquilizers or narcotics, and malnutrition.

In patients whose course is not complicated by severe cerebral edema, there is usually an early improvement in neurologic function. If some voluntary movement is preserved, there is a good chance for return of more. When function improves rapidly after the onset, the outlook for a good recovery is excellent. A slow return of function over weeks or months is associated with a less complete recovery. If flaccid paralysis is present from the onset with no return of increased muscle tonus over 30 to 60 days, the outlook for recovery is poor, because a gradual change from flaccidity to spasticity always precedes the advent of voluntary movement. Significant sensory loss impairs the chances of recovery of motor function. With brainstem infarction, the course is usually one of gradual improvement if the infarct is localized in the lateral medullary area. Symptoms of nausea, diplopia, and ataxia lessen and eventually disappear. Although some residual impairment of eye and extremity movement may be detected on examination, such patients often have little physical limitation. It is important to realize that recovery from cerebral infarction with impaired neurologic function may continue for as long as one to two years.

PROGNOSIS

About one fourth to one fifth of patients with either thrombotic or embolic cerebral infarction die with their first attack. This figure varies somewhat with the cause of the infarction and especially with other factors such as age, cardiac status, and the degree of neurologic disability. The mortality rises sharply with increasing age; for patients over the age of 70 with cerebral infarction from atherosclerotic thrombosis or emboli the initial mortality is nearer 50 per cent. Patients with marked neurologic defects, coma, or extensive vascular disease elsewhere have an initial mortality of nearly 50 per cent. Infarction of the ventral portions of the brainstem after basilar artery occlusion, especially with quadriplegia, carries a poor outlook, although good medical and good nursing care may preserve a vegetative existence for long periods.

The prognosis with cerebral infarction is better in younger patients, in those with the least evidence of vascular disease at other sites, especially cardiovascular disease, and in those who do not have hypertension, diabetes, or severe neurologic defects.

About one fifth of patients who survive a cerebral infarction from atherosclerotic vascular disease suffer another cerebrovascular accident within the next 12 to 24 months. However, the most significant limiting factor on survival is not recurrent stroke but cardiovascular disease. Thus in the Cornell-Bellevue series, fully half of the patients who survived the initial cerebral infarction died at a later date from myocardial infarction or cardiac failure.

Recurrence of cerebral infarction is common with cerebral emboli. In the New York Hospital series about 22 per cent of patients with cerebral emboli suffered recurrences, and nearly all the patients had more than one embolus if extracerebral sites were included. There is a strong chance that each cerebral recurrence will cause death or further neurologic disability.

TREATMENT

General. Treatment of cerebral infarction has four goals: to preserve life, to limit the amount of brain damage, to lessen disability and deformity, and to prevent recurrences.

The treatment program designed to preserve life is similar to that outlined for all seriously ill patients with neurologic illness. Efforts are directed toward maintaining a clear airway, an adequate fluid, electrolyte, and caloric intake, and an adequate urine output. Constant care is required to protect the skin from ischemia and necrosis resulting from pressure. Such a program is necessary for the obtunded or comatose patient, and must often be continued for the remainder of his life.

In patients with hemispheric infarction *cerebral edema* can impair consciousness and vital function early in the course of the illness. When cerebral edema subsides, the patient may again be able to cough, swallow, and voluntarily move paretic parts. A variety of measures can often temporarily reduce the brain swelling and carry the patient through a period of severe difficulty. Hypertonic urea solution, 1 to 1.5 grams per kilogram of body weight given intravenously, rapidly reduces cerebral edema and causes a marked diuresis. The effect is transient, and a rebound effect attributed to recurrence

of swelling has been reported. Hypertonic invert sugar, mannitol, has been used with similar results except that less rebound has been reported. One and one half to 2 grams per kilogram of body weight is given intravenously in a 20 per cent solution. In patients with cerebral infarction and brain edema this therapy is reserved until there is a serious threat to life with declining brainstem function, for the benefits are transient, and most patients can be carried through periods of depressed consciousness with careful nursing care alone. Although glucocorticoids such as methylprednisolone are often dramatically effective in improving patients with brain edema from primary and metastatic brain tumor, they have been found in carefully controlled studies to be ineffective in reducing cerebral edema after infarction.

Several agents have been utilized to increase cerebral blood flow in an effort to decrease the amount of ischemic tissue and limit the extent of cerebral infarction. Nearly all known agents that produce vasodilatation, including aminophylline, papaverine, tolazoline hydrochloride, nicotinic acid, and histamine, have been used without clear evidence of success in cerebrovascular disease. The only agent that produces effective vasodilatation in cerebral vessels is carbon dioxide. Although it has been used to treat acute stroke, there is no evidence that it reduces the neurologic defects.

Treatment for the late acute and convalescent phase of a stroke is directed toward lessening deformity and disability, a goal that requires daily passive exercise of paretic parts to prevent joint fixation and to maintain normal muscle and tendon length. Some increase in muscle tone with spasticity invariably accompanies hemiplegia and tends to be most marked in the flexor muscles in the upper extremities and in the extensor muscles in the lower extremities. If this increase in tone in one muscle group over another persists and cannot be overcome by voluntary movement, daily passive movement of weakened or paralyzed parts through the full range of motion must be carried out by a nurse, physician, physiotherapist, or member of the family to prevent muscle and tendon contracture that may be nearly impossible to correct later on.

Rehabilitation. After cerebral infarction, *programs of retraining and rehabilitation should begin as soon as there is no longer evidence of increasing infarction.* Stabilization of the neurologic findings for 12 to 24 hours with some evidence of improvement is usually sufficient evidence to permit a start. Rehabilitation programs have as their goal the retraining of the remaining functions for maximal effectiveness. Although a few patients do require and benefit from special hospital facilities for rehabilitation, most such programs can be carried out on medical services without the aid of extensive equipment. An internist or general physician who is interested in rehabilitation can direct programs of activity and exercise, and can achieve results in rehabilitating hemiplegic patients that are nearly as effective as those of specialized centers.

An active program of rehabilitation begins by increasing the patient's tolerance to sitting and standing, which is impaired both by weakness and by changes in the sense of balance. Patients are allowed to sit up and then stand for increasingly long periods, beginning with five to ten minutes. During this period daily active and passive exercises of weakened extremities are carried out. When patients begin standing they need firm support and often splinting or bracing of the knee on the weakened side; marked quadriceps weakness may even demand a long leg brace. Ambulation is one of the main goals of rehabilitation. Gait training should begin when the patient can comfortably stand for 15 to 20 minutes without fatigue, and the support of parallel bars or a walker should be depended upon at first. After ambulation has started, it may be necessary to brace the foot to avoid the foot drop and supination that commonly occur after hemiplegia. At the same time that the patient is relearning to walk he should be trained in developing new skills with his unaffected arm and improving the strength and function in the paretic arm. This is done by an active program of exercise and by observing and retraining the patient in the activities of daily living such as eating, dressing and undressing, and personal hygiene. More complete details of programs of rehabilitation are outlined in other sources such as Covalt (1965) and can be followed by patients and their families under the direction of the physician. Usually, the maximal effect is gained in six to eight months, but some patients continue to show improvement over periods lasting as long as two years. Passive exercise must be continued indefinitely for severely paralyzed patients if contractures are to be avoided.

For patients with cerebral infarction who have mild to moderate dysphasia, speech therapy may be helpful. With severe dysphasia, therapy is rarely able to restore usable speech.

PREVENTION

The probability of an asymptomatic individual developing an atherosclerotic cerebral infarction has been analyzed by the Framingham study. The risk of developing stroke is increased in either sex and at any age by hypertension, diabetes, electrocardiographic evidence of heart enlargement, hypercholesterolemia, and cigarette smoking. The risk is higher with more than one of these factors operant and increases with the age of the individual. At the moment, the only factor which, if altered, is clearly related to a reduced risk of cerebral infarction is hypertension. In view of this, careful control of blood pressure in hypertensive individuals emerges as an important factor in prevention of signs and symptoms of cerebral ischemia. For management of hypertension, see Ch. 564.

Prevention of recurrent attacks and of cerebral infarction in patients with transient ischemic attacks and prevention of recurrent infarction in patients with cerebral atherosclerosis and cerebral emboli are the goals of much of the currently recommended treatment for stroke. Two methods to achieve this have been extensively evaluated: anticoagulation and surgical correction of arterial obstruction.

Anticoagulant Drugs or Surgery in Transient Ischemic Attacks. *Anticoagulant therapy* was introduced to treat transient ischemic attacks after its use in myocardial infarction suggested a beneficial action. A controlled study of anticoagulants in transient ischemic attacks indicates that as long as patients receive anticoagulants and their prothrombin times are kept at two to two and a half times the normal value, they have fewer ischemic attacks and less chance of having a cerebral infarction. As a result, anticoagulants are now generally accepted as effective in treating patients with transient ischemic attacks. The question is, which patients should receive the

anticoagulants and for how long? The natural history of attacks is variable; attacks often stop spontaneously; some varieties carry a better prognosis than others. Even admitting these differences, anticoagulants should be given to the patients with transient ischemic attacks who do not have contraindications to their use. They should be continued for six months to one year and then gradually discontinued. If transient ischemic attacks recur, they should be given again. The management of patients on anticoagulants is discussed in Ch. 543 to 545.

Drugs which inhibit platelet aggregation have been used to reduce platelet emboli as a cause of transient ischemic attacks. These agents include aspirin, dipyridamole, sulfinpyrazone, and cyproheptadine. Use of these agents has been shown to reduce the frequency of transient ischemic attacks, especially amaurosis fugax, and they are now being extensively evaluated to determine their effect on reducing strokes in patients with transient ischemic attacks.

Surgical correction of extracranial arterial obstruction has been extensively tried in the United States in treating patients with transient ischemic attacks. Most carefully evaluated series show that transient ischemic attacks are relieved after surgical removal of the obstruction and that chances of cerebral infarction are reduced. Patients with transient ischemic attacks who have evidence of an ulcerated atherosclerotic plaque should undergo surgical removal of this source of cerebral emboli. If skilled, experienced surgeons are unavailable or referral is impossible for other reasons, anticoagulants are the treatment of choice. Patients with transient ischemic attacks in whom arteriography demonstrates no surgically correctable lesion are best treated with anticoagulants.

Anticoagulant Drugs or Surgery in Progressing Stroke or Stroke-in-Evolution. Anticoagulants have been shown by Carter to significantly reduce mortality and morbidity among patients with stroke-in-evolution. Such situations are emergencies and, unless specifically contraindicated, anticoagulation must begin with heparin and must be continued with coumarin derivatives. Anticoagulants are usually given for four to six weeks. Surgical correction of an arterial obstruction for the patient with progressing stroke has sometimes been attempted as a means of reducing neurologic disability, but with poor results, except in those patients in whom it can be demonstrated that showers of emboli from an ulcerated atherosclerotic plaque in the carotid artery are the cause of the progression.

Anticoagulant Drugs or Surgery in Completed Stroke. For the patient with an already completed stroke, there is no clear treatment for preventing recurrences. Most series of patients with completed stroke studied by angiograms illustrate the widespread nature of atherosclerotic obstructive vascular disease. Intra- and extracranial vessels are commonly affected simultaneously and impose limiting factors on the successful outcome of surgical correction of extracranial arterial defects. A controlled evaluation of surgical therapy in this group of patients has been carried out and shows that surgical correction of an isolated carotid stenosis in patients with a mild neurologic defect is effective in reducing future mortality and morbidity. Surgical correction of arterial obstruction in patients with severe neurologic defects or with evidence of extensive atherosclerotic disease and occlusion does not reduce future mortality or morbidity.

Anticoagulants, given for one to four months, are

useful during the acute and early convalescent period after a cerebrovascular accident to prevent pulmonary emboli in paralyzed, bedridden patients. The use of anticoagulants has also been recommended on a long-term basis for prevention of recurrent stroke. However, most studies of this problem indicate that there is no benefit from this form of treatment and that the complication rate is too high to warrant its use. Anticoagulation, therefore, can be recommended only for highly selected patients after cerebral infarction.

Anticoagulant Drugs in Cerebral Embolization. Anticoagulants greatly reduce the mortality and morbidity associated with recurrent embolization, and patients with a well established diagnosis of cerebral embolus should be placed on these drugs if there are no contraindications. If the source of emboli is rheumatic heart disease, anticoagulants are given continuously. When emboli follow myocardial infarction, treatment is usually given for one year. Coumarin anticoagulants are used and should be started immediately after the diagnosis has been made and the lumbar puncture has revealed bloodless cerebrospinal fluid.

Patients with cerebral emboli who have atrial fibrillation are often considered for conversion to normal sinus rhythm. This may be valuable in increasing cardiac output, but does not clearly reduce the chance of recurrent cerebral emboli.

General management of anticoagulant therapy is outlined in Ch. 543 to 545.

Hemorrhagic complications from anticoagulants are serious in about 2 to 4 per cent of patients and fatal in 2 per cent. Minor bleeding does not require that the medication be discontinued, but with serious bleeding it should be. Minor surgical procedures can be undertaken safely in most patients on anticoagulants if the prothrombin time is slightly lowered.

Heparin is the anticoagulant of choice for the initial treatment of patients with progressing stroke.

Patients with transient ischemic attacks, progressing strokes, or established strokes who also have hypertension should be treated with antihypertensive medication. Studies of patients with atherosclerotic cerebrovascular disease and hypertension show that when the blood pressure is returned to normal or nearly normal levels the recurrence rate and mortality rate of stroke are reduced. Hypertension, depending on its severity, should be continuously treated with reserpine, chlorothiazide, or hexamethonium, and the blood pressure should be maintained as nearly normal as possible.

To sum up the prophylaxis of strokes: Patients with transient ischemic attacks should be treated with anticoagulants. If arteriography indicates significant extracranial vascular disease, especially ulceration of an atherosclerotic plaque, and experienced surgical care is available, the patient should be offered this form of treatment. Patients with completed strokes are not likely to benefit from any prophylactic treatment. If they are to remain bedridden for long periods, anticoagulants help to reduce the chances of pulmonary embolism.

HYPERTENSIVE ENCEPHALOPATHY

Hypertensive encephalopathy is an uncommon, acute neurologic syndrome characterized by headache, nausea and vomiting, convulsive seizures, transient focal neurologic defects, retinal artery spasm, papilledema, stupor, and coma. The cerebrospinal fluid pressure and protein content are commonly elevated. The syndrome is encountered in patients with longstanding hypertension. Its occurrence is associated with sudden marked increases in blood pressure from various causes, including malignant hypertension, eclampsia, and glomerulonephritis.

The mechanism by which hypertension causes neurologic dysfunction is believed to be acute cerebral vasospasm causing cerebral ischemia and edema. Similar changes have been observed in hypertensive rats.

Mild transient focal neurologic defects can be encountered in this syndrome. When neurologic defects are severe and sustained, the correct diagnosis is more likely to be cerebral ischemia or cerebral hemorrhage. When the blood urea nitrogen is above 100 mg per 100 ml, hypertensive encephalopathy can be difficult to distinguish from uremia, or can blend into that state.

The outlook for patients with hypertensive encephalopathy has been greatly improved with the use of antihypertensive medication, and temporary recovery is now frequent. The appearance of the syndrome, however, is usually associated with the end-state phases of advanced hypertensive vascular disease.

Hypertensive encephalopathy is a medical emergency, and treatment should be given to rapidly lower the blood pressure, for this is the only effective way to eliminate the symptoms. Initial treatment should be intramuscular reserpine, 2 to 5 mg per day. Blood pressure will begin to fall in two to three hours after administration of reserpine, and it can be maintained at desired levels with daily injections. Care must be exercised to avoid cerebral ischemia from hypotension. Permanent medical therapy must be instituted to maintain the blood pressure at more nearly normal levels, utilizing hydrochlorothiazide, reserpine, or alpha methyldopa (see Ch. 564).

PROGRESSIVE SUBCORTICAL ENCEPHALOPATHY

Progressive subcortical encephalopathy, described by Binswanger, is a rare disorder that occurs in patients with hypertension and atherosclerotic vascular disease. Progressive dementia, seizures, and focal neurologic signs characterize the clinical picture. The diagnosis is usually made at necropsy; the brain shows atrophy mainly in the temporal and occipital regions and patchy demyelination in the white matter of the hemispheres.

Carter, A. B.: Cerebral Infarction. New York, Pergamon Press and the Macmillan Company, 1964.
Kannel, W. B., et al.: Risk factors in stroke due to cerebral infarction. Stroke, 2:423, 1971.
McDowell, F. H. (ed.): Treatment of Strokes. *In* Modern Treatment. New York, Harper & Row, 1965, pp. 15–24, 84–92.
McDowell, F. H., and Brennan, R. W. (eds.): Cerebral Vascular Disease. Transactions of the Eighth Princeton Conference, 1972. New York, Grune & Stratton, 1973.
Millikan, C. H.: Reassessment of anticoagulant therapy in various types of occlusive cerebrovascular disease. Stroke, 2:201, 1971.
Toole, J. F., Moossy, J., and Janeway, R. (eds.): Cerebrovascular Disease. Transactions of the Seventh Princeton Conference, 1970. New York, Grune & Stratton, 1971.
Vinken, P. J., and Bruyn, G. W.: Handbook of Clinical Neurology. Vols. 11 and 12: Vascular Diseases of the Nervous System. New York, American Elsevier Publishing Company, 1972.

380. INTRACRANIAL HEMORRHAGE

DEFINITION

Intracranial hemorrhage, or apoplexy, comprises about one tenth of all acute cerebral vascular illness. Regardless of cause, intracranial hemorrhage is a serious illness with a high rate of mortality. At the bedside the physician can only suspect the diagnosis, which must be confirmed by finding blood in the cerebrospinal fluid or by the demonstration of a hematoma at surgery. The causes of intracranial hemorrhage are numerous, and the clinical pictures are similar regardless of the cause. It helps to understand the clinical problem better if one remembers that nontraumatic bleeding within the cranium takes one of four separate anatomic courses and that these produce three relatively distinct clinical pictures:

1. Bleeding emanating from vessels on the surface of the brain and limited to the cerebrospinal fluid–filled space between the pial and arachnoid membranes is called *subarachnoid hemorrhage.*
2. *Subarachnoid hemorrhage with intracerebral extension* occurs when the sudden force of bleeding from a surface vessel also penetrates into the brain itself; signs and symptoms of both the subarachnoid and the parenchymal lesions result.
3. Bleeding from ruptured vessels within the substance of the brain is called *intracerebral hemorrhage.* This may remain isolated therein as a *cerebral hematoma.*
4. Intracerebral hemorrhage may extend through brain tissue to the ventricles or subarachnoid space, causing signs and symptoms of both the parenchymal and the subarachnoid lesions.

ETIOLOGY

Bleeding from ruptured arteries is the usual source of intracranial hemorrhage, although veins also may bleed. The accompanying table lists the common causes.

Arterial Aneurysms

Berry Aneurysms. These are small, round, or saccular berry-shaped dilatations that form characteristically at arterial bifurcations at or near the circle of Willis. Their cause is uncertain, for aneurysms are not familial and they are rarely found in infants. They arise, however, from what are thought to be congenital defects in the media of cerebral vessels. The wall of an aneurysm is thin, composed usually only of intima and subintimal connective tissue. Muscle or elastic tissues may be evident at the origin of the aneurysmal sac from its parent vessel, but these tissues thin out and disappear as the

Causes of Intracranial Hemorrhage

1. Arterial aneurysms
   a. *"Congenital" berry aneurysms*
   b. *Acquired arterial aneurysms*
      (1) Fusiform aneurysms
      (2) Mycotic aneurysms
2. Arteriovenous (A-V) anomalies
3. Hypertensive vascular disease
4. Vascular lesions associated with primary or metastatic brain tumors
5. Systemic bleeding diatheses
6. Undetermined and miscellaneous causes

sac enlarges. Most aneurysms are less than 1 cm in diameter; a few, however, dilate to as much as 2 to 5 cm. As the aneurysm enlarges, it may develop a narrow neck or may remain broadly attached to the vessel wall.

Most berry aneurysms, approximately 85 per cent, develop around the anterior portion of the circle of Willis, arising from the internal carotid, the posterior communicating, the middle cerebral, the anterior communicating, or the anterior cerebral artery, as shown in Figure 8. The most common site is the point of junction of the posterior communicating artery and the internal carotid. About 15 per cent of aneurysms arise from the vertebral-basilar artery system. Multiple aneurysms are found in about one of every six patients. Not all aneurysms bleed, and some are found incidentally at postmortem examination. Occasionally, they become so large that they compress adjacent cerebral tissue or cranial nerves, and, rarely, they enlarge sufficiently to cause a clinical state that simulates brain tumor.

What makes an aneurysm rupture at any given instant is not clear, although several factors seem important. These lesions gradually enlarge with time under the stress of the arterial blood pressure. They are more frequent in patients who are hypertensive, and their incidence is high in subjects with coarctation of the aorta and polycystic renal disease, both of which cause early hypertension. Atheromatous plaques form in their walls, and clots line the aneurysms, but whether either of these conditions increases the chance of rupture is problematic. Probably a change in the blood pressure is the single final event that precipitates perforation of the sac.

Fusiform Aneurysms. These spindle-shaped dilatations along the course of an artery, usually the basilar, sometimes the carotid artery in the cavernous sinus, are due to atherosclerosis. The resulting elongated and tortuous dilatation may be large enough to compress adjacent cranial nerves or the brain itself. Hemorrhage from such an aneurysm is unusual, but characteristically damages the brain fatally when it does occur.

Mycotic Aneurysms. Mycotic aneurysms are produced

Internal carotid artery
Anterior communicating artery
Anterior cerebral artery
Middle cerebral artery
Posterior communicating artery
Posterior cerebral artery
Superior cerebellar artery
Paramedian arteries
Circumferential artery
Anterior inferior cerebellar artery
Basilar artery
Vertebral artery
Posterior inferior cerebellar artery
Anterior spinal artery

Figure 8. The more common sites of berry aneurysm. The size of the aneurysm at the various sites is directly proportional to the frequency at that site.

by septic emboli associated with bacterial endocarditis. A local necrotic vasculitis occurs at the site where the embolus lodges and results in thinning and dilatation of the vessel wall, which may eventually rupture. Such lesions tend to be multiple, and they are the only aneurysms found distally in the smaller branches of the middle cerebral artery.

Arteriovenous Anomalies or Cavernous Angiomas

Arteriovenous anomalies or cavernous angiomas are tangled, interconnected networks of vessels in which arterial blood passes directly to venous drainage without intervening capillaries. These lesions tend to be supplied by more than one parent cerebral artery, and they range in size from the microscopic to a huge cavernous network large enough to cover most of one cerebral hemisphere or to occupy an entire lobe of the cerebellum. The vessels in an A-V anomaly are themselves malformed so that some structurally resemble arteries, others veins. Since these vessels are usually thin-walled, circulating blood at arterial pressure distends and often eventually ruptures them, with a resultant subarachnoid hemorrhage, intracerebral hemorrhage, or both. Even without hemorrhage, large A-V malformations expand, and the neural tissue adjacent to the anomaly characteristically suffers an uneven pressure necrosis, causing progressively more abnormal neurologic signs of epilepsy. Hemorrhage can destroy all clinical evidence of a malformation of microscopic size and make antemortem diagnosis impossible.

Hypertensive Vascular Disease

Hypertension causes thickening and fibrinoid degeneration of the cerebral arterioles. Red cells can be found free in the perivascular spaces around many of the vessels, and microaneurysms have been described along the arteries since the time of Bouchard and Charcot in the nineteenth century. What part each of these abnormalities contributes to the eventual necrosis and rupture is still debated, although most contemporary pathologists view the fibrinoid degeneration as most important.

When hemorrhage occurs, it usually results from rupture of small arteries in the substance of the brain. This may occur anywhere; it is most common in the cerebrum and least common in the cerebellum and brainstem. In the cerebral hemispheres, small branches of the middle cerebral artery penetrating the region of the basal ganglia are most susceptible, and the lenticulostriate artery has even been termed "the artery of cerebral hemorrhage." In the brainstem, hemorrhages arise from paramedian perforating branches of the basilar more often than they do from the long circumferential branches of either the basilar or the vertebral arteries.

Hemorrhage in Brain Tumors

Hemorrhage may occur in either primary or metastatic lesions, usually in rapidly growing tumors with a large amount of vascular overgrowth. This complication is perhaps most common in glioblastoma multiforme and metastatic neoplasms from the lung. Among the more benign tumors pituitary adenomas have a tendency to cause apoplexy. Of the total number of cerebral hemorrhages, however, those from tumor contribute but a small fraction.

Bleeding Diatheses and Miscellaneous Causes

Leukemia, thrombocytopenia, and the ingestion of excessive amounts of anticoagulants all predispose to cerebral hemorrhage. In some patients it is difficult or impossible to establish what caused a cerebral hemorrhage. As mentioned, in some cases the hemorrhage may have erased the malformation. A hemorrhagic cerebral infarct can be so liquefied that it resembles a primary hemorrhage. However, with the increasing use of cerebral angiography, more and more intracranial aneurysms and malformations are being demonstrated in all age groups as the cause of intracranial hemorrhage.

PATHOLOGY AND PATHOGENESIS

Subarachnoid Hemorrhage. Subarachnoid hemorrhage most commonly comes from rupture of a berry aneurysm, less commonly from an A-V anomaly or a mycotic or fusiform aneurysm. Blood suddenly released in this manner has several deleterious effects, each contributing to the seriousness of the disease. The sudden high pressure jet raises the intracranial pressure and sometimes acts like an acute concussion, causing sudden unconsciousness or, occasionally, rapid brain displacement and death. Blood is also a noxious agent, particularly as it hemolyzes and breaks down into its pigments. It irritates blood vessels, meninges, and the brain itself. Meningeal irritation causes the characteristic headache of subarachnoid hemorrhage, and later, within hours or days, the blood produces a sterile meningitis. This hemogenic meningitis itself becomes a source of considerable disability, for it not only causes subjective discomfort and systemic toxicity but leads to meningeal exudation, thickening, and scarring that can impair cerebrospinal fluid absorption and cause subacute or chronic communicating hydrocephalus. Moreover, the blood may irritate the underlying brain so as to evoke adverse descending autonomic discharges, causing hypertension and cardiac arrhythmias.

In addition to the brain destruction caused by the physical action of the hemorrhage, ischemic changes and infarction of brain tissue are found in as many as two thirds of patients dying from subarachnoid hemorrhage. The ischemia and infarction have been attributed to vascular spasm or vessel wall edema, and they are encountered most commonly in the area of the brain supplied by the artery with the ruptured aneurysm. Evidence for arterial spasm in subarachnoid hemorrhage comes from angiographic studies showing segmental vessel narrowing that correlates with a high incidence of clinical and pathologic evidence of cerebral infarction. The causative mechanism is believed to be a combination of the irritating effect of free blood plus vessel injury. During surgery, mechanical stimulation of cerebral arteries causes significant and sustained vessel narrowing. Presumably, vascular spasm has a potentially protective action in reducing the amount of bleeding from a ruptured artery. Why in some instances it lasts long enough and is severe enough to reduce distal cerebral blood flow to the point of ischemia and neural death is unknown. The possibility that persistent vessel narrowing may be due to edema of the vessel wall and not spasm needs consideration.

Extension of bleeding into the brain occurs in about half of all surface aneurysms and in nearly all A-V anomalies. The complication is particularly likely when the bleeding site lies close to cerebral tissue, as is true with aneurysms of the anterior communicating or anterior cerebral arteries, which are interposed between the frontal lobes, or of branches of the middle cerebral artery, which are buried within the sylvian fissure. Rupture from the anterior communicating vessel tends to damage one or both frontal lobes, and rupture of middle cerebral artery aneurysms tends to lacerate the temporoparietal or posterior frontal lobes.

Intracerebral Hemorrhage. Intracerebral hemorrhage is most often caused by hypertensive vascular disease or ruptured aneurysm, less often by a bleeding arteriovenous malformation. The path that the blood takes with these lesions and the amount of bleeding are somewhat unpredictable. Some hemorrhages dissect the brain along fiber tracts, destroying relatively little brain tissue along the way. Others damage considerable amounts of neural tissue in the region of bleeding. All hemorrhages enlarge the brain and evoke cerebral edema. When the enlargement occurs rapidly, it displaces cerebral structures laterally across the midline under the falx and downward through the tentorium cerebelli, with resulting brainstem compression. Such a course of events is often fatal; at postmortem examination smaller areas of bleeding are found in the midbrain and pons in addition to the massive intracerebral hemorrhage. These secondary brainstem lesions have been attributed to venous obstruction and ischemia from transtentorial herniation.

Small intracerebral hemorrhages can remain entirely confined within the brain substance. Occasionally, the hematoma absorbs fluid, and this plus the surrounding edema can create the clinical picture of an expanding new growth. More often, however, the fluid is resorbed, and the remaining cavity shrinks almost to the point of disappearance.

Most large cerebral hemorrhages rupture into the subarachnoid space, the ventricular system, or both. Although serious consequences have been attributed to this course of events, it is likely that the large size of the hemorrhage causes the disastrous clinical effects rather than the fact that bleeding penetrated into the cerebrospinal fluid spaces.

CLINICAL MANIFESTATIONS OF INTRACRANIAL BLEEDING

Subarachnoid Hemorrhage. Subarachnoid hemorrhage has as its most common initial symptom a sudden violent headache. Initially the headache is usually described as an excruciating, intense, aching pain. Later it becomes dull and throbbing but remains severe, and most patients describe it as the most intense headache they have ever experienced. Even if it is at first localized, it soon becomes generalized, and frequently patients complain of severe neck and back pain. The initial localized headache is due to vascular distortion and injury. The later generalized headache is due to meningeal irritation from blood in the subarachnoid space.

Localization of headache at the onset is helpful in determining the site of the bleeding. Headache that begins in the back of the head suggests a posterior fossa origin of bleeding, and headache that begins in the anterior part of the head suggests a supratentorial bleeding source. If the initial headache is localized to one side, bleeding usually has occurred from a vessel on that side.

Other symptoms include dizziness, vertigo, vomiting, drowsiness, sweating and chills, stupor, and loss of consciousness.

Shortly after the onset of symptoms, the patient may lose consciousness for a few moments. With massive subarachnoid hemorrhage and intracerebral extension, the patient may lapse into and remain in coma until death. In some instances of subarachnoid hemorrhage death may be sudden and is related to intraventricular hemorrhage and sudden intense transtentorial herniation and brainstem compression. When hemorrhage is confined to the subarachnoid space or when intracerebral extension of bleeding is minor, consciousness is regained in a few minutes to a few hours. Delirium and lethargy often follow and may persist for as long as two weeks; severe mental clouding, delirium or coma usually indicates severe bleeding and brain damage.

Patients with subarachnoid hemorrhage usually complain of neck stiffness; this does not appear immediately in most patients but begins with the onset of the meningeal inflammatory reaction 6 to 12 hours later. When neck stiffness is evident shortly after the onset of symptoms, it is ominous and suggests that the meninges in the posterior fossa are stretched by beginning herniation of the cerebellar tonsils into the foramen magnum.

Although subarachnoid hemorrhage does occur during sleep, it most commonly occurs when patients are engaged in their usual activities. Many patients have reported that headache began during activity such as straining at stool, heavy lifting, or coitus.

Convulsions may occur, usually at onset, but sometimes during the acute phase of the illness. When present, they almost invariably indicate that the site of bleeding is in the anterior or middle fossa.

On examination the most conspicuous sign is marked neck rigidity and pain on attempting head movement. The most common localizing neurologic abnormality is pupillary inequality or paresis of vertical and medial movements of one eye that follows oculomotor nerve compression by aneurysms of the internal carotid artery.

Lateralizing neurologic signs, such as hemiparesis or hemiplegia, hemisensory defects or hemianopia, indicate either an intracerebral extension of bleeding or vascular spasm. The distribution of signs of neurologic dysfunction, particularly at onset, may be helpful in localizing the site of bleeding. Marked hemiparesis and severe hemisensory defects suggest bleeding from an aneurysm on the middle cerebral artery in the sylvian fissure. Unilateral oculomotor paresis with ptosis, diplopia, and mydriasis suggests that the bleeding source is from the region of the posterior communicating artery where it joins the internal carotid artery. This junction lies in close approximation to the oculomotor nerve as it passes from the posterior to the middle fossa. Bilateral paresis of the extremities suggests that the bleeding site is near the anterior cerebral-anterior communicating artery junction and suggests extension of bleeding into both frontal lobes. Paresis or sensory impairment present from onset is most likely to be caused by intracerebral extension of bleeding, whereas neurologic signs developing later are more often due to arterial spasm.

Examination of the optic fundi in patients with subarachnoid hemorrhages may reveal smooth rounded hemorrhages near the optic nerve head, "subhyaloid hemorrhages." They are often unilateral and, when present on one side, indicate the side of the bleeding. They are venous in origin and result from sudden increase in intracranial venous pressure at the time of the intracranial bleeding.

Fever caused by the hemogenic aseptic meningitis is common in patients with subarachnoid hemorrhage, appearing usually one to three days after onset and reaching 38 to 39° C (100.4 to 102.2° F). Greater elevations of body temperature usually suggest intraventricular or intracerebral extension of bleeding. Subsequent elevations of temperature during the course of the illness may suggest recurrent bleeding, but they are more often related to intercurrent infections.

Rupture of an Arteriovenous Anomaly. The symptoms and signs of a subarachnoid hemorrhage from a ruptured A-V anomaly are identical to those from a ruptured aneurysm, because both blood into the subarachnoid space or into the brain tissues. Bleeding into surrounding brain is common for a ruptured A-V anomaly, and symptoms and signs are like those of intracerebral hemorrhage from other causes. Seizures may occur at the onset of bleeding and are nearly always focal in pattern. The diagnosis of arteriovenous anomaly is suggested by a history of pre-existing focal seizures or focal neurologic signs and of recurrent, always unilateral, vascular headache, each of which occurs in about a third of the patients. Rupture of arteriovenous anomalies is more frequent at a younger age than is rupture of aneurysms, so that a history of focal seizures in a young patient with subarachnoid hemorrhage makes the diagnosis of arteriovenous anomaly particularly likely.

When the patient with an arteriovenous malformation is examined, in addition to signs of meningeal irritation and focal neurologic defects, careful auscultation may disclose an audible bruit over the eyes or skull. Although bruits may be present with either arteriovenous anomalies or aneurysms, they are more common with the former.

Intracerebral Hemorrhage. When intracranial hemorrhage occurs directly into the substance of the brain, the onset of symptoms is usually abrupt. Severe headache, nausea, and vomiting occur and sometimes precede other signs of a neurologic deficit or loss of consciousness by several hours. These early symptoms are the result of an acute increase in intracranial pressure. Focal neurologic dysfunction follows, with hemiplegia or hemisensory defects; this results from disruption or distortion of the main motor and sensory pathways in the cerebrum. Loss of consciousness within minutes after the onset occurs in more than one third of patients and indicates a large hemorrhage, intraventricular bleeding, or both. Among patients who are not initially in coma, half deteriorate with decline of awareness and eventually lapse into coma. With the progressive decline in consciousness, patients may show neurologic signs at first, indicating functional decortication and later indicating decerebration. This sequence follows herniation of the brain through the tentorial space with secondary brainstem compression.

In patients who retain consciousness but have motor or sensory deficits, it can be difficult to differentiate intracerebral hemorrhage from cerebral infarction until the cerebrospinal fluid is examined and found to be bloody. In about 20 per cent of patients, the intracerebral hemorrhage is circumscribed, and the fluid never becomes bloody. In these instances, except for the higher incidence of headache with intracerebral hemorrhage, it may be impossible to differentiate intracerebral hemorrhage from cerebral infarction.

The clinical picture produced by intracerebral hemorrhages at various sites is often characteristic and may enable an accurate localization of bleeding.

Capsular or Putamen Hemorrhage. Intracerebral bleeding into the region of the internal capsule causes abrupt flaccid hemiplegia, loss of sensory perception, and homonymous hemianopia. Capsular hemorrhages in the dominant hemisphere produce aphasia. When the hemorrhage is large, loss of consciousness promptly follows. With small hemorrhages changes are less severe. Paralysis is usually more prominent than sensory impairment, and paralysis of gaze to the side opposite the hemorrhage may be found.

Thalamic Hemorrhages. Hemorrhage into the thalamus also produces abrupt motor deficits, but in addition an impairment of all modalities of sensory perception is common and more prominent than deficits in motility or the visual fields. Consciousness is less likely to be lost with a thalamic than with a capsular hemorrhage. Thalamic hemorrhages are associated with distinct disturbances in eye movements. Patients commonly show paralysis of upward gaze. At rest, their eyes deviate downward and laterally and they are unable to look up on command or reflex. The pupils may be unequal and react poorly to light. There may be partial oculomotor palsy with ptosis and loss of convergence. The mechanism that causes the gaze palsy is compression of the region of the posterior commissure and the adjacent upper brainstem nuclei. Because the disturbances in gaze gradually clear, actual tissue destruction from extension of the hemorrhage into this area is probably not the cause of the defect.

Cerebellar and Brainstem Hemorrhage. Parenchymal hemorrhage in the posterior fossa can occur either in the cerebellar hemispheres or in the brainstem (usually pons). With intracerebellar hemorrhage, the patient may experience sudden severe occipital headache, diplopia, nystagmus, and ataxia. Examination reveals miosis, conjugate gaze palsy, and irregular respiration. In some subjects, these symptoms and signs may be present for several hours before any loss of consciousness; in others, loss of consciousness is immediate. When warning symptoms occur, the diagnosis can often be made from the clinical examination alone, and prompt evacuation of the hematoma can be lifesaving. Hemorrhage into the brainstem causes immediate impairment of consciousness, irregular breathing, pinpoint pupils, and quadriplegia followed by a rapid decline to death.

LABORATORY FINDINGS IN INTRACRANIAL BLEEDING

Cerebrospinal Fluid Examination. Intracranial hemorrhage can be diagnosed ante mortem with certainty only when blood is found in the cerebrospinal fluid or in the brain substance at operation. Lumbar puncture can be safely carried out on most patients suspected of having intracranial hemorrhage, but should be done with caution when there is evidence of impaired consciousness or a progressive decline in awareness and focal neurologic defects. These signs indicate both extensive brain damage and the possibility of brainstem compression. With suspected intracerebral hemorrhages and hematoma, there is always the possibility of tentorial herniation, which may be precipitated or accentuated by changes in cerebrospinal fluid pressure after puncture. In such instances lumbar puncture is best postponed until after other studies have been carried out.

Examination of the cerebrospinal fluid shortly after

the onset of intracranial bleeding (1 to 24 hours) reveals red cells with a constant red cell count in sequential samples. The supernatant fluid of a centrifuged specimen will have a pink color owing to the presence of oxyhemoglobin. The fluid reacts positively with benzidine. Cerebrospinal fluid examined after 24 hours will begin to show, in addition, a yellowish coloration (xanthochromia) caused by the degradation of oxyhemoglobin to bilirubin. This intensifies over a period of several days and usually reaches peak intensity at 36 to 48 hours after the onset of bleeding.

Bloody fluid caused by a traumatic lumbar puncture is indicated by the absence of pink or yellow discoloration of the centrifuged supernatant cerebrospinal fluid, i.e., not xanthochromic, by failure to obtain a positive benzidine test for hemoglobin in the supernatant fluid, and by a decreasing red cell count in sequential samples of the fluid.

The white cell count in the CSF, when determined shortly after bleeding, will be commensurate with the amount of bleeding—usually one white cell for every 1000 red cells. When the white cell count is made on specimens collected 12 hours or more after the onset of bleeding, it may be elevated. This increase in white cells is caused by the inflammatory reaction in the meninges and may reach levels as high as 500 per cubic millimeter. Early in the course of the inflammatory reaction the cells may be polymorphonuclear leukocytes and lymphocytes; later, the cells are all lymphocytes.

An exudative reaction accompanies intracranial hemorrhage, and the cerebrospinal fluid protein is usually elevated to levels around 100 mg per 100 ml or more. During fresh bleeding, for each 10,000 red cells in the fluid, the protein is said to rise 15 mg per 100 ml. Protein elevations are maximal eight to ten days after bleeding and decline thereafter. The cerebrospinal fluid pressure is often elevated to levels of 200 to 300 mm (of CSF) with subarachnoid hemorrhage. Elevations may be much higher, 300 to 500 mm with large intracerebral hemorrhages. The white count in the peripheral blood can be elevated to levels up to 15,000, and some patients have a transient albuminuria and glycosuria.

Arteriography. It is often impossible on clinical grounds alone to distinguish between a bleeding aneurysm, a bleeding A-V anomaly, or intracerebral bleeding of unknown cause. Once the clinical diagnosis of intracranial hemorrhage has been made, cerebral arteriography is necessary to demonstrate the cause and site of bleeding. Thus if the patient is a satisfactory operative risk, arteriography should be performed as soon as possible with the hope that specific treatment can be instituted.

Arteriography is most useful in demonstrating aneurysms and A-V anomalies. In patients with suspected ruptured aneurysm, cerebral angiograms will demonstrate the aneurysm in over 80 per cent of instances. They may also indicate whether the aneurysm can be approached surgically. In addition to the aneurysm, the angiogram may reveal distortion of the usual vessel patterns near the aneurysm, indicating a hematoma, and frequently there will be arterial narrowing. The technical details of arteriography are discussed elsewhere; however, the physician should see to it that the intracranial branches of both the right and left carotid arteries are visualized to determine whether more than one aneurysm is present. When more than one aneurysm is present, it is often difficult to determine which one rup-

tured. Points that are helpful are that the bleeding aneurysm is often irregular in outline and, in the surrounding area, there may be distortion of other vessels, suggesting a local hematoma, or the nearby vessels may show narrowing. Local hematoma is the most reliable evidence of bleeding. If an aneurysm is not seen in the carotid arterial tree, the vertebral and basilar arteries and their branches should be visualized. The demonstration of an aneurysm on the distal branches of the middle or anterior cerebral arteries is almost diagnostic of mycotic aneurysm.

Arteriovenous anomalies are readily demonstrated in cerebral angiograms, as the usually large flow of blood through these structures produces a characteristic picture of early arterial filling and venous drainage of the anomalous vessels.

Intracerebral hemorrhage often can be visualized on cerebral angiograms. Shift of midline vessels, widening of the space between the anterior and middle cerebral arteries, and downward or upward displacement of the middle cerebral branches are helpful evidence. However, roughly a quarter of small hematomas (20 to 30 per cent) escape detection by angiograms.

When hemorrhage has occurred into a cerebral neoplasm, angiograms help in demonstrating vascular changes suggestive of tumor. In addition to vessel distortion and shift of midline vessels, abnormal vessels in the tumor may fill with contrast media and produce a so-called "tumor stain."

PROGNOSIS

Ruptured Aneurysm. Subarachnoid bleeding from a ruptured aneurysm is extremely serious; the mortality rate is 45 per cent for each major attack, and there is a high risk of recurrence. Among those who succumb to bleeding, about one third do so within the first 48 hours, another one third within the next month, and the remainder from later major recurrences. Recurrence strikes about one patient in three, with the maximal danger during the first two weeks after the initial bleeding, when about 60 per cent of all rebleeding occurs. However, some patients bleed during the third and fourth weeks and about 20 per cent have late recurrences, most of which are within the first six months after leaving the hospital. Fatal recurrences have been reported as long as 20 years after the initial bleeding, and there is no way to predict which patient will have a recurrence of bleeding or when he is likely to have it. The high mortality and the frequency of recurrence make accurate statements of prognosis impossible for individual patients. In general, the longer a patient survives after the initial bleeding, the less are his chances of recurrence. Data submitted to the National Co-operative Study of Subarachnoid Hemorrhage indicate that if a patient with subarachnoid hemorrhage is alive one week after onset, the chance of his surviving five more weeks is 65 per cent. If he lives two weeks without recurrence, he has a 76 per cent chance of living four more weeks. Patients 20 to 50 years of age have a better chance of survival than those over 60. As might be expected, patients with the least neural damage and the least impairment of consciousness have the best chance of survival.

Ruptured A-V Anomaly. The prognosis for bleeding from arteriovenous anomalies is better than for aneurysm. The initial mortality is about 25 per cent and the possibility of recurrence less than that. Because of their location and the tendency to bleed into brain tissue, the neurologic disability among survivors of bleeding A-V anomalies tends to be high. Seizures with A-V anomalies are common before bleeding, and patients who do not have seizures often develop them after bleeding.

Hypertensive Vascular Disease. The prognosis for intracerebral hemorrhage from hypertensive vascular disease is poor; the over-all mortality is more than 50 per cent. Mortality is highest with hemorrhage into the ventricle or when severe brain edema causes temporal lobe herniation with resultant compression of tho midbrain. The initial mortality rises with the age of the patient. It is about 40 per cent for patients in the 40 to 60 age range, 50 per cent in patients over 60, and 80 per cent in patients over 70. Patients who are in coma when first seen have a mortality rate of 70 to 100 per cent. Recurrence of intracerebral hemorrhage is uncommon, but tissue destruction and displacement at the time of bleeding cause serious neural damage and residual neurologic dysfunction. Patients with small intracerebral hemorrhages usually are left with only slight disability.

TREATMENT

The treatment of intracranial hemorrhage has three goals: preserving life, reducing disability, and preventing recurrence. Treatment directed toward preservation of life is similar for all causes of intracranial hemorrhage and for most other life-threatening neurologic illnesses. During the acute phase of intracranial hemorrhage, the patient should be in bed for as long as the symptoms of headache, stiff neck, and prostration require. Rebleeding is unlikely with ruptured A-V anomaly and hypertensive vascular disease, and a patient with one of these disorders need not be kept in bed for a long period once he feels well enough to get up. Just when to mobilize the patient with subarachnoid hemorrhage from intracranial aneurysm is a question more difficult to answer. Four to six weeks of bed rest is usually recommended, because this is the period of maximal danger from rebleeding. Recurrent hemorrhage has been noted to occur with straining at stool and with other activity, and rest in bed is believed to lessen the chances for potentially dangerous activity.

When the patient is in coma or has impaired consciousness after intracranial hemorrhage, meticulous care must be taken to maintain an adequate airway, blood pressure, and fluid and electrolyte balance. The skin and eyes must be protected from pressure and irritation. The urinary bladder should not be allowed to become distended from urinary retention. These are common problems for all patients with neurologic illness and depressed consciousness; they are discussed more fully elsewhere.

Patients with intracranial hemorrhage who are conscious usually complain of severe headache and stiff neck. They also frequently are restless and delirious. Analgesics such as codeine sulfate by mouth or codeine phosphate intramuscularly in doses of 60 mg may be needed as often as every two hours to relieve headache; in most instances this also relieves restlessness. Other narcotics for analgesia should be avoided because they depress respiration. *Delirium may persist for as long as two weeks.* No specific treatment is indicated, but having a member of the family present at all times and reducing

examinations and procedures to a minimum greatly reduce the patient's anxiety and restlessness.

Initially, patients with intracranial hemorrhage should not take fluid or food by mouth for 24 to 48 hours because of the danger of vomiting and aspiration. Subsequently, it is best to give clear fluids for another 24 to 48 hours and then a soft diet. During the period of restricted fluid and food intake, intravenous fluids should be given in the usual physiologic quantities.

Constipation must be avoided. When patients require codeine for relief of pain, mild laxatives or stool softeners should be given if the patient is able to take medication by mouth. Otherwise, small enemas should be given every other day.

When the blood pressure is elevated, it should be returned to nearly normal levels, particularly in patients with bleeding from intracranial aneurysms. This should not be done rapidly, however, because of the risk of precipitating a hypotension-induced cerebral ischemic infarct. Methyldopa or reserpine orally or parenterally is usually an effective antihypertensive.

Ruptured Aneurysm. Prevention of recurrent bleeding from aneurysms is the primary goal of treatment and, in view of the close approximation of recurrent bleeding to the initial hemorrhage, should be attempted as soon as possible. Thus angiograms to identify the source and site of bleeding should be made as soon as practicable, once the diagnosis of intracranial hemorrhage has been made. Similarly, if the aneurysm is believed to be amenable to surgical therapy, this is performed as soon as the patient's condition allows. Patients with no depression of consciousness, who are under 60 and normotensive, who have no evidence of arterial spasm on angiograms, and who have minimal neurologic deficits are considered good surgical risks and can be treated surgically immediately if this form of therapy is indicated for the particular aneurysm. Patients with depressed levels of consciousness or coma or with major neurologic deficits are very poor candidates for surgery; operative mortality in this group is extremely high; operation, if indicated, should be postponed until improvement occurs. Patients over the age of 60 who are hypertensive and who have arterial spasm on angiograms also are poor operative risks, and surgery should be delayed until their condition improves.

The possibility that rebleeding is related to lysis of a clot plugging the aneurysmal sac has been suggested. Agents which inhibit the enhanced intrathecal fibrinolytic state that often follows subarachnoid hemorrhage are being evaluated to see if they decrease the chances of rebleeding. These agents include epsilon-aminocaproic acid and p-aminomethylbenzoic acid. Epsilon-aminocaproic acid must be given in large quantities, 20 to 36 grams per day intravenously, to be effective. Studies indicate that it is useful in the prevention of rebleeding.

Surgical therapy is directed toward removal of the aneurysm or control of the bleeding by a direct surgical attack or toward decreasing the blood pressure in the feeding arterial tree by ligation of a proximal artery. Not all aneurysms can be treated surgically.

Some forms of surgical therapy are more suitable than others. In the past six years, several clinics and hospitals have worked together in a cooperative study to determine the type of surgery most suitable for a particular bleeding lesion. It has been concluded, through carefully controlled studies in the United States and England, that aneurysms arising from the internal carotid artery at the junction with the posterior communicating artery should be treated surgically, the procedure of choice being ligation of the common carotid artery in the neck or direct surgical attack on the aneurysm in good-risk patients.

The controlled studies indicate that patients with anterior cerebral artery aneurysms probably do not benefit from surgery and may actually do worse. However, some surgeons still believe that, in properly selected patients, surgical correction of an aneurysm of the anterior cerebral or anterior communicating artery is beneficial.

The outcome of surgical treatment of middle cerebral artery aneurysms is more uncertain. In the controlled treatment series, direct surgical attack provided better results in male patients, whereas women with middle cerebral aneurysms fared less well with surgery than when treated conservatively. The explanation of this difference appears to be that women are more prone to cerebral infarction after surgery than men. In addition, women have smaller, more fragile aneurysms that make surgery more difficult.

Aneurysms on the vertebral basilar vascular tree are difficult to reach surgically. The most successful surgery reported has been for aneurysms arising from the vertebral artery near the branching of the posterior inferior cerebellar artery.

Current surgical techniques include a large number of methods for dealing with ruptured aneurysms. Most of the carefully controlled treatment trials have utilized either common carotid ligation or clipping or tying of the neck of the aneurysm or its feeding vessels. To reinforce the aneurysm and prevent recurrent bleeding, plastic coating and gauze wrapping have been utilized, but their superiority over other methods of surgical treatment has yet to be proved.

If the patient is not suitable for surgical treatment or if surgery must be delayed, a program of medical treatment should be instituted as outlined above.

Arteriovenous Anomaly. Surgery for A-V anomalies require the tying of feeding vessels or the amputation of a portion of the brain containing the anomaly. The latter treatment is curative if the whole A-V malformation can be removed, but it is limited to those instances in which the anomaly lies entirely in or on the occipital pole or the frontal pole. The chance of neurologic disability associated with removal of A-V anomalies in other sites is usually too great to justify surgical therapy unless major disability had been present before bleeding.

Ligation of vessels feeding the anomaly has been recommended, but no carefully controlled evaluation of this form of surgical therapy has been done. Carotid ligation to reduce the blood pressure in the anomaly is also believed to reduce the chance of recurrent bleeding. Recently, artificial embolization with plastic spheres introduced into the feeding arteries has been reported to be successful in obliterating the anomaly.

Fortunately, the chance of recurrent bleeding with arteriovenous anomalies is less than with aneurysm. Also, bleeding carries a relatively low mortality, so that for most patients with arteriovenous anomaly and intracranial hemorrhage, medical management identical to that described for ruptured aneurysm is the treatment of choice. The frequency of disability and mortality associated with surgical treatment are too high to justify its use except in highly special instances. Convulsive seizures are common with arteriovenous anomalies and should be treated with anticonvulsants as outlined in Part X, Section Sixteen.

Intracerebral Hemorrhage. Cerebral hemorrhage is a severe disease and one for which there is no satisfactory form of treatment. The immediate medical treatment was outlined earlier. It must include meticulous attention to the problems imposed by impaired consciousness and abrupt neurologic disability.

Whether and when to operate on cerebral hemorrhage is a recurrent question, and efforts have been made in this direction for years, although generally with poor results. Recently, McKissock and his colleagues in England carried out a carefully controlled evaluation of surgical treatment of acute cerebral hemorrhage caused by hypertensive disease, in which they showed that patients treated surgically fared less well than those treated conservatively. No matter what the treatment, patients in deep stupor or coma from intracerebral hemorrhage rarely survive. For patients who survive the initial cerebral insult and become stable clinically, removal of a persistent encapsulated hematoma may lessen neurologic disability and hasten improvement.

Surgical removal of an intracerebral hematoma caused by bleeding from a ruptured aneurysm has been no more encouraging than when hypertensive vascular disease causes the hemorrhage. Patients with intracerebral hematoma from ruptured aneurysm are usually in coma and have severe neurologic dysfunction; survival in these circumstances is unlikely.

Removal of an intracerebral hematoma caused by bleeding from a ruptured A-V anomaly has been recommended for patients with neurologic disability. The results are difficult to appraise objectively, but surgical treatment has its best chance of offering relief if the patients have become stable clinically and have a well localized, encapsulated hematoma causing symptoms and signs of a mass lesion.

Patients who recover from intracerebral hemorrhage should begin programs of rehabilitation as soon as the effects of acute brain damage have subsided. Such a program begins with passive exercise of the paretic extremities to help avoid contractures and progresses to active exercises as voluntary movement returns. The program is as outlined under Treatment in Ch. 379.

Dinsdale, H. B.: Spontaneous hemorrhage in the posterior fossa. Arch. Neurol., 10:200, 1964.

McKissock, W., Richardson, A., and Taylor, J.: Primary intracerebral hemorrhage. A controlled trial of surgical and conservative treatment in 180 selected cases. Lancet, 2:221, 1961.

McKissock, W., Richardson, A., and Walsh, L.: Anterior communicating aneurysms. A trial of conservative and surgical treatment. Lancet, 1:873, 1965.

McKissock, W., Richardson, A., and Walsh, L.: Middle-cerebral aneurysms. Further results in the controlled trial of conservative and surgical treatment of ruptured intracranial aneurysms. Lancet, 2:417, 1962.

Pool, J. L., and Potts, D. G.: Aneurysms and Arteriovenous Anomalies of the Brain: Diagnosis and Treatment.. New York, Hoeber Medical Division, Harper & Row, 1965.

Sahs, A. L., Perret, G. E., Locksley, H. B., and Nishiotia, H.: Intracranial Aneurysms and Subarachnoid Hemorrhage. Philadelphia, J. B. Lippincott Company, 1969.

Toole, J. F., Moossy, J., and Janeway, R.: Cerebral Vascular Diseases. Transactions of the Seventh Princeton Conference, 1970. New York, Grune & Stratton, 1971.

Toole, J. F., Siebert, R. G., and Whisnant, J. P.: Cerebral Vascular Diseases. Transactions of the Sixth Princeton Conference, 1968. New York, Grune & Stratton, 1971.

Walton, J. N.: Subarachnoid Hemorrhage. London, E. & S. Livingstone, Ltd., 1956.

Section Twelve. INFECTIONS AND INFLAMMATORY DISEASES OF THE CENTRAL NERVOUS SYSTEM AND ITS COVERINGS

381. INTRODUCTION

Philip R. Dodge

The seriously ill patient with symptoms and signs of disease of the central nervous system and evidence of leptomeningeal inflammation presents a challenging diagnostic and therapeutic problem. Of crucial clinical significance is the determination of whether the involvement of meninges is primary, as in bacterial meningitis, or secondary, as in a variety of parenchymatous and parameningeal infections (e.g., encephalitis, brain abscess, subdural empyema). Central to this clinical problem is some degree of pleocytosis. Various bacteria, fungi, rickettsiae, viruses, and parasites may excite such a cerebrospinal fluid response. In addition, a similar reaction may be produced by a variety of noninfectious processes, including chemical irritation, hypersensitivity responses, and, occasionally, tumors. Elsewhere in this text many of the specific diseases that evoke an inflammatory response in the central nervous system and meninges are discussed. In this section emphasis will be placed on a systematic clinical approach to differential diagnosis and on the manner in which functions of the nervous system are deranged by such inflammatory processes.

382. AIDS TO DIAGNOSIS IN INTRACRANIAL AND INTRASPINAL INFLAMMATORY DISEASE

Philip R. Dodge

CEREBROSPINAL FLUID EXAMINATION

Because diagnosis rests in many instances on the cerebrospinal fluid findings, the importance of a carefully performed lumbar puncture and of meticulous study of the cerebrospinal fluid cannot be overstressed. The cerebrospinal fluid findings characteristic of various inflammatory diseases of the central nervous system and meninges are outlined in Tables 1 and 2. Measurement of the initial pressure should be part of every cerebrospinal fluid examination. In the presence of high pressure, just enough fluid should be removed slowly to allow for an adequate examination. Jugular compression (Queckenstedt's test) should be avoided except in cases of suspected spinal cord compression. Deeply yellow (xanthochromic) fluid derives its color primarily from

TABLE 1.   Initial Cerebrospinal Fluid Findings in Suppurative Diseases of the Central Nervous System and Meninges

	Pressure (mm H$_2$O)	Leukocytes per cu mm	Protein (mg per 100 ml)	Sugar (mg per 100 ml)	Specific Findings
Acute bacterial meningitis	Usually elevated; average, 300	Several hundred to more than 60,000; usually few thousand; occasionally less than 100 (especially meningococcal or early in disease); polymorphonuclears predominate	Usually 100 to 500, occasionally more than 1000	Less than 40 in more than half the cases	Organism seen on smear usually; recovered on culture in more than 90% of cases
Subdural empyema	Usually elevated; average 300	Less than 100 to few thousand; polymorphonuclears predominate	Usually 100 to 500	Normal	No organisms on smear or by culture unless concurrent meningitis
Brain abscess	Usually elevated	Usually 10 to 200; rarely fluid is acellular; lymphocytes predominate	Usually 75 to 400	Normal	No organisms on smear or by culture
Ventricular empyema (rupture of brain abscess)	Considerably elevated	Several thousand to 100,000; usually more than 90% polymorphonuclears	Usually several hundred	Usually less than 40	Organism may be cultured or seen on smear
Cerebral epidural abscess	Slight to modest elevation	Few to several hundred or more cells; lymphocytes predominate	Usually 50 to 200	Normal	No organisms on smear or by culture
Spinal epidural abscess	Usually reduced with spinal block	Usually 10 to 100; lymphocytes predominate	Usually several hundred	Normal	No organisms on smear or by culture; may enter abscess on L.P. and get pus
Thrombophlebitis (often associated with subdural empyema)	Often elevated	Few to several hundred; polymorphonuclears and lymphocytes	Slightly to moderately elevated	Normal	No organisms on smear or by culture
Bacterial endocarditis (with embolism)	Normal or slightly elevated	Few to less than 100; lymphocytes and polymorphonuclears	Slightly elevated	Normal	No organisms on smear or by culture
Acute hemorrhagic encephalitis	Usually elevated	Few to more than 1000; polymorphonuclears predominate	Moderately elevated	Normal	No organisms on smear or by culture

TABLE 2. Comparative Cerebrospinal Fluid Findings in Nonsuppurative Meningitis

	Pressure (mm H_2O)	Leukocytes per cu mm	Protein (mg per 100 ml)	Sugar (mg per 100 ml)	Specific Findings
Tuberculous	Usually elevated; may be low with dynamic block in advanced stages	Usually 25 to 100, rarely more than 500; lymphoyctes predominate except in early stages when polymorphonuclears may account for 80% of cells	Nearly always elevated, usually 100 to 200; may be much higher if dynamic block	Usually reduced; less than 50 in $3/4$ of the cases	Acid-fast organisms may be seen on smear of protein coagulum (pellicle) or recovered from inoculated guinea pig or by culture
Cryptococcal	Usually elevated; average, 225	0 to 800; average, 50; lymphocytes predominate	Usually 20 to 500; average, 100	Reduced in more than half of cases; average, 30; often higher in patients with concomitant diabetes mellitus	Organisms may be seen in India ink preparation and on culture (Sabouraud's medium); will usually grow on blood agar; may produce alcohol in CSF from fermentation of glucose
Syphilitic (acute)	Usually elevated	Average 500; usually lymphocytes; rarely polymorphonuclears	Average, 100; gamma globulin often high with abnormal colloidal gold curve	Normal (reduced rarely)	Positive reagin test for syphilis; spirochete not demonstrable by usual techniques of smear or by culture
Sarcoid	Normal to considerably elevated	0 to less than 100 mononuclear cells	Slight to moderate elevation	Normal	No specific findings
Tumor	Usually elevated; may be considerably so	0 to several hundred mononuclears	Elevated often to high levels	Normal or greatly reduced; (low in $3/4$ of carcinomatous meningitis cases)	Neoplastic cells may be identified on smear, by Millepore filter technique or by tissue block
Viral	Normal to moderately elevated	5 to few hundred; but may be more than 1000, particularly with mumps or echovirus 9; lymphocytes predominate but may be more than 80% polymorphonuclears in first few days	Frequently normal or slightly elevated; less than 100; may show greater elevation in recovering stages (particularly poliomyelitis)	Normal (reduced rarely)	Viral agent may be recovered in tissue culture, embryonated egg or animal inoculation

bilirubin pigment. In the absence of prior hemorrhage, this is most frequently associated with high concentrations of protein, and is often seen with impaired cerebrospinal fluid circulation. Intense bilirubin staining of the cerebrospinal fluid may also occur in jaundiced patients with meningitis (as in Weil's disease).

As few as 200 to 300 leukocytes per cubic millimeter will impart an opalescence to the fluid, and fluid containing thousands of cells will be turbid. The fluid should be examined promptly for cells in a counting chamber, and an accurate differential count should be performed on a stained smear of the sediment after centrifugation. In the event of a traumatic lumbar puncture, care must be exercised to ensure that an underlying pleocytosis is not missed. A gram-stained smear for bacteria should be studied. Quellung and agglutination reactions with type-specific antisera may provide an almost certain, immediate etiologic diagnosis when *D. pneumoniae, N. meningitidis, or H. influenzae* organisms are responsible for meningitis. Whenever tuberculous meningitis is a consideration, a Ziehl-Neelsen or Kenyon stain should be performed on the sediment and on the protein coagulum or pellicle that frequently forms on standing. The India ink technique may outline *C. neoformans* in cases of cryptococcal meningitis (torulosis). The finding of budding forms of the yeast in cerebrospinal fluid will help distinguish cryptococci from lymphocytes, with which they may be confused even by experienced observers; however, confirmation by culture is always necessary.

The cerebrospinal fluid should be cultured whenever leukocytes are found or when an inflammatory process is suspected. A variety of media (blood agar, chocolate agar, thioglycollate broth) and various environmental conditions (reduced oxygen tension, increased CO_2 tension) are used routinely. Special media should be employed for the recovery of fungi or *M. tuberculosis*. The latter may also be injected into guinea pigs. Tissue culture techniques and inoculation of mice and embryonated eggs are used for virus isolation.

The concentration of protein in the cerebrospinal fluid increases whenever there is interference with the blood-CSF barrier, as occurs with inflammation. In bacterial, tuberculous, mycotic, and carcinomatous meningitis the glucose concentration in the cerebrospinal fluid is commonly reduced (hypoglycorrhachia). Although the mechanism of hypoglycorrhachia is incompletely understood, the high metabolic activity of rapidly growing cells, phagocytosis, and impaired glucose transport may all be involved. The gamma globulin concentration may be disproportionately increased in certain inflammatory disorders such as syphilis, subacute inclusion body encephalitis, and certain demyelinating disorders (postinfectious encephalomyelitis, multiple sclerosis). In addition to the time-honored tests for syphilis reagin, a new immunologic test applicable to the CSF is countercurrent immunoelectrophoresis. This is a reliable and simple test which permits identification of certain bacterial antigens within an hour or so of a diagnostic lumbar puncture.

RELATIONSHIP OF CEREBROSPINAL FLUID FINDINGS TO ANCILLARY CLINICAL AND LABORATORY DATA

An immediate etiologic diagnosis is possible only when the responsible agent is identified. However, the clinical and cerebrospinal fluid data can help to exclude certain clinical entities early in the diagnostic study. For example, when the symptoms and signs reflect involvement of the meninges and there is no evidence of cerebral or spinal cord disease, primary meningitis is probable. If, in addition, the cerebrospinal fluid contains about 100 or so lymphocytes, a normal quantity of sugar, and an only slightly elevated protein concentration, then bacterial, including tuberculous, and cryptococcal meningitis are less likely, and some form of aseptic meningitis should be suspected. (However, it should be emphasized that the cerebrospinal fluid sugar may be normal on initial examination of patients with tuberculous meningitis and may be reduced in samples obtained subsequently. It should also be appreciated that on occasion the cerebrospinal fluid glucose may be reduced in aseptic meningitis.) A history of exposure to mumps and manifest parotitis make a diagnosis of mumps meningitis probable. On the other hand, the same findings in the CSF in a patient recovering from varicella, especially if there are symptoms and signs of cerebellar ataxia, suggest a diagnosis of postinfectious (varicella) encephalitis. In addition to primary meningeal disease, parameningeal infections can produce cerebrospinal fluid abnormalities similar to those just described. The coexistence of a progressive dysphasia, superior quadrantanopsia, and hemiparesis on the right side and a history of a chronic draining left ear should immediately direct the physician's attention to the diagnosis of a left temporal lobe abscess. Unfortunately, however, a definite diagnosis cannot be made from either the initial clinical or cerebrospinal fluid findings in many cases. Every attempt should be made to amplify the immediate and remote history, including epidemiologic data. One should search for foci of infection adjacent to or remote from the meninges. The extent of the dysfunction of the nervous system should be defined by repeated neurologic examinations and by laboratory studies. In addition to culturing the cerebrospinal fluid, blood cultures should be obtained, because bacteremia is present in about half the cases of primary bacterial meningitis, and similar cerebrospinal fluid changes may occur in bacterial endocarditis. Secretions of the upper and lower respiratory tracts should also be cultured for bacteria and fungi. Enteroviruses cause aseptic meningitis and encephalitis, and recovery of these agents from the stools of patients may aid in establishing the diagnosis. The development of specific neutralizing and complement-fixing antibodies will help confirm the diagnosis. Acute phase sera should be obtained on admission, and a convalescent serum sample obtained two to three weeks later. A fourfold rise in complement-fixing or neutralizing antibody titer is usually evidence of a recent infection with that agent.

Roentgenograms of the skull, sinuses, chest, or spine may be helpful in establishing a diagnosis by disclosing a related focus of disease. An electroencephalogram or isotope scan may direct attention to a region of the brain that clinically is relatively silent. Roentgenographic contrast studies (myelography, pneumoencephalography, ventriculography, and angiography) have their place in diagnosis, but are reserved for the more precise localization of a focal mass lesion that has already been suspected on clinical grounds. Occasionally the clinician must resort to a tissue biopsy; for example, the granulomatous lesions of sarcoidosis may be demonstrated in a lymph node or liver biopsy, and trichina, toxoplasma, or

an unusual arteritis may be identified in microscopic sections of muscle tissue. Biopsy of the meninges or brain should be resorted to only rarely, but will at times help to establish the diagnosis in an obscure case. The pathologic findings in herpes, subacute sclerosing panencephalitis, and acute necrotizing hemorrhagic encephalitis are histologically specific enough to permit an exact diagnosis. Whenever tissue is obtained for routine histologic study, appropriate methods for the recovery of an infective agent should also be employed.

383. PARAMENINGEAL INFECTIONS
Morton N. Swartz

The three major localized intracranial suppurative lesions are *cerebral abscess, subdural empyema,* and *cerebral extradural abscess.* Of paramount importance in their early recognition and subsequent management is an understanding of the nature of the predisposing suppurative conditions and of the portals by which infection has spread intracranially. Not only must these conditions be distinguished from one another but they must also, from a therapeutic viewpoint, be clearly distinguished from meningitis caused by bacteria or other infective agents.

CEREBRAL ABSCESS

Definition. Brain abscess represents a poorly or sharply delineated suppurative process of brain substance, resulting from extension from adjacent foci or from hematogenous spread.

Incidence. Despite the introduction of effective antimicrobial therapy, the over-all incidence of brain abscess has not changed significantly over the past two decades (about 7 per 1000 neurosurgical operations). It is seen approximately one fifth as frequently as bacterial meningitis in a large general hospital.

Predisposing Factors. More than one third of intracerebral infections are a consequence of an adjacent primary focus of infection: middle ear, mastoid, paranasal sinuses, face or scalp and skull (osteomyelitis, compound fracture with wound contamination, or craniotomy wound infection). Another one third or so are a consequence of bronchiectasis, lung abscess, empyema, skin infections, acute bacterial endocarditis, or congenital heart disease with right-to-left shunt. In the remainder of brain abscesses an underlying cause cannot be determined.

Subacute and Chronic Middle Ear Infection and Mastoiditis. Over one third of all brain abscesses stem from ear and sinus infection. Infection usually spreads from the ear by either of two routes: direct extension to the roof of the tympanic cavity or mastoid bone (osteomyelitis) and then through the meningeal covering of the brain, or by extension along veins of the inner ear through diploic vessels of the skull and through intracranial venous channels into the substance of the brain. Thrombophlebitis of the pial vessels and dural sinuses, by impairing cerebral circulation, may cause infarction of brain tissue and facilitate development of local infection. The temporal lobe and cerebellum adjacent to the ear and mastoid are the most common sites of otogenic abscess.

Infections of the Paranasal Sinuses. Frontal and sphenoid sinuses are most frequently implicated in "rhinogenic" brain abscess of the frontal and temporal lobes, respectively. Infection may erode the sinus wall and invade the brain directly or, as with otogenic infection, may spread by way of veins communicating with the cavernous sinus and brain.

Infections of the Face and Skull. Intracranial spread of infection from the face or nose to the frontal lobe occurs by way of a septic thrombophlebitis. Compound fractures of the skull may result in brain abscess, particularly when the dura and brain are lacerated, leaving a nidus of bone or foreign body in the devitalized tissue. Occasionally the original traumatic episode has seemed trivial and has been overlooked. Several cases of brain abscess caused by a pencil point introduced through the orbit have been reported. Brain abscess may complicate stereotactic surgery and ventriculovascular shunts.

Etiology. A wide variety of microorganisms cause brain abscesses, and a careful attempt to establish a bacteriologic diagnosis should be made in every case. A gram-stained smear of purulent material should be studied at the time of surgery, and aerobic and anaerobic cultures, as well as cultures for fungi, should be obtained. In about 20 per cent of brain abscesses cultures are sterile. In about 25 per cent, most often when there is a contiguous extracerebral focus, two or more microbial species are isolated.

Various streptococci (either anaerobic or non-group A strains) and *Staphylococcus aureus* are the most frequently isolated organisms. Pneumococcus, formerly a leading cause of brain abscess, is only rarely incriminated today. Species of the Enterobacteriaceae (*E. coli*, Proteus, Klebsiella) are sometimes isolated. Anaerobic bacteria (particularly streptococci and Bacteroides) are frequently found. Rarely Actinomyces, *Nocardia asteroides*, and other fungi may be recovered from an abscess cavity. Of interest is the frequent association of pulmonary alveolar proteinosis with pulmonary and occasionally cerebral nocardiosis. *Hemophilus aphrophilus* and the fungus *Cladosporium trichoides* rarely infect human beings, but when they do, they show a curious affinity for the central nervous system.

When *Entamoeba histolytica* causes brain abscess, there are associated lesions of the liver or lung in virtually every case. In Central and South America and parts of Europe and Asia cerebral cysticercosis (usually solitary cysts containing the larval form of the pork tapeworm *Taenia solium*) should be considered in patients presenting with symptoms of brain tumor. In the racemose form of disease, obstructive hydrocephalus results from the growth of cysts in the third or fourth ventricle. The clinical picture may suggest a diagnosis of pseudotumor cerebri. Very rarely the brain is the site of echinococcal cysts and the solitary or multiple granulomas of schistosomiasis.

Pathology. Abscesses resulting from direct spread of infection are found in the brain adjacent to the primary extracerebral site; those resulting from retrograde venous propagation are often located at some distance from the primary focus in the distribution of the nearest venous sinus. Thus, for example, cerebellar abscess from otitis media is the result of spread of infection from the middle ear to its deep venous drainage into the trans-

verse sinus, and thence medially into the veins draining the anterior superior portion of the ipsilateral cerebellar hemisphere. Metastatic abscesses are usually found in the distribution of the middle cerebral artery.

Initially, the site is edematous and infiltrated with polymorphonuclear leukocytes. The lesion is poorly demarcated at this stage and represents a local suppurative encephalitis. Usually within two weeks of onset the center undergoes liquefaction necrosis. The surrounding zone of fibroblasts becomes progressively thicker and contains more collagen; this constitutes the wall of the abscess, and astrocytes proliferate in the adjacent cerebral tissue. Multiple satellite abscesses may develop and frequently communicate with the principal cavity. Since abscess cavities usually spread through the central white matter, they often extend to and through the ventricular wall, producing the dire complications of ventricular empyema and meningitis. Brain abscess seldom if ever results from primary bacterial meningitis. Coincidental occurrence of brain abscess and meningitis is usually related to intraventricular leakage of the abscess. In support of this view, the three most common organisms in primary pyogenic meningitis (pneumococcus, *H. influenzae*, and *N. meningitidis*) occur only rarely as the cause of brain abscess.

Clinical Manifestations. *Age Incidence.* Brain abscesses are most common in the second to fifth decades, but may occur at any age. They are rare in infancy, even in patients with congenital heart disease.

General Features. The natural history of brain abscess consists either of a subacute to acute febrile illness with headache accompanied or followed by localizing neurologic symptoms, or of a "stroke-like" or tumor-like development of focal signs and symptoms in which evidence of infection is lacking. A history of fever at the time of invasion of the brain by the infective agent may be elicited; but a third of patients will lack a history of fever and remain afebrile under observation. Blood cultures are usually sterile except in those with an underlying acute bacterial endocarditis.

Headache, the most frequent initial symptom of brain abscess, may develop suddenly or insidiously while the attention of the patient and physician is directed toward the primary infection of ear, sinus, or lung. The development of unexplained headaches in a child with congenital cyanotic heart disease should be regarded as due to abscess until proved otherwise. The headache may be localized to the side of the abscess, but it is often generalized and increases in severity as the infection progresses. Heightened intracranial pressure, manifested by nausea, vomiting, drowsiness, bradycardia, confusion, and stupor, is common. Papilledema is a relatively late finding that is recognized in a minority of cases. The increased intracranial pressure may result in signs of sixth- and, less often, in those of third-nerve palsy. They are often false localizing signs, because the abscess may be remote from the cranial nerves. Although, pathologically, brain abscess progresses through several phases, there is no clear correlation with the clinical course of most patients. In some patients, usually those with metastatic brain abscesses, the illness runs a fulminating course, ending fatally in 5 to 15 days. In most, however, the course is considerably prolonged, and a diagnosis of cerebral neoplasm is often suspected.

Specific Neurologic Syndromes. TEMPORAL LOBE ABSCESS. Most temporal lobe abscesses are secondary to ear infection. Involvement of the dominant temporal lobe may produce a nominal (inability to name objects) or Wernicke's (inability to read, write, or understand spoken words) aphasia. Homonymous upper quadrantic or hemianopic field defects may occur. The only motor deficit may be a slight contralateral faciobrachial monoparesis. Herniation of the temporal lobe through the tentorium may develop precipitously and cause a homolateral third-nerve paralysis, coma, and bilateral pyramidal tract signs.

CEREBELLAR ABSCESS. Cerebellar abscesses are almost exclusively otogenic. Increased intracranial pressure, suboccipital headache, and stiff neck may be the only manifestations. The patient may stagger and veer to the side of the lesion. Impaired coordination of extremities on the same side, with poor performance of rapid, alternating movements and with intention tremor, may be present. Nystagmus is frequent and usually coarser when the gaze is directed to the side of the abscess. Associated diseases of the inner ear may contribute to the unsteady gait and nystagmus, and may produce vertigo. Seizures do not occur with abscesses restricted to the cerebellum.

FRONTAL LOBE ABSCESS. Frontal lobe abscesses are most commonly associated with disease of the frontal or, less frequently, the ethmoid sinuses. Drowsiness, inattention, disturbed judgment, and impaired intellectual functions are common; the findings may suggest a psychiatric diagnosis. Mutism and increased grasp, suck, and snout reflexes are often present. In about a fourth of cases focal or generalized convulsions occur; deviation of the head and eyes to the side opposite the lesion is a common pattern of seizure. When the abscess is large or in the posterior frontal region, a contralateral hemiparesis usually develops. Rarely, dysphasia results from a lesion on the dominant side.

PARIETAL LOBE ABSCESS. Parietal lobe abscesses are usually hematogenous but large otogenic temporal lobe abscesses may extend to the parietal lobe. Impaired position sense, two-point discrimination, and stereognosis are characteristic signs of an anterior parietal lobe abscess. Focal sensory and motor seizures occur. Homonymous hemianopia, visual inattention (often demonstrated by bilateral simultaneous stimulation of visual fields), and impaired opticokinetic nystagmus are encountered with more posterior and deep lesions. Dysphasia is a feature of inferior parietal lobe abscess on the dominant side. When the posterior parieto-temporo-occipital region is affected, there may be impaired recognition of fingers, difficulty in differentiating left from right, acalculia, and agraphia (Gerstmann's syndrome).

BRAIN ABSCESS PRESENTING AS "ACUTE MENINGITIS." Occasionally patients with brain abscess present signs of meningitis, including fever, headache, stiff neck, and pleocytosis; focal neurologic signs are usually in evidence also. The syndrome is most often due to leaking of the abscess into the lateral ventricle. Massive rupture into the ventricle is a catastrophic event, with high fever, shock, and coma, and should be easily recognized. Pleocytosis with cell counts of more than 30,000 per cubic millimeter and reduced sugar concentrations are usual. Bacteria can often be seen on Gram stain and can be grown on culture.

In some patients with a similar clinical picture organisms are not found, and the syndrome may represent the phase of "bacterial encephalitis." The important point to be stressed is that one should be alert to the possibility of a brain abscess in any patients with chronic ear or sinus disease who develop meningitis. These patients often improve on treatment of the meningitis only to develop evidence of an intracranial mass lesion one or two weeks later as encapsulation of the abscess progresses.

Laboratory Diagnosis. Modern neuroradiologic techniques presently provide the preferred and safest first step in laboratory diagnosis. When the diagnosis is suspected on clinical grounds and preliminary x-rays of chest, skull, sinuses, and mastoids are completed, brain scanning should be the next step; it will be abnormal in 75 to 80 per cent of cases. Once the abscess has localized, cerebral angiography is generally diagnostic, but in some instances the avascular areas of the abscess can be mistaken for neoplasm.

The EEG in brain abscess is localizing in the great majority of cases, showing high voltage slow waves and, occasionally, sharp discharges over the margins of the abscess.

The cerebrospinal fluid may require examination when meningitis is suspected, but lumbar puncture should be approached cautiously when clinical signs point to a mass lesion already being present. Cerebrospinal fluid pressure is commonly 200 to 300 mm H_2O, but may be considerably higher, particularly in the presence of intraventricular rupture. The cell count varies from a few to several hundred, with lymphocytes predominating. In cases of intraventricular rupture of the abscess, cell counts may be in excess of 50,000 or 100,000 (mainly neutrophils). Also, cell counts of several thousand, with neutrophils predominating, may occur during the early phase of brain abscess ("bacterial encephalitis"). The sugar level is not reduced unless there is a simultaneous suppurative meningitis. The protein may be increased up to several hundred milligrams per 100 ml.

Treatment. Early diagnosis and prompt antimicrobial treatment are crucial. Some workers use mannitol to reduce brain edema. Surgery is usually required once acute cerebral inflammation and edema are brought under control, and consists of initial aspiration of the abscess cavity, followed in some cases by excision at a later time, or primary total excision of the abscess. The method employed depends, to some extent, on the site of the lesion and the state of the patient, but whenever feasible, primary excision is probably preferable.

Since in brain abscesses penicillin-susceptible organisms predominate, 10 million to 20 million units of penicillin per day intravenously should be started prior to operation. If there is reason to suspect an organism not susceptible to penicillin, e.g., gram-negative bacilli from a chronic ear infection, then chloramphenicol or similar drugs should be given concurrently. One of the semisynthetic penicillins, e.g., oxacillin, should be used if a penicillin-resistant Staphylococcus is suspected. The antimicrobial therapy should be modified as necessary at the time of operation, based on examination of a gram-stained smear and culture of the abscess.

Mortality from brain abscess remains high (40 per cent) despite antimicrobial and surgical treatment. Residual neurologic damage is frequent, and seizures are a significant sequela (up to 70 per cent) so that all patients should receive anticonvulsants for 24 months.

SUBDURAL EMPYEMA

Definition. The designation subdural empyema (less accurately termed a subdural abscess) refers to a collection of pus in the potential space between the dura and the arachnoid. It usually results from extension of infection from primary foci in the ears or sinuses. It is an infrequent complication of intracranial surgery, and may rarely represent a metastatic infection from a remote focus.

Incidence. Subdural empyema is about one fifth as common as brain abscess. Its prevalence has not changed in the past two decades.

Predisposing Factors and Pathologic Features. More than half the cases of subdural empyema develop in patients with chronic paranasal sinus infection, usually frontal. An acute exacerbation of the sinusitis just prior to the development of the subdural infection is common. Osteomyelitis of the frontal bone and an epidural abscess often accompany subdural empyema. Chronic otitis media and mastoiditis result in subdural empyema less often than formerly. Postoperative infection, penetrating wounds, infection in subdural hematomas, bacteremia, pulmonary infection, and (very rarely) bacterial meningitis are other sources of subdural empyema.

Infection spreads from the sinuses or mastoid by direct erosion of bone and dura or through infected veins. Thrombosis of cortical veins is observed in 90 per cent of fatal cases. Once pus forms in the subdural space it spreads widely over the convexity of the hemisphere and mesially along the falx. Rarely, the exudate extends beneath the falx to the opposite side. Purulent subarachnoid exudate is usually present immediately subjacent to the subdural exudate.

Etiology. Streptococci, often non-group A or anaerobic strains, are implicated most commonly, but a wide variety of gram-negative organisms are also found. Postoperative infections are usually due to *Staphylococcus aureus*.

Clinical Manifestations. The symptoms and signs of antecedent sinusitis, otitis, or osteomyelitis often blend into those of subdural empyema. Swelling and erythema of the tissues overlying the primary infection may be prominent, and percussion of the underlying bone may evoke considerable pain. In the early stages, pain or headache is mild and is limited to the area over the subdural infection. As the illness progresses, headache becomes generalized and severe; concomitantly high fever, chills, vomiting, and nuchal rigidity develop. Progressive obtundation, culminating in coma within 48 to 72 hours, occurs in untreated cases. Focal or generalized seizures and hemiparesis are common. Sensory deficits and visual field defects and dysphasia also occur. Although these signs are in part attributable to the compressive effects of a mass lesion, the associated thrombophlebitis of cortical veins and the consequent infarction of cerebral tissue are probably of equal importance. In the late stages, the intracranial pressure is severely increased, but papilledema is rare except in chronic cases in which the clinical course has been modified by antimicrobial therapy. Without treatment, death usually occurs within a few days of onset of focal neurologic signs.

Laboratory Diagnosis. The cerebrospinal fluid pressure is elevated, and the fluid characteristically contains a few hundred to a thousand or more neutrophils, a normal amount of sugar, and no organisms. Roentgenograms of the skull may show destructive changes in the frontal or mastoid bones. Carotid angiography and/or burr hole examination are diagnostic and distinguish subdural empyema from brain abscess.

Treatment. The patient with a subdural empyema requires prompt and adequate surgical drainage by multiple burr holes or craniotomy. Surgical treatment of the accompanying sinusitis, frontal osteomyelitis, or mastoiditis is a secondary consideration and is usually postponed until the acute intracranial infection has subsided. Vigorous systemic therapy with penicillin (10 million to 20 million units daily) and/or other antimicrobials, depending on the background of the case, is begun before surgery and continued until the infection has been completely controlled. The results of smear and culture of pus obtained at the time of operation may dictate changes in the antimicrobial regimen. Bacitracin or other antimicrobial drugs are commonly instilled into the subdural space at the time of operation and for a variable period thereafter.

CEREBRAL EPIDURAL ABSCESS

Epidural abscess is usually secondary to mastoiditis, sinus infection, osteomyelitis of the skull, skull fracture, or infection of an operative wound. Etiologic and pathogenetic considerations are identical to those described for subdural empyema. The close adherence of the dura to bone limits the size of the epidural abscess. It often represents granulations rather than a frankly purulent collection. Rarely, an extensive destructive osteomyelitis of the frontal bone ("Pott's puffy tumor") may be associated with an epidural abscess.

Diagnosis may be difficult. The patient is not as ill as with a subdural empyema, and the size of the collection is rarely sufficient to produce focal neurologic signs or increased intracranial pressure. Fever, pain, and tenderness over the affected area are the common manifestations. In most cases the cerebrospinal fluid is sterile, and contains few cells (lymphocytes predominating) and a normal concentration of sugar. Many times the diagnosis is made incidentally at the time of sinus or mastoid surgery or when intracranial surgery is performed for an associated subdural empyema or brain abscess. Some cases of epidural abscess are probably cured by antimicrobial therapy alone. Spread of infection from the mastoid along the ridge of the petrous bone may result in a small epidural granuloma or abscess that gives rise to a homolateral sixth-nerve palsy and temporoparietal pain from involvement of the sensory fibers of the fifth nerve (Gradenigo's syndrome).

THROMBOPHLEBITIS AND THROMBOSIS OF MAJOR VENOUS SINUSES

Cortical Thrombophlebitis. The syndrome of cortical thrombophlebitis characteristically appears some three to ten days after the onset of bacterial meningitis. The signs include a secondary rise in temperature, focal or generalized seizures, and focal neurologic deficits, such as a hemiparesis. In some instances at least, the underlying phlebitis has its inception earlier and is the basis for many of the seizures and signs of focal cortical disease encountered in the early stages of meningitis. Treatment includes continuation of the antimicrobial therapy and anticonvulsants. Anticoagulant drugs have no established place in therapy. In most cases the process is limited in extent and the patient recovers, but, when the process is widespread, substantial neurologic deficits and death may result.

MAJOR DURAL SINUS THROMBOSIS

Thrombosis of the large dural sinuses may occur in meningitis, may complicate epidural or subdural abscesses, or may develop during the intracranial spread of infection from extracerebral veins. (For spontaneous sinus thrombosis, see Ch. 379.) The thrombotic process may spread to connecting sinuses and cortical veins. Abscess formation within the thrombosed vessel may result in septicemia and infected emboli that travel to distant sites. The cavernous, lateral, and superior sagittal sinuses are most frequently involved.

Cavernous Sinus Thrombosis. Infection can spread to the cavernous sinus through venous channels by three routes: (1) from lesions of the upper half of the face through the facial veins communicating with the angular and superior ophthalmic veins, (2) from infections of the sphenoid and posterior ethmoid sinuses, inferiorly, and (3) from the ear, posteriorly. The initiating infection is usually an intranasal or facial furuncle, acute sinusitis, or an infection of the ear or mastoid. The widespread use of antimicrobial drugs in the treatment of superficial infections has markedly reduced the incidence of this disease. The majority of infections are due to *Staphylococcus aureus,* particularly in the presence of nasal furuncles.

Clinical Manifestations. The general clinical features are those of severe systemic infection: chills, fever, headache, nausea, lethargy, marked polymorphonuclear leukocytosis, and bacteremia. The specific findings are unilateral initially but become bilateral as the process extends to the opposite cavernous sinus via the connecting circular sinus. They include, in the case of infections about the face, unilateral edema of the forehead, eyelids, and base of the nose, as well as proptosis and chemosis—all caused by obstruction of the ophthalmic vein as it enters the cavernous sinus. The superficial veins over the forehead may be distended. The retinal veins become engorged or even thrombosed. Retinal hemorrhages and papilledema occur but may be late manifestations. Involvement of the ophthalmic branch of the fifth nerve produces pain in the eye, photophobia, and hyperesthesia of the forehead. Partial or even complete paralysis of the ocular muscles develops as a result of involvement of the third, fourth, and sixth cranial nerves as they pass through the sinus. The pupils are usually dilated but may be small; the pupillary reactions are often lost.

In infection spreading by the inferior route (e.g., sphenoid sinusitis) the process may be less acute initially. A meningeal reaction commonly occurs, usually without organisms in the cerebrospinal fluid, but pyogenic meningitis sometimes occurs. Rarely, infarction and abscess of the pituitary complicate septic cavernous sinus thrombosis.

Differential diagnosis includes other causes of proptosis, especially orbital cellulitis, abscess, or acute carotid-cavernous fistula. Retinal hemorrhages, papilledema, and palsies of cranial nerves innervating extraocular muscles rather than general restriction of ocular movement from the mechanical effects of orbital swelling are useful differential points.

Lateral Sinus Thrombosis. Thrombosis of the lateral sinus is almost always a complication of acute or chronic otitis media, of mastoiditis, or of cholesteatoma formation. Rarely, infection may spread in a retrograde fashion from a focus in the neck or from a tonsillar abscess. Streptococci, predominantly group A, and staphylococci have been implicated most frequently. The clinical manifestations include chills, fever, and signs of increased intracranial pressure. Pain, venous engorgement, and edema behind the ear may result from associated involvement of the mastoid emissary vein and may extend into the neck over the jugular vein. Papilledema is common; it may be unilateral as a consequence of extension to the cavernous sinus on that side. A generalized increase in intracranial pressure is more frequent with occlusions of the right lateral sinus, which is commonly larger and more important for venous drainage than the left. Convulsive seizures and obtundation occur, but focal neurologic findings are rare except when the thrombophlebitis extends into cortical veins over the convexity of the hemisphere. Rarely, ninth-, tenth- and eleventh-nerve palsies develop, presumably owing to involvement of the jugular bulb and related venous channels.

Cerebrospinal fluid pressure is elevated, and the fluid contains several to many hundred leukocytes (lymphocytes predominating) but no bacteria.

Superior Sagittal Sinus Thrombosis. The superior sagittal sinus is less commonly involved in septic thrombosis than are the lateral and cavernous sinuses. Infection may spread from the lateral or cavernous sinuses, from the pelvis by way of the vertebral veins, from a primary meningitis, or from a contiguous osteomyelitis and peridural infection. If thrombosis is restricted to that portion of the sinus anterior to the rolandic veins, and there is no associated involvement of cortical veins, then the process is usually asymptomatic. Thrombosis of the posterior portion of the sinus results in increased intracranial pressure; at times there are engorgement of scalp veins and edema of the forehead. Extension of the inflammatory process into the cortical veins results in infarction of the underlying cortex. Focal seizures, which alternately involve one and then the other side of the body, are characteristic. Because the superior and mesial surfaces of the cerebral hemispheres are particularly liable to infarction, weakness and sensory changes are frequently more prominent in the legs. However, hemiparesis, homonymous hemianopia, aphasia, and paresis, or conjugate deviation of the eyes may occur.

The cerebrospinal fluid findings are similar to those in lateral sinus thrombosis. A suspected diagnosis of major venous sinus thrombosis can often be confirmed by angiographic study.

Treatment of Dural Sinus Thrombophlebitis. Appropriate antimicrobial drugs in high dosage and surgical drainage, with removal of infected bone and extradural or intrasinus abscess, constitute proper treatment for major sinus thromboses. Ligation of the jugular vein in lateral sinus thrombosis to prevent spread of infected emboli is usually not necessary. Because of the frequent involvement of penicillinase-producing staphylococci, the use of semisynthetic penicillins (nafcillin, oxacillin) or the combination of penicillin and methicillin is warranted until cultures are reported. Since infarction of cerebral tissue from venous thromboses tends to be hemorrhagic, anticoagulants are not employed. The prognosis for recovery is reasonably good when optimal treatment is given, although there are frequently residual neurologic symptoms and signs.

CEREBRAL MANIFESTATIONS OF BACTERIAL ENDOCARDITIS

Neurologic symptoms or signs occur in about 30 per cent of patients with bacterial endocarditis, and a patient may present as a diagnostic neurologic problem. The neuropathologic findings of subacute bacterial endocarditis (usually due to *Streptococcus viridans)* are distinct from those of acute bacterial endocarditis (see Ch. 192). Diffuse embolic infarctions, with a variable and usually limited inflammatory response about involved blood vessels and adjacent meninges, constitute the major neurologic findings in subacute bacterial endocarditis. Pyogenic brain abscess and purulent meningitis do not occur. The clinical picture can resemble that of diffuse encephalitis, or there may be focal signs such as hemiplegia and hemianopia. The cerebrospinal fluid contains modest numbers of polymorphonuclear leukocytes (sometimes red cells as well) and a normal concentration of sugar; bacteria are absent. Subarachnoid hemorrhage may result from rupture of a mycotic aneurysm.

In acute bacterial endocarditis caused by invasive pyogenic organisms (usually *Staphylococcus aureus*), brain abscess (usually small and multiple), acute purulent meningitis, and embolic infarction of cerebral tissue may occur.

Cerebral Abscess

Ballantine, H. T., Jr., and Shealy, C. N.: The role of radical surgery in the treatment of abscess of the brain. Surg. Gynecol. Obstet., 109:370, 1959.
Garfield, J.: Management of supratentorial intracranial abscess: A review of 200 cases. Br. Med. J., 2:7, 1969.
Gates, E. M., Kernohan, J. W., and Craig, W. M.: Metastatic brain abscess. Medicine, 29:71, 1950.
Heineman, H. S., and Braude, A. I.: Anaerobic infection of the brain. Am. J. Med., 35:682, 1963.
Matson, D. D., and Salam, M.: Brain abscess in congential heart disease. Pediatrics, 27:772, 1961.
Samson, D. S., and Clark, K.: A current review of brain abscess. Am. J. Med., 54:201, 1973.
Swartz, M. N., and Karchmer, A. W.: Infections of the central nervous system. *In* Balows, A., et al. (eds.): Anaerobic Bacteria. Role in Disease. Springfield, Ill., Charles C Thomas, 1974.

Subdural Empyema

Conrood, D., and Dans, P. E.: Subdural empyema. Am. J. Med., 53:85, 1972.
Hitchcock, E., and Andreadis, A.: Subdural empyema: A review of 29 cases. J. Neurol. Neurosurg. Psychiatry, 27:422, 1964.

Cerebral Manifestations of Bacterial Endocarditis

Jones, H. R., Siekert, R. E., and Geraci, J. E.: Neurologic manifestations of bacterial endocarditis. Ann. Intern. Med., 71:21, 1969.
Kerr, A., Jr.: Subacute Bacterial Endocarditis. Springfield, Ill., Charles C Thomas, 1955, Chap. V, p. 92.
Ziment, I.: Nervous system complications in bacterial endocarditis. Am. J. Med., 47:593, 1969.

Thrombophlebitis and Thrombosis of Major Venous Sinuses

Brown, P.: Septic cavernous sinus thrombosis. Bull. Hopkins Hosp., 109:68, 1961.
Kalbag, R. K., and Woolf, A. L.: Cerebral Venous Thrombosis. London, Oxford University Press, 1967.
Krayenbuhl, H.: Cerebral venous and sinus thrombosis. Clin. Neurosurg., 14:1, 1967.
Ray, B. S., and Dunbar, H. S.: Thrombosis of the superior sagittal sinus as a cause of pseudotumor cerebri: Methods of diagnosis and treatment. Trans. Am. Neurol. Assoc., 75:12, 1950.

384. SPINAL EPIDURAL INFECTIONS

Philip R. Dodge

Definition. Spinal epidural infections consist of purulent or granulomatous collections contained within the spinal epidural space and overlying or encircling the spinal cord, roots, and nerves. Infection may be localized or may extend widely, at times involving the length of the spinal canal. In one large series an average extent of 4.3 bony segments was reported.

Incidence. This is a rare type of infection, less than one twentieth as common as bacterial meningitis. Although persons of any age are susceptible, it occurs most frequently in young adults.

Etiology and Pathogenesis. *Staphylococcus aureus* is involved in more than 90 per cent of cases, but group A streptococci, other streptococci, pneumococci, Brucella, Salmonella, and various other gram-negative organisms may be responsible. *M. tuberculosis* is an important cause of chronic epidural infections in areas where tuberculosis is prevalent; occasionally fungi and parasites may be recovered from epidural granulomas. There is a primary infective site remote from the spine in most cases. This usually involves the skin, and furuncles, boils, and cellulitis are the common underlying infections. Less often infections of the upper respiratory tract, genitourinary system, or bone may be responsible. Hematogenous or lymphatic spread of infection to the highly vascular epidural space is postulated. Occasionally the responsible organism may be cultured from the blood. Minor injury to the back frequently antedates the symptoms of epidural abscess, and trauma may in some way determine the site of infection. The lack of restraining fibrous tissue in the epidural fat allows the infection to spread caudally and rostrally, and epidural abscesses may extend into the extraspinal tissues; in contrast, the dura is rarely penetrated. In less than half the cases the spine and adjacent soft tissues are primarily affected, and the infection spreads secondarily to the epidural space. Only in tuberculous infections is primary osteomyelitis the rule. Epidural abscess may rarely complicate a lumbar puncture, myelogram, or spinal operation.

Pathology. The purulent material or granulomatous tissue is usually most abundant over the posterior aspect of the spinal cord. When the primary lesion is in a vertebral body, intervertebral disc, or some other anterior structure, the abscess may be predominantly ventral. Epidural abscess occurs most commonly in the thoracic region, but may develop at any level of the spinal axis. The lesion may be purulent or granulomatous.

The mechanism of neural dysfunction in spinal epidural abscess is uncertain. Since the lesion occupies space, direct compression of spinal cord, roots, and nerves is a prime consideration, but the small size of many epidural abscesses, in association with severe impairment of neural function, demands consideration of other possibilities. The most plausible of these and the one for which there are some supporting facts is a vasculitis with secondary venous and arterial occlusions resulting in infarction of neural tissues.

Clinical Manifestations. Heusner has divided the clinical picture into four phases: spinal ache, root pain, weaknesses (voluntary muscles, sphincters, sensibilities), and paralyses.

Spinal Ache. The spinal ache, characteristically maximal at the level of the major pathologic process, soon spreads axially and may also include the paravertebral regions. Restricted movement of the spine, especially in the anteroposterior plane, is common. A functional or even a structural scoliosis may develop. The spines overlying the disease process are tender to percussion; pain so induced may be exquisite, particularly when there is vertebral caries. Signs of sepsis (fever, leukocytosis) are prominent, except in the more chronic cases. The diagnosis is rarely made at this stage.

Root Pain. Within two or three days (acute cases) nerve roots inevitably become encased by the purulent material, and radicular pains develop. Meningeal signs are present in most cases, and headache is a common symptom. At times reflex activity at the level of the involved segment may be depressed. An erroneous diagnosis of "neuritis" or "shingles" is frequently made, but at this stage of illness the combination of clinical symptoms and signs should permit an accurate diagnosis.

Weaknesses. The characteristic feature of this phase of the illness is progressive impairment of neural functions below the level of the lesion, the exact syndrome depending upon the site of maximal damage. If the abscess overlies the spinal cord, spastic weakness, heightened reflexes, and a sensory level over the trunk are to be expected. There may be urinary urgency and incontinence. Abscesses in the lumbosacral region exert their effects on spinal roots and nerves, giving rise to dysesthesias in dermatomes supplied by the implicated nerves, along with appropriate pareses and depressed stretch reflexes. Pain is usually excruciating and nuchal rigidity extreme. The skin and soft tissues overlying the abscess may be swollen, warm, and red. High fever and signs of systemic toxicity are often present.

The diagnosis may be made as late as this with reasonable anticipation that prompt laminectomy and drainage of pus or removal of granulomatous tissue will effect considerable if not total recovery.

Paralyses. Within hours or at most a few days, severe or even total paralysis of nervous functions below the site of the lesion supervenes. Immediate surgical treatment is mandatory at this stage. Procrastination may vitiate the effect of any subsequent therapeutic measures, for enduring paralyses are usual if the patient remains paraplegic for more than a few hours. When an epidural abscess remains unrecognized and untreated, death occurs in 25 to 33 per cent of cases.

It is axiomatic that the foregoing analysis of the clinical features of subdural abscess is arbitrary and somewhat artificial, because the various stages may merge one into the other. Yet, considered in this way the early stages are stressed and the importance of prompt diagnosis and treatment is underscored.

Differential Diagnosis. Spinal epidural abscess demands consideration in the patient with sepsis, back pain, and even minimal neurologic symptoms and signs. Confirmatory evidence may be obtained by tapping the epidural space with an ordinary spinal needle. This is most safely done in the lumbar area. Gentle suction is applied with a small (2 ml) syringe while slowly advancing the needle. If no purulent material is obtained, the stylet should be replaced in the needle and the subarachnoid space entered. The cerebrospinal fluid is characteristically clear and xanthochromic. It may be acellular,

but more often a few cells or a moderate pleocytosis (lymphocytes predominating) will be found. Normal sugar content and elevated cerebrospinal fluid protein are the rule (several hundred to more than 2000 mg per 100 ml). A partial or complete manometric block below the lesion is found in most cases.

An acute viral, postinfectious, syphilitic, or necrotizing myelitis may produce a neurologic syndrome similar to that seen in stage 4 of a spinal epidural abscess, and may be associated with symptoms and signs of infection and cerebrospinal fluid pleocytosis. There may be back pain in acute myelitis, but the duration of illness is compressed in time. Furthermore, xanthochromic cerebrospinal fluid and manometric block are unusual in myelitis. They are seen, however, in progressive adhesive arachnoiditis, which may be confused with subacute or chronic epidural infections. Spinal caries, demonstrable by roentgenography in less than 20 per cent of cases of spinal epidural abscess, suggests the correct diagnosis. In questionable cases a myelographic study will confirm the presence of a space-occupying intraspinal lesion. Rarely, malignant tumors, especially lymphomas that lodge in the epidural space, may present with fever, backache, neurologic signs, and spinal block. Chronic epidural abscess in which evidence of an inflammatory disease is meager or wanting will, on occasion, be confused with the more benign intraspinal tumors.

Treatment. Prompt laminectomy with drainage of purulent material or removal or granulomatous tissue and the administration of appropriate antimicrobial drugs constitute proper therapy. The antimicrobials must be continued in high doses for a minimum of six weeks when pyogenic osteomyelitis is present.

Heusner, A. P.: Nontuberculous spinal epidural infections. N. Engl. J. Med., 239:845, 1948.
Hulme, A., and Dott, N. M.: Spinal epidural abscess. Br. Med. J., 1:64, 1954.

385. TRANSVERSE MYELITIS OR MYELOPATHY

Philip R. Dodge

Transverse myelitis refers to a clinical syndrome in which there is evidence of complete or partial loss of neurologic funtions below a lesion which pathologically usually has a limited longitudinal dimension in the spinal cord. Thoracic and cervical segments are most frequently involved. Although inflammation is implied, it should be appreciated that evidence for this is frequently lacking, and thus the term transverse myelopathy is preferred by many neurologists.

Etiology. As a syndrome rather than a disease, the spectrum of specific causes is broad (see accompanying table). However, the cause remains unknown in the majority of patients presenting with the typical clinical findings.

Prevalence. No precise epidemiologic data are available. Although rare in general medical practice, the syndrome is not uncommonly encountered in a neurologic setting. Sixty-seven cases (44 adults and 23 children) were encountered over a 25-year period at the Columbia Presbyterian Medical Center in New York. Males and females are affected about equally. Altrocchi,

Diseases Which May Present as an Acute or Subacute Transverse Myelitis or Myelopathy

I. Myelitis due to viruses
   A. Poliomyelitis
   B. Coxsackievirus
   C. Herpes zoster
   D. Rabies
   E. B virus myelitis
   F. EB virus
II. Myelitis of unknown etiology
   A. Demyelination myelitis (acute multiple sclerosis)
   B. Postinfectious or postvaccinal myelitis
   C. Necrotizing myelitis (? myelopathy)
III. Myelitis secondary to inflammatory diseases of the meninges
   A. Syphilitic myelitis
      1. Acute meningitis
      2. Meningovascular spinal syphilis
      3. Tabes dorsalis
      4. Gummatous meningitis, including chronic spinal pachymeningitis
   B. Pyogenic or suppurative myelitis
      1. Subacute or chronic meningomyelitis
      2. Abscess of the spinal cord
      3. Subdural abscess
      4. Acute epidural spinal abscess or granuloma
   C. Tuberculous myelitis
      1. Pott's disease with spinal cord compression
      2. Tuberculous meningomyelitis
      3. Tuberculoma of the spinal cord
   D. Miscellaneous
      1. Parasitic and fungal infections producing an epidural granuloma, localized meningitis, or meningomyelitis
      2. Idiopathic meningomyelitis (chronic adhesive arachnoiditis)
IV. Myelopathies
   A. Vascular
      1. Anterior spinal artery occlusion
      2. Dissecting aneurysm with occlusion of major radicular arteries
      3. Arteritis, e.g., polyarteritis nodosa, lupus erythematosus
      4. Malformations
   B. Nutritional deficiencies

who reported on this experience, excluded compressive lesions, serious trauma, radiation myelopathy, those with evidence of concomitant cerebral involvement, and those thought to probably have multiple sclerosis.

Pathology. The pathology of myelitis or myelopathy includes varying degrees of destruction affecting either white or gray matter or often both, usually in an asymmetrical fashion with this irregular pattern of involvement persisting over the longitudinal extent of the lesion. Patchy destruction frequently involves several segments of the spinal cord but may be even more extensive. Demyelination, neuronal injury, and incomplete or complete necrosis of neural tissue have been described and may at times be associated with inflammatory cells, macrophages, or proliferation of astroglia. The form of the reaction is probably related to the duration of the disease and its cause. Thickening of small arteries and veins within or adjacent to the parenchyma of spinal cord has been prominent in only a few of the recorded cases. Because death rarely occurs in the acute stage of the illness today, recent reports characteristically lack postmortem studies employing modern histochemical and cytologic techniques.

Clinical Manifestations. The onset is usually abrupt, with the neurologic deficit evolving from the initial symptoms to maximal disability within hours to a few days or occasionally a few weeks. A premonitory history of an upper respiratory or other infection or minor trauma is reported in about 25 per cent of cases. The earliest symptoms are (1) muscle weakness, usually involving the lower limbs, (2) sensory aberrations, (3) back discomfort, or (4) root pain, all occurring with about equal frequency. Signs may be asymmetrical, but bilateral involvement of the spinal cord is invariable at some time in the course of disease. Bladder and bowel dysfunction are nearly universal as paresis of the limbs and sensory disturbances progress.

The degree of paraparesis is variable, but moderate to severe weakness of the legs obtains in about two thirds of patients. Weakness may affect the arms in as many as one quarter of patients. Sensory loss is also seen in approximately two thirds of reported cases, pain and temperature being more often affected than position and vibratory sensation. Segmental paresthesias and dysesthesias may occur. Stretch reflexes are often lost in the acute stage of the disease but become exaggerated later. Babinski signs are usual. Meningeal signs are encountered in up to one third of patients. There is fever in about one half of patients, although this may be referable to complicating infections of lung or urinary tract.

The cerebrospinal fluid findings are extremely variable even during the acute stage of the disease. In some patients the CSF may be acellular with only a slight rise in the protein concentration, but there may be several hundred or a thousand or more leukocytes, often with a predominant polymorphonuclear reaction in the acute state. The protein concentration may be elevated to several hundred milligrams per 100 ml, and the percentage of gamma globulin can be increased significantly. The sugar content is typically normal. Spine radiographs are unrevealing, as is myelography, except in rare instances when spinal cord swelling is extreme, impeding the flow of dye. In such instances there can also be a manometric block.

Diagnosis. Although the diagnosis of transverse myelitis or myelopathy can be suspected on clinical grounds, it is incumbent upon the physician to consider first those diseases which demand specific and prompt treatment. Spinal epidural abscess can mimic closely transverse myelitis, although the course of the latter condition is usually more rapid. Contrast myelography should be performed if there is any question about the diagnosis. The risk of this procedure is minimal, and the danger of missing a compressive suppurative lesion which should be treated by surgery is of overriding concern. Intraspinal neoplasms and other compressive tumors will also be excluded by myelography except in those rare instances in which an acutely inflamed, swollen cord may mimic an intra-axial mass. Syphilis, especially the meningovascular form, may mimic nonspecific myelitis and deserves immediate treatment. The treatable nutritional myelopathies evolve more slowly and have a pattern of spinal cord involvement which is more diffuse. Other evidence of vitamin B_{12} deficiency or of pellagra should make exclusion of these disorders relatively easy. A vascular nevus at the segmental level of the spinal cord lesion should signal the possibility of an intraspinal vascular malformation which can be defined by selective spinal cord angiography. Every effort should be made to establish the diagnosis of specific viral infections by appropriate cultural and serologic means. A diagnosis of multiple sclerosis may become obvious only when lesions of the central nervous system disseminated in time and space appear.

Treatment. There is no specific treatment for transverse myelitis or myelopathy of unknown cause. The efficacy of pharmacologic doses of the glucocorticoids is unproved but might be considered, particularly if there is evidence of swelling of the spinal cord. Prevention or appropriate treatment for the complications of paraplegia is criterial.

Prognosis. Proper supportive care, including therapy for complicating infection, prevention of pressure sores, and attention to urinary tract function, renders the prognosis for survival excellent. According to Altrocchi, one third of patients make a good or complete recovery, one third do moderately well, and a poor recovery characterizes the course in the other third. Lipton and Teasdall found similar results. Recurrent neurologic problems are rare among the survivors.

Altrocchi, P. H.: Acute transverse myelopathy. Arch. Neurol., 9:112, 1963.

Greenfield, J. G., and Turner, J. W. A.: Acute and subacute necrotic myelitis. Brain, 62:227, 1939.

Hoffman, H. L.: Acute necrotic myelopathy. Brain, 78:377, 1955.

Lipton, H. L., and Teasdall, R. D.: Acute transverse myelopathy in adults. Arch. Neurol., 28:252, 1973.

386. SYPHILITIC INFECTIONS OF THE CENTRAL NERVOUS SYSTEM

Philip R. Dodge

A general exposition of *T. pallidum* infection is presented in Ch. 246. The following presentation is restricted to a discussion of neurosyphilis.

Although the spirochete invades the nervous system and its coverings during the early weeks of infection in nearly every case, neurosyphilis develops in less than 10 per cent of untreated cases.

Pathology. Involvement of the leptomeninges is an essential feature of all forms of neurosyphilis. A meningitis of varying severity and extent is present in every case of active neurosyphilis regardless of the neurologic syndrome. The cerebrospinal fluid reflects this involvement. Even in cases of *asymptomatic neurosyphilis,* in which the presence of syphilis reagin constitutes the sole abnormality, rare postmortem examinations have disclosed definite meningeal inflammation and ependymal granulations. Similarly, in chronic tabes dorsalis with negative cerebrospinal fluid examination, evidence of prior active meningeal disease will be revealed by pathologic study.

Postmortem study of a few cases of acute *syphilitic meningitis* has shown a meningeal inflammatory reaction in which lymphocytes and plasma cells predominate. Cellular aggregates collect about blood vessels, and evidence of early arteritis may be found, although cerebrovascular accidents are rare in this stage of the disease. Reactive fibrosis of the leptomeninges, especially about the base of the brain, is also seen. This accounts for the cranial nerve palsies and for impaired cerebrospinal fluid circulation that can result in increased intracranial pressure. A granular ependymitis is commonly present, and, rarely, this may obstruct cerebrospinal fluid flow through the aqueduct.

In so-called *meningovascular syphilis,* which is typically a more chronic disorder occurring months or a few years after the primary lesion, the inflammatory response is usually less acute and meningeal fibrosis more prominent. As the name suggests, there is an associated arteritis (usually small vessels) that predisposes to arterial occlusion and consequent infarction of neural tissue. When larger arteries become occluded, infarction of brain or spinal cord may be extensive. In some cases damage to regions of neural tissue adjacent to meninges occurs without obvious vascular occlusions.

The neurologic syndromes of so-called parenchymatous syphilis (*tabes dorsalis, optic atrophy, general paresis*) also are due in part to this meningeal affection and in part to the direct invasion of neural tissue by the spirochete. In tabes dorsalis extension of the meningeal inflammatory reaction to the dorsal roots leads ultimately to their destruction and to secondary atrophy of sensory nerve fibers that ascend in the dorsal funiculi of the spinal cord. On gross inspection the dorsal roots appear gray and atrophic, and the dorsal aspect of the spinal cord appears wasted. Myelin sheaths are damaged as well, and demyelination of dorsal columns is easily demonstrated by appropriate stains. Involvement of anterior roots with resultant amyotrophy occurs also but is exceedingly rare. Why the syphilitic process shows a predilection for dorsal roots is unknown.

Treponema pallidum has been demonstrated only rarely in the spinal cords of patients with tabes dorsalis, and direct invasion by the spirochete is probably of little clinical and pathologic importance. In optic atrophy, also, it is probably the contiguous leptomeningitis that is primarily responsible for damage to visual fibers, and those in the periphery of the nerve are most often affected. Direct invasion of the optic nerve by the spirochete may produce additional damage, but the spirochete has been demonstrated in the optic nerve very infrequently.

In general paresis there are, on gross examination, meningeal thickening, atrophy of cerebral tissue (especially of frontal and temporal lobes), and enlargement of ventricles; a granularity of the ependymal surface is consistently present. Microscopically, diffuse destruction and loss of neurons, especially in the cortex, are found, and special stains may demonstrate a heavy infestation with *Treponema pallidum.* Reactive gliosis is often extreme, pleomorphic microglia being characteristically abundant. Inflammation of the meninges is prominent, and varying degrees of arteritis can be anticipated. Collections of subependymal astroglia account for the granularity noted grossly.

Focal *granulomatous accumulations* (gummas) are rare, but may occur in the meninges and extend into the parenchyma of the central nervous system. More diffuse granulomas of the dura (hypertrophic pachymeningitis) assume significance when they compress neural structures, especially the spinal cord.

CLINICAL SYNDROMES IN NEUROSYPHILIS

Asymptomatic Neurosyphilis

As the term suggests, the patient lacks symptoms or signs of neurologic disease, although pathologic involvement of the meninges and possibly of the nervous system parenchyma is implied. The diagnosis rests on the finding of cellular, chemical, or immunologic abnormalities of the cerebrospinal fluid. This is the most common form of neurosyphilis and constituted about 30 per cent of cases in one large neurosyphilis clinic. With adequate treatment (see Treatment) the development of neurologic symptoms can be prevented in most cases.

Symptomatic Neurosyphilis

Meningitis

Symptoms and signs of an acute meningitis are encountered only rarely by physicians, an incidence of less than 2 per cent among syphilitic patients being reported from one general hospital series. It seems likely that some patients with mild or even moderate symptoms go unnoticed. Symptomatic syphilitic meningitis usually occurs during the early weeks or months of infection, often during the period of the secondary rash or concurrently with a mucocutaneous relapse in a patient previously but inadequately treated. The illness is usually of less than a month's duration, but symptoms may persist for longer periods. Headache, vomiting, malaise, and irritability are prominent symptoms. Kernig and Brudzinski signs develop. Occasionally, confusion, delirium, seizures, and cranial nerve palsies (seventh and eighth nerves most common) occur. Argyll Robertson pupils are not part of the constellation of findings in acute syphilitic meningitis. Acute syphilitic hydrocephalus with evidence of increased intracranial pressure, including papilledema, may lead to confusion with other inflammatory and neoplastic conditions. But the diagnosis should not be difficult if the physician considers the possibility of syphilis. The cerebrospinal fluid will always contain an increased number of white blood cells (average about 500 per cubic millimeter — usually mononuclear, rarely polymorphonuclear), elevated total protein (average, about 100 mg per 100 ml), normal sugar concentrations (reduced rarely), and syphilitic reagins. An abnormal gold-sol (Lange) curve will be found in 70 per cent of cases. The serologic tests for syphilis are usually but not always positive.

The response to therapy is generally prompt and gratifying, although an occasional patient will subsequently develop some other form of neurosyphilis.

Meningovascular Syphilis

Although the incidence of this form of neurosyphilis is difficult to ascertain, a figure of 3 per cent of syphilitic patients has been recorded. As with the other forms of neurosyphilis, men are more often affected than women (3:1). Patients with meningovascular syphilis present most commonly from two to ten years after the primary lesion. Symptoms and signs of meningitis are lacking, although headache is a frequent complaint. The major neurologic abnormalities result from the arteritis and consequent arterial thromboses. The neurologic deficits may develop slowly as the circulation through small vessels becomes compromised, or there may be an abrupt loss of function consequent upon occlusion of a major vessel. The specific syndromes depend upon the distribution of infarction within the brain or spinal cord. The patient may develop hemiplegia, hemisensory defect, dysphasia, or homonymous hemianopia. Involvement of the cortex accounts for seizures in a small percentage of cases. Various spinal cord syndromes have been described. A transverse myelopathy can be expected to produce varying degrees of paraparesis, sensory loss, and impaired function of bladder and bowel. Infarction of the anterior two thirds of the cord, with resultant paraplegia and loss of pain sensation below the lesion, follows occlusion of the anterior spinal artery. Sensory functions subserved by the posterior columns are usually preserved. Asymmetric infarction of one half of the spinal cord will result

in weakness and impairment of light touch and position sense on that side and diminished pain and temperature sensation on the opposite side below the anatomic lesion (Brown-Séquard's syndrome).

Some abnormality of the cerebrospinal fluid is always found in meningovascular syphilis. A lymphocytic pleocytosis (few to 100 cells per cubic millimeter) and/or an elevated protein concentration is characteristic. The globulin content is often elevated; this is reflected in an abnormal Lange curve. Syphilitic reagins are nearly always present in the cerebrospinal fluid as well as in the blood.

The progress of meningovascular syphilis can usually be halted by specific treatment, but the degree of functional recovery depends upon the extent and location of the infarcts and upon the many complex physiologic factors that condition recovery in cerebrovascular disease of any type.

General Paresis
(Dementia Paralytica, General Paralysis of the Insane)

This dread complication of syphilis makes its appearance from 2 to 30 (usually 10 to 25) years after the primary lesion. It occurs more often in men than in women (3:1), and 89 per cent of cases occur between the ages of 30 and 60 years. In one large series about 60 per cent of patients presented with simple dementia, and less than 20 per cent displayed manic symptoms and megalomania. Often faulty judgment, impaired memory (recent memory affected first), disturbed affect (depression or euphoria), or paranoia suggests the presence of a serious mental disturbance. This behavioral change will be especially noticeable when the afflicted individual has been a competitive member of society. Delusions and hallucinations occur less often but, when present, prompt a quick referral to the physician. The patient himself may complain of "nervousness," but characteristically lacks insight into the nature of his difficulty. Fine or coarse tremors, often affecting facial muscles and tongue, are present in about two thirds of the patients with fully developed general paresis. Abnormal pupillary responses, including Argyll Robertson pupil (see Tabes Dorsalis, below), impassive facies, slurred or dysarthric speech, exaggerated stretch reflexes, and extensor plantar responses are additional neurologic signs. Convulsions occur in 10 per cent of patients, and strokes secondary to vasculitis are also seen. When symptoms and signs of tabes dorsalis accompany those of paresis, the designation taboparesis is used.

The cerebrospinal fluid is always abnormal, containing in excess of 5 white blood cells per cubic millimeter (mononuclear) in 85 per cent of untreated cases, and more than 30 cells per cubic millimeter in about a fourth of cases. An elevated total protein concentration (greater than 50 mg per 100 ml) of cerebrospinal fluid can be anticipated in 75 per cent, and a level of 100 mg per 100 ml or higher in about 20 per cent of cases. An elevated gamma globulin level accounts for the first zone colloidal gold (Lange) curve, e.g., 5554433211, which is frequently found in general paresis. Nearly every patient will have a positive reagin test for syphilis in the cerebrospinal fluid, and in more than 90 per cent of cases the blood serologic test will also be positive. Incomplete, prior treatment may modify but will not restore to normal the cerebrospinal fluid.

General paresis, once established, evolves rapidly, and

patients soon become disabled mentally, socially, and, in the late stage, physically. The term general paralysis of the insane derived from observations of patients helpless and bedridden in the terminal stages of the disease. Untreated general paresis is universally fatal, usually within three years.

If the disease is recognized early and treated vigorously, about 80 per cent of patients will return to some form of work, but only in about one half will complete recovery be achieved. There is little hope of a satisfactory result when treatment is delayed until the patient is demented, incontinent, and bedridden.

Tabes Dorsalis
(Locomotor Ataxia)

Tabes dorsalis develops in less than 5 per cent of patients with untreated syphilis, and symptoms usually become manifest 10 to 20 years after the primary infection. Rarely, there is a latent period of 30 or more years. Men are more often affected than women.

Dysfunction of affected posterior roots accrues slowly, and symptoms develop insidiously. Impaired joint position sense frequently results in stumbling and difficulty in walking, especially in the dark when visual compensation is imperfect. As the disease progresses, this sensory ataxia worsens, and a broad-based gait is assumed. Profound hypotonia, secondary to a lack of modulation of muscle tension by afferent fibers, is expressed frequently in a slapping gait. Paresthesias usually appear early in the disease but may be ignored by the patient until the appearance of lightning pains. These pains are characteristic of tabes dorsalis but are in no way specific, because they occur in other diseases affecting dorsal roots, e.g., diabetic neuropathy. Lightning pains develop in at least 75 per cent of patients and may appear in any area of the body, although they are most common in the lower extremities. Some patients insist that they are more troublesome when the barometric pressure is low. They may be described as sharp, burning, or aching. However, sharp jabs of pain are characteristic. These may be mild or excruciating, and frequently flit from one region to another. At times they are so transitory that by the time the patient has made the natural move to rub or massage the involved part, pain has disappeared. For a period of hours or days one spot will seem particularly vulnerable, but then the site of attack shifts to another place. Involvement of thoracoabdominal nerve roots gives rise to visceral pains *(gastric or visceral crises)*, which may simulate intrinsic visceral disease and may lead to unnecessary surgery; in one series an estimated 25 per cent of tabetic patients had undergone operation for tabetic pain. The converse is also true: on rare occasions visceral pain has been ascribed to tabes dorsalis and suppurative appendicitis, or a ruptured peptic ulcer has gone undiagnosed. As the disease advances, pain sensation may be so dulled that recurrent trauma is unnoticed by the patient and indolent ulcers of the skin develop; the toes and balls of the feet are especially vulnerable. Weight-bearing joints and adjacent bone, deprived of pain sensation, are destroyed by the constant trauma of use in 5 to 10 per cent of tabetic patients (Charcot joints).

Unless general paresis coexists, as it does in a small percentage of cases *(taboparesis)*, tabetic patients are mentally normal. Optic atrophy complicates tabes dorsalis in about 10 per cent of cases or occurs as an isolated disorder. Pupillary abnormalities, including meiosis, irregularity, poor responsiveness to light and mydriatics, but retained reaction in accommodation (Argyll Robertson pupils), are present in most cases of tabes dorsalis. Involvement of other oculomotor functions is occasionally seen. Hypotonia, ataxia, and broad-based gait can usually be demonstrated. Affection of the sensory arc of the myotatic reflexes accounts for the greatly diminished or absent stretch reflexes. The Achilles reflex is affected most constantly. The plantar responses are normal in most cases of uncomplicated tabes dorsalis. Loss or diminution of position and vibratory sensation is found in every case. Increased swaying when the eyes are closed and the patient is standing with foot together (Romberg's sign) results from the impaired position sense. Variable degrees of hypesthesia and hypalgesia in a root distribution can be anticipated but may be difficult to plot. Isolated areas of hypalgesia (Hitzig zones) are sometimes found. Delayed perception of a pain stimulus (from one to several seconds) often can be demonstrated. Impaired deep pain sensation may account for a dramatic lack of responsiveness to squeezing of the Achilles tendon or testicles. Because of involvement of sacral nerve roots, functions of the urinary bladder and bowel are impaired in up to one third of cases; overflow incontinence and constipation develop. Impotence is a major complaint in the male. Characteristically a cystometrogram shows an absence of, or reduction in, the normal muscular contractions of the bladder in response to filling; the patient may be unaware of a volume in excess of 500 ml. Hydronephrosis and pyogenic infection are common complications of a hypotonic bladder.

Early in the course of tabes dorsalis, the serologic tests for syphilis are, as a rule, strongly positive. The cerebrospinal fluid may reflect the meningeal inflammatory process with pleocytosis, an elevated total protein, and a positive reagin test. Late in the disease, especially after some antisyphilitic treatment, the serologic tests may be negative (in 25 to 50 per cent of cases), and even the cerebrospinal fluid is negative in up to 20 per cent of cases.

The course of tabes dorsalis is unpredictable, and the response to antisyphilitic therapy is variable. In general, patients who have had symptoms for a few months or at the most a few years, with significant cerebrospinal fluid abnormalities and no prior therapy, are most likely to improve with treatment. Patients with far-advanced disease and severe degeneration of dorsal roots and who suffer from the painful complications will not benefit significantly from antisyphilitic therapy. At least partial relief of pain may be achieved by analgesics, but when narcotics are used the risk of addiction is significant. Recently, some benefit has been reported with diphenylhydantoin (Dilantin) treatment (200 mg per square meter per day). Recourse to spinal cordotomy and other surgical measures to relieve pain should be deferred until all medical measures have failed. Urologic assistance may be required to deal effectively with the tabetic uropathies, and surgery may be required for management of penetrating ulcers of the skin and Charcot joints.

Optic Atrophy

Visual impairment in syphilis may result from iritis, choreoretinitis, increased intracranial pressure (consecutive optic atrophy), or primary optic atrophy. Optic atrophy occurs in 1 per cent of patients with untreated syphilis and is five times more common in males than in females. It is stated that blacks are more prone than whites to optic atrophy, whereas the reverse is reported in other forms of neurosyphilis.

Because the outer portions of the optic nerve are first affected, the visual impairment tends to be peripheral in the early stages. Ultimately, however, the papillomacular bundle lying in the center of the nerve becomes involved, and impaired visual acuity and central and paracentral scotomas develop. It has been estimated that, without treatment, 50 per cent of patients will be blind in two years and 90 per cent in ten years. One eye is typically affected before the other. Optic pallor is usually present by the time symptoms appear, but in the early stages it is recognizable only by the reduced vascularity. A chalk-white disc with sharp margins and prominent lamina cribrosa constitute the fully developed appearance of optic atrophy. The optic atrophy of syphilis is indistinguishable from that caused by other diseases of the optic nerve in which there has been no antecedent papillitis or papilledema. The cerebrospinal fluid is abnormal in most patients with active disease of the optic nerve. Intensive antisyphilitic therapy may arrest the disease process and preserve what vision remains, but return of vision already lost should not be anticipated.

Gumma

This rare complication of syphilis usually declares itself as an intracranial or intraspinal mass lesion and behaves in every way as a slowly growing neoplasm. The correct diagnosis may be suspected from a positive serologic test for syphilis or from cerebrospinal fluid abnormalities. Frequently, however, the diagnosis is not made until the patient is operated upon, and histopathologic studies are made. Removal of the tumor mass, supplemented by antimicrobial therapy (see Treatment), should alleviate symptoms and prevent spread of the disease.

Congenital Neurosyphilis

Syphilis acquired by the fetus from an infected mother after the first trimester of pregnancy tends to be a fulminant disease. Miscarriages and stillbirths are common, and a wide spectrum of clinical manifestations may be recognized in the infant or child who survives. *Neurosyphilis* develops in an estimated 10 to 20 per cent of infants and children with congenital syphilis. *Asymptomatic neurosyphilis* may be diagnosed in the early months or years of life by doing routine cerebrospinal fluid examinations on children of syphilitic mothers. But, as with acquired neurosyphilis, symptoms and signs develop only after a latent period that, in the case of *juvenile paresis*, may be as long as 20 years. More often symptoms first appear late in the first decade or during adolescence. Clinical syndromes and cerebrospinal fluid findings mirror those found with the acquired disease except that *tabes dorsalis* is exceedingly rare and *choreoretinitis* more common. Hydrocephalus, cranial nerve palsies (eighth cranial nerve especially), and seizures may complicate congenital syphilitic meningitis, and syphilis should be remembered as a cause of cerebrovascular accidents in children. Previous studies emphasize that more than a third of all children presenting with juvenile paresis have been retarded mentally since early life. Although mental retardation is very likely due to other factors in some cases, such statistics emphasize the vulnerability of the developing nervous system to syphilitic infection.

Other non-neurologic stigmata of congenital syphilis include dental deformities (Hutchinson's teeth), saddle nose, frontal bossing of the skull, saber shins, and interstitial keratitis (usually developing during the second decade). These signs are not seen in acquired syphilis. Fortunately, the current practice of doing routine serologic tests on all pregnant women and on infants of syphilitic mothers has all but eliminated congenital neurosyphilis in many areas of the world. In this regard it should be remembered that the mother can acquire syphilis at any time during pregnancy and that negative serologic studies obtained early do not exclude the possibility that they might become positive later in the course of pregnancy. In some institutions blood from the umbilical cord is routinely tested for the reagin of syphilis.

Early and intensive treatment of infants with congenital syphilis materially reduces the morbidity (see Treatment) from neurologic complications. Unhappily, results from even optimal treatment of patients with juvenile paresis remain poor.

TREATMENT

Penicillin is the preferred drug for treating neurosyphilis. Reasonable therapy for adults with all forms of neurosyphilis, except general paresis, is a total dose of procaine penicillin G of 9 to 12 million units given over two to three weeks. A total dose of 18 to 24 million units administered over the same period of time is used to treat patients with general paresis. For children, approximately one half of the adult dose is employed, and one quarter of the adult dose is given to infants. We prefer to treat patients with active neurosyphilis in hospital (mandatory in general paresis), but this is not always feasible. When outpatient treatment is necessary, an initial dose of 3 million units of long-acting penicillin (benzathine penicillin G, Bicillin) should be given. The sole use of benzathine penicillin G at weekly intervals in doses equivalent to those presented above has been advocated by some in the treatment of neurosyphilis. It must be stressed that these therapeutic regimens are empirical. Nevertheless, they are reasonable and have stood the test of time. The author suspects that early diagnosis of syphilitic infection is far more critical than the precise dosage and the time course of therapy.

Alternative drugs include the tetracyclines and chloramphenicol (3 to 4 grams per day for 15 days), but they should be reserved for cases in which there is a clearly proved allergy to penicillin. Sensitivity to penicillin should not be confused with the Jarisch-Herxheimer reaction, which occurs within a few hours of the first injection of the drug in 50 per cent or more of patients (see Ch. 246). During therapy, neurologic symptoms and signs may exacerbate temporarily – notably in paresis – presumably because of the Jarisch-Herxheimer reaction.

Clarke, E. G., and Danbolt, N.: The Oslo study of the natural history of untreated syphilis. J. Chronic Dis., 2:311, 1955.
Green, J. B.: Dilantin in the treatment of lightning pains. Neurology, 11:257, 1961.
Hahn, R. D., et al.: Penicillin treatment of general paresis (dementia paralytica) – Results of treatment in 1086 patients, the majority of whom were followed for more than 5 years. A.M.A. Arch. Neurol. Psychiat., 81:557, 1959.
Hooshmand, H., Escobar, M. R., and Kopf, S. W.: Neurosyphilis. A study of 241 patients. J.A.M.A., 219:726, 1972.
Idsøe, O., Guthe, T., and Willcox, R. R.: Penicillin in the treatment of syphilis. Geneva, Bull. WHO, Supplement to Vol. 47, 1972.
Merritt, H. H., Adams, R. D., and Solomon, H.: Neurosyphilis. New York, Oxford University Press, 1946.
Montgomery, C. H., and Knox, J. M.: Antibiotics other than penicillin in the treatment of syphilis. N. Engl. J. Med., 261:277, 1961.

Section Thirteen.   VIRAL INFECTIONS OF THE NERVOUS SYSTEM

387.   INTRODUCTION

Richard T. Johnson

Viral infections of the nervous system, in general, represent uncommon but important complications of systemic infections. With a few exceptions such as rabies or B virus (*herpes simiae*), nervous system infections are caused by agents which often infect man. Some of these viruses, such as polioviruses and arthropod-borne encephalitis viruses, cause clinically significant disease only on the rare occasion when the nervous system is involved. Others, such as herpes simplex and mumps virus, are frequent causes of mild disease that assumes a more serious form when the central nervous system is infected.

Experimentally, viruses have been shown to invade the nervous system by centripetal growth or movement in peripheral nerves, by penetration across the olfactory mucosa, or by a viremia. In man most viruses which infect the nervous system spread to the brain and meninges from blood, although neural spread appears to be important in rabies, B virus, and varicella-zoster virus infections. The infrequency of nervous system involvement can be attributed to a variety of host defense mechanisms, including cellular and humoral responses, interferon production, anatomic barriers of nonsusceptible cells, and the activity of the reticuloendothelial system which clears viruses from the blood. Youth, severe nutritional deficiency, and defects of cellular immunity have been shown to increase the risk of nervous system infection with some viruses, but in the majority of patients the factors which have permitted central nervous system invasion are not evident.

Viral infections of the nervous system can lead to diverse clinical signs and symptoms, varied clinical courses, and protean pathologic changes. This diversity can be explained by the following two principles: (1) the varied cell populations of the nervous system have different susceptibilities to different viruses; and (2) viral infections can have varied effects on susceptible cells. If infection is limited to the meninges covering the nervous system, then signs of headache, fever, stiff neck, and CSF pleocytosis (i.e., meningitis) may be the only clinical manifestations. If the infection spreads to the parenchymal cells of the brain, in addition to signs of meningeal irritation, there may develop a depression of the state of consciousness, seizures, focal neurologic deficits, or increased intracranial pressure (i.e., encephalitis). Some viruses cause even more selective involvement of specific cell populations in the brain and spinal cord and thus evoke characteristic clinical symptoms and signs. For example, in poliovirus infections the selective vulnerability of anterior horn cells leads to a characteristic clinical finding of acute meningitis with lower motor neuron paralysis. On the other hand, rabies virus infections in animals tend to spare the cortical neurons involved in most types of encephalitis and infect neurons of the limbic system. Therefore, instead of obtundation, seizures, and motor or sensory deficits, the infected animal shows alertness, loss of timidity, aberrant sexual behavior, and aggressive activity. This selective infection of cells of the limbic system appears to be a diabolic adaptation of the rabies virus to specific cell populations, so that the clinical disease in animals can drive the host to transmit the virus to another host by biting. Glial cell populations may also be selectively involved, such as in progressive multifocal leukoencephalopathy in which virus infection and cell lysis appear limited to the oligodendrocytes, causing a slowly progressive demyelinating disease.

The virus-cell interaction may be quite varied. There may be *acute lysis* of the infected cell, transformation of the cell with production of neoplasm, or *chronic infection* causing cellular dysfunction, cellular degeneration, or no abnormality. In acute viral infections the clinical and pathologic abnormalities may result either from an acute viral destruction of cells, as in acute viral meningitis or encephalitis, or from the host's immunologic response to the infection, as has been postulated in postinfectious encephalomyelitis. A *latent infection* is a virus-host relationship in which the virus remains present in some form in the host without giving rise to any signs of infection, but which can, when some trigger mechanism comes into play, emerge as an acute infectious process. This appears to occur in herpes zoster and possibly in some cases of herpes simplex encephalitis. *Chronic viral infections* are those in which there is an ongoing active infection, which may give rise to a somewhat irregular or unpredictable course extending over many months or years. Chronic inflammatory disease of the central nervous system is seen with fetal infections by rubella and cytomegaloviruses. In these indolent infections virus can be recovered for long periods of time postnatally and may or may not cause continuing or evolving clinical signs of disease. *Slow infections* have a more predictable course than chronic infections. They are defined as infections with an incubation period lasting for months to years, followed by a protracted but predictable clinical course ending in death. Slow viral infections of the nervous system in man include kuru, Creutzfeldt-Jakob disease, subacute sclerosing panencephalitis, and progressive multifocal leukoencephalopathy (see Ch. 398 to 403).

388.   HERPES ZOSTER

Richard T. Johnson

Herpes zoster is an acute viral infection of sensory ganglia and the corresponding cutaneous areas of innervation. The disease is characterized by localized pain along the distribution of the nerve and a vesicular skin eruption over a single or adjacent dermatomes. The disease is due to the same virus that causes chickenpox (varicella) and is thought to represent an acute localized recrudescent infection by the varicella virus that has remained latent in the sensory ganglia since the primary attack of chickenpox. Herpes zoster is also called shingles or zona.

Etiology. The varicella or varicella-zoster virus is a herpesvirus. The virus core measures 45 to 50 mμ and contains deoxyribonucleic acid. This is surrounded by a capsid with a diameter of 50 to 100 mμ and an outer envelope, giving a total diameter of the virion of 150 to 250 mμ. The virus is naturally pathogenic only for man, although chickenpox has been seen in anthropoid apes in zoos. There is some evidence of experimental transmission of the virus to several species of monkeys. The virus can be grown in a variety of cell cultures of human and primate origin but not in nonprimate cells. The virus is avidly cell-associated and can usually be transmitted in the laboratory only by the inoculation of infected cells, although the virus is stable in a cell-free form in the vesicular fluid. Morphologically, varicella virus resembles herpes simplex virus, with which it shares some common antigens, but it is markedly different from herpes simplex virus in its inability to infect nonprimates and nonprimate cell cultures and in its loss of infectivity in most cell-free preparations.

Incidence. Herpes zoster occurs at a rate of three to five cases per thousand persons per year. The attack rate increases with age. The disease is rare in childhood and is most frequently seen in persons over the age of 50 years. It is estimated that half the people reaching 85 years of age have suffered from at least one attack of herpes zoster. Rates are higher in persons with malignancies, particularly those involving the reticuloendothelial system.

Epidemiology, Pathogenesis, and Pathology. It has long been recognized that chickenpox may develop after exposure to a patient with herpes zoster, although this is less likely than development of chickenpox after exposure to chickenpox. In contrast, zoster rarely develops after exposure to chickenpox or other cases of zoster. These observations are supported by the epidemiologic findings that chickenpox is a seasonal disease occurring mainly in the winter and spring and occurs in epidemic proportions every two to four years. In contrast, zoster is not a seasonal disease, and there is no increase in incidence during the years of chickenpox epidemics. There is, in fact, some evidence that the incidence of zoster decreases slightly during years when there are large numbers of cases of chickenpox.

The precise pathogenesis of herpes zoster is unknown, but the following hypothesis is widely accepted. Chickenpox is transmitted from man to man by respiratory spread, and in the susceptible person the virus is probably disseminated throughout the body by a viremia. Infection of the skin occurs through the blood, and vesicles develop most prominently over the face and trunk. It is postulated that virus then spreads centripetally via sensory nerve fibers to the sensory ganglia, where it becomes latent in some form within the neurons or stellate cells. This latency of varicella virus in ganglia has not been documented in man or laboratory animals, but the recent demonstration of latency of herpes simplex virus in sensory ganglia has added credence to this hypothesis for varicella virus. Virus replication is later activated. In some cases activation is associated with the development of malignancy, local x-irradiation, immunosuppressive therapy, trauma, treatment with arsenicals, neurosyphilis, or tumor entrapment of the dorsal root ganglia or nerve root. Nevertheless, in most patients, there is no obvious exciting cause, and it is thought that the decline of immunity with age and the lack of exposure to children with chickenpox may promote reactivation. When virus multiplies in the ganglia, an active ganglionitis develops, causing pain along its sensory distribution. Virus is then thought to pass down the nerve and multiply again in the skin, causing characteristic clusters of vesicles. The localized zoster lesions are most common over trigeminal or thoracic dermatomes corresponding to the areas of major eruption during the antecedent chickenpox infection. The more rapid secondary immune response may prevent hematogenous dissemination. Resolution and limitation of the rash of herpes zoster do not correlate well, however, with the development of antibody but appear to correlate with the collection of inflammatory cells and the presence of interferon in the vesicular fluid. This theory of pathogenesis is consistent with the occurrence of the disease with increasing age or development of malignancy, the lack of seasonal association with chickenpox, the observation that pain usually precedes the skin eruption, the dermatomal localization of the lesions of herpes zoster, and the pathology and patterns of distribution of herpes zoster.

Pathologic studies of herpes zoster have shown an acute ganglionitis with an intense inflammatory response, cell necrosis, and occasionally hemorrhages within the ganglia. In addition, there is inflammation in the adjacent segments of the cord or brainstem which is predominantly unilateral, more prominent in gray matter, and involves the posterior more than the anterior horns. A mild leptomeningitis is generally found which is most intense over the segments of involvement. Inflammation in the roots distal to the ganglia is also present, representing a true peripheral mononeuritis.

In the skin innervated by the nerve there is degeneration of the basal and deep prickle cell layers of the epidermis. Ballooning degeneration of these cells causes the formation of the intradermal vesicles. Giant cells and eosinophilic intranuclear inclusions are found in the base of the vesicles.

Clinical Manifestations. The eruption of herpes zoster is often preceded by malaise and fever for two to four days. Pain or dysesthesia along the segmental dermatome also precedes the rash usually for four to five days. The pain is often a superficial tingling or burning sensation, but may vary from severe deep pain, suggesting appendicitis, cholecystitis, or pleurisy, to very mild itching. The pain may be intermittent or constant. Tenderness or hypesthesia may be detected along the dermatome on examination during this pre-eruptive stage. The cutaneous lesions present first as small, red macules which rapidly vesiculate, becoming tense, clear vesicles on an erythematous base. On about the third day, the vesicular fluid becomes turbid as inflammatory cells collect within the vesicles. Within five to ten days, the vesicles dry and crusts develop. However, in severe cases the vesicles may become confluent with a gangrenous appearance, and healing may be delayed for many weeks. During the course of the rash, there is usually enlargement of the regional lymph nodes, and there is often spread of a few vesicles to adjacent dermatomes but seldom to the other side of the body. The pain or dysesthesia usually persists for one to four weeks, but approximately 30 per cent of the patients over the age of 40 have pain that persists for months to years. This postherpetic neuralgia is more common in the elderly when there has been a prolonged period of pain prior to cutaneous eruption and a more severe rash.

Although herpes zoster may occur over any sensory nerve distribution, the thoracic dermatomes are the sites in over two thirds of cases. Cranial nerve involvement is next in frequency, and this tends to be more severe, with greater pain, frequent signs of meningeal irritation, paralysis, and sometimes involvement of the mucous membranes. The ophthalmic division of the trigeminal nerve is the most common site of cranial involvement, accounting for 10 to 15 per cent of all cases of herpes zoster. Fortunately, the eye is usually spared, but occasionally a keratoconjunctivitis develops. With ophthalmic zoster it is not uncommon to have involvement of oculomotor function, with extraocular muscle weakness, ptosis, and paralytic mydriasis. The fourth and sixth cranial nerves may also be involved, indicating that the infection is not confined to the trigeminal ganglia and its ophthalmic fibers, but may involve the brainstem and other nerve roots. The association of vesicles in the external ear and ipsilateral facial palsy (Ramsay Hunt's syndrome) was originally ascribed to infection of the geniculate ganglia. This localization of zoster may be accompanied by hearing loss, vertigo, loss of taste, or vesicles on the tongue, and probably represents involvement of multiple cranial ganglia and the associated localized encephalitis and neuronitis.

Since the primary lesion of herpes zoster is in the nervous system, the cerebrospinal fluid commonly shows a pleocytosis and elevation of protein, even when clinical signs of meningeal irritation or encephalomyelitis are absent. Not infrequently, the peripheral mononeuritis or local encephalomyelitis may cause muscle paralysis and atrophy in the area of the segmental rash. Acute urinary retention and hemidiaphragmatic paralysis have also been seen. Signs of major central nervous system infections with herpes zoster are rare, but cases of acute transverse or ascending myelitis, disseminated encephalitis, and acute cerebellar ataxia have been described.

Zoster sine herpete is typical pain in an appropriate sensory area which is not followed by the development of the characteristic vesicles. Whether some of the common transient intercostal pains represent activation of varicella virus in ganglia without spread to the skin is a matter of speculation. An antibody response to varicella virus has been demonstrated in the absence of a rash in patients with transient facial pain resembling trigeminal neuralgia and in patients with facial palsy (Bell's palsy). However, these are rare occurrences, and the vast majority of cases of trigeminal neuralgia and Bell's palsy are not associated with serologic evidence of activation of the varicella or any other known viral infection.

Cutaneous dissemination is rare, occurring in less than 2 per cent of the cases. Dissemination is more common in patients with underlying malignancies, and about one quarter of the patients with Hodgkin's disease show a progressive spread of vesicles beyond the original one or two dermatomes of involvement. Such cutaneous dissemination, however, generally does not progress for more than six days, and spontaneous recovery occurs in most patients.

Diagnosis. Characteristic development of pain and vesicular eruptions over single or adjacent dermatomes served by a segmental or cranial nerve branch usually presents no problem in differential diagnosis. However, similar zosteriform lesions can be caused by herpes simplex virus in infants.

Diagnosis can be confirmed by the demonstration of multinucleated giant epithelial cells with intranuclear inclusions in Giemsa-stained scrapings from the base of an early vesicle. Virions can also readily be found in vesicular fluid by electron microscopic examination. However, neither of these tests differentiates zoster from herpes simplex virus infections, although they can be helpful in differentiating zoster or chickenpox from smallpox infections. Varicella and herpes simplex virus infections can be differentiated by fluorescent antibody staining of cells in scrapings from vesicles.

Virus can be isolated from vesicular fluid and, in some cases, from cerebrospinal fluid by inoculation of fluid onto cultures of human or primate cells. Serologic diagnosis can also be made, but in human sera some cross-reactions are found with herpes simplex virus, so that simultaneous serologic tests should be carried out against both viruses.

Treatment. Little can be done to treat the acute eruption of herpes zoster other than symptomatic application of powder or calamine lotion to the rash and the use of analgesics for the pain. A variety of previously advocated treatments such as protamide, vitamins, x-irradiation, vasodilators, antimicrobials, and gamma globulin have proved to be useless. In a controlled study corticosteroids have been shown not to affect the rate of healing of skin lesions but to shorten the period of the acute pain. This benefit must be weighed against the potential hazard that corticosteroids may promote dissemination. One study has indicated that 5-iodo-2'-deoxyuridine (IUDR) in dimethylsulfoxide applied topically to the lesions shortens the healing time and the duration of pain, but IUDR without the dimethylsulfoxide is of no value, and dimethylsulfoxide is not available for general use in the United States.

Recently, systemic cytosine arabinoside, a drug inhibitory against DNA virus replication in vitro, has been advocated for the control of severe and disseminated herpes zoster infections. However, in a placebo-controlled study, cytosine arabinoside was found to actually prolong the duration of dissemination in some patients compared to the placebo group. This adverse effect of cytosine arabinoside appeared to be related to its depression of antibody response, delay in vesicle interferon appearance, and possibly its effect on the cellular immune response.

Postherpetic Neuralgia. The development of prolonged postherpetic neuralgia after recovery from herpes zoster presents a difficult problem in management. Although this pain usually abates over a period of months to years, it is very refractory to the usual analgesics. Application of cold to the area by use of an ethyl chloride spray may give some transient relief. Tranquilizers or sedatives can sometimes be of help, and tricyclic antidepressants (amitriptyline) in combination with substituted phenothiazines have been effective in relieving pain in some cases. Local injection or section of the nerve root is of no value, and narcotics should be avoided because of the problem of addiction. In the most severe cases when pain persists over long periods, the use of transcutaneous peripheral nerve stimulation or even cordotomy may be considered (see Ch. 349).

Prognosis. There is a popular misconception that herpes zoster does not recur. However, zoster does not give immunity to further attacks, and the likelihood of a second attack is about the same as, if not slightly greater than, that of having suffered the first. Most patients recover uneventfully, although severe vesiculation may lead to permanent scarring. Scarring of the cornea after ophthalmic involvement may result in permanent visual impairment. Motor paralysis of the local nerves recovers to adequate function levels in over 75 per cent of cases.

Even in patients with severe encephalomyelitis, the mortality rate appears to be less than 10 per cent, and permanent sequelae are rare. The prognosis, however, must be more guarded in those patients who have underlying neoplastic disease, in which both the disease and the chemotherapeutic agents used in the treatment of neoplasms may increase the possibility of cutaneous and visceral dissemination.

Prevention.   No vaccine is available for varicella virus. Chickenpox can be modified if gamma globulin is given after exposure, and sera obtained from patients recuperating from herpes zoster can totally prevent chickenpox in children if given within 72 hours of the time of exposure. This zoster immune globulin is recommended for children on immunosuppressive therapy or with leukemia who have been exposed to chickenpox or herpes zoster. Similar measures are not recommended for disabled adults exposed to chickenpox or to zoster, although contact should be avoided in the adult patient with a compromised immune system, because it is in this group that occasional cases of zoster have been thought to be related to exposure to chickenpox or zoster.

Hope-Simpson, R. E.: The nature of herpes zoster: A long-term study and a new hypothesis. Proc. R. Soc. Med., 58:9, 1965.

Juel-Jensen, B. E., MacCallum, F. O., Mackenzie, A. M. R., and Pike, M. C.: Treatment of zoster with idoxuridine in dimethyl sulphoxide. Results of two double-blind controlled trials. Br. Med. J., 4:776, 1970.

McCormick, W. F., Rodnitzsky, R. L., Schochet, S. S., and McKee, A. P.: Varicella-zoster encephalomyelitis. Arch. Neurol., 21:559, 1969.

Stevens, D. A., Jordan, G. W., Waddell, T. F., and Merigan, T. C.: Adverse effect of cytosine arabinoside on disseminated zoster in a controlled trial. N. Engl. J. Med., 289:873, 1973.

Taub, A.: Relief of postherpetic neuralgia with psychotropic drugs. J. Neurosurg., 39:235, 1973.

Taylor-Robinson, D., and Caunt, A. E.: Varicella virus. Virol. Monogr. 12. New York and Vienna, Springer-Verlag, 1972.

389.   VIRAL MENINGITIS AND ENCEPHALITIS

Dorothy M. Horstmann

Definitions.   The term *viral meningitis* is used to describe a syndrome characteristic of acute viral infections of the central nervous system manifested by signs of meningeal irritation, cerebrospinal fluid pleocytosis, and a short, uncomplicated course. In *viral encephalitis* the brain is involved in the inflammatory process; it is a more serious disease than viral meningitis, being commonly characterized by disorientation, alteration in consciousness, tremors, convulsions, coma, and, in a significant number of patients, death. Both syndromes can be induced by a variety of different viruses.

Etiology.   *Aseptic Meningitis.*   At present a specific cause can be established in up to two-thirds of the cases of presumed viral origin. The relative frequency and importance of the many agents which have been implicated vary in different parts of the world. In the United States and in temperate climates generally, the *enteroviruses* are the most common causes, accounting for approximately 75 per cent of cases in which a cause is established. The agents most frequently associated with meningitis are echovirus 4, 6, and 9; coxsackievirus A 7 and 9; and coxsackievirus B 1 to 5. In all, more than 60 enteroviruses have been identified. Not all have yet been associated with meningitis; but in view of the frequent

TABLE 1.   Viruses Associated with Acute Infections of the Central Nervous System in the United States

Enteroviruses
  Polioviruses
  Coxsackievirus A
  Coxsackievirus B
Arboviruses (arthropod-borne)
  St. Louis
  Eastern equine
  Western equine
  Venezuelan equine
  California
  Powassan
Mumps virus
Measles virus
Rubella virus
Herpesviruses
  Herpesvirus hominis
  Varicella-zoster virus
  Epstein-Barr virus
  Cytomegalovirus
Viruses associated with respiratory illness
  Adenoviruses
  Influenza
Lymphocytic choriomeningitis virus
Encephalomyocarditis virus
Rabies virus
Hepatitis viruses (?)

additions from among previously known and newly recognized members of this family of agents, the list can be expected to grow. *Mumps virus* is the next most frequent cause of aseptic meningitis; *herpes simplex* and *adenoviruses* (mainly types 1, 2, 3, 5, and 7) and *lymphocytic choriomeningitis* viruses are infrequently responsible; rarely, the syndrome may be seen as a complication of *infectious mononucleosis* (Epstein-Barr virus), *herpes zoster,* and possibly *viral hepatitis.* Aseptic meningitis associated with the *arthropod-borne* group of viruses follows the geographic distribution of these agents, which is dependent upon specific arthropod vectors.

Encephalitis.   In not more than a third of the cases can a specific viral agent be identified as the cause (Table 2). The geographic distribution of the viruses involved is similar in both aseptic meningitis and encephalitis, but their relative importance is different. Thus mumps virus accounts for more reported cases of encephalitis than any other agent; the arboviruses are also prominent, whereas enteroviruses are infrequently recovered from patients with this syndrome. Herpes simplex virus is a significant cause, both in primary infections and in reactivation of latent infections which involve the central nervous system (see Ch. 390). Encephalitis may also occur with influenza, adenovirus, and other respiratory infections, and rarely lymphocytic choriomeningitis (LCM), toxoplasmosis, infectious mononucleosis, and herpes zoster. When it occurs in association with measles, chickenpox, and rubella, it has been commonly believed to be of the postinfectious type rather than the result of a primary viral invasion, but recent evidence suggests that in mumps and measles encephalitis both mechanisms may be involved in some cases. Rubella meningoencephalitis occurs occasionally in infants with congenital rubella; it is caused by direct viral invasion and tends to be chronic.

Epidemiology.   In the United States some 4000 to 6000 cases of aseptic meningitis and approximately 2000 cases of encephalitis are reported annually; however,

TABLE 2. Reported Cases of Encephalitis by Cause—United States, 1967–1971*

| Year | Total Number | Arbo-viruses | Entero-viruses | Herpes Simplex | Associated with Childhood Diseases | | | | Associated with Respiratory Infection† | Other Known Causes‡ | Unknown Causes |
					Mumps	Measles	Varicella	Rubella			
1971	1891	150	45	54	310	69	54	3	17	10	1179
1970	1950	110	52	37	288	27	46	7	9	14	1360
1969	1917	108	31	29	218	35	48	3	7	20	1418
1968	2283	130	66	35	408	19	69	6	17	23	1510
1967	2368	83	26	30	849	62	77	7	2	14	1218

*From Center for Disease Control, U.S. Public Health Service, Neurotropic Virus Disease Surveillance Reports, 1969–1973.
†Includes infections due to influenza, *M. pneumoniae*, and adenoviruses.
‡Includes infections due to lymphocytic choriomeningitis, varicella-zoster, Epstein-Barr virus, and cytomegalovirus.

these represent only a fraction of the total number, because marked under-reporting is the rule. Both syndromes, whether of known or unknown cause, have their peak incidence in the period from July through October, but sporadic cases may be seen at any time during the year. In temperate climates, aseptic meningitis caused by enteroviruses occurs most characteristically in small or large outbreaks during the summer and autumn, whereas in tropical and semitropical areas there is no striking seasonal incidence. Children are more frequently affected than adults; but in some epidemics caused by enteroviruses which have been absent from circulation for long periods, as many as 50 per cent of cases have been in individuals over 15 years of age. The agents are often widely disseminated in the population, giving rise chiefly to inapparent infections or minor febrile illnesses. Spread is primarily by contact with an infected person, and the healthy individual with an inapparent infection is as infectious as the frank case. Dissemination is greatest in areas of poor sanitation with a high density of preschoolchildren, who are the most frequent virus spreaders. Although one enterovirus type tends to be dominant and to account for the bulk of illness at any given time and place, it is not unusual during epidemic or endemic periods to find several agents circulating at the same time, causing similar illnesses, including meningitis. *Mumps meningitis* and *meningoencephalitis* follow the epidemiologic pattern of mumps infections generally, with the highest incidence in winter and spring. On rare occasions, they appear in epidemic form, without accompanying parotitis. *Lymphocytic choriomeningitis* is a relatively uncommon disease, occurring in the late autumn and winter. The infection is endemic in the common house mouse, *Mus musculus,* and is probably spread to man through dust or food contaminated by mouse excreta. *Adenovirus* and *herpes simplex meningitis* and *encephalitis* occur sporadically in children as primary infections spread by contact; encephalitis caused by herpes virus also occurs in older individuals as a reactivation of latent infection.

Infections caused by the arthropod-borne viruses (arboviruses) occur in epidemics during summer and fall, causing a range of illness which includes minor febrile episodes, aseptic meningitis, and, more characteristically, encephalitis. In the United States, California virus has recently been a prominent cause of this disease in children living in rural areas of the north-midwestern part of the United States, and Powassan virus has been recovered sporadically from cases in the northeast. Eastern equine encephalitis virus is found predominantly along the East and Gulf coasts, and western equine usually occurs west of the Mississippi River. St. Louis encephalitis is endemic in California and parts of the southwest; it has occurred in epidemic form in widely separated urban and suburban areas of New Jersey, Florida, and Texas. In 1971, Venezuelan encephalitis virus moved up from Mexico through Texas and the southern United States, causing epidemics in humans and in horses. Most cases of encephalitis reported in the United States each year (60 to 75 per cent) are of unknown cause. These occur the year round, but there is a concentration in summer and fall, paralleling the pattern of arbovirus and enterovirus infections.

Pathogenesis and Pathology. Like the epidemiology, the pathogenesis of the two syndromes varies with the nature of the infecting agent. The general pattern for enteroviruses is thought to be similar, the sequence being primary multiplication in the alimentary tract, spread to regional nodes, a viremic phase, and eventual invasion of the central nervous system. There is evidence that in enterovirus infections in humans as well as in experimentally infected primates, viremia precedes the onset of illness by several days and has usually disappeared by the time neurologic signs appear. In mumps, LCM, primary herpes simplex, and arbovirus encephalitis, the agents probably reach the central nervous system through the bloodstream, after initial multiplication in extraneural tissues. Spread by neural pathways occurs in rabies and herpes zoster, and possibly secondarily in certain other infections in which the blood-borne route is the major one.

Since *aseptic meningitis* is not a fatal disease, the extent of the pathologic lesions in the central nervous system is not accurately known, but is presumed to be limited mainly to the meninges. However, in the experimental disease induced in monkeys by poliovirus, neuronal lesions are commonly found in the precentral gyrus of the cerebral cortex (and the brainstem and spinal cord), indicating that the difference between aseptic meningitis and encephalitis is merely one of degree and concentration of nerve cell damage. In *encephalitis,* the meninges are also involved in an inflammatory reaction, but the most significant lesions are neuronal. The brain and cord are swollen and congested, and histologic examination of the brain parenchyma reveals changes in the neurons, ranging from slight alterations in the nuclei and cytoplasm to complete necrosis and neuronophagia. The involved areas contain polymorphonuclear leukocytes and microglia, and there is marked perivascular cuffing. The distribution of lesions tends to be characteristic for given agents or groups of agents, although, with the exception of poliomyelitis, it is usually not possible to distinguish between the various viruses on the basis of pathology alone. In arbovirus infections the lesions may be widely distributed, often involving the entire cerebral cortex, cerebellum, brainstem, and spinal cord. Fatal mumps encephalitis is rare, but in a recently reported case acute inflammatory lesions and necrosis attributed to direct viral action were revealed, along with demyelination characteristic of postinfectious encephalitis.

Clinical Manifestations. *Viral Meningitis.* Whatever the specific viral cause, the symptoms and signs are similar to, and not readily distinguished from, the pattern of aseptic meningitis of other causes. The onset is commonly abrupt. The most constant features are severe headache, fever, and stiff neck; other symptoms may occur, including sore throat, nausea and vomiting, listlessness, drowsiness, vertigo, pain in the back and neck, photophobia, paresthesias, myalgias, abdominal pain, and chills or chilly sensations. With certain echo- and coxsackievirus infections a striking skin eruption may appear. In general the severity of symptoms increases with the age of the patient. Although sudden onset is characteristic, in some patients there is a prodromal nonspecific "minor illness," followed by several days of well-being before the reappearance of fever and the development of signs of central nervous system involvement. This occurs most commonly with poliovirus infections in young children, but may be associated with other enteroviruses and with lymphocytic choriomeningitis.

On physical examination there are few findings. The temperature is elevated (38.5 to 40°C), but the patient does not appear as ill as one with bacterial meningitis. Neck and back stiffness are the only neurologic signs in the typical case; Kernig and Brudzinski signs are sometimes positive. Nuchal rigidity may be minimal and apparent only in the last degrees of neck flexion. The deep tendon reflexes are normal or hyperactive. Transient weakness (rarely frank paralysis) has been noted with the coxsackievirus B group, coxsackievirus A 7, and certain echoviruses, notably 7 and 9. *Rash* is encountered chiefly in young children. It has been a prominent feature of certain epidemics in which aseptic meningitis has also occurred, including outbreaks associated with echovirus 4, 6, 9, and 16 and coxsackievirus A 9 and 16; rash has also been observed occasionally with many other enterovirus types. The eruption usually appears with the fever and lasts four to five days (in severe cases, eight or nine days). Characteristically it is maculopapular, discrete, erythematous, and nonpruritic. The lesions may be confined to the face and neck or may spread over the chest and extremities and sometimes involve the palms and soles. At times the rash is petechial (echovirus 9) or vesicular (coxsackievirus A 9 and A 16), but the character is not constant, and a single virus type may induce any of the various forms of eruptions, even during the same epidemic. An *enanthem*, consisting of grayish white dots on the buccal mucosa, has been described in as many as one third of the patients in certain outbreaks caused by echovirus 9, but only occasionally with the other types (echovirus 6 and 16).

Viral Encephalitis. The characteristic signs of encephalitic involvement include mental confusion, delirium, stupor, convulsions, and coma. The onset of the disease may be sudden or gradual, with chills, fever, headache, lethargy, dizziness, vomiting, and stiffness of the neck. A prodrome consisting of headaches, fever, vague aches and pains, and sometimes sore throat may last for several days before the more typical neurologic signs appear. The severity of the clinical picture varies with the etiologic agent and the site and extent of the neuronal lesions. Mumps is commonly associated with a relatively benign meningoencephalitis in which the clinical picture is one of aseptic meningitis with the addition of mild encephalitic signs. Encephalitis caused by arboviruses (Ch. 144 to 152) may also be mild, particularly in infections with California virus, or the disease may be ushered in with severe headache, vomiting, hyperpyrexia, twitchings, tremors, convulsions, disorientation, and drowsiness followed by coma. There may also be ataxia caused by cerebellar involvement, as well as hyperactive reflexes, spasticity, and weakness of the extremities if the neurons of the spinal cord are attacked. In herpes simplex encephalitis, the illness is frequently catastrophic; convulsions are common, and signs suggesting a space-occupying lesion of the temporal lobe may be present. Variations in severity from mild to rapidly fatal may also occur when the disease is associated with other agents, as well as in the two thirds or more cases presumed to be of viral origin, although implication of a specific agent is not possible.

Laboratory Findings. *Viral Meningitis.* The blood count is commonly within normal range, but leukopenia or moderate leukocytosis without marked shift to the left may be present. The cerebrospinal fluid findings are diagnostic: the fluid is clear, with an elevated cell count ranging from 10 to 3000 or more cells per cubic milliliter, most frequently 30 to 300; no organisms are seen when the stained sediment is examined microscopically. Early in the disease the cells may be predominantly polymorphonuclear, but within a few hours there is a shift, with 80 to 90 per cent or more being lymphocytes. In contrast to bacterial meningitis, the glucose content is normal, although transient depression below 40 mg per 100 ml may be encountered early in the course, particularly in mumps meningitis. The protein level is normal or moderately elevated. The height of the cell count bears no fixed relation to the severity of the disease or to signs of meningeal irritation such as neck stiffness. The number of cells tends to return to normal within a few days, except in mumps and echo 9 meningitis, in which pleocytosis may persist for seven to ten days, often after nuchal rigidity has disappeared.

Viral Encephalitis. In encephalitis the peripheral white cell count is usually moderately elevated, but in eastern equine encephalitis marked leukocytosis as high as 60,000 cells with 90 per cent polymorphonuclears has been reported. Cerebrospinal fluid findings are commonly similar to those in viral meningitis, although in some cases the fluid may be entirely normal.

Diagnosis and Differential Diagnosis. *Viral Meningitis.* Recognition of the aseptic meningitis syndrome is not difficult except in young infants who frequently do not have the classic signs of meningeal irritation. There are a number of clinical and epidemiologic features which may suggest the viral agent involved, but a specific etiologic diagnosis can be established only in the laboratory. With enterovirus infections, virus isolation is the usual means of accomplishing this; serologic identification based on antibody rises is impracticable because of the multiplicity of virus types. Enteroviruses are readily isolated from fecal specimens and throat swabs, and coxsackie- and echoviruses (in contrast to polioviruses) may be found in the cerebrospinal fluid in

50 per cent or more of cases associated with these agents. Adenoviruses and herpes simplex virus can be recovered from the same sources as enteroviruses, except that herpes virus is very rarely found in the cerebrospinal fluid. Both blood and cerebrospinal fluid are sources of lymphocytic choriomeningitis virus. Infections caused by mumps, lymphocytic choriomeningitis, and the arthropod-borne viruses are usually diagnosed serologically (rising titers of complement-fixing, neutralizing, or hemagglutination-inhibiting antibodies), although virus isolation is also possible, if more difficult.

DIFFERENTIAL DIAGNOSIS OF CLINICAL EVIDENCE. A careful analysis of the history is most likely to suggest the correct etiologic diagnosis. The season of the year, the presence or absence of an epidemic, and the geographic location (particularly with respect to the arthropod-borne viruses) should be considered. In the United States, epidemics are most often associated with enteroviruses, whereas sporadic cases are likely to be induced by mumps, herpes simplex virus, adenoviruses, or other agents. In the summer and fall, leptospiral meningitis enters into the differential diagnosis, for it has the same seasonal incidence as enterovirus infections. In an epidemic in which there are many patients with paralysis, a relatively high percentage of aseptic meningitis cases will be due to polioviruses. In family epidemics caused by coxsackie- and polioviruses, most infections are inapparent, with only a single individual exhibiting overt illness such as meningitis. By contrast, with certain echoviruses (particularly echo 4, 6, and 9) it is common to find that all members of the family have recently experienced some febrile episode with or without meningeal signs.

The age and sex of the patient are also helpful. Mumps meningitis is much more common in males than in females (at least 3:1), and a similar but smaller difference has been noted in meningitis caused by enteroviruses in individuals under 20 years of age. Herpes simplex meningitis is seen primarily in young infants and in adults. Lymphocytic choriomeningitis occurs in the 20- to 40-year age group; mumps, adenovirus, and enterovirus meningitis affect chiefly children and young adults.

The appearance of parotitis, salivary gland enlargement, or orchitis in patients with aseptic meningitis strongly suggests mumps, but occasionally orchitis has been noted with coxsackievirus B infections and infectious mononucleosis; lymphocytic choriomeningitis virus has been isolated from a patient with meningitis, orchitis, and parotitis. The presence of pleurodynia (with or without orchitis) in a patient with aseptic meningitis is characteristic of coxsackievirus B infection, but occurs on rare occasions with echoviruses also.

CEREBROSPINAL FLUID FINDINGS. An immediate practical problem in dealing with a patient who is thought to have viral meningitis is to exclude the presence of leptospirosis or a bacterial infection which might be susceptible to antimicrobial therapy. A stained smear of the cerebrospinal fluid sediment should be examined carefully for microorganisms, which can usually be detected if the infection is a bacterial one. The question of a bacterial cause arises particularly in cases in which polymorphonuclear leukocytes are predominant in the cerebrospinal fluid and especially if the total count is high, i.e., more than 1000. If the cerebrospinal fluid is examined very early in the course of viral meningitis, the finding that 60 to 85 per cent of cells are polymorphonuclears is

not unusual, but the pattern then shifts rapidly to approximately 90 per cent lymphocytes; a repeat lumbar puncture after 12 to 24 hours will thus help clarify the diagnosis. In meningitis caused by echo 9 virus, moderate predominance of polymorphonuclears may persist for a week or more. Echo 9 viral meningitis has been associated with unusually high cell counts (occasionally 6000 to 8000) in the cerebrospinal fluid. Relatively high counts, i.e., between 500 and 1000 cells, are also characteristic of mumps and lymphocytic choriomeningitis.

SIMULATION OF BRAIN ABSCESS OR BACTERIAL MENINGITIS. Confusion with meningococcal and other bacterial meningitis may also arise in echo 9 or other enterovirus infections, particularly if there is a petechial rash. The milder clinical course, the absence of significant papilledema, the lower cerebrospinal fluid cell count and normal glucose, and the peripheral blood picture usually indicate a viral infection. However, meningococcal meningitis presents occasionally with the clinical picture and laboratory findings of aseptic meningitis; the correct diagnosis is established only when meningococci are recovered from the cerebrospinal fluid. If reasonable doubt exists, the case should be treated as one of purulent meningitis until this has been excluded by appropriate cultures. *Inadequately treated bacterial meningitis* and mechanical irritation of the meninges caused by *brain abscess* (or other intracranial lesions) may also produce an aseptic meningitis syndrome. The possibility of a silent brain abscess is suggested by a history of recent pneumonia, chronic pulmonary infection, congenital heart disease, bacterial endocarditis, otitis media, or infection of the paranasal sinuses. *Tuberculous meningitis* in its early stages is another possibility. Aseptic meningitis caused by *neurosyphilis* may present as an acute illness, although the course is more typically subacute, with papilledema, cranial nerve palsies, and little or no fever.

OTHER FORMS OF ASEPTIC MENINGITIS. Among other causes of aseptic meningitis, the presence of severe sore throat, generalized lymph node enlargement, mild icterus, and a transient rash are compatible with *infectious mononucleosis*. *Leptospirosis* is to be considered in areas in which the infection is common and when there is a history of exposure to dogs, guinea pigs, and particularly rats, which excrete the agent in their urine. Wild rodents are also the probable source of infections with *encephalomyocarditis virus*, which may rarely be associated with typical aseptic meningitis. Involvement of the meninges may also occur in leukemia, Hodgkin's disease, metastatic carcinoma, and cat scratch disease.

Viral Encephalitis. As in viral meningitis, epidemiologic characteristics often point to one or another group of agents. Diseases of the central nervous system besides bacterial meningitis that may be confused with viral encephalitis include tuberculoma, toxoplasmosis, leukemia, primary or metastatic malignancies, and brain abscess. Skull films, electroencephalography, brain scan, and a pneumoencephalogram may be required to exclude these conditions. In the case of tuberculoma, a chest film and tuberculin skin test are helpful. In Reye's syndrome, i.e., encephalopathy and fatty degeneration of the liver occurring in children, the clinical picture is dominated by vomiting, convulsions, and coma. This diagnosis is suggested by the presence of hypoglycemia and deranged liver function tests; the disease usually follows a respiratory infection, notably influenza B, chickenpox, or other viral illness (See Ch. 397). Rabies is a rare disease in the

United States, but it may begin with the symptoms and signs of encephalitis (see Ch. 393).

Both *aseptic meningitis* and *encephalitis* occur in association with infections caused by *Mycoplasma pneumoniae*. They have been reported with increasing frequency, and, as with other syndromes caused by this agent, are seen most often in the fall of the year, primarily in individuals under 20 years of age. The neurologic signs are usually preceded by the characteristic respiratory illness, but nervous system involvement may be the only evidence of infection. The severity of the clinical picture varies widely; coma, seizures, and decorticate posturing may occur in the more severe cases. The cerebrospinal fluid findings are variable, but elevated protein and cell counts with a predominance of lymphocytes are usual at some time during the course; the glucose content is normal. A striking feature is that complete recovery is the rule, although this may require many months in those with extensive involvement. *M. pneumoniae* meningitis and encephalitis can be differentiated from viral central nervous system infections by demonstration of rises in antibody (by complement fixation or metabolic inhibition) and by the presence of high cold agglutinin titers. The agent can be cultured from the throat, and its recovery from the cerebrospinal fluid has recently been reported.

Treatment. There is no specific therapy for viral meningitis or encephalitis, nor is there evidence that steroids are beneficial. Bed rest, adequate fluid intake, and symptomatic treatment are indicated as in any acute febrile illness. In encephalitis, supportive therapy is of prime importance. Respiratory distress may require the use of a respirator. Tracheostomy is essential for comatose patients and for those who require mechanical aids for respiration and who also have problems with pooling of pharyngeal secretions. If secondary bacterial infection develops after tracheostomy, appropriate antimicrobial therapy should be instituted. Attention to fluid and electrolyte balance and to bladder function is essential. Urinary retention usually requires either intermittent or chronic catheterization, and infection is therefore common. The prophylactic use of antimicrobials for prevention of either respiratory or urinary tract infections is not effective and promotes the emergence of resistant organisms.

Prognosis. Aseptic meningitis caused by viruses is a self-limited disease, complete recovery occurring in 3 to 5 days in mild cases, and in 7 to 14 days in the more severe ones. Mortality rates and sequelae from encephalitis depend on the agent involved, the severity of the illness, and the age of the patient. Herpes simplex encephalitis results in death in up to 50 per cent of patients, and survivors are frequently severely damaged. Among the arboviruses, eastern equine and western equine infections are accompanied by significant mortality and neurologic sequelae in survivors, particularly children. Few deaths occur from California encephalitis, but minor sequelae follow in approximately 15 per cent of patients. In encephalitis caused by mumps or enteroviruses other than poliovirus, death is rare, as are residual neurologic deficits. In cases presumed to be viral but of unknown cause, the over-all mortality is approximately 15 per cent, but is higher in young children and in those over 40 years of age.

Balfour, H. H., Siem, R. A., Bauer, H., and Quie, P. G.: California arbovirus (La Crosse) infections. I. Clinical and laboratory findings in 66 children with meningo-encephalitis. Pediatrics, 52:680, 1973.

Casals, J., and Clarke, D. H.: Arboviruses: Group A. *In* Horsfall, F. L., and Tamm, I. (eds.): Viral and Rickettsial Infections of Man. 4th ed. Philadelphia, J. B. Lippincott Company, 1965, p. 583.
Clarke, D. H., and Casals, J.: Arboviruses: Group B. *In* Horsfall, F. L., and Tamm, I. (eds.): Viral and Rickettsial Infections of Man. 4th ed. Philadelphia, J. B. Lippincott Company, 1965, p. 606.
Feigin, R. D., and Shackelford, P. G.: Value of repeat lumbar puncture in the differential diagnosis of meningitis. N. Engl. J. Med., 289:571, 1973.
Gunderman, J. R., and Stamler, R.: Follow-up study of acute encephalitis residuals. Clin. Pediatr., 12:4, 1973.
Jamieson, W. M., Kerr, M., and Sommerville, R. G.: Echo type-9 meningitis in East Scotland. Lancet, 1:581, 1958.
Johnson, R. T., and Mims, C. A.: Pathogenesis of viral infection of the nervous system. N. Engl. J. Med., 278:23, 84, 1968.
Johnstone, J. A., Ross, C. A. C., and Dunn, M.: Meningitis and encephalitis associated with mumps infection. A 10-year survey. Arch. Dis. Child., 47:647, 1972.
Lepow, M. L., Coyne, N., Thompson, L. B., Carver, D. H., and Robbins, F. C.: A clinical epidemiologic and laboratory investigation of aseptic meningitis during the four-year period 1955–1958. I. Observations concerning etiology and epidemiology. N. Engl. J. Med., 266:1181, 1962. II. The clinical disease and its sequelae. Ibid., 266:1188, 1962.

390. HERPES SIMPLEX ENCEPHALITIS

J. Richard Baringer

Definition. Adult encephalitis caused by herpes simplex virus is usually encountered as a sporadic illness, the consequence of infection by the antigenically distinct type 1 herpes simplex virus. Recently it has become apparent that most if not all of the cases previously designated as acute necrotizing encephalitis are related to infection by this virus. Electron microscopic examination of tissues from a number of these cases has revealed characteristic herpes simplex virus particles.

In newborn infants, herpes simplex virus encephalitis is seen as a consequence of maternal genital herpes infection. Usually the infection is due to type 2 herpes simplex virus, but some cases are related to infection by type 1 virus. The type 1 adult infection remains confined to the central nervous system, whereas in newborns the process is commonly disseminated in a variety of other organs, and the virus may be recovered from blood and cerebrospinal fluid. Type 2 virus may also occasionally produce a meningitis or polyradiculitis in adults, frequently in association with genital infection by the same strain.

Rarely the related B virus of monkeys has been incriminated as a cause of encephalitis in humans, usually as a result of accidental transmission of the virus to laboratory workers or attendants. This condition in humans is notable for its high mortality.

Incidence. Because of the difficulty in establishing the diagnosis of herpes simplex encephalitis by currently available means, the precise incidence of the condition is unknown. It has been estimated that 4000 cases may occur in the United States each year. Herpes simplex virus probably causes fewer cases than either mumps or the arthropod-borne viruses. However, the considerable mortality and morbidity resulting from herpes simplex virus infection rank it as the most common cause of sporadic viral encephalitis with severe sequelae. In view of the tendency for some infections to undergo spontaneous resolution and the difficulty in establishing the virologic diagnosis, it is possible that herpes simplex virus may be a more frequent cause of mild encephalitic illness than is currently recognized.

Etiology. Herpes simplex virus is a large, 180 mμ, enveloped deoxyribonucleic-acid-containing virus which is antigenically related to B virus of monkeys but antigenically quite distinct from other herpesviruses. Herpes simplex virus has man as its natural host. It is known for its ability to cause recurrent cutaneous and oral or genital mucosal lesions. Recently it has been demonstrated that the virus commonly remains latent in trigeminal ganglion tissue of humans.

Early observations in man and animals suggested that various strains of herpes simplex virus behaved differently in regard to their ability to produce disease. Subsequent work has demonstrated that there are at least two distinct serotypes of herpes simplex virus (types 1 and 2) which differ not only antigenically but also in distribution. Type 1 is commonly isolated from oral and cutaneous lesions above the waist and from sporadic adult cases of herpes simplex encephalitis, whereas type 2 strains are commonly associated with genital infections and cutaneous lesions below the waist. Exceptions to these general rules are not uncommon. The two strains differ in several other respects. Type 1 has a slightly lower DNA density, produces smaller pocks on chick chorioallantoic membrane, produces a higher yield of virus in most tissue culture systems, possesses slightly less neurovirulence for mice and rabbits, and is slightly more sensitive to idoxuridine in tissue culture systems.

Pathogenesis. Many aspects of the pathogenesis of herpes simplex encephalitis in adults caused by type 1 virus are poorly or incompletely understood. Although most such infections appear to have resulted from a primary infection with the virus, in several cases a previous history of recurrent cutaneous or oral herpes simplex lesions has been obtained. Rare cases have been reported in patients whose immune systems were compromised by disease or immunosuppressive drugs, but most cases are encountered in previously normal adults.

In adults, there is usually no evidence of involvement of other viscera. Within the cerebrum the pathologic process has a characteristic bilateral distribution, necrotic and hemorrhagic lesions being most prominent in the hippocampus, amygdala and medial temporal lobe, orbital surface of the frontal lobe, insular cortex, and cingulum. The distribution is usually asymmetric. The posterior portions of the cerebrum, the cerebellum, the brainstem, and the spinal cord are characteristically spared. Histologically, the lesions are characterized by severe necrosis of all elements of the tissue. The presence of eosinophilic intranuclear inclusions in neurons, oligodendrocytes, and astrocytes is suggestive but not diagnostic of herpes simplex encephalitis. There is a brisk inflammatory reaction, consisting of mononuclear cells and lymphocytes and usually a mild to moderate meningeal exudate. Small hemorrhages within the lesions and on the pial surface are common.

The route by which the virus produces nervous system involvement has been the subject of much speculation. The consistent involvement of portions of the brain subserving olfactory functions has suggested that the virus may enter the nervous system by way of olfactory mucosa whence it may travel along the olfactory tract to reach the brain. The ability of herpes simplex virus to travel within nerves has long been recognized, but there is little evidence from human studies to indicate that the olfactory bulb or tract is uniformly or even commonly involved in cases of herpes simplex encephalitis. The possibility that the nervous system involvement might be the consequence of a viremia and a special affinity or susceptibility of neurons in the limbic system to hematogenous virus has also been considered, but there is little evidence from human or experimental data to support this hypothesis. Futher information concerning the pathogenesis of the disease awaits careful studies of the distribution of lesions and virus in human cases of herpes simplex encephalitis.

Clinical Manifestations. Encephalitis caused by type I herpes simplex virus is a sporadic disease of the nervous system which often has devastating effects and a fairly characteristic clinical course. It is uncertain whether or not the virus also causes a mild form of encephalitis, because the laboratory tests necessary to provide a definitive diagnosis are seldom feasible in patients with benign illness.

In contrast to other viral encephalitides in the United States, herpes simplex encephalitis is nonepidemic. In its severe form, the disease produces a combination of nonspecific signs and symptoms of an acute encephalitis plus focal manifestations of damage to the limbic system and frontal lobes. The onset in some patients is abrupt, with headache, fever, delirium, and, often, generalized or focal convulsions. Few illnesses can produce so much neurologic devastation in so short a time; within hours of the onset some patients may lose consciousness or undergo progressive unilateral or bilateral motor weaknesses.

Alternatively, the disease may have a subacute course. Behavioral changes have often been seen as early signs of disease and at times have prompted admission to psychiatric facilities. Some patients experience olfactory or gustatory hallucinations, presumably as a consequence of the focal involvement of temporal lobe structures. In others memory is impaired out of proportion to other cognitive functions, reflecting the bilateral involvement of the hippocampal system. Seizures are common and may take the form of generalized, focal motor, temporal lobe, or occasionally myoclonic phenomena. Involvement of larger or deeper portions of the cerebrum is signaled by the appearance of hemiparesis, conjugate deviation of the eyes, or aphasia. The illness characteristically undergoes fluctuation in its intensity, and such fluctuation may help in distinguishing herpes simplex encephalitis from involvement of the cerebrum by tumor or abscess.

The type 2 herpes virus, which is the major cause of fatal disseminated herpes infections in the newborn, causes more benign neurologic disease in adults. This virus in adults has been associated with aseptic meningitis and with radicular pain, often over lower lumbar and sacral dermatomes. The pain may mimic symptoms of a herniated intravertebral disc but is often temporally associated with the eruptions of genital herpes.

Diagnosis. The diagnosis of herpes simplex encephalitis rests upon clinical suspicion confirmed by laboratory data.

The cerebrospinal fluid (CSF) findings are of considerable importance. In most cases there are up to 500 cells per cubic millimeter, with lymphocytes or mononuclear cells predominating. Occasional cases, confirmed by isolation of the virus from the brain, have lacked cells in the CSF. Red cells in the CSF and/or xanthochromia may be frequently encountered; this reflects the hemorrhagic nature of the lesions. The CSF protein concentration is commonly elevated, but this does not serve to distinguish the process from a number of other affections.

Although the CSF sugar is usually within the normal range, several cases have been encountered in which the sugar is low.

Recent reports of the identification of herpesvirus antigen by fluorescent antibody study of cells in the CSF suggested a specific and convenient way of confirming that the illness is due to this virus. Further experience will be necessary before it is certain that such procedures correctly identify cases of herpes simplex involvement of the nervous system. Attempts to isolate virus from the cerebrospinal fluid have usually been unrewarding.

Serologic tests for confirmation of the diagnosis have frequently been employed, but have several inherent disadvantages. Comparison of acute and convalescent titers is of little practical value in the management of the acutely ill patient. Furthermore, fluctuations in the titer of antibody to herpes simplex virus are commonly encountered as a reaction to a variety of stimuli. Less than fourfold increases in titer do not necessarily signify recent herpes simplex virus infection; conversely in some confirmed cases of herpes simplex virus encephalitis, the titers have failed to rise. Recently, attempts have been made to confirm the presence of active herpes simplex infection by the use of a complement requiring neutralizing antibody in serum or by passive hemagglutinating antibodies in the CSF. The utility of these tests which require specialized and somewhat complicated techniques must await further experience with them from a variety of laboratories.

The electroencephalogram is virtually always abnormal, although the abnormality may not be specific. Diffuse slowing accentuated in one or both temporal lobes and the appearance of sharp waves or spikes in temporal areas are findings consistent with the diagnosis. Several cases have been associated with relatively specific, periodic sharp and slow wave complexes; such findings are highly suggestive of the disease, but their absence does not exclude it.

Brain scans frequently reveal unilateral or bilateral uptake of the tracer substance, a reflection of the increased permeability of vessels in the lesions. Cerebral arteriography usually demonstrates an avascular mass in the temporal lobe with or without shift of midline structures.

A certain diagnosis of herpes simplex encephalitis requires the use of cerebral biopsy. This is a technique which has several limitations and also some considerable hazard, and it should be performed only in major medical centers possessing the necessary facilities for proper processing of the tissue. The limitations arise from the fact that the encephalitic process is often confined to the medial and undersurfaces of the temporal and frontal lobes, so that biopsy of the lateral or superior portions of temporal or frontal lobes or other portions of the brain may fail to demonstrate the process or identify the agent. The time at which the biopsy is performed is of additional importance. Herpes simplex virus disappears from neural tissue within a short time and cannot be recovered thereafter by ordinary techniques. Thus the biopsy should be performed as early as possible in the course of the illness, and the tissue should be subjected to histologic study, fluorescent antibody study, electron microscopy and viral culture. If the tissue is fixed in Bouin's solution for histology, intranuclear inclusions are stained to better advantage and can be more easily recognized than with formalin-fixed tissue. Fluorescent antibody study has the advantages of relatively great sensitivity for detection of viral antigen, and specificity for the virus when appropriate controls are included. In addition, the test may be completed within a few hours after the tissue is removed. Electron microscopy is less sensitive because of the inherent sampling problems. Viral culture offers the most sensitive method for recovery of virus from nervous system tissue. The technique of inoculating trypsinized cells from the biopsy tissue onto indicator cultures may offer a better opportunity for recovery of virus than does inoculation of clarified suspension of homogenized brain.

Among conditions which must be distinguished from herpes simplex encephalitis, cerebral abscess presents the most difficult problem. Fever, headache, and seizures are all seen in cases of cerebral abscess, and these features do not serve to differentiate abscess from herpes encephalitis. The presence of another site of pyogenic infection, especially in sinus or mastoid, should alert the clinician to the possibility of abscess. However, unusual psychiatric changes or an isolated disorder of memory are less common in cerebral abscess than in herpes, and abscesses usually produce more focal and fewer diffuse signs than herpes. Cerebrospinal fluid changes may be quite similar; there is some tendency for the protein to be higher and the cell count lower in cases of abscess than in encephalitis. In doubtful cases, the arteriogram, electroencephalogram, and brain scan are more apt to reflect the bilateral pathology in encephalitis, and periodic high voltage sharp waves which appear and disappear over a few days are characteristic of encephalitis but are not a feature of abscess. Sometimes proper diagnosis is not reached until after craniotomy, but this is usually in patients in whom the diagnosis of encephalitis has not been given sufficient preoperative consideration.

The distinction between herpes encephalitis and a pyogenic or tuberculous meningitis is somewhat easier because of the prominence of meningeal signs, the more regular lowering of the CSF glucose, the presence of organisms, and the lesser frequency of focal signs in the latter conditions. Distinction between herpes simplex encephalitis and the postinfectious encephalitides may be difficult and rests with the history of one of the common viral exanthems or mumps in the weeks preceding the onset of the cerebral disorder. Cerebral neoplasm can usually be distinguished by its more slowly progressive course, by the absence of fever and of CSF findings suggestive of encephalitis, and by the appearance on scan and arteriographic studies.

Treatment. The difficulties in establishing the diagnosis of herpes simplex encephalitis, the infrequency with which cases are seen at any one medical center, and the great variation in course from one case to another have thwarted attempts to arrive at a reasonable evaluation of treatment. In any given case there is considerable uncertainty concerning the stage in the evolution of the disease at which treatment is instituted. In addition, recent improvements in supportive treatment may tend to invalidate comparisons between series of cases.

Since the original reports of the efficacy of idoxuridine (IUDR) in the treatment of herpetic keratitis in rabbits and humans, individual reports involving single or small numbers of patients have appeared in which IUDR has been used to treat human encephalitis caused by herpes simplex virus. IUDR, a thymidine analogue, presumably exerts its antiviral effect by becoming incorporated into the viral DNA, thus producing a fraudulent molecule which cannot be replicated. Although the experience of some has suggested that the drug is effective, others have found less convincing evidence of its efficacy; to this must be added the known tendency for the disease to subside spontaneously. Side effects of the drug include stomatitis, alopecia, and bone marrow depression with leukopenia and thrombocytopenia. The evaluation of the efficacy of IUDR on herpes simplex encephalitis in humans must await the results of carefully controlled large-scale studies now in progress.

Recently cytosine arabinoside (Ara-C), a pyrimidine nucleoside, has been shown to possess activity against herpes simplex virus both in tissue culture and in studies with herpes simplex keratitis in animals. Although the drug has the practical advantages of being readily available and easily solubilized and there is more experience with its use, it retains some of the toxic effects of IUDR, including granulocytopenia and thrombocytopenia. Experience with Ara-C in treatment of herpes simplex encephalitis is limited to a few largely favorable reports. Further carefully controlled experience with the use of both of these antiviral drugs will be necessary to determine their efficacy in man; at present their use must be regarded as experimental.

It has been suggested that corticosteroids may be helpful in the management of herpes simplex encephalitis in man on the basis of a close temporal association between administration of the steroids and improvement in neurologic function. Although the use of steroids for their antiedematous effect may be appropriate in the patient with brain swelling and impending tentorial herniation, this effect must be weighed against the potential for corticosteroids to enhance the spread and delay the clearing of herpes and virus from lesions. Further data bearing upon this topic are necessary; in the meantime it would seem reasonable to use steroids in situations in which brain swelling seems to be a critical factor threatening the patient's life; an attempt to discontinue their use should be made as soon as is feasible.

Prognosis. Because of the very great difficulty in establishing the diagnosis of herpes simplex encephalitis with certainty, as well as the tendencies for biopsy to be performed in more seriously ill patients and for cases to be reported only if they are confirmed by biopsy or autopsy, the outcome of herpes simplex encephalitis is quite difficult to predict. Published reports from many sources suggest that an over-all mortality of between 30 and 70 per cent is to be expected and that among survivors severe sequelae are common, including prominent impairment of memory. A few reports, however, emphasize that nearly complete recovery is possible even without any specific treatment.

Adams, H., and Miller, D.: Herpes simplex encephalitis: A clinical and pathological analysis of twenty-two cases. Postgrad. Med. J., 49:393, 1973.

Craig, C. P., and Nahmias, A. J.: Different patterns of neurologic involvement with herpes simplex virus types 1 and 2: Isolation of herpes simplex virus type 2 from the buffy coat of two adults with meningitis. J. Infect. Dis., 127:365, 1973.

Dayan, A. D., and Stokes, M. I.: Rapid diagnosis of encephalitis by immunofluorescent examination of cerebrospinal fluid cells. Lancet, 1:177, 1973.

Gilbert, D. N., Johnson, M. T., Luby, J. P., and Sanford, J. P.: Herpesvirus hominis type 1 encephalitis treated with cytarabine, an unresolved problem in encephalitis. Medicine (Baltimore), 52:331, 1973.

Johnson, K. P., Rosenthal, M. S., and Lerner, P. I.: Herpes simplex encephalitis: The course of five virologically proven cases. Arch. Neurol., 27:103, 1972.

Johnson, R. T., Olson, L. C., and Buescher, E. L.: Herpes simplex virus infections of the nervous system: Problems of laboratory diagnosis. Arch. Neurol., 18:260, 1968.

Nolan, D. C., Lauter, C. B., and Lerner, A. M.: Idoxuridine in herpes simplex virus (type 1) encephalitis: Experience with 29 cases in Michigan, 1966 to 1971. Ann. Intern. Med., 78:243, 1973.

Rappel, M.: The management of acute necrotizing encephalitis: A review of 369 cases. Postgrad. Med. J., 49:419, 1973.

Sarubbi, F. A., Sparling, P. F., and Glezen, W. P.: Herpesvirus hominis encephalitis: Virus isolation from brain biopsy in seven patients and results of therapy. Arch. Neurol., 29:268, 1973.

Shope, T. C., Klein-Robbenhaar, J., and Miller, G.: Fatal encephalitis due to herpesvirus hominis: Use of intact brain cells for isolation of virus. J. Infect. Dis., 125:542, 1972.

391. CYTOMEGALOVIRUS INFECTIONS

James B. Hanshaw

Definition. Cytomegalic inclusion disease (CID), generalized salivary gland virus disease, cytomegaly, and inclusion disease are synonyms for an illness caused by cytomegalovirus infection. Although frequently an inapparent infection, it is a cause of fetal encephalitis with irreversible damage to the central nervous system. Disease also occurs in patients on immunosuppressive therapy and others subject to opportunistic infections. The virus has been associated with a mononucleosis-like illness in previously well patients and in individuals receiving transfusions of blood.

Etiology. Cytomegalovirus (CMV) infection is caused by a species-specific agent with the physiochemical and electron microscopic characteristics of a herpesvirus. It was isolated in human fibroblastic tissue culture in the mid-1950's from infants with CID as well as from the adenoid tissue of schoolage children. A cytopathic effect was noted in tissue culture which was characterized by large intranuclear inclusions. The propagation of the virus provided the basis for the development of specific serologic tests.

Epidemiology. Cytomegalovirus infection is worldwide in distribution. The prevalence of complement-fixing antibodies is especially high in communities where crowding and poor living conditions are extant. Although approximately 50 per cent of women in the childbearing age group are seropositive, this may vary from 20 to 90 per cent. Approximately 4 per cent of pregnant women excrete the virus in the urine. In the several studies that have been done in this country and in the United Kingdom, 0.5 to 1.5 per cent of newborns are virus positive. Thus cytomegalovirus is the most common known fetal infection. In some countries infection occurs in the majority of infants at some time during the first year of life. In the United States complement-fixing antibody is present in approximately 5 to 15 per cent of infants from 6 to 24 months of age.

Pathogenesis and Pathology. Cytomegalovirus does not induce a highly communicable infection. Thus a substantial number of individuals remain susceptible to the infection in adult life. The virus has been isolated from saliva, the upper respiratory tract, urine, milk, cervical secretions, semen, feces, and circulating lymphocytes. Virus is probably transferred by intimate contact with an infected individual or by infusion of blood from an asymptomatic blood donor. Nursing personnel working on infant wards and newborn nurseries do not have a higher prevalence of complement-fixing antibody than women in the general population. There is evidence that the placenta itself is infected with the virus prior to transmission to the fetus.

The symptomatic newborn is rarely without neutralizing, complement-fixing, and immunofluorescent IgM antibodies in the cord serum. The presence of specific IgM antibody is of value in differentiating maternal from fetal antibody because of the failure of maternal macroglobulin to pass the placental barrier. Antibody in the serum of the congenitally infected infant does not prevent the persistence of virus excretion for years after birth. The precise mechanism of this remarkable persistence is not known.

Among adults undergoing immunosuppressive therapy after renal homotransplantation, over 90 per cent develop an active cytomegalovirus infection if they have cytomegalovirus antibody prior to surgery. Approximately half of the seronegative patients subsequently become infected on immunosuppressive therapy.

Cytomegalovirus infection tends to be focal in character with spread of the virus from cell to cell. Infected cells may be greatly enlarged and contain eosinophilic intranuclear and basophilic cytoplasmic inclusions.

Clinical Manifestations. *Congenital Infection.* The most frequently encountered signs of the infection in symptomatic newborns are hepatosplenomegaly, jaundice, purpura, microcephaly, cerebral calcifications, and chorioretinitis—in approximate order of decreasing frequency. Any one of these signs may occur alone. A petechial rash on the first day of life is suggestive of CID. Occasionally there are no physical findings other than increased irritability or a general failure to thrive. Some infants have repeated respiratory infections. The incidence of various congenital abnormalities in infants with CID is increased. These include clubfoot, inguinal hernia, strabismus, high-arched palate, microcephaly, and deafness. There have been reports of associated congenital heart disease, but this coexistence may be coincidental.

The major complications of congenital cytomegalovirus infection relate to central nervous system sequelae. There is little evidence that extraneural involvement of viscera such as the liver, spleen, kidney, or lungs results in any permanent damage to these organs. Blindness is associated with macular chorioretinitis or optic atrophy. Deafness may be complete or limited to the higher frequencies. Spastic quadriplegia or hypotonia are common manifestations in severely affected infants. Psychomotor function may range from the vegetative state with no meaningful communication to milder abnormalities with minimal effect on speech, behavior, and motor coordination.

Acquired Infection. Cytomegalovirus acquired after birth is often inapparent but may also produce respiratory symptoms with pneumonia, paroxysmal cough, petechial rash, hepatomegaly, and splenomegaly. Central nervous system disease caused by infection acquired after birth has not been frequently demonstrated, although there are reports of associated myoclonic seizures in infants and infectious polyneuritis. Chorioretinitis has been documented after acquired infection.

Hepatomegaly and mildly abnormal liver function tests are found in well individuals excreting CMV in the urine as well as in patients with cytomegalovirus mononucleosis. The latter patients may experience malaise, fever, chills, myalgia, sore throat, headache, anorexia, and abdominal pain. On physical examination,

pharyngeal edema without exudate, lymphadenopathy, and splenomegaly may be present. Atypical lymphocytosis is common. Some patients have maculopapular rashes, especially if ampicillin is administered, and abnormal serologic reactions, including cold agglutinins, antinuclear antibody, and cryoimmunoglobulins, have been described. An illness similar to cytomegalovirus infection has been described in patients who have received blood transfusions. This condition, referred to as posttransfusion mononucleosis, occurs two to four weeks after the administration of blood.

Acquired cytomegalovirus infection has also been associated with autoimmune hemolytic disease, ulcerative lesions of the gastrointestinal tract, post-transplantation pneumonia, and thrombocytopenic purpura.

There is equivocal evidence that the mild liver dysfunction associated with acquired CMV infection is capable of progressing to chronic hepatitis, granulomatous hepatitis, or cirrhosis of the liver. Children with chronic hepatitis or chronic liver disease may have a higher prevalence of active infection, but the relationship of this infection to the pathogenesis of chronic liver disease is uncertain. For the majority of CMV infections acquired after birth, recovery is without significant complications. Patients with CMV mononucleosis may experience recurrent or protracted periods of malaise, pharyngitis, and cervical adenopathy.

Diagnosis. *Congenital Infection.* The diagnosis of congenital infection is usually not suspected at birth, because 90 per cent of infected infants are asymptomatic. The presence of infection (not necessarily disease) can be established by (1) virus isolation in human fibroblastic tissue culture from the urine, blood, upper respiratory tract, or biopsy material; (2) demonstration of cytomegalovirus 19S antibody in the cord or neonatal serum; (3) persistent cytomegalovirus complement-fixing or hemagglutination-inhibition antibody beyond the sixth month of life; or (4) demonstration of large nuclear inclusion-bearing cells in the urine sediment at birth.

Differential Diagnosis of Congenital Infection. TOXOPLASMOSIS. Cytomegalovirus infection resembles toxoplasmosis in striking detail. Toxoplasmosis, however, is more likely to be associated with microphthalmia, *scattered* cerebral calcifications, hydrocephalus, and chorioretinitis. The demonstration of specific toxoplasma antibody titers persisting beyond six months of age or the presence of toxoplasma IgM antibody is tantamount to isolation of the organism.

RUBELLA. Congenital CMV and congenital rubella may be difficult to distinguish in the neonatal period. Both can be associated with a purpuric rash, jaundice, microcephaly, and deafness. The presence of central cataracts, however, is strong presumptive evidence for rubella. If these are associated with a congenital heart lesion, the probability of rubella is high. Specific laboratory tests for rubella virus, rubella 19S antibody, or serial hemagglutination-inhibition antibody tests are required for a definitive diagnosis.

HERPESVIRUS HOMINIS (HERPES SIMPLEX). *Herpesvirus hominis* infection is usually transmitted to the infant during labor and has its onset in the second week of life. The disease is often fulminant in character and may present as a meningoencephalitis, pneumonitis, or undiagnosed vesicular rash. The virus is readily isolated from vesicular lesions (see Ch. 390).

BACTERIAL SEPSIS. Infants with bacterial sepsis usually are more lethargic than infants with CID and rarely have a petechial rash. Although the diagnosis rests on a positive blood culture, the decision to treat with antimicrobial drugs must be made on the basis of the early clinical findings.

Acquired Infection. The diagnosis of cytomegalovirus infection in a patient with mononucleosis-like symptoms can be established by virus isolation as described above. Serologic determinations, such as the presence of specific immunofluorescent IgM antibody or a fourfold rise or decline in complement-fixing antibody, must be interpreted with more caution than in the newborn period because of cross-reactions with other cell-associated herpesviruses, and a tendency for CF antibody to fluctuate widely in normal subjects. Patients with cytomegalovirus mononucleosis are always heterophil antibody negative.

INFECTIOUS MONONUCLEOSIS. Cytomegalovirus mononucleosis may be difficult to distinguish from heterophil antibody-negative infectious mononucleosis, because both conditions occur in young adults and both have atypical lymphocytosis, anginal symptoms, abnormal liver function tests, splenomegaly, and fever. In addition, the cytomegalovirus IgM (FA) test is positive in cytomegalovirus and infectious mononucleosis, presumably because Epstein-Barr virus (EB virus) and cytomegalovirus share common antigens. A patient with cytomegalovirus mononucleosis usually has virus in the urine, upper respiratory tract, and peripheral lymphocytes. EB virus antibody can be measured by an indirect immunofluorescence technique. The complement-fixation tests for EB virus and CMV are specific for each agent.

SERUM AND INFECTIOUS HEPATITIS. A jaundiced patient with CMV mononucleosis may clinically resemble one with infectious or serum hepatitis. A serum glutamic oxaloacetic transaminase level above 800 units is unusual for CMV infections at any age and common in icteric infectious hepatitis. Both conditions may be associated with mild atypical lymphocytosis. Jaundice in an adult is far more unusual in CMV infections than in infections with the hepatitis viruses. A history of recent contact with a jaundiced person is strong evidence in favor of infectious hepatitis. Serum hepatitis (SH) antigen may be detected in the serum of many patients with serum hepatitis.

Prognosis. *Congenital.* The prognosis is guarded for completely normal psychomotor development in an infant with symptoms of CID at birth. Approximately 75 per cent or more usually have some central nervous system sequelae. Although asymptomatic infants discovered on routine surveys have a more favorable outlook, there is evidence that approximately 50 per cent of infants with cytomegalovirus IgM in the cord serum have detectable CNS sequelae five years after birth. Unilateral or bilateral deafness may become apparent after the second year of life. The absence of cytomegalovirus IgM antibody in the cord serum and a birth weight above 3000 grams are favorable prognostic signs.

Acquired. Although acquired cytomegalovirus infections are usually benign, they may be life-threatening in a patient subject to opportunistic infection. This usually is manifest as a progressive pneumonitis but may take the form of a hemolytic anemia, purpura, gastrointestinal ulceration, hepatitis, pericarditis, and rarely encephalitis.

Treatment. There is no satisfactory treatment for cytomegalovirus infections. The use of corticosteroids, gamma globulin, and antiviral drugs such as deoxyuridine, floxuridine, cytosine arabinoside, and adenine arabinoside have been reported with equivocal, beneficial, or no effect on the clinical course. These reports are difficult to evaluate because of the small numbers of individuals treated, the multiple factors operating simultaneously, and the variability of virus excretion in individuals tested at different times.

Prevention. It is not possible to prevent cytomegalovirus infection at present. Handwashing and gown technique should be used in working with patients with cytomegalovirus infection in a hospital setting. Usually this is ineffectual because of the difficulty the physician has in making the diagnosis. Almost everyone in a given population will acquire CMV at some decade in life. The infection cannot be prevented by a live or killed vaccine, although this approach is under active investigation.

Benyesh-Melnick, M.: Cytomegaloviruses. *In* Lennette, E. H., and Schmidt, N. J. (eds.): Diagnostic Procedures for Viral and Rickettsial Infections. 4th ed. New York, American Public Health Association, Inc., 1969, pp. 701–732.

Hanshaw, J. B.: Congenital cytomegalovirus infection: A fifteen-year perspective. J. Infect. Dis., 123:555, 1971.

Jordan, M. C., Rousseau, W. E., Stewart, J. A., Nobel, G. R., and Chin, T. D. Y.: Spontaneous cytomegalovirus mononucleosis: Clinical and laboratory observations in nine cases. Ann. Intern. Med., 79:153, 1973.

Plummer, G.: Cytomegaloviruses in man and animals. *In* Melnick, J. L. (ed.): Progress in Medical Virology. Basel, S. Karger, 1973, pp. 92–125.

Weller, T. H.: The cytomegaloviruses: Ubiquitous agents with protean clinical manifestations. N. Engl. J. Med., 285:203, 267, 1971.

392. ACUTE ANTERIOR POLIOMYELITIS

Fred Plum

Definition. Acute poliomyelitis is a highly contagious viral disease which ranges in severity from inapparent infection to overwhelming paralytic illness and death. The illness may take a number of forms. An *inapparent infection* consists of an invasion by poliovirus that produces an antibody response but no systemic symptoms. An *abortive infection* produces transient nonspecific symptoms of a minor illness without central nervous system involvement with a rise in antibody. In *nonparalytic poliomyelitis,* the major illness develops with signs and symptoms of central nervous system invasion and meningitis but no paralysis. *Paralytic poliomyelitis* consists of the major illness, often with a biphasic pattern, associated with flaccid weakness in one or more muscle groups, the result of the attack by the virus on the somatic motor and autonomic neurons of the spinal cord and lower brainstem.

Initially endemic in character, poliomyelitis became epidemic during the first half of this century, especially in the highly developed countries of Western Europe and North America. Since the advent of effective vaccines in the 1950's, major epidemics have disappeared, but minor outbreaks have reappeared in groups of nonimmunized children and in specific areas such as the American-Mexican border.

Etiology. The polioviruses are small enteric viruses of the picornavirus group. The virus is naturally infectious only for selected primates, particularly man, and has no other known natural reservoir. Poliovirus can be classified immunologically into three distinct types. Infection with type I, type II, and type III confers immunity against subsequent infection with the same type, but cross-immunity from type to type is minimal, a fact reflected by well documented cases of second attacks of poliomyelitis. Occasionally cases of an acute paralytic illness clinically are caused by coxsackie- and echoviruses (see Ch. 126 to 136).

Epidemiology. The virus of poliomyelitis is worldwide, and the infection is spread largely if not entirely by human contact. Naturally occurring poliomyelitis epidemics tend to be both geographically localized and seasonal in nature. In nonepidemic areas with poor sanitation and largely unvaccinated populations, the illness is mainly confined to infants and children ("infantile paralysis"). In these areas, children come in contact with fecal-borne virus during the early months of life. Such children have a high infection rate with all three types of virus. Presumably they get some protection from maternal antibody, and there is very little serious illness. Under the circumstances, a large percentage of the population develop antibodies early in life and, despite repeated exposures, become immune from epidemic spread. However, once sanitation improves and infant mortality falls in a region, the average age incidence progressively rises, with a concomitant increase in the number of paralytic cases. Prior to the extensive use of preventive vaccines, as many as 35 per cent of affected patients in the northeastern United States were over 14 years old.

Individual epidemics are predominantly the result of a single virus type, although different types of virus may attack the same community in successive years. During epidemics, poliovirus can be recovered readily from the pharynx, nasopharyngeal secretions, and stools of both patients with clinical cases and those with inapparent infection. The ratio of inapparent infection to disease ranges from 50 to 1 to 500 to 1. Thus inapparent infections are by far the largest reservoir for transmission.

Pathogenesis and Pathology. Naturally occurring poliomyelitis infection is transmitted by human contact. Poliovirus enters the body through the alimentary tract and multiplies in the oropharynx and lower intestinal tract. No symptoms accompany this early proliferative stage. From the alimentary canal, the virus disseminates to regional lymph nodes with subsequent viremia which corresponds to the early, nonspecific phase of the abortive illness. With inapparent and abortive attacks, although viremia occurs, the virus apparently fails to penetrate the barriers of the central nervous system.

Both virus and host factors influence whether poliomyelitis virus invades the central nervous system and the severity of CNS involvement. Different strains of the virus vary widely in virulence. Host factors are perhaps even more important. Recent evidence indicates that susceptibility to paralytic poliomyelitis in man is genetically determined. The conclusion stems from studies in tissue culture in which poliovirus was found able to infect only hybridized human cells that contained on their surface a receptor that made it possible for the virus to attach. The sensitive cells contained chromosome 19, whereas resistant hybrids did not, implying that chromosome 19 contains the gene for the receptor. Age, excessive physical activity during the prodromal illness, and pregnancy all unfavorably influence the severity of paralysis. Local injections received during the preceding six weeks appear to increase the risk of paralysis in the injected extremity, and previous tonsillectomy enhances the risk of bulbar poliomyelitis. Inapparent and abortive poliomyelitis infections presumably never invade the nervous system at all, because these tissues undergo no pathologic changes when such mild illnesses are induced in experimental primates. In nonparalytic and paralytic cases, the distribution of lesions in the neural parenchyma is roughly similar, although the intensity of the changes increases proportionately to the degree of paralysis. No one knows just what factors govern the special susceptibility of the motor gray matter and the distribution of the virus along the neuraxis in any given patient. However, in paralytic cases, the spinal cord gray matter is diffusely affected, appearing reddened, swollen, and congested, particularly in the anterior horns; the involvement in some fatal cases commonly extends rostrally to the hypothalamus and thalamus. Lesions in the cerebral cortex are confined to mild alterations of the motor area. Microscopically in regions of maximal damage there are marked perivascular cuffing and diffuse infiltrates of mononuclear cells. The anterior horn cells of the spinal cord and the motor nuclei of the lower brainstem show abnormalities ranging in severity from mild chromatolysis and pericellular infiltration to total destruction. Small areas of necrosis commonly dot regions of intense inflammation. Ouside the anterior horns, the inflammatory reaction sometimes spreads into the intermediate horn of the spinal cord; posterior column demyelination and neuronolysis of dorsal root (sensory) ganglia are rare but well documented. In the brainstem, severe abnormalities can be found in the vestibular nuclei, the roof nuclei of the cerebellum, and especially that part of the reticular formation which regulates autonomic, respiratory, and circulatory functions.

Chronically active neural lesions do not follow poliomyelitis, although collections of lymphocytes may remain in devastated anterior horns for two years or more after the acute illness. In patients dying of motor neuron disease several years after poliomyelitis (see below), the pathologic changes have a degenerative rather than inflammatory character.

Outside the nervous system, pathologic changes of myocarditis may be found. Complications and secondary effects of the illness produce abnormalities in the lungs, gastrointestinal tract, urinary tract, bones, and muscles.

Cerebrospinal Fluid. The cerebrospinal fluid (CSF) in poliomyelitis is characterized by pleocytosis, a moderate increase in protein content, and normal values for sugar and electrolytes. The pressure is not significantly elevated. As many as 10 per cent of patients may have an initially normal fluid, but persistently negative findings are rare.

The white cell counts range from 5 to 10 to as many as 3000 per milliliter in acutely ill patients (more than 1 to 2 lymphocytes per milliliter of CSF is abnormal in a carefully examined fluid). Polymorphonuclear cells predominate at first but give way to a lymphocytosis within 72 hours. The concentration of sugar is not lowered. The initial protein content ranges between 30 and 100 mg per 100 ml, values over 150 mg per 100 ml being unusual. After the first week of the disease, however, the CSF protein often rises to 100 to 150 mg per 100 ml or even more, and by this time the cell count often has returned to normal.

Clinical Features.   One would not suspect that a systemic infection was caused by poliovirus unless the virus invaded the nervous system. Furthermore, once central nervous system invasion has taken place, the severity of the naturally occurring disease still has wide limits. Poliovirus will cause a relatively mild attack of aseptic meningitis in one patient, whereas the most fulminating acute paralytic and encephalitic processes will be encountered in another infected with the same virus and during the same epidemic. The illness of poliomyelitis often pursues a bimodal course. The early stage is the time of viremia and dissemination of virus in the tissues. The later phase reflects the effects of later damage to the cells of the nervous system. Nothing specific characterizes the early illness of poliomyelitis; vague malaise, low-grade fever, muscular aching, and sometimes headache are accompanied by coryza or moderate gastrointestinal difficulties with anorexia, sometimes nausea, and, often diarrhea. This prodromal phase may subside in one to three days or can progress directly into the major illness. If it subsides, three to ten or more days may pass during which the individual feels healthy, only to fall ill again, this time usually with even more severe symptoms.

Nonparalytic Poliomyelitis.   The major illness progresses with more severity and intensity. As a rule, moderate nonspecific malaise develops first, often with a sense of muscular aching or stiffness that may lead to unwise exercise to "work off" the discomfort. Generalized headache appears early and is usually nonthrobbing. Children may have coryzal upper respiratory symptoms. In contrast, anorexia, nausea, diarrhea, constipation, and sometimes vomiting are frequent in adolescents and adults. Chilliness is frequent, but shaking chills are rare. Other visceral symptoms are also prominent; many patients have insomnia as well as excessive and localized sweating. Some report urinary hesitancy or retention even before paralysis develops elsewhere.

As the illness progresses, *muscle pain* becomes prominent, usually antedating paralysis. (Meningeal irritation, involvement of the brainstem reticular formation, and direct inflammation of sensory structures are all present and are potential causes of muscle pain and shortening.) Patients also complain of a deep-seated low back discomfort that repeated changes in position fail to alleviate. Occasionally, frank *muscle twitching and cramping* develop in the early stages of the illness, and *diffuse fasciculations* can be seen.

Fever ranges between 38.5 and 40° C. The pulse is elevated commensurately, usually between 100 and 120 per minute. Most patients have mild hypertension. Patients with poliomyelitis usually look acutely ill. Their skin is flushed, and the lips of those with severe illness may show a dark cherry hue, associated with circumoral pallor. There is usually some facial sweating, and sweating in localized dermatomes or restricted bodily parts may be intense. Many patients are restless and express great anxiety, even at a stage when the diagnosis has not been made and paralysis has not set in. The pathogenesis of these feelings of agitation and fear is a matter of speculation. Along with the diffuse autonomic changes of the early stages of the illness, the psychologic symptoms may reflect the widespread involvement of the brainstem reticular formation or hypothalamus.

A stiff neck and back along with tight hamstring muscles are usually prominent in the early stages of nonparalytic or preparalytic disease. The muscles may be diffusely tender, and cutaneous hyperesthesia is often complained of. Early in the illness, muscle stretch reflexes are often hyperactive.

Paralytic Poliomyelitis.   Paralysis in poliomyelitis may develop with overwhelming rapidity, proceeding from barely detectable weakness to tetraplegia in but a few hours, or it may pursue a more indolent course in which additional weaknesses appear over a four- or five-day period. Rarely this indolent progression may last for as long as 10 to 12 days. In general, the more rapid the early progression, the more severe the eventual involvement.

The virus has a predilection for large motor neurons, with weakness about large joints usually being noted first. Spread of the disease from this point shows no consistent pattern; although there is a tendency for adjacent spinal and brainstem segments to be involved together, paralysis is nearly always asymmetric and at times may be widely scattered in distribution. The lower extremities and lower trunk are involved most frequently, whereas upper extremities and cranial nerves are seriously paralyzed less often. These general incidences are of no help in predicting how the individual case will progress.

Poliomyelitis causes flaccid paralysis. After an initial brief period during which local stretch reflexes may be heightened, the involved part becomes toneless and inert. The stretch reflexes become reduced, and then disappear. Fasciculations are inconstant and transient, and the paralyzed part is initially painless. Indeed, in the first few days of the paralytic disease the absence of soreness or stretch pain usually stands in sharp contrast to the earlier discomfort and the marked degree of weakness that ensues. Sensory loss does occur in acute poliomyelitis, but it is extremely rare, and in most instances the finding of reduced sensation indicates some other illness.

Bulbar Poliomyelitis.   Cranial nerve paralysis may develop at any time. When bulbar palsy initiates the paralytic disease, it is a dangerous sign, for the progress of paralysis seldom halts in less than four to five days. With bulbar poliomyelitis certain signs herald trouble. During the early hours, agitation and fear may become pronounced. Delirium is prone to occur at night. Fulminating bulbar polioencephalitis can produce stupor, acute excitement, or myoclonic twitches. Nystagmus on the extremes of gaze is frequent and carries no serious significance. More severe forms of ophthalmoplegia with opsoclonia or even total external ophthalmoplegia are usually limited to fulminating cases. The pupils, if they show any abnormality at all, tend to be constricted. Funduscopic abnormalities are absent during the acute stage of the disease.

Abnormalities in the rest of the motor cranial nerves are more common than those in the oculomotor nerves. Trismus may precede paralysis of the jaw. Facial paralysis is usually restricted to one or more muscles and rarely extends to produce a total facial diplegia. Paralysis of swallowing is the most frequent abnormality in cranial nerve function. Many such patients later show little or no residual pharyngeal weakness, implying that the acute dysfunction results from involvement of the integrating center for swallowing in the reticular formation of the medulla.

In addition to impaired swallowing, involvement of other somatic motor functions of the vagus is frequent. Muscle paralysis of the larynx creates the danger of respiratory obstruction. Total aphonia is rare, but laryngeal involvement may be so severe that the voice sounds are limited to hoarse cries. Vagal autonomic disturbances occur much more often than do actual cranial skeletal muscle paralyses, and include anorexia during the acute phase as well as vomiting in many subjects. Constipation is almost invariable both during the acute illness and for several weeks thereafter. Diarrhea is rarely persistent.

Autonomic Abnormalities. Many autonomic abnormalities complicate acute poliomyelitis. Hypertension and excessive sweating have already been mentioned. Over 50 per cent of adults suffer at least transiently from bladder paralysis with acute urinary retention. Sialorrhea and bronchorrhea are usually profuse in patients with severe bulbar disease. Indeed, the autonomic instability in such individuals is sometimes overwhelming and can progress into fulminating elevations of blood pressure, tachycardia, and fatal pulmonary edema. Cardiac arrhythmias are frequent with bulbar poliomyelitis and consist of partial heart blocks, wandering cardiac pacemakers, supraventricular tachycardias, or auricular flutter. Electrocardiographic tracings on such bulbar cases usually show abnormalities in the configuration of the T waves.

Differential Diagnosis. Poliomyelitis is singular in producing an acute febrile illness with headache, stiff neck, and asymmetric, flaccid, multifocal, and progressive muscle paralysis. However, unless poliomyelitis invades the nervous system, it cannot be differentiated clinically from many other viral diseases producing myalgia or influenza-like symptoms. Similarly, aseptic meningitis can be caused by mumps, coxsackieviruses and echoviruses that can be identified only by tissue culture or serologic studies (see Ch. 132). Bacterial or fungal meningitides can usually be separated from nonparalytic poliomyelitis by their characteristic cerebrospinal fluid alterations, including the reduction of sugar.

Many diseases may mimic some phase of poliomyelitis. However, those in which muscle pain is combined with weakness and fever provide the greatest difficulty in diagnosis. Of non-nervous system diseases, osteomyelitis or acute arthritis may sometimes produce focal pain and paresis. Here, the non-neurologic nature of the illness is usually evident within a few hours, and the CSF is normal. *Acute polyneuritis* can be differentiated by the presence of sensory changes in approximately 80 per cent of cases. Furthermore, patients with polyneuritis are seldom systemically ill or febrile, and the CSF rarely shows a persistent or significant pleocytosis. Protein elevations in the CSF above 100 mg per 100 ml are frequent in polyneuritis but unusual in polio. Paralysis in poliomyelitis usually lacks the symmetry which characterizes polyneuritis. *Epidemic neuromyasthenia* (benign myalgic encephalomyelitis, Iceland disease) has many clinical similarities to early poliomyelitis. It is characterized by insidious onset, headache, fever, diffusely aching and tender muscles, and the development of muscular weakness in approximately one quarter of the cases. The disease comes in epidemics, predominantly affects adolescents and young adults, and produces considerable emotional instability and lassitude. However, the cerebrospinal fluid is normal, and sensory paresthesias as well as mild sensory loss are often prominent. Paresis fails to progress to severe paralysis, and stretch reflexes are preserved. Viral, bacterial, and serologic studies have thus far failed to identify a cause for this obscure illness.

The course of *acute viral encephalitis* usually differs sharply from poliomyelitis. Although headache and some stiff neck are present in encephalitis, such patients usually have drowsiness, lethargy, convulsions, or mental changes. There may be pupillary changes, ophthalmoplegia, or spastic pareses, but lower motor neuron involvement is absent. The cerebrospinal fluid often is normal in acute encephalitis. Specific neutralizing antibodies can be detected in the blood within seven to nine days after attacks of equine, St. Louis, or herpes simplex encephalitis.

Acute porphyria is characterized by a symmetric motor polyneuropathy and sometimes has an abrupt onset with diffuse peripheral pain. However, fever is usually lacking and there is no CSF pleocytosis. Patients with porphyria often have a history of recurrent attacks, abdominal pain, and prominent psychiatric disturbances. Appropriate urine studies will usually demonstrate porphobilinogen.

Hysteria will occasionally present a difficult clinical picture. This may be particularly the case when the subject has had direct contact with paralytic poliomyelitis or during an epidemic. The hysteric has a normal cerebrospinal fluid and rarely looks severely ill. Hysterical paralyses commonly involve an entire body part rather than selective muscles, and reflex loss is rarely commensurate with weakness. Autonomic changes are seldom prominent in hysteria. Finally, in the face of paralysis persisting for more than three to four weeks, electromyographic studies in the hysteric will fail to detect the expected presence of motor unit degeneration.

Treatment. There is no specific treatment for the poliomyelitis viral infection. Patients with known or suspected acute anterior poliomyelitis are best kept at bed rest and should be hospitalized if signs of nervous system involvement are detected. Since there is no prognostic value in knowing the exact extent of the weakness until progression has ceased, serial studies of muscle function can be restricted to pertinent examinations of bulbar function, respiration, and circulation. Patients with paralytic and nonparalytic poliomyelitis are most comfortable if placed on a firm bed with the back and head supported. A low head pillow helps relieve neck pain, and a thin pad placed beneath the small of the back minimizes lumbar discomfort. Footboards to support the weight of bedclothes help to prevent foot drop.

During the acute illness, aspirin and other non-narcotic analgesics should be used for pain relief. Narcotics and sedatives, with the exception of small and occasional doses of codeine, are dangerous and should be avoided. Hot packs provide comfort to painful muscles and should be gently laid on with minimal manipulations. More vigorous physical therapy should be deferred to the convalescent phase, although the joints should be moved passively through their full range of motion in an effort to prevent contractures.

Patients should be on liquid or minimal diets until their appetite returns. If necessary, parenteral fluids totaling 2000 to 2500 ml should be given in order to maintain a high fluid intake and counteract the risks of immobilization. Either indwelling or intermittent catheterization can be employed to deal with urinary retention, parasympathomimetic drugs not being of much help at this stage.

Complications. The acute complications of poliomyelitis result mainly from the effects of damage to motor neurons and autonomic centers in the upper spinal cord and the brainstem. *Swallowing paralysis* is common in bulbar poliomyelitis and is treated by a combination of withholding oral intake and postural drainage. If respiratory failure coexists, tracheostomy should be performed. *Respiratory failure* can result either from paralysis of the muscles of breathing (peripheral failure) or from damage to the respiratory centers in the medulla oblongata (central failure). Peripheral respiratory failure is characterized by a falling vital capacity and a progressively increasing respiratory rate with shallow breathing. Central failure is characterized by a progressive slowing and irregularity of the respiratory rhythm, with intermittent periods of apnea, especially when drowsy or asleep. The treatment in either instance is the early and effective use of artificial respiration. *Cardiovascular complications* in poliomyelitis include hypertension, centrally induced arrhythmias, pulmonary edema, and shock, all of which are practically confined to patients with fulminating bulbar disease. Rarely, cardiac arrhythmias may persist for years after the severe attack. The management of circulatory problems in poliomyelitis is similar to their management in other diseases.

During convalescence from acute poliomyelitis *urinary tract complications* are common, almost all catheterized patients developing infections and many of the severely paralyzed ones subsequently developing urinary calcium phosphate stones caused by the combination of skeletal demineralization and the alkaline, infected urine. Treatment should include effective antimicrobial therapy, and stones should be prevented by maintaining a high fluid intake and turning severely paralyzed subjects so that gravel drains from the posterior renal calyces. Other complications are less frequent. Papilledema occurs in 5 to 10 per cent of patients during convalescence and has no serious significance. An equal number of patients develop an unexplained but usually reversible increase in various muscle weaknesses as late as three to four weeks after the acute disease. A more severe complication is *late motor neuron disease after poliomyelitis.* This is the uncommon but well documented occurrence of clinically typical progressive muscular atrophy or amyotrophic lateral sclerosis developing 30 to 40 years after acute paralytic poliomyelitis. The frequency of the occurrence is several times that of spontaneous motor neuron disease and strongly suggests an association between the two illnesses. The pathogenesis is unknown.

Prognosis. At the peak of the acute illness it is impossible to predict accurately how much recovery will take place. Less than 10 per cent of patients with paralytic poliomyelitis die when treated with modern methods. Only a few fail to recover significant strength during convalescence. It can generally be estimated that muscle groups which function partially at the end of the acute illness will recover considerably. Recovery or improvement in areas of total paralysis is less certain.

Muscle strength recovers through three mechanisms: recovery of partially damaged anterior horn cells; hypertrophy and increased strength in the muscle fibers of residual undamaged motor units; and peripheral branching from the axons of intact motor cells, the branches reinnervating muscle fibers in denervated motor units. Recovery of partially damaged anterior horn cells appears to provide the greatest return, the maximal rate of recovery usually occurring in the first three to four months after acute illness. Significant improvement in strength is unusual after the end of the first year, and

improvement after this time is largely a matter of learning to use existing strength with greater skill. Muscles that show no voluntary motion at all by three months after the illness only rarely later develop functional usefulness.

Increased neuromuscular excitability is sometimes a more or less permanent residuum of poliomyelitis. Such patients experience diffuse muscle cramping on exercise or night cramps in the legs. They may be troubled by muscle tremulousness on exercise, and some have hyperactive stretch reflexes but not spasticity or pathologic reflexes. Many patients who have partially denervated muscles have fasciculations at least intermittently, and these are sometimes so prominent and enduring as to suggest active motor neuron disease. In most instances, such fascicular activity is benign and unaccompanied by any progression of weakness over the years.

Prevention. Natural infection from any of the three types of poliovirus induces lifelong immunity to the specific infecting strain. Proper vaccination with either the killed- or the live-virus vaccine appears to achieve a similar result and has largely eliminated epidemic poliomyelitis from the developed countries of the world.

Widespread use of poliovirus vaccines since 1955 has resulted in the virtual elimination of paralytic poliomyelitis from the United States. Paralytic poliomyelitis declined from 18,308 cases in 1954 to 17 cases in 1971 and 29 cases in 1972. A national survey in 1971 showed that 77 per cent of individuals 1 to 19 years old had received at least three doses of oral or inactivated poliovirus vaccine. Nevertheless, low immunization rates still prevail in certain disadvantaged population groups, and these represent the principal populations at future risk of paralytic disease.

Both live attenuated virus vaccines which are taken orally and inactivated virus vaccines which must be injected parenterally are effective in creating immunity against poliomyelitis. Because it is easier to administer and supervise, trivalent oral poliomyelitis vaccine has almost completely replaced both the inactivated and monovalent vaccines in this country. Oral poliomyelitis vaccine produces an immune response like that induced by natural poliovirus infection, and a primary series of three adequately spaced doses will produce immunity against the three poliovirus types in well over 90 per cent of recipients. Very rarely, paralysis has occurred in recipients of oral polio vaccine or in their close contacts within two months of administration. The estimated frequency of this complication is 1 case per 5 million doses distributed.

The desirable time to immunize against poliomyelitis is in infancy, when the three-dose series should start at 6 to 12 weeks of age, with the second dose 6 to 8 weeks later and the third 8 to 12 months after that. In older persons, a similar program may be given at any time, and when circumstances demand it, the third dose may be given as early as six weeks after the second. Routine immunization is not recommended for adults residing in the United States. In the event of an epidemic outbreak of poliomyelitis (two or more cases caused by the same virus type in a circumscribed population), immunization with either trivalent or homotypic monovalent oral poliovirus vaccine is recommended for all persons over six weeks of age who have not been completely immunized or whose immunization status is unknown.

In general, vaccination is contraindicated for patients with abnormal immune states caused by disease or drugs. Single booster doses of trivalent oral poliovirus vaccine are recommended for children just entering school and for persons traveling to a high risk area or having an occupational hazard such as employment in hospitals or medical laboratories.

Grist, N. R., and Bell, E. J.: Enteroviral etiology of the paralytic polio-myelitis syndrome. Arch. Environ. Health, 21:382, 1972.

Horstmann, D. M.: Lagging immunity of our children. N. Engl. J. Med., 285:1432, 1971.

Miller, D. A., et al.: Human chromosome 19 carries a poliovirus receptor gene. Cell, in press.

Mulder, D. W., Rosenbaum, R. A., and Layton, D. P.: Late progression of poliomyelitis or forme fruste amyotrophic lateral sclerosis? Mayo Clin. Proc., 47:756, 1972.

Paul, J. R.: A History of Poliomyelitis. New Haven, Yale University Press, 1971.

Plum, F., and Olson, M. E.: Myelitis and myelopathy. In Baker, A. B., and Baker, L. H. (eds.): Clinical Neurology, Vol. 3. New York, Harper & Row, 1973, Chap. 36, pp. 2–20.

Sencer, D. J., et al.: Supplement. Collected recommendations of the Public Health Service Advisory Committee on Immunization Practices. U.S. Department of Health, Education, and Welfare. Morbidity and Mortality Weekly Report, Vol. 21, No. 25, June 24, 1972.

393. RABIES
(Hydrophobia, Lyssa)

Hilary Koprowski

Definition. Rabies is an acute infectious disease of the central nervous system to which all warm-blooded animals and man are susceptible. The virus, frequently present in the saliva of an infected host, is usually transmitted by bites, by licks, and occasionally by the respiratory route. The disease is characterized by a profound dysfunction of the central nervous system and ends almost invariably in death.

History. Rabies is one of the oldest diseases of man. First mention of it dates to the twenty-third century B.C., when it was referred to in the pre-Mosaic Eshunna Code. In the Americas, rabies as a bat-transmitted disease fatal to man was probably first described in the sixteenth century. Since 1753, when it was first recorded, its presence has been evidenced throughout the North and South American continents.

In 1971, 73 countries in the world reported rabies. In most countries, dogs were the main source of bite wounds or other human contact that required treatment. Cats were the second most frequent source of exposure to rabies, with rats, squirrels, foxes, jackals, cattle, and bats a main source in several countries. On the basis of species, the total number of rabid animals reported was as follows: dogs, 35,370; cats, 3737; foxes, wolves, and jackals, 6057; bats, 500; mongooses, 273; farm animals, 12,766; and others, 4767.

The total number of human deaths from rabies reported in 1971 was 769, as compared to 770 in 1970. However, 920,084 were reported to have received antirabies treatment in 1971 as compared to 448,512 in 1970. In 1971, antirabies treatment resulted in 42 paraplegic accidents, including four deaths; out of 16,779 who received the combined serum-vaccine protection against rabies, there were 1532 cases of serum sickness.

Etiology, Host Range, and Experimental Infection. Virus recovered in nature, the so-called *street virus,* is characterized by extremely variable, usually long incubation periods and by its ability to invade salivary glands as well as central nervous tissue. The term *fixed virus* is used for strains of rabies that have been adapted to laboratory animals by means of serial intracerebral passages. Fixed virus is characterized by a short incubation period (usually four to six days) and by its apparent inability to multiply in salivary glands. Prolonged cultivation of some strains of rabies virus in the developing chick embryo or in tissue culture has resulted in modification to the point of complete loss of pathogenicity for animals injected extraneurally.

The physicochemical properties of the virus are shown

TABLE 1. Specific Biologic Activities, Gross Chemical Composition, and Some Physical Properties of Purified Rabies Virus

Property	Observation
Specific infectivity	1×10^{10}–5×10^{10} PFU/mg protein
Specific hemagglutinating activity	10^4 HAU/mg protein
Specific complement-fixing activity	5×10^3 CFU/mg protein
Gross chemical composition	22% lipids 3% carbohydrates 1% RNA 74% protein
Protein composition	Four major proteins, one of which is glycoprotein and the other phosphoprotein
Sedimentation coefficient	600 S
Buoyant density in sucrose solution	1.17 grams per cm³
Genome	Single-stranded RNA, 4.6×10^6 daltons molecular weight

PFU = Plaque-forming unit.
HAU = Hemagglutinating unit.
CFU = Complement-fixing unit.

in Table 1. In addition, the virus is readily inactivated by sunlight, ultraviolet irradiation, formalin, 50 to 70 per cent alcohol, and 0.1 to 1.0 per cent quaternary ammonium compounds, bichloride of mercury, and strong acids. It is relatively resistant to phenol. In aqueous solutions, its thermal death point is reached at 56° C after an exposure of one hour. It survives desiccation from the frozen state, and rabies-infected tissue may be stored successfully at 4° C in 50 per cent glycerol saline or kept frozen at temperatures below −20° C.

All warm-blooded animals are susceptible to rabies. It is principally a disease of mammals, including bats. The virus is also pathogenic for birds, but to a lesser degree than for mammals. As far as we know, the disease is not transmissible by insects or arthropods. It has been found in all parts of the world, in all climates and seasons. The virus apparently cannot invade the body through intact skin, and is supposedly harmless when ingested; however, infection through unabraded mucosa seems possible. An airborne infection occurring in caves inhabited by rabid bats has been described.

Rabbits, guinea pigs, mice, and hamsters are most commonly employed for experimental infection. Hamsters are remarkably susceptible to intramuscular infection with street virus, but intracerebral injection of mice is usually employed for diagnostic purposes.

Epizootics of rabies occur in any climate during any season of the year. Wars and mass movements of men and animals favor the geographic spread of the disease. Man becomes an accidental host upon exposure to the infected saliva of the biting animal, and wild animals are often sources of human rabies. The attack rate in man, after exposure, depends to a certain extent on the location and on the severity of the inflicted wounds. Head and neck bites lead to a higher incidence of infection than bites on other parts of the body. The bites of rabid wolves are apparently very dangerous; an attack rate of

47 per cent was observed in 32 persons who were bitten by the same animal and did not receive antirabies treatment in time to be of any protective value.

Pathology. At autopsy, the brain is friable, edematous, and congested; the convolutions are broad and flattened. Severe vascular congestion of the white and gray matter may extend to the medulla and the spinal cord. Virus-infected salivary glands are usually soft and swollen. On microscopic examination of the central nervous system, the nonspecific findings consist of hyperemia, perivascular and perineuronal infiltration with mononuclear cells, and considerable neuronal degeneration. Mononuclear cell infiltration of periacinal interstitial tissue accompanied by degeneration of acinar cells may be observed in the parotid and sublingual and submaxillary salivary glands.

In the absence of Negri bodies (see below), the lesions are indistinguishable from those observed in some of the other viral encephalitides. The exact nature of the virus-host relationship is unknown.

Incubation. The incubation period in man varies from ten days to over twelve months. As minor and seemingly insignificant contacts with rabies virus in the saliva of an animal not obviously sick at the time of exposure are sometimes forgotten, claims of extended incubation periods (one to two years) have to be critically evaluated. In dogs, signs of rabies may appear after an incubation period of ten days to several months.

The length of the incubation period is related to the amount of virus introduced at the time of exposure and to the severity of the laceration. The site of the original exposure does not seem to affect the duration of the incubation period.

Clinical Manifestations. *Dogs.* In dogs the prodromal phase of the disease lasts two to three days and consists of fever, anorexia, and, very frequently, a change in the tone of the bark. However, these signs are often so slight that only a trained observer may note them. The animal's disposition is altered, and symptoms give way to the excitation phase, usually lasting three to seven days, during which time the animal grows unnaturally restless and agitated. General tremor owing to stimulation of the muscular system appears frequently. In the furious type of the disease, agitation intensifies as the illness progresses. The animal, erratic and aggressive, growls and barks constantly. It will grab viciously at any object or animal encountered. At this stage, an unrestrained animal sometimes leaves home and travels great distances, inflicting damage on other animals and humans along the way. Convulsive seizures are often observed, and the animal may become completely paralyzed. In many cases, however, the excitation phase predominates until the time of death.

In the paralytic type of rabies, the excitation phase may be slight or totally absent, and the disease is characterized only by the paralytic syndrome. Paralysis of the lower jaw, accompanied by excessive salivation, appears as an early symptom, and the animal acts as though it were choking on a foreign body. Paralysis of the muscles of phonation may lead to loss of the bark. As the disease progresses, paralysis of the posterior extremities sets in, followed by general paralysis and death. The time from the onset of the disease to the death of the animal ranges from one to eleven days. On the other hand, dogs may die suddenly without noticeable signs of illness.

Man. In man, the prodromal phase is marked by fever, anorexia, headache, malaise, nausea, and sore throat. *Abnormal sensations around the site of infection,* such as intermittent pain, tingling, or burning, are of diagnostic significance. Extreme stimulation of the general sensory system is manifested by hyperesthesia of the skin to temperature changes and to drafts, and by acute sensitiveness to sound and light. Other symptoms include increased muscular tonus, prompt gag and corneal reflexes, dilation of pupils, and increased salivation.

As the disease progresses, spasmodic contractions of the muscles of the mouth, pharynx, and larynx on drinking—and later at the mere sight of fluid—are observed in the majority of cases. This dysfunction of deglutition gave the disease its common name, *hydrophobia,* or fear of water. Spasms of respiratory muscles and convulsive seizures leading to opisthotonos also may occur. The pulse is very rapid. Periods of irrational and often maniacal behavior are interspersed with those of alertness and responsiveness. Paralysis of the muscles of phonation may lead to hoarseness or loss of voice.

The excitation phase may remain predominant until the time of death. However, in many cases it gives way shortly before death to cessation of muscle spasms, to hyporeflexia or areflexia, and to general paralysis of the flaccid type.

In rabies in man *resulting from vampire bat infection,* the excitation phase is almost totally absent, and the disease is characterized by ascending paralysis without hydrophobia. Without an adequate history of exposure, clinical diagnosis of this type of infection may be difficult.

Diagnosis. Profound dysfunction of the central nervous system, accompanied by impairment in deglutition, in persons who either were exposed to a bite or lick of any animal or may have recently visited caves harboring bats, facilitates the clinical diagnosis. Isolation of virus from saliva obtained in the course of the disease and from brain tissue obtained at autopsy, followed by proper identification of the agent by means of neutralization test, will confirm the diagnosis. Syrian hamsters, rabbits, guinea pigs, and, preferably, suckling mice are used for diagnostic purposes. Demonstration of rabies virus antigen in smears of brain tissue obtained from either patient or animal (preferably brainstem, cerebellum, or Ammon's horn) by means of specific staining with antibody coupled with fluorescein isothiocyanate is of diagnostic significance. The presence of intracytoplasmic inclusion bodies in the neuron (Negri bodies) is pathognomonic, but their absence does not exclude the diagnosis of rabies, as the presence of virus may be demonstrated by other means.

Prognosis. Although inapparent infection with street virus may be induced artificially in laboratory animals, and although animals have recovered completely after exhibiting signs of the disease, there is only one case reported of the recovery of a human from rabies after showing unmistakable signs of disease. In all other reported cases, the disease proved fatal to humans.

Treatment. *General Considerations.* Confinement and observation of the biting animal, preferably under the supervision of a veterinarian, for a period of not less than ten days for dogs and cats, is one of the most important steps in deciding whether an individual has been exposed to rabies. Biting wild animals should be sacrificed and their brain tissue examined properly by immunofluorescent staining. Treatment of severely exposed persons should be started without awaiting results of the laboratory diagnosis. If the absence of rabies infection in the biting animal is reported, treatment may be stopped.

Local Treatment of Wounds. Since the most effective available mechanism of protection against rabies is the elimination of the virus at the site of infection, all bite wounds, as well as scratches and other abrasions exposed to licks of animals, should be treated immediately by thorough cleansing and adequate mechanical flushing of the wound with soap solution followed by treatment with substances such as 40 to 70 per cent alcohol, tincture or aqueous solutions of iodine, or 0.1 per cent quaternary ammonium compounds, which are lethal to rabies virus. If debridement is necessary, infiltration with local anesthetics is not contraindicated. Bite wounds should *not* be sutured immediately. After determination of sensitivity to antirabies serum, the serum should be used in local application upon the wound.

Preliminary application of antimicrobial drugs is of no value as a prophylactic measure. However, antitetanus treatment and local application of antiseptics and antimicrobials should be instituted if indicated.

Indications for Specific Treatment. These are summarized in Table 2, prepared by the Expert Committee on Rabies of the World Health Organization. Emphasis is placed on the condition of the biting animal at the time of exposure and during the ensuing ten days. It is assumed that the saliva of an animal that is not obviously ill at the time of exposure may be infectious during a maximal period of five days preceding the appearance of clinical signs of the disease.

Passive-Active Immunization. Passive-active immunization by the administration of antirabies serum of animal or human origin and immunogenically potent vaccine in repeated doses is the most effective protective specific treatment of the exposed persons. Because of the existence of various vaccine preparations, no emphasis is placed on the use of any special type of vaccine, provided it meets the standard potency requirements and is known to induce antibodies in humans.

Administration of Preventive Treatment. The administration of preventive treatment may give rise to local allergic reactions, to serum sickness (if combined serum-vaccine therapy was used), and to nervous system reactions caused by the presence of nervous tissue in most of the vaccines. These occur most frequently during a repeated course of protective treatment. Treatment should be interrupted if signs of dysfunction of the central or peripheral nervous system are observed. *Avian embryo vaccines* and vaccines prepared from brains of suckling mice, rats, or rabbits are less apt to induce allergic reactions and have been used for preventive treatment in man. Many problems can be avoided if treatment is given only when specifically indicated (Table 2). All courses of vaccine should include booster doses at 10, 20, and 90 days after the regular course of vaccine.

Treatment Once Clinical Signs Are Apparent. Although no specific therapeutic measures are available to save the life of a person exhibiting symptoms of the disease, the survival of one patient with human rabies indicates that all the tools of modern medicine should be used in the attempt to save the patient's life. These therapeutic measures should consist of (1) starting treatment immediately after signs of rabies appear; (2) placing the patient in the intensive medical care unit in a quiet environment, with constant monitoring to prevent cardiac failure; (3) using sedatives for the relief of anxiety and pain; (4) performing a tracheostomy and applying artificial breathing to maintain respiratory function; (5) using curare-like drugs to alleviate spastic muscular contractions if they occur; and (6) instituting intravenous perfusions and administering diuretics to assure proper hydration and diuresis. *Note:* Since rabies virus may be present in the saliva of the patient exhibiting signs of the disease, all attending personnel should be protected against contamination through the use of goggles, masks, and rubber gloves.

Pre-exposure Immunization. Effective immunization with three injections of a potent antirabies vaccine given at five- to seven-day intervals, followed by a booster injection one month after the last dose, is important for persons engaged in veterinary practice, experimental surgery involving handling of dogs and cats, spelunking, dog catching, or any other activity involving unusually high risk of exposure. The vaccine used should be free from paralytic factors, and the vaccinated person should be bled one month after the last vaccination to check his sera for the presence of antirabies antibodies. Such persons upon exposure may be given one booster dose of a

TABLE 2. Specific Systemic Treatment

| Nature of Exposure | Status of Biting Animal Irrespective of Previous Vaccination | | Recommended Treatment† |
	At Time of Exposure	During 10 Days*	
I. Contact, but no lesions; Indirect contact; no contact	Rabid	—	None
II. Licks of the skin; scratches or abrasions; minor bites (covered areas of arms, trunk, and legs)	(a) Suspected as rabid‡	Healthy	Start vaccine; stop treatment if animal remains healthy for five days*§
		Rabid	Start vaccine; administer serum upon positive diagnosis and complete the course of vaccine
	(b) Rabid; wild animal¶ or animal unavailable for observation		Serum + vaccine
III. Licks of mucosa; major bites (multiple or on face, head, finger, or neck)	Suspect‡ or rabid domestic or wild animal,¶ or animal unavailable for observation		Serum + vaccine; stop treatment if animal remains healthy for five days*§

*Observation period in this chart applies only to dogs and cats.
†See Explanatory Notes.
‡All unprovoked bites in endemic areas should be considered suspect unless proved negative by laboratory examination (brain FA).
§Or if its brain is found negative by FA examination.
¶In general, exposure to rodents and rabbits seldom if ever requires specific antirabies treatment.

potent vaccine. Persons without antibody should receive full treatment if re-exposed to rabies.

Control Measures. Although the presence of rabies-infected bats in the Northern Hemisphere presents a difficult problem for rabies control, most human exposure can be prevented by the use of control measures that will rid an area of enzootics or epizootics of rabies.

The following measures should be applied in an efficiently organized rabies control program conducted by public health authorities: control of the canine population (registration, restraint, elimination of stray dogs), reduction in number of susceptible dogs by mass vaccination, reduction in number of wildlife species that are a reservoir of the virus, and continuous educational campaigns for the general public.

Explanatory Notes to Table 2. Practice varies concerning the volume of vaccine per dose and the number of doses recommended in a given situation. In general, the equivalent of 2 ml of a 5 per cent brain tissue vaccine, or the dose recommended by the producer of a particular vaccine, should be given daily for 14 consecutive days. To ensure the production and maintenance of high levels of serum-neutralizing antibodies, booster doses should be given at 10, 20, and 90 days after the last daily dose of vaccine in *all* cases.

Combined serum-vaccine treatment is considered by the Committee as the *best* specific treatment available for the postexposure prophylaxis of rabies in man. Experience indicates that vaccine alone is sufficient for minor exposures. Serum should be given in a single dose—40 IU per kilogram of body weight for heterologous serum, and 20 IU for human antirabies gamma globulin; the first dose of vaccine is inoculated at the same time as the serum but at another site. Sensitivity to heterologous serum must be determined before its administration.

Treatment should be started as early as possible after exposure, but in no case should it be denied to exposed persons arriving late.

In areas in which antirabies serum is not available, full vaccine therapy, including three booster inoculations, should be administered.

Expert Committee on Rabies: Sixth Report. WHO Techn. Rep. Ser., No. 523, 1973.

Hattwick, M. A. W., Weis, T. T., Stechschulte, C. J., Baer, G. M., and Gregg, M. B.: Recovery from rabies. A case report, Ann. Intern. Med., 76:931, 1972.

Hummeler, K., and Koprowski, H.: Investigating the rabies virus. Nature, 221:418, 1969.

Johnson, H. N.: Rabies. *In* Horsfall, F. L., Jr., and Tamm, I. (eds.): Viral and Rickettsial Infections of Man. 4th ed. Philadelphia, J. B. Lippincott Company, 1965.

Kaplan, M., and Koprowski, H. (eds.): Laboratory Techniques in Rabies. 3rd ed. Geneva, World Health Organization, 1973.

ENCEPHALITIC COMPLICATIONS OF VIRAL INFECTIONS AND VACCINES

Donald Silberberg

394. INTRODUCTION

Acute disseminated encephalomyelitis may be associated with banal viral diseases or may follow immunization. Postrabies vaccinal encephalomyelitis resembles acute disseminated encephalomyelitis, but specifically follows immunization against rabies. Reye's syndrome seems to be related to banal viral infections, but has distinctive features. Despite some points in common, these entities are best considered separately.

395. ACUTE DISSEMINATED ENCEPHALOMYELITIS

Definition. Acute disseminated encephalomyelitis (postinfectious encephalomyelitis, postvaccinal encephalomyelitis, acute perivascular myelinoclasis, acute hemorrhagic leukoencephalitis) is an acute or subacute disease of the central nervous system which most commonly occurs after viral infections that do not normally affect the nervous system, or as a complication of immunization. Involvement of the brain and spinal cord may be widespread, or may be limited to discrete areas, such as optic nerves (optic neuritis, papillitis) or a single spinal cord level (transverse myelitis). Acute disseminated encephalomyelitis is characterized by varying degrees of perivenous mononuclear cellular infiltration and demyelination.

Etiology and Pathogenesis. Predisposing factors to acute disseminated encephalomyelitis include exposure to measles, mumps, varicella, rubella, influenza, infectious mononucleosis, smallpox, and poorly characterized upper respiratory infections. Similar disease has been associated with pertussis, tetanus, streptococcal infections, and mycoplasma pneumonia. Acute disseminated encephalomyelitis also follows immunization against smallpox, rabies, influenza, and tetanus. Disease occurring after immunization is often termed postvaccination encephalomyelitis, and the central nervous system disease which may follow immunization against smallpox with attenuated vaccinia virus is termed postvaccinal encephalomyelitis.

The neurologic complications of childhood viral diseases usually occur 4 to 18 days after the appearance of a skin rash or other systemic signs. However, it is important to recognize that encephalomyelitis can occur before, concomitant with, and even in the absence of systemic signs of viral infection.

The pathogenesis of acute disseminated encephalomyelitis may be viewed as the direct consequence of viral infection, as an immune disorder, or as the result of interaction of these two mechanisms. Historically an immune pathogenesis was considered first because of the histopathologic resemblance of acute disseminated encephalomyelitis to postrabies vaccine encephalomyelitis and to experimental allergic encephalomyelitis (see Ch. 396).

There have been few attempts to recover an infectious agent from the central nervous system of patients with acute disseminated encephalomyelitis using modern virologic techniques. Measles virus was isolated from the brain of a patient with postmeasles acute disseminated encephalomyelitis, using co-cultivation techniques. The patient's neuropathologic abnormalities included the typical histologic features of acute disseminated encephalomyelitis. Long after vaccination, vaccinia virus was isolated from the cerebrospinal fluid of a number of patients without neurologic symptoms, suggesting that persistent virus may play a role in postvaccinal encephalomyelitis. Mumps virus may be isolated from cerebrospinal fluid during the first few days of systemic illness in over half the patients.

At present no definite direct evidence exists for primarily immune pathogenesis of human acute disseminated encephalomyelitis, except for the form that follows rabies immunization (see Ch. 396).

Incidence. Approximately 30 per cent of the reported cases of encephalitis in the United States are associated with childhood diseases. Published reports from Great Britain indicate that deaths caused by acute disseminated encephalomyelitis exceed deaths from known encephalitis viruses. The incidence of neurologic complications may vary from epidemic to epidemic, but is approximately 1:1000 cases in measles, 1:5000 in rubella, 1:800 in scarlet fever, and probably exceeds these figures in pertussis. The fact that abnormalities in the electroencephalogram occur in approximately 50 per cent of neurologically uncomplicated cases of measles suggests that asymptomatic involvement of the nervous system is common. A variety of neurologic complications occur in approximately 1 per cent of patients with infectious mononucleosis, but acute disseminated encephalomyelitis is rare. In general, males are affected somewhat more frequently than females, approximating a ratio of 2:1 in some series. Infants younger than two years of age and the elderly are rarely affected; the age incidence reflects the age incidence of the precipitating disease.

Mumps resembles lymphocytic choriomeningitis in its central nervous system involvement. An increase of cells in cerebrospinal fluid is very common in neurologically asymptomatic children with mumps. As many as 18 per cent of patients with mumps have convulsions, and signs of meningeal irritations are frequent. Despite this, the incidence of acute disseminated encephalomyelitis associated with mumps remains very low.

Postvaccinal encephalomyelitis, which is practically unknown in infants under two years of age, occurred in 17 of 800,000 people who were vaccinated during the 1962 epidemic of smallpox in South Wales, suggesting an over-all incidence of approximately 1 in 50,000 vaccinations. Several other series report similar figures. There is a greater incidence of postvaccinal complications after primary vaccination than after revaccination, with the highest incidence among children of school age (3 per 100,000). A long interval between primary vaccination and revaccination increases the incidence.

Pathology. The basic lesion in acute disseminated encephalomyelitis is the presence of mononuclear cells around small veins, chiefly in white matter, but to a lesser extent in gray matter as well. This is accompanied by varying degrees of perivenous demyelination. Individual lesions are scattered and rarely coalesce to give large lesions. Severe cases may include destruction of axons and nerve cell bodies, serous exudate, fibrin impregnation of vessel walls, polymorphonuclear infiltration, and hemorrhages. The inclusion of hemorrhages as well describes acute hemorrhagic leukoencephalitis.

Clinical Manifestations and Course. Acute disseminated encephalomyelitis usually begins with fever, headache, vomiting, and drowsiness. This is quickly followed by depressed consciousness and often coma. Irritability, behavior disturbances, and convulsions are common. Ataxia, involuntary movements, paralyses of one or more extremities, visual impairment, or other focal neurologic signs occur, often accompanied by signs of meningeal irritation. Lesions restricted to the optic nerves producing optic papillitis or retrobulbar neuritis occur. The duration of symptoms varies from a few days to weeks and sometimes months.

Myelitis predominates in approximately 10 per cent of instances of acute disseminated encephalomyelitis. The lesion may affect only one cord level (transverse myelitis), or may progress to involve the entire spinal cord, producing successive backache, urinary retention, paraparesis, paraplegia, quadriplegia, and bulbar signs.

The cerebrospinal fluid may be normal or may show increased pressure and pleocytosis up to 1000 cells per cubic millimeter. The cell counts usually range from 15 to 250. Most cells are mononuclear, although polymorphonuclear cells may predominate during the first several days of illness. Approximately 60 to 70 per cent of patients with neurologic complications have pleocytosis, but over 10 per cent of patients with neurologically uncomplicated exanthemata also have pleocytosis. Cerebrospinal fluid protein may be normal. It is rarely elevated to more than 100 mg per 100 ml. The CSF changes have no prognostic significance and no relation to the type or severity of neurologic disorder.

The electroencephalogram is almost always diffusely abnormally slow. Interestingly, the EEG is reportedly abnormal in 50 per cent of neurologically asymptomatic patients with measles.

Neurologic manifestations may precede signs of systemic infection by up to ten days or follow signs of systemic infection by up to 24 days. The average latent period is about five days. The occurrence and severity of neurologic symptoms appear to bear no relation to the severity of the systemic disease.

The immediate and long-term prognosis varies somewhat with the individual virus. Encephalitis associated with rubella, measles, and mumps has a somewhat higher mortality (20 to 50 per cent) than in scarlet fever (13 per cent) or varicella (10 per cent). Sequelae are most common in scarlet fever (45 per cent) and measles (35 per cent), and less so in varicella (20 per cent) and rubella (2 to 5 per cent). The clinical sign which correlates best with prognosis is the level of consciousness.

Diagnosis. Identification of acute disseminated encephalomyelitis is not difficult when neurologic symptoms are preceded by a recognizable viral illness. Differential diagnosis includes acute infectious encephalitis and acute multiple sclerosis. Encephalitis caused by neurotropic viruses is almost always accompanied by increased cells and protein in the cerebrospinal fluid, which are often lacking in acute disseminated encephalomyelitis. Fever and meningeal signs are rare in multiple sclerosis. Correct diagnosis in the absence of precipitating illness may depend entirely on direct virus isolation from all possible sites and by serum antibody determinations during the course of the illness in an attempt to detect evidence of a virus infection. Fatal cases provide the opportunity for attempts at direct recovery of virus.

Treatment. Corticosteroid therapy appears to produce improvement in some patients with acute disseminated encephalomyelitis. However, no controlled studies have been feasible because of the low frequency of cases, and there is no convincing evidence to support the use of steroids in the absence of increased intracranial pressure. Appropriate measures to reduce increased intracranial pressure, including intravenous mannitol, high doses of corticosteroids, and hyperventilation, may be required to sustain life during severe acute illness. Appropriate symptomatic support includes reduction of fever with aspirin, the use of anticonvulsants and antimicrobial drugs when indicated (such as for pneumonia), and management of fluid and electrolyte balance.

Prevention. Initial smallpox vaccination during infancy reduces the danger of postvaccinal disease. The use of measles, mumps, and pertussis vaccines to induce active immunity to these diseases will reduce the frequency of acute disseminated encephalomyelitis.

396. POSTRABIES VACCINAL ENCEPHALOMYELITIS

The production of neurologic disease is a dreaded complication of immunization against rabies. Postrabies vaccinal encephalomyelitis resembles acute disseminated encephalomyelitis in its clinical manifestations and histology but is related to the presence of nervous system antigen in the vaccine rather than to the presence of virus.

It seems clear that the risk of developing postrabies vaccinal encephalomyelitis is proportional to the amount of brain tissue in the vaccine. The over-all incidence of postvaccinal encephalomyelitis varies from 1 in 2000 to 1 in 9000 of those receiving brain-containing vaccines. Practically no cases occur in young children, but as many as 1 per cent of young adults (20 to 40 years) developed encephalomyelitis after immunization with neural vaccines. The incidence after immunization against rabies with vaccines prepared in avian embryos is low, approximating 1 in 50,000.

With rare exceptions in which live rabies virus was accidentally introduced with vaccines, the pathogenesis of postrabies vaccinal encephalomyelitis seems to be immunologic. The low incidence and the age-related incidence strongly suggest that immune responsiveness plays a role in disease production. In addition, an experimental disease which is very similar histologically, experimental allergic encephalomyelitis (EAE), can be induced in a variety of animals by injection of homologous or heterologous brain tissue or myelin basic protein.

Postrabies vaccinal encephalomyelitis may be divided into encephalitic and myelitic forms. Both are distinguished by widely spread foci of demyelination and cellular infiltration throughout white and gray matter, but more pronounced in white matter. Brain lesions (encephalitic form) tend to be larger, and many are periventricular as well as perivenous. These lesions resemble plaques of multiple sclerosis very closely. More acute lesions are distinguished by perivenous mononuclear cell invasion. Axis cylinders are spared in most instances. The myelitic form resembles acute disseminated encephalomyelitis more closely, with smaller scattered areas of perivenous demyelination and cellular infiltration.

The interval from the last injection to the onset of symptoms averages 15 days with the myelitic form, and about 35 days with the encephalitic form. Headache, fatigue, and changes in mental function commonly precede the appearance of such focal neurologic signs as visual disturbance, hemiplegia, or paraplegia. Progression of neurologic signs and symptoms may proceed for days or weeks. Mortality is approximately 20 per cent, but most cases were reported before the availability of corticosteroids which may increase survival. Permanent sequelae occur, including changes in mentation or behavior.

If any signs of the possible development of postrabies vaccinal encephalomyelitis develop during a course of immunization against rabies, immunization should be stopped. High doses of corticosteroids may be effective in reducing the morbidity of the acute process once postvaccinal encephalomyelitis has started. If a neural vaccine has been used, immunization can be continued with avian embryo vaccine.

Immunization against rabies should be undertaken only when it is reasonably certain that there has been a bite by a rabid animal. Vaccines prepared in avian embryos carry the least risk of producing postvaccinal encephalomyelitis.

397. REYE'S SYNDROME

Definition. Reye's syndrome describes an acute and often fatal encephalopathy of childhood that is characterized by acute brain swelling associated with hypoglycemia and fatty infiltration and dysfunction of the liver. Reye's syndrome may follow a variety of common viral infections.

Etiology and Pathogenesis. Reye's syndrome has been reported after infections with influenza B, varicella, adenovirus type 3, coxsackievirus A and B, reovirus, echovirus, herpes simplex, and parainfluenza. Viral infection is suggested as the initiating factor by recovery of virus from a few patients, by the frequency of varicella as the prodromal illness in sporadic cases, and by the reported increased incidence concurrently with outbreaks of influenza B infection in two epidemiologic studies. The pathogenic relationship between virus infection and the encephalopathy and hepatic injury is unknown.

It is possible that the encephalopathy is secondary to metabolic effects of the hepatic lesion. The combination of hypoglycemia and ammonia retention, together with other abnormalities of intermediary metabolism, may be sufficient to produce the coma and cerebral edema which occur. The early occurrence of mitochondrial abnormalities in liver suggests that induction of a partially reversible mitochondrial injury may be instrumental in the evolution of Reye's syndrome. It is not known whether similar changes in brain mitochondria occur concomitantly.

Incidence. Reye's syndrome occurs in children 6 months to 15 years of age. Approximately 500 cases have been reported. Large series have been described from Australia, Canada, Thailand, and the United States. It occurs both as a sporadic, rare disease, and in minor outbreaks in a particular area. It is a leading cause of death in children one to six years old in Thailand.

Pathology. Marked cerebral edema occurs, with or without anoxic neuronal changes and neuronal degeneration, but with no cellular infiltration or demyelination. The liver is swollen and orange to pale yellow. Fatty infiltration occurs initially as diffuse small vacuoles in the periportal areas, and spreads to cause massive involvement in fatal cases. Electron microscopic examination of liver biopsy specimens shows swollen pleomorphic mitochondria and small droplets of triglycerides in hepatocytes. Fat deposition also occurs in the renal tubules and in the myocardium.

Clinical Manifestations and Course. Typically, Reye's syndrome starts with an upper respiratory infection or mild gastrointestinal disturbance. A symptom-free interval of hours to several days is followed by persistent vomiting and then by delirium and coma. Convulsions are common. Hyperpnea or irregular deep respiration is common. There are no meningeal or focal neurologic signs. Decerebrate posturing may occur as increased intracranial pressure supervenes. Mild to moderate hepatomegaly is the only clinical suggestion of hepatic involvement, and even this is lacking in 50 per cent of cases.

Hypoglycemia, with decreased cerebrospinal fluid glucose, is common in children of less than five years, but is rarely found in older children. Cerebrospinal fluid protein is normal. Elevation of serum transaminases, hyperammonemia, and prolongation of the prothrombin time reflect hepatic damage. Bilirubin levels rise in a minority of patients. Hypocapnia, hyponatremia, hypokalemia, and ketosis are common. Elevation of plasma free fatty acid levels have been present whenever sought.

Deepening coma leading to death occurs in 25 to 80 per cent of patients. More recent reports indicate the lower mortality rates, perhaps because of improved management or because milder cases are being diagnosed. Severe neurologic sequelae, such as mental impairment, seizures, or hemiplegia, occur in some survivors.

Diagnosis. The diagnosis of Reye's syndrome is suggested by the clinical manifestations described above. Biopsy or autopsy demonstration of fatty infiltration of the liver can be considered as a confirmatory abnormality.

Treatment. Treatment is empirical. Hypoglycemia, acidosis, and electrolyte disturbances should be corrected. Enemas, neomycin and low protein intake as employed in hepatic encephalopathy are commonly used. Peritoneal dialysis and exchange transfusions have been used to correct refractory metabolic abnormalities and to correct clotting factor deficiencies. Corticosteroids, mannitol, and hyperventilation may be used to reduce intracranial pressure.

Alvord, E. C.: Acute disseminated encephalomyelitis and "allergic" neuroencephalopathies. *In* Vinken, P. J., and Bruyn, G. W. (eds.): Handbook of Clinical Neurology. New York, American Elsevier Publishing Company, 1970, Vol. 9, pp. 500–571.

Miller, H. G., Stanton, J. B., and Gibbons, J. L.: Para-infectious encephalomyelitis and related syndromes. Quart. J. Med. 25:426, 1956.

Mowat, A. P.: Encephalopathy and fatty degeneration of viscera. Arch. Dis. Child., 48:411, 1973.

Reye, R. D. K., Morgan, G., and Baral, J.: Encephalopathy and fatty degeneration of the viscera: A disease entity in childhood. Lancet, 2:749, 1963.

Shiraki, H.: The comparative study of rabies post-vaccinal encephalomyelitis and demyelinating encephalomyelitides of unknown origin with special reference to the Japanese cases. *In* Bailey, O. T., and Smith, D. E. (eds.): The Central Nervous System: Some Experimental Models of Neurological Diseases. Baltimore, Williams & Wilkins Company, 1968, pp. 87–123.

ter Mullen, V., Käckell, Y., Müller, D., Katz, M., and Meyermann, R.: Isolation of infectious measles virus in measles encephalitis. Lancet, 2:1172, 1972.

SLOW INFECTIONS OF THE NERVOUS SYSTEM

Richard T. Johnson

398. INTRODUCTION

Recently, slow viral infections have been related to several chronic and subacute neurologic diseases in which clinical signs of infection are lacking and in which the pathologic changes are those of degenerative or demyelinative processes. The term slow infection was originally coined in the veterinary literature to describe several transmissible diseases of sheep. Two of these sheep diseases, *scrapie* and *visna,* are the prototypes of slow infections of the nervous system. Both these diseases are transmissible. After inoculation of sheep with tissue from an affected sheep, there is a latent period of one to four years during which the sheep appear well. This is followed by the insidious onset of neurologic signs which progress without fever from one to six months and lead inevitably to death. Scrapie is clinically characterized primarily by ataxia and visna by progressive paralysis. Pathologically the diseases are very different. The lesions of scrapie are confined to the nervous system, where there is marked proliferation of astrocytes and the degeneration of neurons with vacuolization of their cytoplasms. Inflammation and primary demyelination are not present. By contrast, central nervous system lesions of visna are characterized by marked inflammation and demyelination. The agents responsible for these two slow infections of sheep are also very different. The scrapie agent has been transmitted to a variety of other animals, but the agent does not cause cytopathic changes in cell culture, and no virus-like particles have been found in infectious tissue by electron microscopy. The infectivity of this tissue remains remarkably stable on exposure to physicochemical treatments which inactivate classic viruses. Furthermore, animals naturally or experimentally infected with scrapie fail to develop any evidence of an immune response against the agent. In contrast, the visna virus is an enveloped RNA virus. Although transmissible from sheep to sheep, it has not been transmitted to other animals but can be grown in a variety of tissue cultures. Of the four slow infections of the human central nervous system described below, kuru and Creutzfeldt-Jakob disease resemble scrapie pathologically, and the agents responsible for these diseases have properties similar to those described for the scrapie agent. Therefore scrapie, kuru, and Creutzfeldt-Jakob disease have been classified together as the subacute spongiform encephalopathies. Subacute sclerosing panencephalitis and progressive multifocal leukoencephalopathy, like visna, are due to classic viruses. These viruses have been visualized by electron microscopy, are antigenic in natural and experimental hosts, and can produce rapid cytolytic infection in some cell cultures even though they are capable of causing slow infections in man.

399. KURU

Kuru is an endemic disease of Melanesian tribal people inhabiting a remote area of the Eastern Highlands of central New Guinea. The disease has been seen only among the Fore linguistic group and several neighboring groups with whom the Fore have intermarried. However, within this limited area, kuru, until recently, was the most common cause of death. The disease predominantly affected adult women, but children over age five were also affected but without sexual predilection. Adult males were least involved. The disease begins insidiously with unsteadiness of stance and gait. A progressive symmetrical cerebellar ataxia develops over a period of months and follows a relentless, afebrile course until the patient is unable to make the slightest movement without violent ataxic tremors. Late in the course of the disease, abnormalities of extraocular movement and mental changes develop. The disease invariably leads to death in three to six months. Extensive laboratory examinations have failed to show any abnormalities, and the cerebrospinal fluid remains normal. Pathologic changes are confined to the brain where there is a marked increase of astrocytes and degeneration of neurons with vacuolization. The brain is diffusely affected, but the findings are most prominent in the cerebellum and pons and, to a lesser degree, in the hypothalamus and basal ganglia. Inflammation is not found.

Because of the similarities between kuru and scrapie in terms of epidemiology, clinical progression, and pathologic changes, brain tissue from patients dying of kuru was inoculated into a variety of primates for long-term observations. After incubation periods of 18 months to 4 years, a similar disease developed in chimpanzees, and this disease has subsequently been transmitted from chimpanzee to chimpanzee and to several other species of primates. The agent can be transmitted with serial dilutions, proving that it replicates within the primate host. However, like scrapie, the agent of kuru has not been seen by electron microscopy, does not induce cytopathic changes in cell culture, is resistant to physical and chemical treatments that usually inactivate viruses, and fails to evoke a demonstrable immune response in man or experimentally infected primates.

In recent years, there has been a striking decline in the incidence of kuru, particularly among children, in whom the disease has essentially disappeared. This decreasing incidence has been coincident with the suppression of cannibalism in this primitive culture, and there is considerable circumstantial evidence indicating that kuru was transmitted during the practice of ritual cannibalism.

400. CREUTZFELDT-JAKOB DISEASE

Creutzfeldt-Jakob disease is an uncommon form of rapidly progressive dementia accompanied by myoclonus and other neurologic signs. The disease usually develops between ages 40 and 65, is worldwide in distribution, and usually occurs sporadically, although a few familial cases have been reported. The dementia develops rapidly, so that deterioration from day to day or week to week is evident. Myoclonic jerks usually develop early in the disease, and often massive symmetrical myoclonic jerks of the limbs occur when the patient is startled by unexpected light or sounds. Pyramidal tract signs, cerebellar ataxia, visual disturbances, and muscle wasting with fasciculations are common but inconstant features. The disease is inexorably progressive, usually reducing the patient from good health to total helplessness or death in less than a year. The cerebrospinal fluid shows no abnormality; but the electroencephalogram becomes abnormal early in the disease, showing diffuse slowing with superimposed bursts of sharp waves.

Neuropathologic findings include diffuse loss of cortical neurons with a remarkable increase in fibrous astrocytes. Vacuoles are present in neurons and astrocytes, and this may give a spongiform appearance to the cerebral cortex. Inflammatory reactions and inclusion bodies are absent. Thus, despite clinical and epidemiologic differences, the pathologic findings in Creutzfeldt-Jakob disease are very similar to those of kuru and scrapie.

A similar disease develops in chimpanzees inoculated with brain tissue of most patients with Creutzfeldt-Jakob disease after an incubation period of about one year. The chimpanzees developed somnolence, ataxia, tremor, fasciculations, and intermittent jerking of the extremities. The pathologic changes in the brains resembled those of Creutzfeldt-Jakob disease. The disease has also been transmitted from chimpanzee to chimpanzee, to a variety of other primates, and to the domestic cat. Little information is available on the agent of Creutzfeldt-Jakob disease, but the absence of virus-like particles on electron microscopic examination of infectious tissues, the failure to demonstrate cytopathic changes in cell cultures, and the absence of a demonstrable immune response suggest that the agent is similar to those causing kuru and scrapie.

The natural mode of transmission is unknown, but the development of the disease in primates inoculated with brain tissue from several familial cases has raised the possibilities that the familial cases of disease may be dependent on genetically determined susceptibility to a common agent, vertical transmission, or common environmental or dietary factors in families.

401. SUBACUTE SCLEROSING PANENCEPHALITIS (Dawson's Encephalitis, Subacute Inclusion Body Encephalitis)

This is an uncommon, subacute encephalitis that usually occurs in children or young adults between the ages of 4 and 20 years. The onset is usually insidious and is characterized by deterioration in school work and behavioral disorders. This is followed in weeks or months by overt mental deterioration and neurologic signs, the most characteristic of which is myoclonus. The disease usually terminates after a third stage of stupor, blindness, dementia, and decorticate rigidity, which may last months to several years. Characteristically, the cerebrospinal fluid is under normal pressure and shows no pleocytosis, but an increased concentration in gamma globulin results in a first zone colloidal gold curve. During the stage of active myoclonus, the electroencephalogram usually shows a typical pattern of general suppression of activity, with periodic (8 to 15 seconds) synchronous bursts of high-voltage slow and sharp waves. The clinical course is usually characterized by progressive deterioration, but occasionally an apparent arrest of the disease process or even transient clinical improvement is seen.

Although the disease follows a protracted afebrile course, a viral cause has long been suspected because of the pathologic changes. Perivascular infiltrates of mononuclear cells are characteristic, and eosinophilic intranuclear inclusion bodies are found in neurons and glial cells. Because of these inclusions, a herpesvirus was long suspected of being the etiologic agent. However, electron microscope studies of cerebral biopsies show virus-like particles resembling the nucleocapsids of the measles-distemper group of paramyxoviruses. Astonishingly high levels of antibodies against measles virus can be demonstrated in the serums of most patients, and measles virus antigen is present in the brain. Nevertheless, the isolation of measles-like viruses from brains of patients with subacute sclerosing panencephalitis is difficult, requiring the establishment of cell cultures from brains of patients with the disease and subsequent co-cultivation of these cultures with other cells. The measles virus associated with the disease is apparently defective.

The pathogenesis of subacute sclerosing panencephalitis is obscure. This disease bears little resemblance clinically or pathologically to the fulminating forms of measles virus infections, in which virus dissemination may lead to giant-cell pneumonia. Furthermore, it is quite distinct from parainfectious encephalomyelitis that occasionally complicates measles virus infections, in which acute neurologic disease occurs and perivascular demyelination is found in the brain and spinal cord. Epidemiologic studies have shown that subacute sclerosing panencephalitis is more common in males than females, in children of rural than of urban origin, and in patients with a history of measles during the first two years of life. These findings suggest that environmental factors and presence of residual transplacental passive immunity may play roles in inducing defective infection or precipitating disease.

Treatment of patients with antiviral agents and synthetic interferon inducers has been attempted, but without definite beneficial effects. It is not yet evident whether or not the measles vaccine has altered the incidence of the disease.

402. PROGRESSIVE MULTIFOCAL LEUKOENCEPHALOPATHY

This is a rare demyelinating disease of the central nervous system. It usually develops in patients having pre-existing disorders of the reticuloendothelial system such as leukemia, lymphoma, or sarcoidosis, but has also developed in patients immunosuppressed therapeutically or after organ transplantation. Although the underlying systemic disorder may be of long standing, the neurologic abnormalities develop rather suddenly and follow a subacute progressive course until death. The findings usually suggest multifocal disease. Abnormalities of motor function, sensation, vision, or speech are common, and dementia frequently develops. The cerebrospinal fluid shows little if any abnormality, and the electroencephalogram shows only nonspecific slowing. Pathologic lesions in the brain consist of multiple foci of demyelination in various stages of evolution. Oligodendrocytes are depleted within the foci, but surrounding the foci they are enlarged and contain eosinophilic intranuclear inclusions. The astrocytes within the demyelinated areas are often bizarre and contain mitotic figures. Inflammatory cells are usually not prominent.

The presence of the inclusion bodies and the occurrence against a background of disorders associated with impaired immunologic responses led to speculation that the disease might be caused by a viral infection. Electron microscopic examination in almost all cases has shown particles in the oligodendrocyte inclusions resembling small papovaviruses. Two small deoxyribonucleic acid viruses related to simian-virus 40 have been isolated from brain tissue of patients dying from progressive multifocal leukoencephalopathy. The JC virus, a new human

papovavirus to which the majority of people have antibody since childhood, appears to be the causative agent in most cases. Viruses antigenically indistinguishable from simian-virus 40 have been related to two cases. Neither of these viruses has been associated with any disease in man except progressive multifocal leukoencephalopathy. Therefore progressive multifocal leukoencephalopathy apparently results from opportunistic infection of the brain by normally nonpathogenic agents. The viruses appear to selectively infect and lyse oligodendrocytes, the glial cells which maintain the myelin sheaths, and cause demyelination. The disease occurs in patients with impaired cellular immune responses, but it is not known whether this disease represents a primary infection of an immunologically incompetent patient or whether it represents a reactivation of a latent or persistent papovavirus infection.

Evaluation of possible therapeutic agents has not been possible because of the rarity of cases and the infrequency of diagnosis during life.

403. OTHER NEUROLOGIC DISEASES

Since viruses can cause disease after a long incubation period, can produce disease with a subacute or relapsing course, and can give rise to noninflammatory pathologic changes, the possible role of slow or latent viral infection in a variety of neurologic diseases has been entertained.

In several chronic or relapsing inflammatory diseases of the nervous system, a viral cause has been suspected. *Chronic focal epilepsy* (epilepsia partialis continua, Kozhevnikov's epilepsy) is, in some cases, associated with a chronic focal inflammatory process in the brain. In the Soviet Union, this has been thought to represent a persistent focal infection with tick-borne viruses after acute encephalitis; and in several Soviet laboratories, tick-borne encephalitis virus has been isolated from surgically removed cerebral epileptogenic foci. No viruses have been isolated from similar cases in other countries. Chronic focal epilepsy can be a manifestation of focal disease processes such as neoplastic, vascular, or traumatic lesions, but chronic infection may play a role in some cases.

Recurrent acute meningitis or encephalitis occurs in three clinical syndromes of unknown cause in which latent viral infection has been suspected. *Mollaret's meningitis* is a rare, recurrent meningitis characterized by repeated attacks of headache, fever, and nuchal rigidity. Each attack is abrupt in onset and lasts for two to three days; the patient is entirely well between episodes. During attacks, the cerebrospinal fluid may contain large numbers of both polymorphonuclear and mononuclear cells and also large, poorly staining "epithelial cells," characteristic but not pathognomonic of this disease. More severe recurrent neurologic involvement can occur in *Behçet's syndrome* and in the *Vogt-Koyanagi-Harada syndrome*. Behçet's syndrome is a chronic disease characterized by recurrent oral and genital ulcers and inflammatory ocular lesions, usually taking the form of acute recurrent iritis. In about one quarter of the patients neurologic signs develop, consisting either of cranial nerve palsies, focal seizures, hemiparesis, or other focal signs or of severe depression of consciousness, coma, or meningeal signs, suggesting more diffuse neurologic involvement. Neurologic deficits usually remit and relapse but may be progressive. Neuropathologic findings include meningeal inflammatory reactions, perivascular inflammation, and focal areas of necrosis. The Vogt-Koyanagi-Harada or uveoencephalitic syndrome is characterized by depigmentation of skin and hair, inflammatory ocular lesions (usually consisting of iridocyclitis or exudative retinal detachment), and meningitis. Unlike Behçet's syndrome, neurologic involvement occurs in all cases, often precedes the ocular inflammation, and usually consists only of headache, nuchal rigidity, and a mononuclear cell pleocytosis. However, transient decrease in hearing and tinnitus may accompany the meningitis, or a severe encephalitis may develop, leaving permanent neurologic deficits. Neuropathologic findings have consisted only of a chronic arachnoiditis. Reports have been made of isolations of unidentified viruses from patients with Mollaret's, Behçet's, and Vogt-Koyanagi-Harada syndrome; but none of these claims have been entirely convincing. An allergic cause has also been postulated in each of these disorders, and consequently treatment with corticosteroids has been advocated.

Considerable interest in a possible viral cause of *multiple sclerosis* has been stimulated by epidemiologic data that indicate the role of a common exposure factor, serologic studies showing higher antibody levels against measles virus in patients with multiple sclerosis, obser-

vation of viral-like particles in brains, and unconfirmed claims of virus isolations. These data are still inconclusive. A notion that Parkinson's disease might have a viral cause has been entertained ever since the observation was made that a form of parkinsonism was a frequent sequela of encephalitis lethargica (von Economo's disease). Similarly, the possible role of a slow infection in amyotrophic lateral sclerosis and in a variety of other demyelinating and degenerative diseases has also been postulated. Although the spectrum of neurologic disease that can be potentially attributed to slow, latent, or chronic viral infections has greatly broadened in recent years, evidence is still scant for incriminating a transmissible agent in these chronic neurologic diseases.

Detels, R., Brody, J. A., McNew, J., and Edgar, A. H.: Further epidemiological studies of subacute sclerosing panencephalitis. Lancet, 2:11, 1973.

Freeman, J. M.: The clinical spectrum and early diagnosis of Dawson's encephalitis. Pediatrics, 75:590, 1969.

Johnson, R. T., and Herndon, R. M.: Virologic studies of multiple sclerosis and other chronic and relapsing neurological diseases. Prog. Med. Virol., in press.

Lampert, P. W., Gajdusek, D. C., and Gibbs, C. J., Jr.: Subacute spongiform virus encephalopathies. Scrapie, kuru, and Creutzfeldt-Jakob disease: A review. Am. J. Pathol., 68:626, 1972.

Narayan, O., Penney, J. B., Jr., Johnson, R. T., Herndon, R. M., and Weiner, L. P.: Etiology of progressive multifocal leukoencephalopathy: Identification of papovavirus. N. Engl. J. Med., 289:1278, 1973.

Roos, R., Gajdusek, D. C., and Gibbs, C. J., Jr.: The clinical characteristics of transmissible Creutzfeldt-Jakob disease. Brain, 96:1, 1973.

Section Fourteen. NUTRITIONAL DISORDERS OF THE NERVOUS SYSTEM

Pierre M. Dreyfus

404. INTRODUCTION

Malnutrition, undernutrition, and the deficiency of specific nutrients such as vitamins are known to affect normal function of some parts of the central and/or the peripheral nervous system. It is well established that an isolated or combined deficiency of vitamins B_1, B_6, B_{12}, niacin, pantothenic acid, and perhaps riboflavin can be associated with a variety of neurologic disorders. However, despite increasing knowledge regarding the role of these vitamins in general metabolism, the specific mechanisms by which a deficiency state affects the normal development and function of the nervous system remain essentially unknown.

Most of the neurologic disorders discussed in this section, although commonly associated with chronic alcoholism, have also been described in malnourished, chronically debilitated, nonalcoholic patients. The inveterate drinker is frequently the victim of a primary nutritional deficiency which alters the normal metabolic activity of the nervous system. During periods of heavy drinking, the chronic alcoholic patient may change the composition of his diet, sharply decreasing vitamin and other essential nutrient intake, because of decreased appetite. Vitamin absorption, intestinal transport, tissue storage, utilization, and conversion to metabolically active forms may be curtailed while the need for many vitamins and essential nutrients increases. In addition to causing ab-

normal vitamin metabolism, the prolonged and abusive intake of alcohol leads to a somewhat unusual and extreme state of nutritional imbalance characterized by an excess of carbohydrate, fatty acid, cholesterol, glycerol, glycogen, and calories combined with a severe deficiency of B vitamins and other essential nutrients. The chronic alcoholic patient may also suffer from a secondary nutritional deficiency which may be the result of a chronic illness, such as infection, anemia, or blood loss, which increases his over-all metabolic demands.

The various nutritional syndromes described in this section may present separately in relatively pure form, but more frequently they occur together in varying combinations, some more prevalent than others. It is not known why, under seemingly identical circumstances, one nutritionally depleted patient develops one or several neurologic syndromes whereas another emerges essentially unscathed. Basic constitutional and genetic differences combined with as yet unknown metabolic factors may underlie the individual response of patients to malnutrition and the chronic ingestion of alcohol.

Nutritional disorders of the nervous system are associated with one or more biochemical lesions which invariably antedate the appearance of symptoms and signs and histopathologic changes. These diseases all share the common neuropathologic attributes of other metabolic disorders of the nervous system by virtue of their predilection for specific areas or parts of the nervous system and because of the bilateral symmetry of the lesions.

405. NUTRITIONAL POLYNEUROPATHY (Dry Beriberi, Alcoholic Neuropathy)

Clinical Manifestations. Nutritional polyneuropathy, the most common of all the nutritional diseases of the nervous system, is characterized by progressive weakness and muscle wasting of varying degrees, involving, symmetrically, the legs more than the arms and the distal muscles more than the proximal ones. Weakness may be almost imperceptible or so severe that the legs are virtually paralyzed and the hands useless. Motor signs and sensory manifestations most frequently occur concomitantly. Abnormalities of sensation are usually striking. Patients complain of aching, coldness, hotness, deadness, numbness, prickliness, and tenderness, most commonly in the calves, on the plantar surfaces of the feet, and in the fingers. Deep pressure or light touch may be extremely unpleasant. In the most severe cases, the muscles become wasted, atrophic, flabby, and tender, and the skin may be dry, red, and shiny. Excessive perspiration of feet and hands is occasionally noted. The deep tendon reflexes, which may be exaggerated in some patients at the onset of the illness, are usually greatly diminished or totally abolished. The sensory loss is symmetrical, most severe distally, and diminishes gradually over more proximal parts; all modalities are involved, some more than others. On rare occasions, severe burning, shooting, lightning, or "electric" types of pain can occur in the absence of clear-cut signs of neuropathy. The term "burning feet syndrome" has been applied to this variety of neuropathic disorder. This syndrome has been encountered in inmates of prison camps, chronic alcoholics, and patients undergoing dialysis for chronic renal failure. In rare instances, nutritional polyneuropathy may be accompanied by vertigo, deafness, hoarseness, dysphagia, and amblyopia.

The mode of evolution and the severity of nutritional polyneuropathy can be quite variable. Usually the onset is insidious, and the progression is slow. Sometimes the course is rapid and abrupt, crippling the patient in a matter of weeks. Recovery requires months and is sometimes incomplete. A temporary worsening of paresthesias and of weakness may follow the start of therapy. In early or mild cases, a prolonged nerve conduction velocity may be the only objective manifestation of the disease. Examination of the cerebrospinal fluid reveals a normal level or a very slight elevation of the protein content.

Pathology. The salient pathologic changes suggest segmental demyelination of peripheral nerves involving distal parts to a greater degree than proximal ones. Occasionally dorsal root ganglia reveal a loss of nerve cells, and axonal reaction may be seen in some of the anterior horn cells of the spinal cord. In patients afflicted with hoarseness and dysphagia, degeneration of the vagus nerve and of the paravertebral sympathetic chain has been observed. It has been speculated that in nutritional polyneuropathy, primary axonal degeneration or a process of "dying back" results in destruction of both the axon and myelin sheaths in the periphery of the largest and longest nerve fibers.

Pathogenesis and Treatment. Nutritional depletion probably alters the normal metabolism of peripheral nerves in several different ways. Both experimental and clinical studies support the view that a deficiency of several of the B vitamins can result in neuropathy. Certain neuropathies respond to the administration of thiamin alone. Recent studies have shown decreased levels of thiamin in the blood, urine, and muscles of patients afflicted with alcoholic neuropathy. Prior to nutritional replenishment, the activity of blood transketolase is usually reduced, and blood pyruvate levels, measured before and after the administration of glucose, may be elevated. The fact that biochemical evidence of thiamin deficiency in nutritional polyneuropathy cannot always be obtained is explained by the slow evolution of this disorder. Whereas the biochemical lesion antedates all clinical manifestations of neuropathy, the latter linger on for many months after the metabolic insult has been removed. A deficiency of pyridoxine has also been blamed for nutritional polyneuropathy. A neuropathic disorder has been observed in patients who were given desoxypyridoxine, a metabolic antagonist of vitamin B_6. The neuropathy that develops in the course of isoniazid (isonicotinic acid hydrazide, INH) therapy can be reversed by pyridoxine alone. Isoniazid causes a deficiency of the essential cofactor pyridoxal phosphate by interfering with phosphorylation of the vitamin. Pyridoxal phosphate is an essential cofactor for a number of enzymatic reactions known to participate in protein metabolism. The specific role of these enzymatic reactions in the metabolism of peripheral nerves remains to be defined. A deficiency of pyridoxal phosphate results in the inadequate synthesis of nicotinic acid from tryptophan. Reduced blood levels of nicotinic acid and nicotinamide have been measured in some patients with nutritional polyneuropathy. Pantothenic acid deficiency may also be involved in the production of some forms of nutritional polyneuropathy. It has been claimed that the administration of pantothenic acid relieves the burning feet syndrome, regardless of its cause.

406. WERNICKE-KORSAKOFF SYNDROME

Of all the disorders of the central nervous system associated with the protracted and abusive intake of alcohol and nutritional depletion, Wernicke's disease and Korsakoff's psychosis are the most frequent. The term "cerebral beriberi" has sometimes been applied to these conditions.

Clinical Manifestation. *Wernicke's disease* is characterized by disturbed ocular motility, ataxia, impaired mentation, and, occasionally, polyneuropathy. The patient may complain of diplopia and unsteadiness of gait, but is usually unaware of his deficit. On examination, bilateral weakness or paralysis of the external recti muscles and paralysis of lateral conjugate gaze are common. Horizontal nystagmus is almost always present, although it sometimes cannot be elicited until abducens function has improved. Vertical nystagmus, particularly on upward gaze, is frequently present. Occasionally there are ptosis, complete paralysis of eye movements, miosis and, very rarely, unreactive pupils. The ataxia, which is almost always present, affects stance and gait primarily. It may be so slight that only special tests for cerebellar function betray its existence. When it is severe, the patient cannot stand or walk without help. Advanced polyneuropathy usually masks cerebellar ataxia. Intention tremor is less common and tends to affect the legs more than the arms. Scanning speech is a rarity. A mild to severe mixed sensory-motor polyneuropathy exists in at least 50 per cent of cases. When first seen, the patient with Wernicke's disease may display symptoms and signs attributable to alcohol withdrawal: i.e., delirium, tremulousness, confusion, agitation, hallucinosis, altered sense perception, and autonomic overactivity. More often, he lacks spontaneity, is apathetic, listless, indifferent, disoriented in time and place, and tends to misidentify objects and people around him. Dull mentation, impaired retentive memory, and general lack of grasp are more common than drowsiness or unconsciousness. With improved nutrition and supplemental thiamin the patient becomes more alert, more attentive, and more readily testable. He may then display a characteristic amnestic confabulatory syndrome known as *Korsakoff's psychosis*. In addition, the patient with Korsakoff's psychosis reveals a number of abnormalities of cognitive function. He may have a great deal of difficulty in forming visual and verbal abstractions. His capacity to shift from one mental set to another and his ability to learn are defective. Perceptual function and concept formation are affected. However, the most prominent and serious mental abnormality seen in Korsakoff's psychosis is the disordered memory function that renders some patients incapable of performing any but the simplest tasks. Recent retentive memory and the ability to learn newly presented material are strikingly impaired. An extensive retrograde amnesia covering a variable period of time is also common. Finally, the patient confabulates and fabricates fictitious stories. Confabulation is by no means unique to Korsakoff's psychosis and tends to disappear in the chronic stages of the illness.

Features of Wernicke's disease and Korsakoff's psychosis are frequently encountered in the same patient. In many instances of Korsakoff's psychosis, slight, residual nystagmus and ataxia may be detected years later. The Wernicke-Korsakoff syndrome may be complicated by other stigmata of chronic malnutrition, including cirrhosis of the liver, anemia, and mucocutaneous lesions of various types. Many patients suffer from postural hypotension, dyspnea, and tachycardia, but full-blown beriberi heart disease is rare. The Wernicke-Korsakoff syndrome usually begins abruptly. Some degree of recovery is the rule, except in the most advanced cases and in those complicated by other illnesses. During the acute stage of the disease the mortality may be as high as 17 per cent. The ocular manifestations, except for nystagmus, respond promptly and dramatically to vitamin therapy. Ataxia improves more slowly, and incomplete recovery occurs in over half the patients; complete recovery from Korsakoff's psychosis occurs in less than one third of patients. The recovered patient usually shows permanent amnesia for the acute phase of the illness.

Pathology. The pathologic alterations that affect the cerebrum and the brainstem are remarkably constant. They almost always involve structures in a bilaterally symmetrical manner. Lesions are invariably seen in the mamillary bodies and the terminal fornices. Lesions in the periaqueductal region of the midbrain, in the floor of the fourth ventricle, in the vicinity of the dorsal motor nucleus of the vagus, and in the anterior superior parts of the cerebellar vermis probably account for the paralysis of gaze, nystagmus, and ataxia. The lesions involving thalamic nuclei (anteromedial, lateral dorsal, and pulvinar) and the hypothalamus and those seen in the mamillary bodies and fornices may underlie some of the psychologic abnormalities, particularly the amnestic syndrome. Microscopically, the lesions consist of necrosis of both nerve cells and myelinated structures. A striking glial reaction involves the center of the lesion. Both endothelial proliferation and hemorrhages are found, but the latter are usually fresh and may represent a nonspecific, terminal change. In the vermis of the cerebellum the principal changes consist of a loss of Purkinje cells and gliosis of the molecular layer of the cortex.

Pathogenesis. There is now an overwhelming body of evidence that favors a specific lack of vitamin B_1 (cocarboxylase) as the main nutritional factor in the Wernicke-Korsakoff syndrome. Most patients give a history of inadequate nutrition and weight loss. Other stigmata of malnutrition, such as loss of subcutaneous fat and skin turgor, mucocutaneous manifestations, and an enlarged liver, are frequent. Clinical studies have shown that the continued intake of alcohol is not followed by aggravation of symptoms, provided adequate nutritional repletion is undertaken promptly. Thiamin alone, given orally or parenterally, can dramatically reverse some of the symptoms and signs. Victor and Adams maintained patients with Wernicke's disease on either glucose or a boiled rice diet containing no vitamins for brief periods, then gave them B vitamins selectively. Ophthalmoplegia, apathy, listlessness, and inattentiveness began to improve within a few hours and cleared completely within a few days after thiamin had been added to the regimen. Nystagmus and ataxia diminished, but Korsakoff's psychosis did not improve significantly. Other B vitamins were ineffective. The improvement of neurologic signs can be closely correlated with levels of blood transketolase activity, which are reduced prior to thiamin administration and increase toward normal with clinical improvement, sometimes within four to five hours after the injection of 25 to 50 mg of thiamin.

Although most commonly associated with chronic alcoholism, Wernicke-Korsakoff syndrome has been observed in clinical settings totally unrelated to abusive drinking. It has been described as a complication of chronic hemodialysis, pernicious vomiting of pregnancy, thyrotoxicosis, and gastric carcinoma.

407. NUTRITIONAL AMBLYOPIA
(Tobacco-Alcohol Amblyopia, Nutritional Retrobulbar Neuropathy)

Clinical Manifestations. A remarkably uniform and stereotyped disorder of vision is encountered occasionally in persons who are chronically undernourished. Characteristically it evolves slowly and subacutely, the mode of onset of symptoms being much the same from patient to patient. Visual impairment usually starts insidiously and reaches a maximum in several weeks to months. Blurred or dim vision, difficulty in reading, photophobia, and retrobulbar discomfort on moving the eyes are the common presenting complaints. On examination, the patient has bilaterally symmetrical central, centrocecal, or paracentral scotomata. Ophthalmoscopic changes are restricted at first to slight redness of the temporal margins of the optic discs; minimal pallor is observed at a later stage. Often, no abnormality is visible. The peripheral visual fields are usually intact. The visual disorder is, to a large extent, reversible with improvement of nutrition.

Pathology. The pathologic change in nutritional amblyopia consists of bilaterally symmetrical loss of myelinated fibers in the central parts of the optic nerves, chiasm, and optic tracts, corresponding in location to the papillomacular bundle. In severe cases, the retina loses macular ganglion cells, probably secondary to the "zonal" destruction of medullated fibers in the retrobulbar parts of the optic nerve.

Pathogenesis. This type of visual disturbance has been encountered in undernourished populations all over the world. It is commonly seen during famine, and among civilian and military prisoners of war. It is endemic in certain parts of Africa, Asia, and South America. Among the more privileged populations in the western world, the syndrome is seen in persons chronically addicted to alcohol or, occasionally, to tobacco, who neglect their nutrition. A similar syndrome also occurs as a complication of vitamin B_{12} deficiency and diabetes mellitus, as well as in patients treated with isoniazid for tuberculosis. This visual disorder accompanies other neurologic syndromes believed to have a nutritional cause, such as *Strachan's syndrome,* in which amblyopia is combined with paresthesias of the feet, hands, trunk, and, occasionally, face, loss of reflexes, dizziness, deafness, hoarseness, spasticity, ataxia, and a variety of mucocutaneous lesions (genital dermatitis, corneal degeneration, glossitis, and stomatitis). In the chronic alcoholic patient, amblyopia may occur in conjunction with Wernicke's disease, cerebellar degeneration, Marchiafava-Bignami's disease, and peripheral neuropathy. In recent years, a nutritional deficiency rather than a toxicity has been held responsible for so-called tobacco-alcohol amblyopia. Detailed clinical and pathologic studies fail to distinguish this type of amblyopia from nutritional amblyopia. In clinical experiments, patients with amblyopia continued their usual consumption of alcohol and tobacco, but ate an adequate diet supplemented by B vitamins. All showed some recovery of visual acuity and a reduction in the size of the scotomata. As yet, the metabolic aberration or specific vitamin deficiency responsible for the development of amblyopia has not been defined. A lack of vitamin B_{12}, thiamin, riboflavin, and pyridoxine or a failure in the detoxification of cyanide present in tobacco smoke has been implicated in the genesis of the syndrome. Except for isolated findings of reduced serum vitamin B_{12} levels, the abnormal urinary excretion of methylmalonic acid and low levels of blood transketolase activity, no specific biochemical abnormalities have been reported in cases of amblyopia.

Treatment. Treatment with oral or parenteral B vitamins and improved nutrition are usually followed by improvement, depending upon the severity of the amblyopia and its duration before therapy is instituted.

408. CEREBELLAR CORTICAL DEGENERATION

Cerebellar cortical degeneration, or parenchymatous cerebellar degeneration, has often been referred to as alcoholic cerebellar degeneration, although well documented instances of cerebellar cortical degeneration have occurred as a result of chronic nutritional depletion not attributable to alcohol. This disorder can be set apart from all other known forms of acquired or familial cerebellar degeneration because of the uniformity of the clinical and pathologic manifestations. The clinical and pathologic findings are discussed in Ch. 431 to 440.

A substantial body of evidence favors the contention that cerebellar degeneration is due to nutritional factors. The history of chronic alcoholic patients is admittedly unreliable, yet most admit improper eating habits. Many patients with cortical cerebellar degeneration give a history of progressive weight loss before the onset of their symptoms. Signs of malnutrition are common, and the cerebellar syndrome frequently occurs in conjunction with cirrhosis and other nutritional complications of alcoholism. Furthermore, a number of nonalcoholic patients develop cortical cerebellar degeneration in the setting of other diseases associated with nutritional depletion, such as pellagra, amebiasis, and protracted vomiting. In general, improved nutrition and supplementary B vitamins result in some degree of improvement of ataxia.

409. CENTRAL PONTINE MYELINOLYSIS

Central pontine myelinolysis is a relatively rare disease characterized by demyelination of the central portion of the pons. It was described originally in patients afflicted with chronic alcoholism and malnutrition but has since been encountered in nonalcoholic patients who were nutritionally deprived. The illness affects adults mainly, but has been reported in children; males and females are equally afflicted. Although the precise clinical course has not yet been defined, the principal neurologic abnormalities are progressive weakness of facial muscles and tongue, causing severe impairment of speech and deglutition. In a number of cases, pseudobulbar phenomena such as emotional lability and pathologic crying have been noted. Quadriparesis at the onset of the illness usually leads to a flaccid and areflexic quadriplegia with Babinski signs. Lack of response to painful stimuli and absence of corneal reflexes are said to be common. Urinary incontinence, decerebrate posture, and respiratory paralysis have been reported in isolated cases. The illness evolves rapidly over a period of two to three weeks, usually ending in coma and eventual death; slow and partial recovery has been observed in rare instances. Examination of the cerebrospinal fluid is unremarkable.

Pathologic examination reveals a focus of demyelination, variable in size and extent, involving the center of the basal portion of the mid and upper pons. Axis cylinders, nerve cells, and blood vessels are relatively well preserved. An appropriate glial and phagocytic reaction is seen within the lesions. Vascular or inflammatory changes are absent. The clinical symptoms and signs depend upon the size of the lesion and, in general, correlate with its anatomic localization.

The pathogenesis of this curious disorder has been much debated, toxic and nutritional factors being the causes most frequently cited. The lesion has been found at postmortem examination in patients suffering from alcoholism, other forms of chronic malnutrition, neoplasia, renal disease, hepatic insufficiency, and a variety of infectious processes. To date, no biochemical data have been obtained.

410. MARCHIAFAVA-BIGNAMI DISEASE

Marchiafava-Bignami disease is among the rarest disorders complicating chronic alcoholism. Few cases have been examined in detail, and it is difficult to state the precise nature of the clinical manifestations. The disease affects males of middle age predominantly. The course is variable; it may evolve over a period of a few days or several months. Complete recovery, although rare, has been documented. The patients are agitated, confused, and have hallucinations (visual, auditory, and gustatory), disturbance of memory, negativism, impaired judgment, and progressive dementia. Neurologic symptoms and signs suggest bilateral involvement of frontal lobes and include disturbance of language, gait and motor skills, seizures, incontinence, rooting, grasping, sucking, and delayed initiation of action. Tremulousness of the hands and dysarthria have been reported.

Pathologically, Marchiafava-Bignami disease is characterized by symmetrical zones of demyelination affecting the central parts of the corpus callosum, beginning in the most anterior parts and extending caudally. Similar changes affect the central parts of the anterior commissure, the optic chiasm and tracts, and, in severe cases, the central white matter of the frontal lobes. In zones of demyelination, axis cylinders tend to be preserved. Occasionally, there are extensive tissue destruction and cavitation. The degree of glial reaction in these areas depends on the chronicity of the process.

Originally, it was assumed that the disease occurred exclusively in males of Italian descent who consumed excessive amounts of crude red wine. The illness has since been encountered in patients of varied ancestry, some of whom were addicted to other types of alcoholic beverages. The characteristic pathologic changes of Marchiafava-Bignami disease have been encountered in conjunction with Wernicke's disease and nutritional amblyopia as well as in malnourished, nonalcoholic patients. It is probable that Marchiafava-Bignami disease is yet another example of a nutritionally determined disease entity characterized by symmetrical and zonal demyelination.

411. VITAMIN B$_{12}$ DEFICIENCY

Definition.   Insufficient absorption of vitamin B$_{12}$ from the gastrointestinal tract can result in a subacute degeneration of the spinal cord, optic nerves, cerebral white matter, and peripheral nerves. Although the neurologic manifestations of vitamin B$_{12}$ deficiency are frequently associated with a macrocytic anemia (pernicious anemia), the latter is not always present. Neurologic symptoms develop in approximately 80 per cent of patients between the ages of 25 and 75 years afflicted with pernicious anemia. They rarely occur as a result of secondary vitamin B$_{12}$ deficiency complicating fish tapeworm *(Diphyllobothrium latum)* infestation, sprue, vegetarianism, or gastrointestinal surgery. (This subject is also dealt with in Ch. 731.)

Clinical Manifestations.   Symptoms and signs of spinal cord involvement *(combined system disease)* constitute the most common neurologic manifestations, and their mode of onset and progression is remarkably uniform. Symmetrical progressive paresthesias of the feet or hands in the form of numbness, tingling, burning, tightness and stiffness, and a feeling of generalized weakness constitute the most frequent initial symptoms. Vague asthenia and lameness progress to a measurable weakness and stiffness of the legs and an unsteadiness of gait that tends to be worse in the dark. The lower limbs may give way unexpectedly. The hands may be stiff and clumsy. When untreated, the illness progresses slowly and relentlessly. Spasticity, ataxia, and paraplegia ensue, often followed by bowel and bladder dysfunction. In the early stages of the disease, examination of the patient often reveals a few objective changes, but eventually signs of disturbed peripheral nerve and posterior and lateral column function become readily apparent. Diminution or loss of position and vibratory sense involves the legs, the hands, and, occasionally, the trunk, and tends to be pronounced. Pain, temperature, and tactile sensation are sometimes blunted over the distal parts of the legs in a pattern suggestive of peripheral nerve involvement. The motor examination reveals weak and, later, spastic legs and extensor plantar responses. The activity of the deep tendon reflexes is variable and appears to depend upon the severity of the illness. The knee jerks are often hyperactive and the ankle jerks absent. In advanced cases, all stretch reflexes may be diminished or absent, but may return when vitamin therapy has been promptly instituted. Psychologic symptoms range from apathy, irritability, and suspiciousness to confusion and dementia, and at times are the presenting neurologic abnormality. On rare occasions, failing vision caused by symmetrical centrocecal scotomata may be the presenting neurologic symptom of vitamin B$_{12}$ deficiency.

Pathology.   The lesions associated with subacute combined degeneration involve in sequence the posterior columns, the lateral columns, and the cerebral white matter. The earliest visible change consists of swelling of individual myelinated nerve fibers in small foci. These lesions subsequently coalesce into large, irregular, spongy, honeycomb-like zones of demyelination. Fibers with the largest diameter are predominantly affected. Axis cylinders tend to be spared. Myelin destruction frequently begins in the cervical and upper thoracic segments of the cord, spreading axially to involve other segments. The cerebral white matter is affected last. The large fibers of the peripheral nerves may show minimal loss of myelin.

Diagnosis. A number of diseases other than vitamin B_{12} deficiency affect the posterior and lateral columns of the spinal cord, the most important being multiple sclerosis, tumors, cervical spondylosis, syphilitic meningomyelitis, and familial spastic paraplegia. These entities can usually be differentiated from one another clinically, but ancillary examinations such as myelography and special tests involving the cerebrospinal fluid may be necessary to establish a correct diagnosis. In B_{12} deficiency of the nervous system, the cerebrospinal fluid is usually normal. The electroencephalogram is often abnormal. The serum vitamin B_{12} content correlates well with the severity of the neurologic impairment and is invariably low in untreated cases. The Schilling test, using radioactive cyanocobalamin, is always positive, and gastric achlorhydria can be demonstrated in almost every instance. Blood and bone marrow examinations are of limited value, particularly when the patient has been treated with folic acid, which corrects the anemia but not the neurologic manifestations. The urinary excretion of methylmalonic acid, an intermediary metabolite in the conversion of propionic acid to succinic acid, is a sensitive indicator of vitamin B_{12} deficiency, but its relation to the lesions in the nervous system is as yet unknown.

Pathogenesis. The pathogenesis of the neurologic manifestations of vitamin B_{12} deficiency is unknown, although it probably differs from the biochemical lesion affecting the hematopoietic system, because the neurologic manifestations are independent of the anemia and may appear when folic acid corrects the anemia. The specific biochemical role of vitamin B_{12} in the nervous system has not yet been elucidated. It is an essential cofactor for at least two enzyme systems which exist in mammalian tissue, including brain: (1) methylmalonyl-CoA isomerase, which converts methylmalonyl-CoA to succinyl-CoA, a step in the utilization of propionic acid, and (2) methylfolate-H_4 methyltransferase, which is responsible for the synthesis of methionine from homocysteine. In experimentally induced vitamin B_{12} deficiency, the activity of both of these enzyme systems is reduced in brain. These enzymes may be essential to the maintenance of the myelin sheath. Recently it has been shown that sural nerve specimens obtained from patients with pernicious anemia incorporate radioactively labeled propionate into abnormal fatty acids that have been identified as C_{15} branched-chain and C_{17} odd-chain acids. The presence of these abnormal fatty acids may explain, in part, the structural changes observed in central and peripheral myelin. An experimental approach to the pathogenesis of the neurologic manifestations of vitamin B_{12} deficiency in animals has been hampered by the absence of white-matter lesions in deficient animals.

Treatment. Prompt initiation of therapy is of the utmost importance, because the early neurologic manifestations can be rapidly and completely reversed. The greatest degree of improvement is achieved in patients treated within three months of onset of symptoms, although variable degrees of amelioration can be attained after longer untreated periods (six to twelve months). In the first two weeks, daily intramuscular injections of 50 μg of cyanocobalamin, or an equivalent amount of liver USP, should be administered. During the next two months, 100 μg of cyanocobalamin should be injected twice a week. For the remainder of his life, the patient should receive a minimum of 100 μg intramuscularly every month to prevent a relapse that might be caused by metabolic stress such as systemic illness or surgery. The administration of oral vitamin preparations containing folic acid must be avoided for patients with pernicious anemia, because folic acid may actually precipitate neurologic complications.

Denny-Brown, D.: Neurological conditions resulting from prolonged and severe dietary restriction. Medicine, 26:41, 1947.

Dreyfus, P. M., and Geel, S. E.: Vitamin and nutritional deficiencies. *In* Albers, R. W., Siege, G. J., Katzmann, R., and Agranoff, B. W. (eds.): Basic Neurochemistry. Boston, Little, Brown & Company, 1972, p. 517.

Gyorgy, P., and Pearson, W. N.: The Vitamins. New York, Academic Press, 1967.

Mayer, R. F., and Garcia-Mullin, R.: Peripheral nerve and muscle disorders associated with alcoholism. *In* Kissin, B., and Begleiter, H. (eds.): The Biology of Alcoholism. New York, Plenum Press, 1972, Chap. 2.

Pant, S. S., Asbury, A. K., and Richardson, E. P., Jr.: The myelopathy of pernicious anemia—a neuropathological reappraisal. Acta Neurol. Scand., 44 (Suppl. 35), 1968.

Victor, M.: The effects of nutritional deficiency on the nervous system. A comparison with effects of carcinoma. *In* Brain, R. L., and Norris, F. H., Jr. (eds.): The Remote Effects of Cancer on the Nervous System. New York, Grune & Stratton, 1965.

Victor, M., and Adams, R. D.: The effects of alcohol upon the nervous system. Am. Res. Ment. Dis. Proc., 32:526, 1953.

Victor, M., Adams, R. D., and Collins, G. H.: The Wernicke-Korsakoff Syndrome, Philadelphia, F. A. Davis Company, 1971.

Wolstenholme, J. E. W.: Thiamine Deficiency: Biochemical Lesions and Their Clinical Significance. Boston, Little, Brown & Company, 1967.

Section Fifteen.

THE DEMYELINATING DISEASES

Labe C. Scheinberg

412. BIOLOGY OF MYELIN

Demyelination or myelin breakdown may be a secondary feature of many disorders of the nervous system such as infections, intoxications, degenerations, vascular lesions, trauma, or deficiency states. However, what concerns us here are the demyelinating diseases, in which the myelin is primarily affected. These have as a common feature the selective involvement of the myelin sheaths with relative sparing of the axons. The distribution of the lesions is random and the cause is unknown. Electrophysiologic studies of the axon have not been made in these diseases; the criteria for the functional and structural integrity of the axon are usually those established by light microscopy. Recently biopsy material of chronic areas of demyelination in the cerebral cortex and subcortical white matter has been studied by means of electron microscopy. These areas reveal denuded axons, vacuolization of the endoplasmic reticulum of oligodendrocytes, fibrous astrocytosis, and evidence of remyelination.

The devastating consequences of myelin breakdown indicate the vital importance of this structure. Recent work has provided much new information about the formation, structure, chemistry, and metabolism of myelin. There is also much new information about its pathology, and many studies have been made of experimental demyelinating disorders.

The neuroglia, namely the oligodendrocyte and astrocyte, are now recognized as more than supporting elements in the brain. They appear to participate in myelin formation, transport of material to the neurons, and the maintenance of the neurons' ionic environment.

The formation of myelin in both the central and peripheral nervous system follows a similar pattern. Central myelin is formed by an extension of the external plasma membrane of the oligodendrocyte wrapping the axons, whereas peripheral myelin is formed by the extension of the Schwann cell membrane. This wrapping produces a structure comprised of layers of concentric, tightly packed membranes of uniform thickness. If one examines the C fibers of the peripheral nerve with the electron microscope, one sees the axon-myelin relationship in its simplest form. The individual membranes of the Schwann cell and the axon membrane of the C fiber each represent "unit membranes," which are equivalent to the plasma membranes of the cells. The unit membrane of the Schwann cell or oligodendrocyte closes upon itself to form the major and minor period lines of myelin. The internal surface becomes apposed to form the dark major line, and the external surfaces give rise to the interaperiod line. The results of studies employing x-ray diffraction, electron microscopy, and lipid analyses suggest that each unit membrane consists of a sandwich of a bimolecular lipid leaflet between parallel layers of hydrated protein, in close contact with the polar groups of the lipids. The lipids that make up this leaflet appear to be interdigitated molecules of cerebroside, phospholipid, and cholesterol. Detailed chemical analysis of myelin reveals protein (primarily proteolipid protein) 22 per cent of dry weight, and lipid 78 per cent of dry weight. The lipids are in approximately equal molar ratios of cholesterol and phospholipids with about one half as much galactolipid. The lipids in the myelin sheath, once deposited at the time of its formation, undergo little subsequent turnover. The biologic half-life of cholesterol in myelin is about one year, compared to about ten days in other biologic membranes.

The myelin sheath is a compact, highly organized membrane structure that must be regarded as one of the more permanent tissue elements of the body. However, myelin should not be considered as metabolically inactive, because white matter accounts for about 30 per cent of total cerebral oxygen consumption and the glial cells utilize about two thirds of this.

THE DEMYELINATING DISORDERS

413. INTRODUCTION

The foregoing considerations suggest that demyelination must be considered as a basic disorder of the oligodendrocyte or the Schwann cell. To consider demyelina-tion solely as myelin breakdown, ignoring the fact that the myelin lamellae are an integral part of the parent glial cell, may be contradictory to the pathogenesis. The etiologic agent may attack either the perikaryon of the glial cell or its plasma membrane to produce demyelination.

Prior to a consideration of the pathogenesis of demyelinative disorders, one must make some attempt to classify the varied primary disorders of myelin. In 1957 Poser suggested classification into two basic types. One, a so-called "myelinoclastic" or demyelinating type, includes disorders in which myelin forms normally to a certain age and then for unknown reasons breaks down. This includes the most common demyelinating disease, multiple sclerosis, and also acute disseminated encephalomyelitis and certain other disorders. The other, the "dysmyelinative" type, includes disorders in which a presumed familial inborn error of metabolism results in defective myelin formation. The category includes the so-called leukodystrophies or some of the diffuse scleroses and lipidoses of the nervous system and the aminoacidurias resulting from genetic enzymatic disorders.

Pathogenesis. In most demyelinating disorders, the cause remains unknown. Demyelination is the typical response of white matter to noxious stimuli not severe enough to cause complete necrosis of the tissue, and almost any infectious, nutritional, vascular, or toxic disorder can result in demyelination. At present there is insufficient evidence to incriminate any one cause. Some workers interpret present evidence as supporting most strongly an allergic basis for most of the primary demyelinating disorders, with genetic and geographic factors influencing susceptibility, whereas others favor a viral cause based on epidemiologic, electron microscopic, and tissue culture studies. Autoradiographic studies in experimental allergic encephalomyelitis, using tritiated precursors of DNA, RNA, and protein, have shown a rise in circulating plasma-like cells prior to onset of neurologic signs. Supernatant from cultures of these cells produces demyelination in tissue culture of rat cerebellum similar to that produced by serum from multiple sclerosis patients.

The strongest stimulus for suspecting allergic factors in the pathogenesis of the demyelinating diseases lies in the similarity of their pathologic changes to those of rabies encephalomyelitis. Rivers and co-workers in 1933 showed that multiple injections of normal rabbit brain tissue in monkeys resulted in encephalomyelitis with lesions similar to those seen in rabies postvaccinal encephalomyelitis. This was followed by the extensive investigations of Kabat, Wolf, and co-workers in the 1940's, who demonstrated that experimental allergic encephalomyelitis (EAE) could be produced in monkeys by a few injections of adult homologous, heterologous, or autologous central nervous system tissue mixed with paraffin oil and killed mycobacteria (Freund's adjuvant). White matter appeared more encephalitogenic than gray, whereas peripheral nerve and fetal (unmyelinated) brain were ineffectual as encephalitogens. EAE is not transferable to other animals by serum, although the serum contains complement-fixing antibodies to brain. The pathologic change is primarily in the white matter of the central nervous system, with perivascular and meningeal inflammation and demyelination. These findings are in many instances indistinguishable from those in certain human demyelinating disorders.

This pioneering work has been followed by genetic, immunologic, biochemical, and ultrastructural investigations. It has been shown that there are variations in susceptibility to EAE among various species and strains within species. Other workers have successfully transferred EAE by means of sensitized lymphoid cells in isologous (inbred) strains. Finally, workers have found that serum from EAE animals or from some patients with multiple sclerosis causes destruction of myelin in cultures of transplanted brain tissue.

The nature of the encephalitogen in EAE has been extensively studied, and most work indicates that it is a basic protein of myelin (Kies and Alvord, 1965). Specifically sensitized lymphocytes are found in immunofluorescence studies to take up this myelin protein. The demyelination in EAE has recently been shown in electron microscopic studies to be a result of the phagocytosis of oligodendroglial cells and dissolution of the myelin lamellae by mononuclear cells.

The relationship of EAE to the spontaneous demyelinating disorders is still conjectural. Since the brain lacks a lymphatic drainage, myelin antigens are inaccessible to the body's reticuloendothelial system. It is plausible to assume that in certain situations the body could produce myelin autoantibodies (cellular or humoral) that would react with central nervous system myelin and produce demyelinating lesions. How the normally inaccessible myelin autoantigens reach the antibody-forming site and under what circumstances this occurs are still unknown.

The other major theory on the etiology of multiple sclerosis based on epidemiologic studies is that it is of viral origin related to exposure in late childhood or early adolescence. Higher familial incidence is consistent with exposure in early life, whereas twin studies suggest little if any genetic influence. Family and migration studies of individuals who have moved from high risk areas to low risk areas suggest a latency period of 3 to 23 years between exposure and clinical onset.

The role of a myxovirus was first suggested by the finding of significantly higher concentrations of measles antibodies in patients with multiple sclerosis. Recently paramyxovirus-like particles have been found as intranuclear inclusions in the macrophages about acute lesions in multiple sclerosis autopsy and biopsy material. Using tissue culture techniques, paramyxovirus has been isolated from the brains of patients with multiple sclerosis.

414. ACUTE NECROTIZING HEMORRHAGIC ENCEPHALOMYELITIS

This is a rare and fulminant variant of demyelinating disease that often progresses to death in days or weeks. The disease is characterized by a rapid course, fever, headache, convulsions, progressive change in state of consciousness from drowsiness to coma, nuchal rigidity, and hemiplegia or quadriplegia. The cerebrospinal fluid examination reveals a pleocytosis up to several thousand white blood cells that are predominantly polymorphonuclear leukocytes, and an elevated protein content. On pathologic examination, there are large foci of hemorrhagic necrosis of white matter. Although most patients succumb within a few weeks, there are rare alleged reports of recovery. There appears to be an experimental allergic model of this disorder with similarities on histologic examination. The only therapy that can be offered is supportive, though ACTH and corticosteroids should be tried.

415. ACUTE DISSEMINATED ENCEPHALOMYELITIS

Occasionally acute neurologic symptoms may occur without apparent preceding infection. The clinical picture is dependent on the location of the lesions and may include the symptoms and signs of meningitis, encephalitis, myelitis, or any combination of the preceding. Some cases blend indistinguishably into chronic, typical multiple sclerosis and so may represent the initial acute attack of that disease. Other cases may be uniphasic, and the patient may recover with or without neurologic residua and have no further attacks. Only prolonged follow-up with a recurrence or progression of symptoms can enable one to diagnose acute multiple sclerosis and exclude acute disseminated encephalomyelitis.

416. MULTIPLE SCLEROSIS

Definition. Multiple or disseminated sclerosis is the most common demyelinating disorder. It is usually pleomorphic and difficult to define completely in the absence of specific diagnostic tests. There are a number of well recognized and readily diagnosed syndromes, but borderline cases may be difficult to categorize clinically and pathologically. Generally it is chronic and relapsing, but fulminating attacks occur and as many as 30 per cent of

---

TABLE 1.   Primary Disorders of Myelin

A. Demyelinating (myelinoclastic or leukoencephalopathic): breakdown of normally constituted myelin
  1. Postimmunization encephalomyelitis (smallpox and rabies vaccination, other immunizations)
  2. Parainfectious encephalomyelitis (postinfectious, postexanthematous, etc.)
  3. Acute necrotizing hemorrhagic encephalomyelitis (rare)
  4. Multiple sclerosis (disseminated sclerosis) and possible variants, including:
    a. Acute disseminated encephalomyelitis
    b. Optic and retrobulbar neuritis
    c. Transverse myelitis, including necrotizing myelopathy
    d. Neuromyelitis optica (Devic's)
    e. Transitional sclerosis
  5. Diffuse sclerosis (Schilder's cerebral sclerosis)
  6. Concentric sclerosis (Balo's) (rare)
  7. Progressive multifocal leukoencephalopathy (viral)
  8. Subacute sclerosing panencephalitis (viral)
  9. Central pontine myelinolysis (nutritional deficiency?) (see Ch. 409)
  10. Progressive subcortical encephalopathy (Binswanger's disease, vascular)
B. Dysmyelinating (leukodystrophic): Failure to form normally constituted myelin, possibly secondary to genetically determined errors of myelin anabolism
  1. Simple storage type (metachromatic leukodystrophy, glial insufficiency type of sulfatidosis)
  2. Sudanophilic type (Pelizaeus-Merzbacher disease)
  3. Globoid cell type (Krabbe's disease)
  4. Spongy degeneration of white matter (spongy sclerosis or Canavan's disease)
  5. Other lipidoses (Tay-Sachs disease, Gaucher's disease, gargoylism, etc.)
  6. Aminoacidurias (phenylketonuria, maple syrup urine disease, etc.)

patients tend to progress steadily from the onset. The symptoms and signs reflect involvement of central myelin, but occasionally symptoms are typical of neuronal or gray-matter involvement. Multiple sclerosis is a disease of the central white matter with "lesions separated in time and space."

Incidence.   The prevalence of multiple sclerosis in the United States varies from about 10 per 100,000 in the South to 60 per 100,000 in the North, with similar prevalence and distribution in Europe. The disease affects males and females about equally. About 67 per cent of cases begin between the ages of 20 and 40 years and 95 per cent between 10 and 50 years.

Populations residing between latitudes 40° N and 40° S (tropical and subtropical zones) have a low risk of multiple sclerosis. With a few notable exceptions, all populations residing north of this latitude in North America and Europe are at higher risk. Other exceptions to these generalizations are found in other parts of the world; e.g., a low incidence is reported in the Union of South Africa and in Japan. Efforts have been made to correlate these geographic variations with dietary intake, temperature, solar radiation, and geomagnetic latitude, without success. Racial factors seem to play little part in the United States, because the incidence in blacks is almost the same as in whites.

Genetic studies have contributed indirectly to theories on the etiology of multiple sclerosis. There are occasional reports of a greater family incidence than could be expected by chance, but these fail to exclude the common effects of environmental factors. A purely hereditary basis seems to be excluded by concordance studies in identical twins.

Pathology.   The external surface of the brain and cord generally shows no abnormality. Occasionally there is atrophy of the optic nerves, and rarely there is focal or generalized atrophy of the cerebral hemispheres. Acute large lesions may cause swelling of the cord. Rarely there may be sufficient focal swelling of the cerebrum to give the appearance of a neoplasm in roentgenologic contrast studies.

Cut sections of the brain or spinal cord reveal numerous scattered, grayish, well defined lesions that are slightly depressed and vary in diameter from a few millimeters to a few centimeters. These are found throughout the white matter of the brain, optic nerves, and spinal cord and occasionally extend into gray matter. The number of lesions is usually greater than would be expected from the clinical picture.

Microscopic abnormalities depend on the age of the lesion. Acute lesions show an infiltration of microglial phagocytes and mononuclear cells about vessels, as well as scattered in the lesion itself. The myelin sheaths are affected to varying degrees, from partial to complete destruction, with relative sparing of axons, glia, and other structures. In more severe lesions there may be total destruction of tissue and cyst formation. As the lesions become chronic, there is a proliferation of glial cells and fibers to give the typical "sclerotic plaque." The axons in these areas may be preserved or destroyed.

Aggravating Factors.   An *infective process* (upper respiratory infection, "influenza," urinary tract infection, gastroenteritis, etc.) is said to precede the initial attack or a relapse of multiple sclerosis in 10 to 40 per cent. *Immunizations* are without apparent effect on the course of the disease, and any exacerbations seen following these are probably coincidental.

Many workers have stated that *pregnancy* aggravates the disease, but this is open to question. The disease and pregnancy occur in the same age group, and although some studies show a higher incidence in married childbearing women, more attacks occur during the puerperium than during pregnancy itself. The physician must consider many nonmedical factors when advising on this problem. Pregnancy is generally considered nondeleterious to the course of multiple sclerosis in any patient who has had no attack in two years.

There seems to be no clear-cut association of attack or relapse with surgical procedures, and indications for *surgery* in patients with multiple sclerosis should be judged solely on their merit.

Trauma has likewise been incriminated in an almost anecdotal manner, but there is no statistical evidence to support a relationship between peripheral trauma and the onset or relapses of multiple sclerosis. There is a tendency for patients to associate trauma with the onset of an attack or relapse, but in many cases it is more likely that the trauma resulted from the disability of multiple sclerosis. Similarly, *emotional stress* has been incriminated as a precipitant of attacks or relapses of multiple sclerosis. This is difficult to substantiate, but it is reasonable to assume that cerebral changes in multiple sclerosis make it difficult for the patient to cope with emotional stress.

Certain diagnostic procedures such as lumbar puncture, pneumoencephalography, cerebral angiography, and myelography have been implicated in the worsening of symptoms in multiple sclerosis. However, these

TABLE 2.   Frequency of Occurrence of First Symptom of Multiple Sclerosis in Cases Proved by Clinical Study and Autopsy

Symptom	Autopsy (Carter et al.) (46 Cases)	Autopsy (Poser) (111 Cases)	Clinical Diagnosis (Carter et al.) (539 Cases)
	per cent	*per cent*	*per cent*
Weakness	42	39	54
Diplopia, impaired vision	35	32	21
Tremor, ataxia, incoordination	20	6	19
Paresthesias	13	16	32
Pain	11	1	—
Sphincter impairment	11	1	7
Dizziness or vertigo	7	1	8
Changes in muscle tone	7	—	—
Facial pain	2	—	—
Mental changes	2	2	—
Seizures	—	—	3

procedures are performed usually in patients whose disease is progressing or soon after an attack or relapse. They should be performed in cases in which there are serious questions whether a neoplasm exists in the nervous system, and not simply in frustration because "there's nothing else to be done."

Clinical Manifestations. The clinical picture of multiple sclerosis is pleomorphic, but there are usually sufficient typical features to enable one to diagnose the disorder in the absence of a specific diagnostic test or without extensive "excluding" diagnostic procedures. The disease is chronic, often characterized by exacerbations and remissions, with evidence of multiple lesions in central white matter occurring in young adults without other systemic disorders. The symptoms of central white matter involvement are usually those of supranuclear weakness, incoordination, paresthesias, and visual complaints. Other symptoms and signs that are more characteristic of lesions in gray matter, e.g., aphasia, seizures, fasciculations, and neurogenic atrophy, are rare. Mental changes have an intermediate incidence and affect perhaps 30 per cent of patients.

The onset may be acute, with symptoms appearing within minutes to hours, or it may be insidious, with gradual, slow progression of symptoms over a period of months.

The frequency of occurrence of the first symptom of multiple sclerosis is given in Table 2.

The weakness usually begins or is most prominent in the lower extremities, but the upper extremities may be involved. When both lower extremities are involved, there are usually accompanying urinary complaints such as urgency or frequency. The weakness may be minimal, or there may be a total paralysis. There are usually upper motor neuron signs such as spasticity, hyperreflexia, and pathologic reflexes.

Visual complaints include blurring of vision with a central scotoma and decreased visual acuity or diplopia with extraocular paresis and nystagmus.

The incoordination is seen as ataxia or clumsiness and intention tremor of the upper extremities. Often a combination of spastic-ataxic gait is seen.

The paresthesias may involve any or all of the extremities. Usually there is impairment of vibratory sense and position sense in the lower extremities, whereas cutaneous sensation is relatively spared.

The typical clinical course of multiple sclerosis is one of exacerbations and remissions over a period of years,

with increasing neurologic deficits caused by an increasing number of disseminated lesions. Less frequent are (1) an acute, severe course progressing to death in a few days or weeks; (2) a chronic, progressive course over a period of years; and (3) a benign form with relatively few presenting symptoms and signs and long-lasting remissions. In middle age the insidious onset of a progressive spastic paraparesis is often seen as the major clinical manifestation, particularly in women.

Multiple sclerosis is sometimes divided into clinical types, depending upon which portion of the neuraxis is most involved, e.g., spinal, cerebral, brainstem-cerebellar, or mixed. The most common form is spinal with prominent features of spastic paraparesis, lower extremity paresthesias, and urinary complaints. The brainstem-cerebellar variety with prominent visual complaints, cranial nerve signs, nystagmus, vertigo, and incoordination is also common, but the cerebral form with mental changes and hemiparesis and hemisensory changes is uncommon.

Although most cases may be classified as one of these forms early in the course, almost all patients appear to have a mixed type of involvement after about 15 years.

In Table 3 may be noted the frequency of various symptoms and signs of multiple sclerosis in clinical and autopsy series reported by Carter et al. and by Poser.

Certain uncommon symptoms and signs such as nausea, vomiting, facial pain, seizures, dysphagia, atrophy, hearing loss, tinnitus, and changes in states of consciousness occur in 2 to 10 per cent of cases. Signs such as internuclear ophthalmoplegia are highly characteristic of multiple sclerosis; headache and aphasia are rare.

Laboratory Data. Abnormal findings in multiple sclerosis are usually confined to the cerebrospinal fluid. In the acute disease, there may be a mild mononuclear pleocytosis of as much as 200 to 300 cells per cubic millimeter, but usually less than 40. The protein content is usually normal or slightly elevated (50 to 100 mg per 100 ml); values higher than this are rare. The gamma globulin content is elevated in about two thirds of the cases and, correspondingly, there is often an abnormal colloidal gold curve (first or second zone), accompanied by a negative serologic test for syphilis.

The electroencephalogram may be mildly abnormal in about two thirds of cases, revealing either focal or generalized abnormalities.

Diagnosis. Because of the pleomorphic nature of the disease, it is often necessary to exclude many other

TABLE 3.   Frequency of Occurrence of Symptoms and Signs in Course of Multiple Sclerosis

	Carter et al. (46 Cases)	Poser (111 Cases)
	per cent	*per cent*
Weakness (symptom or sign)	89	96
Abnormal movements	67	
Abnormal reflexes (absent superficials, Babinski signs, or hyperreflexia)	99	95
Sphincter and genital difficulties	78	82
Visual disturbance (symptom or sign)	100	85
Nystagmus (any type)	85	70
Disc pallor, atrophy, decreased acuity	75	85
Third nerve impairment (and internuclear ophthalmoplegia)	67	
Tremor, ataxia	93	79
Impaired vibration and position sense	81	58
Impaired touch, pain, temperature sense	35	35
Mental changes (symptom or sign)	61	45
Paresthesias	44	65
Pain	42	19
Vertigo or dizziness	18	15

neurologic disorders. Most often one must consider spinal cord, brainstem or cerebellar tumors, degenerative diseases such as the spinocerebellar degenerations, and combined system disease.

The fact that multiple sclerosis has a remitting nature in many instances and the dissemination of symptoms and signs should indicate that one is not dealing with an expanding lesion involving the nervous system. If all the symptoms and signs can be explained by a single lesion, then one should assume that the condition is not multiple sclerosis. If the patient complains of headache, seizures, or progressive focal neurologic signs, which are uncommon in multiple sclerosis, and if these are accompanied by abnormalities such as increased cerebrospinal fluid pressure, roentgenographic changes in the skull or spine, and marked elevation of cerebrospinal fluid protein, then one must proceed further to exclude a neoplasm. This can be done in most cases by a neuroroentgenologic procedure such as myelography, pneumoencephalography, cerebral angiography, or computerized transaxial tomographic scan. Vascular disease, particularly that involving the brainstem, can be confused with multiple sclerosis in middle-aged patients. In some of these cases only prolonged follow-up reveals the true diagnosis.

Certain degenerative disorders of the nervous system can be confused with multiple sclerosis. However, the former tend to have a family history, to be slowly progressive without remission, and to confine themselves to systems, e.g., cerebellar, extrapyramidal, or motor system. In the differential diagnosis of spastic paraparesis of middle age, one should consider, respectively, motor neuron disease (amyotrophic lateral sclerosis), cervical spondylosis, or spinal cord tumor. The first has no sensory abnormalities, and the latter two both have characteristic roentgenologic abnormalities. Combined systemic disease can be excluded in most cases by hematologic studies and gastric analysis.

Treatment.   There are several aspects to the management of multiple sclerosis. The first is the possible benefit to be gained from ACTH or corticosteroids during acute exacerbations. Many authorities advise a course of three to four weeks of therapy with suitable precautions against complications, and some recent controlled studies have shown that this treatment has some benefit in the acute symptom complex. There are no indications for long-term maintenance therapy on ACTH or corticosteroids, and the risks outweigh any possible benefit. Preliminary studies with other immunosuppressive agents indicate that the course of the disease may be stabilized with fewer exacerbations. From a consideration of the pathology it is unreasonable to expect alleviation of symptoms that have been static for many months.

The second aspect is the general management of the patient. During acute exacerbations, especially severe ones, there may be some benefit from bed rest, although the demoralizing effects of prolonged immobilization must be avoided. The prevention of complications, especially genitourinary infections, bedsores, contractures, and flexor spasms, requires adequate nursing care, physiotherapy, and occasionally more specific measures such as rhizotomy, tenotomy, antimicrobials, and other indicated measures. Exhausting physiotherapy with active exercises offers no benefit and may even be harmful. Certain other measures such as unnecessary catheterization have serious consequences and should be avoided.

The third aspect of patient care is the management of long-term disabling illness with an unpredictable course. Initially there arises the question of informing the patient, and this must be dealt with on an individual basis after considering the emotional makeup of the patient and his family, the patient's responsibilities, and other factors. This is particularly important in relation to pregnancy. The route of delivery is an obstetrical decision.

One must encourage and support the patient to remain active and yet protect him from constantly seeking untried and potentially harmful therapies or unnecessary diagnostic tests and operations.

Prognosis.   In the early stages of the disease it is not possible accurately to predict the course, although certain symptoms seem to indicate a better prognosis. Monosymptomatic and acute symptoms lasting hours to weeks tend to give a better prognosis than polysymptomatic or slowly progressive manifestations. Cranial nerve, visual, and sensory symptoms carry a better prognosis for remission or a benign course than do motor or cerebellar symptoms. More than half the cases remit after an initial attack, but one cannot predict the next attack. The remission of certain symptoms, e.g., retrobulbar neuritis, may be so complete as to make the clinician doubt the history.

Within the first five years after onset, about 70 per cent of patients are able to be employed, although with occasional interruptions in some cases. By the end of ten years this drops off to 50 per cent. At the end of 20 years 35 per cent are still employed, with minor interruptions, and about 20 per cent of patients succumb to complications of the disease by this time. The major disabilities are spasticity, disturbances of coordination, and disturbance in bladder and bowel function.

Life expectancy varies considerably, ranging from a few weeks to over 50 years regardless of whether one considers hospitalized, severe cases or the more benign forms. The average life expectancy is from 13 to more than 25 years after onset. The cause of death is often an intercurrent infection, usually respiratory or genitourinary.

417. POSSIBLE MULTIPLE SCLEROSIS VARIANTS

OPTIC AND RETROBULBAR NEURITIS

Optic neuritis is a term used to describe involvement of the optic nerve as a result of inflammation, demyelination, or degeneration. When the site of the lesion is intraocular, ophthalmoscopy reveals papilledema and the terms *papillitis* or intraocular neuritis are employed. *Retrobulbar neuritis* indicates involvement of the orbital or intracranial optic nerve behind the eye. There is often a predilection for the papillomacular bundle, producing a characteristic central scotoma but usually with minimal or absent ophthalmoscopic abnormalities in the acute stage.

Optic neuritis has many known causes, such as nutritional deficiency, intoxications (tobacco, alcohol), local inflammatory conditions (sinusitis, meningitis, orbital infections), and metabolic diseases (diabetes mellitus, pernicious anemia, other vitamin deficiencies). Once these have been excluded, demyelinating disease must be considered as a likely cause. In several large series of patients who presented with retrobulbar neuritis and were followed for many years, 15 to 30 per cent later developed other manifestations of multiple sclerosis. Conversely, about 50 per cent of patients with multiple sclerosis exhibit symptoms of optic neuritis at some time during the course of the disease.

Both optic and retrobulbar neuritis are characterized by an abrupt or progressive loss of vision that is rarely total and is usually unilateral. Associated with the visual loss may be pain in and around the eye that is accentuated by ocular movement. There may be tenderness on palpation of the eyeball. Visual testing reveals decreased acuity and central or paracentral scotomas. In *intraocular neuritis* or *papillitis*, the optic disc appears inflamed, and there may be hyperemia, blurred margins, and even elevation. A few hemorrhages may be seen in the retina adjacent to the disc. In *retrobulbar neuritis* the ophthalmoscopic picture is normal, but the features are otherwise similar to those of optic neuritis.

It is essential to differentiate optic neuritis from papilledema associated with increased intracranial pressure or other conditions. Papilledema is almost always bilateral, and vision is usually well preserved until late in the course. The disc elevation is usually greater in papilledema, and the only visual field defect is an enlarged blind spot. In optic neuritis the cerebrospinal fluid pressure is almost always normal, and there may be other findings indicative of multiple sclerosis.

Optic and retrobulbar neuritis may be treated with ACTH or corticosteroids. However, almost complete spontaneous recovery often occurs, and the benefits of therapy are difficult to assess.

The prognosis in a single attack of optic or retrobulbar neuritis is usually good. There may be complete recovery, or there may be residual visual field defects, temporal pallor of the discs, or optic atrophy. The visual acuity may be further impaired with subsequent attacks, but complete visual loss is rare.

ACUTE TRANSVERSE MYELITIS

Acute transverse myelitis may appear as the initial event in a subsequently typical form of multiple sclerosis, or it may develop during the course of the disease. The findings include complete or partial paralysis of both legs or of all four limbs, variable sensory loss, and bladder and bowel involvement. The condition is described in detail in Ch. 385.

Subacute necrotizing myelopathy is often associated with vascular malformations of the spinal cord or thrombophlebitis (Foix-Alajouanine syndrome). In acute necrotizing myelopathy there is hemorrhagic necrosis of the spinal cord without any associated vascular malformation. Such cases, which are rare, show a rapidly ascending motor and sensory paralysis with polymorphonuclear cells in the cerebrospinal fluid, and death may occur in weeks or months.

NEUROMYELITIS OPTICA (DEVIC'S DISEASE)

This clinical syndrome is characterized by acute transverse myelitis and optic neuritis. It may be considered to be a variant of multiple sclerosis and may occur as the initial illness or later during the course of the disease. There may be sudden loss of vision in both eyes, with central scotoma or sudden onset of paraplegia with sensory loss. The ocular involvement may be due to optic or retrobulbar neuritis, and the transverse myelitis may be partial or complete. Days or weeks may elapse between the onsets of the two symptom complexes. In severe cases the motor symptoms tend to be permanent, but otherwise the course, laboratory data, and treatment are similar to those of multiple sclerosis.

TRANSITIONAL SCLEROSIS

Transitional sclerosis is probably a pathologic variant of multiple sclerosis in which the disseminated plaques tend to become confluent, creating large areas of myelin loss. Clinically these cases are indistinguishable from cases of typical multiple sclerosis. Transitional sclerosis probably represents an intermediate pathologic form between multiple sclerosis and Schilder's cerebral sclerosis.

418. DIFFUSE SCLEROSIS

There is a group of progressive neurologic disorders of young patients who manifest severe neurologic deficits of various types and progressive visual and mental deterioration. In three publications from 1912 to 1924, Schilder described three cases of diffuse disease of white matter that he proposed grouping under the name *encephalitis periaxialis diffusa* (now called Schilder's disease). Actually, Schilder had described three distinct entities, and these, plus cases subsequently described, are of three types: (1) the myelinoclastic group, closely related to multiple sclerosis, referred to hereafter as Schilder's cerebral sclerosis; (2) the leukoencephalitides, which are probably of viral origin; and (3) the dysmyelinating group or leukodystrophies, which are probably due to genetically determined enzymatic defects.

SCHILDER'S CEREBRAL SCLEROSIS

The demyelinative disorders in this group are related pathologically to multiple sclerosis. The characteristic lesions are large, bilateral areas of demyelination in the cerebral hemispheres with preservation of the subcortical "U" fibers, a relative sparing of the axons, and a replacement gliosis. Recent lesions show a perivascular inflammatory reaction. Swelling of the cerebral hemispheres in acute, fulminant cases may rarely cause increased intracranial pressure and may mimic brain tumor. In more chronic lesions there is a suggestion of confluence of smaller plaques to make the large areas of demyelination. In some cases there are, in addition, randomly scattered small lesions in other areas of the central nervous system, and these have been called "diffuse-disseminated sclerosis" or transitional sclerosis. These cases may represent an intermediate form of the same process, diffuse sclerosis representing one extreme whereas multiple sclerosis represents the other.

The disease may occur at any age, but unlike multiple sclerosis the majority of cases begin in childhood. About half the cases begin prior to the age of 10 years, and three fourths begin before the age of 20. The disease is relatively rare; fewer than 50 autopsied cases have been reported. Both sexes are equally involved.

The onset is usually insidious but may be acute. It is usually slowly progressive, but there may be successive bursts to simulate the course of multiple sclerosis. A typical presenting picture is of insidious mental deterioration with loss of recently acquired intellectual achievements, and this progresses slowly to dementia. Many patients develop aphasia, apraxia, and dysarthria. Various psychiatric syndromes may be manifested. Visual loss with cortical blindness is characteristic, and auditory complaints with cortical deafness may follow involvement of the cortical radiations. Motor symptoms such as hemiparesis may be prominent, and seizures of various types tend to appear during the course. Other neurologic symptoms and signs such as vertigo, ataxia, nystagmus, paraplegia, or extraocular palsies are less frequent.

The course varies from days to many years, with an average duration of about three years. Terminally patients are severely demented and often in a decerebrate state.

Laboratory findings are usually abnormal only in the cerebrospinal fluid and electroencephalogram. The CSF pressure may be elevated, and there may be mild pleocytosis and elevation of protein content. The gamma globulin content is usually abnormal. The EEG findings vary from paroxysmal discharges to focal slowing. Patients with increased intracranial pressure may have misleading indications of a mass lesion in encephalographic or angiographic studies. There is no specific therapy.

BALO'S CONCENTRIC SCLEROSIS

Some cases of demyelinating disease have an unusual concentric arrangement of the demyelinating lesions of the cerebrum. Balo gave these the name *encephalitis periaxialis concentrica*. This rare entity probably represents a variant of Schilder's cerebral sclerosis.

419.   LEUKODYSTROPHIES

This group includes heredofamilial diseases in which normal myelin is probably not formed because of some genetically determined enzymatic defect. The classification is not completely satisfactory; the group tends to merge with the lipidoses of the nervous system, so that authorities differ in their classifications. Only further elucidation of the enzymatic defects of myelin metabolism in these disorders will lead to a satisfactory classification.

METACHROMATIC LEUKOENCEPHALOPATHY

These are otherwise known as the glial insufficiency forms or the sulfatide lipidoses. This group includes those cases in which large amounts of metachromatic material accumulate in the central nervous system. The disease is inherited as an autosomal recessive and begins in the first ten years of life, usually with gait disturbances, convulsions of various types, hypotonia, ocular palsies, and dysarthria. There are coarse tremors of the extremities and, terminally, severe mental deterioration and spasticity or rigidity.

The cerebrospinal fluid protein is usually elevated (100 to 200 mg per 100 ml), and metachromatic material (staining red with toluidine blue) can be found in the urinary sediment. The metachromatic material also collects in the kidney, liver, gallbladder, spleen, or peripheral nerves, and biopsy confirms the diagnosis. Gallbladder function studies may be abnormal. The course is one of progressive neurologic deterioration leading to death in one to four years, although some patients have survived 10 to 20 years. Some cases may begin later in childhood and run a more protracted course. The disorder is one of the more common leukodystrophies and can often be diagnosed in life. There is no therapy.

SUDANOPHILIC LEUKODYSTROPHY
(Pelizaeus-Merzbacher Disease)

This is a very rare, familial leukodystrophy, predominantly of males. The pathologic changes consist of extensive diffuse demyelination in the cerebral hemispheres and cerebellum. The disease appears to be transmitted as a sex-linked recessive and begins in early life with a slowly progressive course. Disturbances of coordination such as intention tremor, gait disturbances, dysarthria, spasticity, abnormal movements, and mental deterioration occur. The illness lacks pathognomonic features, but the predominant progressive cerebellar symptoms in a male with a positive family history should make one suspect the entity. It runs a course of several years or more before fatal termination. There is no therapy.

GLOBOID CELL LEUKODYSTROPHY
(Krabbe's Disease)

This rare familial type of leukodystrophy begins in infancy and rapidly progresses to death. The typical pathologic feature is the deposition of cerebrosides in globoid cells of the brain. These may be glial or another type of macrophage. The cases described by Krabbe began at about four months of age with seizures, spastic quadriplegia, abnormal startle responses, cortical blindness, and optic atrophy, and progressed rapidly to death in one or two years. The protein in the cerebrospinal fluid is usually elevated. There is no therapy.

SPONGY DEGENERATION OF WHITE MATTER
(Canavan's Disease)

In this rare familial leukodystrophy there is widespread demyelination accompanied by microscopic vacuolation that gives rise to a spongy appearance. It appears to be transmitted as an autosomal recessive and seems to be most common among Jews. Usually it begins early in infancy with atonia of the neck muscles, spastic paraplegia, severe mental retardation, optic atrophy, abnormal reflexes, and enlargement of the head. Laboratory studies, except for skull roentgenograms showing enlargement, are usually normal. Death usually occurs at about 18 months of age. There is no therapy.

LIPIDOSES OF THE CENTRAL NERVOUS SYSTEM

These comprise disturbances of metabolism that result in an increase of lipids in the brain. Included are amaurotic idiocy, or Tay-Sachs disease (gangliosidoses) (see below); Niemann-Pick disease (sphingomyelin) (see Ch. 777); Gaucher's disease (cerebrosides) (see Ch. 776); and Hurler's disease (mucopolysaccharides) (see Ch. 934).

The dividing line is by no means sharp between the dysmyelinating diseases, characterized by faulty myelin formation, and the lipid storage diseases, characterized by the accumulation of lipid-staining materials within nerve cell bodies. The distinction is further blurred by the fact that demyelination also occurs in many of the lipidoses, particularly amaurotic idiocy.

Amaurotic idiocy, or cerebromacular degeneration, can have an infantile (Tay-Sachs), late infantile (Bielschowsky), or juvenile (Batten-Spielmeyer-Vogt) onset. The Tay-Sachs variety is found chiefly among children of Jewish descent and has a recessive genetic pattern. The incidence of the other forms is genetic recessive and nonracial. All three are characterized by a progressive decrease in vision leading to complete blindness within one to two years. Concomitantly, there is a progressive and usually severe dementia combined with convulsions and advancing weakness, leading eventually to the patient's being bedridden with paralysis. Diagnosis in all three forms depends upon the characteristic clinical combination of dementia and blindness plus, in the Tay-Sachs and Batten-Spielmeyer-Vogt varieties, either a cherry-red or red-purple discoloration, respectively, marking the area of macular degeneration in the retina. An adult form (Kufs') has also been recognized. This group of late onset neuronal storage disorders without organomegaly is characterized by seizures, pigmentary degeneration or cherry-red spot changes in the retina, pyramidal signs, basal ganglia signs, cerebellar signs, and dementia. The problem remains whether these disorders are examples of identical or different genetically determined enzymatic defects of the nervous system. Clinicopathologic changes are not diagnostic. Rectal biopsy disclosing fat-packed ganglion cells in Meissner's plexus provides morphologic confirmation of the diagnosis.

Adams, J. M., and Imagawa, D. T.: Measles antibodies in multiple sclerosis. Proc. Soc. Exp. Biol. Med., 111:562, 1962.

Carter, S., Sciarra, D., and Merritt, H. H.: The course of multiple sclerosis as determined by autopsy proven cases. Am. Res. Nerv. Ment. Dis. Proc., 28:471, 1950.

McAlpine, D., Lumsden, C. E., and Acheson, E. D.: Multiple Sclerosis. A Reappraisal. London, E. & S. Livingstone Ltd., 1965.

Miller, H. G., Stanton, J. B., and Gibbons, J. L.: Parainfectious encephalomyelitis and related syndromes. Quart. J. Med., 25:427, 1956.

Poser, C. M.: Recent advances in multiple sclerosis. Med. Clin. North Am., 56:1343, 1972.

Prineas, J. W.: Paramyxovirus-like particles associated with acute demyelination in chronic relapsing multiple sclerosis. Science, 178:760, 1972.

Raine, C. S., Powers, J. M., and Suzuki, K.: Acute multiple sclerosis. Confirmation of "paramyxovirus-like" intranuclear inclusions. Arch. Neurol., 30:39, 1974.

Vinken, P. J., and Bruyn, G. W. (eds.): Multiple Sclerosis and Other Demyelinating Diseases. Handbook of Clinical Neurology, Vol. 9. Amsterdam, North-Holland Publishing Company, 1970.

Wolfgram, F., et al. (eds.): Multiple Sclerosis: Immunology, Virology and Ultrastructure. New York, Academic Press, 1972.

Section Sixteen.   THE EPILEPSIES

Gilbert H. Glaser

Definition and Prevalence. Epilepsy is derived from the Greek *epilepsia* meaning a "taking hold of" or "a seizing." It refers to the many types of recurrent seizures produced by paroxysmal excessive neuronal discharges in different parts of the brain that can be due to a variety of cerebral and general bodily disorders. Designation of "the epilepsies" as symptom complexes, therefore, is more appropriate, and the term encompasses convulsions or convulsive disorders with loss of consciousness as well as nonconvulsive seizures with only slight changes in conscious awareness.

An accurate epidemiology of the epilepsies is difficult, but various studies indicate an over-all incidence of between 0.5 and 1.0 per cent in general populations involving all age groups. The experience of a single seizure is more common, especially in early childhood, but recurrence is necessary for the diagnosis of an epilepsy.

Pathogenesis. *Basic Mechanisms of Epileptic Discharge.* Given the sufficient and proper electrical and chemical stimuli, abnormal discharges and seizures can arise in even the normal brain. Certain regions of the brain are particularly sensitive to seizures, having a low threshold and a high susceptibility. These include particularly the motor cortex and the structures within the limbic system. The temporal lobe and its deeper nuclear aggregates, the amygdala and hippocampus, are especially susceptible; their vascularity is vulnerable to compression, and the tissues themselves are especially sensitive to biochemical disturbances. It sometimes is difficult to separate cause from effect in temporal lobe lesions, because morphologic abnormalities in these regions may result when a severe seizure produces secondary vascular insufficiency and hypoxia.

Factors related to age and development are important in the genesis of the epilepsies, and brain lesions acquired during the perinatal period often mature and produce clinical epileptic phenomena only years later. Certain seizure types such as massive spasms are more common in infants; petit mal seizures appear in childhood rather than later in life. This is reflected by different electroencephalographic patterns associated with seizures in infancy and childhood, compared with those in older age groups. The immature brain also is more susceptible than that of the adult to biochemical disturbances such as hypoxia, hypocalcemia, hypoglycemia, and hyponatremia. The occurrence of seizures with high fever is almost confined to early childhood. The periodicity of epilepsy correlates with sleep or menstrual cycles in some patients.

Seizures may be *focal,* arising from an abnormal focus or a number of foci, or *generalized from the onset,* seemingly without focal origin. However, generalization throughout the brain of an initially focal paroxysmal discharge may occur so rapidly that the focal origin can be obscured, and the attacks of many patients with fixed cerebral lesions and *secondary or symptomatic seizures* are in this category. It is still uncertain whether generalized seizures, such as some idiopathic grand mal convulsions and the brief seizures of petit mal absence (see below), develop immediately as generalized cerebral discharges involving specific pathways, or whether initially a localized discharge occurs. Convulsions caused by metabolic disturbances such as water intoxication, hypocalcemia, or hypoglycemia may be considered examples of those generalized from the onset. In these instances, the initial detonation starting the seizure is believed to be in the subcortical mesodiencephalic nonspecific reticular systems, with diffuse propagation bilaterally into the cerebral cortex. The rapid loss of consciousness that first occurs and the marked memory disturbance after the seizure can be related to this spread.

Hughlings Jackson concluded many years ago from clinical observations that most seizures develop from a focus or aggregate of abnormally excitable neurons, and many studies since his time have supported this hypothesis. It is postulated that the nerve cells of patients with epilepsy contain intrinsic intra- and extracellular metabolic disturbances which produce excessive and prolonged depolarization of the membrane, producing a defect in the recovery process after excitation. The cortical regions containing such cells generate shifts in slow or standing wave potentials as a result of abnormal electrical activity arising in the region of neuronal dendrites. The neurons in the abnormal, epileptic focus are a hyperexcitable aggregate, and they tend to discharge paroxysmally. Clinical seizures develop if the discharge propagates along neural pathways or if sufficient local recruitment occurs. The abnormal discharges, once initiated, spread through essentially normal brain; the manifestations of the particular seizure then depend upon both the focus of origin and the region of the brain subsequently involved in the propagated discharge. In certain cases, seizures may be provoked by various sensory stimuli ("reflex" or sensory-induced epilepsy), especially flickering light or visual patterns and sound. At other times, peripheral sensory stimulation has been found to arrest the development of a seizure.

The metabolic environment of epileptogenic neurons is most important in the genesis of attacks, and many metabolic disturbances may be associated with seizures. For example, a balance of electrolytes is required to maintain the resting potential of the neuronal membrane. An alteration in membrane permeability with an increased, intraneuronal sodium content could be a significant change preceding seizure discharge. Initiation and maintenance of neuronal hyperexcitability have been related to increases in extraneuronal potassium. Depletion of available calcium ions upsets membrane stability and causes oscillations; conversely, an increase in calcium has a depressant, anticonvulsive effect. Both hypoxia and hypoglycemia deprive neurons of basic substrates, allowing insufficient energy for the maintenance of appropriate ionic gradients. However, if effects of excessive muscle metabolism and apnea during generalized convulsive seizure activity are eliminated, such seizures do not induce cerebral hypoxia; actually, cerebral blood flow increases to meet cerebral oxygen demands in this state.

An excess of excitatory transmitter, such as acetylcholine, produces repetitive discharges and seizure activity. This may be induced experimentally by anticholinesterase drugs, but it is not found significantly in naturally occurring epilepsy.

The coenzyme function of pyridoxal phosphate is directly involved in the metabolic pathway of gamma-aminobutyric acid, which has neuronal inhibitory activity. Experimental alterations of this system can be produced by such substances as the antimetabolite methoxypyridoxine and the hydrazides, but pyridoxine deficiency seizures occur only rarely and in infants. Isoniazid toxicity occurs with an overdosage by this mechanism.

Etiology. It is customary to divide epilepsy into two categories, *idiopathic* and *symptomatic or acquired.* A diagnosis of idiopathic epilepsy is made when no specific cause is found; in acquired epilepsy the cause can be determined by available diagnostic procedures. Present techniques fail to uncover a specific structural or biochemical cause of epilepsy in up to 75 per cent of patients.

Idiopathic Epilepsy. Idiopathic epilepsy has been designated as *genetic,* with the implication that a transmitted predisposition for seizures is present. A family history of seizures exists in high incidence for some groups of seizures, particularly those with an onset in early life. The relatives of patients with idiopathic epilepsy have a 3 to 5 per cent incidence of epilepsy, six to ten times that in the ordinary population. There is also an increased incidence of electroencephalographic abnormality in the relatives of seizure patients, particularly in monozygotic twins, in whom the incidence of concordant abnormalities may exceed 20 per cent. Since epilepsy may be but a symptom associated with other neurologic abnormalities, an inheritance pattern for a specific cerebral disease must be considered in some cases. There are also a number of indirect factors, such as cerebral birth trauma resulting from a narrow maternal pelvis, that tend to produce seizures in families.

Acquired Epilepsy. Most diseases or structural abnormalities of the brain may be associated with seizures. *Congenital malformations* induced chromosomally or otherwise, such as microgyria, porencephaly, and hemangiomas, have a varying incidence of associated epilepsy, depending upon the intensity of the abnormality and possibly on more general genetic factors. Maternal infection, as by rubella, can produce multiple cerebral abnormalities, and severe toxemia of pregnancy also can affect the fetus. Perinatal difficulties causing *birth trauma* and *asphyxia* are relatively common causes of cerebral damage and later epilepsy.

Acute, subacute, and chronic infections of the brain and its coverings, such as meningitis, encephalitis, and abscess, cause seizures, both during the active process and later as healing leaves cerebral scars. Acute viral encephalitis often causes seizures, and convulsions, caused by cerebral tuberculomas (more often by tuberculous meningitis) remain common in certain countries such as India. Cysticercosis and schistosomiasis have specific geographic distributions and are frequent causes of seizures in highly endemic areas.

Febrile convulsions commonly accompany nonspecific infections in infants and young children and are to be distinguished from direct infection of the nervous system. The seizure usually accompanies a high rise in fever in an otherwise neurologically normal child. However, at least 30 per cent of these children may develop epilepsy later without fever. Sometimes febrile convulsions precipitate status epilepticus, which, in turn, contributes to permanent cerebral damage. The deep temporal lobe structures are particularly sensitive to these effects; the lesions occurring therein may later produce a temporal lobe–psychomotor seizure state.

Head injury is a major cause of acquired epilepsy, the seizures occurring both in the acute phase and as a chronic residual. The incidence of epilepsy after head injury is difficult to determine, because of the great variability of injury. General surveys report an incidence of up to 10 per cent after closed-head injury and between 30 and 40 per cent after open-head injuries, seizures developing in most cases within three years. The seizure incidence is highest when the wound is severe, when the dura is penetrated, and when the injury involves the rolandic or parietal regions.

Brain tumors are an important cause of seizures, particularly in adults, but it has been difficult to ascertain the relative incidence of brain tumor within the large population of epileptics. Between 30 and 40 per cent of all patients with cerebral tumors have seizures, especially if the tumor is supratentorial. The seizure is apt to be focal and, in 15 to 20 per cent of cases, is the first symptom. The brain tumors most likely to cause seizure are astrocytomas, meningiomas, and metastatic neoplasms, especially those from the lung.

Cerebral vascular disease is a relatively common cause of seizures, particularly in the older age groups. The attacks may result either from localized vascular insufficiency and secondary ischemic hypoxia or from a chronic residual scar, left after thrombosis, embolism, or hemorrhage. Episodes of loss of consciousness owing to diminished cerebral blood flow may progress into seizures, as in severe states of carotid sinus sensitivity and Adams-Stokes syndrome caused by heart block. Seizures appear in up to 20 per cent of patients with the various collagen disorders, i.e., systemic lupus erythematosus and periarteritis nodosa, and are the result of small vascular lesions involving the brain.

Various *allergic reactions* may be related to single seizures, but usually not recurrent epilepsy. Convulsions have been reported after immunizations, in drug sensitivity reactions, and after insect bites.

Certain generalized *cerebral degenerative and demyelinating diseases* carry a significant incidence of seizures; in multiple sclerosis this is 5 per cent, and patients with Alzheimer-Pick dementia may experience generalized and myoclonic seizures. The complex cerebral lesions of tuberous sclerosis often produce seizures, including infantile massive spasms. The cerebral lipidoses, such as Tay-Sachs disease, may cause generalized and myoclonic seizures.

Toxic and metabolic disorders are an important cause of seizures since treatment may be directed quite specifically. Seizures are prominent during withdrawal from chronic drug intoxications, particularly from barbiturates (and other sedatives and tranquilizers), and from alcohol. Seizures developing in association with alcoholism usually appear within 48 hours after cessation of drinking and may precede delirium tremens. Carbon monoxide intoxication and other forms of hypoxia may cause seizures. Lead poisoning has been a common cause of convulsions in young children. Water intoxication or excessive hydration, with hemodilution, can produce seizures, again especially in the young. Other pertinent metabolic causes are pyridoxine deficiency, phenylketonuria, hypocalcemia (with or without hypoparathyroid-

ism), porphyria, and hypoglycemia. Hypoglycemia may be a complication of the treatment of diabetes or may accompany islet cell tumors of the pancreas and other endocrine disturbances such as hypopituitarism. Seizures, especially myoclonic, are common in acute and chronic renal insufficiency but are relatively unusual in hepatic failure. Secondarily induced magnesium deficiency, such as that after severe gastrointestinal fluid loss, has been implicated in the production of seizures.

It is likely that, in many patients, several factors combine to produce attacks: a genetically determined predisposition, an increased cerebral excitability related to a general metabolic disturbance, the presence of a focal brain lesion or a tendency to vascular insufficiency, and a triggering disturbance such as an emotional crisis or an excessively flickering light. Each patient, therefore, must be evaluated from many different aspects in order to establish causation on different levels and to develop appropriate total therapy.

Clinical Manifestations. The classification of seizures employed here is based, whenever possible, on a combination of clinical manifestations and electroencephalographic correlates.

Generalized Seizures (Grand Mal or Major Convulsions). The major tonic-clonic seizures have many causes and arise in all age groups. These seizures usually start with a *prodromal phase* that lasts minutes or even hours, with a change in emotional reactivity or affective responses, such as increasing anxiety or depression, often difficult to recognize. More commonly, the specific onset of the seizure is the *aura,* a brief experience directly related to the locus of origin of the seizure. Frequently experienced auras are a sense of fear, a peculiar epigastric sensation welling up into the throat, an unpleasant odor, various visual and auditory hallucinations, and strange sensations in an arm or leg. At times, localized movements of an extremity or portions of the face precede the onset of the general convulsion. The *convulsion* itself occurs with sudden vocalization (the "epileptic cry"), loss of consciousness, tonic extensor rigidity of the trunk and extremities, then clonic movements, a brief cessation of respiration, cyanosis, and then heavy, stertorous breathing. Incontinence of urine and feces occurs; there is often biting of the tongue and cheeks in the clonic phase. After some minutes, the excessive motor activity ceases, breathing becomes more normal, and consciousness gradually returns. Frequently a *postictal state* appears, characterized by confusion, general fatigue, headache, and, at times, certain specific, residual neurologic signs such as hemiparesis or monoparesis, sensory disturbances, and dysphasia. Automatic behavior may be present. As with the aura, these postictal phenomena have significance with regard to possible focal origins of the generalized seizure. The postictal paralysis, sometimes called "Todd's paralysis," ordinarily lasts for several minutes to hours after the seizure. In general, there is amnesia for a generalized seizure with the exception of possible recollections of the prodromal phase or the aura.

The designation *fragmentary seizure* is given to the occurrence of brief components of the generalized complex. For example, only auras may appear and may or may not be followed by abortive tonic movements or loss of consciousness. Such fragments occur particularly during therapy with anticonvulsant drugs and reflect incomplete control.

Grand mal seizures vary in their frequency from once

or twice yearly to many times daily; 20 per cent of patients may have only nocturnal seizures. In women the seizures may appear cyclically with or immediately before the menstrual periods, and the incidence may increase or decrease with pregnancy, being increased by toxemia and water retention.

The *electroencephalographic (EEG) patterns associated with generalized seizures* during the attack are difficult to distinguish from movement artifact. Between attacks, the EEG often contains paroxysms of bilateral, essentially synchronous, 4- to 7-cycle-per-second discharges from all areas, interspersed with nonspecific patterns of high amplitude spikes and slow waves. A paroxysmal or slow wave discharge localized to one region of the scalp suggests that a focal cerebral lesion may be present. Between seizures up to 25 per cent of patients have an electroencephalogram within the normal range.

Petit Mal (Absence Attack). The petit mal seizure is a specific form of minor epilepsy, consisting of a sudden brief lapse of consciousness, usually lasting no longer than 30 seconds, more commonly 5 to 10 seconds. Petit mal almost always appears in childhood, with onset usually between the ages of three and ten. Its incidence diminishes during postpuberty, and persistence into adult life after the age of 30 is rare. Usually, no specific cause is found. In rare instances a specific brain lesion such as a vascular calcified tumor of the frontal lobe or diffuse cerebral lipidosis has been reported with petit mal seizures, but the EEG was seldom entirely characteristic.

Clinically, the patient with petit mal has a sudden cessation of activity and stares blankly, making no movements, except at times a 3 per second blinking of the eyelids, a slight deviation of the eyes and head, or brief minor movements of the lips and hands. The end of the spell is equally abrupt. More complex behavioral disturbances or postictal confusion or drowsiness suggest another type of minor seizure such as psychomotor automatism rather than petit mal. The attacks of petit mal can be as few as a flurry every several days to as many as 100 or more per day. As the frequency increases, the repeated absences sometimes produce difficulties in continuing motor tasks and in learning. The designation *petit mal status* or absence state refers to many attacks occurring close together for minutes to hours and producing confusion and disorientation.

The electroencephalographic correlate of the petit mal or absence seizure is a rhythmic 3-cycle-per-second spike and wave discharge appearing synchronously from all scalp regions both during and between seizures. Usually, a discharge of more than a few seconds' duration is associated with a clinical absence. The characteristics of the seizure and the typical electroencephalographic discharge have led to these seizures being designated as "centrencephalic," implying an origin in the centrally placed, "integrating," mesodiencephalic regions of the brain. Experimentally, there is evidence to support this hypothesis, although direct confirmation in the human is inconclusive.

Akinetic Seizure. The term akinetic attack is applied to a generalized seizure associated with loss of consciousness and simple falling. It may be accompanied by an absence and minor movements, but generally there is a marked diminution of postural tone with falling and, often, self-injury. Afterward, the reappearance of normal posture and mental clarity is common, although there may be a brief period of confusion. Electroencephalogra-

phically, there is a diffuse abnormality with slow wave discharges or atypical spike waves, often slower than 3 per second.

Myoclonic Seizures. These are characterized by sudden involuntary contractions involving an integrated response of a single muscle or several muscle groups, producing relatively simple arrhythmic jerking movements about a single joint or several joints, or of a segment of the body. The jerks may exist as an independent entity, as a phenomenon preceding and building up to a generalized grand mal convulsion or as an accompaniment to petit mal absences in children. Myoclonic attacks are often sensitive to sensory stimulation and may be precipitated or accentuated by sound or light, by change in posture, by movement of an extremity, by drowsiness, or by an emotional upset. Myoclonic jerks occur as a normal phenomenon in normal subjects during drowsiness.

Myoclonus Epilepsy. The myoclonus epilepsy of Unverricht refers to generalized myoclonus and mental deterioration secondary to a diffuse degenerative metabolic disorder of undetermined origin. Other forms of myoclonus appear in diseases of cerebral lipid metabolism, in subacute encephalitis, and with rare forms of cerebellar disease. A severe myoclonus appearing in the first 18 months of life and associated with general cerebral deterioration is called *infantile massive spasms* or jackknife seizures. In this condition, the infant develops severe flexion spasms of the head, neck, and trunk and extension of the legs and arms. Some known causes of this disorder are phenylketonuria, tuberous sclerosis, and Down's syndrome, but in most instances neither a biochemical nor an anatomic abnormality can be found.

The *electroencephalographic correlates of the myoclonic seizure* are variable, depending on the severity of the seizure state; in mild instances, generalized, synchronous slow spike and wave complexes or sharp and slow wave elements occur intermittently, with relatively clear electroencephalographic patterns interspersed. Infantile massive spasms are commonly associated with *hypsarhythmia*, which consists of more or less continuous, nonsynchronous, asymmetric discharges of spike and sharp wave elements along with slow waves from all regions.

Focal or Partial Seizures. Involvement of a specific region of the brain may be manifested by characteristic signs and symptoms. They are typical of acquired epilepsy, although occasionally no definite morphologic lesion is found. As indicated above, a focal onset seizure can occasionally spread extremely rapidly to become generalized, but in seizure states specifically classified as focal or partial, the attack usually remains limited. There often is a disturbance of consciousness or awareness with varying degrees of amnesia, but total loss of consciousness occurs only with general spread.

Lesions involving any of the motor regions of the brain, but particularly the so-called motor cortex, produce focal motor seizures. The classic *jacksonian motor seizure,* caused by a lesion sharply localized in a specific region of the motor cortex, begins as a repetitive movement of a distal portion of an extremity, such as the fingers or toes, and then spreads by a march of the clonic contractions up the extremity toward the trunk. Such a seizure usually remains limited to the extremity, but it may spread to the rest of the ipsilateral side, the face, and the contralateral side. Occasionally, these seizures begin at the corner of the mouth and are associated with masticatory movements and speech disturbances. Other focal motor seizures involve gross movements of the arms or legs without the classic jacksonian march. *Adversive seizures* produce turning movements of the head, eyes, and trunk toward the side opposite the cerebral lesion, which is usually in the prefrontal cortex.

Focal seizures originating from the *supplementary motor area* of the mesial frontal supracingulate cortex are not common; they are characterized by gross body movements, especially raising of the contralateral arm with the head turning toward that arm, rhythmic bilateral arm and leg movements, and repetitive speech, usually of syllables, not words. Occasionally, speech is slowed or totally inhibited during such a seizure. Other experiences are peculiar sensations in the abdomen, generalized flushing, and palpitations.

Focal sensory seizures caused by a lesion involving the sensory cortex may be jacksonian with a march of abnormal sensations such as numbness and tingling spreading up an extremity. Other sensory areas of the cerebral cortex produce more complex seizures with paroxysmal visual, auditory, olfactory, gustatory, and vertiginous components in varying degrees of organization. As with other types of focal attacks, the pattern of onset is often the most accurate guide to the locus of an abnormal cerebral lesion.

Autonomic seizures are produced by focal lesions in the regions of the brain associated with autonomic representation, namely the deep temporal, limbic, and diencephalic (hypothalamic) areas. Many autonomic symptoms are associated with other focal or generalized seizures, but they also appear in attacks more or less by themselves, as paroxysms of abdominal pain, sweating, piloerection, incontinence, salivation, and, rarely, fever.

Psychomotor (temporal lobe, limbic system) epilepsy is due to seizure activity involving the temporal lobe, its deeper nuclear masses (the amygdala and hippocampus), and their associated limbic system structures. Psychomotor epilepsy is common in both children and adults and occasionally coexists with grand mal seizures. Evidence of an acquired lesion is found in more than half the patients, with a frequent history of trauma at birth or, later, encephalitis or neoplasm. Some patients with psychomotor seizures are found to have focal frontal or occipital lobe lesions, but even with these there is evidence that the discharges produce their eventual manifestations by propagation through temporal-limbic lobe structures.

Psychomotor-temporal-limbic seizures are manifested by an initial aura of anxiety and visceral symptoms, especially by a peculiar epigastric sensation welling up into the throat. An alteration in consciousness follows, associated with many varied, complex feeling and thinking states, as well as automatic somatic and autonomic motor behavior. Activity is first arrested or suspended, then simple movements ensue, such as chewing, swallowing, sucking, lip smacking, and aimless twistings of the arms and legs. Automatisms then appear which are of varying complexity and involve either partially purposeful or inappropriate and bizarre behavior. Usually, the automatism is stereotyped, but, despite this, the movements usually interplay with the environment, and occasionally they appear to be determined in part by psychologic factors. The activities in this phase of the seizure may merge into normal behavior. The complex attack beginning with unpleasant olfactory hallucinations caused by lesions of the mesial portions of the temporal

lobe, the uncus, was specifically called an uncinate seizure by Jackson, who also described the "dreamy" and confused state of the patient. Visceral manifestations are common in young patients, who experience hunger, nausea, vomiting, and abdominal pain as well as urinary incontinence. Destructive aggressive behavior occasionally occurs but usually is not goal-directed. Affective disturbances may be present, particularly expressions of fear, anger, and depression. Occasionally, prolonged fuguelike states with running or wandering may last many minutes. During some psychomotor-temporal lobe seizures, patients experience hallucinations, visual or auditory as well as interpretive illusions involving their own bodies or the immediate environment. These symptoms frequently are associated with ideational blocking and forced thinking as well as peculiar feelings of familiarity called "déjà vu" and "déjà pensée." Amnesia is usually present.

ELECTROENCEPHALOGRAPHIC CONCOMITANTS OF FOCAL SEIZURES.   These are represented by discharges of slow waves, spikes, and sharp and slow complexes localized over the particular cerebral region involved. Frequently, the abnormalities are bilateral but asynchronous, representing transmission and diffusion of the abnormal discharge from one hemisphere to its mirror point on the other. At times, deeply situated lesions produce only minimal or no significant alteration in the ordinary electroencephalogram recorded from the scalp.

Status Epilepticus.   The rapid repetitive recurrence of any type of seizure without recovery between attacks is called status epilepticus. The term is usually applied to attacks of generalized epilepsy in which the patient remains unconscious and in continuous seizures, with tonic and clonic fluctuations, incontinence, severely disturbed breathing, high fever, excessive sweating, and elevation of blood pressure. Such status may last for hours, even days, and requires emergency medical treatment because of the possible dangers of cerebral damage, thought to be due to ischemic anoxia (or "consumptive" hypoxia) and cardiac and renal failure. The onset of status epilepticus can be spontaneous, but frequently withdrawal from anticonvulsant medication or a too rapid shift of medication is the precipitating cause.

Focal motor seizures may appear in continuous fashion, lasting many hours; this state has been called *epilepsia partialis continua.*

Petit mal status is associated with sustained 3-cycle-per-second spike-wave discharges in the electroencephalogram. The patient is in a state of confusion, has a continuously dazed expression, and has minor movements around the lips or in the arms and legs. *Psychomotor* or *temporal lobe status* also occurs, but less frequently. Such patients are found in a confused state with persistent, inappropriate, bizarre complex behavior patterns lasting over many hours, occasionally associated with fluctuating visceral symptoms.

The Interseizure State.   A patient with a progressive cerebral degenerative disease, an extensive cerebral malformation, a severe encephalitis, or an expanding brain tumor may develop changes in behavior and intellectual functioning, primarily because of the underlying structural lesions and not directly because of any seizures that might be present. However, in the past much attention has been paid to the possibility of a specific personality distortion in epileptic patients. Most patients subject to seizures have normal behavior and intellectual functions between attacks and adjust appropriately to society, often excelling. In some instances, however, severe emotional problems do develop, usually in response to environmental restrictions. *Neurotic, maladjusted behavior* occurs, along with obsessional, particularly religious, preoccupations. Often, under these circumstances, the seizures increase and become more difficult to control.

An undetermined number of patients with frequent recurrent generalized seizures, especially status epilepticus, or with recurrent psychomotor temporal-limbic seizures, develop continuing *defects in intellectual function*. Psychologic tests reveal persistent impairments of concentration and attention, memory lapses, word-finding distortions, subtle losses in the ability to associate, and perceptual difficulties. It is possible that prolonged subclinical seizure activity contributes to these disturbances.

More severe personality disturbances, ranging all the way to *psychosis with schizophrenic manifestations,* complicate the interseizure course of a few patients with either psychomotor or severe grand mal epilepsy. The psychotic reactions often have psychologic precipitating factors; occasionally, they follow control of the actual seizures by medication, and these instances may be related, in part, to a reaction to the drug. The symptoms include paranoid, depressive, and hallucinatory reactions, catatonic disorders, flattening of the affect, and severe obsessional states. The patients suffer marked difficulty in concentration and disorientation of time sequences. Defects in memory are present and are accompanied by abnormalities in perception as well as difficulties in word finding, in calculating, and in analyzing the thought content of written material. However, the patients usually attempt to maintain contacts with reality, and major withdrawal is not present, in contrast to most examples of spontaneous schizophrenic illness. Diffuse electroencephalographic abnormality, with either bilateral temporal lobe involvement or diffuse spike wave paroxysms, accompany some of these clinical phases, but with others, the electroencephalogram remains normal.

Diagnosis in Epilepsy. The patient with epilepsy should receive a thorough diagnostic evaluation to determine causative factors and precipitating circumstances. This requires a thorough history, a detailed medical and neurologic physical examination, and selected laboratory investigations, with particular reference to blood chemistry tests, cerebrospinal fluid analysis, electroencephalography, and special roentgenologic studies. Every effort should be made to identify a specific medical illness or a focal cerebral lesion.

History. The history must contain a detailed description of the attacks to help establish the fact of recurrent seizures. As much recollection as possible should be obtained from the patient, particularly of experiences of the aura and the onset of the seizure. The patterning or course of events during and after the seizure should be documented, especially by eyewitness accounts, with special attention to any phenomena that might possess localizing significance. Information should be sought as to the various circumstances under which seizures occur, such as the time of day or night, the frequency of attacks and how medication influences them, their relationship to the menstrual cycle, pregnancy, food intake, sound or light stimulation, intake of alcoholic drinks, or psychologic stresses. All symptoms of neurologic disturbances should be described, such as headache, hemiparesis, hemisensory disturbances, dysphasia, visual difficulties, or vertigo.

The *past medical and developmental history* is of great aid in establishing the cause. Information should be obtained concerning pregnancy, delivery, the neonatal period, the developmental neurologic milestones, head injuries, and reactions to immunizations and the various childhood illnesses such as measles, mumps, and chickenpox. The occurrence of any severe illness with delirium or coma that might be considered an encephalitis should be inquired about, as well as any exposure to toxic substances. Drug intake needs particular investigation, particularly with adults suspected of taking barbiturates or tranquilizer drugs. One must inquire into the patient's social development and behavior in and out of the family setting, his intellectual performance at school, and his vocational adjustments and performance. Any alteration in these phases of existence should be related to seizure occurrence, to the interseizure state, and to the possible effects of medication.

A *family history* of susceptibility to seizures may delineate a significant number with a history of febrile seizures in early childhood as well as of generalized and focal seizures extending into later life. The family history may reveal not only genetically determined cerebral disorders associated with seizures but also other neurologic abnormalities as well.

The *general medical history* can reveal evidence of pertinent cardiovascular disease, blood dyscrasias, and metabolic and endocrine disorders; a seizure may be the first manifestation of a cerebral metastasis or of a generalized vascular disease.

Clinical Examination. In most patients with seizures, physical examination fails to disclose significant physical or neurologic abnormalities. Nevertheless, a thorough general examination is warranted; careful examination of the skin, for example, may produce the diagnosis in cases of tuberous sclerosis, neurofibromatosis, or cerebral hemangioma. Examination of the lungs provides evidence for consideration of metastatic tumor or abscess; evaluation of the peripheral circulation and blood pressure gives an indication of the possibility of the various types of cerebral vascular lesions or aids in differentiating between syncope and seizure.

The *neurologic examination* serves two purposes: to elicit signs of any general neurologic disorder and to determine whether or not focal signs of a localized cerebral lesion are present. A neurologic examination is particularly valuable at the time of, or shortly after, a seizure if it reveals a transitory hemiparesis or related signs.

A battery of *psychologic tests* can aid the evaluation of both intellectual capabilities and psychologic adjustments. Simple tests of memory and perception are part of the regular neurologic examination. For more complete studies, the most useful tests include the Wechsler Intelligence Scale (especially the Kohs block test), the memory scales, the Bender-Gestalt, the Rorschach, and the Thematic Apperception tests. Attention should be paid to the patient's performance during these tests as well as to the actual scores.

Laboratory Investigations. Each patient with recurrent seizures, no matter the age, should be examined with certain laboratory investigations at least once and more often if changes develop in seizure patterns or neurologic signs. At different ages certain tests are more apt to produce results leading to specific etiologic diagnosis. Additional studies are necessary to evaluate the general health of the patient and follow the potentially toxic effects of medication.

There are no abnormal laboratory findings associated directly with seizure activity except electroencephalographic discharges. Urine analysis is necessary to determine the state of kidney function; if abnormal, a specific renal disorder may be present, and certain drugs cannot be administered. Similarly, a complete blood count is necessary. Severe seizure states such as status epilepticus may be associated with proteinuria, leukocytosis, and fever as secondary manifestations. In certain instances, special blood chemistry studies are warranted, such as the blood sugar for the diagnosis of suspected hypoglycemia and in the evaluation of a diabetic with epilepsy, and the serum calcium determination for infants and young children with seizure states. Evaluation of fluctuations in serum electrolytes and acid-base balance is necessary to study both children and adults with disorders of the kidney, liver, heart, and lungs. Serologic tests help to diagnose past infections.

The *cerebrospinal fluid* is apt to be normal in all constituents and pressures, except in the minority of patients who have specific neurologic disease. After severe seizures, there may be a slight increase in the cerebrospinal fluid protein and white cell count. In structural neurologic disorders with seizures, the protein and/or pressure may be elevated persistently, and the specific diagnosis then depends on other tests, such as contrast roentgenologic studies. Chronic nervous system infection can be associated with an increase in the white cell count of the cerebrospinal fluid; occasionally, a cerebral tumor may be revealed by neoplastic cells in the fluid.

Roentgenograms of the skull and chest must be taken of all patients. The film of the skull may reveal asymmetry caused by early injury or maldevelopment, abnormal calcifications, shift of the calcified pineal, or signs of increased intracranial pressure. The chest film potentially detects pulmonary infection or tumor and aids in evaluating the cardiac status. Roentgenologic studies of the intracranial contents employing contrast media are extremely useful diagnostic procedures if employed at the proper time, but must be selected with care because of their morbid potential. Such procedures are considered when a focal intracranial lesion is suspected. *Ventriculography* is the procedure of choice when there is increased intracranial pressure, particularly when a lesion is suspected in the posterior fossa. Ordinarily, when the pressure is normal, a fractional *pneumoencephalogram* gives more information about a lesion occupying space within the skull or distorting the ventricular or subarachnoid systems. Pneumoencephalography also discloses focal brain atrophy as reflected by selective enlargements of important specific space such as the temporal horns. *Cerebral arteriography* is useful for patients with or without evidence of increased pressure and can demonstrate localized abnormal vascular patterns in neoplasms as well as intracranial hematomas, vascular malformations, and the location of vascular occlusions.

Radioactive isotopic brain scanning may be of use. A negative brain scan often eliminates the immediate necessity for performing a contrast roentgenologic procedure, whereas an abnormal study requires further investigation.

Electroencephalography. The various electroencephalographic correlates of the different types of seizures have been described. The electroencephalogram is an indicator of a certain kind of cerebral activity determined by recording electrodes upon the scalp. This is important to realize, because electroencephalograms from up to 25 per cent of patients with seizures are normal; yet, abnormal discharges are disclosed in many of these same patients by depth electrodes recording from deeper cerebral structures such as the amygdala and hippocampus. The electroencephalogram, therefore, has limited diagnostic applications and must be correlated with other information from the various physical and neurologic examinations. It can be utilized to confirm the presence of a seizure disturbance, particularly if paroxysmal discharges are recorded during and correlated with a seizure. An example of this specificity is that up to 85 per cent of children with petit mal will have the typical 3-cycle-per-second spike and wave discharges both during and between seizures and, in many instances, these discharges can be precipitated during the recording by overventilation and light stimulation.

In other instances of epilepsy, the electroencephalogram contains generalized, nonspecific slow wave discharges that merely indicate the presence of cerebral dysfunction, but not a definite seizure disorder. Focal slow wave abnormalities in the electroencephalogram suggest a localized structural lesion and ordinarily lead to further investigations. Finally, in certain forms of focal epilepsy, the electroencephalogram may show focal discharges of spikes, sharp waves, and complex components indicative of the epileptogenic nature of the focus. Yet, in some of these instances, such an abnormality might be transmitted, the basic discharging focus being elsewhere.

In most laboratories of electroencephalography the test procedure involves recording in the waking state and during voluntary overventilation. Additional attempts are usually made to provoke generalized and focal paroxysmal discharges by means of sleep, sensory stimulation with light and occasionally sound, and sometimes by utilizing certain metabolic and pharmacologic adjuvants.

The recording of the electroencephalogram during sleep is useful in the attempt to demonstrate focal temporal lobe discharges in patients with psychomotor–temporal lobe epilepsy. In adults, such discharges are increased during sleep in up to 75 per cent of patients, but the results in children are less definitive, the increase occurring in only 30 per cent. In many patients, sleep produces increased bilateral appearance of abnormal temporal discharges. The use of sphenoidal electrodes is occasionally of some help in lateralizing temporal lobe discharge, particularly when patients are being evaluated for surgical therapy. At times, barbiturate-induced fast wave activity is found to be diminished on the side of the involved temporal lobe. Photic stimulation identifies patients with light-sensitive epilepsy and, occasionally, produces lateralized discharges in patients with a sensitive focus. There have been many attempts to alter the electrical activity of the brain in susceptible patients by inducing metabolic changes, such as hydration after an injection of Pitressin. Various stimulant drugs have been used, such as Metrazol and Megimide. All these methods, particularly the use of the drugs, may produce paroxysmal discharges as well as clinical seizures, usually generalized. However, attempts to measure seizure discharge threshold have been unsuccessful because of great variability, and many normal subjects respond with seizures to these procedures. Accordingly, these methods are not recommended for general use in the diagnosis of epilepsy. Occasionally, it may be important in the evaluation of a specific patient to study in detail the phenomena of the seizure and to determine focal components either in the electroencephalogram or clinically. In selected cases, this can be accomplished by the administration of a controlled dose of a seizure-producing drug.

The use of the electroencephalogram in following patients with epilepsy is limited, because in many instances some degree of electroencephalographic abnormality persists even though seizures are controlled. This is most often the case in patients with psychomotor–temporal lobe epilepsy and least often in children with petit mal and myoclonic seizures.

Differential Diagnosis. The diagnosis of epilepsy has profound implications, medically and psychologically, as it affects the total life situation of the patient and his family. Consequently, careful attention must be given to make this diagnosis positively and specifically, and to differentiate it from other disturbances that produce somewhat similar abnormalities of neurologic function that are not seizures.

Consciousness may be disturbed episodically by inadequate cerebral blood flow in attacks of *cerebrovascular insufficiency* or of *syncope* of various types, particularly the vasodepressor form. Disturbances of cerebral circulation affect older persons especially, and such patients generally suffer other evidence of hypertension and cerebral arteriosclerosis. Periodic blackouts and recurrent confusional states are manifestations of basilar artery insufficiency, as are other episodic signs of brainstem and cerebellar dysfunction. Patients with carotid arterial insufficiency characteristically experience transitory hemiparesis and hemisensory disturbances along with dysphasia, but the clonic movements of a paroxysmal disorder usually are absent. The electroencephalographic findings of paroxysmal discharge do not occur with cerebrovascular disease although, at times, bilateral rhythmic discharges are observed related to vascular lesions of the upper brainstem. The differential diagnosis is sometimes difficult and may require arteriographic confirmation of a vascular lesion as well as the usual evaluation of the history and general medical state of the patient.

Syncopal episodes may resemble akinetic or brief motor seizures; prolonged syncope can progress into a convulsion resulting from the persistence of cerebral ischemia and hypoxia. The patient with syncope usually has indications of disturbed vasomotor reactivity with excessive sweating, pallor, and tachycardia. Specific precipitating factors often are present such as fear or other psychologic upset. The confusion, headache, and drowsiness that occur after a generalized seizure usually do not appear in syncope. The electroencephalogram during simple syncope consists of diffuse asynchronous slow waves without paroxysmal or focal discharges.

Certain *psychogenic disorders* resemble epileptic states and can be difficult to differentiate. Hysterical "seizures" not only occur as independent problems, but also complicate the course of a limited number of patients with known seizures, the combination being called "hysteroepilepsy." The clinical problem is difficult to unravel because of the interrelationships between the actual seizure and the reactive psychologic disturbance. The hysterical seizure is not associated with neurologic signs of reflex abnormality and, during it, the electroencephalogram contains no paroxysmal discharges. The pattern of hysterical seizures is often bizarre and not a stereotyped tonic-clonic movement sequence. Self-injury is an unusual result of the seizure, and the postictal states of confusion, headache, and drowsiness are absent. Hysterical or psychotic fugue disturbances and dissociative reactions must be distinguished from psychomotor–temporal lobe seizures. The diagnosis of an hysterical seizure state requires careful psychiatric evaluation because of the severe neurotic process involved.

Treatment. Treatment of the epilepsies must take into account not only the patient and his disorder, but his family and general life situation. Much depends on the diagnostic evaluation and the finding of specific causes whenever possible that can be treated directly. This is clearly defined in instances in which metabolic disturbance is obvious, such as hypoglycemia and hypocalcemia, or when an operable cerebral tumor is found. However, in many cases of acquired epilepsy, the basic cause of the seizure cannot be treated directly. Seizures may continue in patients even after removal of a brain tumor because of scarring, or when the tumor is found to be inoperable or incompletely removable. The diagnosis of an acquired epilepsy after head injury or encephalitis usually does not lead to specific therapy. Only a limited number of patients with post-traumatic epilepsy are satisfactory candidates for surgical removal of a localized meningocerebral scar. The administration of anticonvulsant drugs is necessary, therefore, for the majority of patients.

Medical Therapy. There are many available anticonvulsant drugs, as shown in the accompanying table. None is capable of achieving total seizure control in all patients, but careful selection and utilization in each case often leads to optimal results. Each physician should learn to use a number of these drugs well and to recognize disturbing side effects as early as possible. Periodic blood counts, urinalyses, and liver function tests are necessary with certain drugs.

The basic mechanisms of anticonvulsant drugs are not definitely known. Most of the drugs are neuronal depressants with certain variations in action. The hydantoin drugs reduce the synaptic activity of post-tetanic potentiation; the oxazolidine (methadione) drugs decrease nerve transmission during repetitive stimulation. The drugs are believed to increase the stability of excitable neuronal membranes by acting upon electrochemical characteristics involved in ion permeability and membrane polarization. Such stabilizing effects would decrease the activity of the hyperexcitable neuronal aggregates in an epileptogenic focus and prevent the spread of discharge through normal neuronal circuits.

The anticonvulsant drugs are administered to achieve the desired effect of seizure control and must be built up in dosage while not producing untoward toxic reactions. It is best to start with one drug of choice, but usually a single drug is not totally effective, and a second is necessary. Two drugs might be needed initially for patients with two different types of seizure such as grand mal and petit mal. This occurs fairly frequently (from 25 to 50 per cent in some series, especially in adolescents [see Lennox, 1960]). The process may require weeks of adjustment and, during this time, the patient's or parent's cooperation in reporting effects on seizure frequency or side-reactions is most important. Determination of anticonvulsant blood levels, i.e., diphenylhydantoin, phenobarbital, primidone, may be very helpful in identifying patients who are obtaining unsatisfactory control be-

Anticonvulsant Drugs: Dosage, Indications, and Toxic Effects

Bromides
Daily dosage:	1.0 to 3.0 grams for adults; not recommended for children
Indications:	All types of seizures, especially grand mal and psychomotor; may be combined with hydantoins
Toxic effects:	Drowsiness, dulling, rash, psychosis; rarely used now

Celontin
Dose:	0.3 gram capsules
Daily dosage:	Children: 0.6 gram; adults: 1 to 1.5 grams
Indications:	Petit mal, psychomotor seizures, myoclonic seizures, massive spasms
Toxic effects:	Ataxia, drowsiness; rarely, blood dyscrasias

Dexedrine (dextroamphetamine)
Dose:	5 mg tablets; 5 mg, 10 mg, and 15 mg long-acting Spansules
Daily dosage:	Children: 5 to 15 mg; adults: 15 to 30 mg
Indications:	To counteract sedative effects, hyperkinetic behavioral disturbances in children, narcolepsy
Toxic effects:	Anorexia, irritability, sleeplessness

Diamox (acetazolamide)
Dose:	250 mg tablets
Daily dosage:	Children: 0.75 to 1.0 gram; adults: 1.0 to 1.5 grams. Use intermittently; tolerance occurs
Indications:	As an adjuvant in all types of seizures, especially those in females related to menstrual cycles
Toxic effects:	Anorexia, acidosis, drowsiness, numbness of extremities; rarely, blood dyscrasias

Dilantin (diphenylhydantoin)
Dose:	0.03 gram and 0.1 gram capsules; 0.05 gram tablets; 0.1 gram delayed action capsules; 0.025 gram per ml suspension; 0.1 gram in oil, capsules; 0.25 gram ampules for parenteral use
Daily dosage:	Children: 0.15 to 0.3 gram; adults: 0.3 to 0.6 gram. Effective blood level 10 to 20 μg/ml
Indications:	Grand mal, psychomotor and focal seizures; most useful in combination with phenobarbital or primidone
Toxic effects:	Rash, fever, gum hypertrophy, gastric distress, diplopia, ataxia, hirsutism (young females); drowsiness, uncommon; megaloblastic anemia (due to secondary folic acid deficiency); lymphadenopathy

Mebaral (mephobarbital)
Dose:	0.03 gram, 0.1 gram tablets
Daily dosage:	Children: 0.06 to 0.3 gram; adults: 0.3 to 0.6 gram
Indications:	Grand mal, petit mal, psychomotor, focal seizures; similar to phenobarbital; most useful in combination with hydantoins
Toxic effects:	Drowsiness, irritability, rash

Mesantoin (methylphenylethylhydantoin)
Dose:	0.1 gram tablets
Daily dosage:	Children: 0.1 to 0.4 gram; adults: 0.4 to 0.8 gram
Indications:	Grand mal, psychomotor, and focal seizures
Toxic effects:	Rash, fever, drowsiness, ataxia, gum hypertrophy (less than Dilantin), neutropenia, agranulocytosis

Milontin (methylphenylsuccinimide)
Dose:	0.5 gram capsules; 250 mg per 4 ml suspension
Daily dosage:	Children: 0.25 gram to 1.5 grams; adults: 2.0 to 4.0 grams
Indications:	Petit mal, myoclonic and akinetic seizures; occasionally psychomotor seizures
Toxic effects:	Nausea, dizziness, rash, hematuria (may be nephrotoxic)

Mysoline (primidone)
Dose:	0.05 gram, 0.25 gram tablets; 250 mg per 5 ml suspension
Daily dosage:	Children: 0.25 gram; adults: 0.75 to 2.0 grams. The daily dosage should be built up very slowly. Effective blood level range 5 to 15 μg/ml
Indications:	Grand mal, psychomotor and focal seizures; occasionally, petit mal; useful in combination with Dilantin
Toxic effects:	Drowsiness, ataxia, dizziness, rash, nausea, leukopenia (rare)

Paradione (paramethadione)
Dose:	0.15 gram, 0.3 gram capsules; 0.3 gram per ml solution
Daily dosage:	Children: 0.3 gram to 1.8 grams; adults: 1.2 grams to 2.4 grams
Indications:	Petit mal, myoclonic and akinetic seizures, massive spasms, occasionally psychomotor seizures (in children); often useful in combination with Dilantin and phenobarbital; somewhat less effective and less toxic than Tridione
Toxic effects:	Rash, gastric distress, visual symptoms (glare, photophobia), neutropenia, agranulocytosis

Peganone (ethylphenylhydantoin)
Dose:	0.25 gram, 0.5 gram tablets
Daily dosage:	Children: 0.5 gram to 1.5 grams; adults: 2.0 to 3.0 grams
Indications:	Grand mal, psychomotor and focal seizures
Toxic effects:	Similar to those of Dilantin but less frequent; may be substituted for Dilantin, but is generally less effective

Phenobarbital
Dose:	0.015 gram, 0.030 gram, 0.060 gram, 0.1 gram tablets; 4 mg per ml elixir
Daily dosage:	Children: 0.045 gram to 0.1 gram; adults: 0.1 gram to 0.3 gram. Effective blood level range 15 to 30 μg/ml
Indications:	All seizure states: grand mal, petit mal, psychomotor and other focal; most useful in limited dosage in combination with other drugs such as Dilantin
Toxic effects:	Drowsiness, dulling, rash, fever; irritability, and hyperactivity in some children

Phenurone (phenacemide)
Dose:	0.5 gram tablets; 0.3 gram enteric-coated tablets
Daily dosage:	Children: 0.5 gram to 2.0 grams; adults: 1.5 grams to 3.0 grams
Indications:	May be effective in all types of seizures, especially psychomotor–temporal lobe seizures, should be used only in very resistant cases
Toxic effects:	A highly toxic drug, producing liver damage, agranulocytosis, psychotic reactions, and rashes

Tridione (trimethadione)
Dose:	0.15 gram tablets; 0.3 gram capsules; 0.15 gram per 4 ml solution
Daily dosage:	Children: 0.3 gram to 1.8 grams; adults: 1.2 grams to 2.4 grams. Effective blood level range 10 to 30 μg/ml
Indications:	Petit mal, myoclonic and akinetic seizures, massive spasms; often useful in combination with Dilantin and phenobarbital
Toxic effects:	Rash, gastric distress, visual symptoms (glare, photophobia) neutropenia, agranulocytosis, nephrosis

Zarontin (ethosuximide)
Dose:	0.25 gram capsules
Daily dosage:	Children: to 0.75 to 1.0 gram; adults: 1.5 grams. Effective blood level range 40 to 80 μg/ml
Indications:	Petit mal seizures (now the drug of choice); used with Dilantin in mixed seizure states
Toxic effects:	Blood dyscrasias (pancytopenia, leukopenia) unusual; dermatitis, anorexia, nausea, drowsiness, dizziness

The following drugs may be used in the emergency treatment of status epilepticus:

Diazepam (Valium):	2.5 to 10 mg intravenously
Sodium phenobarbital:	0.25 to 0.50 gram intravenously
Sodium amytal:	0.25 to 0.50 gram intravenously
Paraldehyde:	3.0 to 5.0 ml intravenously (diluted in 10 to 20 ml saline)
Dilantin sodium (parenteral):	0.25 gram intravenously or intramuscularly (to 0.5 gram per 24 hours in patients previously receiving this drug or as much as 1.0 to 1.5 in previously untreated patients). *Caution:* Dilantin intravenously must be given slowly in 0.05 gram increments to avoid vasodepression

---

General anesthetics such as ether, Avertin, and xylocaine have a limited usefulness in the treatment of status epilepticus. Careful nursing and attention to fluid and electrolyte balance, airway, cardiac and renal functions, and temperature control are essential in the over-all management of status epilepticus.

cause they either fail to take the drug or metabolize it abnormally. Frequent and rapid shifting or replacement of drugs is to be avoided. Following blood levels in each individual patient and adjusting medication dosage into the therapeutic range have significantly improved seizure control as well as increased our understanding of overdosage and toxic effects.

Diphenylhydantoin metabolism is impaired in patients with acute and chronic liver disease, resulting in elevations of blood levels when standard doses of the drug are taken. By contrast, in the presence of uremia, the blood level of diphenylhydantoin is reduced; however, apparently adequate amounts of the drug unbound to plasma protein may be achieved with administered low dosage.

There also is increasing evidence that other drugs can alter the rate of diphenylhydantoin metabolism induced in liver microsomal enzymes so as to lead to an increase in diphenylhydantoin blood levels even to toxicity (see Ch. 20). These drugs include isoniazid, bishydroxycoumarin, phenyramidol, disulfiram, methylphenidate, diazepam, chlordiazepoxide, phenylbutazone, chlorpromazine, prochlorperazine, and some estrogens. Carbamazepine and ethanol have been reported to lower diphenylhydantoin blood levels. On the other hand, diphenylhydantoin has been reported to lower blood levels of digitoxin, bishydroxycoumarin, metyrapone, and DDT. Diphenylhydantoin also has been found to stimulate enzymes which rapidly turn over endogenous or exogenously administered adrenocorticosteroids; this has resulted, in some instances, in increased adrenocorticotrophic and cortisol production by negative feedback effects.

A specific anticonvulsant drug for each type of seizure is not available. However, there is one major therapeutic division; petit mal absences respond best to either succinimide or oxazolidines (methadiones). These drugs are not effective in the treatment of major generalized (grand mal) or focal cerebral seizures, nor are the hydantoins (used in grand mal and other seizures) effective in petit mal. It is stated that the drugs used in the therapy of petit mal may worsen a generalized seizure state, but this has not been proved.

Generalized grand mal and focal motor seizures are best treated by diphenylhydantoin sodium and phenobarbital. Initially, either drug may be administered to patients who have infrequent attacks, but generally the combination of diphenylhydantoin and phenobarbital produces the most effective seizure control. The average dose of diphenylhydantoin is 0.3 to 0.4 gram per day, usually administered as 0.2 gram in the morning after breakfast and 0.2 gram after dinner. The dosage of phenobarbital is initially 60 mg at bedtime, with 30 mg increments over the day, up to three times daily, if necessary, limited by the unwanted sedative effect.

Patients with psychomotor–temporal lobe epilepsy are often more difficult to control. Many trials of different agents and different doses may be necessary in these cases; the best results are to be expected with diphenylhydantoin and either phenobarbital or primidone. Although in some clinics the two latter drugs are used together, primidone is partially converted to phenobarbital, and their sedative effects combine to make such administration difficult. It is most important with primidone to start therapy with small doses, such as 125 mg, increased at weekly intervals to reach a maximal dosage of 0.75 gram for children or 1.0 to 2.0 grams per day for

adults. If untoward side effects to diphenylhydantoin occur, substitution with the less reactive Peganone is sometimes successful, although this drug has less anticonvulsant effect. Mesantoin and phenacemide are used only for the most difficult cases and even then with extreme care because of their high degree of toxicity.

Acetazolamide is an adjuvant to the treatment of any type of seizure. It seems to have a general effect upon hyperexcitable cerebral neurons because of its properties of inhibition of carbonic anhydrase and production of acidosis. Because tolerance develops, the drug should be administered intermittently. It is occasionally useful, for example, in helping to control seizures appearing periodically in females at the time of menstruation. Under these circumstances, acetazolamide is administered for a week prior to and during menses.

The results of drug therapy are difficult to predict. With careful attention to individual details and general management, most patients with occasional generalized and psychomotor seizures achieve either complete or nearly complete reduction of seizures. Satisfactory or complete control can be achieved in most children with petit mal absences. However, each group of patients, especially those with grand mal and psychomotor epilepsy, contains a refractory number who suffer from troublesome side effects of drugs and from increasing psychologic and sociologic difficulties as the years go by.

In a relatively small but significant number of patients under treatment with diphenylhydantoin and occasionally phenobarbital-related drugs, a paradoxical increase in seizures occurs, along with depressed mentation and increased electroencephalographic abnormalities. The blood levels of the drugs are usually in a "toxic" range, but not always, and other signs of "toxicity," such as nystagmus and ataxia, may not be present. Reduction of anticonvulsant drug dosage, in these instances, leads to a diminution of seizure activity and clearing of mental functions.

When to stop drugs for a patient whose seizures are completely controlled is a recurrent question. Some authorities recommend cautiously withdrawing anticonvulsants if patients have been free of attacks for two years, but in relatively few cases can drugs be withdrawn without seizures recurring even after symptom-free periods of three to five years. Thus continued treatment is indicated for most adults with grand mal and psychomotor epilepsy. The electroencephalogram may remain abnormal in clinically seizure-free patients, indicating persistent seizure potentiality, but even in patients with normal electroencephalograms drug withdrawal may be unsuccessful. Yet, in the management of some patients, it is understandable that a calculated risk of drug withdrawal be considered if this represents a psychologic achievement of great magnitude. Under these circumstances, the drug should be withdrawn carefully with small decrements over many weeks. Drug elimination may be carried out more successfully in children with controlled petit mal, particularly because there is a natural tendency for the absences to diminish with age and maturity.

A presentation of drugs used in the medical treatment of epilepsy is given in the accompanying table in alphabetical order, with statements concerning dose administration, indications for different seizure types, and toxic effects.

Adrenocorticotrophic hormone (ACTH) and adrenocortical steroids are now used in the treatment of massive spasms in infancy associated with the "hypsarhythmic" electroencephalogram. Such therapy is administered after primary causes of massive spasms, such as phenylketonuria, have been excluded. Although initial improvements in the spasms and the electroencephalogram may occur, the prognosis is poor, particularly with regard to the mental deterioration accompanying this condition. Nothing is known about the mechanism of action of the hormones in this disorder; this is somewhat paradoxical because these hormones are known to raise cerebral excitability and precipitate seizures in older persons and in experimental situations.

Dietary Treatment. In general, there are no dietary restrictions for the patient with epilepsy, nor is there a specific diet capable of aiding most patients. However, a diet high in fat content producing significant ketosis, the *ketogenic diet,* occasionally is helpful in treating young children, particularly those with intractable petit mal and generalized motor seizures. Anticonvulsant drugs usually have to be continued, and the diet is difficult to maintain because it is unpleasant.

Psychologic Therapy and Sociologic Management. Many basic problems in the over-all life adjustments of the patient need additional management even though drugs can achieve significant control of seizures. In many cases, the coexistence of seizures and personality problems requires a combination of medical anticonvulsant therapy and psychologically oriented management.

The sedative properties of anticonvulsant drugs usually are not used directly. The so-called tranquilizing drugs have limited usefulness in the management of seizure patients; chlordiazepoxide (Librium) and diazepam (Valium) may reduce disturbed behavior, particularly in children. The phenothiazine drugs have variable effects; an alerting phenothiazine, fluphenazine, is of some use in controlling abnormal behavior in certain patients with psychomotor seizures. However, other drugs in the chlorpromazine group are known to provoke seizures and paroxysmal discharges in the electroencephalogram.

There is often a direct interplay between emotional disturbances and clinical seizure activity. Some patients in a state of psychologic turmoil experience increased seizures and require greater amounts of anticonvulsant drugs. The subsequent achievement of psychologic adjustment decreases the frequency of seizures and lessens the drug requirement. This needs to be developed in various ways, depending on the patient's age and his family and social circumstances. Family understanding is of primary importance, because the child with seizures has to live, insofar as possible, as a normal person within home and school settings. A great problem, still to be overcome, is the stigma attached by society to the diagnosis of epilepsy, and the lack of understanding that not only exists among people in general but is reflected by various restrictive legal practices. Most children with seizures are able to attend schools and vocational programs successfully; most adults with controlled seizures are capable of developing productive careers and engaging in the activities that are so much a part of our culture, such as marriage, childbearing, obtaining an education, driving an automobile, traveling from country to country, and working with appropriate safeguards, protected by insurance and worker's compensation programs. Only a relatively small number of patients require a protected environment, such as that in schools

or colonies specifically developed for epileptic patients. Even these no longer should be institutions where many hundreds or thousands of epileptic patients are kept in essentially custodial care. "Colonies" with schools, homelike units, and small villages exist in Great Britain, Holland, and Denmark and take care of relatively small numbers of patients (up to a few hundred at most in each), involved in intensive programs of medical therapy, psychologic management, education, and vocational training. From these places increasing numbers of adequately controlled patients are sent out into the general community, where they live well adjusted and productive lives.

Only a few occupations are contraindicated for patients with seizures. These include activities of potential danger to either the patient or others, such as work requiring unprotected climbing to great heights and utilizing heavy power equipment or dangerous chemical substances.

Informal and formal psychotherapeutic measures can be undertaken in order to reduce emotional disturbances. The role of the family physician is all-important in these considerations. Often he alone can judge the problems that exist in a family, school, or social setting. His understanding and guidance help both the patient and his family to overcome the feelings of despair, anxiety, fear, and self-consciousness that otherwise interfere with the normal adjustments of everyone involved. It is only when anxieties and depressive tendencies develop into more severe reactions, associated with paranoid states, increased withdrawal, and excessive obsessional tendencies, that more intensive psychiatric treatment becomes necessary. Occasionally, brief periods of hospitalization help in the evaluation of the intensity of the psychologic disturbance and any associated intellectual difficulties that may interfere with the patient's performance. Drug schedules may be revised at the same time, under controlled conditions.

Even the child with epilepsy and behavioral disorder can be cared for best if he attends a regular school in an understanding environment and is associated with a clinical outpatient service in which the physician and social service department work together with both the child and the family. It is becoming less necessary to arrange for either home tutoring or the placement of such children into schools or other facilities for the maladjusted.

Surgical Therapy. The patient with a potentially remediable lesion, such as a brain tumor, usually is considered for operation, whatever the state of the seizures. Surgical intervention for the removal of a focus of abnormal discharge is appropriate only for selected patients who have focal epilepsy that remains intractable after intensive medical therapy. A constant focally discharging area should be confirmed by serial electroencephalographic studies, and the region of brain considered for excision must be such that the patient will not be left afterward with a severe speech, memory, or other disabling neurologic deficit.

Patients so evaluated usually do not have gross space-occupying lesions, but the epileptogenic region eventually excised may contain a small tumor, a vascular lesion, or a scar secondary to trauma or previous encephalitis. The surgical approach has been utilized particularly for patients with focal motor and psychomotor–temporal lobe seizures. Even though many patients are considered for surgical therapy, relatively few are chosen, and the numbers of patients so treated are still only in the hundreds the world over. In carefully selected series, about half the patients enjoy significantly improved control of seizures postoperatively, although this sometimes merely represents less anticonvulsant drug requirement. In some patients, generalized seizures appear instead of previous psychomotor–temporal lobe attacks. A small number experience relief from severe personality disturbances, particularly aggressive psychotic behavior, but this is an uncertain effect, and surgical intervention usually is not primarily directed toward this. Bilateral operations on the temporal lobe have been of limited success and have produced severe memory disturbances.

Cerebral hemispherectomy has been accomplished in a small number of carefully selected children with severe infantile hemiplegia, intractable convulsions, and behavior disturbances. Improvement in the seizures and behavior has occurred despite the persistence of motor and sensory neurologic disability.

Much more must be learned about the natural history of the epilepsies in order to evaluate thoroughly the different therapies. Adequate seizure control can be achieved now for most patients. The drugs involved are increasingly less toxic, but anticonvulsant medication remains essentially nonspecific and is directed against mechanisms of neuronal hyperexcitability that are little understood. A relatively small number of cases not responding to other management can be selected for surgical intervention. It is hoped that combined physiologic and biochemical studies of disturbed cerebral and bodily functions in the epilepsies will lead eventually to more rational and effective therapy.

Epilepsia (Journal of the International League Against Epilepsy), H. Gastaut. G. H. Glaser, M. Lennox-Buchthal (eds.). Raven Press, New York.
Gowers, W. R.: Epilepsy and Other Chronic Convulsive Disorders: Their Causes, Symptoms and Treatment. London, J. & A. Churchill, 1881. Reprinted by Dover Publications, New York, 1964.
Jasper, H. H., Ward, A. A., and Pope, A.: Basic Mechanisms of the Epilepsies. Boston, Little, Brown & Company, 1969.
Lennox, W. G.: Epilepsy and Related Disorders. Boston, Little, Brown & Company, 1960.
Lennox-Buchthal, M. A.: Febrile convulsions. A reappraisal. Amsterdam, Elsevier Scientific Publishing Company, 1973.
Penfield, W. G., and Jasper, H. H.: Epilepsy and the Functional Anatomy of the Human Brain. Boston, Little, Brown & Company, 1954.
Schmidt, R. P., and Wilder, B. J.: Epilepsy Contemporary Neurology Series Monograph No. 2. Philadelphia, F. A. Davis Company, 1968.
Woodbury, D. M., Penry, J. K., and Schmidt, R. P. (eds.): Antiepileptic Drugs. New York, Raven Press, 1972.

Section Seventeen.   INTRACRANIAL TUMORS AND STATES CAUSING INCREASED INTRACRANIAL PRESSURE

Robert A. Fishman

420.   INTRACRANIAL TUMORS

Intracranial tumors include neoplasms, both benign and malignant, and other space-taking lesions of chronic inflammatory origin that develop in brain, meninges, or skull. Their clinical manifestations are diverse and vary greatly according to tumor type and location. Errors in diagnosis are relatively common because the clinical manifestations of tumor may simulate a variety of neurologic disorders. Brain tumors occur at any age; they are common in children under ten, but have their peak incidence in the fifth and sixth decades of life. Race, occupation, and history of trauma have not been established as predisposing factors in the occurrence of intracranial tumors. Genetic factors are relevant, however, to the occurrence of a few tumor types, e.g., hemangioblastoma and neurofibromatosis.

Classification and Pathology.   A great number of tumor types have been variously classified. Most classifications include (1) primary tumors originating in brain, (2) meningeal tumors, (3) vascular tumors, (4) pituitary tumors, (5) congenital tumors, (6) adnexal tumors, (7) metastatic tumors, and (8) granulomas and parasitic cysts.

Primary Brain Tumors.   The largest group of primary brain tumors are the gliomas, composed of malignant glial cells. These include the following:

GLIOBLASTOMA MULTIFORME.   These most malignant gliomas are composed of very undifferentiated cells. Complete surgical removal is impossible. The average life expectancy is 12 months. They have a very rapid growth rate and are characterized by much tissue necrosis and brain edema.

ASTROCYTOMA.   Astrocytomas are composed of astrocytes that infiltrate the brain and are often associated with cysts of varying size. They are generally slow growing and may occasionally run a course of many years or even decades. They may infiltrate normal brain widely but with relatively little effect on brain function early in the illness. Complete surgical excision of cystic astrocytomas of the cerebellum may be possible, particularly in children, but in most other instances their marked invasiveness of brain prevents complete removal. Astrocytomas may undergo malignant change, and a highly malignant glioblastoma may develop within a relatively benign astrocytoma.

OLIGODENDROGLIOMA.   Oligodendrogliomas, composed of oligodendroglial cells, are similar in behavior to astrocytomas and are distinguishable only on histologic study.

EPENDYMOMA.   Ependymomas are derived from ependymal cells. They arise from the walls of the ventricular system, filling or obstructing the ventricles and invading adjacent tissues. They are malignant and cause death in about three years.

MEDULLOBLASTOMA. Medulloblastomas develop from a primitive cell within the cerebellum. They are chiefly tumors of childhood but can occur in older patients. They are highly malignant and frequently metastasize throughout the subarachnoid space to involve the cerebrum or spinal cord.

Meningeal Tumors. The most important tumor arising in the meninges is the *meningioma,* which may invade the adjacent bone as well as compressing and distorting the brain. It is slow growing, well circumscribed, often highly vascular, and may be calcified. It is benign, and complete removal is often possible unless the tumor involves critical structures.

Vascular Tumors. Tumors composed of vascular elements include the arteriovenous malformations (angiomas) and hemangioblastomas. The angiomas are congenital malformations composed of an abnormal collection of blood vessels of adult structure. They are present from birth but slowly enlarge and may not cause symptoms for many years. They may compress normal brain, may bleed intracerebrally or into the subarachnoid space, may be manifest only as a source of seizures, or may be an incidental finding at autopsy. Hemangioblastomas are true neoplasms composed of primitive vascular elements that may be quiescent for many years or may enlarge very slowly. They are most commonly found in the cerebellum but occur also in the cerebrum. Cerebellar hemangioblastoma may be associated with angiomatosis of the retina and cysts of the kidney and pancreas (the von Hippel–Lindau syndrome).

Pituitary Tumors. Pituitary tumors may arise from chromophobe, eosinophil, or basophil cells of the anterior pituitary. Of these, chromophobe adenomas are the most common. Chromophobe adenomas are nonfunctioning tumors that give symptoms by compression of the normal pituitary gland as well as the optic chiasm, the hypothalamus, and the adjacent brain with their suprasellar growth. Eosinophilic adenomas give rise to hyperpituitarism, acromegaly in adults, and gigantism in children, but do not generally compress suprasellar structures unless the tumor is mixed with chromophobe elements. Basophil adenomas are small and, although associated with Cushing's syndrome, are not responsible for symptoms by compression of adjacent tissues. *Craniopharyngiomas* derived from Rathke's pouch may be intrasellar or suprasellar in location, may compress the pituitary and optic chiasm, and are similar in effect to the chromophobe adenoma. They are frequently calcified and often contain cysts filled with thick, lipid-laden fluid.

Congenital Tumors. These tumors develop from congenital rests and include craniopharyngiomas of the pituitary, chordomas, dermoids, and teratomas. Chordomas are composed of cells derived from the embryonic notochord. They are midline and usually arise on the clivus, posterior to the sella. They grow slowly, but are highly invasive, and their total extirpation can seldom be accomplished. Dermoids and teratomas may occur anywhere in the central nervous system, particularly near the midline, adjacent to the ventricular system, or at the distal end of the cord. They tend to become symptomatic during the first decade of life, but may be silent for many years.

Adnexal Tumors. These tumors include those origi-

nating within the pineal body and those derived from the choroid plexus, the choroid papilloma. Pinealomas are rare tumors that cause symptoms by compressing the aqueduct, resulting in obstructive hydrocephalus and giving paralysis of vertical gaze by involvement of the pretectum of the midbrain. They may compress the hypothalamus and give rise to precocious puberty or diabetes insipidus. Choroid plexus papillomas are benign lesions that may cause intraventricular bleeding. They may cause increased intracranial pressure by obstructing the ventricular system or, it has been suggested, by excessive formation of cerebrospinal fluid.

Metastatic Tumors. Metastatic tumors constitute 10 to 25 per cent of brain tumors. They may originate from almost any primary tumor, most commonly those of breast and lung, but also from neoplasms of the gastrointestinal and genitourinary tracts, bone, thyroid, or nasal sinuses. They may be single or multiple, well encapsulated or diffuse, spread by extension from adjacent tissues or hematogenously. They may occur as a late manifestation in widespread carcinomatosis or as the first manifestation of an unrecognized primary visceral malignancy.

Granulomas and Parasitic Cysts. Granulomas affecting the nervous system include those associated with tuberculosis, mycotic infection, sarcoidosis, parasitic infestation, and syphilis. *Tuberculoma* may present as a solitary mass lesion within the brain; although rare in the United States, it is common in some areas, including Central and South America. Tuberculoma usually develops without evidence of tuberculous meningitis, although evidence of pulmonary tuberculosis is common. Favorable results with surgical excision and antituberculosis therapy have been reported. *Toruloma* is the most common mycotic granuloma affecting brain. This is usually associated with some evidence of meningeal involvement as well. The *granulomas of sarcoidosis* have been reported to occur in the brain; there is usually evidence of meningeal or posterior pituitary involvement, although the evidence for systemic sarcoid may be minimal. *Cysticercosis,* caused by the larvae of *Taenia solium* or *Taenia saginata,* may be responsible for single or multiple cerebral masses. This is seen chiefly in South America and in the Middle East and India. *Syphilitic gummas* are extremely rare, but have been reported, presenting like slow-growing cerebral gliomas.

Pathophysiology. Intracranial tumors give rise to focal disturbances in brain function and to increased intracranial pressure. Focal manifestations occur because brain is compressed or infiltrated by tumor, because the blood supply of the region is compromised, resulting in tissue necrosis, and because of cerebral edema. Tumors may be located either within or outside brain parenchyma, i.e., intra-axial or extra-axial in location. Brain dysfunction is generally greatest with rapidly growing, infiltrative intra-axial tumors, e.g., glioblastoma, because of marked infiltration, compression, and necrosis of brain. Cyst formation within tumors also compresses adjacent normal brain. Cerebral edema about tumors increases the neurologic deficit. In edema, the water and sodium content of the brain are increased owing to their accumulation in the extracellular space and in glial cells. Extra-axial tumors, e.g., meningioma, which slowly compress brain, may reach great size with few, if any, clinical signs.

Tumors cause a generalized increase in intracranial pressure when they reach sufficient mass, because of the fixed volume of the intracranial cavity. Obstruction of the ventricular system also increases intracranial pressure and causes hydrocephalic dilatation of the proximal ventricles and thinning of the cerebral hemispheres. Tumors that obstruct the intracranial venous sinuses also cause increased intracranial pressure. Complete compensation with very little or even no rise in pressure can occur with slowly growing neoplasms, but with rapidly growing malignant tumors, increased intracranial pressure is an early sign. Increased intracranial pressure becomes life threatening when there is sufficient displacement of brain to cause herniation of the uncus or cerebellum. In *uncal herniation,* the most medial gyrus of the temporal lobe, the uncus, is displaced inferiorly by a hemispheric mass through the tentorial notch, thus causing compression of the midbrain, which results in depression of consciousness and ipsilateral or bilateral dilated and fixed pupils owing to compression of the third nerve. In *cerebellar herniation,* the tonsils are displaced downward through the foramen magnum by a posterior fossa mass, causing compression of the medulla and respiratory arrest. Characteristic vasomotor changes ensue with increased intracranial pressure, only if rapid or severe. These include *progressive bradycardia* caused by vagal slowing of the heart; *systemic hypertension,* which occurs as the intracranial pressure begins to approach arterial diastolic pressure, inducing medullary ischemia and compensatory systemic vasoconstriction; and, finally, *central respiratory failure.* Any degree of CO_2 retention will further increase intracranial pressure because of its cerebrovasodilator effects, and therefore adequate ventilation with maintenance of a clear airway is essential for the patient with increased intracranial pressure. (Drugs such as morphine, which depress respiration sufficiently to raise arterial CO_2 levels, are therefore contraindicated.)

Clinical Manifestations. The natural history of intracranial tumor is characterized by insidious onset and progression of focal or general neurologic deficits, or both. Many tumors have rather characteristic manifestations that point to the diagnosis (see below). There is great variation, depending upon location and rate of growth. Occasionally symptoms may be explosive in onset, suggesting a vascular lesion, and there may also be variations in course, suggestive of a remission. The symptoms and signs of intracranial tumor are discussed below.

Headache. Headache is a major but not invariable symptom of intracranial tumor. Patients with extensive tumors may not complain of headache, particularly if they have slowly growing infiltrative tumors (astrocytoma) or slowly growing extra-axial tumors (such as meningiomas, acoustic neuromas, or pituitary tumors). Similarly, when tumors interfere with the higher intellectual functions, headache may not be reported. Tumors give rise to headache by displacement of the pain-sensitive structures within the cranial cavity. Rarely, tumors give rise to a chronic meningeal inflammatory response that also may be responsible for pain. The problem of headache with brain tumor is discussed more extensively in Ch. 350.

Mental Changes. Mental changes may occur either early or late in the history of brain tumor, depending upon tumor location. Subtle evidence of personality change may be the first manifestation of a mass in the cerebral hemispheres, particularly involving the frontal lobes. This may take several forms. The symptoms may be chiefly affective, simulating an involutional depression. Some patients develop confusional states, at times associated with episodes of bizarre behavior. The most common mental changes are progressive impairment of abstraction, recent memory and judgment, and a shortened attention span (see Ch. 326 to 331). However, some patients, particularly those with slowly growing neoplasms in the right (nondominant) hemisphere, may harbor huge tumors with only minimal impairment of intellect. Drowsiness progressing to stupor and coma accompanies severely increased intracranial pressure.

Disturbances of Speech. Various forms of aphasia occur with neoplastic involvement of the dominant hemisphere. The aphasic disorders are insidious in their development, and minor disturbances may be overlooked or erroneously attributed to psychologic factors. The various discrete forms of apraxia and agnosia may occur in evolution of the tumor syndrome, and may be the initial symptom in otherwise well persons.

Papilledema and Vision. The presence of the characteristic ophthalmoscopic appearance of papilledema suggests increased intracranial pressure; however, the funduscopic findings may be indistinguishable from those of optic neuritis or pseudopapilledema. Pseudopapilledema is a congenital change in the funduscopic appearance of the disc that simulates the swelling associated with increased intracranial pressure. Differential points include the late loss of visual acuity in increased intracranial pressure as opposed to early and more severe visual loss in optic neuritis. Visual acuity is generally unaffected in pseudopapilledema. Episodes of *amaurosis fugax,* fleeting moments of dimming vision, may be associated with a marked degree of papilledema and are a dangerous warning sign of potential loss of vision. The visual fields in true papilledema or pseudopapilledema may show enlargement of the blind spots. Disturbance of vision in patients with intracranial tumor also can be caused by extraocular muscle palsies, disturbances of the central visual pathways (see below), and disorders of visual interpretation, as in the alexias and visual agnosias. Uniocular papilledema with contralateral optic atrophy occurs characteristically, with subfrontal tumors that cause optic atrophy by direct involvement of the nerve and papilledema in the opposite eye owing to increased intracranial pressure. The fundi may not reveal papilledema despite very elevated intracranial pressure; this may be attributable to glaucoma when present, but may also occur for unexplained reasons.

Diplopia and Hemianopia. Diplopia with brain tumors is due to involvement of one or both sixth cranial nerves, either directly by the tumor or, more commonly, indirectly because of generalized increase in intracranial pressure (see False Localizing Signs, below). Third-nerve palsy may be due to involvement of the superior orbital fissure by meningioma, although the nerve may be involved by a variety of other lesions anywhere along its course. Hemianopias result from involvement of the visual pathways. Lesions affecting the optic chiasm, most notably originating in or near the pituitary, give rise to bitemporal hemianopia. Lesions of the optic tract, optic radiation, or occipital cortex give rise to contralateral homonymous hemianopias. Lesions of the anterior temporal pole characteristically cause a contralateral homonymous, superior quadrantopsia.

Ataxia and Hemiplegia. Unsteadiness in walking may occur with tumor in various intracranial sites.

Lesions affecting the midline cerebellum cause a characteristic truncal ataxia with lateralized ataxia of the extremities if the cerebellar hemispheres are also involved. Disease in the frontal lobes may give rise to unsteadiness in walking, an apraxia of gait, which may simulate cerebellar truncal ataxia. Drug intoxication caused by diphenylhydantoin or barbiturates may potentiate ataxia. Tumors of the hemisphere characteristically cause contralateral spastic hemiparesis; initially the signs may be so minimal as to be easily overlooked.

Sensory Disturbances. Hemisensory defects occur with intracranial tumors affecting the contralateral sensory pathways. The primary sensory modalities of touch, pain, temperature, and proprioception are impaired when the thalamus or the ascending spinothalamic pathways are involved. Tumors of the parietal sensory cortex cause loss of cortical sensory functions that results in impairment of sensory localization, two-point discrimination, graphesthesia, stereognosia, and position sense. Tumors of the thalamus may be manifested by episodes of pain affecting the contralateral side of the face or body. Tumors of the cortex may cause focal sensory seizures with a jacksonian march; these may be reported as an aura before a grand mal seizure. Pain in the face occurs with tumors affecting the base of the skull, particularly those arising in the nasopharynx and paranasal sinuses. Tumors affecting the trigeminal nerve may give rise to paroxysms of pain in the face simulating trigeminal neuralgia (tic douloureux), but unlike the latter there is also some loss of facial sensation.

Seizures. Seizures may serve as the first clinical manifestation of brain tumor, or may occur at any time in the course of the illness. The types include classic grand mal seizures and various forms of focal seizures. Typical petit mal is probably never due to neoplasm; minor seizures with brain tumor that at first may resemble petit mal generally are, in fact, either fragmentary grand mal seizures or a variety of psychomotor attack. With any cerebral seizure, it is extremely important to note its aura or the pattern of its onset, for this often provides a reliable indicator of the location of the neoplasm. Focal motor and sensory seizures may be limited to one region of the body or may progress (jacksonian seizures) to involve the entire body. Lesions in the temporal lobe characteristically give rise to psychomotor seizures. These may be associated with olfactory hallucinations (uncinate fits), disorders of visual or auditory perception, experiential attacks such as déjà vu and various types of automatic behavior, for which the patient is generally amnesic (see Part X, Section Sixteen). The onset of convulsions in an otherwise healthy subject over the age of 20 without history of convulsions raises the possibility of an expanding lesion. This possibility is greater if focal signs can be detected in the neurologic examination; if so, additional specialized neurologic diagnostic studies are warranted.

Nausea and Vomiting. Nausea and vomiting occur as a result of direct or reflex stimulation of the emetic center of the medulla. This is most likely to occur in association with increased intracranial pressure, particularly with displacement of the brainstem owing to herniation or the presence of bleeding into the cerebrospinal fluid. The vomiting may occur without preceding nausea and may be projectile. Brain tumor is not suggested by the occurrence of nausea and vomiting alone, i.e., there are invariably other clinical manifestations of the tumor. Antiemetic drugs, e.g., the phenothiazines, inhibit this type of centrally induced vomiting.

Stiff Neck. Signs of meningeal irritation may occur in brain tumor, as a manifestation of cerebellar herniation through the foramen magnum, because of the effects of bleeding into the subarachnoid space, or with meningeal involvement. Cervical rigidity may be striking but Kernig's sign is generally absent (see Tumors of the Cerebellum, below).

Vasomotor and Autonomic Changes. These occur as ominous late signs. They include bradycardia and hypertension, as described above. Apnea generally precedes cardiac arrest in fatal cases. Autonomic manifestations of brain tumor include gastric ulceration (Cushing's ulcer), which may present as a massive gastrointestinal hemorrhage. This may occur with mass lesions anywhere in the intracranial cavity. (The use of adrenocortical steroids in the management of patients with brain tumor may further increase this hazard.) Fever may also occur in patients with mass lesions in the absence of pulmonary, urinary, or other infection, because of a central disturbance, presumably of hypothalamic origin. Hyperthermia is not uncommon just prior to death, but hypothermia may also occur. Fever commonly accompanies the presence of blood in the subarachnoid space. This may occur with rapidly growing neoplasms or as a result of surgery. Disturbances of sweating may occur, lesions of hypothalamus and brainstem giving rise to contralateral signs of sympathectomy.

Metabolic Manifestations. The complex interrelationships between the hypothalamus and the anterior and posterior pituitary may be deranged with intracranial tumors, giving rise to various systemic metabolic disorders. These include diabetes insipidus, inappropriate secretion of antidiuretic hormone, hypopituitarism, and precocious puberty (see Ch. 834, 805, 831, and 858, respectively).

False Localizing Signs. These may occur with increased intracranial pressure or with shift of intracranial structures. The most common such sign is unilateral or bilateral lateral rectus palsy due to sixth-nerve compression. This need not imply neoplastic involvement of the nerve, for it frequently occurs as a pressure palsy of the nerve resulting from increased intracranial pressure itself. Signs of hemiplegia can occur ipsilateral to the tumor owing to compression of the opposite cerebral peduncle on the tentorium; i.e., hemiplegia need not be contralateral to the mass. There are relatively silent areas in brain, wherein tumors reach large size with relatively little clinical deficit; these are the right frontal and temporal lobes. This must be considered in evaluating patients with the syndrome of increased intracranial pressure without localizing signs (see below).

Diagnosis. Patients suspected of having an intracranial tumor require complete medical evaluation to establish the relationship of the neurologic findings to possible coexisting systemic disease. Appropriate laboratory studies should be obtained to search for a primary systemic neoplasm, e.g., lung, breast, gastrointestinal, genitourinary, or thyroid malignancies. The major neurologic diagnostic techniques are described below.

Skull Roentgenograms. The films should be examined for the following: (1) changes suggestive of increased intracranial pressure, (2) bone destruction, (3) bony thickening or hyperostosis, (4) abnormal vascular channels, (5) abnormal calcifications, (6) the shape of the sella turcica, (7) the position of the pineal if calcified, and (8) the relationship of the skull to the cervical spine in suspected platybasia, basilar impression, and related disorders (see Ch. 424).

Characteristic roentgenographic changes may occur with chronically increased intracranial pressure as a result of pressure atrophy of bone, which produces a beaten-silver appearance in the cranial vault, decalcification of the clinoid processes, and separation of the sutures in children. Bone destruction is characteristic of metastatic neoplasms arising from distant organs and of directly invasive tumors that arise in the paranasal sinuses and nasopharynx. Focal hyperostosis of the skull, i.e., thickening of the inner or outer tables of the skull, or both, with increased calcification, is characteristic of meningioma. Generalized thickening of the skull occurs with Paget's disease. Hyperostosis frontalis interna, localized bilateral thickenings of the inner table of the skull, is generally considered an incidental finding without clinical significance. The vascular markings of the skull, which accompany arterial and venous channels, vary greatly in the normal subject. Focal enlargements of the markings occur characteristically with meningioma involving adjacent meninges and skull. Abnormal calcifications characteristically occur in very slowly growing primary neoplasms (astrocytoma, oligodendroglioma, craniopharyngioma, meningioma), in arteriovenous malformations, in aneurysmal walls, and in the glial nodules associated with tuberous sclerosis. Calcifications may also occur in the gliotic walls of old abscesses, in hemorrhagic cavities, and in granulomas of cerebral toxoplasmosis. Displacement of the pineal laterally more than 2 mm is pathologic, and this or a shift superiorly or inferiorly suggests the presence of a space-taking lesion.

Electroencephalography. The electroencephalogram is useful in screening for possible brain tumor. Focal changes, particularly slowing in frequency of the record, are common with tumors in the cerebral hemispheres. Rapidly growing tumors with adjacent cerebral edema are more likely to evoke focal changes than are slowly progressive tumors with only minimal clinical manifestations, and with the latter the record may be entirely normal. The electroencephalogram is often normal with posterior fossa neoplasms.

Cerebrospinal Fluid. Examination of the cerebrospinal fluid (CSF) for pressure, protein, sugar, cell count, cultures, serologic tests, and cytologic analysis is often helpful in the diagnosis of intracranial tumor. The incidence of abnormalities varies with the stage of the illness and the site and nature of the neoplasm. The fluid is crystal clear unless the protein exceeds about 150 mg per 100 ml or unless bleeding has occurred. With slowly growing neoplasms the intracranial pressure will remain normal, less than 200 mm, until late in the illness, whereas in rapidly growing tumors increased pressure may be an early manifestation. Jugular compression for the Queckenstedt test is contraindicated in patients who are suspected of having brain tumor. A protein content greater than 100 mg per 100 ml is frequently associated with rapidly growing tumors near the ventricles or subarachnoid space. With slowly growing tumors, the protein may be normal despite the presence of a huge mass. Of the posterior fossa neoplasms, acoustic neuroma commonly results in marked elevation of the protein, 100 to 500 mg per 100 ml. The fluid is normal in most patients with brainstem gliomas. The cell count is elevated from 5 to 100 white cells per cubic millimeter in about one third of the cases, and may exceed 1000 white cells, particularly when the tumor involves the ventricular wall and has undergone necrosis. Malignant cells may be detected with suitable techniques. The glucose content is normal with brain tumor, apart from patients with diffuse neoplastic involvement of the meninges, when it is characteristically reduced to levels below 40 mg per 100 ml; in some cases this may be the sole abnormality, although commonly 10 to 100 mononuclear cells are seen, and with special cytologic techniques malignant cells may be detected.

Lumbar puncture may be hazardous; it is *contraindicated* in critically ill patients with clinical signs of incipient herniation because the removal of fluid from the lumbar sac may increase the degree of *pre-existing* herniation of the temporal lobe or of the cerebellar tonsils.

Roentgenographic Contrast Studies. Pneumoencephalography by the lumbar route, *ventriculography,* and *arteriography* are of major importance in the diagnosis and localization of brain tumor. Lumbar pneumography delineates the ventricular system and the subarachnoid space and thus may reveal the presence of a mass lesion. In ventriculography, air is injected via burr holes in the skull directly into the lateral cerebral ventricles; this may prove necessary for patients with increased intracranial pressure, in whom the lumbar route is deemed hazardous, and for patients in whom there is nonfilling of the ventricular system by the lumbar route. Cerebral angiography may yield much information concerning the location and size of a tumor. Major advances in neuroradiology have established angiography as the most useful of the contrast studies. The vascular patterns of the tumor, arterial, capillary, and venous, may give indications of its histology. The decision as to which contrast technique is most likely to give maximal information in any patient depends upon the specific circumstances of the diagnostic problem in question and must be resolved individually. Some patients need more than one such study.

Noninvasive Radiographic Procedures. Various scanning techniques have become available that permit the recording of the radioactivity present over regions of the skull after intravenous administration of radioiodinated human serum albumin, technetium, and other gamma emitters. The isotope may enter more rapidly and in greater concentration into the tumor and its adjacent area of edema because of the greater permeability of the capillaries and adjacent cellular membranes. The isotope scan does not readily differentiate between focal changes caused by neoplasm, sepsis, or infarction, and is often negative with slowly growing tumors. A recent development in this field is *computerized axial tomography,* which accurately outlines both normal and abnormal intracranial structures without the necessity to employ contrast materials. Although presently available only in a few major centers, the technique promises to add greatly to accurate and safe diagnosis of brain tumor and other lesions.

Echoencephalography. This technique is useful in determining the position of midline structures, i.e., whether there is a shift of the intracranial contents. This is particularly valuable in patients without a calcified pineal. Although the technique gives no information regarding the cause of a shift, it is a useful screening device for patients with suspected mass lesions.

Ancillary Laboratory Tests. Audiometry and vestibular tests are necessary in evaluating patients with suspected tumor of the eighth nerve, and visual fields are valuable in assessing lesions of the visual system.

Tumor Syndromes. *Tumors of the Skull.* Benign osteomas rarely reach a size sufficient to compress underlying brain; generally these can be extirpated. Malignant tumors arising in the paranasal sinuses or nasopharynx directly invade the base of the skull and cause chronic facial pain and multiple cranial nerve involvement. Tumors of the glomus jugulare (nonchromaffin paraganglioma) arise near the jugular bulb and often lead to progressive deafness and a bloody discharge in the external auditory canal. Other lesions that give roentgenographic evidence of bone destruction and that must be differentiated include Paget's disease, Hand-Schüller-Christian disease, eosinophilic granuloma, and cholesteatoma (epidermoids).

Diffuse Meningeal Neoplasia (Neoplastic Meningitis). Carcinomas, gliomas, sarcomas, melanomas, and lymphomas may diffusely infiltrate the leptomeninges and subarachnoid space to produce a syndrome of chronic meningitis, which may simulate chronic meningitis caused by fungi, tuberculosis, sarcoidosis, and meningovascular syphilis. Common manifestations include headache, mental changes, cranial nerve palsies, areflexia, and minimal if any signs of meningeal irritation. The cerebrospinal fluid findings generally will establish the diagnosis. The pressure is usually normal; sugar content may be below 45 mg per 100 ml and as low as 10 mg per 100 ml; protein content is normal or elevated; cell count reveals from 5 to several hundred mononuclear cells; cultures are negative; cytologic studies may reveal malignant cells. The diagnosis may not be apparent at autopsy because gross lesions are generally absent, and microscopic sections are needed to verify the diagnosis.

Tumors of the Cerebral Hemispheres. Tumors affecting the cerebral hemispheres are characterized by progressive focal neurologic deficits and, commonly, by generalized or focal convulsive seizures. Hemispheric tumors involving any lobe may be associated with contralateral hemiplegia; when located in the parasagittal region the paralysis is greater in the leg than in the arm. Tumors of the frontal lobes are also characterized by early impairment of intellectual function. Tumors in the parietal region cause contralateral cortical (interpretive) sensory deficits, impairment of primary sensation, and homonymous hemianopia. Tumors in the occipital region also cause contralateral homonymous hemianopia plus disorders of visual interpretation. Tumors in the temporal lobe, in the nondominant hemisphere, are relatively silent apart from contralateral superior quadrantopsia. Tumors of regions adjacent to the sylvian fissure of the dominant hemisphere give rise to aphasic disorders; anterior lesions in the frontal lobe cause expressive aphasia, posterior lesions in the parietal region cause the receptive aphasias, and lesions in the superior temporal gyrus cause anomic aphasia.

Tumors of the Cerebellum. The common tumors of the cerebellum include medulloblastomas, which affect the midline vermis most commonly in childhood, and tumors of the cerebellar hemisphere, chiefly gliomas and metastatic tumors. Early manifestations of tumor of the midline vermis include truncal ataxia on tandem walking and symptoms of increased intracranial pressure. Tumors of the cerebellar hemisphere cause ipsilateral limb ataxia as an early manifestation. Tilting of the head to one side may be an early sign as well. Stiffness of the neck is often seen in posterior fossa neoplasms as an early sign of herniation.

Brainstem Tumors. These intrinsic tumors of midbrain, pons, and medulla are most commonly gliomas. The initial symptoms are those of cranial nerve dysfunction, most commonly affecting the extraocular muscles (nuclear or internuclear ophthalmoplegia), chewing and swallowing, as well as the long tracts, ascending and descending. Headache and other manifestations of increased intracranial pressure occur late in the course. The cerebrospinal fluid is often normal.

Pituitary Tumors. The earliest symptoms may be those of endocrine disturbances (see above) or may be due to effects on the visual system. Frontal headache may be an early symptom, as well as progressive bitemporal hemianopia caused by chiasmatic involvement. Pituitary tumors may invade the sphenoid sinus and thus permit the development of bacterial meningitis. The cysts associated with craniopharyngioma may release lipid-laden fluid into the subarachnoid space, thus causing bouts of sterile meningitis.

Optic Nerve Glioma. Gliomas may develop in the intraorbital, retro-orbital, or chiasmatic region of the optic nerve, the first of these being the most common location. These tumors usually occur in early childhood with uniocular loss of vision as the most common presenting symptom. Proptosis is seen in about one third of cases. Uniocular optic atrophy or papilledema may be noted. Roentgenographic evidence of enlargement of the optic foramen is common. The tumor is most often a slowly growing astrocytoma and may be associated with neurofibromatosis.

Acoustic Neuroma (Cerebellopontine Angle Tumor). These neurofibromas (schwannomas) of the eighth nerve begin within the auditory canal or in the subarachnoid space. They are slowly growing and characteristically cause progressive tinnitus and nerve deafness. The vestibular portion is more seriously involved than the acoustic portion, and in patients who do not have a dead labyrinth on caloric testing, the diagnosis is suspect. There are few symptoms referable to loss of vestibular function. A mild sensation of giddiness or unsteadiness is common, but recurrent episodes of vertigo are very rare in acoustic tumors. Adjacent cranial nerves are also commonly involved, particularly the fifth, sixth, and seventh nerves. Large tumors cause ipsilateral cerebellar signs and manifestations of increased intracranial pressure. Meningiomas of the cerebellopontine angle may give a similar clinical picture without, however, enlargement of the auditory canal on roentgenograms of the skull.

Metastatic Tumors. The clinical pictures that result from metastatic neoplasms are very variable, depending on the site and number of metastases and their rate of growth. The diagnosis is readily made in patients with evidence of widespread metastatic disease who then develop focal neurologic signs. However, frequently the metastatic tumor may become symptomatic in brain with few if any manifestations of systemic malignant disease. Therefore patients with an apparently single intracranial mass lesion should be studied for a hidden neoplasm.

Differential Diagnosis. A wide variety of neurologic diseases may simulate brain tumor because they are also characterized by progressive focal neurologic signs or signs of increased intracranial pressure. Some of the more common problems in differential diagnosis are considered in the following paragraphs.

Syndrome of Increased Intracranial Pressure Without Localizing Signs. A major diagnostic problem is seen in the patient who presents with increased intracranial pressure manifested by headache and papilledema and who is otherwise apparently normal. The many diagnostic possibilities (see Ch. 422) include extra-axial neoplasms that obstruct the ventricular system, such as tentorial meningioma and pinealoma, and intraventricular tumors like ependymoma and glioma. Some patients have the syndrome of aqueduct stenosis, generally a manifestation of congenital forking (see Ch. 423). Tumors of relatively silent areas like the right frontal and temporal lobes must be excluded. Arteriography and ventriculography and/or lumbar pneumography are generally required to establish the diagnosis.

Tumor vs. Vascular Disease. The differential diagnosis between tumor and vascular disease is generally made on the basis of history: most tumors have an insidious onset and progress slowly, but most vascular lesions characteristically have an abrupt onset. However, some neoplasms such as glioblastoma or metastatic tumors may have a very abrupt onset, most often caused by bleeding into the tumor. Also, the stepwise progression ("stuttering onset") of hemiplegia in some patients with vascular disease of the extracranial portions of the internal carotid and vertebral arteries and, at times, of the intracranial arteries, may pose diagnostic uncertainty. Careful analysis of the history, the laboratory studies, and observation of the patient's course will clarify the diagnosis.

Tumor vs. Chronic Subdural Hematoma. The clinical picture in these patients simulates an expanding hemispheric mass: e.g., headache, drowsiness, papilledema, hemiparesis. About one third of patients with chronic subdural hematoma provide no significant history of head injury. The differential diagnosis can be made almost always with arteriography.

Tumor vs. Demyelinating Diseases, Multifocal Leukoencephalopathy. The more common forms of multiple sclerosis do not usually simulate expanding intracranial lesions. There are occasional cases of acute multiple sclerosis or Schilder's disease that may simulate a progressive hemispheric deficit. Diagnostic difficulty also may be encountered in patients with another disorder of white matter, multifocal leukoencephalopathy, which has been reported in association with the lymphomas and malignant disease arising in lung and other organs. In this disorder, multiple foci of demyelination are associated with electron microscopic evidence of viral infection. Clinically, there are signs of multiple lesions in the brain that can simulate metastatic disease. However, despite clinical evidence of multiple lesions and rapid progression, signs of increased intracranial pressure are absent. Although the diagnosis may be suspected, pathologic confirmation is necessary and usually comes only after death.

Tumor vs. Presenile Dementia. Progressive development of an organic dementia in middle age may be caused by many diseases, including frontal or bifrontal neoplasms. Tumors most likely to present with dementia include frontal and subfrontal tumors (olfactory groove meningioma and tumors of the corpus callosum, "butterfly glioma"). Roentgenographic contrast studies may be necessary to establish the diagnosis. A CSF protein greater than 100 mg per 100 ml favors tumor over the degenerative dementias.

Tumor vs. Abscess, Granuloma. Encapsulated brain abscess and the granulomas associated with cysticercosis may simulate brain tumor. Cysticercosis must be considered in any patient in an endemic area having signs of a cerebral mass lesion. An eosinophilic pleocytosis in the cerebrospinal fluid favors cysticercosis. Differentiation between tumor and abscess may be particularly difficult because patients with encapsulated brain abscess generally do not have systemic manifestations of infection (fever, leukocytosis), and the primary source of infection may be obscure. The cerebrospinal fluid may show little, if any, inflammatory change. The correct diagnosis of abscess or granuloma may not be made until surgery is performed.

Tumor vs. Epilepsy. The common occurrence of convulsive seizures with intracranial tumors requires consideration of this diagnosis when patients develop seizures (apart from true petit mal, which is never due to brain tumor). This is particularly true of patients in whom seizures first develop after the age of 20. The occurrence of transient focal neurologic signs in the postictal state (Todd's paralysis) favors the presence of a structural lesion as basis for the attacks. It is estimated that about 20 per cent of patients who develop seizures after the age of 20, who do not have post-traumatic seizures, will in time be shown to have intracranial tumors. The likelihood of a brain tumor diminishes with the passage of years if focal signs do not appear. There are differences of opinion as to how far one should proceed with diagnostic tests in a patient otherwise normal, with onset of seizures after the age of 20, particularly with regard to the indications for contrast studies. The occurrence of focal seizures, a focal neurologic deficit on clinical examination, or focal EEG slowing all increase the likelihood of the presence of tumor; in the absence of any of these, air study or arteriography is generally unrewarding.

Treatment. *Surgical Therapy.* Total surgical removal without sacrifice of normal cerebral tissue is possible only with tumors that are extra-axial in location, such as some meningiomas, osteomas, neurofibromas, and pituitary tumors. Total surgical extirpation of the primary tumors of brain, glioblastomas, and the less malignant gliomas, is not possible, although there are rare exceptions, e.g., cystic astrocytomas of the cerebellar hemisphere. Complete surgical removal of angiomas may be possible. Therefore it is essential to establish the precise location and tumor type to allow optimal therapy. Surgical attack on primary brain tumors may be helpful as palliative therapy, e.g., internal decompression or partial removal of tumor and edematous brain may relieve headaches and prolong useful life, particularly if the tumor is cystic and in the nondominant frontal or temporal lobes. There is no absolute rule for the surgical treatment of metastatic tumors. In some patients with major symptoms caused by an apparent single brain tumor without widespread systemic disease, surgical excision may offer useful palliation.

Radiotherapy. The gliomas may have a high degree of sensitivity, and x-ray therapy is generally indicated for palliation. Although biopsy and tissue diagnosis are highly desirable prior to instituting radiotherapy, a specimen is not always obtainable, particularly when the tumor is located in an inaccessible area like the brainstem. In such cases, diagnosis must be made on clinical and roentgenographic grounds. Unfortunately, the response of the gliomas to radiation is often brief, and recurrent growth supervenes. Chromophobe adenomas of the pituitary are generally radiosensitive, and radiotherapy is often the treatment of choice unless there is a rapidly progressive threat to vision, in which case surgical therapy is indicated.

Supportive Measures. Anticonvulsant drugs are indicated for patients with a history of convulsive seizures and for patients who have had intracranial surgery. Diphenylhydantoin, 300 to 500 mg per day, and phenobarbital, 30 to 60 mg three times a day, are common dosages. Higher dosages of these and other anticonvulsant drugs may be necessary for seizure control. The use of hypertonic intravenous solutions such as 30 per cent urea or 25 per cent mannitol to lower intracranial pressure has a limited place in management of patients with increased intracranial pressure. This is chiefly for very acute situations while the patient awaits neurosurgical intervention. Adrenal corticosteroids, such as dexamethasone, in high dosages help to reduce cerebral edema associated with brain tumors, particularly in the postoperative period and during radiotherapy; gastrointestinal bleeding, however, is a potential complication. Dosages of dexamethasone of 22 mg in the first 24 hours are recommended. The administration of parenteral fluids must be planned carefully when hydrating patients with increased intracranial pressure, because intravenous infusion of 5 per cent glucose in water can result in a significant increase in intracranial pressure. This danger can be avoided by use of normal saline, 5 per cent glucose in saline, or 5 per cent glucose in 0.42 per cent saline. The phenothiazines may be used as antiemetic agents for patients with severe vomiting. These drugs are depressants and must be used cautiously. Parenteral administration of caffeine transiently reduces intracranial pressure (it causes cerebral vasoconstriction and reduces cerebral blood flow) and may be useful in controlling brain tumor headaches. A variety of chemotherapeutic agents for the treatment of brain tumor are under active study, but their value has not yet been established.

Dastur, H. M., and Desai, A. D.: A comparative study of brain tuberculomas and gliomas based upon 107 case records of each. Brain, 88:375, 1965.

Dixon, H. B. F., and Lipscomb, F. M.: Cysticercosis: An Analysis and Follow-up of 450 Cases. Medical Research Council Special Report, Series No. 299. London, Her Majesty's Stationery Office, 1961.

Jelsma, R., and Bucy, P. C.: Glioblastoma multiforme: Its treatment and some factors affecting survival. Arch. Neurol., 20:171, 1969.

Richardson, E. P.: Neurologic effects of cancer. In Holland, J. F., and Frei, E. (eds.): Cancer Medicine. Philadelphia, Lea & Febiger, 1973.

Rubinstein, L. J.: Tumors of the Central Nervous System. Atlas of Tumor Pathology. Second series. Fascicle 6. Washington, D.C., Armed Forces Institute of Pathology, 1972.

Samson, D. S., and Clark, K.: A current review of brain abscess. Am. J. Med., 54:201, 1973.

Zulch, K. J.: Brain Tumors. Their Biology and Pathology. 2nd ed. New York, Springer Publishing Company, 1965.

421. RADIATION INJURY OF THE NERVOUS SYSTEM

Radiation injury of the nervous system occurs as a complication of x-ray therapy wherein tissue dosage has been excessive. Signs of injury may appear within hours or days of high-dosage irradiation in laboratory animals; in man, with the doses used therapeutically, the onset is delayed. Characteristically, a progressive neurologic deficit develops after a latent period of many months or years after the termination of radiotherapy. This complication occurs when irradiation has been directed at neoplasms of the brain or at other tumors in the head and neck. The spinal cord is also subject to injury from excessive radiation, whether directed at a primary cord tumor or at tumors overlying the spine and paraspinal regions, e.g., tumors of the thyroid or mediastinum. Peripheral nerves are relatively radioresistant but are injured also by high doses.

Pathology. The response of the central nervous system to ionizing radiation can be recognized in three phases: an acute phase of meningoencephalitis, a period of apparent normalcy, and a period of late nerve cell damage, demyelination, and vascular change. The lesions in the nervous system attributed to irradiation are extensive in both white and gray matter. There are hyaline thickenings in the walls of blood vessels that may partially or completely occlude the lumen. There is a variable degree of cellular necrosis and degeneration of myelin. Astrocytosis and thickening of the leptomeninges are common. The long latent period between the time of irradiation and the onset of progressive signs is poorly understood; it has been attributed to progressive ischemia caused by gradual narrowing of the vascular lumen. Latent radiation effects in skin are readily attributable to vascular and connective tissue damage; this lends weight to the primary importance of the vascular injury in the brain, although it is likely that neuronal degeneration is not due to progressive ischemia alone. It has been suggested that autoimmune mechanisms play a role in the tissue damage that develops after a latent period.

Dosages. The precise tissue dosage that will induce radiation injury is uncertain. The minimal dose in Lindgren's series of 71 cases that produced pathologic evidence of brain necrosis was 4500 to 5000 roentgens, with delivery through medium-sized fields over a period of 30 days. The spinal cord is vulnerable to somewhat lower doses; radiation myelopathy has been reported after 4000 r in 28 days directed toward the mediastinum. Boden has defined the tolerance of the brainstem and spinal cord from a review of his own material. With small treatment fields of 10 by 7 cm or less, tissue doses up to 4500 r in 17 days or their biologic equivalent seem to be tolerated by the cord and brainstem. With large fields, a tissue dose of 3500 r is considered as the maximal tolerance dose to the brainstem and cord. There is considerable biologic variation in susceptibility of normal tissue to radiation damage, and precise definition of the effects of various dosages on normal tissue is difficult.

Clinical Manifestations. When radiotherapy has been administered to tumors close to, but sparing, the brain and spinal cord, the development of a focal neurologic deficit after a latent period raises the possibility of radiation injury. After radiotherapy to brain or spinal cord tumors, clinical improvement that persists for one to five years with subsequent regression suggests the possibility of late radiation damage to normal nervous tissue. A transient form of radiation myelopathy is not uncommon; its major manifestation is the occurrence of Lhermitte's sign 2 to 37 weeks after radiation. Symptoms most often appear about a year after irradiation. The onset is insidious, and the rate of subsequent progress is unpredictable. The process may become arrested or may progress to cause a major cerebral hemispheric deficit or complete functional spinal cord transection. The clinical differentiation between radiation injury and recurrent tumor growth may be very difficult and uncertain pending pathologic confirmation at autopsy, and both may be coexistent. A repeated roentgenographic contrast study may help in differentiation. There is no specific therapy for radiation injury of the nervous system.

Boden, G.: Radiation myelitis of the brain-stem. J. Fac. Radiol., 2:79, 1950.
Coy, P., Baker, S., and Dolman, C. L.: Progressive myelopathy due to radiation. Can. Med. Assoc. J., 100:1129, 1969.
Lindgren, M.: On tolerance of brain tissue and sensitivity of brain tumours to irradiation. Acta Radiol. (Stockholm), (Suppl. 170):1, 1958.
Locksmith, J. P., and Powers, W. E.: Permanent radiation myelopathy. Am. J. Roentgenol., 102:916, 1968.
Reagan, T. J., et al.: Chronic progressive radiation myelopathy. J.A.M.A., 203:106, 1968.

422. BENIGN INTRACRANIAL HYPERTENSION
(Pseudotumor Cerebri)

Definition. Benign intracranial hypertension (BIH) describes the syndrome of increased intracranial pressure in which intracranial mass lesions, obstruction of the cerebral ventricles, intracranial infection, and hypertensive encephalopathy have been excluded. It has also been termed pseudotumor cerebri, serous meningitis, and otitic hydrocephalus. BIH includes a heterogenous group of disorders in which a number of different etiologic factors have been identified, although in most cases the cause and pathogenesis of these syndromes are poorly understood. They are termed "benign" because spontaneous recovery generally occurs; however, serious threats to vision may occur.

Clinical Manifestations. The presenting symptoms are headache and disturbance of vision. The headache is often worse on awakening and is aggravated by coughing and straining. It is often relatively mild and may be entirely absent. The most common ocular complaint is visual blurring, a manifestation of papilledema. Some patients complain of brief, fleeting movements of dimming or complete loss of vision, occurring many times during the day (amaurosis fugax), at times accentuated or precipitated by coughing and straining. The ominous symptom indicates that the patient's vision is in serious jeopardy. Visual loss may be minimal despite severe chronic papilledema, including retinal hemorrhages; however, blindness rarely may develop very rapidly—in less than 24 hours. Visual fields characteristically show enlargement of the blind spots, and may show constriction of the peripheral fields and central or paracentral scotoma. Diplopia caused by unilateral or bilateral sixth nerve palsy may develop as a result of increased intracranial pressure. The neurologic examination is otherwise normal. A major clinical point is that patients with BIH commonly look well; that is, their appearance and apparent well-being belie the ominous appearance of the papilledema.

Pathophysiology. The signs and symptoms of BIH are due to the effects of increased intracranial pressure; pressures between 300 and 600 mm are frequent. The intracranial pressure is normally between 50 and 180 to 200 mm of water as measured in the lumbar sac or ventricles with the patient in the lateral recumbent position. This pressure is dependent upon the pressure-volume relationships within the intracranial and spinal cavities. The intracranial cavity contains about 1400 ml of brain, 75 ml of blood, and 75 ml of CSF, and an additional 75 ml in the spinal subarachnoid space. The CSF pressure is directly dependent upon the intracranial venous pressure; changes in the latter pressure are readily transmitted to the CSF, and thus a sustained increase in intracranial venous pressure may result in the syndrome of chronically increased intracranial pressure. The intracranial pressure is largely independent of the systemic arterial pressure, and it is normal in essential hypertension; however, it falls with acute systemic hypotension and rises acutely with very acute increases in systemic blood pressure, e.g., with the administration of vasopressor drugs or in the syndrome of acute hypertensive encephalopathy. Increased intracranial pressure also accompanies increased cerebral blood flow resulting from CO_2 retention, as in acute asphyxia or with chronic pulmonary insufficiency. In patients with BIH apart from those with obstruction of the intracranial venous system and chronic pulmonary insufficiency, the mechanism of the increase in intracranial pressure is unknown. Two different kinds of changes have been noted on pneumoencephalography. The first has been normal air studies except for narrowed, slitlike ventricles and little air in the cortical subarachnoid space, which has been interpreted to mean that the brain volume is increased owing to "edema." The second has been normal air studies apart from normal or enlarged ventricles with an excessive amount of air in the cortical subarachnoid spaces, implying an increased volume of CSF. It is not clear whether these differences represent separate entities or whether the differences can be attributed to variation in time, i.e., the first type may develop into the second type after sufficient time has elapsed. Although cerebral edema has been suspected, there are few clinical manifestations of cerebral dysfunction in these patients to denote any functional changes as a result of the edema.

There are new methods available that permit measurement of the rates of formation and of removal of CSF in man, but to date these have not been applied to patients with this syndrome. (The only disease in which there is any evidence in favor of a pathologic increase in CSF formation is papilloma of the choroid plexus.) The calculation of the Ayala index at lumbar puncture, an old clinical guide to the volume of CSF, favors an increased CSF volume in many patients with BIH.

$$\text{Ayala index} = \frac{\text{Final pressure}}{\text{Initial pressure}} \times 10 \text{ ml removed.}$$

5.0 to 7.0 is normal. Values greater than 7.0 denote increased CSF volume; values less than 5.0 denote decreased CSF volume.) The index is almost always increased in patients with benign intracranial hypertension. Although there are clinical correlations between various endocrinopathies (see below), the mechanism wherein the adrenal, parathyroids, ovaries, or anterior pituitary might affect brain or CSF volumes is obscure.

Etiologic Factors and Associated Disorders (Table). *Intracranial Venous Sinus Thrombosis.* Increased intra-

Benign Intracranial Hypertension: Etiologic Factors and Associated Disorders

1. Intracranial venous sinus thrombosis
   a. Mastoiditis and lateral sinus thrombosis
   b. After head trauma
   c. Pregnancy and postpartum
   d. Oral progestational drugs
   e. "Marantic" sinus thrombosis
   f. Cryofibrinogenemia
2. Endocrine dysfunction
   a. Obesity and menstrual irregularities
   b. Pregnancy and postpartum (without sinus thrombosis)
   c. Menarche
   d. Addison's disease
   e. Hypoparathyroidism
3. Drugs and toxins
   a. Adrenal steroids and steroid withdrawal
   b. Female sex hormone
   c. Vitamin A
   d. Tetracycline and nalidixic acid
4. Hematologic disorders
   a. Iron deficiency anemia
   b. Infectious mononucleosis
   c. Wiskott-Aldrich syndrome
5. Pulmonary encephalopathy
   a. Paralytic hypoventilation
   b. Pulmonary emphysema
   c. Pickwickian syndrome
6. High cerebrospinal fluid protein
   a. Spinal cord tumors
   b. Polyneuritis
7. Miscellaneous
   a. Roseola infantum
   b. Sydenham's chorea
   c. Familial
8. Idiopathic

cranial pressure as a result of occlusion of the intracranial venous sinuses occurs as a consequence of otitis media with extension of the infection into the petrous bone and to the wall of the lateral sinus. This syndrome has been termed otitic hydrocephalus. It occurs as a complication of both acute and chronic infection; at times the evidence for otitis media is minimal and readily overlooked. The sixth cranial nerve may also be involved, giving rise to diplopia on lateral gaze. Thrombosis of the superior longitudinal sinus may occur as a consequence of relatively mild closed head injury and may give rise to a pseudotumor syndrome. (Occlusion of this sinus that drains both cerebral hemispheres is more likely to result in hemorrhagic infarction in the cerebrum as the thrombosis extends into the cerebral veins, giving rise to bilateral signs. In such cases, the course is frequently fulminant and the prognosis guarded, although occasionally complete recovery may occur.) Aseptic or primary thrombosis of the superior longitudinal sinus may also be responsible for a pseudotumor syndrome. This develops as a complication of pregnancy and has been reported to occur during the first two to three weeks post partum, at the end of the first trimester of pregnancy, and with the use of oral progestational drugs. A disorder of the blood clotting mechanism has been suggested as basis for these events during the postpartum period, although this has not been substantiated. Sinus thrombosis occurs as a complication of cachexia ("marantic" thrombosis), and in association with cryofibrinogenemia.

Endocrine Dysfunction. The most common association is the occurrence of BIH in women with a history of menstrual dysfunction. The women are frequently moderately to markedly overweight (without evidence of alveolar hypoventilation). Menstrual irregularity is common, often with amenorrhea. Galactorrhea is a rare associated symptom. The histories usually emphasize excessive premenstrual weight gain. Endocrine studies thus far have not revealed any abnormalities of urinary gonadotrophins or estrogens, and the pathogenesis is unknown. BIH has been reported as a complication of Addison's disease, improvement occurring with replacement therapy. The mechanism is obscure. Hypoparathyroidism may present with evidence of increased intracranial pressure. The presence of hypocalcemic seizures or cerebral calcifications roentgenographically may further complicate the clinical picture. Increased intracranial pressure disappears with replacement therapy.

Drugs and Toxins. BIH has been reported in patients treated with adrenal corticosteroids for prolonged periods. Many of the patients have been children with allergic skin disorders or asthma. The syndrome is more likely to occur when the steroid dosage is reduced, suggesting that relative adrenal insufficiency might have been present, but this has not been substantiated. BIH has been reported in women taking oral progestational drugs when angiography has excluded sinus thrombosis. BIH has been reported in otherwise healthy adolescents taking huge doses of vitamin A for the treatment of acne. Doses as low as 25,000 units per day orally have been noted to cause headache and papilledema; there is rapid improvement after cessation of the therapy. The syndrome is said to have occurred in Arctic explorers who consumed polar bear liver, a great source of the vitamin. A few cases of BIH, manifested by bulging fontanelle and papilledema, have been reported in children after the administration of tetracycline or nalidixic acid. The mechanisms involved are obscure. Spontaneous rapid recovery occurs when the drugs are stopped.

Hematologic Disorders. Papilledema and increased intracranial pressure have been attributed to severe iron deficiency anemia, with striking improvement after treatment of the anemia. The mechanism presumably is dependent upon the marked increase in cerebral blood flow that accompanies profound anemia. BIH occurs with infectious mononucleosis and the Wiskott-Aldrich syndrome, but its mechanism is not known.

Pulmonary Encephalopathy. BIH can be a major complication of chronic hypoxic hypercapnia caused by paralytic states such as muscular dystrophy and cervical myelopathy, as well as of obstructive pulmonary disease and the pickwickian syndrome. The mechanism is dependent upon the chronic increase in cerebral blood flow resulting from the anoxemia and carbon dioxide retention.

High Spinal Fluid Protein. BIH occurs rarely with spinal cord tumors and polyneuritis without any evidence of pulmonary insufficiency. Papilledema and headache have disappeared with treatment of the spinal lesion. The mechanism may involve the effects of a very high CSF protein upon CSF absorption at the arachnoid villi, both in the cranial and spinal subarachnoid spaces.

Idiopathic. One of the more common forms of BIH is its occurrence in otherwise healthy subjects in the absence of any of the etiologic factors described above. Both sexes are involved and the occurrence is most often between the ages of 10 and 50 years. These cases represent the idiopathic form of BIH; its pathogenesis is a mystery. There are rare case reports of BIH with roseola infantum and Sydenham's chorea in which the mechanism is unknown.

Diagnosis. The patient with headache and papilledema without other neurologic signs must be considered to have an intracranial mass, ventricular obstruction, or intracranial infection until proved otherwise. Although the diagnosis of BIH may be suspected by the appearance of apparent well-being and by the history of some of the associated features listed above, the diagnosis is essentially one of exclusion dependent upon ruling out the more common causes of increased intracranial pressure. Brain tumor, particularly when located in relatively silent areas such as the frontal lobes or right temporal lobe or when obstructing the ventricular system, may be manifest only by headache and papilledema. Patients with chronic subdural hematoma, without history of significant trauma, may present in the same way. Diagnostic evaluation requires skull films, electroencephalography, and arteriography and/or air studies (see Ch. 420). Lumbar puncture is necessary in these patients, but is generally deferred until arteriography has revealed that the ventricular system is normal in size and location. Laboratory studies regarding possible hypoadrenalism or hypoparathyroidism may be rewarding in rare cases of these disorders that present with the pseudotumor syndrome. The cerebrospinal fluid pressure is elevated, between 250 and 600 mm, but the fluid is otherwise normal. The protein content is generally low normal, and lumbar CSF protein levels below 15 mg per 100 ml are common, suggesting that such patients have increased rates of CSF absorption. The electroencephalogram is normal in BIH. Pseudopapilledema may be a source of diagnostic confusion. It is a developmental anomaly of the fundus wherein the ophthalmologic appearance may be indistinguishable from that of the true papilledema; there is elevation of the optic disc, but exudates or hemorrhages are absent. The visual acuity is normal, although visual fields may show some enlargement of the blind spots. The unchanging appearance of the fundus in subsequent examinations favors the diagnosis of pseudopapilledema, as does the finding of normal CSF pressure on lumbar puncture.

Treatment. In patients with lateral sinus thrombosis caused by chronic infection in the petrous bone, surgical decompression is often indicated. When the pseudotumor syndrome is a manifestation of hypoadrenalism or hypoparathyroidism, replacement therapy is indicated. Vitamin A intoxication disappears when administration of the vitamin is stopped. Anticoagulation therapy has been recommended for patients with dural sinus thrombosis; however, for patients with extension of the clot into cerebral veins with infarction of tissue, anticoagulation is hazardous because it increases the likelihood of hemorrhagic infarction.

The idiopathic form of BIH and its occurrence in patients with menstrual disorders and obesity require individualized management. This syndrome is self-limited in most cases, and after some weeks or months spontaneous remissions occur, making evaluation of therapy difficult. In rare instances, the illness may last as long as two years. In the very obese, weight reduction is recommended. The use of daily lumbar punctures has been advocated to lower pressure to normal levels by removing sufficient fluid; 15 to 50 ml of fluid may be required, but its value is dubious. Subtemporal decompression has been widely used in the past. This procedure may be necessary for patients with serious threat to vision caused by pressure, although its efficacy has been questioned in a number of reports. The use of dexamethasone has been advocated because it minimizes cerebral edema of diverse causes. However, many patients with BIH appear to have a large volume of CSF and adrenal steroids have uncertain effects on CSF volume or the rate of CSF formation. Acetazolamide has been used because this carbonic anhydrase inhibitor has been shown to reduce CSF formation. Digoxin has been suggested for the same reason. Hypertonic intravenous solutions (20 per cent urea or 25 per cent mannitol) to lower intracranial pressure can be used in acute situations when there is rapidly failing vision, while one awaits neurosurgical intervention; however, prolonged dehydration therapy is impossible because of its deleterious systemic effects. The use of oral glycerol has the disadvantage of high caloric intake for obese patients. Management of these patients is difficult and requires the attention of neurologists and neurosurgeons experienced in these problems.

Feldman, M. H., and Schlezinger, N. S.: Benign intracranial hypertension associated with hypervitaminosis A. Arch. Neurol., 22:1, 1970.

Greer, M.: Benign intracranial hypertension. I. Mastoiditis and lateral sinus obstruction. II. Following corticosteroid therapy. III. Pregnancy. IV. Menarche, V. Menstrual dysfunction. Neurology, 12:472, 1962; 13:439, 670, 1963; 14:569, 668, 1964.

Lysak, W. R., and Svien, H. J.: Long-term follow-up on patients with diagnosis of pseudotumor cerebri. J. Neurosurg., 25:284, 1966.

Miller, A., Bader, R. A., and Bader, M. E.: The neurologic syndrome due to marked hypercapnia with papilledema. Am. J. Med., 33:309, 1963.

Neville, B. G. R., and Wilson, J.: Benign intracranial hypertension following corticosteroid withdrawal in childhood. Br. Med. J., 3:554, 1970.

423. HYDROCEPHALUS

Definitions. Hydrocephalus is a pathologic state characterized by dilatation of the cerebral ventricles with an increase in volume of cerebrospinal fluid (CSF), almost always caused by an obstruction in the circulation of this fluid. In children, prior to fusion of the cranial sutures, there is enlargement of the skull. Hydrocephalus must be distinguished from other causes of macrocephaly in infancy, including subdural hematoma. In older subjects, cranial enlargement cannot occur. Hydrocephalus is termed "active," i.e., progressive and associated with increased intraventricular pressure, or "arrested" when the intraventricular pressure has returned to normal and is no longer a stimulus for ventricular enlargement. These forms of hydrocephalus are distinguished from hydrocephalus ex vacuo, which is characterized by an increase in the volume of CSF under normal pressure that is compensatory to a primary atrophy of the brain. "Normal" pressure occult hydrocephalus refers to the syndrome of ventricular dilatation associated with inadequacy of the subarachnoid spaces without evidence of increased intracranial pressure (see below).

Etiology and Pathophysiology. There are three possible mechanisms for the development of hydrocephalus: overproduction of CSF, defective absorption of CSF, and obstruction of the CSF pathways. *Overproduction* of the fluid has not been documented, although it may occur with the rare papilloma of the choroid plexus. *Defective absorption* of the CSF at the arachnoid villi, where the fluid passes through valvelike structures to enter the venous sinuses, may occur with subarachnoid hemorrhage, meningitis, and with a very high CSF protein. *Obstruction* of the CSF pathways, which results in dilatation of the channels proximal to the site of obstruction, is the most common underlying mechanism in both the hydrocephalus of infancy and in adults. When the block is within the ventricular system, the process is termed *non-communicating hydrocephalus,* whereas *communicating hydrocephalus* describes ventricular dilatation in which there is free flow of fluid and air between the ventricular system and the spinal subarachnoid space. Communicating hydrocephalus is characterized by extraventricular obstruction of the CSF pathways, most commonly in the subarachnoid spaces about the brainstem at the incisura of the tentorium or in the subarachnoid spaces about the cerebral hemispheres, or both. Ventricular dilatation develops in hydrocephalus because the intraventricular pressures (both the mean pressure and the pulsatile pressures, synchronous with cardiac systole) are pathologically increased; these give rise to a transmural pressure gradient across the cerebral mantle sufficient to cause characteristic compression of the adjacent white matter that has a loss of protein and lipid but an increase in water and sodium content. The magnitude and duration of the transmural pressure gradient necessary to induce ventricular dilatation have not been well defined. These changes may be reversible if surgical therapy can successfully relieve the increased intraventricular pressure (see below).

The major causes of obstruction in the CSF pathways that produce hydrocephalus are neoplasms, congenital malformations, and post-traumatic and postinflammatory lesions.

Neoplasms most likely to give rise to hydrocephalus are those that arise within or adjacent to the ventricular system and obstruct the flow of CSF. These include gliomas and ependymomas of the third and fourth ventricles and of the aqueduct (see Ch. 420). Congenital malformations give rise to hydrocephalus by causing a variety of obstruction, the most common being "forking" or stenosis of the aqueduct. This may give rise to symptoms early in life, or manifestations may be absent until adulthood. Congenital malformations of the craniovertebral junction also may be associated with hydrocephalus (see Arnold-Chiari Malformation in Ch. 424). Most frequently, hydrocephalus is related to postinflammatory or post-traumatic obstruction of the basilar cisterns, particularly in the region of the tentorium. In infancy, this follows intracranial bleeding at the time of birth, at times unrecognized, or episodes of bacterial meningitis or toxoplasmosis. These processes lead to progressive fibrosis of the subarachnoid pathways at the base of the brain, with subsequent obstruction. In adults, postinflammatory hydrocephalus may develop with or after purulent, tuberculous and mycotic meningitis or with cysticercosis, and also may follow subarachnoid hemorrhage caused by trauma or ruptured congenital aneurysm.

Clinical Manifestations. The major signs and symptoms of hydrocephalus are those of increased intracranial pressure (see Ch. 420). In infancy, this is manifest by a greater than normal growth rate and size of the head and by distended scalp veins; in severe cases there is downward displacement of the eyes and mental retardation. Although the head size (occipitobregmatic circumference) in comparison with the chest circumference is of importance, repeated observations of the *rate* of head growth are more significant. Additional information can be obtained from measurements of the anterior fontanelle, as active hydrocephalus does not occur in conjunction with a closing fontanelle. On the other hand, a fontanelle enlarging from month to month is evidence for increased intracranial pressure, and further investigations are warranted.

In older children and adults, the major manifestations include headache, diplopia caused by sixth nerve palsy, papilledema, visual blurring, nausea, and vomiting. Thus occult hydrocephalus that is due to a benign process must be differentiated from intracranial mass lesions, including tumor without localizing signs and chronic subdural hematoma, as well as from the various forms of benign intracranial hypertension and the chronic meningitides, including fungal meningitis, sarcoidosis, and diffuse meningeal neoplasia (carcinomatous meningitis).

Occult "Normal Pressure" Hydrocephalus. In recent years, a new syndrome has been delineated as occult "normal pressure" hydrocephalus. Typically, there is a gradual development over weeks or months of a mild impairment of memory with mental and physical slowness which progresses insidiously to a severe dementia with unsteady gait and urinary incontinence. The patients are usually headache-free and have no signs of increased intracranial pressure, e.g., they have normal fundi and normal CSF pressure at lumbar puncture. Pneumoencephalography reveals enlarged ventricles and a lack of filling of the subarachnoid space over the hemispheres. Isotope cisternography (intraspinal injection of RISA with serial scanning of the skull) has revealed a pathologic reflux of the isotope into the ventricular system with delayed and inadequate visualization of the cortical subarachnoid space. Some patients have a previous history of head injury or subarachnoid bleeding; in others, the cause is obscure. Striking improvement in the mental state and gait has been noted to follow ventriculoatrial or other shunting procedures. This treatable syndrome is uncommon but must be differentiated from the more frequent forms of organic dementia as discussed in Ch. 326 to 331.

Diagnosis. Detailed neurologic study is necessary to determine the cause of increased intracranial pressure and ventricular dilatation. Skull films show characteristic signs of increased intracranial pressure in young children; the signs in adults are generally less striking and may be absent. Electroencephalograms may be normal or may demonstrate bilateral slowing of nonspecific nature. Carotid angiography will show displacement of the arteries and veins characteristic of ventricular enlargement. Air contrast studies are essential to establish the diagnosis of hydrocephalus in most cases. Ventriculography via a parietal burr-hole or lumbar pneumoencephalography, or both, will reveal the degree of ventricular enlargement, the presence of obstructive lesions in the cerebrospinal fluid pathways, and the adequacy of the subarachnoid spaces about the brainstem, base, and cerebrum. Precise neuroradiologic analysis is essential to establish the diagnosis. The cerebrospinal fluid pressure is characteristically, but not invariably, increased in the cerebral ventricles and lumbar sac. The protein content is generally normal; elevated protein levels favor an underlying neoplastic process in the absence of bleeding or chronic meningitis.

Treatment. The treatment of hydrocephalus is surgical; it is directed toward reducing the volume and pressure of cerebrospinal fluid by bypassing obstruction. A wide variety of shunting procedures have been used. The choice of procedure will depend upon technical factors and the skill and experience of the operating surgeon. If the block exists in the third ventricle, aqueduct, or fourth ventricle (as with intraventricular tumors or with "aqueduct stenosis"), the Torkildsen procedure is often employed (ventriculocisternal shunt), wherein a catheter is placed from one or both lateral ventricles over the occiput into the cisterna magna to enable normal CSF reabsorption into the intracranial venous sinuses. In patients with communicating hydrocephalus, direct shunting of the ventricular fluid into the venous system is generally used, particularly the ventriculoatrial shunt wherein the fluid exists from the ventricle through a valved tube, which extends into the superior vena cava and right atrium of the heart. There are many variations of these procedures in use, including shunting to other body cavities, e.g., ventriculopleural, ventriculoureteral, and ventriculoabdominal shunts. Infections and recurrent obstruction of the shunt are common complications of the various shunting procedures, and the results of treatment particularly in young children are frequently discouraging. Acetazolamide, a carbonic anhydrase inhibitor, reduces the rate of formation of CSF; but there is no convincing evidence that it is useful in the management of the various forms of hydrocephalus. Some hydrocephalic children will have spontaneous arrest and may function within the normal range with only a prominent forehead and large hat size as residual defects. Shunting procedures have established occult "normal pressure" hydrocephalus as a treatable dementia.

Benson, D. F., Le May, M., Patten, D. H., and Rubens, A. B.: Diagnosis of normal pressure hydrocephalus. N. Engl. J. Med., 283:609, 1970.

Milhorat, T. H.: Hydrocephalus and Cerebrospinal Fluid. Baltimore, Williams & Wilkins Company, 1972.

Ojemann, R. G., Fisher, C. M., Adams, R. D., Sweet, W. H., and New, F. P. J.: Further experience with the syndrome of "normal" pressure hydrocephalus. J. Neurosurg., 31:279, 1969.

Wolinsky, J., Barnes, B. D., and Margolis, M. T.: Diagnostic tests in normal pressure hydrocephalus. Neurology, 23:706, 1973.

424. ANOMALIES OF THE CRANIOVERTEBRAL JUNCTION, SPINE, AND MENINGES

A wide variety of neurologic syndromes are associated with morphologic anomalies in the region of the foramen magnum of the skull that are due to distortion of the brainstem, cervical cord, and cerebellum. The most common of these are: (1) Arnold-Chiari malformation, (2) fusion of the cervical vertebrae (Klippel-Feil syndrome), (3) basilar impression and platybasia, and (4) spina bifida and meningocele. These defects may occur singly or together, with or without clinical symptoms. Symptoms result from compression, distortion, or malformation of adjacent neural structures. These are most often congenital lesions, but acquired defects caused by bone disease or neoplasms of this region may give rise to similar syndromes.

ARNOLD-CHIARI MALFORMATION

This congenital anomaly is characterized by downward displacement of the cerebellum through the foramen magnum of the skull and by similar caudal elongation of the medulla. These cases can be divided into two major types, the infantile and the adult.

Infantile Form. The infantile form is commonly associated with other midline defects such as spina bifida and meningocele, hydrocephalus caused by aqueductal or fourth ventricular obstruction, and other congenital malformations of the brain and cord. The infantile form of the Arnold-Chiari malformation usually presents itself because of hydrocephalus in the early months of life, with evidence of spina bifida or frank paraparesis resulting from myelomeningocele. Therapy is directed toward surgical relief of the hydrocephalus with a ventricular shunting procedure and repair of the meningomyelocele. Prognosis is poor for patients with extensive defects.

Adult Form. The malformation may be asymptomatic until adult life, when there is the onset of symptoms and signs of damage to the cerebellum, lower cranial nerves, pyramidal tracts, and posterior columns. The presenting signs may be due to hydrocephalus secondary to obstruction of the cerebrospinal fluid pathways or to coexisting syringomyelia of the cervical spinal cord and medulla (see Ch. 423 and 452). Commonly, there is evidence, clinical or roentgenographic, of fusion of the cervical vertebrae, platybasia, or basilar impression. The Arnold-Chiari malformation in adults may simulate syndromes produced by tumors near the foramen magnum and by multiple sclerosis. Surgical enlargement of the foramen magnum and decompression of the cervicomedullary junction are beneficial in selected cases.

CONGENITAL FUSION OF CERVICAL VERTEBRAE
(Klippel-Feil Syndrome)

Fusion of one or more of the cervical vertebrae is a congenital malformation that may be an asymptomatic finding, detected only with roentgenograms of the cervical spine; malformation of the atlas and axis may coexist. Multiple fusions and condensation of vertebrae result in shortening of the cervical spine, which produces a characteristic appearance of a short, thick neck, head set low on the shoulders, and limitation of neck movements.

Coexisting abnormalities are common, including undescended scapula (Sprengel's deformity), platybasia, basilar impression, Arnold-Chiari malformation, and other "dysrhaphic" disorders such as syringomyelia and meningomyelocele. Clinical evidence of spinal cord involvement is most likely to be due to coexisting syringomyelia. "Mirror movements" may occur with the Klippel-Feil syndrome, and other anomalies of the craniovertebral junction and high cervical cord, in which voluntary movements of one upper extremity are involuntarily imitated by the other upper extremity. Surgical decompression may be indicated if there is evidence of spinal cord compression.

BASILAR IMPRESSION AND PLATYBASIA

Basilar impression refers to abnormal invagination of the cervical spine into the base of the posterior fossa of the skull. The diagnosis is made from lateral roentgenograms of the skull when there is excessive protrusion of the tip of the odontoid process of the axis above Chamberlain's line, that is, a line drawn from the back of the hard palate to the posterior margin of the foramen magnum. Other radiologic criteria are also useful. *Platybasia* refers to flattening of the base of the skull, wherein lateral roentgenograms of the skull reveal flattening of the angle between the orbital plates of the anterior fossa and the clivus, the sloping anterior floor of the posterior fossa. The angle is normally 135 degrees, and becomes 145 degrees or more in platybasia. Platybasia alone is asymptomatic.

These malformations, which commonly coexist or may exist alone, are usually developmental in origin, and there may be hereditary transmission. Occasionally, these deformations of the base of the skull may result from metabolic bone diseases such as rickets, osteitis deformans, osteomalacia, or osteogenesis imperfecta. The congenital form may be associated with the Klippel-Feil syndrome, Arnold-Chiari malformation, and other congenital malformations of the atlas and axis, such as fusion of the atlas to the base of the skull, malpositioning of the odontoid process, or atlantoaxial subluxation. Minor degrees of deformity of the base of the skull give rise to no symptoms. The neck appears shortened, and its movements may be limited. With more severe invagination, there may be signs of impaired function of the cerebellum, lower cranial nerves, pyramidal tracts, and posterior columns. Syringomyelia and syringobulbia may also be present. Increased intracranial pressure may develop owing to obstruction of the foramina of the fourth ventricle and the basal cisterns. The clinical manifestations must be differentiated from those caused by neoplasms in the region of the foramen magnum and multiple sclerosis. When neurologic signs are progressive, surgical decompression of the posterior fossa and upper cervical cord may be indicated.

SPINA BIFIDA AND MENINGOCELE

Various malformations of the meninges and spinal cord result from developmental defects in the closure of the bony canal. Although many of these are obvious at birth, some may not be symptomatic until adult life. The classification of these defects would include the following: (1) *Complete rachischisis*, in which the bony vertebral arches are missing in the lumbar region, the cord is undeveloped or aplastic, and the nerve elements have no covering. (2) *Meningomyelocele*, an obvious soft tissue saccular mass which extends over the lumbosacral spine. The cerebrospinal fluid may leak from a defect which may be responsible for bacterial meningitis. (3) *Meningocele,* a bony defect in the spine associated with a meningeal diverticulum covered by atrophic skin. The spinal cord and roots are generally not involved and there may be no associated neurologic defect. (4) *Spina bifida occulta*, a defect in the bony arches in the lumbar region often discovered incidentally on roentgenographic examination. In most cases, neither cord nor roots are involved. The overlying skin may be the site of a tuft of hair, a pilonidal dimple, or a dermal sinus, which is continuous with the subarachnoid space. The latter may serve as a portal of entry for recurrent bouts of meningitis. It should be sought in all patients presenting with bacterial meningitis. These malformations may be associated with Arnold-Chiari malformation and with hydrocephalus. There may also be evidence of syringomyelia. The neurologic deficit varies with the degree of involvement of the spinal cord, conus medullaris, and cauda equina. In adults the chief manifestation may be a neurogenic bladder and defective anal sphincter. Asymptomatic spina bifida requires no therapy. Dermal sinuses, when responsible for bacterial meningitis, require surgical excision. In patients with neurologic deficits, attempts at surgical correction may be indicated.

Appleby, A., Foster, J. B., Hankinson, J., and Hudgson, P.: The diagnosis and management of the Chiari malformations in adult life. Brain, 91:131, 1968.

Bharucha, E. P., and Dastur, H. M.: Craniovertebral anomalies (a report on 40 cases). Brain, 87:469, 1964.

Greenberg, A. D.: Atlanto-axial dislocations. Brain, 91:655, 1968.

Gunderson, C. H., Greenspan, R. H., Glaser, G. H., and Lubs, H. A.: The Klippel-Feil syndrome: Genetic and clinical re-evaluation of cervical fusion. Medicine, 46:491, 1967.

McRae, D. L.: Bony abnormalities at the cranio-spinal junction. Clin. Neurosurg., 16:356, 1969.

Section Eighteen. NONMETASTATIC EFFECTS OF CANCER ON THE NERVOUS SYSTEM

Jerome B. Posner

When patients with systemic cancer develop nervous system dysfunction, metastasis is usually the cause. However, cancer also exerts deleterious effects on the nervous system in the absence of direct metastatic involvement. Recognition of these nonmetastatic neurologic complications can prevent inappropriate and perhaps harmful therapy directed at a nonexistent metastasis. Since at times the nervous system symptoms precede the discovery of the cancer, they can also lead the physician to the diagnosis of an otherwise occult neoplasm.

An almost bewildering variety of neurologic disorders have been ascribed to effects of systemic cancer, as shown in the accompanying table. Many of these bear only an indirect nutritional or metabolic (e.g., hepatic coma) relationship to cancer and are discussed elsewhere in this book. The term "remote effects of cancer on the nervous system" as used in this section applies to nervous system dysfunction of unknown cause occurring in association with cancer (see accompanying table). The classification is similar to that of Brain and Adams (see Brain and Norris), but progressive multifocal leukoencephalopathy is not included because its cause (a viral infection by a papovavirus) is known.

Remote effects of cancer on the nervous system are uncommon. Croft and Wilkinson found remote effects in 96

Nonmetastatic Effects of Systemic Cancer on the Nervous System

I. "Remote effects," cause unknown
 A. Brain and cranial nerves
  1. Dementia
  2. Bulbar encephalitis
  3. Subacute cerebellar degeneration–opsoclonus
  4. Optic neuritis
 B. Spinal cord
  1. Gray matter myelopathy
   a. "Amyotrophic lateral sclerosis"
   b. Poliomyelitis-like syndrome
  2. Subacute necrotic myelopathy
 C. Peripheral nerves and roots
  1. Dorsal root ganglionitis
  2. Sensorimotor peripheral neuropathy
  3. Acute polyneuropathy, "Guillain-Barré" type
 D. Neuromuscular junction and muscle
  1. Polymyositis and dermatomyositis
  2. "Myasthenic" syndrome
II. Metabolic encephalopathy
 A. Destruction of vital organs
  1. Liver (hepatic coma)
  2. Lung (pulmonary encephalopathy)
  3. Kidney (uremia)
  4. Bone (hypercalcemia)
 B. Elaboration of hormonal substances by tumor
  1. "Parathormone" (hypercalcemia)
  2. "Corticotrophin" (Cushing's syndrome)
  3. Antidiuretic hormone (water intoxication)
 C. Competition between tumor and brain for essential substrates
  1. Hypoglycemia (large retroperitoneal tumors)
  2. Tryptophan (carcinoid)
III. Infections (usually associated with lymphomas)
 A. Parasites
  1. Toxoplasma cerebral abscess
 B. Fungi
  1. Meningitis (cryptococcosis)
  2. Encephalitis (aspergillus, mucormycosis)
 C. Bacteria
  1. Meningitis (*Listeria monocytogenes*)
 D. Viruses
  1. Herpes zoster (radiculitis, myelitis, encephalitis)
  2. Progressive multifocal leukoencephalopathy
IV. Vascular disease
 A. Intracranial hemorrhage (secondary to bleeding disorders)
  1. Subdural hematoma
  2. Subarachnoid hemorrhage
  3. Intracerebral hemorrhage
 B. Cerebral infarction
  1. Thrombotic (due to "disseminated intravascular coagulation")
  2. Embolic (tumor emboli, marantic endocarditis)
V. Effects of therapy
 A. Steroids
  1. Myopathy
  2. Psychosis
 B. Chemotherapy
  1. Central effects (asparaginase encephalopathy)
  2. Peripheral effects (vinca alkaloid neuropathy)
 C. Radiation
  1. Encephalopathy
  2. Myelopathy
  3. Neuropathy

of 1465 patients, an incidence of 6.6 per cent, but a rather ill-defined weakness and wasting of proximal muscles associated with diminished deep tendon reflexes accounted for two thirds of their patients. The incidence varied according to the type of cancer, with ovary (16.4 per cent) and lung (14.2 per cent) leading the list. Rectal (0.5 per cent) and uterine (1.3 per cent) cancer rarely caused remote effects. Since carcinoma of the lung is much more common than ovarian carcinoma, about half of all their patients with remote effects had lung cancer, usually of the oat cell type. Shy and Silverstein found a 3.5 per cent incidence of "neuromyopathy" in 1500 patients with cancer. In patients with hematologic malig-

nancies, the incidence of "remote effects" was 2.2 per cent; polyneuropathy was the most common syndrome, and polymyositis next. My experience is that "remote effects" are less common than the aforementioned series suggest, and the diagnosis should never be accepted until a thorough evaluation has excluded metastatic or other nonmetastatic (e.g., infection, vascular disease) causes of neurologic dysfunction.

The etiology and pathogenesis of these disorders are unknown; suggestions for their cause have included autoimmune reactions, viral infections, toxins secreted by the tumor, and nutritional deprivation. It is possible that different mechanisms are responsible for the several types of remote effects. Although the neurologic disorders described below are separated into anatomic categories, there is often an overlap. This is particularly true of the dementias, which are often lumped together with brainstem, cerebellar, and spinal cord lesions as "carcinomatous encephalomyelitis," and of myopathy and peripheral neuropathy associated with cancer, often called "carcinomatous neuromyopathy." The latter term was also applied by Brain to all the remote effects of cancer on the nervous system.

BRAIN AND CRANIAL NERVES

Cerebrum. Dementia, with or without other neurologic signs, characterizes about 40 per cent of patients with remote effects of carcinoma. The dementia is insidious in onset and progressive. There is usually a striking loss of recent memory and an alteration of the affect, either anxiety or depression. Generalized seizures are prominent in some patients, and others have a fluctuating confusional state mimicking metabolic encephalopathy. When other abnormal neurologic signs are present, they usually point to brainstem, cerebellar, or peripheral nerve involvement (see below). The electroencephalogram in the demented patients is diffusely slow, and there are sometimes 10 to 40 lymphocytes per milliliter in the cerebrospinal fluid and a slight elevation of the protein.

Pathologically, there are two main groups: In some patients, particularly those who also have subacute cerebellar degeneration, bulbar encephalitis, or carcinomatous neuropathy (q.v.), no significant pathologic changes can be found in the cerebrum despite clinical dementia. Other patients demonstrate widespread cerebral neuronal loss with perivascular collections of lymphocytes, particularly in the temporal lobes (limbic encephalitis) or the thalamus.

The etiology of the dementing illness is unknown, but the inflammatory changes have led some to propose that a virus is responsible. The differential diagnosis includes metastatic disease of the brain or meninges, fungal or parasitic infections of the brain, a metabolic encephalopathy, and multifocal leukoencephalopathy. In the first three, focal cerebral signs other than dementia are present, and appropriate contrast and cerebrospinal fluid studies support the diagnosis of infectious or metastatic disease of the brain. Metabolic encephalopathy can usually be diagnosed by appropriate laboratory tests, as indicated in Ch. 320. The presence of a progressive dementia in middle age accompanied by cerebellar, brainstem, or peripheral nerve dysfunction but no other focal cerebral signs suggests carcinomatous dementia. There is no treatment for the dementias associated with carcinoma.

Bulbar Encephalitis.   Henson et al. have reported a few patients with brainstem dysfunction and usually dementia, which develops insidiously or subacutely and is progressive. The brainstem signs include vertigo, nystagmus, dysphagia, ophthalmoplegia, and at times ataxia and extensor plantar reflexes. The pathologic changes, predominantly in the lower pons and medulla, are those of neuronal loss and perivascular lymphocytic cuffing. The lymphocytic infiltration is responsible for the term encephalitis. The cause is unknown, and there is no effective treatment.

Cerebellum.   Subacute cerebellar degeneration represents about 3 per cent of the remote effects of cancer but has a clinical picture sufficiently characteristic to suggest strongly that cancer is present even if the neurologic symptoms predate the appearance of the tumor. There is a subacute onset of bilateral and symmetrical cerebellar dysfunction, the patient being equally ataxic in arms and legs. Severe dysarthria is usually present, but nystagmus is generally absent or mild. Many patients have neurologic signs pointing to disease outside the cerebellum: extensor plantar responses are common; tendon reflexes may be either diminished or exaggerated; and dementia occurs in about half. The cerebrospinal fluid is usually normal, but there may be as many as 40 lymphocytes and an elevated protein content. The disease, which is usually associated with either carcinoma of the lung or of the ovary, precedes the discovery of the neoplasm by periods of from weeks to three years in more than half the patients, and it tends to run a progressive course over six to eight weeks, rendering the patient severely disabled. Characteristic pathologic changes consist of diffuse loss of Purkinje cells in all areas of the cerebellum with lymphocytic cuffs around blood vessels. There is often additional neuronal degeneration of brainstem nuclei and subthalamic structures as well. This illness can be distinguished from cerebellar metastases by the symmetry of its signs and the absence of increased intracranial pressure, and from alcoholic-nutritional cerebellar degeneration because dysarthria and ataxia in the upper extremities are prominent in the carcinomatous cerebellar degenerations, and are usually mild or absent in the alcoholic variety. The hereditary cerebellar degenerations rarely run so rapid a course. There is no treatment for this disorder, and its cause is unknown. There is no evidence that treatment of the tumor reverses the neurologic disability.

Another, less common, cerebellar syndrome is that of opsoclonus (spontaneous, conjugate, chaotic eye movements most severe when voluntary eye movements are attempted). Opsoclonus is frequently associated with cerebellar ataxia and myoclonus of the trunk and extremities. It has been reported in adults as a remote effect of cancer, but is more common in children as a remote effect of neuroblastoma. In children, the neurologic symptoms respond to adrenocorticosteroid therapy and to removal of the tumor.

Optic Nerves.   Acute optic neuritis is a rare remote effect of cancer which may precede the discovery of the cancer by months or years. The disease is bilateral, acute or subacute in its onset, and associated with decreased vision, central scotomas, and papilledema. The cerebrospinal fluid is normal, and vision usually does not improve. Pathologically, there is widespread demyelination of the optic nerves with relative preservation of the axis cylinders and occasional perivascular cuffings with lymphocytes. The illness cannot be distinguished from the optic involvement which is a common accompaniment of meningeal carcinomatosis except by examination of the cerebrospinal fluid, which in meningeal tumor usually reveals increased protein and decreased glucose concentrations and the presence of malignant cells. Treatment of the acute optic neuritis with corticosteroids is not helpful.

SPINAL CORD

Two rare but distinct myelopathies complicate cancer. The first, which involves spinal gray matter (particularly anterior horn cells), has clinical and pathologic findings at times indistinguishable from amyotrophic lateral sclerosis, except that the patients with cancer are usually older and suffer a more indolent course. Alternatively, the course may be subacute, more like poliomyelitis, but with sensory changes. In these patients, there are inflammatory changes in the spinal gray matter as well as neuronal loss. Rarely, gray matter myelopathies with clinical courses resembling syringomyelia or autonomic insufficiency (q.v.) complicate systemic cancer. The second myelopathy is that of a subacute necrotic destruction of the spinal cord in which both gray and white matter are affected to an equal degree. Clinically, there is a rapidly ascending sensory and motor loss, usually to midthoracic levels, the patient becoming paraplegic and incontinent within hours or days of the onset of symptoms. The neurologic symptoms often precede the discovery of the neoplasm, and the illness is clinically and pathologically indistinguishable from idiopathic subacute necrotic myelopathy. Since epidural spinal cord compression from metastatic tumor or arteriovenous spinal cord anomalies may present similar clinical signs, a myelogram is essential to the diagnosis. In addition to the two aforementioned entities, many patients with carcinomatous cerebellar degeneration develop extensor plantar responses, mild sensory changes, and reflex asymmetries and weakness associated with degenerations of long tracts and anterior horn cells of the spinal cord. However, spinal cord symptoms do not predominate in these patients.

PERIPHERAL NERVES

Three types of peripheral nerve disorders occur in association with cancer. Characteristic of carcinoma is a subacute sensory neuropathy (dorsal root ganglionitis) marked by loss of proprioception and cutaneous sensory modalities with relative preservation of motor power. The illness sometimes precedes the appearance of the carcinoma and progresses over a few months, leaving the patient with a moderate or severe disability. The cerebrospinal fluid protein is usually elevated. Pathologically, there is destruction of posterior root ganglia with perivascular lymphocytic cuffing. There is wallerian degeneration of sensory nerves. Many of the patients have inflammatory and degenerative changes in brain and spinal cord as well. The entity is rare; in one series no examples were found on examination of 1476 patients with cancer. The illness is of interest, however, both because it is almost pathognomonic of cancer and because four such patients have been reported to have complement-fixing antibodies to brain tissue in their plasma. These findings suggest an autoimmune disorder, but the exact pathogenesis is unknown. There is no treatment.

More common than sensory neuropathy is a distal sensorimotor polyneuropathy characterized by motor weakness, sensory loss, and reflex absence distally in the extremities. Croft et al. subdivided their 33 patients with cancer and sensorimotor polyneuropathy into three groups: (1) a mild neuropathy often occurring in terminal patients (10 patients), (2) a more severe subacute or acute neuropathy at times preceding discovery of the cancer (15 patients), and (3) a remitting or relapsing neuropathy (8 patients). The illness is pathologically characterized by both segmental demyelination and wallerian degeneration of sensory and motor peripheral nerves. Dorsal root ganglia are never involved to the same degree that they are in the purely sensory neuropathy. Pathologically and clinically, the sensorimotor neuropathy is indistinguishable from nutritional polyneuropathies as well as those associated with uremia and other metabolic defects. Indeed, some have suggested that the late or terminal polyneuropathy may be due to nutritional deprivation associated with cancer. Its etiology, however, is not clear, and it does not respond to treatment with vitamins and other nutritional supplements.

A polyneuritis clinically and pathologically indistinguishable from acute postinfectious polyneuropathy (Guillain-Barré syndrome) also complicates cancer, but the association may be coincidental because both acute polyneuropathy and carcinoma are common illnesses.

NEUROMUSCULAR JUNCTION AND MUSCLES

Neuromuscular Junction. *Myasthenia gravis* is associated with thymomas but not other systemic tumors. However, Lambert and Eaton described a *"myasthenic syndrome"* occurring predominantly in men over 40 and associated with intrathoracic tumors in 70 per cent of the patients (see Brain and Norris). The patients complain of weakness and fatigability of proximal muscles, particularly of the pelvic girdle and thighs. The cranial nerves and respiratory muscles are involved less. In addition, patients complain of dryness of the mouth, impotence, pain in the thighs, and peripheral paresthesias. On examination there is weakness of the proximal muscles, but strength increases over several seconds of a sustained contraction. The deep tendon reflexes are diminished or absent. The diagnosis is made by electromyographic studies in which repeated nerve stimulations at rates above ten per second cause a progressive increase in the size of the muscle action potential (exactly the opposite of the effect of myasthenia gravis). The neuromuscular defect in this illness is believed to be deficient release of acetylcholine. The illness responds poorly to anticholinesterase drugs, but does respond to guanidine hydrochloride given in doses of 35 to 50 mg per kilogram per day. There is no direct relationship between treatment of the tumor and change in the myasthenic syndrome.

Muscle. Typical *polymyositis* and/or *dermatomyositis* may appear as a remote effect of cancer. About 20 per cent of patients with this disorder have cancer, and although polymyositis is considerably more common in women, the illness is more commonly associated with cancer in men over the age of 50. In at least 60 per cent of males over 50 with polymyositis, a cancer either can be found when the disease develops or will appear within a few months or years. The clinical picture is indistinguishable from that of dermatomyositis or polymyositis. Pathologically there may be two groups: one with the typical inflammatory lesions of polymyositis, and one with little inflammation but severe muscle necrosis. The latter group may suffer an explosive clinical course. The patients respond somewhat less well to corticosteroid therapy than do those with dermatomyositis unaccompanied by cancer, although improvement with steroid treatment does occur in some.

MUSCLE WEAKNESS

A small number of patients with cancer complain of weakness and fatigability which seems worse than can be accounted for by their cancer alone. The weakness is usually proximal and produces particular difficulty in climbing stairs and getting out of low chairs. Ankle reflexes may be diminished or absent. Further neurologic evaluation does not yield findings diagnostic of one of the remote effects of cancer described above. Brain and his colleagues have labeled this entity a "neuromyopathy" because its exact anatomic locus is unclear, but Hildebrand and Coers have suggested that it is a nonspecific accompaniment of cachexia and systemic illness. The cause and treatment of the weakness are unknown, but a recent report by Sloane and Truong suggests that some of the patients have mild neuromuscular transmission disorders of the "myasthenic syndrome" type and respond to guanidine HCl.

Brain, R., and Norris, F. H., Jr.: The Remote Effects of Cancer on the Nervous System. New York, Grune & Stratton, 1965.

Croft, P. B., and Wilkinson, M.: The course and prognosis in some types of carcinomatous neuromyopathy. Brain, 92:1, 1969.

Curries, S., Henson, R. A., Morgan, H. G., and Poole, A. J.: The incidence of the nonmetastatic neurological syndromes of obscure origin in the reticuloses. Brain, 93:629, 1970.

Henson, R. A., Hoffman, H. L., and Urich, H.: Encephalomyelitis with carcinoma. Brain, 88:449, 1965.

Hildebrand, J., and Coers, C.: The neuromuscular junction in patients with malignant tumors. Brain, 90:67, 1967.

Section Nineteen. INJURIES OF THE HEAD AND SPINE

Russel H. Patterson, Jr.

425. INJURIES OF THE HEAD

Trauma claims over 110,000 lives each year in the United States and ranks in frequency as a cause of death after heart disease, cancer, and stroke. Head injury accounts for death in 70 per cent of cases and surpasses all other causes in persons between the ages of 1 and 35. Good management can benefit many of these patients, but often responsibility for their care falls first on someone who lacks formal training in the field of cerebral trauma. This need not be a disadvantage if the physician follows a few simple principles of management based on an understanding of the pathophysiology of the injury. Properly prepared, he can recognize the indications for specialized diagnostic procedures and possible surgery.

Pathophysiology. The scalp, hair, skull, and bones of the face protect the brain from trauma by absorbing energy from blows to the head. When struck by a blow of moderate velocity, the calvaria bends inward, but a few centimeters away the skull bends outward, and linear fractures radiate toward and away from the point of impact. A blow of higher kinetic energy may comminute or penetrate the skull to cause a depressed fracture.

Beneath the point of impact intracranial pressure may increase for a few milliseconds to as much as 5000 mm Hg, and low or even negative pressure can be recorded simultaneously in the brain at the opposite side of the skull. Cavitation occurs in the brain in regions of low pressure, which accounts for many contrecoup injuries. The pressure gradients distort the brain, which attempts to flow toward the foramen magnum, inducing shear stresses in the brainstem and upper cervical spinal cord. Other shearing forces, induced by rapid acceleration and deceleration of the head, tear axonal processes; this is manifest pathologically by chromatolysis in the cell body of the neuron and microglial proliferation in the white matter associated with abnormalities of the myelin sheath. These changes may not be visible macroscopically at autopsy but account for widespread dysfunction in the cerebral hemispheres, basal ganglia, and brainstem.

The brain and skull respond at different rates to forces of acceleration and deceleration produced by a blow which results in mass movements of the brain. Sharp and irregular surfaces inside the cranial cavity such as the orbital surface of the frontal fossa, the sphenoid ridge, the falx, and the tentorium lacerate and contuse the moving brain. Rotational forces shear nervous tissue around arterioles and result in parenchymal hemorrhages; fragile cerebral veins draining into the dural venous sinuses may tear and fill the subdural space with blood. Fractures that divide meningeal arteries or major venous sinuses commonly cause bleeding in the epidural space.

After brain injury cerebral blood flow may decrease in some areas owing to vasospasm, whereas in other areas the arterioles dilate and lose their capacity to regulate flow in response to change in arterial blood pressure. Loss of the normal autoregulatory mechanism accompanies many, but by no means all, severe head injuries. The resulting dilation of the vascular bed combines with cerebral edema and any hematoma that might be present to increase the intracranial pressure. The elevated intracranial pressure fluctuates rhythmically and, in cases of severe injury, periodically may rise further to levels of 50 to 100 mm Hg for 15 to 20 minutes. These additional pressure elevations, known as *plateau waves*, are often associated with a transient deterioration in neurologic status.

Cerebral contusions and lacerations accompany 90 per cent of severe nonpenetrating injuries. Blood stains the cortical surface and subarachnoid space over both cerebral hemispheres, areas of hemorrhage are found in the brain parenchyma, and clots form in the subdural and epidural spaces. Edema further crowds the contents of an unyielding cranium. The swollen cerebrum displaces the uncus of the temporal lobe through the tentorial notch to compress the oculomotor nerve and the midbrain. Continued pressure obstructs the posterior cerebral artery and basilar vein, inducing ischemia and augmenting edema.

The supratentorial structures generally are most susceptible to damage from head trauma because a heavy layer of muscle protects the contents of the posterior fossa. But should the effects of an injury swell the cerebellum, the tonsils herniate downward through the foramen magnum to compress the medulla while the vermis pushes upward through the apex of the tentorial notch to squeeze the vein of Galen against the corpus callosum, which is backed by the rigid falx.

Increased intracranial pressure causes constriction of the peripheral vascular bed, bradycardia, and increased return of venous blood to the heart. The left ventricle of the heart may be unable to increase cardiac output sufficiently to prevent the development of high pressure in the left atrium and pulmonary edema. Even in the absence of pulmonary edema, pulmonary arteriovenous shunts may open in response to both the increased blood flow in the pulmonary artery and increased sympathetic tone in the pulmonary vascular bed. The consequence is frequently arterial hypoxemia even if the patient's ventilation is adequate to maintain normocapnia or hypocapnia. If the tongue or secretions obstruct the airway, hypoxia develops in association with hypercapnia. Hypercapnia augments cerebrovasodilatation and causes a further increase in intracranial pressure with the grave consequences outlined above. In addition, blood flow may be shunted to one area of the brain through a portion of the vascular bed that is dilated and of low resistance, thereby reducing circulation to other areas that become relatively ischemic.

Hemorrhages are found about the pituitary gland and hypophyseal stalk in about two thirds of patients dying of craniocerebral trauma. Necrosis of the anterior lobe is present in more than a fifth of cases and has been attributed to shock, swelling of the gland, and obstruction of the portal vessels. The consequence may be some combination of diabetes insipidus, absence of thirst, and hypoadrenalism producing a varied picture of abnormal fluid and electrolyte metabolism which can range from hypernatremia to water intoxication.

CONCUSSION

Concussion is a clinical term that may be defined as loss of consciousness after an injury to the head without macroscopic damage to nervous tissue. Recovery is usually prompt after less severe injuries, but long periods of unconsciousness or death may occur, and amnesia for events before and after the accident is common. Concussion implies that contusions and lacerations of the brain have not accounted for the symptoms, but the diagnosis must be presumptive except in occasional fatal cases studied at autopsy. Information about the pathophysiology of concussion therefore is derived largely from experiments with animals.

How an injury to the head causes unconsciousness is not entirely clear. Transmitted pressure gradients and rotational forces distort the brainstem, but bilateral injury to the cerebral hemispheres may be equally important. Changes in the brainstem probably account for the apnea and bradycardia that immediately follow the blow as well as for the unsteadiness and giddiness with change in position of which patients often complain for a time. Amnesia, forgetfulness, irritability, fatigue, and impaired memory are attributed to neuronal damage in the cerebrum, although long persistence of these vague symptoms after cerebral trauma may be hard to evaluate, particularly if a lawsuit is unsettled.

Microscopic changes in the brain after a concussive blow are observed in the neurons and glia within a few hours. Some cells may recover, but others do not, and thus permanent damage to the nervous system occurs. Psychologic tests and neurologic examination may not reveal evidence for the loss of a relatively few neurons, but the effects of repeated small injuries are cumulative as the dull, querulous behavior of the punchdrunk fighter testifies.

EVALUATION OF THE ACUTE HEAD INJURY

The diagnosis of an intracranial clot may be difficult and often depends on the demonstration of an increasing neurologic deficit. Consequently, the initial examination of the patient assumes importance as a baseline for subsequent observations.

Details of the accident suggest what parts of the brain may be injured. The duration of unconsciousness is a rough index to the severity of the injury; even brief unconsciousness is evidence of enough damage to merit hospitalization and careful observation. The neurologic examination is repeated at intervals to detect any change in consciousness, breathing, pupillary diameter, motor strength, speech, or vision, which may signal the presence of an expanding intracranial mass.

The blood pressure, pulse, respirations, and temperature should be recorded frequently after an injury to the head. However, the classic response to increasing intracranial pressure of bradycardia and arterial hypertension may not occur, and any instability of vital signs implies a change in intracranial homeostasis.

Continuous monitoring of intracranial pressure by a ventricular catheter can be of substantial value in following patients with acute head injury. The appearance of plateau waves (described earlier) may signal the need for the lowering of intracranial pressure either by the drainage of ventricular fluid or by the administration of an osmotic diuretic.

As death after trauma is usually due to failure of the respiratory and circulatory centers, the physician must be particularly alert to the early signs of damage to the brainstem. Coma may result from extensive injury to both cerebral hemispheres, but stupor that progressively deepens usually results from distortion of the brainstem caused by an enlarging clot or progressively edematous brain. The evolution of these signs of dangerous rostral-caudal deterioration is emphasized later in this discussion. Grave signs, however, are fixed pupils, impaired oculovestibular responses, and decerebrate posturing.

If edema or a clot herniates the temporal lobe through the tentorial notch, the uncus compresses the ipsilateral third cranial nerve, and the pupil first dilates, then fixes to light. Occasionally the contralateral third nerve is first affected, but eventually both nerves are paralyzed, and both pupils dilate. Later, when sympathetic centers in the midbrain are damaged, the pupils may contract to become fixed in midposition. Treatment, to be fully effective, must reverse the process before this advanced stage.

Sometimes retinal hemorrhages follow intracranial bleeding, or an occluded venous sinus causes papilledema, but mydriatics alter pupillary responses and for this reason should not be used to obtain a better view of the ocular fundus.

Diagnostic Procedures. *Roentgenograms.* Roentgenographic examination of the skull should be performed without undue delay in all cases of injury to the head. Fractures of the calvaria are generally visible, but most basilar fractures are obscured in the bony detail. The presence of skull fracture is reason enough to admit a patient to the hospital after an injury even if he appears to have sustained no brain damage. Roentgenograms perhaps will reveal an indriven fragment of bone, a displaced pineal gland, or intracranial air if a fracture through a paranasal sinus tears the dura and arachnoid. The patient is a likely candidate for an intracranial blood clot if fracture is found which crosses a venous sinus or meningeal artery.

Lumbar Puncture. Lumbar puncture is helpful in the differential diagnosis of coma because the cerebrospinal fluid is commonly xanthochromic after being centrifuged in cases of trauma. However, if a good history is available, lumbar puncture is better avoided because in a patient with an edematous brain or an intracranial clot the withdrawal of fluid can precipitate transtentorial or foramen magnum herniation.

Echoencephalography. A shift of the midline structures of the brain caused by edema or hematoma can be identified by a displaced pineal gland on roentgenograms of the skull or by echoencephalography if the gland is uncalcified. After evacuation of a clot, the displaced midline structures return to their normal position unless the clot reaccumulates. The absence of a shift does not necessarily mean that an intracranial clot is not present; bilateral subdural hematomas are common and may cause transtentorial herniation of the temporal lobes without shift of the midline structures.

Electroencephalography. The electroencephalogram

is rarely helpful in the management of acute injury to the head. An abnormal tracing is common immediately after the trauma and tends to improve as recovery takes place. In cases of chronic subdural hematoma the electroencephalogram may be of value if low voltages and abnormal wave forms are recorded from the scalp overlying the hematoma.

Radioactive Scan. Chronic subdural hematomas are often well demonstrated by the radioactive scan technique. In acute injuries a scan is less helpful because the study does not differentiate space-occupying lesions from contused areas of brain.

Cerebral Angiography. Angiography is widely used in evaluating trauma to the head, and in some cases, such as subdural hematoma, the films are almost diagnostic. The procedure is not without danger, particularly when the circulation to a region of the brain is already impaired by an injury. Consequently, angiography is best reserved for patients in whom progressive deterioration or focal signs such as hemiparesis raise suspicion that a blood clot may be present.

Burr Holes. Burr holes placed in the skull can be used to diagnose and treat subdural and epidural hematoma. The advantages of the procedure lie in low risk and speedy evacuation of the clot if the patient's condition is rapidly worsening. Unfortunately, a subdural hematoma in an unusual location may escape detection unless the burr holes are judiciously placed, and a parenchymal hematoma will not be revealed by inspection of the surface of the brain. Angiography remains the most useful diagnostic tool in head trauma. Diagnostic burr holes are reserved for emergencies or occasions when angiography is not available.

Air Encephalography. Air encephalography provides less information than angiography in patients with trauma and carries more risk because of the possibility that a change in pressure relationships in the head may precipitate an unfavorable shift in the brain with serious consequences. As a result, air studies are employed infrequently in the management of head injury.

MANAGEMENT OF ACUTE HEAD INJURY

Although it sometimes accompanies a severe head injury, hypovolemic shock is rarely the consequence of moderate head trauma or a scalp laceration. Consequently, a patient with a head injury who is in shock deserves investigation for a source of an occult hemorrhage, such as a pelvic fracture with retroperitoneal bleeding. Scalp lacerations are best repaired in the emergency room before roentgenograms are obtained in order to control bleeding and to prevent infection. This is the time to initiate baseline observations of vital signs and neurologic status and to examine the patient for associated injuries of the skeleton, viscera, and soft tissues. Prophylaxis against tetanus is administered, as are antimicrobial agents if open fractures are present.

Respiration. A number of steps may be taken to reduce edema in the brain after an injury. The most important is the establishment of an adequate airway. Hypoxia and hypocarbia have grave consequences on cerebral homeostasis as outlined earlier. If a stuporous patient is unable to clear his own airway, the trachea should be intubated.

Blood gases should be monitored even in patients who appear to be respiring adequately, because pulmonary edema and shunting in the lung, described above, may result in low values of arterial Po_2 that the administration of oxygen can correct. When spontaneous respirations cease, even if cardiac action continues, death is inevitable, and mechanical ventilation is unavailing.

Opiates and sedatives are avoided for patients with injuries to the head. These drugs further depress an already damaged nervous system, impair respirations, and increase stupor. Urinary retention often accounts for restlessness in drowsy patients and is readily treated by catheterization.

Blood and Fluid Replacement. Motor vehicle accidents commonly result in multiple injuries. Hypovolemic shock occurs and is best treated by the ordinary measures except that the head-low position is avoided if the brain is damaged. Elevation of the extremities increases the return of blood to the heart without contributing to cerebral edema.

Cerebral swelling is increased when hypotonic fluids are administered. Five per cent dextrose in water becomes hypotonic as the sugar is metabolized, and therefore should not be given in large quantities. Isotonic saline is less hazardous because sodium chloride passes the blood-brain barrier poorly. Consequently, fluids are mildly restricted for patients with brain injury, and more saline is employed than in ordinary practice.

Patients with head injury sometimes develop inappropriate secretions of antidiuretic hormone with consequent water intoxication, even if fluids are replaced with care. The resulting symptoms of stupor and seizures are often mistakenly attributed to extensive parenchymal damage. Water intoxication is confirmed by demonstrating a serum sodium of 120 mEq per liter or less. The primary treatment consists of restricting water and perhaps giving small amounts of intravenous 5 per cent saline.

Occasionally trauma damages homeostatic centers in the hypothalamus so that diabetes insipidus results. A patient who is alert ordinarily will drink enough to prevent dehydration. However, if osmoreceptor mechanisms are also disturbed or the subject is in stupor with a lack of thirst, serum hyperosmolarity with high electrolyte levels occurs if adequate fluids are not administered. Replacement of water, restriction of salt, and administration of Pitressin are indicated until the condition corrects itself, as it usually does.

Severe injuries to the brain are sometimes associated with impaired renal function despite the absence of shock, or a reaction to blood transfusion, or other common causes of damage to the renal tubules. Characteristically the output of urine remains good, but the specific gravity is fixed at 1.010, albuminuria is present, and the sediment contains red cells, white cells, and casts. Death from renal failure may occur in spite of treatment. The mechanism of the renal damage is not entirely clear, but stimulation of certain cortical areas and destructive lesions in the hypothalamus cause similar renal lesions in laboratory animals.

Osmotic Diuretics. By administering a hypertonic solution it is possible to establish an osmotic gradient across the blood-brain barrier that removes water from the brain and reduces cerebral edema. Drugs that penetrate the brain slowly are employed, such as a 30 per cent solution of urea in 10 per cent invert sugar or 20 per cent mannitol given intravenously or glycerin given by mouth.

The administration of an osmotic diuretic often stabilizes or improves the neurologic status of a patient who is deteriorating rapidly after a head injury. The beneficial effects, if observed, are only temporary, but respite even for an hour or two may be enough to perform angiography or emergency burr holes. If the patient is sufficiently ill to warrant the use of osmotic diuretics, his state is serious enough to deserve prompt and vigorous management. Any temporary improvement that might follow their use should not lull the physician, because the patient's neurologic status once again may worsen rapidly when the drug effect wears off.

During the first several days after injury, osmotic diuretics may also be of value to treat episodes of neurologic deterioration of the sort associated with the plateau waves of increased intracranial pressure. They also are helpful in controlling the cerebral edema that sometimes follows removal of a compressive hematoma.

Steroids. Steroids effectively reduce cerebral edema and are used when intracranial pressure persists for several days, a circumstance that limits the utility of the osmotic diuretics. Doses equivalent to more than 1000 mg of cortisone daily are employed; dexamethasone, which has less salt-retaining property, is frequently prescribed in doses of 16 to 40 mg daily. The incidence of pituitary necrosis after severe head injury ranges around 25 per cent, which is an additional reason to administer steroids. However, the hoped-for benefits are often unrealized because extensive structural brain damage is present.

COMPLICATIONS OF HEAD INJURY

Cranial Nerve Injury. Damage may occur to the cranial nerves as they exit from the skull. Among the more common complications, anosmia and blindness are often permanent in contrast to extraocular palsies and facial paralysis, which usually improve.

Depressed Fractures. The incidence of epilepsy is 30 per cent or more after depressed fractures and penetrating wounds, but the risk is reduced if the fracture is elevated, and fragments of bone and other foreign bodies are promptly removed. As seizures may occur even if the site of fracture is remote from the motor areas of the cerebral cortex, all depressed fractures should be elevated except possibly a small depression over a major venous sinus. If a laceration of the scalp overlies a depressed fracture, antimicrobial agents are administered to prevent the occurrence of osteomyelitis and intracranial infection.

Debridement of a depressed fracture or penetrating missile wound often leaves an unsightly cranial defect that a properly executed cranioplasty will correct. The current use of synthetic material such as tantalum, acrylic plastic, and stainless steel has simplified this operation and improved its cosmetic results. Some have thought that cranioplasty both ameliorates such subjective symptoms as headache and giddiness and reduces the frequency of convulsive seizures, but properly controlled studies do not bear this out.

Basilar Skull Fracture and Cerebrospinal Fluid Fistula. Because they are often not visible on skull roentgenograms, basilar fractures are usually diagnosed by clinical signs such as anosmia, Battle's sign, bilateral periorbital ecchymoses, and the drainage of blood or cerebrospinal fluid from the nose or ears. Cerebrospinal fluid can be distinguished from a mucoid nasal discharge by testing for sugar, which can be done conveniently with the paper test strips used in urinalysis. Patients with cerebrospinal fluid fistulas should be treated prophylactically with antimicrobial agents to prevent meningitis until the leak stops, as it does in 75 per cent of cases of rhinorrhea and almost all cases of otorrhea. The ear or nose should not be probed or packed, and sealing of the leak may be hastened by repeated lumbar punctures in which 30 ml or more of cerebrospinal fluid is withdrawn. A fistula which persists more than 10 to 14 days demands surgical repair.

Epilepsy. The incidence of epilepsy after head injury varies with the severity of the injury to the brain. Seizures occur in 40 per cent of patients who sustain penetrating missile wounds, but follow only 10 per cent of the blunt injuries characteristic of civilian life. Depressed skull fracture is associated with an increased incidence of epilepsy, which reaches 40 per cent if accompanied by evidence of severe brain damage such as traumatic amnesia lasting more than 24 hours. Elevation of the depressed fracture, debridement of the wound, and prevention of the infection can reduce this toll.

The first convulsive seizure occurs within the first week after injury in 95 per cent of cases. These early seizures are typically focal motor in type and many do not recur. Late epilepsy, meaning seizures which occur after the first week, has a more ominous prognosis. It is treated by anticonvulsants. Fortunately in many patients the attacks decrease in frequency as the years pass and ultimately stop in half the cases. A persistent, debilitating convulsive disorder can sometimes be improved by surgical excision of the epileptogenic focus.

Intracranial Hematomas. Both increasing edema and an enlarging hematoma cause neurologic signs that progress. As the two are difficult to distinguish, progressive signs are a justifiable reason in any patient to search for a clot by angiography or trephination of the skull.

Epidural Hematoma. Although small amounts of blood are often found in extradural space after fracture of the skull, large hematomas are uncommon, occurring in only 1 or 2 per cent of injuries to the head. Despite their rarity, epidural hematomas are important because they are potentially fatal, yet proper treatment is followed by recovery with little or no neurologic deficit if the brain has not sustained other injuries.

Epidural hematomas most frequently occur in the temporal region from a tear in the middle meningeal artery but are sometimes found in the frontal parietal, occipital, and suboccipital areas. Typically, a patient receives a blow on the temple that results in transitory unconsciousness. After a lucid interval of a few minutes or hours the expanding clot causes headache, drowsiness, contralateral hemiparesis, and paralysis of the ipsilateral third cranial nerve. Signs of decompensation of the brainstem soon follow, and death results.

The classic case is easily recognized but not often encountered. The patient may relate that the blow was light and unconsciousness brief. His prompt recovery and normal roentgenograms apparently substantiate the unimportance of the injury. Yet an epidural hematoma may be present and may reach a critical size some hours later, and death may ensue if the patient has been sent home with inadequate observation.

Variations from the typical pattern are common. An associated serious brain injury may cause the patient to remain stuporous without the lucid interval, or symptoms may be delayed several days if the bleeding is slow or intermittent. Progressive coma without localizing signs is the rule with clots over the cerebellum, and occasionally occurs with supratentorial clots. At times a hematoma is missed at operation, especially in children in whom the dura adheres to the suture lines of the skull and restricts the spread of blood over the convexity.

About 40 per cent of patients with epidural hematoma die or are permanently incapacitated. Because the hematoma often occurs in patients with other severe injuries to the brain, some morbidity doubtless is inevitable. But the gratifying recovery that may follow surgery justifies a meticulous evaluation of every patient with severe head injury in a search for this infrequently occurring intracranial clot.

Subdural Hematoma. Subdural hematomas are conveniently divided into categories of acute, subacute, and chronic, which differ in both symptomatology and prognosis. A subdural hematoma is called acute when a rapid progression of symptoms leads to its discovery within hours or a day or two after the injury. Prospects for recovery depend on the severity of the associated brain damage. The fatality rate is 90 per cent in patients whose symptoms warrant operation within 12 hours of injury, but the outlook is much improved if the need for surgery is evident only after several days have passed.

Chronic Subdural Hematoma. Chronic subdural hematoma in adults usually occurs after the age of 50 and often in alcoholics because of their unsteadiness and frequent falls. With age the brain shrinks away from the dural lining of the skull and leaves a space that can fill with blood if a fragile vein should tear. The trauma that initiates the bleeding is often trivial and even forgotten when symptoms commence several weeks later. Headache occurs in 90 per cent of cases. Even if a confused patient denies it, the family may testify to his earlier complaints of pain or to his increased consumption of aspirin. Fatigue and irritability are followed insidiously by drowsiness, urinary incontinence, and stupor, which may be attributed erroneously to a natural deterioration in senescence. Hemianopsia, hemiparesis, or pupillary abnormality are observed in less than half the cases. Lumbar puncture usually reveals normal pressure, but in 50 per cent of cases the fluid is xanthochromic. Bruises about the head are frequently present, but a fracture of the skull is identified in only one third of cases, and a calcified pineal is displaced in only one fifth.

The patient usually deteriorates at an irregular rate. Intervals of substantial improvement interrupt the gradual decline and give hope of recovery, but sudden decompensation and unexpected death may occur.

Small clots may be tolerated or occasionally resorbed, but a persistent mass causes edema and irreversible anoxic-ischemic demyelination of the underlying brain. Subdural hematomas are therefore best treated by surgical drainage. The diagnosis, when suspected, is readily confirmed by arteriography or trephination. The results of treatment are good except that irreversible effects of pressure on the brain may leave a noticeable defect in mentation after recovery, particularly in elderly patients. If treatment is delayed until stupor signals dysfunction of the brainstem, evacuation of the clot and the administration of steroids and osmotic diuretics may be unable to reverse progressive transtentorial herniation that results in death.

Intracerebral Hematoma. Scattered petechial hemorrhages are commonly observed in fatal injuries to the brain, but large parenchymal hematomas occur in only 1 to 2 per cent of cases and are usually located in the frontal or temporal lobes or, less frequently, in the occipitoparietal region or cerebellum. The diagnosis is difficult because stupor from associated concussion or contusions may mask the focal neurologic signs produced by the hematoma. The mass is best demonstrated by arteriography, after which it can be removed through a small craniotomy. The results of surgery are often disappointing because the hemorrhage has destroyed sufficient cerebral tissue to leave a substantial neurologic deficit.

Vascular Complications. A blow to the head may rupture the carotid artery within the cavernous sinus and establish a *carotid-cavernous sinus fistula.* The arterial pressure dilates the tributaries of the sinus such as the orbital veins, with the result that the eye protrudes and pulsates, a bruit is usually heard, and chemosis and extraocular palsies occur. Altered arterial circulation to the eye causes loss of vision and, eventually, blindness. If the fistula is small, the symptoms may progress slowly, but spontaneous cure is uncommon. Repair by a direct approach through the cavernous sinus is not often attempted because of the threat of serious bleeding and injury to the nerves supplying the extraocular muscles. Ligation of the carotid artery in the neck or trapping of the fistula by proximal and distal ligation of the carotid artery is sometimes successful. Good results have been obtained by embolizing the fistula with bits of muscle floated up from the carotid bifurcation in the neck, possibly after first ligating the internal carotid artery intracranially just beyond the cavernous sinus in order to prevent the muscle embolus from migrating into the anterior or middle cerebral artery.

Trauma about the head occasionally leads to *thrombosis of the internal carotid artery* in the neck, resulting in hemiplegia. Less frequently, *thrombosis of the middle cerebral artery* by a dissecting aneurysm accounts for an unexpected paralysis several days after the injury.

Depressed fractures may cause *occlusion of the superior longitudinal sinus,* blocking venous drainage from the cerebral hemispheres and thereby raising intracranial pressure and causing the rapid appearance of papilledema and hemorrhages in the ocular fundus. Patients display paralysis of both lower limbs and often of one or both upper limbs.

Infection. Osteomyelitis of the skull, meningitis, and abscesses of the brain occasionally complicate open injuries of the head, and may recur for years after the injury. Antimicrobial therapy and proper debridement of the wound greatly reduce the incidence of these infectious complications.

Cerebral Swelling. Enthusiasm for aggressive surgery to cope with cerebral edema in patients with serious head injury waxes and wanes. Current interest lies in the removal of large areas of the skull and opening the dura to allow room for brain swelling, particularly in young patients with advanced signs of transtentorial herniation. Good results are sufficiently infrequent to leave the merit of such surgery in doubt.

Cerebral Fat Embolism. Fat embolism is an infrequent complication observed after severe trauma in which a long bone is fractured, or occurs occasionally with just extensive soft tissue injury. Symptoms start between 12 and 48 hours after the accident; a frequent history is that a patient has remained comatose after general anesthesia to reduce a fractured extremity. Cerebral symptoms and signs consist of rapidly progressive stupor often associated with extensor plantar responses and decerebrate posturing but with preservation of pupillary responses. Petechiae may appear on the chest and in the conjunctivae; dyspnea, tachypnea, and cyanosis are evidence that the lungs are affected. The diagnosis is best made by bedside examination, but the finding of fat globules in urine and sputum can lend laboratory support to the clinical impression.

Although cerebral fat embolism has an ominous prognosis, some patients recover even after long periods of coma. Treatment consists of taking measures to prevent shock and hypovolemia, providing ventilatory support, and perhaps administering steroids to reduce cerebral edema. The value of intravenous ethanol or of anticoagulation with heparin, which have been suggested, remains to be seen.

Prognosis in Severe Head Injuries.   The young are more likely to recover from the effects of severe head injury than are adults. Patients between 20 and 50 years old who remain in coma for as long as two weeks rarely make a good recovery, whereas patients less than age 20 sometimes recover from coma lasting several weeks. The presence of nonpurposeful motor responses to noxious stimuli in young patients in coma is an unfavorable sign, and in patients over age 30, the combination of abnormal motor responses and coma makes recovery unlikely.

After head injury some patients remain in a *persistent vegetative state* that also has been called the *apallic syndrome,* or *coma vigil* or *akinetic mutism* if the patient appears alert but is unresponsive to his environment. At autopsy, multiple lesions are likely to be present throughout the brain, with the most consistent pathologic changes to be found in the periaqueductal gray matter of the rostral brainstem. Unfortunately, it is not possible to predict with certainty soon after injury which survivors will persist in a vegetative state. This often obligates the physician and the family to embark on supportive treatment which results in the great cost and heartache that accompany prolonged coma.

Less severely damaged patients profit from intensive care in a rehabilitation center where their physical, emotional, and social disabilities receive appropriate attention. Recovery from the injury continues for a long time, even several years. Ultimately 80 per cent can be returned to work, but others remain handicapped by permanent neurologic defects. Even some who appear to make a good recovery have subtle defects in memory, concentration, and comprehension which prevent their achieving their expected potential at work. Others manifest distressing psychopathology ranging from mildly asocial behavior through psychosis or dementia.

426. INJURIES OF THE SPINE

General Considerations.   The first morphologic changes in the spinal cord after injury are observed in the microvasculature of the gray matter and in the myelin sheaths of the white matter. Small hemorrhages occur in the gray matter within an hour, spinal cord blood flow falls,

and hypoxia develops. Catecholamines are released at the site of injury and appear to contribute hemorrhage and necrosis. Based on these observations, a variety of experimental treatments are now under study. These include longitudinal myelotomy to permit the injured spinal cord to swell, the administration of drugs such as corticosteroids and osmotic diuretics to prevent edema, epsilon-aminocaproic acid to inactivate proteolytic enzymes, and compounds such as reserpine to inactivate catecholamines.

The Cervical Spine.   Forced flexion of the cervical spine often compresses the vertebral bodies, dislocates a vertebra forward on the one below, and interlocks the articular facets. Either the squeeze between the upper lamina and the lower body or displaced fragments of bone or intervertebral disc then compress the spinal cord. A prolapsed intervertebral disc does not usually damage the cord in a flexion injury unless the force is sufficient to cause a fracture-dislocation as well.

Flexion injuries tend to block circulation in the branches of the anterior spinal artery as the result of either direct pressure or injury to the radicular or vertebral arteries in the intervertebral foramen. The resulting ischemic injury is most severe in the central portion of the spinal cord. Actual thrombosis of the anterior spinal artery is rarely observed.

Hyperextension of the neck, on the other hand, buckles the ligamentum flavum forward, pinching the cord, especially if an arthritic spur bridges the interspace anteriorly. Several centimeters of the central portion of the cord can be damaged by such an injury even though roentgenograms of the spine remain normal. The upper limbs are left weaker than the lower, and a variable loss of sensation occurs with relative sparing of touch, position, and vibration sense. Bleeding into the central cord (hematomyelia) may complicate the injury and has similar clinical effects.

Patients with injury to the cervical spine must be handled carefully to prevent an unfavorable shift of the fracture-dislocation from further damaging the spinal cord. A conscious patient usually gives warning of his plight, but the possibility of an unstable spine is easily overlooked if the patient is unconscious. A gentle pull on the head in line with the spine is advisable to keep traction on the neck whenever the patient is moved. Spine boards to which the head and trunk can be strapped commonly are used to protect the spinal cord when removing a patient from a wrecked automobile. If one is not available, a bulky wrapping about the neck which supports the chin and occiput will help reduce motion that might be dangerous. A firm board or a door makes a better litter than a sagging canvas stretcher that flexes the neck. Roentgenograms are best obtained on the litter to avoid the manipulation of a transfer to the x-ray table.

The primary treatment of fracture-dislocation of the cervical spine is traction with tongs or wires inserted in the skull to achieve and maintain the reduction. The pull should be in the line of the spine, and weights exceeding 30 pounds should be used with care to prevent a sudden shift from causing further damage.

After reduction is obtained, traction can be continued for six weeks, after which the patient is ambulated in a collar that is worn for three months. An acceptable alternative that shortens the period of immobilization is to perform an operation at which loose fragments of bone and disc are removed and the vertebral bodies fused anteriorly. Atlantoaxial dislocations are characteristically unstable and are appropriately treated by early fusion of the first three cervical vertebrae.

The Thoracolumbar Spine. Hyperflexion in a fall characteristically causes compression of one or more vertebral bodies between T12 and L3. Unless neoplasm or osteoporosis has softened the bone, a heavy direct blow is needed to fracture the midthoracic vertebrae.

Hyperextension, plaster jackets, and operation were formerly used in an often futile effort to restore a normal roentgenographic appearance to the fractured spine. At present the deformity of a stable fracture is accepted and treated by bed rest until the pain subsides; this is followed by progressive ambulation. The occasional unstable fracture-dislocation requires open reduction and fusion.

Surgical Decompression. Whether surgical decompression restores function to a traumatized spinal cord is a matter of controversy. Here the initial neurologic examination assumes importance because almost no patient with complete loss of motor power and sensation that persists more than 24 hours ever regains much useful function regardless of treatment. Examination should include the testing of perianal sensation, and current clinical research includes efforts of record electrical activity in the cerebral cortex when sensory nerves below the level of the lesion are stimulated. If either a trace of motor activity or persistent sensation confirms that the cord has been only partially interrupted, surprising improvement may take place and may continue as long as two years, even without surgery.

All agree that the rare patient who shows progression of the neurologic defect after an injury should have a decompressive operation. Surgical debridement and closure prevent a spinal fluid fistula in open fractures, and possibly damaged nerve roots of the cauda equina benefit from decompression. At present many patients with fracture-dislocation of the cervical spine are operated upon by the anterior approach to achieve decompression of the cord and fusion of the vertebral bodies. The results are difficult to assess because of the relatively good prognosis without surgery when the damage to the cord is incomplete, and a conservative approach is usually justified.

Dresser, A. C., Meirowsky, A. M., Weiss, G. H., et al.: Gainful employment following head injury. Arch. Neurol., 29:111, 1973.

Jennett, B., Teather, D., and Bennie, S.: Epilepsy after head injury. Residual risk after varying fit-free intervals since injury. Lancet, 2:652, 1973.

Kornblum, R. N., and Fisher, R. S.: Pituitary lesions in cranio-cerebral injuries. Arch. Path., 88:242, 1969.

Leech, P. J., and Paterson, A.: Conservative and operative management for cerebrospinal fluid leakage after closed head injury. Lancet, 1:1013, 1973.

Lewin, W.: Vascular lesions in head injuries. Br. J. Surg., 55:321, 1968.

Maloney, A. F. J., and Whatmore, W. J.: Clinical and pathological observations in fatal head injuries. Br. J. Surg., 56:23, 1969.

Ommaya, A. K., Grubb, R. L., Jr., and Naumann, R. A.: Coup and contrecoup injury: Observations on the mechanics of visible brain injuries in the rhesus monkey. J. Neurosurg., 35:503, 1971.

Osterholm, J. L.: The pathophysiological response to spinal cord injury. The current status of related research. J. Neurosurg., 40:5, 1974.

Overgaard, J., Christensen, S., Hvid-Hansen, O., et al.: Prognosis after head injury based on early clinical examination. Lancet, 2:631, 1973.

Raynor, R.: Severe injuries of the cervical spine. Treatment by early anterior interbody fusion and ambulation. J. Neurosurg., 28:311, 1968.

Symposium on head injuries. Clin. Neurosurg., 19:1, 1972.

Weiss, G. H., and Caveness, W. F.: Prognostic factors in the persistence of posttraumatic epilepsy. J. Neurosurg., 37:164, 1972.

Weisz, G. M., and Barzilai, A.: Nonfulminant fat embolism: Review of concepts on its genesis and physiopathology. Anesth. Analg. (Cleve.), 52:303, 1973.

427. SEVERE SPINAL CORD DYSFUNCTION AND PARAPLEGIA

Many disorders, including spinal trauma, neoplasms, acute myelitis, poliomyelitis, and multiple sclerosis, can result in extensive spinal paralysis and cause similar problems in care and in the management of complications.

Antimicrobial agents and improved medical care have greatly reduced the mortality among patients with paraplegia or other forms of extensive spinal paralysis. Life expectancy is related to the severity of the neurologic deficit. Patients who are partially paraplegic have a mortality which approaches the normal population; partial quadriplegia carries a mortality twice normal, complete paraplegia four times the normal, and complete quadriplegia twelve times the normal.

Prognosis. The degree of independence that a paraplegic achieves largely depends on how many muscle groups escape paralysis. The lower the spinal level of the injury or disease, the more skills a well motivated patient can develop if good care prevents the complications of muscle spasm, decubitus ulcers, and infection of the urinary tract.

An understanding of how much recovery is possible sets goals and supplies a yardstick with which to measure progress during rehabilitation. The patient with a complete or extensive lesion of the spinal cord just below C5 retains innervation of the neck musculature and some of the shoulder girdle. He is unable to move in bed, and becomes easily fatigued because of poor respiratory reserve, but he may be able to feed himself with special equipment. With lesions of the lower cervical cord, function of more muscles of the upper limb is preserved; thus the patient is able to roll over, sit up, propel a wheelchair and possibly learn a job at home that does not require strength and dexterity of the hands. He depends upon an attendant for most of his needs.

High levels of thoracic spinal cord injury leave a functional upper limb, but the trunk is unstable, and intercostal breathing is not possible. The patient can transfer to and from a wheelchair, but even with bracing cannot develop a useful gait. Lower thoracic injuries, which leave a strong pectoral girdle and good respiratory reserve, permit the patient to be independent in all his daily activities. Bracing is still cumbersome, and ambulation is generally not practical.

Patients with lesions at T12 to L3 can usually walk in long leg braces and even negotiate stairs, but depend heavily on wheelchairs. Even with an injury below L3 a patient may sometimes use a wheelchair because such acts as arising from the sitting position, climbing steps, and standing for prolonged periods are difficult.

Emotional Aspects. Severe depression may accompany the realization that paralysis and partial dependency are permanent. Progress in rehabilitation is slowed, and recently learned skills may be temporarily lost, but emotional support from the hospital staff does much to reduce the depth and length of the depression. The environment of a center where others face and overcome similar hurdles also bolsters the morale of the paraplegic.

Cardiorespiratory System. Injuries in the cervical

region paralyze the intercostal muscles and leave only diaphragmatic respiration. Exercise quickly results in dyspnea, so that the usefulness of a hand-driven wheelchair or braces for walking is limited.

Interruption of motor pathways in the cervical spinal cord isolates the thoracic sympathetic centers from higher control. Consequently, the patient cannot constrict peripheral arteries when he sits or stands. Blood pools in the limbs and viscera, thus reducing venous return to the heart, and even elastic supports cannot adequately compensate. Venostasis in the lower limbs also accounts for a higher incidence of pulmonary embolus in paraplegics who are confined to bed.

Gastrointestinal System and Nutrition. Paralytic ileus commonly follows spinal injury or acute poliomyelitis for a few days. In treatment oral feedings should be omitted until bowel activity returns. If abdominal distention occurs, a nasogastric tube is advisable to decompress the intestinal tract.

Most paraplegics eventually begin to defecate without an enema. However, fecal impactions are frequent in patients with acute spinal paralysis, so that stool softeners, gentle laxatives, or low enemas may be needed at first. As recovery progresses, a regular dietary schedule and adequate fluids are important to achieve spontaneous evacuation. Some patients initiate reflex evacuation by abdominal massage or digital stimulation of the rectum.

Adequate nutrition is imperative for recovery but is difficult to attain, particularly for patients confined to bed. A diet high in protein and calories helps repair injured tissue and prevent bedsores. A reasonable goal at first is 2000 to 2500 calories daily, although this may have to be lowered later to avoid obesity. During the early months the daily calcium intake should be kept below 0.5 gram to minimize the likelihood of urinary calculus. Transfusions to correct anemia and low blood volume in poorly nourished patients are often beneficial.

Skin. Decubitus ulcers are a serious problem for paraplegics and can occur in any paralyzed, immobilized patient who is neglected. The danger of an anesthetic region is that it tolerates continuous pressure without the pain that ordinarily prompts a shift in position. After about two hours of immobility, ischemic changes begin in the subcutaneous tissue and are manifested by erythema of the overlying skin. Repeated ischemic insults are followed by ulceration.

Bedsores can be prevented by turning the patient at least every two hours, protecting reddened skin from further pressure, and maintaining adequate nutrition. Alternating air mattresses and rotating frame beds help to vary pressure points but are not by themselves guarantees against ulcers forming over the occiput, heels, trochanters, and sacrum. The weight of bedding is sometimes sufficient to erode the tips of the toes. Plaster casts over anesthetic areas may ulcerate the skin, and even supporting braces are dangerous.

Bedsores that heal with scar tissue remain particularly vulnerable to pressure. Therefore the most satisfactory coverage of a sizable decubitis ulcer is obtained by rotating pedicle tissue into the defect after trimming off any underlying bony prominence.

Musculoskeletal System. Many operations and mechanical devices have been used to compensate for paralyzed muscles. Crutches, braces, or wheelchairs restore mobility. An automatic lift enables anyone to transfer a patient from bed to chair. Bracing or surgery can reconstruct the loss of pinch between the thumb and index finger and thus allow the patient to feed and shave himself.

Kyphosis or lordosis is a grave consequence of the unequal pull of partially paralyzed muscles that distorts the growing spine of a child. Spinal fusion halts progression of such deformity, and often can correct a moderate curvature. Good results have been reported with internal fixation of the spine to avoid the complications of plaster immobilization.

Although a certain amount of muscle spasm may help a paraplegic to support the trunk or to position an extremity, painful or recurrent spasms that forcibly flex or adduct the lower limbs interfere with sitting and ambulation and thus prevent rehabilitation. As flexor spasms are reflex responses, the first step is to remove sources of noxious, afferent stimuli such as infection of the bladder and bedsores. If these measures plus physical therapy fail, more drastic procedures may be required, such as myelotomy, excision of the distal end of the spinal cord, anterior rhizotomy, subthecal injections, peripheral neurotomy, or division of muscles and tendons. Any procedure that increases the neurologic deficit of an already paralyzed subject is undesirable. Accordingly, division of spastic muscles and tendons or a myelotomy that disconnects the afferent sensory input from the efferent limb of the spinal reflex is appropriate if motor or sensory function is present. Subthecal alcohol, anterior rhizotomy, or excision of the cord is suitable only for those who have no useful spinal cord function.

Urinary Tract. Renal calculi, pyelonephritis, and hydronephrosis are the major causes of death in paraplegics and are sources of considerable disability in patients with lesser paralysis. These renal complications follow incomplete emptying of the bladder, which initially necessitates catheterization. Secondary infection and vesicoureteral reflux follow. These complications can be minimized by providing a low calcium diet, intermittently turning patients soon after the onset of paralysis, forcing fluids to achieve 1500 to 2000 ml of daily urine output, and treating culturally proved urinary tract infections promptly—but not prophylactically—with antimicrobial drugs. During recovery, nearly all patients with poliomyelitis and about 80 per cent of paraplegics become able to void without catheterization. Patients with poliomyelitis regain essentially normal bladder function. In paraplegics with high lesions of the spinal cord, reflex micturition occurs, mediated through the distal spinal segments. If an injury has destroyed sacral roots, suprapubic pressure may be necessary to empty the bladder.

Regaining spontaneous voiding after spinal injury is always difficult. In many patients a fluid intake of 3000 to 4000 ml daily and either intermittent catheterization or intermittent clamping of an indwelling catheter may establish spontaneous, automatic voiding. Intermittent catheterization using aseptic technique has given the best results as the urine remains sterile in three quarters of patients; if a catheter is left indwelling, one of the Gibbon type is preferred to the more irritating Foley. Some may need a transurethral resection of obstructing tissue at the bladder neck. If there is spastic hypertrophy of the bladder, especially with vesicoureteral reflux, satisfactory voiding usually cannot be obtained without partially interrupting the reflex arc. If there are no undesirable muscle spasms of the lower limbs, graded sacral rhizotomy is the most satisfactory procedure for enabling some patients to master bladder training. Myelotomy, as described earlier, is useful in managing patients with disabling spasticity of both the bladder and lower limbs. The more extensive procedures will also relieve autonomic hyperreflexia manifested by unpleasant episodes of sweating, hypertension, and headache triggered by contraction of bladder, bowel, or skeletal muscle. Recently, electrical stimulation of the conus medullaris to induce micturition has shown some promise, although the stimulus may also induce unwanted motion of lower limbs and penile erection.

Even patients who have apparently established satisfactory micturition may have slowly progressive hydronephrosis that, if unrecognized, will eventually cause death. Consequently, all patients should be evaluated periodically by intravenous pyelography. Progressive renal damage is an indication for urinary diversion, usually by implantation of the ureters into an ilial conduit.

Bosch, A., Stauffer, S., and Nickel, V. L.: Incomplete traumatic quadriplegia. A ten year review. J.A.M.A., 216:473, 1971.
Grimes, J. H., Nashold, B. S., and Currie, D. P.: Chronic electrical stimulation of the paraplegic bladder. J. Urol., 109:242, 1973.
Guttman, L.: Spinal cord injuries, comprehensive management and research. Oxford, Blackwell Scientific Publications, 1973, p. 696.
Kottke, F. J., Kubicek, W. G., Olson, M. E., and Hastings, R. H.: Studies on the parameters of cardiovascular performance of quadriplegic patients. Arch. Phys. Med. Rehabil., 44:635, 1963.
Laitinen, L., and Singounas, E.: Longitudinal myelotomy in the treatment of spasticity of the legs. J. Neurosurg., 35:536, 1971.
Long, C., II, and Lawton, E. B.: Functional significance of spinal cord lesion level. Arch. Phys. Med. Rehabil., 6:249, 1965.
Wilcox, N. E., and Stauffer, E. S.: Follow-up of 423 consecutive patients admitted to the spinal cord centre, Rancho Los Amigos Hospital, 1st January to 31st December, 1967. Paraplegia, 10:115, 1972.

Section Twenty.   DEGENERATIVE AND HEREDOFAMILIAL DISEASES OF THE CENTRAL NERVOUS SYSTEM

Donald J. Reis

MOTOR NEURON DISEASE

428.   INTRODUCTION

The motor neuron diseases are a group of disorders of the motor system of unknown cause whose principal pathology is a degeneration of lower motor neurons in spinal cord and brainstem. Clinically, several distinctive syndromes can be recognized on the basis of heredity, age of onset, and course and associated signs, particularly of upper motor neuron dysfunction. These syndromes are amyotrophic lateral sclerosis, progressive muscular atrophy, including the infantile, juvenile, and adult forms, and the Mariana type of amyotrophic lateral sclerosis. In the absence of any knowledge of the cause of the disorders, a clinical classification is useful, particularly because each nosologic entity tends to be true to type. However, cases intermediate to the major groups are occasionally found so that in "atypical" cases classification may be difficult.

429.   AMYOTROPHIC LATERAL SCLEROSIS

Definition.   Amyotrophic lateral sclerosis is a chronic progressive disease of the nervous system of unknown cause. It is usually sporadic but rarely familial, and is characterized pathologically by degeneration of motor neurons in the spinal cord and the lower brainstem, and often of Betz cells in the motor cortex. Clinically, it appears in its usual form as a disturbance in motility, reflecting dysfunction of both lower and upper motor neurons.

Pathology.   On gross inspection, the most obvious abnormality of the spinal cord is thinning of the ventral roots and reduction of the size of the cervical enlargement. In the brain, atrophy of the hypoglossal nerve and occasionally of the precentral gyrus is evident. Microscopically, there is a diffuse pallor of myelin staining, most noticeable in the lateral columns of the spinal cord, the bulbar pyramids, and the anterior limb of the internal capsule. Loss or degeneration of neurons occurs in the ventral horns and in the nuclei of some cranial nerves. The motor nucleus of the trigeminal nerve and nuclei of the facial and hypoglossal nerves are particularly involved. Affected muscles show the typical features of neurogenic atrophy with intermingling of small, atrophic muscle fibers and fibers of normal size. The structure and staining of the affected fibers are preserved until late in the disease when they finally disappear, leaving residual clumps of hyperchromatic sarcolemmal nuclei. Myopathic changes may sometimes be observed as well.

Clinical Manifestations.   Amyotrophic lateral sclerosis is a disorder of later life with a peak incidence in the fifth and sixth decades. It is slightly more common in men than in women and is found in all races and on all continents. For reasons unknown it has a higher incidence in patients afflicted many years earlier with poliomyelitis. It has been estimated that in the United States there are about 3000 new cases occurring annually and a total of about 8000 to 10,000 persons afflicted with the disease at any given time. The clinical picture of the disorder reflects the underlying pathologic changes of the lower and upper motor neurons. Lower motor neuron dysfunction causes weakness and wasting of the afflicted muscles. An additional consequence of the disease process may be a spontaneous irregular discharge of motor neurons, reflected peripherally by irregular twitchings in the distribution of one or several motor units. This is termed fasciculation. Fasciculations may be observed as continuous movements of portions of muscles anywhere in the body and may be perceived by the patient. Characteristically, fasciculations are widely distributed, extending beyond the territory of a single nerve root or peripheral nerve, and are ominous when associated with weakness. Involvement of the upper motor neuron leads to spastic rigidity, augmented deep tendon reflexes, and extensor plantar responses. When the corticobulbar tracts are involved bilaterally, the syndrome of *pseudobulbar palsy* may ensue. In this state, voluntary swallowing, tongue movements, or facial mimicry may be impaired. In addition, the patient may have episodes of inappropriate crying or laughing which are often provoked by an innocuous stimulus and are dissociated from feelings of excessive sadness or mirth.

There are several clinical variations of the disease that depend upon the regional distribution and the relative involvement of lower and upper motor neurons. Most commonly the disease presents in the distal muscles of the upper limb. The anterior horn cells in the cervical region are the first affected, and this leads to the appearance of wasting and fasciculation in the upper limbs which is particularly obvious in the small muscles of the hand. Involvement of both lateral and medial thenar groups leads to the thumb falling into the plane of the palm of the hand—the "simian hand." Although bilaterally symmetrical in later stages, the disease may be unilateral or even hemiparetic early in its course. As the disease progresses, proximal muscles and then muscles of the trunk and bulb become weak. In some cases involvement of motor units in the leg may be the earliest sign of the disease. The disease may present as footdrop, which is confused in its earliest stage with palsy of the lateral peroneal nerve. As the signs of lower motor neuron dysfunction are progressing, some associated signs of upper motor neuron disease become evident, particularly in the lower extremities.

Less commonly, bulbar signs may predominate in the early stages of the disease, producing the syndrome of *progressive bulbar palsy.* The muscles of the palate, pharynx, and tongue are most commonly affected. Jaw movement and facial expression are impaired somewhat later. Extraocular movements are rarely involved in the disease. Involvement of the hypoglossal nucleus is an early sign, resulting in a slurring dysarthria and weakness of tongue movements. As the disease progresses, the tongue, small and shriveled, lies immobile but fasciculating in the floor of the mouth. The palatal and pharyngeal musculature becomes weak, and aphagia, nasal speech, and regurgitation of liquids result. Later there is often wasting of the facial muscles, especially the orbicularis oris, which may be coupled with the signs of pseudobulbar palsy. Usually some signs of involvement of upper or lower motor neuron innervation of the trunk and limbs are evident in later stages of the disease.

Rarely, the disease may present as a progressive spastic paraparesis in which the evident signs of the disorder can be attributed to dysfunction of the upper motor neuron. This form of the disease has sometimes been called *primary lateral sclerosis.* At this stage it is not possible to make the diagnosis of amyotrophic lateral sclerosis, and full investigation, particularly to exclude spinal cord compression, is mandatory. If there is no evidence of denervation, it is probably not amyotrophic lateral scle-

rosis. Only the subsequent development—perhaps a number of years later—of fasciculations, of electromyographic evidence of denervation, or of the characteristic pattern on muscle biopsy permits the proper diagnosis to be made with certainty. By then, the disease is no longer confined to the upper motor neuron.

Despite the massive involvement of upper and lower neurons of the cortical spinal system, there are no adventitious movements, signs of cerebellar dysfunction, sensory disturbances, or involvement of sphincteric function. In a few patients dementia may occur.

Diagnosis. In making the diagnosis of amyotrophic lateral sclerosis the only laboratory test of value is electromyography. A sampling of affected muscles will reveal a reduction in the number of motor units active on contraction, as well as fasciculations and fibrillation potentials which represent the electrophysiologic consequence of denervation. Nerve conduction velocities are normal until advanced stages of the disease. There are no characteristic chemical changes in the blood or the cerebrospinal fluid. Serum creatine phosphokinase activity may be elevated. A muscle biopsy is useful in distinguishing between a neurogenic and amyopathic process. However, the histologic findings in muscle are nonspecific for any neurogenic atrophy.

Differential Diagnosis. Because of the bleak prognosis of amyotrophic lateral sclerosis, it is imperative that all efforts be made to establish with certainty the diagnosis of the disease. The disease can be diagnosed without difficulty when presenting in its most typical form as progressive, painless, diffuse muscle weakness with atrophy, fasciculations, and an associated spasticity, enhanced stretch reflexes, and extensor plantar responses. In the earliest stages, when presenting as a more localized disease, it is necessary to distinguish amyotrophic lateral sclerosis from other conditions which may produce lower motor neuron dysfunction, particularly when signs of corticospinal tract involvement are evident. When presenting as localized wasting of muscles, particularly in the hand, the disease must be distinguished from *lesions of peripheral nerves.* Mononeuritis or multiple mononeuritis will have a distribution characteristic of the involved nerve or nerves, reduced or absent deep tendon reflexes, and sensory abnormalities in the territory of the sensory innervation of the nerve. The metabolic polyneuritides, such as diabetic polyneuritis, tend to involve the feet before the hands, and sensory abnormalities are common. Conduction velocity in those peripheral nerves that can be tested is commonly abnormal in these conditions. Polyneuritis of the Guillain-Barré variety will have a more rapid onset; it is unassociated with fasciculations and is usually accompanied by elevation of the cerebrospinal fluid protein. *Compression of the brachial plexus by cervical rib* may present itself with weakness and wasting of intrinsic muscles of the hand. The relatively static and localized nature of the disease, the presence of pain, and confirmatory roentgenographic evidence of bony abnormalities will establish the diagnosis. Compression of cervical or lumbar *nerve roots* by osteoarthritic spurs or a herniated intravertebral disc may result in painless wasting, and in limb muscles is often associated with fasciculations. A differential diagnosis from amyotrophic lateral sclerosis in this condition may be further complicated by evidence of spasticity in the extremities, occurring as a result of extradural compression of the spinal cord by bony ridges of the vertebra. Pain, sensory abnormalities, a fixed location of the defect, and localized EMG abnormalities, as well as the characteristic roentgenographic changes of the vertebral column, may help to establish this diagnosis. However, in some cases the differential diagnosis may be extremely difficult and may only be resolved by following the evolution of the disease. *Epidural compression* of the spinal cord by tumor, by arachnoidal thickening secondary to syphilis or other infectious processes of the meninges, or in cervical spondylosis may lead to segmental weakness, atrophy, and long tract signs in the legs. Most such lesions cause pain, and the fixed nature of the lower motor neuron disorder and the evidence on myelography of a compressive lesion of the cord can usually establish the diagnosis. *Intramedullary* lesions of the spinal cord, including tumors or syringomyelia, usually interrupt segmental reflex arcs and also produce sensory signs. The sensory loss may occasionally be of the dissociated type with selective loss of pain sensation and preservation of touch and deep sensibilities over several segments. When presenting as *bulbar palsy,* myasthenia gravis can be diagnosed by appropriate pharmacologic tests. The syndrome of *primary lateral sclerosis* is most commonly due not to amyotrophic lateral sclerosis, but to multiple sclerosis or spinal cord compression. Investigation of such a case must include careful cerebrospinal fluid examination and myelography. The diagnosis of motor neuron disease becomes established only when signs of lower motor neuron involvement are unequivocally demonstrated. *Benign fasciculations* or myokymia is a troublesome but innocuous syndrome of migrating or static fasciculations of skeletal muscles. It may be localized, often to one eyelid, or it can be more generalized. It is common in younger patients. The distinguishing feature in the differential diagnosis in that weakness or wasting of muscles does not occur with benign fasciculations. However, the overt fasciculations may alarm both the patient and unwary physicians, and may sometimes lead to a misguided clinical diagnosis of amyotrophic lateral sclerosis. However, such patients lack EMG evidence of muscle denervation. Degeneration of the lower motor neuron may occasionally occur as a remote effect of cancer on the nervous system, and is discussed in Part X, Section Eighteen.

Course and Prognosis. Amyotrophic lateral sclerosis almost always has a dismal prognosis. In most cases death occurs within three to four years after the onset of symptoms. There are atypical cases in which the condition may appear to become arrested with little or no progression of symptoms over many years. In general the prognosis is worse when the initial symptoms are bulbar; survival in these cases seldom exceeds two years. Inability to handle secretions and weakness of the respiratory muscles are the predisposing causes of the usual terminal event, bronchopneumonia.

Treatment. The absence of any treatment that could influence the course of motor neuron disease only increases the physician's responsibility for the symptomatic care of these patients. In advanced cases, tracheostomy may be indicated to prevent the patient from drowning in his own secretions. Tube feeding or gastrostomy may prolong survival.

THE MARIANA FORM OF AMYOTROPHIC LATERAL SCLEROSIS

In the early 1950's it was discovered that the Chamorro Indians in the Mariana Islands had an unusually high incidence of a disease very similar in both its clinical and pathologic features to amyotrophic lateral sclerosis. Subsequent studies have demonstrated that this disease deviates from the classic form of amyotrophic lateral sclerosis (1) clinically, by its appearance at a generally younger age and its more prolonged course, and (2) pathologically, by the presence, in most cases, of neurofibrillary changes and granulovacuolar bodies, an uncommon finding in sporadic cases. Of particular interest is the fact that 10 per cent of patients with the Mariana form of amyotrophic lateral sclerosis show evidence, in the course of the disease, of either dementia or extrapyramidal types of motor dysfunction, particularly parkinsonism. At present it has not been conclusively determined whether the disease is truly genetic or is caused by environmental factors.

430. THE PROGRESSIVE MUSCULAR ATROPHIES

PROGRESSIVE MUSCULAR ATROPHY OF INFANCY
(Werdnig-Hoffmann Disease)

Definition. Infantile progressive muscular atrophy is a heredofamilial disorder of early onset and progressive course, characterized pathologically by degeneration of anterior horn cells and bulbar motor nuclei, and clinically by signs of disease of the lower motor neuron.

Etiology. The cause is unknown. However, the disorder is genetically determined and transmitted as an autosomal recessive trait.

Clinical Manifestations. The disease may begin in utero or in early or even late infancy. The features that draw attention to the disease are profound hypotonia and absence of volitional movements in an infant. An observant mother may note a lack of intrauterine movements, and soon after birth the infant, though bright and alert, is seen to lie immobile. The legs lie abducted and externally rotated at the hips and flexed at the knees. The arms hang limply at the sides. A few feeble movements may occur in the distal parts of the extremities. With handling the hypotonia is revealed. It may be so marked that when supported under the arms, the infant tends to slip through the examiner's hands. Painful stimuli are clearly appreciated, but there is little, if any, movement of withdrawal. The deep tendon and superficial reflexes are uniformly absent as a consequence of denervation. The limbs do not appear unduly thin, because the wasting of the muscles may be obscured by normal infant fat. Within a few months, weakness of the respiratory muscles leads to a characteristic retraction of the ribs on inspiration, and such accessory muscles as remain are brought into play. The disease spreads to involve the hypoglossal nuclei, and typical fasciculations of the tongue are observed. If life is prolonged beyond a year, contractures may occur, but death often supervenes before their advent. Less commonly, the paucity of movement is noted toward the end of the first year of life or even later when the child fails to stand or to talk at a normal age. In these cases the disease may be limited to the lower limbs, and the course may be slow. In general, the older the child at the onset of the disease, the more gradual its evolution. The natural rate of maturation of movement patterns may exceed the rate of destruction of anterior horn cells, so that apparent improvement occurs. Rarely, after development of paralysis, contractures, and wasting, the progress of the disease is apparently arrested for years. The occurrence of anterior horn cell disease during intrauterine life may result in *arthrogryposis multiplex congenita,* a clinical syndrome of multiple congenital contractures of the extremities that may also be caused by congenital muscular dystrophy, developmental defects of the spinal cord, intrauterine polyneuritis, or any disease which produces joint immobilization prenatally.

Differential Diagnosis. The diagnosis of the infantile form of progressive muscular atrophy is made on the basis of muscle biopsy and electromyographic findings, in addition to the clinical features of the disease. Generalized hypotonia may occur in a number of other disorders of infancy and lead to the syndrome of the "floppy infant." Malnutrition, chronic diseases, and lipidosis may all manifest hypotonia, which is also occasionally seen in retarded children. A small number of cases may be due to congenital myopathy, central core disease of muscle, or polyneuritis. In *benign congenital hypotonia,* unlike progressive muscular atrophy, there are spontaneous movements of the limb and reflexes that may be preserved. Recovery or improvement is the rule, and muscle biopsy shows no abnormality.

JUVENILE FORM OF PROGRESSIVE MUSCULAR ATROPHY
(Kugelberg-Welander Disease)

The juvenile form of progressive muscular atrophy may be inherited as an autosomal recessive or an autosomal dominant trait, and it has pathologic features similar to infantile spinal muscular atrophy. Indeed the presence of both diseases in members of a single family suggests that they may be variants on a continuum of motor neuron diseases.

Clinical Manifestations. The onset of the disease usually occurs in two peaks, in the preschool years or in adolescence. With an early onset there is no clear distinction from cases of infantile spinal muscular atrophy of late onset. When appearing in adolescence the clinical manifestations of the disease can be strikingly similar to those of the limb girdle form of muscular dystrophy. The initial complaint is usually clumsiness in walking. The gait is waddling and lordotic, and the child has difficulty rising from the lying position. There are weakness and wasting of the proximal muscles of the legs and pelvic girdle, with relative preservation of the distal musculature. Weakness of the arms usually does not appear until several years later and is also proximal. Muscles innervated by the cranial nerves are often spared, with the exception of the sternomastoid. Fasciculations, when evident, help to establish the diagnosis as neurogenic. Deep tendon reflexes are impaired or lost in proportion to the muscular atrophy. Mental and sensory functions are unimpaired. Skeletal abnormalities, such as scoliosis, a high arched palate, or pes cavus, are sometimes seen. The course is long, and a number of patients are still able to walk more than 20 years after the onset of the disease. Many patients enjoy a normal life span despite this ailment.

Diagnosis. The diagnosis of neurogenic atrophy rather than muscular dystrophy can be made on the basis of the clinical history and of electromyographic and muscle biopsy findings characteristic of disease of the lower motor neuron.

ADULT FORMS OF PROGRESSIVE MUSCULAR ATROPHY

A number of patients have been described with progressive muscular atrophy with onset in adult life. The disorder may occur spontaneously or can be inherited as an autosomal dominant, recessive, or sex-linked trait.

Clinical Manifestations. In the familial form there is some interfamilial variation in the disease. In general, the disorder presents as progressive weakness, which may begin either proximally or distally, or rarely with preponderant involvement of the scapuloperoneal muscle groups. Bulbar involvement is variable. Weakness, atrophy, fasciculations, reduction or disappearance of deep tendon reflexes in the affected muscles, and the preservation of sensation are characteristic in this disorder as in other progressive muscular atrophies. Unlike amyotrophic lateral sclerosis, the course is prolonged and the prognosis generally favorable.

Diagnosis. The diagnosis of progressive muscular atrophy in the adult is clearly established when it presents as a familial disorder with clinical, electromyographic, and biopsy evidence of lower motor neuron disease. It is distinguished from rare familial forms of amyotrophic lateral sclerosis by the absence of any evidence of corticospinal tract disease, specifically spasticity, enhanced deep tendon reflexes, and extensor plantar responses. Sporadic cases of progressive muscular atrophy occur, although uncommonly, and present difficult diagnostic distinctions from amyotrophic lateral sclerosis early in the disease. The absence of both upper motor neuron dysfunction and a prolonged course marks these cases as different from that of the typical patient with amyotrophic lateral sclerosis. However, until a cause is found, it will not be possible to know whether such cases represent a separate disease or cases of amyotrophic lateral sclerosis with an uncommonly prolonged course.

Bobowick, A. R., and Brody, J. A.: Epidemiology of motor-neurone diseases. N. Engl. J. Med., 288:1047, 1973.
Dubowitz, V.: Infantile muscular atrophy, a prospective study with particular reference to a slowly progressive variety. Brain, 87:707, 1964.
Fenichel, G. M.: The spinal muscular atrophies. *In* Norris, F. H., Jr., and Kurland, L. T. (eds.): Motor Neuron Diseases. New York, Grune & Stratton, 1969, p. 122.
Kugelberg, E., and Welander, L.: Heredofamilial juvenile muscular atrophy. Arch. Neurol. Psychiatry, 75:509, 1956.
Kurland, L. T., Choi, N. W., and Sayre, G. P.: Implications of incidence and geographic patterns on the classification of amyotrophic lateral sclerosis. *In* Norris, F. H., Jr., and Kurland, L. T. (eds.): Motor Neuron Diseases. New York, Grune & Stratton, 1969, p. 28.

THE SPINOCEREBELLAR DEGENERATIONS
431. INTRODUCTION

The spinocerebellar degenerations are a group of closely related neurologic disorders, usually heredofamilial, but not infrequently sporadic, which manifest themselves clinically as progressive disorders of gait, posture, equilibrium, and movement. Pathologically they are

The Spinocerebellar Degenerations*

A. Spinal forms
 1. Friedreich's ataxia
 2. Roussy-Levy syndrome
 3. Hereditary spastic paraplegia
 4. Bassen-Kornzweig syndrome

B. Spinocerebellar forms
 1. Hereditary spastic ataxia
 2. Subacute spinocerebellar degeneration (carcinogenic)

C. Cerebellar forms
 1. Olivopontocerebellar atrophy
 2. Cerebello-olivary degeneration
 3. Parenchymatous cerebellar degeneration (nutritional-toxic)
 4. Bassen-Kornzweig syndrome
 5. Dyssynergia cerebellaris myoclonica

*Modified from Greenfield.

characterized by a simple neuronal atrophy, affecting primarily the cerebellar cortex and peduncles, the inferior olivary nuclei, and the long motor and proprioceptive tracts of the spinal cord. Degeneration of the cerebral cortex, basal ganglia, anterior horn cells, and optic and peripheral nerves is sometimes associated, producing appropriate symptoms. The rich variety of signs and symptoms in this heterogeneous collection of disorders — over 50 "syndromes" may be found in the literature — reflect differences in the regional patterns of distribution of lesions as well as in age of onset and course. Certain neuropathologic and clinical forms of spinocerebellar degeneration are found more commonly than others. These have been recognized as single disease entities. However, even in families with the purest of clinical syndromes, some members may have a clinical disorder typical of another symptom complex. Because of intrafamilial variations in the clinical and pathologic manifestations, the spinocerebellar degenerations have been viewed as a continuum of inherited diseases linking the degenerative disorders of peripheral nerve at one extreme to those of the cerebral cortex at the other. The cause of this group of diseases is unknown. In the absence of any identifiable biochemical defects it is not possible to state whether the varying clinical pictures are due to different biochemical abnormalities or just represent a different expression of a common metabolic defect. A useful clinicopathologic classification of the spinocerebellar degeneration, modified from Greenfield, is presented in the accompanying table.

432. FRIEDREICH'S ATAXIA

Definition. Friedreich's ataxia is a heredofamilial disease of early onset. It is characterized pathologically by degeneration of the lateral corticospinal tract and the posterior columns and the spinocerebellar pathways in the spinal cord, and clinically by progressive ataxia, nystagmus, absent or diminished deep tendon reflexes, and extensor plantar responses.

Etiology. The disease is transmitted as an autosomal recessive, and rarely as a dominant trait, with equal incidence in both sexes.

Pathology. The disease predominantly affects the posterior columns and peripheral nerves, where there is a selective degeneration of the large primary sensory neurons, the spinocerebellar tracts, and the lateral corticospinal tracts. Degeneration of the axis cylinders and their myelin sheaths with gliosis occurs. In the posterior columns, the degeneration is most obvious in the middle root zone. There may be associated loss of nerve cells in the dorsal root ganglia, and less commonly in the retinal ganglion cell layer. There are often diffuse fibrosis and focal degeneration of the myocardium.

Clinical Manifestations. Friedreich's ataxia usually presents in the first decade of life as an abnormality of gait. At first, stumbling and awkwardness are seen, but as the disease progresses, the gait becomes markedly ataxic, with superimposed truncal titubation. Unsteadiness remains the most prominent and disabling symptom throughout the course of the disease. Later, ataxia in the arms and a progressive ataxic disorder of speech become evident. Words are unevenly scanned and syllables explosively uttered. As the disease progresses, the patient becomes confined to a chair and is unable to feed himself, and speech becomes unintelligible. Examination discloses signs referable to the three primary neuronal systems involved. Degeneration of the spinocerebellar pathways results in a profound ataxia of all extremities. Until its final stages, the disease is most pronounced in the lower limbs. Impairment of function of the posterior columns leads to a loss of position sense, particularly in the lower extremities, which may further aggravate the ataxia. Corticospinal tract dysfunction is indicated by extensor plantar responses. Spasticity is not a feature of the disease. Weakness, as a consequence of combined cerebellar and pyramidal tract dysfunction, is evident. Deep tendon reflexes at the ankle are usually lost; those in the arms are diminished, but those of the knees may be retained for considerable periods. Choreic and pseudoathetoid movements are sometimes observed. Nystagmus is almost invariably present and is usually horizontal, but vertical nystagmus is occasionally seen. Involvement of other neuronal symptoms occurs rather commonly. Primary optic atrophy and, rarely, retinitis pigmentosa are sometimes seen in afflicted members of some families. Intellectual impairment is not uncommon and can be progressive. Loss of anterior horn cells in cervical and lumbar enlargements of the spinal cord may, in rare cases, lead to distal wasting of the extremities, suggesting a link to familial amyotrophic lateral sclerosis. Skeletal defects are commonly associated. Pes cavus with clawing of the toes may be evident before ataxia develops, and is thought by some to be caused by muscle imbalance. Kyphoscoliosis is usual as the disease develops. Cardiac abnormalities, including cardiac enlargement, murmurs, and congestive failure, are well recognized and may cause the patient's death. Bundle branch block, complete heart block, and inversion of the T wave are the common electrocardiographic abnormalities. Patients with this disease have an unusually high incidence of diabetes mellitus.

Course and Prognosis. The usual course of Friedreich's ataxia is steadily progressive. Although some patients with mild forms of the disease may live a normal life span, it is more common for the disease to run a progressive, downhill course. Total disability occurs within five to ten years in most cases, and death from intercurrent infection, cardiac failure, or, rarely, from complications of associated diabetes usually occur sometime in the third or early part of the fourth decade. There is no specific treatment, and therapy is primarily effected through symptomatic treatment of the cardiac or metabolic abnormalities. However, in patients with very slowly evolving disease, physical therapy may offer useful training to help the patient compensate for his progressive motor impairment.

Laboratory tests are of little specific value in establishing the diagnosis. The cerebrospinal fluid, on examination, is usually normal. Electromyography may demonstrate signs of denervation in patients in whom anterior horn cell disease is evident. Nerve conduction velocity may be impaired. The differential diagnosis between Friedreich's ataxia and multiple sclerosis must be made in patients with a sporadic form of the disease characterized by late onset and minimal skeletal abnormalities. The principal features by which the two diseases may be distinguished are the progressive course and the absence of deep tendon reflexes in Friedreich's ataxia.

433. THE ROUSSY-LEVY SYNDROME
(Hereditary Areflexic Dystaxia, Hereditary Ataxia with Muscular Atrophy)

This disease is transmitted as an autosomal dominant trait. It is characterized by the development in childhood of an unsteadiness of station and gait, associated with a general loss of deep tendon reflexes, club foot, and kyphoscoliosis. A static tremor of the hands may be a prominent sign. There is occasionally some evidence of wasting of muscles of the legs and small muscles of the hand. Nerve conduction velocities may be reduced. It differs from Friedreich's ataxia in that nystagmus and dysarthria are absent, sensation is usually preserved, and there is a tendency for this syndrome to remain static or evolve slowly throughout life. However, since this particular combination of symptoms has been reported in relatives of patients with pure forms of both Friedreich's ataxia and peroneal muscular atrophy, some have considered the disease an intermediate between these two disorders.

434. HEREDITARY SPASTIC PARAPLEGIA

Definition. This is a rare, genetically determined disease transmitted as an autosomal dominant, and, less commonly, as an autosomal recessive or sex-linked recessive trait. It is characterized pathologically by degeneration in the spinal cord of the corticospinal tracts and dorsal columns, and occasionally of other spinal tracts as well, and clinically by the onset in early life of progressive spasticity.

Clinical Manifestations. The disease is more common in males than in females. Its onset is gradual and usually occurs in the first decade of life, but may occur later. The disease is characterized by a progressive bilateral and symmetrical spastic impairment of gait. Weakness of dorsiflexion of the feet results in the toes being dragged along the ground in a scissor gait. The patient has difficulty in climbing stairs because of weakness and rigidity of hip flexors. There is evident

spasticity in extensor muscles with increased deep tendon reflexes and extensor plantar responses. Sensory disturbances are absent. Involvement of the bladder, upper limb, and bulbar musculature, when present, occurs late. The course may extend over many decades. Rarely, families have been described in which affected members, although presenting in early life with spastic paraplegia, have later developed wasting of the small muscles of the hand with lesser involvement of the peripheral musculature of the legs. Additionally such subjects usually have mild sensory loss of the modalities of touch-pressure, vibration, and joint position. The characteristics of the EMG in such patients suggest an axonal degenerative process. The distribution of this wasting, so suggestive of that of peroneal muscular atrophy, and the occasional association of pes cavus, scoliosis, and nystagmus indicate the close tie of this syndrome to the other spinal cerebellar degenerations. In the sporadic case the disease must be distinguished from multiple sclerosis and progressive muscular atrophy.

435. HEREDITARY SPASTIC ATAXIA
(Sanger-Brown's and Marie's Ataxia)

Definition. Hereditary spastic ataxia, a usually heredofamilial disease, is characterized pathologically by atrophy of the cerebellum, cell loss in the dentate and olivary nuclei, and degeneration of the spinocerebellar tracts, and clinically by progressive ataxia associated with spasticity.

Clinical Features. This is an uncommon form of spinocerebellar degeneration. It is usually hereditary with several clinical and pathologic variants. Clinically and pathologically, these variants represent an intermediate between Friedreich's ataxia, which is principally spinal, and olivopontocerebellar degeneration, primarily a cerebellar disease. The age of onset varies according to the pedigree, and often may not occur until the fifth and sixth decades of life. The disease consists of a mixture of ataxia and spasticity. The onset is most usually characterized by ataxia of gait, which may progress to incoordination of the upper extremities. There may be associated optic atrophy, ptosis, diplopia, and extraocular muscle palsies. Deep tendon reflexes are preserved and are often hyperactive, and ankle clonus and extensor plantar responses are frequently seen. In some patients spasticity may be the prominent finding. Unlike Friedreich's ataxia, nystagmus and abnormalities of the skeleton are usually absent. Dementia may sometimes be prominent. Phenotypic variation of the disease within a family may be striking.

Course and Prognosis. The course, although progressive, is often slow so that impairment may be delayed over many years. There is no specific therapy.

436. OLIVOPONTOCEREBRAL ATROPHY

This disorder, first described by Déjérine and Thomas in 1900, is characterized by the onset in late life of a progressive disorder of cerebellar function. The disease, when hereditary, is inherited as either an autosomal dominant or recessive trait. It is often sporadic.

Pathology. There is loss of the Purkinje cell layer, which may be limited to the lateral lobes of the cerebellum or may involve the vermis only slightly. In addition, there is atrophy of the middle cerebellar peduncle and pontine nuclei. In a number of cases loss of pigmented cells in the substantia nigra has been seen. In rare cases, there is degeneration of the corticospinal and spinocerebellar pathways in the spinal cord and of ganglion cells in the retina.

Clinical Manifestations. The clinical syndrome is characterized by the development in late middle life of slowly progressive cerebellar deficiency. This includes a cerebellar ataxia of trunk and limbs, dysmetria, action tremor, impairment of rapid rhythmic alternating movements, dysarthria, and sometimes a static tremor of the head and trunk. Nystagmus is usually absent. Volitional movements are usually unimpaired, and the deep tendon reflexes are usually normal, although loss of ankle jerks and an occasional extensor plantar response are sometimes seen. A number of patients may display signs of an extrapyramidal nature, including rigidity, bradykinesia, and a parkinsonian tremor. A progressive dementia may also be associated. Infrequently, retinal degeneration leads to blindness. The diagnosis is made clinically, laboratory findings usually being normal. The course of the disease is progressive, incapacitation usually occurring within five to ten years after the onset of clinical signs. There is no specific therapy.

437. CEREBELLO-OLIVARY DEGENERATION
(Holmes Type of Hereditary Ataxia, Late Corticocerebellar Atrophy)

Cerebello-olivary degeneration is a rare form of spinocerebellar degeneration, characterized pathologically by atrophy of the cerebellum and shrinkage of the medulla and pons, and histologically by the almost complete disappearance of Purkinje cells diffusely throughout the cerebellum, with atrophy of the inferior and accessory olivary nuclei. The disorder is usually familial and inherited as an autosomal dominant trait. It is characterized by the onset, in early middle life or even later, of a progressive cerebellar syndrome, with gait ataxia, action tremor, dysmetria, dysarthria, and static tremor of the trunk and head. Deep tendon reflexes are normal, and the plantar responses are flexor. Nystagmus may occur late in the course of the disease. There are no visual, sensory, or skeletal disturbances. The diagnosis is made clinically. There is no specific therapy.

438. BASSEN-KORNZWEIG SYNDROME
(Acanthocytosis, Abeta-lipoproteinemia)

In 1950, Bassen and Kornzweig described a heredofamilial disease inherited as a recessive trait, in which a progressive ataxic disturbance of gait in childhood (simi-

lar in its clinical symptoms to Friedreich's ataxia) was associated with thorny erythrocytes (acanthocytes) and a marked diminution in the serum β-lipoproteins. These children usually first develop celiac disease with fatty stools as the presenting symptom. Somewhat later the patient becomes progressively more unsteady. The neurologic abnormalities include kyphoscoliosis, cerebellar ataxia, and distal sensory loss, involving especially dorsal column functions. Bilateral ptosis, paresis of extraocular muscles, and retinitis pigmentosa have been reported. The relationship among the abnormal erythrocytes, the absence of β-lipoprotein, and the neurologic syndrome remains to be determined. This disorder is also discussed in Ch. 817 and in Part XIV, Section Three.

439. PARENCHYMATOUS CEREBELLAR DEGENERATION

Degeneration of cerebellar neurons, particularly of the Purkinje cells, may result in an acute, subacute, or chronic cerebellar syndrome. The disease usually occurs in late middle life, and is sporadic. Pathologically, there is atrophy of the cerebellum which can be demonstrated microscopically to be due to disappearance of Purkinje cells in atrophic areas, to the reduction of the granular and molecular cells, and to some reduction of the white matter. No changes in the brainstem nuclei are seen. The etiology of the syndrome is multiple, the most common cause being prolonged and excessive intake of alcohol. This form of cerebellar degeneration occurs in chronic alcoholics, and its onset is usually subacute. Maximal disability is reached over weeks or months, and if the patient is abstinent the disorder may stabilize. The usual symptom is unsteadiness, which on examination may be demonstrated to be due to severe cerebellar impairment of the lower extremities. The gait is slow and lurching, and on heel-knee-shin tests there is an evident ataxia of the legs. The arms are usually mildly affected, if at all, and nystagmus and dysarthria are usually mild or absent. Pure cerebellar degeneration may sometimes occur in association with carcinoma of ovary or lung. Heat strokes and intoxication with some heavy metals, particularly with organic mercuric compounds and lead, may also result in isolated degeneration of the cerebellum.

440. DYSSYNERGIA CEREBELLARIS MYOCLONICA
(Familial Myoclonus and Ataxia)

This rare disease of children and young adults is both sporadic and familial and is characterized by myoclonic jerks, epilepsy, and progressive cerebellar ataxia. Postmortem examination has shown degeneration of the dorsal columns and atrophy of the dentate nucleus and the superior cerebellar peduncle. When familial, the inheritance appears to be by an autosomal dominant with incomplete penetrance.

Bell, J.: Hereditary ataxia and spastic paraplegia. Treasury of Human Inheritance. Vol. IV, Part 3. London, Cambridge University Press, 1939.

Boyer, S. H., Chisholm, A. W., and McKusick, V. A.: Cardiac aspects of Friedreich's ataxia. Circulation, 25:493, 1962.

Gach, J. V., Adriange, M., and Franck, G.: Hypertrophic obstructive car-
    diomyopathy and Friedreich's ataxia. Am. J. Cardiol., 27:436, 1971.
Gilbert, G. J., McEntee, W. J., and Glaser, G. H.: Familial myoclonus and
    ataxia. Neurology, 13:365, 1963.
Greenfield, J. G.: The Spino-cerebellar Degenerations. Springfield, Ill.,
    Charles C Thomas, 1954.
Konigsmark, B. W., and Weiner, L. P.: The olivopontocerebellar atrophies:
    A review. Medicine, 49:227, 1970.
Oelschlager, R., White, H. N., and Schimke, R. N.: Roussy-Levy syn-
    drome. Acta Neurol. Scand., 47:80, 1971.
Podolsky, S., and Sheremata, W. A.: Insulin-dependent diabetes mellitus
    and Friedreich's ataxia in siblings. Metabolism, 19:555, 1970.
Schwartz, J. F., Rowland, L. P., Eder, H., Marks, P. A., Osserman, E. F.,
    Hirschberg, E., and Anderson, H.: Bassen-Kornzweig syndrome: defi-
    ciency of serum β-lipoprotein. Arch. Neurol., 8:438, 1963.
Sperling, M. A., Hengslenberg, F., Kunis, E., Kenny, F. M., and Drash,
    A. L.: A-betalipoproteinemia: Metabolic, endocrine and electron-
    microscopic investigations. Pediatrics, 48:91, 1971.
Victor, M., Adams, R. D., and Mancall, E. L.: A restricted form of
    cerebellar cortical degeneration occurring in alcoholic patients. Arch.
    Neurol., 1:579, 1959.

441. SYRINGOMYELIA

Definition. Syringomyelia is a chronic disease of the
spinal cord, characterized pathologically by cavitation of
the spinal cord with gliosis and clinically by a mixture of
segmental and suprasegmental motor and sensory abnormalities and trophic disturbances. When a syrinx
occurs in the brainstem, the disease is called *syringobulbia.*

Etiology. The cause of syringomyelia is unknown.
Several theories have been proposed to explain its pathogenesis, but none are entirely satisfactory. Because of
the common association of syringomyelia with other congenital abnormalities of the neuraxis and skeleton, the
most popular hypotheses have attributed the disease to
developmental anomalies. One hypothesis has suggested
that the disease is due to abnormal closure of the neural
tube; another, that it results from the persistence of
ependymal cell rests which later proliferate and cavitate. A third, based on the frequent association of intramedullary vascular malformations, vascular neoplasms, and gliomas with syrinxes, is that focal ischemia
within the spinal cord resulting from abnormalities of
the microcirculation is pathogenic. Finally, a theory first
elaborated by Gardner and since modified by others has
proposed that the cavitation is hydrodynamic in origin
and is caused by distention of the central canal by ventricular fluid displaced caudally from the fourth ventricle as a consequence of atresia of the foramina of
Luschka and Magendie.

Pathology. On gross inspection the spinal cord may
appear normal, enlarged, or flattened in its anteroposterior axis, depending upon the size and state of the
syrinx. The syrinx itself, when intact, is filled with clear,
slightly yellow serous fluid. The walls of the cavity are
irregular, and consist of degenerated neural and neuroglial elements. The cavity is usually surrounded by
gliosis, composed for the most part of glial fibers. Abnormal blood vessels with hyalinized walls may sometimes
be seen. There is usually secondary degeneration and
demyelination of long ascending and descending tracts of
the spinal cord and brainstem as a result of extension of
the syrinx. The syrinx most commonly runs over several
segments in the cervical cord. It may extend into thoracic segments for a varying distance and may even terminate at lumbar levels. The cavity often begins in the
gray matter adjacent to the central canal, and tends, as
it enlarges, to interrupt the decussating fibers and destroy neurons in the dorsal and ventral horns. Within
the thoracic cord, the cavity is commonly seen in the dorsal horns, and may affect the intermediolateral cell column, producing autonomic deficiencies. Syrinxes of the
lumbar cord are uncommon. *Syringobulbia* is associated
with cavitation that is usually slitlike and often in communication with the fourth ventricle. Bulbar syrinxes
commonly involve several cranial nerve nuclei, notably
the descending root of the trigeminal nerve, and the solitary, ambiguous, and hypoglossal nuclei. They also may
involve the medial longitudinal fasciculus, the pyramidal tract, and the medial lemniscus. Extensions into the
pons are rare. A *secondary syrinx* consisting of central
cavitation of the spinal cord and sometimes associated
with gliosis may occur as a result of chronic arachnoiditis, spinal tuberculosis, or meningeal or vascular syphilis. It may also be found after trauma of the spinal
cord, the cavitation gradually extending many cord segments above or below the lesion and leading, clinically,
to a post-traumatic myelopathy.

Clinical Manifestations. The clinical manifestations of
syringomyelia depend upon the localization and size of
the lesion. The disease most commonly presents in the
second decade, but sometimes the onset may be delayed
until the patient is in his sixties or seventies. In its most
usual form the signs and symptoms of the disease are
referable to a *syrinx in the cervical cord.* The presenting
symptoms are often wasting and weakness in the muscles of the upper extremity, associated with mild burning
dysesthesias and loss of pain sensation distally in the
arms. There are sometimes complaints of weakness of
the legs, and bowel and bladder symptoms. On examination the patient may have Horner's syndrome as a consequence of interruption of the sympathetic pathways in
the spinal cord. Nystagmus resulting from damage to the
spinal projections of the medial longitudinal fasciculus
may also be seen. Muscle weakness in the upper extremity is usually associated with obvious atrophy, and
frequently involves the small muscles of the hand. If the
syrinx has extended into the corticospinal tract,
weakness and spasticity in the lower extremities are evident. At the level of the lesion, the deep tendon reflexes
may be absent or reduced. Because of the interruption of
the second order afferent fibers arising from cells in the
dorsal horn and crossing to the contralateral ventrolateral spinothalamic tracts, there may be a dissociated
segmental type of sensory loss, often in a shawl- or
capelike distribution over the shoulders, upper trunk,
and arms. In this zone, light touch, vibration, and deep
sensibility are preserved with a striking absence of pain
and temperature sensation. When the lesion has extended to include the dorsal columns or the spinothalamic pathways, there are appropriate sensory abnormalities in the trunk and lower extremities. Trophic changes,
particularly involving the hands, are common. Their
pathogenesis is not known, but may in part be related to
the absence of pain sensation and to the interruption of
vasomotor outflow to the limb. Unfelt burns from cigarettes or light bulbs may lead to tissue destruction and
severe scarring. Cyanosis, hyperkeratosis, and thickening of subcutaneous tissues may result in puffy, swollen
fingers. True hypertrophy of body parts may occur. Traumatic osteoarthropathy (Charcot's joint) is common.
Sometimes the distal phalanges may atrophy and be lost

painlessly, a condition known as Morvan's disease. The common clinical features of *lumbosacral syrinxes* are atrophic weakness of the lower limbs, loss of deep tendon reflexes, dissociated anesthesia, and fecal and urinary incontinence. If the lesion lies high in the lumbar cord, it may be associated with an extensor plantar response. Trophic changes of the lower extremity, particularly club foot deformities, are common. In *syringobulbia* the syrinx formation in the medulla may be unassociated with the syrinx in the cervical cord. Common findings in this disorder are atrophy of the tongue, nystagmus, impairment of pain and temperature sensation on one side of the face, dysphonia, and respiratory stridor. In addition, sensory and spastic motor abnormalities of the extremities may be seen.

There are many associated findings in syringomyelia. Papilledema may result from an associated hydrocephalus. Skeletal abnormalities are common and include cervical rib, spina bifida, premature closures of the skull, Klippel-Feil syndrome, basilar impression, and kyphoscoliosis. The association of syringomyelia with intramedullary gliomas or vascular tumors has long been recognized.

Diagnosis.   The diagnosis may often be made clinically by the observation of muscular atrophy and weakness, dissociated sensory loss, trophic changes, and long tract signs attributable to a lesion in the cervical cord. The laboratory findings in this disorder are nonspecific. The cerebrospinal fluid may be under increased pressure as a result of an associated hydrocephalus. A mild pleocytosis or increased protein in the cerebrospinal fluid may sometimes be seen. Elevated cerebrospinal fluid protein is more commonly associated with intramedullary gliomas or cysts. Electromyography may reveal evidence of denervation in affected muscles. Roentgenographic evidence of bony deformities may be helpful. Pantopaque x-ray myelography may sometimes give evidence of a swollen syrinx. Gas myelography has proved useful in distinguishing a syrinx from an intramedullary cyst.

Differential Diagnosis.   Syringomyelia must be differentiated from tumors of the spinal cord or cervical ribs, other bony anomalies, amyotrophic lateral sclerosis, multiple sclerosis, and tabes dorsalis. Intramedullary tumors of the cord, which produce comparable symptomatology because of a similar location, and extramedullary tumors, which can sometimes simulate an intramedullary lesion by compressing the anterior spinal artery, can often be differentiated from syringomyelia by myelography. Cervical rib may be identified roentgenographically, although the fact that this abnormality may be associated with a syrinx sometimes complicates the differential diagnosis. Amyotrophic lateral sclerosis is never associated with sensory abnormalities. Multiple sclerosis can be differentiated by its remitting course and by the fact that muscular wasting, trophic changes, and dissociated sensory abnormalities are uncommon. Tabes dorsalis can be differentiated by the serology and by a different pattern of sensory loss.

Course and Prognosis.   The course of syringomyelia is variable, but is usually protracted over many years. In some patients there may be gradual deterioration; in others, changes may occur in a stepwise fashion. In some patients, after an initial attack, the disease may appear to have become arrested. In syringobulbia, death from respiratory paralysis may sometimes occur.

Treatment.   At present there is no satisfactory treatment for syringomyelia. Some surgeons recommend decompression of the syrinx, but the therapeutic results have been at best doubtful.

Barnett, H. J. M., Botterell, E. H., Jousse, A. T., and Wynn-Jones, M.: Progressive myelopathy as a sequel to traumatic paraplegia. Brain, 89:159, 1966.
Ellertson, A. B.: Semiologic diagnosis of syringomyelia related to roentgenologic findings. Acta Neurol. Scand., 45:385, 1969.
Gardner, W. J.: Hydrodynamic mechanism of syringomyelia: its relationship to myelocele. J. Neurol. Neurosurg. Psychiatry, 28:247, 1965.
McIlroy, W. J., and Richardson, J. C.: Syringomyelia. A clinical review of 75 cases. Can. Med. Assoc. J., 93:731, 1965.
Netsky, M. G.: Syringomyelia. A clinicopathological study. Arch. Neurol., 70:741, 1953.
Williams, B., and Weller, R. O.: Syringomyelin produced by intramedullary fluid injection in dogs. J. Neurol. Neurosurg. Psychiatry, 36:467, 1973.

NEUROCUTANEOUS SYNDROMES

442. MULTIPLE NEUROFIBROMATOSIS (Von Recklinghausen's Disease)

Multiple neurofibromatosis is a congenital defect of the ectoderm, usually heredofamilial, characterized by cutaneous pigmentation and multiple tumors of the spinal and cranial nerves and skin. The cutaneous and osseous manifestations of the disease are described in Ch. 921. Tumors of the peripheral nerve are most characteristic, and occur as nodules along the course of the nerve or nerve roots, usually without interfering with nerve conduction. Occasionally diffuse involvement of the nerve trunk in its distal branches produces a plexiform neuroma which, when it occurs, is particularly common in the cervical and occipital regions. Other tumors of the nervous system, particularly meningiomas and gliomas, are often associated. Neurofibromas may undergo sarcomatous degeneration. The signs and symptoms of neurofibromatosis depend upon the localization and rate of growth of the tumors. When lying within the spinal canal, they may produce a syndrome of spinal cord compression. Cranial nerve tumors are often found. When tumors of the eighth nerve are bilateral, they are almost invariably a manifestation of neurofibromatosis, and optic nerve gliomas are frequently associated with that disease. Tumors of other cranial nerves may occur, particularly the trigeminal vagus, and hypoglossal.

443. TUBEROUS SCLEROSIS (Epiloia, Bourneville's Disease)

Definition.   Tuberous sclerosis is a congenital disease characterized by the presence of congenital tumors and malformations of the brain, skin, and viscera, and clinically by epilepsy and mental retardation.

Etiology.   The disease is both sporadic and heredofamilial and is probably inherited through a single dominant trait.

Pathology. The brain, although usually normal in size, is studded by many small nodules or tubers. These are firm, and occasionally calcified. Sometimes they distort the normal configuration of gyri and may project into the cerebral ventricles, where they present as characteristic "candle gutterings." Microscopically, the tubers are composed of nests of glial fibers and abnormal ganglion cells. They may undergo gliomatous degeneration or develop into meningiomas. Glial tumors of the retina (phakomas) and gliomatous tumors of the nerve head and optic tract are also found in some cases. Adenoma sebaceum, the characteristic skin lesion, is a small firm tubercle often found over the nose and cheeks. They are rarely present at birth, but usually develop during the first decade toward puberty. Although tending to cluster over the bridge of the nose and the cheeks, they may be found elsewhere over the head. In addition, a variety of other polyps, subcutaneous nodules, pigmented warts, and café-au-lait spots similar to those of von Recklinghausen's disease are found. Hypopigmented macules may be the earliest cutaneous manifestations. Mesodermal tumors of the kidney, liver, pancreas, lung, and thyroid gland are seen, along with rhabdomyoma of the heart.

Clinical Manifestations. The presenting symptom of this disease is usually epilepsy, which appears in the first few years of life. The attacks may present as minor or focal seizures, but in time generally progress to major motor convulsions. Mental retardation is usually noticed during the early years of life and may vary in degree, differing in no way from mental retardation from any other cause. Some patients, however, may have normal I.Q.'s. The adenoma sebaceum usually appears toward the end of the second or the beginning of the third year of life as small, lightly pigmented, shiny papules that appear vascular. They may first appear on the malar areas, but as they proliferate they become confluent and more deeply pigmented, and extend in a butterfly distribution over the nose and cheeks. The retinal lesions are flat, white or gray, round or oval areas, and are present in almost half the patients. Subungual fibromas on the toes or fingers may be seen but most commonly not until after puberty. Patients with mild or partial forms of the disease are not uncommon.

Diagnosis. The clinical triad of seizures, mental retardation, and adenoma sebaceum will establish the diagnosis. Roentgenographic examination of the skull may often reveal scattered calcifications in areas of increased or decreased density in the skull vault. Pneumoencephalography may sometimes demonstrate the tubers projecting into the ventricles.

Course and Prognosis. The disease is usually progressive. The outlook in individual cases, however, depends on the severity of the mental impairment and the frequency and intensity of seizures. It must be emphasized that the three cardinal features of the disease may occur singly or in any combination with varying degrees of severity in members of the same family. Often the defects are progressive, and death occurs in the second decade of life. The development of gliomatous changes in the brain may also shorten the course of the disease, as may progressive pulmonary insufficiency from pulmonary tumors. Sudden death from rhabdomyoma of the heart may occur.

Treatment. The treatment is the same as that for epilepsy with appropriate measures for the mental retardation. Institutionalization is sometimes indicated.

444. STURGE-WEBER-DIMITRI DISEASE
(Encephalotrigeminal Angiomatosis)

The Sturge-Weber-Dimitri disease is characterized by a unilateral, port-wine, facial nevus usually confined to the distribution of the first and occasionally the other divisions of the trigeminal nerve, together with a capillary hemangioma of the ipsilateral cerebral cortex. The full clinical picture consists of the nevus, a contralateral hemiparesis, smallness of the affected limbs, epilepsy — often consisting of jacksonian seizures beginning in the paralyzed limbs — ipsilateral exophthalmos, angiomas of the retina, and some degree of mental retardation. Incomplete manifestations of the disease may be observed, and there is great variability in the severity of the retardation, the frequency of the seizures, the profoundness of the hemiplegia, and the extent of the cutaneous abnormalities. Extensive linear calcification of the cortex often occurs in parallel lines, and, when visible roentgenographically, may help to establish the diagnosis. The films may also show hemiatrophy of the skull reflecting the maldevelopment of the underlying cerebral hemisphere. The cause of the disease is unknown, and there is no evidence of hereditary transmission. The diagnosis can be made clinically without difficulty.

445. VON HIPPEL – LINDAU DISEASE

This is a rare, usually heredofamilial disease, consisting of a hemangioblastoma of the brain (usually in cerebellum, but occasionally elsewhere) in association with an angioma of the retina and, less commonly, cysts of the pancreas, kidneys, and other viscera and a pheochromocytoma. The disease is inherited as an autosomal dominant trait. Its onset usually occurs in the third decade of life with symptoms referable to the retinal or cerebral tumors. The angioma of the retina (von Hippel) is usually peripheral, and is supplied by a large, entering artery and drained by a single vein. Hemorrhages, exudates, and papilledema may occur in association with the lesion. The hemangioblastoma is usually a solitary cystic vascular tumor. It is most commonly localized to the cerebellum, but may occur in the medulla, brainstem, or spinal cord. The hemangioblastoma of the cerebellum presents with the usual signs of cerebellar deficiency. The protein content of the cerebrospinal fluid tends to be unusually high, and a polycythemia of unknown cause is commonly associated. However, it should be emphasized that the majority of cases of proved cerebellar hemangioblastoma present no evidence of von Hippel–Lindau disease. The diagnosis is established in patients with a positive family history by the onset of retinal or brainstem symptoms. Diagnosis of a tumor in the brainstem is made by the usual roentgenographic methods of pneumoencephalography or angiography. Early recognition of cerebellar tumors in afflicted members of the family is important, for early surgical resection may effect a cure.

446. ATAXIA TELANGIECTASIA
(Louis-Bar Syndrome)

Ataxia telangiectasia is a heredofamilial disease manifested by ocular and cutaneous telangiectasia, a progressive cerebellar ataxia, and various immunodeficiencies which are discussed in Ch. 69. This rare disease is linked clinically and pathologically with both the neurocutaneous syndromes and the hereditary ataxias.

The neuropathologic changes of the disease consist of widespread atrophy of the cerebellar cortex, with loss of Purkinje cells and thinning of the internal granular layer. There is chronic neuronal degeneration of the dentate and inferior olivary nuclei, as well as demyelination affecting particularly the posterior columns of the spinal cord.

The onset of the disease is usually marked by the appearance in infancy of the cerebellar ataxia first noted as the child begins to walk. The gait is reeling and wide based. The loss of equilibrium persists, and is later aggravated by the onset of limb ataxia. At about the age of four, telangiectasia appears, first being noted in the bulbar conjunctiva and then spreading over the malar surfaces in a butterfly distribution, on the ears, the palate, along the neck, and in the antecubital and popliteal fossae. Occasionally, café-au-lait spots are seen. Patients also suffer from sinusitis and frequent pulmonary infections. As the disease progresses, other neurologic signs, including opsoclonus, choreoathetoid movements, and, rarely, myoclonic jerks, may be observed. The disease is slowly progressive, and patients rarely live beyond the age of 25.

Aguliar, M. J., Kamoshita, S., Landing, B. H., Boder, E., and Sedgwick, R. P.: Pathological changes in ataxia-telangiectasia. J. Neuropathol. Exp. Neurol., 27:659, 1968.

Alexander, G. L.: Sturge-Weber syndrome. *In* Vinken, P. J., and Bruyn, G. W. (eds.): The Phakomatoses. New York, American Elsevier Publishing Company, 1972, pp. 223–240.

Bundey, S., and Evans, K.: Tuberous sclerosis: A genetic study. J. Neurol. Neurosurg. Psychiatry, 32:591, 1969.

Canale, D. J., and Bebin, J.: Von Recklinghausen's disease of the nervous system. *In* Vinken, P. J., and Bruyn, G. W. (eds.): The Phakomatoses. New York, American Elsevier Publishing Company, 1972, pp. 132–162.

Donegani, G., Grattarola, F. R., and Wildi, E.: Tuberous sclerosis. *In* Vinken, P. J., and Bruyn, G. W. (eds.): The Phakomatoses. New York, American Elsevier Publishing Company, 1972, pp. 340–389.

Dwyer, J. M., Hickie, J. B., and Garvan, J.: Pulmonary tuberous sclerosis. Quart. J. Med. (N.S.), 40:115, 1971.

Grossman, M., and Melmon, K. L.: Von Hippel–Lindau disease. Von Recklinghausen's disease of the nervous system. *In* Vinken, P. J., and Bruyn, G. W. (eds.): The Phakomatoses. New York, American Elsevier Publishing Company, 1972, pp. 241–259.

McFarlin, D. E., Strober, W., and Waldmann, T. A.: Ataxia-telangiectasia. Medicine, 51:581, 1972.

Section Twenty-One. MECHANICAL LESIONS OF THE NERVE ROOTS AND SPINAL CORD

Albert J. Aguayo

447. SYMPTOMS OF NERVE ROOT AND SPINAL CORD COMPRESSION

Certain diseases result in compression of the nerve roots or spinal cord within the spinal canal. In general the symptoms and signs that accompany such intraspinal lesions may be classified into two groups: radicular syndromes caused by spinal root injury, and myelopathy caused by compression of the spinal cord; but a combination of both syndromes is also common.

RADICULAR SYNDROMES

Compression of nerve roots causes pain, paresthesia, sensory loss, weakness, atrophy, and reflex changes which are confined to a radicular anatomic distribution. A single nerve root can be compressed, as in most cases of intervertebral disc protrusion, but several roots are often involved in arachnoiditis or when there is neoplastic invasion of the spinal canal.

The pain caused by root compression is experienced in the overlying spine, deep in certain muscles, or along the cutaneous distribution of the injured root *(dermatome)*. This pain is often influenced by movement and increases with strain. Radicular pain is usually unilateral, but some intraspinal lesions, by compressing roots bilaterally, can give rise to pain in both limbs or on both sides of the thorax or abdomen. The most common sensory symptoms are hypesthesia and paresthesia, both of which may be described by patients as numbness. These sensory symptoms are usually accompanied by sensory impairment in the distribution of the compressed root or roots. Because of the more extensive overlapping of adjacent innervation for touch, this sensory loss is better outlined by testing responses to pinprick than to light touch.

Muscles supplied by roots that originate from the same spinal cord segment constitute a *myotome*. Because most muscles are supplied from more than one segmental level, compression of a single root causes different degrees of weakness and atrophy in different muscles. The effects of a root lesion on a muscle ultimately depend on the importance of the innervation provided by the injured root; weakness of certain muscles within a particular myotome may be difficult to elicit, whereas other muscles may be severely affected. For example, although fibers from the L5 root innervate approximately 30 different muscles in the lower limb, severe changes after

TABLE 1.   Clinical Findings in the Four Most Common Radicular Syndromes

Root	Usual Distribution of Pain	Principally Affected Muscles	Sensory Loss	Muscle Stretch Reflexes Affected
C6	Neck, parascapular, lateral aspect of arm and forearm	Biceps, brachioradialis, wrist extensors and flexors	Radial border of forearm, thumb	Biceps and/or brachioradialis may be diminished
C7	Neck, parascapular, posterolateral arm, dorsum of forearm	Triceps, wrist, finger flexors and extensors	Dorsum of forearm; index and middle fingers	Triceps
L5	Low back, buttock, lateral thigh, dorsum of foot	Dorsiflexors of foot and toes	Anterolateral aspect of lower leg, dorsum of foot	Usually none, but ankle jerk may be diminished
S1	Low back, buttock, posterior thigh	Calf muscles, plantar flexors	Outer edge of foot and sole	Ankle jerk

compression of this root may be clearly apparent in only two: the extensor hallucis longus and extensor digitorum brevis muscles.

Muscle stretch reflexes are diminished or absent when reflex arcs are interrupted by root compression. At the levels at which they can be clinically tested, reflex changes have an important localizing value (Table 1).

Differentiation between symptoms caused by nerve root and peripheral nerve lesions must follow anatomic guides (see figure and Table 2). In radiculopathy, as mentioned above, weakness and atrophy of muscles occur within a myotome. In a neuropathy, weakness and reflex changes are confined to the anatomic distribution of the nerve, and sensory deficits do not fully correspond to individual dermatomes. Differentiation is made easier when the affected muscles are supplied by different nerves (e.g., the deltoid and biceps may be weak in lesions of the C5 root; these muscles are supplied by different nerves: axillary and musculocutaneous nerves, respectively). Because of the proximity of roots and spinal cord within the spinal canal, both structures may be compressed together. Associated signs of spinal cord compression are not a feature in peripheral neuropathies except in rare disorders such as familial hypertrophic neuropathy, in which pathologically enlarged roots may encroach upon the spinal cord (Symonds and Blackwood).

Schematic representation of dermatomes and peripheral nerve sensory areas:
1. Trigeminal 1st division
2. Trigeminal 2nd division
3. Trigeminal 3rd division
4. Greater auricular nerve
5. Branches from cervical plexus
6. Axillary nerve
7. Radial nerve
8. Medial brachial cutaneous nerve
9. Musculocutaneous nerve
10. Median nerve
11. Ulnar nerve
12. Lateral femoral cutaneous nerve
13. Femoral nerve
14. Saphenous nerve
15. Peroneal nerve
16. Sural nerve

SPINAL CORD COMPRESSION

The clinical symptomatology depends on the speed of compression, the transverse and longitudinal extent of the lesion, the functional role of the compressed level of the spinal cord, and the cause of compression.

The spinal cord accommodates to slow forms of compression such as occur with meningiomas and neurofibromas. As a result these tumors in their early stages may cause few symptoms and signs. However, an acute intervertebral disc protrusion or an epidural hematoma will result in rapid impairment of function with severe paralysis, sensory loss, and loss of bladder and bowel control.

The effects of compression may be limited to only a portion of the transverse area of the cord. When one half of the spinal cord is injured at levels higher than the tenth thoracic level, the symptoms and signs that follow are designated the *Brown-Séquard syndrome*. Such patients have spastic weakness, exaggerated muscle stretch reflexes, and an extensor plantar response (Babinski sign) all on the same side as the lesion. Joint position and vibration sense are decreased ipsilaterally, but pain and temperature are impaired on the opposite half of the body. The contralateral loss of pain and tempera-

TABLE 2.   Peripheral Nerve and Radicular Innervation of Muscles

Upper Limb:

Nerves	Radicular Innervation					
	C-4	C-5	C-6	C-7	C-8	T-1
Suprascapular	– –Supraspinatus– –					
Axillary	– –Deltoid– – – – –					
Musculocutaneous	– –Biceps– – – – – – – –					
Median			– –Flexor carpi radialis– –			
				– – – –Flexor pollicis longus– –		
				– –Flexor digitorum– –		
				– –Abductor pollicis longus– –		
				– –Opponens pollicis– – – –		
Ulnar				– –Flexor carpi ulnaris– – – –		
				– –Opponens digiti quinti– –		
				– –Abductor digiti quinti– – – –		
				– –Interossei– – – – –		
Radial			– –Triceps brachialis – – – – – – – – – –			
		– –Brachioradialis– –				
			– –Extensor carpi radialis– –			
			– –Extensor carpi ulnaris– –			
			– –Extensor digitorum longus– –			

Lower Limb:

Nerves	Radicular Innervation						
	L-1	L-2	L-3	L-4	L-5	S-1	S-2
Gluteal	– –Iliopsoas– – – – –						
Femoral					– –Gluteus maximus– – – – –		
Obturator		– – – – – – – – –Quadriceps femoris– –					
Sciatic		– –Adductors– – – – –					
C. Peroneal					– – – –Hamstrings– – – – –		
			– –Tibialis anterior– –				
Tibial			– –Extensor digitorum brevis– –				
					– – – –Gastrocnemius– –		
			– –Abductor hallucis– –				
					– –Abductor digiti quinti– –		

ture sensation is due to crossing of spinothalamic fibers subserving these modalities. Spinothalamic fibers are somatotopically arranged within the ventrolateral columns of the spinal cord, with fibers originating at lower levels lying most laterally. Because of this anatomic organization, extrinsic compression tends to first produce symptoms well below the site of the lesion, the level of sensory impairment gradually ascending as the compression affects deeper parts of the spinal cord. Conversely, because deep-seated lesions may spare superficially arranged fibers, sensation may be normal in the lower dermatomes in patients with intramedullary lesions (sacral sparing).

In addition, intramedullary lesions may give rise to sensory dissociation with loss of pain and temperature sensation and relative preservation of touch. This occurs when mainly crossed fibers are interrupted by a central cord lesion (commissural or syringomyelia-like syndrome). In addition, by predominantly disturbing postural sensibility, cord compression may cause ataxia.

LEVELS OF INTRASPINAL COMPRESSION

Foramen Magnum and Upper Cervical Spine.   Compression at this level may cause symptoms resulting from spinal cord, nerve root, or intracranial involvement. Pain in the neck and back of the head is the most common and earliest sign. The pain is made worse by head movement, particularly nodding. There may be weakness and atrophy of muscles of the neck and shoulder girdle with spasticity in the lower limbs. Paresthesia and sensory deficits may also occur in the oc-

cipital head region (C2 dermatome) and the neck (C3 dermatome). Radicular-like motor and sensory signs may even extend to involve the hands (C6 to C8 segmental level); this extension to the mid- and lower cervical cord has been thought to be due to impaired circulation from compression of spinal vessels. Tumors of the foramen magnum may also extend intracranially and cause increased intracranial pressure, cerebellar dysfunction, nystagmus, trigeminal sensory loss, and atrophy of the tongue.

The most common causes of compression at the craniocervical junction are bony abnormalities which result in basilar invagination, dislocation of the atlantoaxial and atlanto-occipital joints, and neoplasms, meningiomas in particular.

Cervical Region.   Compression at this level characteristically produces segmental and radicular signs in the upper limbs combined with long tract signs in the lower extremities.

There is loss of power and bulk in muscles of the shoulder girdle and arms. The biceps, brachioradialis, or triceps jerks mainly depend on the integrity of the C5, C6, or C7 reflex arcs, respectively, and may be diminished or absent. In addition, there can be "inversion" of the brachioradialis reflex; tapping the tendon of this muscle elicits a brisk reflex contraction of the hand and finger flexor muscles and not a normal flexion and supination of the forearm. This unusual response is due to efferent interruption of the segmental reflex arc; the spread of the response and hyperreflexia at lower spinal levels results from pyramidal tract involvement.

When sensory symptoms extend along the radial border of the forearm and thumb ("numb thumb"), they suggest involvement of the C6 cord segment or nerve root. Symptoms in the index and middle fingers point to C7, and sensory impairment in the ring and little fingers suggest C8. Lesions at the cervicothoracic junction can cause unilateral Horner's syndrome which can be associated with wasting of the small muscles of the hand and a sensory deficit on the ulnar border of the hand and forearm (C8, T1).

The most common causes of compression at this level are cervical spondylosis and protrusion of an intervertebral disc, but intramedullary and extramedullary tumors also occur.

Thoracic Region. Compression is suggested by the finding of normal upper limbs and spasticity in the legs. When thoracic radicular symptoms are present, a more precise localization is possible. It is useful to remember that the projection of the thoracic segments coincides with that of the intercostal spaces. Important landmarks are the level of the nipples for the fourth thoracic, the xiphoid process for T7, and the umbilicus and groin for T10 and T12, respectively. Patients will often complain of a tight, bound feeling which usually coincides with the compressed root or segment. In addition, intercostal muscles may be wasted. In low thoracic lesions the umbilicus may elevate when the patient, in the supine position, raises his head against resistance (Beevor's sign).

Common causes of compression at the thoracic spine level are metastatic tumors, meningiomas, and neurofibromas. Intervertebral disc protrusions are comparatively rare at this level.

Lumbosacral Region. *Lower Spinal Cord.* There is a close relation between the segments in the lower cord and the roots that form the cauda equina. As a result, pain, sensorimotor signs in the lower limbs, and loss of sphincter control can result from the involvement of either cord or roots. It is seldom that a discrete spinal cord segmental lesion can be clinically identified at this level. When they occur, lesions at the first lumbar segment usually cause referred pain to the groin, and there may be loss of the cremasteric cutaneous reflex, weakness of hip flexion, and spasticity in the lower legs. A compression localized at L2 and L3 may give rise to weakness of the quadriceps and adductors of the thigh, loss of knee jerks, brisk ankle reflexes, and bilateral Babinski signs. Involvement of L5 and S1 results in weakness and atrophy of the peroneal, calf, and intrinsic foot muscles. Knee jerks may be present, but, because the lower segmental reflex arcs are interrupted, ankle jerks and Babinski signs cannot be elicited.

Normal power in the legs, preservation of knee and even ankle jerks, but loss of sensation in the perianal and genital (saddle) area, together with impaired bladder and bowel control, are characteristic of lesions that involve the lower sacral segments. When this localization is suspected, sensory function over the buttocks must be carefully examined, and rectal sphincter tone should be tested.

Cauda Equina. Compression of nerve roots forming the cauda equina is difficult to differentiate from signs caused by involvement of the lower segment of the spinal cord. In cauda equina compression, dull, aching pain may be experienced in the sacrum or perineum or can radiate to the legs in a sciatic distribution. Symptoms depend on the level of compression and number of motor and sensory roots affected. Often there is atrophic, areflexic paralysis combined with asymmetrical bilateral radicular sensory impairment. Sensory dissociation does not occur. Progression of signs is usually slow, and loss of bladder and bowel control may occur late.

Presumably because of interference with blood supply to the roots of the cauda equina by compression, some patients with a narrowed lumbar spinal canal experience transient radicular signs or pain in the calf muscles when walking or after prolonged standing. This syndrome has been named intermittent claudication of the cauda equina.

The most important cause of single or multiple root compression at the low lumbar and sacral level is an intervertebral disc protrusion. Cauda equina compression occurs in congenital spinal stenosis and lumbar spondylosis, Paget's disease, and achondroplasia. Ependymomas, teratomas, and lipomas may constrict the lower segments of the cord and cauda equina. Tabes dorsalis, diabetic neuropathy, and other lesions affecting peripheral nerves to the lower limbs must be differentiated from lesions compressing the lumbosacral roots.

Aids to the Investigation of Peripheral Nerve Injuries. London, Her Majesty's Stationery Office, 1960.

Haymaker, W.: Bing's Local Diagnosis in Neurologic Diseases. 15th ed. St. Louis, C. V. Mosby Company, 1969.

Keegan, J. J., and Garett, F. D.: The segmental distribution of the cutaneous nerves in the limbs of man. Anat. Rec., 102:409, 1948.

Klenerman, L.: Cauda equina and spinal cord compression in Paget's disease. J. Bone Joint Surg., 48B:365, 1966.

Rewcastle, N. B., and Berry, K.: Neoplasms of the lower spinal canal. Neurology (Minneap.), 14:608, 1964.

Symonds, C. P., and Blackwood, W.: Spinal cord compression in hypertrophic neuritis. Brain, 85:251, 1962.

448. LABORATORY AIDS TO INVESTIGATION

To localize and establish the nature of lesions causing intraspinal compression, several diagnostic tests may be used. Roentgenographic investigations are the most important, but electrophysiologic techniques, radioisotope scanning, and cerebrospinal fluid examination are also helpful.

ROENTGENOGRAPHIC METHODS

Roentgenographic investigation should begin with plain films of the suspected site of spinal cord or root compression. Frontal, lateral, and oblique views are required for examination of the cervical spine; frontal and lateral views are generally satisfactory for visualization of the thoracic and lumbosacral spine. Lateral films of the cervical spine in flexion and extension are needed if recurrent subluxation is suspected. In certain situations, tomography may be necessary to define a bone lesion more precisely.

Plain films of the spine should be systematically examined, noting the number, shape, density, and alignment of the vertebrae and the contour of the pedicles, the size of the intervertebral foramen, the size and shape of the spinal canal, the width of the disc spaces, and the presence of abnormal soft tissue shadows or calcifications. The anteroposterior depth of the spinal canal is a particularly important measurement. Sagittal diameters of less than 10 mm at any level of the cervical spine usually indicate spinal cord compression; bony compression of the cord is also possible with canals measuring 10 to 13 mm but improbable if measurements are greater than 13 mm. Increases in the transverse diameter of the spinal canal may be associated with thinning of the pedicles and are seen with syringomyelia or intramedullary tumors. Narrowing of the spinal canal with compression of the spinal cord or roots may occur in spondylosis, achondroplasia, and Paget's disease.

Plain x-rays of the vertebral column may suggest certain specific conditions. Dumbbell-shaped neurofibromas which enlarge the intervertebral foramen will become readily apparent in such x-rays. Congenital anomalies of the vertebral bodies are at times associated with intraspinal teratomas or lipomas. Bone caries suggests an infectious process such as tuberculosis, typhoidal infection, or brucellosis. Vertebral bone destruction by infection often involves the intervertebral discs; conversely, tumor metastases to the vertebral column spare the discs.

When surgical treatment is contemplated, radiopaque *oil myelography* by lumbar or cisternal injection is required for precise localization. In expert hands, *air myelography* is also a useful tool for the assessment of spinal cord size and for a diagnosis of small tumors. *Spinal angiography* is a specialized technique necessary for the detailed investigation of tumors and vascular malformations.

SCANNING AND ELECTROMYOGRAPHY

Bone scanning after radioisotope injection may be helpful if metastases are suspected as a cause of bone destruction. However, fractures, infection, and ankylosing spondylitis may also cause increased radioisotope uptake.

Electromyography is useful for the localization of intraspinal lesions affecting the motor unit at the anterior horn cell or the nerve root levels, as noted in Ch. 358.

CEREBROSPINAL FLUID EXAMINATION

Cerebrospinal fluid examination rarely provides specific diagnostic information about compressive spinal cord or root lesions. Therefore because satisfactory myelograms are difficult to obtain in patients who have had lumbar puncture in the preceding week, cerebrospinal fluid examinations are usually best performed at the time of myelography. In general, the examination of cerebrospinal fluid may suggest certain diagnostic possibilities. Xanthochromic fluid is seen with intraspinal hemorrhage or block of cerebrospinal fluid circulation. Intraspinal bleeding may originate from vascular malformations, ependymomas, or melanomas. Inflammatory cells indicate an infectious process or chemical meningitis caused by a ruptured teratoma or dermoid cyst. Tumor cells may be identified in the cerebrospinal fluid of patients with carcinomatous infiltration of the meninges.

In the absence of a block in the circulation of cerebrospinal fluid, elevations of CSF protein over 60 mg per 100 ml suggest other intraspinal lesions than an intervertebral disc protrusion or spondylosis. Spinal fluid blocks are best established by myelography; because ir-

reparable damage to the spinal cord may result from displacement of an intraspinal mass after pressure changes resulting from jugular compression (Queckenstedt test), this procedure should not be done if spinal cord compression is suspected.

Aguilar, J. A., and Elvidge, A. R.: Intervertebral disc disease caused by the Brucella organism. J. Neurosurg., 18:27, 1961.
Ambrose, G. B., Alpert, M., and Neer, C. S.: Vertebral osteomyelitis. A diagnostic problem. J.A.M.A., 97:101, 1966.
Charkes, N. D., Sklaroff, D. M., and Young, I.: A critical analysis of strontium bone scanning for detection of metastatic cancer. Am. J. Roentgenol. Radium Ther. Nucl. Med., 96:647, 1966.
DiChiro, G., and Doppman, J. L.: Differential angiographic features of hemangioblastomas and arteriovenous malformations of the spinal cord. Radiology, 93:25, 1969.
Elsberg, C. A., and Dyke, C. G.: Diagnosis and localization of tumors of the spinal cord by means of measurements made on x-ray films of vertebrae and the correlation of clinical and x-ray findings. Bull. Neurol. Inst., 3:359, 1934.

449. MANAGEMENT OF PATIENTS WITH SUSPECTED NERVE ROOT OR SPINAL CORD COMPRESSION

The specific management of intraspinal compression of nerve roots or cord depends on the suspected diagnosis, the severity of the symptoms, and the extent of the neurologic signs.

Conservative Management Aimed at Reducing Pain and Preventing Future Recurrences.   Patients in this category have acute localized pain in the spinal or paraspinal region with or without peripheral radicular radiation; they do not have neurologic deficits indicative of spinal cord or severe root compression. The most likely diagnosis is an acute intervertebral disc protrusion, and with time complete recovery can usually be anticipated. This approach is particularly justified when there is no history of similar previous episodes and when the pain follows minor trauma, effort, or strain.

Patients may stay at home and should rest on a firm bed and make no physical effort. Analgesics and muscle relaxants are given for symptomatic relief. When pain subsides, exercises aimed at strengthening the muscular support of the spinal column may help prevent recurrences.

Plain x-rays of the involved segment of the spine help ascertain changes in the vertebral bodies or discs. Initially, however, these investigations can be deferred if the patient is in considerable pain.

Conservative Management Aimed at Deciding If the Course of Intraspinal Root Compression Is Progressive. Acute pain may be accompanied by signs of moderate sensory or motor deficit in a root distribution. Such signs are represented by some loss of strength, paresthesia, and mild sensory impairment or a loss of muscle stretch reflexes. If these signs worsen or do not subside after a trial of conservative treatment, admission to hospital should be arranged to assure immobilization and rest and to arrange further investigations.

Management Aimed at Possible Surgical Decompression. This approach is indicated for patients showing signs of spinal cord compression. It is also advisable for patients with nerve root compression if there is intractable or severe recurrent pain or if there are signs of severe neurologic deficit, particularly marked weakness and muscle atrophy. These patients should be admitted to hospital for investigation. If there are no contraindications to surgery, myelography should be performed to establish a diagnosis and determine the site and extent of compression. If indicated, operative treatment should soon follow.

Prompt Investigation and Surgical Decompression. This approach is required for patients who rapidly develop spinal cord or cauda equina compression. A particular emergency is represented by impaired bladder or rectal control. Patients should be immediately admitted to hospital to undergo only those investigations which enable a localization of the lesion. Such investigations usually include plain films of the spine and an emergency myelogram. In the course of these investigations, patients should be kept fasting to allow for immediate anesthesia if surgical intervention is decided upon.

SPECIFIC DISORDERS THAT CAUSE NERVE ROOT OR SPINAL CORD COMPRESSION

450.   INTERVERTEBRAL DISC PROTRUSION

Each intervertebral disc consists of fibrocartilage and has a soft center, the nucleus pulposus, surrounded by thicker fibrous tissue, the anulus fibrosus. The nucleus pulposus constitutes most of the disc substance in the young, but with age it loses volume and resilience. When, during effort or trauma, the disc is suddenly compressed and the nucleus pulposus is caused to protrude through the anulus, fragments of disc may be extruded into the spinal canal. The herniated disc is usually directed toward the spinal canal because the anulus and longitudinal ligament are thinner posteriorly. Disc disease is more common in the cervical and lumbar spine where there is greater mobility; in the thoracic spine, where movement is limited, disc herniations are rare.

The signs and symptoms of disc herniation result from compression of pain-sensitive structures within the spinal canal, including nerve roots or the spinal cord itself. Posterolateral disc herniations tend to involve individual nerve roots at the intervertebral foramina, whereas central protrusions may compress the spinal cord or cauda equina. Commonly the compressed root approximately corresponds to the level of the protruded disc, but this may not be the case in the lumbosacral region where several roots can be compressed by a single disc. Furthermore, extruded disc material may move several centimeters along the dural sac and compress roots situated below the site of disc rupture.

Clinical Manifestations.   Pain is the main symptom of an intervertebral disc protrusion. It is usually severe and accompanied by local reflex contraction of paraspinal muscles. Other symptoms and signs depend upon the localization of the protruded disc.

Herniated Cervical Discs.   Cervical disc herniations occur most frequently at the fifth and sixth interspaces with fewer protrusions at C4 and C7 interspaces. Symptoms are often precipitated by sudden twisting, hyperextension, or hyperflexion of the neck. The pain may radiate to the shoulder and parascapular region and usually has a boring, aching quality. If nerve roots are compressed below the midcervical level, pain may extend into the upper extremity. Movements of the neck, but particularly hyperextension and tilting toward the affected side, are limited by pain. Symptoms caused by compression of the C6 and C7 roots are summarized in Table 1, Ch. 447. More rarely cervical disc protrusion results in cord compression. In such patients, long tract signs which develop below the level of the lesion are mainly due to involvement of the corticospinal tract.

Herniated Lumbar Discs.   The most common disc protrusions are in the low lumbar region and affect the L5 and S1 roots (Table 1). There is often a poorly localized low backache (lumbago), and pain may radiate into the buttocks, thigh, and lower leg (sciatica). The pain is generally severe and follows effort, such as lifting. In some patients, however, the pain may be spontaneous; occasionally sensory and motor deficits caused by disc herniation occur in the absence of pain. In most patients, the radiation of pain is unilateral; when there is a central disc protrusion, however, pain may occur in both lower extremities.

On examination patients show straightening of the normal lumbar curvature, and the pelvis may be tilted away from the side of the protrusion. Paraspinal muscles and vertebral spinous processes are tender to palpation. Straight leg raising (Lasègue's maneuver) on the side of compression is limited by back pain. In addition, the pain can occur with raising of the opposite leg ("crossover pain"). There may be tenderness on palpation of the sciatic notch.

Cord compression occurs when disc herniation occurs higher than the first lumbar intervertebral space. Compression of several of the roots of the cauda equina is more common, however, and gives rise to pain, asymmetric bilateral sensory and motor changes, and even to loss of sphincter control. Occasionally, bladder control may be lost in the absence of other symptoms.

Diagnosis.   The symptoms of an intervertebral disc protrusion must be differentiated from those caused by arthritis of the spine and other bone and joint diseases. Neuropathies caused by entrapment, neuralgic amyotrophy, and diabetic neuropathy may enter the differential diagnosis because they may present with localized pain, sensory, and motor deficits.

Plain x-rays of the spine reveal narrowing of disc spaces in less than half the patients. In the cervical spine, oblique views are necessary to establish whether there is a reduction in the size of intervertebral foramina. Myelography should be performed only when the cause of compression is doubtful or when surgical treatment is contemplated. Disc protrusions are evidenced by myelography as a filling defect at the level of the interspace. Obliteration of the root sleeve by a protruded disc may also be demonstrated by this procedure. The cerebrospinal fluid protein may be normal or increased; in the absence of complete block of cerebrospinal fluid circulation, protein values are usually below 60 mg per 100 ml.

Treatment. Patients presenting with acute pain should be treated with analgesics, muscle relaxants, rest, and immobility. A cervical collar or a lumbar brace may reduce mobility, and rest in bed on a hard mattress is often helpful. If improvement follows such measures, usually no investigations other than plain x-rays of the spine are necessary. If pain and other symptoms persist after a period of rest, hospitalization must be considered to ensure immobilization. Intractable pain, persistent disability, or development of progressive sensory or motor signs of radicular compression requires consideration of surgical treatment. Prompt operative treatment is mandatory when signs of progressive cord involvement or impairment of bladder or rectal sphincter control develop.

Recurrent symptoms after discoidectomy may be due to arachnoiditis or to a recurrent intervertebral disc prolapse. In addition the possibility that a herniated disc may have been associated with another type of intraspinal disease must be considered.

Fisher, R. G.: Protrusions of thoracic disc. The factor of herniation through the dura mater. J. Neurosurg., 22:591, 1965.
Kessler, L. A., and Stein, W. Z.: Posterior migration of a herniated disc. Radiology, 76:104, 1961.
Love, J. G., and Emmett, J. L.: "Asymptomatic" protruded lumbar disc as a cause of urinary retention. Mayo Clin. Proc., 42:249, 1967.
Love, J. G., and Schorn, V. G.: Thoracic disc protrusions. J.A.M.A., 191:627, 1965.
Scott, P. J.: Bladder paralysis in cauda equina lesions from disc prolapse. J. Bone Joint Surg., 47B:224, 1965.
Spanos, N. C., and Andrew, J.: Intermittent claudication and lateral lumbar disc protrusions. J. Neurol. Neurosurg. Psychiatry, 29:273, 1966.
Spurling, R. G.: Lesions of the Lumbar Intervertebral Disc. Springfield, Ill., Charles C Thomas, 1953.
Spurling, R. G.: Lesions of the Cervical Intervertebral Disc. Springfield, Ill., Charles C Thomas, 1956.

451. MYELOPATHY AND NERVE ROOT COMPRESSION DUE TO SPONDYLOSIS

Spondylosis refers to degenerative changes in the spine which may be neurologically asymptomatic or may cause symptoms by compression of nerve roots or spinal cord.

Spondylotic changes consist of intervertebral disc narrowing, osteophyte formation, and thickening of spinal ligaments. These changes most frequently involve the cervical or lumbar spine and are rare in the thoracic region. The term spondylosis is not generally used to describe acute protrusion of intervertebral discs, although the two conditions may be associated.

Pathogenesis. Spondylosis presumably results from the "wear and tear" of repeated spinal movement. Although more than one half of people older than 50 years of age have cervical spine osteophytes, associated neurologic symptoms and signs are much less frequent. The single most important factor in the development of clinical manifestations caused by spondylosis is the size of the spinal canal. If the canal is congenitally narrow, the spinal cord or roots may be compressed by relatively small osteophytes or ligamentous hypertrophy; on the other hand, a wide spinal canal may accommodate extensive spondylotic changes without causing appreciable neurologic signs of compression.

When the cervical spinal cord is compressed by osteophytes from the vertebral bodies or by thickening of the posterior longitudinal ligament and ligamentum flavum, symptoms and signs may follow trauma caused by neck movement or from impairment of spinal cord circulation. The cauda equina may also be injured in lumbar spondylosis. At both the cervical and lumbar levels, nerve roots are compressed by degenerative changes in bone and soft tissues adjacent to the intervertebral foramina.

Clinical Manifestations. *Cervical Spondylosis.* The most important symptoms and signs of cervical spondylosis are due to spinal cord (cervical myelopathy) and root (cervical radiculopathy) compression.

Cervical Myelopathy. Cervical myelopathy commonly develops insidiously, but symptoms may be precipitated by minor trauma. Sensory abnormalities are usually less striking than signs of disturbed motor function. Spastic paresis, clonus, and hyperreflexia in the legs as well as extensor plantar responses are the most common neurologic signs of this myelopathy.

In the upper limbs, there may be segmental muscle weakness and atrophy, as well as loss of muscle stretch reflexes, particularly if there is an associated radiculopathy. Vibration sense may be diminished in the lower limbs, but loss of joint position sense or pain and temperature sensation is uncommon. As a rule, bladder and bowel control are normal in patients with cervical myelopathy.

Cervical Radiculopathy. Cervical radiculopathy may occur in the absence of cervical myelopathy. Various radicular syndromes may develop, depending on the particular root affected. In the cervical spine the most common radiculopathies are those of the C6 and C7 root (Table 1, Ch. 447).

Pain and limitation of neck movement are common in cervical spondylosis, and some patients may present with occipital headaches.

Diagnosis. X-rays of the cervical spine confirm the presence of cervical spondylosis. However, there is a high incidence of asymptomatic spondylotic changes, and careful clinical correlation is required for interpretation of such radiologic findings. To prove the diagnosis of cervical spondylotic myelopathy, the anteroposterior diameter of the cervical canal must be measured. If this measurement is less than 10 mm, there is almost certain cord compression. The extent of compression can best be determined by myelography which also shows soft tissue changes in spondylosis. Oblique x-ray views demonstrate narrowing of the intervertebral foramina.

Prognosis and Treatment. Because of wide variations in the natural course of cervical spondylotic myelopathy, it is difficult to assess the relative merits of conservative and surgical management. Recent advances in surgical techniques have been accompanied by more effective relief of spinal cord compression in patients with advancing or rapidly progressing disability. Other patients can usually be managed effectively with analgesics, muscle relaxants, and cervical immobilization.

LUMBAR SPINAL STENOSIS DUE TO SPONDYLOSIS

In addition to compression of individual nerve roots by osteophytes encroaching upon intervertebral foramina, spondylosis of the lumbosacral spine may significantly reduce the size of the spinal canal. In such circumstances, spinal canal stenosis may cause injury to the cauda equina.

The pathogenesis of neurologic symptoms in patients with lumbar stenosis is similar to that in other bone diseases resulting in shallow lumbar canals, namely, congenital spinal stenosis, achondroplasia, and Paget's disease. In all these disorders, further narrowing by osteophytes, disc herniation, or ligamentous hypertrophy may give rise to compression of the cauda equina.

Clinical Manifestations. The only symptom in patients with lumbar spinal stenosis may be backache after prolonged standing or effort. Signs of single or multiple root compression may develop gradually or have a sudden onset. These radicular symptoms are similar to those of intervertebral disc herniation and other causes of lumbosacral nerve root compression. Patients with lumbar spinal stenosis may suffer acute compression of the cauda equina after minor trauma or when subjected to prolonged hyperextension as during anesthesia for certain surgical procedures.

Intermittent Claudication of the Cauda Equina. Intermittent claudication of the cauda equina is a rare syndrome which may present in association with narrowing of the spinal canal. Typically, symptoms and signs are evoked or accentuated by walking and disappear soon after stopping. In other patients symptoms follow prolonged standing. In both varieties of intermittent claudication of the cauda equina, roots are compressed within a narrow spinal canal. The onset of symptoms has been explained by postulating that transient additional spinal narrowing is caused by the lordotic posture adopted during walking and standing. Patients usually present with pain in the low back and legs and may show weakness and sensory symptoms. During examination signs of motor and sensory deficit, as well as diminished reflexes, may be temporarily elicited by asking the patient to walk until symptoms reappear.

The absence of signs of vascular insufficiency in the iliofemoral and other arteries to the lower extremities helps differentiate claudication caused by compression from that which results from primary vascular disease.

Diagnosis. The diagnosis of lumbar spinal stenosis requires radiologic demonstration of a narrow lumbar canal and myelographic confirmation of cauda equina compression.

Treatment. In advanced lumbar spinal stenosis, progressive signs of individual root or cauda equina compression can be relieved by surgical decompression.

Crandall, P. H., and Batzdorf, U.: Cervical spondylotic myelopathy. J. Neurosurg., 25:57, 1966.

Ehni, G., et al.: Significance of the small lumbar spinal canal: Cauda equina compression syndromes due to spondylosis: (Parts I to V). J. Neurosurg., 31:490, 1969.

Stoltmann, H. F., and Blackwood, W.: The role of the ligamenta flava in the pathogenesis of myelopathy in cervical spondylosis. Brain, 87:45, 1964.

Turnbull, I. M.: Microvasculature of the human spinal cord. J. Neurosurg., 35:141, 1971.

Waltz, T. A.: Physical factors in the myelopathy of cervical spondylosis. Brain, 90:395, 1967.

Wilkinson, M. (ed.): Cervical Spondylosis. Its Early Diagnosis and Treatment. Philadelphia, W. B. Saunders Company, 1971.

452. SPINAL CORD TUMORS

Depending upon their anatomic relation to the dura mater, tumors affecting the spinal cord may be classified as *extradural tumors,* which usually arise in the bone of the spinal column or within the extradural space; *intradural extramedullary tumors,* which lie between the dura mater and the spinal cord; and *intramedullary tumors,* which arise within the substance of the cord itself. The relative incidence in a general hospital population is approximately 50, 40, and 10 per cent, respectively.

EXTRADURAL TUMORS

Such tumors are usually manifested by symptoms and signs of spinal cord compression and are most often caused by extradural bone metastases. Common primary sources are carcinomas of the lung, breast, kidney, and prostate; less frequent sources are the gastrointestinal tract and thyroid gland. Spinal extradural compression may also occur in multiple myeloma, sarcomas, or lymphomas. Most metastases give rise to localized compression, but a few, particularly lymphomas and sarcomas, may extensively infiltrate the epidural space.

Pain resulting from bone destruction or root compression is the first symptom in over 90 per cent of patients with extradural tumors. It is usually dull, constant, and localized, is made worse by movements of the spine or pressure over the vertebral spinal processes, and is often exacerbated by bed rest. Radicular symptoms usually follow the local pain and are often bilateral. Pain alone is usually present for weeks or months before signs of spinal cord dysfunction develop; but once spinal cord signs appear, they usually progress rapidly over a few days or weeks to produce, if untreated, complete paralysis. More rarely, compression develops acutely, because of pathologic collapse of an infiltrated vertebral body or from hemorrhage within the metastasis. In either event, spastic weakness and loss of vibration and joint position sense below the level of the lesion are the first spinal cord signs to develop, whereas disturbances of bladder and/or bowel control generally occur late.

Radiologic changes are present on the plain x-ray films of most patients with malignant extradural metastases. Signs vary from osteoporosis to frank destruction of bone. When ordinary x-ray films of the spine are normal, evidence of bone involvement may be provided by radioisotope scanning. A definitive diagnosis of malignant extradural metastasis, however, can be made only by myelography, which must be carried out promptly if there is clinical suspicion of spinal cord compression, no matter what the plain radiograms reveal.

As a rule the cerebrospinal fluid protein is elevated, but there are no malignant cells. The CSF glucose is normal, in contrast to the decreased levels often seen in patients with carcinomatous invasion of the subarachnoid space.

Because metastatic tumors are a frequent cause of spinal cord compression in adults, this possibility should always be considered in patients with signs or symptoms of compression. In particular, the lungs and breasts should be carefully examined as sources of a possible primary malignancy. Anemia, bone pain, mediastinal enlargement, hepatomegaly, or splenomegaly all suggest metastatic disease or lymphomas. Bone x-rays, serum electrophoresis, testing for Bence Jones protein in the urine, and bone marrow examinations are all of help in diagnosing multiple myeloma.

Hormones, radiotherapy, and/or chemotherapy are used in the treatment of most metastatic tumors involving the spine. Surgical decompression is indicated when such therapy is ineffective or when there are signs of rapidly progressing compression of the cord. Whatever form of treatment is chosen, it must be begun promptly and be vigorous, because if neurologic signs are mild, the chances of maintaining or improving neurologic function are better.

INTRADURAL EXTRAMEDULLARY TUMORS

The two most important tumors in this category are meningiomas and neurofibromas, which together account for almost two thirds of all primary intraspinal neoplasms. Less common tumors are teratomas, arachnoid cysts, some lipomas, and meningeal invasion by carcinoma.

Meningiomas show a high incidence among middle-aged women. They are usually single, relatively small, and located posterior or lateral to the spinal cord. Excluding those that occur in the region of the foramen magnum, approximately 90 per cent are found in the thoracic region. Signs of spinal cord compression develop insidiously so that an ataxic, spastic syndrome, which superficially resembles subacute combined degeneration of the spinal cord, may result. Moderate localized or segmental pain is presented in only 50 per cent of patients and is the central symptom in only 20 per cent. Tenderness on percussion of the vertebral spinous processes may be present. Tumors of the foramen magnum are particularly difficult to diagnose. Spastic ataxia and nystagmus are often early symptoms and may suggest multiple sclerosis rather than tumor. With tumor there may be pain or sensory loss in the C2 distribution, and the CSF protein is elevated.

X-rays may show bone erosion or calcification within a meningioma (4 per cent). Myelography is required for a precise localization of intraspinal meningiomas. In tumors of the foramen magnum a routine myelogram may be negative; therefore if such a tumor is suspected, myelography must be done in the supine as well as in the prone position to localize high, posteriorly placed tumors.

Neurofibromas arise from dorsal nerve roots, affect both sexes equally, occur at all ages, and may be present at any level of the spinal canal. Neurofibromas may extend extradurally but may also arise from within the substance of the spinal cord. In some cases the tumors are part of a generalized neurofibromatosis. A small percentage of neurofibromas undergo sarcomatous changes and become invasive or metastasize.

Patients with intraspinal neurofibromas often give a history of longstanding radicular pain, and this symptom usually long precedes any sign of cord compression. When neurofibromas extend on either side of an intervertebral foramen, they may adopt a dumbbell or hourglass shape. X-rays, including oblique views of the spine, may often show enlargement of a foramen and thinning of the adjacent pedicle. The degree of radiographic change may be out of proportion to the presenting symptoms. When the intraspinal portion of the tumor is small in comparison to the extraspinal, the latter may grow to such a large size that it is palpable externally even when there are few signs of cord compression.

As with meningiomas, the cerebrospinal fluid protein is almost always elevated. Myelography is essential for precise localization. A complete recovery usually follows the early surgical removal of both meningiomas and neurofibromas.

INTRAMEDULLARY TUMORS

Most of these tumors arise from constituent cells of the spinal cord. Ependymomas are the most common, followed by astrocytomas, glioblastomas, and oligodendrogliomas. In addition, vascular tumors (hemangioblastomas), lipomas, and even metastases may occur as intramedullary tumors.

Ependymomas arise at all levels of the spinal cord but have a preference for the caudal region. They represent more than two thirds of the tumors of the conus medullaris and are even more common as causes of tumors of the filum terminale. Ependymomas may extend through several segments of the spinal cord; in rare instances the entire length of the cord is involved. Syringomyelia may develop in association with these and other intramedullary tumors. Spontaneous hemorrhages into ependymomas and hemangioblastomas occur and may give rise to sudden pain and neurologic deficit. Excluding glioblastomas and metastases, most intramedullary tumors have a slow progression. Radicular signs are not an early manifestation. Dull, localized aching pain, muscle weakness or atrophy, impotence in males, and sphincter disturbances in both sexes are common early symptoms. Intramedullary tumors affecting the cervical or thoracic cord may cause sensory dissociation with predominant pain and temperature impairment. In such cases the sacral dermatomes are usually spared. Rarely, increased intracranial pressure with headache and papilledema is the first sign of spinal tumor. The symptoms result from hydrocephalus, believed to result from blocking of CSF absorptive pathways by elevated CSF protein.

Longstanding intramedullary tumors may cause radiologically visible widening of the spinal canal and erosion of the pedicles. Contrast myelography usually demonstrates an enlarged spinal cord. In the lumbosacral region tumors may present as a pedunculated mass involving the cauda equina. Tumors of the filum terminale may be mobile and be a source of confusion for myelographic localization.

Successful surgical removal of intramedullary tumors is sometimes possible. Operative success is particularly high with ependymomas and hemangioblastomas, but recurrences may occur; gliomas respond poorly to any form of treatment, and lipomas are technically difficult to remove.

Davis, R. A., and Washburn, P. L.: Spinal cord meningiomas. Surg. Gynecol. Obstet., 131:15, 1970.

Harries, B.: Spinal cord compression. Br. Med. J., 1:611, 673, 1970.

Posner, J. B.: Neurological complications of systemic cancer. Med. Clin. North Am., 55:625, 1971.

Thomas, J. E., and Miller, R. E.: Lipomatous tumors of the spinal canal. Mayo Clin. Proc., 48:393, 1973.

White, W. A., Patterson, R. H., Jr., and Bergland, R. M.: Role of surgery in the treatment of spinal cord compression by metastatic neoplasm. Cancer, 27:558, 1971.

453. SPINAL ARACHNOIDITIS

Spinal arachnoiditis results from a low grade inflammation of the spinal meninges with formation of fibrous adhesions and loculation of cerebrospinal fluid. The changes extend throughout the length of the subarachnoid space or may be confined to a few segments. The adhesions may compress roots or the spinal cord itself.

Arachnoiditis may result from spinal surgery or spinal anesthesia and, more rarely, from myelography. It can be a late complication of subarachnoid hemorrhage, syphilis, tuberculosis, or other bacterial or parasitic spinal meningitides. In some cases no cause is found.

The development of symptoms and signs is insidious, the earliest symptoms usually reflecting multiple root involvement. This is particularly true if the adhesions extend into the lumbosacral spinal region, thereby involving the cauda equina. Pain is common and may be unrelated to movement; sensory symptoms usually exceed motor deficit. Signs of cord compression gradually develop and may progress to paraplegia; in other cases the disease process spontaneously arrests.

The diagnosis of spinal arachnoiditis depends upon the clinical course, as well as on examination of the cerebrospinal fluid and myelography. The CSF protein is elevated, and there may be pleocytosis. On myelography there are spotty, irregular collections of oil and an impairment of the flow of contrast material in the subarachnoid space.

When a specific infectious agent is identified, appropriate chemotherapy is indicated. Surgical exploration may provide histologic evidence as to the diagnosis, but laminectomy and removal of adhesions are not always beneficial for the relief of spinal and root compression.

Davidson, S.: Cryptococcal spinal arachnoiditis. J. Neurol. Neurosurg. Psychiatry, 31:76, 1968.

Guidetti, B., and LaTorre, E.: Hypertrophic spinal pachymeningitis. J. Neurosurg., 26:496, 1967.

Seaman, W. B., Marder, S. N., and Rosenbaum, H. E.: The myelographic appearance of adhesive spinal arachnoiditis. J. Neurosurg., 10:145, 1953.

Weiss, R. M., Sweeney, L., and Dreyfuss, M.: Circumscribed adhesive spinal arachnoiditis. J. Neurosurg., 19:435, 1962.

Wise, B. L., and Smith, M.: Spinal arachnoiditis ossificans. Arch. Neurol., 13:391, 1965.

454. ARTERIOVENOUS MALFORMATIONS AND OTHER VASCULAR LESIONS OF THE SPINAL CORD

Vascular malformations may be present on the surface of the spinal cord or within its substance. They may thus give rise to subarachnoid hemorrhage, intramedullary hemorrhage (hematomyelia), or both. Rarely, a spinal epidural hematoma results from such bleeding. The sudden development of partial or complete transverse myelopathy is the most common form of onset. This is manifested by paralysis, sensory impairment, and loss of sphincter control. If there is bleeding into the subarachnoid space, pain in the neck and back and other signs of meningeal irritation occur. Sudden headache, neck stiffness, and blood in the cerebrospinal fluid may be mistakenly attributed to hemorrhage of intracranial rather than intraspinal origin.

Arteriovenous malformations may also compress the spinal cord or give rise to hemodynamic changes that result in spinal ischemia. Distortion and compression of the cord by enlarged, abnormal vessels occur only gradually, and patients present with slowly progressive symptoms of spinal cord dysfunction. In some patients transient exacerbation of symptoms may occur in association with menstrual periods or pregnancy, but in others exacerbations occur spontaneously.

Complete or partial recovery of function can follow episodes of spinal cord ischemia or even small hemorrhages. The unchanging localization of the attacks and the prominence of pain help to differentiate those symptoms caused by arteriovenous malformations from other recurrent neurologic disorders such as multiple sclerosis. In some patients a spinal bruit may be heard by auscultation over the site of the malformation.

Cavernous angiomas of the spinal cord are vascular hamartomas which may be associated with cysts and tumors in other organs or with hemangioblastomas of the cerebellum. Retinal vascular changes (von Hippel–Lindau syndrome) and cutaneous vascular nevi may be associated with spinal vascular malformations. The presence of these associated signs lends support to the assumption that, in a patient who presents them, spinal symptoms may be due to a vascular malformation.

Intraspinal bleeding caused by vascular malformation must be differentiated from bleeding that occurs as a complication of hemorrhagic diathesis, anticoagulant therapy, or collagen diseases such as polyarteritis nodosa. In these conditions, however, there are usually signs of a more general disorder, cutaneous hematomas or other skin lesions, hematuria, or abnormal laboratory investigations.

In most patients with vascular malformations presenting with acute symptoms, examination of the cerebrospinal fluid reveals body or xanthochromic fluid, but, when there has been no recent bleeding, the only finding may be an elevated protein. Plain x-rays of the spine may show erosion, coexistent vertebral hemangiomas, or calcification within the spinal canal. On myelography, serpentine streaks within the column of oil may reveal the site of the vascular malformation. Angiography with regional catheterization of radicular vessels is a necessary preliminary to surgical treatment. Advances in microsurgery have increased considerably the chances for a satisfactory removal of spinal vascular malformations.

Antoni, N.: Spinal vascular malformations (angiomas) and myelomalacia. Neurology, 12:795, 1962.

Fine, R. D.: Angioma racemosum venosum of spinal cord with segmentally related angiomatous lesions of skin and forearm. J. Neurosurg., 18:546, 1961.

Henson, R. A., and Parsons, M.: Ischaemic lesions of the spinal cord: An illustrated review. Quart. J. Med., 36:205, 1967.

Matthews, W. B.: The spinal bruit. Lancet, 2:1117, 1959.

Taylor, J. R., and Van Allen, M. W.: Vascular malformation of the cord with transient ischaemic attacks. J. Neurosurg., 31:576, 1969.

455. SPINAL EPIDURAL HEMATOMA

Bleeding into the spinal epidural space may occur spontaneously but is more commonly associated with trauma, bleeding diathesis, or vascular malformations. It is a particular risk in patients receiving anticoagulants. The hemorrhage usually originates in the epidural venous plexus, and the hematomas tend to collect over the dorsum of the thoracic dura mater. Epidural hematomas vary in size, but the larger ones cause spinal cord compression. The clinical picture is characterized by the sudden onset of severe, localized back pain. Cord compression, when it occurs, results in the rapid development of flaccid paralysis, sensory loss, and impaired bladder and bowel control. The sudden onset of signs of cord compression in a patient on anticoagulants should allow few doubts as to the likelihood of a spinal epidural hematoma.

In epidural hematomas the cerebrospinal fluid may be clear or very slightly hemorrhagic.

Emergency surgical evacuation of the hematoma is essential. Although myelography is of great help in the diagnosis and localization of epidural hematomas, this and other investigations should not take the place of prompt surgical intervention in order to avoid irreversible spinal cord damage.

Bidzinski, J.: Spontaneous spinal epidural hematoma during pregnancy. Case report. J. Neurosurg., 24:1017, 1966.

Jacobson, I., McCabe, J. J., Harris, P., and Dott, N. M.: Spontaneous spinal epidural hemorrhage during anticoagulant therapy. Br. Med. J., 1:522, 1966.

Markham, J. W., Lynge, H. N., and Stahlman, G. E. B.: The syndrome of spontaneous spinal epidural hematoma. Report of three cases. J. Neurosurg., 26:334, 1967.

Section Twenty-Two. DISEASES OF THE PERIPHERAL NERVOUS SYSTEM

Peter James Dyck

456. BIOLOGY OF THE PERIPHERAL NERVOUS SYSTEM

Peripheral nerves are made up of bundles of nerve fibers whose cell bodies lie within the ventral gray horn of the spinal cord (motor fibers), within the dorsal root ganglion (sensory fibers), and within autonomic ganglia. Myelinated and unmyelinated fibers are surrounded by longitudinally directed collagen fibrils (endoneurium). A bundle of fibers (a fascicle) is surrounded by a tough sheath (the perineurium) made up of neuroepithelial cells and collagen. Between the fascicles and surrounding them is the epineurium.

Peripheral nerves receive their blood supply along their length from various regional blood vessels. Anastomatic arteries, which lie in the epineurium, are formed by the branches from regional arteries. Only the arterioles penetrating the perineurium are thought to be end-arteries. Because of the nature of the blood supply, large-artery disease, unless extensive, does not usually cause infarction within the nerve, but small-artery and arteriolar disease may do so. The collateral blood supply also explains why a peripheral nerve may be undercut for long distances and placed into a new bed without becoming infarcted.

The peripheral nervous system includes all the cranial nerves (except the olfactory and the ocular) from their point of exit from the brainstem to their termination. It further includes all segmental nerve roots from their point of exit from the spinal cord; dorsal root ganglia; autonomic ganglia; mixed spinal nerves; brachial, lumbar, and sacral plexuses; and peripheral nerves. A knowledge of the anatomic arrangement of these structures is essential for adequately assessing the signs of motor, sensory, and autonomic dysfunction in disease of the peripheral nervous system. Since portions of both motor and sensory neurons lie within the spinal cord, it is apparent that diseases of these neurons may affect both the central and the peripheral nervous systems.

The electron microscope has clarified the nature of the structure of myelinated and unmyelinated fibers. Both myelinated and unmyelinated fibers are clothed along their length by a series of Schwann cells of neuroectodermal origin. Unmyelinated fibers, first described by Remak, usually occur in clusters. In transverse sections, individual fibers may be seen occupying invaginations of the Schwann cell cytoplasm; but they remain extracellular. Myelinated fibers in their development also extend into invaginations of Schwann cell cytoplasm, but in addition—either by rotation of Schwann cells or by differential growth—wrap Schwann cell membrane around themselves to form myelin. Especially from the x-ray diffraction and electron microscopic studies of nerve, it is now known that myelin is layered Schwann cell membrane and that nodes of Ranvier are constituted by abutment of two Schwann cells along a fiber.

There is evidence that certain macromolecules, such as enzymes and various proteins, are synthesized in the cell body and flow down the axis cylinder. In addition, Schwann cells have a trophic influence on the axis cylinder.

A lower motor unit is the anterior horn cell (including its axon and terminal branches) and the muscle fibers it innervates. Primary sensory units might be thought of as the nerve cell within the dorsal root ganglion which innervates a small region of skin by its peripheral axon and terminal branches. Its central axon makes connections within the spinal cord.

From the work of Gasser and Erlanger, it is known that if a peripheral nerve is laid on a series of electrodes in the appropriate environment, a rapidly conducted wave (usually called the A-α potential) evoked by low-voltage stimulation of large myelinated fibers can be detected. As the voltage is increased, other deflections appear that correspond to groups of small myelinated fibers (A-δ) and finally of unmyelinated fibers (C fibers). The modality of sensation lost in diseases of primary sensory neurons usually falls into one of three types: (1) selective decrease or loss of touch-pressure, two-point discrimination, and perception of joint position and motion, with preservation of pain and temperature sensation, from selective loss of large myelinated fibers; (2) sensory loss inverse to that just mentioned, from loss of unmyelinated and small myelinated fibers; and (3) loss of all sensory modalities, from loss of all groups of fibers.

457. PATHOLOGY OF THE PERIPHERAL NERVOUS SYSTEM

Pathologic changes in peripheral nerve tissue can be divided broadly into interstitial and parenchymatous. Interstitial pathologic changes arise outside the nerve and Schwann cells and may damage these cells secondarily. Usually in interstitial neuropathies the initial change is in the supporting tissue of the nerve or in its blood vessels. Examples of such neuropathies are amyloidosis, necrotizing angiopathy, and acute, chronic, and relapsing inflammatory polyradiculoneuropathy. In parenchymatous neuropathies the nerve and Schwann cells are primarily affected from various causes such as inherited metabolic diseases, toxic substances, deficiency states, and other metabolic diseases. Examples of parenchymatous neuropathies are those caused by alcohol, lead, arsenic, diphtheria, and metachromatic leukodystrophy.

Two histologic features of especial importance in peripheral nerve disease are, respectively, the formation of linear rows of myelin ovoids and myelin balls (wallerian degeneration or axonal degeneration) and the focal absence of myelin with preservation of the axis cylinder along the length of myelinated fibers (segmental demyelination). Linear rows of myelin ovoids and balls are formed in distal nerve fibers after crush or transection of nerve fibers. In parenchymatous neuropathy similar linear rows of myelin ovoids and balls are seen, but no mechanism of acute transection has been demonstrated, and the electron microscopic abnormalities of axis cylinders are not identical to wallerian degeneration. For these reasons a distinction should be made between the terms wallerian degeneration consequent to transection and the histologic changes of acute axonal degeneration. Segmental demyelination is usually interpreted as evidence of Schwann cell disease. Actually, however, segmental demyelination may also occur secondary to axis cylinder atrophy and degeneration. In many neuronal disorders such segmental demyelination and remyelination are clustered on degenerating fibers, especially at the distal aspect of the neuron. When demyelination and remyelination occur repetitively on fibers, "onion bulb" formations and increased collagen are formed. These characteristics of hypertrophic neuropathy therefore are found to varying degrees in a variety of neuropathies.

Although in many parenchymatous neuropathies the main symptoms, signs, and morphologic changes suggest involvement of the distal processes of the peripheral nervous system neurons only, this reflects more generalized disease of these neurons. Recently, peripheral nerve biopsy has been used to evaluate selected patients with peripheral neuropathy. Nerve biopsy, especially in patients with mild neuropathy, is often followed by a disagreeable or painful numbness and with a small region of sensory loss. The procedure should be done sparingly and only at centers which can adequately evaluate the tissue.

Fascicular or whole biopsy of such nerves as the sural may provide diagnostic information in leprosy, amyloidosis, angiopathic vasculopathy, inflammatory polyradiculoneuropathy, and various lipidoses. It may provide unequivocal evidence of the presence and of the type and severity of fiber degeneration. A subclinical or mild neuropathy may be recognized by good histologic evaluation of nerve biopsy tissue even when clinical examination and nerve conduction and electromyography are normal. Furthermore, an examination of teased-out fibers helps to identify the exact type of neuropathy. Nerve biopsy tissue may be studied electrophysiologically by recording the compound action potential, thus giving information not only about A-α fibers (which are also studied in vivo) but also about A-δ and C fibers. Nerve biopsy tissue may also be utilized for biochemical studies of lipids and of transport of such substances as dopamine beta hydroxylase.

458. MANIFESTATIONS OF PERIPHERAL NEUROPATHY

The hallmarks of peripheral neuropathy are muscle weakness with or without atrophy, sensory changes, autonomic manifestations, or mixtures of these, all in the appropriate anatomic distribution. Conventionally, peripheral neuropathy is considered to be a disorder of the peripheral nerves that affects predominantly the distal muscles of the extremity, and is associated with sensory loss of all modalities, which also is greatest distally and shades off to normal in more proximal regions of extremities. Although this is a common clinical pattern, not all neuropathies conform to it. Some polyradiculoneuropathies (for example, the Guillain-Barré syndrome) affect the ventral roots and varying amounts of the posterior roots and peripheral nerves, producing weakness in axial and proximal limb muscles as well as in the distal limb muscles. In other diseases such as Friedreich's ataxia or in subacute combined degeneration, the dorsal root ganglia neurons (in addition to other CNS structures) are particularly affected. In some maladies such as metachromatic leukodystrophy or Krabbe's disease, the central nervous system manifestations so dominate the clinical pattern that the disorder in nerve may be overlooked unless one subjects the nerve to histologic examination or measures its conduction velocity.

Patients with neuropathy may not have symptoms or may attribute them to other disease. Commonly the patient with an inherited neuropathy or a chronic neuropathy has no symptoms, or attributes them to a past accident or poliomyelitis. The insidious development of many neuropathies allows for accommodation to the disease. Motor symptoms in such patients are usually described as clumsiness of gait, difficulty in picking up the toes in walking, frequent tripping or stumbling, or inability to perform some ordinary act such as combing the hair, turning a key in a lock, or fastening a safety pin. Some patients notice muscle atrophy, but in chronic neuropathy many of them do not—presumably because the development is so gradual.

Patients with sensory nerve involvement may have symptoms of tightness, burning, jabbing, searing, pricking, tingling, and numbness. These are particularly common in the neuropathies associated with diabetes mellitus, vitamin deficiency, vasculitis, arsenic intoxication, and sprue. In other neuropathies, the predominant symptoms are not of pain or discomfort but rather of a decrease or loss of function, evident as inability to locate a pill in the mouth or to recognize a comb in the pocket, or as unsteadiness in walking owing to kinesthetic loss. Patients with a very slow course tend to have fewer symptoms. Patients with acute axonal degeneration of small and large fibers tend to have discomfort, whereas those with segmental demyelination predominantly usually have little if any. Loss of sympathetic nerve function, such as occurs in such diseases as diabetes mellitus and amyloidosis, results in postural hypotension, loss of sweating, and bladder and bowel incontinence.

459. DEFINITION, DIFFERENTIAL DIAGNOSIS, AND CLASSIFICATION OF PERIPHERAL NEUROPATHY

The cells of the peripheral motor nerves lie in the anterior horn of the spinal cord or in autonomic ganglia, and the cells of sensory fibers lie in the dorsal root ganglia. Many diseases that start in the peripheral nerve sooner or later affect the perikaryon (cell body)

and vice versa, so that peripheral neuropathies, anterior horn cell diseases, radicular sensory disorders, and even diseases of the dorsal columns have a certain biologic overlap. This chapter arbitrarily gives attention to conditions in which the peripheral nerve is heavily affected. The relations among these several disorders can be seen by examining the accompanying table.

In evaluating a patient with possible peripheral nerve disease, it is first necessary to establish that there is disease of the peripheral nerves. In some cases the clinical symptoms, the diffuse muscle weakness and atrophy, and the sensory loss may unequivocally suggest a disorder of peripheral nerves. In patients with only muscle weakness and atrophy with either no or equivocal sensory loss, it may be difficult to decide whether the disease is neurogenic or myogenic, but there are three types of study that may help. (1) Concentrations of such serum enzymes as phosphocreatine kinase and the transaminases are often elevated in muscle disease but are usually normal or only slightly elevated in neurogenic muscular atrophy. (2) A particularly helpful study is determination of the conduction velocity of nerves and electromyography. In disease of muscle, conduction velocity of nerves should be normal, unless spuriously decreased by low temperature or by pressure palsies from the patient's remaining in bed for a long time. Conduction velocities may be normal in neurogenic muscle atrophy as well, but in this situation the characteristics of the

Classification of Peripheral Neuropathy

I. Mononeuropathy and plexus neuropathies
  A. Cranial nerves
  B. Peripheral nerves
    1. Physical injury
    2. Entrapment neuropathies
      a. Carpal tunnel syndrome
      b. Tardy ulnar nerve palsy
      c. Acute radial nerve palsy
      d. Acute and tardy peroneal nerve palsy
      e. Tarsal tunnel syndrome
      f. Meralgia paresthetica
      g. Thoracic outlet syndrome
    3. Mononeuropathy multiplex
    4. Plexus neuropathy
      a. Brachial plexus neuropathy
      b. Lumbar and sacral plexus neuropathy

II. Multiple neuropathy
  A. Associated with malnutrition and vitamin deficiency
    1. In alcoholism
    2. In malnutrition
    3. In pellagra
    4. In celiac disease
    5. In pernicious anemia
    6. In postgastrectomy condition
  B. Associated with carcinoma and other malignancy
    1. Primary sensory neuropathy with carcinoma
    2. Mixed neuropathy with carcinoma
    3. Peripheral neuropathy with lymphoma
  C. Associated with mesenchymal disease and with necrotizing arteritis
  D. Associated with diabetes mellitus
  E. Associated with drugs and toxins
    1. Heavy metals
      a. Lead
      b. Arsenic
      c. Thallium
      d. Mercury
      e. Copper, antimony, and zinc
    2. Organophosphate compounds (TOCP)
    3. Industrial poisons
    4. Drugs
  F. Neuropathy associated with hormonal disturbances
  G. Neuropathy associated with possible immunologic disorders

    1. Acute inflammatory polyradiculoneuropathy of the Guillain-Barré-Strohl type
    2. Chronic and relapsing inflammatory polyradiculoneuropathy
    3. Serum neuropathy
  H. Neuropathy associated with infection
    1. Diphtheria
    2. Leprosy
  I. Neuropathy associated with inborn errors of metabolism (hereditary disorders)
    1. Predominant involvement of lower motor neurons
      a. Hereditary proximal motor neuropathy
        Infantile
        Juvenile
        Adult
      b. Hereditary distal motor neuropathy
      c. Hereditary scapuloperoneal motor neuropathy
      d. Hereditary fascioscapulohumeral motor neuropathy
      e. Motor neuron disease
      f. Progressive bulbar paresis of childhood
    2. Predominant involvement of primary sensory neurons
      a. Inherited sensory neuropathy, Type I (dominantly inherited sensory radicular neuropathy)
      b. Inherited sensory neuropathy, Type II (recessively inherited congenital sensory neuropathy)
      c. Inherited sensory neuropathy, Type III (Riley-Day syndrome)
      d. Inherited sensory neuropathy, Type IV
      e. Angiokeratoma corporis diffusum (Fabry's)
    3. Involvement of lower motor or primary sensory neurons and other systems
      a. Spinocerebellar degeneration
      b. Friedreich's ataxia
      c. Spastic paraplegia with peroneal muscular atrophy
      d. Hypo-β-lipoproteinemia (Bassen and Kornzweig)
      e. Hypo-α-lipoproteinemia (Tangier disease)
      f. Hereditary motor and sensory neuropathy, Types I–VII
      g. Acute intermittent porphyria
      h. Dominantly inherited amyloidosis (Portuguese)
      i. Dominantly inherited amyloidosis (Indiana)
  J. Associated with peripheral vascular disease
  K. Associated with uremia
  L. Of unknown cause

electromyographic examination may be distinguishing (see Ch. 358). (3) Biopsy of muscle or nerve. The diagnostic usefulness of these methods of examination varies considerably in different clinics, primarily because of differences in the experience of the persons doing the studies. Neither enzyme tests nor electrophysiologic studies ever provide a specific diagnosis, and the muscle and nerve biopsies do so only infrequently.

A second differential to be made is between disorders of peripheral nerve and disorders of central nervous system disease. In peripheral disorders, muscle weakness is usually associated with atrophy, denervation in electromyographic studies, decrease or absence of the tendon reflexes, and a pattern of sensory loss compatible with disease of multiple nerves. In central lesions muscle weakness is usually unaccompanied by atrophy, tendon reflexes are hyperactive with corticospinal and corticobulbar tract signs, and sensory loss is of the type seen in spinal cord or cerebral hemisphere disease.

Probably the most satisfactory method of classifying the peripheral neuropathies would be based on etiology. Unfortunately, however, the precise etiologic factors for most neuropathies are unknown. Additionally, the diagnosis of many other neuropathies depends entirely on an association with a disease, such as diabetes mellitus, carcinoma, or uremia.

Neuropathies may also be classified by the anatomic site of involvement: cranial neuropathy and peripheral neuropathy, mononeuropathy (single nerves) and multiple neuropathy (multiple nerves), radiculopathy (roots), and plexus neuropathy (brachial, lumbar, or sacral plexus). They may be classified as motor, sensory, and autonomic neuropathy, depending on the predominant type of fiber involvement. On the basis of their rate of progression, neuropathies may be divided into acute, subacute, and chronic categories. In general, they may further be divided into those associated with diffuse low conduction velocity of peripheral nerves (a velocity less than 60 per cent of the mean for normal nerves probably signifies a demyelinating type of fiber degeneration), and those in which the conduction velocities are borderline or only slightly reduced but in which there is other electrophysiologic evidence of fiber degeneration (probably an axonal type of fiber degeneration). Another classification is based on the nature of the sensory loss: in one type there is a selective loss of touch-pressure, two-point discrimination, and joint position, indicating involvement of large myelinated fibers; in another type there is a selective loss of pain and temperature sensation and of autonomic function, indicating loss of unmyelinated fibers; and in a third type there is loss of all sensory modalities, indicating loss of all groups of fibers. Pathologic classifications are based on the nature of the fiber degeneration (wallerian, axonal degeneration, segmental demyelination) or site of pathologic changes, as well as on the specific histologic pattern (vasculitis, granulomatous reaction, hypertrophic neuropathy, amyloidosis, and specific infective organism).

MONONEUROPATHY AND PLEXUS NEUROPATHIES

460. CRANIAL NERVES

Olfactory. Anosmia is most often the result of local disease in the nasal passageways, skull fracture, or brain tumor and is usually reported by the patient as a defect in taste.

Optic. Any visual field defect is a serious matter and demands thorough investigation. Permanent visual impairment or blindness can occur because of unnecessary delay in the diagnosis and treatment of benign and removable compressive lesions such as meningiomas, craniopharyngiomas, cholesteatomas, and chromophobe adenomas. Intrinsic lesions of the optic nerves, such as occur in multiple sclerosis, tend to produce scotomas, whereas compressive lesions like tumors and carotid aneurysms predispose to monocular and binasal or bitemporal visual field defects. Homonymous field defects are usually the result of lesions of the optic pathways posterior to the chiasm, generally as the result of lesions involving the brain itself.

Oculomotor, Trochlear, and Abducens. The motor nerves to the eye may be damaged by a variety of diseases anywhere in their long course from brainstem to orbit. Tumor, aneurysm, and temporal lobe herniation often cause oculomotor palsy, usually with pupillary involvement. A slightly dilated pupil and sluggish response to light may be early, subtle signs of third-nerve compression. Either purulent or granulomatous meningitis may impair third- or, more commonly, sixth-nerve function. Increased intracranial pressure may cause unilateral or, especially, bilateral abducens palsy.

Loss of normal eye movement can be a difficult diagnostic problem. The rapid onset of oculomotor palsy associated with pain around or behind the eye immediately suggests diabetic mononeuropathy, migraine, or intracranial aneurysm. However, in as many as one third of such cases no satisfactory cause is found. The pupil is usually dilated with aneurysm and migraine, but not in diabetes or in the idiopathic types. Aneurysm is frequently, but not always, accompanied by hypertension and subarachnoid hemorrhage. A history of typical headache, previous ocular palsy, and occurrence in childhood favors migraine. Diabetic ophthalmoplegia occasionally also includes the sixth nerve and may occur with only mild glucose intolerance; improvement usually begins within three to five weeks, though diplopia persists until motor balance is nearly perfect. Occurrence of other neurologic deficits, along with impaired ocular motility, is common with aneurysm or tumor, and is expected with a midbrain infarct. *Myasthenia gravis* can affect extraocular muscles as an isolated symptom and should be considered, especially when the weakness differs from typical cranial nerve patterns, is inconstant, includes eye opening and closing, does not involve the pupil, and is bilateral.

Abnormalities of pupillary size, shape, and reaction are not confined to third-nerve injuries. The *Argyll Robertson pupil* is small, irregular, usually bilateral, responds to convergence accommodation but not to light, and responds poorly to mydriatics; it is common with neurosyphilis and rare with diabetes. The pupils of diabetics are often unequal and may be completely nonreactive. *Adie's myotonic pupil* may cause confusion. It reacts only slowly to light or accommodation convergence, but constricts to fresh 2.5 per cent mecholyl instilled in the conjunctival sac, whereas a normal pupil does not.

Bilateral external ophthalmoplegia of rapid or sudden onset occurs with four diseases, all of which are potentially serious and demand prompt treatment: *acute myasthenia gravis, acute thiamin deficiency with Wer-*

nicke's syndrome, botulism, and *acute idiopathic cranial polyneuropathy.*

Trigeminal. Impairment of function peripherally in the sensory components of the trigeminal nerve may result from a variety of neoplastic and inflammatory processes. Divergence of the third division from the first and second, which pass forward through the cavernous sinus, frequently allows precise localization.

Trigeminal neuralgia is described in Ch. 349.

Facial. Brain injury above the facial nucleus usually spares the brow and forehead muscles because they are bilaterally represented at higher nervous levels; injury to the facial nerve at, or peripheral to, its nucleus paralyzes all the ipsilateral facial muscles. An intrapontine lesion causing facial weakness usually also affects abducens nerve function. As the facial nerve leaves the pons and enters the internal auditory meatus along with the acoustic nerve, it also carries fibers for lacrimation, salivation, and taste. As the nerve descends through the petrous bone, fibers to the lacrimal glands branch off first, then salivary and taste fibers depart in the chorda tympani and cross the middle ear. Only motor fibers to the face emerge from the stylomastoid foramen. Thus the syndrome of seventh nerve damage varies according to the site of injury. Acoustic neurinomas and other tumors of the cerebellopontine angle often involve the facial nerves, as do infections and neoplasms of the meninges.

Bell's palsy is a peripheral facial weakness of unknown cause and rapid onset, occasionally attended by aching pain about the angle of the jaw or behind the ear. Recent work has shown that the point of nerve conduction block is usually in the vicinity of the internal auditory meatus. Retraction of the angle of the mouth and eye closure are impaired, and the forehead is smooth on the affected side. Taste perception on the anterior part of the involved half of the tongue may be distorted. Rarely, hyperacusis results from paralysis of the stapedius muscle. Recovery usually begins within a week, and three of four patients fully recover over a period of several weeks. Occasionally, some permanent deficit remains after a protracted course. In these cases, distressing facial spasms may accompany voluntary facial movement. Adrenal corticosteroids begun near the onset of the illness and continued for seven to ten days may favor a more rapid and complete recovery.

Herpes zoster affecting the geniculate ganglion produces a severe facial paralysis that is associated with a painful eruption within the external ear canal. This, often referred to as the *Ramsay Hunt syndrome,* may also involve the auditory nerve.

Chronic facial hemispasm affects middle-aged or older women somewhat more commonly than men, with spontaneous, unilateral, frequent, sudden, strong, brief contractions of part or all of the facial musculature. The condition usually begins with the orbicularis oculi muscle and, over many years, spreads to involve more of the face. The cause is not known, but a slowly progressive, degenerative condition of the facial nucleus in the pons has been postulated. Relief can be obtained by alcohol injection or section of the facial nerve, but it must be weighed against the facial paralysis necessarily produced.

Auditory. Disturbances of eighth nerve function are discussed in Ch. 351 and 352.

Glossopharyngeal, Vagus, and Spinal Accessory. The glossopharyngeal and vagus nerves supply sensory and motor innervation to the pharynx. They may be involved by tumor or aneurysm along with the spinal accessory nerves in their common exit through the jugular foramen. Hoarseness and asymmetric elevation of the soft palate result from lesions of the vagus nerve, and weakness and atrophy of sternocleidomastoid and superior trapezoid muscles result from disruption of the spinal accessory.

Glossopharyngeal neuralgia is described in Ch. 349.

Hypoglossal. This motor nerve to the tongue is rarely involved in its peripheral course. Atrophy and fasciculation of the ipsilateral half of the tongue are seen, and the tongue deviates toward the affected side upon protrusion.

461. PERIPHERAL NERVES

Physical Injury. Spinal nerves, plexuses, and peripheral nerve trunks may be injured by traction, compression, contusion, and laceration. Nerves may be damaged by electricity and radiation. Fractured bones may lacerate or compress nerves. Excessively tight casts or tourniquets may damage nerves by direct compression or by ischemia. Injection of penicillin or other medications into the sciatic nerve can cause serious injury. In Sunderland's textbook (1968) details on these and other nerve injuries are presented.

Entrapment Neuropathies. Peripheral nerves may be injured by compression or ischemia at points where they pass through rigid anatomic canals or beneath tight fascial bands. Such injury occurs more readily when inflammation or degeneration develops in adjacent joints and tendons (as may happen in rheumatoid arthritis, myxedema, and acromegaly), and when the nerves lie in shallow grooves allowing them to be compressed or repeatedly traumatized.

Carpal Tunnel Syndrome. In the carpal tunnel syndrome the median nerve is compressed as it passes through the canal made by the carpal bones and ligament. Some cases are idiopathic, and, in these, surgeons report a flattening of the median nerve just distal to the crease of the wrist and either thickening of the ligament or, more commonly, noninflammatory thickening of the synovia of the flexor tendons. The median nerve may be compressed within the carpal tunnel by a ganglion or by degenerative joint and synovial changes from rheumatoid arthritis, myxedema, and acromegaly.

This common disorder especially affects women. Pricking numbness and pain in the fingers and hands, coming on especially during the night and relieved by changing the position of the hands (shaking them), are characteristic. It is uncommon for patients to localize the numbness to the exact cutaneous distribution of the median nerve. Furthermore, the aching discomfort that may accompany the numbness may extend up the arm. Atrophy of the muscles innervated by the median nerve (for example, the thenar muscles) is not an early sign. In many cases it is possible to reproduce the painful numbness by holding the wrist in extreme flexion for a short period *(Phalen's sign).* Also a burst of tingling may occur when the skin over the nerve at the wrist is percussed *(Tinel's sign).* There may be sensory loss in the distribution of the median nerve, though more frequently none is detected.

An important confirmatory test can now be done in most electromyographic laboratories. It consists in determining the time from stimulation of the median nerve at a point above the carpal ligament to the appearance of the thenar muscle action potential. Similarly, one can determine the time from stimulation of digital fibers to the obtaining of an action potential in electrodes overlying the median nerve above the carpal ligament. In the carpal tunnel syndrome, the latency of both responses is usually prolonged.

Since the carpal tunnel syndrome may be brought on by an excess of gardening, ironing, sewing, crocheting, or similar activity, relief may follow their discontinuance. Immobilization of the wrist during the hours of sleep with a posterior splint of forearm and hand may give relief. Injections of corticosteroid preparations beneath the carpal ligament sometimes help. Treatment for an associated disease (myxedema, rheumatoid arthritis, acromegaly) may effect an improvement. However, in most instances the treatment of choice is surgical section of the carpal ligament, which usually provides almost immediate relief.

Tardy Ulnar Nerve Palsy. The ulnar nerve may be injured at the elbow, especially in persons with a shallow ulnar groove, those who rest their weight on their elbows excessively, and those who are cachectic and lie in bed.

Contrary to the finding in the carpal tunnel syndrome, muscle weakness and atrophy characteristically predominate over sensory symptoms and signs, possibly because the ulnar nerve at the elbow has relatively fewer sensory fibers than the median nerve at the wrist. Characteristically, the patient notices atrophy of the first dorsal interosseous muscle or difficulty in performing fine manipulations. There may be numbness of the small finger and contiguous half of the proximal and middle phalanges of the ring finger and ulnar border of the hand. Treatment consists in prevention of further injury. A doughnut cushion for the elbow may be helpful. Mobilizing and transplanting the nerve to a position in front of the median epicondyle may prevent further progression of the disorder.

Acute Radial Nerve Palsy. The radial nerve may be compressed against a hard edge or surface after digesting an excess of alcohol or sedatives (Saturday night palsy) or may be compressed for excessive periods by the weight of the head of another (bridegroom's palsy). With time, complete recovery may be expected.

Acute and Tardy Peroneal Nerve Palsy. The common peroneal nerve is vulnerable where it crosses the head of the fibula, and can be injured when a person falls asleep in the sitting position with the knees crossed. A more chronic form occurs in cachectic patients who lie for prolonged periods with the legs externally rotated. In this disorder, dorsiflexion of the foot at the ankle and extension of the toes are weak, but usually little or no sensory loss is found over the lateral surface of the leg and on the dorsum of the foot.

Tarsal Tunnel Syndrome. In fractures of the ankle, compression of the posterior tibial nerve may occur, resulting in pain and numbness of the sole of the foot.

Meralgia Paresthetica. Fat people wearing tight corsets, people wearing gun belts, and people with pendulous abdomens may develop superficial paresthesia and burning discomfort in the distribution of the lateral cutaneous nerve of the thigh. Presumably the trouble results from compression of this nerve as it passes beneath the inguinal ligament.

Thoracic Outlet Syndrome. Formerly, paresthesias of the fingers were frequently attributed to compression of the brachial plexus by a cervical rib or a tight scalene anterior muscle. However, most such patients prove to have either a cervical disc or carpal tunnel syndrome.

Mononeuropathy Multiplex. The term "mononeuropathy multiplex" implies that a process involves several individual peripheral nerves in different regions of the body. Characteristically, the disorder begins with pain, paresthesias, or weakness in the distribution of a peripheral nerve which progresses to a maximal deficit within a few hours to several days. Other nerves become affected within days. The nerves of the lower extremities are affected more often than those of the upper, and signs are usually asymmetric. After the initial involvement the disorder may improve, relapse, or deteriorate. This type of neuropathy is a common manifestation of polyarteritis nodosa, but is also encountered in diabetes mellitus, rheumatoid arthritis, disseminated lupus erythematosus, and scleroderma.

The pathologic changes in most instances affect the interfascicular arteries of nerves, which may show degeneration of the media, fragmentation of the internal elastic lamina, thickening of the intima, and infiltration of the media and adventitia by mononuclear cells and polymorphonuclear cells (especially eosinophils). At necropsy arterioles with an occluded lumen may be widespread along the length of the nerve. Regions of fiber degeneration do not coincide with these occluded vessels, but begin in isolated central regions of fascicles at watershed zones of poor blood supply. For the ulnar and median nerves these zones are at mid-upper arm; for the peroneal and tibial nerves they are at midthigh. Because of separation and recombination of fascicles at more distal levels of the nerve, degenerating fibers in a section from the nerve taken distal to these regions of fiber degeneration may contain in many of its fascicles degenerating fibers that come from the same circumsected origin.

Plexus Neuropathy. *Brachial Plexus.* The brachial plexus can be injured by traction, penetrating wounds, or compression. *Acute nontraumatic brachial plexus neuropathy* is a disorder of unknown cause. Antecedent needle injections into shoulder muscles, intercurrent infections, and an allergic basis have been suggested as possible etiologic factors. Typically this disorder begins with aching pain in the lateral aspect of the shoulder or, less often, in the region of the elbow or arm. Muscle weakness develops within a few hours or days, and atrophy follows; sensory loss is usually minimal and is restricted to a small patch in the cutaneous distribution of the axillary nerve. The upper brachial plexus is much more commonly affected than the lower, and therefore the weakness and atrophy are more often located in the region of the shoulder. In mild cases, improvement begins in a few weeks, and clinical recovery is complete within months. More characteristically, improvement does not begin for several months and may not be complete for years. Recently it has been shown that the likelihood of eventual complete or almost complete recovery is good. Sometimes, as improvement on one side occurs, the other brachial plexus becomes affected. Careful examination by electromyography may reveal much more extensive involvement of nerves as expected from the clinical examination. The cerebrospinal fluid is usually normal. There is no known treatment.

Lumbar and Sacral Plexus and Roots. Under the term *femoral neuropathy,* a disorder has been described which in many cases arises from the lumbar plexus.

Many such cases occur in association with diabetes, but sometimes no associated illness is found. Pain centered in the thigh and extending to the medial side of the leg may herald the onset of muscle weakness and atrophy, which usually develops rather rapidly over the next week. If the onset is abrupt and the neurologic signs are restricted to the distribution of the femoral nerve, an infarction of that nerve is a possibility. Careful examination and electromyography, however, often indicate that the condition is more widespread. Such studies often indicate that multiple lumbar and sacral roots are affected with or without involvement of lumbar and sacral plexuses (in reality a lumbosacral radiculoplexus neuropathy). The cerebrospinal fluid protein may be elevated. Although recovery may not occur before months or years have passed, the prognosis is good.

Occasionally, patients with lumbosacral plexus neuropathy present with the symptoms of sciatica, which differs from that caused by disk disease in the lack of a history of injury, the lack (usually) of marked back symptoms, and the clinical and electromyographic evidence of involvement of multiple roots and the negative myelogram. Although marked muscle weakness and wasting may occur, the outlook is usually favorable. The cause, pathology, and treatment are unknown.

MULTIPLE NEUROPATHY

462. NEUROPATHY ASSOCIATED WITH MALNUTRITION AND VITAMIN DEFICIENCY

The common feature of these disorders is deficiency of one or more essentials in the diet owing either to inadequate intake (as in alcoholism, hyperemesis of pregnancy, food fads, and starvation) or failure of absorption (as in pernicious anemia, sprue, or gastrointestinal cancer). The pathologic changes in the peripheral nerves are similar in that distal axons of large fibers are affected first and more severely than proximal parts. Rows of myelin breakdown products are seen along peripheral nerves. At the dorsal root ganglion level there may be some slight decrease in the number of neurons. The posterior columns may show some demyelination. Ordinarily the conduction velocities of the nerves are not markedly abnormal. These disorders are also discussed in Ch. 404 to 411.

463. NEUROPATHY ASSOCIATED WITH CARCINOMA AND OTHER MALIGNANCY

In malignancy, peripheral nerves may be affected by direct implantation, by compression against bony structures, and by remote unknown mechanisms (see Part X,

Section Eighteen). Sites at which peripheral nerves may be compressed are the foramina of exit of the segmental nerves, the retroperitoneal space, and the nasopharynx. Neuropathy in a patient with malignancy may also develop from drugs used in treatment, as from vinca alkaloids in treatment of lymphoma.

Mixed Neuropathy with Carcinoma. Mixed sensory motor neuropathies have been found in association with carcinoma of the bronchus, gastrointestinal tract, thyroid, ovary, and other organs. Whether this is a specific association or is due to nutritional effects is still unknown.

Peripheral Neuropathy with Lymphoma. Peripheral neuropathies have been found in association with multiple myeloma and various leukemias and lymphomas. The lack of pain and the symmetry of the disorder are usually interpreted as indicating that the peripheral nerve involvement is a remote effect and not due to direct invasion. However, such invasion has been demonstrated in a few cases, particularly when meticulously searched for. The treatment for the neuropathy is the treatment for the primary tumor.

464. NEUROPATHY ASSOCIATED WITH MESENCHYMAL DISEASE AND NECROTIZING ANGIITIS

The neuropathy associated with these disorders is usually a mononeuropathy multiplex as described above. However, in a small percentage of cases the onset is that of a symmetrical multiple neuropathy. With the latter presentation, the correct category of disease is suggested by the painful nature of sensory symptoms and the associated signs of multiple tissue involvement.

465. NEUROPATHY ASSOCIATED WITH DIABETES MELLITUS

It is now known that most patients with diabetes mellitus have some dysfunction of the peripheral nerves, and that even those who are asymptomatic may have an abnormality of conduction velocity. The neuropathies fall into two types: mononeuropathy, involving single cranial nerves such as the oculomotor or large single peripheral nerves and plexuses, as described in Ch. 460 and 461, and polyneuropathy, as described here.

Pathology. Neither the pathogenesis nor the pathology of diabetic neuropathy is fully understood. The greater amount of atherosclerosis of limb vessels of diabetic patients probably does not account for the neuropathy. If the polyneuropathy is due to ischemia, it is more likely to be due to a specific angiopathy involving small arteries or arterioles. Thickening of the basement membranes of such vessels has been described. It is not clear whether the observed segmental demyelination is due to ischemia or to deranged metabolism selectively affecting Schwann cells, or whether it is secondary to nerve fiber change.

Clinical Manifestations. Many diabetics have asymptomatic polyneuropathy. Symptomatic polyneuropathy is typically a symmetric, distal sensorimotor neuropathy occurring in elderly patients with mild diabetes. Sensory symptoms in the toes and feet predominate and include numbness, burning paresthesia, and stabbing pains. The soles of the feet are often excessively sensitive to tactile or painful stimuli, rendering walking unpleasant. In the majority of patients with diabetic neuropathy, touch-pressure, vibration, and joint position sensations are predominantly affected, presumably because of a greater involvement of large myelinated fibers. If the loss of position sensation is severe, locomotor ataxia develops (pseudotabes diabetica). The ataxia is worse in the dark. Those patients with much discomfort are usually found to have loss of pain sensation, temperature sensation, and autonomic function, presumably owing to loss of small myelinated and of unmyelinated fibers. The disorder usually develops insidiously and may remain static or progress over the course of many years. It is unlikely to remit, as are the femoral, lumbar, and lumbosacral radiculoplexus, and oculomotor neuropathies. It has not been established that good control of the blood sugar with insulin or with oral hypoglycemic agents prevents the development or results in improvement of symptomatic neuropathy. Charcot joints, although rare, do occur. Disturbances of intestinal motility, loss of hair, and shiny tight dry skin are attributable to autonomic nerve damage.

One clinical variant of the neurologic complications of diabetes has been called diabetic amyotrophy. Older males with recent substantial weight loss are said to be predominantly affected. Bilateral asymmetric proximal weakness of the lower limbs, with anterior thigh pain, myalgia, and muscle wasting, is seen. Some have extensor plantar responses. Based on the characteristics of the electromyographic examination, patients with the aforementioned symptoms usually can be shown to have involvement of multiple lumbar nerve roots or of the lumbar or sacral plexus. The relatively abrupt onset and good prognosis exclude spondylosis as a cause. Most of the cases described under this term would probably fall under the previously described category of femoral neuropathy, which in reality is a lumbosacral radiculoplexus neuropathy.

The protein concentration of the cerebrospinal fluid in diabetic neuropathy is often elevated from 50 to 400 mg per 100 ml.

Treatment. It is the current practice to maintain good control of the blood sugar in order to prevent or improve neuropathy in spite of the lack of evidence of such prevention or improvement. There is a suggestion from some reports that repeated hypoglycemic attacks may hasten the onset or worsen the existing neuropathic state. To prevent trophic ulcers of the feet in patients with loss of pain and temperature sensation, good foot care and special shoes are needed.

466. NEUROPATHY ASSOCIATED WITH DRUGS AND TOXINS

Many drugs and toxins can damage peripheral nerves, and new agents constantly join the list. Publicity, legislation, and education have reduced the frequency of poisoning by some of the older chemicals.

Heavy Metals. Peripheral neuropathy has been reported in association with lead, arsenic, thallium, mercury, copper, antimony, and zinc. However, only the first two occur with any frequency.

Lead poisoning was formerly a common occurrence, but is becoming rare. Lead ingestion or inhalation may occur among farm workers using insecticides (for example, arsenate of lead), among painters using lead paint, among children who chew lead-containing paint from cribs and walls, among factory workers burning batteries or working with white lead, and among persons who drink beer or water stored in lead-lined containers or sent through lead pipes. Upper abdominal colic, joint pain, peripheral neuropathy, and encephalopathy develop. The encephalopathy is particularly characteristic of toxicity in children. The neuropathy is mainly motor and asymmetric, beginning in the upper extremity with wrist drop and weakness of the extensor muscles of fingers.

The peripheral nerves in lead neuropathy undergo axonal degeneration and segmental demyelination. The normal amount of lead in the urine ranges from 0.00 to 0.06 mg per liter. For a diagnosis of lead poisoning the value should be at least twice this. (See Ch. 29.)

Arsenic has been a favorite choice for homicide. Arsenic poisoning has also resulted from drinking illegal alcohol ("moonshine") and from eating food sprayed with insecticides. It is manifested by vomiting and other gastrointestinal symptoms, a scaly exfoliating rash, and evidences of neuropathy. White lines in the fingernails (Aldrich-Mees lines) may provide a diagnostic clue.

Arsenic poisoning produces a mixed motor and sensory neuropathy which is symmetric and distal and affects the lower extremities preferentially. The nerve fibers undergo an axonal type of degeneration. Diagnosis is made by identifying increased levels of arsenic in the nails, hair, or urine. (See Ch. 28.)

Thallium neuropathy has the clinical features of arsenic neuropathy but is associated with loss of hair.

Organophosphate (Triorthocresylphosphate) Compounds. Widespread ingestion of fluid extract of ginger in the United States in 1930 was followed by thousands of cases of severe polyneuropathy, mostly motor and distal in distribution. It was established that adulteration with triorthocresylphosphate was responsible and, since that time, periodic outbreaks have occurred traceable to adulterated cooking oil. Usually, stolen motor oil has been sold for cooking purposes. The neuropathy is delayed 10 to 14 days after poisoning. Imperfect recovery is the rule. Years after the acute poisoning, spastic paraparesis emerges, indicating that damage to the spinal cord occurs but is not immediately apparent because of the severe neuropathy. There is no effective treatment.

Industrial Poisons. Trichlorethylene, an anesthetic agent, is also a powerful solvent used in industry. In toxic amounts, it produces multiple cranial nerve palsies and trigeminal nerve analgesia. Particularly in Japan, n-hexane, an organic solvent used in printing, extraction of vegetable oil, and cleaning, has been associated with peripheral neuropathy. Acrylamide is a chemical that is pumped into soil to render it waterproof. In both man and animals, it produces peripheral neuropathy by an axonal type of degeneration of myelinated fibers. A recent outbreak of peripheral neuropathy in Japan was traced to the eating of fish which contained an excessive content of organic mercury.

Drugs. Many medicaments can produce numbness in

distal extremities and neurogenic weakness, including isoniazid, diphenylhydantoin sodium, nitrofurantoin, and the vinca alkaloids. Arsenic in Fowler's solution, mercury in various antisyphilitic preparations, and gold in treatment for rheumatoid arthritis also can produce peripheral neuropathy. The medication clioquinol, used frequently in Japan for nonspecific gastrointestinal disturbances, has now been implicated in subacute myelo-opticoneuropathy (SMON). Dosages of 1 gram or more per day for a period of one week or longer may lead to abdominal colic and numbness of the feet. Prolonged use may lead to severe neuropathy, spasticity, and optic atrophy.

467. NEUROPATHY ASSOCIATED WITH HORMONAL DISTURBANCES

Myxedema and acromegaly both predispose to the syndrome of the carpal tunnel. In myxedema a more diffuse peripheral neuropathy may occur.

468. NEUROPATHY ASSOCIATED WITH POSSIBLE IMMUNOLOGIC DISORDERS

ACUTE INFLAMMATORY POLYRADICULONEUROPATHY
(Postinfectious Polyneuritis, Guillain-Barré-Strohl Syndrome)

Etiology.   The cause is unknown, although a similar illness has been produced in animals by inoculating extracts of peripheral nerve plus adjuvants. This, plus the characteristic postinfectious timing, has led many workers to postulate an autoimmune mechanism.

Pathology.   The pathologic changes bear some resemblance to those of experimental allergic neuritis. There are foci of mononuclear cells in the roots and in the peripheral nerves, and these are associated with segmental demyelination. Proximal slowing of conduction velocity may be seen in about a third of the cases. In others the low conduction velocities are more generalized.

Clinical Manifestations.   Many, but not all, patients give a history of a banal, nonspecific, febrile illness, usually respiratory, preceding the neurologic disorder by 10 to 21 days. The polyneuropathy usually begins insidiously and without fever, malaise, nausea, or prostration. In most instances, motor weakness is predominant. A few patients suffer muscle pain or, occasionally, stiff neck. Weakness may start in the face or hands but is most common in the lower extremities, and always is bilateral, though sometimes asymmetrical. The motor paralysis is flaccid and has a considerable tendency to ascend the body *(Landry's ascending paralysis)* and to involve both the trunk and upper limbs. Less frequently, paralysis affects the face, the muscles of swallowing, or the oculomotor muscles. About 5 per cent of patients develop urinary retention. Sensory symptoms and signs affect 90 per cent of patients. Paresthesias usually begin in the toes and fingers, and may spread proximally, but

demonstrable sensory deficits are usually modest. Variant onsets are common, and weakness may begin in the upper limbs or even in the oculomotor muscles. Progression may cease at any point in the course. Once weakness reaches its maximum, a plateau occurs that lasts for several days to several weeks, depending on the individual. After this, improvement begins and continues for weeks or, rarely, many months. About one patient in 20 develops papilledema.

An acute inflammatory polyradiculoneuropathy of dorsal roots may produce the sensory counterpart of the same illness that affects ventral roots (usually called the Guillain-Barré-Strohl syndrome). Like the predominantly motor form, the development of the sensory disorder can be acute or subacute, the maximal deficit developing over days to a few weeks. The disorder may first be heralded by lancinating pain. Subsequently pain may continue, but its quality may turn into a more constant hyperpathia. Additional symptoms may come from sensory ataxia. The sensory loss sometimes persists—possibly because the perikarya of cells have been irreversibly damaged. Areflexia, cutaneous sensory loss, and absence of compound nerve action potentials from afferent fibers of median, ulnar, and sural nerves are characteristic.

The classic cerebrospinal fluid findings are of a normal pressure with an elevated protein concentration but without increased numbers of leukocytes. However, many exceptions exist, and the protein concentration may be normal at any time in the course of the illness, particularly at the onset. Rarely, a mild lymphocytosis is discovered in the cerebrospinal fluid at the outset of the disease.

The prognosis for full recovery from paralysis is good but not invariable, and perhaps one of ten patients is left with muscle weakness of some degree. Without mechanical ventilation, there is 10 to 20 per cent mortality, the result of respiratory and vasomotor failure. Thus, upon first encounter with the patient, even one in whom weakness may be slight and distal, the physician must anticipate a possible need for a respirator and vasopressor agents within a day or so.

Treatment.   Adrenal steroids have been widely used to treat severe cases, but there are no controlled studies by which to judge their effectiveness, and it is difficult to know whether they are beneficial. Skilled nursing care is imperative, as is the availability of an intensive care unit to manage potential respiratory insufficiency. Full convalescence may require months, and a few patients suffer recurrent bouts of weakness and a relapsing course that may go on for years.

CHRONIC AND RELAPSING INFLAMMATORY POLYRADICULONEUROPATHY

This disorder may be the same as the preceding one, except that possibly the pathogenic mechanisms persist, and so the disorder continues. Typically, the onset is much more protracted, and the disease is more prolonged; but the symptoms are symmetric and predominantly motor. In some patients spontaneous remissions and relapses occur. When sensory loss is present, it affects the modalities of touch-pressure, joint position, and vibration in particular. Occasionally papilledema develops, but usually without headaches or focal cerebral disorders. In addition, a tremor with the features of essential tremor may develop. The cerebrospinal fluid protein is elevated and without cells. Conduction velocities are usually diffusely low. In nerve biopsies, segmental demyelination and remyelination are evident. In some cases, corticosteroids bring a remission; in others they worsen the disorder. Controlled studies to determine the long-term beneficial and adverse effects of corticosteroids in this condition have not been done.

SERUM NEUROPATHY

The use of antitetanus serum is sometimes associated with a diffuse and severe peripheral neuropathy, but more often it has the characteristic features of a brachial plexus neuropathy.

469. NEUROPATHY ASSOCIATED WITH INFECTION

Diphtheria is commonly complicated by paralysis of the nasopharynx and oculomotor and ciliary muscles. More widespread cranial polyneuropathy is uncommon. Paralysis of the extremities and trunk can also occur, usually appearing later and sometimes with cutaneous rather than the pharyngeal infection. The disease is discussed fully in Ch. 205.

Leprosy causes a characteristic peripheral neuropathy resulting from invasion of nerves by *M. leprae*. The neuropathy, in which selective pain and temperature loss are often striking, is discussed along with other manifestations of the disease in Ch. 245.

470. DISORDERS OF PERIPHERAL SENSORY NEURONS

Patients with disorders of peripheral sensory neurons characteristically suffer from pain, cutaneous injury from lack of sensation, unsteady movement from kinesthetic sensory loss, or combinations of these. Frequently they also have autonomic dysfunction. The nature of these symptoms and the kind of sensory loss correspond reasonably well with the populations of fibers affected. Thus it is generally true that patients with loss of pain and temperature sensation and with autonomic impairment have degeneration, particularly of unmyelinated and of small myelinated fibers, whereas patients with loss of touch-pressure sensation have degeneration of large myelinated fibers of cutaneous nerves. The nature of the sensory loss, particularly early in the course of the disorder, may be of help in differential diagnosis. In advanced disease this selectivity of involvement by fiber size tends to be lost.

Mild degrees of these disorders can be difficult to recognize, because clinical methods of determination of sensation are imprecise and nerve conduction studies have only recently been applied to their analysis.

Acquired disorders of sensory neurons include those of herpes zoster (see Ch. 388), acute inflammatory polyradiculoneuropathy (Guillain-Barré-Strohl syndrome) (see Ch. 468), and carcinomatous neuropathy (see Ch. 463).

Hereditary Sensory Neuropathy, Type I.   Hereditary sensory neuropathy, Type I, is a dominantly inherited sensory radicular neuropathy. It has been variously described as perforating ulcers of the feet, mutilating acropathy, lumbosacral syringomyelia, acrodystrophic neuropathy, and hereditary sensory radicular neuropathy. Great variability in severity of involvement is commonplace. Sensory loss is usually much more severe over the feet and legs than in the hands and forearms, and some patients have lancinating pains. Pain and temperature sensation are affected more than touch-pressure sensation, and sensory ataxia is not a feature. Loss or decrease of sweating usually corresponds to the region of sensory loss. Nerve conduction of motor fibers is usually normal, but it is usually not possible to record compound action potentials of afferent fibers. Denervation may be seen in foot and leg muscles. The ankle tendon reflex may be absent. Life expectancy is probably normal in most cases. The treatment is described below. Late in the disorder, perforating ulcers of the foot may develop, especially when there has been poor foot care. In kinships, signs such as pes cavus, hammer toes, plantar calluses, inability to walk on heels, and sensation loss of acral parts of lower limbs point to the affliction.

Hereditary Sensory Neuropathy, Type II.   This is a recessively inherited disorder, also called congenital sensory neuropathy, which usually manifests itself in infancy or childhood with a mutilating acropathy characterized by paronychia, whitlows, ulcers of the fingers and plantars of the feet, and frequently unrecognized fractures of the extremities. Sensory loss affects all types of cutaneous and sometimes kinesthetic sensation and is most marked distally in all four limbs. Tendon reflexes are usually absent. Sweating loss usually occurs over the distal limbs. Nerve action potentials of afferent fibers of cutaneous and limb nerves cannot be detected. Pathologically, there is an almost complete absence of myelinated fibers from the cutaneous nerves of the distal lower limb with preservation of decreased numbers of unmyelinated fibers. Treatment is discussed below.

Hereditary Sensory Neuropathy, Type III (Dysautonomia of Riley-Day).   Familial dysautonomia is a recessively inherited disorder of Jewish infants and children. It affects peripheral autonomic neurons, peripheral sensory neurons, peripheral motor neurons, and probably other central nervous system neurons. Characteristics are an onset in infancy, premature death, a history of poor feeding, repeated episodes of vomiting and pulmonary infections, and autonomic disturbances. The last-named include defective lacrimation, defective temperature control, skin blotching, excessive perspiration, hypertension, and postural hypotension. There are also insensitivity to pain, areflexia, corneal insensitivity, and an absence of the fungiform papillae of tongue. In infants the symptoms reported by mothers are poor sucking, poor swallowing, failure to thrive, lack of tears, and unexplained fevers. At an older age one notes delay in development, stunted growth, corneal abrasions, kyphoscoliosis, clumsiness, excessive sweating, and blotching of skin, with emotion and lack of pain from stimuli usually considered painful. Evidence for involvement of peripheral neurons comes from the observed hyporeflexia and the finding of a decrease of unmyelinated fibers of cutaneous nerves. An abnormality of catecholamine metabolism has been demonstrated.

Hereditary Sensory Neuropathy, Type IV.   In this recessively inherited sensory neuropathy insensitivity to pain, anhidrosis, and mental retardation are found. This disorder has been attributed to an abnormality of differentiation of the neural crest.

Angiokeratoma Corporis Diffusum (Fabry's). This rare disorder, described in Ch. 918, is characterized by angiokeratomas, impaired renal function, and small purple to black spots distributed especially over the lower trunk and buttocks along segmental lines. Typically, patients have pain and numbness in the limbs but no motor symptoms. A deposition of glycolipids in the cell bodies of peripheral sensory neurons and a decrease in the number of small neurons of spinal ganglia and of unmyelinated and small myelinated fibers have been observed and may be important in explaining the painfulness of the disorder.

Treatment of Insensitive Hands and Feet. Persons with pain and temperature insensitivity of hands and feet are vulnerable to many injuries which potentially can result in a chain of events, including ulceration, cellulitis, lymphangitis, osteomyelitis, and osteolysis. These events are seen particularly in the disorders of leprosy, inherited amyloidosis, and other inherited and acquired neuropathies with this type of sensory loss. Congenital neuropathies with such sensory loss are particularly difficult to manage, because they occur at an age when it is difficult to obtain the cooperation of the patient. The goal in treatment is to prevent the onset of tissue damage or, when it has occurred, to promote healing and prevent further damage. Persons with such sensory loss should not engage in most forms of manual labor or perform repetitive tasks with hands and feet which can cause bruising. Repeated inspection of feet and hands is necessary. Any bruise or ulcer should be taken seriously and, if on the foot, one should stop weight bearing until healing has occurred. Shoes should be wide and well constructed. The inside of the shoes must be inspected before the foot is placed inside in order to remove retained objects or nails. The feet of such patients should be soaked in lukewarm water for 15 minutes twice a day and lightly covered with petrolatum lotion so that the moisture in the softened skin is retained.

471. INHERITED DISORDERS OF PERIPHERAL MOTOR, SENSORY, AND AUTONOMIC NEURONS

In this group of disorders, the predominant involvement is of peripheral motor neurons. The disorders are usually inherited, are usually progressive, and usually have signs which are symmetrical. Neurons of similar structure and function are affected. The pathologic features are nonfocal, and the nature of the fiber degeneration is that of an axonal atrophy and degeneration. Although an inborn error of metabolism probably underlies these disorders, for the most part this has not been elucidated.

Hereditary Motor and Sensory Neuropathy, Type I (Hypertrophic Neuropathy Type of Peroneal Muscular Atrophy). This is a fairly common, mild, dominantly inherited variant of peroneal muscular atrophy. Affected persons may have no symptoms or signs, but yet be known to have the disorder by their position in the kinship and by characteristic low conduction velocities of all nerves.

Pathologically the disorder affects myelinated fibers predominantly, producing segmental demyelination and remyelination and varying degrees of onion-bulb formation (the hallmark of hypertrophic neuropathy). An actual loss of myelinated fibers probably occurs.

In kinships with the disease an affected person may be recognized by high arches of the feet, hammer toes, curled-up toes (with convexity upward), frequent corns or calluses, and a high-stepping, awkward gait caused by paresis of the dorsiflexor muscles of the ankle and instability of the ankle joint. Persons with greater weakness may have weakness and wasting of the intrinsic hand muscles and weakness of the plantar flexor muscles of the ankles. Ankle joint instability makes it difficult for such persons to stand still. The amount of muscle atrophy is usually not great. Typically, the tendon reflexes are reduced or absent, disappearing successively from the Achilles tendon, the quadriceps, and the upper extremity. Sensory loss is mild, affecting the modalities of touch-pressure, two-point discrimination, and joint position and motion in the distal parts of the extremities. Clinical enlargement of peripheral nerves may be detected in about one fourth of the cases. Some members of kinships have, in addition to the clinical features mentioned, a tremor of the head and outstretched hands which is indistinguishable from essential tremor (Roussy-Levy syndrome). Foot ulcers occur in occasional persons with this disorder. Osteomyelitis and mutilation of the feet develop only if the ulcers are neglected. There is no specific treatment. Corrective surgery should be reserved for those affected persons who develop ulcers at pressure points owing to excessively high arches and for those with excessive inversion of the foot. Foot-drop springs or braces may be used to elevate the toes in walking and to stabilize the ankle. When foot ulcers develop, a program of ulcer debridement and rest in bed should be begun immediately. Weight-bearing should not be resumed until the ulcer is completely healed. Then shoes should be fitted which have sufficient width, an adequate arch support, and a fit that distributes the weight to all parts of the foot.

Hereditary Motor and Sensory Neuropathy, Type II (Neuronal Type of Peroneal Muscular Atrophy, Charcot-Marie-Tooth Disease). This dominantly inherited disorder begins in the second decade of life or later. Not uncommonly it begins in the fifth or sixth decade. Symmetric muscle weakness with atrophy begins in small foot muscles, peroneal, long toe extensor, and ankle dorsiflexor muscles. Pes cavus and hammer toes may or may not be associated with the weakness. Initial symptoms include inability to pick up the toes in walking, instability of the ankle, difficulty in standing still in one position, and visible atrophy of muscles. Some patients tend to stand with their feet spread apart, and shift the position constantly to maintain balance. Others tend to stand with their knees bent to lock the ankles. Later weakness of small hand muscles may make such acts as unlocking a door with a key, unscrewing the top of a glass jar, or buttoning difficult. The muscle atrophy of the lower limbs may be typical of peroneal muscular atrophy, with a greater degree of atrophy in the distal aspect of thigh muscles and with much atrophy of leg muscles. Most frequently tendon reflexes are diminished or absent in the lower limbs. Touch-pressure, joint position, and vibration sensation are mildly decreased distally in lower limbs. Conduction velocities of motor fibers are within the limits of normal in upper limbs and only slightly reduced in lower limbs.

Sporadic cases similar in every way to the above are seen. These cases may be a different disorder or the same disorder in which the inherited nature has not been detected. However, Charcot-Marie-Tooth disease is genetically and morphologically entirely distinct from either Friedreich's ataxia or spastic paraplegia with peroneal muscular atrophy, disorders discussed in Ch. 432 and 434.

These patients can often be helped significantly by leg braces that stabilize the ankle joint. Their use permits these patients to stand still without losing their balance for such acts as shaving.

Hereditary Motor and Sensory Neuropathy, Type III (Recessively Inherited Hypertrophic Neuropathy). This is a rare disorder transmitted as an autosomal recessive trait and beginning in infancy. The children learn to walk late, have great difficulty in walking even at their best point of neuromuscular development (ages 8 to 12), and are usually in wheelchairs by the age of 20 years. The patients are usually short, and most have a severe, symmetrical, sensory motor neuropathy affecting predominantly the distal extremities with enlarged peripheral nerves. Some weakness of proximal muscles of the extremities usually is present also. Sometimes there are associated miosis and nystagmus. The conduction velocity of motor and sensory fibers of peripheral nerves is among the lowest determined in electromyographic laboratories. Pathologically, marked segmental demyelination and remyelination are found in myelinated fibers; unmyelinated fibers are not decreased in number but are probably affected also. A systemic biochemical abnormality involving ceramide hexoses and their sulfates has been found. No specific treatment is available.

Hereditary Motor and Sensory Neuropathy, Type IV (Recessively Inherited Hypertrophic Neuropathy with Excess of Phytonic Acid; Refsum's Disease). This rare progressive or relapsing disorder is inherited as an autosomal recessive trait and is due to the inability of affected subjects to alpha-oxidize ingested phytanic acid. Clinical manifestations usually begin in the second decade with night blindness and constriction of the visual fields owing to an atypical retinitis pigmentosa. Additionally, symptoms caused by a distal sensorimotor neuropathy develop, as well as an ataxia which is thought to be greater than that accounted for by kinesthetic loss. Ichthyosis, skeletal abnormalities, and sudden death in the third or fourth decade from involvement of the heart all provide evidence of systemic extraneural involvement. The cerebrospinal fluid protein is usually markedly elevated. Pathologically, the peripheral nerves contain evidence of segmental demyelination and remyelination and onion-bulb formation. Pathognomonic is the occurrence of 3,7,11,15-tetramethylhexadecenoic acid (phytanic acid) in the serum, red blood cells, liver, heart, kidneys, and skeletal muscles. Treatment consists of withholding dietary phytols (chlorophyll-free diet); if begun early it can result in dramatic improvement.

Hereditary Spastic Paraplegia with Motor and Sensory Neuropathy, Type V. Symptomatic onset and severity of this dominantly inherited disorder are extremely variable. Difficulty in walking and running because of stiffness is the usual manifestation. The progression is slow, and life expectancy is probably normal. The most prominent changes consist of a spastic, scissoring gait, hyperreflexia, and Babinski signs. However, careful examination usually gives evidence of involvement of lower motor and peripheral sensory neurons.

Hereditary Motor and Sensory Neuropathy with Optic Atrophy, Type VI. In this very rare dominantly inherited disorder, there is optic atrophy in addition to peroneal muscular atrophy.

Hereditary Motor and Sensory Neuropathy with Retinitis Pigmentosa, Type VII. This disorder has many of the features of the syndrome described by Refsum, but elevated plasma phytanic acids are not found.

472. AMYLOIDOSIS

Dominantly Inherited Amyloidosis (Portuguese). Amyloid neuropathy has been noted most often in countries surrounding the Mediterranean Sea, although kinships are sometimes encountered in the United States, Japan, and other countries. The disorder usually begins in the late second or third decade with loss of the sensations of pain, cold, and heat in the lower extremities accompanied by anhidrosis and, sooner or later, loss of sphincter control. Males become impotent. Nerve biopsy studies disclose selective loss of small myelinated and unmyelinated fibers, accounting for the selective sensory loss. Subsequently other fibers are also affected so that sensory loss becomes more generalized, and motor weakness and atrophy develop. The disorder progresses relentlessly to death, usually in the fourth or fifth decade. Amyloid deposits may be found in many tissues, including peripheral nerve, muscle, vitreous of the eye, and many other organs.

Dominantly Inherited Amyloidosis (Indiana). In contradistinction to the Portuguese type of dominantly inherited amyloidosis, the symptoms of the Indiana type usually begin in the upper extremities, and may suggest the diagnosis of carpal tunnel syndrome. Eventually, a more generalized neuropathy develops.

473. NEUROPATHY ASSOCIATED WITH PERIPHERAL VASCULAR DISEASE

Besides the vasculitis previously described in polyarteritis nodosa and other collagen diseases, there are alterations produced in the peripheral nerves by atherosclerosis of larger vessels. Patients who experience claudication when walking or who have evidence of peripheral gangrene may also have a distal sensory and motor neuropathy that appears to be due to inadequate blood supply and infarction of nerves. All sensory modalities are affected, and there may be burning, pricking, and jabbing pains in the feet. Depending on the site and distribution of vascular involvement, the neuropathy may be symmetric or asymmetric.

474. NEUROPATHY ASSOCIATED WITH UREMIA

Particularly since the development of dialysis programs for the treatment of chronic renal disease, severe peripheral neuropathy has appeared in many patients with uremia, affecting approximately one half of the patients receiving dialysis. This neuropathy is mixed motor and sensory, symmetric, and more severe in the distal parts. Bladder and bowel disturbances are unusual. The pathogenesis is unknown. Frequent and apparently adequate dialysis does not always produce a remission, but with successful kidney transplantation the peripheral nerve function returns toward normal.

Asbury, A., Victor, M., and Adams, R.: Uremic polyneuropathy. Arch. Neurol. 8:413, 1963.

Austin, J.: Recurrent polyneuropathies and their corticosteroid treatment. Brain, 81:157, 1958.

Cooke, W., and Smith, W.: Neurological disorders associated with coeliac disease. Brain, 89:683, 1966.

Croft, P., Urich, H., and Wilkinson, M.: Peripheral neuropathy of sensorimotor type associated with malignant disease. Brain, 90:31, 1967.

Denny-Brown, D.: Primary sensory neuropathy with muscular changes associated with carcinoma. J. Neurol. Neurosurg. Psychiatry, 11:73, 1948.

Dyck, P., and Lambert, E.: Lower motor and primary sensory neuron diseases with peroneal muscular atrophy. I. Neurologic, genetic, and electrophysiologic findings in hereditary polyneuropathies. Arch. Neurol., 18:603, 1968.

Dyck, P., and Lambert, E.: Lower motor and primary sensory neuron diseases with peroneal muscular atrophy. II. Neurologic, genetic, and electrophysiologic findings in various neuronal degenerations. Arch. Neurol., 18:619, 1968.

Dyck, P., and Lambert, E.: Dissociated sensation in amyloidosis. Compound action potential, quantitative histologic and teased-fiber, and electron microscopic studies of sural nerve biopsies. Arch. Neurol., 20:490, 1969.

Engel, W., Dorman, J., Levy, R., and Fredrickson, D.: Neuropathy in Tangier disease. Arch. Neurol., 17:1, 1967.

Lovelace, R., and Horwitz, S.: Peripheral neuropathy in long-term diphenylhydantoin therapy. Arch. Neurol., 18:69, 1968.

Moress, G., D'Agostino, A., and Jarcho, L.: Neuropathy in lymphoblastic leukemia treated with vincristine. Arch. Neurol., 16:377, 1967.

Nickel, S., et al.: Myxedema neuropathy and myopathy. A clinical and pathological study. Neurology (Minneap.), 11:125, 1961.

Raff, M., Sangalang, V., and Asbury, A.: Ischemic mononeuropathy multiplex associated with diabetes mellitus. Arch. Neurol., 18:497, 1968.

Steinberg, D., Mize, C. E., Herndon, J. H., Fales, H. M., Engel, W. K., and Vroom, F. O.: Phytanic acid in patients with Refsum's syndrome and response to dietary treatment. Arch. Intern. Med., 125:75, 1970.

Sunderland, S.: Nerves and Nerve Injuries. Edinburgh and London, E. and S. Livingstone Ltd., 1968.

Swanson, A. G., Buchan, G. C., and Alvord, E. C., Jr.: Anatomic changes in congenital insensitivity to pain. Arch. Neurol., 12:12, 1965.

Thomas, P., and Lascelles, R.: The pathology of diabetic neuropathy. Quart. J. Med., 35:489, 1966.

Tyler, H.: Neurological complications of dialysis, transplantation and other forms of treatment in chronic uremia. Neurology (Minneap.), 15:1081, 1965.

Wiederholt, W., Mulder, D., and Lambert, E.: The Landry-Guillain-Barré-Strohl syndrome or polyradiculoneuropathy. Historical review, report on 97 patients, and present concepts. Mayo Clin. Proc., 39:427, 1964.

Section Twenty-Three.   DISEASES OF MUSCLE AND NEUROMUSCULAR JUNCTION

Lewis P. Rowland

475.   INTRODUCTION

Definitions. Muscles can be weakened by many different disorders. When muscles become weak, they may waste away. Until recently it has been conventional to ascribe the varied causes of weakness and wasting to neurogenic and myopathic disorders, a fundamental distinction originally made a century ago when diseases were defined by pathologists. In the neurogenic disorders, the brunt of pathologic change was seen in the motor neuron or peripheral nerve; changes in muscle were less pronounced or could be attributed to secondary effects of denervation. In the myopathic disorders, on the other hand, the histopathologic changes in muscle were of different type and there was little abnormality in nerve cell or peripheral nerve.

Pathologic criteria, however, have limitations when one is dealing with living people. Muscle biopsy is possible, but there is no way of obtaining a sample of the spinal cord. Other criteria were therefore introduced to separate neurogenic and myopathic disorders: clinical and genetic characteristics, electromyography, nerve conduction velocity, and assay of serum activity of sarcoplasmic enzymes. Together, these criteria have provided a reasonably consistent basis for continued separation of those syndromes characterized by weakness into neurogenic and myopathic groups.

The concept, however, has been shaken in recent years. Denervation and cross-innervation studies of fast and slow muscles have shown that physiologic and biochemical characteristics of muscle are under neural control. A new kind of electrophysiologic evidence has been adduced to indicate a neurogenic cause for the muscular dystrophies, long held to be the prototype of myopathy. Unsurprisingly, there is confusion. Nevertheless, the traditional separation of neurogenic and myopathic disease may be more than an editorial convenience and will be perpetuated in this section.

Because of these conceptual problems, an air of vagueness pervades the language used to describe neuromuscular diseases, and the same words have different meanings to different authorities. It is not mere nit-picking to attempt definitions; the ideas are important. It is therefore appropriate to define some of the more prevalent words before going on with this discussion.

The word *atrophy* means, literally, "lack of nourishment." It has come to mean wasting of muscle, or loss of muscle bulk from any cause, and it is also used to denote single muscle fibers that are smaller than normal when viewed microscopically. But when used in the name of a disease, it always implies that the muscle wasting is secondary to a neural disorder, e.g., infantile spinal muscular atrophy, progressive spinal muscular atrophy, or peroneal muscular atrophy. To avoid ambiguity, it is therefore appropriate in examining patients to use "wasting" rather than "atrophy" to describe diminution in muscle bulk unless the cause is known to be neurogenic. *Myopathies* include disorders characterized by weakness that is not due to emotional or neurogenic cause. Some authors speak of "primary" or "secondary" myopathies but there is little evidence that any muscle disease is really "primary," in the sense that there is an abnormality in muscle and nowhere else. In some myopathies, as in thyrotoxic myopathy, the fundamental disorder is elsewhere, and this could be true even in genetically determined diseases. The *dystrophies* are a subgroup of myopathy with two special characteristics: they are genetically determined, and the weakness is progressive. There are other genetic disorders of muscle in which the weakness seems to be stationary, and some in which progressive weakness is not the dominant symptom (transient attacks of weakness in periodic paralysis, cramps, and myoglobinuria in some glycogen diseases, or myotonia); other names are given to these conditions individually.

DIFFERENTIATION OF NEUROPATHIC AND MYOPATHIC DISEASE

When muscles are sick, they are usually weak. Few other symptoms result; sometimes muscles ache (myalgia); sometimes they relax with difficulty (myotonia); sometimes they shorten abruptly and painfully (cramp or contracture). Weakness is the most common symptom of muscle disease, but it is also the symptom that results from neurogenic diseases affecting corticospinal pathways, motor neurons, or peripheral nerves. The differential diagnosis of muscle disease is therefore a problem in distinguishing myogenic from neurogenic causes. Corticospinal disorders have characteristic signs that immediately identify them, and therefore they do not often enter into this differential diagnosis. Disorders of the lower motor neuron or peripheral nerve may be difficult and sometimes impossible to separate from muscle disease. In this kind of neurogenic disorder and in myopathies, weakness, wasting, and depression of myotatic reflexes are common to both groups. Neurogenic disorders are apt to affect distal muscles primarily, whereas myopathic disorders are more likely to affect proximal muscle, but there are so many exceptions that this is an unreliable guide. (Distal myopathy is rare but does occur; proximal weakness is not so rare in motor neuron disease or peripheral neuropathy.) Twitching of muscle is probably a reliable guide to motor neuron disease, but it is not yet definitely excluded as a myopathic sign. The combination of active reflexes in a limb with weak, wasted, and twitching muscles is almost pathognomonic of amytrophic lateral sclerosis, especially if there are also Babinski signs. Sensory loss and an increased protein content of the cerebrospinal fluid are reliable guides to peripheral neuropathy, but once it is established that there is a peripheral neuropathy, it may be difficult or impossible to state whether there is also a concomitant myopathy. Because of these ambiguities in clinical diagnosis, increasing attention has been directed to three laboratory aids: serum enzymes, electromyography and nerve conduction velocities, and muscle biopsy. Some syndromes are virtually defined by electromyography: distal myopathy and "juvenile muscular atrophy simulating muscular dystrophy."

Serum Enzymes. Several different enzyme activities are increased in the serum of patients with X-linked dystrophies and polymyositis, whereas they are not increased in neurogenic diseases. It is often stated that determination of creatine phosphokinase (CPK) activity is the "best" because it is the most sensitive. This enzyme is significantly increased in almost all muscle diseases, but it is, if anything, too sensitive; it picks up all the myopathic cases, but it is sometimes also increased in neurogenic disease. Other serum enzyme levels, e.g., SGOT or lactate dehydrogenase, LDH, and others, do not rise so much in myopathies, but neither do they give falsely positive reactions in neurogenic disorders. For this reason, it is useful to couple determinations of CPK with SGOT or LDH in evaluating individual cases. CPK has one other considerable advantage: it is not present in erythrocytes or liver and is therefore normal in serum contaminated by hemolysis or in patients with liver disease.

Electromyography. Needle electromyography, the amplification of action potentials from muscle, has been refined to a very useful technique. Normal muscle is electrically silent at rest, and patterns of potentials evoked by voluntary contraction have been analyzed in terms of frequency, duration, and amplitude of individual motor unit potentials. In denervated muscle, there is spontaneous activity (fibrillations from single muscle fibers or fasciculations from motor units), the number of potentials during a voluntary contraction is reduced, and the duration of potentials is increased. In myopathic disorders, there is usually no spontaneous activity, there is no reduction in the number of potentials under voluntary control, and the potentials are reduced in duration. These signs are usually reliable, but in some cases the results are equivocal, and there may be features of both a neurogenic and myopathic disorder.

Nerve Conduction Velocities. The speed of conduction along motor nerves can be recorded accurately, and slowing of conduction is a reliable guide to neuropathy. A normal conduction velocity, however, does not exclude a nerve lesion.

Muscle Biopsy. The features of neurogenic and myopathic diseases can usually be differentiated in a muscle biopsy, especially when one utilizes the new techniques of the rapid examination of frozen tissue and the application of histochemical methods. The electron microscope has opened new approaches that are still in the process of refinement. Only a few diseases can be definitively identified by muscle biopsy: periarteritis nodosa, trichinosis, sarcoidosis, and most (but not all) cases of glycogen storage disease. The congenital myopathies are best identified by histochemical and other special procedures.

In most cases, the results of all these special studies are consistent, one with the other. In some cases, however, the results are conflicting, and problems of classification remain.

Dubowitz, V., and Brooke, M. H.: Muscle Biopsy: A Modern Approach. Philadelphia, W. B. Saunders Company, 1973.
Hausmanowa-Petrusewicz, I., and Jedrzejowska, H.: Correlation between electromyographic findings and muscle biopsy in cases of neuromuscular disease. J. Neurol. Sci., 13:85, 1971.
Lenman, J. A. P., and Ritchie, A. E.: Clinical Electromyography. Philadelphia, J. B. Lippincott Company, 1970.
McComas, A. J., Sica, A. E. P., and Campbell, M. J.: "Sick" motoneurones. A unifying concept of muscle disease. Lancet, 1:321, 1971.
Rowland, L. P.: Are the muscular dystrophies neurogenic? Ann. N.Y. Acad. Sci., 228:244, 1974.

INHERITED DISEASES

476. MUSCULAR DYSTROPHIES

Definition. Muscular dystrophies are inherited myopathies, characterized primarily by progressively severe weakness.

Etiology. Although it is generally believed that inherited diseases must be due to a missing or structurally abnormal protein (either an enzyme or a structural protein), this abnormality has not been identified in any form of dystrophy. Indirect evidence implicates the muscle membranes in several forms, but this hypothesis cannot now be put to direct test. Pathologic and biochemical abnormalities can be detected in muscle, and there is no clear evidence of neural abnormality in traditional terms. It is conceivable, however, that the funadmental abnormality is in another organ (such as the liver or bowel) and that the muscular abnormalities are secondary. Some authors have postulated a debatable vascular cause, one of chronic and relative ischemia.

Classification. No classification of the muscular dystrophies is entirely satisfactory, but the application of clinical and genetic analysis provides the best approach at present. The classification in the accompanying table is based upon the clearly identifiable features of Duchenne dystrophy, facioscapulohumeral dystrophy, and myotonic muscular dystrophy. Limb-girdle dystrophy is probably not a single disease, but merely encompasses cases that do not fall into the other categories.

Incidence. None of the muscular dystrophies are common. Incidence rates vary from 5 per million births for facioscapulohumeral dystrophy to about 250 per million births for Duchenne dystrophy. Many cases seem to be sporadic; the mutation rate of Duchenne dystrophy is high, 7×10^{-5}, and about two thirds of the cases appear sporadically, with no other affected individual in the family.

Pathology. Pathologic abnormalities are restricted to skeletal muscle, sometimes involving cardiac muscle. The brain, spinal cord, and peripheral nerves are devoid of histologic change, although some authors have implicated the brain because of a seemingly high incidence of mental retardation in children with Duchenne dystrophy. Terminal pneumonia may cause changes in the lungs, and there may be a variety of associated diseases not directly linked to the dystrophy. In myotonic muscular dystrophy, however, baldness and testicular atrophy are integral parts of the disease in men, and corneal opacities affect both sexes.

The abnormalities in muscle seem to involve all fibers in random fashion. Early, there is scattered evidence of necrosis and regeneration, with prominent variation in fiber size, including many fibers much larger than normal. Later, fibers disappear, to be replaced by fibrous connective tissue and fat. "Pseudohypertrophy" is probably due to both "true" hypertrophy (large fibers) and

Classification of Human Muscular Dystrophies

	Duchenne Dystrophy	Facioscapulohumeral Dystrophy	Limb-Girdle Dystrophy	Myotonic Dystrophy
Genetic pattern	X-linked, recessive	Autosomal, dominant	Autosomal, recessive	Autosomal, dominant
Age at onset	Before age 5	Adolescence	Adolescence	Early or late
First symptoms	Pelvic	Shoulders	Pelvic	Distal; hands or feet
Pseudohypertrophy	+	0	0	0
Predominant weakness, early	Proximal	Proximal	Proximal	Distal
Progression	Relatively rapid; incapacitated in adolescence	Slow	Variable	Slow
Facial weakness	0	+	0	Occasional
Ocular, oropharyngeal weakness	0	0	0	Occasional
Myotonia	0	0	0	+
Cardiomyopathy	0 or late	0	0	Arrhythmia, conduction block
Associated disorders	None (?mental retardation)	None	None	Cataracts; testicular atrophy and baldness in men
Serum enzymes	Very high	Slight or no increase	Slight or no increase	Slight or no increase
Prevalence (per million population)	38	5	20	25
Incidence (per million births)	251	5	47	—
Mutation rate	9×10^{-5}	5×10^{-7}	3×10^{-5}	10×10^{-6}

increased accumulations of fat and connective tissue. In myotonic dystrophy, unusual figures form "ring fibers" (with one fiber running at right angles, encircling the other fibers in the same bundle) and "sarcoplasmic masses," or accumulations of sarcoplasm that are free of myofilaments. However, these abnormalities occur occasionally in other diseases and are not pathognomonic of myotonic dystrophy. In Duchenne dystrophy, the myocardium may be affected by similar changes at autopsy, but cardiac symptoms are rarely evident in life, a discrepancy that has been attributed to the sedentary life imposed upon the patients by advanced muscular weakness. Myopathic changes in the heart are common in myotonic dystrophy. There is no good evidence that smooth muscle is affected in any form of dystrophy. Ultrastructural investigations have not provided any clues to the initial lesion. Disruption of myofibrillar structure, alterations of mitochondria, and degeneration of tubules and sarcoplasmic reticulum all seem to proceed together.

Clinical Manifestations. The symptoms and signs of all forms of the muscular dystrophies are related to weakness alone, except that additional systems are involved in myotonic dystrophy. In other forms, the symptoms depend upon the distribution of weakness and the age at onset. In *Duchenne dystrophy* weakness is primarily proximal at onset, and symptoms begin early. By definition, girls are not affected. There are no symptoms in the first year of life, but walking may be somewhat delayed beyond 18 months. Once the child walks, some abnormality is usually evident to an experienced observer (either a parent with a previously affected child or a skilled physician). The boys tend to waddle when they walk, or walk on their toes, or fall frequently and have difficulty rising. They are probably never able to run, because they have difficulty raising their knees. These symptoms become more evident as the children grow older, and even the most unsuspecting parent becomes aware of some abnormality by age five, or teachers sometimes may be the first to recognize the difficulty when the child starts school. Some cases are averred to start between ages five and ten, but these must be exceptional. It is difficult to examine individual muscles of a young child, but the waddling gait, the typical method of rising from the ground by "climbing up" himself (Gowers' sign), enlargement of calf or other muscles, and inability to run are characteristic. Myotatic reflexes may be normal at first, but by three years the knee jerks are usually lost, and later the ankle jerks disappear. As the child grows there are two countervailing influences; increased growth and coordination may compensate temporarily for the concurrent progressive weakness and wasting, but the disease always wins. There is increased difficulty walking. Going up grades or stairs first requires aid, then becomes impossible. Weakness of the trunk muscles leads to increased lordosis and a protuberant abdomen. Then the arms become weak. Finally, in early adolescence, the child becomes unable to walk. This is inevitable, but may be accelerated by a period of inactivity after an injury or an orthopedic operation. Contractures appear, at first in the feet, as the gastrocnemius muscles tighten. When the child stops walking, flexion contractures limit motion of the knees, and scoliosis becomes more a problem with prolonged sitting. Ultimately respiration becomes shallow and the child is increasingly subject to pulmonary infection. Sooner or later, one of these infections is fatal, usually in the third decade. Although muscles are ravaged from the neck down, the cranial

muscles are entirely spared, an apparently important clue to the nature of the disease, but presently uninterpretable. Congestive heart failure and abnormalities of cardiac rhythm are rare.

Becker dystrophy has manifestations similar to those of Duchenne dystrophy, but the onset is later in childhood or in adolescence, and the tempo is slower and more variable. This form may also be devastating, but some patients are able to function, albeit with limitations, well into adult life. The clinical similarities include pseudohypertrophy of calf muscles. However, it is clear that although the two forms are similar, they are genetically separate; there are no mildly affected individuals in typical Duchenne families, nor are children affected severely in Becker families.

The manifestations of *limb-girdle dystrophy* are also similar because weakness of muscles of the pelvic girdle usually initiates the syndrome, but symptoms start in late childhood or adolescence. Girls are affected as often as boys, and pseudohypertrophy is rare. Waddling gait, difficulty in walking and climbing, and frequent falls are common. Occasionally, symptoms may begin in the shoulder girdle. In either case, there is usually weakness in all four limbs by the time the patient seeks medical attention. The severity, age at onset, and rate of progression vary considerably, suggesting that this category contains more than one disease.

Facioscapulohumeral dystrophy is distinct. Symptoms vary in severity so that some affected individuals never have any disability (but can be recognized by the signs), whereas others become incapacitated early; there are all grades in between. The first symptoms are apt to be related to difficulty in raising the arms or to prominence of the scapulae. Weakness of the legs may affect pelvic girdle muscles, or equally prominent weakness of the anterior tibial muscles may lead to a steppage gait. Truncal weakness may lead to prominent scoliosis. The face is always involved on examination; the perioral muscles may be more affected than those of the upper face, but ultimately patients develop difficulty in closing the eyes. The sternal head of the pectoral muscle is affected earlier than the clavicular head, a selectivity that can be detected on testing the individual muscles, and leads to a peculiar appearance of the axillary folds when the arms are dependent, because the anterior axillary fold of normal people is formed by the sternal portion of the pectoral muscle. Winging of the scapulae can be seen when the patient leans against a wall with the arms extended, and the weakness of shoulder girdle muscles leads to an unusual appearance because, viewed from the front, the superior margin of the scapula is higher than the clavicle.

Myotonic muscular dystrophy diverges from the preceding types in several respects. (1) The distribution of weakness differs in that cranial muscles are often affected and limb weakness is initially more marked in distal muscles. Thus weakness of the hands (as in twisting bottle caps or using tools) precedes shoulder weakness, and footdrop or steppage gait precedes symptoms of pelvic muscle weakness. *Ptosis, facial weakness,* and *dysarthria* are signs not seen in the other forms of dystrophy. Moreover, there is almost always selective weakness of the sternomastoids. The masticatory muscles either are poorly developed or waste early (even when not symptomatically weak), causing a characteristic facial appearance. The long, lean look has led physicians to use several callous descriptive phrases that are best not perpetuated. (Among the more foolish designations is "myopathic facies," but the facial appearance of a patient with myotonic dystrophy differs from facioscapulohumeral dystrophy or from myasthenia gravis.) (2) Myotonia, or difficulty in relaxation, may be symptomatic, and after a firm grip the patient may have difficulty letting go. Myotonia may cause other symptoms in patients with mytonia congenita (see below), but in the dystrophy only the hands are affected by this kind of stiffness. Myotonia of grip may be evident on examination, and can also be elicited by percussing the thenar eminence. In normal persons this evokes a rapid twitch, whereas in patients with myotonia, a sustained contraction of the adductor pollicis muscle persists for several seconds, only gradually relaxing. Similar responses to percussion may be elicited uncommonly in other limb muscles, but can often be seen in the tongue. Although myotonia is a dramatic sign and a symptom that can be relieved by drugs, it is not the symptom that causes the major disability in myotonic dystrophy; weakness is the problem. (3) Other systems are involved in this pleomorphic disorder; cataracts appear sooner or later in all patients, and are sometimes the only sign of the disease; most of the men (but not the women) have frontal baldness; testicular atrophy affects most of the men, but often after they have sired children to perpetuate the disease (there is no definite evidence of gonadal insufficiency in affected women); the basal metabolic rate is often low, but other tests of thyroid function are normal (extrathyroidal hypometabolism). The incidence of diabetes mellitus may be increased. (4) Conduction defects are common in the electrocardiogram, and may lead to clinically significant arrhythmia or congestive heart failure.

Certain rare forms of muscular dystrophy are named after the prominent manifestations. *Ocular dystrophy* is a slowly progressive disorder in which ptosis of the eyelids and progressive immobility of the eyes are the cardinal features. The pupils are spared, and both eyes are usually affected symmetrically so that diplopia is uncommon (but may occur). Other muscles of the head, neck, and limbs may also be affected, varying from family to family. This syndrome raises problems of definition; some cases probably are myopathic in origin, but this kind of ophthalmoplegia is often associated with other manifestations that are clearly neurogenic (such as spinocerebellar degeneration or peripheral neuropathy). The final distinction as to the origin of the ophthalmoplegia is often difficult or impossible to make because the ocular muscles normally differ so much from limb muscles that signs of myopathy in muscle biopsy or electromyography are not valid in studying them. In some, but not all, patients with myopathic ophthalmoplegia, structural and biochemical abnormalities may be found in limb muscles. Abnormally large mitochondria are present in increased numbers; this can be seen dramatically in electron microscopy, and the numbers are sufficient to stain fibers red in the trichrome stain for light microscopy, leading to the appellation "ragged red fibers." In these cases there is apt to be an accumulation of glycogen, but the biochemical cause of this has not been ascertained.

Distal myopathy, as the name implies, affects distal leg and hand muscles first. It is probably the rarest form of dystrophy, and can be identified only by characteristic signs of myopathy in electromyography and muscle biopsy.

In the *scapuloperoneal syndrome* distal weakness in the legs resembles that of neurogenic peroneal muscular atrophy, but sensory loss is lacking, and there is proximal weakness in the shoulder girdle very similar to that of facioscapulohumeral dystrophy. Some of these cases are myopathic and some seem to be neurogenic as distinguished by electromyography, muscle biopsy, and serum enzymes. In either case, autosomal dominant inheritance and a relatively slow progression seem characteristic.

Diagnosis. The clinical picture of Duchenne dystrophy is so characteristic that it entails little diagnostic confusion. In its first stages, some children are merely regarded as clumsy, and some receive orthopedic care because of toe-walking; otherwise the diagnosis becomes obvious. As noted, the trait is transmitted as a sex-linked recessive, and once a case is recognized, members of the family rapidly detect the signs in subsequently affected youngsters. Once a family is known, affected individuals can be identified in the neonatal period because the serum enzymes are already markedly abnormal. Limb-girdle and facioscapulohumeral dystrophy must be differentiated from neurogenic diseases, from congenital myopathies, and from polymyositis, as will be discussed below. Myotonic dystrophy may be confused with endocrine disorders or, because of the distal weakness, with neuropathy or amyotrophy, or with hypothyroidism or gonadal disorders. Ocular myopathy must be differentiated from myasthenia gravis; this is usually not a problem because there is no fluctuation of symptoms in the myopathy, and the weakness does not respond to cholinergic drugs. The differential diagnosis of the dystrophies depends also upon the age of the patient. In childhood and adolescence, the major problems involve peroneal muscular atrophy (Charcot-Marie-Tooth) and "muscular atrophy simulating muscular dystrophy" (Wohlfart-Kugelberg-Welander). In adults, amyotrophic lateral sclerosis is the major problem. At all ages, polyneuritis must be considered.

Treatment. There is no specific treatment for the weakness of any form of dystrophy. Physical medicine, exercises, splints, braces, and corrective orthopedic surgery are applied in different centers with varying degrees of enthusiasm. Some therapeutic activists claim that walking can be prolonged into late adolescence in Duchenne dystrophy. They may be correct, but it is difficult to prove. The most poignant decisions concern the use of antimicrobial drugs or supported respiration for young men paralyzed from the neck down and with no hope of ultimate recovery. The myotonia of myotonic dystrophy can be relieved by diphenylhydantoin (0.3 to 0.6 gram daily), quinine (0.3 to 1.5 grams daily), or procainamide (4 to 6 grams daily), but this is rarely the problem, and nothing can be done for the weakness. Cataracts are treated surgically upon appropriate indication, and cardiac arrhythmias or congestive heart failure are managed accordingly.

Prophylaxis. Genetic counseling offers the only possibility to control muscular dystrophy at present. Carriers of Duchenne dystrophy may often but not always be identified by abnormally increased serum enzyme activity (higher than normal, but not as high as in affected boys). In some centers, antenatal detection of sex allows selective prophylactic abortion. There is presently no way to determine whether a male fetus is affected, however. Birth control ought to be effective in dominantly inherited diseases such as facioscapulohumeral and myotonic dystrophy, but since many cases are mild, the families go on interminably. The high rates of mutation do not encourage optimism that genetic restriction can be the ultimate goal.

Caughey, J. E., and Myrianthopoulous, N. C.: Dystrophia Myotonica and Related Disorders. Springfield, Ill., Charles C Thomas, 1963.

Dyken, P. R., and Harper, P. S.: Congenital dystrophia myotonica. Neurology, 23:465, 1973.

Emery, A. E. H., Watt, M. S., and Clacl, E. R.: The effects of genetic counseling in Duchenne muscular dystrophy. Clin. Genet., 3:147, 1972.

Gardner-Medwin, D., Pennington, R. J., and Walton, J. N.: The detection of carriers of X-linked muscular dystrophy genes. J. Neurol. Sci., 13:459, 1971.

Research Committee, Muscular Dystrophy Group (eds.): Research in Muscular Dystrophy. London, Sir Isaac Pitman & Sons, Ltd., 1969.

Rowland, L. P.: Muscular dystrophies. DM, November 1972, p. 1.

Walton, J. N.: Disorders of Voluntary Muscle. 2nd ed. Boston, Little, Brown & Company, 1969.

477. CONGENITAL MYOPATHIES

Definition.   These are rare diseases characterized by weakness that is usually relatively mild but persists throughout life, either progressing slowly or remaining stationary.

Etiology.   The cause is not known. A few of these disorders are familial and are suspected of having a genetic basis, but so many cases are sporadic that other causes are not excluded, and there are no clear clues.

Pathology.   These diseases are defined in terms of pathology, and most of them have been delineated within the past 15 years since the introduction of histochemical techniques to study muscle biopsy. The names of the diseases reflect the predominant anatomic disorder.

In *central core disease,* the central portion of the muscle fiber appears rather amorphous, in contrast to the fibrillar appearance of the surrounding normal portion. In cross-section, the central portion appears blue when stained with Gomori's trichrome, in striking contrast to the red periphery. The central areas lack all oxidative enzyme activity, and there are no mitochondria in this region. In *nemaline myopathy or rod myopathy,* small threadlike or rod bodies are scattered throughout the fiber. The rods are barely visible in conventional hematoxylin and eosin stains, but can be seen readily in phase contrast or with the trichrome stain. In electron microscopy the structures seem to originate in the Z-band, and circumstantial evidence suggests that they are composed of tropomyosin. *Myotubular myopathy* designates the appearance of myofibers that resemble a stage in the early development of fetal muscle, with nuclei located centrally rather than at the periphery and surrounded by a halo of apparently empty space. Because the pathogenesis of this appearance is uncertain, some investigators prefer the name *centronuclear myopathy.* In other disorders mitochondria have appeared abnormal, either in number (too many) or size (too large), often associated with accumulations of lipid droplets.

Clinical Manifestations.   Although designated "congenital," these diseases are only exceptionally symptomatic in the first year of life, except that the onset of walking may be delayed. Later, the symptoms of proximal limb weakness become evident: waddling gait, difficulty in climbing stairs, frequent falls, and scoliosis. Later, there may be weakness of the arms. There are few clinical clues to each specific histologic abnormality. Among the nemaline cases there have been skeletal abnormalities (kyphoscoliosis, pigeon breast, pes cavus, high palate, and an unusually elongated face). In two families with myotubular disease, ophthalmoplegia was present as well as limb weakness. Central core and mitochondrial disorders have not been assciated with distinctive clinical signs other than proximal limb weakness. In two unrelated patients, similar morphologic alterations of mitochondria were found in muscles of patients with nonthyroidal hypermetabolism; these disorders were neither familial nor congenital, however, and hypermetabolism has not been a manifestation of the congenital disorders. In none of the structurally defined congenital myopathies, therefore, is it possible to link the morphologic abnormality to a biochemical or physiologic cause of the weakness.

Diagnosis.   Proximal limb weakness in a young child is usually myopathic in origin, but must be distinguished from the neurogenic Wohlfart-Kugelberg-Welander syndrome and from polyneuritis. Myopathic abnormalities in the EMG, an abnormal family history, an incidence in girls, and especially the histologic abnormalities define the individual entities. The serum enzymes may be normal or slightly increased. In some clinics most cases of apparently congenital myopathy fail to meet the specific histologic criteria, showing only nonspecific myopathic changes in biopsy. There is no better designation for these cases than "congenital myopathy," but it is likely that there is more than one cause.

In infancy, the major cause of weakness is a form of motor neuron disease (Werdnig-Hoffmann disease). Among infants with multiple congenitally fixed joints (arthrogryposis multiplex), some prove to have myopathic disease as defined by muscle biopsy and electromyography. In some cases, neonatal difficulty in swallowing is followed by delayed onset of walking, possibly persistent weakness, obesity, childhood diabetes, mental retardation, and a characteristic facial appearance (Prader-Willi syndrome), but there is no abnormality on muscle biopsy or electromyogram.

Treatment and Prognosis.   There is no specific treatment for any of these disorders. Physical therapy and orthopedic corrective measures are of value. There are too few cases to generalize about the course of these illnesses; most seem to be mild and nonprogressive, but occasional cases are more severe.

Afifi, A. K., Ibrahim, M. Z. M., Bergman, R. A., Haydar, N. A., Mire, J., Bahuth, N., and Kaylani, F.: Morphologic features of hypermetabolic mitochondrial disease. J. Neurol. Sci., 15:271, 1972.

Bharucha, E. P., Pandya, S. S., and Dastur, D. K.: Arthrogryposis multiplex congenita. J. Neurol Neurosurg. Psychiatry, 35:425, 1972.

Dubowitz, V.: The Floppy Infant. London, Spastics International Medical Publications, 1969.

Hall, B. D., and Smith, D. W.: Prader-Willi syndrome: A résumé of 32 cases. J. Pediatr., 81:286, 1972.

Hefferman, L. P., Rewcastle, N. B., and Humphrey, J. G.: The spectrum of rod myopathies. Arch. Neurol., 18:529, 1968.

Kinoshita, M., and Cadman, T. E.: Myotubular myopathy. Arch. Neurol., 18:265, 1968.

478. MYOTONIA CONGENITA (Thomsen's Disease)

Definition.   Myotonia congenita is a disorder characterized by difficulty in relaxation of skeletal muscle after forceful contraction, present from early childhood.

Incidence.   This is one of the rarest of all muscular disorders.

Etiology.   There are occasional sporadic cases, but most are inherited in a pattern corresponding to an autosomal dominant trait. In a few families, the disease seems to be autosomal recessive. The biochemical fault is not known, but the muscle membrane is electrically unstable and tends to fire repetitively. The abnormality must be inherent within the muscle, because myotonic phenomena may be elicited after all neural influences are abolished by spinal anesthesia, block of motor nerves by local anesthesia, or blockade of the neuromuscular junction by intra-arterial injection of d-tubocurarine. Myotonia is abolished, however, by the intramuscular administration of procaine. That the membrane is abnormal is suggested by the myotonia that occurs in otherwise normal individuals taking diazacholesterol, a substance that interferes with the biosynthesis of cholesterol. How this affects the membrane, however, is not known, and membranes of other organs are not functionally altered.

Clinical Manifestations. The difficulty in relaxation in this disorder, in contrast to that in myotonic dystrophy, is widespread. Difficulty in relaxing the grip may lead to prominent and sometimes embarrassing symptoms. Ocular muscles may also be affected, so that the eyes seem momentarily "stuck" in one position, or the eyelids may remain closed after forceful closure. Sometimes oropharyngeal muscles are affected, with difficulty in speaking or swallowing. Startle reactions may induce stiffness of the legs, thwarting sudden attempts to catch a bus or run from home plate. There is no weakness, and one unexplained characteristic is the unusual muscular development of many patients, causing a Herculean appearance, and perhaps related to involuntary and repeated isometric exercise. The myotonia can be elicited by tapping any muscle in severely affected cases. Reflexes are unaltered.

Diagnosis. The major problem is in distinguishing these patients from those with myotonic muscular dystrophy. Here the only symptoms and signs are related to myotonia. There is no weakness, no cataract, no baldness, no gonadal atrophy. Some authors have described "transitional cases," but these are probably patients in families with myotonic muscular dystrophy who are only mildly affected and show only myotonia before the other manifestations. There may be some weakness in families with the rare autosomal recessive form of myotonia congenita. In general, families with myotonia congenita breed true.

Treatment. Drug therapy is effective. For many years, quinine was the staple treatment in doses of 0.3 to 1.5 grams daily. Recently, diphenylhydantoin has proved equally effective and less apt to cause disagreeable side effects in therapeutic doses of 0.3 to 0.6 gram daily. Should this fail, procainamide may also be used, in doses of 4 to 6 grams daily, but this drug is prone to cause drug-induced lupus erythematosus.

Landau, W. M.: The essential mechanism in myotonia. Neurology, 2:369, 1952.
Lipicky, R. J., Bryant, S. H., and Salmon, J. H.: Cable parameters, sodium, potassium, chloride and water content, and potassium efflux in isolated external intercostal muscle of normal volunteers and patients with myotonia congenita. J. Clin. Invest., 50:2091, 1971.

479. FAMILIAL MYOGLOBINURIA

Most cases of myoglobinuria are sporadic, and they will be described in Ch. 484. Some persons, however, have repeated attacks from early childhood, suggesting some genetic fault, and sometimes more than one individual in a family is affected. Some of these familial cases are due to lack of muscle phosphorylase or phosphofructokinase. They can be recognized by the ischemic work test in which contracture is induced and venous lactate fails to rise. (See Ch. 809). In one family, an abnormality of fatty acid oxidation associated with attacks of myoglobinuria was shown to be due to lack of carnitine palmityl transferase deficiency. Several families have been studied, however, in which glycogen metabolism was normal, and contracture could not be induced. The genetic abnormality in these patients has not been identified.

DiMauro, S., and DiMauro, P. M.: Muscle carnitine palmityltransferase deficiency and myoglobinuria. Science, 182:929, 1973.
Rowland, L. P., DiMauro, S., and Bank, W. J.: Glycogen storage diseases of muscles. Problems in biochemical genetics. Birth Defects, 7:43, 1971.

480. FAMILIAL PERIODIC PARALYSIS

Definition. Periodic paralysis is characterized by recurrent attacks of flaccid weakness usually associated with abnormally high or low serum potassium concentrations. Many cases are familial. In sporadic cases the abnormality may be secondary to identifiable aberrations of potassium metabolism.

Etiology and Pathogenesis. Familial cases are distributed in a pattern consistent with autosomal dominant inheritance. Hypokalemia during attacks was the first metabolic abnormality to be recognized, with no loss of potassium in urine. It was therefore presumed that potassium shifted from extracellular to intracellular compartments, especially muscle. This has been difficult to prove, and the anticipated hyperpolarization of the muscle membrane potential has not been substantiated by direct measurement with intracellular electrodes. Abnormalities of glucose metabolism have been suspected, because attacks can be precipitated by infusions of glucose and insulin, by eating a large meal, or by administration of epinephrine. However, biochemical studies have failed to pinpoint the abnormality.

During the past two decades it has been recognized that the serum potassium tends to rise in some patients, and attacks in these individuals are induced by the ingestion of potassium. This variety is therefore called "hyperkalemic periodic paralysis," and is generally considered to be the mirror image of the hypokalemic type, with potassium presumably shifting out of muscle and into blood during attacks. Why this should happen is not clear, but at least in the hyperkalemic type there are alterations of the intracellular potential in the direction required by theory. There are clinical differences between the two forms of periodic paralysis, but there are so many areas of overlap and so many common features that it is difficult to decide just how many genetically distinct forms there really are.

Pathology. In both forms of periodic paralysis there may be vacuoles within muscle fibers. These may be numerous or scanty, and it is not clear that they are more frequent in paralyzed muscle. Most electron microscopists believe that the vacuoles are derived from the sarcoplasmic reticulum, but others think they originate in the T-system in areas of necrotic muscle. Glycogen seems to be increased in amount in ultrastructural studies, but the results of biochemical analysis have been inconsistent. There is no evidence that other organs are affected in either form of the disease. The heart is usually spared pathologically.

Clinical Manifestations.   There are clinical differences between the two forms. In the hypokalemic variety, attacks tend to start in late childhood or adolescence, frequently occur at night, are apt to be severe, and last for a day or more. In the hyperkalemic variety, attacks start at an early age, occur much more frequently, tend to be milder, and may last minutes or hours. Moreover, patients with hyperkalemic periodic paralysis usually have some evidence of myotonia, which is rarely symptomatic and often limited to percussion myotonia of the tongue. Lid-lag and Chvostek's sign are identified with the hyperkalemic type. These clinical distinctions may break down in application to individual cases and are therefore only crude guides. Moreover, many features are common to both types: a dominant pattern of inheritance, a susceptibility to attacks during periods of rest after vigorous exercise, the ability to ward off attacks by mild exercise after a mild attack has begun, persistent weakness between attacks, vacuoles in muscle, a lack of clear relation between the serum potassium concentration and the severity of paresis, the induction of local weakness by cooling, and protection against attacks by acetazolamide. Some patients are affected by attacks in which the serum potassium may be either high or low.

Typical attacks start with weakness of the legs that ascends to the arms. Cranial muscles are affected in severe attacks only, and respiratory insufficiency is exceptional. The attacks may be mild and brief, or severe and prolonged, with all gradations in between. During severe attacks, the myotatic reflexes are lost, and the muscles are electrically inexcitable. Attacks are rarely apoplectic in onset and usually take an hour or more to develop, except that attacks beginning in sleep may be fully developed when the patient awakes. Paresthesias and myalgia may be prominent at the onset, or may be completely lacking. Some patients are aware of oliguria during the attack and of diuresis afterward.

The serum potassium is in the range of 2.5 to 3.5 mEq per liter in hypokalemic attacks, and 5.0 to 7.0 mEq per liter in the hyperkalemic type. Between attacks serum potassium values may be normal. The electrocardiogram is altered as would be predicted from the serum values, with low T waves in hypokalemia and peaked T waves in hyperkalemia.

Patients with hyperkalemic periodic paralysis may have mild symptoms attributable to myotonia, especially of the hands. When individuals in a family are studied, some may be found to have myotonia without any history of periodic paralysis.

In both types of the disease, there may be persistent weakness between attacks, most often proximal, sometimes distal. In the past this has been attributed to a permanent "myopathy," but experience with acetazolamide therapy indicates that even longlasting weakness may be reversible, regardless of pathologic changes in muscle. A few patients with intermittent normokalemic or hyperkalemic paralysis have had persistent cardiac arrhythmia, especially bigeminy, and bouts of ventricular tachycardia. The cardiac disorder is neither temporally related to attacks of limb weakness nor related to serum potassium content.

Diagnosis.   Periodic paralysis can be recognized by the history of typical attacks; no other disease causes this pattern of recurrent weakness. In myasthenia gravis, weakness may come and go, but less abruptly and with a duration of weeks rather than hours or days; remissions are less frequent so that it is less "periodic." Polymyo-

sitis may be transient, but episodes are rarely shorter than several weeks or months. Attacks of myoglobinuric weakness could conceivably be confusing if the pigmenturia were not recognized, but myalgia and malaise are so prominent that is rarely mistaken for periodic paralysis. Hysterical attacks might be confusing.

If the patient is seen during the attack and the serum potassium is abnormal, other causes of hypo- or hyperkalemia must be considered. Low serum potassium concentrations with paralysis are also encountered in hyperaldosteronism, potassium-losing nephritis, potassium depletion caused by laxative abuse, diuretics, or diarrhea, and thyrotoxicosis. *Thiazide* and *thalidone diuretics* are in such widespread use nowadays that these drugs are likely to be an increasingly frequent cause of hypokalemic weakness; in one series, about 25 per cent of randomly chosen patients receiving these drugs had serum potassium contents below normal. Hyperkalemia is most often due to renal insufficiency, but may also occur in adrenal insufficiency, after administration of spironolactone, or as a manifestation of aldosterone deficiency.

The signs of these other disorders usually provide appropriate diagnostic clues. A family history of periodic paralysis is useful in diagnosis, but apparently sporadic cases may be indistinguishable from the familial disorder. If the patient is not having a spontaneous attack when studied, the only way to distinguish the two forms is to provoke an attack. The techniques to be described have been used in numerous centers with many patients, without serious complications. But induced attacks may be frightening to patient and physician, and should be left to experienced investigators. Facilities for supported respiration should be immediately available. Appropriately informed consent is mandatory. Because of the uncertainty of clinical distinction, it is advisable to start with glucose (100 grams) given intravenously in one hour, with 20 units of regular insulin either in the infusion or given subcutaneously. Hypoglycemic symptoms should be anticipated, and the electrocardiogram should be monitored. Hypokalemia is induced as the blood sugar falls, usually within one hour after the infusion is completed. If an attack is induced, it can be terminated with administration of 7 to 10 grams of potassium chloride (KCl) by mouth. Whether or not an attack is induced by glucose and insulin, but especially if it is not, the patient should then be challenged with potassium. This poses delicate problems because it is not clear how much potassium constitutes an adequate challenge. We start with 3 grams of KCl by mouth. If this fails we gradually increase the dose on successive days to a maximum of 8 or 10 grams. Patients with hyperkalemic paralysis have attacks with serum potassium levels between 5 and 8 mEq per liter.

Other members of the family should be investigated clinically and electromyographically for evidence of myotonia.

Treatment.   Acute attacks of hypokalemic paralysis are best treated with oral KCl, 5 to 10 grams. Relief of weakness usually commences within 30 minutes but may take several hours, and some attacks are peculiarly refractory. Hyperkalemia may be relieved by infusions of glucose and insulin. Chlorothiazide and calcium gluconate have also been reported to be effective. In severe attacks, weakness may persist even after the serum potassium has returned to normal concentrations.

The traditional method used to protect patients

against hypokalemic paralysis was, until recently, a low-sodium diet supplemented by oral KCl, or perhaps by spironolactone or dexamethasone. Then, acetazolamide in small doses, sometimes only 250 per mg daily, sometimes more, was found to be effective prophylaxis in the hyperkalemic type. Subsequently, it was found that similar doses of acetazolamide were equally effective in the hypokalemic variety, so a single drug is beneficial in both forms. How it exerts this effect is not known. The best-known effects of this compound relate to its ability to inhibit carbonic anhydrase, but muscle lacks this enzyme, and no definite systemic effects of the drug have been recognized in the doses used, but metabolic acidosis may be responsible.

Gordon, R. M., Green, J. R., and Lagunoff, D.: Studies on a patient with hypokalemic familial periodic paralysis. Am. J. Med., 48:185, 1970.

Griggs, R. C., Engel, W. K., and Resnick, J. S.: Acetazolamide treatment of hypokalemic periodic paralysis: Prevention of attacks and improvement of persistent weakness. Ann. Intern. Med., 73:39, 1970.

Pearson, C. M., and Kalyanaraman, R.: Periodic paralyses. In Stanbury, J. B., Wyngaarden, J. B., and Frederickson, D. S. (eds.): The Metabolic Basis of Inherited Disease. 3rd ed. New York, McGraw-Hill Book Company, 1972, pp. 1180–1203.

Satoyashi, E., Murakami, K., Kowa, H., Kinoshita, M., and Hishiyama, Y.: Periodic paralysis in hyperthyroidism. Neurology, 13:746, 1963.

Zierler, K. L.: Speculations on hypokalemic periodic paralysis. Am. J. Med. Sci., 266:131, 1973.

481. MYOSITIS OSSIFICANS

This rare disorder is most dramatic in its consequences, producing the "stone man" of circus sideshows. Symptoms usually begin in early childhood, with transient and localized swellings of the neck and back. Ultimately there is progressive rigidity of the neck, trunk, and limbs. Palpable plates are discernible beneath the rigid parts. Severely affected patients may be able to stand and walk, and yet be totally unable to bend so that they must be raised from bed with assistance. The bars beneath the skin are visible roentgenographically. Microscopically, muscle is replaced by bone and connective tissue. Whether the primary disorder is in the fibroblasts (leading to abnormal ossification) or in the muscle itself is not resolved. Muscle biopsy early in the disease may show widespread necrosis and inflammation, but serum enzymes are not always elevated, nor is the electromyogram always myopathic. Few cases are familial, but the disorder is believed to be inherited because digital abnormalities are almost always present in both the patients and other members of the family in a pattern suggesting an autosomal dominant inheritance. Microdactyly commonly affects the great toe, and clinodactyly (curved digits) may affect the hands. There is no detectable systemic abnormality of calcium and phosphate metabolism, and there has been no effective therapy, but recent reports suggest that administration of disphosphonates may prevent the deposition of bone. Once bone is formed, however, these drugs are ineffective.

Bassett, C. A. L., Donath, A., Macagno, F., Preisig, R., Fleisch, H., and Francis, M. D.: Diphosphonates in the treatment of myositis ossificans. Lancet, 2:845, 1969.

Lutwak, L.: Myositis ossificans progressiva. Am. J. Med., 37:269, 1964.

SPORADIC DISORDERS

482. DERMATOMYOSITIS AND POLYMYOSITIS

The main discussion of these conditions is found in Ch. 80. However, the concept of polymyositis is central to the analysis and concepts of acquired myopathies of adult life, and thus it is appropriate to review some of the problems here.

Definition. These conditions are usually considered together, but this practice may prove imprudent. *Dermatomyositis* is a recognizable syndrome of unknown cause, characterized by a rash and myopathy, both with distinctive clinical features. The name is derived from the inflammatory cellular response that is usually found in skeletal muscle, but lymphocytic infiltration is not present in all cases. This lack causes problems in defining *polymyositis,* a disorder presumably identical with dermatomyositis but without the rash. There probably is such a disease, because the rash of dermatomyositis may be so mild that it could be overlooked by parents or inexperienced clinicians, and there are patients with no history of rash who develop subcutaneous calcinosis, implying that the skin had been involved even without visible dermatitis. But once the rash is taken away, an essential sign of dermatomyositis is withdrawn, and it becomes impossible to define polymyositis as the same condition. Polymyositis, therefore, is a syndrome, probably of diverse causes, and is identifiable by the following set of diagnostic criteria.

Diagnosis. At the outset it should be noted that the diagnosis of dermatomyositis is a clinical diagnosis, depending upon the characteristic rash and muscular weakness. In some patients the features of scleroderma may also be prominent, warranting the name "sclerodermatomyositis." But there is no overlap with lupus erythematosus or periarteritis nodosa, and the visceral lesions of these conditions do not occur in dermatomyositis.

Problems arise when there is no rash. The syndrome must be differentiated from the dystrophies by lack of family history, onset after age 35 (because no familial limb-girdle dystrophy starts so late), rapidity of onset in weeks or months rather than years, spontaneous improvement (which does not occur in dystrophy, by definition), distribution of weakness affecting cervical and cranial muscles, or systemic symptoms such as arthralgia or Raynaud's syndrome. The muscle biopsy ought to be crucial, but inflammatory lesions may be lacking in dermatomyositis, and may occasionally be seen in dystrophies; severe inflammation, when present, supports the diagnosis of polymyositis, but lack of leukocytic infiltration does not exclude the diagnosis. The electromyogram is helpful, but, again, not distinctive; there are the usual features of myopathy with the additional evidence of irritable muscle (increased insertional activity and some spontaneous activity). Serum enzymes tend to be high. There may also be an increased erythrocyte sedimentation rate, increased serum gamma globulin concentration, or a positive latex fixation test for rheumatoid factor. But there are no antibodies to muscle. Evidence of lymphocytes sensitized to muscle may be demonstrable, but this has not yet attained diagnostic reliability.

The problem of diagnosis is best exemplified by a patient with limb weakness commencing at age 40 and evidence of myopathic disease in muscle biopsy and EMG. Search must be made for the known causes of muscle disease, to be discussed below. If none is found, the diagnosis of exclusion is polymyositis, no matter what the laboratory data show or do not show. That this residual group is all due to one disease seems unlikely, not only because there is clinical heterogeneity, but also because if there are so many known causes of the syndrome, there are some others still to be recognized. Because inflammatory cells are not always seen in the muscle biopsy, some authorities eschew the word "polymyositis" and prefer "myopathy of unknown cause." This, at least, identifies the problem, but for the present "polymyositis" seems to be entrenched. Clinicians should recognize, however, that "polymyositis" is no more a specific diagnosis than "headache," "polyneuritis," or "convulsive disorder," terms that also imply inadequately defined syndromes of diverse etiology.

483. OTHER ACQUIRED MYOPATHIES

Proximal limb weakness in patients with no rash, with or without inflammatory lesions in muscle, and with or without increased serum enzyme activity, occurs in several disorders. These may be considered diseases associated with polymyositis or causes of polymyositis. To identify these disorders, appropriate diagnostic tools must be utilized.

Carcinomatous Myopathy. Muscle weakness without rash may occur in patients with carcinoma of the lung or of any other primary site. Myeloma, macroglobulinemia, and other gammopathies may also be associated with myopathy. The tumor itself may or may not be symptomatic, and treatment of the tumor may or may not affect the muscular symptoms.

Collagen Diseases. Proximal limb weakness may occur in the course of systemic lupus erythematosus, progressive systemic sclerosis, rheumatoid arthritis, and, rarely, periarteritis nodosa or giant cell arteritis. In these circumstances, the myopathy is treated as part of the general disorder.

Endocrine Disease. Thyrotoxic myopathy is a well-recognized syndrome. Usually there is clinical evidence of hyperthyroidism, but not always ("apathetic hyperthyroidism"). Signs of hypermetabolism are especially apt to be lacking in elderly patients. This myopathy inevitably disappears when the patient is rendered euthyroid by treatment. Similarly, weakness may complicate hypothyroidism. Another muscle syndrome of hypothyroidism is Hoffmann's syndrome, a peculiar difficulty in relaxing muscles that lack the characteristic electromyographic abnormalities of myotonia and is therefore called "pseudomyotonia," but may appear similar clinically. This, too, disappears with appropriate replacement therapy. Infants with cretinism may have unusually well developed muscles but not the disorder of relaxation.

Hyperparathyroidism and hyperadrenocorticism may also be responsible for weakness that looks like any other proximal myopathy. Surprisingly, because asthenia has so long been regarded as prominent, Addison's disease seems not to be a cause of this syndrome. Weakness may be part of hyperpituitarism, but acromegalic features always overshadow the myopathy.

Myalgia, with or without weakness, may be a prominent symptom in patients with osteomalacia, and the muscular disorder may respond dramatically to administration of vitamin D.

Infections. Structures resembling viral particles have been seen with the electron microscope with polymyositis, and sometimes there are acute myopathic disorders in individuals with influenza or encephalomyelitis, but no specific virus has been isolated from these cases. Muscle may be affected by a variety of organisms, but the only one of practical importance in the differential diagnosis of acute or subacute myopathy is trichinosis. Toxoplasmosis may affect muscle in the course of a syndrome that looks like severe infectious mononucleosis with adenopathy, rash, mucosal lesions, and hepatomegaly. In tropical countries, trypanosomiasis and schistosomiasis are important causes of muscle involvement.

Sarcoidosis. In muscle clinics, sarcoidosis is recognized as a significant cause of polymyositis. Usually there is other evidence of the disease, but sometimes the first symptoms are due to weakness, and in a few cases only muscle seems to be involved. Myalgia may be severe in these patients.

Drugs. A variety of drugs used to treat more common disorders may themselves cause muscular weakness, especially triamcinolone and other fluorinated adrenal steroids (but probably all steroids), vincristine, chloroquine, bretylium, and guanethidine. Repeated injections of narcotics and other drugs may lead to fibrosis of muscle that simulates a diffuse myopathy.

Alcoholic Myopathy. The clearest myopathic disorder in alcoholic persons is acute myoglobinuria. Some of these individuals, and some who never have an attack of pigmenturia, also suffer from proximal limb weakness, especially affecting the legs. The serum creatine phosphokinase is often elevated. The problem in some of these patients, however, is that they also suffer from the typical polyneuritis of alcoholism, and it then becomes difficult to prove that the muscular weakness is not also secondary to a neurogenic disorder. Too few patients have been evaluated to know whether abstinence and a good diet will reverse the persistent weakness. Chronic hypokalemia from any cause may be associated with the syndrome of polymyositis: weakness of relatively abrupt onset, muscle necrosis in biopsy, and high serum enzymes. This is most commonly seen in patients taking thiazide diuretics, but may also occur in hypokalemic states caused by chronic diarrhea. Hypokalemia may also contribute to some cases of alcoholic myopathy. (Other acquired disorders of potassium metabolism are discussed under Diagnosis in Ch. 480).

Byers, R. K., Bergman, A. B., and Joseph, M. C.: Steroid myopathy. Report of five cases occurring during treatment of rheumatic fever. Pediatrics, 29:26, 1962.
Dawkins, R. L., and Mastaglia, F. L.: Cell-mediated cytotoxicity to muscle in polymyositis. Effect of immunosuppression. N. Engl. J. Med., 288:434, 1973.
Frame, B., Heize, E. G., Block, M. A., and Manson, G. A.: Myopathy in primary hyperparathyroidism. Ann. Intern. Med., 68:1022, 1968.
Hall, W. H.: Proximal muscle atrophy in adult celiac disease. Am. J. Dig. Dis., 13:697, 1968.
Mastaglia, F. L., Gardner-Medwin, D., and Hudgson, P.: Muscle fibrosis and contractures in a pethidine addict. Br. Med. J., 4:532, 1971.
Perkoff, G. T.: Alcoholic myopathy. Ann. Rev. Med., 22:125, 1971.
Scarpalezos, S., et al.: Neural and muscular manifestations of hypothyroidism. Arch. Neurol., 29:140, 1973.
Silverstein, A., and Siltzbach, L. E.: Muscle involvement in sarcoidosis. Arch. Neurol., 21:235, 1969.
Trojaborg, W., Frantzen, E., and Andersen, I.: Peripheral neuropathy and myopathy associated with carcinoma of the lung. Brain, 92:71, 1969.

484. SPORADIC MYOGLOBINURIA

Definition. Sporadic myoglobinuria comprises a group of disorders characterized by injury of muscle and excretion of myoglobin in the urine. *Rhabdomyolysis* has been proposed as a more precise term, but it is used to mean "myoglobinuria," and therefore is of dubious value.

Pathogenesis. Myoglobin may be released from muscle whenever there is extensive and rapid destruction. Sometimes the cause is evident, as in the *crush injuries* of World War II when individuals were pinned beneath the timbers of buildings destroyed in bombing raids. Similar pressure injuries may occur in comatose persons who lie on one side without moving for prolonged periods. This kind of injury is perhaps more apt to occur when there are other causes of *metabolic depression;* for instance, in coma after suicidal ingestion of barbiturates or carbon monoxide intoxication, or prolonged unconsciousness in the snow. A similar effect may be induced by *arterial occlusion* by tourniquet or embolism, or even by prolonged knee-chest posture under anesthesia.

In other patients, the cause is less discernible. In every series of patients with myoglobinuria, a disproportionate number are *alcoholics,* but why this should occur is not known. Sometimes there has been exposure to a known *membrane toxin,* such as the bite of the Malayan sea snake. In some addicts, heroin itself seems to cause myoglobinuria. Or there may be *metabolic alterations* that do not ordinarily cause this kind of trouble, such as diarrhea with hypokalemia; potassium depletion caused by diuretics, amphotericin, or licorice; diabetic acidosis; or systemic infection with fever. In many attacks, however, not even these clues prevail.

The most common cause of myoglobinuria is probably unusually *vigorous exercise* by an otherwise normal person. Most cases have been reported by military physicians, and local designations include such titles as the "squat-jump syndrome." Some cases are attributed to "march hemoglobinuria." When large numbers of recruits endure these tortures, a certain number will have attacks of myalgia followed by pigmenturia. Why these individuals have attacks and others are spared is not clear, but this seems to be a "normal" variation. In civilians, cases have been caused by the excess muscular activity of an initiation rite into a club or fraternity, and isolated attacks have occurred after the vigorous muscular activity induced by succinylcholine before it achieves relaxation. In *malignant hyperthermia,* there is a rapid rise in temperature, widespread muscular rigidity, hyperkalemia, and metabolic acidosis, with a fatal outcome in about 75 per cent. The offending agents are usually halothane and succinylcholine. Increased serum activities of sarcoplasmic enzyme are the rule, and often there is myoglobinuria. The intense muscular contraction may be the proximate cause of myoglobinuria in this syndrome, but the widespread metabolic disorder probably contributes. Spontaneous convulsions and electroconvulsive therapy have also been followed by myoglobinuria. If an individual is subject to repeated attacks, it may be suspected that there is some kind of undiscovered genetic defect, although the only ones recognized now are deficiencies of phosphorylase, phosphofructokinase, or carnitine palmityl transferase.

Clinical Manifestations. In attacks other than those caused by local crushing or arterial occlusion, the clinical picture is similar. Affected muscles are apt to be the ones subject to greatest physical strain (the legs in squat-thrusts, the arms after chinning or push-ups, the arms and legs after wrestling matches). The muscles ache, may be swollen, and are weak. Sometimes there is so much edema that local vascular abnormalities are suspected. There may be fever and considerable malaise. Symptoms persist for several days even though pigmenturia rarely lasts more than 48 hours. Recovery may be gradual. Cranial muscles are rarely involved, and although respiratory failure is uncommon it is a hazard. The most important threat to life is renal injury secondary to excretion of heme. There may be red cells or myoglobin in the urine as well as casts. Oliguria is followed by azotemia and hyperkalemia. This may be treated by appropriate measures.

Diagnosis. The diagnosis of myoglobinuria can be made on clinical grounds and with relatively simple tests, but precise identification of the pigment depends upon biochemical analysis. The urine may appear red-brown because of hemoglobin, myoglobin, or porphyrins. The latter would not give a positive test with benzidine (or other heme-reacting reagents), and would not give a positive Watson-Schwartz test for porphobilinogen. Besides, the neurologic disorder of porphyria is neuropathy, not an acute myopathy. If the urine gives a positive test for heme and contains no or few erythrocytes, the pigment is either myoglobin or hemoglobin. If it is hemoglobin, the serum would be pink (after a hemolytic reaction), whereas the color of the serum in myoglobinuria is normal. (This distinction depends upon the affinity of serum haptoglobin for hemoglobin and not for myoglobin. Hemoglobin is not excreted until haptoglobin is saturated by visible amounts of the pigment, whereas myoglobin is excreted at much lower concentrations.) Furthermore, in attacks of myoglobinuria, the muscular weakness and myalgia are distinctive, and serum enzymes are greatly increased, whereas they are not in hemolysis. Positive identification of myoglobin can be achieved by several tests: absorption spectrophotometry is direct and simple, but in many laboratories the most convenient method is electrophoresis on starch gel or cellulose acetate. In the future, immunochemical methods are apt to gain favor. In all patients presenting in coma, especially after drug ingestion or carbon monoxide intoxication, it is important to check the urine for heme pigment and to assay serum for sarcoplasmic enzyme activity because of the possibility of a crush syndrome; if recognized, mannitol diuresis may prevent renal injury.

Treatment. If there is no renal injury, myoglobinuria is not threatening. The hazards of renal injury are not directly correlated to the amount of pigment excreted, and other factors are probably involved. Once an attack starts, it is useful to encourage excretion of dilute urine, and some authorities still favor alkalinizing agents although it has not been clearly demonstrated that these treatments protect the kidneys. Few patients are left with residual weakness, but in some the syndrome is characterized by prolonged weakness punctuated by attacks of myoglobinuria.

Gordon, R. A., Britt, B. A., and Kalow, W. (eds.): International Symposium on Malignant Hyperthermia. Springfield, Ill., Charles C Thomas, 1973.

Greenberg, J., and Arneson, L.: Exertional rhabdomyolysis with myoglobinuria in a large group of military trainees. Neurology, 17:216, 1967.

Kagen, L. J.: Immunologic detection of myoglobinuria after cardiac surgery. Ann. Intern. Med., 67:1183, 1967.

Rowland, L. P., and Penn, A. S.: Myoglobinuria. Med. Clin. North Am., 56:1233, 1972.
Vertel, R. M., and Knochel, J. P.: Acute renal failure due to heat injury: An analysis of ten cases with a high incidence of myoglobinuria. Am. J. Med., 43:435, 1967.

485. MYASTHENIA GRAVIS

Definition. Myasthenia gravis is usually defined as a state of abnormal fatigability. This definition has the merit of being consistent with the characteristic electrophysiologic disorder found in patients with this condition, but there are serious disadvantages. "Normal" fatigue is not defined, muscles weakened from any cause are apt to fatigue more readily than normal, and myasthenic muscle may be completely paralyzed (especially ocular muscles), with no signs of fatigue. Moreover, emphasis on fatigue has led to the treatment of many psychoneurotic patients with cholinergic drugs. An alternative definition has therefore been proposed:

"Myasthenia gravis is a disease characterized by weakness that has special characteristics: predilection for ocular and other cranial muscles; tendency to fluctuate during brief periods of observation (in the course of a single day) or for longer periods (remissions and exacerbations); with no signs of neural lesion, and partial reversibility by the administration of cholinergic drugs."

Etiology. The cause of myasthenia gravis is not known. Several disorders tend to occur more frequently in patients with myasthenia gravis, such as hyperthyroidism or other thyroidal disorders, and a significant number of patients with myasthenia gravis have thymomas. But neither in these situations nor in others has a causal relationship been proved. Whether or not there is a significant association with "autoimmune" diseases remains to be proved; rheumatoid arthritis and systemic lupus erythematosus have been reported in patients with myasthenia gravis, but the statistical significance of these associations is uncertain.

Several lines of evidence suggest an immunologic disorder in myasthenia gravis. Thymomas occur in about 15 per cent of all patients, more often in patients older than 40 years. Germinal centers are seen frequently in the thymus glands of patients who have no tumor. Infiltration of muscle by monocytes is characteristic, especially in perivascular collections called lymphorrhages. Antibodies to muscle can be demonstrated by immunofluorescent techniques in approximately a third of all patients with myasthenia, and in almost all patients with concomitant myasthenia and thymoma. However, the nature of the antigen that elicits these antibodies is uncertain, and it seems quite clear that the antibodies are not responsible for the symptoms of myasthenia. Thus antibodies may be present in patients with thymoma who have no evidence of myasthenia. There is no correlation between the presence of antibodies in serum and the appearance of transient neonatal myasthenia, and the concentration of serum antibodies does not correlate with the severity of symptoms. Finally, physiologic evidence indicates a disorder of neuromuscular transmission in myasthenia, and the antibodies react with proteins in the myofiber, but not at the neuromuscular junction. The significance of these human antibodies is therefore uncertain. The possibility that lymphocytes are sensitized to some component of muscle is currently being evaluated. No one has yet succeeded in designing a fully reproducible experimental model of the disease by immunologic techniques; however, injections of muscle and thymus may produce an experimental disorder, and injections of acetylcholine receptor from electric eel have induced a myasthenic state in rabbits.

Neuromuscular Disorder. The symptoms of myasthenia gravis resemble those of curare intoxication. This observation led to the use of curare antagonists in the treatment of myasthenia gravis. All effective therapies have been derived from this initial observation, and all drugs currently in use are inhibitors of the enzyme cholinesterase. These drugs also partially repair a physiologic defect that can be detected in patients by relatively simple techniques. When the ulnar nerve of normal individuals is stimulated at rates of 25 per second or less, the action potential of the hypothenar muscles is sustained at a constant amplitude. In patients with myasthenia, however, there is a rapid decline in the height of the evoked potentials. If the patient is then given neostigmine, the amplitude of the evoked potentials is restored to normal. This pattern could be consistent with either excessive cholinesterase activity, inadequate release of acetylcholine, or blockade of the junction by some curare-like compound. Microelectrode studies have been performed upon intercostal muscle fibers of patients with myasthenia (after excision of these muscles, they can be studied in vitro with the most advanced techniques). Investigations of this nature suggest that the basic defect is a reduced amount of acetylcholine released in each quantum from the motor nerve terminal. This could be caused by either some defect in the binding of acetylcholine or the presence of a "false transmitter," but how the defect comes about is not known.

Incidence and Prevalence. The prevalence of myasthenia gravis is about 33 per million population and the annual incidence about 2 to 5 per million. Translated into the experience of a busy 1000-bed general hospital, about 20 new cases are encountered each year, or about the same incidence as for lupus erythematosus. Cases occur in all decades of life, most frequently at about age 40. Among young adults, the disease affects women about three times more frequently than men. Among children and older persons, however, there is no sexual predilection.

Pathology. Pathologic changes in myasthenia gravis are limited to muscle and thymus. Skeletal muscles may appear completely normal, but there are often collections of lymphocytes around blood vessels. In some cases there is evidence of degeneration of muscle fibers, and the inflammatory cellular response may be more extensive. Rarely, similar lesions are encountered in the myocardium. The thymus gland is often abnormal. Encapsulated tumors (thymoma) occur in about 15 per cent of the cases, almost all after age 30. In about 25 per cent of these tumors there is evidence of local invasion, but distant metastases are virtually unknown in patients with myasthenia, and the local invasiveness is not a cause of symptoms. Lymphocytic proliferation, in the form of germinal centers, is seen in the thymus glands of almost all other patients, but sometimes the gland appears normal, and in some older individuals the gland is so involuted that it cannot be found. Patients dying of this disease usually have some pulmonary disorder (edema, atelectasis, infection) but this is secondary to the terminal events. Patients with myasthenia may live long enough to develop a carcinoma of any organ, but it has not been shown that myasthenia occurs more frequently in patients with cancer than might be expected on the basis of chance.

Clinical Manifestations. The symptoms of myasthenia gravis are all due to weakness. The most common presenting symptoms relate to weakness of eye muscles, ptosis, or diplopia. At the onset these symptoms may last only a few days, then disappear, only to return weeks or months later. Ptosis frequently varies even in the course of a single day. Diplopia may be noted in particular directions of gaze. Difficulty in chewing, dysarthria, and dysphagia are other common initial symptoms. Limb weakness is perhaps more often proximal in accentuation, so that patients have difficulty climbing stairs or rising from chairs, or have difficulty lifting heavy objects or raising the arms overhead. However, distal weakness is not uncommon, and the initial symptoms may be related to the strength of the hands or fingers. Selective respiratory weakness is most unusual. There is no alteration of consciousness, no pain, and, in untreated patients, no cramps or muscular twitching. Difficulty in eating and swallowing may lead to considerable loss of weight, but there is no specific wasting of muscle except in patients with severe chronic weakness.

On examination, evidence of weakness of the appropriate muscle groups is found. If any sensory abnormality is found, there must be some other disorder, alone or in combination with myasthenia. Similarly, hyperactive reflexes and Babinski signs imply some other disorder, as does the complete loss of reflexes. Weakness is responsible for all the signs of myasthenia. Ptosis may be unilateral or bilateral. The patient may experience diplopia even when there is no obvious weakness of the ocular muscles; more often, there is weakness of several muscles in a pattern that cannot be explained by disorder of a particular ocular motor nerve and is not usually symmetrical in the two eyes. In addition, there is frequently weakness of eye closure because of paresis of the orbicularis oculi. Muscles of the lower face are involved later. Lingual and palatal weakness are evident in patients with dysarthria. A nasal twang and indistinct speech imply that dysarthria has facial, lingual, palatal, and, sometimes, respiratory components. In advanced cases, patients support the chin with one hand to help them talk, a maneuver that seems almost pathognomonic of myasthenia. Neck weakness may be mild or severe enough to cause difficulty in holding the head erect. Limb weakness may be mild or so severe that the patient cannot walk or even turn in bed. Respiratory weakness does not occur alone; ventilatory insufficiency occurs only in severely affected patients and usually in generalized disease, but some patients with oropharyngeal weakness may be unable to breathe unassisted even though limb muscles are strong. Even though weakness fluctuates, a normal neurologic examination is inconsistent with the diagnosis of myasthenia gravis if the patient is symptomatic at the time.

SPECIAL FORMS OF MYASTHENIA

Neonatal Myasthenia. Infants born to myasthenic women may have a transient syndrome of weakness. The most prominent symptom is difficulty in sucking and swallowing. This may be the sole manifestation, or there may also be noticeable reduction in spontaneous movement and in the vigor of the baby's cry. Only rarely is there respiratory difficulty, but unrecognized neonatal myasthenia has been fatal in exceptional cases. The condition can be identified by the intramuscular injection of neostigmine (0.1 to 0.25 mg), followed by improved sucking, a louder cry, better response to the Moro reflex, and

stronger spontaneous movements. Small doses of cholinergic drugs may be administered therapeutically, but more often all that is needed is a nasogastric tube to ensure adequate nutrition. Symptoms subside within a week, or at most, a month.

Congenital Myasthenia. Myasthenia gravis may commence at any age. But there are some children who seem to have had ophthalmoplegia from birth, with or without other signs of myasthenia. Although presumably congenital, this disorder rarely causes concern in the first year of life. It is only later, when the ophthalmoplegia is recognized, that the parents state the child's eyes have always been that way. There may be a disproportionate number of familial cases among children with congenital myasthenia; ophthalmoplegia occurs in almost all of them, and there may be somewhat less tendency for crisis and remission. Otherwise, there are no characteristics that distinguish this syndrome from myasthenia at any other age.

Thyrotoxicosis. About 5 per cent of patients with myasthenia have thyrotoxicosis at some time. Usually the two disorders occur simultaneously, but sometimes hyperthyroidism is evident for weeks or months before there are myasthenic symptoms. Only rarely does myasthenia come first, long before the thyrotoxicosis, and patients who appear euthyroid do not ordinarily have laboratory evidence of thyroid overactivity. Treatment of the two disorders is directed according to the usual indications for each. (There is still talk of a "seesaw" relationship, the myasthenia worsening if the patient is rendered euthyroid; this may have been a consideration years ago when surgery was the only treatment for hyperthyroidism, but it is not important now.)

Diagnosis. In almost all cases the diagnosis of myasthenia is obvious from the history and examination. The diagnosis is immediately confirmed by the response to cholinergic drugs. For adults, 1 ml of edrophonium (10 mg) is given by vein intermittently; after injection of 2 to 3 mg, specific muscle groups are evaluated. If there is no response within 30 seconds, the injection is continued to a total of 6 mg and the patient is evaluated once again. If there is still no response, the remainder is given, a total of 10 mg. This drug is preferred when cranial muscles are being tested because the response is prompt and dramatic. Cranial weakness cannot be simulated voluntarily, and placebo injections are therefore not necessary. If it is desired to evaluate limb strength, the injection of neostigmine has advantages because the effect lasts longer, permitting more leisurely testing. The adult dose is 1.5 mg intramuscularly, and it is usually combined with atropine, 0.5 mg, to avoid the muscarinic symptoms of abdominal cramps and sweating. When limb strength is evaluated, it is sometimes advisable to evaluate placebo responses by giving the atropine 30 minutes before the neostigmine. In all cases of myasthenia gravis there is some response to these drugs, but the response is sometimes slight, and the test may have to be repeated on several occasions to provide convincing evidence.

To provide confirmatory evidence in some cases, the electromyographic response to ulnar nerve stimulation may be studied. The characteristic decline in amplitude of the evoked potential is usually seen in affected muscles, but the response may be normal when the disease is restricted to the eyes. Rarely, it is desirable to administer d-tubocurarine, a drug to which myasthenics are unusually sensitive. There are hazards in the administration of this drug, however, and it should probably be left to research centers; d-tubocurarine should never be given without appropriate precautions to support respiration.

No other laboratory tests provide diagnostic information, but it is useful to perform a standard series of studies. Thymomas can almost always be identified in standard roentgenograms of the chest, supplemented by oblique views. Laminagrams rarely provide more information, and there is little need for thymic venography or mediastinal pneumography as practiced in some centers. Thyroid function should be tested in all myasthenics, and it is useful to evaluate immunologic disorders by serum protein electrophoresis, LE cell preparation, latex fixation test for rheumatoid factor, and antinuclear antibodies. Tests for muscle antibodies or lymphocyte sensitivity are performed in special centers.

The differential diagnosis of myasthenia includes most of neurology, but a few conditions require special consideration. Probably the most frequent error in diagnosis concerns patients with emotional fatigue states and hysterical weakness. There are no cranial muscle symptoms in these patients (except globus hystericus), whereas cranial muscles are involved in virtually all myasthenics. Their symptoms are not those of weakness but of exhaustion, and in tests of strength against resistance there is apt to be marked variation in effort, or dramatic giving way. The diagnosis of myasthenia may be mistakenly made in a patient with botulism. As the discovery of botulism calls for urgent action, for both patient and eating companions, the physician should be aware of this diagnostic pitfall whenever he first sees a patient with apparent myasthenia gravis (see Ch. 23). Amyotrophic lateral sclerosis and peripheral neuropathy may be confused with myasthenia when these disorders affect cranial muscles, but signs indicative of a neurogenic disorder distinguish them from myasthenia. Polymyositis may be confusing, but ocular muscle paresis is not found. There is some debate about the specificity of the therapeutic effect of cholinergic drugs, but for practical purposes it may be taken that an authentic (not placebo), convincing (not equivocal), and reproducible (not seen by one examiner only) effect is found only in myasthenia gravis.

Treatment. *Cholinergic Drug Therapy.* The major drugs used to treat myasthenia gravis are inhibitors of cholinesterase, neostigmine, and pyridostigmine. Another drug, ambenonium, is also used in some clinics, but has no special advantages. It is best to use only one drug; there is no benefit from combinations of two or more. Neostigmine is provided in 15 mg tablets, and pyridostigmine in 60 mg tablets; these are essentially interchangeable. The choice of drug is arbitrary because there is no evidence that the maximal benefit achieved by one is more than that of the other. Most patients, but not all, prefer pyridostigmine because it is less apt to cause abdominal cramps and diarrhea, and it is less apt to cause noticeable peaks and valleys of strength. But these advantages have never been proved objectively, and some patients do very well with neostigmine. Pyridostigmine is also provided in a slow-release capsule (Timespan) of 180 mg, said to provide 60 mg immediately and the remainder in 8 to 12 hours. Some clinicians use the prolonged-action preparation throughout the day, but because of uncertainties of release, it seems advisable to use this only at bedtime for patients who would otherwise have to awaken at night or who are very weak on waking in the morning. (For patients who cannot swallow pills, both drugs may be administered parenterally, and pyridostigmine may be given as a syrup. The intramuscular dose is about one tenth of the oral dose, and the intravenous dose is one thirtieth of the oral dose.) Decisions about optimal dosage are sometimes difficult. Some authorities advocate the use of edrophonium to evaluate oral drug therapy; a test dose of 2 mg is given intravenously. If the patient improves, oral therapy has been too little. If there is aggravation of weakness, oral therapy has been too much. If there is no change, oral therapy has been just right. But other authorities find this test an unreliable guide. If edrophonium is not used, there is nothing but clinical observation to guide the therapist. For mild cases, two tablets of either neostigmine or pyridostigmine three times daily, with meals, is useful. If there is inadequate response, the dose may be increased, first by shortening the interval between doses, then by increasing the quantity of drug with each dose. Problems arise because these drugs never completely reverse symptoms. Therefore the dose should be increased only so long as there is clear-cut response, and it should not be increased beyond the amount giving some perceptible benefit.

The question of proper dosage is important because overtreatment itself can cause weakness; cholinesterase inhibitors may cause a depolarizing block at the neuromuscular junction. How often this happens is a matter of debate among experts, but that it can happen is unquestionable.

Because drugs currently available have limited effect, the search for better agents continues. Drugs advocated as "adjuvants" include potassium chloride, ephedrine, and guanidine; they may have some effect in individual patients, but their true value is unproved.

Steroids and Immunosuppressive Drugs. The use of adrenocorticosteroid drugs in myasthenia has had a curious history. For almost 15 years after the introduction of these agents, they were viewed with skepticism. Then, after a favorable report at an international symposium in 1965, there was an avalanche of confirmations, none the result of controlled trial. These papers appeared in such rapid succession and included such a variety of doses and combinations that it is difficult to make precise recommendations. Corticotrophin (ACTH) is given in short courses (100 units daily or more for 10 to 14 days), sometimes followed by maintenance therapy, 100 units weekly. Because significant worsening may precede the anticipated improvement, this treatment is best reserved for patients with severe myasthenia who already have a tracheostomy in place. Prednisone has been given in doses of 80 to 100 mg daily for variable periods, then gradually tapered. Most recently alternate-day treatment, 100 mg every other day, has been favored, but some investigators omit cholinergic drugs and some continue them. Whether this form of treatment will avoid the steroid-induced weakness or the long-term ill effects of steroids remains to be seen. Other investigators start with small amounts of prednisone and gradually increase. Whether steroid treatment should be used before or after thymectomy is another undecided variable.

A reasonable program starts with thymectomy for patients who are significantly disabled despite cholinergic drug treatment. If there is no further improvement promptly after thymectomy, prednisone is used, 100 mg every other day, for an indefinite period. Because of the possible worsening, the introduction of prednisone should be done with the patient in the controlled setting of a hospital equipped with respiratory care facilities.

The mechanism of action of steroids in myasthenia is not known, but current theories favor an immunosuppressive role. More specific immunosuppressive drugs such as azathioprine, methotrexate, or cyclophosphamide have also been used. There is no indication that these drugs are any better than prednisone, and evaluation of them is probably best performed in research centers.

Surgical Treatment. Thymectomy is followed by significant improvement in about two thirds of patients with myasthenia and no tumor. Patients with thymoma fare worse whether the tumor is excised or not. Chest surgeons, anesthesiologists, and respirator units for postoperative care are now so skillful that the risks of operation are almost negligible, and recent attempts to remove the gland through an incision in the neck rather than by splitting the sternum should reduce the morbidity considerably. Because not all patients improve, and because it is difficult to predict which patients will benefit, there is still some uncertainty in the selection of patients. Some recommend the operation for all patients who are incapacitated in daily living for more than six months despite adequate drug therapy. In preparing patients for operation, their usual oral dosage is continued until the day of operation, then stopped. Endotracheal intubation is used for all patients with oropharyngeal weakness, and intermittent positive pressure breathing is used in the postoperative period. The endotracheal tube may have to be replaced by tracheostomy after a few days, but often tracheostomy can be avoided. Specific drug therapy is withheld for several days, until fever subsides, and then started again at a level of one half or less of the preoperative dose.

Crisis. Patients with myasthenia gravis may suddenly develop difficulty breathing, severe enough to require artificial ventilation. This may be induced by systemic infection or major surgical procedures, but often there is no apparent cause. Patients with oropharyngeal weakness are especially liable to this threat, perhaps because of aspiration. Whenever there is doubt about the need for a tracheostomy, it is best to err on the side of caution and perform it. Increasingly, however, endotracheal intubation is being used for short periods of respiratory support, obviating the need for tracheostomy. The insertion of a cuffed tube makes intermittent positive pressure breathing feasible, and also reduces the hazard of aspiration. Patients are best transferred to a respiratory intensive care unit. Cholinergic drugs are stopped. After several days, usually after fever (an almost inevitable concomitant of crisis and tracheostomy) has started to subside, drugs may be started once again, at half the precrisis dosage. The cause of crisis is not clear, but it is usually transient, and will subside if the patient can be kept alive. The mortality rate of crisis was formerly about 50 per cent, but since the advent of intensive care units, only about 10 per cent die, and these are mostly elderly patients with complicating cardiac and renal disease.

Some patients require assisted ventilation for prolonged periods, some longer than one year. For these patients, trial programs of ACTH or prednisone seem advisable.

Prognosis. The course of myasthenia is variable. The disease may be restricted to ocular muscles for many years, with no threat to life. Other patients are disabled to a variable degree by oropharyngeal or limb weakness, and a few are crippled. Crisis occurs in about 25 per cent of the cases. The over-all mortality is probably about 15 per cent, and although myasthenia itself was formerly the main hazard, intercurrent and unrelated disease is now more often the cause of death.

Elmqvist, D., Hofmann, W. W., Kugelberg, J., and Quastel, D. M. J.: An electrophysiological investigation of neuromuscular transmission in myasthenia gravis. J. Physiol., 174:417, 1964.

Fields, W. S. (ed.): Myasthenia gravis. Ann. N. Y. Acad. Sci., 183:3, 1971.

Flacke, W.: Treatment of myasthenia gravis. N. Engl. J. Med., 288:27, 1973.

Harvey, A. M.: Myasthenia gravis: The first 100 years in perspective. Trans. Am. Clin. Climatol. Assoc., 82:149, 1970.

Namba, T., et al.: Corticotropin therapy in myasthenia gravis: Effects, indications, and limitations. Neurology, 21:1008, 1971.

Osserman, K. A., and Genkins, G.: Studies in myasthenia gravis: Review of a twenty-year experience in over 1200 patients. Mt. Sinai J. Med. N.Y., 38:497, 1971.

Papatestas, A. E., et al.: Studies in myasthenia gravis. Effects of thymectomy. Am. J. Med., 50:465, 1971.

486. EATON-LAMBERT SYNDROME
(Myasthenic Syndrome)

Definition. Eponyms are in disfavor these days, but they are still useful when there is no other satisfactory name for a syndrome and when the eponym pays homage appropriately, without arguments of priority. This syndrome qualifies on both counts. The originators regarded it as "myasthenic" because of a disorder of neuromuscular function, but there are so many important differences from myasthenia gravis that this term may be confusing. The syndrome is defined essentially in terms of electromyography. In the Eaton-Lambert syndrome, the amplitude of the muscle action potential evoked by stimulation of its nerve is markedly reduced, and with repetitive stimulation the action potential is augmented.

Pathogenesis. The first cases were all associated with oat-cell carcinoma of the lung, but cases have been found with other tumors, other diseases, and sometimes with no complicating disorder. Microelectrode studies indicate that the defect is due to impaired release of acetylcholine at the nerve terminals. How the tumor effects this syndrome is not known.

Clinical Manifestations. The first evidence of the Eaton-Lambert syndrome may be prolonged apnea after curarization for surgery. Formal testing with d-tubocurarine also indicates that patients are unduly sensitive. Other patients may have symptoms of limb weakness, but cranial muscle weakness is never prominent. The response to cholinergic drugs is usually equivocal at best. Pain in the limbs may be prominent. Movements may be peculiarly slow. In tests of strength it may seem as though the patient gets stronger with continued effort. Myotatic reflexes are frequently depressed.

Diagnosis. The signs listed above diverge sufficiently from myasthenia to avoid confusion; only limb weakness and curare sensitivity are similar. The remainder of the syndrome resembles polymyositis, and polyneuritis would also have to be considered. The diagnosis is made by electromyography.

Treatment. Under a variety of experimental conditions, guanidine promotes the release of acetylcholine. It was therefore a logical choice to treat this rare syndrome, and the drug is effective in daily doses of 35 mg per kilogram of body weight, given orally. This drug may suppress bone marrow, and appropriate precautions should be taken.

Eaton, L. M., and Lambert, E. H.: Electromyography and electric stimulation of nerves in diseases of motor unit: Observations in myasthenic syndrome associated with malignant tumors, J.A.M.A., 163:1117, 1957.
Elmqvist, D., and Lambert, E. H.: Detailed analysis of neuromuscular transmission in a patient with myasthenic syndrome sometimes associated with brochogenic carcinoma. Mayo Clin. Proc., 43:689, 1968.

487. UNUSUAL CAUSES OF NEUROMUSCULAR BLOCK

Botulism and *tick paralysis* are described in Ch. 23 and 51. Both cause a syndrome of flaccid quadriplegia with paresis of cranial muscles, and must be differentiated from polyneuritis, myasthenia gravis, and periodic paralysis. In neither is there a sensory disorder, but autonomic fibers may be affected in botulism, especially pupilloconstrictor fibers (resulting in a dilated, fixed pupil). The physiologic disorder in both syndromes is impaired release of acetylcholine from motor nerve terminals. The electromyogram in botulism may resemble that in the Eaton-Lambert syndrome, an observation that may be diagnostically important. Guanidine has been used with benefit to treat botulism and might also be effective in tick paralysis. Supportive therapy (tracheostomy and assisted respiration) is mandatory in severe cases. Tick paralysis is reversed by removal of the organism.

Several *aminoglycoside antimicrobial drugs* interfere with the release of acetylcholine, and may cause clinical syndromes in man. The offending drugs include neomycin, streptomycin, colistin, polymyxin, and kanamycin. The most common manifestation is postoperative apnea without other evidence of paralysis. This is most apt to occur in patients with renal failure, presumably with unusually high blood levels of the antimicrobial drug. In occasional cases, however, there may be flaccid quadriplegia. Administration of calcium and guanidine may be helpful, but the essence of management is supportive treatment and use of a safer antimicrobial.

Cherington, M., and Ryan, D. W.: Botulism and guanidine. N. Engl. J. Med., 278:931, 1968.
de Jesus, P. V., Slater, R., Spitz, L. K., and Penn, A. S.: Neuromuscular physiology of wound botulism. Arch. Neurol., 29:425, 1973.
McQuillen, M. P., Cantor, H. E., and O'Rourke, J. R.: Myasthenic syndrome associated with antibiotics. Arch. Neurol., 18:402, 1968.

488. SYNDROMES OF MUSCULAR OVERACTIVITY: CRAMPS AND RELATED DISORDERS

Cramps, caused by painful, abrupt shortening of muscle, affect almost everyone at some time or other. Electromyographic investigation indicates that motor units fire at a rate of about 300 per second, much higher than the most vigorous voluntary contraction. It is presumably the high rate of discharge that causes the palpable muscle tautness and the pain. Anyone who has had more than one cramp knows that the pain can be relieved by stretching the affected muscle, or by massage. The stimulus responsible for cramps is not known; relief by stretching suggests that some central mechanism is involved, since this is the stimulus for receptors in muscle that inhibit discharge of the motor neuron to the same muscle. Certain conditions are known to be associated with a propensity to cramps: denervation (especially amyotrophic lateral sclerosis), pregnancy, and electrolyte disorders (especially water intoxication and hyponatremia). Some people are more susceptible than others for reasons which are not known. Sometimes cramps occur only at night, and can be prevented by quinine sulfate, 0.3 gram orally at bedtime. Sometimes cramps occur frequently during the day, occasionally so often that the individual is effectively crippled. Diphenylhydantoin, 0.3 to 0.6 gram daily, may be helpful to these patients, but some are resistant to this and to other drugs that may be tried, including diazepam and procainamide.

Tetany is a special form of cramp, identified by its predilection for flexor muscles of the hand and fingers, its association with laryngospasm, and its relationship to hypocalcemia. Tetany can be painful. It differs from other cramps electromyographically because of the characteristic rhythmic grouping of discharging potentials.

Contracture is the term reserved for the painful shortening of muscles in glycogen storage diseases, in which the muscles are electrically silent although maximally shortened.

Myokymia has been used to describe a variety of apparently different disorders characterized by cramps in association with spontaneous twitching of muscle. In some cases there are prolonged trains of spontaneous potentials, whereas in others there is grouping of potentials. Some of these patients have difficulty in relaxing grip, but, unlike myotonia, the muscular activity is abolished by neuromuscular blocking agents, indicating a neural rather than a muscular origin. Hyperhidrosis is prominent in some patients and is secondary to the increased muscular activity.

Continuous shortening of the muscle would lead to abnormal postures and abnormally increased resistance to passive movement. These abnormalities, of course, are often due to central neurologic disorders. In recent years, however, an increasing number of patients have been described because of fluctuating rigidity of axial and limb muscles. For want of a better name, and lacking understanding of the pathogenesis, this has been called the *stiff man syndrome.* The diagnosis requires that there be no signs of cerebral or spinal cord disease, and there must be continuous electromyographic activity despite authentic attempts to relax. Ordinary cramps may be superimposed upon the persistent stiffness. Diazepam, 30 to 60 mg daily, may bring dramatic relief.

A variety of other names have been applied to these syndromes, including *quantal squander, armadillo disease, neuromyotonia,* and *continuous muscle fiber activity.* Some cases of brief duration may be related to mild cases of tetanus. It will take some time to sort out the variety of causes. If these unusual forms can be analyzed, we may yet understand why an otherwise normal individual occasionally has a cramp.

Editorial: Writer's cramp. Br. Med. J., 1:67, 1972.
Garner-Medwin, D., and Walton, J. N.: Myokymia with impaired muscular relaxation. Lancet, 1:127, 1969.
Geschwind, N.: Skeletal muscle cramps. J. Clin. Pharm. Therap., 5:859, 1964.
Gordon, E. E., Januszko, D. M., and Kaufman, L.: A critical survey of stiff man syndrome. Am. J. Med. 42:582, 1967.
Layzer, R. B., and Rowland, L. P.: Cramps. N. Engl. J. Med., 285:31, 1971.
Wallis, W. E., Van Poznak, A., and Plum, F.: Generalized muscular stiffness, fasciculations and myokymia of peripheral nerve origin. Arch. Neurol., 22:430, 1970.

Part XI
RESPIRATORY DISEASE

489. INTRODUCTION

M. Henry Williams, Jr.

In recent years, there have been dramatic changes in the field of chest medicine. New techniques, advances in therapy, and awareness of new diseases have changed and greatly increased the demands upon the knowledge and skill of both internist and pulmonary specialist.

Major advances have been made in the treatment of tuberculosis. Modern chemotherapy has led to substantial decrease of morbidity and mortality and has made it possible to treat the disease successfully on an ambulatory basis. Nevertheless, tuberculosis remains prevalent in the large cities, and it is apparent that many social and personal factors are important in its pathogenesis and in response to therapy. In treating tuberculosis the physician must concern himself with the frequently coexistent problems of alcoholism, drug addiction, and, particularly, failure of the patient to take prescribed medication regularly and for a sufficient period. Because the treatment of tuberculosis belongs rightfully within the province of the internist, because it should be treated as an infection in general hospitals instead of in sanatoriums, and because it still ranks as a major cause of undiagnosed febrile, pulmonary, or hematologic disease, the practicing physician must be thoroughly familiar with its manifestations and with the principles of therapy. This disease is discussed in detail in Ch. 227.

Pneumonia also remains a common problem in medical practice, and the mortality among patients sick enough to be hospitalized is still distressingly high, despite antimicrobial therapy. Pneumococcal infection is the most common cause of pneumonia, but infections with Staphylococcus, Klebsiella, and other organisms are sufficiently frequent and the proper choice and use of antimicrobial drugs is so important that the physician must be familiar with the clinical features of the different infections (see Ch. 175, Ch. 179 to 183 inclusive, Ch. 188, and Ch. 195).

In particular, he must be skilled in obtaining and interpreting sputum smears so as to institute appropriate therapy at the earliest possible moment and to avoid the use of unnecessary drugs.

Lung cancer and chronic obstructive pulmonary disease (COPD), discussed in detail in Ch. 540 and Ch. 502 to 507, respectively, have both emerged as major health problems during the past two decades. Treatment is far from satisfactory for either. The physician can provide some measure of comfort to the patient with COPD, can successfully treat life-threatening episodes of ventilatory failure, and by discriminating radiographic study can select an occasional patient whose cancer can be resected. Nevertheless, hope for cure of these diseases is bleak, and efforts must be directed at prevention, especially by combating cigarette smoking.

The interstitial pneumonias and alveolar proteinosis are some of the newly described diseases with which the physician must now be familiar, and they are discussed in Ch. 520. Sarcoidosis, particularly as manifested by asymptomatic hilar adenopathy, has emerged as an extremely common disease, rivaling tuberculosis in prevalence in many places. Although sarcoidosis commonly involves the lung and hilar lymph nodes, it can involve any organ of the body; it is discussed in Ch. 102.

The organization of Part XI has been based partly on common anatomic features (bellows, airways, air spaces, lung parenchyma, pleura, and pulmonary circulation) and partly on common clinical features (irritants and neoplasm). Major emphasis is placed on principles of pathophysiology; diseases which have been well studied and which illustrate important principles have received special emphasis.

Evaluation and treatment of respiratory disease requires an understanding of pulmonary physiology and of the meaning and value of tests of pulmonary function. Section One (Ch. 490 to 497), which concerns pulmonary structure and function, is not a complete exposition of anatomy and physiology, but it is designed to build on a framework of basic knowledge and to relate the basic material to clinical phenomena. The purpose of Section One is to emphasize pulmonary physiology as it relates to clinical medicine, to refresh the reader about important physiologic principles, and to bridge the gap between the basic text and the clinical problem. In addition to understanding how the lung works, the physician should know when and why to perform various tests. Serial studies of arterial blood gas composition are essential to the appropriate management of ventilatory failure; measurement of peak expiratory flow provides useful, moment-to-moment evaluation of the patient with asthma; spirographic measurement is as much a part of the evaluation of the chest patient as an electrocardiogram is part of the evaluation of the cardiac patient; and a measurement of diffusing capacity may be the only clue to the presence or extent of diffuse interstitial pulmonary disease. Abnormalities of pulmonary function have differing degrees of therapeutic urgency. Arterial oxygen unsaturation is a potentially lethal condition which requires treatment, whereas impaired diffusion is seldom of consequence to the patient, but knowledge of its presence is vital for accurate diagnosis and prognosis.

A number of clinical problems and diagnostic techniques cut across the material presented here and elsewhere. The emergence of respiratory failure as a common problem requiring skilled, intensive therapy warrants a separate chapter on the subject (Ch. 507), but it is also a serious complication of many types of neuromuscular disease, and is discussed in Part X as well as here under COPD. Hemoptysis is a significant clinical entity requiring appropriate diagnostic study and management (see Ch. 227, 516, and 540). The physician must be familiar with the specific physical findings in each illness, but today it is even more important to have a working familiarity with the x-ray film of the chest. Every patient with pulmonary disease should have an anteroposterior, lateral, and apical lordotic film, and the physician should know when to request oblique views, tomograms, bronchograms, and angiograms and how to evaluate localized and diffuse densities when they are present. Specialized procedures, such as needle biopsy of lung and pleura and, now, bronchoscopy, are important tools for the chest physician, who should also be aware of the value, limitations, and risks of bronchography, me-

diastinoscopy, and thoracic surgery. As in all medicine, the risk and discomfort of a thoracic diagnostic procedure must be balanced carefully against the likelihood of obtaining useful and important information.

Section One. STRUCTURE AND FUNCTION

490. INTRODUCTION

M. Henry Williams, Jr.

The primary function of the lung is the exchange of respiratory gases—the elimination of carbon dioxide and the uptake of oxygen. The actual gas exchange occurs in the alveoli and is governed by the physical laws which govern the diffusion of gases. In order for gas exchange to occur and for arterial blood gas composition to be maintained at normal, the alveolar gas composition must be kept constant and normal despite the continuing extraction of oxygen and addition of carbon dioxide. This is achieved by periodic ventilation of the alveolar gas with fresh air containing 21 per cent oxygen and essentially no carbon dioxide. Closely related to this primary function is the maintenance of a normal partial pressure of oxygen and of carbon dioxide in the arterial blood. For this system to operate successfully, all the blood perfusing the tissues must come from the lung, and all the blood leaving the tissues must be pumped to the lung for repletion of oxygen and removal of carbon dioxide.

Since all the blood leaving the cells is pumped through the lungs, the pulmonary cells and capillaries are subject to assault by a variety of potentially noxious materials: blood clots, foreign proteins, and other toxins. Mechanisms must be present to deal with these insults. Likewise, the air which ventilates the alveoli may contain organic and inorganic materials which are capable of producing disease, and the lung must maintain an effective defense against these invaders. In addition, the lung itself is an organ that must remain viable and maintain itself by cellular replication and other metabolic functions. Although the following chapters are organized around consideration of the primary, gas-exchanging function of the lung, mention will be made of important metabolic functions as well as of the structural characteristics of the system which are essential to its proper functioning.

In studying pulmonary function, physiologists have developed a battery of tests which have proved useful to the physician. Sometimes these tests provide direct and critical insight into pathophysiologic processes; they often shed light on the ways in which the primary function of the lung is faulty, but even more often provide quantitative information of clinical significance even when the over-all function of the system remains adequate to maintain normal arterial blood gas composition.

491. VENTILATORY FUNCTION

M. Henry Williams, Jr.

LUNG VOLUMES, PLEURAL PRESSURE, AND THE RESPIRATORY CYCLE

The most obvious and easily measured aspect of pulmonary function is ventilatory function. Inspiration con-

sists in the enlargement of the thorax by contraction of the diaphragm and intercostal muscles. By forceful contraction of inspiratory muscles, it is possible to inspire considerably more air than the tidal volume. Chest expansion is limited largely by the structural, fibrous restraints within the lung parenchyma. Measurement of the *total lung capacity* (TLC), the volume of air in the lung at the end of a maximal inspiration, provides useful clinical information. In some patients with emphysema, destruction of lung tissue and reduced resistance to lung expansion is associated with an increased TLC. Reduction of the TLC results from imperfect function of the thoracic bellows (chest deformity, pleural disease, muscle paralysis), from increased resistance of the lung to stretch (pulmonary fibrosis), or from diseases in which air-containing tissue is replaced by abnormal tissue (inflammation, neoplasia, or granulomatous disease).

Expiration is largely the result of the passive recoil of the lung which becomes greater as the lung is stretched by an inspiration. The tendency of the lung to collapse is counterbalanced by the tendency of the thoracic cage to enlarge. As the lung empties and gets smaller, its elastic recoil becomes less, whereas the outward recoil of the thorax increases. When these opposing forces become equal, expiration ends. The lung volume at which this occurs, the *functional residual capacity* (FRC), is determined by the mechanical properties of the lung and the thorax. Increased retractive force of the lung or decreased retractive force of the thorax causes reduction of the FRC, whereas reduced retractive force of the lung or increased retractive force of the thorax leads to an increase of the FRC. The inherent tendency of the lung to collapse at all volumes above residual is responsible for the negative intrapleural pressure, the magnitude of

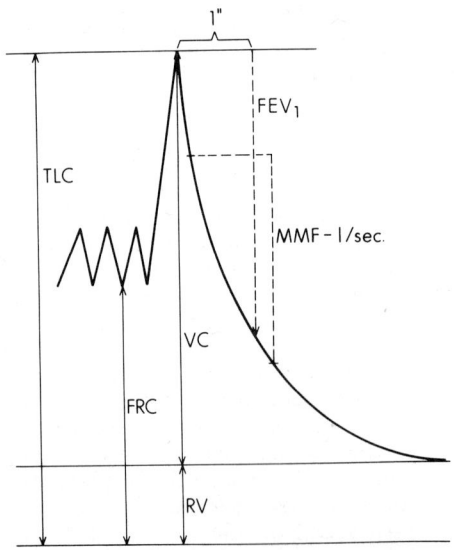

Schematic representation of lung volumes and a maximal forced expiration with depiction of one-second forced expiratory volume (FEV₁) and maximal midexpiratory flow rate (MMF).

which is directly proportional to the lung volume. Normally the pleural pressure is minus 2 cm H_2O at FRC, decreasing to minus 6 cm H_2O at the end of an inspiration and to less than minus 20 cm H_2O at TLC. Although the pleural pressure is always negative, the alveolar pressure is atmospheric at the end of inspiration and of expiration. During inspiration, enlargement of the thorax generates additional negative intrapleural pressure which, transmitted to the alveoli, causes air to enter the lung. The opposite occurs during expiration when the tendency of the chest to collapse makes the intrapleural pressure less negative and the alveolar pressure positive so that air leaves the lung.

By forceful contraction of expiratory muscles, additional air can be expelled from the lung. Forced expiration is limited by airway closure, by loss of lung recoil, or by weakness of the muscles of expiration. Generally, however, an increase of residual volume (RV), the volume of air left in the lung after maximal expiration, signifies airway obstruction. The *vital capacity* is the maximal volume of air expired from full inspiration and is one of the oldest and most useful indices of pulmonary function. It is determined by the total lung capacity and by the degree to which the lung can be emptied. The vital capacity is reduced in patients whose respiratory muscle strength is abnormal, in patients in whom the lung is rendered indistensible by fibrous tissue or by chest wall deformity, in patients whose air-containing tissue is replaced by tumor or inflammatory disease, and in patients with obstructive disease leading to complete occlusion of airways at an increased residual volume.

EXPIRATORY FLOW RATES AND LUNG MECHANICS

The dimensions of the conducting system through which air must move in and out of the lung are so large that inspiration and expiration can be accomplished easily and quickly. In various types of obstructive pulmonary disease, the airways become so narrow as to limit the rate of air flow into and out of the lung. This impairment is easily assessed by spirometry, which involves recording inspiration and expiration as the patient breathes in and out of a cannister or bellows (see accompanying figure). Obstruction to air flow is particularly obvious during expiration, both because the diameters of the airways narrow as lung volume becomes smaller and because the positive intrapleural pressure which tends to drive air from the lungs during a forced expiration also tends to collapse the conducting airways. As a result, attention is generally focused on air flow during a forced expiration. Useful indices of airway obstruction include the *timed vital capacity,* the percentage of the total which can be expired in one, two, and three seconds (normally at least 70, 85, and 95 per cent), and the volume of air expired in the first second, the *forced expiratory volume* (FEV_1), or during the middle half of expiration, the *maximal midexpiratory flow rate* (MMF: normal 2 to 4 liters per second). Patients with chronic obstructive pulmonary disease always have an MMF below 1 liter per second, and generally below 0.5 liter per second. In these patients the MMF is relatively constant and little improved by administration of a bronchodilator. In patients with bronchial asthma, the MMF may or may not be very low, and when low generally increases with therapy.

The *peak expiratory flow rate* (PEFR) is a very simple and convenient method of evaluating ventilatory function, particularly when one wishes to obtain frequent serial measurements, as in asthma. The PEFR is measured by having the patient inspire maximally and then expire as forcefully as possible into a portable meter which registers the maximal velocity of air flow. Since this is achieved early during the forced expiration, the patient need not empty his lungs completely, but he must fill his lungs at the start and employ maximal expiratory effort. Normally, the PEFR exceeds 400 liters per minute, and in asthma associated with such severe airway obstruction as to cause death from asphyxia the PEFR is less than 80 liters per minute. In general, asthmatic patients with a PEFR less than 120 liters per minute should be considered seriously ill and in need of constant medical attention.

The presence of audible rhonchi and wheezes signifies turbulent air flow, suggesting the presence of obstructive disease, and the physician can obtain a semiquantitative index of the problem by timing the duration of a forced vital capacity by listening over the larynx. By measuring intrapleural (esophageal) pressure, and simultaneously recording the air flow at the mouth, the physiologist can obtain more precise measurements of respiratory mechanics. *Lung compliance,* defined as change of volume per change of pressure, is an index of the mechanical properties of the lung, and *airway resistance,* defined as the pressure required to generate flow through the airways, is an index of the dimensions of the tracheobronchial tree. Both these measurements vary with lung volume, the lung becoming stiff (less compliant) as it is inflated and the airways becoming wider and less resistant to flow as the lung volume increases. Although these measurements provide interesting information, a study of expiratory flow rates and vital capacity generally provides adequate clinical assessment of restrictive and obstructive disease so that the more precise measurements are seldom necessary.

INSPIRATORY FLOW RATE

Fixed narrowing of airways, particularly of the extrathoracic trachea and larynx, produces just as much impedance to inspiration as to expiration. Lesions such as vocal cord paralysis and tracheal stenosis characteristically cause similar reductions of inspiratory and expiratory flow rates and are easily detected on spirometry. Patients with this type of obstruction may be surprisingly asymptomatic, since dyspnea in obstructive pulmonary disease appears to result from the extreme narrowing and closure of airways that occur during expiration, and a fixed degree of obstruction may cause significant increase of the work of inspiration without extreme expiratory limitation. This may result in hypercapnia, predominantly related to the inspiratory work cost of breathing, and measurement of inspiratory flow rates is strongly indicated in the patient with unexplained elevation of the arterial P_{CO_2}.

MINUTE VENTILATION

Measurements of the lung volumes, expiratory flow rates, and lung mechanics provide useful information about the respiratory system. They do not, however, indicate whether or not the minute ventilation is normal. Patients with severe abnormality of lung volumes or mechanics may or may not have reduced ventilation. The effectiveness of ventilatory function must be considered in terms of the purpose of the minute ventilation, which is to add oxygen to the alveolar air and to remove carbon dioxide in accordance with the metabolic needs of the body. The ventilation is regulated to meet these metabolic needs by maintaining a normal alveolar gas composition: a P_{CO_2} of 40 mm Hg and a P_{O_2} of 100 mm Hg. Increased metabolic rate, as in fever or muscular exercise, is matched by an appropriate increase of ventilation so that alveolar gas composition remains constant. Under a variety of conditions, to be discussed subsequently, ventilation may not be maintained at the appropriate level, resulting in increase of alveolar P_{CO_2} and a decrease of alveolar P_{O_2}. It should be emphasized that the alveolar P_{CO_2} and the arterial P_{CO_2}, which are essentially identical, actually measure the effectiveness of ventilation. Hypercapnia indicates that ventilation is reduced, and hypocapnia means that ventilation is increased in relationship to metabolic needs.

The alveolar P_{O_2} also reflects the level of ventilation, a high P_{O_2} indicating hyperventilation and a low P_{O_2} hypoventilation. Hyperventilation will cause the alveolar P_{O_2} to be elevated about as much above 100 mm Hg as the P_{CO_2} is reduced below 40 mm Hg, and in hypoventilation the P_{O_2} will be as much below 100 mm Hg as the P_{CO_2} is above 40 mm Hg. However, alveolar gas is often neither uniform nor measurable, and assessment of hypoventilation is best based on arterial blood measurements. Since many abnormalities can cause reduction of arterial P_{O_2} but not hypercapnia, adequacy of ventilation is best assessed by the arterial P_{CO_2}.

Although the clinician may form some conclusions about ventilatory function by listening to the breath sounds generated by movement of air in and out of the lungs and by observation of the movement of the chest cage, these observations are grossly inexact, and accurate assessment of total ventilation requires a measurement of tidal volume and respiratory rate. Evaluation of the adequacy of the ventilation, which depends upon the size of the physiologic dead space (see Ch. 493) as well as the minute ventilation, requires a measurement of arterial P_{CO_2}.

ALVEOLAR VOLUME

Although gas exchange actually occurs across the walls of individual alveoli, the basic unit of the lung is now considered to be the acinus, the alveolar ducts and alveoli supplied by a terminal bronchiole. This unit of respiratory function is ventilated with each inspiration, and the air spaces are so small as to allow practically instantaneous diffusion of gases within the unit so that alveolar gas composition is essentially uniform throughout. Indeed, alveolar "ventilation" is largely the result of diffusion of gas molecules within the small airways and alveoli, and is not due to mass movement of air much beyond the large bronchi. Only a small portion of the lung volume within the acinus is actually turned over with each breath. The existence of a large alveolar volume, even at the end of a maximal expiration, may be considered to be a homeostatic adjustment to the fact that gas exchange across the alveolar capillaries is continuous, whereas ventilation is discontinuous—fresh air

enters the alveoli only during inspiration. If the volume of the unit were not large compared to the amount of gas exchanged, the alveolar P_{O_2} would fall and the alveolar P_{CO_2} would rise from the end of one inspiration until the beginning of the next, and there would be large fluctuations of arterial blood gas composition. Thus one may consider that the function of the lung volume is to maintain constancy of the alveolar and arterial blood gas composition throughout the respiratory cycle.

RESPIRATORY CONTROL

Respiration serves several purposes, including metabolic gas exchange, communication, and heat regulation. In addition, the respiratory system is endowed with a number of protective reflexes, some of which influence the respiratory rate and depth; others induce coughing, sneezing, and yawning. The principal integration and regulation of these several functions are achieved by respiratory neurons located in the medulla oblongata and lower pons. This "respiratory center" is, in turn, influenced by structures at higher levels of the nervous system as well as by changes in its local chemical environment. In the metabolic regulation of ventilation, priority is awarded to the maintenance of a normal P_{CO_2}. Increased arterial P_{CO_2} leads to increase of the P_{CO_2} within tissue fluids and, hence, to a decreased pH within the chemosensitive neurons of the respiratory center. This is followed by increased respiratory activity. The resultant increase of ventilation causes decreased P_{CO_2} and, hence, decreased respiratory drive. This feedback control system maintains the arterial P_{CO_2} within narrow limits unless there is gross disturbance of the effector system (the lungs and the chest cage) or of the respiratory center itself. In addition, chemosensitive arterial receptors respond to hypercapnia, to an increased hydrogen ion concentration, and to hypoxia, the last accounting for the mild hyperventilation which exists at altitude or in subjects with hypoxemia. This is generally considered to be an emergency mechanism, and it plays little part in normal regulation of ventilation. A variety of reflex pathways also exist in lungs and other tissues which directly or indirectly affect respiration. Of these the most important clinically are afferent stimuli from pulmonary vessels stretched by pulmonary hypertension or from lungs stiffened by edema, fibrosis, or granulomatous disease.

Increased respiratory drive in excess of CO_2-determined stimulation leads to increased ventilation and hypocapnia. Decreased respiratory drive causes hypoventilation and hypercapnia and is usually the result of depressant drugs or impaired mechanical performance of the lung and chest bellows so that extra muscular effort is needed to achieve a given minute ventilation.

A clear distinction should be made between hyperventilation and dyspnea. The latter is the patient's *subjective awareness* of respiratory discomfort. This symptom, which is present in many diseases, may have as its physiologic basis an inappropriate shortening of respiratory muscle fibers in response to respiratory need. Respiratory need is determined by all the chemical and nervous stimuli to respiration and cannot be measured. However, one can measure the mechanical properties of the lung and ascertain that excessive muscular effort is being spent on the act of ventilation or that excessive ventilation is indeed taking place, in which case the patient might be "entitled" to dyspnea. But beyond that, the subjective nature of the symptom, attenuated and amplified by emotional factors, precludes quantitative assessment.

492. ABNORMALITIES IN RESPIRATORY CONTROL

Fred Plum

Neurologic or neuromuscular disorders frequently produce breathing abnormalities. Diseases of the cerebrum or upper brainstem commonly induce disturbances in the respiratory rate and rhythm which do not interfere with gas exchange. Diseases of the lower brainstem, spinal cord, nerve, or muscles can produce respiratory failure, and this is often the most serious aspect of such illnesses.

Abnormal Respiratory Rhythms in Neurologic Disease. The abnormal, irregular breathing rhythm of medullary disease is discussed below.

Patients with disease at upper pontine or low midbrain levels sometimes show *central neurogenic hyperventilation.* Such patients are usually in stupor or coma, and their metronomically regular hyperpnea must be distinguished from the other causes of hyperpnea listed in Table 1.

Cheyne-Stokes respiration is a regularly oscillating pattern of respiratory rhythm in which hyperpneic and apneic periods alternate, one full cycle requiring twice the circulation time. Usually such periodic breathing reflects bilateral neurologic damage at subcortical or diencephalic brain levels. Occasionally, particularly when the hyperpneic phase is brief and the apneic phase relatively long, periodic breathing can be a manifestation of severe lower brainstem injury at pontine levels.

Respiratory Failure in Neurologic Disease. Neurologic or muscular disease may cause either peripheral or central respiratory failure.

Peripheral respiratory failure results when the skeletal musculature of the diaphragm, chest wall, abdomen, and neck becomes so weakened that the chest bellows cannot move sufficient air to ventilate the lungs. Potential causes of peripheral respiratory failure are listed in Table 2; those that are most frequent or tend to create medical emergencies are marked with an asterisk.

The symptoms of peripheral respiratory failure depend partly upon which muscles are affected first. Patients suffering progressive paralysis of chest wall or abdomen

TABLE 1. Conditions Causing Hyperpnea with Stupor or Coma

Respiratory Alkalosis	Metabolic Acidosis
Central neurogenic hyper-ventilation:	Diabetic coma
Brainstem infarcts	Uremia
Secondary brainstem compression	Ingested organic acids
	Methyl alcohol
Severe hypoglycemia	Ethylene glycol
Acute anoxia	
Hepatic coma	
Salicylate poisoning (adult)	
Sepsis	

TABLE 2. The Neurologic Causes of Respiratory Failure

A. *Peripheral*

  I. Diseases of the respiratory muscles
    Progressive muscular dystrophy
    Myotonic muscular dystrophy
    Polymyositis
  II. Diseases and disorders of the myoneural junction
    Myasthenia gravis*
    Botulism*
    Anticholinesterase poisons* (parathione, DFP etc.)
    Hypersensitivity to curare in patients with pseudomyasthenia (malignancy)
  III. Peripheral neuropathies
    Guillain-Barré syndrome*
    Diphtheria
    Acute intermittent porphyria
  IV. Anterior horn cell diseases
    Poliomyelitis*
    Amyotrophic lateral sclerosis
  V. Lesions of the spinal conducting pathways
    High cervical trauma*
    Acute myelitis
    High spinal compression or malignancy

B. *Central*

  I. Infections
    Encephalitic poliomyelitis
    Postexanthematous or disseminated encephalomyelitis
  II. Trauma, brainstem hemorrhage, or neoplasm (rare)
    Craniovertebral abnormalities
  III. Drug depression
    Barbiturates
    Opiates
    Other depressants

may have few symptoms until their diaphragms are involved, at which time no respiratory reserves are left. On the other hand, patients whose diaphragms are paralyzed first may feel breathless almost immediately. Those who need to cough may become incapacitated rapidly if they lose their abdominal muscles. These considerations imply that whenever faced with the diseases listed in Table 2, the alert physician must evaluate respiratory function, using serial vital capacity measurements to estimate the quantitative functional impact of paralysis. Gross indices of respiratory function such as attention to respiratory rate, inspecting the apparent magnitude of chest expansion, and checking for dyspnea usually are unreliable. Patients with acute peripheral respiratory failure almost never become anoxemic or hypocarbic until ready to collapse, so that therapy, to be effective, must be started before cyanosis appears or abnormalities appear in blood gases.

Central respiratory failure results when the respiratory integrating neurons in the medulla oblongata become damaged or diseased. Common causes are listed in Table 2. Central respiratory failure produces defects in the respiratory rate and rhythm, and symptoms usually evolve through progressive stages. At first, a subtle respiratory irregularity appears, which is most pronounced during drowsiness or rest. Patients may report that it is impossible to sleep or that they must concentrate on the breathing act. By this time, the pattern of breathing may be frankly irregular. In those with drug-induced depression, the respiratory rate is slow and the volume shallow; intermittent, irregular apneic periods may occur. Respiratory sensitivity to carbon dioxide is reduced, and anoxia or CO_2 retention may develop unless treatment is instituted. By this point, progressive failure and decompensation are usually rapid.

The treatment of respiratory failure is artificial respiration. There are many satisfactory respirators. Both the "iron lung" and positive-pressure types create intrapulmonary pressures that cyclically exceed external pressures on the chest. However, individual models vary widely, and the physician would do well to familiarize himself with available devices before trying to use them in emergencies. When treating respiratory failure, careful and constant attention is required to see that the airway is unobstructed. If there is any doubt, tracheostomy should be performed.

Bendixin, H. H., Egbert, L. D., Hedley-Whyte, J., Laver, M. B., and Pontoppidan, H.: Respiratory Care. St. Louis, C. V. Mosby Company, 1965.
Campbell, E. J. M., Agostini, E., and Newsom Davis, J.: The Respiratory Muscles. London, Lloyd-Luke, 1970.
Plum, F.: The neurologic integration of behavioral and metabolic control of breathing. In Porter, R. (ed.): Ciba Foundation Symposium: Breathing. Hering Breuer Centenary Symposium. Boston, Little, Brown & Company, 1970.

493. CONDUCTING AIRWAYS

M. Henry Williams, Jr.

The airways leading to the acini are tubes which branch by irregular dichotomy and provide increasing surface area at each branching. As a result, the highest resistance to flow through the conduction system occurs in the major bronchi and trachea, the smaller airways actually contributing relatively little resistance to airflow. Narrowing of the large bronchi has more effect on expiratory air flow than a similar narrowing of peripheral bronchioles, and a patient must develop widespread occlusive disease of peripheral airways before symptoms of chronic obstructive disease develop.

The airways are designed to conduct tidal volume in and out of the alveoli, and their size must represent a compromise between a large surface for conducting air with little resistance and a minimal dead space, the latter being that portion of the inspired air which remains in the airways and is not available for gas exchange. Normally about a third of each breath is so wasted. The *physiologic dead space* is measured by relating the expired to the arterial carbon dioxide tension, the difference between the two being essentially a measure of the amount of dead space air which dilutes the alveolar gas to form the expired air. Measurement of physiologic dead space is useful in determining total ventilatory requirements of a patient. The measurement also has clinical value, since an increase of physiologic dead space rarely stems from increased volume of the conducting airways but, rather, reflects ventilation of alveoli which are not perfused with blood. Air going to such units remains unaltered in composition and is wasted ventilation. The physiologic dead space is extremely variable, even in a single subject, but is closely related to the tidal volume, and the ratio of dead space to tidal volume (V_D/V_T) is essentially constant. This ratio is normally less than 0.30, and increase or decrease signifies worsen-

ing or improvement of matching of ventilation to perfusion.

Because, as mentioned above, inspired air contains a variety of inorganic and organic pollutants which may settle anywhere along the tracheobronchial tree, mechanisms must be present to remove these potential pathogens from the lungs. The bronchial mucus, secreted by goblet cells and mucous glands, serves this function. The mucus is propelled up the tracheobronchial tree by the constant beating of cilia. Any material which settles on the airways, or is brought there by alveolar macrophages, is carried up this mucous escalator to the mouth and is expectorated or swallowed. Normally, about 100 ml of mucus is produced per day, and this amount is greatly increased in those exposed to air pollution, particularly cigarette smoke. Excessive secretion of mucus, which is accompanied by morphologic evidence of hypertrophied mucous glands, is the cardinal symptom of chronic bronchitis.

494. ALVEOLAR STRUCTURE AND FUNCTION

M. Henry Williams, Jr.

DIFFUSION

The actual process of gas exchange takes place in the 300 million alveoli. The alveolar wall consists of a thin epithelial lining separating the air space from the pulmonary capillary. The design of the structure provides maximal exposure of circulating blood to alveolar gas over some 80 square meters of surface area and through a minimal layer of separating tissue. This permits such rapid diffusion of gases that, in normal subjects, there is no discernible difference between the partial pressure of oxygen in the alveolar air and in the blood leaving the alveolar capillary. In patients with extensive loss or thickening of this diffusion surface, by emphysema or inflammatory disease respectively, diffusion may be imperfect, leading to measurable reduction of the end-capillary P_{O_2}. It is rare for this impairment to be so severe as to cause detectable unsaturation of arterial blood. As carbon dioxide is 20 to 30 times as "diffusible" as oxygen, hypercapnia is never a result of diffusion impairment. Although diffusion is rarely a cause of blood gas abnormality, measurement of the *diffusing capacity* of the lung is a very useful index of pulmonary structure and function. In many patients with diffuse lung disease, reduction of the diffusing capacity may be the only indication that parenchymal disease is present, and the measurement provides useful information about prognosis and the effects of therapy.

METABOLIC FUNCTION

The alveolar walls are not dry, but are lined by a complex substance, *surfactant*, which has the property of reducing surface tension, particularly at small lung volumes when the high surface tension would tend to collapse the small alveoli into larger units with correspondingly lower internal pressure. This surfactant is undoubtedly important in maintaining stability of alveolar structure and in preventing atelectasis, but the role of surfactant deficiency in human disease is uncertain. The surface-active material is apparently synthesized by alveolar lining cells, one of the many metabolic functions of the lung that are essential to maintenance of its functional integrity.

VENTILATION-PERFUSION RELATIONSHIPS

One of the extraordinary features of pulmonary function is the correspondence between ventilation and circulation in individual lung units. Although there is considerable variation of ventilation to various parts of the lung, the upper lobes receiving less than the lower, normally there is, in general, a matching of perfusion so that the well-ventilated units receive more circulation than those that are poorly ventilated. This is very important, since ventilation of nonperfused lung would be wasted dead-space ventilation, and perfusion of nonventilated lung would, in effect, constitute a right-to-left shunt of venous blood through the lung. Imbalance of ventilation and perfusion is common in chronic pulmonary disease and, indeed, represents the major cause of arterial unsaturation (see Ch. 497). A number of mechanisms provide for the matching of ventilation and diffusion. It is likely that an alveolus of normal size represents the least resistance to blood flow so that alveoli which are collapsed and nonventilated because of complete obstruction, or which are overexpanded because of partial obstruction, hinder blood flow and so are correspondingly poorly perfused. In addition reduction of the oxygen tension in the alveolar air is capable of causing vasoconstriction which prevents perfusion of poorly ventilated alveoli. Likewise, reduction of the P_{CO_2} in the alveoli elicits bronchial constriction, tending to reduce the alveolar ventilation to a unit of lung which has been deprived of circulation. These mechanisms are imperfect in extreme disease but are valuable contributors to normal pulmonary function.

OXYGEN AND CARBON DIOXIDE TRANSPORT

The function of the lung is to maintain an appropriate alveolar environment with respect to oxygen and carbon dioxide and to permit the rapid diffusion of oxygen into the blood and of carbon dioxide from the venous blood into the alveoli. Maintenance of cellular function by provision of adequate oxygen supplies and carbon dioxide removal also depends upon the transport function of the blood.

Most of the carbon dioxide is carried in the form of bicarbonate (HCO_3), which is in equilibrium with carbonic acid (H_2CO_3). The concentration of the latter is determined by the concentration of CO_2 in the blood, which is, in turn, dependent upon the P_{CO_2}. These relationships are discussed in more detail in Ch. 805.

Although a little oxygen is dissolved in blood (approximately 0.3 ml per 100 ml), most of the oxygen is bound to hemoglobin, which has the unique property of combining with large amounts of oxygen when the P_{O_2} is high and of releasing oxygen as the P_{O_2} falls. At a normal arterial P_{O_2} of 100 mm Hg and in the absence of anemia,

approximately 20 ml of oxygen is carried in 100 ml of blood. In the tissues, where the oxygen tension is lower, substantial quantities of oxygen are given up to the cell. Furthermore, the oxyhemoglobin dissociation curve has the additional feature of a flat, upper portion so that there can be considerable reduction of arterial oxygen tension before appreciable hypoxemia develops.

495. PULMONARY CIRCULATION

M. Henry Williams, Jr.

PRESSURE FLOW AND RESISTANCE

The pulmonary circulation is unique in two important respects: the entire cardiac output passes through the lung, and the function of this circulation is to replenish the blood with oxygen rather than to deliver oxygen to metabolically active tissue. The pulmonary artery and its branches are so capacious as to offer minimal resistance to blood flow and to permit passage of blood through the large alveolar capillary network with a pressure head only one fifth of that required to pump blood to the rest of the body. Since there is no need to vary blood flow in the lung with the metabolic needs of competing tissues, the muscular arterioles which are present in the other organs of the body are not needed here. Another characteristic of the pulmonary circulation is its enormous capacity for expansion. Doubling of cardiac output by muscular exercise or of the blood flow through one lung by occlusion of the contralateral pulmonary artery is associated with relatively little increase of pulmonary artery pressure because the total cross section area of the pulmonary vascular bed expands in response to a small rise of intraluminal pressure. In acute experiments, 75 per cent of the pulmonary vascular bed must be obstructed before pulmonary hypertension develops, and the presence of severe pulmonary hypertension implies the existence of widespread vascular disease.

REGIONAL CIRCULATION

Because of the low pressure in the pulmonary artery, variation of hydrostatic pressure caused by gravity has a relatively large effect on the perfusion pressure at the apex and the base of the lung. At the top of the lung, the pressure inside the small arteries may actually be less than the atmospheric pressure within the alveoli, so that the vessels are totally occluded and there is no blood flow. At the bottom of the lung, the hydrostatic pressure is large, and blood flow is correspondingly great. The gravitational effects on the lung volume also tend to divert more ventilation to the lower lung zones than to the upper. This is due to the fact that the pleural pressure is less negative at the bottom of the lung than at the top. As a result, at FRC the upper lobes are under greater stretch, are larger and less compliant, so that they fill less with a given inspiratory change of pleural pressure than do the less expanded and more compliant lower lobes.

A number of isotope techniques have been developed

for studying regional circulation through the lung, of which the most widely used is lung scanning with I^{131}-labeled microaggregates of albumin. Aggregates of albumin are injected into the pulmonary circulation where they embolize functioning capillaries and are detected by appropriate scintillation counting. Albumin aggregates do not embolize areas of lung not perfused with blood; hence these appear as nonradioactive areas on the lung scan. Such filling defects are encountered in patients who have suffered pulmonary embolization or in patients in whom areas of the pulmonary circulation have been obstructed because of inflammation, collapse, or even overinflation, as in bronchial asthma.

BRONCHIAL CIRCULATION

The main nutritive circulation to the lung is provided by the systemic blood brought by the bronchial arteries. As a result, total occlusion of a pulmonary artery does not necessarily lead to necrosis of pulmonary tissue, or even to x-ray changes so long as the bronchial circulation remains intact. The bronchial circulation assumes clinical importance when it becomes excessive, as in chronic suppurative lung disease (bronchiectasis) or after interruption of the pulmonary artery circulation. An expanded bronchial circulation represents a flow load on the left ventricle which pumps blood round and round through the affected pulmonary tissue, and an expanded bronchial circulation is a rare cause of left ventricular failure. Of greater importance is the fact that these systemic vessels are a potential source of serious hemoptysis. Modern techniques of angiography have made it possible to visualize the main bronchial arteries radiographically after injection of contrast material.

PULMONARY HYPERTENSION

As mentioned, significant elevation of the pulmonary artery pressure implies the presence of severe obstruction to the pulmonary circulation. This subject is considered in detail in Ch. 546 to 550.

496. DISABILITY EVALUATION

M. Henry Williams, Jr.

PULMONARY FUNCTION TESTING

As is the case with dyspnea, disability evaluation can only be partially aided by pulmonary function testing because of the importance of subjective factors. The physician can learn whether or not an abnormality which might limit performance is present, but he cannot say that it does or will. For example, patients with apparently similar degrees of severe obstruction to airflow show marked variation in their exercise capacity.

In normal subjects, physical activity is limited largely by cardiac rather than by pulmonary performance. Even at maximal exercise, the limits of ventilation are not reached, and there is no decrease of arterial oxygen tension, implying that total pulmonary performance is perfectly adequate. Theoretically, severe obstruction of airways or severe stiffening of the lungs might make it impossible to achieve levels of adequate ventilation commensurate with the high metabolic rate induced by heavy exercise, but one rarely encounters patients in whom exercise is actually associated with worsening hypercapnia and hypoxemia. In practical terms, there is a rough correlation between the severity of obstructive airway disease and extent of disability so that a patient with a maximal midexpiratory flow rate (MMF) of 1 liter per second may be expected to be unable to do heavy work and a patient with an MMF of 0.2 liter per second can probably do no more than walk slowly on the level. Likewise, when the vital capacity is reduced to 1 liter by severe restrictive lung disease, the effort to achieve more than a slight increase of minute ventilation, such as that induced by slow walking, may become intolerable.

Disability is not synonymous with disease. Extensive involvement of the lung by metastatic disease or with granulomatous disease, as in sarcoidosis, may be associated with little impairment of pulmonary function because of preservation of large areas of normal lung. On the other hand, diffuse microscopic alteration of the alveolar capillary membrane may lead to sufficient impairment of oxygen diffusion as to result in arterial unsaturation, particularly with exercise, and to sufficient stiffening of the lung as to make breathing difficult on mild effort. It may be important for the physician to know that an inhaled pollutant, such as beryllium, has led to extensive lung disease which may be evident only by measurement of the diffusing capacity; but this need not imply that the patient has limited ability to work. A careful assessment of the type and extent of lung disease and evaluation of whether or not the disease has led to mechanical impairment of the respiratory system and/or to blood gas abnormalities at rest or on exercise are the essential ingredients of disability evaluation.

PREOPERATIVE EVALUATION

A special type of disability evaluation is represented by the patient who is being considered for pulmonary resectional surgery. In performing this evaluation, the physician must first determine whether or not the resected tissue is functioning, since nonfunctioning tissue can be removed with relative impunity. Isotope studies of regional ventilation and perfusion now make this estimation possible. Indeed, if it is determined that an area of lung is ventilated but not perfused, resection may be of benefit in that this tissue is of no value to the patient, and its ventilation actually represents wasted effort. Likewise, a perfused but nonventilated lung contributes to hypoxemia and is of little value to the patient.

Since, as in the case of the pulmonary circulation, there is a tremendous reserve of pulmonary function available for ventilation and for gas diffusion, large amounts of pulmonary tissue may be resected from a normal individual without causing hypoxemia or even respiratory discomfort. Often, however, one must decide whether a patient with restrictive or obstructive lung disease is capable of withstanding removal of some functioning lung tissue, generally in connection with cancer surgery. One useful guide is a study of exercise tolerance. If a patient can sustain exercise requiring twice the normal resting oxygen consumption, one can anticipate that he could tolerate removal of half his functioning lung. Calculation of the extent to which the lung to be resected is contributing to gas exchange, most easily based on studies of regional perfusion with lung scan coupled with measurements of ability to increase oxygen uptake with exercise, permits a reasonable assessment of whether or not surgery can be carried out. Other evidence of severe functional impairment may represent compelling contraindications to surgery. Most physicians feel that a patient with resting hypercapnia represents enough of a risk to preclude a thoracotomy. Likewise, pulmonary hypertension, at rest or after balloon occlusion of the segment of lung to be resected, is considered a contraindication to surgery. Beyond that, although severe obstructive or restrictive diseases represent relative contraindications to surgery, assessment must be made on the basis of the patient's general health, age, and vigor and of the indications for operation.

497. HYPOXEMIA

M. Henry Williams, Jr.

HYPOXIA

Tissue hypoxia occurs when the supply of oxygen to the cells is inadequate to meet metabolic needs. The two general causes of hypoxia are reduction of blood flow and reduction of oxygen concentration within the blood. Reduction of blood flow may be localized, as in occlusive arterial disease, or general when the cardiac output is reduced. Arterial oxygen concentration may be diminished if there is impairment of the transport function of the blood. Impaired transport is most commonly the result of anemia, and the oxygen-carrying capacity is reduced in direct proportion to the reduction of hemoglobin concentration. Reduced transport also results from replacement of normal hemoglobin by abnormal hemoglobin such as methemoglobin or carbon monoxide hemoglobin. Heavy smokers may have as much as 10 per cent of their hemoglobin combined with carbon monoxide instead of with oxygen, and they are at a further disadvantage in that the carbon monoxide hemoglobin affects the oxygen dissociation curve of the remaining hemoglobin so that there is interference with release of oxygen to the tissues. Impaired transport also occurs when the amount of oxygen in the arterial blood is reduced because the oxygen tension is reduced. Reduced arterial oxygen tension and saturation is always, with the exception of right-to-left intracardiac shunts, the result of impaired pulmonary function.

ARTERIAL UNSATURATION

Reduced arterial oxygen saturation may, if severe, be evident clinically as cyanosis of the skin or mucous membranes. Since mild degrees of arterial unsaturation are not detectable as cyanosis and since cyanosis can result from any condition which will lead to increased amounts of reduced hemoglobin in the capillaries, such as polycythemia and reduced blood flow, accurate assessment of the arterial oxygen saturation requires its measurement. Since arterial oxygen unsaturation may be an important cause of tissue dysfunction and since it also has clinical implications concerning the type and extent of pulmonary disease present, the measurement should be carried out routinely in patients in whom hypoxemia is suspected to be present.

Hypoxemia may result from four types of impairment of pulmonary function: reduced alveolar ventilation, impaired diffusion of oxygen, right-to-left shunts, and abnormal ventilation-perfusion relationships. Two or more of these abnormalities often coexist in a given patient.

Alveolar hypoventilation is characterized by hypercapnia out of proportion to hypoxemia. Reduction of alveolar ventilation causes proportional increase of arterial Pco_2 and reduction of arterial Po_2, but the flat portion of the oxygen dissociation curve of hemoglobin permits substantial reduction of arterial Po_2 before the arterial oxygen saturation falls appreciably. Thus a patient with an arterial Pco_2 elevated from 40 up to 80 mm Hg would have significant respiratory acidosis, but the concurrent reduction of the arterial Po_2 from 100 to about 50 mm Hg would be associated with only mild arterial unsaturation of little clinical significance. Alveolar hypoventilation may occur after overdosages of drugs, in acute paralytic disease of muscles, or, rarely, in individuals with isolated abnormality of the respiratory center (alveolar hypoventilation syndrome), but it is associated most commonly with severe obstructive pulmonary disease, which leads to hypoxemia for other reasons.

The diffusing capacity of the lungs for oxygen is so large that even during heavy exercise the arterial oxygen tension is only slightly lower than the alveolar oxygen tension, and the diffusing capacity must be severely reduced by disease before arterial oxygen unsaturation develops. When hypoxemia is present because of impaired diffusion, as in advanced pulmonary fibrosis, it is characteristically exaggerated by exercise and is not accompanied by hypercapnia.

Right-to-left shunts produce hypoxemia in direct proportion to the magnitude of the shunt, and they are found most commonly in patients with intracardiac defects. Since the venous carbon dioxide tension is only 6 mm higher than the arterial, even a large shunt leads to little elevation of the arterial Pco_2. A 50 per cent shunt would cause the arterial Pco_2 to be increased by only 3 mm Hg, whereas the oxygen saturation would be substantially reduced because of the much lower venous oxygen saturation.

Mismatching of ventilation and perfusion is the most important cause of hypoxemia. Arterial unsaturation results from the fact that well-perfused but poorly ventilated alveoli have a very low oxygen tension and the blood leaving these alveoli contains low concentrations of oxygen. Since these alveoli are relatively well perfused, they contribute large amounts of blood to the total cardiac output and, hence, cause substantial reduction of arterial oxygen saturation. Hypercapnia is also a feature of this condition, but is mitigated by the fact that alveoli which are excessively ventilated but underperfused contain correspondingly low concentrations of carbon dioxide, and the blood coming from these alveoli tends to counterbalance the CO_2-rich blood from underventilated alveoli. There is no similar compensation for oxygen because the extra ventilation does not serve to increasse the oxygen saturation above the normal 98 per cent.

OXYGEN THERAPY

Most types of hypoxemia are corrected completely and easily by oxygen breathing. Inspiration of air containing a higher than normal concentration of oxygen will lead to an increase of the oxygen concentration in all the ventilated alveoli. Thus if a patient breathes 31 per cent oxygen instead of 21 per cent oxygen, the inspired air will contain an oxygen tension which is 70 mm Hg higher than normal, and all except the very poorly ventilated alveoli will have an oxygen tension which is elevated by approximately 70 mm Hg. This will more than suffice to raise the oxygen tension to a level capable of saturating the hemoglobin passing through these alveoli whether the hypoxemia is due to total alveolar hypoventilation, regional hypoventilation, or impaired diffusion. Hypoxemia caused by a right-to-left shunt will not be corrected fully by this treatment since the inspired oxygen fails to affect the blood passing through the shunts. Inspiration of 100 per cent oxygen will have some effect on arterial oxygen saturation because it will dissolve an extra 2 volumes per cent of oxygen in the blood which does circulate through ventilated lung. This will increase the arterial oxygen saturation 10 per cent in a patient with a normal hematocrit.

Knowledge of arterial blood gas composition during air and oxygen breathing makes possible an accurate assessment of the type of pulmonary malfunction which is causing hypoxemia, and it also provides an indication of the severity of the disease. Since high concentrations of oxygen increase the tendency for atelectasis to develop and adversely affect the metabolic functions of the lung, the physician should use as little additional inspired oxygen as necessary to correct hypoxemia. Measurement of the arterial oxygen saturation is the proper guide to rational oxygen therapy.

ACCLIMATIZATION

One of the extraordinary adaptations of which man is capable is the acclimatization to chronic hypoxia. Whereas acute reduction of arterial oxygen saturation to 70 per cent in a normal subject is associated with gross evidence of cerebral dysfunction and slightly lower levels of saturation will cause death, patients with chronic hypoxia, due either to chronic pulmonary disease or to prolonged residence at high altitude, are capable of normal function with an arterial oxygen saturation as low as 25 per cent. Some of this acclimatization results from polycythemia, which increases the oxygen-carrying power of the blood and from a change in the oxygen-combining character of hemoglobin, which releases oxygen more readily to the tissues. Arteriolar dilation and increased cardiac output permit a more rapid flow of blood and oxygen to the tissues. A fundamental and major adaptation undoubtedly resides in the expansion of the capillary network throughout the body. This brings the oxygen in the capillaries nearer to the cells and makes possible the diffusion of oxygen into the cells even though the partial pressure of oxygen in the capillaries is very low.

Bates, D. V., Macklem, P. T., and Christie, R. V.: Respiratory Function in Disease. 2nd ed. Philadelphia, W. B. Saunders Company, 1971.

Briscoe, W. A.: The current status of pulmonary function tests. Arch. Environ. Health, 16:531, 1968.

Comroe, J. H. Jr., Forster, R. C., DuBois, A. B., Briscoe, W. A., and Carlsen, E.: The Lung. Clinical Physiology and Pulmonary Function Tests. 2nd ed. Chicago, Year Book Publishers, 1962.

Howell, J. B. L., and Campbell, E. J. M. (eds.): Breathlessness. Philadelphia, F. A. Davis Company, 1966.

Hugh-Jones, P., and Campbell, E. T. M. (eds.): Respiratory physiology. Br. Med. Bull., 19:1, 1963.

Liebow, A. A., and Smith, D. C. (eds.): The Lung. Baltimore, Williams & Wilkins Company, 1968.

Section Two. THE DIAPHRAGM

J. B. L. Howell

The diaphragm is the most powerful muscle of inspiration and is responsible for the major part of the tidal volume in quiet breathing. Developmentally, the mesodermal partition which separates the thoracic and abdominal cavities, the septum transversum, is invaded by premuscular tissue derived principally from the fourth cervical myotome, and forms the muscular diaphragm. The motor nerve supply is bilateral and is derived from the third, fourth, and fifth cervical segments via the phrenic nerves. Sensory fibers are also derived from the lower six or seven intercostal nerves.

Congenital Defects. The posterolateral foramen of Bochdalek and less commonly the anterior foramen of Morgagni, owing to persistence of the pleuroperitoneal canal, may be the sites of herniation of abdominal viscera into the thoracic cavity. Herniation may also occur through normal foramina, especially the esophageal opening (see Ch. 635).

Paralysis of the Diaphragm. Paralysis of the diaphragm may occur from interruption of its nerve supply, from muscular atrophy, or temporarily from diaphragmatic pleurisy. Unilateral diaphragmatic paralysis is usually the result of phrenic nerve interruption in the

mediastinum by bronchial carcinoma or other tumors. Unilateral or bilateral diaphragmatic paralysis occurs in high cervical cord injuries, motor neuron disease, paralytic poliomyelitis, infectious polyneuritis (Landry-Guillain-Barré syndrome), or peripheral neuritis associated with diphtheria, tetanus, measles, typhoid, and rheumatic fever; or it may occur after antitetanus serum injection into the deltoid region as part of a cervical radiculitis. Phrenic crush or section was once used therapeutically in the treatment of pulmonary tuberculosis; it may still occur inadvertently during cervical sympathectomy.

Congenital atrophy, called *eventration*, of one half of the diaphragm is a rare and usually symptomless finding on routine roentgenography; its prevalence is about 1 in 12,000. It is more common on the left side. Its main significance is that it may be confused with the potentially more sinister phrenic paralysis. Occasionally, left-sided eventration is associated with mild dyspepsia.

Phrenic paralysis causes elevation of the affected hemidiaphragm, which shows paradoxic movement on sniffing, the basis of its fluoroscopic diagnosis.

The main disturbance of pulmonary function tests in

diaphragmatic paralysis is reduction in the vital capacity, especially when the patient is supine. Symptoms are orthopnea and difficulty in inspiration. Arterial oxygen saturation may be reduced, but hypoventilation does not occur.

Inflammation of the Diaphragm. Inflammation of the diaphragm and its serous surfaces may occur in viral infections, e.g., epidemic pleurodynia, or as extensions of pneumonia, pleurisy, or peritonitis. The clinical significance is that of the underlying condition, except that diaphragmatic, like thoracic wall, pleurisy may cause pain referred to the abdomen or to the shoulder, leading to diagnostic confusion.

Rupture of the Diaphragm. Rupture of the diaphragm is due to trauma, especially when associated with abdominal compression injuries. Direct trauma to the chest may also be responsible. On the right side, the liver may herniate into the thorax. The diagnosis should be suspected when roentgenographic features of paralysis of a hemidiaphragm follow thoraco-abdominal injury, especially if breathlessness is disproportionately severe.

Myotonia Dystrophica and Hemiplegia. The diaphragm may also be involved as part of generalized muscular disease in myotonia dystrophica. Unless extremely severe, spirometry, resting ventilation, and the ventilatory response to CO_2 are normal; however, sedatives readily induce respiratory depression. In hemiplegia, diaphragmatic movement is in a normal direction. Chest movements are reduced on voluntary breathing maneuvers, but not when breathing is stimulated by CO_2. This indicates that although supramedullary innervation of the respiratory muscles is bilateral, it is not symmetrically represented.

HICCUP

Hiccup is an involuntary spasm of the inspiratory muscles followed by abrupt closure of the glottis which is responsible for the characteristic sound. Normal subjects may experience hiccup, especially after eating or drinking, but it may also be a symptom of disease. It may occur in conditions which irritate vagal nerve endings in the abdomen or thorax. These include gastritis, peritonitis, pleurisy, pericarditis, and mediastinitis. It may occur in lateral brainstem ischemia (Wallenberg's syndrome), and as a very troublesome symptom in uremia when it is also thought to have a central origin. When no cause is found, the psyche may be blamed, but there is no evidence to support this. In most instances, hiccup is a short-lived symptom and can sometimes be induced to stop by a variety of maneuvers such as taking a deep breath, breath holding, or drinking cold water. Rebreathing from a paper bag may sometimes help. If symptoms still persist, chlorpromazine, 25 to 50 mg intravenously, may be successful. In the small number of cases in which hiccup has proved resistant to these simple measures, local anesthesia of one of the phrenic nerves has been successful, block of the left nerve usually being tried first.

Section Three. THE CHEST WALL

J. B. L. Howell

498. SCOLIOSIS

Definition. Scoliosis means lateral curvature of the spine which may occur in the lumbar, thoracolumbar, or thoracic regions. The higher the location of the scoliosis in the vertebral column, the greater the likelihood of severe deformity and of disturbance of cardiopulmonary function (heart failure of the hunchback). Lumbar scoliosis is relatively benign. Thoracic scoliosis is associated with rotation of the spine and prominence of the posterior angles of ribs which form the hump or gibbus, and gives rise to the hunchback appearance. Although commonly called kyphoscoliosis, forward angulation of the spine or kyphosis is usually not the major component of kyphoscoliosis; indeed marked lumbar or cervical lordosis is characteristic.

Etiology and Mechanism. Four types of scoliosis are recognized. The largest group is *idiopathic,* developing in childhood and forms 80 per cent of all scoliosis. When idiopathic scoliosis occurs in infancy, boys predominate in the ratio of 6 to 4, and the curvature is usually to the left; when it occurs in adolescence, girls predominate in the ratio of 9 to 1 and the curvature is usually to the right.

Congenital scoliosis results from a variety of developmental abnormalities, including hemivertebrae, fused vertebrae, spina bifida, and absent ribs. Other congenital abnormalities are commonly associated. *Paralytic* scoliosis resulting from poliomyelitis is especially likely to cause deformity and disability owing to the associated muscular paralyses.

Genetic abnormalities may be due to autosomal dominant conditions such as neurofibromatosis, osteogenesis imperfecta, Marfan's and Ehlers-Danlos syndromes, or autosomal recessive conditions, including Morquio's disease, Hurler's syndrome, and diatrophic dwarfism. The mechanism of the deformity is probably a combination of abnormal bone growth, usually in the vertebrae, and altered distribution of muscular forces. The importance of each factor will vary according to the type of scoliosis. The degree of deformity varies between individuals and at different ages. In one series, two thirds of the patients with thoracic idiopathic scoliosis had curvature of the spine greater than 70 degrees, and in over a fourth it was greater than 100 degrees. Scoliosis may also follow fibrotic disease of the lungs and pleura, e.g., tuberculous empyema. This is not as severe as the scoliosis that may develop in the aforementioned varieties, and cardiopulmonary disturbances are due largely to the thoracic disease.

Clinical Manifestations. Deformities with less than 70 degrees of angulation rarely cause symptoms other than those due to their psychologic effects. When more severe deformities interfere with pulmonary function the first symptom is breathlessness on exertion. With progression of the deformity or with superadded bronchitis, disturbance of pulmonary function increases, and arterial hypoxia develops; breathlessness now becomes more severe. If ventilatory failure supervenes, more severe cyanosis and signs of congestive cardiac failure develop. These findings are similar to those of chronic cor pulmonale developing in association with chronic obstructive bronchitis; however, symptoms of morning chest tightness and bronchial irritability are not present in scoliosis unless bronchial disease coexists. Abnormal physical signs are those associated with congestive cardiac failure, but allowance must be made in their elicitation and interpretation for the deformity and displacement of the viscera.

Laboratory Tests. In all patients with significant deformity, total lung capacity, vital capacity, and residual volume are reduced in relation to the degree of deformity. The FEV_1/VC is essentially normal. Airway resistance in relation to lung volume is normal or slightly raised. Maximal breathing capacity is particularly reduced in paralytic scoliosis. In patients with mild deformity, Sa_{O_2} is normal. With increasing severity, Sa_{O_2} becomes reduced while Pa_{CO_2} first remains normal; but when congestive cardiac failure develops Sa_{O_2} is reduced further, Pa_{CO_2} is elevated, CO_2 sensitivity is reduced, and polycythemia may develop. Intrapulmonary gas mixing and diffusing capacity are usually not markedly abnormal. The electrocardiogram may show evidence of right ventricular hypertrophy. Interpretation of the chest film may be very difficult owing to the distortion of the bony cage and displacement of the thoracic contents.

Mechanism of Cardiorespiratory Failure. The deformity of the bony thoracic cage reduces its capacity; it also impairs the action of the inspiratory muscles, resulting in reduced total lung capacity and its component volumes. The work of breathing is increased largely because of increased elastic resistances in the chest wall and altered mechanical advantage of the muscles. This results in more rapid shallow breathing which increases dead space ventilation and causes arterial unsaturation. Initially, over-all alveolar ventilation is maintained, but with progression of the deformity the work of breathing and arterial desaturation are further increased, and alveolar hypoventilation develops in association with impaired ventilatory response to CO_2. Hypoxemia becomes more severe, resulting in polycythemia and increased pulmonary vascular resistance. This, together with the reduction in the pulmonary vascular bed resulting from the low lung volumes, causes pulmonary hypertension and congestive cardiac failure. The end result is similar to the cardiorespiratory failure of primary alveolar hypoventilation, and of chronic obstructive bronchitis ("blue bloater" form).

Pathologic Conditions of Lungs and Heart in Scoliosis. Characteristically, the lungs are small and may appear atrophic; areas of atelectasis are common. Emphysema is not a feature. When the deformity has arisen in infancy, hypoplasia of the air spaces and vascular bed may be found. In patients dying with cardiorespiratory failure, there is usually right ventricular hypertrophy as well as other evidence of pulmonary hypertension.

Prognosis. The factors which influence the progression of minor degrees of scoliosis in childhood are poorly understood. In some it may disappear, but in others, apparently similar, rapid deformity may develop. Cardio-

pulmonary abnormalities are most likely with thoracic deformities, especially when due to muscular paralysis and when the deformity has occurred in infancy and early childhood rather than later in life.

Treatment. *Prophylaxis.* Progress of the deformity is usually preventable by a Milwaukee brace (frame) in growing patients with idiopathic curves of less than 50 degrees. With more severe curves operation may be required to reduce the curvature. At best about 50 per cent reduction in the curvature may be obtained, but there is no general agreement on the best surgical procedure. Prevention and treatment of recurrent bronchitis (see Ch. 503) is important as the pulmonary damage is additive to the effects of the deformity.

Cardiopulmonary Failure. The treatment of acute cardiopulmonary failure is similar to that provided in chronic obstructive bronchitis (see Ch. 503). It includes the treatment of bronchial infection and retained secretions with antimicrobial drugs and physiotherapy, controlled administration of oxygen, venesection for polycythemia, and diuretics. Chronic cardiopulmonary failure requires attention to bronchial toilet, diuretics, and digitalis, and repeated venesection to maintain the hematocrit below 55 per cent. Surgical correction of the deformity at this late stage is not feasible; surgery is usually restricted to the prevention of paraplegia if early signs of spinal cord damage appear. A period of assisted ventilation may be necessary for acute cardiorespiratory failure, but intubation may be difficult owing to the marked cervical lordosis. Intermittent positive pressure inspirations have caused increased lung compliance, but the effect lasted only up to three hours, and the clinical significance, if any, has not been assessed.

499. ANKYLOSING SPONDYLITIS

Ankylosing spondylitis results in bony ankylosis of posterior intervertebral, costovertebral, and sacroiliac joints; there is also ossification of the spinal ligaments and the margins of the intervertebral discs. As a result, the bony thoracic cage becomes rigid and immobile, and respiratory movement becomes increasingly dependent upon diaphragmatic movement. It was once thought that respiratory illnesses were unduly common in this condition, but this has been shown not to be the case. Respiratory symptoms are not common, and pulmonary function shows few abnormalities. In the most severely affected patients, the vital capacity and maximal breathing capacity may be reduced to approximately two thirds of normal. Total lung capacity remains normal, but the residual volume and functional residual capacity are increased, suggesting that the chest is fixed in an inspiratory position. Diffusing capacity for carbon monoxide is reduced only in the most severely affected group. At autopsy, the lungs are normal.

DEFORMITIES OF THE ANTERIOR CHEST WALL

Three types of deformity are recognized: depression of the sternum (pectus excavatum or funnel chest), prominence of the sternum (pigeon chest), and depression of the rib cage anterolaterally in the region of the sixth rib (Harrison's sulcus). Of these deformities, only the first-named may cause any disturbance of cardiopulmonary function.

Pectus excavatum is a congenital abnormality of the anterior chest wall in which the sternum is depressed, being most marked just above the xiphisternal junction, with symmetrical or asymmetrical prominence of the ribs on either side. Occasionally, the xiphoid may project backward as a xiphoid horn. The cause of this deformity is uncertain; some believe that it is due to excessive diaphragmatic traction on the lower sternum, but others believe it is secondary to displacement of the heart into the left hemithorax. Symptoms are not common and appear to be of cardiac origin. They include breathlessness on exertion, precordial pain, palpitation, and dizziness; rarely congestive cardiac failure has been reported. The electrocardiogram may show arrhythmias and changes suggestive of ischemia, but there is no supporting evidence of myocardial disease. Hemodynamic studies have rarely demonstrated restriction of ventricular filling similar to that which occurs with constrictive pericarditis. It is unlikely that disturbed pulmonary function ever plays any part in the disability. Tests are usually normal, but with very severe deformity the vital capacity and maximal breathing capacity may be reduced. Surgical correction has been reported to afford immediate symptomatic benefit, although there is a high incidence of recurrence of the deformity. Surgery is contraindicated if there are serious psychiatric manifestations.

500. PRIMARY OR IDIOPATHIC ALVEOLAR HYPOVENTILATION

Definition. The term primary or idiopathic alveolar hypoventilation denotes a rare clinical syndrome occurring in patients with normal pulmonary and thoracic cage mechanics in whom the primary abnormality is alveolar hypoventilation. It is sometimes referred to as Ondine's curse. The syndrome is characterized by symptoms of headache, drowsiness, or somnolence, exertional dyspnea, and signs of cyanosis and congestive heart failure.

Etiology. The causes of this syndrome are not known. Resistances to breathing and respiratory muscular power are essentially normal, which distinguishes it from hypoventilation occurring in chronic bronchitis, in neuromuscular disorders, in skeletal abnormalities of the thorax, e.g., kyphoscoliosis, or in extreme obesity. Associated central nervous system disorders, such as the sequelae of encephalitis, neurosyphilis, and mental retardation with or without epilepsy, have been reported in over half the patients, but no specific lesions have been found in the region of the respiratory center at autopsy. Alveolar hypoventilation has also been reported in a small proportion of patients after bulbar poliomyelitis, sometimes many years after apparent recovery, and it seems likely that in these patients central nervous system disease is responsible.

Incidence and Prevalence. Primary or idiopathic hypoventilation is a rare disease; it was first described in 1955, and since then fewer than 50 cases have been reported. The majority of patients have been between 30 and 50 years, with a preponderance of males.

Clinical Manifestations. Symptoms have usually been present for many years, but occasionally the presentation has been more acute, usually in response to a respiratory infection or after surgical anesthesia. The dominant symptoms include breathlessness on exertion, drowsiness, or even somnolence suggesting narcolepsy. When the symptoms are severe, the patient is cyanosed, the face being dark and suffused, sometimes with chemosis; tachycardia, raised jugular venous pressure, hepatomegaly, and peripheral edema are present. Crepitations at the bases are common. Clinical evidence of cardiac enlargement, pulmonary hypertension, and right ventricular hypertrophy is commonly present. Periodic breathing and snoring may be prominent during sleep. Laboratory findings include raised Pa_{CO_2} (55 to 75 mm Hg), usually with good compensation of the respiratory acidosis; there is arterial desaturation (70 to 80 per cent), mainly resulting from ventilation-perfusion abnormality, and the hematocrit is usually greater than 60 per cent. The ventilatory response to inhaled CO_2 is markedly depressed and, in one recent report, to hypoxia as well. The vital capacity may be slightly reduced, but the FEV_1/VC ratio is normal. Physiologic dead space ventilation is increased.

Diagnosis. The aforementioned findings in the absence of other disorders of the lungs and thorax are highly suggestive of idiopathic alveolar hypoventilation. This diagnosis is supported if the patient can temporarily restore the blood gas tensions to normal by a period of voluntary hyperventilation. Differential diagnosis includes other causes of congestive cardiac failure, cyanosis, polycythemia, and somnolence, the most common being chronic obstructive bronchitis ("blue bloater" form) and cyanotic congenital heart disease; the syndrome may also be confused with primary polycythemia or narcolepsy. Severe metabolic alkalosis caused by prolonged vomiting, as in anorexia nervosa or chronic pyloric stenosis, may be accompanied by severe hypoventilation. It is not certain whether the cardiorespiratory failure of extreme obesity is an essentially different disorder or not.

Pathology. No specific disease has been found in the central nervous system. In two patients substantial increase in the number and size of capillaries was found at autopsy in the floor of the fourth ventricle, reticular substance, periaqueductal region, mamillary body, and hypothalamus. There was no evidence of neuronal loss. There are usually right ventricular hypertrophy and evidence of chronic pulmonary hypertension. Thromboses of large branches of the pulmonary artery with pulmonary infarcts are common.

Pathogenesis. The primary abnormality in primary alveolar hypoventilation is impaired responsiveness of the respiratory center to carbon dioxide, leading to ventilatory failure. As a result of this reduced CO_2 sensitivity, the center is unable to increase its motor output to the inspiratory muscles by the normal amount when alveolar ventilation is reduced by increased resistances to breathing. Although the normal subject will double or treble the resting power (rate of work) of the inspiratory muscles in response to a rise in the Pco_2 of only 1 mm Hg, these patients are unable to do so even with a rise in

Pco_2 of 20 to 30 mm Hg. Consequently, normally trivial events like acute bronchitis or increase in body weight may cause profound underbreathing, with further elevation of alveolar Pco_2 and fall in alveolar Po_2. Because of altered ventilation-perfusion relationships which accompany underbreathing, Pa_{O_2} is reduced even further until it becomes the dominant ventilatory stimulus and stabilizes ventilation at a new reduced level. Administration of oxygen is likely to be harmful by reducing or removing ventilatory drive, increasing hypercapnia, and leading to increased drowsiness or even unconsciousness. A similar response may follow small doses of sedatives or narcotics, and a number of cases have been recognized for the first time by this striking response. The hypoxemia causes polycythemia, increased pulmonary vascular resistance, and increased cardiac output, resulting in pulmonary hypertension, right ventricular hypertrophy, and systemic venous congestion. Although most patients have various degrees of ventilatory failure, some patients with this syndrome maintain alveolar ventilation at virtually normal levels, alveolar Pco_2 and Po_2 being only slightly abnormal, providing that they do not have respiratory obstruction. It is the failure to maintain adequate alveolar ventilation in the face of increased mechanical hindrance that characterizes the syndrome.

Mechanism of Impaired Sensitivity of the Respiratory Center to Carbon Dioxide. Reduced CO_2 sensitivity is not peculiar to this syndrome. It has been reported in association with a wide range of disorders, including chronic bronchitis and airway obstruction, scoliosis and kyphoscoliosis, obesity, and brainstem disorders; it also occurs as a normal event during sleep. Experimentally, reduced CO_2 sensitivity has been observed in man after vagal blockade and narcotic drugs, and has been thought to occur during partial curarization. The control of breathing is a complex process involving the integration of a variety of sensory inputs from mechanical and chemical receptors, and of motor outputs to the ventilatory apparatus. Theoretically, control may be impaired at any of a number of points, and it is possible that in different diseases interruption of normal control mechanism occurs at different sites. It is generally believed that the abnormality in primary alveolar ventilation is in the central nervous system, but its nature is unknown.

Treatment. Treatment of congestive cardiac failure usually improves the ventilatory failure as well. Oral diuretic therapy with, for example, chlorothiazide, 1 gram, or furosemide, 40 to 80 mg daily; venesections to reduce the hematocrit to between 50 and 55 per cent; and digoxin or digitoxin will reduce pulmonary congestion and peripheral edema, with improvement in arterial Pco_2 and Po_2 (see Ch. 541). Sometimes, when these measures are not successful, a short period of artificial or assisted ventilation to reduce the arterial Pco_2 and raise Po_2 may be followed by prompt diuresis. Cuirass ventilators permit ventilation to be assisted without endotracheal intubation, and in some patients regular artificial ventilation at night in a cuirass ventilator may maintain them in an improved state. Attempts to increase ventilation with acetazolamide, progesterone, aminophylline, and analeptics have not been successful. Instruction in voluntary increased breathing and electrophrenic stimulation with surface electrodes have been successful in the short term only. All other abnormalities likely to hinder breathing, e.g., bronchitis, asthma, and obesity, should be treated as effectively as possible. If upper airway obstruction occurs during sleep (see Ch. 501) despite weight reduction and withdrawal of all central nervous system depressant drugs, tracheostomy should be considered.

Prognosis. There is insufficient information at present to estimate the prognosis with accuracy. Without effective treatment of congestive cardiac failure, the prognosis is very poor. With treatment, patients may continue in reasonable health for several years, requiring only intermittent therapy for acute pulmonary infections and venesections if polycythemia becomes severe. One patient has been reported to have maintained normal arterial Pco_2 for nine months after three years of continuous hypercapnia and repeated episodes of ventilatory and cardiac failure; this was attributed to voluntary increase in ventilation.

501. CARDIORESPIRATORY FAILURE OF EXTREME OBESITY

Cardiorespiratory failure similar to that of primary alveolar hypoventilation has been described in association with extreme obesity, the average weight being approximately 325 pounds. The similarity in appearance and behavior of these patients to the description of the fat boy, Joe, in *Pickwick Papers,* has led to this association being termed the pickwickian syndrome. The main symptoms are breathlessness on exertion and somnolence. Apart from obesity, the physical signs and physiologic abnormalities are similar to those in idiopathic alveolar hypoventilation. Periodic breathing is common during sleep. Prominent cyanosis, tachycardia, raised central venous pressure with cardiac dilatation, functional tricuspid incompetence, hepatomegaly, and peripheral edema may be observed. Investigations reveal diminished total lung capacity and its component volumes, decreased lung compliance, and increased airway resistance at functional residual capacity owing to the low lung volume. Physiologic dead space is increased. Arterial saturation is reduced to about 80 per cent; this is due partly to underbreathing but mainly to increased venous admixture. The Pco_2 is usually 60 to 70 mm Hg. Ventilatory response to CO_2 is markedly reduced. Cardiac output is normal or increased; there is pulmonary hypertension usually of the order of 75 systolic and 30 diastolic in mm Hg. There may also be systemic hypertension, which is common in obesity. With voluntary overbreathing patients can restore the blood gases to normal.

Pathogenesis. The mechanism of the cardiorespiratory failure associated with obesity is obscure. First, it has been attributed to the increased work of breathing which occurs in obesity. Two observations make this unlikely; only a minority of patients with this degree of obesity develop the syndrome, and small amounts of weight reduction of the order of 25 pounds may be associated with marked improvement. Second, this syndrome may be essentially similar to the idiopathic alveolar hypoventilation syndrome, obesity being either a fortuitous association or the result of an underlying central nervous system lesion, e.g., in the hypothalamus, which is responsible for both features. Against this are reports of the restoration of normal ventilatory control in those patients in whom weight has been restored to normal. Third, a combination of increased respiratory work resulting from obesity and low sensitivity to carbon dioxide, which occurs in a proportion of normal people, may initiate a vicious circle of events. Thus gross obesity may cause a small reduction in ventilation with increase in Pco_2 and arterial unsaturation; this leads in turn to further reduction in CO_2 sensitivity, further underbreathing, and more severe arterial unsaturation and the development of congestive cardiac failure. This increases respiratory work and causes further ventilatory failure. A sequence of events such as this would explain the reversibility of the condition, but at present insufficient knowledge is available concerning the range of CO_2 sensitivity in these patients when nonobese. Recently a small number of cases have been reported in which intermittent asphyxia caused by collapse of hypotonic pharyngeal muscles occurred during sleep; the resulting hypoxia caused arousal and prevented the patient from reaching deep sleep. Permanent tracheostomy resulted in marked clinical improvement, including disappearance of somnolence.

Treatment. Weight reduction and the measures described under idiopathic alveolar hypoventilation, i.e., diuretics, venesection, digitalis, and antimicrobial drugs, as well as attention to bronchial toilet result in marked reduction in ventilatory failure and circulatory abnormalities, and improvement in the ventilatory responsiveness to CO_2. Uncontrolled administration of oxygen is likely to cause severe underbreathing and CO_2 narcosis. If pharyngeal obstruction is present and persists despite weight reduction and withdrawal of CNS depressant drugs, tracheostomy may be necessary.

Diaphragm, Scoliosis, and Ankylosing Spondylitis

Bergofsky, E. H., Turino, M., and Fishman, A. P.: Cardiorespiratory failure in kyphoscoliosis. Medicine, 38:263, 1959.

Borgeskov, S., and Raahave, D.: Long-term result after operative correction of funnel chest. Thorax, 26:74, 1971.

Fluck, D. C.: Chest movements in hemiplegia. Clin. Sci., 31:383, 1966.

Gacad, G., and Hamosh, P.: The lung in ankylosing spondylitis. Am. Rev. Respir. Dis., 107:286, 1973.

Gillam, P. M. S., Heaf, P. J. D., Kaufman, L., and Lucas, B. G. B.: Respiration in dystrophia myotonica. Thorax, 19:112, 1964.

McCredie, M., Lovejoy, F. W. J. R., and Kaltreider, N. L.: Pulmonary function in diaphragmatic paralysis. Thorax, 17:213, 1962.

Nordwall, A.: Studies in idiopathic scoliosis. Acta. Orthop. Scand. (Suppl. 150), Copenhagen, 1973.

Wachtel, F. W., Ravitch, M. M., and Grishman, A.: The relation of pectus excavatum to heart disease. Am. Heart J., 52:121, 1956.

Idiopathic Hypoventilation Syndrome and Obesity

Burwell, C. S., Robin, E. D., Whaley, R. B., and Bickelman, A. G.: Extreme obesity associated with alveolar hypoventilation—A pickwickian syndrome. Am. J. Med., 21:811, 1956.

Proceedings of a Symposium: Hypersomnia with Periodic Breathing, Rimini, May, 1972. *In* Bull. Physiopathol. Respir. (Nancy), 1972. This reference contains many papers on primary alveolar hypoventilation and the cardiopulmonary syndrome of obesity.

Severinghaus, J. W., and Mitchell, R. A.: Ondine's curse. Failure of respiratory center automaticity while awake. Clin. Res., 10:122, 1962.

Section Four. AIRWAY OBSTRUCTION

GENERALIZED AIRWAY OBSTRUCTION: CHRONIC OBSTRUCTIVE LUNG DISEASE

502. INTRODUCTION

J. B. L. Howell

The term chronic obstructive lung disease embraces a number of clinical syndromes of varying etiology and pathology, with the common feature of increased hindrance to the flow of air out of the lungs resulting from an intrapulmonary pathologic condition. In some, airflow obstruction is intermittent, and the clinical presentation is one of asthma; in others, airflow obstruction is continuous, often associated with chronic bronchitis or emphysema or both, and the clinical presentation varies depending upon the degree to which the pulmonary condition results in disturbance of pulmonary and circulatory function. In recent years, considerable advances have been made toward understanding the basic pathophysiology of airflow obstruction and of gas exchange in these various conditions; many studies have correlated the clinical features, pulmonary pathology, and disturbances of pulmonary function. It is now possible to recognize a number of different patterns of disorder within the ill-defined group called chronic nonspecific lung disease, which includes simple chronic bronchitis and chronic obstructive disorders associated with chronic bronchitis, emphysema, and allergic disorders of the bronchi.

Ultimately, an etiologic classification of generalized obstructive disorders of the lungs may be possible, but at present, knowledge is incomplete and classification depends largely on differences in clinical presentation supplemented by what is known about their mechanism and pathology.

503. CHRONIC BRONCHITIS

J. B. L. Howell

Definition. Chronic bronchitis is characterized by increased mucous secretion by the tracheobronchial tree, resulting in cough productive of mucus present at some time of the day for at least three months of two consecutive years. It may be diagnosed on this history providing that a localized pulmonary cause such as bronchiectasis, tuberculosis, or tumor has been excluded. The definition is often interpreted less rigidly to include those with chronic or recurrent cough productive of sputum of unspecified duration. It is therefore a clinical diagnosis made solely upon the history. It has a close pathologic counterpart in an increase in the mucus-secreting glands and goblet cells of the bronchial mucosa.

Etiology and Epidemiology. The United Kingdom has the highest recorded mortality attributed to chronic bronchitis in the world. It is 4 to 5 times that of Western Europe and more than 15 times that of Scandinavia and the United States.

Factors predisposing to chronic bronchitis have been identified from epidemiologic studies carried out mainly in Europe and North America. Cigarette smoking has been shown to be the most important single factor; because of its almost overwhelming effect, the contributions of other factors have been partly obscured. Studies comparing the prevalence of chronic bronchitis in urban and rural communities, in workers in different occupations and of different social classes, have shown that, in addition to cigarette smoking, air pollution, dusty occupations, poorer social and economic circumstances, and, especially, increasing age all lead to a higher prevalence of chronic bronchitis. An indication of the magnitude of these factors can be seen from recent statistics of death rates attributable to chronic bronchitis in England and Wales. The standard mortality rate (SMR) was six times greater in males living in a heavily air-polluted area of the industrial Northwest of England compared with a South coast holiday resort. It was five times greater in the lowest social class (Class V) compared with social class I. Recent reduction in air pollution in certain areas in North America and Europe has already been associated with a reduction in the prevalence of chronic lung disease. The effect of occupation is shown by an approximately tenfold increase in SMR in coal miners and laborers compared with clergymen, teachers, and doctors.

There is mounting evidence that during childhood environment is important in influencing both the frequency of lower respiratory tract infections and the ventilatory capacity. In recent epidemiologic studies in the United Kingdom, peak flow rates were found to be significantly lower in children living in areas of high air pollution and were further reduced in those with a past history of bronchitis or pneumonia. The prevalence of acute bronchitis in children is similarly increased by air pollution and also by cigarette smoking; it has been reported also to be more common among children of smokers than of nonsmokers. These influences in childhood probably play an important part in the development of chronic bronchitis and obstructive lung disease in adult life, a view which is supported by the observation that deaths attributed to this cause are higher in male immigrants from Europe to the United States of America than in native-born males. In addition, a history of lower respiratory tract illness occurring under the age of two years has recently been shown to be more important than social class or air pollution in influencing the tendency to winter bronchitis in young adults; but current smoking habits had an even greater effect. As only a proportion of individuals exposed to adverse provoking factors develop chronic bronchitis, other factors which make the individual more susceptible to their effects and which might be termed endogenous must exist, although we have little information about them in most instances.

There are two special circumstances about which more is known. First, the genetically determined abnormality of mucus production, mucoviscidosis, impairs bronchial clearance and protective mechanisms leading to recurrent or, more commonly, chronic bronchial infection. Second, and more common, bronchial allergies may themselves increase secretion of mucus by direct stimulation of the glands, or alternatively, cause increased liability to bronchial infections.

Pathology and Pathogenesis. In the majority of patients with chronic productive cough, mucous gland hyperplasia and increased numbers of goblet cells, especially in the smaller bronchioles, are present. The degree of mucous gland hyperplasia and hypertrophy may be expressed as the ratio of the thickness of the mucous glands to thickness of the bronchial wall between cartilage and epithelium (Reid index) and is normally between 0.14 and 0.36. In chronic bronchitis the ratio is increased; for example, in patients with symptoms of five years' duration or longer, the ratio was found to be from 0.41 to 0.79. In the epithelium increased numbers of goblet cells and areas of squamous metaplasia reduce the numbers of ciliated cells. Scanning electron microscope studies have revealed unsuspected marked irregularities of the bronchial surface even in the absence of gross infection. If infection is present, the bronchial wall is infiltrated with inflammatory cells and congested by dilated capillaries and lymphatics, and, if severe, small abscesses may form. Healing of these more severe infections may lead to fibrosis and deformity of the bronchial wall: bronchitis deformans, stenosans, or obliterans; or bronchiectasis. The combination of increased bronchial mucus, fewer cilia, and irregularities of the bronchial wall impairs the rate of mouthward movement of mucus, and the bronchial protective mechanisms are therefore less effective.

Normally the trachea and bronchi yield no bacteria on culture, but in chronic bronchitis a variety of organisms may be isolated, and pus cells may be seen on microscopy. The organisms include those which are normally commensals in the oropharynx and recognized pathogens such as *D. pneumoniae* and *H. influenzae.* Any factors which further impair the clearance mechanisms or other defenses against infection may lead to the development of acute purulent bronchitis. This is presumably a common mechanism of the recurrent "winter" bronchitis to which these patients are prone, although in a number of cases various respiratory viruses, especially respiratory syncytial virus and *Mycoplasma pneumoniae,* have been isolated. Many exacerbations are not associated with recognizable infecting agents. When resulting from an allergic cause, a purulent appearance of the sputum may be due not to bacterial infection with pus cells but to heavy infiltration with eosinophils.

Diagnosis. The diagnosis of chronic bronchitis is made on the history. Confirmation of the associated pathologic changes of mucous gland hyperplasia may be made by bronchial biopsy, but this is a research, not a routine, procedure. Bronchography may reveal dilated enlarged ducts of hypertrophied glands, and the bronchi themselves may be irregular, giving a "concertina" appearance.

Clinical Manifestations. The productive cough of chronic bronchitis is often not regarded as abnormal and is dismissed as a "smoker's cough." The patient expectorates mucus each morning shortly after rising and may produce only a few pieces of mucoid sputum at times during the remainder of the day. This stage is called *simple chronic bronchitis.* However, two other manifestations may occur, and standard terminology has been recommended by the Chronic Bronchitis Committee of the Medical Research Council of Great Britain. First, the sputum may become purulent, either continuously or for at least a part of the day, usually in the morning; this is termed *chronic or recurrent mucopurulent bronchitis.* Second, airflow obstruction may develop, the condition becoming *chronic obstructive bronchitis,* which will be discussed in more detail later. All forms of chronic bronchitis may be subject to acute exacerbations with increased volumes of sputum with or without purulence. These acute exacerbations frequently follow a head cold, exposure to smog, or other irritants.

Treatment. *Simple Chronic Bronchitis.* A careful history to establish the likely role of smoking, occupational hazard, or presence of allergies must be taken. The patient must be urged to stop smoking, and realization that only a minority will succeed should not deter the attempt. Most patients are unlikely to change occupations, and the physician must not lightly advise it without also considering the social and economic circumstances of the patient. Chronic bronchitis occurring in a nonsmoker is unusual; it should raise the suspicion of bronchiectasis, or of an allergic cause. Mucoviscidosis is a much less common cause of chronic bronchitis. In the relatively small number of patients in whom there is suspicion of allergy, the diagnosis is strengthened by the finding of eosinophils in the sputum or blood or both; attempts to identify the allergen by history and skin testing then may be worthwhile. (For treatment of bronchial allergies, see Ch. 505.)

Mucopurulent Bronchitis. In addition to the aforementioned measures, administration of the appropriate antimicrobial drug may be successful in removing evidence of infection. Occasionally, despite administration of the whole range of antimicrobials, the infection persists. This usually implies structural damage to the bronchi, possibly with bronchiectatic areas and grossly impaired bronchial clearance. In some such patients, infection is due to organisms such as *P. aeruginosa,* Proteus, and *E. coli.* (For management of the last-named group of infections, see Ch. 181 to 183).

In nonhospital practice, it is not necessary or feasible to obtain sputum culture during each acute exacerbation. Treatment should be started with a minimum of delay and is best achieved by self-administration at the earliest sign of infection of either tetracycline, 500 mg four times a day, or ampicillin, 500 mg four times a day, for seven to ten days. The patient must be instructed that, should his condition not improve within 48 hours, or deteriorate within this time, he should seek medical advice without further delay.

A variety of other antimicrobials may be used. These are usually variants of tetracycline or penicillin. If the patient is intolerant of these drugs or the organisms are resistant, cephalothin, clindamycin, erythromycin, or trimethaprim with sulfamethoxazole may be substituted. Tetracycline is particularly effective in mycoplasma infections. In infections with *H. influenzae,* ampicillin, 1 gram every six hours for seven to ten days, is particularly effective when started in the acute phase, and may reduce the frequency of subsequent exacerbations. Chloramphenicol, 250 to 500 mg four times a day, is very effective, but fear of blood dyscrasia has limited its use to situations in which delay in using an effective drug would be very dangerous, e.g., in association with ventilatory failure.

Long-Term Antimicrobial Therapy for Mucopurulent Chronic Bronchitis. In controlled studies, long-term treatment with oxytetracycline, 2 grams daily, did not affect the frequency of acute exacerbations but reduced the

duration of illness. Pneumonias were less frequent but did occur; there was no change in the frequency of isolation of *H. influenzae.* Superinfection with drug-resistant bacteria was not found to be a problem. Equally good results have been obtained from prompt intermittent therapy, and most physicians consider that unless the frequency of recurrences is so great that virtually continuous therapy is being given, individual therapy of exacerbations is the method of choice.

Chronic Obstructive Bronchitis. The special additional features of management in patients with chronic obstructive bronchitis are considered later.

Prognosis. Reduction in cough and sputum may be expected if the provoking irritant can be removed, and some regression of the histologic changes has been recorded. Mortality depends largely on whether generalized obstructive changes develop in the bronchi.

Prevention. Chronic bronchitis is usually a preventable disease. Education in the dangers of cigarette smoking, control or elimination of dusty atmospheres in occupations with known hazards, and prompt effective treatment of bronchial infections in childhood are measures that would reduce chronic bronchitis to a minor disorder. Although the medical profession has a leading role to play in alerting the public to the dangers, in the last analysis it is the community as a whole which must provide the solutions. There is one exception: recognition of allergic factors and their elimination or effective treatment comprise one area in which the physician alone is responsible.

Air Pollution and Health. Summary and Report on Air Pollution and Its Effects on Health by the Committee of the Royal College of Physicians of London on Smoking and Atmospheric Pollution. London, Pitman Medical and Scientific Publishing Company, Ltd., 1970.

American Thoracic Society: Chemoprophylaxis of chronic bronchitis. A Statement by the Committee on Therapy. Am. Rev. Respir. Dis., 104:776, 1971.

Bates, D. V.: Air pollution, chronic bronchitis and emphysema. Am. Rev. Respir. Dis., 105:1, 1972.

Colley, J. R. T.: Respiratory disease in childhood. Br. Med. Bull., 27:9, 1971.

Ferris, B.: Chronic bronchitis and emphysema. Classification and epidemiology. Med. Clin. North Am., 57:637, 1973.

Holland, W. W., Bennett, A. E., and Elliot, A.: Factors influencing the onset of chronic respiratory disease. Br. Med. J., 2:205, 1969.

Medical Research Council Report of the Committee on Etiology of Chronic Bronchitis: The definition and classification of chronic bronchitis for clinical and epidemiological purposes. Lancet, 1:775, 1965.

Reid, L.: Emphysema with chronic bronchitis. *In* Pathology of Emphysema. London, Lloyd-Luke, 1967, Chap. 12, p. 158.

Report to Medical Research Council—The value of chemoprophylaxis and chemotherapy in early chronic bronchitis. Br. Med. J., 1:1317, 1966.

504. BRONCHIECTASIS

J. B. L. Howell

Definition. The Greek word "ectasia" means widening; hence bronchiectasis means widening of the bronchi. There are no symptoms or signs directly related to widening of the bronchi. However, to the clinician, bronchiectasis usually means more than the anatomic lesion; it includes in addition the chronic or recurrent bronchial infection and hypersecretion of mucus which usually accompanies it.

Etiology. The causes of bronchiectasis are varied and their relative frequency has changed since the introduction of antimicrobial drugs and the control of pulmonary tuberculosis. In the prechemotherapy era, the most common causes of bronchiectasis were postbronchopneumonic atelectasis and pulmonary tuberculosis. Aspiration of a foreign body, pulmonary complications of surgery, pertussis, and measles were also responsible, but in approximately 25 per cent of cases no cause could be identified. Since the advent of antimicrobial drugs the incidence and the problems in management of bronchiectasis have become much less. It now occurs mainly after the pneumonias that may complicate pertussis or measles, although all the previous causes may still occasionally be responsible. Bronchiectasis secondary to infected obstructive atelectasis resulting from bronchial neoplasm is being seen more frequently. So-called congenital bronchiectasis is probably the result of infections and collapse in infancy, but bronchiectasis associated with chronic sinusitis and situs inversus (Kartagener's syndrome) is probably truly congenital. Mucoviscidosis may also result in widespread bronchiectasis, the ectatic regions sometimes tending to extend more centrally. Bronchiectasis localized to a proximal region of a segmental bronchus, with normal bronchial distribution distal to it, is sometimes seen with pulmonary aspergillosis when the bronchial wall is infiltrated and weakened by the fungus.

Pathogenesis. The caliber of intrapulmonary bronchi depends upon a balance between the inward acting forces of the connective tissues of the bronchial wall and the outward traction of surrounding lung tissue. An increase in outward traction is insufficient to cause dilatation; weakening of the wall resulting from chronic inflammation must also occur. Both these factors may occur after obstructive atelectasis with chronic infection; the atelectasis tends to increase traction and the chronic infection causes damage to the connective tissue and bronchial smooth muscle. Irregular dilatation of the bronchus and damage to the epithelial lining interfere with bronchial drainage; secretions are retained and chronic bronchial suppuration becomes established.

Pathology. Bronchiectasis usually affects segmental bronchi and may involve one or more segments, a lobe, or rarely a whole lung. It is often distributed in patches over a number of segments, and is frequently bilateral. The regions most frequently involved are the basal segments, right middle lobe, and lingula. Upper lobe bronchiectasis is usually secondary to tuberculosis.

The affected bronchus may become dilated into thick-walled sacs, *saccular bronchiectasis,* cyst-like spaces, *cystic bronchiectasis,* or may cause irregular widening over the affected length to form *fusiform* or *cylindrical bronchiectasis.* In saccular bronchiectasis approximately only four generations of bronchi, widely dilated and distorted, can be identified; the distal generations of bronchi and alveoli are usually obliterated by inflammatory tissue and fibrosis. In fusiform bronchiectasis, the distal bronchi are occluded with mucus and pus but are usually not obliterated. Extension of infection to the pleural surface causes pleurisy and adhesions to the chest wall. Histologically, some bronchi are infiltrated with lymphocytes and have lymphoid nodules in their walls; mucus-secreting glands and cells are prominent. This is likely in children with fusiform bronchiectasis of lower lobe bronchi. In saccular bronchiectasis particularly, the walls of the sacs are fibrous and contain granulation tissue in places lined with metaplastic squamous epithelium. The normal structures of the bronchial walls are destroyed. The bacterial flora is similar to that of chronic muco-

purulent bronchitis. The usual commensals of the nasopharynx are present, and *H. influenzae,* pneumococci, and staphylococci may also be found. Sometimes various species of spirochete, the fusiform bacilli, and other anaerobic bacteria are present and are largely responsible for the offensive fetor (see Ch. 211).

Clinical Manifestations. The clinical manifestations of bronchiectasis are dominated by the chronic infection and hypersecretion of mucus in the ectatic bronchi. *Cough* productive of copious purulent sputum, occurring especially with changes of posture, is the classic symptom. In a minority of cases, infection is minimal (dry bronchiectasis), and recurrent hemoptysis associated with episodes of infection is the major symptom.

In the heavily infected extensive case, the sputum may have a fetid odor and volumes of 400 to 500 ml daily may be seen. After adequate drainage and control of infection this may be reduced to a few milliliters a day. Hemoptysis is common and occasionally may be profuse. Coexisting chronic sinusitis, especially of the maxillary antrum, is common, but its relationship to the bronchiectasis is uncertain. *Chest pain* usually occurs as a result of pleurisy during an infective episode, but occasionally there may be a continuous ache in the region of the bronchiectasis. Shortness of breath on exertion and edema of the ankles may occur when the bronchiectasis is complicated by chronic cor pulmonale. General symptoms caused by chronic infection include tiredness, fatigue, and, in children, stunted growth. Sometimes, bronchiectasis is entirely without symptoms and is a fortuitous finding on routine chest roentgenography or on physical examination.

The physical signs depend on the extent and degree of purulence of the bronchiectasis and on whether generalized obstructive bronchial changes have developed.

If the bronchial changes are extensive and associated with airway obstruction, the patient may be dyspneic and cyanosed. With extensive purulent bronchiectasis the fingers are clubbed. There may be flattening of the thorax and the mediastinum may be deviated to the side of the lesion. Movement is diminished, tactile fremitus is reduced, and there may be dullness to percussion. Breath sounds may be bronchial in quality over consolidated segments. Crepitations occur over affected regions and have a characteristic coarse character, well expressed by the term "leathery" crepitations; they do not clear but may be altered by coughing.

Complications. These include recurrent pneumonia, hemoptysis, lung abscess, brain abscess, empyema, pyopneumothorax and, if longstanding, amyloid disease. The frequency of these has been greatly reduced with the improved management of bronchiectasis.

Disturbance of pulmonary function is more frequent in bronchiectasis than is generally realized but is due mainly to the associated generalized bronchitis. In a recent study, increased airway resistance and residual volume—total lung capacity ratio and reduced maximal breathing capacity were present in over half the patients. Physiologic dead space—tidal volume ratio and nitrogen washout, indicating alteration in the distribution of inspired gas, was abnormal in the majority. However, arterial oxygen saturation below 90 per cent and slightly raised arterial P_{CO_2} was seen in only 10 to 15 per cent. These disturbances of pulmonary function were rarely severe but increased in proportion to the number of segments involved. The effects of cylindrical and saccular bronchiectasis on pulmonary function tests were similar. The persistence of *H. influenzae* was correlated with a lower maximal breathing capacity, but no deterioration was observed over a period of three years in any of these patients irrespective of whether *H. influenzae* was eliminated from the sputum by antimicrobial drugs. The rate of deterioration is related to the frequency of lower respiratory infections.

Diagnosis. The clinical diagnosis may be confirmed by roentgenography, and the chest roentgenogram is nearly always abnormal in some respect. Increased, coarse-meshed lung markings are seen in over half the patients. Evidence of lobar atelectasis occurs particularly in young patients; a honeycomb appearance is less common. Sometimes with saccular and cystic bronchiectasis, ring shadows with fluid levels are present. The diagnosis, extent, and location of the bronchiectasis is established by *bronchography* in which a radiopaque oil is introduced into the trachea and allowed to spread evenly through the tracheobronchial tree, followed by chest roentgenograms in the anteroposterior, lateral, and right anterior oblique positions. It is inadvisable to fill both sides at one examination if there is evidence of impaired pulmonary function. If a primarily endobronchial cause of the bronchiectasis is suspected, bronchoscopy must be performed. A microcytic anemia, neutrophil leukocytosis, and an elevated erythrocyte sedimentation rate, all due to chronic infection, may be present.

There is a spectrum of chronic purulent disease of the bronchi, ranging from mucopurulent bronchitis with little ectasia at one end to gross bronchiectasis at the other. In certain intermediate cases therefore the categorization is arbitrary.

Treatment. *Medical.* After identification of the affected segment or segments, a rational program of postural drainage can be introduced, usually twice or thrice daily. In selected cases of basal bronchiectasis, drainage throughout the night by elevation of the foot of the bed may be beneficial. After improvement has occurred, postural drainage should be continued routinely even if it is unproductive of sputum during drainage; the secretions are often moved and coughed up later. Antimicrobial drugs appropriate to the sputum culture should be administered for a limited course, but should not be administered continuously because of possible superinfection, although admittedly this rarely seems to occur. With adequate postural drainage, sputum should be reduced to small quantities daily even though it remains purulent. The drugs should be reserved for acute exacerbations when they should be administered with minimal delay. The choice of drug regimen is the same as in the treatment of chronic bronchitis and is discussed in Ch. 181 to 183 and Ch. 503.

Surgical. If bronchography shows localized unilateral bronchiectasis which is causing sufficient symptoms to be troublesome, usually as a socially disturbing productive cough, surgical removal of the affected segment or lobe should be considered, providing that over-all lung function is adequate. Rarely, bilateral disease may be treated in this way. Sequential resections for recurring disease will result in a greater loss of lung function than if the diseased segments had been removed at one point in time. Prognosis is poorer with left lobe bronchiectasis owing to frequent recurrence in the lingula. The best results are obtained with unilateral bronchiectasis affecting patients less than 30 years old.

Incidence and Prevalence. There is little recent information about the prevalence of bronchiectasis. It has

been estimated to affect 1.3 per 1000 persons, but certainly significant clinical problems arising from this cause are becoming rare. Cylindrical bronchiectasis is reported to complicate bronchopneumonia in approximately 4 per cent of cases.

Prognosis. The prognosis has altered substantially since the introduction of antimicrobial drugs. With good control of infection, either by medical or surgical treatment, life expectancy is normal. If extensive suppuration cannot be controlled, the outlook is poor, and it has been estimated that approximately one third will die within ten years. The development of chronic airway obstruction is a serious complication and affects prognosis accordingly.

Cherniak, N. S., and Carton, R. W.: Factors associated with respiratory insufficiency in bronchiectasis. Am. J. Med., 41:562, 1966.
Gudbjerg, C. E.: Bronchiectasis—Radiological diagnosis and prognosis after operative treatment. Acta Radiol. (Suppl. 143), 1957.
James, U., Brimblecombe, F. S. W., and Wells, J. W.: The natural history of pulmonary collapse in childhood. Quart. J. Med., 25:121, 1956.
Perry, K. M. A., and Holmes Sellers, T. (eds.): Chest Diseases. London, Butterworth, Ltd., 1968.
Prolonged antibiotic treatment of severe bronchiectasis. Clinical Trials Committee of the British Medical Research Council. Br. Med. J., 2:255, 1957.

505. ASTHMA: ACUTE REVERSIBLE AIRWAY OBSTRUCTION

J. B. L. Howell

Definition. Asthma has proved difficult to define. It is not a disease entity, but one form of clinical presentation of bronchial disorder associated with airway obstruction. It is characterized by marked changes in bronchial caliber occurring over short periods of time, either spontaneously or in response to treatment.

Because the degree of reversibility of bronchial narrowing may vary widely from complete to barely measurable, it is not possible, nor even desirable, to define asthma in more quantitative terms. The term merely describes that end of the spectrum of reversibility of bronchial narrowing at which the changes both in the bronchi and in the clinical state of the patient are unequivocal. Many cases are encountered in which the variability in the caliber of the bronchi and in the state of the patient is such as to make categorization as asthma uncertain. However, the management of the individual patient does not require that this uncertainty be resolved; it is the cause and mechanism by which the disorder is produced that must be recognized if effective therapy is not to be withheld. Most patients with this clinical entity have an allergic basis for their bronchial disorder. Nevertheless, other nonallergic mechanisms are sometimes responsible so that the presence of asthma is not in itself unequivocal evidence of the presence of an allergic disorder.

Mechanism and Etiology. In asthma, there is a continuous state of hyper-reactivity of the bronchi, during which exposure to a wide variety of bronchial irritants will precipitate an asthmatic attack.

Bronchial Hyper-reactivity. In normal subjects, inhalation of histamine or carbachol may cause small increases in airway resistance. By contrast, the bronchi of patients with asthma are highly reactive and show marked bronchoconstriction in response to these substances. This phenomenon is termed *bronchial hyper-reactivity*. Bronchial hyper-reactivity has also been shown to occur with a variety of nonspecific irritants such as dusts and cold air. This reaction is not restricted to asthmatic patients; it may also occur in many patients with chronic bronchitis and chronic airflow obstruction. It may sometimes be seen in normal subjects, especially for short periods after an acute tracheobronchial infection. This state of hyper-reactivity may be reversible; in subjects with seasonal grass-pollen asthma, hyper-reactivity increases during the pollen season whether attacks are occurring or not. In children with perennial asthma, removal from an urban environment to the Swiss Alps has been followed by progressive reduction in the degree of hyper-reactivity; appropriate therapy with sodium cromoglycate may also have the same effect. In subjects with hyper-reactivity associated with nonallergic states, e.g., chronic bronchitis, clinical observation of the effects of removal of inhaled irritants such as smoking or moving to a less polluted environment suggests that some degree of reversibility is possible.

At least two types of mechanism are involved in hyper-reactivity. The bronchoconstriction induced by cold air, for example, is blocked by atropine, indicating that a nervous reflex is involved. By contrast, the actions of histamine and So_2 are less affected by atropine, and the mechanism resides partly in the tissues. The nature of the changes in allergic or nonallergic states is not known.

Bronchial Irritants. A number of "trigger factors" may cause hyper-reactive bronchi to constrict. Although the end-result of their action is similar, it is important clinically to decide whether they act by inducing an allergic reaction or by some other mechanism, because specific therapy is available only for the allergic type.

Allergic or Presumed Allergic Factors. Allergic or presumed allergic factors are involved in most cases of asthma. They may induce either bronchial hyper-reactivity or trigger attacks, or both. The most common and best recognized reaction is the immediate (Type I) reaction in which antigen combines with reaginic antibody (IgE) present on the surface of bronchial mast cells, causing their degranulation and release or formation of a number of "spasmogens." In some patients, possibly as many as 20 per cent, the reaginic antibody appears to be an IgG. The spasmogens include histamine, slow-reacting substance of anaphylaxis (SRS,A), bradykinin, rabbit aorta contracting substance, and possibly 5-hydroxytryptamine which cause increased mucus secretion, edema, and bronchial muscle contraction. Common antigens include grass and tree pollens, mold spores, fungi including Aspergillus, animal dander, and house dust mite (*Dermatophagoides pteronyssinus*). Food allergies, e.g., to eggs, shellfish, and chocolate, may cause asthma but are more likely to cause urticaria.

After exposure, airway obstruction develops over minutes, and the immediacy of the response may enable the patient to recognize the relationship between exposure and attack. This contrasts with a different type of late allergic reaction (Type III) in which there is a delay, usually of 6 to 12 hours, between exposure and the development of airway obstruction. The late reaction involves circulating precipitating antibodies, and has been found to occur with a variety of antigens, e.g., Aspergillus,

Contrasting Features of Extrinsic and Intrinsic Asthma

	Extrinsic	Intrinsic
Age of onset	Childhood or young adulthood	Middle age
Family history of allergies	Positive	Negative
Nasal symptoms	Hay fever	Nasal polyps
Aspirin sensitivity	Not a feature	Significant association
Skin tests	Positive	Negative
IgE levels	Raised	Normal

house dust mite, *B. subtilis* in the manufacture of biologic detergents. With some antigens, e.g., Aspergillus and house dust mite, both immediate and late reactions may occur in the same individual.

In some individuals, often in those in whom asthma has occurred for the first time in middle age, there may be no evidence of an IgE-mediated mechanism. IgE levels are normal, and skin tests to a wide range of antigens are negative. Because of this, their asthma is often called "intrinsic." However, in many cases sputum eosinophilia and response to sodium cromoglycate and/or steroid therapy suggest underlying allergic reactions. Some workers have denied any fundamental difference between intrinsic and extrinsic asthma, believing that if only the appropriate antigen were used for testing, all asthmas would be found to be extrinsic in origin. However, there are other features which indicate differences between the two types, as listed in the accompanying table. A clear-cut separation as suggested by this table is not always evident, but there can be little doubt that the distinction between the two types is a valid one. It does not necessarily follow that these are two diseases. It is also well recognized that some patients with extrinsic asthma in childhood may develop intrinsic asthma in middle age.

Physical or Chemical Irritants. Irritants such as inert dusts, sulfur dioxide, and other atmospheric pollutants are often responsible for asthma; for example, so-called Tokyo-Yokohama asthma is believed to be due to the high levels of atmospheric irritants in these cities, acting on individuals with pre-existing bronchitis or asthma. A number of industrial chemicals, for example, aluminum solder flux and toluene diisocyanate (TDI), a chemical widely used in the plastics industry, may induce asthma, almost certainly on an allergic basis.

Psychologic and Nervous Factors. Psychologic stress and conditioned reflexes have been shown to be important in precipitating attacks in subjects with bronchial hyper-reactivity, presumably through an exaggerated response to efferent autonomic nervous activity. Effective drug therapy may remove or override these influences, but if this fails, "verbal deconditioning" as reported by Moore (1966) should be considered for intractable cases. Hypnosis probably has little place.

Physical Exertion. Although the immediate effect of brief exercise may be to induce bronchodilatation in an asthmatic subject, many patients experience chest tightness and breathlessness if exercise is prolonged for several minutes; this may be especially noticeable after stopping the exercise. It is due to bronchoconstriction and is particularly common in children and young adults with mild asthma. The mechanism is uncertain and may be caused by different factors in different people. Hyperventilation with a lowering of PCO_2 or release of a circulating bronchoconstrictor substance during exercise has been suggested, but neither mechanism will explain all cases. The response is usually not blocked by the administration of atropine, but isoproterenol and cromolyn sodium are effective in the majority, the latter suggesting that mast cell degranulation may be the final common pathway. Occasionally exercise-induced attacks are the only clinical manifestation of asthma for years before spontaneous attacks begin to occur.

Infections. Respiratory infections, especially viral, are commonly associated with attacks of asthma. Whether this represents an allergic reaction to the infecting agent or is merely a nonspecific response of hyper-reactive bronchi to the infection is uncertain. There is still no firm evidence that chronic infections such as chronic sinusitis, tonsillitis, or dental sepsis are a cause of asthma in those patients in whom clear evidence of allergy is lacking (intrinsic or "infective" asthma). Lack of correlation between exacerbations of asthma and degree of activity of infection, together with failure of removal of infected foci or of long-term antimicrobial therapy to influence the course of the disease, casts doubt on the relevance of this mechanism. Skin tests to bacterial antigens are usually negative, but this may merely mean that an immediate Type I allergic reaction is not involved; delayed skin reactions to killed bacterial antigens have been reported in many patients with intrinsic asthma.

Pathology. Pathologic studies of asthma are largely related to the lungs of patients who die in status asthmaticus. The lungs are voluminous, and the smaller bronchi are largely occluded by mucous plugs. Histologically, large numbers of eosinophils are present in the bronchial walls together with varying numbers of lymphocytes and neutrophils and plasma cells. Hypertrophy of bronchial mucous glands and bronchial smooth muscle is usual; shedding of the epithelium is common.

Clinical Manifestations. Asthma occurs characteristically as episodes which may last from a few minutes to several days with a wide range of severity; between attacks the patient is well. Frequently asthma begins in childhood, and in about 30 per cent of the cases it is associated with eczema. Asthma may be particularly troublesome once the child begins school, possibly because of additional emotional stress and respiratory tract infections. Exercise-induced asthma may prevent the child from participating in games. It is at this stage that the etiologic role of psychologic factors is likely to be overrated; instead they should be recognized as only one of several possible provoking factors. Parental anxiety is especially likely to be blamed but only leads to even greater stress if not dealt with sympathetically. Alternatively, asthma may appear for the first time in middle age or later, sometimes after a lower respiratory tract infection. In some patients, especially with intrinsic asthma, there is a gradual change in the character of the disorder. Attacks become less frequent and less severe, but the degree of recovery between them is less complete. The patient develops chronic narrowing of the bronchi with airflow obstruction, and his capacity for physical

exertion is progressively reduced. This chronic airway obstruction is usually associated with chronic cough and sputum (chronic bronchitis) and liability to episodes of purulent bronchitis.

The Attack of Asthma. The attack may begin within minutes of exposure to antigen and may or may not be associated with symptoms of hay fever. Alternatively, it may be precipitated by exertion, irritants, emotional stress, excitement, or infection; often there is no known precipitating factor. The patient experiences a sensation of chest tightness, with coughing and wheezing, which increases in severity. Dyspnea may become severe, and expiration is usually felt to be more difficult than inspiration. If untreated, the attack may last a variable time from a few minutes to several hours, but the prompt inhalation of an aerosol of isoproterenol or similar substance may abort the attack.

In some patients, attacks occur only at night, usually between 2 and 4 A.M., and in older subjects may then be mistaken for left ventricular failure. Nocturnal attacks may occur sporadically for months or years before also occurring during the day.

In a severe attack, the patient is extremely dyspneic, orthopneic, and often cyanosed. He is agitated and may be confused. He is often most comfortable sitting forward with his arms leaning on some support, a point to remember when asking the patient to lean back on the pillows to be examined. There is indrawing of the soft tissues of the neck, and the accessory muscles are active. Retraction of the sternomastoid muscle has been reported to be the only consistent accompaniment of severe asthma. The chest is overinflated with diminished hepatic and cardiac dullness to percussion, and respiratory movement is reduced. The larynx is pulled downward and the lower lateral rib cage inward with inspiration. High pitched, sibilant rhonchi, often associated with coarse crepitations in some areas, occur during inspiration as well as expiration. It is important to remember that when airflow obstruction becomes extreme, rhonchi may disappear. The pulse is rapid and blood pressure is normal. Pulsus paradoxus may be present, and indicates at least a 60 per cent reduction in the FEV_1; unlike the situation in pericardial tamponade, there is no associated engorgement of the cervical veins on inspiration. The sputum is usually viscid and difficult to expectorate; it may contain branched white bronchial casts and spirals of condensed mucus up to a few millimeters long, so-called Curschmann's spirals. A purulent appearance is commonly due to infection but may be due solely to the presence of large numbers of eosinophils. If the attack has been present for many hours or days without remission despite treatment, the patient has "status asthmaticus." This is often associated with signs of exhaustion and dehydration. Tachycardia is the rule, and, if greater than 130 per minute, indicates severe hypoxemia. Rarely, in patients with very prolonged severe airflow obstruction, edema of the feet and ankles may occur without other clinical evidence of heart failure.

The severity of an attack of asthma is often misjudged. Disturbance of consciousness, general exhaustion, marked pulsus paradoxus, any elevation of the PCO_2, very low FEV_1, pneumothorax, and pneumomediastinum are signs of great severity and indicate need of urgent effective therapy.

Laboratory Tests. Vital capacity, FEV_1, and FEV_1/VC ratio are diminished. Residual volume is increased, and, if airflow obstruction is severe and prolonged, total lung capacity may also be increased. Airway resistance is markedly increased. Arterial Po_2 is reduced owing to disturbed ventilation-perfusion relationships. An FEV_1 of less than 1 liter is almost always associated with reduction in arterial Po_2, and in status asthmaticus the arterial Po_2 may reach alarmingly low levels but is usually above 50 mm Hg. In moderate asthma, the Pco_2 is often low, indicating hyperventilation. Any elevation of the Pco_2 is of grave significance, for it indicates that the resting ventilation is virtually the maximum of which the patient is capable and that further increase in airway resistance, or reduction in drive to breathe, either through exhaustion or because of the use of sedatives or opiates, may be rapidly lethal. During recovery, symptoms disappear when the FEV_1 is still less than 50 per cent of predicted normal; signs disappear between 60 and 70 per cent. The Pa_{O_2} may not return to normal between attacks owing to persisting ventilation-perfusion disturbances.

The peripheral blood often shows eosinophilia. A slight polymorphonuclear leukocytosis is not uncommon. Microscopy of the sputum reveals eosinophilia and also long narrow crystals, Charcot-Leyden crystals, which are believed to be derived from eosinophils and with which they are always associated. The chest roentgenogram usually shows signs of overinflation, but occasionally patchy radiopacities may be present. These are particularly common in association with aspergillosis. Heart size is normal.

Prognosis and Prevalence. It is usual for attacks to become less frequent and severe during middle and late adolescence, and they may disappear completely. Approximately 50 per cent of children with asthma will become symptom free before adult life, and only 5 to 10 per cent continue to have severe disability, this unfortunate outcome being more likely when asthma has begun in infancy in association with eczema. This presumably reflects their greater tendency to develop hypersensitivity reactions. Often those not wholly symptom free in adulthood will experience only occasional mild attacks at infrequent intervals, but sometimes severe attacks may recur years or decades later. In adult asthmatics of the intrinsic type, followed for at least 15 years, Rackemann found that 22 per cent were symptom free, 44 per cent were improved, 33 per cent were unimproved, and 3 per cent had probably died of their asthma. Sinusitis and nasal polyps were more common in the unimproved group. There is general agreement that deaths are most common in patients with severe disabling chronic symptoms.

Asthma occurs in approximately 1 to 2 per cent of the population. There is a higher prevalence in childhood which varies between countries, as follows: Sweden, 0.73 per cent; United Kingdom, 3.8 per cent; United States, 6.9 per cent; and Australia, 11 per cent. Asthma occurs more frequently in boys up to ten years of age, and the ratio becomes even wider during adolescence. Severe childhood asthma is much more common among boys.

Between 1959 and 1966, the death rate from asthma in the United Kingdom in the age group 5 to 34 years increased threefold from 0.7 to 2.2 per 100,000, and this rise corresponded with increased sales of pressurized bronchodilator aerosols. Asthma then accounted for 7 per cent of all deaths in persons 10 to 14 years old. A study of the possible causes was initiated, but the "epidemic" rapidly declined, and by 1969 the death rate was only slightly higher than it had been ten years earlier.

Fifty-two deaths in the age group 5 to 34 years were analyzed. Below 15 years there were four males to each female death, but over 30 years females predominated. Death was unexpected in 79 per cent, about one third being judged by their doctors not to have been severely ill. Eighty-one per cent died at home or on the way to hospital. There was no evidence to incriminate excessive use of pressurized aerosols. Indeed, the duration of the final attack was considerably longer in those who had used their aerosols excessively compared with those who had not. It was noted that the "epidemic" of asthma deaths had not occurred in countries like the United States, where a concentrated form of pressurized aerosol was not available; but epidemiologic studies, particularly in Australia, do not support the hypothesis that the concentrated aerosol was responsible for the "epidemic." Severe reactions have been recorded resulting from hypersensitivity to penicillin, aspirin, indomethacin, and radiopaque contrast media.

Differential Diagnosis. States of increased ventilation may be confused with asthma. These include severe metabolic acidosis, e.g., "renal" asthma, hyperventilation syndrome, and pulmonary embolism in which bronchospasm may also occur. Airflow obstruction with wheezing also occurs in certain patients with left ventricular failure, and inhalation of isoproterenol may give temporary relief. Paroxysmal nocturnal dyspnea caused by left ventricular failure may be confused with asthma. Large airway obstruction, e.g., laryngeal carcinoma and tracheal growths or compression from lymph nodes, may sometimes cause confusion, but inspiratory stridor should indicate the mechanism. Asthma may sometimes occur in association with other disorders of immunologic mechanisms; in association with polyarteritis nodosa, marked eosinophilia is characteristic. Carcinoid tumors are a rare cause of asthmatic attacks associated with flushing.

Management of Asthma. Obviously the most direct form of management of the patient with asthma is to terminate the exposure to responsible allergens or irritants. This may give complete relief and is most likely to be effective with occupational exposures or specific sensitivities, e.g., to animal dander. If avoidance of the allergen is not feasible, attempts may be made to *hyposensitize* the patient by injections of graded doses of the antigen at regular intervals. This is believed to induce IgG antibody, which competes for the antigen and prevents it from reaching IgE-sensitized mast cells. This procedure, which is particularly successful for hay fever, is less successful for the relief of asthma, although sometimes dramatic success occurs with complete relief of symptoms for varying periods up to several years. Further courses of antigen injection may not be so successful. It is not possible to predict which patients will benefit, and therefore it is always worth trying in patients with continuing disability whenever other methods of treatment have failed.

Reversal of the Asthmatic Reaction. Acute exacerbations of asthma may be promptly relieved by inhalation of 0.1 mg of isoproterenol, or 0.1 ml of 1:1000 epinephrine subcutaneously or 1:100 by nebulizer. Longer-acting beta-adrenergic drugs, such as orciprenaline, salbutamol, and terbutaline, are available in some countries as pressurized aerosols. The latter two are largely beta-2 (bronchial) stimulators and have relatively little effect upon the heart. All tend to cause a further small reduction in the Pa_{O_2}, but there is no unequivocal evidence that this is dangerous; if necessary, it can be corrected by oxygen administration. Unfortunately, the more severe the asthmatic reaction, the less is the response to these drugs, and the shorter their duration of action. It is in these circumstances that repeated doses are taken at short intervals and the danger of overdosage is present. In some individuals, a rebound bronchoconstriction occurs as the bronchodilator effect wears off.

For continuous symptoms, the most successful drugs are those which stimulate β-adrenergic receptors. Ephedrine, 15 to 30 mg, may be given twice or three times daily. This should be first given in low dosage as it may cause palpitation and tremor and, in the elderly male, urinary retention. Other effective drugs are isoproterenol, 5 to 20 mg sublingually as required, aminophylline, 100 to 300 mg three times a day, and salbutamol, 2 to 4 mg, terbutaline, 5 mg, aminophylline, 100 to 300 mg three times a day, or orciprenaline 20 mg four times a day. Aminophylline is liable to cause gastric irritation, but there are several proprietary chemical analogues which are better tolerated. Nocturnal symptoms may be relieved by suppositories of aminophylline, 360 mg rectally on retiring at night. In persistent asthma, potassium iodide, 0.6 gram three times a day after meals, is often valuable in thinning tenacious sputum.

Although the aforementioned drugs are often given in combination, they should be first administered singly and with caution to patients with heart disease, hypertension, and hyperthyroidism. Antihistamines are rarely of much value in asthma and may cause drowsiness, but because of occasional successes should be considered in special situations.

Suppression of Allergic Reactions. If the asthmatic response is not controlled by simple measures, suppression of the allergic reaction should be attempted. Three types of drugs may be employed: corticosteroids, corticotrophin (ACTH), and cromolyn sodium. The mode of action of *corticosteroids* in asthma is uncertain. They will not suppress the acute asthmatic response to inhaled antigen but are effective in suppressing clinical extrinsic and intrinsic asthma in most cases. It has been suggested that they reduce the inflammatory reaction and may therefore act mainly by reducing edema and mucous secretion as well as bronchial hyper-reactivity. A large number of different corticosteroid preparations are available, each with different dosage schedules. For simplicity, dosages will be described for prednisone or prednisolone; dosages of other preparations should be adjusted accordingly.

ACUTE ATTACK. *For the treatment of an acute attack* comparatively large doses, 30 to 60 mg daily, may be given for a few days with safety, and after relief has been obtained reduction in dosage at a rate of 5 mg daily is usually possible without early recurrence. The occasional use of large doses of prednisone in this way is without significant risk of side effects except in patients with peptic ulceration in whom gastrointestinal bleeding may be induced. In children, as many as 15 courses of steroids have been given in a year without any detectable side effects developing.

CONTINUOUS SYMPTOMS. For continuous symptoms which recur during or shortly after the course of corticosteroids administered as described above, there are two alternative forms of dosage, continuous or intermittent.

CONTINUOUS THERAPY. An initial dose of prednisolone is given sufficient to produce effective, rapid suppression of symptoms, for example, 10 mg three times a day (range usually 20 to 60 mg daily). When definite improvement has occurred (usually within four days) the daily dosage may be reduced by 2.5 mg (half tablet) daily (or at longer intervals if experience indicates). When the daily dosage is down to 15 mg daily (that is, one to two weeks after start), reduction by 1 mg once or twice weekly may be continued until either symptoms begin to recur or it has been found possible to discontinue treatment. If troublesome symptoms recur while reducing dosage, the daily dose may be increased by 3 to 5 mg, and the procedure restarted.

INTERMITTENT THERAPY. Treatment is given for one to three days with the lowest dose of corticosteroids which will permit them to be omitted for a similar period without return of symptoms. The patient will usually find a dosage below which reduction is always followed by recurrence of symptoms.

Whether the intermittent or the continuous regimen is being used, superimposed acute exacerbations should be treated promptly with a large increase in dosage for a few days; then a progressive reduction may be followed as before.

Corticotrophin, natural or synthetic, may be used in place of corticosteroids for continuous symptoms. By using depot preparations, a satisfactory regimen of intermittent injections can usually be achieved. Initially, 1 mg of depot ACTH may be given daily and reduced to once weekly. The need for reducing the dose to the minimum which will maintain adequate control is the same as for oral corticosteroids. Corticotrophin has been reported to cause less retardation of growth in children than oral corticosteroids. Suppression of pituitary secretion of ACTH may occur and abrupt cessation of therapy may lead to acute adrenocorticoid insufficiency. Allergic reactions have occurred to the natural hormone, and a case of sensitivity to the synthetic preparation has recently been reported.

Recently, beclomethasone dipropionate and betamethasone 17-valerate, widely used for topical therapy in dermatology, have been prepared in pressurized aerosol form and shown to be effective substitutes in many patients for oral corticosteroid therapy without causing suppression of the hypophysial-pituitary-adrenal (HPA) axis. The usual initial dose is 100 μg every six hours, slowly reducing to minimal requirements. In patients already receiving long-term oral therapy in moderate dosage (e.g., less than 15 mg per day), it may be possible to substitute completely with an aerosol preparation, but care must be taken that hypocorticism caused by existing HPA suppression is not induced by too rapid withdrawal of oral steroid. Sometimes troublesome allergic rhinitis and eczema may recur as systemic steroid effects are reduced, and may require reinstitution of some oral therapy. The only side effect reported to date is an increased incidence of oral and laryngeal candidiasis which may occur in up to 10 per cent of patients.

CROMOLYN SODIUM (SODIUM CROMOGLYCATE). Cromolyn sodium, a bis-cromone derived from khellin, is a new type of compound used for prophylaxis of allergic asthma. When inhaled prior to antigen provocation challenge in sensitized subjects, it has the unique property of inhibiting the development of the immediate (Type I) asthmatic reaction. It is effective only when inhaled. Cromolyn sodium acts by stabilizing mast cells; it does not prevent antigen and reaginic antibody from combining but prevents the combination from triggering the degranulation of mast cells and thereby releasing spasmogens. Cromolyn sodium also inhibits the late (Type III) precipitin-mediated asthmatic and febrile reactions to inhaled house dust, Aspergillus, avian, and other proteins. In a recent study of subjects in whom both Types I and III reactions occurred after exposure to Aspergillus or house dust, prior inhalation of cromolyn sodium inhibited both reactions, whereas corticosteroids inhibited only the late (Type III) reaction. Cromolyn sodium does not possess anti-inflammatory or bronchodilator properties and does not antagonize histamine, SRS(A), bradykinin, serotonin, or prostaglandins F_{2alpha} and E_1. It may possess alpha-adrenergic blocking properties, but these also may be mediated through its effects upon the mast cell membrane.

Because of its mode of action, cromolyn sodium is used to prevent rather than treat attacks. Despite extensive trials there are still no firm criteria for the selection of patients who will benefit. Young patients with strong evidence of allergy are most likely to respond, about 80 per cent showing worthwhile improvement. Recent work has shown that patients who do not respond to cromolyn sodium may possess IgG rather than IgE mediated allergic reactions. Up to two thirds of older patients with "intrinsic" asthma are likely to benefit to some extent. In general, clear evidence of allergic factors, e.g., seasonal history, positive skin tests, sputum and/or blood eosinophilia, or the presence of exercise-induced asthma, especially if inhibited by cromolyn sodium, make benefit from cromolyn sodium likely; associated chronic bronchitis and irreversible airway obstruction make improvement less likely.

Improvement may be reflected in a number of ways such as reduction in the number of attacks, reduced cough and sputum, and reduced bronchodilator and corticosteroid requirements. These changes may sometimes occur without corresponding improvement in the results of spirometry.

In a group of patients already receiving continuous corticosteroid therapy, cromolyn sodium permitted an average reduction of steroid dosage of 40 per cent in approximately two thirds of cases; it was rarely possible to discontinue corticosteroids. The only known side effect is irritation of the throat by the dry powder.

Cromolyn sodium is prepared as a powder in capsules containing 20 mg of drug dispersed with lactose, and is inhaled through a specially designed turbo-inhaler (Spinhaler). For patients in whom the dry powder induces irritation of hyper-reactive bronchi, a preparation containing 0.1 mg of isoproterenol is available in the United Kingdom only. The usual dose schedule is inhalation of the contents of one capsule (20 mg) four times a day, but this may be adjusted to the minimal dose that maintains suppression of symptoms.

IMMUNOSUPPRESSIVE THERAPY. Immunosuppressive therapy similar to that used in tissue or organ transplantation has been used in attempts to suppress the allergic reaction in asthma. In a small number of trials using azathioprine, chlorambucil, and methotrexate in chronic severe asthma, conflicting results have been reported, and their value has yet to be determined.

Status Asthmaticus. The majority of patients with asthma improve rapidly after admission to hospital, administration of corticosteroids, and bronchodilator therapy. Subcutaneous epinephrine should not be administered because the patient may already have taken large doses of isoproterenol before admission. Sedatives are po-

tentially dangerous and are absolutely contraindicated if the Pco_2 is raised; with lesser degrees of severity, their cautious use may be helpful. When improvement is delayed, particular attention must be paid to humidification of the inspired air, preferably by an ultrasonic nebulizer, although occasionally this aerosol is itself a bronchial irritant. Oxygen may be administered freely since CO_2 sensitivity is not impaired. Hydration of the patient must be maintained, with intravenous fluids if necessary. Occasionally hypovolemia is present and requires more rapid rehydration.

Intravenous hydrocortisone, 100 to 200 mg, may be repeated hourly if necessary, and some workers advocate even higher dosage up to 1 gram repeated as necessary. However, gastrointestinal hemorrhage has been reported on such a regimen. If severe respiratory acidemia is present, intravenous sodium bicarbonate, 50 to 100 mEq, may be beneficial. Serial measurement of Pa_{CO_2} and Pa_{O_2} is helpful in monitoring ventilatory status and oxygen therapy.

A decision which is often difficult is that of when to use *assisted ventilation.* This is made on the basis of the overall state of the patient, with particular attention to whether he is becoming exhausted, is unable to cooperate in bronchial toilet, or if the Pa_{CO_2} is rising progressively. It should not be made on any arbitrary level of Pa_{CO_2} or Pa_{O_2}. Endotracheal intubation has replaced tracheostomy in this situation; in addition to assisting ventilation, it enables bronchial toilet to be improved if necessary by direct instillation of 5 to 10 ml of warmed saline a few minutes prior to tracheal suction. (For discussion of the general question of acute respiratory failure, see Ch. 507.)

Altounyan, R. E. C.: Changes in responsiveness to histamine and atropine as a guide to diagnosis and evaluation of therapy in obstructive airway disease. *In* Proceedings of a Symposium on Disodium Cromoglycate in Allergic Airways Disease. London, Butterworth & Co., Ltd., 1970.

Bernstein, L., Siegel, S. C., Brandon, M. L., Brown, E. B., Evans, R. R., Feinberg, A. R., Friedlander, S., Krumhelz, R. A., Hadley, R. A., Handelman, N. I., Thurston, D., and Yamate, M.: A controlled study of cromolyn sodium sponsored by the drug committee of the American Academy of Allergy. J. Allerg. Clin. Immunol., 50:235, 1972.

Brompton Hospital/Medical Research Council Collaborative Trial: Long-term study of disodium cromoglycate in treatment of severe extrinsic or intrinsic asthma in adults. Br. Med. J., 4:383, 1972.

DeVries, K., Booij-Noord, H., Goei, J. T., Grobler, N. J., and Orie, N. G. M.: Inhalation tests. The influence of nonspecific irritants on the airways. Acta Allergol. (Kbh), (Suppl. 8):131, 1967.

D'Souza, M. F., Pepys, J., Wells, I. D., Tai, E., Palmer, F., Overell, B. G., McGrath, I. T., and Megson, M.: Hyposensitization with *Dermatophagoides pteronyssinus* in house dust allergy: A controlled study of clinical and immunological effects. Clin. Allergy, 3:177, 1973.

Jones, R. S.: Assessment of respiratory function in the asthmatic child. Br. Med. J., 2:972, 1966.

McFadden, E. R., Kiser, R., and deGroot, W. J.: Acute bronchial asthma. Relations between clinical and physiologic manifestations. N. Engl. J. Med., 288:221, 1973.

McNeill, R. S., Nairn, J. R., Millar, J. S., and Ingram, C. G.: Exercise-induced asthma. Quart. J. Med. (N.S.), 35:55, 1966.

Moore, N.: Behaviour therapy in bronchial asthma: A controlled study. J. Psychosom. Res., 9:257, 1965.

Pepys, J.: Asthma. Br. J. Hosp. Med., 7:709, 1972.

Porter, R., and Birch, J. (eds.): Identification of Asthma. Ciba Foundation Study Group No. 38. Edinburgh and London, Churchill-Livingstone, 1971.

Rackemann, F. M., and Edward, M. C.: Asthma in children. N. Engl. J. Med., 246:815, 1952.

Rebuck, A. S., and Read, J.: Assessment and management of severe asthma. Am. J. Med., 51:788, 1971.

Sodium cromoglycate (cromolyn): A review of its mode of action, pharmacology, therapeutic efficiency and use. Drugs, 1974.

Szentivanyi, A.: The beta adrenergic theory of the atopic abnormality in bronchial asthma. J. Allerg. Clin. Immunol., 42:203, 1968.

506. CHRONIC AIRWAY OBSTRUCTION

J. B. L. Howell

Chronic airway obstruction denotes an alteration in the mechanical properties of the lungs characterized by poorly reversible increased hindrance to expiratory airflow; it is usually but not necessarily accompanied by increased resistance to inspiration. It occurs mainly in association with primary disorders of the lungs such as chronic bronchitis, emphysema, and asthma, but rarely may complicate systemic disorders such as polyarteritis nodosa. The two main abnormalities responsible for this obstruction are, first, generalized narrowing of the bronchi and, second, destruction of the pulmonary parenchyma. An understanding of the interaction of these two factors is important in order to appreciate the significance of the abnormalities involved and the nature of the disability experienced by the patient.

MECHANISMS OF AIRWAY OBSTRUCTION

During inspiration, the inspiratory muscles lower alveolar pressure, and air flows into the alveoli at a rate which depends upon the caliber of the bronchi. During expiration, recoil of stretched elastic tissues expels air from the lungs by raising intra-alveolar pressure above mouth pressure. The rate of flow depends upon the pressure difference and the resistance of the airways. In normal subjects, this mechanism is sufficient to meet ventilatory needs even under conditions of severe exercise. In subjects with increased resistance to airflow, elastic recoil alone may not be sufficient to achieve the ventilation required, and active expiratory muscular efforts may be made. However, the increased intrathoracic pressure which results from this expiration muscle effort introduces a new factor in expiratory airflow, a tendency to compression of the large airways. *The key to understanding this new factor is that elastic recoil of the lung alone is responsible for raising intrabronchial pressure above intrathoracic pressure.* Providing that the pressure within the bronchi is higher than intrathoracic pressure, there is no airway compression. However, when expiratory airflow is increased in subjects with raised airway resistance or diminished elastic recoil of the lungs, the greater pressure drop along the bronchial tree may cause the pressure inside the trachea and large bronchi to fall below the surrounding intrathoracic pressure, and these structures will be compressed unless there is sufficient rigidity in their walls to resist it. Once compression occurs, no amount of further effort will increase airflow because the pressure within the bronchi cannot be increased without simultaneously increasing the surrounding pressure. In this way, compression which usually occurs in the larger segmental or main-stem bronchi forms a flow-limiting mechanism (often called a Starling resistor), and determines maximal rate of expiratory airflow. This mechanism cannot operate during inspiration; the rate of inspiratory airflow is always effort-dependent.

The maximal rate of expiratory airflow will therefore be reduced by (1) increased resistance to airflow due to structural narrowing or increased tone; (2) decreased elastic recoil of the lung parenchyma; and (3) decreased rigidity of larger airways.

Increased Airway Resistance. Increased airway resistance may be due to increased secretions; thickening of the wall of the airways caused by infiltration, edema, or glandular hypertrophy; or constriction resulting from smooth muscle contraction or fibrosis; deformity of the bronchi may also contribute. The dominant mechanism varies in different circumstances. When associated with chronic bronchitis, there are both narrowing of the smaller bronchi and increased mucus, sometimes causing plugging. When emphysema is also present, there are both narrowing and a slight loss in the number of airways, with an increased tendency to mucus plugging. The role of infection is doubtful; it has not been possible to establish a correlation between the rate of progression of airway obstruction and the frequency of infective bronchial episodes, although during acute infections airway obstruction is temporarily increased. In some areas, complete occlusion of bronchi requires that ventilation of distal areas be by collateral channels, thereby increasing airway resistance. It is possible that narrowing of chronic airways may involve increased smooth muscular tone at least in the initial stages before irreversible structural changes develop. Two observations suggest that some process additional to the results of chronic inflammation and fibrosis may be involved. First, hyper-reactivity of the bronchi is a feature of most patients with narrowing of the small airways; second, airway resistance is reduced, albeit to a small degree, after administration of isoproterenol and atropine aerosols.

Decreased Rigidity of the Walls of Larger Airways. A diminished rigidity of the trachea and bronchi is a common feature of chronic mucopurulent bronchitis. In itself, it is not responsible for reducing maximal expiratory airflow but predisposes toward airway compression when the other factors are present.

Diminished Elastic Recoil: Emphysema

The most important cause of diminished elastic recoil is emphysema. This word is derived from the Greek word meaning "an inflation" and was introduced by Laennec to describe the overinflated and partially destroyed state of the lung "vesicles." Unfortunately, many workers later adopted this term for the clinical syndrome of breathlessness, cough, and sputum with which emphysema is often associated. This resulted in confusion because a similar clinical picture may occur without emphysema. *There is now general agreement to restrict the use of the word emphysema to its original meaning as a pathologic term.* The most generally accepted definition at present is that agreed on by the World Health Organization (1961): "Emphysema is a condition of the lung characterised by increase beyond the normal in the size of air spaces distal to the terminal bronchiole, with destructive changes in their walls." There is still difference of opinion whether dilatation caused by distention without destruction should be included in the definition.

Destructive changes and dilatation may be restricted to the respiratory bronchioles (centriacinar or centrilobular emphysema), or may be more extensive with destruction of the whole of the acinus (panacinar emphysema), involving both air spaces and vascular bed. These may coalesce or distend to form bullae and cysts. Changes restricted to the periphery of the acinus (paraseptal emphysema) are never extensive and are without functional significance.

Gradual stretching but not rupture of lung tissue occurs with age (senile emphysema) and with longstanding overdistention as in severe chronic airway obstruction or status asthmaticus. Rupture of connective tissue requires weakening or destruction of the connective tissue; but until Eriksson reported in 1965 that the electrophoretic alpha$_1$ globulin peak, of which alpha$_1$ antitrypsin (AAT) is the major component, was absent in some patients with emphysema, little was known about the factors responsible. The substance AAT is a nonspecific inhibitor of proteolytic enzymes such as trypsin, elastase, skin collagenase, thrombin, and bacterial and leukocyte proteases, and is normally responsible for 90 per cent of the total serum trypsin inhibitory capacity. The degree of plasma protease inhibitory activity depends upon the inheritance of certain genes. The normal gene is termed Pi^M, the gene associated with the lowest level of inhibitory activity is Pi^Z, and other genes, e.g., Pi^S, have lesser degrees of deficiency. The homozygous ZZ phenotype has marked deficiency, whereas the heterozygous ZM phenotype and the homozygous SS have intermediate levels. Eriksson originally thought that only the homozygous (ZZ) state developed emphysema and that this was rare. It is now known that the heterozygous state with intermediate levels of inhibitory activity may also show an increased incidence of emphysema, and in one recent series 26 per cent of patients with emphysema showed some degree of inhibitor deficiency. The characteristics of emphysema associated with AAT deficiency are its development at an earlier age (mean age for homozygotes and heterozygotes 45 and 57 years, respectively) and its tendency to be more severe in the basal regions. Diminished basal perfusion on lung scan is strongly supportive of the likelihood of its presence.

These findings have suggested a possible etiology for emphysema. Proteolytic enzymes are released in the lungs at sites of inflammation and leukocyte breakdown but are normally limited in their action by the serum inhibitors. Deficiency of inhibitors may permit a greater degree of proteolysis of lung parenchyma causing emphysema. Although bronchial infection and inhaled irritants may cause widespread low-grade acinar inflammation, the localization of centriacinar emphysema to the upper parts of the lobes is explained by increased alveolar wall tension at these sites owing to gravitational effects. Basal panacinar emphysema in AAT deficiency may be related to the reported sequestration of leukocytes in the lungs, especially at the bases, with failure to inhibit leukocyte proteases. In support of this concept, emphysema has been produced experimentally by inhalation of extracts of leukocytes in animals. The importance of this hypothesis is that all types of emphysema are seen as an imbalance between proteolysis and protease inhibition. This may occur either because of increased protease production in otherwise normal individuals or because of deficient protease inhibition.

Extensive emphysema may be a major factor in limiting the maximal rate of expiratory airflow by reducing elastic recoil. The reduction in recoil is not due to alteration in the properties of the elastic fibers themselves; it is due largely to the increased size of the affected air spaces, occupying a larger proportion of the thorax and allowing less room for distention of the normal parts of the lung. This is reflected in a reduction of the maximal intrathoracic pressure which may be developed at full inspiration from the normal of 20 to 30 cm of water to as low as 3 to 5 cm of water.

Diagnosis of Emphysema During Life. There are no clinical stigmas of emphysema, and the diagnosis cannot easily be made during life because it requires evidence of the pathologic lesion. Extensive emphysema, especially centrilobular, may be present without roentgenographic abnormality. The presence of emphysema may be inferred from the chest roentgenogram if it shows reduction in the caliber and number of the peripheral branches of the pulmonary artery, usually associated with increased transradiancy of the lung field. This is the most reliable radiologic sign. Other abnormalities such as low, flat diaphragm and increased retrosternal space, although commonly present, are actually evidence only of overinflation of the lungs.

CLINICAL FEATURES OF CHRONIC AIRWAY OBSTRUCTION

Typically, the patient with chronic airway obstruction is a male cigarette smoker, between 50 and 60 years old, who may or may not have a long history of chronic bronchitis with recurrent winter bronchitis. His cardinal symptom is breathlessness on exertion, often with wheezing; it is worse in the morning, associated with a sensation of tightness until he has expectorated the night's accumulation of sputum. Intolerance of sudden exposure to cold air or smoky atmospheres which induce coughing, tightness, and breathlessness (bronchial irritability) is usually present when dyspnea is of sufficient severity to interfere with everyday activity. Similar symptoms may be precipitated by involvement in argument or other emotional situations. There is often orthopnea, along with shortness of breath on stooping. These features are attributable to disturbance of the bronchi and are common to nearly all patients with chronic airway obstruction. However, in some patients varying degrees of disturbance of pulmonary gas exchange may occur, leading to a wider range of clinical presentation; some patients have little evidence of disturbances of cardiopulmonary function, but others become cyanosed and edematous.

Professor Dornhorst of London caught the clinical imagination when he described the extremes of this range as "pink and puffing" and "blue and bloated." A number of studies have correlated these presentations with pulmonary pathology and pulmonary function disturbances, leading to the introduction of other descriptive terms, for example, emphysematous or bronchitic, "fighters or nonfighters," Type A or Type B. It must be emphasized that these are not two distinct diseases but the extremes of a range of presentation; some patients intermediate in type might well be called "blue puffers."

Type A, Emphysematous Type, "Pink Puffers"

This patient is severely breathless on exertion. He is underweight, his appearance often suggesting hyperthyroidism. The mucous membranes are pink; there is no finger clubbing. The chest is overinflated, and the accessory muscles are prominent. Cardiac and hepatic dullness are diminished or absent, and resonance extends down to the region of the eleventh to twelfth rib posteriorly. The larynx and trachea are pulled down with each inspiration. On auscultation, breath sounds are quiet, expiration is prolonged, and forced expiration induces fine sibilant rhonchi. The forced expiratory time (the time taken to deliver the forced vital capacity) is prolonged beyond four seconds.

The apex beat is usually impalpable, but pulsation is often seen and felt in the epigastrium where the heart sounds are also heard best. The chest roentgenogram confirms the overinflated state of the chest and usually shows roentgenographic evidence of emphysema. The cardiac shadow is long and narrow.

Laboratory Findings. Total lung capacity, residual volume, and residual volume–total lung capacity ratio are increased. The vital capacity, FEV_1, and the FEV_1/VC ratio are reduced. Other indices of airflow obstruction such as peak flow rate and maximal midexpiratory flow rate are also reduced. Pa_{CO_2} is normal and Pa_{O_2} may be slightly reduced. The transfer factor (diffusing capacity) for carbon monoxide is reduced.

Many of these patients have little increase in inspiratory airway resistance, expiratory airflow obstruction being dominated by *reduced pulmonary elastic recoil.* Flow limitation may be present even during quiet breathing in severe cases, and is best seen when flow-volume curves of the lung are displayed. CO_2 sensitivity is characteristically normal or near normal, and this together with the reduction in ventilatory capacity accounts for the severe exertional dyspnea.

Pathology. Panlobular emphysema is the dominant pathologic lesion in most cases. Mucous gland hyperplasia and hypertrophy may or may not be present. The heart is usually normal.

Type B, Bronchitic Type, "Blue Bloaters"

Typically, the history can be considered in three stages. First, there is a long history of chronic bronchitis with recurrent mucopurulent exacerbations. At this stage there may be no reduction of exercise capacity, although spirometry may reveal reduction in maximal ventilatory capacity. The second stage usually merges gradually with the first as the reduction in ventilatory capacity progresses to the stage at which shortness of breath on exercise becomes noticeable. Sometimes, as in Type A, this may develop relatively suddenly after an acute infective exacerbation. Usually, before shortness of breath becomes very severe, the third stage begins when the patient notices ankle edema, at first in the evenings but gradually becoming more marked and persistent.

Characteristically, the patient is well covered with a plethoric appearance. He is cyanosed at rest with warm extremities. The chest is overinflated but usually less so than in Type A. The signs of increased airway obstruction may be similar to those of Type A, but breath sounds are usually well heard and rhonchi and basal crepitations may be prominent; expiration is prolonged. The forced expiratory time is prolonged. There may be cardiac enlargement, right ventricular hypertrophy, raised jugular venous pressure, and hepatic enlargement together with edema. These signs often become more prominent during an acute exacerbation.

Laboratory Findings. Although the type B patient may have severe airway obstruction, it is not uncommon for the airway obstruction to be relatively mild (FEV_1, 1 to 1.5 liters) even though the Pco_2 is raised. Total lung capacity is usually normal, but residual volume is raised.

There is arterial desaturation of varying degree, but not often lower than 80 per cent. Secondary polycythemia occurs with the more severe degrees of desaturation. The Pa_{CO_2} is raised, usually less than 55 mm Hg in the early phases of the illness, but may progress to severe ventilatory failure with Pa_{CO_2} 65 to 75 mm Hg. This is usually well compensated but with higher levels of Pco_2 may fall below pH 7.35. During acute exacerbations more severe changes may develop.

Airway resistance is increased during both inspiration and expiration. Diffusing capacity may be normal if emphysema is slight; CO_2 sensitivity is depressed. The latter is not usually measured as a routine procedure, but can readily be observed if a rebreathing method for measuring Pco_2 is used.

The chest roentgenogram shows good bronchovascular markings with thickening of bronchial walls, but characteristically there is no roentgenographic evidence of emphysema. The heart is usually enlarged. The electrocardiogram may show evidence of right ventricular hypertrophy. In acute exacerbations, Kerley B lines, indicating edema of interlobular septa, may be seen; in addition to pulmonary hypertension, cardiac catheterization may reveal raised left ventricular end-diastolic pressure, indicating left ventricular failure. A raised blood urea is common during an acute exacerbation; this is temporary and is corrected when the patient improves.

Pathology. The lungs usually show a combination of centrilobular and panacinar emphysema, but centrilobular emphysema is the more prominent. Occasionally emphysema is absent, but mucous gland hyperplasia is said to be present always. The right ventricle is usually hypertrophied, and there may be evidence of hypertensive changes in the pulmonary artery. Thrombosis of branches of the pulmonary artery is common.

Mechanism and Significance of Differences Between the Type Extremes of Clinical Prototypes

The "pink puffer" may be regarded as an otherwise normal subject with severe reduction of ventilatory capacity resulting from the development of a flow-limiting mechanism. The pulmonary pathology does not lead to gross disturbance of ventilation-perfusion relationships, and arterial blood gas composition is virtually normal, at least at rest. Ventilatory control mechanisms are intact. By contrast, the "blue bloater" has, in addition to airflow obstruction, gross disturbance of ventilation-perfusion relationships and impairment of CO_2 sensitivity of the respiratory center. The ventilation-perfusion abnormality leads to a chain of abnormalities, beginning with arterial hypoxemia and followed by polycythemia, pulmonary hypertension, right ventricular hypertrophy, and systemic venous congestion with edema. The mechanism of impaired CO_2 sensitivity of the respiratory center is unknown; it leads to chronic ventilatory failure with hypercapnia and impairs the ability to maintain ventilation in the face of increased airway resistance.

DIAGNOSIS OF CHRONIC AIRWAY OBSTRUCTION

Clinical Diagnosis. When dyspnea is associated with symptoms of bronchial irritability and morning tightness, it strongly suggests that airway obstruction is responsible. Although rhonchi are highly suggestive, they may be absent even with severe airway obstruction. *Prolonged expiration and forced expiratory time are the only reliable signs of airway obstruction.*

Etiologic Diagnosis. A history of heavy smoking or occupational exposure to dust often suggests the causative mechanism. Radiographic evidence of emphysema in a younger person, especially basal, raises the possibility of alpha$_1$ antitrypsin deficiency. Occasionally, a striking improvement follows administration of corticosteroids or cromolyn sodium (see Ch. 505), suggesting that allergic factors are causing or contributing to the disability. *It is important never to overlook this treatable possibility; its presence is suggested if chest tightness tends to recur during the day, if there is nocturnal dyspnea, and especially if there is sputum and/or blood eosinophilia.* If there is any doubt, a therapeutic trial of these drugs should be given, but it is sometimes difficult to separate specific from general effects of corticosteroids.

Assessment of Severity of Airway Obstruction. Simple clinical assessment of the severity of airflow obstruction and reduction in ventilatory capacity may be obtained from the vital capacity and FEV$_1$, or from peak flows. More detailed measurements are seldom needed for initial clinical assessment. The following are rough correlations between FEV$_1$ and physical activity. If the FEV$_1$ is greater than 1.5 liters, the subject can usually undertake moderate exercise. With an FEV$_1$ between 1.0 and 1.5 liters, the subject can usually undertake light activity but is somewhat short of breath on hurrying or climbing stairs. With an FEV$_1$ below 1.0 liter, he is usually breathless on slight exertion, although there are wide differences according to clinical type and personality. If the degree of disability grossly exceeds the severity of the airway obstruction, other causes of shortness of breath should be sought. These include heart disease, pulmonary hypertension, anemia, thyrotoxicosis, and metabolic acidosis. An important but often overlooked cause is a psychologic disturbance. This diagnosis should be suspected if attacks of breathlessness also occur at rest and are associated with symptoms of hyperventilation, i.e., dizziness and paresthesia. This reaction tends to occur in patients with strong obsessional traits associated with an anxiety reaction or depression; the three most common precipitating factors are bereavement, illness or fear of illness, and resentment; less commonly it is an hysterical reaction.

Detection of Early Changes. Macklem has pointed out that because of the very low resistance of small bronchioles, considerable pathologic changes may be present without causing a significant increased airway resistance. Thus, doubling the resistance or halving the number of the peripheral airways will result in only a 10 per cent increase in over-all airway resistance, because this region normally contributes only 10 per cent of the total. This raises problems in the early detection of airway disease. Measurements reflecting airway resistance are relatively insensitive, and it is now considered that abnormalities in the distribution of inspired gas (single breath N$_2$ test), increased closing volume, or the demonstration of frequency dependent compliance are more likely to reveal early peripheral bronchial disease.

TREATMENT OF AIRWAY OBSTRUCTION

Despite ignorance of basic causes of chronic airway obstruction, it is nevertheless possible to reduce the effects of these disturbances by attention to detail in management.

Removal of Irritants and Treatment of Infection. Removing atmospheric irritants and stopping cigarette smoking may cause a gradual reduction in the volume of mucus and the degree of hyper-reactivity of the bronchi and a moderate decrease in airway obstruction. One of the most potent irritants is bronchial infection, and this should be eradicated or minimized by appropriate antimicrobial therapy.

Bronchodilatation. Oral and aerosol bronchodilator drugs as discussed in Ch. 505 may be helpful. However, more prolonged bronchodilatation in subjects without an allergic cause for their bronchial narrowing can sometimes be achieved with an aerosol of atropine methonitrate (0.04 mg). Its action is slower in onset, and for this reason commercial preparations combine isoproterenol or its variants and atropine.

Bronchial Toilet and Mucolytics. Attention to humidification of inspired air and active bronchial toilet with physiotherapy may induce considerable improvement in airway obstruction. Inhalation of mucolytic drugs such as acetylcysteine may occasionally be helpful, but in allergic subjects hypersensitivity reactions have been recorded. Bromhexine (8 mg three times a day) by disrupting the mucopolysaccharide fibers of noninfected sputum aids expectoration and in controlled studies has been shown to improve airway obstruction.

Respiratory Stimulants. Oral analeptics, e.g., amiphenazole, 100 to 200 mg thrice daily, and prethcamide, 400 mg three or four times daily, have been advocated for the treatment of chronic ventilatory failure. They may result in transient slight reduction in Pco$_2$, but there is no evidence that they afford clinical benefit. Acetazolamide, 250 to 500 mg, or dichlorphenamide, 50 to 100 mg twice a day, has been reported to improve the breathlessness of some patients with airway obstruction. These carbonic anhydrase inhibitors may cause reduction in Pco$_2$ up to 8 to 10 mm Hg, but this fall does not correlate with subjective improvement. Paresthesia, headache, and general malaise may occur as side effects which disappear rapidly on stopping the drug.

Circulatory Management. The use of diuretics, e.g., chlorothiazide, 0.5 to 1.0 gram, furosemide, 40 to 80 mg orally from twice weekly to daily, has greatly improved management of edematous patients. Adequate diuresis may cause considerable improvement in pulmonary gas exchange and mechanisms. Daily administration requires supplements of potassium (600 to 1200 mg four times a day). Alternatively, amiloride, triamterene, or spironolactone may be effective without the need of potassium supplements. Digoxin or digitoxin should be given only if clearly indicated because of the risk of inducing ventricular arrhythmias (see Ch. 541). These drugs should not be used during acute respiratory failure; routine monitoring of patients admitted to hospital with chronic obstructive lung disease recently showed an incidence of arrhythmia of 89 per cent, with 57 per cent requiring specific therapy; there was no correlation between the occurrence of arrhythmia and the Pa$_{CO_2}$, Pa$_{O_2}$, or pH. If the hematocrit is raised above 55 to 60 per cent, repeated venesection should be used to reduce the hematocrit to about 55 per cent.

Oxygen Therapy. This has been used in two ways: first, intermittently during exercise and in the recovery phase. Portable oxygen cylinders which provide small supplements of O$_2$ in the inspired air are available, but self-consciousness in wearing the equipment often deters patients from using them. Second, long-term oxygen therapy has been studied in patients with the Type B, "blue bloater" form of the disease and has been shown to reduce the severity of the circulatory abnormalities, at least in residents of Denver at 5000 feet. Its value at lower altitudes is unproved, and clinical trials are presently in progress.

Surgery of Emphysema. Removal of large localized emphysematous bullae or regions may reduce airway obstruction by permitting increased inflation of the remaining lung tissue and therefore increased elastic recoil. Selection of suitable patients is difficult; the best results have been obtained after removal of a single large cyst or when emphysematous changes have been in lower rather than in upper lobes. When tests of over-all function suggest widespread emphysema, improvement after bullectomy is less likely.

PROGNOSIS IN CHRONIC AIRWAY OBSTRUCTION

The prognosis in chronic airway obstruction is related to the severity of the lung disease; it is worse when airway obstruction is severe, when the diffusing capacity is markedly reduced, and when cor pulmonale is, or has been, present. It is worse at altitude than at sea level, presumably because of the greater hypoxemia. The length of history and the age of onset of symptoms are not related to mortality.

In a group of patients with chronic bronchitis with or without airway obstruction in London, 54 per cent died within ten years; 57 per cent of these died of respiratory causes, and 8 per cent died of bronchial carcinoma. The prognosis of 200 patients with airway obstruction has been studied in more detail in a group of patients in Chicago. The severity of ventilatory impairment, resting pulse rate, and mixed venous Pco_2, were the most predictive of poor survival. The conclusions were that if there is no resting tachycardia, chronic hypercapnia, or severe impairment of diffusing capacity, a five-year survival may be expected in 80 per cent of cases when the FEV_1 exceeds 1.2 liters; in 60 per cent when FEV_1 is close to 1 liter; and in 40 per cent when the FEV_1 is below 0.75 liter. If the factors listed initially are present, the survival figure is reduced by 25 per cent.

The development of weight loss is of bad prognostic significance. Intensive treatment with bronchodilator aerosols or with antimicrobial drugs is without influence on the rate of deterioration of airflow obstruction. Advances in therapy in the past 15 years have not improved survival rates after the onset of cor pulmonale, approximately two thirds of the patients being dead at five years in one series.

ACUTE RESPIRATORY FAILURE

The greatest risk to the life of a patient with chronic airway obstruction is the development of an acute increase in bronchial secretions and airway obstruction which occurs in response to an acute bronchial infection or on exposure to irritant atmospheres such as smog. In patients of the "blue bloater" type, a rise in Pco_2 will almost certainly occur; it is unusual in the "pink puffer" patient, in whom an elevation of Pco_2 implies very severe airway obstruction unless unwise sedation has been given. If Pco_2 rises above 50 mm Hg or Pa_{O_2} falls below 60 mm Hg, respiratory failure is said to be present. It is very unusual for the Pco_2 to exceed 80 mm Hg because of the concomitant development of hypoxemia. Higher values generally imply the prior administration of oxygen.

Management of this life-threatening situation requires appreciation of three things. First, the acute situation has been caused largely by increased secretions and increased airway obstruction. Second, the immediate danger is hypoxemia. Third, hypercarbia and acidemia, if present, may cause clouding or even loss of consciousness and an inability by the patient to cooperate in his therapy.

The assessment of the patient therefore requires the following two immediate decisions: Can the patient raise the secretions by coughing? And does the patient need oxygen?

Ability to Raise Secretions by Coughing. Ability of the patient to raise the secretions by coughing can only be ascertained by instructing the patient to cough; the response to this is the most useful single physical sign in this situation. If he is unable to do so unaided, skilled physiotherapy may yet be successful, especially if effective humidification can be achieved. Administration of aminophylline, 250 mg intravenously over three to five minutes, may enable an effective cough to be produced. If the patient is too drowsy to cooperate, he may be roused sufficiently by this treatment or by the administration of nikethamide, 500 to 1000 mg intravenously, or some equivalent analeptic. There is no place in this situation for continuous intravenous analeptics unless combined with intensive chest physiotherapy.

The expectoration of even a few pieces of sputum may result in dramatic improvement. If the patient cannot raise secretions despite all efforts, there is no alternative but bronchoscopy and tracheal suction or, preferably, endotracheal intubation with regular tracheal suction and a period of assisted ventilation. Tracheostomy should be avoided unless prolonged assisted ventilation becomes necessary.

Oxygen Need. The presence of severe hypoxemia does not *necessarily* mean that tissue damage is occurring because increased perfusion may transport sufficient oxygen to the tissues to permit aerobic metabolism to continue. It has been shown that an arterial Po_2 even below 30 mm Hg can be adequate for tissue oxygenation *providing that a good circulation is maintained;* but usually Pa_{O_2} values below this level are associated with evidence of tissue hypoxia in the form of lactic acidosis and raised serum transaminase levels. Because of the steep slope of the hemoglobin dissociation curve for oxygen at these levels, relatively small increases in inspired oxygen will move the patient away from the brink of tissue hypoxia.

The *danger* of administration of high concentrations of oxygen is that by correcting hypoxemia, the main source of ventilatory stimulation will be removed, thus converting a conscious, cyanosed patient capable of cooperation into a pink unconscious patient in whom secretions accumulate and in whom intubation and assisted ventilation become mandatory. With care, the cautious administration of oxygen in inspired concentrations of 24 to 28 per cent, e.g., using a Venturi device, will increase arterial oxygen tension sufficiently without seriously reducing ventilatory drives in the majority of patients. With improvement in ventilatory capacity, progressive increases in oxygen concentrations will be tolerated.

The absolute indications for oxygen may be taken as, first, evidence of poor peripheral circulation, i.e., poor volume pulse, low blood pressure, poor capillary filling; and second, an arterial Po_2 below 30 mm Hg. In practice, when arterial Po_2 levels may not be available, it is advisable to administer 24 to 28 per cent O_2, e.g., using a Venturi device, to all patients and to measure Pco_2 serially. If the Pco_2 does not rise more than a few millimeters over the next one to two hours, it may be possible to increase the concentration of oxygen further. If adequate improvement in Pa_{O_2} cannot be achieved by these means without causing a progressive rise in Pa_{CO_2}, then assisted ventilation must be considered.

Other Therapeutic Measures. While these more urgent measures are being instituted the sputum should be obtained for culture. A broad-spectrum antimicrobial drug should be started, e.g., tetracycline, 500 mg four times a day, or ampicillin, 500 mg four times a day orally or parenterally, unless there are clinical indications for a different drug. A diuretic, e.g., furosemide, 40 to 80 mg intravenously, should be given if there is any evidence of pulmonary congestion or peripheral edema. Digitalis should be given with caution in the acute severely hypoxemic state because of the danger of inducing a ventricular dysrhythmia.

Prophylaxis. In view of the seriousness of acute exacerbations, advice about minimizing their occurrence should be given. The patient and his relatives should be warned of the signs of acute exacerbation and the need for attention to bronchial toilet and prompt antimicrobial therapy. A patient with previous history of respiratory failure should be admitted to hospital without delay if no rapid improvement occurs. Influenza vaccination should be administered annually.

Bates, D. V., Macklem, P. T., and Christie, R. V.: Respiratory Function in Disease. 2nd ed. Philadelphia, W. B. Saunders Company, 1971.

Burns, B. H., and Howell, J. B. L.: Disproportionately severe breathlessness in chronic bronchitis. Q. J. Med., 38:277, 1969.

Burrows, B., and Earle, R. H.: Prediction of survival in patients with chronic airway obstruction. Am. Rev. Respir. Dis., 99:865, 1969.

Burrows, B., Fletcher, C. M., Heard, B. E., Jones, N. L., and Wootliff, J. S.: The emphysematous and bronchial types of chronic airways obstruction. Lancet, 1:830, 1966.

Cotes, J. E.: Lung Function: Assessment and Application in Medicine. 2nd ed. Oxford and Edinburgh, Blackwell Scientific Publications, 1968.

Filley, G. F., Beckwitt, H. J., Reeves, J. T., and Mitchell, R. S.: Chronic obstructive bronchopulmonary disease. II. Oxygen transport in two clinical types. Am. J. Med., 44:26, 1968.

Hogg, J. C., Macklem, P. T., and Thurlbeck, W. M.: Site and nature of airway obstruction in chronic obstructive lung disease. N. Engl. J. Med., 278:1355, 1968.

Lane, D. J., Howell, J. B. L., and Giblin, B.: Relation between airways obstruction and CO₂ tension in chronic obstructive airways disease. Br. Med. J., 3:707, 1968.

Lieberman, J.: Alpha₁-antitrypsin deficiency. In Symposium on Chronic Respiratory Disease. Med. Clin. North Am., 57:691, 1973.

Matsuba, K., and Thurlbeck, W. M.: Disease of the small airways in chronic bronchitis. Am. Rev. Respir. Dis., 107:552, 1973.

Nash, E. S., Briscoe, W. A., and Cournand, A.: The relationship between clinical and physiological findings in chronic obstructive disease of the lungs. Med. Thorac., 22:305, 1965.

Oswald, N. C., Medvie, V. C., and Waller, R. E.: Chronic bronchitis: A ten year follow up. Thorax, 22:279, 1967.

Pride, N. B., Barter, C. E., and Hugh-Jones, P.: The ventilation of bullae and the effect of their removal on thoracic gas volumes and tests of over-all pulmonary function. Am. Rev. Respir. Dis., 107:83, 1973.

Tarkoff, M. P., Kueppers, F., and Miller, W. F.: Pulmonary emphysema and alpha₁-antitrypsin deficiency. Am. J. Med., 45:220, 1968.

Uses and Dangers of Oxygen Therapy. Report of a Sub-Committee of the Standing Medical Advisory Committee. Edinburgh, Her Majesty's Stationery Office, 1969.

507. RESPIRATORY FAILURE AND ITS MANAGEMENT

James P. Smith

Definitions. *Respiratory insufficiency* indicates impaired ability of the lungs to eliminate carbon dioxide or to take up oxygen. The condition may be obvious at rest or may be manifested only by inability of the patient to meet increased demands of exercise. Respiratory insufficiency has progressed to *respiratory failure* when serious abnormalities of the arterial blood gases are present at rest.

Respiratory failure is characterized by an arterial carbon dioxide tension (Pa_{CO_2}) in excess of 50 mm Hg or an arterial oxygen tension (Pa_{O_2}) of 60 mm Hg or less. Normal or only slight abnormalities of the blood gases may be present until the immediate preterminal stages of widely different disorders, including neuromuscular respiratory paralysis and pure emphysema. In these and other disorders the clinical signs of respiratory insufficiency indicate treatment before the appearance of serious blood gas changes.

Etiology and Classification. The causes of respiratory failure are multiple and often coexist in the individual patient. The classification in the accompanying table identifies five groups of disorders according to the anatomic component of the breathing apparatus which has been primarily damaged. The table also separates the causes of failure based on the characteristic alteration in Pa_{CO_2} and Pa_{O_2} which they produce. *Ventilatory failure* is distinguished by carbon dioxide retention, and is always accompanied by hypoxemia, as long as air without supplemental oxygen is breathed (hypercapnic-hypoxemic respiratory failure). *Oxygenation failure* consists purely in hypoxemia with initially low Pa_{CO_2} (hypocapnic-hypoxemic respiratory failure).

Ventilatory failure is characteristic in neurologic disorders, in respiratory muscle disease, in other chest bellows conditions, and in chronic obstructive pulmonary disease.

Oxygenation failure is usual in infiltrative diseases of the lung, both diffuse and localized, in pulmonary vascular disorders, and in the extrapulmonary conditions which cause secondary respiratory failure. When extremely severe, oxygenation failure has been variously termed "shock lung," "wet lung," or "adult respiratory distress syndrome."

Pathophysiology. The essential difference between *ventilatory failure* and *oxygenation failure* is the occurrence in the former of CO_2 retention.

Hypercapnia in disorders of the central and peripheral nervous systems and the respiratory muscles is caused by simple alveolar hypoventilation and is accompanied by a necessary reduction in Pa_{O_2}, which is proportional to the increase in Pa_{CO_2} (see Ch. 491). Most commonly, *ventilatory failure* is due to chronic obstructive pulmonary disease (COPD), and the development of hypercapnia is more complex than over-all alveolar hypoventilation (West, 1971). Moreover, hypoxemia observed during ventilatory failure in COPD is much more severe than predicted from the Pa_{CO_2}. This "extra" reduction in Pa_{O_2} is caused by gross disturbances in ventilation–blood flow relationships ($\dot{V}_A/\dot{Q}$), which occur early

Causes of Respiratory Failure

I. Disorders of the central nervous system:
  A. Drug intoxication
      Sedatives (barbiturates, glutethimide)
      Tranquilizers (phenothiazines, meprobamate)
      Analgesics (opiates, e.g., morphine, heroin, methadone)
      Anesthetic gases
  B. Vascular disorders and hypoperfusion states
      Brainstem infarction
      Brainstem hemorrhage
      Postcardiac arrest
      Shock
  C. Trauma to the brainstem
      Head injury
      Increased intracranial pressure
  D. Infection
      Encephalitis (viral)
      Bulbar poliomyelitis
  E. Miscellaneous
      Primary alveolar hypoventilation (with or without obesity)
      Myxedema
      Status epilepticus

II. Disorders of the peripheral nervous system and respiratory
      muscles:
  A. Anterior horn cell and peripheral nerve disorders
      Guillain-Barré syndrome
      Poliomyelitis
      Amyotrophic lateral sclerosis
      Other polyneuritides
  B. Myoneural junction disorders
      Myasthenia gravis
      Tetanus
      Curariform drugs (succinylcholine, curare, polymyxin,
      Coly-Mycin, streptomycin, kanamycin)
      Anticholinesterase drugs (insecticides, neostigmine)
  C. Muscular disorders
      Polymyositis
      Muscular dystrophies
      Myotonia

III. Disorders of the chest wall and pleura:
  A. Scoliosis
      Congenital
      Idiopathic
      Paralytic (postpolio)
      Miscellaneous (post-thoracic surgery, post-tubercular,
      Marfan's syndrome, von Recklinghausen's disease)

These disorders produce *ventilatory failure;* hypoxemia
precedes carbon dioxide retention

_____

  B. Chest trauma
      Flail chest
      Multiple rib fractures
      Post-thoracotomy
  C. Pleural disorders
      Massive effusions
      Tension pneumothorax
      Massive fibrosis

IV. Intrinsic pulmonary disorders:
  A. Airway obstruction
      Chronic obstructive pulmonary disease (chronic bronchitis,
      emphysema, asthma)
      Acute obstruction (foreign body, acute epiglottitis and
      laryngitis, inhalation burns, noxious gases)

These disorders produce *either ventilatory or oxygenation failure;*
ventilatory failure is more common

_____

  B. Alveolar and interstitial disorders
      Pneumonia (lobar, aspiration, interstitial)
      The granulomatoses and fibroses
      Pulmonary edema (left ventricular failure)
      Lymphangitic metastases
  C. Vascular disorders
      Embolic disease (thrombo-, fat, tumor)
      Obliterative vasculitis (primary pulmonary hypertension,
      scleroderma)

V. Extrapulmonary disorders leading to pulmonary disease:
      Hepatic failure, shock, renal failure, acute pancreatitis,
      peritonitis, sepsis, postcardiopulmonary bypass, and
      post-traumatic states (extrathoracic injuries and surgery)

These disorders produce *oxygenation failure;* hypercapnia is
usually a preterminal event

_____

in chronic bronchitis and emphysema and during attacks of asthma.

The lungs in oxygenation failure are also characterized by $\dot{V}_A/\dot{Q}$ disturbances with regions of poorly or nonventilated alveoli. When perfusion continues through such areas, the issuing capillary blood has relatively high Pco_2 and low Po_2. But by way of contrast to COPD, hyperventilation of the relatively large volume of alveoli remaining normal in the disorders causing *oxygenation failure* is sufficient to offset the increment of Pco_2. However, the amount of oxygen which is added by hyperventilation to hemoglobin already normally saturated is limited by the shape of the oxyhemoglobin dissociation curve (see accompanying figure). This is never sufficient to counter the contribution of deoxygenated blood to the arterialized stream; thus low Pa_{O_2} results. Equally or perhaps more important in the genesis of hypoxemia in cases of very *severe oxygenation failure* (shock lung, wet lung, adult respiratory distress syndrome) is the impediment to oxygen diffusion which results from invasion of the interstitium by edema, inflammatory cells, fibrosis, granuloma, or tumor cells. Yet even in these cases with extreme hypoxemia, hyperventilation, sustained by hypoxic stimulation of the peripheral chemoreceptors and by stimulation of the respiratory centers via stretch receptors in the alveoli and chest wall, maintains normal or low Pa_{CO_2}.

Respiratory acidosis, acute or chronic, is typical of *ventilatory failure.* Not infrequently, however, the administration of diuretic agents to patients with *chronic ventilatory failure* without adequate chloride replacement may impose a *metabolic alkalosis.* Caution is necessary to avoid too rapid reduction of chronic hypercapnia by mechanical ventilation, especially in these circumstances, because myoclonus, seizures, coma, and dangerous cardiac arrhythmias may result. *Oxygenation failure* is characterized initially by *respiratory alkalosis.* In addition, a metabolic contribution to alkalosis may obtain from diuretic therapy, vomiting, gastric tube drainage, or multiple blood transfusions. The appearance of *metabolic acidosis* resulting from hypoxia, shock, sepsis, or renal failure is a dire and often preterminal complication of both *ventilatory* and *oxygenation* failure. The pathophysiologic bases and the clinical signs and symptoms associated with these important disturbances of acid-base equilibrium are discussed in Ch. 805. The important cardiovascular disorders, including pulmonary hypertension, cor pulmonale, and left ventricular failure, which commonly exist during respiratory failure are discussed in Ch. 546 to 550.

Clinical and Laboratory Evaluation. *Clinical Phenomena.* In respiratory failure the clinical indicators of disturbances in blood gases and pH are unreliable. Even a low order of suspicion of hypoxemia or hypercapnia

OXYGEN-HEMOGLOBIN DISSOCIATION CURVE

The clinical importance of a low Pa_{O_2} is determined by the reduction in arterial oxygen content it produces. Oxygen content in turn is dependent on hemoglobin concentration and the arterial oxygen saturation (Sa_{O_2}%); i.e., oxygen content = grams of hemoglobin × 1.34 ml oxygen × Sa_{O_2}%. Note that a decrease in Pa_{O_2} from 95 to 50 mm Hg causes only a 10 per cent decrease in Sa_{O_2} and O_2 content. However, at 50 mm Hg, a small reduction in Pa_{O_2}, as may occur with a minor decrease of alveolar ventilation, produces a sharp fall of Sa_{O_2} and content. *Arterial hypoxemia* then causes *tissue hypoxia* at some indefinite point over the steep portion of the curve and before the lethal limit of 30 per cent Sa_{O_2}. Moderate arterial oxygen unsaturation (75 to 85 per cent) is acceptable during treatment of respiratory failure, provided that tissue oxygen is adequate. The latter is generally assessed as follows: tissue oxygen = $\frac{\text{cardiac output} \times \text{arterial } O_2 \text{ content}}{\text{tissue } O_2 \text{ consumption}}$. Successful therapy of respiratory failure requires attention to all elements of this expression.

should prompt laboratory confirmation. Maximal information about the initial severity of respiratory failure is obtained if Pa_{CO_2}, Pa_{O_2} or Sa_{O_2}, and pH are measured before treatment is initiated. The inspired oxygen concentration (Fi_{O_2}), respiratory frequency (f), tidal volume (V_T) and whether breathing is spontaneous or supported by mechanical ventilation should be recorded. Often it is necessary to sample the arterial blood and to begin treatment before the history, physical examination, and other laboratory investigations are completed.

History taking should be directed at determining rapidly the nature of the disorder underlying the respiratory failure and the acute precipitating event. The precipitating event may be obvious in patients with an asthmatic attack, trauma, airway burn, or confessed drug overdose; however, concealed drug overdose, minor infection in chronic lung disease, or excessive transfusion during surgery may be detected only after meticulous questioning or search of the medical record. A history of taking narcotics, tranquilizers, or other respiratory depressants should be sought in all patients.

The level of consciousness manifested by the patient indicates the severity of failure. Mental cloudiness, apathy, headache, and depressed tendon reflexes comprise the classic "CO_2 narcosis syndrome," but diffuse myoclonus, asterixis, and papilledema may also be observed with hypercapnia. When the brain is hypoxic, irritability, insomnia, and impaired judgment usually precede delirium, convulsions, or coma. Bradypnea (f<10) is characteristic of central nervous system damage or depression by drugs, whereas tachypnea (f>20) occurs in failure from most other causes. The excursion of the chest bellows and diaphragm as evaluated by percussion and palpation gives some index of ventilatory ability. Auscultation of the neck and chest can detect obstruction of the upper airway, pneumothorax, pleural rub or effusion, or rales and wheezes in the lower air-

ways. In chronic obstructive pulmonary disease wheezes may not be heard because of diminished airflow until the patient is directed to increase his depth and rate of breathing. This maneuver is also useful in other causes of *ventilatory failure,* because an increase in breath sounds suggests that alveolar ventilation might be improved by continued verbal or tactile stimulation without resorting to immediate mechanical ventilation. Rales and rhonchi are produced by bronchopulmonary infection in patients with *ventilatory failure* and by pulmonary edema causing *oxygenation failure.* These conditions must be differentiated, because treatment with high concentrations of oxygen and morphine is appropriate in some cases of pulmonary edema, but it may be lethal in hypercapnic subjects.

Examinations of the cardiovascular system may demonstrate systolic hypertension, flushed skin, and warm extremities which suggest the presence of hypercapnia, whereas hypotension implies severe acidemia, marked hypoxia, or a nonpulmonary disorder such as sepsis, hemorrhage, or low cardiac output. Cyanosis appears with reduction of peripheral blood flow and as a late sign of arterial hypoxemia, not appreciated by most observers until Sa_{O_2} is less than 75 per cent.

Laboratory Evaluation. Minimal laboratory survey of patients with acute respiratory failure includes complete blood count, urinalysis, measurement of blood urea nitrogen or serum creatinine and serum electrolytes, electrocardiogram, chest x-ray, vital capacity (VC), some measure of air flow, i.e., one-second forced expiratory volume (FEV_1), or peak expiratory flow rate (PEFR), and determinations of arterial blood gases. The hemoglobin determination may identify anemia and the potential for increase of blood oxygen content by transfusion, or it may reveal erythrocytosis secondary to chronic hypoxemia. If polycythemia is severe (HCT > 60 per cent), therapeutic phlebotomy is warranted once oxygenation is adequate. The leukocyte count varies among the disorders causing failure, but it is usually normal during bronchial infection in patients with chronic obstructive pulmonary disease. A normal urinalysis and a normal serum creatinine exclude a renal contribution to acidosis. The importance of chloride and potassium levels has been discussed previously. The *electrocardiogram* during respiratory failure may be normal, or it may identify cardiac arrhythmia, right or left ventricular hypertrophy, or myocardial infarction. The chest roentgenogram can identify the presence of pneumonia, pleural effusion, pneumothorax, atelectasis, fibrosis, and pulmonary edema. The chest film is usually normal in neuromuscular disorders and is frequently normal or unchanged during acute ventilatory failure in patients with asthma or chronic bronchitis. Bedside measurements of vital capacity and FEV_1 or PEFR are useful in quantitating the extent of ventilatory impairment and changes with treatment. Decrease of FEV_1/VC per cent or PEFR suggests obstruction caused by chronic bronchitis, emphysema, or asthma. A reduced vital capacity without airway obstruction indicates a restrictive ventilatory defect caused by neuromuscular disease, diffuse pulmonary infiltration, massive pleural effusion, or other causes. Additional laboratory studies are selected according to the underlying cause and precipitating event of failure. Gram stain and culture of the sputum are indicated in all patients suspected of having a pulmonary infection. Monitoring of central venous pressure is a useful guide when correcting disturbances of fluid balance. A flow-directed pulmonary cardiac catheter can be used to monitor pulmonary artery pressure and pulmonary "wedge" pressure when it is considered necessary to assess pulmonary vascular dynamics and left ventricular performance.

TREATMENT OF ACUTE RESPIRATORY FAILURE

General Approach

Acute respiratory failure is prevented by identifying patients at risk, promptly starting ambulatory treatment, and immediately hospitalizing patients with respiratory insufficiency. This medical emergency is best managed in a respiratory intensive care facility. Such units, when staffed by specially trained physicians and nurses, permit close patient monitoring and the appropriate use of the many therapeutic modalities now available.

Immediate life-saving measures, such as establishing a patent airway and ensuring adequate ventilation and oxygenation, often must be implemented before the cause or the severity of the physiologic derangements is known in detail.

The upper airway is cleared by suctioning or manual removal of debris and secretions from the nose and mouth. Tactile and verbal stimulation of somnolent patients is employed to achieve a more wakeful state and to induce cough for clearing the lower airway. In patients with impairment of swallowing or severe obtundation, an oropharyngeal airway should be installed to facilitate suctioning and to prevent obstruction by the tongue. *Immediate endotracheal intubation* is indicated when the oropharyngeal airway appears inadequate or when the patient is comatose. An oral or nasal endotracheal tube with an inflatable cuff provides ready access for suctioning, prevents aspiration, and secures a reliable airway for mechanical ventilation if required. The cuff is pretested for leak and maintained in the inflated state to prevent aspiration of upper airway secretions. Periodic deflations for five minutes every two hours and use of minimal inflation pressure reduce injury to the tracheal mucosa. Meticulous attention to sterile techniques minimizes the risk of introducing bronchopulmonary infection when the airway is suctioned. With proper care, an endotracheal tube can be kept in place without being changed for several days.

Emergency tracheostomy is performed for obstruction of the airway at or above the level of the larynx (e.g. maxillofacial injury, laryngeal edema, foreign body), whereas in all other conditions it is deferred until the later care of respiratory failure. *Elective tracheostomy,* performed over the cuffed endotracheal tube in the operating room or intensive care unit with oxygenation and ventilation assured, is indicated when secretions are unmanageable or when mechanical ventilation is required for longer than one week.

Artificial ventilation is necessary in patients with apnea or obviously inadequate minute ventilation. This is accomplished by mouth-to-mouth breathing or a self-inflating bag-mask combination while the need for a mechanical respirator is assessed. A respirator is required for patients who remain apneic or fail to increase minute ventilation after several minutes of emergency ventilation. Other indications for mechanical ventilation vary greatly according to the disorder causing failure; these are considered below. Once the decision to employ a respirator is made, endotracheal intubation is required. *Attempts to provide prolonged mechanical ventilation by a face mask are ineffective and hazardous.* Essential features of any mechanical respirator include (1) reliable delivery of a preselected tidal volume despite changes in the patient's airway resistance and pulmonary compliance; (2) accurate control of the inspired oxygen concentration over the full range of 21 to 100 per cent; (3) efficient humidification; and (4) effective safeguards to prevent bacterial contamination. Other desirable features include the ability of the machine to provide periodic large tidal volumes ("sighs"), positive end-expiratory pressure, in-line nebulization of medication, and the "assist" and "controlled" modes of breathing. In the "assist" mode, inspiration is initiated by the patient and tidal volume is supplemented by the respirator. With "controlled" ventilation, both rate and depth are imposed by the apparatus; this mode of ventilation is preferred because it eliminates the patient's respiratory work and establishes adequate inspiratory time for delivery of the tidal volume. A machine setting of 12 to 20 cycles per minute and an inspiratory-to-expiratory-time ratio of 1:2 or 1:3 are acceptable for most adults. A longer time for expiration minimizes the increase in intrathoracic pressure and consequent decrease of venous return and cardiac output. Tidal volume settings and the inflation pressures required for their delivery should be varied according to the size of the patient and the specific disorder causing respiratory failure.

Oxygen is indicated whenever hypoxia is suspected, and this therapy should be started before arterial blood gas results are available. The initial oxygen concentration should be selected according to the cause of the failure.

When chronic obstructive pulmonary disease is likely and the patient is not in coma, 24 to 28 per cent oxygen is used to achieve adequate arterial saturation without inducing underventilation from complete loss of hypoxic ventilatory drive. Controlled low-dose oxygen is also suitable for immediate treatment of conscious patients with other causes of *ventilatory failure* and chronic hypercapnia, e.g., scoliosis and the primary hypoventilation syndromes. Although not all patients with chronic hypercapnia demonstrate reduction of ventilation with oxygen administration, those at risk cannot be readily identified. It is therefore safest to initiate treatment with an $F_{I_{O_2}}$ of 24 per cent, increasing to 28 to 35 per cent if there is failure to promptly achieve an Sa_{O_2} of 75 to 85 per cent. When *ventilatory failure* is associated with coma or one of the other indications for mechanical ventilation listed above, oxygen is delivered by the respirator and poses no threat of underventilation at any $F_{I_{O_2}}$.

In conscious patients suspected of having *oxygenation failure,* an initial oxygen dosage of 30 to 40 per cent is appropriate. These concentrations are approximated by nasal cannulas with oxygen flow rates of 4 to 6 liters per minute, but more closely by Venturi-type masks. A much higher $F_{I_{O_2}}$ may be necessary in the treatment of severe *oxygenation failure;* concentrations between 40 and 100 per cent can be provided by several available bag-mask appliances with a nonrebreathing reservoir. Oxygen toxicity of the lung which is both dose- and time-related is a complication of prolonged therapy with $F_{I_{O_2}}$ above 40 per cent.

Neurologic Disorders

Drug overdose is the most important central nervous system cause of *ventilatory failure.* When respiratory depression by opiates (heroin, methadone, morphine) is suspected, a specific pharmacologic antagonist (naloxone HCl, 0.4 mg intravenously) is administered immediately and repeated at two- to three-minute intervals two or three times if necessary. With other drug intoxications (e.g., barbiturates), the nonspecific analeptic respiratory stimulants (e.g., nikethamide) have limited value, and serious side effects, especially seizure, may accompany their use.

Techniques for the care of the airway and the indications for endotracheal intubation in drug-induced and other neuromuscular causes of *ventilatory failure* are discussed above. In addition, the subject of abnormalities in the neurologic control of respiration is considered in Ch. 492.

In both neurologic and respiratory muscle disease, changes in the arterial blood gases are late and insensitive indications of impending ventilatory disaster. The time to institute mechanical ventilation, except in the obvious instance of apnea or grossly inadequate minute ventilation, is identified by changes in physical signs and vital capacity. Commonly the earliest signs of ventilatory insufficiency appear during sleep when Pa_{CO_2} rises and when the conscious effort to breathe, which may be a critically important ventilatory drive in neuromuscular disease, is eliminated. Rapid shallow breathing, the depth of which cannot be augmented on command, characterizes peripheral nervous system and respiratory muscle impairment. Dyspnea is usually prominent, and the patient frequently complains of air hunger before significant changes in minute ventilation occur. Total ventilation is maintained by the rapid rate, but dead space ventilation is favored. When the patient is exhausted, rapidly progressive hypoventilation supervenes. This sequence is prevented by serial measurements of vital capacity as a progressive decrease of VC long precedes the development of hypercapnia. Preparations for mechanical ventilation should be made when VC is less than one half of predicted, and use of a respirator should be considered when VC is one third of the predicted value. If alveolar hypoventilation and hypoxemia of a degree requiring therapy ($Sa_{O_2} < 75$ to 85 per cent) are demonstrated in acutely progressive neuromuscular disease, the patient has already been too long without mechanical support of ventilation.

Since the distribution of ventilation, airway resistance, and lung compliance are generally normal in patients with neurologic or respiratory muscle disease, the minute ventilation required from a mechanical respirator is predictable from conventional nomograms. Similarly, because ventilation/perfusion relationships and diffusion capacity are also typically normal, unless pneumonia or aspiration has occurred, an $F_{I_{O_2}}$ of 25 to 30 per cent is usually sufficient to maintain Pa_{O_2} and Sa_{O_2} at normal values. An important and common exception to these modest ventilatory and oxygenation requirements, however, is *heroin or methadone pulmonary edema*. Typically, the patient is in coma with pinpoint pupils, deep cyanosis, apnea or bradypnea, and hypotension. Pink, foamy edema fluid is present in the mouth, airway, and lungs, causing reduced lung volume, severe ventilation/perfusion disturbances, and abnormalities of diffusion. Acute hypercapnia, profound hypoxemia, and combined respiratory and metabolic acidosis result. Successful therapy requires endotracheal intubation, immediate mechanical ventilation with large tidal volumes, and minute ventilation of three or more times that predicted. Initially, an inspired oxygen concentration of 60 to 100 per cent is necessary to achieve adequate Sa_{O_2}; the oxygen concentration is lowered as rapidly as possible to avoid oxygen toxicity. Sodium bicarbonate may be required to correct the metabolic component of the acidosis, and rapidly acting diuretics may facilitate clearance of the edema. Temporary support of blood pressure with vasopressor agents may occasionally be necessary, but hypotension, shock, and the other clinical features of this dramatic syndrome are most effectively reversed by correction of the hypoxia and acidemia.

Chronic Obstructive Pulmonary Disease

Acute ventilatory failure in chronic obstructive pulmonary disease often develops insidiously, and consciousness remains relatively well preserved. Common precipitating events include bronchopulmonary infection, congestive heart failure, and injudicious administration of high-dose oxygen, sedatives, or tranquilizers to hypercapnic subjects.

Treatment of acute failure is guided by the patient's level of consciousness rather than the arterial blood gas values. Conscious patients should receive (1) controlled low dose oxygen, (2) intensive nursing care, and (3) general supportive measures without mechanical ventilation.

The objective of controlled low dose oxygen is prompt restoration of Sa_{O_2} to 75 to 85 per cent. This is achieved in the majority of patients with 24 per cent $F_{I_{O_2}}$; increasing to 28 or 35 per cent only as necessary minimizes the risk of oxygen-induced depression of ventilation. The appropriate Venturi-type mask is the most reliable device for delivering oxygen in this low range; nasal cannulas at low flow rates with close monitoring of the blood gases are preferred by some physicians. When adequate Sa_{O_2} is established, time becomes available for intensive nursing care and general supportive measures to reverse the disturbances that led to acute failure.

Intensive nursing care is both one of the most important facets of treatment and the most difficult to ensure. During early treatment, techniques to reduce airway obstruction and improve the patient's level of consciousness are performed by a specially trained nurse assigned to the bedside. Secretions are often cleared by demanding the patient to cough and to breathe deeply and by striking the chest with a flat hand. The nurse also assists the patient with nebulizers that deliver bronchodilator aerosols, and she suctions the lower airway in precomatose patients. Verbal and tactile stimulation may be constantly required to increase alertness and ventilatory effort in the initial hours of care. Later, the patient is permitted to sleep for periods to avoid exhaustion and further hypercapnia.

Antimicrobials, bronchodilator drugs, diuretics, digitalis, and electrolyte preparations are administered to combat infection, reverse airway obstruction, improve heart failure, and correct metabolic disturbances. Bronchopulmonary infection is assumed to be present during *acute ventilatory failure* secondary to chronic obstructive pulmonary disease. In the absence of specific pneumonia and if the usual mixed bacterial floras are present in the sputum, treatment is begun with ampicillin or tetracycline. Bronchodilator drugs should also be tried in most patients. Aerosols of these drugs should be delivered by nebulizers that require minimal patient effort. For this purpose, conventional intermittent positive pressure breathing (IPPB) machines designed as respirators are best avoided, because they often produce fatigue and have not been demonstrated to be more effective than simple devices which employ a fluidic principle or other means to generate an aerosol. Solutions of 0.3 to 0.5 ml of 1:200 isoproterenol, or 0.5 ml of a mixture of isoetharine and phenylephrine diluted with 2 to 3 ml of saline may be given every two to six hours. Careful monitoring and caution in the use of these drugs are required to avoid cardiac arrhythmias. Orally or parenterally administered bronchodilators may be used in addition to aerosols. Of the xanthine derivatives, aminophylline by intravenous infusion or rectal suppository (250 to 500 mg every four to six hours), is most effective during severe failure. During convalescence, oral preparations of aminophylline alone or in combination with ephedrine sulfate may be useful.

Corticosteroids, unless specifically contraindicated, are used in all cases of asthma producing *ventilatory failure*. The equivalent of 60 to 80 mg of prednisone daily in divided doses is usually adequate in nonsteroid-dependent asthmatics, but much higher doses (to 1000 mg per day) have been recommended for patients already receiving these drugs. In chronic bronchitis and emphysema, corticosteroids are reserved for patients with intractable wheezing or those in whom the sympathomimetic effects of the other bronchodilator agents are not acceptable. An effective diuretic (furosemide, 40 to 120 mg intravenously) is indicated whenever edema is present. The value of a diuretic in patients without overt edema or signs of cor pulmonale is controversial, but its use has been recommended to eliminate occult increases in extravascular lung water and thereby to improve gas transfer.

Administration of adequate amounts of fluids facilitates clearance of tenacious secretions, but excessive parenteral fluids may precipitate or worsen cor pulmonale. It should be emphasized that patients with chronic hypercapnia and cor pulmonale who have received diuretics before the development of acute ventilatory failure are frequently depleted of potassium and chloride. Replacement of these ions, especially chloride, is recommended from the outset of therapy.

Digitalis is useful in cor pulmonale, but initiation of the drug early in *acute ventilatory failure* is hazardous and usually unnecessary. In patients who have already been given digitalis, maintenance on the drug is continued after severe hypoxemia has been relieved.

Conservative therapy with controlled low dose oxygen, intensive nursing care, and general measures is successful in most patients with *acute ventilatory failure* secondary to chronic obstructive pulmonary disease. Endotracheal intubation and mechanical ventilation are reserved for the small number of patients (10 per cent) with untreated ventilatory failure who present in coma and for those in whom conservative therapy either fails to provide adequate Sa_{O_2} or is associated with marked respiratory acidosis, shock, or coma. Endotracheal tubes are well tolerated for several days; performance of a tracheostomy is not likely to improve the outcome in patients with ventilatory failure secondary to COPD that is not corrected during respirator care for seven or more days. Mechanical ventilation is best achieved with a volume-cycled respirator operating in the "controlled" mode. Requirements for minute ventilation in this group cannot be predicted without reference to the Pa_{CO_2}, but tidal volume and rate should initially be set to deliver twice the minute ventilation needed as predicted from the patient's size. The immediate objectives of mechani-

cal ventilation are to produce normal pH rather than normal Pa_{CO_2} and normal Sa_{O_2}. Normal Sa_{O_2} can usually be achieved with an $F_{I_{O_2}}$ of 35 to 40 per cent delivered by the respirator. Continuous mechanical ventilation is provided until the patient is fully conscious, the cardiovascular system is stable, and acid-base and electrolyte abnormalities are corrected. Complications of mechanical ventilation in addition to overcorrection alkalosis include gastrointestinal hemorrhage, local tracheobronchial injury from the tube or suctioning, and bronchopulmonary infection. Sedation and antacids may reduce the risks of gastrointestinal hemorrhage, and meticulous suctioning technique and cleaning of the respiratory equipment reduces the risk of injuring and contaminating the airway. Procedures for weaning patients from the respirator are not within the scope of this discussion; the general management of patients with chronic obstructive pulmonary disease and chronic hypercapnia may be found in Ch. 506.

Oxygenation Failure

The provision of adequate oxygen to the tissues without producing oxygen toxicity of the lungs is the main therapeutic goal in *oxygenation failure* (hypocapnic-hypoxemic respiratory failure). Concomitantly, other measures should be applied to reverse the underlying disorder. When hypoxemia is moderate (Pa_{O_2}: 45 to 60 mm Hg) and specific therapy is initiated early, as in bacterial pneumonia, 35 to 40 per cent $F_{I_{O_2}}$ (oxygen delivered by nasal cannulas, 6 liters per minute or Venturi mask) usually suffices. However, severe and progressive hypoxemia (Pa_{O_2}: 20 to 45 mm Hg), sometimes resistant to all forms of oxygen therapy, may be encountered with fulminant pneumonia and a wide variety of other clinical disorders (table). Typically with *severe oxygenation failure* ("shock lung," "wet lung," "adult respiratory distress syndrome") there are tachypnea and hyperventilation yet progressive hypoxemia despite administration of oxygen in increasing concentrations, decreased pulmonary compliance, and advancing opacification of the lungs in the chest films. Pathologically, interstitial pulmonary edema, fibrin accumulation, alveolar hemorrhage, and hyaline membrane formation are prominent. In some disorders (bacterial and viral pneumonia, hypersensitivity alveolitis, acute pancreatitis, uremia, pulmonary edema), the syndrome evolves steadily, whereas in other conditions (trauma, shock, respiratory burns, postcirculatory perfusion states) there is characteristically a latent period from the initial insult to the onset of *severe oxygenation failure*.

Preventive and early treatment measures in *severe oxygenation failure* include (1) prompt treatment of pneumonia, (2) avoidance of excessive parenteral fluid or blood transfusion, (3) early use of diuretics when an increase in extravascular lung water is suspected, (4) rapid correction of hypotension and shock, (5) use of ultrafilters during transfusion to prevent particulate matter from lodging in the pulmonary microcirculation, and (6) restriction of $F_{I_{O_2}}$ to 40 per cent to avoid oxygen toxicity.

The risk of lung damage notwithstanding, an $F_{I_{O_2}}$ as high as 100 per cent may be necessary to sustain life once *severe oxygenation failure* has developed. Many causes of this syndrome are accompanied by circulatory insufficiency, which further compromises tissue oxygenation; thus the acceptable levels of Pa_{O_2}, and Sa_{O_2} are higher than in hypoxemic states with normal circulation. The decision to increase $F_{I_{O_2}}$ above 40 per cent is made on the basis of clinical deterioration, including signs of cerebral hypoxia, with apprehension, disorientation, and poor cooperation with therapy, and blood gas measurements indicating severe and progressive hypoxemia. High-dose oxygen (50 to 100 per cent) delivered by a bag-mask with a nonrebreathing reservoir can be given to increase Pa_{O_2} and gain time for either the natural evolution of the underlying disorder or additional treatment to improve blood and tissue oxygenation. The time required for irreversible pulmonary damage to result from oxygen toxicity is unknown but is probably less than 72 hours with 100 per cent O_2. During this limited "safe" time, tissue oxygenation may be improved using one or a combination of the following measures: (1) increase of Pa_{O_2} by mobilization of pulmonary edema with a potent diuretic; (2) increase of arterial oxygen content by restoration of hemoglobin to normal levels with transfusion of red cells or whole blood; (3) increase of oxygen delivery by improving cardiac output and blood pressure (depending on the primary disorder and its complications, this may require either an increase or decrease in plasma volume or the use of vasoactive or cardioactive drugs); and (4) decrease of oxygen utilization by elimination of fever with antipyretics and hypothermia. Corticosteroids in large doses (methylprednisolone, 1.0 gram or more daily) have been recommended for this stage of *severe oxygenation failure*, but their use is controversial and may be hazardous in primarily infectious disorders.

Mechanical ventilation is indicated in *severe oxygenation failure* when the underlying cause is potentially reversible, $F_{I_{O_2}}$ has been in the toxic range but for less time than causes irreversible lung damage, and Pa_{O_2} and Sa_{O_2} remain inadequate. Commonly at this stage, consciousness is depressed and the rapid, shallow breathing no longer sustains hyperventilation as indicated by change in Pa_{CO_2} from low to a normal value. Extensive, bilateral opacification of the lungs with a mixed interstitial and alveolar pattern ("white lung") is typically seen radiographically. The appropriate time for endotracheal intubation and takeover ventilation is difficult to determine, but it should occur before the appearance of metabolic acidosis, shock, bradycardia, severe hypercapnia, or cardiac arrest. Ventilation is "controlled" (see General Approach, above) to eliminate respiratory muscle work and to improve the distribution of the inspired gas. A central respiratory depressant (morphine sulfate, 4 to 8 mg intravenously initially) or a neuromuscular blocking agent (pancuronium bromide, 0.04 to 0.1 mg per kilogram initially) may be required for intubation and subsequently to relax the patient and eliminate competition with the respirator. These agents may induce hypotension, and their use in shock is hazardous. During the initiation of mechanical ventilation and for a short period of stabilization thereafter, 100 per cent oxygen is delivered by the respirator to minimize the risk of hypoxia. Thereafter, $F_{I_{O_2}}$ is reduced as rapidly as is compatible with maintenance of satisfactory Sa_{O_2}. The application of positive end-expiratory pressure (PEEP) using 5 to 15 cm H_2O has been shown to increase Pa_{O_2} and allow reduction of $F_{I_{O_2}}$ to safe levels in patients in whom this was previously not possible. PEEP should be used cautiously, since cardiac output may fall, especially in hypovolemic patients, because of the increased mean intrathoracic pressure; despite an increase of Pa_{O_2}, oxygen delivery to the tissues is thereby worsened. Once $F_{I_{O_2}}$ is reduced to 40 per cent, the lung is no longer at risk of oxygen toxicity, and the outcome is largely determined by the response of the primary disorder.

In a small but important number of patients, despite mechanical ventilation with PEEP, no reduction below 100 per cent $F_{I_{O_2}}$ is possible. In these patients, the use of extracorporeal supplementation of oxygenation with a membrane oxygenator and pump has achieved limited success.

Filley, G. F.: Pulmonary Insufficiency and Respiratory Failure. Philadelphia, Lea & Febiger, 1967.
Moore, F. D., Lyons, J. H., Jr., Pierce, E. C., Jr., Morgan, A. P., Jr., Drinker, P. A., MacArthur, J. D., and Dammin, G. J.: Post-Traumatic Pulmonary Insufficiency. Philadelphia, W. B. Saunders Company, 1969.
Petty, T. L., and Ashbaugh, D. G.: The adult respiratory distress syndrome. Clinical features, factors influencing prognosis and principles of management. Chest, 60:233, 1971.
Smith, J. P.: Respiratory failure and its management. *In* Holman, C. W., and Muschenheim, C. (eds.): Bronchopulmonary Diseases and Related Disorders. Hagerstown, Md., Harper & Row, 1972, pp. 694-727.
Smith, J. P., Stone, R. W., and Muschenheim, C.: Acute respiratory failure in chronic lung disease: Observations on controlled oxygen therapy. Am. Rev. Respir. Dis., 97:791, 1968.
Sykes, M. K., McNicol, M. W., and Campbell, E. J. M.: Respiratory Failure. Oxford and Edinburgh, Blackwell Scientific Publications, 1969.
West, J. B.: Causes of carbon dioxide retention in lung disease. N. Engl. J. Med., 284:1232, 1971.
Williams, M. H., Jr., and Shim, C. S.: Ventilatory failure: Etiology and clinical forms. Am. J. Med., 48:477, 1970.

LOCALIZED AIRWAY OBSTRUCTION

J. B. L. Howell

508. INTRODUCTION

The causes of localized airway obstruction may be grouped as endomural, intramural, and extramural. Endomural causes include bronchial secretions and aspirated foreign bodies; intramural causes include benign and malignant neoplasms, edema, and fibrous strictures; extramural causes are mainly due to enlargement of lymph nodes and other structures which cause airway compression. The effects of obstruction vary according to its location and whether it is complete or partial.

Laryngeal Obstruction. Laryngeal obstruction may be caused by laryngeal spasm, carcinoma, partial paralyses of the vocal cords, or collapse of the cartilaginous elements of the larynx as in rheumatoid arthritis or polychondritis.

Tracheal Obstruction. Tracheal obstruction is uncommon. Foreign bodies either impact in the larynx or descend beyond the bifurcation. Tracheal carcinoma, benign cylindroma, and amyloid tumors are rare. An increasingly common cause is tracheal stricture after tracheostomy or endotracheal intubation. It occurs at the site of the cuff or lower end of the tube and, if severe, may cause marked airway obstruction both during inspiration when it is associated with stridor and during expiration when a Starling resistor mechanism may operate (see Mechanisms of Airway Obstruction in Ch. 506). Surgical excision may be required.

External compression of the trachea may occur from goiter, thymic tumors, or neoplastic lymph nodes. Such pressures initially cause an irritating nonproductive cough but may progress to severe obstruction with stridor.

Localized Bronchial Obstruction. Localized bronchial obstruction does not cause interference with resting airflow unless it is severe; it is more likely to cause infection distally by interfering with mucous flow. When obstruction is nearly complete, overdistention of the distal lung tissue (obstructive emphysema) may occur; complete obstruction results in atelectasis.

509. ATELECTASIS

Definition. Strictly, the word atelectasis means imperfect expansion, and pathologists often use the term in this sense to describe the failure of expansion of the lungs at birth. In clinical practice, it usually implies airlessness in lung which had once been normally aerated.

Etiology and Pathogenesis. Airlessness of lung tissue may arise in two ways. First, alteration in the alveolar surfactant material by increasing alveolar surface tension may permit alveoli to deflate completely, thus expelling the air through the bronchial tree. This occurs in the lungs of premature infants and contributes to the *respiratory distress syndrome of the newborn*. Damage to alveolar surfactant is believed to occur in oxygen toxicity when multiple atelectases and sometimes massive collapse may develop. Surfactant may also be reduced after severe pulmonary edema. Second, when a bronchus is occluded, e.g., by secretions, foreign body, or neoplasm, continued perfusion of the distal alveoli results in absorption of the air (absorption atelectasis). Alternatively, when the lung is permitted to relax to its minimal volume by large quantities of air or liquid in the pleural cavity, as in pneumothorax or pleural effusion, collapse of the small bronchi or bronchioles occurs. The final removal of air is again by absorption into the perfusing blood, but the atelectasis is termed "relaxation atelectasis."

Absorption of alveolar gas occurs because the total pressure of the gases in mixed venous blood is less than that in the alveoli since, in its passage through the tissues, oxygen tension falls by approximately 60 mm Hg and is replaced by a rise in carbon dioxide tension of only 4 to 6 mm Hg. The absorption of air takes a few hours because of its poorly soluble nitrogen content; if the subject has been breathing pure oxygen, absorption may be complete within a few minutes. After relaxation atelectasis, the lung tissue remains undamaged, and reinflation with normal function is said to be possible after prolonged airlessness. With obstructive atelectasis, obstruction may interfere with bronchial toilet and lead to infections, abscesses, and fibrosis.

Clinical Manifestations. Atelectasis of one or more pulmonary segments is a common complication of acute tracheobronchial infections and is diagnosed usually as a result of chest roentgenograms. The atelectatic areas usually disappear with recovery from the generalized bronchitis without any specific therapy. The sudden development of atelectasis in larger segments of lung, e.g., a lobe or even a whole lung, may cause severe symptoms of dyspnea and chest pain associated with cyanosis, and, if very large, with sweating and peripheral circulatory failure. This is common in the postoperative period, especially with upper abdominal operations. A similar picture may be seen with foreign body inhalation. Over a period of a few hours, the symptoms often subside as the circulation through the atelectatic area is reduced. Lobar or segmental atelectasis resulting from bronchial neoplasm is often symptomless presumably because of its slow evolution. Segmental or lobar atelectasis may occur in patients with mild asthma, and is attributed to obstruction by secretions; however, atelectasis is an uncommon finding at autopsy in status asthmaticus. Atelectasis may also be a component of pulmonary infarction resulting from embolism. Plate atelectases have been described in drug addicts who administer their drugs intravenously.

Physical signs depend upon the size of the atelectatic area. If large enough, chest movement and tactile fremitus are diminished, the mediastinum is deviated toward the affected side, the percussion note is impaired, and breath sounds are characteristically absent. Atelectasis is confirmed by roentgenography, but unless the cause is obvious, bronchoscopy is indicated. Aspiration of occluding material may occasionally be possible through the bronchoscope.

Treatment. Treatment of atelectasis is directed at the underlying cause. For conditions requiring medical treatment, antimicrobial drugs and chest physiotherapy are given. Specific therapy of the atelectasis is seldom indicated, most conditions resolving spontaneously. When associated with bronchiectasis, the treatment is the same as for bronchiectasis. In relaxation atelectasis, removal of fluid from the pleural cavity usually causes re-expansion, often associated with transient precordial pain and violent coughing.

Lemoine, J. M.: L'atelectasie pulmonaire. Étude critique. Bronches, 17:109, 1967.

510. RIGHT MIDDLE LOBE SYNDROME

The right middle lobe bronchus is especially prone to involvement during primary tuberculosis because its origin is surrounded by a ring of lymph nodes draining both the middle and lower lobes of the right lung. Enlargement of these nodes readily compresses the narrow bronchus, causing atelectasis; extension of the infection into the bronchial wall leads to subsequent stricture with the eventual development of bronchiectatic changes distally. In later life, these changes may lead to recurrent infection, and the combination of recurrent pneumonic illness, hemoptysis, and right middle lobe atelectasis has been given the name of right middle lobe syndrome.

However, post-tuberculous bronchostenosis is only one of the causes of this syndrome. Other causes include chronic suppuration, foreign body, and bronchial neoplasm. Full investigation including bronchoscopy is essential; if the cause remains uncertain, thoracotomy should be considered.

Albo, R. J., and Grimes, O. F.: The middle lobe syndrome: A clinical study. Dis. Chest, 50:509, 1966.
Brock, R. C., Cann, R. J., and Dickinson, J. R.: Tuberculous mediastinal lymphadenitis in childhood. Guy's Hosp. Rep., 87:295, 1937.

Clements, J. A., and Tierney, D. F.: Alveolar instability associated with altered surface tension. In Handbook of Physiology, Section 3: Respiration. Baltimore, Williams & Wilkins Company, 1965, p. 1565.
Graham, E. A., Burford, T. H., and Mayer, J. H.: Middle lobe syndrome. Postgrad. Med., 4:29, 1948.
Hinshaw, H. C.: Diseases of the Chest. 3rd ed. Philadelphia, W. B. Saunders Company, 1969, pp. 241 et seq.
Hutcheson, S., and Guerrant, J. L.: Atelectasis in asthma. A report of five cases and a review of the literature. Va. Med. Mon., 94:629, 1967.
Lindskog, G. E., and Spear, H. C.: Middle lobe syndrome. N. Engl. J. Med., 253:489, 1955.
Rahn, H.: The role of N$_2$ gas in various biological processes with particular reference to the lung. Harvey Lectures Series, 55:173, 1959–1960.

Section Five. ABNORMAL AIR SPACES

Richard V. Ebert

511. GIANT BULLOUS EMPHYSEMA (Vanishing Lung)

Lungs examined at autopsy frequently contain small blebs or bullae. These are most commonly found in older men. Bullae are air-containing structures resembling cysts but with a wall which is trabeculated and not lined with epithelium. The lesion is derived from the terminal air spaces of the lung, and the trabeculae represent remnants of the blood vessels and fibrous tissue of the lung. Similar lesions occurring just beneath the visceral pleura are called blebs. Occasionally these lesions may be of great size and give rise to a characteristic appearance on the chest roentgenogram. These giant bullae may or may not be associated with generalized emphysema of the lung.

Large solitary bullae are occasionally observed. The lesion is usually not associated with symptoms and pulmonary function studies may reveal no abnormality. If the bulla becomes huge, it may produce dyspnea and impair pulmonary function. The term "anepithelial air cyst" has been used to describe these lesions.

More commonly, multiple large bullae are found. These may be confined to one lobe or to one lung, or they may involve both lungs. They usually occur in the upper lobes. The lesions are commonly seen in relatively young persons, being found in approximately 1 in 1000 routine roentgenograms of the chest. The patient may be asymptomatic. If the lesions are large or if there is associated generalized emphysema, the patients may complain of exertional dyspnea. Physical examination may reveal increased resonance to percussion and diminished breath sounds over the involved area. Pneumothorax is a common complication. The bullae rarely become infected or filled with fluid. On the chest roentgenogram the area involved is devoid of lung markings. The wall of the lesion is extremely thin and may not be visible. This has given rise to the term *vanishing lung*. The roentgenographic appearance can be easily confused with a pneumothorax. Pulmonary function studies are variable because the lesions may be either well ventilated or poorly ventilated and because there may be generalized emphysema that is not visible on the roentgenogram. There may or may not be adequate expansion of the remaining normal lung. If the lesions are not accompanied by diffuse pulmonary emphysema, the usual findings are a relatively normal vital capacity, a considerable increase in functional residual capacity, a normal or only slightly impaired maximal breathing capacity and rate of expiratory air flow, and normal blood gases. With very large bullous lesions there may be more severe impairment of pulmonary function. Finally, some patients present the typical clinical picture of chronic obstructive lung disease, and in addition demonstrate giant bullous lesions on roentgenography.

The therapy of giant bullae is surgical excision, but there is little reason to remove these lesions if the patient is asymptomatic. Occasionally, repeated pneumothorax may be an indication for surgery. A difficult problem is presented by those patients who are symptomatic. The dyspnea may be related to diffuse pulmonary emphysema rather than to the bullae. In this case removal of the bullae will be of little or no benefit. In certain patients, however, the bullae may be important in the production of symptoms. This occurs if the bullae interfere with the function of the remaining normal lung. If the bullae reach sufficient size to occupy much of the thorax, the intrathoracic pressure may not be sufficiently negative to expand the remaining lung. The normal portion of the lung may be partially atelectatic and poorly ventilated. Removal of the bullae may lead to significant improvement. Careful evaluation of the chest x-ray and of pulmonary function is necessary for a proper decision as to the need for surgery.

Boushy, S. F., Kohen, R., Billig, D. M., and Heiman, M. J.: Bullous emphysema. Clinical, roentgenologic and physiologic study of 49 patients. Dis. Chest, 54:327, 1968.
Pride, N. B., Barter, C. E., and Hugh-Jones, P.: The ventilation of bullae and the effect of their removal on thoracic gas volumes and tests of over-all pulmonary function. Am. Rev. Respir. Dis., 107:83, 1973.

512. LUNG CYSTS

The classification of lung cysts is somewhat confusing, since any air-containing structure in the lung can enlarge and form a cyst or cavity. There is tension on the wall of all air-containing structures in the lung because the pressure within fluctuates about atmospheric pressure, whereas the intrathoracic pressure is negative. If there is obstruction to the egress of air from a cyst or cavity, the pressure within may be considerably in excess of atmospheric pressure. The tension on the wall of a sphere such as a lung cyst is proportional to both the pressure difference across the wall and to the radius of curvature. For this reason a thin-walled cyst or cavity in the lung tends to continue to enlarge.

Thin-walled cavities may form in the lung as a result of destruction of lung substance and formation of a communication with a bronchus. Such cavities may be seen in pulmonary tuberculosis, the pulmonary mycoses, and lung abscess. These are called cavities and not cysts, but their appearance on the roentgenogram may be similar to that of lung cysts. Cystlike lesions can also form in bronchiectasis.

Belcher, J. R., and Siddons, A. H. M.: Air-containing cysts of the lung. Thorax, 9:38, 1954.

513. BRONCHOGENIC CYSTS

These cysts arise from the bronchi, as indicated by the name. It is thought that in most instances they are caused by a congenital defect. The cyst is lined with epithelial cells. The wall of the cyst may contain glands, smooth muscle, and cartilage. The cysts may be located in the lungs or mediastinum.

The patient with a bronchogenic cyst may be asymptomatic. Symptoms are usually the result of secondary infection and consist of a productive cough, hemoptysis, and fever. The roentgenographic appearance is variable. The cyst may contain only air or may be filled with fluid. In the latter case the cyst may be confused with a solid tumor of the lung. The cyst may have an air-fluid level, in which case it is often mistaken for a lung abscess. The treatment of symptomatic lung cysts is surgical removal.

Congenital cysts in the lower lobe of the lung may be associated with an anomalous artery arising from the aorta near the diaphragm. This complex developmental abnormality is called *intralobar bronchopulmonary sequestration*. A knowledge of this abnormality is of some importance because the artery may be inadvertently cut during surgery, with serious hemorrhage.

514. HONEYCOMB LUNG

Honeycomb lung describes a pathologic state in which the lung contains many small cystic structures that are several millimeters in diameter. These cysts are derived from the bronchioles and are lined by epithelium. Fibrous tissue and smooth muscle are found about the cysts. Honeycomb lung has been described in association with eosinophilic granuloma, rheumatoid lung disease, and idiopathic interstitial pulmonary fibrosis. It occurs in association with advanced fibrosis and represents the end stage of the disease. A similar pathologic lesion may be found in association with tuberous sclerosis.

The major symptom is dyspnea. Spontaneous pneumothorax is a common complication. The chest roentgenogram reveals a fine or coarse reticular appearance. Small rounded translucencies may be seen.

Heppleston, A. G.: The pathology of honeycomb lung. Thorax, 11:77, 1956.

515. ACQUIRED CYSTS

As mentioned above, any air-containing structure in the lung can enlarge and form a cyst or cavity. Lung abscess as a cause of such cavities is discussed immediately below. The other necrotizing lung diseases are considered in Ch. 178 to 183, Ch. 211, and Ch. 227.

516. LUNG ABSCESS

Definition. Lung abscess is a suppurative infection of the lung resulting in destruction of lung parenchyma with the formation of a cavity containing fluid and air.

Etiology. *Aspiration of infectious material* into the lung is the most common cause of lung abscess (primary lung abscess). A history of an episode of stupor or unconsciousness is often obtained. This is most commonly the result of excessive drinking. Careful inquiry will reveal that a high proportion of persons with lung abscess are chronic alcoholics. Other causes of unconsciousness predisposing to aspiration lung abscess are convulsive seizures, anesthesia, diabetic coma, ingestion of large amounts of sedatives, and various neurologic lesions. The infected material aspirated is usually from the mouth. Most people with lung abscess will be found to have periodontal disease with accumulation of infected materials about the teeth and gums. Lung abscess is rare in an edentulous person. Aspiration of infected materials during surgery on the oral cavity or tonsils was common at one time, but is rare now because of improvements in anesthetic techniques. Aspiration is common in cancer involving the upper respiratory passages or esophagus.

As might be anticipated, the pus from a primary lung abscess contains a mixture of bacteria. Cultures performed on material aspirated from an abscess cavity prior to the use of antimicrobial drugs may demonstrate gamma streptococci, diphtheroids, and a variety of anaerobic organisms.

Pneumonia caused by *Staphylococcus aureus* or Klebsiella may be complicated by abscess formation. Primary pneumococcal pneumonia is rarely associated with abscess formation. Treatment of patients with therapeutic agents which interfere with the normal body defenses, such as high doses of corticosteroids or the chemotherapy for cancer, predisposes to necrotizing pneumonia with abscess formation. In many hospitals lung abscesses occur almost exclusively in patients with terminal cancer.

Bronchial obstruction may lead to a lung abscess. The obstructing lesion is most commonly a bronchogenic carcinoma but may be a foreign body or an enlarged lymph node causing compression of a bronchus.

Metastatic lung abscess may result from septic emboli

secondary to right-sided bacterial endocarditis or pelvic thrombophlebitis. Lung abscess may occur in association with septicemia.

Rare causes of lung abscess include amebic abscess of the lung, melioidosis, glanders, actinomycosis, and nocardiosis.

Incidence and Prevalence. The exact incidence of lung abscess has not been determined. Recent reports indicate that five to ten instances of primary lung abscess are seen each year in a large general hospital. The disease was more common prior to the introduction of antimicrobial drugs. Lung abscess occurs as a terminal event in a variety of illnesses.

Pathogenesis. The sequence of events to be described is thought to be the mechanism of formation of lung abscess in those cases in which aspiration of infected material is the initiating agent. Although this mechanism of abscess function cannot be proved in every case, there is a large body of circumstantial evidence in its support.

When infected material is aspirated into the tracheobronchial tree, it lodges in a small bronchus in the dependent portion of the lung. As aspiration usually occurs in the supine position, the posterior segment of the upper lobe and the superior segment of the lower lobe are most commonly involved. Pneumonia develops in the surrounding tissue. The critical event is the formation of a cavity. This occurs as a result of necrosis and liquefaction of the pneumonic lung. The cavity is created when this liquid is discharged into the bronchus. For the lung parenchyma to be disrupted the collagen and elastic framework of the lung must be destroyed. The frequent finding of fragments of elastic tissue in the sputum is evidence of this destruction. The exact means by which liquefaction necrosis occurs is not known. It has been suggested that thrombosis of small vessels leads to ischemia of the pneumonic area. The liquefaction and destruction of the connective tissue framework of the lung must result from the liberation of proteolytic enzymes.

Clinical Manifestations. Patients with primary lung abscess often give a characteristic history. The illness begins with fever, sweats, malaise, loss of appetite, and loss of weight. After a few days or weeks a productive cough develops. The amount of sputum increases until several hundred milliliters is produced daily. The patient and his associates may note a foul odor to the sputum. Some patients give a history of suddenly coughing up large amounts of foul sputum. Hemoptysis occurs in about 40 per cent of the cases. Pleuritic chest pain may occur. In some cases the characteristic abundant foul sputum may be absent. This is most commonly seen in patients receiving antimicrobial drugs. Careful questioning of both the patient and his relatives may elicit a history of a period of unconsciousness or of excessive use of alcohol. When lung abscess complicates pneumonia caused by Staphylococcus or Klebsiella, the symptoms are those of a severe pneumonia. Abscess formation is detected on the chest roentgenogram.

The patient with lung abscess usually appears acutely ill and is febrile. Periodontal disease is often present, and infected material may be seen about the teeth and gums. Examination of the lung most commonly shows fine or medium moist rales over the involved area. Dullness and change in breath sounds may or may not be detected. Clubbing of the fingers is seen in about one fourth of the patients.

In primary lung abscess the sputum is usually copious, forms several layers on standing, and has a putrid odor.

Occasionally the sputum is scanty or absent. Culture of the sputum will reveal the specific organism if the abscess is caused by Staphylococcus or Klebsiella. In lung abscess resulting from aspiration, a mixed flora is found. In patients receiving penicillin a variety of gram-negative organisms may be cultured. The important anaerobic organisms described earlier are not cultured by the routine methods used in most clinical laboratories.

The diagnosis of lung abscess is usually made on roentgenography. A cavity containing fluid surrounded by alveolar infiltrate is found. A fluid level in the cavity can usually be demonstrated and can be confirmed by roentgenograms taken in different body positions. Approximately one third of the abscesses related to aspiration are found in the posterior segment of the right upper lobe. Other common locations are the superior segments of the right and left lower lobes and the posterior segment of the left upper lobe. With treatment the surrounding pneumonic infiltrate may rapidly disappear and fluid may no longer be seen if good drainage is obtained. Ultimately a thin-walled cavity is left. In most cases this will eventually disappear.

Complications. Empyema with or without bronchopleural fistula may complicate lung abscess. This usually occurs in the neglected cases, and rarely is seen once antimicrobial therapy has been started. If therapy of lung abscess is begun weeks or months after the onset of the disease, complete healing may not occur, and a residual thick-wall cavity remains. Scarring may be associated with local bronchiectasis. Recurrent infection may occur and lead to prolonged disability. Other complications are rare. Brain abscess and amyloidosis are almost never seen with present methods of therapy.

Diagnosis. The tentative diagnosis is made from the appearance of the chest roentgenogram, and particularly from the presence of a cavity with an air-fluid level. Differentiation from other diseases simulating lung abscess is made by analysis of the history, examination of the sputum, and careful study of serial roentgenograms after initiation of therapy.

The most common mistake in diagnosis is the confusion of bronchogenic carcinoma and primary lung abscess. Bronchogenic carcinoma can simulate lung abscess in two ways. A true lung abscess can develop peripheral to the obstructed bronchus, or a large tumor can undergo necrosis and cavitate. The latter event usually occurs with a squamous cell bronchogenic carcinoma but may occur with metastatic carcinoma. The diagnosis of an obstructing carcinoma can usually be made by bronchoscopy. Diagnosis of a peripheral cavitating carcinoma is difficult, and bronchoscopy is usually of no aid. The diagnosis may be suspected if the predisposing factors to an aspiration abscess are absent, if the sputum is not foul, if the location of the abscess is in the anterior portion of the lung, if the wall of the abscess is irregular, and if there is failure to respond to therapy. Examination of the sputum for neoplastic cells may be helpful. The diagnosis can be established in selected cases by the introduction under fluoroscopic control of a specially designed bronchial brush into the cavity. Tissue for histologic examination and culture can be obtained.

The differentiation of lung abscess from pulmonary tuberculosis is less difficult. Tuberculosis has a more insidious onset and less systemic symptoms. The sputum is not foul. The cavity usually does not contain a fluid level. Examination of the sputum for tubercle bacilli by microscopy and culture should always be done and will establish the diagnosis. Cavitating fungal infection of the lungs, such as histoplasmosis or coccidioidomycosis, can usually be distinguished from lung abscess without difficulty.

An infected lung cyst may simulate a primary lung abscess. Differentiation may be made by a careful history and by the lack of severe systemic symptoms or foul sputum. The wall of the cavity as seen by x-ray is thin and not surrounded by an area of pneumonitis. Previous films may show an air-containing cyst. Occasionally a bulbous lesion containing fluid may be seen in an area of resolving pneumonia and may be mistaken for a lung abscess.

Other lesions occasionally simulate lung abscess. At times an uninfected infarct of the lung will cavitate. Cystic bronchiectasis may be confused with lung abscess. There is a history of long-standing chronic cough, and the cavities are usually multiple and basal in location. Echinococcus cyst of the lung is extremely rare in the United States. Rheumatoid nodules and the lesions of Wegener's granulomatosis may cavitate, but are readily differentiated from lung abscess.

Treatment. The cornerstone of therapy in lung abscess is the administration of the appropriate antimicrobial drug in adequate dosage for a sufficiently long period. In abscesses complicating pneumonia caused by Staphylococcus or Klebsiella, the drug should be chosen on the basis of the susceptibility of the organism isolated from the sputum. In aspiration lung abscess, however, a variety of organisms are isolated. Moreover, the important anaerobic bacteria may not be cultured. Nevertheless, on an empirical basis penicillin in large doses has been found to be highly effective and is the antimicrobial drug of choice.

As a definable syndrome, primary lung abscess is usually quite readily distinguishable from the cavitation so prominent in the pneumonias produced by klebsiellae, staphylococci, or tubercle bacilli (for treatment of these three diseases see Ch. 182, 195, and 227). Moreover, selection of the proper drug therapy for primary lung abscess is quite a different type of medical judgment from that involved in selecting drugs for microbial diseases produced by a single clearly identifiable agent. In lung abscess the choice must be based on knowledge of the pathogenesis of the condition rather than on the identity of the microbial species isolated from the sputum. The latter, more often than not, have no etiologic significance or, at the very least, their relationship to the disease is by no means assured. Whether this syndrome of lung abscess is wholly microbial in origin and, if so, whether only a single microbial species is involved has not been established. Several lines of evidence, including the rarity of lung abscess in the edentulous person and the similarity of the flora in peridental and pulmonary abscesses, indicate that anaerobic microbes are significantly involved. Recent studies of secretions obtained by transtracheal aspiration, using special methods of culture, have revealed the constant presence of anaerobic bacteria in untreated primary lung abscess. *As a practical matter, lung abscess can be regarded as a cavitating pneumonia caused by anaerobic microbes.*

Since penicillin is known to maintain its effectiveness in anaerobic environments and is demonstrably of high effectiveness in lung abscess, it represents the major drug for the treatment of this condition. Five to ten million units of crystalline penicillin daily by continuous

intravenous drip may be used initially. After improvement has occurred, 600,000 units intravenously every four to six hours can be substituted. Therapy should be continued until the lesion heals or until continued improvement fails to occur. This usually requires four to six weeks. An alteration in the bacterial flora of the sputum with penicillin therapy is to be expected, but change to another antimicrobial drug should not be made unless there is clear evidence that penicillin is ineffective. Clindamycin may be used in those individuals with primary lung abscess allergic to penicillin and those failing to respond to an adequate course of penicillin therapy. Postural drainage facilitates emptying of the cavity and may be useful early in the course of therapy.

Surgery is no longer performed early in the disease. The usual indication for surgical intervention is a residual thick-walled cavity persisting after antimicrobial therapy. Thin-walled cavities or cystic lesions need not be removed and will often heal spontaneously. Residual lesions requiring surgery usually occur in patients in whom antimicrobial therapy has been delayed or was inadequate.

Barnett, T. B., and Herring, C. L.: Lung abscess. Initial and late results of medical therapy. Arch. Intern. Med., 127:217, 1971.
Bartlett, J. G., Gorbach, S. L., Tally, F. P., and Finegold, S. M.: Bacteriology and treatment of primary lung abscess. Am. Rev. Respir. Dis., 109:510, 1974.
Bernhard, W. F., Malcolm, J. A., and Wylie, R. H.: The carcinomatous abscess. A clinical paradox. N. Engl. J. Med., 266:914, 1962.
Flavell, G.: Respiratory tract disease. Lung abscess. Br. Med. J., 1:1032, 1966.
Perlman, L. V., Lerner, E., and D'Esopo, N.: Clinical classification and analysis of 97 cases of lung abscess. Am. Rev. Respir. Dis., 99:390, 1969.

517. UNILATERAL HYPERLUCENT LUNG

Unilateral hyperlucent lung is discovered by roentgenography of the chest. One lung is translucent as compared with the other. The vascular markings of the hyperlucent lung are diminished, and the pulmonary artery may be inconspicuous. Fluoroscopy demonstrates a shift of the mediastinum away from the involved lung on expiration. Dilatation and irregularity of the small bronchi are visible on bronchograms. Histopathologic examination of the diseased lung demonstrates an extensive bronchitis and bronchiolitis. The alveoli may be enlarged, but typical destructive emphysema is not usually found. The pulmonary artery is present. One theory of pathogenesis is that a severe pulmonary infection occurred in childhood, with consequent altered development of the lung.

The patient usually gives a history of productive cough. Dyspnea and hemoptysis may be present. Breath sounds are often diminished over the affected lung, and rales may be heard. The perfusion and ventilation of the involved lung are impaired. This can be demonstrated by obtaining an image of the lungs with a scintillation camera following the administration of radioactive xenon.

Treatment consists of management of infection. Surgery is not usually performed.

Hamilton, C. R., Jr., Ballinger, W. F., II, and Cader, G.: The unilateral hyperlucent lung syndrome. Bull. Hopkins Hosp., 123:222, 1968.

Section Six. DIFFUSE LUNG DISEASE

Richard V. Ebert

518. INTERSTITIAL LUNG DISEASE

The normal alveolar wall is made up of capillaries, connective tissue, and thin alveolar epithelium. A network of delicate collagen, reticulin, and elastic fibers gives strength and support to the tissue. Coarser and more abundant connective fibers surround the alveolar ducts, bronchioles, and small bronchi. Except for the lobular septa there is surprisingly little fibrous tissue in the peripheral portions of the lung. A group of diseases is associated with cellular infiltration and increase in fibrous tissue in the walls of the alveoli. The cause of many of these diseases is unknown. All are associated with similar roentgenographic findings and have similar symptoms and physiologic findings.

ROENTGENOGRAPHIC, CLINICAL, AND PHYSIOLOGIC FEATURES

Roentgenographic Findings. The changes in the lungs are diffuse and consist of fine mottling and reticulation. Early in the disease the change may be subtle and can be readily overlooked. Later the shadows may be dense. Annular shadows may appear, giving a honeycomb appearance. In contrast to alveolar disease the vascular shadows persist and may be accentuated.

Clinical Manifestations. The major symptom is exertional dyspnea. This begins insidiously and in the early stages may be disregarded by the patient. The symptoms are usually progressive, and ultimately ordinary activities become limited by shortness of breath. In the advanced form of the disease dyspnea may be present at rest. Wheezing is not present, but a dry cough is common. Purulent sputum is not seen unless there is secondary bronchitis. Examination of the lungs may reveal no abnormal findings, or crackling fine rales may be observed over the lower portions of the lung. Clubbed fingers are common in diffuse interstitial pulmonary fibrosis. Cyanosis and evidence of right heart failure occur in the terminal phase of the illness.

Physiologic Features. The pulmonary function is usually altered. The changes in function differ from those in obstructive lung disease, there being no evidence of impairment of expiratory air flow. The breathing is rapid and shallow. The total pulmonary ventilation is increased both at rest and on exercise. The vital capacity and total lung capacity may be normal but are usually reduced to a variable degree. The maximal breathing capacity is normal or only slightly reduced, and the ratio of the volume of air forcibly expelled in one second to the vital capacity is normal. The diffusing capacity for carbon monoxide is reduced, and the reduction parallels the severity of the disease. In the milder forms of the disease the oxygen saturation of the hemoglobin of the arterial blood may be normal at rest and on exercise. In more severe disease the oxygen saturation is mar-

kedly decreased on exercise and may be abnormal at rest. The carbon dioxide tension of the arterial blood is normal or decreased. The basis for these changes in pulmonary function is complex. Capillaries are obliterated and alveoli destroyed by fibrosis. Some alveoli have thickened walls, and others are normal. Contrary to common opinion the alveolar capillary membrane is usually not thickened. These changes in the structure of the lung result in alterations in the mechanical properties of the lung and in gas exchange. The compliance of the lungs is reduced, resulting in an increased work of breathing. The irregular distribution of pathologic changes in the lung produces regional differences in ventilation-perfusion ratios, resulting in inadequate oxygenation of blood leaving certain regions of the lung (venous admixture).

CAUSES OF INTERSTITIAL LUNG DISEASE

Diffuse Interstitial Fibrosis. In 1944 Hamman and Rich described a group of patients with intense dyspnea, cyanosis, and right heart failure. The disease was rapid in its course, only a few months elapsing between the onset of symptoms and death. The lungs at autopsy showed thickening of the alveolar walls with edema, fibrin deposition, and cellular infiltration, together with extensive interstitial proliferation of fibrous tissue. The term Hamman-Rich syndrome was used to describe this clinical and pathologic entity. Subsequently it was found that there was a larger group of patients with diffuse thickening and fibrosis of the alveolar walls who exhibited a more prolonged clinical course. The term idiopathic diffuse interstitial fibrosis or fibrosing alveolitis has been used to describe these patients. Although no specific cause has been found, the presence of rheumatoid factor or antinuclear factor in the serum of a number of these patients has raised the question of whether this is an autoimmune disease.

Approximately 1 to 2 per cent of patients with *rheumatoid* arthritis will have diffuse interstitial fibrosis. Most of these have a high titer of rheumatoid factor in the blood. Approximately 20 per cent of patients with diffuse interstitial fibrosis in whom there are no joint changes have an elevated titer of rheumatoid factor in their blood. Diffuse interstitial fibrosis associated with rheumatoid arthritis or with rheumatoid factor in the blood does not differ from the idiopathic type of fibrosis. A peculiar type of fibrosis involving the upper portion of the lung and associated with cyst formation has been described in ankylosing spondylitis. This differs from diffuse pulmonary fibrosis complicating rheumatoid arthritis, and is not usually associated with a positive test for rheumatoid factor.

Diffuse interstitial fibrosis is also found to occur in association with *scleroderma* and less frequently with dermatomyositis. The fibrosis in scleroderma is not accompanied by a cellular reaction. The changes are usually more marked at the bases of the lungs.

Lymphoid Interstitial Pneumonia. The pathologic findings consist of extensive infiltration of the interstitial tissue of the lungs with mononuclear cells. The pathologic changes may be confused with those of lymphoma of the lung. Lymphoid interstitial pneumonia is often associated with alterations in the plasma gamma globulins and may be associated with Sjögren's syndrome or Waldenström's macroglobulinemia.

Eosinophilic Granuloma. Eosinophilic granuloma of the lung may produce clinical and roentgenologic findings which are indistinguishable from those in diffuse interstitial fibrosis. Bone lesions may or may not be demonstrable. (For further description see Ch. 108).

Idiopathic Pulmonary Hemosiderosis. Idiopathic pulmonary hemosiderosis is described in Ch. 520. In severe cases interstitial fibrosis of the lungs develops, and may resemble roentgenographically the other types of diffuse fibrosis.

Chemical and Physical Irritants. Chemical and physical irritants may lead to interstitial fibrosis (see Ch. 521 to 538).

Extrinsic Allergic Alveolitis. Diseases such as farmer's lung, bagassosis, and pigeon breeders' disease produce an interstitial inflammatory reaction and may lead to interstitial fibrosis (see Ch. 533).

Drug Reaction. Certain drugs such as nitrofurantoin, busulfan, methotrexate, bleomycin, and hexamethonium may produce interstitial edema which may be followed by diffuse interstitial fibrosis.

Sarcoidosis. Sarcoidosis involving the lung may lead to a diffuse interstitial involvement of the pulmonary parenchyma. Initially the lesions are granulomas, but later fibrosis may be present. The roentgenologic appearance of the lung may simulate diffuse interstitial fibrosis. The hilar lymph nodes are usually but not always enlarged (see Ch. 102).

Tuberculosis and Fungal Diseases of the Lungs. Tuberculosis and fungal diseases of the lungs may lead to a diffuse interstitial lesion with granuloma formation. Miliary tuberculosis results from hematogenous spread of the tubercle bacilli. Early in the illness the lesions may not be visible on chest roentgenography. Later diffuse fine miliary densities are seen. Healing occurs with chemotherapy, and the patient is usually left with no functional disability. Histoplasmosis may also give a diffuse granulomatous lesion of the lung. Healing is often associated with multiple small areas of calcification of the lung.

Neoplasm. Lymphangitic spread of primary or metastatic carcinoma of the lung may produce the clinical picture of interstitial lung disease. Occasionally, lymphoma involving the lung may present similarly.

DIAGNOSIS

The appearance of the chest roentgenogram usually establishes the pulmonary lesion as interstitial in character. The differentiation of the various interstitial lesion may be difficult. Inquiry should always be made regarding exposure to various dusts. This should include a review of the various jobs held during a lifetime of work. Special emphasis should be placed on possible exposure to silica or asbestos. Physical examination may give evidence of rheumatoid arthritis or scleroderma. Enlarged lymph nodes may be discovered and on biopsy show the lesions of sarcoid. Bone x-rays may demonstrate the lesions of eosinophilic granuloma or sarcoid.

Serologic studies, including tests for rheumatoid factor and complement fixation tests for histoplasmosis and blastomycosis, should be done.

In spite of careful study, a group of patients remain in whom diagnosis is obscure. Most of these will fall into the category of diffuse interstitial fibrosis of unknown cause. A much smaller group will have eosinophilic granuloma or one of the other granulomatous diseases. A firm diagnosis in these doubtful areas can be established only by lung biopsy. This need not be done in every case but should be strongly considered if there is any question of the clinical diagnosis being correct.

TREATMENT

Treatment will depend on the cause of the interstitial lesion. Idiopathic diffuse interstitial fibrosis is often treated with corticosteroids. Immunosuppressant drugs have also been used. The best results have been reported in patients treated in the early stages of the disease. Results are difficult to evaluate, as no controlled clinical trials have been carried out.

The course of idiopathic pulmonary fibrosis is variable. The disease is fatal in a few months in some patients, and may continue with only slow progress for many years in others. Development of hypoxemia at rest usually means that the end of life is approaching. Cor pulmonale with right heart failure often follows and leads to death. A few patients die with alveolar cell carcinoma.

Fraire, A. E., Greenberg, S. D., O'Neal, R. M., Weg, J. G., and Jenkins, D. E.: Diffuse interstitial fibrosis of the lung. Am. J. Clin. Path., 59:636, 1973.

Liebow, A. A., and Carrington, C. B.: Diffuse pulmonary lymphoreticular infiltrations associated with dysproteinemia. Med. Clin. North Am., 57:809, 1973.

Livingstone, J. L., Lewis, J. G., Reid, L., and Jefferson, K. E.: Diffuse interstitial pulmonary fibrosis. A clinical, radiological, and pathological study based on 45 patients. Quart. J. Med., 33:71, 1964.

Nagaya, H., and Siecker, H. O.: Pathogenetic mechanisms of interstitial fibrosis in patients with serum antinuclear factor. Am. J. Med., 52:51, 1972.

Sharp, J. T., Sweaney, S. K., and Van Lith, P.: Physiologic observations in diffuse pulmonary fibrosis and granulomatosis. Am. Rev. Respir. Dis., 94:316, 1966.

Walker, W. C., and Wright, V.: Pulmonary lesions and rheumatoid arthritis. Medicine, 47:501, 1968.

519. DIFFUSE ALVEOLAR DISEASES OF THE LUNG

ROENTGENOGRAPHIC, CLINICAL, AND PHYSIOLOGIC FEATURES

A variety of diseases may lead to replacement of air in the alveoli and alveolar ducts by fluid. The alveoli may be filled by edema fluid (pulmonary edema), by inflammatory exudate (pneumonia), by blood (pulmonary infarct, bleeding from bronchi and aspiration, Goodpasture's syndrome), by exudate containing a high lipid content (alveolar proteinosis, lipoid pneumonia), or by cancer tissue (alveolar cell carcinoma). The roentgenographic appearance of the lungs is similar in all of these and can usually be differentiated from the changes pro-

duced by interstitial lung disease. The shadows form a
homogeneous density with fluffy ill-defined edges. The
infiltrates tend to obliterate the vascular markings, and
at times an air bronchogram may be seen. In chronic
lesions a pattern related to filling of acini is seen at the
edge of the lesion. This is a rosette-like density measuring several millimeters in diameter.

The clinical manifestations of alveolar disease will
depend on the nature of the underlying lesion, the duration of the disease, and the extent of involvement. Cough
and dyspnea are the two major symptoms. Fever may or
may not be present. If the cough is productive, examination of the sputum grossly and with the microscope may
cast light on the nature of the alveolar lesion. The sputum in pulmonary edema is thin, and white or pink in
color. The sputum in pneumonia is tenacious and purulent, and may contain blood. The sputum in pulmonary
hemorrhage consists of pure blood. The degree of dyspnea is related to the acuteness of the lesion and the
amount of lung involved. Diffuse pulmonary edema or
pneumonia will be associated with rapid, shallow, labored breathing at rest. A chronic alveolar lesion such as
alveolar proteinosis may result only in exertional dyspnea.

The physiologic changes will also be dependent on the
extent of the lesions and whether they are acute or
chronic. The vital capacity will be reduced. The change
in blood gases will depend on whether blood flows
through the capillaries of the involved alveoli or not.
Blood often continues to flow through areas of lung involved by acute lesions, with resultant shunting of unoxygenated blood into the pulmonary venous system. In
more chronic lesions the blood flow from the pulmonary
artery into the involved area is diminished or absent.
The decrease in oxygen saturation of the arterial blood
will be dependent on the magnitude of the shunt. If the
shunt is large, hypoxia will persist while the patient is
breathing high concentrations of oxygen. With massive
filling of alveoli with fluid, death occurs from hypoxia in
spite of oxygen administration. Hypoxia may also result
from alteration in the ventilation-perfusion ratio in alveoli adjacent to the lesion. These alveoli may be poorly
ventilated and well perfused, resulting in inadequate
oxygenation of blood in the pulmonary capillaries. Administration of oxygen will correct this type of hypoxia.
In alveolar disease the carbon dioxide tension of the arterial blood remains low or normal until massive involvement of the lung occurs.

Felsen, B.: The roentgen diagnosis of disseminated alveolar diseases. Semi-
nars Radiol., 2:3, 1967.
Goodman, N.: Differential diagnosis of pulmonary alveolar infiltrates. Am.
Rev. Respir. Dis., 95:681, 1967.

520. CAUSES OF DIFFUSE ALVEOLAR DISEASE

PULMONARY EDEMA

Mechanism of Formation of Edema of the Lungs. The formation of edema in the lungs bears a certain similarity
to the formation of edema in the subcutaneous tissues. In
both instances the forces involved are the same, namely,

the hydrostatic pressure in the capillaries, the colloid
osmotic pressure of the plasma and interstitial fluid, and
the interstitial fluid pressure. There are, however, major
differences in the anatomy of the tissues and the hemodynamics in the two locations which lead to differences
in the mechanism of formation of edema.

The anatomy of the lung is designed to permit efficient
exchange of gas between the alveoli and the pulmonary
capillaries. The alveolar septa are made up largely of
capillaries. Between the capillaries is a very small
amount of connective tissue, including ground substance, collagen, and elastin fibers. The plasma in the
capillaries is separated from the air in the alveolus by a
thin membrane consisting of capillary endothelium,
basement membrane, and alveolar epithelial cells. There
is more abundant connective tissue about the bronchi
and blood vessels and in the interlobular septa. The pulmonary capillary pressure is below 10 mm Hg in normal
human beings. As a result, the difference between pulmonary capillary pressure and colloid osmotic pressure
of the plasma is large and creates a force tending to move
fluid into the capillary. Another important force is
created by the surface tension at the fluid-air interface in
the alveoli. This force is related to the radius of curvature of the alveoli and the surface tension. The latter is
influenced by a lipid on the surface of the alveolar wall
(surfactant). The effect of this force is to make the interstitial fluid pressure negative.

Recent experimental work has elucidated the mechanism of formation of pulmonary edema. As a result of alteration in the hydrostatic forces or increase in capillary
permeability to protein, fluid moves from the capillary
into the interstitial space in the alveolar septum. As the
interstitial fluid increases, it moves into the connective
tissue about the blood vessels and bronchi and into the
interlobular septa. Lymphatic flow is increased and removes some of this fluid. If the interstitial fluid continues to accumulate, fluid dissects between the capillary endothelial cells and the adjacent basement
membrane, resulting in damage to the capillary wall. Finally, fluid moves through the alveolar epithelium into
the alveolus. This fluid contains plasma protein and
often fibrinogen and red cells.

Roentgenogram. The chest roentgenogram mirrors
the pathologic changes. During the phase of interstitial
edema linear shadows may be seen (Kerley's A and B
lines) which represent edema of the septa of the lungs.
There may be thickening and loss of definition of the
shadows of the vessels. A perihilar haze may be seen. In
some circumstances the edema may remain interstitial
and not progress to intra-alveolar edema. Intra-alveolar
edema results in confluent shadows of uniform density.
These may be diffuse, confined to the lower portion of the
lung, or seen at the hila of the lungs (butterfly pattern).
Occasionally the shadows are unilateral.

Symptoms and Signs. During the period of development of interstitial edema there is intense suffocating
dyspnea, and the breathing is rapid and shallow. A
severe attack of paroxysmal nocturnal dyspnea resulting
from left ventricular failure exemplifies the symptoms of
interstitial edema. During the attack the patient is in the
sitting position and breathing rapidly and in a labored
manner. His face gives evidence of apprehension and is
sweating. He may have difficulty in talking because of
the urge to continue breathing. In spite of the intense
dyspnea, examination of the lungs may fail to demonstrate rales, and the roentgenogram may not show intra-

alveolar edema. If interstitial edema has been present for some time as in mitral stenosis, the patient may be free of dyspnea at rest, although exertional dyspnea is present.

With the development of intra-alveolar edema the patient continues to be severely dyspneic at rest and may cough up white or pink frothy sputum. Examination of the lungs reveals numerous moist rales. Cyanosis may be present if the edema is severe. If formation of edema fluid continues, the patient drowns in the edema fluid.

Alterations in Pulmonary Function. The rapid shallow breathing characteristic of developing pulmonary edema is believed to be related to neurogenic stimuli arising from receptors in the alveolar septa. As a result of the abnormal stimulus to ventilation, the carbon dioxide tension of the arterial blood is decreased. With interstitial edema the oxygen saturation of the arterial blood may show little change, but with the development of alveolar edema hypoxia occurs. The oxygen tension of the arterial blood may fall to extremely low levels in severe diffuse intra-alveolar edema in spite of the administration of high concentrations of oxygen. Increase in the carbon dioxide tension of the arterial blood may be present at this stage. A decrease in the pH of the arterial blood is common in severe pulmonary edema. This may be caused by metabolic acidosis related to increased lactic acid production as well as by carbon dioxide retention. Death results from hypoxia.

Edema of the lung leads to changes in the mechanics of ventilation. The vital capacity is decreased, and the course of pulmonary edema can be followed by repeated use of this simple bedside measurement. The total lung capacity is also reduced. This reduction is associated with a change in the elastic properties of the lung. A greater change in intrapleural pressure is required to produce a given volume change in the lung (decrease in compliance of the lung). This in turn leads to an increase in the work of breathing. With early edema there is usually no change in the resistance to air flow in the lung. Later, obstruction to flow of air may result from fluid in the bronchi. Occasionally this obstruction is severe and associated with wheezing, giving rise to the term cardiac asthma.

Causes of Pulmonary Edema. *Increase in Pulmonary Capillary Pressure.* This is the most common cause of pulmonary edema. The usual mechanism is failure of the left ventricle with rise in left ventricular end diastolic pressure. Hypertension, aortic valve disease, and acute myocardial infarction are common causes of acute failure of the left ventricle. Mitral stenosis leads to elevation in pulmonary capillary pressure by obstructing blood flow to the left ventricle. As a consequence the edema of the lungs is often chronic and interstitial in character. Mitral stenosis may also be associated with acute intra-alveolar edema usually precipitated by severe exertion or a sudden increase in heart rate.

The pulmonary capillary pressure may be elevated by an increase in blood volume. A general increase in blood volume is accompanied by an increase in pulmonary blood volume, which in turn leads to an elevation in pulmonary vascular pressures. Administration of large amounts of blood may precipitate pulmonary edema in a normal person. More commonly, the administration of blood or salt solution leads to pulmonary edema in an individual with previous disease of the heart or kidney. Great care must be taken in administering blood or saline to a person with a history of left ventricular fail-

ure, as small amounts of fluid may precipitate pulmonary edema. A combination of left ventricular failure and increase in blood volume may produce pulmonary edema in patients with severe chronic anemia who are receiving blood transfusions.

Pulmonary edema complicating renal disease involves fluid overload and left ventricular failure. If the patient is oliguric, as in acute tubular necrosis or acute glomerulonephritis, and receives excessive fluid orally or intravenously, the blood volume increases, and pulmonary edema may occur. Often hypertension is present and predisposes to left ventricular failure. In chronic renal disease left ventricular failure plays an important role in the formation of pulmonary edema. Uremic pneumonia is thought to be a form of pulmonary edema occurring in patients with severe renal insufficiency.

Pulmonary edema may complicate intracranial lesions. The most common cause is marked increase in intracranial pressure secondary to head injury or spontaneous intracranial hemorrhage. It has also been described in association with brain tumors and following generalized convulsive seizures. The mechanism of production of the edema is not completely understood, but is thought to be related to reflex effects on peripheral circulation and heart with massive peripheral vasoconstriction.

High altitude pulmonary edema is a poorly understood disorder. It occurs in those recently arrived at high altitude who have engaged in vigorous exercise. The clinical picture is similar to other types of pulmonary edema. Recovery is the rule with suitable treatment and evacuation to lower altitudes. The pathogenesis is believed to be related to the effect of hypoxia on the pulmonary vascular bed. Pulmonary edema may complicate self-administration of large doses of heroin or methadone. The mechanism of production of this type of edema may relate to hypoxia secondary to respiratory depression.

Lowered Colloid Osmotic Pressure of Plasma. Pulmonary edema is rarely caused by diminution in the concentration of plasma proteins unless other predisposing factors are present. In the nephrotic syndrome there may be massive peripheral edema, yet the lungs remain free of fluid. In edema of the lungs produced by massive infusion of saline, the lowered plasma proteins contribute to edema formation. This is particularly true if the plasma proteins have been depleted by hemorrhage. In renal disease decrease in the concentration of plasma proteins may be one of several factors contributing to pulmonary edema.

Negative Intrapleural Pressure. Sudden re-expansion of the lung by the rapid removal of large amounts of pleural fluid may result in unilateral pulmonary edema. Edema may also result from the rapid expansion of a lung collapsed by a pneumothorax. The edema is thought to result from the application of a large negative intrapleural pressure to the lung.

Increased Capillary Permeability. Certain gases when inhaled into the lungs damage the pulmonary capillaries and increase the permeability of the capillary wall to protein. Among these gases are phosgene, chlorine, and nitrogen dioxide. The latter may result from fermentation of corn in a closed space (silo-filler's disease). Certain herbicides such as paraquat may cause pulmonary edema.

Pulmonary edema may occur as an idiosyncratic reaction to certain drugs. Drugs reported to cause increased capillary permeability with edema include hexamethonium, nitrofurantoin, busulfan, and methotrexate. Pulmonary edema has been reported after a single blood transfusion as a result of hypersensitivity.

Pulmonary edema may complicate septic shock. It may also occur in patients being resuscitated from severe shock associated with nonthoracic trauma. The pathologic findings in the *shock lung* consist of focal areas of atelectasis as well as interstitial and alveolar edema. The mechanism of production of these pathologic changes in the lung is not well understood. Among the factors involved may be damage to the pulmonary capillaries and overzealous administration of intravenous fluids in the treatment of shock.

Certain pneumonias resemble pulmonary edema. Fulminating pneumonia may occur with influenza virus infection, and death may occur in 24 hours. The alveoli are filled with edema fluid, fibrin, red blood cells, and mononuclear cells. The pneumonia associated with *Pneumocystis carinii* infection is more chronic. The alveoli contain a foamy amorphous exudate.

There is considerable evidence that the administration of a high concentration of oxygen for long periods of time will cause damage to the pulmonary capillaries. It has been known for many years that damage to the lungs of animals could be produced by the prolonged administration of pure oxygen at atmospheric pressure. More recently interstitial edema and hyaline alveolar membranes have been described in patients receiving high concentration of oxygen in association with mechanical ventilation. During life there is a progressive fall in the oxygen tension of the arterial blood in spite of continuing high concentration of oxygen in the inspired air.

Treatment. The treatment of pulmonary edema consists of general measures and therapy specific for the underlying cause. Examples of specific therapy are digitalis for left ventricular failure, appropriate treatment of arrhythmias, and the use of antihypertensive drugs in heart failure precipitated by severe hypertension.

Morphine will produce dramatic relief of symptoms if administered during the interstitial phase of edema or in the early stages of alveolar edema. The pattern of breathing may return to normal, and apprehension is relieved. Morphine is of special value in attacks of pulmonary edema resulting from acute left ventricular failure. The drug is given subcutaneously in a dose of 15 mg. If rapid action is desired or shock is present, it may be given intravenously. The administration of morphine to patients with chronic obstructive lung disease under the mistaken impression that pulmonary edema is present should be avoided at all costs. Morphine should also be avoided in the late stages of pulmonary edema when respiration is depressed because of severe hypoxia.

Oxygen should be administered, as hypoxia may be present. In mild pulmonary edema an adequate concentration of oxygen in inspired air can be obtained with a nasal catheter. A high concentration of oxygen may be required in severe pulmonary edema. If pulmonary edema fails to respond to usual treatment and if hypoxia persists in spite of the use of oxygen, consideration should be given to intubation with an intratracheal tube and the application of intermittent positive pressure using positive end expiratory pressure (PEEP). Positive pressure breathing decreases cardiac output, inhibits the movement of fluid into the alveoli, and prevents the terminal airways from closing. The latter effect is believed to be the most important. The use of high concentrations of oxygen for prolonged periods of time in the treatment of pulmonary edema should be avoided, as further damage to pulmonary capillaries may ensue.

Reduction in pulmonary blood volume is imperative in pulmonary edema associated with high pulmonary capillary pressure. This can be accomplished by pooling blood in the extremities or by venesection. Placing the patient in the sitting position with legs dependent will pool blood in the legs. Additional blood can be pooled by the application of venous tourniquets to the upper thighs. Venesection of 500 to 700 ml of blood is particularly useful in those cases in which the attack of pulmonary edema has been precipitated by administration of blood or the excessive use of intravenous fluids. Diuretics have also been found valuable. Ethacrynic acid given intravenously in a dose of 50 mg will produce a prompt massive diuresis with consequent reduction of blood volume.

Aberman, A., and Fulop, M.: The metabolic and respiratory acidosis of acute pulmonary edema. Ann. Intern. Med., 76:173, 1972.

Fishman, A. P.: Pulmonary edema. The water-exchanging function of the lung. Circulation, 46:390, 1972.

Fishman, A. P.: Shock lung—a distinctive nonentity. Circulation, 47:921, 1973.

Heitzman, E. R., and Ziter, F. M.: Acute interstitial pulmonary edema. Radiology, 98:291, 1966.

McMahon, S. M., Halprin, G. M., and Sieker, H. O.: Positive end-expiratory airway pressure in severe arterial hypoxemia. Am. Rev. Respir. Dis., 108:526, 1973.

Robin, E. D., Cross, C. E., and Zelis, R.: Pulmonary edema. N. Engl. J. Med., 288:239, 292, 1973.

PULMONARY ALVEOLAR PROTEINOSIS

In pulmonary alveolar proteinosis the microscopic appearance of the lungs is typical. Large groups of alveoli are filled with a proteinaceous material containing a high concentration of phospholipid. The material gives a positive reaction with periodic acid–Schiff stain. A few large cells containing stainable lipid are present in the alveoli and along the alveolar septa. The septa themselves are remarkably normal. It is thought that the lipid material in the alveoli is derived from granular pneumocytes and may be related to surfactant.

Symptoms consist of gradually progressive dyspnea and a productive cough. Physical examination of the lungs may be normal. The roentgenogram reveals bilateral diffuse soft densities seen most commonly at the hila or bases of the lungs. The vital capacity is reduced to a variable degree. The maximal breathing capacity is normal or slightly reduced. The oxygen saturation of the hemoglobin of the arterial blood may be normal or reduced. Complicating infection occurs. Fungal infection is common, Nocardia being the most frequent offending organism. The disease may remain stable for considerable periods of time and spontaneous improvement may occur, but it is eventually fatal in about one third of the patients.

Pulmonary alveolar proteinosis must be differentiated from diseases of the heart with pulmonary edema and from the pulmonary fibroses, pneumoconioses, sarcoidosis, and fungal infections of the lung. *Pneumocystis carinii* infection can present with a similar clinical picture and similar pathologic findings. Lung biopsy is usually necessary to clarify the diagnosis.

Various methods of treatment have been attempted. These include the use of proteolytic enzymes and pulmonary lavage; of these, lavage appears to be the most promising. One lung is irrigated at a time using several liters of saline. The washings contain material with a high lipid content similar to that seen in the alveoli.

Davidson, J. M., and Macleod, W. M.: Pulmonary alveolar proteinosis. Br. J. Dis. Chest, 63:13, 1969.
Pulmonary alveolar proteinosis—editorial. Br. Med. J., 1:395, 1972.
Ramirez-R., J., and Harlan, W. R.: Pulmonary alveolar proteinosis. Nature and origin of alveolar lipid. Am. J. Med., 45:502, 1968.
Rosen, S. H., Castleman, B., and Liebow, A. A.: Pulmonary alveolar proteinosis. N. Engl. J. Med., 258:1123, 1958.

DESQUAMATIVE INTERSTITIAL PNEUMONIA

The tissue response in desquamative interstitial pneumonia consists of proliferation and desquamation of large alveolar cells with slight thickening of the walls of the distal air spaces.

Patients with this disease complain of cough and shortness of breath, which is gradually progressive. Rales may or may not be heard on physical examination of the chest. The roentgenogram demonstrates a ground-glass appearance in the basilar portion of the lungs. Diagnosis must be made by lung biopsy. The course is chronic, the lesions persisting for months or years. Steroids are said to have a beneficial effect.

There is some question whether this entity is distinct and separate from diffuse interstitial fibrosis (fibrosing alveolitis). Cases are seen which are intermediate between the two entities with varying degrees of alveolar wall thickening and varying numbers of cells in the alveoli. There is evidence that patients with typical desquamative interstitial pneumonia may develop interstitial fibrosis after several years.

Gaensler, E. A., Goff, A. M., and Prowse, C. M.: Desquamative interstitial pneumonia. N. Engl. J. Med., 274:113, 1966.
Liebow, A. A., Steer, A., and Billingsley, J. G.: Desquamative interstitial pneumonia. Am. J. Med., 39:369, 1965.
Scadding, J. G., and Hinson, K. F.: Diffuse fibrosing alveolitis (diffuse interstitial fibrosis of the lungs). Correlation of histology at biopsy with prognosis. Thorax, 22:291, 1967.

LIPOID PNEUMONIA

Lipoid pneumonia can be exogenous or endogenous in type. In the exogenous variety mineral oil or animal fats are introduced into the lung by aspiration. A common cause is the use of nose drops with a mineral oil as a base. The oil has ready access to the larynx and trachea when applied through the nose. Another cause is the habitual use of mineral oil to regulate bowel movements. In certain persons the mineral oil is aspirated into the trachea and lungs. This is most commonly seen in the elderly in whom the protective reflexes may be dulled. Animal fats may be introduced into the lungs in chronic disease of the esophagus where regurgitation of food occurs. Achalasia of the esophagus is often associated with a chronic pneumonitis as a result of aspiration (see Ch. 635).

In pneumonia caused by mineral oil the earliest reaction is phagocytosis of the oil by alveolar macrophages. The alveolar walls become thickened, and there is an increase in fibrous tissue. Lymphocytes and globules of oil are seen in the interstitial tissue. Ultimately extreme fibrosis of the involved area of the lung occurs.

The endogenous form of lipoid pneumonia consists of a chronic inflammatory process involving a segment or lobe of the lung. The alveoli contain large mononuclear cells with a vacuolated cytoplasm. These cells are also found in the walls of the alveoli. Lymphocytic infiltration and fibrosis of the alveolar walls are present. The lipid present in the lesion is cholesterol. This type of pneumonitis not infrequently occurs secondary to an obstructed bronchus. Occasionally it is present without evident cause.

The symptoms of lipoid pneumonia are extremely variable. The patient may be virtually asymptomatic and the lesion be detected on a routine chest film, or productive cough and dyspnea may be present. The earliest roentgenographic change is the presence of an alveolar type of infiltrate. An acinar pattern may be visible at the periphery of the lesion. Later evidence of fibrosis is present, and there may be contraction of the involved area of the lung. In the exogenous form of the disease the lesions are usually seen in the basilar or posterior segments of the lung.

An important method of diagnosis is the demonstration of oil-containing macrophages in the sputum. The sputum should be collected before breakfast and after cleansing the mouth. Appropriate fat stains should be used. In some cases bronchial brushing or biopsy may be necessary to establish the diagnosis.

There may be difficulty in differentiating lipoid pneumonia from bronchogenic carcinoma. The failure to demonstrate an obstructed bronchus is of great importance in diagnosis. The history of aspiration and the lack of tumor cells in the sputum or in specimens obtained by bronchial brushing of the involved area confirm the diagnosis of lipoid pneumonia.

There is no specific treatment except prevention of aspiration of oil or fat. If symptoms are troublesome and persistent or if the diagnosis is in doubt, resection of the segment or lobe involved should be considered.

Miller, A., Bader, R. A., Bader, M. E., Teirstein, A. S., and Selikoff, J.: Mineral oil pneumonia. Ann. Intern. Med., 57:627, 1962.
Padula, R. T., and Stayman, J. W., Jr.: Chronic interstitial pneumonia: Cholesterol type. Review of the literature and report of two cases. J. Thorac. Cardiovasc. Surg., 54:272, 1967.
Wagner, J. C., Adler, D. I., and Fuller, D. N.: Foreign body granulomata of the lungs due to liquid paraffin. Thorax, 10:157, 1955.
Weill, H., Ferrans, V. J., Gay, R. M., and Ziskind, M. M.: Early lipoid pneumonia. Roentgenologic, anatomic and physiologic characteristics. Am. J. Med., 36:370, 1964.

GOODPASTURE'S SYNDROME AND IDIOPATHIC PULMONARY HEMOSIDEROSIS

Goodpasture's syndrome is a rare disease characterized by repeated episodes of hemorrhage into the pulmonary alveoli associated with glomerulonephritis. The presenting symptoms are hemoptysis and dyspnea. Roentgenographic examination of the lungs demonstrates fluffy infiltrates in both lungs. An iron deficiency anemia is present, and the urine contains albumin, red blood cells, and casts. The course of the disease consists of remissions and exacerbations. Repeated episodes of hemoptysis and pulmonary infiltration occur. Progressive impairment of renal function is common, and uremia often results. The disease has a poor prognosis, and recovery is rare. There is no specific therapy. The pathology of the disease is of great interest. Red blood cells and hemosiderosin-containing macrophages are in the alveoli. The alveolar septa may be thickened with an increase in collagen. A proliferative type of glomerulonephritis is found in the kidneys. An important finding is the presence of gamma globulin and complement in the basement membrane of the renal glomeruli and of the pulmonary alveoli demonstrated by immunofluorescence. Globulins eluted from lung tissue react with glomerular basement membrane. These findings suggest that antibodies against kidney and lung basement membrane are important in the pathogenesis of the disease.

The pulmonary lesions of *idiopathic pulmonary hemosiderosis* bear considerable similarities to those of Goodpasture's syndrome, but no renal lesion is present. The disease occurs most commonly in children, but may occur in young adults. The earliest symptom is hemoptysis. This is associated with transient confluent infiltrates seen on chest roentgenography. The hemoptysis and pulmonary infiltrates come and go. Pallor develops which can be ascribed to an iron deficiency anemia. The patient ultimately develops chronic dyspnea. The chest roentgenogram now may show a reticular appearance with fine stippling. Biopsy of the lung will demonstrate hemosiderin-laden macrophages in the alveoli and an increase in interstitial fibrous tissue. Hemosiderin-containing macrophages can also be found in the sputum. Massive hemoptysis is not uncommon and may lead to death.

The mortality with both syndromes is high. Death in Goodpasture's syndrome may occur after a relatively brief period of time and results from uremia or from pulmonary hemorrhage. Corticosteroids and immunosuppressive agents have been used in therapy, but the results have not been dramatic. Bilateral nephrectomy followed by renal transplantation has been performed in Goodpasture's syndrome with some success.

Koffler, D., Sandson, J., Carr, R., and Kunkel, H.: Immunologic studies concerning the pulmonary lesions in Goodpasture's syndrome. Am. J. Path., 54:293, 1969.
McCombs, R. P.: Diseases due to immunologic reactions in the lungs (second of two parts). N. Engl. J. Med., 286:1245, 1972.
Proskey, A. J., Weatherbee, L., Easterling, R. E., et al.: Goodpasture's syndrome. A report of five cases and review of the literature. Am. J. Med., 48:162, 1970.
Repetto, G., Lisboa, C., Emparanza, E., et al.: Idiopathic pulmonary hemosiderosis. Pediatrics, 40:24, 1967.
Weiss, E. B., Earnest, D. L., and Greally, J. F.: Goodpasture's syndrome. Case report with emphasis on pulmonary physiology. Am. Rev. Respir. Dis., 97:444, 1968.

ALVEOLAR MICROLITHIASIS

Alveolar microlithiasis is a rare disease characterized by the presence of round calcified bodies in the alveoli. The origin and exact nature of these bodies are not known. The disease develops in young adults, and multiple cases may be seen in a family. It is most commonly discovered by examination of a routine roentgenogram of the chest. The appearance of the lungs is characteristic. Fine miliary calcific densities are distributed throughout the lung. The lesions are most prominent at the bases of the lung. The shadows may coalesce, giving a uniform density in portions of the lung. Early in the disease the patient is asymptomatic. Later dyspnea and cough are present. The course is prolonged over many years, and death occurs from pulmonary insufficiency.

Fulechon, F. J. D., Abboud, A. T., Balikian, J. P., and Nucho, C. K. N.: Pulmonary alveolar microlithiasis. Lung function in five cases. Thorax, 24:84, 1969.
Sears, M. R., Chang, A. R., and Taylor, A. J.: Pulmonary alveolar microlithiasis. Thorax, 26:704, 1971.

Section Seven.   PHYSICAL AND CHEMICAL IRRITANTS

Margaret R. Becklake

521.   INTRODUCTION

Man, in taming his environment, in developing his complex industrial society, and, more recently, in pursuit of his hobbies, has become increasingly exposed to a wide variety of materials which may act as chemical and physical irritants to his lungs. The industrial physician is sensitized to the need for a detailed occupational history. However, in many communities working men and women first seek medical advice from their personal physician who may easily fail to recognize an occupational exposure because it occurs in a small plant, using experimental materials, or in the processing as a secondary user of dangerous products whose hazards are not appreciated. Thus *a work history should always be exhaustive* and should cover every job ever held, even part-time or vacation jobs, together with the materials handled directly or indirectly, as well as safety measures recommended on the job and information about the health of co-workers. Place of residence is also impor-tant, as well as the occupation of other family members, because exposure may be only indirect.

Thus today *occupational lung disease* covers the reaction of the lung to *a variety of physical and chemical irritants,* extending beyond those conditions originally described by the term *pneumoconioses,* which refers to lung diseases consequent to the inhalation of dust, in keeping with its Greek derivation. Originally applied only to inorganic (mineral) dusts, it has subsequently been extended to cover organic (biologic) "dusts" as well, because exposure to the latter is also frequently occupational. However, these biologic "dusts" act as neither physical nor chemical irritants, but as stimulants to the subject's immune mechanisms. A large number of variants of the term have been coined to describe specific occupations at risk or specific dust diseases, and probably serve more to confuse than to clarify.

The classification of lung irritants outlined in the accompanying table, although it implies more precise understanding of mechanisms of lung response than is justified by current knowledge, does provide a working and essentially practical approach for diagnosis.

Physical and Chemical Irritants: Working Classification of Their Pulmonary Effects

Agent	Effect on the Lung	Produced by	Circumstances of Exposure, Including Occupation at Risk
Inorganic dusts	1. Noncollagenous pneumoconioses	Carbon, tin, iron, coal, graphite	Mining, welding
	2. Collagenous pneumoconioses		
	a. Nodular	Silica	Hardrock mining, sandblasting
	b. Diffuse	Asbestos, fume and fine silica	Mining, all secondary users of asbestos in industry
		Beryllium	Fluorescent light industry, space industry
	c. Complicated	An altered tissue response to a usually nonfibrogenic dust	Progressive massive fibrosis in coal miners
	3. Neoplasia	Asbestos, radioactive dusts	Asbestos mining, milling, and manufacturing; uranium mining
Organic "dusts"	1. Asthma-like reactions	Enzymes of *B. subtilis,* western red cedar	Manufacturers of detergents; wood workers and processors
	2. Delayed, eventually irreversible, airway obstruction	Cotton, hemp, flax, jute	Processors of vegetable fiber, particularly the carding of cotton
	3. Extrinsic allergic alveolitis	Spores of fungi, e.g., *Thermopolyspora polyspora*	Haymaking, sugar cane picking or processing the residue; mushroom and malt growing; maple bark stripping, etc.
	4. Chronic (lipoid) interstitial pneumonia	Blackfat tobacco (Guyana)	Smoking
Chemicals	1. Asthma-like reactions	Complex salts of platinum, aluminum soldering flux	Platinum refining
		Toluene diisocyanate (TDI)	Manufacturing and home use of polyurethane plastics
	2. Chemical bronchitis	TDI in heavier doses	Ditto
		SO_2	Pulp and paper mills
		NH_3	Refrigeration
	3. Chemical pulmonary edema	NO_2, phosgene	Silo filling, fire fighting
		Paraquat	Accidental ingestion of weed killer
Radiation	Pneumonitis	X-radiation	Medical treatment

INORGANIC DUSTS

522. DOSAGE, CLEARANCE, AND CELLULAR REACTION

Although a heavy inorganic dust load may produce some acute reversible obstruction in airways, the main biologic effects of inorganic dusts depend on their retention in the lungs of man for long periods of time, measured usually in years, not months. It has been suggested that any mineral dust, if relatively insoluble and not immediately toxic, can produce a pneumoconiosis when inhaled in sufficient quantities. The physician is probably better advised to adopt this oversuspicious attitude to mineral dusts than to fail in recognizing old as well as new pneumoconioses.

Human lungs have been aptly called *"size-selective dust samplers."* Airborne dust, when inspired into the lung, undergoes a process of separation based on size and falling rate. Likewise, breathing patterns and minute ventilation affect penetration and deposition. Over 80 per cent of larger particles (6 μ and over) impact on the mucous lining of the larger airways to be removed, usually quite rapidly (i.e., within hours), by ciliary escalation; however, some particles of considerable length, e.g., asbestos fibers up to as much as 100 μ in length, may penetrate as far as terminal respiratory units. Small dust particles penetrate more deeply, but only the fine particles (below 2 μ) penetrate the alveolar spaces.

The retention rate is about 40 per cent in the 2 to 1 μ size, and higher for those below 0.2 μ (see Fig. 1).

Since the respiratory bronchioles and alveoli are lined with surfactant, not mucus, dust particles settling here are removed by alveolar phagocytosis; dust-laden phagocytes migrate toward the alveolar ducts and terminal bronchioles; if not extruded into the airways they may penetrate into lung interstitium and lymphatics. Furthermore, clearance mechanisms may be provoked, i.e., mucus and surfactant production, ciliary activity, and

Figure 1. Deposition rate of particles in the human lung in the nose and supraglottic structures (URT) and in the tracheobronchial tree and lung parenchyma (LRT) in relation to aerodynamic diameter, a measurement which refers to the actual diameter in the presence of water vapor which may exceed the particle size in dry air. (Courtesy of Professor Paul Morrow, University of Rochester, N.Y.; reproduced from Lee, D. H. K. [ed.]: Environmental Factors in Respiratory Disease. New York, Academic Press, 1972.)

endocytosis all increase, in response to the inhalation of irritants, particularly if exposure is intermittent. Heavy doses, on the other hand, may overwhelm the removal mechanisms, and their efficiency may also be reduced by associated pollutants, either industrial or personal (tobacco smoke).

The *lung tissue response to inorganic dust* has been likened to the color spectrum to emphasize the variety in the type of response and its intensity, ranging from noncollagenous dust deposits to intense collagen fibrosis. The nature of the tissue response is thought to depend on the physicochemical properties of the dust as well as on its antigenic properties. It is almost certainly dose related, the consequence of the integrated personal exposure less the integrated clearance over the years, and probably relates to how long the dust has been resident in the lung. Other factors which may influence the response are the presence or absence of infection, and possible synergistic or antagonistic effects of other respirable materials in the environment. Finally, although dust dose is probably the most important factor determining the lung response, individual susceptibility undoubtedly plays a role.

The nodular pneumoconioses, either noncollagenous or collagenous, are caused by the relatively insoluble dusts, and the diffuse pneumoconioses by relatively soluble dusts.

523. DIAGNOSIS, LUNG FUNCTION, AND DISABILITY IN THE INORGANIC DUST PNEUMOCONIOSES

The *diagnosis* of the inorganic dust pneumoconioses depends on the characteristic changes in the chest roentgenogram, *provided that the subject in question has had a suitable history of dust exposure.* In other words, there may be no physical signs and no impairment of physical performance, even in the presence of marked radiographic changes. In no other field therefore is the quality of the chest radiograph more important, and the technique used should be appropriate; e.g., low kv to define pleural calcification, high kv to define the pulmonary parenchyma and noncalcified pleural changes. In addition, use of standard films in conjunction with the UICC/Cincinnati Classification of Radiographic Appearances of the Pneumoconioses (1970) will improve the accuracy of film interpretation. In the absence of an exposure history, it may be necessary to resort to *mediastinal node biopsy* or to *open* or *needle lung biopsy* to establish a diagnosis. However, the pathologic findings may also be inconclusive, because lung tissue has only a limited number of response patterns and a given response may be evoked by several stimuli, e.g., irritants and infections. Thus adequate tissue samples should be sent for chemical assay and mineralogic study with x-ray diffraction as well as histopathology. The electron microprobe may ultimately allow precise characterization of mineral in very small tissue samples, or even in the single ferruginous (asbestos) body. Since most pneumoconioses develop as a consequence of occupational exposure, *precise evaluation of disability* is frequently called for, with a view to establishing compensation; hence, the many studies of pulmonary function in pneu-

moconiosis. However, the interrelationship between the dyspnea and measurable disturbance of static or dynamic pulmonary function has not yet been satisfactorily defined in pneumoconiosis, or, indeed, in lung disease in general. To date, the most acceptable theory is that *dyspnea* is felt when the respiratory effort (either minute volume or muscular effort) for a given task is greater than the subject habitually experiences. In health there exists a tremendous reserve of cardiopulmonary function, indicated by the capacity to increase O_2 consumption (going from rest to maximal exercise) by a factor varying from 20 in the young athlete to perhaps 10 in the middle-aged man. In its early stages pneumoconiosis may produce only very minor measurable changes in function, affecting performance at high levels of exercise only, and this may well be interpreted by the subject as the natural consequence of aging. As the condition progresses, dyspnea may be more easily related to demonstrable changes in lung function. In the following chapters, an attempt is made to describe the usual clinical picture and lung function findings in the different pneumoconioses in their different stages of development. *In evaluating the individual case,* however, *there is no substitute for the detailed study of pulmonary function at rest and on effort,* with a view to determining performance at an average aerobic workload (such as many jobs demand) and possibly to determine maximal aerobic work capacity. This information can then be interpreted in the light of industrial history, dust exposure (quality and quantity), medical history (in particular, previous and present heart and lung disease), and appropriate laboratory investigations.

In a case of industrial lung disease, the physician's responsibility to his patient does not cease until he has assured himself that the case has been referred to the correct local authority in charge of industrial safety. This is important, not only from the point of view of the individual patient who may merit compensation because of already evident disease, but also from the point of view of others working in the same environment whose future health might be ensured by early and adequate preventive action.

524. NONCOLLAGENOUS INORGANIC DUST PNEUMOCONIOSES

Examples. Examples include *coal workers' pneumoconiosis; siderosis* in welders; *pneumoconiosis* in hematite and magnetite miners; *stannosis* in tin miners; *baritosis* in barium miners; *pneumoconiosis* in *chromite* and *china clay miners,* and in workers with *Fuller's earth.*

Pathogenesis and Mechanisms. The dusts mentioned above are those which elicit a virtually noncollagenous response in the lung; hence the diseases associated with such exposure have been called the *"benign" pneumoconioses.* The dusts concerned can accumulate in large amounts, usually in phagocytes which accumulate in the alveolar spaces or penetrate the interstitial pulmonary tissue to collect as discrete macules, or as thick sheaths of cells around the respiratory bronchioles. Although considerable amounts of dust (up to 20 grams) may be recoverable from the lungs at autopsy, only small amounts of fibrous tissue develop in these macules, usually in a radial rather than a concentric fashion. The intensity of the fibrosis, never marked, is thought to be related to quartz contamination in the dust, and variations in quartz content probably explain such regional differences as exist, for example, among the dust macule of the Welsh soft coal miner, the more fibrous macule of his counterpart in Belgium, and the *stellate "mixed dust" nodule* of the foundry worker. In addition, the radiodensity of the nodules appears to be related to their iron content, endogenous iron accumulating around dust as it does around other foreign bodies. In time the respiratory bronchioles around the dust foci dilate, perhaps because of the local traction of the dust-encased bronchioles on the surrounding lung parenchyma, and a characteristic form of *focal proximal acinar emphysema* develops, involving primarily the respiratory bronchioles.

The pathologic changes of generalized emphysema may also be seen in lungs which are affected by these nodular pneumoconioses, particularly when the nodulation is of the smaller variety (pinhead rather than micronodular). Such changes occur more frequently and to a more disabling degree (leading to pulmonary hypertension and right heart failure) in certain geographic areas, e.g., the iron mines of Lorraine and the coal mines of Belgium. Finally, pulmonary emphysema has been shown to occur more frequently in the lungs of miners than in the lungs of the nonmining population, even in the absence of pneumoconiosis, thus strengthening the evidence that dust exposure, particularly in the cigarette smoker, is an important factor contributing to the development of chronic obstructive lung disease.

Clinical Manifestations. The term "tattooing" of the chest roentgenogram has been applied to this group of *"benign" noncollagenous nodular pneumoconioses,* because even in the presence of diffuse radiologic nodular densities symptoms and signs of chest disease are rarely present. Likewise, most tests routinely used to evaluate pulmonary function such as measurements of lung volume, flow rates, diffusing capacity at rest, and even the pulmonary mechanics, have been found to be within the normal limits in keeping with the histology of the dust macules. However, abnormalities of gas exchange (reflected in increased A-a O_2 differences) have been shown to exist. These changes, demonstrable at rest and exaggerated during effort, presumably reflect regional inequalities in ventilation vis-à-vis perfusion. Such changes probably do not impair function enough to cause symptoms, and disability affecting performance, if present, is usually attributable to chronic obstructive airway disease.

Epidemiology and Prognosis. The prevalence rate of simple pneumoconiosis varies very much from operation to operation, even within the same industry; for example, rates range from 58 to 253 per 1000 underground workers in the coal mining industry of Great Britain, and from 100 to 400 per 1000 working coal miners in various American pits. In small uncontrolled operations prevalence may well be higher. These differences are thought to be related to the dust exposure levels, and prevalence usually falls dramatically as dust control becomes effective, e.g., in the Dutch coal miners rates fell from 270 to 160 per 1000 working miners over a seven-year period.

In addition to the pathologic evidence quoted above, there is also epidemiologic evidence that the prevalence of chronic obstructive lung disease (as measured by questionnaire or simple ventilatory tests, or both) is in-creased in coal miners and that this is related to their occupation since dose relationships have been shown. However, other factors which influence its prevalence include environment (e.g., in some areas bronchitis appears to be as common among miners' wives as among the miners themselves) and cigarette smoking, since miners are frequently heavy smokers. Thus attributability is a taxing and difficult problem for compensation commissions, especially as the noncollagenous nodular pneumoconioses in this group do not usually per se produce significant disability.

It is *unusual* for these pneumoconioses *to develop for the first time or to progress after exposure has ceased,* but this does occur. Likewise, the disappearance of radiologic changes after removal from exposure, though unusual, has been described, and is in keeping with animal experiments showing that dust nodules are not static structures but are the site of continuing phagocytic activity. Life expectancy does not appear to be affected by the presence of these "benign" pneumoconioses, especially if exposure stops and they are not complicated by obstructive lung disease.

525. COLLAGENOUS INORGANIC DUST PNEUMOCONIOSES OF THE NODULAR TYPE

Examples. Examples of these disorders include *classic silicosis of hardrock miners* and of *granite workers* and *cutters;* and silicosis in *iron and steel workers* and *sandblasters,* in the *pottery industry,* in industries using *silica flour,* and in those processing *bentonite.*

Pathogenesis and Mechanisms. If the dusts of carbon and coal represent those at the low end of the response spectrum, free crystalline silica dust represents the opposite end, with its almost unique biologic capacity to evoke a powerful fibrogenic tissue response. Reaction to silica appears to start with an alteration of the lung macrophages, though by what mechanism is not fully understood; neither a mechanical nor a simple solubility theory fully explains the biologic findings. There is support for the view that damaged macrophages release altered cell material which is antigenic and which activates the reticuloendothelial system. A fibroblastic reaction follows (peribronchiolar, perivascular, or both) which leads to the accumulation of hyaline material at the site of the macrophage collections, and ultimately to the development of the *characteristic fibrous silicotic nodule* made up of layers of whorled connective tissue, like an onion. Extensive and marked fibrosis may be present in the lungs at autopsy with only relatively small amounts of dust (up to 10 grams, of which perhaps half is silica). Involvement of the hilar and mediastinal lymph nodes is common, occasionally with *egg-shell calcification,* whereas abdominal nodes are occasionally affected. In nature, free crystalline silica occurs almost exclusively as quartz; however, other free crystalline silicas, e.g., crystobalite, tridymite, though rare in natural geologic formation, may be formed from quartz in steelmaking and in other high-heat smelting processes, and probably have a more powerful silicosis-producing action than quartz.

Conglomerate silicosis is the result of the matting together by fibrosis of silicotic nodules, frequently associated with caseous areas, which often but by no means always show conclusive histologic evidence of tuberculosis. These changes account for the right heart strain, hypertrophy, and failure which may develop subsequently, perhaps as a consequence of the pulmonary vascular bed's being reduced by the fibrosis and tissue loss and associated emphysematous changes in the adjacent lung. A reversible element in the pulmonary hypertension may also be present, related perhaps to hypoxia or hypercapnia or both.

Clinical Manifestations. Even in nodular silicosis (in which the radiologic lesions are fibrous nodules, not collagenous dust macules, as in the "benign" pneumoconioses) there may be no clinical manifestations, and no apparent impairment in pulmonary function. The proportion of cases without signs and symptoms is probably only about 20 per cent, in contrast to about 90 per cent in the "benign" pneumoconioses of equivalent radiologic category.

The first complaint in nodular silicosis is commonly *shortness of breath,* brought on by moderate, and then progressively less, exercise until it is present at rest. This symptom is probably due to the increased muscular work required to ventilate incompliant lungs and is aggravated by increased minute ventilation to offset impaired gas exchange. Lung volumes are reduced as the nodular disease becomes more widespread. However, miners who smoke may present with the symptoms, signs, and classic lung function pattern of chronic obstructive lung disease, even though the radiologic pattern is primarily that of diffuse nodular pneumoconiosis.

When *complicated pneumoconiosis* develops *on a background of classic silicosis,* the symptoms, signs, and clinical presentation usually represent a progression from an already symptomatic state, and the diagnosis is made from the chest radiograph which shows a conglomeration of existing lesions, usually in the upper mid-zones, often bilateral, with eventual progression to the characteristic bilateral "angels' wings" shadows. The lung function pattern may suggest restrictive disease but frequently shows a pattern characteristic of obstructive disease, or there may be a mixed picture. Infection with *M. tuberculosis* is more likely to be demonstrable in conglomerate silicosis than in the progressive massive fibrosis of coal workers, and is more likely to behave and progress as in the nonsilicotic lung with constitutional symptoms (see below). Right heart strain and failure may complicate the picture, particularly if chronic bronchitis and emphysema are present.

Epidemiology and Prognosis. Prevalence rates vary from operation to operation, depending chiefly on the efficiency of dust control. Thus in the Witwatersrand gold mining industry, rates fell from 40 per 1000 underground miners in the 1920's to less than 10 per 1000 in the 1950's, and the average period of mining service prior to diagnosis rose from 10 to 23 years over this period. However, the simple silicosis of gold miners is undoubtedly a less benign disease than the simple pneumoconiosis of coal miners, despite the fact that it does not appear to affect life expectancy. Thus figures for Sweden indicate that, after withdrawal from exposure, x-ray changes never regress but progress in the majority of cases (Fig. 2). The prevalence of chronic obstructive lung disease does not appear to be occupationally related to classic silicosis, other than can be accounted for by a man's smoking habits.

526. COLLAGENOUS INORGANIC DUST PNEUMOCONIOSES OF THE DIFFUSE TYPE

Examples. These pneumoconioses include *asbestosis* in mining, milling, manufacturing, and all the secondary industrial uses of asbestos; *aluminosis,* as in shaver's disease; *talcosis* in miners and millers of talc; and *chronic beryllium disease of the lung.*

Pathogenesis and Mechanisms. Asbestos, the most important mineral in this group, occurs in several forms: *chrysotile* (a magnesium silicate, occurring as long, white, flexible fibers), the chief asbestos of commerce, mined primarily in Canada and the U.S.S.R. as well as in Italy and in Southern Africa; and the *amphiboles,* iron silicates (occurring as brittle fibers such as amosite, anthophyllite, and blue crocidolite) mined in South Africa, Australia, and Finland. Exposure occurs in mining and milling, and in the manufacture of a wide variety of the commodities used by modern man. *Asbestos cement products,* such as tiles and pipes, account for 70 per cent of production; and *insulation materials,* including floor tiles, for another 10 per cent; the rest is used in *paper, friction materials* (car brake and clutch linings), and *textiles* for use as protection against heat in industry and in homes.

The extent to which asbestos fibers penetrate the lung in all likelihood depends on their physical properties, the curly fibers of chrysotile being more likely to impinge on the mucus blanket than the short straight amphibole fibers. Some fibers appear to penetrate the interstitium

Figure 2. Rate of progression of different pneumoconioses after removal from dust exposure. The figures are based on five occupational groups of Swedish workers (each containing a minimum of ten cases) followed for 15 years after dust exposure ceased. (From Bruce, T., Nystrom, A., and Ahlmark, A. L.: Scand. J. Resp. Diseases, Supp. 63, 1968.)

directly and remain there, perhaps undergoing chemical and physical degeneration but nevertheless visible in much greater profusion than was ever suspected before the use of electron microscopy in their detection. Other fibers become engulfed by macrophages, and still others, but probably only a very small proportion, become enveloped in a smooth protein film which becomes iron-impregnated, giving rise to the typical drumhead, golden-brown *asbestos bodies,* a process also attributed at least in part to macrophage action. The pleura also appears to be a target organ, and *pleural reactions* to exposure include *effusion* (often bloody); dense, fibrous, *adhesive pleurisy; plaques* and *calcification* involving parietal rather than visceral pleura; and malignancy in the form of *mesothelioma* (see below).

It is not known which fibers are, or become, fibrogenic; nor is their precise mode of action known. Fibers deposited in alveolar structures elicit a cellular reaction similar to *desquamative alveolitis;* others at the level of the respiratory bronchiole produce an appearance of *bronchiolitis obliterans;* a third reaction is characterized by *interstitial edema* going on to *collagenization.* Nonspecific antinuclear antibodies may accelerate the fibrosis once it has started, and it eventually becomes confluent, obliterating air spaces and replacing them with cystic spaces lined by flattened epithelium *("honeycomb" lung).* Other mineral dusts which produce this pattern of diffuse fibrosis are talc, diatomaceous earth, and some of the very fine silicas currently used in industry, particularly if the exposure is heavy. *Caplan's syndrome* (see below), though more frequently recognized in coal workers, may be seen in relation to exposure to asbestos, silica, and probably most dusts.

Generalized pulmonary fibrosis may also be found in *chronic beryllium disease* of the lung, a manifestation of systemic poisoning with this mineral rather than a pneumoconiosis. The early signs are characterized by chronic interstitial pneumonitis, which is frequently granulomatous. The granulomas may vary from loose collections of histiocytes to large circumscribed granulomas, often containing giant cells with various inclusion bodies, indistinguishable histologically from sarcoidosis. The end result is frequently fibrosis of varying severity. Diagnosis can be made with certainty only by isolation of the element beryllium in tissues or body fluids. There is often a very long period of latency, up to 30 years, and initial exposure may only have been indirect, so that cases related to the manufacture of fluorescent light in the United States during World War II continue to be reported today, even though the use of beryllium in the fluorescent lamp industry ceased in 1949. Although its modern uses, particularly those concerned with space exploration, appear to be better controlled, physicians should remain vigilant because new cases continue to be added to the U.S. Beryllium Registry at the Massachusetts General Hospital.

Clinical Manifestations. These are no different from those of diffuse pulmonary fibrosis, whatever the underlying cause. In some subjects *dyspnea* is the first symptom, brought on at first by considerable exertion and then by progressively less effort, until it is eventually present at rest. In other subjects, an *irritating dry cough* precedes the awareness of shortness of breath, often by many years. With the progress of the disease, the cough may become productive, and *spells of chest pain* may be associated with the coughing. When the condition is advanced, there are usually diffuse basal rales, but these may also occur early before radiologic evidence of lung changes. The lung signs may be modified by the presence of pleural thickening or calcification. Respiratory failure may only appear late in the course of the disease, with pulmonary hypertension, right heart strain, and right heart failure. Nor is the victim of these diffuse pneumoconioses immune from the attack by general atmospheric pollutants—in particular, cigarette smoking—which may encourage the development of chronic bronchitis and bronchiectasis and increase the risk of bronchial neoplasm.

The *established case of asbestosis* is associated with changes in pulmonary function characteristic of restrictive lung disease, i.e., small volumes, impaired gas exchange with reduced diffusing capacity, and hyperventilation on effort and eventually at rest. The earliest function changes in response to asbestos dust exposure appear to be reduced vital capacity and increased exercise ventilation, tests which may eventually prove useful in the longitudinal surveillance of exposed workers. In addition, the function changes of chronic obstructive lung disease are not infrequently seen, particularly in workers who smoke.

In certain parts of the world, e.g., Finland, *pleural calcification* may appear as the only manifestation of exposure to asbestos, and less commonly to talc and mica. It is rarely seen under 20 years of industrial exposure, and neighborhood cases are seen with diminishing frequency as the circumferential distance of the place of residence from the industry increases.

Epidemiology and Prognosis. The *attack rate of asbestosis* varies in different industries (probably in relation to the heaviness of exposure) from under 10 per cent of working miners in open mining, as in Quebec, up to over 70 per cent in men with over 20 years' exposure in the insulation and construction industries.

The epidemiology of *population exposure to asbestos* has been established from the search for asbestos bodies in lung scrapings or extruded lung fluid in routine autopsies. Positive results are reported in many parts of the world, ranging from 1 per cent in rural Scotland to over 50 per cent in Finland, the site of the world's oldest known asbestos deposits. Insofar as the lung is an accumulator over time, and the world's use of asbestos is increasing dramatically, it is not surprising that this percentage is increasing in adults in London; New York studies by contrast report between 50 and 60 per cent both in recent and in 1934 autopsy material. It must be emphasized that the presence of *ferruginous bodies* (as experts now urge that they be called) indicates exposure, not disease. Nor are they specific for asbestos, because other types of fibers, e.g., glass, wool, cotton, talc, may constitute their core, and the lung probably uses this method to "inactivate" a large variety of inhaled particles. However, their presence in the sputum should alert the physician to the possibility of asbestos-related disease.

527. NEOPLASIA ASSOCIATED WITH EXPOSURE TO INORGANIC DUSTS

Asbestos. Exposure to asbestos increases the attack rate (probably in a dose-related fashion) of *bronchial carcinoma,* particularly and perhaps only in smokers, suggesting a synergism between carcinogens. The presence of asbestosis increases the risk, and some reports indicate that neoplasia will develop in 50 per cent of patients with already established asbestosis. Exposure to asbestos dust is also associated with increased risk of *gastric neoplasia*, presumably because of dust swallowing. Finally a rare tumor, *mesothelioma of the pleura and/or peritoneum*, occurs with greater frequency not only in industrially exposed populations, but also in association with indirect exposure, often after a long latent period, e.g., neighborhood exposure as a child 40 years before.

Although all types of asbestos fiber are implicated in the increased incidence of neoplasia, the order of increase varies, being on the whole higher for those engaged in processing and using than for those engaged in mining or milling. To what extent these differences are attributable to dust dose, fiber type, changes in physical and chemical properties with processing, and/or contamination by cocarcinogens remains to be determined.

Airborne Radioactive Particles. An increased number of deaths from lung cancer have been observed in American uranium miners, the risk being related to the radiation dose with a preponderance of small cell cancers. Increased deaths from lung cancer have also been observed in miners handling other materials, thought to be noncarcinogenic, in whom exposure has occurred to mine air contaminated by radon decay products from the ore-bearing rock or mine water, e.g., fluorspar miners of St. Lawrence, Newfoundland, and hematite miners in Cumberland, England.

Whether or not a neoplasm is occupation associated makes no difference to the outcome as far as the individual patient is concerned; *recognition of this association* on the part of the attending physician may, however, be important both from the patient's point of view (if there is a question of compensation) and from the point of view of the patient's working colleagues, since index cases serve to direct attention to occupational hazards.

528. COMPLICATED PNEUMOCONIOSIS

Examples. Examples of the complicated pneumoconioses include *progressive massive fibrosis of coal workers* and *Caplan's syndrome*.

Pathogenesis and Mechanisms. Most inorganic dust pneumoconioses can advance to progressive massive fibrosis whether or not exposure continues. Thus, although initially the response to dust exposure may be a macrophage reaction producing a noncollagenous response with little effect on the lung architecture, years later the same lung tissue may react to the same dust with severe fibrosis which obliterates and destroys all anatomic structure. The lesions of *progressive massive fibrosis in coal workers* (PMF) consist of dust irregularly mixed with bundles of coarse, hyaline collagen fibers. Few blood vessels and air passages are seen, but the persistence of internal elastic lamellae suggests that they have been obliterated by invading fibrous tissue. Sclerosis of the vessel walls and intimal thickening at the periphery of the lesions are common. At autopsy histologic and/or bacteriologic evidence of tuberculosis is found in about half the cases, even though in only a small proportion is it possible to recover tubercle bacilli in the sputum during life.

Several mechanisms may be operative in the development of complicated pneumoconiosis, of which infection by *M. tuberculosis* and/or atypical mycobacteria is probably the most frequent (the recovery rate of organisms both in life and at autopsy increases with increasing effort and has exceeded 50 per cent in some autopsy series). Other factors are the overwhelming of clearance mechanisms by lung dust; aseptic necrosis owing to interference with blood supply; significant silica contamination of the coal dust; and, finally, reaction on an immunologic basis, perhaps caused by liberation of antigenic material from macrophages damaged by dust. A comparable mechanism in the susceptible individual is thought to occur in *Caplan's syndrome*. Caplan observed an association between rheumatoid arthritis and a particular radiologic picture, characterized by well-defined opacities 0.5 to 5 cm in diameter, widely distributed and developing rather more suddenly than progressive massive fibrosis, often on a background of slight or no pneumoconiosis. Some lesions eventually cavitate, then shrink, perhaps with calcifications, and may later become incorporated into a mass radiologically indistinguishable from progressive massive fibrosis. Histologically, the rheumatoid nodule is distinguished by wide concentric bands of necrotic collagen separated by bands of dust, with a peripheral zone of active inflammation and a well-marked arteritis in the adjacent vessels. Caplan's syndrome, though first recognized and most frequently seen in coal miners, has been described in workers in foundries, asbestos, potteries, sandblasting, and boiler scaling.

Clinical Manifestations. In coal workers, the appearance of progressive massive fibrosis usually marks the onset of symptoms and signs of lung disease. The first symptom is commonly *dyspnea* on heavy effort, and subsequently at lesser work loads until it becomes evident at rest. The changes in function initially suggest loss of functioning volume, followed by a generalized restrictive lung disease. The symptom of cough does not appear to be more common in the earlier stages of complicated pneumoconiosis than in simple pneumoconiosis. *Melanoptysis* (sudden coughing up of a moderate amount of jet black fluid) is not uncommon, and frequently relates to cavitation. *Chest pain,* dull and aching, and diffusely located, is common, and there is an increasing tendency to *acute purulent bronchitis.* Pulmonary hypertension and right heart hypertrophy, leading ultimately to *right heart failure,* is present in many instances, with the usual symptoms and signs. When infection with *M. tuberculosis* appears to be the factor precipitating the development of the complicated pneumoconiosis, it is seldom accompanied by the usual systemic symptoms, i.e., fever, weight loss, and hemoptysis.

When the chest roentgenogram suggests Caplan's syndrome (see above), serum tests for rheumatoid factor are positive in 80 per cent of cases, whereas arthritis, already present in about 50 per cent of cases, may develop in others only after a delay of several years.

Epidemiology and Prognosis. Attack rates of progressive massive fibrosis in Welsh coal miners increase from 1 per cent in the lowest category of simple pneumoconiosis to 30 per cent in advanced simple pneumoconiosis, and appear to be highest in the younger men working on heavier jobs. Rheumatoid pneumoconiosis occurs in 2 to 6 per cent of United Kingdom coal miners affected by pneumoconiosis, and should be suspected when PMF develops suddenly in an individual with minimal or no pneumoconiosis. Prevalence rates of PMF relate to the prevalence of pneumoconiosis in that industry concerned (which, in turn, relates to dustiness), as well as to the prevalence of tuberculosis. It is therefore somewhat disappointing to find that vigorous antituberculosis measures in coal-mining communities have not reduced attack rates of progressive massive fibrosis as dramatically as hoped.

529. TREATMENT AND PREVENTION OF THE INORGANIC DUST PNEUMOCONIOSES

Treatment. There is *no specific treatment for the simple nodular or diffuse inorganic dust pneumoconioses.* The medical management of associated chronic obstructive lung disease and right heart failure and pulmonary heart disease is the same whether or not it coexists with pneumoconiosis (see Ch. 507). Progression of the condition, particularly to complicated pneumoconiosis, appears to depend as much on past as on subsequent exposure. Thus the physician faces the difficult question of *whether he should advise the individual patient to find other employment.* A reasonable decision must be based on an accurate knowledge of what determines progression of simple pneumoconiosis and the attack rates of complicated pneumoconiosis in the particular operation concerned. Such knowledge is accumulating in the larger industries which can mount well-planned research operations, e.g., the coal mining industries in Great Britain, Germany, and the United States, but cannot necessarily be applied to other situations, e.g., a welder in a small local plant. In general, most physicians, when faced with such a problem, permit continued employment, with the proviso that regular medical surveillance be available.

Likewise, in *complicated pneumoconiosis,* medical management is concerned with treatment of the complications. When active tuberculous infection or even a positive skin test to PPD can be demonstrated, appropriate chemotherapy should be instituted (see Ch. 228). However, controlled clinical trials do not support the routine use of tuberculosis chemoprophylaxis in all cases. Since complicated pneumoconiosis is invariably accompanied by disability, often associated with right heart failure, most patients with complicated pneumoconiosis will have already left the industry concerned. Opinion is divided on the advisability of withdrawal from exposure if the patient is still so occupied.

Dust Control. Inorganic dust pneumoconioses cannot be treated effectively, but they can be prevented, and *prevention* means, essentially, *dust control.* Attack rate increases with exposure, and there is a dust dose–disease relationship. Thus *control should be at an epidemiologic level,* aiming at controlling the exposure of the community at risk, not at a personal level with the use of masks or respirators which should be regarded only as temporary until the environment has been controlled. Dust can seldom be completely eliminated from industrial operations. However, disease could be controlled if the mini-

mal exposure which produces health effects in a given industry were known. It is possible to envisage a future in which, using cumulative ongoing records of each worker's exposure, operations could be planned so that no worker would be likely to exceed the exposure known to produce disease within his working life. Such an ambitious scheme, already under way in the West German coal mining industry, is likely to be set up only in large industries able to mount extensive research programs. However, for smaller industries, it is quite valid to assert that *less dust means less disease;* definitions of low-risk levels of exposure for different dusts (threshold limit values) are annually revised by bodies such as the American Conference of Governmental Industrial Hygienists and provide general reference standards. There is, however, room for much more definitive action than has occurred in the past on the part of the treating physicians, communities, and governments concerned.

Tuberculosis Control. Medical attention should be directed toward reducing the attack rates of complicated pneumoconiosis and silicotuberculosis. All subjects with pneumoconiosis are at a higher risk in terms of tuberculosis than the general population; in addition the circumstances of employment may favor infection, e.g., recruitment of workers from populations in which infection with tubercle bacilli occurs relatively late in life. Case finding and control of tuberculosis should thus be of a particularly high standard in populations exposed to an inorganic dust hazard; at the very least this should include the annual chest roentgenogram. Finally, gastrectomy for peptic ulcer should be avoided in subjects with pneumoconiosis, because this increases the chance of developing PMF much in the same way that it constitutes a risk factor in developing active tuberculosis.

Prophylactic Substances. Studies in laboratory animals have indicated that certain substances (ferric oxide, iron, coal, aluminum, and more recently poly-2-vinyl-pyridine-N-oxide or PVNO) inhibit the biologic effects of silica dust. Of these materials only aluminum has received a trial in man when it was introduced into the gold mines of Ontario in 1943; however, no conclusive evidence on its effectiveness has come out of this experience, and this type of prophylaxis is a sorry substitute for proper environmental dust control. A therapeutic trial of PVNO has been started in West German coal miners, and a prophylactic trial may be undertaken in the future.

ORGANIC "DUSTS"

530. FACTORS INFLUENCING REACTIONS TO INHALED ORGANIC "DUSTS"

The inorganic "dusts" referred to here include fungal spores, components of plants, and a wide variety of other biologic material. Unlike the inorganic dusts, the effects of which are related primarily to exposure dose, the effects of exposure to inorganic "dusts" appear to depend to a major extent on the reactivity of the subject, atopic individuals usually showing both immediate and delayed responses (attributed to Type I and Type III allergy, respectively) and nonatopic individuals usually showing delayed responses only (attributed to Type III allergy). The list of organic "dusts" generated in industrial and commercial operations and capable of producing *asthma in the atopic individuals* is virtually limitless, and such subjects frequently withdraw voluntarily from an occupation involving exposure. Treatment of such patients is on an individual basis (see Ch. 505). However, with the relatively heavy exposures which occur in certain industrial and other commercial processes often involving large numbers of workers, *many nonatopic individuals* may also be affected, and the term *organic dust pneumoconioses* has come into use to underline their occupational association. Evaluation of the individual patient should therefore be made in terms of the following three factors considered by Pepys to be of prime importance in determining an individual's response: (1) his immunologic reactivity (whether or not atopic, since this may determine the approach to treatment); (2) the nature of the inhaled antigen, including particle size, which will influence its penetration in the respiratory tract; and (3) the nature and circumstances of exposure (obtained by careful history taking).

531. ASTHMA-LIKE REACTIONS TO ORGANIC "DUSTS"

Examples. Examples include asthma in workers exposed to the enzymes of *B. subtilis* in the manufacture of detergents and asthma in workers with Western red cedar *(Thuja plicata).*

Pathogenesis and Mechanisms. Reactions to these occupational exposures occur usually within months of first exposure in the case of the enzymes, but often only after years in the case of *Thuja plicata.* The nonatopic individual is as much at risk as the atopic individual. In the case of *detergent workers who are atopic,* bronchial provocation tests invariably elicit a dual response, i.e., immediate and late (within hours), attributed to Type I (IgE-mediated) and Type III (precipitin-mediated) hypersensitivity, respectively. In *nonatopic workers* (usually the majority of the factory personnel), the immediate effects may be irritant rather than allergic, but there is growing evidence that the late effects are precipitin mediated (see Ch. 505). Skin reactions are positive in about half the workers, but do not distinguish the symptomatic from the nonsymptomatic.

Clinical Manifestations. In sensitized workers, symptoms follow exposure within minutes and include chest tightness, cough, and wheezing, with audible rhonchi. Without bronchodilators, the symptoms subside slowly over about four hours, to be followed by the development of *dyspnea, wheezing,* and *rhonchi,* and the general symptoms of headache, malaise, and muscle pains at about six hours. *Nocturnal exacerbations of wheezing* are also characteristic and have been attributed to inhibition of endogenous regulatory mechanisms, and their association with a daytime occupational exposure can easily be missed. There is no present evidence of chronic effects, but the manufacture of these detergents is too recent to be certain that such effects may not occur, particularly because animal exposures, admittedly to much higher doses, have produced diffuse emphysema. A case of

chronic granulomatous lung disease attributed to the inhalation of cedar sawdust has been reported.

Treatment and Prevention. Sensitized individuals should be removed from exposure. However, since some 50 per cent of exposed workers appear to become sensitized, control must be environmental. In some instances this has been achieved by coating the enzyme particles to increase their size (from 0.5 to 1.0 mm), thus reducing the chance that they will be inhaled into smaller airways.

532. AIRWAY OBSTRUCTION (DELAYED, EVENTUALLY IRREVERSIBLE) DUE TO ORGANIC "DUSTS"

Examples. Examples include *byssinosis* in association with the processing of *cotton* (particularly spinning), *flax,* and *soft hemp dusts*; *jute* may be implicated; sisal probably is not.

Clinical Manifestations. An acute response to cotton dust may occur at first exposure or only after many years of exposure; the term *byssinosis* usually refers to the latter, and, again, the nonatopic individual appears to be as much at risk as the atopic one. The diagnosis is made on the basis of a characteristic symptom pattern in a subject with suitable exposure. Symptoms are *cough, tightness in the chest,* and *breathlessness,* occurring at first only occasionally on the first day of the working week (Grade $1/2$), then regularly on Monday morning (Grade 1), then persisting beyond Monday (Grade 2), and finally, after several years, persisting throughout the week (Grade 3), when it is indistinguishable from nonindustrial chronic obstructive lung disease. There are no specific radiologic changes. Attack rates may reach over 90 per cent of exposed populations; a family history of atopy, with hypersensitivity to inhaled histamine, is unusual; immediate skin reactions to cotton dust are infrequent. Cigarette smoking increases the risk and severity of the disease. In the nonsymptomatic worker, dust exposure may result in small decreases in airway conductance, suggesting a nonspecific effect on major airways. By contrast in the worker with the *Monday morning dyspnea* of byssinosis, exposure causes a reduction in forced expiratory flow rates and vital capacity with effects on flow volume curves which can be improved by isoproterenol inhalation. Antihistaminic drugs may also improve the flow rates in byssinosis without necessarily affording subjective relief, a finding pointing to the probable importance of small airway involvement. Pretreatment with orciprenaline, antihistamines, and ascorbic acid appears to diminish the biologic response to cotton dust.

Pathogenesis and Mechanisms. It is thought that some fraction of the offending dusts (probably the protein fraction) causes the nonantigenic release of histamine and perhaps of other pharmacologically active substances; these reduce the caliber of large and/or small airways, the site of action perhaps being related to dust size and site of maximal deposition. Whether the histamine release is entirely nonantigenic, as originally proposed, or whether there is an antigenic component to the reaction, as recently proposed, has not been determined. Information on the long-term effects comes from the few published autopsy reports in which chronic bronchitis and emphysema were noted, together with occasional "ferruginous" bodies containing what was assumed to be cotton fibers; in addition, the lungs contain somewhat increased amounts of nonspecific dusts, probably carbonaceous. A single report of extensive fibrosis with plasma cell infiltration suggests an immunologic background for the disease, indicating the need for further study.

Epidemiology. Attack rates of byssinosis vary widely, usually, though not invariably, in relation to exposure levels; in some instances plant modernization has even led to increased environmental dust. Reported rates for Egyptian workers vary from 0 to 90 per cent; for Swedish, Dutch, and British workers, about 50 per cent; and for American workers, up to 30 per cent; whereas a study of retired rural Spanish workers shows a high prevalence of chronic disease. There are no data on the rate and inevitability of progression from Grade I (essentially reversible) to Grade III (essentially irreversible) disease. However, it is not insignificant; indeed the recognition of byssinosis resulted from the observation of increased mortality and morbidity rates for cardiovascular and respiratory disease in certain Lancashire cotton workers.

Prevention. Present efforts to control byssinosis are directed toward dust control by means of environmental engineering, and its success depends on defining as accurately as possible the dust levels which constitute risk in respect of particle size and number in relation to toxic properties of the dust concerned. However, a recent study of cotton workers under controlled dust exposures has shown that *preprocessing the cotton* by autoclaving diminished by tenfold the incidence of the biologic response. Thus dust control of the future may well be a source intervention as envisaged many years ago by Schilling. Medical aspects of prevention include a *pre-employment examination* (to eliminate those with pre-existing lung disease and those who show a marked response to dust) and *regular medical surveillance,* because this may be one of the few industrial exposures in which progression to chronic disease may be halted by removal from exposure at any early clinical stage of the disease.

533. EXTRINSIC ALLERGIC ALVEOLITIS

Examples. Examples of this disorder include *farmer's lung, bagassosis* in sugar cane workers, *mushroom-worker's lung, maplebark-stripper's lung, suberosis* of cork workers, *sequoiosis,* and *malt-worker's lung.*

Pathogenesis and Mechanisms. The term *extrinsic allergic alveolitis* is used to describe reactions produced in the gas-exchanging tissues of the lung, usually of nonatopic individuals, after inhalation of spores of a number of different fungi. It is thought to occur when the spores penetrate the alveoli in sufficient numbers initially to sensitize (with the production of serum precipitins) and subsequently to elicit an alveolitis. The reaction is thought to be a Type III or Arthus one on the basis of its time relationship to exposure, its correlation with the presence of serum precipitins and delayed skin reactions, and its inhibition by corticosteroid drugs. The presence of precipitins, however, is not decisive, and it is presumed that a critical balance between antigen exposure and antibody production is necessary for the formation of

the damaging antibody-antigen complexes to occur which mediate the inflammatory and probably also the granulomatous response. Identification of the major source of allergen in *farmer's lung* (the spores of the thermophilic actinomyces, *Micropolyspora faeni* and *Thermoactinomyces vulgaris,* found in moldy hay) has led to the recognition of an increasing number of diseases of similar origin and of certain unusual exposure risks, e.g., contamination of air conditioner systems with spores; undoubtedly more will be documented in the future. The main examples currently recognized are *bagassosis,* from the spores of *T. sacchari* in moldy bagasse (sugar-cane residue used in the production of hard board, acoustic, and other thermal boards); *mushroom-worker's lung,* usually from the spores of both *T. vulgaris* and *M. faeni,* two of some 20 fungi found in mushroom compost; *malt-worker's lung* from the spores of *Aspergillus clavatus* and *A. fumigatus* in moldy barley and malt dust; *maplebark-stripper's lung,* from the spores of *Cryptostroma corticale; sequoiosis* from the spores of *Pullularia pullulans; cheese-washer's lung* from the spores of *Penicillium casei;* and *suberosis* from moldy cork dust. All these spores are of the order of 6 μ or less in size, but there is evidence that spores up to 10 μ may penetrate the lung in adequate numbers to elicit alveolitis. In addition, a number of heterologous serum proteins are implicated, e.g., those of avian origin occurring in bird droppings, causing *bird-breeder's lung,* and disease caused by antigens of insect origin, e.g., wheat weevil.

Lung biopsy in the early stages shows changes attributable to a foreign body reaction resulting from the cellular removal and sequestration of large antigen-antibody complexes, rather than implicating an additional Type IV allergy. The changes may resolve completely or may, particularly if associated with recurrent exposures, go on to fibrosis, which may also involve the organization of endobronchial exudates with bronchiolitis obliterans.

Clinical Manifestations. After a variable period of exposure, symptoms usually develop within six to eight hours of re-exposure, commonly appearing in the evening after a day's work with the particular spore source. *Fever, chills, malaise,* and generalized nonpleuritic *chest pain* are characteristic, together with a dry irritant *cough* productive of scanty sputum, and respiratory distress. *Weight loss* is common. On clinical examination in the acute stage, rales are heard, often less widespread than anticipated, and rhonchi are not usually prominent. The chest roentgenogram, though sometimes normal, usually shows a widespread interstitial pattern of a reticular nature, occasionally with fine, nodular shadows, which may become confluent. Pulmonary function measurements are in keeping with the location of the disease in alveoli and small airways, i.e., volumes are reduced, gas exchange is impaired, but expiratory flow rates are usually normal. Only occasionally does an obstructive function pattern predominate.

In the absence of further exposure, clinical, radiologic, and function changes usually resolve fully, or there may be minor residual changes; these, however, recur with re-exposure. A *chronic form* appears to follow the superimposition of repeated acute episodes, particularly if the initial acute episode is not severe (usually because spore dose is lower) and the victim is not aware of its association with his occupation. In these individuals the chest film is more suggestive of a diffuse pulmonary fibrosis, sometimes complicated by cystic changes and associated with appropriate effects on lung function. The long-term complications include pulmonary hypertension, right heart strain, and failure.

Diagnosis and Treatment. Diagnosis during the acute attack is made on the basis of a characteristic clinical pattern, providing that there is a suitable exposure history. The chest film and lung function tests may add confirmatory evidence. A high percentage of patients have positive serologic tests (such as the demonstration of precipitins, double diffusion tests, and immunoelectrophoresis) in the acute episode, but the number diminishes with time thereafter. Taken on their own, however, positive reactions are evidence of exposure rather than evidence of disease. In subjects seen in remission, in whom serologic tests are negative, the *cautious use of provocation tests* involving inhaled aqueous extracts of the appropriate allergen is suggested; these result in symptoms and in reduction of forced expiratory volumes and VC several hours after the challenge. The diagnosis of the chronic case may be more difficult because of its nonspecific character, particularly if there have been no acute episodes which are clearly exposure related.

In the treatment of the acute episodes, the usual general measures are advised, together with adrenal corticosteroids which, in some cases, produce very satisfactory remissions, though it is uncertain whether they can always prevent progression to fibrosis. Avoidance of reexposure is of prime importance to prevent repetitive episodes with progression to chronic form.

Epidemiology and Prevention. It is difficult to estimate attack rates in undefined exposed populations (as, for instance, in self-employed farmers). Furthermore, attack rates vary with spore dose, and this again will vary with the seasonal conditions predisposing to moldy hay, bagasse, or sequoia dust as the case may be. Bagassosis, once considered a rare entity, has been reported in half the workers in a Puerto Rican factory, and on another occasion in 10 per cent of employees of a West Indian plant.

Prevention at an epidemiologic level, i.e., by removal of exposure hazards, is not easy, because the conditions favoring spore formation occur only intermittently. Spraying with 2 per cent propionic acid, an inexpensive fungicide, has been suggested. Nor is the prevention at the individual case level practicable, since masks appear to be capable only of reducing, not of wholly excluding, particles of small size such as the 1 μ spores of *M. faeni*. Furthermore, the increased resistance to breathing on exercise imposed by even the best mask limits their regular use. The only safe course is to ensure that the subject who has suffered one acute episode avoid altogether any further exposure, a drastic recommendation which may involve a farmer, for instance, in giving up his means of livelihood.

534. CHRONIC INTERSTITIAL (LIPOID) PNEUMONIA

Example. Blackfat tobacco smokers' lung.

Pathogenesis and Mechanism. In Guyana, a high prevalence of diffuse interstitial pulmonary fibrosis in older individuals, recognized for at least 25 to 30 years, has recently been shown to be due to a chronic interstitial lipoid pneumonia, the consequence of many years of smoking blackfat tobacco. Blackfat tobacco is unusual in that certain oils are added to the leaf during processing, and smoking causes these to distil over into the lungs. Lung biopsy has shown the lipid to be present in alveolar phagocytes, lying free in alveoli or in collections in the interstitium in a peribronchiolar or subpleural location where they evoke first a cellular and eventually (if the dose is large) a collagenous response, with lesions resembling those of liquid paraffin granulomas. The end result is a diffuse interstitial fibrosis and vasculitis, with deposits of lipid and black material in the walls of blood vessels and in the interstitium. Immunologic studies have for practical purposes excluded hypersensitivity to the suspected agent, teichoic acid, and extrinsic allergic alveolitis as the background of the chronic interstitial fibrosis.

Clinical Manifestations. The symptoms are cough, dyspnea, and rather striking weight loss, with eventually pulmonary heart disease, in subjects with a long history (usually 20 to 30 years) of blackfat tobacco smoking. Basal crepitations are characteristic, and wheezing is unusual except during superimposed infection. Radiologic changes are those of diffuse interstitial fibrosis, whereas the pulmonary function changes are unusual in that an obstructive profile predominates in a diffuse pulmonary fibrosis.

Treatment, Epidemiology, and Prevention. Treatment, essentially palliative, is not different from that of other chronic interstitial lung diseases. Giving up smoking blackfat tobacco is apparently no guarantee that symptoms will not develop in the future. The steady decline in blackfat tobacco smoking in Guyana suggests that this local health problem is also on the decline. However, *recognition that inhaled additives to tobacco* can produce *long-term effects* of a *low-grade inflammatory type* on the lungs is of great importance to physicians the world over who are concerned with the health effects of tobacco smoking.

CHEMICAL IRRITANTS

535. CHEMICALS CAUSING ASTHMA-LIKE REACTIONS

Examples. Those affected include workers with *toluene di-isocyanate* (TDI) and other isocyanates used in the application of certain lacquers and resins and in the manufacture of polyurethane foams for cushioning, insulation, and soft toys; and *cable jointers* using certain aluminum soldering flux. *Platinosis* (describing rhinorrhea, asthma, and urticaria) results from exposure to complex platinum salts in refineries.

Pathogenesis and Mechanisms. From carefully controlled occupational-type provocation tests monitored by measurements of forced expiratory volumes, it has been shown that immediate, late, and dual asthmatic reactions occur in workers sensitized to the chemical vapors, fumes, and dusts listed above. The presence of reaginic and precipitating antibodies against platinum salts and against TDI in symptomatic subjects suggests an immunologic basis (Types I and III allergy) for these reactions, and others may well come to light in the future. Furthermore, it seems likely that Type I reactions occur in the atopic worker who is exposed, and Type III reactions in the nonatopic worker. These reactions, which may follow exposure to very low doses, should be distinguished from the well recognized irritant effects of the same chemicals in higher doses and other chemicals discussed subsequently. Thus sensitization to isocyanate vapors may occur at very low exposure levels (0.003 parts per million) which is well below the threshold limit value of 0.02 ppm, which is again below the level at which the irritant effects of isocyanates are seen.

Clinical Manifestations. Symptoms of asthma, immediate and/or late and often nocturnal, develop after periods varying from one week to several months after first exposure and if possible should be distinguished from those of high dose irritation, of which eye, nose, and throat irritation are the most common. Symptoms subside after removal from exposure, and function may return to normal within days or weeks. However, re-exposure regularly results in recurrence, often more violent. The number of people who become sensitized varies and may be related to exposure level (estimated at 4 per cent in a well-controlled plant and 100 per cent in a poor one). Most exposed persons show some reduction in expiratory flow rates during working hours, a change eliminated by the oral administration of an aminophylline compound.

Diagnosis and Treatment. Diagnosis depends on a high degree of suspicion particularly when symptoms occur predominantly at night, and can be confirmed using carefully controlled occupational-type provocation tests as suggested by Pepys. These can be carried out only under hospital supervision with monitoring of forced expiratory flow tests, together with observation of the effects of isoproterenol and dichromoglycolate on the reactions. Objective demonstration of sensitization is important, because it calls for removal from exposure with potential financial and other hardships for the worker. The suggestion that long-term exposure leads to chronic obstructive lung disease should be followed up, because it has been estimated, for example, that workers exposed to TDI number between 50,000 and 100,000 in the United States alone.

536. CHEMICAL BRONCHITIS

Examples. Those affected include workers exposed to sulfur dioxide (SO_2) in the *pulp and paper industry*; *refrigeration workers* exposed to ammonia (NH_3); and *chemical workers* exposed to sulfurous acid (H_2SO_3) and chlorine (Cl_2).

Pathogenesis and Mechanisms. The acutely irritant effects of these gases and mists can probably be attributed to their high solubility; of the physiologic gases, CO_2 is the most soluble (56.7 vols per cent in water at 37° C at 1 atmosphere); however, equivalent values for SO_2 (280 vols per cent), Cl_2 (257 vols per cent), and NH_3 (139 vols per cent) indicate their very much greater solubility. Accidental inhalation of high concentrations results in rapid solution in the mucous membranes of the upper airways with the formation of irritant compounds, e.g., H_2SO_3 from SO_2, NH_4OH from NH_3, HCl from Cl_2. The initial irritation causing *bronchorrhea* is rapidly followed by sloughing and a *frank necrotizing bronchitis*. If exposure is prolonged or unduly heavy, the lower respiratory tract becomes exposed, with the development of an *acute chemical pulmonary edema*. Recovery may be complete. However, residual mucosal scars and submucosal thickening are not uncommon, particularly if the mucosal sloughs were deep and secondary infection prominent. Acute chemical irritation may also result from the *aspiration of vomited or regurgitated material high in HCl content*, an event more common in the frail and elderly than is generally supposed, or in relation to blunting of the gag reflex as in anesthesia, head injuries, and alcoholic or other intoxications. If the aspirate is chiefly water or saline in small amounts, absorption is quick and the consequences usually slight. Large food particles on the other hand may obstruct large or small airways.

Clinical Manifestations. When exposure to a chemical irritant is heavy, clinical manifestations are invariably immediate, the patient is alerted to his exposure, and he makes every effort to remove himself therefrom. *Conjunctivitis, irritation* and *burning* in the *mucosa* of the mouth and throat, *cough, laryngitis, laryngospasm,* and *difficulty in breathing* are in keeping with the usual site of damage, i.e., upper respiratory tract, and coarse *rhonchi* are a characteristic physical finding, often with profound *mucorrhea*, which may be bloodstained. More profound *dyspnea* usually implies alveolar involvement resulting from either chemical edema or aspiration of bronchial sloughs. These complications can frequently be suspected from chest roentgenograms and may result in profound impairment of pulmonary blood gas exchange with *severe arterial hypoxemia* and a low arterial CO_2 tension. Nausea, vomiting, and stupor may complicate the picture.

If the patient survives the acute event, complete recovery is usual. However, some patients may be left with chronic bronchitis or saccular bronchiectasis or both, sometimes of considerable severity, with residual effects on pulmonary function.

Chronic irritation from long-term exposure to low doses, e.g., SO_2, as in city air pollution, Cl_2, as in chlorine plants, may perhaps be more important in terms of community health, particularly in relation to the etiology of chronic obstructive lung disease.

Treatment. *Acute chemical bronchitis* and *acute chemical pulmonary edema* are *medical emergencies*. In the acute phase, survival depends on maintaining airway patency and adequate oxygenation. To aspirate sloughs, it may be necessary to employ intubation, lavage with saline, using modest amounts only (10 ml at a single flush), and even bronchoscopy. Controlled oxygen administration is usually necessary, and frequently must be supplemented with positive pressure respiration, assisted in mild cases, controlled in the severe ones. Corticosteroids, thought to modify the acute inflammatory reaction at the gas-exchanging surface, should always be given in the presence of pulmonary edema and indeed are recommended by some in all cases of exposure on a prophylactic basis. Heavy initial doses should be reduced as the clinical picture improves. Infection should be controlled by the use of antimicrobial drugs.

537. CHEMICAL PULMONARY EDEMA

Examples. Chemical pulmonary edema can result from exposure to *oxides of nitrogen* such as may occur in freshly filled silos (*silo-filler's disease*); welding in poorly ventilated spaces; misfires in blasting operations carried out in closed spaces (e.g., mines); burning of N$_2$-containing materials in closed spaces; *exposure to phosgene* after its liberation from many chlorinated substances, e.g., carbon tetrachloride in fire extinguishers; or *accidental ingestion of the herbicide paraquat.*

Pathogenesis and Mechanisms. The immediate clinical effects of exposure of the oxides of nitrogen and phosgene may be mild, but a severe, chemical pulmonary edema, often fatal, may develop after a *delay of several hours to several days.* The physicochemical processes underlying this delay are not fully understood. If the acute event is not immediately fatal, healing by fibrosis may lead to the development of *bronchiolitis fibrosa obliterans,* usually four to eight weeks after initial exposure, often with a fatal result. Autopsy studies show widespread organization of exudates, primarily located in the terminal bronchioles; atelectasis is not seen, however, presumably because of the collateral ventilation now recognized to be extensive in man.

Acute chemical pulmonary edema of delayed onset (one to three days) may also follow the *accidental ingestion of the herbicide paraquat* (1,1'-dimethyl-4,4'-dipyridilium), a common constituent of commercial weed-killers. Thus the acute effects of this poison, which also include acute oral, esophageal, hepatic, and renal damage, become evident only after a delay of several days, i.e., after the peak blood levels and at a time when most of the material has been excreted. These characteristics have earned it the name of the "hit and run" poison, and once the pulmonary damage starts, it invariably runs a relentless course to death within weeks from respiratory failure caused by a *diffuse progressive pulmonary fibrosis* and replacement of gas-exchanging tissue by cystic changes. Its mechanism of action is unknown, but it has been suggested that the primary action is to inactivate or depress formation of surfactant.

Clinical Manifestations. Immediate effects of exposure to the oxides of nitrogen and phosgene, which may include cough, chest irritation, and sputum, are often so mild that the victim may even fail to report to the first-aid post, only to return from hours to several days later with the symptoms, signs, and chest roentgenogram of *acute, severe, pulmonary edema.* Hence it is reasonable to suggest observation in hospital for 48 hours after possible exposures (e.g., for firefighters who have been inside burning buildings), perhaps even giving steroid therapy if suspicion of exposure is strong. In the mild case of edema, symptoms may escape attention, changes on the chest film at the most may be equivocal, and the diagnosis depends on the finding of coarse rales, sometimes lasting over a short period only, with a transient hypoxemia. Clinical management has been discussed above; in cases of frank, severe edema, steroid therapy should probably be prolonged for six to eight weeks to cover the period when the subacute complication of bronchiolitis obliterans is likely to develop. This complication, probably avoidable if steroid therapy is given early, should be suspected when symptoms recur or appear at three to six weeks, and generally responds to steroid therapy.

Management of a patient known to have ingested paraquat should include heroic measures to prevent absorption. In laboratory animals bentylol and/or Fuller's earth by mouth has been shown to inactivate the material more effectively than charcoal. Forced diuresis and hemodialysis are recommended once blood levels have risen. There is some evidence that corticosteroids may be effective in the treatment of the pulmonary edema, and that O$_2$ therapy should be used with the utmost caution, experimental work indicating that it potentiates the action of the poison.

Epidemiology. Large-scale heavy exposure to, for instance, oxides of nitrogen occurs only in relation to mass disasters, e.g., in the Cleveland clinic fire in 1929 owing to the burning of stored x-ray film, and in the Cocoanut Grove fire in Boston in 1943 owing to the burning of nitrogen-containing plastics. Many modern plastics no longer contain nitrogen. However, in most fires involving domestic buildings in which wood is used, circumstances exist in which these fumes could be evolved, and three or four cases are seen annually in most city hospitals.

538. RADIATION

Increased use of x-irradiation in the treatment of cancer of the breast and of various intrathoracic organs led to the recognition that the lungs themselves may be affected by this procedure. It is thought that the *acute changes,* which may come on within weeks of the onset of treatment up to six months after its cessation, include an alveolar cellular reaction followed by desquamation and in some instances by hyaline membrane formation. Focal necrosis of the bronchial mucosa may develop as a result of damage to capillary endothelium with subsequent necrosis and vascular occlusion. These changes may resolve or go on to loss of lung volume, sometimes of marked degree, occurring rather suddenly, and usually ascribed to fibrosis, shrinkage, and hyalinization, particularly if there has been infection. Studies in animals suggest, however, that the loss of volume may, on occasion, be due to atrophy and that the hyalinization may be in part due to autohypersensitivity, the consequence of new cell antigens formed as a result of the ionizing radiation.

There may be no clinical manifestations of *radiation pneumonitis* even in the face of definite radiologic changes. The most common symptom is a persistent, hacking dry cough. Fever, some dyspnea, and weakness may be seen, and the symptoms of radiation esophagitis are common. On physical examination the effects of radiation on the skin of the thorax are usually evident; rales and a friction rub may be found. The chest film characteristically reveals regional or diffuse haziness, and pulmonary function tests indicate a restrictive pattern. Spontaneous remission over weeks is frequent. Recommended therapy includes steroids (to lessen the chances of healing by fibrosis) and anticoagulants (to lessen the ischemic effects of small-vessel thrombosis commonly seen at autopsy), though the value of these measures has not been conclusively demonstrated (see Ch. 543 to 545). When *radiation fibrosis* supervenes, clinical presentation will depend on how much functioning lung tissue is lost and on the function in the remaining lung. Respiratory failure, pulmonary hypertension, and right heart failure may all follow.

Some authors suggest that there is a parenchymal reaction to ionizing radiation of the thorax in 100 per cent of cases so exposed, that some degree of pneumonitis is common if not invariable, though symptoms occur in a small percentage of these cases only, and that progression to radiation fibrosis is rare. Factors thought to affect the attack rate include total dose as well as the time over which it is given, and the technique of application. Clinically important reactions are unusual at total doses below 2000 rads and invariable above 6000 rads. The age of the patient, the chest wall thickness, and the presence of complicating disease may also be important. Individual factors remain to be identified, however, since identical doses can be harmless to one person and cause a severe reaction in another.

Inorganic Dusts

Becklake, M. R.: Pneumoconioses. *In* Handbook of Physiology, Respiration II. Baltimore, Williams & Wilkins Company, 1965, Chapter 71, p. 1601.
Biological effects of asbestos. Ann. N.Y. Acad. Sci., 132:338, 1965.
Bruce, T.: Occupational diseases of respiratory system. Scand. J. Resp. Dis., 63(supp.):73, 1968.
Coalworkers' pneumoconiosis. Ann. N.Y. Acad. Sci., Vol. 200, 1972.
Fitzgerald, M., Carrington, C. B., and Gaensler, E. A.: Environmental lung disease. Med. Clin. North Am., 57:593, 1973.
Hatch, T. F., and Gross, P.: Pulmonary Deposition and Retention of Inhaled Aerosols. New York, Academic Press, 1964.
Leading article: Asbestos → lung cancer → mesothelioma. Lancet, 1:815, 1973.
Selikoff, I. J., Bader, R. A., Bader, M. E., Churg, J., and Hammond, E. C.: Asbestosis and neoplasia. Am. J. Med., 42:487, 1967.
Stoeckle, J. D., Hardy, H. L., and Weber, A. L.: Chronic beryllium disease: Long-term follow-up of sixty cases and selective review of the literature. Am. J. Med., 46:545, 1969.
Walton, W. (ed.): Inhaled Particles and Vapours. III. Surrey, England, Unwin Bros. Ltd., Gresham Press, 1971.

Organic Dusts

Bouhuys, A., Gilson, J. C., and Schilling, R. S. F.: Byssinosis in the textile industry. Arch. Environ. Health, 21:475, 1970.

Hearn, C. E. D.: Bagassosis: An epidemiological, environmental and clinical survey. Brit. J. Industr. Med., 25:267, 1968.
Hogg, J. C., Macklem, P. T., and Thurlbeck, W. M.: Site and nature of airway obstruction in chronic obstructive lung disease. N. Engl. J. Med., 278:1355, 1968.
Merchant, J. A., Kilburn, K. H., and O'Fallon, W. M.: Byssinosis and chronic bronchitis among cotton textile workers. Ann. Intern. Med., 76:423, 1972.
Miller, G. I., Ashcraft, M. T., Beadnell, H. M. S. G., Wagner, J. C., and Pepys, J.: The lipoid pneumonia of blackfat tobacco smokers in Guyana. Quart. J. Med., 160:457, 1971.
Nicholson, D. P.: Extrinsic allergic pneumonias. Am. J. Med., 53:131, 1972.
Schilling, R. S. F.: Byssinosis in cotton and other textile workers. Lancet, 2:261, 319, 1956.

Chemical Irritants

Bates, D. V., Macklem, P. T., and Christie, R. V.: Respiratory Function in Disease. 2nd ed. Philadelphia, W. B. Saunders Company, 1971, pp. 389–398.
Connor, E. H., DuBois, A. B., and Comroe, J. H.: Acute chemical injury of the airways and lungs. Anesthesiology, 23:538, 1962.
Leading article: Poisoning from paraquat. Br. Med. J., 3:690, 1967.
Morrow, P.: Adaptations of the respiratory tract to air pollutants. Arch. Environ. Health, 14:127, 1967.
Moskowitz, R. L., Lyons, H. A., and Cottle, H. R.: Silo-filler's disease: Clinical, physiological and pathological study of a patient. Am. J. Med., 36:457, 1964.
Peters, J. M., and Murphy, R. L. H.: Pulmonary toxicity of isocyanates. Ann. Intern. Med., 73:654, 1970.
Royal Society of Medicine: Symposium on isocyanates. Proc. R. Soc. Med., 63:365, 1970.
Walton, M.: Industrial ammonia gassing. Br. J. Ind. Med., 30:78, 1973.

Radiation

Fraser, R. F., and Paré, J. A. P.: Diagnosis of Diseases of the Chest. Vol. II. Philadelphia. W. B. Saunders Company, 1970, pp. 1076–1085.
Smith, J. C.: Radiation pneumonitis: A review. Am. Rev. Respir. Dis., 87:647, 1963.

Section Eight. NEOPLASMS OF THE LUNG

Alvan R. Feinstein

539. INTRODUCTION

The benign or malignant clinical consequences of pulmonary neoplasms do not depend on histologic type alone. Their biologic behavior is demonstrated by their site, dissemination, and functional effects. All are important. For example, a histologically "benign" tumor can become lethal by leading to such complications as exsanguinating hemoptysis, pneumonia, or lung abscess. Conversely, a histologically "malignant" tumor may not be fatal if it grows slowly enough to be found and removed before it disseminates. Uncommonly, a slow-growing carcinoma may be undetected during life and first found at necropsy after the patient has died of some other disease.

Tumors of the lung can arise from any part of the trachea, bronchi, bronchial tree, pulmonary parenchyma, or pleura. Although larger bronchi are the most common sites of primary lung tumors, only about 25 per cent of the tumors are central enough to be seen at bronchoscopy.

The lung is a frequent site of metastasis from carcinomas originating elsewhere, particularly in the kidney, thyroid, breast, testis, or intestine. The cellular types and biologic behavior of the metastases in the lung usually depend on the characteristics of the primary tumor. When multiple lesions are found on a chest roentgenogram, an extrapulmonary tumor can be suspected; when the lesion is solitary in an asymptomatic patient, its differentiation from a primary lung tumor may be difficult and is sometimes resolved only after surgical exploration.

Carcinomas are the most common type of primary lung neoplasm. Among 757 primary lung tumors diagnosed consecutively in adults at a single medical center in the United States, 708 were carcinomas, 18 were bronchial adenomas, 10 were hamartomas, 8 were pleural mesotheliomas, and 3 were primary tracheal tumors. The remainder consisted of 2 teratomas, 2 fibromas, 2 lymphosarcomas, 1 fibrosarcoma, 1 sarcoma, 1 neurofibroma, and 1 Hodgkin's disease. These patterns and ratios of occurrence are similar to those reported in England and in Israel. The proportion of different cellular types in primary carcinomas will vary at any medical center, in part reflecting differences in the histologic criteria used by the pathologist. In general, squamous cell tumors are the most common, followed in frequency by anaplastic tumors and adenocarcinomas. No current scheme of histologic classification is used universally, however, and diverse discrepancies have been reported in reclassifications of the same tumor.

Bronchial adenomas, which are particularly common in women, usually have a central location. With slow growth of the tumor, bouts of pulmonary infection or small hemoptyses may occur repeatedly for a long time before the patient seeks medical attention. Peripheral tumors are often detected before they become symptomatic, particularly in countries where diagnostic roentgenograms are readily available. A routine roentgenogram may show an unexpected circumscribed shadow that is often called a "coin lesion" if it happens to present in coinlike size and shape. *Hamartomas* of the lung are usually peripheral and are often found by surgical exploration of such a symptomatically silent coin lesion. *Adenocarcinomas* tend to be peripherally located, whereas most other types of primary carcinoma are central. *Mesotheliomas* arise in the pleura and produce clinical manifestations related to pleural effusion or invasion of the chest wall.

Aside from these morphologic distinctions, neoplasms of the lung show no constant correlations between histologic type and clinical manifestations. Primary carcinoma, as the predominant neoplasm in this group of tumors, will be the topic of the remainder of this discussion.

540. PRIMARY CARCINOMA OF THE LUNG

Occurrence. The occurrence rate of cancer of the lung is difficult to estimate because the annual statistics for a particular population depend on the likelihood of a correct diagnosis being established in members of the population who have the disease. The opportunity to establish a correct diagnosis has sharply increased in recent years, with the frequent use of chest roentgenograms and with the availability of such diagnostic techniques as bronchoscopy, biopsy of affected structures, and cytologic examination of sputum and other fluids. These better methods of diagnosis lead to the detection of many cases of lung cancer today that might have been unrecognized years ago. During the past few decades, the occurrence rates of lung cancer have risen markedly, particularly in countries where the cited diagnostic aids are available and in general use.

In addition to these distinctions, several other features of diagnostic selectivity tend to cloud the epidemiologic picture. Patients referred to medical centers for specialized modes of therapy, such as thoracic surgery, high voltage radiotherapy, and new chemotherapeutic agents, may not reflect the true distribution of lung cancer in that community or in other regions. Certain cancers formerly regarded as metastatic have been called primary in the past few decades, after pathologists recognized that nonbronchogenic lung cancers can arise peripher-

ally and disseminate widely to other parts of the body. The opportunity for cancer to develop is enhanced by the increased life span of people who formerly might have died at a young age because of microbial diseases that today are prevented or cured by sanitation, vaccination, and the various agents of modern therapy.

For all these reasons, cancer of the lung is now diagnosed more frequently than ever before. The epidemiologic significance of the increase is difficult to evaluate, but the clinical significance of this increased occurrence rate is that lung cancer is now perhaps the most commonly recognized form of carcinoma in man.

Etiology and Prevention. No single cause for lung tumors has been identified. Although cigarette smoking has been generally accepted as a major factor, particularly for squamous cell tumors, tobacco has had a less striking role in undifferentiated tumors, and has not been proposed as a cause of human adenocarcinomas and other forms of lung neoplasia.

Among the other agents variously invoked as contributory factors in causing lung cancer are atmospheric fumes and pollution (among urban dwellers), airborne radiation (among uranium miners), and proliferating scar tissue (in patients with previous pulmonary infections). Inhalation of asbestos fibers appears to have a dose-related role in the lung cancers found in asbestos workers, and has been suspected as a cause of mesotheliomas. Genetic factors may be implicated by reports that relatives of lung cancer patients have a higher death rate from lung cancer than matched controls.

The Spectrum of Clinical Patterns. It is not possible to describe a set of clinical signs and symptoms that could be considered as typical of the disease and illness produced by lung cancer. This problem occurs because a lung cancer, by metastasis or by other mechanisms, can affect the structure or function of almost any system in the body. Consequently, the following discussion is intended to identify and indicate the relative frequency of the major phenomena that occur with lung cancer and to describe how this knowledge can be used in the diagnosis of that disease.

The functional disorders can be "direct" effects, caused by the physical presence of the tumor at the involved site, or "indirect" effects, occurring without anatomic dissemination of tumor to the affected site or system.

Some of the effects are *pulmonic,* arising from the affected lung, pleura, or chest wall. Others are *extrapulmonic,* arising more remotely from involvement of the mediastinum or of regions beyond the thorax. The extrapulmonic effects can be *systemic* or *metastatic,* or both. It is the fact that these different manifestations of cancer of the lung can occur alone or in various combinations that gives the disease its wide, protean spectrum with many different patterns of appearance.

The clinical spectrum of lung cancer according to the presence or absence of any of the described pulmonic, systemic, and metastatic features is best seen in the form of a Venn diagram (see accompanying figure). The numbers in each subset of this diagram indicate the proportionate distribution of these clinical features at the time of diagnostic detection of lung cancer in 1032 consecutive patients. The most common pattern of appearance was the combination of pulmonic and systemic symptoms, which were present in 340 patients. Of the other patients in this series, 271 had pulmonic symptoms only, 196 had a combination of pulmonic, systemic, and metastatic features, 70 were asymptomatic, 34 first pre-

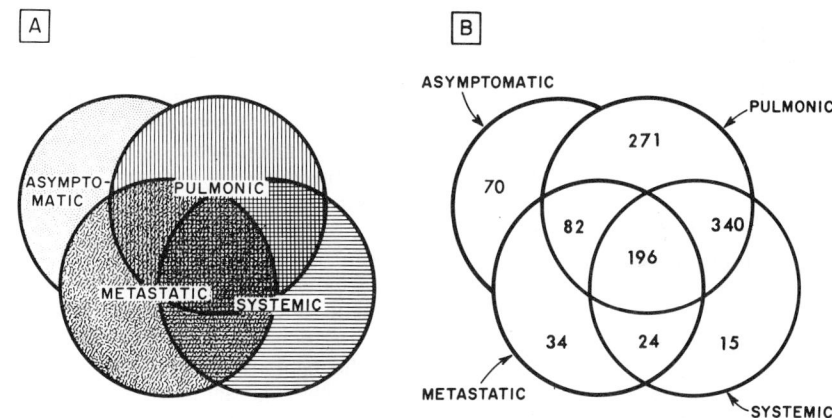

The clinical spectrum of lung cancer. The three main circles of the Venn diagram in part *A* are shaded to demonstrate sets of patients with pulmonic, systemic, or metastatic manifestations, as described in the text. The overlap of the circles produces seven subsets, in which these manifestations are present alone or in various combinations. An eighth subset, containing asymptomatic patients, is appended at the upper left of the diagram. Part *B*, for which the shading is removed, demonstrates the number of patients in each of these subsets at the time of clinical detection of lung cancer in 1032 cases.

sented only with metastatic features, and the remaining cases were distributed as shown.

Diagnosis. As shown in the figure, patients with lung cancer frequently seek medical attention after development of a cough, often with hemoptysis and with an associated infection or chest pain. Anorexia and weight loss may also be present, and the chest roentgenogram almost always shows an abnormal shadow or shadows.

Although no single pattern of clinical and roentgenographic features is either characteristic or pathognomonic for diagnosis, certain manifestations are particularly suspicious. Lung cancer is suggested clinically by the combination of hemoptysis, weight loss, and clubbing of the fingers in a patient who has no evidence of infection, congenital heart disease, or previous lung disease. The roentgenographic findings that most suggest lung cancer are (1) a mass arising in the hilar area; (2) an apparently pneumonic infiltrate that persists long after improvement of concomitant clinical symptoms; (3) a mass that obstructs a bronchus, usually demonstrated by tomography; and (4) a localized peripheral or coin lesion that shows no calcium in tomographic views. All of these and other clinical and roentgenographic manifestations associated with lung cancer can also be produced by such diseases as tuberculosis, various chronic pneumonias, granulomas, and other entities.

In diagnosis, therefore, the patient's signs and symptoms serve mainly to suggest the presence of a pulmonary lesion. The existence and extent of the lesion can be shown by roentgenography, which can also be used to detect lesions in asymptomatic patients. To specify the identity of any pulmonary lesion, however, requires additional tests. It is necessary to exclude causes other than cancer, and to provide cytologic or histologic evidence of the neoplasm. Many microbial or circulatory causes of lung lesions can be identified by appropriate examination of sputum or blood, although their demonstration does not exclude the possible coexistence of an underlying lung cancer.

Papanicolaou smears of the sputum are often positive in patients with primary carcinoma, particularly if special techniques are used to induce sputum when it is absent, and particularly when the tumor is centrally located. Peripheral cancers may not communicate well with the bronchial tree or may not exfoliate enough cells to yield positive results on cytologic examination. In these circumstances, the tests of sputum may produce "false negative" results; a rare "false positive" may occur in patients who have chronic bronchial inflammation rather than cancer.

Bronchoscopy is useful both for grossly visualizing the tumor (when possible) and for obtaining bronchial specimens for histologic or cytologic examination. Most other pathologic specimens used for the diagnosis of lung cancer are obtained by biopsy of metastatic sites or from the fluid of a neoplastic pleural or pericardial effusion. A favorite location of metastasis for lung cancer is the mediastinal and supraclavicular lymph nodes. Mediastinoscopy and biopsy of the scalene nodes are often done to obtain histologic evidence when none is otherwise available, and also to exclude metastasis, although a scalene node biopsy is seldom positive for tumor unless the node is palpably enlarged.

In some instances, when no other cytologic evidence is obtainable, needle biopsy of a peripheral lung lesion may disclose the tumor. More often, however, when diagnostic tests have failed to reveal the identity of the lesion disclosed by x-ray, exploratory thoracotomy is performed. Because the risk is low, surgical thoracic exploration is now a common diagnostic procedure in these circumstances. A benign tumor, granuloma, or a metastasis from a "silent" primary site may sometimes be found, but just as often a lung cancer is discovered in a still curable state. Among patients with "operable" lung cancer, about 70 per cent do not have a specific histologic diagnosis established until thoracotomy.

Correlation of Anatomic, Functional, and Clinical Manifestations. The direct and indirect effects of lung cancer can produce a variety of anatomic, clinical, and other manifestations.

Pulmonic Manifestations. Irritation of bronchial mucosa by tumor or by inflammation adjacent to the tumor may cause a change in the pattern of a chronic cough or may produce a wholly new cough. Hemoptysis of bright red blood, flecks of blood, or "rusty" sputum may be due to vascular invasion or to pneumonia developing behind the tumor. Occasionally, the tumor may occlude enough of a large bronchus to make the patient notice a respiratory wheeze.

An obstructed bronchial lumen may cause retention of secretions, predisposing to parenchymal infection. If the lumen is completely obstructed, the distal parenchyma may become atelectatic. Although roentgenographically apparent atelectasis may be asymptomatic, parenchyma that is infected or inflamed may produce all the classic clinical, bacteriologic, and roentgenographic manifestations of a pneumonia. With conventional treatment of the pneumonia, the patient may have a conventional symptomatic and bacteriologic response, but the roentgenogram may fail to clear because of the underlying neoplasm. In this circumstance, the "unresolved pneumonia" becomes the clue that leads to further tests and discovery of the tumor. A lung abscess can sometimes be produced at the site of such a pneumonia, although an alternative cause of lung abscess is necrosis of the interior of a large tumor.

As a parenchymal manifestation, dyspnea is the direct result of metastasis when the tumor either replaces large amounts of parenchymal tissue or, more commonly, invades the pleural surface, causing an effusion that reduces the space available for ventilation. In many other circumstances, however, dyspnea may be indirect, occurring because (1) parenchymal inflammation extending to the pleura initiates a pleural effusion, (2) the primary tumor may locally obstruct the trachea or carina, or (3) the amount of secondary parenchymal inflammation or atelectasis may be great enough to impair ventilation in a patient whose respiratory reserve had been reduced—by chronic lung disease or by poor cardiac compensation—before the tumor developed.

Involvement of *the pleural surface* can produce inspiratory chest pain, the physical findings of an effusion, or dyspnea if the effusion is massive. When pleural involvement is due to the inflammatory extension of pneumonia developing behind the primary tumor, the pleural fluid is often pink or bloody. Another form of indirect pleural involvement, usually associated with serous effusion, occurs when the primary tumor obstructs appropriate vascular and lymphatic channels draining the pleura. In both these indirect circumstances, the pleural fluid contains no tumor cells. In other circumstances, however, the pleura can be directly invaded via contiguous spread from a peripherally located tumor or by lymphatic metastases from a tumor in the bronchus. A neoplastic pleural effusion is seldom clinically different from one that is inflammatory or hydrostatic, but the fluid is more likely to be bloody and will usually contain cancer cells.

Although pleural involvement is the most common single cause of chest pain in lung cancer, inspiratory chest pain may also occur when a peripheral tumor extends through the pleura to the chest wall, involving muscle, bone, or both. Rib invasion may alternatively occur as a distant metastasis from a central tumor. Chest pain that lacks inspiratory accentuation can develop with invasion of an upper rib, sternum, or thoracic vertebra. The tumor may sometimes extend beyond the vertebra or rib to involve a thoracic nerve, with pain in the anatomic distribution of the nerve.

Extrapulmonic Manifestations. The many possible extrapulmonic manifestations of lung cancer include *systemic features,* which are often indirect, and *metastatic features,* which are due to direct spread of tumor to the affected site.

SYSTEMIC MANIFESTATIONS. Anorexia may occur indirectly because of persistent infection, pain, or other discomforts of the pulmonic features just cited. With decreased food intake, the patient may then lose weight and become easily fatigued. Alternatively, however, anorexia and other digestive disturbances can be the direct result of hepatic, peritoneal, or other intra-abdominal metastases.

Hypertrophic pulmonary osteoarthropathy, i.e., clubbing of the fingers and/or pain in the articular extremities of long bones, can occur with either central or peripheral tumors of the lung. They may sometimes be the earliest or the only clinical clues that suggest the presence of a lung cancer. The clubbing has no physical differences from the clubbing sometimes found in congenital heart disease, chronic lung disease, and other non-neoplastic entities. Careful criteria are often needed to distinguish "curving" of the nail bed from true clubbing.

The osteoarthropathy is actually a "periostopathy" and, when present, involves the distal third of a long bone, commonly in the leg. The bone becomes exquisitely tender to pressure, and an associated synovitis may make the subcutaneous tissues swollen and the joint painful on movement. Although the articular surface of the neighboring joint is not affected, the clinical manifestations may be attributed to arthritis until the periosteal changes are noted roentgenographically. By palpating tenderness in the bone well beyond the region of the joint, the clinician can suspect osteoarthropathy before the radiologist finds it. The mechanisms of clubbing and of hypertrophic osteoarthropathy are unknown. The manifestations may be improved by vagotomy or by direct treatment that removes or shrinks the primary tumor.

With the availability of modern laboratory techniques, many "hormonal" effects, although not common, have been reported with almost any type of lung tumor, most often with "oat cell" cancers. So many different systems have been involved that lung cancer seems to have the occasional capacity either for acting like an auxiliary pituitary gland or for producing other nonpituitary hormonal effects.

When a patient with lung cancer has an endocrine problem resulting from a *decrease* in hormone, the cause is usually destruction of the glandular site by metastasis. An *increase* in hormone may represent one of the functional "endocrinopathies" that can produce adrenal hyperfunction, inappropriate antidiuresis, hypercalcemia, or the carcinoid syndrome (see Ch. 869 and 870). The hypersecretive endocrine problems can often occur without metastasis and can sometimes be the first evidence of the tumor.

The weakness often associated with lung cancer was long regarded only as a nonspecific systemic effect until the discovery in recent years that many instances of weakness were due to *neurologic lesions,* occurring without metastasis and presumably caused by a secretory product of the tumor. The lesions can include cortical cerebellar degeneration, peripheral neuropathies, encephalomyelitis, and various myopathic syndromes.

METASTATIC MANIFESTATIONS. *Hoarseness* occurs when tumor impinges on the mediastinal portion of the recurrent left laryngeal nerve. The subsequent paralysis of the left vocal cord is demonstrated at laryngoscopy (or bronchoscopy).

The superior vena cava syndrome can be produced by metastases in mediastinal nodes. Lung cancer today is the most common cause of the suffusion and brawny edema that occur in the face, neck, or upper arms as a consequence of compression or invasion of the superior vena cava.

Involvement of the esophagus by lung cancer in the mediastinum can produce the same clinical pattern of *dysphagia* noted in esophageal carcinoma.

Although *myocardial involvement* is rare in lung cancer, direct invasion of the pericardium is more common. Neoplastic cells found in a bloody pericardial effusion may sometimes be the first evidence of the cancer.

Carcinomas arising in the apex of the lung—*superior sulcus tumors* (sometimes called Pancoast tumors)—can invade adjacent bone or the nerve bundles that pass through the thoracic inlet. Involvement of the first or second rib can produce local pain; involvement of the brachial plexus can produce sensory or motor disturbances in the arm; and involvement of the sympathetic nerve chain can produce Horner's syndrome on the affected side.

EXTRATHORACIC MANIFESTATIONS. Cancer of the lung can metastasize to any structure of the body. The brain has been a distant metastatic site so commonly that pulmonary examination is often performed to exclude metastasis from a lung cancer in any adult suspected of having a primary brain tumor.

Among the other diverse extrathoracic metastatic manifestations of lung cancer are pathologic fractures of bone, the development of multiple cutaneous nodules, enlargement of the liver, hypoadrenalism caused by metastatic replacement of the adrenal glands, diabetes mellitus resulting from destruction of the pancreas, gastrointestinal bleeding from metastasis to small bowel, jaundice from metastasis to periportal nodes, ascites from peritoneal invasion, and various peripheral neurologic manifestations from metastasis to vertebrae or to spinal cord.

Prognosis and Treatment. Therapeutic procedures in lung cancer begin with the diagnostic and epidemiologic effort to detect the tumor in a premetastatic state, suitable for surgical resection. The effort depends on the hope that symptomatic patients will seek medical aid promptly and that asymptomatic patients, not under medical surveillance, will be found by widespread use of routine roentgenography of the chest.

This hope of "early discovery" followed by surgical cure, which currently seems to be the most effective form of therapy, is often thwarted by diverse biologic behavior in the rate and direction of growth of the cancer. Symptomatic patients with a rapidly growing tumor may seek medical aid promptly but may already have metastases. Conversely, the initial symptoms of a slowly growing tumor may be so mild and unprovocative that a long time elapses before the patient decides to see a physician; yet the lesion may still be curable by surgical resection despite the apparently "late" treatment. Among asymptomatic patients with no previous roentgenograms, a shadow found unexpectedly in a routine film often represents a slowly growing curable tumor. If the shadow is found on the *subsequent* film of an asymptomatic patient, the increment of size in the interval between "negative" and "positive" film helps denote the rate of growth of the tumor; and for a rapid-growing tumor, even an "early" asymptomatic discovery may sometimes come too "late."

Because the clinical course and outcome of lung cancer depend on its diverse patterns of behavior, the disease does not have a single, clearly demarcated natural history. The differences in survival of different subgroups are shown in Table 1, in which 1032 consecutive patients with lung cancer are classified according to the evidence

TABLE 1. Six-Month Survival Rates in 1032 Patients with Lung Cancer

Symptomatic Stage	Anatomic Stage			Totals
	Localized	Regional	Distant	
Asymptomatic	36/43 (84%)	19/25 (76%)	1/2 (50%)	56/70 (80%)
Pulmonic	90/114 (79%)	59/139 (42%)	7/18 (39%)	156/271 (58%)
Systemic	66/110 (60%)	76/194 (39%)	13/51 (25%)	155/355 (44%)
Metastatic	9/28 (32%)	55/144 (38%)	23/164 (14%)	87/336 (26%)
Totals	201/295 (68%)	209/502 (42%)	44/235 (19%)	454/1032 (44%)

present at the time of diagnostic detection, before a therapeutic decision was carried out. The symptomatic manifestations are cited in four stages of ascending severity. The anatomic stage before treatment is classified as *localized* if none of the available roentgenographic or microscopic evidence showed spread of tumor; *regional,* if the spread was confined to the mediastinum or same hemithorax as the primary lesion; and *distant,* for contrathoracic or ultrathoracic dissemination. The six-month survival rates are shown, regardless of therapy, for the 12 symptomatic-anatomic subgroups and for the totals in each category of staging.

The varying rates of survival in Table 1 indicate the diverse behavior of the disease. Less than half (44 per cent) of the 1032 patients in the entire series survived for six months or more. Among subgroups, the six-month survival rate was 26 per cent (87 of 336) in patients found with symptomatic evidence of metastasis, and 41 per cent (175 of 429) in the six subgroups of patients whose regional or distant spread was not accompanied by metastatic symptoms. On the other hand, of the 267 patients who had neither symptomatic nor anatomic evidence of metastasis, 72 per cent (192) survived six months. Within the anatomically localized group, the survival rates showed a distinctive prognostic gradient according to the associated symptoms. The rates were highest (84 per cent) in the asymptomatic patients; 79 per cent in those with pulmonic symptoms only; and 60 per cent in the systemic group. The symptomatic stages were associated with analogous survival gradients within the other two anatomic stages.

These biologic distinctions must be borne in mind for selecting and evaluating different modes of therapy. Unless patients are analyzed according to both morphologic and clinical features, the compared populations will not be similar, and many triumphs attributed to therapy may actually be due to unrecognized aspects of the neoplasm's biologic behavior. Table 2 contains quantitative evidence of the selective prognostic "bias" with which therapy is chosen. The patients in Table 2 are classified according to the same arrangement used in Table 1, but the rates show the relative frequency with which patients were regarded as "operable," with performance of exploratory thoracotomy and possible surgical resection. The highest rates of choice for thoracotomy in Table 2 occurred in those patients who, as noted earlier in Table 1, had the best prognostic expectations.

TABLE 2.   Rate of Selection for Thoracotomy in 1032 Patients with Lung Cancer

Symptomatic Stage	Anatomic Stage			
	Localized	Regional	Distant	Totals
Asymptomatic	37/43 (86%)	13/25 (52%)	0/2 (0%)	50/70 (71%)
Pulmonic	92/114 (81%)	55/139 (40%)	0/18 (0%)	147/271 (54%)
Systemic	75/110 (68%)	70/194 (36%)	7/51 (14%)	152/355 (43%)
Metastatic	7/28 (25%)	16/144 (11%)	2/164 (1%)	25/336 (7%)
Totals	211/295 (72%)	154/502 (31%)	9/235 (4%)	374/1032 (36%)

Conversely, the lowest rates of thoracotomy occurred in patients with the worst prognoses.

These differences in case selection may demonstrate the skill with which surgeons choose relatively "healthy" patients for thoracotomy, but they also reveal that the surgically treated group had a major prognostic advantage over patients assigned to other modes of treatment. These natural prognostic distinctions must also be contemplated when the results of different forms of surgery are evaluated in the operable group or when different forms of radiotherapy and/or chemotherapy are appraised in patients whose tumor was not resected. For example, among all patients with surgical resection of the cancer, the five-year survival rate was 25 per cent (69 of 279); but the rate ranged from 34 per cent (12 of 35) in the asymptomatic, localized group, to 22 per cent (23 of 104) in patients with systemic symptoms, to 0 per cent (0 of 14) in those with metastatic symptoms. The results of different forms of surgical resection will obviously depend on the kinds of patients chosen for operation.

Similarly, among all patients with nonresected tumors (i.e., inoperable and/or surgically explored but not excised), the six-month survival rate was 31 per cent (237 of 753). This rate ranged, however, from 66 per cent (27 of 41) among patients with localized tumors and with no metastatic or systemic symptoms to 13 per cent (22 of 163) when symptomatic and anatomic evidence of distant metastasis was present. The neglect of these and other clinical distinctions can be an important source of ambiguous, misleading, or controversial results whenever one mode of therapy is compared against another without regard to the major pretherapeutic prognostic differences that can occur in subsets of patients with "unresected" or "inoperable" lung cancer.

As for specific considerations in choice of treatment, a morphologic prerequisite to surgical resection is location of the tumor at a resectable site, i.e., not in the trachea or carina. A functional prerequisite is the ability of the patient to tolerate both the operation itself and the subsequent reduction in functioning lung tissue. For the resection, some surgeons routinely perform pneumonectomy and radical dissection of mediastinal nodes regardless of the apparent gross extent of the tumor. Other surgeons — hoping to preserve as much normal lung tissue as possible — confine resection to the smallest amount of lung in which the tumor appears grossly con-

tained. At operation, some surgeons may decide against resection of primary tumor if metastatic deposits are adjacent to the aorta, pericardium, or other critical mediastinal structures; other surgeons remove both the primary tumor and any deposits that do not actually invade the adjacent structures. A "palliative" resection of the primary tumor is sometimes performed despite apparent "incurability" in order to relieve hypertrophic pulmonary osteoarthropathy or lung abscess.

Irradiation may be used before or after surgery or when surgery is unfeasible. By "shrinking" a juxtacarinal lesion or mediastinal nodes, irradiation may sometimes permit subsequent surgery in a previously "inoperable" case. Radiotherapy is particularly valuable for pain caused by bony metastasis and for alleviating such symptoms as osteoarthropathy, superior vena cava syndrome, and vocal cord paralysis. Malignant pleural effusions are sometimes treated by instillation of nitrogen mustard radiotherapeutic or other chemotherapeutic substances.

Antineoplastic chemotherapy is usually reserved for widely disseminated tumors beyond help by either surgery or irradiation. In the panorama of available agents, adrenocortical steroids or nitrogen mustard have often had transiently good results with the superior vena cava syndrome and in cutaneous metastases. No antineoplastic agent has been consistently successful in metastatic cancer, but new agents are constantly becoming available. Cyclophosphamide has sometimes been beneficial, and adriamycin may prove useful.

Supportive care is needed to help the patient maintain good nutritional intake. Rhizotomy or cordotomy can be attempted for pain relief when other measures have failed, and narcotics or sedatives should be used liberally in appropriate circumstances. Such complications as infections and hormonal imbalances require appropriate treatment.

Many rapidly growing tumors produce death within six months. A patient who survives more than six months, however, is likely to have a slowly growing tumor. For such patients the best therapeutic attitude, even when metastases are present, is to regard the cancer as a chronic incurable disease for which a great deal can still be done. By maintaining an attitude of hope, by suitable attention to remediable or improvable situations, and by attention to the personal aspects of clinical care, the physician can often prolong useful life, prevent needless suffering, or permit death to come, when it must, in circumstances of tranquility and dignity.

Boucot, K. R., Cooper, D. A., Weiss, W., and Carnahan, W. J.: The natural history of lung cancer. Am. Rev. Respir. Dis., 89:519, 1964.

Carbone, P. P. (moderator): Lung cancer: Perspectives and prospects. Ann. Intern. Med., 73:1003, 1970.

Feinstein, A. R.: A new staging system for cancer and a reappraisal of "early" treatment and "cure" by radical surgery. N. Engl. J. Med., 279:747, 1968. See also Ann. Intern. Med., 61:127, 1964; Nature, 209:241, 1966; and Amer. Rev. Respir. Dis., 101:671, 1970, and 107:790, 1973.

Garland, L. R., Coulson, W., and Wollin, E.: The rate of growth and apparent duration of untreated primary bronchial carcinoma. Cancer, 16:694, 1963.

Kreyberg, L.: Histological lung cancer types. Acta Pathol. Microbiol. Scand., Suppl. 157, 1962.

LeRoux, B. T.: Bronchial Carcinoma. Edinburgh, E. & S. Livingstone, Ltd., 1968.

Selawry, O. S., and Primack, A. (eds.): First International Workshop for Therapy of Lung Cancer. Cancer Chemotherapy Reports, Part 3, Vol. 4, No. 2, 1973.

Watson, W. L. (ed.): Lung Cancer. A Study of Five Thousand Memorial Hospital Cases. St. Louis, C. V. Mosby Company, 1968.

Section Nine. DISEASES OF THE PLEURA

John H. McClement

INTRODUCTION

The pleura, a serous membrane of mesodermal origin, covers the lung, the chest wall, the diaphragm, and the mediastinum. It is a closed sac which encloses the pleural space and separates the lung from adjacent structures. The visceral pleura designates that portion of it which covers the lung; the remainder is the parietal pleura. The parietal pleura receives its blood supply from the systemic circulation, whereas the visceral is supplied by the pulmonary circulation. The normal pleural space contains no gas and only a small amount of serous fluid. During quiet breathing, the elastic recoil of the lung produces a subatmospheric pressure (-4 to -10 cm H_2O) in the pleural space.

Pleural pain and signs and symptoms secondary to collections of fluid and gas in the pleural space are principal indicators of pleural disease.

Pleural pain originates in the parietal pleura; stimulation of the visceral pleura does not cause pain. Typically, pleural pain is sharp, aggravated by respiration and thoracic motion, and relieved by splinting of the involved area. When it arises from the pleura of the chest wall, the pain is referred to the chest wall overlying the involved area; pain arising from the pleura of the central portion of the diaphragm is referred to the posterior part of the shoulder area; pain from the costal portions of the diaphragm is referred to adjacent parts of the chest wall and abdomen.

The formation and removal of pleural fluid are dependent on those forces which regulate the exchange of fluid into and out of capillary beds, and on lymphatic drainage. The hydrostatic pressure in the pleural capillaries (Pc), the hydrostatic pressure in the pleural space (Ppl), the oncotic pressures of the plasma (OPp) and the pleural fluid (OPpf), and the permeability of the pleural capillaries (K) are the factors which regulate the transport of fluid (F) into and out of the pleural capillaries. According to Starling's law of transcapillary exchange, this can be expressed as follows:

$$F = K(Pc - OPp) - (Ppl - OPpf)$$

The visceral pleura is supplied by arterioles from the low pressure pulmonary arterial system, whereas the parietal pleura is supplied by the higher pressure systemic arteries. There is evidence that the permeability (K) of the visceral capillaries is less than that of the parietal pleura. Normally a balance of these forces favors absorption of fluid by the visceral pleura at about the same rate it is formed. However, all these forces may be altered by disease, and the removal of fluid may be slowed or its formation increased. An increase in capillary permeability (K) from inflammation, a decrease in the oncotic pressure of the plasma proteins (OPp) from hypoalbuminemia, and an increase in the hydrostatic pressure in the pulmonary capillaries (Pc) are the common alterations that lead to pleural fluid collections. Uncommonly a decrease in the hydrostatic pressure in the pleura (Ppl) from a collapsed and nonexpandable lung will cause effusion. Protein, red blood cells, and particulate matter are removed from the pleural space by the pleural lymphatics. The absorption and transport of pleural fluid by way of the lymphatics is increased by diaphragmatic and intercostal activity. Decrease in this activity or obstruction of local or distant lymphatic channels may prolong or prevent reabsorption of pleural fluid.

METHODS OF EXAMINATION IN PLEURAL DISEASE

History and Physical Examination. Pleural pain and shortness of breath are the symptoms which most often call attention to pleural disease. A dry, irritating, nonproductive cough may sometimes accompany the pleural pain. Shortness of breath may sometimes be caused by severe pleural pain, but usually indicates the presence of fairly large amounts of intrapleural fluid or gas. Early in the course of pleural inflammation a friction rub may be heard over the involved area. As fluid forms, the friction rub and the pain disappear, and dullness to percussion and diminished breath sounds on auscultation appear. At the upper limits of pleural fluid, egophony is sometimes elicited. Pleural disorders for the most part arise from derangements in cardiac, hepatic, or renal function which lead to increased collections of fluid, or by extension of disease from adjacent structures such as the lung, mediastinum, chest wall, esophagus, or the upper abdomen. Evidence of disease in these structures must be searched for in the history and physical examination.

Radiologic Examination. Up to 300 ml of fluid may be present in a pleural space and not be apparent on the usual upright chest x-ray film. Small amounts of fluid may sometimes be suspected, especially on the left side, from the presence of a density or apparent widening of the diaphragmatic shadow as it is seen between the gas-containing stomach and the lower limits of the lung. Decubitus films taken with the involved side dependent may also sometimes make small amounts of fluid apparent on the x-ray film. With larger amounts of fluid the characteristic density of pleural fluid with its curvilinear upper border appears. However, if pleural fluid occurs in a pleural space in which previous inflammatory disease has produced adhesions, the distribution of the fluid may produce varied shadows. The x-ray shadows of pleural fluid are characteristically adjacent to the chest wall; rarely fluid will collect in or become encapsulated in one of the interlobar fissures and produce a pattern similar to a parenchymal pulmonary tumor.

Examination of Pleural Fluid. A detailed chemical, bacteriologic, and cytologic analysis of all pleural fluids aspirated is essential in patients in whom the diagnosis is not completely clear. Analysis for total protein and lactic acid dehydrogenase (LDH), a complete blood count with a differential count, cultures for bacteria including mycobacteria, a Gram-stained smear, and a search for malignant cells should be carried out initially on virtually all pleural fluids. Glucose, amylase, fat, and cholesterol measurements may also sometimes be indicated. The specific gravity of pleural fluid was once recommended as a measurement that would help differentiate between exudates and transudates. Because the specific gravity depends almost entirely on the protein content of the pleural fluid, and because it is a measurement that is frequently inaccurate, it can usually be omitted if an accurate measure of protein content is available.

The differentiation of pleural transudates and exudates is most helpful diagnostically and can usually be accomplished from examination of pleural fluid. Transudates are those fluids which occur in response to a decrease in the oncotic pressure of plasma, an increase in hydrostatic pressures in the pleural capillaries, or a decrease in intrapleural pressure. Exudates result from infections or from inflammatory or neoplastic processes which alter the permeability of pleural capillaries. Characteristically, transudates have a low protein content, a low specific gravity, and few white blood cells, whereas exudates have a high protein, high specific gravity, and increased numbers of white blood cells. Arbitrary limits have been chosen to separate transudates and exudates (e.g., total protein more than 3.0 ml per 100 ml and specific gravity greater than 1.015). Unfortunately, when these arbitrary limits are tested in patients who have pleural fluid in which the cause is certain, both transudates and exudates are sometimes misclassified. Light and his associates have examined the cellular and chemical characteristics of pleural fluid from patients in whom a definite diagnosis could be established. On this basis they were classified as transudates or exudates. The three measurements which they found most reliable in differentiating transudates and exudates were the pleural fluid to serum protein ratio (greater than 0.5 in exudates), the level of LDH (greater than 200 IU in exudates) and the ratio of pleural fluid to serum LDH (greater than 0.6 in exudates). Although white blood counts greater than 10,000 per cubic millimeter are usually found only in exudates and counts of greater than 2500 per cubic millimeter suggest that the fluid is an exudate, counts below 2500 per cubic millimeter do not distinguish transudates from exudates.

Chylothorax refers to the presence of chyle in the pleural space and results from trauma to or obstruction (most often by a neoplastic process) of the thoracic duct or some other major intrathoracic lymphatic. Chylous pleural effusions are characteristically milky in appearance and have a high fat content which can be identified both microscopically and chemically. The protein content is usually about half that of plasma.

Milky-appearing pleural collections may also occur late in the course of tuberculous pleural effusion, in the pleural effusions of rheumatoid lung disease, and in other chronic effusions from the accumulation of cholesterol and cholesterol crystals in these fluids. Chemical analysis of such fluids will show a high cholesterol content and a low fat content and distinguish them from chylous effusions.

Pleural Biopsy. Biopsy of the pleura with a Cope or Abrams needle is indicated in nearly every patient in whom the diagnosis is not clear, and who has sufficient pleural fluid to make this a safe procedure. Material from the biopsy should be submitted not only for histologic examination, but also for culture for tubercle bacilli. Pleural biopsy has been particularly useful in establishing the diagnosis of tuberculous pleurisy and malignant neoplastic implants in the pleura.

SIMPLE HYDROTHORAX

Pleural fluid collections occur more often as a result of cardiac, hepatic, or renal disease than from inflammatory or malignant disease of the pleura. These fluid collections most often result either from increases in hydrostatic pressures in the pleural capillaries, from a decrease in the oncotic pressure of the plasma, or from a combination of these factors. There is some exchange of fluid between the peritoneum and the pleura through the diaphragmatic lymphatics, and in patients with ascites this mechanism may result in pleural collections. Clinically these fluid collections are usually identified by physical examination, from x-rays of the chest, or, if they are large, from the appearance of dyspnea. They occur much more frequently on the right side than on the left. Pleural fluid in patients with simple hydrothorax will have those characteristics of a transudate which have been described. Because the parietal pleura is thin and uninvolved, pleural biopsy often fails to yield any identifiable pleural tissue. The treatment of these pleural collections is the treatment of the underlying disease, and pleural aspiration should be used therapeutically only if these measures fail and dyspnea requires relief.

PULMONARY EMBOLISM AND PULMONARY INFARCTION

Pulmonary embolism frequently produces pleural manifestations. In patients with pulmonary embolism, confirmed by pulmonary angiography, more than half will have a clinically detectable pleural effusion. The pleural effusion does not appear immediately and is usually identified more than 24 hours after the embolic event. The pleural effusion is an exudate and sometimes has moderate numbers of red blood cells; however, it is usually a clear amber fluid. Unless repeated embolization occurs, the pleural fluid disappears as the pulmonary infarction resolves.

PLEURAL EFFUSIONS WITH PNEUMONIA: EMPYEMA

Inflammation of the adjacent pleura occurs in most patients with pneumonia whatever the cause. Bacterial pneumonia frequently has clinically significant pleural involvement; in most pneumonias caused by viruses and mycoplasma, pleural disease is not clinically prominent.

The extent of pleural inflammation in bacterial pneumonia varies widely from case to case. There may be minor inflammation which produces pleural pain with clinically undetectable amounts of fluid, and which leaves no clinical residue; or large collections of grossly purulent fluid containing large numbers of bacteria (empyema) resulting in marked pleural fibrosis and fibrothorax. In practice one encounters patients who produce a continuum between these two extremes. Treatment of these effusions depends largely on the severity and intensity of the pleural inflammation, but is primarily the treatment of the associated pneumonia with appropriate antimicrobial drugs. The less intense small serous effusions with relatively small numbers of white blood cells and few organisms will usually respond to drug treatment alone. With larger collections of fluid and more white blood cells, aspiration by means of closed drainage through an intercostal tube may speed resolution and lead to smaller pleural residues. With grossly purulent fluid and larger numbers of bacteria, surgical rib resection and open dependent drainage may be necessary. Infrequently pleural inflammatory disease leads to persistent massive fibrous entrapment of the underlying lung even after the infection has been controlled. A so-called fibrothorax results; the affected lung has its volume greatly decreased; ventilation and perfusion are reduced; there is a shift in the mediastinum toward the entrapped lung, and overdistention of the contralateral lung occurs. In such cases surgical decortication may free the entrapped lung and restore pulmonary function.

TUBERCULOSIS OF THE PLEURA

Definition. Localized tuberculosis of the pleura probably occurs in most patients with pulmonary tuberculosis. It is usually clinically inapparent, but does result in pleural adhesions over the involved area.

Tuberculosis of the pleura with pleural effusion and without apparent pulmonary tuberculosis is the principal or first clinical manifestation of tuberculous disease in a few patients. Characteristically it is a febrile illness, accompanied by a serous pleural effusion. Although the acute illness, even if untreated, usually subsides in a few weeks with resorption of the fluid, it is very frequently followed by pulmonary tuberculosis or some other form of tuberculosis. Roper and Waring found that 65 per cent of patients with serofibrinous pleurisy who did not receive antituberculous chemotherapy developed tuberculosis during the next five years. Thus recognition of the tuberculous cause is of great importance. Infrequently pleural effusions that are grossly purulent and contain large numbers of tubercle bacilli are encountered; such cases are designated as tuberculous empyema.

Epidemiology. Tuberculous pleurisy with effusion can occur at any age but occurs most often in older children and young adults. It usually occurs soon after tuberculous infection, and is uncommon in patients who are known to have had tuberculous infection for a long time.

Pathology and Pathogenesis. Tuberculosis of the pleura in nearly all cases results from extension of disease from the lung. Extension from tuberculosis of adjacent bones or lymph nodes is rare. Usually this extension from the lungs results only in localized pleural disease, and pleural effusion is not significant. In an occasional patient there is a massive outpouring of pleural fluid, and tuberculous infection is generalized over the visceral and parietal pleura. Myriads of typical tubercles stud the pleural surfaces. The immunologic reasons why some patients have this acute, widespread disease whereas others have only insignificant localized disease are not known. In a few weeks the acute reaction subsides, the pleural fluid decreases and then disappears, and fibrous adhesions between the visceral and parietal pleura form. Infrequently the fluid persists, becomes more purulent, and has increased numbers of tubercle bacilli; a chronic tuberculous empyema is established, which may persist for many years. Perhaps because the adjacent subpleural area is richly supplied with lym-

phatics, there is easy access for the dissemination of tubercle bacilli. In any case the subsequent development of tuberculosis in the lung and in other organs is a common event after untreated tuberculous pleurisy with effusion.

Clinical Manifestations. The onset of tuberculous pleurisy with effusion is usually fairly sudden and acute. Sharp, fairly severe pleural pain is the most common first symptom. It is usually unilateral, made worse by breathing, and relieved by splinting the affected area. It is sharpest and most painful for the first few days, and then with the outpouring of pleural fluid it becomes duller and gradually subsides. Shortness of breath which is sometimes severe results from large collections of pleural fluid. Fever, which is sometimes as high as 39 to 40° C, is usually present in the first two or three weeks, and gradually subsides. Physical examination and x-ray examinations will identify the presence of variable amounts of fluid. In the typical case the parenchymal focus in the lung from which the disease originated is not apparent radiologically.

Diagnosis. The diagnosis of tuberculous pleurisy should be considered in every patient with a pleural effusion; should be strongly suspected if this is accompanied by skin reactivity to 0.0001 mg of PPD; and should be presumptively diagnosed if, in addition, the fluid has the characteristics of an exudate and another diagnosis cannot be firmly made. Fortunately, methods for making the diagnosis of pleural tuberculosis have improved to such an extent that, if they are all used in a concerted fashion before treatment is started, the number of cases in which only a presumptive diagnosis must be made is small. Tubercle bacilli can be cultured from pleural fluid in up to 20 per cent of cases, from the sputum in a similar number, and from pleural biopsy material in over 60 per cent of cases. Typical tuberculous granulation tissue is seen in over 60 per cent of pleural biopsies from cases of tuberculous pleurisy. Although none of these methods are diagnostic in all cases, if they are used together, bacteriologic or histologic evidence of tuberculosis will be found in most cases.

Congestive heart failure, metastatic carcinoma involving the pleura, pulmonary infarction, and the effusions of bacterial pneumonia are the most commonly encountered conditions from which tuberculous pleurisy with effusions must be differentiated. Pleural mesothelioma, subdiaphragmatic abscess with an associated pleural effusion, rheumatoid pleural disease, and disseminated lupus erythematosus are less common conditions that may resemble tuberculous pleurisy.

Treatment. The treatment of tuberculous pleurisy is the prolonged administration of isoniazid and at least one other antituberculous drug and is the same as that for pulmonary tuberculosis (see Ch. 228). Surgical decortication to free a lung trapped by pleural adhesions (fibrothorax) after chemotherapy has controlled the infection is rarely necessary. With prompt and adequate chemotherapy, pleural residues are usually minor and do not benefit from surgical correction.

NEOPLASMS OF THE PLEURA

Metastatic Carcinoma. Implants of metastatic carcinoma of the pleura are, especially in older age groups, a common cause of pleural effusions. Carcinomas of the lung and breast are the tumors that most commonly extend to the pleura, but almost any carcinoma can have this complication. If the primary tumor has already been identified, the diagnosis is usually quickly made. If the pleural effusion is the first indication of the tumor, the diagnosis may not be so apparent. Characteristically the pleural effusions of malignant implants in the pleura are not accompanied by fever, the fluid is an exudate and often contains a large number of red blood cells, and the course is marked by the continued outpouring of fluid. The diagnosis can be established by finding malignant cells in the pleural fluid, by the presence of tumor in the parietal pleura on pleural biopsy, or by open surgical biopsy of the pleura.

Treatment is aimed at preventing the accumulation of fluid in the pleural space and eliminating the need for repeated thoracenteses for the relief of dyspnea. Obliteration of the pleural space may be produced by the instillation of various irritating substances (e.g., atabrine, nitrogen mustard, cyclophosphamide, radioactive gold), followed by aspiration of the fluid to assure that the visceral and parietal layers are opposed. The insertion of an intercostal tube attached to suction is sometimes used for continuous aspiration after the irritating material has stimulated an inflammatory response.

Mesothelioma. Pleural mesotheliomas may be either localized or diffuse. The localized tumor, the so-called fibrous mesothelioma, is relatively benign, may grow to a very large size, is sometimes cured by surgical resection, but does have a tendency to recur. The diffuse mesothelioma is a highly malignant tumor which involves the pleura widely and produces massive encroachment on the pleural space with fluid and tumor. Formerly this was believed to be a very rare tumor. It is now being seen with increased frequency, and its association with exposure to asbestos has been established (see Ch. 527).

Other Pleural Tumors. Benign tumors of the pleura include lipomas, fibromas, vascular tumors, and pleural cysts. Primary malignant tumors of the pleura other than mesotheliomas include various sarcomas. They are all very uncommon.

Pleural effusions from intrathoracic lymphoma are not uncommon and apparently can result either from direct involvement of the pleura or from intrathoracic lymphatic obstruction. Chylothorax is sometimes seen when there is lymphatic obstruction.

SPONTANEOUS PNEUMOTHORAX

The pleural space normally does not contain gas, and if gas is instilled into the pleural space, it is absorbed. The total pressure of dissolved gases in venous blood is 54 mm Hg less than the atmospheric pressure which is transmitted to the pleura. This negative gradient keeps the intact pleural space gas free. Air may enter the pleural space through either the chest wall or the lung. Trauma to the chest wall or lung, medical procedures that permit the entry of air through the chest wall or that puncture the lung, and the spontaneous entry of gas from a ruptured emphysematous bleb are the most common causes of pneumothorax. The rupture of lung abscesses and tuberculous cavities into the pleura are less common causes. Spontaneous pneumothorax occurs in at least two distinct populations: the young, tall, otherwise healthy male, and the older person with underlying and usually clinically apparent chronic obstructive pulmonary disease or some other disease that has produced pulmonary fibrosis and localized emphysema.

Clinical Manifestations. Pleural pain and shortness of breath are the principal symptoms of spontaneous pneumothorax. The severity of the shortness of breath may vary from insignificant to very severe and depends on the amount of gas in the pleural space and the amount of underlying pulmonary disease which is present. Physical examination of the chest will sometimes show increased resonance to percussion over the affected side, but a decrease in the intensity of the breath sounds is a more definite and discernible sign. If the pneumothorax is large and there is a marked increase in intrapleural pressure, a shift in mediastinal structures away from the affected side may be detected. The chest x-ray will show air in the pleural space and the amount of collapse of the lung which has occurred.

Diagnosis. The possibility of spontaneous pneumothorax should be considered whenever there is the sudden onset of shortness of breath and particularly when it is accompanied by chest pain. It is a diagnosis which is usually made easily when it occurs in an otherwise healthy person and when the clinical findings which have been enumerated are present. The diagnosis is occasionally missed when it occurs in an asthmatic, a patient with obstructive pulmonary disease, or in other patients who have some other disease that seems to explain their shortness of breath. Because it can be lethal in such patients if untreated, the possibility of its occurrence should be kept prominent.

If a vessel in the lung or chest wall is torn when a pneumothorax occurs, a hemopneumothorax may result. When the chest x-ray shows the presence of fluid as well as air, this possibility should be considered, and a thoracentesis should be performed. Massive intrapleural bleeding is uncommon, but if present it requires surgical correction.

Treatment. The treatment of pneumothorax is concerned with its immediate and acute management, and with the prevention of recurrences.

The methods used in the early management of spontaneous pneumothorax will depend on the size and cause of the pneumothorax, the presence or absence of complicating pulmonary disease, and whether the leak between the lung and the pleura is closed or continuing. If the pneumothorax has occurred in a young healthy person, is small (e.g., 10 to 15 per cent), is causing few or minimal symptoms, and does not increase during the first 12 hours of observation, it requires no treatment. However, the fact that it has indeed resorbed should be confirmed by chest x-ray about two weeks later. In a similar patient with a larger pneumothorax, and especially if there is significant shortness of breath, the gas may be removed by inserting a small venous catheter through a thoracentesis needle and aspirating the intrapleural gas. This simple method will usually succeed in patients who do not have underlying pulmonary disease and who do not have a continuing leak. If there is significant pulmonary disease, pleural adhesions, or evidence of a continuing bronchopleural fistula, a larger intercostal tube should be inserted and attached to an underwater seal. The relief of an increasing and positive pressure—a *tension pneumothorax*—by prompt decompression is occasionally lifesaving. If there is a significant continuing leakage of air or evidence of respiratory insufficiency, continuous suction is required. If the lung cannot be reexpanded or there is continued leakage for more than a few days, an open thoracotomy with resection and closure of the bronchopleural fistula may be required.

Recurrence. Spontaneous pneumothorax may recur once or many times over several years after the first episode. Recurrences may be on the same side or the opposite side. The possibility of recurrence can be greatly reduced or eliminated by surgical treatment. Surgical treatment includes the resection of blebs and bullae if they are sufficiently localized to permit this and the obliteration of the pleural space. The removal of the parietal pleura, the application of irritating substances to the pleura, and the scarification of the pleura followed by intrapleural suction are methods which are used to obliterate the pleural space.

MISCELLANEOUS PLEURAL DISEASES

The pleura is involved in a great variety of systemic diseases and in diseases of the lung and adjacent structures.

Collagen Vascular Diseases. Systemic lupus erythematosus and rheumatoid arthritis are the collagen vascular diseases in which pleural effusions are most often encountered. In rheumatoid arthritis pleural effusions are usually seen in older men in whom the arthritis is of long duration. The fluid is an exudate and characteristically has a very low glucose content.

Pancreatitis. Pleural effusions secondary to acute and chronic pancreatitis are occasionally encountered. They may occur in either pleural space, but are more common on the left. There is often an associated pancreatic pseudocyst. The fluid is an exudate, may have extremely high amylase content (500 to 50,000 units per milliliter), and characteristically has a higher level of amylase than the serum.

Asbestosis. Inhalation of asbestos dust commonly leads to pleural disease. Serous pleural effusion, pleural fibrosis, pleural calcification, and pleural mesothelioma are all complications of asbestos dust exposure.

The pleural effusion of asbestos exposure is commonly bilateral and frequently recurrent; the fluid is usually an exudate and is often serosanguineous. Pleural effusion is often accompanied by clinically apparent parenchymal fibrosis, but can occur in the absence of obvious asbestosis. Duration and intensity of exposure to asbestos can vary widely.

Pleural fibrosis is a common accompaniment of pulmonary asbestosis and has been identified in up to 14 per cent of cases of asbestosis. Like pleural effusion it may be seen in patients who do not have evident parenchymal fibrosis.

Pleural calcification is common among asbestos workers and has been found in more than 10 per cent of workers with prolonged exposure. It is often bilateral, predominantly involves the basilar portions, is primarily in the parietal pleura, and usually occurs only after lengthy exposures to asbestos.

Although pleural mesothelioma has been reported to follow these more benign forms of pleural disease from asbestos, it is an uncommon complication.

Meigs' Syndrome. Ascites, pleural effusion, a benign fibroma, or fibroma-like ovarian tumor, with cure of the ascites and pleural effusion by removal of the tumor, is a syndrome that Meigs called attention to in 1934. It is an uncommon cause of pleural effusion, but many cases of the syndrome have been reported. Most often the fluid is found in the right pleural space, but it can be present in either or both pleural spaces. The fluid is usually a clear transudate, but exudative fluids and serosanguineous collections have been reported. The amount of fluid in both the pleural and peritoneal spaces is variable, and in some cases the amount of ascites has been quite small. The mechanism for the formation of the pleural and peritoneal fluid has not been completely explained, but it is suggested that somehow the fibroma causes the ascites which is then transported to the pleural space by diaphragmatic lymphatics. Because this uncommon condition can be cured by pelvic surgery, it should be considered in women with pleural effusion of obscure origin, especially if there is evidence of concurrent ascites and pelvic disease.

Subdiaphragmatic Abscess. Pleural effusion and pleurodiaphragmatic pain, particularly on the right side, are common manifestations of a subdiaphragmatic abscess, and are frequently the first indicators of the location of the infection. The pleural effusion is most often a serous exudate, and the organism in the subdiaphragmatic abscess is often not found in the pleural fluid. Amebic infection from the liver may also extend through the diaphragm and cause a pleural exudate, which is characteristically purulent and chocolate-colored and may contain amebae.

Besson, L. N., Ferguson, T. B., and Burford, T. H.: Chylothorax. Ann. Thorac. Surg., 12:527, 1971.

Black, L. F.: The pleural space and pleural fluid. Mayo Clin. Proc., 47:493, 1972.

Bruneau, R., and Rubin, P.: The management of pleural effusions and chylothorax in lymphoma. Radiology, 85:1085, 1965.

Gaensler, E. A., and Kaplan, A. I.: Asbestos pleural effusions. Ann. Intern. Med., 74:178, 1971.

Killen, D. A., and Gobbel, W. G., Jr.: Spontaneous Pneumothorax. Boston, Little, Brown & Company, 1968.

Light, R. W., MacGregor, M. I., Luchsinger, P. C., and Ball, W. C., Jr.: Pleural effusions: The diagnostic separation of transudates and exudates. Ann. Intern. Med., 77:507, 1972.

Meigs, J. V.: Fibroma of the ovary with ascites and hydrothorax — Meigs' syndrome. Am. J. Obstet. Gynecol., 67:962, 1954.

Mellins, R. B., Levine, O. R., and Fishman, A. P.: Effects of systemic and pulmonary venous hypertension on pleural and pericardial fluid accumulation. J. Appl. Physiol., 29:564, 1970.

Scharer, L., and McClement, J. H.: The isolation of tubercle bacilli from needle biopsy specimens of parietal pleura. Am. Rev. Respir. Dis., 97:466, 1968.

Selikoff, I. J.: The occurrence of pleural calcification among asbestos insulation workers. Ann. N.Y. Acad. Sci., 132:351, 1965.

Szucs, M. M., Brooks, H. L., Grossman, W., Banas, J. S., Meister, S. G., Dexter, L., and Dalen, J. E.: Diagnostic sensitivity of laboratory findings in acute pulmonary embolism. Ann. Intern. Med., 74:161, 1971.

Yeoh, C. B., Hubaytar, R. T., Conklin, E. F., Simpson, D. G., and Ford, J. M.: Spontaneous pneumothorax: Treatment with small lumen polyethylene tube. New York State J. Med., 70:779, 1970.

Part XII
CARDIOVASCULAR DISEASES

541. HEART FAILURE

Alfred P. Fishman

The heart is part of an elaborate circulatory apparatus that is designed to serve two major functions: (1) in the usual course of events, to provide the tissues with sufficient blood (carrying oxygen, substrates, and nutrients) for their metabolic needs, both at rest and during activity; and (2) as a temporary expedient, to reapportion the cardiac output according to the physiologic priorities of the moment, e.g., muscular exercise, heat loss, digestion. The same regulatory mechanisms that satisfy physiologic priorities in health also serve to protect vital organs, e.g., the heart and brain, when cardiac output is seriously compromised.

As a pump, the heart is remarkable not only for its capacity to adjust rapidly to metabolic need and to varying loads, but also for its durability. Unfortunately, it is also vulnerable to a wide array of congenital, metabolic, inflammatory, and degenerative disorders that affect its muscular walls, its linings, its valves, and particularly its nutrient vessels, i.e., the coronary arteries. Some cardiac disorders, such as arteriosclerosis of the small coronary arteries, progress slowly and insidiously, and their disease takes a lifetime to become clinically evident. Others, such as bacterial infection of the aortic valve, are often dramatic in onset and catastrophic in their consequences.

In general, signs and symptoms of heart disease are of two different kinds: those referable to the heart itself, such as pain and palpitation, and others that are extracardiac and originate in congested circulatory beds and hypoperfused organs. Considered out of context, each extracardiac manifestation may be disappointingly nonspecific. For example, breathlessness is a common symptom that is shared by disorders of the heart, the lungs, and the brain. Nonetheless, when breathlessness develops in a patient with left heart disease in association with other evidence of congested and edematous lungs, and grows worse when the patient lies flat, there is little question that the patient is suffering from left heart failure.

Subsequent chapters in Part XII will deal with individual cardiac disorders. The present chapter will be concerned with heart failure, a final common pathway for many of the diverse etiologies and pathogenic mechanisms that will be discussed subsequently.

GENERAL ASPECTS

Heart failure may be considered in clinical, physiologic, or biochemical terms. In the clinic, "heart failure" refers to a distinctive constellation of symptoms and physical signs that has emerged in a patient with an underlying cardiac disorder. The hemodynamic counterpart at that time is an inability of the heart to match its output to the metabolic needs of the body (determined as O_2 consumption) even though filling pressures of the heart are adequate. The biochemical equivalent is not as certain as the hemodynamic, but appears to involve defective conversion by the heart muscle of chemical energy to mechanical work.

By convention, the designation "heart failure" is used as a synonym for myocardial failure. Consequently, heart failure is concerned with a myocardium that is performing inadequately because of either overload or intrinsic disorder. This stipulation automatically excludes syndromes in which the seat of the difficulty is in abnormalities of the heart valves or pericardium or excessive heart rates—each of which can compromise the circulation even though the cardiac muscle is normal.

Disproportion between hemodynamic load and myocardial capacity to cope with it initiates the sequence that culminates in heart failure. In general, the heart tolerates volume overloads better than pressure overloads. For example, *volume* overload of the left ventricle produced by aortic insufficiency may exist for years without causing distress; in contrast, *pressure* overload from aortic stenosis generally elicits signs and symptoms of heart failure much earlier. Sustained overloads are also accommodated better than acute overloads. Thus chronic mitral regurgitation caused by rheumatic heart disease may last for years without signs of heart failure, whereas the acute mitral regurgitation produced by a ruptured chorda tendinea is apt to precipitate a disastrous syndrome of heart failure.

The myocardium responds differently to volume and pressure loads. Volume overloads generally elicit dilatation followed by hypertrophy; conversely, pressure overloads characteristically elicit hypertrophy until late in the natural history when dilatation supervenes. Primary myocardial disease generally elicits both dilatation and hypertrophy.

Categories of Heart Failure

In the clinic, the type of heart failure is generally identified by its durations (acute or chronic), initiating mechanisms, the ventricle that is primarily affected, the characteristic clinical syndrome, and the underlying physiologic derangements.

Acute vs. Chronic Heart Failure. The manifestations of heart failure usually begin insidiously, blurring at the outset with those of the underlying cardiac disorder and continuing gradually into a chronic state. However, the syndrome may also begin acutely, as after myocardial infarction. Between these extremes of acute and chronic heart failure are many instances of subclinical heart failure in which a successful cardiotonic program, coupled with self-restriction of activity by the patient, minimizes signs and symptoms even though cardiac performance remains seriously compromised. On the other hand, it is not uncommon for the course of chronic heart failure that is nicely controlled to be punctuated by bouts of acute heart failure that stem either from lapses in therapy or from progression of the underlying heart disease.

Both acute and chronic heart failure elicit compensatory adjustments. These include increase in peripheral vascular resistance, redistribution of blood flow, and increase in erythropoietic activity. But the adaptive mechanisms differ strikingly in type, degree, and intensity, and even in direction. For example, *acute* distention of the left atrium generally promotes a sodium-poor diuresis, whereas *chronic* distention of the left atrium elicits salt and water retention. This distinction between acute and chronic heart failure must be borne in mind when attempting to relate observations on experimental heart failure in animals to the clinical syndrome of chronic heart failure in man, because experimental heart failure is generally acute in onset, is fulminating in course, and is generally ended abruptly by the death of the animal.

Initiating Mechanisms. Each initiating mechanism generally imposes its own distinctive stamp upon the clinical syndrome. Thus rheumatic heart disease leads to a different constellation of symptoms and signs from that of hypertensive heart disease; in turn, both have a different natural history from cor pulmonale. Indeed, even a single etiology, arteriosclerosis, may have distinctly different consequences; progressive narrowing and gradual occlusion of *peripheral* branches of the coronary arteries may be so covert that the characteristic shortness of breath and undue fatigue of left ventricular failure may be misinterpreted as evidence of the general physical decline of advancing age. Conversely, abrupt closure of a major coronary artery, as a consequence of thrombosis superimposed on an arteriosclerotic plaque, may elicit massive myocardial necrosis, followed by extensive myocardial scarring and unremitting heart failure.

Left vs. Right Heart Failure. With rare exception, one ventricle fails before the other. Because of the prevalence of cardiac disorders which overload or damage the left ventricle, e.g., coronary arteriosclerosis and hypertension, heart failure usually begins with the left ventricle. Breathlessness, the key clinical expression of pulmonary congestion and edema, is the most common initial complaint. Conversely, when the right ventricle fails, systemic venous congestion and peripheral edema generally predominate. Left ventricular failure is the most common cause of right ventricular failure, and breathlessness often improves as right ventricular output falls and pulmonary congestion diminishes.

The mechanism by which left ventricular failure causes the right ventricle to fail is not entirely clear, although pulmonary (venous and arterial) hypertension from the failing left ventricle and the continuity of heart muscle around both ventricles are undoubtedly involved. In contrast to the accepted sequence of left ventricular failure followed by right ventricular failure, it is still debated whether isolated right ventricular failure inevitably elicits left ventricular failure. The latter association is difficult to prove because of the frequent coexistence of independent and unrelated left ventricular disease in patients with right ventricular failure.

The combination of combined left and right ventricular failure, in which evidences of systemic and pulmonary venous hypertension predominate, is traditionally referred to as "congestive heart failure." This is a colloquialism that conveys the image of severe physical incapacity, breathlessness, distended neck veins, hepatic engorgement, and troublesome peripheral edema. But it

also highlights clinical features that can be measured at the bedside: a high venous pressure, a prolonged circulation time, and a diminished vital capacity, all of which improve as the patient gets better.

Backward vs. Forward Heart Failure. Somewhat reminiscent of the fable about the blind men and the elephant is the vintage controversy about "backward" versus "forward" heart failure. "Backward failure" calls attention to the damming up of blood in the veins proximal to the failing ventricle and attributes to this venous congestion a critical role in the evolution of the syndrome of heart failure; "forward failure" assigns the same pivotal role to a decrease in cardiac output and underfilling of the arterial tree. In reality this distinction is meaningless, because it is inevitable in a closed circuit that the inability of the heart to sustain its output (forward failure) and the pooling of blood on the venous inflow side (backward failure) must go hand in hand.

Low vs. High Output Failure. Cardiac catheterization in man has made it possible to sort myocardial failure according to the level of the cardiac output. This practice has served at least three purposes: (1) to separate, on clinical and physiologic grounds, a type of myocardial failure ("high output failure") in which the circulation remains vigorous and the extremities remain warm despite venous congestion, edema, and a lower cardiac output than existed prior to the heart failure; (2) to emphasize that the level of the cardiac output and the circulatory adjustments during myocardial failure are, to large extent, a consequence of the cardiac output that existed prior to heart failure; and (3) to relate etiology and clinical evidences of heart failure to the state of the circulation: the more common causes of heart failure—arteriosclerosis, hypertension, myocardial disease, valvular disease, and pericardial disease—tend to be low output states; less common causes, such as hyperthyroidism, Paget's disease, anemia, beriberi, arteriovenous fistula, tend to be high output states. But the hemodynamic hallmark of cardiac failure remains the same regardless of the level of cardiac output at rest: an inability of the heart to increase its output (or stroke volume or stroke work) as end-diastolic volume (as well as pressure) is increased (see Frank-Starling Principle, below).

The separation into "high" and "low" output failure is concerned with the clinical manifestations, rather than the causes, of myocardial failure. But it is also a hemodynamic frame of reference to which the anatomist and the biochemist can relate the myocardial origins of heart failure. For example, "high output" failure probably has different biochemical bases from "low output" failure. Nor are all types of "low output" or "high output" failure apt to have the same biochemical origins. For example, it is unlikely that the "high output" failure of a peripheral arteriovenous fistula has the same anatomic or biochemical beginnings and evolution as the "high output" failure of severe anemia or malnutrition.

Congestive Failure vs. Congested State. Overfilling of both venous circulations, without myocardial failure, is the hallmark of the "congested state." It may be induced by rapid infusions; it may also occur in the course of "hyperkinetic" circulatory states as diverse as severe anemia and peripheral arteriovenous fistula. Similar but less dramatic venous congestion may also complicate Paget's disease or beriberi. In each of these situations, venous hypertension may arise from a combination of an expanded venous volume and heightened venomotor tone, rather than from heart failure.

It is true that persistence of a "hyperkinetic" congested state may, in time, cause the heart muscle to fail from overwork. The onset of myocardial failure may then be difficult to detect on clinical grounds, because the hyperkinetic circulation persists and the congestion may be only slightly increased during myocardial failure. Accordingly, the transition from the congested state to congestive heart failure may be difficult to detect on clinical grounds alone. But when heart failure does supervene, cardiac catheterization will disclose an inadequate increase in cardiac output during exercise as well as a considerable increase in cardiac output after digitalis. Fortunately, identification of the transition from a "congested state" to "congestive heart failure" is of greater theoretical than practical importance, because therapeutic measures, such as the administration of diuretics and the replacement of particular nutrients, e.g., thiamin in beriberi, are effective in both situations. However, digitalis will exert an important therapeutic effect once the myocardium has failed, whereas it is clinically useless when administered to a heart that is coping well with an overfilled circulation.

Subcellular Bases for Contraction

With each beat, the heart develops force and expends energy. Electrical activity at the cell surface activates the contractile machinery. Connecting the electrical activity at the surface and the contractile machinery within the muscle cell is the sarcoplasmic reticulum which plays a critical role in the release and uptake of calcium during contraction and relaxation.

For the development of the contractile force, heart muscle depends on interactions among contractile proteins, the hypothetical "elastic components" with which they are connected in series, and the constraining bounds within which the contractile elements function. The contractile proteins are contained within sarcomeres, repeating units that comprise the individual muscle fibers (myofibrils). Within the sarcomere, the contractile proteins are arranged in two orderly groups of myofilaments, one consisting of myosin, the other predominantly of actin. Holding the contractile apparatus at bay are two modulator proteins, troponin and tropomyosin. Delivery of calcium to troponin from the sarcoplasmic reticulum and sarcolemma sets the contractile process into motion.

To account for changes in the length of heart muscle during contraction and relaxation, the sliding filament hypothesis of Huxley is generally invoked: during contraction, the thin actin filaments slide past the thicker myosin filaments to shorten the sarcomere; the entire muscle cell follows suit. Conversely, during relaxation, the sarcomeres and the muscle cell resume their initial lengths as the original actin-myosin relationships are restored. Nearby mitochondria generate energy for the contractile machinery by oxidative phosphorylation of free fatty acids and glucose supplied by the circulation.

The tension that is developed in cardiac muscle during contraction depends on actin-myosin relationships. Projecting from the myosin filaments are cross-bridges. Before activation, these bridges are not attached to actin filaments. Upon activation, the cross-bridges on the myosin filaments lock into receptor sites on the actin filaments, thereby developing the force that leads to contraction. As the muscle shortens, the cross-bridges disengage and slide along the actin filament, like a pawl on a ratchet, to engage other sites. Depending on the number of cross-bridges that are interlocked at the same time, different tensions will be developed.

In addition to these subcellular elements that are directly involved in the contractile process, there appears to be a subcellular beta sympathomimetic system that can enhance the inotropic state. Although an increase in intracellular calcium is involved, the precise mechanism is unclear.

Evidence exists that for the sarcomere, as for the whole heart (see Frank-Starling Principle), the tension developed during contraction is directly related to its initial length. This correspondence implies that, for the whole heart, stretching increases the ability of its individual contractile elements to develop force. Also, since stretching does not affect the rate of interaction of active sites, elongation of cardiac muscle fibers before contraction should not affect the velocity of the subsequent contraction. These considerations underlie many current notions about cardiac contractility. But it is still unclear whether the ultrastructural-physiologic correlations are real or simply models for eliciting a new kind of reflection about an exceedingly complicated problem.

PATHOPHYSIOLOGIC INTERPLAY

Each ventricle functions as a separate muscular pump supplied by its own booster pump (atrium). The two ventricles empty in unison, simultaneously dispatching their respective contents: the right ventricle sending blood to the lungs for arterialization, the left ventricle sending arterialized blood to the rest of the body for metabolic purposes. In the normal heart, at least 50 per cent of the end-diastolic volume is ejected with each beat. Much of the ejection force is the result of the inherent properties (fiber-length and inotropism) of the myocardium. But a wide range of adaptability to the everchanging metabolic needs of daily life is provided by a superimposed series of extrinsic neurohumoral adjustments which, in daily life, modify and obscure the intrinsic inherent properties of the heart muscle.

Each ventricle, as with any man-made machine, is endowed with a finite capacity for stress, strain, and repair. The two ventricles also have somewhat different designs in keeping with their different long-range functions as pumps. The rate of obsolescence of each ventricle depends on the wear and tear to which it is subjected, its supply of nutriments and substrates, and its continuing state of good health. Before birth, both ventricles are taxed equally, because they bear the same pressure loads. After birth, as pulmonary arterial pressure falls, the right ventricular burden decreases and its walls thin. Consequently, other influences remaining equal, the durability of right ventricular performance is destined from birth to exceed that of the left ventricle. The brighter prospects of the right ventricle for longevity in performance are intensified by the greater vulnerability of the left side of the heart to disease and to disorders in its blood supply.

Chronic Compensatory Mechanisms

Two principal mechanisms mark the progression from normal myocardial performance to myocardial failure: hypertrophy and dilatation.

Hypertrophy.   An increase in the muscle mass of a ventricle takes time to develop. It involves increased protein synthesis in response to mechanical overload or dilatation. The common denominator for these two mechanisms may be the Laplace relationship (Fig. 1) which indicates that an increase in wall tension (stress) follows an increase in pressure or radius. Early in hypertrophy, muscle mass and capillary vessels increase proportionately and the contractile properties of the myocardium are preserved. But later, the inotropic behavior becomes abnormal and the capacity of the myocardium to synthesize adrenergic transmitter decreases. Indeed, once hypertrophy begins, the myocardium has been eased on to the road to failure.

In the depressed inotropic state associated with hypertrophy, circulatory function is maintained for a long while by the combination of the increase in muscle mass, the Frank-Starling mechanism (Fig. 2), and augmented sympathetic stimulation. But as the myocardial inotropic state continues to deteriorate, perhaps after intrinsic catecholamine stores have been depleted, circulatory compensation can no longer be maintained. Resting cardiac output then falls and filling pressures increase, leading to the clinical and hemodynamic manifestations of overt congestive heart failure.

Dilatation. Progressive and persistent dilatation marks the transition between ventricular hypertrophy and failure. For a long while, dilatation may serve as a compensatory mechanism, increasing the contractile force of the heart by way of the Frank-Starling relationship. But dilatation gradually becomes inadequate to maintain stroke output.

Several different mechanisms seem to be involved in the ultimate inability of the dilated heart to maintain its output: (1) slippage and rearrangement of sarcomeres during progressive dilatation; as a result, they neither produce a coordinated contraction nor are properly stretched to enhance contractility as the heart dilates further; (2) high wall tension in accord with the law of Laplace (Fig. 1); as the volume of the ventricle increases so that its wall tension for a given pressure in the ventricular cavity during contraction is greater than normal, the myocardial oxygen consumption increases accordingly; (3) protracted maintenance of high wall tension during contraction; in contrast to the normal heart, in which the wall tension decreases in the course of systole, wall tension remains high in the dilated heart; (4) high energy requirements coupled with an inefficient

conversion of chemical to mechanical energy; despite the decrease in stroke output, the dilated heart does more internal work and has a higher myocardial oxygen consumption than does the normal heart. Because of these limitations, chronic enlargement is an inefficient and ill-fated mechanism for achieving sustained improvement in cardiac performance.

Assessment of Cardiac Performance

With respect to evaluating cardiac performance, the heart may be regarded from three points of view: as a pump; as a muscle; and as a component of the circulation. Hemodynamic measurements are used to characterize its behavior as a pump: cardiac output, stroke output, stroke work, stroke power, ventricular end-diastolic pressure, ejection fraction, and ventricular end-diastolic volume. To ascertain its behavior as a muscle, principles of muscle mechanics are applied. Its adequacy as a component of the circulation is reflected in the derangements that result from the low cardiac output, the redistribution of blood flow among tissues and organs, organ hypoperfusion, and venous congestion.

Heart as a Pump: Hemodynamics

By the time the heart fails, a variety of mechanisms are operating to bolster its flagging performance. In contrast to the inappropriately low cardiac output, the blood pressure generally remains normal or even increases.

Cardiac Output. At each level of activity, in health and disease, a complicated interplay automatically adjusts the extent of shortening of myocardial fibers and, consequently, the stroke volume and the cardiac output. Four principal determinants set the stroke volume: preload (end-diastolic volume), afterload (impedance to ventricular emptying during systole), the inotropic characteristics of the heart, and the coordinated pattern of contraction. A fifth determinant, the heart rate, sets the cardiac output (stroke volume times heart rate). For practical purposes, three of these five principal determinants of cardiac output—preload, afterload, heart rate—are quantifiable. The fourth, the pattern of contraction, can be evaluated qualitatively. But the fifth, inotropic state, remains difficult to determine except when distortions are so gross that they can be detected at the bedside or visualized by fluoroscopy.

Relationships among these determinants are not fixed; they play greater or lesser roles, depending on the state of the heart. Thus when the inherent contractility (inotropic state) is impaired, stroke output and cardiac output may be maintained by ventricular dilatation (Frank-Starling mechanism). This flexible arrangement limits the value of cardiac output as a measure of cardiac contractility (inotropic state) to situations in which preload, afterload, and heart rate can be held constant. Unfortunately, this degree of control of loading conditions and heart rate is easier to achieve in the experimental laboratory than in clinical situations.

Indicator-dilution techniques are now widely used for the bedside determination of cardiac output. The normal range in adults at rest is between 2.5 and 3.6 liters per minute per square meter. A decrease in cardiac output at rest represents a late stage in abnormal cardiac performance. Failure to increase cardiac output during exercise occurs much earlier. Thus in normal subjects exercising in a supine position, the increase in cardiac output

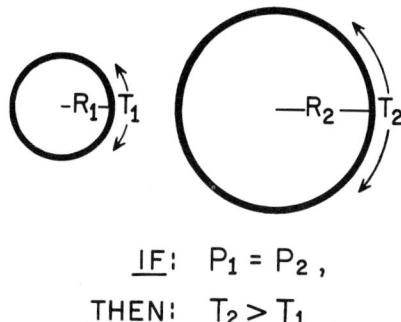

$$\text{IF: } P_1 = P_2 ,$$
$$\text{THEN: } T_2 > T_1$$

Figure 1. An illustration of the Laplace equation (T = P × R). The mean tension in the wall of the heart during systole (T) is directly proportional to the product of the mean radius (R) and the mean transmural pressure (P) that the wall is supporting. Dilatation of the heart ($R_2 > R_1$) at the same pressure ($P_1 = P_2$) is associated with an increase in wall tension ($T_2 > T_1$).

exceeds 600 ml per minute for each 100 ml increase in oxygen consumption. Lower values indicate abnormal cardiac performance. In heart failure, the arteriovenous difference for oxygen is abnormally wide, resulting almost entirely from the low oxygen content of venous blood returning to the heart rather than from impaired oxygenation in the lungs.

During exercise, heart rate and cardiac output increase as linear functions of oxygen consumption. This is true during both supine and upright exercise, but for any level of exercise the cardiac output is appreciably lower in the upright position. These increases in cardiac output are accomplished principally by acceleration of the heart rate rather than by increase in the stroke volume. In heart failure, cardiac output is even more dependent on heart rate, both at rest and during exercise.

Ventricular End-Diastolic Pressure. Inadequate ventricular emptying during systole leads to an increase in the residual volume of blood in the ventricle after systole, and thereby to an increase in end-diastolic ventricular volume. Since end-diastolic ventricular volumes are difficult to measure, end-diastolic ventricular pressures are generally substituted, thereby taking advantage of the predictable relationship between diastolic pressure and volume in the ventricle as long as the compliance of the ventricular wall remains normal. Accordingly, if ventricular compliance can be assumed to be normal, an end-diastolic pressure in the *left* ventricle greater than 12 mm Hg is a sign of depressed myocardial function; correspondingly, a value greater than 10 mm Hg in the *right* ventricle is abnormal. It is rather simple to estimate the right ventricular end-diastolic pressure by measuring the central venous pressure; the left ventricular end-diastolic pressure is more difficult to estimate because of its inaccessibility. However, in the absence of mitral obstruction or of an increase in pulmonary vascular resistance, pulmonary arterial diastolic pressure may be used to obtain an estimate of left ventricular end-diastolic pressure. Similar information can be obtained from a pulmonary wedge pressure.

Frank-Starling Principle. The Frank-Starling principle describes the force of contraction, generally measured as

the work done by the ventricle per beat, as a function of ventricular end-diastolic volume. The end-diastolic volume (initial fiber length) depends in large measure upon the venous return. According to the Frank-Starling relationship, ventricular function curves may be determined by successively increasing venous return, thereby increasing the volume of blood in the ventricle at the end of diastole and the subsequent stroke output (Fig. 2).

The shape and position of the ventricular function curve are modified by autonomic nervous activity. Figure 2 illustrates the displacement of the curve produced by sympathetic nervous activity or the administration of norepinephrine. It also illustrates the effects of heart failure in displacing the curve. It is noteworthy that the failing heart operates on a lower curve instead of slipping over the hump of a single curve onto a descending limb; digitalis relocates the position of the curve toward normal. Although a descending limb has been described in experimental heart failure and occasionally in human subjects with diffuse myocardial disease who have been subjected to physical stress, ventricular function curves in man generally do not show a descending limb.

In the normal heart, the Frank-Starling mechanism operates chiefly to match the stroke outputs of the two ventricles. But in heart failure this mechanism plays an important role in sustaining the cardiac output.

Ejection Fraction. Normally the ratio of stroke volume to left ventricular end-diastolic volume (determined angiographically) ranges from 0.56 to 0.78. A reduced ejection fraction suggests a decrease in myocardial performance.

Systolic Time Intervals. Simultaneous recording of the electrocardiogram, phonocardiogram, and carotid arterial pulse allows indirect bedside appraisal of cardiac function. By this combination of recordings, total electromechanical systole is subdivided into left ventricular ejection time and the pre-ejection period. In patients with abnormalities of myocardial contractility—even before overt congestive heart failure—pre-ejection time usually lengthens, whereas ejection time shortens (the normal ratio of pre-ejection time to left ventricular ejection time is 0.35 ± 0.04 SD). This noninvasive technique is most useful in chronic coronary artery disease, arterial hypertension, and the cardiomyopathies. It does not distinguish between inotropic state and other mechanical determinants of contractility, particularly loading of the ventricle. Disturbances in conduction, valvular disease, and other unanticipated disorders may invalidate the determinations.

Heart as a Muscle

The contractile performance of the heart depends on two essential components: fiber length (Frank-Starling mechanism) and the inherent contractility (inotropic state) of the muscle.

Contractility. Increase in sympathetic nervous activity provides the major inotropic effect for the normal heart (in conjunction with increase in heart rate and venous tone). In contrast to the Frank-Starling mechanism, the increase in force and velocity of contraction is accomplished without corresponding increase in fiber length (end-diastolic ventricular volume).

Inotropic State. Clinicians would welcome an objective index of myocardial contractility in which the inotropic state (intrinsic contractility of the muscle) could be measured independent of change in the length of

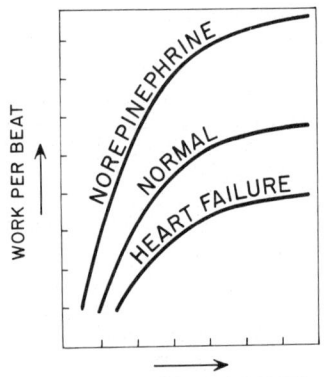

Figure 2. Hypothetical Frank-Starling relationships for different states of myocardial contractility. Enhanced contractility, as after sympathetic nervous stimulation or the administration of norepinephrine, moves the normal curve toward one in which more stroke work is done at lower filling pressures. In heart failure, as contractility is progressively impaired and the heart continues to dilate, the relationship is displaced to a lower curve instead of slipping along a single curve on to a descending limb.

myocardial fibers (Frank-Starling relationship). This would be useful in three different ways: (1) to examine the effects on the myocardium of an acute intervention, such as the administration of digitalis, (2) to determine consecutive changes in the inotropic state of the myocardium in the same individual during the evolution of heart failure and in response to treatment; and (3) to compare the inotropic state in different individuals.

Unfortunately, distinction between the effects of fiber length and of intrinsic contractility is difficult to accomplish for the heart. The main obstacle stems from the strong influence of mechanical loading conditions on hemodynamic measurements. Thus a change in either the preload (length of ventricular fibers at end-diastole) or the afterload (force developed in ventricular muscle during systole) can modify ventricular performance greatly without affecting its intrinsic inotropic state. Another complication is the inability of conventional hemodynamic measurements to take heart size into account so that comparisons of contractility in hearts of different size are generally unreliable.

Because changes in mechanical loading conditions confuse determinations of inotropic state, attempts are being made (1) to make these determinations under constant conditions of mechanical loading (constant diastolic volume, aortic pressure) and heart rate, (2) to devise methods for determining inotropic state that are insensitive to loading conditions, or (3) to interpret hemodynamic values in terms of a change in inotropic state when loading conditions can be adequately discounted. But when determinants of mechanical performance other than inotropic state cannot be discounted—which is usually the case—more independent indices of contractility have been sought, particularly the rate of rise in ventricular pressure in the pre-ejection phase of ventricular contraction and force-velocity relationships.

Rate of Increase in Intraventricular Pressure (dp/dt). Several indices of dp/dt are being used. In practice, dp/dt is determined electronically as the first derivative of the ventricular pressure. For comparative purposes, measurements are generally made at some preselected point(s) in the cardiac cycle, e.g., at 40 mm Hg. Often the value for dp/dt is further standardized by reference to some common denominator; e.g., peak dp/dt may be divided by total pressure instead of being used as dp/dt, per se. At present, application in man of the dp/dt determinations is handicapped by the need for extraordinarily high fidelity recording systems and by the difficulty in reproducing loading conditions. Although it holds considerable promise for comparisons of contractile performance in a single patient before and after intervention, it has little prospect for comparing different hearts. Attempts to obtain a related kind of information by using an end-catheter velocity gauge to determine the rate at which blood is ejected into the aorta are promising but are still in their infancy.

As in the case of pressure, the rate of development of wall tension is also decidedly abnormal in heart failure. Moreover, in contrast to the normal heart in which wall tension decreases during systole, wall tension in heart failure remains high throughout systole so that both the velocity and the degree of shortening are abnormal.

Velocity of Contraction. The use of the velocity of contraction as a measure of contractility involves the force-velocity relationship originally developed by A. V. Hill for skeletal muscle. According to this relationship, the velocity of shortening in skeletal muscle is inversely

related to the magnitude of the tension that the muscle develops, i.e., the greater the load that the muscle is obliged to lift during contraction, the slower its speed of shortening. In skeletal muscle, this relationship is a hyperbolic one, the intercept on the velocity axis being called V_{max} (velocity at zero force), whereas the intercept on the force axis (force at zero velocity) is called P_0.

Applying this relationship to the myocardium (Fig. 3), the position of the force-velocity curve would be affected both by a change in end-diastolic fiber length (initial stretch or preload) and by a change in inherent inotropic activity. But the effects would be different. Thus a change in the degree of initial stretch of the heart muscle, and presumably in the number of active sites at which the chemical reactions of contraction can occur, would modify the total force that the muscle develops; in Figure 3, this change would shift the horizontal, but not the vertical, intercept (P_0). In contrast, a change in inotropic activity by cardiotonic agents, on the one hand, or myocardial failure, on the other, would be expected not only to affect the horizontal intercept (total force) but also to displace the force-velocity curve with respect to the vertical axis (rate of force-generating processes). Indeed, the original observations on skeletal muscle even suggested that an ideal measure of contractility might be obtained by extrapolating the force-velocity relationships to the vertical axis (V_{max}), thereby determining the maximal velocity of shortening that would exist at zero load. Although it is acknowledged that P_0 is length dependent, the claim has been made that for heart muscle V_{max} is independent of length. Unfortunately, the latter claim has not been substantiated; consequently, V_{max} does not automatically distinguish between effects of Frank-Starling relationship and changes in inotropic state.

It should be stressed that the assessment of force-velocity relations in the human heart is still empirical and in its infancy. Serious reservations have been expressed about the relevance of the ultrastructural model, which depicts contractile elements in series with elastic elements, to heart muscle. At present, the assessment of force-velocity relations is a technical feat which involves a combination of cineangiography, high fidelity

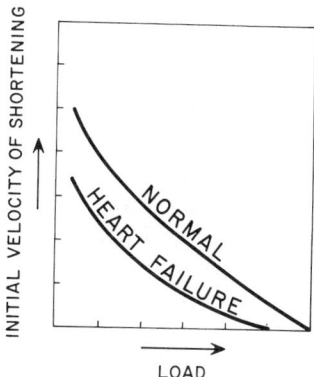

Figure 3. Hypothetical representation of force-velocity changes in heart failure. Under special conditions of loading, the position of the force-velocity curve is determined by the inotropic state of the myocardium. The force-velocity relationship shifts as shown during heart failure, decreasing both the velocity of shortening at any given load and the maximal developed tension. V_{max}, which may be obtained by extrapolation to the vertical axis, is not shown, because the interpretation of this extrapolation is uncertain. (Modified from Braunwald, E., Ross, J., Jr., and Sonnenblick, E. H.: Mechanisms of Contraction of the Normal and Failing Heart. Boston, Little, Brown & Company, 1968.)

recording of ventricular pressures, and an assumed geometric model of the ventricular cavity as a basis for relating wall stress to the velocity and extent of shortening. But these practical limitations should not obscure the conceptual values of the new approaches to contractility. Moreover, even though direct determinations of force-velocity relationships have yet to be made on the human heart in failure, there is little reason to doubt that in the human heart, as in the isolated papillary muscle, myocardial failure will prove to be associated with a decrease in both the force and the velocity of myocardial contraction.

Finally, although the experimental techniques described in this chapter for determination of inotropic state are invasive, elaborate, and expensive, they not only promise fresh insights into myocardial contractility but may also pave the way for noninvasive, bedside techniques by providing reliable standards of reference and calibration as well as a bank of useful empirical information about myocardial performance.

Relaxation and Distensibility. Although most studies of ventricular performance during heart failure have centered around the contraction phase, the course of the relaxation phase (diastole) influences the pattern of the subsequent cardiac contraction. The filling of the ventricle during diastole depends not only on the time available but also on the pattern of relaxation. Relaxation consists of two components: an active one, which promotes relaxation by way of intrinsic mechanisms; and a passive one, arising from extension of the fibers by the inflowing blood. Incomplete relaxation would be expected not only to increase the filling pressure of the heart but also to dissipate energy. In the normal heart, the active and passive components appear to work synergistically to minimize losses in chemical energy. But in heart failure the viscous and elastic properties of the heart muscle seem to change so that there is a diminished resistance to filling (decreased "impedance") and an increased extent of ventricular expansion on filling (increased "compliance"). Thus not only the velocity and duration of relaxation but also changes in the physical properties of the muscle seem involved in heart failure.

Energetics. The heart does work and expends energy during contraction. The principal determinants of myocardial oxygen consumption are the tension developed in the ventricular wall during systole (a function of systolic pressure and ventricular volume), the heart rate, and the inotropic state (contractility) of the ventricular muscle; of less importance is the stroke volume. Myocardial wall tension is described by the Laplace relation which relates pressure, radius, and wall thickness.

For its contraction, the heart depends on the conversion of the chemical energy of oxidizable substrates into the mechanical energy of muscular contraction. ATP participates in this process as the principal store of energy released by oxidation; its breakdown by myosin ATPase is the principal way by which chemical energy is transformed into mechanical energy. ATP resynthesis in the myocardium is accomplished chiefly through oxidative phosphorylation. The rate of ATP breakdown and the quantity of energy used by the myocardium depend chiefly on the tension that is developed in the myocardial fibers rather than on the degree of shortening or the work done; this developed tension causes the ventricular walls to contract and the blood to be ejected. From a biochemical point of view, the muscle of a ventricle has failed when its generation of free energy, or its utilization of that energy in the process of contraction, is insufficient for the circulatory load which it has to handle.

Unfortunately, the biochemical basis for heart failure is not yet settled. But it is now clear that there are no consistent defects in energy metabolism or in protein synthesis. The investigative focus at present is on excitation-coupling and the role of calcium in the contractile process.

Heart as Component of Circulation

As the overburdened ventricle fails, it elicits venous hypertension and slowed circulation, and sets into motion peripheral mechanisms to sustain blood pressure and cardiac output.

Venous Hypertension. With the onset of failure, the ventricle fails to empty properly during systole so that the volume of blood left in the ventricle after contraction increases, i.e., ejection fraction decreases. An increase in diastolic pressure in the ventricles and in the atrium and veins that lead to the ventricle accompanies the increase in ventricular volume. Several other elements contribute to the venous hypertension: (1) heightened venomotor tone; (2) expansion of the blood volume as a consequence of sodium retention by the kidney; and, on occasion, (3) regurgitation of blood from ventricle to atrium as the atrioventricular valve becomes incompetent either from ventricular dilatation of from improper closure during an arrhythmia.

Slowed Circulation. The circulation time depends on the cardiac output and the volume of blood interposed between the sites of sampling and injection. Should either ventricle fail, the time for a tracer substance to pass from the site of intravenous injection to the site of detection will be prolonged. For example, in left heart failure, the arm-to-tongue circulation time, measured by using Decholin as a tracer, will be prolonged beyond the normal limits of 10 to 15 seconds; delay of the tracer in traversing the pulmonary circulation and dilated left heart, as well as excessive dilution of the tracer by the enlarged intervening blood volume, contributes to the delay. Similarly, the arm-to-breath circulation time measured after the intravenous injection of ether will be prolonged in right heart failure. By relating the circulation times to the central venous pressure, it may be possible to establish at the bedside which ventricle has failed. For example, in left heart failure, central venous pressure and ether circulation time will be normal, whereas Decholin time will be prolonged.

Peripheral Mechanisms to Sustain Cardiac Output and Blood Pressure. In order to sustain the cardiac output, to apportion it selectively, and to maintain the systemic arterial blood pressure, a variety of peripheral mechanisms are activated.

Autonomic Nervous System. Normally, a four- or fivefold increase in oxygen consumption elicits a doubling of the cardiac output. When the increase in cardiac output cannot keep pace with the level of activity, distribution of blood flow is altered to defend vital areas, e.g., brain and heart. The autonomic nervous system is deeply involved in this rearrangement of the circulation. It also contributes to activation of the mechanisms for retaining sodium and water.

Peripheral vasoconstriction and tachycardia are the hallmarks of the usual forms of heart failure. Paradoxically, despite a generalized increase in sympathetic nervous activity, norepinephrine stores in the heart muscle are depleted because of defective local synthesis. Consequently, the failing heart, denied local adrenergic support for its inotropic and chronotropic responses, is obliged to rely on norepinephrine delivered to it by the blood from the adrenal medulla and the peripheral vasculature. Pharmacologic agents, such as guanethidine, which further deplete the heart of its catecholamines, aggravate heart failure. In many respects, the performance of the human heart that has failed resembles that of both the "denervated" heart and the isolated heart-lung preparation that Starling used. The role that the parasympathetic nervous system plays in heart failure is ill defined, but evidence does exist to indicate that its contribution to the control of heart rate and baroreceptor activity is impaired.

PERIPHERAL VASOCONSTRICTION. Peripheral arteriolar and venoconstriction, mediated by heightened sympathetic nervous activity, are essential compensatory mechanisms in heart failure. The extent to which accumulation of sodium and water in the arteriolar wall contributes to increased arteriolar resistance is as yet unclear. Selective arteriolar vasoconstriction helps not only to sustain the blood pressure but also to preserve function in critical organs. The pattern of selective vasoconstriction, in turn, influences the cardiac output by determining the total peripheral resistance to cardiac emptying.

Selective venoconstriction promotes venous return by transfer of returning blood to the central veins. Although peripheral venoconstriction may contribute importantly to the increase in central venous pressure, the major determinant is myocardial incompetence in coping with the venous return.

REDISTRIBUTION. In order to maintain oxygen delivery to vital organs (brain and myocardium) during heart failure, blood flow is diverted by heightened sympathetic nervous activity from skin, kidneys, splanchnic viscera, and muscle. At first the redistribution of blood flow among organs occurs during activity or stress, i.e., as cardiac output fails to increase appropriately for the increment in metabolism; later it operates also at rest. The mechanism for diversion is the balance between sympathetic innervation and local metabolism: the circulations to skin, kidney, splanchnic organs, and skeletal muscle are richly innervated, and these viscera have low metabolic rates; sympathetic nervous vasoconstriction easily overrides local metabolites. In contrast, the circulations to brain and myocardium are poor in alpha-adrenergic receptors; these organs, with high oxygen consumption, produce ample metabolic dilators to counterbalance heightened sympathetic activity.

In the normal subject during exercise, as need for heat dissipation increases, cutaneous hyperemia develops. In contrast, the patient in heart failure fails to develop cutaneous hyperemia despite increasing need for heat dissipation. The net effect is that the patient in heart failure, suffering from a low cardiac output during exercise, preserves blood pressure and blood flow to vital organs by paying the penalty of impaired heat loss as well as inadequate blood flow to exercising muscles.

VALSALVA MANEUVER. An abnormal response to the Valsalva maneuver, in which intrathoracic pressure is maintained at approximately 40 mm Hg for 10 to 12 seconds, is a useful test for left heart failure. The autonomic nervous system, operating in conjunction with the expanded volume of blood in the left side of the heart and pulmonary venous system, contributes to the abnormal response. During strain, the normal subject manifests a characteristic decrease in blood pressure and pulse pressure and increase in heart rate; when straining stops, the blood pressure, pulse pressure, and bradycardia "overshoot." In contrast, the patient in left heart failure demonstrates a "square wave response" of blood pressure: at the start of straining, blood pressure increases abruptly, stays high during the maneuver, and drops precipitously after the maneuver, without overshoot. Throughout the procedure there is little or no change in pulse pressure and no tachycardia. The lack of reflex changes stems from the failure of stroke output or arterial pulse pressure to change during the straining phase, so that no reflex changes are elicited in peripheral vessels.

Salt and Water Retention. As the patient slips into heart failure, the reduction in cardiac output is associated with a decrease in renal blood flow and glomerular filtration rate, and with a redistribution of blood flow within the kidneys. These hemodynamic changes undoubtedly contribute to the sodium and water retention of heart failure, but in different ways and to different degrees according to the stage of heart failure. Early in heart failure, when filtration rate is decreased, much of the sodium retention is attributable to the decrease in the filtered load of sodium presented to the tubules for reabsorption. Later on, humoral factors, predominantly hyperaldosteronism and a group of extra-adrenal, sodium-retaining influences ("factor III") predominate.

There is little doubt that disturbed hemodynamics are importantly involved in the release of the humoral factors. Thus a large role is currently envisaged for diminished baroreceptor stimulation in the renal afferent arterioles or a decrease in the sodium load passing the macula densa, or both, in activating the renin-angiotensin-aldosterone mechanism. In addition, baroreceptor effects arising in the distended left atrium or underfilled arterial tree may affect renal hemodynamics and the renin-angiotensin-aldosterone system. Other reflexes engaged in the intense sympathetic activity of heart failure may also be involved. Clearly, the hemodynamic-neurohumoral interplay that results in sodium and water retention is complex and incompletely understood. On the other hand, awareness of the important role of hyperaldosteronism in the genesis of sodium and water retention has provided new approaches to the therapy of heart failure using aldosterone antagonists.

Not only urine but also sweat and saliva are sodium poor. But the underlying mechanisms are different. Antidiuretic hormone is not directly involved in the genesis of the edema of heart failure.

The expansion of the circulating blood volume contributes to sustaining the cardiac output and the perfusion of vital organs. Rarely is the expansion in blood volume marked, usually ranging from 10 to 20 per cent in moderately severe heart failure to 30 to 50 per cent in severe, refractory heart failure. But even modest expansion helps to augment the ventricular end-diastolic volume, thereby improving ventricular performance by way of the Frank-Starling principle. Unfortunately, the high end-diastolic volume and pressures promote the formation of edema by raising capillary pressures in the circulation behind the failing ventricle. At a time when circulation blood volume may be increased by 20 per cent, the extravascular fluid volume may have doubled.

CLINICAL MANIFESTATIONS OF HEART FAILURE

The signs and symptoms of heart failure depend on the ventricle that has failed and the duration of the failure. The clinical syndrome of left ventricular failure is dominated by *symptoms* of pulmonary congestion and edema. In contrast, right ventricular failure is dominated by *signs* of systemic venous congestion and peripheral edema. Fatigue and weakness are common in both types of heart failure.

Left Ventricular Failure

Symptoms

Complaints of respiratory discomfort or distress dominate the symptoms of left ventricular failure. They vary with position, stress, and activity. They are often associated with physical signs of disturbances in the lungs or in respiratory control mechanisms.

Dyspnea. Like pain or anxiety, dyspnea is subjective and difficult to quantify. Because breathing is ordinarily automatic and effortless except after strenuous exertion, the complaint of breathlessness may signify anything from awareness to distress. Dyspnea during modest exertion is usually the first symptom of left heart failure. Usually dyspnea is associated with increased rate of breathing (tachypnea).

The physiologic basis for the sensation of dyspnea remains unclear. Both lungs and the chest muscles may contribute. Thus interstitial edema in the vicinity of the pulmonary capillaries stimulates juxtacapillary receptors ("J-receptors"), thereby reflexly setting a pattern of rapid, shallow breathing; associated with this abnormal pattern is an increase in the work and oxygen cost of moving the stiff lungs. However, this increased amount of work on the lungs is done in the face of diminished blood flow to the respiratory muscles, a consequence of the diminished cardiac output and redistribution of blood flow. Consequently, the disproportion between work done by the respiratory muscles and the supply of blood delivered to them may contribute to fatigue of the respiratory muscles and to the sensation of dyspnea. Sensory elements within the respiratory muscles may also contribute to respiratory discomfort by registering the disproportion between the inordinate amount of energy that is being spent by muscles and the amount of ventilation that they produce.

Although precise mechanisms for dyspnea remain uncertain, its occurrence in left heart failure clearly depends on the increase in the blood and water content of the lungs at the expense of the air volume. Ventilation increases as the air volume is progressively encroached upon, and, as the minute ventilation approaches the maximal ventilatory capacity, the likelihood of dyspnea increases.

Orthopnea. Progressive, and often urgent, dyspnea that occurs soon after lying flat is designated as orthopnea; it is relieved by sitting up. The physiologic basis for orthopnea is the augmented venous return from the lower extremities and splanchnic bed to the lungs that results from redistribution of gravitational forces in the supine position and the reabsorption of diurnal edema. In the patient with heart disease, orthopnea is reliable evidence of left ventricular failure. In contrast, the dyspnea of chronic lung disease or musculoskeletal disorders is rarely aggravated by lying flat.

The patient learns to avoid respiratory distress at night by supporting head and thorax by two or more pillows. In severe heart failure, orthopnea may force the patient to sleep upright in a chair rather than in bed. In some patients with extensive coronary artery disease and left ventricular failure, orthopnea occurs only in the left lateral position; the mechanism for this is unclear.

Cough and expectoration are common in left heart failure, presumably a consequence of reflexes from the congested lungs and bronchi. The patient may also manifest an orthopneic cough which has the same significance as orthopnea, and is presumably the consequence of venous congestion and edema of the tracheobronchial walls. In some patients, precordial distress may substitute for breathlessness in the supine position. This "nocturnal angina" is also somehow related to the mobilization of water from the tissues to the circulation when the patient goes to bed.

Paroxysmal Nocturnal Dyspnea. A bout of urgent respiratory distress, verging on suffocation, may rouse the patient unexpectedly from sleep and cause him to seek relief desperately, either by sitting up or by rushing to the open window to breathe "fresh air." Respiration may be labored and wheezing, hence the designation "cardiac asthma." The episodes represent intolerable aggravation of pulmonary congestion and edema during sleep in the supine position. A combination of dulling of the respiratory center to sensory input from the lungs during sleep and increase in venous return to the lungs makes it possible for pulmonary venous congestion and edema to accumulate to the point of precipitating the frightening episode of breathlessness.

Acute Pulmonary Edema. In an acute episode of left ventricular failure, such as that which follows myocardial infarction, the inability of the left ventricular myocardium to handle the blood that the competent right ventricle is delivering to it may result in an abrupt increase in pulmonary venous and capillary pressure, followed by flooding of the interstitial spaces and alveoli. If the edema is confined to the interstitial spaces of the lungs, an increase in respiratory frequency because of stiff lungs would be expected to produce alveolar hyperventilation and respiratory alkalosis; conversely, once free fluid enters the terminal bronchioles and mounts the respiratory tree, respiratory acidosis may occur because of imbalances between alveolar ventilation and alveolar blood flow (ventilation-perfusion inhomogeneities).

Pulmonary edema may begin with a cough, with wheezing, or with breathlessness. Often there is a sense of oppression in the chest. At first, except for the abnormal breathing pattern and the evidences of heart disease, there may be few physical signs. In time, as free fluid enters the distal airways, rales become audible, most marked in the dependent parts of the lungs, but extending upward as the attack worsens. In a severe attack, the patient is pale, sweating, cyanotic, obviously gasping for breath, and usually producing frothy sputum which may be blood tinged.

Hemoptysis. Rusty sputum, laden with heart failure cells (alveolar macrophages containing hemosiderin), occurs frequently in severe left heart failure. Frankly bloody sputum is generally a sign of pulmonary infarction. In severe pulmonary edema caused by left ventricular failure, the frothy fluid that pours from the bronchial tree is often pink, i.e., blood tinged, owing to the escape of red cells into the alveoli from the congested minute vessels of the lungs.

Cheyne-Stokes Respiration. Some patients with severe heart failure display periodic breathing characterized by alternate periods of apnea and hyperventilation. Cyclic changes in arterial blood gas tensions accompany this waxing and waning of the ventilation: during apnea, the arterial Po_2 reaches its peak, whereas the arterial Pco_2 reaches its nadir. At the same time, alveolar gas tensions are exactly opposite: the alveolar Po_2 reaches its peak during hyperpnea; the alveolar Pco_2 reaches its nadir during hyperpnea. This discrepancy between arterial and alveolar gas tensions has been attributed to the fact that changes in arterial blood gases *cause* the swings in ventilation, whereas the changes in alveolar gas tension are the *consequences* of the changes in ventilation. The critical role of the arterial blood gases stems from the prolonged circulation time between the lungs and the respiratory centers in the brain. This slowing of the circulation exposes the central respiratory control mechanisms to arterial blood that differs in gaseous composition from that in pulmonary venous blood. In essence, because of slowing of the circulation, negative feedback is delayed. As expected, the longer the circulation time, the longer the cycles of hyperventilation and apnea. The neurologic and cerebrovascular changes of old age predispose to Cheyne-Stokes breathing.

Physical Signs

In addition to being breathless, the patient is generally pale, a bit dusky, and sweaty. His handshake is cold because of peripheral vasoconstriction. The heart rate is rapid and the pulse pressure is narrow, with a modest increase in diastolic blood pressure. If only the left ventricle has failed, the neck veins are not distended.

The Heart. Enlargement of the heart is usually evident to inspection and palpation of the apical impulse and is confirmed by roentgenologic and radiographic examination. Angina pectoris is not a manifestation of heart failure, nor is palpitation common unless overzealous administration of digitalis and diuretics has occasioned digitalis toxicity. As the left ventricle fails and pulmonary venous pressure increases, pulmonary arterial pressure also increases, and the heart sound attributable to pulmonary valve closure increases in intensity. Also, as the left ventricle dilates, the mitral valve leaflets fail to appose properly, resulting in mild mitral incompetence.

Gallop Rhythm. The advent of a third heart sound during diastole in an adult with heart disease signifies the advent of heart failure. The fixed sequence of the two normal sounds and the abnormal third sound, in conjunction with an increase in heart rate, is responsible for the characteristic cadence of a gallop rhythm. The third heart sound ("S-3 gallop") occurs early in diastole during the state of rapid ventricular filling. This ventricular gallop presumably originates in the vibrations of the ventricular walls as the rapidly inflowing blood is abruptly arrested; this extra sound, normal in young children and in young adults, is generally a reliable sign of ventricular failure in the middle-aged or elderly patient with heart disease.

A gallop rhythm may also originate in the atrial contribution to ventricular filling. This atrial or "S-4 gallop" is not unique for heart failure, because it may reflect diminished ventricular compliance resulting from hypertrophy or ischemia rather than myocardial failure. If a patient with a fourth heart sound develops heart failure, a third sound appears to cause a quadruple rhythm. If the heart rate is rapid or the P-R interval is prolonged, the atrial and ventricular gallop sounds summate ("summation gallop"). In the candidate for heart failure, summation gallop has the same implication as other diastolic gallop rhythms, particularly if it persists as the heart is slowed.

Pulsus Alternans. In patients with heart disease, particularly if the cause is hypertension, cardiomyopathy, or coronary arteriosclerosis, the appearance of alternating strong and weak beats, even though the fundamental rhythm remains regular, heralds the onset of heart failure. This pulsus alternans may be detected by palpation or by sphygmomanometry. It often follows an extrasystole. Rarely is this mechanical alternans associated with electrical alternans. The mechanism for pulsus alternans has been attributed to alternations in fiber length (ventricular end-diastolic volume) or to alternating increase and decrease in the number of contractile units, or to both.

The Lungs. A characteristic consequence of interstitial edema and pulmonary venous congestion is tachypnea. As left heart failure progresses, interstitial edema is succeeded by alveolar edema and fluid in the terminal bronchioles, particularly at the lung bases. Accordingly, bilateral basal rales are common in moderate failure of the left ventricle.

Electrocardiogram

Abnormalities in the electrocardiogram arise from the underlying cardiac disorder and from therapeutic agents, e.g., digitalis and diuretics, rather than from heart failure, per se.

Radiologic Aspects

The x-ray can be exceedingly helpful in the diagnosis of left ventricular failure. Typically, the cardiac silhouette is enlarged, often assuming telltale configurations that are determined by the underlying disorder. In contrast to the normal, in which pulmonary *arteries* are prominent in the lower lung fields, pulmonary vasculature is prominent at the apices, reflecting pulmonary *venous* hypertension and redistribution of blood flow because of edema and fibrosis at the bases. Enlarged hilar shadows accompany the prominent pulmonary veins in the upper lung fields.

Prominent septal lines, particularly near the costophrenic angles (Kerley's lines), indicate the presence of interstitial edema. The advent of alveolar edema is signaled by a generalized clouding of the lung fields. Pleural effusion may occasionally occur in left heart failure, but is much more apt to occur in biventricular heart failure. Evidence of interstitial and alveolar edema often lessens or disappears when right ventricular failure supervenes. However, hydrothorax generally persists. A widened shadow of the superior vena cava may provide reliable evidence of right ventricular failure and systemic venous congestion.

Pulmonary Function Tests

Traditionally, the course of overt failure of the left ventricle, particularly the response to treatment, has been followed by consecutive determinations of vital capacity. This is an insensitive measure, usually associated with decrease in compliance and occasionally with increase in airway resistance. Recently it has been shown that earlier in the course of pulmonary edema—presumably when the excess fluid is still confined to the interstitial space around alveoli and terminal airways (less than 2 mm in diameter)—expiratory flow rates at *low lung volumes* are reduced and peripheral airways tend to close prematurely during expiration, trapping gas within the lungs and disturbing the distribution of alveolar gas with respect to pulmonary capillary blood. This has led to a variety of tests (e.g., "closing volumes") which are designed to detect premature closure and resultant maldistribution of air—presumably by interstitial edema—long before compliance falls and total resistance of airways increases. During recovery there is usually a delay before expiratory flow rates and closing volumes return to normal, even though left atrial pressure is again within normal limits. The basis for the persistent abnormalities is presumably the gradual removal of interstitial edema from the vicinity of the small airways and blood vessels.

Associated with the high closing volume is evidence of ventilation-perfusion abnormalities manifested by widening of the alveolar-arterial ΔP_{O_2} and a decrease in arterial P_{O_2} caused by "venous admixture." Nonetheless, arterial oxygen saturation is generally near normal unless independent lung disease is present. Along with the decrease in arterial P_{O_2} is a widening of the arterial venous difference in O_2 content owing to the increased extraction of oxygen in the tissues. Arterial CO_2 tension remains normal or low unless free fluid enters the terminal airways in the course of pulmonary edema. Abnormally high values for CO_2 tension indicate that considerable free fluid has made its way into the airways.

Right Ventricular Failure

Clinical Manifestations

Isolated failure of the right ventricle is uncommon, generally a consequence of cor pulmonale secondary to intrinsic lung disease. More often, right ventricular failure is a sequel to left ventricular failure. In right ventricular failure, neck veins are distended and fill from below; the engorged liver may be tender to gentle pressure, and compression causes a surge of blood into the neck veins (hepatojugular reflux). In time, when both ventricles have failed, evidence of right ventricular failure may dominate the scene; but continuing dyspnea and rales attest to the persistence of left ventricular failure, and the continuing low cardiac output is manifested by signs of increased sympathetic nervous activity and of organ hypoperfusion.

Weakness may be marked and is occasionally associated with anorexia, weight loss, and malnutrition ("cardiac cachexia"). Not only severe heart failure, but also digitalis, diuretics, and electrolyte disturbances are generally involved in the genesis of this cachectic state.

Cyanosis. Bluish discoloration of the skin and mucous membranes is designated as cyanosis. It is due to an abnormal concentration of reduced hemoglobin (more than 5 grams per 100 ml) in the subpapillary venous plexus of the skin. In right heart failure, the congested venules, containing blood from which considerable oxygen has been extracted because of the slow flow, account for the cyanosis. In left heart failure, cyanosis is usually caused

by a complication, e.g., pneumonia, unless overt pulmonary edema is present.

Abnormal Heart and Lungs. Although the breathlessness of the left ventricular failure may be somewhat relieved by right heart failure, usually some dyspnea persists along with tachypnea and basal rales. Severe right heart failure (and dilatation) may produce tricuspid valvular insufficiency, thereby contributing to systemic venous engorgement. The murmur of tricuspid insufficiency is distinguished from that of mitral insufficiency by its location (lower left border of sternum) and by its tendency to increase during inspiration. Hydrothorax, generally unilateral, is more common than in isolated left ventricular failure.

Systemic Venous Congestion. Distention of systemic veins is a hallmark of right heart failure. Several different mechanisms contribute to its genesis: (1) the inability of the failing right ventricle to cope adequately with the venous return; (2) the increase in the quantity of blood contained in the large systemic veins; and (3) increased venomotor tone, resulting from heightened sympathetic nervous activity. The increase in systemic venous pressure underlies the hepatomegaly, splenomegaly, and peripheral edema that characterize right heart failure. Less apparent are the congestion and edema of the gastrointestinal tract that the systemic venous hypertension produces.

Pressure in the superficial jugular vein is a useful index of right atrial pressure and, with experience, may be reliably estimated from the height of the fluid column distending the cervical vein. Normally, the cervical veins are flat in the erect position, whereas in right heart failure they are prominent and distended, usually with a level that pulsates. Functional tricuspid insufficiency, complicating dilatation of the right heart, distorts the normal venous pulse by increasing its v wave. Usually superficial venous distention precedes the onset of hepatomegaly and peripheral edema. Occasionally, compression of the abdomen over the liver (hepatojugular reflux) is necessary to display the increased blood volume in the venous system.

Liver. The liver is usually enlarged and palpable in right heart failure, often in association with mild abdominal discomfort, and generally somewhat tender to compression. In severe right heart failure, particularly if the onset is acute, constraint of the swollen liver by its tight capsule may cause right upper quadrant pain. Tricuspid insufficiency accompanying right ventricular dilatation may cause synchronous pulsations in neck veins and liver. Splenomegaly is uncommon except in prolonged congestion of the liver. Rarely is the enlarged spleen tender from congestion per se.

Early in hepatic congestion, sensitive liver function tests, such as the handling of Bromsulphalein, are apt to be abnormal, and modest increases in the concentrations of cellular enzymes in serum, such as glutamic oxaloacetic transaminase (SGOT) increases in serum bilirubin, are not uncommon. The hyperbilirubinemia consists of a combination of quick- and slow-reacting bilirubin, presumably a consequence of decreased oxygen delivery to the liver arising from hypoperfusion and venous hypertension. But jaundice is uncommon unless hepatic congestion is associated with longstanding pulmonary congestion and, often, with pulmonary infarction.

If cardiac output is severely curtailed and liver congestion is marked and protracted, hypoglycemia may occur, presumably owing to depletion of glycogen stores in the liver and increased formation of lactic acid from glucose because of hypoxia. During physical activity, hepatic blood flow in heart failure decreases further, resulting in a marked decrease in aldosterone breakdown, thereby furthering sodium retention.

Repeated bouts of right heart failure elicit atrophy and necrosis of liver cells in the vicinity of the central veins and stimulate extensive fibrosis ("cardiac cirrhosis"). Many months of reduced hepatic blood flow and high venous pressures are required for this reaction, which may result in a shrunken, fibrotic liver difficult to distinguish from posthepatitic cirrhosis. Hepatic coma is a rare, preterminal complication of severe hepatic congestion and fibrosis.

Extracellular Fluid Compartments. In normal subjects, the fluid compartments of the body are held remarkably constant as the result of an automatic interplay among *intake* (governed by thirst and appetite), *transcellular exchanges* of fluid and electrolytes (governed by passive and active mechanisms), and *excretion* (regulated mainly by the kidneys). In heart failure, this automatic balance tends to be upset mainly because of inordinate retention of salt and water by the kidneys. The result is an isosmotic expansion of the extracellular fluid in which the circulating blood volume shares. It is conceivable that early in heart failure the conservation of salt and water may serve a useful purpose by expanding the blood volume either to sustain venous return to the failing heart or to relieve the arterial baroreceptors from undue stimulation as the cardiac output fails. But this teleologic explanation does not apply when the myocardium can no longer respond to increased filling pressures and volumes, and the retention of salt and water only aggravates congestion and edema.

The distribution of the excess extracellular fluid varies from patient to patient. In the patient who is up and about, edema accumulates in the feet and ankles under the influence of gravity; in the bedridden patient, the fluid shifts to the sacral region. Low tissue pressure, as around the back of the ankle, predisposes to localization. The level of colloid osmotic pressure and the integrity of the lymphatic system also influence the distribution of the excess fluid.

Subcutaneous Edema. Dependent edema, manifested as swelling of feet or ankles, developing gradually during the day and subsiding by morning, is a characteristic feature of right heart failure. Invariably, it is anteceded by systemic venous congestion, but after diuresis subcutaneous edema may linger even though systemic venous hypertension has been relieved by the reduction in venous blood volume. Usually a gain in weight precedes clinical evidence of edema. If edema is allowed to persist, complications such as low-grade cellulitis may occur. The combination of edema and slowed venous flow predisposes to thrombosis and to pulmonary embolism. The massive pitting edema of the lower extremities that was commonly seen before the advent of potent diuretics is now rarely encountered except in instances of gross neglect.

Hydrothorax. It is so uncommon for hydrothorax to complicate isolated failure of the right ventricle, that the association of pleural effusion and cor pulmonale should lead to search for an independent mechanism for the pleural effusion, e.g., pulmonary infarction. On the other hand, as indicated previously, it is quite common in combined heart failure (right and left). The pathogenesis of hydrothorax involves impaired removal of water from the pleural space because of high venous pressures in both the pulmonary and systemic circulations, thereby not only compromising transcapillary exchange of water in the pleura but also impeding lymphatic drainage. Hydrothorax contributes to dyspnea not only by encroaching on the air volume but also reflexly, probably by stimuli from lungs and chest wall. Pulmonary infarction may cause pleural effusion in two ways: by direct contiguity of the infarcted area of the lung and the pleural space, or by aggravation of heart failure.

Ascites. Clinically evident excess of free fluid in the abdominal cavity is designated as ascites. It is a late manifestation of right heart failure, generally associated with marked systemic venous hypertension, severe peripheral edema, and hydrothorax. It occurs most frequently in patients with tricuspid valvular disease (or with constrictive pericarditis). Portal and hepatic venous hypertension, coupled with high pressure in the systemic veins draining the peritoneum, seem to be involved in the etiology of ascites; but retention of salt and water is a fundamental prerequisite for ascites to occur. Usually ascites is first noticed by the patient as a gradual increase in abdominal girth. But in severe right heart failure, it may cause anorexia, abdominal discomfort, or pain.

Pericardial Effusion. In severe and persistent heart failure, abnormal quantities of transudate may accumulate in the pericardial sac. Rarely does fluid accumulate to the level of tamponade.

Anasarca. Massive right heart failure may cause excess fluid to accumulate everywhere in the body, most conspicuously in subcutaneous tissues and abdominal and thoracic cavities. Because of the influence of gravity, face and arms are spared until preterminally.

Gastrointestinal Tract. The bowel wall shares in the systemic venous congestion and edema. These changes rarely interfere with absorption of drugs or foods unless heart failure is extreme. In severe congestive heart failure, anorexia, nausea, and vomiting may occur from reflex, central, or local causes. Occasionally, when right heart failure is severe, a protein-losing enteropathy may develop.

Brain. Neurasthenia, headache, and insomnia are common in heart failure. Usually these manifestations are attributed to a combination of a modest diminution of cerebral blood flow and triggering mechanisms, e.g., dyspnea contributing to insomnia. Cerebral manifestations are more frequent when the reduction in cerebral blood flow is superimposed on antecedent cerebrovascular disease, e.g., arteriosclerosis, or personality disorder. Severe heart failure is often associated with irritability, restlessness, and difficulty in fixing attention, particularly in older persons. Preterminally, stupor and coma may develop. The possibility exists that central nervous abnormalities may be enhanced by the delivery to the brain of abnormal products elaborated by remote organs (liver, endocrines, gastrointestinal tract) that suffer deranged metabolism during heart failure as a result of congestion and hypoperfusion.

Kidney. Oliguria occurs in both right and left heart failure but is much more striking in the latter. As the heart improves, urinary output increases. The urine is poor in sodium but has a high specific gravity (1.020 to 1.030). Azotemia is common but generally moderate except when intrinsic renal disease is present or after vigorous diuresis. The combination of azotemia and high specific gravity is distinctive for heart failure (and dehydration) and contrasts with the low specific gravity of intrinsic renal disease. Proteinuria is common but rarely severe—usually less than 1 gram per day. A variety of casts accompany the proteinuria. Renal function, as determined by clearance techniques, is only slightly depressed except in severe right heart failure of long standing.

Other Manifestations.   In severe congestive heart failure, the accumulation of edema may obscure the gradual loss of tissue mass. Often this tissue wasting is associated with *weakness*. In extreme instances, *cachexia* may develop. At this late stage, the patient is usually suffering from anorexia, gastrointestinal upsets, anemia, and electrolyte upsets. Part of the picture undoubtedly stems from organ hypoperfusion and congestion, but often a large contribution has been made by overvigorous use of diuretics and digitalis.

Anxiety.   It is not surprising that patients with organic heart disease become anxious. Indeed, anxiety is a regular feature by the time the heart fails. But not always is it an easy matter to distinguish between cardiac complaints as manifestations of anxiety or of the cardiac disorder. Part of the difficulty stems from the nonspecific nature of complaints, such as breathlessness, especially if the patient does have organic heart disease. The difficulty is compounded if the patient misinterprets or exaggerates his symptoms unconsciously. For example, the severely anxious patient may hyperventilate to the point of alkalosis, producing the characteristic lightheadedness, cold hands, and tingling fingers of hypocapnia, reduced cerebral blood flow, and peripheral vasoconstriction, thereby reinforcing his view of the organic nature of his breathlessness. Palpitation is also commonly misinterpreted by the patient suffering from anxiety as a telltale sign of organic heart disease.

The standard approach for the physician is the separate assessment of the organic versus the psychosomatic aspects of the heart disease. Particularly helpful in this regard are excessive or inconsistent complaints for the extent of the cardiac disease. Not infrequently, hemodynamic measurements may be required to settle the role of organic heart disease in producing the clinical symptoms.

CLINICAL MANAGEMENT

General Measures

The aim of treatment in heart failure is to arrest and reverse the pathogenic sequence that led to the clinical signs and symptoms. The response to treatment of the more common types of heart failure, i.e., hypertensive and arteriosclerotic, is often dramatic. But each relapse marks another milestone on the road to refractory heart failure, not only by signaling progressive deterioration of the myocardium, but also because intensified and protracted treatment enhances the prospect for eliciting the toxic manifestations of the therapeutic agents.

Increasing Cardiac Output.   In most forms of chronic heart failure, the cardiac output can be made to increase by decreasing the cardiac load, by improving myocardial contractility, or by a combination of the two. In the patient with severe bradycardia associated with heart failure, acceleration of the heart rate by cardiac pacing may cure heart failure that would otherwise be refractory. Conversely, severe tachycardia must be arrested if filling times of the ventricles are too greatly curtailed by the abbreviated diastole.

Decreasing the Work of the Heart.   The excess load on the heart may be in the form of pressure, e.g., arterial hypertension, or volume, e.g., the physiologic expansion of the blood volume in late pregnancy. Lightening the load is prerequisite for a successful cardiotonic program. In recent years, serious attention has been paid to decreasing the pressure load during heart failure by administering vasodilator agents. But rarely is specific antihypertensive therapy necessary unless hypertension antedated the heart failure and persists after heart failure is relieved. If hypertension led to heart failure, small doses of ganglionic blocking agents may be helpful.

Rest is an effective way to decrease the cardiac burden in conventional types of heart failure. Rest must be both physical and mental; after recovery from an acute bout of heart failure, a new life style of lessened activity may be required as part of the cardiotonic program. Reassurance is essential, because anxiety automatically augments metabolic activity and induces peripheral arterial constriction. Should reassurance prove inadequate, sedatives or tranquilizers (such as chloral hydrate, 0.5 to 1.0 gram, phenobarbital, 15 to 30 mg, or diazepam, 2 to 10 mg, taken orally three times per day and at bedtime) may be needed to promote mental ease, particularly as the patient improves and grows restless. Narcotics are rarely needed in heart failure unless pulmonary edema has generated intolerable anxiety. Excessive sedation, to the point of immobilizing the patient, enhances the risk of venous thrombosis and embolism, particularly in the elderly.

In left heart failure, the sitting or semisitting position, either in bed or in a chair, usually relieves tachypnea and dyspnea. Oxygen by nasal catheter (4 to 6 liters per minute) also seems to make the patient more comfortable even though hypoxemia is generally mild in heart failure. Finally, mental rest is impossible if urinary retention and constipation are unattended.

It is remarkable how often the proper use of rest as the initial step in treatment will promote a vigorous diuresis, slow the heart rate, and relieve dyspnea, thereby allowing a more leisurely use of other cardiotonic agents, such as digitalis and diuretics. On the other hand, if metabolic demands remain high, as during undetected thyrotoxicosis or fever, heart failure may prove refractory to the conventional cardiotonic program until the thyroid overactivity is curtailed.

Acute Pulmonary Edema

Treatment of the acute pulmonary edema of left ventricular failure is begun with the patient in the sitting position, thereby draining the upper portions of his lungs of excess fluid. Meperidine, 50 mg, or morphine, 10 to 15 mg, is administered intravenously for restlessness or dyspnea. These agents seem to act primarily by relieving anxiety and agitation. Morphine is the traditional agent, but distressing side effects, such as nausea, vomiting, and urinary retention, have detracted from its popularity. Dramatic and immediate relief may be accomplished by reducing venous return to the right heart; this may be done by one or two small phlebotomies (250 ml of blood), by rotating tourniquets (releasing one at a time for five minutes every half hour), or by intermittent positive pressure breathing which raises pleural pressure, thereby impeding venous return. A rapid-acting diuretic, ethacrynic acid or furosemide, is administered intravenously. Even though arterial oxygenation may be near normal, high concentrations of humidified oxygen, 50 to 100 per cent, are frequently used empirically to relieve dyspnea, restlessness, and confusion. Severe hypotension is a contraindication to phlebotomy and to assisted ventilation.

Digitalis (digoxin or lanatoside C, 1.0 mg) may be administered intravenously if the patient has had none during the preceding two weeks. However, the urgency for intravenous injection of digitalis has decreased considerably since the advent of potent, rapid-acting diuretics. An exception to this generalization is the attack of pulmonary edema precipitated by a bout of tachycardia which can be slowed by digitalis, e.g., paroxysmal atrial fibrillation. In this instance, digitalis relieves the heart failure primarily because of its effect on slowing atrioventricular conduction, and consequently the ventricular rate, rather than because of its inotropic effect on the heart. In ectopic tachycardias, it may be necessary to resort to DC electroshock in order to restore normal heart action and tolerable heart rates.

Face to face with a patient in pulmonary edema, the physician often feels compelled to apply a battery of strenuous measures in rapid succession or simultaneously. Especially for patients in poor condition, this treatment may be worse than the disorder which is usually self-limited once the upright position has been assumed, mental rest accomplished, and a potent diuretic administered. As soon as the crisis is over, a more conventional cardiotonic program is begun, and a search is made for the cause of the left heart failure as well as for the mechanism that precipitated the episode.

The role of left heart failure in producing high-altitude pulmonary edema is not clear. Prompt recovery usually follows bed rest, descent to lower altitude, and the administration of oxygen.

Inotropic Agents: Digitalis

Although immediate therapeutic agents for coping with the acute episode of heart failure may not include digitalis, once the crisis is over, lasting improvement almost invariably requires the use of digitalis glycosides. Unfortunately, establishing the proper dose of digitalis is not always straightforward, because optimal doses vary somewhat from patient to patient and with associated clinical disorders. Moreover, unless standard brands of predictable potency are prescribed, tablets may vary considerably in effectiveness. Finally, the concomitant administration of other, apparently unrelated, medications may lead to drug interactions which interfere with the effects of the digitalis.

Drug Interactions. Multiplicity of drugs is the rule in modern therapy. Some drugs are deliberately prescribed in combinations, either to reinforce a desirable therapeutic effect or to avoid an untoward side effect. A familiar example of this practice is the combination of digitalis, a potassium-losing diuretic, and potassium supplements for the treatment of heart failure; the dosage of each is individualized to achieve maximal inotropic effect on the heart and to relieve circulatory congestion. But other drugs, such as sleeping pills and anticoagulants that are administered concomitantly for subsidiary or unrelated purposes, may interact and decrease the effectiveness of the cardiotonic program.

There are several ways by which one therapeutic agent can influence the effects of another. Among these are (1) chemical interaction (cholestyramine, a cholesterol-lowering, ion-exchange resin, impedes absorption of digitoxin [and, to a much lesser extent, of digoxin] by binding in the intestine); (2) competition for binding sites on plasma proteins (digitoxin and ethacrynic acid compete for albumin); (3) induction of drug-metabolizing enzymes (phenobarbital and phenylbutazone enhance the metabolism of digitoxin by hepatic microsomal enzymes); and (4) enhanced excretion (polar metabolites of digitoxin are eliminated more rapidly in urine and bile than is digitoxin per se). In conventional dosages, few of these interactions seem to be clinically significant even though cholestyramine has been advocated in treating digitoxin intoxication. But they do introduce an element of unpredictability into standard therapeutic programs, and they do urge caution whenever medications are either added to or deleted from a stable therapeutic regimen.

Related to the concept of drug interaction is the broader concept of drug-biologic interaction which determines how drugs act. This broader concept includes reactions between the pharmacologic agent and some biologic aspect of the living subject. For example, digitalis effects depend heavily on ion fluxes at ultrastructural membranes; changes in ionic composition and behavior are known to modify the clinical influence of digitalis. Or the physiologic state of the patient may shape the response: acidosis blunts the effectiveness of norepinephrine; the administration of a conventional dose of a ganglionic blocking agent, when sympathetic vasomotor tone is high because of vigorous diuresis and depletion of blood volume, may precipitate circulatory collapse.

The concept of drug-biologic interaction is complicated by individual variability in responsiveness to drugs. Part of this variability is undoubtedly inherited; part is immunologic; most remains to be explained.

Digitalis: General Aspects. Digitalis improves the contractility of the failing myocardium regardless of the type of heart failure, the rate, or the rhythm. After digitalis has been given in effective doses and myocardial contractility has increased, the heart shrinks in size, cardiac output increases, end-diastolic volume and pressure decrease, venous pressure normalizes, and evidences of peripheral vasoconstriction, circulatory congestion, and organ hypoperfusion disappear. In the reordering of the circulation that follows relief of congestive heart failure, blood that had been sequestered in the splanchnic venous bed is redirected to the systemic veins by appropriate adjustments in vascular tone, thereby helping to sustain the improved cardiac output.

Molecular Bases. Although the full picture of how the digitalis glycosides improve cardiac contractility is not yet clear, they do seem to act by altering surface and intracellular (sarcoplasmic reticulum and mitochondria) membranes so that they release calcium ions more readily. Another manifestation of a change in cellular membrane characteristics caused by the glycosides is inhibition of the Na^+-K^+-ATPase activity. However, it is unsettled whether this interference with ATPase, as well as the associated decrease of sodium pumping into the cell, is directly related to the inotropic effect of the glycosides.

Effect on Inotropic State. In low output heart failure, digitalis increases the cardiac output and restores the end-diastolic pressure in the left ventricle to normal.

This is a consequence of increased myocardial contractility. A similar effect on contractility occurs in the normal myocardium, but the cardiac output does not increase because of a direct vasoconstricting effect of digitalis on the peripheral resistance vessels. But in low output heart failure in which sympathetic nervous activity is consistently high, restoration of the cardiac output by digitalis reflexly diminishes sympathetic tone, thereby overriding the direct vasoconstricting effects of digitalis on the vessels. These distinctions underscore the unique property of digitalis glycosides as inotropic agents because of their ability to improve myocardial contractility in heart failure without simultaneously eliciting antagonistic effects, such as peripheral vasoconstriction (or tachycardia).

Myocardial Oxygen Consumption. The increase in the strength of contraction produced by the digitalis glycosides increases the oxygen consumption of the myocardium in the normal heart. But this tendency is neutralized in the failing heart which responds to glycosides by shrinking in volume, thereby reducing wall tension and its associated oxygen consumption. Accordingly, the increase in contractility produced in the dilated failing heart is generally accomplished with no increase in myocardial oxygen consumption.

Catecholamine Depletion. Although reduction in cardiac catecholamines is a feature of chronic heart failure, this depletion leaves unaffected the positive inotropic effects of the digitalis glycosides.

Coronary Circulation. In the normal unanesthetized animal, ouabain elicits coronary vasoconstriction. Unfortunately, nothing is known about the behavior of the coronary circulation in response to digitalis during heart failure.

Systemic Circulation. Digitalis elicits an increase in cardiac output, thereby reducing the reflex vasoconstriction of the low output state. But because of the direct constrictor action of cardiac glycosides on vascular smooth muscle, there is apt to be a brief period of increase in systemic arterial pressure, particularly if large doses of cardiac glycosides are administered intravenously.

Choice of Digitalis Preparation. Five digitalis preparations are in common use today in the United States: digitalis leaf, digoxin, digitoxin, deslanoside (Cedilanid-D), and ouabain. Their basic pharmacologic actions on the heart and their toxic-therapeutic ratios are quite similar. But they do differ considerably with respect to the rate and degree of absorption from the intestine and both the onset and duration of action.

Digoxin and digitoxin have replaced digitalis leaf for chronic oral administration; ouabain and deslanoside, as well as digoxin, are administered intravenously. Digitoxin is not as satisfactory an intravenous agent, because it is relatively slow in reaching its peak effect. Digitalis leaf is gradually disappearing from use, because it varies in potency, requires bioassay for standardization, and has no therapeutic advantage over digitoxin which is its principal constituent.

Traditional practice in digitalization has relied on a preliminary loading phase to achieve a therapeutic level, followed by maintenance dosage to sustain a balance between intake and elimination. Accordingly, the preset loading dose is administered over a period of one to three days (Table 1), providing enough digitalis to load body stores and to compensate for daily elimination. Unless a desperate situation—such as a life-threatening cardiac arrhythmia—calls for acute digitalization, slow digitalization is preferable. Indeed, if there is no hurry, continued administration of the maintenance dose, without a loading dose, has proved to be a practical way to achieve digitalization.

Dosages listed in Table 1 are intended to indicate orders of magnitude rather than precise schedules. Dosage is determined individually according to the nature and severity of the heart disease, the clinical setting, the use of other drugs such as potassium-losing diuretics, and continued observation of the patient's response.

Oral Preparations. Digoxin and digitoxin have replaced digitalis leaf for chronic oral administration.

DIGOXIN. The maintenance dosage of digoxin is determined by a balance between renal excretion, dose, and absorption. Ordinarily, between 75 and 90 per cent of an oral dose is absorbed. Digoxin is lipid soluble and absorbed from the small intestine by diffusion. Some variation in absorption may occur, depending on the solubility of digoxin molecules in the intestinal fluids. Variability in absorption may also result from different preparations of digoxin. Consequently, once a digoxin preparation from one manufacturer has proved effective, changes should be avoided.

Digoxin is excreted primarily by the kidney, and most of the drug appears unchanged in the urine. When fully digitalized, the concentration of digoxin in serum is approximately 1 per cent or less of total body stores of digoxin. If renal function is normal, approximately one

TABLE 1.   Administration of Common Cardiac Glycosides

| Preparation | Digitalization | | | Cardiotonic Effects | | Blood Levels | |
	Loading Dose* (mg/24 hrs)	Initial Dose† (mg)	Maintenance Dose (mg)	Onset of Activity (min)	Peak Effect (hrs)	Steady State Therapeutic Level¶ (mg/ml)	Half-Life (hrs)
Digoxin (oral)	2.5	1.0	0.25	60–120	1–3	1.5	36
Digitoxin (oral)	1.2	0.75‡	0.1	30–120	4–6	17	96–144
Deslanoside (IV)	1.6	0.8§	–	10–30	1–2	–	33
Ouabain (IV)	0.25	0.25§	–	3–10	0.5–2	0.5	21

(These values are examples to illustrate orders of magnitude.)

*Total quantity to be administered in 24 hours for therapeutic effect.
†Assuming no prior digitalis during previous two weeks.
‡The same dose may be administered intravenously if urgent digitalization is required.
§When feasible, switch to oral maintenance doses of digoxin or digitoxin.
¶On conventional maintenance doses.

TABLE 2. Features of Cardiac Glycoside Preparations in Common Use

Preparation	Source	Usual Route of Administration*	Gastrointestinal Absorption	Protein Binding†	Principal Route of Elimination
Digoxin	*Digitalis lanata*	Oral	75–90%‡	23%‡	Kidneys
Digitoxin	*Digitalis purpurea*	Oral	90–100%	97%	Liver; kidney for metabolites
Deslanoside	*Digitalis lanata*	Intravenous	Erratic	—	Kidneys
Ouabain	*Strophanthus gratus*	Intravenous	Erratic	0	Kidneys

(These values are examples to illustrate orders of magnitude.)

*All can be administered intravenously.

†Affinity for protein (albumin) determines rate of urinary excretion and persistence in body.

‡Varies according to preparation. Different tablets differ in bioavailability of digoxin.

third of the body stores is eliminated per day; the maintenance dose replenishes this daily loss. The half-life of digoxin in serum is approximately the same in normal subjects and in patients with heart failure, averaging one and one half days. However, the half-life is prolonged in renal failure. The serum level of digoxin in renal insufficiency is directly related to the creatinine clearance and inversely to the concentration of urea nitrogen in the blood (BUN). Formulas have been devised to take these relationships into account, recognizing that, in contrast to the normal daily elimination of one third of body stores of digoxin, the anuric patient eliminates about one seventh. Accordingly, the anuric patient will require one half or less of the usual maintenance dose.

Only 5 per cent of digoxin in serum is bound to protein. Its polar structure accounts for the difference between its concentration and that of digitoxin (nonpolar) in the serum (Table 2).

Without an initial loading dose, patients receiving digoxin orally reach a steady state in the serum, reflecting equilibrium between body stores, intake, and elimination in about one week. The steady state level in serum is approximately 1 per cent or less of total body stores of digoxin. Body stores are related to lean body weight, because digoxin does not accumulate in fat or interstitial fluid. In an adult patient, body stores are generally of the order of 0.01 mg per kilogram of body weight. Rarely are body stores required greater than 0.02 mg per kilogram of body weight. Therefore for a 70 kg patient, digitalization usually requires a minimal dose of approximately 0.7 mg. Should this digitalizing dose be exceeded in order to achieve better control of the clinical state, the prospects for toxicity will increase accordingly.

The essential features in using digoxin therapeutically are summarized in Table 1. Because of its short half-life, a single dose per day will cause a wide swing in serum concentration (and in body stores, including the heart) before the next dose is administered. In practice this swing is often unimportant; but, if desirable, its magnitude may be reduced (and therapeutic control improved) by administering one half the daily dose at 12-hour intervals. Many clinicians use digoxin for intravenous as well as oral administration, because its hemodynamic and biologic properties are comparatively well understood, and dosages are relatively easy to adjust.

DIGITOXIN. This agent is widely used for chronic administration. It differs importantly from digoxin in its metabolism and its slow rate of elimination; the main route of elimination is by metabolism in the liver, only a small fraction being eliminated by the kidney.

Digitoxin is completely absorbed after oral administration so that oral and intravenous dosages are identical. Body stores and digitalizing doses are approximately the same, but maintenance doses are quite different because of different rates of elimination. Approximately 12 per cent of body stores of digitoxin is eliminated per day in patients with normal renal function. The usual body store is estimated to be of the order of 0.8 mg in a 70-kg adult. Therefore the daily maintenance dose is generally 0.1 mg per day (0.12 × 0.8 mg). Because of its slow dissipation and elimination, serum levels of digitoxin vary less from hour to hour than do digoxin levels. But the drug accumulates insidiously so that maintenance doses established at the onset often prove to be toxic in time.

In contrast to digoxin, digitoxin has a strong avidity for albumin so that 97 per cent in plasma is nondialyzable. This combination is a critical factor in limiting glomerular filtration and excretion of digitoxin by the kidneys. After an oral dose of 1.0 mg, 50 per cent of the inotropic effect is reached in one hour; 85 to 100 per cent is achieved in four hours and sustained for the rest of the day. The average half-life is approximately five days. Digitoxin enters into an enterohepatic cycle. Between 30 and 60 per cent of the 1.0 mg dose is eliminated in the feces and urine, the larger fraction generally in the urine. The remainder is metabolized, primarily to digoxin, which is eliminated in the urine. Digoxin is preferable to digitoxin in renal or hepatic insufficiency.

Intravenous Preparations. As a rule, these are reserved for life-threatening situations. These include acute heart failure complicating a bout of atrial fibrillation with rapid ventricular rate, fulminating pulmonary edema as a complication of left ventricular failure, and the onset of heart failure or a serious arrhythmia during surgery. As a rule, the larger the dose of the glycoside, the more apt it is to create problems, particularly arrhythmias, of its own.

An intravenous bolus of a digitalis preparation may elicit a bout of hypertension, particularly if the dose is large, e.g., 1.0 mg of digoxin. The increase is generally of the order of 20/10, and the effect is generally short lived. But it may suffice to overburden the failing heart and to aggravate the situation until it subsides and is succeeded by the inotropic effect. Hypertension is rarely a problem if the intravenous dose is modest and administered slowly.

OUABAIN. This is the traditional digitalis preparation for intravenous use. It is a pure crystalline substance that is unsuitable for oral use because of erratic absorption from the gastrointestinal tract. Its latency after intravenous injection is exceedingly brief (less than five minutes); it is rapidly eliminated so that it is not suitable for maintenance of digitalization. The initial intravenous dose is 0.25 to 0.3 mg, administered slowly. An additional 0.15 or 0.3 mg may be repeated after 24 hours.

DESLANOSIDE. This preparation is identical with digoxin except for the addition of a glucose residue. It is gradually replacing ouabain in popularity for intravenous use. Its digitalizing effect appears in 10 to 30 minutes after intravenous injection, reaches peak effect in one to two hours, and regresses in 24 hours. For rapid intravenous digitalization, the full 1.6 mg may be given at once, or, preferably, 0.8 mg may be followed by another 0.8 mg, either in four hours or in divided doses, at two- to four-hour intervals for two to three additional doses. Maintenance of digitalization is preferably done by oral digoxin or digitoxin. But, if necessary, 0.4 mg may be given intravenously or intramuscularly at 8- to 12-hour intervals.

DIGOXIN. For rapid digitalization, 0.5 mg is given initially, followed by 0.25 mg every two to four hours as needed, but taking care to avoid exceeding a total dose of 2 mg in 12 hours. As soon as practical, the oral route is substituted for the intravenous route.

Diagnostic Preparations. ACETYLSTROPHANTHIDIN. This is a partial synthetic which, because of its exceedingly rapid onset of action and dissipation, has been advocated more as a diagnostic test for adequacy of digitalization than as a therapeutic agent for heart failure. In practice, repeated injections of the substance (0.25 mg in 5 ml of glucose and water) are made until toxic or therapeutic effects are observed. Because it is potentially dangerous, other diagnostic tests are being investigated.

Guides to Proper Dosage of Digitalis. A major problem in using digitalis for its inotropic effect is the threat of inducing arrhythmias by virtue of its other effects on the heart (Fig. 4). On the other hand, if rapid atrial fibrillation coexists with heart failure, slowing of the ventricular rate, a consequence of slowed atrioventricular conduction, has proved to be a practical guide to digitalis

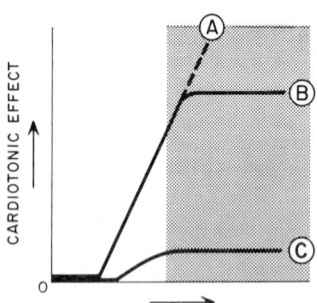

SERUM CONCENTRATION OF GLYCOSIDES

Figure 4. Hypothetical effects on contractility elicited by increasing doses (and serum concentrations) of digitalis. Once the inotropic effect of the digitalis preparation begins, it is unlikely that it will continue indefinitely as in A. Instead, it is likely that beyond a certain point the inotropic effects will taper to a plateau despite increasing serum concentration. When this plateau will occur depends on the capability of the heart to respond; a left ventricle that is suffering its first bout of failure is apt to manifest an excellent inotropic response for small increments in serum concentration before the plateau is reached (B). On the other hand, a spent heart that has suffered multiple myocardial infarctions may only manifest a sluggish inotropic response from the start and plateau early despite enormous increments in serum levels of glycoside (C). The shaded area is intended as a reminder of the increasing likelihood of serious arrhythmias as serum glycoside levels continue to increase.

dosage. Fortunately, slowing of the heart rate when atrial fibrillation coexists with heart failure also provides a rough measure of the inotropic effect (and of serum levels of the glycoside). On the other hand, when heart failure coexists with a normal sinus rhythm, slowing of the heart is a treacherous index of inotropic effect. Digitalis toxicity is common if large doses are administered in the attempt to slow the sinus tachycardia, particularly if a mechanism such as pulmonary emboli, infection, or hyperthyroidism is operating to sustain the rapid heart action.

The clinician now has available several different and effective digitalis preparations. Although none of these have any intrinsic advantage over the others with respect to myocardial contractility, they vary considerably with respect to speed of action, time course of effectiveness, and rates of elimination. Because of the ever-present prospect of digitalis toxicity, before starting to administer digitalis it is important to know whether digitalis, in any form, has been taken during the preceding week or two. Longer may be required if renal failure is present, particularly if digoxin was used. It cannot be overemphasized that the intravenous administration of a bolus of a digitalis preparation to a patient who has recently taken digitalis may precipitate ventricular tachycardia or fibrillation.

Clinical manifestations and the electrocardiogram are the key guides to dosage. As the circulation improves and signs and symptoms of heart failure abate, conventional dosage schedules are tailored to individual needs. The usual changes in the S-T segment and in the T waves produced by digitalis merely indicate that appreciable quantities of digitalis have been taken but provide no measure of dosage or efficacy. On the other hand, digitalis toxicity may first be manifested by electrocardiographic changes of abnormal conduction and of ectopic pacemakers.

Prophylactic. The perennial question of administering digitalis prophylactically, especially before surgical procedures, is again being discussed. This practice requires the administration of a preset dose without conventional criteria for distinguishing between adequacy versus toxicity. Therefore uncertain guidelines for safe administration are coupled with questionable therapeutic benefits. Compounding this uncertainty is the prospect of hypoxia and electrolyte imbalance during surgery. Because of the availability of digitalis preparations that do act rapidly and effectively, there seems to be little basis at present for prophylactic digitalization.

Digitalis Toxicity. Digitalis preparations are among the most dangerous, as well as the most useful, of current medications. The incidence of cardiotoxicity is staggering—of the order of 10 to 20 per cent in hospitalized patients receiving conventional doses of digitalis—and mortality from digitalis cardiotoxicity is estimated to run into the thousands per year.

Several different reasons account for much of this morbidity and mortality. (1) The narrow margin between therapeutic and toxic doses; this predisposes to digitalis toxicity during ordinary use but enhances its prospects when dosages are increased in the attempt to deal with increasing congestive heart failure. (2) The heavy reliance on slowing of heart rate and clearance of circulatory congestion as indices of improved contractility; this practice works well in atrial fibrillation but may be disastrous in normal sinus rhythm. (3) The ease with which changes in the clinical situation can derange stability of control; among the more common upsetting influences are electrolyte disturbances (particularly hypopotassemia), acute myocardial ischemia, upset acid-base balance, hypoxemia, renal impairment, autonomic nervous imbalances, other drugs, and infection. (4) Incomplete understanding by the physician of the distinctions in the clinical pharmacology of the various digitalis preparations; for example, differences in the renal handling of digoxin and digitoxin must be taken into account when choosing the proper glycoside in patients with renal insufficiency.

Recognition. The electrocardiogram is generally the final arbiter of digitalis cardiotoxicity. But three categories of clinical clues direct attention to the electrocardiogram: (1) the appearance of central nervous system evidence of digitalis toxicity, particularly anorexia and aversion to food; (2) a change in the arrhythmia, including unusual slowing or acceleration of the heart rate; and (3) regularization of the heart rate in the patient with atrial fibrillation while taking maintenance doses of digitalis.

Although serum levels are now quite popular as indices of digitalis toxicity, the lack of close correspondence between serum levels of glycosides and moderate cardiotoxicity in individual patients has kept alive interest in other tests to evaluate myocardial sensitivity to digitalis. These include the acetylstrophanthidin tolerance test, which is dangerous and should be reserved for experts. Among the more recent and innocuous is the salivary electrolyte test which relies on increases in the concentration of calcium and potassium in the saliva as an index of digitalis toxicity. This test is as yet empirical, because the mechanism for the increase in the concentration of these electrolytes is unknown. The practical value of this test remains to be established.

Digitalis cardiotoxicity is primarily a matter of arrhythmias. As might be expected from the diverse effects of digitalis on the heart, the arrhythmias are generally nonspecific. However, the coincidence of depressed atrioventricular conduction and stimulation of ectopic pacemakers is virtually unique for digitalis toxicity. This combination accounts for arrhythmias characterized by simultaneous rapid atrial rates and slow ventricular responses, for escape beats, and for nonparoxysmal junctional tachycardia. For example, atrial tachycardia with atrioventricular block, generally precipitated by overzealous administration of potassium-losing diuretics, is characteristic, although not specific, for digitalis toxicity. Even more distinctive is atrioventricular dissociation with junctional rhythm, in which two pacemakers operate independently above and below the intervening area of atrioventricular block. In atrial fibrillation, the advent of serious digitalis toxicity may be signaled by regularization of the ventricular rate because of acceleration of an ectopic focus below a high degree of atrioventricular block.

The usual cause of death in digitalis toxicity is ventricular fibrillation. Rarely does it appear unexpectedly. More often, it is presaged by multifocal premature contractions and runs of ventricular tachycardia. Consequently, premature ventricular beats that appear after digitalis has been started or during maintenance therapy have to be regarded as serious warnings of toxicity, particularly if they are multifocal in origin and if there is bigeminy involving premature beats that are bizarre in appearance. Rarely do ventricular arrhythmias occur

without other evidence of digitalis intake, including the characteristic ST-T deformations, disturbances in atrial ventricular conduction, and atrial arrhythmias.

Treatment. The mainstay for treating digitalis cardiotoxicity is to stop the digitalis and to discontinue diuretics that contributed to hypokalemia. There is no specific antidote. Fortunately, most digitalis-induced arrhythmias are arrested by stopping digitalis. Thus junctional rhythms without excessive ventricular rates or evidence of ventricular irritability are generally treated without specific medication or intervention. But if the arrhythmia is characteristic of ventricular irritability or if it has caused hemodynamic upset in the form of hypotension, heart failure, and pulmonary edema, medical intervention is mandatory.

Potassium is the agent of choice for suppressing digitalis-induced automaticity. But because it slows conduction through the myocardium and specialized conduction tissues, thereby potentiating the depression produced by digitalis, it must be used with extreme caution when atrioventricular block is severe. In the latter case, the introduction of a temporary perivenous cardiac pacemaker may prove useful in tiding the patient over the period needed to eliminate the excess digitalis, particularly if antiarrhythmic drugs are to be used to suppress ectopic atrial or ventricular beats.

If the arrhythmia has produced no crisis, if renal function is adequate, and if there is no hyperkalemia, potassium salts (4 to 6 grams of potassium chloride per day) may be administered orally. On the other hand, if the situation is deteriorating rapidly because of ectopic beats or uncontrollable tachycardia, potassium salts may be administered intravenously. Continuous electrocardiographic monitoring is mandatory during intravenous administration. The combination of continuous monitoring and careful intravenous titration of the arrhythmia is generally safer than is oral administration. The usual preparation for intravenous use contains 40 mEq of potassium in a 500 ml solution of 5 per cent glucose in water; this is administered slowly, e.g., at a rate of 40 mEq per hour. This may be repeated, if necessary, for up to three doses. Hypotension may limit the amount of potassium that can be given by vein. The electrocardiogram is monitored throughout, recognizing that high plasma concentrations of potassium may per se cause death through cardiac depression, arrhythmias, or arrest. The characteristic changes in the EKG are disappearance of the P wave, widening of the QRS complexes, changes in the S-T segments, and tall, peaked T waves.

Antiarrhythmic drugs which decrease ventricular automaticity by slowing diastolic depolarization, such as procainamide, lidocaine, propranolol, and diphenylhydantoin, are effective but must be used cautiously. Procainamide is useful when potassium fails to control the arrhythmia or if potassium is contraindicated because of uremia or hyperkalemia. It also has the advantage of sustained action if digitalis toxicity should persist. But it runs the risk of hypotension, depression of contractility, and producing AV block.

Lidocaine (1 to 2 mg per kilogram in one to two minutes by intravenous injection or as continuous infusion) has been used to control premature ventricular beats and ventricular tachycardia resulting from digitalis. It produces an effect within 45 to 90 seconds which is dissipated within 20 minutes. It has the advantage over procainamide of not causing hypotension. Doses less than 750 mg per hour are rarely associated with significant toxic effects, i.e., neurologic disorders and convulsions.

Diphenylhydantoin has been advocated for the treatment of digitalis-induced arrhythmias because it does not depress atrioventricular conduction. It is administered intravenously at a rate of 5 to 10 mg per kilogram over a 5- to 15-minute period. Propranolol, quinidine, and chelating agents are also being used. Electroconversion by DC shock, which has proved to be remarkably effective in controlling many arrhythmias, is a desperate measure of last resort in digitalis-toxic arrhythmias because of the likelihood of producing uncontrollable paroxysmal ventricular arrhythmias.

Blood Levels.   The pharmacologic effectiveness of most drugs depends on concentration at the site of action. Dosage may be a poor guide to this effective concentration because of biologic unpredictability with respect to absorption from the gastrointestinal tract, patterns of distribution throughout the body, and in rates of metabolism and excretion. In general, it is anticipated that concentration of a drug in the blood (serum or plasma) will relate better to therapeutic consequences, including toxicity, than will dosage.

In recent years, as a result of advances in radioimmunoassay technology, determination of serum concentrations of some cardiac glycosides became practical and available as well as reliable, accurate, and specific. The application of these tests to patients taking digitalis preparations (digoxin, digitoxin) has shown that the frequency and severity of toxic effects increase progressively as serum concentrations exceed therapeutic levels.

But some overlap in concentrations does occur, particularly in the zone between toxic and therapeutic levels. Moreover, occasionally there is a complete disparity between serum concentration and clinical consequences. These divergences are not unexpected because of the multiplicity of physiologic, pathologic, and biochemical influences that can modify the response to a given concentration of glycoside in the serum (and at the site of action): e.g., hypokalemia, acid-base disturbances, hypoxemia, interaction with other drugs, hypoproteinemia, acquisition of tolerance. But the exceptions do emphasize that serum concentrations must be interpreted critically in the light of the clinical setting.

Currently, determination of serum concentration of a digitalis glycoside is most useful in patients who are suspected of digitalis toxicity but are unable to provide an accurate account of digitalis dosage. It also has a place in guiding dosage in candidates for digitalis toxicity, e.g., heart failure complicated by renal insufficiency or by violent biochemical and physiologic perturbations, as after cardiac surgery. At the other extreme, determination of serum concentration may indicate that refractory heart failure may simply be a consequence of inadequate dosage.

Digitalis in Acute Myocardial Infarction.   As a general rule, digitalis is the drug of choice for myocardial failure. Since some degree of left ventricular failure is characteristic of acute myocardial infarction, it might seem reasonable to afford high priority to digitalis in the therapeutic program. Although this generalization still applies to *severe* heart failure during acute myocardial infarction, particularly if the heart is enlarged, the value of digitalis in less urgent degrees of left ventricular failure during acute myocardial infarction is much less certain.

The dilemma stems from the noninfarcted myocardium. If the noninfarcted ventricle has failed, considerable improvement is to be expected from the inotropic effects of digitalis; conversely, if the noninfarcted ventricle is normal, the inotropic effect will be of little consequence, particularly when compared to the inotropic effects of circulating catecholamines that the acute crisis has promoted. The possibility also exists that, even if digitalis does enhance contractility of the noninfarcted area, the net effect on cardiac performance may not be impressive because of the paradoxical motion of the infarcted area during cardiac contraction.

In addition to these uncertainties concerning enhanced contractility, the threat exists that digitalis may promote ventricular irritability in the peri-infarcted, ischemic zone of the myocardium, thereby predisposing to ectopic foci and uncontrollable ventricular arrhythmias. This likelihood is accentuated by a variety of other concomitant influences that predispose to ventricular arrhythmias: increased sympathetic activity, hypokalemia, and hypoxemia (to which excess sedation may contribute).

These reservations, plus the availability of effective diuretics to clear pulmonary congestion and edema during the first few days of an acute myocardial infarction, encourage extraordinary circumspection in using digitalis during the acute episode. On the other hand, if heart failure persists after the acute crisis—because of either extensive scarring or unremitting hemodynamic overload—digitalis is clearly required because the myocardium has failed globally. Moreover, should atrial fibrillation with a rapid ventricular response complicate acute myocardial infarction early or late in its course, digitalis may be lifesaving. For other supraventricular arrhythmias, which generally require larger doses of digitalis and may even prove refractory, antiarrhythmic agents or electrical conversion are preferable during the phase of increased ventricular irritability.

Other Inotropic Agents: Sympathomimetic Amines. Although fashions in diuretics continue to change, no inotropic agent has as yet been found to compete with digitalis. Substitutes have been sought among the sympathomimetic amines which also stimulate the myocardium but differently from digitalis. The qualifications that have been sought include effectiveness after oral administration, improved contractility in conjunction with peripheral vasodilatation, increased renal excretion of sodium, and a greater increase in coronary blood flow than in myocardial oxygen consumption. Three catecholamines have been singled out for close scrutiny because of their ability to stimulate the heart and to decrease peripheral resistance: epinephrine, isoproterenol, and dopamine. Unfortunately, none of these is on a clinical par with digitalis: all three provoke tachycardia; epinephrine decreases the elimination of sodium by the kidney, whereas isoproterenol usually has no effect on sodium excretion; dopamine has to be given intravenously, acts briefly, and causes undesirable increments in systemic arterial pressure.

Glucagon, a polypeptide hormone produced chiefly by the α cells of the pancreas, attracted considerable attention for a while as a possible adjunct for the patient in refractory heart failure who can tolerate no more digitalis. Like the catecholamines, glucagon presumably exerts its cardiotonic effects by activating adenyl cyclase. It has been given by continuous intravenous infusion (2 to 4 mg per hour for 10 to 13 days) and by injections of large single doses (10 to 25 mg). In these doses, the major side effect was nausea; abnormalities in blood sugar levels were uncommon. Unfortunately, enthusiasm for this agent has begun to wane because of recent evidence that the effects of glucagon on myocardial contractility are far less consistent in chronic heart failure than in the normal heart.

Cardiac Assist Devices. In some clinics, attempts have been made to gain temporary respite for the heart in acute refractory failure, using devices which share the load for hours to days while the heart recuperates. The most popular methods are (1) venoarterial bypass, which assists the heart by diverting blood from the heart and returning it by a pump to the arterial tree, and (2) counterpulsation, which is synchronized with the heart beat to modify aortic pressure by rhythmically changing either the blood volume in the aorta, using an external pump, or the capacity of the aorta, using an intra-aortic balloon. All methods aim to reduce the external work of the heart, the developed tension, and the myocardial oxygen consumption while improving coronary perfusion. Technical problems have restricted the use of these appliances in man to desperate circumstances (e.g., cardiogenic shock) and for as brief a period as possible. As yet, there are exceedingly few long-term survivors.

Diuretics

Inordinate retention of salt and water, followed by expansion of the plasma and the interstitial tissue compartments of the extracellular fluid volume, is a hallmark of congestive heart failure and is responsible for many of its symptoms. Consequently, elimination of the excess salt and water and contraction of the extravascular fluid volume by diuresis are essential for the successful treatment of heart failure.

"Dry" Weight. The use of diuretics entails two separate problems: elimination of excess fluid, and the maintenance of edema-free ("dry") weight. In the hospital, where the patient is at rest and salt intake is precisely controlled, low dosages of diuretics may suffice to maintain dry weight. Out of the hospital, where the patient engages in various degrees of exercise, and salt intake is neither readily monitored nor controlled, larger doses may be needed. However, continued use of large doses of diuretics inevitably leads to serious derangements in electrolyte balance, often predisposing to digitalis toxicity by way of hypokalemia. Consequently, once the urgent need for brisk diuresis has passed—as during an episode of acute pulmonary edema—the optimal cardiotonic program relies heavily on digitalis and salt restriction and depends on diuretics as an ancillary measure.

Salt and Water Restriction. Restriction of sodium intake should be directed not only at sodium chloride per se but also at sodium-containing medications, e.g., antacids. Restriction of water intake is rarely necessary except after the use of potent diuretics which predispose to hyponatremia and water intoxication. In mild heart failure, salt intake is generally restricted to less than 3 grams per day; in severe congestive heart failure, intake of less than 0.5 gram per day is often needed to promote diuresis and to reduce the blood volume and venous pressure. Overzealous sodium restriction in conjunction with potent sodium-losing diuretics, particularly in the elderly or in others with impaired renal function, may lead to weakness, oliguria, and azotemia.

The Sodium Control System. The major diuretics increase the rate of sodium excretion by the renal tubule. As indicated previously, the tubule is the end organ of an elaborate control system that is influenced by hemodynamic and neurohumoral mechanisms. For some mysterious reason, the control system seems to be reset in heart failure so that an expanded extracellular fluid volume, usually a stimulus to diuresis, coexists with antidiuresis. Nonetheless, despite this reset, it is possible to modify the handling of sodium by intervening at several different sites in the control system.

The diuretics that will be considered interfere with the control system by modifying the reabsorption of sodium, with its accompanying anions and water, by the end organ, the renal tubule (Fig. 5). Five distinct categories of diuretics are in common use (Table 3). Each affects tubular reabsorption somewhat differently, and each produces its own characteristic abnormalities in electrolyte pattern, hydration, and acid-base balance. These abnormalities represent the pharmacologic consequences of effective drug action. When carried to extremes, or when effects interact, they are responsible for the toxicity of these different diuretics.

Thiazides. Because of their effectiveness by mouth, their reliability, and their relative freedom from toxicity if administered circumspectly, the benzothiadiazine drugs are usually the diuretics of choice in cardiac edema. The prototypes of this group are chlorothiazide and hydrochlorothiazide (Table 4). *Acute* administration promotes the urinary excretion of sodium, chloride, and potassium without consistent change in urinary pH or bicarbonate excretion. The predominant diuretic effect (natriuresis and chloruresis) has been localized to inhibi-

Figure 5. Schematic representation of a nephron, indicating predominant sites of action of the five groups of diuretics. Carbonic anhydrase inhibitors exert predominant effects on the proximal tubule. The potassium-retaining diuretics affect the distal nephron. The major diuretic effect of the thiazides is at a site of urine dilution in the cortical portion of the ascending limb of the loop of Henle. Ethacrynic acid, furosemide, and the organomercurials act chiefly on the loop of Henle, affecting both the diluting and concentrating segments to achieve potent diuretic effects.

TABLE 3.　Diuretic Agents in Heart Failure

Type of Diuretic	Effect on Kidney		Effect on Electrolytes		Toxic Manifestations	Special Features
	Principal Site of Action	Mechanism	In Urine	In Blood		
Thiazides (chlorruretic sulfonamides)	Ascending limb of loop of Henle; distal tubule	Interference with dilution of urine	Increased excretion of Na, Cl, K	Hypochloremic alkalosis; hypokalemia	Nausea; vomiting; skin rashes; hyperuricemia; hypercalcemia; hyperglycemia; azotemia	Loss of effectiveness and hypokalemia are common on continued administration
Ethacrynic acid*	Ascending limb of loop of Henle; distal tubule; probably proximal tubule	Interference with dilution and concentration of urine	Increased excretion of Na, Cl, HCO₃, K, H	Hypochloremic alkalosis; hypokalemia; hyponatremia	Hypotension; contraction alkalosis; hyperuricemia; hypercalcemia; azotemia; hyperglycemia; hearing loss	Causes renal vasodilatation; effective in renal insufficiency, systemic acidosis or alkalosis; potent diuresis often followed by rebound
Organomercurials	Proximal and/or distal tubule	Decrease of isosmotic reabsorption	Increased excretion of Na, Cl, H	Hypochloremic alkalosis	Mercury intoxication; sudden death (after IV injection); occasional agranulocytosis	Inactivated by hypochloremic alkalosis; hazardous in oliguria
Potassium-sparing†	Distal tubule	Aldosterone antagonism for Na-K exchange	Decreased excretion of K and H; slight increase in Na, Cl, HCO₃	Hyperkalemia	Generally nontoxic; GI upset; gynecomastia; rare agranulocytosis	Synergistic with thiazides and ethacrynic acid; avoid in renal insufficiency and in hyperkalemia
Carbonic anhydrase inhibitors	Proximal tubule	Inhibition of enzyme involved in acidification of urine	Increased excretion of Na, K, HCO₃; decrease in H	Hyperchloremic acidosis; hypokalemia	Generally nontoxic; mild GI and mental upsets; occasional sulfonamide idiosyncrasy	Not very potent and loses effectiveness in a few days

*Furosemide (Lasix), a nonthiazide sulfonamide, has practically the same indications and effects despite its different chemical structure.
†Spironolactone (Aldactone) operates as a competitive inhibitor of endogenous aldosterone; triamterene and amiloride are noncompetitive inhibitors and produce the characteristic effects on the urine even though aldosterone is absent.

TABLE 4. Administration of Diuretics

	Example	Relevant Chemical Structure	Preferred Route of Administration	Usual Range of Daily Dosage	Suggested Pattern of Administration
Thiazides	Chlorothiazide (Diuril)	Benzothiadiazine derivative	Oral	500 mg × 2–4	Standard type of diuretic to start treatment; few days on, few days off to avoid refractoriness and serious electrolyte disturbances
Ethacrynic acid*	Ethacrynic acid (Edecrin)	Ketone derivative of aryloxyacetic acid	Oral or IV*	50 mg × 2–3	Reserve for serious or refractory edema
Organomercurials	Meralluride (mercuhydrin)	Theophylline plus organic mercurial	IM	2 ml	Adjunct diuretic or for moderately rapid response in hospital
Potassium sparing†	Triamterene (Dyrenium)	Pteridine derivative	Oral	200 mg	Continuous administration in conjunction with more potent potassium-losing diuretics; do not use with potassium supplements
Carbonic anhydrase inhibitors	Acetazolamide (Diamox)	Sulfanilamide derivative	Oral	250 mg × 4–6	Episodic as booster diuretic; useful before injection of organomercurial for chloride-retaining effect

*Furosemide and ethacrynic acid may be given intravenously as well as by mouth. For ordinary use, however, furosemide is administered as a single oral dose in the morning. In an urgent situation (pulmonary edema), furosemide, as well as ethacrynic acid, may be administered intravenously (50 mg). Intravenous administration should not be administered at less than six-hour intervals.

†Spironolactone (Aldactone), 75 to 100 mg per day, is commonly used as a potassium-sparing diuretic. In refractory heart failure doses of 100 to 600 mg per day have proved helpful.

tion of sodium absorption at a diluting site in the distal nephron (Fig. 5). Although there is also a carbonic anhydrase-inhibiting effect, it is generally insignificant until large daily doses are reached (of the order of 2000 mg per day). Kaliuresis depends on an increase in the quantity of sodium delivered to the distal nephron. Intravenous administration of chlorothiazide is uricosuric, whereas chronic administration results in hyperuricemia. The mechanisms responsible for the paradoxical uric acid effects are still unclear.

Hypokalemia is particularly apt to arise after intensive diuresis with thiazides or after prolonged thiazide therapy. Supplementary doses of potassium may then be required. Several generalizations have proved useful as practical guides to therapy. Acute hypokalemia that is modest in degree is managed by diet; if diet fails to correct the hypokalemia, supplementary doses of potassium may be required. Potassium chloride is generally the agent of choice for oral supplementation, because hypochloremic metabolic alkalosis usually accompanies diuretic-induced hypokalemia. For severe hypokalemia, intravenous infusions are used. To prevent hypokalemia during chronic administration of potassium-losing diuretics, aldosterone inhibitors are useful.

Certain precautions merit attention in applying these guides to therapy. Potassium salts administered orally in any form cause gastric irritation. This side effect is generally tolerable, especially in the hospital, where potassium chloride can be safely given in liquid form after meals. Prolonged administration of potassium salts, particularly if enteric coated, is particularly hazardous because of the high incidence of intestinal ulceration, perforation, and peritonitis, often followed by intestinal stenosis and obstruction. No matter how administered, excessive doses of potassium are apt to lead to hyperkalemia. This likelihood is enhanced in older persons who often have slight renal impairment, especially if an aldosterone inhibitor is given concomitantly.

Ethacrynic Acid and Furosemide. These are the most potent natriuretic agents currently available. Both are

organic acids but otherwise are quite different chemically. Furosemide is a sulfonamide–anthranilic acid derivative related to the thiazide diuretics, whereas ethacrynic acid is a ketone derivative of aryloxyacetic acid (Table 4). Like the thiazides, they are effective orally and are rapid acting. They exert powerful diuretic effects by inhibiting both the renal diluting and concentrating mechanisms in the ascending limb of the loop of Henle (Fig. 5). Ethacrynic acid is without appreciable effect on carbonic anhydrase, whereas furosemide does elicit modest anti-carbonic anhydrase activity.

Ethacrynic acid, administered orally, exerts its effects in 30 minutes and continues to act for six to eight hours; administered intravenously, it acts within a few minutes, reaching its peak activity in one hour. Both agents elicit a marked increase in urine flow containing large quantities of sodium and chloride (of the order of 20 to 30 per cent of the filtered load). Kaliuresis is consistent and appreciable. In conventional doses, neither drug consistently increases bicarbonate secretion or modifies urine pH. But chronic administration of ethacrynic acid promotes hydrogen loss in a bicarbonate-free urine, i.e., produces metabolic alkalosis.

A cardinal virtue of these agents (in contrast with thiazides and carbonic anhydrase inhibitors) is their lack of effect on filtration rate or renal plasma flow unless sodium depletion occurs. This lack of direct hemodynamic effect is fortunate, because a decrease in filtration rate interferes with their action; conversely, increase in filtration rate, as by intravenous administration of mannitol or albumin, enhances their effects. At peak effect, both agents decrease renal vascular resistance.

Ethacrynic acid and furosemide remain effective despite gross electrolyte disturbances and hypoalbuminemia. If pushed, either may cause hyponatremia, volume depletion, fall in blood pressure, fall in urine volume, azotemia, and water retention. Because of the upsets in the electrolyte concentrations which they induce, other diuretics are preferred for maintenance treatment. They are most valuable in three situations: in acute pulmonary edema (25 to 50 mg intravenously), in severe or refractory heart failure, or when renal function is impaired (because they increase renal blood flow). Both agents produce "contraction alkalosis," i.e., an increase in plasma bicarbonate consequent to the decrease in extracellular fluid volume that follows excretion of a large volume of bicarbonate-poor urine. The metabolic alkalosis that follows hydrogen depletion and "contraction" predisposes to alveolar hypoventilation through its depressant effects on respiratory control mechanisms.

Organomercurial Diuretics. Until the advent of potent oral diuretics, the organomercurials, generally a combination of an organic mercurial and theophylline, were the diuretic agents of choice in heart failure. Now they are generally reserved for parenteral administration in hospital. After administration of a maximally effective dose intravenously, large (and approximately equal) amounts of sodium and chloride are eliminated in the urine. The normal subject is apt to eliminate 10 per cent of the filtered load, whereas the individual that has been primed to the stage of hyperchloremic acidosis by prior administration of ammonium chloride may eliminate up to 20 per cent of the filtered load. Bicarbonate excretion does not increase, and urinary acidity persists during the diuresis. The effect on potassium excretion is variable and generally small, depending on prior rates of excretion. Generally they tend to decrease potassium.

Like ethacrynic acid and furosemide, the organomercurials exert an important inhibitory effect on sodium reabsorption in the loop of Henle, impairing both the diluting and concentrating mechanisms. In Figure 5, the organomercurials are shown as acting predominantly on the distal tubule, beyond the predominant sites of action of the thiazides, ethacrynic acid, and furosemide. However, these distinctions are far from absolute. Theophylline-containing mercurials usually elicit transient increases in filtration rate, but this effect is generally neutralized by volume concentration if diuresis is effective.

The organomercurials are almost invariably administered intramuscularly. After intramuscular injection, the onset of action is in one to two hours, reaching a peak in six hours, and lasting for 12 to 24 hours. Early in treatment, a brisk diuresis and natriuresis occur. But with continued use, refractoriness may result, generally for one of two reasons: (1) the onset of a hypochloremic hypokalemic alkalosis (with fairly normal sodium levels); responsiveness may then be restored by administering ammonium chloride; or (2) the advent of a low-salt syndrome in which sodium as well as chloride levels in the serum are severely depressed; this state responds to water restriction.

Aldosterone Antagonists. A characteristic feature of chronic heart failure is high circulating levels of renin and aldosterone. Aldosterone, either by providing energy for active transport or by increasing permeability, enhances the movement of sodium through the distal tubular cell, from lumen to interstitium. Water follows passively. In addition to promoting sodium reabsorption, aldosterone also increases potassium excretion by a mechanism that is not entirely clear but is more than an ion-exchange mechanism. In heart failure the hyperaldosteronism causes continuing sodium retention, whereas potassium excretion remains normal, i.e., no hypokalemia. Aldosterone antagonists interfere with these actions, causing potassium retention and sodium excretion.

Three agents are available: spironolactone, triamterene, and amiloride (MK-870). Spironolactone is most popular; amiloride is not yet available for general use. Although all three act by competing for receptor sites in the distal tubule, the intimate mechanisms involved in electrolyte secretion may be quite different. The major site of action of spironolactone is in the distal tubule, in the region of the aldosterone-stimulated secretion of hydrogen and potassium. It is a specific competitive inhibitor of aldosterone and has no action if aldosterone is absent. It promotes natriuresis, water loss, and potassium retention by depressing aldosterone-dependent sodium-potassium exchange in the distal tubule. It is only effective in the presence of high levels of mineralocorticoid activity; it is devoid of effect after adrenalectomy. Conversely, triamterene (Table 4) and amiloride are noncompetitive inhibitors that inhibit potassium and hydrogen ion excretion even if aldosterone is absent. Their mechanism of action is unclear. Although these natriuretic agents are far less potent than the thiazides, ethacrynic acid, furosemides, and the organomercurials, they have the extraordinary advantage for prolonged use of continuing effectiveness, minor electrolyte derangements, and the virtual absence of toxicity as long as hyperkalemia is avoided. These agents are unique in that they are given without interruption, because, in contrast to the thiazides, ethacrynic acid, and furosemide, they do not lose effectiveness in a few days nor do they cause violent electrolyte upheavals.

Spironolactone is expensive but effective. Oral doses, ranging from 50 to 600 mg per day, are well tolerated for months. A few days may elapse before its action becomes apparent. It is currently being used primarily to potentiate the effects of the more powerful diuretics, particularly if potassium depletion is a serious consideration.

Carbonic Anhydrase Inhibitors. These agents are effective by mouth. They elicit an increase in excretion of bicarbonate, sodium, and potassium and an increase in urine pH. The most striking increments are in bicarbonate and potassium. By interfering with carbonic anhydrase activity in the kidney, they inhibit hydrogen ion secretion primarily in the proximal and distal portions of the nephron, exerting lesser effects on the loop of Henle, i.e., little effect on urinary diluting or concentrating mechanisms.

The prototype of this group is acetazolamide (Table 4). It is a weak diuretic and loses its effectiveness as hyperchloremic metabolic acidosis develops because of diminished hydrogen ion excretion (usually in 48 hours). Like ammonium chloride, this class of diuretics is particularly valuable in patients with high serum bicarbonate, as occurs in cor pulmonale or metabolic alkalosis. They are valuable in preparing for a mercurial diuresis because of the hyperchloremic acidosis that they produce. This group also enhances natriuresis produced by thiazides, ethacrynic acid, and furosemide. A contraindication for its use is severe acidosis, as from renal failure or hepatic insufficiency.

Special Diuretics. This is a miscellaneous group of agents that are used with extreme caution and under special conditions. For example, osmotic diuretics such as mannitol and albumin, which expand the circulating blood volume, have the potential for increasing the renal blood flow and for blocking the reabsorption of sodium and water at the proximal tubule. However, in heart failure they entail the risk of circulatory overload and pulmonary edema.

Combinations. There are two main reasons for introducing a combination of diuretics into a cardiotonic program: to avoid serious electrolyte upsets that are bound to occur if the powerful primary diuretics are administered without pause, in large dosage, for long periods; and to stimulate diuresis when the prevailing cardiotonic program no longer suffices to prevent edema. In either case, the net diuretic effect of the combination will be determined by a wide variety of influences: the respective sites of action on the renal tubule of each agent, the extent of competitive inhibition at common receptor sites, the dose-response curves of the individual drugs, strategic timing of the administration of one agent with respect to the other, and the acid-base and electrolyte balances at the time that the agents are given.

A currently popular duo of diuretics is a potassium-sparing agent (triamterene or spironolactone) that is taken daily and a thiazide that is taken intermittently (e.g., for four days of each week). In time, the thiazide may be succeeded by ethacrynic acid or ethacrynic acid may be given sporadically as needed to sustain the edema-free state. On occasion, particularly in the hospital, a mercurial diuretic (after prior acidification) may prove helpful in overcoming a resistant state of edema. In contrast to the foregoing, other combinations hold little promise for success. Thus the combined use of acetazolamide and a mercurial diuretic is not apt to be exceedingly effective, because, by preventing acidification of the urine, the carbonic anhydrase inhibitor is apt to block, rather than to enhance, the diuretic effect of the mercurial.

The same general principles govern the use of combinations of diuretics in the treatment of refractory edema. This troublesome state is now relatively uncommon because of the advent of powerful primary diuretics, particularly furosemide and ethacrynic acid, coupled with a better understanding of the sites of action of the auxiliary diuretics. On the other hand, refractory edema may again become tractable by reversing electrolyte and acid-base imbalances that have been produced by unremitting administration of the primary diuretics for long periods. As a working principle, resistance to diuresis is overcome by deliberate selection of agents that act on different parts of the tubule. This approach presupposes that digitalis dosage is optimal. On occasion, aminophylline, by its inotropic effect, may reinforce the diuretic action of a thiazide or ethacrynic acid. Clearly, many opportunities exist for the physician to devise original sequences and combinations of diuretics. However, a restraining influence is imposed by the complicated interplay that is to be expected, not only between the diuretic agents per se, but also within the broad context of a deranged internal environment that generally is a feature of the state of refractory edema.

Refractory Edema. This is a state of edema that resists conventional cardiotonic and diuretic measures. Before embarking on an endless train of drug combinations, the patient should be carefully re-evaluated for either a complication or an underlying disorder that has been overlooked: a surgically correctable disorder, such as mitral stenosis or constrictive pericarditis; a medical disorder, including hyperthyroidism, anemia, pulmonary emboli, bacterial endocarditis, persistent infection, and arrhythmias; inappropriate or excessive diuretic therapy that elicits serious disturbances in blood volume and electrolyte composition, digitalis toxicity, and water intoxication; physical overactivity; excessive salt intake and renal disease; sodium-containing medicaments, such as antacids, or agents such as reserpine, propranolol, and guanethidine which depress the myocardium to the point of failure.

Complications. A variety of disturbances may complicate effective diuretic therapy. These include hypotension and vascular collapse from rapid, massive diuresis; sodium depletion, usually the consequence of prolonged and effective diuretic therapy in conjunction with excessive water intake; hypokalemia from uninterrupted use of diuretics, predisposing to digitalis toxicity; hyperkalemia from injudicious administration of aldosterone antagonists and potassium supplements; metabolic alkalosis, either from a massive excretion of a bicarbonate-poor urine or from a combination of increased hydrogen ion excretion in the urine and alveolar hypoventilation as produced by ethacrynic acid or potassium depletion; and hyperuricemia after prolonged administration of small doses of the thiazides, ethacrynic acid, and furosemide, which share an inhibiting effect on uric acid excretion. In predisposed individuals, the hyperuricemia of prolonged diuretic therapy may precipitate an episode of gout. The thiazides, and occasionally furosemide, may precipitate diabetes which is rarely severe.

General Comments. In treating heart failure, rarely is there a desperate need to restore everything to normal at once by vigorous diuresis. The temptation to restore the patient immediately to dry weight and to free him of breathlessness and congestion must be tempered by the penalty of dehydration and severe electrolyte disturbances. The more leisurely the diuretic therapy, the more durable and tolerable the relief.

The ability of these potent diuretics to elicit dramatic diuresis has led to their abuse. Thus without direct inotropic effect on the heart, a single injection of ethacrynic acid can effect a decrease in blood volume, a decrease in intracardiac filling pressures, an increase in cardiac output, and clear edema. But ethacrynic acid is rarely advisable as the mainstay of therapy unless edema is refractory and less drastic measures have proved ineffective. Only when coupled with a full cardiotonic program can judicious control of heart failure be maintained, particularly if the underlying heart disease is progressive and severe complications of diuretic therapy are to be avoided.

Cherniack, N. S., and Longobardo, G. S.: Cheyne-Stokes breathing. In Physiology in Medicine. N. Engl. J. Med., 288:952, 1973.

Dollery, C. T., George, C. F., and Orme, M. L'E.: Drug interaction in cardiovascular disease. Prog. Cardiology, 1:31, 1972.

Fishman, A. P.: Pulmonary edema. The water-exchanging function of the lung. Circulation, 46:390, 1972.

Fishman, A. P., and Richards, D. W. (eds.): Circulation of the Blood. Men and Ideas. New York. Oxford University Press, 1964.

Goldberg, M.: The renal physiology of diuretics. In Berliner, R. W., and Orloff, J. (eds.): Handbook of Physiology—Renal Physiology. Washington. American Physiological Society, 1973.

Lee, K. S., and Klaus, W.: The subcellular basis for the mechanism of inotropic action of cardiac glycosides. Pharmacol. Rev., 23:193, 1971.

Marshall, R. J., and Shepherd, J. T.: Cardiac Function in Health and Disease. Philadelphia. W. B. Saunders Company, 1968.

Mason, D. T., Zelis, R., and Wikman-Coffelt, J. (eds.): Symposium on congestive heart failure. Am. J. Cardiol., 32:395, 1973.

Noble, M. I. M.: Problems concerning the application of concepts of muscle
    mechanics to the determination of the contractile state of the heart.
    Circulation, 45:252, 1972.
Ross, J., Jr., and Peterson, K. L. (editorial): On the assessment of cardiac
    inotropic state. Circulation, 47:435, 1973.
Smith, T. W., and Haber, E.: Digitalis. N. Engl. J. Med., 289:945, 1010,
    1063, 1125, 1973.

542. SHOCK

Alfred P. Fishman

GENERAL FEATURES

Circulatory shock ("shock") is a life-threatening state in which vital processes are profoundly depressed because of inadequate organ blood flow. Often the interval between the onset of shock and death is less than 48 hours. The circulatory inadequacy may stem from a large decrease in cardiac output, in venous return to the heart, or in peripheral vascular resistance. Of these three potential mechanisms, a considerable decrease in venous return, as after massive hemorrhage, is most common. Not uncommon is acute enfeeblement of the left ventricle after extensive myocardial infarction. Rarely does shock *begin* with massive peripheral vasodilation. On the other hand, peripheral vasodilation invariably complicates prolonged circulatory inadequacy and often is responsible for the fatal outcome.

A diverse assortment of initiating mechanisms (Table 5) can set into motion the sequence culminating in shock. Since each mechanism registers its own distinct imprint on the final picture, the clinical manifestations of shock can vary greatly. But certain features occur quite regularly, particularly if shock is advanced or progressing: arterial hypotension (see below); a decrease in cardiac output sufficient to elicit signs of organ hypoperfusion; metabolic acidosis; and a need for therapeutic intervention to sustain cerebral, cardiac, or renal function at levels compatible with life.

The longer shock lasts, the worse the prognosis. In time, a stage of refractory shock may be reached in which the peripheral circulation continues to dilate despite intense sympathetic nervous activity and vigorous therapy; at the same time, cardiac output falls progressively because of inadequate venous return and inadequate blood flow to the myocardium. The nature of refractory shock is still unsettled, particularly with respect to the role of toxins in producing the fatal outcome. Many toxic factors have been proposed. Most of these are held to arise in splanchnic organs (liver, spleen, pancreas, intestine), from which they are distributed throughout the body by blood and lymph, exerting their principal noxious effects on heart, lungs, microcirculation, and reticuloendothelial system.

Organ Hypoperfusion. The common denominator in shock is cellular dysfunction and death from organ hypoperfusion. This "cellular hypoperfusion" compromises the delivery of metabolic nutriments, substrates, and oxygen to cells and allows metabolic end products to accumulate, thereby deranging intracellular and extracellular environments, disturbing energy pathways, and disordering cellular function. The decrease in blood flow does not affect all organs and tissues equally: first deprived are the nonvital tissues of the gastrointestinal tract, muscle, connective tissue, and skin; only later do the kidneys, liver, heart, lungs, and brain become ischemic. One clinical manifestation of organ hypoperfusion is the lower skin temperature than rectal temperature, caused by cutaneous vasoconstriction; another is oliguria, reflecting diminished renal blood flow.

Arterial Hypotension. A decrease in arterial blood pressure used to be considered a sine qua non for the clinical diagnosis of shock. This stricture no longer applies, because blood pressure in shock may vary considerably, depending on initiating mechanism, severity of shock, duration, and complications. Early in traumatic or hemorrhagic shock, if anxiety is high and pain is intense, blood pressure may be high because of an outpouring of catecholamines into the circulation. This is a treacherous phase, for the hypertension is apt to be fleeting and followed by a precipitous drop in blood pressure. Oppositely, blood pressure inevitably falls to hypotensive levels before death. Between these two extremes are areas of critical clinical importance. A modest decrease in arterial blood pressure, of the order of 10 to 20 mm Hg, quite common at the start of shock, generally represents success of compensatory mechanisms, at least transiently, in stabilizing the circulation; frank arterial hypotension (systolic blood pressure less than 80 mm Hg) signals that shock is progressing and that compensatory mechanisms are proving inadequate. From the point of view of therapy, a more favorable prognosis is to be anticipated from early recognition and intervention than from relying on definite hypotension as the indication for therapy.

The significance of hypotension in shock depends largely on the concomitant state of vasomotor activity. Clinically the assessment of vasomotor activity is generally quite simple: low blood pressure in conjunction with warm hands and good urine flow indicates vasodilation and good cardiac output; hypotension, cold hands, and oliguria represent intense vasoconstriction. Interpretation of these findings in terms of prognosis may vary according to etiology, duration, and severity of the shock. Warm hands may occur early in septic shock when opportunity for successful treatment is at its peak. Later on in septic shock, warm hands may reflect paralysis of

TABLE 5.   Categories of Shock

Type	Etiology
Medical:	
1. Hypovolemic shock: decrease in blood volume by loss of blood, plasma or extracellular fluid	Hemorrhage, burns, vomiting, diarrhea, metabolic acidosis, Addisonian crisis, heat exhaustion
2. Septic shock	Bacteremia, endotoxemia
3. Cardiogenic shock	Myocardial infarction
4. Shock from inadequate cardiac filling	Severe tachycardia
Surgical:	
1. Shock from inadequate cardiac filling	Pericardial tamponade, tension pneumothorax
2. Shock from acute cardiac defects	Ruptured valve cusp or chorda, perforated ventricular septum
3. Shock from mechanical obstruction in central circulation	Massive pulmonary embolus, ball-valve thrombus of mitral valve

arterioles and opening of arteriovenous shunts in the skin before death. Conversely, persistence of warm hands and good urine flow in cardiogenic shock after acute myocardial infarction raises the prospects for reversibility.

When peripheral vasoconstriction is intense, the sphygmomanometer may give artificially low values in shock because of the low cardiac output and the narrow pulse pressure. Consequently, many clinics use arterial cannulation to follow the course of the blood pressure during shock. The cannula affords the additional advantage of providing blood samples for the determination of arterial oxygen tension and pH.

Individual Clinical Syndromes. The diverse etiologic agents in shock are sorted in Table 5 according to medical versus surgical management. Only those amenable to medical management will be considered in this chapter. Moreover, this chapter will not deal with states of circulatory inadequacy that mark the end of chronic cardiac disability, such as prolonged heart failure or myocarditis, in which the spent myocardium is no longer capable of improving its performance.

HYPOVOLEMIC SHOCK

Depletion of the blood volume by hemorrhage, trauma, or burns may produce shock. At least 1 liter of blood must be withdrawn from a healthy man before signs of shock appear; these disappear if the blood is returned at once. Trauma to skeletal muscles may also cause shock as blood escapes into the muscles. Extensive burns produce shock because of loss of plasma from the denuded surface. Despite these individual differences, the net effect is hypovolemia. Prompt restoration of the blood volume after hemorrhage restores the circulation to normal. However, extensive burns or trauma to muscle are generally more difficult to manage because the effects of depleted blood volume are complicated by the products of local infection and dead tissue.

The blood volume may be depleted by ways other than direct loss of blood or plasma from the bloodstream. The same end result may be produced by vomiting, diarrhea, intestinal obstruction, diabetic acidosis, and Addison's disease, all of which cause severe loss of water and electrolytes.

The patient who has just experienced a massive hemorrhage is restless and agitated, dimly aware that he is the victim of a calamity but not quite clear about its nature. Organ hypoperfusion is evident in the pallor, oliguria, and disordered cerebration. He asks for water but becomes nauseated after a few sips. The pulse is rapid and thready. The arterial blood pressure is low, and the pulse pressure is narrow. In essence, he is manifesting the consequences of a decrease in cardiac output, heightened sympathetic nervous activity, and redistribution of blood flow.

Pathophysiology. The clinical syndrome is a consequence of an acute decrease in venous return → low cardiac output → arterial hypotension → baroreceptor stimulation → sympathetic nervous activation (including release of epinephrine and norepinephrine) → nonuniform organ perfusion.

The microcirculation of the skin and viscera contains alpha receptors and responds therefore to the increase in circulating catecholamines by vasoconstricting. In turn, the viscera that are poorly endowed with alpha receptors, i.e., brain, heart, and muscle, receive a disproportionately large fraction of the cardiac output. Moreover,

since heart and muscle contain beta receptors that are also stimulated by the circulating catecholamines, the heart exhibits inotropic and chronotropic effects in conjunction with arteriolar and venular dilatation. The cerebral circulation, which has neither alpha nor beta receptors, does not vasoconstrict.

As a result of the low cardiac output and nonuniform vasoconstriction, blood flow slows in the affected vascular beds and formed elements in the blood tend to clump. Cells become damaged and die, releasing lactic acid and enzymes, such as lactic dehydrogenase and glutamic oxaloacetic transaminase, into the blood; coagulation mechanisms are disturbed. If hypoperfusion persists, irreversible metabolic changes in the cells may preclude restoration. Consequently, early treatment of shock is mandatory.

For comparable decrements in cardiac output, the patient in shock is almost invariably worse off than the patient in chronic left ventricular failure. In large measure this clinical discrepancy stems from the acuity of onset and the initiating mechanisms. Thus the same hemodynamic abnormality may operate differently in the two states: the high atrial pressure of *chronic* ventricular failure is characteristically associated with antidiuresis, whereas *acute* elevation of left atrial pressure elicits a diuresis. The left atrial receptors involved in these responses are currently under intensive study. Another important modifying influence is expansion of the blood volume during chronic heart failure as a consequence of salt and water retention by the kidneys; this compensation is lacking in shock.

Peripheral Vascular Resistance. Because of generalized arteriolar constriction, peripheral vascular resistance is generally high in hypovolemic shock. Calculations of peripheral vascular resistance, expressed as the ratio of drop in blood pressure across the systemic circulation to the cardiac output, are commonly advocated as guides to therapy in hypovolemic shock. Usually the ratio is increased, a consequence of heightened sympathetic nervous activity and of increase in circulating catecholamines. But rarely does this calculation provide a more reliable guide to treatment than do the clinical appearance of the patient, the warmth of the skin, the level of blood pressure, the rate and fullness of the pulse, and the urine output. Moreover, because of the nonuniform effects of heightened sympathetic activity, such calculations often tend to obscure the complicated and heterogeneous engagement of the different systemic vascular beds in the different types of shock.

Oxygen Delivery. In addition to the slowed circulation, which impairs oxygen delivery to tissues, disturbances in acid-base balance upset erythrocyte metabolism, including that of the organic phosphate, 2,3-diphosphoglyceric acid (2,3-DPG), thereby increasing the affinity of hemoglobin for oxygen and hindering oxygen delivery to the tissues.

The Heart. In shock that is simply due to an acute decrease in venous return, the heart is rarely seriously affected unless hypotension persists at levels that are insufficient to sustain coronary arterial blood flow, i.e., less than 70 to 80 mm Hg. Toxins from splanchnic viscera may also contribute to depressed contractility when hypotension is prolonged. One potentially toxic substance has been designated "myocardial depressant factor." It is a peptide which is released from the pancreas during hypotension from any cause. During splanchnic hypoperfusion consequent to systemic hypotension, splanchnic tissues release lysosomal hydrolases which not only exert a negative inotropic action on the heart but also sensitize the myocardium to the myocardial depressant factor from the pancreas.

Shock Lung. Early in shock, unless the tracheobronchial tree or chest is abnormal, the lungs generally pose no clinical problem: alveolar ventilation is usually high, and even though there may be some imbalance in alveolar ventilation-perfusion relationships, arterial hypoxemia and hypocapnia are slight and generally insignificant. But as shock continues and grows worse, pulmonary performance deteriorates. Arterial hypoxemia then becomes more marked, principally because of continued blood flow through airless lungs. This situation may be aggravated by narcotics and sedatives which depress alveolar ventilation, by inspissated bronchial secretions which block ventilation in perfused parts of the lungs, by oxygen toxicity which damages the alveolar-capillary membrane, and by overtransfusion which causes pulmonary edema.

Entirely different from this *progressive* deterioration in pulmonary performance in the course of refractory shock is the entity of "shock lung" (or "wet lung" or "Da Nang lung") which has been applied to the syndrome of respiratory failure that interrupts recovery from circulatory collapse. The typical sequence of shock lung was popularized during the Vietnam war: a soldier who experiences severe *nonthoracic* injury, blood loss, and hypotension during combat; successful resuscitation, using tourniquets, transfusions, and opiates on the battlefield; prompt evacuation to a sophisticated medical facility for more deliberate management and recovery; and then, a few days later, the unexpected interruption of convalescence by progressive respiratory distress and failure.

Only a few who reached the hospital in Da Nang developed shock lung. But in them, the clinical syndrome was unmistakable; interruption of convalescence by the insidious onset (over days) of rapid shallow breathing, breathlessness, and productive cough; somewhat later, rales and wheezes; finally, refractory cyanosis. Paralleling this clinical sequence, x-ray examinations showed enlarging interstitial and alveolar infiltrates that continued to extend and to coalesce until the entire lung was enveloped in a diffuse haze. Enriched oxygen mixtures and assisted ventilation became less and less effective in achieving tolerable levels of oxygenation. Finally, death occurred from respiratory insufficiency, often complicated by circulatory collapse. At autopsy the morbid anatomy was stereotyped; vascular congestion, interstitial and alveolar edema, and focal atelectasis ("congestive atelectasis"). Other anatomic changes were common but not quite as consistent: hemorrhage in the interstitial spaces and alveoli, vascular thrombi, fat emboli, fibrin deposits, and hyaline membranes.

The physiologic picture of shock lung observed in Vietnam held no surprises: its features were reduced compliance and arterial hypoxemia. In part, the reduced compliance reflected stiffening of the lungs by congestive atelectasis; the extent to which loss of surfactant contributed was, and still is, enigmatic. The progressive arterial hypoxemia (without hypercapnia) was shown to represent increasing "venous admixture," evidence of continuing blood flow through parts of the lungs which were functionless in gas exchange.

Unfortunately, many of the links that relate injury and resuscitation on the battlefield to respiratory insufficiency during convalescence are missing. Those that have been proposed include damage to hypoperfused areas of the lungs during the hypotensive episode, endotoxinemia, fat emboli, release of injurious fatty acids and proteolytic agents, discharge of leukocyte lysosomes in the pulmonary capillaries, and disseminated intravascular coagulation or microemboli. There is also the haunting prospect that therapeutic measures which are lifesaving on the battlefield may be involved in the subsequent respiratory distress during convalescence. Thus overzealous administration of liquids immediately after injury, particularly of crystalloid solutions, predisposes to pulmonary congestion and edema. Also, if bank blood was administered, thrombi may have embolized the lungs, thereby contributing to congestive atelectasis. Even the hospital provides opportunity for inflicting lung damage by way of injudicious administration of enriched oxygen mixtures and oversedation. Once the syndrome is full blown, distinctions between cause and effect tend to become blurred as self-perpetuating mechanisms become operative.

The designation "shock lung" has carried over from Vietnam to civilian life and has been applied indiscriminately to a wide variety of adult respiratory distress syndromes. Favoring this practice is the stereotyped "congestive atelectasis" found at autopsy. However, the high mortality from "shock lung" has stimulated reevaluation of the civilian disorders in the hope of elucidating unique etiologies and pathogenetic mechanisms at which specific therapeutic measures may be directed.

The Liver. Blood flow through the liver increases early in shock but decreases later on. Accompanying the decrease in hepatic blood flow is a sequestration of blood in the splanchnic venous bed. As hepatic blood flow decreases, the effectiveness of the liver in detoxification and in performing its metabolic activities decreases. Consequently, organic acids accumulate in the blood. The metabolic acidosis is associated with hyperglycemia and hyperkalemia and the release of toxic products from splanchnic viscera.

The Kidneys. Oliguria (less than 25 ml per hour) and anuria are common, particularly if systemic arterial hypotension is marked; prerenal azotemia may also be prominent. As the circulation is restored and blood pressure increases, urinary output improves and the azotemia disappears. But if severe hypotension and renal vasoconstriction have persisted for hours, particularly in patients who have abnormal pigments from hemolysis or muscle trauma in the blood, irreversible injury to the kidneys may occur from tubular necrosis.

SEPTIC SHOCK

Septic shock is a state of circulatory collapse associated with toxicity that results from the spread of bacteria and/or their products throughout the body from a focus of infection. A wide range of microbial organisms can elicit septic shock. Chief among these are the common gram-positive and gram-negative pathogens. But even relatively avirulent microorganisms can produce the syndrome of circulatory collapse if sufficient numbers enter the bloodstream for dissemination. Before the days of antimicrobial drugs, gram-positive organisms, including the Staphylococcus, Streptococcus, Pneumococcus, and *Clostridium perfringens* (septic abortion), were common invaders of the bloodstream; the shock then seemed to originate in the primary infection rather than in the bacteremia. But in recent years, gram-negative organisms have emerged as the principal basis for shock associated with sepsis. All gram-negative bacteria—Escherichia, Klebsiella, Pseudomonas, Proteus, Bacteroides—contain a complex lipopolysaccharide, called endotoxin, in their cell walls. In contrast with gram-positive shock, bloodstream invasion by endotoxin seems to elicit the shock.

Endotoxin Shock. Endotoxin shock is a subset of septic shock. It is a complication of a gram-negative infection associated with the death of the bacteria and the consequent release of endotoxin from their walls. Some investigators believe that the action of endotoxin is primarily via an immune response involving complement. Within the bloodstream endotoxin combines with complement of leukocytes, and activates latent systems, to produce a variety of agents, including sympathomimetic amines (epinephrine, norepinephrine, histamine), that derange the control of circulation. Other vasoactive substances, including kinins, are also present, as well as enzymes released from cellular lysosomes. In addition, there are serious aberrations in the coagulation mechanism, resulting in intravascular coagulation with the consumption of fibrinogen and the production of hemorrhage.

The most common organisms involved in endotoxin shock reside in the human intestinal tract. In the elderly male, endotoxin shock usually follows urethral instrumentation for prostatism. In many adults, it is associated with infections of the urinary tract, gastrointestinal tract (including peritonitis), or biliary tree; often endotoxin shock follows trauma and manipulation (including surgery) of these areas.

Clinical Manifestations. Since septic shock is a complication of bloodstream invasion from a focus, the clinical manifestations reflect both the underlying disorder and the sepsis. The patient is cold, pale, often cyanotic, and oliguric; hypotension is the rule, but it is usually not as marked as after hemorrhage, trauma, or burns. The death rate from endotoxin shock is high, and most patients die if pulmonary complications, particularly "shock lung," appear.

Pathophysiology. Both the associated disorder and the endotoxinemia contribute to the cardiovascular and pulmonary disorders. The endotoxin molecule has no direct depressant effect on the myocardium. Arterial blood pressure is generally near normal, but different mechanisms may be operative: high or normal cardiac output associated with a decrease in peripheral vascular resistance or low cardiac output associated with an increase in peripheral vascular resistance. Hemodynamic combinations may vary with time, but predominant vasodilatation generally supervenes.

The vasodilatation of septic shock has been attributed to fever, bacterial toxins, and the generation of vasodilator substances (including histamine and kinins) and metabolic end products evoked by endotoxin. But despite extensive peripheral vasodilation, these patients also manifest organ hypoperfusion and heightened sympathetic nervous activity: cold fingertips indicate activation of alpha-adrenergic sensitive beds; oliguria suggests that renal blood flow has decreased even though the cardiac output may be high. Catecholamines, released into the circulation in response to stress, not only contribute to local vasoconstriction but also exert direct inotropic effects on the heart.

Lactic acidosis is common, partly attributable to organ hypoperfusion. Its presence should be suspected when a considerable decrease in serum bicarbonate concentration is accompanied by an increase in unmeasured anions ("anion gap"). An increasing anion gap is a bad prognostic sign that signals need for a prompt reappraisal of therapy. In contrast to the metabolic acidosis of hemorrhagic shock, early endotoxin shock is often associated with a high pH and evidence of a mixed respiratory alkalosis and metabolic acidosis. As shock persists and the lungs become involved in the picture of "shock lung," venous admixture increases because of ventilation-perfusion inhomogeneities. Intravascular coagulation may produce the syndrome of disseminated coagulation, afibrinogenemia, and hemorrhage. The coup de grâce in septic shock may be delivered by a generalized Shwartzman phenomenon (intravascular coagulation, deposition of fibrin in glomeruli, and bilateral renal cortical necrosis).

CARDIOGENIC SHOCK

Cardiogenic shock refers to a combination of heart failure and shock that follows extensive myocardial infarction (more than 40 per cent of left ventricular muscle). Evidence of shock, particularly of organ hypoperfusion and hypotension, predominates over that of left ventricular failure. Approximately 15 per cent of patients hospitalized for acute myocardial infarction develop cardiogenic shock. Mortality from cardiogenic shock is high, averaging about 80 per cent in different coronary care units.

Clinical Manifestations. The full-blown picture is characteristic. A patient who has suffered a recent myocardial infarction develops signs of a falling cardiac output, peripheral vasoconstriction, and organ hypoperfusion. Mentation is disturbed; the patient is restless; the skin becomes cold and clammy, and beads of perspiration appear on the head and neck. A persistent tachycardia develops in association with weak peripheral (femoral) pulses. Auscultatory blood pressure (including pulse pressure) decreases.

Of great importance is the urine output. As long as it remains high, the patient may recover without therapy. Conversely, if oliguria appears and progresses in conjunction with evidence of peripheral vasoconstriction, therapy to restore the circulation is mandatory. Delay in starting treatment may be crucial, because the syndrome may cascade precipitously, within hours, from premonitory signs to death.

At the outset, the lungs are often free of rales, because pulmonary edema is confined to the interstitial spaces. However, the increase in respiratory frequency produced by the stiff lungs will elicit respiratory alkalosis. If shock progresses, hypocapnia will become associated with a low pH as metabolic acidosis supervenes. Oxygenation of arterial blood is generally well maintained at the outset but may be compromised in time as venous admixture increases. Consequently, an arterial cannula is valuable in early cardiogenic shock not only for monitoring blood pressure but also for serial sampling to detect the advent of metabolic acidosis and of impaired arterialization.

Occasionally, generalized vasodilation ("warm-handed shock") may dominate the course of cardiogenic shock, usually without apparent reason. The arterial blood pressure decreases, the cardiac output is normal or nearly normal, and the renal blood flow and urine volume remain within the normal range; there is no evidence of organ hypoperfusion. There is neither acidosis nor an increase in the "anion gap" or in lactic acid in blood. The prognosis is generally better than in those patients who manifest hypotension and intense vasoconstriction after myocardial infarction.

Mechanisms other than massive myocardial damage may elicit a shocklike syndrome after acute myocardial infarction: arrhythmias (bradycardia or tachycardia); long-lasting effects of pharmacologic agents, such as propranolol, administered before the episode of infarction; rupture of a necrotic area (papillary muscle, septum, or free wall). Each of these influences requires individual consideration and attention.

Pathophysiology. Cardiogenic shock in the course of acute myocardial infarction is characterized by left ventricular failure, low cardiac output, and arterial hypotension. The damaged left ventricular wall, high left atrial pressure, pulmonary venous congestion, and pulmonary edema initiate one set of reflexes that modify the circulation through remote organs, including kidney and muscles. A different set of reflexes results from the decrease in cardiac output and in filling of the arterial tree. Consequently, it is not surprising that hemodynamic patterns may range from intense peripheral vasoconstriction, as usually occurs in hemorrhagic shock, to mixtures of vasoconstriction and vasodilatation, as may occur in septic shock. But despite these variations, the consistent feature is organ hypoperfusion signaled by oliguria, pale skin, and disturbed mentation. That the kidney can still respond by vasodilating can be shown by a brisk diuretic response to furosemide administered intravenously.

Because of the limited capacity of the cerebral and coronary beds for autoregulation, their blood flow depends largely on the aortic pressure. With respect to cardiogenic shock this dependence is critical, because a decrease in coronary arterial blood pressure entails the prospect of extending the myocardial infarct and of compromising further the performance of the residual viable muscle. Consequently, persistent hypotension enhances the prospects for irreversible cardiac damage and unremitting cardiogenic shock.

That indirect methods for determining arterial blood pressure are unreliable in patients with decreasing cardiac output and peripheral vasoconstriction has been amply demonstrated in cardiogenic shock. Therefore intra-arterial pressure should be monitored directly in patients with early signs of cardiogenic shock. A suitable pressure transducer and a recording or monitoring device are essential for the bedside monitoring. If this electronic system is not available, the physician bases his assessment of arterial pressure on the strength of the femoral pulses and on his indirect assessment of the adequacy of coronary and cerebral perfusion.

SHOCK FROM INADEQUATE FILLING

Excessively rapid heart rates sharply curtail diastolic filling, thereby decreasing cardiac output. In many respects, the clinical picture resembles that of acute pericardial tamponade or acute tension pneumothorax which restrict filling of the heart by mechanical obstruction to venous inflow rather than by excessive heart rate. Success in treatment depends on controlling the arrhythmia.

OTHER HYPOTENSIVE STATES

Acute Disorders

These disorders include the syndromes of vasomotor paralysis and syncope. They differ from shock in etiology, duration, clinical course, and prognosis.

Vasomotor Paralysis. This syndrome represents paralysis of arterioles and is usually manageable. The clinical picture is diametrically opposite to that of hypovolemic shock in which sympathetic vasomotor tone is high. On the other hand, it does share some features of the picture of peripheral vasodilation that occurs frequently in septic shock and occasionally in cardiogenic shock.

The prototype of this syndrome is the massive vasodilatation and circulatory collapse induced by a severe blow to an unguarded abdomen (e.g., a blow to the solar plexus). The same effect can be elicited by spinal anesthesia or by giving vasodilator agents during hypovolemia or anaphylaxis. The onset of hypotension is often precipitous, and proper treatment usually arrests the disorder in minutes.

Treatment of vasodilated hypotension begins with volume expansion, on the assumption that the *effective,* rather than the *actual,* circulating blood volume has been reduced by vasodilatation. But should volume expansion fail to provide prompt relief, vasoconstrictors, such as levarterenol or metaraminol, are in order.

Syncope. A precipitous decrease in systemic arterial blood pressure may produce a transient loss of consciousness, or syncope. The drop in blood pressure may be due to an abrupt decrease in cardiac output or to sudden vasodilatation. The syncope stems from inadequate delivery of oxygen and glucose to the brain as a consequence of the decrease in cerebral blood flow that accompanies the drop in blood pressure.

Syncope is distinguished from shock by the loss of consciousness, by its brief duration, and by its prompt reversal once the initiating mechanism is removed. Any episode of severe hypotension that lasts for more than a few seconds can elicit syncope (see Ch. 353). The most familiar example is the common episode of fainting.

The common faint (vasovagal or vasodepressor syncope) stems from a sudden and precipitous fall in peripheral resistance, probably involving both arterioles and veins, unaccompanied by the increase in cardiac output that usually follows peripheral vasodilatation. The usual setting is one of intense emotional stress, often when the discomfort or anxiety is relieved. Thus it occurs in blood donors after only small quantities of blood have been withdrawn, in subjects with indwelling arterial needles who experience gnawing, dull pain at the puncture site, and in anxious subjects who realize suddenly that they are not about to be harmed. The upright subject feels light-headed, becomes pale, breaks into a cold sweat, complains of nausea, and abruptly passes out. The heart rate slows, and arterial pressure falls precipitously. The cardiac output shows only a slight decrease or remains unchanged from the precollapse level. Vasodilatation is marked in skeletal muscles, but the compensatory increase in heart rate and cardiac output fails to materialize because of intense parasympathetic discharge. The syndrome usually ends abruptly when the subject lies or falls down. Smelling salts usually help. Atropine is rarely needed.

Chronic Disorders

Two states of arterial hypotension, one benign and the other incapacitating, also pertain to the function of the autonomic nervous system in regulating the circulation.

Chronic Arterial Hypotension. Many persons maintain a blood pressure of 90 systolic and 60 diastolic for a lifetime without dire results. Indeed, systemic hypotension predisposes to longevity. They differ from the hypotensive patient in shock in that the low blood pressure is not associated with evidences of intensified sympathetic nervous activity or organ hypoperfusion.

Orthostatic Hypotension. In normal individuals, an elaborate system of cardiovascular reflexes prevents pooling of blood in the periphery when the upright posture is assumed. Central to these mechanisms is the carotid sinus reflex which constricts arterioles and venules and increases heart rate and myocardial contractility. Mechanical pumping by leg muscles and release of neurohumoral substances (catecholamines, renin, and angiotensin) are also involved in maintaining the blood pressure.

Disturbances in the autonomic nervous system (see Ch. 377) that interfere with the cardiovascular reflexes may elicit postural hypotension and syncope. Thus orthostatic hypotension generally represents a chronic inadequacy of the sympathetic nervous contribution to the control of the circulation.

TREATMENT

Mortality from hypovolemic types of shock has decreased dramatically because of prompt administration of blood, plasma, plasma substitutes, and saline solutions. But mortality from septic and cardiogenic shock remains at 70 per cent or higher. Consequently, it is much more difficult to be categorical about managing cardiogenic and septic shock than hypovolemic shock.

Five separate components enter into the planning of therapeutic regimens: initiating mechanisms, duration of shock, level of autonomic nervous activity, state of the peripheral circulation, and performance of the myocardium. The importance of each of these components varies according to the nature of the shock. For example, effective treatment of septic shock is impossible without control of bacterial infection. Also, prolonged shock of any cause is apt to be associated with depressed myocardial contractility and a refractory peripheral circulation even though sympathetic nervous activity is intense.

The crux of any program for treating shock is early detection and prompt intervention. An essential determinant of prognosis is the health of the patient before the onset of shock. A patient who has an underlying debilitating disease or has been receiving anticancer medications may be incapable of recovering from the episode that precipitated shock.

General Measures

Among the general measures that may promote recovery are several simple maneuvers: (1) proper positioning, generally supine in hypovolemic and endotoxin shock and partially upright in cardiogenic shock; (2) judicious relief of pain and restlessness, using morphine (15 mg) or meperidine (100 mg) administered intravenously, while avoiding excess analgesia and narcosis that predispose to arterial hypotension; (3) withholding food, allowing sips of water for thirst, in order to minimize the prospects of vomiting and aspiration; (4) adequate oxygenation accomplished as simply as possible, e.g., oxygen by nasal catheter; and (5) prevention of acidosis, e.g., by restoring circulating blood volume and blood pressure and, if necessary, by administering sodium bicarbonate intravenously, in order to maintain peripheral vascular responsiveness to endogenous and exogenous catecholamines.

Once incipient shock is recognized, a central venous catheter is introduced for the administration of fluid and medications, for blood sampling, and for measuring right atrial pressure. Should shock materialize, steps are immediately taken for intensive treatment. Blood is withdrawn for typing and cross-matching. The electrocardiogram is monitored for early detection of arrhythmias. If the patient is oliguric or anuric, a urinary catheter is placed for reliable determinations of urine flow. A cannula introduced into a peripheral artery will provide not only serial determinations of blood pressure but also blood samples for Po_2 and pH. From the outset, attention is paid to adequate ventilation. If arterial Po_2 falls below 60 to 70 mm Hg, tracheal intubation and assisted ventilation are required to maintain tolerable levels of oxygenation.

Once these general measures—volume replacement and provisions for monitoring—have been instituted, a decision has to be reached concerning priorities: continued transfusions to replenish the decreased circulating blood volume; use of autonomic agents to change the calibers of systemic blood vessels; or cardiotonic agents, such as digitalis, to improve cardiac performance.

Replenishment of the Circulating Blood Volume. In shock associated with hypovolemia, intravenous administration of fluids is clearly the first line of treatment. If blood has been lost, it should be replaced. The aim is to restore arterial blood pressure to tolerable levels rather than to original levels, e.g., systolic pressure of 90 to 100 mm Hg rather than 120 or 130 mm Hg. Crystalloid solutions, such as isotonic saline or glucose, may serve as temporary expedients while matching blood is obtained. More lasting support for the circulation is provided by macromolecular agents, particularly the dextrans of low viscosity and molecular weight (about 40,000), which remain longer in the circulation. Care is taken when blood substitutes are administered to avoid excess hemodilution. Except in states of hypofibrinogenemia and bleeding dyscrasias, low molecular weight dextran is remarkably free of side effects. It is usually administered intravenously as a 6 per cent solution, either in physiologic saline or glucose solution. Five hundred milliliters generally expands the blood volume by an average of approximately 1200 to 1800 ml; the effect is over in a few hours because of its loss via the kidneys unless an additional slow infusion is administered. If oliguria persists during the infusion, the plasma volume may be overexpanded, and pulmonary edema may be precipitated. Colloidal solutions of albumin (25 grams in 100 ml of 0.9 per cent saline) are as effective but much less available. Albumin is preferable to plasma because it does not entail the risk of hepatitis.

The therapeutic goal in the administration of fluids is the re-establishment of an adequate circulating volume and a near-normal distribution of blood flow among organs and tissues without severely upsetting the electrolyte balance. If treatment has to be prolonged, different sequences and combinations of fluids are generally needed, depending on whether the problem is to maintain electrolyte balance, to provide energy, or to combat acidosis. Assuming the judicious selection of fluids, the key clinical guides for administration of adequate amounts of fluid intravenously are clearing of the sensorium, improved circulation to the skin, restoration of the arterial blood pressure, slowing of the heart rate, and increase in urine flow. Unfortunately, consecutive determinations of blood volume have proved to have little practical value as guides to fluid replacement because of the changing natures of most kinds of shock and the inevitable delays that are involved between the times of sampling, the analysis, and the final reporting.

The clinical state of intense peripheral vasoconstriction and organ hypoperfusion, manifested by the cold, clammy skin, thready pulse, and oliguria, clearly calls for intravenous fluids. Arterial blood pressure, governed by an elaborate baroregulatory apparatus, is a complicated guide to fluid replacement. Indeed, overzealous attempts to restore arterial blood pressure to preshock levels are responsible for many attacks of frank pulmonary edema, especially if the left ventricle has been damaged previously.

Currently, central venous pressure is the popular guide to fluid replacement. Its determination involves the measurement of blood pressure in a large intrathoracic vein close to the heart. Normally, this value is of the order of −2 to +5 cm of water. Unfortunately, like the arterial blood pressure, the value may be difficult to interpret, because central venous pressure is a function not only of blood volume but also of venous tone, of the competence and distensibility of the right ventricle, of heart rate, and of intrathoracic pressure. The interpretation of central venous pressure as a guide to fluid administration is even more complicated when vasopressors are being administered, because they raise venous pressure by local effects on venous walls. The greatest value of central venous pressure is in hypovolemic shock in which the myocardium generally performs well. Conversely, it is potentially misleading in cardiogenic shock in which the competent right ventricle responds to an increase in venous return by flooding the lungs with blood that the damaged left ventricle cannot handle.

In hypovolemic and septic shock, the central venous pressure is used as follows: fluids are administered intravenously in an attempt to increase the arterial blood pressure and the urine output without driving the central venous pressure to abnormally high levels (to more than 10 to 15 cm of water). A modest increase in central venous pressure, e.g., to 15 cm of water, may prove necessary during intravenous infusions in order to sustain the cardiac output, particularly if shock is protracted. But should the central venous pressure start mounting abruptly, a state of overtransfusion has been reached and the right ventricle is assumed to have failed.

In cardiogenic shock in which the competence of the left heart is in question, the pulmonary arterial diastolic pressure may be used as an approximate index of left ventricular end-diastolic pressure and as a more meaningful guide for the intravenous administration of fluids than is the central venous pressure.

Autonomic Agents. Endogenous catecholamine levels in the blood are generally high throughout the course of shock, often continuing to increase as shock grows refractory. Moreover, a wide variety of sympathomimetic amines are currently being used to supplement endogenous levels when shock either has failed to respond

to administration of fluids or has reached the stage where fluid overload is in prospect. By exerting their effects on alpha or beta receptors, their actions are excitatory, inhibitory, or a combination of the two. Alpha-excitatory drugs, such as methoxamine (Vasoxyl) cause vasoconstriction; beta-excitatory drugs, such as isoproterenol (Isuprel), relax vascular smooth muscle while exerting positive inotropic, chronotropic, and dromotropic effects on the myocardium. Norepinephrine (levarterenol) exerts both alpha and beta effects and is particularly useful in producing vasoconstriction in conjunction with inotropic and chronotropic effects on the myocardium. Metaraminol can serve the same purpose if the stores of catecholamines in myocardium and vascular smooth muscle are not depleted; it has the advantage over norepinephrine of avoiding local injury and necrosis should leakage occur from a misdirected needle at the site of infusion.

Opinions vary concerning the proper use of vasoactive agents in managing shock. In general, vasoconstrictors constitute first-line drugs that are used in early forms of shock if response to volume expansion is delayed or inadequate. Vasodilators, on the other hand, are generally reserved for shock that is refractory to fluids and in which vasoconstriction is intense. When central venous pressure is high, vasodilators (e.g., phentolamine, isoproterenol) usually increase cardiac output and renal blood flow, raise blood pressure, promote diuresis, and relieve peripheral vasoconstriction. Unless central venous pressure is high, vasodilators are apt to promote deterioration in the clinical state. Resort to vasodilators underscores the common experience that excessively high levels of circulating catecholamines may impede recovery. Consequently, fluids remain the mainstay of therapy for shock, and when vasopressors are given, doses are kept as small as possible.

Despite divergent views and incomplete data, it is possible to distill a few general principles for the use of autonomic agents in treating the common types of shock in which sympathetic activity is high: (1) Vasoconstrictive and inotropic agents, such as norepinephrine, are most likely to be effective if the blood volume is normal or somewhat expanded. (2) Since increasing the level of arterial blood pressure by vasoconstrictors generally increases flow to the brain and heart at the expense of flow to other organs, such as the kidneys, the use of any one of these agents should be as brief and in as small a dose as possible. (3) Acidosis, a regular concomitant of severe shock, lessens the effectiveness of vasoconstrictive agents such as norepinephrine, leading to larger doses and increasing side effects. (4) Vasodilators seem to be in order when volume expansion and intense peripheral vasoconstriction have proved ineffective. (5) Prolonged and severe oliguria that has resisted both volume expansion and the administration of vasoconstrictors during shock may respond to diuretic agents that elicit renal vasodilation, such as furosemide, thereby helping to prevent serious renal injury. (6) Massive doses of adrenocortical steroids, such as hydrocortisone, may be useful in states of bacteremic shock and merit trial in other instances of refractory shock; they have a mandatory role in preventing shock in those patients on maintenance doses of steroids for systemic illness, e.g., rheumatoid arthritis, who are about to be subjected to the stress of anesthesia or surgery.

Oxygen Therapy. It has been noted above that patients in shock are candidates for a wide variety of pulmonary disorders, including atelectasis, pneumonia, and pulmonary edema; the prospects for these grave complications to occur increase as shock persists. Early in shock, when abnormalities in pulmonary performance are generally mild, administration of oxygen by nasal catheter generally suffices. But should shock be severe and protracted, patients may require tracheal intubation and assisted ventilation to relieve labored breathing and to improve alveolar ventilation. Since the use of mechanical respirators to improve gas exchange entails the risk of aggravating shock by impeding venous return, particularly if blood volume is depleted, assisted ventilation in shock should be undertaken only by experts.

Cardiotonic Agents. Even though the normal myocardium may suffer somewhat in early shock from being hypoperfused, rarely is it sufficiently compromised to require the support of digitalis. More justifiable is the administration of digitalis in protracted shock if the heart has previously been damaged by disease or by aging. Even then, extraordinary care is required in digitalization because of the potentiating effects of acidosis, hypoxia, and electrolyte disturbances in severe shock on the production of ventricular arrhythmias and conduction disturbances by digitalis.

In cardiogenic shock, digitalization is apt to be helpful only if evidence can be accrued that the noninfarcted part of the ventricle has failed. Digitalis therapy is then undertaken cautiously, while monitoring the electrocardiogram carefully for arrhythmias.

Intravascular Coagulation. Defects in coagulation are common in shock, but bleeding is uncommon. Despite the tendency to intravascular aggregation and clotting disorders, none of these seem to require anticoagulant therapy. Improvement in the circulation suffices to correct these deficiencies.

Specific Measures

Special attention should be called to certain therapeutic measures that are used in septic and cardiogenic shock.

Septic Shock. Elimination of the cause of sepsis is of cardinal importance in treating septic shock. Intensive treatment on several fronts must be started as soon as the diagnosis is made. While the blood pressure is being sustained by intravenous infusions—usually plasma, dextran, crystalloids, or blood if the hematocrit is low—and possibly by pharmacologic agents, it is critical to administer the proper antimicrobials as soon as blood cultures have been taken. Since most cases of septic shock in a general hospital are due to gram-negative bacilli, it is reasonable to institute antimicrobial therapy with Escherichia, Klebsiella, Pseudomonas, and Enterobacteriaceae in mind, e.g., with an aminoglycoside (gentamicin or kanamycin) and a cephalosporin (cephalothin).

If there is a likelihood of a complicating bacteremia with penicillinase-producing staphylococci, nafcillin or oxacillin should be added.

This regimen can be modified after the results of blood cultures are known, e.g., by adding clindamycin if a gastrointestinal strain of bacteroides is identified or carbenicillin if pseudomonas infection and severe neutropenia coexist (see Ch. 214).

Often the patient relapses after a brief period of response to intravenous fluids. This is presumably due to continuing intravascular stagnation and extravascular fluid loss. Massive doses of glucocorticosteroids (e.g.,

hydrocortisone, 50 to 150 mg) have been proved helpful, particularly if used early in septic shock. Presumably, the corticosteroids correct the defects produced by endotoxin: restore the normal microcirculation by vasodilation, stabilize cell walls to prevent release of vasoactive and proteolytic substances, and decrease adhesiveness of blood cells and platelets. Other vasodilating agents (e.g., phenoxybenzamine) are currently under trial, but there is no great optimism about their therapeutic prospects.

Cardiogenic Shock. Patterns for treating cardiogenic shock after myocardial infarction have been set by coronary intensive care units in which extensive monitoring of blood pressures and of the electrocardiogram are routine. The patient is positioned semiupright, a compromise between the need for cerebral blood flow and the threat of pulmonary edema. The ideal way to support the blood pressure in cardiogenic shock is to increase the cardiac output and to decrease the peripheral resistance. Patients in cardiogenic shock who have only a modest increase in left ventricular pressure often improve after cautious expansion of the circulating blood volume or cautious administration of inotropic agents. Since fluid overload is particularly undesirable after myocardial infarction, failure to restore blood pressure to tolerable levels by volume expansion is generally followed by the administration of vasopressor agents.

In cardiogenic shock the use of inotropic agents, chiefly isoproterenol and levarterenol, is done cautiously, realizing that although the increase in blood pressure does increase coronary blood flow, it does so at the cost of increasing cardiac work and oxygen demand. Hopefully the increased coronary flow will offset the increased work. Unfortunately, this goal is often elusive, and myocardial anoxia may be intensified, leading to extension of the myocardial damage that originally caused the shock. Rarely does isoproterenol have any advantage over levarterenol as the initial catecholamine in cardiogenic shock; not only may it fail to raise the blood pressure if the direct inotropic effects on the heart are neutralized by peripheral vasodilation, but it is also likely to evoke troublesome arrhythmias. Dopamine has staunch advocates because of its vasodilating effects on the kidney, but it is generally reserved as an alternative for levarterenol or isoproterenol. New vasoactive and inotropic agents continue to be tried. But at the moment it seems that cautious administration of levarterenol holds the brightest prospect for restoring the blood pressure unless the patient is already maximally vasoconstricted; isoproterenol is then generally tried. As prerequisites for administering catecholamines, hypoxemia should be corrected and arterial pH should be restored to normal. Disturbances in cardiac rhythm should be handled promptly, with care taken to avoid interventions and drugs that depress myocardial function.

Medical therapy in cardiogenic shock is directed toward maintaining coronary blood flow and preventing extension of the myocardial infarct. Should medical measures prove ineffective, mechanical circulatory assistance is currently being tried in some medical centers. The widest experience has been gained with the intra-aortic balloon pump which requires little surgery and offers circulatory assistance by way of counterpulsation. The limited long-term survival rate after balloon-pumping alone has encouraged the use of coronary revascularization procedures, particularly aortic–coronary artery bypass grafts, to restore myocardial blood flow on an emergency basis. These surgical procedures are complicated, requiring preoperative coronary angiography and left ventriculography while the heart is being assisted mechanically. The role of surgical measures in cardiogenic shock remains to be established.

Fishman, A. P.: Shock lung. A distinctive non-entity. Circulation, 47:921, 1973.

Forscher, B. K., Lillehei, R. C., and Stubbs, S. S.: Shock in Low- and High-Flow States. Amsterdam, Excerpta Medica, 1972.

Guyton, A. C., and Jones, C. E.: Central venous pressure: Physiological significance and clinical implications. Am. Heart J., 86:431, 1973.

Hershey, S. G., Del Guercio, L. R. M., and McConn, R. (eds.): Septic Shock in Man. Boston, Little, Brown & Company, 1971.

Lefer, A. M.: Blood-borne humoral factors in the pathophysiology of circulatory shock. Circ. Res., 32:129, 1973.

Lluch, S., Moguilevsky, H. C., Pietra, G., Shaffer, A. B., Hirsch, L. J., and Fishman, A. P.: A reproducible model of cardiogenic shock in the dog. Circulation, 39:205, 1969.

Swan, H. J. C.: Power failure of the heart in acute myocardial infarction. In Likoff, W., Segal, B. L., and Insull, W., Jr. (eds.): Arteriosclerosis and Coronary Heart Disease. New York, Grune & Stratton, 1973.

THROMBOEMBOLIC DISEASES

Sol Sherry

543. INTRODUCTION

Thrombosis is the formation from the constituents of the blood of a solid mass or plug in the heart or blood vessels. The thrombus which forms may be dislodged in whole or in part to another vascular site; when this occurs the thrombus or its fragment is referred to as an embolus. Collectively the states associated with such thrombi or emboli are referred to as the thromboembolic diseases or disorders, and when viewed together they represent a leading cause of serious illness and death in the Western world; furthermore, their importance is likely to grow with increasing longevity. This chapter is concerned with only one form of the thromboembolic disorders, i.e., peripheral venous thrombosis and its major complication, pulmonary artery embolism. The thromboembolic disorders involving the heart, brain, systemic arteries, and selected veins, e.g., hepatic, portal, and renal, are considered elsewhere in the text.

Alterations in blood flow, damage to the vessel wall, and changes in the coagulability of the blood have been stressed as the major factors responsible for thrombus formation in vivo. To these we need add the formed elements (notably the platelets) and fibrinolysis. The interplay among these factors, whose importance varies with the circumstances, controls the initiation and the dynamics of thrombus growth. *In the arterial system*, a vascular lesion is generally accepted as the most frequent primary cause of an acute thrombotic event, and the latter is viewed as an exaggeration of the normal hemostatic response to vascular injury. Thrombi originate adjacent to lesions in arterial walls, and each is composed primarily of a large white head containing platelets and some fibrin; a variable amount of fresh clot then extends from this white head. It is postulated that platelets adhere to the exposed microfibrils and collagen fibers at the site of vascular injury, e.g., fissured or ul-

cerated atheromatous plaque. After adherence and in response to a continuing stimulus, platelets release certain constituents like ADP (adenosine diphosphate) which stimulate platelet aggregation and the formation of a platelet mass. Subsequently, there is activation of the clotting mechanism; this results in formation of fibrin within the the platelet head (so as to stabilize it) and the superimposition of a fresh clot.

The pathogenesis of *venous thrombosis* is less well understood, except when there is direct injury or infection of the vein wall which leads to a thrombus much like that in an artery. However, in most instances, thrombus formation takes place in the absence of a demonstrable vascular lesion, because the venous intima, unlike the arterial, is much less exposed to injury from high fluid pressure or atherosclerosis. Furthermore, in contrast to the arterial, the venous thrombus is composed primarily of a red, gel-like mass similar to a test tube blood clot; a white platelet head is either inconspicuous or absent. Most venous thrombi are postulated to be initiated through local activation of the clotting mechanism with the insular accumulation of thrombin. The latter then triggers both fibrin formation and platelet aggregation and accounts for the successive layers of fibrin coagulum and platelets (lines of Zahn) commonly observed histologically in growing venous thrombi. Local activation of the clotting mechanism is believed to arise as a consequence of two considerations: (1) the presence in the general circulation of activated enzymatic components of the clotting reactions consequent to recent or ongoing tissue damage, trauma, or necrosis and possibly in association with impaired inhibitory or clearing mechanisms; and (2) stasis, which serves to sustain the action of the activated enzymatic clotting factors, as in the animal model developed by Wessler. In this model, immediately after the systemic injection of early activated components of the clotting mechanism (either in purified form or as serum), isolation of a venous segment by ligatures or clamps, so as to effect stasis, results in rapid formation of a thrombus in situ; thrombosis is not seen in the freely flowing circulation and is markedly delayed in the isolated venous segment of control animals.

Venous thromboembolism is a frequent, important, and challenging clinical problem and a particularly frustrating one, because in most instances it can be prevented. In the United States it is estimated that 250,000 cases of deep vein thrombosis are diagnosed yearly, but this is only a fraction of the total because most are silent. Pulmonary embolism, the main complication of thrombosis in the deep veins of the lower extremity, is currently estimated to cause 50,000 deaths yearly; furthermore, the morbidity and mortality of other diseases are significantly influenced when a pulmonary embolism occurs.

544. THROMBOPHLEBITIS AND PHLEBOTHROMBOSIS

The presence of a thrombus in a vein is referred to clinically as thrombophlebitis or phlebothrombosis. Adherence to the vein wall incites an inflammatory reaction with local symptoms, and because of the associated phlebitis the process is referred to as thrombophlebitis. When the thrombus is poorly adherent and extends primarily into the free-flowing circulation, local symptoms of phlebitis may be minimal or absent, and the process may be referred to as phlebothrombosis. Since the two states are, for the most part, identical and subject to the same complications, little virtue attaches to such a clinical differentiation; hereafter only the term thrombophlebitis will be used.

Etiology, Risk Factors, Pathogenesis, and Prevalence. Mutliple causes probably initiate venous thrombosis. Injury to the vessel wall by mechanical trauma, infection, chemical irritants, or the process of thromboangiitis obliterans is responsible for some cases, particularly the superficial variety.

In most instances, stasis with slowing of blood flow and venous distention appears to be the major predisposing factor, e.g., in the venous thrombi which frequently complicate the use of constricting garments, and in such clinical conditions or states as the hyperviscosity syndromes (including polycythemia vera), severe obesity, varicose veins, postoperative and postpartum states, trauma (particularly when extensive or involving fractures of the pelvis or femur), acute myocardial infarction, heart failure, hemiplegia, debility, and cachexia. Long periods of cramped sitting, e.g., in travel or watching television, or in fact any state involving partial or complete immobilization, particularly in the older age group, because of the loss of the normal pumping action of the leg muscles, is subject to an increased incidence of venous thrombosis. The risk of stasis-mediated as well as other forms of venous thrombosis is increased when there has been a previous episode of thrombophlebitis or pulmonary embolism.

Alterations in blood components have received much attention, but a "hypercoagulable state," i.e., one predisposing to thrombus formation, has defied simple description. Rather, it is recognized that many disorders of the blood may be associated with predisposition to venous thrombosis. These include thrombocythemia as well as certain thrombocytopathies, particularly those involving shortened survival and increased platelet functional activities (adhesion, aggregation, and coagulant properties), dysfibrinogenemias, accelerated thromboplastin generation, constitutionally elevated levels of plasma factors V and VIII, heightened antifibrinolytic activity, and decreased antithrombin III activity.

Finally, many other clinical conditions are associated with an increased incidence of thrombophlebitis, but the responsible factors have not been adequately elucidated. These include ulcerative colitis, malignancies of all types (possibly more so of the pancreas), homocystinuria, and prolonged administration of large doses of estrogens or estrogen-containing oral contraceptive agents. The presence of a "migratory thrombophlebitis" should cause suspicion of an underlying malignancy, collagen disease, thromboangiitis obliterans, or polycythemia vera. When thrombosis occurs without evidence of a known predisposing factor or associated clinical condition, the term *idiopathic* thrombophlebitis may be used.

Thrombosis in veins occurs most commonly in the deep and superficial veins of the lower extremities. Deep leg vein thrombi usually begin in the soleal arcade of the calf muscles where they may resolve, organize, extend, or trigger additional thrombi at independent sites. As long as the thrombus remains limited to the soleal veins, no significant clinical problem is posed. However, once extension into the major deep vessels of the leg occurs, or additional thrombi appear at other sites in the major deep veins, the patient is at significant risk for one or

more complications (circulatory obstruction, valve damage, pulmonary embolism). When extension occurs from the soleal vessels, the thrombus extends proximally into larger vessels, frequently progressing to involve the popliteal, superficial femoral, common femoral, and iliac veins. More rarely the inferior vena cava is also affected. Thrombi originating in the major deep veins usually begin at the base of valve pockets and then extend either up along the vein wall or into the flowing circulation, or they may completely obstruct the entire vascular lumen. When the latter occurs, retrograde thrombosis as well as continued proximal growth is likely.

Next in frequency to thrombi in the deep leg veins are thrombi in the pelvic venous network, the right cardiac chambers, and the veins of the upper extremities. However, thrombi may occur in any veins (retinal, cerebral, renal, hepatic, portal, mesenteric) and contribute significantly to disease of the organ system involved.

Until recently, data on the incidence and frequency of leg vein thrombi were inadequate, because most of these are inapparent clinically. In studies in which leg vein dissections were carried out post mortem, the incidence was shown to be very high, varying from 27 to 80 per cent, depending on the nature of the series and the extent of the dissection; in most, the incidence ranged from 44 to 65 per cent. This incidence did not appear to depend on sex or clinical diagnosis, for the likelihood of thrombosis was similar in patients dying of medical, surgical, and traumatic causes. The most important factors influencing the frequency of leg vein thrombosis appeared to be the duration of bed rest and advancing age, although other factors undoubtedly contributed to those incidence figures.

With the advent of the ^{125}I labeled fibrinogen leg-scanning technique, important epidemiologic and prevalence data are being obtained on leg vein thrombi appearing during life and in nonfatal situations. For example, in Kakkar's study of 469 consecutive patients aged 40 or over, undergoing elective surgery, 28 per cent developed deep vein thrombosis; older patients undergoing major operations had an incidence of over 50 per cent. Half the thrombi developed within the first 24 hours postoperatively, and the remainder occurred three to seven days after surgery; in one third of the patients, the thrombi were bilateral. The incidence in other conditions was as follows: fractured hips, 75 per cent of pertrochanteric and 34 per cent of subcapital femoral neck fractures; retropubic prostatectomy, 50 per cent; acute myocardial infarction, 38 per cent; stroke, 60 per cent in the hemiplegic lower extremity; gynecologic patients over 30 years of age and undergoing major abdominal or vaginal surgery, 18 per cent; and obstetric patients during the puerperium, 4 per cent. Probably the highest risk is in patients undergoing reconstructive or total hip replacement.

In over 90 per cent of the patients undergoing thrombosis, leg vein thrombi appear first in the veins of the calf; one fifth of these soleal thrombi extend proximally into the major deep vessels of the leg and thigh; of the latter, half embolize. In acute myocardial infarction, in which the over-all incidence of leg vein thrombosis is approximately 30 per cent, 6 per cent of patients may be expected to develop thrombi in the major deep vessels of the leg or thigh, and in 3 per cent the illness will be complicated by an acute pulmonary embolism; the risk of leg vein thrombosis, extension, and embolization, however, is doubled in patients in the older age group who develop shock or congestive heart failure with their infarction.

Clinical Manifestations and Diagnosis. Thrombophlebitis occurs suddenly or gradually. Superficial thrombophlebitis is not difficult to diagnose, because the thrombosed vessel can usually be felt beneath the skin as a tender cord, and the lesion may be accompanied by a surrounding area of localized inflammation. With more extensive use of the venous route both for therapy and drug abuse, the incidence of this form of thrombophlebitis has increased sharply. Although usually benign, a significant number of patients may become infected, e.g., after the use of contaminated equipment or when intravenous catheters have been left in situ for periods of more than 48 hours, and this may lead to a serious septic state.

Deep vein thrombophlebitis is much more difficult to diagnose, because it may or may not be accompanied by local (pain and tenderness) and systemic (fever) symptoms; these occur in only 20 to 30 per cent of patients. In the absence of local findings, the diagnosis should be suspected when there is a "doughy" feeling or an unexplained increase in the circumference of the limb and the presence of *Homans' sign* (pain in the calf and/or popliteal space on dorsiflexion of the foot). The *sphygmomanometer cuff pain test of Lowenberg* may also prove useful, particularly when carried out during ambulation. A blood pressure cuff around the involved part of the extremity is slowly inflated to 200 mm Hg and then deflated. During inflation, discomfort is normally experienced at or above 160 mm Hg. In venous obstructive disease, discomfort or tenderness is evident at a lower level (60 to 150 mm Hg). The test may often be positive when other symptoms and signs are absent, but it is not sufficiently specific to be considered diagnostic. The most useful noninvasive diagnostic techniques are the *augmented Doppler ultrasound examination* and *electrical impedance phlebography* with a thigh cuff. However, these tests are positive only when the major deep veins are obstructed; they do not detect thrombi limited to the soleal veins. *Venography* is the most specific for diagnostic purposes, but it has limitations; it is expensive, may require a cut-down, and cannot be interpreted properly unless all the deep veins, including the soleal vessels, are filled adequately; there is also the possibility (still unresolved) that the large amounts of dye used in the procedure will aggravate an underlying thrombophlebitis.

Unless the patient has local complaints, the signs of venous thrombosis are often overlooked until the occurrence of pulmonary embolism calls attention to the limbs. Therefore special attention should be paid to the possibility of venous thrombi in all patients who are predisposed, and frequent observations should be made in older patients immobilized for any period of time.

Local tenderness in the calf and pain on forced dorsiflexion of the foot should suggest involvement of the deeper branches of the popliteal vein. Edema and mottled cyanosis will be present when the superficial femoral vein is affected; these findings are absent when adequate collateral channels exist. When the disease extends to involve the common femoral and iliac veins, edema and cyanosis of the leg may develop rapidly, often with diminished pulsation of the femoral artery. When associated perivenous inflammation and pelvic lymphatic involvement accompany thrombosis of the iliac vein, the swelling can be massive and result in a "milk leg" or *phlegmasia alba dolens*. In a particularly serious form of deep vein thrombosis called *phlegmasia cerulea dolens,* cyanosis and swelling of the extremity are associated with a disappearance of the arterial pulses; the leg becomes cold; gangrene appears imminent and may follow. This is associated with massive venous occlusion involving the deep, superficial, and intercommunicating veins so that there is almost total outflow obstruction; the rapid rise in tissue pressure compromises the arterial inflow and produces the picture of combined arterial and venous occlusive disease.

Damage to the venous valves resulting from an extensive episode or repeated attacks of deep vein thrombophlebitis may cause venous stasis and insufficiency; this leads to chronic edema, fibrosis, pigmentation, and trophic ulceration in the limb. The eventual deformity in this *postphlebitic syndrome* may be extreme and disabling. However, the most frequent and serious complication of thrombophlebitis is pulmonary embolism, a subject discussed in Ch. 545.

Prophylaxis. Stasis should be eliminated whenever possible, particularly in the older patient. This includes the wearing of elastic or supportive hose in the presence of varicose veins; avoidance of long periods of cramped sitting and of constricting garments about the abdomen and lower extremities; and the use of appropriate measures during periods of immobilization or illness or after surgery, trauma, or fracture. The value of elastic hose during periods of immobilization is very limited, as are foot and leg exercises, even when carried out frequently and in the elevated position. More effective are physical devices which ensure repeated calf muscle contraction or intermittent pulsation of the leg veins. Early but active ambulation is to be encouraged after illness, surgery, or trauma. Whether the elimination of contaminants by filtering parenteral fluids during their administration will reduce the risk of thrombophlebitis is being evaluated.

Iatrogenic thrombophlebitis can be minimized by avoiding prolonged use of intravenous catheters or administration of hypertonic or chemically irritating solutions.

Prophylactic therapy with anticoagulants is to be considered in high risk groups, i.e., those most likely to develop venous thrombi and pulmonary embolism. Included in this category are patients over the age of 50 who will be bedridden or immobilized for long periods of time as a result of extensive fractures, particularly of the femur, or other forms of trauma, debilitating disease, cardiac failure, myocardial infarction, or surgery, particularly hip arthroplasty. The pharmacologic basis for the use of anticoagulation in the prevention of venous thrombotic disease is sound, and its effectiveness in reducing thromboembolic complications after fractured hips or extensive trauma, during the postoperative state, and after acute myocardial infarction has been established in several series of observations. When indicated, anticoagulant therapy should be instituted immediately; it can be carried out solely with *oral agents (coumarin or indandione compounds),* for although these agents take several days to induce an appropriate antithrombotic state, the danger period for pulmonary embolism usually begins somewhat later. Anticoagulation should be continued until full mobilization is completed, because the risk of thrombosis remains as long as stasis exists. Such anticoagulation is not a contraindication to surgery or other procedures. Surgery can be performed without much danger either before or shortly after the institution of anticoagulant treatment, because hemostasis is not impaired for several days; later, in the more chronically anticoagulated patient, surgery can be undertaken after reduction of the level of anticoagulation with careful attention to wound hemostasis. Nevertheless, despite its proved value, physicians have been reluctant to use such prophylactic anticoagulant therapy except in cases of recurrent thrombophlebitis or pulmonary embolism; cited are the hazard of bleeding and the difficulties in maintaining adequate anticoagulation in older patients. Some of these difficulties can be avoided by elimination of a loading dose and recognition of the various factors which influence drug responsiveness (see below).

Infusion of *dextran* 40 or 75 (500 to 1000 ml on day of surgery, 500 ml daily for next five days) can also be used to prevent postoperative thrombophlebitis, presumably by increasing blood flow and preventing surface interactions. However, although effective, it provides little advantage over anticoagulants, because it also enhances the risk of bleeding and is tolerated poorly in individuals with impaired cardiac reserve.

The most promising development in the prevention of deep vein thrombi in immobilized patients is administration of small doses of *heparin*, i.e., 5000 units twice a day subcutaneously into the abdominal wall during periods of high risk. This regimen maintains circulating heparin blood levels at a fraction of that ordinarily achieved with conventional therapeutic doses as used in the treatment of established thrombosis (see below), and does not significantly affect the Lee-White clotting time and activated partial thromboplastin time; nor does it enhance the risk of bleeding. However, there is sufficient circulating heparin to activate enough heparin cofactor (antithrombin III) to block the action of earlier activated enzymes of the clotting reaction (notably Xa and IXa). In several trials, prophylactic therapy with low dose heparin has strikingly reduced the incidence of venous thrombosis occurring postoperatively (except after femoral fractures and hip arthroplasty) and after acute myocardial infarction as measured by ^{125}I labeled fibrinogen scanning. Should trials currently underway also reveal a significant reduction in pulmonary embolism, this mode of prophylaxis is likely to receive widespread acceptance.

The use of *platelet function inhibitors*, e.g., *aspirin, dipyridamole,* and *sulfinpyrazone,* for the prevention of deep vein thrombosis remains unclear; however, sulfinpyrazone (600 to 800 mg daily) has been found useful in reducing the incidence of arteriovenous shunt thrombosis in patients undergoing chronic renal dialysis, and in decreasing the frequency of attacks in patients with recurrent thrombophlebitis who are refractory to coumarin therapy. When sulfinpyrazone is used with coumarin, the dose of the latter should be lowered because of occupation by sulfinpyrazone of coumarin-binding sites.

Treatment. *General Measures.* Acute superficial thrombophlebitis is most often self-limited, unless infected, and usually responds promptly to analgesics, bed rest, warm moist packs, and elevation of the affected limb. Pulmonary embolism is a rare complication unless there is also involvement of the deep venous system. Antimicrobial drugs are not indicated except in septic phlebitis, in which the choice of agent depends on the organism responsible for the infection.

Acute deep vein thrombophlebitis must be managed more aggressively because of the tendency of these thrombi to extend, embolize, and produce serious venous obstruction and damage to venous valves (a postphlebitic insufficiency syndrome occurs in about 5 per cent of those with an ascending thrombophlebitis). In addition to the local measures described above, the objectives of treatment are to prevent further disease and, if indicated, to remove the obstructing thrombus.

Anticoagulants. Currently the principal therapeutic agents for the prevention of further extension and embolization are the anticoagulants, and with their use alone most cases can be managed successfully and without complication. In the absence of contraindications (bleeding diathesis, hemorrhagic lesion, malignant hypertension, known allergy to heparin) anticoagulation should be instituted immediately with heparin, for it is the most effective of the agents available and induces an immediate antithrombotic state.

Heparin can be administered intravenously or by the intramuscular and subcutaneous routes. Based on control of antithrombotic effects, the intravenous route is most often recommended, particularly for the first several days of therapy. Because of local pain and frequent hematomas, intramuscular injections are the least desirable. Even with the intravenous route, dosages and regimens vary. Continuous intravenous infusions of heparin, although requiring special care in administration, are becoming the preferred mode of therapy; control of dosage is easier and, more important, evidence is accumulating that bleeding complications can be reduced significantly. A suggested procedure is to begin with a loading dose of 75 IU per pound of body weight, followed by a sustaining infusion of 10 IU per pound per hour through an indwelling plastic catheter placed above the antecubital fossa. Subsequent dosage is adjusted to maintain the activated partial thromboplastin time at twice normal (range $1\frac{1}{2}$ to $2\frac{1}{2}$); with Lee-White clotting times, the range is 2 to $2\frac{1}{2}$ times normal). If the intermittent injection technique is employed, it is suggested that 60,000 IU be given during the first day (e.g., 10,000 units every four hours) and that, beginning on the second day, dosage be regulated by coagulation determinations; one hour before the next injection, the activated partial thromboplastin time or Lee-White clotting time should be at the level recommended above for sustaining infusions.

Once the dose requirement has been established, the clotting time may be checked once daily at an appropriate time to exclude possible increase or decrease in the anticoagulant effect and to allow for variations in heparin requirement during the course of therapy. Not infrequently, patients in whom thrombosis is occurring require more heparin in the first 24 to 48 hours of treatment than several days after the institution of therapy. Heparin therapy is recommended for periods of seven to ten days before relying solely on oral anticoagulation with coumarin drugs; this will ensure the most potent antithrombotic state and allow the underlying thrombus to become firmly fixed to the vessel wall.

"Burning fingers" and an occasional allergic reaction may be seen with heparin (osteoporosis and alopecia are additional adverse effects associated with long-term administration), but the primary risk in heparin therapy is bleeding. In one series it was as high as 50 per cent in women over the age of 60; usually the incidence is of the order of 5 to 8 per cent. This risk can be reduced by better control of the anticoagulant state, eliminating aspirin and aspirin-containing compounds, and avoiding intramuscular injections and invasive procedures. When significant bleeding occurs, heparin in the circulation can be immediately neutralized with protamine sulfate; the latter reacts with heparin stoichiometrically and on a milligram per milligram basis. Protamine is administered slowly intravenously after dilution in physiologic saline in an amount equivalent to half the last dose of heparin but not in excess of 100 mg. For this calculation 100 units of heparin can be taken to represent 1 mg.

Oral anticoagulation with *coumarin* (or, less popularly, *indandione*) compounds should be instituted several days before the discontinuation of heparin therapy. It should be continued for six weeks to six months, unless the phlebitis is associated with immobilization, in which case the drug should be continued until full physical activity is resumed. If thrombi recur when anticoagulants are discontinued, the treatment should be resumed, and long-term therapy may be necessary. Patients with known recurrent episodes of phlebitis may require prophylactic anticoagulant therapy extending over years.

The action of coumarin compounds is indirect, i.e., the induction of a hypocoagulable state, in contrast to the action of heparin as an immediate activator of antithrombin III. At present, the aim of therapy is to reduce the level of the prothrombin complex factors (factors II, VII, IX, and X) to approximately 20 per cent of normal and sustain it there. (Antithrombin III levels are increased during coumarin administration and may contribute to the antithrombotic effect.) This is achieved by regulating dosage so as to prolong the one-stage prothrombin time test to one and a half to two times the control time by the Quick test. Levels of two and a half times or greater are associated with an increased incidence of bleeding, and levels of less than one and a half times the control may not be effective.

There is little difference in the onset of effect or smoothness of control among the various coumarin derivatives, and vitamin K_1 is equally effective in counteracting their action. Because factor VII of the various vitamin K dependent factors (II, VII, IX, and X) has the shortest half-life, it is depressed most quickly by coumarin therapy. However, the rapid depression of factor VII does not provide good antithrombotic protection but does enhance the risk of bleeding. Accordingly, previous regimens involving the use of a loading dose are being employed less frequently. A suggested regimen is to give warfarin, 10 to 15 mg daily, until the desired effect on the prothrombin time is achieved and the dose adjusted to maintain that level. Individualization of dosage is essential, because a variety of drug interactions, other pharmacologic considerations, and metabolic factors influence the sensitivity and response to the coumarin compounds. *Drugs to be avoided during warfarin therapy* include aspirin, phenylbutazone, oxyphenbutazone, and indomethacin, and the following have been shown to potentiate its effect: anabolic steroids, certain antimicrobials (particularly chloramphenicol and those which affect the intestinal bacterial flora), chloral hydrate, clofibrate, disulfiram, ethacrynic acid, glucagon, mefenamic acid, methylphenidate, quinidine, quinine, and sulfinpyrazone. Those agents which inhibit the prothrombinopenic effect of warfarin include barbiturates, corticosteroids, cholestyramine, ethchlorvynol, glutethimide, griseofulvin, haloperidol, meprobamate, and oral contraceptives. Also, older patients, particularly women, are more sensitive to warfarin, as are individuals suffering from febrile illnesses, malnutrition, steatorrhea, and hepatic or pancreatic disease, as well as those in the im-

mediate postoperative state. Increased resistance to warfarin is associated with hyperlipidemia and hyperuricemia. Warfarin also interferes with the metabolism of other drugs; it enhances the action of diphenylhydantoin, chlorpropamide, and tolbutamide.

In patients being switched from heparin to warfarin therapy, a period of overlap is necessary because of the delay in the antithrombotic effect of the coumarin. A suggested procedure is to give warfarin, 10 to 15 mg daily for two to three days, until the desired therapeutic range for the prothrombin time is achieved; then, while continuing maintenance warfarin therapy, heparin dosage is progressively reduced over another three- to four-day period before discontinuation. Since prothrombin times are influenced by the presence of heparin, such assays should be carried out on blood specimens with a normal or near normal activated partial thromboplastin time; for patients on sustaining infusions of heparin, this may require the in vitro addition of protamine.

Bleeding is a significant hazard, with oral anticoagulation occurring in 3 per cent or more of patients on long-term therapy; vitamin K_1 in doses of 5 to 10 mg is usually corrective. Long-term therapy should not be undertaken unless a reliable laboratory is available and the patient's cooperation can be assured. Individuals on such therapy should avoid contact exercise, aspirin, and aspirin-containing compounds, and should be observed carefully even after slight trauma (subdural hematoma in the aged is often an unsuspected complication of coumarin therapy). Invasive procedures, including needle biopsies and spinal taps, are to be avoided unless the prothrombin time is first restored to or near the normal range. Other adverse effects are minimal; probably of most interest is the occasional appearance of skin necrosis and the rare "purple toe syndrome." Contraindications to coumarin therapy are similar to those previously mentioned for heparin and, in addition, pregnancy. Not only has coumarin administration been shown to increase teratogenicity in animals during the first trimester but, unlike heparin, it crosses the placental barrier and can produce fetal hemorrhage. The use of coumarins also should be avoided, when possible, for patients with severe liver disease or advanced renal insufficiency.

Other Antithrombotic Agents. Low molecular weight *dextran* infusions, based on their ability to improve flow rates by expanding plasma volume and to inhibit platelet adherence and aggregation, have been recommended by some as a useful adjunct in the management of acute thrombophlebitis. In contrast to its proved value in prevention, the efficacy of such therapy for thrombophlebitis remains to be established; at present there is little justification to have dextran infusions replace anticoagulant therapy. Also, there is considerable interest in the use of defibrinating agents; the most promising agents in this respect are the highly purified fraction *(Arvin)* obtained from the venom of the Malayan pit viper, and *Defibrase.* It remains to be established whether these agents will have advantages over heparin.

Surgical Therapy. Surgical procedures may be helpful in the management of some cases of thrombophlebitis; *proximal interruption of venous flow* can be employed to prevent embolization, and thrombectomy to relieve obstruction. The surgical procedures of choice to protect adequately against pulmonary embolization from the lower extremities and pelvis are inferior vena caval ligation, plication, or the insertion of an appropriate filter or umbrella. The last-named can be accomplished transvenously and does not require abdominal surgery. Each procedure has its adherents, and all but the first obviate the difficulty of sudden acute fluid sequestration with hypovolemia and impaired venous return, an event which may be tolerated poorly by people with underlying heart disease. Since all these procedures are usually followed by retrograde thrombosis, and consequently carry a significant incidence of distressing sequelae, both immediate and late, and do not permanently protect (large collaterals develop in several months and may provide a new route for embolization), they are not given consideration except in the presence of pulmonary embolism, or when pulmonary embolism has been known to occur in the past and there is a contraindication to the use of anticoagulant therapy.

Thrombectomy, including the use of Fogarty and similar types of catheters, has been employed successfully in the management of occasional cases of phlegmasia cerulea dolens. However, since this procedure is often followed by venous rethrombosis as well as complicating the subsequent use of anticoagulation, it is currently indicated only for those patients in whom acute fluid sequestration and high tissue tension sufficiently jeopardize the arterial circulation as to threaten the survival of the limb.

Thrombolytic Therapy. Clot-dissolving agents ultimately should prove useful as adjuncts in the management of deep vein thrombophlebitis, for they provide the only medical means for directly lysing a thrombus already formed. The most useful agents for thrombolytic therapy are *streptokinase* and *urokinase,* activators of the naturally occurring human fibrinolytic enzyme system. Streptokinase is a secretory product of the hemolytic Streptococcus and can be produced readily in large quantities and relatively inexpensively for therapeutic purposes. Its major disadvantage is its antigenicity; this poses problems in dosage and, more important, in retreatment should thrombosis recur. Urokinase, a normal constituent of human urine, is nonantigenic and simpler to use therapeutically, but more expensive. Although originally prepared from urine, currently it is being processed from the culture medium of fetal kidney tissue cells. Both agents are given intravenously; for thrombophlebitis, a suggested procedure for streptokinase is to give 250,000 units as a loading dose over a 20- to 30-minute period, followed by a sustaining infusion of 100,000 units per hour for 48 to 72 hours; with urokinase, 2000 units per pound of body weight is given as a loading dose, followed by a sustaining infusion of the same amount per hour for 24 to 48 hours. Heparin therapy is instituted at the termination of the fibrinolytic therapy so as to prevent rethrombosis. Although both agents when used in appropriate dosage are capable of lysing large thrombi in the deep leg veins, the intense fibrinolytic state has a propensity to induce bleeding. Consequently, current recommendations are to limit their use to those patients with extensive occlusions of the major deep veins of the extremity or with a rapidly ascending thrombophlebitis or pulmonary embolism. If lower doses of these agents can be shown to be effective and safe when combined with anticoagulants, as now under test, they may prove an important adjunct to the management of all cases of deep vein thrombosis.

Both urokinase and streptokinase are still under evaluation in the United States and neither is as yet commercially available. The only available preparation, human fibrinolysin, is in reality a mixture of steptokinase and human plasmin. At the dosages recommended by the manufacturer, the fibrinolytic activity induced in the patient is extremely variable, and currently little enthusiasm exists for use of this material for thrombolytic purposes.

Follow-up Therapy. When the systemic symptoms and signs of thrombophlebitis have subsided and the involved limb is pain free and nontender, the patient can begin walking with the leg supported by elastic stockings, unless such activity is followed by return of symptoms. After walking has been resumed, the patient should be advised to elevate the extremity above heart level for several half-hour periods a day. Elastic stockings should be worn until measurement of the extremity reveals no accumulation of edema fluid. Early and persistent therapy is important to prevent development of the postphlebitic syndrome. Once the brawny swelling and induration of the postphlebitic limb have occurred, they may be relieved somewhat by long periods of elevation, elastic compressions, vigorous massage, special exercises and mechanical devices, providing that there has been no recent recurrence of phlebitis. Gross deformities, ulcerations, and persistent or repeated infections may ultimately require one or more surgical procedures.

545. PULMONARY EMBOLISM AND INFARCTION

Definition. Pulmonary embolism is the impaction in the pulmonary vascular bed of a previously detached thrombus or foreign matter. Its major complication, pulmonary infarction, is the necrosis of lung parenchyma resulting from interference with blood supply. Since pulmonary embolism is the more common event, is not invariably accompanied by infarction, and has distinguishing features of its own, this chapter will be devoted primarily to pulmonary embolism; however, discussion of pulmonary infarction will be included as indicated.

Etiology. Pulmonary embolism is a complication, not a primary disease; therefore its etiology is considered in terms of the nature and source of the offending embolus. Almost all pulmonary emboli originate as thrombi; on occasion nonthrombotic materials such as amniotic fluid, fat, air, bone marrow, or tumor may embolize to the lung.

Venous thrombi in the deep veins of the lower extremities are the most common source for pulmonary emboli, accounting for 80 to 90 per cent. Another important source for pulmonary embolization is thrombi in the pelvic veins and prostatic plexus. Prostatic vein thrombosis may accompany malignant disease of the prostate but more frequently follows prostatic surgery. In the female, thrombosis in the pelvic veins may follow parturition or surgery; a particularly severe form, with frequent and protacted embolization, may complicate septic abortion. Pulmonary emboli may also arise from the right heart and are seen in association with cardiac failure, atrial fibrillation, myocardial infarction, the primary cardiomyopathies, and bacterial endocarditis (involving the tricuspid or pulmonic valves). Thrombi in the right heart frequently embolize and are said to account for approximately 25 per cent of pulmonary emboli among cardiac patients.

The factors controlling detachment of the whole or part of a venous thrombus into the general circulation are even less well understood than thrombus formation itself; frequently such thrombi will break away without apparent cause. It was formerly believed that embolization occurred more frequently with phlebothrombosis, but evidence to support this concept is lacking, and symptomatic thrombophlebitis is often complicated by embolization. Of more importance are the location of the vessel (embolism is rare from a superficial vein but very frequent from the iliofemoral vein), the presence of a free floating tail, and factors which acutely change pressure relationships in veins or suddenly increase venous blood flow; these include straining at stool, exertion, and ambulation after a long period of immobilization.

Once a thrombus is released into the venous circulation, it is usually carried rapidly through the great veins and right heart into the pulmonary arteries, except under those circumstances in which the embolus is shunted, through a patent foramen ovale or other defect, into the left heart and systemic circulation (paradoxical embolization). However, even this latter condition tends to occur most frequently after a bout of pulmonary embolism, for the associated pulmonary hypertension predisposes to paradoxical embolization.

Incidence and Prevalence. Pulmonary embolism with or without infarction is a common disorder and a most important cause of morbidity and mortality. It is frequently misdiagnosed. Next to pneumonia, it is the most common acute pulmonary lesion seen in hospitalized patients today. Thirty per cent of pulmonary emboli occur in cardiac patients, another 30 per cent occur among medical noncardiac patients (particularly among the aged), and most of the remainder occur postoperatively. Immobilization, venous disease, and prior cardiopulmonary disease are the factors most frequently predisposing to pulmonary embolism. The over-all incidence of pulmonary embolism in general autopsy series ranges from 5 to 14 per cent, but the incidence is considerably higher (25 per cent) in institutions for the care of the aged, and highest (30 to 45 per cent) among cardiac patients. The incidence of pulmonary embolism appears to have increased progressively over the past several decades.

Embolism to the main pulmonary artery or its primary branches so as to occlude acutely the major portion of the circulation through the lungs, although less frequent than embolism of smaller vessels, is the third most common cause of sudden death (5 per cent) among hospitalized patients. It occurs in about 3 per cent of general autopsy series, but with antemortem diagnosis of only one in eight.

Embolism to medium-sized vessels, i.e., lobar and segmental vessels, is observed approximately three to five times more frequently in autopsy series than is embolism of the major vessels; but since the former is commonly not fatal and is often recurrent, the actual incidence of acute episodes is relatively much greater. Furthermore, in contrast to embolism of the major vessels, the presence of medium-sized emboli at autopsy can be considered only incidental in two thirds of the cases; in the other third, the clinical features are such as to suggest some relation to the fatal termination. Pulmonary infarction complicates embolism of medium-sized arteries in less than 25 per cent of cases. In cardiac patients, the incidence of infarction after such embolism is considerably increased; in one autopsy series, more than 90 per cent of the lungs of cardiac patients with emboli were found to have areas of infarction.

Embolism to small-sized vessels, i.e., subsegmental arteries and their branches, probably occurs with great frequency, but the incidence is difficult to assess. As an isolated and focal lesion, such embolization has little clinical significance, for it usually is not large enough to produce a macroinfarction, and in routine autopsies the lesion is likely to be overlooked unless there are associated thrombi in the larger vessels. However, multiple small emboli scattered throughout the lungs are frequently observed in association with thrombotic occlusions of larger vessels; under these circumstances they contribute significantly to the impairment of pulmonary circulation and associated morbidity. Miliary small vessel occlusion is also the major cause of morbidity when nonthrombotic emboli, such as fat, amniotic fluid, air, or nitrogen, are involved.

Pathology. Pulmonary emboli may be single or multiple and vary in size from microscopic particles to large saddle emboli that completely occlude the pulmonary artery and its major branches. In addition, a large embolus may break up during passage through the heart or upon impaction and not only obstruct a major vessel but further embolize into one or more smaller branches in both lung fields. Also, there is evidence that, subsequent to impaction, emboli may shift or further fragment into previously unobstructed pulmonary vessels.

With occlusion of the main pulmonary artery or of both its primary branches, or when there is extensive involvement of medium-sized vessels so as to cut off the major portion of the pulmonary arterial circulation, there is acute mechanical obstruction to pulmonary blood flow; the pulmonary artery is distended by the presence of both clot and blood, the right ventricle is acutely dilated, the peripheral veins are engorged, and the liver is congested. Acute infarction rarely occurs; either the lung parenchyma is fairly normal or there is moderate atelectasis, usually explained by the loss of surfactant, and edema. Although the low incidence of acute infarction is possibly attributable to the rapidity with which death occurs (90 per cent of the deaths from acute pulmonary embolism occur within the first two hours), other factors are probably responsible for this phenomenon. In 40 per cent of the cases there is evidence of previous embolization and infarction.

Emboli which pass beyond the pulmonary artery and its major branches tend to impact the arteries of the lower lobes, more often the right than the left. Embolism to other lobes is much less frequent; combined, they account for only 25 per cent of cases. The more frequent involvement of the lower lobes is believed to be due to the fact that these areas lie in the more direct stream of the pulmonary arteries.

When *infarction* occurs, it spreads to involve a pleural surface, either peripheral or interlobar. The infarcted area is airless and hemorrhagic; the hemorrhage is both interstitial and alveolar. Because of the associated pleuritis, hypoventilation, and pre-existing disease, there may be surrounding atelectasis and edema as well. Although occlusion of the larger medium vessels, e.g., interlobar arteries, tends to be associated with infarcts of larger size, the relation between size of vessel occlusion and infarction is a poor one; other factors appear to be more critical in determining the presence and size of the infarct. By roentgenography, infarcts are poorly visualized on the first day. Thereafter they usually appear as humped, wedge-shaped, or, less commonly, rounded shadows. When they occur near the bases, considerable diaphragmatic elevation and restriction of motion may be observed. In 30 to 40 per cent of cases, infarcts are associated with a variable amount of *pleural effusion* that may be serous, serosanguineous, or frankly hemorrhagic; usually the specific gravity is in the range of 1.014 to 1.017 (protein, 3 to 3.5 grams per 100 ml) and there is mild to moderate increase in cell content.

Some shadows clear rapidly (two to three days) on roentgenographic examination and have been referred to as "incomplete" infarcts; however, it is likely that this clearing represents reventilation of an atelectatic or congested area occasioned by the embolic occlusion rather than true resolution of an infarct. "Complete" infarcts clear slowly over a two- to three-week period, ending as an area of linear fibrosis.

Mechanisms of Disease, Including Pulmonary Infarction. Emboli lodging in the pulmonary arterial tree acutely reduce the circulation distal to the site of obstruction. Potentially, the effects are fourfold: (1) less blood proceeds through the pulmonary circuit to the left heart and systemic circulation; (2) there is a damming back of blood behind the mechanical obstruction; (3) hemorrhagic necrosis of the ischemic area may occur; and (4) pulmonary function is impaired (pulmonary capillary perfusion and diffusion; later, ventilation may be compromised as well).

Except for the occurrence of infarction, which must be considered as a localized or focal disorder, the average person is believed capable of withstanding considerable obstruction of the pulmonary arterial bed without serious consequences to the vascular dynamics; in normal animals, a 60 to 70 per cent obstruction is usually well tolerated. Nevertheless, exceptions occur, particularly in the presence of underlying heart disease, when less extensive occlusions may elevate pulmonary arterial pressure or significantly reduce pulmonary venous outflow and when pulmonary circulation has been previously impaired by disease or prior embolization.

With a large occlusion of the main pulmonary artery or its primary branches, the effects are acute and primarily mechanical: rapidly rising pulmonary artery pressure, failure of the right ventricle, cyanosis, venous engorgement, and hepatic congestion. The consequences of impaired pulmonary venous return are sharp reduction in left ventricular filling, diminished cardiac output, reduced coronary and cerebral blood flow, hypoxia (also caused by pulmonary blood shunting), dyspnea, pallor, tachycardia, and hypotension, often progressing quickly to shock and death. Sudden dyspnea and retrosternal pain are frequently the most prominent initial complaints; the dyspnea is believed to be due to anoxia, apprehension, and stimulation of Hering-Breuer and other reflexes; the angina is usually attributed to acute coronary insufficiency, but direct stimulation of sensory nerves in the wall of a rapidly distending pulmonary artery may also play a significant role.

The effects of embolization to medium-sized vessels depend on the number, size, and distribution of the emboli and the prior state of the lung and circulation. Several patterns may be observed. (1) There may be no observable effects; a transient episode of dyspnea may be the only clue to its occurrence. (2) The picture may be predominantly one of pulmonary infarction with hemoptysis, pleuritic chest pain, friction rub, and abnormal roentgenographic shadows. Often, however, some ele-ments of this pattern may be absent, notably the hemoptysis or the evidence of pleural involvement. (3) There may be an acute picture similar to, but frequently not as severe as, that seen with embolization of the main pulmonary artery or its primary branches, in which pattern the primary difficulty is one of extensive and sudden compromise of the pulmonary arterial circulation but here by multiple emboli or recurrent embolization; it may or may not be complicated by infarction. (4) There may be a chronic and insidiously developing syndrome of cor pulmonale from progressive pulmonary hypertension that has evolved slowly after repeated episodes of embolization with or without infarction. This is often superimposed and obscured by the presence of other underlying chronic disease.

Controversy exists concerning the factors that acutely compromise the pulmonary circulation when emboli impact in medium-sized or smaller vessels. Some hold that vasoconstriction (pulmonary and perhaps coronary), mediated through reflexes from occluded arterioles or by the local release of serotonin or other vasoactive substances, plays an important role. It seems probable, however, that the continuing effects of most pulmonary emboli are primarily mechanical; when a major segment of the circulation is organically occluded, pulmonary hypertension and decreased venous outflow result. The suggestion has been made, and experimental studies have been cited to support the concept, that idiopathic pulmonary hypertension and pulmonary arteriosclerosis may result from repeated small pulmonary emboli.

The mechanism of pulmonary infarction is poorly understood. It does not result from ligation of pulmonary vessels and is unusual after embolization in animals with normal lungs; however, it does occur with great frequency in the congested, infected, or hypoventilated lung. Currently the best working hypothesis is that when medium-sized embolization occurs, enhancement of the circulation through the bronchial artery collaterals and bronchopulmonary vascular anastomoses distal to the embolus ordinarily serves to sustain the lung. However, in the presence of congestion or other conditions that predispose to local intrapulmonic circulatory stasis, augmentation of the collateral circulation is delayed or its benefits voided, and infarction occurs.

Hemorrhagic necrosis of the lung tissue and the overlying pleural inflammation are responsible for the characteristic clinical features of pulmonary infarction. The former accounts for the hemoptysis, cough, and fever; the latter for the pleural friction rub and pain. Since both lung tissue and the visceral pleura are devoid of sensory nerves, infarcts that do not extend to the outer surface of the lung to involve the parietal pleura do not cause pleural pain. When pain is present, it usually occurs over the ribs in the axillary region, but occasionally it may appear in the abdomen along the costal margin, or, when there is involvement of the parietal diaphragmatic pleura, in the shoulder or neck. The mechanism of the pain has usually been attributed to friction over an inflamed pleura, but an alternative explanation that may better explain its features (accentuation only on inspiration) is tension exerted during inspiration on those sensitized nerve ends of the parietal pleura that are attached to the intercostal muscles.

Clinical Manifestations.   The manifestations of *massive pulmonary embolism* (defined for clinical purposes as occlusion of 50 per cent or more of the pulmonary arterial circulation and representing approximately one third to one half of the suspected cases) may include sudden dyspnea; tachypnea; cyanosis; precordial or substernal oppressive pain, occasionally with radiation to shoulders and neck; evidences of right-sided cardiac dilatation and failure; tachycardia; restlessness; anxiety; syncope, occasionally with convulsions; and hypotension.

With massive embolism, death may be sudden or may occur over a period of several hours. In the latter instance, shock with vascular collapse becomes prominent. In an additional 2 to 3 per cent of patients, death may be delayed from one to several days; but when blood pressure spontaneously returns to normal, recovery is likely (unless the course is complicated by recurrence or an underlying disease). The physical signs noted include pulsation in the second left interspace, accentuation of P_2, a pseudo- or pleuropericardial friction rub, systolic or diastolic murmurs in the second left interspace, and interscapular bruit, S_3 or S_4 gallop rhythm, increased cardiac dullness to the right, distended neck veins, increased venous pressure with an hepatojugular reflex, and enlarged liver. Dislodgment of a large obstructing embolus may be associated with the dramatic transient appearance of a "red arterial wave" suddenly passing over a pallid cyanotic face.

Serial *electrocardiograms* reveal transient changes in most patients (85 per cent), but the pattern is extremely variable. The most frequent initial finding is T wave inversion (40 per cent). The electrocardiographic signs of acute cor pulmonale ($S_1Q_3T_3$, complete right bundle branch block, P pulmonale, or right axis deviation) are present in only 25 per cent of patients; left axis deviation is observed more frequently than right axis deviation. Rhythm disturbances (most commonly, premature ventricular beats) are observed in 10 per cent, as is a pseudoinfarction pattern. Patients with prior cardiopulmonary disease have a greater frequency of arrhythmias, conduction disturbances, and QRS changes; patients with extensive embolization demonstrate more QRS, RST, and T wave changes. In general, little change occurs during the first 24 hours, but after five to six days the QRS, primary RST segment, and T wave abnormalities begin to disappear. Roentgenographically, massive pulmonary embolism may result in the appearance of a large pulmonary arterial shadow that terminates abruptly; in some cases the ischemia may produce radiolucency of portions of the lung field (Westermark's sign).

With *submassive embolism*, i.e., occlusion of less than 50 per cent of the pulmonary circulation and usually involving the medium-sized or smaller vessels, the clinical manifestations may vary from a transient episode of dyspnea or the sudden or insidious worsening of an underlying pulmonary or cardiac disease, to the full-blown picture described for massive embolism (submassive embolism in patients with prior embolism or severe underlying cardiopulmonary disease frequently presents with the findings usually attributable to massive embolism); however, when pulmonary infarction occurs, its manifestations may also be superimposed.

The manifestations of *pulmonary infarction* are usually less dramatic. They vary in intensity from silent to those characterized by pleuritic chest pain, hemoptysis, cough, moderate dyspnea, fever, tachycardia, pleural friction rub, areas of dullness or flatness on percussion, and diminished breath sounds, occasionally with tubular breathing and rales. The leukocyte count is usually elevated, the sedimentation rate is accelerated,

and, subsequently, the serum bilirubin and serum lactic dehydrogenase levels rise. Roentgenographic examination may show typical humped or wedge-shaped shadows; on occasions the lesions are rounded or indistinguishable from pneumonic infiltrates. At other times, a pleural effusion may be the only clue to an underlying infarct. The average patient with pulmonary infarction runs a moderately febrile course for a few days, which is followed by clearing of roentgenographic and physical signs in one to three weeks.

Diagnosis. Despite the introduction of such diagnostic aids as pulmonary isotopic and ventilation photoscanning and selective pulmonary angiography, the diagnosis of pulmonary embolism with or without infarction is accurately made in no more than 50 per cent of cases when compared to autopsy findings. Frequently the diagnosis is overlooked because the disorder appears in the guise of congestive heart failure or pneumonia rather than as a distinctive syndrome; furthermore, the cardinal features do not occur with any great regularity. In half the patients subsequently proved to have recurrent infarction, no evidence of phlebitis, pleural pain, pleural friction rub, or hemoptysis is present, and in any one episode the incidence of each of these is less than 20 per cent. Thus in the absence of classic features, the diagnosis must be made on the basis of a high index of suspicion followed by confirmatory laboratory findings.

Pulmonary embolism with or without infarction should be suspected in all cases of chest pain of unknown cause, atypical pleural effusion, or bronchopneumonia. The possibility of this complication should also be considered in any patient who has a proved or suggestive history of a previous episode (present in 25 per cent of cases), in groups at high risk for deep vein thrombosis, and, most carefully, in critically ill patients with congestive heart failure; the incidence among the last-named group approaches 50 per cent and is much higher among those who exhibit unexplained fever or the *triad of tachycardia, digitalis toxicity, and edema unresponsive to diuretic therapy.*

Actually, the presence of one or more of the following symptoms, signs, or laboratory findings should raise the possibility of pulmonary embolism for consideration: sudden or increased dyspnea, tachypnea, cough, or cyanosis; substernal or pleuritic chest pain; hemoptysis; phlebitis; acute right-sided failure or sudden worsening of congestive heart failure; shock; pulmonary consolidation; pleural friction rub; roentgenographic evidence of pulmonary infiltration, elevated diaphragm, large areas of increased radiolucency, or pleural effusion; unexplained arrhythmias or electrocardiographic changes, particularly when the latter is indicative of acute right-heart strain or dilatation; pulmonary function studies indicating an increased ventilatory dead space, i.e., reduction in the mean alveolar carbon dioxide tension in the presence of a normal or nearly normal arterial carbon dioxide tension; or unexplained fever, leukocytosis, elevated erythrocyte sedimentation rate, serum bilirubin, lactic dehydrogenase, and fibrinogen/fibrin split products (normal levels of fibrinogen/fibrin split products and fibrin monomer are rare in pulmonary embolism).

The most reliable *screening procedures* for excluding an acute pulmonary embolism are pulmonary isotopic photoscanning with technetium-labeled microspheres or macroaggregates of human serum albumin, and an arterial Po_2 determination; a negative four-positional (anterior, posterior, and both laterals) lung scan virtually eliminates acute embolism, and it is rare when the arterial Po_2 is 90 mm Hg or above.

Confirmation of the diagnosis can often be achieved through the use of either selective pulmonary angiography or pulmonary isotopic photoscanning; on occasion, both techniques will be necessary. Since selective *pulmonary angiography* provides direct visualization of the vascular tree, it is the more definitive of the two procedures, and is the choice for establishing the diagnosis of pulmonary embolism. However, there are limitations to its usefulness. It is expensive and requires a skilled team; catheterization of the pulmonary artery is associated with some morbidity; the technique does not distinguish between new and old emboli; the subsegmental and smaller vessels are not visualized adequately; and there may be errors in interpretation unless the angiographer is experienced and strict criteria are used.

Pulmonary isotopic photoscanning has the advantages of convenience and lack of significant morbidity, and allows for repeated observation in following the course of the patient. However, unlike pulmonary arteriography, photoscanning does not visualize the pulmonary arterial tree; rather, it is a measure of the distribution of blood flow or pulmonary capillary perfusion, and defects in perfusion may be misinterpreted as to cause, especially in the presence of any underlying pulmonary lesion, e.g., infiltrates, blebs, cysts, emphysema, an acute asthmatic attack, or alterations in perfusion as a result of previous or associated disease. Since the scan is not specific for pulmonary embolism, perfusion defects should be characterized as to whether they are segmental or not and only interpreted as having a high, medium, or low probability of being due to an embolism. Although emphysema may also be responsible for high probability perfusion defects, the differential diagnosis can usually be resolved by a radioactively labeled xenon ventilation scan, because such a scan is unaffected by pulmonary embolism, at least for a period of five days. Pulmonary isotopic photoscanning is most useful for demonstrating and quantitating the perfusion defect of a pulmonary embolism when the chest roentgenogram is normal; it may also be diagnostic by revealing multiple perfusion defects (indic-·ative of multiple pulmonary embolism) when only an isolated infiltrate or lesion is present roentgenographically. Resolution of the perfusion defect after an embolism occurs progressively (50 per cent in two weeks), and this, too, may be useful diagnostically. It is noteworthy that patients with underlying cardiac disease have an impaired resolution rate.

Acute pulmonary embolism may be most readily confused with acute myocardial infarction, pulmonary edema, acute asthma, atelectasis, pericarditis, spontaneous pneumothorax, ball-valve thrombus in the left atrium, dissecting aneurysm, and pulmonary artery thrombosis. The last-named condition occurs rarely as a primary form of obscure cause or as a complication of a partially obstructing embolus, invading tumor, narrowed vascular lumen, or atherosclerotic plaque.

The differential diagnosis of pulmonary infarction includes pneumonia, pleurisy, other forms of pleural effusion, neoplasm, acute upper abdominal conditions, and the various causes of pulmonary hemorrhage. During resolution, an occasional infarct may slough out, leaving a thin-walled cavity which may be confused with an abscess.

To distinguish between an infarct and pneumonia may be difficult, yet this question arises frequently. Findings that are helpful in pointing to the diagnosis of infarct are a history or the presence of one of the preconditions of infarct, e.g., recent surgery, trauma, cardiac disease, previous venous disease, or pulmonary embolism; an extremely rapid appearance of roentgenographic abnormalities from the time of the first respiratory symptom; illness that seems disproportionately mild in relation to the extent of the pulmonary involvement or leukocytosis; and relative lack of cough or lack of preceding respiratory disease.

A spontaneous form of pulmonary infarction occurs in sickle cell disease, in the mixed sickle cell hemoglobinopathies, or in persons with sickle cell trait who are exposed to high altitude.

Treatment. *General Measures.* Supportive treatment for the usual acute embolism should include bed rest, an analgesic or narcotic (preferably meperidine hydrochloride [Demerol]) for pain and apprehension, and oxygen as indicated. The administration of antimicrobial drugs to prevent bacterial disease of the lungs is not indicated unless a septic infarct is suspected. All sudden effort should be avoided, especially straining at stool. Stool softeners and colonic lavages may prove useful. Pleural effusions may require aspiration, particularly if dyspnea is progressive. Digitalization is indicated if cardiac failure appears or worsens, but usually is of little benefit.

In more severe cases, continuous oxygen therapy should be employed, and positive pressure oxygen may prove particularly useful when pulmonary edema is present. Cardiac arrhythmias, which occur in 10 per cent of cases, should be treated appropriately. If shock occurs, fluids and isoproterenol should be given. Intravenous fluids should be monitored by central venous pressure measurements but maintained below 150 mm saline to prevent pulmonary edema. For hypotension, isoproterenol, because of its inotropic effect on the heart, is the agent of choice. It should be given intravenously slowly, usually at a rate of 2 μg per minute to sustain the systolic blood pressure at about 100 mm Hg (preferably at 120 mm Hg in previously hypertensive patients). Aminophylline, 250 to 500 mg (by suppository, intramuscularly, or by slow intravenous administration), may prove useful, particularly when dyspnea is prominent or pulmonary edema is present. Venesection may be dangerous, however, because of impaired left ventricular filling. The value of pulmonary vasodilators, e.g., papaverine, and bronchodilators, e.g., atropine, is still highly controversial.

Anticoagulants. In the absence of contraindications, heparin therapy should be instituted immediately in all patients with pulmonary embolism to lessen the danger of a recurrent and frequently fatal embolic accident (when heparin allergy is present, anticoagulation should be instituted immediately with coumarin compounds). Hemoptysis from pulmonary infarction is not a contraindication to anticoagulant therapy. The regimen for heparin therapy and subsequent oral coumarin anticoagulation is as described under the treatment of thrombophlebitis. Aspirin and aspirin-containing compounds should be avoided because of the increased risk of bleeding. Coumarin therapy is continued for six weeks unless there is a chronic disease, e.g., cardiac failure, that predisposes to repeated venous thrombus formation; under these circumstances anticoagulant therapy should be continued for prolonged periods.

Thrombolytic Agents. When available, these will

provide an important adjunct to the management of the more seriously ill patient with pulmonary embolism. Clinical trials have demonstrated that urokinase and streptokinase lyse pulmonary emboli extensively, reduce the hemodynamic abnormalities, improve pulmonary capillary perfusion, and increase gas exchange. These effects are observed fairly rapidly and are most striking in patients with massive embolism. Regimens as described previously for thrombophlebitis also should reduce significantly the need for surgical embolectomy, particularly when the therapy is combined with temporary cardiac bypass to tide the patient over the most critical period. Whether local perfusion of the agent directly into the pulmonary artery has any advantage over intravenous administration remains to be established. At present, thrombolytic agents are not indicated for the treatment of submassive embolism when stable vital signs are present; in the absence of complications, the patient is destined to recover and there is little need to increase the risk of bleeding. *Arvin,* the defibrinating agent, may also prove to be of benefit in the managment of acute pulmonary embolism, but its advantage over heparin remains to be established.

Surgical Therapy. Inferior vena caval ligation, plication, or the insertion of a filter or umbrella should be reserved for those patients in whom anticoagulants are contraindicated, must be discontinued, or whose disease for one reason or another cannot be successfully managed with this form of therapy. Since these procedures carry a significant incidence of sequelae, they are not indicated unless there has been massive embolism or there is evidence of recurrent embolization (a minor recurrence is observed in about 10 per cent of patients during the first few days of heparin therapy, and should not be considered as a failure of anticoagulant therapy unless the episode is significant clinically or continues to recur during adequate levels of anticoagulation).

Surgical embolectomy may be lifesaving in critically ill patients. However, this procedure requires cardiac bypass, and because of the condition of the patients, the mortality in patients treated with surgical embolectomy is still very high. At present, the indication for embolectomy is limited to patients with angiographic evidence of massive embolism of the main pulmonary artery or its primary branches and with sustained peripheral hypotension despite the use of appropriate supportive measures. Pulmonary embolectomy may also be considered for patients who have survived a massive embolism but in whom pulmonary hypertension resulting from the presence of an accessible embolus is leading to the development of cor pulmonale.

Prognosis. The prognosis of pulmonary embolism is difficult to establish because the clinical diagnosis is frequently obscure. Of those who succumb, approximately 90 per cent die immediately or within the first two hours. Another 2 to 3 per cent die of protracted shock during the next 48 hours. Once stable vital signs are established, subsequent mortality approximates 7 per cent and is usually attributable to recurrent embolism or adverse effects on an underlying cardiopulmonary disease. The likelihood of a fatal episode is increased with succeeding embolic attacks and, most important, in the presence of a significant impairment of cardiopulmonary reserve. The greatest hope for the management of this problem is prevention.

Unfortunately, such measures as the use of elastic stockings or bandages, leg exercises for immobilized pa-

tients, and early ambulation postoperatively have not greatly affected the high incidence of pulmonary embolism; nevertheless, the intelligent use of such measures, and particularly of the more recently developed mechanical devices which enhance blood flow, is to be encouraged. In addition, serious consideration should be given to the use of anticoagulants for all patients predisposed to thrombus formation. When used carefully, anticoagulants have significantly reduced the incidence of pulmonary embolism after fracture of the femur and in cases of congestive heart failure. This form of therapy should not be undertaken lightly, because the hazards, in any specific case, may outweigh the benefits to be derived. Low-dose heparin, should it prove successful, will obviate this problem.

Anticoagulation also has an important role to play in the *prevention of arterial embolism.* Coumarin therapy is useful in avoiding systemic embolization from endocardial mural thrombi in the left ventricle, e.g., after acute transmural infarction, and in the left atrium, e.g., in rheumatic mitral disease or during an electrical conversion of an arrhythmia. For acute myocardial infarction, coumarin therapy should be administered to those at high risk for such embolic episodes; the high risk factors include age over 60, previous myocardial infarction, shock, congestive heart failure, and evidence of large transmural infarction as judged by the levels of serum enzymes, fever, leukocytosis, sedimentation rate, and the extent of the electrocardiographic abnormalities. Therapy should be initiated at the onset of the illness and continued for a period of four weeks. Patients with rheumatic mitral disease with a nonseptic embolus (anticoagulants are contraindicated in subacute bacterial endocarditis) should be maintained on long-term anticoagulation or until surgical correction of the lesion. For individuals undergoing electrical conversion of an arrhythmia, coumarin therapy should be initiated two to three weeks prior to attempting reversion to a sinus rhythm in all patients with previous emboli or evidence of mitral stenosis; in other situations the need for anticoagulation should be considered and evaluated on an individual basis.

Coumarin anticoagulation is less effective for the prevention of platelet emboli such as may occur from prosthetic heart valves and in the transient ischemic attack syndrome. Better results are being obtained for the former condition when coumarin anticoagulation is combined with antiplatelet agents, e.g., sulfinpyrazone (800 mg daily) or dipyridamole (400 mg daily). For the transient ischemic attack syndrome, sulfinpyrazone alone appears to be yielding good results (aspirin, 1.2 grams daily, is also under study).

Medical therapy of an acute embolic event with antithrombotic agents is as described under the management of thrombophlebitis and pulmonary embolism.

Anticoagulants in acute myocardial infarction. Results of a cooperative clinical trial. J.A.M.A., 225:724, 1973.

Basu, D., Gallus, A., Hirsh, J., and Cade, J.: A prospective study of the value of monitoring heparin treatment with the activated partial thromboplastin time. N. Engl. J. Med., 287:324, 1972.

Coon, W. W., Willis, P. W., III, and Keller, J. B.: Venous thromboembolism and other venous disease in the Tecumseh Community Health Study. Circulation, 48:239, 1973.

Foster, C. S., Genton, E., Henderson, M., Sherry, S., and Wessler, S. (eds.): The epidemiology of venous thrombosis. Milbank Memorial Fund Quarterly, 50 (1), Part 2:9, 1972.

Gallus, A. S., Hirsh, J., Tuttle, R. J., et al.: Small subcutaneous doses of heparin in prevention of venous thrombosis. N. Engl. J. Med., 288:545, 1973.

Genton, E.: Guidelines for heparin therapy. Ann. Intern. Med., 80:77, 1974.

Hume, M., Sevitt, S., and Thomas, D. P.: Venous Thrombosis and Pulmonary Embolism. Cambridge, Mass., Harvard University Press, 1970.

Kakkar, V. V., Howe, C. T., Flanc, C., and Clarke, M. B.: Natural history of postoperative deep vein thrombosis. Lancet, 2:230, 1969.

Koch-Weser, J., and Sellers, E. M.: Drug interaction with coumarin anticoagulants. N. Engl. J. Med., 285:547, 1971.

McIntyre, K. M., and Sasahara, A. A.: The hemodynamic response to pulmonary embolism in patients without prior cardiopulmonary disease. Am. J. Cardiol., 28:288, 1971.

O'Reilly, R. A., and Aggeler, P. M.: Studies on coumarin anticoagulant drugs. Institution of warfarin therapy without a loading dose. Circulation, 38:169, 1968.

Paraskos, J. A., Adelstein, S. J., Smith, R. E., et al.: Late prognosis of acute pulmonary embolism, N. Engl. J. Med., 289:55, 1973.

Sasahara, A., Hyers, T. M., Cole, C., et al. (eds.): The urokinase pulmonary embolism trial. Circulation, 47 (Supplement II): II-5, 1973.

Stein, M., and Moser, K. M. (eds.): Pulmonary Thromboembolism. Chicago, Year Book Medical Publishers, 1973.

PULMONARY HYPERTENSION

Daniel S. Lukas

546. INTRODUCTION

Morphologically and physiologically, the circulation of the lungs differs from that of all other organs. Although the entire cardiac output passes through the lungs, a mean pressure in the pulmonary artery only one ninth of the pressure in the aorta is needed to sustain this flow. Under a wide variety of physiologic circumstances, simple adjustments of the pulmonary vascular bed minimize increases of pulmonary arterial pressure. Because many diseases of the heart and lungs can seriously compromise this regulatory capacity, pulmonary hypertension is a common clinical phenomenon. In some disorders elevations of pulmonary arterial pressure are acute and episodic, whereas in others the pulmonary hypertension is chronic and progressive.

The mechanisms producing pulmonary arterial hypertension in the major categories of disease are sufficiently different to warrant separate consideration and are best appreciated in the context of the normal structure and function of the pulmonary circulation.

THE NORMAL PULMONARY CIRCULATION

Structure. The pulmonary arterial tree consists of three distinct types of arteries that differ from each other in the composition of their walls and in size. The elastic arteries include the main pulmonary artery, its major branches, and arteries with external diameters greater than 1.0 mm. The muscular pulmonary arteries range in diameter from 0.1 to 1.0 mm. The smallest pulmonary arteries, the arterioles, have diameters less than 0.1 mm. The walls of all three types of arteries are much thinner than those of systemic arteries, and aside from the main pulmonary artery and its branches, these vessels have no strict anatomic counterparts in the systemic vascular bed.

The media of the main pulmonary artery and the elastic arteries contains a small amount of smooth muscle, collagen, and elastic fibers that are short, irregularly branching, and fragmented in appearance. The media of the aorta, in contrast, is 1.5 to more than 2 times thicker, and its elastic fibers are long, unbranching, and distributed in parallel fashion.

The muscular pulmonary arteries are closely apposed to the bronchioles and alveolar ducts. They have a large lumen and a thin wall that is composed of an intima and a thin media of concentrically oriented smooth muscle fibers bounded by internal and external elastic laminae.

The arterioles differ vastly from those of the systemic circuit, because they contain no muscle except at their point of origin. They consist of an endothelium, a single elastic lamina, and a scanty adventitia.

The pulmonary capillaries are the most prominent structural component of the alveolar walls, in which they form an extensive, interlacing network that is separated from the alveolar air by the lining cells of the alveoli and their basement membrane. The total surface of the capillaries that is available for gas exchange in adults has been estimated to comprise 60 to 70 square meters.

The pulmonary venules are thin-walled structures histologically indistinguishable from the arterioles. The structure of the veins is less ordered than that of the muscular arteries. The media, which is not bounded by well-defined elastic laminae, blends indistinguishably with the adventitia, and both contain smooth muscle and fragmented elastic fibers. The main venous trunks acquire a layer of cardiac muscle before they enter the left atrium. The venules and veins, unlike the arteries, do not course with the bronchial tree but are lodged in the septa that separate lobules and segments of the lung.

The bronchial arteries wind in spiral fashion around the bronchi and anastomose extensively with each other in and around the walls of the airways. They also form vasa vasorum in the adventitia of the elastic and larger muscular pulmonary arteries. Evidence that the two arterial systems intercommunicate in the normal lung is inconclusive. The bronchial veins, however, normally form numerous, small anastomotic channels with the pulmonary veins.

It is of considerable significance that the pulmonary arteries in the fetus and newborn differ structurally from those of the adult and do not attain their final form until the sixth to twelfth month of postnatal life. In the newborn, the media of the main pulmonary artery is as thick as that of the aorta and contains numerous, tightly packed, long, elastic fibers that are fairly uniform in thickness and are arranged in parallel fashion as in the aorta. Progressively after birth, the media diminishes in thickness, and the elastic fibers become fragmented, irregularly shaped, randomly distributed, and less densely packed, until they assume the full adult appearance. The muscular pulmonary arteries in the newborn resemble small systemic arteries. Typically, the wall contains a wide media composed of circularly oriented smooth muscle, and its thickness exceeds the diameter of the lumen. Rapid increase in luminal and external diameters and thinning of the media occur during the first sixth months of life. The arterioles at birth are surrounded by dense connective tissue and their lumina are barely patent. Their wall:lumen ratio likewise rapidly diminishes in the first few months of life.

During the early days of the postnatal period, the mean pulmonary arterial pressure is two or more times greater than that of the adult and may be high enough to reverse flow through the ductus arteriosus. The pulmonary arterial pressure declines to normal adult values within the first month, well before the metamorphosis of the pulmonary vasculature has been completed.

Hemodynamics. The average normal pressure in the pulmonary artery at rest is 19/6 mm Hg (systolic/diastolic) with a mean pressure of 11 mm Hg. Normally at rest, the systolic pressure does not exceed 25 mm Hg, and the mean pressure is not greater than 15 mm Hg. Mean pressures in the large pulmonary veins and left atrium are essentially identical, ranging from 3 to 8 mm Hg, with an average of 5 mm Hg. Thus a pressure gradient from the pulmonary artery to the large pulmonary veins of only 6 mm Hg is sufficient to sustain a blood flow in the normal adult at rest of approximately 6.0 liter per minute. These values are eloquent testimony to the low resistance offered to the flow of blood by the thin-walled and capacious pulmonary vessels. Calculated in the conventional manner as the mean pressure gradient divided by flow, the normal pulmonary vascular resistance is 1.0 mm Hg per liter per minute, or 80 dyne sec cm^{-5}, a value only 7 per cent of the normal systemic vascular resistance. The linear distribution of resistance in the pulmonary vascular bed is uncertain, but measurements in dogs indicate that the pulmonary arteries are responsible for approximately half the total resistance, the pulmonary capillaries for 30 per cent, and the veins for 20 per cent.

Several observations testify to the capacity of the pulmonary vascular bed to accommodate increases in blood flow with disproportionately small increases in pressure. During exercise, two- to threefold increases in cardiac output are associated with increments of only 25 to 50 per cent in mean pulmonary arterial pressure, but the pressure doubles when the output rises to four to five times the resting value. Large left-right shunts through an atrial septal defect that commonly triple the pulmonary blood flow are tolerated for many years with no more than slight elevations of pulmonary arterial pressure. After pneumonectomy or occlusion of either main branch of the pulmonary artery by a balloon catheter and in patients with congenital absence of a main branch of the pulmonary artery, the pulmonary arterial pressures remain within the normal range at rest if the perfused lung is normal.

Augmentation of pulmonary blood flow is facilitated and concomitant changes in pressure are minimized by several mechanisms that combine to expand the net cross-sectional area of the pulmonary vessels and thereby decrease the resistance they offer to the flow of blood. One of these mechanisms relates to the effect of changes in intravascular pressures on the caliber of the vessels. It has been demonstrated that increases in pulmonary arterial pressure well within the normal operational range are associated with large decreases in pulmonary vascular resistance and that the resistance declines further with the addition of a 2 to 3 mm Hg rise in left atrial pressure. The vessels are also subjected to the deforming effects of the pressures that surround them. The total pressure that acts on the vascular wall is the transmural pressure, or the difference between the intravascular and perivascular pressures. Some uncertainties exist regarding perivascular pressures in the lungs, but for vessels that are not intrinsic components of the alveolar structure, perivascular pressure is considered to approximate pleural pressure; for intra-alveolar vessels, the alveolar pressure has been regarded as the

extravascular pressure. Since the vessels that account for the major fraction of the pulmonary vascular resistance are exposed to the normally negative pleural pressure, their transmural pressures exceed the hydrostatic pressures within them.

During exercise, the more negative pleural pressures generated to augment tidal volume increase the transmural pressure gradients acting on the extra-alveolar vessels, thereby stretching them open further and decreasing their resistance to flow. Pressure changes within the pleura and the lungs can profoundly affect the pulmonary vasculature. For example, when intrapleural and alveolar pressures are greatly increased, as during a Valsalva maneuver, pulmonary vascular transmural pressures fall, some vessels collapse, and the resistance rises markedly.

Primarily because of gravitational effects on regional intravascular pressures, the lungs are not evenly perfused. In the erect position, the height of the blood column from the apices of the lungs to the midpoint of the left atrium is sufficient to reduce pressures within the pulmonary arteries at the apex almost to zero and decrease the transmural pressures of the pulmonary capillaries and veins in these regions to less than zero. Consequently, the vascular bed in the apices is not open, whereas at the bases of the lungs the vessels are subjected to the distending effects of the overlying column of blood and all are patent. These regional differences in vascular resistance produce a progressive decrease in regional blood flow within the lungs from base to apex, and in the upright position blood flow per unit volume of lung is eight times greater at the base than at the apex. At some point below the apices of the lungs, the transmural pressures of the arteries and the arterial limbs of the alveolar capillaries are high enough to maintain patency of the vessels, but the pressure within the venous segment of the capillaries or the venules is less than or just equals the perivascular pressure. The collapsible vascular segments in this region behave like sluices; they are either barely open or closed, and flow of blood through them no longer depends on the pressure gradient between the arterial and venous limbs but varies directly with the pressure difference between the arterial end of the segment and the pressure surrounding the collapsed segment. These hemodynamic conditions have been compared to those of a waterfall.

With increases in pulmonary flow, small changes in intravascular pressures open previously closed or partially collapsed vessels, thus expanding the size of the vascular bed and further lowering resistance to flow. This recruitment of small vessels and capillaries partly explains the increase of pulmonary diffusing capacity that occurs during exercise.

The volume of blood contained by the pulmonary vessels of an average size adult is approximately 400 to 500 ml, 70 to 100 ml of which is in the pulmonary capillaries. Because of its geometric complexity and the probably nonuniform dimensional rearrangements that the pulmonary vascular bed undergoes with changes in volume, the interrelationships among resistance, pressures, flow, and blood volume in the vessels of the lungs are far from simple. It is clear that the distensibility of the pulmonary arterial tree is much greater than that of the systemic arteries, and that this partially accounts for its lower resistance to flow. The large pulmonary veins, however, are less compliant than the major systemic venous segments. Also, the compliance of the small pulmonary vessels is not uniform; the capillaries are less distensible than the arteries and veins. In one study of normal subjects during an exercise that evoked an almost twofold increase in cardiac output, the pulmonary blood volume increased by only 27 per cent, mean pulmonary arterial pressure increased slightly, and pulmonary vascular resistance fell. The pulmonary vasoconstriction produced by hypoxia is associated with a decrease in pulmonary blood volume, despite the increase of pressure in the elastic pulmonary arteries.

The compliance of the pulmonary vessels is finite, and changes in the volume of blood in the lungs do produce changes in vascular pressures. For example, the intense constriction of the systemic vessels that sometimes occurs after injury to the brain (*Cushing reflex*) results in systemic hypertension, displacement of blood from the systemic circuit into the lungs, and marked pulmonary venous and pulmonary arterial hypertension.

Whereas the systemic vessels are closely regulated by the autonomic nervous system and respond to a wide variety of endogenous compounds and drugs, adjustments of the pulmonary vascular bed appear to result almost entirely in response to physical forces. The pulmonary arteries are supplied with autonomic nerves, and there is experimental evidence in animals that the larger pulmonary arteries can be reflexly induced to stiffen, but reflex control of the pulmonary circulation has not been convincingly demonstrated in man. Similarly, many pharmacologic agents considered on the basis of experiments in animals to exert a vasoconstrictor action on the pulmonary arteries (norepinephrine, epinephrine, and serotonin) or a vasodilator effect (bradykinin, isoproterenol, and acetylcholine) have been shown to have either little or no direct action on the normal human pulmonary vascular bed. Because these compounds profoundly affect the systemic circulation and may alter pulmonary mechanics, the changes in pulmonary vascular pressures and resistance that are observed after they are administered are mainly secondary consequences of their actions elsewhere.

Hypoxia. Ample evidence of several types indicates that hypoxia directly constricts the pulmonary bed and elevates the pulmonary vascular resistance by direct action on the muscular pulmonary arteries, which are separated from the inner surface of the small airways by only 0.1 mm. The mechanism of this effect is not completely understood, but there is evidence that the smooth muscle cells of the pulmonary arteries, unlike those of systemic arteries, lose intracellular potassium and gain sodium when exposed to low oxygen tension; consequently, their transmembrane potential falls to levels close to the threshold for discharge, and the frequency of muscular contraction increases. A recent study suggests that prostaglandins E and F synthesized in the lung may mediate the vasoconstriction.

The vasoconstrictor response to hypoxia is greatly potentiated by increases in blood hydrogen ion and is almost abolished by alkalosis. The hypoxic reflex serves a useful local regulatory function by limiting blood flow to underventilated pulmonary segments and thereby restores the regional ventilation-perfusion ratio to normal, but when the hypoxia is generalized, the response is far from beneficial. Inhalation of 12 per cent oxygen at sea level (Po$_2$: 91 mm Hg) promptly results in twofold increases of pulmonary vascular resistance and pulmonary arterial mean pressure, with no increase in cardiac output or left atrial pressure.

Pulmonary Arterial Pressure at High Altitude. Chronic exposure to the hypoxia of high altitude produces a sustained increase in pulmonary arterial pressure. The average values of pulmonary arterial pressure in natives of Morococho, Peru, which is at 14,900 feet above sea level (Po$_2$: 80 mm Hg), are 41/15 mm Hg (systolic/diastolic), with a mean pressure of 28 mm Hg at rest and 77/40 (mean: 60 mm Hg) during exercise. Their right ventricles are hypertrophied, and their small pulmonary arteries are thicker and contain increased amounts of smooth muscle, which extends farther down into the smallest vessels than normally. After two years of residing at sea level, the pulmonary arterial pressures of these people fall to normal values at rest but still rise to abnormal values with exercise.

Studies of the pulmonary circulation in residents of Leadville, Colorado (altitude: 10,200 feet; Po$_2$: 100 mm Hg), have emphasized the considerable individual variation in the reactivity of the pulmonary vasculature to chronic hypoxia. The average mean pulmonary arterial pressure at rest in one group of subjects was increased to 25 mm Hg, but it varied from 10 to 45 mm Hg, and in one 15-year-old woman the pressure rose to 105 mm Hg during exercise. This subject's pressure became normal after she had resided at sea level for 11 months.

The individuality of the response to hypoxia is further emphasized by the occurrence of acute pulmonary edema at high altitudes in susceptible persons who are otherwise normal. The pathogenesis of the pulmonary edema, which responds promptly to inhalation of oxygen, has not been fully elucidated, but it is not due to left ventricular failure, and pulmonary venous constriction has not been proved to be the cause. It occurs at altitudes greater than 9000 feet in persons who have not previously been exposed to altitude as well as in residents at high altitude within 12 to 36 hours after returning from even a brief sojourn at a lower level. Such persons are liable to recurrence of pulmonary edema with each transition from low to high altitude. Studies of susceptible subjects have revealed hyper-reactivity of their pulmonary vessels to hypoxia. Their pulmonary hemodynamics and pulmonary function were normal at sea level, but at 10,000 feet after a day of exposure to the altitude and a period of vigorous activity at higher altitude, despite the maintenance of normal pulmonary wedge pressures and no evidence of pulmonary edema, their pulmonary arterial pressures were two to three times greater than those of normal subjects at the same altitude.

In many disease states affecting the pulmonary circulation, including those not producing alveolar hypoxia, individual variations in pulmonary vascular reactivity are common, and the spectrum of physiologic and structural abnormalities of the pulmonary vessels in each condition is usually wide.

547. PRIMARY PULMONARY HYPERTENSION

Primary pulmonary hypertension is a disease of unknown cause characterized by marked increase in the pulmonary vascular resistance and pulmonary arterial pressure. Despite exhaustive search while the patient is alive, or at autopsy, no evidence can be found of underlying diseases known to produce pulmonary arterial hypertension, such as congenital or acquired heart disease, pulmonary disease, disorders of respiration, and systemic diseases that affect the pulmonary vessels.

Incidence. Primary pulmonary hypertension is uncommon. In one series of 10,000 patients with heart disease, it was found in only 17. Among reported cases, the patients ranged in age from 1 to 68 years, but most were 20 to 40 years old. There were three times as many women as men; most of the women were in their early thirties and had borne children. The disease is known to occur in a familial form. Among the 14 families reported, 22 female members and 12 males were affected. In six families, apparent parent-to-offspring transmission was documented, and in one kindred five members of three generations manifested the disease. The mode of genetic transmission is uncertain. In five families, the mother and either a daughter or a son were affected; in the other family, the father and his son and daughter died of the disease.

Pathology. In all patients, the pulmonary arteries show structural abnormalities characteristic of hypertensive pulmonary vascular disease usually of the most advanced degree (Grades 4 to 6 of Heath and Edwards). The walls of the muscular arteries and arterioles are greatly thickened, and their lumina are markedly narrowed and even obliterated. The smooth muscle in the media of the muscular arteries is hypertrophied and extends well down into the arterioles, which normally do not have a distinct media. In the arterioles and extending back to the smaller muscular pulmonary arteries less than 0.3 mm and occasionally those as large as 0.5 mm, marked cellular proliferation and fibrosis of the intima are seen. In some of the vessels, the intimal proliferation is concentric, shows an onion-layering appearance, and encroaches evenly on the lumen; in others, the masses of protruding fibrous tissue are unevenly distributed and create an eccentric, irregularly shaped lumen. The fibrous tissue contains elastic fibrils and eventually assumes a hyaline appearance.

Although the media attains a thickness equivalent to 30 per cent of the external diameter of the small arteries in some areas, in other areas the media is atrophied and the vessels dilated. Such generalized dilatations of the arterial wall are often found at and downstream from an occluded segment of a small muscular artery or arteriole and upstream from occlusions in the medium-sized arteries.

In addition to the generalized dilatations, localized dilatations that form morphologically complex, saccular structures develop from the walls of the smallest muscular arteries and arterioles. One of these structures, known as a plexiform lesion, is characterized by a thin-walled sac protruding from the wall of the vessel. The sac frequently contains a thrombus, over which an area of cellular intimal tissue has proliferated to form a complex, plexiform pattern. An overlying layer of fibrous tissue is continuous with the intimal proliferative layer of the artery. In other dilatation lesions, groups of thin-walled, cavernous vessels arise from thin-walled branches of muscular arteries, or occluded arteries give rise to veinlike branches that have been misinterpreted as arteriovenous anastomoses. Because of their thin walls, the vessels of dilatation lesions are subject to rupture and are associated with focal collections of hemosiderin-laden macrophages in the pulmonary tissue.

In the most advanced stage of hypertensive pulmonary vascular disease (Grade 6), fibrinoid necrosis occurs in the media of some of the muscular arteries. The necrotic muscle produces an inflammatory reaction consisting of polymorphonuclear leukocytes and some eosinophils that may invade all layers of the vessel. The necrotizing arteritis may destroy the entire vessel or only a segment of it, and thrombi are found in the lumina of some of the affected arteries.

The elastic pulmonary arteries, especially the main trunk and its branches, are greatly dilated, but the walls are thick. The media shows an increase in muscle mass that in the main pulmonary artery causes the thickness of the media to approximate or exceed that of the aortic media. The elastic fibers in the media are fragmented, irregularly shaped, and arranged in a loose network characteristic of the adult pulmonary artery. This configuration of the elastic tissue is evidence that the pulmonary hypertension was acquired rather than present at birth, because in patients with congenital heart diseases that produce pulmonary arterial hypertension from birth, the elastic fibers of the main pulmonary artery retain their fetal form and appear like those in the aorta. The media contains an excess of acid mucopolysaccharides that can accumulate in cystic fashion. A few atheromas are often found in the intima of the main pulmonary arteries; in occasional patients, they are numerous and scattered throughout the intima of all the elastic arteries.

The capillaries, veins, and parenchyma of the lungs are normal.

The right ventricle is extensively hypertrophied and dilated, and the ring of the tricuspid valve is often dilated. The right atrium is also dilated, and in a few patients, the foramen ovale is patent. The systemic arteries are usually free of significant abnormalities, although James has reported the occurrence of fibrous lesions in the intima of the small arteries of the sinus node in patients with primary pulmonary hypertension.

Etiology and Pathogenesis. None of the several theories proposed for the pathogenesis of primary pulmonary hypertension has been verified. Amniotic fluid embolization of the pulmonary arteries has been suggested as a cause because of the preponderance of young women among patients with the disease, some of whom experienced their first symptoms after pregnancy. Congenital defects in the pulmonary arteries, such as medial aplasia or failure of the pulmonary arteries to undergo normal transformation from their fetal form, have been suggested; however, the appearance of the elastic fibers in the media of the main pulmonary artery of patients with primary pulmonary hypertension indicates that the hypertension was not present from birth, as would be expected if the pulmonary arteries maintained their thick-walled, fetal form. The theory of medial aplasia holds that the areas of dilatation and thinning of the media observed in the muscular arteries represent congenital defects of the media and that the intima over these areas is subject to the development of intimal proliferation that then acts as the primary obstructive lesion. This explanation neglects the fact that all patients with primary pulmonary hypertension do not manifest dilatation lesions or defects of the media other than hypertrophy.

The occurrence of Raynaud's disease in some patients with primary pulmonary hypertension has prompted the speculation that the hypertension is due to vasospasm or to involvement of the pulmonary arteries by a systemic disease of a collagen, autoimmune, or allergic variety. Pulmonary vascular lesions and marked pulmonary hypertension are the predominant abnormalities in rare patients with lupus erythematosus, scleroderma, or sarcoidosis, but other stigmata of these diseases are evident during life or at autopsy. Neurogenically or humorally induced spasm of the pulmonary arteries is an attractive possibility, especially because these vessels in a few patients manifest medial hypertrophy with only slight abnormalities of the intima, but the hypothesis lacks support. Alveolar hypoxia, a potent pulmonary vasoconstrictor, is not present in these patients, and there is no history of residence at altitude, although an occasional patient may first experience symptoms during an excursion to a region several thousand feet above sea level.

The possibility that primary pulmonary hypertension is the consequence of multiple pulmonary emboli is most difficult to deny. Recurrent, small emboli to the lungs are often "silent" and can eventually produce marked increase in pulmonary arterial pressure and a clinical and physiologic syndrome identical to that of primary pulmonary hypertension. It is also often difficult to distinguish between the two conditions by examination of the vasculature of the lungs, because the small pulmonary arteries in widespread pulmonary embolization often exhibit the medial hypertrophy and intimal proliferation of hypertensive pulmonary vascular disease, and recanalized, fibrotic emboli in the small arteries can resemble occlusive intimal lesions. Differentiation of the two conditions depends on identification in the embolic disease of intraluminal thrombi, recent or old, throughout the pulmonary arteries, especially in the larger elastic arteries, and absence of dilatation lesions and necrotizing arteritis, which do not occur in the embolic disorder.

The practical difficulty in discriminating between pulmonary hypertension of the primary type and that caused by recurrent pulmonary embolization can be illustrated by the author's experience with 14 patients who after extensive study were considered to have primary pulmonary hypertension. Nine of these came to autopsy, and no cause for the hypertension other than the pulmonary vascular lesions of primary pulmonary hypertension was found in five. All five were women 32 to 33 years of age, except for one who was 44. In the other four patients, multiple thromboemboli were present in the pulmonary arteries. Two of these were men age 37 and 60 years, and two were women, 48 and 53 years of age. This and other reported experiences suggest the likelihood of an embolic cause of unexplained pulmonary hypertension in patients older than 40 years, especially if they are men. These data were collected before the widespread use of oral contraceptives, and it is conceivable that the proportion of young women with thromboembolism among patients with cryptic pulmonary hypertension may be modified in the future.

Whatever the cause, it appears that once pulmonary hypertension is established, the media of the pulmonary arteries reacts by progressive hypertrophy of its smooth muscle mass, probably as a consequence of increased arterial wall tension and work. The intima subsequently responds to the elevated pressure by proliferation, perhaps as the arterioles do in systemic hypertension. Thus each structural response of the pulmonary arterial tree leads to further compromise of its patency, further elevation of pressure, and the eventual development of the highest grades of hypertensive pulmonary vascular disease.

Pathologic Physiology. The cardinal hemodynamic ab-

normality is marked increase in the pulmonary vascular resistance with no evident physiologic cause. The resistance is usually 12 to 18 times normal and in the range of the systemic vascular resistance, and in an occasional patient it exceeds the systemic resistance. In one series, the average pulmonary arterial systolic pressure was approximately 110 mm Hg and the mean pressure approximately six times normal. During exercise the pulmonary vascular resistance remains fixed, and the pulmonary arterial pressures rise further. At rest and during exercise, the pulmonary wedge and left atrial pressures are normal. In contrast, the right ventricular end-diastolic and right atrial pressures are usually greatly increased. In some patients, the cardiac output is normal at rest, but more often it is only 50 to 60 per cent of normal and fails to increase appropriately with exercise. As the function of the right ventricle declines under its enormous afterload, cardiac output dwindles further, and evidences of tricuspid regurgitation may appear. Because of the small stroke volume, systemic arterial systolic and pulse pressures are frequently low.

The arterial oxyhemoglobin saturation is usually normal at rest and during exercise, but a few patients display mildly (91 to 92 per cent) and rarely substantially diminished (less than 90 per cent) saturation. Slight reduction in arterial carbon dioxide tension reflects the hyperventilation that commonly exists.

Infusion of tolazoline or acetylcholine into the pulmonary artery has been observed to produce slight to moderate decrease of pulmonary vascular resistance and pulmonary arterial pressure in some patients. Inhalation of oxygen has little effect.

Clinical Manifestations. These are the direct result of the physiologic and anatomic disturbances produced by the disease. Dyspnea during exertion, closely intertwined with fatigue and weakness, is a universal symptom. An oppressive substernal sensation and even frank angina are commonly experienced during effort, although this symptom, which is most likely the result of right ventricular ischemia, can occur in some patients in the form of recurrent and exceedingly disturbing episodes at rest. Syncope on exertion is an ominous sign because patients with primary pulmonary hypertension are subject to sudden death. There is evidence that an abrupt fall in cardiac output secondary to acute right ventricular failure or arrhythmia is the essential mechanism producing the syncopal attacks. Rupture of the flimsy walls of localized arterial dilatation lesions probably accounts for the intermittent minor hemoptyses experienced by some patients. An occasional patient may experience hoarseness related to compression of the left recurrent laryngeal nerve by the enlarged left pulmonary artery.

Overt signs of right ventricular failure develop in many patients before death and initially respond to digitalis and diuretics, but within a short period of time become increasingly more difficult to control. Because of the marked and fixed obstruction to flow in the pulmonary vessels and severe impairment of right ventricular function, the cardiac output is not only low but does not increase on demand to meet peripheral needs. Consequently, systemic arterial pressure can fall precipitously and fatally during anesthesia; after vasodepressor drugs, such as barbiturates; with physiologic stresses, such as fever and hemorrhage; and during diagnostic procedures, such as cardiac catheterization and angiocardiography. Because of the enormous obstruction to blood flow in the lungs, resuscitation from cardiopulmonary arrest is usually unsuccessful.

The patient usually appears normally developed and in good nutritional state. Occasionally the nail beds are slightly cyanotic, but the peripheral origin of the cyanosis is demonstrated by its disappearance after rubbing the digits. Clubbing is absent. Its presence should promptly suggest other causes of the pulmonary hypertension. Depending on the state of right ventricular function, the jugular veins may be distended; almost invariably, they show a prominent and sustained atrial contraction wave ("a" wave). If right ventricular failure and dilatation are advanced, the systolic wave of tricuspid regurgitation can also appear. The carotid arterial pulse is usually small.

The heart may be of normal size or considerably enlarged to the left and right. In contrast to the localized and unimpressive apical impulse, the heave associated with vigorous contraction of the hypertrophied right ventricle can be seen and felt along the left sternal border. Especially in patients with thin-walled and long chests, the prominent systolic pulsation of the enlarged main pulmonary can be seen and palpated for several centimeters to the left of the sternal border in the second left intercostal space. In almost every patient, a loud, sharp, pulmonic ejection sound can be heard and often felt. The second sound is usually closely split (0.02 to 0.03 sec), but in some patients the splitting may be wider (0.04 to 0.05 sec) and may vary relatively little during the respiratory cycle. The sound of pulmonic valvular closure is invariably accentuated in intensity, sharp or ringing in quality, and often palpable. Murmurs may be absent, but in many patients a systolic ejection murmur that is rarely harsh is heard in the third left interspace and extends well up along the left sternal border over the pulmonary artery. The diminuendo, medium-high-pitched murmur of pulmonic valvular regurgitation is audible in the third and fourth left interspaces in patients whose main pulmonary artery is very large, and is most easily detected with the patient erect and his chest held in full expiration. Either an atrial gallop sound (fourth sound) or an early diastolic gallop sound (third sound) or both are often heard over the lower right ventricle; increase in their intensity with inspiration signifies that they are generated in the right heart. When both gallop sounds are present, they can create the auditory illusion of a mitral diastolic rumble, an illusion that is enhanced by the early ejection sound, which may be misidentified as the loud closure sound of a stenotic mitral valve. A systolic murmur of tricuspid regurgitation that increases with inspiration may be heard in the fourth and fifth intercostal spaces along the left sternal border; it occasionally radiates well toward the apex if the tricuspid valve has been displaced to the left by a very enlarged right atrium and right ventricle. The usual signs of right ventricular failure and systemic venous congestion may be present.

Early in the course of the disease, the only abnormality in radiograms of the chest is enlargement of the main pulmonary artery and its major branches. Hypertrophy of the right ventricle is first manifested by its encroachment on the retrosternal space in lateral films and by a globular appearance of the heart in the posteroanterior projection. The heart is seldom massively enlarged, but the right ventricle may be sufficiently hypertrophied and dilated to displace the heart posteriorly, thereby creating some difficulty in assessing the size of the left ventricle. The right atrium usually appears rounded in frontal view, and eventually it and the superior vena cava dilate well into the right chest. The lung fields appear normal or slightly avascular, and the normal size of the small pulmonary arteries contrasts sharply with the dilated central arteries, which can attain considerable size. The pulmonary veins and left atrium are normal in size.

The electrocardiogram invariably reveals evidences of right ventricular hypertrophy, usually of the type associated with a systemic arterial systolic pressure in the ventricle. The mean QRS axis is at 90 degrees or more to the right. Lead V_1 shows an R wave of 1.0 to 1.5 mV with a small S wave, and the T waves in leads V_1 and V_2 are inverted. The P waves are tall (greater than 0.25 mV) and peaked in leads II, III, and aV_f; in V_1 the P wave is upright, peaked, narrow, and associated with a long PR segment. Higher grades of right ventricular hypertrophy are reflected by increasing amplitude of the R wave in V_1 and V_2, prominent S waves in the left precordial leads, and depression of the S-T segment and increasingly negative and coved T waves in V_1 and V_2 and even V_3.

Polycythemia occurs in some patients late in the course of the disease despite a normal or only slightly decreased arterial oxyhemoglobin saturation.

Diagnosis. Although the diagnosis of primary pulmonary hypertension can be made on the basis of the clinical, radiographic, and electrocardiographic manifestations, it is very difficult in some patients to be certain on these grounds alone that an underlying lesion of the heart, such as septal defect, cor triatriatum, or silent mitral stenosis, does not exist. It is especially difficult to exclude multiple pulmonary emboli or a systemic disease as the fundamental disorder. Cardiac catheterization should be performed to establish the diagnosis and to demonstrate that a congenital defect or mitral stenosis is not present. In pulmonary angiograms, filling defects or occlusions of the larger elastic pulmonary arteries are certain signs of pulmonary thromboemboli that are not found in primary pulmonary hypertension. Large areas lacking radioactivity in the lung fields in radioisotopic perfusion scans of the lungs constitute further evidence of the presence of embolic obstruction of large pulmonary arteries.

Because death of patients with primary pulmonary hypertension has been reported to occur during cardiac catheterization and angiocardiography, considerable judgment and care must be exercised in performing these studies and determining how extensive they should be. The general state of the patient, the blood pressure, and the electrocardiogram should be meticulously monitored throughout the procedure and for some time afterward. Arrhythmias and frequent ectopic beats should be promptly suppressed; significant falls in blood pressure should be immediately corrected with an infusion of norepinephrine to maintain perfusion of the right ventricular myocardium. Many patients with primary pulmonary hypertension have undergone these essential diagnostic studies without complication.

The appropriate laboratory tests, including skin biopsy to exclude scleroderma and lupus erythematosus, should be performed in all patients with primary pulmonary hypertension, especially those who manifest Raynaud's phenomenon. Sarcoidosis involving the pulmonary arteries almost exclusively and producing pulmonary hypertension is exceedingly rare and has only recently been reported. The author has also observed one such sponse of the pulmonary arterial pressure and pulmonary vascular resistance to infusion of tolazoline or inhalation of oxygen as a means of identifying a vasospastic component of an increased resistance.

Except in occasional infants with lower grades of hypertensive pulmonary vascular disease, the pulmonary vascular resistance does not usually fall after closure of an atrial or ventricular septal defect, and although the patient may be greatly benefited by the procedure, some degree of pulmonary hypertension persists.

Stenosis of Pulmonary Arterial Branches. Although multiple coarctation-like, congenital stenoses of the large branches of the pulmonary artery produce an increase in pressure only in the pulmonary arterial segments upstream from the stenotic regions, the malformation in some patients raises the systolic pressure in the main pulmonary artery and right ventricle to 70 or 80 mm Hg and can create difficulty in diagnosis. The lesions can occur in isolated form, but they often coexist with supravalvular aortic stenosis or an atrial septal defect. The total obstructive effect is usually slight, and the systolic pulmonary arterial pressure is increased to only 35 to 40 mm Hg at rest. The stenoses generate a continuous murmur or simply a systolic murmur that can be heard over the upper right or left precordial region. The diagnosis is conclusively established by an angiogram of the pulmonary arteries.

PULMONARY EMBOLI

Thrombi, globules of fat, and particulate matter of amniotic fluid can embolize the pulmonary arteries and produce acute pulmonary hypertension. The pathophysiologic basis for the hypertension is described in Ch. 543 to 545. Repeated embolization of the pulmonary arteries by thrombi (see Ch. 543 to 545 and Ch. 547) schistosomal ova (see Ch. 296), tumors, and cotton fibers and foreign matter contained in some drugs illicitly administered by vein cause chronic, progressive pulmonary hypertension by their primary obstructive effects and by the subsequent development of hypertensive pulmonary vascular lesions. In addition, schistosomal ova and particulate foreign matter evoke a granulomatous inflammatory reaction in the intima and walls of the arteries.

Although fragments of several types of cancer can embolize the pulmonary arteries after the tumor has invaded the liver or the inferior vena cava, the propensity of choriocarcinoma (chorioepithelioma) to metastasize in this manner deserves special consideration. Choriocarcinoma may remain undetected for several years after pregnancy, but soon after it originates it can invade the inferior vena cava and repeatedly discharge fragments of tissue into the pulmonary circulation. These embolic episodes may give rise to symptoms and signs of acute pulmonary embolization, or they can be clinically silent. The consequent obstruction of the larger pulmonary arteries can be extensive and give rise to marked pulmonary hypertension before the tumor invades the walls of the pulmonary arteries and appears in the lung fields.

Choriocarcinoma should be suspected in a woman who has had a recent pregnancy or even one a few years previously and has repeated bouts of pulmonary embolization or unexplained pulmonary hypertension. An increased concentration of human chorionic gonadotrophin and the demonstration of multiple occlusions of the pulmonary arteries by angiography confirm the diagnosis. The tumor is exquisitely sensitive to methotrexate, actinomycin D, and 6-mercaptopurine, and complete cure has been achieved in 50 per cent or more of patients by administration of these agents.

COLLAGEN AND MULTIPLE SYSTEM DISEASES

Pulmonary hypertension caused by the pulmonary arterial lesions of scleroderma, lupus erythematosus, and sarcoidosis has been discussed in Ch. 547. The clinical features and diagnosis of these diseases are presented in Ch. 79, 81, and 102, respectively. It is worth emphasizing that the pulmonary hypertension and its secondary effects may rarely be the only clinically apparent manifestations of these disorders. Hemodynamic studies of patients with scleroderma have demonstrated the high frequency of increases in pulmonary vascular resistance and slight pulmonary hypertension without involvement of the pulmonary parenchyma by the disease.

549. LEFT ATRIAL AND PULMONARY VENOUS HYPERTENSION

Elevation of pulmonary venous pressure is the most common cause of pulmonary arterial hypertension. Most frequently, left atrial and pulmonary venous hypertension are the result of dysfunction of the left ventricle characterized by impairment of its contractile state, decrease in its compliance, or both. Even in the absence of clinical signs of left ventricular failure, left ventricular end-diastolic pressure can be elevated, at first only with physical exertion or stress; later, as ventricular function becomes more impaired, it is chronically increased even at rest. Twofold increases in left atrial, pulmonary venous, and pulmonary arterial pressures are common. During episodes of acute left ventricular failure, pressures in the pulmonary veins and capillaries rise to levels exceeding 25 mm Hg.

The state of left atrial function is a significant determinant of the degree of left atrial and pulmonary venous hypertension. A properly timed, vigorous atrial contraction will generate a considerably increased left ventricular end-diastolic pressure without the need for much increase in left atrial pressure during the rest of diastole, but when the pumping function of the left atrium is lost because of atrial arrhythmia or left atrial failure, its pressure throughout diastole becomes greater. Thus for a given level of ventricular end-diastolic pressure, mean pressures in the atrium and the entire pulmonary vascular circuit are higher in the presence of left atrial failure or arrhythmia, such as atrial fibrillation, than in the presence of normal atrial function.

Disorders of the mitral valvular apparatus are another frequent cause of left atrial hypertension. In general, stenosis of the mitral valve and stenosis combined with regurgitation produce more severe degrees of left atrial hypertension than does mitral regurgitation alone. Nevertheless, in certain patients with chronic, marked mitral regurgitation caused by rheumatic valvular disease or rupture of the chordae tendineae, high-grade hypertension can occur in the left atrium, pulmonary veins, and pulmonary artery.

Less common causes of obstruction at the mitral valve are left atrial myxoma and left atrial ball-valve thrombus. A ball-valve thrombus almost invariably occurs with pre-existing mitral stenosis. A myxoma, which is tethered by a stalk attached to the atrial septum in the region of the fossa ovalis, produces left atrial hypertension by obstructing blood flow through the mitral orifice in diastole, but it can also pass through the mitral valve and obstruct left ventricular outflow. Other tumors of the left atrium can obstruct the mitral valve and may also grow into and obstruct the main pulmonary veins.

Cor triatriatum, a congenital anomaly in which an abnormal diaphragm with one or more small perforations partitions the pulmonary venous outflow region from the main left atrial chamber, mimics mitral stenosis in its effects on the pulmonary circulation. However, it is often not associated with a diastolic murmur and can thus escape clinical detection. Although cor triatriatum and left atrial myxoma are rare, their recognition is of great importance because they can be completely corrected by appropriate surgical procedures.

Mediastinal collagenosis with constriction of the extrapulmonary veins and diffuse pulmonary veno-occlusive disease are rare causes of pulmonary venous hypertension. The etiology of the latter disease, which occurs predominantly in women, is unknown. The small and medium sized pulmonary veins are narrowed and occluded by thrombi and fibrous tissue without evidence of inflammation in the venous walls. The clinical picture resembles that of primary pulmonary arterial hypertension; however, because of increased pressure in the pulmonary capillaries, radiographic evidence of pulmonary congestion and edema are present. The disease leads relentlessly to death in a few weeks to five years after the onset of symptoms.

Pulmonary Circulation in Mitral Stenosis

The physiologic and anatomic modifications of the pulmonary circulation induced by various degrees of chronic pulmonary venous hypertension are well illustrated by the extensive observations that have been made in patients with mitral stenosis. When the mitral orifice is only slightly restricted, left atrial pressure and intravascular pressures throughout the pulmonary circuit may be normal when the patient is at rest, but they exceed normal values with exercise or during other states accompanied by augmentation of cardiac output, such as fever, anemia, pregnancy, thyrotoxicosis, and hypermetabolism of other causes. Tachycardia alone, by abbreviating diastole, requires the generation of a higher left atrial pressure to maintain cardiac output through the stenotic valve. At this stage, as in animals with acutely produced mitral stenosis not severe enough to cause pulmonary edema, the modest vascular hypertension dilates the small pulmonary vessels and produces a decrease in their resistance to flow. In these circumstances, the increase in pulmonary arterial pressure is less pronounced than the increase in pulmonary venous and left atrial pressures.

In moderate and severe mitral stenosis with valvular orifice areas less than 1.5 sq cm, left atrial mean pressure at rest is often in the range of 25 to 30 mm Hg and rises with slight exercise to values of 40 to 55 mm Hg,

especially if cardiac output increases substantially. Even if the pulmonary vascular resistance is normal, the pronounced pulmonary venous hypertension causes the mean pressure in the pulmonary artery to exceed normal values by three- to sixfold. In most patients, however, pulmonary vascular resistance is greater than normal, resulting in an increase of pulmonary arterial pressure that is disproportionately greater than that caused by the left atrial hypertension alone.

The range of abnormality of pulmonary vascular resistance in mitral stenosis is wide. In one series of 180 patients, the resistance was two or more times greater than normal in 67 per cent of the patients. In 11 per cent, the resistance and consequently the pulmonary arterial pressure equaled or exceeded systemic arterial values. Patients with such advanced disturbances usually have very severe mitral stenosis and appear also to have a predisposition to advanced alterations in the pulmonary arteries in response to hypertension in the pulmonary veins and arteries that is not shared by other patients whose mitral obstruction and left atrial hypertension are equally pronounced. The clinical features of such patients resemble in many respects those of patients with primary pulmonary hypertension. A mitral diastolic murmur may not be audible, mainly because the cardiac output is greatly diminished as the result of the pulmonary vascular restriction and marked right ventricular dysfunction. Normal sinus rhythm persists in many of them despite the advanced mitral stenosis. Unlike patients with primary pulmonary hypertension, however, they do not experience frequent syncope.

In mitral stenosis, structural lesions are present in all segments of the pulmonary vascular bed. The pulmonary veins are dilated, and their walls are greatly thickened by medial hypertrophy and proliferation of the intima. In some patients, numerous anastomoses develop between the pulmonary and bronchial veins. These anastomotic channels form submucosal varicosites in the bronchi that can rupture and produce brisk hemoptysis when the left atrial pressure rises acutely.

The basic anatomic expression of increased hydrostatic pressure in the pulmonary capillaries is dilatation and engorgement of these vessels with edema of the alveolar walls and leakage of edema fluid into the alveolar spaces. Measurements made by the simultaneous injection of isotopically labeled water and a nondiffusible indicator into the pulmonary artery of patients with mitral stenosis and with pulmonary venous hypertension of other causes have demonstrated expansion of the interstitial pulmonary water volume directly related to the increase in left atrial pressure. At left atrial pressures of 25 to 30 mm Hg, the extravascular water volume is three or more times normal. Increased transport by the lymphatics is reflected by dilatation of these vessels. When the pulmonary capillary pressure exceeds values of 20 mm Hg, which is on the threshold of plasma protein osmotic pressure, the lymphatic vessels and the edematous interlobular septa at the bases of the lungs become sufficiently radiopaque to appear as short lines extending horizontally to the pleura (Kerley B lines) in radiograms of the chest.

Rupture of alveolar capillaries and pulmonary venules leads to scattered microhemorrhages and subsequent hemosiderosis. When the edema is of long standing, it promotes the development of interstitial fibrosis in the alveolar walls and the surrounding parenchyma most marked in the bases of the lower lobes and the lower segments of all lobes. These regional differences attest to the gravitational augmentation of capillary pressure and the greater and more persistent edema in the dependent regions of the lungs. In these regions, the alveolar septa are greatly thickened and the pulmonary capillaries are compressed or obliterated. Rarely, the fibrotic regions become ossified and appear as small calcified nodules scattered throughout the lower lung fields.

The small pulmonary arteries manifest the medial hypertrophy, proliferation and fibrosis of the intima, increased wall thickness, and diminished internal diameter characteristic of hypertensive pulmonary vascular disease; however, dilatation lesions and necrotizing arteritis that are the hallmarks of the most advanced grades of pulmonary vascular disease are very rarely found. Also, in contrast to the hypertensive pulmonary vascular disease associated with congenital heart disease and primary pulmonary hypertension, the distribution of the arterial lesions is not uniform throughout the lungs. The arteries in the lower lobes are most affected and show the greatest restriction of their lumina; even in the upper lobes, in which the larger arteries are dilated and the small arteries are relatively spared, the vascular lesions are more prominent in the lower segments. As a consequence of the pattern of distribution of the vascular abnormalities and probably because of the more pronounced interstitial fibrosis in the lower lobes, blood flow is preferentially directed to the upper zones of the lungs and away from the lower zones, resulting in reversal of the normal ratio of perfusion between the two zones. The ratio of upper zone perfusion to lower zone perfusion can be as large as 4:1 in contrast to the normal ratio of 1:8. The degree to which perfusion of the upper zones exceeds that of the lower regions is directly related to the height of the pulmonary venous pressure. The ratio also increases directly with the pulmonary vascular resistance, but when the resistance attains values in the range of the systemic vessels, the ratio decreases toward normal, probably because of more widespread distribution of the vascular abnormalities.

Pulmonary embolization and infarction are exceedingly frequent in mitral stenosis and in one series were found at autopsy in approximately one third of the patients who had manifested moderate to severe pulmonary arterial hypertension during life. These occlusions and their secondary effects on the parenchyma of the lung undoubtedly contribute to the restriction of the pulmonary vascular bed.

The main pulmonary artery and its central branches are dilated, and their intima often contains atherosclerotic plaques. The cross-sectional diameter of these vessels increases directly with the pulmonary arterial pressure. When the internal diameter of the main pulmonary artery is 4.0 cm or more, the murmur of pulmonic regurgitation (Graham Steell murmur) commonly appears.

Some insight into the mechanisms producing the pulmonary arterial hypertension and the relative roles of the various vascular disturbances in the genesis of the increased pulmonary vascular resistance is offered by observations of the hemodynamic changes that occur after successful mitral valvotomy or replacement of the mitral valve by a prosthetic valve with a functionally adequate orifice. In almost all patients whose left atrial pressure is lowered by the surgical procedure, the pulmonary vascular resistance decreases and the decline in pulmonary arterial pressure is consequently even greater than that

of the pulmonary venous pressure. Substantial decreases in pulmonary vascular resistance have been observed as early as two days after surgery and have been attributed to dilatation of muscular pulmonary arteries that had been reflexly induced to constrict by the pulmonary venous hypertension. However, failure of the resistance to fall immediately after the surgical procedure despite the decrease in left atrial pressure has been interpreted as indicating that interstitial and perivascular edema exert a cardinal role in the pathogenesis of the increased resistance and that resolution of the edema lags behind the fall of pulmonary venous pressure. In the ensuing weeks and months, the pulmonary vascular resistance often decreases further; even in patients whose preoperative values exceeded systemic vascular resistance, the arterial pressure and vascular resistance in the lungs can eventually attain values only slightly in excess of normal. The most striking changes occur in patients whose left atrial pressures postoperatively at rest and during exercise are normal or only slightly greater than normal. Evidence is now available that regression of the medial hypertrophy and intimal proliferation in the small pulmonary arteries is responsible for the progressive decline of the vascular resistance, but the way in which the pulmonary venous hypertension initiated the development of the structural abnormalities in the pulmonary arteries remains uncertain.

550. PULMONARY DISEASES AND DISORDERS OF RESPIRATION

Constriction of the pulmonary arteries by hypoxia and destruction or restriction of the pulmonary vascular bed are the two basic mechanisms that operate to increase the pulmonary arterial pressure in diseases of the lungs and disorders of the respiratory system. Primary alveolar hypoventilation is an example of a condition in which the disturbances in gas exchange alone initiate the pulmonary hypertension; but in most diseases of the lungs, anatomic restriction of the pulmonary vessels alone in the early stages of these diseases usually increases pulmonary arterial pressure only slightly because of the enormous reserve capacity of the pulmonary vasculature. By the time that the disease process has obliterated enough of the vessels to produce high-grade pulmonary hypertension, structural damage of the pulmonary parenchyma is sufficiently advanced to result in marked disturbances in gas exchange. In most pulmonary diseases therefore both mechanisms are operative.

Since diseases of the lungs and respiratory system are described in Part XI, only those features of significance in the production of pulmonary hypertension, its consequences, manifestations, and treatment are considered here.

Pathologic Physiology. In *chronic obstructive pulmonary disease,* loss of pulmonary capillaries accompanies the loss of alveoli. Some muscular arteries adjacent to terminal bronchioles may show intimal fibroelastosis of sufficient extent to obliterate their lumina. The media of the muscular arteries is slightly thickened, but these vessels and the arterioles show few of the changes characteristic of hypertensive pulmonary vascular disease.

The loss of pulmonary vessels is tolerated with little or

no increase of pulmonary arterial pressure at rest, although the pressure does rise to abnormal levels when pulmonary blood flow is augmented by exercise. In such patients, defects in distribution of ventilation and perfusion within the lungs and reduction in diffusing capacity exist but are not severe enough to cause hypercapnia and more than slight hypoxemia. With increase in the extent of hypoventilated but perfused pulmonary segments, marked hypoxemia develops and the pulmonary arterial pressure rises in direct proportion to the degree of oxygen unsaturation of systemic arterial blood. The hypercapnia that accompanies more widespread alveolar hypoventilation does not appear to affect the pulmonary arteries directly, and its effect on blood pH is minimized by concomitant increase in plasma bicarbonate concentration. Acidosis, arising as the consequence of sudden increase in carbon dioxide tension or failure of the buffering capacity to keep pace with the hypercapnia, potentiates the pulmonary vasoconstrictor response to the hypoxia and further raises the pulmonary arterial pressure.

The greater afterload to ejection of blood created by the increased pulmonary vascular resistance and pulmonary hypertension is met by hypertrophy of the right ventricle. Since the pulmonary arterial mean pressure at this stage is usually no more than twice normal, the right ventricle does not fail until a bronchopulmonary infection or some other event aggravates the bronchial obstruction and the disturbances in gas exchange and produces marked, generalized alveolar hypoventilation. Under such circumstances, as much 80 per cent of the cardiac output perfuses underventilated alveoli, and the arterial oxyhemoglobin saturation falls to values of 40 to 80 per cent; the arterial carbon dioxide tension rises to 60 or 80 mm Hg, and the arterial pH falls to values as low as 7.20. Renal blood flow and glomerular filtration decrease; the excretion of sodium and water diminishes, and the extracellular volume expands. The consequent increase in blood volume is augmented by hypoxia-induced polycythemia of variable degree. The end-diastolic pressure of the right ventricle increases and raises the pressure in the right atrium and systemic veins. The contractile function of the right ventricular myocardium is progressively depressed, and the right ventricle dilates and fails. Several studies have demonstrated that left ventricular function, if it was previously normal, is not disturbed by these events, and that left atrial and pulmonary venous pressures remain within the range of normal.

The relative pathogenic role of each physiologic disturbance in producing the sudden increase in pulmonary arterial pressure in this complex state has been difficult to assess. Correction of the hypoxemia or the acidosis while the failure persists reduces the pulmonary arterial pressure, but it remains considerably elevated. Phlebotomy does not promptly lower the pulmonary arterial pressure. In some patients, because of infection and hypermetabolism, the cardiac output is higher than in the prefailure period, but in many patients the cardiac output is subnormal.

It is striking that as the manifestations of acute respiratory insufficiency and congestive right ventricular failure resolve with appropriate treatment, the pulmonary arterial pressure gradually falls and, together with the systemic arterial oxyhemoglobin saturation, finally returns to its prefailure values. It is difficult to avoid assigning a cardinal role to hypoxia in the pathogenesis of

the marked pulmonary hypertension and the overt cor pulmonale.

During recurrent acute exacerbations of respiratory failure, and occasionally as the result of pulmonary thromboembolism to which these patients are prone, signs of increased pulmonary hypertension and right ventricular failure reappear. Eventually these manifestations and the disturbances in gas exchange do not respond fully to treatment, and the cor pulmonale becomes chronic.

In *fibroproliferative and chronic inflammatory diseases of the lungs,* the pulmonary vascular bed is compromised in many ways. In the diffuse interstitial disorders that affect the alveolar walls, such as *sarcoidosis* and other granulomatous diseases, the *Hamman-Rich syndrome, scleroderma, polymyositis, berylliosis, asbestosis, lymphangitic carcinomatosis, radiation fibrosis,* and *idiopathic pulmonary hemosiderosis,* the alveolar capillaries are compressed or obliterated. In massive pulmonary fibrosis caused by *silicosis* or coal miner's *pneumoconiosis,* the fibrotic nodules develop in proximity to muscular and small elastic arteries, and as they enlarge, they engulf and obliterate these vessels.

In all these disorders, increasing disruption of parenchymal structures and fibrosis cause progressive distortion, obstruction, and obliteration of pulmonary vessels. With the development of pulmonary hypertension, the medial hypertrophy and intimal proliferation of hypertensive pulmonary vascular disease are superimposed.

Early in the course of the pulmonary disease, as for example in the interstitial disorders of the lung, pulmonary hypertension may be only slight at rest despite marked restriction of lung volume, but the pressure usually rises steeply with exercise. Similarly, hypoxemia is only mild at rest, but the arterial oxygen saturation usually falls during exercise. With diminution of pulmonary diffusion capacity, the development of marked maldistribution of alveolar ventilation and perfusion, and increase in the extent of intrapulmonary arteriovenous shunting, oxygenation of arterial blood is progressively impaired, pulmonary arterial pressure rises further, and the right ventricle fails. Episodic exacerbations of failure are often precipitated by respiratory infections as in obstructive pulmonary disease, but reduction of pulmonary arterial pressure with treatment is less impressive, and once right ventricular failure occurs, it usually becomes chronic. The highest grades of chronic pulmonary hypertension secondary to pulmonary disease are found in fibrotic diseases of the lungs.

In bronchiectasis, tuberculosis, and other chronic inflammatory diseases of the lungs, extensive intercommunications can develop between the bronchial and pulmonary arteries; occasionally, the mammary and intercostal arteries participate in the formation of the anastomoses. The bronchial collateral flow through these channels is usually small, but in a rare patient it is large enough to constitute a significant left-right shunt that increases the pulmonary blood flow, further elevates the pulmonary arterial pressure, and taxes the left ventricle.

Alveolar hypoventilation pronounced enough to produce hypoxemia and hypercapnia, secondary constriction and hypertension in the pulmonary arteries, and right ventricular failure is encountered in a group of disorders characterized by a *defective ventilatory apparatus.* The fundamental defect exists in the chest bellows, as in *kyphoscoliosis, marked obesity,* and *neuromuscular diseases* that affect the respiratory muscles, or in the respiratory control centers, as in hypoventilation of central nervous origin *(Ondine's curse)*. The lungs and pulmonary vessels are intrinsically normal except in patients with severe kyphoscoliosis, whose pulmonary vascular bed is restricted by the inordinately small dimensions of the lungs and in whom concomitant bronchiectasis, areas of atelectasis, and bronchopulmonary infections are common.

Regardless of the nature of the basic defect in this group of diseases, alveolar ventilation not only is diminished at rest, but also fails to increase normally with exercise and increased metabolic demand, which consequently accentuates the hypoxemia and hypercapnia. In patients with these disorders, as well as in those with primary lung diseases who have had bouts of hypercapnia, the sensitivity of the chemoreceptors to both carbon dioxide and hypoxemia is progressively impaired, and the loss of ventilatory response to these stimuli enhances the propensity to the development of cor pulmonale. A respiratory infection commonly precipitates the development of marked pulmonary hypertension and right ventricular failure.

Clinical Manifestations and Diagnosis. Pulmonary disease is usually readily identified by the history, the physical findings, and radiograms of the chest, but clues to the presence and severity of pulmonary hypertension may be masked by the pulmonary disease. In some patients, the classic signs of pulmonary hypertension described in Ch. 547 may be present, but in others, especially those with chronic obstructive disease, the cardiac sounds are barely audible or are obscured by adventitious pulmonary sounds, and enlargement of the right ventricle and main pulmonary artery cannot be detected with certainty. Despite considerable pulmonary hypertension, the sound of pulmonic valvular closure may not be audibly accentuated.

The patient with right ventricular failure typically presents a history of a recent respiratory infection followed by exacerbation of his usual respiratory symptoms and progressive dyspnea. He presents the appearance and physical signs of a patient with acute pulmonary insufficiency. Cyanosis is usually marked, especially in the presence of polycythemia, but often it is not impressive despite pronounced decrease in the arterial oxyhemoglobin saturation. If hypercapnia exists, drowsiness and the other central nervous system manifestations of hypercapnia may be evident. The jugular veins are distended and are further engorged by applying pressure over the enlarged, usually tender liver. Edema of the lower extremities may be present. The cardiac rate is rapid, and an early diastolic gallop sound may be audible over the mid-left precordium.

Radiograms usually reveal a prominent main pulmonary artery and enlargement of its main branches; but if the pulmonary hypertension is not marked or has not been sustained for a prolonged period of time, these vessels may appear normal in size. Especially in patients who have manifested chronic cardiac failure, the right ventricle and the right atrium are grossly enlarged. In other patients with obvious failure, the cardiac dimensions seem surprisingly normal, but serial films will often show diminution in the size of the right ventricle and right atrium with recovery from the failure.

The electrocardiographic manifestations of right ventricular hypertrophy are also modified by lung disease; even in patients with considerable pulmonary hyperten-

sion and right ventricular hypertrophy, the usual criteria considered diagnostic of hypertrophy and enlargement of the right ventricle are often not present. Large S waves in the precordial leads as far to the left as V_5 or V_6, a small rS or rSR' complex in V_1, negative T waves in the right precordial leads, a vertical or slight rightward displacement of the mean QRS axis in the frontal plane, and peaked P waves in the limb leads (P pulmonale) may be the only signs that the right ventricle is hypertrophied. These electrocardiographic alterations may not be present if the pulmonary arterial pressure is not two or more times greater than normal at rest. Regression of these electrocardiographic features in the course of recovery from an episode of respiratory failure often permits a retrospective appreciation of their significance. Atrial arrhythmias, especially flutter and fibrillation, and ventricular premature contractions are common in patients with acute respiratory insufficiency and cor pulmonale.

The findings of a reduced oxyhemoglobin saturation, diminished oxygen tension and pH and elevated carbon dioxide tension in the arterial blood, increase in plasma bicarbonate, and polycythemia support the diagnosis of pulmonary hypertension caused by pulmonary disease or respiratory disorder. Studies of pulmonary function are useful in defining the disorder, monitoring the effects of treatment, and assessing the probability that cor pulmonale will develop. Primary alveolar hypoventilation of central origin as the cause of pulmonary hypertension and congestive cardiac failure may go undetected without measurements of arterial blood gases and studies of the ventilatory response to carbon dioxide. In some patients with cardiac murmurs or evidence of left ventricular enlargement, the issue of whether the pulmonary hypertension is primarily due to the pulmonary disease or is secondary to an intracardiac lesion or left ventricular dysfunction may sometimes be resolved only by hemodynamic and angiographic studies. Pulmonary disease does not protect the patient from the development of coronary arteriosclerosis or systemic hypertension, which may compromise left ventricular function. The left ventricle may also be directly affected by scleroderma, polymyositis, sarcoidosis, certain forms of muscular dystrophy, and obesity.

Treatment. Treatment must be simultaneously directed at improving the function of both the lungs and the heart. The specific measures to be used are described in Part XI. When cardiac failure appears, a cardiac glycoside and a diuretic, such as hydrochlorothiazide or furosemide, should be administered. Losses of body potassium during diuresis should be replaced, but because of pre-existing disturbances in potassium balance and impairment of renal function, serum potassium should be closely monitored as a guide to such replacement. The hypoxemia, hypercapnia, acidosis, and electrolyte imbalances appear to predispose the heart of patients with cor pulmonale to arrhythmias and to the toxic effects of cardiac glycosides. Daily maintenance doses larger than 0.1 mg of digitoxin or 0.25 mg of digoxin should be used with caution, and manifestations of digitalis intoxication should be watched for. Correction of hypoxemia by inhalation of oxygen in concentrations that do not depress alveolar ventilation is a cardinal feature of therapy during an acute episode of failure, and chronic administration of oxygen may be indicated to control pulmonary hypertension in patients with marked chronic hypoxemia. Because polycythemia enhances the tendency to develop thromboemboli and increases viscosity of the blood and consequently the resistance to its flow, periodic phlebotomy is indicated to maintain the hematocrit at 50 per cent in patients with marked polycythemia.

Prognosis. The development of pulmonary arterial hypertension and right ventricular failure in patients with pulmonary disease is a serious complication, but its prognostic significance depends on the underlying disorder. With appropriate treatment, the patient with chronic obstructive pulmonary disease may survive repeated bouts of cardiac and pulmonary failure over the course of many years. In patients with pulmonary fibrosis, the course after the onset of cardiac failure is variable but generally much shorter.

Bergofsky, E. H., and Holtzman, S.: A study of the mechanisms involved in the pulmonary arterial pressor response to hypoxia. Circulation Res., 20:506, 1967.

Blount, S. G., Jr., and Grover, R. F.: Pulmonary hypertension. *In* Hurst, J. W., and Logue, R. B. (eds.): The Heart. Arteries and Veins. 2nd ed. New York, McGraw-Hill Book Company, 1970, p. 1126.

Enson, Y., Giuntini, C., Lewis, M. L., Morris, T. Q., Ferrer, M. I., and Harvey, R. J.: The influence of hydrogen ion and hypoxia on the pulmonary circulation. J. Clin. Invest., 43:1146, 1964.

Harris, P., and Heath, D.: The Human Pulmonary Circulation. Its Form and Function in Health and Disease. Baltimore, Williams & Wilkins Company, 1962.

Tsagaris, T. J., and Tikoff, G.: Familial primary pulmonary hypertension. Am. Rev. Respir. Dis., 97:127, 1968.

Yu, P. N.: Pulmonary Blood Volume in Health and Disease. Philadelphia, Lea & Febiger, 1969.

CONGENITAL HEART DISEASE

Joseph K. Perloff

551. INTRODUCTION

Definition. *Congenital* is a Latin derivative from "con," together, and "genitus," born. However, the simple implication that congenital heart disease merely means "present at birth" requires qualification. The natural history begins before birth, because most anomalies compatible with six months of intrauterine life permit live offspring at term. A "congenital" anomaly originating in the developing fetus is often considerably modified, at least physiologically, by the dramatic circulatory adjustments at birth; it may then take weeks, months, or even years for the anomaly to evolve into the prototype pattern recognized as the "typical" clinical picture. Both physiologic and structural changes may subsequently continue. The ductus in a premature infant sometimes remains widely patent for months, finally closing spontaneously, leaving the baby with a normal heart. A ventricular septal defect that delivers a large left to right shunt in infancy may gradually develop progressive infundibular pulmonic stenosis, so that years later the physiologic and the clinical picture resembles classic cyanotic Fallot's tetralogy. A congenital bicuspid aortic valve that is functionally normal at birth may take two, three, or more decades to stiffen, calcify, and present as overt aortic stenosis. Accordingly, congenital heart disease should not be viewed narrowly as a static group of anatomic defects present at birth, but instead as a dynamic group of anomalies that originate in fetal life and

change during the course of postnatal natural histories. Certain defects that are not "anatomic" in the gross morphologic sense are considered congenital, such as congenital complete heart block, whereas others that are "anatomic," such as the aortic root disease of Marfan's syndrome are, by convention, generally not dealt with as congenital.

Incidence, Changing Population, and Role of the Internist and Medical Cardiologist. The prevalence of congenital heart disease has little meaning unless certain preconditions are considered. An impression of over-all prevalence can be derived from 1970 population figures when 3,718,000 live births were registered in the United States. An estimated 28,000 infants were born with congenital heart disease, i.e., 0.8 per cent. About half died within the first year, leaving 14,000 survivors. Thus well in excess of 20,000 infants with congenital heart disease are probably born annually in the United States. Both over-all incidence and incidence of specific defects vary according to patient age (neonate, infant, child, adolescent, young adult, older adult) and according to whether figures are derived from living subjects or necropsy material. A further distinction must be made between incidence based upon *natural* history and the incidence modified by *palliative* or *corrective surgery*. It is now possible to perform palliative or corrective surgery on almost all congenital cardiacs, even the most complex. Survival patterns are affected, often profoundly. We are therefore confronted with a changing population of congenital heart disease. Recent decades of intense diagnostic and therapeutic effort have resulted in survival of larger numbers of adolescents, postadolescents, and adults with congenital defects of the heart or circulation. Accordingly, postpediatric congenital heart disease is increasingly represented not only by anomalies with a natural tendency for long survival, but also by those in which palliative or corrective surgery has been successfully employed. Operation not only increases life expectancy in anomalies with a natural tendency for long survival, but may also permit increasing numbers of patients with disorders hitherto fatal in infancy or childhood to reach postadolescence or even adulthood. Intelligent long-term management requires an understanding of both the preoperative anomaly and the effects of surgical repair. *Thus congenital heart disease from the point of view of patient care should be considered not only in terms of age of onset, but also in terms of the age range that potential survival now permits.* Such patients require specialty care, be it by a pediatric cardiologist who extends an interest to older subjects or by a medical cardiologist who has a satisfactory comprehension of congenital cardiac disease. By the same token, it is no more important for the pediatrician to provide primary general pediatric care for the infant or child with congenital heart disease than for the internist to provide primary general medical care for the late teenager and adult with these malformations.

Etiology. Congenital heart disease is etiologically multifactorial, the result of a complex interplay between genetic and environmental factors. These determinants in part include heredity, chromosomal defects, teratogens, prematurity, altitude at birth, sex, and maternal age.

Some tendency exists for congenital heart disease to run in families. There is an increased incidence of defects in the offspring of propositi. Distribution and incidence are difficult to ascertain, because survival into the reproductive age is a necessary requirement for transmission. Atrial septal defect commonly permits adult survival, and can be not only familial but recurrent through a number of generations. Parents who in childhood experienced spontaneous closure of ventricular septal defects may live to adulthood and produce offspring with ventricular septal defects. There is also the prospect that increasing numbers of operated congenital cardiacs will reach childbearing age and produce a higher incidence of offspring with congenital defects of the heart or circulation. About 2 per cent of siblings of propositi have congenital heart disease. If one of a nonidentical twin pair has a congenital cardiac anomaly, the incidence in the co-twin is about the same as for sibs in general, but about 25 per cent of identical twins with congenital heart disease have affected co-twins with a high probability of identical defects.

Certain abnormal chromosome patterns are associated with predictable types of congenital cardiac disease, although chromosomal abnormalities per se are uncommon in the general population of congenital cardiacs. Down's syndrome (trisomy 21) has a high incidence of endocardial cushion defects, and about 50 per cent of patients with complete endocardial cushion defects have trisomy 21. Typical Turner's syndrome (phenotypic female with XO) occurs with coarctation of the aorta; trisomy 18 occurs with right ventricular origin of both great arteries; the Holt-Oran syndrome heightens suspicion of ostium secundum atrial septal defect, and the Ellis–van Creveld syndrome predicts common atrium.

The role of *teratogens* at critical times in fetal development is epitomized by the effects of thalidomide taken by the pregnant mother. Maternal rubella (German measles) during the first trimester increases the risk of offspring with patent ductus arteriosus and stenosis of the pulmonary artery and its branches.

Ventricular septal defect and patent ductus arteriosus are relatively common in *premature infants*. It has been postulated that the expected intrauterine time of ventricular septal closure is not limited to early fetal life but sometimes continues through gestation into the postpartum period. Delayed closure of the ductus arteriosus is more likely to occur in premature infants in whom the duct may remain patent for as long as four to six months after birth. Incompletely developed cholinergic innervation and reduced constrictor response to oxygen of the premature ductus may in part account for this.

The *altitude at birth* is another factor affecting the occurrence of congenital heart disease. Persistence of the ductus arteriosus is six times as frequent in people born at high altitudes as in those born at sea level. Reduced oxygen tension in ambient air at high altitudes may provide inadequate stimulus for ductal constriction even if cholinergic innervation of the ductal wall is well developed.

Parental age has been considered an etiologic factor. There is no evidence that paternal age plays a role, but *maternal age* has been called into question. Late maternal age (immediate premenopausal) seems to increase the risk of Fallot's tetralogy.

Sex distribution has been a point of interest in congenital diseases of the heart and circulation. The bicuspid aortic valve is predominantly a male disease. In fact, aortic valve disease in general has a strong male prevalence. The male-to-female ratio in ventricular septal defect with aortic regurgitation is twice as high as in uncomplicated ventricular septal defect. Aortic atresia is almost exclusively a disease of male infants. On the other hand, patent ductus arteriosus predominates in females (sex ratio of 2 or 3:1). Female predominance in ostium secundum atrial septal defect is estimated to be as high as 3.5:1, and females predominate in partial endocardial cushion defects. Congenital aneurysms of sinuses of Valsalva carry a male-to-female ratio of 4:1. A similar male-to-female ratio occurs in complete transposition of the great arteries, with a range of 2 to 4:1.

Physiologic Adaptation after Birth. The concept has been underscored that congenital heart diseases are not static in time, but change anatomically and functionally during the course of their natural histories. The most spectacular change in this context occurs at birth. A given congenital cardiac defect may exist in harmony with the fetal circulation, but is confronted with dramatic circulatory changes at birth that alter this harmony to widely varying degrees. It is therefore appropriate to examine briefly the principal immediate and delayed circulatory alterations at birth and in the neonatal period. The immediate changes consist of (1) a colossal fall in pulmonary vascular resistance associated with expansion of the lungs; (2) a pronounced rise in systemic vascular resistance associated with elimination of the low resistance placental circulation; (3) a fall in blood flow to the right atrium owing to abolition of umbilical venous return; (4) an abrupt rise – as much as tenfold – in pulmonary blood flow, which is promptly translated into a rise in left atrial volume and pressure; (5) functional closure of the valve of the foramen ovale caused by the rise in left atrial and the fall in right atrial pressure; and (6) constriction of the ductus arteriosus at about 12 hours after birth in response to an increase in systemic arterial Po_2. Several important delayed changes complete the picture. The thick-walled fetal pulmonary arterioles are designed to meet the full force of systemic right ventricular pressure the instant the lungs expand. After this need has been met, the fetal arterioles involute during the first two months of life. As respiration is established at birth, there is a marked rise in alveolar and systemic arterial oxygen tension to which pulmonary arterioles are exquisitely sensitive, setting the stage for dilatation and anatomic involution. A possible effect of bradykinin in this regard should also be mentioned. In addition, the larger pulmonary arteries may also play a role – though much less – in determining the total drop in pressure across the lungs after birth. Maturational changes may affect the neonatal disparity in size between the main and branch pulmonary arteries as well as the angulation at the origins of the right and left branches; both these factors have been held responsible for a physiologic drop in pressure distal to the pulmonary trunk. The third important delayed change relates to the fetal right ventricle, which slowly loses its relative thickness during the first year of life. Adaptive hypertrophy is an expected feature of the fetal right ventricle, which ejects at systemic pressure via the ductus arteriosus. After birth, with the stimulus of right ventricular afterload eliminated, there is a gradual reduction in its thickness relative to septum and left ventricle. The thick neonatal right ventricular wall does not undergo regression; it merely does not increase its thickness as rapidly as the left in the growing infant.

These physiologic adaptations of the normal heart to the events at birth are remarkable in their own right. It is no surprise that congenital defects of the heart or circulation will, to varying degrees, interact with or be modified by adaptations to extrauterine life. A few examples suffice. At one end of the spectrum is the ductus arteriosus, which is a normal part of the fetal circulation. However, when the fetal ductus remains widely patent after birth, the neonatal fall in pulmonary vascular resistance establishes a left to right shunt; pulmonary blood flow increases, and the left ventricle is volume overloaded and may fail under the burden. What was a normal structure in the fetus becomes a potentially hazardous congenital defect after birth. At the other end of the spectrum, aortic atresia is a case in point. This anomaly is characterized by an atretic aortic valve, a rudimentary left ventricular cavity, and a rudimentary or atretic mitral valve. The left atrium has no effective exit, but in the fetus this is not a serious handicap, because flow into the left atrium via the lungs is negligible and right to left flow across the foramen ovale is not vital. Accordingly, survival to term is the rule, because systemic venous blood received by the fetal right heart is pumped into the systemic circulation via the fetal ductus, bypassing the left heart. However, at birth, the lungs expand and pulmonary blood flow suddenly and dramatically increases, abruptly delivering a large volume into a left atrium that has no effective outlet, because forward flow through the left ventricle is totally obstructed by the atretic mitral and/or aortic valves. Temporary survival depends upon decompression of the left atrium via a herniated valve of the foramen ovale. Death follows in short order. An intermediate case in point is large ventricular septal defect which, although abnormal, does not disturb the fetal circulation, because it allows right ventricular blood to enter the aorta in a fashion analogous to the fetal ductus. However, after birth, a fall in pulmonary vascular resistance establishes a left to right shunt which may significantly disturb the postnatal circulation. Subsequently, the pulmonary vascular resistance may rise again and, in a decade or more, reverse the shunt (Eisenmenger's complex).

The principle to be extracted from these examples is clear. The anatomy and physiology of the heart and circulation in congenital heart disease change with the passage of time from the fetus, to the dramatic changes at birth, to further changes in the infant, child, adolescent, and adult survivor. Some of these changes result in neonatal death; others express themselves gradually over weeks, months, years, or decades. A satisfactory comprehension of the clinical manifestations of congenital heart disease requires that these patterns be taken into account.

Diagnosis. Clinical diagnosis of congenital heart disease can represent the epitome of clinical logic. The pathologic anatomy should first be clarified to shed light on the resulting physiologic derangements. The question can then be asked: "What clinical manifestations result from these anatomic and physiologic derangements?" The stage is then set for the clinical diagnosis, which depends upon a synthesis of information derived from the history, the physical signs, the electrocardiogram, the x-ray, and the laboratories (noninvasive and cardiac catheterization). Similarly, the physical diagnosis consists of a synthesis of its own five parts, namely, physical appearance, the arterial pulse, the venous pulse, precordial movements and palpation, and auscultation. Maximal data should be extracted from each clinical source, relating the information from one source to that from another. A simple principle emerges—on the one hand, depth; on the other, synthesis. Each step should advance

our thinking and narrow the diagnostic possibilities. By the end of the clinical appraisal, untenable considerations should have been abandoned, diagnostic *possibilities* retained for due consideration, and high priority *probabilities* brought into sharp focus.

Diagnostic thinking benefits from the devices of anticipation and supposition. Anticipate what the next step holds, and less will be missed. Once tentative conclusions have been drawn from the history, it is useful to pause momentarily and ask, "If these assumptions are correct, what can I expect the physical examination to show? What specific points might I anticipate in the electrocardiogram or x-ray in order to support or refute the conclusions based on the history?" The device of *anticipation* not only helps achieve a synthesis of each step with the next but also serves to heighten interest as the clinical assessment progresses. The device of *supposition* lends itself to the clinical classification of congenital heart disease proposed in Table 1. As clinical information becomes available, it can be directly related to this classification so that orderly thinking begins apace. For example, we can ask, "*Suppose* this were a *congenital* cardiac defect in an *acyanotic* patient with a *left to right shunt;* which if any of the malformations in this category are appropriate to the information thus far at hand?" By simply asking, "Suppose this were so, what is likely to follow?" one is permitted the dual advantages of thoughtful consideration without inflexible commitment.

Diagnostic information is best handled within the framework of an orderly classification (Table 1) which was selected because it is practical and clinical and can be effectively used irrespective of which of the five sources of diagnostic information one is dealing with. The classification is based essentially on the answers to five simple questions: *(1) Is the patient acyanotic or cyanotic? (2) Is pulmonary arterial flow increased or not? (3) Does the malformation originate in the left or right heart? (4) Which is the dominant ventricle? (5) Is pulmonary hypertension present or absent?* It is not even necessary to ask all five questions for each patient. If the answer to question 1 is "acyanotic," only two additional questions need be posed, namely, "Is a shunt absent or present" (i.e., is pulmonary arterial flow increased or not?), and if a shunt is absent, "On what side of the heart does the malformation originate, left or right?" (Table 2). On the other hand, if the answer to question 1 is "cyanotic," three additional questions need be asked. First, "Is pulmonary arterial flow increased or not?" If the answer is "normal" or "decreased," we need ask, "Which is the dominant ventricle?" and "Is pulmonary hypertension present or absent?" (Table 3).

To illustrate, begin with an acyanotic patient (Table 4). If the answer to question 2 is negative (acyanotic without shunt), then we must ask, "Does the malformation originate in the left or right heart?" (Table 2). Now move step by step through the heart in the direction of blood flow (Table 4). If the malformation originates in the right heart, is it at the level of the venae cavae, right atrium, tricuspid valve, right ventricular inflow, right ventricular outflow, pulmonary artery and its branches, or pulmonary arterioles? Similarly, if the malformation originates in the left heart (Table 5), is it at the level of the pulmonary veins, left atrium, mitral valve, left ventricular inflow, left ventricular outflow, aortic root (supravalvular) or thoracic aorta? If the answer to question 2 is that pulmonary arterial blood flow

TABLE 1. A Clinical Classification of Congenital Heart Disease*

General

Innocent or normal murmurs
Congenital complete heart block
Congenitally corrected transposition of the great arteries
Congenital positional anomalies of the heart—the cardiac
malpositions

Acyanotic without a Shunt

Malformations originating in the left heart
1. Aortic stenosis
   a. Valvular
   b. Discrete subvalvular
   c. Muscular subvalvular
   d. Supravalvular
2. Coarctation of the aorta
3. Congenital mitral incompetence
   a. Endocardial cushion defect
   b. Congenitally corrected transposition of the great arteries
   c. Primary endocardial fibroelastosis
   d. Anomalous origin of the left coronary artery from the
      pulmonary artery
   e. Miscellaneous (double orifice mitral valve, congenital perfora-
      tions, accessory commissures with anomalous chordal inser-
      tion, congenitally short or absent chordae, cleft posterior
      leaflet, Marfan's syndrome, etc.)
4. Primary endocardial fibroelastosis
5. Congenital obstruction to left atrial flow
   a. Cor triatriatum
   b. Mitral stenosis
   c. Pulmonary vein stenosis
6. Congenital aortic incompetence
Malformations originating in the right heart
1. Pulmonic stenosis
   a. Valvular
   b. Infundibular
   c. Supravalvular (stenosis of the pulmonary artery and its
      branches)
   d. Subinfundibular
2. Idiopathic dilatation of the pulmonary artery
3. Congenital pulmonary valve incompetence
4. Primary pulmonary hypertension
5. Ebstein's anomaly of the tricuspid valve
6. Hypoplastic right ventricle

Acyanotic with a Shunt (Left to Right)

Shunt at atrial level
1. Atrial septal defect (isolated)
   a. Ostium secundum
   b. Ostium primum
   c. Sinus venosus
2. Atrial septal defect with mild pulmonic stenosis
3. Total anomalous pulmonary venous connection with low
   pulmonary vascular resistance
4. Partial anomalous pulmonary venous connection with intact
   atrial septum
5. Atrial septal defect with mitral stenosis (Lutembacher's syndrome)
Shunt at ventricular level
1. Ventricular septal defect (isolated)
   a. Infracristal
   b. Supracristal
   c. Muscular
   d. Endocardial cushion location
2. Ventricular septal defect with mild pulmonic stenosis (acyanotic
   Fallot's tetralogy)
3. Ventricular septal defect with right ventricular origin of both
   great arteries
4. Ventricular septal defect with congenitally corrected transposition
   of the great arteries
5. Ventricular septal defect with aortic incompetence
6. Ventricular septal defect with left ventricular to right atrial shunt
7. Ventricular septal defect with complete interruption of the aortic
   arch

Shunts between aortic root and right heart
1. Coronary arteriovenous fistula
2. Ruptured sinus of Valsalva aneurysm
Shunt at aorticopulmonary level
1. Patent ductus arteriosus
2. Aorticopulmonary septal defect
3. Anomalous origin of the left coronary artery from the
   pulmonary artery
4. Truncus arteriosus with large pulmonary arteries and low
   pulmonary vascular resistance
Shunts at more than one level
1. Complete endocardial cushion defect (complete persistent common
   atrioventricular canal)
2. Ventricular septal defect with patent ductus arteriosus
3. Ventricular septal defect with atrial septal defect

Cyanotic with a Shunt (Right to Left)

Increased pulmonary blood flow
1. Complete transposition of the great arteries
2. The Taussig-Bing anomaly (right ventricular origin of both great
   arteries with supracristal ventricular septal defect or right
   ventricular aorta with biventricular pulmonary trunk)
3. Truncus arteriosus with large pulmonary arteries
4. Total anomalous pulmonary venous connection
5. Single ventricle with low pulmonary resistance and no
   pulmonic stenosis
6. Common atrium
7. Fallot's tetralogy with pulmonary atresia and increased
   bronchial arterial flow
8. Tricuspid atresia with large ventricular septal defect and no
   pulmonic stenosis
Normal or decreased pulmonary blood flow
Dominant left ventricle
   a. Tricuspid atresia
   b. Ebstein's anomaly with right to left interatrial shunt
      (mechanical dominance)
   c. Pulmonary atresia with intact ventricular septum and
      diminutive right ventricle
   d. Congenital vena caval to left atrial communication
   e. Single ventricle with pulmonic stenosis and noninversion of
      the infundibulum
   f. Large pulmonary arteriovenous fistula in infancy
Dominant right ventricle
Normal or low pulmonary arterial pressure
   a. Pulmonary stenosis or atresia with ventricular septal defect
      and right to left shunt (cyanotic Fallot's tetralogy)
   b. Pulmonic stenosis with right to left interatrial shunt
   c. Complete transposition of the great arteries with severe pul-
      monic stenosis and large ventricular septal defect
   d. Pulmonic stenosis with right ventricular origin of both great
      arteries
   e. Pulmonic stenosis with single ventricle and inversion of the
      infundibulum (electrical dominance)
   f. Pulmonary atresia with intact ventricular septum and dilated
      right ventricle
   g. Truncus arteriosus with hypoplastic or absent pulmonary
      arteries
Normal or nearly normal ventricles
   a. Pulmonary arteriovenous fistula
   b. Congenital vena caval to left atrial communication
Elevated pulmonary arterial pressure (pulmonary hypertension)
1. Ventricular septal defect with reversed shunt (Eisenmenger's
   complex)
2. Patent ductus arteriosus or aorticopulmonary septal defect with
   reversed shunt
3. Atrial septal defect with reversed shunt
4. Right ventricular origin of both great arteries with high
   pulmonary vascular resistance
5. Hypoplastic left heart (aortic atresia, mitral atresia, complete
   interruption of the aortic arch)
6. Complete transposition of the great arteries with high pulmonary
   vascular resistance
7. Single ventricle with high pulmonary vascular resistance
8. Total anomalous pulmonary venous connection with pulmonary
   venous obstruction

*Modified from Perloff, J. K.: The Clinical Recognition of Congenital Heart Disease. Philadelphia, W. B. Saunders Company, 1970.

TABLE 2

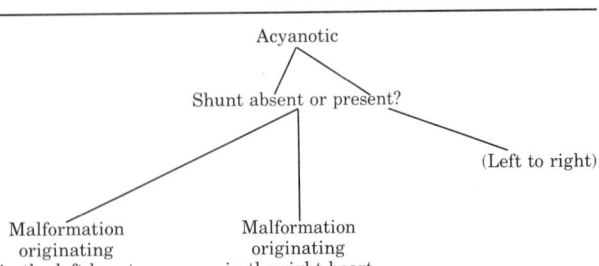

TABLE 4

Acyanotic without a shunt, malformation originating in the right heart. Start proximally (venae cavae) and end distally (pulmonary arteries):

1. Venae cavae
2. Right atrium
3. Tricuspid valve
4. Right ventricular inflow
5. Right ventricular outflow
6. Pulmonary artery and branches
7. Pulmonary arterioles

is increased, then the shunt by definition is left to right, because cyanosis is absent. We can then methodically consider the origin of the shunt and the chamber or vessel that receives it. Again, move step by step through the heart in the direction of blood flow, i.e., shunts at atrial level, ventricular level, from aortic root to right heart, or from aortic arch to pulmonary artery (Table 6).

Next, consider cyanotic patients (Table 3). If pulmonary arterial blood flow is increased, there are for all practical purposes, a total of eight possibilities, but only the first four are likely (Table 1, cyanotic with a shunt, increased pulmonary blood flow). If pulmonary arterial flow is normal or decreased, and the left ventricle is dominant, there are a total of six possibilities, only two of which are likely, i.e., tricuspid atresia or Ebstein's anomaly of the tricuspid valve (Table 1). If the right ventricle is dominant, question 5 must be asked, "Is pulmonary hypertension present or absent?" If pulmonary hypertension is present (Table 7), again, move step by step through the heart in the direction of blood flow; i.e., is one dealing with a pulmonary hypertensive right to left shunt at atrial, ventricular, or great vessel level? If pulmonary hypertension is absent (Table 8), this necessarily implies obstruction to outflow into the pulmonary bed, i.e., normal or low pulmonary arterial pressure with high right ventricular pressure. In practical terms, the probabilities are two, pulmonic stenosis with right to left shunt at either atrial or ventricular level.

In dealing with the history, physical examination, electrocardiogram, x-ray, and diagnostic laboratories, it is worthwhile briefly to call attention to a few points especially appropriate to congenital heart disease. In the history, questions should include the pregnancy, for example, maternal exposure to teratogens such as rubella in the first trimester, or the altitude at which the patient was born. Maternal age may be important. Details of a

cardiac murmur—the detection of which often heralds the diagnosis of congenital heart disease—should be precise regarding onset and intensity. Was the murmur present at birth (newborn nursery), or was it first detected in early infancy, adolescence, or young adulthood? Was the murmur always readily heard irrespective of patient cooperation (conspicuous murmur), or was it absent at times, difficult to hear, or believed to be unimportant? Was a new murmur even commented upon (ventricular septal defect with subsequent aortic regurgitation)? Cyanosis should similarly be defined precisely according to time of onset, degree, and distribution. A history of squatting in a cyanotic patient is classic information suggesting Fallot's tetralogy. Patterns of growth and development should be established. It is worth recalling that the clinical manifestations of congestive heart failure differ in infants, older children, and adults. Family history of congenital cardiac disease may shed light on the defect in the patient, especially if kinship is close. Susceptibility to lower respiratory infections suggests large left to right shunts. Neck pulsations (arterial or venous) may provide useful clues. A history of infective endocarditis calls attention to a relatively limited number of defects.

Physical appearance should consider the presence of certain *somatic* congenital defects that are associated with specific types of congenital *cardiac* anomalies, such as *mongolism* (endocardial cushion defect), *Turner's syndrome* (coarctation of the aorta), *peculiar facies and dentition* associated with supravalvular aortic stenosis and pulmonary artery stenosis, the *Holt-Oram syndrome* (defects in the atrial septum), the *Ellis–van Creveld syndrome* (common atrium), or trisomy 18 (double outlet right ventricle).

The arterial pulses should be compared in the upper and lower extremities (coarctation of the aorta), but the brachials should also be palpated (cyanotic male infant with absent brachials and present femorals may mean aortic atresia). Right and left arterial pulses should be compared (increased pulse pressure in the right carotid and brachial arteries in supravalvular aortic stenosis). The jugular venous pulse deserves special attention as soon as the patient is old enough to permit such observa-

TABLE 3

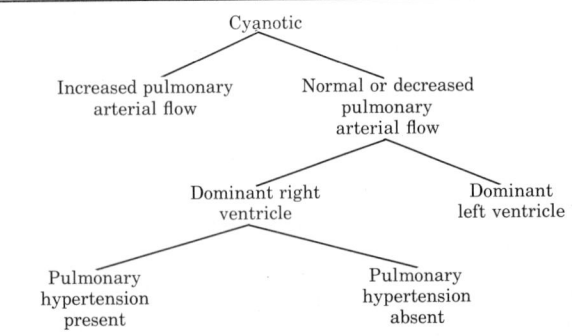

TABLE 5

Acyanotic without a shunt, malformation originating in the left heart. Start proximally (pulmonary veins) and end distally (aorta):

1. Pulmonary veins
2. Left atrium
3. Mitral valve
4. Left ventricular inflow
5. Left ventricular outflow
6. Thoracic aorta

TABLE 6

Acyanotic with a shunt. Where is the left to right communication, i.e., where does it originate and what chamber or vessel receives the shunt? Start proximally and end distally:

1. Atrial level
2. Ventricular level
3. Great vessel level (aortic root, aortic arch)

TABLE 8

Cyanotic with normal or decreased pulmonary arterial flow, dominant right ventricle, and no pulmonary hypertension.

1. Pulmonic stenosis or atresia with right to left shunt at ventricular level.
2. Pulmonic stenosis or atresia with right to left shunt at atrial level.

tion (the short neck of the infant usually makes examination difficult or impossible). Percussion is useful in establishing visceral positions (cardiac and hepatic dullness and gastric tympany) to avoid missing a congenital positional anomaly. Palpation should carefully define each precordial movement according to chamber or vessel of origin, avoiding vague, meaningless terms such as point of maximum impulse. During auscultation, designations such as pulmonary area, aortic area, or mitral area should be avoided, because they assume normal topographical anatomy of the heart, i.e., situs solitus without transposition of the great arteries and without ventricular inversion, assumptions which cannot be made, especially in the context of congenital heart disease. Simple descriptive terms should be used, such as apex, left or right lower, mid or upper sternal border, and the like. Murmurs should be precisely characterized, especially their timing in the cardiac cycle, with systolic murmurs classified as early, mid, late or holosystolic; diastolic murmurs as early diastolic, mid-diastolic or presystolic; and the continuous murmur defined as one that begins in systole and continues without interruption through the second heart sound into all or part of diastole.

The 12-lead surface electrocardiogram should be supplemented by leads V_3R and V_4R, and a vectorcardiogram is often necessary to clarify complex electrocardiograms.

Technically satisfactory plain films of the chest in the posteroanterior, lateral, right and left oblique positions with barium have for all practical purposes replaced cardiac fluoroscopy except for the detection of intracardiac calcium. The noninvasive technique of *echocardiography* is a valuable source of diagnostic information that is available repeatedly and without risk. Cardiac catheterization and angiocardiography should be an extension of clinical judgment, a judgment which should decide not only which patients should be selected for study, but also which type of investigation is most appropriate for a given subject. Accurate diagnosis depends upon synthesis of the broad range of clinical data with results of carefully planned and well-executed laboratory studies.

Scope of These Chapters. Survival in congenital heart disease results from natural selection or from surgical intervention. These chapters will emphasize those defects with a natural tendency to survive beyond the pediatric age group. Such emphasis is appropriate for a text-

TABLE 7

Cyanotic with normal or decreased pulmonary arterial flow, dominant right ventricle, and pulmonary hypertension. Where is the right to left shunt? Start proximally and end distally.

1. Atrial level
2. Ventricular level
3. Great vessel level

book of medicine. It must be stated, however, that congenital cardiac disease is a continuum from birth to adult life and that the only way to understand the patterns of postpediatric survival is to have dealt at some point with the same disorders in the infant and young child. The following categories will be considered: (1) *common* congenital cardiac defects in which postpediatric survival is expected; (2) *uncommon* congenital cardiac defects in which postpediatric survival is expected; (3) *common* congenital cardiac defects in which postpediatric survival is exceptional; and (4) *uncommon* congenital cardiac defects in which postpediatric survival is exceptional. Congenital cardiac anomalies (common or uncommon) in which postpediatric survival is unknown will not be considered. Chief emphasis will be placed on the common or uncommon anomalies with *expected* postpediatric survival. The common or uncommon defects with exceptional postpediatric survival will be touched upon more briefly to provide necessary perspective. It should be borne in mind, however, that as time goes on more and more congenital cardiacs beyond the pediatric age group will be postoperative; this is only as it should be.

552. COMMON CONGENITAL CARDIAC DEFECTS IN WHICH POSTPEDIATRIC SURVIVAL IS EXPECTED

FUNCTIONALLY NORMAL BICUSPID AORTIC VALVE

The frequency of congenitally bicuspid aortic valves—functionally normal, stenotic, and/or incompetent—may approach 2 per cent of the population. If this figure is correct, it would mean that the bicuspid aortic valve is not only the most frequent congenital anomaly of the heart or great vessels, but that the most common congenital cardiac defect in man manifests itself in the *postpediatric population*. The typical bicuspid aortic valve consists of two commissures and two cusps. One cusp, generally the larger, contains a low ridge or raphe ("false commissure"), adjacent to the aortic wall but not reaching the edge of the leaflet. If the free edges of a congenital bicuspid aortic valve are sufficiently redundant to permit unimpeded forward flow (no systolic gradient) yet not redundant enough to cause malapposition in diastole (little or no aortic regurgitation), then the bicuspid aortic valve is said to be "functionally normal." The natural history of such a valve is variable. A bicuspid aortic valve that functions normally at birth may continue to do so throughout life and be found as an incidental necropsy finding in late adult life. However, the same valve may take three unfavorable courses. The first is the tendency to become thickened, fibrotic, calcified, and stenotic during early or mid-adult life. Second, infective endocarditis may convert a functionally benign lesion into the catastrophic mechanical fault of severe aortic regurgitation. Third, the larger of the two cusps may progressively evert or prolapse, causing progressive aortic regurgitation that ultimately can be severe. It is not yet known what determines which of these courses a given functionally normal congenitally bicuspid valve will take.

Clinical recognition of a functionally normal bicuspid aortic valve can be suspected especially in teenagers and young adults. Innocent systolic murmurs in this age group, except for infraclavicular radiation of the innocent brachiocephalic systolic murmur, are not heard at the right base. Accordingly, a short, somewhat impure Grade I to II midsystolic murmur at the right base in a child, adolescent, or young adult is suspect. If that murmur is introduced by an ejection sound and if careful auscultation detects the soft murmur of aortic regurgitation, the clinical diagnosis reaches a high degree of probability. Physical interventions that increase aortic pressure (squatting, isometric tension with clenched fists) increase the audibility of the soft murmur of aortic regurgitation. Suspicion is always greater in the male, because the congenital bicuspid aortic valve, whether functionally normal or not, is predominantly a male disease. If clinical suspicion is high, an argument can be made for verification by thoracic aortography, because the bicuspid aortic valve is highly susceptible to infective endocarditis and appropriate antimicrobial prophylaxis must be recommended.

CONGENITAL VALVULAR AORTIC STENOSIS

Congenital obstruction to left ventricular outflow can be *valvular, subvalvular,* or *supravalvular.* The most common type is valvular and is usually characterized by narrowing of a bicuspid valve which can be intrinsically stenotic from birth or can become stenotic after progressive thickening and calcification (see above). Unicommissural unicuspid aortic valves are relatively common causes of intrinsically stenotic aortic valves at birth but, like the congenital bicuspid valve, sometimes exhibit delayed obstruction owing to thickening and rigidity.

Congenital valvular aortic stenosis is much more common in males, with a sex ratio approximating 4 or 5:1. If the obstruction is present at birth, the murmur is likely to date from the newborn nursery. On the other hand, the functionally normal congenital bicuspid aortic valve usually goes undetected in infancy or childhood, but may subsequently generate the prominent murmur of aortic stenosis in the second, third, or fourth decade. Angina and effort syncope arouse suspicion of aortic stenosis in acyanotic young patients with a history of dyspnea, fatigue, and either a prominent cardiac murmur dating from infancy or a murmur appearing in the second, third, or fourth decades. Cerebral symptoms can be subtle, consisting of nothing more than mild giddiness or lightheadedness, especially with effort. On the other hand, recurrent syncope is dangerous and heralds sudden death even in childhood or adolescence. Inappropriate sweating sometimes occurs and increases with the advent of cardiac failure. Infective endocarditis is a serious complication of congenital valvular aortic stenosis; all varieties are susceptible. The pulse pressure is small, and there are a slow rate of rise, a sustained peak, and a gentle collapse when obstruction is severe.

Precordial palpation reveals a left ventricular impulse that varies from normal (mild stenosis) to the strong, sustained heaving movement of the hypertrophied left ventricle with severe obstruction. Presystolic distention of the left ventricle implies increased force of left atrial contraction, and is good evidence in young adults that the obstruction is significant. The thrill of aortic stenosis may be trivial or absent with mild obstruction or with severe obstruction and advanced heart failure. The typical aortic stenotic thrill radiates upward and to the right, is maximal in the second right interspace, and is readily detected in the suprasternal notch and over both carotids. In some patients the thrill is confined to the apex or, if the heart is small, to the lower left sternal edge where the atypical location can be misleading. In addition to the thrill, the sharp impact of an ejection sound can often be palpated at the apex in congenital valvular aortic stenosis.

An ejection sound is a characteristic although not invariable feature of congenital valvular aortic stenosis. The sound is caused by abrupt upward movement of the dome-shaped or truncated stenotic valve and implies good valve motion. In adults calcification may impair valve mobility so that the ejection sound diminishes or vanishes. The aortic stenotic murmur begins after the first sound (or with the ejection sound), rises in a crescendo to a systolic peak, and declines in a decrescendo to end before the aortic component of the second sound. The quality at the right base is harsh, rough, and grunting, especially when loud. Although configuration, length, and loudness do not necessarily relate to the degree of obstruction, the longer and louder the murmur and the later its systolic peak, the greater the likelihood of severe obstruction. However, an unimpressive midsystolic murmur—or none at all—may occur in severe aortic stenosis with advanced heart failure or in adults with increased anteroposterior chest dimensions. The right basal location and radiation of the murmur of valvular aortic stenosis are related to the upward and rightward direction of the high velocity jet within the ascending aorta. The second heart sound should be judged with regard to the intensity of the aortic component and the presence, degree, and type of splitting. In congenital valvular aortic stenosis with mobile valve, the aortic component of the second sound is well preserved even in the presence of significant obstruction. Prominent inspiratory splitting usually (but not invariably) means mild obstruction, because the duration of left ventricular ejection is not prolonged by that standard. *Paradoxical* splitting is a sign of severe obstruction and generally indicates that the duration of left ventricular ejection is appreciably prolonged. However, the majority of patients with aortic stenosis exhibit a second sound that is single or closely split through a wide range of severity.

A soft murmur of aortic regurgitation may be heard with congenital valvular aortic stenosis but is more common with discrete subvalvular aortic stenosis because of cusp distortion (see below). A fourth heart sound in aortic stenosis is the acoustic counterpart of presystolic distention of the left ventricle and is likely to mean appreciable obstruction. However, after age 40, the fourth heart sound is not a reliable sign of severity, because there is an age-related incidence.

Electrocardiographic estimates of severity should be made with caution, because mild valvular aortic stenosis occasionally occurs with left ventricular hypertrophy, and severe obstruction occasionally exists with a normal electrocardiogram. Occasionally sudden death occurs in patients with severe congenital aortic stenosis and normal electrocardiograms. Although these points must be kept in mind, they should not obscure the value of the scalar tracing. The best electrocardiographic index of appreciable obstruction is the combination of both voltage and repolarization criteria for left ventricular hypertrophy, especially in preadolescent patients. In congenital valvular aortic stenosis the x-ray features are poststenotic dilatation of the aorta with a relatively convex, globular left ventricular contour. In adults, aortic calcification is presumptive evidence of valvular obstruction and must be sought with the aid of an image intensifier.

Despite considerable clinical sophistication, cardiac catheterization and angiocardiography are generally required to be precise about the morphologic type and severity of congenital valvular aortic stenosis. If clinical evidence strongly points to mild obstruction, diagnostic intervention may be deferred, the risk of postoperative endocarditis far exceeding the risk and benefits of surgery. When clinical findings point to severe obstruction, diagnostic investigation should precede selection for surgery. If valvular obstruction is severe and the patient is *asymptomatic,* surgical intervention depends in large part on the morphologic type of obstruction. In relatively young patients with mobile congenital bicuspid aortic valves intrinsically stenotic at birth because of commissural fusion, direct repair provides excellent results at low risk. Severe valvular aortic stenosis in the *symptomatic* patient — especially with angina or syncope but without significant congestive heart failure — is appropriately selected for surgical intervention even if this means valve replacement. The more severe the left ventricular dysfunction, the smaller the gradient, the smaller the ejection fraction, the higher the surgical risk, and the poorer the results.

COARCTATION OF THE AORTA

The basic anatomic defect is a localized deformity of the media manifested by a curtain-like infolding that eccentrically narrows the aortic lumen. The zone of coarctation is characteristically located distal to the origin of the left subclavian artery at or just beyond the insertion of the ligamentum arteriosum. Occasionally coarctation is situated at or just proximal to the left subclavian artery so that the orifice of that vessel is in the low pressure zone.

Nearly 25 per cent of patients with coarctation of the aorta have bicuspid aortic valves which may be functionally normal or may take one of the courses described above. The most important noncardiac anomaly is an aneurysm of the circle of Willis which may remain clinically silent or may announce itself by rupture.

Aortic coarctation occurs predominantly in males. After early infancy, these patients are usually asymptomatic when the malformation is first diagnosed. Serious symptoms are relatively uncommon before age 15 years, but it is uncommon for symptoms to be absent beyond age 30. The majority of patients live to adult life, but only a minority reach age 40, and only 10 per cent live beyond age 50. The longest survival was recorded in 1828 by Reynaud in his account of coarctation in a 92-year-old man. Discovery of systemic hypertension provides the initial suspicion unless the brachial and femoral pulses are palpated. A number of minor symptoms such as headache, spontaneous epistaxes, and leg fatigue sometimes occur. The major symptoms are related to four complications: congestive heart failure, rupture of the aorta or dissecting aneurysm, infective endocarditis or endarteritis, and cerebral hemorrhage. The incidence of cardiac failure is highest in early infancy or after the third decade and can develop in adults previously devoid of symptoms related to the malformation. Rupture of the aorta or dissecting aneurysm occurs most frequently in the 20's and 30's. The rupture originates either in the proximal ascending aorta or in a postcoarctation aneurysm. Infective endocarditis or endarteritis occurs most commonly on the peculiarly susceptible bicuspid aortic valve; endarteritis at the site of coarctation occurs less frequently. Cerebral hemorrhage, the fourth major complication, is usually due to rupture of an aneurysm of the circle of Willis. In the pregnant female with coarctation, blood pressure fluctuations are similar in direction to those of uncomplicated pregnancy. The incidence of toxemia is lower in women with coarctation than in pregnant women with other forms of hypertension, intracranial hemorrhage is not more likely to occur, and cardiac failure seldom develops. However, pregnancy does increase the risk of rupture of the aorta, especially at the end of the third trimester. Furthermore, the bacteremia that accompanies labor and delivery can cause endocarditis or endarteritis.

The physique in coarctation is at times especially good, and an athletic appearance of the chest and shoulders contrasts with narrow hips and thin legs. Coarctation of the aorta can sometimes be suspected because of the characteristic physical appearance of *Turner's syndrome,* namely, a female with short stature, webbing of the neck, absent or scanty pubic and axillary hair, wide-set nipples, low hairline, small chin, and wide carrying angle of the arms.

Abnormal differences in upper and lower extremity arterial pulses are the clinical hallmarks of coarctation of the aorta. Diagnostic differences in arm and leg blood pressures should be based upon systolic and not diastolic levels. These pressure differences between arm and leg are exaggerated by exercise, which can therefore be a useful adjunct in confirming mild coarctation. The level of upper extremity blood pressure must be interpreted according to the patient's age. A blood pressure that is normal in an adult may be hypertensive in a child. As patients with coarctation grow older, the systolic pressure rises relatively more than the diastolic, so the pulse pressure increases. Such patients may exhibit conspicuous, forceful carotid and suprasternal pulsations resembling aortic regurgitation, which may coexist. In addition, the subclavian arteries can sometimes be seen pulsating below the clavicles. Collateral vessels are seldom obvious and must be specifically sought by having the patient stand and bend forward with the arms hanging at the sides. The examiner inspects the back, particularly around and between the scapulae, using a tangential light source to expose the subcutaneous collaterals in shadowed relief. The retinal arteries may be tortuous and narrowed, but hypertensive retinopathy is rare.

The right and left brachial arteries should also be simultaneously compared by palpation and blood pressure determination. An absent or relatively small left brachial pulse means that the coarctation is at or just proximal to the left subclavian artery. In aortic stenosis with coarctation, the brachial arterial pulse (and pressure) may be relatively normal rather than hypertensive, whereas the femoral pulses are diminished or absent. Conversely, aortic regurgitation increases the femoral pulse, especially in mild coarctation, so the clinical diagnosis of the combined defects may be overlooked.

Precordial palpation detects a left ventricular impulse that varies from normal to the sustained heaving impulse of ventricular hypertrophy. A dilated ascending aorta can cause a visible and palpable systolic impulse at the right base. Suprasternal thrills are relatively frequent in uncomplicated coarctation, but precordial thrills are seldom present without coexisting aortic stenosis.

An aortic ejection sound increases suspicion of coexisting bicuspid aortic valve, although such sounds may arise in the dilated aortic root. Coarctation of the aorta is associated with systolic, diastolic, or continuous murmurs. Systolic murmurs originate from arterial collaterals, the coarctation itself, and the bicuspid aortic valve. Collateral systolic murmurs are distributed widely over the thorax. There is a tendency for these murmurs to be especially conspicuous along the left sternal border (the left internal mammary artery). Collateral murmurs are crescendo-decrescendo in shape and delayed in onset because of origin in vessels distant from the heart. The coarctation itself is responsible for a localized midline posterior murmur, the level of which is related to the site of coarctation. With mild coarctation, the posterior systolic murmur is relatively short; as the degree of obstruction increases, the murmur gets longer and may extend well into diastole, becoming "continuous." The most common diastolic murmur is aortic regurgitation, a useful sign of coexisting bicuspid aortic valve.

Isolated *right* ventricular hypertrophy is for all practical purposes confined to infants in the first six months with heart failure and reactive pulmonary hypertension. In uncomplicated coarctation, left ventricular hypertrophy is manifested by both voltage and repolarization criteria. However, prominent S-T segment depressions with deeply inverted T waves seldom occur with uncomplicated coarctation and suggest coexisting aortic stenosis.

The x-ray provides considerable information regarding both the diagnosis and the anatomic variations of coarctation of the aorta. Notching of the ribs results from collateral flow through dilated, tortuous, pulsatile *posterior* intercostal arteries. The notches typically appear as irregular, scalloped areas on the undersurfaces of the posterior ribs. The *anterior* ribs are spared because the anterior intercostal arteries do not run in costal grooves. Notching seldom appears before six or seven years. When the coarctation is located *distal* to the left subclavian artery, collateral circulation fails to develop on the left side; *unilateral* notching appears in the *right* posterior ribs. In older children or adults, the lateral x-ray may show *retrosternal* notching caused by dilated tortuous internal mammary arteries. In classic coarctation of the aortic isthmus, the hypertensive ascending aorta is dilated. Aortic dilatation *distal* to the zone of coarctation (poststenotic enlargement) produces a recognizable leftward convexity of the descending thoracic aorta. When this sign is accompanied by the convex shadow of a dilated left subclavian artery, the two convexities form a typical "figure 3" in the frontal projection.

Cardiac catheterization and angiocardiography define the anatomic features of coarctation, including the collateral circulation, but as a rule they are not necessary for a secure clinical diagnosis upon which a therapeutic decision can be based. If there is clinical suspicion of coexisting bicuspid aortic valve, the inclination to perform thoracic aortography is increased, because the diagnosis gives insight into the postoperative natural course and the need for continued prophylaxis for infective endocarditis. The presence of all but mild coarctation warrants consideration for surgical correction. There is still a consensus that optimal age for correction awaits the seventh year. On the other hand, selection of patients for elective repair at earlier ages has progressed, because subsequent recurrence of coarctation has been shown to be negligible when correction is done in early childhood. In fact primary repair in small infants with persistent heart failure is now selectively and successfully accomplished. In older patients, risk of technical complications during surgical correction increases. Irrespective of the quality of the repair, the risk of infective endocarditis on a coexisting bicuspid aortic valve is not diminished, and we do not know whether the risk of intracranial hemorrhage (berry aneurysm) is affected. Although the incidence of heart failure continues to rise during the fourth decade in unoperated coarctation, after age 40 there appears to be an even chance of death from incidental causes. In those surviving to this age, the efficacy of correction becomes debatable. Furthermore, long-term analyses of patients after surgical correction of coarctation of the aorta have revealed a high incidence of premature cardiovascular disease despite adequate surgical repair. Particularly disturbing in this regard are the data on unexplained late postoperative hypertension.

PULMONIC STENOSIS

Congenital obstruction to right ventricular outflow can be valvular, subvalvular, or supravalvular. *Valvular* pulmonic stenosis, the most common variety, is characterized by a conical or dome-shaped valve with a narrow outlet at its apex. Three raphes extend from the small central opening to the wall of the pulmonary artery, although separate leaflets cannot be identified. Rarely, valvular pulmonic stenosis is caused by myxomatous dysplasia of the valve.

The functional consequences of valvular pulmonic stenosis are related to the resistance to right ventricular outflow. Males and females are equally affected. Early discovery of the murmur is the rule, because the anatomic and physiologic conditions necessary for its production are present at birth. Survival into adulthood is relatively common. The tendency for the valve to grow in proportion to body size may in part account for this. However, with advancing age fibrous thickening and even calcification may reduce valve mobility and increase the degree of obstruction.

Familial occurrence is not a feature of the history of ordinary valvular pulmonic stenosis, but a convincing family history may occur with valvular pulmonic stenosis caused by myxomatous dysplasia.

Subjective complaints tend to increase with age, although equivalent degrees of stenosis may handicap one patient in childhood and yet leave another relatively unlimited in the fourth decade. An appreciable number of patients with moderate to severe stenosis are virtually symptom free well into the postpediatric age group. Dyspnea and fatigue are the most common symptoms.

These complaints tend to remain absent as long as the right ventricle can maintain a normal stroke volume at rest and augment its output with effort. Right ventricular failure is the single most common natural cause of death. Patients with valvular pulmonic stenosis sometimes experience giddiness, lightheadedness, or frank syncope, especially with effort. Children as well as adults occasionally have chest pain resembling myocardial ischemia. Some patients with severe pulmonic stenosis may be subjectively aware of giant A waves in the jugular venous pulse, especially during effort or excitement. These patients are susceptible to infective endocarditis.

Infants with isolated typical valvular pulmonic stenosis may appear remarkably healthy, with good fat deposits and chubby round faces. Even older patients may have faces that are wide, full, or even bloated, with highly colored cheeks. Turner's syndrome with small stature, shield chest, and web neck is occasionally associated with valvular pulmonic stenosis. *Myxomatous dysplasia* causing valvular pulmonic stenosis may be associated with slow body growth and abnormal facies (triangular face with hypertelorism, ptosis of the eyelids, and low-set ears).

The jugular venous pulse exhibits an A wave that generally gets progressively larger as the degree of obstruction increases. Exercise and excitement augment these A waves. In addition, powerful right atrial contraction may be associated with presystolic pulsation of the liver. An increase in the height of the V wave occurs with the advent of right ventricular failure and tricuspid regurgitation.

Thrills mirror the location and intensity of accompanying murmurs (see below). In valvular pulmonic stenosis, the thrill is maximal in the second or occasionally third left interspace, radiating upward and toward the left, because the intrapulmonary jet is directed toward the left pulmonary artery. A right ventricular systolic impulse is an important physical sign of pulmonic stenosis and, when absent, the diagnosis should be in doubt. The location of the parasternal right ventricular impulse can sometimes be related to the level of obstruction, because the transmitted systolic movements originate in the high-pressure zone proximal to the stenosis. Presystolic distention of the right ventricle is caused by forceful contraction of the right atrium and is typically accompanied by a large jugular venous A wave.

An ejection sound is a characteristic feature of valvular pulmonic stenosis and serves an important function in identifying this form of obstruction. The pulmonic ejection sound is high pitched, sharp or clicking, and maximal in the second left interspace, often selectively decreasing during inspiration. An ejection sound is not present in valvular pulmonic stenosis caused by myxomatous dysplasia.

The systolic murmur of typical valvular pulmonic stenosis is maximal in the second left interspace, although it may be just as loud in the third. The lower location may be related to secondary subvalvular hypertrophy. The murmur, like the thrill, radiates upward and to the left, and when loud may be heard in the suprasternal notch and at the base of the neck, especially on the left. Loudness per se is not necessarily an index of severity, although as a rule intensity tends to vary directly with the degree of obstruction. However, the magnitude of obstruction is a major determinant of the *duration* of right ventricular ejection which, in turn, determines the *length* of the systolic murmur. A soft, symmetrical murmur, peaking late in systole and extending well beyond aortic closure, is a feature of severe obstruction.

The intensity of the pulmonic component of the second sound varies from normal to inaudible as severity increases. However, the *timing* of the pulmonic component is more important than intensity in assessing the degree of obstruction. A relatively slight increase in expiratory splitting, with normal intensity of the pulmonic component, is evidence of mild stenosis, whereas a marked increase in splitting with a faint or absent pulmonic component is evidence of severe obstruction.

The electrocardiogram commonly shows tall, peaked P waves. The QRS axis in the frontal plane shifts to the right, the degree of right axis deviation tending to vary directly with right ventricular pressure. The severity of pulmonic stenosis corresponds fairly well to the R/S ratios in V_1 and V_6 and to the height of the R wave in V_1. In mild pulmonic stenosis an rSr' pattern in V_1 is sometimes difficult to distinguish from normal. In severe pulmonic stenosis, leads V_1 and V_3R exhibit tall monophasic R waves, and lead V_6 shows an rS pattern. Between these extremes all gradations exist. In severe pulmonic stenosis, deeply inverted T waves that curve upward on the downstroke and that extend beyond V_2 are typical and assume greater significance when accompanied by ST segment depressions. Upright T waves occur with increased right ventricular pressure in young children, and upright T waves in the right precordium are the only electrocardiographic signs of right ventricular hypertension in some children with mild pulmonic stenosis.

The x-ray evaluation of valvular pulmonic stenosis should concentrate on (1) the peripheral (interpulmonary) vascular pattern, (2) the main pulmonary artery and its branches, and (3) the size and contour of the right ventricle and right atrium. The pulmonary vascular pattern is normal even in severe valvular stenosis until the output of the right ventricle falls. Poststenotic dilatation of the pulmonary trunk is characteristic and is often accompanied by conspicuous enlargement of the left branch. Poststenotic dilatation is not a feature of myxomatous dysplasia of the valve. Calcification of the congenitally stenosed pulmonary valve is rare, although examples have been reported. The left anterior oblique view is best for defining the contour of right ventricular enlargement even though a prominent right atrial sweep may be seen in the posteroanterior projection. A conspicuous increase in right heart size is almost always a sign of severity, especially at an early age. Cardiac catheterization and angiocardiography permit definitive diagnosis of the level, morphologic type, and severity of obstruction to right ventricular outflow. However, patients with typical trivial to mild valvular pulmonic stenosis can be identified with such clinical confidence that further diagnostic investigation is generally not required. But in this group, clinical distinction from idiopathic dilatation of the pulmonary trunk may be difficult or impossible.

In typical valvular pulmonic stenosis, surgical repair is probably indicated for all patients with resting gradients of 50 mm Hg or more, although a single determination may be misleading, because gradients vary considerably with cardiac output. The risk of operative repair in typical valvular pulmonic stenosis is low, and technical results are excellent. Postoperative pulmonary regurgitation often occurs, but as a rule it is mild and is a small price to pay. Occasionally, in very severe valvular pulmonic stenosis, secondary hypertrophic subpulmonic stenosis may require infundibular resection. This intervention is relatively uncommon, and its value is still debated; it should not be taken lightly, because right ventriculotomy is necessary.

ATRIAL SEPTAL DEFECT

Atrial defects are designated according to their sites in the septum: (1) in the region of the fossa ovalis (ostium secundum); (2) inferior to the fossa, i.e., between the fossa and the inferior vena cava; (3) in the upper part of the atrial septum (sinus venosus); (4) in the lower part of the septum (ostium primum); and (5) in the position normally occupied by the coronary sinus. The most common variety to be dealt with here is generally referred to as *ostium secundum defect.*

The physiologic consequences of an atrial septal defect depend chiefly upon the magnitude and duration of the shunt and upon the behavior of the pulmonary vascular bed. Two mechanisms have been proposed to explain the left to right shunt. First, in infancy the right and left ventricles have similar distensibility characteristics and hence should have similar end-diastolic volumes. As pulmonary vascular resistance falls in the neonatal period, the right ventricle ejects into a low resistance bed and would be expected to have a larger ejection fraction than the left. During the subsequent diastole the volume received by the right ventricle would increase, and a left to right shunt would therefore be established. Second, as the pulmonary arterioles involute, the relatively thick-walled neonatal right ventricle becomes thinner and offers less resistance to filling than the left. Conditions become appropriate for augmenting flow from left atrium across the defect. This may in part explain the relative infrequency of pulmonary hypertension in young people with atrial septal defect. Pulmonary hypertension is rare in infants and children with uncomplicated atrial septal defects and does not reach its peak incidence of about 14 per cent until early adult life.

In ostium secundum atrial septal defect the female-to-male ratio ranges from 2 to 3.5:1. Family history is important, because these defects not only can be familial, but also may recur through a number of generations.

Atrial septal defects often go unrecognized for years, because symptoms may be trivial or absent and physical signs subtle. The relatively soft pulmonic midsystolic murmur is easily overlooked in restless or crying children and may be mistaken for an innocent murmur in both children and young adults. In apparently healthy normal adults, atrial septal defect is often first suspected because of a routine chest x-ray. Life expectancy is shortened, although adult survival is the rule, and some may live to an advanced age. Survival is more limited in young adults who develop pulmonary hypertension, but even in them the span of life appears to average more than 40 years. It is not rare to find atrial septal defects in patients beyond age 70 years. Death may be unrelated to the defect; but when a relationship exists, cardiac failure is the most common natural cause. Since the natural history of uncomplicated ostium secundum atrial septal defect spans the childbearing age and since the majority of such patients are female, it is important to note that pregnancy is usually well tolerated. After the third or fourth decade, complications generally arise, and practically all patients who survive to the sixth decade are

symptomatic. Effort dyspnea and fatigue are most frequent. Older patients with large left to right shunt atrial septal defects may experience not only effort dyspnea but also orthopnea. In the presence of decreased lung compliance caused by longstanding large left to right shunts, the work of breathing is greater in the supine than in the sitting position.

Infective endocarditis is rare in isolated ostium secundum atrial septal defect, a rarity attributed to the absence of jet lesions or turbulence because of low velocity flow across the interatrial communication.

Older patients with ostium secundum atrial septal defects deteriorate chiefly on two accounts. First, degenerative diseases such as coronary artery disease or systemic hypertension cause the left ventricle to become less distensible, so a larger volume of left atrial blood preferentially flows across the defect, adding to the work of an already overloaded right ventricle. The second problem is the advent of atrial arrhythmias — fibrillation, flutter, or paroxysmal atrial tachycardia. After the fourth decade atrial arrhythmias increase in frequency and represent one of the most serious complications.

Physical appearance of adults with ostium secundum atrial septal defect is generally normal, but children often exhibit delicate, frail, or gracile builds, with weight affected more than height. A left precordial bulge is common and is often associated with Harrison's grooves. A distinctive appearance that heightens suspicion of an ostium secundum atrial septal defect is the *Holt-Oram syndrome.* The thumb is hypoplastic, with an accessory phalanx that gives it a "crooked" appearance. Apposition of the thumb with other digits is difficult, and in some cases the thumb is rudimentary or absent.

The jugular venous pulse in ostium secundum atrial septal defect may show A and V waves of equal heights, because the two atria are in communication. Pulmonary hypertension results in an increased force of right atrial contraction and a dominant A wave which may reach giant proportions.

Precordial movement and palpation characteristically detect a right ventricular impulse that is hyperdynamic and relatively brief in duration. This pattern occurs because the left to right shunt distends the right ventricle in diastole, and the chamber then contracts vigorously into a low resistance pulmonary bed. The dilated pulmonary trunk is often palpable in the second left interspace. A systolic thrill in the second left interspace indicates either a very large shunt or coexisting valvular pulmonic stenosis. In the presence of pulmonary hypertension, the right ventricular impulse becomes sustained and less dynamic, and presystolic distention may result from an increased force of right atrial contraction.

The "first heart sound" at the left sternal edge and apex may be split and the *second component* relatively loud. It has been variously proposed that the loud second component originates in the tricuspid valve or represents a pulmonic ejection sound. The location favors the former, although the two mechanisms may coexist. The typical murmur of atrial septal defect results from rapid ejection of a large right ventricular stroke volume into a dilated pulmonary trunk. The murmur is usually Grade 3 or less, maximal in the second left intercostal space, beginning after the first heart sound, crescendo-decrescendo in shape, peaking in early or midsystole, and ending well before both components of the second heart sound. The septal defect itself is, with rare exception, acoustically silent. A murmur exceeding Grade 3 is likely to mean an unusually large shunt or associated valvular pulmonic stenosis. In slightly built patients, widely distributed thoracic systolic murmurs can sometimes be heard in the right chest, axilla, and back because of rapid flow through peripheral pulmonary arteries in low resistance, high-flow atrial septal defects.

A hallmark of atrial septal defect is the behavior of the second heart sound. The aortic and pulmonic components are widely and persistently split and exhibit little or no change in the degree of splitting with respiration or Valsalva's maneuver. The relative loudness of the two components is usually normal, although at times the second component is increased despite little or no pulmonary hypertension. Proximity of the dilated pulmonary trunk to the chest wall and the brisk elastic recoil of the distended pulmonary trunk may account for this.

Two types of diastolic murmurs occur in atrial septal defect with left to right shunt. One is mid-diastolic and is caused by torrential flow across the tricuspid valve, indicating a sizable left to right shunt. The second diastolic murmur is rare and is due to pulmonary regurgitation in the absence of pulmonary hypertension; a very large pulmonary trunk is probably responsible.

Atrial septal defect with pulmonary hypertension exhibits auscultatory signs that differ considerably from the foregoing. The pulmonic midsystolic flow murmur is replaced by a softer, shorter midsystolic murmur caused by ejection of a normal stroke volume into a dilated pulmonary trunk. Tricuspid flow murmurs vanish. Typical pulmonic ejection sounds appear, especially in the second left interspace, and exhibit characteristic respiratory variation in intensity. The pulmonic component of the second heart sound becomes progressively louder, although fixed splitting persists as long as a significant left to right shunt exists. With abolition or reversal of the shunt, the pulmonic component becomes very loud, and the wide fixed split disappears. A *Graham Steell murmur* may develop. The holosystolic murmur of tricuspid regurgitation appears when the pressure load of pulmonary hypertension results in right ventricular failure. Since the right ventricle occupies the apex in atrial septal defect, the tricuspid murmur is heard at that site and mistaken for the murmur of mitral regurgitation.

After the third decade *atrial arrhythmias* increase, with atrial fibrillation the most common, but atrial flutter and paroxysmal atrial tachycardia also occur. When right atrial P waves are present, they generally manifest themselves by peaking in lead II rather than by an increase in amplitude. The QRS duration is usually upper limits of normal with a tendency to increase with age. As QRS duration increases, the pattern resembles complete right bundle branch block, but this rarely develops before the fourth decade. Depolarization is typically clockwise, with q waves in inferior leads and a vertical QRS axis. These electrical directions are important, because they distinguish ostium secundum defects from ostium primum defects in which the axis is directed upward and to the left and depolarization is counterclockwise (see below).

An electrocardiographic sign of atrial septal defect is the rSr' complex in right precordial leads. This feature is believed to stem from localized hypertrophy of the crista supraventricularis, depolarization of which causes the terminal electrical forces to be directed superiorly, to the right, and anteriorly. These terminal force patterns do not result from interference of electrical impulses

through the right bundle branch. In fact, the sequence of ventricular activation is normal, so the term "incomplete right bundle branch block" is inappropriate. With the advent of pulmonary hypertension, the right ventricular free wall thickens and lead V_1 exhibits an increase in the amplitude of the R' wave together with a gradual decrease in the depth of the S wave.

The *chest x-ray*, especially in postadolescents and adults, is often distinctive. The lung fields show increased pulmonary arterial vascularity that generally extends to the periphery. The combination of a small aorta and a markedly dilated pulmonary trunk with disproportionate enlargement of the right branch can be striking. With the advent of pulmonary hypertension, peripheral pulmonary vascularity is replaced by relatively clear lung fields, the pulmonary trunk and its proximal branches get still larger, and the right branch presents as a huge inverted comma with an abrupt cutoff that makes the contrast between the large central vessels and the clear lung field stand out in bold relief. In an occasional older subject, the main pulmonary artery and its branches dilate aneurysmally and calcify.

Right atrial enlargement is ordinarily seen as a rightward convexity in the posteroanterior projection. Although radiographic signs of left atrial enlargement are occasionally found in adults, this is rarely so in children. Dilatation of the right ventricle is an expected feature, resulting in a convex lifted apex that usually forms an acute angle with the diaphragm. Dilatation of the outflow tract sometimes causes relatively smooth continuity or even a hump-shaped appearance below the enlarged pulmonary trunk. In the left oblique projection the right ventricle casts a rather typical convex anterior shadow.

Although uncomplicated ostium secundum atrial septal defect in the young is among the most easily diagnosed congenital malformations of the heart, the same anomaly may be most misleading in some adults. Mitral stenosis with pulmonary hypertension comes under suspicion because of dyspnea, orthopnea, atrial fibrillation, an increased V wave in the jugular venous pulse, a right ventricular impulse, a loud first heart sound, a delayed pulmonic component of the second sound that is mistaken for an opening snap, a tricuspid flow murmur mistaken for a mitral diastolic murmur, vascular peripheral lung fields believed to represent pulmonary venous congestion, and a cardiac silhouette that exhibits dilatation of the pulmonary trunk and occasionally of both right and left atria. Similarly, mitral regurgitation may be suspected because the holosystolic murmur of tricuspid regurgitation is heard at the apex which is occupied by the right ventricle. A delayed pulmonic component of the second sound followed by a tricuspid flow murmur may be mistaken for the opening snap and the mid-diastolic murmur of coexisting mitral stenosis. In older subjects, coronary artery disease, systemic hypertension, atrial arrhythmias, or inverted left precordial T waves may cloud the issue. A catalogue of these misleading clinical points makes impressive reading, but it is rare to be confronted with all of them at once. However, even when the entire clinical picture is considered, the correct diagnosis may remain uncertain, although clues generally emerge to provide the background for an intelligently planned laboratory study.

Echocardiography has been a major step forward in the noninvasive diagnosis of atrial septal defect, defining not only the expected large right ventricular dimensions but, more important, the paradoxical motion of the interventricular septum. Normally, the interventricular septum moves *away* from the anterior chest wall during systole, behaving as part of the left ventricle. In ostium secundum atrial septal defect (volume overload of the right ventricle), the septum moves *toward* the anterior chest wall in systole, functioning as part of the right ventricle.

Cardiac catheterization is generally employed even in patients in whom the clinical diagnosis is not in doubt. Such an intervention provides precise preoperative quantitative data that set the stage for comparative postoperative assessment. In addition to quantification of the shunt and confirmation of intracardiac pressures, there are a number of other reasons why cardiac catheterization is undertaken. An attempt should be made to separate ostium secundum from sinus venosus atrial septal defects which clinically are usually indistinguishable. Patients with pure ostium secundum atrial septal defects sometimes exhibit mitral leaflet prolapse—especially posterior—analogous to the systolic click—late systolic murmur syndrome. This movement can be detected by left ventricular angiography or echocardiography and need not be accompanied by auscultatory signs. Theoretically, such patients are at risk of infective endocarditis whether the atrial septal defect is repaired or not.

Patients with high flow, low resistance uncomplicated ostium secundum atrial septal defect (pulmonary to systemic flow ratios of at least 2:1) should be electively repaired, optimally in childhood. At this age, surgical risk is minimal, and delay always gives rise to concern over postoperative residua, especially resolution of dilatation and hypertrophy of the right ventricle. There has been some debate regarding surgical correction in older patients (beyond age 40), but current experience has shown that patients in the fifth, sixth, or even seventh decades with relatively low resistance–high flow ostium secundum atrial septal defects benefit from surgical repair which can be undertaken at comparatively low risk. What is still more encouraging is that older patients benefit at an acceptable risk despite the presence of moderate pulmonary hypertension and cardiac failure, provided there is still a sizable left to right shunt. In an occasional patient, irrespective of age, in whom pulmonary resistance has reached or exceeded systemic so that the left to right shunt has been abolished, operative repair is contraindicated.

PATENT DUCTUS ARTERIOSUS

Patent ductus arteriosus represents persistence of the normal fetal vascular channel between the pulmonary artery and the aorta. The pulmonary orifice of the ductus is located immediately to the left of the bifurcation of the pulmonary trunk. The aortic end of the duct usually arises just beyond the origin of the left subclavian artery. A patent ductus is apt to be largest at its aortic insertion, exhibiting the shape of a truncated cone, because the tendency to close begins at the pulmonary arterial end. The ductus arteriosus in full-term infants normally undergoes an initial stage of *functional* closure, followed by a later stage of *anatomic* closure. At the end of a week the ductus is generally no more than probe patent, and by four to eight weeks anatomic closure is usually established.

The physiologic consequences of persistent patency of the ductus arteriosus depend upon the size of the communication and the level of pulmonary vascular resistance. When the ductus is small, the pulmonary arterial pressure remains normal; the left to right shunt and hemodynamic burden are insignificant despite continuous aortic to pulmonary flow across the ductus. When the duct is large, aortic pressure is transmitted directly into the pulmonary trunk, so pulmonary hypertension exists with pressure overload of the right ventricle. Under these circumstances the direction of flow through the ductus depends upon the relative resistances in the pulmonary and systemic beds. If the pulmonary resistance is appreciably lower than systemic, a sizable left to right shunt exists, with volume overload of the left heart together with pressure overload of the right. If the pulmonary resistance is appreciably higher than systemic, left to right flow through the ductus is abolished, leaving a pure right to left shunt and pure pressure overload of the right ventricle. The vast majority of patients with isolated patent ductus arteriosus, literally 95 per cent, have left to right shunts with pulmonary arterial pressures considerably below systemic. Only 5 to 7 per cent have very high pulmonary vascular resistances with exclusive right to left shunts.

For all practical purposes the history in patent ductus arteriosus does not begin at birth, because the diagnosis is not entertained in the newborn nursery. The mother is likely to report that her infant was examined as a newborn and pronounced normal. As the neonatal pulmonary vascular resistance falls, a left to right shunt is established, the ductus murmur emerges, and the diagnosis becomes apparent. Patent ductus arteriosus predominates in females, with a sex ratio as high as 3:1. The female preponderance is even greater in older patients with this anomaly. Family history is important, because patent ductus tends to recur in siblings. The prenatal history also deserves comment, especially regarding maternal rubella in the first trimester. Patent ductus arteriosus (together with pulmonary artery stenosis) is the most common congenital cardiac defect in the offspring of mothers who have had rubella in the first trimester. Birth weight in uncomplicated patent ductus is normal but in the rubella syndrome low birth rate is common, and there is failure to thrive even though the shunt is small and cardiac failure absent. Another interesting point in the history is the *altitude* at which the patient is born. It has been estimated that persistence of the ductus arteriosus is six times as frequent in patients born at high altitudes as in those born at sea level, and there is a tendency for such patients to develop pulmonary hypertension. The physical appearance in patent ductus may be one of underdevelopment, owing to a large shunt, cardiac failure, and recurrent respiratory infections. In addition, maternal rubella results not only in patent ductus and low birth weights, but also in poor growth irrespective of the size of the duct. Differential cyanosis and clubbing occur when pulmonary vascular resistance exceeds systemic so that unoxygenated pulmonary arterial blood flows through the ductus and enters the aorta distal to the left subclavian artery; this unoxygenated blood goes to the lower body so that the toes will be cyanosed and often clubbed.

A wide pulse pressure is an important physical sign of patent ductus with large left to right shunt. Diastolic flow from aortic root into pulmonary artery lowers the aortic diastolic pressure, whereas the large left ventricular stroke volume caused by the left to right shunt results in elevation of aortic systolic pressure.

Precordial impulses are normal with small patent ductus. A moderately large ductus causes isolated volume overload of the left heart; the left ventricular impulse is moderately dynamic, the right ventricular impulse is unimpressive, and a continuous thrill with systolic accentuation is present in the first or second left intercostal space. A large ductus with appreciable left to right shunt results in marked volume overload of the left ventricle with pulmonary hypertension; the left ventricular impulse is hyperdynamic, and a heaving right ventricular impulse appears. If a thrill is present, it is more likely to be systolic. When flow through the ductus is reversed, pulmonary hypertension exists without volume overload of the left ventricle. Palpation detects a right ventricular and pulmonary arterial impulse, a loud pulmonic component of the second sound, but the ductus thrill is absent and a left ventricular impulse is trivial or absent.

Auscultation is virtually diagnostic when the classic murmur of uncomplicated patent ductus arteriosus rises to a peak in latter systole, continues without interruption through the second sound, and then declines in intensity during the course of diastole. High velocity flow through a small duct results in a relatively soft high-frequency continuous murmur. The larger ductus is likely to cause a loud, noisy "machinery" murmur, accentuated in latter systole and punctuated with "eddy" sounds. The ductus murmur is typically loudest in the first or second intercostal space or just beneath the left clavicle. With progressive elevations in pulmonary vascular resistance, the classic murmur is shortened, always beginning with the diastolic portion, and is finally abolished, to be replaced by auscultatory and phonocardiographic signs of pulmonary hypertension per se. Such patients present with a pulmonic ejection sound, a short pulmonic midsystolic murmur, a single or closely split second heart sound, and a loud pulmonic component of the second sound followed by the Graham Steell murmur of pulmonary regurgitation. Under these circumstances the diagnosis of patent ductus arteriosus cannot be made on auscultatory grounds. Differential cyanosis may be the key.

The electrocardiogram can be entirely normal when the ductus is small. Variations from normal depend upon the degree and duration of volume overload of the left heart and pressure overload of the right.

In the x-ray, the ductus can sometimes be seen in the frontal projection as a separate convexity between the aortic knuckle and the pulmonary trunk. In older patients calcium is occasionally identified in the ductus; this should be sought in the frontal, left oblique, and lateral projections. A large left to right shunt *without* appreciable pulmonary hypertension results in varying degrees of pulmonary plethora while the pulmonary trunk and its branches increase in size. The ascending aorta is normal in infants but tends to enlarge in older children or adults. Volume overload of the left heart results in left ventricular dilatation and left atrial enlargement. The increase in left atrial size is usually mild to moderate but can occasionally be marked. Right atrial and right ventricular dilatation develop when pulmonary arterial pressure is elevated in patent ductus with left to right shunt. In infants and young children, a sizable patent ductus arteriosus with left to right shunt and pulmonary hypertension is often associated with congestive heart failure and appreciable cardiomegaly; all four chambers contribute to the cardiac silhouette.

When flow through the ductus is reversed (suprasystemic pulmonary vascular resistance), a different radiologic picture emerges. The left ventricle and the left atrium are normal in size, and the right ventricle is hypertrophied but not conspicuously dilated. The pulmonary trunk and its main branches enlarge, but the ascending aorta tends to be normal, and the peripheral pulmonary vasculature is normal or reduced.

The typical patient with uncomplicated patent ductus in childhood, adolescence, or early adult life can be confidently diagnosed clinically and does not, as a rule, require cardiac catheterization for preoperative confirmation. However, the sick infant with congestive heart failure and large left to right shunt should be investigated preoperatively, not only to confirm the clinical suspicion of patent ductus but also to determine the presence or absence of coexisting anomalies, especially ventricular septal defect. Also requiring diagnostic investigation are those patients (generally postadolescent) with increased pulmonary vascular resistance, in whom the degree of left to right shunt must be firmly established before division of the ductus is recommended.

For all practical purposes typical patent ductus presenting in childhood is uniformly corrected by surgical division. A number of variations in therapeutic judgment are required, however. Since persistent patency of the ductus with *delayed* spontaneous closure is frequent in premature infants, there is a tendency to delay surgery in such patients because of the prospect of spontaneous closure within several months. On the other hand, large patent ductus is a relatively common cause of congestive heart failure in acyanotic infants, and generally requires operative intervention which may take the form of ligation rather than division. After the first year of life most patients with patent ductus are asymptomatic. Division of the ductus in such patients not only carries a low risk but also results in complete anatomic and physiologic correction. The tendency to wait until the child is at least five years old has been modified in most centers so that the disorder in younger children is now corrected. The adult poses a more complex problem. The simplest decisions in the adult group are in patients — generally women — with large left to right shunt, relatively low resistance patent ductus in which the duct is not calcified. These should be surgically divided once the diagnosis is established. Calcification of the patent ductus increases the risk, but, if the shunt is large, operation is still advisable. When pulmonary resistance has exceeded systemic, abolishing the left to right shunt, patients are inoperable. A difficult decision occurs in the occasional adult with a very small patent ductus that is hemodynamically insignificant. The question is a comparison of the risk of infective endocarditis as opposed to the risk of surgery. Each case requires individual judgment. If there has been a previous episode of infective endocarditis and the patient expresses concern regarding recurrence, surgical correction should be advised. If there has been no previous episode of infective endocarditis and the patient is reluctant to undergo thoracotomy, operation should be deferred.

VENTRICULAR SEPTAL DEFECT WITH PULMONIC STENOSIS
(Fallot's Tetralogy)

This combination encompasses a wide anatomic, physiologic, and clinical spectrum. Two elements of the tetralogy are of prime importance, namely, pulmonic stenosis and large ventricular septal defect with right ventricular pressure at systemic levels. Large ventricular septal defect with mild to moderate pulmonic stenosis is looked upon as *acyanotic* Fallot's tetralogy; large ventricular septal defect with severe pulmonic stenosis and right to left shunt as *classic cyanotic Fallot's tetralogy;* and large ventricular septal defect with complete pulmonic stenosis as *Fallot's tetralogy with pulmonary atresia.* It is wise to remain flexible, however, and use appropriate *anatomic* designations instead of, or coupled with, the eponym, to serve the cause of clarity.

In classic cyanotic Fallot's tetralogy, a *large* ventricular septal defect approximates the size of the aortic orifice. The aorta may be entirely left ventricular in origin, or biventricular to varying degrees, but the aortic wall maintains anatomic continuity with the anterior mitral leaflet. Pulmonic stenosis can be located in the pulmonary trunk, pulmonary valve, infundibulum, or subinfundibular zone, although typically the obstruction is infundibular. Pulmonary atresia can be viewed as the ultimate expression of pulmonic stenosis and therefore the most severe form of Fallot's tetralogy. With pulmonary atresia, the pulmonary circulation is supplied chiefly by large bronchial collateral arteries.

The degree of obstruction to right ventricular outflow does not always remain constant but may progress with the passage of time. When life expectancy is prolonged by an anastomotic operation, the patient may develop progressive narrowing of the zone of stenosis until complete closure (atresia). Furthermore, infundibular stenosis can progress sufficiently to reverse the interventricular shunt. Accordingly, a single patient may exhibit a broad spectrum of severity ranging from mild stenosis with large left to right shunt to marked obstruction with reversed shunt.

A number of *additional congenital cardiac malformations* have a tendency to occur in patients with Fallot's tetralogy: (1) right aortic arch, (2) persistent left superior vena cava, (3) hypoplasia, stenosis, or absence of a pulmonary artery, (4) absence of the pulmonary valve, (5) incompetence of the aortic valve, and (6) a coronary arterial anomaly consisting of right coronary arterial origin of the left anterior descending coronary artery.

The *physiologic consequences* depend upon three variables, namely, the degree of pulmonic stenosis, the size of the interventricular communication, and, to a lesser extent, the systemic vascular resistance. These variables can best be understood by beginning with the idea of a large ventricular septal defect upon which increasing degrees of pulmonic stenosis are imposed. When the stenosis is mild, the shunt is entirely left to right, and the condition closely resembles large isolated ventricular septal defect with increased pulmonary blood flow and volume overload of the left heart. As the degree of obstruction increases, the left to right shunt diminishes. When the resistance offered by the obstruction equals systemic resistance, the shunt is balanced. As the stenosis increases still further, a right to left shunt is established, because it becomes easier for the right ventricle to eject into the aorta than into the pulmonary trunk. Since right ventricular blood under these circumstances preferentially enters the aorta, blood flow through the lungs is reduced and the left heart underfilled. When the stenosis is complete (pulmonary atresia), the entire right ventricular output is ejected through the ventricular septal defect into the aorta. No matter how severe the pulmonic stenosis, the right ventricle decompresses into the aorta via the large ventricular septal defect, so right ventricular systolic pressure does not exceed systemic. The magnitude of right ventricular systolic overload is then determined by *aortic* pressure.

The *history in typical Fallot's tetralogy* generally dates from the neonatal period because of detection of a murmur or cyanosis. Arterial unsaturation is usually obvious by three to six months. When an infant is born with very severe pulmonic stenosis or atresia, cyanosis dates from birth, and the murmur is relatively inconspicuous. A history of *squatting for relief of dyspnea* has long been a hallmark of Fallot's tetralogy. In addition, Taussig clearly described the preference for certain other postures, such as the knee-chest position, sitting with the legs drawn underneath, or lying down. A history of right ventricular failure is rare in classic Fallot's tetralogy. The neonatal right ventricle is well equipped to pump at systemic pressures, and is seldom called upon to do more, because the ventricular septal defect permits direct decompression into the aorta. A number of other complications may occur in the natural history, such as recurrent cerebral hypoxia that can lead to brain damage and mental retardation, cerebral venous sinus thromboses, cerebral embolism, or brain abscess. Death from brain abscess is twice as frequent in cyanotic Fallot's tetralogy as in any other form of congenital cardiac disease. Infective endocarditis sometimes occurs on the zone of pulmonic stenosis. There are two chief determinants of long survival: a moderate degree of pulmonic stenosis that permits adequate but not excessive pulmonary blood flow with little or no cyanosis, and pulmonary stenosis that evolves gradually enough to permit the formation of a well developed collateral circulation.

After age four, most cyanotic children with congenital heart disease have Fallot's tetralogy. This malformation is also present in the largest number of *cyanotic adults* with congenital heart disease.

The physical appearance of the majority of patients with either classic cyanotic Fallot's tetralogy or pulmonary atresia reflects small size and physical underdevelopment. When Fallot's tetralogy occurs with little or no cyanosis, the physical appearance is generally normal.

Knowledge of the brachial arterial systolic pressure allows an accurate bedside estimate of the gradient in cyanotic Fallot's tetralogy. Since right ventricular systolic pressure is the same as systemic, the gradient across the zone of stenosis is simply the difference between the brachial arterial systolic pressure and the estimated pulmonary arterial systolic pressure (15 to 25 mm Hg).

The jugular venous pulse in classic cyanotic Fallot's tetralogy is seldom elevated, and the A wave is normal or nearly so, because the right ventricle maintains its neonatal capability of ejecting at systemic pressures without extra help from its atrium.

Precordial movement and palpation in classic Fallot's tetralogy detect a right ventricular systolic impulse that is quiet and usually located inferior to the third left intercostal space because of the stenosed infundibulum. The right ventricle ejects at systemic pressures without an appreciable increase in the vigor of contraction and without dilating. In cyanotic Fallot's tetralogy, especially in the presence of pulmonary atresia, a right aortic arch is relatively frequent, and its pulsation can be detected at the right sternoclavicular junction.

The auscultatory signs mirror the pathologic physiology of cyanotic Fallot's tetralogy. The incidence of aortic ejection sounds varies inversely with the degree of obstruction; the more hypoplastic the pulmonary trunk, the larger the aortic root. The systolic murmur in cyanotic Fallot's tetralogy originates at the zone of stenosis and not across the ventricular septal defect. The murmur tends to be maximal in the third left interspace, because obstruction is usually infundibular. The length and loudness of the murmur (and accompanying thrill) are of considerable importance in estimating the severity of obstruction. A loud, long murmur extending up to the aortic component of the second sound means that an appreciable amount of blood is being ejected into the pulmonary trunk. As resistance at the zone of stenosis rises, there is an increase in the right to left shunt and a reciprocal fall in pulmonary blood flow; the murmur gets shorter and softer. When obstruction is complete (pulmonary atresia), the pulmonic stenotic murmur vanishes altogether and is replaced by a soft midsystolic murmur caused by ejection into the dilated aorta. A continuous murmur is an auscultatory sign of pulmonary atresia because of flow through bronchial collateral circulation. The pulmonic component of the second heart sound is typically inaudible in cyanotic Fallot's tetralogy and pulmonary atresia, but when cyanosis is mild or absent a soft delayed sound can sometimes be detected. When a large ventricular septal defect is associated with mild pulmonic stenosis, the auscultatory signs resemble those of uncomplicated ventricular septal defect, although the murmur tends to have midsystolic accentuation (a combination of the ventricular septal defect and pulmonic stenotic murmurs) and there is likely to be moderately wide splitting of the second heart sound.

The *electrocardiogram* is another useful index of the physiologic spectrum encompassed by ventricular septal defect with pulmonic stenosis. Since the force of right atrial contraction is not appreciably increased, P waves of right atrial enlargement are absent about half the time. The mean QRS axis in the frontal plane is rarely to the right of 150 degrees so that right axis deviation takes the form of a dominant S wave in lead I but dominant R waves in leads II and III. In the precordial leads, a tall monophasic R wave is usually confined to lead V_1 with rS complexes in the remaining chest leads. In the left precordial leads, q waves are conspicuous by their absence in classic cyanotic Fallot's tetralogy, because the left ventricle is underfilled. When the shunt is balanced, right ventricular pressure remains at systemic levels, so the electrocardiogram continues to exhibit right ventricular hypertrophy as described. However, the left heart is no longer underfilled, so left precordial leads exhibit well developed R waves and small q waves. When a large ventricular septal defect appears with mild pulmonic stenosis, the electrocardiogram resembles that of isolated ventricular septal defect with right ventricular hypertension.

The *x-ray* in ventricular septal defect with pulmonic stenosis shows vascular markings that are normal or increased when a large defect exists with a balanced or left to right shunt. More severe obstruction to right ventricular outflow diverts more right ventricular blood into the aorta, so that pulmonary blood flow falls and lung vascularity diminishes. In adults, these oligemic lungs may have an emphysematous appearance. In cyanotic Fallot's tetralogy the pulmonary artery segment is characteristically represented by a *concavity*. The aortic arch size varies inversely with the pulmonary trunk. In pulmonary atresia the aorta receives the entire output from both ventricles, so the rightward sweep and knuckle are especially prominent. A right aortic arch occurs in 20 to 30 per cent of patients with cyanotic Fallot's tetralogy, the incidence increasing with the severity of pulmonic stenosis, so that a right arch is most frequent with pulmonary atresia. In typical cyanotic Fallot's tetralogy the left atrium and left ventricle are normal or small because the left heart is underfilled; the right atrium and right ventricle cope with systemic pressures without dilating, so the cardiac size is normal or nearly so. In pulmonary atresia, however, the cardiac silhouette tends to be larger, especially in older subjects. The configuration of the heart has long been a subject of interest in cyanotic Fallot's tetralogy because of the distinctive boot-shaped appearance caused by a combination of concentric hypertrophy of the right ventricle, an abnormally small left ventricle, a relatively horizontal ventricular septum, and a concave pulmonary artery segment. In Fallot's tetralogy with little or no cyanosis (balanced or bidirectional shunt), the right ventricle remains concentrically hypertrophied, but the left ventricle is not underfilled. The cardiac apex is more likely to be smooth and rounded. When a large ventricular septal defect exists with mild pulmonic stenosis, the x-ray in many ways resembles that of large isolated ventricular septal defect except that the size of the pulmonary trunk may be comparatively small.

The *echocardiogram* serves a useful purpose in identifying continuity between posterior aortic wall and the anterior mitral leaflet, confirming Fallot's tetralogy rather than right ventricular origin of both great arteries. Cardiac catheterization and angiocardiography are important in characterizing the morphology of the right ventricular outflow tract, in identifying the location of the ventricular septal defect, and in ruling out right ventricular origin of both great arteries. Intracardiac repair is technically a lesser problem in the patient with large ventricular septal defect, left ventricular aorta, and acquired pulmonic stenosis, even if the stenosis is severe enough to have reversed the shunt.

Large ventricular septal defect with biventricular aorta and hypoplastic right ventricular outflow tract is far more difficult to repair (classic cyanotic Fallot's tetralogy). Primary intracardiac repair (total correction) is the treatment of choice and can be accomplished even in infancy. Nevertheless, shunt operations (Waterston or Blalock) are appropriately applied in cyanotic symptomatic infants, especially those less than one year old. A previous shunt operation does not materially add to the risk of complete repair. After age five and certainly after age eight, complete repair should be employed, with few exceptions. Similarly, total correction can be undertaken in adults without anticipation of significantly greater operative mortality. Postoperative "complete right bundle branch" is expected after right ventriculotomy. The long-term effects of a patch for relief of outflow obstruction are still to be assessed.

553. UNCOMMON CONGENITAL CARDIAC DEFECTS IN WHICH POSTPEDIATRIC SURVIVAL IS EXPECTED

Situs Inversus. The term "situs inversus" refers to an organ arrangement the reverse of normal (mirror image dextrocardia). Situs inversus is often accidentally discovered on a routine chest x-ray or physical examination, because the malposition is likely to occur with an otherwise normal heart. Such patients experience normal longevity and hence fall into age groups that are susceptible to acquired cardiac disease. Pain of myocardial infarction may be referred to the *right* chest and pain of acute appendicitis to the *left* lower quadrant. Palpation and percussion identify the cardiac apex and stomach on the right and the liver on the left; the left ventricular impulse forms the apex. The heart sounds are louder in the right chest, and splitting of the second sound is detected in the second right intercostal space. The electrocardiogram shows negative P, QRS, and T waves in lead I; the complexes in lead aVR and aVL are the reverse of normal, and right precordial leads resemble those normally recorded from the left chest. The x-rays are the exact mirror image of normal, so that the reader must identify the symbols on the film that designate left and right. The aortic arch and stomach bubble are on the right, together with the cardiac apex.

Dextroversion of the Heart. This term applies when thoracic and abdominal viscera are in normal position but the cardiac *apex* is on the *right* (right thoracic heart). In early fetal life the cardiac apex begins on the side opposite to that which it ultimately occupies. When the apex remains on the right while the aortic arch, left atrium, and stomach are in their normal left-sided positions, the term "dextroversion" is used. Dextroversion of the heart is likely to be detected because of other congenital cardiac anomalies which almost invariably coexist. The most common of these are congenitally corrected transposition of the great arteries (see below), pulmonic stenosis, and ventricular or atrial septal defect. Palpation and percussion identify the cardiac apex and liver on the right with the stomach on the left (normal abdominal situs with right thoracic heart). Heart sounds and murmurs are louder on the right. The electrocardiogram shows upright P waves in lead I, because the atrial situs is normal. Prominent R waves or RS complexes are recorded from the right chest, whereas the left chest leads exhibit small septal q waves and small r waves. The x-ray shows the aortic arch and stomach bubble on the left but the apex on the right; the heart retains its peculiar silhouette whether or not the film is reversed.

Congenital Complete Heart Block. This is a straightforward diagnosis by electrocardiogram. The AV block is likely to be congenital if the slow heart rate existed from infancy (or in utero) and if the QRS configuration exhibits a "supraventricular configuration," i.e., a normal sequence of ventricular excitation. If liberal use were made of the electrocardiogram in infants and children with inappropriately slow heart rates, few cases of congenital heart block would be missed. The conduction defect is generally discovered accidentally in otherwise healthy asymptomatic children, or an alert obstetrician may detect a slow fetal heart rate. The arterial pulse is inappropriately slow for age, the upstroke brisk, the pulse pressure wide, and the rhythm regular. The jugular venous pulse shows intermittent "cannon waves" (right atrial contraction against a closed tricuspid valve), with independent A waves occurring at rates faster than the carotid pulse. The left ventricular impulse is dynamic (large stroke volume). The first heart sound varies in intensity from booming to soft, and there are short midsystolic basal flow murmurs, soft intermittent

fourth heart sounds, and intermittent summation sounds. The x-ray may show mild cardiac enlargement related to increased diastolic filling (slow heart rate). The slow rate, regular rhythm, intermittent cannon waves, and variation in intensity in the first heart sound are a diagnostic combination.

Congenitally Corrected Transposition of the Great Arteries. In this anomaly there is a right to left interchange of the ventricles and their respective AV valves. Right atrial blood flows across an AV valve that is morphologically mitral into a venous ventricle that is morphologically left, and then into the pulmonary trunk. Left atrial blood flows across an AV valve that is morphologically tricuspid into an arterial ventricle that is morphologically right, and then into the aorta. Since the pulmonary trunk springs from an anatomic left ventricle and the aorta from an anatomic right ventricle, the term "transposition of the great arteries" is appropriate. Since right atrial blood finds its way into the pulmonary trunk (across a mitral valve and through an anatomic left ventricle) and since left atrial blood finds its way into the aorta (across an anatomic tricuspid valve and through an anatomic right ventricle), the "transposition" can be considered "congenitally corrected." Hemodynamic consequences of congenitally corrected transposition depend chiefly upon the presence of *associated defects,* the most common of which are (1) incompetence of the left AV valve which is tricuspid and deformed by Ebstein's anomaly (see below), (2) ventricular septal defect, and (3) disturbances in AV conduction. Theoretically, *uncomplicated* congenitally corrected transposition (a rarity) should cause little or no physiologic disturbance. However, even when the malformation is uncomplicated, "spontaneous" failure of the systemic ventricle tends to occur before the fourth decade, although a few patients live longer. The unanswered question is the durability of an anatomic right ventricle as a systemic pump, i.e., whether a right ventricle subjected to systemic work loads will fail for that reason alone.

Idiopathic Dilatation of the Pulmonary Trunk. The malformation is characterized by congenital dilatation of the main pulmonary artery and occasionally its branches in the absence of anatomic or physiologic cause. Patients are asymptomatic, and physical appearance, arterial pulse, and jugular venous pulse are entirely normal. Palpation of the precordium may detect a pulmonary arterial impulse but no right ventricular impulse. Auscultation detects a characteristic pulmonic ejection sound that introduces a soft, short pulmonic midsystolic murmur and generally normal splitting of the second heart sound. The electrocardiogram is normal. The chest x-ray is also normal except for a conspicuous convexity caused by the dilated pulmonary trunk.

Congenital   Discrete   Subvalvular   Aortic   Stenosis. Discrete subvalvular aortic stenosis is usually characterized by a circumferential fibrous collar that encircles the left ventricular outflow tract and attaches to both the ventricular septum and the anterior mitral leaflet. The fibrous collar is located so close to the aortic leaflets that they may be mildly incompetent. The arterial pulse is similar to that of valvular aortic stenosis. The systolic thrill is maximal in the first or second right interspace with radiation into the neck. The left ventricular impulse is sustained, and presystolic distention with an accompanying fourth heart sound may be present. *An aortic ejection sound is typically absent.* The midsystolic stenotic *murmur* is rough and noisy, and its location and radiation correspond to the thrill. The sound of aortic valve closure is normal or reduced; a soft early diastolic murmur of aortic regurgitation is relatively common. The electrocardiogram is indistinguishable from other forms of discrete aortic stenosis. In the x-ray, the ascending aorta is usually normal, although slight to moderate dilatation may occur.

Precise characterization of the level and degree of obstruction requires cardiac catheterization and angiocardiography. Echocardiography sometimes detects relatively normal systolic opening of at least two leaflets. Discrete subvalvular aortic stenosis is amenable to direct surgical repair, although it should be remembered that the aortic leaflets are often distorted and that care must be taken not to damage the anterior mitral leaflet to which the subvalvular fibrous collar is attached.

Supravalvular Aortic Stenosis. This malformation is characterized by a segmental hourglass-shaped narrowing immediately above the aortic sinuses. Occasionally there is tubular hypoplasia of the ascending aorta. Associated mental retardation is presumptive evidence that the aortic stenosis is supravalvular. Under these circumstances stenosis of the pulmonary artery and its branches almost always coexists. Physical appearance is sometimes sufficiently typical to permit these diagnoses to be entertained at a glance: small chin, large mouth, malformed teeth, abnormal bite, and retarded growth. The brachial and carotid arterial pulses are sometimes asymmetrical, with the pulse pressure and rate of rise conspicuously greater on the right. The left ventricular impulse is similar to other forms of discrete aortic stenosis. An aortic ejection sound is typically absent, and the midsystolic stenotic murmur tends to be more conspicuous in the first right intercostal space with disproportionate radiation to the right neck. The aortic component of the second sound is normal or soft, and the murmur of aortic regurgitation is rare. The electrocardiogram is similar to those of valvular or discrete subvalvular aortic stenosis. The x-rays are distinguished by one chief feature—not only is poststenotic dilatation of the aorta absent but the ascending aorta is usually undersized. Precise diagnosis of morphology and severity requires cardiac catheterization and angiocardiography. Surgical repair, although possible, is difficult and at times untenable, especially with tubular hypoplasia of the ascending aorta.

Subvalvular Pulmonic Stenosis. The location can be either infundibular or, rarely, subinfundibular. Discrete infundibular stenosis generally results from localized narrowing of the entrance to the outflow tract, beyond which the infundibulum may be somewhat dilated. Subinfundibular stenosis, a rare variety of right ventricular outflow obstruction, may be caused by hypertrophy of either abnormal muscle groups or normal bulbar muscle. Subvalvular pulmonic stenosis is uncommon as an isolated anomaly and is generally associated with ventricular septal defect. Isolated infundibular pulmonic stenosis can be suspected if the right ventricular impulse does not reach the third left interspace, if the murmur and thrill are maximal in the fourth interspace, if an ejection sound is absent, and if the x-ray shows a nondilated pulmonary trunk, a right aortic arch, and a local indentation at the site of the ostium or the infundibulum. Cardiac catheterization and angiocardiography delineate the level of obstruction, its morphologic type, and the degree of severity. It must be borne in mind that surgical correction requires right ventriculotomy, so operative risk is greater than with valvular pulmonic stenosis.

Supravalvular Pulmonic Stenosis (Stenosis of the Pulmonary Artery and Its Branches). This defect results from narrowing of the pulmonary trunk, its bifurcation, or its primary or peripheral branches; it may be unilateral or bilateral, single or multiple. Stenosis of the pulmonary artery and its branches causes hypertension in the proximal pulmonary trunk, whereas the converse is true with valvular or subvalvular obstruction. Isolated stenosis of the pulmonary artery and its branches exhibits the following features: murmurs, sometimes discovered in early life but sometimes inconspicuous or even absent in infants and young children; an occasional history of maternal rubella with low birth weight, physical and mental underdevelopment, cataracts, and deafness; familial occurrence; occasional hemoptysis from rupture of thin-walled poststenotic aneurysms; or the distinctive appearance associated with supravalvular aortic stenosis (see above). Auscultatory signs include absence of an ejection sound, normal intensity and splitting of the second heart sound, and left basal midsystolic murmurs with peripheral murmurs of nearly equal intensity in the axillae and back. X-rays show little or no dilatation of the pulmonary trunk but may reveal clusters of poststenotic dilatations of intrapulmonary vessels. Cardiac catheterization and angiocardiography establish the severity and define the anatomic pattern and distribution. Stenosis of the pulmonary artery and its branches is not currently amenable to surgical repair except in the occasional patient with isolated obstruction confined to a discrete zone within the pulmonary trunk.

Congenital Pulmonary Valve Regurgitation. Healthy, asymptomatic individuals may be found to have cardiac murmurs and dilatation of the pulmonary trunk on routine chest x-rays. When congenital pulmonary regurgitation accompanies *idiopathic dilatation of the pulmonary trunk,* the clinical features are those of idiopathic dilatation (see above) plus the characteristic diastolic murmur described below. Regurgitation caused by *structural abnormalities of the valve itself* results in the following picture. Palpation detects a right ventricular impulse that becomes progressively more dynamic as the degree of incompetence increases. Systolic expansion of the pulmonary trunk may impart an additional impulse in the second left intercostal space. Auscultation reveals a characteristic diastolic murmur maximal in the second or third left interspace, medium to low in frequency, crescendo-decrescendo in shape, delayed in onset, short in duration, and louder during inspiration. A midsystolic pulmonic flow murmur may be heard; the second sound can be normal or widely split and the pulmonic component soft or inaudible. The electrocardiogram is generally normal or exhibits volume overload of the right ventricle with an rSr' pattern in lead V_1. The x-ray shows moderate dilatation of the pulmonary trunk and occasionally of the right ventricle.

Ebstein's Anomaly of the Tricuspid Valve. Displaced, fused, malformed portions of tricuspid valvular tissue project into the right ventricular cavity. The portion of the right ventricle underlying the adherent tricuspid valvular tissue is thin and functions as a receiving chamber analogous to the right atrium ("atrialized right ventricle"). Abnormal function of the right heart is related to three derangements: the malformed tricuspid valve, the "atrialized" portion of right ventricle, and the reduced capacity of the pumping portion of the right ventricle. Ineffective emptying of the right atrium may result in an appreciable increase in right atrial volume and a right to left shunt through a foramen ovale or an atrial septal defect, although most are acyanotic. Tricuspid regurgitation caused by the malformed leaflets adds to the hemodynamic burden. However, Ebstein's anomaly is compatible with a relatively long and active life, because there is a considerable range of severity. The majority of patients survive into the second, third, or fourth decade, but fewer than 5 per cent live beyond age 50.

Ebstein's anomaly can generally be diagnosed clinically. Bouts of paroxysmal rapid heart action—especially in cyanotic subjects—raise the index of suspicion. A key to the clinical recognition of Ebstein's malformation with right to left shunt is the combination of cyanosis with normal or diminished pulmonary blood flow and a functionally dominant left ventricle (see Table 1). A right ventricular impulse is conspicuously lacking, although the infundibulum may be palpable. A large jugular venous V wave is lacking despite tricuspid regurgitation because of the large size of the right atrium. The murmur of tricuspid regurgitation is either absent or early systolic, because tricuspid regurgitation occurs with normal or low right ventricular systolic pressure. The murmur is usually rough, scratchy, and of medium frequency, tending to be maximal over the region of the displaced tricuspid valve, i.e., further toward the cardiac apex. Third and fourth heart sounds commonly cause triple or quadruple rhythms. Short mid-diastolic or presystolic murmurs occur, especially when the P-R interval is prolonged, which is often the case. Type B Wolff-Parkinson-White electrocardiograms are noteworthy, and, in the context of cyanotic congenital heart disease, are likely to mean Ebstein's anomaly. The electrocardiogram otherwise shows prominent right atrial P waves and generally right bundle branch block but no right ventricular hypertrophy. The chest x-ray may have a relatively characteristic appearance with normal or clear lung fields, small vascular pedicle, and a globular cardiac silhouette caused by rightward convexity of the enlarged right atrium and leftward convexity of the infundibulum.

Congenital Pulmonary Arteriovenous Fistula. This defect is believed to be caused by abnormal development of pulmonary arteries and veins from a common vascular complex. The fistula consists of either one or more relatively large vascular trunks or of a thin aneurysmal sac or a tangle of distended tortuous vascular channels. The arterial supply is derived from one or more abnormal branches of the pulmonary artery. Drainage is almost always through anatomically recognizable dilated pulmonary veins. Such connections are truly *pulmonary* arteriovenous. The physiologic consequences depend chiefly on the amount of unoxygenated blood delivered through the right to left shunt. As a rule the shunt is large enough to result in cyanosis but small enough to cause no significant hemodynamic burden. These fistulas are usually discovered in healthy young adults who are found to have abnormal densities in routine chest x-rays or who exhibit cyanosis or hereditary hemorrhagic telangiectasia. Dyspnea and fatigue are mild even in the presence of conspicuous cyanosis. Intermittent hemoptysis may punctuate the history. Recurrent bleeding also occurs from nose, mouth, or lips from the telangiectasia, and members of the family may have similar complaints.

Cerebral symptoms include dizziness, vertigo, paresthesias, faintness, visual aberrations, speech disturbances, headache, extremity weakness, mental confusion, and convulsions, although the mechanisms are unclear. Physical appearance is characterized by cyanosis and clubbing, together with small ruby patches (telangiectasia) on the face, tongue, lips, skin and nail beds, and nasal or oral mucous membranes. Thoracic auscultation may detect delayed systolic murmurs or occasionally continuous murmurs with systolic accentuation, usually located over the lower lobes or the right middle lobe. The murmurs are generally less than Grade 3 and may get louder with inspiration or Müller's maneuver and softer with expiration or Valsalva's maneuver. The lung fields show densities that may be single or multiple, unilateral or bilateral, and small or large; they are typically located in the lower lobes or right middle lobe. The opacities are homogeneous, rounded or lobulated, fairly well demarcated, and attached to the hilus by bandlike shadows that represent dilated vessels entering and leaving the fistula. The size of a mass tends to decrease with Valsalva's maneuver and increase with Müller's maneuver. In simple terms, pulmonary arteriovenous fistula is a cause of cyanosis with normal ventricles (see Table 1). The combination of cyanosis and telangiectasia with normal electrocardiogram and normal cardiac silhouette is distinctive in its own right, and conclusive when the fistulas cause shadows in the films.

Lutembacher's Syndrome. This syndrome generally consists of a congenital atrial septal defect upon which acquired mitral stenosis is superimposed. A large atrial septal defect has an ameliorating effect upon mitral stenosis, which in turn aggravates the hemodynamic effects of the interatrial communication. Left atrial pressure is relatively low, and symptoms of pulmonary venous congestion are attenuated. Atrial fibrillation is relatively common, and the systemic arterial pulse may be small owing to a decrease in left ventricular stroke volume. The jugular venous pulse may exhibit a prominent A wave in the absence of pulmonary hypertension, because the left atrial pressure is transmitted into the right atrium. The right ventricular impulse tends to be especially dynamic. Auscultation does not readily detect the telltale signs of mitral stenosis which as a rule are incomplete or absent altogether. The pulmonary flow murmur is prominent, because a large right ventricular stroke volume is ejected into a dilated pulmonary trunk. The electrocardiogram shows P waves of combined atrial enlargement, although left atrial P waves need not occur; evidence of right ventricular hypertrophy is common. The x-ray exhibits pulmonary plethora without pulmonary venous congestion; the right atrium and right ventricle are conspicuously dilated, and the pulmonary trunk may reach a remarkable size. Lutembacher's syndrome is more common in females, because this sex predilection exists for both isolated atrial septal defect and isolated mitral stenosis.

Common Atrium. This relatively rare variety of interatrial communication is the result of complete or virtual absence of the atrial septum. The right-sided portion of the common chamber has anatomic features of a *right* atrium and receives both venae cavae and the coronary sinus. The left-sided portion has anatomic features of a left atrium and receives the pulmonary veins. Absence of the septum means that the septum primum is deficient so that elements of the endocardial cushion malformation coexist, especially a cleft anterior mitral leaflet with or without mitral regurgitation. Appearance of the Ellis–van Creveld syndrome heightens suspicion. The clinical picture resembles large atrial septal defect, with the following exceptions: (1) symtpoms begin earlier and are generally more severe; (2) cyanosis exists without sufficient pulmonary hypertension to account for its presence; (3) the physical signs are those of atrial septal defect in which a large left to right shunt persists despite the presence of cyanosis (cyanosis with shunt vascularity; see Table 1); (4) the P wave axis tends to shift leftward, because there is absence of the upper or sinus venosus portion of the atrial septum with absence of a left sinus node), and the QRS shows left axis deviation resembling endocardial cushion defect; and (5) the chest x-ray resembles a large atrial septal defect in which pulmonary arterial blood flow is increased even though cyanosis is present.

Congenital Coronary Arteriovenous Fistula. Here both coronary arteries arise from the aorta, but a fistulous branch of one communicates directly with a cardiac chamber or the pulmonary trunk. The right coronary artery is more frequently involved than the left. However, the *drainage* site is of greater clinical importance than the vessel of origin. Ninety per cent of coronary arterial fistulas drain into the right heart (arteriovenous). Most of these enter the right atrium, coronary sinus, or right ventricle, whereas relatively few enter the pulmonary trunk. Congenital coronary arteriovenous fistula should be considered when an asymptomatic acyanotic child or young adult is found to have an atypically located precordial continuous murmur that is relatively soft and "superficial"; the suspicion is heightened when the murmur does not peak around the second heart sound but instead is louder in either systole or diastole. The precordial location is determined by the chamber or vessel that receives the fistula and not by the vessel of origin. In young patients with small fistulas, an "atypical" continuous murmur is likely to be the only clinical abnormality. Larger flows acting over longer periods of time can result in the following pictures. When the fistula enters the *right atrium* or *coronary sinus,* precordial palpation detects both left and right ventricular impulses; the continuous murmur tends to be louder in systole and maximal along the right sternal border, over the lower sternum, or close to the lower left sternal edge; volume overload of both ventricles may be seen in the electrocardiograms; the x-ray shows increased pulmonary arterial flow. When the communication drains into the body of the *right ventricle,* palpation detects right and left ventricular impulses; the continuous murmur is louder in either systole or diastole and is maximal along the mid- to lower left sternal border or subxiphoid area; volume overload of both ventricles may be seen in the electrocardiogram; the x-rays exhibit increased pulmonary arterial flow. When the pulmonary artery receives the fistula, palpation detects only a left ventricular impulse; the continuous murmur is usually indistinguishable from patent ductus arteriosus in both configuration and location; volume overload of the left ventricle may appear in the electrocardiogram; the x-ray may show increased pulmonary arterial flow.

Congenital Aneurysms of the Sinuses of Valsalva. Sinuses of Valsalva are three small dilatations in the wall of the aorta immediately above the attachments of each aortic cusp. More than 90 per cent of congenital aneurysms originate in the right or noncoronary sinus and project into the right ventricle or right atrium. The typical aneurysm begins as a blind pouch or diverticulum; the entire sinus is not dilated, but instead the aneurysm projects as a finger-like or nipple-like extension with a perforation at its tip. Acute rupture of a large aneurysm creates a dramatic clinical picture; a previously healthy young adult, generally male, develops sudden chest pain, dyspnea and a loud continuous murmur, bounding arterial pulse, and relentless cardiac failure that follows a period of temporary improvement. The arterial pulse resembles that of aortic regurgitation, the jugular venous pulse is elevated, and dynamic biventricular impulses are palpable. The continuous murmur is maximal below the third intercostal space along the right or left sternal border or over the lower sternum. The murmur is usually louder in either systole or diastole and does not peak around the second heart sound as in patent ductus. The electrocardiogram is likely to show biatrial P waves and left ventricular or combined ventricular hypertrophy. The chest x-ray indicates increased pulmonary arterial flow which may be obscured by pulmonary venous congestion, dilatation of both ventricles, and enlargement of the right and occasionally the left atrium. Small perforations sometimes progress slowly and at first go unnoticed. Such patients come to attention because continuous murmurs are detected. Occasionally, unruptured aneurysms are discovered because of accompanying to-and-fro or diastolic murmurs, or because of heart block or myocardial ischemia resulting from coronary arterial compression by the aneurysm.

Cardiac catheterization and angiocardiography are usually definitive. Such studies must be undertaken, because ruptured congenital aneurysms of the sinuses of Valsalva are amenable to complete correction by relatively simple intracardiac repair.

Vena Caval to Left Atrial Connection. Isolated drainage of a vena cava into the left atrium is a rare anomaly, but its presence can be suspected with a high degree of accuracy. The malformation is a form of cyanotic congenital heart disease without right ventricular hypertrophy (see Table 1). Cyanosis dates from early life, but cardiac symptoms are absent or nearly so. A right ventricular impulse is absent, whereas the left ventricle is normal or slightly thrusting. There are no significant murmurs. The electrocardiogram is usually normal but occasionally exhibits left ventricular hypertrophy. The x-ray reveals a normal cardiac silhouette, normal or diminished pulmonary blood flow, and perhaps the shadow of a persistent left superior vena cava.

554. COMMON CONGENITAL CARDIAC DEFECTS IN WHICH POSTPEDIATRIC SURVIVAL IS EXCEPTIONAL

Ventricular Septal Defect. The most common variety of ventricular septal defect lies below and posterior to the crista supraventricularis in the region of the membranous septum. Variations in size of ventricular septal defects deserve special comment. The normal growth of the heart is most rapid in the first two years of life, during which the ventricular septal defect remains about the same in size or enlarges less rapidly than the rest of the heart. Accordingly there is a tendency for the *relative* size of the defect to diminish. This tendency occasionally results in complete spontaneous closure. Ventricular septal defects are seldom seen after the fourth decade, not because patients have succumbed but probably because their communications have spontaneously closed or diminished to the point that they are clinically unrecognizable. The physiologic consequences of isolated ventricular septal defect depend chiefly on the size of the defect and the pulmonary vascular resistance. Both variables may change with time, and the physiologic and clinical manifestations vary accordingly. A small defect causes little or no functional disturbance, because the shunt is negligible and the pressures in the right heart are normal. With moderately large defects, the left to right shunt increases and, up to a point, occurs with little or no elevation in pulmonary arterial pressure. In such patients the physiologic derangements are essentially due to volume overload of the left heart. A large defect (equal to or greater than aortic orifice size) results in equalization of systolic pressures in the two ventricles. The amount of flow into the pulmonary and systemic beds then depends on their relative vascular resistances. Three regulatory mechanisms affect the volume and direction of the interventricular shunt and the level of pulmonary arterial pressure in infants born with large ventricular septal defects: first, the pattern taken by the pulmonary vascular resistance; second, the relative decrease in size that the defect undergoes, especially in the first two years of life; and third, the development of obstruction to right ventricular outflow, i.e., acquired infundibular pulmonic stenosis.

A *small ventricular septal defect* is ordinarily suspected because of a prominent holosystolic parasternal murmur in a patient in whom cardiac evaluation is otherwise normal. The murmur is generally absent at birth but is readily detected at the first well-baby examination. With passage of time, if the size of the defect decreases, the holosystolic murmur becomes softer, shorter, and higher pitched and is usually early systolic prior to complete closure. Similarly, *very small defects* are associated with soft, localized high frequency early systolic murmurs. *Large ventricular septal defects* with appreciable left to right shunts cause congestive heart failure in infancy, with retarded growth and development, recurrent lower respiratory infections, diaphoresis, and malaise. Physical examination reveals an elevated jugular venous pressure, hyperdynamic biventricular impulses, a harsh holosystolic left parasternal murmur accompanied by a thrill, an apical mid-diastolic flow murmur, and normal or wide splitting of the second heart sound with a relatively prominent pulmonic component. The electrocardiogram exhibits biatrial and biventricular hypertrophy with volume overload of the left ventricle. The x-ray shows pulmonary plethora, a large pulmonary trunk, a normal ascending aorta, dilatation of both ventricles, and often dilatation of the left and right atria as well. Spontaneous improvement is related to a reduction in left to right shunt caused by a decrease in the size of the defect, especially in the first year, by an increase in pulmonary vascular resistance, or by acquired infundibular pulmonic stenosis.

In *large ventricular septal defect with reversed shunt (Eisenmenger's complex)*, cyanosis ordinarily dates from childhood, although not from birth. Effort dyspnea occurs without left ventricular failure. The jugular venous pulse is usually normal and the precordium quiet, with moderate right ventricular and pulmonary arterial impulses. There are auscultatory signs of pulmonary hypertension but *no murmur of ventricular septal defect*. The electrocardiogram shows right ventricular hypertrophy with little or no evidence of volume overload of the left heart. The x-ray exhibits normal or decreased pulmonary vasculature, a relatively normal cardiac silhouette, moderate dilatation of the pulmonary trunk, and normal aortic arch (see Table 1).

In patients with typical small ventricular septal defects, the clinical diagnosis is so evident and the physiologic consequences are so benign that cardiac catheterization and angiocardiography are not necessary, and such patients should be followed expectantly. They are, however, at risk of infective endocarditis. Patients with *large* ventricular septal defects, especially those with clinical evidence of pulmonary hypertension, should be investigated to determine the presence and degree of the left to right shunt, the pulmonary arterial pressure and vascular resistance, and the angiographic location of the defect or defects.

Large ventricular septal defect with congestive heart failure in infancy is a special problem that will not be dealt with here. Beyond infancy, patients with ventricular septal defects and pulmonary to systemic flow ratios in excess of 1.5 to 1.7:1 should have elective correction. If the pulmonary to systemic flow ratio is less than 1.5:1 because the defect is small, the benign functional consequences do not warrant the risk of operative repair. If a similar flow ratio is the result of *high pulmonary resistance* with *large* ventricular septal defect, operative risk is high and results are poor, because little or no beneficial effect on the pulmonary resistance follows elimination of such a small shunt.

Ventricular Septal Defect with Aortic Regurgitation. Here the murmur of the ventricular defect is usually known from infancy. Between the ages of three and eight years a *new* murmur appears, together with the gradual development of bounding arterial pulses and a dynamic left ventricular impulse. The combined murmurs are *not* continuous but are holosystolic and early diastolic. The electrocardiogram and x-ray may show left ventricular hypertrophy and enlargement out of proportion to what would be expected on the basis of the estimated size of the left to right shunt. As time goes on, the ventricular septal defect may decrease in size and the aortic regurgitation will progressively worsen. Survival to adult life occurs, although cardiac failure eventually develops because of progression of the regurgitation.

Endocardial Cushion Defect. The endocardial cushions of the embryo contribute to the development of the mitral and tricuspid valves and to the growth and convergence of the atrial and ventricular septa. Defects therefore include varying combinations of anomalies in these four contiguous parts of the heart. Three general categories are recognized, namely, complete endocardial cushion defect, partial or incomplete endocardial cushion defect, and transitional forms. In the complete variety, separate atrioventricular valves do not exist as such. There is a common AV valve in a canal formed by an atrial septal defect above and a ventricular septal defect below. The partial or incomplete form is represented by an ostium primum atrial septal defect and a cleft mitral valve. Transitional forms represent intermediates between complete and partial or incomplete endocardial cushion defects. Less commonly, any one of the four component lesions occurs as an isolated anomaly. The physiologic consequences depend upon the presence and degree of the various combinations of the four anatomic components. The following remarks will relate to partial endocardial cushion defects in which postpediatric survival is possible.

An ostium primum atrial septal defect with cleft mitral valve occurs more frequently in females than males. The physical signs resemble those of ostium secundum atrial septal defect except that the left ventricle occupies the apex and is accompanied by the holosystolic murmur of mitral regurgitation. Congestive heart failure may begin in childhood, especially when marked mitral regurgitation exists with a large left to right shunt. Growth and development are poor and lower respiratory infections frequent. If mitral regurgitation is relatively mild and the left to right shunt moderate, symptoms may be delayed for one or two decades. The incompetent left atrioventricular valve is susceptible to infective endocarditis, and mongolism occurs, but not so frequently as with complete endocardial cushion defects. The electrocardiogram is important, because the frontal plane consists of counterclockwise depolarization with left axis deviation, with precordial leads that show the rSr' pattern of expected volume overload of the right ventricle. In persistent ostium primum with cleft but competent mitral valve, this electrocardiogram is the only distinguishing clinical feature from ostium secundum defect.

The most important laboratory study in identifying endocardial cushion defect is a left ventricular angiocardiogram in the frontal projection which shows a characteristic "goose neck" deformity of the outflow tract caused by the cleft anterior mitral cusp and its abnormal chordal arrangements. Surgical repair in partial endocardial cushion defect is limited chiefly by the degree of mitral regurgitation rather than the presence of the atrial septal defect.

Tricuspid Atresia.   In this disorder tricuspid valvular tissue cannot be identified. A small imperforate dimple is found on the floor of the right atrium, but no direct pathway exists between right atrium and right ventricle. The only outlet for the right atrium is an interatrial communication which can take the form of a fossa ovale or an atrial septal defect. Variations beyond the mitral valve form the basis of Edwards' anatomic classification from which physiologic inferences can be drawn and clinical expressions of tricuspid atresia understood. According to this classification, tricuspid atresia occurs either with or without transposition of the great arteries and, in each category, with no pulmonic stenosis, with pulmonic stenosis, or with pulmonary atresia. Pulmonary blood flow is the key determinant of longevity. Longevity is greatest when pulmonic stenosis of just the right degree exists so that blood flow to the lungs is favorably regulated. When the great vessels are normally related, the subpulmonic obstruction is generally marked, and most patients die in the first year. Nevertheless, occasional examples of survival have been recorded from the second through the fifth decade, with one exceptional survival to age 57. When the great vessels are *transposed,* coexisting pulmonic stenosis is more likely to permit longer survival. In isolated cases in this category patients have lived into the second, third, and fourth decades, and one died at age 56. The key to the clinical diagnosis of tricuspid atresia is the presence of cyanosis, normal or diminished pulmonary blood flow, and a dominant left ventricle (see Table 1). The electrocardiogram shows right atrial P waves with left axis deviation and adult progression of the QRS in the precordial leads. Definitive diagnosis is achieved by angiocardiography. Palliative surgery is possible through (1) creation of an atrial septal defect in those patients with a foramen ovale, or (2) a shunt operation to improve pulmonary blood flow. More recently, blood from the right atrium has been directed through a conduit to the pulmonary arteries, permitting the right atrium to act as a pumping chamber for the pulmonary circulation.

Complete Transposition of the Great Arteries.   According to Elliott and Edwards: "In complete transposition, there are two ventricles. . . . The aorta, with the coronary arteries arising from it, takes origin from the right ventricle, while the pulmonary trunk takes origin exclusively from the left ventricle. Both atrioventricular valves are patent and have the corresponding structure of the right and left sided atrioventricular valves of the normal heart. The connections of the systemic, pulmonary and coronary veins are normal." Survival in complete transposition requires the presence of some means of blood exchange between the pulmonary and systemic circulations which exist in parallel rather than in series, as in hearts with nontransposed great arteries. Connections between the greater and lesser circulations may take the form of interatrial communication, ventricular septal defect, or patent ductus arteriosus. The pathologic physiology of complete transposition of the great arteries depends largely upon three variables: the types of communications that join the pulmonary and systemic circulations, the resistance to flow through the pulmonary bed, and the pressure gradients between the communications that join the greater and lesser circulations. As a general rule, complete transposition of the great arteries is characterized as a congenital cardiac anomaly that exists with cyanosis and increased pulmonary blood flow (see Table 1). Life expectancy is best when the anomaly exists with large ventricular septal defect *and* pulmonic stenosis sufficient to exert a favorable regulation of pulmonary blood flow, so that flow is adequate to prevent serious hypoxia but not great enough to cause left ventricular failure. Even so, the large majority of patients with complete transposition of great arteries die within the first year, often within the first months. Isolated examples of unusual longevity have been recorded into the second, third, or fourth decade; one patient aged 56 years at autopsy was believed to have complete transposition. Definitive diagnosis is by angiocardiography. Two physiologic corrective operations are currently applied. The Mustard operation redirects venous inflows, whereas the Rastelli operation achieves redirection of ventricular outflows.

555. UNCOMMON CONGENITAL CARDIAC DEFECTS IN WHICH POSTPEDIATRIC SURVIVAL IS EXCEPTIONAL

Anomalous origin of the left coronary artery from the pulmonary trunk is characterized by normal origin of the right coronary artery from the aorta and anomalous origin of the left coronary artery (LCA) from the pulmonary trunk. The aberrant left coronary artery is relatively small and thin walled, resembling a venous channel, whereas the right coronary artery is dilated and tortuous, especially in patients who reach adult life. Myocardial ischemia is a serious problem. The ischemic derangement is not due to the fact that only *one* coronary artery originates from the aorta, but is due to direct flow from the right coronary artery to the LCA through intercoronary anastomoses which bypass the capillary bed. Thus the anomalous left coronary artery flows retrograde into the pulmonary artery but does not receive blood from it.

In the natural history of this anomaly, three general patterns emerge: serious symptoms in early infancy with death before one year; early illness followed by improvement so that by childhood symptoms may be absent or nearly so; and absence or virtual absence of early symptoms with survival into adulthood. About 15 or 20 per cent of individuals with anomalous origin of the LCA reach adulthood, but relatively few survive through the fourth decade, although one of the first known patients with this anomaly was a 50-year-old woman. The intercoronary anastomoses often result in a continuous murmur, and the myocardial ischemia results in papillary muscle dysfunction with mitral regurgitation. The electrocardiogram is important, because at a relatively early age deep Q waves appear in leads I and aVL. Definitive diagnosis is by cardiac catheterization and angiocardiography. A left to right shunt from right coronary through intercoronary anastomoses to anomalous LCA into the pulmonary trunk is identified. Selective coronary arteriography (injection into the right coronary) traces this pathway and provides specific anatomic diagnosis. Two surgical interventions have been applied. In infancy, ligation of the anomalous left coronary artery interrupts retrograde flow and improves capillary circulation. In older children or adults, the left subclavian artery or the internal mammary artery or a saphenous vein graft can be directly anastomosed to the left coronary artery, which is then ligated at its origin from the pulmonary artery.

Cor triatriatum is characterized by drainage of the pulmonary veins into an accessory left atrial chamber that lies proximal to the true left atrium. The distal compartment communicates with the mitral valve and contains the left atrial appendage and the fossa ovalis. The fibrous or fibromuscular diaphragm that partitions the left atrium contains one or more openings, the size of which determines the degree of left atrial obstruction. Cor triatriatum is therefore a congenital anomaly that is acyanotic without a shunt, with the malformation originating in the left heart (see Table 1). Severe cor triatriatum is ordinarily detected in infants or young children, but symptoms may not begin until adolescence or adulthood. Patients with mild obstruction may be entirely asymptomatic. The functional consequences are analogous to those of mitral stenosis with elevated pulmonary venous and pulmonary arterial pressures. However, the auscultatory signs of mitral stenosis are lacking, and enlargement of the left atrial appendage is absent, because that structure is in the distal low pressure compartment. It is wise to consider cor triatriatum in postadolescents with clinical signs of obstruction to left atrial flow but without signs of mitral stenosis. The diagnosis is materially assisted by echocardiography that detects normal movements of anterior and posterior mitral leaflets, and by angiocardiography which, with pulmonary arterial injection of contrast material, defines the zone of obstruction as dye opacifies the left heart. Surgical intervention can completely remove the partition and relieve the left atrial obstruction.

Total anomalous pulmonary venous connection (TAPVC) applies to a condition in which all venous blood from both lungs enters the right atrium directly or through one of its tributary veins. The four anomalously connecting pulmonary veins emerge individually from the lungs and either enter the right atrium directly or, more often, unite in the mediastinum to form a confluence which joins the right atrium via (1) the coronary sinus; (2) an anomalous vertical vein or left superior vena cava that connects the left innominate vein to the right superior vena cava; or (3) the right superior vena cava, directly or via the azygos vein. In the right atrium, there is mixing of systemic and pulmonary venous blood, part of which enters the left heart via an atrial septal defect and most of which enters the right ventricle and low-resistance pulmonary bed. Accordingly, TAPVC can be classified as a cyanotic congenital anomaly with increased pulmonary arterial blood flow (see Table 1). The clinical picture in many ways resembles isolated atrial septal defect with large left to right shunt except for cyanosis, which varies from clinically subtle to marked. However, the patient is likely to be male, and symptoms generally begin in early childhood, although some patients reach adult life with surprisingly little disability. The jugular venous pulse may exhibit a large A wave because of pulmonary hypertension. Palpation and auscultation are similar to atrial septal defect with large left to right shunt, but signs of pulmonary hypertension are more likely to coexist. Similarly, the electrocardiogram shows right atrial and right ventricular hypertrophy. The x-ray may resemble atrial septal defect with large left to right shunt, but there is one distinctive picture. When the pulmonary veins communicate with the left innominate vein via a left vertical vein or left superior vena cava, the heart may exhibit a "figure of 8" appearance. The upper part of the figure of 8 is the left vertical vein on the left and the dilated right superior vena cava on the right. The lower part is the cardiac silhouette itself, i.e., dilated right atrium and right ventricle.

Diagnosis is established by cardiac catheterization and angiocardiography; the latter defines the specific connecting pathways. Surgical correction can be achieved, especially when the confluence of pulmonary veins can be anastomosed directly to the left atrium and the vascular channel to the systemic venous bed divided.

Right ventricular origin of both great arteries and "double outlet right ventricle" are synonymous terms for a congenital malformation in which the pulmonary artery arises in its normal position but the aorta arises wholly from the right ventricle. A ventricular septal defect provides the left ventricle with its only outlet. Pulmonic stenosis may or may not coexist. Right ventricular origin of both great arteries can exist with a ventricular septal defect inferior or superior to the crista supraventricularis. In double outlet right ventricle with infracristal ventricular septal defect and no pulmonic stenosis, two steps help in clinical diagnosis. The first step involves recognition of large ventricular septal defect with left to right shunt and pulmonary hypertension. Since both great vessels originate from the right ventricle, pulmonary arterial pressure is by definition systemic. It is a good rule to consider double outlet right ventricle in all patients who present with the picture of large left to right shunt pulmonary hypertensive ventricular septal defect. The second step in the clinical diagnosis consists of the following additional points: (1) a QRS that exhibits left axis deviation and counterclockwise depolarization, and (2) mild to moderate cyanosis with increased pulmonary arterial blood flow in the presence of persistent murmur of ventricular septal defect. It can be seen that the clinical diagnosis depends chiefly on left axis deviation in the presence of a pulmonary hypertensive ventricular septal defect with a large left to right shunt. Favorable adjustments in pulmonary vascular resistance sometimes regulate pulmonary blood flow so that, even though increased, it is not excessive. Under these circumstances longevity is improved; patients occasionally survive into young adulthood, and one underwent successful surgical correction at 53 years of age.

In right ventricular origin of both great vessels with supracristal ventricular septal defect, the defect lies just beneath the pulmonary valve. At times the pulmonary artery straddles the defect. This anomaly, called the *Taussig-Bing complex,* is a diagnostic consideration in patients with increased pulmonary blood flow and cyanosis from birth or early infancy. Radiologic, electrocardiographic, and physical signs of pulmonary hypertension are obligatory. In the presence of patent ductus arteriosus (which often coexists) and high pulmonary vascular resistance, a distinctive type of reversed cyanosis occurs in which the toes are less cyanotic than the fingers, because oxygenated blood from the left ventricle is ejected into the pulmonary trunk and then through the ductus into the descending aorta, whereas unsaturated right ventricular blood is ejected into the aortic root and brachiocephalic vessels. It is a good rule to consider the Taussig-Bing anomaly in patients who appear to have Eisenmenger's complex but in whom cyanosis dates from birth or early infancy.

Right ventricular origin of both great vessels occurs with all grades of pulmonic stenosis (mild to severe to complete, i.e., pulmonary atresia). The ventricular septal defect is usually infracristal if pulmonic stenosis coexists. Double outlet right ventricle with mild to moderate pulmonic stenosis resembles ordinary large ventricular septal defect with equivalent pulmonic stenosis except for three points: (1) the electrocardiogram may exhibit counterclockwise depolarization with left axis deviation; (2) the murmur of ventricular septal defect may persist despite pulmonic stenosis; and (3) there is a tendency for cyanosis to develop in the presence of increased pulmonary blood flow.

Right ventricular origin of both great vessels with severe pulmonic stenosis closely resembles cyanotic Fallot's tetralogy and should be considered whenever the clinical diagnosis of cyanotic Fallot's tetralogy is entertained. Clinical distinction between the two is difficult or impossible, although some points favor double outlet right ventricle: (1) auscultatory evidence of a holosystolic murmur at the lower left sternal edge despite the presence of cyanosis (obligatory left to right shunt through the ventricular septal defect); (2) palpable left ventricular impulse in this context; and (3) electrocardiogram showing small q waves in leads I and aVL and relatively broad slurred S waves in leads I, aVL, and V_{5-6}. The echocardiogram may assist in identifying lack of continuity between the posterior aortic wall and anterior mitral leaflet, because in double outlet right ventricle there is no continuity between the anterior mitral leaflet and the wall of either great vessel. Definitive diagnosis is angiographic. Corrective surgery is technically feasible, although it is more complex than with closure of isolated large ventricular septal defect or with repair of Fallot's tetralogy.

Truncus arteriosus is a congenital anomaly in which a single great artery leaves the base of the heart through a single semilunar valve. The truncus is situated just above a ventricular septal defect, receives blood from both ventricles, and gives rise to the coronary arteries and to the pulmonary and systemic circulations. No remnant of the second semilunar valve is present. Truncus arteriosus with large pulmonary arteries may occur with cyanosis and pulmonary plethora (see Table 1). Both pulmonary branches may arise from a short main pulmonary artery that emerges from the truncus, or the two pulmonary arterial branches may arise directly from the truncus. Truncus with absent pulmonary arteries is debatable and is physiologically analogous to pulmonary atresia with ventricular septal defect.

The outlook is better when there is an appropriate increase in pulmonary vascular resistance or relatively small pulmonary arteries, either mechanism advantageously controlling pulmonary blood flow and delaying death from cardiac failure. Occasional patients with favorably regulated pulmonary circulations have survived into the third or fourth decade, and one died at the age of 43 years. However, postpediatric survival is rare, especially with truncus arteriosus and large pulmonary arteries.

Definitive diagnosis of truncus arteriosus is by angiocardiography. Physiologic correction is feasible, employing an operation which joins the two pulmonary arteries to the outflow of the right ventricle with an aortic homograft.

Single ventricle refers to a rare congenital anomaly in which there are two atria but only one ventricular chamber that receives both the mitral and tricuspid valves. The usual type is a morphologic left ventricle with a small outlet chamber that represents the infundibular portion of the right ventricle. The infundibulum represents a subdivision of the single left ventricle, not a separate ventricular chamber. The great arteries are almost always transposed. If the infundibulum is situated at the right basal aspect of the heart, this arrangement is called "noninversion"; if the infundibulum is situated at the left basal aspect of the heart (corresponding to its expected location with congenitally corrected transposition), this arrangement is termed "inversion." Pulmonic stenosis may or may not coexist. Single ventricle without pulmonic stenosis occurs with increased pulmonary blood flow, and hence is an anomaly exhibiting cyanosis with pulmonary plethora (see Table 1). In single ventricle with high pulmonary vascular resistance, cyanosis is conspicuous and pulmonary blood flow is normal or diminished (see Table 1). Single ventricle with pulmonic stenosis is an anomaly exhibiting cyanosis with normal or diminished pulmonary blood flow (see Table 1).

This malformation has also been referred to as *cor triloculare biatriatum,* which merely means that there is a three-chambered heart with two atria. Clinical diagnosis is difficult, and definitive diagnosis depends upon cardiac catheterization and angiocardiography. Surgical intervention is palliative, and consists of either banding the pulmonary trunk to limit pulmonary plethora or providing a shunt operation to improve pulmonary blood flow in patients with critical pulmonic stenosis or atresia.

Carter, J. B., Sethi, S., Lee, G. B., and Edwards, J. E.: Prolapse of semilunar cusps as causes of aortic insufficiency. Circulation, 43:922, 1971.

Davis, J. E., Cheitlin, M. D., and Bedynek, J. L.: Sinus venosus atrial septal defect: Analysis of 50 cases. Am. Heart J., 85:177, 1973.

de la Cruz, M. Z., Anselmi, G., Romero, A., and Monroy, G.: A quantitative and qualitative study of the ventricles and great vessels of normal children. Am. Heart J., 60:675, 1960.

Edwards, J. E., Carey, L. S., Neufeld, H. N., and Lester, R. G.: Congenital Heart Disease. Philadelphia, W. B. Saunders Company, 1965.

Feigenbaum, H.: Echocardiography. Philadelphia, Lea & Febiger, 1972.

Gault, J. H., Morrow, A. G., Gay, W. A., and Ross, J., Jr.: Atrial septal defect in patients over age 40 years. Clinical and hemodynamic studies and the effects of operation. Circulation, 37:261, 1968.

Higgins, C. B., and Mulder, D. G.: Tetralogy of Fallot in the adult. Am. J. Cardiol., 29:837, 1972.

Higgins, I. T.: The epidemiology of congenital heart disease. J. Chronic Dis., 18:699, 1965.

Maron, B. J., Humphries, J. O., Rowe, R. D., and Mellits, E. D.: Prognosis of surgically corrected coarctation of the aorta. A 20-year postoperative followup. Circulation, 47:119, 1973.

Nadas, A. S., and Flyer, D. C.: Pediatric Cardiology. 3rd ed. Philadelphia, W. B. Saunders Company, 1972.

Nora, J. J.: Multifactorial inheritance hypothesis for the etiology of congenital heart disease. Circulation, 38:604, 1968.

Perloff, J. K.: Pediatric congenital cardiac becomes a postoperative adult. The changing population of congenital heart disease. Circulation, 47:606, 1973.

Perloff, J. K.: The Clinical Recognition of Congenital Heart Disease. Philadelphia, W. B. Saunders Company, 1970.

Polani, P. E., and Campbell, M.: An aetiological study of congenital heart disease. Ann. Hum. Genet., 19:209, 1955.

Roberts, W. C.: The congenitally bicuspid aortic valve. Am. J. Cardiol., 26:72, 1970.

ACQUIRED VALVULAR HEART DISEASE

John Ross, Jr.

556. INTRODUCTION

Before considering the characteristic features and treatment of each acquired valvular heart lesion, it will be useful to consider broad differences in the physiologic effects of these lesions and to suggest a general diagnostic approach to the patient with valvular heart disease. It will also be worthwhile to discuss the indications for cardiac catheterization, as well as the general considerations that enter into a decision to recommend surgical treatment.

GENERAL PHYSIOLOGIC EFFECTS OF VALVULAR HEART DISEASE

The consequences of stenosis or regurgitation of the heart valves may be considered in relation to their direct effects on the cardiac chamber that must compensate for the valvular lesion by undergoing hypertrophy or dilatation, and their secondary effects on intravascular pressures and blood flow in the aorta, pulmonary vascular bed, and systemic veins. When a semilunar valve of the heart (aortic or pulmonic) is stenotic or regurgitant, or when an atrioventricular valve (mitral or

tricuspid) is regurgitant, the primary burden is placed upon the adjacent *ventricle*. With aortic stenosis and regurgitation, important secondary effects occur in the aortic pressure pulses, and with mitral regurgitation there are major secondary effects on the pulmonary venous bed. When an atrioventricular valve is stenotic, the primary burden is placed on the *atrium*, and secondary effects are prominent on the adjacent venous bed; in tricuspid stenosis, for example, there are right atrial overload and secondary elevation of pressure in the systemic veins. These general consequences of stenotic and regurgitant valvular lesions are summarized in the accompanying figure.

Aortic stenosis places an overload on the left ventricle during systole, a pressure gradient being developed to overcome the obstruction at the aortic valve (see figure). This leads to progressive hypertrophy of the left ventricular wall without an increase in chamber volume. Aortic regurgitation, in contrast, places a volume overload on the left ventricle during diastole. This leads to an augmented forward stroke volume into the aorta which, in turn, causes a substantial increase in the systolic pressure in the aorta and left ventricle, an increase in left ventricular volume, and moderate hypertrophy of the left ventricular wall. An excessive oxygen consumption by the left ventricle occurs in aortic stenosis because of the hypertrophy and increased pressure required to drive blood across the narrowed valve, and myocardial oxygen consumption also is increased to some degree in aortic regurgitation because of the large stroke volume and the increased systolic pressure in the aorta. In addition, there is a low diastolic aortic pressure available for coronary artery perfusion in aortic regurgitation and a low aortic pressure relative to left ventricular pressure in severe aortic stenosis (see figure), which can lead to imbalances between coronary blood flow and myocardial oxygen demands. Angina pectoris is therefore common in both these conditions. Both aortic stenosis and regurgitation, in time, lead to left ventricular myocardial dysfunction.

Mitral regurgitation also places a diastolic volume overload on the left ventricle, but it differs importantly from aortic regurgitation in that the regurgitant leak occurs during ventricular systole and takes place into a relatively low pressure chamber, the left atrium (see figure). The ventricular chamber dilates to allow the increased total stroke volume (forward plus backward flow), but the ventricular systolic pressure is not elevated, wall hypertrophy is only moderate, oxygen demands are not greatly augmented, and coronary artery perfusion pressure is normal. Therefore this lesion, when it develops slowly, tends to be well tolerated, and left ventricular myocardial dysfunction develops late in the course of the disease. Mitral stenosis does not place an overload on the left ventricle; rather, obstruction at the mitral valve overwhelms the capacity of the atrial booster pump to maintain forward blood flow, and progressive elevation of left atrial pressure ensues (see figure).

The secondary effects of these valvular lesions on the arterial and venous beds are many. As mentioned above, the reduced aortic pulse in aortic stenosis and the wide aortic pulse pressure with low diastolic pressure in aortic regurgitation have important effects on coronary artery perfusion. In addition, when valvular lesions are sufficiently severe, or when left ventricular myocardial failure supervenes, the forward cardiac output becomes

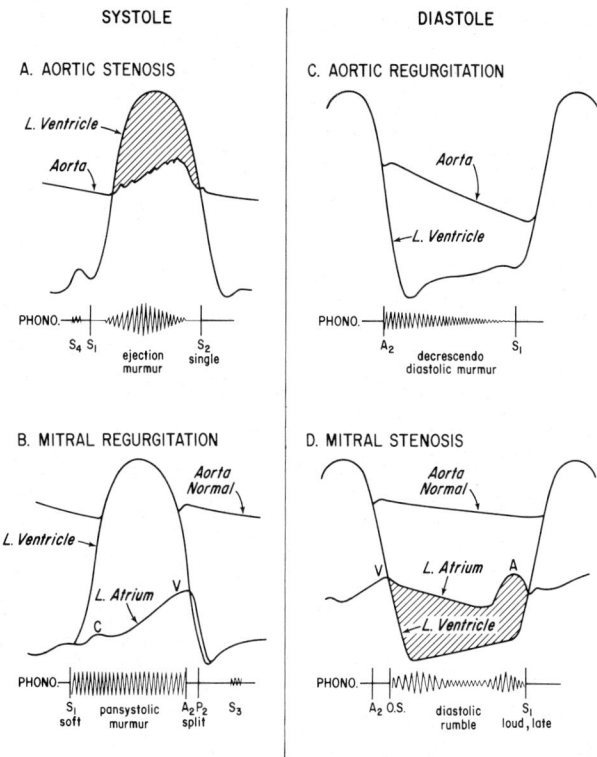

Diagrams of pressure tracings and phonocardiograms in valvular heart disease. The left-hand panels illustrate systole; the right-hand panels, diastole.

A, Pressure tracings in the aorta and left ventricle in aortic stenosis. The shaded area indicates the pressure gradient between left ventricle and aorta. The presystolic (A wave) in the left ventricle is shown, which correlates with the atrial diastolic gallop (S_4) on the phonocardiogram (Phono.). The murmur follows the time course of the pressure gradient during ventricular ejection, and the prolonged left ventricular ejection time results in a single second heart sound (S_2).

B, Pressure tracings in the aorta, left ventricle, and left atrium in mitral regurgitation. (Similar events occur in the right atrium, jugular venous pulse, and right ventricle in tricuspid regurgitation.) A prominent V wave is visible in the left atrium, and the pansystolic murmur on the phonocardiogram persists as long as there is a pressure gradient from left ventricle to left atrium across the leaking mitral valve. The A_2P_2 interval is more widely split than normal because of a shortened left ventricular ejection time in severe mitral regurgitation. The rapid filling wave in the left ventricle and left atrium is illustrated, which is often accompanied by a ventricular diastolic gallop (S_3).

C, Pressure tracings in the aorta and left ventricle in aortic regurgitation. There is a widened arterial pulse pressure with a rapidly falling aortic diastolic pressure. On the phonocardiogram the decrescendo diastolic murmur can be seen to follow the time course of the diminishing diastolic pressure gradient from the aorta to the left ventricle across the leaking aortic valve.

D, Pressure tracings in the aorta, left ventricle, and left atrium in mitral stenosis. (Similar events occur in the right atrium, jugular venous pulse, and right ventricle in tricuspid stenosis.) The left atrial pressure is elevated and the pressure gradient between left atrium and left ventricle during diastole is indicated by the shaded area. The slow fall in left atrial pressure after the V wave (slow Y descent) indicates obstruction to left atrial emptying, and the prominent A wave of left atrial contraction is not transmitted to the ventricle. The dumbbell-shaped diastolic rumble of mitral stenosis in the presence of normal sinus rhythm follows the time course of the pressure gradient, which is greatest early and again late in diastole. It can be seen how an increase or a decrease in the height of the left atrial pressure will move the mitral opening snap (O.S.) closer to or farther from, respectively, the aortic closure sound (A_2); similarly a higher left atrial pressure will result in a later and louder first heart sound (S_1).

reduced, the arterial pulse weakens, and there is reflex systemic vasoconstriction with cool extremities and peripheral cyanosis. Such signs constitute evidence of *"forward" cardiac failure.* The effects of *"backward" cardiac failure* in the presence of left-sided valvular lesions are due to left atrial and pulmonary venous hypertension, and they are reflected in the lungs and the right heart. In mitral stenosis, obstruction to left atrial emptying leads to left atrial hypertension, distention of the pulmonary veins, interstitial edema of the lung, reactive pulmonary arteriolar constriction, and eventually pulmonary arterial hypertension. However, the same sequence of effects can also occur when aortic stenosis becomes extremely severe, or when left ventricular myocardial dysfunction becomes significant in the presence of aortic valve disease or mitral regurgitation. The common denominator under these conditions is marked elevation of the left ventricular diastolic pressure, and late in the course of each of these left-sided valvular lesions left atrial and

pulmonary venous hypertension, lung congestion, and pulmonary arterial hypertension can also occur, as in mitral stenosis.

Once severe pulmonary hypertension develops, the resulting pressure overload on the right ventricle may then result in secondary right ventricular failure, tricuspid regurgitation, and right atrial hypertension. This, in turn, leads to congestion of the systemic venous bed and the peripheral tissues (liver, abdomen, and extremities). Tricuspid stenosis alone can produce such effects, the right atrial hypertension being caused by mechanical obstruction at the tricuspid valve.

APPROACH TO THE PATIENT WITH VALVULAR HEART DISEASE

Five basic steps in the evaluation of a patient with acquired valvular heart disease should be taken in a logical sequence: (1) the history, (2) the physical examination, (3) the chest roentgenogram (usually with multiple views and barium swallow), (4) the electrocardiogram, and (5) other special tests (phonocardiogram, echocardiogram, cardiac catheterization). The patient is often seen initially, of course, because of an abnormal finding in one of these areas (cardiac murmur, abnormal electrocardiogram, unusual chest x-ray).

History. The clinical course of patients with each major type of acquired valvular lesion tends to be rather characteristic, and often the findings to be encountered on physical examination can be predicted on the basis of a careful history alone. Thus in mitral stenosis the earliest symptoms are those due to episodic left atrial hypertension and pulmonary congestion, occurring particularly when the heart rate is rapid during exercise, and during intermittent atrial fibrillation or tachycardia. Such symptoms often begin in early adult life, and the dyspnea increases as the mitral valve narrowing progresses and reaches a critical degree. In contrast, patients with aortic stenosis or regurgitation, or mitral regurgitation, tend to develop dyspnea in relation to the duration and severity of the overload on the left ventricle. In acquired isolated aortic stenosis, there is often a long period without symptoms while the stenosis progresses and left ventricular hypertrophy increases; this is followed by a rather abrupt downhill course over four or five years, beginning at age 55 or 60, as the compensatory mechanisms are exhausted. The average downhill course in patients with chronic rheumatic aortic regurgitation tends to be less precipitous than that of aortic stenosis after symptoms begin, taking place over seven or eight years, but it usually begins somewhat earlier in life. On the other hand, in chronic mitral regurgitation the onset of symptoms is gradual and deterioration tends to be slow owing to the relatively favorable loading conditions on the left ventricle, discussed above.

These average clinical courses represent those of patients who experienced rheumatic fever in childhood, or who develop progressive stenosis of a congenitally bicuspid aortic valve. Departures from the typical patterns occur when, for example, coronary artery disease leads to angina pectoris in the presence of mild aortic stenosis, or when mitral regurgitation occurs acutely as a consequence of chordal rupture or papillary muscle dysfunction associated with coronary heart disease. Such deviations from the usual history should arouse the suspicion of a nonrheumatic etiology of valve dysfunction, or of other associated disease.

Physical Examination. In examining the heart, it is well to develop an ordered approach, commencing with careful inspection of the neck veins, palpation of the carotid arteries, and inspection and palpation of the precordium. Palpation of the carotid arteries may be highly useful, for example, in differentiating aortic stenosis caused by valvular obstruction from that caused by hypertrophic subaortic stenosis. Estimation of the jugular venous pressure (which, with practice, can be done reliably within 1 or 2 cm H_2O) and examination of the contour of the jugular venous pulse waves carry great importance, because these veins provide direct clues to events occurring in the right atrium. The jugular veins therefore serve as an "external manometer," and the characteristically slow downslope of the jugular venous pulse (Y descent) associated with tricuspid stenosis (see figure) or the dominant V wave of tricuspid regurgitation, may suggest organic tricuspid valve involvement.

The jugular venous pulse waves often disclose atrial arrhythmias, or provide a clue to the presence of pulmonary hypertension and right ventricular hypertrophy, evidenced by a prominent venous A wave.

Auscultation of the heart is of course the key to an accurate diagnosis in valvular heart disease. An orderly sequence for listening should be developed, each area being examined first for normal or abnormal heart sounds and then for cardiac murmurs. Simultaneous palpation of the carotid artery and observation of the neck veins should be used as aids in the proper timing of the heart sounds and murmurs. By listening first at the aortic area, the aortic component of the second heart sound can be readily identified; the intensity of the pulmonic closure sound and its movement with respiration can then be assessed at the pulmonic area. As one moves down the left sternal border with the diaphragm of the stethoscope, the opening snap of mitral stenosis may be revealed even before the murmur is heard at the apex, or the high-pitched blowing murmur of aortic regurgitation may be audible. The tricuspid and mitral areas should then be examined for the characteristics of the first heart sound. Sometimes a very loud first heart sound alerts the examiner to the possibility of mitral stenosis, whereas mitral regurgitation leads to a reduction in the intensity of the first heart sound at the apex (see figure).

The duration and intensity of the murmurs of valvular heart disease occur with, and tend to follow, the time course of pressure gradients between two adjacent cardiac chambers or between a chamber and its great vessel. Thus the diamond-shaped systolic murmur ("ejection" murmur) of aortic stenosis increases and decreases as the pressure gradient, and the velocity at which blood is forced across the narrowed aortic orifice rises and falls (see figure); this type of murmur does not occur during isovolumetric ventricular contraction and relaxation, and therefore begins well after the first heart sound and ends before the second sound. The decrescendo murmur of aortic regurgitation occurs as the diastolic pressure gradient between the aorta and the left ventricle gradually falls during left ventricular filling (see figure). The holosystolic (pansystolic) murmur of mitral or tricuspid regurgitation begins with the first heart sound and persists as long as active ventricular contraction maintains a positive pressure gradient from the ventricle to the passively filling atrium (see figure). The duration and intensity of the diastolic rumbling murmurs of mitral or tricuspid stenosis closely follow the diastolic pressure gradient across the valve from atrium to ventricle (see figure). Presystolic accentuation of the murmur during the A wave of atrial systole tends to disappear when atrial fibrillation occurs, and if the stenosis is mild the pressure gradient and the murmur may disappear midway during diastole. It also can be seen from the figure why the first heart sound is both late and loud in mitral stenosis, the left ventricle contracting rapidly and forcefully by the time it has built up sufficient pressure to close the mitral valve, and why the interval between the aortic closure sound and the mitral opening snap becomes progressively shorter as left atrial pressure rises.

Finally, it is important that changes in body position and certain other maneuvers become a regular part of the complete physical examination in a patient with valvular heart disease. The murmur of mitral stenosis may not be heard until the patient is placed in the left lateral decubitus position; the same position may be required to move the left ventricle sufficiently close to the chest wall to allow a ventricular diastolic gallop to be appreciated. The diagnosis of mitral stenosis should also not be excluded until a brief period of muscular exercise, or an isometric handgrip, has been performed to accentuate the murmur by increasing the heart rate and cardiac output, thereby augmenting the pressure gradient across the mitral valve. The handgrip maneuver tends to increase aortic pressure as well, and it is useful for augmenting a left ventricular gallop, or for accentuating the murmur of aortic regurgitation. The faint murmur of mild aortic regurgitation may also be detected only when the patient leans forward and breathes out completely. Sometimes the standing position is required to bring out the murmur of hypertrophic subaortic stenosis; the Valsalva maneuver is also useful for accentuating this murmur and for diminishing the murmur of valvular aortic stenosis.

Chest Roentgenogram. As mentioned above, the jugular venous pulse provides a "direct access" route to the right atrium and allows estimation of the right atrial or systemic venous pressure. The pulmonary veins, of course, are inaccessible to physical examination, and therefore the chest roentgenogram is relied upon heavily to aid in detecting left atrial and pulmonary venous hypertension. Often, when there is left atrial hypertension, enlargement of the upper lobe pulmonary veins reflects redistribution of pulmonary blood flow, with reduced perfusion of the lung bases relative to the upper lobes (reversing the normal pattern in the upright posture), and there are signs of interstitial pulmonary edema (such as the Kerley B line) which usually precede the development of pulmonary (intra-alveolar) edema.

Oblique, overpenetrated views of the heart with barium swallow provide valuable information in evaluating valvular heart disease. Left atrial enlargement may be evidenced in the frontal view by a round "double density" or by elevation of the left main-stem bronchus in the frontal view, but it also may be detected only in the right anterior oblique view as a discrete, posterior displacement of the barium-filled esophagus. This view is also useful for identifying right ventricular enlargement in patients suspected of having pulmonary hypertension. The left anterior oblique projection is the most reliable for detecting enlargement of the left ventricle. Other clues to the location of valvular heart lesions include poststenotic dilatation of the aorta in valvular aortic stenosis or calcification in a heart valve. Sometimes the latter is detected only by image intensification fluoroscopy.

The Electrocardiogram. In acquired valvular heart disease, the electrocardiogram should be carefully scrutinized for signs of chamber enlargement. Left atrial enlargement may be the only electrocardiographic sign of isolated mitral stenosis in the patient with sinus rhythm, and this single sign disappears when atrial fibrillation occurs. The presence or absence of left ventricular hypertrophy is of importance in considering the hemodynamic severity of aortic stenosis and in assessing the degree of mitral regurgitation; in the patient with mitral stenosis who has an apical systolic murmur, the presence of left ventricular hypertrophy may indicate that associated mitral regurgitation is of significance. The suspicion of associated coronary heart disease or myocardial disease may be raised by a bundle branch block pattern or by evidence of a previous myocardial infarction. Prominent (septal) Q waves associated with left

ventricular hypertrophy can also occur with hypertrophic subaortic stenosis. Right axis deviation or right ventricular hypertrophy suggests significant pulmonary hypertension. Sometimes the vectorcardiogram is employed to confirm the presence or absence of myocardial infarction or ventricular hypertrophy.

Special Laboratory Tests. Short of cardiac catheterization (discussed below), two other noninvasive tests are highly useful in the precise diagnosis of acquired valvular heart disease: the *phonocardiogram* and the *echocardiogram.*

The *phonocardiogram* is of value particularly for ascertaining the timing of normal and abnormal heart sounds. Recorded with the heart sounds are the indirect carotid pulse wave, which substitutes for the arterial pressure tracing; the indirect jugular venous tracing, which resembles the atrial pressure pulse; and the apex cardiogram, which corresponds roughly to the diastolic left ventricular pressure pulse. For example, a mitral opening snap can be identified by its close relation to the onset of left ventricular filling on the apexcardiogram, and its precise timing in relation to the aortic closure sound can be determined from the carotid pulse wave (see figure). A prolonged left ventricular ejection time and a single second heart sound are often associated with the abnormal carotid pulse wave of severe aortic stenosis (see figure). The phonocardiogram is not particularly useful for detecting soft cardiac murmurs; these are better identified by careful auscultation at various locations and by the several maneuvers described above.

The *echocardiogram* can aid considerably in reaching an accurate clinical diagnosis. Thus the characteristically abnormal pattern of anterior mitral valve leaflet motion can be demonstrated in mitral stenosis, or the fluttering movement of this leaflet associated with a diastolic Austin-Flint murmur can be identified. The echocardiogram may show posterior mitral leaflet prolapse when mitral regurgitation is associated with the click-murmur syndrome or with papillary muscle dysfunction. The characteristic anterior movement of the mitral leaflet during systole and echocardiographic identification of septal hypertrophy have simplified the diagnosis of hypertrophic subaortic stenosis. The applications of echocardiography are many, and the technique is finding increasing application in the study of cardiac diseases of all types.

DECISIONS CONSIDERING CARDIAC CATHETERIZATION AND OPERATION

Cardiac catheterization is rarely necessary for the *diagnosis* of valvular heart disease. An accurate diagnosis can usually be accomplished by careful application of the approaches described above, including the use of special noninvasive techniques such as echocardiography when necessary. Therefore cardiac catheterization and angiography are generally reserved until the patient is considered a potential candidate for a corrective operation. Of course there are some occasions when cardiac catheterization is used to make a definitive diagnosis, such as in differentiating angina pectoris caused by aortic stenosis from that resulting from associated coronary atherosclerosis, or in the differential diagnosis of pulmonary hypertension. In the latter situation, it is clearly important not to make a diagnosis of primary pulmonary hypertension until mitral valve obstruction has been carefully excluded by hemodynamic studies.

Prior to considering a surgical procedure, cardiac catheterization is usually undertaken for several purposes: (1) To determine whether the valve lesion (stenosis or regurgitation) is sufficiently severe to make it likely that surgical correction will relieve symptoms. (2) To assess carefully the degree of left ventricular myocardial dysfunction or failure associated with aortic valve lesions and mitral regurgitation. (3) To detect significant associated lesions, such as unexpectedly severe mitral regurgitation or aortic stenosis in a patient with mitral stenosis. (4) To study the coronary circulation, particularly in older subjects or in patients with aortic valve disease in whom symptoms may be due primarily to coronary heart disease rather than the valvular lesion. (5) To assess the relative significance of myocardial and valvular disease in patients with recurrent symptoms after previous cardiac surgery.

Once appropriate information has been assembled concerning the mechanical severity of the valve defect, the degree of involvement of the left ventricular myocardium, the severity of any associated coronary artery disease, and possible complicating illnesses (such as diabetes mellitus, liver disease, anemia, or thyroid disease), a decision concerning the advisability of a cardiac operation can be undertaken. Such a decision must also be based upon knowledge in several other important areas:

1. The risk to the patient's life of the proposed operation versus the risk of medical management alone. Operative risk is related to the nature of the surgical intervention required. Must a valve prosthesis be inserted, or is a commissurotomy possible? Is more than one valve involved? Is there associated coronary artery disease that will require a myocardial revascularization procedure? The patient's age and the presence of associated noncardiac illness also influence the operative risk.

2. The usual natural course of the valve lesion and the long-range outlook after operation. Knowledge of the natural history as well as the likely course after operation is important. For example, once significant symptoms begin in patients with aortic stenosis, the downhill course is usually rapid and the risk of *not* operating outweighs that of the surgical procedure. The average downhill course is somewhat slower after the onset of symptoms in patients with aortic regurgitation, but the degree of secondary left ventricular myocardial dysfunction must be considered, and operation should be undertaken before myocardial disease becomes irreversible. A similar consideration applies in patients with chronic mitral regurgitation, but their more gradual downhill course allows a more leisurely decision concerning the proper time for surgical intervention. The probable finite limitations in the life span of the various valvular prostheses should be taken into account before recommending operation in a young patient who has only moderate limitation of activity.

3. The social setting. This must be considered carefully, for in the final analysis the expected benefits of the operation must be judged in relation to the patient's age, occupational needs, family responsibilities, and expectation of substantially improved longevity and functional capacity.

557.   MITRAL STENOSIS

Etiology and Pathology.   Stenosis of the mitral valve in the adult usually develops as a sequel to rheumatic fever;

only rarely is it caused by such malformations as congenital cor triatriatum (see Ch. 555) or left atrial myxoma. It is the most common single valvular lesion to follow acute rheumatic fever, accounting for over half the patients with chronic rheumatic heart disease. About two thirds of the subjects are female.

The rheumatic mitral valve shows fibrosis and thickening of the cusps, with partial fusion of the commissures; in patients with longstanding disease, leaflet fusion may produce restriction of the mitral orifice to as little as 0.5 sq cm. There are thickening and shortening of the chordae tendineae, and there may be heavy calcium deposits in the valve. The left ventricle is generally normal in size and weight unless there is associated mitral regurgitation or disease of the aortic valve, but the left atrium is enlarged and thick walled. Microscopic examination of the myocardium often shows evidence of old rheumatic myocarditis (Aschoff bodies). In the lungs, there is thickening of the muscular walls of the pulmonary arterioles and venules with intimal proliferation, and in the late stages of mitral stenosis there is diffuse hemosiderosis (primarily disintegrated hemoglobin within alveoli), and there may be interstitial fibrosis and pulmonary infarction.

Pathologic Physiology.   The primary physiologic abnormality in mitral stenosis is mechanical obstruction to emptying of the left atrium produced by the narrowed valve orifice. Left ventricular function is usually normal, and therefore the defect in mitral stenosis stands in marked contrast to that of mitral regurgitation, or of aortic valve disease, in each of which a chronic overload is placed in the left ventricle.

When the mitral valve orifice is only mildly reduced, the mean left atrial pressure and filling of the left ventricle remain normal at rest. However, the rate of blood flow across the mitral valve is dependent not only on the orifice area of the valve and the driving pressure gradient (from left atrium to left ventricle), but also on the *time* available for flow across the mitral valve during diastole. With an increase in heart rate, the duration of left ventricular systole shortens only slightly, and tachycardia therefore occurs mainly at the expense of diastolic filling time per minute. Hence patients with mild mitral stenosis generally experience their earliest symptoms only during severe exertion, or with the onset of rapid atrial fibrillation. With exertion, both the normal tachycardia of exercise and the increased cardiac output lead to an increased left atrial pressure, whereas with atrial fibrillation and an uncontrolled ventricular rate the increased rate alone leads to a left atrial pressure elevation because of compromised filling time per minute.

With increased narrowing of the mitral orifice, the mean left atrial pressure becomes somewhat elevated at rest (over 12 mm Hg), but as the mitral orifice is reduced to below 1 sq cm the resting cardiac output can be maintained only at the expense of a markedly elevated left atrial pressure (often in excess of 20 mm Hg), in which the high pressure gradient forces blood across the narrowed orifice at high velocity. In this stage of the disease, the increased left atrial pressure and critically narrowed mitral valve often lead to pulmonary edema. Although pulmonary edema theoretically should occur when the pulmonary venous pressure exceeds about 30 mm Hg, higher levels have occasionally been recorded without its occurrence. This may be related to thickening of the alveolar-capillary membrane, which has been noted in the lungs of patients with mitral stenosis.

As the disease progresses, the elevated pressure in the pulmonary veins leads to pulmonary artery hypertension. When pulmonary hypertension becomes persistent at rest, it reflects two major factors: first, the elevated left atrial pressure is transmitted retrogradely and requires an increased pressure head in the pulmonary artery to drive blood forward; and second, pulmonary arteriolar vasoconstriction occurs. This vasoconstriction is accompanied in time by organic changes, mainly intimal proliferation and medial thickening in the walls of the small pulmonary arteries. At this stage, the pulmonary vascular resistance becomes elevated, which in turn leads to a reduction in the resting cardiac output. This sequence tends to limit any further increase in the left atrial pressure, which may even fall somewhat as the cardiac output becomes diminished. Symptoms of pulmonary venous congestion and pulmonary edema often diminish at this stage. In late mitral stenosis, pulmonary hypertension may become extreme, with the systolic pressure in the pulmonary artery equal to or exceeding that in the systemic arterial bed. Even with less marked elevations in pulmonary arterial pressure, the right ventricular end-diastolic volume and pressure become elevated, and this may lead to functional tricuspid regurgitation. Finally, signs of right ventricular failure appear with peripheral venous congestion.

Clinical Manifestations. *Symptoms and Clinical Course.* After one or more attacks of rheumatic fever in childhood, there is a latent period averaging about 12 years before mitral stenosis becomes clinically manifest, symptoms and signs usually first becoming apparent in young adulthood. There is commonly then a relatively long period (five to eight years) of mild to moderate symptoms as the scarring and obstruction at the valve gradually progress.

The earliest manifestation of mild to moderate mitral stenosis is dyspnea caused primarily by the increased cardiac output and tachycardia of exercise, leading to transient elevation of left atrial pressure, as discussed above. Elevation of the left atrial pressure causes pulmonary venous hypertension, increasing lung stiffness and the work of breathing, and thereby leads to the subjective sensation of dyspnea. As the disease progresses, orthopnea at night commences as a result of redistribution of the peripheral blood volume into the central circulation and of peripheral resorption of fluid caused by the supine posture. Coughing, particularly at night, may also be a troublesome symptom. Dyspnea eventually becomes extreme with minimal activity, and hemoptysis may occur owing to rupture of dilated endobronchial vessels, which appear to form collateral channels between the pulmonary and bronchial venous systems. The hemoptysis, consisting of bright red blood which can accumulate in sufficient quantities to cause atelectasis, usually subsides with bed rest and sedation with opiates; most commonly it occurs in patients who do not have severe elevation of the pulmonary vascular resistance. An increased number of pulmonary infections may occur, perhaps related to the interstitial pulmonary edema present in this stage of the disease, and other factors such as severe emotional stress, sexual activity, and fever with tachycardia may acutely worsen the patient's symptoms.

Significant left atrial enlargement develops as the left atrial hypertension becomes persistent, and atrial premature beats, paroxysmal atrial tachycardia, or atrial fibrillation commonly occur. The sudden onset of atrial fibrillation with rapid ventricular rate may precipitate acute pulmonary edema when the obstruction at the mitral orifice is of sufficient severity. Eventually, sustained atrial fibrillation supervenes, requiring control of the ventricular response with digitalis. Intermittent atrial fibrillation, in particular, may be associated with peripheral embolic phenomena, and the incidence of emboli in patients with chronic atrial fibrillation is substantial. As the left atrium enlarges and stasis occurs, thrombus formation is most frequent within the left atrial appendage, and adherent clots have been found at operation in this location in about 30 per cent of patients. Small emboli may break loose to become lodged in the renal, splenic, or cerebral circulations, and the effects of such emboli, causing a convulsion or perhaps a renal infarction, sometimes provide the initial symptom in a patient with mitral stenosis. Coronary artery embolization with myocardial infarction has also been reported. Sometimes a large embolus to the brain results in serious and permanent sequelae, and saddle embolus in the aorta has been encountered on a number of occasions. Infrequently a thrombus within the left atrium may become sufficiently large to obstruct a pulmonary vein, leading to localized unilateral pulmonary edema, and rarely a pedunculated "ball-valve thrombus" can be formed which mimics the findings of left atrial myxoma (see below).

As mitral stenosis progresses further, the pulmonary vascular resistance rises, tending to limit flow across the pulmonary bed; with the associated diminution of pulmonary venous hypertension, hemoptysis and pulmonary interstitial edema diminish. Thus in patients with longstanding, severe mitral stenosis, dyspnea on exertion and orthopnea often become less prominent, and fatigue now predominates. The development of functional tricuspid regurgitation may result in a further drop in the cardiac output and some reduction in the pulmonary artery pressure. In this stage of the disease weakness and signs of right heart failure become extreme, and abdominal discomfort with hepatomegaly, ascites and peripheral edema dominate the clinical picture. Pulmonary embolus with pulmonary infarction are common late complications.

Physical Findings. The patient (usually a female) with severe mitral stenosis may exhibit peripheral cyanosis and a "mitral facies" (blue-tinged with malar flush), and often there is some degree of emaciation. In such advanced cases, peripheral edema and ascites may also be evident.

The peripheral arterial pulses are typically small, and the blood pressure is normal or low. The jugular venous pulse is initially normal in the presence of moderate mitral stenosis, but as pulmonary hypertension develops, the mean venous pressure is increased and the A wave becomes prominent owing to right ventricular hypertrophy and elevation of the right ventricular end-diastolic pressure. In the presence of atrial fibrillation, there is a dominant V wave in the jugular veins.

In patients with mitral stenosis without pulmonary hypertension, palpation of the precordium may be unremarkable except for the presence of a diastolic thrill localized just inside the left ventricular apex. The apical impulse is otherwise normal, and the heart is not enlarged. In patients with pulmonary hypertension, there is a right ventricular lift in the left parasternal area, and the bulging pulmonary artery segment and pulmonic closure sound may be palpable at the upper left base if the mean pulmonary arterial pressure is in excess of 50 mm Hg.

On auscultation, the first heart sound is generally loud, snapping in quality, and somewhat delayed. These features occur because the left atrial pressure is elevated, and additional time is required for the left ventricle to build up sufficient pressure to close the mitral valve; the rate of change of left ventricular pressure (dP/dt) is rapid by that time, which results in the more forceful than normal mitral valve closure. The aortic closure sound is normal, but a mitral opening snap follows the second sound, the snap being audible at the lower left sternal border and the apex. A general correlation exists between the severity of mitral stenosis and the timing of the opening snap, necessitating careful evaluation of the interval between aortic closure and the opening snap. As the left ventricular pressure declines during the isovolumetric relaxation period after aortic valve closure, eventually it falls below the left atrial pressure and the stenotic mitral valve then snaps open. The higher the left atrial pressure, the closer this event must occur in relation to aortic closure (A_2). This time interval (the so-called A_2-OS interval) tends to be long (0.10 second or more) in patients with mild mitral stenosis and mean left atrial pressures below 15 mm Hg, whereas in patients with severe mitral stenosis and mean left atrial pressures of 20 mm Hg or more, the interval is usually shorter (less than 0.09 second). As might be expected, however, the interval will vary considerably with the heart rate. If the heart rate is below 100 and the interval 0.07 second or less, the mitral stenosis is usually of significant degree.

The opening snap is followed immediately by a low-pitched *diastolic rumble* resulting from turbulent flow across the stenotic mitral orifice. The murmur is usually localized to an area about 2 cm in diameter near or just inside the left ventricular apex in the fourth or fifth left intercostal space, and it is best brought out by positioning the patient in the lateral decubitus position. The mitral rumble is loudest in early diastole; it diminishes somewhat as the pressure gradient between left atrium and left ventricle falls, and, in patients with sinus rhythm, it then becomes loud (presystolic accentuation) as the left atrium contracts to again raise the pressure gradient (see figure in Ch. 556). When the stenosis is mild, the diastolic murmur may not be audible until the patient is placed in the lateral decubitus position *after* performing mild exercise or during a handgrip maneuver, when the cardiac output and heart rate are increased, thereby augmenting the pressure gradient across the valve. In the presence of atrial fibrillation, presystolic accentuation disappears; when the ventricular rate is slow, the murmur may occur only in the early and middle phases of long diastolic periods, because given sufficient time the left atrial and left ventricular pressure will come into equilibrium. In patients with severe mitral stenosis and a very low cardiac output, the murmur may be unusually difficult to appreciate. It is most important therefore to position the patient properly and to listen carefully over a wide area of the left chest for the well localized murmur, as well as to carry out the aforementioned exercise maneuvers. When such precautions are taken, "silent" mitral stenosis will be encountered rarely. Occasionally the murmur is inaudible when massive right ventricular enlargement places the left ventricle far posteriorly from the chest wall.

Individuals with "pure" mitral stenosis have a small fixed orifice, and it is not uncommon to hear a soft systolic murmur at the cardiac apex, which represents a trivial mitral regurgitant leak. When a louder pansystolic murmur at the left ventricular apex is accompanied by a third heart sound, by left ventricular enlargement on physical examination, or by electrocardiographic signs of left ventricular hypertrophy, the associated mitral regurgitation is undoubtedly of significance. In the patient with severe pulmonary hypertension, when a very large right ventricle fills the anterior chest and displaces the left ventricle posteriorly, the murmur of tricuspid regurgitation can mimic that of mitral regurgitation. The systolic murmur of tricuspid regurgitation is ordinarily heard best at the lower left sternal border; it increases with inspiration, and is not heard in the axilla or over the spine posteriorly, features which serve to distinguish it from the murmur of mitral regurgitation. With severe pulmonary hypertension the high-pitched, early diastolic blowing murmur of pulmonic regurgitation (the Graham Steell murmur) may also be audible. This murmur, heard best at the left sternal border, is usually indistinguishable from that of mild aortic regurgitation.

Diagnosis. *Electrocardiogram.* In patients with moderate mitral stenosis and sinus rhythm, the electrocardiogram may show only left atrial enlargement, with a notched and prolonged P wave in the limb leads and an increased negative component of the P wave in lead V_1. When there is atrial fibrillation, patients with rheumatic heart disease tend to show coarse fibrillation waves, presumably owing to the thickened atrial wall and enlarged chamber volume, a finding which contrasts with the fine fibrillatory waves often found in patients with coronary heart disease.

In severe mitral stenosis with pulmonary hypertension, the electrocardiogram often shows right axis deviation, and voltage criteria for right ventricular hypertrophy are sometimes present. Evidence of left ventricular hypertrophy in a patient with mitral stenosis generally indicates accompanying aortic valve disease or significant associated mitral regurgitation.

Roentgenographic Features. Minimal enlargement of the left atrium may be the only radiographic abnormality in patients with moderate mitral stenosis. It may be apparent only with barium swallow, the right anterior oblique view showing best the localized, posterior displacement of the barium-filled esophagus. As the disease progresses, left atrial enlargement becomes distinct, and this chamber is visible as a large round "double density" in the center of the cardiac shadow on the frontal view. The left main-stem bronchus is elevated by the enlarged left atrium (the angle formed by the bronchus with a central, vertical line increasing to more than 45 degrees), and enlargement of the left atrial appendage results in straightening of the left heart border.

As left atrial and pulmonary venous hypertension develop, there is a redistribution of the pulmonary vascularity in the lung fields. Initially, in the upright posture the normal, relative avascularity of the upper lobes is lost, and the pulmonary vascular pattern appears equal in the upper and lower lungs. In later stages of the disease, vascularity in the upper lobe vessels is increased. Redistribution of the pulmonary vascular pattern generally occurs when left atrial pressure exceeds 15 mm Hg, and evidence of interstitial pulmonary edema commonly appears when the mean left atrial pressure at rest exceeds 20 mm Hg. Interstitial edema may be evidenced by *Kerley's B lines,* transverse linear densities about 1 cm in length and located at the lung bases laterally above the diaphragm, representing engorged septal lymphatic vessels. Acute pulmonary edema is reflected by typical butterfly densities in the hilar regions.

As pulmonary hypertension develops, the pulmonary artery segment becomes enlarged, the peripheral pulmonary arteries become dilated, and enlargement of the right ventricle and right atrium is evident. With longstanding pulmonary hypertension a diffuse reticular pattern in the lung fields may result from pulmonary hemosiderosis. Calcification in the mitral valve should be searched for, using image intensification fluoroscopy. The presence of calcification makes it less likely that the valve will prove amenable to valvuloplasty.

Echocardiography.   Reflected ultrasound to confirm the presence of mitral stenosis and to estimate its severity has found increasing application. The echo recorded from the mitral leaflets exhibits characteristic features in the presence of significant mitral stenosis, the degree of the abnormality correlating in general with the severity of stenosis. Thickening of the anterior and posterior leaflets can often be identified, and there is a reduced anterior excursion of the leaflet during diastole. Both the anterior and posterior leaflets move forward with diastole as the domed, stenotic valve opens (in a normal valve, the posterior leaflet opens in an opposite direction to the anterior leaflet). Because of the persistent pressure gradient from left atrium to left ventricle, the normal posterior floating motion of the anterior mitral leaflet during mid-diastole does not occur; the leaflet is held open in an anterior position and moves only slowly posteriorly. This posterior motion (the so-called E to F slope) is reduced to less than 12 mm per second with severe mitral stenosis (normally it is 40 mm per second or more).

The detection of characteristic moving echoes from behind the mitral valve can indicate the presence of left atrial myxoma or a ball-valve thrombus.

Pulmonary Function Tests.   Patients with longstanding mitral stenosis generally have a reduced pulmonary compliance owing to elevation of the left atrial pressure and interstitial pulmonary edema. The vital capacity, total lung capacity, maximal breathing capacity, and oxygen uptake per unit of ventilation may be reduced, and abnormalities of ventilation-perfusion relations are often seen as well.

Cardiac Catheterization.   In the young patient with obvious features of pure mitral stenosis and marked symptoms, cardiac catheterization is not performed in some centers prior to operation. On the other hand, when there is uncertainty about the severity of the stenosis in relation to the level of symptoms, cardiac catheterization should be performed to document objectively the degree of valve narrowing, and to calculate the orifice area. At cardiac catheterization, the typical patient with significant mitral stenosis will exhibit an elevated mean pulmonary artery wedge pressure. If a satisfactory wedge pressure tracing cannot be obtained, transseptal left atrial puncture is often performed. If the patient is in sinus rhythm, the forceful left atrial contraction produces a dominant A wave in the tracing, and there is a slow fall in the pressure after the V wave (reduced rate of the Y descent), reflecting obstruction to left atrial emptying during diastole. The left ventricular end-diastolic pressure is usually normal (below 12 mm Hg). The pressure gradient from left atrium to left ventricle is high early in diastole, falling progressively as left ventricular filling occurs, but the gradient is again increased late in diastole by left atrial contraction (see figure in Ch. 556). In patients with atrial fibrillation, the V wave is dominant and left atrial pressure continues to fall throughout diastole until the onset of ventricular systole.

The *mitral valve orifice area* can be calculated if both the cardiac output and the pressure gradient are known. By the Gorlin formula, the valve orifice area is directly proportional to the flow across the valve per second of diastole and is inversely proportional to the square root of the pressure gradient. In simple terms, this means that if the flow doubles, the pressure gradient will quadruple. Because of this nonlinear relation, measurement of the left atrial or wedge pressure alone can be misleading in assessing the severity of the mitral stenosis. Thus if the cardiac output is unusually high, an elevated left atrial mean pressure may give a false picture of the severity of the stenotic lesion; if it is low, a moderate left atrial pressure elevation may belie the presence of severe stenosis. Also, if the heart rate is abnormally rapid or slow and a shorter or longer diastolic filling time is available, the left atrial mean pressure may not reflect accurately the size of the mitral orifice. The area of the normal mitral valve is about 4 sq cm. Mitral stenosis is generally considered mild when the calculated orifice area is over 1.2 sq cm, moderate when it is between 1.2 and 0.9 sq cm, and severe when it is below 0.8 sq cm. Thus an area of 1.1 sq cm or less is usually considered to represent stenosis of sufficient severity to warrant operation.

Left ventriculography usually shows the left ventricle to contract normally, with a normal end-diastolic volume. It also provides information concerning the degree of thickening and fusion of the chordal attachments of the mitral valve, the pliability of its leaflets, and the degree of associated mitral regurgitation. All these factors, together with the presence or absence of valve calcification, weigh in the decision of whether to perform closed or open mitral valvuloplasty, or whether to recommend replacement of the valve with a prosthesis.

In older patients, selective coronary arteriography is indicated to search for significant coronary vascular disease. Cardiac catheterization will also document the severity of any associated aortic valvular disease; in patients with recurrent systemic emboli, a pulmonary angiogram may verify the presence of a left atrial thrombus.

Differential Diagnosis.   Clinical findings of pulmonary hypertension should raise the suspicion of mitral stenosis. *Primary pulmonary hypertension* usually occurs in young females; it is associated with hyperventilation, chest pain, fatigue and dyspnea, and effort syncope, but with a relative paucity of objective physical findings. Whenever this diagnosis is considered, mitral stenosis and left atrial myxoma, treatable causes of left atrial and pulmonary hypertension, should be excluded by measurement of left atrial pressure directly or from an adequate pulmonary arterial wedge pressure. *Pulmonary hypertension caused by severe chronic lung disease* usually presents no diagnostic difficulty; but sometimes patients are given a diagnosis of ordinary bronchial asthma, when in fact their wheezing is due to mitral stenosis with left atrial hypertension ("cardiac asthma").

The murmur of rheumatic mitral stenosis may be mimicked by that resulting from a *left atrial myxoma.* However, with the latter lesion there may be other abnormal diastolic sounds, and the murmur may disappear when the patient's position is altered. In addition, symptoms can vary with changes in body position, syncope may occur, and there is usually an elevated sedimentation rate, anemia, fever, or other evidence of systemic disease. Echocardiography may detect the left atrial myxoma. In the young patient, *congenital cor triatriatum* (a rare malformation consisting of a fibrous partition within the left atrium above the mitral valve) may be considered.

The diastolic rumble which occurs in the presence of severe aortic regurgitation, the *Austin Flint murmur,* may be attributed to organic mitral stenosis. This murmur is typically ushered in by a ventricular diastolic gallop (S_3) rather than an opening snap, and it is loudest in mid-diastole. Amyl nitrite inhalation decreases this murmur by lowering diastolic aortic pressure, but the reflex tachycardia and increased cardiac output increase the murmur of mitral stenosis. Echocardiography is particularly helpful in differentiating the Austin Flint murmur from that of mitral stenosis by detecting a characteristic fluttering motion of the anterior leaflet during diastole as its motion is affected by the regurgitant jet.

In the older patient, *atrial septal defect* is occasionally mistaken for mitral stenosis. In atrial septal defect, the tricuspid closure sound is loud, the widely split second heart may mimic the opening snap of mitral stenosis, and the rumble of excessive flow across the tricuspid valve may be confused with the murmur of mitral stenosis. The murmur of mitral stenosis diminishes with inspiration, in contrast to this murmur and the murmur of tricuspid stenosis, which increase.

Treatment. *Medical Management.* In the patient with mild mitral stenosis and few symptoms, restriction of strenuous activity may result in many years of comfortable existence. If the patient is under 40 years of age, monthly Bicillin injections or oral penicillin (sulfonamides may be used in the allergic patient) are advisable to prevent infection with the beta-hemolytic Streptococcus and recurrence of acute rheumatic fever (see Ch. 191). In addition, antimicrobial drugs in therapeutic doses should be recommended prior to and after dental procedures or surgical manipulations, particularly those on the genitourinary tract, to prevent bacterial endocarditis (see Ch. 192).

In patients with moderate symptoms, limitation of activity should be combined with *sodium restriction* and/or administration of a *diuretic* agent. There is little rationale for the use of digitalis in patients with sinus rhythm, because left ventricular function is normal and this agent has no effect on exercise-induced tachycardia. *When atrial fibrillation occurs* for the first time, one or more attempts at *electrical reversion of the rhythm,* followed by maintenance with oral quinidine, are generally indicated. When mitral stenosis is significant, however, permanent atrial fibrillation will generally supervene in time, despite such therapy. In the presence of chronic atrial fibrillation, *digitalis* should be administered to maintain the ventricular rate at an acceptable level both at rest and during moderate exertion. In patients who are particularly sensitive to digitalis, the addition of a *beta-adrenergic blocking agent* (such as propranolol) in small doses may result in very effective control of the ventricular response. Moreover, during acute stress, such as a pneumonia, patients with atrial fibrillation may develop a rapid ventricular response caused by enhanced atrioventricular conduction con-

sequent to excessive sympathetic nervous discharge; under these circumstances the addition of a beta-adrenergic blocking agent to digitalis may allow effective reduction of the ventricular rate in a safer manner than with high doses of digitalis alone. When the ventricular rate is refractory to digitalis in the absence of acute stress, or when signs of heart failure are out of proportion to the degree of mitral stenosis, hyperthyroidism should be suspected. Obvious signs of thyrotoxicosis may be masked in the presence of cardiac disease; but if such hyperthyroidism is detected and treated, symptoms caused by mild mitral stenosis may disappear.

In patients who have suffered a systemic embolus originating from the left atrium, long-term *anticoagulation* with Coumadin derivatives has been shown to be effective in preventing recurrence. Minor neurologic episodes, or a frank convulsion, often provide the earliest sign of systemic embolization. Emboli also may occur to the legs, or to the mesenteric artery (causing abdominal and bowel necrosis), and prompt surgical treatment with embolectomy is required. If systemic embolization recurs while the patient is on adequate anticoagulant therapy, a mitral valve operation with removal of left atrial clot may be recommended for the patient with somewhat milder mitral stenosis, or with less marked symptoms than are usually required for an elective operation.

When pregnancy occurs in a patient with mitral stenosis, symptoms frequently develop for the first time or intensify. Such symptoms become most severe during the second trimester, when increased cardiac output and blood volume are maximal, and a substantial period of hospital treatment may be required. Generally, such symptoms diminish during the third trimester, and only rarely is a mitral commissurotomy necessary during pregnancy.

Once severe symptoms begin in the patient with tight mitral stenosis (New York Heart Association [N.Y.H.A.] Class III), the average mortality in patients treated medically approaches 30 per cent at five years. In severely limited patients (Class IV), the outlook without operation is extremely poor, less than 20 per cent of patients being alive after five years if data gathered prior to the cardiac surgical era are considered. Surgical treatment has greatly altered this outlook.

Surgical Treatment. In the typical younger patient with symptoms on normal activity (N.Y.H.A. Class II) and findings of pure mitral stenosis, the decision of whether to recommend operation is usually reached by considering the individual in his desired activity setting. In the patient with significant mitral stenosis who has had a complication such as a systemic embolus and who develops symptoms on ordinary exertion, operation is usually recommended. In the older patient in functional Class II who has evidence of mitral valve calcification on x-ray and physical findings suggesting a thickened and immobile mitral leaflet (soft first heart sound and reduced or absent opening snap), or in whom significant associated mitral regurgitation is suspected, a waiting period until symptoms are more severe is justified, because mitral valve replacement with a prosthesis will undoubtedly be necessary. In patients with symptoms on less than normal activity (N.Y.H.A. Class III) or at rest (Class IV), the outlook without surgical treatment is poor and the indication for operation is clear.

The presence of severe pulmonary hypertension was considered at one time to represent a relative contraindication to operation, but more recent studies have indicated that even marked elevations of the pulmonary vascular resistance invariably regress postoperatively. Some reduction in the pulmonary vascular resistance occurs within a few hours postoperatively. In most patients studied by cardiac catheterization six months to one year after operation, the pulmonary artery pressure and pulmonary vascular resistance have returned to normal or near normal levels, provided the left atrial pressure is normal.

Surgical practices differ somewhat as to the type of procedure performed in the patient with mitral stenosis. Closed mitral valvulotomy by opening the valve commissures with the finger, inserted through the left atrial appendage, sometimes combined with the use of a mechanical dilator passed through the left ventricular apex, is still employed by some surgeons without the use of cardiopulmonary bypass (heart-lung machine). In many centers, open mitral commissurotomy is now carried out even in the uncomplicated patient, the left atrium being opened with the patient on cardiopulmonary bypass and the mitral stenosis relieved by blunt and sharp dissection under direct vision. The operative risk of such a mitral valvuloplasty is now about equal to that of cardiopulmonary bypass alone (under 4 per cent). This approach also allows removal of any clot that may be present within the left atrium. If significant mitral regurgitation is produced by the attempted valvuloplasty, it is then possible to proceed readily with replacement of the mitral valve by a ball-valve or other prosthesis.

The late results of valvuloplasty have been poor when there is significant mitral regurgitation, or if there is calcification with severe shortening and thickening of the chordae tendineae and immobilization of the mitral valve leaflets. When the valve exhibits such unfavorable anatomic signs, it is replaced with a prosthetic device. The average operative mortality for valve replacement ranges between 6 and 10 per cent.

After a valvuloplasty, the average patient experiences 8 to 12 years of symptomatic relief, but a second operation is often necessary (usually mitral valve replacement). The late results of mitral valve replacement have been generally favorable, with improved life expectancy and relief of symptoms. Long-term anticoagulation is required for many types of prosthetic devices.

558. MITRAL REGURGITATION

Etiology and Pathology. A wide spectrum of disease processes can result in mitral regurgitation, although rheumatic involvement is by far the most common cause. Rheumatic mitral regurgitation occurs more commonly in males, in contrast to mitral stenosis, and the murmur is commonly heard during or soon after the acute rheumatic episode, again in contrast to the relatively late development of the murmur of mitral stenosis. In chronic rheumatic disease, the left ventricle is generally dilated and the wall thickened, there is left atrial enlargement, and the mitral valve exhibits mild, diffuse scarring of the leaflets associated with some thickening of the chordae tendineae. The finding of associated aortic valve disease favors a rheumatic cause.

Other forms of mitral regurgitation include rupture of one or more chordae tendineae, most commonly resulting from bacterial endocarditis, but also sometimes attributed to rheumatic disease, trauma, or unknown causes. Papillary muscle dysfunction is usually secondary to necrosis or fibrosis of one or both papillary muscles owing to coronary artery disease, mitral regurgitation resulting from poor contraction of the muscles, and systolic eversion of the mitral leaflets. In acute myocardial infarction, rupture of a papillary muscle causes sudden, severe mitral regurgitation (see Ch. 567). Mitral regurgitation caused by ballooning with prolapse of the posterior leaflet during systole, or to abnormally long chordae, the so-called *"floppy valve syndrome,"* sometimes is inherited, and increased acid mucopolysaccharide deposits may be found in the valve. Congenital mitral regurgitation can occur as an isolated condition, but more commonly it accompanies such lesions as ostium primum atrial septal defect or Marfan's syndrome in which the valve may resemble that found in the floppy valve syndrome, but is associated with other stigmata.

Mitral regurgitation also occurs as a secondary phenomenon in patients with idiopathic hypertrophic subaortic stenosis, as discussed subsequently. In primary myocardial disease, mitral regurgitation may be secondary to massive dilatation of the left ventricle and the mitral anulus. Acquired, heavy calcification of the mitral anulus, which typically occurs in elderly women, is sometimes associated with significant mitral regurgitation.

Pathologic Physiology. With insufficiency of the mitral valve of the type found in chronic rheumatic heart disease, regurgitation of blood from the left ventricle into the left atrium commences as soon as the left ventricular pressure during early systole exceeds that in the left atrium, and persists until the left ventricular pressure falls below the left atrial pressure. Therefore the regurgitation is pansystolic, commencing with the first heart sound and often ending with or just after the second heart sound, and at the peak of the atrial V wave. The prominent V wave in the left atrial pressure pulse is due to the normal inflow of blood from the pulmonary veins (when the mitral valve is ordinarily closed) which is augmented by the regurgitant leak.

An important physiologic characteristic of mitral regurgitation relative to the function of the left ventricle is that this lesion provides a relatively low impedance pathway for blood to exit from the left ventricle, pressure in the left atrium being lower than that in the aorta. The pressure in the left ventricle tends to fall more abruptly than normal late in ventricular systole because of the leak, and the average afterload or active tension in the wall of the left ventricle is thereby reduced. This effect favors increased shortening of the myocardial wall because of the inverse relation between force and fiber shortening (and velocity), and the ratio of stroke volume to end-diastolic volume (ejection fraction) may therefore be normal or even high in mitral regurgitation. In addition, although myocardial oxygen consumption is greatly enhanced by lesions which cause increased systolic pressure work or augmented wall tension, it is little affected by the increased volume load imposed by mitral regurgitation. These favorable mechanical loading conditions and the minimal effect of this lesion on oxygen consumption help to explain the prolonged clinical course observed in many patients with chronic mitral regurgitation.

In chronic mitral regurgitation the diastolic volume of the left ventricular chamber becomes increased because of ventricular dilatation and increased muscle mass. The increased diastolic ventricular size allows delivery of a much larger than normal *total* stroke volume during systole (forward stroke volume plus the regurgitant volume), but with a normal extent of shortening of each unit of the enlarged left ventricular circumference. When left ventricular myocardial function is not impaired, the left ventricular end-diastolic pressure is normal or only slightly elevated, and the forward cardiac output is well maintained. Under these conditions, the *mean* left atrial pressure may be minimally elevated, because the exaggerated V wave occurs only briefly during the cardiac cycle. There is no impairment of left atrial emptying into the left ventricle and hence little or no rise in mean left atrial pressure during exercise.

With longstanding, severe mitral regurgitation, left ventricular myocardial contractility is eventually depressed. When this happens, the extent of shortening of the left ventricular wall become reduced, the residual volume in the left ventricle at the end of ejection increases, the ejection fraction falls, and the end-diastolic volume and left ventricular end-diastolic pressure rise. The latter, in turn, leads to elevation of the mean left atrial pressure and subsequently to pulmonary hypertension. Left atrial hypertension also occurs when there is some associated narrowing of the mitral valve. The mechanism of pulmonary hypertension in mitral regurgitation resembles that in mitral stenosis, and in later stages elevations of the pulmonary vascular resistance as severe as those seen with mitral stenosis have been encountered.

The aforementioned description encompasses most patients with chronic rheumatic mitral regurgitation, but there are unusual physiologic manifestations seen late in the course of chronic disease or with acute mitral regurgitation, such as that caused by ruptured chordae tendineae. In the former category is the finding of giant left atrium with low mean left atrial pressure and greatly reduced cardiac output. This syndrome appears to be due to a combination of poor left ventricular function, with reduced forward cardiac output and diminished regurgitant volume, as well as to a capacious and compliant left atrium, which absorbs the regurgitant leak with little change in the pressure. At the other extreme is the situation in sudden, severe mitral regurgitation. In this setting, the left atrium is small, distended, and noncompliant, and the large regurgitant leak produces a giant V wave which can reach 70 to 80 mm Hg (so-called "ventricularization" of the left atrial pressure pulse). Severe pulmonary hypertension and reduced forward cardiac output accompany such marked, acute regurgitation.

Clinical Manifestations. *Symptoms and Clinical Course.* As mentioned earlier, the mean left atrial pressure may not be significantly elevated at rest in patients with mitral regurgitation in whom the left ventricle is compensated, and, unlike mitral stenosis, there is little increase in left atrial pressure during exercise or with tachycardia. Therefore the earliest symptom in mitral regurgitation is often exertional fatigue, which reflects inability to maintain a normal forward cardiac output to supply the exercising skeletal muscles. Mild symptoms of this type may persist for many years without significant dyspnea or pulmonary congestion.

Later in the course of severe chronic mitral regurgitation, with the onset of early left ventricular failure, the ventricular end-diastolic pressure increases, left atrial hypertension develops, and dyspnea on exertion and orthopnea occur. However, paroxysmal nocturnal dyspnea and acute pulmonary edema are distinctly unusual in this condition. With the onset of pulmonary hypertension, right heart failure accompanied by venous distention and peripheral edema may occur. Atrial fibrillation is a common complication, but left atrial thrombi are relatively unusual, and systemic emboli occur much less commonly than with mitral stenosis.

Chronic mitral regurgitation is the best tolerated of the lesions involving the left side of the heart. Frequently, patients remain relatively asymptomatic for 10 or 20 years, even in the presence of severe regurgitation, and it is not uncommon for patients to respond well to medical therapy for an additional 10 years or more before progressive left ventricular failure causes serious progressive difficulty and death. This long clinical course undoubtedly reflects in part the favorable loading conditions of this lesion on the left ventricle, as discussed earlier. It seems likely that a sizable number of patients with only moderate mitral regurgitation never experience serious difficulty and may have a normal life expectancy.

Physical Findings. When mitral regurgitation is severe, the peripheral pulse is sharp and abbreviated, owing to lack of sustained forward stroke volume in the face of the regurgitant leak. The jugular venous pulse is normal unless there is pulmonary hypertension or tricuspid valve disease. Atrial fibrillation is frequently present.

On palpation of the precordium, the left ventricle is enlarged, the apex beat is hyperactive and displaced laterally, and frequently there is a systolic thrill at the apex. In the lateral decubitus position, a rapid outward movement in early diastole (rapid filling wave) may be palpable. If pulmonary hypertension is present, there is a right ventricular lift. When the left atrium is markedly enlarged and the mitral regurgitation is severe, expansion of this chamber during systole may push the right ventricle and pulmonary artery out against the chest wall in the third and fourth left interspaces during late systole, a finding which may be confused with right ventricular enlargement.

The characteristic feature of mitral regurgitation in chronic rheumatic disease is a high-pitched *pansystolic murmur* at the cardiac apex which is transmitted to the left axilla (see figure in Ch. 556). If the lesion is severe, it is accompanied by four other findings: (1) soft first heart sound, (2) loud ventricular diastolic gallop (third heart sound), (3) short early diastolic rumble, which accompanies the rapid inflow of blood to the left ventricle, and (4) wide splitting of the second heart sound caused by early closure of the aortic valve. The last-named finding is caused by shortening of the left ventricular ejection time consequent to the regurgitant leak.

Although the murmur of mitral regurgitation is usually pansystolic, variations may be heard. When mitral regurgitation is due to papillary muscle dysfunction, the murmur begins well after the first heart sound and may have a crescendo-decrescendo quality. These characteristics result from posterior herniation of the mitral leaflet as the papillary muscles fail to contract normally late during ventricular systole. In the *click-murmur syndrome,* late ballooning of the mitral leaflets into the left atrium also occurs, but caused by intrinsic mitral valve disease. In this condition the late systolic murmur may be ushered in by one or more midsystolic clicks. In sudden, severe mitral regurgitation, sinus rhythm is often preserved and there may be a loud fourth heart sound, a most uncommon finding in chronic mitral regurgitation. When a giant left atrial V wave accompanies acute mitral regurgitation, the murmur may occur early in systole; but it is short and terminates before the end of systole, because the left ventricular pressure and massive left atrial V wave equalize near or even before the time of aortic valve closure.

Diagnosis. *Electrocardiogram.* In patients with mild to moderate mitral regurgitation the electrocardiogram may be normal; but with longstanding moderate disease or with severe regurgitation, the electrocardiogram usually shows left ventricular hypertrophy and atrial fibrillation. Typically, there is evidence of a so-called diastolic overload pattern, with upright T waves and voltage criteria for left ventricular hypertrophy. Right ventricular hypertrophy may develop in the late stages of the disease when there is pulmonary hypertension. If sinus rhythm is present, left atrial enlargement may be evident.

In the "click-murmur syndrome" S-T segment and T wave abnormalities may be seen; in the familial form, the QT interval may be prolonged. Evidence of old or recent myocardial infarction may be seen with papillary muscle dysfunction caused by coronary heart disease.

Roentgenographic Features. The left ventricle and left atrium are usually enlarged. Occasionally, the left atrium is of giant size and can extend well into the right chest. The left ventricle is observed to contract vigorously on fluoroscopy, and systolic expansion of the left atrium may be striking. The presence of calcium in the mitral valve suggests some degree of associated mitral stenosis. If left atrial hypertension is marked, the findings in the lung fields resemble those of mitral stenosis.

Echocardiography. The echo from the mitral valve leaflets can be particularly useful in detecting abnormal posterior prolapse of one or both mitral leaflets into the left atrium during systole. This distinctive echocardiographic pattern may allow a definitive diagnosis in the *click-murmur syndrome* or papillary muscle dysfunction.

Cardiac Catheterization. Cardiac catheterization is indicated prior to considering cardiac surgery in order to confirm the presence of severe regurgitation, assess the degree of left ventricular myocardial dysfunction, exclude associated coronary artery disease, and assess the severity of any associated valvular lesions.

The severity of mitral regurgitation can be estimated by cineangiography, with injection of contrast medium into the left ventricle. The backward regurgitation of contrast medium into the left atrium during ventricular systole is readily apparent, and it is also possible to calculate the diastolic volume of the left ventricle, the total stroke volume, and the ejection fraction. If the forward cardiac output and forward stroke volume are calculated by the Fick method, when the regurgitation is severe the regurgitant volume per beat may be well in excess of the forward stroke volume.

An elevated V wave in the left atrium (peak of the V wave over 20 mm Hg) may be detected on the pulmonary artery wedge pressure tracing, or from direct measurement by transseptal puncture, with relatively normal mean left atrial pressure. The increased V wave is followed by a rapid pressure fall (the Y descent) as the ventricle relaxes, the mitral valve opens, and an excessively rapid inflow of blood (forward plus regurgitant volume) crosses the mitral valve in early diastole (see

figure in Ch. 556). Even with pure mitral regurgitation, there is often a pressure gradient across the mitral valve in early diastole, reflecting functional mitral stenosis in the presence of increased flow. A normal, simultaneous rise in left atrial and left ventricular pressures then ensues later in diastole, with no pressure gradient.

With the onset of left ventricular dysfunction, the ventricular end-diastolic pressure increases, the ratio of stroke volume to ventricular end-diastolic volume (ejection fraction) falls to less than 55 per cent, and the forward cardiac output diminishes. At this stage of the disease, pulmonary hypertension of moderate degree is generally present.

Differential Diagnosis. Several conditions may produce a systolic murmur resembling that of mitral regurgitation. The thrill and murmur of *ventricular septal defect* are pansystolic, but their location at the lower left sternal border is characteristic. The murmur of *tricuspid regurgitation* may be heard well to the left of the sternum whenever the right atrium and right ventricle are markedly enlarged, but the prominent V waves in the jugular venous pulse and the characteristic increase in intensity of the murmur with inspiration should help differentiate this lesion from mitral regurgitation.

When the jet of mitral regurgitation caused by a leak through the posterior mitral leaflet strikes the interatrial septum, the murmur is heard well in the aortic area, and it may be confused with the murmur of aortic stenosis. However, the murmur of mitral regurgitation increases when systemic arterial pressure is raised (as with the handgrip maneuver), and it decreases when the systemic arterial pressure is lowered (as with amyl nitrite inhalation), whereas opposite responses tend to occur in aortic stenosis.

The ejection type of murmur associated with *idiopathic hypertrophic subaortic stenosis* may be well heard at the apex, as well as at the left sternal border. The characteristic increase of this murmur with the Valsalva maneuver should provide a point of differentiation.

Treatment. *Medical Management.* In the absence of significant symptoms, the only therapeutic measures necessary are *antimicrobial prophylaxis* against streptococcal infections in the younger patient with a history of rheumatic fever and antimicrobial prophylaxis against bacterial endocarditis with dental or surgical procedures. With the onset of fatigue, dyspnea, or atrial fibrillation, the use of *digitalis* is indicated both to control the ventricular rate and to improve the contractile function of the left ventricle. Frequently, even in patients with severe mitral regurgitation, the use of an oral diuretic and digitalis, together with reduced sodium intake, will serve to maintain the patient in a comfortable status for a number of years.

Surgical Treatment. Surgical treatment is generally indicated when symptoms of severe fatigue or dyspnea occur on less than normal activity (N.Y.H.A. Class III or IV), despite appropriate medical management. Such symptoms generally indicate the onset of significant left ventricular myocardial disease. Obviously, in reaching the decision to recommend operation, the prolonged natural course of this disease should be kept in mind, and the low incidence of serious complications such as acute pulmonary edema, systemic emboli, and sudden death should be considered. Nevertheless, it is desirable to recommend operation prior to the development of irreversible left ventricular myocardial disease, and the persistence of significant symptoms while the patient is maintained on adequate medical therapy is generally considered to presage the onset of this process.

Occasionally, the surgical repair of a ruptured chorda or of a deficient posterior leaflet is possible. Almost always, however, in rheumatic and other forms of mitral regurgitation, replacement of the valve with a prosthesis is necessary. The average operative mortality is 6 to 10 per cent for this procedure, and with most types of valve prostheses, there is need for prolonged anticoagulant therapy. Sudden, severe mitral regurgitation is not well tolerated and generally requires early surgical intervention.

559.   AORTIC STENOSIS

Etiology and Pathology.   There is evidence that a congenitally bicuspid aortic valve is present in more than one half of adult patients with isolated aortic stenosis, most of the remainder being of rheumatic cause. Although the bicuspid valve is frequently not stenotic in early life, this malformation sets up abnormal stresses within the valve, leading to progressive fibrosis and thickening, with eventual immobility of the leaflets and calcification. This sequence may take many years, and the typical patient presents with findings of significant stenosis in the sixth decade of life. Three quarters of patients with isolated valvular aortic stenosis in adult life are male. The varieties of congenital aortic stenosis as they present in childhood and adolescence are discussed in Ch. 552. When aortic stenosis is due to rheumatic heart disease, the sex distribution is relatively equal, and frequently there is evidence of associated mitral valve involvement. With rheumatic disease, the aortic valve is tricuspid and shows fusion of one or more commissures and scarring and thickening of the leaflets; calcification may also be present. Acquired aortic stenosis may also occur in elderly subjects as a degenerative process without fusion of the commissures, stenosis resulting from heavy deposition of calcium within the valve leaflets. When calcification of the aortic valve is marked, the calcium may extend into the anulus and even into the upper portion of the ventricular septum, leading to involvement of the bundle of His or the left bundle branch.

When aortic stenosis is significant, the left ventricle shows concentric hypertrophy with marked thickening of the left ventricular wall, and there is poststenotic dilatation of the ascending aorta. The left atrium is usually normal unless there has been left ventricular failure.

Pathologic Physiology.   The earliest physiologic response to obstruction at the aortic valve, as in acute experimental constriction of the ascending aorta, is to cause an increased left ventricular diastolic volume and pressure and compensatory use of the Frank-Starling mechanism. Consequent to the more forceful contraction, the systolic left ventricular pressure is elevated and a pressure gradient is created across the aortic valve, forcing blood across the narrowed orifice at high velocity. The chronic effect of longstanding systolic pressure overload on the left ventricle is to induce hypertrophy of the ventricular wall, a compensatory process which tends to maintain the force or tension in the wall at relatively normal, without substantial enlargement of the left ventricular cavity. (Wall tension, or stress, is directly re-

lated to systolic pressure but inversely proportional to wall thickness, and the increased pressure load is distributed over a larger number of muscle fibers.) The stroke volume is generally well maintained by these mechanisms until very late in the disease. Even when the pressure gradient across the aortic valve is quite large, the compensatory left ventricular hypertrophy, coupled with a forceful left atrial contraction, serves to maintain the cardiac output at normal. This strong left atrial "booster pump" generates a prominent presystolic wave in the pressure tracings, leading to an elevated end-diastolic pressure in the hypertrophied and noncompliant ventricle (often near 20 mm Hg). However, elevation of the end-diastolic pressure by this mechanism does not indicate left ventricular failure, and the mean left atrial pressure is maintained at relatively normal.

It should be recognized that a significant gradient is not produced across the aortic valve until the valve orifice is narrowed substantially, by more than 60 per cent of its normal area. A murmur may be created by turbulent flow in the absence of a pressure gradient; but as the stenosis progresses beyond this critical point, an increasing systolic pressure gradient develops between the left ventricle and aorta.

With the increased heart rate which accompanies muscular exercise, diastole is primarily abbreviated, and therefore more time is available per minute for systolic ejection. Hence the aortic valve gradient does *not* tend to increase during exercise, despite an augmented cardiac output, and the left ventricular end-diastolic pressure and mean left atrial pressure may also remain unchanged. This finding is in marked contrast to the situation in mitral stenosis, when filling occurs during diastole and less time is available for flow during exercise.

The arterial pulse pressure is usually narrow when there is significant aortic stenosis, and an important accompanying effect is a tendency toward reduction of the diastolic aortic pressure. The perfusion pressure available to the coronary circulation is therefore diminished. In addition, the oxygen demands of the left ventricle are increased because of the hypertrophy and the need to maintain an elevated systolic pressure in the ventricle (often well over 200 mm Hg in severe aortic stenosis). Heart rate, as well as pressure development, is an important determinant of myocardial oxygen consumption, and the increased heart rate during exertion, together with a limitation of coronary perfusion pressure, can lead to an imbalance between oxygen supply and demand in the left ventricle. Thus *angina pectoris* is common in aortic stenosis in the absence of coronary artery disease. Transient myocardial ischemia in the hypertrophied heart may also explain, at least in part, the tendency toward *sudden serious arrhythmia* which can lead to sudden death. Likewise, this mechanism, perhaps coupled with transient hypotension caused by momentary inability to maintain cardiac output (such as may occur with sudden assumption of the upright posture), may have a role in the *syncopal attacks* which sometimes mark the clinical course of patients with aortic stenosis.

Longstanding pressure overwork by the hypertrophied left ventricle in aortic stenosis eventually leads to evidence of myocardial disease with inability of the heart muscle to maintain normal basal contractile processes, often associated with some degree of myocardial fibrosis. With the onset of left ventricular dysfunction, the degree of emptying becomes reduced. This, in turn, leads to an increased residual ventricular volume and elevation of the end-diastolic volume, with a further increase in the end-diastolic pressure. Elevation of the left atrial mean pressure then ensues, with the onset of orthopnea and exertional dyspnea through the same mechanisms discussed in Ch. 557. In the late phases of myocardial failure, pulmonary hypertension develops and cardiac output falls.

Clinical Manifestations. *Symptoms and Clinical Course.* Usually there is a latent period of many years, during which aortic stenosis is present and progressing in severity but symptoms are absent. When congenital aortic stenosis is severe, symptoms may occur in childhood, but typically they begin in middle or late life. If there is associated mitral valve disease in patients with rheumatic aortic stenosis, particularly mitral stenosis, the onset of symptoms may be much earlier and may lead to earlier detection of the associated aortic lesion. The three cardinal symptoms of aortic stenosis are (1) angina pectoris, (2) syncope, and (3) symptoms caused by left ventricular failure.

The pathophysiology of *angina pectoris* in aortic stenosis, an imbalance between oxygen supply and demand, is discussed above. It may mimic in every way the exertional chest pain which occurs in patients with coronary artery disease. In the older patient, the *coexistence* of coronary heart disease should be considered. Thus even when the aortic stenosis is moderate, or when stenotic lesions in the coronary vessels are moderate, increased oxygen utilization by the myocardium may lead to angina pectoris. Angina pectoris is often the first symptom in patients with aortic stenosis, and in the young patient it usually indicates severe obstruction to left ventricular ejection.

Syncope is sometimes the initial symptom in patients with aortic stenosis. This may be due to a transient arrhythmia such as atrial or ventricular tachycardia. The tendency of the hypertrophied ventricle to develop transient ischemia undoubtedly makes it more susceptible to ventricular fibrillation or ventricular tachycardia. Other mechanisms for syncope may consist of a transient fall in blood pressure during or immediately after exercise, or upon abruptly assuming the upright posture; such mechanisms are related to transient inability of the left ventricle to maintain a normal forward cardiac output, as discussed earlier, or are perhaps associated with metabolic or reflex peripheral vasodilatation. So-called presyncope may also occur, in which the patient experiences a transient graying out or loss of vision.

One of the major problems in the patient with hemodynamically significant aortic stenosis is the occurrence of *sudden death,* which is occasionally the first sign of the disease. In postmortem studies of patients who have died from aortic stenosis, death was sudden in about 15 per cent. It should be recognized, however, that most of these patients had significant symptoms, and that only 3 to 4 per cent of the patients who die do so without prior symptoms. The mechanism of sudden death is unclear, but it may be due to serious arrhythmia or mechanisms similar to those occurring with syncope.

With longstanding pressure overload, and increasing obstruction at the aortic valve, *left ventricular myocardial dysfunction* eventually develops. The earliest symptom of left ventricular dysfunction is usually orthopnea, caused by elevation of the left atrial mean pressure. Mild dyspnea on exertion may then ensue, which progresses to dyspnea on minimal exertion. In the late stages of aortic stenosis, pulmonary edema or evidence of pulmo-

nary hypertension with right ventricular failure and peripheral edema may occur.

The onset of atrial fibrillation in patients with aortic stenosis is uncommon, but when it occurs in the absence of mitral valve disease it is ominous. Usually it indicates an elevated mean left atrial pressure with left atrial distention. Because of the loss of left atrial contribution to ventricular filling, further elevation of the mean left atrial pressure, fall in the cardiac output, and severe cardiac failure may ensue.

The onset of symptoms in a patient with significant aortic stenosis has real importance, because the subsequent course is generally downhill. Although earlier mortality figures based on retrospective clinical analyses of patients with aortic stenosis may be modified somewhat by the advent of modern diuretic, antiarrhythmic, and antimicrobial therapy, the typical course after symptoms begin remains relatively short. Thus the average life expectancy in an adult patient after the onset of congestive heart failure is 18 months to 2 years; after the onset of angina pectoris it is about 5 years; and when syncope begins it is about 6 years, although survivals as long as 18 to 20 years after onset of syncope have been reported. The natural history in the patient with severe stenosis who has few or no symptoms has not been clearly established.

Complications of aortic stenosis include *bacterial endocarditis,* which has been estimated to occur in as many as 25 per cent of patients during their lifetime. Rarely, hemolytic anemia has been seen in patients with severe calcific aortic stenosis, presumably owing to local blood trauma at the valve, and perhaps also to intrinsic red blood cell abnormalities. Systemic emboli have been reported as a result of calcium or fibrin particles breaking loose from the aortic valve.

Physical Findings. The primary findings on physical examination can be related to three features: abnormal ejection of blood into the arterial bed, turbulent flow and prolonged ejection across the stenotic aortic orifice, and left ventricular hypertrophy. Physical findings reflecting all three phenomena can generally be detected in hemodynamically significant aortic valve obstruction; but despite their helpfulness, such signs do not always predict accurately the degree of stenosis in the individual patient.

The patient with aortic stenosis is typically not debilitated or wasted, the cardiac output being well maintained until late in the course of the disease. The mean jugular venous pressure is generally normal, although the A wave may be prominent in patients with hemodynamically significant aortic stenosis, presumably because of septal hypertrophy with decreased right ventricular compliance. The carotid pulse is small, the upstroke is delayed, and a systolic thrill may be felt in the carotid vessels. The blood pressure is usually low-normal, with narrowing of the pulse pressure, but in elderly patients having reduced compliance (increased stiffness) of the aortic wall and arteries it is not unusual to find an elevated *systolic* blood pressure, even in the presence of significant aortic stenosis. However, marked systemic hypertension with a substantial diastolic pressure elevation is not encountered in the presence of severe aortic stenosis.

On palpation of the precordium, there is a systolic thrill at the aortic area, the apex beat is enlarged, and there is a sustained apical impulse. A presystolic atrial impulse may be palpable at the apex in the lateral decubitus position. The first heart sound is usually normal, and the aortic component of the second heart sound is diminished. Often, the second heart sound is single owing to a prolonged left ventricular ejection time; or aortic valve closure may even follow pulmonic valve closure, leading to paradoxical splitting of the second heart sound (decreased splitting during inspiration) (see figure in Ch. 556). The *systolic murmur* of aortic stenosis is crescendo-decrescendo in quality, is loudest at the aortic area, is transmitted to the carotid arteries, and is also audible at the apex. Being ejection in type, the murmur begins well after the first heart sound and ends before the second heart sound. In the presence of severe aortic stenosis, the murmur is long and peaks in mid- or late systole. Frequently there is an atrial diastolic gallop (fourth heart sound), which reflects both reduced compliance of the thickened left ventricular wall and forceful left atrial contraction. This gallop is best heard in the left lateral decubitus position.

When aortic stenosis is mild, there tends to be less delay of the carotid upstroke, the duration of ventricular ejection may be normal, and the second heart sound splits normally with respiration. The systolic murmur tends to be less intense and shorter, peaking early in systole. It should be appreciated, however, that in the late stages of aortic stenosis, when cardiac failure and low cardiac output supervene, the murmur of aortic stenosis may also become markedly diminished in intensity. Under these circumstances, the left ventricle is generally substantially enlarged, and there are symptoms and signs of cardiac failure.

It is not uncommon to hear a soft, early diastolic blowing murmur at the left sternal border caused by mild aortic regurgitation, even in patients with severe aortic stenosis. This small leak occurs because of the small, fixed orifice. The murmur of associated mitral stenosis should be searched for carefully, particularly in female patients with aortic stenosis, because the association of these two obstructive lesions serves to diminish the physical findings of each. When mitral and aortic stenosis coexist, the cardiac output tends to be reduced, the severity of aortic stenosis may be underestimated, and the murmur of mitral stenosis may be difficult to appreciate.

Diagnosis (see table). *Electrocardiogram.* In both children and adults, a normal electrocardiogram is rarely found in the presence of significant aortic stenosis. In children under 10 or 12 years of age, the degree of left ventricular hypertrophy on the electrocardiogram tends to relate to the degree of obstruction, but in adults relatively marked degrees of left ventricular hypertrophy are sometimes seen in mild or moderate obstruction. Typically, the electrocardiogram shows voltage criteria for left ventricular hypertrophy, with associated S-T segment and T wave changes and left atrial enlargement. Occasionally, intraventricular conduction delay or left bundle branch block is seen, particularly late in the course of the disease, and atrial fibrillation is a late and relatively uncommon problem. Complete heart block has been reported in some patients resulting from extension of aortic calcification into the conduction system.

Roentgenographic Features. There may be little or no over-all cardiac enlargement, but when aortic stenosis is significant some degree of left ventricular enlargement is usually discernible, with straightening of the left heart border, downward displacement of the left ventricular apex, and overlapping of the spine by the left ventricular shadow at 60 degrees of rotation in the left anterior oblique view. In the presence of left ventricular failure, the chamber is enlarged and the left atrium is also usually dilated, causing posterior displacement of the barium-filled esophagus. When significant left atrial enlargement is seen, however, it should always raise the suspicion of associated mitral stenosis. Poststenotic dilatation of the ascending aorta is common in the frontal view, and calcification of the aortic valve should be searched for on the plain roentgenogram. However, image intensification fluoroscopy may be necessary for detection of mild valve calcification. In the presence of left ventricular failure, there is evidence of pulmonary venous engorgement and interstitial pulmonary edema.

Cardiac Catheterization. In patients who have symptoms, cardiac catheterization is carried out to determine whether the degree of mechanical obstruction at the aortic valve is sufficient to warrant surgical treatment. It is important to measure both the systolic pressure gradient between left ventricle and aorta (see figure) and the cardiac output at the time of left heart catheterization because of the nonlinear relation between the pressure and flow across the stenotic orifice, the orifice area being directly related to flow and inversely proportional to the square root of the pressure gradient (see Ch. 557). Thus if the cardiac output is reduced by 30 per cent, the pressure gradient will fall by about 50 per cent and the severity of the stenosis will be underestimated if the pressure gradient alone is relied upon. For example, when myocardial failure is responsible for a reduced resting cardiac output, the peak gradient from left ventricle to aorta may be below 50 mm Hg, even in the presence of marked aortic valve narrowing.

When the cardiac output is normal, with relatively mild aortic stenosis the aortic valve orifice area is between 0.75 and 1.5 sq cm in the adult (normal area 2.5 sq cm), and the systolic pressure gradient across the aortic valve is small. When aortic stenosis is moderate, the orifice area is 0.5 to 0.75 sq cm and the peak pressure gradient usually exceeds 50 mm Hg. With very severe or "tight" aortic stenosis, the orifice area is 0.5 sq cm or less, there may be a left ventricular systolic pressure in excess of 250 mm Hg, and transvalvular pressure gradient is often over 100 mm Hg. The right heart pressures are normal, unless there is left ventricular failure which can produce pulmonary hypertension. Simultaneous measurements should be made of the pulmonary artery wedge pressure and the left ventricular pressure to exclude associated mitral stenosis.

It is important that selective left ventricular angiography be carried out to document the functional status of the left ventricle. Such a study will indicate whether or not the left ventricular end-diastolic volume is elevated and the ejection fraction reduced to below 55 per cent, factors which bear on the operative risk in the individual patient. In older patients, it is also important that selective coronary arteriography be performed. Lack of appreciation of significant coronary artery lesions can lead to difficulty during surgical treatment, and coronary revascularization procedures are sometimes carried out at the time of the aortic valve replacement.

Phonocardiography. Recording of heart sounds and the external carotid pulse wave may help in assessing the severity of aortic stenosis by documenting the presence or absence of a single second heart sound, paradoxical splitting, or a prolonged ejection time. A slow rising carotid pulse wave and the characteristics of the ejection murmur can also be documented.

Differential Diagnosis. An ejection murmur at the aortic area and lower left sternal border can be heard in the patient with *idiopathic hypertrophic subaortic stenosis,* although the murmur is generally poorly transmitted to the carotid vessels and has other special features (see Ch. 560). The key differentiating points between this lesion and valvular aortic stenosis are shown in the accompanying table.

In the younger patient who has a murmur suggesting congenital aortic stenosis, other locations for the lesion (supravalvular, subvalvular membrane) should be considered. Occasionally the murmur of papillary muscle dysfunction or ruptured chordae tendineae, caused by mitral regurgitation through the posterior leaflet, can mimic the murmur of aortic stenosis. The mitral regurgitant jet impinges on the interatrial septum, which is directly contiguous to the posterior wall of the aorta, leading to transmission of the murmur to the aortic area; however, this murmur tends to transmit poorly to the carotid arteries; it increases with isometric handgrip and diminishes with amyl nitrite inhalation, whereas the murmur of aortic stenosis will behave in an opposite manner with these two maneuvers.

Treatment. *Medical Management.* The adult patient with findings suggestive of moderate aortic stenosis and no symptoms may be followed carefully, although cardiac catheterization is sometimes done to be certain of the severity of obstruction. In such patients, very strenuous physical exertion, such as competitive athletics, should be prohibited in order to minimize risk of sudden death. Antimicrobial prophylaxis for dental or surgical procedures is advised to prevent the development of bacterial endocarditis. In children or adolescents with congenital aortic stenosis who are suspected of having severe obstruction, cardiac catheterization is generally advised even when they are without symptoms.

Early symptoms of orthopnea or mild dyspnea may respond temporarily to digitalis, sodium restriction, and diuresis. However, as soon as significant symptoms appear (angina, syncope, or symptoms of left ventricular failure), the adult patient should usually be sent for cardiac catheterization and coronary arteriography, and consideration should be given to early operation.

Surgical Treatment. In children or young adult patients with congenital aortic stenosis, surgical treatment is generally advocated even in the absence of significant symptoms if the obstruction is severe, because the risk of operation appears to be lower than the risk of sudden death. The bicuspid valve in the young patient is generally favorable for a valvuloplasty, and clinical improvement may be experienced for a number of years.

In the adult patient with symptoms and significant narrowing of the aortic orifice (less than 0.75 sq cm) or peak systolic pressure gradient over 50 mm Hg with normal cardiac output, aortic valve replacement, using a prosthesis or a graft, is carried out, using cardiopulmonary bypass. In patients with severe associated coronary artery disease, saphenous vein bypass grafting may also be performed. If there is associated severe mitral valve disease, double valve replacement is sometimes necessary.

The question whether the adult patient with documented, hemodynamically severe aortic stenosis but with few symptoms should be operated upon is not settled at present. The risk of aortic valve replacement is now between 5 and 10 per cent in many centers, but whether the risk of sudden death in asymptomatic patients over a period of several years approaches this figure is unknown. Therefore older patients are referred for operation if they have significant symptoms.

Differential Diagnosis in Aortic Stenosis

	Valvular Aortic Stenosis	Idiopathic Hypertrophic Subaortic Stenosis
Carotid pulse	Delayed	Rapid and bifid
Systolic murmur, location	Second right ICS, neck and apex	LLSB and apex
Effect of Valsalva maneuver	Murmur decreased	Murmur increased
Aortic closure sound	Soft	Normal
Systolic ejection click	Common when valve not calcified	Rare
Diastolic murmur of aortic regurgitation	Common	Rare
Electrocardiogram	LVH	Marked LVH; deep Q waves (septal in origin); left atrial enlargement
Chest roentgenogram	Normal heart size	Cardiomegaly (left ventricular); left atrial enlargement
Poststenotic dilatation of aorta	Present	Absent
Calcium in aortic valve	Present	Absent

LLSB = Lower left sternal border; ICS = intercostal space; LVH = left ventricular hypertrophy.

560. IDIOPATHIC HYPERTROPHIC SUBAORTIC STENOSIS

Definition. Idiopathic hypertrophic subaortic stenosis (IHSS) is synonymous with the terms muscular subaortic stenosis and hypertrophic obstructive cardiomyopathy. Because all patients with this form of left ventricular hypertrophy do not exhibit hemodynamic obstruction within the left ventricular outflow tract, the more general term asymmetric septal hypertrophy is sometimes used.

Etiology and Pathology. Hypertrophy of the muscular wall of the left ventricle is particularly prominent in the region of the interventricular septum. The septum may be several times as thick as the free wall, and abnormalities in the direction of fibers and in the connections between myofilaments have been demonstrated by electron microscopy in the septal region. In cases in which obstruction is present, the anterior leaflet of the mitral valve is thickened, probably secondary to contact with the hypertrophied septum, and the chordae tendineae may be thickened and elongated. The aortic valve is normal.

An autosomal dominant mode of inheritance has been recognized in some patients with this disease. When echocardiography is used to identify enlargement of the interventricular septum in individuals without other physical findings, it has been claimed that in the great majority of instances this pattern of inheritance can be documented in the relatives of patients who have evident disease.

Pathologic Physiology. Although hypertrophy of the left ventricular wall is most marked in the region of the interventricular septum, hypertrophy also is present elsewhere in the ventricle, and reduced ventricular compliance leads to increased resistance to ventricular filling from the left atrium. The left ventricular end-diastolic pressure is usually elevated in patients with or without obstruction. There is a prominent atrial contraction wave, and the mean left atrial pressure may be somewhat elevated.

The hallmark is variable obstruction to left ventricular ejection below the aortic valve, in the ventricular outflow tract. There is a pressure gradient between the body of the left ventricle and the outflow tract, and the obstruction has been shown to result from abnormal forward movement of the anterior mitral valve leaflet during systole. This leaflet forms the posterior wall of the ventricular outflow tract; when the leading edge of the anterior mitral leaflet meets the hypertrophied septum during ejection, obstruction is produced. This malposition of the anterior mitral valve leaflet probably results largely from lateral displacement of the papillary muscles by the enlarged interventricular septum, and the abnormal position produces some mitral regurgitation as well.

Because of the dynamic nature of the obstruction, the pressure gradient tends to develop progressively during the course of each cardiac systole. There is no obstruction initially, leading to the sharp, early arterial upstroke, but the arterial pulse falls rapidly as the obstruction develops. The pressure gradient may also be variable over time, and can be altered by a variety of interventions. Influences which alter left ventricular volume, systemic arterial pressure (which affects the distending pressure in the outflow tract during systole), or the force of muscular contraction change the caliber of the muscular outflow tract and affect the degree of obstruction. For example, the Valsalva maneuver or assumption of the upright posture produces a decrease in venous return, a fall in arterial pressure, and reflex tachycardia, all of which reduce ventricular volume and outflow tract size. The associated reflex increase in contractility further augments the degree of obstruction with these maneuvers, and the pressure gradient across the outflow tract increases.

Clinical Manifestations. *Symptoms and Clinical Course.* Patients may be detected because of a long-standing heart murmur, sometimes first noted in childhood. In patients with severe left ventricular hypertrophy and outflow tract obstruction, the chief symptoms resemble those of valvular aortic stenosis: angina pectoris (which may be atypical in character), syncope, and manifestations of left ventricular failure. Angina pectoris results from an imbalance between oxygen supply and demand in the hypertrophied ventricle (see Ch. 559) and is usually exertional in nature. However, patients with this disease may experience prolonged, severe chest pain mimicking that of myocardial infarction, undoubtedly related to increased oxygen demand consequent to the elevated left ventricular systolic pressure and marked ventricular hypertrophy. Symptoms caused by

pulmonary congestion and low cardiac output may occur, in part related to the reduced left ventricular compliance and impaired left atrial emptying which characterize this disease, as well as to severe obstruction. However, all these symptoms, including sudden death, also occur in patients without significant obstruction. The clinical picture in such patients can resemble that of a generalized cardiomyopathy.

The course tends to be variable, particularly in patients with mild to moderate symptoms, and periods of spontaneous improvement may be noted. With severe obstruction the disease may be progressive, death usually being due to congestive heart failure. Tachyarrhythmias and atrial fibrillation are poorly tolerated complications, and may lead to severe hypotension. Bacterial endocarditis, once considered rare, has recently been reported in between 5 and 10 per cent of cases.

Physical Findings. The jugular venous pulse generally exhibits a prominent A wave, owing to reduced right ventricular compliance. The carotid pulse is sharp, and when a gradient is present across the outflow tract, the pulse is bisferious with a secondary tidal wave. The left ventricular apex is displaced laterally, in the lateral decubitus position a presystolic apical impulse can usually be felt, and sometimes there is a double impulse during systole as well. With significant obstruction, a systolic thrill may be felt at the lower left sternal border.

On auscultation, there is a low-pitched systolic ejection murmur at the lower left sternal border, which is also heard at the apex but transmits poorly to the base and is not transmitted to the carotid arteries or the left axilla. Sometimes there is a separate pansystolic murmur at the cardiac apex associated with mitral regurgitation. If a murmur is absent in an individual without obstruction at rest, it may be induced by the Valsalva maneuver. If the murmur is present, it can be markedly augmented during the Valsalva maneuver, and it is greatly diminished or disappears after release of the Valsalva maneuver. The murmur of hypertrophic subaortic stenosis may also be increased by having the patient suddenly assume the upright posture, and it may be abolished by squatting.

Diagnosis (see table in Ch. 559). *Electrocardiogram.* A normal electrocardiogram is very rare in the presence of this disorder. Usually there is evidence of left ventricular hypertrophy, which is often striking, with secondary S-T segment and T wave changes. Left atrial enlargement is common. In addition, the hypertrophied septum frequently leads to enlarged initial QRS forces, and prominent "septal" Q waves may be seen in leads II, III, AVF, AVL, or the precordial leads. These changes often resemble those of previous myocardial infarction. There also may be prominent R waves in the limb or right precordial leads. In about 10 per cent of patients, there is a short P-R interval and a partial delta wave, suggestive of a variant of the Wolff-Parkinson-White syndrome. An intraventricular conduction delay is sometimes seen, and left bundle branch block occurs occasionally.

Roentgenographic   Features. The   plain   chest roentgenogram shows left ventricular enlargement, often with a bulge along the lateral wall of the left ventricle in the frontal view, and left atrial enlargement is frequent. The aorta is small, and there is no poststenotic dilatation. There is no calcification in the aortic valve.

Phonocardiogram. When obstruction is present, the indirect carotid pulse wave shows a characteristic sharp upstroke followed by a tidal wave. The murmur is of the ejection type, beginning after the first heart sound and ending before the second sound, and varying intensity of the murmur with provocations can be documented by the phonocardiogram.

Echocardiogram. Ultrasound provides the most useful noninvasive method for diagnosis. In patients with obstruction, the tracing shows an abnormal systolic anterior movement of the mitral valve leaflet. In addition, there is disproportionate thickness in the region of the interventricular septum, as compared to the posterior free wall.

Cardiac Catheterization. The characteristic finding in hypertrophic subaortic stenosis is a pressure gradient within the outflow tract of the left ventricle, the pressure being high in the left ventricular chamber and reduced in the outflow tract, with no pressure gradient across the aortic valve. It is important to measure the elevated systolic pressure in the *inflow tract* of the left ventricle just in front of the mitral valve, because when the catheter is entrapped in the apex, artifactually high ventricular systolic pressures may be measured. Usually the left ventricular end-diastolic pressure is elevated to 20 mm Hg or more owing to a large presystolic wave in the left ventricle, reflecting a large A wave in the left atrium.

If there is no pressure gradient across the outflow tract at rest, or if the gradient is small, it may be increased by having the patient perform a Valsalva maneuver. This decreases venous return, augments heart rate, and increases left ventricular contractility, all of which serve to narrow the outflow tract further and enhance the gradient. In fixed, valvular aortic stenosis the pressure gradient diminishes during the Valsalva maneuver. In addition, an infusion of isoproterenol or administration of amyl nitrite may bring out the pressure gradient, although these agents also will increase the gradient in valvular aortic stenosis.

The pressure gradient tends to diminish markedly during the systemic arterial pressure overshoot after the release of the Valsalva maneuver in hypertrophic subaortic stenosis, and the pressure gradient may be greatly reduced or abolished by infusion of a pressor agent such as methoxamine, or by administration of propranolol. All these maneuvers tend to increase left ventricular volume and reduce contractility and heart rate, thereby widening the outflow tract and decreasing the obstruction.

A characteristic sign, which helps differentiate this lesion from valvular aortic stenosis, is the alteration of pulse pressure in the beat after a ventricular extrasystole. In hypertrophic subaortic stenosis, the systemic arterial *pulse pressure decreases* during this beat, the increased force of contraction produced by postextrasystolic potentiation leading to a narrower outflow tract, increased obstruction, and fall in stroke volume. In valvular aortic stenosis, however, the stroke volume increases and the pulse pressure is augmented. Although 25 to 30 per cent of patients exhibit a small pressure gradient across the right ventricular outflow tract caused by septal bulging, in a few patients a subvalvular pressure gradient may be quite marked on the right side.

Left ventricular angiography shows characteristic findings. There is enormous hypertrophy of the interventricular septum, often with marked distortion of the shape of the left ventricular cavity, and with lateral tilting of the papillary muscles. During systole, the mitral valve can be visualized as it is held forward in an abnormal position, obstructing the left ventricular outflow tract. Mitral regurgitation, usually moderate, occurs beneath this displaced leaflet and is best seen in the oblique or lateral view.

Differential Diagnosis. The murmur of hypertrophic subaortic stenosis may be confused with that of valvular aortic stenosis, but a number of differences in the physical examination, x-ray, and electrocardiogram clarify the diagnosis (see table in Ch. 559).

The systolic murmur is also frequently mistaken for that of mitral regurgitation alone, or of papillary muscle dysfunction. The Valsalva maneuver may be useful in differentiating these murmurs, and the echocardiogram will show characteristically different movements of the anterior mitral valve leaflet. The occurrence of angina pectoris and Q waves in the electrocardiogram sometimes causes a mistaken diagnosis of coronary heart disease.

Treatment. *Medical Treatment.* Beta-adrenergic blocking agents, such as propranolol, have been shown to acutely reduce the pressure gradient at cardiac catheterization in patients with hypertrophic subaortic stenosis. Chronic oral administration of these agents may relieve angina pectoris, and they appear to be particularly effective in patients with latent obstruction. Propranolol also tends to slow the heart rate and improve ventricular filling, and syncope may be relieved. Digitalis and nitroglycerin tend to increase the obstruction; they should be used with caution or avoided.

Atrial fibrillation is poorly tolerated by patients with hypertrophic subaortic stenosis because of loss of the atrial contribution to ventricular filling, and the noncompliant left ventricle then requires an elevated mean left atrial pressure to maintain an adequate diastolic ventricular volume. In addition, if the ventricular response is rapid in atrial fibrillation (or if atrial tachyarrhythmias occur), the hypertrophied left ventricle relaxes poorly and hypotension with pulmonary congestion may result. Therefore such arrhythmias should be promptly terminated by appropriate drugs or electrical reversion.

If the patient with hypertrophic subaortic stenosis becomes hypotensive, the use of isoproterenol will increase the obstruction and generally worsen the patient's condition. Therefore drugs of choice are peripheral vasoconstrictor agents, such as methoxamine or phenylephrine.

Surgical Treatment. Operation is usually reserved for patients with severe symptoms and marked outflow tract obstruction. The most widely used surgical procedure consists of resecting a portion of the hypertrophied left ventricular outflow tract, the septum being approached through the aorta and aortic valve. In some centers, simple myotomy with division of the fibers of the outflow tract has also resulted in relief of the obstruction. These operations have generally been successful, often producing complete or nearly complete relief of the left ventricular pressure gradient, but operative mortality has ranged between 10 and 20 per cent. Replacement of the mitral valve with a prosthesis in order to remove the posterior component of the obstruction (the anterior mitral valve leaflet) has been used with some success, but the complications associated with insertion of a prosthetic device limit the application of this approach.

561. AORTIC REGURGITATION

Etiology and Pathology. Aortic regurgitation is usually the result of rheumatic fever, but it has been described as a complication of an increasing number of systemic diseases (see below). A careful history may be of substantial help in ascertaining etiology. In chronic aortic regurgitation of rheumatic etiology, the aortic valve leaflets are scarred, thickened, and retracted and do not close during diastole. With longstanding disease, marked dilatation of the ascending aorta and the aortic anulus may add further to the insufficiency. Combined aortic stenosis and regurgitation are most frequently associated with rheumatic disease, but can also be seen in the late stages of a congenitally bicuspid valve. Aortic regurgitation may be associated with the most marked enlargement and hypertrophy of the left ventricle encountered in valvular heart disease. Approximately 70 per cent of patients with predominant aortic regurgitation are male.

Isolated congenital aortic regurgitation has rarely been reported as a consequence of a bicuspid aortic valve, but congenital aortic regurgitation can occur as a complication of discrete subvalvular stenosis which produces secondary thickening and insufficiency of the aortic leaflets. In younger children, ventricular septal defect may be complicated by prolapse of an aortic valve leaflet, thereby causing aortic regurgitation.

Acquired aortic regurgitation occurs in association with the following conditions: (1) *Syphilis,* which causes scarring and degeneration of the media and intima of the ascending aorta, resulting in part from disease of the vasa vasorum. There can be an aneurysm in the ascending aorta and dilatation of the aortic anulus, with thickening of the aortic leaflets, as well as narrowing of the coronary ostia caused by syphilitic involvement of the aortic intima. (2) *Ankylosing spondylitis,* in which associated medial disease of the aorta results in significant aortic regurgitation. (3) *Rheumatoid arthritis;* degeneration of the aortic valve leaflets and the ascending aorta have been described. (4) *Marfan's syndrome,* in which loss of elastic tissue and connective tissue degenerative changes can lead to marked dilatation of the aorta and aortic anulus with severe aortic regurgitation. (5) *Hurler's syndrome,* or mucopolysaccharidosis, which may be accompanied by significant aortic regurgitation. (6) *Severe systemic hypertension,* which can be associated with aortic dilatation and relative aortic insufficiency; other complications associated with hypertension, such as ascending aortic aneurysm or dissecting aneurysm, may also cause aortic regurgitation. (7) *Bacterial endocarditis,* which usually occurs on a deformed valve, and can lead to rapid progression of aortic regurgitation or to fenestration of the leaflets.

Pathologic Physiology. The physiologic defect in aortic regurgitation is retrograde leakage of blood from the aorta into the left ventricle during diastole. This results in low diastolic aortic pressure and increase in the end-diastolic volume of the left ventricle. The amount of blood ejected during systole is abnormally large, because it consists of the normal stroke volume plus blood regurgitated during the previous diastolic period. In severe aortic regurgitation the amount of blood regurgitated per beat may equal or even exceed the forward stroke volume. The initial compensation to this volume overload on the left ventricle is by the Frank-Starling

mechanism (increased end-diastolic volume), and in mild aortic regurgitation there is increased systolic emptying as well, with little chronic dilatation of the ventricle. As regurgitation becomes more severe, the left ventricle slowly dilates, and new sarcomeres are laid down both in parallel and in series in the left ventricular wall during the process of dilatation and hypertrophy. This compensatory mechanism allows the enlarged left ventricle to deliver a greater stroke volume, but with normal shortening of each unit of the enlarged circumference.

The pathophysiology of aortic regurgitation somewhat resembles the volume overload of mitral regurgitation, but there are two important differences. (1) The increased forward stroke volume is delivered into a high impedance system (the aorta), and because the total forward stroke volume is increased, the left ventricular and aortic systolic pressures are elevated (sometimes to 160 mm Hg or higher). This, together with the increased size of the left ventricular chamber, leads to pressure as well as volume overloading and a somewhat elevated myocardial oxygen consumption. (2) The lowered diastolic aortic pressure tends to impair coronary artery perfusion. Normally the coronary blood flow occurs during diastole; with the reduced diastolic pressure which accompanies aortic regurgitation, coronary blood flow may become inadequate either during exercise or when heart rate and hence the diastolic pressure become very low, as during sleep. The increased myocardial oxygen consumption coupled with relative underperfusion of the coronary bed may lead to an imbalance between oxygen supply and demand. Thus unlike patients with mitral regurgitation, patients with severe aortic regurgitation commonly develop *angina pectoris* in the absence of coronary artery disease.

With adequate left ventricular myocardial contractility the ejection fraction of the left ventricle (ratio of stroke volume to end-diastolic volume) is maintained at normal (over 55 per cent), the forward cardiac output is normal, and left ventricular end-diastolic pressure may remain nearly normal despite ventricular dilatation. However, because longstanding overload leads to myocardial damage and depression of contractility, the extent of wall shortening during ejection tends to diminish, the residual volume in the left ventricle rises, and the end-diastolic pressure in the left ventricle becomes elevated. Indeed, in the late stages of severe aortic regurgitation the diastolic pressure in the aorta and that in the left ventricle may reach equilibration near the end of diastole, leading to an abbreviation of the murmur. Occasionally, "preclosure" of the mitral valve even occurs, leading to a dissociation between the rising left ventricular diastolic pressure and the left atrial pressure, which remains at a lower level. This situation may occur in sudden severe aortic regurgitation, such as with bacterial endocarditis, when sufficient time has not elapsed for ventricular dilatation and hypertrophy to occur. Such mitral valve preclosure may be audible as a snapping sound in mid- to late diastole.

In the late stages of aortic regurgitation the cardiac output decreases, and the left ventricular end-diastolic pressure becomes further elevated because of myocardial failure. The mean left atrial pressure then rises, leading to decreased pulmonary compliance and interstitial edema, and acute pulmonary edema occasionally occurs.

Clinical Manifestations. *Symptoms and Clinical Course.* The typical patient with rheumatic aortic regurgitation has experienced acute rheumatic fever in childhood, and a period of about ten years then follows during which the severity of the regurgitant lesion progresses. Marked aortic regurgitation may become apparent by age 18 or 20, and there often follows a period of compensation during which the patient is asymptomatic, despite the presence of severe regurgitation. Occasionally during this stage of the disease, palpitations caused by transient atrial arrhythmias, headache caused by the high systolic blood pressure during exercise, or subjective sensations resulting from cardiac hyperactivity may be noted. Studies in children followed for many years after developing severe aortic regurgitation indicate that even after 20 years about 25 per cent of the individuals with this lesion remained asymptomatic. However, the average duration of the latent or asymptomatic period in severe aortic regurgitation is about ten years.

The earliest symptoms are usually due to the onset of left ventricular dysfunction or to coronary insufficiency. Mild dyspnea on exertion is noted as a result of elevation of the left ventricular end-diastolic and mean left atrial pressures during exercise. The length of time between onset of this symptom and death of the patient averages seven to ten years, although it should be recognized that many of these data were derived before the advent of modern diuretic therapy and rheumatic fever prophylaxis. Angina pectoris usually begins somewhat later, postdating the onset of dypsnea by two to three years. It may occur during exertion, and may or may not respond to nitroglycerin. Angina pectoris can also be atypical and occur at rest or at night, presumably caused by low heart rate which can lead to very low diastolic aortic pressure and inadequate coronary perfusion during long diastolic periods. The onset of severe nocturnal angina associated with profuse sweating, particularly in young patients, can portend a poor prognosis.

Once left ventricular decompensation begins, patients with severe aortic regurgitation usually tolerate infections poorly. They may experience severe congestive heart failure, and they are also at some risk of unexpected death. There are no clear-cut figures on the incidence of sudden death in patients with severe aortic regurgitation; although not as common as in aortic stenosis, it is by no means rare and probably results from sudden ventricular arrhythmia. In the late stages of severe aortic regurgitation, orthopnea and paroxysmal nocturnal dyspnea occur, and eventually symptoms and signs of right ventricular failure may supervene.

The natural history in the other forms of aortic regurgitation depends largely on the rapidity with which the lesion develops and on its severity. Patients with aortic regurgitation caused by syphilis may exhibit a course resembling that of rheumatic disease, although it usually begins later in life. With acute regurgitation such as that in bacterial endocarditis, there is insufficient time for chronic compensation to occur, and the clinical course may be fulminating. Under these circumstances, severe intractable left ventricular failure may develop.

Physical Findings. The diastolic pressure determined by sphygmomanometry correlates generally with the severity of the regurgitant leak, although in some patients there is severe regurgitation with diastolic pressure as high as 60 mm Hg. A diastolic sound over the artery is usually audible down to 0 mm Hg when regurgitation is severe, but the level at which the diastolic sound muffles corresponds reasonably well to the directly measured aortic pressure at the end of diastole, deter-

mined by a needle within the artery. The systolic arterial pressure is elevated. Characteristic clinical features caused by the large stroke volume and rapid runoff of blood from the aorta consist of *head bobbing* (a nodding motion of the head with each systole, which may be visible from a considerable distance), *visible pulsations of the carotid arteries,* a *Corrigan or water-hammer pulse* (sharp upstroke with collapsing quality), *Quincke's sign* (on light compression of the fingernail, alternate blushing and blanching are visible in the nailbed with each cardiac cycle), *pistol shot sounds* on auscultation with a stethoscope over the femoral arteries, and *Duroziez' murmur* (a to-and-fro bruit over the femoral artery, using slight compression with stethoscope diaphragm). Palpation of the carotid arteries may reveal a bisferious or bifid pulse, particularly if there is some associated aortic stenosis.

On palpation of the precordium, a diastolic thrill may be felt at the lower left sternal border, and a systolic thrill is palpable at the aortic area, the jugular notch, and the carotid arteries. The left ventricle is enlarged, the apex is displaced laterally, and the apex beat is hyperkinetic with marked retraction during systole.

The first heart sound may be normal or slightly reduced; the aortic component of the second heart sound is diminished or inaudible in the presence of severe regurgitation. Frequently, a loud third heart sound is audible at the apex, and there may also be a fourth heart sound. The most characteristic feature of the lesion is a decrescendo, blowing *diastolic murmur* at the left sternal border in the third and fourth intercostal spaces (see figure in Ch. 556). In the presence of mild aortic regurgitation, this murmur is high pitched, soft, and heard only in early diastole; it may be appreciated only with the patient in an upright position, leaning forward, and with held expiration. With a more severe regurgitant leak, the murmur may have a somewhat rougher quality and may last throughout diastole. Late in the course of severe aortic regurgitation, or with acute aortic regurgitation, the diastolic murmur may be shortened by equilibration of aortic pressure with markedly elevated left ventricular end-diastolic pressure before the end of diastole; occasionally, a snapping sound caused by mitral valve "preclosure" is audible (see above). In patients in whom the aortic regurgitation is due primarily to aneurysmal dilatation of the ascending aorta or to enlargement of the aortic anulus, as in Marfan's syndrome, the diastolic murmur may be loudest to the *right* of the sternum, thereby providing a clue to the cause.

Invariably, when aortic regurgitation is severe, there is a systolic ejection murmur at the aortic area which is transmitted to the jugular notch and carotid arteries. This may be very loud even in the presence of pure aortic regurgitation, reflecting the extremely large stroke volume delivered across a deformed aortic valve, but usually there is little or no pressure gradient from left ventricle to aorta during systole. Frequently in the presence of severe aortic regurgitation, an *Austin Flint diastolic rumble* is audible at the apex. Although true mitral stenosis may accompany aortic regurgitation of rheumatic origin, the Austin Flint rumble is characterized by its onset with a third heart sound; it is loudest in mid-diastole and often exhibits some presystolic accentuation. The Austin Flint murmur is probably due not only to interference with opening of the anterior mitral leaflet by the regurgitant jet, but also to a more rapid rise in the left ventricular than the left atrial diastolic pressure. The effect is to prevent full opening of the normal mitral leaflets during diastole, leading to turbulent flow across the mitral orifice (see Ch. 557, Differential Diagnosis).

Sometimes, in the late stages of aortic regurgitation when left ventricular dilatation and failure are present, a holosystolic murmur of relative mitral regurgitation may be audible at the cardiac apex. Signs of pulmonary hypertension and right ventricular enlargement may also be encountered in the late stages of the disease.

Diagnosis. *Electrocardiogram.* The electrocardiogram usually shows left ventricular hypertrophy, sometimes of marked degree, with associated S-T segment and T wave changes. Left atrial enlargement may also be present, particularly when the left ventricular end-diastolic pressure becomes elevated. When myocardial disease develops, left axis deviation, intraventricular conduction defects, or left bundle branch block may occur. Atrial fibrillation is a late and relatively uncommon complication.

Roentgenographic Features. The major findings are enlargement of the left ventricle and aorta with vigorous pulsations of the ascending aorta on fluoroscopy. The left ventricular enlargement is characterized by a downward and lateral displacement of the left ventricular apex, the left ventricle being particularly prominent and overlying the spine in the left anterior oblique view. With severe aortic regurgitation, left atrial enlargement may be apparent on the right anterior oblique view with barium in the esophagus. When aortic regurgitation is associated with aortic root disease, the ascending aorta may be markedly dilated or aneurysmal, although sometimes the major dilatation takes place posteriorly and may not be visible on the plain chest film. Occasionally, calcium is seen in the aortic valve, and calcification in the ascending aortic wall is characteristic of syphilitic involvement.

Echocardiography. By the use of ultrasound, calculation of the diameter of the aortic root and of left ventricular chamber size may be feasible. In addition, in the presence of an Austin Flint rumble there is a characteristic fluttering motion of the anterior mitral leaflet during diastole caused by the impinging aortic regurgitant jet. This finding, together with absence of mitral valve thickening and normal excursion of the posterior leaflet, provides evidence against organic mitral stenosis.

Cardiac Catheterization. It is generally desirable to perform cardiac catheterization prior to undertaking cardiac surgery in order to characterize the status of left ventricular myocardial function and to exclude associated lesions. Supravalvular injection of contrast medium into the aortic root often provides adequate radiographic visualization of the left ventricle and the anatomy of the ascending aorta, and also allows assessment of the severity of the aortic regurgitation. The systolic, left ventricular, and aortic pressures are moderately elevated; there may be a slight systolic pressure gradient across the aortic valve and a low diastolic aortic pressure (see figure in Ch. 556); a normal or moderately elevated left ventricular end-diastolic pressure (less than 20 mm Hg) is encountered when left ventricular myocardial function is maintained, and the forward cardiac output is normal. There may be an early diastolic gradient across the mitral valve from the pulmonary artery wedge or left atrial pressure tracing to the left ventricle; this is probably related to the rapid early rise of left ventricular diastolic pressure and impaired opening

motion of the anterior mitral leaflet consequent to the aortic regurgitation. Simultaneous recordings of this nature should exclude the presence of associated organic mitral stenosis, in which there is usually a pressure gradient throughout diastole. In longstanding aortic regurgitation there is elevation of the calculated left ventricular end-diastolic volume (in excess of 90 ml per square meter), with or without an elevation of the left ventricular end-diastolic pressure.

A reduced ejection fraction, an impaired forward cardiac output, and marked elevation of the left ventricular end-diastolic pressure all indicate depressed left ventricular myocardial function, which may increase the operative risk. Under these conditions, the left ventricular and aortic diastolic pressures may become equal late in diastole at a pressure of 35 to 40 mm Hg, or even higher. It is under the latter circumstances that early closure of the mitral valve can occur (see above), leading to a higher pressure in the left ventricle than in the left atrium in the last portion of diastole. Finally, selective coronary arteriography should be carried out in older patients to search for significant coronary artery disease.

Differential Diagnosis. When mild aortic regurgitation is associated with mitral valve disease, the aortic pulse pressure may be normal and the early diastolic blowing murmur may be confused with that of pulmonic regurgitation (Graham Steell murmur). If severe mitral valve disease with pulmonary hypertension is present, it may not be possible to make this differentiation on physical examination; but when aortography is performed, such a murmur has been shown to be due most commonly to aortic regurgitation. Handgrip, which increases aortic pressure, augments the murmur of aortic regurgitation but usually does not affect that of pulmonic regurgitation.

Treatment. *Medical Management.* In marked aortic regurgitation, some restriction of physical exertion is advisable to reduce the likelihood of sudden arrhythmia. In the younger patient with a history of rheumatic fever, prophylaxis against streptococcal infection is indicated, and the use of antimicrobial drugs to prevent bacterial endocarditis during and after dental or surgical procedures is important at all ages. Patients with syphilitic aortic regurgitation should receive a full course of treatment with penicillin.

In the patient with angina pectoris, nitroglycerin is not always effective, but it may be worth a cautious trial; it should be recalled, however, that nitroglycerin causes peripheral arterial vasodilatation and may lower the aortic diastolic pressure even further. With the onset of dyspnea or orthopnea (symptoms of early left ventricular failure), the use of digitalis, sodium restriction, and diuretics when necessary can result in substantial improvement, and consideration for operation can sometimes be postponed.

Surgical Treatment. Once signs of left ventricular failure become significant, the course of the disease tends to be downhill. Although the natural course is not as abrupt as that in aortic stenosis, the life expectancy averages only about seven years after onset of significant symptoms. When dyspnea or angina becomes troublesome on less than ordinary activity (N.Y.H.A. Class III) despite optimal medical management, surgical treatment should clearly be considered.

An additional factor in selecting the appropriate time for operation is the finding that in some patients, despite hemodynamic improvement after aortic valve replacement, left ventricular dilatation and myocardial dysfunction may persist. Therefore it is desirable that surgical treatment be undertaken prior to the onset of such irreversible left ventricular disease. It may be hoped that improved noninvasive methods eventually allow detection of this potential problem before permanent changes occur.

Sudden, severe aortic regurgitation is poorly tolerated, and the average life expectancy is short. Therefore surgical treatment should usually be undertaken promptly.

In the great majority of patients, replacement of the diseased aortic valve with a prosthesis is necessary. In some patients with marked dilatation of the aortic root and aneurysm formation, aortic valve replacement is combined with replacement of a portion of the ascending aorta.

562. TRICUSPID VALVE DISEASE

TRICUSPID STENOSIS

Tricuspid stenosis is rare as an isolated lesion. Almost always it accompanies rheumatic involvement of other cardiac valves, and it is of clinical significance in only about 5 per cent of patients with rheumatic heart disease. Seventy to 80 per cent of patients with tricuspid stenosis are female, and most often they have accompanying disease of both the mitral and aortic valves. *Rare causes* of tricuspid stenosis include *carcinoid heart disease, endomyocardial fibroelastosis, congenital malformations,* and obstruction from a *right atrial myxoma.*

The primary abnormality in tricuspid stenosis, like that in mitral stenosis, is mechanical obstruction to atrial emptying. This results in an elevated right atrial pressure and a pressure gradient across the tricuspid valve during diastole. It is important to measure simultaneous pressures in the right atrium and right ventricle at cardiac catheterization, because signs of peripheral venous congestion may occur with substantially lower pressure gradients (less than 10 mm Hg; often only 3 or 4 mm Hg) than are observed with mitral stenosis. Generally, the cardiac index is reduced substantially.

Tricuspid stenosis should be suspected particularly in the patient who has signs of multivalve disease and severe right-sided venous congestion but no evidence of marked pulmonary hypertension. The patient may also be relatively free of signs and symptoms of pulmonary venous congestion, despite the presence of mitral valve stenosis. This feature may be due to a limiting effect of this lesion on the cardiac output (a protective effect of the tricuspid stenosis) which may prevent sudden augmentation of blood flow into the pulmonary vascular bed. Such an effect would help explain the unusually prolonged clinical course seen in some patients with tricuspid stenosis.

On physical examination, the mean jugular venous pressure is elevated, and in patients with sinus rhythm there is a very sharp, prominent A wave which reflects right atrial contraction against the stenotic valve. There is a characteristic slow fall in the jugular V wave (delayed Y descent), caused by the obstruction to right atrial emptying and the resulting slow fall in right atrial pressure during diastole (see figure in Ch. 556).

On palpation of the precordium, the right ventricle is not enlarged, and a diastolic thrill may be palpable at the lower left sternal border. The diastolic murmur of tricuspid stenosis will often be missed unless specifically searched for at that location. It resembles that of mitral stenosis, having a low-pitched rumbling quality often beginning with a tricuspid valve opening snap (somewhat later than a mitral opening snap), and an early diastolic decrescendo murmur is followed by presystolic accentuation if sinus rhythm is present. A characteristic feature in differentiating the murmur from that of mitral stenosis is augmentation in the intensity of the tricuspid rumble during *inspiration,* or during the *Müller maneuver* (attempted inspiration against a closed glottis). This augmentation is due to the transitory increase in right atrial filling and tricuspid valve flow, which results from the negative intrathoracic pressure. Both these maneuvers diminish the murmur of mitral stenosis. There may be an associated abnormal increase in the venous pressure during such inspiration in tricuspid stenosis. When atrial fibrillation is present, the murmur is even more difficult to detect, because it may occur only in early diastole and can be confused with the murmur of pulmonic regurgitation.

The electrocardiogram, if sinus rhythm is present, exhibits peaked P waves in leads II and V_1, evidence of right atrial enlargement, but atrial fibrillation is often present. There is no evidence of right ventricular hypertrophy. On the chest roentgenogram, in addition to the findings caused by associated valvular lesions, there is enlargement of the right atrium.

Surgical treatment is not indicated for mild tricuspid stenosis, but if it is severe or if the patient must undergo operation for a mitral valve lesion, surgical treatment may be undertaken. The tricuspid valve is usually not favorable for valvuloplasty, and most often a tricuspid valve prosthesis is inserted. Sometimes the tricuspid stenosis is not detected prior to a mitral valve operation, and is recognized only when unexpected signs of right-sided congestion develop postoperatively.

TRICUSPID REGURGITATION

Tricuspid regurgitation, like tricuspid stenosis, is usually associated with rheumatic disease of other cardiac valves, particularly the mitral. It may occur as an organic lesion, usually combined with some degree of tricuspid stenosis, or more commonly it is a functional lesion secondary to right ventricular dilatation with severe pulmonary hypertension. Such functional tricuspid regurgitation usually occurs late in the course of mitral valve disease. Other forms of severe pulmonary hypertension, such as the Eisenmenger reaction in congenital heart disease or pulmonary hypertension caused by chronic lung disease, can also cause functional tricuspid regurgitation. Rheumatic involvement of the tricuspid valve can result in tricuspid regurgitation when the right ventricular systolic pressure is normal, although most frequently such organic lesions are of a mixed variety, with both stenosis and regurgitation. Isolated tricuspid regurgitation can occur congenitally (as in Ebstein's malformation), and progressive tricuspid regurgitation caused by traumatic damage to the valve has been reported after crush injuries of the chest. The normal tricuspid valve can serve as a focus for bacterial endocarditis, particularly in drug addicts.

Tricuspid regurgitation constitutes a leakage of blood retrograde into the right atrium during right ventricular systole, which places an augmented volume load on the right ventricle. The pathophysiology resembles that of mitral regurgitation but involves the right heart. In mild tricuspid regurgitation, when the right ventricular end-diastolic pressure is not elevated, the right atrial mean pressure is normal and the V wave may not be particularly prominent. As the right ventricular and mean right atrial pressures rise in the presence of more severe regurgitation, the V wave becomes increased. If the right ventricle fails, the right ventricular diastolic and mean right atrial pressures rise, and the V wave becomes markedly enlarged.

Examination in severe tricuspid regurgitation may show the V wave in the jugular venous pulse high in the neck, with the patient in the upright position. Sometimes the height of the venous pressure may be difficult to discern, because the mean pressure may exceed 20 cm of water, and the top of the column may not be visible even in the sitting position. Systolic hepatic pulsations may be present, and there may be marked hepatomegaly, ascites, and peripheral edema. In tricuspid regurgitation secondary to severe pulmonary hypertension, there is a palpable pulmonary artery segment in the second left interspace, and a markedly accentuated pulmonic closure sound is evident. With severe tricuspid regurgitation, there is a thrill over the lower left sternal border and lower sternum, and an enlarged right ventricle is palpable along the left sternal edge and in the subxiphoid region. A pansystolic murmur is heard near the lower left sternal border and lower sternum, transmitted to the right sternal edge or the subxiphoid region. An early diastolic rumble caused by increased blood across the tricuspid valve flow may be audible; when there is organic involvement of the tricuspid valve by rheumatic disease, a longer diastolic murmur caused by associated tricuspid stenosis may be present. A characteristic feature of the murmur of tricuspid regurgitation is its augmentation during inspiration *(Carvallo's sign)*, and the murmur can also be increased by the Müller maneuver (see Tricuspid Stenosis, above). These maneuvers lead to decreased intensity of a mitral regurgitant murmur.

There is electrocardiographic evidence of right ventricular hypertrophy, and atrial fibrillation is usually present in severe tricuspid regurgitation. Enlargement of both the right atrium and the right ventricle is evident on the chest roentgenogram.

The *treatment* of tricuspid regurgitation, if moderate and secondary to severe pulmonary hypertension, is conservative. Generally, the patient will respond to medical measures aimed at the left-sided valvular disease (sodium restriction, diuresis, digitalis). When aortic or mitral valve surgery is undertaken, such functional tricuspid regurgitation generally disappears gradually after relief of the left-sided lesion, as the pulmonary hypertension regresses. Occasionally, plication of the tricuspid valve anulus is done in patients with functional tricuspid regurgitation who are undergoing operation on other cardiac valves. If the functional tricuspid regurgitation is very severe, or if organic disease of the tricuspid valve is present in the absence of severe pulmonary hypertension, replacement with a prosthesis is necessary.

563. PULMONIC VALVE DISEASE

PULMONIC REGURGITATION

Regurgitation at the pulmonic valve most commonly accompanies severe pulmonary hypertension caused by left-sided valvular heart disease. The murmur is high pitched, decrescendo in quality, and best heard at the lower left sternal border. It may be indistinguishable from the murmur of mild aortic regurgitation; however, it should be noted that by far the most common cause of such a murmur in the patient with rheumatic valvular heart disease is aortic regurgitation. Isolated congenital pulmonic regurgitation with a normal pulmonary arterial pressure occurs rarely, and in this situation the murmur occurs later in diastole, is lower in pitch, and may be confused with the murmur of tricuspid stenosis. Pulmonic regurgitation with a normal pulmonary artery pressure can also occur in association with bacterial endocarditis on a normal pulmonic valve, particularly in drug users. Occasionally, if antimicrobial therapy is unsuccessful in this condition, excision of the pulmonic valve has been used to eradicate the source of infection, and this procedure does not appear to result in serious hemodynamic difficulties.

PULMONIC STENOSIS

Pulmonic stenosis usually occurs as a congenital malformation and is discussed in Ch. 552. Occasionally, acquired subpulmonic stenosis occurs in association with hypertrophic subaortic stenosis, owing to bulging of the interventricular septum into the right ventricular chamber. Rarely an intrapericardial tumor can compress the main pulmonary artery or right ventricular outflow tract, resulting in a pressure gradient between the right ventricle and the pulmonary artery.

Braunwald, E., Lambrew, C. T., Rockoff, S. D., Ross, J., Jr., and Morrow, A. G.: Idiopathic hypertrophic subaortic stenosis. I. A description of the disease based upon an analysis of 64 patients. Circulation, 30:Suppl.4:213, 1964.

Cohen, L. S., Gault, J. H., and Ross, J., Jr.: Mitral regurgitation. *In* Barondess, J. A. (ed.): Diagnostic Approaches to Presenting Syndromes. Baltimore, Williams & Wilkins Company, 1971, p. 1.

Dexter, L., and Werko, L. (eds.): Evaluation of Results of Cardiac Surgery. American Heart Association Monograph, No. 22, New York, 1968; also: Circulation 37 and 38 (Suppl. V), V-1, 1968.

Hancock, E. W., and Fleming, R. R.: Aortic stenosis. Quart. J. Med., 29:209, 1960.

Kirklin, J. W., and Karp, R. B.: Surgical treatment of acquired valvular heart disease. *In* Hurst, J. W. (ed.): The Heart. 3rd ed. New York, McGraw-Hill Publishing Company, 1974, p. 971.

Pluth, J. R., and McGoon, D. C.: Current status of heart valve replacement. Mod. Concepts Cardiovasc. Dis., 43:65, 1974.

Rees, R. J., Epstein, E. J., Criley, J. M., and Ross, R. S.: Haemodynamic effects of severe aortic regurgitation. Br. Heart J., 26:412, 1964.

Ross, J., Jr., Braunwald, E., Gault, J. H., Mason, D. T., and Morrow, A. G.: On the mechanism of the intraventricular pressure gradient in idiopathic hypertrophic subaortic stenosis. Circulation, 34:558, 1966.

Salazar, E., and Levine, H. D.: Rheumatic tricuspid regurgitation, the clinical spectrum. Am. J. Med., 33:111, 1962.

Sanders, C. A., Harthorne, J. W., De Sanctis, R. S., and Austen, W. G.: Tricuspid stenosis: A difficult diagnosis in the presence of atrial fibrillation. Circulation, 33:26, 1966.

Segal, J., Harvey, W. P., and Hufnagle, C.: A clinical study of one hundred cases of severe aortic insufficiency. Am. J. Med., 21:200, 1956.

Wood, P.: An appreciation of mitral stenosis. Parts I and II. Br. Med. J., 1:1051, 1113, 1954.

564. ARTERIAL HYPERTENSION

W. S. Peart

Definition. A statement that a given arterial pressure is above normal requires a knowledge of the range of normality. For a true definition of a raised arterial pressure, such as is used in epidemiologic studies, a rise above the mean of a population studied under standard conditions is usually used. It is easy to say that an arterial pressure of 120 systolic, 80 diastolic in mm of mercury is normal from the age of 15 years on and that an arterial pressure of 250 systolic, 150 diastolic in mm of mercury is abnormal at any age. The intermediate ranges are decided somewhat arbitrarily. In clinical practice this is of little help. It is wise when there is some doubt not to state either that hypertension exists or that it does not exist, but to substitute observation over a period of time to make sure that casual arterial pressure readings are consistently on the higher side of what is usually encountered in a completely normal subject. Again, it must be realized that single readings taken with a sphygmomanometer under varying circumstances may not reflect the usual arterial pressure in a given person. Measurements taken with automatic apparatus over 24-hour periods have shown considerable lability of pressure in many persons. This does not mean that high casual pressures may not be harmful, but in an individual case it must not be readily assumed that they are, because in these days of intensive therapy and investigation a great deal depends on this decision.

There are thus the two approaches: epidemiologic, which may have to depend upon isolated single readings of large populations that give information only about the range of casual readings, and the clinical approach, in which other factors have to be taken into account. It seems quite clear that most manifestations of disease in patients with raised arterial pressure are the consequences of, or are made worse by, the presence of raised pressure. This applies, for example, to the incidence of atheroma and other vascular disease. There is no doubt either that the higher the arterial pressure, whether systolic or diastolic, the higher the morbidity and mortality, and there is a distinct quantitative relation between these factors in many population studies. The fact that some patients withstand high arterial pressures without showing very many significant changes in their vascular systems compared with other patients with lower pressures and more serious vascular diseases does not invalidate this thesis. One individual's blood vessels may be of better quality than another's.

Some patients have mainly a rise in systolic arterial pressure. This particularly applies to the elderly, in whom such figures as 200 systolic, 90 diastolic in mm of mercury are not uncommon. It is likely that this mainly systolic hypertension represents increasing rigidity of the aorta and main vessels with less effect on the arterioles. There are all gradations from rise of the diastolic pressure with a relatively small rise in the systolic pressure to rise in the systolic pressure with a relatively smaller rise in the diastolic pressure. Too much has been made of the greater importance of diastolic hypertension in morbidity. It is highly likely that rise in the mean pressure is of greatest importance whatever way it is produced.

Measurement of Arterial Pressure. The ordinary sphyg-

momanometric method of measuring has been shown to be subject to considerable error. This has emerged in epidemiologic studies of distribution of arterial pressure and must be taken into account clinically, particularly in following the results of treatment. Quite apart from the influence of arm circumference, so that those with fat upper arms have higher recorded pressures than those with thin arms for the same true direct intra-arterial measurements, observer error creeps in. Many observers show conspicuous digit preference in measuring the arterial pressure, and this can make 10 mm of mercury difference in one reading. It should now be agreed that the diastolic pressure is the point at which the Korotkoff sounds become muffled and not where they disappear. To reduce observer bias, an essential goal in epidemiologic or drug treatment studies, automatic or concealed measurement instruments have been introduced. The importance of observer bias cannot be overemphasized; it is best brought out when the examining doctor, after an initial reading which he considers too high, makes the patient recumbent for a variable period so that the pressure then falls below some cutoff point which he regards as normal. This maneuver is often used when a great deal depends on the measurement, such as an insurance policy or a job. It is self-deception and not in the best interests of the patient.

Causes of Hypertension. In most cases of hypertension (high arterial pressure) it is impossible at present to establish a cause. These cases, probably about two thirds of all those seen, are called "essential" or "idiopathic" hypertension. Fortunately, inroads are continually being made into this majority as greater knowledge accrues about disorders known to cause raised arterial pressure. These may be classified as follows:

I. Nonrenal causes
   A. Adrenal cortical overactivity
      1. Cushing's syndrome: Overproduction of hydrocortisone and corticosterone
      2. Conn's syndrome: Overproduction of aldosterone
      3. Pseudohermaphroditism: Overproduction of androgenic steroids
      4. Deoxycorticosterone production due to enzyme defect
   B. Adrenal medullary overactivity
      1. Pheochromocytoma: Overproduction of epinephrine, norepinephrine, and occasionally other amines such as hydroxytyramine
   C. Pregnancy
      Although pregnancy exacerbates the effects of underlying renal disease, the arterial pressure may be raised without any obvious renal disease as part of the "toxemia of pregnancy" syndrome.
   D. Coarctation of the aorta
      Although the coarctation has to take place above the level of the renal arteries for hypertension to exist, no conclusive evidence of renal involvement has yet been provided.
   E. Miscellaneous
      1. Ovarian tumors of varying histologic type: Overproduction of various steroid hormones similar to those in Cushing's syndrome is sometimes seen.
      2. Porphyria during acute attacks
      3. Lead poisoning during acute phase
      4. Raised intracranial pressure, more usually of acute onset, as with subarachnoid hemorrhage
      5. Administration of monoamine oxidase inhibitors followed by cheese ingestion
      6. Licorice, usually used for peptic ulcer treatment
      7. Contraceptive pill
II. Renal causes
   Practically all renal diseases known have been associated with hypertension. Important examples are:
   A. Acute and chronic glomerulonephritis
   B. Pyelonephritis
   C. Diabetic kidney
   D. Polyarteritis nodosa
   E. Polycystic disease
   F. Hemangiopericytoma (renin-producing tumor)

The probable link is interference with blood supply to the kidney, best exemplified by renal artery stenosis due to atheroma, extrinsic bands, or fibromuscular disease.

Incidence and Prevalence. In a given population group there is no comprehensive information about the distribution of causes. Attempts have been made to define this in selected groups of the population. It has been found, for example, by population study in both Wales and Jamaica, that there is a similar incidence of symptomless bacilluria in some subjects with hypertension, but whether cause or effect is uncertain. It is not known how many patients have atheromatous renal artery stenosis or fibromuscular hyperplasia of the renal arteries, or even chronic glomerulonephritis. To completely exclude a renal cause of hypertension requires considerable investigation in depth, including pyelography, arteriography, and renal biopsy, and even with such aids the presence of occult pyelonephritis as a scattered disease of the kidney may be missed. It still seems likely, however, that the bulk of cases picked up in epidemiologic surveys will have no known cause at present with the most intensive of our investigations. The prevalence varies widely in different parts of the world and among various races. For example, blacks in Georgia have a very high incidence of hypertension, as do coastal dwellers in northern Japan. The black population in various parts of Africa may also have a high incidence of hypertension, and although environmental factors, especially dietary ones like salt as in Japan, have been incriminated, the evidence is weak and incomplete. In some areas hypertension is very uncommon, as in many isolated island communities (for example, the Gilbert Islands), and studies of such groups moving to "civilized" environments show a rise of pressure.

Epidemiology. Much effort has been devoted to the epidemiology. Most of the studies depend upon casual arterial pressures taken under reasonably standard conditions, and the results show certain definite features. In general, arterial pressure in urban communities rises with age. The tendency is less marked or nonexistent in some communities, for example, the Gilbert Islands and northern Kenya, and does not seem to be associated with obvious disease but rather with body build and calorie intake. The rise applies to both the systolic and diastolic pressures in both males and females, although the rise in females is greater from the age of 30 to 40 years. This difference in the female has been noted in widely separated populations in different parts of the world. There is a quantitative likeness in the arterial pressure of blood relatives. Despite the common occurrence of hypertension in certain families, over-all there is no evidence of a common dominant genetic inheritance but rather of multiple factors. Environment as well as genetic inheritance has a common role in families. For example, the husbands of multiparous women in a study in South Wales had a lower than average arterial pressure, as did their wives. Unexpected correlations of this sort emerge in epidemiologic studies. Another is the higher incidence of hypertension among the relatives of subjects with hypertension and pyelonephritis. Nevertheless, identical twins may develop severe hypertension at about the same age even though they have spent their lives apart.

Pathology. Certain changes are common to all forms of hypertension and may properly be regarded as due solely to the level of arterial pressure. Other changes are peculiar to each cause of high arterial pressure, and they will be considered separately. In nearly all diseases associated with hypertension, the malignant phase may follow, so that a complicated picture resulting from the presence of the disease and the effects of malignant hypertension may be seen. Despite occasional suggestions to the contrary, the best evidence points to the malignant phase (necrotizing or accelerated phase) of hypertension as being mainly related to the absolute height of the mean pressure or the rate of rise of the mean pressure. Efforts to segregate malignant hypertension as a peculiar disease in its own right have been unrewarding, and the fact that some patients have all the evidence of malignant hypertension at mean pressures lower than other patients who have been withstanding higher pressures for many years does not disprove this general thesis. In any study of a large number of patients, those with malignant hypertension have a higher arterial pressure than those without. The manifestations of malignant hypertension in pathologic terms are acute vascular changes with fibrinoid necrosis in arterioles. The brunt of the damage is borne by vessels in the kidney, pancreas, mesentery, adrenal, and retina. It is rarely seen in voluntary muscle, and no cause can be suggested for this type of distribution. Since the kidney is always involved in all forms of hypertension, it is often difficult to be sure of the difference between primary change causing the hypertension and secondary damage because of the hypertension. It is reasonably certain that there is a primary disease in the kidney when the changes are most clearly seen in the glomeruli, as in glomerulonephritis, disseminated lupus erythematosus, amyloidosis, and diabetes. The glomerular changes with interference of blood flow lead to tubular atrophy, and in those cases in which the blood pressure is elevated, the most common changes are initially hypertrophy of the muscular wall of the afferent arteriole; next, hyalinization; and finally, in the malignant phase, intimal hyperplasia of the onion skin variety, which occurs also in slightly larger arteries, as well as the definitive fibrinoid arteriolar necrosis. All the elements of the blood, including cells, may be demonstrated in these lesions. Since this may resemble a vasculitis, the suggestion that it is part of an immunologic disorder has been made, but this is unlikely because the lesions heal readily with reduction of pressure. The occurrence of microangiopathic hemolytic anemia, with reduction of all formed elements in the blood, and the occurrence of platelets and fibrin on the damaged arterioles, with the potentiality of rapid decrease in renal function, are similarly reversible by rapid reduction of arterial pressure. In the larger arteries within the kidney, from the interlobar to the arcuates, hypertension causes intimal thickening, replication of the internal elastic lamina, and fibrosis with atheromatous deposits, sometimes in a very uniform manner but often as a nodular process. It is thought that this change, when it occurs in the apparently normal kidney, may be responsible for perpetuation of hypertension when the opposite abnormal kidney, the seat of pyelonephritis or involved by renal artery stenosis, is removed. The signs of ischemic change are best seen when the main renal artery is stenosed. The kidney volume shrinks; the glomeruli are crowded but generally appear normal; the juxtaglomerular apparatus in the afferent arteriole and the cells surrounding close to the macula densa of the distal convoluted tubule hypertrophy, sometimes grossly, and become hypergranulated, whereas the tubules between the glomeruli are atrophic and the interstitium may be expanded or fibrotic. The opposite kidney may show all the signs of hypertensive change previously described. The effects of acute narrowing of the arteriolar lumen on the performance of the relevant organs are seen, so that, in the case of the kidney, diminution of function with proteinuria, microscopic hematuria, and even frank hematuria occur. In the retina, exudation and hemorrhage caused by small infarcts, and papilledema associated with a raised intracranial pressure, which is of uncertain origin, are the main features. When this process occurs in the brain, various disturbances result, according to the part of the brain affected; fits and unconsciousness are not rare and are given the clumsy name of hypertensive encephalopathy. Arteriolar spasms may underlie some of these attacks as opposed to cerebral edema, previously implicated, and full recovery may occur. Because the impact may be apparently greater in some organs than in others, it is possible to find fibrinoid necroses in renal biopsies without any characteristic change in the retina. The converse is perhaps less common. In most untreated cases this disorder runs its course to death within two years of diagnosis. The features it shares with all other hypertensive manifestations are those due to the increased load put upon the heart and the blood vessels in different territories. A main finding is the increased incidence of atheroma, both experimentally and pathologically. The increased pressure leads to hypertrophy of the left ventricle and a tendency to angina pectoris and myocardial infarction. The increased load on the left heart leads to raised pulmonary venous pressure, pulmonary edema, raised pulmonary artery pressure, and congestive cardiac failure. The increased pressure in the vessels to the brain leads to a high incidence of strokes caused by cerebral hemorrhage, thrombosis, and subarachnoid hemorrhage. The site of these is probably the arterial microaneurysms originally described by Charcot. Vascular damage in the kidney leads to renal failure. It must be emphasized again that all these manifestations may be linked quantitatively with the level of arterial pressure. There is no doubt that in such conditions of acute onset as acute glomerulonephritis and eclampsia, the manifestations of malignant hypertension, particularly in the brain and retina, may appear at lower pressures and may seem more florid in the presence of renal failure. The latter, however, is not essential to the appearances, for example, of multiple cotton wool exudates and hemorrhages. It is likely that the rate of rise of pressure at least in part governs the severity of the signs.

The Mechanisms of Hypertension. *Circulatory Pattern.* The major factors controlling the arterial pressure are the cardiac output and the total peripheral resistance. If the cardiac output rises, the arterial pressure will rise unless there is a corresponding drop in the peripheral resistance. Most peripheral resistance occurs in the arterioles and is governed by contraction of their muscular walls. A given level of arterial pressure depends on the interplay between these two major factors and, in order to describe the pattern of the circulation, it is necessary to be able to say what the peripheral resistance is and in which part of the body the major changes are occurring. Although it has been claimed that changes in cardiac output are responsible for rises in pressure and may even ultimately lead to persistent high arterial pressure, the evidence for this is weak. In most cases of high arterial pressure, either experimental or in man, the one uniform feature is a raised peripheral resistance. The cardiac out-

put in most cases of established hypertension in man is within normal limits. Theoretically, it might be thought that to know the particular pattern of peripheral resistance could give important clues to the cause of high arterial pressure. In only one form of high arterial pressure is there a very distinctive pattern, and this is pheochromocytoma. Epinephrine and norepinephrine, the amines most commonly released by these tumors, are particularly potent as vasoconstrictors in the skin. Measurements of skin blood flow show very low levels in such patients, unlike other causes of high arterial pressures. Removal of the tumor is followed by a rise in skin flow. If there were a wide variety of different agents raising the arterial pressure by increasing the peripheral resistance in various territories, certain characteristic patterns might emerge. However, in either renal hypertension or hypertension of unknown origin, the pattern is strikingly the same, so that the distribution of resistance is much the same from patient to patient. Admittedly, simultaneous measurements of flow in different parts of the body have not been done. Certain organs show the increased resistance most, the kidney and splanchnic area in particular. The general impression is, however, of a widely distributed increase of peripheral resistance in every tissue and organ of the body except the voluntary muscles.

Increased Cardiac Output. There are a few situations in which increased cardiac output seems to play an important role in raising the arterial pressure: renal failure, toxemia of pregnancy, and acute glomerulonephritis. Most studies have been made of patients with renal failure; these patients are particularly susceptible to fluid load, and the arterial pressure may rise abruptly when the patients are overloaded with water.

Cause of Rise in the Peripheral Resistance. This is uncertain in most cases of hypertension except those associated with high plasma levels of norepinephrine and epinephrine or renin and angiotensin, as in pheochromocytoma or hemangiopericytoma of the kidney. Hypertension itself causes changes in peripheral resistance in the sense that at a high arterial pressure the vessels contract, whereas lowering the arterial pressure causes decreased contraction. This is presumably a direct effect of pressure on the smooth muscle of the arteriolar wall, leading not only to contraction but also to hypertrophy, as was first shown by Folkow and his colleagues (1958). At one extreme, Borst (1963) has claimed that the sequence may be retention of salt and water caused by a renal fault, rise in the cardiac output, rise in arterial pressure to enable the kidney to excrete the salt and water, and secondary contraction of peripheral arterioles, leading to further rise in arterial pressure. Others believe that there is a primary cause for a rise in peripheral resistance, leading inevitably to a rise in arterial pressure. Guyton has emphasized the importance of correlating the many factors, including blood volume, cardiac output, peripheral resistance, the nervous system, and hormonal influences in terms of homeostatic mechanisms. The following major fields require deeper discussion.

Hypertension Associated with Retention of Water and Salt, with or without the Action of Adrenocortical Steroids. The best example, mentioned before, is of the patient with renal failure who tolerates fluid load badly and who is incapable of adjusting cardiac output and peripheral resistance so as to maintain his arterial pressure at normal levels. Removing body fluid by dialysis and lowering the salt intake will control this high arterial pressure in most instances. Even here another renal factor is revealed by the further lowering of arterial pressure brought about in this type of patient by total nephrectomy prior to renal transplantation. In some patients it is the only way in which the arterial pressure may be controlled, and these patients have some of the highest levels of renin activity, angiotensin, and aldosterone yet observed, which is of obvious importance. It was in animals that the condition of "renoprival hypertension" was described, but from closer studies made recently it seems that the hypertension that develops without kidneys is most likely to be due to increased sensitivity to salt and water overload with a rise in cardiac output. One of the experimental links of hypertension with salt and water metabolism is the observation that salt feeding in the rat leads to hypertension and also to renal damage, particularly if deoxycorticosterone (DOCA) is administered subcutaneously. Dahl and his colleagues have shown that there are salt-sensitive and salt-insensitive strains of rats, so that the possibility exists of a genetic factor acting in conjunction with an environmental one to produce high arterial pressure. The high incidence of hypertension and cerebral hemorrhage in northern Japan may be related, because there is a high salt intake in that area, but the exact mechanism is uncertain. In Cushing's syndrome with excess secretion of cortisol from hyperplastic adrenals, hypertension may be very severe and is associated with sodium and water retention as well as increased potassium excretion. The condition may be cured by removal of the suprarenals. It is still not certain whether there are other adrenal steroids capable of raising the arterial pressure, although since every patient with severe Cushing's syndrome does not have hypertension, it is at least suggestive.

Renal Hypertension. That the kidney is directly and primarily responsible for some cases of raised arterial pressure is shown by the successful cure of hypertension by unilateral nephrectomy when one of the two kidneys is diseased. Among the many renal diseases known to be associated with curable hypertension, pyelonephritis, tuberculosis, carcinoma, and, perhaps most important, obstruction to the main renal artery by atheroma or fibromuscular hyperplasia need to be mentioned. The link seems to be interference with blood supply to the kidney. Similar arguments can be applied to bilateral disease. Recent work has made much clearer the way in which the kidney raises the arterial pressure, and this includes experimental hypertension produced by a clip on the renal artery, first successfully accomplished by Goldblatt and his colleagues (1934).

Following are some of the major ways in which the kidney may be associated with elevation of the arterial pressure.

Failure to Excrete or Destroy an Extrarenal Pressor Substance. This has been partly touched on in the discussion of renoprival hypertension, in which the emphasis was on extracellular fluid volume sensitivity, but certain experimental observations suggest that some metabolic function of the kidney might be important apart from its effect on extracellular fluid volume. The hypotensive effect of introducing a normal kidney into the circulation of an animal with hypertension caused by a renal clip and the way in which a kidney with normal blood supply yet deprived of excretory function by a ureteric tie prevents the rise in pressure caused by a clip on the opposite renal artery point to this suggestion. The

ready reversal of renal stenosis hypertension both in man and in animals by removal of the obstruction, even with hypertension of long duration, argues against a very potent extrarenal pressor system.

Failure to Produce a Vasodilator. The hypothesis that the kidney has its main effect on the arterial pressure by providing a vasodilator to keep the arterial pressure down and that hypertension may be due to a failure of vasodilator production has received much recent study. Various extracts, particularly of the medulla of the kidney, have appeared to lower the arterial pressure on injection into animals. Some of these substances are prostaglandins, mainly of the E series, and they have been shown to appear in renal venous blood when the circulation to the kidney is reduced. It is uncertain whether they play a part in general hemodynamic changes in any form of renal hypertension, and the same uncertainty surrounds a possible local role in the renal circulation, particularly of the medulla.

Increased Response of a Normal Pressor Mechanism. An obvious candidate for this role is the sympathetic nervous system and its higher neural centers. If the kidney produced some substance that increased the over-all activity of the sympathetic system, this might be reflected in high arterial pressure. The main substance which has been shown to stimulate the vasomotor centers in the brain as well as facilitate the action of the sympathetic nervous system peripherally is angiotensin. Studies of norepinephrine metabolism have advanced considerably, and it is now possible to get a better estimate of the degree of activity of the sympathetic nervous system since it was discovered that not only norepinephrine but also dopamine beta hydroxylase is released into the circulation as a result of sympathetic activity. The latter substance, unlike norepinephrine, may not be taken up again after discharge, and therefore its plasma level, taken in conjunction with that of norepinephrine, may reflect sympathetic activity. Higher levels of both substances have been reported in hypertension.

Another way in which an increased response in the body could occur would be for the arterioles to respond more markedly than usual to a normal stimulus. For example, if the degree of contraction produced by a given dose of norepinephrine were markedly increased, then a state of high arterial pressure might follow. In hypertension, renal or otherwise, the degree of response to norepinephrine and angiotensin is not easy to quantitate in terms of the familiar log dose-response curve in comparison with a normal situation, so that the apparent decreased response in severe hypertension may be caused by the responses being tested at the top of the curve; although there is no positive evidence of this, the possibility has not been excluded.

Decreased Response of Baroreceptors. The view has been proposed that the fault in hypertension may lie in the baroreceptors and that by an alteration in their response the arterial pressure is allowed to rise to a higher level. Both in man and in animals it has been shown that the baroreceptor can be affected so as to permit a rise of pressure, and changes in stretch of the aortic wall at the root and arch produced experimentally have been associated with such a rise. It is clear that the baroreceptor mechanism in the carotid sinus is easily modified and seems to respond only to change or rate of change in pressure, so the depressor mechanism rapidly becomes reset at higher levels of arterial pressure and operates again only when the arterial pressure is even further elevated. There is need for much greater knowledge of baroreceptors, both central and peripheral in man, and merely to consider the carotid sinus is inadequate.

Renin-Angiotensin System. The development of better methods of measuring renin activity and angiotensin in plasma, especially by sensitive and specific radioimmunoassay methods, makes it possible to assign a role in various physiologic and pathologic situations, especially related to hypertension.

ANATOMY. Renin is stored in granules in the modified smooth muscle cells of the afferent arteriolar wall to the glomerulus, contiguous with the macula densa of the ascending limb of the loop of Henle (Goormaghtigh apparatus).

RELEASE OF RENIN. There are beta receptors within the kidney, stimulation of which governs renin release. Catecholamines, e.g., isoproterenol, epinephrine, and norepinephrine, which stimulate these receptors, liberate renin, whereas stimulation of alpha receptors seems to inhibit release, as does the use of beta blockers like propranolol. It may be that the sympathetic nerve endings close to the juxtaglomerular apparatus may act through the beta receptor. The way in which diuretics like furosemide release renin is not clear, but it is thought that altered sodium concentration in the urine may act as a stimulus, perhaps through the macula densa. In the normal animal or man, renin is released readily by changing from the supine to the erect posture and by sodium deprivation or blood volume depletion; it seems to be released readily by stimuli leading to autoregulation of renal blood flow. The quickest inhibitor of renin release is angiotensin itself, and longer-term effects are brought about by mineralocorticoid excess, e.g., of aldosterone. The way in which the latter inhibition occurs is unclear.

FUNCTIONING OF THE SYSTEM. Renin is probably released in a protein-bound form which reacts with substrate to produce first the decapeptide angiotensin I, which is mainly converted to the pressor octapeptide angiotensin II by cleavage of the two C-terminal amino acids in passage through the lung as well as other sites. Both peptides are readily cleared from the circulation by various tissues and readily destroyed by peptidases.

ACTIONS OF ANGIOTENSIN. Although angiotensin I has some actions of its own, the operation of the system mainly depends on angiotensin II. This peptide is the most potent direct smooth muscle vasoconstrictor known. It also raises the arterial pressure by a direct action on vasomotor centers in the brain, especially the hindbrain, and is known to facilitate sympathetic ganglionic transmission as well as the final sympathetic nerve ending effect. In some species it will liberate epinephrine from the adrenal medulla. The effect of vasoconstriction varies in different organs, but in the kidney, since it tends to reduce renal blood flow, it acts as an antidiuretic agent. Its other major action is in stimulating production of aldosterone from the adrenal cortex, and in different physiologic and pathologic situations it acts as a major but not unique stimulus.

ROLE IN HYPERTENSION. The first point to establish is that the actions of angiotensin are much influenced by electrolyte and water balance. For this reason it is possible to have very high levels of renin and angiotensin in the circulation of subjects with quite normal arterial pressure, as, for example, in cirrhosis of the liver with ascites, in Addison's disease, or in women taking contraceptive pills. Conversely, it may well be true that without too much elevation of the level, an expansion of intravascular volume and sodium retention markedly increases arterial pressure. Simple estimation of renin activity and angiotensin does not allow very precise definition of their action.

HIGH RENIN GROUP. In both human and experimental hypertension it has become clear that when the renin and angiotensin levels are high, reduction will usually lead to a fall of pressure. Good examples are bilateral nephrectomy in patients with terminal renal failure in whom intensive hemodialysis has failed to lower the pressure; the inhibition of renin release by beta-blocking drugs, e.g., propranolol, in malignant hypertension; and the reduction of arterial pressure in experimental renal clip hypertension by competitive angiotensin analogues (sarcosyl-1-alanine-8-octapeptide) or high titer angiotensin II antibodies.

LOW RENIN GROUP. Soon after the discovery by Conn (1961) of primary hyperaldosteronism caused by small tumors of the zona glomerulosa in the adrenal cortex, removal of which cured the hypertension and returned the high plasma and total body sodium, low plasma and body potassium, and high plasma aldosterone and secretion rate to normal, it was discovered that these patients had very low plasma renin activity and angiotensin levels which were difficult to elevate by any of the usual stimuli but which responded to spironolactone, an aldosterone antagonist. There followed the discovery that as many as 20 per cent of patients with hypertension had low plasma renin values. Most of these patients do not have excess mineralocorticoid; but in addition to increased aldosterone, some may have increased deoxycorticosterone or some other steroid, e.g., 18-hydroxydeoxycorticosterone, but the evidence is less convincing. Many of these patients have unexplained hyperplasia of the zona glomerulosa. The elaborate methods needed to distinguish patients with definite tumors from the others indicate some of the difficulties, but definition of the tumor by venography or by radioisotope scanning techniques shows that anatomy still has a place. Surgery is useless unless the patient has been shown to have a convincing drop of arterial pressure after administration of spironolactone in a dose of 300 mg daily for one month.

HYPERTENSION IN PREGNANCY. In patients in whom the arterial pressure rises without subsequently proved underlying renal disease, plasma renin and angiotensin levels tend to fall rather than rise, and although aldosterone production rises in pregnancy, there is also a fall with the development of hypertension.

RENIN-PRODUCING TUMOR (HEMANGIOPERICYTOMA). After the first description by Robertson and his colleagues (1967) of a patient with high arterial pressure, low plasma potassium, high aldosterone levels, and a small tumor on the outside of the renal cortex with a high content of renin, several other such patients have been reported. Such patients represent the clearest examples of the effects of overproduction of renin, because they are cured by removal of the tumor.

Clinical Manifestations. The symptoms and signs are usually secondary to effects on blood vessels in the various organs and tissues or to the increased load borne by the heart.

Cerebral. Headache is common, and the early morning occipital headache with stiffness of the neck, sometimes awakening the patient from sleep, commonly associated with vomiting attended by relief, is almost diagnostic of hypertension. Many patients have headache only on Saturday or Sunday mornings when they sleep later. The mechanism of this typical headache is uncertain. It is not closely related to the level of arterial pressure, and many patients with severe hypertension never experience it, but it is uncommon at diastolic pressures less than 120 in millimeters of mercury. It is most likely to be related to changes in cerebrospinal fluid pressure, as in patients with cerebral tumors. Various other forms of headache are associated, but are not diagnostic of hypertension. *Giddiness* short of true vertigo is a common complaint. Although disturbances in the balancing mechanisms are suggested by this, no direct evidence can be offered. *Personality changes* are not uncommon with the severe forms of hypertension and are presumably secondary to vascular damage. Some of these can be reversed by lowering the arterial pressure effectively; for example, ill-defined symptoms of anxiety may disappear. With extreme vascular disease, of course, *fits,* including jacksonian epilepsy, *minor strokes,* and *cerebral deterioration,* all occur. The experimental demonstration that the blood vessels in the brain may contract vigorously in response to high arterial pressure must obviously be related to these manifestations collected under the term *hypertensive encephalopathy,* quite apart from any more permanent vascular change induced by hypertension.

Thoracic. Angina pectoris is common and that it is linked to the high pressure and not necessarily to pure narrowing of coronary arteries is demonstrated by its alleviation on lowering the arterial pressure by drugs. An early symptom is *shortness of breath* on effort. This presumably is due to a change in the physical properties of the lung, leading to the sensation of dyspnea. This is often ascribed to left ventricular failure but perhaps more accurately should be attributed to a rise in left atrial pressure and consequently in pulmonary venous pressure. This process may occur acutely at night when the patient has been recumbent and asleep for, usually, about two hours. The typical attack of *cardiac asthma* ensues in which the patient has to sit up, gasping for breath. He dangles his legs over the edge of the bed and may get up and sit by an open window until his breathing is restored to normal. In extreme cases, frank pulmonary edema occurs and may be recognized by the coughing up of pink, frothy sputum. Listening over the chest reveals crackling sounds of all degrees from fine to coarse, depending on the degree of edema, and even wheezing noises may be produced, leading occasionally to confusion with so-called bronchial asthma. Acute lowering of the pressure by drugs alleviates these attacks dramatically. A surprising and unexplained feature is the fact that when the patient resumes his slumbers, he is very rarely reawakened by a second attack.

Because of the increased tendency to vascular disease, *myocardial infarction* may be superimposed on angina or may occur without warning. This may in some patients lead to a permanent cure of the hypertension, presumably because of reduced cardiac output. After a period in which there has been shortness of breath on effort and cardiac asthma, right-sided heart failure may follow, with improvement in the shortness of breath and cardiac asthma but with the other consequences of congestive cardiac failure. Some patients who have had few or no previous symptoms present for the first time in *congestive cardiac failure.* No convincing explanation has been offered for this, but perhaps the response of the pulmonary vasculature in some patients is different, so that the symptoms of left heart failure are minimized until the load on the right heart produces its own failure.

Vascular. The peripheral arteries may be observed to be either occluded in part or conspicuously tortuous. In this respect, a curly right carotid is common, as are tortuous brachial and radial arteries. The heart may show obvious hypertrophy of the left ventricle with an apex outside the midclavicular line, forcefully lifting the ribs above it. Auscultation of the heart typically reveals a presystolic triple rhythm heard usually best between the apex and the sternum. This disappears with successful treatment of the hypertension. The second sound in the right second space is loud and may have a distinctly twangy quality. Otherwise, in the absence of secondary cardiac disease, the sounds are unremarkable.

A rare observation is the presence of *pulsus alternans,* occasionally appreciated by variation in the strength of alternate beats at the wrist. Pulsus alternans may be observed more easily on taking the arterial pressure with a sphygmomanometer; the apparent rate of the pulse doubles as the pressure is slowly decreased. This again may be abolished by lowering the arterial pressure. The presence of failure of all types may be readily recognized from the rales in the lungs or the raised venous pressure, edema, hepatic enlargement, and congestive failure.

Bleeding from unexpected sites occurs in the higher ranges of arterial pressure. Nosebleeds, in the absence of uremia, and hemospermia are not rare.

In addition to the vascular disease already mentioned, involvement of the blood vessels to the legs is perhaps most commonly indicated by the complaint of *intermittent claudication.* This feature may, in fact, be made worse when the arterial pressure is lowered, since the usual cause is a block in the arteries somewhere between the external iliac and the popliteal.

A rare cause of *absent or delayed femoral pulses* is coarctation of the aorta. Although this is often diagnosed in childhood, it may present in young adults. It is fairly easily recognized clinically by the pulse changes. The collateral vessels are clearly seen and felt around the posterior scapular margin and the intercostal spaces, particularly on the back. In the other main vessels, the most striking occurrence is dissecting aneurysm through the media, which is practically always associated with hypertension in the older age group. Aneurysmal dilatation of other vessels and the rupture of berry aneurysms within the skull indicate other types of strain imposed on the vascular system.

Ocular. Patients commonly present with *vascular manifestations in the eye,* and bilateral or unilateral blurring of vision or scotoma is common. In the malignant phase, the changes include papilledema, in which characteristically the swelling is in the retina around the disc and encroaches on the edge, eventually involving the whole; a small, circumscribed so-called "hard" exudate, often arranged like grains of salt, between the disc and the macula; the "cotton-wool" exudate commonly associated with acute rise of arterial pressure as in acute glomerulonephritis and eclampsia, but especially florid in uremia; the typical macular fan or star figure of white lines of exudate between the nerve fibers leading from the macula; and hemorrhages, both linear and round. Papilledema is occasionally unilateral without hemorrhages or exudates, and, conversely, hemorrhages and exudates of all varieties may occur without papilledema; yet all are associated with this accelerated phase. Less severe changes are tortuosity in the arteries and nipping of the veins so that they are distended distally from crossings. Actual white sheathing of the arteries from the disc may be seen, as well as variations in caliber. Spontaneous variations in caliber have been reported in severe hypertension, but this must be an extremely rare observation. One of the most common retinal changes is segmental venous thrombosis, usually starting in the vessels on the temporal side of the retina and clearly occurring at a point of arteriovenous crossing. Central venous obstruction is another similar manifestation. Less common are central retinal arterial obstruction and, perhaps surprisingly, segmental arterial obstruction.

Renal. The symptom resulting purely from hypertension and not related to the underlying renal disorder is increased *nocturnal frequency.* This may be an early manifestation of hypertension, usually occurring when the diastolic pressure is 120 in mm of mercury or more, and it may be alleviated by lowering the arterial pressure by any means. In severe hypertension of recent onset, diuresis may be extreme and associated with increased water, sodium, and potassium loss, leading to thirst, weakness, and cramps. Longstanding hypertension with vascular damage to the kidneys leads to all the secondary consequences of renal failure and ultimately to uremia.

Special Investigations. *Urine.* The presence of protein in the urine is a most important sign in hypertension. It may indicate the presence of the malignant phase, congestive cardiac failure, or a primary renal disease causing hypertension. When proteinuria is associated with glycosuria and ketones, a diabetic kidney, as in the Kimmelstiel-Wilson syndrome, may be present. Alternatively, glycosuria with very little proteinuria may raise the suspicion of a pheochromocytoma with associated hyperglycemia. Examining the centrifuged deposit may reveal the red cells and red cell casts typical of acute glomerulonephritis, polyarteritis nodosa, or the malignant phase of hypertension. Pus cells and motile bacteria characterize urinary infection and point to pyelonephritis. Greater precision is given to the diagnosis of chronic pyelonephritis with sterile urine by quantitative demonstration of the increased rate of cellular excretion, particularly when further stimulated by intravenous injections of prednisolone.

If proteinuria persists, it may be impossible to decide the underlying renal disease without percutaneous renal biopsy and light or electron microscopy. The presence of chronic glomerulonephritis, lupus erythematosus, and other renal diseases causing hypertension may readily be shown by this procedure. It is of much less help in the absence of proteinuria.

One other striking feature of the urine in hypertension is persistent alkalinity in the presence of potassium deficiency, which is most important because it points to hyperaldosteronism. The presence of an inappropriately high potassium excretion for the level of plasma potassium is further evidence of hyperaldosteronism. Estimation of the catecholamine content of the urine, including the free amines epinephrine and norepinephrine, together with measurements of their metabolic products, vanillylmandelic acid and the metanephrines, adds precision to the diagnosis of pheochromocytoma. A simple test of renal function is failure to raise the specific gravity above 1.010 or the osmolality above 500 mOsm per liter after overnight water deprivation.

Blood. The level of blood urea gives only a rough indication of renal performance, because it is much influenced by dietary protein, and a better estimation, particularly in following the results of treatment, is that of creatinine clearance, which is still probably the most reliable and easily repeated of the tests of renal function. Electrolyte patterns have become of very great importance and are essential to the investigation of any case of hypertension. A low potassium and high bicarbonate point to hyperaldosteronism, and if associated with a higher than normal sodium level, they are strongly suggestive. The most common cause, however, of low plasma potassium and raised bicarbonate is previous administration of a thiazide or similar diuretic. With a suspicion of hyperaldosteronism, either primary or secondary, the use of radioactive isotopes to measure total exchangeable sodium which is high and potassium which is low, is often helpful. Measurement of plasma and urinary levels of aldosterone by radioimmunoassay has provided a practical procedure in suspected cases, although the posture of the patient and the sodium balance when the blood or urine is collected require careful standardization to avoid misleading results. Failure to suppress aldosterone production by DOCA administration points to autonomy either of the tumor or of the zona glomerulosa itself. Epinephrine and norepinephrine in the blood can now be measured either by a double isotope technique, which is laborious, or more readily by radioimmunoassay, but the diagnosis of pheochromocytoma is best made upon urinary excretion of catecholamine derivatives. Plasma renin activity and angiotensin levels will be considered later.

Feces. The sodium and potassium content in the stools reflects the function of the colonic wall which is under the influence of mineralocorticoids like aldosterone. Increased aldosterone activity promotes sodium reabsorption and potassium excretion, altering the sodium-to-potassium ratio. A real advance was the finding that the electrical potential between the skin and the colonic wall is influenced by mineralocorticoid action, and that with increasing sodium reabsorption the difference increases (Edmonds and Godfrey, 1970). This can be used in a quantitative manner as a simple clinical procedure to indicate the action of aldosterone, especially when combined with changes induced by the aldosterone antagonist spironolactone.

Chest Roentgenogram. In the roentgenogram of the chest, signs purely related to the hypertension and not to its cause are increased size of the heart, particularly the left ventricle, and increased vascularity of the lung fields caused by pulmonary venous congestion, often with edema, shown initially by small horizontal lines in the costophrenic angles ("B" lines) before the typical hilar butterfly shadows develop. The heart may not appear obviously enlarged according to ordinary roentgenologic criteria, even though enlargement is clinically obvious by the thrust of the left ventricle. Special signs occur in coarctation of the aorta, in which the notching of the lower margin of the rib by the collateral intercostal arteries is diagnostic.

Electrocardiogram. Even with well marked hypertension, the electrocardiogram may show no definite changes, but probably the most reliable evidence of left ventricular hypertrophy is high voltage in the precordial leads. Left axis deviation is common, and depression of the S-T segments and T wave inversion over the lateral chest leads are usually present in a well established case of severe hypertension. This is often termed "left ventricular strain pattern," but it is uncertain whether this is on an ischemic basis, particularly as it may merge with the changes of ischemia resulting from coronary artery disease.

Intravenous Pyelography. Using this technique, it is possible to pick out those patients with a nonfunctioning kidney and those in whom the clubbed calices and the irregular outline of the scarred kidney point to pyelonephritis. Dilatation of the pelvicaliceal system points to the need to look for obstruction in the urinary tract, because, particularly when associated with infection, this type of obstruction from the urethra upward can be a cause of hypertension. Naturally stone or calcification in the kidney can be seen and may be relevant to the hypertension. It is worth examining the pelvic films carefully for evidence of iliac arterial calcification. On pyelography the delayed appearance on one side of a small volume system in rapid sequence films taken at 1-minute intervals up to 5 minutes, together with increased contrast of dye in the later films up to 20 or 30 minutes, is typical of renal artery obstruction, especially when associated with a smaller kidney. Retrograde ureteric pyelography is used only when obstruction is either apparent or suspected and caliceal anatomy is indistinct. The use of high dose intravenous pyelography has reduced the frequency and need for retrograde examination. The size and shape of the kidney may be better appreciated by the use of tomography, which, when combined with intravenous pyelography, will not only give better indication of these factors, but may also show tumors in the renal areas.

Arteriography. In the search for renal causes of hypertension, arteriography is used only when surgical intervention is intended should an appropriate renal disorder be discovered. The clearest pictures are given by selective catheterization of each renal artery, with a final aortogram to pick up multiple arteries, one of which may be stenosed. Small scars or poor cortical filling can be seen by this technique as well as major blocks in the main renal arteries. Cysts show as avascular round filling defects, and tumors, such as hypernephromas, as areas of increased and irregular vascularity. Renin-producing tumors (hemangiopericytoma) are shown on the outer edge of the cortex and appear as filling defects. Pheochromocytomas can be demonstrated as round or ovoid vascular blush areas by using aortography under the protection of epinephrine-blocking drugs (phentolamine).

Venography. The adrenal veins may be catheterized selectively, the right with difficulty from the wall of the cava, and the left via the renal vein. The anatomy of the gland can be shown by retrograde dye injection, and tumors may be demonstrated. This technique is also used for collecting blood from the renal vein for assay of renin and the adrenal vein for assay of corticosteroids.

Renography. Most information is gained by comparing the curves of radioactivity obtained from the two kidneys simultaneously after the administration of ^{131}I hippuran. This gives quantitative information about individual renal function which is extremely useful in relation to vascular and parenchymal disease as well as obstructions in the urinary tract. Combined with scanning techniques, either instantaneous using a gamma camera, or slowly using a scintillation scanner, information about both function and morphology can be gained. Development of technetium-labeled compounds enables the gamma camera to be used for external tests of individual renal function by steadily improving methods.

Divided Renal Function Studies. Divided renal function tests, in which the urine is collected through separate ureteric catheters and the composition is compared, are the ultimate tests of renal function, despite their technical difficulties, but are being superseded by improvements in radioisotope renography. For example, in stenosis of the main renal artery, water reabsorption increases markedly, leading to increased concentration but reduced clearance of such filtered substances as creatinine, inulin, and para-aminohippuric acid (PAH). The sodium concentration in contrast drops markedly. In parenchymal disease, as for example pyelonephritis, the water reabsorption is reduced and the concentration, as well as the clearance, of inulin, creatinine, and PAH drops, and the sodium concentration may be higher than or no different from that on the normal side. As a preliminary to surgery of the kidneys, such tests are essential.

Essential (Idiopathic) Hypertension. Hypertension for which no recognizable cause can be found is called essential or idiopathic. It should be emphasized that even if a known cause appears to exist—for example, renal disease—an etiologic relationship has not been established conclusively. Frequently the removal of an apparently diseased kidney is not followed by a fall in arterial pressure. (In some cases, secondary damage in the vascular system or opposite kidney may account for this.)

A great deal of controversy has gone on over the role of inheritance in hypertension. The most reasonable position on the basis of data now available seems to be that many factors, predominantly environmental but also inherited, lead to similar arterial pressures in members of certain families. In some families there is perhaps a stronger inherited tendency than in others; for example, twins have been described who developed malignant hypertension at about the same age while in different environments. The tendency to develop high arterial pressure certainly seems to be present at an early age and long before high arterial pressure itself is present. This is shown by the effects of pregnancy. In some women a high arterial pressure may occur for which no cause can be discovered; the arterial pressure may drop after pregnancy and may rise again later in life. They usually come from families with a history of high arterial pressure.

No consistent factor in hypertension of unknown origin has yet emerged that tells us anything about mechanism apart from these few clues.

Prognosis and Treatment. The outlook for a patient with high arterial pressure may in general be quantitatively related to the level of arterial pressure. The higher the pressure, the lower the survival rate over any period. This has been shown repeatedly in population studies. In an attempt to differentiate the outlook for various patients with hypertension, the terms *benign* and *malignant hypertension* have been used; the latter is also called the *accelerated* or *necrotizing phase* to describe both the rapidity of the course and the fibrinoid arteriolar necroses that define the histologic condition. The term "benign" should be abandoned, because it is a poor description for a condition that leads to death by stroke, myocardial infarct, and renal failure. It is easier from the epidemiologic viewpoint in describing large populations to give a quantitative prognosis, but in the individual patient seen for the first time the wise clinician takes account of all the variable factors discussed previously that may influence a particular value measured on the sphygmomanometer. This analysis, of course, influences his decision about whether the patient needs treatment or not.

There is no doubt in malignant hypertension that, unless the arterial pressure is successfully lowered, the patient will be dead usually within two years. It has been shown many times that it is possible to prolong life well over ten years by successful medical or surgical treatment of this phase of hypertension. Now that controlled trials of treatment in less severe grades of hypertension have been carried out, it is clear that improvement in outlook is conferred by successful treatment. In these cases, the prognosis depends on many factors, such as the presence of obvious vascular disease in major organs and the level of arterial pressure in relation to age. Although malignant hypertension may arise abruptly in a patient with previously normal pressure, it commonly supervenes after many years of moderately severe hypertension and seems clearly related to a rise over some months. Adequate treatment keeps this sort of patient out of this dangerous situation. The treatment depends in part on whether a potentially curable cause has been found. The curable causes of hypertension include pheochromocytoma, Cushing's syndrome, Conn's syndrome, renin-producing tumor, coarctation of the aorta, unilateral renal disease, and, occasionally, bilateral renal disease caused by surgically correctable renal artery stenosis. By "cure" in these cases is meant that the arterial pressure is returned to a completely normal level after operation.

Philosophy of Investigation and Treatment. *The first decision* a physician has to make is whether the arterial pressure as measured is too high for the individual, considering both the circumstances of the measurement and any of the other factors that can influence a single arterial pressure reading. *Time is on the side of the physician,* and repeated measurements under similar conditions, weeks or months apart, are often necessary to determine this point in the absence of any obvious signs of the effects of hypertension. It is also good to take the pressure three times in succession at one visit, because it is striking in many patients that the second and third pressures are lower when the stimulus of the initial cuff tightening has worn off. Measurements made over 24 hours by portable apparatus have shown how variable a pressure may be and how it may only be elevated when being measured by the physician. The next decision to be made after deciding that the arterial pressure is too high is given by the answer to the question, *"Am I seeking a cure or merely alleviation?"* Clearly in a young person with severe hypertension and no evidence of vascular disease, a cure is always sought. In a patient of 65 years with evidence of vascular disease of considerable degree, the answer may well be alleviation. In the first place this means that all the investigations that are currently available will be used to obtain a diagnosis, whereas in the second, one will be content with a few investigations useful in the management but concentrating on treatment by drugs. This is a good rule for other conditions than hypertension. The next important therapeutic rule is to make sure that the *symptoms complained of are caused by hypertension* and that the treatment by drugs

is not going to cause more trouble than the underlying condition. Too many elderly patients in their seventies with pressures of 190 systolic, 90 diastolic in mm of mercury are treated with potent hypotensive drugs for symptoms of giddiness caused by positional changes or for headaches as a manifestation of anxiety or depression that have nothing to do with hypertension, and are made much worse. Age needs no additional therapeutic hazards, and when treatment is indicated the arterial pressure should be brought down gently.

With severe hypertension it is unusual to be able to control the pressure by one major drug alone. A diuretic is needed in at least two thirds of the cases.

There is no particular "best" drug for the treatment of high arterial pressure. One of the mysteries of high arterial pressure is the way in which some patients respond well to one drug, some to another, without any other obvious difference between the patients. It is best to become accustomed to the actions and side effects of a small variety of drugs and to use them on all the patients who need treatment, exploiting each one to the full or to the limit of side effects before adding the adjunct or shifting to a new major drug. In the higher range of drug dose in which side effects accrue, multiple therapy is to be encouraged and not sneered at. Some patients do better, for example, on alpha-methyldopa plus guanethidine plus chlorothiazide than on either of the main drugs alone. There is now emerging the possibility of selecting more appropriate drugs for particular patients from studies of plasma renin levels. Some patients with high levels respond to inhibitors of renin release like propranolol, whereas some in the low renin group respond best to an aldosterone antagonist like spironolactone, or even to a thiazide.

Curable Hypertension. Once the rarities such as pheochromocytoma, coarctation of the aorta, Cushing's syndrome, and renin-producing tumors have been considered, two less rare conditions are of great interest because of the problems posed.

RENAL ARTERY STENOSIS. Once clearly diagnosed, prediction as to success of either nephrectomy or reconstructive arterial surgery depends upon other factors. It is best to be under 40 years with fibromuscular hyperplasia of one renal artery on the left side and a high peripheral plasma renin activity or angiotensin level with a higher concentration of renin in venous blood from the affected kidney than from the other side, and with a PAH clearance on the normal side that is well above 200 ml per minute. This enables the surgeon to bring down the splenic artery distal to the stenosis with the knowledge that if the blood flow can be restored satisfactorily, the arterial pressure will be lowered and not maintained, for example, by disease in the opposite kidney. The plasma renin activity is useful in conjunction with clear evidence of ischemia determined by pyelography, renography, and divided renal function studies. By contrast, it is bad to be over 40 years with an atheromatous block and other evidence of atheromatous vascular disease elsewhere as, for example, in the coronary arteries, and an absence of the criteria noted above.

CONN'S SYNDROME. Although initially primary hyperaldosteronism associated with a single tumor of the suprarenal cortex was believed to be easily identified by the presence of hypokalemia, moderate hypertension, raised plasma aldosterone or aldosterone secretion, and a suppressed plasma renin activity, it has now become clear that there are patients with all these criteria who have bilateral hyperplasia of the suprarenal cortex and whose hypertension is not cured by adrenalectomy. It is not even true that all patients with undoubted tumors of the zona glomerulosa have their arterial pressure brought down to normal levels after removal, even though evidence of hyperaldosteronism may disappear. As with most other conditions causing hypertension, there is a variable percentage of patients whose arterial pressure either does not fall at all or does not completely return to normal after operation (for example, pheochromocytoma); presumably secondary changes maintain the hypertension. In general the criteria of curable hypertension associated with an aldosterone adenoma are suppressed plasma renin level which fails to rise in the upright posture on a low sodium diet and injections of furosemide; high aldosterone plasma level resistant to lowering by DOCA administration; increased colonic potential difference reversed by spironolactone; low plasma potassium (less than 3.4 mEq per liter) and total body potassium; and plasma sodium usually above 142 mEq per liter with increased total body sodium. Anatomic demonstration of the tumor by venography, isotope localization with external scanning, or high aldosterone-to-cortisol ratios in adrenal venous blood complete the arduous diagnostic path.

Medical Treatment. From the results in large series of patients medically treated for hypertension, there is no doubt that morbidity and mortality are both reduced so long as the arterial pressure has been consistently lowered. Symptoms and signs both improve, as shown, for example, by the early relief of angina and the diminution in cardiac size roentgenographically. The occurrence of a cerebrovascular stroke in hypertension is an indication for lowering the pressure in order to lessen the risk of further stroke, because it is clear that a major reduction in mortality rate in treated hypertension is due to stroke prevention. Only occasionally in the older age group when the pressure has been reduced too quickly do signs of reduction of cerebral blood flow occur. Similarly, the presence of renal damage with hypertension is usually an indication for lowering the pressure to minimize further deterioration. The creatinine clearance may drop for a short time on lowering the arterial pressure but usually rises again, often to higher levels than at the outset if successful treatment is maintained. This temporary drop must not be used as an argument for lessening the vigor of treatment, and this is also true of intermittent claudication in which the condition will often improve.

The *drugs used in treatment* have known major actions as well as a number of others that are not altogether well defined. It is fair to say that very few of the drugs in current or in past use have had their action of lowering the arterial pressure completely explained. Various types of drugs are used, as follows:

Ganglion Blockers. The best example of these is hexamethonium. The basic chemical structure of this drug has been altered in various ways to produce substances of more desirable properties that are capable of predictable absorption by mouth and predictable duration of action. Acting on parasympathetic and sympathetic ganglia, these agents produce a widespread blockade, leading to changes in peripheral resistance and in venous tone, so that part of their action, seen best with the patient in the standing position, is due to venous pooling and diminished cardiac output. Most of these drugs will lower the arterial pressure in many patients, particu-

larly in the standing or sitting position. The major undesirable side effects are dryness of the mouth, paralysis of ocular accommodation, constipation, and impotence.

Pempidine tartrate may be used in a dose of 5 mg three times a day, which may be increased by 5 mg on each dose. This is probably the best of this type of drug for oral use. It should not be used in patients with distinct uremia (blood urea nitrogen over 50 mg per 100 ml), because paralytic ileus is a real risk. This drug, because of its quick onset of action and relatively short duration, is best given three times daily. The paralysis of ocular accommodation may be overcome by the use of pilocarpine hydrochloride 0.5 per cent eye drops. There is now very little place for this type of drug except as an adjunct in a very severe and resistant hypertensive patient.

Sympathetic Blockers. These have largely replaced the ganglion blockers, and either deplete or interfere with catecholamine metabolism at nerve endings or centrally. A prototype is *guanethidine,* which is concentrated in the postganglionic sympathetic fibers and interferes with the release of norepinephrine from the nerve endings. It also clearly has central effects, shown by the sleepiness and depression produced in some patients. Like the ganglion blockers, these agents produce a fall in pressure, mainly with the patient in the standing position, and, because of the sympathetic blockade, a distinct slowing in heart rate is seen. The major side effects are tiredness, peculiar muscular achings affecting the thighs and upper arms, shortness of breath, giddiness and postural hypotension on exercise owing to failure of vasoconstriction, diarrhea, and occasional impotence after failure of ejaculation.

Guanethidine sulfate in a starting dose of 10 to 25 mg daily is recommended. The full effects of the drug take a few days to become apparent, so that increases of dose (5 mg) should not be made more frequently than about every four or five days. Since it has a prolonged action, it need only be given once daily.

Bethanidine is like guanethidine in its actions but is quicker in onset and shorter in duration of action and has the merit of not causing diarrhea. The initial dose is 10 mg three times daily.

Debrisoquine sulfate has few central effects psychologically, does not cause diarrhea, and has a prolonged action. The starting dose is 10 mg twice daily.

Reserpine (various extracts of *Rauwolfia serpentina*) depletes nerve endings and organ stores of norepinephrine and epinephrine. It can be useful as long as a dose of 0.5 mg daily is not exceeded; beyond this amount, its major side effect of depression, even to suicide, becomes common. It is best used in a dose of 0.25 mg daily in conjunction with a thiazide diuretic, and even then the physician must remember that depression may slowly occur after several apparently trouble-free months; this can be reversed by removing the drug.

Alpha-methyldopa, among its other actions, serves as a competitive substrate for dopa decarboxylase on the route of production of norepinephrine via dopamine. It has marked central effects with tiredness and depression. Patients commonly seem to escape from its effects after some months of treatment. The starting dose is 250 mg either twice or three times daily, with a warning to the patients that they will feel extremely sleepy for the first few days, but that this usually wears off. The dose may be increased slowly as with guanethidine; because of its sedative action, it is well to begin by increasing the night dose. Occasional cases of jaundice and hemolytic anemia have been reported. In higher doses, especially if renal or brain damage is present, a state like akinetic parkinsonism may occur.

Propranolol hydrochloride is different from the aforementioned group in that it is mainly a beta blocker and acts not only on blood vessels, but also on the heart. It perhaps lowers the supine pressure relatively more than the other group of drugs and, apart from its beneficial effect in angina pectoris, it may provoke cardiac failure in those patients with a poor myocardium. The starting dose is 40 mg twice daily for one week, increasing to 80 mg twice daily, and so on. Its main interest now lies in its use in the high renin group of hypertensive patients, and some of these patients are very responsive when the renin levels are effectively suppressed. Another important side effect is shortness of breath on effort or asthma; it should never be used when this is present, and it should be remembered that the wheeziness may take some time to become troublesome.

Pargyline hydrochloride is a monoamine oxidase inhibitor, has a marked central effect, and is often useful in the depressed patient with hypertension. Like all other drugs of this type, it is dangerous if the patient is not warned about taking cheese, yeast and beef extracts, and heavy red wine, all of which may provoke severe hypertension and cerebral hemorrhage. Nevertheless some patients do well.

Adjuvant Drugs. Various drugs are used mainly as adjuvants to these main lines of treatment. They include hydralazine hydrochloride (starting dose 20 mg three times daily), whose mode of action is obscure, and phenoxybenzamine hydrochloride (starting dose 10 mg three times daily), which antagonizes the action of norepinephrine or epinephrine on the vessel wall but is surprisingly ineffective by itself.

Diuretics. In any case of severe hypertension, one of the previously described drugs is usually used in conjunction with a diuretic. The addition of a diuretic increases the hypotensive action and may make possible the use of a smaller dose of the major drug. The most commonly used are the thiazide derivatives, and there is nothing to choose between any of them. For example, chlorothiazide, 0.5 gram daily, is an adequate adjuvant, but has largely been replaced by smaller dose derivatives. The maximal adjuvant action is between two and four times the basic dose. Most doctors give potassium supplements because of the fear of potassium depletion. In general this is quite unnecessary, and a plasma potassium of 3 mEq per liter is not usually associated with any symptoms. Symptomatic hypokalemia in a patient on thiazides needs investigation for possible hyperaldosteronism. The initial mode of action is probably by sodium depletion and reduction in plasma volume, but action still continues when the plasma volume and sodium have been repleted, probably by diminished peripheral resistance. If it is nevertheless wished to give potassium, combined tablets should not be given, because small gut ulceration and stricture occur. Slow-release tablets of potassium chloride are safer. The thiazides may also occasionally precipitate diabetes mellitus, and more commonly gout and light-sensitive rashes. Although it was initially thought that only mild cases of hypertension would respond to a thiazide, experience has shown that quite severe cases may often respond to a thiazide alone; and if there is no particular urgency, then it is worth using, for example, 25 mg of hydrochlorothiazide twice daily. The full effect may take three to six weeks to be demonstrated but is undoubted. Furosemide in a dose of 40 to 80 mg daily is often used instead of a thiazide, but the very rapid diuresis may prove inconvenient.

Spironolactone. Although this can also be used as an adjuvant, it has a place of its own quite apart from its use in lowering the arterial pressure of patients with definite Conn's syndrome. In a dose of 25 mg twice daily, it can be introduced and the dose increased. It must be taken after meals, because otherwise it may cause nausea; it is contraindicated in peptic ulcer which it may cause to bleed. In some males it causes gynecomastia; in fewer females, interference with the menstrual cycle occurs, presumably because of its estrogenic effects. In the presence of renal failure, it should be used cautiously because of the elevation of plasma potassium it causes. Given together with a thiazide, it can provide smooth, well controlled, and symptomless control of hypertension. Suitable treatment is hydrochlorothiazide, 25 mg, spironolactone, 25 mg, each twice daily, or a combination tablet of spironolactone, 25 mg, and hydroflumethiazide, 25 mg, twice daily. Unless there is urgency, this is an excellent approach to the treatment of even severe hypertension. The combination which may well replace this treatment is that of a thiazide with amiloride. The latter is a potent, potassium-sparing diuretic which antagonizes potassium loss by a thiazide; together they can be very effective.

Treatment of Acute Pulmonary Edema and Hypertensive Encephalopathy. Two situations in hypertension demand emergency treatment in which it is essential to bring the arterial pressure down as rapidly as possible. The first is pulmonary edema caused by left ventricular failure, and the second is the state of fits and unconsciousness called hypertensive encephalopathy. In the first, if the patient is overloaded with fluids as in acute glomerulonephritis, the best form of treatment is to reduce the extracellular fluid volume, either by bleeding or by dialysis, although even with quite marked degrees of renal failure, the intravenous injection of furosemide, 40 to 400 mg, usually provides a rapid and dramatic diuresis without notable toxicity. It is always worth trying first, especially when there is doubt about the patient's fluid balance. If there is no obvious fluid overload, the dyspnea may be relieved by use of pentolinium tartrate in a dose starting at 1.5 mg intramuscularly and increasing until the pressure is brought down. The patient should, if possible, be sitting up for this procedure. Good results have been obtained with other drugs such as reserpine (5 mg intramuscularly), alphamethyldopa as an intravenous injection (50 mg per ml, total 250 mg), guanethidine sulfate as an intramuscular injection (25 mg), and sodium nitroprusside by continuous intravenous infusion (25 to 400 μg per minute); in a particular patient it may be necessary to try various of these in sequence. Relief of symptoms can be speedy. It is dangerous to use guanethidine sulfate intravenously, because the release of norepinephrine raises the arterial pressure even higher. Diazoxide (300 mg intravenously) given as a rapid injection produces flushing, nausea, and occasionally vomiting; nevertheless it can usually prompt a fall in arterial pressure within 15 minutes which may last 12 to 24 hours before a further injection is needed. Its mode of action is unknown. If given over a long period, it may cause hyperglycemia and frank diabetes, and even occasional pancreatitis. It is best in fulminating hypertension, but given by the oral route (starting dose, 40 mg three times daily) it has been very effective in patients with hypertension complicating renal impairment when the commonly used remedies have failed. Long-term treatment demands vigilance for the development of diabetes.

Typical Drug Dosages. Pempidine, 5 to 20 mg three times daily; guanethidine, 10 to 100 mg daily; bethanidine, 10 to 30 mg three times daily; debrisoquine, 10 to 80 mg twice daily; reserpine, 0.25 to 0.5 mg daily; alpha-methyldopa, 250 mg twice daily to 750 mg three times daily; propranolol, 40 to 160 mg two to three times daily; pargyline, 10 to 25 mg twice daily. To each of these drugs in moderate to severe hypertension, hydrochlorothiazide, 25 to 50 mg or equivalent thiazide is added daily.

Combined therapy in severe resistant hypertension: e.g., alpha-methyldopa, 250 mg three times daily, guanethidine, 25 mg daily, and hydrochlorothiazide, 25 mg daily. Debrisoquine, 20 mg twice daily, propranolol, 40 to 80 mg twice daily, and hydrochlorothiazide, 25 to 50 mg daily. Aldomet, 250 mg twice daily, propranolol, 40 to 80 mg twice daily, and hydrochlorothiazide, 25 to 50 mg daily. It is possible to replace hydrochlorothiazide with another diuretic such as Lasix, 40 to 80 mg daily, or spironolactone, 25 to 50 mg daily. Although combination treatment reduces side effects of each of the main drugs, some combinations have particular although occasional complications. The most important to recognize are dreaming and hallucinations, as well as muscle ache even to the point of severe pain, on combinations of the guanethidine group with propranolol.

Conclusion. Finally, the main aim of treatment is that the patient should live a more comfortable life than before treatment. The patient with diarrhea, impotence, tiredness, and a normal arterial pressure is not a therapeutic triumph. To treat hypertensive subjects requires patience, perseverance, optimism, and a belief that the drugs can be manipulated in most cases to lower the arterial pressure while keeping the patient comfortable.

Aldosterone in Clinical Medicine. Copyright by Searle & Company, San Juan, Puerto Rico. New York, Medcom, Inc., 1972.

Britton, K. E., and Brown, N. J. G.: Clinical Renography. London, Lloyd-Luke (Medical Books) Ltd., 1971.

Conn, J. W.: Aldosteronism and hypertension: Primary aldosteronism versus hypertensive disease with secondary aldosteronism. Arch. Intern. Med., 107:813, 1961.

Gross, F. (ed.): Antihypertensive Therapy, Principles and Practice. Proceedings of the Symposium held in Siena, Italy, June 28 to July 3, 1965, sponsored by CIBA. Berlin and Heidelberg, Springer-Verlag, 1966.

Leishmann, A. W. D.: Merits of reducing high blood pressure. Lancet, 1:1284, 1963.

Page, I. H., and Bumpus, F. M. (eds.): Handbook of Experimental Pharmacology. Volume XXXVII: Angiotensin. Berlin and Heidelberg, Springer-Verlag, 1973.

Page, I. H., and McCubbin, J. W. (eds.): Renal Hypertension. Chicago, Year Book Medical Publishers, 1968.

Peart, W. S.: Hypertension and the kidney. *In* Black, D. A. K. (ed.): Renal Disease. 3rd ed. Oxford, Blackwell Scientific Publications, 1972, p. 705.

Pickering, G. W.: High Blood Pressure. 2nd ed. London, J. & A. Churchill, Ltd., 1968.

Pickering, G. W.: The Nature of Essential Hypertension. London, J. & A. Churchill, Ltd., 1961.

Quinn, E. L., and Kass, E. H.: Biology of Pyelonephritis. Henry Ford Hospital International Symposium. Boston, Little, Brown & Company, 1960.

Robertson, P. W., Klidjian, A., Harding, L. K., Walters, G., Lee, M. R., and Robb-Smith, A. H. T.: Hypertension due to a renin-secreting renal tumor. Am. J. Med., 43:963, 1967.

Rose, G. A., and Blackburn, H.: Cardiovascular Survey Methods. Geneva, World Health Organization, 1968.

Stamey, T. A., and Good, P. H.: Diagnostic tools in the evaluation of renal vascular disease. *In* Brest, A. N., and Moyer, J. H. (eds.): Hypertension: Recent Advances—The Second Hahnemann Symposium on Hypertensive Disease. Philadelphia, Lea & Febiger, 1961, p. 189.

Symposium: Arterial hypertension. Arch. Intern. Med., 133:911, 1974.

Symposium: Primary hyperaldosteronism. Arch. Intern. Med., 123:113, 1969.

Veterans Administration Cooperative Study Group on Antihypertensive Agents: Effects of treatment on morbidity in hypertension. II. Results in patients with diastolic blood pressure averaging 90 through 114 mm Hg. J.A.M.A., 213:1143, 1970.

CORONARY ARTERY DISEASE

Thomas Killip

565. THE PROBLEM: ATHEROSCLEROSIS

Atherosclerosis is a disease of large and medium-sized arteries characterized by fatty deposits and thickening of the intima with disruption of the media. The aorta, its large branches such as the iliac, femoral, and carotid vessels, and the arteries supplying the heart and brain are commonly affected. Characteristically atherosclerosis progressively or abruptly interferes with blood flow; it is the leading cause of death in the United States. Deaths caused by vascular disease, specifically myocardial infarction and stroke, are more numerous than the next two leading causes, cancer and accidents, combined. Myocardial infarction and sudden death are the most common causes of vascular death. Acute myocardial infarction is responsible for 35 per cent of the deaths in the United States in males between the ages of 35 and 50. At present, a North American male has a 1 in 5 chance of having a myocardial infarct or sudden death before the age of 60. Data from many sources indicate that clinical events resulting from coronary artery disease are being recognized with increasing frequency and that the incidence has been rising for several decades.

Pathology. The advanced atherosclerotic lesion is pleomorphic and consists of accumulations of lipid, smooth muscle, fibroblasts, products of coagulation, and neovascularization in the intima of medium-sized coronary arteries. Eventually the lesion obstructs nutrient flow with consequent chronic or sudden ischemia or infarction. Although accumulation of lipid, largely cholesterol, is characteristic, proliferation of smooth muscle and fibroblasts, not normally present in the intima or media of mammalian arteries, comprises the so-called "complicated" lesion. As the focal atherosclerotic lesion increases in size, it becomes unstable. Rupture of the plaque into the lumen, intimal dissection of microscopic hematoma, or formation of thrombi and subsequent recannulation occur. Such events probably contribute to changes in the clinical state of the patient with chronic vascular disease being associated, for example, with transient cerebral ischemic attacks or unstable angina pectoris.

It is generally assumed that the atherosclerotic process begins with the *fatty streak,* a yellowish plaque visible when the affected artery is exposed. Fatty streaks have been observed in youngsters dying accidentally in the first decade. Prevalence increases rapidly with age.

The yellow streak consists of lipid deposits found mainly within intimal smooth muscle cells. How the lesion progresses from the benign fatty streak found in many mammalian species to the complex, obstructive changes of advanced atherosclerosis unique to man is unknown.

Also observed in infancy and childhood are mesenchymal lesions in the intima which show fibromuscular hyperplasia, increase in ground substance, some lipid, and disorder of elastic fibers. These lesions, found especially at bifurcations, are thought by some workers also to be precursors of atherosclerosis, but this view is not generally accepted.

Many epidemiologic surveys have demonstrated a convincing relationship between the level of dietary cholesterol, saturated fat intake, and vascular disease. How hyperlipidemia accelerates lipid deposition in the arterial system is not clear. Of the serum lipoproteins only the largest, chylomicrons, cannot pass through the endothelium into the arterial wall. In general the composition of the atheroma reflects plasma lipid content. It has been suggested that low density lipoproteins, which are characteristically found in the plaque, induce proliferation of smooth muscle cells altered to accumulate lipid. Injury to the endothelial barrier exposes the atheromatous material in the plaque to circulating platelets. This is known to induce platelet clumping and thrombus formation, leading to further damage of the vessel wall and obstruction.

Anatomy. Atherosclerosis of the coronary artery is found in the proximal segments of the medium-sized vessels, especially at branching points. Grossly the disease is segmental, although microscopic examination in advanced cases invariably reveals diffuse involvement. Lesions occur only in the vessels distributed over the surface of the heart. For reasons unknown, atheroma is not found in the penetrating or muscular branches which turn into the myocardium at right angles to the surface. Although much has been written about small vessel disease and ischemia, it is important to emphasize that the small intramuscular branches of the coronary arterial system are not involved in atherosclerosis. Small vessel involvement is said to occur in patients with diabetes mellitus, but this cannot be universally demonstrated. It is common, however, in association with various forms of muscular dystrophy.

Risk Factors. Numerous epidemiologic and clinical surveys during the past several decades have identified a series of risk factors which significantly increase the likelihood that coronary artery disease will become clinically evident. The variety of major and minor factors so far identified suggest that coronary artery disease and to the same extent cerebral vascular disease are multifactorial conditions whose probability is controlled by genetic, metabolic, anatomic, and environmental factors.

The risk of myocardial infarction increases progressively with *age* but is lower for *women* than for *men* until the sixth decade. The Framingham study and others have shown a clear association between the presence and severity of *hypertension* and occlusive vascular events. A recent Veterans Administration study revealed that persistent mild hypertension, defined as a diastolic pressure from 105 to 115 mm Hg after three days of hospitalization, was associated with increased risk of stroke and heart attack. Furthermore, treatment significantly lowered the risk of vascular disease. Curiously, although many studies have shown that reduction in occurrence of stroke is associated with effective treatment of hypertension, the same cannot be said for myocardial infarction, at least during the first three years of treatment. Although a relationship between hypertension and acceleration of atherosclerosis is well accepted, the failure to reduce the incidence of myocardial infarction after treatment emphasizes the important role of other factors in the perpetuation of the sclerotic process, once initiated.

There is overwhelming evidence that one of the most significant risk factors for atherosclerosis is elevation of *blood lipids.* This factor is most prominent in younger patients and decreases with age. An elevated blood cholesterol, of the Type IIA lipoproteinemia according to the Fredrickson et al. classification (see Ch. 817), is associated with a premature risk of extensive coronary artery disease and early myocardial infarction. Individuals, presumably homozygous for a Type II lipoproteinemia, have been reported with extraordinary high blood cholesterol and fatal myocardial infarction before age 20. A curious lesion, supervalvular aortic stenosis caused by a cholesteroloma, has also been described secondary to marked hypercholesterolemia. Elevation of triglyceride levels also carries an increased risk of myocardial infarction, whether with high cholesterol or normal cholesterol. Elevated triglyceride is frequently carbohydrate induced and associated with diabetes mellitus.

About 30 per cent of the survivors of myocardial infarction have elevated blood lipids. Among male survivors under age 40, the incidence in one study was 60 per cent. Diabetes, obesity, and hypertension are more common in those having elevated triglycerides than in those with normal blood lipids or elevation of cholesterol alone.

After an extensive survey of the relatives of patients surviving myocardial infarction, Goldstein concluded that five forms of hyperlipidemia were present: (1) a nongenetic, sporadically occurring hypertriglyceridemia, reflecting exogenous factors; (2) polygenic hypercholesterolemia, probably influenced by complex genetic and environmental interactions; and three types of monogenic hyperlipidemia: (3) familial hypercholesterolemia; (4) familial hypertriglyceridemia; and (5) an increase in both cholesterol and triglycerides, termed familial combined hyperlipidemia. Characteristically, familial hypercholesterolemia (Type II) was accompanied by early occurrence of arcus cornealis and tendinous xanthomas which could be recognized in childhood. There was no consistent relationship between the lipoprotein pattern according to the Fredrickson classification, and the apparent genetic disorder. This suggests that although the Fredrickson classification is useful clinically, it does not necessarily reflect a basic description of the genetic influences controlling lipid metabolism in patients with coronary artery disease. Goldstein estimated that in Seattle one in 150 individuals is a carrier of genes predisposing to one of the three described heritable lipid disorders.

Cigarette smoking is a prime risk factor for symptomatic coronary artery disease in the United States and Great Britain, but curiously this has not been shown to be the case in continental Europe. The tobacco, paper, and various chemicals used in the preparation and preservation of the product vary widely over the world. Such factors and their response to combustion may influence the health risk of tobacco.

Which components of the cigarette adversely affect the

cardiovascular system is subject to debate. *Nicotine* has well known vasospastic properties and releases endogenous catecholamines. This is not generally believed to be the culprit, however. Smokers have distinctly higher levels of *carbon monoxyhemoglobin* (COHb) than nonsmokers. Excessive concentration of COHb has many potential adverse effects, including reduction of available hemoglobin and a shifting of the oxyhemoglobin dissociation curve to the left. This reduces availability of oxygen in the capillary. According to Fahri, an increase in COHb concentration in blood from a normal 1 to 2 per cent to 5 to 6 per cent requires a 20 per cent increase in coronary blood flow to prevent ischemia, a requirement that could not be achieved in many patients with coronary artery disease. Increased exposure to carbon monoxide reduces exercise tolerance and decreases the threshold for pacing-induced angina in patients with coronary artery disease. Such effects have been shown under carefully controlled laboratory conditions, and also in patients with angina being driven along a Los Angeles freeway during rush hours! The possibility that carbon monoxide is an important factor in the hazard of cigarette smoking could explain the observation that, unlike the risk of cancer of the lung, the increased risk for myocardial infarction of the smoker falls rather rapidly to that of the nonsmoker after the habit is discontinued.

In addition to the so-called risk factors of dietary fat, hyperlipidemia, hypertension, and smoking discussed above, many other influences of possible importance have been identified. The association between *diabetes mellitus* and premature vascular disease, including myocardial infarction, is well known. Diabetes is commonly accompanied by hypertriglyceridemia, but how a disease expressed as glucose intolerance accelerates atherosclerosis is not understood.

Although often identified as a primary risk factor, *obesity* is not per se associated with an increased risk of coronary artery disease when coexisting hypertension or diabetes mellitus is taken into account. An increased incidence of coronary artery disease has been associated with certain *blood types,* the *hardness* of drinking water, and *hyperuricemia.* Individuals with blood types A, B, and AB have a higher incidence of myocardial infarction and angina pectoris than patients with blood type O. Communities whose residents drink *hard water* have lower death rates in general, and specifically for coronary artery disease, than do similar communities whose residents consume soft water. Water softness is a reflection of total rainfall; mortality rates in various communities have been inversely related to this factor also. That elevation of *blood uric acid* is almost as significant a marker for risk of coronary artery disease as cholesterol has long been recognized. How this factor operates is not known. Recently, excess drinking of *coffee* has been reported in patients discharged from hospital with a diagnosis of acute myocardial infarction.

Considerable debate, at times more emotional than rational, has centered on the role of *exercise* in reducing the risk of coronary disease. Vigorous exercise several times a week is postulated to enhance the growth of coronary collaterals by increasing ventricular work and myocardial oxygen demand. Many reports suggest that subjects who regularly exercise have a lower incidence of coronary events than those who are more sedentary. Although there is little doubt that such individuals may have an enhanced sense of well-being, unfortunately little of the data stands up to close scrutiny. Coronary artery disease is a slow multifactorial process developing over decades prior to clinical recognition. This, together with the difficulty of changing life styles and patterns of physical activity, makes the design of prospective studies especially difficult. It has been said that marathon running, for example, is the answer to coronary artery disease. Who ever saw an obese, hypertensive, marathon runner who was a heavy smoker? One well designed British study found that in men recording vigorous exercise during routine weekly activity, the risk of developing coronary artery disease was about one third that of a comparable group who did not. Vigorous exercise included swimming, four hours of heavy work, one hour of rapid walking in the country, or climbing 500 or more stairs a day.

Goldstein, J. L., Hazzard, W. R., Schrott, H. G., Bierman, E. L., and Motulsky, A. G.: Hyperlipidemia in coronary heart disease. J. Clin. Invest., 52:1533, 1544, 1569, 1973.
Gordon, T., and Kannel, W. B.: Premature mortality from coronary heart disease. J.A.M.A., 215:1617, 1971.
James, T. N.: Anatomy of the coronary arteries in health and disease. Circulation, 32:1020, 1965.
Kannel, W. B., Castelli, W. P., Gordon, T., and McNamara, P. M.: Serum cholesterol, lipoproteins and the risk of coronary heart disease. Ann. Intern. Med., 74:1, 1971.
Maugh, T. D., II: Coffee and heart disease: Is there a link? Science, 181:534, 1973.
Morris, J. N., Chave, S. P. W., Adam, C., Sirey, C., and Epstein, L.: Vigorous exercise in leisure-time and the incidence of coronary heart disease. Lancet, 1:333, 1973.
Ross, R., and Glomset, J. A.: Atherosclerosis and the arterial smooth muscle cell. Science, 180:1332, 1973.
Ross, R. S.: Pathophysiology of coronary circulation. The Sir Thomas Lewis lecture of the British Cardiac Society. Br. Heart J., 33:173, 1971.
Wissler, R. W.: Development of the atherosclerotic plaque. Hospital Pract., 8:61, 1973.

566. ANGINA PECTORIS

Definition. Angina pectoris is a clinical syndrome caused by inadequate oxygenation of the heart, characteristically precipitated by exertion, and relieved by rest or sublingual nitroglycerin.

Historical. Although there were several earlier reports, the condition since known as angina pectoris was masterfully described by William Heberden in 1772 in a paper entitled "Some Account of a Disorder of the Breast." The word angina refers to the sensation of strangling and anxiety which accompanies an attack. Heberden pointed out that the condition is common; that the seizure occurs while walking, especially uphill or after a meal; that the uneasiness vanishes with standing still; that prior to an attack the subjects appear perfectly well; that the pain is in the sternal area but may go to the left arm; that males past 50 are the most common victims; and that sudden death may terminate an attack.

Clinical Manifestations. *Pain.* The discomfort of angina may vary from mild to most intense. It may persist as a vague ache, and although the patient is aware of the sensation, he may continue his activities. On the other hand, once started, angina may rapidly build up to the point of intolerance, forcing the victim to stop and seek immediate relief. The pain of angina is usually not as severe as the intense precordial crushing sensation associated with acute myocardial infarction. It is usually described as pressing, boring, or gripping. The patient may feel as though a weight is on his chest. The chest feels tight, and there is often a sensation of heavy breathing. It may be difficult at times to determine whether the patient is complaining of angina, dyspnea, or both. This confusion may be partly explained by the striking alterations in ventricular function, including a sharp and reversible rise in left ventricular filling pressure, which accompany an attack of angina. Many sufferers, in describing angina, will make a fist as they grope for words to describe the discomfort. This gesture is a helpful clue.

The pain is characteristically a deep, visceral sensation—dull, aching, or heavy. Some patients do not refer to it as pain; rather they describe it as an ache or a vague awareness of discomfort. Sharp, fleeting sensations are not typical of angina. Pattients who complain of lightning pains in the anterior chest usually have some other process. Although the patient may feel that his chest is tight or squeezed so that his breath is restricted, the pain is not exaggerated by inspiratory movements. It is not searing, knifelike, or hot.

Angina may be attributed to indigestion. In some patients the sensation felt in the epigastrium is described as burning. It may be accompanied by considerable abdominal distress, including bloating and belching. The need to belch during an attack is common, and this may even give relief. Symptoms of peptic ulcer, hiatus hernia, or gallbladder disease are not uncommon in the age group suffering from angina. Clinicians have long recognized that these upper gastrointestinal conditions may precipitate attacks of angina pectoris. Intermingling of gastric and cardiac symptoms does not ease the diagnostic task.

The reaction to angina is highly variable. Those with mild discomfort may ignore the sensation and carry on normal activities, whereas others may manifest an acute fear of death. Often a strong element of denial makes obtaining an accurate history of the frequency, nature, and intensity of angina difficult. Patients with severe forms may limit activity to avoid triggering another attack. A careful history with emphasis in the frequency of attacks, the number of nitroglycerin tablets consumed, and the level of daily physical activity should enable the physician to recognize the true intensity of the condition.

The discomfort of angina is characteristically substernal. It is not felt on the surface of the chest, but may be located beneath the upper, middle, or lower portions of the sternum. Most commonly it is described in the midsternal region. The pain may also be felt beneath the precordium. It is important to emphasize that angina is seldom felt in the region of the cardiac apex. A complaint of pain localized to the apex described as "in the heart" will usually be a manifestation of a noncardiac condition. The pain may radiate widely. Typically the sensation is felt in the left arm and shoulder. It may radiate from the substernal region as intensity increases, or it may be felt predominantly in the arm, with minimal or no chest component. Usually the discomfort radiates down the medial side of the arm and may go to the fingers. Occasionally it may radiate down the right arm or both arms. A relationship between the intracardiac localization of myocardial ischemia and the pattern of pain radiation has not been established. The pain may radiate to the back, neck, or jaw, or discomfort may be localized in the intrascapular area. Occasionally, it is felt in the upper or lower abdomen. In all the areas of remote pain, the sensation retains the deep and aching character of visceral pain.

Precipitating Factors. Angina is characteristically episodic and triggered by *physical activity.* A patient may be able to predict discomfort by a specific act, for example, climbing a flight of stairs, but in other patients the effort of exertion is variable. Walking may be tolerated, but climbing a small hill may precipitate an attack. Angina is frequently induced by a heavy meal, especially if followed by exertion. Some patients are forced to change their habits and eat several small meals to avoid discomfort. Cold weather is especially prone to produce angina. Sometimes the first contact with cold air on leaving a warm room is sufficient, even though the patient is standing still. Many patients are able to walk indoors and perform labor, although they cannot do the same outdoors without discomfort.

Emotion is a well-known trigger for angina. An argument, a tense encounter, an anxiety-producing situation, or sexual excitement may induce pain. Angina may occur when the patient is resting quietly, seemingly without stimulation *(angina decubitus).* It is thought to imply more severe disease and to have a worse prognosis than other forms. Most instances of angina decubitus are probably triggered by emotion.

Nocturnal angina may be troublesome. In this form the patient has awakened from an apparently sound sleep with angina. It is important to differentiate this condition from nocturnal dyspnea secondary to left ventricular failure, which is usually due to redistribution of interstitial water and resultant increase in plasma volume in the recumbent position. On occasion congestive failure may precipitate angina in the patient with myocardial insufficiency and inadequate coronary blood flow. It has been shown that nocturnal angina is frequently preceded by a dream in which the subject is emotionally stimulated or is exercising. The dreams are often accompanied by striking increases in respiration, heart rate, and blood pressure. In one reported example the subject dreamed he was riding a bicycle uphill, and awoke with angina.

Although most individuals will stop exertion with the onset of angina, some will carry on and "walk through" the pain. There are typically three patterns of response if exertion continues with angina. In some patients the angina eventually subsides, and physical activity can continue without discomfort. In others the pain persists, is of only moderate intensity, does not progress, and the patient is able to tolerate the level of discomfort. He continues his activity. In a third group, however, the pain becomes progressively intense and forces the subject to obtain relief by rest or medication. Most patients fall into the last category.

Duration and Relief. Anginal pain usually persists no more than three to five minutes. The duration is somewhat variable, depending on the stimulus triggering the attack. When the pain is related to exertion, such as walking, it characteristically subsides, becoming progessively less severe, if the sufferer promptly stops and rests. Most patients with angina have pain only a few times a week. Since angina characteristically occurs with exertion, especially after meals or in cold weather, many patients learn to modify their daily activity to avoid pain. To evaluate severity of symptoms the careful historian determines not only the frequency of attacks but also the pattern of daily physical and emotional effort.

Spontaneous angina decubitus or angina developing during emotional tension may be especially severe in intensity and duration. Such episodes tend to persist for 10 to 15 minutes or longer and to be of agonizing intensity. The blood pressure may rise to an extraordinary degree, with development of striking diastolic hypertension during these attacks.

Some patients with clear-cut angina complain of long periods of chest discomfort lasting an hour or more. The sensation tends to be low grade, almost at the threshold of awareness. The patient equates the sensation with angina, describing it as an ache or an annoyance, but carries on his normal activities. Exertion or emotion may precipitate a full-blown attack. It seems likely that the complaint reflects a mild, chronic myocardial ischemia. Its presence is usually a sign of advanced coronary artery disease with multiple vessel involvement. It may or may not be relieved by nitroglycerin.

Usually the characteristics of angina are reasonably constant for the individual patient. The type of stimulus, whether emotional or physical, and the intensity, frequency, radiation, and duration of the pain are fairly regular from one attack to another. Any change in pattern causing an increase in symptoms should be viewed with grave suspicion. Increase in frequency, intensity, or duration or any lowering of the threshold for triggering the pain may presage an impending coronary syndrome, also termed *unstable angina pectoris.* Both the physician and the patient should be aware of the significance of an increase in symptoms. This subject is discussed in more detail later.

Causes of Pain. Many theories have been proposed in an attempt to explain the mechanism of cardiac pain. It is most likely directly related to metabolic changes caused by ischemia. Electrocardiographic abnormalities may precede awareness of pain or may occur in absence of pain, suggesting that an accumulation of active substances to some threshold necessary to cause pain is occurring. Such substances might be H^+, K^+, and possible components of the kallikrein system. There are two networks of sensory nerve fibers in the heart: a perivascular network encircling the coronary arteries, and fibers running beside the vessels and terminating between muscle bundles. Presumably the latter are stimulated by the ischemic process.

The pain of angina pectoris and that of myocardial infarction are similar in quality. The pain of infarction tends to be more intense, and may persist for several hours. Prolonged pain implies continued ischemia, not infarction. Once death of myocardium has occurred, pain is no longer present. One explanation for the occasional sudden improvement in previously stable angina is infarction of the chronically ischemic area.

Ischemic cardiac pain and the pain of intermittent claudication presumably have a similar mechanism. Both are described as deep, visceral sensations. Both occur with increased muscular work and are relieved by rest. Both are usually secondary to obstructive vascular disease.

The nerve pathways from the myocardium travel through the superficial and deep cardiac plexus, and the thoracic cardiac nerves to the first four or five thoracic ganglia. They enter the spinal cord via the white rami of corresponding thoracic segments. Cord segments D1 to D5 also receive pain fibers from the precordium, the medial portion of the anterior surface of the arm, and the forearm. Convergence within a common anatomic pathway of nerve impulses doubtless accounts for the characteristic radiation of the pain of angina pectoris.

Physical Findings. Between attacks, patients who suffer from angina may or may not have signs of organic heart disease. During an angina episode the patient usually becomes apprehensive. He may begin to sweat. Often he will press hard on the sternum with his hands. If he has had previous experience with the medication, he is anxious to take a nitroglycerin tablet as quickly as possible.

During the attack the heart rate usually rises. The blood pressure is frequently elevated, occasionally to alarming levels. Heart sounds may become more distant. The apical impulse may be more diffuse. Careful inspection and palpation of the precordium may reveal a localized systolic bulging or a paradoxic movement, a reflection of segmental myocardial ischemia producing a localized area of noncontracting myocardium. The second sound may become paradoxically split during angina so that the components close during inspiration and widen during expiration. This reversal of the normal splitting is thought to reflect a more prolonged left ventricular ejection time during the ischemic episode, because normally the aortic valve closes before the pulmonic valve.

A *fourth heart sound (S_4)* is extremely common in patients with ischemic heart disease, especially during an attack of angina. It is so common that its absence could be interpreted as evidence against the diagnosis. Curiously this sign was usually overlooked until recently. An excellent technique for recognizing an S_4 is first to identify the A wave in superficial neck veins and then to auscultate in the appropriate areas, using a bell while watching the jugular A wave. The S_4, whether of right- or left-sided origin, will be heard synchronous with the A wave. If this technique is followed, many an apparent first heart sound will be recognized as actually an S_4.

In some patients a *systolic murmur* may appear in the region of the cardiac apex during angina. Characteristically the murmur begins in mid- or late systole after the first sound. It is rather shrill and not exceptionally loud. This murmur is ascribed to papillary muscle dysfunction secondary to localized ischemia. If the papillary muscles are involved in the ischemic process, they become incapable of holding against left ventricular pressure during systole. During the latter half of systole, the mitral valve is forced open, and regurgitation occurs. The condition is often self-limited, for the murmur may not be detected when the patient is free of pain.

Careful observation and examination of the patient during an attack of chest pain may be extremely rewarding. Detection of abnormal cardiac findings and the disappearance of the findings with the subsidence of the complaints may help considerably in establishing the diagnosis.

Electrocardiogram. It must be emphasized that the resting electrocardiogram may be entirely within normal limits in the patient who has clear-cut and indisputable angina pectoris. The electrocardiogram is more likely to be normal when the syndrome first begins. Perhaps 20 to 30 per cent of patients first experiencing angina have a normal electrocardiogram on initial examination. Neither the extent nor the distribution of coronary artery disease can be predicted from a normal electrocardiogram. In one study 16 per cent of a group of patients with greater than 50 per cent obstruction of the three major coronary arteries, as determined by selective angiography, had completely normal electrocardiograms. Of patients with total obstruction of one or more major coronary arteries, 53 per cent had abnormal Q waves, suggesting old myocardial infarction, but 5 per cent had a completely normal resting electrocardiogram.

Chronic Changes. The presence of chronic electrocardiographic abnormality does not establish a diagnosis of angina. These changes may indicate the presence of organic heart disease. The chronic abnormalities that may be present include evidence of left ventricular hypertrophy, S-T segment and T wave change, bundle branch block, or pathologic Q waves, suggesting old myocardial infarction. Abnormalities of the S-T segments or T waves in the electrocardiogram are frequently nonspecific, and one must avoid overinterpretation. It is important to know whether the patient is receiving digitalis, which will reduce T wave amplitude and produce an S-T segment depression in most leads. In the normal person the effects of digitalis may be difficult to detect in the electrocardiogram, and consist largely of some decrease in amplitude of the T wave and a very slight S-T segment depression. In the patient with organic heart disease, on the other hand, digitalization may produce more striking changes. T waves may become inverted, and S-T segments markedly depressed. A pattern of "left ventricular strain" may appear when

prior to digitalis the electrocardiogram was essentially normal.

Scarring, owing to small infarcts, may cause abnormalities of the T waves and S-T segments. Patchy fibrosis is said also to produce high frequency alterations in the QRS complex. A characteristic "ischemic" sign is said to be a flat S-T segment depression from the end of the QRS complex to the onset of the T waves. Since there are many variations of S-T segment depression and the changes are usually nonspecific, it is impossible to utilize the electrocardiogram obtained in the absence of pain to confirm the diagnosis of angina pectoris.

Significant Q waves suggesting old myocardial infarction are helpful in confirming a diagnosis of coronary artery disease. Bundle branch block patterns may be difficult to evaluate. Right bundle branch block is perhaps a more benign lesion, in terms of diagnostic implications and prognosis. Blockage of the right bundle causes a delay of terminal QRS forces, and hence does not interfere with the recognition of abnormal Q waves of myocardial infarction. It is generally held that left bundle branch block implies disease of the left ventricle, either fibrosis or coronary artery disease. The abnormality in blockade of the left bundle is a prolongation of the initial QRS vector and a change in direction. Hence the pattern

Figure 1. Electrocardiogram recorded in a 57-year-old man during an episode of angina pectoris. *Top,* During the attack. *Bottom,* After pain had spontaneously subsided. The electrocardiogram shows extensive abnormality of the S-T segments and T waves. During angina the elevation of the S-T segments in several leads and especially V₂-V₅ is characteristic of that seen in variant or Prinzmetal's angina. The electrical location of these changes suggests epicardial ischemia of the area of myocardium supplied by the left anterior descending coronary artery. The tracing obtained after angina is abnormal.

Figure 2. Physiologic changes during spontaneous angina pectoris in a 53-year-old man. The patient was able to grade the intensity of angina on a scale of 0, "no discomfort," to 10, "worst pain ever." Figure shows from top, lead 2 of electrocardiogram, brachial arterial pressure recorded directly; lead V₃ of electrocardiogram, one-second time marker, grade of angina, and time in minutes. Arterial pressure before onset of angina is 135/90 mm Hg, and heart rate is 60 beats per minute. One minute before onset of sensation of heaviness in chest, heart rate and arterial pressure have increased moderately, and slight S-T segment depression has appeared, best seen in V₃. During the next five minutes intensity of angina progressively increases, electrocardiographic changes are more marked, and blood pressure and heart rate increase. When angina is most severe, arterial pressure has risen to 210/135 mm Hg. After sublingual administration of nitroglycerin, angina is relieved within 90 seconds. Arterial pressure falls coincident with improvement of symptoms.

of old or recent infarction may be obscured in the presence of left bundle branch block by the absence of expected Q waves.

Acute Changes. An acute, self-limited, and reversible abnormality of the electrocardiogram may be recorded during an attack of angina. The electrocardiogram is abnormal in virtually all patients during angina, provided that sufficient observations with appropriate leads are obtained. The recording of an electrocardiogram continuously during an attack of chest pain may be of inestimable value in establishing the diagnosis. During angina there are dramatic changes in the so-called "ischemic" pattern, in the repolarization waves of the electrocardiogram, the S-T segment, and the T waves. Sometimes QRS changes may also appear. The R wave may increase or decrease in height, and Q waves may appear temporarily. Intraventricular conduction disturbances or bundle branch block occasionally develop. Usually the most striking electrocardiographic change during an acute attack of angina is the S-T segments and T waves. The T waves may flatten and invert. If already inverted, they may become upright. "Ischemic" S-T segments, consisting of depression of 0.1 mv or more, may appear. At times the depression is truly striking, reaching 0.4 mv or more.

In some patients the S-T segments become markedly elevated in leads with upright R waves. The changes resemble those seen in the so-called "hyperacute" stage of myocardial infarction, but promptly subside after the pain is relieved. If infarction were present, the electrocardiographic abnormality would gradually evolve rather than rapidly return to the control tracing. S-T segment elevation probably represents dominant ischemia in the subepicardial layer, whereas the more typical S-T segment depression is an expression of subendocardial circulatory and metabolic change.

Exercise Tolerance Tests. An objective assay of the cardiovascular response to exercise is an important tool in the diagnosis and evaluation of patients with suspected or known coronary artery disease or angina pectoris. The purpose of exercise is to increase body oxygen consumption and augment myocardial work. In the subject with coronary artery disease the increased cardiac oxygen demand thus induced may exceed the available supply, thereby producing myocardial ischemia as reflected in the electrocardiogram.

The *two-step exercise test of Master* is gradually being replaced by the more carefully controlled *treadmill* or *bicycle ergometer tests.* In these procedures the work of exercise is gradually increased with close electrocardiographic monitoring until fatigue, chest pain, rapid heart rate, or positive electrocardiographic changes are achieved. An important concept in exercise testing is based on the observation that the maximal heart rate during exercise can be related to maximal oxygen consumption. Under conditions of stress, the ability to transport oxygen to the tissues is a reflection of the adequacy of cardiac function and is expressed as the product of heart rate × stroke volume × arteriovenous oxygen difference. During exercise there is a general linear relationship between heart rate and oxygen uptake by the body. Thus the adequacy of an exercise test may be judged by the heart rate achieved during stress.

Maximal heart rate attained during exercise declines with age. Tables are available relating predicted maximal heart rate during exercise to sex and age. Since exercise testing to maximal heart rate is often followed by a prolonged sense of fatigue or uneasiness and might be dangerous to the patient with significant coronary artery disease, testing is usually limited in many laboratories to achieving 80 to 90 per cent of the predicted value.

The ability to attain maximal exercise in patients with angina pectoris is often limited by dyspnea, fatigue, greatly reduced endurance, or chest pain. In advanced coronary artery disease the normal increase in cardiac output, stroke volume, and even arteriovenous oxygen difference may be greatly restricted. Exercise thus may induce evidence of severe left ventricular dysfunction which is not necessarily responsive to administration of digitalis.

In the patient with coronary artery disease, an episode of myocardial ischemia induced during exercise is usually associated with the development of significant electrocardiographic abnormalities during or after the exercise. Although studies during exercise are few, the changes interpreted as "ischemic" are accompanied by evidence of anaerobic myocardial metabolism with excess lactate concentration in the coronary sinus during angina induced by pacing or isoproterenol infusion. It is not necessary to induce angina to precipitate the electrocardiographic change. The electrocardiographic patterns observed are similar to those described earlier as occurring during an episode of angina pectoris.

The hallmark of an abnormal "ischemic" electrocardiographic response to exercise is S-T segment depression or development of an S-T segment vector essentially opposite in direction to the mean QRS vector. Although many criteria have been proposed, most authorities would agree that S-T segment depression of 0.5 to 1.0 mv is of borderline significance, but that depression of greater than 1.0 mv is definitely abnormal. Significant arrhythmia or rate-related bundle branch block is also interpreted as evidence of a positive or abnormal test. These findings, however, do not necessarily reflect coronary artery disease but may be due to primary conduction abnormality.

It is important to bear in mind two essential points. First, the demonstration that a patient has an abnormal electrocardiographic response to exercise does not prove that his chest complaint is angina unless the symptom recurred during exercise and was associated with characteristic electrocardiographic change. Second, a diagnosis of ischemic heart disease owing to coronary artery abnormality as a result of a positive exercise test is inferential. Many conditions such as valvular heart disease, myocardiopathy, and diseases of the small coronary arteries may be associated with a positive test. A syndrome, discussed in greater detail below, has been described as occurring mostly in young women, and is characterized by an angina-like pain, abnormal electrocardiographic exercise tolerance test, and normal coronary arteriogram. In some patients excessive hyperventilation during exercise is associated with changes in the cardiogram, especially T wave inversion. The abnormality is apparently related to increased blood pH and decreased plasma potassium. It may be prevented by breathing 5 per cent carbon dioxide during the test and by administration of potassium salts intravenously.

The results of an exercise tolerance test must be interpreted with caution. The implications of a diagnosis of ischemic coronary artery disease are so important that there must be continued awareness of the possibility of a false positive result. The frequency of a positive maximal exercise test in normal subjects increases with age. Bruce found 12 per cent positives in the fourth decade, 18 per cent in the fifth decade, and 22 per cent in the sixth and seventh decades. What percentage of these subjects have coronary artery disease is not known. A recent study found that 65 per cent of a large group of patients with known coronary artery disease (greater than 70 per cent obstruction of one vessel determined angiographi-

cally) in whom an interpretable result was obtained had a positive treadmill test. The rate of false positivity was 8 per cent. The frequency of positive tests increased with the number of coronary arteries obstructed. Generally, greater degrees of S-T segment depression were correlated with more extensive disease. Eighty-nine per cent of patients with typical angina pectoris had significant coronary artery disease, but only 58 per cent had a positive exercise test.

Although the exercise tolerance test is a potentially dangerous manuever in a patient with severe ischemic heart disease, relatively few serious accidents have been reported. The test is contraindicated when the resting cardiogram is unstable or suggests acute ischemia or infarction. Patients with crescendo angina or frequent, severe attacks of pain, or those in whom a diagnosis of myocardial infarction is suspected should not be exercised. The test should be performed only when a defibrillator and appropriate emergency drugs are immediately available.

Pathogenesis. According to current understanding, angina pectoris develops when cardiac work, and hence myocardial oxygen need, is greater than the ability of the coronary arterial system to supply oxygen per unit time. Angina can be precipitated by an increase in cardiac work and hence oxygen need, or, conversely, angina may occur after a decrease in the oxygen supply secondary to obstruction of coronary flow or a reduction of arterial oxygen content. It most commonly results when cardiac work and hence myocardial oxygen need exceed the available oxygen supply because coronary blood flow to certain regions is restricted. Obstruction of coronary flow owing to coronary atherosclerosis is the most common anatomic finding in the presence of angina. Other conditions which greatly increase cardiac work, such as aortic stenosis, hypertrophic subaortic stenosis, and aortic regurgitation, may be associated with angina despite anatomically normal coronary arteries.

Oxygenated arterial blood is supplied by the two main coronary arteries. Coronary blood flow occurs mainly during diastole because the systolic contraction of the ventricles so increases the resistance in the coronary tree that nutrient flow is largely blocked. An adequate coronary blood flow is therefore dependent on adequate diastolic pressure. When the aortic diastolic pressure drops abruptly, as in aortic regurgitation, coronary blood flow may be severely diminished.

The oxygen content of blood obtained in the coronary sinus is the lowest in any vein draining a major organ. Usually the coronary sinus blood oxygen content, saturation, or Po_2 varies but little despite marked variations in cardiac work. Increase in myocardial oxygen consumption is met not by increased extraction from arterial blood but by increased coronary blood flow. Coronary vascular resistance is rather precisely adjusted, by mechanisms largely under metabolic control, to regulate blood flow in relation to oxygen need. Although reflex control of the coronary vasculature may be demonstrated experimentally, it is probably not an important factor in man. Many metabolites, including ADP, are vasodilators. Berne has suggested that transient excess of ADP when myocardial oxygen need increases is an important control of coronary blood flow. Thus when cardiac work and oxygen utilization increase, coronary vascular resistance falls, permitting an increase in coronary blood flow and oxygen delivery. Conversely, when oxygen demand falls, coronary vascular resistance rises, and coronary blood flow and oxygen delivery decline. Implicit in the mechanism is the maintenance of relatively constant coronary sinus oxygen levels, because changes in extraction of oxygen from arterial blood are relatively minor.

Changes in arterial Po_2, as influenced by hypoxia or abnormal ventilation, may lessen myocardial oxygenation. It has been suggested that increased affinity of hemoglobin for oxygen, which would increase the oxyhemoglobin saturation or content for a given Po_2, may precipitate myocardial ischemia. A number of hemoglobin variants with abnormal affinity for oxygen are now known, but their relation to ischemic heart disease has not been clarified.

Carbon monoxide may be important in myocardial ischemia. It has an affinity for hemoglobin 200 times that of oxygen, and displaces oxygen from the hemoglobin molecule; thus a given level of carbon monoxyhemoglobin reduces the blood oxygen content that can be reached even by breathing 100 per cent oxygen. The effect of carbon monoxyhemoglobin in the threshold for angina during pacing and traveling on an urban highway was discussed in Ch. 565.

Under normal conditions, myocardial metabolism is

entirely aerobic, there being little capacity to maintain normal function anaerobically. A wide variety of substrates are utilized as fuels, depending on availability. These include free fatty acids, glucose, ketones, lactate, and pyruvate. Under ischemic or anaerobic conditions, glycolysis is activated through the Embden-Meyerhof cycle to derive high energy phosphate. The rate-limiting enzyme is phosphofructokinase. In mammalian hearts relatively little glycogen is available during anaerobiosis. In these circumstances pyruvate becomes the hydrogen acceptor, substituting for oxygen, and lactate is produced.

The most useful metabolic index of myocardial ischemia is demonstration of myocardial lactate production via coronary sinus sampling during angina or myocardial stress. Myocardial stress may be induced by pacing the heart at a rapid rate or by intravenous infusion of isoproterenol, which increases both heart rate and myocardial contractility, thus increasing oxygen need. Production of lactate with myocardial stress generally indicates a 90 per cent or greater occlusion of a major coronary artery.

It is difficult to obtain precise metabolic data during an episode of myocardial ischemia or angina in man. Certain animal experiments are pertinent, however. When coronary blood flow is gradually reduced but cardiac work is kept constant, a sequence of events may be identified. Myocardial extraction of oxygen is near maximal initially, so that coronary sinus Po_2 falls little. Coronary vascular resistance declines progressively to reach a low plateau. Further reduction in blood flow and hence oxygen delivery is followed by metabolic and physiologic evidence of ischemia. The myocardium switches from lactate extraction to lactate production. Coronary sinus blood pH falls. Potassium loss from the myocardium is detected. Electrocardiographic abnormalities appear, and the S-T segments are depressed. Ventricular performance begins to deteriorate, and left ventricular filling pressure and left atrial pressure rise.

In man, during spontaneous angina pectoris or ischemia induced by exercise, pacing, or isoproterenol, metabolic and functional changes can be detected similar to those described in animals. Lactate is produced, and potassium efflux occurs. The electrocardiogram becomes abnormal, and frequently left ventricular diastolic pressure rises. The increase in left ventricular filling pressure and hence pulmonary venous pressure probably explains the not uncommon association of dyspnea with angina in many patients.

The major determinants of myocardial oxygen consumption are heart rate, systolic tension or pressure, and contractility. In the occasional patient whose angina is made worse by digitalis, increased myocardial oxygen demand secondary to the effect of digitalis on the contractile mechanism has been postulated. Any mechanism by which heart rate, ventricular systolic pressure, or contractility is increased may induce angina. Studies during exercise or cardiac pacing have shown that patients with angina will predictably develop metabolic or electrocardiographic signs of ischemia or pain when cardiac work reaches a given value for the individual patient. Thus the level of cardiac work required to induce angina is usually reproducible under laboratory conditions.

Studies during spontaneous angina at rest have shown that the subjective awareness of pain is usually preceded by increase in heart rate and rise in blood pressure. In

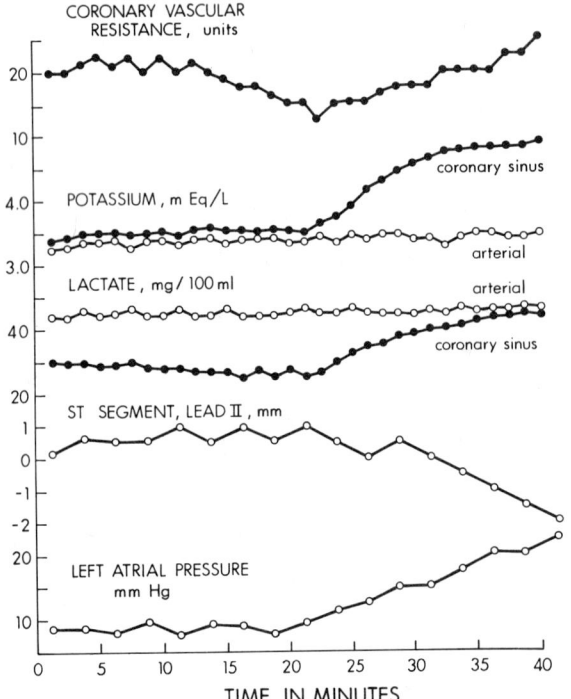

Figure 3. Physiologic and metabolic changes in experimental myocardial ischemia. A cannula is inserted into the left coronary artery, and myocardial blood flow is measured. Serial blood samples are obtained from an artery and the coronary sinus. The electrocardiogram and ventricular pressures are recorded continuously. Nutrient flow through the left coronary artery is progressively reduced in this experiment in a dog, and a series of sequential changes occurs. Coronary vascular resistance declines and reaches a minimum at 20 minutes. When coronary resistance reaches a low point, the following changes occur: onset of potassium efflux into the coronary sinus; change of myocardial metabolism from lactate utilization to lactate production; appearance of S-T segment depression in the electrocardiogram; and development of progressive rise in left ventricular filling left atrial pressure. Thus in this experiment, myocardial ischemia develops when reduction of coronary vascular resistance can no longer compensate for deficient coronary blood flow. With the onset of ischemia, there are progressive changes in myocardial cell membranes and metabolism, in the electrocardiogram, and in the function of the left ventricle. (After Case.)

some patients electrocardiographic changes appear one to three minutes before the pain, suggesting a buildup of metabolic substances prior to stimulation of pain receptors. Blood pressure usually continues to rise as the ischemic attack progresses. If the angina is not relieved by medication, the blood pressure, both systolic and diastolic, may rise to alarming levels. I have observed levels as high as 200 systolic, 150 diastolic in a patient who was normotensive between attacks.

The rise in systemic blood pressure and increase in heart rate during angina represent a potentially disastrous bio-feedback system: the higher the blood pressure and the faster the heart rate, the greater the unmet myocardial oxygen need. In patients who become severely hypertensive during angina, prompt treatment with vasodilators such as nitroglycerin or amyl nitrite is mandatory. Narcotics such as morphine will frequently relieve the pain, but usually do not lower the pressure significantly. Careful evaluation of the patient with prolonged, excruciating angina will often reveal paroxysmal hypertension, presumably in association with the pain. Adequate treatment of the pressor response will ease the angina in most instances.

The cause of the rise of blood pressure in angina is not established. It does not appear to be related to adrenocortical function. It is not initially due to pain, because the pressure usually begins to rise before pain is perceived. Although a pheochromocytoma has on occasion been suspected, there is no evidence that it is due to abnormal adrenocortical function. A chemoceptor supplied from the left descendens coronary artery has been described in dogs, and the possibility of pressor reflexes triggered by the metabolic insult of rapidly increasing local ischemia is intriguing.

The mechanism by which exposure to cold induces angina has been elucidated by recent studies. During such exposure, arterial pressure and peripheral vascular resistance reflexly rise. Cardiac work may be suddenly and sharply increased, thus inducing an ischemic attack. The exposed skin of the face is an important cold receptor triggering this reflex. This susceptibility of the face to cold may be an atavistic expression of the diving reflex found in aquatic mammals and birds. The wearing of a face mask in cold weather may reduce the frequency of angina.

Pathology. Coronary artery disease with atherosclerosis of major vessels is the most common cause of angina pectoris. Pathologic studies in patients who die almost invariably reveal extensive atherosclerosis. Blumgart showed many years ago in postmortem perfusion studies that the patient with angina has occlusion of at least one major coronary artery. Coronary arteriography has demonstrated that angina is almost invariably associated with a significant obstruction of a major coronary artery. At autopsy, the myocardium frequently also shows small scars and areas of fibrosis. This observation suggests that patients with angina may have multiple small and clinically silent myocardial infarcts.

Any condition which obstructs coronary flow or increases cardiac work may be associated with angina. *Syphilitic aortitis* is often complicated by angina, because the inflammatory process may constrict the coronary ostia. Patients with hemodynamically significant *aortic stenosis* are especially susceptible; indeed the onset of angina is an important symptom implying poor prognosis. Its presence should suggest careful evaluation of the severity of the obstructive lesion, and surgical in-

tervention should be considered. Three factors contribute to the association between angina and aortic stenosis. First, the obstructive lesion markedly increases cardiac work because of increased left ventricular systolic pressure, especially during exercise. Second, excrescences from the degenerative process of calcific aortic stenosis may obstruct the coronary ostia or cause coronary emboli. Third, patients with aortic stenosis tend to be males in the sixth or seventh decade when concomitant coronary artery disease is not uncommon.

Occasionally nonsyphilitic *aortic regurgitation* is complicated by angina. Although flow work, high cardiac output, is less costly in terms of oxygen requirement than pressure work, systolic pressure in severe aortic regurgitation is quite high. The ventricle is enlarged because of the very large stroke volume, and wall tension is increased. Diastolic pressure is correspondingly low. Coronary blood flow which occurs predominantly in diastole is reduced, and ischemic attacks may occur.

Angina is a complication of *hypertrophic subaortic stenosis.* The myocardium in this condition may be massively hypertrophied. Angina appears to be related to the markedly increased pressure – work and left ventricular wall tension – associated with this condition, because usually the coronary arteries are large and patent.

Angina is said to complicate advanced *mitral stenosis.* It is frequently difficult to separate anamnestically a sensation of chest tightness owing to acute dyspnea from that of angina. In my experience, patients with mitral stenosis and classic symptoms of angina have had concomitant coronary artery disease. It is possible that angina may reflect right ventricular ischemia in some patients with advanced pulmonary vascular change secondary to mitral stenosis.

Angina may be associated with severe *right ventricular hypertension* in congenital heart disease such as severe pulmonic stenosis, primary pulmonary hypertension, or tetralogy of Fallot. The *so-called hypercyanotic angina* or pain of pulmonary arterial hypertension is most likely right ventricular angina. There is no convincing evidence that distention of the pulmonary arteries is painful.

Anemia, hyperthyroidism, and *hypothyroidism* may be complicated by angina. In most instances there is severe pre-existing coronary atherosclerosis. The patient with myxedema may present a special problem. Restoration of a euthyroid state with thyroid medication may precipitate severe angina. There is a significant risk of acute myocardial infarction or sudden death if excessive doses of thyroid are used. Most authorities recommend a prolonged treatment period with small increments of thyroid.

Angina and Normal Coronary Arteries. Since the advent of coronary arteriography, a syndrome of angina pectoris with anatomically normal coronary arteries has been recognized. This variant amounts to 5 to 10 per cent of patients referred for arteriography. The condition occurs predominantly in young women. In some cases the history suggests classic angina. In others the story is less clear, and the physician may be uncertain about the true diagnosis, but a diagnosis of "atypical" angina is suggested. Attacks may be precipitated by exercise or emotion, but often occur spontaneously. Since current techniques for coronary arteriography can visualize vessels no smaller than 1 mm, it has been postulated that the syndrome reflects small vessel disease. Pathologic evidence is not available to support this thesis. It is also likely that a significant number of these patients do not have angina at all, and that the "atypical" pain is not cardiac in origin.

Despite the doubts raised above, there is a small group of patients who have a typical syndrome of angina pectoris and anatomically normal coronary arteries as revealed by angiography.

It is possible that occasionally obstruction of the coronary arteries is overlooked through failure to obtain high quality films or multiple views. Injection of the dye after administration of nitroglycerin may be necessary to ensure that no local obstruction exists in the coronary tree. Lactate production during stress has been observed in some of the patients with normal coronary anatomy and angina. Many patients are heavy smokers, and coronary spasm not caused by catheter trauma has been convincingly demonstrated in a small number of patients.

Raynaud's phenomenon is rarely found in association with this syndrome. Increased affinity of hemoglobin for oxygen or local metabolic abnormality has also been postulated, but confirmation is lacking.

Diagnosis. Angina pectoris is a clinical diagnosis, largely dependent on the history. In some cases the diagnosis may be established by direct observations during an attack. In the vast majority of patients, however, the diagnosis is evident to the experienced physician from the history alone, and confirmatory tests are not needed.

The electrocardiogram may be utilized to confirm the diagnosis. In doubtful cases the recording of typical electrocardiographic "ischemic" changes, as described earlier, during an attack of pain will often be diagnostic. However, use of exercise tolerance tests with electrocardiographic recording to confirm the presence or absence of angina is frequently unsatisfactory. Occurrence of pain, the patient's actual complaint, is uncommon. As discussed earlier, it is important that the test be standardized and closely monitored. A positive test, in the absence of pain, does not confirm the presence of angina. It does suggest, however, the presence of ischemic or coronary artery disease.

The response to nitroglycerin may be utilized as a critical diagnostic test. Angina pectoris is characteristically relieved in from 90 seconds to 3 minutes after sublingual administration of nitroglycerin. Failure of the symptom to be relieved promptly by nitroglycerin should cast suspicion on the diagnosis of angina. Many patients have a poor sense of timing, and cannot accurately describe the duration of an attack or the quickness of relief after medication. It is important to emphasize to the patient the necessity for accurate information before drawing the conclusion that nitroglycerin is not useful and therefore that the diagnosis is in doubt.

Coronary Arteriography. Visualization of coronary anatomy is achieved by coronary arteriography. The technique most widely used involves selective cannulation with a specially shaped catheter that is passed to the aortic root from the brachial or femoral artery. Use of the brachial artery usually requires a cut-down and incision of the vessel. After repair of the vessel, loss of the brachial pulse should occur in less than 5 per cent of patients. Utilization of larger vessels such as the femoral artery permits a percutaneous technique, as described by Seldinger, in which the vessel is punctured with a needle and a guide wire inserted. The needle is then withdrawn and a catheter advanced over the guide wire to the desired location. The wire is then withdrawn, and the catheter is flushed with heparinized saline or other fluid.

The coronary arteriogram is obtained when radiopaque dye is injected into the coronary ostia. Usually the pictures are recorded on 35 mm cine film. Several injections are filmed in various oblique views so that all vessels may be observed in multiple projections. In doubtful cases arteriograms are obtained before and after administration of nitroglycerin. The resulting vasodilation may reveal areas of obstruction not previously recognized.

Several studies have shown good correlations between the coronary arteriogram and postmortem findings. A properly performed and technically correct coronary arteriogram is believed to satisfactorily represent the anatomic configuration at the time of study. Coronary atherosclerosis is recognized by narrowing, beading, or occlusion of the arteries. Vessels as small as 1.0 mm may be demonstrated with good technique. Collateral vessels may be seen bridging obstructed areas or providing retrograde filling of a proximally obstructed artery.

At the time of the examination further information may be obtained by injecting dye into the left ventricle to obtain a left ventriculogram, and also by measurement of left ventricular end-diastolic pressure. Although the latter is influenced by many factors, including the stiffness of the ventricle, elevated levels suggesting compromised ventricular performance are frequently observed in patients with severe coronary artery disease. Myocardial contractility and size may be evaluated by scrutiny of the ventriculogram. The ejection fraction, the ratio of the volume of blood ejected during systole to the volume remaining at end-systole, may be calculated. Normally, approximately 50 to 60 per cent of the end-diastolic volume is ejected with each beat. Smaller fractions suggest myocardial disability and increased residual volume. Areas of abnormal contractility, termed *dyskinesia* or *akinesia,* owing to old scar or infarction may be observed.

The primary indication for coronary arteriography, including ventriculography, is to determine the location and extent of disease in patients being considered for coronary artery surgery and revascularization procedures. Other indications are being applied by many groups but remain controversial. They include investigation of certain electrocardiographic abnormalities such as bundle branch block or T wave inversion, especially in individuals with job security problems (e.g., airline pilots); after myocardial infarction or ischemic events in younger patients; and evaluation of a positive exercise test in the absence of symptoms.

Coronary angiograms are frequently performed to evaluate the cause of atypical chest pain. The procedure cannot establish the presence of angina; nevertheless, in some patients with incapacitating chest pain the finding of a normal coronary arteriogram can provide helpful reassurance. Attention can then be directed to symptomatic management and search for other causes of pain.

Complications of the procedure include precipitation of angina, dissection of a coronary artery, acute myocardial infarction, and asystole or ventricular fibrillation. Asystole usually responds to a blow on the chest. Atropine in several doses intravenously (0.3 to 1.0 mg) is a useful preventive in susceptible subjects. Immediate DC precordial shock usually reverts ventricular fibrillation. To be successful the shock must be applied within a few seconds of the onset of fibrillation. Mortality from coronary arteriography is approximately 0.1 to 0.5 per cent *in skilled hands.* Morbidity is largely related to complications of the arterial puncture or cut-down. Myocardial infarction may occur as a complication. The incidence depends on patient selection but should be less than 0.5 per cent.

Differential Diagnosis. Many conditions cause pain in the chest, but few if any truly mimic angina pectoris. The syndrome of angina is so characteristic in the majority of patients that errors in diagnosis are usually the result of careless history taking. In obtaining an accurate history, it is best first to allow the patient to describe his problem in his own way, and then to amplify the story by a series of questions.

Diseases of the gallbladder and gastrointestinal tract, chest wall disorders, abnormalities of the cervicodorsal spine, and pulmonary conditions may cause discomfort in the chest. Costochondral separation may be a source of confusion, but it is readily diagnosed by demonstration of exquisite point tenderness at one or more costochondral junctions on the anterior chest. Evaluation of the role of peptic ulcer disease, gallbladder abnormality, or hiatus hernia may be troublesome. Many patients with angina suffer from one or more of these conditions. It may be difficult to recognize that the patient actually has two or more complaints. Clinical experience supports the view that disease of the upper gastrointestinal tract may exacerbate angina. In some cases removal of a diseased gallbladder reduces the incidence of angina. In many patients symptoms of hiatus hernia trigger angina, especially at night; treatment with antacids and elevation of the head of the bed may give relief. Electrocardiographic changes have been reported during gallbladder attacks or symptoms from hiatus hernia. Usually these are nonspecific S-T segment or T wave changes. They probably reflect the presence of coronary artery disease and represent an abnormal response to fever or tachycardia. Reflex changes have also been postulated as causative.

Treatment. An effective plan of treatment must be based on a thorough understanding of the severity and intensity of the patient's complaint. The physician should explore carefully the circumstances in which angina occurs. Often, minor adjustments in the patient's activity will reduce the frequency of attacks. Angina often occurs repeatedly during the same activity. Avoidance of that specific activity or administration of nitroglycerin before onset will usually reduce symptoms. Should an attack occur, most patients will stop, rest, and administer a nitroglycerin tablet. Some will ignore the discomfort and continue their exertion. Progressive increase in intensity of pain usually forces the subject to stop. Occasionally the pain will improve despite continued activity. Although the development of angina usually indicates significant obstruction of one or more vessels by coronary atherosclerosis, it is important to emphasize the generally good prognosis in patients with stable angina. The patient should be encouraged to report any change in the pattern of angina promptly to his physician.

Association of angina and moderately severe depression is not uncommon. Angina may remind the patient that he is growing older, and that his activity is becoming restricted. Physician and patient should take an optimistic and realistic point of view. With appropriate therapy and some adjustment of the daily living pattern, activity may be nearly normal. Angina may persist for many years. During this time the patient may continue to work and to enjoy recreation and normal family relationships. There may be considerable anxiety, especially on the part of the spouse, about sexual activity. The patient may reasonably be encouraged to continue those activities as long as they do not precipitate disturbing symptoms.

An essential component of management of the patient with angina is recognition by both patient and physician of the importance of identified risk factors followed by a firm outline of proposed therapy.

The evidence for an adverse effect of *smoking* on the natural history of coronary artery disease is overwhelming. Patients with coronary artery disease and angina pectoris should be urged in the strongest terms to cease smoking. Many patients who develop angina are overweight. Reduction of body mass to more normal values may be associated with clinical improvement. Significant *hypertension* should be brought under control. It is frequently useful to treat even mild diastolic hypertension, levels of 90 to 100 mm Hg, with an agent such as hydrochlorothiazide, 50 mg daily. In older patients systolic pressure may be increased because of increased vascular stiffness. Although this systolic hypertension may increase left ventricular work, treatment of systolic blood pressure elevation of itself is not usually recommended unless the condition is severe.

Occasionally angina is a manifestation of left ventricular failure; treatment of the heart failure may produce dramatic improvement. The onset of exertional dyspnea prior to the perception of pain is a clue suggesting the possibility that it is precipitated by left ventricular failure. Nocturnal angina may be a manifestation of heart failure. Rarely digitalis intensifies angina, and the drug must be discontinued. Rapid paroxysmal arrhythmia may precipitate angina even in the absence of coronary artery disease. Usually, however, angina in the presence of arrhythmia in the older patient indicates coronary atherosclerosis. Treatment aimed at prevention of the arrhythmia may forestall chest pain.

Drug Therapy. IMMEDIATE TREATMENT. *Nitroglycerin* (glyceryl trinitrate sublingual tablets) in doses of 0.15 to 0.60 mg sublingually is the single most effective agent for treatment of the acute episode in most cases. With the exception of amyl nitrite, no other agent can approach it in general usefulness. Onset of action begins in one and a half to three minutes. Relief is usually dramatic and immediate. Occasionally the patient will take a second dose a few minutes after the first for complete effect. A large number of tablets may be ingested daily with few side effects. A fullness or pounding in the head is common, but most patients tolerate this well. An occasional patient will refuse to continue the medication because of intolerable headache. Because the drug is an effective peripheral vasodilator, the individual should first test its effectiveness while sitting or lying to avoid the possibility of syncope. Nitroglycerin may lose its potency unless stored in tightly sealed glass containers. It is good therefore to advise the patient to keep small amounts only in plastic or other types of small, portable containers.

Nitroglycerin is a potent smooth muscle vasodilator. After administration, a decline in coronary vascular resistance and an increase in coronary blood flow can be demonstrated in laboratory animals and normal man. In the past it was thought that the drug relieved angina by its direct action on the coronary vascular tree. Sublingual administration of the drug probably has little primary influence on coronary vascular resistance or coronary blood flow in patients with advanced coronary artery disease. It may have an effect in small vessels, however, and the possible role of spasm of large vessels, even in the presence of extensive disease, has attracted renewed interest. Injection of nitroglycerin directly into coronary ostia in diseased vessels causes a fleeting increase in coronary flow as revealed by disappearance curves of radioactive krypton or xenon. Therapeutic effectiveness of nitroglycerin results from a complex interaction of direct cardiac and indirect systemic effects. After use of sublingual nitroglycerin there is a fall in systemic blood pressure and decrease in systemic vascular resistance. The great veins dilate, causing pooling of venous return, and cardiac output declines. The net result is a marked decrease in cardiac work. Since angina results from an imbalance between oxygen demand and oxygen delivery, any mechanism that restores a more favorable relationship by either increasing delivery (coronary blood flow) or reducing demand (cardiac work) should be helpful. Current evidence strongly suggests that an important aspect of nitroglycerin's dramatic effectiveness is its ability to rapidly reduce cardiac work, thus reversing myocardial ischemia in patients with abnormalities of the coronary arteries.

Amyl nitrite is an extremely potent vasodilator that was first used in the treatment of angina more than 100 years ago. The drug is extremely volatile; it is contained in small, 0.3 ml ampules which are crushed, and the vapor is briefly inhaled. It has a strong, clinging odor, and is best used in a room with good ventilation. Because of its potency, the drug should be applied only when the patient is lying down. The ampule is crushed and wafted under the nose two or three times. A deep breath or two is generally all that is needed to obtain an effect. If the drug is administered by a second person, caution is advised to avoid inhalation of too much drug.

Amyl nitrite causes profound peripheral arterial vasodilation. Blood pressure falls precipitously with adequate dosage. In contrast to nitroglycerin, acute administration has relatively little measurable effect on the great veins, and venous pooling is not marked. For this reason cardiac output increases considerably after inhalation of the drug. Because of these effects on peripheral resistance and flow, amyl nitrite has been utilized to evaluate certain heart murmurs, such as those associated with aortic stenosis or mitral regurgitation, and to reveal the characteristic pressure pulse in hypertrophic myocardial disease. After use of amyl nitrite, the murmur of aortic stenosis is accentuated because of the increased cardiac output, whereas the murmur of mitral regurgitation declines in intensity because of the marked drop in peripheral resistance.

The use of amyl nitrite is currently unfashionable. It is, however, extremely effective in the occasional patient with severe, persistent angina and concomitant hypertension with high levels of diastolic pressure. The hypertension may be secondary to the ischemia. In some patients with angina complicated by hypertension, amyl nitrite is the only consistently effective form of therapy.

DRUGS GIVEN TO LESSEN THE FREQUENCY OF ATTACKS. Long-acting nitrites are said to provide relief of angina throughout the day by virtue of sustained blood levels of active substances. These include *erythrityl tetranitrate* (10 to 30 mg), *pentaerythritol tetranitrate* (10 to 20 mg), and *isosorbide dinitrate* (5 to 30 mg) taken three or four times daily. Although large amounts of these drugs are dispensed and many physicians and patients are satisfied with their usefulness, objective evidence of signifi-cant prolonged clinical effect is lacking. Evaluation of the treatment of angina is difficult, because the response to therapy is often highly subjective and depends on the patient's assessment of his own symptoms. A skillful physician with positive transference from the patient may be extremely effective in managing angina, but aside from the acute effects of nitroglycerin and amyl nitrite, the role of other agents such as long-acting nitrites has been difficult to measure. A recent study of several so-called long-acting nitrites found that improvement in exercise tolerance in patients with angina persisted for only about one hour after administration of drug.

Sedation is a useful adjunct to therapy in many instances. Neither phenobarbital nor any of the many available tranquilizers have specific cardiac action in small dosage, but they may reduce anxiety and fearfulness. Alcohol in moderation may be helpful for some patients. In patients with a major component of depression, antidepressant agents such as imipramine, amitriptyline and methylphenidate may be useful.

Propranolol, a beta-adrenergic blocking agent, is effective in selected patients for reducing the frequency and severity of angina. Stimulation of the sympathetic nerves to the heart or infusion of isoproterenol intravenously increases cardiac rate and augments contractility, or the strength and velocity of the cardiac contraction. These functions are specifically blocked by propranolol, which is an important adjunct in the medical treatment of angina pectoris. Approximately two thirds of patients offered a therapeutic trial of the drug are significantly improved with a reduction in frequency and severity of angina.

Propranolol reduces heart rate and decreases myocardial contractility. Studies in man have shown that administration of the drug is associated with a fall in cardiac output and reduction in maximal dp/dt. Left ventricular and end-diastolic pressure may rise. The normal response to exercise is blunted so that the anticipated increase in heart rate and cardiac output is limited. During exertion left ventricular end-diastolic pressure in patients on propranolol may increase, suggesting impairment of myocardial function. Propranolol may induce heart block or severe bradycardia and should be used cautiously in patients with known atrioventricular conduction disturbance. The drug is contraindicated in patients with advanced forms of heart block, such as a greatly prolonged P-R interval, intermittent atrioventricular block with dropped beats, or complete heart block. As discussed subsequently, heart failure may be induced or worsened by propranolol therapy.

During treatment with propranolol, both at rest and during exercise, the product of heart rate and blood pressure (termed the *double product*) is reduced when compared to the pretreatment state at comparable levels of oxygen consumption. For a given amount of exercise, systolic pressure, heart rate, and cardiac output are lower after the drug. Tissue oxygen requirement is met by increased extraction, so atrioventricular oxygen difference across the body is higher. Thus the patient with angina treated with propranolol is able to perform more useful muscular work and to get about more before developing symptoms.

The mechanism of action of propranolol is related to its myocardial depressant effects. Myocardial oxygen need is largely controlled by systolic pressure, contractility, and heart rate. Since propranolol reduces all three, oxygen demand is lower after administration of the drug.

The drug does not increase coronary blood flow or oxygen delivery; indeed these may actually decline.

The dose of propranolol required for clinical effectiveness varies. Many patients respond well to 80 to 160 mg per day, but larger doses are sometimes needed. In treating patients with propranolol, it is best to begin with a low dose, 10 to 20 mg four times daily, and continuously increase the dosage if the drug is well tolerated in an attempt to achieve the desired therapeutic effect. Excessive dosage may induce decreased exercise tolerance owing to marked fatigue. Patients may develop heart failure on high doses of the drug, and it is common practice to administer digitalis and even mild diuretics such as hydrochlorothiazide, 25 to 50 mg daily, with appropriate potassium replacement before beginning propranolol. In some patients severe bradycardia or the development of heart block necessitates withdrawal of treatment. Propranolol is an extremely potent agent, and it must be used with caution under medical supervision. The myocardial depressant action of the drug can be demonstrated in the individual patient by noninvasive techniques. Left ventricular pre-ejection period, analyzed from the indirect carotid pulse and the phonocardiogram, is prolonged. Serial echocardiograms show an increase in width of the left ventricular minor axis after drug administration. Postural hypotension and aggravation of bronchial spasm in patients with asthma are occasional troublesome side effects.

Propranolol has many complex actions. Serum drug levels do not correlate with therapeutic effectiveness. This is not surprising for a blocking agent and probably indicates that those factors classified as "sympathetic tone" and the resting level of ventricular function are highly variable. Propranolol in vivo shifts the oxyhemoglobin dissociation curve to the right. The drug also reverses in vivo the increased aggregatability of platelets frequently observed in patients with angina. It appears to act by restoring the second stage of platelet clumping to normal. Propranolol also has a quinidine-like effect on the transmembrane action potential and is thus an antiarrhythmic. There is experimental evidence also that the drug protects myocardial glycogen stores during stress, thus increasing ability of the heart to sustain anaerobic metabolism during hypoxia or ischemia. Whether the pharmacologic effects of the drug other than its myocardial depressant action contribute to its therapeutic effectiveness in patients with angina is moot.

Surgical Treatment. Many surgical procedures have been advocated to provide additional coronary blood supply or relieve obstructed vessels. Most have been abandoned after an initial wave of enthusiasm for the lack of objective evidence of improvement and symptoms or favorable alteration of prognosis. Implantation of an internal mammary artery into a myocardial tunnel (Vineberg procedure) with various modifications was recently popular among surgeons. When the artery is implanted in an ischemic area, a network of fine anastomotic vessels gradually develops. Full development and clinical improvement usually require several months. Success varies, but angiography reveals neovascularization. Pacing studies have shown reversal of lactate production in selected cases. An acute myocardial infarction may complicate the procedure. This event could explain the immediate benefit which is sometimes observed.

During the past five years many thousands of *coronary bypass* surgical procedures have been performed in the United States in patients with coronary artery disease. There is now little doubt that this procedure is capable of providing a sizable increase in coronary blood flow around an area of coronary arterial obstruction. The procedure is technically possible because most significant obstructive lesions are segmental and proximal. Furthermore, experience has shown that a bypass graft from the aorta can be successfully anastomosed to a coronary artery as small as 1 mm in diameter. Postoperative angiograms are often impressive and have shown that the anastomoses function and provide an immediate increase in blood flow to large areas of the myocardium.

Indications for surgical revascularization of the heart focus predominantly on the relief of angina. Surgery may be considered in the patient with frequent episodes of angina which seriously hinder normal activity and are not satisfactorily responsive to medical therapy. The "ideal" candidate is one who has severe angina, risk factors that are responsive to medical treatment, proximal obstruction of major coronary arteries with good distal "run-off," normal heart size, and normal left ventricular function. The decision regarding surgery should be made by consultation between physician and surgeon. The patient's interests are best served when he is evaluated first by a physician who works closely with a cardiac surgical group and who has a continuing experience in the pre- and postoperative management of patients undergoing cardiovascular surgery.

In good risk patients, surgical mortality in the hands of experienced teams should be 3 to 5 per cent or less. Mortality is inversely related to cardiac function. Evidence of previous myocardial infarction or ventricular dysfunction sharply increases the operative risk. Congestive heart failure is not considered an indication for a bypass procedure. It is claimed by some workers that the poor ventricular contractility, elevated end-diastolic pressures, and low ejection fraction (stroke volume/end-diastolic volume) in some patients with recurrent ischemia is reversed after a successful bypass procedure. The debate on this point continues, but the author does not yet find the evidence convincing.

Recent reports suggest that after one year 65 to 80 per cent of patients undergoing surgery have complete or very good relief of angina pectoris. Approximately 85 per cent of the vein grafts remain functional after one year. Frequently an internal mammary artery will be anastomosed when technically feasible to the anterior descending coronary vessel; one-year patency rates of 95 per cent for this procedure have been reported.

After a successful bypass operation, work performed during maximal exercise is significantly increased in the patient with coronary artery disease. Appropriate dosage of propranolol has only a modest effect in comparison. Improvement in exercise tolerance has been directly related to continued patency of the bypass graft. Indeed, serial exercise testing may be utilized to assess the efficacy of the procedure. Sudden sharp reduction in exercise tolerance suggests closure of the shunt.

A troublesome problem in evaluating the bypass procedure is the apparent high *risk of myocardial infarction.* One study suggested that in the early postoperative period over 60 per cent of patients undergoing bypass had an increase in blood level of creatinine phosphokinase activity identified as myocardial in origin by electrophoresis. In contrast, less than 5 per cent of patients undergoing aortic valve replacement had such a rise. Clinical evidence of myocardial infarction postoperatively is much lower. Early reports suggested an incidence of about 20 per cent. More recently a frequency of 8 to 10 per cent has been encountered, utilizing the development of new Q waves on the postoperative electrocardiogram as criteria for diagnosis. It has been suggested that some of the electrocardiographic changes indicating new infarction are actually old infarction now revealed by the improved blood supply to an ischemic area and the generation of previously hidden QRS vector forces. A perioperative myocardial infarction could explain improvement of angina in some patients postoperatively, but would not be associated with improved maximal exercise performance.

Availability of bypass surgery is a significant therapeutic advance in the management of angina pectoris caused by coronary artery disease. Much remains to be learned before its value is fully understood. Although carefully selected patients may anticipate low surgical mortality and a good chance for relief of symptoms, the long-term effects are not yet known. How long the grafts will continue to function and whether the procedure prevents myocardial infarction or alters the prognosis in patients with angina are important questions that will require many years to answer satisfactorily.

Prognosis. Heberden wrote: "The termination of the angina pectoris is remarkable. For if no accident intervenes but the disease goes on to its height, the patients all suddenly fall down and perish almost immediately." In fact this gloomy prognosis is incorrect. An unwarranted emphasis on premature and sudden death complicating angina pectoris influences medical practice even today, particularly the impetus for newer forms of surgical treatment.

In a pioneering study, Richards, Bland, and White reported a 25 year follow-up of 500 patients with angina pectoris who entered the survey between 1920 and 1931. Annual mortality rate was slightly more than 4 per cent; 50 per cent of the patients were dead in about 12 years. Women had slightly better survival than men, an observation that has been repeatedly made. More recent workers have emphasized the adverse effect of risk factors. A Health Insurance Plan of New York study reveals an average of 1.4 per cent annual mortality in males with angina, no history of myocardial infarction, and normal electrocardiogram and blood pressure. In contrast, annual mortality in those who also had evidence of systolic hypertension was 7.4 per cent. With an abnormal electrocardiogram the risk was 8.4 per cent per year. If both factors were present, the risk was 12 per cent per year. The Framingham study has shown similar results.

Prognosis in angina pectoris is also related to the extent of coronary disease determined angiographically. Stenosis of only a single major vessel seems to have a good prognosis. An average annual mortality of 3 per cent per year has been reported in single-vessel disease unless the anterior descendens is completely occluded, in which case the mortality is approximately doubled. Annual mortality in two-vessel disease has been reported as 6 per cent, and in three-vessel disease, about 10 per cent.

Increased recognition of adverse clinical factors combined with precise anatomic and physiologic characterization in selected patients has greatly improved our understanding of prognosis in angina pectoris. Data derived from a number of clinical studies have provided a clear description of the "natural history" of angina pectoris under conservative medical management. Each ad-

dition to accepted treatment must be compared to the yardstick of prognosis as currently described. This admonition applies no less to medical than to surgical therapeutic innovations.

Variant Angina. In 1959 Prinzmetal called attention to a form of angina characterized by pain at rest and S-T segment elevation which subsides after the attack. The electrocardiogram during pain resembles that of acute myocardial infarction. Arrhythmia is not uncommon. Since most patients with angina have pain during exercise accompanied by S-T segment depression, he termed the syndrome variant angina. With the advent of routine oscillographic monitoring for patients with chest pain, variant angina has been recognized with increasing frequency.

In the laboratory animal or, as is occasionally observed, during coronary arteriography in man, occlusion of a large coronary artery produces prompt S-T segment elevation. Prinzmetal postulated that variant angina reflected organic obstruction of a major coronary artery accompanied by spasm. In exercise-induced angina and in most cases of decubitus pain, cardiac work usually increases sharply before pain and there is S-T segment depression. These EKG changes are believed to reflect subendocardial ischemia, because this layer is most vulnerable to the decreased coronary flow when left ventricular wall tension rises. Exercise performance in variant angina may be normal.

Arteriography in variant angina usually reveals high grade obstruction of a major coronary vessel. However, in some patients, with recurrent and striking changes in the electrocardiogram, the coronary angiogram has been normal. In a small number of patients with variant angina, coronary spasm not caused by catheter trauma has recently been convincingly demonstrated. It is likely that a combination of spasm and severe organic obstruction may be present in some. The prognosis in variant angina is less favorable. A high incidence of myocardial infarction and sudden death has been reported. The results of bypass surgery have been disappointing.

Aronow, W. S.: Management of stable angina. N. Engl. J. Med., 289:516, 1973.

Braunwald, E.: Determinants of myocardial oxygen consumption (Thirteenth Bowditch Lecture). Physiologist, 12:65, 1969.

Fischl, S. J., Herman, M. V., and Gorlin, R.: The intermediate coronary syndrome. Clinical, angiographic, and therapeutic aspects. N. Engl. J. Med., 288:1193, 1973.

Fulton, M., Lutz, W., Donald, K. W., Kirby, B. J., Duncan, B., Morrison, S. L., Kerr, F., Julian, D. G., and Oliver, M. F.: Natural history of unstable angina. Lancet, 1:860, 1972.

Oliva, P. B., Potts, D. E., and Pluss, R. G.: Coronary arterial spasm in Prinzmetal angina. N. Engl. J. Med., 288:745, 1973.

Parker, J. O., West, R. O., Case, R. B., and Chiong, M. A.: Temporal relationships of myocardial lactate metabolism, left ventricular function, and S-T segment depression during angina precipitated by exercise. Circulation, 40:97, 1969.

Reeves, T. J., Oberman, A., Jones, W. B., and Sheffield, L. T.: Natural history of angina pectoris. Am. J. Cardiol., 33:423, 1974.

Swan, H. J. C., Chatterjee, K., Corday, E., Ganz, W., Marcus, H., Matloff, J., and Parmley, W.: Myocardial revascularization for acute and chronic coronary heart disease. Ann. Intern. Med., 79:851, 1973.

567. ACUTE MYOCARDIAL INFARCTION

Definition. Acute myocardial infarction is a clinical syndrome resulting from deficient coronary arterial flow to an area of myocardium with eventual cellular death and necrosis. It is characterized by severe and prolonged precordial pain similar to, but more intense than, that of angina pectoris, and signs of myocardial damage, including acute electrocardiographic changes and a rise in level of certain serum enzymes.

Etiology and Pathology. Atherosclerosis of the coronary arteries is the common denominator in the overwhelming majority of patients with acute myocardial infarction. Although it is attractive to view acute myocardial infarction as the direct result of a sudden obstruction of a major coronary artery, this is not always the case. Infarction without occlusion and occlusion without infarction may be observed pathologically. An occlusion may result from an acute thrombosis, subintimal hemorrhage, or rupture of an atheromatous plaque which may initiate clot formation.

The development of coronary artery thrombi apparently depends on the time and mechanism of death. Clots in the coronary arteries have been observed in approximately 25 per cent of patients who die suddenly. Patients who survive myocardial infarction for several hours or days and then die from heart failure or cardiogenic shock manifest a high incidence of coronary thrombi; an incidence of up to 60 or 70 per cent has been reported. Often the thromboses appear younger than the associated infarction, suggesting that the myocardial damage caused the clot. In a recent report ^{125}I-labeled fibrinogen was administered to seven patients with acute myocardial infarction who subsequently died. A coronary thrombus was found in all seven at autopsy. In six the entire clot was radioactive; in the seventh there was a central portion of the thrombus without radioactivity.

Significant coronary artery disease can usually be demonstrated in the vessel directly supplying the area of infarction. Extensive collateral development may make correlation of precise myocardial and vascular relationships difficult. In the presence of collaterals, an acute arterial occlusion may not produce ischemia or infarction. If an area is dependent on collateral flow, on the other hand, a remote occlusion or a change in the balance of vascular resistance may cause infarction of an area considerably removed from the source of difficulty.

The possibility that evanescent platelet agglutination may precipitate myocardial infarction has recently attracted interest. Platelets adhere to collagen and basement membrane, and these structures may be exposed in injured vessels. Injured platelets release adenosine diphosphate and other factors which accelerate agglutination and clumping. It has been shown experimentally that injection of adenosine diphosphate causes platelet aggregation within the coronary arteries. The peripheral platelet count falls. Although platelet thrombi can be observed on microscopic sections shortly after injection of the adenosine disphosphate, the clumps are no longer apparent after ten minutes. Acute myocardial infarction can be recognized pathologically in two hours, and yet by this time the coronary arteries are not obstructed. The theory that platelets may play a role in the development of acute myocardial infarction or angina pectoris remains an intriguing but as yet unproved possibility.

A myocardial infarct is termed *transmural* when it extends from endocardium to epicardium and *nontransmural* when the necrosis does not reach the inner or outer surface. A *subendocardial* infarct involves the endocardial and subendocardial layers. In general, trans-

mural infarcts tend to be larger and are associated with more severe complications of ventricular dysfunction. Subendocardial infarcts may also be quite extensive, and are associated with occlusive disease of all three of the major coronary arteries. Since the subendocardial layer is subjected to the greatest amount of wall tension, subendocardial infarcts may result from prolonged hypotension or shock owing to noncardiac causes, and may complicate hemorrhage, anesthesia, or extensive surgical procedures.

Acute myocardial infarction is predominantly a disease of the left ventricle and the interventricular septum. Occasionally the infarct extends into the right ventricle, and the atria may also be involved. Atrial infarcts are usually not diagnosed during life; current electrocardiographic criteria are unreliable. Primary infarction of the right ventricle with severe right heart failure and tricuspid regurgitation in absence of left ventricular involvement has been described. The extent and location of the infarct depend upon the causative factors, the extent of coronary artery disease, the presence of collateral blood supply, and whether previous infarctions have occurred.

Other Causes. Coronary embolization may complicate bacterial endocarditis or left atrial thrombosis, resulting in acute infarction or sudden death. Embolization of calcified excrescences may occur in aortic stenosis. Myocardial infarction without coronary obstruction may complicate aortic stenosis if coronary perfusion pressure drops, with syncope or hypotension, when ventricular systolic work is maintained at a high level because of the fixed obstruction. Acute myocardial infarction secondary to arteritis has been described in periarteritis nodosa and acute hypersensitivity syndromes. In Marfan's syndrome, cystic necrosis of the media may involve the coronary arteries as well as the aorta. In acute aortic dissection, the separation may extend to the base of the aorta and occlude a major coronary artery. Electrocardiographic changes suggesting subendocardial ischemia or necrosis may be observed after prolonged surgical procedures, often with extensive blood loss and replacement, or secondary to hypotension or shock from a variety of causes. Coronary arteriography after recovery from myocardial infarction has revealed a small number of patients with perfectly normal coronary anatomy and no recognizable cause for the acute event.

Clinical Manifestations. The outstanding characteristic of acute myocardial infarction is severe, prolonged pain. The pain is similar to that of angina, but is more intense and persists much longer. It is usually present for at least half an hour, but may last for many hours. Nitroglycerin affords no relief or only temporarily abates the attack. The pain is usually relieved by administration of opiates, although repeated doses may be required.

The pain is described as pressing or crushing, like a deep ache inside the chest. Often patients will press on the sternum or state that it feels as though there were a great weight on the chest, such as a rock or someone sitting on it. The pain is a deep visceral discomfort, and is seldom described as sharp or stabbing. The radiation of pain is similar to that of angina; it may be felt in the right or left arm but usually the left, in the elbow and down to the fingers, in the jaw, in the back, or in the upper epigastric area. Although the symptoms have never occurred before, many patients will state that they are having a heart attack. Intense fear of impending death or doom is common. If pulmonary edema and cardiogenic shock are early complications, the pain may be obscured.

Although the typical patient with acute infarction presents with severe pain, the range of response is wide. The pain may be brief and not severe. Occasionally, an electrocardiogram will reveal evidence of acute or recent infarction without a history of pain. Patients who have associated gastrointestinal disease, such as peptic ulcer, hiatus hernia, or gallbladder disorders, may have difficulty separating the pain of infarction from that of other conditions. In patients with pre-existing angina pectoris, infarction may be heralded by a more intense episode of pain that is unrelieved by nitroglycerin or rest. Should the infarction precipitate acute pulmonary edema, the pain often becomes a minor complaint. Acute arrhythmia, especially heart block or ventricular tachycardia, may be the presenting sign. Atrioventricular dissociation is relatively common in diaphragmatic-inferior infarctions, and the first symptom may be weakness or syncope owing to marked bradycardia. Patients with severe coronary artery disease may develop myocardial infarction secondary to any prolonged circulatory disorder such as heart failure, hypertension, or arrhythmia. Sometimes it is difficult to be certain which came first, the circulatory disorder or the acute infarction.

In patients who survive to be hospitalized for acute infarction, prodromata are common. Several studies have shown that approximately two thirds of the hospitalized patients have prodromal symptoms, almost always ischemic cardiac pain, prior to the acute infarction. Prodromata are characteristically recurrent and crescendo in nature. The pain is more easily triggered, lasts longer, and is more intense than usual. Prodromata are more common in patients with angina. Any change in the pattern of previously stable angina pectoris should be viewed as possibly a forewarning of impending acute infarction. Infarcts occurring after prodromal symptoms are more likely to be anterior than posterior-inferior and nontransmural than transmural.

Physical Findings.   The patient with acute infarction is usually restless, apprehensive, and in severe pain. His color may be poor, the face ashen, and the nailbeds cyanotic. Sweating is frequent, and the skin is cool. Examination of the lungs may reveal normal findings; alternatively there may be signs suggesting early heart failure or acute pulmonary edema. The heart sounds are often distant and muffled. Paradoxical splitting of the second sound has been described but is seldom detected. A fourth heart sound is almost universally present. Auscultation may reveal a soft murmur, suggesting mitral regurgitation. The pulse may be thready and the blood pressure reduced. Careful examination provides the physician with an evaluation of myocardial performance, but it can neither establish nor deny the possibility of a diagnosis of acute infarction.

Laboratory Findings.   Routine laboratory examinations reveal abnormalities compatible with necrosis of tissue. The *temperature* is usually elevated for the first three to five days after acute infarction. The rise is usually modest, but occasionally the temperature becomes quite high, up to 40° C. Rarely, continued high fever, apparently caused by myocardial necrosis, threatens survival. Measures to reduce the temperature, including cooling baths and cold blankets, may be necessary.

Leukocytosis occurs regularly, but usually persists no longer than five days to a week. White counts of 12,000

to 15,000 cells per cubic millimeter with a shift to the left are usual. Counts above this level should be viewed with suspicion and possible complications assiduously sought.

Serial analysis of activity in blood of a variety of *enzymes* normally found in muscle cells is of great value in establishing the diagnosis of acute myocardial infarction. Necrosis of as little as 1 gram of myocardium will result in detectable serum enzyme rise. If the enzyme activity is not elevated in a patient suspected of having acute infarction, it is assumed that no infarction occurred or that the tissue damage was so small that it could not be recognized by current techniques. Proper interpretation of serum enzyme patterns requires measurement of enzyme activity for several days after the presumed acute infarction.

Serum creatine phosphokinase (CPK), an enzyme occurring in high concentration in heart, skeletal muscle, and brain, rises rapidly, reaching peak levels approximately 24 hours after acute myocardial infarction. Serum activity returns to normal within 72 hours. Three CPK isozymes have been identified by electrophoresis. Each is a dimer composed of two subunits of the M or B type. Brain contains BB, skeletal muscle MM, and myocardium MM and MB. Serial analysis of CPK is extremely useful in the diagnosis of acute myocardial infarction if the patient is seen within a few hours of symptoms.

Glutamic oxaloacetic transaminase (GOT) is an enzyme present in high concentration in myocardium, skeletal muscle, liver, brain, and kidney. Normal serum activity is 20 to 40 Frank-Karmen units, or 30 to 60 international units. After myocardial infarction, serum activity rises, reaching a peak in 48 to 72 hours, and gradually falling to normal by five days. Providing that liver necrosis secondary to decreased splanchnic blood flow has not also occurred, peak levels correlate with the extent of myocardial damage. Levels of over 300 Frank-Karmen units are usually associated with extensive infarction complicated by heart failure or shock. Serum GOT activity increases also in a wide variety of disorders associated with hepatic necrosis, including central necrosis of the liver, heart failure, hypotension, or shock. Narcotics such as morphine and, to a lesser extent, meperidine may cause a rise in serum activity, presumably secondary to spasm of the sphincter of Oddi. It is often useful to obtain serum glutamic pyruvic transaminase, an enzyme found predominantly in liver, to evaluate possible hepatic contribution to elevated serum GOT activity.

Lactic dehydrogenase (LDH) is found in a variety of tissues, and elevations of serum activity are usually not specific for a diagnosis of myocardial infarction.

Electrocardiogram.   The electrocardiogram is extremely useful in evaluating a tentative diagnosis of acute myocardial infarction, providing that the tracing is interpreted with full knowledge of the wide variety of nonspecific factors which may induce abnormality. The hallmark of acute transmural infarction is the appearance of Q waves of sufficient amplitude and duration to be termed significant. It has been said that changes may not occur for two to five days after infarction in some patients, but this seems unlikely. Late appearance of EKG abnormality usually indicates that an impending infarction syndrome finally culminated in infarction and death of cardiac tissue. During the early state of infarction the S-T segments are markedly elevated in those leads depicting the area of infarction, with reciprocal S-T segment depression elsewhere. As the infarct evolves electrically, the S-T segments become depressed and the T waves inverted. Varying degrees of abnormality persist, although in some patients recognition of healed transmural infarction from the EKG may be difficult.

In nontransmural and subendocardial infarction, abnormalities in the EKG are primarily in the S-T segments and T waves. The S-T segments may be elevated, but are usually depressed in leads reflecting the area of infarction, and the T waves are usually inverted. Interpretation of the EKG may be difficult because of the nonspecific nature of the S-T segment and T wave change. Serial tracings over several days may be helpful, especially if the abnormalities progressively improve toward the preinfarction pattern.

Diaphragmatic or inferior infarctions are reflected in leads 2, 3, and AVF. Anterior-septal infarctions influence leads V_2 to V_4, whereas anterior-lateral infarctions involve leads V_3 to V_6. Strictly posterior infarctions are recognized by changes in V_1 and V_2. Subendocardial damage usually results in development of an S-T and T vector opposite in direction to the mean QRS vector. Left bundle branch block frequently obscures the recognition of acute infarction because of the abnormal initial QRS vector, but right bundle branch block does not. In some patients the first EKG is diagnostic. In others serial tracings and blood enzyme analysis are necessary to detect changes compatible with the diagnosis.

Diagnosis. The diagnosis of acute transmural myocardial infarction is straightforward when the patient presents with severe, crushing precordial pain lasting 30 minutes or more and the electrocardiogram reveals characteristic Q waves and S-T segment elevation of the "hyperacute" stage. Myocardial infarction, however, has a wide range of clinical manifestations, and recognition of the acute episode may be difficult.

Diagnosis is based on a clinical triad: (1) prolonged cardiac pain, more severe and longer lasting than angina; (2) abnormal electrocardiograms with a progressive evolution of pattern; and (3) rise and fall in serum enzyme activity. At least two of these should be present to support the diagnosis. In some patients pain either

does not occur or is not recognized as representing a serious illness. Denial is an important component of the initial response to the symptoms of acute infarction in many patients, making interpretation of the history difficult. As with angina, the pain may be ascribed to indigestion or other gastrointestinal complaint. When acute infarction is a complication of a surgical procedure, anesthesia, trauma, or other disease such as gastrointestinal hemorrhage, hypertension, or shock, pain may be absent. The diagnosis is then suspected from changes in the electrocardiogram, and may be corroborated by serial analysis of blood enzyme activity.

In acute transmural infarction the electrocardiogram is usually diagnostic when obtained within a few hours of symptoms. Interpretation of the electrocardiogram in nontransmural or subendocardial infarction may be difficult. Frequently the tracing was previously abnormal, and changes in the S-T segments or T waves may not be marked. The electrocardiogram may be surprisingly unrevealing in some patients with one or more previous infarctions and extensive atherosclerosis of the three major coronary vessels. Presumably the widespread yet discrete abnormalities cancel each other out on the surface electrocardiogram.

Serial assay of blood enzyme activity is most useful when the clinical story is not helpful or is imprecise. However, intramuscular injection of many drugs, including narcotics, will increase serum CPK and GOT, causing potential errors in diagnosis. Acute abnormality of the electrocardiogram followed by resolution toward normal coupled with a characteristic rise and fall of enzyme activity will usually be diagnostic. There are many situations in which it is not possible to prove or disprove the diagnosis of acute infarction, yet the wise decision may be to treat the patient as though infarction had occurred.

Differential Diagnosis. The most frequent problem is determining whether the patient has had a prolonged attack of *angina* or an infarction. Electrocardiographic abnormalities usually develop during angina, but revert to the previous pattern when the pain subsides. Fever and leukocytosis are not present. The serum enzymes do not rise after angina pectoris. Persistent electrocardio-

Figure 4. Large myocardial infarction with chronic heart failure. Electrocardiogram from a 66-year-old man obtained seven weeks after hospitalization for acute myocardial infarction. He had previously been in excellent health without known risk factors for cardiovascular disease. His hospital course was complicated by ventricular tachycardia, heart failure, low blood pressure, fatigue, and lassitude. Intensive treatment with antiarrhythmics, digitalis, and diuretics was required. Convalescence was prolonged. Eight weeks after the acute event, he developed an abdominal abscess from a perforated appendix and died suddenly. Electrocardiogram shows evidence of extensive transmural anterior and inferior diaphragmatic myocardial infarction.

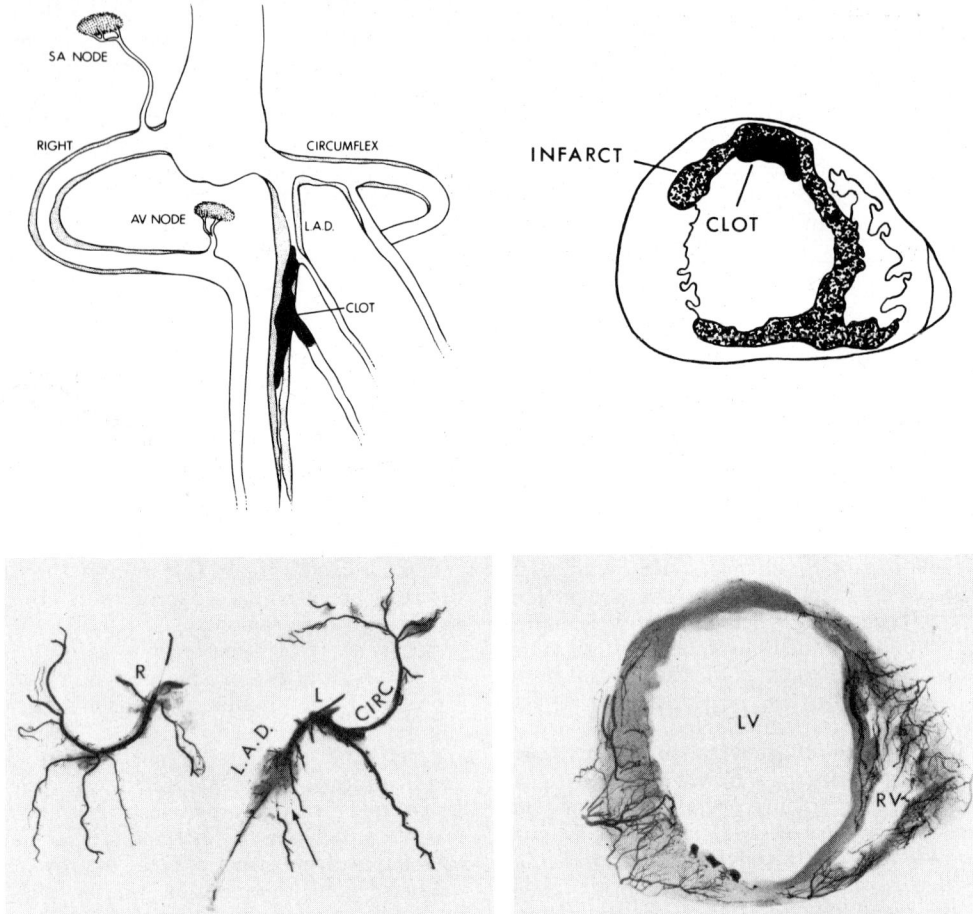

Figure 5. Large myocardial infarction with chronic heart failure. Diagrams and postmortem roentgenograms of major coronary vessels and coronal section of ventricles, obtained at autopsy from patient described in Figure 4. Coronary arteries were injected with a barium mixture and heart was fixed in formalin. Large coronary arteries were then dissected free, ventricles sectioned, and X-ray exposures obtained. Coronary artery disease in right, circumflex, and first diagonal branch of anterior descending artery is minimal. However, there is extensive involvement of left anterior descending artery with complete obstruction caused by thrombosis. Area of infarct involves anterior, septal, and posterior wall of left ventricle and septum and posterior segment of right ventricle. A mural thrombosis was present in left ventricle. Forty-four per cent of left ventricular mass was destroyed in the infarction. Extent of damage suggests continued cardiac disability had patient survived. (Courtesy of D. Alonso, M.D.)

graphic abnormality after a severe attack of angina suggests that subendocardial or nontransmural infarction has developed, especially if accompanied by changes in serum enzyme activity. Although great reliance is often placed on assay of serum enzymes, it seems likely that small, discrete infarctions may occur without detectable rise in enzyme activity.

Acute *pericarditis* may be mistaken for acute myocardial infarction. The pain of pericarditis is often made worse by deep inspiration. Relief is obtained by sitting up and leaning forward. The hallmark of pericarditis is a precordial friction rub which characteristically has three components: presystolic, early diastolic, and systolic. Faint rubs with only one or two components are often missed or mistaken for soft murmurs. The electrocardiogram in acute pericarditis shows moderate S-T segment elevation initially with upright T waves. Later the S-T segment may be slightly depressed and the T waves become inverted. Q waves do not occur in pericarditis.

Pulmonary embolus may cause chest pain and electrocardiographic changes, but the pleuritic pain is seldom suggestive of myocardial infarction. The electrocardiogram in pulmonary embolus may reveal an S_1, S_2, S_3 pattern, complete or incomplete right bundle branch block (usually evanescent), or clockwise rotation of the precordial pattern, suggesting right ventricular overload.

Other conditions which may be confused with myocardial infarction include ruptured aortic aneurysm, acute aortic dissection, acute pneumothorax, gallbladder disease, pneumonia, and acute arrhythmia. Errors in diagnosis can frequently be ascribed to inadequacies of the history and physical examination or overinterpretation of nonspecific changes in the electrocardiogram.

Unstable Angina.   Onset of recurrent episodes of ischemic pain or worsening of pre-existing angina is termed unstable angina. Evaluation of symptoms is particularly troublesome when prolonged pain occurs at rest, not infrequently at night, and is accompanied by transient electrocardiographic changes. This constellation of symptoms has also been called the *"intermediate syndrome," "preinfarction angina,"* or the *"impending coronary syndrome."* There is considerable controversy about prognosis and management. Recently advocates of early coronary arteriography and subsequent urgent surgical revascularization have been especially vocal.

A prospective study from Edinburgh by Oliver, Julian, and associates suggests that the prognosis is not as guarded as has been thought. Of 167 patients who developed unstable angina and were followed for several months, sudden death occurred in only 3 and acute myocardial infarction in 23. During the same period in the population under survey, about 70,000 persons at risk, there were 79 cases of sudden death and 110 of myocardial infarction. Sixty per cent of the patients with myocardial infarction had preceding unstable angina, but only a fourth of these sought medical aid. It would appear then that the major risk of unstable angina is infarction; denial or failure to recognize important symptoms is a serious problem.

Because current data are insufficient to evaluate medical or surgical therapy for unstable angina pectoris, a carefully designed random study of treatment is being carried out under the auspices of the National Institutes of Health. At this writing more than 100 patients have been randomized. No therapeutic advantage for either treatment is yet apparent, but several observations are pertinent. Angiography can be performed in unstable angina with little increase in risk. Surgical mortality is less than 10 per cent; myocardial infarction is the principal hazard occurring in both the medical and the postsurgical groups. Medical therapy generally consists of bed rest, oxygen, sedation, anticoagulants (usually), treatment of heart failure or arrhythmia, and propranolol. The results of this important study are being awaited with keen interest.

Complications. *Sudden Death.* Sudden, unexpected fatality is a common complication of acute myocardial infarction. It is currently believed that as many as 50 per cent of patients with acute infarction do not survive to reach a hospital. Early death is not related to the severity of the infarction and is most likely to occur in the

first four to six hours after onset, the frequency decreasing exponentially thereafter. Observations from monitoring units suggest that the mechanism is ventricular fibrillation in most cases, although acute heart block may be the initial arrhythmia in some.

Frequently patients do not seek medical attention until several hours after the onset of pain. The major cause of delay is failure to appreciate the significance of symptoms and denial that a problem exists. Physicians may err in evaluation of the complaint. Hospital emergency rooms, often oriented to treatment of trauma, may not move the patient into a coronary treatment system with sufficient rapidity after arrival. Cardiac arrest in the patient waiting to be evaluated for chest pain is all too common.

Arrhythmia. More than 90 per cent of patients hospitalized with acute infarction have arrhythmia, especially during the first 72 hours. Some of these are trivial, some are potentially life threatening, and some have such immediate consequences that their mere recognition should impel prompt, vigorous therapy. Abnormal rhythms may affect cardiac performance by adversely influencing ventricular rate, altering the sequence of atrial and ventricular contraction, or initiating depolarization from an abnormal focus. Of greatest importance clinically is the ventricular rate. In general if the ventricular rate is reasonable (60 to 110 beats per minute) and well tolerated, treatment of an abnormal rhythm may not be urgent. On the other hand, if the ventricular rate is either too fast or too slow, prompt correction is usually indicated. Patients with myocardial damage often have fixed stroke volumes so that minute volume, or cardiac output, is dependent upon heart rate. If the heart rate is too slow, cardiac output may fall.

A sinus rate greater than 110 beats per minute is often an ominous sign. *Sinus tachycardia* may reflect a low stroke volume or impending shock. If evidence of heart failure is present, the rate may slow after cautious ad-

Figure 6. Crescendo angina and sudden death. Electrocardiogram obtained 24 hours before death from a 58-year-old man with stable, infrequent angina for four years. Risk factors included moderate obesity, hypertension, and history of moderate smoking. Three months previously he was hospitalized after a prolonged bout of chest pain, but a diagnosis of myocardial infarction could not be established. After this, he had progressively severe angina, including nocturnal attacks requiring several sublingual nitroglycerin tablets for relief. He was hospitalized for evaluation. Blood pressure was 125/75 mm Hg. The heart was normal on examination without evidence of failure. He continued to have intermittent episodes of chest pain at rest after hospitalization, but there was no objective evidence of myocardial infarction. On the morning of the fourth day of hospitalization he was found dead in bed. The electrocardiogram shows nonspecific S-T segment depression in most leads. The prominent R wave in leads V_1 and V_2 suggests the possibility of an old "strictly posterior" myocardial infarction.

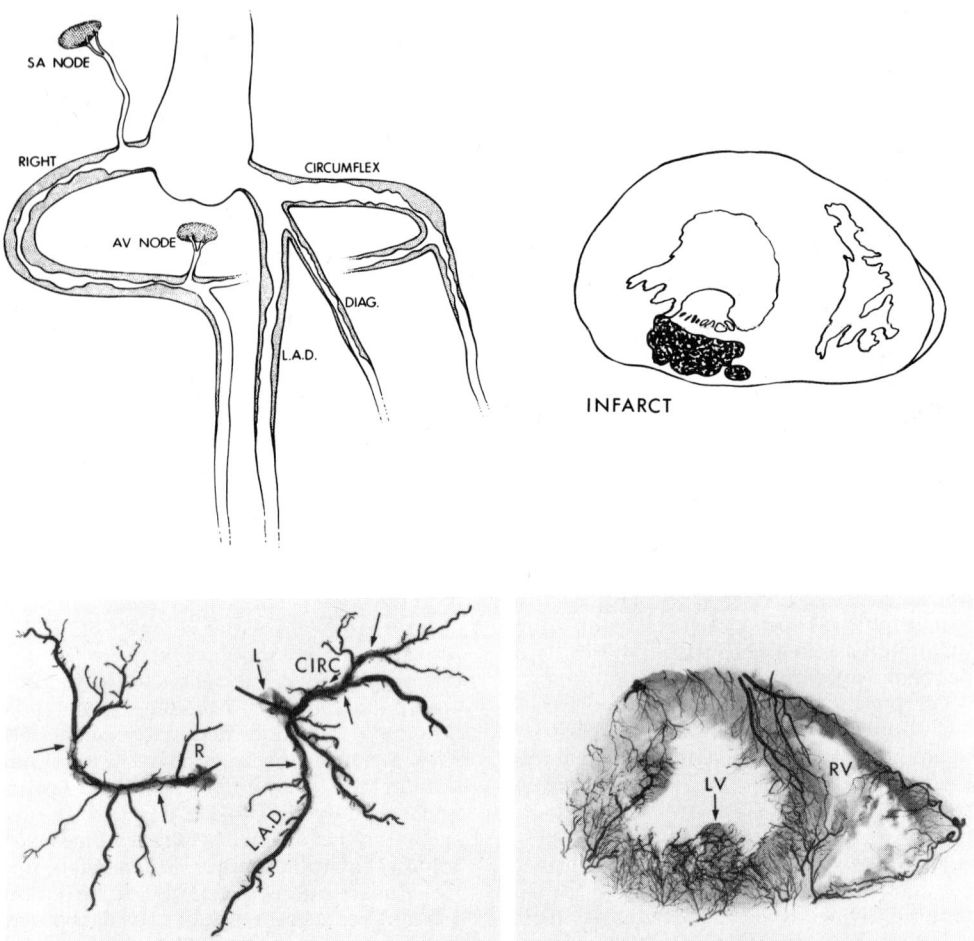

Figure 7. Crescendo angina and sudden death. Diagrams and postmortem roentgenograms of major coronary vessels and coronal section of ventricles obtained at autopsy from patient described in Figure 6. There is advanced disease of the three major coronary arteries but no complete occlusion. Neovascularization (arrow) in posterior wall of left ventricle indicates old (months) scar from myocardial infarction which was confirmed histologically. Posterior location confirms electrocardiographic interpretation. Although extent of heart disease is obvious, precise cause of death could not be determined from autopsy. (Courtesy of D. Alonso, M.D.)

ministration of digitalis. *Sinus bradycardia* occurs in 10 to 15 per cent of patients with acute infarction. Presumably it is a reflection of sinus node dysfunction secondary to alteration of blood supply, although reflex "vagotonia" has been postulated. Bradycardia is usually an early complication and lasts but a few hours. It is commonly associated with inferior wall infarction.

Arrhythmia of atrial or nodal (junctional) origin may reflect atrial infarction, the development of heart failure, hypokalemia, digitalis excess, or a combination of factors. *Atrial premature beats* are often the forerunner of sustained atrial dysrhythmia. *Atrial tachycardia* is uncommon in myocardial infarction. *Atrial fibrillation* or *flutter* occurs in about 10 per cent of patients and has a marked tendency to spontaneous reversion followed by relapse within minutes.

Prolongations of the P-R time *(first-degree block)* and Wenckebach phenomenon *(second-degree block)* are due to disorders of conduction in the region of the AV node. They are frequent complication of inferior-diaphragmatic infarctions (electrocardiographic changes in leads 2, 3 AVF) and reflect disturbance of blood supply to the AV node from the posterior surface of the heart. This form of block is almost always temporary, and improves after a few hours or a day or two. In inferior-diaphragmatic in-

farctions the normal sinus and the AV nodal pacemaker may discharge at approximately the same rate. The dominant pacemaker oscillates between the two nodes, producing AV dissociation depending on their respective rates. The QRS complex is normal in form, and the ventricular rate is usually above 55. This arrhythmia is not a form of heart block, because the normal conduction pathways will be utilized whenever a sinus node impulse arrives in the region of the AV node after ventricular repolarization. Specific treatment is not required.

Complete heart block is a dangerous and potentially lethal complication of acute myocardial infarction. It is usually associated with a large, anterior infarction. The mortality is approximately 50 per cent. In the form known as Mobitz type II, AV block develops suddenly without previous prolongation of the P-R interval or dropped beats. Direct recordings of the electrocardiogram from the bundle of His indicate that this conduction disturbance is almost always caused by bilateral bundle branch block. Prior conduction abnormality, such as right or left bundle branch block or marked by left axis deviation, is usually present. When complete heart block complicates acute infarction, the ventricular response is usually slow, and the QRS complexes are wide and bizarre. About half the patients with pre-existing bundle branch block develop acute heart block as a complication of myocardial infarction. The incidence is especially high with the QV₁-RBBB pattern. Some authorities advocate the placement of a temporary pacemaker-electrode in the right ventricle in all patients with pre-existing bundle branch block because of the danger of developing bilateral bundle branch block.

Ventricular premature beats are common in acute myocardial infarction, occurring in about 75 per cent of monitored patients. Premature beats are important because they may initiate ventricular tachycardia or ventricular fibrillation if sufficiently premature to strike the vulnerable period of the diastolic repolarization phase of the cardiac cycle. The vulnerable period occurs during the latter portion of the relative refractory period, and coincides with the ascending limb of the T wave. The more closely coupled a ventricular premature beat is to the preceding normal beat, the more likely it is to initiate tachycardia or fibrillation.

Ventricular tachycardia, defined as three or more consecutive ventricular beats, and *ventricular fibrillation* occur in about 10 per cent of patients hospitalized with acute infarction. When the rate in ventricular tachycardia is slow, the arrhythmia is usually well tolerated. With fast rates, however, the circulation rapidly deteriorates, requiring immediate emergency treatment. Ventricular tachycardia may progress to ventricular fibrillation. Fibrillation is usually heralded by preceding ventricular premature beats or tachycardia. In some instances, termed *primary* fibrillation, the arrhythmia develops suddenly without warning ectopic beats. Primary fibrillation is probably an important factor in sudden death, because its incidence is greatest in the early hours after infarction.

Physiologic Changes. Acute myocardial infarction induces regional abnormalities in cardiac contraction and adversely influences function of the heart as a whole. The left ventricle is primarily involved. Malfunction of the right ventricle is usually secondary to left ventricular failure but may occasionally reflect right ventricular infarction. In general the degree of left ventricular dysfunction reflects the extent of myocardial damage. The larger the infarct, new or old, the greater the hemodynamic abnormality. Infarction of even a small mass of myocardium is accompanied by significant increase in left ventricular filling pressure. With larger infarcts the increased filling pressure is often accompanied by signs of overt congestive failure. Damage involving more than 40 per cent of left ventricular mass is complicated by hypotension, low cardiac output, and cardiogenic shock.

It is useful to classify patients according to the presence or absence of *clinical evidence of left ventricular failure.* Mortality and the extent of hemodynamic abnormality vary directly with the severity of heart failure. Patients in Class I, no clinical evidence of heart failure, have hemodynamic performance which is essentially normal when compared with that of age-matched controls. Left ventricular diastolic pressure, however, ranges from normal (less than 12 mm Hg) to as high as 30 mm Hg without pulmonary congestion. Hospital mortality is 5 per cent owing to arrhythmia or cardiac rupture.

Class II patients have clinical evidence of mild left ventricular failure with reduced intensity of heart sounds, a third heart sound, and pulmonary rales. Left ventricular filling pressure is consistently increased;

there is sinus tachycardia; stroke volume and cardiac output are reduced. Blood pressure is usually normal or slightly reduced, and peripheral vascular resistance is increased. Hospital mortality averages about 17 per cent.

Class III is defined as *pulmonary edema.* Mean left ventricular diastolic pressure is 25 mm Hg or higher, severe sinus tachycardia is the rule, and cardiac output is sharply reduced. Blood pressure may be normal or low. Mortality is 25 to 30 per cent.

Class IV, *cardiogenic shock,* develops in about 10 per cent of hospitalized patients, on the average some ten hours after the acute infarction. Shock is characterized by hypotension and signs of inadequate peripheral circulation; including cold skin, mental confusion, peripheral cyanosis, decreased urine flow, and tachycardia. Hemodynamic studies reveal marked arterial hypoxia and low stroke volume and cardiac output. A cardiac index of 1.0 liter per minute per square meter, a level barely able to support life, is not uncommon. Cardiac work is low; this factor can be related to prognosis. Progressive acidosis caused by accumulation of lactic acid is frequent. Pathologic studies have shown that fatal cardiogenic shock is characteristic of massive infarction. A combination of fresh and old scar, involving 40 per cent or more of ventricular mass, is found. Frequently also there is evidence of recent extension or reinfarction, events which have usually not been recognized clinically. Despite intensive treatment, mortality in cardiogenic shock averages about 85 per cent.

Hypoxia. Reduced arterial oxygen tension is a common complication of myocardial infarction. Po₂ in Class I patients is normal. Po₂ is reduced in classes II to IV. The degree of arterial unsaturation can be related to the clinical severity of heart failure and to the degree of elevation of left ventricular filling pressure. In one study, Po₂ in cardiogenic shock averaged 40 mm Hg, a value consistent with that observed in normal subjects at an elevation in excess of 10,000 feet. The arterial hypoxia reflects increased intrapulmonary venoarterial shunting secondary to the elevated pulmonary venous pressure and interstitial water accumulation in the lungs. Serial analysis of arterial Po₂ while the patient is breathing room air and an enriched oxygen mixture is extremely useful in management of myocardial infarction, because it provides an indirect assay of left ventricular function. Provided that primary pulmonary disease does not complicate the picture, effective treatment and recovery from the cardiac problem are accompanied by a return of arterial Po₂ to normal.

Embolism. Both systemic and pulmonary emboli may complicate myocardial infarction. Use of anticoagulants and less restrictive bed rest with attention to movement of the extremities have reduced the frequency of these hazards. Incidence of clinically recognizable episodes is currently extremely low. Pulmonary emboli from the right heart tend to be small and nonfatal, whereas those from the deep veins may be massive and cause sudden death. Systemic emboli have their source in the mural thrombi which form on the endocardium of the infarcted left ventricle.

Insufficiency of the Mitral Valve. Mitral regurgitation complicating acute infarction is usually caused by dysfunction of the papillary muscles, secondary to the ischemic process. However, it is usually not functionally significant. Heikkila reported that 30 per cent of patients with acute infarction develop murmurs of mitral insufficiency detected by repeated, daily auscultation. The murmur is usually soft and blowing, is heard at the apex, and may be holosystolic or confined to the latter half of systole. Rupture of the papillary muscle may precipitate acute and intractable pulmonary edema. The murmur is loud and holosystolic, and is usually accompanied by a systolic apical thrill. Differentiation clinically from rupture of the ventricular septum may not be easy. In the patient with refractory heart failure, emergency replacement with an artificial mitral valve may be indicated.

Cardiac Rupture. Rupture of the heart occurs in about 5 per cent of fatal cases. It is the only complication of acute infarction that is more common in women than in men. Rupture develops in transmural infarction, usually within the first ten days. Death is caused by acute hemopericardium and tamponade. The condition is characterized clinically by sudden loss of blood pressure without arrhythmia. Sinus tachycardia often persists for several minutes, although the patient is unresponsive. Occasionally the rupture is sealed by the pericardium, and survival for several months is possible.

Rupture of the interventricular septum is heralded by the appearance of a loud systolic murmur with a thrill along the left sternal border. It is seven to ten times more common than rupture of a papillary muscle. The dynamic effects depend on the size of the tear and volume of left to right shunt. Numerous reports attest to the success of surgical repair of acquired ventricular septal defect in selected cases.

Weakening of the Ventricular Wall. Aneurysm of the left ventricle results from scarring and thinning of the ventricular wall after transmural infarction. When large, the aneurysm bulges outward during systole, and this paradoxical movement may be appreciated by careful palpation of the precordium. Large aneurysms are often lined with clot, and systemic embolus is a hazard. Occasionally aneurysm of the left ventricle may be recognized on a chest film when the bulge is especially prominent. Localized disorder of ventricular contraction is common after myocardial infarction. Angiography frequently reveals unsuspected aneurysm or areas of ventricular akinesia. When the area of disordered contraction is large, the ventricle is dilated and the ejection fraction (stroke volume/end-diastolic volume) is reduced. Surgical removal of the dyskinetic muscle, often with bypass grafting to diseased coronary vessels, may improve cardiac function in selected cases.

Postinfarction Syndrome. A postinfarction syndrome, *Dressler's syndrome,* has been described, occurring a week or more after acute infarction and characterized by pericarditis with pleuritis and pleural effusions. This condition is similar to the postpericardiectomy syndrome observed after cardiac surgery. It responds dramatically to moderate doses of corticosteroids.

Treatment. The aims of treatment are (1) to make the patient comfortable, (2) to reduce the demands on the heart by maintaining the patient at rest during the healing phase, (3) to prevent complications, or (4) to treat them. Recent experiments suggest that a fifth aim, preservation of ischemic myocardium and limitation of infarct size may be feasible.

Prehospital Management. The majority of deaths from acute myocardial infarction occur before hospitalization is achieved. Two factors, a high incidence of life-threatening arrhythmia in the first few minutes or hours after the acute event, and the ubiquitous problem of misinterpretation or denial of symptoms, contribute to the early death rate. Intensive efforts to provide mobile coronary care with rapid diagnosis, treatment, and transport to hospitals have been reported from several major urban areas. Although these units have enthusiastic supporters, a careful study from Stockholm suggests that they will have little impact on survival without intense public education, because the major component of delay is failure of the victim to seek help in time.

The principles of early treatment are rapid diagnosis, alleviation of pain and apprehension, and stabilization of heart rhythm and blood pressure. Frequent ectopic ventricular beats usually respond to 50 to 100 mg of lidocaine given intravenously. Intramuscular injection of 400 mg of lidocaine will achieve a therapeutic blood level in 5 minutes and be effective for 45 minutes or more. Emergency treatment of bradycardia has become controversial. Profound slowing of heart rate and hypotension will often respond to 0.5 to 2.0 mg of atropine given intravenously in divided doses. Moderate slowing with heart rates of 60 to 65 beats per minute and an adequate blood pressure may be treated expectantly. In laboratory animals injection of atropine and the resultant increase in heart rate have been shown to enlarge the area of infarction after coronary occlusion. The administration of drugs without precise electrocardiographic control is not without hazard. In the acute situation the physician or nurse must judge what is in the best interest of the patient. Once the situation is stabilized, the patient should be transported to a hospital with adequate monitoring and resuscitative facilities.

In-Hospital Care. Serious complications of acute myocardial infarction cannot be properly managed outside the hospital. Treatment of the patient in a coronary care unit with appropriate monitoring facilities and trained personnel has reduced mortality in hospital by 30 to 50 per cent. In the well-run coronary care unit at present, hospital mortality for unselected patients with acute myocardial infarction averages 12 to 18 per cent. Despite the wide variety of electronic monitoring instruments available, the only body function which has been shown to be useful to monitor routinely and continuously is the rate and rhythm of the heart as revealed by the electrocardiogram. It is now well accepted practice to train nurses and other personnel to interpret the electrocardiogram and initiate therapy for abnormal rhythm, because the physician is only intermittently in attendance on the patient.

About a third of patients routinely admitted for coronary care will have no serious complications and recover uneventfully. Were it possible to identify these patients with low risk, hospitalization could be avoided and home care advised. Pantridge has suggested that patients hospitalized with acute myocardial infarction without significant arrhythmia and S-T segments and T wave changes only which return to normal within 48 hours can be promptly discharged to convalesce at home. A study from Bristol, England, reported that hospital mortality and home mortality in unselected patients with acute myocardial infarction were similar. It is clear, however, that both the extent of infarction and the interval from acute onset to medical intervention influence mortality and the decision to treat at home. Continued studies of the effectiveness of home treatment in selected patients will be viewed with great interest. General clinical status, suitability of home environment, and availability of medical help will affect the outcome. In the United States at present, hospitalization and monitoring in a coronary care unit for the first few days of illness are the recommended treatment for acute myocardial infarction.

Environment. The patient should be put to bed in a quiet, calm area. Rest and relaxation should be sought. Most patients prefer a single room, although this may not always be possible. Light should be subdued and noise kept to a minimum. Usually visitors are restricted during the first few days of illness. Radio, newspapers, and television are reduced to a minimum. A clock and a calendar provide the patient with considerable security and prevent a sense of isolation.

Pain and Apprehension. Morphine sulfate, 8 to 15 mg parenterally, is usually effective for pain or restlessness. In severe cases, it may be necessary to repeat the drug in smaller dosages every three to four hours. Morphine depresses respiration, reduces myocardial contractility, and is a potent vasodilator. Hypotension, which can usually be overcome by elevation of the lower extremities, or bradycardia, responsive to atropine, may develop. Meperidine, 50 to 100 mg, is also useful, although not as effective as morphine. Since intramuscular injections may elevate serum enzyme activity (CPK, GOT) and confuse diagnostic interpretation, injection into the abdominal panniculus has been recommended. The patient who is confused and restless may be suffering from cerebral dysfunction or delirium owing to heart failure or shock. It is wise therefore to be cautious in administering narcotics, especially in repeated doses.

Mood changes with apprehension are common. It is important to have a well trained, sympathetic nursing staff under the direction of an understanding physician to interpret and explain the illness and treatment. Specific treatment with barbiturates, chlordiazepoxide (Librium) or diazepam (Valium), may help.

Bowel Function. Maintenance of reasonably normal bowel function and avoidance of straining at stool are important aspects of treatment. An effective therapy is milk of magnesia, 30 ml twice daily. Dioctyl sodium sulfosuccinate (Colace), 100 mg twice daily, may be added if necessary. This program usually produces a satisfactory evacuation in midmorning. Milk of magnesia combined with cascara tends to cause bloating, cramps, and excessive flatus, as does Colace when used alone.

Smoking. Admission to a coronary unit is one of the most effective deterrents to smoking. The physician should not fail to take advantage of this opportunity.

Bed Rest. Traditional treatment has overemphasized the value of bed rest. Strict bed rest is reasonable for the first three or four days. If no serious complication develops, the patient may then be allowed modified bed rest with some activity, sitting in a chair. Use of a bedside commode is much appreciated. In an uncomplicated infarction, after a few days of chair rest, progressive ambulation may begin, to prepare the patient for discharge about three weeks after the acute attack. At home activity is gradually increased, and the patient may anticipate returning to work in six to ten weeks.

Bladder. Urinary retention resulting from bladder neck obstruction is not uncommon in older patients during prolonged bed rest. If urinary retention is suspected, the physician should not hesitate to insert an indwelling catheter with aseptic technique. After the cardiac problem has improved, definitive therapy may be undertaken if necessary.

Diet. Acutely ill patients usually have little appetite, although modest amounts of tastily prepared food may be appreciated. Usually the patient is offered a soft diet, moderately reduced in calories, 1500 to 1800, and in sodium, 2 to 3 grams (87 to 130 mEq) as soon as he wishes to eat. A number of adequate salt substitutes are available. Salt intake and the variety of food may be liberalized after the first week if no evidence of heart failure has been detected. For the overweight patient, close supervision of the convalescent period may offer an opportunity for weight reduction.

Oxygen. Hypoxia secondary to increased pulmonary venous hypertension and left ventricular dysfunction in myocardial infarction has been discussed previously. Administration of oxygen may (1) increase arterial Po_2 and (2) increase oxygen tension in the ischemic myocardium bordering the infarcted zone, thus perhaps reducing the size of infarction. Despite uncertainty about the importance of oxygen therapy, it seems reasonable to provide an atmosphere of increased oxygen to most patients during the first few days, utilizing either the Venturi mask or nasal cannula. The loose-fitting Venturi mask is comfortable and efficient. Models are available which deliver 28, 35, or 40 per cent oxygen. An oxygen tent is inefficient and expensive.

Anticoagulation. At present, with emphasis on the treatment of heart failure, early ambulation, reduced sedation, and limb movement in bed, it is apparent that the morbidity is low and the mortality essentially nil from thromboembolism complicating myocardial infarction. There is no evidence to suggest that anticoagulants influence the course of the infarction itself. The decision to use anticoagulants is largely elective. Their use should be based on the patient's past history, the quality of the supporting laboratory, and the experience of the physician with anticoagulant drugs. Recent phlebitis or embolism favors treatment. History of ulcer, bleeding tendency, signs of pericarditis, or hemorrhage would argue against anticoagulation. The most commonly used agents are Coumadin derivatives. Heparin is indicated only occasionally when thrombosis or embolism appears as a life-threatening complication.

Arrhythmia. Recognition and management of arrhythmia in acute myocardial infarction is based on a thorough understanding of electrophysiology and electrocardiography. The reader is urged to consult Ch. 569 and 570 before proceeding.

SINUS BRADYCARDIA. Reduction of the heart rate below 55 owing to failure of the normal sinus mechanism may be accompanied by evidence of low cardiac output, development of heart failure, or hypotension. Intravenous atropine, 0.5 to 1.0 mg, is usually effective. Occasionally 2.0 mg may be required. Atropine is not practical for long-term maintenance. Repeated use of the drug is limited by occasional central nervous system effects, urinary retention, and the rare precipitation of acute glaucoma. Overdosage may cause unpleasant tachycardia with consequent adverse effect in infarct size. Slowing of the sinus rate is usually temporary. Occasionally the condition persists as a manifestation of the "sick sinus syndrome," and temporary pacing with an electrode inserted into the right atrium or right ventricle is required.

ATRIAL ARRHYTHMIA. Frequent atrial premature complexes are often the harbinger of atrial fibrillation or flutter. They usually respond to digitalis. If atrial flutter and fibrillation are well tolerated, without hypotension or heart failure, they are best treated with digitalis to control the ventricular rate. If complications develop or the patient is not tolerating the arrhythmia well, DC precordial shock should be employed. Supraventricular arrhythmias are frequently recurrent, but after the acute illness subsides, spontaneous reversion is the rule.

ATRIOVENTRICULAR BLOCK. An important guide to therapy of heart block is the ventricular rate. In atrioventricular dissociation with an escape junctional rhythm, the QRS configuration is usually normal and the heart rate is well maintained. This is also true in the Wenckebach phenomenon (second degree block, Mobitz Type I). Thus treatment may be expectant. However, when there is intermittent atrial capture of the ventricle with unexpected dropped beats or complete AV block with a slow idioventricular rate characterized by wide QRS complexes (Mobitz type II), therapy is usually required. An intravenous infusion of isoproterenol may be immediately effective. Isoproterenol, 0.4 to 1.0 mg, is dissolved in 500 ml of 5 per cent glucose in water and carefully administered intravenously by slow drip. The rate of infusion and the concentration of the drug should be adjusted according to the ventricular response. Isoproterenol may induce both atrial and ventricular arrhythmia, and its use requires constant, close medical supervision.

Temporary transvenous pacemaking with an electrode catheter in the right ventricle is an effective form of therapy for a slow ventricular rate. The electrode should be activated by a battery-powered demand-type pacemaker. *Heart block* in acute myocardial infarction is almost always self-limited. Established heart block after recovery from infarction is rare. Thus if a satisfactory ventricular rate can be maintained for a few days, conduction will almost invariably resume through normal pathways, and the pacemaker catheter can then be withdrawn.

Sudden *complete heart block,* Mobitz Type II, is usually due to bilateral bundle branch block. Fifty per cent of patients with right or left bundle branch block prior to acute infarction develop bilateral bundle branch block during the acute illness. Patients with left bundle branch block have a high frequency of ventricular fibrillation. Despite widespread use of pacemakers for treatment or on standby, the mortality when complete heart block complicates myocardial infarction remains high, averaging 50 per cent.

VENTRICULAR PREMATURE BEATS; UNSUSTAINED VENTRICULAR TACHYCARDIA. The appearance of more than three ventricular premature beats per minute or bursts of ventricular contractions requires urgent treatment. In ischemia or infarction they may be forerunners of cardiac arrest, and prompt, aggressive treatment may forestall a catastrophe. The most effective and rapidly acting agent currently available is lidocaine hydrochloride intravenously in doses of 50 to 100 mg by rapid injection (bolus). The dose may be repeated in three to five minutes to achieve the desired result, obliteration of extrasystoles. When the ectopic beats have disappeared after bolus injection, a constant intravenous drip of lidocaine may be administered and the drip rate adjusted to maintain an infusion rate of 1.0 to 5.0 mg per minute. The infusion rate may be gradually reduced after several hours if there is no recurrence, and may be discontinued in 24 to 36 hours. Recurrence of extrasystoles may require extra immediate doses of lidocaine followed by an increase in the infusion rate.

Lidocaine is a local anesthetic, and it may cause sensations of body numbness or tingling or twitching of the face muscles. Large doses often cause drowsiness. Convulsions occasionally occur with excessive dosage, especially in the presence of cerebral anoxia.

If lidocaine is not effective, procainamide or quinidine sulfate may be required. Diphenylhydantoin every four to eight hours is also occasionally effective. In refractory situations, overdrive suppression with a temporary pacemaker may be tried. Overdriving shortens electrical diastole and suppresses the tendency for ectopic beats to develop.

VENTRICULAR TACHYCARDIA AND VENTRICULAR FIBRILLATION. These two arrhythmias are considered together, because ventricular tachycardia often precedes and degenerates into ventricular fibrillation. If blood pressure is maintained without circulatory collapse in the presence of ventricular tachycardia, 100 mg of lidocaine may be administered rapidly intravenously. If there is no effect within three to five minutes, DC precordial shock is applied. If blood pressure is not maintained and the patient develops clinical cardiac arrest, immediate treatment with precordial shock is mandatory.

VENTRICULAR FIBRILLATION. The proper therapy of this arrhythmia is immediate defibrillation. If the defibrillator is available, time is wasted attempting to ventilate the patient or attempting closed-chest cardiac massage. In older patients there are approximately 60 seconds in which to administer an effective shock and revert ventricular fibrillation to normal rhythm before the development of serious metabolic disturbance or brain damage. "Thump version," delivery of a sharp blow to the precordium, may be attempted for ventricular tachycardia or fibrillation. In the well run coronary care unit, defibrillation for unexpected cardiac arrest can frequently be applied by the trained nurse within 30 seconds of onset.

ASYSTOLE. Sudden, unexpected asystole is uncommon in acute infarction. Most often it is the culmination of a gradual decline in cardiac function in severe heart failure or shock. A series of thumps on the chest or closed chest cardiac massage may restore cardiac action. If an electrode catheter is in place or can be rapidly inserted, artificial pacemaking may be effective.

Pulmonary Edema. The initial manifestation of acute infarction may be sudden development of pulmonary edema. The aims of therapy are to improve cardiac function, reduce airway resistance and the work of breathing, and increase arterial oxygen tension. If the blood pressure is well maintained, the patient is propped into a sitting position. Morphine sulfate, 8 to 15 mg parenterally, is effective. Oxygen is administered, preferably by mask, in high concentration. If the patient can tolerate a tightly fitting mask, oxygen under positive pressure or with positive pressure on exhalation is useful, because the increased intrathoracic pressure impedes venous return and lowers ventricular filling pressures. Blood pressure should be carefully followed, because positive pressure inhalation is contraindicated in hypotension or shock. Rotating tourniquets impound a significant portion of the circulating blood volume in the extremities and are extremely useful. Tourniquets should be applied to three limbs tightly enough to inhibit venous return yet permit transmission of the arterial pulse, and should be rotated every 20 minutes.

Digitalis is usually not necessary in the immediate

treatment unless the condition has been precipitated by acute supraventricular arrhythmia, especially rapid atrial fibrillation or flutter. The drug is usually indicated for long-term management, and may be necessary in refractory cases. Furosemide, 40 to 80 mg, and ethacrynic acid, 50 to 100 mg, are potent diuretic agents which will initiate diuresis within 15 minutes of intravenous administration. Both are frequently used in patients with pulmonary edema. They also increase venous capacitance and have been shown to sharply reduce left ventricular filling pressure before diuresis commences. Other measures include phlebotomy of 300 to 500 ml or more, administration of aminophylline as a suppository (0.5 gram) or intravenously in a slow infusion in a dosage of 250 to 500 mg.

Heart Failure. Congestive heart failure is fairly common in acute myocardial infarction, occurring in approximately two thirds of hospitalized patients. Early signs of pulmonary congestion may be treated with diuretics or reduction of salt intake. There is strong experimental and clinical evidence to support the view that the infarcted heart has increased sensitivity to the toxic effects of digitalis. Digitalis should not be withheld when clearly indicated but should be given in smaller dosages than usual. Serum potassium level should be followed closely. Additional digitalis can always be given in cases of need. It is impossible to remove an excess.

Many different digitalis preparations are available, but it is best to avoid administration of more than one agent to a patient, as judgment about the level becomes exceedingly difficult. *Digoxin* is useful; it is rapidly absorbed and excreted with a serum half-life of about 30 hours; hence dosage depends upon frequency and route of administration. In patients who are acutely ill, the author prefers intravenous administration, as there is certainty about the time and amount given. A reasonable schedule is 0.5 mg initially intravenously, followed by 0.25 mg in six hours, followed by 0.125 mg in six hours. The total dose is conservative, but this schedule will usually avoid any problem of digitalis intoxication. For oral dosage 0.5 mg is given, followed by 0.25 mg at 6 and 12 hours, and then a maintenance schedule of 0.25 mg is given daily thereafter. *Ouabain,* available only in an intravenous preparation, has been advocated by some authorities in the treatment of heart failure complicating acute myocardial infarction. This drug has the same physiologic half-life as digoxin, and a convenient dosage schedule is as follows: 0.4 mg intravenously as an initial dose, followed by 0.1 to 0.2 mg every two hours for two or three additional doses. A detectable effect occurs within 20 minutes, with a peak action at about 2 hours.

Hypotension. If blood pressure falls, yet the patient remains alert and warm, has an adequate urine output, and is not in shock, management may be expectant. A treatable cause should be sought. The fall in blood pressure may be caused by drugs, particularly sedatives, or narcotics such as morphine. If hypotension is due to peripheral venous pooling, elevation of the lower extremities is an effective measure. Occasionally the fall in blood pressure is a reflection of reduced blood volume, and ventricular filling pressures are low. This has been observed in patients previously treated for acute pulmonary edema who then become hypotensive after brisk diuresis. The most common precipitating factor is use of potent diuretic agents such as ethacrynic acid or furosemide.

Thus when blood pressure falls, a venous pressure of less than 80 mm of saline or wedge pressure (obtained with a balloon-tipped floating catheter of the Swan-Ganz type) of less than 12 mm Hg suggests the possibility of hypovolemia. Infusion of 100 ml increments of half-normal saline or low molecular weight dextran is initiated, with careful monitoring of the ventricular filling pressure. If blood pressure increases with little or no change in venous or wedge pressure, hypovolemia is indeed present. Some patients may receive 2 or 3 liters of fluid before filling pressure increases. However, if filling pressures rise promptly as the fluid is infused, it is unlikely that hypovolemia is a contributing factor to the hypotension.

Cardiogenic Shock. The patient in shock has a systolic blood pressure less than 90 mg Hg, is usually restless, and has reduced mental awareness, cyanosis, oliguria (less than 20 ml per hour) or even anuria, and cool, moist extremities. As discussed earlier, cardiac function is severly deranged. The function of the heart as a pump is inadequate to support life. Myocardial oxygenation is insufficient, and the heart produces lactate. Progressive metabolic acidosis is a hallmark of shock, and arterial pH should be measured frequently. Mortality remains high. Autopsy almost invariably reveals massive myocardial infarction with extensive coronary artery disease.

Treatable causes such as cardiac tamponade, hypovolemia, or serious arrhythmia should be sought and vigorously managed. Tamponade may be suspected when hypotension or shock is accompanied by marked distention of the neck veins or very high venous pressure. To evaluate the possibility of hypovolemia, central venous or wedge pressure should be measured, and, if low, the response to volume replacement, as described above, carefully evaluated.

Treatment of cardiogenic shock is unsatisfactory. Isoproterenol increases myocardial oxygen demand and induces lactate production in the ischemic heart. Its overall effect in cardiogenic shock is deleterious and it is contraindicated. Norepinephrine increases peripheral vascular resistance, improves myocardial contractility, and may decrease lactate production. Despite extensive use and many eloquent testimonials, convincing evidence that infusion of norepinephrine improves mortality in cardiogenic shock is lacking. Administration of so-called alpha-blocking agents such as phenoxybenzamine or phentolamine or of large doses of adrenal corticosteroids has been advocated. Although these are apparently effective in certain types of experimental shock, there is no evidence supporting their effectiveness in cardiogenic shock secondary to acute myocardial infarction. Support of the circulation with an intra-aortic counterpulsating balloon effectively reverses myocardial lactate production, reduces left ventricular filling pressure, and increases cardiac output and coronary blood flow. Unfortunately the device does not much improve survival when applied to patients with established shock. Early use of the device when cardiac work has acutely fallen and before clinical manifestations of shock appear may be helpful. A variety of devices for applying counterpulsation externally are being developed but await critical testing.

Emotional Aspects. Anxiety, denial, and depression are almost universal in the patient with myocardial infarction. Anxiety is most prominent during the first 24 hours, when pain, fear, close medical attention, and hospitalization are intensely experienced. Denial and unrealistic evaluation of symptoms may confuse interpretation of a potentially serious illness during the first few hours or days after onset of ischemic pain.

By the third day of illness, the emotional impact of the situation, knowledge of cardiac injury, and fear of disablement engender a normal sequence of reactions characterized by *depression*. It is important for the physician and nurse to recognize that depression is almost invariable in the patient with acute myocardial infarction. Treatment with an early rehabilitation program should begin no later than the third day after hospitalization, the usual time of onset of depression. Overemphasis on bed rest and inactivity is a focus for depression and causes rapid physical "deconditioning." Beginning after the third or fourth day, the value of a thorough explanation of the illness, outline of a positive rehabilitation program, and discussion of the depression and misconceptions about illness cannot be overemphasized. It is important to include the family in these discussions. The wise physician is aware that once the acute phase of illness is passed, his most important tasks are management of depression, rehabilitation, and institution of a reasonable long-term preventive program.

Rehabilitation. Bed rest for more than a short period is deleterious. Rapid "deconditioning" results in a decrease in work capacity, an increase in heart rate during effort, and orthostatic hypotension. Depression and feelings of helplessness are intensified by bed rest. The need for prolonged bed rest or hospitalization is being vigorously re-examined. Certainly bed rest should not be prescribed without good cause. Experiments in home care in Bristol, England, suggest that some patients will do well without hospitalization. A Boston study showed that patients without complications discharged after two weeks suffer no more morbidity than those with prolonged hospitalization. Even earlier discharge has been advocated for rapidly resolving T wave infarcts.

In the patient without complications passive exercise can begin after three or four days, about the time chair rest becomes appropriate. By a week after the infarct, slow walking about, daily toilet activities, and nonstressful paperwork can commence. Current evidence suggests that the uncomplicated patient may be discharged after two to three weeks. A gradual increase in physical activity is outlined to cover the next three to six weeks at home. The majority of patients can return to former occupations from six to twelve weeks after the acute infarction. Many factors such as age, extent of myocardial injury, presence of arrhythmia or heart failure, occupation, and personal ambition will modify the rehabilitation program.

Resumption of sexual activity is of concern to patient and spouse, although the subject may not be directly broached. Folklore emphasizes a hazard of sudden death during coitus. Hellerstein points out that the risks are greatly exaggerated. The oxygen cost of sexual activity in middle-aged men with spouse of long standing is equivalent to moderate exercise such as walking briskly or climbing one or two flights of stairs. Generally, sexual activity may be resumed in parallel with other normal moderate physical exertions.

Experimental Therapy. Patients with myocardial infarction who die from heart failure or shock have less viable myocardium at autopsy than those who die from arrhythmia. Pathologic studies suggest that reinfarction or extension may be more common than is currently recognized clinically. After recovery, cardiac performance, especially during stress, may be importantly influenced by the mass and distribution of nonischemic, normally functioning myocardium.

In a significant series of experiments, Moroko and Braunwald have demonstrated a direct relationship between reduction of the area of acute myocardial ischemia after coronary occlusion and alteration of myocardial oxygen need or delivery. Reduction of oxygen requirement is correlated with a decrease in the extent of ischemia or infarction. Thus increase in coronary perfusion or reduction of afterload with vasodilators was associated with a smaller infarction. Infusion of potassium-insulin-glucose mixtures also limited myocardial damage. Whether this resulted from metabolic, osmotic, or other effects is not known. Hyaluronidase also had a protective effect. Conversely, factors which increased cardiac work, such as tachycardia or digitalis and glucagon in the nonfailing heart, increased the apparent ischemic area.

The possibility of controlling myocardial work and hence reducing infarct size has attracted widespread interest. Clinical data supporting this concept are not yet available. Careful study in man appears to be justified, but will be dependent on development of satisfactory methods to measure infarct size. Imaging techniques, CPK curve analysis, and precordial S-T segment mapping are being applied in many centers with varying success. The importance of clinical testing is illustrated by the difficulty in evaluating the usefulness of potassium-insulin-glucose preparations which were introduced as "polarizing" solutions in the mid-1960's. Many clinical studies have been performed. Few have been able to withstand close scientific scrutiny, and no clear-cut evidence of benefit is yet available.

Prognosis. Mortality is greatest during the first few hours, before most patients reach a hospital. The risk declines rapidly from onset of the acute attack. Studies from both Belfast and Edinburgh have revealed essentially the same findings: 50 per cent of the deaths from acute myocardial infarction occur within the first 2 hours and 15 minutes after the onset of the illness. Approximately three fourths of all deaths occur within the first 24 hours. The majority of the early deaths are sudden, owing to electrical instability of the heart, and are not necessarily related to the size of the infarct or the development of heart failure.

Reliable data for total mortality outside and inside the hospital in acute myocardial infarction are difficult to obtain. Oliver observed that 42 per cent of all patients under 70 died during the first four weeks. At the end of six months the total mortality was 49 per cent. The greatest risk was incurred by women age 60 to 69, in whom the mortality was 52 per cent at four weeks and rose to 59 per cent after six months.

The patient who is admitted to hospital has already survived a considerable risk. Prognosis after recovery depends upon many factors, including age, history of previous infarctions, presence of diabetes, presence of heart failure, mental attitude, type of employment, and employment policies. Patients who have survived ventricular fibrillation and successful resuscitation have an excellent prognosis in the absence of heart failure. Persistent heart failure and frequent ventricular ectopic beats warrant a guarded prognosis. If cardiac function is well maintained six weeks after acute infarction, most patients are able to return to previous employment and a full range of normal activity. Serial evaluation of left ventricular size with a calibrated roentgenogram exposed at end-diastole at known lung volume is of considerable prognostic value. During almost one year of follow-up in one study, 8 per cent of postinfarct patients with normal heart volume died. In those with enlarged hearts, mortality was threefold higher and functional status significantly more impaired.

Alonso, D., Scheidt, S., Post, M., and Killip, T.: Pathophysiology of cardiogenic shock. Quantification of myocardial necrosis, clinical, pathologic and electrocardiographic correlations. Circulation, 48:588, 1973.
Case, R. B., Nasser, M. G., and Crampton, R. S.: Biochemical aspects of early myocardial ischemia. Am. J. Cardiol., 24:766, 1969.
Coronary Drug Project Research Group: Prognostic importance of premature beats following myocardial infarction. Experience in the Coronary Drug Project. J.A.M.A., 223:1116, 1973.
Epstein, S. E., Goldstein, R. E., Redwood, D. R., Kent, K. M., and Smith, E. R.: The early phase of acute myocardial infarction: Pharmacologic aspects of therapy. Ann. Intern. Med., 78:918, 1973.
Erhardt, L. R., Lundman, T., and Mellstedt, H.: Incorporation of 125I-labelled fibrinogen into coronary arterial thrombi in acute myocardial infarction in man. Lancet, 1:387, 1973.
Fillmore, S. J., Gumaraes, A. C., Scheidt, S. S., and Killip, T.: Blood-gas changes and pulmonary hemodynamics following acute myocardial infarction. Circulation, 45:583, 1972.
Hackett, T. P., and Cassem, N. H.: The psychological adaption of myocardial infarction patients to convalescence. Heart and Lung, 2:382, 1973.
Heikkila, J.: Mitral incompetence as a complication of acute myocardial infarction. Acta Med. Scand. (Suppl.) 475:1–139, 1967.
Hellerstein, H. K., and Friedman, E. H.: Sexual activity and the post coronary patient. Arch. Intern. Med., 125:987, 1970.
Hutter, A. M., Sidel, V. W., Shine, K. I., and DeSanctis, R. W.: Early hospital discharge after myocardial infarction. N. Engl. J. Med., 288:1141, 1973.
Killip, T.: Management of arrhythmias in acute myocardial infarction. Hosp. Practice, 7:131, 1972.
Maroko, P. R., and Braunwald, E.: Modification of myocardial infarction size after coronary occlusion. Ann. Intern. Med., 79:720, 1973.
Nyquist, O.: Shock complicating acute myocardial infarction. Acta Med. Scand. (Suppl.) 536:1–72, 1972.
Scheidt, S., Ascheim, R., and Killip, T.: Shock after acute myocardial infarction: A clinical and hemodynamic profile. Am. J. Cardiol., 26:556, 1970.
Scheidt, S., Wilner, G., Fillmore, S., Shapiro, M., and Killip, T.: Objective haemodynamic assessment after acute myocardial infarction. Br. Heart J., 35:908, 1973.
Scheidt, S., Wilner, G., Mueller, H., Summers, D., Lesch, M., Wolff, G., Krakauer, J., Rubenfire, M., Fleming, P., Noon, G., Oldham, N., Killip, T., and Kantrowitz, A.: Intra-aortic balloon counter pulsation in cardiogenic shock. Report of a co-operative clinical trial. N. Engl. J. Med., 288:979, 1973.
Sobel, B. E., and Shell, W. E.: Serum enzyme determinations in the diagnosis and assessment of myocardial infarction. Circulation, 45:471, 1972.
Solomon, H. A., Edwards, A. L., and Killip, T.: Prodromata in acute myocardial infarction. Circulation, 40:463, 1969.
Weinblatt, E., Shapiro, S., Frank, C., and Sager, R.: Prognosis of men after first myocardial infarction: Mortality and first recurrence in relation to selected parameters. Am. J. Public Health, 58:1329, 1968.
Wilson, C., and Pantridge, J. F.: ST-segment displacement and early hospital discharge in acute myocardial infarction. Lancet, 3:1284, 1973.
Wolk, M. J., Scheidt, S., and Killip, T.: Heart failure complicating acute myocardial infarction. Circulation, 45:1125, 1972.

568. SUDDEN DEATH

Unexpected, rapid demise in the apparently healthy individual has recently been recognized as a major health problem. Considerable information has accumulated describing sudden death in a variety of circumstances. The perplexing problem of unexpected crib death is well known to the pediatrician. A familial syndrome of deafness, prolonged Q-T interval, and sudden death has been described. The Dalmatian coach hound suffers from a similar condition. Sudden death during or after exertion in aortic stenosis and idiopathic hypertrophic subaortic stenosis (asymmetrical septal hypertrophy, hypertrophic obstructive cardiomyopathy) is an ever-present, though statistically small, threat. Noncardiac in origin but responsive to emergency treatment is the "restaurant arrest" syndrome secondary to aspiration of a large bolus of meat with rapid asphyxia, usually associated with excess alcohol intake.

Instantaneous (a few minutes) and sudden (hours) unexpected death in the adult has been repeatedly shown to be associated with coronary artery disease in the overwhelming majority. Extensive coronary disease is the almost invariable autopsy finding in instantaneous death; evidence of acute infarction or coronary thrombosis is rare. When death occurs within a few hours of onset of symptoms, the incidence of coronary thrombosis and myocardial infarction is significantly higher.

Evidence from several epidemiologic surveys indicates that the majority of individuals who die suddenly have antemortem signs, symptoms, or significant risk factors suggesting coronary artery disease. Particular attention has focused on abnormalities of the electrocardiogram. Evidence of left bundle branch block, left axis deviation with right bundle branch block, left ventricular hypertrophy, or old infarction is associated with increased risk of sudden death. In the patient with coronary artery disease, a single ventricular premature complex recorded during routine electrocardiography or the detection of ten ventricular extrasystoles per 1000 beats is reported to increase the risk of sudden death seven- to tenfold! Despite recognition of some risk factors, there is unfortunately no information yet available on effective preventive therapy.

Many individuals who die suddenly can be resuscitated if trained personnel are available. High risk areas in hospital are the emergency room, cardiac and intensive care units, operating room, and recovery room. A long-term survival rate of 20 per cent after resuscitation has been reported from a general hospital with an intesive staff educational program. Most sudden deaths occur outside the hospital and are usually secondary to ventricular fibrillation. If life can be supported with mouth-to-mouth ventilation and closed-chest cardiac massage, defibrillation with recovery is possible.

The experience of the Seattle, Washington, community under the leadership of Alvarez and Cobb is testimony to what can be accomplished in prehospital emergency care. A system based on a rapid (two- to five-minute) response time by the fire department paramedics trained to a near-physician capability, resuscitation and defibrillation on the spot, and intense public education has proved remarkably effective. During three years, in a community of about 500,000 persons, 202 patients with cardiac or respiratory arrest outside a hospital were treated in the field, brought to a hospital, and subsequently discharged home. Seventy per cent had ventricular fibrillation. Several important observations have developed from this experience: Survival is nil if arrival of the rescue team occurs more than five minutes after the call is placed. Over 20 per cent of the successful resuscitations were initiated by lay bystanders. (Approximately 20 per cent of the Seattle population has been instructed in cardiopulmonary resuscitation.) The rate of survival has improved steadily with increasing experience and is currently about 22 per cent.

Long-term outlook in those survivors with evidence of myocardial infarction is good. When EKG criteria alone were used to diagnose acute transmural infarction, mortality after two years was 14 per cent. The survivor with no evidence of myocardial infarction has a high probability of suffering cardiac arrest again. Mortality after two years in those without infarctions was 43 per cent. These observations suggest that cardiac arrest not caused by acute myocardial infarction is likely to recur and may well be related to problems of conduction and arrhythmia in the presence of coronary artery disease without recognized ischemia.

Physicians, nurses, rescue squads, and paramedical personnel have an important obligation to maintain technical skills in cardiopulmonary resuscitation, because they may be called upon to provide or supervise emergency support of life at any time. The gratifying Seattle experience challenges medical leadership in many another community.

Cobb, L. A., and Alvarez, H.: Medic I: The Seattle system for management of out of hospital emergencies. Proceedings of National Conference in Standards for Cardio-Pulmonary Resuscitation and Emergency Cardiac Care. National Research Council, 1974.
Coronary Drug Project Research Group: Prognostic importance of premature beats following myocardial infarction. Experience in the Coronary Drug Project. J.A.M.A., 223:1116, 1973.
Eller, W. C., and Hangen, R. K.: Food asphyxiation—restaurant rescue. N. Engl. J. Med., 289:81, 1973.
Fraser, G. R., Froggat, P., and James, T. N.: Congenital deafness with electrocardiographic abnormalities, fainting attacks and sudden death: A recessive syndrome. Quart. J. Med., 33:361, 1964.
Friedman, M., Manwaring, J. H., Rosenman, R. H., Donlon, G., Ortega, P., and Grube, S.: Instantaneous and sudden deaths. Clinical and pathological differentiation in coronary artery disease. J.A.M.A., 225:1319, 1973.
Fulton, M., Lutz, W., Donald, K. W., Kirby, B. J., Duncan, B., Morrison, S. L., Kerr, F., Julian, D. G., and Oliver, M. F.: Natural history of unstable angina. Lancet, 1:860, 1972.
Kuller, L., Lilenfield, A., Fisher, R.: Sudden and unexpected deaths in young adults. J.A.M.A., 198:158, 1966.

CARDIAC ARRHYTHMIA

Anthony N. Damato

569. INTRODUCTION

Normally, the pacemaker of the heart is the sinoatrial (SA) node, which is an elongated structure (1.5 cm in length) located at the junction of the superior vena cava and the lateral border of the right atrium. In 55 per cent of cases the SA node receives its blood supply from the right coronary artery, and in 45 per cent of the cases, from the left circumflex artery. Cells of the SA node possess the property of automaticity which is responsible for the spontaneous rhythmicity of the heart beat. Automatic or pacemaker cells undergo spontaneous diastolic depolarization (phase 4 depolarization) in contrast to nonautomatic or working myocardial cells which maintain a steady diastolic or resting potential. When an automatic cell achieves threshold potential, it undergoes depolarization and serves as the excitatory or depolarizing stimulus for adjacent cells. Increasing the rate of diastolic depolarization of sinoatrial nodal pacemaker cells increases the heart rate and vice versa. The property of spontaneous diastolic depolarization can also be found in certain cells of the atrium, atrioventricular

(AV) junction, bundle branches, and Purkinje network, but not in ordinary working myocardial cells. These specialized cells serve as latent or potential pacemakers of the heart, and their rate of spontaneous diastolic depolarization is normally less than that of the sinoatrial node. However, if sinus node function is depressed, latent pacemaker activity can emerge and establish an escape rhythm. At other times, certain stimuli such as digitalis excess, ischemia, or hypoxia can enhance the rate of spontaneous diastolic depolarization of latent pacemakers beyond that of normal sinus node automaticity, which then results in an ectopic rhythm.

The transmission of impulses from the sinus node to the ventricles occurs along specialized conducting tissue which includes the AV node, the bundle of His (also called the common AV bundle), the right bundle branch, the left bundle branch, including its fascicular divisions, and the subendocardial Purkinje network. The bundle of His, bundle branches, and Purkinje network are commonly referred to as the His-Purkinje system or the ventricular specialized conducting system. In addition, three internodal connecting pathways (anterior, middle, and posterior internodal tracts) have been described which originate from the sinus node region and insert into different parts of the AV node. Fibers from these internodal pathways also spread in various degrees from the right to the left atrium. It has been suggested by some investigators that transmission of the sinus node impulse to the AV node and between the atria is along these specialized and preferential pathways and not by radial spread alone. Internodal pathways have also been invoked to explain some cases of short P-R interval in which it is suspected that an atrial impulse either partially or completely bypasses the AV node during its conduction to the ventricles.

The AV node lies beneath the right atrial endocardium, anterior to the os of the coronary sinus, and above the insertion of the septal leaflet of the tricuspid valve. The human adult AV node measures between 5 and 7 mm in length, and its deep surface abuts the central fibrous body of the heart. Anteriorly, the AV node is directly continuous with the bundle of His. Most of the fibers of the internodal tracts, mentioned above, enter the superior and posterior margins of the AV node, and a smaller number of fibers enter along its lateral margin. Conduction velocity within the AV node is slow (0.05 meter per second), which accounts in part for the normal physiologic AV delay that is reflected in the P-R interval. In most human hearts, the AV node receives its blood supply from the right coronary artery, which explains the association of AV nodal conduction abnormalities seen in some cases of inferior or diaphragmatic myocardial infarctions.

The anterior and deep part of the AV node becomes the common AV bundle or bundle of His in which the muscle fibers are arranged in parallel. The bundle of His penetrates the collagenous central fibrous body and lies on the upper margin of the muscular interventricular septum. At the posterior margin of the membranous interventricular septum the common bundle gives off a relatively wide left bundle branch which courses over the left side of the interventricular septum. The left bundle branch divides into anterior and posterior fascicles which enter the anterior and posterior papillary muscles, respectively. In addition, fibers from the left bundle insert directly into the interventricular septum. On the right side of the heart, the common bundle continues as a slender right bundle branch which courses over the interventricular septum and enters the anterior papillary muscle. Peripheral arborization of the right and left bundle branches constitutes the Purkinje network. In contrast to the AV node, the velocity of conduction throughout the His-Purkinje system is more rapid, being within the order of 1.0 to 3.5 meters per second.

The AV node and the proximal portion of the bundle of His are in close anatomic relationship to the tricuspid and mitral valve rings. In addition, the distal part of the bundle of His and the proximal portions of the bundle branches lie in close proximity to the noncoronary artery aortic cusp. These anatomic relationships of the AV conducting system are important to bear in mind, because inflammation, fibrosis, or calcification of the valve rings or central fibrous body may cause different types of AV block.

The P-R interval represents a combination of intra-atrial, AV nodal, and His-Purkinje conduction times. Unfortunately, the electrical activities of the sinus node, AV node, bundle of His, bundle branches, and subendocardial Purkinje network are not recorded by the surface electrocardiogram. Figure 1 presents in a schematic way the electrical events occurring during the P-R interval. The sinus node generates an impulse prior to the inscription of the P wave. As the atrial muscle is being depolarized (P wave), the sinus node impulse enters the AV node. Conduction within the bundle of His, bundle branches, and subendocardial Purkinje network occurs during the P-R segment. The QRS complex represents depolarization of the ventricular muscle.

It has become possible to record electrical activity of the bundle of His in man, using an electrode catheter which is fluoroscopically positioned in the region of the tricuspid valve. The electrode catheter records a low atrial electrogram (A), a His bundle deflection (H) which appears as a bi- or triphasic deflection within the P-R segment, and a ventricular electrogram (V) (Fig. 2). His bundle recordings permit division of the P-R interval into two subintervals, namely the A-H and H-V intervals. The A-H interval represents an approximation of AV nodal conduction time, and the H-V interval represents conduction time within the His-Purkinje system. Normal values for A-H and H-V intervals have varied slightly as reported by different investigators, but in

Figure 2. Tracings from top to bottom are as follows: surface EKG; a recording from the high right atrium (HRA); His bundle electrogram recording (HBE); and time lines (T) at 10 and 100 msec. A = Low atrial electrogram; H = His bundle electrogram; V = ventricular electrogram. During sinus rhythm the sequence of activation is from the high to low atrium. During retrograde conduction across the AV node, the sequence of atrial activation is reversed; the low atrial electrogram precedes the high atrial electrogram.

general are 60 to 140 msec and 30 to 55 msec, respectively. Bundle of His recordings provide a more precise method of localizing sites of AV conduction delay and block which may occur proximal to, within, or distal to the bundle of His. In addition, bundle of His recordings provide an accurate method for determining whether beats are of supraventricular or ventricular origin. Beats of supraventricular origin are preceded by His deflections with H-V intervals which are normal or greater than normal. In general, beats of ventricular origin are not preceded by His deflections.

570. ARRHYTHMIAS

SINUS ARRHYTHMIA

Sinus arrhythmia is characterized by irregular changes in the sinus rate which most often occur in relationship to the phases of respiration. The sinus rate increases at end inspiration and decreases at end expiration. The respiratory changes in sinus rate are believed to result from changes in vagal tone. Sinus arrhythmia is a normal phenomenon seen more frequently in children and young adults and tends to become less pronounced with increasing age. Electrocardiographically the P wave configuration is normal but may show slight changes in shape. The P-P intervals show cyclical increases and decreases in relation to the phase of respiration, whereas the P-R intervals remain fairly constant. Sinus arrhythmia requires no treatment.

SINUS BRADYCARDIA

Sinus bradycardia has been arbitrarily defined as a sinus rate of less than 60 per minute. It is a normal finding in a significant number of young healthy adults and is the expected finding in well trained athletes. Sinus bradycardia may result from administration of drugs such as digitalis, propranolol, morphine, reserpine, and prostigmine. Normal sinus rates return when these

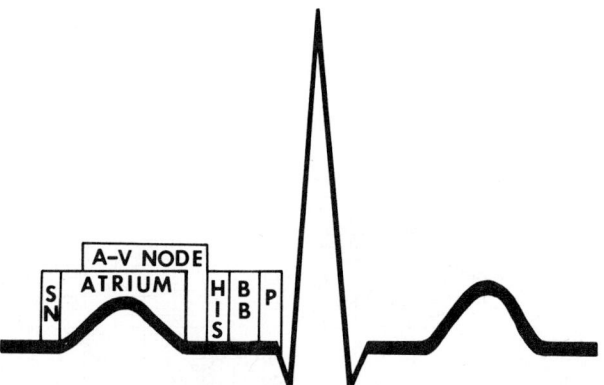

Figure 1. Schematic representation of the sequence of AV conduction in relationship to the P wave, P-R segment and QRS complex. SN = sinus node impulse; AV node = atrioventricular node; HIS = His bundle; BB = bundle branches; P = subendocardial Purkinje system. (Modified from Hoffman, B. F., and Singer, D. H.: Prog. Cardiovasc. Dis., 7:226, 1964.

drugs are withdrawn. A temporary sinus bradycardia may occur during acute diaphragmatic myocardial infarction. Usually, sinus bradycardia is associated with normal AV conduction (1:1 AV response with a normal P-R interval). In older patients AV block may signify depression of both sinus and AV nodes. Sinus bradycardia at rates of 40 per minute or less should raise the possibility of a 2:1 sinus node exit block, which is a rare phenomenon (see Fig. 4).

In general, sinus bradycardia requires no treatment. In most cases, the sinus rate shows a normal acceleration in response to exercise, atropine, or other appropriate stimuli. An inappropriate response to such stimuli raises the possibility of the sick sinus syndrome. If symptoms such as lightheadedness, syncope, congestive heart failure, or angina pectoris are the result of a low resting heart rate or inappropriate acceleration of the heart rate during stressful situations, a permanent ventricular pacemaker should be inserted.

SINUS TACHYCARDIA

For adults, sinus tachycardia is defined as a sinus rate in excess of 100 per minute. Most often, sinus tachycardia represents a normal physiologic response to stressful situations such as exercise, fright, emotional upset, fever, congestive heart failure, and hypotension. Under these conditions, the increase in sinus rate is generally associated with a normal or less than normal P-R interval, because the sympathetic stimuli causing sinus node acceleration also enhance AV nodal conduction. Vagolytic drugs, such as atropine, can also produce a sinus tachycardia. The treatment for sinus tachycardia is that of the underlying condition. Carotid sinus pressure will produce a temporary and incomplete slowing of the sinus rate which quickly returns to original levels. If sinus tachycardia is the result of congestive heart failure, digitalis will slow the sinus rate as the failure improves. However, digitalis will be ineffective in sinus tachycardias from other causes such as fever or thyrotoxicosis.

SICK SINUS SYNDROME

The sick sinus syndrome (SSS) refers to a variety of electrocardiographic abnormalities which result from dysfunction of the sinoatrial node. Included in SSS are the following:

1. Persistent, severe, or unexpected sinus bradycardia. At times, sinus bradycardia may alternate with episodes of supraventricular tachyarrhythmias, and this combination has been termed the bradycardia-tachycardia syndrome.

2. Sinoatrial block or exit block not related to drug therapy.

3. Sinus arrest (cessation of sinus rhythm) for short or long intervals, during which time either no escape rhythm arises or an atrial, junctional, or ventricular rhythm emerges.

These electrocardiographic abnormalities result because (1) the sinus node fails as an impulse generator, or (2) the sinus node impulse is delayed or blocked in its conduction out to the atrial muscle. Often, patients with SSS have an associated AV block or intraventricular conduction abnormality. The most commonly encountered symptoms in SSS are lightheadedness, dizziness, syncope, convulsions, dyspnea, fatigue, and angina pectoris.

Sinus Bradycardia

Sinus bradycardia may be the initial manifestation of SSS, and consequently not all sinus bradycardias are benign. SSS should be suspected when sinus bradycardia occurs in a symptomatic patient or is an inappropriate response to the clinical environs, such as during exercise, fever, pain, or congestive heart failure. Failure of the sinus rate to increase after atropine administration should raise the possibility of SSS, and further observations are indicated.

Bradycardia-Tachycardia Syndrome

The bradycardia-tachycardia syndrome is included in the spectrum of SSS and is characterized by sinus bradycardia alternating with episodes of atrial tachycardia, atrial fibrillation, or atrial flutter. The atrial tachycardia may be ectopic in origin or may result from AV nodal re-entry (Fig. 3). Symptoms may be related to either slow or rapid heart rates or both.

Treatment. Sinus bradycardia as a manifestation of SSS is generally, although not always, unresponsive to pharmacologic treatment. If belladonna alkaloids, atropine, or sympathomimetic amines are ineffectual in speeding up the sinus rate and the patient is symptomatic from the slow heart rate, a permanent ventricular pacemaker should be inserted. In the bradycardia-tachycardia syndrome the therapeutic problem is compounded by the fact that not only are agents such as procainamide and quinidine often ineffectual in controlling the atrial tachyarrhythmias, but these drugs may aggravate the sinus bradycardia. Likewise, digitalis,

Figure 3. Bradycardia-tachycardia syndrome. After two sinus beats (rate, 45 per minute), two ectopic atrial beats occur, the second of which initiates an AV nodal re-entrant tachycardia. The initial part of the tachycardia shows aberrant ventricular conduction.

which can effectively slow the ventricular response during a period of supraventricular tachycardia, may also worsen the bradycardia. The most effective therapy to date has been the insertion of a permanent ventricular pacemaker by which the ventricular rate can be controlled and pharmacologic agents more safely administered to control the atrial arrhythmia.

SINOATRIAL BLOCK

The tissue surrounding the sinoatrial node normally imposes a conduction delay between the sinus node impulse and depolarization of the atrial myocardium. Disturbances in conduction of the sinus node impulse can take the form of first, second, or third degree SA block, all of which constitute uncommon manifestations of the clinical spectrum of SSS. Because of the inability to record the sinus node impulse in man, the diagnosis of SA block is an inferential one based primarily on the behavior of the P waves.

First Degree SA Block

In the first degree SA block the sinus node impulse is conducted more slowly out to the atrial myocardium. However, the clinical diagnosis of uncomplicated first-degree SA block cannot be made, because each sinus impulse elicits a P wave and the degree of delay is not reflected in the EKG recording.

Second Degree SA Block

Second degree SA block, like second degree AV block, has been classified into types I and II.

Type I Second Degree SA Block

In type I second degree SA block, sinoatrial conduction is of a Wenckebach type in which there is progressive conduction delay until a sinus node impulse fails to elicit a P wave. Like AV nodal Wenckebach cycles, the increment of SA conduction delay decreases throughout the cycle so that the P-P intervals progressively shorten prior to the dropped P wave. The P-P interval encompassing the dropped P wave is less than twice the P-P interval preceding the absent P wave.

Type II Second Degree SA Block

In type II second degree SA block, a sinus P wave is intermittently and unexpectedly dropped. The resultant pause is equal to twice the normal P-P interval. Atrial extrasystoles, which are hidden in the T wave and followed by a near compensatory pause, may simulate a type II SA block. In 2:1 SA block the normal sinus rate is halved. The resultant bradycardia is indistinguishable from the usual variety of sinus bradycardia unless an abrupt spontaneous doubling of the heart rate occurs (Fig. 4). Atrial bigeminy in which the ectopic P waves are masked by the T wave may simulate 2:1 SA block.

Third Degree SA Block

In third degree SA block, all the sinus impulses are blocked and there is absence of P waves. After a period of arrest, a subsidiary pacemaker located in the atrium, AV junction, or ventricles usually emerges as an escape rhythm. Third degree SA block is indistinguishable from sinus node arrest in which the pacemaker cells fail to generate impulses (Fig. 5).

ABERRATION

Ventricular aberration is defined as an alteration in the sequence of ventricular activation which results whenever an impulse of supraventricular origin is asynchronously conducted within the His-Purkinje system. Aberration results because a supraventricular impulse enters the His-Purkinje system during its refractory period. For atrial impulses the determinants of aberration include (1) the degree of prematurity of the atrial impulse; (2) the cycle length (R-R interval) preceding the premature atrial impulse; (3) the speed of AV nodal conduction; and (4) the state of recovery of excitability of the His-Purkinje system. In general, the more premature an atrial impulse, the greater the tendency for aberration to occur. Fast or relatively rapid AV nodal conduction enhances the possibility of aberration, because the premature atrial impulse can be delivered to the His-Purkinje system during its refractory period. However, at very close coupling intervals, aberrant ventricular activation may disappear if the premature atrial impulse encounters sufficient AV nodal delay that its arrival time within the His-Purkinje system is delayed and the latter is no longer refractory.

A direct relationship exists between cycle length (R-R interval) and refractoriness within the His-Purkinje system. Refractoriness of the His-Purkinje system increases with longer R-R intervals and decreases as the R-R interval shortens. A long R-R interval preceding a sufficiently premature atrial beat favors aberration, whereas de-

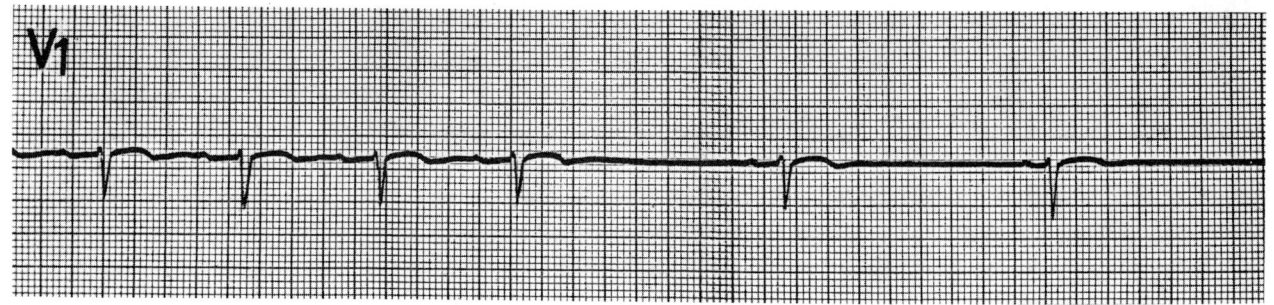

Figure 4. 2:1 SA exit block. The sinus rate is suddenly halved.

Figure 5.   Third degree SA block. After three sinus beats, the sinus node impulse either fails to be generated or to exit from the sinus node. An AV junctional pacemaker emerges, followed by resumption of sinus rhythm. During the AV junctional rhythm, the QRS complexes are similar to those of sinus origin.

creasing the preceding cycle length may abolish aberration.

Aberrant conduction involving the right bundle branch is seen more commonly than aberration involving the left bundle branch. Given the right conditions, aberrant ventricular activation can occur in normal or abnormal hearts and therefore it is not of itself a sign of heart disease. Aberrant conduction of consecutive beats during a supraventricular tachycardia can mimic a ventricular tachycardia. Examples of aberrant conduction of supraventricular impulses are shown in Figures 3, 6, 8, 9, 11, and 29.

ATRIAL EXTRASYSTOLES

Atrial extrasystoles are premature depolarizations of the atria resulting from impulses which originate in ectopic foci located anywhere within the atria. Atrial extrasystoles are also referred to as premature atrial beats, premature atrial contractions, or premature atrial systoles.

Atrial extrasystoles result in P waves (P′) which are different from sinus P waves. These differences, which may be marked or subtle, are due to an altered sequence of atrial activation resulting from an ectopic origin of the depolarizing impulse.

Atrial extrasystoles may have a constant or inconstant coupling interval to the preceding sinus beat and can occur in a bigeminal or trigeminal sequence. Three or more consecutive atrial extrasystoles occurring at a rate of 100 per minute or greater constitute an ectopic atrial tachycardia.

Atrial extrasystoles occurring late in the diastolic period may be associated with little or no AV conduction delay, in which case the P-R interval will be the same as or close to that of the sinus beats. Extrasystoles of greater prematurity are almost always associated with an increased P-R interval (relative to sinus beats), which may be due to conduction delay within the AV node, His-Purkinje system, or both.

Atrial extrasystoles may result in normal or aberrant ventricular activation, the determinants of which are discussed above. Aberrant ventricular activation may mimic premature ventricular extrasystoles if the premature atrial P′ wave is not recognized or is obscured within the T wave of the preceding QRS complex (Fig. 6). Atrial extrasystoles which are not conducted to the ventricles may block within the AV node or His-Purkinje system. A nonconducted atrial extrasystole may result in prolongation of the P-R interval of one or more subsequent sinus beats—a phenomenon which is called concealed conduction.

Figure 6.   The third, sixth, and ninth P waves (P′) are atrial extrasystoles which occur with trigeminal regularity. The first and third atrial extrasystoles are aberrantly conducted to the ventricles. The second atrial extrasystole is blocked.

Atrial extrasystoles generally invade and prematurely depolarize the sinus node pacemaker, causing a reset of the sinus cycle which is reflected in the pause that follows the atrial extrasystole. If the delay in the appearance of the postextrasystolic sinus beat equals the prematurity of the atrial extrasystole, the pause is said to be compensatory. In a fully compensatory pause, the sum of the pre- and postextrasystolic R-R intervals equals two sinus cycle lengths. Complete compensatory pauses are uncommonly associated with atrial extrasystoles. More often, one sees postextrasystolic pauses which are incompletely compensatory; that is, the sum of the pre- and postextrasystolic pauses is less than two sinus cycles. Occasionally, one may see significant suppression of sinus node automaticity after an extrasystole.

Atrial extrasystoles are common and may occur in completely normal individuals or may be associated with various types of organic heart disease. They may presage atrial fibrillation, atrial flutter, ectopic atrial tachycardias, or AV nodal re-entrant tachycardias. Very often, patients are unaware of the presence of infrequent atrial extrasystoles, and no special treatment is required. The patient may complain of "skipped beats" and "palpitations" which are the result of the pause and forceful ventricular contraction that follow the extrasystole. Mild sedation and abstinence from alcohol, tobacco, or caffeine may be all that is required to treat occasional extrasystoles which produce mild symptoms. Quinidine sulfate is used to treat atrial extrasystoles which cause disturbing symptoms, foreshadow other atrial arrhythmias, or are unabated by conservative measures.

ATRIAL FIBRILLATION

Atrial fibrillation is a frequently encountered cardiac arrhythmia which commonly occurs in association with some form of organic heart disease. Most cases of atrial fibrillation are associated with arteriosclerotic heart disease, followed in frequency by rheumatic and hypertensive heart diseases. A high incidence of this rhythm disorder is seen in patients with thyrotoxicosis. The greater tendency for enlarged atria to fibrillate may explain the frequent occurrence of atrial fibrillation in patients with congestive heart failure and mitral valvular disease. Atrial fibrillation, usually paroxysmal in nature, can occur in apparently healthy individuals who have no detectable evidence of associated heart disease.

The exact mechanism(s) underlying the development of atrial fibrillation is uncertain. Many of its characteristics are compatible with re-entry of multiple activation fronts. However, the fact that atrial fibrillation is frequently induced by premature atrial extrasystoles suggests that alterations in automaticity also play a role in the mechanism of this arrhythmia. Factors which favor the development and perpetuation of atrial fibrillation include frequent atrial extrasystoles, increased vagal tone, and an increase in atrial muscle mass wherein significant differences in conduction and refractoriness exist in adjacent fibers. Atrial fibrillation can be precipitated by a single atrial extrasystole which occurs in the so-called vulnerable period of the atrial cycle. At sinus cycle lengths the atrial vulnerable period has been estimated to be between 180 and 300 msec after a sinus P wave.

Electrocardiographic Features. Atrial fibrillation is characterized by absence of P waves and an irregular ventricular response. Normal sinus P waves are replaced by irregular chaotic and rapid atrial impulses occurring in excess of 400 per minute. The presence or absence of P waves is best observed in leads II and V_1. Atrial fibrillation has been described as "coarse" when the baseline of the electrocardiogram presents rapid, irregular fibrillatory (f) waves of varying amplitude, and "fine" when practically no atrial activity is detected. In untreated and uncomplicated atrial fibrillation, the irregular and rapid ventricular response is generally between 110 and 160 per minute, and most or all of the QRS complexes are of normal configuration for that patient (Fig. 7).

Concealed conduction within the AV node is the major determinant of the irregular R-R cycles during atrial fibrillation. The inherent capacity of the AV node to accept and transmit impulses to the ventricles is exceeded by the rapid, irregular atrial rate in atrial fibrillation. Consequently, many atrial impulses are blocked or concealed within the AV node, thereby altering its state of refractoriness which in turn affects the conduction of subsequent impulses. Impulses which exit from the AV node and enter the His-Purkinje system almost invariably result in a ventricular response. Uncommonly is the His-Purkinje system the site of concealment. Digitalis, propranolol, or increased vagal tone increases the degree of concealment or block within the AV node and thereby slows the ventricular response. The irregular R-R intervals during atrial fibrillation predispose to the occurrence of aberrant intraventricular conduction. In atrial fibrillation the distinction between aberrant conduction and ventricular ectopy is an important one which unfortunately is made more difficult because of the absence of P waves. The diagnosis of aberrant conduction is favored (80 per cent of the time) if the beat in question (1) has a right bundle branch block pattern, (2) terminates a short cycle which is preceded by a long cycle, and (3) has initial

Figure 7.   Untreated atrial fibrillation. There is absence of P waves with an irregular ventricular rate.

Figure 8. Atrial fibrillation with aberrant ventricular conduction. The R-R intervals are indicated above. The first four beats are the patient's normal QRS complexes with H-V intervals of 55 msec. The last four beats result from supraventricular impulses which are aberrantly conducted with a left bundle branch block pattern. The increase in H-V interval of 80 msec reflects conduction delay in the right bundle also.

vector forces which are the same as known supraventricular beats. No single criterion or combination of criteria provides absolute evidence for the origin of any beat. The distinction can be made with bundle of His recordings. In atrial fibrillation with a rapid ventricular response, aberration may persist for many consecutive cycles and may simulate ventricular tachycardia (Fig. 8). The occurrence of aberrant conduction during digitalis administration for atrial fibrillation is not a contraindication to continued use of the drug. In fact aberration usually disappears when the desired effect of ventricular slowing is achieved with digitalis. On the other hand, ventricular ectopy may signify digitalis toxicity or the presence of an additional dysrhythmic problem.

Treatment. Treatment of atrial fibrillation depends upon the urgency of the situation. If the irregular rapid ventricular response is causing severe dyspnea, hypotension, congestive heart failure, or severe anginal pain, conversion to normal sinus rhythm by DC countershock is the treatment of choice. DC countershock is contraindicated if it is suspected that digitalis intoxication is the cause of atrial fibrillation, which is uncommon. In less urgent situations, ventricular slowing is achieved with digitalis. Digoxin, 0.5 mg, is given intravenously and followed by a second dose in one half to one hour. If the ventricular rate is slowed (80 to 100 per minute), maintenance therapy of 0.25 mg digoxin per day is started. If the ventricular rate is not slowed within 2 hours of the initial dose, 0.25 mg digoxin is given every 3 to 4 hours until the desired effect is obtained. Infrequently, digitalis may convert atrial fibrillation to sinus rhythm.

Once the ventricular rate is under control, consideration is given as to whether conversion to sinus rhythm is indicated. Conversion should not be attempted in those patients who have longstanding chronic atrial fibrillation, or in whom previous conversions have been unsuccessfully maintained. In some patients with severe heart disease, the loss of atrial contribution to the cardiac output may be significant, and conversion to sinus rhythm is necessary in order to avoid intractable heart failure. Patients with atrial fibrillation of recent onset should be converted to sinus rhythm, using either DC countershock or quinidine sulfate. The maintenance dose of digitalis should be withheld for 1 to 2 days prior to DC countershock.

ATRIAL FLUTTER

Atrial flutter is characterized by a rapid, regular atrial rate between 220 and 350 beats per minute. However, there is no universal agreement about which range of atrial rates specifically defines atrial flutter and separates it from an ectopic atrial tachycardia. There can be an overlap in the lower ranges of atrial rate; some ectopic atrial tachycardias may achieve atrial rates of 220 beats per minute, whereas some cases of atrial flutter may be associated with rates of less than 220 beats per minute. Atrial flutter is almost always associated with some form of organic heart disease (coronary artery disease, cor pulmonale, rheumatic valvular disease), and rarely does it occur in normal healthy individuals. Digitalis is rarely a cause of atrial flutter. Clinical symptoms associated with atrial flutter are related primarily to the ventricular response. Atrial flutter with a 3:1 or 4:1 AV conduction ratio may result in no symptoms, and the patient may be unaware of any dysrhythmia. On the other hand, during a 2:1 or a varying AV conduction ratio, the patient may experience palpitations, shortness of breath, anginal symptoms, or congestive heart failure.

Electrocardiographic Features. The following are the commonly found electrocardiographic features associated with atrial flutter: (1) the atrial rate is between 220 and 350 beats per minute; (2) the P waves are broad, bizarre atrial deflections which have been termed F waves; (3) leads II, III, and AVF show a "sawtooth effect with absence of an isoelectric period between flutter waves." One flutter wave appears to be merging directly with the next. The "sawtooth" effect may be absent in lead I and left-sided chest leads (V_5,V_6); (4) in most cases of atrial flutter, atrial activation is in a caudocranial direction; and (5) some degree of AV block exists which may be fixed, alternating, or variable. Many of the characteristic features associated with atrial flutter are presented in Figure 9.

A 1:1 AV response in atrial flutter is very uncommon, because atrial rates of 220 or greater generally exceed the inherent transmission capacity of the AV node. The presence of atrial flutter with a suspected 1:1 AV response should raise the possibility of an accessory or anomalous AV pathway such as exists in the Wolff-Parkinson-White syndrome. Conduction ratios of 2:1 or 4:1 are more commonly observed. Effective vagotonic maneuvers such as carotid sinus pressure temporarily

Figure 9. Atrial flutter with varying degrees of AV block. In the middle of the tracing, a period of high degree AV block occurs, during which time the atrial flutter waves are more easily identified. The second to the sixth beats after the long pause are aberrantly conducted with a right bundle branch block pattern.

increase the degree of AV block, permit a more positive identification of the atrial flutter waves, and do not significantly affect the atrial flutter rate. At times an increase in vagal tone which causes a shortening of atrial refractory period may convert atrial flutter to atrial fibrillation. By a similar mechanism, digitalis may convert atrial flutter to fibrillation.

Treatment. Direct current countershock is very effective in converting atrial flutter to sinus rhythm and is often the treatment of choice. Conversion can be achieved with low energy discharges. Direct current countershock is certainly the treatment of choice when the ventricular response is rapid and the patient is symptomatic.

Digitalis and quinidine sulfate are the primary drugs used in the treatment of atrial flutter. Depending upon the urgency of the situation, digitalis may be given intravenously or orally. Its main function is to increase the degree of AV nodal block and to slow the ventricular rate. Rarely does digitalis convert atrial flutter directly to sinus rhythm; it may, however, convert flutter to atrial fibrillation, whereupon withdrawal of digitalis may re-establish sinus rhythm or atrial flutter may resume. Once the ventricular rate is controlled with digitalis, quinidine sulfate is given orally to convert the atrial flutter to sinus rhythm. It is preferred not to give quinidine initially without first digitalizing the patient, because quinidine may slow the atrial flutter, enhance AV nodal conduction, and precipitate dangerously rapid ventricular rates. If digitalis and quinidine are the primary therapies and prove to be unsuccessful, cardioversion by direct current countershock can be used but only after digitalis has been withheld for several days, because countershock and excessive amounts of digitalis may precipitate more serious ventricular dysrhythmias.

PAROXYSMAL ATRIAL TACHYCARDIA

Paroxysmal atrial tachycardia (PAT) is a relatively common arrhythmia. Two forms are recognized which differ in etiology, underlying mechanism, and therapeutic approach. One form of PAT results from sustained reciprocation or re-entry within the AV node, and the other results from ectopic atrial foci.

PAT Due to Sustained Reciprocation or Re-entry Within the AV Node

This form of atrial tachycardia is the more common of the two. It is seen in all age groups and frequently occurs in the absence of any clinically detectable heart disease. Characteristically, these tachycardias begin and terminate abruptly. During the tachycardia the patient may be keenly aware of a rapid heart rate and may complain of a fluttering within the chest or palpitations. Other associated symptoms include dyspnea, lightheadedness, or diaphoresis. Syncope may occur upon termination of the tachycardia if a sufficiently long pause follows prior to re-establishment of sinus rhythm or the occurrence of an escape beat. In patients with coronary artery disease, episodes of PAT may produce angina pectoris and significant S-T segment depression.

Electrocardiographic Features. Sustained re-entry within the AV node is almost always initiated by an atrial extrasystole. It is uncommon for this type of tachycardia to be precipitated by a ventricular extrasystole. If an atrial extrasystole encounters sufficient antegrade delay within the AV node (as indicated by a prolonged P-R or A-H interval), the impulse may at some point enter a nonrefractory pathway within the AV node and may be retrogradely transmitted back to the atria. If the retrogradely conducted impulse finds the antegrade pathway recovered, it may re-enter it, and the sequence is repeated, resulting in sustained reciprocation and a paroxysmal atrial tachycardia (Fig. 10).

During the reciprocating tachycardia, the atria are retrogradely activated. The P waves are inverted in leads II, III, and AVF and most often occur during the inscription of the QRS complex or the S-T segment. In some cases the retrograde P waves are located on the descending limb of the T wave or within the T-P segment and thereby mimic an ectopic atrial tachycardia with first degree heart block. The rate of these tachycardias is generally between 150 and 250 per minute. Aberrant conduction may occur for the first few beats or may persist for the entire episode of the tachycardia (Fig. 11). If aberration persists throughout the duration of the tachycardia, differentiation from ventricular tachycardia may be difficult.

Perpetuation of a reciprocating tachycardia depends primarily upon a balance of refractoriness and conduction between the reciprocating limbs within the AV node. Consequently, any intervention which alters AV nodal conduction or refractoriness can terminate these tachycardias. Abrupt termination of these tachycardias can be achieved by increasing vagal tone with carotid sinus massage, gagging, Valsalva maneuvers, or raising the blood pressure. Propranolol and digitalis, both of which increase AV nodal conduction and refractoriness, have been used successfully to treat AV nodal reciprocating tachycardias.

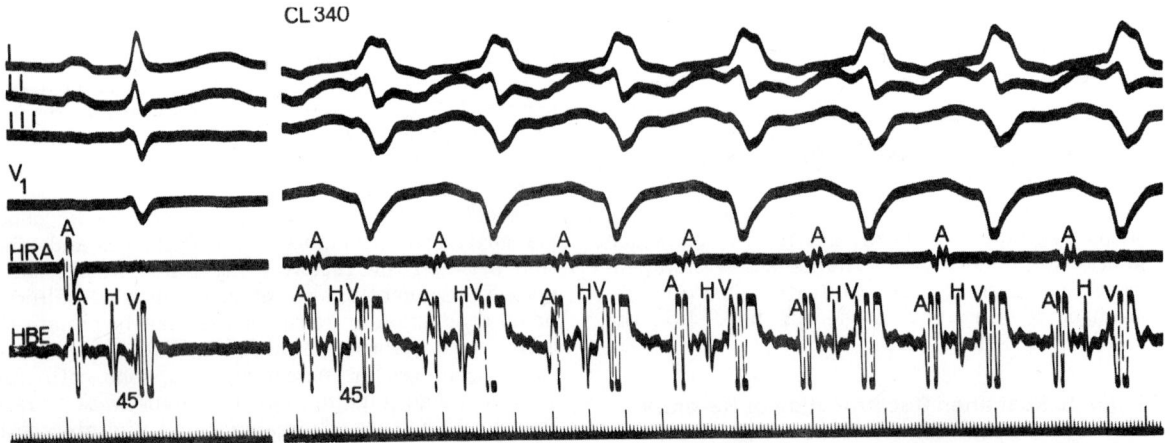

Figure 10.   Re-entry within the AV node resulting in a paroxysmal atrial tachycardia. In panels A and B, the tracings from top to bottom are as follows: electrocardiographic leads 2 and V$_1$, a high right atrial electrogram (HRA), His bundle electrogram (HBE), and time lines at 10 and 100 msec. In each panel the first two beats are of sinus node origin with upright P waves in lead 2, a high to low sequence of atrial activation, AV nodal conduction time of 165 msec, and His-Purkinje conduction time of 45 msec. In panel A, a premature atrial depolarization (P′ or A$_2$), introduced 300 msec after the last sinus beat (A$_1$), is conducted within the AV node with a delay of 380 msec; after activation of the ventricles, sinus rhythm resumes. In panel B, a slightly earlier atrial extrasystole (P′ or A$_2$) encounters greater AV nodal delay as indicated by an A-H interval of 440 msec, which for this patient was sufficient to initiate an AV nodal re-entrant or reciprocating tachycardia at a cycle length of 520 msec. Note that the sequence of atrial activation is from the low to the high right atrium and the P waves are inverted in lead 2. Atrial activation during the reciprocating tachycardia is indicated by P* on the surface EKG's and by Ae on the intracardiac recordings. The lower part of panel B depicts the events in the form of a ladder diagram.

Figure 11.   Aberrant conduction during PAT. The first panel depicts a normal sinus beat. The second panel illustrates aberrant conduction of a left bundle branch type during AV nodal re-entry which was initiated by a single atrial extrasystole. Note the low to high sequence of atrial activation during the PAT and the normal H-V interval (45 msec) associated with the aberrant beats.

V₁

P P

Figure 12. Digitalis-induced atrial tachycardia with 2:1 AV block.

Prophylactic therapy should be directed toward eliminating atrial extrasystoles, which are the most frequent initiating cause. For this purpose quinidine sulfate is given orally every four to six hours. Digitalis may be added to the therapeutic regimen if required.

Ectopic Atrial Tachycardia

Areas within the atria but outside the sinus node can serve as the pacemaker of the heart. Depolarization of the atria by an ectopic atrial pacemaker in excess of 100 beats per minute constitutes an ectopic atrial tachycardia. The atrial rates of most ectopic tachycardias are between 150 and 220 per minute. The tachycardias may be sustained for long periods of time or occur in paroxysms lasting seconds to hours. Ectopic atrial tachycardias can occur in all forms of heart disease. They may occur in association with digitalis toxicity, chronic obstructive lung disease, or enlarged diseased atria, or may be associated with no apparent heart disease.

Electrocardiographic Features. In ectopic atrial tachycardias the configuration of the P waves is different from that of sinus beats. If all the ectopic P waves are of the same size and shape, it is called unifocal ectopic atrial tachycardia. A multifocal ectopic tachycardia is one in which the ectopic atrial impulses arise from different parts of the atria, and consequently the configuration of P waves varies.

Depending upon the atrial rate and the capacity of the AV node to transmit impulses to the ventricle, ectopic atrial tachycardias may be associated with 1:1 AV conduction with normal or prolonged AV conduction times, AV nodal Wenckebach cycles, or 2:1 AV block. Digitalis toxicity is a frequent cause of rapid unifocal ectopic atrial tachycardias with 2:1 AV block (Fig. 12). Multifocal ectopic atrial tachycardias are frequently associated with chronic obstructive lung disease or marked atrial disease and may precipitate atrial fibrillation (Fig. 13).

The differentiation between paroxysmal atrial tachycardias caused by AV nodal re-entry from a unifocal ectopic tachycardia may at times be difficult. Tachycardias associated with inverted P waves in leads II, III, and AVF favor re-entry within the AV node as the mechanism but do not exclude a rhythm of ectopic origin. Upright P waves in these same leads strongly suggest an ectopic tachycardia. If the configuration of the P waves during the tachycardia is the same as the initiating atrial extrasystole, ectopy is favored, especially if the P waves are upright in leads II, III, and AVF. If the initiating atrial extrasystole is upright in II, III, and AVF and inverted in these same leads during the tachycardia, re-entry is likely. Abrupt termination of the atrial tachycardia by carotid sinus massage or an electrically induced atrial extrasystole favors a mechanism of AV nodal re-entry. These maneuvers generally produce a temporary slowing or pause in the ectopic atrial tachycardia, followed by resumption of its inherent firing rate.

Treatment. The treatment of digitalis-induced ectopic atrial tachycardias is withdrawal of the cardiac glycoside and administration of potassium supplements. Treatment of ectopic tachycardias in patients with chronic obstructive lung disease should first be directed toward correcting hypoxemia, hypercapnia, or acid-base or other metabolic imbalances, which frequently are present and are the initiating cause of these rhythm disturbances. Ectopic atrial tachycardias of other causes should be treated with either quinidine or procainamide.

VENTRICULAR EXTRASYSTOLES

Ventricular extrasystoles (ventricular premature beats, contractions, or systoles) are a common occurrence in patients with and without heart disease. In young healthy individuals, the incidence varies between 0.5 and 2.0 per cent. They may be caused by emotional stress, tobacco, alcohol, caffeine, anoxia, sympathomime-

L2

Figure 13. Multifocal atrial tachycardia. Note changing configuration of P waves.

Figure 14. Ventricular bigeminy. A single premature ventricular extrasystole is coupled at a constant interval to each sinus beat.

tic drugs, or exercise. They are associated with all forms of heart disease and occur frequently (up to 80 per cent) in patients with acute myocardial infarction. Digitalis excess is a common cause of ventricular extrasystoles, especially if hypokalemia is present. Patients with occasional or even frequent ventricular extrasystole may be completely unaware of their presence. On the other hand, some patients complain of "pauses," "palpitations," or "thumping" in the chest.

Electrocardiographic Features. Ventricular extrasystoles are characterized by wide QRS complexes (0.12 sec) with S-T and T wave changes. They may occur early or late in the cardiac cycle and very often have a constant coupling interval to the preceding sinus beat. The coupling interval is considered constant if the variation is within 0.08 sec (80 msec). A single ventricular extrasystole occurring after each sinus beat is referred to as ventricular bigeminy (Fig. 14). The term trigeminy refers to repeat cycles of either two sinus beats followed by a single extrasystole or one sinus beat followed by two consecutive ventricular extrasystoles.

Recurrent ventricular extrasystoles which always exhibit the same QRS morphology are referred to as unifocal in origin (arising from the same ectopic focus), whereas recurrent extrasystoles of different morphologies are termed multifocal in origin. Ventricular extrasystoles can arise anywhere within the bundle branch–Purkinje network. Extrasystoles arising from the left side of the conduction system result in QRS complexes which resemble right bundle branch block

patterns, and those arising from the right side result in QRS complexes resembling a left bundle branch block pattern. Infrequently, extrasystolic impulses may arise high in one of the bundle branches, close to the bundle of His, and conduct with slight asynchrony down both bundle branches, resulting in narrow QRS complexes.

Most ventricular extrasystoles occur late in the cardiac cycle, i.e., after completion of the T wave of the preceding sinus beat, and are frequently coupled to the preceding sinus beat by a fairly constant interval. Less commonly, ventricular extrasystoles occur in early diastole, near the peak of the T wave or on its descending limb. This has been called the R on T phenomenon; it may reflect a very serious situation, because extrasystoles occurring near the so-called vulnerable period of the ventricle may lead to ventricular tachycardia or ventricular fibrillation.

Ventricular extrasystoles may be associated with various types of retrograde conduction patterns. The more common of these patterns include the following:

1. Complete retrograde conduction may occur across the AV conducting system, resulting in premature retrograde depolarization of the atria with inverted P waves in leads II, III, and AVF.

2. The extrasystolic impulse may retrogradely block within the AV node. This may result in the phenomenon of retrograde concealed conduction in which the next sinus impulse either is blocked or conducts with a P-R interval longer than sinus beats (Fig. 15).

3. During prolonged retrograde AV nodal conduction

Figure 15. Retrograde AV nodal concealed conduction caused by a ventricular extrasystole. Note absence of His deflection preceding the second QRS complex. The ventricular extrasystolic impulse retrogradely penetrates the AV node and leaves it partially refractory to the second sinus P wave, which is conducted with a longer P-R interval. The delay in conduction is localized to the AV node, as indicated by an A-H interval of 145 msec compared to normal values of 112 msec.

delay, the extrasystolic impulse may reciprocate within the AV node and return to the ventricles, producing a ventricular echo beat (see Fig. 19).

4. Very premature extrasystolic impulses may retrogradely block within the His-Purkinje system. This type of retrograde conduction pattern cannot be determined from the electrocardiogram.

Treatment. The treatment of ventricular extrasystoles depends upon their cause, the underlying cardiac condition, severity of symptoms, their frequency, the coupling interval, and whether they are unifocal or multifocal in origin.

Ventricular extrasystoles which are related to emotional upsets, tobacco, alcohol, or sympathomimetic drugs may require only reassurance, mild sedation, or abstinence. Withholding of digitalis therapy for one or more days, in conjunction with oral potassium supplements, may be all that is necessary to treat extrasystoles caused by excess digitalis.

Ventricular extrasystoles occurring during an acute myocardial infarction require antiarrhythmic therapy. Therapy is urgently indicated if the extrasystoles have a close coupling interval, occur at a rate of five or more per minute, or are multifocal in origin. Irrespective of the underlying cardiac condition, antiarrhythmic therapy is indicated for ventricular extrasystoles which demonstrate the R on T phenomenon, are multifocal in origin, or occur consecutively in pairs.

VENTRICULAR TACHYCARDIA

Three or more consecutive beats occurring at rates greater than 100 per minute and arising from a focus located below the bundle of His constitute an episode of ventricular tachycardia. Most ventricular tachycardias occur at rates between 120 and 180 beats per minute; they may occur in paroxysms lasting a few seconds to several minutes or may persist for hours or days. Ventricular tachycardia is almost always associated with some form of organic heart disease, the most common being arteriosclerotic, rheumatic, and hypertensive heart diseases. As many as 50 per cent of patients with acute myocardial infarction may have one or more episodes of ventricular tachycardia of varying duration. Toxic doses of digitalis are a common cause of ventricular tachycardia. Other precipitating causes of paroxysmal ventricular tachycardia include hypoxia, hypokalemia, exercise, drugs (such as epinephrine, quinidine, and procainamide), cardiac catheterization of either the right or left heart, and anesthetic agents (cycloproprane, chloroform). Ventricular aneurysms may be the cause of recurrent or drug-resistant ventricular tachycardias.

Paroxysmal ventricular tachycardia has been reported to occur in young patients (less than 30 years old) in whom no evidence of heart disease could be detected. In this group, some attacks have been demonstrated to occur during exercise or emotional stress, implying a relationship between increased sympathetic tone and the ventricular dysrhythmia. In other patients, no precipitating factor could be demonstrated.

Electrocardiographic Features. In ventricular tachycardia, the QRS complexes are wide (0.12 sec or greater) and bizarre, recurring regularly at rates over 100 per minute (usually 120 to 180). Since the pacemaker is located below the bundle of His (i.e., within the bundle branches or Purkinje network), ventricular tachycardia is characterized electrophysiologically by the absence of a His bundle electrogram preceding the onset of ventricular activation. The bundle of His is retrogradely activated, and although in most cases it is not discernible, it is located within the ventricular electrogram. Initiation of the tachycardia may begin with a premature ventricular beat occurring close in time to the peak of the T wave of a preceding sinus beat; at other times, the initiating beat is located at the end of or after inscription of the T wave. Once initiated, ventricular tachycardia may be continuous for long periods of time or intermittent with one or more sinus beats interspersed (Fig. 16).

Often, it is extremely difficult to define the pattern of atrial activity during episodes of ventricular tachycardia from standard electrocardiographic tracings. Esophageal or intra-atrial recordings can be quite helpful in defining the frequency of atrial activity and its relationship to the QRS complexes.

During ventricular tachycardia, the atria may be dissociated from the ventricles, in which case independent P waves will be observed. At other times, various degrees of retrograde capture of the atria will occur (1:1, 2:1 retrograde Wenckebach cycles) (Fig. 17). If discernible, the P waves would be inverted in leads II, III, and AVF during retrograde activation of the atria.

An important and sometimes difficult clinical problem is the differentiation of supraventricular tachycardia with aberration from ventricular tachycardia. A comparison of Figures 11 and 17 demonstrates the value of His bundle recordings in making this distinction. In the former, a His deflection with a normal or greater than normal H-V interval precedes ventricular activation, whereas in the latter there is absence of a His electrogram preceding ventricular activation.

Figure 16. A short episode of a unifocal ventricular tachycardia interspersed between periods of sinus rhythm.

Figure 17. Ventricular tachycardia showing a left bundle branch block pattern and 1:1 retrograde conduction. Note the absence of a His deflection preceding ventricular activation. A retrograde His deflection can be seen within the ventricular electrogram. A low to high sequence of atrial activation occurs during retrograde atrial depolarization. The last beat is a sinus beat which occurs after spontaneous termination of the tachycardia. These results should be compared with those of Figure 11.

From the electrocardiographic point of view the presence of fusion beats during a sustained tachycardia provides strong supportive evidence that the rhythm in question is of ventricular origin. Fusion beats refer to partial activation of the ventricles by both supraventricular and ventricular impulses. During ventricular tachycardia, fusion beats may result because the atria are dissociated from the ventricles, and a sinus impulse occurring at an appropriate time in the cardiac cycle penetrates the AV conducting system and partially activates the ventricles; or during retrograde Wenckebach cycles, the impulse may reciprocate within the AV node and return to the ventricles, resulting in partial activation of that chamber. Complete activation or capture of the ventricles by either of the aforementioned mechanisms may terminate the tachycardia for one or more cycles, during which time sinus beats may appear, after which the tachycardia usually resumes.

A diagnosis of ventricular tachycardia is favored if one can discern independent atrial activity at a rate slower than the ventricular rate. On the other hand, supraventricular tachycardia with aberration is favored if carotid sinus pressure or other vagal maneuvers abruptly terminate the tachycardia.

Treatment. The choice and urgency of treatment for ventricular tachycardia depends on a number of factors, including its cause, the age and general condition of the patient, the severity and type of the underlying heart disease, blood pressure, and the state of consciousness. Causative factors such as hypoxia, hypokalemia, or other metabolic imbalances must be recognized and corrected.

DC countershock and drug therapy are the two commonly used methods for treating ventricular tachycardia. DC countershock is generally reserved for emergent situations in which the ventricular dysrhythmia is continuous or causes profound hemodynamic disturbances, or when drug therapy is ineffective. DC countershock is not the preferred treatment for ventricular tachycardias caused by digitalis toxicity.

Lidocaine is the most commonly used drug for the conversion of ventricular tachycardia to sinus rhythm. It is administered intravenously as a 100 mg bolus which can be repeated in two to three minutes if the initial injection is totally or partially ineffective. After suppression of the arrhythmia, lidocaine may be given as a continuous intravenous drip of 1 to 3 mg per minute. Occasionally, higher concentrations (4 mg per minute) are required. Approximately, 90 per cent of ventricular tachycardias can be suppressed at lidocaine blood levels of 2 to 4 μg per milliliter. The more common side effects of lidocaine include drowsiness, paresthesias, decrease in auditory acuity, agitation, and convulsions. Since lidocaine is metabolized by the liver, lower doses of the drug may cause side effects in patients with hepatic dysfunction.

Intravenous procainamide is also highly effective in the treatment of ventricular tachycardia. The drug can be administered at a rate of 25 to 50 mg per minute until either the tachycardia is terminated or 1000 mg has been administered. Most ventricular tachycardias are suppressed at blood concentrations of 4 to 8 μg per milliliter. Occasionally, higher concentrations are required. Continued suppression of the tachycardia can be achieved by a continuous intravenous drip at a rate of 2.5 mg per minute. Procainamide, like most antiarrhythmic drugs, may cause significant hypotension after intravenous administration, especially if the underlying myocardial dysfunction is severe. At other times, the arrhythmia is the cause of a lowered blood pressure which improves when normal sinus rhythm is restored.

If lidocaine and procainamide are ineffective in controlling the arrhythmia, one can use diphenylhydantoin, propranolol, or quinidine sulfate. On occasion, a combination of drugs is required.

If ventricular tachycardia is associated with an underlying complete or high degree of AV block, an electrode catheter should be positioned within the right ventricular cavity and endocardial pacing initiated immediately upon terminating the ventricular tachycardia with drug therapy. This is required because effective drug therapy may suppress all idioventricular pacemaker activity and ventricular asystole may ensue.

ACCELERATED IDIOVENTRICULAR RHYTHMS

Accelerated idioventricular rhythms (AIVR) is a term applied to ectopic ventricular rhythms with rates intermediate between idioventricular escape rhythms (30 to 40 per minute) and ventricular tachycardia (120 to 180 per minute). Most frequently the rates are between 75 and 100 per minute. Accelerated idioventricular

Figure 18. Accelerated idioventricular rhythm which begins just prior to the fourth sinus P wave. The rates of the sinus node and idioventricular pacemakers are nearly identical, thereby resulting in a period of isorhythmic AV dissociation.

rhythms are commonly associated with myocardial infarction or digitalis toxicity. Current thinking holds that AIVR represents an enhancement of the normal escape rhythm of latent ventricular pacemakers. Like other ventricular rhythms, the QRS complexes are bizarre and wide (0.12 sec). The rate of the AIVR is usually close to that of the sinus rate, and consequently it becomes manifest when sinus rhythm is slowed by increasing vagal tone (carotid sinus massage) or premature atrial extrasystoles, or when some degree of AV block develops. AIVR usually begins late in the cardiac cycle, and it may start with a fusion beat (Fig. 18). If dissociation between the atria and ventricles is present, fusion beats may occur frequently. If 1:1 retrograde conduction occurs, the AIVR may persist for long periods of time (Fig. 19). In some patients, episodes of AIVR (75 to 100 per minute) and ventricular tachycardia (120 to 180 per minute) coexist. Treatment of AIVR is the same as that of ventricular tachycardia. Also, acceleration of the sinus rate by atropine or atrial pacing can and usually does suppress AIVR.

BIDIRECTIONAL TACHYCARDIA

Bidirectional tachycardia is an infrequently encountered arrhythmia which is characterized by (1) rapid regular rate of 140 to 180 beats per minute, (2) alternating rightward and leftward axis shifts in the frontal plane, and (3) a constant right bundle branch block pattern in lead V_1. Most bidirectional tachycardias occur in the presence of severe myocardial disease and digitalis toxicity and are associated with a poor prognosis. Two different mechanisms have been proposed to explain the electrocardiographic pattern of bidirectional tachycar-

dia. One suggested mechanism is that bidirectional tachycardia originates from a supraventricular tachycardia in which there is permanent aberrant conduction within the right bundle branch along with alternating aberrant conduction in the two divisions (anterior and posterior fascicles) of the left bundle branch. The other mechanism, confirmed by His bundle recordings, indicates that bidirectional tachycardia results from an ectopic focus located in the left ventricle, which would account for the permanent right bundle branch block pattern observed (Fig. 20). It is as yet unclear whether the alternating rightward and leftward axis shift is the result of alternating routes of ventricular activation by a single ectopic left ventricular focus or alternating discharge of two separate left ventricular foci. The treatment of bidirectional tachycardia is withdrawal of digitalis and administration of potassium and an antiarrhythmic agent such as lidocaine or diphenylhydantoin.

VENTRICULAR FIBRILLATION

Ventricular fibrillation consists of rapid, disorganized, multifocal depolarizations of the ventricular myocardium. The absence of rhythmic coordinated muscular contractions produces a loss of the pumping action of the heart and causes a precipitous fall of the blood pressure to zero levels and unconsciousness. Ventricular fibrillation is most often seen in patients with significant underlying cardiac disease, especially ischemic heart disease. It may also occur in patients without clinical or pathologic evidence of heart disease. It may accompany digitalis toxicity, especially if hypokalemia or other metabolic imbalances are present. Quinidine sensitivity or

Figure 19. Accelerated idioventricular rhythm associated with retrograde Wenckebach type conduction to the atria. The sixth ventricular impulse re-enters within the AV node and is antegradely conducted back to the ventricles, resulting in a ventricular echo beat (seventh QRS complex).

Figure 20. Bidirectional ventricular tachycardia. The first six QRS complexes show a persistent RBBB pattern in lead V_1 and alternating left and right axis deviation in lead 2. The ventricular origin of these beats is indicated by absence of a His deflection preceding the QRS complex. Ventricular activity is dissociated from atrial activity. The last beat shows a normally conducted atrial impulse with normal A-H and H-V intervals. (From Kastor, J. A., and Goldreyer, B. N.: Circulation, *48*:897, 1973. Copyright 1973, American Medical Association.)

toxicity may also be the cause of ventricular fibrillation. Ventricular extrasystoles occurring within the so-called vulnerable period of the ventricles (R on T phenomenon) may initiate ventricular fibrillation (Fig. 21).

The treatment of ventricular fibrillation must be prompt and decisive. The patient must be ventilated and defibrillated, using DC countershock at 400 watt-seconds.

AV DISSOCIATION

AV dissociation is a general term which describes any rhythm in which the atria and ventricles are independently activated by different pacemakers discharging at similar or dissimilar rates. The atria may be activated by either the sinus node or an ectopic atrial pacemaker, whereas the ventricles may be under the control of either a junctional or an idioventricular pacemaker. AV dissociation may occur with an essentially intact AV conduction system and may be of short duration, lasting for one or a few cardiac cycles, or it may persist for much longer periods. AV dissociation may be caused by (1) acceleration of a junctional or idioventricular pacemaker (Fig. 18), (2) slowing of an atrial pacemaker accompanied by an escape rhythm located in either the AV junction or ventricles, or (3) SA or AV block accompanied by an escape rhythm (Fig. 5).

Isorhythmic AV dissociation is one type of dissociated rhythm in which (1) the atria and ventricles are controlled by independent pacemakers discharging at equal or nearly equal rates, and (2) the P waves remain in close proximity to the QRS complexes; they may precede, occur simultaneously with, or follow the QRS complex. An example of isorhythmic AV dissociation in which the ventricles come under control of a junctional pacemaker is shown in Figure 22. As the atrial cycle length increases, the ventricles come under control of a junctional pacemaker, and the P waves which remain under control of the sinus node appear to be "marching" into the QRS complex. The P wave may appear to the right of the QRS complex and maintain a fixed R-P relationship, during which time the atria may remain under control of the sinus node or be retrogradely activated by the junctional pacemaker. After a variable period of time, acceleration of the sinus rate occurs, the P waves reappear in front of the QRS complex, and sinus rhythm is re-established. Sinus acceleration results from changes in baroreceptor activity, consequent to changes in arterial pressure or the effect of right atrial stretch, or both. Acceleration of the sinus rate is dependent upon the magnitude of these accelerating influences and the responsiveness of the sinus node.

JUNCTIONAL RHYTHMS

Traditionally, AV nodal rhythms have been described as arising from the upper, middle, or lower portions of the AV node. This classification has been based primarily on the relationship of inverted P waves (leads II, III, AVF) to the QRS complex. In upper AV nodal

Figure 21. Ventricular fibrillation initiated by a rapid burst of ventricular activity (arrow).

Figure 22. Isorhythmic AV dissociation. After the first five sinus beats, the sinus rate slows and an AV junctional pacemaker emerges, starting with the sixth QRS complex. The atria continue to be activated by the sinus node, and the P waves are obscured within the QRS complex. In the bottom strip, accelerating forces cause an increase in the sinus node rate and sinus rhythm is re-established.

rhythms the inverted P wave precedes the QRS complex, whereas in middle or lower AV nodal rhythms the P wave occurs simultaneously with or follows the QRS complex, respectively. It has been recommended that the terms "junctional" or "AV junctional rhythms" replace that of "AV nodal rhythms," because (1) experimentally it has been difficult to consistently and convincingly demonstrate pacemaker activity (phase 4 depolarization) in all three regions of the AV node and (2) pacemaker activity in other areas of the heart (coronary sinus, left atrium, and bundle of His) can result in electrocardiographic patterns similar to those ascribed to AV nodal rhythms.

AV junctional rhythms are primarily escape rhythms with rates usually in the range 40 to 70 per minute. They become manifest if there is (1) significant sinus slowing, (2) AV block, or (3) SA block. If the discharge rate of the sinus node falls below that of a subsidiary junctional pacemaker, as may occur during sinus bradycardia or after premature discharge of the sinus node by an extrasystolic impulse, an area within the AV junction can take over as the pacemaker of the heart. In similar fashion, an escape junctional rhythm can emerge when sinus node impulses fail to conduct to surrounding atrial myocardium such as occurs in SA block (Fig. 5). Escape junctional rhythms also occur during AV block in which supraventricular impulses block in the AV node and proximal to the site of a junctional pacemaker (see Fig. 35). In complete AV block in which the nonconducted atrial impulses block below the bundle of His, the escape rhythms are located below the AV junction (idioventricular pacemaker). AV junctional rhythms result in QRS complexes which are similar to those of sinus rhythm.

ventricular tachycardias is known as the Lown-Ganong-Levine syndrome. The mechanisms responsible for both the short P-R interval and the tachycardias have remained obscure. Several theories, based primarily on anatomic considerations, have been proposed to explain the short P-R interval. The most popular theory centers about the presence of specialized internodal pathways by which atrial impulses can partially or completely bypass the AV node. Recent electrophysiologic studies, using His bundle recordings and atrial pacing techniques, have shown that most cases of short P-R interval are associated with AV nodal conduction times which are at the lower range of normal values. The A-H intervals were 60 to 80 msec, whereas H-V intervals were between 30 and 55 msec. In addition, in most patients when the right atrium was stimulated at progressively increasing rates, the expected A-H interval increases were qualitatively similar to, but quantitatively less than, that observed for subjects with normal P-R intervals. In only an occasional patient with a short P-R interval was the A-H interval found to be less than 60 msec or did the A-H interval not increase as the paced atrial rate was increased. These limited data suggest that most cases of short P-R interval are due to an abbreviated AV nodal conduction time which could be due to (1) atrial impulses partially bypassing the AV node (? specialized internodal tracts), (2) an anatomically small AV node, (3) preferential intranodal pathways, or (4) a combination of these. In only occasional patients are the electrophysiologic data compatible with a complete bypass of the AV node, accounting for the short P-R interval. It should be pointed out that prolonged periods of isorhythmic AV dissociation can mimic a short P-R interval with normal QRS complexes. Studies to date have shown that AV nodal re-entry is a common mechanism for the paroxysmal supraventricular tachycardias in this syndrome.

SYNDROME OF SHORT P-R INTERVAL, NORMAL QRS COMPLEXES, AND SUPRAVENTRICULAR TACHYCARDIAS
(Lown-Ganong-Levine Syndrome)

The syndrome of short P-R interval (0.12 sec or less), normal QRS complexes (0.10 sec), and paroxysmal supra-

WOLFF-PARKINSON-WHITE SYNDROME

The electrocardiographic pattern of the Wolff-Parkinson-White syndrome is characterized by a short P-R interval (less than 0.12 sec) and a widened QRS

Figure 23. Wolff-Parkinson-White syndrome, showing Type A QRS complexes. The delta wave can be seen in almost all leads. The precordial leads resemble a right bundle branch block pattern. In leads 2, 3, and AVF the delta wave produces a Q wave which mimics a diaphragmatic myocardial infarction.

complex, starting with an initial delta wave. This abnormal electrocardiographic pattern occurs in approximately 0.1 to 0.4 per cent of routine tracings. A significant number of patients exhibiting this pattern have episodes of supraventricular tachycardia. Other terms used to describe this phenomenon include anomalous AV excitation, ventricular pre-excitation, and accessory AV conduction.

Over the years, many hypotheses have been put forth to explain the electrocardiographic findings in this syndrome. Currently, there is anatomic as well as electrophysiologic evidence indicating that atrial impulses pre-excite the ventricles via accessory bypass tracts composed of myocardial fibers which connect the atria and ventricles. These bypass tracts are referred to as bundles of Kent. Atrial impulses are simultaneously conducted to the ventricles via the normal AV nodal His-Purkinje conducting system and the accessory pathway. AV con-

Figure 24. The first two QRS complexes show a Wolff-Parkinson-White type of ventricular excitation in which the delta wave (d) in leads II and III mimics a diaphragmatic myocardial infarction. Atrial impulses are also conducted along the AV nodal His-Purkinje system; bundle of His activation occurs at about the time of the onset of the delta wave. The third P wave (A₂) is premature and finds the accessory pathway refractory. Exclusive conduction along the AV nodal His-Purkinje system results in normal ventricular activation, followed by a re-entrant supraventricular tachycardia. Note the absence of electrocardiographic evidence of myocardial infarction.

Figure 25. Type B QRS complexes of the Wolff-Parkinson-White syndrome in which the precordial leads resemble a left bundle branch block pattern.

duction via the latter results in shortening of the P-R interval, and pre-excitation of the ventricle produces the delta wave. In most cases, the QRS complex in the Wolff-Parkinson-White syndrome represents fusion activation, the delta wave being an expression of ventricular excitation via the accessory pathway, and some part of the remaining portion of the QRS the result of excitation via the normal AV nodal His-Purkinje conducting system. If significant delay or block exists within the AV nodal His-Purkinje pathway, the QRS complex may represent one of total pre-excitation. Alternatively, if AV nodal conduction time is shortened, as may occur with increased sympathetic tone or during an isoproterenol infusion, activation of the ventricles by the AV nodal His-Purkinje system is increased and the QRS tends toward normalization. Anomalous AV excitation may be always present during sinus rhythm, or it may intermittently alternate with periods of normal activation. At times, anomalous AV excitation may mimic the electrocardiographic pattern of a myocardial infarction (Fig. 23). Bundle of His recordings in conjunction with atrial pacing techniques can establish the correct diagnosis (Fig. 24).

The syndrome has been divided into two major groups, types A and B. In type A the accessory bundle crosses the AV sulcus on the left side, causing pre-excitation of the base of the left ventricle. The vector of the delta wave is directed anteriorly in all precordial leads (upright in V_1 V_6), and the QRS pattern resembles right bundle branch block pattern (Fig. 23). In type B, the accessory bundle pre-excites the lateral margin of the right ventricle and the initial delta forces are directed leftward and posteriorly, producing a biphasic or negative delta wave in V_1 and QRS complexes resembling the left bundle branch block pattern (Fig. 25). Intermediate forms of these two major categories exist. Early activation of the base of the left ventricle in type A Wolff-Parkinson-White syndrome and of the lateral margin of the right ventricle in type B Wolff-Parkinson-White syndrome has been confirmed by epicardial mapping studies performed at the time of cardiac surgery.

Supraventricular Tachycardias in Wolff-Parkinson-White Syndrome

Between 25 and 70 per cent of patients with Wolff-Parkinson-White type QRS complexes have episodes of supraventricular tachycardia, and most of these appear to be re-entrant in nature. However, it should be noted that atrial tachycardias which are ectopic in origin may also occur in these patients. Most re-entrant tachycardias occurring in the patients with the Wolff-Parkinson-White syndrome have normal QRS complexes with long P-R intervals and are initiated by premature atrial beats. Less commonly are re-entrant tachycardias associated with pre-excitation type QRS complexes.

There are two possible mechanisms to explain re-entrant supraventricular tachycardias with normal QRS complexes in patients with the Wolff-Parkinson-White syndrome. If a closely coupled premature atrial beat finds the accessory pathway refractory to antegrade conduction, it may traverse the AV nodal His-Purkinje conducting system (usually with some delay) and activate the ventricles, producing a normal QRS complex. If sufficient time has elapsed to permit recovery of excitability of the accessory pathway, retrograde conduction back to the atria will occur via the accessory pathway. If, after atrial activation, the AV nodal His-Purkinje conducting system has recovered, activation of the ventricles will follow and a self-sustaining re-entrant tachycardia will result. Alternatively, a re-entrant supraventricular tachycardia with normal QRS complexes could be initiated by a premature ventricular beat which was retrogradely blocked within the His-Purkinje AV nodal conducting system but which retrogradely activated the atria via the accessory pathway. Recovery of excitability of the AV nodal His-Purkinje conducting system would allow antegrade conduction to ventricles to follow retrograde activation of the atria; if the process is repetitive, a sustained tachycardia with normal QRS complexes will result.

The second mechanism involved in producing re-entrant supraventricular tachycardias with normal QRS complexes is one in which reciprocation or re-entry occurs only within the AV node; the accessory pathway, although present, is not utilized in the re-entrant process. This type of re-entry is the same as that occurring in patients who have paroxysmal atrial tachycardia without Wolff-Parkinson-White complexes.

Re-entrant supraventricular tachycardias with pre-excitation type QRS complexes result when antegrade conduction occurs via the accessory pathway and the impulse is retrogradely returned to the atria via the AV nodal His-Purkinje pathway.

A potentially life-threatening situation may occur in patients with the Wolff-Parkinson-White syndrome who develop atrial fibrillation. Rapid irregular activation of the ventricles via the accessory pathway exclusively or both pathways simultaneously may lead to ventricular fibrillation.

Treatment.   Most re-entrant tachycardias associated with the Wolff-Parkinson-White syndrome respond to vagotonic maneuvers such as carotid sinus stimulation, the Valsalva maneuver, eyeball pressure, or elevation of blood pressure. Increased parasympathetic tone alters the re-entrant pathway by increasing refractoriness and delaying conduction within the AV node. Similarly, digitalis and propranolol can terminate re-entrant tachycardias by the same mechanism. DC countershock is reserved for those tachycardias which (1) are resistant to vagotonic maneuvers and require excessive amounts of drug therapy, or (2) are associated with very rapid ventricular responses. If, during atrial fibrillation, excitation of the ventricles occurs in part or totally through the accessory AV pathway, DC countershock should be applied immediately in order to avoid the possibility of ventricular fibrillation.

Prophylactic therapy should be directed at suppressing atrial extrasystoles which are a very common initiating cause of re-entrant tachycardias in the Wolff-Parkinson-White syndrome. Quinidine sulfate should be given for this purpose. In some cases quinidine given in combination with digitalis or propranolol is more effective. Less commonly, when ventricular extrasystoles are the initiating cause of the re-entrant tachycardias, procainamide is the drug of choice.

A small percentage of patients with the Wolff-Parkinson-White syndrome have frequent severe episodes of supraventricular tachycardia which, in addition to causing disabling symptoms, are resistant to control by drug therapy alone. An operative procedure has been devised for surgically interrupting the anomalous atrioventricular bypass tract which in some reported cases has effectively terminated the recurrence of tachycardias. Surgical therapy in these very selective patients requires that the region of the anomalous bypass tract be localized by epicardial mapping studies.

DISORDERS OF AV CONDUCTION
First Degree Heart Block

In adults a P-R interval of more than 0.20 sec constitutes electrocardiographic evidence of first degree heart block which most commonly (90 per cent or more) is due to conduction delay occurring within the AV node. First-degree heart block in the presence of normal QRS complexes is almost always due to AV nodal conduction delay, an example of which is presented in Figure 26. Bundle of His recordings reveal that the A-H interval was prolonged at 310 msec and His-Purkinje conduction time was within normal limits at 39 msec.

Drugs such as digitalis and propranolol cause P-R prolongation by delaying conduction within the AV node. Neither drug affects conduction within the His-Purkinje system to any significant degree. The A-H interval returns to normal when these drugs are discontinued. At times, first degree AV nodal block may alternate with periods of type I second degree AV block or 2:1 AV block. In general, no specific treatment for first degree AV block is required. In most patients an increase in sympathetic tone, such as occurs during exercise or vagal blockade by atropine (0.5 to 1.0 mg intravenously), causes a decrease in the A-H interval concomitant with an increase in sinus rate so that 1:1 AV conduction is maintained.

His-Purkinje Delay

Less commonly, first degree heart block is due solely to conduction delay within the His-Purkinje system. Figure 27 is an example of P-R prolongation and right bundle branch block in which AV nodal conduction (A-H interval) is within normal limits and His-Purkinje conduction time (H-V interval) is markedly prolonged at 90 msec. The presence of a prolonged H-V interval is almost always associated with a bundle branch block pattern or widened QRS complex. However, not all patients with a bundle branch block pattern have prolonged H-V intervals. A prolonged H-V interval (greater than 60 msec) in the presence of a bundle branch block pattern usually indicates that there is conduction delay within the contralateral bundle. In asymptomatic patients, no specific treatment is required.

AV Nodal Plus His-Purkinje Conduction Delay

First degree AV block may be due to conduction delays in both the AV node and His-Purkinje system.

Figure 26.   First degree heart block due to AV nodal delay.

Figure 27. First degree heart block due to a prolonged H-V interval (90 msec) in a patient with right bundle branch block.

Intra-His Bundle Delay

Conduction delay occurring within the bundle of His itself can cause a prolongation of the P-R interval. However, this is an uncommon cause of first degree heart block.

Second Degree AV Block

Second degree heart block has been classified into two types. Type I second degree heart block (Wenckebach phenomenon, Mobitz type I AV block) is electrocardiographically characterized by a progressive prolongation in the P-R interval preceding a nonconducted atrial beat. After the nonconducted P wave, the P-R interval is shorter. Type II second degree AV block (Mobitz II) is electrocardiographically characterized by a constant P-R interval preceding an unexpected nonconducted atrial impulse.

Type I Second Degree AV Block

The electrocardiographic pattern of type I second degree AV block can result from Wenckebach type conduction occurring within (1) the AV node, (2) the bundle of His itself, or (3) the bundle branch–Purkinje system. Delay in the AV node is by far the most common cause (more than 90 per cent) of type I AV block. The next most common site is the bundle branch–Purkinje system, and the least common is the bundle of His itself.

Classically the AV nodal Wenckebach phenomenon is depicted as one in which the greatest increment in P-R interval occurs with the second beat of the Wenckebach cycle and thereafter progressively diminishes. This re-

sults in a decreasing R-R interval in the presence of increasing P-R intervals. Some AV nodal Wenckebach cycles do not follow this classic pattern, and the greatest increment in P-R interval may occur with the last conducted beat. Also, one may observe little or no change in the P-R interval for several beats throughout the cycle.

Figure 28 is an example of type I second degree AV block resulting from progressive conduction delay and block within the AV node. Type I AV block in the presence of normal QRS complexes is almost always AV nodal in origin. At times, the second beat of the Wenckebach cycle may be aberrantly conducted to the ventricles. Aberrant conduction is favored by the fact that the nonconducted atrial impulse of the preceding Wenckebach cycle results in a long R-R interval. In a 3:2 AV nodal Wenckebach cycle, aberrant conduction of every second beat may simulate a ventricular bigeminy, especially if the P wave of the aberrant beat is obscured by the T wave of the preceding QRS complex (Fig. 29).

Type I AV block occurring within the AV node may be associated with inferior wall myocardial infarctions or excessive digitalis administration, and in both of these situations the block is generally reversible. Small doses of atropine, which enhances AV nodal conduction, usually re-establish 1:1 AV conduction. However, in some cases atropine may increase the sinus rate without appreciably affecting AV nodal conduction, and higher degrees of AV block (2:1, 3:1) may result. In type I AV block of AV nodal origin, the ventricular rate is seldom slow enough to warrant aggressive drug therapy or temporary right ventricular endocardial pacing.

The electrocardiographic pattern of type I second degree AV block can also result from Wenckebach type conduction occurring within the His-Purkinje system, as

Figure 28. Type I second degree AV block due to progressive conduction delay and block within the AV node.

Figure 29. A 3:2 AV conduction during type I second degree AV block within the node, in which every second beat of the Wenckebach cycle is aberrantly conducted with a right bundle branch block pattern.

illustrated in Figure 30. During 3:2 AV conduction in the presence of a fixed right bundle branch block pattern, a small increase in the P-R interval precedes a nonconducted P wave. The H-V interval increases from an initially abnormal value of 60 msec to 100 msec, indicating progressive conduction delay within the left bundle branch and the third P wave blocks within the His-Purkinje system. Patients exhibiting the findings illustrated in Figure 30 will also have intermittent periods of high degree (e.g., 2:1, 3:1) AV block within the His-Purkinje system, which accounts in part for their symptoms of fatigue, dizziness, and even syncope. Also, these patients almost invariably go on to develop complete AV block within the His-Purkinje system.

In the presence of a fixed bundle branch block pattern, the distinction, based solely on the EKG tracings, between type I second degree AV block occurring within the AV node and that of His-Purkinje origin may be quite difficult. In general, although not always, the increase in P-R interval from the first to the last of the conducted beats is significantly less in a His-Purkinje Wenckebach cycle than in an AV nodal Wenckebach cycle. However, when AV nodal Wenckebach type conduction is superimposed on a pre-existing first degree AV nodal block, the difference in P-R interval changes from the first to the last of the conducted beats may be of the magnitude seen with His-Purkinje Wenckebach cycles.

The least common site for the occurrence of Wenckebach type conduction is within the bundle of His itself (Fig. 31). This phenomenon is characterized by the re-cording of two His deflections (H and H′), which signifies intra-His bundle conduction delay. As the P-R interval increases, the H-H′ interval increases, and the nonconducted atrial impulse of the Wenckebach cycle is followed by only a single His deflection (H).

Type II Second Degree AV Block (Mobitz II)

Type II second degree AV block occurs less commonly than type I; it is almost always associated with a bundle branch block pattern and is a forerunner to complete AV block. The AV conduction ratio may be 3:2, 4:3, 5:4, and so forth, and the P-R intervals preceding the nonconducted atrial beat are constant. His bundle recordings have consistently demonstrated that the site of block is within the His-Purkinje system. Figure 32 is a typical example of type II second degree AV block; a left bundle branch block pattern is present, and 3:2 AV conduction progresses to 2:1 AV block. The third P wave, which is unexpectedly blocked within the His-Purkinje system, is preceded by constant P-R intervals. A prolonged H-V interval of 76 msec in the presence of left bundle branch block indicates that a significant conduction delay also existed in the right bundle branch system.

In patients with type II second degree AV block, acceleration of the atrial rate by atropine, exercise, or atrial pacing generally leads to an increase in the degree of AV block within the His-Purkinje system. Lightheadedness, dizziness, fatigue, syncope, convulsions, and congestive heart failure are common symptoms and signs associated

Figure 30. Type I second degree AV block within the His-Purkinje system.

Figure 31. A 3:2 AV conduction and Type I second degree AV block occurring within the bundle of His itself. The H-H′ interval increases from 25 to 55 msec, and the third P wave, which is followed by only an H deflection, blocks within the bundle of His.

Figure 32. Type II second degree AV block in a patient with left bundle branch block and 3:2 AV conduction which progressed to 2:1 AV block. The third P wave is blocked within the His-Purkinje system.

Figure 33. 2:1 AV nodal block in a patient with normal QRS complexes.

Figure 34. Patient with left bundle branch block and 2:1 AV nodal block. Both the A-H and H-V intervals (155 and 65 msec, respectively) of the conducted beats are prolonged.

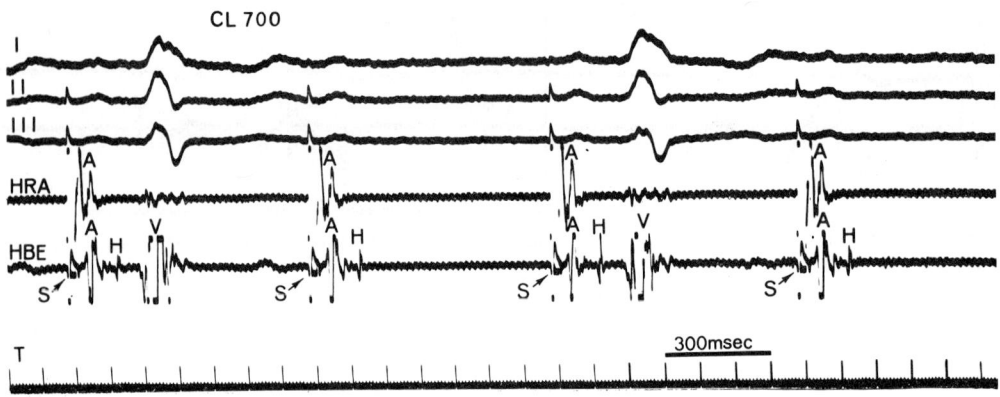

Figure 35.   Patient with left bundle branch block and 2:1 AV block within the His-Purkinje system. Each of the nonconducted atrial impulses is followed by a His deflection. The H-V intervals of the conducted beats are prolonged.

with type II AV block. The demonstration of type II AV block requires that a permanent ventricular pacemaker be inserted, because this form of block almost always progresses to complete AV block within a relatively short period of time.

During complete AV block, atrial impulses continue to block within the His-Purkinje system, and the ventricles come under the control of an idioventricular pacemaker discharging at a rate of 35 to 50 per minute (see Fig. 37). It is not unusual for patients with type II AV block which progresses to complete AV block to demonstrate 1:1 retrograde conduction during ventricular pacing at a rate faster than the sinus rate. This is called unidirectional block.

2:1 AV Block

Like all other forms of AV block, 2:1 AV block may result from lesions in the AV node, bundle of His, or bundle branch–Purkinje system.

A fixed 2:1 AV block in the presence of normal QRS complexes is almost always due to AV nodal block, and the nonconducted P waves are not followed by bundle of His deflections (Fig. 33). The P-R interval of the conducted atrial impulses may be normal or prolonged. Uncommonly, 2:1 AV block with normal QRS complexes is due to block within the bundle of His itself. Each of the nonconducted atrial impulses is associated with a bundle of His deflection, and the P-R intervals of the conducted beats are normal.

In 2:1 AV block with a bundle branch block pattern, the localization of block by electrocardiographic record-

ings alone is difficult. In our experience, block within the His-Purkinje system is slightly more common than AV nodal block. The two forms of block are illustrated in Figures 34 and 35.

Third Degree AV Block

Third degree AV block (also referred to as complete AV block) may result from lesions located in the AV node, bundle of His, or bundle branch–Purkinje system.

In third degree AV nodal block (Fig. 36), atrial impulses are blocked within the AV node. The bundle of His usually emerges as the subsidiary or escape pacemaker, activating the ventricles at a rate of 40 to 60 per minute. Each QRS complex is preceded by a single His bundle deflection, and in general both the QRS complex and H-V intervals are the same as prior to the occurrence of AV block. Patients with complete AV nodal block and a junctional pacemaker (bundle of His) may remain asymptomatic for relatively long periods of time, and therefore the mere presence of complete AV block is not an indication for pacemaker therapy. Junctional pacemakers generally increase their discharge rate in response to exercise or after administration of atropine.

Complete AV block within the bundle of His itself is characterized by nonconducted atrial impulses which are followed by a His bundle deflection (H) and QRS complexes which are preceded by His bundle deflections (H'). The QRS complexes may be normal or abnormal and the H'-V intervals normal (30 to 55 msec) or greater than normal. It is believed that the junctional pacemaker is located within the bundle of His but distal to the site of

Figure 36.   Third degree AV block. Atrial impulses are blocked within the AV node and dissociated from the ventricles. The latter come under control of a bundle of His pacemaker. H-V interval of 47 msec is within the normal range.

Figure 37. Third degree AV block within the His-Purkinje system. Nonconducted atrial impulses are followed by His bundle deflections. The wide QRS complexes come under control of a subjunctional pacemaker and are not preceded by bundle of His deflections.

block. These patients may not demonstrate acceleration of their ventricular rates in response to exercise or atropine. This would not be surprising if the process which caused the intra-His bundle block also affected the autonomic innervation of the common bundle. In these cases of determination for pacemaker, therapy depends upon the patients' symptoms.

Complete AV block distal to the bundle of His is characterized by nonconducted atrial impulses which are followed by His bundle deflections and abnormal QRS complexes which are not preceded by His bundle deflections (Fig. 37). The subsidiary pacemaker is located somewhere within the bundle branch–Purkinje system, and its discharge rate is generally between 35 and 50 per minute. These patients are almost always symptomatic (fatigue, dyspnea, dizziness, syncope, congestive heart failure) and require permanent ventricular pacemaker therapy.

Simulated Type II Second Degree AV Block

The electrocardiographic pattern of type II second degree AV block can be simulated when subtle increases in AV nodal delay are superimposed on a pre-existing first degree AV nodal block, as shown in Figure 38. During sinus rhythm and first degree heart block caused by AV nodal delay, the fourth P wave appears unexpectedly blocked and preceded by constant P-R intervals. However, His bundle recordings at rapid paper speeds (150 mm per second) reveal that a slight increase in the A-H interval preceded the fourth P wave which is blocked in the AV node. The electrophysiologic findings are consistent with a type I second degree AV block of the AV node and not a type II block within the His-Purkinje system. Small increases in AV nodal conduction can result from either spontaneous fluctuations in vagal tone or changes in the P-P cycle length. It is apparent that the small

changes in AV nodal conduction, depicted in Figure 38, would not be appreciated on standard EKG recordings at paper speeds of 25 mm per second. Thus caution should be exercised in making the diagnosis of type II AV block in the presence of an underlying first degree AV block. However, the fact that the patient had normal QRS complexes would argue against the diagnosis of type II AV block, because the latter is generally associated with bundle branch block patterns. In addition, atropine may help in distinguishing the site of block. In type I AV block, atropine shortens the P-R interval and 1:1 AV conduction is established at a faster sinus rate. In type II block, atropine would have a tendency to increase the degree of AV block at a faster sinus rate, because atropine does not directly effect conduction within the His-Purkinje system.

Functional or Physiologic AV Block

At sinus rates of 60 to 100 per minute, the spontaneous occurrence of various types of AV block usually represents an abnormal response of the AV conducting system. On the other hand, acceleration of the atrial rate in resting subjects, such as may occur with atrial flutter, with an ectopic atrial rhythm, or during electrical stimulation of the atrium, can result in various degrees of AV block which may be considered physiologic or functional in nature. Normally, the autonomic nervous system mediates a fine balance between atrial rate and AV nodal conduction. During exercise or other stressful situations, sympathetic stimulation simultaneously increases sinus rates and enhances AV nodal conduction so that there occurs little or no change in the P-R interval. During nonsympathetically mediated increases in atrial rate, the capacity of the AV node to transmit impulses to the ventricles is exceeded and a functional AV nodal block ensues.

Figure 38. Subtle AV nodal Wenckebach type of conduction simulating type II second degree AV block. The P-P intervals are constant. During 4:3 AV conduction, the A-H interval increases only 15 msec prior to the fourth P wave being blocked in the AV node.

PERICARDITIS*

Patrick J. Hogan

571. INTRODUCTION

Inflammation of the pericardium results in deposition of inflammatory cells over the serosal surface and, depending on the cause, a variable amount of serous, fibrinous, purulent, or hemorrhagic exudate. The character, amount, and rate of formation of this exudate determine whether acute fibrinous pericarditis, pericardial effusion, cardiac tamponade, or constrictive pericarditis will develop. The pericardium is involved by a variety of etiologic agents, but rarely is it the sole structure reflecting underlying disease (see accompanying table). The diagnosis of pericarditis is consequently incomplete until the clinician has determined the precise cause with its relatively predictable subsequent clinical course and specific therapeutic demands.

572. ACUTE FIBRINOUS PERICARDITIS

Clinical Manifestations. The most reliable signs of acute pericarditis are chest pain, friction rub, and elec-

---

*The assistance of Dr. Henry D. McIntosh in the preparation of this chapter is gratefully acknowledged.

Classification of Pericardial Disease

I. Inflammatory
  A. Acute pericarditis
    1. Nonspecific (idiopathic)
    2. Infectious
      a. Viral (coxsackievirus, echovirus, cytomegalovirus, influenza, Epstein-Barr)
      b. Bacterial
      c. Tuberculous
      d. Mycotic (histoplasmosis, actinomycosis, nocardia)
      e. Other (protozoal, mycoplasmal, spirochetal)
    3. Associated myocardial infarction
    4. Traumatic
      a. Penetrating or nonpenetrating injury to thorax
      b. Postmyocardial infarction syndrome
      c. Postpericardiotomy, postcardiotomy
    5. Connective tissue disorders (systemic lupus erythematosus, progressive systemic sclerosis, rheumatoid arthritis, rheumatic fever)
    6. Allergic and hypersensitivity diseases (serum sickness, penicillin, drugs)
    7. Metabolic disorders (uremia, myxedema, gout)
    8. Physical and chemical agents
      a. Postirradiation
      b. Postanticoagulation
  B. Chronic pericarditis
    1. Chronic pericardial effusion
    2. Chronic adhesive pericarditis
    3. Chronic constrictive pericarditis
II. Neoplastic
  A. Benign (teratoma, fibroma, angioma, lipoma)
  B. Malignant
    1. Primary (mesothelioma, sarcoma)
    2. Secondary (lung, breast, other)
    3. Leukemia and lymphoma
III. Congenital
  A. Pericardial cysts and diverticula
  B. Complete or partial absence of pericardium

---

trocardiographic (EKG) changes. Pericardial *pain* is usually abrupt, sharp, and severe, with a wide area of radiation to the neck, back, and left shoulder and, rarely, to the arm. Characteristically, it is parasternal, exacerbated by deep inspiration and recumbency, and relieved by sitting or leaning forward. The severity, location, and radiation of the pain may be strikingly similar to that of myocardial infarction, although, in the young, its epigastric location can suggest an acute abdominal disorder. Chest pain may be constant, trivial, or even totally absent, as is often the case in later stages of tuberculous or uremic pericarditis. Most patients are dyspneic and febrile, and complain of malaise, weakness, chills, or other symptoms reflecting the primary disorder.

On physical examination these patients appear anxious and restless, and are either sitting or leaning forward. They are generally febrile and tachycardic, particularly so with idiopathic and suppurative pericarditis. Heart sounds are of normal intensity unless muffled by large effusions. *Friction rubs,* the hallmark of pericarditis, result from inflammation of the pericardial surface, and are often well localized to the lower left parasternal area where they may be palpable (*pericardial fremitus*). These "grating" or "leathery" high frequency sounds exhibit marked changes in intensity, timing, and duration, and vary with phases of respiration and body position. Roughly half are augmented or are equally loud in inspiration and hence often confused with pleural or pleuropericardial rubs. Typically, rubs consist of three or two components, less often of one. The ventricular systolic component is generally the loudest; it may extend throughout systole, and is easily confused with adventitious sounds or systolic murmurs. The persistence of a rub longer than two to three weeks suggests a uremic, tuberculous, or neoplastic origin.

Laboratory studies reflect systemic reaction to pericardial inflammation and often suggest or confirm the presence of the primary underlying disease. Myocardial enzymes are normal or only slightly elevated. X-ray may demonstrate evidence of the primary disease; a pericardial effusion can be appreciated once 200 ml or more of fluid has collected. Electrocardiographic abnormalities are seen in 90 per cent of patients with acute pericarditis, but pathognomonic serial changes are observed in less than 50 per cent of such patients. Characteristically, in standard and lateral precordial leads, there is an initial S-T segment elevation, often with an upward concavity, that persists for a few days to several weeks. As the subepicardial muscle injury subsides, the S-T segment elevation disappears, the P-R segments may become displaced, and the T waves diminish and progressively invert owing to repolarization delay. The notched or inverted T waves generally return to normal by three months, but may be persistent in conditions that cause adhesive or constrictive pericarditis. Absence of Q waves and reciprocal S-T segment depression, plus the notable concavity of the upward S-T segment elevation, helps make the important electrocardiographic differentiation between acute pericarditis and myocardial infarction. Rhythm disturbances, predominantly atrial fibrillation or flutter, are seen in 10 per cent of patients with pericarditis, most likely a consequence of the proximity of the sinus node to the inflamed pericardium.

Differential Diagnosis. The diagnosis can be made with considerable certainty when a young man suddenly develops chest pain, later exacerbated by inspiration and relieved by sitting forward, and demonstrates a loud friction rub and characteristic serial EKG changes without Q waves, with normal serum myocardial enzymes, and with a normal or rapidly enlarging cardiac silhouette on chest x-ray. More commonly, the differentiation of pericarditis from myocardial infarction, dissecting aneurysm, pneumonia, pulmonary emboli, pleurisy, pneumothorax, mediastinitis, intercostal neuralgia, and acute pericardial fat necrosis may not be immediately apparent. Once the diagnosis of pericarditis has been established, the clinician must then attempt to determine the cause with its specific prognostic and therapeutic implications.

573. INDIVIDUAL VARIETIES OF PERICARDITIS

IDIOPATHIC (NONSPECIFIC) PERICARDITIS

Despite the prevailing suspicion of a viral, autoimmune, or hypersensitive cause, this clinical syndrome by definition remains of questionable and presumably diverse origin. The diagnosis is made only after carefully excluding known causes of acute pericarditis. Acute idiopathic pericarditis is largely a disease of males in the third or fourth decade, although it is certainly seen over a wide spectrum of ages and in females. A history of preceding upper respiratory infection can be elicited in one third to two thirds of these patients. They generally note a sharp, "sticking," retrosternal pain, often of maximal intensity within 24 hours, that is markedly influenced by respiratory changes. The majority of these previously healthy individuals are usually mildly toxic, but a few have high fevers. A transient rub is present, more often than not with a small serous pericardial effusion. Moderate leukocytosis is common; leukopenia and anemia are rare. Pneumonitis and pleural effusions are noted on x-ray one third of the time, occasionally accompanied by evidence of congestive heart failure. The EKG is nearly always abnormal, consistently demonstrating the typical evolutionary changes of pericarditis. The major symptoms of this syndrome generally respond to bed rest and analgesics, and usually resolve by one to three weeks. A quarter of these patients suffer recurrences of their symptoms months to years later with a generally shorter and less severe course. Rare fatalities have been reported to be due to cardiac tamponade, occasionally precipitated by anticoagulation. Although an occasional patient will have a protracted course, development of constrictive pericarditis is decidely rare and should raise the possibility of an underlying tuberculous or collagen-vascular process.

VIRAL PERICARDITIS

The consistent recovery of certain enteroviruses from cardiac tissue in perimyocarditis strongly suggests a pathogenic correlation. Although other viruses have been isolated, for practical purposes viral carditis is mainly associated with coxsackievirus infection, primarily type B and rarely type A. Systemic manifestations of viral disease such as myalgias and arthralgias are common and accompany the typical pain, fever, and friction rub. Rubelliform rash or lymphadenopathy may be present. Pleural effusions are very frequent, and pleurodynia is present 25 per cent of the time. An en-

larged cardiac silhouette is the rule, and congestive heart failure has been noted in perhaps a quarter of these patients. The increased incidence of conduction disturbances, occasional transient Q waves, and higher myocardial enzyme elevations reflect the more significant myocardial involvement seen with viral pericarditis. A fourfold rise in neutralizing antibody titer or isolation of the virus in tissue culture confirms the diagnosis. Treatment of viral pericarditis is essentially the same as for idiopathic pericarditis, namely rest and analgesics; steroid therapy should be reserved for clearly refractory patients, particularly in life-threatening situations. The immediate prognosis depends on the degree of accompanying myocarditis.

PERICARDITIS OF ACUTE MYOCARDIAL INFARCTION

Pericarditis complicates acute myocardial infarction in one of five cases. Large effusions are exceptional and suggest an underlying diffuse pericarditis, whereas hemorrhagic effusions suggest the ominous complications of myocardial rupture or excessive anticoagulant therapy. Pericardial pain or friction rubs generally occur during the second to fourth day, rarely as early as the first or as late as the tenth day. These transient rubs are limited in extent, and are best appreciated at the apex or medial to the sternum. Fever and tachycardia may coincide with the rub, or may continue on from the time of the initial infarction. This self-limited process usually requires little therapy other than analgesics and occasionally anti-inflammatory agents such as aspirin or indomethacin; steroids are rarely needed. To avoid the development of cardiac tamponade or hemopericardium, anticoagulants should be withheld in the presence of a diffuse rub or with evidence of a large or enlarging effusion or ventricular aneurysm.

POSTCARDIAC INJURY SYNDROME

The common association of fever, pericarditis, and pleuritis that follows a latent period after injury to the heart or thorax has prompted many investigators to consider that the postmyocardial infarction syndrome, postpericardiotomy syndrome, post-traumatic pericarditis, and even idiopathic pericarditis may be subsets of a syndrome with a common pathogenic basis. Trauma or injury of some kind to the pericardium, myocardium, or both appears to be essential; the possibility of reactivation of latent virus infections is proposed by some. The common association of elevated titers of heart antibodies with serositis and arthritis is supportive, if indirect, evidence for an immunologic cause. However, these antibodies may represent a nonspecific response to traumatized or infarcted tissue.

Postmyocardial Infarction Syndrome
(Dressler's Syndrome)

In 1 per cent of cases of myocardial infarction, pericarditis develops late, has a prolonged course, or recurs. This syndrome normally develops 2 to 12 weeks after the infarction. Pericardial pain precedes or occurs simultaneously with the prolonged, recurrent fever that characterizes this disorder. Pericardial and pleural effusions are common, as is patchy pneumonitis. Tamponade is rare. The EKG may be helpful if typical features of pericarditis are present, but this is unusual. The characteristic pain, friction rub, and fever occurring several weeks to months after a myocardial infarction in the presence of pleural effusion and pneumonitis help make the necessary differentiation from pulmonary emboli or recurrent or extending myocardial infarction. The symptoms generally respond to analgesics, anti-inflammatory drugs, and reassurance; however, steroids may be required. Once instituted, it is often difficult to avoid rebound of symptoms when steroids are tapered. Anticoagulants are contraindicated once this diagnosis is made, because of the more diffuse pericarditis and extensive effusion seen with this disorder.

Post-thoracotomy-Pericardiotomy Syndrome

Approximately 10 per cent of post-thoracotomy patients will develop a delayed febrile response one week to several months after surgery, with signs and symptoms of pericarditis and often with pleural or pericardial effusion. Typically, the pain, fever, rub, and effusion follow a benign and self-limited course. The timing of this syndrome demands close scrutiny to rule out more significant postoperative complications such as pulmonary infarction, atelectasis, or hemopericardium. Bed rest, sedation, and analgesics are important adjuncts to therapy. Steroids effect prompt cessation of symptoms but must be used with particular caution in this setting in which infections are commonplace. This syndrome recurs often and on occasion has persisted intermittently for periods of several years.

COLLAGEN VASCULAR DISEASES AND PERICARDITIS

Systemic Lupus Erythematosus

Lupus pericarditis accounts for less than 5 per cent of all types of pericarditis, yet it may be clinically evident in up to 40 per cent of documented cases of systemic lupus erythematosus (SLE). Pericarditis may precede the more common signs and symptoms of lupus by a considerable time period, often resulting in a misdiagnosis of rheumatic or idiopathic pericarditis. This diagnosis is facilitated by the demonstration of a positive lupus preparation or antinuclear antibody test in serum or more rarely in the pericardial fluid itself. These patients generally respond to steroids, often needed in large doses for prolonged periods. Aside from an increased incidence of congestive heart failure, there is no apparent prognostic significance to the development of pericarditis in SLE over and above that of the primary disease process.

Rheumatoid Arthritis

Clinical evidence of acute pericarditis is uncommon in patients with rheumatoid arthritis (RA), but surgical and postmortem specimens indicate that a nonspecific fibrinous inflammation resulting in adhesive pericarditis has occurred in one of two RA patients. Pericarditis is typical of the extra-articular features of rheumatoid arthritis, in that it occurs in patients with significant, well documented peripheral arthritis, usually having

subcutaneous nodules and high titers of rheumatoid factor. Fever, leukocytosis, anemia, and an elevated sedimentation rate give evidence of the active inflammatory process commonly associated with the development of pericarditis. Friction rub is normally present, and signs of pleural effusion and congestive failure are not uncommonly detected. The fluid in rheumatoid pericardial effusion, like that of rheumatoid pleural effusion, is characterized by a markedly low concentration of glucose, elevated LDH enzymes, elevated gamma globulin, and decreased hemolytic complement and complement components. Cytologic examination may demonstrate giant round or oval multinucleated cells, thought by some to be pathognomonic of this disorder. Rheumatoid pericarditis is a low-grade inflammatory process that usually pursues a short course and requires minimal therapy. Steroids predictably reverse the pericardial symptoms of these patients, but may have little or no effect on the articular symptoms. Rare cases of rheumatoid pericarditis have developed into constrictive pericarditis despite steroid intervention.

UREMIC PERICARDITIS

Formerly regarded as a sign of imminent death, pericarditis is now an expected manifestation of uremia. The introduction of hemodialysis has significantly altered the natural history, clinical features, and therapy of uremic pericarditis. Previously, other symptoms and signs of uremia overshadowed the infrequent chest pain, insignificant friction rubs, rare nonspecific EKG findings, and small fibrinous effusions that characterized uremic pericarditis. Now, the 10 to 15 per cent of patients who develop uremic pericarditis while on hemodialysis complain of significant pain and fever, have loud friction rubs, and manifest large, often hemorrhagic, pericardial effusions with pronounced EKG changes and rhythm disturbances. These patients are often hypotensive during dialysis, have frequent arrhythmias, and have cardiomegaly on x-ray, with elevated venous pressure with or without evident pericardial effusion. Heart failure and pulmonary congestion are not uncommon and give evidence of the severity of underlying myocardial damage that occurs with uremic pericarditis. The precise cause of both fibrinous and hemorrhagic pericarditis in uremia remains obscure. The level of renal function does not differentiate between those patients who will or will not develop pericarditis or hemorrhagic effusion. The apparent protection afforded by more intense hemodialysis suggests that dialyzable compounds play an etiologic role in the development of this syndrome. Cardiac tamponade and subsequent constriction are seen with increased frequency after the institution of hemodialysis, presumably reflecting the increased bleeding tendency and qualitative platelet abnormalities of chronic uremia and technical anticoagulation problems of the hemodialysis procedure. It is vital to recognize the development of these syndromes and not attribute a falling glomerular filtration rate (GFR) to terminal renal failure, rather than to an altered cardiac output resulting from pericardial disease which may be correctable. The development of uremic pericarditis is an indication for initiating or increasing hemodialysis. This therapeutic technique will prevent the occurrence or reoccurrence of pericarditis in two thirds of uremic patients. Recurrent pericarditis and effusion, particularly with hypotension or evidence of tamponade, requires at least pericardiocentesis, but more often will require pericardiectomy.

PURULENT PERICARDITIS

Pyogenic pericarditis demands early recognition and specific, aggressive therapy to avoid its lethal consequences. The clinical signs of pericarditis may significantly postdate the initial infection, may be overshadowed by the primary focus, or may be altered by intervening antimicrobial therapy. Purulent pericarditis generally occurs as a consequence or complication of other diseases, particularly mediastinal or pulmonary infection. Pneumonia, empyema, or other thoracic infections most commonly invade the pericardium by direct extension, often after penetration of the thorax and pericardium during surgery or by trauma. Septicemia from distant skin, soft tissue, or bone infections is less often responsible for this syndrome, and subdiaphragmatic abscesses rarely so. Pericarditis occurs more than 10 per cent of the time in fatal bacterial endocarditis, and may accompany myocardial abscesses. Dyspnea, fever, tachycardia, and chest pain are prominently present in adults. Cardiomegaly is frequent, often with muffled heart sounds and pulsus paradoxus, attesting to the usual presence of an accompanying significant effusion. A friction rub or classic EKG pattern is absent in more than half of these patients and should not impede a diagnostic and often therapeutic pericardiocentesis. Appropriate antimicrobial drugs and surgical drainage have led to gratifying results. *Pneumococcal* pericarditis, formerly the prototype of purulent pericarditis, is now rarely seen, and is nearly always due to untreated pneumonia or associated empyema. *Staphylococcal* pericarditis, often hospital acquired, usually arises from a remote focus of infection, and pursues a devastating clinical course. It is renowned for complicating a variety of surgical procedures, particularly open heart surgery. Gram-negative organisms, including Pseudomonas, Proteus, *E. coli,* and Klebsiella, involve the pericardium, especially in the immunosuppressed patient. Meningococcus, with or without meningitis, and gonococcus can infect the pericardium in the untreated patient, often with massive effusion. The systemic mycoses *histoplasmosis, actinomycosis, and aspergillosis* have caused purulent pericarditis, but more often result in a granulomatous reaction, occasionally with resultant constrictive pericarditis. *Amebiasis* of the left lobe of the liver has involved the pericardium by simple contiguity or by direct rupture into the pericardial space. Creation of a pericardial window with pleural drainage or pericardiectomy is mandatory with purulent pericarditis and usually eliminates the possibility of constrictive pericarditis developing subsequently.

TUBERCULOUS PERICARDITIS

Tuberculous pericarditis occurs in 5 to 10 per cent of tuberculous patients. It accounts for up to one tenth of all cases of acute pericarditis and a significantly larger percentage of cases of constrictive pericarditis. It shares with the other forms of pericarditis a characteristic male predominance, usually appearing between the second and sixth decade, but is peculiar in its racial predisposition, occurring perhaps 10 to 12 times more commonly in blacks than in whites. The pericardium may appear as the sole or primary site of tuberculous involvement, but it is probably always secondary to tuberculous infection elsewhere. Obvious pulmonary or pleural tuberculous manifestations are detected in half these patients. In nearly all clinically recognized cases, there is retrograde tuberculous extension from pleural, pulmonary, or mediastinal lymph nodes. The onset of symptoms may be sudden, but generally these symptoms occur insidiously. Unexplained cardiomegaly may be the initial indication of disease, and dyspnea, cough, and chest pain are common, particularly with large effusions. High spiking temperatures are noted in the acute phase, but more commonly low-grade fever, weakness, fatigue, night sweats, and transient arthralgia are noted. It is not rare for patients with this disease to present initially with symptoms of constrictive pericarditis or cardiac tamponade.

The diagnosis is established by determining that pericarditis exists in the presence of pulmonary or extrapulmonary tuberculous lesions. The absence of x-ray evidence of tuberculosis by no means excludes this diagnosis. Under optimal circumstances it is possible to culture the mycobacterium, or to verify the diagnosis by pericardial biopsy in about half the patients in which the condition is suspected. Nevertheless, tuberculous pericarditis should be high on the list of diagnostic possibilities if a positive tuberculin reaction is present with evidence of pericarditis, particularly with weight loss, fever, night sweats, and massive or rapidly occurring sanguineous or hemorrhagic effusion. Triple therapy with isoniazid, streptomycin, and rifampin or ethambutol is required for 18 to 24 months. Most authorities recommend a brief trial of steroids to decrease the toxic manifestations of this disease and to diminish inflammatory exudation. If symptoms of constriction persist for six weeks, or if there is no evidence of chemotherapeutic response by six months, these patients should undergo pericardiectomy.

574. PERICARDIAL EFFUSION

Pericardial effusion can occur with any variety of acute pericarditis, or can accompany hepatic, renal, or cardiac failure or other conditions complicated by anasarca. Rarely the effusion may persist for many years, and such patients have been misdiagnosed as having chronic congestive heart failure. Chronic effusion has been associated with a variety of systemic disorders such as myxedema, collagen diseases, and chronic anemia. Some cases are idiopathic, with the pericardial fluid having markedly elevated protein and excessive "cholesterol" crystals.

Pathophysiology. The sudden accumulation of even a few hundred milliliters of blood in the pericardium may impair cardiac filling to the point of arterial hypotension, syncope, or sudden death. In contradistinction, several liters of fluid may gradually accumulate in myxedema or tuberculous or idiopathic pericarditis and may fail to elicit recognizable signs or symptoms. Other determinants of the physiologic response to pericardial effusion include the type of fluid, the size and compliance of the pericardial sac, the functional competence of the underlying myocardium, and the status of the visceral pericardial lymphatics and right heart venous drainage.

Physical Findings. The clinical detection of less than 200 to 300 ml of pericardial fluid in the absence of cardiac compression may be impossible. Larger amounts of fluid, especially if rapidly acquired, can be determined reliably by physical examination. Such patients are anxious, dyspneic, tachycardic, and diaphoretic and often assume the upright position. Depending on the compression caused by the pericardial accumulation, the pulses may be normal, depressed, or paradoxical; the neck veins may be normal or elevated. The heart sounds are of normal intensity, and friction rubs are commonly heard despite the presence of large effusion. Repeated examination, particularly in the prone position, may disclose muffling of the heart sounds. The cardiac apical impulse may be weak or absent; its detection medial to the left border of cardiac dullness is diagnostically helpful. A distinctive flatness to percussion that extends laterally beyond the apex or to the right of the sternum, that extends to the lower half of the sternum, or that expands to the second or third left intercostal space on recumbency is similarly a useful sign. Another helpful, if uncommon, indicator of pericardial effusion is the development of an area of dullness under the angle of the scapula generally associated with bronchial breath sounds, referred to as *Ewart's sign.* This sign is due to compression of the lung and can occasionally result from marked cardiomegaly.

Laboratory Studies. The *EKG* may be normal or, more commonly, may demonstrate nondiagnostic changes. The association of low QRS voltage and pericardial effusion has long been appreciated. It is not an invariable finding, but any diminution of voltage in patients with acute pericarditis suggests the development of an effusion. With large effusions and tachycardia, a regular alternating QRS voltage may be recorded (*electrical alternans*). This is thought to result from the oscillatory movements of the heart cushioned from mediastinal and pulmonary restraints by the pericardial effusion. Total electrical alternans of both P and QRS waves is seen only with very large effusions, usually with cardiac tamponade. The most reliable and earliest *radiologic sign* of pericardial effusion is the demonstration of an abrupt, symmetrical increase in the cardiac silhouette on serial roentgenograms, especially in the absence of congested lung fields. The normal contour of the left heart border may straighten, or the right cardiophrenic junction may bulge convexly. With widening and obliteration of the outline of the great vessels and general loss of angular curves, the heart assumes a characteristic "pear" or "flask" configuration. The *fluoroscopic* demonstration of decreased ventricular pulsations is helpful, and is quite specific if these pulsations are totally absent. The demonstration of the epicardial fat line well inside the cardiac contour with image intensification is another indication of the presence of pericardial fluid. All these roentgenographic signs are helpful but are rarely totally definitive in distinguishing pericardial effusion from cardiac hypertrophy, dilatation, or variations of the normal cardiac silhouette. Conclusive differentiation between them often requires the use of some form of contrast: positive contrast with angiographic techniques, negative contrast with carbon dioxide, or gamma-emitting radioisotopes. *Echocardiography* has proved to be a safe, simple technique that permits accurate diagnosis and monitoring of pericardial effusions. When fluid separates the ventricular epicardium from the posterior or anterior pericardium, a distinctive motionless echo interface can be detected. The echo-free space between the epicardium and pericardium roughly estimates the amount of peri-

cardial effusion. The echocardiogram can supply additional information relating to cardiac size and contractility. Most centers now initially use this diagnostic mode and resort to further angiographic verification when echoes are technically difficult or the results confusing.

575. CARDIAC TAMPONADE

Etiology. When intrapericardial pressure rises sufficiently to impede ventricular filling and myocardial contractility, cardiac compression or *tamponade* exists. Essentially anything that causes pericardial inflammation or injury can result in tamponade, depending on the tempo and duration of the inciting process. Overwhelming exudation from pyogenic, tuberculous, or neoplastic pericarditis, or the exuberant transudation of lupus, rheumatic, or even idiopathic pericarditis has caused tamponade. More commonly, tamponade occurs with the sudden development of intrapericardial hemorrhage or the transformation of a pre-existing effusion into hemopericardium. Contusion, laceration, or rupture of the heart or great vessels, hemorrhagic complications of uremic or neoplastic pericarditis, and the excessive administration of anticoagulants have all led to cardiogenic shock from tamponade.

Pathophysiology. The presence of large pericardial effusions in the absence of cardiac compression may cause no hemodynamic impairment; but once the pericardium becomes indistensible, further increments of fluid cause severe restriction of diastolic expansion by the myocardium. Pericardial compression of the right atrium interferes with venous inflow, resulting in a back-up or pooling of venous blood causing elevated central venous pressures. Both ventricles are similarly compromised by decreasing compliance, with elevated end-diastolic pressures and reciprocally depressed end-diastolic volumes resulting in decreased stroke volumes and cardiac output. Compensatory tachycardia and vasoconstriction may initially support the circulation; but once the fluid accumulation proves inexorable, the stroke volume decreases further and the elevated heart rate alone becomes insufficient to maintain cardiac output. In the face of escalating tachycardia with decreased diastolic filling periods, lowered aortic pressures, and increasing compression on the myocardium and coronary vessels, coronary insufficiency and eventual myocardial necrosis become inevitable, resulting in decreased myocardial performance and an even further decreased stroke volume. The unsupported venous pressure then falls and diastolic filling substantially decreases, causing this vicious cycle to perpetuate itself, leading eventually to total circulatory collapse.

Physical Findings. The dramatic appearance of patients with tamponade should impress the clinician with the necessity for rapid diagnosis and decisive therapy. When first seen, these patients may be comatose and in profound shock, particularly in cases of acute hemopericardium; but more often they appear anxious, pale or cyanotic, and dyspneic, sitting or leaning forward and often giving a history of antecedent pericarditis. Such patients are characteristically hypotensive, with marked venous distention and no evidence of cardiac enlargement (Beck's triad), and usually demonstrate paradoxical pulse and narrowed pulse pressure.

Pulsus paradoxus is defined as a drop in systolic blood

pressure of more than 10 mm Hg on quiet inspiration. Demonstration of this pulse deficit at the bedside can be a valuable clue to the presence of cardiac compression, particularly if accompanied by elevated venous pressures that distend or fail to collapse on inspiration. Virtually always present with cardiac tamponade, this sign is similarly seen in some cases of constrictive pericarditis. With normal inspiration there is a decrease in intrathoracic pressure, and the right heart pressures decline accordingly with the lowered intrapleural pressure. This results in augmented right ventricular filling by virtue of the increased gradient between the extrathoracic veins and the right chambers of the heart. Coincident with the more negative intrathoracic pressure, there is a redistribution of blood to the more compliant pulmonary veins and left atrium at the expense of decreased filling of the less compliant left ventricle. These mechanisms account for the physiologic lowering of both systolic and pulse pressure during inspiration when intrapleural pressure is minimal. With the development of cardiac tamponade, these normal respiratory variations become amplified and acquire pathologic significance. As the right ventricle distends during inspiration with tamponade, there is competition for the limited available space in the pericardium, resulting in an intrapericardial pressure rise with subsequent compromise of the left ventricular output and systemic arterial pressure. Other factors of varying significance include inspiratory descent of the diaphragm, causing traction in the already taut pericardium; heightened inspiratory pooling of blood in the lungs and right heart, accounting for decreased left ventricular ejection; and interference by the tense pericardial sac with the transmission of intrathoracic pressures to the left ventricle, resulting in a decreased effective filling pressure with pooling of the blood in the pulmonary veins. This sign is not pathognomonic of pericardial tamponade and is more commonly associated with obstructive airway disease. Prominent engorgement of neck veins should suggest cardiac tamponade and help distinguish it from other conditions of shock. Inspiratory augmentation of cervical venous waves and the precipitous pulse collapse of these veins are further evidence of tamponade. The lung fields are surprisingly clear, with Ewart's sign occasionally observed. Percussion and palpation of the heart are typically unremarkable, whereas with auscultation the heart sounds are often distant or frankly muffled, with a notable absence of gallops or murmurs. Diastolic sounds and friction rubs are generally not heard. Liver tenderness and enlargement may be the initial signs of tamponade. Manual compression of the liver with cervical venous distention (positive *hepatojugular reflux*) is further indirect evidence of tamponade. Ascites may be prominent with chronic tamponade, but edema is rarely noted in either acute or chronic tamponade.

Laboratory Studies. Cardiac tamponade is primarily a clinical diagnosis, and laboratory studies, although they may be supportive, are of secondary value and are rarely diagnostic in themselves. EKG findings are usually nonspecific, but occasionally demonstrate typical changes of acute pericarditis. S-T segment changes that revert after pericardiocentesis suggest that tamponade was present, causing subendocardial ischemia. Electrical alternans and low QRS voltage are suggestive, but do not help differentiate effusion from tamponade. Total electrical alternans of the P, QRS, and T waves is said to be virtually diagnostic of acute tamponade. In view of the fact that

acute tamponade can be produced by small effusions that are radiologically indistinct, a normal-sized cardiac silhouette in no way excludes this diagnosis. Fluoroscopy or angiography may document an effusion in a majority of patients, but does not distinguish effusion from tamponade.

Pericardiocentesis. Pericardiocentesis becomes mandatory when tamponade causes hypotension, pulse pressure less than 20 mm Hg, central venous pressure greater than 20 cm H_2O, pulsus paradoxus greater than 50 per cent of the pulse pressure, or shock. The subxiphoid-subcostal approach is preferred as a safe, anatomically well defined position which avoids the pleural space and is more likely to yield small amounts of dependent pericardial fluid. A large-bore, short-beveled needle attached to the precordial or exploring lead is advanced, with continuous EKG monitoring, upward under the rib cage and medially toward the right shoulder until fluid is returned. Should inadvertent contact with the atria or ventricle be made, cardiac pulsations can be felt and indicated electrocardiographically by S-T segment elevation or runs of premature atrial or ventricular contractions. It is vital to recognize myocardial puncture in order to avoid myocardial or coronary laceration, air embolism, catastrophic arrhythmias, or excessive aspiration of intravascular fluid in an already hemodynamically compromised patient. Once the aspiration needle has been correctly positioned, enough fluid should be removed to demonstrate at least overt hemodynamic improvement, often a quantity as small as 50 to 100 ml. This fluid should always be submitted for culture and cytologic examination.

Treatment. All patients with acute pericarditis or effusion require repeated physical examinations with serial x-rays and careful monitoring of vital signs for manifestations of cardiac tamponade. If aspiration attempts prove unsuccessful or fail to relieve the tamponade, surgical exploration with pericardiectomy or creation of a pericardial window should be undertaken without delay, especially in situations of trauma or after cardiac surgery. If the pericardial fluid cannot be evacuated immediately, the circulation must be stabilized by the maintenance and expansion of venous blood volume. Vasopressors and digitalis are often ineffective in this setting, but isoproterenol has been consistently helpful, provided the heart rate is sufficiently slow and the central venous pressure well maintained.

576. CONSTRICTIVE PERICARDITIS

Recovery from pericarditis can be complicated by the development of chronic pericardial effusion, adhesion, or constriction.

Adhesive pericarditis may develop between the visceral and parietal pericardium, the pericardium and myocardium, or the pericardium and neighboring mediastinal structures. Adhesive pericarditis, by and large, causes negligible circulatory disturbances. *Constrictive pericarditis* ensues once the adherent layer of the pericardium becomes thickened and fibrosed to the extent of myocardial encasement and impairment of diastolic filling. Although constrictive pericarditis was formerly considered to be a common sequela of tuberculosis, more recent surveys have been unable to identify any consistent etiologic agent. Pyogenic pericarditis, particularly staphylococcal or pneumococcal, often results in subacute and chronic constrictive pericarditis, as does idiopathic and viral pericarditis. Trauma to the heart, neoplastic invasion or irradiation of the pericardium, and uremia, all conditions associated with hemorrhagic pericarditis, have been associated with the development of this syndrome.

Pathophysiology. Many factors contribute to the altered physiology of constrictive pericarditis, not the least of which being the degree and location of fibrosis interfering with ventricular diastolic filling. Usually the restrictive scar tissue involves both ventricles equally, resulting in a typical "small, quiet" heart. On occasion it may selectively surround a single ventricle, atria, great vessels, or vena cava. Such patients may have compensatory enlargement of the heart, particularly if there is some associated myocardial or valvular disease. Persistence of this syndrome after surgical failure to adequately liberate each ventricle emphasizes how hemodynamically significant localized pericardial constriction can be. Variable myocardial fibrosis and disuse atrophy accompanying pericardial fibrosis add to the hemodynamic burden imposed by impaired diastolic filling.

Clinical Manifestations. Signs and symptoms suggestive of right heart failure develop in this syndrome, predictably in young or middle-aged adults of either sex, who often have a recent or remote history of pericarditis. Some patients complain of relatively acute exertional dyspnea, abdominal swelling, or peripheral edema occurring over a matter of weeks to months. Other patients notice the insidious progression of weakness and fatigability, slight breathlessness, epigastric discomfort, or a tendency for fluid retention occurring over many years. Abdominal swelling and discomfort caused by tender hepatomegaly and accumulated ascitic fluid are prominent features of this syndrome that usually antedate and overshadow any peripheral edema. Subtle signs of left heart failure, such as dyspnea occurring only with exertion, or gradually increasing orthopnea, are often elicited and generally tend to be progressive. Paroxysmal nocturnal dyspnea and pulmonary edema are not usual features of this syndrome.

The cervical veins are obviously engorged and highlight the cardiogenic origin of the ascites, hepatomegaly, and edema that generally bring this disorder to medical attention. Careful examination of the swollen jugular venous pulse reveals a marked diastolic collapse or prominent "Y" descent. The magnitude and volume of the arterial pulse are normally decreased; pulsus paradoxus is not common. Examination of the lungs may reveal modest pulmonary congestion and, generally at some stage of the disease, signs of pleural effusion. Sometimes there is an early diastolic tap or shock caused by the rapid inflow of blood against an indistensible ventricle. On auscultation the heart sounds may be distant, with mid- to late systolic clicks frequently heard. A loud snapping, apical, high-pitched diastolic sound (pericardial knock), occurring 0.09 to 0.12 second after aortic valve closure, helps confirm this diagnosis. This sound coincides with the "Y trough" and palpable diastolic shock, reflecting termination of rapid inflow of blood by the sudden pericardial impediment to the dilating ventricle. Prominent, tender hepatomegaly, ascites, and splenomegaly have more than once caused the erroneous diagnosis of hepatic cirrhosis.

Laboratory Studies. Characteristic but nondiagnostic electrocardiograms are present in nearly all cases of chronic constrictive pericarditis. The EKG most commonly demonstrates decreased QRS voltage, flattened or inverted T waves, broad or notched P waves, and, often, right axis deviation. These changes usually persist after pericardiectomy and are undoubtedly attributable to subepicardial fibrosis and myocardial atrophy. Electrical alternans does not occur in the absence of a significant effusion. Arrhythmias are seen 40 per cent of the time, with atrial fibrillation most consistently recorded. The heart on chest x-ray may appear small, normal, or slightly enlarged. Fluoroscopy typically reveals diminished cardiac pulsations, dilated superior vena cava, abrupt, early diastolic dilatation, and straight left and right heart borders, with a small to absent aortic knuckle. *Pericardial calcification* signifies the presence of pericardial adhesion but not necessarily constriction. Although not pathognomonic, this valuable sign can be detected in over 75 per cent of the cases of chronic constriction if carefully sought. Angiography may delineate the presence of a thickened, rigid atrial wall, slowed circulation, and possible right or left atrial enlargement. The *echocardiographic* confirmation of diminished ventricular volumes, enlarged atrium, and thickened, immobile posterior wall with impaired contraction affords corroborative evidence of pericardial constriction. Hepatic function tests, particularly the Bromsulphalein test, become abnormal with progressive, passive liver congestion. Hypoalbuminemia, normal or elevated globulins, and albuminuria, as well as other results associated with protein-losing enteropathy, can accompany this syndrome. At cardiac catheterization the right atrial pressure is invariably elevated and is usually equaled by that of the left atrium, as well as the right and left ventricular end-diastolic, pulmonary artery diastolic, and wedge pressures. Prominent atrial "X" and "Y" descents result in a distinctive "M" or "W" pressure tracing. Right ventricular pressures reflect an abrupt termination of this "Y" descent by an early diastolic dip with a rapid rise to an elevated diastolic pressure plateau, notably more than a third that of the pressure recorded at end-systole. This "square root" pattern with its high end-diastolic pressure and compromised stroke volume is duplicated, as expected, in left ventricular pressure tracings. The cardiac output is usually normal at rest, and there is diminished response to exercise. Similar hemodynamic changes have been recorded with severe myocardial failure, usually biventricular, from a variety of causes. Differential diagnosis can be difficult at times.

Treatment. The definitive treatment of constrictive pericarditis consists of adequate surgical decortication. Symptoms or signs of excessive fatigue, dyspnea, edema, or ascites and evidence of depressed cardiac output, impaired diastolic filling, or hepatic congestion are indications for surgical intervention. Ideally this should be performed before obliteration of the pericardial space has occurred; before hepatic dysfunction, protein-losing enteropathy, or nephrotic syndrome has developed; and before the myocardium and great vessels become inextricably fibrotic and calcified. Surgical results, previously dismal, have improved substantially to an expected 10 to 12 per cent perioperative mortality and 5 per cent late mortality. Factors that determine the surgical outcome include the duration of the disease, age of the patient, character of the constrictive tissue, atrial fibrillation, ability to establish a cleavage plane at the time of surgery, and, most important, the presence and degree of cardiomyopathy or dilatation. Patients who have had pericarditis for a long time, with marked myocardial atrophy from longstanding constriction, may experience only minimal improvement, or may require very long recuperative periods.

Bishop, L. H., Jr., Estes, E. H., Jr., and McIntosh, H. D.: The electrocardiogram as a safeguard in pericardiocentesis. J.A.M.A., 162:264, 1956.

Comty, C. M., Cohen, S. L., and Shapiro, F. L.: Pericarditis in chronic uremia and its sequels. Ann. Intern. Med., 75:173, 1971.

Cortes, F. M. (ed.): The Pericardium and Its Disorders. Springfield, Ill., Charles C Thomas, 1970.

Dressler, W.: The postmyocardial infarction syndrome. A report on forty-four cases. Arch. Intern. Med., 103:28, 1959.

Ellis, K., and King, D. L.: Pericarditis and pericardial effusion. Radiol. Clin. North Am., 9:393, 1973.

Feigenbaum, H.: Echocardiographic diagnosis of pericardial effusion. Am. J. Cardiol., 26:475, 1970.

Fowler, N.: Cardiac Diagnosis. New York, Harper & Row, Publishers, 1968, p. 593.

Franco, A. E., Levine, H. D., and Hall, A. P.: Rheumatoid pericarditis. Ann. Intern. Med., 77:837, 1972.

Holt, J. P.: The normal pericardium. Am. J. Cardiol., 26:455, 1970.

Koontz, C. H., and Ray, C. G.: The role of Coxsackie Group B virus infections in sporadic myopericarditis. Am. Heart J., 82:750, 1971.

Schepers, G. W.: Tuberculous pericarditis. Am. J. Cardiol., 9:248, 1962.

Shabetai, R., Fowler, N. O., and Guntheroth, W. G.: The hemodynamics of cardiac tamponade and constrictive pericarditis. Am. J. Cardiol., 26:480, 1970.

Spodick, D. H.: Acute cardiac tamponade. Pathologic physiology, diagnosis, and management. Progr. Cardiovasc. Dis., 10:661, 1967.

Spodick, D. H.: Chronic and Constrictive Pericarditis. New York, Grune & Stratton, 1964.

Spodick, D. H.: Diagnostic electrocardiographic sequences in acute pericarditis. Circulation, 48:575, 1973.

Thadani, U., Chopra, M. P., Aber, C. P., and Portal, R. W.: Pericarditis after acute myocardial infarction. Br. Med. J., 2:135, 1971.

Wood, P.: Disease of the Heart and Circulation. 3rd ed., Philadelphia, J. B. Lippincott Company, 1968, p. 762.

DISEASE OF THE MYOCARDIUM

Wallace Brigden

577. INTRODUCTION

General Considerations. Many diseases of the heart are initiated by mechanical faults concerned with valve defects, deprivation of fuel supplies, or increased cardiac work. The myocardium, although showing remarkable reserves, is eventually secondarily affected in these conditions, and its failure often finally determines the course of events. These chapters are concerned with those rather less common conditions which are primarily localized in the myocardium leading to defective muscle function and its final failure.

These primary myocardial diseases are probably much more common than is generally recognized. Their true incidence is unknown, because serious investigation into these disorders has developed only in the last two or three decades. Furthermore, diagnostic errors are common not only because physical signs are often inconspicuous, but also because symptoms and signs may suggest one of the more well known disorders which affect the heart of man. The incidence of primary myocardial diseases is greatly affected by socioeconomic and geographical factors, and it happens that primary myocardial diseases are most common in developing parts of the world such as central Africa where sophisticated medical care with modern diagnostic methods is thinly spread.

Innumerable terms have been used for these disorders, but most are unsatisfactory and must remain so until the etiologic processes are fully understood. Primary myocardial disease indicates a process often of obscure etiology which is localized in the myocardium; cardiomyopathy indicates a somewhat wider range and includes processes which, although dominantly affecting the myocardium, may be of a generalized nature. Myocarditis, in keeping with usage of the suffix, should be restricted to disorders of an infectious or inflammatory nature. Myocardosis is an unsatisfactory term sometimes used to embrace all the noninflammatory processes. Classification is as unsatisfactory as terminology and for similar reasons. However, it is apparent that the myocardium may be damaged by any of the known disease processes which affect man; thus genetic, infective, metabolic, nutritional, and immunologic disorders may be found among the causes of cardiomyopathy. It would be rational, in such a classification, to include muscle disease resulting from vascular disorders, but habit and the magnitude of the problem have naturally led to isolation and separate consideration of coronary disease. However, there are rare cases of diffuse small vessel coronary occlusion which result in diffuse myocardial fibrosis causing clinical features which resemble other forms of cardiomyopathy. The following features concern primary myocardial disease in general.

Clinical Manifestations. The primary myocardial diseases present in diverse ways and their clinical features depend on the site, extent, and nature of the myocardial disorder and consequent disturbance of hemodynamics. Almost any of the symptoms and signs of heart disease (and any combination thereof) which arise in the whole field of heart disease may occur in the cardiomyopathies.

Dyspnea is the most common symptom. All forms are met, but since most myopathies dominantly affect the left ventricle, orthopnea and nocturnal asthma are common. *Syncope* is especially likely to occur in those forms of myocardial disease which cause heart block and paroxysmal arrhythmia; it may also result from effort when there is outflow tract obstruction (see Ch. 578), as in other obstructive disorders of the cardiovascular system. *Cardiac pain* is not common, but when it occurs an erroneous diagnosis of coronary disease is often made. True angina is a feature of idiopathic hypertrophic subaortic stenosis (see Ch. 578). Myocarditis, possibly when associated with pericarditis, may cause prolonged cardiac pain. Hepatic pain arising and increasing during effort may superficially resemble angina pectoris. *Palpitation* from frequent extrasystoles or other arrhythmia is common, especially in the familial forms, in alcoholic cardiomyopathy, and in myocarditis. Occasionally a primary muscle disorder may masquerade as an innocent paroxysmal tachycardia in the early stages of the disease process.

Physical examination and cardiovascular investigation may show any one of a number of dynamic disturbances which depend on the site and nature of the pathology. These may be classified in various ways. A division into congestive, constrictive, and hypertrophic (including obstructive) types, depending on the dominant hemodynamic derangement, has been suggested. From increasing experience with these conditions, it is clear that although there are such clear-cut hemodynamic disorders, there is also much overlap. However, the hypertrophic obstructive type is sufficiently discrete to be considered a separate and possibly single disease entity (see Ch. 578).

Chronic hypokinetic heart failure (congestive type) occurs in many forms of primary myocardial disease, but is probably most common in postinflammatory cardiomyopathy, active myocarditis, and familial cardiomegaly. The heart is very large and relatively "quiet" on fluoroscopy, and lung fields are often clear owing to right ventricular failure. All signs point to a chronic low cardiac output. At *necropsy* the heart weight is usually well above average, but the ventricular wall may appear thinner than normal because of the great dilatation. Macroscopic appearances of the muscle vary from normality to patchy fibrosis, and even large areas of damage may be found. Mural thrombi in varying stages of organization are common.

"Constrictive" forms of cardiomyopathy are not uncommon and cause confusion with constrictive pericarditis. This disorder is produced by restriction of ventricular filling because of diminished compliance of thick abnormal muscle or because of obstruction at the atrioventricular valves by masses of ventricular myocardium, or by massive endocardial thrombi and fibrosis (see Endomyocardial Fibrosis in Ch. 583). However, in many cases of cardiomyopathy the resemblance to constrictive pericarditis is relatively superficial. The venous pressure is high, an early diastolic sound is usual, and the right ventricular pressure curve shows a sharp early diastolic dip coincident with the *y* descent and a late diastolic plateau of the JVP. The *x* descent of the venous pulse (or RA pressure pulse) is usually shallow in primary myocardial disease in contrast to constrictive pericarditis. Furthermore, the electrocardiogram in constrictive cardiomyopathy usually shows a very abnormal QRS-T, whereas in constrictive pericarditis the QRS tends to remain near normal. However, the greatest diagnostic difficulty arises in some forms of endomyocardial fibrosis when the bulk of the muscle mass may be relatively normal, resulting in a nearly normal QRS complex. Calcification of the pericardium is absent, but difficulty may arise when there is myocardial or endomyocardial calcification. Cardiac amyloidosis and the African form of endomyocardial fibrosis often cause features of the constrictive syndrome.

Burch, G. E. (ed.): Cardiomyopathy. *In* Cardiovascular Clinics, Vol. 4. Philadelphia, F. A. Davis Company, 1972.
Goodwin, J. F.: Clarification of the cardiomyopathies. Mod. Concepts Cardiovasc. Dis., 41:41, 1972.
Mattingly, T. W.: Clinical features and diagnosis of primary myocardial disease. Mod. Concepts Cardiovasc. Dis., 30:677, 683, 1961.

578. HYPERTROPHIC CARDIOMYOPATHY

A group of patients have primary myocardial disease which is essentially of a hypertrophic nature. This hypertrophy may be of such magnitude that it causes dynamic derangement of an *obstructive nature* which may embarrass inflow to, or outflow from, either ventricle. The clinical features, laboratory findings, and pathologic changes are sufficiently uniform to justify consideration of this condition as a single disease entity variously known as *asymmetrical hypertrophy, idiopathic hypertrophic subaortic stenosis,* and *hypertrophic obstructive car-*

diomyopathy. The cause is unknown, but in at least 30 per cent of patients there is a strongly positive family history of the same disease.

Pathology. Necropsy shows great ventricular hypertrophy which is often asymmetrical, and the ventricular cavity tends to be obliterated. The heart weight is always above normal and often greatly so. Diffuse fibrosis may be apparent, but large areas of fibrosis are not usually seen. The microscopic picture is of a bizarre arrangement of large muscle fibers separated by connective tissue. Fibrosis is common in the center of the muscle bundles. Using histochemical methods and electron microscopy, Pearse found widespread dystrophy of grossly hypertrophic muscle fibers accompanied by glycogen storage and mitochondriosis. There are also abnormal shortness of myofibers, proliferation of connective tissue with functional hyperplasia of arterioles and capillaries, and a proliferation of sympathetic nerve fibers (sympathosis) with consequent noradrenosis. At the electron microscopic level there is a close resemblance of cardiomyopathic fibers to normal atrial fibers; thus there is a possibility that developmental abnormality lies behind the syndrome. However, the proliferation of the sympathetic nerves may indicate a primary role of the autonomic nervous system.

Etiology. It is clear that many patients with hypertrophic obstructive cardiomyopathy have familial cardiomyopathy (see Ch. 579); however, in many cases there is no evidence of a familial disorder. A real division into familial and nonfamilial groups is supported by a different sex incidence which appears to be equal in the familial form, whereas males predominate in the nonfamilial forms. Furthermore, sudden death is much more common in the familial disease. It is possible that obstructive features may develop in any condition causing extreme ventricular hypertrophy associated with long survival. Thus it appears to be most common in congenital cardiomyopathy. Its rare appearance in such conditions as hypertensive heart disease and aortic valve disease is possibly due to the limited "natural history" imposed by other factors such as coronary disease.

Clinical Manifestations. The clinical features and diagnosis of this condition are discussed in Ch. 560.

Natural History. Many patients are apparently asymptomatic for many years. Even those with severe symptoms may undergo a period of remission, and symptoms may remain unchanged over a long period. Prognosis is difficult, but it appears to be less serious than might be anticipated from the severity of symptoms and signs. Sudden death is most likely to occur in the familial form and may occur in asymptomatic patients as well as in incapacitated ones.

Treatment. There is no effective treatment, but longterm medication with propranolol is under investigation. Restriction of physical activity should be advised as this may provoke arrhythmia, and it is known that the pressure gradient is increased by effort. A prolonged rest with sodium restriction or thiazide diuretics may help those with dyspnea or other evidence of heart failure. Digitalis is not advisable. Beta-adrenergic blocking drugs should be beneficial, but long-term results of treatment with these drugs are not available. *Surgical treatment* is indicated for patients with serious progressive symptoms from obstruction. Operative relief by resection of obstructing muscle or myotomy can be consistently accomplished even in severely ill patients, and survivors show striking symptomatic and hemodynamic improvement. Complete heart block is sometimes a complication of the operation, and postoperative left bundle branch block is usual though not invariable, but is not essential for a good result.

Braunwald, E., Lambrew, C., Morrow, A., Pierce, G., Rockoff, S. D., and Ross, J.: Idiopathic hypertrophic subaortic stenosis. Circulation (Suppl.), 1964.
Spodick, D. H.: Hypertrophic obstructive cardiomyopathy. Cardiovasc. Clin., 4:133, 1972.

579.   FAMILIAL CARDIOMYOPATHY

Some forms of primary myocardial disease are perhaps best regarded as congenital cardiomyopathy. These include so-called *idiopathic familial cardiomegaly, obstructive cardiomyopathy* (idiopathic hypertrophic subaortic stenosis), some forms of *endocardial fibroelastosis,* and certain hereditary neuromuscular disorders which also involve the myocardium.

Familial cardiomyopathy may be a single disease entity which presents in a variety of ways, including hypertrophic obstructive disorder (see Ch. 578), congestive cardiac failure, and dysrhythmia. In some cases there is evidence of inheritance as a mendelian dominant, and transmission appears most commonly through the female parent, possibly because males die at a younger age; but there is no evidence of sex linkage. Birth order is not important, as most pedigrees suggest an erratic distribution in the family. It has been suggested that this may be the same disease as the cardiomyopathy associated with familial muscular dystrophies and ataxias, but the history of families with primary cardiomyopathies does not generally reveal other members with neuropathy. However, cardiomyopathy may be apparent before the development of neurologic features in Friedreich's ataxia and in myotonia, and a few families affected by neuropathy have been reported with some members having cardiomyopathy alone. It has also been suggested that familial heart disease is a result of intrauterine myocarditis from an infection such as toxoplasmosis, but the evidence for this is poor. Organisms have not been found in the myocardium in familial cardiomegaly, although inflammatory reactions have been reported, and, on a priori grounds, it is unlikely that latent infection could persist through many generations, or be transmitted through the male as it is in some affected families.

At necropsy the heart is often very large, and heart weights tend to be greater in this condition than those found in other cardiomyopathies. Histologic examination shows giant fibers with vacuolation and varying amounts of fibrous tissue. Electron microscopy and histochemistry show interesting and possibly specific features at least in the variety presenting as subaortic obstructive myopathy.

The symptoms of familial cardiomyopathy include palpitation from arrhythmia, giddy attacks and syncope, either from arrhythmia or after effort in obstructive cardiomyopathy, and dyspnea from varying degrees of heart failure. The age at onset of symptoms is variable, but it is usually between 5 and 30 years. Pregnancy may precipitate heart failure in the last trimester or early in the puerperium, thus leading to an erroneous diagnosis of "puerperal cardiomyopathy." Sudden death in pre-

viously asymptomatic individuals is not uncommon and has been recorded in most writings on the subject. Various arrhythmias have been described in this condition, including atrial fibrillation, atrial flutter, multiple ventricular extrasystoles, and heart block.

As in other cardiomyopathies the electrocardiogram is not specific, but gross conduction defects, left ventricular preponderance, and widespread Q waves are common. Radiology provides no special evidence in diagnosis, but some degree of cardiomegaly is usual, the left ventricle being most commonly affected. The left atrium is selectively enlarged when mitral valve regurgitation is a feature as in some cases. Angiography may show the characteristic appearance of left ventricular outflow tract obstruction in a minority; in others there is ventricular dilatation.

There is no specific treatment for familial cardiomyopathy. Arrhythmias are usually difficult to control. However, the poor prognosis of patients in heart failure may be considerably improved by prolonged rest, a low salt regimen, thiazide diuretics, and indefinite restriction of physical activity. Considerable reduction in heart size may be achieved by these means. Surgical treatment may be indicated when there is dominant left ventricular outflow obstruction (see Ch. 578).

Emanuel, R.: Familial cardiomyopathies. Postgrad. Med. J., 48:742, 1972.
Whitefield, A. G. W.: Familial cardiomyopathy. Quart. J. Med., 30:119, 1961.

580.   INFLAMMATORY OR INFECTIVE CARDIOMYOPATHY (Myocarditis)

The term "myocarditis" should be restricted to inflammatory disease of the myocardium. Clinicians have been reluctant to diagnose myocarditis, but there is no doubt that the myocardium may be damaged in many different infections of viral, rickettsial, bacterial, protozoal, and even metazoal origin. Myocarditis is mainly incidental in the course of a generalized infection and remains relatively unimportant. However, it may dominate the clinical picture and determine the outcome of the disease, and sometimes it appears to be "isolated" with no evidence of generalized infection. Fatal heart failure and sudden death may result from severe myocarditis, but most attacks are probably subclinical or mild and are easily overlooked by the unwary. The long-term effects of such infection may lead to myocardial damage and fibrosis, but such sequelae are difficult to investigate and prove. It is probable that idiopathic myocardial hypertrophy, diffuse myocardial fibrosis, subendocardial fibrosis, and idiopathic cardiomyopathy are in some instances the residue of previously unrecognized acute or subacute myocarditis. Such sequelae may follow any type of myocardial inflammation.

Fiedler's myocarditis is not a specific disease, and the eponym should be dropped. The lesions found in the heart muscle in hypersensitivity diseases, serum sickness, diseases of connective tissue, hypokalemia, and many other states without evidence of an infectious inflammatory nature are not classified here as myocarditis.

Clinical Manifestations.   Clinical manifestations include almost the whole range of symptoms and signs found in heart disease. They clearly depend on the nature of the infection, the severity and site of the myocardial damage, the resistance of the host, the capacity of the damaged myocardium to recover, and other associated factors such as anemia, nutritional status, and the presence or absence of pre-existing cardiovascular disease.

In acute cases substernal discomfort and even pain (possibly caused by accompanying pericarditis) are common. Dyspnea will depend on the degree of damage to left ventricular function. The most frequent physical signs of myocarditis are tachycardia, dysrhythmia, gallop rhythm, and evidence of developing congestive cardiac failure. The electrocardiogram provides good evidence of myocardial damage; it may show evidence of myocarditis before enlargement of the heart is seen on x-ray or before physical signs of abnormality appear.

Viral Myocarditis. Poliomyelitis, measles, mumps, viral pneumonias, encephalitis, infectious hepatitis, psittacosis, choriomeningitis, influenza A, rabies, varicella, and infectious mononucleosis may be complicated by myocarditis, but proof of direct viral invasion is almost invariably lacking. However, during the past decade there have been many reports of *Coxsackie Group B* myocarditis in infants and children, and, as in suckling mice, it was thought that the virus was especially cardiotropic at this age. Coxsackie myocarditis does not produce a specific histologic picture, but interstitial edema, infiltration with mononuclear cells, and areas of myocardial necrosis are usual. The criteria for the diagnosis of a Coxsackie myocarditis, apart from the evidence of myocardial disease, are the isolation of the virus from blood, feces, or throat swabbings, and the demonstration of a rising titer of neutralizing antibodies against the virus recovered from a patient. Pericarditis is the most common manifestation of Coxsackie carditis in adults.

Myocarditis is a common feature in *poliomyelitis* and its prevalence probably varies in different epidemics. Histologic examination may show capillary dilatation and perivascular infiltration with lymphocytes and polymorphonuclear leukocytes, and in some cases the myocardial fibers are necrotic. The lesions are similar to those found in influenza A infection and are probably produced by the direct invasion of the poliomyelitis virus which has been recovered from human heart muscle by transfer to monkeys. Some myocardial damage may be due to the anoxia which occurs in most cases prior to death.

Although many filterable viruses—possibly all of those which cause disease in man—may cause myocarditis, it is probable that other factors which impair myocardial metabolism make the myocardium susceptible to infection. Pre-existing disease, anoxia, digitalis, steroids, alcohol, and electrolyte disturbances are possible determinants. Indeed, it has been shown in laboratory animals that those procedures which reduce the supply of oxygen to the heart result in a high incidence of myocardial lesions in laboratory animals infected with Virus III. Furthermore it is possible that in some viral diseases the mechanism of heart damage may concern biochemical disturbances, lesions of the central nervous system, or autoimmune reactions rather than direct viral invasion.

Bacterial Myocarditis. Bacterial myocarditis rarely if ever occurs in isolation. The incidence of pyogenic myocarditis has fallen with the use of antimicrobials for all bacterial infections. Myocarditis associated with bacterial endocarditis remains an important component of the disease—indeed, late-developing heart failure after cure of the infection is in some cases due to myocardial damage rather than to increased valve disease.

The most important effect of specific bacterial infection is by an indirect action of which rheumatic carditis and diphtheritic myocarditis are the well known common examples. Streptococcal fever may cause a myocarditis (other than rheumatic); diffuse parenchymatous and focal interstitial reactions have been observed. Although clinical evidence may suggest that recovery is complete, it is possible that healing may result in fibrosis which, with hypertrophy, appears as a chronic cardiomyopathy many years later.

Diphtheritic Myocarditis. Diphtheritic myocarditis, although now uncommon, remains the most serious sequel of diphtheritic infection, and is responsible for more than half the deaths from diphtheria. Myocardial cells are primarily damaged, but an interstitial reaction occurs which may be a nonspecific response to muscle death. The clinical picture varies in intensity, and in severe cases the development of hypokinetic failure or severe hypotension carries a bad prognosis. The electrocardiogram shows various abnormalities. Conduction defects are especially common, and complete heart block may lead to Adams-Stokes syndrome.

Toxoplasma Myocarditis. Toxoplasmosis may involve the heart in both its congenital and acquired forms. The organism has been observed in heart muscle in the acquired generalized form and, although myocarditis is usually part of the generalized illness, it may be the presenting and dominant feature of the disease. There are several well documented fatal cases of toxoplasmic myocarditis, the diagnosis being proved by finding the organism on histologic examination or by inoculation of heart muscle into a mouse. It has been suggested that some cases of familial cardiomyopathy are due to toxoplasmosis; pregnancy may reactivate toxoplasmosis in the mother, resulting in fetal infection. It is thus clear that in cases of subacute myocarditis, familial cardiomegaly, or isolated chronic cardiomyopathy, the possibility of toxoplasmosis should be considered although proof is generally unobtainable.

Trichinosis. It is known that the heart muscle may be infected in trichinosis. The parasite may be seen in heart muscle, but this is unusual even in cases in which there has been evidence of myocarditis in life. Trichinosis may be mistaken for rheumatic fever because of arthralgia, fever, epistaxis, and electrocardiographic abnormalities; ventricular ectopic beats are common. These signs of myocarditis may disappear with the administration of corticotrophin or cortisone, which probably suppresses the inflammation after invasion by the larvae which later became encysted.

Trypanosomiasis. The myocardium may be damaged in both the acute generalized and chronic forms of infection with *Trypanosoma cruzi* (Chagas' disease). Interstitial myocarditis and even extensive necrosis of muscle may be found in the acute form. Chagas' disease should be regarded as an essentially cardiotropic infection by the trypanosome. The acute form occurs mainly in infants and children, and the heart is affected in most cases. In chronic cases, arrhythmias and conduction defects are especially common. Sometimes chronic lesions of the heart are associated with megaesophagus, and men between 20 and 50 are more often affected than women. As in other forms of myocarditis, it is probable that the healing process is associated with fibrosis and hypertrophy of undamaged muscle, although even in chronic cases some degree of inflammatory reaction persists.

Giant Cell Myocarditis. Giant cells occur in the granulomas caused by tuberculosis, syphilis, and some fungal infections, but there seems to be a distinct form of giant cell myocarditis unassociated with these conditions. This rare disease affects young adults and affects the sexes equally. An acute onset of heart failure is followed by a rapidly deteriorating fatal course. At necropsy only the heart is affected. The myocardium shows a lymphocytic reaction with occasional eosinophils and a variable number of multinucleate giant cells. The etiology is quite obscure, and there is no known specific treatment.

Treatment. The management of acute myocarditis concerns the causal disease process (if known) and the heart disease per se. The former is dealt with in the appropriate chapters of this book. From the cardiac point of view, absolute rest is indicated for any form of active myocarditis, and rest should be continued until clinical and laboratory evidence indicates that active myocarditis has subsided. Heart failure demands treatment by routine methods as soon as the most minimal evidence appears. A slight elevation of venous pressure, the presence of a gallop sound, or venous congestion on x-ray is an indication for the use of a thiazide diuretic, and a maintenance dose of digitalis should be given providing that there is no electrocardiographic sign of developing heart block. A light diet with sodium restriction is an obvious requirement. Adrenal corticosteroids have a favorable effect in myocarditis associated with rheumatic fever and other hypersensitivity forms of myocarditis, but indications for their use in isolated myocarditis and the infectious forms mentioned above are not clear. However, because occasional favorable effects have been observed, a trial is indicated when activity of the myocarditis is not subsiding with rest or when a life-threatening deterioration develops.

Burch, G. E., and DePasquale, N.: Viral Myocarditis. Cardiomyopathies. Ciba Foundation Symposium, 1964, p. 376.
Case Records of the Massachusetts General Hospital: Giant cell myocarditis. N. Engl. J. Med., 287:296, 1972.
Dilling, N. V.: Giant cell myocarditis. J. Pathol., 71:295, 1956.
Gore, I., and Saphir, O.: Myocarditis. Am. Heart J., 34:827, 1947.
Webster, R. H.: Cardiac complications of infectious mononucleosis. Am. J. Med. Sci., 234:62, 1957.
Wenger, N. K.: Infectious myocarditis. Cardiovas. Clin., 4:167, 1972.
Whitehead R.: Isolated myocarditis. Br. Heart J., 27:220, 1965.

581. NUTRITIONAL CARDIOMYOPATHY

The association of myocardial disease and malnutrition has been recognized for a long time. Several distinct but overlapping syndromes have been described, and it is probable that multiple factors are involved in most cases. Mixed vitamin deficiencies, repeated infection and infestation, disturbed immunologic mechanisms, anemias, hypoproteinemia, hypomagnesemia, and hypokalemia are some known factors, and no doubt there are many unknowns which may cause disturbed myocardial function. Thus exact pathogenesis remains obscure in most cases.

In Africa two distinct syndromes of nutritional heart disease have been recognized. A *form of hypokinetic heart failure occurs in the Bantu,* which is reversible when an adequate mixed diet is given, although in the most seriously affected patients deterioration continues in spite of treatment. At necropsy there are hepatic cirrhosis and patchy fibrosis in the heart without hydropic change. A second form occurs in *kwashiorkor* which is due to protein deficiency in the growing child after weaning, and, as in other severe nutritional disorders, recovery occurs when the condition is treated early enough.

Beriberi causes the most well known form of nutritional cardiomyopathy, but this disease is relatively rare among the more affluent peoples of the world. Beriberi heart disease, although occurring in alcoholics, is perhaps the least common form of myocardial disease associated with alcohol. It has been known for a long time that not all patients with beriberi have a hyperkinetic circulatory state; indeed some investigations have shown that chronic myocardial disease with hypokinetic heart failure is more common. Some confusion arises here from the use of the term "beriberi," which should be restricted to patients with a hyperkinetic circulatory state and with a clear response to thiamin.

Potassium deficiency may cause cardiomyopathy. Myocardial damage and patchy necrosis result in some animals from being fed potassium-deficient diets. Similar abnormalities have been found in man; after chronic potassium deficiency extensive myocardial fibrosis has been found in the absence of coronary disease. A low potassium level should be corrected completely if permanent myocardial injury is to be avoided.

Alcoholic Cardiomyopathy. Perusal of case histories presented in the many papers on noncoronary myocardial disease reveals a frequent mention of alcohol, sometimes ignored by the authors. A causal relation has, however, long been recognized, with varying degrees of conviction, by many writers. It is now clear that there is an association in some patients between a longstanding high consumption of alcohol and the development of cardiomyopathy.

Adult males are most commonly affected, and three clinical syndromes which depend on the dominant derangement of circulatory function at any one time have been recognized. *Cardiac beriberi* (thiamin-responsive disease) is the least frequent and least serious disorder, occurring especially in very heavy beer drinkers (not averse to spirits as well) who have an additional adverse nutritional status for economic, psychiatric, or gastrointestinal reasons. Therapeutic response to vitamin B_1 and withdrawal of alcohol is effective, but relapse occurs on resumption of previous habits. A chronic myocardial fault may be indicated by persistent abnormality in the electrocardiogram. *Arrhythmia*—especially atrial fibrillation—with or without varying degrees of heart failure is probably the most common mode of presentation in alcoholic cardiomyopathy. The ventricular rate tends to be fast, and multifocal ventricular ectopies are common. Fast heart rates, frequent ventricular extrasystoles, cardiomegaly, and abnormal QRS-T complexes in the electrocardiogram distinguish the condition from so-called idiopathic atrial fibrillation. Treatment with digitalis, diuretics, and conversion of the rhythm meets with varying degrees of success. Reasonable health may be maintained if total abstinence is observed, especially when the development of an arrhythmia with accompanying palpitation draws attention to alcoholic heart disease before irreversible damage has been done.

A few patients present with *hypokinetic heart failure,* cardiomegaly, and electrocardiographic evidence of severe myocardial disease. Response to treatment is poor, and an episodic downhill course is usual.

The electrocardiogram in alcoholic cardiomyopathy shows a wide range of abnormality as in other forms of myocardial disease. A normal or nearly normal electrocardiogram strongly supports a diagnosis of beriberi heart disease. There is a fairly close correlation between the degree of cardiographic abnormality and the severity of the myocardial disease as judged by heart size and response to treatment. Mild polycythemia, which is probably a response to low-grade chronic cardiac insufficiency, and low serum cholesterol levels, probably the result of dietary replacement by ethanol, are common findings. Differential diagnosis may be difficult. "Silent" coronary occlusion, "fallen" hypertension, and thyrotoxicosis (because of tremor, atrial fibrillation, tachycardia, and low cholesterol) are common errors.

Necropsy shows moderate left ventricular hypertrophy and small areas of macroscopic fibrosis. Microscopically there are scattered small areas of muscle degeneration, showing fibrosis or recent necrosis with a slight cellular reaction. The histochemical findings show an accumulation of neutral lipid in the myocardial fibers and varying degrees of mitochondrial damage. These findings are nonspecific and indicate a process of chronic myocardial degeneration, the end result of which is cell death and healing by fibrosis. There is some evidence that electron microscopy may show more specific features.

It is clear that there is some causal relationship between a high consumption of alcohol and myocardial disease, but the pathogenesis of the lesion and the nature of individual susceptibility remain obscure. The following theories merit consideration: (1) That alcohol acts as a direct myocardial toxin; however, there is little evidence for this and it would not explain great variation in individual and organ susceptibility. (2) That alcohol exhausts thiamin and resources, but few patients are helped by thiamin therapy, and the clinical features are unlike those of thiamin depletion. (3) That alcohol causes hypomagnesemia and thence hypokalemia; certainly histologic appearances are similar to those produced by hypokalemia, which may be associated with magnesium depletion known to occur in some alcoholics. (4) That alcoholic injury to the myocardium provides conditions for viral invasion. (5) That myocardial necrosis caused by alcohol in one way or another initiates an autoimmune process which is self-perpetuating; however, none of the usual clinical features of hypersensitivity are found.

Cobalt-Beer Cardiomyopathy. A fulminating form of heart failure in heavy beer drinkers was first described in Quebec and subsequently in other cities, notably Omaha and Minneapolis. This curious syndrome, which appeared between 1964 and 1967, has been shown to be due to the addition of trace amounts of cobalt (0.5 to 1.5 ppm) to certain beers as a foaming agent. This condition differs from chronic alcoholic cardiomyopathy in the abrupt onset and severity of heart failure; indeed, cardiogenic shock soon caused fatality in some patients. Polycythemia and pericardial effusion are common features. The mortality for the acute illness seems to be between 15 and 20 per cent. Most survivors have evidence of continuing myocardial disease, although a few appear to make a complete recovery.

Examination of the myocardium from necropsy or biopsy material shows abnormalities of myofibrils, mitochondria, and sarcoplasmic reticulum. Significantly the swollen mitochondria contain particles of a cobalt protein complex. It seems probable that the cardiotoxicity of cobalt is conditioned by previous myocardial injury from alcohol or protein malnutrition, or both.

Treatment. Total abstinence is indicated. A first attack of heart failure should respond well to routine measures, but relapse is inevitable unless rest is prolonged and alcohol avoided altogether. When there is atrial fibrillation, an attempt at conversion by DC countershock after treatment of heart failure, and under anticoagulant therapy, should be made. Excellent recovery, even in patients with longstanding heart failure and cardiomegaly, has been achieved by prolonged bed rest under sanatorium conditions.

Alexander, C. S.: Cobalt beer cardiomyopathy. Am. J. Med., 53:395, 1972.
Brigden, W.: Alcoholic cardiomyopathy. Cardiovasc. Clin., 4:187, 1972.
Burch, G., Walsh, J., Ferrans, V., and Hibbs, R.: Prolonged bed rest in the treatment of the dilated heart. Circulation, 32:852, 1965.
Morin, Y. C., Foley, A. R., Martineau, G., and Roussel, J.: Quebec beer drinkers' cardiomyopathy, 48 cases. Can. Med. Assoc. J., 97:881, 1967.

582. CARDIAC AMYLOIDOSIS

Cardiac amyloidosis usually appears in primary amyloid; it also occurs in some 15 per cent of patients with myelomatosis, and accounts for between 5 and 7 per cent of all forms of isolated noncoronary myocardial disease in adults. The sexes are equally affected. Small amounts of amyloid may be found in perhaps 2 per cent of elderly hearts (in patients over age 60), but cardiac amyloidosis of sufficient severity to cause death from heart failure is a relatively rare disease; however, some 50 per cent of patients with primary amyloidosis die of heart failure.

Pathology. At necropsy the heart weight is usually moderately increased. Any structure in the heart may be the site of amyloid deposition, and the amount may vary from an occasional small nodule or vascular cuff to almost total replacement of the myocardial mass. The pericardium is frequently affected, and small nodules may be seen on its surface. Occasionally both layers are diffusely thickened and gray. Histologic examination may show perivascular amyloid in the small vessels of the epicardial fat. In patients who have died from heart failure, the greatest amount of amyloid is found in the myocardium, both atria and ventricles being frequently affected. The muscle is curiously stiff, and presumably this diminished compliance of the ventricular mass is the main factor in creating the hemodynamic features of restricted ventricular filling which closely resemble those of constrictive pericarditis. Histologically the muscle cells appear surrounded by rings of amyloid apparently deposited on the cell surface or in the perivascular reticulum of the interstitium. In most severely affected hearts the muscle fibers appear atrophic, necrotic, completely replaced by amyloid, or actually transformed into amyloid substance. Hypertrophic fibers, presumably responsible for the increased heart weight, may be seen in less damaged areas. The valves are occasionally affected.

Clinical Manifestations. Most patients with cardiac amyloidosis are over 50 years old, and the sex distribution is about equal. The majority present with insidious heart failure, although occasionally palpitation or syncope resulting from arrhythmia may be the first symptom. Cardiac pain may occur, and when it is associated with the finding of abnormal Q waves in the cardiogram, an erroneous diagnosis of coronary disease may be made. Effort dyspnea is the most common symptom, but it may be conspicuously absent in patients with the "constrictive" syndrome, which occurs when both sides of the heart are equally affected. Paroxysmal nocturnal dyspnea develops when disease mainly affects the left side of the heart. Uneven deposition of amyloid within the heart may affect the clinical features. Thus deposition in papillary muscle and the mitral valve may cause left atrial enlargement and even a mitral diastolic murmur, although murmurs are absent in most cases. Arrhythmia, including atrial fibrillation and nodal and ventricular extrasystoles, and various degrees of heart block are not uncommon. Deposition of amyloid in the lung parenchyma and small vessels may increase dyspnea from heart failure, and possibly cause obstructive pulmonary hypertension.

Diagnosis is helped by finding evidence of amyloid in other organs. Macroglossia and infiltration of the base of the tongue may cause difficulty in speaking and swallowing. Cutaneous manifestations are important from the diagnostic point of view and include purpura, papules, and localized nodular deposits. The central nervous system is usually unaffected, but a few patients have presented with minor degrees of peripheral neuropathy. Hoarseness may be due to amyloid infiltration of the larynx, and biopsy of a vocal cord nodule has led to correct antemortem diagnosis. Although clinical evidence of renal disease is uncommon in patients with dominant cardiac amyloidosis, the kidneys are affected in about one third of cases at necropsy. Diarrhea, meteorism, and gastrointestinal bleeding may result from gastrointestinal amyloid, but this is rare in primary cardiac amyloid.

The electrocardiogram is always abnormal in clinically significant cardiac amyloid. The findings, although not specific, are perhaps more suggestive of the nature of the underlying disease than in most other forms of cardiomyopathy. P waves are often small, and the P-R interval may be prolonged. The most characteristic abnormalities are low voltage of the QRS-T complex, especially in the frontal plane leads, and abnormal Q waves indicating extensive myocardial disease. Both forms of bundle branch block have been reported, and T waves are almost invariably flat or inverted. Cardiac catheterization may show great elevation of both right and left atrial pressures as in other forms of severe myocardial failure. Restricted ventricular filling (probably owing to diminished compliance of ventricular myocardium) and diminished contractility result in low arterial pulse pressures and a low cardiac output. As a reasonably accurate assessment of hemodynamic status can be made at the bedside, there seems little indication for cardiac catheterization, for the findings are not specific. Confirmation of diagnosis is best obtained by biopsy of some accessible part that appears to be affected, but even a "positive" specimen may be misinterpreted or missed because of the variable tinctorial character of amyloid. The Congo red test is positive in less than 50 per cent of the patients in whom it has been performed. Hypoproteinemia and hyperglobulinemia (moderate increase in alpha-2 and gamma-fractions) support a diagnosis of amyloid, but as serum protein studies are abnormal in only 15 per cent of cases they do not provide much help in diagnosis.

The outlook for patients with clinical cardiac amyloidosis is uniformly bad. Progressive heart failure usually leads to death in less than two years. Rest, digitalis, and diuretics may improve heart failure temporarily, but the response is mostly unsatisfactory. Various treatments have been suggested, including large doses of liver, ascorbic acid, corticotrophin, and coritisone, but none has been clearly effective.

Brigden, W.: Cardiac amyloidosis. Prog. Cardiovasc. Dis., 7:142, 1964.
Buerger, L., and Braunstein, H.: Senile cardiac amyloid. Am. J. Med., 28:357, 1960.

583. OTHER CARDIOMYOPATHIES

Endomyocardial Fibrosis. Minor degrees of endocardial fibrosis are common in myocardial disease but this should not be confused with an obscure cardiopathy which occurs commonly in tropical Africa and sporadically elsewhere. It is characterized by extensive endocardial and subendocardial fibrosis. The disease appears to be a specific entity, but its etiology remains unknown. Indirect evidence suggests that it is of an infectious nature, the organism or its vector being responsible for the geographical distribution of the disease (Parry). Malnutrition is not likely to be a factor, for this disease occurs in well-fed Africans, and it has been seen in well nourished expatriates from Africa residing in the United Kingdom.

At necropsy the cavities of either or both ventricles are partially obliterated by dense fibrous tissue which may be organized into a dense white thick lining. Fibrous tissue may bind papillary muscles and chordae to the posterior wall of the ventricle, producing gross mitral reflux.

The clinical manifestations are varied and depend on which ventricle is most severely affected. Insidious heart failure of a "constrictive" type results from uniform biventricular disease. Dominant left ventricular disease may present with symptoms of left ventricular failure with or without severe mitral reflux. A few patients develop severe reactive pulmonary hypertension which dominates the clinical picture. Pure right ventricular disease is not uncommon, and its features have been described by Abrahams (1962). Ascites and hepatomegaly without peripheral edema are usual, the jugular venous pressure is very high, and roentgenography shows an aneurysmal right atrium.

There is no specific treatment. Routine treatment of heart failure may delay the inevitable deterioration which occurs in this extraordinary disease.

Löffler's Fibroplastic Endocarditis. See Ch. 108.

Sarcoidosis. See Ch. 102.

Peripartum Cardiomyopathy (Puerperal Myocarditis). Peripartum cardiomyopathy is probably not a single disease entity. It describes a condition of heart failure arising in the last trimester of pregnancy or the puerperium and is due to idiopathic myocardial disease. It is unrelated to toxemia of pregnancy but may be difficult to differentiate from "silent" pulmonary thromboembolism; however, the heart failure tends to be mainly of left ventricular origin. It is probable that the late stages of pregnancy and/or the metabolic effects of involution in the puerperium in some unknown way have an adverse effect on hitherto asymptomatic myocardial disease. Clinical recovery is usual, but the electrocardiogram usually reveals the continuation of myocardial disease. Furthermore, subsequent pregnancies are likely to be followed by heart failure. No specific treatment is known.

Myocardial Disease and Neurologic Disorders. Friedreich first recorded that the heart was affected in the congenital neurologic disorder named after him. This finding has since been amply confirmed; indeed, some have considered that the disease is as much an affection of the heart as of the nervous system. The left ventricular myocardium is the site of degenerating fibers, interstitial fibrosis, and hypertrophy. The electrocardiogram may be abnormal in infancy before neurologic features appear. Furthermore, the author of these chapters has seen cardiomyopathy without neurologic manifestations in a man whose several adult siblings suffered from ataxia. Arrhythmias and congestive cardiac failure are the usual outcome.

Myocardial disease also occurs in association with the *myotonic dystrophies.* Cardiac manifestations may arise at any time in the natural history of the disease, and arrhythmia is the most common presenting feature.

Boyer, S. H., Chisholm, A. W., and McKusick, V. A.: Cardiac aspects of Friedreich's ataxia. Circulation, 25:493, 1962.

Burch, G. E., and Walsh, J. J.: Postpartal heart disease. Arch. Intern. Med., 108:817, 1961.

Emanuel, R.: Cardiomyopathy and neuromyopathic disorders. Proc. R. Soc. Med., 65:939, 1972.

Parry, E., and Abrahams, D.: The natural history of endomyocardial fibrosis. Quart. J. Med., 34:383, 1965.

Perloff, J.: Cardiomyopathy associated with heredofamilial neuromyopathic diseases. Mod. Concepts Cardiovasc. Dis., 40:23, 1971.

584.　TUMORS OF THE HEART

Primary tumors of the heart are rare but important, because the majority may be cured by surgery. *Myxomas* are the most common; they are benign in the oncologic sense, but malignant insofar as they cause death by obstruction or embolism. *Rhabdomyoma, fibroma,* and *lipoma* are other very rare benign tumors. Malignant *sarcomas* are also rare and may arise from any part of the heart or pericardium.

Myxomas are of special interest not only because they are the most common and can be cured, but also because of their clinical features, which mimic other diseases and pose difficult problems in diagnosis. They may occur at any age. Myxomas arise from atrial endocardium, most commonly in the left heart, and produce features resulting from obstruction, a generalized systemic disturbance, or peripheral embolism. Obstruction at the atrioventricular valves may cause signs resembling mitral or tricuspid stenosis, but because these tumors may move, the symptoms and signs characteristically vary from time to time. Acute transient obstruction may be caused by a change in posture, leading to syncope, and there may be a periodic change in venous congestion of the lung. Occasionally the mitral valve cusps may be kept open in systole, leading to an erroneous diagnosis of valvar mitral reflux. In one patient we have seen the development of severe pulmonary hypertension presumably caused by chronic obstruction of pulmonary veins. Systemic symptoms probably resulting from an abnormal immunologic response to the tumor may sometimes dominate the clinical picture. They comprise vague aches and pains, low-grade fever, anemia, raised sedimentation rate, and abnormal serum proteins. When present, these features may lead to an erroneous diagnosis of bacterial endocarditis or collagen disease. Sudden embolism of a major artery may be the presenting feature, and diagnosis has been made on histologic examination of emboli removed at emergency surgery. Right atrial myxomas may produce signs of tricuspid valve obstruction or recurrent pulmonary emboli and polycythemia. We have seen one with features resembling rheumatoid arthritis and anemia which disappeared after successful removal of the tumor.

The diagnosis of myxoma depends first on the physician's being sensitive to the possibility in a patient with unexplained dyspnea, hints of mitral valve disease without hard evidence, and/or the systemic features mentioned above. Thereafter a firm diagnosis may be readily established by echocardiography and selective angiocardiography; the former shows characteristic echos behind the valve leaflet, whereas the latter is confirmatory in showing an atrial filling defect. Occasionally these tumors develop calcification which may be seen on x-ray.

Treatment is by removal under cardiopulmonary bypass. Successful surgery is followed by rapid resolution of the mechanical and immunologic features.

Metastatic tumors in the heart are much more common than primary ones. Various necropsy series in malignant disease place the incidence between 10 and 20 per cent. Bronchial cancer accounts for one third; breast and esophageal neoplasms are other common sources. Pericarditis with effusion is the usual mode of presentation; indeed, this occasionally provides the first evidence of malignant disease.

Goodwin, J. F.: Diagnosis of left atrial myxoma. Lancet, 1:464, 1963.

Hambling, S. M.: Metastatic cancer to the heart. Circulation, 22:474, 1960.

Hudson, R. E. B.: Tumours of the heart. *In* Cardiovascular Pathology. Vol. 2. London, Edward Arnold, Ltd., 1965, p. 1563.

Selzer, A., Sakai, F. J., and Popper, R. W.: Protean manifestations of tumors of the heart. Am. J. Med., 52:9, 1972.

DISEASES OF THE AORTA

J. Willis Hurst

585.　ELONGATION AND KINKING OF THE AORTA

Medial sclerosis (*Mönckeberg's sclerosis*) is one of the most common disease processes affecting the larger arteries. In this condition the media shows varying degrees of loss of muscular and elastic tissue along with calcification.

The cause of medial sclerosis is not known, but it begins in middle life and increases with advancing age. The abnormality of the media causes the vessels to elongate and is responsible for the firm and tortuous nature of the temporal, brachial, and radial arteries observed in some middle-aged and most elderly people. This process in itself does not lead to occlusion or rupture of a vessel. The disease may be associated with atheromatous changes in the media, which, of course, may lead to more serious complications.

The decrease in elastic and muscular elements of the media, with or without calcification, causes systolic hypertension. The aorta, as well as the visible peripheral

Figure 1. Posteroanterior *(A)* and lateral *(B)* roentgenograms of the chest showing an "elongated" aorta with pseudocoarctation.

arteries, becomes long and tortuous. The abnormality and the medical calcification may be detected on a roentgenogram of the chest. The elongated aorta may simulate an aneurysm. The esophagus tends to follow the course of the aorta because it is bound intimately to it. Accordingly, when the aorta takes an unusual course because of the effects of medial sclerosis, the barium-filled esophagus will be seen to do the same when viewed under the fluoroscope or on the roentgenogram of the chest. The unusual path taken by the esophagus in such cases may simulate posterior displacement of that structure by the heart.

The aortic arch may elongate until it becomes kinked or folded downward in the region of the ligamentum arteriosum. The condition is called *pseudocoarctation.* There may be mild obstruction in rare cases (Fig. 1). This abnormality can resemble mediastinal tumor. An aortogram may occasionally be needed for its identification.

Elongation of the aortic arch combined with similar changes in the brachiocephalic arteries may cause pulsating masses in the base of the neck which simulate aneurysms. This is most commonly found on the right side. Arteriography usually reveals twisting, coiling, or looping of the innominate, subclavian, or common carotid artery. This is sometimes called the *innominate loop.* Once diagnosis is established, the lesion has little significance, but it may rarely result in some deviation of the esophagus or trachea which produces annoying, though not disabling, symptoms.

Robbins, S. L.: Pathology. Philadelphia, W. B. Saunders Company, 1967, pp. 578 ff.

586. ANEURYSM OF THE AORTA

Definition. An aneurysm is a localized or diffuse enlargement of an artery. When one or all of the layers of the aorta make up the sac of the aneurysm, it is called a *true aneurysm.* When the aorta is injured by trauma or infection, a pulsating hematoma may develop owing to destruction of the wall of the vessel. Perivascular clot and connective tissue make up the wall of the enlargement, and the condition is called a *false aneurysm.* A *saccular aneurysm* has a pouchlike appearance and appears to be a sac attached to the side of the aorta. A *fusiform aneurysm* is spindle-shaped and involves the entire circumference of the aorta. The terms *saccular* and *fusiform* are used for clinical designation, whereas the terms *true* and *false* are pathologic designations.

Etiology. Aneurysms of the aorta may be due to atherosclerosis, syphilis, medial cystic necrosis, trauma, infection (mycotic aneurysm), and congenital vascular disease. The discussion dealing with atherosclerotic and syphilitic aneurysms of the aorta will make up the major portion of this chapter. Inasmuch as dissecting aneurysm, traumatic aneurysm, mycotic aneurysm, and aneurysms of the sinuses of Valsalva have many unique features, they will be discussed separately.

Pathogenesis. Although the pathologic processes associated with production of aortic aneurysm are varied, certain factors are common to all. The media of the normal aorta must remain intact in order for the aorta to withstand the systolic blood pressure. When the media is damaged, there is progressive dilatation at the weakened area and an aneurysm gradually develops. Once an aneurysm develops it tends to increase gradually in size, being restrained only by blood clots and scar tissue; hence, there is the likelihood that the aneurysm may finally rupture.

Incidence. The incidence of aneurysms at autopsy is approximately 2 per cent. The majority of aortic aneurysms are found in patients between 40 and 70 years of age, and the incidence is higher in men than in women. Syphilitic aneurysms of the arch of the aorta are still found, but are fortunately decreasing in frequency. Today most aneurysms of the aorta seen in the United States are due to atherosclerosis, regardless of location, even those of the ascending aorta.

Clinical Manifestations. The signs and symptoms depend upon the size and location of the aneurysm. Venous distention and edema of the face, neck, and shoulders may develop when an aneurysm compresses the superior vena cava. Impingement on the trachea and bronchi may produce cough and dyspnea, and compression of the esophagus can produce dysphagia. An aneurysm may impair the function of the recurrent laryngeal nerve and cause hoarseness. A syphilitic aneurysm of the first portion of the aorta may erode the sternum (Fig. 2). Severe pain may occur when a syphilitic aneurysm of the arch and early descending aorta erodes the vertebra and ribs. Death may be the result of hemorrhage into the trachea, bronchi, pleural space, or pericardium. An atherosclerotic aneurysm of the abdominal aorta may cause no symptoms until rupture occurs. The patient or his physician may discover the aneurysm because of a pulsating mass in the abdomen. The aneurysm may cause pain in the upper portion of the abdomen, the lower portion of the back, the groin, and occasionally in the testicles. The mechanism of such pain may be associated with rupture, sudden enlargement, or a small leak into the retroperitoneal space. The pulsating mass, usually felt without difficulty, may extend from above the umbilicus into the pelvis. The mass may be nontender and movable, but tends to become tender and fixed when there has been recent symptomatic enlargement.

A thoracic aortic aneurysm can usually be identified on posteroanterior and lateral roentgenograms of the chest. The pulsation of the mass can be studied during fluoroscopic examination. Pulsations may be absent, however, because thrombosis in the aneurysm may prevent movement. Since some solid tumors located adjacent to the heart appear to pulsate, it is occasionally necessary to resort to aortography in order to differentiate an aortic aneurysm from a tumor. An abdominal aneurysm can often be identified in the ordinary roentgenogram of the abdomen (particularly in the lateral view) because calcification of the aortic wall is frequently present. Aortography may be needed to establish the diagnosis.

Figure 2. Lateral roentgenogram of the chest showing the erosion of the sternum by a syphilitic aortic aneurysm.

Prognosis and Complications. Aortic aneurysm is a serious disease with poor prognosis. According to Estes, one third of patients with atherosclerotic aneurysm of the abdominal aorta die within a year after the diagnosis is made. Three fourths of the patients die within five years after diagnosis, usually from rupture. Kampmeier's study of aneurysms of the thoracic aorta indicated that the average duration of life, after the onset of symptoms, was six to eight months, and De Bakey found that over 90 per cent of patients with aneurysms of the thoracic aorta died within five years.

Aneurysm results in increased lateral pressure, so that the natural history of an aneurysm in the body cavity is one of progressive though highly variable expansion. Rupture is almost inevitable if the patient survives long enough. Patients with aneurysm, however, usually have significant coexisting diseases which modify this outlook. Thus many patients do die of causes other than rupture of the aneurysm with exsanguination. Nevertheless, because the aneurysm is potentially lethal, it is correct to recommend aneurysmectomy in most instances. Naturally, the threat of rupture is greater when the aneurysm is larger. An appropriate dividing line appears to be a transverse diameter of 6 cm. Complications with smaller aneurysm are infrequent except for the fact that smaller ones usually become larger. Turbulence in an aneurysm results in platelet and fibrin thrombi which are a source of peripheral arterial emboli.

Treatment. There is no medical treatment for aortic aneurysms. The discovery of an aortic aneurysm forces one to consider resection of the lesion and replacement by a plastic prosthesis. When an aneurysm of the abdominal aorta is found and the patient has no other recognizable disease, surgical resection is usually possible; the operative mortality is less than 5 per cent in many medical centers. When the patient is older than average, say in the eighth decade of life, or when there is clear evidence of heart, cerebrovascular, renal, or other serious disease, the operative mortality may be 25 per cent or more. It is obvious also that, if such a patient survives the operation, his life expectancy will be less than that of a normal person because of the underlying disease. Generally speaking, then, aneurysms of the abdominal aorta that have a transverse diameter of 6 cm or greater should be surgically resected regardless of symptoms. Aneurysms of the abdominal aorta that are smaller than this must be carefully observed for change in size. Resection should not be attempted for asymptomatic lesions if the patient has associated disease that will shorten his life anyway or will greatly increase the operative risk. The mortality of untreated ruptured aneurysm is 100 per cent. Accordingly, if the aneurysm has actually ruptured or if symptoms suggest that rupture may be imminent, operation should be attempted even though the operative risk is high.

Surgical treatment of aneurysms of the thoracic aorta carries a higher operative mortality rate than that for aneurysm of the abdominal aorta. Even in expert hands the operative mortality is about 30 per cent. A saccular aneurysm can at times be resected at its neck and the wall of the aorta repaired. Fusiform aneurysms are more difficult to resect. The mortality varies with the location of the aneurysm. Although it is possible to resect an aneurysm of the entire aortic arch, the death rate from the procedure is very high. Techniques have been developed that prevent cardiac strain and provide blood to the heart, brain, spinal cord, and kidneys, while the aorta is occluded, using extracorporeal circulation, temporary bypass shunts, and hypothermia. The prognosis of thoracic aneurysm is so grave that one is forced to consider resection of the lesion despite the high operative mortality. Accordingly, if resection seems technically possible and no serious associated disease precludes the procedure, an attempt should be made.

De Bakey, M. E.: Surgical treatment of the diseases of the aorta and arteries. *In* Hurst, J. W. (ed.): The Heart. 3rd ed. New York, McGraw-Hill Book Company, 1974, p. 1666.
De Bakey, M. E., et al.: Aneurysm of abdominal aorta: Analysis of results of graft replacement therapy one to eleven years after operation. Ann. Surg., 160:622, 1964.
Estes, J. E., Jr.: Abdominal aortic aneurysm: A study of 102 cases. Circulation, 2:258, 1950.
Lord, J. W., Jr., and Imparato, A. M.: The abdominal aortic aneurysm. Its importance to the internist. J.A.M.A., 176:93, 1961.
Szilagyi, D. E., et al.: Contribution of abdominal aortic aneurysmectomy to prolongation of life. Ann. Surg., 164:678, 1966.

DISSECTING ANEURYSM

Definition. Dissecting aneurysm of the aorta is really a dissecting hematoma. Blood enters the wall of the aorta and splits the media of the vessel.

Etiology and Pathology. Medial cystic necrosis is usually considered to be the abnormality responsible for dissecting aneurysm. Actually the problem is complex, because dissecting aneurysm may occur when medial cystic necrosis is absent or slight, or, on the other hand, medial cystic necrosis may be found without dissection. The cause of medial cystic necrosis is not known. It is considered by some to be a nonspecific change in the aorta in response to hemodynamic stresses. The disease process is usually most severe in the ascending aorta and decreases progressively toward the distal aorta, but may be extensive throughout the aorta and major vessels.

Dissecting aneurysm and rupture of the aorta can be produced experimentally by feeding growing rats. *Lathyrus odoratus* (sweet pea) meal, which contains B-aminopropionitrile. The rats develop skeletal abnormalities and medial degeneration of the aorta.

Dissecting aneurysm is common in *Marfan's syndrome.* This condition is characterized by severe medial cystic necrosis, which, like the remainder of the syndrome, is genetically determined. In fact, some persons with dissecting aneurysm may appear normal, yet are found in a family group whose other members have typical Marfan's syndrome. In addition, the incidence of dissecting aneurysm seems to be increased in patients with skeletal deformities, e.g., scoliosis, pigeon breast, and funnel depression of the thorax.

The relation of *hypertension* to dissecting aneurysm is not clear. Although hypertension is frequently associated with dissecting aneurysm, it is notable that the younger the patients in a series, the larger is the proportion without hypertension. Some believe that hypertension, by increasing hemodynamic stresses on the aorta, accelerates the development of medial cystic necrosis.

Dissecting aneurysm may occur during *pregnancy;* many case reports are available emphasizing this point. Patients with *coarctation of the aorta* may die of dissecting aneurysm. Dissecting aneurysm has also been reported to be associated with *aortic stenosis* and with *myxedema.*

Atheromatous disease of the aorta is not the direct cause of medial cystic necrosis, although the two diseases may occur together. Occasionally bleeding into the media of the aorta may originate at the edge of an atheromatous ulcer. Syphilis is not the cause of medial cystic necrosis, and the syphilitic process does not prevent dissection in situations in which both diseases occur together. Other lesions, such as an aortic abscess, may initiate dissection of the aorta.

De Bakey classified dissecting aneurysm into three types. Type I begins as a transverse tear in the intima of the ascending aorta and extends distally for a variable distance. Type II is said to be present when the dissection is confined to the ascending aorta. Type III is used to signify the condition when the process begins distal to the arch vessels. When the dissection proceeds distal to the intimal tear it may also involve the branches of the aorta and may re-enter the lumen of the aorta some distance from the origin. (This can produce a double-barreled aorta). Occasionally an intimal tear is absent; this has led to speculation that an intramural hematoma developed because the vasa vasorum ruptured as a result of medial cystic necrosis. Some have extended the reasoning to state that the intimal tear itself occurred because the media supported it so poorly. Braunstein's study refutes this idea and supports the concept that dilatation and hypertension promote the intimal tear by increasing the tension on the intima of the aorta.

Incidence. Dissecting aneurysm of the aorta is far less common but far more serious than myocardial infarction. Men are affected twice as often as women except in the advanced age groups. The peak incidence is in the fourth to seventh decades. Type I dissection is more common than Type III dissection, and Type II is comparatively rare.

Clinical Manifestations. The clinical features and prognosis associated with dissecting aneurysm are determined by the anatomic derangement which characterizes the three types of the condition. Dissecting aneurysm is frequently mistaken for and treated as myocardial infarction. It can be misdiagnosed as pulmonary embolism. In view of the fact that the arteries supplying blood to the brain and cord, the abdominal viscera, and the extremities branch off the aorta, it must be borne in mind that dissecting aneurysm can mimic cerebrovascular accident, acute abdominal crises, or peripheral vascular occlusions. The following points are useful in differential diagnosis:

Pain. Although the majority of patients with dissecting aneurysm of the aorta have chest pain, it is now clear that some do not. Painless dissection occurs especially with Marfan's syndrome. It must be remembered that a severe neurologic deficit, caused by the dissection, may prevent the patient from giving a history of pain. The patient usually experiences severe anterior chest pain, however, and it is for this reason that the condition is frequently misdiagnosed as myocardial infarction. Dissecting aneurysm should be considered under the following circumstances: when the chest pain is excruciating and when considerable morphine is needed for relief; when the pain is maximal at the onset rather than gradually increasing, as it frequently does with myocardial infarction; when the pain radiates to the back or predominates in the back; when the pain is widespread and radiates to the abdomen, legs, head, and neck; and when the pain shifts to a lower level in the body as the dissection extends.

Pain may be the only manifestation of the condition in patients with Type II dissection, whereas patients with Types I and II are likely to have pain plus other physical abnormalities.

Level of Blood Pressure.   Although the patient may have the appearance of being in shock, with anxiety, pallor, sweating, tachypnea, and tachycardia, the blood pressure is elevated in most patients with dissecting aneurysms. This occurs because many patients have hypertension prior to the catastrophic event and there may be an increase in blood pressure during dissection as a result of severe pain. In addition, the heart may function well in such circumstances, unlike myocardial infarction, in which a portion of the myocardium is destroyed. Marked elevation of systemic blood pressure is more common in patients with Type III dissection as compared with those with Type I dissection. Shock levels of blood pressure are seldom observed in patients with Type III dissection but may be seen in 20 per cent of patients with Type I dissection.

Arterial Pulsations.   The carotid, brachial, radial, and femoral arteries must be palpated repeatedly for change in pulsation. Absence or inequality of pulsations is an important clue and indicates arterial occlusion. The degree of pulsation may vary from hour to hour because of arterial spasm. When signs and symptoms of peripheral arterial occlusion occur within a few hours after chest pain, dissecting aneurysm should be considered rather than myocardial infarction, because an embolic episode resulting from infarction is delayed until several days after the onset of chest pain. Alteration of the pulsation of the various arteries is more common in patients with Type I dissection than in those with Type III dissection.

Aortic Regurgitation.   The murmur of aortic regurgitation may be heard in about one third of patients with dissection of the aorta. It is more common in patients with Type I dissection. Aortic regurgitation occurs because the integrity of the aortic ring is altered and because the support of the aortic valve cusps may be destroyed. On rare occasions a peculiar fluttering sound can be heard in diastole, probably caused by a piece of the intima vibrating in the bloodstream during diastole. Chest pain followed by the development of aortic regurgitation should suggest dissecting aneurysm.

Pulsation of the Sternoclavicular Joint.   Pulsation of the right or left sternoclavicular joint may be noted in dissecting aneurysm. This unusual pulsation can also be produced by other types of aortic aneurysms. A rare cause of right sternoclavicular pulsation is an anomalous right aortic arch.

Neurologic Abnormalities.   Neurologic abnormalities are common and result from decreased blood flow to the brain and cord associated with shock or obstruction of the arteries by the dissecting hematoma. Neurologic complications are more often associated with Type I dissection. Coma, hemiplegia, confusion, and visual disturbances may occur. Weakness and even paralysis of the lower extremities may be caused by ischemia of the spinal cord or ischemia of the legs. The weakness may be associated with pain, paresthesia, and sensory and reflex changes in the extremities. Severe chest pain accompanied by severe weakness of the lower extremities should always suggest the possibility of a dissecting aneurysm.

Abdominal Findings.   When abdominal symptoms predominate in a patient with dissecting aneurysm, laparotomy may be performed because of the diagnosis of "acute abdomen." At operation, the bowel, gallbladder, or other organs are found to be ischemic or blood is found leaking into the abdominal cavity.

When the renal arteries are involved, hematuria, suppression of urine flow, and the aggravation of hypertension by renal ischemia may result.

Cardiovascular Findings.   A pericardial friction rub may be noted. Such a finding does not invariably mean that the aorta has dissected into the pericardial space, because a rub may occur when the beads of blood surrounding the injured vasa vasorum of the ascending aorta leak into the pericardial space. (The pericardium encloses a small part of the aorta). Neck veins may be distended because of superior vena caval obstruction or because of bleeding into the pericardial space with subsequent cardiac tamponade. The latter is almost always followed by death. The precordial thrust may be large and sustained because of left ventricular hypertrophy owing to previously existing hypertension. Aortic regurgitation has already been mentioned. The electrocardiogram may show left ventricular hypertrophy, nonspecific S-T and T changes, rhythm disturbances, and pericarditis. Dissection of the coronary arteries may cause myocardial infarction and death.

Roentgenographic Findings.   Enlargement of the aortic shadow is the most common roentgenographic sign of dissecting aneurysm (Fig. 3). Unfortunately the roentgenogram must be made with the patient recumbent because of his critical state. Bedside techniques for roentgenography of the chest produce considerable distortion of the heart and great vessels, thereby making accurate interpretation of a wide upper mediastinum difficult. Progressive enlargement of the aorta over a period of days or weeks may be noted. Occasionally the width of the aortic wall may be identified if intimal calcification is present, thereby marking the internal limit of the aortic wall. When a hematoma is present, the wall thickness is greater than the normal 2 to 3 mm. In many instances aortography may be needed to determine the presence and extent of dissection (Fig. 4). Modern aortographic techniques have assisted in clarifying the clinical spectrum of this condition. The identification of Type III dissection has improved considerably since the development of aortography.

Figure 3. Roentgenogram of chest showing a wide aorta due to a dissecting aneurysm.

Figure 4. Aortogram showing a "double lumen" aorta secondary to dissecting aneurysm.

Laboratory Findings. Leukocytosis may develop in a few hours and may reach 25,000 cells per cubic millimeter. Anemia may develop, and hyperbilirubinemia may occur occasionally. Urinalysis may show erythrocytes, albumin, casts, and gross hematuria because of renal artery occlusion.

Prognosis. Dissection of the aorta is a serious disease and is usually fatal within hours or days. The natural history of dissecting is poorly understood, and this fact makes it difficult to assess therapeutic intervention. In one report (Lindsay and Hurst) of 62 patients, the initial and long-term survival was far better in patients in whom the ascending aorta was spared by the disease process. No patients in this series in whom the ascending aorta (Type I) was involved survived more than 3 weeks, whereas 8 of 19 patients whose disease began distal to the arch of the aorta (Type III) were known to survive 6 to 69 months.

Death is usually due to hemopericardium and cardiac tamponade, hemothorax, hemomediastinum, retroperitoneal hemorrhage, myocardial infarction, shock, neurologic abnormalities, congestive heart failure, renal failure, and, rarely, gangrene of the bowel.

Treatment. The treatment of patients with dissecting aneurysm is unsatisfactory. Pain must be relieved with opiates, blood should be replaced when needed, and oxygen may be administered. Anticoagulants are absolutely contraindicated. Wheat, Palmer, et al. have pioneered in the use of drugs to reduce the arterial blood pressure and pulsatile forces in patients with dissecting aneurysm. Trimethapan, guanethidine, α-methyldopa, and parenteral reserpine may be used to lower the systolic blood pressure to 100 to 120 mm of mercury as quickly as possible. It may not be possible to use such therapy when the blood pressure is already low, when ventricular arrhythmias are present, or when oliguria is present. Propranolol hydrochloride can be used to diminish the force of ventricular contraction and pulsatile force of aortic flow. It may be used alone or with other agents in doses of 1.0 mg intramuscularly every four to six hours. After the acute phase is over, oral medication may be used. This drug produces little change in arterial

pressure and may be quite useful in normotensive patients with aortic dissection and in the long-term management. It is now clear that this form of treatment decreases the degree of pain, may decrease the extent of dissection, and favorably alters the mortality rate.

Operation is not indicated during the acute stages of disease because the risk is prohibitive, although it is occasionally attempted if a limb appears to be dying from lack of blood supply or if there appears to be a slow leak from the aorta. After several days, when the dissection is presumed to be no longer progressing, operation may be considered. On rare occasions the dissection may be well localized, and excision with aneurysmorrhaphy may be possible. A re-entry passage may be created into the true lumen of the descending aorta, and the false lumen can be obliterated by suture. When possible, it seems wise to use some form of excisional therapy and aortic replacement with the use of left atriofemoral bypass perfusion, external bypass graft, or hypothermia. Aortic regurgitation has occasionally been corrected by means of a Starr-Edwards ball-valve prosthesis. The operative mortality experienced by the De Bakey team is about 25 per cent. Follow-up observations for more than five years reveal that many vascular problems have occurred in the group of survivors.

The treatment of dissecting aneurysm is now being studied in many medical centers. The trend in therapy seems toward a combination of drug therapy and surgical therapy. Unfortunately the treatment remains unsatisfactory.

Braunstein, H.: Pathogenesis of dissecting aneurysm. Circulation, 28:1071, 1963.

De Bakey, M. E., Henley, W. S., Cooley, D. A., Morris, G. C., Crawford, E. S., and Beall, A. C.: Surgical management of dissecting aneurysms of the aorta. J. Thorac. Cardiovasc. Surg., 49:130, 1965.

Hirst, A. E., Johns, V. J., Jr., and Kime, S. W., Jr.: Dissecting aneurysm of the aorta. A review of 505 cases. Medicine, 37:217, 1958.

Lindsay, J., Jr.: Diseases of the aorta. *In* Hurst, J. W. (ed.): The Heart. 3rd ed. New York, Mc-Graw-Hill Book Company, 1974, p. 1586.

Lindsay, J., Jr., and Hurst, J. W.: Clinical features and prognosis in dissecting aneurysm of the aorta: A reappraisal. Circulation, 35:880, 1967.

Lindsay, J., Jr., and Hurst, J. W.: Drug therapy of dissecting aortic aneurysms: Some reservations. Circulation, 37:216, 1968.

Lindsay, J., Jr., and Hurst, J. W.: Dissecting aneurysm of the aorta. J.A.M.A., 217:1533, 1971.

Shuford, W. H., Sybers, R. G., Weens, H. S., Lindsay, Jr., and Hurst, J. W.: Aortographic findings in dissecting aneurysm of the aorta. Am. J. Cardiol., 24:111, 1969.

Wheat, M. W., Jr., Palmer, R. F., Bartley, T. D., and Seelman, R. C.: Treatment of dissecting aneurysms of the aorta without surgery. J. Thorac. Cardiovasc. Surg., 50:364, 1965.

TRAUMATIC ANEURYSM

Injury of the aorta may be caused by penetrating wounds or by blunt trauma. Damage to the thoracic aorta may be produced by injuries that do not produce rib fractures. The most common cause of such injuries is automobile, motorcycle, and helicopter accidents.

Ruptures and tears with subsequent aneurysm formation are usually found at points where the aorta is relatively fixed in position—just distal to the origin of the left subclavian artery at the site of the ligamentum arteriosum, and in the ascending aorta just beyond the aortic valve. When a severe accelerative or decelerative force is sustained, the remainder of the aorta moves more freely than the fixed points, producing an injury to the vessel. An injury to the aorta that tears all layers of the aorta causes death, but when the tear involves only the intima it may cause only a hematoma in the media or, on rare occasion, a dissecting aneurysm.

A small leak from the aorta may cause mediastinal hemorrhage, which may be diagnosed by the mediastinal widening in chest roentgenograms. An aortogram should be done promptly if aortic rupture is suspected. When immediate surgery is not carried out, repeat roentgenograms of the chest should be made in such cases in order to detect the appearance of aortic aneurysm, which may become visible in a few days to several weeks. The aneurysm may be noted first on a routine chest film made years after the injury.

Resection is usually indicated for traumatic aneurysms of the aorta. Since this type of aneurysm is not necessarily related to other diseases, the general vascular status in patients is frequently good. Accordingly, the operative risk for the resection of traumatic aneurysms is less than it is for other kinds of aneurysms.

An unexplained aneurysm, discovered on x-ray of the chest, in the region of the left subclavian artery may be the result of old trauma.

De Bakey, M. E., and Crawford, S. E.: Surgical considerations of acquired diseases of the aorta and major peripheral arteries. I. Aortic aneurysms. Mod. Concepts Cardiovasc. Dis., 28:557, 1959.
Goyette, E. M., Blake, H. A., Forsee, J. H., and Swan, H.: Traumatic aortic aneurysms. Circulation, 10:824, 1954.
Symbas, P. N.: Traumatic rupture of the aorta. Ann. Surg., 178:6, 1973.
Symbas, P. N.: Traumatic injuries of the heart and great vessels. Springfield, Ill., Charles C Thomas, 1972.

MYCOTIC ANEURYSM

Myocotic aneurysm of the aorta may be associated with bacterial endocarditis, septicemia, or the extension of a neighboring abscess into the aortic wall. Perdue and Smith have emphasized that patients in the older age group may have mycotic aneurysms at the site of atherosclerotic ulceration or aneurysm of the aorta. Microscopic examination of the vessel wall shows inflammatory cells and destruction of tissue. The offending organisms include streptococci, staphylococci, and salmonellae.

Mycotic aneurysm or suppurative arteritis caused by salmonellae is being recognized more frequently than before. Sower and Whelan have reported that three types of vascular lesions may be produced by salmonellae: (1) a diffuse suppurative arteritis with rupture and the development of a saccular or false aneurysm; (2) a focal arteritis with the formation of a mycotic aneurysm and rupture; or (3) a secondary infection superimposed upon a pre-existing arteriosclerotic aneurysm. A normal vessel can be involved when an infected embolus becomes lodged on its wall, or organisms gain access to the vessel wall through the vasa vasorum. The vessels involved in many of the reported cases have had pre-existing lesions, including dissecting aneurysm, atherosclerosis, and syphilis.

Once a mycotic aneurysm of the aorta has developed, surgical resection offers the only possibility of cure, and prolonged antimicrobial therapy must be provided.

Allen, E. V., Barker, N. W., and Hines, E. A.: Peripheral Vascular Diseases. 3rd ed. Philadelphia, W. B. Saunders Company, 1962.
Perdue, G. D., Jr., and Smith, R. B., III: Surgical treatment of mycotic aneurysms. South. Med. J., 60:848, 1967.
Sower, N. D., and Whelan, T. J.: Suppurative arteritis due to salmonella. Surgery, 52:851, 1962.

ANEURYSMS OF THE SINUSES OF VALSALVA

An aneurysm of one of the sinuses of Valsalva may be due to syphilitic aortitis, bacterial endocarditis, medial cystic necrosis, or a congenital defect. The lesion is described in Ch. 553.

587. SYPHILIS OF THE AORTA

Syphilis is described in Ch. 246. The discussion here is confined to its effect on the aorta (and the heart). Aneurysm of the aorta caused by syphilis has been described in Ch. 586.

Pathology. Although syphilitic myocarditis, gummas of the myocardium, and syphilitic involvement of the coronary arteries are known to occur rarely, it is safe to assume that the aorta is always involved in cardiovascular syphilis. Syphilitic aortitis begins with perivascular inflammation of the vasa vasorum in the adventitia. Treponemas subsequently invade the media via the lymphatics, producing medial inflammation and destruction. The ensuing fibrous proliferation results in intimal wrinkling and the characteristic "tree bark" appearance. It seems likely that many of the lesions of the aorta just described are secondary to changes that have occurred in the vasa vasorum that result in a diminished blood supply to the aorta itself. As a rule, the pathologic process is limited to the thoracic portion of the aorta. Gummatous lesions of the aorta may occur, but they are not common.

Clinical Manifestations. Uncomplicated syphilitic aortitis is difficult to diagnose during life. There are no reliable clinical signs that allow one to make a diagnosis. The majority of patients who have had inadequate treatment of syphilis during its early stages show syphilitic aortitis at autopsy. Diagnosis of uncomplicated aortitis is not based on signs and symptoms.

Syphilitic aortitis may lead to *dilatation of the aorta*. This almost always occurs in the ascending portion, and no symptoms are produced by it. There are no clearly diagnostic physical findings. It has long been said that the second heart sound is accentuated and has a tambour-like quality when there is syphilitic aortitis. Dilatation of the aorta secondary to systemic hypertension or atherosclerosis can also be associated with a loud second heart sound. Since these diseases are far more common than dilatation of the aorta caused by syphilis, the sign is not of diagnostic value. Dilatation of the ascending aorta may produce a nonspecific systolic murmur in the aortic area. Visible and palpable pulsations in the upper parasternal region may be noted. When there is moderate dilatation or aneurysmal formation of the ascending aorta, pulsation of the right or left sternoclavicular joints may be detected (see Fig. 2). When the ascending aorta is dilated, the upper parasternal dullness may be wider than normal.

Dilatation of the ascending aorta may be detected at fluoroscopic examination of the heart and aorta and on roentgenograms of the chest utilizing the oblique positions. Unfortunately, it is not easy to state when the aorta has attained definitely abnormal size. The width of the root of the aorta can be studied far more adequately by angiocardiography. This is not always needed, but it may occasionally be justified. The surest sign of syphilitic aortitis is calcification of the early portion of the ascending aorta (Fig. 5). About one fifth of the cases of

Figure 5. Lateral roentgenogram of chest showing calcification of the early portion of the aorta. This type of calcification is characteristic of atherosclerosis superimposed on syphilitic aortitis.

The surgical correction of aortic regurgitation with the use of a prosthetic aortic valve is discussed in Ch. 561.

Syphilitic aortitis may cause *narrowing of the ostia of the major arterial branches* of the thoracic aorta. There may be diminished pulsation of the carotid arteries, and the blood pressure and pulsations of the upper extremities may be altered (see Ch. 591). Narrowing of the coronary ostia, when mild, causes no symptoms. Angina pectoris in patients with syphilitic aortitis is usually due to a combination of factors, including narrowed coronary ostia, the hemodynamic effects of aortic regurgitation, the increased demand of associated left ventricular hypertrophy, congestive heart failure, and associated coronary atherosclerosis. Angina pectoris in this clinical setting may be more severe and less responsive to nitroglycerin than usual. Myocardial infarction is an uncommon autopsy finding in patients with cardiovascular syphilis, but prolonged chest pain and sudden death are not rare. It is not wise to make a diagnosis of isolated coronary ostial disease caused by syphilis with no other evidence of syphilitic aortitis. Coronary atherosclerosis is so common that it is likely to be the cause of angina pectoris in such cases.

Rimsa, A., and Griffith, G. C.: Trends in cardiovascular syphilis. Ann. Intern. Med., 46:915, 1957.

syphilitic aortitis have the sign. The calcification is actually due to the atherosclerosis of the aorta. Ordinarily calcification of the intima of the aorta caused by atherosclerosis is seen roentgenographically in the aortic knob. The atherosclerotic process seems to increase in the root and ascending portion of the aorta where the syphilitic process is most severe. Calcification of the early portion of the aortic arch may also occur in patients with giant cell arteritis of unknown cause.

Aortic regurgitation, the most frequent complication of syphilitic aortitis, is mainly due to the dilatation of the aortic ring. The syphilitic process also extends into the base of the valve leaflet. The result is separation of the valve commissures and deformity of the cusps. This deformity, plus the dilated aortic ring, produces aortic regurgitation. Aortic stenosis never develops as a result of syphilis, and a systolic murmur in such patients is due to "turbulent" blood flow.

Aortic regurgitation caused by syphilis usually appears between the ages of 35 and 50. Men have the condition far more often than women. It occurs in about half of all cases of cardiovascular syphilis. The murmur of aortic regurgitation may be louder to the right of the mid-sternal area than to the left. An Austin Flint murmur is commonly heard at the apex. The cooing diastolic murmur caused by a retroverted aortic cusp may occur.

The signs and symptoms of aortic regurgitation caused by syphilis depend upon the degree and duration of the abnormality. Symptoms and signs of heart failure are likely to ensue within three to four years after aortic regurgitation is discovered. Heart failure may develop gradually or may be heralded by acute pulmonary edema. Therapy may be beneficial for a time and a few patients survive more than a decade after heart failure has developed, but the majority do not live more than a few years. Sudden and unexpected death may occur in patients with severe aortic regurgitation.

Treatment. The treatment of heart failure is discussed in Ch. 541.

588. THROMBOSIS OF THE TERMINAL AORTA

Thrombosis of the terminal aorta may occur suddenly or may develop gradually, usually on atheromatous lesions. Most often it occurs in males between the ages of 40 and 65, although it has occurred at a younger age.

Sudden thrombosis of the terminal aorta may simulate embolic obstruction when the aortic lumen has been almost normal in size prior to the formation of the clot (see Ch. 589). If sudden thrombosis is superimposed on a partially obstructed aorta, the signs and symptoms may be less severe because collateral circulation has had time to develop prior to the acute thrombosis. Pain and weakness of the lower extremities may occur after sudden thrombosis of the aorta. The pain may radiate to the lower back and inguinal regions. The arterial pulses below the obstructed area are absent. The legs may be pale, mottled, cyanotic, or white, and signs of shock may be present. It may be impossible to differentiate a saddle embolus to the aortic bifurcation from sudden thrombosis of the terminal aorta. When a heart lesion is present that could be the source of an embolus, the diagnostic scale tips in that direction.

When thrombosis of the aorta occurs with normal aortic lumen, the outlook is poor. The treatment is similar to that of saddle embolus. When thrombosis of the aorta occurs in a partially occluded aorta with a better collateral circulation, the outlook may be somewhat less grave. Surgical resection and grafting of the occluded portion of the aorta is usually indicated as an emergency procedure.

Gradual thrombosis of the terminal portion of the aorta has been called *Leriche's syndrome.* This condition differs from sudden occlusion of the aorta and is far more common. The patient feels distress produced by walking and relieved by rest. The discomfort develops in the thighs, hip region, or buttocks and represents intermittent claudication at a high level. Sexual impotence is a frequent associated symptom in male patients. The arterial pulses are absent or decreased in the lower extremities. Feeble pulsations are sometimes found when collateral circulation has developed to a moderate degree. Bruits may be heard over the abdominal aorta and over the iliac and femoral arteries. Atrophy of leg muscles may develop in time. Many patients with Leriche's syndrome have good nutrition of the skin of the extremities because of the adequate collateral circulation that develops when the vascular obstruction is high. In fact, the good prognosis with regard to limb survival should be emphasized. Some patients do have coldness, pallor, cyanosis, trophic changes of the legs, and rarely, gangrene of the feet, but it is likely that the smaller peripheral vessels are also diseased when these signs of arterial insufficiency are present. Many cases of Leriche's syndrome are misdiagnosed as osteoarthritis of the lumbosacral spine or hip, ruptured intervertebral disc, or bursitis of the hip. The majority of these patients die as a result of cerebral or coronary atherosclerosis. Rarely, the renal arteries may become occluded by cephalad extension of the aortic thrombus.

Aortography is not usually needed to make the diagnosis of thrombosis of the aorta. It is useful, however, in determining the site and extent of the obstruction, estimating the collateral circulation, and determining the amount of disease in the distal vessels. The modern contrast media and newer techniques have made aortography much safer than formerly.

The usual conservative therapy for chronic occlusive peripheral vascular disease is indicated. Surgical treatment is indicated when the intermittent claudication is severe enough and disabling enough to justify the mortality and morbidity risk of such treatment. Recognizable cerebral, coronary, and other serious diseases are usually contraindications to operation. Three operative procedures are utilized; thromboendarterectomy, excision with graft replacement, and bypass graft. The operative risk reported by De Bakey is only about 2.5 per cent, and relief of symptoms and restoration of pulses were obtained in 96 per cent of cases. Operation on the aorta of course does nothing to prevent the complications of cerebral and coronary atherosclerosis in these patients.

De Bakey, M. D., and Crawford, S. E.: Surgical considerations of acquired diseases of the aorta and major peripheral arteries. III: Atherosclerotic occlusive vascular disease. Mod. Concepts Cardiovasc. Dis., 29:571, 1960.
Juergens, J. L., Barker, N. W., and Hines, E. A.: Arteriosclerosis obliterans: Review of 520 cases with special reference to pathogenic and prognostic factors. Circulation, 21:188, 1960.
Leriche, R., and Morel, A.: The syndrome of thrombotic obliteration of the aortic bifurcation. Ann. Surg., 127:193, 1948.
Massarelli, J. J., Jr., and Estes, J. E.: Atherosclerotic occlusion of the abdominal aorta and iliac arteries: A study of 105 patients. Ann. Intern. Med., 47:1125, 1957.
Perdue, G. D., Long, W. D., and Smith, R. B., III: Perspective concerning aorto-femoral arterial reconstruction. Ann. Surg., 173:940, 1971.

589.   EMBOLISM AT THE BIFURCATION OF THE AORTA

An embolus lodging at the bifurcation of the aorta is called a *saddle embolus*. Perhaps no more than 5 per cent

of all systemic arterial emboli lodge at this point; but when one does, a true emergency is created.

Large emboli almost always originate in the heart. In patients with rheumatic heart disease who have mitral valve disease and a dilated left atrium, left atrial clots may be the source of emboli. Emboli are more often associated with mitral stenosis than with mitral regurgitation. They occur with higher frequency when there is atrial fibrillation rather than normal sinus rhythm. The presence of heart failure does not seem to increase the frequency of emboli from this source. Occasionally an embolus seems to be related to a change in cardiac rhythm from atrial fibrillation to normal sinus rhythm. An embolus may follow mitral valve surgery. A large, friable, left ventricular thrombus may develop secondary to myocardial infarction, and it may break off and be swept by the blood to the bifurcation of the aorta, where it lodges. This has occurred with decreasing frequency since anticoagulants have been used in the treatment of myocardial infarction. Emboli can occur from such a source a week or several weeks after the myocardial infarction. The presence of heart failure increases the possibility of left ventricular thrombosis and peripheral emboli in such cases. The emboli related to bacterial endocarditis are usually too small to cause a saddle embolus. Rarely an embolus may arise from the systemic veins and pass through an atrial septal defect into the systemic arteries. Thrombi in aortic aneurysms or on ulcerated atherosclerotic lesions of the aorta may be the source of emboli.

Although a rather large clot is required to produce a saddle embolus, the clot need not be as large as the aorta itself. Edema of the aortic wall and intense arterial spasm of the involved collateral vessels occur very quickly after an embolus. These factors, along with secondary thrombosis, can convert a partial block into a complete one.

Clinical Manifestations.   Pain in the legs usually develops suddenly, but may come on gradually. Abdominal or sacral pain may occasionally predominate. Paresthesia, anesthesia, and muscular weakness of the lower extremities may follow the pain or may develop without pain. The clinician must be alert when a patient with reason for peripheral arterial embolus complains that his leg has "gone to sleep." The skin of the lower extremities may be cold, pale, mottled, or cyanotic. Pulsations of the femoral, popliteal, posterior tibial, and dorsalis pedis vessels are usually not felt. Saddle embolus of the aorta must be differentiated from thrombosis of the terminal aorta and thrombophlebitis with associated severe arterial spasm.

It should be emphasized that more distal peripheral emboli may proceed or follow the embolus to the bifurcation of the aorta.

Patients with saddle block embolus frequently die or lose a limb unless embolectomy can be performed promptly. Even with surgical intervention the mortality is high, especially when the embolus occurs subsequent to myocardial infarction. The technique described by Cranley et al., using an "embolectomy catheter" with a balloon, has been employed with moderate success. Heparin should be administered as soon as the diagnosis of arterial embolism is made. Heparin and drugs useful for long-term anticoagulation should be used postoperatively. At times, cardiac valve abnormalities should be corrected surgically when they are thought to be responsible for the intracardiac thrombi.

Cranley, J. J., Krause, R. J., Strasser, E. S., Hafner, C. D., and Fogarty, T. S.: Peripheral arterial embolism: Changing concepts. Surgery, 55:57, 1964.

Crave, C.: Embolism to the bifurcation of the aorta. N. Engl. J. Med., 258:359, 1958.

Deterling, R. A.: Acute arterial occlusion. Surg. Clin. North Am., 46:587, 1966.

Fogarty, T. J., and Cranley, J. J.: Catheter technic for arterial embolectomy. Ann. Surg., 161:325, 1965.

Whitman, E. J., and McGoon, D. C.: Surgical management of aorto-iliac occlusive vascular disease. J.A.M.A., 179:923, 1962.

590. THE AORTA AS A SOURCE OF MICROEMBOLI

Perdue and Smith have emphasized that disease of aorta may be a source of atheromatous microemboli. They report that fragmentation of atheromatous plaques or dislodgment of debris from aneurysm or ulcerated areas in the aorta and larger arteries may cause distal emboli of various sizes. The small arterioles may be obstructed by the particles themselves or by an inflammatory response to cholesterol crystals and subsequent thrombosis and fibrosis.

Autopsy reports have indicated that renal lesions (with or without the acute development of hypertension), acute pancreatitis, and gastrointestinal ulceration and bleeding can be the result of microemboli. When multiple organs are involved, the clinical picture may resemble that of collagen disease.

Cerebral and retinal emboli may be associated with multiple system emboli. Atheromatous emboli to the extremities may simulate primary occlusive disease of the peripheral arteries. An embolic cause is suggested when myalgia and muscle tenderness occur in association with skin changes of lividity, necrosis, and ulceration with or without evidence of associated occlusive arterial disease. Some clinical investigators have concluded that a search for cholesterol crystals in random muscle biopsy may assist one in identifying the exact cause of the occlusive disease.

The microemboli may occur spontaneously, but may also occur when a diseased aorta is manipulated at the time of surgery or after catheter aortography.

Heparin and corticosteroids have been used in some patients with microemboli to the extremities. At times an aortogram is indicated in an effort to find the origin of the emboli. The recognition and treatment of surgically curable lesions eliminates the primary sources and prevents recurrences.

Crane, C.: Atherothrombotic embolism to lower extremities in arteriosclerosis. Arch. Surg., 94:96, 1967.

Haygood, T. A., Fesset, W. J., and Strange, D. A.: Atheromatous microembolism simulating polymyositis. J.A.M.A., 203:135, 1968.

Perdue, G. D., Jr., and Smith, R. B., III: Atheromatous microemboli. Ann. Surg., 169:954, 1969.

591. THE AORTIC ARCH SYNDROME

The term "aortic arch syndrome" is given to a group of disorders leading to occlusion of the vessels arising from the arch of the aorta. (The term "pulseless disease" is often used synonymously with the term "aortic arch syndrome.") The disease may be due to nonspecific arteritis (*Takayasu's disease*). It may be due to the obstructive lesions found in arteries associated with *supravalvular aortic stenosis*. Years ago *syphilitic arteritis* was a common cause of the obstructive lesions of the vessels arising from the aortic arch. Today the majority of patients seen in the United States with pulseless disease are in the middle and older age groups, and the pathologic lesion causing the occlusive disease of the arteries is almost invariably *atherosclerosis*. The signs and symptoms associated with obliterative disease of the vessels arising from the arch of the aorta are predictable when one considers the blood supply of the brain, eyes, face, and arms.

The rare disease known as *Takayasu's disease* has been observed as early as age 11 and as late as age 64. The diagnosis is usually made during the third decade of life. For unexplained reasons, most patients with the syndrome are females. Reports from many countries prove that the condition is not confined to Japan, as it was once thought to be. The clinical features include vertigo; syncope; convulsions; aphasia; headache; transient cerebral ischemia resulting in hemiplegia or hemiparesis; absence of palpable carotid arteries on one or both sides; transient episodes of blindness; amblyopia; rapidly developing cataracts; retinal atrophy or pigmentation; photophobia; optic atrophy; atrophy of the iris; sluggish blood flow in the retinal vessels; decreased intraocular arterial pressure; muscular atrophy of the face; thin pigmented skin of the face; ulcerated nose and palate; claudication of muscles of mastication; decreased or absent audible blood pressure in the arms and increased blood pressure in the lower extremities (hence the term "reversed coarctation"); diminished or absent subclavian, brachial, and radial pulses; decreased to absent blood pressure in arms and legs; claudication of upper extremities; palpable collateral arteries in the neck and intercostal spaces; rib notching; and continuous murmurs in the neck and upper chest. Calcification of the intima of the ascending aorta, aortic regurgitation, angina pectoris, and myocardial infarction may occur. The blood pressure in the aorta may be quite high for several reasons, and yet the blood pressure as measured in the extremities may be low. This multitude of symptoms and signs can be kept in mind if one remembers that they are associated with ischemia of the brain, eyes, face, and upper extremities. Leukocytosis and elevated sedimentation rate are common.

Histologically the lesions are characterized by an arteritis of all layers of the involved vessels with giant cell infiltration and obliteration of the lumen. The pathologic process is usually limited to the innominate, subclavian, and carotid arteries as well as the coronary ostia. It has also been observed to involve the thoracic and abdominal aorta and the mesenteric arteries.

Patients with this syndrome usually die of cerebral ischemia or heart disease. No figures are available to indicate the average length of life after onset of the disease. After the onset of symptoms, patients have lived from 1½ to 14 years. Long-term anticoagulant treatment has been recommended in an effort to prevent arterial thrombosis. Surgical treatment, including endarterectomy, local resection, and vessel grafts, may be applicable in suitable cases.

Cheitlin, M. D., and Carter, P. G.: Takayashu's disease. Unusual manifestations. Arch. Intern. Med., 116:283, 1965.

Judge, R. D., Currier, R. D., Gracie, W. A., and Figley, M. M.: Takayasu's arteritis and the aortic arch syndrome. Am. J. Med., 32:379, 1962.

Kalmansohn, R. B., and Kalmansohn, R. W.: Thrombotic obliteration of the branches of the aortic arch. Circulation, 15:237, 1957.

Shimizu, K., and Sano, K.: Pulseless disease. J. Neuropathol. Clin. Neurol., 1:37, 1951.

Vinijchaikul, K.: Primary arteritis of the aorta and its main branches (Takayasu's arteriopathy): A clinicopathologic study of eight cases. Medicine, 43:15, 1967.

592. RHEUMATOID AORTITIS

Aortitis may be recognized in a small percentage of patients with rheumatoid arthritis. A rheumatoid etiology for aortic regurgitation is especially likely when there is rheumatoid spondylitis, uveitis, or psoriasis. Complete heart block may occur when the atrioventricular conduction tissue in the heart is involved by the disease process. Heart failure may result from the aortic regurgitation. When the murmur of aortic regurgitation develops during an exacerbation of rheumatoid arthritis, particularly in the presence of uveitis, it is considered to be diagnostic of rheumatoid aortitis and aortic valve disease. Aortic regurgitation caused by rheumatoid aortitis and aortic valve disease is differentiated from syphilitic heart disease when the serologic tests for syphilis are negative and when the murmur occurs at an early age in a patient with rheumatoid arthritis.

Although the clinical features of rheumatoid aortitis and aortic valve disease are similar to the findings in rheumatic heart disease, the pathologic findings are more distinctive. The cusps of the aortic valve do not fuse at the commissures as they do in rheumatic aortic valve disease. Plaquelike lesions of the aortic intima near the valve commissures found in rheumatoid aortitis have not been observed in rheumatic fever. The lesions in the aorta usually do not extend beyond the ascending portion of the vessel. The entire clinical and pathologic picture forces one to support the idea that rheumatoid aortitis is a specific complication of rheumatoid arthritis.

When surgical treatment for aortic regurgitation is deemed necessary in patients with rheumatoid spondylitis, the newest surgical techniques, including the placement of a Starr-Edwards prosthetic valve, can be utilized. A cardiac pacemaker may be needed for heart block.

Clarke, W. S., Kulka, J. P., and Bauer, W.: Rheumatoid aortitis with aortic regurgitation; An unusual manifestation of rheumatoid arthritis (including spondylitis). Am. J. Med., 22:580, 1957.

Cobbs, B. W., Jr.: Clinical recognition and medical management of rheumatic heart disease and other acquired valvular disease. In Hurst, J. W. (ed.): The Heart. 3rd ed. New York, McGraw-Hill Book Company, 1974, p. 826.

Graham, D. C., and Smythe, H. S.: The carditis and aortitis of ankylosing spondylitis. Bull. Rheum. Dis., 9:171, 1958.

593. OTHER CAUSES OF AORTITIS

Aortitis may develop in association with a variety of conditions. These include scleroderma and Hodgkin's disease.

Giant cell arteritis may involve the aorta and produce the aortic arch syndrome, aneurysm of the ascending aorta, aortic regurgitation, and dissecting aneurysm. This condition is being recognized with increasing frequency.

Behçet's syndrome, consisting of mouth and genital ulcerations, blindness, central nervous system involvement, thrombophlebitis, and arterial involvement, may be associated with aortic aneurysms.

Austin, W. G., and Blennerhassett, J. B.: Giant cell aortitis causing an aneurysm of the ascending aorta and aortic regurgitation. N. Engl. J. Med., 272:80, 1965.

Fraumeni, J. F., Jr., Herweg, J. C., and Kissane, J. M.: Panaortitis complicating Hodgkin's disease. Ann. Intern. Med., 67:1242, 1967.

Hills, E. A.: Behçet's syndrome with aortic aneurysms. Br. Med. J., 4:152, 1967.

Hunder, G. G., Ward, L. E., and Burbank, M. K.: Giant-cell arteritis producing an aortic arch syndrome. Ann. Intern. Med., 66:578, 1967.

Roth, L. M., and Kissane, J. M.: Panaortitis and aortic valvulitis in progressive systemic sclerosis (scleroderma). Am. J. Clin. Pathol., 41:287, 1964.

594. CONGENITAL ANOMALIES OF THE AORTA

A right aortic arch may occur as an isolated and asymptomatic abnormality. It may produce pulsation of the right sternoclavicular joint and is usually identified on the chest roentgenogram. The anomaly may be associated with other cardiovascular defects. For example, 25 per cent of patients with tetralogy of Fallot and truncus arteriosus and 5 per cent of patients with tricuspid atresia have the aortic arch on the right side.

The right subclavian artery may arise from the descending aorta (*aberrant right subclavian artery*). The anomaly may be unassociated with other abnormalities, but an association with tetralogy of Fallot has been reported. The vessel passes posterior to the esophagus and for this reason is usually identified by observing an indention of the barium-filled esophagus during fluoroscopy. This anomaly is occasionally associated with a large aneurysmal diverticulum of the aorta (*Kommerell's diverticulum*). An aberrant right subclavian artery is found in approximately 1 per cent of routine barium studies of the esophagus. It is almost always asymptomatic but has been claimed to cause dysphagia on rare occasions. Aneurysmal dilatation and rupture of an aberrant subclavian artery have been reported.

A number of vascular anomalies of the aortic arch may contrive to encircle the esophagus and trachea and produce a *vascular ring*. Although many varieties of rings are possible, the two common types are *double aortic arch* and *right aortic arch with retroesophageal segment with a left-sided ligamentum arteriosum*. Vascular rings may produce noisy respiration, brassy cough, recurrent pulmonary infections, and dysphagia during early life. Infants may be more comfortable with the neck hyperextended. The vascular abnormality may be suspected in a routine roentgenogram of the chest if the air column of the trachea is constricted at the proper location. More often the condition is identified by fluoroscopic examination of the barium-filled esophagus. More exact delineation of the vessels can be accomplished by aortography (Fig. 6). When obstructive lesions are severe, surgical correction is indicated.

Atresia of the aortic arch may be the cause of heart failure during the first few days of life. In fact, heart failure at this age is a clue to the diagnosis. Death usually occurs in a few days to weeks. On rare occasions pulmonary arteriolar disease protects the lungs and prolongs survival time. The atretic area is usually located be-

Figure 6.   Angiocardiogram showing double aortic arch.

tween the left common carotid artery and the ductus arteriosus. Arterial unsaturation is found in the lower extremities.

Supravalvular aortic stenosis may be misdiagnosed as ordinary valvular aortic stenosis. This less common condition occasionally occurs as a familial trait and is characterized by unusual facies, occasional mental retardation, a pressure difference in the two arms (lower in left arm), obstructive lesions of the vessels arising from the aortic arch (including obstruction of the coronary arteries), associated pulmonary stenosis, multiple pulmonary artery stenoses, and hypercalcemia, in addition to the murmur of aortic obstruction. Surgical correction of this condition is not entirely satisfactory since multiple abnormalities may be present.

COARCTATION OF THE AORTA

This is described in Ch. 552.

Blake, H. A., and Manion, W. C.: Thoracic arterial arch anomalies. Circulation, 26:251, 1962.
Brinsfield, D. E., and Wedwards, F. K.: Clinical recognition and medical management of congenital heart disease. *In* Hurst, J. W. (ed.): The Heart. 3rd ed. New York, McGraw-Hill Book Company, 1974, p. 683.
Stewart, J. R., Kincaid, O. W., and Edwards, J. E.: An Atlas of Vascular Rings and Related Malformation of the Aortic Arch System. Springfield, Ill., Charles C Thomas, 1964.

594a.   TUMORS OF THE AORTA

Primary malignant tumors of the aorta may present a clinical picture suggesting herniated nucleus pulposus, renal colic, peripheral vascular disease, coarctation of the aorta, or Leriche's syndrome. The tumor may originate in the arch of the aorta or thoracic aorta but may originate in the thoracoabdominal aorta or abdominal aorta. The tumors, which may be spindle cell sarcoma, giant cell sarcoma, malignant endothelioma, fibromyxosarcoma, or leiomyosarcoma, metastasize widely to the kidney, spleen, vertebra, mesentery, skin, and pleura.

Hypertension, which may begin abruptly, has occurred in about a quarter of the patients.

The medical and surgical management of patients with malignant tumors of the aorta is quite limited, and death usually occurs a short while after the first symptoms appear.

Stevenson, J. E.: Primary malignant tumor of the aorta. Am. J. Med., 51:555, 1971.

DISEASES OF THE PERIPHERAL VESSELS

Jay D. Coffman

595.   PERIPHERAL VASCULAR DISEASES DUE TO ORGANIC ARTERIAL OBSTRUCTION

ARTERIOSCLEROSIS OBLITERANS

Definition.   Arteriosclerosis obliterans is caused by arteriosclerotic narrowing or obstruction of large and medium-sized arteries supplying the extremities; symptoms and signs are produced by ischemia.

Etiology.   The etiology of arteriosclerosis is discussed in Ch. 723.

Incidence.   Arteriosclerosis obliterans is the leading cause of obstructive arterial disease of the extremities after age 30. The lower extremities are involved most commonly; the superficial femoral artery is affected by stenosis or obstruction in approximately 90 per cent of patients. The aortoiliac and popliteal areas are the next most common sites. The greatest incidence of superficial femoral and more distal arterial disease occurs in the seventh decade, but aortoiliac disease has its peak a decade earlier. The disease is more common in males than in females, especially before the menopause (about 9:1). Patients with diabetes mellitus develop arteriosclerosis obliterans more frequently and at an earlier age than nondiabetics. Diabetics have the same incidence of femoropopliteal disease but a greater frequency of vessel involvement between the knee and ankle than nondiabetics. In patients with isolated aortoiliac disease, high plasma cholesterol and total lipids are frequent findings, but diabetes mellitus is not.

Pathology.   It should be emphasized that the stenotic or occlusive process is usually segmental, for surgical therapy depends on this characteristic; however, the intima also displays widespread arteriosclerotic changes proximal and distal to the segmental lesion. Although the occlusive or stenotic lesions causing symptoms are usually proximal to the knee, the incidence of lower leg arterial occlusions is high (45 per cent in some surveys) and rises steeply with increasing age. Of the vessels in the calf, the posterior tibial artery is most often affected. A specific lesion of arteriolar and capillary endothelial proliferation has been described in diabetes by some investigators but has not been found by others. In patients with diabetes the development of indolent ulcers in the presence of adequate pulses may be due to diabetic neuropathy and not to small vessel disease.

Pathophysiology. Symptoms and signs are produced by inadequate oxygenation of the tissues distal to the arterial lesion, secondary to the decrease in blood flow or pressure at rest or during exercise. Large and medium-sized arteries must have a decrease in cross-sectional area of 70 to 90 per cent before a decrease in blood flow or pressure occurs at rest; during exercise a 60 per cent decrease may suffice. The critical stenosis diameter which decreases flow or pressure is dependent on the velocity of flow and therefore the peripheral resistance; the length of the stenotic segment has a lesser effect. Factors affecting peripheral resistance are discussed below. In patients who develop ischemic symptoms only during exercise, the calf blood flow may be normal at rest; however, during exercise the blood flow may stop or be abnormally slow. The decreased blood pressure in the artery distal to the obstructing lesion allows the force of the contracting muscle during exercise to partially or completely obstruct arterial flow. Also, if full vasodilatation (reactive hyperemia) is produced in an involved limb, the total blood flow is usually much less than in the normal limb.

Although all the vessels of a system contribute to its total resistance, the arterioles and precapillary sphincters are of greatest importance. Peripheral resistance is regulated reflexly by the sympathetic nervous system and locally by the formation of vasodilator metabolites. Activity of the sympathetic nervous system usually causes cutaneous vasoconstriction, thereby increasing peripheral resistance. This normal activity, i.e., reflex vasoconstriction when exposed to cold, can be harmful to an ischemic extremity. Removal of vasoconstrictor activity in an extremity results in vasodilatation. Blood vessels in skeletal muscle also are affected by sympathetic activity but only to a very limited extent during exercise when vasodilator metabolites are active.

Blood supply to the limb distal to an obstructing or stenotic arterial lesion is via collateral blood vessels. Most of these collaterals are present in the normal limb but unused until an obstruction occurs; many appear almost immediately after an acute arterial occlusion, but others form more gradually over a period of months. Little is known concerning the reactivity of the collateral vessels in man; in animals, exercise and systemic blood pressure elevation decrease collateral vessel resistance, whereas a decrease in systemic blood pressure increases collateral vascular resistance. Blood flow can be increased through collateral vessels in man by raising the systemic blood pressure.

Clinical Manifestations. The most common symptom of arteriosclerosis obliterans is *intermittent claudication* (intermittent limping). The patient experiences cramping pain, tightness, numbness, or severe fatigue in the muscle group being exercised. The amount of exercise producing the pain is relatively constant in each patient, and the pain is relieved promptly by rest. In a few patients, pain may disappear on further walking, perhaps because of an unconscious slowing of gait. Intermittent claudication is most frequent in the calf muscles because femoral artery disease is so common. However, even in more proximal lesions (aortoiliac disease) the calf is the most common site of claudication because these muscles do the most work in walking. Low back, buttock, thigh, and foot claudication may also occur; the site of the symptoms localizes the obstructing lesion proximally.

Rest pain is the other important symptom of obstructive arterial disease. Rest pain is a grave sign indicating that the blood supply is not sufficient even for the small nutritional requirements of the skin. It may be localized to one or more toes but often has a stocking distribution. The latter distribution means that ischemic neuritis is not usually the cause of rest pain. Rest pain is worse at night and is relieved somewhat by dependency and by cooling.

Other symptoms of arteriosclerosis obliterans include coldness, numbness, paresthesias, and color changes in the involved extremity.

Examination of the patient with intermittent claudication reveals diminished or absent pulses below the site of obstruction. Although the dorsalis pedis pulse may be absent congenitally in more than 10 per cent of people, the posterior tibial pulse is absent in only 2 per cent, and both pulses in approximately 0.5 per cent. If pulses are palpable in the presence of an obstructive lesion, exercise will make the pulses disappear; this is often a valuable diagnostic test. If pulses cannot be detected with the fingertips, an oscillometer is often useful. The oscillometer gives a qualitative measure of the pulse beneath a blood pressure cuff. It will reveal pulsations in the presence of edema and obesity when vessels are too deep to be palpated, and sometimes when vasospasm rather than complete obstruction is present. Marked differences in oscillometric readings between two limbs at symmetrical positions or between different levels on the same limb are important. The second important part of the examination is to listen with the stethoscope over the aorta and peripheral arteries. The presence of a systolic or continuous bruit indicates a proximal obstructive or stenotic lesion; a continuous bruit denotes a very low diastolic pressure distal to the obstruction and therefore an inadequate collateral blood flow.

Examination may also reveal signs of ischemia. Distal to an arterial obstruction, the limb is often cool when compared with the proximal part of the same extremity or the symmetrical part of the opposite extremity. Skin temperature may vary widely in health, and even profound coldness, if present in all extremities, particularly in a cool environment, may be physiologic. Severe coldness that persists in a warm environment is usually abnormal, and, if unilateral, definitely abnormal. A warm extremity with normal color but absent pulses means collateral blood flow is adequate. The involved extremity may also show color changes: pallor, owing to a markedly decreased blood flow; cyanosis, caused by a diminution in blood flow not sufficient to cause blanching of the skin; rubor, a persistent red or reddish-blue discoloration of a cold extremity secondary to persistent dilatation of the cutaneous capillaries and venules owing to injury from anoxemia. Trophic changes may develop: the subcutaneous tissue becomes puffy and thickened; the skin becomes dry, atrophic, shiny, and tightly drawn with an absence of hair; and the toenails become hard, brittle, thickened, ridged, and deformed. Indolent ulceration and gangrene indicate severe local ischemia. Ischemic ulcers on the toes, and sometimes over the anterior and lateral lower calf, are usually quite painful and sensitive.

Isolated aortoiliac disease (Leriche's syndrome) produces a characteristic picture. Intermittent claudication of the low back, buttock, thighs, or calves may be present. Global atrophy of the limbs and pallor of the legs and feet are frequent findings. Other trophic changes are usually absent; if present, concomitant femoropopliteal disease is often found. Hypertension may be present in the upper extremities; impotence has been emphasized as a symptom but is not frequent. All pulses are usually absent in the legs, but weak femorals may be felt if the collateral circulation is well developed or if the occlusive process is only partial. A systolic murmur is often heard over both femoral arteries and lower abdomen.

Diagnosis. By careful palpation of pulses and auscultation for bruits, the diagnosis and site of obstruction or stenosis are easily determined in most patients. The presence of coldness, discoloration, and trophic changes indicates the degree of ischemia. A triad of tests can be used to evaluate the degree of ischemia and collateral circulation. With the patient supine, the involved limb is raised to a 45 degree angle. Normally the plantar surface remains pink; pallor indicates a deficient blood supply. If pallor occurs only after ankle exercise, the circulation is not as compromised. Then the patient sits up quickly, allowing the extremities to assume a dependent position, and flushing and filling of the veins of the feet are timed. Flushing should occur immediately; veins should fill in about 10 seconds. Flushing and venous filling times of greater than 20 and 30 seconds, respectively, denote a severely ischemic limb with inadequate collateral circulation. These tests should be performed in a warm room to rule out vasospasm; varicosities invalidate the venous filling time. The use of a Doppler to measure systolic blood pressure in the dorsalis pedis and posterior tibial arteries with the pneumatic cuff on the thigh and then at the ankle is especially helpful in diagnosing obstructive disease (the pedal pressures should be equal to or higher than the brachial artery pressure) and its site. A pressure less than 30 mm Hg indicates very severe ischemia and often presages gangrene.

The presence or absence of calcification by x-ray of the extremities is usually meaningless. *Arteriography* may be necessary if the diagnosis is in doubt. It is always performed if surgery is being considered to reveal the exact location and extent of the obstructive lesion and the collateral circulation. In doubtful cases, an exercise test may be performed while blood flow is measured by the disappearance of a radioisotope (^{131}I, ^{133}Xe) from the involved muscle. During exercise the disappearance rate either stops or is abnormally slow in claudicators compared with that in normal subjects. The postexercise disappearance rates are also usually abnormal in obstructive arterial disease. Postexercise or postischemic flow can also be measured with a plethysmograph, but there is some overlap of values between claudicators and normal persons. A variety of equipment has been used to demonstrate the small, rounded pulse with a slow upstroke and downstroke and absent dicrotic notch, or to show the decrease in systolic pressure below an obstructing or stenotic lesion. These tests can be valuable, but it is important that the "normal ranges" are first established for the particular combination of methods or procedures used.

Intermittent claudication may occur in *severe anemia* and in *McArdle's syndrome;* both are easily distinguished from arteriosclerosis obliterans by the presence of normal pulses. The pain of *arthritis* may radiate to the thighs or calves, but is present at rest and not usually worse with exercise. *Arterial embolism* pain does not develop as insidiously as arteriosclerotic ischemic symp-

toms. In occasional patients with *lumbar disc, spinal canal, or cauda equina disease,* pain may occur only with exercise; also vasospasm may be intense so that distal pulses cannot be felt. Usually neurologic signs are present or appear with exercise. Even large vessel pulsations may disappear in patients taking *vasoconstrictive drugs* (see Ergotism and Methysergide Toxicity in Ch. 596); patients should be carefully questioned concerning the use of these drugs.

Ischemic ulcers resulting from arteriosclerosis obliterans must be differentiated from ulcers that occur in patients with hypertension *(Hines' ulcers).* In hypertensive ischemic ulcers, pulses in the leg and foot are normal, and signs of ischemia are absent elsewhere in the extremity. The hypertensive ulcer is most commonly located on the lateral aspect of the leg or ankle, but arteriosclerotic ulcers are usually on the toes. Hypertensive ulcers are more common in females and are extremely painful. They begin as a purplish plaque which develops into a hemorrhagic bleb; the bleb then ulcerates, leaving a lesion with purplish red margins.

Prognosis. Often intermittent claudication is the first symptom of generalized arteriosclerotic vascular disease, and most patients die eventually from myocardial infarctions or cerebrovascular accidents. Seventy to 90 per cent of patients with femoral artery disease remain stable in their symptoms or improve over a nine-year follow-up period. If diabetes mellitus is present, the prognosis is grave, for progression of the disease almost always occurs. The prognosis after surgical revascularization appears good in large vessel (aortic or femoral artery) disease.

Treatment. If the patient has only intermittent claudication with a normal-appearing limb, he should be treated conservatively. He will be able to walk farther without pain if he slows his gait and loses excess weight. Tobacco should never be used in any form, for it causes cutaneous vasoconstriction via the sympathetic nervous system. The patient is advised to exercise frequently to the development of pain but to rest until the pain totally disappears. It is hoped that exercise will stimulate further growth of collateral blood vessels, but proof is lacking for this point. Although studies are not yet available to demonstrate that treatment of the common forms of hyperlipoproteinemias (Types 2 and 4) will prevent or improve arteriosclerotic lesions, they may be a contributing factor and should be sought and treated if present (see Ch. 819). Patients should protect their limbs from cold or trauma; careful attention to keep the skin scrupulously clean, dry, and soft is important. Even minor infections such as the dermatophytoses may produce problems. Toenail trimming should be done regularly and with care.

If the claudication is found to be progressively worse over a six-month to two-year observation period, if it interferes seriously with the patient's daily activity, or if even minor ischemic symptoms such as numbness or paresthesias are present, *surgery* should be considered. Since the lesion is often localized and segmental, restoration of circulation beyond segmental stenotic or obstructive areas by graft bypass or thromboendarterectomy is the treatment of choice. Currently autogenous saphenous vein grafts are used most frequently because the incidence of thrombosis is less than with grafts made of synthetic materials. Often patch grafts are used on one portion of the vessel. Thromboendarterectomy is performed when there is minimal medial and adventitial involvement of the artery by the sclerotic process. Bypass grafts are favored over excision and graft replacement, because collateral circulation is not destroyed with the bypass method. Before a grafting procedure can be performed, arteriography must be done to determine that there are patent vessels below the obstruction ("good runoff"). However, connection of a graft to an "isolated" popliteal segment (no calf vessels patent) may produce good results with healing of trophic lesions. Vein grafts have been connected to distal arteries in the lower calf and foot in attempts to save ischemic, even gangrenous, feet. In patients with aortoiliac disease who cannot undergo major surgery, subcutaneous axillofemoral or, if one femoral is patent, femorofemoral grafts have been a very successful innovation. In patients with more than one obstructing lesion in the vessels supplying an extremity, correction of the most proximal obstruction often produces relief of symptoms. The success of a surgical attack on involved vessels is proportional to the size of the vessel involved; aortoiliac operations have a 90 per cent or better success rate; femoropopliteal, 70 to 80 per cent; and posterior tibial artery, 50 per cent.

If surgery cannot be performed because of poor runoff or other serious disease, and rest pain or gangrene is present, rest in bed is essential. The affected extremity should be kept 20 to 30 degrees below the horizontal, for the dependent position increases blood flow and pressure and occasionally is the only position the patient can tolerate. If edema is present, the extremity should be kept horizontal but never elevated. External local warmth, if used at all, is best applied by means of a thermoregulated cradle kept at a temperature below 38° C (100.4° F). Direct application of external heat should never be used, because ischemic tissue blisters and burns at much lower temperatures than normal tissue. Rest pain may require the use of aspirin, phenobarbital, propoxyphene (Darvon), pentazocine (Talwin), or even narcotics. Ulcers caused by ischemia are treated the same as rest pain; warm saline soaks should be used to keep the ulcer open, moist, and clean. Enzymatic debridement is not advised because of possible local allergic reactions. If infection is present, the appropriate systemic and local antimicrobial drug should be used as determined by culture and sensitivity tests.

Preganglionic lumbar sympathectomy may be performed to increase skin blood flow when ulcers, rest pain, or small areas of gangrene are present. Before surgery, it must be demonstrated that the sympathetic nervous system is intact in the extremity, especially in diabetics in whom peripheral neuropathy sometimes produces an autosympathectomy. To assess sympathetic activity in an extremity, plethysmographic foot blood flow, toe pulse, or skin temperature may be measured before and after a procedure to remove sympathetic activity. Methods used to remove sympathetic activity are (1) a warm environment, (2) local anesthesia of sympathetic ganglia, (3) local anesthesia of appropriate mixed nerves, (4) spinal anesthesia, or (5) autonomic blocking agents. An increase in the parameter being measured after one of these procedures indicates that a sympathectomy may be beneficial. Sweating of the involved extremity is also an indication of sympathetic activity. Although superficial ulcers often heal after the operation, sympathectomy alone rarely improves intermittent claudication.

Arteriosclerotic *gangrene* often necessitates *amputation* of the limb. In the presence of gangrene with ascending infection (advancing lymphangitis, fever, and leukocytosis), antimicrobial chemotherapy is indicated. Prompt amputation must be considered, because the efficacy of the antimicrobial agents may be limited by the ischemia of the affected tissues and by local necrosis. The level of amputation is determined by palpable pulses and the presence of warm viable tissue of good color. The percentage of patients who become ambulatory after amputation is much higher with below-the-knee than above-the-knee operations.

Vasodilator drugs and agents are widely advertised but have little, if any, place in the treatment of arteriosclerosis obliterans. They are consistently ineffective in relieving intermittent claudication but may increase muscle or skin blood flow at rest in some patients. The efficacy of drugs with prolonged vasodilator action depends upon the degree to which structural disease has rendered the peripheral arteries rigid and incapable of dilatation; it has yet to be shown that they are active on the collateral vessels. Vasodilator drugs often lower systemic blood pressure so that flow to the ischemic limb may be decreased; even intra-arterial administration has been shown to decrease foot flow in some patients.

Long-term anticoagulation has also been recommended for treatment of arteriosclerosis obliterans, but conflicting results have been reported. Fibrinolytic therapy with intravenous streptokinase has been evaluated for chronic arterial occlusive disease, and a few patients, especially those with a recent onset of symptoms, have benefited.

Coffman, J. D.: Peripheral collateral blood flow and vascular reactivity in the dog. J. Clin. Invest., 45:923, 1966.

Coffman, J. D., and Mannick, J. A.: An objective test to demonstrate the circulatory abnormality in intermittent claudication. Circulation, 33:177, 1966.

Coffman, J. D., and Mannick, J. A.: Failure of vasodilator drugs in arteriosclerosis obliterans. Ann. Intern. Med., 76:35, 1972.

Cooke, T. D. V., and Lehmann, P. O.: Intermittent claudication of neurogenic origin. Can. J. Surg., 11:151, 1968.

Davis, R. C., O'Hara, E. T., Mannick, J. A., Vollman, R. W., and Nasbeth, D. C.: Broadened indications for femorofemoral grafts. Surgery, 72:990, 1972.

Gaskell, P., and Becker, W. J.: The erect posture as an aid to the circulation in the feet in the presence of arterial obstruction. Can. M. Assoc. J., 105:930, 1971.

Levy, R. I., Fredrickson, D. S., Shulman, R., Bilheimer, D. W., Breslow, J. L., Stone, N. J., Lux, S. E., Sloan, H. R., Krauss, R. M., and Herbert, P. N.: Dietary and drug treatment of primary hyperlipoproteinemia. Ann. Intern. Med., 77:267, 1972.

Mannick, J. A., and Coffman, J. D.: Ischemic Limbs. New York, Grune & Stratton, 1973.

Schadt, D. C., Hines, E. A., Jr., Juergens, J. L., and Barker, N. W.: Chronic atherosclerotic occlusion of the femoral artery. J.A.M.A., 175:937, 1961.

Verstraete, M., Vermylen, J., and Donati, M. D.: The effect of streptokinase infusion on chronic arterial occlusions and stenoses. Ann. Intern. Med., 74:377, 1971.

THROMBOANGIITIS OBLITERANS
(Buerger's Disease)

Definition. Thromboangiitis obliterans is an obliterative vascular disease or syndrome, probably inflammatory in type, affecting chiefly the peripheral arteries and veins. Identified first as endarteritis obliterans (von Winiwarter, 1879), it was described more fully and given its present name by Buerger (1908).

Incidence. All races are subject to thromboangiitis obliterans, but the greatest incidence is in the Ashkenazic Jews, of whom 20 in 100,000 develop the disease compared with 7 or 8 per 100,000 in the general population. The disease is also common in the Orient. The incidence of the disease in the United States has decreased markedly in the last two decades. Men are affected far more frequently than women, in a ratio of about 75 to 1. Thromboangiitis obliterans has been observed at all ages but occurs most frequently between 20 and 45.

Etiology. Although many agents, toxic and infectious, have been suggested, no etiology has received general acceptance. Cigarettes are used moderately or excessively by many, but not all, patients with thromboangiitis obliterans and have been thoroughly investigated as a causative agent, for smoking aggravates the disease. An increased skin sensitivity to tobacco has been reported by some investigators but not found by others. The higher carboxyhemoglobin levels observed in smokers have been proposed as an etiologic factor by increasing the affinity of hemoglobin for oxygen. Recent research has been directed at a thrombotic etiology; the thromboplastin generation test has been reported abnormal, and higher levels of heparin precipitable fraction of fibrinogen in plasma have been found in patients with thromboangiitis obliterans than in normal persons or patients with arteriosclerosis obliterans. A rise in adhesive platelet counts has also been described in the disease and apparently correlates with tobacco smoking.

Considerable skepticism has been expressed that this disease is an entity different from arteriosclerosis occurring in young people. Evidence has been presented that its clinical and pathologic pictures are specific; however, it may be a syndrome with more than one cause.

Pathology. The lesions are segmental in that diseased sections of arteries or veins are separated by normal areas. In the acute stage cellular proliferation of the intima is accompanied by the formation of red thrombi in small and medium-sized vessels, but the internal elastic lamina usually remains intact. Polymorphonuclear leukocytes, lymphocytes, and giant cells infiltrate all coats of the artery and extend into the thrombus. The formation of sterile microabscesses within the thrombi is a specific finding in this disease. Additional segments of artery or vein are involved acutely at intervals from days to years; hence, a single long artery may exhibit many stages, ranging from the acute picture to dense scar formation. Late stages cannot be distinguished pathologically from arteriosclerosis obliterans.

Pathophysiology. The disease is characterized by alternating periods of activity and quiescence. Depending upon the time relation between the developing occlusion and compensation by collateral circulation, the onset and course vary from insidious to fulminant. Usually occlusion gradually outstrips the developing collateral circulation, and definite peripheral ischemia brings the patient under medical care within one to four years after the first mild symptoms appear. The disease often has an initially more active course of six to twelve years, and then advances much less rapidly; at this stage it is very difficult to differentiate from arteriosclerosis obliterans.

Clinical Manifestations. The typical patient with thromboangiitis obliterans is a young male who smokes cigarettes, presents symptoms of peripheral vascular ischemia, and may have a history of thrombophlebitis. The lower extremities are affected most commonly, and the most frequent presenting complaint is persistent coldness of the limbs. The upper extremities are involved in more than 70 per cent of patients (sometimes without symptoms), the digital arteries being affected more frequently than the ulnar or radial. Raynaud's phenomenon, hyperhidrosis, and ulcers of the digits are common.

In comparison with other vascular diseases, the pain is often excruciating. Migratory thrombophlebitis may precede or accompany arterial involvement and occurs in approximately 40 per cent of patients. Tender, red, elevated areas about 1 cm in diameter appear suddenly in the skin near the valves of small, superficial veins and gradually disappear during two to three weeks, to be followed after irregular intervals by new lesions. Other symptoms and signs (intermittent claudication, rest pain, ulcers, gangrene) are the same as in arteriosclerosis obliterans except that femoral artery disease is less frequent and aortoiliac, rare. Thromboses of the mesenteric, coronary, cerebral, and renal arteries have been described but are uncommon.

Diagnosis. The diagnosis may be suspected when a young male presents with peripheral vascular insufficiency and thrombophlebitis, but it can be definitely proved only by biopsy of an active lesion. The age group, sex, thrombophlebitis, frequent involvement of upper extremities, Raynaud's phenomenon, and normal blood cholesterol and glucose tolerance test help differentiate the disease from arteriosclerosis obliterans. Arteriography can be helpful in demonstrating normality of vessels between lesions, absence of atheroma, a characteristic tree root configuration of the collateral vessels around the point of abrupt occlusion, and asymptomatic involvement of the upper extremities. Since Raynaud's disease is rare in men, affects the upper extremities more severely, and does not obliterate arterial pulsation at the wrist or ankle, it should not be confused with Raynaud's phenomenon in thromboangiitis obliterans. Migratory thrombophlebitis without symptoms or signs of arterial involvement cannot be diagnosed as thromboangiitis obliterans unless histologic proof is obtained.

Prognosis. The prognosis for life is good, but amputation of extremities is common, especially in the fulminant form. In the late stages, the prognosis and course are similar to arteriosclerosis obliterans.

Treatment. The treatment is the same as that outlined for arteriosclerosis obliterans, but it is imperative that tobacco never be used in any form. Nicotine produces transient vasoconstriction and probably favors extension of the disease. Bilateral preganglionic sympathectomy has been advocated for established, gradually advancing thromboangiitis obliterans, especially if vasospasm is prominent. This major operation is not indicated in mild cases responding well to medical treatment or in advanced cases with massive gangrene. Opinion is still divided concerning the usefulness of sympathectomy in this disease. In thromboangiitis obliterans resistance to infection is fairly high and collateral circulation usually good, so that minor amputations may be performed more safely than in arteriosclerotic gangrene.

Astrup, P., Hellung-Larsen, P., Kjeldsen, K., and Mellemgaard, K.: The effect of tobacco smoking on the dissociation curve of oxygen hemoglobin. Scand. J. Clin. Lab. Invest., 18:450, 1966.

Barker, N. W.: Diagnosis and treatment of thromboangiitis obliterans (Buerger's disease). Minnesota Med., 39:303, 1956.

Craven, J. L., and Cotton, R. C.: Haematological differences between thromboangiitis obliterans and atherosclerosis. Br. J. Surg., 54:862, 1967.

Goodman, R. M., Elian, B., Mozes, M., and Deutsch, V.: Buerger's Disease in Israel. Am. J. Med., 39:601, 1965.

McKusick, V. A., Harris, W. S., Ottesen, O. E., Goodman, R. M., Shelley, W. M., and Bloodwell, R. D.: Buerger's disease: A distinct clinical and pathologic entity. J.A.M.A., 181:5, 1962.

Wessler, S., Ming, S. C., Gurewich, V., and Freiman, D. G.: A critical evaluation of thromboangiitis obliterans. N. Engl. J. Med., 262:1149, 1960.

Williams, G.: Recent views on Buerger's disease. J. Clin. Pathol., 22:573, 1969.

ARTERIAL EMBOLISM

Definition. Fragments of centrally located thrombi or atheromatous material may embolize and occlude large or small peripheral blood vessels.

Etiology. Emboli usually originate from mural or valvular thrombi in the left side of the heart (atrium or ventricle), less commonly from an atheromatous ulcer in the aorta or a more peripheral artery, and from thrombi in aneurysms. Paradoxical emboli originate from the right side of the heart and pass through a patent foramen ovale. Most emboli occur in association with myocardial infarction, atrial fibrillation, mitral valve disease, chronic congestive heart failure, or endocarditis. With the advent of surgical replacement of heart valves, prostheses have become a common source of emboli.

Pathophysiology. Emboli lodge at bifurcations of arteries and at narrowed arteriosclerotic areas. The most common site is at the junction of the femoral artery with the profunda femoris; emboli at the origin of the iliac arteries from the aorta (*saddle emboli*) are also frequent. The embolus stops blood flow through the artery and is followed within a few hours by secondary progressive arterial thrombosis below and sometimes above the point of obstruction. Secondary vasospasm has been assumed to be an important factor causing ischemia of the affected extremity, but convincing experimental evidence has not been presented to support this theory. The amount of muscle and skin ischemia that occurs depends on the degree of collateral circulation development.

Pathology. Emboli from the heart or aneurysms show the same pathology as the parent thrombi. Emboli lodged in arteries usually organize by the ingrowth of connective tissue, and later recanalization may occur. However, fragmentation of the embolus before organization is not uncommon with fragments lodging in more distal vessels. Emboli that originate from friable, ulcerated atheromatous lesions produce either large vessel obstruction by amorphous debris or arteriolar and capillary blockage by a variable combination of cholesterol crystals and lipoid material. The cholesterol crystals incite an inflammatory response which leads to fibrosis and complete vessel obstruction.

Clinical Manifestations. In approximately half of patients, there is the sudden onset of severe pain in the extremity distal to the site of embolization. The other cases have an insidious beginning over one to several hours; numbness and paresthesias may precede the pain. Pain is present in 80 per cent of patients and may become excruciating within one or two hours, particularly if the patient exercises the limb. Paresthesias occur in about 60 per cent of cases, and 20 per cent develop muscular weakness or actual paralysis. With an aortoiliac embolus, fainting, nausea, vomiting, and abdominal pain may precede a shocklike state.

Examination of the involved extremity reveals pallor and coldness, sharply demarcated distal to the site of embolization, viz., at the inguinal ligaments or sometimes as high as the umbilicus in saddle embolus, at the lower third of the thigh in femoral artery embolus, and at midcalf in popliteal artery embolus. Arterial pulses are absent below the embolus by palpation or oscillometry. In the arms, because of the easy palpability of the brachial artery, the site of embolus lodgment can be determined by the disappearance of the pulse. Occasionally there is tenderness directly over the embolus in an artery. The extremity may also show collapsed veins, decreased to absent reflexes and sensation, and weakness and paralysis. Later the initial pallor changes to a blotchy cyanosis. If collateral circulation is good, the extremity soon shows signs of improvement in color and temperature, but muscle tenderness and pitting edema may develop. If the collateral circulation is inadequate, massive gangrene follows with bleb formation, spotty vermilion discoloration of the skin, and mummification.

Large emboli from thrombi or amorphous atherosclerotic debris show the aforementioned picture. Smaller emboli may produce only local digital cyanosis with or without pain. Atheromatous microemboli (cholesterol crystals and lipoid material) may produce sudden leg pain, tender muscles, cool legs with pulses, petechiae, livedo reticularis, and plaquelike reddened elevations of the skin. Pedal pulses may disappear later in this syndrome. The spontaneous appearance of painful dusky discoloration of a toe or toes in the presence of pulses should suggest atheromatous microembolism.

Diagnosis. The diagnosis of embolization is not difficult in the patient with the acute onset of a painful, ischemic extremity who demonstrates a source for embolus formation. Acute arterial thrombosis can be distinguished from an embolus only by the presence or absence of underlying etiologies; absent or decreased arterial pulsations in the opposite limb support a diagnosis of acute thrombosis. Patients with acute iliofemoral thrombophlebitis sometimes have no palpable pulses in the affected extremity and may show signs resembling those of arterial embolus. Detection of a feeble pulse by oscillometry, distended veins, and massive edema of the extremity helps rule out embolus. In patients with symptoms and signs of embolization or microembolization and normal pulses, angiography must be performed to look for ulcerative atherosclerotic lesions or aneurysms in the proximal large vessels. Microembolization is often confused with polymyositis or polyarteritis nodosa; muscle biopsy may be necessary to demonstrate the cholesterol crystals.

Prognosis. The prognosis in acute arterial embolization depends on several factors, including size of vessel affected, age of patient, collateral blood supply, and speed of treatment. The larger the artery involved, the worse the prognosis without treatment. Gangrene is much more common after the age of 60 years, probably because of concomitant arteriosclerotic involvement of the blood vessels and collaterals. The development of collateral circulation is very important, for sufficient collaterals may save a limb without treatment. The presence of patent companion vessels, e.g., around the elbow, gives a favorable outlook. The earlier an embolus can be removed surgically, the better the prognosis for survival of the severely ischemic limb.

With any method of treatment, the mortality in most studies is usually greater than 20 per cent, owing to the underlying disease and recurrent embolization to vital areas. The incidence of embolus recurrence is very high. After either medical or surgical treatment, limb incapacity from muscle fibrosis with tendon shortening or intermittent claudication is common.

Treatment. Although embolectomy should restore the normal physiology and is strongly recommended in the surgical literature, conservative medical management often gives as good end results. The exception is emboli at the aortic bifurcation, when surgery is the optimal treatment. When the patient is first seen, treatment should be instituted to improve blood flow to the extremity, and a vascular surgeon should be immediately called in consultation. Anticoagulation with heparin should be started at once to prevent thrombus formation below and above the embolus, and further embolization (long-term anticoagulation is usually indicated to prevent recurrent emboli). Early studies indicate that thrombolytic therapy with streptokinase may be valuable in acute embolization in about one third of patients; such therapy is given intravenously and must be followed by adequate anticoagulation (see Ch. 545). The limb should be positioned in 15 degree dependency and adequate analgesics given to relieve the pain. The affected limb should be kept comfortably warm, as in a thermoregulated (30 to 34° C, 86 to 93.2° F) cradle, and the body and uninvolved extremities warmed in an effort to produce reflex vasodilatation in the involved limb. Every precaution should be taken to prevent burning during heat application; ischemic limbs burn at much lower temperatures than normal limbs. Lumbar sympathetic block by paravertebral injection of procaine or xylocaine has been recommended to relieve vasoconstrictor tone and vasospasm if present; if used it should be performed before anticoagulation.

If conservative medical therapy is not effective in greatly improving the extremity in two to four hours and the underlying condition of the patient will allow surgery, embolectomy is indicated. Early diagnosis is essential as the greatest success with embolectomy is within eight to ten hours of the incident. In recent years, embolectomy has been performed longer than 48 hours after the acute insult with some success, although less than with earlier operations. Muscle tenderness and edema often occur after embolectomy and may be mistakenly diagnosed as thrombophlebitis. In cases presenting with gangrene, amputation is usually necessary. In atheromatous embolization or emboli from aneurysmal thrombi, surgical attack on the proximal lesion may be successful in preventing further emboli.

Amery, A., Deloof, W., Vermylen, J., and Verstraete, M.: Outcome of recent thromboembolic occlusions of limb arteries treated with streptokinase. Br. Med. J., 4:639, 1970.
Baird, R. J., and Lajos, T. Z.: Emboli to the arm. Ann. Surg., 160:905, 1964.
Eliot, R. S., Kanjuh, V. I., and Edwards, J. E.: Atheromatous embolism. Circulation, 30:611, 1964.
Haygood, T. A., Fessel, W. J., and Strange, D. A.: Atheromatous microembolism simulating polymyositis. J.A.M.A., 203:423, 1968.
Jacobs, A. L.: Arterial embolism in the limbs. Edinburgh, E. & S. Livingstone, Ltd., 1959.
Silverblatt, C. W., Wasserman, F., and Wolcott, M. W.: Pulmonary artery embolism and paradoxical embolization. Arch. Intern. Med., 107:105, 1961.
Szekely, P.: Systemic embolism and anticoagulant prophylaxis in rheumatic heart disease. Br. Med. J., 1:1209, 1964.
Wessler, S., Sheps, S. G., Gilbert, M., and Sheps, M. C.: Studies in peripheral arterial occlusive disease. III. Acute arterial occlusion. Circulation, 17:512, 1958.

PERIPHERAL ARTERITIS AND GANGRENE IN SYSTEMIC INFECTIONS

Symptoms and signs of peripheral vascular disease, mild or severe, appear occasionally as complications in bacterial, viral, rickettsial, and fungal infections. Bacterial arteritis and abscess of the wall of an artery are uncommon complications of bacterial endocarditis and septicemias and may lead to hemorrhagic lesions or aneurysm formation. The rickettsial diseases, especially typhus and Rocky Mountain spotted fever, may cause endothelial proliferation of the arterioles, capillaries, and venules followed by degeneration and necrosis of the media; thrombosis of larger arteries may occur rarely. In infectious arteritis with direct vascular involvement, signs of subacute or acute arrest of peripheral blood flow occur with necrosis of skin and sometimes massive gangrene. However, peripheral ischemia may be transitory and, in large part, vasospastic. Gangrene of the extremities may follow acute infectious conditions, such as pneumonia and gastroenteritis, especially in children; the cause is unknown.

Tuberculosis of the peripheral arteries is rare, but occasionally metastatic infection or embolism produces panarteritis or endarteritis with fully developed tubercles in thrombosed vessels. Direct involvement by extension from adjacent tuberculous lesions, although common in centrally located vessels, is rare in the extremities.

Syphilis may diminish peripheral circulation by producing periarteritis, obliterative intimal hyperplasia, or panarteritis, but the media is much less affected than in the large arteries. True gummas have been found in the vessels of gangrenous limbs. Peripheral vascular complications of syphilis are more common in men than in women. Peripheral ischemia, vasospastic or organic, appears insidiously or suddenly, but gangrene is rare. Active antisyphilitic therapy usually arrests the acute progress of the disease and relieves vasospasm, but organic occlusion remains.

Collins, R. N., and Nadel, M. S.: Gangrene due to the hemolytic Streptococcus—a rare but treatable disease. N. Engl. J. Med., 272:578, 1965.
Derick, C. L., and Hass, G. M.: Diffuse arteritis of syphilitic origin. Am. J. Path., 11:291, 1935.
Koten, J. W.: Peripheral gangrene in infancy and childhood. Br. Med. J., 3:798, 1967.
Learmouth, G. E.: Gangrene of the lower extremities complicating scarlet fever. Can. Med. Assoc. J., 15:69, 1925.
Slaughter, W. H.: Symmetrical gangrene of malarial origin. J.A.M.A., 86:1607, 1926.

SHIN SPLINTS AND ANTERIOR TIBIAL COMPARTMENT SYNDROMES

The anterior tibial compartment is a closed space in which the muscles and blood vessels are surrounded by nonexpanding fascia and bone. Swelling of the tissues in this compartment can cause mild to severe complications.

Shin splints is a frequently encountered syndrome of pain and discomfort in the lower anterior part of the leg after repetitive, unusual exertion. The syndrome is presumably a result of ischemia from an abnormally high tissue pressure compressing the blood vessels. It often occurs in athletes or dancers early in the season. The pain in the front of the legs occurs during or after exercise and is only slowly relieved by rest. Tenderness is most frequent at periosteal attachments of the muscles to the tibia or interosseous membrane. Mild swelling and a slight rise in local skin temperature may be present. When the pain is reproduced by repeated dorsiflexion of the foot against resistance, the anterior tibial muscles become very hard and bulge prominently; a pulsation may become visible over the front of the legs. Arterial pulses are normal. Treatment consists of rest of the muscles, supportive strapping, and a program of graduated exercise.

The *acute anterior tibial compartment syndrome* is a

rare condition caused by the rapid onset of ischemic necrosis of muscles in the anterior tibial space. Swelling of the muscles compresses muscles, nerves, and blood vessels. The cause is unknown, but there is usually a history of excessive exertion. A dull, aching pain which becomes progressively severe is the major symptom; it is unrelieved by rest and sometimes by analgesics. Extreme tenderness is present over the entire anterior tibial compartment, and the fascia rapidly becomes tense and boardlike. The skin becomes glossy, erythematous, and edematous as muscle necrosis occurs; a slight fever and leukocytosis may be present. Loss of dorsiflexion of the great toe and foot then occurs, and sensation may be lost between the first and second toes (deep peroneal nerve compression). The dorsalis pedis pulse may be present or absent. Treatment must be immediate and involves surgical decompression of the anterior tibial compartment by fasciotomy. If treatment is delayed, complete necrosis of the muscles occurs with a resultant permanent footdrop.

A *chronic anterior tibial compartment syndrome* also has been described with pain similar to intermittent claudication in the front of the lower leg on severe exertion but not with ordinary walking. The discomfort disappears with rest. Tenderness is present over the entire compartment when the pain occurs; arterial pulses are normal. The syndrome is thought to be due to an abnormally small compartment. Treatment is usually unnecessary, but a fasciotomy will relieve the symptoms.

French, E. B., and Price, W. H.: Anterior tibial pain. Br. Med. J., 2:1290, 1962.
Leach, R. E., Zohn, D. A., and Stryker, W. S.: Anterior tibial compartment syndrome. Arch. Surg., 88:187, 1964.
Slocum, D. B.: The shin syndrome. Am. J. Surg., 114:875, 1967.

596. PERIPHERAL VASCULAR DISEASE DUE TO ABNORMAL VASOCONSTRICTION OR VASODILATATION

RAYNAUD'S PHENOMENON AND DISEASE

Definition. Raynaud's phenomenon is a syndrome characterized by paroxysmal, bilateral ischemia of the digits induced by cold or emotional stimuli and relieved by heat.

Etiology. Raynaud's phenomenon may be secondary to an underlying disease or anatomic abnormality, but the most common cause is *Raynaud's disease,* which is of unknown etiology. It is less common before puberty and after age 40 but may occur at any age. Women are affected more frequently than men (5:1). Raynaud concluded from his early studies (1862, 1874) that excessive sympathetic activity was responsible for the attacks, but Lewis found that the digital vessels were abnormally reactive to local cold. Since ischemic attacks can still be induced after sympathectomy, it may be concluded that there is a local fault in the blood vessels in Raynaud's disease which is aggravated by the normal degree of reflex sympathetic nervous activity. However, about a dozen cases of Raynaud's phenomenon associated with pulmonary hypertension have been reported, suggesting that a neurohumoral mechanism may be operative in causing both syndromes.

Raynaud's phenomenon may occur in occlusive arterial disease (thromboangiitis obliterans, arteriosclerosis obliterans, arterial emboli), collagen disease (especially scleroderma), after trauma (pneumatic hammer disease, injuries to pianists or typists, after gangrene from any cause), drug intoxication (ergot, methysergide), blood dyscrasias (cryopathies, cold hemagglutinins), and neurogenic lesions (thoracic outlet compression syndromes, poliomyelitis, syringomyelia, causalgia). In Raynaud's phenomenon from secondary causes, the syndrome is caused usually by irritation of the sympathetic nerves, pathologic alterations in the small blood vessels, or sludging and agglutination of red blood cells.

Pathologic Physiology. The paroxysmal ischemia of the digits is due to constriction of the digital and palmar or plantar arteries; initial pallor indicates that vasoconstriction involves the small cutaneous vessels. Later the digital capillaries and venules become dilated, and the slowed blood flow allows the hemoglobin to release more of its oxygen, producing cyanotic, cold digits. When the vasoconstriction is relieved, blood flow increases greatly (reactive hyperemia), imparting a red color to the previously ischemic digits. Total and capillary fingertip blood flow are smaller in patients with Raynaud's phenomenon and disease than in normal subjects. With a cooling stimulus, patients show a significant decrease in fingertip capillary flow not seen in normal subjects.

Pathology. In the early stages of the disease, the blood vessels are histologically normal. Later, in progressive cases, the intima is thickened and the muscular coats of the arteries are hypertrophied. Eventually thrombosis of small arteries may occur and focal gangrene of the digital tips may form, although elsewhere the arteries are still histologically normal or show only slight hypertrophy.

Clinical Manifestations. In typical Raynaud's phenomenon, the fingers of both hands blanch on exposure to cold and then may turn cyanotic; sometimes only cyanosis occurs. During recovery, a bright red color (reactive hyperemia) replaces the cyanosis. During the ischemic phase, the digits are cold, numb, and covered with perspiration. In the reactive hyperemia phase, throbbing pain, tingling, swelling, and a rise in skin temperature are found. The digits are affected to different levels in each patient (sometimes extending to the wrist), but the terminal phalanges are always most severely involved. Initially, attacks may be unilateral and involve only one or two digits, but they soon become bilateral and may be induced by emotional upsets as well as by cold exposure.

In Raynaud's disease, the onset is usually gradual with attacks only in the winter. Attacks may be rare, or they may occur several times a day; they may last a few minutes in mild cases to two hours or more in severe cases. They end spontaneously or can be terminated by immersing the hands in warm water. Between episodes, the digits are normal or, in severe cases, mildly cyanotic.

The hands alone are affected in half the cases, hands and feet in the remainder; nose, cheeks, ears, and chin are affected much more rarely. The course of the disease varies; after onset it may persist indefinitely in mild form, improve spontaneously, or become more severe. In the small number of cases that are progressive, the attacks become more frequent, persist during the summer, and last longer; finally, mild cyanosis may be present constantly.

Trophic changes appear in progressive cases, usually one to four years after onset. The fingers become thin and tapering and their skin smooth, shiny, less mobile, and eventually tightly stretched (sclerodactyly). The nails grow slowly and are ridged or curved. Recurrent infections, blisters, and small areas of local cutaneous gangrene appear on the fingertips, but gangrene of a whole digit is rare. The gangrenous areas are extremely painful and, on healing, leave tiny depressed scars.

Diagnosis. Criteria which should be present in patients with Raynaud's phenomenon in order to diagnose Raynaud's disease include (1) absence of any disease or anatomic abnormality to which paroxysmal digital ischemia might be secondary; (2) digital pallor or cyanosis occurring in intermittent attacks, induced by cold or emotion and followed by recovery with reactive hyperemia; (3) symmetrical or bilateral involvement of digits; and (4) gangrene, if present, usually limited to small areas of skin. Previously, presence of symptoms for two years with no evidence of an underlying cause had been considered a fifth diagnostic point; however, Raynaud's phenomenon may precede the diagnosis of scleroderma by 12 years. It is probably unsafe to diagnose the idiopathic disease in the presence of an elevated sedimentation rate or minor symptoms or signs suggestive of an underlying disease (arthralgias, telangiectasis). Raynaud's phenomenon is diagnosed by discovering an underlying disease or condition known to cause attacks.

Raynaud's disease and phenomenon are distinguished from acrocyanosis by the intermittency of attacks. The cyanotic, cold, and edematous limb affected by poliomyelitis or other diseases causing paralysis is also persistent in nature. The cause of sudden "bilateral gangrene of the digits" (Lewis), which appears rarely in children or young adults without previous attacks of discoloration and without cold exposure, is unknown. The fingers, toes, nose, and ears become permanently cyanotic, and within a few days gangrene develops in the distal phalanges of one or more fingers, often symmetrically and bilaterally. The gangrene is extensive and is due to sudden thrombotic occlusion of the final end branches of the digital arteries. The relationship of this syndrome to Raynaud's disease is uncertain, although typical cyclic color changes may appear during the healing stage.

Prognosis. Mild cases of Raynaud's disease improve slowly or remain stationary for years, and the attacks, being few and avoidable, are merely an inconvenience. In a large series of cases, the disease caused no deaths and very little disability; amputations of terminal phalanges were necessary in only 0.4 per cent, and the phenomenon improved or disappeared in 46 per cent. The progressive form, with recurring infection and local gangrene, becomes increasingly painful and disabling, usually despite treatment, but only rarely results in the loss of more than the distal phalanges. The prognosis for secondary Raynaud's phenomenon depends on the underlying cause. Generalized scleroderma and rheumatoid arthritis, which are frequently associated with Raynaud's phenomenon, may produce extreme deformity and disability.

Treatment. Mild cases of Raynaud's disease with infrequent attacks limited to cold exposure, and without trophic changes or gangrene, may be relieved by reassurance, sedatives or tranquilizers, and protection from cold exposure. Smoking has been shown to produce cutaneous vasoconstriction, and the use of tobacco should therefore be avoided. Rauwolfia products in continued small oral doses (reserpine, 0.25 to 0.5 mg daily) will often decrease the severity and frequency of attacks. If necessary, a vasodilator drug (tolazoline long-acting tablets, 80 mg every 12 hours) can be added to the therapeutic regimen. The addition of thyroid substances and androgens has been recommended but helps little, if any.

Vasoconstrictor tone caused by sympathetic nervous system activity is an important factor in bringing on and maintaining attacks of digital ischemia, whether or not the local arteries are abnormally reactive to cold. Removal of vasoconstrictor impulses by regional sympathectomy may be of benefit for the progressive type of Raynaud's disease with indolent ulcers or local gangrene. The success of the sympathectomy depends upon the extent to which the normal capacity for vasodilatation is preserved, as shown by the vasodilator response to body warming or sympathetic ganglion nerve block with lidocaine. In early Raynaud's disease of the lower extremities, lumbar sympathetic ganglionectomy gives complete relief of symptoms. For the upper extremity, preganglionic cervicodorsal sympathectomy is the operation of choice but usually is of temporary (six months to two years) benefit.

The treatment of Raynaud's phenomenon secondary to an underlying disease or anatomic abnormality is directed at the secondary causes. Sympathectomy is of little or no benefit in scleroderma or arthritis but may be helpful in Raynaud's phenomenon secondary to pneumatic hammer disease or causalgia (reflex sympathetic dystrophy).

Baddeley, R. M.: The place of upper dorsal sympathectomy in the treatment of primary Raynaud's disease. Br. J. Surg., 52:426, 1965.
Coffman, J. D., and Cohen, A. S.: Total and capillary fingertip blood flow in Raynaud's phenomenon. N. Engl. J. Med., 285:259, 1971.
Farmer, R. G., Gifford, R. W., Jr., and Hines, E. A., Jr.: Raynaud's disease with sclerodactylia: a follow-up of seventy-one patients. Circulation, 22:13, 1961.
Gifford, R. W., Jr., and Hines, E. A., Jr.: Raynaud's disease among women and girls. Circulation, 16:1012, 1957.
Guntheroth, W. G., Morgan, B. C., Harbinson, J. A., and Mullins, G. L.: Raynaud's disease in children. Circulation, 36:724, 1967.
Lewis, T., and Pickering, G. W.: Observations upon maladies in which the blood supply to digits ceases intermittently or permanently, and upon bilateral gangrene of digits; observations relevant to so-called "Raynaud's disease. Clin. Sci., 1:327, 1934.
Mannick, J. A., and Coffman, J. D.: Ischemic Limbs. New York, Grune & Stratton, 1973.
Winters, W. L., Jr., Joseph, R. R., and Learner, N.: "Primary" pulmonary hypertension and Raynaud's phenomenon. Arch. Intern. Med., 114:821, 1964.

ACROCYANOSIS

Acrocyanosis (Croq, 1896; chronic acro-asphyxia, Cassirer, 1900) is a symmetrical cyanosis of the hands and, less commonly, the feet with few or no symptoms and no complications.

Etiology and Pathology. It is primarily a vasospastic disturbance of the smaller arterioles of the skin of unknown cause, but is probably due to local cold sensitivity. When compared with normal digits, acrocyanotic digits have a heightened arteriolar tone at average room temperature. Secondary dilatation of the capillaries and the subpapillary venous plexus occurs, and the slower blood flow allows the hemoglobin to release a greater part of its oxygen content, accounting for the blue color. Acrocyanosis occurs without special age or sex incidence, and may be associated with various endocrine disorders or asthenias as well as with certain anxiety states. No specific pathology has been described.

Clinical Manifestations. Patients usually present with an unevenly blue and red discoloration of the skin which may extend from the digits to the wrists and ankles but is most intense distally. The digits are also persistently cold and sweat profusely. Puffiness of the digits and mild hypesthesia may be present, but other trophic changes are rare. The cyanosis is intensified by cold or emotional upsets and is relieved by warmth.

Diagnosis. Acrocyanosis can be distinguished from Raynaud's disease by the persistent nature of the discoloration. The presence of normal arterial pulses rules out obstructive arterial disease. Since the discoloration is limited to the hands and feet and disappears when the extremities are warmed, it should not be confused with various types of generalized cyanosis.

Treatment. Except for reassurance, treatment is usually unnecessary. Possible endocrine abnormalities should be investigated. To prevent reflex sympathetic vasoconstriction, general body protection from cold, as well as local measures, helps to decrease the intensity of the discoloration. For cosmetic reasons, vasodilator drugs (tolazoline long-acting tablets, 80 mg every 12 hours, or nicotinyl alcohol, 50 mg every 6 hours) may be used. Sympathectomy is helpful but seldom warranted.

Elliot, A. H., Evans, R. D., and Stone, C. S.: Acrocyanosis: A study of the circulatory fault. Am. Heart J., 11:431, 1936.

Larsson, Y.: The vasoconstrictor tone of the cutaneous arterioles in acroasphyxia, hypertension, and in the cold pressor test. Acta Med. Scand. (Supp. 206), 130:146, 1948.

Lewis, T., and Landis, E. M.: Observations upon the vascular mechanism in acrocyanosis. Heart, 15:229, 1930.

Lottenbach, K.: Vascular response to cold in acrocyanosis. Helv. Med. Acta, 33:437, 1966.

ERGOTISM AND METHYSERGIDE TOXICITY

Definition. Intense vasoconstriction of small and large blood vessels, producing symptoms and signs of peripheral vascular ischemia, may result from the ingestion of ergot or methysergide.

Etiology. Ergotism results from the use of ergot-containing drugs or the ingestion of bread made from rye or wheat infected with the ergot fungus (*Claviceps purpurea*). It formerly occurred in epidemic form, but is now seen only sporadically (due to the fungus), or after the repeated administration of ergotamine (Gynergen, Cafergot) for migraine or pruritus or of ergot in abortion. Methysergide is a synthetic serotonin antagonist useful in the treatment of migraine headaches. Approximately 7 per cent of patients develop peripheral vascular symptoms or signs with methysergide ingestion, usually after large doses, although as little as 1 mg has caused symptoms in some patients.

Pathophysiology and Pathology. Both drugs induce large and small blood vessel vasoconstriction. Ergot induces vasoconstriction by a direct action on vascular smooth muscle and can lead to secondary intimal hyperplasia and thrombosis. Gangrene may result if thrombosis occurs. The pathology of methysergide toxicity is unknown as is the mode of action, but it does potentiate the effect of catecholamines on blood vessels.

Clinical Manifestations. *Acute ergotism* produces diarrhea, colic, and vomiting, followed by headache, vertigo, paresthesias, convulsive seizures, and occasionally gangrene of the digits, nose, and ears. It is rarely seen with the drug ingestion. In *chronic intoxications,* intermittent claudication, muscle pains, numbness, coldness and pallor of the digits, and even Raynaud's phenomenon may

occur. Examination reveals only cool, pale digits or mottling of the skin with normal or decreased arterial pulsations; however, complete absence of medium- and large-vessel pulsations in the extremities may occur. Gangrene may develop in the severe cases. A similar picture of peripheral vascular ischemia may follow methysergide ingestion. Abdominal angina, angina pectoris, and cerebral ischemic symptoms have also been caused by these drugs. Methysergide has been implicated as an etiologic agent in periureteral or retroperitoneal fibrosis which can extrinsically obstruct arteries and veins.

Diagnosis. The diagnosis is made from the history of drug ingestion associated with symptoms and signs of peripheral ischemia. Arteriography characteristically shows diffuse or segmental narrowing of large arteries and often very constricted distal vessels with collateral vessels present. Arteriosclerosis obliterans, Raynaud's disease, and acrocyanosis are differentiated from ergotism and methysergide toxicity by the history of drug ingestion and by arteriography.

Prognosis. The prognosis is excellent if gangrene has not appeared before treatment and if drug administration is stopped.

Treatment. Treatment involves anticoagulation to prevent thromboses and the use of vasodilators, e.g., tolazoline, 25 mg, intra-arterial or intravenous, to counteract the vasoconstriction. Body warming is recommended to produce reflex vasodilatation in the involved extremities, but is often unsuccessful as is vasodilator drug therapy. With avoidance of the offending drug, the vasoconstriction usually subsides in one to three days. Sympathetic nerve block or sympathectomy may be necessary in pregangrenous or gangrenous cases.

Cranley, J. J., Krause, R. J., Strasser, E. S., and Hafner, C. D.: Impending gangrene of four extremities secondary to ergotism. N. Engl. J. Med., 269:727, 1963.

Graham, J. R.: Methysergide for prevention of headache. N. Engl. J. Med., 270:67, 1964.

Rackley, C. E., Mengel, C. E., Pomerantz, M., and McIntosh, H. D.: Vascular complications with use of methysergide. Arch. Intern. Med., 117:265, 1966.

Richter, A. M., and Banker, V. P.: Carotid ergotism. Radiology, 106:339, 1973.

ERYTHROMELALGIA
(Erythermalgia)

Definition. Erythromelalgia (Mitchell, 1872) is a rare syndrome of paroxysmal, bilateral vasodilatation of the feet and, less often, the hands, associated with burning pain, increased skin temperature, and redness of the skin.

Etiology and Pathology. The cause is unknown. It has occurred as an hereditary affliction. Increased blood flow is usually present, but symptoms may occur in a limb in which the arteries are occluded by a blood pressure cuff. Therefore it is thought that there is a hypersensitivity of the skin to heat or tension. No uniform pathologic condition has been found, but data are scarce. The syndrome occurs without special age or sex incidence.

Clinical Manifestations. The patient with erythromelalgia complains of attacks of bilateral burning pain, superficial or deep, involving circumscribed areas on the soles or palms, the entire foot or hand, or even the whole extremity. The attacks follow stimuli that normally induce only physiologic peripheral vasodilatation or engorgement such as local heat, a warm environment, exercise, standing, or simple dependency of the extremity. The onset is gradual, and symptoms may remain mild for years or may become so severe and continuous that total disability results. Examination during an attack (which may be produced by exposure to a 32 to 36° C environment) usually reveals that the affected skin is hot and red and often sweats profusely; arterial pulsations are normal. Trophic changes, gangrene, and ulceration do not occur, but swelling may be present.

The syndrome may be either idiopathic or secondary to *polycythemia vera* or *hypertension.* The condition may precede the polycythemia by as long as 12 years. Secondary erythromelalgia occurs more commonly in an older age group, is more often unilateral, and produces pain of lesser intensity than idiopathic erythromelalgia.

Diagnosis. Arteriosclerosis obliterans may produce localized and often unilateral burning pain and redness but, unlike erythromelalgia, is not associated with normal pulses or a rise in skin temperature. Neuritis, infectious ganglionitis, and poisoning by thallium, lead, or arsenic may produce painful peripheral hyperemia. Chronic inflammatory states produce in the skin a "susceptible state" with diminished capillary and arteriolar tone. Burning pain (erythralgia, Lewis) is then induced by mild grades of heat, cold, friction, and congestion that leave normal skin unaffected. A temporary reactive vasodilatation of the cutaneous vessels also normally occurs after prolonged exposure to cold in response to a histamine-like substance liberated by local tissue damage (Lewis). This is easily distinguished from erythromelalgia by the history.

Treatment. Attacks can be avoided or aborted by rest, elevation of the extremity, and cold applications. Aspirin (0.6 gram orally) quickly relieves pain in some cases, and the remarkable response is of diagnostic value. Vasoconstrictor agents such as ephedrine (25 mg orally) may be useful; methysergide (1 to 4 mg orally) has also produced relief. Even vasodilator agents (isoproterenol, nitroglycerin) have been reported to be helpful. Contrast baths, using heat below the threshold for pain, often afford considerable but temporary relief. Severe attacks require liberal doses of sedatives, and the therapy is generally unsatisfactory. Occasionally section or alcohol injection of peripheral nerve is required; sympathectomy has been successful in the treatment of three cases.

Prognosis. The prognosis in idiopathic erythromelalgia is guarded, because the severe pain may become disabling. Prognosis of secondary cases depends on the underlying disease; treatment of polycythemia often relieves the symptoms.

Babb, R. R., Alarcon-Segovia, D., and Fairbairn, J. F., II: Erythermalgia. Review of 51 cases. Circulation, 29:136, 1964.
Catchpole, B. N.: Erythromelalgia. Lancet, 1:909, 1964.
Cross, E. G.: The familial occurrence of erythromelalgia and nephritis. Can. Med. Assoc. J., 87:1, 1962.
Lewis, T.: Clinical observations and experiments relating to burning pain in extremities and to so-called "erythromelalgia" in particular. Clin. Sci., 1:175, 1933.
Telford, E. D., and Simmons, H. T.: Erythromelalgia. Br. Med. J., 2:782, 1940.

597. PERIPHERAL VASCULAR DISEASES DUE TO EXPOSURE TO COLD

Exposure to cold induces vasoconstriction by a direct action on blood vessels and also by reflex sympathetic nervous system activity. Cold application to the forehead or to one extremity stimulates vasoconstriction in all extremities. The decreased blood flow and local anoxia may lead to tissue damage, depending on the degree and duration of exposure and the susceptibility of the patient.

Even brief exposure to nonfreezing cold is followed in sensitive persons by an exaggerated and prolonged type of reactive vasodilatation, low-grade edema, and tingling pain. Similar exposure in more susceptible patients produces pronounced edema of the angioneurotic or urticarial type on exposed areas; even mucous membranes may be involved on ingesting cold substances. A systemic reaction with increased pulse rate, decreased blood pressure, flushing of the face, and even syncope may accompany the edema. After swimming in cool water, this reaction has proved fatal in some instances. Familial cases of cold urticaria have been described; this is a milder condition not affecting mucous membranes. A histamine-like substance has been shown to be released and is measurable in the urine in about 50 per cent of patients. The passive transfer of cold urticaria has been demonstrated with both IgE and IgM fractions of patients' serum. Diagnosis is made by exposure of a hand or arm to 12 to 14° C (53 to 57° F) water; edema will develop during or after exposure. Antihistamines or cyproheptadine (Periactin, 4 mg three times a day) may be of use in the treatment of cold sensitivity, but protection of the patient from cold exposure is most important.

Tindall, J. P.: Cold urticaria. Postgrad. Med., 50:133, 1971.
Wanderer, A. A., and Ellis, E. F.: Treatment of cold urticaria with cyproheptadine. J. Allergy Clin. Immunol., 48:366, 1971.
Wanderer, A. A., Maselli, R., Ellis, E. F., and Ishizaka, K.: Immunologic characterization of serum factors responsible for cold urticaria. J. Allergy Clin. Immunol., 48:13, 1971.

IMMERSION FOOT
(Trench Foot)

Definition. Immersion foot is due to prolonged exposure of the extremities to water; syndromes characterized only by painful, swollen feet or hands to the more serious manifestations of muscle necrosis, ulceration, and gangrene may result.

Etiology. Although prolonged exposure (greater than 48 hours) to dampness or water is the important factor in the production of immersion foot, immobility and dependency of the lower extremities, constricting garments, chilling of the body, trauma, exhaustion, or dehydration, and, in some instances, semistarvation with deficient intake of protein and vitamins are often contributing causes. Two types, cold water and warm water (tropical) immersion foot, exist and present different clinical pictures. The combination of wetness plus cold (not necessarily freezing) temperatures produces the most serious condition.

Pathophysiology. The factors causing cold water immersion foot tend to decrease blood flow to the extremities. Vasoconstriction is caused by direct and reflex cold stimulation; actual cellular damage and the ensuing hyperemia are important in producing the clinical and pathologic picture. Persistent local anoxia leads to tissue necrosis and injures the capillary walls. Capillary filtration increases remarkably, and plasma and protein pass freely into the interstitial tissue, producing a tense edema. The resultant increased viscosity of the blood leads to stasis and occlusion of small vessels. The local anoxia may also produce wallerian degeneration of the nerves in the affected area.

Warm water immersion foot is thought to be caused by waterlogging and swelling of the stratum corneum together with abrasion from footwear. *Pseudomonas aeruginosa* can usually be cultured from the affected areas and may contribute by digesting human callus with its proteolytic enzymes.

Pathology. The early pathologic picture of the cold type has not been studied. In late stages, a nonspecific picture of vascular occlusion, desquamation of skin, deep fibrosis, and superficial gangrene is seen. The nerves may be embedded in contracting fibrous tissue, and fibrosis of the media of arterioles and venules is present. The pathologic features of the severe, warm-water type are a lymphocytic infiltration, diapedesis of red blood cells, and swelling and proliferation of the endothelial lining of capillaries in the upper dermis.

Incidence. Cold water immersion foot is common in most wars and is seen in training camps where appropriate conditions exist. Non-Caucasians are thought to be more susceptible to the disease, perhaps on the basis of acclimatization.

Clinical Manifestations. At the time of rescue from sea, or when first seen in trench warfare, cold water immersion foot often presents as pulseless, cold, red feet with a sock distribution of hypesthesia or anesthesia. The condition may develop insidiously with only numbness, paresthesias, and slight swelling as long as the tissues are supported by boots or shoes. As soon as the support is removed, edema, tingling, itching, and severe pain occur. The skin later becomes mottled yellow, blue, or black. This is called the prehyperemic stage and lasts a few hours to a few days. A hyperemic stage follows, characterized by red, hot, dry feet, burning paresthesias, and intense pains, shooting or stabbing in nature. Pulses are now bounding. Edema increases with formation of blisters, which may weep serous fluid and then slowly heal. In severe cases, muscle weakness and wasting, ulcerations, and gangrenous patches develop. Gangrene is often superficial, and the necrotic skin sometimes sheds in large pieces, leaving healthy skin beneath. Even in the absence of gangrene, extensive exfoliation is common. This stage lasts one to ten weeks, depending on the grade of initial injury.

The recovery stage (posthyperemic) blends indistinguishably with the hyperemic stage; there is a return of vascular tone with restoration of normal skin color and temperature. Recovery may be complete in mild cases within two to five weeks, but severe cases often require three to twelve months. A few patients show late sequelae such as sensitivity to cold with Raynaud's phenomenon; general or marginal hyperhidrosis; paresthesias that are increased by warmth, dependency, or exertion; rigid toes caused by fibrosis of muscles; contracted joints in the feet and toes; or painful, indolent ulcers of the digits or their stumps.

Warm water immersion foot presents with painful and extremely tender feet, especially over pressure areas. Wrinkled, white, convoluted plantar surfaces and even maceration are seen on examination in the mild syndrome. In the more severe cases, one also finds pronounced erythema and edema of the ankles and dorsal aspects of the feet; fever and femoral lymphadenopathy may occur. During healing, these patients develop diffuse ecchymoses, vesicles, and a maculopapular rash.

Symptoms and signs subside within a week, usually leaving no residua.

Prophylaxis. Drying of the feet overnight is the best method to prevent immersion foot. Avoidance of constricting clothing, prolonged dependency, or immobility; frequent rest periods; and several changes of clothes and boots will also help. If these conditions are impractical, application of silicone grease once a day will reduce the incidence of the affliction.

Treatment. In the prehyperemic stage bed rest and body warming are important. It is probably best to keep the extremities at heart level until pulses are present. Treatment of the hyperemic stage consists of complete bed rest, cooling of the hyperemic tissues to control pain and edema, keeping the body warm, elevation of the extremities above heart level, and correction of dietary deficiencies. If cleansing is necessary, light washing with dilute hexachlorophene solution may be used. Infected tissue and epidermophytosis should be treated with appropriate agents. For cooling, it may be sufficient to expose the extremities to room air, but sometimes electric fans with water sprays or ice bags are needed. With cooling, pain is usually relieved in a few hours, but in some instances it is necessary to discover an optimal temperature, because too low a temperature may again produce pain. Analgesics must be used. Tobacco smoking is prohibited. The patient is ready to walk when edema does not occur on dependency.

Sympathectomy has not been helpful in the hyperemic stage but appears to improve late sequelae such as chronic painful ulcers, persistent vasospasm, and hyperhidrosis.

The treatment of warm water immersion foot involves bed rest with extremity elevation until edema and pain entirely disappear. Other measures are usually unnecessary; the symptoms and signs disappear in one to seven days.

Allen, A. M., and Taplin, D.: Tropical immersion foot. Lancet, 2:1185, 1973.
Clayton, A. J. W.: Twenty-one cases of immersion foot. Med. Ser. J. Canada, 23:857, 1967.
Lange, K., Weiner, D., and Boyd, L. J.: The functional pathology of experimental immersion foot. Am. Heart J., 35:238, 1948.
Montgomery, H.: Experimental immersion foot; review of physiopathology. Physiol. Rev., 34:127, 1954.
White, J. C.: Vascular and neurologic lesions in survivors of shipwreck. I. Immersion foot syndrome following exposure to cold. II. Painful swollen feet secondary to prolonged dehydration and malnutrition. N. Engl. J. Med., 228:211, 1943.

CHILBLAIN AND PERNIO

Chilblain and pernio (*erythrocyanosis*) occur commonly in patients, especially females, with a history of cool limbs in summer as well as winter. The etiologic and pathogenic factors are unknown, but the disease is seen only in cold, damp climates. However, it is much more frequent in England than in areas of the United States with comparable climates.

Acute chilblain occurs on the dorsum of the digits, hands, or feet as localized, warm, red, intensely pruritic swelling that may disappear spontaneously in a few days. Pernio is probably the same disease but involves the lower parts of the legs, especially in women who, because of their mode of dress, do not adequately protect their legs from cold weather. Rarely, indolent lesions, dull red or violaceous, proceed to painful bleb formation.

The blebs contain blood-stained serous fluid and often lead to ulcer formation.

In some patients exposed repeatedly to cold, recurrent and chronic lesions, often appearing in crops, may develop. The lesions are erythematous and ulcerative and may leave residual scarring, fibrosis, and atrophy of the skin and subcutaneous tissues. The disease is more active during the cooler months and subsides in warm weather. Bilateral and symmetrical parts of the extremities are involved. This state is called chronic chilblain or pernio (erythrocyanosis frigida crurum).

Treatment is nonspecific. Corticosteroid creams may be used for itching and inflammation, antimicrobials for sepsis. Reserpine (0.25 mg orally daily) has been reported to ameliorate the disease.

Eskell, J.: Reserpine in the treatment of chilblains. Practitioner, 189:792, 1962.

Lewis, T.: Observations on some normal and injurious effects of cold upon the skin and underlying tissues. II. Chilblains and allied conditions. Br. Med. J., 2:837, 1941.

McGovern, T., Wright, I. S., and Kruger, E.: Pernio: A vascular disease. Am. Heart J., 22:583, 1941.

Thomas, E. W. P.: Chapping and chilblains. Practitioner, 193:755, 1964.

FROSTBITE

Definition. Frostbite is due to freezing of tissues which may result in damage to skin, muscle, blood vessels, and nerves.

Etiology. Superficial freezing of tissues evidently begins when the temperature of deeper tissues reaches about 10° C (50° F). During the Korean War, most cases of frostbite occurred at −6.5° C (20° F) or below, after 7 to 18 hours' exposure. High winds, dampness, and general chilling of the body make frostbite more likely at above-freezing temperatures. Predisposing factors include any type of peripheral vascular insufficiency, improper clothing, exhaustion, and previous cold injury. Lack of acclimatization and geographic origin have also been implicated; the black race is more susceptible to frostbite. Most frostbite is of the slow freezing type, but a rapid frostbite (occurring in a few minutes) takes place at high altitudes with extremely low temperatures and has a predilection for the extremities rather than the face and ears.

Pathophysiology. Whether actual tissue freezing or decreased blood flow from vasoconstriction is most important in producing cell injury is unknown. Damage is probably due to a combination of direct freezing with the formation of extracellular ice crystals, inducing dehydration of cells, and to intense vasoconstriction. The vasoconstriction is due to direct cold exposure of the tissues but may also involve reflex vasoconstriction from chilling of other body areas. The reduced blood flow leads to capillary stasis and arteriolar and capillary thromboses. Capillary permeability is increased and results in edema formation.

Pathology. The pathologic findings vary with the stage of the disease and the depth of tissue affected. In early stages, low-grade vasculitis and inflammation in all tissues are seen. Later the skin is atrophied and may be keratinized, muscle is necrosed and shows waxy degeneration, arterioles and capillaries are thrombosed, and nerves demonstrate fibroblastic proliferation and neurolysis.

Clinical Manifestations. The first indication of frostbite is often a sharp, pricking sensation that draws attention to a yellowish-white, numb area of hardened skin. However, cold itself produces numbness and anesthesia that may allow freezing of tissue without warning. When the freezing is superficial, thawing leads to local reddening and wheal and flare formation. When freezing involves deep tissues, subcutaneous edema occurs with thawing, followed by formation of vesicles and bullae. A hyperemic, reddish zone may be apparent between frozen and normal tissue. As the edema subsides in a day or two, necrosis and gangrene may become evident. However, it may take two to three months before final demarcation between viable and dead tissue can be ascertained. In the healing phase, a black eschar usually covers the area.

The traditional classification of frostbite has been from first to fourth degree, depending on the depth of tissue injury. Since the true extent of tissue damage cannot be judged on initial examination, a simpler classification of superficial and deep frostbite is more practical. The prognosis depends on the depth of freezing, as superficial cases usually have no sequelae, although deep freezing may finally end in amputation.

Prophylaxis. Frostbite is preventable and occurs rarely among those who have been instructed how to protect themselves. Prophylactic measures include observance of each other for signs of frostbite; wearing adequate, loose fitting, dry clothing and mittens; exposure for only brief periods when exercise is not possible; and avoidance of smoking before and during exposure. Feet and socks should be kept dry.

Treatment. Superficial frostbite can be treated immediately by rewarming; affected areas on the face and ears can be warmed with the hands, hands can be placed in the axillae, or frostbitten parts can be warmed on the exposed torso of a partner. Frostbitten areas should not be rubbed with snow or exercised.

Treatment of deep frostbite should be delayed until adequate facilities for rewarming are available. Therapy should always be very conservative, because the depth of tissue damage is difficult to ascertain, sometimes for months. It is best to rewarm the tissues as rapidly as possible in 40 to 44° C water (104 to 111° F). Massage, exposure to too high temperatures, and reactive hyperemia should be avoided because they tend to increase pain and edema. Analgesics usually are needed during rewarming. After rewarming, which usually requires about 20 minutes, the frostbitten area is exposed to room air (21 to 26° C, 70 to 78° F). Although pressure dressings may be used, the open method with sterile surroundings is usually preferred. Vesicles, bullae, and eschars are left untouched. Antimicrobial drugs are indicated if infection is present. Tobacco smoking should be prohibited. Regional sympathectomy has been reported as beneficial, both clinically and experimentally, if performed at an optimal time of 24 to 48 hours after frostbite occurs. Sympathectomy may conserve tissue and lead to earlier demarcation, cessation of pain, and healing of tissue.

Eventual recovery is usually surprisingly good, the black eschar peeling off to leave normal tissue beneath. Sensitivity to cold, paresthesias, and a predilection to repeated frostbite often persist. In severe frostbite, fibrosis of tissue may lead to disability, and gangrenous extremities may require amputation.

Golding, M. R., Martinez, A., DeJong, P., Mendosa, M., Fries, C. C., Sawyer, P. N., Hennigar, G. R., and Wesolowski, S. A.: The role of sympathectomy in frostbite, with review of 68 cases. Surgery, 57:774, 1965.

Lapp, N. L., and Juergens, J. L.: Frostbite. Mayo Clin. Proc., 40:932, 1965.

Meryman, H. T.: Tissue freezing and local cold injury. Physiol. Rev., 37:233, 1957.

Washburn, B.: Frostbite. What it is, how to prevent it, emergency treatment. N. Engl. J. Med., 266:974, 1962.

598. PERIPHERAL VASCULAR DISEASES DUE TO ABNORMAL COMMUNICATIONS BETWEEN ARTERIES AND VEINS

ARTERIOVENOUS FISTULA

Definition. Arteriovenous fistulas are abnormal communications, single or multiple, between arteries and veins by which arterial blood enters the veins directly without transversing a capillary network.

Etiology. Arteriovenous fistulas created to facilitate renal dialysis are the most common fistulas. Acquired arteriovenous fistulas, usually single and saccular, may develop after a bullet or stab wound involving an artery and a contiguous vein. Fistulas of the iliac vessels may occur after surgery for intervertebral disc disease. Congenital fistulas are present from birth and are usually multiple; they result from defects in differentiation of the common embryologic anlage into artery and vein. There is no special sex incidence, and any part of the body may be involved.

Pathophysiology. Arterial blood, following the path of least resistance, flows directly into the vein, bypassing the corresponding capillary bed. The arterial pressure is transmitted to the venous side of the fistula; the distal vein pressure is increased, but the proximal vein pressure may actually be negative during systole owing to the high velocity of blood flow. The elevated venous pressure leads to the development of varicose veins and venous stasis changes in the limb. Increased blood flow makes the tissues near the fistula abnormally warm, and diminished flow distal to the fistula may produce peripheral coldness and trophic changes. Large fistulas impose a burden on the heart; the cardiac output must be increased above normal by an amount proportional to the size of the fistula in order to maintain the general circulation. Total blood volume may be increased. The low peripheral resistance of the involved area tends to decrease diastolic and increase systolic and pulse pressures systemically. Large fistulas may lead to cardiac decompensation. Even the small fistulas created for renal dialysis have been shown to induce a small increase in cardiac output and heart rate with a decrease in peripheral resistance.

Pathology. In the region of the fistula, the intima and media of the involved veins become thickened, and newly developed elastic fibers appear. The arteries show a thinning of their walls with loss of elastic tissue and muscular fibers in the media.

Clinical Manifestations. Patients complain of aching pain, edema, varicosities, or hypertrophied extremities. Occasionally, cardiac symptoms such as palpitation, substernal pain, and dyspnea on exertion are present. Examination reveals tortuous, dilated superficial veins in the extremity, and venous pulsation can be felt unless the fistula is small and deeply placed. In congenital fistulas, the skin temperature is usually elevated locally but decreased distal to the fistulas, although in acquired lesions, the temperature of the digits may be greater than in the opposite normal limb. A bruit and thrill are common over acquired fistulas; the bruit lasts throughout systole and diastole and has a coarse, machinery-like quality. The tissues near the fistula may be tender, edematous, and either red or slightly cyanotic. The circumference of the extremity is increased by edema or true hypertrophy, but bony structures are hypertrophied only if the fistula was present before epiphyseal closure. Stasis pigmentation and chronic indurative cellulitis with or without indolent ulceration may be present distal to the fistula. In contrast to the postphlebitic limb in which ulcers form around the medial malleolus, the ulceration of fistulas may affect the distal parts of the foot. Rarefaction of bone in the extremity may also occur. Temporary compression of the artery supplying a large fistula diminishes the heart rate (*Branham's sign*) and may be a helpful diagnostic sign.

Diagnosis. If the diagnosis cannot be made from the clinical manifestations, other examinations may be helpful. The oxygen saturation of blood removed from fistula veins will be found to be greater than that of blood removed from corresponding veins in the opposite extremity. Arteriography will reveal the lesion, its location, and the number and size of communications. Edema of one or both extremities after surgery for intervertebral disc disease should suggest the possibility of a fistula. Thrombophlebitis and the postphlebitic extremity can be distinguished from fistulas by the oxygen studies and arteriography.

Prognosis. The prognosis of acquired and single congenital fistulas is good after surgical repair. In acquired iliac vessel fistulas, congestive heart failure develops in two thirds of patients, and immediate repair is important. Without surgical repair, which is often not possible in multiple fistulas, the outlook is for a chronically swollen limb with varicosities, stasis pigmentation, and ulceration. Bacterial infection of acquired fistulas occurs but is rare.

Treatment. Single fistulas can be repaired surgically by re-establishing the continuity of the involved artery and vein walls by a variety of procedures (arteriorrhaphy, end-to-end suture, grafting). Ligation of the involved artery and vein leads to a high incidence of arterial and venous insufficiency of the extremity and should be avoided if possible. If the arterial supply depends upon a large anomalous artery, ligation of this vessel, followed by sclerosing injections of the dilated veins, may be effective. Multiple fistulas are much less amenable to surgery. Ulcers, edema, and pain may be relieved by wearing elastic bandages or stockings; pressure on the veins encourages blood flow to follow the arterial pathway. Amputation is required for large inoperable fistulas producing cardiac decompensation or gross deformity.

Binak, K., Regan, T. J., Christensen, R. C., and Hellems, H. K.: Arteriovenous fistula: Hemodynamic effects of occlusion and exercise. Am. Heart J., 60:495, 1960.

Johnson, G., Jr., and Blythe, W. B.: Hemodynamic effects of arteriovenous shunts used for hemodialysis. Ann. Surg., 171:715, 1970.

Lawton, R. L., Tidrick, R. T., and Brintnall, E. S.: A clinicopathologic study of multiple congenital arteriovenous fistulae of the lower extremities. Angiology, 8:161, 1957.

Nickerson, J. L., Elkin, D. C., and Warren, J. V.: The effect of temporary occlusion of arteriovenous fistulas on heart rate, stroke volume, and cardiac output. J. Clin. Invest., 30:215, 1951.

Spittell, J. A., Jr., Palumbo, P. J., Love, J. G., and Ellis, F. H., Jr.: Arteriovenous fistula complicating lumbar disk surgery. N. Engl. J. Med., 268:1162, 1963.

Wakim, K. G., and Janes, J. M.: Influence of arteriovenous fistula on the distal circulation in the involved extremity. Arch. Phys. Med. Rehabil., 39:431, 1958.

GLOMANGIOMA OR GLOMUS TUMOR

Definition.   Glomangioma or glomus tumor designates painful enlargement of a glomus body.

Pathology.   The pathology consists of hypertrophy of the glomus body which contains an arteriovenous anastomosis with its associated smooth muscle coat, nonmyelinated nerve fibers, and connective tissue. Histologically, the lesion is encapsulated, occasionally diffuse but never invasive, and contains numerous epithelioid cells with no inflammatory cells.

Clinical Manifestations.   Glomus tumors are extremely tender but inconspicuous subcutaneous nodules which develop slowly during adult life. Pain may be present before the nodule becomes visible. They are found in various parts of the upper and lower extremities, but most frequently (30 per cent) beneath the fingernail. The diameter of the tumor is usually only a few millimeters. The nodule has a flat or slightly raised surface with reddish-blue to purplish discoloration. Excruciating burning or shooting pain, both local and referred up the extremity, occurs spontaneously or is produced by the slightest pressure. Hyperhidrosis, abnormal vasomotor activity, increased skin temperature, and tissue atrophy in the involved limb may be present. Heat, cold, and even contact with clothing may become intolerable so that protection is required continuously day and night. In glomus tumors beneath nails, a small excavation of the phalanx from erosion by the tumor can often be seen by roentgenography.

Treatment.   Surgical excision leads to complete and immediate relief without recurrence.

Bailey, O. T.: The cutaneous glomus and its tumors—glomangiomas. Am. J. Path., 11:915, 1935.

Cooke, S. A. R.: Misleading features in the clinical diagnosis of the peripheral glomus tumor. Br. J. Surg., 58:602, 1971.

Horton, C., Maguire, C., Georgiade, N., and Pickrell, K.: Glomus tumors: An analysis of 25 cases. Arch. Surg., 71:712, 1955.

599. DISEASES OF THE PERIPHERAL VEINS

THROMBOPHLEBITIS

This subject is discussed in Ch. 544.

VARICOSE VEINS AND THE POSTPHLEBITIC SYNDROME

Definition.   Varicose veins are distended, tortuous veins with incompetent valves. The postphlebitic syndrome denotes the chronically swollen extremity with trophic changes secondary to chronic venous stasis; despite the name, a previous history of thrombophlebitis is often not obtainable.

Etiology.   Varicose veins are considered to be caused either by congenitally defective valves or by a condition that deforms valves or obstructs venous outflow over long periods of time. Varicosities resulting from congenital defects may develop early in life. Thrombophlebitis may lead to the formation of varicosities by deformation or destruction of venous valves and venous obstruction. Pregnancy, ascites, abdominal tumor, excessive weight or height, and prolonged weight bearing are all considered accelerating factors which cause increased venous pressure in the legs, distention of veins, and finally incompetency of valves. A generalized abnormality of the veins has been suggested as a predisposing factor. An increased forearm vein distensibility and a decreased amount of collagen and hexosamine in uninvolved veins have been demonstrated in patients with lower extremity varicosities; however, genetic evidence is not substantial. Since the majority of patients do not have obvious causes and varicose veins are an affliction of Western civilization, other factors in our society have been sought. The constipation associated with the Western countries' low-residue diet has been proposed as a frequent etiologic factor in varicosities. Emphasis is placed on the association of varicosities with hemorrhoids and diverticulosis, as a result of either increased intra-abdominal pressure during bowel movements or local pressure exerted by the bowel on intra-abdominal structures.

Incidence.   Varicose veins are very common, appearing in approximately 40 per cent of women; the incidence is less in men. The saphenous veins in the lower extremities are most frequently affected.

Clinical Manifestations.   The dilated, tortuous, sacculated varices are easily visible. Some patients with extensive superficial varicosities have no other symptoms or signs, but others have aching pain or easy fatigability of the calf muscles and edema after weight bearing. The edema usually disappears with bed rest overnight. Rarely the varicosities are so large that postural hypotension may result from pooling of blood in the lower extremities. When the communicating or deep veins are incompetent, symptoms and signs are more common. Chronic venous insufficiency is manifested by edema, which may later become fibrosed to produce a brawny induration. Extravasation of blood locally may cause a brownish pigmentation; an itchy, eczematoid rash may appear in the area. Finally the skin may ulcerate, producing an indolent, nonpainful lesion, usually above the medial malleolus near a palpable, incompetent communicating vein. This picture of chronic swelling and stasis dermatitis is called the postphlebitic syndrome. Arterial pulses are normal. When the deep venous system is blocked, pain similar to intermittent claudication may rarely occur.

Diagnosis.   The diagnosis can be made from the clinical picture. Retrograde flow of blood past incompetent valves can be demonstrated by the Trendelenburg test and its variations. The leg of the recumbent patient is elevated to empty the veins, and then a tourniquet is applied to occlude the superficial veins. The patient quickly assumes a standing position, the tourniquet is released, and the veins will become distended immediately if back flow is present. If two tourniquets are applied and left in place when the patient stands, filling of the saphenous veins between the tourniquets indicates an incompetent communicating vein. Application of the tourniquets to different levels on the limb can delineate exactly the sites of vein pathology. Venography may be used in doubtful cases or to be certain the deep venous system is patent. In a patient with varicosities and edema, other causes of edema, e.g., cardiovascular and renal disease, should be investigated.

Prognosis. The prognosis for simple superficial varicose veins is good with treatment. Once the postphlebitic syndrome has developed, progressive disability usually can be expected despite treatment.

Treatment. Uncomplicated varicose veins respond well to support with elastic stockings or bandages to prevent progression. Panty girdles should never be worn. Frequent periods of elevation of the extremity above heart level, high ligation with stripping of the saphenous veins, and injection of sclerosing solutions may become necessary to prevent or treat the postphlebitic syndrome. However, since saphenous veins may be needed for arterial (coronary or peripheral) surgery, stripping should be performed only when absolutely unavoidable. Venous stasis ulcers are treated with sponge rubber pressure dressings or gelatin boots; local or systemic antimicrobials are indicated if infection is present. Sometimes the entire fibrosed area must be removed and a skin graft applied to heal an indolent ulcer.

Alexander, C. J.: The theoretical basis of varicose vein formation. Med. J. Aust., 1:258, 1972.

Bauer, G.: Pathophysiology and treatment of the lower leg stasis syndrome. Angiology, 1:1, 1950.

Burkitt, D. P.: Varicose veins, deep vein thrombosis, and haemorrhoids: Epidemiology and suggested etiology. Br. Med. J., 2:556, 1972.

Fegan, W. G.: Conservative treatment of varicose veins. Prog. Surg., 11:37, 1973.

Mullarky, R. E.: The Anatomy of Varicose Veins. Springfield, Ill., Charles C Thomas, 1965.

Thurston, O. G., and Williams, H. T. G.: Chronic venous insufficiency of the lower extremity. Arch. Surg., 106:537, 1973.

Wood, J. E.: The Veins. Boston, Little, Brown & Company, 1965.

600. DISEASES OF THE PERIPHERAL LYMPHATIC VESSELS

Lymph is formed by the transudation of plasma through capillary walls into tissue spaces. The plasma that is not reabsorbed into the venular end of the capillaries is collected by a rich intercellular network of tiny lymphatic vessels. These vessels possess semilunar valves and become larger as they convey lymph to the regional lymph nodes; then the lymph travels through trunk lymphatics to the thoracic duct and finally to the left internal jugular vein. In the extremities, there are superficial and deep lymphatic systems which probably are joined by communicating vessels. The flow of lymph depends on intrinsic, rhythmic contractions of the lymph vessels, muscular contraction, respiratory movements, and, to a certain extent, gravity. The lymphatic vessels are responsive to sympathetic nerve stimulation, but the functional significance of this is not known.

LYMPHEDEMA

Definition. Lymphedema is a form of chronic unilateral or bilateral edema of the extremities caused by the accumulation of lymph secondary to abnormalities or blockage of the lymph vessels or pathologic conditions of the lymph nodes.

Etiology. Primary lymphedema may be a hereditary disease or may occur sporadically. Various classifications exist according to whether the lymphedema is present at birth (*congenital*), appears at or near puberty (*praecox*), occurs after age 35 (*tarda*), or is familial and congenital (*Milroy's disease*). The mode of inheritance is probably dominant but has not been thoroughly investigated. An increased incidence occurs in ovarian dysgenesis syndromes. Primary lymphedema affects females predominantly (about 8:1); the onset of the disease occurs before age 40 in more than 90 per cent of cases.

Secondary lymphedema is most commonly caused by inflammation and follows recurrent lymphangitis (see below). In tropical and subtropical regions, filariasis often leads to lymphedema. Neoplasms are the second most common cause either by invasion or compression of lymph vessels or nodes. Surgical removal of lymph nodes and the fibrosis that follows irradiation may also cause lymphedema. Secondary cases have no special sex incidence and are uncommon before age 40.

Pathology. Examination of primary lymphedematous limbs by lymphangiography has revealed aplasia, hypoplasia, or hyperplasia (varicosities) of the lymphatic vessels. The lymph nodes may also be aplastic or hypoplastic, producing an obstructive type of lymphedema. No specific pathologic picture has been correlated with the current classification system, but the few cases of Milroy's disease examined have revealed aplasia (or absence) of the lymphatic vessels. There is some indication that lymphedema may be part of a generalized defect in lymphatic vessels. Patients with lymphedema have been reported to have chylous pleural effusions, chylous ascites, and even intestinal lymphangiectasis. A syndrome of yellow nails, recurrent pleural effusion, and lymphedema occurs and is believed to be secondary to lymphatic abnormalities in each area. Another familial syndrome of recurrent intrahepatic cholestasis and lymphedema exists, the cholestasis probably being caused by defective hepatic lymphatic vessels. In secondary lymphedema, innumerable small, irregular lymphatics are usually seen beside normal or tortuous, sometimes varicose, vessels.

Clinical Manifestations. Primary lymphedema is usually gradual in onset and asymptomatic; the distal portion of the extremity or whole extremity, or even a portion of the trunk, may increase in size. The edema is soft and pitting at first and disappears with treatment but later becomes firm and nonpitting, and cannot be relieved completely by treatment. At this stage, the skin becomes thickened and resists wrinkling; hair follicles are prominent. The lower extremities are involved most often; about half the patients develop bilateral swelling. The edematous tissue is especially susceptible to episodes of lymphangitis and cellulitis, which add to the deformity.

Secondary lymphedema is seldom bilateral. Lymphedema of the inflammatory type follows recurrent episodes of lymphangitis. Each attack leaves more residual edema after the inflammation subsides. The skin finally becomes thick, coarse, folded, and hard so that the eventual deformity may be extreme (elephantiasis). Secondary lymphedema resulting from neoplasm and other noninflammatory causes produces painless swelling of an extremity. Painless swelling of an extremity in an elderly male must be considered secondary to carcinoma of the prostate until proved otherwise.

Diagnosis. Painless chronic swelling of an extremity suggests the diagnosis of lymphedema. Differentiation from venous insufficiency may be made by the lack of prominent veins, stasis dermatitis, and ulceration; lymphangiography and venography may be necessary. Mixed lymphangiomatous and hemangiomatous malformations that cause enlarged limbs can be diagnosed by the obvious tumor mass. In lipodystrophy, lymphangiography is necessary to delineate the normal lymphatics displaced by the lipomatous masses.

Prognosis. Primary lymphedema usually progresses inexorably to a chronically swollen limb or limbs despite treatment. However, the lymphedema associated with gonadal dysgenesis may disappear spontaneously in months to years. Secondary lymphedema caused by infection may be controlled with adequate treatment. The prognosis is that of the underlying disease in other causes.

Treatment. In primary lymphedema, the most important aim of therapy is to keep the involved extremities free of edema in order to prevent fibrosis and recurrent infection. Frequent elevation of the extremity (including sleeping with the extremity above the heart level), elastic support applying graded pressure from the foot proximally when ambulatory, low sodium diet, and diuretics are usually necessary. Local infection and obvious lesions, such as epidermophytosis, should be eradicated. Surgical attack in advanced cases with fibrosis and resistant edema (Kondoleon operation and its modifications) has produced some relief but is usually disappointing.

Dilley, J. J., Kierland, R. R., Randall, R. V., and Shick, R. M.: Primary lymphedema associated with yellow nails and pleural effusions. J.A.M.A., 204:670, 1968.

Gough, M. H.: Primary lymphedema: Clinical and lymphangiographic studies. Br. J. Surg., 53:918, 1966.

Hall, J. G.: The flow of lymph. N. Engl. J. Med., 281:720, 1969.

Kinmonth, J. B.: The Lymphatics: Diseases, Lymphography and Surgery. Baltimore, Williams and Wilkins Company, 1972.

Sigstad, H., Aagenaes, Ø., Bjorn-Hansen, R. W., and Rootwelt, K.: Primary lymphoedema combined with hereditary recurrent intrahepatic cholestasis. Acta Med. Scand., 188:213, 1970.

Smith, R. D., Spittell, J. A., Jr., and Schirger, A.: Secondary lymphedema of the leg: Its characteristics and diagnostic implications. J.A.M.A., 185:80, 1963.

Stone, E. J., and Hugo, N. E.: Lymphedema. Surg. Gynecol. Obstet., 135:625, 1972.

LYMPHANGITIS

Definition. Lymphangitis is an acute or chronic inflammation, usually pyogenic, of the lymphatic vessels.

Etiology. In the majority of cases of lymphangitis the hemolytic Streptococcus is the infecting agent; second most common is the coagulase-positive Staphylococcus. The bacteria enter the skin via areas of local trauma, trichophytosis, or arterial ischemic or venous stasis ulcers, although a portal of entry cannot always be discovered. Infection then spreads by the lymphatic vessels to the local lymph nodes; an accompanying diffuse cellu-

litis of the extremity is often present. An immune response to previously present bacteria or their products has been postulated as a cause of lymphangitis when an organism cannot be isolated, but proof of this is lacking.

Pathology. Acute, subacute, or chronic inflammation is found in the subcutaneous tissues and regional lymph nodes.

Clinical Manifestations. Attacks of lymphangitis may be ushered in by malaise, headache, nausea, vomiting, and shaking chills followed by fever. Systemic symptoms, however, may not be present. Red streaks appear in the affected extremity, originating at the portal of entry and following the pathway of lymphatic vessels. Regional lymph nodes are usually enlarged and tender. There may be a surrounding area of cellulitis with tenderness and red discoloration in the lower part of the extremity, which is usually swollen with a soft, pitting edema.

Diagnosis. The clinical picture is usually typical and allows the diagnosis to be made easily. A leukocytosis is often present. The inciting organism should be sought by culturing the portal of entry if obvious or by needle puncture of the subcutaneous tissues. A difficult diagnosis to rule out is acute thrombophlebitis, especially when a diffuse cellulitis is present, for symptoms and signs are similar; it is often wise to administer therapy for both diseases simultaneously.

Prognosis. For an initial attack in a limb without underlying disease, the prognosis with treatment is excellent. However, some patients have recurrent attacks, often mild, which can lead to the development of lymphedema. In recurrent cases, the limb may remain somewhat larger after each attack.

Treatment. Systemic antimicrobial drugs should be administered as indicated by culture (and sensitivity studies if necessary). If no organism is cultured, penicillin should be given because the Streptococcus is so commonly the etiologic agent. Drainage of any focus of origin is also extremely important. Adjunctive measures include rest, elevation of the extremity above heart level, and warm wet dressings. Possible fungal infections in the feet and causes of secondary lymphedema should be sought. When attacks subside, elastic support should be worn on the extremity for three months to prevent residual swelling. In recurrent cases, either with or without underlying lymphedema, prophylactic long-term antimicrobial therapy should be instituted. Lymphangitis is especially dangerous in the ischemic tissues of patients with obstructive arterial disease; only under these unfavorable conditions is prompt amputation sometimes required.

Babb, R. R., Spittell, J. A., Jr., Martin, W. J., and Schirger, A.: Prophylaxis of recurrent lymphangitis complicating lymphedema. J.A.M.A., 195:871, 1966.

Edwards, E. A.: Recurrent febrile episodes and lymphedema. J.A.M.A., 184:858, 1963.

Part XIII
RENAL DISEASES

601. INTRODUCTION: ROLE OF THE KIDNEY IN HEALTH AND DISEASE

D. N. S. Kerr

EXCRETION

The prime function of the kidney is to excrete the surplus water and nonmetabolized solute in the diet, as well as the nonvolatile end products of metabolism, in such a manner as to preserve a constant internal environment. The major constituents of the urine are water, urea, sodium, chloride, potassium, phosphate, and creatinine; but several hundred substances can be identified in urine, and the excretion of many minor constituents is essential to health. The minimal urine volume is determined by the osmotic load, of which urea, sodium, and chloride are the main determinants. A subject taking a low protein, low salt diet can survive on a daily urine output of only 200 ml, whereas the steak and salt addict must excrete well over the conventional 500 ml per 24 hours. In a temperate climate a subject with normal renal function can preserve a nearly constant extracellular fluid volume and chemical composition on a sodium intake which can vary one hundred fold, or on a water intake of from less than 1 liter to more than 10 liters per 24 hours.

These extremes of renal function are rarely required in modern living. The average citizen keeps his water intake within narrow limits of 1 to 2 liters per day, and his sodium and protein intake do not vary any more widely from day to day. His kidneys are stressed only occasionally at a celebration night in the bar or during illness involving fever, water deprivation, vomiting, and diarrhea. If his kidneys are slowly destroyed by disease, he may continue to live a comfortable life and hold down a demanding job until about 90 per cent of his excretory function is lost, provided he continues his normal routines and does not challenge his kidneys by dietary aberration, intercurrent illness, or the consumption of medications which contain drugs or electrolytes he cannot readily excrete. Apparently those mechanisms which control excretion in health can be adapted very successfully to achieve the same end while the nephron population is declining. The nature of these control mechanisms and their modification in disease are subjects of intensive research and lively controversy.

Water excretion is controlled mainly by the secretion from the neurohypophysis of antidiuretic hormone, which affects the permeability of the distal tubule. The osmotic load per nephron is a second mechanism controlling water excretion, of particular importance when intake is low. Alteration in glomerular filtration rate (GFR) was once regarded as the first mechanism controlling sodium excretion, but it now seems unlikely that it plays a major part in health. There is some evidence, discussed in Ch. 603, that the patient in chronic renal failure does utilize alterations in GFR to achieve sodium

balance. Aldosterone is a second important control mechanism, but it cannot be responsible for more than the fine control of sodium excretion. The remaining mechanisms controlling the tubular reabsorption of sodium and chloride are still uncertain; they may include the colloid osmotic pressure and hydrostatic pressure of peritubular capillaries and an unidentified natriuretic hormone. These and other possibilities are lumped together in imprecise nephrologic jargon as *"third factor."*

One of the most remarkable adaptations to chronic renal disease is an increase in the proportion of filtered sodium which is excreted in the urine, from the normal 0.5 to 1 per cent up to 20 per cent or more in late renal failure. An increased osmotic load per nephron and suppression of aldosterone secretion may play a part in this adaptation, but much of the change has yet to be accounted for. Presumably "third factor" is altered in the appropriate direction. The feat may not be achieved without some cost. Bricker has suggested that many of the symptoms of renal failure may be the result of overproduction of hormones to achieve such compensation, rather than the effect of more direct mechanisms such as the retention of waste products. He illustrates this "trade-off hypothesis" with an example that is better understood than sodium excretion. Phosphate is retained as glomerular filtration falls, depressing plasma-ionized calcium concentration and stimulating parathyroid hormone secretion. This corrects plasma phosphate until late in the course of renal failure but at the cost of causing osteitis fibrosa. Another effect of increased parathyroid hormone secretion is to produce a renal bicarbonate leak which contributes to "renal acidosis."

There is a limit to the loss of renal function which can be compensated in this manner. In chronic renal disease it is reached when GFR falls to about 10 per cent of normal, at which point symptoms often become prominent even on normal diet and undisturbed routine. When excretory function is lost suddenly, as in bilateral ureteral obstruction, cortical necrosis, or fulminant glomerulonephritis, no compensation is possible, and death may occur within a few days from intoxication with water (convulsions), salt and water (pulmonary edema), or potassium (cardiac arrest). Only if the intake is regulated to prevent these disasters does the patient survive long enough to suffer from the retention of metabolic end products. Which of these waste products harm him and in what way are still topics of which we are surprisingly ignorant. Ultimately any of them would prove toxic; if there were no alternative pathway of excretion it would accumulate until it caused cell death or the patient turned, like Lot's wife, into a pillar of crystallized solute. However, it remains uncertain which of these compounds in practice achieve toxic concentrations in human disease. Even the contribution of urea to the symptoms of uremia is undecided, although it is probably small. Creatinine is declared innocent by almost every commentator even though it accelerates autohemolysis in vitro. Guanidines, phenols, amines, and sulfate have been blamed for some symptoms by some authors. When an alternative, unphysiologic pathway of excretion is provided through the peritoneum or the artificial kidney, small molecules are removed preferentially, and "middle molecules" of molecular weight 300 to 1500 are retained. There is a burgeoning literature attributing uremic symptoms, particularly those in the nervous system, to these unidentified compounds, but the case is far from proved and their role, if any, in unmodified renal failure is largely unexplored.

The glomerulus has only one function—production of glomerular filtrate. *Glomerular disease* is therefore manifest as acute or chronic renal failure or through a leak of protein and cells in the filtrate. *Tubular function* is much more complex, involving many different enzyme systems in active transport. One would therefore expect to find a number of syndromes associated with enzyme deficiencies in the tubules, the result of inherited defects and intoxications. This proves to be the case; many defects of amino acid, dextrose, phosphate and uric acid reabsorption, hydrogen ion excretion, and end-organ responsiveness to individual hormones are recognized. They have provided invaluable insight into renal physiology and are often rewarding conditions to treat, but numerically they make up a very small part of clinical nephrology, compared with glomerular disease and whole nephron failure.

BLOOD FLOW

The kidneys receive a quarter of the cardiac output. Renal blood flow varies little during sedentary activity, but it falls during strenuous exercise, in hypovolemia, and in many pathologic states such as cardiac or hepatic failure. Infusion of vasodilator drugs such as acetylcholine, papaverine, and dopamine increase renal blood flow by up to 100 per cent. Over a wide range of blood flow in these conditions glomerular filtration rate is kept almost constant. This autoregulation has been attributed to balanced control of tone in the afferent and efferent arterioles, maintaining constant glomerular capillary pressure, but it is now apparent that intraglomerular pressure varies appreciably and is balanced by other mechanisms such as compensatory rise in proximal tubular pressure.

Radiokrypton studies show four components in the blood flow pattern through the kidney. There is a fast flow through the outer cortex and progressively slower streams through inner cortex, outer medulla, and papilla. Outer cortical nephrons have short Henle loops and are concerned primarily with excretion; inner cortical nephrons have long loops which maintain the high osmolality of the papilla and permit urinary concentration. Outer cortical ischemia is accompanied by sodium retention, e.g., in prerenal uremia or hepatic failure; renal vasodilatation causes sodium and water loss, e.g., in one phase of endotoxic shock. Alterations in the pattern of renal blood flow do not appear to be important in physiologic control of water and electrolyte excretion, but they probably play an important part in many diseases.

ENDOCRINE FUNCTION

The kidney has at least three endocrine functions: secretion of renin, erythropoietin, and the active metabolites of vitamin D; medullary prostaglandins and unidentified intrarenal hormones may also be important endocrine secretions, but the evidence is inconclusive.

Renin, an enzyme which has been obtained almost pure from the pig, has a molecular weight of about 40,000. It acts on a substrate in plasma to produce the decapeptide angiotensin I which is split by a converting enzyme, mainly in lung capillaries, to form the active octapeptide angiotensin II. Angiotensin II stimulates the adrenal to produce aldosterone, and this appears to be its main physiologic function. It is not the only control mechanism. After bilateral nephrectomy, the output of aldosterone responds to changes in plasma potassium, probably from a direct action on the adrenal, and it rises with a fall in plasma sodium. The latter phenomenon is unexplained. However, in health, aldosterone secretion rate is probably controlled mainly by angiotensin II, and this in turn is determined by the secretion rate of renin, because the supply of substrate, converting enzyme, and angiotensinases is seldom rate limiting. Renin is produced in the juxtaglomerular apparatus, which comprises the macula densa of the distal convoluted tubule, the lacis cells continuous with the mesangium, and specialized cells of the afferent arteriole. Consequently, alterations in tubular fluid composition and/or vascular stretch have been suggested as stimuli for renin secretion. The output of renin is increased by sodium depletion, hypovolemia, stimulation of sympathetic nerves or secretion of catecholamines, adoption of the upright posture, and several drugs, including diuretics and antihypertensives. It is decreased by the administration of mineralocorticoids or beta-blockers. Consequently, withdrawal of drug therapy and controlled conditions of posture and freedom from stress are required for studies of renin in disease.

In concentrations higher than those usually found in the plasma in health, angiotensin II is a powerful vasoconstrictor which has direct actions on the tubule. Hypersecretion of renin is important in at least two disease states: hypertension caused by renal artery stenosis; and the severe hypertension, resistant to sodium and water removal, found in a small minority of patients with bilateral renal disease maintained on regular hemodialysis. After bilateral nephrectomy, loss of renin secretion produces surprisingly few ill effects, but some patients suffer troublesome postural hypotension.

Erythropoietin is a glycoprotein, or proteins, produced in the kidney which stimulates committed stem cells in the bone marrow to produce normoblasts. It has proved very difficult to isolate, assay, label, and study physiologically. Its molecular weight is uncertain, but is probably between 10,000 and 60,000. Its site of origin is equally doubtful, but it can be extracted from both medulla and cortex. Its action is enhanced by normal plasma, and it may, like renin, require a plasma substrate. Erythropoietin output is increased by renal hypoxia, e.g., at high altitudes, in cyanotic heart disease, and in chronic lung disease. Plasma erythropoietin is high in all forms of anemia except that of renal disease. Androgens increase the hemoglobin concentration, partly by stimulating erythropoietin output, and estrogens block the action of erythropoietin. A rare form of polycythemia is associated with overproduction of erythropoietin from renal tumors or cysts, and erythropoietin lack is one of several factors producing the anemia of renal failure. This anemia is aggravated by bilateral nephrectomy, suggesting that even shriveled remnants of kidney produce useful amounts of the hormone.

The kidney is the only organ which converts *25-*

hydroxycholecalciferol to its very active *1,25-dihydroxy metabolite.* The output of this hormone is increased by hypocalcemia, which acts via parathyroid hormone secretion, and by hypophosphatemia; 1,25-HCC stimulates calcium and phosphate absorption from the gut and mobilization from the bones, correcting the plasma calcium and phosphate. Trihydroxy metabolites of vitamin D are also produced in the kidney and may have a similar effect. Osteomalacia is a characteristic feature of severe, longstanding renal osteodystrophy, and it is tempting to attribute this to lack of 1,25-HCC. However, it is not yet certain that 1,25-HCC mediates the healing effect of vitamin D on osteomalacia, and some patients with bilateral nephrectomy have bones which are normal clinically, radiologically, and histologically.

THE CLASSIFICATION OF RENAL DISEASE

This topic has obsessed nephrologists and puzzled students for more than a century. The traditional medical textbook presents a series of diseases, each with a specific etiology, and with pathogenesis, pathology, clinical features, and treatment that proceed from it in logical order. The cause of many renal diseases is unknown, and it is probable that many different etiologic agents can initiate some pathogenic mechanisms, e.g., the formation of immune complexes of the right size to lodge in the glomerular filter. It is therefore necessary to attach to each patient a series of diagnoses at different levels: etiologies, pathogenic mechanisms, pathology (morphologic and functional), and clinical features. The first of these is plural, because two or more factors are often necessary for the development of a renal disease. It is likely that only some individuals have the necessary immunologic constitution to develop glomerulonephritis when exposed to the appropriate organism; and whereas many women (perhaps all) admit bacteria into their bladders, only a minority with impaired defense mechanisms, e.g., refluxing ureters, develop pyelonephritis.

Ideally the nomenclature should indicate at what level a diagnosis has been made. A child with hematuria, oliguria, edema, and hypertension should be labeled as having "acute nephritic syndrome." When the pathology has been confirmed and the streptococcal origin has been demonstrated from a rising antistreptolysin-O titer, he merits the full diagnosis of "poststreptococcal acute glomerulonephritis." Since the pathogenesis of this disease is believed always to involve the formation of immune complex, a pathogenetic diagnosis is unnecessary. However, when a similar syndrome is seen in the absence of streptococcal infection and the role of immune complexes can be inferred from the presence of cryoglobulins in plasma, a fall in serum complement, deposition of complement fractions and immunoglobulins in the glomerulus, and "humps" on the basement membrane, "immune complex nephritis of unknown etiology" is a legitimate title and a pointer to possible therapy.

Logical terminology is cumbersome, and the habits of a lifetime are not easily broken. Consequently the chapters which follow preserve some traditional usages which are not strictly logical. However, in these chapters more space is devoted to the description of clinical syndromes, states of disordered function, and pathogenic mechanisms than to individual diseases.

602. INVESTIGATION OF RENAL FUNCTION

D. N. S. Kerr

The common effects of disease on the function of the renal parenchyma are increased excretion of protein, alteration in the formed elements in the urine, reduction in renal blood flow and glomerular filtration rate, impairment of tubular reabsorption and secretion, alteration in the secretion rates of erythropoietin and renin, and disordered metabolism of vitamin D. Accurate study of these functions is an essential part of renal research, but most of the precise methods are too demanding or too tedious for routine clinical use. Plasma renin and angiotensin assays are employed almost exclusively in the investigation of hypertension. Assay of erythropoietin is still too imprecise and difficult to be of use outside research laboratories, and measurement of plasma 1,25-hydroxycholecalciferol is available in only a few centers in the world. Individual tubular functions, other than concentrating power, are tested in the investigation of renal tubular acidosis, other inherited and acquired tubular disorders, and renal calculous disease, and the appropriate tests are described in the chapters dealing with those subjects.

The study of proteinuria and urine microscopy are important in differential diagnosis. Measurement of glomerular filtration rate has little value in diagnosis, except in distinguishing early renal disease from physiologic states such as postural proteinuria, but is important in following the progress of disease and the response to treatment. Renal blood flow would be of some value diagnostically were it not so difficult to measure. Concentrating ability has been used more as a test for early renal damage than as one of specific tubular function, but in the latter role it has a limited value in differential diagnosis.

Proteinuria. The urine of normal adults contains about 40 to 100 mg of protein per 24 hours during sedentary activity. The very low concentrations in normal urine are difficult to measure accurately, and the mean figure quoted varies widely. Conventionally the upper limit of normal is taken as 150 mg per 24 hours in the ambulant subject and 0.03 mg per minute during short collection periods in recumbency. The most sensitive screening test for urinary protein is the formation of a white cloud on heating filtered urine saturated with sodium sulfate and acidified with a few drops of 3 per cent acetic acid; this detects about 5 to 10 mg per 100 ml as a faint trace. A definite positive with any clinical test therefore indicates a protein concentration higher than the normal should achieve under resting conditions, and "proteinuria" has been accepted as the term to describe excessive proteinuria.

All such screening tests have a considerable observer error. The formation of a cloud with 25 per cent salicylsulfonic acid and the appearance of a green color on paper impregnated with bromophenol blue and a buffer (Albustix, Labstix) are much simpler than the heat test, and this compensates for their slightly lower sensitivity. All three tests give a very crude guide to the concentration of protein, the +, ++, +++, and ++++ corresponding roughly to 30, 100, 300, and 1000 mg per 100 ml in the case of bromophenol blue. However, the middle part of the range has poor reproducibility, and a more accurate test is necessary even for general medical use. A turbidimetric method, using salicylsulfonic acid, can be performed in the ward laboratory, the sample being compared with an albumin standard. It underestimates globulins but is sufficiently accurate for clinical purposes. An automated biuret method is more satisfactory, but interfering substances must be removed for really accurate results.

Normal urinary protein contains at least 30 components, the largest of which is a high molecular weight mucoprotein called *Tamm-Horsfall protein,* which originates in the cells lining the ascending limb of Henle's loop and the macula densa segment of the distal convoluted tubule. Precipitation of this protein in the distal tubule forms the basis of renal casts. Other components include most of the plasma proteins of small molecular weight, with albumin the most prominent, and several proteins derived from the prostate and seminal vesicles. The normal glomerulus has been shown to have a high selectivity, i.e., to filter predominantly small colloid molecules, by studies with graded dextrans.

Increased protein excretion occurs with heavy exertion, fever, heart failure, and operative trauma without any known changes in renal structure or permanent change in renal function. Proteinuria from these sources is usually under 500 mg per 24 hours and rarely over 1 gram per 24 hours; its major component is albumin and its presumed origin, the glomerular filtrate. Proteinuria is detected in about 5 per cent of children and adolescents at school medical examinations; the majority of the "positives" prove to have benign exercise or postural proteinuria. Nearly all adolescents and about 50 per cent of young adults can produce proteinuria by adopting a lordotic position, e.g., bent backward over a chair. The proteinuria may be heavy but has no pathologic significance. A smaller proportion (about 5 per cent) of adolescents and a few young children and young adults develop proteinuria simply from standing erect. During prolonged standing the proteinuria may become quite heavy—up to 14 mg per minute has been recorded—but over 24 hours the loss is usually below 1 gram, rarely exceeds 2 grams, and virtually never causes nephrotic syndrome. This *orthostatic proteinuria* in an adolescent or young adult is nearly always benign and often disappears around the age of 20. However, before making the diagnosis and reassuring the patient, it is important to confirm that the proteinuria consistently disappears on recumbency and that there is no other evidence of renal disease. The patient should be asked to empty his bladder immediately before retiring and to collect a urine sample as soon as he rises on three convenient days. He should collect three afternoon samples for comparison. If there is no proteinuria in the morning samples, proteinuria in some of the afternoon samples, a 24-hour excretion of less than 1 gram, a normal plasma urea and creatinine, and no abnormality in the urine deposit on three careful examinations, a confident diagnosis of benign orthostatic proteinuria can be made.

Lordotic and postural proteinuria are generally attributed to temporary obstruction of the renal venous outflow, but their origin within the kidney is uncertain. The proteinuria is unselective (see below), but glomerular permeability is normally selective as judged by the dextran test, suggesting that some of the larger proteins originate below the glomerulus. However, studies with labeled proteins suggest that most of the protein passes through the glomerulus, and transient changes in the podocytes, similar to those found in childhood nephrosis, have been shown in a few patients with orthostatic proteinuria.

Persistent proteinuria is always pathologic. Even if there is no other evidence of renal disease, biopsy usually reveals glomerular or vascular disease. Pathologic proteinurias can be subdivided by concentrating urine (when necessary) and examining it electrophoretically and by immunologic methods. A characteristic pattern, with only a small proportion of albumin, large components of alpha₁, alpha₂, and beta₁ globulins, and an abnormally high proportion of beta₂ microglobulin, is found in patients with active pyelonephritis, medullary cystic disease, congenital tubular disorders, Wilson's disease, hypokalemic nephropathy, sarcoidosis, some toxic nephropathies, including the Balkan nephropathy, and some forms of transplant rejection. It is referred to as "tubular proteinuria" and rarely exceeds 1 gram per 24 hours. In some forms of myelomatosis, the light chains of the abnormal immunoglobulins, being small enough to pass through the glomerular filter easily, appear in the urine as "*Bence Jones proteinuria.*" All other patterns of proteinuria are attributed to increased permeability of the glomerular filter. The normal glomerulus allows macromolecules to enter the filtrate at a rate proportional to the logarithm of their molecular size (Fig. 1). This relationship still holds approximately when the glomerulus becomes excessively leaky, but the slope of the graph varies according to the disease. In nephrotic syndrome with minimal change (childhood nephrosis) it remains steep, so that only the smaller plasma proteins such as albumin appear in the urine in detectable quantities (Fig. 2). In several diffuse diseases of the glomeruli, including membranous glomerulonephropathy and amyloidosis, the graph is less steep, and very large molecules such as alpha₂ macroglobulin can be detected in the urine. Proliferative glomerulonephritis occupies an intermediate position, but yields rather variable results. This is probably due to the

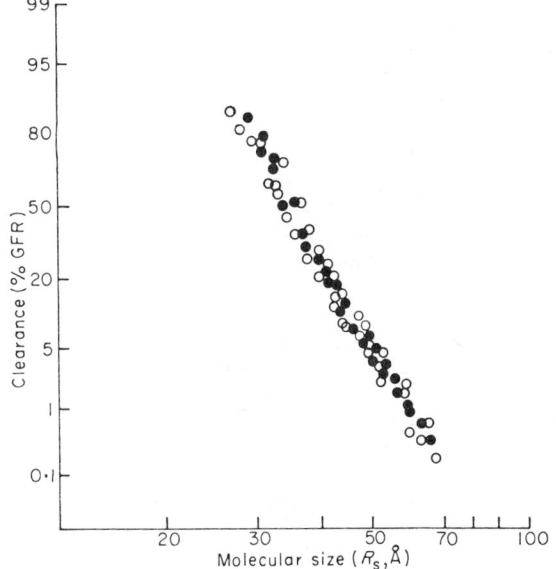

Figure 1. Relationship between the molecular size and the glomerular clearance of large polymers (○ = allyl-dextran; ● = polyvinylpyrrolidone) in normal rabbits. (From Hardwicke, J., et al.: Clin. Sci., 34:509, 1968.)

M = Membranous
P = Proliferative
N = 'Minimal'

Figure 2. Relationship between molecular weight and relative clearance of plasma proteins in the three main types of nephrotic syndrome. (From Blainey, J. D., et al.: Quart J. Med., 34:235, 1959.)

patchy nature of the lesion; tests of selectivity based on proteins in plasma and urine exaggerate the loss of selectivity in this condition, probably because protein is reabsorbed in the tubules of the least affected nephrons. A simplified test for selectivity of proteinuria in which transferrin and IgG or alpha$_2$ macroglobulin are measured in serum and urine with the aid of immunoplates is now a standard laboratory test much simpler than electrophoresis of concentrated urine. Its main value is in the nephrotic syndrome of childhood in which selective proteinuria makes a response to corticosteroids so likely that renal biopsy may often be avoided.

Urine Microscopy.   Midstream urine should be collected at a time when it is likely to be concentrated, using the same precautions as for culture. It should be handled by a constant technique, e.g., by centrifuging 10 ml at 3000 rpm for five minutes and resuspending the sediment in the last 0.5 ml of urine. When many urines are examined, an acceptable alternative is to allow the urine to settle in a test tube for an hour and withdraw the sediment with a Pasteur pipette. A well spread thick drop should be examined under low power for casts and crystals, and a thin film under high power for red cells, white cells, and bacteria and for the exact identification of casts. Red and white cells are often confused under low power even by experienced observers, but the most common error in microscopy is omission of the initial thick drop examination and consequent failure to recognize casts. The microscope must be well maintained and equipped with a variable illuminator and preferably a polarizer. A medium power high enough to permit identification of casts in the thick drop is an added advantage.

Red cells are normally excreted at a rate of about 150 to 300,000 per 24 hours, with an approximate upper limit of 1 million per 24 hours or 1000 per minute in

short collections. Only an occasional red cell should be seen on qualitative microscopy as described above. White cells are excreted at an average of about 70,000 per hour in both sexes, but this applies only to urine entirely free from contamination in the female. If there has been much contamination with vaginal secretion, as indicated by large numbers of squamous epithelial cells, leukocyturia cannot be interpreted unless it is extremely heavy. The upper limit of normal leukocyte excretion is 200,000 per hour, which yields one or two leukocytes per high-power field in qualitative microscopy of a concentrated urine. Leukocytes are difficult to distinguish from nonsquamous epithelial cells from the renal tubules, and the two are usually counted together. The increase in leukocyte excretion after pyrogen injection or prednisolone has been proposed as a test for chronic pyelonephritis, but it is so difficult to obtain noncatheter, timed urine samples from females free from vaginal contamination that it is seldom employed in practice. Qualitative examination for leukocytes is nonetheless of great importance in the detection of urinary infection, renal tuberculosis, and analgesic nephropathy.

Hyaline casts consist of precipitated Tamm-Horsfall protein only; they have a refractive index close to that of urine and are easily missed if the illumination is too high. Up to 10,000 per 24 hours are excreted by normal subjects, but at this rate only a very occasional one is seen even on the thick drop under low power. Numerous hyaline casts are seen in nearly all renal diseases associated with glomerular proteinuria; hyaline casts with few or none of the other varieties described below are seen in benign essential hypertension and nephrotic syndrome with minimal change. Hyaline casts are mainly of roughly constant diameter corresponding to the lumen of the distal convoluted tubule, but short thick casts, formed in the collecting duct, are seen in chronic renal failure and recovering tubular necrosis or glomerulonephritis. Misshapen, long, and branching casts are formed in the late stages of chronic renal diseases, particularly chronic nephritis, reflecting the distorted shape of some nephrons.

Granular casts are speckled or barred owing to the presence of immunoglobulin aggregates in a matrix of Tamm-Horsfall protein. Lightly speckled casts may appear in normal urine after strenuous exercise or during fever; when present in the resting afebrile subject, they nearly always indicate renal pathology but do not point to any particular disease. Densely granular casts, which may appear almost black on microscopy and which are readily confused with red cell casts, are always a sign of disease and are commonly found in active glomerulonephritis, lupus nephritis, malignant hypertension, and renal amyloidosis. Deeply pigmented granular casts are found in association with hemoglobinuria and in the brown urine that is often excreted in the early stages of acute renal failure. Bile-stained granular casts are excreted in large numbers by patients with obstructive jaundice, often without any other evidence of renal dysfunction.

Red blood cell casts have greater diagnostic significance than any other variety. They indicate glomerular bleeding and are excreted in very large numbers in the acute phase of poststreptococcal glomerulonephritis. Smaller numbers are excreted in other forms of glomerulonephritis, notably membranoproliferative nephritis and the focal nephritis of Henoch-Schönlein syndrome and polyarteritis, and in malignant hypertension. They are said to have a reddish tinge, but this is rarely found and is confined to casts with very numerous red cells. Usually they have a greenish tinge under tungsten light. They are readily distinguished from other cellular casts because the red cells are incorporated in the matrix; this can be confirmed by focusing up and down through the cast under medium or high power. *Leukocyte casts* are typical of active pyelonephritis; they are rarely found in chronic pyelonephritis with sterile urine, in which the deposit contains only a few leukocytes if the patient is normotensive. *Epithelial cell casts* are typical of acute tubular necrosis but may be found in active glomerulonephritis, which is often an important differential diagnosis. *Fatty casts,* staining red with Sudan III and showing "Maltese crosses" in polarized light, accompany heavy proteinuria and are probably due to the leakage of lipoproteins through the glomerular filter. Free fat globules and oval fat bodies—degenerate tubular cells in which the "Maltese crosses" of cholesterol esters are best demonstrated—are also typical of nephrotic syndrome.

The recognition of casts is a very important step in establishing the existence of renal disease; they are particularly helpful in the investigation of proteinuria and hematuria, indicating a probable renal cause for the latter. They have a limited usefulness in distinguishing between different renal diseases and have some value in following the activity of disease. The disappearance of red cell casts and dense granular casts from the deposit as malignant hypertension is controlled points to essential hypertension as the primary disease. Once the diagnosis is established, however, cast excretion has little additional prognostic value. Excessive excretion of hyaline and lightly granular casts can continue for decades in inactive disease such as treated essential hypertension, gouty nephropathy, or nonprogressive chronic glomerulonephritis.

Glomerular Filtration Rate. If a substance is filtered at the glomerulus in proportion to plasma water and is not reabsorbed or secreted by the tubule, it can be used to estimate glomerular filtration rate (GFR) because the excretion rate is then determined only by the plasma level and the GFR.

$$\text{GFR (clearance rate of marker substance)} = \frac{\text{excretion rate}}{\text{plasma level}}$$

The one universally accepted marker substance is *inulin,* a mixture of fructose polymers with an average molecular weight of about 5200, but it has the disadvantages of being a variable mixture, of having a low solubility, and of hydrolyzing to fructose during the boiling necessary to dissolve it. The analytic methods for inulin are also difficult. Polyfructosan, with a narrow range of molecular weight and better solubility, is probably superior but less familiar. Any exogenous substance used for measurement of GFR must be infused at a constant rate for long enough to allow complete stabilization of the blood level, and then continued until several urine samples can be obtained of sufficient volume to minimize bladder-emptying errors. Consequently accurate measurement of GFR with inulin, without bladder catheterization, takes four to six hours, and is unsuitable for routine clinical use. The need for urine collection can be eliminated if the constant infusion is continued long enough to ensure that plasma levels are completely stable; the infusion rate is then assumed to equal the urinary excretion rate,

the very small extrarenal loss of inulin being ignored. The technique has some popularity in pediatrics.

Several substances more easily measured than inulin are available; they are not protein bound, are freely filtered, and are little affected by tubular secretion or reabsorption. EDTA labeled with ^{51}Cr is the most popular, but ^{131}iodine labeled inulin and diacetrizoate are also in use. As all these substances have a very low rate of extrarenal excretion, they can be used to measure GFR approximately by a single injection technique. After an initial delay for equilibration in its volume of distribution, the plasma level of the marker substance falls exponentially, and the slope of the line is a measure of GFR. This technique gives a reproducibility of about ±5 per cent using multiple plasma samples, and a little poorer result using an external counter to avoid blood sampling. The method is now provided by many hospital physics departments on a routine basis, and is sufficient for clinical purposes, as the GFR is in any case subject to a diurnal variation of about ±10 per cent, reaching its peak in the afternoon and its trough during the night; it is also readily disturbed by exercise or emotional disturbance.

The most popular rough estimate of GFR is the endogenous *creatinine clearance,* using a 24-hour urine collection and a single plasma sample. If renal function is stable, the plasma sample can be drawn at any time in the collection period, because plasma creatinine varies little during the 24 hours in these circumstances. In outpatient investigation it is even permissible to draw the blood sample a few hours after the end of the collection period. The automated technique used in most hospitals, based on the Jaffé reaction, measures creatinine plus some of the creatinine-like chromogen, but its reproducibility is better than that of the manual methods measuring true creatinine. Even with the automated method there is a high interlaboratory variation in quality control surveys, particularly when the result is close to normal. This reflects the difficulty in measuring plasma creatinine accurately in the normal range. The analytical error alone is of the order of ± 10 per cent, so small changes in creatinine clearance should not be overinterpreted when they are close to normal. Important additional sources of error are loss of urine during defecation, mistiming of collection, incomplete bladder emptying, and washout effects caused by the consumption of diuretics or fluctuations in fluid intake. Careful instruction and good patient cooperation are needed for meaningful results. Two or three consecutive collections are preferable, to compensate for bladder-emptying errors. Creatinine clearance considerably and unpredictably overestimates GFR in nephrotic syndrome, after renal transplantation, and in terminal renal failure, probably because of tubular secretion of creatinine.

The plasma creatinine concentration is determined by the production rate, which is largely a reflection of muscle mass, and the excretion rate, which is roughly proportional to GFR. In a patient whose muscle mass is not changing rapidly, alterations in plasma creatinine are determined almost exclusively by changes in GFR; diet and fluid intake have very little effect. When plasma creatinine is greater than 1.0 mg per 100 ml its estimation presents few difficulties, and it is a much more convenient and reproducible test than creatinine clearance. It is therefore used by most nephrologists as their day-to-day guide to the progress of renal function. The relationship to GFR is hyperbolic; a large change in GFR produces a small change in plasma creatinine close to the normal range, whereas a small change in GFR causes a large change in plasma creatinine in late renal failure.

Although plasma creatinine is of pre-eminent importance in following renal function, it cannot be readily converted into an estimate of GFR, owing to the wide differences in muscle mass between individual patients. This limits its usefulness in confirming normal renal function. A raised plasma creatinine always indicates a depression in GFR, temporary or permanent, but a normal plasma creatinine does not exclude renal disease unless the patient's muscle mass is obviously normal, e.g., the young athlete with exertional proteinuria. The prediction of GFR from plasma creatinine can be improved if allowance is made for age and sex, which are two major determinants of muscle mass. The calculation is particularly useful when drug therapy is required by the patient with renal impairment; an accurate, recent estimate of GFR is usually unavailable, but a plasma creatinine can be obtained within the hour and used to calculate the required dose. A formula for calculating GFR from plasma creatinine, with correction factors, is shown in Table 1. It is only valid if plasma creatinine is stable, and this should be confirmed during the first 12 to 24 hours of drug therapy.

Plasma urea has been used as the main guide to renal function by the majority of general physicians and surgeons at least until the last few years, but it is a poor guide. Under stable conditions of diet, lean body mass, and fluid intake, it has a roughly hyperbolic relationship to GFR in the same manner as plasma creatinine, but the curve is distorted in severe renal failure by a rise in urea clearance relative to GFR (reaching almost 100 per cent when GFR is below 5 ml per minute) and by extrarenal removal of urea. However, these stable conditions are not common in clinical practice, and plasma urea is readily affected by variations in protein intake and in net body catabolism or anabolism caused by trauma, infection, inactivity, refeeding, the anabolic phase after illness, and drug therapy, particularly corticosteroids. It takes about two weeks for the plasma urea to stabilize under constant conditions in the metabolic ward. Plasma urea is affected by fluid intake; it falls during a water diuresis and fluctuates appreciably during the 24 hours under the influence of food and drink. Many laboratories now provide a plasma creatinine result

gratis when a plasma urea is requested, in the hope of educating doctors to use the better estimate of renal function. However, plasma urea retains some usefulness as an index of retention of the compounds produced in response to protein ingestion. The ratio of plasma urea and plasma creatinine has some diagnostic significance. Plasma urea rises preferentially during water or sodium and water depletion, whereas plasma urea and creatinine rise together in established acute renal failure.

Renal Blood Flow.   Renal blood flow can be estimated by dye dilution methods or by the elution curve of radiokrypton if the renal artery and vein are catheterized. These techniques are sometimes employed clinically after renal transplant when fine catheters can be left in the donor organ at operation and kept in situ during the first few weeks. A fall in renal blood flow is probably the first detectable sign of rejection of a homograft. In other situations renal plasma flow is usually measured as the clearance rate of para-aminohippurate (PAH) on the assumption that PAH is both filtered at the glomerulus and secreted by the tubules so that it is cleared almost completely from the plasma in a single passage through the kidney. PAH is easy to measure accurately, and it equilibrates in the body more rapidly than inulin so the performance of PAH clearance is relatively simple. In the normal subject the removal of PAH from blood traversing the kidney is about 92 per cent, which is near enough to the theoretic 100 per cent to make the test useful; it has been employed to show that renal blood flow varies more widely than GFR with exercise and emotion but has about the same and parallel diurnal variation. In renal disease the extraction ratio of PAH may be well below 92 per cent, so PAH clearance cannot be equated with renal plasma flow unless the extraction ratio can be measured simultaneously with the aid of a renal vein catheter—seldom a justifiable clinical procedure.

Glomerular filtration rate and renal blood flow are both related to body size, and surface area has been found to correlate with them most closely in the adult. They are therefore corrected to a standard surface area of 1.73 square meters before comparison with the normal range. This correction is of course unnecessary when they are used serially to follow the progress of disease. In infants under one year the GFR and renal blood flow are low in relationship to surface area, but this is probably a reflection of the high surface area of the infant rather than of a reduced renal reserve. On other criteria, e.g., using body volume as a standard, the GFR reaches adult proportions at about one month. Both GFR and renal blood flow rise in pregnancy, reaching a peak at about 36 weeks, so it is essential to compare results in pregnancy with the normal range for the same stage of gestation. Glomerular filtration rate and renal plasma flow both decline with age. In men, mean GFR falls from about 125 ml per minute at age 40 to about 60 ml per minute at age 90 in a roughly linear manner but with a wide scatter. The fall with age in women is not so well documented and is probably slower. Normal ranges at different ages are illustrated by Wesson.

Urinary Concentrating Power.   The ability to concentrate urine is impaired as the population of nephrons declines with disease, and it is seldom worthwhile testing concentrating power at a GFR less than 20 ml per minute. It is impaired disproportionately by any disease affecting the loop of Henle or the collecting duct. The concentration test has often been described as a sensitive

TABLE 1.   Calculation of Creatinine Clearance
from Corrected Serum Creatinine*

$$\text{Creatinine clearance per 1.73 sq m} = \frac{64.56}{\substack{\text{Corrected} \\ \text{serum} \\ \text{creatinine}}} - 0.55$$

Corrected serum creatinine is calculated by multiplying observed serum creatinine by a correction factor from the table below:

Age (Years)	Males	Females
30	0.68	0.76
40	0.74	0.86
50	0.80	0.97
60	0.87	1.09
70	0.94	1.24
80	1.03	1.40

*Relationship calculated from the data of Nielsen et al., 1973.

index of early renal damage, but the reproducibility is so low and the normal range so wide that it cannot be more than a crude index. To obtain maximal concentration reliably, it is necessary to deprive the patient of fluid for more than 24 hours, which makes the test inapplicable to outpatients and dangerous to those in renal failure. Four simpler tests are therefore used to give a rough idea of concentrating ability. (1) *Early morning urine;* if one or more of several early morning samples, taken without special precautions, have an osmolality over 700 mOsm per liter, it is unlikely that there is an important defect in urinary concentration. (2) The *16-hour test;* fluid is withheld from 4 P.M. and a dry supper administered. The bladder is emptied at 10 P.M. and all samples collected until 8 A.M. Breakfast and morning drinks are not given until 8 A.M. One of the samples should have an osmolality of 700 mOsm per liter or greater. (3) *Pitressin tannate test;* fluid is withheld from 6 P.M.; 5 units of pitressin tannate in oil, well warmed and shaken, is given intramuscularly at 8 P.M.; the bladder is emptied at 10 P.M. and all samples collected until 10 A.M., when a late breakfast is provided. This gives results close to those of a 24-hour fast, the difference being negligible in patients with impaired concentrating ability. (4) The *16-hour test* can be *improved by the administration of a short-acting diuretic* such as furosemide, 40 mg, at the start of fluid deprivation.

Traditionally urine specific gravity has been used as the criterion of urinary concentration, but as it bears an inconstant relationship to osmolality (which is the best measure of the work of concentration), particularly in the presence of proteinuria, glycosuria, and some exogenous substances such as contrast media, it should now be abandoned in favor of osmolality, which can be measured more accurately on a much smaller sample and, with modern instruments, almost as quickly. An osmolality of 700 corresponds roughly to a specific gravity of 1.020.

Heinemann, H. O., Maack, T. M., and Sherman, R. L.: Combined clinical and basic science seminar: Proteinuria. Am. J. Med., 56:71, 1974.

Morrison, R. B. I.: Urinalysis and assessment of renal function. *In* Black, D. A. K. (ed.): Renal Disease. 3rd ed. Oxford, Blackwell, 1973, Chapter 9.

Nielsen, B., Sørensen, A. W. S., Szabo, L., Pedersen, E. A., and Scharff, A.: Kanamycin serum half-life and renal function: Age and sex. Dan. Med. Bull., 20:144, 1973.

Relman, A. S., and Levinsky, N. G.: Clinical examination of renal function. *In* Strauss, M. B., and Welt, L. G. (eds.): Diseases of the Kidney. 2nd ed. Boston, Little, Brown & Company, 1971, Chapter 3.

Spencer, E. S., and Pedersen, I.: Hand Atlas of the Urinary Sediment. Copenhagen, Munksgaard, 1971.

Wesson, L. G., Jr.: Physiology of the Human Kidney. New York, Grune & Stratton, 1969.

603. CHRONIC RENAL FAILURE

D. N. S. Kerr

ETIOLOGY

The major causes of renal failure, and some of the minor ones, are set out in Table 2 in a manner intended to aid differential diagnosis. Diseases in the first group usually present with features of renal disease, although extrarenal manifestations such as tuberculous epididymitis or back pain with retroperitoneal fibrosis may

TABLE 2. A Clinical Classification of the Causes of Chronic Renal Failure

1. Local causes:
Diseases in which the kidneys are predominantly involved and in which the presenting features are usually those of renal disease
    Proliferative glomerulonephritis
    Membranous glomerulonephropathy
    Chronic pyelonephritis
    Tuberculous pyelonephritis
    Renal calculi
    Congenital nephritis
    Polycystic disease
    Medullary cystic disease
    Renal hypoplasia
    Renal tubular acidosis
    Balkan nephropathy
    Upper urinary tract obstruction
        Hydronephrosis
        Retroperitoneal fibrosis
        Neoplasm

2. Lower urinary tract obstruction:
Presenting features often those of bladder dysfunction, but may present in renal failure
    Prostatic enlargement
        Adenoma
        Neoplasm
    Urethral stricture
    Urethral valves
    Bladder neck obstruction
    Neurogenic bladder

3. Systemic diseases and intoxications:
  a. In which renal failure is not infrequently a presenting feature
    Malignant essential hypertension
    Polyarteritis nodosa
    Disseminated lupus erythematosus
    Primary and secondary amyloidosis
    Analgesic overconsumption
    Potassium deficiency
    Hypercalcemia
    Cystinosis
    Oxalosis
    Consumption coagulopathies
        Hemolytic-uremic syndrome
        Thrombotic thrombocytopenic purpura
        Postpartum renal failure
    Lead or cadmium poisoning
  b. In which renal failure is usually a late feature or overshadowed by other manifestations
    Benign essential hypertension
    Atheroma
    Systemic emboli
        Subacute bacterial endocarditis
        Rheumatic heart disease
    Gout
    Diabetes
    Heart failure
    Cirrhosis

provide a clue. Many diseases in Groups 2 and 3a will be identified by involvement of the bladder or of some other system, and most of those in Group 3b should be recognized readily from other features of the disease, although renal failure may occasionally be a presenting feature. If a full history and examination fail to reveal a systemic cause for chronic renal failure, the most likely possibilities are in Groups 1 and 3a.

Selection of the most appropriate diagnostic aids is helped by a knowledge of the relative frequency of the diseases listed in Table 2, some of which are rare. Unfortunately death certification statistics are not a reliable source of this information. They have been repeatedly contradicted by more accurate surveys of living patients, and they provide some information that stretches credulity. An example is shown in Figure 3. The data are from England and Wales, but the trends were observed in many developed countries. Between 1950 and 1966, the reported mortality from urinary infection trebled, and pyelonephritis appeared to displace glomerulonephritis as the leading renal cause of death. This seems improbable at a time when increasingly effective urinary antiseptics were introduced and there was no effective treatment for glomerulonephritis. The anomaly is partly explained by the changing age structure of the population; three quarters of all deaths from urinary infection, but only half those from nephritis and nephrosis, occur after the age of 65. However, the aging population alone cannot account for the dramatic changes reported. The main explanation is probably a change in habits of certification as doctors became more aware of chronic pyelonephritis after the introduction of midstream culture and the campaign against the catheter. The pendulum swung too far and pyelonephritis was overdiagnosed. It is now swinging back and has done so abruptly in Scotland, where a national survey of renal disease led to more accurate diagnosis from about 1969.

An alternative source of information is provided by the annual reports of the transplant and dialysis registries. They give little information on the extremes of life and they are subject to some selection, but they are our best guide to the incidence of disease in children and young and middle-aged adults. European statistics are quoted in Table 3, which shows the relative importance of the main disease in each group; American and Australasian experience is similar. Essential hypertension is certainly underrepresented in these statistics as a cause of renal failure. Malignant hypertension of rapid onset in young adults causes afferent arteriolar necrosis and renal failure, with kidneys of normal size which are not easily confused with those of glomerulonephritis. More slowly progressive severe hypertension causes medial and intimal thickening of interlobular arteries and hyaline degeneration of afferent arterioles which leads to diffuse scarring of the kidney. In its late stages this hypertensive nephrosclerosis may be difficult to distinguish from chronic glomerulonephritis with secondary hypertension. The effects of hypertension merge into those of atheroma, which frequently complicates hypertension but which also occurs in normotensive subjects. Atheroma of the renal arteries may cause renal hypertension, atheroembolism, or thrombosis with infarction,

TABLE 3.   Main Causes of Renal Failure in Children and Young and Middle-Aged Adults*

	Adults (%)	Children (%)
Glomerulonephritis	55.7	52.1
Pyelonephritis	21.2	19.9
Polycystic disease	7.5	2.6
Renal vascular disease	4.4	2.0
Drug nephropathy	2.9	0.2
Congenital nephritis	1.5	6.2
Congenital hypoplasia	1.5	9.3
Other	5.3	7.7

*Data of the European Dialysis and Transplant Registry.

any of which will hasten the decline in renal function. Methods of data collection used by the renal registries discourage these diagnoses, and patients with hypertension or atheroma tend to be misclassified as having glomerulonephritis.

Gout does not figure individually in Table 3, although it is a fairly common disease which is usually accompanied by histologic damage in the kidney and which has been said to terminate in renal failure in 18 to 30 per cent of cases. This is an overstatement based on selected hospital patients. The very few patients with gout who reach dialysis and transplant units do so in middle age, usually beyond the age of 40.

INVESTIGATION OF CHRONIC RENAL DISEASE

Investigation has four objectives: recognition of the primary disease, assessment of the degree of renal failure, detection of any aggravating factors, and exploration of other medical and social problems which may have a bearing on the treatment of renal disease.

Recognition of the Primary Disease. It is the plea of every nephrologist that patients with chronic renal disease be referred early, when pyelography is particularly informative and renal biopsy can be performed without the hazards of uremia, hypertension, and small fibrotic kidneys. At this stage diagnosis of the primary renal disease is usually straightforward and worthwhile. When patients first present in established renal failure, exact diagnosis is more difficult. High-dose pyelography may still provide a good deal of information, but fine details of the calyceal pattern cannot be expected; if renal biopsy is performed, it may be difficult to interpret in an "end-stage kidney." Nonetheless, considerable information can still be obtained, and it is important, even in late renal failure, to recognize several reversible causes and some conditions which will influence later decisions about dialysis and transplantation. Correction of urinary obstruction, removal of calculi, and withdrawal of analgesics from patients with analgesic nephropathy may all arrest a decline in renal function and occasionally reverse it. Retroperitoneal fibrosis often improves, spontaneously or with steroid therapy, after withdrawal of methysergide and is also amenable to surgery. Lupus nephritis reponds to corticosteroid and other immunosuppressive agents, and gouty nephropathy may improve with allopurinol therapy. The demonstration of a normal bladder and competent ureterovesical valves is an important preliminary to transplant in patients with chronic pyelonephritis who may therefore require micturating cystography at a stage when surgery for reflux

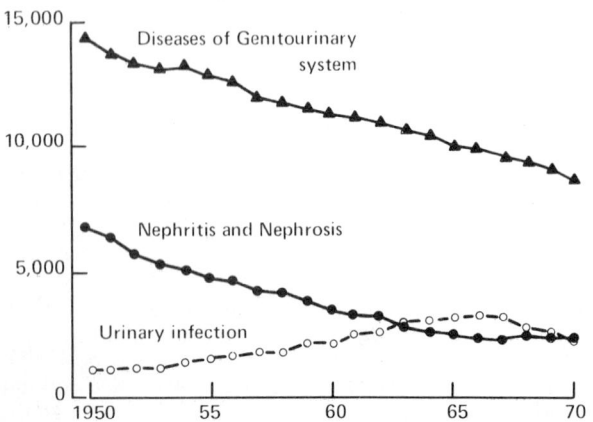

Figure 3. Crude death rate from diseases of the genitourinary tract in England and Wales (population approximately 50 million).

would not otherwise be contemplated. The recognition of oxalosis, cystinosis, and mesangiocapillary nephritis has important implications, because all may recur in a grafted kidney, whereas Fabry's disease may be a specific indication for transplantation, because it replaces the missing enzyme.

The *history* should include a lifelong survey of previous renal complaints, occupations, and drug consumption. Specific inquiry should be made about symptoms suggestive of urinary obstruction and the intake of analgesics, other phenacetin-containing drugs, and methysergide, because these are often overlooked by the patient. The family history should include specific inquiry about renal disease, hypertension and its sequelae, gout, collagenoses, preeclampsia, and deafness. Comprehensive history-taking is aided by a self-administered questionnaire; even experienced clinicians often omit vital questions when relying on memory alone. The facets of physical examination and general medical investigation that may be important compose most of the physician's repertoire. Among the physical signs that should be sought are those indicating longstanding uremia (skin pigmentation and excoriation, a brown arc under the nail margins, tissue-wasting, neuropathy), hypertension (retinopathy, cardiac enlargement), atheroma (peripheral pulses, murmurs in main vessels), disturbed calcium metabolism (band keratopathy, pseudoclubbing, proximal muscle weakness), and collagenoses (joint deformity, arteritic skin lesions).

Investigations should include qualitative tests for glycosuria and hematuria and a quantitative test for proteinuria; pH of early morning urine; urinary microscopy and midstream culture; plasma or serum urea, creatinine, sodium, potassium, chloride, bicarbonate, urate, calcium, phosphate, alkaline phosphatase, total protein, and electrophoresis; and straight roentgenography of the renal tract. Chest roentgenogram, electrocardiogram, serum magnesium, and creatinine clearance should also be included in the initial screening, but not for the sake of differential diagnosis. If the renal size is not obvious from the straight roentgenogram, it is often revealed by tomography. *High dose or infusion pyelography,* with *renal tomograms* and late films up to 24 hours, usually provides some information about the calyceal pattern down to a GFR of about 5 ml per minute and gives an idea of renal size, shape, and quantity of peripelvic fat down to a GFR of about 2 ml per minute. It is particularly helpful in the diagnosis of urinary obstruction and polycystic disease, even at a very late stage in renal failure.

Proteinuria exceeding 3 grams per 24 hours is unusual in chronic pyelonephritis, analgesic nephropathy, benign hypertension, urinary obstruction, calculous disease, renal tubular acidosis, and polycystic disease; it is usual or common in chronic proliferative glomerulonephritis, membranous glomerulonephropathy, amyloidosis, diabetic nephropathy, polyarteritis, disseminated lupus erythematosus, and malignant hypertension. Glomerular proteinuria diminishes as GFR falls, but heavy proteinuria may still be encountered in terminal renal failure, and the consequent derangements of plasma protein may persist for several weeks after the start of regular hemodialysis. Mild hypoproteinemia accompanies fluid overload in many forms of chronic renal disease, but severe hypoproteinemia (below 5 grams per 100 ml), particularly if accompanied by a nephrotic electrophoretic pattern and hypercholesterolemia, strongly suggests

that heavy proteinuria was present in the recent past, even if it is no longer demonstrable.

Red cell *casts in the urinary deposit* in chronic renal failure suggest one of the progressive forms of glomerulonephritis (e.g., crescent nephritis, mesangiocapillary nephritis, the renal lesion of subacute bacterial endocarditis), including the collagenoses or malignant hypertension. Numerous dense granular casts are encountered in these conditions and in amyloidosis and diabetic nephropathy. They are seldom found in chronic pyelonephritis or analgesic nephropathy, in both of which an increased output of white cells is often the only abnormality of microscopy. Hyaline casts predominate in membranous glomerulonephropathy and benign essential hypertension.

Hyperchloremic acidosis accompanies urinary diversion into the bowel. If the lower urinary tract is intact, it should suggest chronic pyelonephritis, analgesic nephropathy, renal tubular acidosis, or polycystic disease, although it may be encountered in other renal diseases. *Hypercalcemia* is occasionally found in secondary hyperparathyroidism, but it should always raise the suspicion that the hypercalcemia is the cause of the renal failure and not vice versa. *Serum electrophoresis* and search for Bence Jones protein in urine will detect most examples of renal failure caused by myelomatosis, but specific immunologic tests for light chains are sometimes required. Immunoelectrophoresis may be required to demonstrate the monoclonal gammopathies that underlie most cases of "primary" renal amyloid—one of the diseases that most frequently elude detection until renal biopsy is performed.

Very large kidneys are typical of obstruction or polycystic disease. Renal failure with *kidneys of normal size* should always alert the clinician to the possibility of acute rather than chronic renal failure, although amyloidosis, crescent nephritis, and membranous glomerulonephropathy may all reach the end stage without much contraction of the kidney. *Small symmetrical kidneys* with preservation of the calyceal pattern are found in many chronic renal diseases, notably most forms of glomerulonephritis. Chronic pyelonephritis is confirmed by *asymmetrical and irregular scarring,* with clubbing and outdrawing of the calyces; in late renal failure, when calyceal detail is poor, a gross increase in peripelvic fat on the tomograms is a helpful sign. Typical findings in analgesic nephropathy are small kidneys with scalloped outlines—sometimes misinterpreted as fetal lobulation—and clubbed calyces corresponding to the sloughed papillae. Rare but diagnostic signs are calcification of papillae and encirclement of separated papillae by contrast medium ("ring sign"). The pyelogram may, however, remain normal until late in the disease. Passage of separated papillae causes attacks of renal colic and may permit firm diagnosis by histologic examination of a soft black "calculus."

Urinary *infection* is still present in about half the patients with chronic pyelonephritis currently seen in renal failure; it is also a common accompaniment of calculous disease, analgesic nephropathy, and lower urinary tract obstruction, but is probably no more common in other renal diseases than in the general population. Nonetheless, all patients with chronic renal disease should be screened for urinary infection by the culture of at least three midstream urines at a time when no antimicrobial drugs are being, or have recently been, administered.

Assessment of the Degree of Renal Failure. An initial measurement of GFR should be made by one of the techniques discussed in Ch. 602. Thereafter serial measurement of serum creatinine is the most useful and practical guide to changes in renal function.

Detection of Aggravating Factors. Glomerular filtration rate may be depressed by hypovolemia from renal sodium loss, vomiting and diarrhea, systemic infections, surgery, trauma, hemorrhage, urinary infection, sudden reduction of longstanding hypertension, rapid rise in blood pressure, and administration of nephrotoxic drugs. The production rate of urea and other metabolic end products may be increased by excessive protein intake, tissue wasting from starvation, infection, trauma and surgery, resorption of hematoma, bleeding into the gut, and administration of corticosteroids or tetracyclines.

These aggravating factors should be sought and corrected in every patient seen for the first time in chronic renal failure, and no subsequent deterioration should be blamed on the primary disease until they have been excluded as contributory factors. When doubt exists, the patient should be kept alive for several weeks, if necessary by peritoneal dialysis or hemodialysis, to provide time for investigation and for his recovery from complications.

Investigation of Other Medical and Social Problems. This is an essential part of the management of any chronic disease, but it is particularly important in chronic renal failure because regular dialysis and transplantation place heavy demands on the patient's physical and social resources. A full social report should be carried out at the time of diagnosis and updated as the need for dialysis becomes imminent, so that such factors as rehousing and home adaptations can be planned well in advance. Family planning should be discussed and sterilization procedures carried out before advanced renal failure adds to their hazards; they are best performed on the affected partner in young couples, because five-year survival on dialysis and transplantation is still of the order of 70 to 80 per cent, so remarriage of the unaffected partner is a considerable possibility. A dental survey should be arranged so that extractions can be performed before intermittent anticoagulation and immunosuppressive therapy become necessary, and regular conservative dental care should be maintained thereafter. Indigestion should be thoroughly investigated and surgery for peptic ulcer considered before transplantation makes corticosteroid therapy essential.

As renal failure advances, regular search should be carried out for the complications discussed below, notably hypertension and its sequelae, neuropathy, myopathy and encephalopathy, pericarditis, bone disease, anemia, sexual dysfunction, and electrolyte disturbances. This tedious and repetitive work can be aided by regular completion of a self-administered questionnaire and a structured physical examination and biochemical screen, guided by a checklist. A problem-oriented summary of all the medical and social problems in the front of the case record is an invaluable adjunct to management.

THE PATHOPHYSIOLOGY OF CHRONIC RENAL FAILURE

Chronically diseased kidneys often support life in comfort until about 90 per cent of their glomerular filtration

has been lost, and they maintain some sort of life until 97 to 99 per cent has gone. This statement applies to most of the conditions listed in Table 2 and is the justification for considering them together. It implies that even in the late stages of disease the kidneys retain some ability to respond to the demands of the body by varying the output of water and important solutes. The most popular explanation for this response of the diseased kidney to physiologic stimuli is the "intact nephron hypothesis."

According to this theory the deformed nephrons seen in histologic preparations and nephron dissections are largely nonfunctional; excretory function is maintained by a remnant of surviving nephrons in which both glomerulus and tubule have escaped irreparable damage. In these nephrons the glomerulus produces an increased volume of glomerular filtrate. Hypertrophy of the tubule enables it to handle this extra filtrate within limits, but the additional solute load causes an osmotic diuresis which has the same effects as a saline or urea diuresis in the normal subject. Urine is produced at a nearly constant rate throughout the 24 hours, at an osmolality which is eventually fixed around 300 mOsm per kilogram (specific gravity, SG, about 1.010) – a state referred to as isosthenuria. This condition becomes established only when the GFR is reduced to about a quarter of normal. It results in nocturia, one of the most common symptoms of early renal failure (but one which often fails to alert the patient to his condition; the accompanying polyuria leads to thirst, and the nocturia is blamed on an increased consumption of fluid in the evenings).

There is substantial evidence in support of the intact nephron hypothesis, and the events outlined in the preceding paragraph probably underlie most of the adaptations to chronic renal failure. However, there are important exceptions. The grotesquely deformed nephrons of polycystic disease retain some excretory function, and the same may apply to other renal diseases. Those conditions in which medullary damage is a prominent feature – particularly chronic pyelonephritis, analgesic nephropathy, and medullary cystic disease – are often characterized by severe polyuria with hypotonic urine, suggesting that many functioning nephrons have lost their concentrating mechanism, and there is other evidence of impaired distal tubular function in these patients. At the other end of the scale are diseases such as rapidly progressive nephritis, in which glomerular damage is widespread and roughly uniform in time, which do not pass through an isosthenuric phase, so that patients may enter the terminal stage of renal failure without ever having experienced nocturia.

Water. Polyuria commonly accompanies isosthenuria. It reaches a peak while the GFR is declining through the range 25 to 5 ml per minute, then gives way to oliguria in the preterminal phase of chronic renal failure, except in a minority of patients with predominant medullary damage who remain polyuric to the end. Thirst is a constant accompaniment of polyuria, and if the patient has free access to water he will usually maintain his water balance with reasonable accuracy. The once popular practice of "pushing fluids" to reduce the plasma urea is unnecessary and potentially dangerous. Thirst is sometimes excessive, because dryness of the mouth is common in late renal failure. This symptom is occasionally due to overbreathing from acidosis, but is usually the result of an unexplained reduction in salivary flow.

Large water loads are excreted more slowly than in

the normal subject; hyponatremia follows their ingestion for several hours; convulsions are occasionally precipitated. Conversely, obligatory water loss through the kidneys is increased, and patients are therefore sensitive to water deprivation, caused by drowsiness or vomiting.

Sodium. The excretion of most solutes can only be varied over a restricted range in renal failure. The patient remains in reasonable health if his intake is adjusted to the ability of his kidneys to excrete, but he faces trouble if it is close to one of the extremes tolerated by normal persons. The hormonal mechanisms which maintain sodium homeostasis in health with remarkably little change in extracellular fluid (ECF) volume become inadequate as renal function declines. Changes in sodium intake produce alterations in ECF, and plasma volume and fluctuations in GFR acquire an important role in sodium homeostasis. A patient with chronic renal failure placed on a very low sodium diet, e.g., the traditional 22 mEq per day, is often unable to reduce his sodium output by hormonal control alone because of the osmotic diuresis in his surviving nephrons. He goes into negative sodium balance and excretes a corresponding volume of water; his extracellular fluid volume, plasma volume, and GFR all fall. This reduces the osmotic load per nephron and permits more avid sodium retention. Sodium balance is re-established at the price of some decline in glomerular filtration rate.

If the patient is now placed on a high-sodium intake, he passes into positive sodium balance, retaining water in proportion, expanding his extracellular fluid volume, and raising his GFR. This increases the osmotic load per nephron until sodium output again equals intake. This new equilibrium is achieved at the price of an expanded extracellular fluid volume, which may be detectable as peripheral or pulmonary edema and which is often interpreted by the clinician as heart failure. Quite often, however, several liters of tissue fluid are accommodated without overt edema; the overloaded subcutaneous tissue conceals the wasting of muscle and fat characteristic of chronic renal failure, giving the patient a false appearance of adequate nutrition, which is rapidly corrected when his surplus fluid is removed at the start of regular dialysis.

A fortunate minority of patients remain normotensive even when grossly edematous, but the majority develop hypertension when their ECF is overexpanded. In the animal with experimental chronic renal failure, the initial event is a rise in cardiac output followed by a compensatory increase in peripheral resistance and a fall in cardiac output; there is accumulating evidence that this sequence of events is followed in man. Soon after the hypertension develops, the events can be reversed by removing the surplus ECF and preventing its reaccumulation by dietary restriction. This is the treatment employed when the patient becomes dependent on regular hemodialysis. Control of hypertension may be followed by the disappearance of any remaining excretory function, which is unimportant at this juncture. At an earlier stage in renal failure the same control of blood pressure can often be achieved with diuretics and low sodium diet, but at the cost of some reduction of GFR. There is therefore no ideal sodium intake for an individual in chronic renal failure; he must often choose between being normovolemic and normotensive with a low GFR or edematous and hypertensive with a higher GFR. In those countries where the majority of young and middle-aged patients will be offered dialysis and transplanta-

tion, it is better to err on the side of sacrificing GFR to blood pressure control; a well-preserved vascular tree is a much better asset than a few extra months of conservative treatment of renal failure.

As GFR declines to a few milliliters per minute, the proportion of filtered sodium excreted in the urine must rise if sodium balance is to be maintained. The normal subject excretes only about 1 per cent of his filtered sodium, but in terminal renal failure some patients lose about 30 per cent of the filtered sodium in their urine—about the same as a normal subject under maximal osmotic diuresis. However, a substantial proportion are unable to approach this theoretic maximum, and they can be maintained in sodium balance only by severe dietary restriction or high-dose diuretic therapy. Their hypertension is accordingly difficult to control, and regular hemodialysis may be required for control of blood pressure before being required on other grounds. Low sodium dieting in this group can be inadvertently vitiated by the use of medicines; indigestion mixtures and antidiarrheal preparations, e.g., magnesium trisilicate mixture NF and kaolin and morphine mixture NF, are the main offenders, providing 20 to 40 mEq of sodium per day at standard dosage.

At the other extreme a minority of patients excrete a high proportion of their filtered sodium even in early renal failure, and are liable to become sodium depleted if they fail to keep up a high dietary intake. The condition is sometimes referred to as "salt-losing nephritis," but it is not a separate pathologic entity. The syndrome may be encountered in analgesic nephropathy, polycystic disease, or occasionally chronic pyelonephritis. The most common cause in childhood and early adult life is probably medullary cystic disease. The patients are often pigmented and may be thought to have Addison's disease. A helpful point in differentiation is the almost invariable presence of hyperchloremic acidosis in those with renal disease. Most of these patients are normotensive and tolerate dietary sodium supplements (usually as sodium bicarbonate or citrate, liberal condiment, and slow-release sodium tablets) without trouble. Postural hypotension is an early sign of inadequate sodium intake, and hypertension or edema indicates an excess. A few unfortunate patients live on a knife edge between sodium depletion and overload, and require careful control. Sodium depletion makes the patient unduly susceptible to potassium intoxication.

Potassium. Hypokalemia is found in a minority of patients with early renal failure. It is usually caused by diuretic therapy, diarrhea, vomiting, or purgation, but is sometimes due to spontaneous potassium loss in the urine. In a very few patients potassium loss is sufficient to cause severe hypokalemia and muscular paralysis. The condition has been called "potassium-losing nephritis," but is not a separate disease; it is an unusual manifestation of chronic pyelonephritis, renal tubular acidosis, ureterosigmoid anastomosis, and very occasionally other renal diseases. Excessive sodium and calcium loss in the urine sometimes coexist. When the potassium leak is an isolated defect, differentiation from Conn's syndrome can be difficult; a hyperchloremic acidosis strongly suggests a renal cause and a complete response to spironolactone an aldosteronoma, but diagnosis has sometimes awaited adrenal exploration.

During most of the course of renal failure most patients maintain normal plasma potassium, and their potassium excretion varies with their intake. As renal failure advances, potassium excretion may exceed the filtered potassium, presumably as a result of increased exchange for sodium in the distal tubule aided by the osmotic diuresis. However, the maximal capacity to excrete potassium is impaired even in early renal failure. An oral or intravenous dose causes an excessive rise in plasma potassium, which is corrected only over an extended period. Dangerous hyperkalemia may therefore follow endogenous release of potassium after hemolysis, trauma, or infection, or its administration medicinally or in stored blood. Deaths have resulted from the use of potassium citrate in chronic urinary infection (in which it is of doubtful value), and care must be exercised in prescribing potassium supplements, amiloride, and spironolactone during diuretic therapy.

Hyperkalemia is common in terminal renal failure; at this stage even dietary ingestion of excess potassium as instant coffee, fruit, fried potatoes, meat, and meat products can be hazardous. Occasional patients complain of muscle weakness or paresthesias when the plasma potassium reaches dangerous levels (over 7 mEq per liter), but the majority are unaware of the condition until cardiac arrest occurs. The only warning signs are those detected by electrocardiography — flattened P wave, widened QRS complex, and peaked T wave.

In patients with a potassium leak, hypokalemia usually reflects severe depletion of total body potassium, but in other situations in renal failure the plasma level is not a reliable guide to body stores. Plasma potassium rises in acidosis and falls rapidly when this is corrected with sodium bicarbonate, without appreciable change in body potassium. Some hyperkalemic patients in terminal renal failure or on regular dialysis have diminished total body potassium, but this may be a reflection of reduced muscle mass rather than cellular potassium deficiency and is not to be regarded as an indication for potassium therapy.

Magnesium. Mild asymptomatic hypomagnesemia is not uncommon in early renal failure. It is due to an increased fecal loss which is accentuated by high calcium diet, because calcium and magnesium compete for the same absorptive mechanism. Hypomagnesemia of more than slight degree is usually due to diuretic therapy.

For most of the course of renal failure serum magnesium is usually normal, but hypermagnesemia appears with increasing frequency when the GFR falls below 30 ml per minute, and is the rule in terminal renal failure. Serum magnesium rises in the presence of acidosis or tissue trauma and is increased by the administration of vitamin D or its analogues; very high levels (over 3.5 mEq per liter) are nearly always due to administration of magnesium salts as antacids, purgatives, or enemas (magnesium is well absorbed from the colon). Little is known about total body magnesium in chronic renal failure, but severe magnesium depletion has been reported in the presence of hypermagnesemia.

Spontaneous hypermagnesemia impairs nerve conduction time but probably plays no part in the development of neuropathy and may even protect against it; it is probably not responsible for any of the symptoms of renal failure. The very high levels (3.5 to over 8 mEq per liter) that have followed magnesium medication or the use of hard water for hemodialysis have produced drowsiness, light coma, muscle weakness, and skin irritation.

Hydrogen Ion. Nonrespiratory acidosis virtually always develops during the progression of chronic renal failure, though it can be reversed temporarily by vomiting. In patients without predominant medullary damage it becomes pronounced only after the GFR falls below about 20 ml per minute. A renal bicarbonate leak can be demonstrated in many patients with chronic renal failure when their plasma bicarbonate level is restored to normal with sodium bicarbonate. When the bicarbonate infusion is stopped, renal excretion of bicarbonate continues until the plasma bicarbonate falls again to its previous level. This resetting of the plasma level at which a bicarbonate leak occurs is also encountered in primary hyperparathyroidism, and it has been attributed to hypersecretion of parathyroid hormone in renal failure.

As renal acidosis progresses, urine becomes more acid, eventually reaching a pH of about 5 — close to the minimum achieved by normal subjects after acid loading. This does not imply normal urinary acidification, as the patient achieves this urine pH at a much lower plasma bicarbonate level than normal. Moreover he excretes a considerably smaller quantity of hydrogen ion at any given urinary pH than normal. This is mainly due to a defect in ammonia production shown by a lower excretion of ammonium. Titratable acidity is normal or slightly reduced for the urine pH, because the main buffers (monohydrogen phosphate and creatinine) are excreted in nearly normal amount until late in renal failure.

It is now possible to calculate with fair accuracy the hydrogen ion produced by a stated diet. It is derived mainly from the oxidation of sulfur-containing amino acids to sulfuric acid, the hydrolysis of phosphate esters to phosphoric acid, the metabolism of purines to uric acid, and the production of intermediary acids during carbohydrate metabolism. Balance studies show that patients in renal failure excrete only about three quarters of their acid production, retaining 10 to 20 mEq of hydrogen ion per day. In spite of this, their plasma bicarbonate level changes very slowly; the extra acid is believed to be neutralized by calcium carbonate in bone. This probably accounts in part for the negative calcium balance in renal failure, and may be a factor in the genesis of renal bone disease.

Respiratory compensation for the acidosis occurs in a predictable manner if there is no lung disease, the uremic subject behaving in the same manner as a normal subject ingesting ammonium chloride. Pa_{CO_2} falls by about 1.2 mm Hg for every 1 mEq per liter fall in plasma bicarbonate. This does not completely correct the blood pH, which falls in a roughly linear relationship to the plasma bicarbonate, reaching the lower limit of normal (7.35) when the plasma bicarbonate is about 15 mEq per liter. In terminal renal failure the plasma bicarbonate falls below 10 mEq per liter and there is deep sighing (Kussmaul) respiration which produces a low Pa_{CO_2}, but blood pH is well below the normal range. Any interference with respiratory compensation by chest infection, pulmonary edema, heavy sedation, or coma leads to a rapid increase in the acidosis, and the plasma bicarbonate then ceases to be a reliable guide to the severity of the condition.

Rapid correction of extracellular acidosis by fast hemodialysis or infusion of sodium bicarbonate is followed by a respiratory alkalosis which persists for up to 24 hours. Bicarbonate diffuses slowly into the CSF, which therefore remains acid and continues to stimulate the respiratory centers on the anterior surface of the medulla, inappropriately lowering the Pa_{CO_2}.

The *genetic forms of renal tubular acidosis* have been divided into a *proximal type,* usually found in infants and caused by incomplete reabsorption of bicarbonate in the proximal tubule, and a *distal type,* caused by inability of the distal tubule to maintain a low pH. In both types, urinary pH remains high (typically over 6.0) in the presence of an acidosis. A distal type of renal tubular acidosis is found in analgesic nephropathy, some cases of chronic pyelonephritis, calculous disease, and polycystic disease, and as a manifestation of tubular damage in Sjögren's syndrome, disseminated lupus, and amyloidosis. Both proximal and distal tubular types are encountered after renal transplantation. In these diseases urinary pH remains higher than in other renal disease at the same level of GFR. The fall in plasma bicarbonate is then accompanied by a rise in plasma chloride which may exceed 110 mEq per liter. Presumably when there is a reduced bicarbonate concentration in glomerular filtrate, some other anion must be reabsorbed with sodium; in early renal failure the readily available anion is chloride. Hyperchloremic acidosis therefore indicates impairment of hydrogen ion excretion greater than would be expected from loss of nephrons alone. A striking hyperchloremic acidosis is found after urinary diversion into the bowel, particularly the sigmoid colon, and is attributed to the action of bowel mucosa on retained urine, compounding the effect of the commonly associated pyelonephritis. When acidosis develops late in renal failure, plasma chloride is usually normal or depressed, the anion concentration being made up by retained sulfate and phosphate.

Calcium and Plasma Phosphate. Renal *calcium excretion* falls early in renal failure, before there is any drop in serum calcium, probably as a reflection of the fall in GFR. However, tubular reabsorption also decreases so that calcium excretion declines more slowly than GFR. In very early renal failure, intestinal absorption of calcium is normal; but as the GFR falls below about half normal, intestinal absorption is progressively impaired, and in late renal failure there may be net intestinal excretion of calcium. At this stage urinary calcium excretion has usually fallen to less than 100 mg per day, but over-all negative calcium balance is usual and is not corrected by regular hemodialysis, in spite of the absence of urinary excretion, unless calcium is effectively infused into the patient by the use of a high calcium dialysate. Positive calcium balance can be restored by the administration of *vitamin D* (1 to 2.5 mg per 24 hours) or its metabolites and analogues *25-hydroxycholecalciferol, 1-alpha-hydroxycholecalciferol* (up to 5 μg per 24 hours), or *dihydrotachysterol* (0.25 mg per 24 hours) by mouth. The natural hormone 1,25-dihydroxycholecalciferol is poorly absorbed by mouth but readily restores positive calcium balance in a dose of 1 to 3 μg per 24 hours by injection. These more potent derivatives of vitamin D are increasingly used in place of the parent compound because they are less subject to storage in body fat and to the "therapeutic overshoot" that results with vitamin D. Normal calcium balance is restored by renal transplantation if renal function is close to normal and steroid therapy is not excessive.

Serum calcium declines in late renal failure, often reaching 6 mg and occasionally 4 mg per 100 ml, when cataract formation is a hazard. The proportion of total serum calcium which is ionized and complexed is increased so that ultrafilterable calcium remains close to normal until serum calcium is depressed below about 8

mg per 100 ml. Even in the presence of very low serum calcium, which must be accompanied by a fall in ionized calcium, tetany is unusual in renal failure. It may be precipitated by the infusion or ingestion of sodium bicarbonate or lactate to correct acidosis, and may then be accompanied by grand mal seizures. However, the common forms of muscle cramp, muscle twitching, and convulsion seen in terminal uremia are probably not related to the serum calcium, and are seldom alleviated by calcium infusion.

Hypercalciuria accompanying the hypercalcemia of parathyroid adenoma, sarcoidosis, and hypervitaminosis D disappears when renal failure develops, but the hypercalciuria of renal tubular acidosis, medullary cystic disease, and other tubular disorders may persist in the presence of renal failure. A high urinary calcium is also found in a minority of patients with medullary damage, usually in association with a sodium leak.

Plasma phosphate remains in the normal range until the GFR has fallen to about 30 ml per minute. This is the result of a normal urinary phosphate excretion in the face of a falling GFR, probably owing to the elevated plasma parathormone level, which in late renal failure reaches about ten times the normal level. The rise in plasma phosphate which occurs in late renal failure bears no constant relationship to the simultaneous changes in serum calcium. Patients on regular hemodialysis maintain nearly stable serum calcium in the face of wide fluctuations in plasma phosphate, and those receiving vitamin D may experience a simultaneous rise in plasma phosphate and serum calcium.

Bone Disease. Bone disease is a clinical problem to about 5 per cent of patients reaching the end stage of chronic renal failure, but radiologic abnormalities can be detected in 30 per cent, and bone histology is abnormal in 90 per cent. Growing children are more susceptible than adults to the development of symptomatic bone disease, and it was in adolescents that "renal rickets" was originally described in the last century. The term is a misnomer, because the resemblance to nutritional rickets is only superficial; bone histology reveals a mixed picture of osteitis fibrosa and impaired ossification of cartilage, with the former often predominating even though radiograms resemble those of rickets. Until recently it was believed that osteomalacia developed early in renal failure to be replaced at a later stage by osteitis fibrosa. It is now apparent that osteitis fibrosa is an almost invariable accompaniment of chronic renal failure unless special measures have been taken to prevent it, whereas osteomalacia develops only in a minority of patients, particularly those with slowly progressive renal failure caused by obstructive uropathy, chronic pyelonephritis, renal hypoplasia, and analgesic nephropathy. It is uncertain whether the underlying disease is important in any other respect, but it has been pointed out that these are diseases with a particular proneness to acidosis.

Secondary hyperparathyroidism, shown by proliferation of both osteoclasts and osteoblasts, scalloping, and bone marrow fibrosis, correlates well with the size and cellularity of the parathyroid glands and with the circulating level of parathyroid hormone. Only when histologic changes are severe do the radiologic signs appear — subperiosteal erosions, best seen in the phalanges; "rugger jersey" spine (density of the upper and lower margins of the vertebrae); "pepper pot" skull, and erosion of the outer ends of the clavicles. Bone pain and pathologic fractures are unusual until radiologic change is far advanced. Metastatic calcification occurs, first in the larger vessels, and then in small peripheral vessels, periarticular tissues, and skin. Rarely an ischemic myopathy results from vascular calcification. Metastatic calcification in the cornea produces band keratopathy, best seen with a slit lamp but often visible with the +30 lens of the ophthalmoscope when viewing from the side. "Red eye"—irritation and conjunctivitis—may accompany conjunctival calcification but is an inconstant symptom.

The main stimulus to the parathyroid glands is phosphate retention which probably acts by temporarily depressing plasma ionized calcium. Plasma parathyroid hormone concentration can be restored to normal and osteitis fibrosa healed by dietary phosphate restriction or administration of aluminum hydroxide gel by mouth. Excessive use of the latter can cause phosphate depletion and produce osteomalacia. Suppression of hyperparathyroidism is aided by administration of oral calcium carbonate (1 to 2 grams, three times a day), but in combination with aluminum hydroxide it readily produces hypercalcemia. Metastatic calcification occurs particularly when the Ca × P concentration product exceeds 70, so regular estimation of serum calcium and phosphate is essential during such manipulations. Serum alkaline phosphatase and hydroxyproline are consistently raised in secondary hyperparathyroidism.

Regular hemodialysis has a variable effect on hyperparathyroidism. In some medical centers the disease slowly heals; in others it progresses, the difference probably reflecting the enthusiasm with which plasma phosphate levels are controlled. After renal transplantation, hyperparathyroidism resolves over a period of 6 to 12 months on biochemical and radiologic criteria, provided that renal function is satisfactory. In a few patients there is persistent hypercalcemia which has been attributed to autonomous "tertiary" hyperparathyroidism. A more likely explanation is that very large parathyroid glands involute slowly, and while they remain large they are not as readily suppressed as normal glands.

Pruritus is common in patients with hyperparathyroidism and is attributed to calcium phosphate deposition in skin. It sometimes resolves with control of plasma phosphate and is regularly relieved by parathyroidectomy.

Osteomalacia is uncommon in the United States but a major problem in some centers in Britain, particularly after the start of regular dialysis. The difference is probably due to variations in sunshine exposure and vitamin D intake which produce borderline vitamin D deficiency in northern Britain in winter. Even though the damaged kidneys cannot make 1,25-dihydroxycholecalciferol, the accumulation of the precursor 25-hydroxycholecalciferol has some antirachitic action and probably protects patients with a high intake or production of vitamin D. Looser zones and pathologic fractures are much more common in osteomalacia than in osteitis fibrosa, and bone pain is a more prominent symptom. Proximal muscle weakness (myopathy) is commonly present.

Osteosclerosis is often shown by bone biopsy on a membrane bone such as the iliac crest and is occasionally seen on radiograms. Since the patients are in negative calcium balance, the sclerosis is presumably caused by redistribution of bone. During regular dialysis there is often a very rapid loss of skeletal calcium, and osteosclerosis rapidly gives way to osteoporosis.

All the lesions of renal osteodystrophy—osteitis fibrosa, osteomalacia, osteosclerosis, and osteoporosis—can occur simultaneously or successively in the same patient.

Trace Elements. Regular hemodialysis has permitted study of the role of trace elements in the manifestations of renal failure. Many trace elements are present in tap water, and they may accumulate in anuric patients exposed to large volumes of dialysis fluid made from raw water. Fatal copper poisoning has resulted from solution of copper pipes by acid dialysis fluid, and zinc uptake has resulted from the use of zinc oxide plaster on coils. During renal failure plasma fluoride may rise to two or three times the range for normal subjects in areas where tap water is fluoridated, and it rises to about 100 times the control value after some years of regular dialysis in these areas. An association with renal bone disease in dialyzed patients has been suggested, but the evidence is not conclusive.

Sulfate. Sulfate is produced from the metabolism of sulfur-containing amino acids and is therefore in approximate proportion to protein ingestion. The plasma sulfate level rises as GFR declines, roughly parallel with plasma urea. Sulfate retention is not the direct cause of any known symptom of renal failure.

Urea and Ammonia. *Urea* diffuses into all body secretions. If the plasma level is very high, it occasionally crystallizes out of sweat, leaving "urea frost" on the skin. The breakdown of urea to ammonia in a dry and crusted mouth is probably the cause of the unpleasant taste and "uremic odor" of terminal renal failure.

In normal subjects about 20 per cent of the daily production of urea is secreted into the gut and broken down by bacteria to ammonia and carbon dioxide. The *ammonia* is reabsorbed and resynthesized into urea in the liver. In chronic renal failure the proportion of urea production removed extrarenally may rise as high as 80 per cent; most of this is probably broken down and resynthesized to urea, as in the normal person. However, ammonia can be used as a substrate for the synthesis of amino acids, and a patient in renal failure who has an adequate supply of essential amino acids, but an over-all protein deficiency, will utilize a considerable proportion of the ammonia released in his gut for protein synthesis; this observation is the basis of the Giordano-Giovannetti dietary regimen. Even in terminal renal failure the large supply of ammonia from the gut does not elevate the blood ammonia level of peripheral blood, which is usually subnormal. However, simultaneous hepatic and renal failure cause a rapid rise in blood ammonia and the early onset of coma.

Urea was long regarded as nontoxic, but the Giovannetti diet, which reduces plasma urea without much change in other plasma constituents, relieves nausea, vomiting, and diarrhea and raises the hemoglobin level. Ammonia released by bacteria from urea in the gastrointestinal tract has been blamed for vomiting, hematemesis, and uremic ulceration of the gut, but there are alternative explanations for these symptoms and signs.

Uric Acid. A rise in plasma urate level begins very early in chronic renal disease, but it is so slight that the level becomes consistently abnormal only when the GFR falls to about 15 ml per minute. This stability of the plasma urate in the face of a normal production rate and a declining GFR is the result of increased distal tubular secretion of urate and increased uricolysis in the gut. In late renal failure there is a further increase in fractional urate clearance so that plasma urate rises less steeply than plasma urea or creatinine. Levels at least as high as those in gout are often encountered in terminal renal failure, but secondary gout is rare except in lead nephropathy, obstructive uropathy, and analgesic nephropathy, or during regular dialysis. Urate crystals are often found in the kidneys of patients with secondary hyperuricemia, and may accelerate the decline in renal function.

Plasma urate correlates much better than plasma urea with the onset of uremic pericarditis, but urate crystals are not found in the inflamed pericardium, and pericarditis is a rare complication of primary gout.

Carbohydrate. More than 50 per cent of patients in late renal failure have *glucose intolerance* as severe as in mild diabetes but with a normal fasting blood dextrose and often without glycosuria. It is not a cause of symptoms unless a large dose of glucose is administered during intravenous therapy, peritoneal dialysis, or hemodialysis, when severe hyperglycemia can be provoked. Fructose, galactose, and sorbitol tolerance are normal, showing that there is no defect in hepatic glycogenesis. Plasma insulin levels are appropriate to blood sugars, or nearly so, and there is a reduced response to injected insulin, implying peripheral antagonism to insulin action. Plasma growth hormone levels are usually normal, and potassium deficiency is only occasionally implicated. Glucose tolerance returns to normal after one or two weeks of adequate dialysis, suggesting the presence of a dialyzable insulin antagonist.

Lipids. Total plasma lipids are raised in late renal failure, mainly owing to a rise in triglycerides; phospholipids and cholesterol are normal or slightly elevated. There is a consistent rise in pre-β lipoproteins. More striking elevation in plasma lipids is found in those who remain nephrotic in renal failure. Hyperlipidemia may act synergistically with hypertension to produce a high incidence of atheroma in older patients with renal failure.

Other Compounds Implicated in Uremia. "Uremia" comprises those symptoms and signs of renal failure which are not explained by water and electrolyte imbalance or hypertension. Most of these features correlate only approximately with the plasma levels of urea, creatinine, uric acid, and other substances that have been thoroughly investigated. Current contenders for the role of "uremic toxins" include *guanidines, amines,* and *phenolic acids.* They are difficult to measure accurately, and it is uncertain whether they correlate with symptoms any more closely than urea, but some of them, e.g., methylamine and methylguanidine, produce convulsions, coma, vomiting, and other uremic symptoms in laboratory animals at concentrations found in uremic plasma. "Middle molecules"—substances of molecular weight 300 to 1800, probably predominantly polypeptides—accumulate in patients on regular hemodialysis, as they are poorly dialyzable through conventional membranes, but they are also present in excess in untreated uremia. They have been blamed for some of the features of renal failure, notably neuropathy and encephalopathy, but without conclusive proof.

Many of the symptoms of renal failure are mimicked by the side effects of drugs that accumulate when GFR is depressed. The claims that "the best thing you can do for a uremic is to stop all his drugs" has a germ of truth.

CLINICAL FEATURES OF RENAL FAILURE AND THEIR TREATMENT

Plan of Management in Irreversible Renal Failure

Patients without extensive vascular disease and with no systemic disease which threatens life should receive conservative management on a moderately restricted (40-gram protein) diet until the first incapacitating symptoms of uremia begin to appear or until working time is lost—usually when the GFR is around 5 ml per minute. Regular hemodialysis should then be instituted until a well-matched cadaver transplant is available. If this plan is followed, these patients sacrifice a few months of independence in increasing discomfort, but escape most of the clinical features listed below and should require therapy only for hypertension and, in some cases, bone disease. Their treatment must be planned well in advance of the crises. An arteriovenous fistula should be inserted many months before it is required so that it is available for dialysis during intercurrent illness and is well developed when required. The blood group, tissue type, and calculated chance of a well matched cadaver donor should be recorded on the case record, because they influence decisions such as the choice of home or hospital dialysis. Home adaptations should be completed before training begins so that a minimum of time is lost from work; the uremic patient has a precarious hold on his employment. The following description applies mainly to those patients for whom definitive treatment is not available.

Skin. Pruritus is common and often distressing. It is particularly associated with secondary hyperparathyroidism, but occurs in the absence of radiologic bone disease; it is sometimes caused by sensitivity to *Candida albicans.* The skin is often dry, flaky, and affected by erythematous and maculopapular rashes which become excoriated with scratching. Pigmentation, which is common in slowly progressive renal failure, is due to melanin and urochromes.

Itching occasionally responds to oral aluminum hydroxide gel. Phenothiazine antipruritics are not very effective, and their cumulation in renal failure causes mental blunting and parkinsonism; oculogyric crises are sometimes misinterpreted as uremic fits. Hydrocortisone cream is useful in areas of skin rash.

Gastrointestinal Tract. Dry mouth, metallic taste, and uremic odor can be helped a little by chewing gum. Anorexia is a common early symptom, progressing to nausea and vomiting. Vomiting is sometimes effortless and unexpected, but in the terminal stage continuous dry retching becomes a distressing feature. The disorder responds to the Giovannetti diet, provided that an anorexic patient can be persuaded to eat it. Preliminary treatment with peritoneal dialysis and intravenous feeding may be required until appetite returns. Antiemetics are of little value in restoring appetite, but they do have a role in controlling the retching of terminal uremics for whom no better treatment is available. Metoclopramide, 10 mg, or prochlorperazine, 10 mg, three times a day may be tried orally, but can be given intramuscularly in the same dosage if necessary. Thiethylperazine, 10 mg, can be given as a suppository. In the last resort, stupor caused by large doses of chlorpromazine is preferable to continuous retching.

Diarrhea is often described as a feature of chronic

renal failure, but it is seldom encountered before the very last stages of the illness unless produced by antihypertensives, antimicrobial drugs, or the high vegetable content of some Giovannetti diets. Constipation is a much more common complaint.

There is probably an increased incidence of hematemesis and melena in uremic patients even before they are subjected to intermittent anticoagulation for hemodialysis. Autopsy used to reveal ulceration of nasopharynx, mouth, stomach, or bowel in about a quarter of all uremics, but these features are now uncommon.

Nutrition and Growth.   Anorexia and vomiting cause inadequate caloric intake, leading to wasting of fat and muscle. Dry, straggly, and depigmented hair is common in malnourished uremics. Gain of weight and improvement in hair texture occur during adequate hemodialysis and, to a lesser extent, during successful Giovannetti dieting.

Children with a GFR below about 20 per cent of normal have impairment of growth and are often below the third percentile for height. Bone age is retarded, and a late growth spurt may occur during adequate dialysis or after transplantation. Loss of height is often accentuated by bone bending owing to renal rickets. Bone growth and gain in height are promoted by high caloric feeding.

Endocrine Function.   The onset of puberty is delayed by several years in children with renal insufficiency. In adults, libido and potency decline in the last few months of the illness in males. Libido is depressed, ovulation suppressed, and amenorrhea common in females. However, contraception is advisable, because pregnancy can occur late in renal failure, and is associated with decline in renal function, increased hypertension, slow fetal growth, and high fetal mortality. As a general guide, pregnancy is hazardous and unlikely to produce a live child if the plasma urea is consistently raised on a normal diet and hypertension is present in the first trimester. It is usually uneventful for mother and child if the renal disease is static or slowly progressive and the plasma urea and the blood pressure are normal at the start of pregnancy. Immunologic tests for pregnancy often give false positives in the presence of proteinuria.

Hypertension.   Hypertension develops at some stage in more than 80 per cent of patients with chronic renal failure. It is associated with sodium and water retention; plasma renin is usually normal except in malignant hypertension. The complications are similar to those of any type of hypertension, but a malignant phase and resistance to drug therapy are more common in renal failure. After the primary disease, hypertension is the most important determinant of survival; it leads to a vicious spiral of declining renal function, further sodium retention, and rising blood pressure. The aim of treatment should be the restoration of normal blood pressure in all postures. This demands persistence and close supervision — weekly outpatient visits for many months in resistant cases.

Methyldopa is a common first choice, in a starting dose of 250 mg twice daily increased every few days. Side effects appear at a lower dose in renal failure than in essential hypertension as it is partly dependent on renal excretion, and depression and drowsiness are common if the dose exceeds 2 grams per day. Many patients are uncontrolled by this dose and require one of the sympathetic blockers — bethanidine, debrisoquine, or guanethidine — all in an initial dose of 10 mg daily and with increments every few days. These drugs all produce incapacitating postural and exercise hypotension if supine blood pressure is restored to normal. It is a salutary experience to check blood pressure of the patient supine, standing, and after exercise at each examination.

Propranolol reduces blood pressure without postural change and suppresses renin secretion. The initial dose is 10 mg three times a day, and it can be increased to 320 mg per day or more. Heart failure or bronchial asthma is occasionally precipitated; bradycardia below 50 per minute calls for a reduction in dose. Oxprenolol is an alternative which may be less likely to cause cardiac failure.

Thiazide diuretics lose their diuretic and probably their antihypertensive — action below a GFR of about 15 ml per minute. Furosemide, bumetanide, and ethacrynic acid in high doses still produce a diuresis down to a GFR of about 3 ml per minute; ethacrynic acid occasionally causes deafness in renal failure. Furosemide is given in an initial dose of 40 to 80 mg daily and is increased until adequate diuresis is obtained. In terminal renal failure a daily dose of 1 to 2 grams may be required. No antihypertensive effect is exerted without a diuresis. Hypokalemia can occur even in renal failure, and potassium supplements may be required; regular estimation of plasma potassium is essential.

Diazoxide is a thiazide derivative without diuretic action which probably lowers blood pressure by direct vasodilatation. It can be given intravenously (200 mg) or orally (200 mg three times a day, increasing as necessary) and has proved very effective in controlling hypertension resistant to all conventional drugs. It causes hyperglycemia and may precipitate frank diabetes mellitus, but this can be controlled with sulfonylureas while diazoxide is continued.

Minoxidil is a new drug with actions similar to those of diazoxide but without the same risk of hyperglycemia; it is not yet available in Britain.

Clonidine (0.1 to 0.5 mg three times a day) has an unexplained action similar to that of methyldopa, with the side effects of drowsiness and dry mouth.

Edema.   Edema may be due to hypertensive heart failure, impaired sodium and water excretion, or nephrotic syndrome. The last should be recognized by the heavy proteinuria, the electrophoretic pattern, and the hyperlipidemia, as it may call for high protein feeding except in late renal failure. Heart failure and salt and water retention are difficult to distinguish, but the treatment is the same — sodium and water restriction plus diuretics if necessary. Cardiac glycosides confer little benefit if rhythm is normal, and are dangerous when plasma potassium is varying, particularly during dialysis which removes potassium faster than the glycosides. If they are employed, the dose should be reduced by about a third to compensate for the loss of renal excretion, but they are best avoided except in atrial fibrillation.

Pulmonary edema is a common complication of renal failure with hypertension; it is characterized by attacks of nocturnal dyspnea, basal crepitations, and "bat's wing" perihilar shadows on chest roentgenograms. After repeated attacks the lung becomes infiltrated with macrophages and the fibrous septa thickened, a condition sometimes called *"uremic lung"* in this situation, but it is essentially the same as the *"hexamethonium lung"* of inadequately treated essential hypertension. Vital capacity, forced expiratory volume, and diffusing capacity are all reduced, particularly the last. Acute pulmonary edema responds rapidly to fluid removal by diuretics, peritoneal dialysis, or hemodialysis.

Pericarditis. Pericarditis was once the harbinger of death. It occurred in about half the patients dying of chronic renal failure, and they seldom survived its onset by more than two months. It is now a sign that dialysis has been delayed or ineffective and calls for urgent treatment.

The onset is usually signaled by pain, which is often felt on the left side of the chest on inspiration for the first few hours, but may be central from the start. Pain is frequently severe, mimicking myocardial infarction, but it may appear after the friction rub and disappear long before it. The friction rub is usually loud, generalized, and palpable, and it may persist when the pericardial cavity contains half a liter of fluid and fatal tamponade is imminent. Tamponade was rare until the 1960's, but became a major cause of death in the early weeks of regular hemodialysis when this was instituted late. The important signs are falling blood pressure and pulse pressure, paradoxic fall in blood pressure with inspiration, cold, poorly perfused extremities, and raised jugular venous pressure. Paradoxic movement of the neck veins is a late and inconstant sign. On chest roentgenogram the typical globular shape of the heart may be seen in first attacks, but recurrent pericarditis produces a dense fibrous parietal pericardium which alters little in shape when fluid accumulates. The effusion can be confirmed by an ultrasonic scan, by superimposing a radioalbumin scan on the chest film or passing a cardiac catheter into the right atrium to demonstrate that the edge of the cardiac shadow is beyond the atrial wall. The fluid should be removed by paracentesis, repeatedly if necessary, and intensive dialysis should be instituted; many authors favor early pericardectomy. Hemorrhagic effusion is the rule in uremia. The hematocrit of the aspirated effusion is usually about half that of circulating blood.

In the acute stage there is a fibrinous exudate over the visceral pericardium. After several attacks, sometimes after a single attack, an adherent pericardium thickens and within a few months to a few years produces constrictive pericarditis, usually without calcification, which must be treated surgically. The whole affected pericardium should be stripped off the heart.

Other Cardiovascular Effects. Deposits of calcium phosphate are found in the heart in severe hyperparathyroidism, and calcium oxalate and urates are deposited after some months of inadequate regular hemodialysis. Sudden cardiac arrest or arrhythmias result from deposition in the conducting tissue.

Anemia. Anemia is so nearly universal in chronic renal failure that a uremic patient with a normal hemoglobin must be presumed to have acute renal failure until proved otherwise. Red cells are normochromic or have a slightly reduced MCHC, about 30 to 31. The major cause is a reduction in plasma erythropoietin level which results in relative hypoplasia of the marrow. The red cell precursors in the marrow are normal or slightly increased, the reticulocyte count, when corrected for red cell count, is one to four times normal, and radioiron transit time through the marrow is normal or reduced; but in each case the level of activity is well below that which occurs in anemia of the same degree from other causes.

Uncommon exceptions to this rule are a few patients with urinary obstruction, renal artery stenosis, and polycystic disease who overproduce erythropoietin and maintain a normal or even increased hemoglobin in early renal failure. Polycystics as a group have significantly higher hemoglobins than other patients with renal failure throughout the course of the illness and into their experience of regular hemodialysis.

Mild degrees of folate deficiency can be demonstrated by leukocyte lobe counts and marrow morphology in a minority of patients in late renal failure, but response to folic acid is slight. Deficiency of folic acid and pyridoxine, which are dialyzable, and deficiency of iron become important after the start of regular hemodialysis.

Uremia may be responsible for some of the marrow hypoplasia. Improvement in erythropoiesis occurs during regular hemodialysis. Bilateral nephrectomy causes fall in hemoglobin, but a stable hematocrit can eventually be maintained.

An important effect of uremia is the occurrence of mild hemolysis. Red cell life is shortened to about half normal when the blood urea exceeds 200 mg per 100 ml. Burr cells, helmet cells, and other misshapen red cells appear in the blood film as uremia increases. An improvement in red cell survival and hemoglobin level occurs when plasma urea is lowered by the Giovannetti diet. Much more striking hemolysis and deformation of red cells occur in malignant hypertension and in association with several diseases that cause renal failure, such as thrombotic thrombocytopenic purpura.

Anemia becomes a major cause of symptoms in uremia only when the hemoglobin falls below about 7 grams per 100 ml. It is then responsible for dyspnea, may precipitate angina and claudication, and produces ejection systolic murmurs, raised cardiac output, and elevated venous pressure.

Two groups of drugs will raise the hemoglobin level in chronic renal failure by a modest 1 to 3 grams per 100 ml. Salts of cobalt probably act by inducing tissue anoxia, and have therefore been condemned as illogical and dangerous; cardiac failure and impaired thyroid function may develop. Androgens and related anabolic steroids increase the hemoglobin level of normal women in small doses and normal men in larger doses. They act on the marrow directly, as well as through an increased output of renal erythropoietic factor. Success has been claimed in the anemia of renal failure in patients of both sexes, with and without kidneys and before and after regular hemodialysis. Testosterone propionate, 150 mg intramuscularly per week, may be given in men, and it may incidentally help to restore flagging libido. Priapism is a risk, particularly in those on overnight hemodialysis. In females nonicterogenic steroids of low androgenicity, such as nandrolone decanoate, 25 mg intramuscularly per three weeks, seldom cause troublesome side effects, and their anabolic effect at least is well established. Patients should be warned to report hair growth and skin thickening, which are reversible, because the voice change which follows them may be permanent.

Transfusion was once the mainstay of treatment. Packed red cells are given in small volume (200 to 500 ml) with particular caution if the patient is hypertensive. The fear that a rise in hematocrit might imperil renal function by reducing renal plasma flow has been dispelled in clinical trial; renal function declines only if heart failure is precipitated by overtransfusion. However, the benefit is short lived; donor cells have the same shortened life span as the patient's own red cells, and erythropoiesis is depressed by even a small transfusion. Transfusion should be avoided if possible, and only blood negative for hepatitis B associated antigen should be used. A hemoglobin level compatible with reasonable activity can be maintained without transfusion during regular hemodialysis if blood losses are kept to a minimum; after successful transplantation the hemoglobin rises to, or even above, normal. Symptomatic anemia in a patient destined for regular dialysis or transplantation is therefore an indication for expediting definitive treatment. Hypersplenism has been described, particularly in patients on regular dialysis. Splenectomy raises hemoglobin and white cell counts.

Bleeding Tendency. A hemorrhagic tendency is common in late renal failure. Epistaxis, menorrhagia, gastrointestinal hemorrhage, and excessive bleeding or bruising after trauma are common manifestations; purpura is unusual. Whole blood clotting time and prothrombin time are usually normal, although deficiencies of factors V and VII are occasionally described. The total platelet count is normal or slightly reduced, and the life span of platelets is normal; but defects of platelet function can usually be detected and are thought to be the major cause of uremic bleeding. The proportion of sticky platelets is reduced, platelet aggregation with ADP impaired, the prothrombin consumption test abnormal, and platelet factor III availability decreased. The bleeding time is often prolonged, but a modification of the Ivy test, using multiple punctures and measurement of blood loss, may be required to demonstrate it. The platelet defect is roughly proportional to plasma urea, is corrected when plasma urea is reduced by dialysis or low protein diet, and can be reproduced in normal persons by feeding urea, but it is not produced by addition of urea to blood in vitro.

Plasma fibrinogen level is usually raised in renal failure, the mean elevation being about 30 per cent, and this is probably responsible for the characteristic rise in erythrocyte sedimentation rate. Plasma fibrinolytic activity is depressed, as indicated by a prolonged euglobulin lysis time, but fibrin degradation products can often be demonstrated in plasma, suggesting excessive intravascular deposition and removal of fibrin. As the kidney is a major source of plasminogen activator, it is tempting to attribute the reduced blood fibrinolytic activity in renal failure to the loss of renal mass, but this is probably not the true explanation, because regular hemodialysis restores the fibrinolytic activity to normal, even after bilateral nephrectomy. Plasma fibrinogen also returns to normal during regular dialysis.

Troublesome bleeding in uremia is best controlled by peritoneal dialysis or hemodialysis with reduced, or regional, heparinization. Infusion of inhibitors of fibrinolysis, such as aminocaproic acid (EACA) in an initial dose of 100 mg per kilogram of body weight over four hours, is helpful if local measures and dialysis fail to control bleeding externally or into the gut. It should be used only in dire emergency for bleeding into the urinary tract or internal cavities because of the risk of producing indissoluble clot.

Infection. Susceptibility to bacterial infection is characteristic of uremia; it is the main cause of death in acute renal failure and a major source of morbidity in chronic renal failure. The neutrophil count is normal and rises normally in response to infection, but the ability of the cells to ingest and kill bacteria is impaired. Total serum immunoglobulins are normal, unless reduced by the primary disease or by heavy proteinuria, and the anamnestic response to antigens such as tetanus toxoid is nor-

mal, but the appearance of antibodies to new antigens is delayed and their titer low, at least in laboratory animals. The Mantoux and similar tests show impairment of delayed hypersensitivity which is not corrected by regular hemodialysis. The circulating lymphocyte count is reduced. The prolonged tolerance of homografts in uremia is further evidence of altered cellular immunity.

Two common and important problems in renal failure are colonization of the nose and other carrier sites by staphylococci, leading to recurrent infection of the operation wounds and arteriovenous shunts, and infection with *Candida albicans*. Both are encouraged by repeated exposure to antimicrobials and the hospital environment, and may reflect this rather than a specific vulnerability of the uremic patient. On the tongue and buccal mucosa, Candida forms painful white plaques which may make eating almost impossible and which are the usual cause of "uremic ulceration of the mouth." It spreads to the esophagus, causing dysphagia and a moth-eaten appearance on barium swallow. In the gut it causes diarrhea, and may produce generalized allergic rashes as well as pruritus ani. In the vagina it causes discharge and pruritus vulvae.

Strenuous efforts should be made to identify the causative organisms before starting antimicrobial therapy and to follow the change in the bacterial flora during treatment. In seriously ill patients it is worthwhile swabbing the usual carrier sites and wounds and culturing sputum, blood, urine, and stool every few days in an effort to keep one jump ahead of the bacteria. Pathogens found in the nose on Monday are likely culprits in a pneumonia or wound infection developing on Friday; their antimicrobial sensitivities can guide therapy during the first 48 hours while the new invaders are being identified.

If the causative organism can be identified, narrow-spectrum antimicrobials should be employed when there is a choice. If broad-spectrum therapy is needed, and in all seriously ill uremics receiving antimicrobials, antifungal agents, e.g., nystatin suspension, 500 mg four times a day, should be given orally to prevent Candida superinfection, and particular care should be taken with mouth toilet. Established Candida infection of mouth and esophagus should be treated with amphotericin lozenges (10 mg) sucked continuously, at a rate of 10 to 20 per day. If response is slow, the lesions should be painted with gentian violet solution, 1 per cent, three times a day.

The loading dose of antimicrobials is unchanged in renal failure, but the size or spacing of maintenance doses must be adjusted to renal function (Table 4). When the drug is wholly dependent on excretion by glomerular filtration, the blood level produced by a standard regimen will vary up and down with the alterations in GFR that commonly occur in the course of infections in renal failure. If the drug has a low margin of safety, e.g., all ototoxic antimicrobials, the dose should be adjusted daily on the basis of blood antimicrobial measurements; these can now be performed in most hospital laboratories, and the results are available within 24 hours, provided that only one or two drugs are used at a time.

Peripheral Neuropathy. Nerve conduction slows with uremia, falling to about half normal in the legs in terminal renal failure; the arms are less affected. The abnormality is gradually reduced during regular hemodialysis and corrected by successful transplant. Hypesthesia of the feet and diminished ankle jerks can often be detected in the most severely affected patients, but they seldom

TABLE 4. Maintenance Dose of Antimicrobials in
Renal Failure

Group 1. Mainly excreted or metabolized by nonrenal routes. Must be
given in normal dosage for therapeutic effect.
Fusidic acid
Chloramphenicol

Group 2. Major pathway of nonrenal excretion or metabolism. Normal
dosage schedule may be used for a day or two, but some reduction in dosage is desirable.

Methicillin	Erythromycin
Cloxacillin	Sulfadimidine
Flucloxacillin	Carbenicillin
Ampicillin	Doxycycline
Amoxycillin	Cephalexin

Group 3. Predominantly renal excretion. Some dosage reduction is
desirable from the start. Space doses (of normal size) more
widely than usual, but not more than 24 hours apart.

Penicillin G	Co-trimoxazole
Cephaloridine	Nalidixic acid
Cephalothin	Isoniazid
Lincomycin	Ethambutol
Clindamycin	Rifampicin

Group 4. Mainly renal excretion and toxic effects during cumulation.
Major adjustment of dosage required; daily monitoring of
blood antibiotic concentration required.

Kanamycin	Vancomycin
Gentamicin	Para-aminosalicylate
Polymyxin B	Amphotericin
Colomycin	
Streptomycin	

Group 5. Contraindicated in renal failure.
Nitrofurantoin
All tetracyclines except doxycycline
Long-acting sulfonamides

cause spontaneous complaint, and severe neuropathy
was rare until the advent of regular hemodialysis. The
first symptom is usually numbness of the toes and feet,
sometimes accompanied by unpleasant tingling and
burning. Ascending anesthesia, areflexia, and muscle
weakness may progress rapidly over a few days or weeks
to quadriplegia. The condition may deteriorate during
the first few weeks of regular hemodialysis, particularly
if rapid fluid removal is necessary; the most disabling
permanent neuropathies have occurred during inadequate hemodialysis. Sural nerve biopsy shows axonal
degeneration and segmental demyelination.

The incidence of fulminant uremic neuropathy varies
between geographic centers. This is partly explained by
local fashions in drug therapy; nitrofurantoin is an important cause of neuropathy in the uremic, and the onset
of symptoms demands a careful review of drug therapy.

The only effective treatment is intensive hemodialysis—30 to 40 hours per week on the Kiil dialyzer or its
equivalent. Multivitamin supplements, including thiamin, pyridoxine, and hydroxycobalamin, are usually
given to protect against any deficiency caused by anorexia, diet, or dialysis, but they have no therapeutic effect. All but the most advanced cases of neuropathy
remit completely within a few months of successful
transplant.

The tingling and numbness of neuropathy must be distinguished from the similar symptoms produced by hypocalcemia, which are usually precipitated by feeding sodium bicarbonate, and from Raynaud's phenomenon.
The latter is common in renal failure, particularly in patients whose hypertension has been controlled by sodium
and water removal.

Myopathy. A proximal myopathy accompanies renal
osteomalacia and may occur with severe osteitis fibrosa.
It may be severe enough to produce a waddling gait and
prevent stair-climbing. Wasting is slight and tendon
reflexes paradoxically brisk. This rare syndrome becomes more common after the start of regular hemodialysis in those centers where bone disease is a major
problem.

Cramps. Muscle cramps in the calves, thighs, and
flexors of the toes are common in early renal failure, particularly at night. They may also occur in the upper
limbs and during the day when they are precipitated by
stretching, awkward posture, or repetitive exercise such
as knitting. They accompany sodium depletion or dehydration through the artificial kidney, and are then relieved by infusion of saline, but they also occur commonly in the absence of any specific electrolyte
abnormality. Nocturnal cramps are alleviated by a
nightly dose of quinine sulfate, 300 mg orally.

Other Nervous and Muscular Symptoms. *Muscle twitching* affects single muscles or groups in late renal failure.
It wakes the patient as he dozes off, and, when severe, interferes with activities such as writing or holding a cup.
Flapping tremor, which is demonstrated by dorsiflexing
the wrist of an outstretched arm, is due to a similar sudden involuntary relaxation of muscle groups. A common
complaint, probably of central origin, is *restlessness of
the limbs,* particularly the legs. The limbs or the whole
body must be moved to relieve an uncomfortable feeling
which the patient finds it hard to describe. The symptom
is at its worst during the first hour after lying down to
sleep. It may be accompanied by a feeling as of insects
crawling under the skin—a sensation so unpleasant that
it may be described as a pain. This dysesthesia and restless limbs may be precursors of a state of extreme hyperexcitability and muscular overactivity, seen at its
worst in patients undertreated by peritoneal or hemodialysis, which is rapidly fatal unless treated by intensive dialysis. As a symptomatic measure, diazepam,
5 to 10 mg intravenously, is effective and may be
repeated every four hours.

Persistent *hiccup* is common in terminal renal failure,
and it occasionally affects a patient at an earlier stage,
exhausting him over the course of a few days. There is no
really effective treatment short of very heavy sedation,
but chlorpromazine, 25 mg orally three times a day, will
sometimes abort an attack.

Insomnia is common and, although sometimes caused
by restless limbs or pruritus, it often persists beyond the
first hour in bed when these are at their worst. It is accompanied by lethargy during the day and may represent reversal of normal sleep rhythm. Recourse to nocturnal sedatives is often necessary; barbiturates,
nitrazepam, and methaqualone are currently most popular and about equally effective. They are given in full
dosage, and all but the longest-acting barbiturates are
well tolerated without troublesome hangover in spite of
the fact that they all depend partly on renal excretion.

Tiredness is almost universal in uremia, although the
level at which it occurs is variable; some patients are active in business with a blood urea over 200 or even 300
mg per 100 ml. Its causes include sleep disturbance, anemia, hypertensive heart failure, muscle weakness, and
drug side effects, but there is probably a specific effect of
uremia that is noticeably relieved by the first one or two
hemodialyses.

Increased *mental fatigability* may begin early in renal

failure and is succeeded by loss of concentration, reduced performance at mental arithmetic and other demanding skills, impaired memory, and in terminal renal failure by drowsiness, disorientation, stupor, and coma. Episodes of toxic psychosis with confusion, hallucinations, delusions, and intervals of insight are particularly associated with infections and pericarditis in late renal failure. Major electroencephalographic changes accompany these severe mental symptoms; spike potentials occur sporadically in bursts, and slow waves come to dominate the recording, the mean frequency falling as low as 2 or 3 per second. Toxic *psychosis* and *confusion* respond to intensive peritoneal or hemodialysis, but some caution must be exercised during initial treatment. A "disequilibrium syndrome" of headache, vomiting, confusion, coma, and convulsions with further deterioration of the EEG occurs when patients with severe uremia are treated by rapid dialysis. It was a common and sometimes fatal problem in the days when hemodialysis was instituted at a blood urea of 400 mg per 100 ml with large membrane area machines. It has almost disappeared from those centers at which dialysis is performed early and at a reasonable pace, and is there encountered almost exclusively in the treatment of already confused patients with chronic renal failure. It is attributed to cerebral edema caused by the removal of osmotically active substances — urea and in some cases sodium and chloride — from the extracellular compartment. A shift in the oxygen dissociation curve resulting from correction of acidosis, causing hypoxia, may be an additional explanation. It can be prevented by using a slow method of dialysis, e.g., peritoneal dialysis, for the first 24 to 48 hours and by inducing a compensatory hyperglycemia. This is achieved by using dialysis fluid with an increased dextrose content and monitoring blood sugar every few hours. The main dangers of the syndrome are convulsions and inhalation of vomitus; anticonvulsants should be given prophylactically and the stomach kept empty with the aid of a gastric tube.

Convulsions. Convulsions can be precipitated in terminal renal failure by a variety of alterations in plasma composition, of which water intoxication is the most common. Intravenous therapy should be planned to correct abnormalities slowly. However, the most important precipitant is severe hypertension, which is responsible for about two thirds of all uremic fits and for nearly all such episodes in early renal failure. Acute hypotension initiates some fits, particularly in the course of hemodialysis. In terminal renal failure convulsions may occur without any obvious precipitant. They are usually of grand mal type, occasionally jacksonian. They often recur in rapid succession, and carry a formidable mortality from asystole or ventricular fibrillation. They are a dire medical emergency and must be controlled rapidly, by anesthetizing the patient and maintaining him on a respirator if necessary. Usually they can be managed less drastically with intravenous diazepam, 10 mg, or sodium amylobarbitone, 125 to 250 mg, repeated every hour or two initially. If fits recur, sedation should be heavy enough to allow the insertion of an intratracheal tube, as it is vital to prevent anoxia; the stomach should be aspirated hourly. Intravenous sodium phenytoin, 200 mg, should be given at the start and may be repeated two or three times in the first 24 hours. Maintenance therapy with phenobarbitone, 60 to 120 mg daily, and sodium phenytoin, 50 to 100 mg three times a day, should be continued until definitive treatment for uremia has begun.

Phenobarbitone and phenytoin accumulate in renal failure, and their blood levels should be checked if the patient develops depression, drowsiness, or mental blunting. Severe hypertension should also be corrected as an emergency. A useful regimen is hydralazine, 20 to 40 mg intramuscularly hourly until the blood pressure is controlled, if an initial test dose of 10 mg is well tolerated. Methyldopate hydrochloride, 250 to 1000 mg every 6 hours by infusion, acts more slowly, reducing blood pressure over 6 to 12 hours. Diazoxide, 200 mg intravenously, is effective within an hour or two.

The brain of a patient dying in uremia shows areas of nerve cell depopulation in addition to the acute neuronal damage, scattered petechiae, and edema attributable to uremia or convulsions. Some permanent decline in cerebral function probably occurs if the patient survives, and one survey suggested an average drop of 10 to 15 per cent in IQ in a group treated by regular hemodialysis. However, the most striking examples of failing intelligence and impoverished personality are seen in hypertensive patients; these probably reflect vascular damage in the brain rather than the effects of uremia.

Ocular Manifestations. The most important changes in the eye are those of *hypertensive retinopathy*. In spite of many references to "albuminuric retinopathy" there are no features that distinguish these changes from those of hypertension in the patient with normal renal function. Visual acuity is usually impaired in the presence of papilledema, and scotomas corresponding to large hemorrhages may be noticed by the patient. Control of hypertension is followed in sequence by the clearing of hemorrhages, resolution of papilledema, and disappearance of exudates, the macular star often persisting for some months after blood pressure is normal. Vision usually returns to nearly normal, but some patients are left with optic atrophy and permanent loss of acuity.

Retinal detachment, usually of globular shape in the lower half of the eye, occurs in patients with severe hypertensive retinopathy, renal failure, and fluid overload; hypertension is probably the most important precipitant, but the condition often resolves spontaneously even if the blood pressure is poorly controlled. It is due to serous effusion below the retina. Resolution is usually complete if hypertension and fluid overload are treated rapidly by dialysis.

"Red eyes" in renal failure are caused by conjunctival vasodilatation and are described above.

Pancreatitis. Pancreatitis is common in renal failure. A modest rise in serum amylase can occur from renal failure alone.

Wound Healing. Wound healing is impaired, and incisional hernia is common. Stitches should be retained for an extra week.

Low Protein Diet. Diet is used solely as a symptomatic measure. It is important that the treatment should be more tolerable than the disease and that it should improve the patient as well as his biochemical data. A common fault is the prescription of diet before it is really needed. The only symptoms consistently relieved are anorexia, nausea, and vomiting, although improvement in mental symptoms, muscle twitching, and pruritus are described often enough to suggest that they are genuine.

With 40 grams of predominantly first-class protein per day a diet can be constructed with a calorie content sufficient for light work which is reasonably attractive to patients with some culinary skill and an adventurous palate. Extra calories for heavy workers can be provided in electrolyte-free carbohydrate supplements such as Hycal or Caloreen which are less sweet than natural carbohydrates and can be disguised in other food.

The diet is much less attractive when simultaneous restriction of sodium, potassium, or water becomes necessary. It is expensive, involves a change from traditional food, and is unacceptable to other members of the family. It is rarely consumed conscientiously unless supported by detailed initial training and prolonged follow-up with dietary counseling by medical staff as well as dietitians. Poorly instructed patients, fobbed off with a diet sheet, merely consume a calorie-deficient, truncated version of their normal diet.

A 40-gram protein diet should be started when symptoms first develop on free diet—a variable point in the course of renal failure, but on average at a GFR of about 10 ml per minute. When these symptoms recur on the 40-gram diet, a diet containing only 18 grams of protein will maintain nitrogen balance after an initial period of nitrogen loss, reduce plasma urea, and relieve many uremic symptoms, if at least two thirds of the protein is first class, providing a high proportion of essential amino acids and sufficient caloric content. This is achieved in the *Giordano* or *Giovannetti diet* by using cereals, from which most of the protein has been removed, as calorie sources and egg with a little milk or meat to provide the protein. This high egg content makes the diet nauseating to some, and acidosis is increased by the metabolism of phospholipids in yolk. Bread and spaghetti made from protein-free flour are stodgy and flavorless. Many modifications have been devised to suit local tastes. Egg white can be baked into the bread to improve its texture. Potatoes have a better amino acid mixture than cereals and can be used without protein extraction, but their potassium content must be reduced by preboiling. With ingenuity the diet can be made just tolerable to most patients with GFR down to 3 ml per minute, but even its conscientious use adds only a few months to the average life span of the patient in renal failure. If facilities for dialysis and transplantation are available, this short respite does not justify the effort involved.

Bennett, W. M., Singer, I., and Coggins, C. H.: Guide to drug usage in adults with impaired renal function. J.A.M.A., 223:991, 1973.

Bergström, J., Furst, P., Josephson, B., and Norée, L. O.: Factors affecting the nitrogen balance in chronic uremic patients receiving essential amino acids intravenously or by mouth. Nutr. Metab., 14:(Suppl., p. 162), 1972.

Blagg, C. R., and Scribner, B. H.: Diet, drugs and dialysis in the management of renal failure. *In* Edwards, K. D. G. (ed.): Drugs Affecting Kidney Function and Metabolism. Basel, Karger, 1972.

Boulton-Jones, J. M., Vick, R., Cameron, J. S., and Black, P. J.: Immune responses in uremia. Clin. Nephrol., 1:351, 1973.

Chantler, C., and Holliday, M. A.: Growth in children with renal disease with particular reference to the effects of calorie malnutrition: A review. Clin. Nephrol., 1:230, 1973.

Coburn, J. W., and Norman, A. W.: Role of the kidney in the metabolism of calciferol (vitamin D). Clin. Nephrol., 1:273, 1973.

Dathan, J. R. E., Johnson, D. B., and Goodwin, F. J.: The relationship between body fluid compartment volumes, renin activity and blood pressure in chronic renal failure. Clin. Sci., 45:77, 1973.

David, D. S.: Dietary treatment of renal failure. Am. Heart J., 86:1, 1973.

Davies, D. L., Schalekamp, M. A., Beevers, D. G., Brown, J. J., Briggs, J. D., Lever, A. F., Medina, A. M., Morton, J. J., Robertson, J. I. S., and Tree, M.: Abnormal relation between exchangeable sodium and the renin-angiotensin system in malignant hypertension and in hypertension with chronic renal failure. Lancet, 1:683, 1973.

DeFronzo, R. A., Andres, R., Edgar, P., and Walker, W. G.: Carbohydrate metabolism in uremia: A review. Medicine (Baltimore), 52:469, 1973.

Goldsmith, R. S., Furszyfer, J., Johnson, W. J., Fournier, A. E., Sizemore, G. W. and Arnaud, C. D.: Etiology of hyperparathyroidism and bone disease during chronic hemodialysis. III. Evaluation of parathyroid suppressibility. J. Clin. Invest., 52:173, 1973.

Hosking, D. J., and Chamberlain, M. J.: Calcium balance in chronic renal failure. Quart. J. Med., 42:467, 1973.

Kodicek, E.: The story of vitamin D. From vitamin to hormone. Lancet, 1:325, 1974.

Massry, S. G., Friedler, R. M., and Coburn, J. W.: Excretion of phosphate and calcium. Arch. Intern. Med., 131:828, 1973.

Milne, M. D. (ed.): Management of renal failure. Br. Med. Bull., 27:No. 2, 1971.

Peacock, M., Gallagher, J. C., and Nordin, B. E.: Action of 1-alpha-hydroxy vitamin D_3 on calcium absorption and bone resorption in man. Lancet, 1:385, 1974.

Popovtzer, M. M., Katz, F. H., Pinggera, W. F., Robinette, J., Halgrimson, C. G., and Butkus, D. E.: Hyperkalemia in salt-wasting nephropathy. Arch. Intern. Med., 132:203, 1973.

Reidenberg, M. M.: Renal Function and Drug Action. Philadelphia, W. B. Saunders Company, 1971.

604. ACUTE RENAL FAILURE

Neal S. Bricker

Definition. Acute renal failure is a clinical syndrome characterized by a sudden decrease in glomerular filtration rate, often to values of less than 1 to 2 ml per minute. Acute renal failure is usually associated with oliguria (urine volumes of less than 400 ml per day), and is always associated with biochemical consequences of the reduction in glomerular filtration rate such as a rise in blood urea nitrogen (BUN), and serum creatinine concentrations. The occurrence of other abnormalities in body fluids such as metabolic acidosis, hyperkalemia, hyperphosphatemia, and hypocalcemia will depend upon the duration and severity of the renal failure, the nature and severity of any underlying injury or disease process, and the nature and intensity of treatment.

Acute renal failure so defined encompasses many different forms of disease with widely varying pathogeneses, natural histories, and prognostic implications. For example, a sudden decrease in glomerular filtration rate may occur in association with profound reduction in effective extracellular fluid volume or fall in blood pressure, and may be readily reversible by volume expansion or blood pressure elevation. More commonly acute renal failure is due to intrinsic disease of the renal parenchyma; but some forms are ultimately (albeit not immediately) reversible, and others are not. Finally, this syndrome may occur in consequence of urinary tract obstruction or occlusion of the renal arteries or veins.

Because of the diversity of etiologic and pathogenetic events which can culminate in acute renal failure; because recognition of the immediately reversible forms of the syndrome can lead to prompt restitution of normal renal function, whereas failure of recognition may lead to persistence of renal failure, increasingly severe manifestations of uremia, and, in some instances, permanent nephron destruction; because the syndrome is so frequently superimposed upon major injuries or serious systemic disease; and because a substantial percentage of patients will survive their disease if therapy is dedicated and skillful, this group of abnormalities stands among the most challenging problems in clinical medicine.

The discussion in this chapter will deal principally with one form of acute renal failure, *acute tubular necrosis.* Other types of the syndrome will be considered, but primarily as they relate to the differential diagnosis of acute tubular necrosis.

Acute tubular necrosis is defined as a special form of

acute renal failure caused by an intrinsic abnormality of the renal parenchyma that is potentially reversible after an interval ranging from several days to several weeks. Although the term acute tubular necrosis may not reflect accurately the basis of the lesion or even its pathologic concomitants, and although other names have been used or proposed (e.g., lower nephron nephrosis, tubulointerstitial nephritis, and vasomotor nephropathy), the designation acute tubular necrosis (or ATN) will be retained in this chapter because it remains the most commonly used expression and because none of the other terms have gained more widespread acceptance. Acute tubular necrosis may follow exposure to a nephrotoxic drug or to a primary extrarenal injury or disease, especially when attended by hypotension; occasionally it may appear without an obvious predisposing abnormality. Most characteristically there is a period of oliguria, followed by gradually increasing rates of urine flow, culminating in a period of polyuria. Recovery of renal function toward the pre-illness level then occurs in patients who survive.

Causes of Acute Renal Failure. *Acute Tubular Necrosis.* NEPHROTOXIC DRUGS OR CHEMICALS. Acute tubular necrosis may follow exposure to a host of different chemical agents, some when administered in therapeutic doses. Sulfonamides and many of the commonly used antimicrobial drugs, including gentamicin, kanamycin, streptomycin, colistin, cephaloridine, amphotericin, bacitracin, neomycin, vancomycin, and polymixin, have been incriminated as the causal agents in the induction of acute tubular necrosis. ATN has occurred after exposure to organic iodonated x-ray contrast media and after the use of the anesthetic methoxyflurane. It may also follow either accidental or intentional exposure to a variety of nephrotoxic agents. Included among these are organic solvents (especially carbon tetrachloride and tetrachloroethylene); ethylene and diethylene glycol; inorganic mercurials and other heavy metals, including bismuth, uranium, lead, and, rarely, organic mercurials; methyl alcohol; and massive doses of salicylates and paraldehyde. This subject is dealt with in greater detail in Ch. 626.

SYSTEMIC INJURY OR ILLNESS. Acute tubular necrosis may follow severe trauma such as crushing injuries or major operative procedures, especially when blood loss and/or hypotension occur. It may occur in association with rhabdomyolysis and myoglobinuria of any cause, including heat stroke and overdosage with heroin and probably intravenous methadone. It may also follow severe febrile illnesses, gram-negative or, less frequently, gram-positive sepsis, profound and sustained lactic acidosis, major losses of extracellular fluid volume, or major translocations of this volume, into gut, soft tissues, and skin (in burns). Acute tubular necrosis may develop in the course of complicated pregnancies, particularly when hemorrhage or hypotension occurs. It may follow an incompatible blood transfusion and, occasionally, intravascular hemolysis resulting from other mechanisms. In most of the foregoing entities, one or more of the following events frequently occurs: (1) profound depletion of actual or effective extracellular fluid volume, (2) hypotension, or (3) hemoglobinuria or myoglobinuria.

ACUTE TUBULAR NECROSIS OCCURRING DE NOVO. Rarely, the disease occurs without known exposure to any nephrotoxic agent and in the absence of a detectable fall in blood pressure, obvious change in circulatory dynamics, loss or translocation or extracellular fluid volume, intravascular hemolysis, or myoglobinuria. Indeed, it may in some instances occur without any apparent predisposing illness or injury and in an apparently healthy individual.

Other Parenchymal Diseases. BILATERAL RENAL CORTICAL NECROSIS. Cortical necrosis may be diffuse or patchy. In the former instance, acute renal failure is severe, and may be characterized by total anuria. In patchy cortical necrosis, the occurrence and severity of the renal failure will depend upon the extent of cortical destruction. Return of enough renal function to support life is unusual (but may occur) in patients with diffuse bilateral cortical necrosis; it is not infrequent in patients with patchy cortical necrosis.

GLOMERULITIS. Severe acute renal failure may be seen occasionally in poststreptococcal acute glomerulonephritis, particularly in the adult. Acute renal failure may also be seen in the acute glomerulitides associated with systemic lupus erythematosus, hypersensitivity angiitis, polyarteritis nodosa, rapidly progressive glomerulonephritis, Henoch-Schönlein purpura, Goodpasture's syndrome, thrombotic thrombocytopenic purpura, the hemolytic-uremic syndrome, and malignant nephrosclerosis. It may also be seen in accelerated scleroderma in which the predominant site of involvement is in the small arterioles of the kidney.

PAPILLARY NECROSIS. Renal papillary necrosis appears classically in patients with diabetes mellitus, urinary tract obstruction (especially when accompanied by severe pyelonephritis), and sickle cell anemia, as well as in patients who have ingested excessive quantities of phenacetin and possibly other analgesic drugs. The severity of the renal failure, as well as the potential for ultimate recovery, will depend upon the number of renal papillae that escape destruction.

END-STAGE CHRONIC RENAL DISEASE. Acute renal failure may occur under two circumstances in patients with chronic progressive renal disease: (1) when the nephron population diminishes below a critical level and oliguria supervenes; and (2) when an acute complicating process (such as extracellular fluid volume depletion, acute glomerulitis, or urinary tract obstruction) results in a sudden but potentially reversible decrement in renal function from the previous steady-state level.

MISCELLANEOUS FORMS OF PARENCHYMAL INVOLVEMENT. Severe *hypercalcemia* may be associated with the rapid onset of acute renal failure. In most instances the rising BUN is accompanied by polyuria rather than oliguria; but occasionally, particularly with extremely high levels of serum calcium, urine volumes may fall to the oliguric range. *Hyperuricemia* can lead to acute renal failure when the plasma levels increase very rapidly and to concentrations in excess of 15 to 20 mg per 100 ml. The renal failure presumably is due to intrarenal obstruction caused by deposition of uric acid precipitates in collecting ducts and the renal papillae. Renal failure may occur during the course of *multiple myeloma*. In some instances this is the result of severe (but reversible) hypercalcemia; the disease may also follow a period of fluid deprivation, usually for purposes of performing intravenous pyelography, in patients with Bence Jones proteinuria. The renal failure is presumed to be due to the inspissation of proteinaceous materials in the tubular lumina. Wheter the x-ray contrast media per se play a role in this form of the disease is not clear. Another cause which is being seen with increasing frequency is *homograft rejection* in transplanted kidneys. Treatment of the rejection often results in reversal of the acute renal failure. However, patients receiving transplanted kidneys, particularly from cadaveric sources, are also prone to the development of acute tubular necrosis.

Occlusion of the Renal Arteries or Veins. Acute interruption of the blood supply to the kidneys may occur after embolization, in situ thrombosis, or dissection of the aorta. For renal failure to occur, virtually the entire nephron population of both kidneys must be deprived of blood supply, and, with the exception of aortic surgery, when "sludge" may flow into both renal arteries during or after release of aortic clamping or extensive atheroembolization, arterial occlusion is an unusual cause of the renal failure. Bilateral renal vein thrombosis is also an unusual cause of the disease, for the involvement must be bilateral (if there are two kidneys), and the luminal occlusion must be complete or virtually complete.

Hemodynamic Alterations (Prerenal Azotemia). Prerenal azotemia is a reversible abnormality characterized by a functional reduction in glomerular filtration rate per nephron. The latter may be secondary to a decrease in mean arterial blood pressure and/or to intrarenal vascular adjustments initiated by marked depletion of effective extracellular fluid volume. This loss may be extracorporeal, or it may represent a sequestration of fluid in areas of the body such as the intestine (after major surgical procedures), or skin bullae (in burns). If prerenal azotemia is not recognized promptly and treated, it may lead to the development of acute tubular necrosis.

Hepatorenal Syndrome. Acute renal failure may occur in the course of severe hepatic failure, usually in association with incipient or overt hepatic encephalopathy. In some instances it is due to acute tubular necrosis; but it may also be due to the hepatorenal syndrome, an abnormality that typically is irreversible. The etiology and pathogenesis of the syndrome are unknown, and there are no characteristic pathologic changes in the kidneys. From a pathophysiologic point of view, the hepatorenal syndrome has functional characteristics (to be described under Pathologic Physiology) which simulate those of prerenal azotemia and clearly differentiate the abnormality from acute tubular necrosis.

Urinary Tract Obstruction. For obstruction of the urinary tract to produce acute renal failure, the obstructing process must interfere with the flow of urine from the vast majority of nephrons. Thus if the obstructing lesion is at or above the ureterovesical junction, it must be bilateral if both kidneys are functioning.

Pathogenesis of Acute Tubular Necrosis. Several theories have been proposed for the pathogenesis of acute tubular necrosis. Each has its proponents, and there are at least some supporting experimental data in animals. But for each, contradictory evidence has also accrued; and for none is there universal acceptance.

The most prominently considered theories are the following: (1) *Obstruction of tubular lumina* secondary to inspissated debris; the debris may be composed of hemoglobin or myoglobin, or of sloughed epithelial cells and protein. (2) *A profound reduction in glomerular filtration rate per nephron,* with or without tubular obstruction. The decrease in glomerular filtration rate would be sufficiently severe to eliminate the great majority of nephrons from the urine-forming group, and would presumably affect the cortical nephrons preferentially. Both

the renin-angiotensin system and an intrinsic change in glomerular permeability have been incriminated in the production of the drastic fall in single nephron glomerular filtration rate; but for the former the data are conflicting, and for the latter the evidence is preliminary and incomplete. (3) *"Back-leak" of tubular fluid into the renal interstitium through areas of discontinuity in the tubular walls.* The accumulation of tubular fluid in the interstitium would result in obstruction of contiguous nephrons. Back-leak could occur with or without nephron obstruction and with or without a decrease in glomerular filtration rate per nephron.

Essential to each of the hypotheses is damage to the tubular epithelial cells. The proponents of tubular obstruction believe that the damaged cells contribute to the luminal occlusion. Proponents of the reduced glomerular filtration rate thesis secondary to activation of the renin-angiotensin system view the damage as impairing sodium reabsorption in proximal tubules. An increase in volume or sodium concentration of tubular fluid reaching the macula densa would follow. The sensors in the macula densa, in turn, would initiate the release of renin from the juxtaglomerular granules, and the renin would lead to high local concentrations of angiotensin. Finally the angiotensin would produce vasoconstriction of the afferent arteriole and a decrease in glomerular filtration rate. A reduction in single nephron GFR secondary to impaired glomerular permeability would also require tubular damage, for, as will be discussed under Pathologic Physiology, a decrease in GFR without any change in the integrity of tubular function should produce the physiologic changes of prerenal azotemia rather than those of acute tubular necrosis. In the "back-leak" hypothesis, damage to the epithelial cells and basement membranes would account for the discontinuity of the tubular walls, and thus the cycling of tubular fluid from nephron lumina into interstitial spaces.

In at least some forms of experimental acute tubular necrosis, there is little evidence of widespread cast formation, of diffuse tubular dilatation, or of increase in intratubular pressure in individual surface nephrons. Thus distal tubular obstruction is not a universal phenomenon. Moreover, direct measurement of glomerular filtration rate in single nephrons indicates that a primary or at least causal reduction in the filtration rate is not universal. Finally in some models, inulin injected directly into proximal tubules has been recovered essentially completely in the urine, thus indicating that back-leak is not universal. The ambiguity, in all probability, relates to the fact that many different techniques have been used to produce acute tubular necrosis in the animal; and there may be differences in pathogenesis among these entities. Hence, it is conceivable that tubular obstruction, reduction in single nephron glomerular filtration rate, and back-leak may contribute either alone or in combination to the pathogenesis of the acute renal failure in the laboratory animal. But acute tubular necrosis in man also arises in a wide spectrum of circumstances and after a multiplicity of different insults; and it is equally conceivable that there is more than one pathogenetic pathway leading to the development of the human disease.

Pathology. On gross examination, kidneys with acute tubular necrosis appear enlarged and swollen. On cut section they exhibit a pale cortex and a dark congested medulla. Microscopically the changes are largely confined to the tubules, and neither the glomeruli nor the vessels show consistent abnormalities. The changes in the tubular epithelia tend to be scattered and nonuniform, and in some cases no abnormalities can be seen on light microscopy. Usually, however, the proximal tubular epithelia tend to appear flattened, and mitotic figures may be seen. Frank necrosis may be observed in the proximal tubule, particularly after exposure to a nephrotoxic agent. The distal tubules appear dilated, and the epithelia are low and basophilic with dense staining nuclei and occasional mitotic figures. Casts of varying types may appear within the distal segments of the nephrons. Tubular basement membranes may be disrupted in scattered areas in non-nephrotoxic acute tubular necrosis, but this change is unusual when the disease is secondary to a nephrotoxic drug. Within several days of the onset of acute tubular necrosis, round cell infiltration and edema of the interstitial spaces occur in most cases. The edema may become quite pronounced in overhydrated patients.

Electron microscopic examination has revealed structural alterations in the mitochondria of tubular epithelial cells, loss of the microvilli in the proximal tubular epithelia, and loss of endoplasmic reticulum; there may also be disruption of continuity of the tubular basement membrane. However, the glomeruli have shown no consistent lesion that could provide a morphologic basis for a decrease in glomerular permeability.

Pathologic Physiology of Acute Tubular Necrosis. With normal renal function, less than 1 per cent of the water filtered at the glomeruli is ordinarily excreted in the urine, and only about 0.5 per cent of the filtered sodium is excreted on an average salt intake. In a typical patient with oliguric acute tubular necrosis, from 10 to 20 per cent of the filtered water and from 5 to 10 per cent of the filtered sodium are excreted. Considering the marked decrease in total kidney glomerular filtration rate, these increased *fractional* excretion rates are appropriate in direction; however, the changes are much less marked than in patients with chronic renal failure. For example, a patient with chronic uremia and a filtration rate of 1 ml per minute may excrete 50 per cent or more of the filtered water and sodium. The consequences of these excretory patterns are as follows: At a glomerular filtration rate of 1 ml per minute, the patient with acute tubular necrosis will typically excrete less than 300 ml of urine and less than 20 mEq of sodium per day, whereas the patient with chronic renal disease may excrete 1 liter or more of urine and as much as 100 mEq of sodium per day.

Two questions about the patterns of salt and water excretion in acute tubular necrosis thus emerge: (1) Are the increments in fractional salt and water excretion regulatory in nature or are they fortuitous consequences of intrinsic damage to the tubular epithelial cells? (2) Why are the responses not greater? Does it take time to build up natriuretic forces in a patient with uremia; or do the functioning nephrons in acute tubular necrosis fail to respond to these forces, either because the tubular epithelial cells are damaged or because single nephron glomerular filtration rate is too low? To date, the answer to these questions is not available. However, the fact that patients with acute tubular necrosis do spontaneously excrete a moderately high percentage of filtered water and filtered sodium (regardless of the mechanism) provides a clear explanation for "nonoliguric" tubular necrosis and for certain of the characteristics of the diuretic phase of the disease.

In most patients with the disease, the glomerular filtration rate (as estimated by endogenous creatinine clearance) drops to values of 1 ml per minute or less. Such patients are oliguric. However, in some patients the drop in the filtration rate is not as severe, and values may not fall below 3 to 5 ml per minute. Urea synthesis will still far exceed urea excretion, and the BUN will rise progressively. Creatinine and phosphate concentrations also will rise, and acidosis and hyperkalemia may develop. The patient thus may develop all the symptoms and signs of acute uremia. However, if 20 per cent of the filtered water is excreted at a glomerular filtration rate of 4 ml per minute, urine flow will be almost 1200 ml per day and sodium excretion may exceed 60 mEq per day. Hence there will exist a seeming paradox wherein the patient will present with stigmata of mounting uremia but with urine volumes that are not reduced, i.e., nonoliguric acute tubular necrosis.

A similar physiologic basis exists for the continued rise of the BUN during the first few days of the diuretic phase of oliguric acute tubular necrosis. If 20 per cent of the filtered water is excreted, urine volumes may exceed 1.5 to 2 liters per day before the glomerular filtration rate becomes high enough to allow for the filtration (and thus the excretion) of an amount of urea equal to that produced. The more catabolic the patient is, the higher must be the filtration rate (and the rate of urine flow) before the BUN will start to decline.

As the GFR increases progressively during the recovery phase of acute tubular necrosis, urine volumes may rise to very high levels. Three factors appear to have a profound influence on the magnitude of the diuresis. The first is the degree to which urea and other endogenous solutes accumulate in the blood during the oliguric phase. If urea is allowed to accumulate in body fluids rather than being removed by repeated dialysis, the retained solute will be excreted as the filtration rate rises toward normal. And because the urine remains isosmotic in acute tubular necrosis, every 300 mOsm of extra solute excreted will obligate the excretion of approximately a liter of water. If the BUN concentration is lowered by 20 mg per 100 ml in a 24-hour period via excretion in the urine, approximately 18 grams of urea (equal to 300 mOsm) will be excreted in a 70-kg man, and this will increase the 24-hour urine volume by about 1 liter.

The second factor that may influence the magnitude of the diuresis is the degree of expansion of extracellular fluid volume. If effective extracellular fluid volume is supernormal, natriuretic forces will be mobilized, and as the diuretic phase proceeds, the nephrons will respond to these forces and excrete an increasing fraction of filtered sodium and water. This phenomenon can lead to a vicious cycle wherein urine volume and solute excretion increase in consequence of fluid volume expansion, and the rate of fluid administration in turn is increased to keep up with the rising urine volumes.

The third factor which will influence importantly the magnitude of the diuresis is the rate of recovery of tubular reabsorptive capacity.

Clinical Manifestations. When there is an inciting event, the onset of acute renal failure follows the insult by an interval varying from hours to as long as two days. The oliguric phase may last from a few hours to three or more weeks, and in some instances it appears not to occur at all. The diuretic phase lasts from a few days to a week or longer. The recovery phase is characterized by a progressive rise in glomerular filtration rate and restoration of renal responsiveness to the volume needs of the organism. With recovery, renal function is restored toward the pretubular necrosis level, but in most patients some permanent nephron loss probably occurs.

The presenting picture is usually that of an oliguric patient with a rising concentration of blood urea and creatinine. If the oliguria has been present for some period of time and if salt and water intake have continued unabated, or if an effort was made to restore normal renal function by overzealous fluid administration, salt and water retention, occasionally of massive proportions, may be present. Hyperkalemia may also be present when the patient is first seen. In untreated patients, the symptoms and signs of uremia may develop rapidly, and if there is an underlying injury or illness, the total constellation of clinical abnormalities will reflect the primary disease plus the superimposed manifestations of advancing uremia.

Uremia in acute tubular necrosis may affect many organ systems. *Gastrointestinal manifestations* include anorexia, nausea, and vomiting; if water must be restricted, thirst may become a disturbing symptom. *Central nervous system manifestations* include asterixis, subtle to overt changes in mentation (including organic psychosis), convulsions, and coma. *Cardiovascular changes* include an increase in cardiac output, presumably resulting from anemia and acidosis and, when present, hypervolemia, an increase in blood pressure in some patients, acute left ventricular failure in patients who are markedly hypervolemic, and pericarditis. Electrocardiographic changes are principally those of hyperkalemia, and may include the successive development of tall peaked tent-shaped T waves, prolongation of the P-R interval, prolongation of the QRS interval, disappearance of P waves, and ultimately disintegration of the electrocardiographic pattern with a so-called sine wave appearance. For any given level of elevation of plasma potassium concentration, the cardiotoxic effects tend to be greater when either severe acidosis or hyponatremia is also present.

Therapy will exercise a profound influence on the clinical course of acute tubular necrosis. If dialysis is performed early and at frequent intervals, the patient may progress through the entire course of his illness with few symptoms or signs attributable to the renal failure and without the burden of severe dietary restrictions. If the patient is treated with optimal conservative therapy, but without dialysis, he will develop progressive manifestations of uremia, and moreover will be required to restrict markedly his fluid intake and protein intake. He also may require special treatment for preventing a dangerous rise in plasma potassium concentration. The diuretic phase will be more exaggerated. *In all instances the clinical course is influenced greatly by the nature and severity of any underlying illness or injury.* Patients with acute tubular necrosis need no longer die of uremia, but many, unfortunately, continue to die of the underlying abnormality that precipitated the renal failure.

During the recovery phase patients not infrequently exhibit reactive mental depression. They also may require a long period of recuperation, particularly if catabolism has been severe. Finally, at the end of the diuretic phase, body weight may be substantially less than the clinical estimate of dry weight. This reflects the fact that lean body mass often decreases far more than is suspected during the course of the illness, and the decrease is masked by unrecognized extracellular fluid volume expansion.

Treatment. The treatment of the renal failure in acute tubular necrosis is best accomplished by early and frequent dialysis. Either peritoneal or hemodialysis may be employed. If hemodialysis is preferred or is required because peritoneal dialysis is contraindicated, an arteriovenous shunt may be placed in an extremity at the beginning of the illness to facilitate dialysis on a daily or every-other-day basis. When frequent dialysis is employed, only modest salt and water restriction is needed, and a moderate amount of protein, e.g., 40 to 60 grams per day, may be allowed in the diet. However, when dialysis is not used on a frequent basis, the amount of water, sodium, and potassium must be regulated carefully so as to minimize chemical and volumetric abnormalities of body fluids.

The standard principles of management in a patient who is not dialyzed repeatedly include fluid restriction sufficient to effect the loss of approximately half a pound of body weight per day. In general this amounts to the administration of 400 to 500 ml of fluid plus the amount lost in the urine and gastrointestinal tract. Excessive fluid administration carries the risk of inducing congestive heart failure and pulmonary edema. If the patient is able to take food by mouth, a diet providing approximately 2000 calories which is potassium and protein free and essentially sodium free is recommended; there are some observers, however, who favor the inclusion in the diet of a small amount of protein (ca. 20 grams per day), containing the minimal daily requirements of essential amino acids. If parenteral alimentation is necessary, it is the general practice to infuse dextrose (at least 100 grams per day) and vitamins; but the caloric requirements may also be partially fulfilled by intravenous fat emulsions. When glucose is administered, it must usually be given as a hyperosmotic solution because of the requirement for fluid restriction. Precautions are required to prevent venous thrombosis and infection of the venous catheter.

Particular attention may be necessary to prevent the development of progressive hyperkalemia. The administration of a potassium-binding resin either by mouth or by enema two to four times daily will generally serve to prevent serious elevations of plasma potassium concentrations.* If marked hyperkalemia is present when the patient is first seen, intravenous glucose and insulin, sodium bicarbonate, or calcium chloride all will protect temporarily against the cardiotoxic effects of potassium. But potassium exchange resins and/or dialysis, both of which remove potassium from the body, should be initiated promptly to prevent the recurrence of hyperkalemia. Metabolic acidosis can generally be corrected and controlled by dialysis. If dialysis is not available, or the acidosis progresses despite dialysis, the administration of $NaHCO_3$ in carefully regulated amounts is indicated to keep the plasma bicarbonate concentration above 15 mEq per liter. Hyponatremia can best be controlled by preventing progressive water retention and can best be corrected by dialysis. *Hyponatremia should not be treated by the administration of hypertonic saline.* Anemia will develop routinely in the course of acute tubular necrosis,

---

*The resin generally used in the United States is a sodium cycle resin (Kayexalate), and in a standard dose of 15 to 60 grams per day over 30 mEq of Na may be released into the gastrointestinal tract. To obviate sodium retention, part or all of the resin may be given as a calcium cycle resin if the latter is available.

and ordinarily no effort should be made to maintain the hematocrit in excess of 20 volumes per 100 ml. If blood transfusion does become necessary because of a progressive fall in hematocrit or cardiovascular complications, packed red blood cells using fresh blood should be employed. In treating hemorrhage, fresh whole blood may be preferable. Hyperphosphatemia may occasionally become very pronounced, and may be attended by the development of hypocalcemia. The latter ordinarily does not produce manifestations of tetany; but if ionized calcium concentrations become reduced inordinately, as may occur if the patient becomes alkalotic from the infusion of bicarbonate in excessive amount or from vomiting, tetany and even seizures may develop. Hyperphosphatemia is best controlled by protein restriction and/or frequent dialysis, but the administration of phosphate-binding gels, e.g., aluminum hydroxide gel, 30 to 60 ml every six hours by mouth may be of great value.

All drugs from antimicrobials to digitalis glycosides must be administered with full knowledge of their route of degradation and excretion. Drugs which are not detoxified, metabolized, or excreted by the kidney may be given in full dosage. But these are the exception rather than the rule. Most drugs, including many antimicrobials, will have to be given in reduced amounts and at prolonged intervals. It is tragic indeed to have a patient recover from acute tubular necrosis only to have a permanent vestibular or auditory defect owing to streptomycin or kanamycin toxicity. Digoxin is the most widely recommended digitalis glycoside, although some authorities prefer digitoxin. If digoxin is employed, a digitalizing dose of 1.5 to 2.0 mg and a maintenance dose of 0.125 mg daily will provide a therapeutic effect without toxicity in most adult patients with acute tubular necrosis.

If the renal failure is treated satisfactorily, the outcome will depend almost entirely upon the natural history of any underlying illness or injury. Thus the intensity of treatment of a surgical wound, an area of necrotic tissue, or a burn should not be diminished because of the existence of acute tubular necrosis; quite the contrary: any delay in appropriate treatment may compromise the patient's chances of survival. Removal of necrotic tissue is, if anything, more urgent in the patient with acute renal failure than in the patient with normal renal function; and surgical procedures, even major ones, are not contraindicated if they are considered to have lifesaving importance. Finally, although prophylactic antimicrobial drugs are contraindicated, infection must be treated promptly with the correct drugs but with prorated dosages. In the same context, careful attention must be given to avoiding the introduction of secondary infection. Thus after the first day of the disease, the use of a bladder catheter solely to monitor urine volumes is not justified, and intravenous catheters should be treated aseptically and never left in place for more than three days. Skin care, with special attention to the prevention of pressure sores, is an essential component of rational and effective therapy.

Differential Diagnosis. The fact that the patient with acute tubular necrosis characteristically excretes a relatively large percentage of filtered salt and water may be very helpful in differentiating the disease from the oliguric states associated with volume depletion, hypotension with a readily reversible decrease in effective filtration pressure, acute glomerulitis, and the hepatorenal syndrome.

As indicated previously, a normal person with normal salt and water intake will excrete less than 1 per cent of his filtered sodium and water. If extracellular fluid volume depletion occurs, the appropriate response is to *decrease* fractional salt and water excretion. If volume losses are profound, the glomerular filtration rate may fall markedly, in which case the patient will present not only with oliguria but with a rising level of BUN and creatinine. Thus he will fulfill the criteria for acute renal failure. But in contrast to the patient with acute tubular necrosis, the patient with volume depletion will typically excrete less than 5 per cent of his filtered water, and may excrete urine which is virtually free of sodium. A similar picture evolves early in the course of a severe glomerulitis and in the hepatorenal syndrome.

The urine/plasma (U/P) creatinine ratio is a readily available test for estimating the fraction of filtered water excreted. The accompanying table compares the U/P ratios with the fractional rate of water excretion. A U/P ratio of 10 indicates that approximately 10 per cent of the filtered water is excreted. A U/P ratio of 5 is equivalent to the excretion of 20 per cent of the filtered water, and a ratio of 2 signifies the excretion of 50 per cent of the filtered water. In acute tubular necrosis, creatinine U/P ratios typically range between 5 and 10, and rarely exceed 20. In extracellular fluid volume depletion, acute glomerulitides, and the hepatorenal syndrome, creatinine U/P ratios typically exceed 10, and often are well above 20. The urinary sodium concentration (U_{Na}) in acute tubular necrosis typically exceeds 20 mEq per liter, and in most patients ranges from 40 to 90 mEq per liter. In volume depletion, acute glomerulitis, and the hepatorenal syndrome, U_{Na} is usually less than 20 mEq per liter, and often is less than 10 mEq per liter. Calculation of the fraction of filtered sodium excreted may also be very helpful. This value is equal to the U/P ratio for sodium divided by the U/P ratio for creatinine and expressed as a percentage. In acute tubular necrosis, 5 per cent or more of the filtered sodium typically is excreted; in volume depletion, acute glomerulitis, and the hepatorenal syndrome, less than 5 per cent and often less than 2 per cent of the filtered sodium is excreted. In chronic end-stage renal disease, the values will depend upon the glomerular filtration rate and the salt intake; but at a GFR of 2 ml per minute and with an average salt and water intake (approximately 7 grams of salt and 1 liter of water per day), about 30 per cent of the filtered salt and water is excreted.

The creatinine U/P ratio, U_{Na}, and the U/P Na U/P creatinine ratio are thus of help in the differential diagnosis of acute renal failure. But there are substantial gray zones where the patterns overlap, and these biochemical values must in all instances be viewed in light of the historical and clinical findings. There are also

The Relationship Between Creatinine Urine/Plasma (U/P) Ratios and the Percentage of Filtered Water Excreted

Creatinine U/P ratio	Per Cent Filtered H₂O Excreted
100	1
50	2
20	5
10	10
5	20
2	50

sources of error in utilizing the biochemical values. One of these is that acute renal failure secondary to volume depletion may progress to acute tubular necrosis; and if the urine examined was produced prior to the advent of acute tubular necrosis, it will be low in sodium and have a high creatinine U/P ratio. Another source of error exists in a patient with true acute tubular necrosis in whom there is a profound stimulus to sodium retention. For example, in acute tubular necrosis associated with burns, the translocation of extracellular fluid into the affected areas results in a striking decrease in effective ECF volume. The patient thus may present with oliguria, a glomerular filtration rate below 1 ml per minute, a creatinine U/P ratio of less than 10, but virtually no sodium in the urine. A low U_{Na} has also been observed in acute tubular necrosis after cardiac surgery and mercury poisoning.

Error in using the creatinine U/P ratio and U_{Na} may also occur in patients with glomerulitis, after the occurrence of compensation but before the filtration rate rises appreciably. After enough salt and water have been retained to expand extracellular fluid volume appreciably, natriuretic forces may be mobilized and fractional reabsorption of sodium (and water) in the urine-forming nephrons may be markedly depressed. Thus creatinine U/P ratios may fall below the 10 to 20 range and U_{Na} may be high. When acute renal failure is superimposed on underlying chronic renal disease, e.g., from volume depletion or acute glomerulitis, the creatinine U/P ratio may remain low, and the U_{Na} high.

Other Aids in Differential Diagnosis. URINE VOLUME. Total anuria is very rare in acute tubular necrosis unless it is due to the ingestion of bichloride of mercury. Total anuria is seen in severe acute glomerulitis, bilateral cortical necrosis, and urinary tract obstruction. If there is a history of an abrupt change in urine volume from very low to high levels in a short period of time, or if there are alternating periods of oliguria and polyuria, obstruction is strongly suggested.

URINARY SEDIMENT. Red blood cell casts are unusual in acute tubular necrosis (but they occur) and are the rule in glomerulitides (but they may be absent). Qualitative measurements of protein in urine in the disease rarely exceed 1 to 2+ in acute tubular necrosis, whereas they often are 3 to 4+ in glomerulitides.

URINE OSMOLALITY. The osmolality of the urine is the same as that of the plasma in patients with tubular necrosis. In patients with severe volume depletion, glomerulitides, and the hepatorenal syndrome, the urine may occasionally be hyperosmotic to the plasma. *Consequently isosmotic urine is not of value in differential diagnosis, although hyperosmotic urine favors volume depletion, acute glomerulitis, and the hepatorenal syndrome, and virtually excludes acute tubular necrosis.*

RESPONSE TO MANNITOL, FUROSEMIDE, OR VOLUME EXPANSION. A limited increase in urine volume may occur in the disease after mannitol infusion, furosemide administration, or volume expansion. However, unless the increase is progressive and is attended by a substantial rise in glomerular filtration rate, repeated administration of either mannitol or furosemide or continuous infusion of a synthetic extracellular fluid solution is contraindicated in patients with acute renal failure of unknown variety. The differential diagnostic implications of a small increase in urine volume and sodium excretion after the administration of potent diuretics such as furosemide are not yet clear; but large incre-

ments in urine volume point away from the diagnosis of acute tubular necrosis.

Prognosis. In uncomplicated cases of acute tubular necrosis, in which there is no serious underlying disease and treatment is optimal, survival rates in excess of 70 to 80 per cent are common. On the other hand, when there is a serious underlying disease or injury, the death rate exceeds 50 per cent, and in severely traumatized patients may exceed 70 per cent. Judging from the experience in the Vietnam war, as contrasted with the Korean war, the speedy evacuation of wounded and rapid treatment of blood loss and shock will substantially reduce the incidence of acute tubular necrosis; but unfortunately once it does develop, the mortality rate among wounded patients requiring hemodialysis remains at about 70 per cent.

Prevention. The likelihood of occurrence of acute tubular necrosis after a given insult is influenced by the composite physiologic adversities. Thus the better the supportive therapy, the lower should be the incidence of the disease. The war experience just cited supports this view.

The role of mannitol in preventing acute tubular necrosis is uncertain. Some observers have favored the view that administration of mannitol to an oliguric patient will confer a substantial degree of protection by eliminating the contribution of luminal obstruction to the disease. However, at the very least, obstruction is not a universal factor in its pathogenesis; moreover, it can be induced in the laboratory animal with myoglobinuria despite the presence of high rates of urine flow per nephron. Mannitol may also increase renal blood flow, and conceivably some protective effect could derive from this. But it seems most reasonable to confine the use of mannitol chiefly to patients in whom there is an increase in the creatinine U/P ratio and a decrease in urinary sodium concentration, but no evidence of hypervolemia. The mannitol should be administered only for a limited period of time and in an amount not to exceed 25 to 50 grams; if no substantial rise in glomerular filtration rate and/or urine flow occurs, its use should not be continued. The role of furosemide in preventing the development of acute tubular necrosis also has not been established, and repeated administration of high doses of this drug is contraindicated.

In patients with extracellular fluid volume depletion and oliguria, volume repletion should be effected as expeditiously as possible. When hypotension exists, this also should be corrected as rapidly as possible. The use of sodium bicarbonate intravenously in patients with intravascular hemolysis is of dubious value.

The early recognition of urinary tract obstruction is of importance not only for the prompt reversal of acute renal failure, but also for the prevention of progressive nephron destruction. When obstruction is suspected in a patient with acute renal failure, either bladder catheterization or unilateral ureteral catheterization should be performed without delay.

Flamenbaum, W.: Pathophysiology of acute renal failure. Arch. Intern. Med., 131:911, 1973.

Franklyn, S. S., and Maxwell, M. H.: Acute renal failure. *In* Maxwell, M. H., and Kleeman, C. R. (eds.): Clinical Disorders of Fluid and Electrolyte Metabolism. New York, McGraw-Hill Book Company, 1972.

Merrill, J. P.: Acute renal failure. *In* Strauss, M. B., and Welt, L. G. (eds.): Diseases of the Kidney. Boston, Little, Brown and Company, 1971.

Muehrcke, R. C.: Acute Renal Failure: Diagnosis and Management. St. Louis, C. V. Mosby Company, 1969.

TREATMENT OF IRREVERSIBLE RENAL FAILURE BY TRANSPLANTATION AND DIALYSIS*

605. INTRODUCTION

Priscilla Kincaid-Smith

Renal transplantation and intermittent dialysis have become established as successful methods of treatment for irreversible renal failure over the last 10 to 15 years. There are few medical reasons for a definitive choice between dialysis and transplantation, and both offer reasonable success rates and good rehabilitation. From the patient's point of view a successful transplant offers a more independent life and avoids anemia, which is the major disadvantage of maintenance dialysis. Furthermore cadaveric transplantation is the only practical approach for a country wishing to accept and treat all medically suitable patients with irreversible renal failure and to avoid the allocation of very considerable financial and medical resources to treatment by dialysis.

An integrated program for patients with irreversible renal failure, utilizing both dialysis and transplantation, has evolved in the last few years. Such an approach is based on an initial choice made by patient and physician together. The medical commitment is to maintain the highest quality of life possible for each patient. Successful transplantation will usually remain the ultimate goal, but dialysis is carried out preferably in such a way that it can continue indefinitely if the need arises. Transplantation is carried out on optimally fit patients and is not regarded as a treatment for "failed" dialysis. Grafts are removed early if function is poor or deteriorating, and immunosuppression is not used to excess. Failed transplants are returned to dialysis to await another transplant should it be indicated. This integrated approach allows maximal use of available cadaver kidneys and in addition achieves an improved patient survival rate. This approach in the last three years at the Royal Melbourne Hospital has resulted in a two-year patient survival of 80 per cent, four fifths of whom have a functioning cadaveric renal transplant.

Progress in clinical transplantation has proved disappointingly slow. Tissue typing assists the selection of living related donors but does not help in the majority of cadaveric donors. Organ preservation is now widely used and allows elective surgery and better preparation and selection of recipients. There has been a worldwide increase in patient survival, particularly in cadaveric transplantation (Table 1). Isolated units and some national programs, for example, that in Australia, report significantly better results than the worldwide experience.

THE PROBLEM OF IRREVERSIBLE RENAL FAILURE IN THE COMMUNITY

The provision of services to the community has recently been reviewed by Kerr. No country has yet reached an equilibrium in providing services for patients with irreversible renal failure in which the number of patients presenting for treatment equals those dying after treatment with dialysis or transplantation. It is notable that in Denmark and Australia, where cadaveric transplantation has been the major goal, twice the number of patients have been accepted for treatment and are alive as in countries where the major effort has gone toward dialysis (Table 2).

The most significant factor in determining the need for facilities is the number of patients presenting for treatment. This number is age dependent, because renal failure is common above the age of 55. The other significant variable is "medical suitability." The criteria for medical acceptance have widened with experience, and there are now few absolute contraindications for either dialysis or transplantation. Estimates of the number of patients requiring treatment have varied from 25 to 75 per million per year, depending on the upper age limit. The figures of 35 per million of the population per year with an upper age limit of 55 and 50 per million per year for patients up to 65 years of age are probably accurate for most communities.

Utilizing published survival data for dialysis and transplantation and making reasonable assumptions in keeping with an integrated program, Kerr has calculated that approximate equilibrium could be achieved after 12 years (Table 3). These figures provide a valuable guide to physicians and administrators in planning the community requirements.

Transplantation costs approximately equal those of home dialysis in the first year but thereafter have been estimated to be a quarter of those of maintenance dialysis at home. Countries with transplantation as the major goal may therefore expect to save about US$500,000 per year per million of population (based on Australian cost estimates applied to Table 3), compared with countries where the major goal is home dialysis.

A program based on cadaveric transplantation is dependent on an adequate supply of donor kidneys and a

---

*The assistance of Dr. T. H. Mathew in preparation of this article is gratefully acknowledged.

TABLE 1. Patient and Graft Survival, 1968 and 1971—Primary Cadaveric Transplants (10th Report of Human Renal Transplant Registry)

	One Year			
	% Living		% Functioning	
1968	58	(58)	46	(39)
1971	68	(88)	46	(69)

Royal Melbourne Hospital data are shown in parentheses.

TABLE 2. Dialysis and Transplant Survivors per Million Population on December 31, 1971*

Country	Population (Millions)	Rate Per Million		
		On Dialysis	With Graft	Total
Denmark	4.9	29	41	70
Australia	12.9	20	38	58
France	50.8	31	6	37
Britain	55.7	21	9	30

*Data from EDTA, 1971 and Australian National Hemodialysis and Transplant Survey.

TABLE 3. Approximate Equilibrium Population of Dialysis and Transplant Patients Expected from Current Survival Rates at Two Different Rates of Admission*

Treatment	Admission Rate 25 Million/Year		Admission Rate 50 Million/Year	
	Annual Cohort	Equilibrium Population	Annual Cohort	Equilibrium Population
Live donor graft	2.5	18	5	35
Home dialysis	18	32	22.5	40
Hospital dialysis	4.5	8	22.5	37
Cadaver graft	20	97	39	189
		155 million†		301 million†

*From Kerr, D. N. S.: Kidney Int., 3:197, 1973; with permission.
†The calculations are based on many simplifying assumptions and should be used only as a rough guide.

reasonable success rate. The Australian experience has proved encouraging in both these areas, with a donor procurement rate of 9 (18 kidneys) per million per year and a two-year graft survival of 62 per cent with primary cadaveric transplants (compared to the Human Renal Transplant Registry report of 46 per cent). Factors contributing to the high donor procurement and graft success rate are discussed below.

PREVENTION OF IRREVERSIBLE RENAL FAILURE

A program which aims to treat irreversible renal failure in the community must include adequate provision for prevention. Irreversible renal failure can be prevented by the application of available methods of treatment to renal disease and improvement of present methods of treatment through research. All major renal units should include facilities for research and for adequate diagnosis and treatment of renal disease and renal failure at all stages. Even by applying present methods of prevention and treatment, the numbers requiring dialysis and transplantation may decrease substantially. Detection and treatment of asymptomatic bacteriuria and hypertension are very likely to reduce the numbers presenting with chronic renal failure. Glomerulonephritis is the most common cause of irreversible renal failure; although treatment of this condition has usually proved ineffective, promising results with newer forms of treatment, including immunosuppression and anticoagulants, have been reported. Analgesic nephropathy, a totally preventable disease, is at present contributing 18 per cent of all patients presenting for dialysis and transplantation in Australia. This disease, which results from prolonged high doses of proprietary "over-the-counter" analgesic drugs, would disappear completely if abuse could be stopped by public education or if such preparations were available only on prescription.

606. RENAL TRANSPLANTATION
Priscilla Kincaid-Smith

The value of renal transplantation in identical twins was established 20 years ago; however, despite the sur-

prising success of some of Hume's cadaver transplants in 1955, many years passed before transplantation became accepted as an effective means of treatment in chronic renal failure. Early deaths were mainly due to immunosuppressive methods, including total body irradiation; clinical success dates from the introduction of azathioprine in 1962. This drug remains the major immunosuppressive agent used in renal transplantation.

SELECTION AND PREPARATION OF PATIENTS

The selection of patients with irreversible renal failure who are suitable for renal transplantation poses few problems if adequate dialysis facilities exist and the invidious situation of competition for places is thus avoided.

Relative contraindications include old age, metastatic carcinoma, psychosis, active infection (e.g., tuberculosis), and severe cerebral, myocardial, or peripheral vascular disease. Patients with diabetes, inactive tuberculosis, coronary artery disease, multisystemic disease such as systemic lupus erythematosus, chronic obstructive lung disease, and peptic ulceration have all had successful transplants.

Age alone is not a contraindication to transplantation, because transplants have been performed in neonates and in those over the age of 80. Patient survival decreases in both low and high age groups. More important than chronologic age is the quality of life which can be achieved by the patient under consideration after a successful graft.

Transplantation in the very young poses problems relating to size of vessels, lack of growth, and difficulties in social adjustment. Dialysis in this age group introduces further problems such as fluid and diet restriction and long hours of dialysis, and does not avoid the problems of growth and social adjustment. Children over age eight who weigh 20 kg or more pose fewer problems; with reduction in dose and the use of alternate-day steroid regimens, growth, sometimes with impressive spurts, has been reported.

In Fabry's disease and cystinosis, transplantation may allow correction or alleviation of specific enzyme defects; however, the success of transplantation in these conditions may be due to improved renal function alone. In the congenital nephrotic syndrome transplantation appears to be "curative," whereas in hyperoxaluria the defect persists and has led to early graft loss.

There is no medical state (except for steroid-related psychosis) for which dialysis is definitely indicated and transplantation not. Advanced vascular disease has been suggested as a contraindication to transplantation, but it is the most common cause of death on dialysis and makes blood vessel access difficult. Reported experience with hyperoxaluria patients on dialysis is poor, and survival in diabetes is worse than with transplantation.

Immunologic sensitization to transplantation antigens may make the selection of a suitable kidney more difficult; but if an appropriate donor can be found, transplantation is not contraindicated.

The patient must be optimally fit at the time of transplantation in order to have every chance of surviving the stresses and complications of surgery, high steroids, and immunosuppression. Hypertension must be effectively controlled, the heart size returned toward normal, calcium and phosphate abnormalities rectified, anemia improved as far as possible, and infection eradicated. Preparatory surgery such as bilateral nephrectomy, ileal bladder construction, and peptic ulcer surgery may be necessary. Careful attention to patient preparation may be a major factor in the increased graft and patient survival rate achieved in Australia.

Bilateral nephrectomy carries a predictable morbidity and mortality and is only indicated when the patient's own kidneys may contribute to subsequent graft failure or death. Atrophic pyelonephritis and persistent active infection, as in some polycystic kidneys and in association with calculi, require bilateral nephrectomy. Patients with anti-GBM antibody mediated glomerulonephritis have been transplanted successfully with kidneys in situ. The case for leaving kidneys intact is compelling in an integrated program which may involve long periods on dialysis. This will significantly minimize anemia and fluid restriction and may permit clearance of "middle molecules" which may be of value.

DONOR PROCUREMENT

An adequate supply of cadaveric donors can be achieved only with cooperation and understanding between the public and physicians. To achieve HL-A phenotype identical and ABO compatible cadaver donors for a pool size of 500 recipients and an average waiting time of six months, Kountz has estimated the necessity for 50 donors per month. This recruitment rate is not an unrealistic target even for large geographic areas, because Australia has consistently recruited one donor per month per 1.5 million of population over the last four years.

Any patients under the age of 65 to 70 years who have basically normal renal function and have no evidence of malignancy (excluding cerebral tumor) are potential donors. Systemic or urinary infection, severe hypertension, and renal disease are not acceptable in the donor. Urine flow must exceed 30 ml per hour up to one hour before death. Despite these liberal criteria, the vast majority of donors have in practice come from patients with head injuries or spontaneous intracerebral vascular catastrophes.

ORGAN PRESERVATION

Although kidneys can be successfully stored by simple flushing with a hyperosmolar solution followed by immersion in saline slush for up to 10 to 12 hours, pulsatile perfusion with oxygenated plasma at 10° C for 24 hours is associated with little deterioration in graft function. The advantages of perfusion are the performance of elective surgery at a time convenient to the patient and to the medical and surgical staff, as well as more detailed cross-matching and tissue typing and better preparation of the patient.

CADAVER VERSUS LIVE DONOR

There is a clear improvement in graft survival rate using living related donors with only one haplotype difference or no difference between donor and recipient. Experience with "HL-A identical" siblings has been very good. If both haplotypes are nonidentical, results are no better than those of cadaveric transplantation, and most units no longer transplant in this situation.

The data in "HL-A identical" siblings are so impressive that the results should be actively pointed out to families for their consideration.

The over-all trend is toward cadaveric transplantation.

HISTOCOMPATIBILITY TESTING

There is now general agreement that a single autosomal gene complex constitutes the major histocompatibility system (HL-A) in man. This system includes at least two closely linked loci (first locus or LA and second locus or Four) whose alleles determine serologically defined antigens. The system also includes other loci which have been detected so far only by in vitro lymphocyte response studies in mixed lymphocyte culture tests. Each individual has four serologically defined antigens, two of which (one LA and one Four locus antigen) are inherited en bloc from each parent. The chromosomal segment carrying these closely linked loci is called a haplotype. Each child receives one haplotype from each parent, and both antigens associated with each parental haplotype are detectable in the child.

Skin and renal grafts in man have verified the importance of the HL-A system in determining histocompatibility, and, as discussed above, HL-A matching allows definite prognostic implications for the living related donor-recipient pair. For the cadaveric situation, however, the multiplicity of antigens (15 of which have now been identified on the first locus and 25 on the second) has meant that in practice it is rare to achieve four antigen (or full house) identity between donor and recipient. With the most frequent phenotypes the chance of finding an HL-A identical donor is approximately 1 in 100, and with the less frequent phenotypes it may be as little as 1 in 100,000. Initial hopes that partial identity, or sharing of one, two, or three antigens by donor and recipient, might also lead to a more favorable graft outcome have not been realized. Most reports suggest that there is a significant difference between four antigen identity and the remainder, but do not show a grade of success relating to antigen identity. In practical terms this has led to the recommendation that tissue typing should not be used as the basis for cadaver kidney distribution except in the case of four antigen identity. This has led to the establishment of large kidney donor sharing programs in order to increase the likelihood of perfect matching; however, the rarity of these matches means that they can make little impact on the over-all results of cadaver transplantation.

The further contribution of HL-A typing to cadaveric transplantation has been its use as a means to detect sensitization to HL-A antigen. Such sensitization may arise through previous blood transfusion, pregnancy, or prior transplantation. The demonstration of donor-specific cytotoxic antibodies in the recipient, referred to as a positive direct cross-match, is generally regarded as a contraindication to transplantation and is associated with a 95 per cent failure rate caused by hyperacute rejection. Poorer results in patients demonstrating non-donor-specific HL-A antibodies (with a negative direct lymphocytotoxicity cross-match) have led to the suggestion that this group of antibody formers may be an immunologically active or "responder" group. The ability of such patients to produce antibodies to blood transfusion may reflect a broader ability to mount a strong immune attack on a future transplant. In this sensitized group, HL-A matching has been shown by some workers to correlate better with graft outcome. Future work may lead to the identification of a responder group in whom only full antigen identity with cadaveric transplantation or identical sibling transplantation should be performed, and of a nonresponder group in whom HL-A typing of donors is unimportant.

PATHOLOGIC FEATURES OF REJECTION

Although intense cellular infiltration is a prominent feature in the unmodified rejection reaction seen in animals, this is not a prominent feature in patients in whom rejection is modified by treatment with steroids and azathioprine. The major lesions seen in renal allografts in man are in the vessels and they involve all blood vessels from the main artery and vein to the glomerular capillaries and intertubular sinusoids.

Polymorphonuclear leukocytes may accumulate within the blood vessels of the allograft within minutes, and so-called "hyperacute" rejection, with very florid thrombotic vascular lesions, may develop within hours or days of grafting. Such patients probably have preformed humoral antibody in their serum which conventional screening methods failed to detect. The vascular lesions of hyperacute rejection are similar to those occurring in acute and chronic rejection. The differences between the three are differences of degree and rate of progress, but the essential pathogenesis of lesions seen in vessels in serial percutaneous biopsies is similar. Platelet and fibrin thrombi may be demonstrated within vessels of all sizes in the acute stages, and the glomerular and vascular lesions seen months or years after transplantation represent the residual lesions that follow these thrombotic lesions. This process of "organization" may result in lesions which resemble atheroma and cause stenosis of the main renal artery. Intimal proliferation causes narrowing of interlobar, arcuate, and interlobular arteries and of arterioles. Glomerular capillaries show changes which closely mimic those of mesangiocapillary glomerulonephritis and make the distinction between late rejection and glomerulonephritis difficult.

Rejection poses the most danger during the first three months; subsequently severe acute rejection is rare, but episodes of rejection may occur as long as several years after transplantation. In a controlled trial, anticoagulation and antithrombotic drugs appear to affect the histologic lesions but have not shown any effect on graft function during the first three years.

NATURAL HISTORY OF PATIENTS WITH RENAL ALLOGRAFTS

Early Course

Although urine flow usually commences promptly with well-prepared live donor kidneys, a period of oliguria is common in cadaveric transplantation. Prompt urine flow will occur if warm ischemic times are kept to less than one hour and cold ischemic time to a minimum. Early good renal function avoids dialysis and facilitates the early diagnosis of rejection, but initial oliguria does not alter the long-term outcome.

In the absence of complications, the patient may be ambulant on the second day and discharged from hospital between the fifth and tenth postoperative days. Daily outpatient attendance for review of renal function and detection of rejection and complications is essential during the first three to four weeks. Visits are gradually reduced in frequency to once a week at three months and once a month at a year and thereafter. Close and intense supervision in the first weeks and months is probably the major factor responsible for higher success rates in some programs.

Return to full activities is achieved in over 90 per cent of patients at about two months, and this coincides with the spontaneous restoration of a normal hemoglobin.

Rejection crises occur in the majority of cadaver transplants and may even occur with identical sibling live donor kidneys. Although a number of techniques such as urinary FDP's, I^{131} fibrinogen uptake, urinary enzyme levels, urine cell counts, hyperchloremia, induced lymphocyte transformation, urinary electrolyte patterns, and scanning techniques have all been suggested to give advance warning of rejection, alteration of renal function as judged by an elevation of the serum creatinine remains the mainstay of diagnosis. The urinary sodium is the only additional test that is reliable, easy to perform, and may precede the rise in creatinine by one to two days. Fever, leukocytosis, local pain, and systemic symptoms are late features and correlate much better with a local complication such as a perirenal hematoma or a urinary leak.

The majority of rejection crises can be reversed by increased steroid dosage, and heparin may be of benefit.

It is important that immunosuppression and steroids should not be pushed to excess with consequent severe morbidity and mortality from infection and marrow depression. Azathioprine should be reduced in dosage when renal function is abnormal rather than increased. Consistent elevation of the serum creatinine above a level of 6 mg per 100 ml after the first four weeks results in high morbidity and mortality and is an indication for graft removal.

The best guide to graft prognosis is percutaneous renal biopsy, which is simple and safe owing to the fixed and superficial position of the kidney. The histologic appearance assists in the diagnosis of the cause of acute functional deterioration and may lead to the diagnosis of renal artery stenosis or obstruction if the histologic features of rejection are not sufficient to account for the deterioration in function.

Early Complications

Persistent Nonfunction of Renal Allograft

If the serum creatinine is not falling a month after transplantation, severe rejection, major vessel thrombosis, or nonviability is likely and the graft should be removed, but obstruction to urine flow must always be excluded, and a biopsy is helpful before the graft is removed.

Urinary Leakage

The incidence of urinary leaks leading to fistula formation or obstruction from a urine collection is only about 5 per cent if careful attention is paid to preserving ureteral blood supply and to surgical technique. Early surgical intervention in established urinary fistula reduces the morbidity from infection, although a fistula will usually close spontaneously in four to six weeks.

Lymphocele

Interruption of lymph channels during graft insertion may lead to lymph collections around the kidney or to fistula formation. Meticulous attention must be paid to ligation of all visible lymph channels at the time of initial operation. Marsupialization of the lymphocele into the peritoneal cavity may be necessary if leakage persists and collections recur.

Urinary Infection

Seventy-five per cent of all patients will have a urinary infection in the first three postoperative months, and in a few it will be recurrent. The patient who refluxes up the transplanted ureter often shows deterioration of function accompanying reflux and is at high risk from septicemia; but in the absence of reflux, infections are easily eradicated by conventional antimicrobial treatment. Preliminary data suggest that reflux in the absence of infection may cause scarring in the transplanted kidney.

Hypertension

Hypertension may be difficult to control during severe acute rejection, and intravenous diazoxide administration may be necessary. The majority of successful cadaveric transplants are hypertensive, but control of the blood pressure is easily achieved. An increase in dose requirements or the development of severe hypertension is an indication for renal arteriography to exclude renal artery stenosis. Tight renal artery stenosis occurring just distal to the anastomosis is common, and correction may cure hypertension and improve renal function.

Other Infections

The patient receiving immunosuppressive agents is particularly liable to develop infections, most especially those fungal and viral infections for which man requires an intact "T" cell lymphocyte population to ensure an adequate resistance. Cytomegalic virus, herpes simplex and zoster, *Pneumocystis carinii*, Listeria, Nocardia, actinomycoses, and other unusual infections may be fatal. Most infections can be treated; early diagnosis, a high index of clinical suspicion, and sophisticated microbiologic facilities are essential for optimal results.

Bacteria are more likely to cause serious infection, and death from an overwhelming septicemia can occur within hours.

Respiratory Distress Syndrome

A syndrome of progressive dyspnea, cyanosis, with or without fine crepitations at the lung bases, an alveolar capillary block, and diffuse mottling and opacity on chest x-ray has been described. Progressive hypoxia with death in one to three weeks from presentation is the rule. The suggestion that this "transplant lung" syndrome is immunologic in origin seems unlikely because path-

ogenic organisms such as *Pneumocystis carinii* and cytomegalic virus are almost always found, and an identical syndrome is seen in immunosuppressed patients without a renal transplant.

Aseptic Necrosis of Bone

This disabling complication usually affects the hip joint and may be bilateral. Its incidence correlates with prolonged or high doses of steroids, rapid reduction of steroid dose, and secondary hyperparathyroidism.

Other Steroid Complications

Any of the well-recognized complications of steroid therapy such as peptic ulceration, diabetes, and cataract formation may develop after transplantation.

Late Course

The long-term prognosis for patients completing one year with normal or near normal renal function is excellent; however, there is a continuing slow rate of loss of grafted kidneys and mortality (see accompanying figure). Slow deterioration of renal function may be due to the chronic rejection, recurrence of glomerulonephritis, or other disease. Vesicoureteral reflux may contribute progressive "atrophic pyelonephritic" lesions in the absence of infection. In some patients the kidney is both histologically and functionally normal five or more years after a cadaver graft.

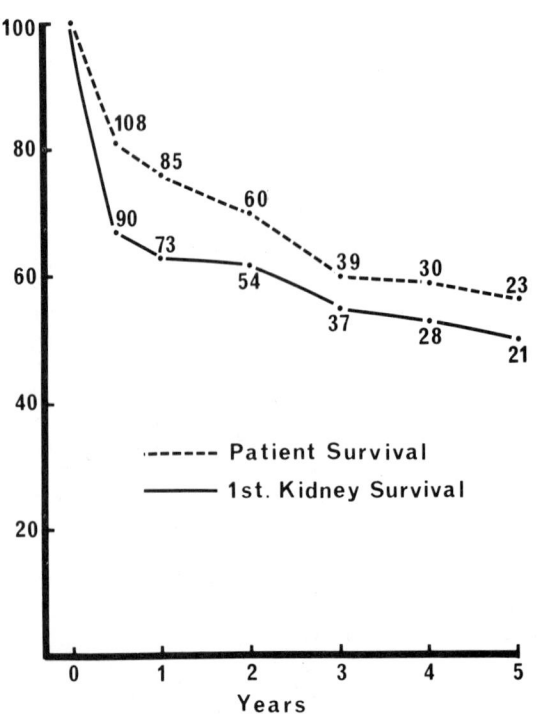

Cumulative survival of patients who received cadaveric renal allografts at the Royal Melbourne Hospital between April 1965 and April 1970. There are no exclusions. Beyond five years, numbers in the groups are small. Few grafts failed between one year and five years after transplantation, even though this figure includes early experience when results were not as good as they are at present.

Chronic Rejection

Progressive ischemia of the kidney caused by the vascular lesions affecting small and large vessels, along with glomerular capillary change identical to that seen in mesangiocapillary glomerulonephritis, characterizes chronic rejection. Deterioration of renal function is slow and occurs over several years. European experience suggests that there is a correlation between chronic rejection and the number of pretransplant blood transfusions.

Recurrent Glomerulonephritis

A true recurrence of an identifiable type of glomerulonephritis is unusual but has been described in focal and segmental hyalinosis, antiglomerular basement membrane antibody-mediated glomerulonephritis, IgA-IgG glomerulonephritis, "dense deposit" disease, and hypocomplementemic mesangiocapillary glomerulonephritis, including lobular glomerulonephritis. Unless a histologic marker is present, it may be very difficult to separate changes caused by rejection from those of glomerulonephritis, particularly as the change is usually of the mesangiocapillary type. Minor degrees of mesangiocapillary change always accompany rejection lesions identical with those of mesangiocapillary "recurrent" glomerulonephritis and may occur in a patient who had chronic pyelonephritis or some other "nonglomerular" cause of end-stage renal failure. Transplantation is not contraindicated in any form of glomerulonephritis, because the incidence of significant "recurrence" is low in the first five years and deterioration in the function of the affected transplant is often slow. Sometimes the same morphologic lesion which recurs progresses much more slowly in the transplanted kidney than it did when it caused renal failure prior to transplantation.

Malignancy in the Transplant Recipient

There is little doubt the the incidence of malignancy is increased significantly in transplanted patients, presumably as a result of immunosuppression. There is a 5 to 6 per cent chance of a cancer's developing within a few years of transplantation. Of reported cases 61 per cent have been epithelial in origin and 39 per cent mesenchymal. Skin, lip, and cervix have been the sites of the most common epithelial tumors, and reticulum cell sarcoma, often of the central nervous system, is the most common mesenchymal tumor. It appears that the risk of cancer is increased by 20 to 40 times. This complication may prove to be a major limiting factor in transplantation.

Treatment

Treatment regimens vary considerably from center to center. Azathioprine and steroids remain the major agents used for immunosuppression, although steroids may be avoided in "identical" sibling grafts, and cyclophosphamide is a reasonable alternative to azathioprine.

Antilymphocyte Sera

Despite the experimental evidence of the effectiveness of antilymphocyte serum, doubt still remains regarding its benefit to graft survival in man. Controlled trials are few; none have shown a statistically significant improvement in survival, and most have failed to demonstrate any difference. The problems of hypersensitivity and thrombocytopenia have been overcome by the use of goat antisera, but concern has been expressed about an increased incidence of exotic infections as a delayed complication. The role of antilymphocyte serum in clinical transplantation awaits clarification by further controlled trials, but it seems unlikely to prove a major advance in transplantation.

Fate of Secondary Transplants

The results of multiple transplantation, particularly with repeated cadaveric donors, have been disappointing. The American College of Surgeons' Renal Transplant Registry (1972) shows a 26 per cent two-year survival. However, isolated units are achieving much better success rates, to as high as 75 per cent graft survival at one year. The major factor is presumably sensitization from the first graft; with careful selection of the second kidney, retransplantation remains justifiable. The avoidance of disparate antigens which were present on the first kidney, particularly HL-A2, careful crossmatching using donor spleen or lymph node cells which increase the sensitivity of the test, and an insistence on three or more shared antigens may increase second graft survival. In an integrated program in which home dialysis is available, the time needed to achieve these requirements in a second donor is not a problem. Splenectomy has now been shown in a large series to be ineffective in prolonging the function of a second transplant.

A. L. G. Therapy and Standardization Workshop. Behring Institute Mitteilungen No. 51, September 1972.

Australian National Renal Transplantation Survey: Second report by a Subcommittee. Med. J. Aust., 2:605, 1971.

Brunner, F. P., Gurland, H. G., Harlem, H., et al.: Combined report on regular dialysis and transplantation in Europe II, 1971. Proc. E.D.T.A., 9:3, 1972.

Kerr, D. N. S.: Provision of services to patients with chronic uremia. Kidney Int., 3:197, 1973.

Kincaid-Smith, P.: The pathogenesis of the vascular and glomerular lesions of renal allografts and their modification by antithrombotic and anticoagulant drugs. Alsian Ann. Med., 19:201, 1970.

Kountz, S. L.: Clinical transplantation—an overview. Transplant. Proc., 5:59, 1973.

Penn, I., and Starzl, T. E.: Immunosuppression and cancer. Transplant. Proc., 5:943, 1973.

Stewart, J. H., Topp, N. D., Martin, S., et al.: The costs of domiciliary maintenance dialysis. Med. J. Aust., 1:156, 1973.

Tenth report of the Human Renal Transplant Registry. J.A.M.A., 221:1495, 1972.

607. DIALYSIS

Constantine L. Hampers

The process of dialysis is based on simple physical concepts. Essentially, it involves the separation of two fluid compartments by a semipermeable membrane which can be viewed as having finite holes. Materials of low molecular weight can cross from one side of the membrane to the other toward decreasing concentration gradients. Larger particles, such as protein molecules and red blood cells, cannot traverse the membrane. In the case of peritoneal dialysis, the "membrane" is the peritoneum which is separating the dialysate fluid (in the peritoneal cavity) from the interstitial fluid surrounding the peritoneal membrane. With hemodialysis, the "membrane" is a synthetic material such as cellophane or cuprophan which separates blood from the dialysis bath.

PERITONEAL DIALYSIS

Peritoneal dialysis is a well-established technique in most general hospitals. Its use, however, is primarily reserved for the treatment of reversible renal failure, and it has not been widely instituted on a repetitive basis for management of the patient with chronic renal failure. However, the development of permanent peritoneal catheters which do not require repeated punctures of the abdomen with each treatment and the ability to produce dialyzing fluid economically have rekindled some interest in long-term maintenance of patients by this means.

The procedure requires insertion of a catheter into the peritoneal cavity, usually in the midline. Where permanent catheters are used, an attempt is made to separate the entrance into the peritoneal cavity by some distance (subcutaneously) from the exit site from the skin. The location of the insertion of the catheter need not necessarily be midline, and under special circumstances it can be placed in almost any area of the abdominal wall. Strict asepsis when inserting the catheter and throughout the entire procedure is of the greatest importance, because peritonitis is the most common complication of peritoneal dialysis. There appears to be an indirect relationship between infection and the fastidiousness of technique utilized in manipulating the catheter.

A "routine" peritoneal dialysis will last between 12 and 48 hours, depending upon the individual needs. One or 2 liters of peritoneal dialyzing fluid (commercially available and containing electrolytes in their proper concentrations) is allowed to run into the peritoneal cavity as rapidly as possible, usually five to ten minutes. The dialysate remains in the abdomen for 15 to 60 minutes ("dwell time") in order for the transfer of solutes to take place. The fluid is then drained out by gravity flow, and the cycle is repeated. This procedure is continued until the desired effect is accomplished. The reason for the variation in dwell time depends upon what one needs to accomplish. The most efficient length of time for the removal of solutes, such as urea or creatinine, is 30 to 60 minutes, and this is the period generally utilized. Automatic cycling machines are available which can be set to adjust the dwell time and reinstill fresh dialysate as required. When peritoneal dialysis is performed for the alleviation of gross overhydration, the dwell time may be considerably shortened, because the transfer of water across the peritoneum is rapid and is accomplished within a few minutes of the instillation of a hyperosmolar (4.5 per cent) glucose solution into the peritoneal cavity.

Some patients have been taught to perform peritoneal dialysis at home. They usually undergo dialysis for 12 to 18 hours twice a week. When maximally automated, this can be done overnight while the patient is asleep. Although some centers have utilized this method repeatedly in the same patient for a period of years, in most hands it has been unsatisfactory. The various prosthetic devices for access to the peritoneum are limited by propensity to infection.

HEMODIALYSIS

Hemodialysis was applied to animals by Abel, Rountree, and Turner, in 1913, with the use of a collodion dialyzing membrane. Its application in clinical medicine, however, was not attempted until the mid-1940's when Willem Kolff, working in Europe, applied the procedure to man. Despite the fact that hemodialysis was successfully utilized for the treatment of acute renal failure for a number of years, it was not applied repetitively for patients with chronic renal failure until the late 1950's. The major breakthrough in its use for the patient with end-stage kidney disease was the development of a prosthetic arteriovenous bypass which could be used for repeated access to the circulation. Prior to this, each dialysis required a fresh arterial and venous cutdown.

The type of access to the circulation has been modified somewhat, and presently there are two methods. Arteriovenous shunts are generally constructed of Teflon connected subcutaneously to a Silastic tube. The Silastic tube exits from the skin and remains extracorporeal. It can be disengaged for attachment to the machine. A second type of access (which is the most popular today) is the arteriovenous fistula. The fistula is made by surgically creating a window between a peripheral artery and vein, usually in the forearm; this results in the arterialization of the peripheral veins. After a few days to a few weeks, the veins become prominent and can be easily identified for venipuncture. Two large needles (15 gauge) are inserted into the arterialized veins with each dialysis. The arteriovenous fistula has the advantage of requiring little foreign material and thereby reduces the risk of infection. In addition, because no prosthetic material of any kind is present between dialyses, it allows the patient more freedom with the use of the extremity and eliminates the possibility of accidental dislodging of the access, as may occur with the shunt.

Arterial venous shunts or fistulas are usually placed in the upper extemity but can, under special circumstances, also be placed in the leg. The life of the access tube is variable, depending on individual patient factors, but some patients have kept the original access for a number of years.

TYPES OF ARTIFICIAL KIDNEYS

A hemodialysis system is composed of two basic units. The first is the exchanger and is that portion of the system in which mass transfer occurs. The basic components are a blood compartment, a dialysate compartment, and an intervening semipermeable membrane. The second portion of the system is a device which functions to deliver fresh dialysate of suitable composition to the exchanger. Exchangers in common clinical use today fall into three basic types: coil, parallel plate, and hollow fiber.

A *coil dialyzer* is constructed from one or more membrane tubes which are concentrically wound with an intervening membrane support. Blood passes through the tubes and the dialysate is pumped through the supporting structure over the outside of the blood conduits. The high velocity of dialysate flow and the turbulence created by the supporting structure are sufficient to reduce the dialysate side fluid film mass transfer resistance to very low levels. By and large, coils are highly efficient devices which may yield a urea dialysance (clearance) of up to 160 ml per minute at a blood flow rate of 200 ml per minute. Coils operate at relatively high pressure, and a blood pump is required for their use.

Parallel plate exchangers were among the earliest dialyzers to achieve clinical use, and a variety of permutations on the basic design have been described. A dialyzing membrane is stretched over a supporting structure. Another membrane is placed on top of the first, and blood ports are placed at either end of the dialyzer between the membranes. Another support is placed on top of the second membrane. Blood flows between the membranes while dialysate flows between the support structures and the membrane. The mass transfer performance of these devices has not been as impressive as that observed with coils. Generally, the number of hours per week required to achieve the same clinical results is longer than with coil devices. Dialysance of urea at blood flow rates of 200 ml per minute is only 120 to 130 ml per minute. Blood flow resistance in parallel plate dialyzers is usually small so that they can be operated without a pump when used in a patient with an arteriovenous shunt.

The *hollow fiber kidney* employs 10,000 to 15,000 fibers with an internal diameter of 200 to 250 μ as a dialyzing surface. From an engineering point of view, this configuration represents an optimal design. The narrow channels allow a minimal blood fluid film resistance and a maximal surface area to blood volume ratio. The device has extremely stable dimensions and is, for all practical purposes, noncompliant. Mass transfer capability approaches that achievable with coil-type devices. The most significant problem with this device is clotting in the hollow fibers.

It should be pointed out that all types of artificial kidneys are adequate and the choice depends on the experience and prejudices of the physician in charge.

SELECTION AND CARE OF THE PATIENT

Many factors enter into the type of treatment to be provided. These include the patient's age, availability of a suitable living kidney donor, patient motivation and ability to cooperate, support for the patient at home, the presence or absence of a spouse and the spouse's occupation, patient intelligence, in some instances financial resources, and, finally but equally important, the patient's own preference. It has been our feeling, as well as that of most others, that the availability of a suitable and willing living donor should make transplantation the treatment of choice for the young and middle-aged. Recognizing the hazards of arbitrary age limits, we nevertheless tend not to recommend transplantation in patients over age 55. There are some, however, who feel that the use of living donors is inappropriate and that transplantation should take place only when cadaveric material is available. In our hands, when a suitable living donor is not available and the patient is seemingly an appropriate candidate for home dialysis, this then becomes the next most preferred method of treatment. In general, dialysis and transplantation should be considered as complementing procedures used together to offer the best type of therapy for each patient. An attempt to separate these procedures into an either/or category is a disservice to the patient.

It is most desirable to select patients for maintenance hemodialysis and transplantation prior to their actual need for therapy. As chronic renal failure develops and the serum creatinine rises to 10 mg per 100 ml or above, it is usually appropriate to plan for dialysis. When patients begin to show signs of being unable to perform adequate business, social, or personal functions because of mounting azotemia, dialysis should be considered. It is clear that the complications of uremia are considerably more difficult to correct than they are to prevent.

Once a patient is selected for a dialysis/transplantation program, access to the circulation needs to be established. In cases in which arteriovenous fistulas are to be utilized, some lead time should be allowed for development of the access. Often a fistula can be created months prior to actual need. In the case of shunts, a few days to a week should be allowed prior to use.

When patients are severely uremic at the time of initial dialysis, complications are more likely to ensue, and considerably more caution should be exercised in treatment. In this setting, peritoneal dialysis may be employed to more gradually correct the uremic syndrome. The most common complication seen with initiation of dialysis is the *"disequilibrium" syndrome*. These manifestations are more likely to appear when the patient has undergone very efficient dialysis; they are most common in the elderly; however, they may occur at any time, even after the most gentle dialyses. The cause of this syndrome is not wholly clear. Available data suggest that a rapid lowering of serum osmolality plays a major role in the neurologic manifestations seen. With an acute reduction in osmolality which may occur with the removal of urea and/or other ions, there may be insufficient time for equal reduction in the cerebrospinal fluid. Because of the slow transport of urea and/or some other as yet unidentified substances across the "blood-brain barrier," an osmotic gradient is produced in which water moves from the blood and extracellular fluid into the central nervous system. A "reverse osmotic effect" is produced, and water moves down the gradient into the central nervous system. The symptoms seen in the patient are headache, nausea, vomiting, restlessness, agitation, rising blood pressure, confusion, and, in severe cases, grand mal seizures. Anticonvulsants may be given prophylactically to patients who are at high risk. Fortunately, the syndrome tends to subside after 12 to 24 hours.

Once a patient has begun dialysis therapy and has been stabilized, the procedure is usually performed on a regular basis three times per week. The number of hours required for each treatment depends on the size of the patient and the type of dialyzer utilized. Some centers dialyze two times per week, but the majority of experience would indicate that this is inadequate.

Where a patient receives his dialysis depends somewhat on long-term plans for transplantation as well as the medical or social factors surrounding him. Most centers agree that a hospital setting is not proper for long-term dialysis. The high cost and acute problems associated with the hospital dialysis unit make it unattractive for long-term care. When the home environment is stable and a suitable family member can cooperate, *dialysis at home* is the treatment of choice. In this situation, a family member is trained to operate the artificial kidney along with the patient, and the pair then perform the treatments in the home setting. The use of home dialysis requires a suitable home atmosphere and an emotionally stable patient and spouse. The advantage, in addition to whatever savings may be effected, is the maximal rehabilitative potential of such an environment.

An alternative to home dialysis is dialysis performed in a *limited care center* or a self-dialysis type of facility. Here, costs can be kept to a minimum while providing the patient his treatment in a noninstitutionalized setting. Limited care facilities are especially useful when the patient need be dialyzed for only a short period of time prior to transplantation. In these instances, even when home dialysis can be performed, it may not be feasible to train the family for only one or two months of dialysis in preparation for transplantation. Home dialysis has also been found unsuitable for programs which deal with disadvantaged communities in which motivation and proper home environment are lacking. The number of patients entering a chronic program who can be successfully treated at home varies, depending, among other things, on location. Estimates run as high as 85 per cent in some middle-class rural areas and as low as 10 per cent in urban ghetto populations.

MEDICAL PROBLEMS OF CHRONIC DIALYSIS

Hematologic. Patients maintained with the artificial kidney invariably show some degree of *anemia*. The degree of anemia varies and may be in some way related to the type of renal disease present. Patients with polycystic kidney disease tend to run higher hematocrits than those with other diseases.

The problems of anemia are compounded in the dialysis patient by some blood loss during the procedure. Loss of red cells left in the dialyzer at the close of the treatment may aggravate the anemia. Similarly, care should be taken to keep the laboratory evaluation of the patient to a minimum, because repeated blood testing can only contribute to the anemia. Since there is some evidence to indicate that, in addition to a lack of production of erythrocyte stimulating factor (ESF), the uremic marrow is unresponsive to the effects of ESF, one might expect that severely uremic patients may be benefited by chronic dialysis. This is the case, and most individuals can be maintained without the need for transfusions even though they do not have normal hematocrits. This must be individualized, however, depending on the accompanying symptoms produced by the anemia. In young patients, hematocrits as low as 12 to 14 vol per 100 ml can be tolerated without difficulty. In the older patient with cardiovascular difficulties, it may be necessary to tranfuse weekly. Since hepatitis can be a significant complicating factor in a hemodialysis unit, decision to use transfusion should be considered carefully.

Peripheral Neuropathy. There has been increasing awareness of peripheral nerve dysfunction in uremia. The neurologic involvement when it occurs is typically symmetrical, beginning distally at the toes and spreading up the leg. Upper extremity involvement, seen only when there is severe lower extremity involvement, develops insidiously and in the majority of patients is manifested solely by reduction in nerve conduction velocity. Only in its severe stages are there clinical symptoms. The neuropathy may cause pain and paresthesias of the lower extremities, marked sensitivity to touch, and a "burning" feeling. Although sensory manifestations of the disease may initially predominate, there may be a significant motor component as well. The presence of peripheral neuropathy is a clear indication for beginning treatment. In addition, peripheral neuropathy has been adjudged by some to be a manifestation and a consequence of inadequate dialysis. A significant percentage of patients referred to maintenance dialysis centers already have demonstrable neuropathy, at least

as measured by nerve conduction velocity. The incidence and severity of neuropathy usually depend upon the timeliness of the referral for dialysis, and neuropathy is much less common when dialysis is instituted three times per week than when the patient is treated only twice a week.

Cardiovascular. *Hypertension* is a common accompaniment of chronic renal failure, and the majority of patients presenting to a dialysis program have elevated blood pressure. Approximately 80 to 85 per cent of these can be managed without antihypertensive medication simply by careful attention to salt and water balance. Ultrafiltration with the artificial kidney and dietary restriction of salt and water are mandatory. Despite fluid control, however, a small number of patients continue with hypertension and require antihypertensive medications. An even smaller group with malignant hypertension cannot be controlled with dialysis and antihypertensive drugs at all. In the latter case, which is generally accompanied by a markedly elevated peripheral renin concentration, bilateral nephrectomy can be curative. Since the renin-angiotensin-aldosterone system has been incriminated in the hypertension associated with renal disease, this beneficial effect of nephrectomy is not surprising. It should be pointed out, however, that bilateral nephrectomy as a treatment for uncontrollable hypertension should be a last resort. Aside from the hazards of the surgical procedure, the anephric state usually complicates the dialysis treatment by imposing stricter dietary fluid controls upon the patient and results in a more severe anemia. Totally anephric patients tend to run lower hematocrits and require more transfusions than do others with their kidneys in situ.

Pericarditis, which is a common manifestation of untreated uremia, may occasionally occur in patients undergoing chronic dialysis. In our experience, pericarditis is usually associated with a stressful situation such as surgery or infection, and we have regarded it as an indication for increasing dialysis time. However, there are a few patients who develop pericarditis despite what is apparently adequate dialysis and without evidence of stress. The importance of pericarditis in dialysis patients, aside from the symptoms they may produce, lies with the potential development of *pericardial tamponade.* Inasmuch as patients are anticoagulated with each dialysis, an inflamed pericardium may bleed heavily, producing tamponade. This can be an emergency which requires pericardiocentesis and, if recurrent, pericardiectomy. If the patients are seen frequently prior to dialysis and a pericardial friction rub is detected, one can adjust the dialysis procedure with regional heparinization and lessen the risk of bleeding.

Congestive heart failure is commonly seen in patients on dialysis and is most often related to volume overload. The problem is most severe in patients with underlying coronary artery disease or hypertension but may occur in anyone who is markedly overhydrated. The physician must work with the dietician to impress upon the patient the importance of dietary control of salt and water.

Skeletal System. There seems little doubt that defective absorption of calcium from the gut is one of the prime factors resulting in the abnormal calcium metabolism of chronic renal failure, and this is not totally corrected with long-term hemodialysis. In addition, deranged metabolism of vitamin D seems to play a major role.

The main circulating form of vitamin D_3 is 25-hydroxycholecalciferol (25-HCC), and this is produced by hydroxylation in the liver from the parent substance. When the plasma calcium is low, 25-HCC is further metabolized in the kidneys to 1,25-dihydroxycholecalciferol (1,25-DHCC); when the plasma calcium is high, it is metabolized to 21,25-dihydroxycholecalciferol. The 1,25 derivative is the most active form of the vitamin so far discovered. After production by the kidneys, it is taken up by the intestines and bones. Therefore the kidneys may be regarded as endocrine organs producing a calcium-regulating hormone at a rate dependent on the serum calcium. Alterations in metabolism of vitamin D or its hydroxylated metabolites in uremia may result in accumulation of structurally related abnormal metabolites which compete with 1,25-DHCC for receptor sites in specific target organs. The end result in bone is decreased or defective mineralization of collagen, probably secondary to maturation arrest of collagen tissue. The combination of defective calcium absorption, abnormal vitamin D metabolism, and hyperphosphatemia accompanying decreased excretory function may all serve to depress serum calcium which in turn stimulates parathyroid hormone secretion. In clinical practice, patients being maintained by dialysis may histologically show osteomalacia, osteitis fibrosa cystica, and/or osteosclerosis.

It seems important to control serum phosphate levels in patients on chronic dialysis in order not to further suppress serum calcium levels, and this is usually done by giving phosphate binders orally. If serum phosphate is excessive, one may see precipitation of calcium salts in ectopic sites such as blood vessel walls or soft tissues.

The vast majority of patients with severe renal failure and almost all individuals who have been maintained with the artificial kidney for a long period show some evidence of parathyroid hyperplasia and histologic evidence of early bone resorption. Fortunately, only a small percentage of these develop clinical abnormalities of bone metabolism which require specific treatment.

It is helpful to divide renal osteodystrophy into two categories: osteomalacia and osteitis fibrosa cystica. Pathologic examination of bone in uremia, however, may show a mixture.

Treatment of the patient with marked parathyroid hyperfunction as manifested by progressive disability seems to be subtotal parathyroidectomy. By removing all but half of the smallest parathyroid gland, one may reverse or at least arrest the progression of hyperparathyroidism. Therapy with vitamin D and calcium in the postoperative period is optional but usually helpful.

In patients with less severe signs of hyperparathyroidism one may attempt to overcome vitamin D resistance by supplementing higher doses of the vitamin along with oral calcium. Dihydrotachysterol along with control of serum phosphate by use of antacids may be effective in preventing further progression of the disease. Further discussion of renal osteodystrophy may be found in Ch. 890.

Infection. Peritonitis is the most common complication in patients being maintained with peritoneal dialysis. Usually physical signs of peritonitis are evident, although they may be modified considerably, depending on the extent of the infection and the severity of the uremia. Gram-negative infections are, in our experience, the most common, although many organisms may be responsible. It is not always necessary to discontinue peritoneal dialysis because of peritonitis. Despite the fact that the catheter is a "foreign body," it is frequently possible to treat the peritonitis with the appropriate antimicrobials instilled into the peritoneal dialyzing fluid (and systemically administered if required) while continuing the dialysis. Salvaging the catheter is particularly important when permanent prosthetic devices are being used.

Infections commonly occur in patients being treated with the artificial kidney, and a whole spectrum of infectious diseases is seen. By all odds the most common site of infection is at the access to the circulation and is usually localized. Patients with arteriovenous shunts (i.e., permanent foreign bodies) have the highest incidence. Infection may also be seen, however, with an arteriovenous fistula. The most common reason for the infection is faulty technique in handling the shunt or fistula. The Staphylococcus is the predominant organism cultured, but, as in peritonitis, a wide range of organisms can be seen. Depending, of course, on the severity of the infection, one need not necessarily remove the access, and the majority of these incidents can be treated with local measures and systemic antimicrobials. We have had the impression that once an access (especially an arteriovenous shunt) is infected, its longevity is limited, but this is difficult to quantitate. Occasionally septicemia may occur from shunts and fistulas and must be treated vigorously. Usually the site of infection is obvious, but occasionally an endarteritis may be present as a site of a "seeding" and is not clinically apparent. In some cases acute or subacute bacterial endocarditis may occur, although this is unusual. In more than 500 patients treated with the artificial kidney over the last five years, we have seen endocarditis only three times. The treatment of this complication is discussed in Ch. 192.

It goes without saying that the responsible organism must be identified in cases of infection and treated appropriately. One must be aware, however, of the limited excretory ability of these patients and how this relates to the use of antimicrobial drugs. Administration should be modified to take into account the lack of kidney function and the dialyzability of the individual drug (see Ch. 268).

One of the most feared problems which may occur in a dialysis unit is *hepatitis*. Every precaution should be exercised to reduce its incidence in both patients and staff. In the United States a survey of a number of dialysis units disclosed the incidence of hepatitis infection for center-based patients and staff to be 4.4 cases and 3.4 cases, respectively, per 100 persons at risk. It is of interest that almost 70 per cent of the hemodialysis patients were anicteric; many would not have been detected if periodic screening for hepatitis B antigen or liver function tests had not been performed routinely. The hemodialysis patient seems to tolerate hepatitis quite well and usually recovers. However, the disease in staff members may be fulminant, and a number of deaths have been reported. It is essential that a hemodialysis unit take every precaution to protect the staff and patients from this infection.

General Comment. No matter how well adjusted or how well dialyzed a patient may be, it must be acknowledged that he is not totally well. In addition to low level uremia and chronic anemia, he is confronted regularly with the time-consuming dialysis, limitations in diet, and whatever hemodynamic instability may be caused by the procedure itself. Despite, this, however, many patients can lead productive and comfortable lives. Some need to change their type of vocation since they are not capable of doing heavy manual labor. Sedentary occupations can be performed quite effectively, however. The patient on dialysis also has to come to grips with the real and psychologic dependence on the machine. Travel is much less available to him, and he must constantly arrange travel schedules with a back-up dialysis facility in mind. There are organizations which do provide dialysis patients with a list of units in various locations, and this has been a great help. In short, life on dialysis, although adequate and productive, is not optimal and is at the very best a compromise. Its use in combination with an active transplantation program offers the patient a number of treatment choices, and seems the best approach. Although, as pointed out, the quality of life achieved with the artificial kidney does not approach that possible with a well-functioning transplanted kidney, differences in mortality and morbidity with both procedures must be considered. In a well-run, carefully monitored dialysis program, the yearly mortality rate may be as low as 5 per cent, and this needs to be measured against the higher mortality rate which may occur with some forms of transplantation. The decision as to which modality or combination of modalities of therapy is employed must be made considering all these factors.

Abel, J. J., Rountree, L. G., and Turner, B. B.: On the removal of diffusible substances from circulating blood by means of dialysis. Trans. Assoc. Am. Physicians, 23:51, 1913.

Bailey, G. L. (ed.): Hemodialysis—Principles and Practice. New York, Academic Press, 1972, p. 496.

Garibaldi, R. A., Forrest, J. N., Bryan, J. A., Hanson, B. F., and Dismukes, W. E.: Hemodialysis-associated hepatitis. J.A.M.A., 225:384, 1973.

Hampers, C. L., Schupak, E., Lowrie, E. G., and Lazarus, J. M.: Long-term Hemodialysis. 2nd ed. New York, Grune and Stratton, 1973.

GLOMERULAR DISEASE

O. M. Wrong

608. INTRODUCTION

Diseases which affect glomeruli display such important features in common that they can usefully be considered together and contrasted with diseases commencing in other parts of the kidney. Numerically, glomerular disease accounts for approximately half of the patients with severe renal disease seen in most communities and over two thirds of the patients accepted for renal replacement by units undertaking intermittent hemodialysis or renal transplantation.

Each glomerulus consists of a complex branching system of capillaries; thus, even though these capillaries are highly specialized, glomerular disease can be regarded as a form of capillary disease. In many forms of glomerular disease small blood vessels in other parts of the body are also diseased, but because the glomerular circulation is particularly vulnerable to pathologic insult the effects of renal damage may dominate the clinical picture. Many glomerular diseases, particularly the inflammations, are the result of antigen-antibody reactions; in others the glomeruli are infiltrated with abnormal deposits, e.g., diabetic renal disease, amyloid, Fabry's disease.

Most forms of glomerular disease are macroscopically diffuse, affecting equally the cortex of both kidneys, and one part of the cortex as severely as another. Con-

sequently the small amount of material which can be removed by percutaneous renal biopsy usually yields a histologic picture which is representative of the kidneys as a whole, and this investigation has been valuable in both diagnosis and study of the natural history of glomerular disease. Histologically glomerular lesions may be *generalized* (i.e., involving all glomeruli), or *focal* (involving only some); within a glomerulus a lesion may be either *diffuse* (affecting the whole glomerulus) or *segmental* (affecting only a portion of the glomerulus). These topographic distinctions are of help in categorizing glomerular disease further.

Proteinuria. Increased loss of protein in the urine, in excess of the 30 to 130 mg per day excreted normally, is almost invariable in glomerular disease; it is a direct result of increased glomerular permeability to plasma proteins caused by the disease process. The amount of protein lost in the urine may be much greater than in other forms of renal disease; losses of more than 3 grams per day are not seen except in glomerular disease, and this finding therefore has great diagnostic value. The main urinary protein is always albumin, but variable amounts of the other plasma proteins are also lost, depending on the type of disease. When urinary protein losses of more than 5 grams a day persist, hepatic synthesis may not be able to increase sufficiently to maintain the serum albumin, and hypoalbuminemic edema may result. The triad of proteinuria, hypoalbuminemia, and edema is known as *nephrotic syndrome,* and is discussed in detail in Ch. 609.

Hypertension. Hypertension may complicate any form of renal disease, but is particularly common and severe in glomerular disease, although even here it is not invariable. It is now known that renal hypertension has at least two causes: (1) increased secretion of renin by the juxtaglomerular apparatus (JGA), and (2) increased extracellular fluid and blood volume caused by diminished renal ability to excrete salt and water, e.g., the "renoprival" hypertension that follows bilateral nephrectomy. Both factors play a part in the hypertension of glomerular disease, but their relative contributions differ from case to case. The JGA may be directly involved or rendered ischemic by the primary disease, and hypertension may be caused by the resultant hypersecretion of renin. When glomerular disease has resulted in renal failure, hypertension analogous to renoprival hypertension may develop simply from failure to excrete salt and water. The development of severe hypertension in glomerular disease is an ominous sign, as it leads to further damage from the effects of high blood pressure on the renal circulation. Prompt control of hypertension is therefore of vital importance in the care of such patients.

Tubular Defects. Evidence of tubular dysfunction occurs early in the clinical course of many types of renal disease, e.g., analgesic nephropathy, polycystic disease, and obstructive uropathy. In such conditions renal acidosis, or renal wasting of sodium or water, may develop when there is still little reduction in glomerular filtration rate. In primary glomerular disease these defects are rarely seen until renal failure develops, with serum creatinine raised above 3 to 5 mg per 100 ml, and even then marked tubular abnormalities are rare. The acidosis is less severe than occurs in tubular syndromes with similar degrees of renal failure, and is not usually hyperchloremic in type. Urinary concentrating ability is impaired, but the defect is usually an obligatory isosthenuria rather than the hyposthenuria seen in some tubular syndromes. Experiments involving dietary sodium depletion have shown that patients with glomerular disease are often unable to reduce urinary losses of sodium as efficiently as normal subjects, but their obligatory losses are usually well below the amounts supplied by their diet, and it is exceptional for a sodium supplement to be required.

In clinical practice use of the aforementioned principles will usually distinguish glomerular disease from other forms of renal disease. However, it is frequently difficult to distinguish between different forms of glomerular disease, even with the assistance of all modern diagnostic laboratory aids. To some extent this is the result of artificial distinctions between so-called disease entities, which may represent merely groups of commonly associated clinical features, rather than the results of distinct etiologic processes. But the problem is also due to the very limited way in which glomeruli can respond to different pathologic insults, which means that the same histologic and clinical picture may result from several different pathologic processes.

609. NEPHROTIC SYNDROME

Definition. In the first half of this century the term *nephrosis,* introduced by Müller in 1905, was widely used in at least two quite different senses: (1) as a descriptive histopathologic term for renal disease without an inflammatory component, and (2) to describe the clinical picture caused by heavy urinary protein losses. Much confusion was caused by this double use, and as a result the word has been largely abandoned. By general agreement the term *nephrotic syndrome* has been adopted for the second of these meanings, and refers to the *clinical association of heavy proteinuria, hypoalbuminemia, and generalized edema.* It is further understood that the

TABLE 1. Causes of Nephrotic Syndrome

Autoimmune forms of primary glomerular disease (see Table 2, Ch. 610)
Glomerular involvement in connective tissue diseases
    Systemic lupus erythematosus
    Polyarteritis
    Anaphylactoid purpura
    Goodpasture's syndrome
    Hemolytic-uremic syndrome
Familial nephritis
Congenital nephrotic syndrome
Glomerular involvement in other systemic diseases
    Quartan malaria
    Schistosomiasis
    Secondary syphilis
    Accelerated hypertension
    Diabetic glomerulosclerosis
    Amyloidosis
Mechanical causes
    Renal vein thrombosis
    Constrictive pericarditis
    Obstruction of inferior vena cava
    Sickle cell anemia
Toxins
    Mercury, organic or inorganic
    Gold
    Allergy to pollen, insect bites, snake venom, plant toxins, vaccines
    Serum sickness
Drug hypersensitivity
    Trimethadione and paramethadione, perchlorate, probenecid, penicillamine, sulfonamides, etc.
Miscellaneous
    Toxemia of pregnancy
    Renal transplant

plasma albumin is low as a result of urinary albumin loss, and the edema is the result of the altered Starling capillary forces caused by the consequent low plasma oncotic pressure. In general these criteria are not fulfilled unless at least 5 grams of protein a day are lost in the urine at some time in the course of the disease and the plasma albumin is less than 3 grams per 100 ml.

The aforementioned definition does not include reference to renal excretory failure, to hypertension, or to hypercholesterolemia. At various times attempts have been made to include one or another of these features as obligatory items in the definition, particularly hypercholesterolemia. However, the advantages of simplicity are lost if the definition includes features not closely linked causally, such as hypertension and renal failure, or of which the mechanism is uncertain, such as hypercholesterolemia.

Etiology. The nephrotic syndrome has many causes. Table 1 shows those that have been fully substantiated. The list includes almost all recognized forms of glomerular disease, and *only* forms of glomerular disease, for urinary protein losses in other forms of renal disease are not gross enough to give rise to hypoalbuminemia. (It has sometimes been claimed that pyelonephritis can give rise to the nephrotic syndrome, but the patients referred to have probably had glomerular disease complicated by pyelonephritis.) The most important items in Table 1 are separately described in the text; in some of the others the glomerular morphology has not been fully established. There is some overlap between parts of the table; thus the nephrotic syndrome caused by various foreign proteins can be due to a proliferative glomerulonephritis or minimal change disease, and that seen in renal transplants may have either a proliferative or a membranous picture. Drug hypersensitivity may cause nephrotic syndrome as part of an allergic vasculitis (sulfonamides), an immune-complex glomerulonephritis (penicillamine), or minimal change disease (probenecid).

Many of the causes listed give rise to transient nephrotic syndrome which in itself is neither a diagnostic nor a therapeutic problem. Persistent nephrotic syndrome, on the other hand, is a major diagnostic and therapeutic problem to all who deal with renal disease. In Europe and North America about 75 per cent of cases are caused by three idiopathic types of glomerular disease — minimal change disease, membranous disease, and the various types of chronic proliferative glomerulonephritis. The frequency of these three types varies between centers, partly because of variations in classification of cases with mixed membranous and proliferative change, but in most centers minimal change disease causes the majority of cases in children and one fifth to one third of adult cases. The proliferative varieties of glomerulonephritis are slightly more common than membranous disease except in elderly men. The main causes of the disease in the remaining 25 per cent of nephrotics who do not have idiopathic glomerular disease are diabetic glomerulosclerosis, amyloidosis, various forms of focal glomerulonephritis (including lupus erythematosus and anaphylactoid purpura), and renal vein thrombosis.

Clinical Manifestations. Generalized edema, often accompanied by ascites and pleural effusions, is the sine qua non of the nephrotic syndrome. The edema is primarily due to the reduced plasma oncotic pressure caused by hypoalbuminemia, but numerous other factors, such as salt intake and mineralocorticoid activity, contribute to its development, and because of these there is no predictable relationship between the amount of edema and the level of the plasma albumin. The sequence giving rise to edema is shown in Figure 1. In children gross edema of the face may develop early in the course of the disease, but in adults the legs are usually most affected. In severe cases the weight of the body may be increased by 50 per cent simply from accumulation of edema fluid.

Hypertension is present in some patients, but its presence depends on the type of glomerular disease. The low plasma volume which results from a very low plasma albumin may occasionally cause severe vascular collapse with hypotension. Protein malnutrition caused by the high urinary losses may lead to muscle wasting (often obscured by the generalized edema) or growth retardation in children. Increased opacity of the nails (*leukonychia*) is often present, and occasionally it is possible to estimate how long the nephrotic syndrome has existed by the position of the discolored area.

Urine may be scanty while edema is accumulating, and contains more than 5 grams of protein a day. The feature of the urinary deposit and degree of renal impairment depend on the underlying glomerular pathology, but transient renal failure may occur from hypovolemia or tubular damage without implying a destructive glomerular disease. Children with nephrotic syndrome

sometimes develop evidence of multiple renal tubular defects, with renal glycosuria, aminoaciduria, and a potassium-losing tendency.

Plasma albumin is invariably reduced below 3.0 grams per 100 ml. The usual value is between 1.0 and 3.0 grams per 100 ml, but occasionally concentrations as low as 0.5 gram per 100 ml are seen; in such cases signs of hypovolemia (particularly postural hypotension) are common, and the edema is often resistant to treatment. The plasma proteins other than albumin may be normal, but electrophoresis often shows a decrease in alpha$_1$ and gamma globulins, and an increase in alpha$_2$ and beta globulins which is mainly due to increases in alpha-glycoprotein and beta lipoprotein. The concentrations of the relatively small molecular weight transferrin and ceruloplasmin are reduced, whereas fibrinogen concentrations are increased.

The other characteristic chemical change in the blood is hyperlipidemia. This involves not only cholesterol, the most easily measured plasma lipid, but all the major lipid components of plasma, including triglycerides and phospholipids. Plasma cholesterol may rise to 1500 mg per 100 ml, but the level of this and of the other lipids varies considerably, even in patients with the same type of nephrotic syndrome. Little prognostic or diagnostic value can be attached to the determination except that marked elevations appear to be less common in lupus erythematosus than in other forms of the nephrotic syndrome. The mechanism of the hyperlipidemia is obscure, but seems intimately linked to the low albumin concentration. Nephrotic hyperlipidemia appears to carry an increased risk of premature generalized atheroma.

Differential Diagnosis. Two complex investigations, *renal biopsy* and *differential protein clearances*, have proved of great value in establishing the morphologic diagnosis in individual cases. Nephrotic syndrome is now one of the main indications for renal biopsy. The diseases that cause the syndrome are nearly always diffuse, so that needle biopsy yields a representative picture. The procedure is not usually technically difficult unless the kidneys are small, which is unusual. Frequently it is possible to base treatment and prognosis on the histologic findings. This matter is discussed under the various disease headings, and will not be further elaborated here.

The diagnostic value of differential protein clearances was largely established by Squire and his colleagues (for references, see under minimal change glomerular disease). The principle is that the abnormal glomerulus in nephrotic syndrome permits the passage of increased amounts of protein, and that the selective pattern of this permeability varies in different diseases. Some glomerular diseases permit only the smaller proteins, e.g., albumin and transferrin, to escape in the urine (selective), whereas in others all the plasma proteins are found (nonselective). A crude idea of glomerular permeability can be obtained by electrophoresis of the urine; a highly selective proteinuria consists almost entirely of albumin with small peaks of alpha$_1$ and gamma globulin, whereas a nonselective proteinuria shows an electrophoretic pattern similar to that of normal plasma. However, electrophoresis is an unsatisfactory method for the study of glomerular selectivity, for the electrical charge and molecular weight of proteins are not closely related, and more satisfactory results can be obtained by measurement of individual proteins. A useful indication of selec-

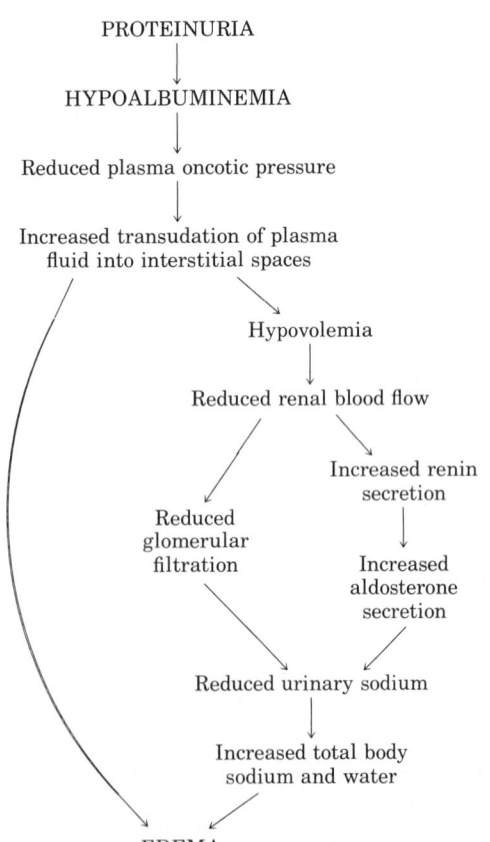

Increased glomerular permeability to
large molecules

PROTEINURIA

HYPOALBUMINEMIA

Reduced plasma oncotic pressure

Increased transudation of plasma
fluid into interstitial spaces

Hypovolemia

Reduced renal blood flow

Increased renin
secretion

Reduced
glomerular
filtration

Increased
aldosterone
secretion

Reduced urinary sodium

Increased total body
sodium and water

EDEMA

Figure 1. Sequence of main events giving rise to edema in the nephrotic syndrome.

tivity, suggested by Cameron and Blandford, is the ratio of the clearance of IgG to that of transferrin; in highly selective proteinuria, values below 0.15 are obtained. The major cause of a highly selective proteinuria is minimal change glomerular disease, which carries a good prognosis and usually responds well to steroids. The forms of nephrotic syndrome likely to be confused with this disease, which have a much worse prognosis and do not satisfactorily respond to steroids, i.e., membranous and proliferative glomerular disease, show poor selectivity in their pattern of protein excretion. There appear to be only two exceptions to the general rule that a highly selective proteinuria indicates a good prognosis, and both are uncommon — congenital nephrotic syndrome, a rare and invariably fatal disease, and occasional cases of renal amyloidosis.

Treatment. *Glomerular Lesion.* Treatment of the underlying glomerular disease of the common causes of nephrotic syndrome will be discussed under specific glomerular diseases. In general it is unsatisfactory, but exceptions will be mentioned as they arise.

Treatment of the Nephrotic Syndrome. Gross edema carries an appreciable morbidity and mortality, mainly from infection and the effects of immobility, and patients appear to be improved both physically and psychologically when treatment leads to its disappearance. But although the cause of the edema is the low serum albumin, there is no practicable way of increasing plasma albumin while urinary protein losses persist. *High protein diets* have been advocated for years; occasionally they cause a marginal increase in plasma albumin, but usually their only obvious effect is to increase urinary protein losses. Moreover, protein is the most costly item of the diet, and many patients are unable to take a high protein diet because of its expense. *Intravenous protein,* given as salt-poor human albumin, is occasionally of value in the treatment of hospital patients with circulatory collapse caused by hypovolemia, or to initiate diuresis in a patient with refractory edema, but it produces a transitory effect and is impractical for long-term treatment.

The most important factor in treatment is the proper use of *diuretics.* Except in cases of profound hypoalbuminemia, or when the syndrome is complicated by severe renal failure, edema can nearly always be controlled by diuretics alone. The diuretic regimen required varies from patient to patient; in general oral agents are best, and it is wise to start treatment with a relatively gentle drug, such as a thiazide, and only use the more powerful diuretics, e.g., furosemide and ethacrynic acid, if initial treatment fails to produce diuresis. Potassium deficiency usually arises in patients given diuretics more than three times a week, and should be prevented by the simultaneous administration of potassium supplements or of potassium-sparing diuretics, such as spironolactone or amiloride; however, in renal failure potassium depletion is seldom a problem, and these measures should be avoided as they can precipitate hyperkalemia. Disappearance of edema can be hastened by combining diuretics with a low sodium intake (as low as 20 mEq per day), but this step is not usually necessary except in advanced renal failure.

Modern diuretics are now so efficient that there is no longer a place for local fluid removal by abdominal paracentesis or Southey's tubes, although occasionally benefit may be obtained by aspiration of pleural effusions if these do not disappear rapidly.

When assessing the progress of a patient with nephrotic syndrome, the most useful guides are the presence or absence of edema, body weight, 24-hour urinary proteins, and serum albumin, and decisions regarding changes in treatment can be taken only with this information. Even when there is no effective treatment for the glomerular lesion per se, it is often found that proteinuria varies spontaneously over a wide range, and it may be possible to reduce or stop the use of diuretics as plasma albumin rises to a level at which edema no longer occurs. When diuretics are required, the mistake must not be made of pushing treatment to the point at which the patient suffers severe postural hypotension, and it may be good judgment to allow mild edema to persist, particularly when the serum albumin is below 1.0 gram per 100 ml.

Nephrotic syndrome is usually a chronic state, and it is wise therefore to encourage patients to follow their normal activities as far as possible. Frequently the physician will be asked about possible risks of pregnancy. The dangers depend largely on the nature of the underlying renal disease and the risk that because of this the pregnancy will be complicated by hypertension and placental insufficiency. Hypoalbuminemic edema does not per se contraindicate pregnancy (although edema frequently gets temporarily worse during pregnancy), and many women with nephrotic syndrome, particularly that resulting from minimal change glomerular disease, have completely normal pregnancies.

Cameron, J. S., and Blandford, G.: The simple assessment of selectivity in heavy proteinuria. Lancet, 2:242, 1966.

Edwards, K. D. G.: Antilipaemic drugs and nephrotic hyperlipidaemia. *In* Edwards, K. D. G. (ed.): Drugs Affecting Kidney Function and Metabolism. Basel, S. Karger, 1972, p. 370.

Robson, J. S.: The nephrotic syndrome. *In* Black, D. A. K. (ed.): Renal Disease. 3rd ed. Oxford, Blackwell Scientific Publications Ltd., 1972, p. 331.

610. GLOMERULONEPHRITIS

Definition. The term "glomerulonephritis" has usually been applied to forms of glomerular disease characterized by an inflammatory reaction, with leukocyte infiltration and cellular proliferation of the glomeruli. However, in recent years it has become clear that most forms of glomerular inflammation are caused by immune injury; this chapter has therefore been expanded to include some types of glomerular disease, e.g., minimal and membranous glomerulopathies, which strictly are not glomerular inflammations at all but also appear to be the results of immune glomerular injury.

Etiology. Repeated attempts to isolate microorganisms from the lesions of glomerulonephritis have failed, and these diseases are not considered to be the direct result of bacterial invasion of the kidneys. It is more difficult to exclude the role of viruses, but at present there is no good evidence that any form of human glomerulonephritis is caused by the presence of viruses in the glomeruli.

The detailed pathogenesis of glomerulonephritis is still obscure, but there is considerable evidence that an antigen-antibody reaction plays a major part in initiating the glomerular lesions in most forms of glomerulonephritis. The evidence can be summarized as (1) demonstration by immunofluorescence and electron microscopy of complexes of antigen-antibody and complement either on or within the glomerular basement membrane in many forms of glomerulonephritis; (2) marked lowering of various fractions of serum complement in many cases; (3) experimental production of glomerular lesions resembling human glomerulonephritis by injections either of antikidney antibodies prepared from other species or of nonspecific antigen or antigen-antibody complexes.

Two main types of immune injury appear to be etiologically important in glomerulonephritis. In the first of these, antibodies are directed against the glomerular basement membrane (anti-GBM nephritis) which becomes the seat of a reaction involving antigen (GBM), antibody, and complement, leading to polymorphonuclear infiltration, cellular proliferation, and fibrin deposition, with eventual crescent formation and obliteration of the glomerular space. Antibody (IgG) and complement can be shown by immunofluorescence to be deposited in a fine continuous line along the basement membrane of every capillary loop (Fig. 2). This type of immune injury appears to account for most cases of Goodpasture's syndrome and some cases of rapidly progressive proliferative glomerulonephritis and renal transplant nephritis.

The second and more common type of immune glomerular injury, immune complex disease (ICD), does not involve antibodies directed against renal tissues. The glomeruli are damaged by immune complexes which arise in the circulation from interaction of antibody with antigens of extrarenal origin. These complexes are deposited in the glomeruli in close relation to the basement membrane. Antigen-antibody complexes arising from relative antigen excess are particularly liable to cause glomerular injury, as they are relatively small and are not removed by the reticuloendothelial system as rapidly as larger complexes. Once deposited in the glomeruli, antigen-antibody complexes activate complement, leading to an acute inflammatory reaction, with polymorphonuclear infiltration and fibrin deposition. Immunofluorescent studies show irregular granular staining for gamma globulin and complement along the basement membrane (Fig. 3), a pattern distinct from the smoothly linear deposition seen in anti-GBM disease (Fig. 2). Under the electron microscope complexes appear as electron-dense masses arising from the basement membrane, usually on

Figure 3. Granular glomerular deposition of IgG in a patient with idiopathic membranous disease. (× 1050.) (Courtesy of Dr. D. J. Evans.)

its epithelial surface. Examples of this type of glomerular disease are lupus nephritis (in which the antigen is DNA), poststreptococcal nephritis (streptococcal antigen), glomerulonephritis with glomerular deposition of Australia antigen, and the nephritis of both quartan malaria and infective endocarditis. However, in most cases of immune complex disease, it has not yet been possible to identify the responsible antigen.

It may eventually prove possible to devise a classification of glomerulonephritis entirely in immunologic terms, but this is not yet practicable. Renal immunology is still in its infancy, and there are many unanswered questions — for example, the role of deficiencies in the immune response of the host, the parts played by complement fixation and cell-mediated immunity, and the importance of damaged renal tissues as antigens promoting a further immunologic reaction. The classification used here (Table 2) is therefore based primarily on clinical and morphologic criteria.

Platelet aggregation in glomerular capillaries and fibrin deposition in the glomerulus and glomerular space occur in inflammatory forms of glomerular disease and potentiate immunologic damage. The presence of fibrin deposition can be suspected from the finding of fibrin degradation products in the urine; when intravascular coagulation is marked, and particularly when the renal disease is part of a generalized small vessel disease, fragmented and distorted red cells may appear in the peripheral blood and occasionally the full picture of a microangiopathic hemolytic anemia, with a lowered platelet count, increased platelet turnover, and reduced plasma fibrinogen.

Figure 2. Linear glomerular deposition of IgG in a patient with Goodpasture's syndrome. (× 1050.) (Courtesy of Dr. D. J. Evans.)

TABLE 2.   Classification of Glomerulonephritis

1. Minimal change glomerular disease
2. Focal glomerulosclerosis
3. Idiopathic membranous glomerular disease
4. Proliferative glomerulonephritis
    a. Acute poststreptococcal glomerulonephritis
    b. Acute glomerulonephritis caused by other infections
    c. Glomerulonephritis in infective endocarditis
    d. Mesangiocapillary glomerulonephritis
    e. Focal glomerulonephritis with recurrent hematuria
    f. Other varieties of proliferative glomerulonephritis
5. Renal involvement in connective tissue diseases

Logical therapeutic attempts to interrupt the immunologic processes responsible for glomerulonephritis, as well as their immediate consequences, have included cytotoxic drugs, such as the nitrogen mustards, cyclophosphamide, and azathioprine, to reduce antibody formation; steroids or other anti-inflammatory agents to reduce the effects of immune injury on the kidney; and anticoagulants to lessen platelet and fibrin deposition. Such rational forms of therapy have in general proved disappointing; the occasional successes are mentioned when appropriate.

Brain, M. C., Dacie, J. V., and Hourihane, D. O.: Microangiopathic haemolytic anaemia: The possible role of vascular lesions in pathogenesis. Br. J. Haematol., 8:358, 1962.

Dixon, F. J.: The pathogenesis of nephritis. Am. J. Med., 44:493, 1968.

Fish, A. J., Michael, A. F., and Good, R. A.: Pathogenesis of glomerulonephritis. *In* Strauss, M. B., and Welt, L. G. (eds.): Diseases of the Kidney. 2nd ed. Boston, Little, Brown & Company, 1971, p. 373.

Germuth, F. G., and Rodriguez, E.: Immune Complex Deposit and Antibasement Membrane Disease. Boston, Little, Brown & Company, 1973.

Peters, D. K.: The kidney in allergic disease. *In* Gell, P. G. H., Coombs, R. R. A., and Lachmann, P. J. (eds.): Clinical Aspects of Immunology. 3rd ed. New York, Oxford University Press, 1974.

MINIMAL CHANGE GLOMERULAR DISEASE
(Lipoid Nephrosis)

Definition. This is a glomerular disease causing heavy proteinuria, characterized by absence of obvious histologic glomerular changes on light microscopy.

The term "lipoid nephrosis" was introduced by Munk in 1913, and refers to the presence of fat bodies in the urine and fatty change in the tubular cells. These changes are now known to be the result of a glomerular protein leak, but with the light microscope it is not usually possible to see glomerular abnormalities, and it was not until the advent of the electron microscope that glomerular changes were shown to be invariably present. Hamburger's suggestion that the term "minimal change" should be used to describe the glomerular lesions has been widely followed.

Etiology, Incidence, and Pathology. The frequent association with allergic conditions such as asthma and sensitivity to foreign proteins, and the dramatic response induced by steroids, have suggested to some that the condition is a form of IgE-mediated immune glomerular injury, but this has not been convincingly demonstrated.

The disease is most common in infancy and childhood, a fact largely responsible for the good prognosis of the nephrotic syndrome in childhood. The peak incidence is between three and four years, but no age is exempt. Males are affected more often than females, in a ratio of 3:2. In adults lymphoma elsewhere in the body, particularly Hodgkin's disease, has sometimes been reported in association with this type of renal disease, but the causal connection between the two conditions has not been explained.

Light microscopy usually shows no glomerular abnormalities, but there may be occasional small areas of glomerular proliferation or adhesions to Bowman's capsule. The tubules usually show protein casts and doubly refractile lipid vacuoles in the cells of the proximal tubule; edema of the interstitium is often present and may cause considerable renal enlargement. The electron microscope invariably shows changes in the glomeruli, consisting of swelling and fusion ("smudging") of the foot processes of the epithelial cells on the outer side of the basement membrane. The basement membrane itself usually has a normal appearance, but sometimes contains small vacuoles or shows irregular thickening.

Until recently the view was widely held that this form of renal disease represented an early form of glomerulonephritis which would eventually show destructive glomerular changes. This view is no longer tenable; serial renal biopsies have shown that the glomerular lesions do not usually progress; indeed, they disappear after a spontaneous or steroid-induced clinical remission. The few patients who do not remit appear to have a different condition to start with—either an early form of membranous glomerulopathy, which should be detected by electron microscopy, or focal glomerular sclerosis (described subsequently) which usually produces a nonselective proteinuria.

Despite the absence of gross changes in the basement membrane on light microscopy, it is likely that the protein leak is the result of change in the basement membrane itself. The change in the foot process is probably caused by the presence of protein within Bowman's space, for identical appearance can be produced in animals by intravenous injection of proteins which cross the glomerular filter. This histologic appearance is also a feature of other forms of glomerular disease with heavy proteinuria, and is in no way specific for minimal change glomerular disease, although here it is the only constant glomerular finding.

The permeability characteristics of the glomerulus in this disease have been well worked out (Squire, Blainey, Hardwicke, and Soothill). The urinary proteins consist almost entirely of the plasma proteins of lower molecular weight, particularly albumin (molecular weight 68,000) and transferrin (90,000), whereas plasma proteins of larger size, such as beta-lipoprotein (molecular weight up to 2,500,000) are almost completely absent. The same pattern of glomerular permeability can be demonstrated after intravenous injection of dextrans of different molecular sizes, when only the smaller molecules are found in the urine. The glomerular protein leak is thus highly selective, whereas in almost all other forms of glomerular disease the leak is nonselective, or poorly selective, in that plasma proteins of every molecular size are found in the urine.

Clinical Manifestations. The most common first symptom is edema, which develops insidiously and often reaches mammoth proportions. Examination at this stage reveals all the characteristics of the nephrotic syndrome: heavy proteinuria (more than 5 grams per day), hypoalbuminemia, and usually hypercholesterolemia. The urine sediment contains hyaline, granular and fatty casts, and occasional red cells; red cell casts are not found. The plasma urea and creatinine are usually normal; however, azotemia is not uncommon in the early stages of the disease, and rarely transitory oliguric renal failure develops—perhaps the result of hypovolemia or obstruction of tubules by protein casts.

The disease has a remarkable tendency to remit. This may take place spontaneously, may follow systemic infections such as measles, or may result from treatment with steroids or cytotoxic drugs. Remissions are usually complete, with disappearance of all signs, but partial remissions with continuing mild proteinuria are also common. Relapses are unfortunately frequent, and may exactly replicate the initial attack. Repeated relapses may occur over a period of many years (over 20 years in one case personally known to the author) without deterioration in renal excretory function or the appearance of destructive changes in the glomeruli.

Treatment. The chief hazard lies in the complications of edema, particularly infection, which have been greatly reduced by modern diuretics and antimicrobial drugs. Before the advent of penicillin, pneumococcal peritonitis was a common cause of death, but this is now very rare. Treatment of edema is discussed in connection with the nephrotic syndrome. Two other hazards of the disease require mention. Hypogammaglobulinemia, owing partly to reduced synthesis and partly to urinary losses of gamma globulin, itself carries a risk of infection; hypercholesterolemia, as in other forms of nephrotic syndrome, may eventually lead to early atheroma and a predisposition to arterial thrombosis.

This is one of the very few forms of glomerular disease in which the underlying glomerular fault can be remedied by treatment. When given steroids or corticotrophin (ACTH), most patients rapidly lose their proteinuria and all other signs, usually within two to six weeks of the start of treatment. Serial renal biopsies have shown that the glomerular foot processes simultaneously return to normal. It is not known how adrenal steroids exert this remarkable effect, and the dose required varies from case to case, usually being in the range of 20 to 60 mg of prednisolone, or equivalent, daily. Relapses often follow withdrawal of steroids, even when the dose has been reduced very gradually.

Treatment with steroids should not be lightly undertaken. It must be realized that this is the only form of nephrotic syndrome which shows a satisfactory response at all frequently, and that this treatment has definite dangers. The diagnosis should not rest on clinical manifestations alone, but should be based on the appearances of renal biopsy and on the finding of a highly selective proteinuria. In children, in whom high doses of steroids are less dangerous, and in whom most cases of nephrotic syndrome are caused by this process, it is justifiable to commence steroids without the evidence of renal biopsy or protein clearances, provided that treatment is gradually withdrawn if no effect is seen within six weeks. Conversely, in a few elderly patients, even those who have been shown by renal biopsy to have the disease, the risks of long-continued steroids, particularly peptic ulcer, may be greater than the risks of nephrotic syndrome, provided that edema can be satisfactorily controlled.

Once a decision is made to employ steroid treatment, it is wise to begin with a high dose, e.g., 60 to 80 mg of prednisolone per day in an adult, or 40 to 60 mg in a child. This should be maintained for three to six weeks and then reduced to a maintenance dose of one half to two thirds the original dose if a satisfactory response (disappearance or marked lessening of proteinuria) occurs; if not, the treatment should be gradually withdrawn. Maintenance treatment should be continued for three to six months; then periodic attempts can be made to reduce dosage further or stop altogether; if clinical relapse occurs, it will be necessary to increase the dose temporarily.

Troublesome side effects of steroids are common, but there is some evidence that they can be prevented or lessened by giving steroids on alternate days, without loss of therapeutic effect. It is unwise to regard complete abolition of proteinuria as the sole aim of treatment, for in some cases this requires an unacceptably high dose of steroids, whereas a much smaller dose will sufficiently

lessen proteinuria to return the plasma albumin to normal and so remove the risk of edema.

The most difficult patients to treat are those who become steroid dependent, relapsing as soon as the dosage is reduced or after intercurrent infections, yet developing severe side effects of steroid overdose. These patients are usually children, in whom retardation of growth is the most troublesome complication. In such cases ACTH may be preferable to steroids, because there is evidence that it has less effect in retarding growth. Alternatively, prolonged remission may be obtained by the use of cytotoxic drugs, of which cyclophosphamide and chlorambucil have been the most successful.

Barratt, T. M., and Soothill, J. F.: Controlled trial of cyclophosphamide in steroid-sensitive relapsing nephrotic syndrome of childhood. Lancet, 2:479, 1970.

Black, D. A. K., Rose, G., and Brewer, D. B.: Controlled trial of prednisone in adult patients with the nephrotic syndrome. Br. Med. J., 3:421, 1970.

Connolly, M. E., Wrong, O. M., and Jones, N. F.: Reversible renal failure in idiopathic nephrotic syndrome with minimal glomerular changes. Lancet, 1:665, 1968.

Farquhar, M.: Ultrastructure of the nephron disclosed by electron microscopy. A review of normal and pathologic glomerular ultrastructure. In Metcoff, J. (ed.): Proceedings, 10th Annual Conference on the Nephrotic Syndrome. New York, National Kidney Disease Foundation, 1959, p. 2.

Hardwicke, J., and Soothill, J. F.: Proteinuria. In Black, D. A. K. (ed.): Renal Disease. 2nd ed. Oxford, Blackwell Scientific Publications, Ltd., 1967, p. 252.

Squire, J. R., Blainey, J. D., and Hardwicke, J.: The nephrotic syndrome. Br. Med. Bull., 13:43, 1957.

FOCAL GLOMERULOSCLEROSIS
(Segmental Hyalinosis)

Definition, Pathology, and Incidence. This form of glomerular disease is characterized by focal and segmental areas of glomerular sclerosis, usually commencing in the juxtamedullary glomeruli and gradually spreading to involve other parts of the kidney, with eventual renal failure. The condition has only recently been demarcated from other varieties of glomerulonephritis. The cause is obscure, but affected glomeruli have been shown to contain deposits of complement and gamma globulin. There is evidence that patients treated by renal transplantation may develop the disease in the transplanted kidney.

Incidence and Clinical Course. The incidence of the disease is unknown, for it is still frequently confused with minimal change glomerular disease, benign recurrent hematuria, and various other types of proliferative glomerulonephritis. It most commonly presents in children or adolescents, with nonselective proteinuria, often gross enough to cause nephrotic syndrome, or recurrent macroscopic hematuria. Renal biopsy may not sample the affected glomeruli, thus giving rise to a false diagnosis of minimal change glomerular disease. No treatment is known to definitely alter the course of the disease, but the progression to renal failure usually takes many years.

Churg, J., Habib, R., and White, R. H. R.: Pathology of the nephrotic syndrome in children. Lancet, 1:1299, 1970.

IDIOPATHIC MEMBRANOUS GLOMERULAR DISEASE
(Epimembranous Nephritis)

Definition. This is a glomerular disease of obscure cause, characterized by thickening of the capillary basement membrane, without cellular infiltration. The condition is often called "membranous glomerulonephritis," but this term is inappropriate inasmuch as there is no histologic evidence of glomerular inflammation.

Etiology, Incidence, and Pathology. The finding of granular deposits of IgG and complement on the thickened basement membrane has led to the suggestion that it is a form of immune-complex disease.

The disease affects all ages, but is most common in adults; males are affected more often than females, particularly in middle age and later life.

Histologically it can be recognized with the light microscope by a more or less uniform thickening of the capillary basement membrane of every glomerulus. This is often obvious in sections stained with hematoxylin and eosin, but is particularly apparent in thin sections (less than 2μ) stained with periodic acid–methenamine–silver. The thickening may be so marked that the capillary lumen is reduced in caliber or obliterated, but there is no increase in glomerular cellularity. Under the electron microscope the basement membrane is thickened, vacuolated, and irregular; arising from its epithelial side, under the fused foot processes of the epithelial cells, are electron-dense granules which can be shown by immunofluorescence (Fig. 3) to contain IgG and complement. These findings are very similar to those in some forms of proliferative glomerulonephritis, except for the absence of a cellular reaction, and the suggestion has been made that this is a similar type of immune-complex disease, but without involvement of cell-mediated immunity.

An association of membranous glomerular disease with malignancy arising outside the kidneys (especially bronchus and gut) has been reported, suggesting that in these cases the renal disease is caused by immune complexes of host antibody and tumor antigen.

The membranous form of glomerular disease is generally believed to be distinct from other forms, not merely a stage in the evolution of another process. This view is supported by serial renal biopsies, which have shown a worsening in the glomerular alterations with time but no real change in nature.

Clinical Manifestations. Membranous glomerular disease usually presents with nephrotic syndrome, less often with asymptomatic proteinuria, renal hypertension, or chronic renal failure. All features of the nephrotic syndrome may be found, but the condition may be distinguished from minimal change glomerular disease by higher average age of patients, frequent presence of hypertension and renal failure, nonselective nature of the proteinuria, and rarity of clinical remission. Microscopic hematuria is slightly more common than in minimal change glomerular disease, but hypercholesterolemia is less frequent.

The disease runs a slowly progressive course; usually many years elapse before renal failure is a serious problem. Very occasionally a fulminant course is followed, oliguric renal failure developing within a few months of onset. No treatment is known to alter the course of the disease, although there have been occasional reports of remission after use of steroid or cytotoxic drugs. It is difficult to evaluate the role of these treatments, and the few properly controlled trials that have been reported have shown no evidence of benefit. Spontaneous clinical remissions occur but are rare, in most cases only temporary and not accompanied by change in the histologic features. When the disease is associated with carcinoma, remission may follow successful removal of the tumor.

Franklin, W. A., Jennings, R. B., and Earle, D. P.: Membranous glomerulonephritis. Long-term serial observations on clinical course and morphology. Kidney Int., 4:36, 1973.

Gluck, M. C., Gallo, G., and Lowenstein, J.: Membranous glomerulonephritis. Evolution of clinical and pathologic features. Ann. Intern. Med., 78:1, 1973.

PROLIFERATIVE GLOMERULONEPHRITIS

Definition. This term strictly covers all diseases in which cellular proliferation affects the glomeruli, but is most conveniently restricted to those in which renal involvement is not part of the vasculitis of systemic disease (e.g., lupus erythematosus).

Etiology. Until quite recently it was widely believed that most cases were poststreptococcal in origin. This view is now clearly recognized as incorrect; it is difficult to know the true proportion, but in adults less than 25 per cent appear to have disease of this cause.

The group is heterogeneous, but immune renal injury probably plays a part in all forms. Some cases of rapidly progressive disease show linear deposition of IgG and complement in the glomeruli, and are probably examples of anti-GBM nephritis. Immune-complex injury appears to be responsible for poststreptococcal nephritis, the nephritis caused by other acute infections and infective endocarditis, and that caused by chronic quartan malaria. In many other cases the immunofluorescent findings are those of immune-complex disease, but the nature of the antigen is unknown. Often patients come to medical attention late in the course of their disease, when evidence of the original immune glomerular injury can no longer be found.

Acute Poststreptococcal Glomerulonephritis

This is the best documented and most understood form of proliferative glomerulonephritis. Although its course is complex and variable, it does demonstrate almost all the possible features of glomerular disease, and therefore has served in the past as the usual starting point and reference in discussing glomerulonephritis. To some extent this emphasis has been unfortunate in that it has tended to delay recognition of the many forms of glomerulonephritis which are unrelated to the Streptococcus and are now becoming relatively more important because of the falling incidence of streptococcal infection. However, the disease is still common enough to deserve emphasis in its own right.

Etiology. In 1836 Richard Bright recognized that acute glomerulonephritis usually followed an infection, particularly scarlet fever. Since then scarlet fever has become much less common, and the incidence of postscarlatina nephritis has likewise fallen. It is now recognized that acute nephritis can follow streptococcal infection in any part of the body, although the pharynx is the usual site, and is unrelated to the production of erythrotoxin by the organism. Only certain strains of Streptococcus are "nephritogenic" (capable of initiating nephritis); all the offending organisms are Group A hemolytic streptococci, and the majority are of Type 12. Other less common nephritogenic strains are Types 1, 4, 25, 41, 49 (Red Lake strain), and 57; the last two have been incriminated in outbreaks of streptococcal pyoderma causing nephritis.

Symptoms of acute glomerulonephritis do not usually develop until 7 to 20 days after the streptococcal infection, by which time the patient appears to have recovered from the local infection. Transitory mild proteinuria and microscopic hematuria are common during the initial streptococcal infection, particularly in persons who subsequently develop clinical nephritis, but it is not clear whether these are the first manifestations of nephritis or merely represent the urinary changes common in any severe infection.

Coincident with the development of nephritis there is a marked reduction in serum complement, apparently caused by its deposition in the kidney. Immunofluorescent studies during the acute stage of the disease show irregular staining for complement and gamma globulin, particularly IgG, within the glomeruli, and electron microscopy reveals electron-dense deposits, corresponding to this immunofluorescence, on the epithelial side of the glomerular basement membrane. These findings indicate that the disease is an immune-complex form of renal injury, but it is not known why only certain strains of streptococci can provide the necessary antigenic stimulus. Antigenic similarities between the glomerular basement membrane and Streptococcus have been demonstrated, but the weight of evidence is against this being a form of anti-GBM nephritis.

Incidence. Acute poststreptococcal nephritis occurs in all parts of the world. Males are affected about twice as frequently as females. No age is exempt, but the disease is particularly common in children and adolescents, perhaps because of the increased risk of acquiring a streptococcal infection from exposure at school. In temperate climates it is most common in winter, when streptococcal infections are at their peak. The relationship of acute nephritis to certain streptococcal strains explains some epidemiologic features of the disease, such as its tendency to cause small epidemics in homes or schools, as well as the variations in incidence in persons known to have had streptococcal infections—from nil with a non-nephritogenic strain to as high as 40 per cent with a strain known to be nephritogenic. By contrast the incidence of rheumatic fever in those with streptococcal infections who have not previously had the disease is fairly constant at 2 to 3 per cent.

Pathology. The disease is rarely fatal, and most knowledge of its pathology comes from material obtained by biopsy. The occasional necropsy has shown symmetrical renal enlargement and pallor of the cortex. Histologically the glomeruli are nearly all similarly affected, with enlargement of the whole glomerulus and marked increase in the number of nucleated cells, consisting mainly of endothelial and mesangial cells and mononuclear leukocytes, although polymorphonuclears may also be found. Epithelial cell proliferation is usually not prominent. The glomerular lobules are swollen and relatively bloodless, with reduced capillary lumina and occasional necrotic and thrombosed capillary loops. The transitory renal failure of the acute phase of the disease is the result of these changes, rather than obliteration of Bowman's space by epithelial crescents.

During resolution the last feature to remain is hypercellularity, most marked in the vicinity of the glomerular stalk or mesangium, which may be detectable several months after apparently complete clinical recovery. This change, though typical of resolving poststreptococcal

glomerulonephritis, does occur in some other forms of proliferative glomerulonephritis, and its presence cannot be regarded as conclusive evidence of an earlier poststreptococcal disease.

Clinical Manifestations. Most patients have a fairly clear history of preceding streptococcal infection. Usually it is a pharyngitis which has been sufficiently severe to keep the patient away from school or work, but occasionally the infection lies elsewhere—for example, an otitis media, a leg ulcer, or a surgical wound. Sometimes the infection can only be demonstrated by a positive bacteriologic culture, or presumed from the finding of a raised antistreptolysin O titer.

The patient has usually recovered from the initial infection when manifestations of nephritis appear, some 7 to 20 days after onset of the original infection. The most common presenting symptom is *edema,* noted particularly in the face on first arising. *Hematuria* is also a common first symptom; usually the urine has a smoky brown color, but occasionally it is frankly blood stained. Less commonly the patient complains of *reduced urine output,* or of bilateral dull *loin pain,* which is probably caused by stretching of the renal capsules.

It is important to note that the edema present at the onset of the disease is invariably caused by fluid retention, which itself is the result of reduced renal excretion of salt and water. In an adult of average size the presence of generalized edema implies a weight gain of at least 5 kg. At this stage patients have not lost enough protein in the urine to develop hypoalbuminemic edema (nephrotic syndrome), although this complication may develop later; nor is there good evidence for the earlier views that the edema of acute nephritis is caused either by increased capillary permeability or by heart failure.

Vague *malaise, nausea,* and *headache* are common in acute nephritis, but fever is unusual, and patients do not usually feel really ill, although often distressed by the appearance of edema. In mild cases they may be quite asymptomatic; the disease may be picked up only by examining the urine of a person known to have had a recent streptococcal infection.

Physical examination usually shows generalized edema and mild hypertension of the order of 140 to 160 systolic, 90 to 110 diastolic. Very occasionally hypertension is severe, with retinal hemorrhages and exudates, papilledema, or hypertensive encephalopathy. In general, the degree of hypertension is in proportion to the amount of edema. Fluid retention, if marked, may lead to the signs of congestive cardiac failure, with cardiac enlargement and triple rhythm, venous engorgement, hepatic distention, and gross pulmonary and systemic edema.

Urinary output is usually reduced, although the reduction is often not noticed by the patient. Complete suppression of urine is rare, and indicates a very severe attack of nephritis; this complication may develop within a few days of the onset, or urinary output may gradually fall to nothing over several weeks. As might be expected, fluid retention is particularly severe in such cases, and unless rigid restriction of sodium and water has been instituted, edema and hypertension are particularly marked. Unless renal function returns rapidly, symptoms of renal failure eventually appear, with nausea and vomiting, twitching and pruritus, acidotic respirations, and progressive anemia.

Urine. Urinary concentration is usually in the range of 350 to 600 mOsm per kilogram (corresponding to a specific gravity of 1.010 to 1.017) when correction is made for a protein content, but appears more concentrated because of the presence of red cells. Moderate quantities of protein are present, and occasionally mild renal glycosuria occurs. The urinary sediment contains large numbers of red cells and leukocytes, particularly the former, and a smaller number of renal tubular cells. Casts, particularly the granular variety, are also present; erythrocyte and hemoglobin casts indicate bleeding from the glomerulus and are particularly helpful in diagnosis.

Laboratory Tests.   Mild renal failure, with plasma creatinine values of 1.5 to 4.0 mg per 100 ml, is very common in the initial stage of the disease. In the rare case of severe renal failure, the biochemical sequelae are similar to those of renal failure from other causes except that hyperkalemia seems particularly common, probably because these patients are usually previously fit and active young people who rapidly lose muscle mass during their illness.

A nephritogenic strain of Streptococcus can be cultured from the pharynx of many patients, except those treated with effective antimicrobial drugs, even when all clinical evidence of local infection has disappeared. Occasionally cultures taken from the throats of other members of the family will reveal the presence of a nephritogenic organism when this can no longer be cultured from the patient's own throat.

The serum antistreptolysin O titer is usually raised, indicating recent streptococcal infection, but the titer may fall rapidly to normal and so pass unnoticed, or it may not rise at all if the streptococcal infection is rapidly aborted by the use of antimicrobials. Unfortunately, as has been pointed out by Rammelkamp, not all nephritogenic strains of streptococci produce streptolysin O (nor do they invariably cause beta-hemolysis in culture), and so detection of the preceding streptococcal infection by this means may be difficult. The serum titer of type-specific antibody to streptococcal M antigen is more difficult to measure, but remains raised for considerably longer after a streptococcal infection (often for years), and has the added advantage of indicating whether an infection was caused by a strain known to be nephritogenic. A marked drop in serum complement is characteristic of acute poststreptococcal nephritis, but this finding is not diagnostic because it may occur in other forms of nephritis, e.g., systemic lupus erythematosus and the nephritis of bacterial endocarditis, and few laboratories can provide the measurement as a routine.

The erythrocyte sedimentation rate is moderately raised. The hemoglobin concentration is usually slightly reduced (to 11 to 12 grams per 100 ml) as a result of dilution.

Course and Prognosis.   Diuresis usually starts 7 to 14 days after the onset of symptoms, and over the space of two days the patient loses edema and hypertension. Renal clearances and the plasma creatinine concentration return to normal, but microscopic hematuria and proteinuria persist longer, and may not disappear for weeks or months. During this period clinical relapses may occur, particularly at the time of other respiratory infections.

Occasionally urinary losses of protein during the first few weeks are sufficiently large to cause hypoalbuminemic edema, which at first reveals itself when renal excretory function improves and the expected diuresis does not materialize. Although the development of nephrotic syndrome is of grave import if it first appears after several months, its rapid appearance at this early stage of the disease does not necessarily carry a bad prognosis, and patients with this syndrome may recover completely within the next few weeks.

It is difficult to ascertain what proportion of patients recover completely, for hospital series are weighted by the more severe cases. Most estimates state that over 90 per cent of children and about 60 per cent of adults eventually make a full clinical recovery. These figures may be unduly pessimistic, because many of the published series have included patients, who, with the benefit of more recent advances of glomerular immunofluorescence and electron microscopy, might not now be classified as having poststreptococcal nephritis.

In the early years of this century, poststreptococcal nephritis in the acute stage caused death in about 5 per cent of patients. Death was usually due to pulmonary edema, the complications of hypertension, or intercurrent infections. Nowadays these complications can usually be prevented, and most fatalities are the result of acute renal failure with anuria or severe oliguria. Patients can be kept alive by peritoneal dialysis or hemodialysis, and many so treated, particularly children, experience return of renal function after days or weeks. If renal recovery does not ensue or is inadequate to maintain life, and renal biopsy shows irrecoverable glomerular damage, they may be treated by intermittent hemodialysis or renal transplantation.

Unfavorable features which suggest that satisfactory recovery will not take place are (1) delayed or absent diuresis; (2) persistent renal failure; (3) persistent hypertension; (4) prolonged or increasing proteinuria, often leading to nephrotic syndrome; (5) a persistently lowered plasma complement; and (6) severe changes in the renal biopsy, particularly obliteration of Bowman's space by epithelial crescents and disappearance of glomerular capillaries.

Patients who recover from acute glomerulonephritis are not immune to second attacks, but these are uncommon because of the development of type-specific antibodies which protect against infection by the original strain of Streptococcus and exert an effect for many years. Some apparent second attacks of acute poststreptococcal glomerulonephritis are in reality exacerbations of a longstanding chronic glomerulonephritis.

Differential Diagnosis.   The condition most easily confused with acute poststreptococcal nephritis is exacerbation of a subacute or chronic glomerulonephritis, with transitory hematuria and further reduction in renal function. Such exacerbations may be precipitated by many different infections, even those caused by viruses, but are particularly common after streptococcal infections; in the absence of previous evidence of renal disease, this situation closely resembles an initial attack of poststreptococcal nephritis. This diagnostic problem is now rather infrequent, probably because of the declining incidence of streptococcal infections.

The transient proteinuria and microscopic hematuria that accompany many severe systemic infections may also be mistaken for poststreptococcal nephritis, but these signs occur at the height of the infection and are not usually associated with other features of renal disease.

It may be difficult to distinguish acute poststreptococcal nephritis from other forms of acute glomerulonephritis, such as Henoch-Schönlein nephritis (which may also be precipitated by a streptococcal infection), systemic lupus erythematosus, the microscopic form of polyarteritis nodosa, recurrent focal nephritis with hematuria, and the nephritis of bacterial endocarditis. Here the physician will be guided by features suggesting systemic involvement and by evidence of recent streptococcal infection. Renal biopsy may also help by showing a glomerular lesion more focal than that of poststreptococcal nephritis.

Less often, acute poststreptococcal nephritis may be confused with primary malignant hypertension, with various forms of hemolytic anemia with hemoglobinuria, or with acute tubular necrosis, particularly when the latter is precipitated by a systemic infection.

Treatment. It has not been convincingly shown that any form of treatment alters the course of the glomerular lesion, but individual manifestations and complications frequently require treatment.

Infection. In the acute stage of nephritis, penicillin is usually given either by mouth or by injection to eradicate any remaining streptococcal infection. This treatment has much to commend it, but there is no evidence that it alters the subsequent evolution of the glomerular disease. Penicillin should also be used prophylactically to treat close contacts, particularly members of the family who may have contracted streptococcal infection from the patient, unless this possibility is excluded by bacteriologic tests. Oral penicillin V (phenoxymethyl penicillin, 250 mg twice a day) is often recommended after attacks of acute nephritis to reduce subsequent respiratory infections which might cause exacerbations of nephritis; if used, it is best continued through the next winter season when streptococcal infections are more widespread. (The question of prophylaxis against streptococcal infections is further discussed in Ch. 190.)

Edema. Fluid retention during the oliguric phase of the disease should be prevented by careful attention to body weight. Salt and fluids should be restricted if edema is present or a weight gain of more than 2 to 3 kg occurs. In these circumstances oral fluids should be limited to no more than 500 ml per day, plus a volume equal to the urine output of the previous day, and dietary sodium should be reduced as far as possible, preferably to 20 mEq per day. If severe edema is already present, or develops despite these measures, a diuresis may occasionally be obtained by oral diuretics, particularly furosemide in doses of 40 to 1000 mg twice a day. Digitalis is ineffective, despite the presence of many classic features of congestive cardiac failure, because the circulatory troubles are due to excess of extracellular fluid, and not to a primary cardiac cause. In the rare case in which fluid overload threatens life and diuresis cannot be obtained by drugs, the excess fluid should be removed by dialysis.

Uremia. There is no convincing evidence that dietary protein influences the course of the glomerular lesion, but early in the disease it is wise to restrict protein intake moderately (40 to 70 grams per day) until it is clear that the patient is not likely to develop renal failure. Patients who do develop severe renal failure should be treated by more drastic protein restriction, with or without some form of dialysis, as described in Ch. 605 to 607.

Hypertension. If fluid retention is carefully controlled, there is usually no need to treat hypertension specifically. But the patient with severe fluid overload may require treatment for hypertensive encephalopathy with convulsions, or retinopathy with failing vision; in these emergencies parenteral hydralazine, reserpine, or diazoxide is the drug of choice.

Other Drugs. Steroids, anticoagulants, and cytotoxic drugs, either alone or in various combinations, have been used in the acute stage of the disease, particularly in patients with severe renal failure, but there is no good evidence that they alter the outcome.

Rest. In the acute stage of the disease bed rest is advisable. The patient does not usually wish to be active, and the recumbent position facilitates diuresis. Once macroscopic hematuria, edema, and hypertension have disappeared and the plasma creatinine has returned to normal, the value of rest is uncertain. Many authorities recommend that bed rest continue as long as proteinuria is diminishing, but there is no evidence that this alters the course of the disease, and it may be impractical or economically disastrous for the patient whose proteinuria persists for months.

Continued Observation. Because of the difficulty in deciding when a patient has recovered from the disease, it is valuable to follow all patients until at least a year after the last clinical evidence of nephritis. Frequent determinations of blood pressure, urinary proteins and sediment, and plasma creatinine and creatinine clearances are the most useful indications of disease activity. The purpose of this follow-up is to observe any exacerbation of the disease, so that renal failure, nephrotic syndrome, or hypertension can be immediately recognized and treated. Acute urinary infections, which are not uncommon in such patients, can also be recognized and treated.

Bright, R.: *In* Osman, A. A. (ed.): Original Papers of Richard Bright on Renal Disease. London, Oxford University Press, 1937.

Dodge, W. F., Spargo, B. H., Travis, L. B., Srivastava, R. N., Carvajal, H. F., Debeukelaer, M. M., Longley, M. P., and Menchaca, J. A.: Poststreptococcal nephritis. A prospective study in children. N. Engl. J. Med., 286:273, 1972.

Heptinstall, R. H.: Pathology of acute glomerulonephritis. *In* Strauss, M. B., and Welt, L. G. (eds.): Diseases of the Kidney. 3rd ed. Boston, Little, Brown & Company, 1971, p. 405.

Levy, J. E., Salinas-Madrigal, L., Herdson, P. B., Pirani, C. L., and Metcoff, J.: Clinico-pathologic correlations in acute poststreptococcal glomerulonephritis. Medicine, 50:453, 1972.

Rammelkamp, C. H., and Earle, D. P.: Pathogenesis of chronic glomerulonephritis. *In* Ingelfinger, F. J., Relman, A. S., and Finland, M.: Controversy in Internal Medicine. Philadelphia, W. B. Saunders Company, 1966, p. 331.

Schwartz, W. B., and Kassirer, J. P.: Clinical aspects of acute poststreptococcal glomerulonephritis. *In* Strauss, M. B., and Welt, L. G. (eds.): Diseases of the Kidney. 3rd ed. Boston, Little, Brown & Company, 1971, p. 419.

Zabriskie, V., Utermohlen, V., Read, S. E., and Fischetti, V. A.: Streptococcus-related glomerulonephritis. Kidney Int., 3:100, 1973.

Acute Glomerulonephritis Caused by Other Infections

Frequently patients with acute glomerulonephritis show no evidence of a preceding streptococcal infection, even though in almost every other way their disease is typical of poststreptococcal nephritis. It is impossible to be sure that any patient has not had a streptococcal infection, and probably many of these patients have had an infection which cannot be detected in retrospect. However, it is now recognized that an acute glomerulonephritis may follow infections caused by microorganisms other than streptococci. It seems likely, from a consideration of the pathogenesis, that an acute immune complex type of nephritis in humans may, like the experimental model, be precipitated by exposure to a variety of foreign proteins, which need not be exclusively of infective origin.

When pneumococcal pneumonia was a common disease, before the advent of antimicrobial drugs, it was frequently reported to be a cause of acute glomerulonephritis. The disease was similar to the poststreptococcal variety, except that the latent interval was shorter and fluid retention and hypertension were less apparent. In most instances the possibility of a complicating streptococcal infection was not adequately excluded, and there must be doubt as to the existence of such an entity.

Acute glomerulonephritis has also been reported after typhoid fever and diphtheria and after many virus infections such as mumps, measles, chickenpox, infective hepatitis, mononucleosis, and infections with echovirus and adenovirus. Although in many instances a complicating streptococcal infection has not been excluded, the number of these reports is so great that it is difficult to accept that they all represent cases of poststreptococcal nephritis. In several recent cases a renal biopsy has been obtained or the patient has come to necropsy, and glomerular changes very similar to those of poststreptococcal nephritis have been found.

The concept of an acute diffuse glomerulonephritis which results from nonstreptococcal infections has thus been established, but it should be emphasized that nephritis is much rarer after these infections than it is after infections with nephritogenic strains of group A streptococci.

The natural history of glomerulonephritis caused by other than streptococcal infections is not fully known. The disease appears to behave like poststreptococcal nephritis in that the majority of patients recover completely, but a few are left with a continuing process with progressive impairment of renal function, which may be complicated by nephrotic syndrome of severe hypertension.

Glomerulonephritis in Infective Endocarditis

The subacute glomerulonephritis that complicates endocarditis has often been regarded simply as a form of acute glomerulonephritis caused by streptococcal infection. This view is misleading for several reasons: (1) The viridans streptococci do not cause nephritis when they invade other parts of the body; (2) it has been increasingly realized, perhaps because of longer survival, that patients with other forms of infective endocarditis (e.g., pneumococcal, *H. influenzae,* and fungal) also develop glomerulonephritis. The usual alternative hypothesis, that the disease is caused by bacterial embolization to the glomeruli, would explain the focal type of glomerulonephritis which is sometimes seen, but not the more usual diffuse glomerulonephritis nor the fact that bacteria cannot be demonstrated in the glomeruli. Recent immunofluorescent and electron microscope studies have shown granular deposits of IgG and complement, and more rarely fibrin, in the glomeruli of patients with diffuse glomerulonephritis associated with endocarditis caused by a variety of organisms, findings strongly suggesting immune-complex disease.

Patients with infective endocarditis do not usually show evidence of glomerulonephritis until they have had infection for several weeks. The condition presents with hematuria and proteinuria, and less frequently with impairment of renal function, which is often first mistakenly attributed to severe cardiac failure and resulting reduced renal perfusion. Hypoalbuminemic edema and hypertension have not been features of most reports. Severe renal failure is seldom seen except in patients in the terminal stages of a prolonged endocarditis.

In most cases the diagnosis presents no difficulty because the symptoms and signs of the underlying endocarditis are prominent. Rarely this is not so, and the disease may be confused with diffuse forms of vasculitis, such as periarteritis or systemic lupus, because of fever and evidence of a systemic disease, necrotic and hemorrhagic skin lesions, or renal biopsy findings of a mixed focal and generalized glomerulonephritis. In such patients the true diagnosis may only be revealed by repeated blood culture, by the finding of splenomegaly, or by evidence of a cardiac lesion.

At present there is insufficient information on the natural history of the glomerulonephritis after successful treatment of the causative endocarditis, but it is unlikely that complete healing occurs in those with extensive glomerular disease.

Gutman, R. A., Striker, G. E., Gilliland, B. C., and Cutler, R. E.: The immune complex glomerulonephritis of bacterial endocarditis. Medicine, 51:1, 1972.

Mesangiocapillary Glomerulonephritis
(Membranoproliferative Glomerulonephritis)

Definition. This disorder is a form of chronic glomerulonephritis, only recently demarcated, in which glomerular mesangial cells are increased and capillary walls are irregularly thickened. There is marked and persistent reduction in serum C3 complement.

Etiology and Pathology. The reduction in complement is more persistent than in other forms of glomerulonephritis, and is not the result of deposition in the glomeruli, as it is unrelated to disease activity and persists after nephrectomy. There is evidence of an alternate pathway of C3 metabolism, caused by an abnormal factor of nonrenal origin (C3 "nephritic" factor, or C3 NeF) which in vitro breaks down C3 by a mechanism which does not involve the normal early components of complement activation. The fact that renal transplants can become affected by the disease suggests that a continuing systemic abnormality, perhaps involving the complement system, is responsible for the nephritis.

Immunofluorescence shows granular deposits of complement and properdin in glomerular capillaries; less often IgG and fibrin can be demonstrated. Histologic examination shows increased thickness of the basement membrane of peripheral glomerular capillaries, with some deposits on the endothelial sides of the basement membrane and narrowing of capillary lumina. Mesangial cells are increased in number, and their proliferation throughout the kidney may give the appearance of a lobular nephritis; there are occasional granulocytes.

Clinical Manifestations. Older children and young adults are most often affected. The disease may present with symptomless hematuria, proteinuria, or nephrotic syndrome, or rarely as an acute nephritis, although there is seldom a prior streptococcal infection. The course is slowly downhill, with episodes of hematuria and nephrotic syndrome, persistent hypocomplementemia, and gradual renal failure, apparently uninfluenced by any treatment. The average duration, from diagnosis to death or maintenance dialysis, is about ten years. In view of reports of involvement of renal homografts by the disease, maintenance dialysis is preferable to transplantation as a form of renal replacement.

Lancet Annotation: Pathways in complement activation. Lancet, 1:473, 1973.

Mandalenakis, N., Mendoza, N., Pirani, C. L., and Pollak, V. E.: Lobular glomerulonephritis and membranoproliferative glomerulonephritis. Medicine, 50:319, 1972.

West, C. D., Ruley, E. J., Forristal, J., and Davis, N. C.: Mechanisms of hypocomplementemia in glomerulonephritis. Kidney Int., 3:116, 1973.

Focal Glomerulonephritis with Recurrent Hematuria
(Essential or Benign Hematuria)

The term *focal nephritis* has often been used in the European literature to designate a form of renal disease characterized by repeated attacks of profuse hematuria after systemic infection, leaving little residual renal damage. The renal lesion is a focal glomerular inflammation, but the disease clinically has little in common with other forms of focal glomerulonephritis, such as the renal lesions of polyarteritis or lupus erythematosus.

Clinical Manifestations. The disease is most common in the second and third decades of life, and affects males much more frequently than females. Rarely other members of the family may be affected. The characteristic features are recurrent attacks of hematuria, which usually start about the age of puberty and continue at the rate of several a year for as many as 20 or 30 years. Attacks may occur without obvious precipitating cause, but most often follow a febrile illness or, less frequently, surgical operation or some strenuous unaccustomed exertion. Unlike poststreptococcal nephritis, hematuria may develop within a few hours of the evidence of systemic infection, and is seldom delayed more than two days; it is often heavier than that which occurs in poststreptococcal nephritis, and may be accompanied by renal pain. There is no constant relationship to group A streptococci or to any particular form of infection. Often the manifestations of the precipitating illness (usually an evanescent pyrexia and myalgia) are so slight that this cannot be diagnosed with certainty.

Even during the attack of hematuria it is unusual for hypertension, renal failure, or edema to develop, although the urinary deposit is characteristic of an acute glomerulonephritis. Renal biopsy discloses focal areas of glomerular proliferation, usually affecting only a segment of a glomerulus here and there. The glomerular lesions are similar to those of Henoch-Schönlein purpura, but are usually less diffuse, and, like them, they show immunofluorescence to IgA. Complement and IgG can also be shown, and the deposits tend to have a mesangial distribution.

Prognosis. At first the urine clears completely after each attack, but in older patients mild proteinuria and microscopic hematuria may persist between attacks. The disorder is usually regarded as benign, because renal failure and hypertension do not commonly develop. However, occasionally these complications develop; more rarely still, the nephrotic syndrome is seen, and in such patients renal biopsy shows that the glomerular lesions, although still focal, have resulted in very severe glomerular destruction.

Management. The history is so distinctive that a diagnosis can usually be made with confidence from this alone. However, it is often valuable to demonstrate the characteristic histology by renal biopsy, either in order to reassure the patient that he has a form of renal disease that does not usually shorten life, or to put an end to repeated urologic investigations performed in an attempt to explain the hematuria.

Patients with the syndrome should be advised to avoid infections or any activities which they know are liable to precipitate an attack. Penicillin prophylaxis, to reduce bacterial respiratory infections, is often tried, but the results have been disappointing. The usual benign course of the condition does not justify routine use of steroids, nor is there any evidence that they influence the disease. Prolonged follow-up is advisable, because the course is not invariably benign and some of the long-term complications (e.g., hypertension and renal failure) require treatment.

Rapoport, A., Davidson, D. A., Deveber, G. A., Ranking, G. N., and McLean, C. R.: Idiopathic focal proliferative nephritis associated with persistent hematuria and normal renal function. Ann. Intern. Med., 73:921, 1970.

Roy, L. P., Fish, R. A., Vernier, R. L., and Michael, A. F.: Recurrent macroscopic hematuria, focal nephritis, and mesangial deposition of immunoglobulin and complement. J. Pediatr., 82:767, 1973.

Other Varieties of Proliferative Glomerulonephritis

Many cases of proliferative glomerulonephritis do not fit clearly into one or other of the categories so far described. Although some are probably poststreptococcal in origin, this is no longer believed to be the cause in most cases.

Extracapillary Glomerulonephritis with Epithelial Crescents (Fig. 4). This type of glomerulonephritis is only rarely of poststreptococcal origin, and is often of anti-GBM type, showing linear glomerular immunofluorescence for IgG and complement. Epithelial proliferation leads to the formation of crescents which fluoresce for fibrin and obliterate Bowman's space. The course is often fulminating, justifying the title "rapidly progressive glomerulonephritis," but occasionally the disease appears to become stationary or only slowly progressive. Children are rarely affected, but the condition is a frequent type of glomerular disease at all other ages.

Clinical presentation is with hematuria, nephrotic syndrome, renal hypertension, or oliguric renal failure. No treatment is known to definitely alter the course of the disease; there is good rationale for the use of anticoagulants to reduce crescent formation, but there is no convincing evidence that they improve survival.

Endothelial Glomerulonephritis. When cells from within the glomerulus (endothelial and mesangial cells) proliferate, the histologic changes are those of a lobular nephritis, with fusion of glomerular capillary loops, but without marked adhesion formation between the visceral and parietal layers of Bowman's capsule (Fig. 5). This pathologic picture is much more common than the extracapillary type of glomerulonephritis, but mixed types are also frequent. Some appear to be the result of a streptococcal infection, but in others this cause can be excluded with confidence.

The usual clinical presentations are with recurrent hematuria, nephrotic syndrome, or renal hypertension. Renal failure is not a prominent early feature, but it eventually develops after months or years as a result of progressive glomerulosclerosis. The disease frequently appears to remain unchanged for long periods, and renal function may even improve spontaneously, particularly in poststreptococcal cases. This is the histologic variety of glomerulonephritis to which the descriptive name *chronic glomerulonephritis* can most suitably be applied.

Although mixtures of types of glomerular disorders occur, in any one patient the renal condition usually runs true to type, the histology as shown by serial biop-

Figure 4. Abundant crescent formation in a 13-year-old girl with rapidly progressive glomerular nephritis. No good history of streptococcal infection was obtained. (H & E; × 150.) (From Heptinstall, R. H.: Pathology of the Kidney. Boston, Little, Brown & Company, 1966.)

Figure 5. Lobular form of glomerular nephritis. (H & E; × 400.) (From Heptinstall, R. H.: Pathology of the Kidney. Boston, Little, Brown & Company, 1966.)

sies retaining its characteristics despite evolution of the disease.

In longstanding proliferative glomerulonephritis there may be little or no remaining cellular proliferation in the glomeruli, many of which are destroyed by fibrosis while the remainder show adhesions and segmental scarring. The atrophy of tubules rendered ischemic by glomerular destruction leads to gross renal shrinkage and distortion of renal architecture. Hypertensive damage, involving arterioles and arteries, is usually present and may lead to further ischemic atrophy. The final picture is difficult to distinguish from end-stage renal disease caused by other types of glomerular disease (e.g., membranous glomerular disease) and can even be confused with diseases which are not primarily glomerular, such as hypertensive nephropathy or chronic pyelonephritis.

Cameron, J. S.: The natural history of glomerulonephritis. *In* Black, D. A. K. (ed.): Renal Disease. 3rd ed. Oxford, Blackwell Scientific Publications, 1972, p. 295.

611. RENAL INVOLVEMENT IN CONNECTIVE TISSUE DISEASES

Many generalized diseases of connective tissue may cause glomerular disease which may be difficult to distinguish, on either clinical or histologic grounds, from other forms of glomerulonephritis.

Systemic Lupus Erythematosus.   Some 50 to 75 per cent of patients with this condition develop renal disease at some time. It is an example of immune-complex glomerular injury, the complexes consisting of DNA (antigen), IgG, and complement. Glomerular involvement takes several forms: (1) segmental areas of glomerulitis, with hypercellularity and thickening of the basement membrane; (2) a membranous type of glomerulopathy without cellular proliferation; and (3) a diffuse proliferative glomerulonephritis with cellular proliferation, areas of glomerular necrosis, and crescent formation. These changes are not specific for lupus erythematosus, but their appearance in a patient with serologic and systemic evidence of that disease is sufficient to establish the cause of the glomerular lesion.

Renal involvement may be manifested clinically as a symptomless proteinuria which remains unchanged for months or years, with nephrotic syndrome, or with a severe progressive acute glomerulonephritis. Once renal failure has developed, the course is usually one of steady deterioration, leading to death in renal failure within a few months unless the patient is put on a renal replacement program. Steroids in high dosage (45 mg or more of prednisolone daily) have long been used in the treatment of active forms of lupus, and there is a strong impression that they produce benefit in the nephritis, although this has never been the subject of a properly randomized clinical trial. Patients with localized areas of glomerulitis appear to do best, whereas there is little evidence of benefit in those with diffuse proliferative glomerulonephritis. Various cytotoxic drugs (especially the nitrogen mustards and azathioprine) have also been used, but the number of patients reported has not been sufficient to decide on the benefit of such treatment.

Periarteritis Nodosa.   Small arteries of the kidney may be affected, leading to macroscopic infarcts of the renal substance, or there may be the microscopic form first described by Davson, Ball, and Platt, in which glomerular arterioles and capillaries are involved, leading to a proliferative glomerulonephritis which closely resembles other types of this disease but usually shows a more segmental pattern.

Although the systemic manifestations of the disease may affect any organ of the body, skin involvement seems particularly common in those with renal disease, and is often manifested as small tender areas, 2 to 4 mm across, representing infarcts in the pulp of the fingers and toes. Subungual splinter hemorrhages, if numerous, may have the same significance. However, it is not uncommon for renal disease to be the sole clinical manifestation of a polyarteritis.

The renal presentation may be that of a repeated renal infarction with local pain and hematuria, of an acute oliguric nephritis, or of chronic glomerulonephritis with proteinuria and steady reduction in renal function. Renal hypertension is common.

Usually the course is progressive deterioration, particularly in those with the microscopic form of the disease. Large doses of steroids appear to halt the progress of the disease in a small proportion of cases, and steroid-induced remissions of several years have been recorded. Rarely the disease appears to become stationary spontaneously, or there may even be temporary periods of improved renal function.

Wegener's Granulomatosis.   This entity is discussed in Ch. 105. The renal lesions may contain small granulomas in relation to blood vessels in glomeruli; otherwise the kidney disease cannot be distinguished from classic polyarteritis.

Although it may be months or years before the syndrome is complicated by renal involvement, the progression of the renal disease is usually rapid once it appears, leading to uremia within a few months. Steroids have been used in treatment, with little effect, but more recently encouraging results have been obtained with cytotoxic drugs, particularly cyclophosphamide, the renal disease either becoming stationary or showing actual improvement. No controlled trial of this treatment has been reported, but the course of the untreated renal disease is so uniformly bad that this treatment is worthy of trial.

Anaphylactoid Purpura (Henoch-Schönlein Syndrome). In anaphylactoid purpura hematuria may be caused by bleeding from the mucosal surface of the ureters, bladder, or urethra. Occasionally, however, anaphylactoid purpura causes a true glomerulonephritis, which clinically resembles a poststreptococcal acute glomerulonephritis. This resemblance is enhanced if the disease follows a streptococcal infection, as is often the case. However, serum complement is not diminished, and renal biopsy shows focal rather than diffuse glomerulonephritis. The glomerular lesions are unusual in that they may show deposits of IgA on immunofluorescence, often accompanied by fibrin. It is generally believed, although the evidence is not convincing, that complete renal recovery is less common than after a poststreptococcal nephritis; but it must be remembered that recurrent attacks of anaphylactoid purpura are common, and the possibility of permanent renal damage may be greater for that reason. The course of the disease in patients whose glomerulonephritis does not resolve completely is very like that of other forms of glomerulonephritis, except that the nephrotic syndrome appears to be less common.

Goodpasture's Syndrome (Lung Purpura and Nephritis). Goodpasture's syndrome is a form of acute progressive glomerulonephritis accompanied by massive capillary hemorrhage into the lungs. The primary cause is unknown, but the glomerulonephritis appears to be caused by circulating anti-GBM antibodies (see Fig. 2) which also react with the basement membrane of the pulmonary alveoli. Histologically the renal lesion is difficult to distinguish from other forms of acute proliferative glomerulonephritis, except that it may initially show focal features. Within a few weeks the glomerular disease usually becomes generalized, with glomerular obliteration by epithelial crescents. The lungs show massive confluent alveolar hemorrhage, identical with that seen in the rare condition *idiopathic pulmonary hemosiderosis;* the pulmonary capillaries show patchy basement membrane changes, but it is usually difficult to see changes gross enough to account for the amount of blood in the alveoli.

No age is exempt, but the disease is most common in the second and third decades, and males are affected three or four times as often as females. The first symptom is usually recurrent hemoptysis, and only after days or weeks do manifestations of nephritis occur, most often hematuria. The pulmonary hemorrhage is often very severe, with symptoms and signs of acute blood loss; after repeated episodes an iron deficiency anemia may appear, owing to a sequestration of large amounts of iron in the lungs as hemosiderin. Occasionally the first manifestations are those of subacute glomerulonephritis, and only after several weeks does pulmonary hemorrhage indicate the presence of a generalized disease.

In most cases the renal lesion progresses rapidly to total glomerular destruction, often passing through a nephrotic phase, and leading to uremia within a few weeks or months of the onset of symptoms. Death may also result from pulmonary hemorrhage, either from asphyxia or acute blood loss. Treatment is usually without influence on the course of the disease, although there have been reports of long remissions after treatment with steroids. Hemorrhage into the lungs sometimes ceases after bilateral nephrectomy, and in cases in which lung hemorrhage is life-threatening this drastic form of treatment, combined with maintenance hemodialysis or renal transplantation, may have to be considered.

Hemolytic-Uremic Syndrome. This affects infants and young children and, less frequently, young adults. It is characterized by thrombocytopenia, microangiopathic hemolytic anemia, and acute progressive renal failure. Histologically the renal lesion is a proliferative glomerulonephritis, less frequently a patchy cortical necrosis.

The hematologic manifestations appear to be secondary to vasculitis, which may be generalized or confined to the glomeruli. Minor degrees of the same blood changes are common in all forms of acute glomerulonephritis, or diffuse small vessel vasculitis, and for this reason many authorities do not accept the hemolytic-uremic syndrome as a separate disease entity, but regard it as a syndrome with many causes, including poststreptococcal nephritis and polyarteritis. However, because the condition has sometimes occurred in small local outbreaks and is much more common in some communities, e.g., Argentina and Chile, than in others, it has been suggested by some that there might be an infective basis.

The condition often starts with evidence of acute gastroenteritis with bloody diarrhea, but whether this is infective or due to vascular lesions in the bowel is uncertain. Fever, pulmonary symptoms, cutaneous purpura, and neurologic features (especially convulsions and coma) are common. It is difficult to ascertain in an individual case whether the diffuse organ involvement is caused by underlying vasculitis or by local hemorrhage resulting from the thrombocytopenia, which is often profound.

Renal involvement is shown by hematuria and the rapid development of oliguric renal failure, without clinical remissions. Milder cases occur, but when renal failure develops it seldom improves; the few recoveries that have been reported have often followed treatment with steroids or heparin.

The Kidney in Systemic Sclerosis (Scleroderma). Although systemic sclerosis may affect the kidney, it is unusual among connective diseases in that it does not cause glomerulonephritis. Instead there is a slowly progressive obliteration of renal arteries of interlobular size or smaller, and of the renal arterioles, morphologically identical to the vascular involvement of other organs. Histologically the vascular changes closely resemble those of malignant hypertension and radiation nephritis. The usual clinical manifestations, if indeed there are any, include mild proteinuria, slowly progressive renal failure, and renal hypertension, which may be severe. Treatment of hypertension may be required, but otherwise there is no treatment for the renal lesion.

Benoit, F. L., Rulon, D. B., Theil, G. B., Doolan, P. D., and Watten, R. H.: Goodpasture's syndrome. A clinicopathologic entity. Am. J. Med., 37:424, 1964.

Clarkson, A., Lawrence, J., Meadows, R., and Seymour, A.: The haemolytic uraemic syndrome in adults. Quart. J. Med., 39:227, 1970.

Lieberman, E.: Hemolytic-uremic syndrome. J. Pediatr., 80:1, 1972.

Meadow, S. R., Glasgow, E. F., White, R. H. R., Moncrieff, M. W., Cameron, J. S., and Ogg, C. S.: Schönlein-Henoch nephritis. Quart. J. Med., 41:241, 1972.

Pollak, V. E., Pirani, C. L., and Schwartz, F. D.: The natural history of the renal manifestations of systemic lupus erythematosus. J. Lab. Clin. Med., 63:537, 1963.

Walker, W. G., Harvey, A. M., and Yardley, J. H.: Renal involvement in myeloma, amyloidosis, systemic lupus erythematosus, and other disorders of connective tissue. *In* Strauss, M. B., and Welt, L. G. (eds.): Diseases of the Kidney. 3rd ed. Boston, Little, Brown & Company, 1972, p. 825.

612. HEREDITARY NEPHRITIS
(Alport's Syndrome)

Definition. Hereditary nephritis is a form of hereditary renal disease, characterized histologically by glomerulonephritis and interstitial nephritis, frequently associated with nerve deafness.

Genetic Aspects and Incidence. The disease is inherited as an autosomal dominant. Males and females are approximately equally affected, but the disease usually takes a more serious form and is manifest at an earlier age in men. Patients with renal disease frequently have nerve deafness, and some members of the family may have deafness with normal renal function. Ophthalmologic defects, such as cataracts and lenticonus, occur less frequently.

Several hundred cases have been reported, but it is very difficult to make the diagnosis in sporadic cases or in families without deafness, and the true incidence is probably many times greater.

Etiology and Pathology. The nature of the underlying defect is unknown. Histologically the renal lesion may be a chronic proliferative glomerulonephritis, often with segmental glomerular lesions; in other patients the glomeruli appear normal, but there is an extensive interstitial nephritis which resembles pyelonephritis or analgesic nephropathy. Most writers have remarked on the fat-laden foam cells in the interstitium, but these are common in other forms of renal disease, and their presence cannot be regarded as diagnostic.

Clinical Manifestations. The first symptom is usually hematuria, often noticed in childhood, and frequently preceded by a systemic infection. Proteinuria is usually present, but is seldom severe enough to cause the nephrotic syndrome. Occasionally frank attacks of pyelonephritis occur, with positive urine cultures. The usual course is slow deterioration in renal function, often with hypertension, leading to renal failure in the third to fifth decade. Nerve deafness can develop at any age; initially it affects high tones predominantly, and may be unsuspected until revealed by audiometry.

Diagnosis. The diagnosis is often difficult because no single known feature of the disease is absolutely diagnostic. The most helpful features are nerve deafness in the patient or immediate relatives and familial renal disease. However, to be convincing, the family history should include more than one generation, for the presence of glomerulonephritis in several sibs might be the result of simultaneous infection with a nephritogenic Streptococcus during earlier childhood. Sporadic cases may be confused with other forms of chronic glomerulonephritis, with the syndrome of focal nephritis and recurrent hematuria described above, or with familial renal tubular defects which are occasionally associated with nerve deafness.

Treatment. No treatment is known to alter the progress of the renal disease, but patients may require treatment for urinary infections, for renal hypertension, or for symptomatic renal failure.

Perkoff, G. T.: Hereditary chronic nephritis. *In* Strauss, W. B., and Welt, L. G. (eds.): Diseases of the Kidney. 3rd ed. Boston, Little, Brown & Company, 1971, p. 1275.

613.   RENAL VEIN THROMBOSIS

Increased renal pressure can give rise to heavy proteinuria alone or to all the manifestations of the nephrotic syndrome. This association has occasionally been reported in constrictive pericarditis, congestive cardiac failure, or thrombosis of the inferior vena cava, but it is more often the result of thrombosis of the renal veins.

There are five main varieties of renal vein thrombosis:

1. Thrombosis of the inferior vena cava with secondary involvement of the renal veins. Usually patients have a history of deep venous thrombosis of the legs or repeated pulmonary emboli. The full clinical picture of inferior vena caval obstruction, with conspicuous superficial and anastomotic veins, takes time to develop and is not always apparent.

2. Renal vein thrombosis associated with pregnancy. The cause of the association is unknown; it may be the result of stasis of the blood in the renal veins, caused by pressure of the gravid uterus, or a manifestation of the thrombotic tendency of pregnancy.

3. Obstruction of the renal veins or inferior vena cava by external pressure or neoplasm. Renal carcinoma, which often grows along the lumen of the renal veins, is one of the common causes in this category.

4. Renal vein thrombosis secondary to primary renal disease. This is the most common type of renal vein thrombosis. The main predisposing factor to thrombosis is probably a reduced renal blood flow. Thrombosis, usually bilateral, starts in the renal vein radicles, and only later extends to the main renal veins, whence parts of the thrombi may break away and cause pulmonary emboli. Although patients with many different types of renal disease are at risk, the condition appears to be particularly common as a complication of renal amyloidosis.

5. Primary renal vein thrombosis. This may complicate acute gastroenteritis, particularly in infants, perhaps as a result of increased blood viscosity caused by saline depletion, or there may be no obvious predisposing cause.

Pathology. When renal vein thrombosis is sudden and complete, as in the primary variety in children, the result is hemorrhagic infarction of the kidney. More often thrombosis is slowly progressive, allowing time for an anastomotic circulation to develop. The kidney is enlarged as a result of interstitial edema. The glomeruli show surprisingly little histologic change, and in some cases are virtually normal or merely enlarged. However, there is usually a mild diffuse thickening of the capillary basement membrane which resembles idiopathic membranous disease, even under the electron microscope, except that the thickening tends to be less marked. The glomerular capillaries are widely patent, and often show margination of leukocytes. There may be considerable tubular atrophy and interstitial cellular infiltration. None of these histologic changes are absolutely specific, and the findings on renal biopsy are not usually diagnostic except on the rare occasion when the biopsy includes a thrombosed vein.

Clinical Manifestations. Local pain and swelling may result from edema of the kidney with stretching of the renal capsule. Other clinical features depend very much on the cause of the thrombosis, but two developments are usual—nephrotic syndrome and renal failure. In patients who already have these features because of primary renal disease, there is sudden deterioration which often enables the diagnosis to be suspected. In patients without primary renal disease the picture is very similar to the insidious onset of the nephrotic syndrome of idiopathic membranous disease, and no doubt many patients are incorrectly so diagnosed; features which should arouse suspicion are severity of the nephrotic syndrome (protein losses of 40 to 80 grams a day may occur), the presence of local pain, coincident development of renal failure early in the course, pulmonary emboli, caval thrombosis, and the finding of marked interstitial edema and cellular infiltration in the renal biopsy.

Radiology may make a significant contribution to diagnosis. Venography of the inferior vena cava may show obstruction to this vein, thrombi protruding into the cava from the orifices of the renal veins, or reduced streaming of blood from the renal veins; when combined with the Valsalva maneuver, in which caval blood usually refluxes into the renal veins, phlebography may reveal obstruction to the main renal veins or filling of an anastomotic venous circulation.

Prognosis. In those with underlying renal disease the outlook for renal recovery is grave, and even with all modern resources these patients usually die unless treated with a renal replacement program.

In those without prior renal disease the prognosis is

less serious, although renal failure, gross nephrotic syndrome, and the risk of pulmonary embolization are all hazards. Fortunately renal function usually improves eventually, because of either recanalization or the development of anastomoses, but further attacks of renal vein thrombosis may occur. Renal hypertension is not usually a problem, but there is a risk of secondary pyelonephritis. In patients who survive, the features of nephrotic syndrome gradually relent, although they may take years to disappear.

Treatment. Nephrectomy is often recommended in acute renal vein thrombosis of childhood when the disease is unilateral; the value of the operation is controversial, but its proponents claim that the removal of the infarcted organ may prevent local infection or hypertension, and may reduce the spread of thrombosis. In adults nephrectomy has not been popular, although it is reasonable to believe that it would cure the nephrotic syndrome in the rare cases of unilateral renal vein thrombosis. The main aspects of treatment are anticoagulation, which needs to be continued for very long periods, treatment of the complicating nephrotic syndrome and renal failure, and, when necessary, the use of some form of dialysis.

Harrison, C. V., Milne, M. D., and Steiner, R. E.: Clinical aspects of renal vein thrombosis. Quart. J. Med., 25:285, 1956.
Rosenmann, E., Pollak, V. E., and Pirani, C. L.: Renal vein thrombosis in the adult. A clinical and pathological study based on renal biopsies. Medicine, 42:269, 1968.

614. RENAL CHANGES IN OTHER SYSTEMIC DISEASES

DIABETES MELLITUS

Although the renal complications of diabetes mellitus include capillary necrosis and pyelonephritis, the most serious and relentlessly progressive lesion is *intercapillary glomerulosclerosis (Kimmelstiel-Wilson lesion)* in which nodular deposits of eosinophilic material arise within the lobules of the glomerular tuft, and are associated with diffuse mesangial thickening, obliteration of the basement membrane, and gradual obliteration of the glomerular capillaries.

Glomerular lesions may be present in the prediabetic state, but it is unusual for them to give rise to clinical features until after the development of overt diabetes, and they are first seen most commonly in patients who have been known to have had diabetes for at least 10 to 15 years. Although the pathogenesis of the lesions is not clear, it seems likely that they are part of a generalized small vessel change which is also responsible for diabetic retinopathy and neuropathy. These three complications of diabetes are often found together; in particular, patients with renal disease almost invariably have retinal complications. There is no good evidence that careful control of diabetes influences the development of the glomerular lesion.

Patients with known diabetes usually have their urine tested frequently, and the first sign of glomerulosclerosis is therefore apt to be proteinuria, which may persist unchanged for years. Sooner or later the proteinuria increases and gives rise to the nephrotic syndrome. From then on the course is more rapidly progressive, with steady deterioration in renal function, leading within months to renal failure, often accompanied by severe hypertension. No treatment is known to alter the course of the renal disease. Patients with end-stage uremia may be kept alive by intermittent hemodialysis, but are often not considered suitable for renal transplantation because of the difficulty experienced in controlling diabetes in patients given large doses of steroids. The nonrenal complications of diabetes, particularly the blindness from proliferative retinitis, are apt to cause difficulties even with maintenance hemodialysis.

Churg, J., and Dolgen, H.: Diabetic renal disease. *In* Strauss, W. B., and Welt, L. G. (eds.): Diseases of the Kidney. 3rd ed. Boston, Little, Brown & Company, 1971, p. 873.

AMYLOIDOSIS

Although systemic amyloidosis exists in several different forms that tend to affect different groups of organs, all forms are liable to attack the kidney, and renal failure is the most common cause of death from amyloidosis.

In the early stages renal amyloid causes considerable renal enlargement, but later the kidneys shrink to normal or subnormal size. The glomeruli and small arteries are the usual sites of deposition; tubules are affected less often. Glomerular involvement histologically resembles that of idiopathic membranous disease, except that the lesions are more nodular and often appear to be on the capillary side of the basement membrane. Renal amyloid usually stains well with Congo red, methyl violet, or thioflavine T; occasionally it does not take up these dyes and then can only be recognized with certainty by the electron microscope, which shows a characteristic fibrillary structure with a periodicity of 80 to 100 Å.

The first sign of amyloid is usually proteinuria, which may persist unchanged for years, but it occasionally disappears temporarily. More severe renal involvement causes nephrotic syndrome or renal failure. It was formerly believed that renal amyloidosis does not cause hypertension; this view is incorrect, although hypertension may be less common than in other forms of glomerular disease. Renal vein thrombosis is a very serious complication of amyloidosis, and should be suspected whenever a patient suddenly develops oliguric renal failure or marked worsening of nephrotic syndrome.

Although it is widely believed that cure or surgical removal of sepsis leads to regression of secondary amyloid, this is not a common event as far as the kidney is concerned, and amyloid may persist or accumulate further despite removal of the cause. Certainly it is not justifiable to submit patients to heroic surgery, which would not otherwise be warranted, simply because of the existence of amyloid. Treatment of nephrotic syndrome and renal failure caused by amyloid follows conventional lines. The value of prophylactic anticoagulants in preventing renal vein thrombosis is uncertain.

Very occasionally patients show a sodium-losing tendency and require a small salt supplement. This feature, so unusual in glomerular disease generally, may here be the result of deposition of amyloid in the adrenal cortex or distal renal tubules. Rarely other tubular syndromes, including nephrogenic diabetes insipidus and renal tubular acidosis, have been encountered in renal amyloidosis with unusually severe tubular involvement.

Patients with severe uremia from amyloidosis are eligible for intermittent hemodialysis, but they may be unsuitable for renal transplantation because of the danger that the steroids and cytotoxic drugs given to suppress transplant rejection lead to a flare-up of the original sepsis.

Triger, D. R., and Joekes, A. M.: Renal amyloidosis—a fourteen year follow-up. Quart. J. Med., 42:15, 1973.

615. BENIGN POSTURAL PROTEINURIA
(Orthostatic Proteinuria)

Benign postural proteinuria is a condition in which proteinuria occurs in the erect or lordotic position but disappears in recumbency, and in which there is no other clinical evidence of renal disease.

The condition—hardly a disease—appears to be most common in children and young adults, particularly men, although to some extent this distribution may be the result of their more frequent urine examinations. The condition is usually discovered at a routine medical examination for employment or medical insurance, and its incidence has been stated to be as high as 2 to 3 per cent in military recruits.

Characteristically the proteinuria cannot be demonstrated by conventional tests (Albustix or salicylsulfonic acid) in urine passed during recumbency, and is therefore absent from the urine passed immediately on waking in the morning, but it reappears after standing or placing the patient in a lordotic position while still recumbent. It is widely believed, though not proved, that subjects with this condition have a more marked lumbar lordosis on standing than the average for the population.

Postural proteinuria has long been regarded as a functional condition in which there is no morphologic abnormality in the kidney. Recent studies by Robinson and his colleagues, and others, have shown that this is untrue, for renal biopsy in a series of cases fulfilling the aforementioned criteria showed histologic glomerular lesions in the majority. A few cases showed glomerular lesions typical of some well-recognized type of glomerular disease, particularly membranous disease, but in most patients the lesions were mild and segmental, and were not sufficiently marked to merit classification as any form of glomerulonephritis. A follow-up examination ten years later showed that no subject had developed overt clinical renal disease, and that 50 per cent had lost their proteinuria, thus confirming the general belief that the condition is benign.

Benign postural proteinuria is clinically important for two main reasons: (1) It may interfere with employment of young subjects on the threshold of their adult life, because of the mistaken belief that their proteinuria is due to serious renal disease; and (2) this diagnosis may be incorrectly made in patients with more sinister types of glomerulonephritis in whom the proteinuria is increased by standing. For these reasons it is wise to submit subjects suspected of the condition to a full clinical examination, with urine microscopy (the deposit is normal in postural proteinuria), determination of creatinine clearance, and intravenous pyelography. Renal biopsy is not indicated unless abnormalities are revealed by the initial investigations. Selective protein clearances are of no value, as they show poor selectivity in this condition.

Robinson, R. R.: Idiopathic proteinuria. Ann. Intern. Med., 71:1019, 1969.
Thompson, A. L., Durrett, R. R., and Robinson, R. R.: Fixed and reproducible orthostatic proteinuria. VI. Results of a 10-year follow-up examination. Ann. Intern. Med., 73:235, 1970.

616. RENAL DISEASE IN PREGNANCY
Thomas F. Ferris

Because pregnancy is occasionally associated with edema, hypertension, and proteinuria, pre-existent renal disease in a pregnant woman has traditionally been viewed with alarm. However, the majority of women with renal disease can, with proper medical care, have an uncomplicated pregnancy. In most women, pregnancy does not worsen renal disease or adversely affect the ultimate prognosis.

GLOMERULONEPHRITIS

The development of *acute glomerulonephritis* during pregnancy usually results in fetal death. Differentiation between acute glomerulonephritis and preeclampsia may be difficult if the disease occurs late in pregnancy, but the presence of microscopic hematuria with cellular and hyaline casts is most consistent with glomerulonephritis. The treatment of the disease is similar to that in the nonpregnant patient, with careful control of blood pressure and fluid balance. The danger of pregnancy in women with *chronic glomerulonephritis* is increased incidence of preeclampsia. When proteinuria is the only manifestation of chronic glomerulonephritis, the incidence of preeclampsia is 35 per cent, with fetal survival around 80 per cent. If azotemia and hypertension precede the pregnancy, the incidence of preeclampsia rises to over 75 per cent, with fetal survival less than 40 per cent. The level of azotemia and hypertension best correlates with the risk of preeclampsia and fetal loss. Control of hypertension throughout pregnancy and careful observation of BUN, creatinine, and uric acid, particularly in the last trimester, are essential for a successful pregnancy. When preeclampsia develops early, termination of the pregnancy is indicated, because there is little chance for fetal survival in this group, and the renal disease may worsen.

PYELONEPHRITIS

Acute pyelonephritis occurs in approximately 1 per cent of pregnant women, but in 30 per cent of women who have bacteriuria greater than 100,000 organisms per milliliter on their first prenatal visit. The incidence of bacteriuria is no greater in pregnancy, but the higher incidence of pyelonephritis is attributable to the dilatation of the urinary tract which occurs with pregnancy and which results in stasis and incomplete emptying. Two thirds of all cases of pyelonephritis during pregnancy can be prevented by treatment of asymptomatic bacteriuria. The relationship between asymptomatic bacteriuria, prematurity, fetal loss, and preeclampsia is unclear, because patients with chronic renal disease are more apt to have bacteriuria.

SYSTEMIC LUPUS ERYTHEMATOSUS

The course of systemic lupus erythematosus is varied during pregnancy. Most patients either have no change or an improvement in the symptoms of the disease. Aggravation of lupus seems to occur more frequently post partum. Whether this is a specific effect of the pregnancy or of demands made on the new mother is unclear. The course of lupus nephropathy during pregnancy is similar to that of chronic glomerulonephritis; patients with hypertension and azotemia preceding pregnancy have an increased incidence of preeclampsia, whereas patients with normal renal function usually have uncomplicated pregnancies.

POSTPARTUM RENAL FAILURE

The rapid development of renal failure has been reported to occur from one to ten weeks post partum with findings at autopsy of malignant nephrosclerosis. Evidence of intravascular coagulation is found in some patients with thrombocytopenia, fibrin degradation products in the serum, and findings on renal biopsy of interarteriolar and interglomerular thromboses. The disease has been termed "postpartum hemolytic-uremic syndrome" by some; its cause may have a relationship to preeclampsia in which fibrin deposits are present in glomeruli and evidence of a consumptive coagulopathy is occasionally seen. There is some evidence that anticoagulant therapy may be of benefit in postpartum renal failure.

TOXEMIA OF PREGNANCY

Toxemia of pregnancy is a disease occurring in late pregnancy, characterized by hypertension, edema, and proteinuria. Historically, convulsions have been the hallmark of toxemia, and the disease has been divided into eclampsia (Greek, eclampsis: a sudden flash) and preeclampsia, based upon whether a convulsion has occurred. Although the presence of convulsions is usually indicative of severe disease, separating toxemia on this basis does not imply different causes, and may have no more validity than separating other hypertensive processes associated with convulsions, e.g., acute glomerulonephritis and malignant hypertension.

Incidence. The disease occurs in 5 to 10 per cent of pregnancies, but the reported incidence depends upon criteria used to make the diagnosis and on the population studied. Hypertension alone has been reported to occur during the first pregnancy in 25 per cent of women in Great Britain. There is a bimodal frequency of the disease, with peak incidences in young primiparous women and in multiparous women over 35. Toxemia is more common with pre-existing renal disease, hypertension, and diabetes, with twin pregnancies, and in black women.

Clinical Manifestations. The usual sequence of manifestations is edema and hypertension followed by proteinuria; occasionally proteinuria precedes hypertension. Because normal pregnancy is characterized by reduction in blood pressure, particularly in the second trimester, blood pressures higher than 130 systolic and 80 diastolic should be considered abnormal during pregnancy. Diastolic hypertension is more striking than systolic with toxemia, and systolic blood pressures greater than 180 to 200 mm Hg usually indicate that preceding hypertensive disease existed. Toxemia typically begins after the thirty-second week of pregnancy, but may occur as early as the twenty-fourth week, particularly in women with pre-existing renal disease or hypertension. It can occur during the first trimester with a hydatidiform mole. Excessive weight gain during pregnancy predisposes to its development, probably through mechanisms similar to those associating obesity with hypertension; but sudden weight gain is caused by edema. The edema is similar to that seen in acute glomerulonephritis, with prominent distribution in the periorbital region, hands, and ankles. Headache, visual disturbances, or midepigastric pain are frequent symptoms. On funduscopic examination, segmental arteriolar narrowing and a wet glistening retina ("retinal sheen") are often seen. The presence of increased light reflex and tortuosity of the arterioles points to hypertensive disease having preceded the toxemia. Retinal hemorrhages and exudates are rare. The spinal reflexes may be hyperactive, and are important parameters to follow in assessing the degree of central nervous system excitability. Proteinuria ranges from trace amounts to levels seen in the nephrotic syndrome, 5 to 10 grams per 24 hours. Microscopic examination of the urine may reveal a few red blood cells, but significant hematuria or pyuria is more consistent with the presence of a primary renal disease. Although reduction in glomerular filtration occurs with toxemia, azotemia is seldom prominent because of the increase in glomerular filtration accompanying pregnancy. The low blood urea nitrogen (9 ± 2 mg per 100 ml) and creatinine (0.75 ± 0.2 mg per 100 ml) in late pregnancy are indicative of this increase, and even with a 50 to 75 per cent fall in glomerular filtration, the blood urea nitrogen and creatinine can remain within the normal range. A disproportionate reduction in urate clearance occurs in toxemia so that hyperuricemia usually precedes the development of azotemia.

Pathogenesis. The cause of toxemia is unknown. Nonspecific changes have been described in the liver, brain, heart, and adrenals, but renal biopsies have demonstrated consistent findings. The glomeruli are swollen, and the glomerular lumen is occluded by cytoplasmic swelling of the endothelial cells. Electron microscopy may reveal focal basement membrane thickening, and immunofluorescent studies have demonstrated fibrin deposits in glomeruli. These glomerular changes are distinctive for toxemia and are not seen in other hypertensive diseases.

The mechanism of the hypertension is unclear. Salt retention, caused by the reduction in glomerular filtration rate, might exacerbate the hypertension but alone would not cause it. The similarity of uterus and kidney in containing both renin and prostaglandins is of interest, because there is clinical evidence to suggest uterine ischemia as a factor in the pathogenesis of toxemia. If renin is involved, the sequence of events resulting in hypertension has not been elucidated. Plasma renin is not elevated in toxemia, but since extracellular fluid expansion and increased sensitivity to angiotensin simultaneously occur, the effect of a specific level of plasma renin on blood pressure is difficult to evaluate. Any explanation of the pathogenesis of toxemia must account not only for hypertension but also for the renal pathology and central nervous system excitability which are disproportionate to the magnitude of the hypertension.

Treatment.   Control of weight gain during pregnancy and the use of diuretics when edema appears reduce the incidence of complete expressions of the disease. With the onset of toxemia, bed rest, salt restriction, diuretics, and sedation constitute the initial therapy. If hypertension does not abate, antihypertensive drugs should be instituted. For immediate control of the blood pressure intravenous hydralazine (Apresoline), 25 to 40 mg in 500 ml dextrose and water, diazoxide, 300 mg, or methyldopa (Aldomet), 500 mg, have been efficacious. Magnesium sulfate has been widely used in toxemia, because it has both a depressant effect upon the central nervous system and a mild antihypertensive action. Barbiturates are useful in controlling central nervous system hyperexcitability, and should be used if convulsions appear imminent. The definitive therapy is termination of the pregnancy, and, provided that the fetus is viable, this should be accomplished as soon as the patient's condition is stable. When fetal size makes viability of concern, control of the disease with antihypertensive drugs and diuretics may allow time for further fetal development. If proteinuria or azotemia persists despite therapy, delivery should be accomplished; there is little evidence that fetal growth occurs in the face of persistent toxemia. Eclampsia is sufficient reason for inducing delivery, because convulsions significantly increase maternal and fetal mortality.

Prognosis.   Maternal death with toxemia is now rare. Blood pressure usually returns to normal within two weeks after delivery, although the proteinuria may persist longer. However, women who develop toxemia have a higher incidence of hypertension in later life, and the role toxemia plays in its development has been a subject of concern and controversy. The unresolved question is whether toxemia causes subsequent hypertension or simply occurs more frequently in women with latent hypertension. In women having toxemia with a multiparous pregnancy, two findings favor an underlying hypertensive diathesis as a factor in the toxemia. First, the incidence of late hypertension is greater after multiparous than primiparous toxemia; indeed, in white women with eclampsia, a higher incidence of late hypertension can be demonstrated only after a multiparous toxemia. Second, the recurrence of toxemia with subsequent pregnancies is over 50 per cent after multiparous toxemia, but only 25 per cent in women developing toxemia with the first pregnancy.

Eastman, N. J. (ed.): Williams Textbook of Obstetrics. 13th ed. New York, Appleton-Century-Crofts, 1966.

Sheehan, H. L., and Lynch, J. B.: Pathology of Toxaemia of Pregnancy. Baltimore, Williams & Wilkins Company, 1973.

617. URINARY TRACT INFECTIONS AND PYELONEPHRITIS

Calvin M. Kunin

Definition.   The phrase urinary tract infection is a broad term used to describe both bacterial colonization of the urine and invasion of structures in any part of the urinary tract. Urine is ordinarily sterile. Colonization of the urine, that is, multiplication of large numbers of bacteria in the urine, is often difficult to distinguish from actual tissue invasion eliciting a host response, because of the frequent tendency of urinary tract infections to exhibit either few or no symptoms. This phenomenon is known as *asymptomatic bacteriuria.* At any given point in time, an individual may have bacteriuria alone, or bacteriuria with silent tissue invasion, or bacteriuria accompanied by signs of inflammation of the bladder *(cystitis)* or kidneys *(pyelonephritis).* Infections of the structures of the urinary tract are usually accompanied by colonization of the urine which bathes the kidney, ureter, bladder, and urethra. Thus bacteriuria is the most common denominator of urinary tract infections. Bacteriuria may be absent, however, when the infected focus is not contiguous with the urine as in early lesions of hematogenous pyelonephritis, when there is marked obstruction of the affected portion of the tract or when it is masked by antimicrobial therapy. Bacteriuria does not necessarily indicate that the patient has pyelonephritis or cystitis. Rather, it is an important and generally reliable laboratory finding that indicates an abnormal situation, reflecting either the presence of, or potential for, infection of the urinary tract. It is an excellent guide to early diagnosis and evaluation of therapy, because signs and symptoms of infection may be absent or disappear without bacteriologic cure.

The term *pyelonephritis* refers to immediate and residual effects of bacterial infection in the kidney. The clinical manifestations are generally conceived of as existing in two forms: *acute pyelonephritis,* an active pyogenic infection, usually accompanied by local and systemic symptoms of infection; and *chronic pyelonephritis,* wherein the principal manifestations are caused by the injury sustained in preceding active infections. Actually, considerable uncertainty exists regarding the relationship between acute and chronic pyelonephritis in patients in whom no structural or neurologic abnormality affecting the urinary tract can be detected. For example, many patients known to have had multiple attacks of acute pyelonephritis show no indication of progression to chronic pyelonephritis even after intervals of many years. Furthermore, comparatively few patients thought to have chronic pyelonephritis give a history of acute infection of the urinary tract. The possibility exists therefore that some cases of the disease we are now calling "chronic pyelonephritis" result from something other than bacterial infection of the kidney. Reasons for this uncertainty include inadequacy of diagnostic procedures for diagnosis of chronic pyelonephritis and erroneous interpretation of bacteriologic findings. A large part of the problem is due to the fact that a variety of other disease states can produce renal lesions that mimic pyelonephritis (see Ch. 618).

The normal urinary tract is free of bacteria except near the external urethral meatus. In both sexes, some organisms are normally present in the distal urethra. These are usually similar to the flora of the skin, and frequently consist of staphylococci and diphtheroids. Urine is a variable culture medium, depending upon pH, tonicity, and its constituents. High concentrations of urea, low pH, hyperosmolality, and products of dietary organic acids are generally unfavorable to bacteria. In addition, the dynamics of urine flow, or washout, and antibacterial properties of the lining membrane of the urinary tract appear to be important defense mechanisms.

The large bowel is considered to be the reservoir of most of the bacteria that invade the urinary tract because of the high frequency of aerobic coliforms found in urinary tract infection. Several possible pathways from the lumen of the intestine to the urinary passages and kidney can be postulated. There has been some dispute regarding their relative importance. The principal possibilities are the hematogenous, the lymphatic, and the "ascending" routes. The "ascending" pathway, involving migration of bacteria from the anus to the periurethral zone and through the urethra to the bladder, is the most favored at present. This route can be demonstrated experimentally, particularly in the presence of obstruction or of a foreign body. It also fits in well with the very much higher rate of urinary infections in the female, whose urethra is shorter than that of the male, and with the marked frequency of urinary infections associated with instrumentation of the urethra and bladder. Clear instances of the hematogenous origin of urinary infection have been demonstrated, particularly in the presence of staphylococcal or gram-negative bacteremia, but these are relatively less common.

Pathology. Knowledge of the pathologic process is meager because uncomplicated acute pyelonephritis does not lead to death. Nevertheless, on the basis of occasional chance opportunities and experiments in animals, it is possible to describe the probable form of the lesion with reasonable assurance. One or both kidneys may be affected. The lining of the renal pelvis and calyces is diffusely inflamed. Infection of the renal substance is usually confined to one or more wedge-shaped areas, the apices being in the medulla. In this zone of acute inflammation there are micro-abscesses, some of which may bulge under the capsule of the kidney, but rarely they rupture into the perinephric area, producing *perinephric abscess.* Collections of polymorphonuclear leukocytes can be seen in and around the lumina of the tubules throughout their length. The glomeruli are usually spared structurally, but may become functionless because the tubular part of the nephron is destroyed. The infectious process tends to remain confined within the originally involved segment of renal tissue and to subside gradually over a period of one to three weeks. As healing takes place, the area contracts, polymorphonuclear leukocytes are replaced by mononuclear cells, and scar tissue is deposited. Eventually a linear scar involving a streak of medulla and corresponding cortical tissue is all that remains. Remnants of glomeruli and tubules filled with a colloid-like material lie in this fibrous matrix.

A considerable amount of work has been done on the pathogenesis of pyelonephritis in laboratory animals. The kidney can be infected either by the intravenous route or by introducing bacteria into the urinary tract; the lesion is the same regardless of the route of inoculation. In order to infect the kidney by way of the bloodstream it is necessary to inject large numbers of bacteria, probably because only a minute proportion of the inoculum is trapped by the kidney. As a general rule, coliform bacteria, although the most common cause of human pyelonephritis, are incapable of infecting a normal kidney, although pathogenic strains of Staphylococcus, enterococcus, occasional strains of Proteus, and rare strains of coliform organisms will do so. In the presence of an obstructive lesion, however, the susceptibility of

the kidney to infection by all these bacteria, including the coliforms, is greatly increased. Obstruction has been produced by introducing artificial calculi into the bladder, by partial or complete ureteral ligation, or by mechanical injury of the kidney. Even small injuries of the medulla caused by needle puncture lead to obstruction of a few collecting tubules and localized susceptibility to infection. Experiments of this kind have demonstrated that bacterial multiplication begins in the medulla and then spreads into the corresponding area of cortex. It is thought, therefore, that infection spreads in retrograde manner from the obstructed collecting tubules in the medulla throughout the nephron. Characteristic wedge-shaped areas of acute pyelonephritis involving both medulla and cortex are also produced when small numbers of bacteria, e.g., 10 to 100 living organisms, are inoculated into the medulla. By contrast, as many as 100,000 coliform bacteria must be inoculated into the cortex in order to establish even local infection. A conspicuous feature of the areas of acute pyelonephritis produced in laboratory animals is lack of tendency for infection to invade neighboring, unobstructed areas of renal parenchyma. The process remains confined to the area of intrarenal hydronephrosis, eventually "burns out," and shrinks to a scar, leaving adjacent kidney unaffected. This seems compatible with acute pyelonephritis in man, wherein there is usually no measurable evidence of even temporary impairment of renal function despite evidence that both kidneys are acutely infected. It is reasonable to presume, therefore, that the disease in man is one of patchy renal involvement, leaving large segments of tissue unaffected. Evidence obtained in animals indicates that the medullary zone is the critical one from the standpoint of pathogenesis of acute bacterial infection. Factors that may be responsible include the following: (1) *Ammonia formation.* Evidence has been obtained that high local concentration of ammonia, as may be present when the body is dealing with an acid load, may be sufficient to inactivate complement, thus rendering ineffective a major defense mechanism against bacterial infection. (2) *Hypertonicity.* The unusual osmolarity in this area of the body may be sufficient to affect the activity of complement and phagocytes, as well as to permit survival of bacterial protoplasts. (3) *Differences in the blood supply.* The blood flow to the medulla is far less than that to the cortex.

Clinical Manifestations. Symptoms of cystitis and urethritis include frequency of urination, burning pain on urination, and passage of cloudy, occasionally blood-tinged urine. The patient may complain of a foul odor to the urine, lassitude, and suprapubic discomfort. Fever and leukocytosis are rarely evident in urinary tract infection confined to the bladder and urethra; as a general rule, their presence should be looked upon as evidence of infection of the upper part of the tract. Nevertheless, absence of fever and leukocytosis does not by any means exclude the possibility of kidney involvement.

The clinical picture of acute pyelonephritis may be characteristic: sudden rise of body temperature to 38.9 to 40.6° C, shaking chills, aching pain in one or both costovertebral areas or flanks, and symptoms of bladder inflammation. Physical examination reveals tenderness in the region of one or both kidneys; at times a tender kidney may be detected by palpation. Laboratory tests show polymorphonuclear leukocytosis, and the urine is laden with leukocytes. Stain of the sediment reveals numerous bacteria, usually gram-negative bacilli, and culture confirms this. In a small proportion of cases blood culture is also positive. There are no signs of impaired renal function or of acute hypertension as is sometimes seen in acute glomerulonephritis.

In the absence of an obstructive lesion of the urinary tract, such as stone or tumor, this illness is self-limited, rarely lasting more than a week or ten days.

The clinical picture just described is easy to recognize and is seldom confused with anything else. Yet there must also be subclinical forms, because typical evidence of previous attacks of acute pyelonephritis is encountered at autopsy in patients lacking a history of symptoms of urinary tract infection. Possibly the size of the area of renal tissue involved in an episode is the determining factor. In addition to the "classic" clinical picture and the subclinical form, acute pyelonephritis at times presents with symptoms that do not point to the urinary tract. Dysuria may be lacking, and there may be no fever. There may only be backache, without demonstrable tenderness in the kidney region. Some patients have pain in either the upper or the lower abdomen, together with symptoms of disturbed gastrointestinal function. Others complain only of general fatigue. Mild anemia may be caused by repeated episodes of acute pyelonephritis. The urine can be free of pus cells or bacteria for brief periods. Repeated urinalyses on succeeding days should, however, always reveal presence of pus cells and bacteria.

Acute urinary tract infection, complicated by pyelonephritis, frequently arises in debilitated patients in hospitals and nursing homes who have been subjected to urethral instrumentation, especially the indwelling catheter. In such people the infection may take a fulminating course, with bacteremia and shock, and can in fact be the terminal event of prolonged illness. Gram-negative sepsis and bacteremic shock are described in Ch. 214.

Course. The symptoms of inflammation of the urinary tract tend to disappear after several days even without bacteriologic cure. Recurrence of symptomatic infection is frequent in this group. Bacteriuria also tends to be highly recurrent. Persistence of fever and leukocytosis strongly suggest the presence of obstruction to flow of urine by stones or other mechanical means or a large renal or perinephric abscess. In the unobstructed female patient, recurrence is usually associated with reinfection with a new bacterial strain. Early recurrence, however, may be due to emergence of bacteria from a partially suppressed focus. Persistent infection with the same organisms should alert the physician to the presence of obstruction, calculus, or neurogenic lesions. Frequent follow-up examination of the patient's urine is essential to the management to be described below.

Concept of Significant Bacteriuria. Bacteriuria literally means the presence of bacteria in the urine. The concept of "significant bacteriuria" was introduced to distinguish between bacteria that are actually multiplying in the urine from contaminants in collection vessels, periurethral tissues, the urethra itself, and gross fecal or vaginal contamination. This separation can be accomplished by knowledge of the site and manner in which the urine is collected from the patient and enumeration of the number of organisms present in the sample. The criterion of 100,000 or more organisms per milliliter of urine for diagnosis of significant bacteriuria is an excellent *operational definition* when the clean voided method is used to collect specimens. It is based on the

finding that contaminants will usually be present at numbers ranging from 1000 to 10,000 per milliliter. Organisms found in urinary tract infections grow well in urine; they usually achieve concentrations of greater than 100,000, and are often in the range of 1 to 10 million per milliliter. With proper instruction and cleansing, and prompt processing or refrigeration of specimens, it is usually not difficult to obtain reliable results by the clean voided method in both males and females. It is emphasized that, because the reliability of the method will differ with experience and care, it is often wise to avoid overdiagnosis by obtaining multiple specimens, particularly in the asymptomatic patient. Thus, survey and screening procedures for bacteriuria generally require two or three consecutive positive specimens, indicating that the patient has "persistent significant bacteriuria." Bacterial counts lower than 100,000 per milliliter may occur in patients with true bacteriuria, but when the clean voided method is used, these counts can only be established as valid when shown to be persistent and when the same species of bacteria and preferably the same serotype can be repeatedly isolated. Bacterial counts are higher when urine is allowed to incubate for some time in the bladder. A first morning specimen is preferred, but is not essential. Low or borderline counts may be due to dilution in a well-hydrated patient.

Aseptic methods of collection of urine such as from the renal pelvis or ureter, or by bladder puncture, *permit the diagnosis of significant bacteriuria regardless of the number of organisms found,* provided that the specimen is not contaminated prior to culture.

Bacteriologic Findings. The species of bacteria most likely to be recovered in individuals with bacteriuria depends, for the most part, upon previous history of infection, receipt of antimicrobial therapy, hospitalization, and instrumentation of the urinary tract. In this respect, the bacterial flora found in individuals with asymptomatic bacteriuria is no different from that in cases of clinically obvious pyelonephritis. Enterobacteriaceae are by far the most common organisms identified. *E. coli* generally accounts for more than 80 per cent of all species recovered in so-called uncomplicated cases, whereas Proteus, Klebsiella, Enterobacter, *Pseudomonas aeruginosa,* enterococci, and *Staphylococcus aureus* are more likely to be found in patients who have had previous infection or instrumentation (the so-called complicated group). Occasionally, organisms such as *Serratia marcescens,* Mima-Herellea, *Candida albicans,* and even *Cryptococcus neoformans* may be significant and produce disease in diabetics and in patients treated with corticosteroids and immunosuppressive agents. Diphtheroids, *Staphylococcus epidermidis,* and microaerophilic streptococci are highly suspect as contaminants. They usually will not be isolated on repeated culture. They should not, however, be dismissed if repeatedly recovered under optimal conditions of collection.

Despite the abundance of anaerobic flora in the gut, they are actually rare in urinary infections, presumably owing to the poor growth of these organisms in urine.

Microscopic Methods. Rapid diagnostic methods are available either by preparation of a Gram stain of unsedimented urine and examination with an oil immersion lens, or by study of the centrifuged urinary sediment for bacteria, employing the high dry objective under reduced light with or without the addition of methylene blue. The Gram stain has been the most widely used of these methods and correlates about 80 to 90 per cent with quantitative culture. Examination of the unstained sediment as prepared for search for formed elements in the urine is very helpful. It is much less time consuming than preparation of a stained slide, and can be done in conjunction with the routine examination for formed elements. This method lends itself particularly well in office practice to assessing the presence of a urinary tract infection. The criterion for a positive sediment is the presence of many (preferably more than 20) obvious bacteria. The presence of marked pyuria can mask bacteria in the sediment. Fresh urine is required, because crystals will also obscure the bacteria. If crystals do form, the urine should be warmed until they dissolve.

Ten or more leukocytes per high-powered field in the centrifuged specimen is usually accepted as representing pyuria. When inflammation of the bladder mucosa is intense, there may be some erythrocytes in the urine, and gross hematuria sometimes occurs. *Proteinuria* is not common in urinary infections.

Epidemiology and Natural History. Extensive epidemiologic studies have provided information of the frequency of bacteriuria in various populations. Bacteriuria in the newborn period has been difficult to define because of problems inherent in collection, but information is being obtained with the widespread use of the bladder puncture method. Infection of the urinary tract in this age group appears to be part of a generalized, life-threatening gram-negative sepsis, and is more common in boys than girls. Symptomatic urinary infections, particularly among girls, are prominent in the preschool years, and are frequently associated with important obstructive or neurogenic lesions. Urologic investigation is extremely valuable in this age group. *It is mandatory in males of any age because of the high frequency of important structural abnormalities* found (valves, malformations, obstructive and neurogenic lesions). The prevalence of bacteriuria among schoolgirls is 1.2 per cent; it is only 0.03 per cent in boys of the same age. The incidence rate in girls is 0.3 per cent per year; it is linear with time throughout the school years and is unaffected by menarche. The cumulative frequency or urinary infection in girls occurring at one time or another during the school years exceeds 5 per cent. Bacteriuria in schoolgirls is independent of socioeconomic status and race, and is not increased in diabetic girls. The prevalence of bacteriuria rises with age, and is increased in lower socioeconomic groups, probably because of limited antimicrobial therapy delivered to this population. Urinary infection is common after marriage. The "honeymoon cystitis" syndrome may be due to either infection or local irritation, and these should be clearly differentiated by culture. Bacteriuria in pregnancy varies from 2 to 6 per cent, depending upon age, parity, and socioeconomic groups. Early detection and treatment of bacteriuria in this age group will prevent the emergence of symptomatic infection. Elderly women may have frequencies of bacteriuria as high as 10 per cent; this rate may rise even higher in hospitalized patients, particularly diabetics. Bacteriuria in the male begins to appear in the "prostate" years, and is often initiated by instrumentation.

Role of Instrumentation. Persistent bacteriuria follows single catheterizations in relatively healthy individuals at a frequency of 1 to 2 per cent; the risk is much higher in the debilitated patient and in males with prostatic obstruction. With open indwelling catheter drainage bacterial colonization exceeds 90 per cent within three to four days. This may lead to life-threatening pyelonephritis and gram-negative sepsis. Fortunately, it is partially avoidable by (1) careful preselection of criteria for catheterization, and (2) use of aseptic closed drainage or antimicrobial bladder rinse during prolonged catheterization. The catheter should be removed as soon as it is no longer needed.

RENAL MEDULLARY NECROSIS
(Renal Papillary Necrosis, Necrotizing Papillitis)

Renal medullary necrosis is a severe complication of pyelonephritis—ischemic necrosis of the renal papilla and adjacent portions of the renal medulla. The lesion is most often, though not invariably, associated with severe acute and chronic pyelonephritis. It is especially common in patients with diabetes and pyelonephritis, about half the reported cases having involved such persons. Obstruction of the urinary tract is also regarded as a predisposing factor, but this may relate only to the aggravating effect of obstruction on infection in the kidney. European clinicians report fairly frequent occurrences of renal medullary necrosis in women who have habitually ingested large quantities of analgesic medicines containing phenacetin for headache. These patients also usually have infection of the urinary tract. The relative roles of infection and phenacetin in the pathogenesis of the lesion cannot be specified with certainty.

Although infection appears to be the most important factor in the pathogenesis of this lesion, there can be little doubt that the peculiarities of blood supply of the medulla must also be factors. This could help to explain the frequent occurrence of the lesion in patients with diabetes and generalized vascular disease, as well as the role of obstruction, which must impair the blood supply of this area.

The zone of necrosis may occur throughout the pyramid from the extreme tip as far proximally as the corticomedullary junction. Eventually this usually sloughs, so that chunks of necrotic tissue often migrate down through the urinary passages.

The clinical manifestations of renal medullary necrosis are intensification of symptoms of pre-existing pyelonephritis. There may be pain in the lumbar region, colicky pain along the ureteral radiation, and hematuria. Fever may be high. Manifestations of gram-negative bacteremia may supervene. This lesion should be considered always in elderly patients with diabetes who show rapid deterioration in clinical status with signs of active pyelonephritis and increasing renal decompensation.

The diagnosis can sometimes be made by finding pieces of renal medullary tissue in the urine sediment. Pyelography may also be of assistance: in addition to the scarring and asymmetry of chronic pyelonephritis, cavities and sinuses in the region of the papillae may be demonstrated.

Therapy is not notably effective, but should be directed toward control of infection and whatever measures can be employed to improve the status of patients who have diabetes mellitus or who are habitual abusers of analgesic medicines.

Management. The therapeutic principles are similar for all urinary infections, including bacteriuria, cystitis, or pyelonephritis. *Recognition and relief of obstruction* *are essential.* Therapy is then directed to sterilization of the urine and careful follow-up to detect recurrence, using significant bacteriuria as a guide. Infections uncomplicated by obstruction or many previous episodes will generally respond to oral therapy with sulfonamides, tetracycline, ampicillin, chloramphenicol, nalidixic acid, cephalexin, co-trimoxazole (trimethoprim plus sulfamethoxazole), or nitrofurantoin. The last-named drug is particularly useful in recurrent infections because of relatively less frequency of emergence of resistant strains. It should not be used to treat systemic infection and is contraindicated in the presence of any degree of azotemia, because adequate concentrations cannot be achieved in the urine under these conditions. Oral preparations of carbenicillin are reserved for Pseudomonas infection. Drugs are selected on the basis of relative cost, side effects, and antimicrobial susceptibility, all of which may be highly variable. Antimicrobial susceptibility tests should be used to guide therapy of recurrent episodes. The initial attack is usually due to *E. coli,* which is sensitive to most of the commonly used agents. It can be treated "blindly" with a sulfonamide, ampicillin, or tetracycline with about equal probability of success. Bacteria should disappear within 24 to 48 hours even if pyuria and symptoms continue. It is important to recognize bacteriologic failure early and change to another drug. Generally, short courses of treatment, from 10 to 14 days, are quite adequate; short-term high-dose therapy, sometimes with parenteral agents such as ampicillin, cephalothin, or gentamicin, may be required in some instances of failure with lower doses or when the patient is too ill to receive an oral agent. Recurrence within a few weeks after treatment is usually due to persistence of the same focus, whereas later recurrence, particularly in females, is more often the result of reinfection. Highly recurrent infections may be managed by either very close follow-up and treatment of each episode or by prophylaxis with nitrofurantoin, cotrimoxazole, or urinary antiseptics such as methenamine mandelate or hippurate. *The last-named agents require an acid urine,* preferably at pH 5.5. This may be achieved by addition of a high protein diet, ammonium chloride, ascorbic acid, or methionine. Methionine is an effective acidifier, but it may have to be given in doses as high as 10 grams per day. The dose can be titrated downward by measuring urinary pH. Prophylaxis should not be given for more than three to six months if at all possible. Cessation of prophylaxis permits reassessment of the patient. Prophylaxis can then be reinstituted if frequent infections recur. Some female patients require only a single dose of nitrofurantoin given at bedtime for effective prophylaxis. The drug must be changed if bacteriuria persists or recurs during treatment. This usually means that an organism insusceptible to the agent is now colonizing the urine.

The patient should be instructed to generously drink fluids and void frequently. Double voiding in patients with vesicoureteral reflux is recommended. Voiding after intercourse is felt to decrease the chance of recurrent infection. *Frequent follow-up to detect silent recurrence* is the key to good management. Quantitative urine cultures ideally should be done once monthly for the first three months after each infection and then at three-month intervals for at least two years. Recurrence even after several years of freedom from infection is not uncommon in females.

Complex urinary infections, that is, those in the pres-

ence of obstructive uropathy, neurogenic bladders, or catheters, are exceedingly difficult to eradicate and may be managed by suppressive therapy with urinary antiseptics *if shown effective,* or simply left alone unless systemic complications develop. Sepsis in these cases is usually precipitated by obstruction which should be promptly relieved. Antimicrobial therapy is discussed in Ch. 214. *Bacteriuria in the aged* is frequent, usually uncomplicated, and highly recurrent. It should not be overzealously treated if simple measures fail, because toxicity and expense of therapy may outweigh the risk of disease.

Beeson, P. B.: Urinary tract infection and pyelonephritis. *In* Black, D. A. K. (ed.): Renal Disease. 2nd ed. Oxford, Blackwell Scientific Publications, 1967.
Bengtsson, U.: A comparative study of chronic non-obstructive pyelonephritis and renal papillary necrosis. Acta Med. Scandinav. (Suppl.), 388, 1962.
Kass, E. H. (ed.): Progress in Pyelonephritis. Philadelphia, F. A. Davis Company, 1965.
Kaye, D. (ed.): Urinary Tract Infection and Its Management. St. Louis, C. V. Mosby Company, 1972.
Kleeman, C. R., Hewitt, W. L., and Guze, L. B.: Pyelonephritis. Medicine, 39:3, 1960.
Kunin, C. M.: Detection, Prevention and Treatment of Urinary Tract Infections. 2nd ed. Philadelphia, Lea & Febiger, 1974.
O'Grady, F., and Brumfitt, W.: Urinary Tract Infection. London, Oxford University Press, 1968.

618.   CHRONIC PYELONEPHRITIS

Solomon Papper

Definition. Chronic pyelonephritis is defined as a chronic disease of the kidney resulting from bacterial infection. It is characterized anatomically by an inflammatory reaction especially involving the interstitium (i.e., chronic interstitial nephritis). The interstitial tissue consists of elongated cells (interstitial cells) and their branching processes, fragments of basement membrane-like material, and collagen. The interstitium is found largely in the medulla and papillae surrounding blood vessels, loops of Henle, and collecting ducts. With time and progression, all elements of the kidney may become diseased: the vessels, the glomeruli, and the tubular structures. At the termination of its course, the anatomic features of chronic pyelonephritis may be indistinguishable from the various glomerulopathies, at which time the general term "end-stage" kidney is sometimes applied.

Chronic renal infection associated with urinary tract obstruction is common. However, there is some debate concerning the prevalence of chronic nonobstructive pyelonephritis. The diagnosis of chronic pyelonephritis without obstruction may have suffered twice from polarized excesses. At one time, the diagnosis was rarely made; most chronic renal diseases were labeled chronic glomerulonephritis. Subsequently, with greater interest in quantitative bacteriology of the urine, a tendency evolved equating chronic interstitial nephritis with pyelonephritis.

The following are some of the reasons suggesting that many, and perhaps most, instances of chronic interstitial nephritis may not be due to bacterial infection: (1) Chronic interstitial nephritis is also seen in other conditions: heavy metal nephropathy, papillary necrosis, analgesic abuse syndrome, Balkan nephropathy, nephrocalcinosis, hyperuricemia, and radiation nephritis, as well as when no cause is apparent; (2) most patients with chronic interstitial nephritis do not have a history of acute infection; (3) apparently few patients with acute pyelonephritis or chronic bacteriuria without obstruction progress to chronic renal disease; and (4) bacterial infection, when present, may not necessarily be a primary event, but rather may be superimposed on interstitial disease of other cause.

In any case, the dilemma of how often chronic, nonobstructive pyelonephritis occurs as a primary disease is still with us. Therefore we divide chronic pyelonephritis into two categories according to the presence or absence of structural and/or functional abnormalities of the urinary tract. This also serves to emphasize the importance of a search for such mechanical abnormalities in patients with bacteriuria, as well as in patients with renal disease of unknown nature.

Pathology. Grossly, the kidneys may appear irregular in outline, giving evidence of underlying scar formation, with normal areas between the scars. This emphasizes the fundamental focal, wedge-shaped nature of the condition. In some instances, the two kidneys differ considerably in size, a circumstance viewed by some authors as more consistent with pyelonephritis than with other forms of interstitial nephritis, but this is not established fact. On microscopic examination, one sees a chronic inflammatory reaction (lymphocytes and plasma cells) of the interstitial tissue with ultimate scar formation. The scarring results in distortion of the tubular structures — some small and some dilated tubules which may be filled with eosinophilic casts ("colloid casts"). The glomeruli, although frequently surrounded by a cuff of fibrosis, are spared until relatively late, when they, too, may sclerose. Vascular involvement is variable, but in patients with hypertension, afferent arteriolar sclerosis is found. In recent years, abnormalities of the papillae, including papillary sclerosis and deformity, have been found. Dilatation of one or several calyces with cortical scar formation directly over the dilated calyx is regarded by some as diagnostic of chronic pyelonephritis as distinguished from other forms of interstitial nephritis.

When structural or functional obstruction is present, there may also be diffuse dilatation of the pelvis and calyces.

As stated, if the lesion of interstitial nephritis is sufficiently advanced and uniform, it may be indistinguishable from glomerulonephritis.

Pathogenesis. The particular predilection of the renal medulla to infection is of interest. This may be a consequence of a relatively low blood flow and medullary hypertonicity. The latter has been shown to inactivate phagocytosis, as well as complement-mediated bactericidal activity. Obstruction of the urinary tract may add to medullary vulnerability to infection.

In patients with urinary tract obstruction, there may be virtually constant renal infection with consequent progressive tissue damage. Obstruction results in increased pressure in the conduit system which in and of itself may result in abnormal structure and function of the kidney.

The mechanism of progression in nonobstructive pyelonephritis is less evident. It is possible that as acutely infected areas heal, scar tissue is formed. The latter may cause destruction of adjacent renal structure, including the development of areas of intrarenal hydronephrosis.

The latter are more susceptible to new infection, and so the process of infection causing scar, which in turn predisposes to infection, may be self-perpetuating and may account for the heterogeneous anatomic appearance of scar tissue, chronic inflammatory reaction, and acute inflammation, as well. Another possible mechanism of continued renal damage with or without persistent bacterial infection has its basis in the observation that bacterial antigen persists in the kidney long after the disappearance of viable bacteria. It is therefore possible that previous asymptomatic renal infection initiates the disease, and persistent bacterial antigens lead to its progression by immunologic mechanisms.

There are some factors other than structural and functional abnormalities in the urinary tract that may predispose to chronic pyelonephritis. Some of these, such as pregnancy and diabetes mellitus, remain unproved, although highly suspect as predisposing features. However, instrumentation, sickle cell trait, and other underlying renal disease are well-established factors.

Clinical Manifestations. *Pyelonephritis with Mechanical Abnormalities of the Urinary Tract.* The major structural and functional alterations in the urinary tract predisposing to chronic pyelonephritis are (1) mechanical obstruction, (e.g., enlarged prostate, congenital malformations, renal calculi), (2) neurogenic bladder, and (3) vesicoureteral reflux (see Ch. 625). In some patients, obstructive symptoms are evident. In others, infection or the uremic syndrome is the only manifestation of obstructive uropathy. Because urinary tract infection is far less likely to be cured in the presence of obstruction and because obstruction itself is potentially destructive, it is critical that every patient with infection have radiographic examination of the urinary tract. In some instances, intravenous urography suffices; in others, special radiographic studies for vesicoureteral reflux and cystoscopy are needed.

Pyelonephritis without Mechanical Abnormalities of the Urinary Tract. It is in this group of patients that the problem of chronic pyelonephritis versus other forms of chronic interstitial nephritis presents itself. As previously stated, even the presence or absence of bacteriuria may not distinguish the nature of the underlying process. Chronic pyelonephritis may be associated with periods of "inactivity" without bacteriuria, whereas, on the other hand, bacterial infection may be superimposed on a renal disorder of different cause. In considering other causes of chronic interstitial nephritis, it is especially important to explore the more treatable ones, e.g., analgesic abuse syndrome, heavy metal nephropathy, and urate nephropathy.

When a patient has a long history of episodes of urinary tract infection, decreased renal function, pyuria, white blood cell casts, and bacteriuria and the pyelogram shows an irregular renal outline caused by cortical scars and caliectasis, the diagnosis of chronic pyelonephritis is established. However, this "classic" picture is present in relatively few patients.

Patients more often present as follows: (1) a urinalysis done for other reasons reveals white blood cells, bacteria, and little protein; (2) the blood urea nitrogen determined as a screening test for other purposes may be elevated in a patient previously not suspected of renal disease; (3) the manifestations of renal functional insufficiency may present insidiously when renal disease has not been suspected, i.e., anorexia, nausea, vomiting, fatigue, weight loss, nocturia, polyuria, and anemia.

Inadequately explained splenomegaly is a common accompaniment of chronic pyelonephritis.

The characteristics of the nephrotic syndrome, i.e., heavy proteinuira and edema, are not features of pyelonephritis.

The relation of hypertension to pyelonephritis remains incompletely resolved. It seems that there are patients with unilateral pyelonephritis whose hypertension is cured by nephrectomy. Whether the mechanism is the same as in renovascular hypertension is not known. It seems agreed that when renal failure develops in patients with chronic pyelonephritis, hypertension often occurs. However, it is conceivable that this is a feature of the renal failure rather than of the disease itself. On the other hand, many patients with chronic pyelonephritis never develop high blood pressure. The matter is further complicated by the higher incidence of urinary tract infection in patients with essential hypertension and nephrosclerosis.

Laboratory. *Urinalysis.* The urine generally has white blood cells, ranging from few to many. Red blood cells may be present, but generally in small numbers. White blood cell casts may be seen. More than a trace to one-plus proteinuria is uncommon, and 24-hour urinary protein is surely less than 3 grams and usually less than 1.5 grams. Bacteria may or may not be present. Glitter cells which are not diagnostic of chronic pyelonephritis may be seen with special stains; these are polymorphonuclear cells containing granules that exhibit brownian movement.

Renal Function. Early in the course of chronic pyelonephritis, even before azotemia develops, the medullary interstitial reaction may result in tubular dysfunction, especially of the loop of Henle and collecting ducts. This may result in (1) a defect in concentrating ability, sometimes with polyuria, (2) sodium wasting, and (3) disturbed urinary acidification. The latter may cause hyperchloremic acidosis.

Later in the course, there are the evidences of generalized functional deterioration, including reduction in glomerular filtration and renal plasma flow, as well as tubular functional impairment. When severe enough, renal failure ensues.

Pyelography. The renal size may be normal early in the course, whereas later small kidneys are characteristic, except when obstruction is present. Classically, the renal outlines are described as irregular because of cortical scar formation, and one or more calyces are blunted, dilated, and distorted. As stated, some authorities regard a dilated calyx with overlying cortical parenchymal scar as unique to chronic pyelonephritis, as distinguished from other varieties of interstitial nephritis. However, there appear to be instances of chronic pyelonephritis in which these features are absent, i.e., the pyelogram may be normal.

Renal Biopsy. Since the lesion of pyelonephritis is not uniformly distributed in the parenchyma, biopsy may be normal. If diseased tissue is obtained, it can only disclose interstitial nephritis, not its cause. However, early enough in the course, biopsy can exclude glomerulonephritis.

Course. If there is a remediable obstructing lesion treated surgically early enough in the course, the disease may not progress. In the absence of structural malformation, the course is extremely variable. The disease may progress very slowly and be asymptomatic for many years. Even when renal failure and azotemia ensue, appropriate care of the body fluids may be associated with a prolonged period of months to years of reasonably comfortable life.

In those patients who have hypertension, vascular complications, especially coronary artery disease and cerebral vascular disease, may determine an unfavorable course before renal failure does.

Treatment. If a remediable obstructing lesion is found, this should be corrected promptly with operative care. If successfully accomplished, antimicrobial agents are more likely to be effective in eradicating infection, and a stable or even improved state may result.

In the absence of obstruction, the approach to antimicrobial treatment described in Ch. 617 should be undertaken.

Hypertension should be treated to prevent vascular complications. If renal failure is already present, antihypertensive therapy must be undertaken with special care, because deterioration of renal function may follow the lowering of blood pressure.

The treatment of renal failure, including nondialytic measures, dialysis, and renal transplantation, is considered in Ch. 603 and Ch. 605 to 607.

Beeson, P. B.: Urinary tract infection and pyelonephritis. *In* Black, D. A. K. (ed.): Renal Disease. 2nd ed. Oxford, Blackwell Scientific Publications, 1967.

Braude, A. I.: Current concepts of pyelonephritis. Medicine, 52:257, 1973.

Freedman, L. R.: Urinary tract infection, pyelonephritis, and other forms of chronic interstitial nephritis. *In* Strauss, M. B., and Welt, L. G. (eds.): Diseases of the Kidney. Boston, Little, Brown & Company, 1971.

Heptinstall, R. H.: Pathology of the Kidney. Boston, Little, Brown & Company, 1966.

Hodson, C. J.: The radiological contribution toward the diagnosis of chronic pyelonephritis. Radiology, 88:857, 1967.

Kincaid-Smith, P., and Fairley, K. F. (eds.): Renal Infection and Renal Scanning. Melbourne, Australia, Mercedes Publishing Services, 1970.

Kleeman, C. R., Hewitt, W. L., and Guze, L. B.: Pyelonephritis. Medicine, 39:3, 1960.

Papper, S.: Clinical Nephrology. Boston, Little, Brown & Company, 1971.

OTHER SPECIFIC RENAL DISEASES
William B. Schwartz

619. THE NEPHROPATHY OF POTASSIUM DEPLETION

Potassium depletion often produces characteristic structural and functional disturbances in the kidney. The changes occur regardless of the cause of the depletion; primary aldosteronism, Cushing's syndrome, renal tubular disorders such as Fanconi's syndrome, and gastrointestinal losses from diarrhea or vomiting can all produce a deficit great enough to induce renal injury. It is not certain how long potassium deficiency must be present before renal abnormalities can occur. Occasionally, renal disease has been recognized in a patient who has been depleted for only several weeks, but in most instances depletion has been present for months or years.

The characteristic histologic changes in the kidney consist of multiple vacuoles in the tubular epithelium, usually most numerous in the proximal convolutions. These vacuoles (which do not contain fat or glycogen) are virtually pathognomonic of the disease. In most patients, however, the tubular abnormalities are less specific and are limited to mild degenerative changes or to diffuse foamy swelling. The glomeruli and blood vessels are usually not involved. Occasionally, despite striking functional abnormalities, the histologic appearance of the kidney is entirely normal.

The most frequent and striking functional abnormality is an inability to concentrate the urine even after prolonged restriction of water or after the administration of vasopressin. Diluting ability, on the other hand, is usually well preserved. The exact nature of the defect in concentrating power in man is not known, but it would appear from studies in animals that inability to establish a normal degree of medullary hypertonicity and reduced permeability of the collecting ducts to water are both important factors.

Many patients have no urinary symptoms, but in some, nocturia, polyuria, and polydipsia are prominent complaints. Occasionally these symptoms are of sufficient severity to suggest the diagnosis of diabetes insipidus. The polyuria and related symptoms probably result from impaired concentrating ability, although it has also been proposed that excessive fluid intake induced by a primary abnormality of the thirst mechanism may contribute.

Examination of the urine may reveal slight proteinuria and cylindruria, but often no abnormalities are found. Tubular excretion of phenolsulfonphthalein and para-aminohippurate is often reduced. Blood urea nitrogen and creatinine concentrations are ordinarily within normal limits or only slightly elevated, but frank azotemia may be induced by complications such as sodium depletion, hypotension, or pyelonephritis. Renal potassium wasting is *not* a feature of the disease; its presence indicates that an underlying disorder of adrenal or renal origin is responsible for the potassium depletion.

Pyelonephritis is said to occur with unusual frequency in patients with the nephropathy of potassium depletion, but, in view of the relative frequency with which pyelonephritis complicates virtually all types of renal disease, it is difficult to attach any special significance to this observation.

In some instances, urinary abnormalities, slight azotemia, and inability to concentrate the urine lead to an erroneous diagnosis of irreversible renal disease such as chronic glomerulonephritis. In other instances, kidney injury resulting from potassium depletion may complicate pre-existing renal disease and contribute to the development of serious renal failure.

Repair of potassium deficiency is usually followed within several months by improvement or correction of renal functional abnormalities. Serial renal biopsies indicate that in most instances the structural abnormalities can be completely reversed within a few months to a year.

Hollander, W., Jr., and Blythe, W. B.: Nephropathy of potassium depletion. *In* Strauss, M. B., and Welt, L. G. (eds.): Diseases of the Kidney. Boston, Little, Brown & Company, 1971.

Schwartz, W. B., and Relman, A. S.: Effects of electrolyte disorders on renal structure and function. N. Engl. J. Med., 276:383, 452, 1967.

620. THE NEPHROPATHY OF HYPERCALCEMIA

Hypercalcemic nephropathy is characterized in its early stages by tubular injury and polyuria, and in its late stages by progressive renal insufficiency. The changes in structure and function of the kidney are similar, regardless of the metabolic disturbance responsible for elevation of serum calcium concentration. The usual causes of hypercalcemic nephropathy are *hyperparathyroidism, sarcoidosis, vitamin D intoxication, excessive ingestion of milk and alkali (milk-alkali syndrome, Burnett syndrome), multiple myeloma, malignant disease,* and, less frequently, *immobilization* (particularly in *Paget's disease*) and *hyperthyroidism.*

The characteristic pathologic changes are in the collecting ducts and in the distal convoluted tubules, the epithelium in both areas showing degenerative changes and often necrosis and calcification. Calcified casts, which form in sites adjacent to tubular injury, lead to obstruction of nephrons with resultant dilatation of proximal segments. In longstanding hypercalcemia, calcification of the interstitium and occasionally of the glomeruli and vessels leads to progressive scarring and loss of renal mass. At this stage hypertension often develops, and the resultant nephrosclerotic changes may come to dominate the histologic picture.

Clinical findings vary with the duration and severity of the hypercalcemia. Moderate elevations of serum calcium concentration produce a clinical picture characterized initially by evidence of tubular dysfunction. Injury to the distal nephron impairs the countercurrent mechanism for concentrating the urine and leads to polyuria and polydipsia. Tubular secretory capacity is affected, as evidenced by impairment of phenolsulfonphthalein excretion. Azotemia develops only after a prolonged period and is a consequence of obstruction of nephrons rather than of primary glomerular injury. The urine frequently contains a small quantity of protein as well as casts, erythrocytes, and leukocytes. Roentgenographic examination of the abdomen may demonstrate *nephrocalcinosis,* which is usually seen chiefly in the area of the renal pyramids. Patients with hypercalcemia are likely to have hypercalciuria and therefore to develop *renal calculi,* often complicated by pyelonephritis.

It is worth emphasizing that, when an elevated serum calcium concentration is found in a patient with renal insufficiency, it should be assumed, at least initially, that the calcium disorder is primary since renal failure with secondary hyperparathyroidism rarely produces hypercalcemia. Hypercalcemia occurs with significant frequency, however, in patients with chronic renal failure who undergo successful renal transplantation; in these patients persistence of the parathyroid hyperplasia characteristic of secondary hyperparathyroidism may lead to a state of *autonomous hyperparathyroidism (tertiary hyperparathyroidism)* and to elevations in serum calcium concentration sufficient to threaten the integrity of a transplanted kidney. Transient hypercalcemia has also been noted as an uncommon finding during recovery from *acute renal failure.*

Hypercalcemic nephropathy is best treated by correcting the underlying metabolic disorder. Removal of a parathyroid adenoma, control of hyperthyroidism, discontinuance of excessive milk and alkali intake, or ambulation of the patient with Paget's disease usually leads to prompt reduction of the serum calcium concentration to normal. Reduction in serum calcium concentration after withdrawal of excessive vitamin D is generally slower, but can be hastened by administration of corticosteroids. Steroids may also be effective in the hypercalcemia of a sarcoidosis, metastatic bone disease, and multiple myeloma.

Severe hypercalcemia (15 to 20 mg per 100 ml) presents a special therapeutic problem because it may produce a syndrome characterized by rapidly progressive renal failure, oliguria, confusion, lethargy, and coma. This syndrome of so-called *hypercalcemic crisis* is seen most frequently in association with hyperparathyroidism and with malignant disease. It usually proves fatal within a short time unless a prompt reduction in serum calcium concentration is effected. As an initial approach to accomplishing such a reduction it is current practice to administer 2 to 3 liters of normal saline intravenously over a period of six to nine hours. The expansion of extracellular volume depresses the proximal reabsorption of calcium and thus increases calcium excretion. The concomitant administration of a diuretic such as furosemide serves to further enhance the excretion of calcium, and to accelerate the fall in serum calcium concentration. When diuretic therapy is employed, fluid balance must be followed closely and saline given in quantities sufficient to avoid contraction of the extracellular fluid; if contraction is allowed to occur, it will enhance calcium reabsorption and lower urinary calcium excretion. Still a further technique for lowering serum calcium concentration is the administration of mithramycin, which exerts its effect by diminishing skeletal resorption. Mithramycin usually produces a marked reduction in serum calcium concentration within one or two days. If hypercalcemia does not respond adequately to other measures, it can usually be quickly controlled by the intravenous administration of inorganic phosphate. Phosphate salts are thought to act both by increasing calcium deposition in bone and by diminishing bone resorption. The usual program of treatment consists of the infusion of 500 ml of a buffered 0.1 molar phosphate solution (1.5 grams of phosphorus) over eight or nine hours. The chief risk attendant on such treatment is that of producing severe hypocalcemia; but, with the regimen described above, such an occurrence is uncommon unless renal failure and a diminished ability to excrete phosphate lead to marked hyperphosphatemia. In the patient with renal insufficiency the period of infusion should generally be extended to 24 hours; serum calcium concentration should be measured several times during this interval.

Phosphate therapy may also be of use for the prolonged management of mild or moderate hypercalcemia that cannot be controlled by therapy directed toward the underlying disease state. For example, in certain patients with malignancies the daily oral administration of 1 to 3 grams of phosphorus (as sodium phosphate) may provide the only effective means of holding calcium concentration at or near normal levels. Whether or not such treatment entails an appreciable risk of producing clinically significant soft-tissue calcification has not as yet been clearly determined.

The prognosis in hypercalcemic nephropathy depends on the severity and chronicity of the renal disease. Renal failure of recent onset induced by acute hypercalcemia is often completely reversible. However, renal insufficiency that has developed gradually in association with chronic hypercalcemia is often little affected by restoration of a normal serum calcium concentration; when improvement occurs, it is likely to be slow, sometimes taking many months. The prognosis is particularly poor if severe hypertension and nephrosclerosis are present. Nevertheless, in every instance of hypercalcemia a vigorous effort should be made to restore the serum concentration to normal in the hope of preserving remaining

renal function or of at least slowing the advance of renal insufficiency.

For additional discussion of hypercalcemia, see Ch. 872.

Epstein, F. H.: Calcium and the kidney. Am. J. Med., 45:700, 1968.

Goldsmith, R. S., and Ingbar, S. H.: Inorganic phosphate treatment of hypercalcemia of diverse etiologies. N. Engl. J. Med., 274:1, 1966.

Massry, S. G., Mueller, E., Silverman, A. G., and Kleeman, C. R.: Inorganic phosphate treatment of hypercalcemia. Arch. Intern. Med., 121:307, 1968.

Schwartz, W. B., and Relman, A. S.: Effects of electrolyte disorders on renal structure and function. N. Engl. J. Med., 276:383, 452, 1967.

Singer, F. R., Neer, R. M., Murray, T. M., Keutmann, H. T., Deftos, L. J., and Potts, J. T.: Mithramycin treatment of intractable hypercalcemia due to parathyroid carcinoma. N. Engl. J. Med., 283:634, 1970.

Suki, W. N., Yium, J. J., Von Minden, M., Saller-Hebert, C., Eknoyan, G., and Martinez-Maldonado, M.: Acute treatment of hypercalcemia with furosemide. N. Engl. J. Med., 283:836, 1970.

621. RENAL TUBULAR ACIDOSIS

Renal tubular acidosis (RTA) is an uncommon disease characterized by a defect either in urinary acidification ("distal" RTA) or in bicarbonate reabsorption ("proximal" RTA). The tubular abnormality in both forms of RTA may occur as either a *primary* or a *secondary disorder*.

DISTAL RENAL TUBULAR ACIDOSIS
(Type 1 RTA)

The characteristic abnormality in distal RTA is an inability of the tubule to establish a normally steep concentration gradient for hydrogen ion between blood and tubular fluid. The cardinal clinical finding is that urine pH, even in the face of severe metabolic acidosis, cannot be reduced to a value of less than 6.0.

Primary distal RTA is a disease of unknown origin that often becomes overt during infancy or early childhood but sometimes first manifests itself in early adult life. In some cases the disease is familial, occurring as an autosomal dominant with a variable degree of expression and greater penetrance in females. There are numerous clinical complications of primary distal RTA, the most notable of which are discussed here.

Osteomalacia: Hypophosphatemia and a high rate of phosphate excretion, i.e., increased phosphate clearance, are typical features of the disease and are often accompanied by roentgenologic evidence of rickets or osteomalacia. The clinical and roentgenologic manifestations are closely similar to those encountered with vitamin D deficiency or with resistance to vitamin D. In addition to the disturbance in phosphate metabolism, an important contributory factor to the development of osteomalacia appears to be the metabolic acidosis. In some patients, osteomalacia produces bone pain as its primary manifestation; in others, the initial clinical difficulty is a disturbance in gait resulting from abnormal skeletal growth.

Hypercalciuria and renal calculi: Hypercalciuria is an almost constant feature of the disease and frequently leads to the formation of renal calculi. A low urinary citrate excretion is thought by some investigators to contribute to the tendency to form stones. Symptoms of renal colic are frequent and may be the first manifestations of the underlying tubular disease. Complications of renal calculi, such as ureteral obstruction or pyelonephritis, are encountered commonly and are often responsible for both secondary renal damage and hypertension. Diffuse calcification of the renal medulla (*nephrocalcinosis*) is a characteristic, though not consistent, roentgenologic finding and at times is an important clue to diagnosis.

Hypokalemia and muscle weakness: Hypokalemia, accompanied by continued renal excretion of potassium (renal potassium wasting), is commonly present. The loss of potassium results from an impaired ability of the distal tubule to secrete hydrogen ion, with the result that a larger than normal fraction of sodium-cation exchange takes place by exchange with potassium. The major deleterious effects of potassium deficiency are on the musculoskeletal system and the kidneys. On occasion severe potasssium depletion may lead to quadriplegia and a clinical picture that closely mimics *familial periodic paralysis* (see Ch. 480). Longstanding potassium deficiency of the magnitude encountered in RTA is also prone to produce *hypokalemic nephropathy* (see Ch. 619).

Renal insufficiency: In the early stages of the disease, kidney function is typically normal or only slightly impaired; but over a period of many years there is usually a progressive loss of function which culminates in severe renal insufficiency. The major factors responsible for renal damage appear, as mentioned earlier, to be obstructive uropathy and pyelonephritis.

Secondary distal RTA is seen in a variety of disease states. It has been noted with particular frequency in *hyperglobulinemic states* (e.g., Sjögren's syndrome, cryoglobulinemia), in *amphotericin B nephropathy*, and after *renal transplantation*. It is also seen as a complication of certain *genetically transmitted systemic diseases* such as Fabry's disease. Few data are yet available on the natural history of secondary distal RTA.

PROXIMAL RENAL TUBULAR ACIDOSIS
(Type 2 RTA)

Proximal RTA is characterized by a defect in proximal bicarbonate reabsorption which increases the delivery of bicarbonate to the distal nephron and thus overwhelms the normal acidifying mechanism. The inherent acidifying capacity of the distal tubule is preserved, however, so that if plasma bicarbonate concentration (and thus filtered load of bicarbonate) is reduced sufficiently to allow nearly complete proximal reabsorption of bicarbonate, urinary pH falls to a level of less than 5.5.

Primary proximal RTA occurs chiefly in male infants and has as its sole clinical manifestations metabolic acidosis and growth retardation. Osteomalacia and nephrocalcinosis do not occur. Treatment with alkali and correction of the acidosis lead to a marked improvement in the rate of growth. Within a few years the defect in bicarbonate reabsorption usually disappears, and alkali therapy can then be safely discontinued.

Secondary proximal RTA is seen in association with multiple abnormalities of tubular function in such genetically transmitted disorders as cystinuria (see Ch. 820) and *Wilson's disease* (see Ch. 945), with the administration of *outdated tetracycline*, and in a variety of metabolic disorders, including *secondary hyperparathyroidism*.

The potassium deficiency in "proximal" RTA has a different cause from that seen in the "distal" form of the disease; in proximal RTA, potassium wasting results not from a defect in distal hydrogen ion secretion but from a flooding of distal exchange sites with sodium bicarbonate and consequent acceleration of sodium-cation exchange.

Treatment of Proximal and of Distal Renal Tubular Acidosis. The treatment of renal tubular acidosis consists of the administration of alkalinizing salts, such as sodium bicarbonate or sodium citrate, in quantities sufficient to restore plasma bicarbonate concentration to normal or nearly normal levels. In "proximal" RTA, in which there may be a gross defect in bicarbonate reabsorption, large quantities of alkali (as much as 5 to 10 mEq per kilogram of body weight per day) are sometimes required in order to achieve this purpose.

Correction of potassium deficiency is also an important therapeutic goal. In nearly all patients with "distal" RTA, correction of acidosis will in itself lead to retention of dietary potassium and repair of the potassium deficit; but in patients with "proximal" RTA, administration of supplemental potassium will usually be required to achieve repair.

If severe bone disease is present, treatment with large doses of vitamin D may be indicated; but if such therapy must be employed, serum calcium concentrations should be followed carefully because of the risk of hypercalcemia. In some patients, hypercalcemia will develop before the goal of restoring serum phosphorus to normal is achieved.

Gill, J. R., Bell, N. H., and Bartter, F. C.: Impaired conservation of sodium and potassium in renal tubular acidosis and its correction by buffer anions. Clin. Sci., 33:577, 1967.
Morris, R. C., Sebastian, A., and McSherry, E.: Renal acidosis. Kidney Int., 1:322, 1972.
Nash, M., Torrado, A. D., Greifer, I., Spitzer, A., and Edelmann, C.: Renal tubular acidosis in infants and children. J. Pediatr., 80:5, 1972.
Rodrigues-Sorianao, J.: The renal regulation of acid-base balance and the disturbance noted in renal tubular acidosis. Pediatr. Clin. North Am., 18:529, 1971.

622. THE NEPHROPATHY OF ACUTE HYPERURICEMIA

Acute uric acid nephropathy occurs as the result of a sudden, marked elevation of serum uric acid concentration in patients undergoing intensive treatment for leukemia or lymphoma. This disorder, though relatively infrequent, is a serious complication that can lead to progressive renal failure, anuria, and death. It can occur with any form of treatment, such as cortisone, radiation, or chemotherapy, that abruptly reduces the number of circulating white cells or diminishes the mass of splenic and lymphoid tissue. The increase in the size of the uric acid pool results primarily from the metabolism of nucleic acid released during the process of cellular destruction. With massive cellular destruction, uric acid concentration occasionally reaches a level as high as 50 to 75 mg per 100 ml.

Severe hyperuricemia is most likely to occur in patients with pre-existing hyperuricemia or in whom there is already some impairment of renal function that restricts the ability to excrete an abnormally large uric acid load. The untoward effects on kidney function result either from obstruction of ureters and pelvis by masses of uric acid or from intrarenal precipitation of uric acid within the collecting ducts and the distal tubules. Deposition in the proximal tubules ordinarily does not occur. The observed pattern of deposition can readily be understood if it is appreciated that at a pH above 7.0, uric acid (pK 5.5) is present almost entirely as the highly soluble urate anion, whereas at a pH of 5 to 6 a large fraction is present as the un-ionized and poorly soluble uric acid. Thus it is only in the distal tubule and collecting duct, where marked acidification of the filtrate takes place, that conversion of urates to uric acid creates a condition favorable to uric acid precipitation. Abstraction of water by the distal nephron and the resulting increase in uric acid concentration in the urine are undoubtedly additional factors favoring precipitation in the tubules and the pelvo-ureteral system.

The single most important consideration in uric acid nephropathy is *prophylaxis*. Until relatively recent years the most effective means of preventing renal injury was through the administration of alkalinizing agents in quantities sufficient to keep the urine pH above 7, the excess uric acid in both tubules and urinary tract thus being maintained in a soluble state. To achieve this goal sodium bicarbonate has to be administered at frequent intervals during the day and a carbonic anhydrase inhibitor (such as Diamox) at bedtime. Now, however, *allopurinol*, a potent inhibitor of xanthine oxidase, provides an even more reliable and physiologic approach to prophylaxis. Allopurinol, by blocking the conversion of hypoxanthine and xanthine to uric acid, prevents a rise in serum uric acid concentration (and in uric acid load delivered to the kidney), even in the face of extensive destruction of neoplastic tissue. When used in doses of 200 to 800 mg per day, it virtually eliminates the hazard of acute uric acid nephropathy.

When a patient presents with the problem of uric acid nephropathy and azotemia, cystoscopy and retrograde examination should be carried out in order to make certain that extrarenal obstruction is not present. If uric acid deposits are found to be blocking the pelvis and ureters, irrigation may serve to relieve the obstruction, but in some instances a pyelostomy will be necessary. In those instances in which obstruction is intrarenal rather than extrarenal, one should attempt to reduce plasma uric acid concentration and to alkalinize the urine in the same fashion as described above in the consideration of prophylaxis.

In some instances, osmotic diuresis with mannitol is helpful in initiating urine flow in the oliguric patient. If such efforts are ineffective, and if anuria or severe azotemia persists, some form of dialysis should be used for the purpose of removing uric acid and dealing with the clinical and chemical manifestations of the uremic state. Despite all these measures, there is a high mortality rate among patients who develop severe hyperuricemic nephropathy, and, as mentioned earlier, prevention of renal damage should always be the primary concern.

DeConti, R. C., and Calabresi, P.: Use of allopurinol for prevention and control of hyperuricemia in patients with neoplastic disease. N. Engl. J. Med., 274:481, 1966.
Frei, E., III, Bentzel, C. J., Rieselbach, R., and Block, J. B.: Renal complications of neoplastic disease. J. Chronic Dis., 16:757, 1963.
Muggia, F. M., Ball, T. J., and Ultmann, J. E.: Allopurinol in the treatment of neoplastic disease complicated by hyperuricemia. Arch. Intern. Med., 120:12, 1967.

623. BALKAN NEPHRITIS

During recent years a chronic and progressive nephritis of unknown cause has been noted in a large percentage of the population living in certain areas of Yugoslavia, Bulgaria, and Rumania. The disease occurs only in small villages located in valleys along river bottom land, and is not seen in neighboring cities or in adjacent foothills or mountains. Approximately one third of the population in the endemic areas has been found to have some evidence of renal disease, such as proteinuria, and between 5 and 10 per cent have been found to have significant azotemia. Several members of the same family are often affected by the disease. Proteinuria occurs in adolescents and in young adults, but azotemia is rarely encountered in patients under the age of 30 to 40 years.

The cause is unknown, and epidemiologic studies to date have not been fruitful. The renal lesion is apparently not the consequence of a previous streptococcal infection, of urinary tract infection, or of the excessive use of analgesics such as phenacetin. It is not related to exposure to toxic agents such as cadmium or lead, or to other factors such as the water supply, nutrition, alcohol intake, or economic status. A curious feature is that people who move out of the affected area in childhood almost never develop the disease, whereas those who move into the area frequently develop renal disease, usually in a period of about ten years. Further studies on various environmental factors are obviously required and are, in fact, in progress.

The kidneys in the patient with the advanced form of the disease are characteristically small, their weight averaging 40 to 60 grams. The most severe atrophy is noted at the outer portion of the cortex, the deeper portions of cortex being more or less spared. From both biopsy and postmortem examination it appears that the primary lesion involves the interstitium and the tubules rather than the glomeruli. Interstitial fibrosis is prominent and there is a minimal infiltration of round cells. Many tubules are atrophied, and the remaining tubules are often hyperplastic and show mitotic figures. The glomeruli are relatively uninvolved and appear to degenerate only late in the course of the disease, apparently as a consequence of the interstitial lesion.

The clinical picture in Balkan nephritis is characterized by an insidious onset, usually without a history of edema or hematuria. The urine is found to contain small quantities of protein, usually not exceeding 1 gram per day; and the sediment is scanty, containing only a few leukocytes and erythrocytes and an occasional cast. It is noteworthy that blood pressure is usually normal, though in a small percentage of cases hypertension has been noted. Diminished concentrating ability occurs early, a finding consistent with the histologic observation that tubular damage is a prominent feature of the disease. Hyperchloremic acidosis gives further evidence that injury to tubules is out of proportion to glomerular injury. Renal failure, once present, generally progresses slowly, usually over a five- or ten-year period, to a fatal termination. There is no specific treatment. The most pressing problem remains that of determining the cause of the disease.

Griggs, R. C., and Hall, P. W.: Investigations of chronic endemic nephropathy in Yugoslavia. *In* Metcoff, J. (ed.): Renal Metabolism and Epidemiology of Some Renal Diseases. York, Pennsylvania, The Maple Press Company, 1964, p. 312.
Hall, P. W., Dammin, G. J., Griggs, R. C., Fajgelj, A., Zimonjic, B., and Gaon, J.: Investigation of chronic endemic nephropathy in Yugoslavia. II. Renal Pathology. Am. J. Med., 39:210, 1965.
Wolstenholme, G. E. W., and Knight, J. (eds.): The Balkan Nephropathy. Boston, Little, Brown & Company, 1967.

624. ANALGESIC NEPHROPATHY

Studies over the last two decades have demonstrated a remarkably high incidence of renal disease among individuals who ingest large quantities of analgesics. Early reports laid the responsibility for analgesic-induced renal damage on phenacetin, but with continued observations it has become apparent that singling out phenacetin as the sole etiologic factor is not justified; phenacetin is typically given as part of pain-relieving compounds containing agents such as aspirin and caffeine, and available evidence suggests that such agents in combination are usually responsible for the development of renal damage.

The circumstantial evidence relating excessive ingestion of analgesics to the development of renal disease is impressive, but there are those who remain unconvinced that there is such an entity as analgesic nephropathy. The skeptics note that not all epidemiologic studies have demonstrated an increased incidence of renal damage among abusers of analgesics; they also note that most investigators have found it difficult to produce renal damage in animals given analgesics in doses equivalent to those consumed by patients. Nevertheless, the weight of the epidemiologic findings strongly supports the view that excessive analgesic intake often does produce kidney disease and, indeed, that it produces disease of a rather characteristic type.

Pathology. The characteristic pathologic findings of analgesic nephropathy consist of interstitial nephritis and extensive papillary necrosis. The interstitial lesion typically consists of round cell infiltration with associated severe tubular atrophy and mild glomerular sclerosis. The mechanism through which the renal lesions are produced remains undefined, but it has been suggested that the primary toxic effect of analgesics is on the papillae and that interstitial damage occurs secondarily. It should be emphasized that papillary necrosis, seen in the absence of pyelonephritis, urinary tract ob-

struction, or diabetes mellitus (see Ch. 617), should strongly raise the possibility of analgesic abuse.

Clinical Manifestations. The typical patient with analgesic nephropathy has taken ten or more analgesic tablets a day for eight to ten years or longer. However, some individuals who have taken as few as five tablets a day for only a few years have also been observed to develop renal injury.

Analgesic nephropathy occurs most commonly in women; in nearly all studies there is a three- to fivefold predominance of females over males. Most patients attribute their intake of medication to headaches or musculoskeletal discomfort, but a considerable number have no somatic complaints and have taken analgesics solely for the psychotropic effects. Even among patients with physical complaints there is a remarkably high incidence of psychoneurotic difficulties, notably depression and anxiety. Most observers believe that emotional problems are a near-constant feature in those who abuse analgesics.

It should be emphasized that some patients with analgesic nephropathy steadfastly deny the use of medications. Thus when the diagnosis is suspected, it may be necessary to speak with the family or local pharmacist in order to obtain accurate historical data regarding drug exposure.

A third or more of patients who abuse analgesics have a history of peptic ulceration or gastritis, and many of these also give a history of gastric surgery. The upper gastrointestinal difficulties are thought to be the consequence of injury to the gastric mucosa produced by continued exposure to analgesic compounds.

Patients with analgesic nephropathy often develop gross hematuria and renal colic, findings almost always accounted for by necrosis and sloughing of renal papillae. Occasionally a sloughed papilla will obstruct the ureter, and fulminant pyelonephritis may ensue; in the patient with pre-existing renal damage this sequence of events often produces a rapid and life-threatening deterioration of renal function.

The physical examination is usually unremarkable

Tomogram of a kidney demonstrating renal papillary necrosis in a patient with analgesic nephropathy. Arrows indicate "ring shadows" in two calyces.

save for the frequent presence of hypertension. Laboratory studies ordinarily reveal mild to moderate anemia, small quantities of protein in the urine, and pyuria. The urine is often sterile even in the face of pyuria, but organisms in significant numbers are found in approximately one third of patients. The finding of pyuria without bacteriuria should itself raise the possibility of chronic interstitial nephritis. Renal function may be normal at the time that the patient is first seen, but in most instances it is already somewhat impaired.

In the patient with moderate or severe kidney disease, x-ray examination by intravenous pyelography almost always demonstrates small kidneys and calyceal clubbing. These findings are indistinguishable from those of chronic pyelonephritis, but when seen in association with evidence of papillary necrosis (such as a "ring sign"), they point strongly towards a diagnosis of analgesic nephropathy (see accompanying figure).

Treatment.   Patients with renal dysfunction who continue to ingest analgesics usually develop progressive renal failure. However, those who discontinue the ingestion of drugs will often, for a period of years, show little further deterioration of function. The stability of function in the face of moderate or severe renal damage is almost unique for analgesic nephropathy. Remarkably, some patients who discontinue analgesics may even demonstrate a significant rise in filtration rate and concomitant striking reduction in plasma creatinine concentration. These prognostic considerations emphasize the importance of dissuading the patient from the continued ingestion of analgesic medications.

Gault, M. H., Rudwal, T. C., Engles, W. B., and Dossetor, J. B.: Syndrome associated with the abuse of analgesics. Ann. Intern. Med., 68:906, 1968.

Linton, A. L.: Renal disease due to analgesics. 1. Recognition of the problem of analgesic nephropathy. Can. Med. Assoc. J., 107:749, 1972.

Murray, R. M., Lawson, D. H., and Linton, A. L.: Analgesic nephropathy; clinical syndrome and prognosis. Br. Med. J., 27:479, 1971.

Nanra, R. S., and Kincaid-Smith, P.: Chronic effect of analgesics on the kidney. Prog. Biochem. Pharmacol., 7:285, 1972.

625.   OBSTRUCTIVE NEPHROPATHY*

Francis P. Muldowney

Back pressure arising from urinary tract obstruction may result in important structural and functional derangements of the kidney, and obstructive uropathy is one of the most frequent etiologic factors in patients presenting with unexplained uremia. Clinical progress may be deceptively slow or viciously accelerated, depending on whether obstruction is incomplete or complete, and especially on whether infection is also present. Since obstruction is clearly a remediable cause of kidney damage, accurate diagnosis and appropriate management assume considerable importance for restoration and preservation of renal function.

Etiology (see accompanying figure). The many causes of obstruction may be considered under three headings: those inside the lumen of the urinary conduit (intraluminal), those within the wall (intramural), and those causing pressure from outside. The accompanying table lists the major causes in each category. In unilateral (nonuremic) cases, the ureteropelvic junction is a common site of obstruction under all three etiologic headings. In bilateral (uremic) cases the most frequent causes are prostatic obstruction and urinary stone, comprising together some 55 per cent, with bladder tumor contributing a further 20 per cent. Retroperitoneal fibrosis is covered in detail in Ch. 107.

Incidence and Prevalence.   Obstructive lesions of the urinary tract have been found in 3.8 per cent of a large series of routine autopsies. Corresponding figures from a population of uremic subjects at autopsy show a rise to fully 25 per cent, including those in whom obstructive uropathy was either a contributory or a major factor. A much higher relative incidence of obstructive versus other causes of renal disease is to be expected in particular at-risk age groups such as infants and children on the one hand (congenital strictures or ureteropelvic dysfunction) or elderly males (prostatic obstruction) on the other.

Pathogenesis and Pathology.   In slowly developing or partial obstruction gross dilatation of the renal pelvis and calyces may occur, especially when the impedance is situated high up—for example, at the ureteropelvic junction. In such cases, the distended sac may accommodate 2 to 3 liters of fluid, with a greatly thinned renal cortex, but clinical manifestations may be few. When infection has supervened, pyonephrosis with total destruction of renal parenchyma is the end result, usually with correspondingly severe clinical manifestations. When obstruction develops rapidly or is complete, distention of the renal pelvis and calyces is much less but intraluminal pressure above the level of obstruction may be very high. Correspondingly severe symptoms of loin pain, caused by distention of the renal capsule, or ureteral colic, caused by repeated ureteric peristaltic waves, are usually present. Occasionally, however, complete obstruction of one ureter may occur with very little evidence of back pressure or dilatation, resulting nevertheless in gradual total loss of renal function on that side if not relieved within four to six months. In general, the degree of renal damage is related to the duration of obstruction. In either situation, the occurrence of infection behind the obstruction, either blood-borne or introduced during diagnostic instrumentation, transforms the clinical picture into an acute pyrexial illness with fever, accompanied by rapid destruction of renal tissue.

Infection is therefore an important determinant of the pathologic, functional, and prognostic picture. In lower urinary tract lesions, infection tends to occur early in the disease but is often relatively slow in progression. In upper urinary tract lesions, infection may not occur until much later but runs a more rapidly destructive course. In either case, the most important factor predisposing to infection is instrumentation of the urinary tract, by bladder catheter, cystoscope, or ureteral catheter.

Clinical Manifestations.   Obstructive nephropathy is one of the most important causes of that ubiquitous nephrologic problem, "unexplained uremia," and, as mentioned above, is present at least as a contributory factor in 25 per cent of such cases at autopsy. All patients presenting with renal failure, or in whom there is abrupt deterioration of renal function unexplained by their primary renal problem, should be carefully screened to exclude onset of obstruction.

*The assistance of Mr. Daniel G. Kelly, F.R.C.S., in the preparation of this manuscript is gratefully acknowledged.

OBSTRUCTIVE NEPHROPATHY — CAUSES

Common sites of urinary tract obstruction.

Equally important is the mode of presentation in the form of recurrent urinary tract infection. Symptoms caused by complicating infection are commonly the presenting complaint with obstructive lesions at all levels. Persistent or recurrent urinary tract infection should always raise the suspicion of an obstructive lesion, even when specific localizing symptoms are absent.

In lower urinary tract lesions, the history of pattern of micturition provides an extremely useful guide to both diagnosis and treatment. Thus, for instance, a subject in whom rectal examination indicates apparently gross prostatic hypertrophy may nevertheless have minimal symptoms of urinary hesitancy or dribbling, and therefore does not merit further instrumentation or operation. On the other hand, a palpably normal prostate may give rise to severe obstructive symptoms by virtue of median lobe enlargement impinging inward on the prostatic urethra. In either case the history is of overriding importance.

Lower urinary tract obstruction — for example, in prostatic hypertrophy — is associated classically with hesitancy in commencing micturition, poor stream of urine, and inability to empty the bladder completely, with resulting stop-and-start urination and postmicturition dribbling. Sudden temporary urinary retention may result from vascular congestion of the prostate, e.g., after alcohol ingestion, with suprapubic pain caused by bladder distention. In chronic cases overflow incontinence from a distended bladder may produce deceptively large urinary volumes and thus cause suprapubic bladder enlargement to be overlooked. *Urine flow may be very large in such cases* owing to the associated defect in urinary concentrating ability producing hypotonicity.

Acute upper urinary tract obstruction of one or both ureters results in severe colicky pain referred to the groin, with associated symptoms of weakness and sweating. Chronic cases caused by gradually developing obstruction at the ureteropelvic junction present with dull pain in the renal angle but little or no severe colic. A minority of cases may obstruct one ureter without overt symptoms, with resulting silent loss of renal function on that side.

In some cases, development of high-renin hypertension or primary erythrocytosis may be the presenting features, leading to discovery of unsuspected unilateral hydronephrosis in, for example, pelviureteric obstruction.

Diagnosis and Differential Diagnosis. Background etiologic factors such as family history of stone (cystinuria), arthritis (primary gout), lymphoma (secondary gout), drug therapy (periureteral fibrosis), diabetes (papillary necrosis), or neurologic disorders such as multiple sclerosis must be considered. Microscopic examination of the urinary sediment may reveal red cells, cystine or uric acid crystals, or rarely fragments of a necrosed renal papilla. Frequently, however, no specific abnormality is found in the urine. Physical examination may disclose loin tenderness or palpable renal swelling; careful supra-

Causes of Obstructive Uropathy

Intraluminal	Intramural	Extramural
Stone	Congenital:	Prostatic obstruction
Bladder tumor	Ureteropelvic dysfunction (10% bilateral)	Ureteropelvic juncture — vessels, bands, etc.
Papillary necrosis (diabetes)	Ureterovesical stricture (simple or ureterocele)	Aortic aneurysm
Clot	Bladder neck obstruction	Periureteral fibrosis
Ureteral tumor	Pinpoint meatus	Retroperitoneal tumor or nodes
	Acquired:	Extraurinary growth (carcinoma of colon, diverticulitis)
	Urethral stricture	Pelvic tumor
	Ureteral stricture (tuberculosis, etc.)	Inadvertent ligature
	Neurogenic bladder dysfunction	

pubic palpation and percussion will show a distended bladder. Rectal or vaginal examination may point to extraurinary growth.

Further investigation may then proceed along two lines—the assessment of glomerular filtration rate; and the definition of anatomic outlines of kidneys, ureters, and bladder. If serum urea or creatinine is normal or only slightly raised, glomerular filtration rate (GFR) reduction even if present will not interfere with radiologic procedures such as intravenous pyelography, which may be pursued utilizing normal dosages of intravenous dye. If plasma urea or creatinine is significantly raised, a more exact measurement of GFR may be made by measuring the disappearance rate of ^{51}Cr labeled EDTA from venous blood. This method circumvents the difficulty of conventional clearance measurements in the presence of temporary anuria or oliguria. Values less than 50 per cent of normal are clearly indicative of *bilateral* renal dysfunction. A "double-dose" of intravenous dye (i.e., 35 to 70 grams of iodine rather than the normal 15 to 30 grams) is needed if GFR is in the range 70 to 25 ml per minute. Below this filtration level, doses of up to 70 grams may be given by slow intravenous infusion. In severely uremic cases, pyelography is best postponed until immediately after dialysis. Utilizing this method, good visualization of the renal tract can be expected in 90 per cent of cases no matter how low the GFR. Retrograde pyelography is therefore almost never necessary. Certain extra precautions must, however, be taken to ensure useful results from intravenous pyelography. In addition to the conventional 5-, 10-, and 20-minute films, repeated late exposures over a period of 24 hours may show delayed nephrotomograms or dilated ureteral outlines. Nephrotomography is particularly useful in the definition of renal size and outline. Postmicturition films when feasible may show incomplete bladder emptying (residual urine) or prostatic encroachment.

While preliminary GFR assessment is taking place, a simple straight roentgenogram of the kidney-ureter-bladder area may give important information. A radiopaque stone may be seen along the line of the ureter, especially at the ureterovesical junction. Nonopaque stone (uric acid) is more difficult to exclude. In either case unilateral renal enlargement may be visible.

In order to obtain the maximal information, it is helpful to study the pyelogram films in a definite sequence, as follows:

Are two kidneys present?

Is there a difference in size?

Is there a delay in appearance of dye on one or other side?

Is there evidence of calyceal or pelvic dilatation?

Is there thinning, deformity, or shrinkage of the renal cortex?

Is there dilatation of the ureter and down to what level?

Is there displacement of the ureter medially (periureteral fibrosis) or laterally (aortic aneurysm or tumor)?

Does the bladder outline show a filling defect or deformity?

Does complete emptying of bladder dye occur after micturition?

Adequate answers to most of these questions can be supplied in 90 per cent of cases. Rarely, resort to cystoscopy may be necessary with or without retrograde ureteral catheterization and pyelography. Owing to the danger of introducing infection, these procedures are performed only when absolutely necessary for establishment of the diagnosis or with a view to operative treatment. If, for instance, prostatectomy has been decided upon, preliminary cystoscopy is essential in order to exclude associated asymptomatic pathology such as bladder tumor, diverticulum, or stone which may be present in 10 per cent of cases.

Treatment. The principles of treatment are to (1) relieve obstruction, (2) prevent infection, and (3) treat infection if present, with antimicrobial choice and dosage according to the degree of reduction of GFR (see Ch. 617). Surgical correction of obstruction is aimed at achieving comfort and preventing further damage to the threatened kidney. Before definitive relief of obstruction is attempted, it may be necessary in severely ill or uremic patients to employ dialysis with or without temporary external diversion of urine. Temporary diversion is useful when some doubt exists as to the ultimate viability of the kidney and when immediate radical relief of obstruction may appear hazardous. In some cases also the exact nature of the obstructing lesion may be in doubt for some time, e.g., whether prostatic enlargement is benign or malignant.

The decision to attempt surgical relief of obstruction must therefore be tempered initially by consideration of the aforementioned factors, and subsequently by other important aspects of the obstructive lesion itself such as its nature, location, and duration. Formerly, nephrectomy was commonly advised for unilateral cases, especially when infected, but such an approach obviously fails to provide for possible partial recovery of function on the affected side. Nephrectomy can now be advised only when extensive renal damage or pyonephrosis indicates an irrecoverable situation, especially when the remaining kidney might become involved in the destructive or infective process.

Urgent surgical relief is indicated for high-level lesions such as ureteric stone which is impacted, i.e., not moving spontaneously over a period of days. An initial attempt at dislodgment by cystoscopy and retrograde ureteral catheterization should be quickly followed, if unsuccessful, by direct open ureterolithotomy, because complicating infection must then be expected. Any other cause of recent *total* ureteral obstruction likewise demands surgical relief in order to restore function. "Recent" in this connection implies within the past four to six weeks or at most within four months, because total obstruction of longer duration is likely to have permanently destroyed the kidney.

Postponement of surgical intervention may be preferable in noninfected patients when obstruction is only *partial,* or when there is reasonable expectation of spontaneous relief. Time thus gained will help the eventual decision, based on the nature of the primary lesion. Even when infection is present, time may be gained in this way during which the response to antimicrobial therapy may be assessed. Such caution is particularly advisable in *lower* urinary tract disease, such as prostatic enlargement, in which eradication of infection may relieve many symptoms originally thought to be obstructive in origin. If significant residual bladder urine volumes (more than 100 ml) persist at this stage, however, surgery is indicated. The presence of infection in *high* urinary tract obstruction is a more urgent indication for surgical relief, because the complication of gram-negative septicemia represents a very serious hazard.

After relief of obstruction, whether by temporary external diversion or by definitive surgery, diuresis follows with rapid return to normal of blood urea and creatinine. The subsequent urinary flow may in some cases achieve massive proportions with considerable loss of solute, suggesting a diuresis of proximal tubular origin. Such a postobstructive diuresis is encountered especially in relatively chronic cases with evidence of increase in body sodium and water stores. Usually the diuresis with negative salt balance is self-limited and represents merely a restoration to normal of the previously expanded extracellular fluid volume and as such it does not require treatment. In a small minority, however, intravenous saline replacement may be necessary in this phase. Falling blood pressure or serum sodium concentration, or the occurrence of a secondary rise in serum urea or creatinine, are indications for fluid replenishment.

Prognosis. Prognosis in obstructive nephropathy depends largely on whether treatment is instituted before irreversible damage has occurred. Without treatment, the subsequent natural history of the disorder is dependent on whether the obstructing lesion is complete or incomplete and unilateral or bilateral, and especially on whether infection is present. Complete blockage with infection can totally destroy the kidney(s) within days. Chronic partial blockage, as for example in congenital pelviureteral obstruction, may be consistent with many years without symptoms, but, if bilateral, is likely to present ultimately in the "unexplained uremia" category.

With treatment, much depends on the duration of obstruction prior to relief, and especially on whether infection has been present. Experimental data suggest that complete obstruction for one week results in a permanent 50 per cent reduction in GFR on the affected side. Obstruction of longer duration is associated with correspondingly more severe permanent damage. After three months gross GFR reduction is seen but with potential for partial recovery. Loss of maximal concentrating and acidifying ability may be a prominent residual tubular defect, but sodium excretion, although relatively high in the basal state, nevertheless responds normally to both volume expansion and mineralocorticoid administration, indicating preservation of tubular function. If the history suggests obstruction for longer than four to six months, recovery of function appears very unlikely. Operative interference is therefore not indicated unless complicating pyonephrosis, severe polycythemia, or developing high-renin hypertension supervenes.

Better, O. S., Arieff, A. I., Massry, S. G., Kleeman, C. R., and Maxwell, M. H.: Studies on renal function after relief of complete unilateral ureteral obstruction of three months' duration in man. Am. J. Med., 54:234, 1973.

Bricker, N. S., and Klahr, S.: Obstructive nephropathy. *In* Strauss, M. B., and Welt, L. G. (eds.): Diseases of the Kidney. 2nd ed. Edinburgh and London, Churchill/Livingstone, 1971.

Kerr, W. S.: Effects of complete ureteral obstruction in dogs on kidney function. Am. J. Physiol., 184:521, 1956.

Keuhnelian, J. G., Bartone, F., and Marshall, V. F.: Practical considerations from autopsies on azotemic patients. J. Urol., 91:467, 1964.

Legrain, M., Bitker, M., and Kuss, R.: Obstructive Nephropathy in Adults. Proc. 3rd Int. Cong. Nephrol. Washington, 2:336, 1966 (New York, Basel and Karger, 1967).

Muldowney, F. P., Duffy, G. T., Kelly, D. G., Duff, F. A., Harrington, C., and Freaney, R.: Sodium diuresis after relief of obstructive uropathy. N. Engl. J. Med., 274:1294, 1966.

Proca, E.: Errors and pitfalls in the management of acute urinary obstruction complicated by uraemia with special reference to stone. Br. J. Urol., 44:9, 1972.

626. TOXIC NEPHROPATHY

George E. Schreiner

Toxic nephropathy is a functional or structural change in the kidney caused by a chemical or biologic product. By extension, the concept is often applied to the renal effects of physiologic substances circulating in abnormal concentrations. This situation obtains in hypokalemic, hypercalcemic, and hyperuricemic nephropathies, which are considered in detail in Ch. 619, 620, and 622. The classification of toxic nephropathy is contained in Table 1, and a partial list of nephrotoxins is shown in Table 2.

The peculiar susceptibility of the kidney to an enormous range of drugs and biologically active materials stems from its huge blood supply relative to weight, its large endothelial vascular surface, its high oxygen consumption and glucose production, the fact that excreted compounds are concentrated along the luminal surface of the nephron, and the fact that many drugs occupy, at least transiently, an intracellular position if they are involved in secretory or reabsorptive transport processes. It is possible that some reabsorbed drugs may be concentrated along with sodium in the hypertonic interstitial tissues of the papillae.

Toxic nephropathy accounts for an appreciable fraction of all reported series of acute renal failure. In the past 15 years at Georgetown Hospital it represents 20 per cent of the total experience with acute renal failure. The most frequently encountered nephrotoxins in the series were carbon tetrachloride, mercury, sulfonamide drugs, radiographic contrast media, analgesics, ethylene glycol, and antimicrobials.

Toxic nephropathy may also account for a significant segment of so-called geographic renal diseases. The World Health Organization has cited some 25,000 cases of an interstitial nephritis that has been reported by various investigators as Yugoslavian, Bulgarian, and Balkan nephritis. This disease has a distribution conforming to specific altitudes and river valleys. Pathologically it resembles a toxic nephropathy, but the specific agent has not been identified. As more sophisticated renal diagnostic techniques are correlated with renal biopsy and histochemistry, it is likely that the number of

TABLE 1. Classification of Toxic Nephropathy

Class 1. Drugs, chemicals, or their metabolites with a reasonably *direct* effect, producing an identifiable morphologic or persisting functional change in the nephron. Model: bichloride of mercury.

Class 2. Compounds producing sensitivity disease identifiable as the *nephrotic* or *nephritic* syndrome in which the initial step may be subtle alteration in the renal cell or alteration of a protein, producing an immune reaction. Model: aminonucleoside nephrosis and nephroallergens producing the nephrotic syndrome.

Class 3. Compounds producing sensitivity reactions of the angiitis or vasculitis type involving the kidney as a vascular organ. Model: sulfa sensitivity.

Class 4. Compounds that may produce *chronic nephrotoxicity,* when the mechanism extends over a period of months or years and the evidence remains largely epidemiologic or circumstantial. Model: lead nephropathy.

Class 5. Compounds that aggravate pre-existing renal disease or predispose to secondary renal disease such as pyelonephritis. Model: diuretics and cathartics predisposing to pyelonephritis via potassium deficiency.

TABLE 2.   A Partial List of Nephrotoxins

Metals: Mercury (organic and inorganic), bismuth, uranium, cadmium, lead, gold, arsine and arsenic, iron, silver, antimony, copper, and thallium

Organic solvents: Carbon tetrachloride, tetrachlorethylene, methyl cellosolve, methanol, and miscellaneous solvents

Glycols: Ethylene glycol, ethylene glycol dinitrite, propylene glycol, ethylene dichloride, and diethylene glycol

Physical agents: Radiation, heat stroke, and electroshock

Diagnostic agents: Contrast agents in high concentration (pyelography and aortography) and bunamiodyl

Therapeutic agents: Antimicrobials: Sulfonamides, penicillin, streptomycin, kanamycin, vancomycin, bacitracin, polymyxin and colistin, neomycin, tetracycline, and amphotericin. *Analgesics:* Salicylates, para-aminosalicylate (PAS), ? phenacetin, phenylbutazone, zoxazolamine, phenindione, puromycin, tridione, paradione

Osmotic agents: Sucrose, mannitol

Insecticides: Biphenyl, chlorinated hydrocarbons

Miscellaneous chemicals: Carbon monoxide, snake venom, mushroom poison, spider venom, nephroallergens, cresol, beryllium, hemolysins, aniline, and other methemoglobin formers

Abnormal concentration of physiologic substances: Hypercalcemia, hyperuricemia, hypokalemia, hypomagnesemia, etc.

recognized nephrotoxins will increase during the next decade owing to both chemicals now in existence and substances still to be produced through the remarkable ingenuity and industry of the organic chemists.

SPECIFIC NEPHROTOXINS

Mercury and Other Heavy Metals

Mercury.   Mercury in various forms acts as a nephrotoxin. Acutely it produces tubular necrosis with renal failure. In organic form or with prolonged exposure it may produce the nephrotic syndrome or chronic renal damage. Frequently encountered mercuric compounds are chloride, iodide, oxide, cyanide, and salicylate. Mercurous compounds include the chloride (calomel), iodide, and oxide salts. Organic mercuric compounds associated with nephrotoxicity include merbromin (Mercurochrome) and the mercurial diuretics.

Epidemiology.   Inorganic mercury poisoning usually occurs by accident, in suicide attempts, or after its use as an abortive agent. Poisoning has occurred in a wide variety of industries, including the manufacture of paint, alloys, and scientific instruments. Agricultural exposures are due to disinfectants and pesticides. Medical poisoning stems from mercurial diuretics, ammoniated mercury ointments, and absorption from the skin of widespread dermatoses, such as psoriasis. Inhalation toxicity may occur. The urinary excretion of inorganic mercury normally ranges from 0.1 to 1 μg per liter. Patients with chronic industrial exposure often excrete amounts in excess of 300 μg per liter. Psoriatic patients have had mercuriuria demonstrated from 500 to 1000 μg per liter.

Clinical Manifestations.   Mercury produces a lingering, bitter, metallic taste that may be followed by a sensation of constriction in the throat, suffocation, substernal burning, esophagitis, gastritis, abdominal pain, nausea, and vomiting. Ulcerations occur on the palate or lips; diarrhea may be blood tinged. Circulatory collapse is signaled by feeble pulse, peripheral vasoconstriction, syncope, and shock with oliguria and anuria. It is important to obtain urine before oliguria sets in. The urine usually shows albumin, epithelial cell casts, erythrocytes, glycosuria, aminoaciduria, and increased mercury

content, particularly in the precipitable fractions. Leukocytosis is the rule.

Pathology.   Mercurial vapor, dust, or liquid dissolves locally on moist surfaces of the mucous membranes. Mercuric salts are well absorbed by the gastrointestinal tract and vagina, and ammoniated mercury by the intact skin. Absorbed mercury is bound quickly to circulating protein, and appears in blood, kidney, liver, heart, brain, and some endocrine organs. Inorganic salts are excreted largely by the colon, kidneys, salivary glands, biliary system, and skin, and organic materials predominantly by the kidney. The most striking pathologic changes occur in the form of granular or vacuolar degeneration of the proximal tubules. Mitotic figures and basophilic cytoplasm may be seen in the early phases of healing. Early calcification of the site of necrosis may occur. In severe cases all segments of the tubule may be involved, and patchy tubulorrhexis may occur. Extrarenal autopsy findings include induration of surface membranes in pharynx, esophagus, and stomach, erosive gastritis, softening of the muscular coat of the intestine, severe colitis, congestion of liver and spleen, degeneration of myocardium, and focal hemorrhages in the cerebral cortex. It appears that mercury initiates cellular destruction by combining with the sulfhydryl groups of protein in the mitochrondrial membrane, leading to the disintegration of mitochondria and necrosis of nuclei and subsequent loss in enzyme activity.

Fourteen cases of acute renal failure caused by mercury have been studied at Georgetown Hospital. The dose expressed as inorganic mercury ranged from 0.4 to 10 grams. Oliguria occurred within the first 48 hours, and persisted for an average of 15 days (range 7 to 22). Tissue necrosis was a catabolic factor, and the BUN increased an average of 31 mg per 100 ml per day during the first week. Thirteen patients required hemodialysis, and three died. None of the patients died who underwent hemodialysis within 48 hours after the ingestion of mercury and the administration of BAL. Six cases of nephrotic syndrome secondary to mercury have been observed.

Treatment.   Prevention is exceptionally important. The use of mercuric salts for douching and surgical irrigation should be discouraged. Bottles should be labeled as poison and should be secured in a safe place. Acute ingestion is a medical emergency. Emesis usually occurs, but if not, the stomach should be emptied with a large lavage tube, and rinsed with egg white or concentrated albumin or medicinal charcoal. A useful lavage solution combines 1 pint of skim milk, 50 grams of glucose, 20 grams of sodium bicarbonate, and three eggs beaten into a mixture. One gram of medicinal charcoal can combine with 850 mg of mercuric chloride. After absorption, BAL (2,3-dimercapropanol) acts as an effective antidote because it appears to compete with biologically important sulfhydryl groups. Injections of 2.5 to 3 mg of BAL per kilogram of body weight should be given every four hours up to six injections, depending on the severity of poisoning. BAL may produce transient nausea, vomiting, diarrhea, burning stomatitis and excessive lacrimation. It is a mild hypoglycemic agent. In severe poisoning large doses of BAL are given immediately, and dialysis is carried out shortly thereafter to remove the mercury-BAL complex; the patient is then re-treated with BAL. Exchange transfusion may also be of value. Patients who remain oliguric should be given the same conservative management as other patients with acute renal failure (see Ch. 604).

Treatment of patients with nephrotic syndrome caused by mercury calls for immediate removal of the agent, administration of adrenocortical steroids, and a regimen similar to that recommended for other patients with the nephrotic syndrome. These patients may be subject to repeated renal damage by mercurial diuretics. Hypersensitivity reactions to mercurial diuretics have included generalized pruritus, urticaria, asthma, exfoliative dermatitis, and sudden death. Cystine, penicillamine, BAL, or other sources of sulfhydryl compounds may be used to augment the treatment of mercury sensitivity and especially ventricular fibrillation, which is the cause of sudden death.

Acrodynia (pink disease) occurs in children throughout the world, and is characterized by irritability, emaciation, stomatitis, and erythema of acral parts. The children have fever, leukocytosis, albuminuria, and mercuriuria from mercury used in teething powder or diaper rinses.

Bismuth. Bismuth toxicity arises chiefly from industrial poisons, antisyphilitic therapy, and soluble bismuth compounds such as the subcarbonate and the mixed thioglycolates. Bismuth may produce either acute renal failure or nephrotic syndrome. Sore mouth, diarrhea, peripheral neuritis, stomatitis, obstructive jaundice, and pigmentation of the gum margins may occur, together with evidence of acute renal failure with hyposthenuria, cylindruria, and the desquamation of renal tubular epithelial cells.

Uranium. Uranium causes proximal tubular necrosis in a distribution similar to that of mercury. Uranium nitrate may produce a central lobular lesion in the glomeruli. Uranium has been implicated in some cases of geographic nephritis.

Cadmium. Cadmium is widely used in the metal plating and industrial chemical industries. Interstitial nephritis may follow chronic exposure, and acute poisoning produces proteinuria and proximal renal damage. The most significant feature of cadmium nephrotoxicity is a peculiar proteinuria, ranging from 70 to 2600 mg per 24 hours. There is a low molecular weight protein (20,000 to 30,000) that precipitates with nitric acid but not with boiling, and migrates as an alpha globulin. Cadmium proteinuria is clinically significant and is best treated by removing the patient from the toxic environment. Cadmium is soluble in acid; acid foods and beverages placed in cadmium-plated containers such as ice cube trays may be a source of poisoning.

Lead. Lead nephrotoxicity has been implicated in severe renal disease produced from the drinking of whiskey made in stills improvised from automobile and truck radiators. In Queensland, Australia, the eating of paint or drinking of rain water from porches painted with lead paint has been found to result in a high incidence of chronic nephritis associated with increased skeletal lead content and increased lead in the urine. Unexposed subjects may excrete about 0.08 mg per liter of lead, and asymptomatic exposed subjects may excrete up to 0.15 mg per liter. Patients with lead poisoning may excrete from 0.15 to 0.30 mg per liter. Lead nephropathy is a predominantly tubular syndrome with renal glycosuria, aminoaciduria, albuminuria, casts, and increased excretion of lead, delta-aminolevulinic acid, coproporphyrin, urobilinogen, urobilin, and bile pigments. Roentgenograms show typically the increased density at the ends of the shafts of the long bones. Ziehl-Neelsen acid-fast, intranuclear inclusion bodies may be seen on renal biopsy.

Treatment of lead nephropathy lies in immediate removal of the subject from the source of exposure. Attempts may be made to increase excretion by such agents as sodium citrate, dimercaprol, and disodium calcium ethylenediamine tetraacetate.

Gold. Gold salts are used in rheumatoid arthritis in the form of gold sodium thiosulfate, sodium aurothiomalate, aurothioglucose, and aurothioglycanide. Cutaneous manifestations of hypersensitivity include urticaria, purpura, itching, maculopapular to exfoliative dermatitis, and polyneuritis. Bone marrow depression may be encountered. Nephrotoxicity is usually heralded by proteinuria and microscopic hematuria. The nephrotic syndrome may supervene. Brun et al. studied the localization of gold in renal biopsies of patients receiving gold therapy. Deposits of the metal were found in the proximal tubules shortly after injection. Subsequently (one to four years) they were localized in the distal tubules. In the interstitial tissues gold was stored in macrophages, and could be demonstrated up to 28 years after the last injection. At Georgetown Hospital four patients with the nephrotic syndrome after gold therapy have been observed. Three subsequently developed laboratory features of systemic lupus erythematosus.

Arsine. Arsine intoxication produces shock, hemoglobinuria, and acute tubular necrosis, which has been successfully treated by hemodialysis.

Arsenic. Arsenic may produce a toxic nephritis leading to oliguria and uremia, aggravated by the dehydration from associated diarrhea. The urine contains albumin, casts, erythrocytes, and leukocytes. Arsenic may be recovered in the dialysate of such patients treated with hemodialysis.

Silver. Silver may produce renal tubular degeneration, with sparing of the glomeruli, interstitial deposits of silver, and interstitial edema. It has been reported in persons who regularly handle photographic developers.

Iron. Acute tubular necrosis has been reported with a mortality rate of 50 per cent in children who accidentally ingest large doses of ferrous sulfate. It is presumably related to the mucosal damage in the gastrointestinal tract, metabolic acidosis, hepatic damage, and shock. Chronic renal failure, interstitial fibrosis, and iron deposition may be seen in hemochromatosis and severe transfusion hemosiderosis. In rabbits saccharated iron oxide produces a nephrotoxic lesion.

Antimony. As used therapeutically for leishmaniasis, antimony can lead to transient oliguric renal failure.

Copper. Copper sulfate ingestion can produce vomiting, dehydration, hypotension, sulfhemoglobinemia, and acute renal failure. Tubular degeneration and necrosis are seen, particularly in the ascending loop and distal convolution.

Thallium. Thallium is used in rat poisons, depilatories, and denaturing agents for alcohol. It causes albuminuria, tachycardia, colic, and a neurologic syndrome.

Solvents

Carbon tetrachloride is used as a cleaning agent, grease solvent and vermifuge, and in fire extinguishers. It is heavier than air. Nephrotoxicity may occur after either inhalation or ingestion. It is aggravated by the simultaneous ingestion of alcohol, even in small amounts. The initial symptoms are irritation at the exposure site, followed by headache, mental confusion, coma, and convulsions. Narcosis, encephalomyelitis, cerebellar degeneration, and optic and peripheral neuritis may occur. Gastrointestinal symptoms are prominent, particularly when the substance has been ingested, and include nausea, vomiting, and abdominal pain. The delayed manifestations are toxic hepatitis with jaundice, tender hepatomegaly with hepatic failure, and a toxic nephropathy with anuric acute tubular necrosis. Renal involvement may be insidious and delayed for as long as a week after exposure. The urine is typical of acute renal failure, with proteinuria, cylindruria, pyuria, hematuria, and desquamation of renal tubular epithelial cells. Bleeding manifestations, particularly scleral and periorbital hemorrhages, epistaxis, and hypoprothrombinemia may be seen. In the Georgetown Hospital experience, the most frequent signs and symptoms encountered were oliguria, nausea and vomiting, hepatomegaly, and abdominal pain. Half or less than half of the patients had bleeding, fever, hypertension, jaundice, rash, edema, ascites, and renal tenderness. Patients were azotemic, but the creatinine/BUN ratio averaged 16 per cent, considerably higher than the 11 per cent ratio in the entire group of acute renal failure. This may reflect some impairment of hepatic urea synthesis. The patients were usually hyperuricemic, hyponatremic, hypokalemic, hypochloremic, hypophosphatemic, and acidotic. Serum glutamic oxaloacetic transaminase was elevated. Hyperbilirubinemia, hyperglycemia, abnormal thymol turbidity, cephalin flocculation tests and elevated or high alkaline phosphatase levels were usual.

Treatment consists of removing the patient from the area of exposure and providing adequate ventilation, gastric lavage, and catharsis. The use of unsaturated oils by mouth has been suggested but not clinically proved to be helpful. People chronically exposed to carbon tetrachloride should be warned about the synergism with alcohol. After hepatic or renal failure has ensued, standard therapy for these complications should be employed. Hemorrhagic phenomena require the judicious use of blood transfusions.

Glycols

Ethylene glycol is commonly encountered in antifreeze solutions. Part of the compound is rapidly converted to oxalic acid, which may be deposited in the kidneys and other organs such as the meninges. In the kidney there is destruction of epithelial cells with preservation of the basement membrane, focal regeneration, and tubules filled with masses of calcium oxalate crystals that are birefringent on polarized light. Nephrons are dilated above the crystalline obstruction. Focal mononuclear cell infiltrates and interstitial edema are also seen.

The clinical events may be divided into three stages: During the first 12 hours central nervous system effects resemble those of ethanol intoxication. In severe poisoning this may include stupor, coma, convulsions, and death. During the second 12 hours the manifestations are predominantly cardiopulmonary, with tachypnea, cyanosis, pulmonary edema, and death in cardiac failure. After the first day the problem is mainly renal injury, with slight pain, tenderness over the kidneys, proteinuria, oliguria, and anuria; death may result from uremia.

Ethylene glycol poisoning is a medical emergency, and should be treated with immediate hemodialysis aimed at removal of the circulating alcohol to diminish the substrate for conversion to glycolic and oxalic acid. Gastric lavage and parenteral solutions of sodium bicarbonate may also be used. After anuria has supervened, the treatment is the same as for acute renal failure in general.

Physical Agents

Radiation nephritis is encountered clinically after radiation of tumors in or near the kidneys. The kidney is said to be the most radiosensitive of all major organs. The major syndromes include acute and chronic nephritis and benign and malignant hypertension. Clinically, radiation nephritis is characterized by proteinuria, hypertension, anemia, cardiomegaly, congestive heart failure, encephalopathy, and chronic uremia. In *acute* cases the mortality rate is about 50 per cent; survivors generally begin to improve within six months from the onset. In *chronic* radiation exposure the nephritis may be manifested only by proteinuria, anemia, hyposthenuria, and slowly progressive decline of renal function. These symptoms may occur as a continuum from the acute disease or may be discovered later in patients who have never presented with an acute syndrome.

Histologic study reveals marked thickening of the renal capsule, hyaline obliteration of the glomeruli, focal necrosis of the fibrinoid or hemorrhagic type, proliferation of Bowman's capsule, pericapsular fibrosis, tubular degeneration and atrophy, diffuse interstitial fibrosis, and fibrinoid necrosis of arterioles. There is a remarkable tendency to development of malignant hypertension and necrotizing arteriolitis.

The treatment is not essentially different from that for acute and chronic nephritis from other causes; the hypertension should be treated vigorously with antihypertensive drugs. When radiation nephritis is unilateral, the resulting hypertension may be benefited by nephrectomy.

Heat stroke may be encountered in hyperthermal industrial environments or military situations in the desert, and acute renal failure may be the dominant manifestation. Lack of acclimatization may be a primary factor in pathogenesis. Hemolysis, shock, hemoconcentration, volume depletion, and hypernatremia have been prominent clinical features. Acute renal failure ensues in up to 10 per cent of the patients who survive heat stroke.

Diagnostic Agents

Contrast media: Iodide is an essential component of all absorbable contrast media. A significant percentage of persons manifest iodine hypersensitivity in the form of urticaria, skin rashes, glottal edema, and occasionally anaphylactoid reactions with shock and acute tubular necrosis. Excluding hypersensitivity, organic iodides are, nevertheless, nephrotoxic. The highest incidence seems to be associated with an oral contrast medium, bunamiodyl (Orabilex), and with other double doses of dehydration techniques that have been used for attempted visualization of diseased gallbladders. Toxicity is also associated with abdominal aortography, especially when high concentrations of contrast material are used by direct rapid injection.

The numerous mechanisms suggested to explain the nephrotoxicity of contrast media have included renal vasoconstriction, erythrocyte agglutination and crenation from hyperosmolar injections, and loss of the dispersing effect of albumin, coagulation defect, and high concentration of the material in the tubular cell of a patient who has impaired hepatic excretion. Experimentally it has been shown that stasis with obstruction to urinary flow potentiates the toxicity.

Pathologic changes follow the particular route of pathogenesis: vasculitis in some cases of iodine hypersensitivity, proteinuria and glomerular damage from vasoconstriction and capillary thrombi, and acute tubular necrosis from shock or direct toxicity to the tubular cell. Recent reports suggest a specific reaction between the myeloma kidney and contrast material. Some may be due to dehydration incurred in preparation for pyelography. McAfee surveyed 13,207 abdominal aortograms and uncovered 12 fatal and 27 serious nonfatal instances of nephrotoxicity. Crawford noted reduced renal function in 50 per cent of patients receiving more than 40 ml of Urokon above the renal artery.

Intravenous pyelography, using less concentrated material, appears to produce fewer complications in even the presence of renal insufficiency. Retrograde pyelography carries the risk of infection from instrumentation and edema of the ureters, producing obstruction, and has been associated with papillary necrosis.

Cholecystography: It has been estimated that more than 100 cases of acute renal failure have been caused by bunamiodyl. The major pathologic finding is tubular necrosis, accompanied by deposition of birefringent green-brown crystals at the base of the tubular epithelial cell that are anisotropic with polarized light. Bunamiodyl is more completely absorbed from the intestine than other cholecystographic media and is therefore delivered in higher concentrations to the kidney, particularly in the presence of liver disease and an abnormal gallbladder. Wennberg recently demonstrated depression of glomerular filtration rate caused by bunamiodyl. Renal failure has also occurred in patients with underlying renal disease subjected to dehydration and specialized techniques of rapid intravenous or double-dose cholecystography.

Therapeutic Agents
(Antimicrobial Drugs)

In the presence of infectious disease and its circulatory consequences, recognition of nephrotoxicity from antimicrobial agents may be difficult. Dehydration, hypotension, vomiting, and allergic reactions may lead to renal failure that is not, properly speaking, direct nephrotoxicity. However, a number of antimicrobials do appear to produce direct renal damage.

Sulfonamide compounds may precipitate in the nephron or calyces, and may be excreted in high concentrations into a urine with a low pH. This can produce sulfonamide concretions, obstructive uropathy, and parenchymal damage from crystals. Occasionally direct tubular necrosis, interstitial nephritis, or necrotizing angiitis may also occur. Other lesions have been reported from acetazolamide.

Streptomycin may produce necrosis of the proximal tubular epithelium, cylindruria, and albuminuria. Since the excretion of streptomycin is predominantly renal, underlying kidney disease may be associated with higher and more toxic blood levels.

Kanamycin has been associated with proteinuria and microscopic hematuria in 10 and 20 per cent of the patients, respectively, at dosage levels of 25 to 50 mg per kilogram per day. Oliguria may develop, and tubular necrosis seems to be aggravated by prior therapy with streptomycin or viomycin.

Bacitracin produces renal tubular necrosis.

Polymyxins A, B, C, D, and E have nephrotic properties of varying severity. Only polymyxin B has received extensive clinical use. It may produce albuminuria, casts, epithelial cells in the urine, decrease in concentrating ability, and tubular degeneration. Polymyxin B accumulates if renal function is impaired or if the dose exceeds 3 mg per kilogram per day. Nephrotoxicity is dose related.

Colymycin (colistin) is chemically similar to polymyxin and has a similar nephrotoxicity.

Neomycin is not normally well absorbed from the gastrointestinal tract. It produces foamy vacuolization of the epithelial lining of the proximal convoluted tubules, and progressive renal failure has been reported after intraperitoneal administration.

Tetracycline accentuates azotemia by its catabolic effect in increasing nitrogen turnover. Deteriorated tetracycline, used after its expiration date, has produced a largely reversible Fanconi type of syndrome consisting of reduced renal function, polyuria, polydypsia, glycosuria, aminoaciduria, hyperphosphaturia, hypercalciuria, hypophosphatemia, hypokalemia, hyperuricemia, and severe metabolic acidosis with debilitating lethargy. Instances have also been demonstrated of heavy Bence Jones proteinuria, transient hyperglycemia, and a macular papular rash. The characteristic lesion is tubular degeneration with desquamation of epithelial cells, granular cytoplasm, vacuolization, hemosiderosis, evidence of reparative epithelial cell regeneration, and pale staining nuclei. Among the degradation products believed to account for the syndrome, two have been biochemically identified as epianhydrotetracycline and anhydrotetracycline. Clinical manifestations may appear in three or four days after ingestion of as little as 10 to 12 capsules.

Amphotericin B is dangerous chiefly because of renal damage. Cylindruria is the first manifestation, and may be accompanied by hematuria, pyuria, and proteinuria. The glomerular filtration rate and renal blood flow may decline by half or more. Maximal concentrating capacity decreases; serum urea and creatinine increase. Therapy may have to be terminated. Examination of kidney tissue shows necrosis and degeneration of proximal and distal tubules with flattened epithelium, regenerative foci, and calcification prominent in casts and interstitial tissue. Thickening of the glomerular basement has been noted in some patients.

Analgesic Abuse
(Phenacetin Nephropathy)

Mixed analgesic preparations are among the most frequently used drugs in medical therapy and self-medication. In 1953 Spuhler and Zollinger noted an increase in interstitial nephritis and a high incidence of medullary necrosis in patients who had abused analgesic therapy. Many such patients have now been reported from Switzerland, the Scandinavian countries, Australia, New Zealand, South Africa, Canada, and the United States. At Georgetown Hospital, nine patients with this

NEPHROPATHY OF ANALGESIC ABUSE

Longcope, W. T., and Leutscher, J. A.: The treatment of acute mercury bi-
    chloride poisoning with BAL (2,3-dimercaptopropanol). Med. Clin.
    North Am., 34:469, 1950.
Luessenhop, A. J., Gallimore, J. C., Sweet, W. H., Struxness, E. G., and
    Robinson, J.: The toxicity in man of hexavalent uranium following in-
    travenous administration. Am. J. Roentgenol., 79:83, 1958.
Maher, J. F., and Schreiner, G. E.: Cause of death in acute renal failure.
    Arch. Intern. Med., 110:493, 1962.
Maher, J. F., and Schreiner, G. E.: The clinical dialysis of poisons. Trans.
    Amer. Soc. Artif. Intern. Organs, 9:390, 1963.
McAfee, J. G.: A survey of complications of abdominal aortography.
    Radiology, 68:825, 1957.
Pendergrass, E. P., Hodes, P. J., Tondreau, R. L., Powell, C. C., and Bur-
    dick, E. D.: Further consideration of deaths and unfavorable sequelae
    following the administration of contrast media in urography in the
    United States. Am. J. Roentgenol., 74:262, 1955.
Rich, A. R.: The role of hypersensitivity in periarteritis nodosa as indicated
    by 7 cases developing during serum sickness and sulfonamide therapy.
    Bull. Hopkins Hosp., 71:123, 1942.
Schreiner, G. E.: Dialysis of poisons and drugs: Annual review. Trans.
    Amer. Soc. Artif. Intern. Organs, 16:544, 1970.
Schreiner, G. E.: The nephrotoxicity of analgesic abuse. Ann. Intern. Med.,
    57:1047, 1962.
Schreiner, G. E., and Maher, J. F.: Toxic nephropathy. Am. J. Med.,
    38:409, 1965.
Schreiner, G. E., Maher, J. F., Marc-Aurele, J., Knowlan, D., and Alvo,
    M.: Ethylene glycol—two indications for hemodialysis. Trans. Amer.
    Soc. Artif. Intern. Organs, 5:81, 1959.
Schwartz, W. B., Hurwit, A., and Ettinger, A.: Intravenous urography in
    the patient with renal insufficiency. N. Engl. J. Med., 269:277, 1963.
Setter, J. G., Maher, J. F., and Schreiner, G. E.: Acute renal failure follow-
    ing cholecystography. J.A.M.A., 184:102, 1963.
Spuhler, O., and Zollinger, H. U.: Die chronischinterstitielle Nephritis. Z.
    Klin. Med., 151:1, 1953.
Strauss, M. B., and Welt, L. G.: Diseases of the Kidney. 2nd ed. Boston,
    Little, Brown & Company, 1971.
Wennberg, J. E., Okun, R., Hinman, E. J., Northcutt, R. C., Greip, R. J.,
    and Walker, W. G.: Renal toxicity of oral cholecystographic media.
    J.A.M.A., 186:461, 1963.
Yow, E. M., Moyer, J. H., and Smith, C. P.: Toxicity of polymyxin B. II.
    Human studies with particular reference to evaluation of renal function.
    Arch. Intern. Med., 92:248, 1953.

entity have been studied, and some of the findings are
summarized in the accompanying figure.

Satisfactory understanding of the pathogenesis of
analgesic nephropathy is lacking. Anti-inflammatory effects, salicylates as uncoupling agents, hypokalemia,
manufacturing contaminants (acetic-4-chloranilid),
methemoglobinemia and sulfhemoglobinemia, sensitivity reactions, and predisposition have all been suggested
as playing a role in the disease. Direct toxicity has not
been demonstrated in animals except when excessive
amounts of phenacetin have been used; similar levels of
aspirin ingestion are fatal. In general, clinical cases
have occurred in which the cumulative ingestion calculated as phenacetin is in excess of 1 kg. Continuing investigation may add more epidemiologic and circumstantial evidence for an association between chronic
interstitial nephritis, renal papillary necrosis, and/or a
unique susceptibility to pyelonephritis of patients who
chronically ingest analgesic mixtures.

Insecticides

Biphenyl is a citrus fungicide that produces polyuria
and focal tubular dilatation resembling small cysts.
Chronic exposure to *DDT* may produce fatty degeneration of the tubular epithelium, and anuria has been
reported following exposure to *chlordane*.

Aye, R. C.: Renal papillary necrosis. Diabetes, 3:124, 1954.
Becker, C. G., Becker, E. L., Maher, J. F., and Schreiner, G. E.: Nephrotic
    syndrome after contact with mercury. A report of five cases, three after
    the use of ammoniated mercury ointment. Arch. Intern. Med., 110:178,
    1962.
Brun, C., Olsen, S., Raaschou, F., and Sorensen, A. W. S.: The localization
    of gold in the human kidney following chrysotherapy. A biopsy study.
    Nephron, 1:265, 1964.
Crawford, E. S., Beall, A. C., Moyer, J. H., and De Bakey, M. E.:
    Complications of aortography. Surg. Gynec. Obstet., 104:129, 1957.
Doolan, P. D., Walsh, W. P., Kyle, L. H., and Wishinsky, H.: Acetylsalicy-
    lic acid intoxication. Proposed method of treatment. J.A.M.A., 146:
    105, 1951.
Freeman, R. B., Maher, J. F., Schreiner, G. E., and Mostofi, F. K.: Renal
    tubular necrosis due to nephrotoxicity of organic mercurial diuretics.
    Ann. Intern. Med., 57:34, 1962.
Frimpter, G. W., Timpanelli, A. E., Eisenmenger, W. J., Stein, H. S., and
    Ehrlich, L. I.: Reversible "Fanconi syndrome" caused by degraded te-
    tracycline J.A.M.A., 184:111, 1963.
Goodman, L., and Gilman, A.: The Pharmacological Basis of Therapeutics.
    3rd ed. New York, The Macmillan Company, 1965.
Lauler, D. P., Schreiner, G. E., and David, A.: Renal medullary necrosis.
    Am. J. Med., 29:132, 1960.

627. RENAL CALCULI

William C. Thomas, Jr.

Renal calculi are concretions consisting of crystals and
a matrix of organic matter. Crystals usually constitute
the predominant portion (> 90 per cent) of the mass of
most calculi, but those occurring as a consequence of
urinary tract infections have a higher proportion of matrix material. Occasionally this latter type of calculus
may be almost devoid of crystals. Renal calculi are to be
distinguished from calcific deposits within the renal
parenchyma. Such deposits occurring at sites of previous
inflammation or degenerative change are designated by
the term "nephrocalcinosis." Elsewhere in the text are
specific presentations of a number of disorders often
complicated by nephrolithiasis; this chapter is largely
limited to a discussion of broadly applicable principles in
the cause and management of renal calculi.

Etiology. *General Factors.* Our knowledge of the
cause of various types of calculi is incomplete, but from
available evidence it appears that a combination of factors rather than any single event is most often responsible for calculus formation. The likelihood and type of
calculous disease is modified by geographic factors, sex,
race, and probably diet. In the United States the incidence is greatest in the Southeast, but there are other
areas of the country where the incidence is also high.
South Africa, portions of India, and Southeast Asia are

regions where calculous disease occurs with unusual frequency. In the Southeastern United States "hard water" has been thought by some to be the important factor favoring calculus formation, but such a correlation fails to explain why calculi are infrequent in other "hard water" regions of the world. In India and Southeast Asia protein-poor, predominantly cereal diets have been considered to be of importance in the development of bladder calculi in children. Although these and other suggested explanations to account for the regional incidence of calculi have some attractiveness, none has sufficient investigative support to warrant complete acceptance.

Recurrent calculi composed of calcium oxalate and phosphate are relatively uncommon in women and rare in blacks of either sex. The disproportionate occurrence of such calculi in white males is unexplained, but holds true even in the high incidence areas of the Southeastern United States and South Africa. Women, however, are more susceptible than men to urinary tract infections. Thus women with magnesium-ammonium-phosphate or calcium-phosphate stones that develop as a complication of infection with urea-splitting organisms outnumber similarly affected men. Certain disorders predisposing to calculus formation, especially hyperparathyroidism, overcome the protective influence of sex or race, and this provides a diagnostic lead when searching for the cause of calculi in white women or blacks.

There is an increased incidence of calcareous renal calculi in patients with small bowel disease or in those subjected to ileal resection. Patients who have undergone jejunoileal anastomosis in an effort to control morbid obesity are especially prone to develop calculi. It is now known that such patients usually have a significant hyperoxaluria as probably the most important factor favoring stone formation. Frequently these patients also have some degree of acidosis, presumably from loss of intestinal bicarbonate, and a consequent decrease in urinary citrate.

Although there is disagreement as to the complete explanation of the hyperoxaluria in patients with small bowel disease, there is good evidence that such patients absorb a larger than usual proportion of dietary oxalate. Also, it has been suggested that malabsorption of bile salts may contribute to the hyperoxaluria in this syndrome through the action of colonic bacteria on glycocholic acid to provide absorbable precursors of oxalate.

Structure and Composition of Calculi. Although all calculi must initially be small, it is the aggregation of crystals and matrix into a dense mass with subsequent growth to macroscopic size that accounts for their medical significance. The crystalline components of calculi are formed from the less soluble crystalloids predominant in the urine. It has not been determined whether the matrix component of all calculi can be formed entirely from nonspecific proteinaceous material and cellular debris present in urine, or is dependent on the presence of specific compounds secreted by cells lining the urinary tract.

Examination of sectioned calculi usually reveals a distinct lamellar and sometimes radially striated organization. In most stones there is a small identifiable nidus around which the bulk of the calculus appears to have formed. In calcium oxalate renal stones, the most common variety, this nidus often consists of calcium phosphate, frequently in hydroxyapatite form. There is evidence that such a nidus may originate within the cells of the renal tubules or collecting ducts or beneath the papillary epithelium. As one means of stone formation, it has been suggested that extrusion of this type of nidus into the renal pelvis may promote apposition of crystals and matrix material from an appropriately constituted urine. There are other data, however, to indicate that the nidus of a stone need not be of specific composition. For example, calcium oxalate bladder stones of children in Southeast Asia regularly contain a core of uric acid crystals.

Crystalloids in Urine. Normal urine contains in solution a number of crystalloids, e.g., calcium, magnesium, phosphate, oxalate, and urate, at concentrations exceeding those achievable in water. The maintenance of this supersaturated state may be attributed to a number of factors. Urea, apparently by its interaction with water, increases the solubility of crystalloids, and the concentrations of sodium, potassium, chloride, and other soluble ions in urine also enhance the solution stability of the less soluble components. Organic acids, especially citrate, that form soluble chelates with calcium and magnesium are additional urinary constituents that promote the solubility of calcium or magnesium salts. One should be aware, however, that the potential of urinary organic acids to chelate metal ions is markedly decreased when urinary pH is low (< 5.0).

In addition to the aforementioned factors that may account in part for the supersaturation of urine, specific inhibitors to the crystallization of calcium salts have been detected in urine and also in serum. A deficiency of these biologic "water conditioners" may be important in determining susceptibility to calculus formation. One of these constituents, inorganic pyrophosphate, has been studied in considerable detail. It is a product of intermediary metabolism and is present in serum at concentrations of 75 to 160 μg per 100 ml. Urinary excretion of pyrophosphate by subjects receiving diets free of dairy products ranges from 4 to 10 mg per day, and, within limits, the amount in urine varies directly with orthophosphate excretion. Although urinary pyrophosphate may be a protective constituent, the amount excreted is the same in calculous and normal subjects and is insufficient to account for the solution stability of calcium salts.

A more potent inhibitor of crystal formation than inorganic pyrophosphate has now been identified in urine. This is a water-soluble, acidic compound of low molecular weight, but of undefined composition. Very small amounts of this compound, especially when acting in concert with citrate, prevent crystallization of calcium salts from highly supersaturated solutions. Observations to date indicate that there is a decreased excretion of this biologic "water conditioner" by patients with idiopathic calcareous calculi, but the data are too limited to assess the importance of this deficiency to the genesis of renal calculi. A number of investigators have observed that calcium-containing crystals form more readily in urine from patients with calcareous calculi than in that from normal subjects. This difference is consistent with a deficiency of inhibitors of crystal formation in the urine of stone formers.

The formation of renal calculi is thought to be dependent on the presence of metastable concentrations of crystalloids, but there must also be a component or nidus promoting the formation and aggregation of crystals. Whatever the initiating event, the growth of most calculi is dependent on the presence in urine of metastable concentrations of crystalloids. Such states of supersaturation may be achieved by various means: by increased excretion of specific crystalloids of limited solubility; decrease in urinary pH which converts urates to less soluble uric acid; or infection with urea-splitting bacteria to release ammonia, which causes an increase in urinary pH and provides a setting for crystallization of magnesium-ammonium-phosphate or calcium phosphate complexes. In addition to increased concentrations of crystalloids or alteration of urinary pH, reduced excretion of those urinary constituents that normally inhibit crystal formation would also induce a metastable state of crystalloids. This latter type of change is possibly of more importance to the development of idiopathic calcareous calculi than is increased excretion of calcium or oxalate.

Diagnosis. The medical history often provides important information. Infection as an etiologic or complicating factor is suggested by a history of fever preceding the initial episode of renal colic. Also, in postpartum women with calculi it is important to ascertain whether urinary tract infection occurred during pregnancy. Is there a family history of calculi? Genetic disorders such as renal tubular acidosis and cystinuria are expected in kindred, but idiopathic calcareous calculi may also occur in families. The occurrence of renal calculi in childhood may indicate the presence of a familial disorder, but infection or anatomic defects are more common causes in this age group. The contributory effect of intestinal disease to calculus formation was mentioned previously. A number of medications have been causally related to renal stone formation, and patients should be questioned about chronic use of medicines, particularly acetazolamide, absorbable alkali, silicates, allopurinol, or large amounts of ascorbic acid. The type of water used and unusual dietary habits are additional items of relevant information.

Clinical Manifestations. Many patients with renal calculi are asymptomatic. Inflammation or infection resulting from calculi may lead to symptoms, but passage of a calculus into the ureter with resulting renal colic is the classic manifestation of calculous disease. Passage of small, sandlike concretions with relatively little pain is not uncommon, particularly with uric acid lithiasis and sometimes in patients with calcium oxalate stones. Gross hematuria, especially in the absence of accompanying renal colic and a demonstrable ureteral calculus, should be regarded with suspicion as possibly indicative of infection or a coexistent neoplasm. Microscopic hematuria, however, is quite regularly present in patients with calculi. The malingerer, feigning renal colic in order to obtain narcotics, may demonstrate considerable ingenuity in developing a symptom complex.

Laboratory Findings. Careful examination of fresh urine provides immediate, valuable information. For example, an acid urine and urate crystals may be present in those with uric acid calculi, and octahedral crystals of calcium oxalate are frequent in patients with oxalate stones. A high urine pH (7.0 or higher) may signify infection or a renal tubular disorder. The presence of bacteria in fresh uncentrifuged urine usually indicates significant infection. As mentioned, microscopic hematuria is usual, and there may be few to many white blood cells. The pH of each freshly voided specimen of the patient's urine should be determined for 24 hours. Appropriately selected pH paper (pH range 4 to 9) is adequate for clinical purposes. If the pH is consistently high and infection is present (values between 8.5 and 9.0 always indicate infection), the pH determinations should be re-

peated after eradication of the infection. In normal persons receiving a regular diet, urine pH will be less than 6.0 at some time during the 24 hours. If this degree of acidity is not achieved, the presence of renal tubular acidosis is likely, and should be confirmed by definitive tests. The occasional patient with uric acid stones may excrete unusually acid urine (pH 4.5 to 5.5), but most uric acid stone-formers do not excrete urine of such acidity.

A qualitative test for cystine should be performed in every patient with radiopaque calculi, and freshly voided, concentrated urine is desired for this analysis. If positive, a quantitative analysis of the 24-hour excretion should be obtained. Although cystinuria is not a rare disorder, only a small proportion of cystinurics develop calculi.

A urine culture is indicated in the evaluation of patients with calculi. Of particular relevance to the problem of stone formation are infections with urea-splitting bacteria. It is pertinent to note that some strains of *E. coli* and staphylococci are capable of splitting urea.

Although of limited clinical value, it is sometimes desirable to know the amount of calcium excreted per 24 hours by patients with radiopaque stones. This is conveniently done by having the patient abstain from dairy products (milk, cheese, and ice cream) for one or two days and then, while continuing the diet restriction, collect urine for one or two 24-hour periods. The calcium ingested with this regimen will usually be less than 300 mg per day, and the amount excreted by normal subjects will be less than 175 mg per 24 hours. With unrestricted diets urinary calcium values may be as much as 300 mg per 24 hours in normal subjects. Urinary calcium is increased in the majority of patients with calcareous calculi, but will be normal in patients whose primary problem is infection. Reliable oxalate analyses are not generally available, but, when possible, urinary oxalate should be measured in patients with calcium oxalate stones. The amount of phosphorus in urine reflects dietary phosphorus, and is a useless measurement unless the amount ingested is accurately known.

In patients with calcareous calculi, serum analyses are required chiefly to establish the presence or absence of hypercalcemic states, particularly hyperparathyroidism or renal tubular acidosis. With the patient in a postabsorptive state, determinations of creatinine, carbon dioxide, chloride, uric acid, phosphorus, and calcium are sufficient. Abnormal values should be confirmed by repetition of the tests. The serum concentrations of bicarbonate and chloride may be normal in patients with mild renal tubular acidosis. Phosphorus concentrations in the sera of patients with idiopathic calcareous calculi are often slightly less than those of normal subjects, and uric acid values are frequently increased.

When the calculus is available, both its central and peripheral portions should be subjected to chemical or crystallographic (by x-ray diffraction) analysis. Much information as to cause and treatment may be gained from this.

Radiologic Findings. A plain film of the abdomen or renal tomography in a patient properly prepared with laxatives is often informative, but contrast urography can also be helpful. Roentgenographic visualization of the urinary tract should not be delayed if an infected patient is suspected of having ureteral obstruction. Uric acid and the rare xanthine calculi are radiolucent and may be large or small. It is not uncommon for a patient with idiopathic calcareous calculi to have stones of mixed composition – uric acid and oxalate, and a relatively small proportion as oxalate will induce radiopaqueness of a predominantly uric acid calculus. Also, it should be realized that patients with gout have an increased incidence of the radiopaque oxalate stones.

Large or staghorn-shaped radiopaque calculi are usually the result of infection and are composed of magnesium-ammonium-phosphate or calcium phosphate, but cystine stones may achieve a similar size and configuration. Detectable laminations are not uncommon in large calculi resulting from infection. Calcium oxalate calculi are usually small (2 to 5 mm in diameter), dense, and frequently multiple. Such calculi in children may indicate the presence of oxalosis. When large (diameter greater than 10 mm), extremely dense (more dense than adjacent bone) stones are present in children or adults, hyperoxaluria should be suspected. The coexistence of nephrocalcinosis and renal calculi is not uncommon as a sequel of infection, but may also indicate the presence of medullary sponge kidneys, renal tubular acidosis, hyperparathyroidism, sarcoidosis, and rarely oxalosis.

Stones are often of mixed composition, particularly when infection has supervened; for example, at the center of a large calculus there may be either a radiolucent area composed of urates or a radiologically dense oxalate stone. The rare calculus consisting largely of matrix material may be barely visible radiologically.

Finally, roentgenographic visualization of the urinary tract may reveal anatomic abnormalities conducive to calculus formation. Obstruction, localized deformity, or medullary sponge kidneys are probably the most common such abnormalities.

Treatment. *General.* Avoidance of dehydration is important in calculous disease of all types, but especially in patients with cystinuria, those with a susceptibility to uric acid concretions, and those with urinary tract infections. To maintain continuously dilute urine usually requires a daily intake of approximately 4 quarts of liquids, which should be distributed throughout the 24 hours. Although dairy products are frequently omitted during test procedures, there are no data to suggest that continued avoidance is beneficial in reducing the incidence or growth of calcareous calculi in man. In contrast to the poor absorption of oxalate from vegetables, many beverages (e.g., tea, beer, fruit juices, cola drinks) contain significant amounts of oxalate in absorbable form. In patients with oxalate stones it is probably wise to limit the intake of these particular liquids to no more than 1 pint daily until the specific role of diet in the pathogenesis of calculi is more fully delineated. In patients with small bowel disease and hyperoxaluria, more stringent reductions in dietary oxalate and correction of any existing acidosis are indicated. The possible usefulness of taurine and cholestyramine in reducing the hyperoxaluria of patients with intestinal disease has not been adequately defined.

Every effort should be made to eradicate infection promptly. In paraplegic patients in whom high incidence of calculi correlates with urinary tract infections, dramatic reduction in stone development has been achieved by prompt and effective treatment of incipient infections. The size of ureteral calculi that can be passed spontaneously is surprising. Therefore it is often wise to delay instrumental intervention until it is certain that the calculus will not be extruded.

Specific. Details regarding the rationale for treatment of patients with cystinuria, renal tubular acidosis, and uric acid calculi are recorded in other parts of the text. Suffice it to say here that if treatment with absorbable alkali is to be instituted, the amount required varies, depending on renal function, but for adults with normal glomerular filtration rates it is usually from 100 to 250 mEq of cation per day regardless of the salt used. For example, with sodium bicarbonate these amounts of cation are provided by 8.4 to 21.0 grams, respectively. Cystinurics to be treated in this manner require the larger amounts because of the need to maintain urinary pH in the range of 8.0. Dosage with alkali should be spaced equally throughout the 24 hours to ensure continuous control of urinary pH.

Patients with single or very infrequent calcareous calculi that are passed without undue difficulty should be advised to drink copious amounts of liquid, but usually need not be considered candidates for continuous medicinal treatment.

Several largely empiric modes of therapy are currently in widespread use for patients with recurrent calcareous calculi. Each of these programs was devised in an effort to modify urine in a way that enhanced the solubility of the least soluble salts. Administration of divided doses of orthophosphates, usually as a neutral mixture of monobasic and dibasic salts, in amounts sufficient to provide 1500 to 2100 mg of phosphorus per 24 hours has been remarkably effective in preventing stone formation in uninfected patients with calcareous calculi of various causes. Diarrhea is the major adverse symptom, but most males can tolerate the aforementioned doses. Amounts of phosphates providing less than 1500 mg of phosphorus are usually ineffective in preventing stone formation in males, but many females are adequately treated with 1200 mg of phosphorus per day. Potassium phosphates may be substituted for sodium salts in patients with hypertension. This form of therapy is contraindicated in patients whose renal function is impaired to the degree that there is inadequate excretion of a phosphate load. Phosphate administration induces an increased excretion of inorganic pyrophosphate, and possibly other phosphorylated inhibitors of crystal formation, and usually causes a modest reduction in urinary calcium. There is uncertainty, however, that these are the changes that account for the prevention of calculus formation by phosphates.

Hydrochlorothiazide administration, 50 mg twice daily, has proved effective in preventing stone formation in a large majority of patients so treated. Thiazides reduce urinary calcium and augment magnesium excretion, but frequently cause symptomatic hypokalemia. Complete replacement of the potassium deficiency may lessen the effectiveness of this form of therapy. In calculous patients with hypertension or in those with a hyperactive intestinal tract, hydrochlorothiazide is probably the therapy of choice. Magnesium oxide has been advocated for patients with oxalate stones on the basis that increased urinary magnesium promotes oxalate solubility, but published experiences with this form of therapy indicate it to be of limited effectiveness. In patients who form two types of stones, e.g., uric acid and calcium oxalate, it is often useful to use both allopurinol and phosphates or hydrochlorothiazide.

Patients with calculi caused by infection are the most difficult to manage. None of the regimens mentioned are effective in such patients. The infection should be treated, but it is difficult to prevent recurrence. In addition to control of infection, treatment directed to reducing the urinary phosphorus to several hundred milligrams per day has been used by a number of investigators. This program requires that the patient avoid dairy products and, to further decrease phosphate absorption, ingest 30 ml of aluminum carbonate gel after each meal and at bedtime. Caution must be exercised to guard against phosphate depletion with this regimen. When infection cannot be eradicated by antimicrobial drugs, surgical removal of calculi, especially if they are large, is advisable.

Boyce, W. H. (ed.): Symposium on renal lithiasis. Urol. Clin. North Am., 1:179, 1974.

Dent, C. E., and Sutor, D. J.: Presence or absence of inhibitor of calcium-oxalate crystal growth in urine of normals and stone-formers. Lancet, 2:775, 1971.

Smith, L. H., Jr. (ed.): Symposium on stones. Am. J. Med., 45:649, 1968.

Stauffer, J. Q., Humphreys, M. H. and Weir, G. J.: Acquired hyperoxaluria with regional enteritis after ileal resection. Ann. Intern. Med., 79:383, 1973.

628. CYSTS OF THE KIDNEY

George E. Schreiner

POLYCYSTIC DISEASE

Polycystic disease is the most prevalent renal cystic disease (Table 1). It is inherited as a dominant, non-sex-linked disease emerging at two prominent age peaks, in infancy and in adult life. Progressive dilatation of renal tubules leads to obstruction, infection, rupture of cysts, bleeding, hypertension, and progressive renal failure. There may be associated anomalies, such as cysts in the liver, pancreas, spleen, or lung, or berry aneurysm of the cerebral vessels. Sporadic cases are found without familial history and scattered through childhood. More often the adult disease emerges after the next generation has already been "planted." The infantile type may be autosomal recessive, but the adult disease is a hereditary dominant. Penetrance is high and rises with increasing age. Clinical surveys in large families usually reveal that half or more of the members are afflicted. In advanced age penetrance for cysts is almost total. However, once present, cysts may vary in signficance to mortality or health.

Embryology.   Nephrogenesis is usually complete by 35 weeks. Theories no longer accepted for the pathogenesis of polycystic disease include fetal papillitis with secondary fibrosis and obstruction, cyst formation as a neoplastic process, congenital syphilis, and fetal interstitial nephritis. Popular theories include (1) "nonunion" of ureteric bud and tubules, (2) noncanalization owing to lack of "organizer," and (3) persistence of primitive nephrons that fail to atrophy. A microdissection study subclassified four types: (1) hyperplasia of interstitial portion of collecting tubules, (2 inhibition of ampullary activity, (3) multiple developmental anomalies, and (4) urethral obstruction. Infantile cysts may be totally isolated; adult cortical cysts are younger, larger, and glomerular and do not connect. Juxtamedullary cysts are older and have entering and exiting tubules. In the medulla the cysts involve collecting ducts and may open to a calyx.

Physiology.   In studying polycystic patients with normal, medium, and low filtration rates, we have found progressive loss of concentrating ability and a salt-losing tendency. Bicarbonate wasting may contribute to systemic acidosis. In an excellent family study (M-M), 10 of 12 noncystic family members had U_{max} greater than 900 mOsm per kilogram (1060 $\pm$ 134). In 11 of 13 family members with cysts but without azotemia, U_{max} was less than 700 mOsm per kilogram (657 $\pm$ 169). Patients with renal failure have osmotic U/P ratios near unity. This is a pitressin-resistant concentrating defect. Dilution capability is preserved. Cyst fluid has variable concentrations of Na, K, H, Cr, PAH, and inulin, indicating entry of solutes into cysts and selective transport of water and solutes out of cysts. Cyst/plasma ratios of Cr are above 1.0 in deep cysts. Concentration of amino acids in cysts may add 50 to 100 mOsm per kilogram. Such osmols have the potential of drawing in water for expansion of cysts. Protein, red cells, bacteria, and cellular debris may be found. Enzymatic breakdown of protein could yield amino acid mOsm.

Incidence (Table 2).   Since early diagnosis is difficult, the clinical incidence varies with the vigor of the diagnostic pursuit. Isotopic scans, ultrasound studies, infusion nephrotomography, and other diagnostic techniques enhance the yield. Measurement of concentrating ability in absence of other causes may be the most sensitive screening test. Yet polycystic disease is still often a surprise diagnosis at autopsy.

Pathology.   The kidneys are enlarged and often asymmetrical. They have a nodular surface produced by projecting cysts that may be filled with watery, serous, hemorrhagic, pustular, or viscid fluid or clear urine. Cut surface reveals the entire parenchyma honeycombed by cysts protruding from various levels. About one fifth of polycystic patients have intracranial aneurysm, and 4

TABLE 1.   Simple Classification of Cystic Disease

1. Polycystic disease
     Infantile (Potter, Type 1)
     Adult (Potter, Type 3)
2. Multicystic disease
3. Multilocular cysts   } (?Potter, Type 2)
4. Simple cysts
5. Medullary cystic disease
6. Medullary sponge kidney
7. Dysplasia
8. Miscellaneous cysts of renal origin
9. Miscellaneous cysts of nonrenal origin

TABLE 2.   Some Representative Incidence Figures

Year	Place	No. Polycystic Cases	Ratio to Autopsies
1897	Kiel	16	1:636
1928	Leningrad	192	1:261
1933	Mayo	9	1:1019
1934	New York	14	1:428
1935	Göttingen	38	1:222
1949	Great Britain	16	1:375
1950	Minnesota	70	1:779
1954	Copenhagen	143	1:773
1955	Mayo	35	1:323
1965	Georgetown	—	1:165

Total = 533 +   Avg. = 1:498

per cent of patients with clinical aneurysms have polycystic disease. Cysts may coexist in liver, spleen, lungs, and pancreas, but are rarely clinically significant. Mild renal cysts may occur in hepatic cystic disease and may be clinically subordinate. Histologically, cysts of various caliber, location, and content may be demonstrated. The internal lining may be flattened or cuboidal and rarely may have papillary projections or glomerular tufts. Recently, it has been shown that interruptions of the elastic laminae of small renal arteries, ruptured arteries, and microaneurysms can be demonstrated in the renal parenchyma. It is not clear whether vessel rupture is cause or effect. Degenerative changes from pressure, calculi and secondary infection may be seen. Many cases of renal carcinoma have been reported in polycystic kidneys. Earlier functional evaluation and renal biopsy studies are needed in polycystic families, because little is known of the natural history of cysts in the presymptomatic decades.

Diagnosis. The *infantile type* is usually diagnosed by palpation of bilateral renal masses, roentgenographic findings, or presentation with uremia. Nausea, vomiting, dehydration, and abdominal distention are the most prevalent. We have one such patient six years old. The small cyst variety is the most difficult to diagnose. The *adult type* may be totally asymptomatic for several decades, with a chance finding on roentgenographic examination or even at autopsy. Segmental disease has been described. Patients with large cysts (greater than 3 cm) have more severe disease, are more symptomatic, and die younger. With progressive enlargement, presenting symptoms include lumbar or abdominal pain (28 per cent), palpable mass (20 per cent), hypertension (17 per cent), bladder symptoms of frequency, urgency, and dysuria (17 per cent), painless hematuria (17 per cent), and painful hematuria (10 per cent). Other patients may present with any of the protean manifestations of uremia. Renal osteodystrophy and hyperparathyroidism are especially prevalent in younger patients. Hypertension and palpable kidneys are present in about three quarters of the patients at the time of diagnosis. Kidneys may grow to a size of 6 kg or more and produce weakness, a dragging sensation, increasing abdominal girth, and the displacement of other organs.

Complications. Many patients with polycystic disease present or die with complications such as vascular accidents from ruptured aneurysms or hypertensive disease, secondary pyelonephritis, infected cysts, perinephric abscess, obstruction, gross hematuria, calcification of cyst wall and formation of urinary calculi, and associated renal carcinoma. Both erythrocytosis and polycythemia have been noted. Dalgaard found calculus and/or colic in 18 per cent of 350 patients. Rarely dystocia has been reported owing to distended abdomen of the fetus from infantile cystic disease. We have seen subdiaphragmatic abscess from ruptured infected cysts and obstructive uropathy reversible by surgical decompression. A family history of polycystic kidneys can readily be obtained in the majority of cases by taking a detailed history and surveying causes of death in siblings with emphasis on cerebral aneurysm and kidney disease. Spurious histories are encountered in families with a pathetic desire to hide the trait. General problems we have encountered include psychologic "block" to family surveys; the problems of marriage, pregnancy, and contact sports; questions of elective surgery and medical procedures; economic problems generating from inability to get life, health, hospital, or disability insurance or to meet medical requirements of a job; and the emotional impact of watching other members of the family die from a known affliction of the observer.

Laboratory Findings. These include albuminuria, hematuria, pyuria, passage of epithelial cells, and all the progressive laboratory findings associated with renal failure. Hyperchloremic acidosis, bicarbonate wasting, and defect in excretion of an acid load may be seen. A salt-losing tendency with dehydration, increasing azotemia, and hyponatremia is much more frequent than in other renal diseases.

Roentgenography. Important roentgenographic findings include enlarged or displaced kidneys with varying densities, loculation, or calcification, elongated pelves, crescentic deformities of calyces (wine-glass sign), hydronephrosis and other obstructive phenomena, and "unfolding" of the calyceal system. The small cyst, infantile type, is best diagnosed by observation of nephrographic phenomena persisting up to 72 hours. This parenchymal opacification results from concentration of iodine in tubular cells and excretion into the lumina of dilated tubules. Less than 10 per cent of polycystic disease is unilateral. Most "unilateral" disease on x-ray is bilateral at autopsy or surgery. Recently infusion nephrotomography and renal angiography have been found useful in differentiating neoplasm from cyst. The renal scan may

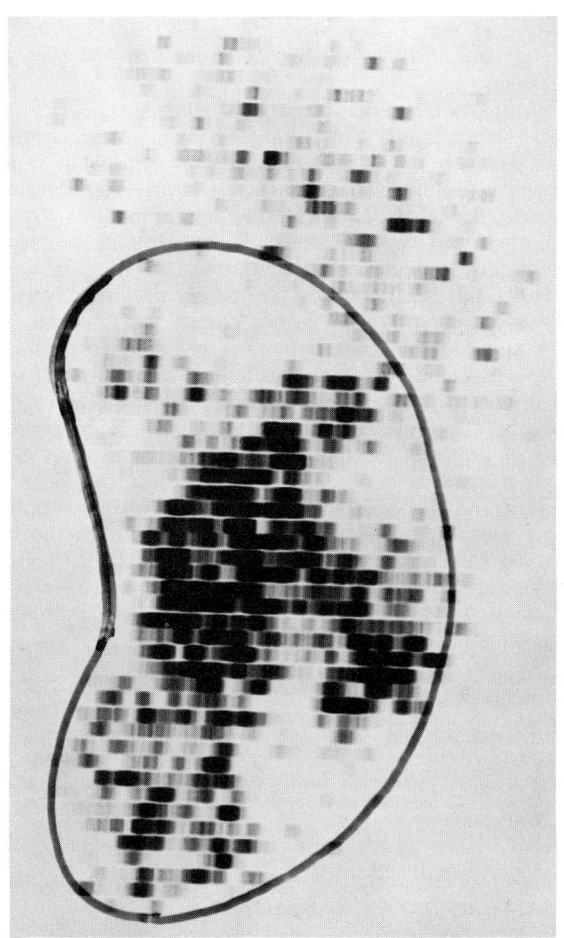

Isotope scan of a kidney; the cystic areas are indicated by areas of diminished or absent radioactivity.

give a characteristic appearance of "holes," as seen in the accompanying figure.

Prognosis. The infantile type is rapidly fatal from uremia or complications. The adult type may be latent and rarely may not interfere with longevity. Progressive cystic disease proceeds to hypertension, uremia, vascular accidents, infections, and death, with the peak mortality in the latter half of the fifth decade. Patients with small cysts (less than 3 cm), without cysts in other organs, or without hypertension tend to live longer. Prognosis can be improved by continuous medical care and treatment of infection and acute obstruction, management of chronic uremia, and avoidance of—or special care during—pregnancy. Polycystic patients often do not tolerate strict salt restriction. The age of diagnosis and the subsequent life expectancy are related. Under 50, one third of males are alive $12\frac{1}{2}$ years later. Over 50, only 14 per cent are alive $2\frac{1}{2}$ years later.

Treatment. The treatment is medical. Marsupialization, bivalving with unroofing, puncture and aspiration, and unilateral nephrectomy have all been tried and have failed. Decompression or heminephrectomy is justified only when extrarenal obstruction is demonstrated. Treatment for infection is as outlined in Ch. 617. Treatment of chronic renal failure and acute renal failure is detailed in Ch. 603 and 604. Bed rest is indicated for hematuria and transfusions for symptomatic anemia of blood loss. In patients suffering recurrent pain from enlarging cysts, we have had some success with the use of acetazolamide, 500 mg daily, as a single dose, or with combinations of acetazolamide and a thiazide diuretic. Strict control of hypertension is essential to halt progression.

Sympathetic understanding of the psychologic problem is important. The diagnosis of polycystic kidneys carries with it the responsibility to conduct a family survey and advise the patient and family members concerning the basic diagnosis, the management of possible complications, and the social concerns of marriage, pregnancy, and choice of occupation.

Hemodialysis has been successfully used for transient exacerbations of renal failure caused by infection, obstruction, dehydration, hyponatremia or hypotension. It may occasionally result in prolonged improvement even in apparently moribund patients. Recent history of a good urinary volume forms a reasonable guide in selection of patients for dialysis. Polycystic patients make good transplant candidates, because the graft does not acquire the disease of the recipient and because immunologic problems are absent. Bilateral nephrectomy is usually indicated before transplantation. Erythrocytosis may follow the relief of azotemia and may be reversed by removal of a cystic kidney, presumably indicating erythropoietin production.

Bialestock, D.: The morphogenesis of renal cysts in the stillborn: A study of microdissection technique. J. Pathol., 71:51, 1956.

Bricker, N. S., and Patton, J. F.: Cystic disease of the kidneys: A study of dynamics and chemical composition of cyst fluid. Am. J. Med., 18:207, 1955.

Dalgaard, O. Z.: Polycystic disease of the kidneys. In Strauss, M. B., and Welt, L. G. (eds.): Diseases of the Kidney. Boston, Little, Brown & Company, 1971, p. 1223.

Gardner, K. D., Jr.: Composition of fluid in twelve cysts of a polycystic kidney. N. Engl. J. Med., 281:985, 1969.

Hatfield, P. M., and Pfister, R. C.: Adult polycystic disease of the kidneys (Potter, type 3). J.A.M.A., 222:1527, 1972.

Martinez-Maldonado, M., Yium, J. J., Eknoyan, G., and Suki, W. N.: Adult polycystic disease: Studies of the defect in urine concentration. Kidney Int., 2:107, 1972.

Osathanondh, V., and Potter, E. L.: Development of human kidney as shown by microdissection. I. Preparation of tissues with reasons for possible misinterpretation of observations. Arch. Path., 76:271, 1963.

Osathanondh, V., and Potter, E. L.: Pathogenesis of polycystic kidneys. Historical survey. Arch. Path., 77:459, 1964. Type 1 due to hyperplasia of interstitial portions of collecting tubules. Arch. Path., 77:466, 1964. Type 2 due to inhibition of ampillary activity. Arch. Path., 77:474, 1964. Type 3 due to multiple abnormalities of development. Arch. Path., 77:485, 1964. Type 4 due to urethral obstruction. Arch. Path., 77:502, 1964.

Safouh, M., Crocker, J. F. S., and Vernier, R. L.: Experimental cystic disease of the kidney: Sequential, functional and morphologic studies. Lab. Invest., 23:392, 1970.

OTHER CYSTS

Serous or *solitary* cysts are thin sacs with flattened epithelium frequent in the lower pole and rarely communicating with a nephron. Congenital in origin, they may grow to 12 liters, produce backache, dragging sensation, palpable mass, obstruction, or urographic abnormality. They may contain blood and calcification. Solutes generally approximate those of plasma water. *Multilocular* cysts have septa or a honeycombed interior. When large they may resemble polycystic disease and may account for some older reports of unilateral polycysts. Comparative features are outlined in Table 3. A few cases of *segmental* cystic disease have been reported with histologic criteria for polycystic disease. *Lymphatic* cysts are found near the hilum and are associated with veins and vascular atresias. They begin 1 to 2 cm in diameter in the newborn but may enlarge. *Diverticula* of pelvis and calyces are associated with infection and obstruction, and they may appear as *cystic dilatations* of the parenchyma. They are suspected by their location. *Perirenal* cysts may follow traumatic extravasation or may be neoplastic. The latter originate in aberrant mesodermal tissue (wolffian or müllerian ducts, lymph channels), are varied in form, are usually unilateral, and are on the left side in females. *Renal hematomas* may liquefy and cavitate. *Angiomas* may produce profuse bleeding over long periods. *Mesenteric* cysts form below the kidney and simulate tumor or cause obstruction. *Dermoid* cysts contain all germ layers and may contain hair, bones, teeth, and other tissues. Infectious erosion of the renal parenchyma or dissolution of infected infarcts in *pyelonephritis* may produce cystlike areas, filled with fluid or pus. *Renal tuberculosis* may produce *caseocavernous abscesses* or ulcerations of the pelvis. Retention cysts of chronic glomerulonephritis are rarely of clinical importance. *Echinococcus cysts* occur from infestation by the larval stage of the dog tapeworm. This is prevalent in

TABLE 3. Characteristics of Cystic Disease

	Polycystic	Multicystic
Hereditary	+	−
Bilateral	+	Rare
Unilateral	Rare	−
Progressive enlargement	+	−
Associated renal anomalies	−	+
In adults	+	−
In children	Rare	+
Functioning cysts	+	−
Communicating cysts	+	−
Measurable renal dysfunction	+	−
Dysplasia	−	+
Normal tissue between cysts	+	−
Thick capsule	−	+

certain sheep-raising countries. The manifestations include tumor, pain, dysuria, hematuria, eosinophilia, and excretion of ova, hooklets, and scolices in the urine. A complement-fixation test may be positive. *Toxoplasma* may produce microscopic pseudocysts in the kidney. *Renal aneurysm* may produce flank pain, hematuria, hypertension, and urographic filling defects. Renal cysts are associated with angiomatous tumors of the cerebellum in *Lindau's disease* and of the retina in *von Hippel-Lindau disease.*

Treatment of most cysts depends on type, location, and manifestation. Known serous and pustular cysts may be aspirated by needle. More often, because of the threat of malignancy, most cysts require surgical exploration and removal. Normal parenchyma should be preserved whenever possible. Erythrocytosis may be reversed by cyst removal, but cysts rarely contain granular cells or significant erythropoietin. They probably stimulate erythropoietin production in nearby tissue. Advances in renal plastic surgery now permit more frequent choices between partial and total nephrectomy. The latter should be avoided in benign conditions.

Boggs, L. K., and Kimmelstiel, P.: Benign multilocular cystic nephroma: Report of 2 cases of so-called multilocular cysts of the kidney. J. Urol., 76:530, 1956.

Hutchins, K. R., Mulholland, S. G., and Edson, M.: Segmental polycystic disease: N.Y. State J. Med., 72:1850, 1972.

Isaac, F., Schoen, I., and Walker, P.: An unusual case of Lindau's disease: Cystic disease of the kidneys and pancreas with renal and cerebral tumors. Am. J. Roentgenol., 75:912, 1956.

Moore, T.: Unilateral cystic kidneys. Br. J. Urol., 29:3, 1957.

Parkkulainen, K. V., Hjelt, L. V., and Sirola, K.: Congenital multicystic dysplasia of the kidney: Report of nineteen cases with discussion on the etiology, nomenclature, and classification of the cystic dysplasias of the kidney. Acta Chir. Scand., Suppl. 244, 1959.

Vertel, R. M., Morse, B. S., and Prince, J. E.: Remission of erythrocytosis after drainage of a solitary renal cyst. Arch. Intern. Med. 120:54, 1967.

UREMIC MEDULLARY CYSTIC DISEASE

Uremic medullary cystic disease, familial juvenile nephrophthisis, and some forms of salt-losing nephritis now appear to be facets of the same disease. There is definite hereditary predisposition exhibiting in various pedigrees as a recessive, a dominant, or an incomplete recessive affecting young children, older children, young adults, and a few rare survivors in the fifth and sixth decades. The majority are in the second and third decades. Male-to-male transmission (? X-linked) has been reported. There is a frequent association with red and blond hair. The disease may present insidiously with pallor, polyuria, anemia, or failure to thrive and grow. Hypotension, salt-wasting, and symptomatic bone disease are frequent. The normochromic anemia is refractory. The urine is deceptively benign, although modest proteinuria is frequent in older patients. Salt wasting is almost the rule. Hypertension is rare. The patients progress inexorably, but at varying rates, into uremia, with any or all of its features. Prominent are hyponatremia, hypochloremia, hypocalcemia, hyperphosphatemia, hyperphosphatasemia, metabolic acidosis and retarded growth. The osteodystrophy may be predominantly rachitic, osteomalacic, hyperparathyroid, or a mixture. Roentgenologic changes include widening of zone of calcification, metaphyseal fraying, decreased bone density, delayed maturation, pseudofractures and deformities, exostoses, localized osteosclerosis, subperiosteal cortical bone erosion, brown tumors, periosteal new bone, and extraosseous calcification—especially

articular (hands, feet), periarticular, and soft-tissue, e.g., cornea, conjunctiva, and kidney. Parathyroid and adrenal hyperplasia and myelofibrosis occur. All tubular defects are distal with impaired concentrating ability, poor response to ADH, impaired acidification, impaired ammonium excretion, salt wasting, and a tendency to hyperkalemia. Infection is rare except after instrumentation. Notably absent are phosphaturia, glycosuria, aminoaciduria, or any disorder of proximal tubular function.

Pathologically, the kidneys are contracted (45 to 100 grams), granular, and lobulated. There are glomerulosclerosis, periglomerular fibrosis, diffuse, severe interstitial fibrosis, tubular atrophy and dilatation, colloid casts, localized lymphangiectasia, and cysts widespread in medulla, but often randomly distributed elsewhere. They vary from 50 mm to 2 cm in diameter. Cut sections from patients with nephronophthisis and medullary cystic disease are indistinguishable. Overemphasis on macroscopic cysts and their anatomy has confused the issue. Goldman et al. have traced 50 members of a family through five generations and found a dominant pattern. Eighteen of 25 persons in the first three generations had either overt renal failure or transmission to offspring. In other families it has been recessive. In some cases there is no family involvement. The cause and progression resemble human toxic nephropathy from a variety of agents, including heavy metals, and the lesions resemble early diphenylamine intoxication in rats. The disease could be an inborn error of metabolism that permits accumulation of a toxic substance, affecting distal tubular development in fetal life or early infancy.

Treatment consists in genetic counseling, management of abnormal physiology such as the salt depletion, treating the full range of defects seen in renal tubular disease, especially osteodystrophy and anemia, and ultimately resorting to the definitive therapy of terminal renal failure—dialysis or transplantation. Patients with renal transplants in place for more than two years have not acquired the defect, indicating that medullary cystic disease is purely renal in origin.

Fanconi, G., Hanhard, E., Albertini, A., von Uhlinger, E., Dolivo, G., and Prader, A.: Die familiare juvenile Nephronophthise (die idiopathische Schrumpfniere). Helv. Paediatr. Acta, 6:1, 1951.

Gielson, N., Heinegard, D., Holmberg, C. G., et al.: Renal medullary cystic disease or familial juvenile nephronophthisis: A renal tubular disease. Am. J. Med., 48:174, 1970.

Goldman, S. H., Walter, S. R., Merigan, T. C., Jr., Gardner, K. D., Jr., and Bull, J. M. C.: Hereditary occurrence of cystic disease of the renal medulla. N. Engl. J. Med., 274:984, 1966.

Herman, R. C., Good, R. A., and Vernier, R. L.: Medullary cystic disease in two siblings. Am. J. Med., 43:335, 1967.

Levin, N. W., Rosenberg, B., Zwi, S., and Reid, F. P.: Medullary cystic disease of the kidney, with some observations on ammonium excretion. Am. J. Med., 30:807, 1961.

Mongeau, J. G., and Worthen, H. G.: Nephronophthisis and medullary cystic disease. Am. J. Med., 43:345, 1967.

Rayfield, E. J., and McDonald, F. D.: Red and blonde hair in renal medullary cystic disease. Arch. Intern. Med., 130:72, 1972.

Strauss, M. B.: Clinical and pathological aspects of cystic disease of the renal medulla. Ann. Intern. Med., 57:373, 1962.

Strauss, M. B., and Sommers, S. C.: Medullary cystic disease and familial juvenile nephronophthisis. N. Engl. J. Med., 277:863, 1967.

SPONGE KIDNEY
(Nonuremic Medullary Cystic Disease)

Sponge kidney, first recognized in 1939, has now been recognized in several hundred patients. It is a congenital anomaly which can be manifested by pain, colic, calculi, recurrent infection, or hematuria; but more often it is asymptomatic and discovered as an incidental finding on roentgenography, biopsy, or autopsy. Branching, radial ducts and cysts are found ramifying from calyces along the pyramids. They may fill on intravenous pyelography, and may *not* fill on retrograde pyelography. Flow is slow, and contrast material hangs behind. They may be uni- or bilateral, segmental, or focal. The roentgenographic appearance has been likened to a sponge, grapes, flowers, and twigs. The cysts are filled with fluid, cellular debris, and concretions. Calcium apatite, carbonate, oxalate, and triple phosphate have been found. Nephrocalcinosis may occur. Hypercalciuria, pyelonephritis, and hypertension may supervene. Distal tubular defects have been noted, but so uncommonly that they may be related to the complications rather than the disease. Similar cysts have been noted in congenital hepatic fibrosis. Reported cases in Ehlers-Danlos syndrome, hemihypertrophy, and congenital pyloric stenosis may be special forms of sponge kidney. The roentgenographic pattern has been seen in two generations of one family and in two siblings, but is generally nonfamilial. The prognosis is related to infection, obstruction, and calculous disease. The asymptomatic form is benign and usually without any counterpart functional disorder. Instrumentation should be avoided.

Abeshouse, B. S., and Abeshouse, G. A.: Sponge kidney: A review of the literature and a report of five cases. J. Urol., 84:252, 1960.

Copping, G. A.: Medullary sponge kidney: Its occurrence in a father and daughter. Can. Med. Assoc. J., 96:608, 1967.

Lagergren, C., and Lindvall, N.: Medullary sponge kidney and polycystic diseases of the kidney: Distinct entities. Am. J. Roentgenol., 88:153, 1962.

MacDougall, J. A., and Prout, W. G.: Medullary sponge kidney: Clinical appraisal and report of twelve cases. Br. J. Surg., 55:130, 1968.

Morris, R. C., Yamauchi, H., Palubinskas, A. J., and Howenstine, J.: Medullary sponge kidney. Amer. J. Med., 38:883, 1965.

629. TUMORS OF THE KIDNEY

George E. Schreiner

Neoplasia of the genitourinary tract accounts for about one fifth of adult tumors and about one quarter of childhood tumors. About 7000 people annually in the United States develop renal cell carcinoma. Renal masses are considered malignant until proved otherwise. Our ignorance of the mechanisms of renal neoplasia parallels our general lack of knowledge of the pathogenesis of unrestrained cell growth. A classification of renal tumors is given in Table 4.

Unending subclassifications of tumors and morphologic grading have generally proved to be a sterile pathologic exercise. Older designations, such as hypernephroma, adenocarcinoma, alveolar carcinoma, and embryonic carcinoma have been dropped in favor of "renal carcinoma" or tumors of epithelial cell origin. Multiple sections often reveal more than one histologic type.

Pathology. Tubular epithelium gives rise to adenocarcinoma. The epithelial lining of the pelvicalyceal system yields transitional cell carcinomas, and immature parenchymal tissue is the source of Wilms' tumor. Carcinoma accounts for 80 per cent of renal malignancy.

TABLE 4.   Classification of Renal Tumors

1. Neoplasms of renal parenchyma
   Benign tumors
      Fibroma
      Adenoma
      Papillary cystadenoma
      Endometriosis
   Epithelial neoplasms
      Renal carcinoma
      Embryonal nephroma (Wilms' tumor, nephroblastoma)
   Mesothelial neoplasms
      Sarcoma
   Neurogenic tumors
      Neuroblastoma
      Schwannoma
      Sympathicoblastoma
2. Neoplasms of the pelvis and calyces
   Papilloma
   Papillary carcinoma
   Squamous cell carcinoma
   Hemangioma
3. Tumors of the renal capsule
   Fibroma
   Fibrolipoma
   Malignant sarcoma
   Angiosarcoma
   Chondroma
4. Perirenal tumors and cysts
5. Tumors metastatic to the kidney

Cell types are *clear* and *granular*. Anatomic staging is as follows: IA—intracapsular tumor; IB—intrarenal but extracapsular (invasion through tumor capsule); II—perinephric microscopic III—perinephric gross; and IV—distant metastases. Renal carcinoma has a male preponderance, with a peak incidence at 45 to 60 years of age. Extension into the renal veins or through the renal capsule offers a bad prognosis (vein invaded—30 per cent five-year survival, versus 60 per cent when the vein is not invaded). Degeneration and calcification are a good prognostic feature. Renal carcinoma may spontaneously regress. A metastatic lesion may regress after removal of primary site, or may occur as late as 20 years after primary removal. Spread is by direct invasion or by vascular and lymphatic channels. Venous occlusion may result from spread of the tumor up the inferior vena cava. Favorite metastatic sites are lungs, liver, bones, and brain. They may be solitary.

Embryonal nephroma (Wilms' tumor) may occur in the fetus or rarely in later life. Seventy-five per cent appear before the age of five; about two thirds occur before two years of age. Eight per cent are bilateral. More than 50 confusing names have been applied to this tumor. It grows rapidly, may approach the weight of the rest of the body, and metastasizes most frequently through the veins to the lungs or through the lymphatics to the periaortic nodes. Widespread metastases in many organs may be seen.

Clinical Manifestations. Since early renal tumors are asymptomatic, diagnoses are achieved by way of accidental or routine diagnostic studies. The classic triad of hematuria, mass, and pain must now be considered a later finding. Fever, leukocytosis, evidence of metastases, abdominal and flank pain, albuminuria, anorexia, weight loss, nausea, and vomiting are the most common symptoms. Even so, in less than half the children with Wilms' tumor is diagnosis achieved within one month of onset of symptoms. Demonstration of hematuria varies with the skill and persistence brought to the urinalysis. Erythrocytes in urine should never be considered a normal finding; suspicion of tumor should become greater during a systemic exclusion of other causes of hematuria. Because of venous extension and vascular spread, examination of patients with nephroma should be cautious, and treatment should be instituted as early as possible. Hypertension has been reported with widely varying incidence in embryonal nephroma; it may not revert on tumor removal. Presumably the tumor produces pressors directly or indirectly via ischemia. Nephroma may simulate or coexist with infantile polycystic disease.

In adult renal cell carcinoma the most prominent manifestations, in order, are hematuria, weight loss, lassitude, flank pain, fever, and abdominal pain. A firm spherical mass may be demonstrable by palpation, or roentgenographic studies may reveal it. Distant metastases may be observed before local signs appear. Notable are "cotton ball" metastases to the lung, osteolytic lesions in the long bones (femur, humerus), and involvement of lymph nodes, liver, adrenals, and contralateral kidney. No organ is exempt; unusual cases have been diagnosed by finding lesions in such places as the eye and vagina. Pelvic angiography and pulmonary fluoroscopy with an image intensifier have revealed asymptomatic metastases unrecognizable by other means.

Unusual Features. Renal carcinoma may present curious features and it has been called the "internist's tumor." These features include large tumor without distortion of the calyceal system, leukemoid reaction with leukocytes ranging up to 100,000 per cubic millimeter, polycythemia, eczematoid dermatitis, hypertension, hypercalcemia, peripheral neuropathy, plasmacytosis, and amyloid disease. Renal carcinoma has emerged as a major consideration in fevers of unknown origin. It may mimic a prolonged septic disease, or it may form an arteriovenous fistula to produce congestive heart failure. Both adult carcinoma and Wilms' tumor have been associated with erythema and polycythemia. Elevated blood and tumor levels or erythropoietin have been reported. Renal carcinomas have polycythemia in 2.3 per cent of cases, and should be considered in the differential diagnosis of polycythemia. We have seen secondary polycythemia, including granulocytosis and thrombocytosis, in a patient with a small renal carcinoma not demonstrable by x-ray. Parathormone-like activity has been reported, with hypercalcemia responding promptly to excision of renal carcinoma. Tumor patients may be hypertensive but are not inordinately so, and renin has not been isolated in a tumor.

Laboratory Findings. In addition to anemia or polycythemia, renal carcinoma characteristically brings about an unusually high sedimentation rate (up to 150 mm per hour). On electrophoresis, serum albumin is reduced, and alpha$_2$ globulin is elevated. A special form of tumor, the clear-cell PAS-positive renal carcinoma, has been associated with evidence of increased glucoprotein synthesis and abnormal serum glucoproteins.

Roentgenographic findings include irregularity of renal margin, multiple calcifications, deformity of infundibulum or calyces, and displacement of the kidney by outward growth. Infusion nephrotomography, mainstream and selective angiography, technetium radioscans, venography, and lymphangiography have vastly improved the early diagnosis. Neovasculature giving a "tumor blush" on arteriography is virtually diagnostic and can separate tumor from cyst. Perinephric insufflation has also been used.

Prognosis and Treatment. Embryonal nephroma was once 90 per cent fatal. The combination of early diagnosis, restriction of palpation, preoperative irradiation, prompt nephrectomy, and postoperative irradiation has dramatically reduced mortality, so that half or more of the patients can survive. Actinomycin D and vincristine have also been used postoperatively. Standard chemotherapy of recurrent disease has generally been ineffective save for sporadic success with progestational agents, androgenic hormones, and, more recently, Lomustine (C-C Nitrosurea). Immunotherapy may hold some promise. Earlier diagnosis and prompt nephrectomy have bettered the former 20 per cent survival in renal carcinoma, but the outlook is still grave. Statistics are confused by the delayed appearance of metastases. Renal carcinoma may stimulate fibrosis such as that seen in periureteral fibrosis. The resulting obstruction can falsely simulate metastases or contralateral spread. The physician who diagnoses or suspects a space-occupying lesion has an urgent obligation to achieve definitive diagnosis and surgery when indicated. There is no infallible way to distinguish clinically between a solitary cyst and a potential malignant disease. Papillary tumors of the renal pelvis yield positive exfoliative cytology in the urine.

Pelvic tumors derive from transitional epithelium and resemble tumors of the urinary bladder. Group I tumors are benign papilloma with excellent prognosis. Group II are noninvasive or focally invasive papillary carcinoma, also favorable. Group III are fully invasive but confined to the kidney and give good surgical results. Group IV spread outside the kidney and pelvis (lymph nodes, bone, liver, and lung) and carry an ominous prognosis. They may occasionally metastasize to unusual sites, including other tumors. About 80 per cent of patients have hematuria, half of it gross. Flank pain or frequency is also found. Pyelography is usually positive. Nephrectomy and ureterectomy are treatments of choice. Renal perfusion pumps used for kidney transplantation have been used for prolonged "open-kidney" surgery with subsequent autotransplant. Cytogenetic studies have revealed karyotypic abnormalities, marker chromosomes, and aneuploidy said to predict greater malignancy in early stages of noninvasive carcinoma of the bladder. The relative risk for coffee drinkers compared to that for nondrinkers is 1.24 for men and 2.58 for women. Transitional tumors occurred in 9 of 104 analgesic abusers and none of 88 pyelonephritic controls.

Bengtsson, U., Angervall, L., Ekman, H., and Lehman, L.: Transitional cell tumors of the renal pelvis in analgesic abusers. Scand. J. Nephrol., 2:145, 1968.

Bottiger, L. E.: Studies in renal carcinoma. I. Clinical and pathologic anatomical aspects. II. Biochemical investigations. Acta Med. Scand., 167:443, 1960.

Burns, W. A., and Kadar, A. T.: Unusual metastases from a transitional cell carcinoma of the renal pelvis and ureter. Med. Ann. D.C., 42:65, 1973.

Clarke, B. J., and Goade, W. J., Jr.: Fever and anemia in renal cancer. N. Engl. J. Med., 254:107, 1956.

Cole, P.: Coffee drinking and cancer of the lower urinary tract. Lancet, 1:1335, 1971.

Editorial: Analgesic abuse and tumors of the renal pelvis. Lancet, 2:1233, 1969.

Falor, W. H.: Chromosomes in noninvasive papillary carcinoma of the bladder, J.A.M.A., 216:791, 1971.

Foot, N. D., Humphreys, G. A., and Whitmore, W. F.: Renal tumors: Pathology and prognosis in 295 cases. J. Urol., 66:190, 1951.

Grabstald, H., Whitmore, W. F., and Melamed, M. R.: Renal pelvic tumors. J.A.M.A., 218:845, 1971.

Johnson, S. H., III, and Marshal, M., Jr.: Primary kidney tumors of childhood. J. Urol., 74:707, 1955.

Rubin, P.: Cancer of the urogenital tract. Kidney: Localized renal adenocarcinoma. J.A.M.A., 204:219, 1968.

Wagle, D. G.: Vagaries of renal cell carcinoma. J. Med. (Basel), 3:178, 1972.

630. MISCELLANEOUS RENAL DISORDERS

George E. Schreiner

Hoxie, H. J., and Coggin, C. B.: Renal infarction: Statistical study of 205 cases and detailed report of an unusual case. Arch. Intern. Med., 65:587, 1940.
Woods, J. W., and Williams, T. F.: Renal infarction. *In* Strauss, M. B., and Welt, L. G. (eds.): Diseases of the Kidney. Boston, Little, Brown & Company, 1971, pp. 789–794.

INFARCTION

Definition. Infarction is the ischemic death of tissue. Total ischemia of the cortical area is better termed *renal cortical necrosis* (see Ch. 604). Bland infarction without reaction is the same as *focal cortical necrosis* and may be seen in trauma, preeclampsia, infectious shock, and in most of the causes of cortical necrosis. The term *renal infarct* is usually applied to the segmental type. These are usually due to *arterial* obstruction such as *embolism* (mural thrombi, cholesterol plaque material, endocarditis), *thrombosis, trauma,* surgical injury, intrarenal *narrowing* (scleroderma, malignant nephrosclerosis), stasis (shock, diabetic acidosis), and sickle cell disease, or to *venous* thrombosis as seen in neoplastic states (hypernephroma, lymphoma), dehydration (infantile diarrhea), septicemia, and hypercoagulable states. In one study of 205 human infarctions, about 77 per cent accompanied a cardiac lesion. The early red lesion evolves rapidly into a central and peripheral dead zone and a marginal area which is presumably the source of the pressor materials that produce the often-accompanying hypertension.

Diagnosis. The diagnosis is suggested by history, flank pain, renal tenderness, transient hematuria and albuminuria, and a space-occupying lesion or change of size or nonfunctioning kidney on pyelography. Total renal infarction with recovery is followed by calcification of the necrotic tissue and hypertrophy of the contralateral kidney. Infarction may produce acute or accelerated hypertension, and should be suspected when that is coupled with history of trauma to the kidney or renal surgery. The hypertension usually peaks at two to three weeks after a single infarction, and may subside as the ischemic tissue progresses to scar formation. Renal infarcts presenting as space-occupying lesions have to be distinguished from cysts and tumors. Nephrograms with "black" areas, scintigrams with "cold" areas, or anomaly in the distribution of dye in the segmental arteriogram may be an aid to diagnosis. Identification of small renal infarcts as embolic phenomena may be the clue that leads to a primary diagnosis, e.g., asymptomatic myocardial infarction.

Heparin perfusion during selective arteriography may have therapeutic benefit.

Treatment. Embolectomy or endarterectomy should be considered as emergency treatment when the blood supply to one kidney is threatened. Aortic repair may be indicated when dissection involves the renal artery. Vascular prostheses with a side arm have also been used to bypass an irreparably damaged renal artery involved in the Leriche syndrome. Anticoagulant therapy may be indicated for a central source of embolization. When diagnostic studies indicate unilateral renal infarct as a cause for accelerated hypertension, surgical intervention may be indicated if the hypertension does not spontaneously ameliorate within two months.

Baum, S.: Renal ischemic lesions. Radiol. Clin. North Am., 5:543, 1967.
Halpern, M.: Acute renal artery embolus: A concept of diagnosis and treatment. J. Urol. 98:552, 1967.

CHYLURIA

Chyluria is lymph in the urine. The entity has been known since Hippocrates. Biochemically the urine contains a colloidal suspension of fat in molecular form, albumin, lecithin, cholesterin, fibrinogen, and soaps producing a milky or creamy appearance resembling lactescent serum. The major component is usually triglycerides. The proteinuria may be sufficient to meet criteria of the *nephrotic syndrome.*

Parasitic (tropical) chyluria is caused by *Filaria sanguinis-hominis (W. bancrofti). Nonparasitic chyluria* is due to a rupture of a lymphatic into the collecting system resulting from observation of lymphatics anywhere between the intestines and the thoracic duct. Specific causes include tumors, fibrosis, pregnancy, and trauma. Pyelonephritis may be associated.

Milky urine, intermittent (postural) or constant, is the major sign. It may be mistaken for pyuria. Milky urine is stable, containing 2 to 4 per cent fat, and does not exhibit fat droplets on microscopy. Retrograde pyelography may demonstrate pyelolymphatic backflow. Oral fats labeled with Sudan 3 or isotopic ^{131}I will appear in the urine. Ether will extract both chyle and the label.

Major items to be differentiated are lipiduria and pyuria. *Lipiduria* has fat droplets that rise to the top on centrifugation. It may be associated with fractures, eclampsia, diabetes, phosphorus, arsenic, and carbon monoxide poisoning.

Primary treatment is identification and removal of the obstruction. A low fat diet reduces chyluria.

Caserta, S. J.: Description of chyluria: Report of a case. N. Engl. J. Med., 255:1239, 1956.
Tuller, M. A., Feuer, M. M., Schapira, H. E., and Ho, Peh-Ping: Recumbent chyluria: Demonstration of unilateral renal-lymphatic communication. Am. J. Med., 33:951, 1962.
Yamauchi, S.: Chyluria: Clinical laboratory and statistical study of 45 personal cases observed in Hawaii. J. Urol., 54:318, 1945.

PNEUMATURIA

Pneumaturia is the passage of gas bubbles in the urine.

In noninfected patients, pneumaturia is usually due to a vesicovaginal or vesicoenteric fistula. Vegetable fibers and fecal contamination may be found in the urine. Such fistulas may be congenital in infants, may result from gross infections or neoplasms, or may follow radical pelvic surgery. Bubbles may also be caused by gas-forming bacteria proliferating in urine. *E. coli, A. aerogenes,* or yeast may be involved. The gas is carbon dioxide. Pneumaturia, although rare, is most frequent in elderly diabetic women.

Bubbling or frothing urine is noted by the patient at the end of micturition or by physician and nurse in the last drainage by catheterization. A gas shadow may be seen in the bladder on roentgenographic study.

Treatment consists of reassuring the patient; finding and repairing the fistula, if present; or treating a specific infection and eliminating glycosuria.

NEPHROPTOSIS

Definition. Nephroptosis is excessive mobility of the kidney. It is to be distinguished from *ectopia,* which is congenital or acquired permanent abnormal placement of the kidney, and *malrotation,* or pivoting of the kidney on its vertical axis, the pelvis and ureter deviating from the normal position. When observing the percutaneous biopsy needle during normal respiratory excursions, most physicians are amazed by the normal mobility of the kidney, which has a fascial attachment to the diaphragm. It is therefore difficult to say how much mobility is "excessive." On palpation the fingers should not be able to slide above the upper pole. On urography the ureteropelvic junction should not descend on standing more than one to one and a half vertebral spaces.

Nephroptosis occurs in about one fifth of adult women and much less frequently in men. There is a right-sided predominance. It is more common in thin, hyperkinetic people.

Pathogenesis. The kidney is held within its normal excursion by its vascular supply (pedicle), its fascia (Gerota) anchored to the diaphragmatic attachments, peritoneal adhesions, intra-abdominal pressure and support of other organs, and its form fit to the lumbar gutter. Nephroptotic kidneys usually have diminished renal fat and poorly developed fascia. A long, thin torso, shallow lumbar gutter, generalized visceroptosis, faulty posture, atrophy of abdominal muscles, and multiple pregnancies may all be contributing causes.

Clinical Manifestations. Nephroptosis is largely asymptomatic, but has been too often made the organic focus for neurotic or hypochondriacal personality. Other than a vague dropping or dragging sensation, specific symptom complexes come from torsion, kinking, ureteral obstruction, infection, and stretching of the vascular pedicle. Recently, orthostatic hypertension and postural hyperaldosteronism (via angiotensin) have been identified with nephroptosis, accounting for 7 of 47 operated patients in one series of renal hypertension. Fibromuscular hyperplasia may accompany the condition. The arteriogram, renin excretion, and aldosterone secretion may be abnormal *only* in the upright position. Recently, we have seen severe orthostatic hypotension (90 to 60/40 to 30 mm Hg) in bilateral nephroptosis. The mechanism could be reduced renin or increased prostaglandins. *Dietl's crisis* is an acute prostrating ureteral colic coming on shortly after assuming the upright posture or after postural fatigue, e.g., in a waitress. The severe pain can be accompanied by nausea, vomiting, hypotension, oliguria, swelling, and tenderness of the kidney. It is relieved by a short period in the Trendelenburg position, followed by horizontal resting, at which time the urine may increase in volume and may contain albumin and erythrocytes. It is thought by some that, in the absence of nephroptosis, Dietl's crisis may occur owing to spasm of the renal pelvis characterized by decreased intrapelvic volume and increased frequency and intensity of peristalsis, analogous to spastic colon.

Diagnosis. Diagnosis is usually made by relating symptoms to posture or occupation and relief by assumption of the horizontal position. Physical examination is performed with the patient in the supine and standing positions, the weight on the leg opposite the side being palpated. Intravenous pyelography in the conventional supine position followed by a view of the upright position is a valuable adjunct. Urinalysis may reveal hematuria and albuminuria from vascular distention or pyuria and bacteria from secondary infection.

Treatment. Reassurance and explanation are the major components of treatment. Weight-gain regimens and exercises to strengthen the abdominal wall may be helpful. Short rest periods in the horizontal position and sensible shoes may work wonders for women whose jobs cause standing fatigue. Often a change of occupation or prolonged rest may be necessary to establish the postural relationship. Patients with recurrent pyelonephritis related to postural fatigue accompanied by ureteral kinking may occasionally benefit from nephropexy. When fibromuscular hyperplasia is present, nephropexy should be combined with arterial repair. The uncomplicated nephroptotic kidney should not be subjected to surgery or used as a psychosomatic crutch.

Derrick, J. R., and Hanna, E.: Abdominal renal mobility and hypertension. Am. J. Surg., 106:673, 1963.
Ginn, H. E., Jr., and Parry, W. L.: Postural hypertension and edema caused by excessive mobility of the kidneys. South. Med. J., 57:735, 1964.

ANOMALIES OF THE GENITOURINARY TRACT

Because of the complex embryologic development of the various specialized structures in the genitourinary tract, developmental mishaps are more common than in any other organ system and affect more than 10 per cent of all humans. Anomalies of the kidney include deviation in number, size, structure, form, and location. In addition, anomalies of the pelvis, ureter, bladder, and urethra may lead to obstruction or infection secondarily involving the kidney.

Kidney. Bilateral renal agenesis, often associated with malformations of the ear, is incompatible with life. Toxic or environmental factors would be most damaging at the fourth week of pregnancy. *Unilateral agenesis (solitary kidney),* which has an incidence of about 0.16 per cent, results from failure of the renal bud, the nephrogenic blastema, or the vascular supply. Arrested development of the wolffian duct results in associated nondevelopment of the rest of the urinary tract on the involved side. No ureteral orifice or ridge is revealed on cystoscopy. Solitary kidney may give rise to anuria when it becomes involved in acute parenchymal disease. As a cardinal principle, the presence of two kidneys should be established before doing any instrumentation or surgical procedure. *Supernumerary kidney,* completely separated and free, is extremely rare. *Fused supernumerary kidney* has an incidence of about 0.025 per cent. *Renal aplasia* may consist of unorganized parenchyma surrounded by fat, and may produce hypertension. *Renal hypoplasia* is generally unilateral and medial in position. In the adult this must be distinguished from renal atrophy secondary to pyelonephritis. Hypoplastic kidneys frequently become infected, demonstrate constant albuminuria, are symmetrically reduced in size, and show small nephrons on biopsy together with atrophic blood vessels. *Renal hypertrophy* may exist congenitally contralateral to a hypoplastic kidney or may be acquired. Functional hypertrophy regularly occurs in transplanted kidneys. *Fetal lobulation* is normal in infants, but persists in about 5 per cent of adults. Fusion of the two kidneys, which is found in about 0.2 per cent of people, may occur at the lower poles, at the lower or upper pole tips *(horseshoe kidney),* at both poles *(doughnut kidney),* throughout *(cake kidney),* or at the contralateral upper and lower poles *(sigmoid kidney)*. The common variety, the lower-pole horseshoe kidney, lies close to the spine, with anterior rotation of the pelves. The vascular supply is almost always anomalous. Surgical separation is sometimes feasible for intractable infection or stone. *Congenital ectopia* (incidence 1 per cent) usually results in a pelvic location for the kidney and has been mistaken for tumor. The position of congenital ectopia is defined by the length of the ureter and vascular supply. In acquired ectopia the ureter and blood vessels were originally of normal length, but upon loss of fascial support the vascular pedicle lengthened and the ureter became redundant. *Malrotation* is frequent in ectopic kidneys. In *crossed ectopia*, the kidney crosses the midline, and lies adjacent to or fused with its mate.

Renal Pelvis. The normal renal pelvis is flask shaped, with upper, middle, and lower major calyces branching into minor calyces. Increase in number of major calyces up to six has been observed. *"Double kidney"* is really double pelvis, and results from the reduplication of the ureteral bud. It is found in about 4 per cent of urograms. The duplication has varying degrees of completion, and may or may not be accompanied by double ureter. *"Spider pelvis"* is a congenitally long, thin pelvis simulating compression. *Congenital hydronephrosis* may result from a variety of conditions present in fetal life. *Extrarenal pelvis* should be considered a normal variant from *intrarenal pelvis*. It becomes important, however, in the pathophysiology of obstructive uropathy.

Blood Vessels. Anomalies of the blood vessels are receiving increased attention because of their possible role in unilateral renal disease with hypertension. They are being discovered with increasing frequency since the advent of the radiohippuran and other radioiodide renograms and increased use of transaortic or retrograde aortography and renal angiography. *Arterial anomalies* include *congenital atresia, tortuosity,* and *aberrant vessels*. Minor anomalies are present in about 25 per cent of people. Renal arteries and veins may derive from the pedicle, aorta, vena cava, adrenals, pancreas, and liver. Anomalous vessels usually involve either pole, and upon crossing the upper portion of the ureter or the ureteropelvic junction may produce obstruction. *Renal artery aneurysm* and intrarenal *arteriovenous fistula* are rare but do occur.

Ureter. Ureteral malformations include agenesis, duplication, triplication, ectopia, ureterocele, herniation, postcaval ureter, aplasia, congenital stricture, congenital valves or folds, hydroureter, diverticula, torsion, kinks, and involvement with aberrant vessels.

Bladder. Malformations of the bladder include agenesis, hypoplasia, reduplication, diverticula, hypertrophy, urachal cysts and fistulas, trigonal folds, and cloaca formation. Vesical neck anomalies are discussed in Ch. 625.

Related Congenital Anomalies. Congenital cysts are discussed in Ch. 628. Malformed ears, particularly asymmetrical, are associated with some genitourinary anomalies. Congenital deficiency of the abdominal musculature is regularly associated with genitourinary problems. Renal anomalies have been described in Marfan's syndrome. Nerve deafness is associated with hereditary nephritis.

Diagnosis. The diagnosis of congenital renal and urinary anomalies is usually made during the course of investigation for other anomalies, as an incidental urographic finding, or when symptoms develop because of infection or obstruction. Most malformed and malrotated kidneys have defects in drainage and are liable to ascending pyelonephritis. Anomalous structures can be mistaken for cysts or tumors and may become significant factors in the course of pregnancy or of surgical procedures on nearby structures. The longest recorded survival in renal agenesis is 39 days.

Benjamin, J. A., and Tobin, C. E.: Abnormalities of kidneys, ureters and perinephric fascia: Anatomic and clinical study. J. Urol. 65:715, 1951.

Campbell, M. F.: Principles of Urology. Philadelphia, W. B. Saunders Company, 1957, Chapter 6.

Smith, E. C., and Orkin, L. A.: Clinical and statistical study of 471 congenital anomalies of kidneys and ureter. J. Urol. 53:11, 1945.

Part XIV
DISEASES OF THE DIGESTIVE SYSTEM

631. INTRODUCTION

Marvin H. Sleisenger

In the chapters that follow, important new ideas and clinical advances in the major diseases and disorders of the gut and liver are presented, and subjects previously treated as isolated topics have been expanded to chapters or important subdivisions of chapters. Among these are an approach to the recognition and differential diagnosis of the acute abdomen (see Ch. 653), diagnosis and treatment of gastrointestinal bleeding (see Ch. 644), vascular diseases of the intestine (see Ch. 658 to 661), and a sizable number of other less common but important diseases of the colon and rectum (see Ch. 670 to 679).

Advances in the technical aspects of diagnosis and management of gastrointestinal disease have been carefully considered. The role of flexible endoscopy, particularly esophagogastroduodenoscopy and colonoscopy, is described. These instruments have greatly influenced the approach to a number of major diseases of the upper and lower intestine, in the areas of both diagnosis and treatment. Appropriately mentioned are the arteriographic techniques which are of immense aid in diagnosis, particularly of diseases which cause massive gastrointestinal bleeding. A description of the usefulness of isotopic scanning and sonographic techniques will also be found.

Therapy for gastrointestinal diseases continues to be nonspecific for many diseases and disorders; however, the number of entities for which specific therapy, replacement type therapy, or symptomatic therapy is effective is growing. For example, it now appears that prolonged therapy with steroids is beneficial for patients with chronic active hepatitis. Instillation of vasoconstrictive substances through arterial catheters or directly into the stomach appears to help in halting massive upper gastrointestinal bleeding; the efficacy of hourly or two-hourly administration of antacids, particularly active aluminum hydroxide gel preparations, although being questioned, seems to be established in therapy for peptic ulcer disease; likewise, administration of these substances to debilitated, postoperative, chronically ill, intubated, or recumbent individuals in prevention of so-called "stress ulceration" is indicated.

Surgical procedures for gastrointestinal disease are an important part of the therapy for complications of peptic ulcer and of chronic inflammatory disease, for cancer and other tumors of the gastrointestinal tract, for calculous biliary tract disease, for portal hypertension, and for complications of acute and chronic inflammation of the pancreas. Of these, peptic ulcer disease is clinically the most important cause for major surgical intervention in gastroenterology. Procedures are evolving which are less mutilative and perhaps more specific for diminishing the vagal influence on gastric secretion while not increasing the possibility of undue antral (gas-trin) influence. Thus the selective vagotomy and the "superselective" vagotomy will be watched very closely and evaluated in terms of a trade-off between reduction in postoperative complications of peptic ulcer surgery and a somewhat increased incidence of recurrence as compared with partial gastrectomy and vagotomy. There is no question that colectomy is a specific procedure for universal ulcerative colitis, especially in view of improved technique for construction of ileostomies, and now clinicians are less and less willing to treat universal colitis indefinitely. In addition, the hazard of carcinomatous degeneration of the bowel in this disease with passing decades is real and affords the physician further reason to intervene surgically. There is no substitute for eradicative surgery for gastrointestinal cancer; radiation and chemotherapeutic agents are relatively ineffective except for some types of squamous cell cancer of the upper gastrointestinal tract.

The usefulness of intensive replacement therapy for patients with malabsorption becomes increasingly evident. Parenteral hyperalimentation for appropriate periods (postoperatively, particularly), followed by frequent supplemental feedings of high calorie substances (medium-chain triglycerides, protein hydrolysates), adequate therapy with both water-soluble and fat-soluble vitamins, and supplementation with calcium and iron, all may maintain these patients in adequate nutritional balance. More specific therapy for this condition may be found in the use of broad-spectrum antimicrobial drugs for those who have bacterial overgrowth.

The newer information concerning the pathogenesis of gallstones is providing the basis for a long-term study of the medical treatment of this disease by administration of a conjugated bile salt, chenodeoxycholate. The rationale is that increasing the cholesterol solubility in bile will not only prevent further crystallization but will also gradually dissolve existing stones. It is too early to tell whether or not the therapy will be effective on a long-term basis, and if continuous therapy will be necessary. Also, the long-term side effects are not yet evaluated. Meanwhile, the mainstay for therapy of symptomatic calculous gallbladder disease is surgery. The question of operation for those with "silent" stones is moot; the majority of observers feel that those under age 60 who are otherwise in good health with asymptomatic stones should undergo cholecystectomy.

Although covered in great detail in Part VIII, the infectious diarrheas are worthy of brief note here. It appears that an increasing number of these infectious organisms cause diarrhea not by virtue of invasiveness or tissue damage but by the elaboration of an endotoxin which, by increasing the concentration of adenylcyclate, leads to the secretion of water and electrolytes into the lumen. This mechanism is also stimulated by the administration of a number of drugs, particularly xanthines, and by endogenously produced substances, particularly prostaglandins.

The clinical pharmacology of the gastrointestinal tract has not changed much since the last edition of this book. The mainstays of therapy for most diseases and disorders of motility and secretion remain antacids, anticholinergics, sedatives, and tranquilizers. Steroids are useful at times for chronic inflammatory disease and for chronic aggressive hepatitis; broad-spectrum antimicrobials are often effective in the bacterial overgrowth syndrome and for Whipple's disease. The clinical usefulness of gastrointestinal hormones or their antagonists is still in the experimental stage and is not yet practicable.

Section One.   DISORDERS OF MOTILITY

Thomas P. Almy

632.   INTRODUCTION

Most gastrointestinal symptoms have as their immediate cause some disturbance of the motility of the gut, and the most common intestinal disorders in clinical practice are those in which disturbed motility is unassociated with a recognizable morphologic or biochemical lesion, i.e., they are "functional" disorders. Much less commonly, the most impressive physiologic and clinical effects of a morphologically definable disease process are disturbances of gut motility, the understanding of which represents the key to effective therapy. These two kinds of disorders are considered together in this section.

Rhythmic contractility is an intrinsic property of the intestinal wall. In the absence of extrinsic nerves or humoral influences, peristalsis is maintained by local reflexes for which the afferents arise in the mucosa, and the efferents include the myenteric ganglia. Extrinsic neural and humoral mechanisms serve to regulate and adapt the intrinsic motility of the gut to the needs of the total organism. A purposeful alternation of propulsive and nonpropulsive patterns of activity, adapted to civilized habits of eating, working, sleeping, and defecating, is referred to as normal intestinal function. The most common and clinically important disorders of intestinal motility occur during periods of stress in persons with normally innervated intestines, when the aforementioned patterns are long sustained as bodily accompaniments of emotional tension.

By contrast certain disorders, such as achalasia, congenital megacolon, and the esophageal disorder in diabetic neuropathy, are based upon permanent defects in integrative mechanisms. The high pressures generated at the sites of colonic and esophageal diverticula appear to result from patterns of disordered motility, the neural basis of which is as yet unclear.

Our knowledge of these disorders has been extended rapidly in recent years through the improvement of methods for the observation and recording of intestinal motility in intact man. The comparison of electromanometric recordings of intraluminal pressure with cineradiographic images of the barium-filled intestine has contributed much to our understanding of mechanisms, and at times has directly aided the diagnosis. The true diagnostic limitations of these methods, however, have not been fully defined.

633.   DISORDERS OF SWALLOWING

Normal deglutition is accomplished by peristaltic movements, triggered by reflexes arising from voluntary contractions of the muscles of the buccal and pharyngeal cavities. The elevation of the tongue and larynx thrusts the food bolus against the posterior wall, raises the pressure in the pharynx, and seals off the aditus of the larynx. A fall in the pressure follows immediately (see Fig. 1) in both the superior (cricopharyngeal) and inferior (vestibular) esophageal sphincters, and a gradient of pressure is established favorable to propulsion of the bolus. The wave of high pressure generated in the pharynx then sweeps progressively downward to the stomach. The reflex pathways subserving this mechanism lie in the fifth, seventh, ninth, tenth, and eleventh cranial nerves, and the effectors include both skeletal muscle (tongue, pharynx, larynx, upper one third of the esophagus) and smooth muscle (lower two thirds of the esophagus). In the latter region the efferent pathway is autonomic and cholinergic, the postganglionic neurons lying in the esophageal wall (Auerbach's plexus). The lower esophageal sphincter or esophagogastric sphincter, although anatomically indistinct, normally

Figure 1. A composite of electromanometric recordings, showing simultaneous pressure changes throughout pharynx and esophagus during a single swallow. Read from left to right; interval between vertical lines = 1 second. P-E Sphincter = pharyngoesophageal sphincter. E-G Sphincter = esophagogastric sphincter or lower esophageal sphincter. (Adapted from Code, C. F.: An Atlas of Esophageal Motility in Health and Disease. Springfield, Ill., Charles C Thomas, 1958.)

presents a functionally important high pressure barrier to the reflux of gastric contents. It is under dual control—a neural mechanism (fast component), comprising cholinergic and alpha-adrenergic stimulatory fibers as well as beta-adrenergic and nonadrenergic inhibitory fibers; and a hormonal mechanism (slow component), which largely determines its tone but permits rapid relaxation and contraction in the act of swallowing. Both exogenous and endogenous gastrin have been shown to increase resting sphincter pressure, whereas secretin, cholecystokinin, and glucagon oppose the action of gastrin. These hormonal effects participate in the important adaptive reactions of the sphincter, which cause it normally to increase its strength of contraction when intra-abdominal or intragastric pressure rises, or when gastric acid secretion is increased.

Difficult swallowing, or *dysphagia,* may result from a defect or disorder in any part of the mechanism outlined above or from mechanical obstruction to the bolus propelled by this mechanism. In other patients a complaint of dysphagia will be found to relate entirely to difficulty in initiating the voluntary act of swallowing or to defects in the reflex coordination of oropharyngeal movements. When dysphagia is due to motor dysfunction, difficulty is experienced with both liquids and solids, whereas, in the presence of a mechanical obstruction or stenosis, the strong peristaltic movements above the lesion serve to propel through it any particle smaller than the stenotic lumen. Thus the patient with an obstructing carcinoma may experience the sudden onset of dysphagia on swallowing a bolus of meat or toast, and, as the lumen progressively narrows, may have to limit his diet to semiliquid and ultimately liquid foods.

Pain on swallowing, if mild, is likely to be incorporated in the experience of dysphagia. Its location often accurately reflects the level of the esophagus principally affected. At times esophageal pain is more severe, outlasts the normal duration of the deglutition, or is dissociated from it in time. Its location is usually substernal, beneath the xiphoid process, and in the episternal notch. It may radiate to the anterior neck and lower jaw, the dorsal spine, the sides of the chest, the shoulders and arms, and the epigastrium. Rarely it may originate in one of these sites. Its quality is most often either crushing or burning. The latter sensation, commonly called *heartburn,* characteristically radiates upward to the neck, and results from inflammation of the mucosa of the lower esophagus usually brought about by reflux of gastric juice.

Esophageal *regurgitation* is a common manifestation of obstructive disorders, and is to be distinguished from vomiting by the absence of nausea, the tendency to occur during or immediately after meals, the lack of digestion of regurgitated food, and the absence of bile or of a sour or bitter taste.

634. DISORDERS OF THE UPPER (PHARYNGOESOPHAGEAL) SEGMENT

The "lump in the throat" is a familiar transitory sensation accompanying fear or acute anxiety. Related is the "globus hystericus," in which a person suffering emotional conflict is incapable of initiating the voluntary movements of deglutition.

In any *disease of the brainstem,* the *cranial nerves,* or the *muscles* of this segment, the coordinated contraction of the pharyngeal musculature and relaxation of the pharyngoesophageal sphincter may fail to develop, with resultant gagging, coughing, and regurgitation of fluids through the nose. The specific cause is usually made obvious by associated symptoms and signs, and may be pseudobulbar palsy, bulbar poliomyelitis, myasthenia gravis, the oculopharyngeal syndrome, dermatomyositis, myotonic dystrophy, or sarcoidosis. This mechanism is important in the causation of the hypopharyngeal (Zenker's) diverticulum (see Ch. 639). The prognosis and treatment are those of the underlying disease.

SIDEROPENIC DYSPHAGIA
(Plummer-Vinson Syndrome, Paterson-Brown-Kelly Syndrome)

Sideropenic dysphagia is a disorder characterized by dysphagia referable to the upper segment, atrophy of the mucous membranes of mouth and pharynx, koilonychia, hypochromic microcytic anemia, hypoferremia, gastric achlorhydria, and stenoses or webs of the upper esophageal mucosa demonstrable by roentgenography or by endoscopy. It occurs mainly in women subsisting on low intakes of iron and vitamins, chiefly those of the B complex. The prognosis is excellent in most cases, but these patients should be observed for later development of carcinoma of the pharynx or esophagus, to which they are unusually susceptible. It is effectively treated with a good general diet, at first soft or semiliquid in consistency, with oral or parenteral iron in the amounts used for iron deficiency anemia and vitamin supplements. Occasionally the stenotic lesions require bouginage.

635. DISORDERS OF THE LOWER (ESOPHAGOGASTRIC) SEGMENT

The motility of the lower esophagus may be altered by diffuse disease of the muscular wall or by disturbances of intrinsic neural mechanisms. In systemic lupus erythematosus and other connective tissue diseases, disordered swallowing is strikingly associated with *Raynaud's phenomenon.* It is commonly seen in *scleroderma* (progressive systemic sclerosis), where it may antedate the appearance of cutaneous changes. In an advanced case the esophagogram reveals dilatation and absent peristalsis, a patulous vestibule allowing free regurgitation of barium from the stomach. In milder instances, and often in the absence of dysphagia, the patient with scleroderma will show defects in peristalsis only while swallowing barium in the recumbent position or when recorded electromanometrically (Fig. 2A). Esophagoscopy may reveal peptic esophagitis, to which acute or chronic blood loss may be due. The therapy is that for regurgitant esophagitis and other aspects of scleroderma.

Figure 2. Electromanometric recordings from lower esophagus and lower esophageal sphincter. *A, Scleroderma.* Note absence of peristalsis; fluctuations in sphincter pressure coincide with inspiration. *B, Diffuse esophageal spasm.* Note extremely large, sustained or repetitive contractions beginning simultaneously at three levels. *C, Achalasia.* Note absence of peristalsis; pressure in the sphincter (here at 34 cm) does not fall on swallowing. (Reproduced from Kelley, M. L., Jr., by permission.)

Healthy persons may fail to generate a primary peristaltic wave, and instead exhibit incoordinate contraction of the lower esophagus after 1 to 10 per cent of swallows. These phenomena may occur after the majority of swallows in elderly persons (presbyesophagus) and in a number of disorders of the nervous system, including multiple sclerosis, amyotrophic lateral sclerosis, parkinsonism, pseudobulbar palsy, and both diabetic and alcoholic neuropathy. In many of these diseases, the esophagogastric sphincter may fail to relax. These defects of neuromuscular activity are seen in exaggerated form in three disorders apparently localized to the esophagus — diffuse spasm, hypertensive esophagogastric sphincter, and achalasia — which appear together or sequentially in the same patient with significant frequency, and hence may be pathogenically related.

DIFFUSE ESOPHAGEAL SPASM
(Corkscrew Esophagus, "Curling")

Particularly in some elderly persons, deglutition may evoke strong, uncoordinated, nonpropulsive contractions of the body of the esophagus (Fig. 2*B*). Although in most instances this condition is asymptomatic, it may induce dysphagia or substernal pain, at times simulating

angina pectoris. On barium swallow, the esophageal lumen appears in the form of an irregular series of concentric narrowings, or a spiral coil (curling, Fig. 3). In some cases the esophagus is abnormally sensitive to methacholine (see Achalasia, below).

This disorder is usually chronic and nonprogressive. Rarely, it is followed by typical achalasia. When required, pain can be prevented or relieved by an anticholinergic agent, e.g., propantheline, 15 to 30 mg three times daily, or isopropamide, 5 to 10 mg twice daily orally. Severe cases may require a long esophagomyotomy for relief of symptoms.

HYPERTENSIVE ESOPHAGOGASTRIC SPHINCTER

In rare instances the resting pressure in the esophagogastric sphincter has been shown to exceed by far the normal upper limit of 40 cm of water. At times of spontaneous or induced emotional conflict, both roentgenographic and manometric studies indicate the occurrence of varying degrees of "spasm" of this sphincter, unassociated with disturbed peristalsis in the body of the esophagus, yet often giving rise to a sensation of obstruction at the xiphoid level. Long persistence

Figure 3. Diffuse esophageal spasm.

of this phenomenon and more severe pain and dysphagia are seen when it is associated with diffuse spasm or hiatus hernia. Treatment is based largely on psychophysiologic principles (see Irritable Colon in Ch. 637) if other lesions have been excluded.

ACHALASIA OF THE ESOPHAGUS
(Cardiospasm, Aperistalsis, Megaesophagus)

Definition. Achalasia is a chronic disorder of motility that leads to obstruction at the level of the lower esophageal sphincter (LES). The previously accepted name, cardiospasm, is inappropriate, because the LES ("cardiac" sphincter) not only is contracted with moderately excessive force but also fails to relax normally (achalasia) on swallowing. Moreover, it is clear that peristalsis fails to progress normally through the lower two thirds of the esophagus.

Prevalence, Epidemiology, and Etiology. Although one of the more common causes of esophageal obstruction, achalasia is a relatively rare disease in medical practice in the United States, where no regional, ethnic, or familial predisposition has been recognized. It develops usually in the third to sixth decades, and is rare in children. No environmental factors of etiologic importance are known.

In Latin America, however, an identical disorder occurs endemically among the poor, chiefly in rural districts, in whom an association with Chagas' disease is suggested by epidemiologic and serologic evidence and by characteristic degenerative changes in the myenteric plexus. In such patients the esophageal disorder is often associated with disturbances elsewhere, such as megaureter or megacolon (see Ch. 273).

Pathology and Pathologic Physiology. The fundamental lesion in achalasia is degeneration of the ganglion cells of the myenteric (Auerbach's) plexus or of the vagal motor nuclei. This varies greatly in degree, at times amounting to complete atrophy and at times being undetectable by ordinary histologic criteria, and appears to be proportional to the duration and severity of the motility disturbance.

Even in those patients without evident structural damage to the ganglia, physiologic abnormalities are demonstrable at any time. In manometric studies the total motor activity in the resting state varies widely; but, consistently on swallowing, a moving peristaltic wave fails to develop in the body, and the LES fails to relax normally (Fig. 2C). Whereas the motility of the normally innervated esophagus is altered by methacholine only when given in subcutaneous doses of 25 mg or more, injection of only 5 to 10 mg in a patient with achalasia is sufficient to induce a strong, sustained, incoordinated, often painful contraction of the body of the esophagus. In accordance with "Cannon's law," stating that a tissue deprived of its autonomic nerve supply is excessively sensitive to the chemical transmitter of the nerve impulse, this is held to be pharmacologic evidence of partial or complete aganglionosis. Recently, the LES in achalasia has been shown to be excessively sensitive to stimulation by gastrin.

With failure of relaxation of the LES on swallowing, food and liquid accumulate in the esophagus until, in the vertical position, the hydrostatic pressure exceeds the resistance of the sphincter, and the contents pass bit by bit into the stomach. The esophagus may be greatly dilated and elongated (Fig. 4), but, if the level of total motor activity is high, may long remain of normal caliber. The wall of the esophagus often becomes greatly thickened, although just above the LES conspicuous thinning or a pseudodiverticulum may appear. With severe retention, the mucosa and submucosa are often

Figure 4. Achalasia. Far advanced changes.

inflamed. Rarely, carcinoma of the lower esophagus appears to be a complication of longstanding megaesophagus. Because patients often lie down before the esophagus empties itself, acute and chronic aspiration pneumonia is a moderately common complication.

Clinical Manifestations. The leading symptom, *dysphagia,* is usually insidious in onset; but in many instances it may begin suddenly and may be intermittent or of variable severity, despite the persistence of the morphologic and physiologic changes in the esophagus. From the beginning, some difficulty will be experienced in swallowing liquids as well as solids. Nevertheless, the patient often learns that he can obtain relief by drinking a liquid after a meal, presumably because the added fluid raises the hydrostatic pressure in the lower esophagus sufficiently to open the sphincter. Substernal *pain* after eating, lasting a few minutes, occurs variably in some patients, apparently because of spasm of the body of the esophagus.

In the more severe and chronic cases, there may be striking *loss of weight* or symptoms of *pneumonia* or lung abscess resulting from aspiration of esophageal contents.

Diagnosis. The symptom of dysphagia should lead promptly to the observation of a barium swallow; in a typical case of advanced achalasia the dilated, elongated, tortuous body of the esophagus, joined by a smooth conical tip to an elongated narrow sphincteric zone, permits easy recognition. Sometimes the disease is suspected because the esophagus produces the shadow of a large paramediastinal mass on plain film of the chest. Even when the esophagus is less strikingly enlarged, fluoroscopic study in the horizontal position will reveal defects in the primary peristaltic wave. Esophagoscopy usually reveals that the sphincter dilates to allow passage of the instrument into the stomach, and thus permits exclusion of an organic stricture. Manometric studies of swallowing and of the response to methacholine (see above) may be of great diagnostic value. In some cases of minimal dilatation of the esophagus, it is impossible to make a clear distinction between achalasia and diffuse esophageal spasm on the clinical and manometric findings.

By these means, achalasia can and must be differentiated from *carcinoma* of the fundus of the stomach or terminal esophagus. In such instances, during endoscopy direct biopsy of the lesion or (better) cytologic study of aspirated contents may reveal neoplastic cells. In *scleroderma* of the esophagus comparable defects in peristalsis are seen in the body of the esophagus, but the LES is most often patent and there is no abnormal sensitivity to methacholine. In *regurgitant esophagitis* the manometric findings are not typical of achalasia, and evidence of regurgitation, of mucosal inflammation, of stricture, or of hiatal hernia is usually obtained by fluoroscopic study, by esophagoscopy, and by measuring the pH of the lower esophageal contents.

Treatment and Prognosis. Initial conservative management is recommended because many patients are able to eat adequately and with minimal distress when freed from stress and emotional tension. The only medication frequently useful is a mild sedative. Anticholinergic drugs, such as atropine sulfate, 0.5 to 1.0 mg, or propantheline, 15 to 30 mg, can prevent or relieve painful spasms of the body of the esophagus, but do not relax the LES. Amyl nitrite inhalation (or glyceryl trinitrite, 0.4 mg sublingually) relaxes the sphincter, but only transiently.

The damage done to the innervation of the esophagus in this disease is, nevertheless, irreversible, and truly effective therapy requires that this be compensated by lasting damage to the sphincter, permitting drainage of the esophagus by gravity. Forcible stretching or rupture of the muscle fibers is accomplished by bougies and other dilators passed and positioned in the sphincter under fluoroscopic control. Although use of the pneumatic or hydrostatic dilators is attended by pain and a small risk of esophageal perforation, lasting relief of dysphagia is obtained in 60 to 80 per cent of patients after one or two treatments. These procedures are recommended for any case of achalasia in which severe dilatation and significant retention are regularly present and in which accurate placement of the dilator is technically feasible.

When adequate dilatation has not been possible or its results have been unsatisfactory, surgical division of the sphincter often becomes necessary. Yet the more radical and successful the destruction of the sphincter, the more likely is the postoperative occurrence of regurgitant esophagitis (discussed later) here worsened by the ineffective clearing of regurgitated material because of defective peristalsis. The most satisfactory compromise appears to be the Heller procedure, in which the muscle of the vestibule is sectioned longitudinally and the mucosa left intact. About 80 per cent of the patients may be expected to remain free from dysphagia, to gain weight, and to escape the symptoms of esophagitis.

Whether the sphincter has been damaged by dilatation or by surgery, measures should be instituted to prevent regurgitant esophagitis. The patient should not lie down for one to two hours after eating, straining and chronic coughing should be controlled; and tight corsets should be discarded.

Cohen, S., Lipshutz, W., and Hughes, W.: Role of gastrin supersensitivity in the pathogenesis of lower esophageal sphincter hypertension in achalasia. J. Clin. Invest., 50:1241, 1971.
Ellis, F. H., Jr., and Olsen, A. M.: Achalasia of the Esophagus. Philadelphia, W. B. Saunders Company, 1969.
Kramer, P.: Progress in gastroenterology: The esophagus. Gastroenterology, 54:1171, 1968.
Leading Article: Esophageal dysfunction in diabetes. Br. Med. J., 2:466, 1969.
Pope, C. E., II: The esophagus, 1967–1969. Gastroenterology, 59:460, 1970.

DIAPHRAGMATIC HERNIA, HIATAL HERNIA, AND REFLUX ESOPHAGITIS
(Regurgitant Esophagitis, Peptic Esophagitis)

Definition. Gaps in the diaphragm resulting from congenital defects, relaxation of supporting tissues, or trauma may permit the stomach, colon, or other abdominal organs to herniate into the chest. *Traumatic hernia* may result in acute chest pain, dyspnea, hiccup, vomiting, and shock, usually in association with other internal injuries; on the other hand, large herniations may result but remain asymptomatic, later to be discovered on routine roentgenographic examinations. *Nontraumatic hernia* may be present at birth or delayed until adult life and may involve (1) the pleuroperitoneal hiatus (foramen of Bochdalek), (2) the gap (usually posterior) left by congenital absence of a portion of the diaphragm, and (3) an anterior substernal opening (foramen of Morgagni). By far the most common and clinically important, however, is (4) *herniation through the esophageal hiatus,* a slitlike opening, bounded by muscle bundles from the right crus of the diaphragm, in which the vestibule of the esophagus is normally located, bound in turn to the inferior surface of the diaphragm by the phrenoesophageal ligament. The clinical manifestations of esophageal hiatal hernia are due in large part to one of its complications, reflux esophagitis. Therefore, although the latter is often seen in the absence of a hernia, these conditions are here described together.

Prevalence and Pathology. The true prevalence of hiatal hernia is not known. Because it is essentially a dynamic process, estimates based on autopsies are too low. In roentgenographic surveys it is extremely common, especially in older women. Peptic esophagitis is the most common benign cause of persistent esophageal pain. In about 75 per cent of instances the hernia is of the *sliding* type, in which the esophagogastric junction lies inside the thorax at the apex of the herniated mass. In these a "short esophagus" exists—the result rather than the cause of the herniation; congenital primary short esophagus is exceedingly rare. In 25 per cent the hernia is *rolling* or *paraesophageal,* in which the apex of the herniated mass is some portion of the greater curvature of the stomach. This has rolled upward, medially and anterior to the sphincter, which may remain in its normal position or may be displaced above the diaphragm. (The latter hernia is often called the *mixed* type.) With the sliding and mixed types, mucosal inflammation may be found in the terminal 1 to 5 cm of the esophagus. Early lesions show edema and vascular engorgement and increased thickness of the basal layers of the stratified epithelium; with advancing disease mucosal erosions, hemorrhage, cellular infiltration, and fibrosis appear. In the end, an elongated, smoothly tapered stricture may be found.

Etiology and Pathogenesis. Normal closure of the esophagogastric sphincter in the face of increases in intra-abdominal pressure is maintained chiefly by the neural and hormonal adaptive mechanisms of the sphincter itself. Earlier emphasis upon the muscular sling provided by the right crus of the diaphragm and upon the short intra-abdominal segment of the esophagus as contributors to the closing mechanism has been offset by convincing evidence that the sphincter can remain competent when totally displaced into the thorax. *Thus the hiatal hernia is no longer considered essential to the production of reflux esophagitis.* The resting pressure and the adaptive increases in pressure in the LES may be reduced by a number of mechanisms which inhibit gastrin release (for example, acid in the pyloric antrum or anticholinergic drugs) or augment the release of secretin or cholecystokinin (for example, fatty meals). For other reasons, smoking and ingestion of alcohol also diminish sphincter tone. On the other hand, any sustained or recurrent influence which increases the intra-abdominal pressure (pregnancy, obesity, ascites, coughing, retching, weight lifting) may determine the frequency and severity of regurgitation and the probability of hiatal hernia formation. The pressures generated within a hernia and the probability of associated reflux esophagitis appear to be the greater, the *smaller* the hernia. Once inflammation occurs in the terminal esophagus, sustained contraction of its musculature raises the local pressure and reflexly diminishes the pressure within the (more distal) sphincter, thus accentuating the reflux.

Reflux esophagitis also occurs in other settings: (1) in prolonged use of intragastric tubes, especially postopera-

tively; (2) after operative disturbance of the diaphragmatic crura or the esophagogastric sphincter; (3) in scleroderma, in which the sphincter is immobilized by inflammation; and (4) in chalasia of infants, in which innervation of the sphincter is retarded. It can occur in the absence of hydrochloric acid or, indeed, of the stomach; it is likely that bile salts have a primary injurious effect. (See Gastroduodenal Syndromes in Ch. 636.)

Hemorrhage in cases of hiatal hernia is believed to arise either from the inflamed esophagus or from the hernial sac itself. Usually it is due to multiple erosions, but when severe it can often be traced to a discrete ulcer in the engorged mucosa of the herniated stomach.

Clinical Manifestations. The majority of hiatal hernias are virtually or wholly asymptomatic, and the most common problem for the physician is to judge whether this condition is in fact responsible for the complaints of the patient. There is no relation between the severity of symptoms and the size of the hernia unless, as some suggest, pain is *inversely* related to size.

In the absence of complications, *pain* usually is described as a dull, early postprandial, retrosternal fullness, disappearing spontaneously after a few minutes to one hour; it is often associated with belching or hiccup. It is often worse on lying down or on exertion after heavy meals; sometimes it radiates to the back, the jaws, the shoulders, and down the inner aspects of the arms, closely simulating angina pectoris. Particularly with large hernias, and with displacement of thoracic structures, there may be dyspnea, palpitation, or cough.

The earliest manifestation of esophageal reflux is usually *heartburn.* It is worse after heavy meals, on lying down, and on bending forward, as in tying a shoe; conversely, it is often improved by sitting or standing upright, by draughts of any liquid, and by ingestion of an effective antacid. With development of true esophagitis the pain becomes more severe, lasts longer, and is worsened by irritating food and drink of all kinds. Still later, dysphagia appears, worse for solid foods, and as it progresses the development of a severe stricture may be indicated by some amelioration of the heartburn.

Hemorrhage may take the form of acute hematemesis and melena or chronic blood loss. In the latter instance, the stools are usually not discolored and are only intermittently positive for occult blood, and the presenting manifestation may be a sideropenic anemia of unknown cause. Neither in acute nor in chronic hemorrhage should hiatal hernia or reflux esophagitis be accepted as the cause until a search has been made for other potential sources.

Diagnosis. The positive diagnosis of hiatal hernia rests usually upon roentgenographic findings or upon such findings considered together with clinical manifestations. With large hernias, the recognition above the diaphragm of a portion of the stomach, marked by its coarse rugae (Fig. 5), is usually simple. Diagnosis of the smaller sliding hernias depends upon precise location of the esophagogastric junction and the demonstration of reflux by fluoroscopy and cineradiography, and is aided by tilting the head downward and by the Valsalva maneuver. Rarely, the displacement of the sphincter upward into the chest may be recognized at esophagoscopy or by manometric techniques.

In the presence of a hiatal hernia or other predisposing cause, the existence of *reflux esophagitis* should be suspected when there is recurrent or persistent heartburn or otherwise unexplained, usually mild, upper gastroin-

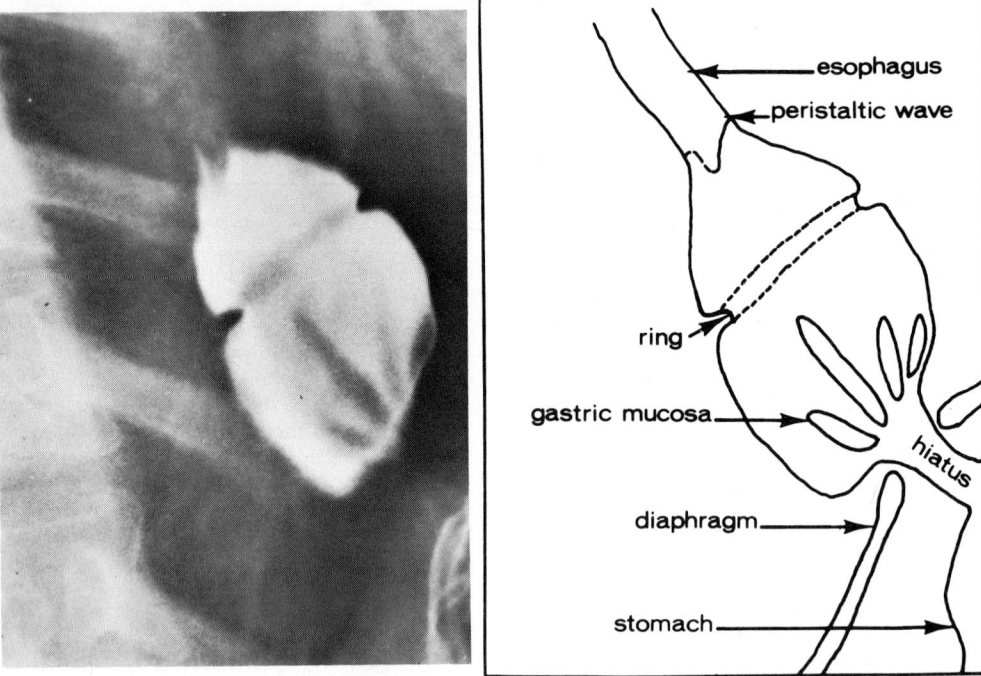

Figure 5. Roentgenogram of a small sliding hiatal hernia, with an associated Schatzki ring (contraction ring).

testinal bleeding. Esophagoscopy and biopsy may reveal epithelial thickening, deep rete pegs, and inflammation of the mucosa, but negative findings do not exclude the diagnosis. Esophagitis may rarely be due to *syphilis* or *tuberculosis,* or, more commonly, to *candidiasis,* particularly in children or debilitated adults with concomitant thrush (see Ch. 266). The regurgitation of gastric juice can be confirmed by aspiration of lower esophageal contents and measurement of its pH, with the patient supine. It may be helpful to infuse into the lower esophagus 0.1N HCl at the rate of 10 ml per minute for 30 to 60 minutes or until pain is experienced (Bernstein test). Reproduction of the pain by this means strongly supports the diagnosis of reflux esophagitis.

Strictures of the lower esophagus resulting from chronic peptic esophagitis must be differentiated from those due to lye or other corrosive poisons, to prolonged intubation, to foreign bodies, or to congenital stenosis or atresia, as well as from carcinoma or achalasia.

As it is capable of causing substernal pain radiating to the shoulders and arms, hiatal hernia may enter importantly into the differential diagnosis of angina pectoris, myocardial infarction, dissecting hematoma of the aorta, gallbladder disease, pancreatitis, and the "splenic flexure syndrome." Patients frequently exhibit two or more of these disorders simultaneously; management therefore requires thorough clinical and laboratory study and judgment based upon careful and repeated inquiry into the setting in which the attacks occur.

Treatment. In the conservative treatment of hiatal hernia, control of symptoms is attempted through the frequent feeding of small meals, the reduction of weight, and the removal of other causes of increased intra-abdominal pressure. Thus efforts are made to control chronic coughing, to reduce effort in defecation, and to eliminate bending forward, as in scrubbing floors or weeding gardens. No food should be taken for three

hours before retiring, and the head of the bed should be elevated 10 inches on blocks. With symptoms of reflux esophagitis, the diet should be reduced in fat content, use of alcohol and tobacco should be interdicted or drastically reduced, and a nonabsorbable antacid such as Maalox or Aludrox should be given in dosage of 15 to 30 ml *immediately* after each feeding. The antacid is used in this instance not so much to buffer gastric acid as to heighten the endogenous release of gastrin. For the same reason, anticholinergics are held to be contraindicated. Except in the presence of esophageal stricture, no restriction of dietary residue is required.

The vast majority of symptomatic cases of hiatal hernia and early reflux esophagitis will be relieved by careful adherence to the aforementioned regimen. Frequent recurrence of substernal pain, heartburn, or dysphagia under these conditions is a clear indication for more radical measures. These are directed at repair of the hernia and the relief of lower esophageal obstruction.

In most instances, surgical reduction of the hernia and reconstruction of the hiatus, performed through either the abdomen or the posterior thorax, is the treatment of choice. If an early esophageal stricture exists, it may be necessary preoperatively to pass metal bougies of gradually increasing diameter over a previously swallowed string as a guide. Because the sacrifice of the esophagogastric sphincter is an invitation to postoperative recurrence of esophagitis, surgical resection of the strictured zone is regarded as a measure of last resort. In recent years the interposition of a loop of jejunum or descending colon between the resected esophagus and the fundus of the stomach has seemed to prevent or delay this complication, but the precise value of this procedure has not yet been determined.

The results of surgical repair are usually excellent in rolling hernias, but only about 80 per cent successful in controlling symptoms of the sliding hernia. With fundoplication and other procedures which firmly anchor the LES within the abdomen, despite present questions as to their rationale, recurrence rates as low as 7 per cent have been reported.

LOWER ESOPHAGEAL RING

In many elderly patients, roentgenographic study of the lower esophagus reveals a symmetrical, annular, shelflike constriction a few centimeters above the diaphragm (Fig. 5). The diameter of the ring may be as small as 5 to 10 mm; yet its detection requires careful fluoroscopy or cineradiography, with the esophagus well distended with barium. It usually lies below the esophagogastric sphincter, at the junction of esophageal and gastric mucosa; it is often associated with hiatus hernia.

In some such patients, attacks of severe lower substernal pain occur acutely on swallowing large and poorly chewed boluses that become lodged in the ring. Relief is afforded in some cases by bouginage and in others by actual cutting of the ring.

Edwards, D. A. W., et al.: Symposium on gastroesophageal reflux and its implications. Gut, 14:233, 1973.
Pope, C. E., II: Reflux esophagitis. In Sleisenger, M. H., and Fordtran, J. S. (eds.): Gastrointestinal Disease. Philadelphia, W. B. Saunders Company, 1973, pp. 430–449.
Schatzki, R., and Gary, J. E.: The lower esophageal ring. Am. J. Roentgenol. Radium Ther. Nucl. Med., 75:246, 1956.
Wilkins, E. W., Jr., and Skinner, D. B.: Medical progress: Surgery of the esophagus. N. Engl. J. Med., 278:824, 887, 1968.

636. DISORDERS OF GASTRODUODENAL MOTILITY

The motility of the stomach and the duodenum may logically be considered together, because these two organs have the common purpose of mixing the food with digestive juices and as the interaction of these two segments is considerable.

On the ingestion of food, initially a small amount is propelled through the stomach into the duodenum, after which the pylorus appears to close and the body of the stomach to dilate progressively as the remainder of the meal enters from the esophagus. After a period of nonpropulsive churning movements, a series of peristaltic waves appears, beginning at or slightly above the antrum and carrying through the pylorus to the second portion of the duodenum. Under normal conditions the stomach is emptied in this manner, after which peristalsis ceases.

The pyloric sphincter is stimulated to contract, and gastric emptying is retarded, by the instillation into the duodenum of fat, of solutions of hydrochloric acid, of hypertonic sodium chloride or glucose, or of amino acids. These effects are believed to be mediated by secretin and cholecystokinin, which stimulate the sphincter when injected intravenously, and the action of which is opposed by endogenous or exogenous gastrin. Thus a form of servomechanism exists, regulating the rate of gastric emptying and, under normal conditions, limiting the regurgitation of duodenal contents into the stomach in the process of digestion.

GASTRODUODENAL SYNDROMES

Disturbances in this motor pattern have been correlated with a number of important digestive symptoms. Vigorous gastric peristalsis in the absence of food has long been associated with normal *hunger*. The sensation of *nausea*, on the other hand, is clearly accompanied by cessation of gastric phasic contractions and simultaneous sustained contraction or spasm of the descending portion of the duodenum. The resulting gradient of pressure and the open pylorus lead to duodenogastric regurgitation, with exposure of gastric and even esophageal mucosa (as the esophagogastric sphincter is often simultaneously relaxed) to the irritant action of bile acids as well as to pancreatic enzymes. This phenomenon can be totally asymptomatic, but in many instances can be correlated with the syndrome of *dyspepsia* (mild epigastric distress, early satiety, abdominal distention, belching, heartburn, and bitter regurgitation). Further, it has been demonstrated to occur with significantly increased frequency in patients with irritable colon, duodenal ulcer, gastric ulcer, and cholelithiasis; and it is considered of probable etiologic significance in chronic gastritis, gastric ulcer, and reflux esophagitis.

Vomiting. Whether or not preceded by nausea, the mechanism of vomiting involves close coordination of visceral and somatic movements. The gastric fundus and corpus are flaccid, the antrum and the proximal duodenum strongly contracted, and the esophageal vestibule (cardia) relaxed. The pharyngoesophageal sphincter is likewise relaxed, the glottis closed, and the larynx and soft palate elevated. At the moment of emesis the diaphragm forcibly descends and the abdominal wall contracts, squeezing the flaccid stomach and causing ejection of its contents. All this activity is triggered by the vomiting center in the floor of the fourth ventricle on chemical, humoral, reflex neural, or psychic stimulation. Persistent vomiting is most readily treated by drugs that depress this center or the vestibular apparatus, or both. The most effective short-term medication is a phenothiazine such as prochlorperazine, 5 to 10 mg (or promethazine, 12.5 to 25 mg) three times a day. For more prolonged use meclizine, 25 to 50 mg daily (or cyclizine, 50 mg), is safer and may be effective.

The Mallory-Weiss Syndrome. This signifies the hematemesis or melena that follows typically upon many hours or days of severe vomiting and retching, and that is traceable to one or several slitlike lacerations of the mucosa, longitudinally placed at or slightly below the esophagogastric junction. These lacerations may extend to or even through the muscularis, with rupture of blood vessels mainly in the submucosa. They are attributed to incoordination of the act of emesis, resulting from fatigue of the vomiting center and consequent forcible distention of the cardiac portion of the stomach while the vestibule remains contracted. Although usually recognized only at autopsy, the characteristic history of hematemesis that follows prolonged vomiting, usually after alcoholic indulgence, may often lead to the detection of these lesions by emergency esophagoscopy. Supportive medical treatment is indicated unless the threat of exsanguination makes emergency surgery mandatory.

Aerophagia. Aerophagia, or the swallowing of air, is

well nigh universal at meal times, though differing widely in degree. Its symptomatic results include belching, epigastric pain or fullness related to distention of the stomach, pain in the right lower quadrant, or in the right or left upper quadrant associated with distention of various parts of the colon, and the passage of flatus by rectum. All these symptoms, or any one of them, may be signified by the term *flatulence* or "gas." As aerophagia is for the most part a compulsive habit and a manifestation of emotional tension, it should be treated as such. The patient's consciousness of the habit can be increased by having him hold a tongue blade between his teeth, thus making swallowing much more difficult.

Acute Gastric Dilatation and Volvulus. Aerophagia may lead to serious overdistention of the stomach under two conditions: (1) during complete or partial *paralytic ileus* (see Ch. 637) after surgery, trauma, or acute medical conditions, when *acute gastric dilatation* may occur; and (2) in *torsion* or *volvulus* of the stomach, in which the most dependent portion of the greater curvature rotates forward, upward, and to the left. Under both conditions the rise in intragastric pressure may lead to increased gastric secretion and congestion of the gastric wall. The upper abdomen on examination is distended and tympanitic; a plain roentgenogram of the abdomen reveals the greatly enlarged gastric air bubble, which in volvulus characteristically presents a broad, smooth upward convexity beneath the left diaphragm.

Milder degrees of distention may give rise only to a feeling of pressure and pain in the epigastrium and left hypochondrium, relieved at times on change of position leading to escape of the gas by belching or, after traversing the intestines, on passage of flatus. In such cases decompression by stomach tube and constant suction of gastric contents should give prompt relief. Prevention of recurrences may demand effective treatment of aerophagia (see above).

In some instances of severe distention or torsion, a large volume of potassium-rich fluid is lost to the gastric lumen from the extracellular space, and the gastric circulation is impaired to the point of necrosis of the gastric wall, with resulting muscular weakness, severe shock, and death if the process is unchecked. In such cases, rapid parenteral repletion of extracellular water and electrolytes, followed by operative intervention, may be lifesaving.

PYLORIC STENOSIS

Definition. Pyloric stenosis, broadly defined, is any obstruction of the pyloric canal. What is commonly called pylorospasm is actually only the failure of relaxation of the sphincter in the absence or diminution of antral propulsive waves. True spasm of the pylorus, especially in adults, is usually associated with nearby duodenal or gastric ulcer or severe gastritis, and is to be differentiated from infiltration of the wall with inflammatory cells, fibrous tissue, or malignant cells.

Congenital hypertrophic pyloric stenosis is an obstructive narrowing caused by thickening of the pyloric muscle, possibly resulting from immaturity of enzymatic mechanisms in its intrinsic ganglion cells. It occurs in up to 3 per 1000 live births, four times more frequently in male than in female infants, and apparently as the expression of a single dominant gene. Never found before the fifth day of life, it is influenced also by multiple environmental factors affecting early infant feeding.

Clinical Manifestations. Typically, an infant between the ages of ten days and three months develops projectile vomiting, constipation, dehydration, and rapid loss of weight. Curiously, the appetite is well preserved, and feeding may be resumed immediately after vomiting. The vomitus may contain blood but no bile. Inspection after a feeding may reveal visible peristaltic waves passing from left to right across the upper abdomen. In many instances a firm tumor mass, 1 to 2 cm in diameter, is felt a few centimeters below the costal margin at the external margin of the right rectus muscle. Roentgenograms after a barium meal indicate gastric dilatation and a symmetrically narrowed, elongated pylorus.

In those patients not treated surgically (see below), attacks of nausea and vomiting occur at intervals for many years, sometimes throughout life. Rarely, such attacks begin in adult life and lead to the discovery of an identical hypertrophy of pyloric muscle.

Treatment. Initially an infant with this disorder is continued on breast milk or a formula yielding soft curds, supplemented with thick cereals. It may be necessary to make up deficits of water and electrolytes parenterally. Traditionally, atropine sulfate (0.06 mg) is given before each feeding, but the value of anticholinergics is not clearly documented. Phenobarbital (8 mg) may be combined to good effect with each dose of atropine. In most instances, as soon as dehydration has been corrected and acid-base balance restored, a Ramstedt operation (pyloromyotomy) should be performed. This requires a longitudinal incision that severs all the circular muscle fibers of the pylorus, leaving the mucosa intact. Although the mortality rate of this procedure is from 1 to 5 per cent, permanent cure is the rule.

In older children and adults, initial treatment of presumed pyloric stenosis should be the same as for peptic ulcer with obstruction (see below). Anticholinergics should not be used. During this interval the possible diagnosis of gastric cancer is studied by cytologic and gastroscopic means, and that of pyloric or duodenal ulcer by repeated roentgenographic examination. Unless the obstruction disappears completely within four to six weeks, it should be relieved surgically by pylorotomy or gastrojejunostomy.

MEGADUODENUM

The term *megaduodenum* is applied to gross dilatation of the duodenum from its upper end to the middle of the transverse portion. No point of true stenosis is to be found. The muscularis is hypertrophic, but the myenteric ganglion cells are damaged or absent. Although physiologic studies are so far lacking, the pathogenic mechanism is considered to be aperistalsis, comparable to the disorder in congenital megacolon, with which it is sometimes associated. A similar phenomenon has been observed in certain cases of South American trypanosomiasis (Chagas' disease), in which megacolon and megaesophagus may also be present.

This form of obstruction of the lower duodenum is to be differentiated from stenosis caused by malignant disease at the same site and from "superior mesenteric ileus," in which the transverse duodenum appears to be compressed between the lumbar vertebrae and the superior mesenteric artery near its origin from the aorta. Treatment is by duodenojejunostomy.

Barnett, W. O., and Wall, L.: Megaduodenum resulting from absence of the parasympathetic ganglion cells of Auerbach's plexus. Ann. Surg., 141:527, 1955.

Carter, C. O.: The inheritance of congenital pyloric stenosis. Br. Med. Bull., 17:251, 1961.

Jones, F. A., and Gummer, J. W. P.: Clinical Gastroenterology. Oxford, Blackwell Publications, Ltd., 1960, pp. 102–117.

Swenson, O.: Pediatric Surgery. 2nd ed. New York, Appleton-Century-Crofts, 1962, pp. 262–270.

637. DISORDERS OF INTESTINAL MOTILITY

Among the significant disorders of intestinal motility, some are adaptive mechanisms of general occurrence among persons under stress. Paralytic ileus and the irritable colon are both here interpreted in this light. These interrelated disorders are presented in the following pages, together with mechanical obstruction of the intestine, so often important in differential diagnosis.

Other disorders are thought to be due to excessive stimulation by humoral agents. These are the metastatic carcinoid syndrome and the diarrhea seen in patients with medullary carcinoma of the thyroid. Still others are known to be related to defects in the efferent cholinergic nerves regulating intestinal motility (megacolon), or thought to result from defects in the afferent limb of intestinal reflex arcs (diabetic pseudotabes; tabes dorsalis).

NORMAL COLONIC FUNCTION

The human colon has two main functions: (1) the absorption of water and crystalloids, and (2) the formation of a reservoir to permit the orderly and convenient evacuation of feces. The daily delivery from the ileum of 0.5 to 1.0 liter of liquid intestinal contents is regulated by the valvelike ileocecal sphincter, the tone of which is diminished by gastrin concurrently with its stimulation of ileal propulsive motility. In the colon the luminal contents are subjected over long periods to slow phasic contractions, kneading or accordion-like movements, which facilitate absorption. During this time the colon is sacculated or haustrated in outline. At long intervals, usually after the ingestion of food, this pattern of motility is replaced by one of mass peristalsis, in which haustra disappear, the proximal portions contract and the distal ones relax, and the entire colon undergoes shortening. In this manner feces are advanced rapidly.

The rectum is usually empty until part of the contents of the sigmoid is forced into it by mass peristalsis. This distends the rectal walls, produces discomfort in the sacral area, and initiates the defecation reflex by which the contraction of skeletal muscles of the abdominal wall and the coordinate relaxation of the anal sphincter assist in the emptying of the terminal colon. Voluntary inhibition of the reflex can be achieved by vigorous contraction of the external sphincter and a thoracic pattern of breathing. With time the walls of the rectum become adapted to the fecal mass; their tension decreases, and the stimulus to defecation subsides until renewed by further additions to the rectal contents.

DIARRHEA

Definition. Diarrhea signifies the passage of excessively liquid or excessively frequent stools. Never a complete diagnosis in itself, its recognition demands careful study to determine its cause. Its duration and course vary widely, depending upon the natural history of the underlying disease.

Etiology. The causes of diarrhea are legion, and are best considered in relation to underlying pathogenetic mechanisms, briefly outlined as follows:

Excessive Intraluminal Volume. In these conditions excessive ingestion of food or fluid is only a minor factor, and fluid accumulations are due chiefly to one of the following:

1. *Decreased absorption of water and solute* (osmotic diarrhea), including that resulting from saline cathartics, lactase deficiency, sprue, postgastrectomy syndrome, and congenital chloridorrhea.

2. *Increased secretion into the lumen,* of which the classic model is cholera. Recent evidence makes clear that the same mechanism is active in infections with enteropathogenic E. coli and other gram-negative organisms, as well as with peptide hormone-producing tumors (medullary carcinoma of thyroid, islet cell tumors). It is mediated by or reproduced by the action of prostaglandins on the production of cyclic AMP by adenyl cyclase in the intestinal epithelium. Abnormal secretion into the colonic lumen is characteristic of diarrhea caused by ileal disease or ileal resection, resulting from the action of excess bile acids on colonic mucosa, as well as of the diarrhea of villous adenoma of the colon or rectum.

Exaggerated Propulsive Motility. Exaggerated propulsive motility, mediated by neurohumoral factors, including acetylcholine, serotonin (5-HT), and prostaglandins, may be an independent and important variable. The most common example is the irritable colon syndrome. Excessive 5-HT, as produced in the malignant carcinoid syndrome, produces hyperperistalsis of the small bowel, with often severe diarrhea (see below). Mild increases in stool frequency occur in thyrotoxicosis. Local increases in intraluminal pressure caused by partial obstruction of the intestine by tumors, strictures, or fecal impactions lead to exaggerated propulsive activity and to diarrhea.

In many inflammatory or neoplastic diseases of the bowel, more than one of these mechanisms are thought to be operative at one time. The main practical advantages in considering them lie in general orientation of differential diagnosis and in utilization of the oral route for repletion of body fluids in cholera-like syndromes.

Differential Diagnosis. The formidable task of identifying the one or the several causes of diarrhea in a given patient can be facilitated by efforts to estimate, in succession, the *location,* the *mechanism,* and the *nature* of the disease process. The location is suggested by the character of the stools and the zone of reference of pain. If each stool is *large* in volume, it may be presumed that the distal colon is reacting as it would to an enema and is itself not diseased, and therefore that the chief site of the disorder is in the proximal colon or small intestine. In such instances, any accompanying pain is usually referred to the periumbilical area or the right lower quadrant. On the contrary, if some stools, though attended by notable urgency, are of *small* size, the conclusion is justified that the distal colon does not tolerate accumulation of a normal amount of feces, and therefore that it is diseased. In such instances, the stool is more likely to contain visible mucus or flecks of blood, and pain is felt in the lower abdomen or the sacral region. With respect to the *mechanism,* osmotic diarrhea should cease if oral intake is interrupted for 24 hours or more. The *nature* of the disease process is estimated from its manner of onset and course over time; history of exposure to toxic, infectious, and allergenic agents; the extent of debility; and the personality and life situation of the patient. The diagnostic study of the patient usually includes sigmoidoscopy, gross and microscopic examination of the stools and cultures for pathogenic bacteria, barium enema, and small bowel x-rays, in the order named. Other useful laboratory tests are mentioned elsewhere under the specific diseases.

Treatment. It is frequently necessary to mitigate the diarrhea or its consequences before the recognition of the true cause permits specific therapy. In most acute infectious diarrheas, the disease is brief, and the diarrhea serves a useful purpose in ridding the body, at least subtotally, of the offending agent. Hence, the first indication is to replace the losses of fluid and electrolytes, usually with infusions of physiologic saline and 5 per cent glucose, guided by measurements of urinary output and plasma volume. Replacement of potassium and further adjustments of acid-base balance are guided by serial determinations of serum sodium, potassium, chloride, and bicarbonates. If oral administration is possible, water, sodium chloride, and glucose should be forced through dilute sweetened fruit juices, tea, and salty broths in sufficient quantity to maintain a urinary output of in excess of 1500 ml per day. Cold liquids and concentrated sweets are poorly tolerated.

Lying flat in bed, with constant use of heating pad or hot water bottle, is usually helpful. Most of the conventional binding agents, such as bismuth, pectins, and kaolin, are of a low order of effectiveness. Aluminum hydroxide gel in large doses (20 to 40 ml four times a day) is often useful. Codeine sulfate, 0.03 to 0.06 gram, or morphine sulfate, 0.008 to 0.015 gram, may be given every three to four hours during acute diarrhea, but will produce severe distention and cramps in most instances. The synthetic opiate, diphenoxylate hydrochloride, carries apparently less risk of addiction and is often effective in doses of 5 to 10 mg three times daily before meals and at bedtime. Camphorated tincture of opium (paregoric) is used in doses of 4 ml after each bowel movement until diarrhea is controlled. In prescribing any of these agents, the physician assumes the responsibility for eventually freeing the patient from dependence upon them.

Fordtran, J. S.: Diarrhea. *In* Sleisenger, M. H., and Fordtran, J. S. (eds.): Gastrointestinal Disease. Philadelphia, W. B. Saunders Company, 1973, p. 291.
Phillips, S. F.: Absorption and secretion by the colon. Gastroenterology, 56:966, 1969.

CONSTIPATION
(With Emphasis on Habitual Constipation or Rectal Constipation)

Definition. Constipation ordinarily signifies the passage of excessively dry stools or the evacuation of the bowels less often than every other day. By many patients, however, the same term is used to refer to a sense of incomplete emptying of the rectum or to the small size of their stools.

Pathogenesis. Inadequate propulsion of feces may result from mechanical obstruction (as in carcinoma of the sigmoid colon), from diminished contractions of the proximal intestine, e.g., paralytic ileus, or from failure of the distal colon to relax, e.g., irritable colon and congenital megacolon. In most instances, however, constipation results chiefly from failure of the defecation reflex (habitual constipation, rectal constipation, or dyschezia).

Early in childhood, despite great variations in the intensity of "toilet training," the habits of defecation become subject to complex patterns of conditioned reflex behavior. Their disruption in adult life is usually associated with major changes in the pattern of living, e.g., travel or going away to school, with intercurrent illness, with emotional tension, or with willful neglect. The mechanical efficiency of defecation may be impaired by the use of high toilet seats, bedpans, or other departures from the primitive squatting position. Weakness of the muscles of the back or of the abdominal wall caused by neurologic disorders or by multiple pregnancies is occasionally an important factor. Failure of relaxation of the anal sphincter may be due to neighboring painful lesions such as anal ulcers or thrombosed hemorrhoids. These are, however, more often a result of the constipation than a cause.

Prolonged retention in the rectum (or rarely in the sigmoid colon) results in excessive dehydration or *impaction* of feces. This may lead to cramping lower abdominal pain and to paradoxical diarrhea, as watery brown stools are passed around the hardened mass. Many patients with constipation complain also of anorexia, bloating, belching, passage of flatus, headache, malaise, weakness, or faintness. Such symptoms are related in part to the attendant disturbances of intestinal motility and in part to the anxiety aroused by the constipation itself.

Diagnosis. In any constipated patient who has not recently been given an enema or a laxative, the finding of more than a few grams of feces on digital examination of the rectum indicates that habitual constipation is present. (Conversely, the usual finding in irritable colon or in megacolon is an empty rectum.) The search for localized anal and rectal lesions should be made carefully with both anoscope and sigmoidoscope. In most instances a barium enema, and in some an upper gastrointestinal roentgenographic series, is indicated to exclude intrinsic intestinal disease. Careful thought should be given to the possible etiologic importance of constipating medications such as opiates, anticholinergics, ganglionic blocking agents, tricyclic antidepressants, and nonabsorbable antacids. Search should be made for systemic diseases such as myxedema, hyperparathyroidism, lead poisoning, scleroderma, and mental depression, of which constipation may at times be the presenting symptom.

Management. The goal of treatment is an empty rectum, or the maximal possible restoration of normal habits of defecation, with minimal disturbance of normal intestinal motility. In bedridden patients, or in others whose daily habits are greatly disrupted, this must be postponed, and an effort is made to avoid fecal impaction by tapwater enemas or mild laxatives at one- or two-day intervals. Any painful anal lesion such as an ulcer or thrombosed hemorrhoid should be treated at once with sitz baths, local anesthesia by ointments or suppositories, and nightly mineral oil. Fecal impactions should be digitally broken, softened by a retention enema of cottonseed oil (150 ml) or dioctyl sodium sulfosuccinate (5 ml of a 1 per cent solution diluted to 90 ml in water), and evacuated by enemas of tapwater or soapsuds.

The cooperation of the patient is enlisted through explanation of the mechanisms of his constipation and of the goal of therapy. He must be persuaded that a daily bowel movement is desirable but not necessary. A large breakfast is prescribed, to contain fruit, cereal, toast or rolls, preserves, and coffee or milk. His diet should be high in vegetable fiber. He is required to sit on the toilet daily within the hour after breakfast, remaining ten minutes, and to distract his attention by a newspaper, magazine, or other device. All previous cathartics or enemas are forbidden; in their place a rounded teaspoon of a hydrophilic colloid (psyllium or agar) is taken with 400 ml of water at bedtime and again on arising. Mineral oil, 15 to 45 ml at bedtime only, may be substituted.

The patient is warned that one to four weeks are required for the achievement of desired results and that his bodily discomfort may in the meantime increase. When relief of this distress is needed, at intervals of two or three days, an enema of tapwater or of prepared hypertonic solutions (Travad, Clyserol, Fleet) is taken after the morning toilet visit. As normal habits are restored, the enemas and mild laxatives are cancelled; they may be recommended for future prophylactic use when the patient's habits of living are again disturbed.

Miner, R. W. (ed.): The colon: Its normal and abnormal physiology and therapeutics. Ann. N.Y. Acad. Sci., 58:293, 1954.

Rakatansky, H., and Kirsner, J. B.: Drugs for gastrointestinal diseases. *In* Modell, W. (ed.): Drugs of Choice, 1972–73. St. Louis, C. V. Mosby Company, p. 321.

IRRITABLE COLON
(Mucous Colitis, Spastic Colon, Unstable Colon, Adaptive Colitis)

Definition.   Irritable colon signifies a variety of disturbances of colonic function that accompany emotional tension and participate in the general bodily adaptation to nonspecific stress.

This disorder is considered to account for more than 50 per cent of all gastrointestinal illness, and ranks with the common cold as one of the leading causes of recurrent minor disability.

Symptoms and Their Mechanisms.   *Abdominal pain* of some degree occurs in most patients. It is usually located in the hypogastrium or left lower quadrant; it is commonly felt in the other quadrants of the abdomen but very rarely in the periumbilical region. In some instances severe pain is felt far laterally over the left costal margin and radiates to the precordium, the left shoulder, and the inner aspect of the left arm (the *splenic flexure syndrome*). In most instances, the pain of irritable colon is relieved by the passage of feces or gas. Hence it is believed to be due to distention or spasmodic contractions of the colon at various points (explaining its variable location). *Constipation* is probably related to heightened nonpropulsive activity (spasm), chiefly in the sigmoid colon, and *gaseous distention* of the proximal colon and *passage of flatus* are commonly associated. *Diarrhea* of varying severity may occur, together with urgency and tenesmus, usually in the morning before and after breakfast. Commonly the *stools are small*, whatever their consistency (hence the term "irritable colon"); they often contain visible *mucus*, or mucus alone may be evacuated with no fecal residues. Diarrhea and myxorrhea appear to represent the motor and secretory response of the colon to exaggerated cholinergic stimulation.

Extracolonic symptoms, often encountered in these patients, emphasize the generalized character of the body's adaptive response. Thus *anorexia, nausea, belching,* and *occasionally vomiting* indicate a concurrent disturbance of gastroduodenal motility. The syndrome of *neurocirculatory asthenia*, including palpitation, shortness of breath, precordial discomfort, and fatigue on mild exertion, is often present. *Headache* is common, and sweating, flushing, faintness, sighing respirations, and hyperventilation may be noted.

Natural History and Pathogenesis.   This disorder may begin at any age, but usually in early adult life or in adolescence. Its course is extremely variable, but in most instances individual episodes of illness can be measured in terms of days, weeks, or months. In many persons the predominant symptoms are pain and constipation, in others painless diarrhea; but irregularly alternating constipation and diarrhea are not uncommon. There is rarely any significant dehydration or loss of weight.

The onset and recurrences of irritable colon usually coincide with periods of life stress and emotional conflict, and the symptoms often disappear spontaneously when these influences abate. Relevant disturbances of colonic function have been observed in the laboratory when emotional conflicts have been induced in patients through stressful interviews (Fig. 6) and have appeared

Figure 6.   *A,* Heightened nonpropulsive contractions of sigmoid colon during stress interview in subject with spastic constipation. (Tandem balloons.) *B,* Reduced phasic activity of sigmoid colon during stress interview in a subject with functional diarrhea. (Single balloon.)

as normal bodily manifestations of emotion, not unlike blushing and weeping. The emotional state accompanying constipation has been described as one of assertive independence, defensiveness, or self-confident resistance to a noxious situation. The attitudes commonly observed with diarrhea are those of dependence, helplessness, and self-reproach. These impressions have been consistent in both clinical and laboratory studies. The pathways by which these reactions are mediated probably include the central and peripheral portions of the autonomic nervous system, as comparable disturbances have been produced transiently by administration of methacholine or neostigmine. It is probable that other chemical mediators, such as serotonin and cholecystokinin and other intestinal hormones, are involved.

Diagnosis. The diagnosis of irritable colon must be based upon (1) the recognition of characteristic symptoms, (2) the exclusion of other disease processes suggested by the symptoms, and (3) repeated and conscientious testing of the hypothesis that the symptoms are related to life and stress and emotional tension. On examination of the patient one commonly finds a palpable, tender sigmoid colon, enlarged areas of tympany over the proximal colon, and proctoscopic signs of mucosal engorgement, spasm, and excessive mucous secretion; yet none of these findings is specific for the disease or is a significant departure from the normal. The condition cannot be diagnosed, but may be suggested, by roentgenographic examination of the colon.

The syndrome of irritable colon may be mimicked very closely by *abuse of cathartics; by specific infections* of the colon such as amebiasis, shigellosis, or lymphogranuloma venereum; by *allergy* to ingested food or drugs; and by intolerance of *specific disaccharides,* particularly lactose. The differentiation from early *ulcerative colitis* or from *carcinoma of the colon* can usually be made by proctoscopy, biopsy, and barium enema. Differentiation from *diverticular disease* may be more difficult, because the symptoms and motor disturbances of the colon in this disease closely resemble those of irritable colon, and the two conditions may coexist or be interrelated (see Ch. 639).

Broadly, irritable colon must be differentiated from all the various causes of abdominal pain, constipation and diarrhea. Of particular note, the pain of *gallbladder disease* may be simulated by gaseous distention of the hepatic flexure, the pain and tenderness of acute or chronic *appendicitis* by distention of the cecum, and the migration of pain to the precordium in the "splenic flexure syndrome" may simulate *angina pectoris* or *myocardial infarction.*

Because of the ubiquity of stress and emotional tension, symptoms of irritable colon may be superimposed upon those of other and more serious diseases, or may reflect the anxiety occasioned by them. Careful consideration of the significance of each process is required, lest a carcinoma go undetected or the removal of a symptomless gallbladder prove useless in the relief of unrelated abdominal distress.

The establishment of a diagnosis of irritable colon on positive grounds depends upon a profound understanding of the social history and personality of the patient. As the process of acquiring this understanding is of both diagnostic and therapeutic value, it is described under the heading of Management.

Management. The recognition of irritable colon as a bodily reaction to stress calls for treatment directed to the patient as a whole rather than to his colon. As in the relief of blushing or weeping, both the environment and the attitudes of the patient must be considered.

At the first visit, the patient is called upon for a brief autobiography, including his relations with parents, marital partner, employers, and others. His speech and expression are observed for evidences of emotion, and topics of special meaning for him are thus usually easily recognized. The several visits required for adequate laboratory investigation and early symptomatic management provide opportunities for further discussion of these topics. Careful note is made of the dates of important events, so that a "life chart" may be constructed, correlating these with the course of bowel symptoms.

After several visits, such a procedure permits the reasonably certain acceptance or rejection of the diagnosis of irritable colon on the positive grounds of coincidence with life stress and correlation with emotional tension. A decision should then be made as to the prognosis and needs for future therapy. Those patients whose episodes of illness appear but *little related in time to easily recognizable stress situations* and who have made a uniformly inadequate adjustment to major personal problems may be considered the "more neurotic" group. The further efforts of the physician are best limited to reassurance regarding the benign character of the illness, manipulation of important environmental factors, explanations to responsible relatives, sympathetic listening, and the conscientious use of placebos.

On the other hand, the "less neurotic" patient who has made a satisfactory adjustment to most life situations, whose bowel symptoms are intermittent and closely related in time to specific difficulties, e.g., new job or marital problem, can often profit by relatively brief and simple psychotherapy in the hands of the general physician. This begins with *reassurance* as to the absence of serious disease and usually a simple explanation of his illness as an expression of emotional tension. He is urged to ventilate his feelings to the physician or members of his family or friends, or to sublimate them through more active and vigorous pursuit of sports, games, or hobbies. He is encouraged to make his own changes in ways of living as a result of the insight acquired.

A patient with irritable colon should be referred to a psychiatrist if his emotional tension is severe and out of proportion to his bowel disorder, if he seems psychotic, if he requires expert manipulation of psychotropic drugs, or if he declares his need of such help.

Concurrently, symptomatic management may be required. The most common problem is habitual *constipation,* which should be treated as outlined above. With *diarrhea* the usual binding agents are ineffective. The most rational therapy is an anticholinergic drug in sufficient dosage to dry the mouth, i.e., propantheline, 15 to 30 mg, or tridihexethide, 25 to 50 mg. This should not be given continuously but in anticipation of the hours of more severe diarrhea, usually in the early morning or just prior to social or business engagements. In some cases, diphenoxylate hydrochloride, 5 mg three times daily before meals and at bedtime, is indicated and is more effective. In view of the chronic and benign nature of the illness, use of opiates, even on a temporary basis, is rarely desirable. Severe abdominal *pain* is best relieved by a hot water bottle or a warm tapwater enema.

Sedatives, tranquilizers, and antidepressants may be required to deal with extreme degrees of anxiety and insomnia. Their use should be guided by the principles set forth in Ch. 321 and 336, and they should not be routinely prescribed for patients with irritable colon. The most convenient "placebo" is tincture of belladonna in doses of 10 to 15 drops in water three times daily before meals.

Prognosis. The "more neurotic" patients, as defined above, may be expected to have symptoms of varying severity, mitigated only temporarily by the solicitude of the physician or favorable life situations. The "less neurotic" should have symptoms at long intervals, reduced in frequency and severity, but rarely abolished, by a high degree of insight and alteration to their environment.

Almy, T. P.: Experimental studies on the irritable colon. Am. J. Med., 10:60, 1951.
Chaudhary, N. A., and Truelove, S. C.: The irritable colon syndrome. Quart. J. Med. (N.S.), 31:307, 1962.
Hislop, I. G.: Psychological significance of the irritable colon syndrome. Gut, 12:452, 1971.

INTESTINAL OBSTRUCTION
(Ileus)

Definition. Intestinal obstruction is broadly defined as any impairment, arrest, or reversal of the normal anad flow of intestinal contents. This concept thus includes obstruction caused by mechanical factors and that caused by failure of peristalsis for reasons of deficient neural stimulation (paralytic ileus) or vascular insufficiency.

Etiology. The majority of severe cases are due to *mechanical factors* that locally occlude the intestinal lumen. The most common of these are extramural, constricting the entire circumference of the gut, and include *hernias* (especially inguinal and femoral), peritoneal *adhesions* caused by previous operations or local inflammatory disease, and *volvulus* (usually of the sigmoid or ileocecal regions). *Mural thickening* resulting from disease or congenital defect of the intestinal wall may narrow or obliterate its lumen; examples are benign and malignant tumors; inflammatory strictures caused by diverticulitis, regional enteritis, or previous operative anastomoses; and congenital atresia or imperforate anus. Least common are *intraluminal* factors, including fecal impactions, meconium, foreign bodies, intussusception, gallstones, and large worms.

Another large group of cases is due to general or regional *failure of peristalsis (adynamic ileus).* This may occur after any abdominal operation and in many severe, acute diseases such as pneumonia and myocardial infarction. It is an impressive feature of many painful conditions in the thoracolumbar area, such as renal and biliary colic, retroperitoneal hematoma, or spinal injuries, but is most severe in the presence of peritonitis. An initially identical picture may result from *ischemia* of the bowel wall caused by *vascular insufficiency.*

In many cases more than one of these mechanisms play a part. Thus, postoperative adynamic ileus may lead to volvulus and subsequent ischemia of the twisted loop. The possible combination of mechanical and physiologic factors calls for periodic reconsideration of the diagnosis in individual cases.

Pathogenesis. Whatever the etiologic mechanism, the immediate effect of ileus is to interrupt the normal pathways of intestinal propulsion and absorption of liquid and gas. *Even in the absence of oral intake,* 7 to 10 liters of water and contained solutes (net flux) enter the upper gastrointestinal tract each day, most of which is to be ab-

sorbed at lower levels. In intestinal obstruction, this cycle is interrupted. Even if vomiting does not occur, this liquid is withdrawn from the body fluid compartments to lie in the intestinal lumen. The result is dehydration, loss from extracellular fluid of sodium and chloride ions, alkalosis, and shift of potassium ion from intracellular to extracellular fluid to compensate for loss of potassium into the gut. Hypovolemia and hypokalemia may lead to acute renal insufficiency, even in the absence of arterial hypotension. Hypokalemia itself further inhibits peristalsis.

Stasis within the gut leads to multiplication of its bacteria, absorption of indoles and other of their metabolic products, and accumulation of gas produced by bacterial action and air swallowing. The resultant distention of the gut leads to dangerous increases in intraluminal pressure, especially in closed-loop obstructions caused by hernia or volvulus, or in complete occlusion of the colon, in which the contents are trapped proximally by the ileocecal valve. Mucosal blood flow is reduced by this increased pressure, as well as by torsion of, or extrinsic pressure upon, the mesenteric vessels. As the gut wall becomes necrotic, plasma proteins and blood exude into the lumen, and bacterial toxins gain access to the peritoneum and the circulating blood.

Mechanical obstruction of the small intestine is usually first indicated by epigastric or periumbilical colicky *pain* and *vomiting.* Early examination of the abdomen may reveal increased tympany but little distention, and the *bowel sounds* are characteristically hyperactive, high-pitched, and coincident with the episodes of pain; the higher the obstruction, the more frequent and severe the pain and the higher the expected pitch of the sounds. Loose stools and flatus may be passed before obstipation sets in. With lower sites of obstruction, distention is more prominent and vomiting may be delayed in appearance, and may resemble dilute feces in odor and appearance—the result of bacterial proliferation related to stasis in the small bowel lumen. In later stages the bowel sounds may become less active, and the development of continuous pain, increasing tenderness to direct pressure and rebound, rigidity of the abdomen, and signs of hypovolemia warn of strangulation of the bowel. Fever is a late and unimpressive feature.

In *paralytic ileus* distention and obstipation are the prominent symptoms, vomiting is less marked, and colicky pain is absent. Early auscultation of the abdomen often reveals absent bowel sounds (none in a period of three minutes or more).

In *colonic obstruction* distention is usually prominent, and pain, often delayed in onset, with less frequent paroxysms, is located either in the hypogastric area (with left colon lesions) or in the epigastrium and right upper quadrant (with disease of the right colon). Bowel sounds are low pitched and less frequent. Vomiting is delayed and often feculent. Rectal examination may reveal unchanged blood or a palpable mass. Previous pelvic surgery, as opposed to abdominal surgery, suggests a colonic rather than a small intestinal site of obstruction. The signs of strangulation (see above) may be evident in the initial examination.

Laboratory Findings. Early in the course, the fluid shifts are manifested by diminished urinary output, fall in serum chloride and potassium, and rise in plasma bicarbonate and pH and in the blood urea nitrogen. As these abnormalities worsen, the hematocrit may rise, and urinary specific gravity and osmolality may become fixed. With strangulation the peripheral leukocyte count rises, far out of proportion to the body temperature.

Early and repeated *roentgenographic examination* of the abdomen is essential. Films taken of the patient in the horizontal position aid in localization of the obstruction in the small or large intestine. Typically, marked gaseous distention of centrally located, horizontal small intestinal loops produces a "ladder" appearance, with no colonic gas. In closed loop obstruction of the colon with a competent ileocecal valve, only the laterally located, haustrated colonic segments are gas filled. With cecal or sigmoid volvulus, characteristically large distended sacs, without mucosal folds, are seen. In paralytic ileus, gas may be found anywhere in the gut, including the stomach and rectum. Films taken in the upright or lateral decubitus positions reveal fluid levels which indicate the degree of accumulation of fluid and gas; the latter is relatively *less* prominent as strangulation develops. Cautious performance of a barium enema, without preparatory cleansing of the bowel, is often indicated in localizing a point of colonic obstruction, but barium or other contrast media should never be given by mouth.

Treatment. The effective management of cases of intestinal obstruction calls for frequent re-evaluation of the status of the patient by clinical and laboratory methods and modification of the therapeutic plan to deal with the changing conditions thus discerned. The cardinal principles of therapy are *replacement* of metabolic losses, *decompression* of the intestine, and *removal of the cause* of obstruction.

Intake of fluid and food by mouth is suspended, and an infusion of equal parts of 0.9 per cent sodium chloride and 5 per cent dextrose in water is begun. As soon as the adequacy of renal function can be estimated or the serum potassium level has been reported, potassium chloride should be added to the infusion and delivered at a rate not exceeding 40 mEq of potassium per hour. An electrocardiogram should be taken before therapy; repeated observation of the T waves and S-T segments can serve, along with repeated determinations of serum potassium and chloride, to gauge the effectiveness of replacement. In the presence of severe dehydration, associated hemorrhage, or signs of strangulation, the central venous pressure, arterial pressure, urinary output, and hematocrit should be monitored, and administration of water, electrolytes, albumin, and whole blood should be adjusted accordingly. When strangulation is suspected, antimicrobial drugs are used in the manner recommended for cases of vascular occlusion.

Decompression of the mechanically obstructed intestine may be largely achieved by nasogastric intubation and constant suction. If this fails, and in all cases of paralytic ileus, the long balloon-tipped intestinal tube (Miller-Abbot or Cantor type) should be passed, with repeated roentgenographic verification of its position. Such a procedure will greatly diminish the symptoms of the patient, but will not benefit his fluid and electrolyte depletion, and may render less clear the signs of strangulation. For this reason, intubated patients must be carefully observed, and, if local tenderness and leukocytosis are not diminished after 24 to 36 hours, surgical intervention is required.

Removal of the cause of ileus requires *operation* in most cases of complete mechanical obstruction and in many cases of severe adynamic ileus. It must be postponed in all instances until dehydration, electrolyte loss, and shock have been overcome; but, in the face of evident strangulation or closed loop obstruction of the colon, it must be accomplished as rapidly as possible. Just before operation, intensive antimicrobial therapy should be started; penicillin, 1 to 2 million units, and streptomycin, 1 gram, should be given in divided doses daily; or ampicillin, 0.5 to 1.0 gram every six hours. The surgical procedure depends upon the findings at laparotomy and the judgment of the surgeon, particularly as to the viability of the bowel.

Some cases of volvulus tend to right themselves on conservative management, permitting later surgery at a time of election, and rare cases of ileocolic intussusception in childhood are relieved by the intracolonic pressure exerted by a barium enema.

Prognosis. The outlook for recovery from intestinal obstruction depends chiefly upon the presence or absence of strangulation and its consequent toxemia, and the presence or absence of renal insufficiency resulting from excessive loss of fluid and electrolytes. These are in turn influenced by the type, location, and degree of obstruction, the existence of related primary disease (such as peritonitis leading to paralytic ileus), and the extent of delay in initiation of effective therapy. For persons recovering from ileus, the outlook for recurrence depends upon the underlying causes; with most patients with mechanical obstruction who recover without emergency operation, the probability of recurrence is so great as to dictate interval elective surgery.

Miller, L. D., Mackie, J. A., and Rhoads, J. E.: The pathophysiology and management of intestinal obstruction. Surg. Clin. North Am., 42:1285, 1962.

Neely, J., and Catchpole, B.: Ileus: The restoration of alimentary-tract motility by pharmacological means. Br. J. Surg., 58:21, 1971.

Silen, W., Hein, M. F., and Goldman, L.: Strangulation obstruction of the small intestine. Arch. Surg., 85:121, 1962.

PSEUDO-OBSTRUCTION OF THE COLON

Pseudo-obstruction is a rare disease of unknown etiology, manifested by episodes of ileus of both large and small bowel. Its usual onset is in early life. Its course is rarely acute, being more commonly a relapsing one over periods of 3 to 20 years. Histologic study of bowel wall reveals mild round-cell inflammation and fibrosis of the mucosa and submucosa, with normal ganglion cells. Motility of the colon and of the upper small bowel is reduced on manometric examination.

The symptoms include poorly localized abdominal cramps, distention, vomiting, mild diarrhea, and some signs of malabsorption. Bowel sounds are reduced, and plain x-rays of the abdomen reveal distended loops with air-fluid levels anywhere in the bowel, including the rectum. The disease is distinguished from scleroderma of the intestine by its earlier onset, absence of skin changes or Raynaud's phenomenon, and lack of striking therapeutic benefit from broad-spectrum antimicrobials.

During acute phases, supportive therapy is provided by nasogastric suction, parenteral fluid replacement, and ampicillin, 4.0 grams per day intravenously. The prognosis for the recurrent form of the disease is poor.

Maldonado, J. E., Gregg, J. A., Green, P. A., and Brown, A. L., Jr.: Chronic idiopathic intestinal pseudo-obstruction. Am. J. Med., 49:203, 1970.

MEGACOLON

The persistent enlargement of all or a long segment of the colon to a diameter greater than 5.5 cm is referred to as *megacolon.* This disorder may be acquired or congenital in origin, and may or may not involve permanent defects in intrinsic innervation of the bowel.

Psychogenic megacolon, or stool-holding, is a common disorder of children after the first year of life. The desire to avoid pain on defecation leads to retention of impacted feces and involuntary soiling. A similar process occurs in adult psychotic patients, mainly with depression, and is complicated by treatment with phenothiazines and tricyclic antidepressants. Treatment is by disimpaction, large and repeated doses of mineral oil, and, in the adult, repeated cleansing enemas.

Similar *acquired colonic dilatation* may accompany the severe constipation of myxedema or lead poisoning, the mural infiltration of scleroderma or amyloidosis, the neurologic deficits of diabetes or parkinsonism, or long-standing incomplete obstruction of the sigmoid or rectum. In *Chagas' disease* (South American trypanosomiasis) megacolon is found as a late complication, owing to destruction of the ganglia of Auerbach's plexus by the tissue reaction to the parasite. The mechanism of this colonic disorder, as well as of its sometimes associated megaesophagus, megaduodenum, or megalobladder, is similar to that of congenital megacolon, as described below.

CONGENITAL MEGACOLON
(Idiopathic Megacolon; Hirschsprung's Disease)

Definition. Congenital megacolon is a chronic disorder of intestinal motility, usually beginning in infancy, characterized by aganglionosis of the distal bowel, and resulting clinically in severe and unremitting constipation.

Etiology and Pathology. Congenital megacolon occurs once in 2000 births, more commonly in male children, and with significantly increased frequency in sibs. The basic lesion is a congenital absence of myenteric ganglion cells in a distal segment of the colon, with neighboring autonomic nerve fibers increased in number or size. The aganglionic segment may be located just inside the anal margin or may extend upward a variable distance into the rectum and sigmoid, or less often as high as the distal ileum. Because its muscle is persistently contracted, it presents a functional obstruction to the passage of feces. This narrow, usually empty segment connects by a short conical portion with a greatly dilated, more proximal segment. The dilated segment has normal myenteric ganglia, hypertrophic muscular coats, and normal propulsive activity; it is usually filled with putty-like feces. Several lines of evidence now suggest that the basic defect is a failure of development of intramural nonadrenergic inhibitory neurons, which migrate downward during embryonic life from a point of entry in the upper esophagus. Megaloureter, megalobladder, Down's syndrome, and cardiac septal defects may be associated congenital anomalies.

Clinical Manifestations. Many patients will have had an episode of intestinal obstruction in the first few days of life. After a remission of several weeks or months there is the gradual return of severe and continuous constipation, sometimes with occasional vomiting. The abdomen progressively enlarges, the costal margin flares, and colonic peristalsis may be plainly visible. Nutrition is poor and growth may be retarded. A mild anemia is common. Neonates and infants may develop pseudo-

membranous enterocolitis or perforation of the colon or the appendix.

Diagnosis. A plain roentgenogram of the abdomen may reveal the fecal retention as a large ovoid mass mottled by small irregular gas shadows. The diagnosis is supported, and differentiation made from acquired megacolon, by demonstration of a distal narrow segment of colon on barium enema, best seen in the lateral position. Pressure studies of the anal canal reveal a failure of the normal relaxation of the internal sphincter on distention of the rectum. Final diagnosis presently requires demonstration of absent ganglia on open biopsy of the wall of the narrowed rectum, performed per anum under general anesthesia. The diagnosis, however, can often be excluded by the finding of submucosal ganglion cells on suction biopsy of the rectum.

Treatment and Prognosis. Except in neonates, the much greater frequency of acquired than of congenital megacolon dictates a trial of therapy (see above) for the former condition before the aforementioned diagnostic measures are instituted.

In a small minority of cases of true megacolon with a very short aganglionic segment near the anus, the colon can be successfully emptied by the daily use of laxatives (magnesia magma, cascara, or senna) and enemas of physiologic saline or soap suds. Rarely, such a patient grows to early adulthood in a fair state of health, but with continuous dependence on these measures.

All the remainder of the cases require surgical relief. The procedure of choice is the resection of the aganglionic segment, with division of the internal anal sphincter and with end-to-end anastomosis of the normally innervated upper colon to the stump of the rectum just inside the anus (Swenson's "pull-through" procedure). Histologic study of the segment removed is necessary to ensure that the anastomosis has been made to normally innervated bowel. If this condition is satisfied, the results are lasting and almost uniformly excellent.

Davidson, M., Kugler, M. M., and Bauer, C. H.: Diagnosis and management in children with severe and protracted constipation and obstruction. J. Pediatr., 62:261, 1963.
Ehrenpreis, T.: Hirschsprung's Disease. Chicago, Year Book Medical Publishers, 1970.
Passarge, E.: The genetics of Hirschsprung's disease. N. Engl. J. Med., 276:138, 1967.
Schnaufer, L., et al.: Differential sphincteric studies in the diagnosis of anorectal disorders of childhood. J. Pediatr. Surg., 2:538, 1967.
Swenson, O.: Congenital megacolon. Pediatr. Clin. North Am., 14:187, 1967.

DIABETIC DIARRHEA

Definition. Persistent or episodic watery diarrhea in patients with diabetes represents a now well-defined functional disorder best referred to as diabetic diarrhea. It occurs infrequently, even among diabetics; its importance lies in the social disability imposed by the symptoms and in the availability at times of striking benefits from therapy.

Etiology and Pathogenesis. This disorder is most frequent among those whose diabetes has been poorly controlled by therapy and is complicated by neuropathy, particularly by other signs of visceral neuropathy, i.e., impotence, urinary incontinence, defects of sweating, pupillary abnormalities, gastric atony, and orthostatic hypotension. Degenerative changes in autonomic ganglia and in dorsal nerve roots have been occasionally observed at postmortem examination. The clinically evident disturbances in motility of the bowel are believed to be associated with defective innervation. The observation of dramatic improvement in some cases with the use of antimicrobial therapy (see below) has indicated that the diarrhea may be due to bacterial overgrowth in the small bowel.

Clinical Manifestations. The diarrhea in this disorder usually occurs in the form of severe and explosive attacks lasting one to a few days each, and separated by periods of either normal bowel function or constipation of variable severity. Less often, diarrhea is continuous. Movements characteristically are associated with great urgency, often waking the patient from sleep, and the penalty for sound sleep is often fecal incontinence. The stools are voluminous, watery, brown, and foul; they only rarely contain gross blood. The attacks are associated with little pain, and usually do not lead to serious dehydration or shock.

Physical examination reveals little except collateral evidence of peripheral or autonomic neuropathy (see above) or of the ocular or vascular complications of diabetes. Gastrointestinal roentgenograms may show atony and delayed emptying of the stomach; the small intestine appears normal in pattern, but passage time may be greatly accelerated or delayed. Chemical examination of the stools may or may not reveal an excess of fat, and the pancreatic juice is normal in volume and enzyme content.

The diagnosis should be suspected whenever explosive watery diarrhea recurs or persists, especially with nocturnal attacks of fecal incontinence. The probability is increased by the finding of neuropathy. The diabetes is not always clinically apparent or previously recognized.

Treatment. Control of the diabetes (maintenance of normal weight through adequate diet and insulin, freedom from ketosis, minimal glycosuria and hyperglycemia) is sufficient to eliminate or substantially diminish the symptoms in about half the cases. Standard medicaments for symptomatic control of diarrhea, including anticholinergics and opiates, are generally ineffective. The tetracyclines have been shown to terminate attacks in a few cases within an hour of the ingestion of a single dose, e.g., tetracycline, 250 mg. When diarrhea occurs frequently or continuously, the same dose may be given once daily or even once weekly (see Part XIV, Section Three).

Prognosis. Even without therapy, this disorder is not progressive in severity, but attacks may be expected to recur with variable frequency over many years or even decades. Severe electrolyte disturbances or dietary deficiencies seldom result. Health and survival are usually limited instead by the other complications of diabetes.

Malins, J. M., and Mayne, N.: Diabetic diarrhea. Diabetes, 18:858, 1969.
Whalen, G. E., et al.: Diabetic diarrhea. Gastroenterology, 56:1021, 1969.

638. GASTROINTESTINAL ALLERGY AND FOOD INTOLERANCE
(Food Idiosyncrasy)

Introduction. The gastrointestinal mucosa is rich in lymphocytes and plasma cells and is exposed to a myriad of potential antigens in food, in drugs and other chemicals, and in microorganisms, resulting in a great variety of antigen-antibody reactions. In addition, it apparently has the capacity to form and react with autoantibodies, as has been postulated in atrophic gastritis. Any and all clinical phenomena resulting from antigen-antibody reactions in the intestinal wall are connoted by the term *gastrointestinal allergy,* and these may include some aspects or some cases of established disease entities of uncertain or variable etiology, e.g., ulcerative colitis. The term *food allergy,* on the other hand, includes all manifestations of hypersensitive reactions to ingested foods, many of which, e.g., urticaria, are in tissues other than the intestine. *Food intolerance* or *food idiosyncrasy* connotes a variety of gastrointestinal disorders attributed in whole or in part to nonallergic mechanisms incited by specific foods or properties of foods.

Pathogenesis and Symptoms. The mucosa is slightly permeable throughout life to whole proteins, but markedly so in the neonatal period, when sensitization of its lymphatic tissue is most likely to occur. Probably as a result of this, many asymptomatic persons have circulating serum precipitins to proteins of cow's milk, hen's eggs, and other foods. Sensitization to chemicals and drugs may occur at any age and may be occult, as when milk from penicillin-treated cows is ingested. In a minority of those sensitized, later exposure to an antigen may give rise to reactions in the gut mucosa characterized pathologically by edema, vascular engorgement, ecchymoses, erosions, excessive mucous secretion, and often spasmodic muscular contractions. The resulting symptoms vary in nature and in time of onset with the segment of gut affected, but commonly include abdominal pain, nausea and vomiting, diarrhea, and mucoid stools. Urticarial eruptions and wheezing may be associated; and in severe cases hematemesis, melena, purpura, arthralgias and prostration may occur. In such acute cases recovery is usually prompt and complete, but in others of more insidious onset the course of symptoms is prolonged and highly variable.

Management. The presumptive diagnosis of intestinal allergy often can be made from a careful history, establishing a consistent temporal relationship between exposure to antigen and onset of symptoms. This impression, the more convincing if a single foodstuff is involved, can be confirmed prospectively by a food diary and notation of the time of symptoms, and then can be tested by elimination and reintroduction of the suspected allergen. The latter is best accomplished without the patient's knowledge, by stomach tube or by admixture with barium given for gastrointestinal roentgenograms, permitting (with suitable controls) observation of the motor effects of contact with the allergen. The gastric or colonic mucosa may be directly viewed by endoscopy after exposure to suspected antigens and to control materials. These methods can give valid information if practiced with great care. Skin tests, levels of serum antibodies, and changes in circulating leukocytes are of little value. According to present evidence, the levels of antibodies in the stool or in intestinal secretions (coproantibodies) more closely reflect antigen-antibody reactions in the gut mucosa, and may be diagnostically useful.

Once an offending antigen is recognized, its removal should constitute effective treatment, provided all sources of the antigen can be identified. Food additives, insecticides, and bread molds are examples of sources often difficult to eliminate. In some conditions, e.g., hypersensitivity to milk protein in ulcerative colitis, reaction to the exogenous antigen may constitute but one of many pathogenic factors in the disease, and the results of total exclusion are of doubtful value.

Differential Diagnosis. The symptoms of gastrointestinal allergy are nonspecific and may be mimicked by a wide range of gastrointestinal disorders, most commonly food poisoning and the irritable colon.

Many other reactions to ingestion of food are based on either nonallergic or questionably allergic mechanisms. The inconsistency in the clinical responses to exposure to the postulated food stimulus is based both on variations in the other influences on intestinal function and on the need for a threshold amount of the offending substance to evoke a clinically evident reaction. Some food idiosyncrasies are clearly *spurious* in that they are not, on repeated careful testing, consistently enough evoked by the suspected food. Intolerance of *roughage* is truly rare, and of probable significance only with marked stenosis of the esophagus, the large or small bowel, an abdominal stoma, or the anus. It should be remembered that food residues constitute only one third to one half of the bulk of the stool. Often certain foods are poorly tolerated because of previous *conditioning,* having been eaten under conditions of anxiety, depression, or disgust. In other instances, *motor disturbances* are brought about by physiologic mechanisms, such as the delayed emptying of the stomach (and feeling of fullness) after a fatty meal, and the osmotically induced distress of the postgastrectomy "dumping" syndrome (see Ch. 643).

Most clearly recognized nonallergic mechanisms of intolerance are related to defects of *digestion* and *absorption.* Gastric achylia may be manifested by a distaste for meat, and pancreatic achylia by steatorrhea on ingestion of fat. Intolerance of wheat, rye, and barley appears to be due to deficiency of a peptidase in the jejunal mucosa (*gluten enteropathy*—see Part XIV, Section Three), and intolerance of milk seems most often due to *deficiency of intestinal lactase* or, in some infants, *sensitivity to cow's milk proteins,* with resulting steatorrhea and severe electrolyte depletion. In the latter instance it is still not clear whether the intolerance is due to hypersensitivity or to defects in peptidase activity. Aside from lactase deficiency, bloating of the abdomen commonly attends the ingestion of beans and other legumes, apparently because of *bacterial fermentation of their nonabsorbable carbohydrates,* such as raffinose. Bloating that follows the eating of onions and cabbage appears to be due to their content of flavone compounds which directly inhibit intestinal motility. Considering the many unknowns in the chemistry of foods, many other nonallergic mechanisms must await discovery.

Sensitivity to cow's milk proteins occurs in about one of every 200 neonates, and is manifested chiefly by watery diarrhea, often with mucus and occasionally with rectal bleeding. There is often a family history of concurrent appearance of eczema, urticaria, or other allergic phenomena. The child fails to gain weight, has edema, and is found to have iron deficiency anemia, eosinophilia, hypoproteinemia, and positive tests for occult blood in the stool. In some infants an acute ulcerative colitis is found, with friable, bleeding, and acute inflamed rectal mucosa. The syndrome is dramatically relieved by elimination of milk and recurs with resumption of milk feedings.

Eosinophilic gastroenteritis is a rare but well defined clinicopathologic entity, in which one or several areas of the bowel, usually the stomach and small intestine, are the sites of infiltration with eosinophils, and in which the patient experiences intermittent nausea, vomiting, diarrhea, and abdominal pain after ingestion of specific foods. There is usually a history of hay fever, asthma, urticaria, or some other allergic disorder; eosinophilia of peripheral blood is common, and skin tests are often positive for suspected allergens. Protein-losing enteropathy, low serum immunoglobulins, and malabsorption are observed in many cases.

In patients with mainly mucosal involvement, upper gastrointestinal x-rays show nodular mucosal surfaces, and multiple suction biopsies of stomach and jejunum reveal a patchy eosinophilic infiltrate, sometimes with villous atrophy. This form must be distinguished from gluten enteropathy, connective tissue disorders, and protozoan or helminthic diseases of the bowel. In others, involvement chiefly of the muscular layers leads to polypoid or infiltrative thickening of the gut wall, the roentgenographic appearance of which resembles carcinoma, lymphoma, or Crohn's disease. *Eosinophilic granuloma* usually presents as an obstructing tumor mass at or near the pylorus in a patient lacking a clear-cut allergic history or a significant eosinophilia. Diagnosis prior to histopathologic examination is virtually impossible. Rarely, subserosal involvement gives rise to ascites with high eosinophil counts in the fluid.

Treatment is first attempted by elimination diet, but often requires temporary or chronic use of corticosteroids (e.g., prednisone, 20 to 30 mg daily for ten days, then tapered or discontinued). The eosinophilic granuloma is excised surgically.

Greenberger, N., and Gryboski, J. D.: Allergic disorders of the intestine and eosinophilic gastroenteritis. *In* Sleisenger, M. H., and Fordtran, J. S. (eds.): Gastrointestinal Disease. Philadelphia, W. B. Saunders Company, 1973, pp. 1066–1082.

Ingelfinger, F. J., Lowell, F. C., and Franklin, W.: Medical progress—gastrointestinal allergy. N. Engl. J. Med., 241:303, 1949.

Klein, N. C., Hargrove, M. D., Sleisenger, M. H., and Jeffries, G. H.: Eosinophilic gastroenteritis. Medicine, 49:299, 1970.

Taylor, K. B., and Truelove, S. C.: Immunological reactions in gastrointestinal disease: A review. Gut, 3:277, 1962.

Waldmann, T. A., Wochner, R. D., Laster, L., and Gordon, R. S.: Allergic gastroenteropathy. N. Engl. J. Med., 276:761, 1967.

639. DIVERTICULA OF THE INTESTINAL TRACT

Saccular outpouchings of the wall of the gut occur at all levels from the hypopharynx to the sigmoid colon and are known collectively as *diverticula.* With the single exception of Meckel's diverticulum, all appear to be acquired herniations of mucosa and submucosa through defects in the muscular layers, often clearly the result of excessive intraluminal pressure (pulsion diverticulum) and sometimes with clear-cut evidence of disordered or incoordinate motor activity in the adjacent bowel.

ESOPHAGEAL DIVERTICULA

Most diverticula of the esophagus occur at one of three locations, and at each of these the lesion has distinctive features.

Hypopharyngeal (or Zenker's) diverticulum is an evagination of the mucosa and submucosa directed posteriorly between the lower margin of the inferior constrictor muscle of the pharynx and the upper border of the cricopharyngeus muscle. It is considered a *pulsion* diverticulum, resulting from sharply localized increase in pressure at this point, when swallowing occurs without perfectly coordinated relaxation of the pharyngoesophageal sphincter. It is usually seen in men over 50 years of age, and enlarges progressively downward to the left of the cervical spine, eventually displacing and compressing the upper esophagus. Symptoms include dysphagia for both liquids and solids; regurgitation with aspiration of food and coughing, chiefly at night; and, ultimately, loss of weight. The sac may sometimes be felt as a mass in the left side of the neck, but is usually first identified on a lateral roentgenogram of the barium-filled pharynx and upper esophagus. Small diverticula usually require no treatment; when dysphagia and weight loss have been severe, the patient should be repleted by tube feeding and the diverticulum surgically resected in one stage, with myotomy of the pharyngoesophageal sphincter.

The *midesophageal* diverticulum is usually located at the level of the bifurcation of the trachea, and extends anteriorly and laterally from the esophagus; its orifice is wide. Its formation is often attributed to the contraction of adherent inflammatory tissue (usually tuberculous lymph nodes), but disordered esophageal motility may also be present. It usually causes no symptoms, and is recognized by its roentgenographic appearance.

The *epiphrenic* diverticulum, rarest of the three, is located a few centimeters above the vestibule and is thought to result from the high pressures of incoordinate contractions in achalasia, diffuse esophageal spasm, or reflux esophagitis. The symptoms and indicated management are usually pertinent to these associated conditions.

GASTRIC DIVERTICULA

Diverticula of the stomach are rare, and are chiefly of two types. The *juxtacardiac* diverticulum, accounting for three fourths of all cases, is found 2 cm below the cardia on the posterior wall of the stomach. Unassociated with any other gastric disease, it is usually asymptomatic but has been incriminated as a cause of recurrent epigastric pain and, rarely, of hemorrhage or perforation. Its identity can be verified on barium x-rays or on gastroscopy by its characteristic location and pliable wall. The *juxtapyloric* diverticulum, accounting for most of the remainder of cases, is the result of pressures resulting from ulceration, inflammation, surgical reconstruction, and the healing of these processes. Differentiation from active ulcer or carcinoma may require gastroscopy, biopsy, and cytologic examination of the gastric contents.

DIVERTICULA OF THE SMALL BOWEL

Diverticula of the small bowel are relatively common, especially in the elderly. Their frequency decreases from the pylorus to the ileocecal junction. Diverticula of the duodenum have been reported in 2 to 22 per cent of unselected cases at autopsy. In most instances they are found on the lesser curvature of the duodenum and the mesenteric border of the jejunum, at the sites of defects in the muscular wall through which major blood vessels (or the common bile duct) penetrate. In the duodenum they more often number but one or a few, whereas in the jejunum they are commonly multiple. Heterotopic gastric or pancreatic tissue is sometimes recognized in their walls. They are usually found as an unexpected and clinically silent abnormality on barium roentgenographic studies. In a minority of patients with duodenal diverticula, abdominal pain, nausea, vomiting, and weight loss may occur without any other explanation. In a few, hemorrhage, obstructive jaundice, perforation, and peritonitis may be seen. The same complications may rarely be observed in jejunal diverticula, wherein bowel obstruction is sometimes due to inflammatory stricture or muscular thickening. Of particular interest is the association of a form of malabsorption syndrome (a variant of the "blind loop syndrome") with jejunal diverticula, in which stasis of intestinal contents has permitted massive bacterial overgrowth (see Part XIV, Section Three). Otherwise, in the absence of complications, no treatment is required; in severely symptomatic cases, surgical resection is warranted.

Meckel's diverticulum is a common developmental anomaly of the ileum, found in 0.3 to 2.0 per cent of the population, and represents the persistence of the stalk of the fetal yolk sac. It may remain attached to the umbilicus by a fibrous cord or (very rarely) by a patent sinus, and is almost always found 2 to 3 feet above the ileocecal junction on the antimesenteric border. Its wall includes all the layers of the intestine, including the muscularis; its mucosa often contains islands of heterotopic gastric, pancreatic, or colonic glands. Although the majority of these pouches are clinically silent, symptoms may arise in a number of ways: (1) intestinal obstruction, with periumbilical cramps and vomiting, may be caused by intussusception or by volvulus around the fibrous attachment to the umbilicus; (2) impaction of intestinal content may lead to inflammation and ischemic necrosis, both pathologic and clinical features closely resembling those of acute appendicitis; and (3) peptic ulceration may result from the secretion of heterotopic gastric glands, including parietal cells, with resulting pain and often perforation or severe hemorrhage in the form of brick red or mahogany stools. In 60 per cent of instances these symptoms occur before the age of ten; hence this anomaly figures importantly in the differential diagnosis of abdominal pain, the acute abdomen, intestinal obstruction, intestinal bleeding, and peritonitis in childhood.

DIVERTICULAR DISEASE OF THE COLON
(Diverticulosis)

The presence of multiple herniations of the mucosa and submucosa of the colon through the circular muscle layer is commonly referred to as *diverticulosis*. This condition, recognizable during life only at laparotomy or on barium roentgenographic studies, probably affects 20 per cent of the American population over the age of 40 years. Although the majority of those harboring diverticula suffer no ill effects or only moderate discomfort, about 20 per cent may develop inflammatory complications (*diverticulitis*) (see Ch. 654). The entire spectrum of disorders associated with these pouches is connoted by the term *diverticular disease of the colon*. These diverticula are easily distinguished from the "wide-mouthed diverticula" of the colon seen in progressive systemic sclerosis (scleroderma).

Prevalence. Both diverticulosis and diverticulitis vary greatly in prevalence in different countries. In North America and northern Europe, the frequency is extremely high, as indicated above; it is approximately 40 times more common than in certain native, nonwhite populations in developing tropical countries. The condition is exceedingly rare below the age of 35, and its prevalence rises steeply as age advances.

Morbid Anatomy and Pathogenesis. A typical diverticulum is a small pouch, the fundus of which measures 3 to 25 mm in diameter, lying beneath the serosa and connected by a narrow neck with the lumen of the colon. It passes through the muscularis at the points of penetration of blood vessels from serosa to submucosa; their close proximity to these vessels is probably a factor in the causation of major hemorrhage in otherwise uncomplicated diverticulosis. In some instances they appear uniformly distributed from cecum to sigmoid, in others virtually confined to the sigmoid and descending colon. Rarely, one or a few diverticula are found in the right colon alone; significantly the rectum, having an intact longitudinal muscle layer, is never involved. In many cases the wall of the distal colon is thrown into many thick, arcuate or concertina-like folds, each consisting of a double layer of thickened circular muscle (myochosis); the taeniae are conspicuously shortened. The diverticula appear at the apices of the small intervening haustra.

Their protrusion is attributed in part to the high intraluminal pressure observed in the affected segments of bowel. Further, the folding of the muscular wall converts the colon into a series of isolated chambers in which high pressures can be confined. In some instances, high pressure and myochosis have been apparently well developed before any significant formation of diverticula, and it is believed that the motility disturbance is the primary change, continuation of which brings about not only herniation of mucosa but also the impaction, vascular congestion, minor necrosis, and perforation which lead to diverticulitis and pericolonic abscess.

Etiology. The cause of the colonic hypermotility is unknown. Such a change is believed to occur in patients with the "irritable colon," and some clinical studies suggest that diverticular disease may be a sequela of that disorder. There appears to be a motor incoordination of the affected segments of bowel, but the neural basis for this has not been recognized by morphologic or physiologic means. The great international variations in prevalence are compatible with the hypothesis that diets high in content of vegetable fiber retard development of diverticula; this is confirmed by dietary experiments on diverticulosis in aged laboratory animals.

Clinical Features. Most commonly, patients experience one or several attacks of griping *pain* in the left lower quadrant or the hypogastrium, lasting one to ten days, with exacerbation after eating. The sigmoid colon in such instances may be felt as a distinct, firm, tender mass. Unless true diverticulitis has developed, rebound tenderness, abdominal rigidity, fever, and leukocytosis are absent. In the intervals between attacks, moderate to severe constipation and a sense of abdominal fullness, relieved by passage of flatus, are commonly reported. Brief episodes of moderate or profuse *rectal bleeding* are not infrequently observed in patients with diverticular disease in the absence of inflammation. These usually cease spontaneously. Chronic low-grade blood loss more commonly arises from areas of diverticulitis, or from some unrelated lesion such as carcinoma or Crohn's disease.

The *diagnosis* of diverticular disease depends chiefly upon the barium enema, although the pockets are readily shown after barium by mouth. The deeply folded wall of the distal colon itself gives rise to the "sawtooth" pattern of the barium outline, and hence this does not constitute evidence for diverticulitis. In view of the high prevalence of diverticula in aged persons, caution must be exercised in attributing rectal bleeding to this source, lest a carcinoma or other more dangerous lesion go undetected.

The *treatment* of early symptomatic diverticular disease is essentially that of the irritable colon with mild constipation. A diet high in fruit and vegetable fiber is recommended, supplied in part by unprocessed bran, 2 teaspoonfuls three times a day with meals, increasing the dose as tolerated. This may be supplemented by the use of hydrophilic colloids, such as agar, psyllium seed, or methylcellulose. Relief of pain may be obtained with anticholinergics, such as propantheline, 15 mg four times daily, or with meperidine, 50 to 100 mg; but opiates are contraindicated because they dangerously elevate intracolonic pressures. Antimicrobial drugs should be reserved for clear-cut cases of diverticulitis.

Patients with demonstrated myochosis of the sigmoid whose painful episodes recur despite vigorous medical therapy may require surgical relief, either by resection of the most affected portion of the colon or by sigmoid myotomy. Both procedures are effective in two thirds or more of the cases.

Almy, T. P.: Diverticular disease of the colon: The new look. Gastroenterology, 49:109, 1965.

Cross, F. S.: Esophageal diverticula: Related neuromuscular problems. Ann. Otol. Rhinol. Laryngol., 77:914, 1968.

Ellis, F. H., Schlegel, J. F., Lynch, V. P., and Payne, W. S.: Cricopharyngeal myotomy for pharyngo-esophageal diverticulum. Ann. Surg., 170:340, 1969.

Horner, J. L.: Natural history of diverticulosis of the colon. Am. J. Dig. Dis., 3:343, 1958.

Nobles, E. R.: Jejunal diverticula. Arch. Surg., 102:172, 1971.

Noer, R. J.: Hemorrhage as a complication of diverticulitis. Ann. Surg., 141:674, 1955.

Painter, N. S., Almeida, A. Z., and Colebourne, K. W.: Unprocessed bran in treatment of diverticular disease of the colon. Br. Med. J., 1:137, 1972.

Reilly, M.: Sigmoid myotomy. Br. J. Surg., 53:859, 1966.

Section Two. PEPTIC ULCER

640. PATHOGENESIS AND PATHOPHYSIOLOGY

Morton I. Grossman

Definition. Peptic ulcer is a sharply circumscribed loss of the tissue lining those parts of the digestive tract exposed to gastric juice containing acid and pepsin. These consist of the lower esophagus, the stomach, the upper intestine (usually only the first part of the duodenum), the small intestine adjacent to a surgically produced connection with the stomach, and those Meckel's diverticula that contain functioning gastric glands.

Pathology. *Acute Lesions.* Acute lesions must be clearly distinguished from chronic ulcers because they are different diseases. Acute lesions are almost always multiple and they are superficial, rarely extending through the muscularis mucosae. Lesions that do not extend through the muscularis mucosae are called erosions, whereas those that do extend through this layer are called ulcers. Thus multiple acute lesions are mainly erosions, but chronic lesions are always ulcers (see accompanying figure).

Chronic Ulcers. When the unqualified term ulcer is used, chronic ulcer is meant. In contrast to acute lesions, chronic ulcers are usually single (figure). About 4 per cent of patients with gastric ulcer and about 20 per cent of patients with duodenal ulcer have two ulcers at the same time. About 40 per cent of patients with gastric ulcer have evidence of past or present duodenal ulcer.

The margins of chronic ulcers are thickened, rounded, and overhanging because of the excavation beneath them. Askanazy was the first to describe the four histologic zones of the ulcer floor: a surface layer of fibrin and pus, a narrow zone of fibrinoid necrosis, a zone of granulation tissue, and a cicatricial or fibrous zone. Chronic ulcers usually destroy the entire muscular coat. During healing a single layer of epithelial cells covers the granulation tissue of the crater floor and then differentiates toward normal mucosa. There is no regeneration of muscle; a permanent scar in the muscular coat marks the site of a healed ulcer.

Gastritis. Chronic gastritis is present in the stomach of almost all patients with chronic gastric or duodenal ulcer. The proximal 80 per cent of the stomach has acid-secreting oxyntic glands; the distal 20 per cent has pyloric glands that produce gastrin but no acid. In patients with duodenal ulcer the gastritis is limited to the pyloric gland area and is mild, seldom showing intestinal metaplasia. In patients with gastric ulcer the extent of the gastritis is correlated with the location of the ulcer. With ulcers near the pylorus the gastritis is usually confined to the pyloric gland area. Most gastric ulcers are located in pyloric gland mucosa at or near the boundary between pyloric and oxyntic glands. The higher the ulcer is located in the stomach, the larger is the extent of the pyloric glands, the more severe is the gastritis, and the more it extends into oxyntic mucosa. The severity and extent of the gastritis do not change with healing of the ulcer. Histologically, chronic atrophic gastritis accompanying gastric ulcer is indistinguishable from the sporadic form common with advancing age but differs from the form associated with pernicious anemia; in the latter the antrum is spared, and antibodies to parietal cells and to intrinsic factor are often present.

Intestinal metaplasia is a common feature of the gastritis associated with gastric ulcer. The converse heterotopia, gastric mucosa in the duodenum, is equally common in patients with duodenal ulcer. In both instances the incidence is related to acid secretion: the higher the level of acid secretion, the greater the incidence of gastric heterotopia in the duodenum; the lower the level of acid secretion, the greater the incidence of intestinal heterotopia in the stomach.

Pathogenesis. Acid and pepsin are required for ulcer formation. Ulcers occur when there is an imbalance between acid-pepsin and mucosal resistance. Increased acid-pepsin secretion, decreased mucosal resistance, or the two acting together are ulcerogenic.

Epidemiology. Peptic ulcer is a common disease, but there is much variation in frequency of occurrence from time to time and from place to place. In male Massachusetts physicians the lifetime prevalence of duodenal ulcer was 7.7 per cent and of gastric ulcer 0.9 per cent. The incidence rates peaked at 3.7 per thousand per year at age 55 to 64 for duodenal ulcer and at 1.4 per thousand per year at age 65 to 74 for gastric ulcer.

Based on the numbers of patients who went to physicians, the ratio of duodenal to gastric ulcers in one study was about 4 to 1 in men and 2 to 1 in women. The ratio of men to women was about 2 to 1 for gastric ulcers and 4 to 1 for duodenal ulcers.

The prevalence of peptic ulcer at autopsy is considerably higher than in clinical studies, probably because many ulcers never cause enough symptoms to lead to diagnosis. In an autopsy series from Leeds, England, the peak prevalence of ulcers plus scars was at ages 46 to 65

Enlarged gastric rugal folds, along with increased gastric secretions, have produced a mottled appearance of the barium in the stomach. Two duodenal ulcers are present (open arrows). Thickened mucosal folds are present in the second portion of the duodenum and in the jejunum. The patient had the Zollinger-Ellison syndrome. (From Goldberg, H. I., *In* Sleisenger, M. H., and Fordtran, J. S. [eds.]: Gastrointestinal Disease. Philadelphia, W. B. Saunders Company, 1973.)

with rates of 27 per cent in men and 15 per cent in women.

In almost all parts of the world morbidity from duodenal ulcer is reported as more common than from gastric ulcer, but deaths from gastric ulcer equal or exceed those from duodenal ulcer. In a few populations, for unknown reasons, gastric ulcer has been reported to be more frequent than duodenal ulcer; examples are fishermen of a village in Norway and Indian miners high in the Peruvian Andes. Mortality rates for gastric ulcer (in number per 100,000 deaths) range from 30 in Japan to 3 in Israel, and for duodenal ulcer from 10 in Scotland to 0.5 in France. Mortality, prevalence, and incidence of new cases all show a higher rate in town than in country. However, high rates have also been reported from areas that are not industrialized such as South India, Assam, South Nigeria, and Uganda.

Duodenal ulcer was a rare disease before 1900. By 1914 it had become common in Europe and North America. The sharp rise in duodenal ulcer was accompanied by a modest increase in gastric ulcer. From 1914 to about 1955 they remained at a relatively constant level and then began to decrease and are still decreasing. Cohort analysis, following all persons born in the same year, shows that death rates steadily increased for cohorts born up to the year 1890, whereas death rates for cohorts born after 1890 steadily decreased.

Environmental Factors. Of the many environmental factors that have been suspected as possible contributing causes of peptic ulcer, the only one that has been adequately studied is smoking. It is clear from all studies on this subject that smokers have more ulcers, both gastric and duodenal, and higher morbidity and mortality rates from their ulcers than nonsmokers. No relation between amount of smoking and ulcer incidence has been found; heavy smokers were not found to have more ulcers than light smokers. The nature of the relation between smoking and ulcer is not understood. Smoking neither stimulates nor inhibits gastric acid secretion but does inhibit pancreatic bicarbonate secretion, and some have suggested that this is related to its ulcerogenic action.

Although a role of diet in ulcer causation is often hypothesized, there is as yet no direct evidence to incriminate either particular diets or elements of diets such as hot spices.

Duodenal ulcer is equally common among all social classes, but ulcer of the body of the stomach is primarily a disease of the poorer economic grades. Despite the persistent myth of the hard-driving executive's proneness to ulcer, occupational differences are in fact small.

Genetic Factors. Genetic factors contribute to both gastric and duodenal ulcer. Gastric and duodenal ulcers are inherited independently. Close relatives of gastric ulcer patients have three times the expected number of gastric ulcers, and close relatives of duodenal ulcer patients have three times the expected number of duodenal ulcers. Concordance for ulcer, that is presence of ulcer in the second twin if one twin has ulcer, is more common in monozygous than in dizygous twin pairs. There is strong evidence that the increased familial incidence of ulcer is due to genetic factors and not simply to a shared environment. For both gastric and duodenal ulcer, the mode of inheritance is polygenic. None of the genes associated with ulcer of the body of the stomach have yet been identified. Duodenal ulcers, alone or with gastric ulcers, and ulcers of the prepyloric part of the stomach show abnormal frequencies of two genes: ABO blood groups and secretor status of blood group substances. Persons with blood group O are 1.4 times as liable to have duodenal or prepyloric ulcer as those with groups A, B, or AB, and persons who are nonsecretors are 1.5 times as liable to these ulcers as those who are secretors. Group O nonsecretors are 2.5 times more liable than secretors of groups A, B, and AB. The excess of group O and nonsecretion is greater in patients with recurrent ulcers after operations than in unoperated patients. The basis for the association of duodenal ulcer with group O and nonsecretion is not yet known.

The group O and nonsecretion factors explain only a small part of the variation in ulcer occurrence. Probably the most important genetic factor in peptic ulcer is the inheritance of acid-peptic glandular mass and the capacity to secrete acid and pepsin that is linked to it; the mode of this inheritance is not yet known.

Psychosomatic Factors. Popular wisdom holds that ulcers are caused by "nerves." At least two notions are implied: (1) that persons who have certain psychic traits are prone to develop ulcers, and (2) that situations that produce psychic tension are likely to bring on ulcers. These are hypotheses awaiting definitive testing. Since it is well established that emotional factors can alter gastric function, it is plausible to hypothesize a role for these factors in ulcerogenesis.

The most complete formulation of the interaction of psychic with other factors is that of Mirsky, whose postulates can be paraphrased as follows. The capacity to secrete acid and pepsin, of which serum pepsinogen level is an index, is genetically determined. Persons genetically endowed with high capacity to secrete acid-pepsin also tend to have a psychic conflict between persistent infantile wishes to be loved and cared for and repudiation of these wishes by their adult sense of shame and pride. Persons who have this combined physiologic and psychic pattern (high acid-pepsin secretory capacity and conflict over dependency wishes) are predisposed to develop duodenal ulcer. Ulcer is most likely to develop when a social event or a series of such events causes an exacerbation of the basic psychic conflict. The mechanism by which the exacerbation of the conflict leads to ulcer is not known, but it probably is not through further increase in acid-pepsin secretion.

Ulcers Caused by Drugs. If all the drugs that cause ulcers when given in massive doses to animals were withdrawn from human use, the pharmacopeia would be noticeably thinner. The drugs that are strongly suspected of being ulcerogenic in man are salicylates, indomethacin, phenylbutazone, and glucocorticoids. Salicylates and indomethacin applied topically break the mucosal barrier to hydrogen ions. This cannot be the sole mechanism by which they produce ulcer in lower animals, however, because they are also ulcerogenic by the parenteral route and do not break the barrier when so given. The mechanism of ulcerogenesis by these drugs is not understood; they do not stimulate acid secretion.

The only drug with a highly incriminating dossier for ulcerogenesis in man is aspirin. It is implicated in peptic disease in two ways. First, there is strong but not conclusive evidence that major bleeding episodes, probably mainly from acute diffuse hemorrhagic lesions, may be provoked by ingestion of aspirin. Second, there is mounting evidence that chronic ingestion of aspirin can cause gastric ulcer. Aspirin-induced gastric ulcers occur in stomachs that do not have the atrophic gastritis that is so characteristic of nonaspirin ulcers.

Peptic Lesions Caused by Stress. The acute diffuse lesions brought on by stress are pathologically and clinically distinct from chronic peptic ulcer. Many different kinds of stress can cause the lesions. Some prominent examples are sepsis, advanced carcinomatosis, shock, severe trauma, surgery, extensive burns (so-called Curling's ulcer), and acute respiratory insufficiency. One category of stress lesions deserves separate mention, namely, those associated with brain injury (so-called Cushing's ulcer). Any kind of acute brain injury, including surgical, traumatic, and cerebrovascular accidents, can cause the lesions. There is good evidence that hypersecretion of gastric acid and pepsin plays a role in stress lesions caused by brain injury, but hypersecretion has not been found in the other kinds of stress lesions. Although ischemia, breaking of the barrier to hydrogen ions, and mucus deficiency have been invoked in the pathogenesis of stress lesions, these are speculations without convincing supporting evidence. Hemorrhage is the main clinical manifestation of stress lesions; perforation occurs occasionally; pain is rare. Stress-related acute gastric lesions are a common life-threatening disease about which little is known.

Association with Other Diseases. The impression that two diseases appear together more frequently or less frequently than would be expected by chance must always be viewed skeptically, because it is easy to draw false conclusions about such associations from studies of nonrandom samples of broader populations. Duodenal ulcer is thought to be more common in patients with chronic obstructive lung disease, hepatic cirrhosis (especially after portacaval shunt), and gastric ulcer in those with rheumatoid arthritis. The evidence for these associations is contradictory, and in no instance is the mechanism for the possible association fully understood. In hepatic cirrhosis hypersecretion caused by a stimulant arising in intestinal mucosa and rendered more effective by bypassing the liver is postulated. In rheumatoid arthritis the ulcerogenic actions of the drugs used for treatment may well be involved.

Patients with hyperparathyroidism have a high incidence of duodenal ulcer. At least a part of this association is due to the occurrence of both parathyroid tumor and gastrinoma in some patients with multiple endocrine adenoma. Since the diagnosis of gastrinoma may not always be obvious, the question of whether patients with hyperparathyroidism without gastrinoma also have an increased incidence of duodenal ulcer must be regarded as unanswered.

Pathophysiology. *Mucosal Resistance.* Since most gastric ulcers and many duodenal ulcers occur in patients who do not have increased gastric secretion, a decrease in resistance of the mucosa to acid-peptic injury is presumably involved. Unfortunately, the factors that determine mucosal resistance have not yet been clearly identified. Some suggested contributory factors include mucosal blood flow, regeneration of epithelium, secretion of mucus, and integrity of the barrier to back-diffusion of hydrogen ions.

Gastric mucosa, like all tissue, requires adequate blood supply to remain intact. Reliable methods for measuring mucosal blood flow in patients with ulcer have not yet been devised. Although impaired blood supply is a theoretical possibility as a contributor to ulcerogenesis, there are no clues suggesting that it is so implicated. This same statement can be made for most factors that have been suggested as being involved in ulcerogenesis.

The epithelium of the entire gastrointestinal tract is rapidly replaced. It is estimated that the surface cells of the human stomach are replaced every four to six days. Good methods for measuring mucosal regeneration rate in man are available, but these have not yet been applied to the study of patients with peptic ulcer. Patients with atrophic gastritis have an increased rate of cell shedding from the gastric surface as measured by the rate of appearance of DNA in gastric washings; this also applies to the atrophic gastritis associated with gastric ulcer.

The notion that mucus somehow protects the mucosa against damage by acid-pepsin is very old and is still widely held, but there is no known biologic or physicochemical basis for such an action. Some sulfated mucosubstances inhibit peptic activity, but these do not occur in human gastric juice or gastric mucosa. The interstices of a gel of mucus are too large to offer significant resistance to diffusion of hydrogen ions or pepsin. The methods presently available have not shown any defects in secretion of mucus in patients with ulcer.

Back-Diffusion. Acid secreted into the gastric lumen diffuses back into the mucosa very slowly provided that the mucosa is normal; the leakback rate is only a few per cent of the maximal rate of acid secretion. This is spoken of as a "barrier" to back-diffusion. A variety of chemical agents, some arising in the body, others ingested, can break this barrier and allow markedly increased rates of back-diffusion of acid. Bile acids are endogenous barrier breakers. Exogenous barrier breakers that are likely to enter the human stomach include alcohol, salicylates, and oxethazaine. To break the barrier the chemical must enter the mucosa. If the agent is ionizable, it must be in its un-ionized lipid-soluble form to enter the mucosa; for example, aspirin must be in acid solution. Manifestations of a broken barrier include decrease in the electrical potential difference across the gastric mucosa and increased bidirectional permeability to sodium with increased accumulation of sodium in the gastric lumen. As acid diffuses through the broken barrier, it causes additional damage manifested by leakage of interstitial fluid and plasma into the gastric lumen and bleeding.

The locus of the barrier to back-diffusion of hydrogen ions is not known. Because Hollander used the term "mucous barrier" and Davenport used the term "mucosal barrier to hydrogen ions," it is commonly assumed that these two are the same barriers. There is no evidence that mucus has anything to do with the barrier to hydrogen ions.

Gastric Acid Secretion. CAPACITY TO SECRETE ACID. The capacity to secrete acid is determined mainly by the number of parietal cells in the gastric mucosa, and this is mainly genetically determined. The capacity to secrete acid can be estimated by measuring the response to a high dose (such that a higher dose would not give a greater response) of a stimulant such as gastrin, pentagastrin, histamine, or betazole, which all give about the same highest attainable response.

Secretory capacity is less in women than in men, a difference partially accounted for by difference in body size. Secretory capacity declines with age, presumably because of increasing incidence of gastritis that destroys acid-secreting cells. These sex and age differences are seen in patients with ulcer as well as in control subjects.

GASTRIC ACID SECRETION IN PATIENTS WITH ULCER.

Normal adults have on average about one billion parietal cells and can secrete about 22 mEq of acid per hour. The corresponding values for duodenal ulcer are 1.9 billion and 42 mEq and for gastric ulcer 0.8 billion and 18 mEq. The variations around the means are very large, so there is much overlap between these groups. However, on average, patients with chronic duodenal ulcer secrete more acid than normal subjects both at rest and in response to stimuli. At all times, day and night, in the fasted and fed states, the acidity of the gastric contents and of the first 5 to 10 cm of duodenum is greater than normal.

REGULATION OF GASTRIC SECRETION IN MAN. Two substances activate the parietal cell to secrete acid: the hormone *gastrin* which reaches the parietal cell by way of the blood, and the neurohumor *acetylcholine* which is released at the parietal cell by the postganglionic endings of the vagus nerves.

Gastrins: Scattered among the mucous cells of the pyloric glands are specialized cells, the G-cells, that produce gastrin and store it in granules.

Gastrin occurs in several molecular sizes. Gastrins with chain lengths of 13, 17, and 34 amino acid residues, designated G13, G17, and G34, have been isolated and chemically identified by Gregory. Each of these occurs in sulfated and nonsulfated forms. Pentagastrin, β-Ala-Trp-Met-Asp-Phe-NH$_2$, a synthetic peptide that contains the last four amino acids of gastrin, is widely used as a stimulant for gastric acid secretion in diagnostic testing.

In antral mucosa the predominant form of gastrin is G17, whereas in blood plasma after eating the most abundant form is G34. The greater abundance of G34 in plasma can be accounted for at least in part by its slower removal; the half-time of G34 is longer than that of G17. A higher blood level of G34 than of G17 is needed to give equal rates of acid secretion.

The richest source of gastrin is antral mucosa. The concentration of gastrin in the mucosa of the upper half of the duodenum is about half that in antral mucosa, and much lower concentrations are found in more distal intestine.

The concentration of gastrin in antral mucosa as measured by bioassay is normal in patients with duodenal ulcer and decreased in patients with gastric ulcer. In patients with duodenal ulcer serum gastrin concentration is normal in the fasting state and greater than normal after feeding.

Patients with gastric ulcer tend to have elevated concentrations of fasting serum gastrin. The increased blood gastrin level is correlated with decreased acid secretion. Dragstedt hypothesized that gastric stasis stimulated gastrin release that in turn caused hypersecretion leading to gastric ulcer. Since the elevated serum gastrin levels seen in some patients with gastric ulcer are associated with decreased acid secretion, Dragstedt's hypothesis is not supported.

All kinds of vagotomy (truncal, selective, proximal gastric) cause an increase in serum gastrin, both fasting and after feeding. Antrectomy causes a modest decrease in fasting serum gastrin level. The serum gastrin response to feeding is absent after Billroth II reconstruction and near normal after Billroth I, indicating that duodenal gastrin is releasable by feeding.

Until the distribution of the various molecular forms of gastrin has been studied in the serum of normal subjects and of patients with duodenal ulcer and gastric ulcer, no definitive conclusions can be drawn about correlation between gastrin and acid secretion and about differences between normal subjects and ulcer patients.

Acetylcholine: Cholinergic nerves supply both parietal cells and antral G cells. These cholinergic nerves are activated both by vagal impulses and by so-called short reflexes that are completed within the wall of the stomach. Vagal activation occurs as a result of stimuli acting in the head (the cephalic phase) and in the stomach (the gastric phase). Cephalic stimuli include chewing, tasting, and swallowing food (as in sham feeding), the sight, smell, or thought of food (conditioned reflex), hypoglycemia induced by insulin, and interference with glucose utilization by nonmetabolizable sugars such as 2-deoxyglucose. Gastric stimuli include distention of the stomach and the action of chemical agents, particularly partially digested protein, on the gastric mucosa. The gastric stimuli initiate both long vagovagal reflexes and short intramural reflexes; the long reflexes are more effective. All these mechanisms, cephalic vagal, gastric long vagovagal reflexes, and gastric short intramural reflexes, activate cholinergic fibers to both parietal cells and gastrin cells. Atropine does not inhibit release of gastrin in response to a meal, so either the cholinergic mechanisms for gastrin release are atropine resistant or there are additional noncholinergic (perhaps nonneural) mechanisms that can fully substitute. Atropine blocks direct vagal stimulation of the oxyntic glands and markedly inhibits the response to gastrin.

The vagus nerve influences gastric secretion in at least three ways: (1) direct cholinergic stimulation of parietal cells, (2) release of gastrin, and (3) sensitizing the parietal cell to stimulation by gastrin and other stimulants. Vagotomy removes that part of the tonic cholinergic background that is vagally dependent and thereby desensitizes the parietal cell to stimulation by gastrin. After vagotomy the highest attainable response to gastrin is reduced and the dose of gastrin needed to get that reduced response is increased. The magnitude and sensitivity of the response to gastrin can be restored to prevagotomy levels by giving a background of a cholinomimetic drug to replace vagal tone. *Thus vagotomy does not reduce the capacity of the stomach to secrete acid but takes away one of the stimulants required to fully activate that capacity.* Antrectomy, removal of the major source of gastrin, reduces the response to vagal stimulation and to other stimulants such as gastrin and histamine. The response cannot be restored to the preantrectomy level by giving a background of gastrin; the mechanism by which antrectomy reduces the capacity to secrete acid is not understood. Antrectomy and vagotomy have additive effects. For example, the highest attainable response to histamine is about 40 per cent of the preoperative level with vagotomy alone, about 50 per cent with antrectomy alone, and about 20 per cent with the two together.

Other factors: Partially digested protein bathing the intestinal mucosa stimulates gastric acid secretion, the intestinal phase. A part of this effect is mediated by antral-type gastrin that is mainly in the first part of the duodenum. Other unidentified humoral agents from the duodenum and jejunum are probably also involved.

Three mechanisms for inhibition of gastric acid secretion are recognized. The first is inhibition of gastrin release by acid bathing the antral mucosa. When antral pH is 1.5 or lower, all forms of gastrin release are almost totally suppressed. The other two inhibitory mechanisms operate from the intestine in response to acid and to fat. Secretin is one inhibitor of acid secretion released by acid, but it is likely that other unidentified hormones and nervous mechanisms are also involved. Fat inhibits acid secretion regardless of the stimulus. The cholecystokinin released by fat inhibits gastrin-stimulated secretion, but other unidentified inhibitors, enterogastrones, are also involved. Secretin and cholecystokinin are weak inhibitors of acid secretion, so they are unlikely to contribute significantly to regulation of acid secretion.

Caffeine and theophylline stimulate gastric acid secretion, an action that may be secondary to inhibition of breakdown of cyclic AMP.

POSTULATED ABNORMALITIES IN ULCER PATIENTS. The increased average rate of secretion in patients with duodenal ulcer could be due to one or more of these factors: (1) increased capacity to secrete, (2) increased responsiveness of acid-secreting cells, (3) increased drive to acid secretion, and (4) decreased inhibition of secretion. These factors are not entirely independent. For example, gastrin not only drives secretion but also stimulates growth of mucosa. Acetylcholine drives secretion and sensitizes to other stimuli; whether it also stimulates growth of mucosa is not known. Of these factors, increased capacity to secrete is the one most clearly involved in the hypersecretion seen in duodenal ulcer. Increased capacity to secrete acid is present long before the duodenal ulcer appears and stays relatively constant during exacerbations and remissions. There is some evidence that increased sensitivity to stimulation is also present, but this cannot be considered as fully established. There is also some evidence for increased drive in the form of greater than normal increments in serum gastrin after feeding, but the relative importance of this factor is not yet clear. Defective inhibitory mechanisms may contribute to hypersecretion. For example, acidification of a test meal causes less suppression of gastrin release and of acid secretion in duodenal ulcer patients than in controls.

Basal acid secretion rate divided by maximal rate can be used as an index of basal "drive." In both duodenal ulcer patients and controls, this fraction increases as basal rate increases, indicating that some unidentified factor other than maximal capacity is a major determinant of high basal rates.

A popular notion holds that the hypersecretion of duodenal ulcer is caused by excessive vagal activity. The only evidence in support of this idea is that the hypersecretion is eliminated by vagotomy. However, since vagotomy decreases the response to all forms of stimulation, the decrease in secretion that follows vagotomy cannot be accepted as proof that vagal overactivity caused the hypersecretion. There is no satisfactory method for measuring vagal "tone."

Impaired release of secretin or impaired capacity of the pancreas to secrete bicarbonate could contribute to the increased duodenal acidity seen in patients with duodenal ulcer. However, there is no convincing evidence for impaired secretin release, and capacity to secrete bicarbonate is actually increased, proportionately to the increased capacity to secrete acid.

In gastric ulcer associated with duodenal ulcer, the secretory pattern tends to be like that of duodenal ulcer. The higher in the stomach the gastric ulcer is located, the lower the secretory capacity; ulcers near the pylorus give secretory patterns like duodenal ulcer, whereas those near the cardia show marked hyposecretion. The decrease in acid secretion in gastric ulcer can be accounted for mainly by the associated gastritis that causes loss of parietal cells, but increased back-diffusion may also contribute.

Pepsins. Seven pepsinogens belonging to two immunochemical groups occur in human gastroduodenal mucosa. Group I pepsinogens are limited to mucous neck cells and zymogen cells of the oxyntic gland area, and Group II pepsinogens are present in these cells and also in the mucous cells of pyloric glands and Brunner's glands. Group I and II pepsinogens are present in blood plasma, but only Group I is found in normal urine.

There is a strong correlation between capacity to secrete acid and capacity to secrete pepsin and also between capacity to secrete acid and pepsin and concentration of pepsinogen in blood. Determination by radioimmunoassay of the concentration of Group I pepsinogens in blood serum is a convenient and accurate method of assessing the secretory capacity for acid and pepsin.

The major stimulants for acid secretion, gastrin and acetylcholine, are also the major regulators of pepsin secretion. The ratio of pepsin to acid is higher in cholinergically stimulated gastric juice (e.g., insulin hypoglycemia) than in that evoked by gastrin. The increase in gastric secretion in patients with duodenal ulcer and the decrease in patients with gastric ulcer involve both acid and pepsin.

Duodenogastric Reflux. Du Plessis (1965) hypothesized that reflux of bile from the duodenum into the stomach may be an important factor in the pathogenesis of gastric ulcer. Patients with gastric ulcer do reflux duodenal contents into the stomach more often and in larger amounts than controls, both in the fasting and fed states, but the overlap between controls and gastric ulcer patients is great. Over the short term this reflux leads to breaking of the gastric barrier to back-diffusion of hydrogen ion, and over the long term it is presumed to lead to gastric atrophy, factors that may make the mucosa less resistant to ulceration. Further studies are needed to assess fully the role of this factor.

Gastric Emptying. Since the stomach shows an exponential pattern of emptying, rate of emptying can best be expressed as a half-time. The half-time for gastric emptying shows wide variation in both ulcer patients and control subjects. There is a tendency for rapid emptying of a mixed meal in patients with duodenal ulcer, but the overlap with normal subjects is great. Some patients with duodenal ulcer or with gastric ulcer have markedly impaired gastric emptying. In most instances this impairment of emptying cannot be accounted for by anatomic narrowing of the gastric outlet, and its pathogenesis is not well understood.

641. DIAGNOSTIC STUDIES AND MEDICAL TREATMENT

Jon I. Isenberg

DIAGNOSTIC STUDIES

Radiography. Radiography is at present the most commonly used technique in the diagnosis of peptic ulcer disease. Ulcers may rarely be visualized on standard abdominal radiograms if air is trapped in the crater.

Barium sulfate suspension is usually used as the radiopaque contrast material for routine gastrointestinal radiography. An absorbable water-soluble contrast agent is used in patients with suspected perforated ulcers. Air contrast films help to define clearly the mucosal pattern of the upper gastrointestinal tract. Delayed films, taken about one hour after ingestion of barium, may demonstrate a collection of barium within an ulcer which was not seen on the initial fluoroscopic examination.

For certainty of diagnosis, the ulcer niche should be seen on more than one x-ray film. When an ulcer is viewed in profile, the niche appears as a collection of contrast material which extends beyond the confines of the gut wall. When the ulcer niche is seen en face, it appears as a puddle of barium, often surrounded by a halo and/or radiating folds to the ulcer. The halo is due to mucosal and submucosal edema surrounding the ulcer.

Ulcers of the esophagus usually occur within the lower half (Fig. 1). Ulcer and diverticulum of the esophagus may have similar radiographic appearances. Esophagoscopy (see below) can distinguish one from the other. The presence of an esophageal ulcer, particularly with an accompanying esophageal stricture, should suggest the possibility that the lower esophagus is lined with columnar epithelium (Barrett's syndrome). Almost all ulcers of the esophagus are visualized on radiography.

The great majority of gastric ulcers (approximately 85 per cent) occur in pyloric gland mucosa at or near the junction with oxyntic gland mucosa. Approximately 85 per cent of gastric ulcers occur on the lesser curvature of the stomach. About 90 per cent of endoscopically visualized gastric ulcers are seen on upper gastrointestinal series.

Gastric ulcers vary in diameter from less than 1 cm to

Figure 2. A benign ulcer of the lesser curvature is surrounded by an ulcer collar—the broad lucent band resulting from edema at the ulcer orifice. Gastric mucosal folds radiate from this mass of edema. (From Goldberg, H. I., *In* Sleisenger, M. H., and Fordtran, J. S. [eds.]: Gastrointestinal Disease. Philadelphia, W. B. Saunders Company, 1973.)

Figure 1. B. H., a 44-year-old housewife with intermittent dysphagia for four years and burning midepigastric pain, recurring after meals and during the night, for eight months. Esophagoscopy revealed chronic esophagitis with stricture; biopsies did not demonstrate neoplasia. The roentgenogram demonstrates an ulcer crater in the esophagus. Antacid therapy facilitated healing, and the dysphagia subsided.

greater than 10 cm. Nearly 80 per cent of gastric ulcers are less than 2 cm in widest diameter. When seen in profile, an apparent density surrounds the neck of the ulcer; this is due to an undermined margin of gastric mucosa which produces a narrow ring around part or all of the ulcer (Hampton's line), and often due to a thicker radiodense ulcer "collar" caused by edema and inflammation of the adjacent mucosa (Fig. 2). Although these radiographic changes tend to be more common with benign ulcers, they may rarely be seen in ulcerating gastric cancers.

Gastric ulcers may not be visualized because (1) the ulcer may be shallow and barium may not collect within it, (2) there may be mucus or blood within the ulcer crater, (3) the edematous margins around the ulcer may occlude the mouth of the ulcer, (4) the positions used may not throw it into profile, or (5) the patient may be too large or may be unable to permit adequate radiographic examination.

Approximately 4 per cent of all gastric ulcers seen on gastrointestinal radiograms are malignant. Radiographic features which tend to distinguish benign gastric ulcer from gastric cancer include the following: (1) most benign ulcers extend beyond the confines of the gastric wall, whereas gastric cancers tend to occur within the confines of the gastric wall; (2) benign ulcers tend to be round or ovoid, whereas cancers often are irregular in shape; (3) benign ulcers usually have a smooth base, whereas the base of a cancer may be nodular; (4) the gastric folds radiate to the lip of a benign ulcer, whereas there may be no radiating folds around a cancer, or the folds may be blunted and stop some distance from an ulcerating cancer; and (5) the stomach around a benign ulcer is usually pliable and has normal motility, whereas the wall around a cancer is rigid and has poor motility. Some ulcerating carcinomas may "heal" radiographically. Therefore other studies, such as endoscopy, biopsy, and cytology (see below), are needed to assist in distinguishing benign gastric ulcer from gastric cancer.

Benign gastric ulcers within the body of the stomach may produce infolding of the gastric wall opposite the ulcer. With healing of the ulcer, this cleft or incisura in the gastric contour may persist, producing an "hourglass stomach."

Most duodenal ulcers are located within the duodenal bulb (Fig. 3). However, ulcers may be located in the postbulbar area as well as the more distal duodenum and proximal jejunum. Approximately 85 per cent of endoscopically visualized duodenal ulcers (see below) are seen on upper gastrointestinal series (Fig. 4).

In the absence of a definite ulcer niche, radiographic findings which suggest duodenal ulcer disease include (1) spasm of the duodenal bulb; (2) eccentricity of the pyloric channel; (3) a persistent fold (i.e., incisura) extending across the duodenal bulb; (4) radiographic loss of the superior or inferior fornix of the duodenal bulb; (5) persistent spasm and/or fibrosis of the duodenal bulb, producing a "cloverleaf" deformity; and (6) distortion of the duodenal mucosa, suggesting edema, heterotopic gastric mucosa, or large duodenal folds. It is often difficult, if not impossible, to determine radiographically if there is an active ulcer in a scarred and deformed duodenal bulb. Giant duodenal ulcers (i.e., greater than 2 cm in diameter) may not be radiographically apparent, because they tend to simulate the normal superior or inferior fornix of the duodenal bulb (Fig. 5).

False-positive radiographic findings of duodenal ulcer may be due to ectopic pancreatic tissue with a minor pancreatic duct in the duodenal bulb, regional enteritis involving the duodenum, varicosities of the pancreaticoduodenal vein, carcinoma of the pancreas extending into the duodenum, and pancreatitis or cholecystitis producing inflammation of the adjacent duodenal mucosa.

Endoscopy. In the diagnosis of peptic ulcer disease, endoscopy is valuable in differentiating esophageal ulcer from diverticulum, in defining the bleeding site in upper gastrointestinal hemorrhage (see Ch. 644), in differentiating benign from malignant gastric ulcers, in differentiating recurrent ulcer from surgical deformity, and possibly in patients with x-ray-negative dyspepsia. In a scarred deformed duodenal bulb, duodenoscopy may demonstrate an ulcer not seen on radiographic study.

With the improved endoscopes, almost all ulcers of the esophagus and stomach are visualized, and approximately 85 per cent of radiographically demonstrated duodenal ulcers are seen. Conversely, about 10 to 15 per cent of duodenal ulcer craters seen endoscopically are not demonstrated radiographically. Mucosal lesions such as esophagitis, gastritis, and duodenitis are often not defined on radiographic study but can be diagnosed endoscopically, particularly with the addition of a directed endoscopic biopsy.

Endoscopically a benign gastric ulcer is usually round or ovoid and has a clear whitish base and a hyperemic border; the gastric folds radiate to the edge of the ulcer crater. Gastric cancers are often irregular in shape, have a necrotic hemorrhagic and nodular base, are surrounded by nodularity, and have clubbed folds radiating toward the cancer but stopping short of the ulcerated area. Multiple deep biopsies of the rim or direct brush cytology can often establish a histologic or cytologic diagnosis of cancer.

Secretory Studies. The following generalizations regarding both basal and stimulated acid secretion can

Figure 3. Edematous folds radiate from a pinpoint ulcer of the posterior duodenal wall (arrows). Compression of the duodenal bulb by the radiologist produced the best roentgenographic demonstration of this ulcer. (From Goldberg, H. I., *In* Sleisenger, M. H., and Fordtran, J. S. [eds.]: Gastrointestinal Disease. Philadelphia, W. B. Saunders Company, 1973.)

Figure 4. A small ulcer (arrow) has produced deformity of the duodenal bulb. Flattening of the superior surface of the bulb has resulted from edema and spasm. The superior and inferior recesses of the base of the bulb appear as diverticular outpouchings, so-called pseudodiverticula. (From Goldberg, H. I., *In* Sleisenger, M. H., and Fordtran, J. S. [eds.]: Gastrointestinal Disease. Philadelphia, W. B. Saunders Company, 1973.)

responses; that is, higher doses do not give higher responses.

Since ulcer disease does not occur in the absence of gastric acid—"no acid, no ulcer"—the finding of histamine-fast achlorhydria (i.e., all posthistamine determinations greater than 6) in a patient with radiographic evidence of gastric ulcer strongly suggests the diagnosis of gastric cancer. Unfortunately only about 20 per cent of patients with gastric cancer have histamine-fast achlorhydria. Thus for the differentiation of malignant from benign ulcer, achlorhydria is a highly *discriminative* test (a positive finding usually means cancer) but not a *sensitive* test (a positive finding is infrequent in patients with cancer).

Patients with duodenal ulcer disease tend to secrete more acid than control subjects in response to any stimulus. In about one third of male duodenal ulcer patients maximal acid output is greater than 42 mEq per hour, the upper limit of normal for control subjects. In addition, patients with duodenal ulcer almost always have a maximal acid output of at least 10 mEq per hour. If a lower rate is found, the diagnosis of duodenal ulcer disease becomes suspect. Maximal acid output of less than 10 mEq per hour is an insensitive criterion for absence of duodenal ulcer, because only about one sixth of normal subjects fall in this range.

There is evidence to suggest that duodenal ulcer patients with rates of stimulated acid secretion greater than approximately 45 mEq per hour may have a greater incidence of recurrent ulcer after vagotomy. No convinc-

be made: (1) patients with gastric ulcers of the body of the stomach tend to secrete subnormal amounts of acid; (2) patients with duodenal ulcer, prepyloric ulcer, or gastric plus duodenal ulcer tend to secrete more acid than normal subjects; and (3) patients with gastrin-secreting tumors of the pancreas (i.e., Zollinger-Ellison syndrome) tend to secrete more acid than most patients with duodenal ulcer. These generalizations refer to the "average patient." There is a great deal of overlap between groups.

Average basal gastric acid secretion in normal males and females is approximately 2.5 and 1.3 mEq per hour, respectively, but may range from 0 to 6 mEq per hour. Average basal secretion in patients with gastric ulcer is similar to normal, whereas average basal secretion for males and females with duodenal ulcer is approximately 5 and 3 mEq per hour, respectively. Some patients with duodenal ulcer disease may have no gastric acid at rest, whereas others may have greater than 10 mEq per hour. At rest only about one fourth of patients with duodenal ulcer secrete amounts of acid more than two standard deviations above the mean for normal subjects. Because of the wide overlap of basal secretion, it offers little assistance in the diagnosis of peptic ulcer disease. In most patients with gastrin-secreting tumors of the pancreas, basal secretion tends to be increased (i.e., greater than 10 mEq per hour in the intact stomach and greater than 5 mEq per hour in the postoperative stomach).

After subcutaneous injection of histamine acid phosphate (40 μg per kilogram), betazole (1.5 mg per kilogram), or pentagastrin (6 μg per kilogram), peak acid secretion is similar. These doses produce "maximal"

Figure 5. The arrows outline an oval-shaped, irregular barium collection at the site of the duodenal bulb. Serial roentgenograms demonstrated the same unchanging configuration. A giant duodenal ulcer occupied the entire bulb in the surgical abdomen. (From Goldberg, H. I., *In* Sleisenger, M. H., and Fordtran, J. S. [eds.]: Gastrointestinal Disease. Philadelphia, W. B. Saunders Company, 1973.)

ing correlation between degree of hypersecretion and severity of ulcer disease has been established in patients not operated on.

After vagal denervation of the stomach, insulin-induced hypoglycemia often fails to stimulate gastric acid secretion. The insulin test (0.2 U per kilogram intravenously) has been used to evaluate the effect of vagotomy on gastric acid secretion. If insulin-induced hypoglycemia produces an increase in gastric acid secretion after vagotomy, some vagal innervation to the stomach is assumed to persist but nonvagal mechanisms may also be involved. One year after vagotomy, approximately 50 per cent of patients have a secretory response to insulin. However, only about one of seven patients with an increase in acid secretion after insulin will develop recurrent ulcer disease. Therefore the vast majority of duodenal ulcer patients in whom vagotomy is performed do not develop ulcer recurrence regardless of whether they do or do not respond to insulin. There is a great deal of overlap in the insulin test responses in those with and without recurrence. The insulin test has so little predictive value as to which patients will develop recurrent ulcer that it is of limited practical clinical value.

MEDICAL THERAPY

The four goals of therapy of peptic ulcer disease are to relieve symptoms, to increase the rate of healing, to prevent complications, and to prevent recurrences. Unfortunately, in spite of the multitude of drugs used in the treatment of ulcer disease, there is a paucity of adequately controlled, prospective, double-blind trials in this common disease. The treatment of ulcer disease is therefore in large part empirical. Since the treatment of esophageal, gastric, and duodenal ulcer is similar, the following applies to all forms of acid-peptic disease except when stated otherwise.

Antacids. Antacids are widely used; approximately $110 million are spent on them each year. Surprisingly enough, there are no convincing data indicating that they improve healing, decrease recurrences, or decrease complications. In uncontrolled studies, antacids have been observed to relieve ulcer pain. However, in order to distinguish antacid effect from placebo effect in the therapy of ulcer disease, it is necessary that controlled double-blind prospective studies be conducted. Such clinical studies are currently in progress.

The rationale for the use of antacids in treating ulcer is as follows: (1) ulcer disease does not occur in the absence of gastric acid and pepsin; (2) peptic activity decreases markedly at pH greater than 3.5; (3) the incidence of experimental ulcers in animals can be decreased by antacids; and (4) ulcer disease usually resolves with surgical therapy which decreases gastric acid and pepsin secretion.

Most commercially available antacids consist of mixtures of magnesium, aluminum, or calcium salts. Factors that influence the in vivo efficacy of an antacid include the neutralizing capacity of the antacid, the rate of reaction with acid, the rate of gastric acid secretion, and the rate of gastric emptying.

Sodium Bicarbonate. Sodium bicarbonate is a potent, rapidly acting antacid. It is completely absorbed and so presents the body with a load of sodium and alkali. With normal renal function the body can tolerate the excess alkaline and sodium load. In patients with decreased renal function or salt retention, the alkaline and sodium load may lead to alkalosis and an increase in total body sodium and water. Because sodium bicarbonate is water soluble, it leaves the stomach rapidly, thus producing only transient intragastric alkalization, and therefore it is not used in the treatment of ulcer disease.

Calcium Carbonate. Calcium carbonate is a potent, rapidly acting antacid. In the duodenum most of the calcium is converted into poorly absorbed calcium carbonate, calcium phosphate, and calcium soaps. Less than 10 per cent of the calcium is absorbed from the gut. The advantages of calcium carbonate are that it is inexpensive and potent. Unfortunately calcium-containing antacids may cause hypersecretion or hypercalcemia. Oral calcium produces an increase in acid secretion in the fasting and fed state after a single or repeated dose, and in patients with and without ulcer disease. The increase in acid secretion is probably mediated in part by increased serum gastrin and occurs only after calcium-containing antacids, not with noncalcium antacids.

Repeated oral doses of calcium may produce an increase in serum calcium, phosphate, creatinine, and bicarbonate. Long-term ingestion of calcium carbonate plus sodium bicarbonate may result in the milk-alkali syndrome. This consists of an increase in serum calcium, blood urea nitrogen, serum creatinine, and serum phosphorus, plus systemic alkalosis. If recognized early in a patient with normal renal function, the milk-alkali syndrome may resolve on discontinuing calcium intake. If unrecognized, the milk-alkali syndrome may progress to renal calculi and permanent renal damage. Symptoms of the milk-alkali syndrome include anorexia, malaise, nausea, vomiting, weakness, muscle pain, polydipsia, and polyuria. The symptoms of milk-alkali syndrome are the same as those of hypercalcemia from other causes such as hyperparathyroidism, vitamin D intoxication or metastatic tumors.

Since there are many noncalcium antacids available which do not have the untoward effects of calcium but are effective antacids, some experts believe that calcium-containing antacids should not be used in the treatment of acid-peptic diseases.

Magnesium Hydroxide. Magnesium hydroxide is a potent antacid that reacts rapidly with hydrochloric acid. Magnesium trisilicate reacts with hydrochloric acid more slowly than magnesium hydroxide. Approximately 5 to 10 per cent of the ingested magnesium is absorbed from the gut and excreted by the kidneys. In patients with decreased renal function, serum magnesium level can increase and rarely may produce hypotension and respiratory arrest. Within the gut magnesium salts act as cathartics, so they can seldom be used as the sole antacid.

Aluminum Hydroxide. Aluminum hydroxide reacts with hydrochloric acid to form aluminum chloride. The neutralizing capacity of aluminum hydroxide preparations varies widely; some are ineffective antacids. In the gut aluminum hydroxide and aluminum chloride bind phosphate, producing nonabsorbable aluminum phosphate. Chronic ingestion of aluminum hydroxide can decrease serum and total body phosphate. It is therefore of therapeutic benefit in patients with chronic renal insufficiency and hyperphosphatemia. The adsorptive properties of aluminum hydroxide may decrease absorption of other drugs.

Fordtran found that in vitro buffering capacity correlated well with in vivo postprandial antacid activity. Patients with high levels of gastric acid secretion, "hypersecretors," tend to require larger amounts of antacid than low secretors to achieve a similar degree of neutralization. Because antacids rapidly leave the empty stomach, the effect of antacids in the fasting patient is transient, lasting about 10 to 20 minutes. However, when adequate amounts of antacids are administered one hour after a meal, their effect lasts up to three hours.

At present, antacids are the mainstay of therapy of acid-peptic disease, despite lack of carefully controlled prospective studies on their effect on rate of healing or recurrence rate. In the acutely ill symptomatic patient with ulcer disease, antacids should be given in doses of about 75 mEq (e.g., Maalox, 30 ml; Mylanta II, 18 ml) at hourly intervals during the day and evening, and about 150 mEq at bedtime. When symptoms resolve, antacids are given one and three hours after each meal and at bedtime. Hypersecretors should receive larger doses than those who are not. In patients with sodium retention or hypertension, low-sodium antacids should be given (e.g., Riopan).

Anticholinergic Drugs. Anticholinergics block the action of acetylcholine on postganglionic nerve sites. They are used in the treatment of ulcer to decrease acid and pepsin secretion. They also decrease salivary, bronchial, sweat, and pancreatic secretion and increase heart rate, produce mydriasis, decrease gastric and intestinal motility, and decrease urinary bladder tone and strength of contraction. There is no convincing evidence that any one anticholinergic has a selective action on a specific target.

Standard doses of anticholinergics (i.e., doses which produce dryness of the mouth) decrease basal and histamine or gastrin-stimulated gastric acid secretion by about 50 per cent. Because anticholinergics produce recognizable side effects in addition to decreasing gastric acid secretion, particularly dryness of the mouth, it is difficult to conduct double-blind studies comparing anticholinergic drugs with placebo. In gastric ulcer an anticholinergic (glycopyrronium) improved healing rate and decreased recurrence rate. Some studies suggest that anticholinergics are of value in duodenal ulcer for inducing pain relief and in prevention of recurrence. Other studies conclude that anticholinergics are of no therapeutic value in duodenal ulcer.

If anticholinergics are to be used in the therapy of ulcer disease, they should be prescribed in doses which produce a recognizable effect, such as dry mouth. They should not be used in patients in whom the anticholinergic effect may be harmful, as in patients with glaucoma, prostatism, gastroesophageal reflux, gastric retention, or chronic bronchitis. Anticholinergics probably have their greatest therapeutic effect in ulcer patients with nocturnal pain; a dose at bedtime may be effective in relieving nocturnal pain. Since the greatest amount of acid is secreted in response to a meal, anticholinergics are usually given about 30 minutes before eating.

Diet. Although bland diets have been used in the treatment of ulcer disease for the past 70 years, there is no evidence that a bland diet is more effective than a regular diet in ulcer healing, prevention of complications, or recurrence. During flare-ups of ulcer distress patients often restrict their diets to bland foods. There is no evidence that this reduces symptoms or shortens the attack.

In patients with ulcer disease, hourly milk and cream produced a lower intragastric pH than three regular meals. In addition, excessive milk and cream with antacid may be a factor in the pathogenesis of the milk-alkali syndrome and of atherosclerosis.

There is no evidence that spices in moderate amounts are ulcerogenic or alter the course of ulcer healing or frequency of recurrence. Also, the texture of the diet, soft versus rough, seems to be unimportant in ulcer pathogenesis or therapy. Since caffeine is a stimulant of acid secretion, caffeine-containing beverages (including cola drinks) should probably be excluded from the diet in ulcer patients. Alcohol, by its ability to damage mucosa, may be involved in the pathogenesis of erosions, and alcohol is therefore interdicted in the patient with ulcer disease.

In summary, at present there are no data to support altering the diet of patients with ulcer disease except to discontinue caffeine and alcohol, and to avoid substances which seem to produce symptoms. Also, bedtime snacks which will stimulate acid secretion while the patient is sleeping should be avoided. Food should not be used as an antacid, because the neutralization produced by food is always followed by increased secretion.

Hospitalization. In gastric ulcer hospitalization has been reported to increase the rate of ulcer healing when compared to outpatient management. The cost for prolonged hospitalization is often prohibitive, so it is recommended that patients with suspected or demonstrated gastric ulcer be hospitalized briefly to expedite careful evaluation of the ulcer by radiography, endoscopy with biopsy, and, if available, gastric cytology. Medical therapy can be initiated during hospitalization.

In hospitalized male veterans with gastric ulcer, the recurrence rate in two years was 60 per cent in those who healed slowly (less than 90 per cent in six weeks) and 40 per cent in those who healed more rapidly. Patients with large gastric ulcers, gastric ulcers plus duodenal ulcers, and black veterans tended to have a higher ulcer recurrence rate.

Serial radiograms of a gastric ulcer should be obtained at three- or four-week intervals for a maximum of 12 weeks. The ulcer should completely heal within this period. For those patients in whom the ulcer does not heal, surgery is indicated. Surgery is also recommended for the patient with second or third gastric ulcer recurrences.

The effect of hospitalization on duodenal ulcer has not been carefully studied.

Other Treatments. *Carbenoxolone Sodium.* Carbenoxolone sodium has been shown to increase healing in ambulatory patients with gastric ulcer to a rate comparable to that of inpatients. Carbenoxolone sodium increases the production and viscosity of gastric mucus, and also increases the life span of the gastric mucosal cells. These may be the mechanisms by which it increased gastric ulcer healing rate. Carbenoxolone sodium is structurally similar to aldosterone and therefore produces salt and water retention. The efficacy of carbenoxolone sodium can be maintained while avoiding salt retention with the administration of thiazide diuretics. Structurally similar aldosterone-blocking agents (e.g., aldactone) decrease the efficacy of carbenoxolone.

Sedation. Sedation has not been shown to be of value in the therapy of peptic ulcer disease. It is not recommended for routine use. Some physicians believe, however, that allaying anxiety in such patients may facilitate the recommended treatment program.

Estrogens. Estrogens have been demonstrated to be effective in increasing healing rate in duodenal ulcer,

1208

XIV. DISEASES OF THE DIGESTIVE SYSTEM

but not in gastric ulcer. Since they have untoward effects, particularly in males, they are not recommended.

Interdiction of Smoking. Discontinuing smoking has been shown to increase the healing rate in hospitalized patients with gastric ulcer. The incidence of gastric and duodenal ulcer is greater in smokers than in nonsmokers. Smoking should be discouraged in patients with peptic ulcer disease—not to the extent, however, that anxiety is produced.

Gastric Irradiation. Irradiation of the oxyntic gland portion of the stomach produces a decrease in acid secretion usually lasting less than one year. In some patients prolonged hypochlorhydria is produced. At present, gastric irradiation is employed only in those rare patients who are intractable to medical therapy and in whom surgery carries a prohibitive mortality.

642. CLINICAL AND ENDOCRINE ASPECTS

John H. Walsh

CLINICAL MANIFESTATIONS

Symptoms. In many patients the diagnosis of peptic ulcer disease may be made with reasonable certainty by history alone. Epigastric pain is the cardinal symptom. The location and character of the pain, its temporal pattern, and factors that aggravate or relieve it produce a characteristic clinical picture. It must be recognized, however, that patients may have peptic ulcer without typical symptoms and, conversely, that other patients may have typical symptoms without a demonstrable ulcer.

Location. Typical ulcer pain is epigastric, near the midline. Patients with gastric ulcer tend to localize the pain slightly to the left of midline, and those with duodenal ulcer, slightly to the right. Such subtle distinctions are rarely helpful in individual patients. The pain may be so sharply localized that the patient will indicate its site by pointing with one or two fingers.

Character. The pain may be described as burning, gnawing, cramping, boring, or aching, or as a sensation of pressure, heaviness, or hunger. It may be mild or severe. It may fluctuate in intensity, but, even when described as cramping, it usually comes in waves lasting at least several minutes. The pain is not aggravated by body motion. The difficulty which many patients have in describing the nature of the pain is probably due to its visceral origin.

Temporal Relationships and Pain Relief. The time course of the pain is the most useful feature which differentiates it from pain of other diseases. Usually, ulcer pain appears in clusters of days to weeks, interspersed with pain-free intervals of weeks to months. Thus chronicity and periodicity are typical of ulcer symptoms. The pattern of recurrent attacks may continue for many years without significant change; the pain may become more frequent or severe, or, in a minority of patients, it may diminish and finally disappear after a few years. The old adage "once an ulcer, always an ulcer" is true for the majority of patients with peptic ulcer.

The daily pain pattern roughly parallels the normal time course of gastric acidity. Thus pain is diminished in the early morning, when gastric acid secretion is low,

and after meals, when acid is buffered by food. Pain is increased several hours after each meal, when acid secretion is high and is not buffered by food, and at bedtime. Likewise, measures which reduce intragastric acidity (oral antacids, food, nasogastric suction) typically relieve the pain. In some patients with gastric ulcer, a meal may produce transient worsening of the pain, followed by relief.

During the periods which are free of ulcer pain, the patient usually feels perfectly well.

Associated Symptoms. Nausea and/or excessive salivation may accompany peptic ulcer pain. Anorexia may occur in patients with gastric ulcer. Spontaneous vomiting is an occasional symptom, more commonly associated with gastric than with duodenal ulcers.

These features of ulcer pain are typical of patients with chronic uncomplicated peptic ulcer disease. Some patients may never experience pain and are found to have peptic ulcer disease only after they present with a complication of their disease (see below). Development of a complication may also lead to a change in the character of the pain (see below). Atypical symptoms are common in children and in elderly patients with peptic ulcer disease.

Physical Examination. Epigastric tenderness is frequently present, but is seldom marked, and is nonspecific. In fact, the general physical examination is of little help in establishing the diagnosis of uncomplicated peptic ulcer disease.

Differential Diagnosis. Any disease producing epigastric pain must be differentiated from peptic ulcer disease. Disease of only a few abdominal organs (stomach, liver, gallbladder, and pancreas) produces pain in this area; pain arising from the small intestine, large intestine, and bladder is felt lower in the abdomen. Pain arising in the gastroesophageal region and esophagus is usually felt in the subxiphoid area or retrosternally.

Pain from intrathoracic structures may also be referred to the epigastrium. Pain referred to the epigastric area may predominate in *pleuritis, myocardial infarction,* or *pericarditis.* These diseases are usually not confused with peptic ulcer disease. The pain they produce tends to be acute rather than chronic, constant rather than episodic, not related to meals or relieved by antacids, and usually associated with other pain or symptoms atypical of ulcer disease.

Pain arising from the esophagus (usually from *peptic esophagitis* or *peptic ulcer disease of the esophagus*) may exhibit some features typical of peptic ulcer pain such as temporal relation to meals and relief by antacids. However, lower esophageal pain, although occasionally epigastric, is usually felt as retrosternal "heartburn," and esophagitis is usually accompanied by symptoms of regurgitation of gastric contents which are accentuated by straining or by assuming a horizontal position.

Epigastric pain produced by intra-abdominal diseases not involving the stomach or duodenum can usually be distinguished easily from peptic ulcer disease. *Acute cholecystitis* may produce epigastric pain or pain in the right upper quadrant with rapid onset and duration of hours to days, and is frequently accompanied by tenderness over the gallbladder and fever. Patients will often have a history of previous attacks of biliary colic. *Acute pancreatitis* frequently produces epigastric pain, but the pain usually radiates to the back, and is aggravated by changes in position. Moreover, in either acute cholecystitis or pancreatitis, signs of acute abdominal inflammation (fever, direct and rebound tenderness, abdominal distention, or ileus) are typical and are not found in uncomplicated ulcer disease.

In the United States most gastric ulcers are benign, but the possibility of *malignant gastric ulcer* must be considered in every patient with gastric ulceration. Appropriate studies are discussed in Ch. 641.

Duodenitis. Duodenitis (inflammation of the duodenal mucosa) is frequently found in conjunction with active duodenal ulcer. It may also be found in patients with typical ulcer symptoms but without demonstrable ulcers. Such patients may have gastric hypersecretion, radiologic evidence of coarse duodenal folds, and histologic evidence of mononuclear infiltration and microscopic ulceration. Many patients with duodenitis later develop frank duodenal ulcer disease, and this condition may be a stage in the natural history of ulcer disease in some patients. Symptomatic duodenitis may also arise from eosinophilic or granulomatous infiltration of the duodenum.

Gastritis. In addition to gastritis associated with ulcer disease (see above), several forms of *chronic gastritis* may affect the stomach. Chronic superficial gastritis, atrophic gastritis, and gastric atrophy increase in frequency with age and sometimes are associated with epigastric symptoms but seldom produce any well defined pattern resembling peptic ulcer. Diseases infiltrating the wall of the stomach (carcinoma, lymphoma, granulomatous gastritis caused by Crohn's disease, eosinophilic granuloma, sarcoidosis, tuberculosis, or syphilis) may produce ulcer-like symptoms. Such symptoms are found in about a third of patients with adult hypertrophic pyloric stenosis and are relatively common in patients with Ménétrier's disease (hypertrophic gastropathy associated with protein loss into the gastrointestinal tract). Most of these diseases are rare. Their diagnosis depends on exclusion of peptic ulcer disease and demonstration of characteristic pathology by radiographic, endoscopic, and/or histologic examination.

Functional Dyspepsia. Functional dyspepsia is a syndrome with symptoms resembling many of those found in peptic ulcer disease but with no demonstrable pathologic lesion and with a prognosis free of complications of ulcer disease. Patients with functional dyspepsia have chronic and recurrent symptoms of epigastric distress. Pain-free intervals tend to be of short duration. Antacids frequently produce either partial or complete relief of epigastric pain, but food is likely to aggravate the distress. Often the pain is poorly localized, and the patients frequently complain of "gas." Nausea, vomiting, and pain may occur in the morning before breakfast. Nocturnal pain is encountered less frequently than in ulcer disease. The distinction between functional dyspepsia and peptic ulcer disease may be impossible to make by history alone. This is a diagnosis of exclusion, made only after careful radiographic and endoscopic examinations have excluded the diagnosis of peptic ulcer disease. As with duodenitis, a significant percentage of patients with "functional dyspepsia" will be found to have peptic ulcer disease when followed over a period of years.

ENDOCRINE HYPERFUNCTION AND ULCER DISEASE

Zollinger-Ellison Syndrome. One syndrome in which it has been established without doubt that ulcer disease is caused by hormonal excess is the Zollinger-Ellison syndrome. This syndrome is usually characterized by fulminant peptic ulcer diathesis or occasionally by diarrhea without ulcer, gastric acid hypersecretion, and a gastrin-secreting tumor, usually originating in the pancreas, which causes hypergastrinemia. The role of gastrin in the production of this syndrome was proved by chemical isolation of gastrin from such tumors and by bioassay of gastrin in serum and tumor extracts from patients with the syndrome. Gastrin radioimmunoassay has provided additional information about the pathogenesis of this disease and has permitted identification of many new patients.

The Zollinger-Ellison syndrome occurs in all age groups but is diagnosed most often between the third and fifth decades. The proportion of patients with ulcer disease who have the syndrome is unknown, but it is probably less than 1 per cent.

The predominant symptom is abdominal pain, which may be similar to that of ordinary ulcer disease or may be more severe. Intervals without pain tend to be shorter than in ordinary ulcer disease. Pain is present in more than 80 per cent of patients and usually has been present for a year or more before the diagnosis is established. Other prominent symptoms include diarrhea, vomiting, melena, and hematemesis. Recurrent ulceration after ulcer operation is unfortunately too often the first evidence of the disease. Some patients do not exhibit florid symptoms or may not have marked hypergastrinemia on a single determination and may be difficult to distinguish from those with ordinary ulcers.

In approximately three fourths of patients with the Zollinger-Ellison syndrome, there is an ulcer in the duodenal bulb or immediate postbulbar area. Ulcers in the distal duodenum or proximal jejunum are very suggestive but are found in less than one fourth of patients. Other radiologic features which are helpful in suggesting the diagnosis are hypertrophic gastric folds, increased quantities of gastric juice, dilatation of the duodenum and jejunum and mucosal edema, and irregularity in the small intestine. Occasionally there is a gastric ulcer (see figure in Ch. 640).

The diarrhea associated with the Zollinger-Ellison syndrome is due primarily to massive gastric hypersecretion and can be relieved by nasogastric aspiration or by total gastrectomy. The large amount of acid delivered into the upper intestine causes mucosal damage and increased intestinal motility. In addition, gastrin exerts an effect on the intestinal mucosa, decreasing absorption of salt and water, and also affects intestinal motility. The diarrhea is frequently accompanied by steatorrhea. Responsible factors include inactivation of pancreatic lipase and precipitation of conjugated bile salts at low intraluminal pH as well as direct damage of the mucosa by acid.

The gastrin-secreting tumors, or gastrinomas, responsible for the Zollinger-Ellison syndrome are usually small and may be difficult to find at operation or at postmortem examination. These tumors are most commonly located in the pancreas where they originate in the islets, but they may also originate in the duodenum. Metastasis and occurrence of multiple primary tumors are both common, so that the chances of locating a single benign operable tumor are probably less than one in four. Therefore treatment is total gastrectomy (see below).

Association with Other Endocrine Tumors. Individuals with the Zollinger-Ellison syndrome frequently have other endocrine abnormalities. The most common associated syndrome is hyperparathyroidism, which is found in about 20 per cent of patients with the disease. Hyperparathyroidism greatly affects the gastric secretory pattern in some of these patients. Hypercalcemia has been shown to release tumor gastrin and leads to increased acid secretion. Conversely, correction of hyperparathyroidism by parathyroidectomy may lead to transient or prolonged decreases in serum gastrin and acid secretion and may lead to periods of clinical remission. Other endocrine tumors found in the Zollinger-Ellison syndrome include pituitary, adrenal, ovarian, and thyroid. The abnormality may be carcinoma, single or multiple adenomas, or diffuse hyperplasia. The islet cell tumors may produce other substances such as insulin, glucagon, and ACTH.

A familial form of the Zollinger-Ellison syndrome was first described by Wermer. Several families have been described subsequently. There is autosomal dominant transmission with high but variable expressivity. The same pattern of glandular involvement and pathology is found as in the sporadic cases of multiple endocrine neoplasia.

Diagnosis. The diagnosis of the Zollinger-Ellison syndrome may be suggested by ulcer symptoms refractory to ordinary medical treatment, by radiologic findings, by gastric acid hypersecretion in the presence of ulcer symptoms, by recurrence of ulcer after an ulcer operation, or by the finding of an increased serum gastrin concentration. Gastric secretion is usually found to be excessive. Suspicion should be aroused when basal secretion is greater than 10mEq HCl per hour in an unoperated patient or greater than 5 mEq per hour in a patient with previous gastric surgery for ulcer. Confirmation of the diagnosis in most patients can be made by measurement of fasting serum gastrin concentration, with levels greater than 600 pg per milliliter in the presence of acid hypersecretion virtually diagnostic of the syndrome. In patients with hypersecretion in whom fasting serum gastrin level is equivocal (150 to 600 pg per milliliter), further evidence for the disease may be obtained by demonstration of minimal response of serum gastrin to a protein meal (normal subjects and duodenal ulcer patients show a twofold increase in serum gastrin concentrations after a protein meal) but an exaggerated increase in response to intravenous infusion of calcium and a paradoxical increase in response to intravenous secretin.

Patients with gastric ulcer tend to have moderately increased basal gastrin values, similar to those found in postprandial subjects. Gastric outlet obstruction leads to a moderate increase in basal gastrin which returns toward normal after a few days of gastric aspiration. Some patients with ordinary duodenal ulcer appear to have an exaggerated postprandial release of gastrin. Moderately to markedly increased fasting gastrin is found in many patients with achlorhydria who lack the normal inhibitory mechanism of antral acidification. The syndrome of *isolated retained antrum* after attempted antrectomy and gastrojejunostomy may produce gastric hypersecretion associated with hypergastrinemia. It is not clear whether there is a separate group of patients with hypergastrinemia caused by gastrin cell hyperplasia of the gastric antrum with autonomous release of gastrin not susceptible to acid inhibition.

Treatment. The usual treatment of the Zollinger-Ellison syndrome is total gastrectomy. Under some circumstances a period of medical treatment with anticholinergic drugs and antacids may be justified, especially for patients in whom the diagnosis is not certain and who have had no complications of ulcer disease. If operation is indicated, performance of less than total gastrectomy often leads to recurrent ulceration, frequently in the immediate postoperative period, and is often complicated by bleeding, perforation, and death. Occasionally it is possible to resect a single tumor and cure the disease.

643. COMPLICATIONS AND SURGICAL TREATMENT

James H. Meyer

COMPLICATIONS

Hemorrhage. Hemorrhage afflicts about 15 to 20 per cent of ulcer patients, being two to three times more common than perforation or obstruction. Duodenal ulcers bleed slightly more often than gastric ulcers; duodenal ulcers along the posterior duodenal wall or postbulbar ulcers bleed more frequently than anterior duodenal ulcers. Hemorrhage is usually from a major artery eroded by the ulcer and less commonly from smaller vessels in granulation tissue in the ulcer.

About 25 per cent of patients with bleeding ulcers have never recognized ulcer symptoms previously. In almost all patients hemorrhage is manifested by melena; but three patients in four (fewer with duodenal ulcer) experience hematemesis as well. Diaphoresis, pallor, palpitations, lightheadedness, mental confusion, or syncope are symptoms of associated hypotension which arises either as a direct result of blood volume loss or from a vasovagal reaction to sudden loss of blood.

Other than ulcer, the only common causes of upper gastrointestinal bleeding are acute gastric *mucosal lesions* (diffuse or localized, spontaneous or drug induced) and *esophageal varices.* Less common causes include *bleeding esophagitis, Mallory-Weiss tears, benign* (leiomyoma) or *malignant* (gastric carcinoma, lymphoma) *tumors, eosinophilic gastritis, milk allergy* (in children), and a variety of *rare vascular lesions* (hereditary hemorrhagic telangiectasia, phlebectasia of the jejunum, pseudoxanthoma elasticum, periarteritis, Ehlers-Danlos syndrome). Spontaneous upper gastrointestinal hemorrhage may accompany severe coagulation defects associated with underlying disease or anticoagulant therapy. As a diagnostic tool, the physical examination is helpful primarily in providing clues to bleeding lesions other than peptic ulcer, especially esophageal varices (e.g., hepatosplenomegaly, ascites, jaundice) and vascular abnormalities.

Upper gastrointestinal hemorrhage carries a significant mortality (about 10 per cent in ulcer disease). Therefore any patient experiencing melena, with or without hematemesis or associated symptoms or hypotension, should be hospitalized immediately for further evaluation and treatment. The over-all approach to the patient with upper gastrointestinal bleeding is discussed in Ch. 644.

Treatment. The program of immediate treatment consists of continued resuscitation as needed, reduction of gastric acidity, and continuous evaluation of the patient with the expectancy that surgical intervention may be required to save the patient's life. It is desirable that both physician and surgeon follow the patient's progress from the outset.

Many physicians prefer to treat the patient with continuous nasogastric aspiration as long as bleeding continues. When properly employed (proper tube placement, periodic venting), this procedure empties 90 to 95 per cent of secreted acid from the stomach and is therefore an adequate treatment. The appearance of blood in the gastric aspirate may also serve as an index of recurrent or continued bleeding. Alternatively, the patient may be treated with frequent antacids (see above) either from the outset or after the nasogastric tube is removed when bleeding has stopped. Most physicians prefer not to use anticholinergic drugs during hemorrhage, because these agents obscure signs of recurrent bleeding (they produce sustained tachycardia and diminish hyperactive bowel sounds which often indicate fresh blood in the gut).

If more than 3000 ml of blood is required for resuscitation, mortality increases significantly and is especially high if this quantity of blood is required in the first 48 hours. Emergency surgery is indicated in a patient who requires transfusion at a rate in excess of 3 units per day for the first 24 to 48 hours to maintain a stable circulation, once antecedent losses have been replenished. When bleeding has stopped under medical management but major hemorrhage subsequently reappears in spite of continued treatment, surgery should be undertaken, because it is likely that further medical treatment will not be successful and it is known that continued medical treatment in this situation carries a high mortality. Under these policies 15 to 30 per cent of bleeding ulcer patients will require emergency surgery.

Until recently, the traditional form of emergency surgery has been subtotal gastrectomy, usually with ligation or removal of the bleeding ulcer. Since the early 1960's, surgeons have favored the use of vagotomy plus pyloroplasty with ligation of bleeding vessels, citing lower mortality because of the speed and ease with which this operation can be performed. Retrospective analyses of mortality rates of these two operations in the bleeding patient are to date inadequate to substantiate the superiority of vagotomy plus pyloroplasty. Both operations effectively stop acute bleeding in 92 to 95 per cent of patients who are bleeding from a single, discrete ulcer, but are much less effective in stopping bleeding in patients with multiple stress ulcers.

Prognosis. Death from bleeding ulcer is more frequent in patients over 50 years of age. Bleeding gastric ulcers are more apt to be lethal than bleeding duodenal ulcers for two reasons: (1) patients with gastric ulcers are older than patients with duodenal ulcer, and (2) regardless of age, patients with gastric ulcer tend to bleed more profusely than patients with duodenal ulcer. Most forms of associated cardiovascular disease other than benign hypertension (ischemic or valvular heart disease, cor pulmonale) adversely affect the prognosis, as does any severe associated disease. It is not known whether earlier surgery in these higher risk patients would reduce mortality, because those patients are also the ones with higher operative mortality.

Thirty to 50 per cent of patients surviving the first hemorrhage without operative intervention will hemor-

rhage again; the severity of the subsequent hemorrhage bears no relationship to the severity of the first episode. Continued morbidity (recurrent hemorrhage, intractable ulcer pain, subsequent perforation) is the rule in up to 70 per cent of ulcer patients who have bleeding. It is not clear whether surgery (emergent or elective) in the bleeding duodenal ulcer patient will significantly reduce recurrent bleeding. For the most part this is due to bleeding from recurrence of ulcer after surgery by either of the two procedures.

Impaired Gastric Emptying ("Outlet Obstruction"). This complication is seen in 5 to 10 per cent of ulcer patients. In the majority of cases (80 per cent), it appears as a complication of duodenal ulcer disease, usually of long duration. Gastric ulcers, most frequently prepyloric, are the second most common cause. Although pyloric channel ulcers may cause gastric outlet obstruction, ulcers at this site are infrequent.

In ulcer disease, impaired gastric emptying may develop as the result of narrowing of the lumen by fibrosis and/or inflammatory tumor around the ulcer. However, in many cases gastric motor dysfunction, associated with inflammation around the ulcer or with gradual dilatation of the stomach and stretching of gastric muscle beyond optimal force/length characteristics, plays a dominant role. Impaired gastric emptying is thus potentially reversible to the extent that gastric motor dysfunction can be corrected or that luminal narrowing by inflammation can be reduced with healing.

In the initial phases, mechanical outlet obstruction is usually not complete. However, ingested materials and gastric secretions gradually accumulate to produce gastric dilatation. With gastric dilatation, the patient begins to experience symptoms of constant epigastric fullness and discomfort, anorexia, sitophobia, and nausea. Vomiting (spontaneous or induced) may relieve these symptoms. The whole process tends to develop insidiously over days or weeks. The eventual development of protracted vomiting, usually of copious amounts of undigested food, brings the patient to the physician.

In the typical case the diagnosis is easily made by the history. However, about a fourth of patients with impaired gastric emptying never vomit before seeking medical attention, presumably because they have reduced oral intake to an amount that can be emptied by the partially obstructed stomach. In this minority the diagnosis is usually discovered during an upper gastrointestinal series which reveals a large, dilated stomach filled with solid and liquid material in spite of the customary overnight fast prior to the examination. In most patients physical examination confirms recent weight loss and evidence of dehydration. Abdominal distention and tenderness are rarely noted, and bowel sounds are normal. A gastric succussion splash may be elicited in about half the patients. Diagnosis suspected on the basis of historical and physical findings can be quickly confirmed by the placement of a large-bore orogastric (Ewald) tube; aspiration of 300 ml or more of gastric contents three or more hours after the last meal indicates gastric outlet obstruction.

Patients with gastric outlet obstruction must be hospitalized for treatment. The goals of hospitalization are fourfold: (1) correction of fluid and electrolyte deficits, (2) gastric decompression, (3) intensive ulcer treatment, and (4) surgery if obstruction persists.

In the face of protracted vomiting and no effective oral intake, fluid and electrolyte depletion may be profound.

Extracellular fluid and plasma volume deficits may be reflected by orthostatic hypotension, prerenal azotemia, elevated hematocrit, and abnormally low central venous pressure. Some degree of metabolic alkalosis and hypokalemia is common. The latter may accentuate gastric motor dysfunction. These deficits must be rapidly corrected; they contribute to continued morbidity and may be responsible for increased surgical mortality.

There are two sources of electrolyte losses in the patient with gastric outlet obstruction: (1) hydrochloric acid and lesser amounts of sodium and potassium chloride are lost with the gastric juice which is vomited or aspirated, and (2) considerable amounts of sodium and potassium are lost in the urine. For every H^+ ion lost in the gastric juice, one Cl^- ion is similarly lost and one HCO_3^- ion enters the circulation. During the early phases of obstruction, bicarbonate entering the bloodstream is cleared from the urine as $NaHCO_3$, and chloride losses are minimized by renal tubular reabsorption. At this stage the urine is characteristically alkaline and contains appreciable sodium, but is low in chloride. In effect, the kidney converts an HCl loss from the stomach to a net NaCl loss from the body (Na^+ lost in urine, Cl^- lost in gastric juice), and in this way metabolic alkalosis is minimized. However, as the body's deficit in NaCl mounts, secondary hyperaldosteronism intervenes. As a result, much more filtered Na^+ is reabsorbed by the renal tubules. Some is absorbed in exchange for K^+, and more is absorbed in exchange for H^+ secreted by the tubules. For every H^+ secreted by the renal tubules, one HCO_3^- enters the bloodstream. At this stage the urine is characteristically low in both sodium and chloride, but may contain significant amounts of potassium and may be paradoxically acidic. In effect, the kidney is no longer compensating for gastric losses; H^+ and Cl^- losses from the stomach are now aggravated by H^+ and Cl^- losses from the kidney. Sustained metabolic alkalosis, hypochloremia, and hypokalemia result.

Reversal of this sequence of events is accomplished by infusion of 0.15N NaCl intravenously. Potassium replacement as KCl may be started once an adequate urinary output has been established. Enough saline has to be given (1) to replenish continued gastric losses and (2) to replace antecedent sodium and chloride deficits. The adequacy of this replacement can be judged (1) by the disappearance of orthostatic hypotension and the return of venous pressure to normal, (2) by the reappearance of an alkaline urine with a rising sodium concentration, and (3) by rising chloride concentration in the urine. As these changes are observed, prerenal azotemia, metabolic alkalosis, and hypokalemia should disappear.

In the meantime gastric decompression is instituted to eliminate gastric dilatation and restore motor tone. This is accomplished by continuous nasogastric aspiration once the stomach has been lavaged free of solid debris through a large-bore orogastric tube. Usually a period of 72 hours is adequate to restore gastric tone. Continuous gastric aspiration, by removing secreted gastric acid, is also an effective treatment for active ulcer disease. This treatment thus serves to reduce inflammatory edema around the ulcer and thus may help to relieve the cause of the obstruction. With good management, fluid and electrolyte disturbances will have been corrected by 72 hours as well.

The end of the first 72 hours thus represents a point of reappraisal. If the nature of the obstructing lesion is in doubt at this time, an upper gastrointestinal series may be obtained to establish the diagnosis. This examination will also provide some indication as to how well the preceding treatment has restored gastric emptying. Some physicians assess gastric emptying by the saline load test. If more than 400 ml remains in the stomach 30 minutes after instilling 750 ml of isotonic saline, emptying is impaired. If the stomach does not empty, it is unlikely that further medical treatment will be effective, and surgery should be considered. If emptying is adequate, the patient may be begun on oral liquids and antacids. However, for the next several days continuous assessment of gastric emptying must be performed. If the patient has more than 300 ml of gastric residual at bedtime (four hours after the last intake) or more than 200 ml of residual after an overnight fast, or if the saline load test is abnormal, gastric emptying is still impaired and surgical treatment is indicated.

About 25 per cent of obstructed patients will require surgery by these criteria. Of those who escape surgery in a given episode, 15 per cent will have a recurrent episode of obstruction, frequently requiring surgery.

Perforation.   Any peptic ulcer may eventually erode through the muscular and serosal walls of the viscus in which it is located. If such erosion establishes a communication between the lumen of the viscus and the surrounding body cavity, allowing spillage of luminal contents into this cavity, perforation has occurred. If, on the other hand, the transmural erosion is sealed by surrounding visceral structures or peritoneum before spillage of luminal contents supervenes, the ulcer is said to have penetrated.

Free perforation occurs in about 5 to 10 per cent of ulcer patients. About 90 per cent of these perforations arise from a duodenal ulcer, usually in the anterior duodenal wall. Nine per cent arise from gastric ulcers and the remainder from perforated malignant gastric ulcers or perforated marginal ulcers after subtotal gastric resection. Free perforation is almost always heralded by the sudden onset of intense, usually generalized and constant abdominal pain. Usually these dramatic symptoms follow years of intermittent ulcer-like pain, but in about 25 per cent of patients ulcer pain preceding the perforation will have been noted for less than three months, and 7 per cent of patients with perforation have never recognized ulcer symptoms previously. Perforation may arise at any age (peak incidence is in the fifth and sixth decades), and age-specific rates of perforation increase throughout life, even though ulcer disease generally remits in older life. Elderly patients who perforate frequently do not experience intense symptoms, so the diagnosis may not be appreciated. Ten per cent of patients who perforate hemorrhage simultaneously.

Physical examination usually confirms the diagnosis suspected on historical grounds. Generalized direct and rebound tenderness, boardlike rigidity of the abdominal musculature, and diminished or absent bowel sounds resulting from reflex ileus are signs of generalized peritonitis which accompanies perforation. Swallowed air escaping through the perforation into the abdominal cavity may result in loss of normal hepatic dullness on percussion; this air can be visualized radiographically under the diaphragm on upright or lateral abdominal films in 75 to 80 per cent of patients who have perforated. In the absence of a classic history, signs of generalized peritonitis from perforated ulcer could be ascribed to any abdominal catastrophe (e.g., rupture of a volvulus, diverticulum, gallbladder, or appendix; fulminant pancreatitis). Moreover, escaping luminal contents are occasionally confined to the upper abdomen or lesser sac or are spilled down the right gutter into the right lower quadrant; in these situations signs of peritonitis may be localized rather than generalized, so the condition may be misdiagnosed. In practice, however, the diagnosis of perforated ulcer is made correctly about 90 per cent of the time.

Peritonitis associated with perforation produces dehydration owing to fluid loss into the peritoneal cavity. Leukocytosis and fever also reflect peritonitis, but the latter is not a common sequel to perforation treated quickly. Serum amylase is often elevated as the result of perforation.

Three forms of treatment are available: (1) medical treatment, which consists of carefully monitored continuous nasogastric aspiration to allow the perforation to seal, (2) simple surgical closure of the perforation, and (3) surgical closure of the perforation combined with an operation for the ulcer disease. Medical treatment, *when properly managed,* is as safe and effective as surgical closure. However, surgical closure permits direct inspection of the abdominal cavity at laparotomy, minimizing errors in diagnosis. Consequently, surgical closure is the preferred treatment. Patients who perforate after longstanding ulcer symptoms continue to experience significant morbidity from ulcer disease after simple closure of the perforation. For this reason, most surgeons undertake definitive ulcer surgery at the time of closure of a perforation in patients with a longstanding ulcer history, provided that the patient's condition permits a more extensive procedure.

Penetration. Ulcers which penetrate are usually refractory to medical treatment. Posterior duodenal ulcers are most likely to penetrate. Penetration is heralded by a change in pain pattern. Classically visceral ulcer pain takes on somatic characteristics felt in the back, chest, or lateral abdomen. Often pain becomes constant and is no longer relieved by food or antacids. Some ulcers which penetrate into the head of the pancreas may result in localized pancreatitis and elevation of serum amylase. Definitive treatment for penetrating ulcer is surgical.

SURGICAL TREATMENT

Indications for Elective Surgery for Peptic Ulcer. It is uncertain whether sustained medical treatment can significantly alter the long-term course of ulcer disease. For the relapse-prone patient who experiences significant cumulative morbidity attended with economic loss and periods of absence from his life's pursuits, surgical treatment is an alternative, but unfortunately the operations available are all associated with continued postoperative morbidity in a significant number of patients (see accompanying table). Moreover, although surgery cures the ulcer in 90 per cent or more of patients, no guarantee can be made to the individual patient. For these reasons, the decision to operate electively for intractable ulcer disease must be carefully considered by patient, physician, and surgeon. The problem is to decide whether morbidity under medical management is likely to be greater than that which arises after surgery. Only a few guidelines can be offered to aid this decision.

Duodenal Ulcer. A period of observation under medical supervision is required to judge the virulence of duodenal ulcer disease in any individual patient. A significant number (probably about 25 per cent) of patients will experience only a single episode of duodenal ulceration which responds adequately to medical treatment; clearly these patients do not require surgery. Repeated recurrences more often than biannually indicate that the patient suffers from an unusually virulent form of the disease and that surgical treatment should be considered, but other factors must be taken into account as well. Among these factors is the disability produced by each recurrence. The personality of the patient must also be considered, for there is some evidence that a poorly motivated patient (as evidenced by poor work records antedating the ulcer disease or poor social adjustments) is more likely to experience postoperative morbidity. Only a minority of duodenal ulcer patients present with less equivocal indications for surgery: duodenal ulcers secondary to gastrinomas (see above), penetrating duodenal ulcers (see above), and giant duodenal ulcers. These are frequently refractory to medical treatment and are prone to complications, so surgical treatment is appropriate. Also, the development of one or more complications alters the prognosis; surgery may be required to treat these complications as they arise or may be subsequently elected because the patient has demonstrated, by the development of these complications, that he has virulent ulcer disease.

Gastric Ulcer. A similar line of reasoning applies to the patient with gastric ulcer. Recurrence is common (up to 40 per cent in two years), and morbidity from frequent recurrence is high. However, the problem of gastric ulcer differs from duodenal ulcer in two respects. (1) In gastric ulcer healing poorly under medical treatment, the possibility arises that the lesion is an ulcerated cancer which has escaped detection. Consequently, surgery may be undertaken even during the first occurrence if there is doubt about the nature of the lesion. (2) The patient with gastric ulcer tends to be older and may suffer from diseases associated with aging which alter operative risks and thus may influence the decision concerning surgery.

Outcome of Elective Operation for Duodenal Ulcer in Patients Followed Three to Eight Years*

Operation	Mortality (%)†	Ulcer Recurrence (%)	Postprandial Symptoms (%)‡	Weight Loss	Diarrhea (%)
Subtotal gastrectomy	0–2	2–5	36–40	++	7
Vagotomy and antrectomy	0–2	0–3	34–39	++	20–23
Vagotomy and drainage	0–2	7–9	21–40	+	25–26

*Results compiled from three randomized studies: Br. Med. J., 2:781, 1968; Ann. Surg., 172:547, 1970; and Surg. Gynecol. Obstet., 131:233, 1970.
†In these studies, high risk patients were not included; therefore mortality rates are lower than would be expected from the application of each procedure to all patients (see text).
‡Highest percentage of patients with any of several varieties of postprandial distress.

Types of Surgical Treatment. *Duodenal Ulcer.* Three types of operation are currently employed for duodenal ulcer: (1) *subtotal gastrectomy,* in which 75 to 80 per cent of distal stomach is removed and gastrointestinal continuity is restored by an anastomosis between the gastric remnant and the jejunum; (2) *vagotomy and "drainage,"* a procedure in which the vagus nerves are cut and the outlet of the stomach is widened by either a pyloroplasty or a gastroenterostomy; and (3) *vagotomy and antrectomy,* which consists of cutting the vagus nerves, removing the distal 50 per cent of the stomach, and re-establishing gastrointestinal continuity by gastroduodenostomy or gastrojejunostomy. "Drainage" is performed to obviate gastric stasis, which tends to occur after vagotomy. "Parietal cell vagotomy" is a promising new operation, not yet adequately evaluated, in which the surgeon cuts vagal fibers to only the part of the stomach proximal to antrum; no "drainage" procedure is required.

All three traditional operations are associated with some degree of postoperative morbidity (see table). The procedure of vagotomy and drainage does not require duodenal transection. This avoids postoperative leakage from a suture line through a badly diseased duodenum, a frequent source of postoperative mortality. This advantage of vagotomy and drainage, as opposed to the resective procedures, is not reflected by the table, because in studies presented there vagotomy and drainage was employed whenever operative conditions were not optimal. Nevertheless, it is apparent from the table that any reduced mortality from this procedure is offset by a significantly higher recurrence rate.

Gastric Ulcer. For gastric ulcer, the traditional surgical treatment is distal gastrectomy with gastroduodenostomy. In most instances this resection removes the ulcer; with high gastric ulcers it may be combined with a wedge resection of the ulcer or biopsies of the ulcer margins to ascertain the benignancy of the ulcer. Some have proposed that vagotomy and drainage be used for gastric ulcer. However, gastric ulcer recurrences are more frequent after this procedure than after distal resection.

Chronic Postoperative Morbidity. *Prandial and Postprandial Symptoms. Early satiety* (intense feeling of fullness before finishing a meal, experienced by 36 to 60 per cent of patients) and *bilious vomiting* (in 13 per cent) shortly after eating are complaints encountered after all three operations. The "dumping" syndrome, a symptom complex which includes any or all of the following: nausea, vomiting, abdominal cramps, borborygmi, flatulence, diarrhea, diaphoresis, palpitations, tachycardia, lightheadedness, and flushing, may be experienced while eating or immediately afterward, especially after meals high in sugar content. The syndrome is believed to arise from the rapid entry of hyperosmolar liquids into the gut. It is experienced in mild form by about 20 per cent of operated patients, but is troublesome in only about 7 per cent. Somewhat later postprandially (two to four hours), some patients (about 10 per cent) may experience *hypoglycemia* and symptoms thereof. Such patients exhibit abnormally rapid rises in both serum glucose and insulin concentrations which are thought to be related to rapid entry of glucose into the gut. All three operations accelerate the passage of liquid material into the gut.

These symptoms are usually more prominent in the first month after surgery and diminish as time passes. They may be ameliorated by the use of frequent small feedings taken without liquids and the avoidance of sugar in the diet (sugar is the most osmotically active dietary component).

Nutritional Problems. Some weight loss is common, particularly after resective procedures. Frequently weight loss is associated with reduced caloric intake as the result of early satiety or the desire to minimize postprandial symptoms. However, about a quarter of the patients have mild steatorrhea after these surgical procedures which may also contribute to malnutrition. Anemias occur in 20 to 50 per cent of patients, particularly after resection. Anemias usually appear more than five years after surgery; usually they reflect deficiency in iron, occasionally in folate or vitamin B_{12}. Osteomalacia may appear many years after subtotal gastrectomy.

Recurrent Ulceration. When the ulcer recurs in a duodenum left in continuity with the stomach, as after vagotomy and drainage, symptoms are typical of duodenal ulcer. However, when a recurrent ulcer arises at a gastrojejunal anastomosis ("marginal ulceration"), symptoms may be atypical. Pain frequently occurs in the left upper quadrant but may appear anywhere in the abdomen; marginal ulcers are refractory to medical treatment, frequently bleed, and occasionally perforate. Appropriate treatment is surgical. In patients who have had a subtotal gastrectomy, the treatment consists of a vagotomy. In patients who have had a prior vagotomy without resection, the treatment is antrectomy, often with attempts to cut more vagal fibers.

Postvagotomy Diarrhea. Although diarrhea may be associated with the dumping syndrome after any of the three procedures, a different form of diarrhea is seen in about one in four patients who have had a vagotomy (see table). This diarrhea tends to be episodic, lasting a day or two, and bears no relationship to dietary factors. In only a few patients is diarrhea disabling. For these few patients treatment with opiates or anticholinergics has been tried but has not been uniformly successful. The cause of postvagotomy diarrhea is unknown.

Rare Mechanical Problems. These problems arise almost exclusively in resected patients with gastrojejunal anastomoses. They include stomal obstruction, partial afferent loop obstruction, intermittent jejunal intussusception, gastro- or jejunocolic fistulas, and gastric bezoars.

644. GASTROINTESTINAL BLEEDING

David H. Law

Types of Bleeding. Bleeding may be manifested by *hematemesis* (vomiting of blood, either bright red or brown and precipitated, resembling coffee grounds), by *melena* (the passage of tarry black, sticky stool), or by *hematochezia* (the passage of fresh red blood per rectum). Bleeding, however, may be only occult, with normal-appearing stools which on chemical determination are shown to contain blood.

Degree and Effects of Bleeding. The pathophysiologic effects which result from gastrointestinal blood loss give rise to many of the symptoms and signs which have been shown to be of clinical importance in determining the presence and the severity of bleeding. In large part, however, this response to blood loss is unrelated to the site or cause of the bleeding, depending more upon the *rate* and *extent*.

After acute massive bleeding, typified by loss of greater than 1500 ml or 25 per cent of the circulating blood volume within a period of minutes to hours, cardiac output and systolic blood pressure decrease, followed by decrease in diastolic blood pressure and increased pulse. Blood pressure responses occur first in the form of orthostatic hypotension. Pulse rate seems to be a far less accurate parameter, even at a time when orthostatic hypotension is clearly evident, but it usually does rise. Compensatory vascular responses include constriction of the arterial bed with skin pallor, decreased splanchnic blood flow, and decreased renal blood flow with relative maintenance of cerebral and cardiopulmonary vascular systems. Vascular complications may include acute tubular necrosis, mesenteric vascular insufficiency with bowel infarction, and centrilobular necrosis of the liver. With continued acute blood loss, cerebral blood flow is embarrassed and there may be confusion, progressing to obtundation. Early electrocardiographic changes of T wave flattening or inversion and possibly S-T segment depression document insufficiency of coronary blood flow. Most of the early changes respond to correction of the diminished plasma volume, using blood transfusions or other plasma expanders such as electrolyte solutions or dextrans. If, however, blood loss continues unabated, the secondary effects of *shock*—increasing anoxia, cellular dysfunction, and acidosis—may lead to death. The mortality from massive gastrointestinal bleeding varies from 5 to 50 per cent, depending upon the cause of the hemorrhage and the age and condition of the patient.

More gradual compensatory physiologic mechanisms, including antidiuretic hormone and aldosterone release, act to re-establish intravascular volume, with a resultant drop in hematocrit and hemoglobin concentration. This plasma restoration begins rapidly, and up to one half the total compensation may occur within 8 to 12 hours. However, depending upon the patient's state of hydration, age, ability to resorb fluid lost into the gut, and rate of both oral and parenteral fluid repletion, this process may continue for 48 to 72 hours. For these reasons hematocrit and hemoglobin concentration values may be misleading during acute bleeding episodes. By recognizing these responses, the reduction in blood volume can be estimated and a logical sequence of diagnostic studies outlined to define the source of bleeding.

The degree of blood loss is the single most important parameter to be defined when a patient presents with gastrointestinal bleeding. This will establish the relative emergency of the problem and set the diagnostic and therapeutic pace to follow. Although the clinical history is often nondiagnostic, it will provide useful information in about one third of the cases and should be thoroughly evaluated.

Examination of the patient provides the best means of assessing blood loss based on the responses previously outlined. As a general rule, blood pressure less than 100 mm Hg or a pulse rate exceeding 100 per minute in an otherwise normotensive patient indicates a 20 per cent volume depletion. Associated pallor and/or postural hypotension lends support to this estimate. A pulse rate increase of 20 per minute or orthostatic blood pressure decreases of greater than 10 mm Hg further suggest acute blood loss in excess of 1000 ml.

Localization and Site. In the acute situation, several points of history may be useful in finding the site of bleeding. (1) Hematemesis indicates bleeding from above the duodenal-jejunal junction, whereas passage of red blood per rectum is most frequently associated with a bleeding site below the start of the jejunum and usually from the colon. (2) The onset of hematemesis after forceful vomiting suggests the Mallory-Weiss syndrome or esophageal rupture. (3) Typical abdominal pain may suggest peptic ulcer or reflux esophagitis. (4) Stress ulcers may occur hours to days after trauma, severe burns, or surgical procedures. (5) Associated diseases may suggest the source of gastrointestinal hemorrhage; i.e., alcoholism is associated with bleeding from gastritis and varices; arthritis is associated with salicylate and other drug ingestion which may cause gastritis; diverticulosis may bleed massively; emphysema carries an increased risk for development of peptic ulcer; and cirrhosis and peptic ulcer suggest sources of blood loss. (6) Past surgical procedures may suggest a bleeding site. (7) Medications and toxins (analgesics, adrenocortical steroids, antihypertensives, and alcohol) may be associated with bleeding. Qualitative characteristics of bleeding, such as the presence of clots or bright red, mahogany, or coffeeground material, have little quantitative significance but may help localize bleeding to a given area of the gastrointestinal tract.

The *physical examination,* in addition to demonstrating signs of blood loss, may show associated disease which is pertinent to gastrointestinal bleeding. One should focus particularly on the oral pharynx and skin changes of the upper trunk for the vascular lesions of Osler-Weber Rendu disease or the pigmentary spots of Peutz-Jeghers syndrome. Hepatosplenomegaly, adenopathy, the presence of a rectal mass, and overt congenital anomalies may be found.

Laboratory Studies. Immediate *laboratory* evaluation should include a white blood cell count, hematocrit, hemoglobin, blood urea nitrogen, and evaluation for bleeding diathesis. An abrupt leukocytosis up to 20,000 per cubic millimeter and an outpouring of platelets may be seen with acute hemorrhage. A nasogastric tube should be inserted to estimate the amount and character of blood present, and guaiac tests performed on gastric contents. A hemoglobin level of less than 11 grams per 100 ml and a blood urea nitrogen (BUN) greater than 40 mg per 100 ml, in an otherwise normal patient, indicates a blood loss greater than 1000 ml. Blood in the upper intestine is reflected in an increased level of BUN with essentially no effect on serum creatinine. With cessation of bleeding, the BUN returns to normal within two to three days.

Management. It is important to stress that management of the patient with massive bleeding frequently does not permit the luxury of a thorough diagnostic search. Immediate steps must be taken to minimize morbidity and mortality. The most important single aim in the management of *emergent* bleeding is the maintenance of an adequate blood volume. This requires adequate access to the venous system. With massive bleeding or shock, central venous pressure measurement may be a valuable guide in determining the need for increasing or decreasing subsequent plasma expansion. Simultaneously with typing and cross-matching of blood for transfusion, some form of *plasma expander* should be infused—normal saline, Ringer's lactate or even 5 per cent dextrose solution may be used initially, but dextran or plasma may be more effective while awaiting the arrival of whole blood. After establishment of intravenous access, an intragastric, large-bore tube should be passed. Blood in the gastric aspirate confirms a bleeding site proximal to the ligament of Treitz; however, failure to find blood does not exclude this possibility. If blood is present, one should continuously lavage the stomach with ice water or saline until it is free of clots and returns are clear. In addition to controlling hemorrhage, this may minimize vomiting and monitor the activity of bleeding. The patient with suspected esophageal variceal hemorrhage constitutes a special problem and will be discussed separately.

The use of vasoconstrictor drugs should be considered when bleeding is massive, but great care must be taken in the presence of hypertensive or arteriosclerotic cardiovascular disease. Intravenous infusion over 20 minutes of 20 units of vasopressin, diluted in 100 ml of 5 per cent dextrose in distilled water, may be effective. Direct selective arterial infusion of vasoactive agents (pitressin, epinephrine, or propranolol) may be directed at the bleeding lesion when arteriography identifies the lesion.

Specific Diagnostic Techniques. The clinical decision as to the diagnostic use of endoscopy or x-ray should be based on skills of the immediately available personnel. If peptic ulcer seems the most likely probability after considering all factors, a barium contrast study of the esophagus, stomach, and upper intestine would most likely yield a diagnosis, while minimizing diagnostic risks. Evidence suggesting the Mallory-Weiss syndrome, gastritis, or portal hypertension is an indication for *panendoscopy* as the *initial* diagnostic procedure if a trained physician is available. The availability of a wide selection of flexible fiberoptic instruments for direct visualization of the esophageal, gastric, and duodenal mucosa has greatly enhanced the detection of lesions responsible for gastrointestinal bleeding. It is the most reliable procedure for diagnosing mucosal disorders of the esophagus, stomach, and duodenum. Although skilled endoscopy in the emergent setting can be performed with minimal patient risk and provide vital diagnostic information, it should be emphasized that optimal visualization requires proper timing of the procedure, a clean stomach, and a relaxed, cooperative patient. These conditions are best accomplished when the patient's clinical situation is stable.

Radiologic evaluation must be performed with close cooperation between the primary care physician and a well-informed radiologist with a preplanned course of action and special handling to avoid delays or untoward risks while the patient is away from his room. Cinefluoroscopy and hypotonic duodenography have increased the sensitivity of this procedure, but the latter rarely offers anything in the management of the patient with emergent bleeding.

If routine studies are negative and the rate of blood loss is greater than 0.5 ml per minute, celiac and mesenteric angiography may be useful by showing puddling of contrast agent at the site of hemorrhage within a bowel. When a bleeding lesion is identified, the catheter may be left in place to infuse vasoactive drugs such as pitressin, propranolol, or epinephrine directly into the arterial system feeding the bleeding lesion. This approach, however, requires a skilled, trained angiographer and should be used only in a center equipped for the purpose.

When all the aforementioned studies are nondiagnostic and very active bleeding persists, small intestinal intubation with sequential aspirations of the intestinal content may localize the bleeding site. Barium contrast study may then be performed through the tube to document a lesion at the site of bleeding. This test is most useful for locating obscure bleeding sites between the ligament of Treitz and the ileocecal valve, such as small bowel tumors, ulcers, Meckel's diverticula, or vascular anomalies.

The terminal ileum is often seen during reflux from a barium enema and may show terminal ileitis, an infrequent cause of massive gastrointestinal bleeding. Colonic diverticula are increasingly frequent with age and therefore cannot necessarily be implicated as the cause of bleeding when they are visualized by x-rays. They are, however, a common cause of massive lower gastrointestinal bleeding. In such instances selective inferior mesenteric arteriography may reveal the precise site of hemorrhage.

On occasion emergency surgical intervention must be considered for the patient with shock caused by uncontrollable massive hemorrhage. In addition, certain patients with gastrointestinal bleeding have an increased mortality, suggesting the need for early surgery, such as those who rebleed while hospitalized with good medical management and those older than 60.

In the setting of nonemergent bleeding, a more deliberate plan, involving detailed history, physical examination, and selected special studies, including endoscopy and complete radiologic survey of the gastrointestinal tract, may be undertaken. Since bleeding may not be evident, laboratory data may be necessary to establish bleeding and to define its source. Inspection and chemical tests (i.e., guaiac) of fresh stool are important in assessing the presence and extent of nonemergent gastrointestinal bleeding. Vomitus and gastric and small bowel aspirates, in addition to stools, should be tested for the presence of occult blood in patients suspected of bleeding. When the aforementioned radiologic and endoscopic studies are nondiagnostic and persistent active bleeding is suspected, small intestinal intubation or passage of a weighted umbilical tape that will reach the small bowel may demonstrate the bleeding site.

Portal hypertension with gastrointestinal bleeding constitutes a special problem and is the most critical hazard to patients with portal hypertension. Approximately one third of cirrhotic patients die from this complication. When the patient with massive gastrointestinal bleeding also has portal hypertension, initial management should follow the guidelines noted above. Panendoscopy should be performed to establish that varices are, indeed, the site of blood loss, because up to one fourth of the patients with varices who present with gastrointestinal hemorrhage may be bleeding from another source. Treatment includes esophageal tamponade and initiation of intravenous pitressin, 20 units diluted in 100 ml of isotonic saline or dextrose, over a 20 to 30 minute period, repeated at two-hour intervals as indicated. Regardless of which tube is used for esophageal tamponade, ultimate survival with minimal morbidity depends on close supervision and strict attention to detail of the method. The immediate aim of therapy is to control hemorrhage, and this is possible in the vast majority of cases. Failure to control bleeding by tamponade may indicate that varices are not the source of bleeding. Ultimate therapy to prevent rebleeding is directed at elective surgical decompression of the portal system.

Operative mortality approaches 70 per cent when

emergent surgery is required to control variceal bleeding; therefore optimal prognosis necessitates surgical decompression of the portal bed as an elective procedure. The most important criteria for selecting a successful surgical candidate relate to the patient's age and hepatic function. A serum albumin above 3.0 grams per 100 ml, bilirubin less than 3.0 mg per 100 ml, sulfobromophthalein retention less than 20 per cent, prothrombin time less than four seconds elevated, absence of ascites, and a liver biopsy showing only minimal fatty metamorphosis and absence of alcoholic hepatitis in the presence of cirrhosis are the most important criteria to consider when selecting the ideal surgical candidate. Mortality and morbidity of shunt surgery seem related directly to abnormalities of these parameters reflecting hepatic reserve. Thus after the emergent gastrointestinal hemorrhage has been controlled, an intensive nutritional and rehabilitation program is essential to improve liver function in preparation for surgery. This may require up to three months to achieve maximal benefit.

Bleeding diathesis, although infrequently a cause of massive gastrointestinal hemorrhage, may be present in patients with blood dyscrasias, vascular abnormalities, or multiple systemic diseases which present with gastrointestinal bleeding. When the history, physical examination, or clinical course suggests such a possibility, the sequence of diagnostic studies should include expert hematologic consultation and the appropriate laboratory tests to detect these disorders.

Baum, S., and Nusbaum, M.: The control of gastrointestinal haemorrhage by selective mesenteric arterial infusion of vasopressin. Radiology, 98:497, 1971.

Brick, I. B., and Jeghers, H. J.: Gastrointestinal hemorrhage. N. Engl. J. Med., 253:458, 511, 555, 1955.

Isenberg, J. I., Walsh, J. H., and Grossman, M. I.: Zollinger-Ellison syndrome. Gastroenterology, 65:140, 1973.

Pitcher, J. L.: Safety and effectiveness of the modified Sengstaken-Blakemore tube: A prospective study. Gastroenterology, 61:291, 1971.

Schille, K. F. R., Truelove, S. C., and Williams, D. J.: Hematemesis and melena with special reference to factors influencing the outcome. Br. Med. J., 2:7, 1970.

Sleisenger, M. H., and Fordtran, J. S. (eds.): Gastrointestinal Disease. Philadelphia, W. B. Saunders Company, 1973, Chapters 12–16, 40–43, 50–63.

Section Three.   DISEASES OF MALABSORPTION

Marvin H. Sleisenger

The malabsorption syndrome is a constellation of symptoms and signs that are the result of abnormal fecal excretion of fat (steatorrhea) and of varying degrees of malabsorption of fat-soluble vitamins as well as carbohydrate, protein, minerals, other vitamins, and water.

MECHANISM OF NORMAL ABSORPTION

In view of the wide range of absorption defects that can be involved, each instance of the malabsorption syndrome must be analyzed against the background of the processes of *normal* absorption. Accordingly, a brief review of the processes of normal absorption is presented at this time.

During absorption, the end products of digestion must leave the intestinal lumen, traverse the mucosal cells, enter the terminal branches of the vascular and lymphatic vessels, and thus gain entrance into the general circulation. Two mechanisms, acting separately or together, are important in this process: *active transport* and *simple diffusion*. Both of these are presumed to take place in relationship to a hypothetical cell membrane.

Simple diffusion requires no energy, and is the passage of a molecule across a membrane barrier according to chemical concentration and electrical gradients. (Examples are the absorption of fatty acids, water, and bile salts in the jejunum. *Facilitated diffusion* is like simple diffusion, in that it requires no expenditure of energy, but a carrier mechanism permits a degree of effective transport exceeding that predictable on the basis of simple diffusion alone.) *Active transport* requires metabolic work with expenditure of energy that results in a net movement of substances against a chemical or electrical difference. An important mechanism of active transport systems is the "carrier," which makes possible penetration of the cell membrane. (Examples are the absorption of Ca^{++} and Fe^{++} in the jejunum and Na^+ and bile salts in the ileum.)

Fat Absorption. *Intraluminal Phase.* Sixty to 100 grams of fat are eaten daily by adults, principally as triglycerides containing long-chain fatty acids. This triglyceride must be digested (i.e., hydrolyzed) and solubilized intraluminally before absorption. Absorption, in turn, consists of uptake and transport, both processes requiring normally functioning mucosal cells.

The stomach plays a role in fat digestion. It reduces the size of particles and, by slowly emptying its acid chyme into the duodenum, ensures not only a normal rate of absorption but also an adequate stimulation for the flow of bile and pancreatic juice. *Gastric acid* may also be important in maintaining sterility of the upper small bowel. Heavy growth of the bacterial flora in this segment interferes with fat and vitamin B_{12} absorption (see below).

The initial intraluminal event in the jejunum is hydrolysis of triglyceride into two fatty acids and a residual β monoglyceride by *pancreatic lipase;* this enzyme, contained in high concentration in secreted pancreatic juice, is activated at the alkaline pH of the upper jejunum. Bile, by its emulsifying action, also facilitates hydrolysis.

At a critical concentration, conjugated bile salts, contained in bile provided by contraction of the gallbladder, form small spheres with detergent properties. These are amphipathic molecules with a portion polar and water soluble and a portion nonpolar and fat soluble. The latter resides at the center of the sphere and solubilizes monoglycerides and fatty acids and the fat-soluble vitamins, A, D, and K. This complex is known as a micelle. Di- and triglycerides remain in an oil phase until hydrolyzed to monoglycerides and fatty acids.

Micelle formation may be impaired in several ways: *inadequate hydrolysis* of triglyceride to monoglyceride and fatty acids (as in pancreatic insufficiency); *poor mixing* of pancreatic lipase and triglyceride (after subtotal gastrectomy); or *deficiency of conjugated bile salts* (as in bacterial overgrowth, cholestatic liver disease, or biliary tract obstruction, or after resection of distal ileum).

Cellular Phase. The monoglycerides and fatty acids of micelles cross the membrane, probably by passive diffusion, but the conjugated bile salts pass into the lower small intestine, where they are actively absorbed, and return to the liver for re-excretion into bile. Normally about 95 per cent of the total bile salt pool, 4.0 grams, is reabsorbed during each enterohepatic cycle, and each day the pool is circulated four to six times. Thus only 400 to 600 mg of bile salts are lost in the feces and are normally synthesized in the liver daily.

Although exact figures are not available, a considerable amount of fat may be absorbed in the absence of bile, indicating that the process is not entirely dependent upon micelles. The question of ileal absorption of fat has not been resolved. The rate of absorption of both free fatty acids and glycerides is determined mainly by both chain length and degree of saturation of the fatty acids involved.

The major site for fat absorption is the upper jejunum. For normal function, at least 90 cm of this segment must be free of bacterial overgrowth and must contain normal villi and patent lymphatics. These are the conditions for the uptake and transport of lipid which are phases of fat absorption. Triglycerides (neutral fat) after emulsification with fatty acids and bile salts *may* be absorbed unhydrolyzed, but apparently only in small quantity. Indeed, 80 to 90 per cent of neutral fat is either partly or completely hydrolyzed.

Conjugated bile salts also help to activate intracellular enzymes, which are required for resynthesis of fatty acids and monoglyceride into triglyceride, a necessary step in chylomicron formation; although unconjugated bile salts at high concentrations may appear to inhibit uptake of lipid as well as resynthesis of triglyceride intracellularly, decreased concentration of conjugated bile salts is responsible for diminished uptake and re-esterification. In the mucosal cells, molecules of triglyceride coalesce into large particles which are then coated with small amounts of protein, cholesterol, and phospholipid, thus becoming β-lipoproteins, called chylomicrons. These exit via the base of the cells, enter the lacteals whence they pass into the mesenteric lymphatic system, the thoracic duct, and, finally, the vena cava. Long-chain fatty acids (i.e., 10 or more C atoms) undergo this process. In the mucosal cells some fatty acids are incorporated into phospholipids.

Medium-chain triglycerides, with fatty acids of length C6 to C10, are more completely hydrolyzed than long-chain triglycerides, being split at two positions with release of three medium-chain fatty acids. Also, they form micelles more readily. Thus this lipid is more readily prepared for absorption than the long-chain triglycerides. Unsplit medium-chain triglyceride also appears to be taken up by cells (30 per cent of an oral dose) and is hydrolyzed by mucosal lipase, releasing fatty acids. Further, medium-chain fatty acids pass directly into the portal venous system without re-esterification. This independence of mucosal re-esterification and of the lymphatics is thought to be advantageous in patients with intestinal mucosal disease. Obviously, medium-chain triglyceride may be extremely useful in the therapy of patients with malabsorption syndrome, and its indications and usefulness will be discussed under Treatment (see below, Table 5).

Absorption of *cholesterol* appears to depend upon its separation from protein and release from fatty acid esters through hydrolysis by pancreatic esterase. The intestine also synthesizes cholesterol as well as very low density lipoproteins. Dietary vitamin A, largely in ester form, undergoes hydrolysis in the intestinal lumen to the free alcohol. The absorption of both cholesterol and vitamin A alcohol requires bile salts. Indeed, it now seems likely that absorption of cholesterol and all fat-soluble vitamins is more dependent upon micelle formation than are the hydrolytic products of neutral fat.

Protein and Amino Acid Absorption. Gastric pepsin may partially hydrolyze dietary protein; however, this action is almost entirely due to pancreatic proteolytic endopeptidases such as *trypsin, chymotrypsin,* and *elastase. Trypsinogen,* as well as precursors of the other endopeptidases, is activated by a mucosal enzyme, *enterokinase,* released by presence of food in the duodenum. *Trypsin* is liberated and, in turn, continues to activate trypsinogen as well as the other pancreatic endopeptidases. These substances attack the interior of the protein molecules, yielding oligopeptides which are further split by exopeptidases such as *carboxypeptidase.* Neutral and basic amino acids are released, as well as small peptides, di- to hexa-, in large quantities. These peptides enter the brush border where they are hydrolyzed by peptide hydrolases; some di- and tripeptides, however, enter the cells and are split into their constituent amino acids. Indeed, amino acid absorption is greater after administration of some dipeptides than with equimolar mixtures of amino acids.

Amino acids liberated intraluminally or within the brush border are transported across the cell membrane actively, i.e., by a process which consumes energy. It is Na^+ dependent to a varying degree. Thus neutral amino acids are more dependent and basic amino acids less so. Both types, however, are absorbed rapidly. Other active carriers operate for movement of glycine (which also is transported as a neutral amino acid), hydroxyproline, and proline; and for the dicarboxylic amino acids, aspartic and glutamic. Di- and tripeptides also enter the cells by one or more transport mechanisms. Resynthesis of protein from absorbed amino acids takes place to a limited extent in the mucosa; the liver, however, is the predominant site for such synthesis.

Most amino acids pass quickly into the blood, however, and enter the general "metabolic pool." The liver is the principal organ for their metabolism.

The rate of transport of amino acids is a function of their chemical configuration. Neutral amino acids are moved most rapidly; the principal component responsible for this rapidity is an intact carboxyl group attached to the α carbon, and affinity for an amino acid carrier is enhanced when the α NH_2 is intact and the side chain ("R" substituent) is nonpolar.

Carbohydrate Absorption. Dietary carbohydrate consists of starch and two disaccharides, sucrose and lactose. Amylose and amylopectin are the principal starches—long chains of connected (C_1-C_4) glucose molecules which are split in the duodenum by pancreatic amylase at these 1 to 4 α glucose-glucose linkages. Amylose is cleaved to yield maltose and maltotriose; amylopectin, however, yields molecules, α-limit dextrins, containing some branch points (C_6-C_1) present sequentially in amylopectin which are not split by the enzyme.

Maltose, maltotriose, α-limit dextrins, and other dietary disaccharides, sucrose and lactose, are split further by specific brush border *disaccharidases* into their component hexoses: glucose-glucose, glucose-fructose, and glucose-galactose, respectively.

The rate of absorption of hexoses in descending order is galactose, glucose, fructose. Glucose and galactose are actively transported, and fructose, whose absorption was thought to be "facilitated" by a poorly understood carrier, now appears also to be actively transported. Xylose shares the same transport system with glucose and galactose but not so avidly.

The exact mechanism of transport has not been elucidated. It is clear, however, that phosphorylation plays no role. Transport of glucose and galactose depends upon a process requiring both energy and Na^+. Possibly glucose and Na^+ bind to a carrier protein in the microvilli, and thus glucose moves into the cell. Na^+ then moves out of the cell via the so-called "Na^+ pump" mechanism. Na^+ also increases cellular permeability for glucose, although glucose may be transported at low concentrations of Na^+.

Vitamin B_{12} Absorption. Vitamin B_{12} absorption is dependent upon the presence of intrinsic factor, a glycoprotein (50,000 to 60,000 m.w.) contained in gastric juice. Vitamin B_{12} is bound to intrinsic factor, and the complex in turn is bound to a specific ileal receptor. In some unknown manner, after several hours, vitamin B_{12} becomes "unbound" and passes into the blood. Whether uptake is energy dependent is not settled. Calcium ion is required for uptake of the vitamin B_{12}–intrinsic factor complex as well as a substance in pancreatic juice which somehow facilitates its absorption. Alterations in bacterial flora, such as are observed in the bacterial overgrowth syndrome (see below), lead to decreased absorption of vitamin B_{12} that, in most instances, can be reversed by the administration of broad-spectrum antimicrobial drugs. In some manner these bacteria bind the vitamin B_{12}.

Folic Acid Absorption. Dietary folic acid is in the form of polyglutamate conjugates of pteroylglutamic acid. About 1000 μg, as contained in yeast, liver, and green vegetables, is ingested daily in the Western world. The conjugated substance is water soluble and may be transported by *facilitated diffusion.* The glutamic acid residues are sequentially cleaved in the mucosal cell, yielding biologically active mono- and difolates. These forms of pteroylglutamic acid are then methylated within the mucosa, and the methylated folates, which are active forms, pass into the general circulation.

Water and Electrolyte Absorption. Water and electrolyte absorption takes place in the small intestine. *Water* moves across the membrane passively, i.e., secondary to osmotic gradients. However, under certain circumstances it can move against a gradient without requiring energy. The rate of water absorption in the small gut is five to ten times that in the stomach. To some extent, also, water follows the active transport of glucose and electrolytes, moving with them to maintain isotonicity of intraluminal contents. The small intestine usually absorbs over 7 liters of water per day.

Sodium absorption is an active process and is linked to an exchange with H^+ in both jejunum and ileum. A similar exchange mechanism for Cl' and HCO_3' exists only in the ileum. The sites of these exchanges in the cell are not known, but the exchanges are certainly mediated by carriers. It is also believed from in vitro studies that an Na^+ pump mechanism may be operative. In man, Na^+ transport is enhanced by absorption of glucose in the jejunum, either via this mechanism or by being "dragged" into the cell by the water in which glucose is carried. Some Na^+ also moves passively, i.e., down a gradient across the mucosa. Potassium movement seems to be passive, diffusing from the lumen proximally and into the lumen distally.

The amount of water and sodium absorbed represents the difference between influx from lumen to blood and efflux in the reverse direction. This net flux is diminished by hypertonicity of the intraluminal solution and is increased by hypotonicity. Changes in concentration of sodium in the lumen depend on relative rates of exchange of both sodium and water between blood and lumen.

During diarrhea, sodium concentration increases with increasing stool volume, and beyond 3 liters approaches values close to that of plasma. Conversely, potassium concentration progressively decreases.

Calcium and Iron Absorption. Calcium is absorbed actively in the duodenum. This transport is facilitated by *parathyroid hormone* and by *vitamin D,* and is inhibited by deprivation of this vitamin. The active form of vitamin D involved in the process is a kidney metabolite, *1,25-dihydroxycholecalciferol.* In vivo calcium absorption depends also upon pH and concentration of phosphates and fatty acids. Vitamin D absorption is necessary for calcium absorption, because 1,25-dihydroxycholecalciferol stimulates synthesis of a calcium-binding protein which is a key substance in the active transport of the cation. 1,25-dihydroxycholecalciferol also stimulates Na^+ dependent ATP-ase to release calcium from its binder in the cell.

Iron, 0.5 to 1.0 mg daily, is absorbed *actively,* in an amount sufficient for normal hematopoiesis and five to eight times this amount in people who are iron deficient. Absorption is a two-step process, principally in the duodenum, of uptake and transfer; the former is dependent upon oxidative metabolism. The latter, probably the rate-limit step, involves movement of Fe through the serosa to the circulation where it is bound to a globulin, *transferrin,* which transports it to tissues, particularly the liver. Iron absorption is diminished in chronic infection and by prior administration of large amounts of iron, and apparently is increased in pregnancy as well as iron deficiency. Animal hemoglobin is an important source of iron in the human, and is absorbed most rapidly, followed by Fe^{++}, then Fe^{+++}. After ingestion, hemoglobin is split in the upper gut; heme is readily absorbed, from which iron is split within the cell and passes thence into the circulation where it is bound by iron-binding protein. Some iron is released from heme intraluminally and is taken up directly by the cells.

In human subjects, absorption of inorganic iron depends upon its release from dietary compounds to which it is originally bound. Absorption of both Fe^{+++} and Fe^{++} is enhanced by chelation with ascorbic acid, carbohydrates, and amino acids at the pH of normal gastric juice.

These complexes remain soluble at the alkaline pH of the duodenum where iron is absorbed. Diminished iron absorption is associated with achlorhydria, because an acid pH is needed to solubilize ferric iron for chelation with ascorbic acid and other substances, in which form it is absorbed. Ferrous iron may also, however, be chelated at an alkaline pH. Over-all, iron absorption is regulated by the state of repletion, content of iron in absorbing cells, and factors affecting erythropoiesis. The influence of gastric and pancreatic juice proteins which bind iron is still uncertain.

CAUSES OF THE MALABSORPTION SYNDROME

The principal diseases and disorders that may give rise to the malabsorption syndrome are listed in Table 1. These conditions are discussed in detail in a subsequent portion of this section and are presented only in brief outline at this point. They can be divided conveniently into seven categories, based upon pathologic and pathophysiologic considerations.

CLINICAL MANIFESTATIONS

The signs and symptoms of the malabsorption syndrome include weight loss, anorexia, abdominal distention, borborygmi, muscle wasting, and passage of abnormal stools that are characteristically light yellow to gray, greasy, and soft. In many instances frequent movements are noted, but occasionally there is only one stool per day. In addition, edema, ascites, skeletal disorders, peripheral and circumoral paresthesias, tetany, and, rarely, convulsions may be observed.

The clinical features that result from deficiencies of fat-soluble vitamins include hyperkeratosis follicularis (vitamin A); bleeding, particularly ecchymoses and hematuria (vitamin K); and bone pain or fractures (vitamin D) (Table 2). Deficiencies of the vitamin B complex are manifested by glossitis, cheilosis, muscle tenderness, peripheral neuritis, and dermatitis (Table 2). The symptoms of the malabsorption syndrome may be intermittent or low grade, so that medical attention is not sought for a very long time—more than 35 years in some instances of adult celiac disease. Unfortunately, many of these patients whose malabsorption is mild escape diagnosis and suffer subtle changes for years. They do not exhibit obvious manifestations of malabsorption; they are chronically fatigued, lack drive, and may have symptoms of chronic depression. Further, they may lose weight only during the early months of illness and then will stabilize at a lower level.

In those with more severe malabsorption, the secondary manifestations may often overshadow the intestinal complaints. For example, about 20 per cent of patients with *adult celiac disease* will seek aid for bleeding or for skeletal pain or fractures. In many patients, weakness, fatigue, dyspnea, or dizziness, all caused by anemia, may be the presenting symptoms. Borborygmi and abdominal distention, which increase during the day and are often not relieved by defecation, are among the most common complaints. An extreme degree of such distress is frequently noted in patients with *scleroderma* of the small intestine.

Cramping lower abdominal pain is noted in a large number of diseases of malabsorption, usually preceding loose bowel movements, and thus does not distinguish between the various entities. Persistent or severe cramping pain, periumbilical or right lower quadrant, not relieved by movements is frequently seen in patients with *Crohn's disease* and, with stricturing and obstruction, may become chronic and associated with distention and emesis. Diffuse periumbilical pain is often suffered by patients with *nongranulomatous ileojejunitis, lymphoma, eosinophilic gastroenteritis, radiation enteritis, amyloidosis,* and, occasionally, *adult celiac disease*. Patients with *chronic pancreatitis* usually suffer recurrent deep epigastric pain that radiates to the midback; in patients with *lymphoma* of the small intestine and mesentery, the pain may be cramping (obstruction) or steady and intense (local invasion or spread).

Patients with malabsorption owing to *ischemia* of the small gut often also have periumbilical or midabdominal cramping pains 20 to 30 minutes after meals and often other evidence of widespread arteriosclerosis, or have

TABLE 1.   Classification of Malabsorption Syndrome

I. Category 1: Defective Intraluminal Hydrolysis or Solubilization
   A. Primary pancreatic insufficiency
   B. Secondary pancreatic insufficiency
   C. Deficiency of conjugated bile salts
   D. Bacterial overgrowth (bile salt deconjugation)
      1. Blind loops
      2. Multiple strictures and jejunal diverticula
      3. Fistulas
      4. Postgastrectomy
      5. Scleroderma and pseudo-obstruction
II. Category 2: Mucosal Cell Abnormality and Inadequate Surface
   A. Primary mucosal cell disorders
      1. Disaccharidase deficiency and monosaccharide malabsorption
      2. A-beta-lipoproteinemia
      3. Vitamin B_{12} malabsorption
      4. Cystinuria and Hartnup disease
   B. Small bowel disease
      1. Celiac disease
      2. Whipple's disease
      3. Nongranulomatous ileojejunitis
      4. Allergic and eosinophilic gastroenteritis
      5. Amyloidosis
      6. Small bowel ischemia
      7. Crohn's disease (granulomatous enteritis)
   C. Inadequate surface
III. Category 3: Lymphatic Obstruction
   A. Lymphoma
   B. Tuberculosis and tuberculous lymphadenitis
   C. Lymphangiectasia
IV. Category 4: Infection
   A. Tropical sprue
   B. Acute infectious enteritis
   C. Parasitoses
V. Category 5: Multiple Defects
   A. Subtotal gastrectomy
   B. Distal ileal resection, disease, or bypass
   C. Radiation enteritis
VI. Category 6: Unexplained
   A. Hypogammaglobulinemia
   B. Carcinoid syndrome
   C. Hypothyroidism
   D. Diabetes mellitus
   E. Mastocytosis
   F. Hyperthyroidism and hypoadrenocorticism
VII. Category 7: Drug-Induced Malabsorption
   A. Cholestyramine
   B. Colchicine
   C. Irritant laxatives
   D. Neomycin
   E. p-Amino salicylic acid
   F. Phenindione

TABLE 2. Correlation of Laboratory Data with Absorptive Defects and
Signs and Symptoms of the Malabsorption Syndrome

Clinical Features	Laboratory Evidence	Pathophysiology
Muscle wasting; small stature; edema	↓ Serum albumin	*Impaired protein metabolism* ↓ Absorption ↓ Intake
Skeletal deformity; pain fractures	X-ray: demineralization; collapsed vertebrae	↑ Enteric loss ?Impaired synthesis
Weight loss; pale, bulky stools	↑ Fecal fat ↓ Serum cholesterol, carotene	*Impaired absorption and excess loss of:* Fat
Paresthesias; tetany; + Chvostek; Trousseau; bone pain; fractures	↓ Serum Ca^{++}; ↓ or normal PO_4'''; ↑ alkaline phosphatase; x-ray: Looser's lines, Milkman's fractures; ↑ osteoid seams; ↓ serum Mg^{++}	Fat-soluble vitamins and calcium Vitamin D, calcium, magnesium
Bleeding: ecchymoses, hematuria	↑ Prothrombin time with response to vitamin K	Vitamin K
Hyperkeratosis follicularis	↓ Serum carotene, vitamin A tolerance	Vitamin A
(ANEMIAS / GLOSSITIS) Paresthesias; neuropathy	Macrocytic anemia; megaloblastosis; ↓ serum B_{12} and ↓ absorption B_{12}	Vitamin B_{12}
	Macrocytic anemia; megaloblastosis; ↓ serum folic acid	Folic acid
Koilonychia	Microcystosis, hypochromia; ↓ serum iron and ↓ saturation iron binding protein; ↓ iron in marrow	Iron
Dehydration; nocturia	↓ Plasma volume	Water
Muscle cramps, weakness	↓ Serum Na^+	Sodium
Muscle flaccidity, weakness; ↓ tendon reflexes, arrhythmias	↓ Serum K^+; EKG abnormalities	Potassium
Cheilosis; neuritis; dermatitis, glossitis; muscle weakness	↑ Urinary I3AA, Indican; ↓ serum B_{12}, folic acid	Vitamin B complex; folic acid vitamin B_{12}
Abdominal distention, flatulence; diarrhea	Low to flat oral glucose tolerance curve; ↓ absorption d-xylose; ↓ oral lactose tolerance; ↓ or absent rise of blood glucose after oral sucrose; ↓ or absent rise of blood reducing substances after oral galactose; fluid levels on x-ray; stools: acid pH, + Clinitest	Impaired hydrolysis of disaccharides, particularly lactose and sucrose, or ↓ absorption of monosaccharides and amino acids

chronic atrial fibrillation. Those with *hypogammaglobulinemia* may have other historic evidences of immunoglobulin deficiency (repeated infections, or even symptoms suggesting malignancy). *Eosinophilic gastroenteritis* may be highlighted by a specific "food allergy" or by a history of skin, nasopharyngeal, bronchial, or other allergy. Virulent peptic ulcer disease *(Zollinger-Ellison syndrome)* will usually highlight the history of malabsorption caused by gastric hypersecretion. Diarrhea associated with carbohydrate will be noted from childhood in those with *disaccharidase deficiency* or *monosaccharide malabsorption.* Surgical scars and associated histories will highlight cases of *massive resection, gastrectomy* and *ileal resection, bypass procedures,* and *blind loops.* Those with *enteroenteric* or *enterocolic fistulas* as well as have a long history of inflammatory disease, usually Crohn's disease, or malignancy. Hepatobiliary tract disorders will have features of chronic obstruction of the common bile duct or of chronic intrahepatic disease.

Physical examination may reveal low blood pressure and evidences of malnutrition and multiple vitamin deficiencies: pallor, diffuse brownish pigmentation of the skin but not of the mucous membranes, hyperkeratosis, petechiae or ecchymoses, muscle wasting, edema, abdominal distention, skeletal deformity (particularly kyphosis), positive Chvostek and/or Trousseau signs, glossitis, cheilosis, impaired vibration sense, deep muscle pain, and clubbing of the fingers. In additions, signs of various underlying diseases may be noted: an abdominal mass *(lymphoma, regional enteritis);* fixation or severe limitation of joint movement and thickened skin *(scleroderma);* facial flush and hepatomegaly *(carcinoid syndrome);* puffed facies, bradycardia, and hair loss

(hypothyroidism); proptosis, thyromegaly, tachycardia, and tremor *(hyperthyroidism);* arthritis or skin rashes *(hypogammaglobulinemia)*; nasopharyngeal congestion, skin rash, and wheezing *(eosinophilic gastroenteritis);* butterfly rash and splenomegaly (systemic lupus erythematosus); neurologic impairments *(abetalipoproteinemia);* diminished or absent peripheral arterial pulsations, skin lesions (particularly dermatitis herpetiformis), cataracts, and absent or diminished deep tendon reflexes or other evidences of diabetic neuropathy or retinopathy *(diabetes mellitus);* lymphadenopathy, arthritis, and signs of pulmonary disease *(Whipple's disease);* enlarged tongue and hepatosplenomegaly *(amyloidosis);* urticaria pigmentosa, flushing, pruritus *(mastocytosis).*

The malabsorption syndrome may be fatal, owing to the nature of the underlying disease *(lymphoma, pancreatic carcinoma, progressive scleroderma,* or *granulomatous enteritis)* or to the complications of malabsorption, which include superimposed infection, hypokalemia, or progressive inanition.

PATHOPHYSIOLOGIC BASIS FOR CLINICAL MANIFESTATIONS

In Table 2 may be seen the correlation between various absorptive defects and vitamin deficiencies, the clinical signs and symptoms, and the abnormalities of the routine laboratory tests in the malabsorption syndrome. Rarely does a patient manifest all the findings listed in Table 2, but many patients will exhibit many of them.

Impaired Protein Metabolism: Weight Loss, Edema. Protein metabolism, reflected by decreased muscle mass and lowered serum protein levels, is impaired for several reasons. Synthesis is below normal owing to defective protein absorption. Catabolism or breakdown is accelerated because of inadequate intake and absorption of carbohydrate. Decreased serum albumin may result also from abnormal loss of protein into the lumen of the gut, so-called *protein-losing enteropathy*. Such loss is usually associated with diseases that cause malabsorption by lymphatic obstruction or in which there is an inflammatory mucosal lesion, although it has also been reported in *adult celiac disease* (see below). *Hypogammaglobulinemia*, both congenital and acquired, has also been associated with steatorrhea, but the defective fat absorption cannot be related directly to low plasma globulins. In some instances, impaired hepatic function contributes to lowered serum protein levels.

The emaciation and weakness may be extreme (Fig. 1). The finding of hypotension and diffuse pigmentation makes the picture closely resemble severe *adrenal cortical insufficiency*. Hypokalemia as well as partial atrophy may underlie muscle weakness.

Clinical Effects of Steatorrhea. Excess loss of fat in the stool deprives the body of substantial numbers of calories and contributes greatly to weight loss and malnutrition. Perhaps the irritative effect of unabsorbed long-chain (C18) fatty acids which are hydroxylated contributes to the diarrhea with its severe losses of water, electrolytes, and other nutrients. In addition, binding of calcium by fatty acids contributes to hypocalcemia. Flatulence, fluid in loops of small intestine, and abdominal distention may be related to both diminished fat absorption and excessive carbohydrate fermentation. Failure to absorb fat-soluble vitamins A, D, and K also results in a variety of serious symptoms as recorded in Table 2.

Vitamin D Deficiency: Hypocalcemia and Skeletal Disease in Malabsorption Syndrome; Hypomagnesemia. Low serum calcium results from failure of normal absorption owing both to vitamin D deficiency and to chelation of calcium by unabsorbed fatty acids. Symptoms caused by depression of unbound or "ultrafilterable" calcium of the blood range from paresthesias of extremities and circumoral area to carpopedal and laryngeal spasms and muscle cramps. When levels are extremely low, the patient may even convulse. Clinically, hypocalcemia may be demonstrated by *Chvostek* or *Trousseau signs*. Obviously, the defect in calcium absorption involves more than deficiency of vitamin D, particularly its metabolite, 1,25-dihydroxycholecalciferol, active in calcium absorption, because the return of serum calcium to normal in

patients with adult celiac disease who are on a gluten-free diet is more rapid than may be attributed to the action of this vitamin.

Low levels of serum calcium stimulate parathyroid activity. Increased secretion of parathormone raises the level of blood calcium both by direct effect upon bone and by a renal mechanism. These processes lead to demineralization — *osteomalacia*. Osteomalacia principally affects the spine, rib cage, and long bones, with or without fractures (Milkman's fractures), and may cause extreme pain and disability.

In patients with poor protein nutrition, in part caused by malabsorption or protein-losing enteropathy (see below), particularly postmenopausal women and elderly men, the demineralization process is aggravated by *osteoporosis* or failure to deposit bone matrix.

Hypomagnesemia may also be noted in the malabsorption syndrome, causing symptoms that are identical with those of hypocalcemia. Differentiation is accomplished by the finding of lowered serum magnesium and by disappearance of symptoms only after administration of magnesium chloride or sulfate. Hypomagnesemia may also dramatically reduce the responsiveness of the parathyroids to hypocalcemia. Indeed, correction of magnesium deficiency may be essential to restoration of normal calcium by action of the parathyroid glands.

Vitamin K Deficiency: Bleeding Diathesis in Malabsorption Syndrome. As noted, *bleeding*, particularly subcutaneous, nasal, urinary, vaginal, and occasionally, gastrointestinal, is not uncommon in the malabsorption syndrome and may be the principal symptom. Defects in coagulation result from deficiency of plasma prothrombin owing to impaired absorption of fat-soluble vitamin K.

Vitamin A Deficiency. In the malabsorption syndrome *hyperkeratosis follicularis* may be noted, but *nyctalopia* is very rare.

Manifestations of Abnormal Carbohydrate Absorption. The abnormal carbohydrate absorption results in diminished glycogen stores in liver and muscle. Also, intraluminal fermentation of sugars contributes greatly to abdominal distention and flatulence. Failure to hydrolyze disaccharides, particularly lactose (*disaccharidase deficiency*), results in watery diarrhea as well as these local abdominal complaints (see below).

Anemia. Deficiency of vitamin B_{12} or folic acid may cause a macrocytic anemia with a megaloblastic bone marrow, whereas iron deficiency will cause a microcytic hypochromic anemia. With deficiency of vitamin B_{12}, folic acid, and iron, anemia with mixed features will be present. The former type is seen in *tropical sprue,* after *resection* of, or *disease* in, a large segment of the *terminal ileum;* rarely, in pancreatic insufficiency; in "*primary*" *malabsorption* of *vitamin* B_{12} (defective ileal receptor); and in conditions in which there is bacterial overgrowth in the upper small intestine — "*blind loops,*" *jejunal diverticulosis, enteroenteric* or *enterocolic fistulas,* and *multiple small bowel strictures.* In contrast to pernicious anemia, in these conditions simultaneous feeding of intrinsic factor does not improve vitamin B_{12} absorption. In those cases caused by bacterial overgrowth as well as in tropical sprue, normal absorption of vitamin B_{12} may be restored by oral administration of a broad-spectrum antimicrobial drug — tetracycline, oxytetracycline, or ampicillin (1.0 gram daily) for 10 to 14 days (Table 3). Indeed, a brisk reticulocytosis may be noted in three to four days. Impaired absorption of vitamin B_{12} and mega-

Figure 1. Extreme wasting in a patient with adult celiac disease (nontropical sprue).

TABLE 3. ^{60}Co-Vitamin B$_{12}$ Absorption (Schilling)

Result after:	Pernicious Anemia and Total Gastrectomy	Megaloblastic Anemia Associated with:				
		Adult Celiac Disease*	Blind Loop Syndrome	Primary Malabsorption of Vitamin B$_{12}$	Tropical Sprue	Pancreatic Insufficiency*
	... Absorption ...					
Vitamin B$_{12}$	Low	Low-normal or low	Low	Low	No change	Normal-low†
Vitamin B$_{12}$ + intrinsic factor	Normal	No change	No change	No change	No change	No change
Vitamin B$_{12}$ after antimicrobial therapy	Low	No change	Normal	No change	Normal or low	No change
Vitamin B$_{12}$ after gluten-free diet	No change	Normal	No change	No change	No change	No change
Vitamin B$_{12}$ + bicarbonate	No change	No change	No change	No change	No change	Normal‡
Vitamin B$_{12}$ + pancreatic extract	No change	No change	No change	No change	No change	Normal‡

*Rare in adult celiac disease; very rare in pancreatic insufficiency.
†Rare to be low.
‡Very rare.

loblastosis may also be noted occasionally in patients with *adult celiac disease.*

Folic Acid Deficiency.   Folic acid deficiency may also underlie *megaloblastosis* and *anemia.* As there is often an associated deficiency of vitamin B$_{12}$, diagnosis may be established only by the finding of low serum folic acid levels (less than 5.0 ng), or of a reticulocytic response to administration of minimal daily effective dosage (0.05 to 0.5 mg parenterally). Usually, however, folic acid deficiency is corrected by adequate diet or oral supplementation.

Glossitis and Peripheral Neuropathy.   *Glossitis* and *peripheral neuropathy* can in part be attributed to deficiency of vitamin B$_{12}$. Since combined system disease may be induced or exacerbated by administration of folic acid, *vitamin B$_{12}$ stores in tissues must be replenished before administration of folic acid alone for megaloblastic anemia.*

Impaired Iron Absorption.   Iron absorption may be subnormal except when the malabsorption syndrome is due to uncomplicated pancreatic insufficiency. Most often the iron deficiency is caused by poor absorption owing either to mucosal disease or to inability to release inorganic iron from organic compounds. However, occult blood loss may contribute to the anemia. Iron deficiency anemia is very common in *adult celiac disease* and may be noted also in the later stages of *tropical sprue.* When associated with deficiencies of folic acid and vitamin B$_{12}$, iron deficiency may not become apparent until these substances are repleted. Incorporation of iron into young marrow red blood cells requires both folic acid and vitamin B$_{12}$.

Diminished Absorption of Water and Electrolytes.   Common in the malabsorption syndrome are *dehydration, weakness,* and *hypotension.* Large amounts of water and electrolytes are lost if diarrhea is severe or if stools are very loose or bulky. Absorption of water in adult celiac disease is slower than normal, and diuresis after a water load is delayed. Thus patients with steatorrhea often have nocturia. *Hyponatremia* not caused by renal loss responds readily to administration of sodium, and symptoms of "low salt"—weakness, lethargy, nausea, cramps—rapidly disappear. *Hypokalemia,* if severe, causes muscle flaccidity and cardiac arrhythmias.

Vitamin B Complex Deficiency: Dermatitis, Neuritis, and Cheilosis.   Although *glossitis, neuritis* (peripheral neuropathy), and *dermatitis* in the malabsorption syndrome have been attributed to deficiency of B vitamins, proof of impaired absorption of these substances (vita-

mins B$_1$, B$_2$, and B$_6$) is not at hand. Perhaps deficiency results from metabolic action of abnormal bacterial flora that ordinarily do not inhabit the small bowel. However, conclusive demonstration of this mechanism also is lacking, particularly in *adult celiac disease.* Moreover, administration of vitamin B complex (B$_{1, 2, 6, 12}$) does not always cure the glossitis, which may be partially due to iron deficiency.

DIAGNOSIS

Although the spectrum of clinical symptoms and signs of malabsorption syndrome is broad, those with mild chronic illness display one or more important clinical or laboratory abnormalities. A high index of suspicion of the diagnosis is essential for those with minimal complaints and seemingly normal-appearing stools. Unfortunately, there is no short cut to diagnosis of the syndrome and, equally important, of its underlying cause.

The clues to diagnosis of the malabsorption syndrome are the history, symptoms, signs, and laboratory abnormalities listed in Tables 2 and 3 that relate to malabsorption of fat and other substances, particularly fat-soluble vitamins, proteins, iron, and vitamin B$_{12}$. The average patient will complain of rather bulky, light-colored stools, often with increased frequency (but not necessarily so), abdominal distention, and variable weight loss, and will also show laboratory evidence of impaired absorption. However, special diagnostic attention must be tendered those with subtler histories and findings and especially those who complain principally of bleeding tendency or of some skeletal disability, chiefly pain. Other features commonly seen in many diseases of this syndrome include *hypotension, abdominal distention, diffuse brownish pigmentation,* and *clubbing* of the fingers and toes.

It is not usually difficult to establish solely by clinical examination that the malabsorption syndrome is present. Much more precise information as to *which* absorption defects are present is necessary, however, if the physician is to treat the illness successfully. In large measure, this essential information can be obtained only by the proper use of a number of laboratory procedures.

Laboratory Diagnosis

The pathophysiologic basis for the abnormal findings of the laboratory tests has been described and is presented in Table 2. The particular values of the individual tests in arriving at a diagnosis are considered in Table 4. The essential diagnostic tests, excluding routine blood studies (complete blood count, determination of Ca^{++}, K^+, and prothrombin time), include measurement of 72-hour stool fat and serum carotene, d-xylose absorption, tests of pancreatic function, tests for bacterial overgrowth, roentgenographic study of the small bowel, vitamin B_{12} absorption, and biopsy of the small intestine.

Measurement of Stool Fat: Serum Carotene. Because the most important feature in diagnosis of the malabsorption syndrome is steatorrhea, accurate measurement of fecal fat is extremely important. The only reliable method is the chemical analysis of a 72-hour stool collection, the patient ingesting 80 to 100 grams of fat per day. Normal excretion in these circumstances is 6.0 grams or less per 24 hours (Table 4).

This test is essential for diagnosis, because only in the so-called primary mucosal cell abnormalities (except for abetalipoproteinemia) is fat absorption normal (Table 1). Steatorrhea, however, does not indicate into which category of malabsorptive disorders the patient falls. If fecal fat is elevated, a roentgenographic study of the small intestine as well as a d-xylose test must be performed. Increasingly, small bowel biopsy is being done routinely if pancreatic disease is unlikely. Finally, determinations which reflect bacterial overgrowth (intestinal stasis) are required either when the roentgenographic

studies display a *blind loop, jejunal diverticula, strictures, enteroenteric* or *enterocolic fistula,* or the marked intestinal stasis of *scleroderma,* or when the biopsy is normal.

Depressed levels of serum carotene will usually be found in patients with steatorrhea. This test is useful in "screening" those in whom the malabsorption syndrome is suspected.

d-Xylose Absorption (Table 4). During recent years, absorption of d-xylose, a pentose, has been measured in the study of malabsorption. Twenty-five grams is given orally; if the patient does not vomit, has no delay in gastric emptying, is well hydrated, and has normal kidney function, 4.5 grams or more will be excreted in a five-hour collection of urine. It is absorbed actively like glucose, but its metabolism is not as rapid as that of glucose, and its renal excretion does not depend upon a threshold. As a measure of carbohydrate absorption, it is more reliable than an oral glucose tolerance test. In patients over 60, renal excretion diminishes; in such individuals, as well as in patients with delayed gastric emptying, liver disease with ascites, or renal disease, blood levels are measured and should reach 20 mg per 100 ml in two hours.

Although the fate of about half of the 50 per cent of the 25.0 gram oral load which is absorbed normally is unknown, it is clear that excretion in five hours is significantly diminished (less than 3.0 grams) with intestinal

TABLE 4. Laboratory Tests Commonly Employed to Study Malabsorption

	Normal Values	Malabsorption Syndrome*
Serum:		
Albumin	4.0 to 5.2 grams/100 ml	Diminished
Carotene	0.06 to 0.4 mg/100 ml	Diminished, particularly in small bowel disease
Calcium	9.0 to 10.5 mg/100 ml	Diminished, particularly in small bowel disease
Cholesterol	150 to 250 mg/100 ml	Diminished
Potassium	3.5 to 4.7 mEq/L	Diminished
Magnesium	1.7 to 2.0 mEq/L	Diminished
Vitamin B_{12}	100 to 700 $\mu\mu g$/ml	Diminished, particularly in tropical sprue and bacterial overgrowth
Folic Acid	5 to 21 ng/ml	Diminished, particularly in small bowel disease
Plasma:		
Prothrombin time	Control value	Elevated
Tolerance tests:		
d-Xylose (25 grams orally)	Urinary excretion of 4.5 grams or greater per 5 hours	Diminished in diseases of the mucosa, particularly celiac disease, and in intestinal stasis (normal in pancreatic insufficiency)
Glucose (100 grams orally)	35 mg over fasting plasma level	"Flat curve" in celiac disease and diseases of intestinal wall and in monosaccharide malabsorption
Lactose (50 to 100 grams orally) (2.0 grams/kg in children)	Rise in blood glucose of 20 mg/100 ml	Low to flat curve in primary lactose deficiency, celiac disease, and diseases of the intestinal wall
Sucrose (100 grams orally)	Rise in blood glucose of 20 mg/100 ml	Low to flat in celiac disease and disease of intestinal wall
Vitamin B_{12} (μc ^{60}CO B_{12})	> 7% urine excretion/24 hours	Decreased with intestinal stasis, ileal dysfunction, or resection
Stool fat:		
Chemical determination (80–100 grams fat daily)	< 6 grams/24 hours	Increased
Miscellaneous:		
5-Hydroxyindolacetic acid (urinary excretion)	1.7 to 8.0 mg/24 hours	9 to 20 mg in adult celiac disease; 30 to 600 mg in metastatic carcinoid syndrome
Indole-3-acetic acid (urinary excretion)	Less than 18 mg/24 hours	
Indican (urinary excretion)	Minute amounts of $^{14}CO_2$/4 to 8 hours	Elevated in bacterial overgrowth and ileal dysfunction
Bile acid breath test		

*Usual findings. Some values for serum tests may be normal in some patients, e.g., carotene, calcium, and vitamin B_{12} in pancreatic insufficiency and calcium in tropical sprue.

disease affecting particularly the *jejunum,* after *massive resection,* and in marked *bacterial overgrowth,* presumably owing to bacterial action. The procedure thus serves to separate these patients from those with pancreatic insufficiency and from normal subjects. d-Xylose absorption has occasionally been found to be abnormal in *pancreatic carcinoma* with metastatic involvement of the small intestine.

Normal d-xylose absorption is strong evidence against the diagnosis of *adult celiac disease.* An abnormal result, however, casts strong doubt upon the diagnosis of *pancreatic insufficiency.* The test is also valuable in gauging the effect of therapy when pretreatment values have been low.

Pancreatic Function.   Evaluation of pancreatic function by measurement of volume and bicarbonate concentration of duodenal aspirates after appropriate stimulation or concentration of enzymes after a test meal is in order if the d-xylose test is normal and roentgenographic study of the small intestine is normal or equivocally so. It is clearly indicated if biopsy is normal and there is no other apparent disease or disorder. Subnormal response strongly indicates pancreatic insufficiency or pancreatic ductal obstruction, although normal values do not exclude these possibilities.

Tests for Bacterial Overgrowth.   The increasing clinical importance of bacterial overgrowth as a cause for malabsorption syndrome has stimulated development of tests which directly and indirectly indicate the presence of this condition. It may be present in a large number of diseases in which there is either small bowel stasis or contamination by lower gut organisms. These tests include the *bile salt breath test,* measurement of *urinary tryptophan metabolites,* and direct *culture* of jejunal aspirates.

Bile Salt Breath Test.   The recent introduction of the so-called "bile salt breath test" promises to be enormously helpful in diagnosis of malabsorption caused by diseases or disorders in which bile salt deconjugation is abnormal. These include diseases of bacterial overgrowth and ileal dysfunction (diseased or absent long segment of terminal ileum). In either situation, bacteria (small intestinal in the former situation and colonic in the latter) will deconjugate a significant amount of orally administered ^{14}C glycine-cholate before it is absorbed; the released ^{14}C glycine will be further metabolized by bacterial enzymes to $^{14}CO_2$ which quickly diffuses into the circulation and is breathed out. Normally, only a minute quantity of $^{14}CO_2$ is detectable in four to six hours; however, when bacteria are present in the small gut or bile salt reabsorption by the terminal ileum is subnormal, $^{14}CO_2$ excretion in breath is elevated tenfold or more after ingestion of ^{14}C glycine-cholate.

Tryptophan Metabolites.   The measurement of two urinary metabolites of L-tryptophan, indican and 5-hydroxyindolacetic acid (50HIAA), has been valuable in diagnosis of diseases of bacterial overgrowth and of ileal dysfunction (diseased, bypassed or absent terminal ileum) and of adult celiac disease. Elevated urinary levels of indoxylsulfate (indican) are found in virtually all diseases in which intestinal stasis is present or the terminal ileum is diseased or absent (greater than 100 mg per 24 hours). Return toward normal values may follow administration of broad-spectrum antimicrobials over a one- to two-week period.

The normal range of 5-hydroxyindolacetic acid is up to about 8.0 mg per 24 hours. In *adult celiac disease,* however, the urinary level is elevated — 9.0 to 15.0 mg — reflecting perhaps an increased amount of circulating 5-hydroxytryptamine or serotonin. Treatment with a gluten-free diet restores normal excretion of this substance. Except for the metastatic *carcinoid* syndrome, in which levels are greatly elevated (300 to 500 mg per 24 hours), or *Whipple's disease,* in which an elevated level (15 mg per 24 hours) has been reported in several instances, excretion of this substance is usually normal in the various disorders which may cause the malabsorption syndrome.

The significance of these findings is not clear, but they indicate abnormal metabolism of tryptophan. Most likely this is related in some way to stasis and bacterial overgrowth, but also, as shown by appropriate loading tests with tryptophan, to a deficiency in vitamin B_6, which is necessary for its normal metabolism. The role of indolacetic acid in the pathophysiology of the malabsorption is not known, but there is evidence that it may have a suppressant effect upon the bone marrow.

Culture of Jejunal Aspirates.   Techniques for culture of jejunal aspirates for fastidious anaerobic bacteria (clostridia, fusiforms, bacteroides) are increasingly available for diagnosis of intestinal stasis (bacterial overgrowth). Usually, the upper small intestine appears bacteria free in about one third of normal subjects; in the remainder, gram-positive or facultative anaerobes are present (lactobacilli and enterococci) in concentrations of 10^1 to 10^3 organisms per gram of content. Coliforms may be transiently present but rarely exceed 10^3. Normally, the terminal ileum has concentrations of organisms approaching 10^5 to 10^8 per gram, and these include gram-negative coliforms and bacteroides. In the colon enormous concentrations of anaerobes — bacteroides, lactobacilli, and clostridia — are usually present. When these organisms, particularly bacteroides and lactobacilli (but also clostridia and coliforms), luxuriate in the small intestine, the so-called bacterial overgrowth syndrome results (see Bacterial Overgrowth).

Figure 2. Small bowel series showing postoperative terminal ileum (arrow on left) and ileotransverse colostomy stoma (between arrows on right). Note the blind loop.

Figure 3. Small bowel roentgenographic series in patient (M.S.) with adult celiac disease. *A*, Before treatment. *B*, Six weeks after elimination of gluten from the diet. Note that the severely disordered pattern has improved.

Cultures of aspirates may now be obtained via sterile polyethylene tubes. Precise microbiologic technique for anaerobic organisms must, however, be practiced or the exercise will be futile.

Roentgenographic Studies. Diagnosis of the malabsorption syndrome may be facilitated by recognition of changes in the roentgenograms of the small bowel which point to bacterial overgrowth and include *strictures* or *fistulas, blind loops* usually from previous surgery (Fig. 2), or marked *stasis,* as in scleroderma. Dilatation of the proximal jejunum with "flocculation" and "scattering" of barium, slight coarsening of valvulae conniventes, and rather oddly shaped collections called "moulage," point strongly to *adult celiac disease* (Fig. 3). The factors underlying these changes are not completely understood but include some disturbance of motility or the effect of overproduction of mucus, caused perhaps in both instances by the collection in the gut of irritating substances such as fatty acids. Such changes, but particularly disordered transit and markedly thickened folds, may be noted in *Whipple's disease. Amyloidosis, radiation enteritis, hypoproteinemia, Zollinger-Ellison syndrome,* and *eosinophilic enteritis* may also be responsible. Differential diagnosis of various malabsorption states by roentgenographic examination of the small bowel, however, is often most difficult unless a characteristic finding for an underlying disease (e.g., tumor, stricture, or blind loop) is evident. Some roentgenographic changes associated with *chronic pancreatitis* or *cancer of the pan-*

Figure 4. Jejunal mucosa of patient (F. G.) with adult celiac disease. *A*, Before treatment (60 ×). *B*, Twenty-eight months after elimination of gluten from the diet. Note the regeneration of the villi and the return toward normal of the columnar epithelium (60 ×).

Figure 5. Comparison of dissecting microscopy and light microscopy of jejunal biopsy specimens. *A*, Finger-like villi vs. *B*, normal villous pattern. *C*, Leaflike villi vs. *D*, normal villous pattern. *E*, Convolutions vs. *F*, partial villous atrophy. *G*, "Mosaics" vs. *H*, total villous atrophy. *E* through *H* are specimens from patients with adult celiac disease.

creas include diffuse calcification or displacement of the stomach by a pseudocyst in the former condition and widening of the duodenal loop or distortion or destruction of mucosal folds in the latter (see Ch. 646 and 648).

Vitamin B$_{12}$ Absorption. Vitamin B$_{12}$ absorption is tested after intramuscular administration of 1000 μg by oral administration of radioactive vitamin B$_{12}$ and measurement of the excretion in the urine over a 24-hour period. Greater than 7 per cent of the administered dose should be excreted. The absolute values depend upon dose of labeled B$_{12}$.

Abnormal results are found after *resection* of the *terminal ileum*, extensive and severe *terminal ileal disease,* and *bacterial overgrowth.* It is also abnormal in *pernicious anemia*, after *total gastrectomy,* or in some patients with *pancreatic insufficiency.* Administration of tetracycline, 1 gram daily for two weeks, will usually restore vitamin B_{12} absorption in bacterial overgrowth to normal. On the other hand, administration of the test substance with intrinsic factor will yield a normal result in patients with pernicious anemia and after total gastrectomy, but not after extensive resection of the terminal ileum or in pancreatic insufficiency. In the latter condition bicarbonate or pancreatic extract may be required (see Table 3).

Jejunal Histology. Histologic study of jejunal mucosa obtained by suction biopsy technique has further aided differential diagnosis of the malabsorption syndrome. The procedure is easily performed with one of several available tubes (Rubin tube or Crosby capsule). Prothrombin time must be normal. Characteristic findings have been associated with *celiac disease* in both children and adults and in *tropical sprue, Whipple's disease, amyloidosis,* and *eosinophilic gastroenteritis.* In some instances alterations may be noted in diffuse nongranulomatous *ileojejunitis,* in *lymphoma,* after *gastrectomy,* in *hypogammaglobulinemia* with steatorrhea, in patients with intestinal *lymphangiectasia* associated with protein-losing enteropathy who have dilated lacteals, and in individuals with *radiation enteritis, mastocytosis,* or severe *drug reactions.* Fat-laden epithelial cells are found in *abetalipoproteinemia.* Certain parasites, namely, *Giardia lamblia* and *Coccidioides immitis,* have also been found on biopsy.

A section of normal jejunal mucosa from a specimen obtained by suction biopsy is shown in Figures 4 and 5. The villi are long, delicate, and frondlike; the lining columnar epithelium is regular with basal orientation of nuclei. The crypts are normal, and cellular infiltration of the lamina propria is minimal. Proper interpretation of jejunal histology, it must be emphasized, depends upon correct (perpendicular) sectioning of the specimen, which, in turn, requires correct mounting before fixing.

The jejunal histology in *adult celiac disease and tropical sprue* is strikingly abnormal. In evaluation of small bowel biopsies from such patients, particular attention must be directed to configuration of the villi, morphology of the epithelial cells with their brush border, and the degree of the chronic inflammatory cell infiltration. The severity of changes may be graded from mild to moderate to severe. In the *severe* group (total villous atrophy) the changes consist of complete flattening of the mucosal surface without detectable villi or, at best, only very short and broad villi. Generally, there is a dense infiltration of chronic inflammatory cells and disorganization of the epithelial cells with a sparse brush border (Figs. 4 and 5). In the *mild* group (partial villous atrophy), the villi are formed but still are shorter and broader than normal. In some areas the villi approach normal in all respects. The epithelial cells with brush border generally may be nearly normal and the cellular infiltration is mild. In the *moderate* subdivision (subtotal villous atrophy), changes ranging between those of the mild and severe groups are noted (Fig. 5).

The degree of infiltration of the lamina propria and of alteration of the epithelial cells is proportional to the extent of villous atrophy. The brush border frequently appears intact in the crypts, although it is disorganized and sparse near the midportion and tip of the villus. Although the severity of the lesion varies considerably among patients, the variation within a limited region of the proximal jejunum in a single patient is minimal; however, definite differences between the samples from more distant locations in the same patient have been noted. Total villous atrophy, although characteristic of celiac disease, is not specific. Occasionally, it may be noted in *tropical sprue,* in *lymphoma,* or in *Whipple's disease,* and it has been reported in *diffuse nongranulomatous ileojejunitis* (often "ulcerative"), as well as in patients with *congenital hypogammaglobulinemia* in whom plasma cells are absent in the lamina propria. Some of the last-named will respond to a gluten-free diet and thus have adult celiac disease as well; the same coincidence may be noted in patients with *diabetes mellitus* after *gastrectomy,* and in *Sjögren's syndrome, mastocytosis, jejunal diverticulosis,* and even *cystic fibrosis.*

Changes of this nature have also been noted (but not responsive to gluten elimination) in patients with *eosinophilic gastroenteritis,* in some *parasitoses,* and in *intestinal ischemia, dermatitis herpetiformis, soy bean sensitivity, radiation enteritis, tuberculosis, viral enteritis,* and conditions caused by *colchicine* and *neomycin.* Recently, mild inflammatory cell infiltration of the lamina propria has been noted in biopsies from patients with bacterial overgrowth.

In *Whipple's disease* the diagnosis may be made by the demonstration of macrophages laden with periodic acid–Schiff staining material in lymph nodes or in the lamina propria of the intestinal wall. In addition, total villous atrophy may be noted (Fig. 6). Recent electromicroscopic studies during the active phase of the disease have revealed membranous structures, which may represent an infectious agent outside the macrophages. Deposits of amyloid have been found in the submucosa of the jejunum in patients with *amyloidosis,* particularly within the walls of arterioles.

In the past few years examination of fresh biopsy specimens under the dissecting microscope has yielded information about a number of diseases of the small intestine associated with malabsorption. The normal patterns of *finger-like villi* and *leaflike villi* are seen in Figure 5. The former are jejunal, and the latter are also normally present in the duodenum and upper jejunum. Epithelial convolutions usually indicate disease and, on histologic examination, correspond to *partial villous atrophy.* A most extreme change is noted with total villous atrophy, with *"mosaics"* or *"brain patterns"* as the picture under

Figure 6. Jejunal biopsy from a patient with Whipple's disease. Periodic acid–Schiff stain. Note macrophages laden with stained material in the lamina propria.

the dissecting microscope. Examples of this classification are presented in Figure 5.

DIFFERENTIAL FEATURES AND TREATMENT OF INDIVIDUAL FORMS OF THE MALABSORPTION SYNDROME

Because the presenting clinical picture includes a wide range of symptoms—e.g., bulky stools, flatulence, distention anorexia, weight loss, weakness, glossitis, paresthesias, bleeding, bone pain—a careful history is of extreme importance in differential diagnosis. Particular atten-

tion must be paid to bowel habits in childhood, family history, previous illnesses and surgical operations, and dietary habits (including consumption of alcohol). A history of symptoms commonly associated with diseases that might underlie the malabsorption must be sought. Valuable clues may also be derived from a careful physical examination. In this way diagnosis of *tropical sprue, adult celiac disease, Whipple's disease, hypothyroidism, hyperthyroidism, hypoparathyroidism, scleroderma, lymphoma,* and other malabsorptive disorders may be facilitated.

The malabsorption syndrome must be differentiated from a wide variety of conditions characterized by a bleeding diathesis, by skeletal pain with or without frac-

---

TABLE 5.   Representative Dosages for Agents Used in Management of Patients with the Malabsorption Syndrome

1. CALCIUM
   Oral: Calcium gluconate (91 mg Ca^{++}/gram), 1 to 5 grams three times daily
   Intravenous: Calcium gluconate injection. U.S.P. 10 per cent solution (9.1 mg Ca^{++}/ml), 10 to 30 ml administered slowly intravenously depending upon response
2. MAGNESIUM
   Oral: Magnesium sulfate (8 mEq/gram), 1.0 to 6.0 grams daily in divided dosage
   Intramuscular: (20% sol.) 10 ml two or three times daily
   Intravenous: Magnesium sulfate, 0.5 per cent solution, up to 1000 ml at a rate not faster than 1.0 mEq/minute
3. IRON
   Oral: Ferrous gluconate, 0.6 gram three times daily
   Intramuscular: (Imferon). Must be calculated according to severity of anemia. Detailed instructions accompany preparation.
4. FAT-SOLUBLE VITAMINS
   a. VITAMIN A
      Oleovitamin A capsules, U.S.P. (25,000 units per capsule), 100,000 to 200,000 units daily in severe deficiencies; maintenance, 25,000 to 50,000 units daily.
   b. VITAMIN D
      Synthetic oleovitamin D, U.S.P. (10,000 U.S.P. units vitamin D/gram), 30,000 units daily; increase dosage as necessary to raise serum calcium to normal. Dosage varies considerably depending on response as determined by level of serum calcium and urinary calcium.
   c. COMBINATION A AND D VITAMINS
      Concentrated oleovitamins A and D, U.S.P. (50,000 to 65,000 U.S.P. A units and 10,000 to 13,000 U.S.P. D units/gram) may be used rather than separate preparations.
   d. VITAMIN K
      Oral: Menadione, U.S.P., 4 to 12 mg daily. Vitamin K_1 tablets (Mephyton), 5 to 10 mg daily.
      Intravenous: (Bleeding episodes—acute situations.) Vitamin K_1 (Mephyton), 50 mg ampule. Administer 50 mg slowly over 10-minute period. Repeat in 8 to 12 hours if prothrombin time has not returned to normal.
5. FOLIC ACID, U.S.P. (5 mg tablets)
   Dose: Initial, 10 to 20 mg daily
   Maintenance, 5 to 10 mg daily
6. VITAMIN B_{12} INJECTION, U.S.P. (15 μg/ml)
   Dose: Initial, 30 to 60 μg daily for two to three weeks
   Maintenance, 100 μg monthly
   If combined system disease is present, a more intensive program is indicated.
7. VITAMIN B COMPLEX
   Any multivitamin preparation that contains daily requirements (thiamine 1.6 mg, riboflavin 1.8 mg, and niacin 20 mg). Use two or three tablets daily. Intramuscular preparations are available for severe deficiencies.
8. PANCREATIC SUPPLEMENTS, ORAL
   Recently these agents have been shown to be more effective when given at 6 to 12 regular intervals during the day rather than at meal times.
   a. *Pancreatin*, U.S.P. (0.3 gram tablet), 6 to 18 grams daily.

b. *Viokase* (0.3 gram tablet), 4 to 12 grams daily in divided doses at meals or hourly per day.
   c. *Cotazym* (0.3 gram capsule), 4.0 to 12.0 grams daily, divided doses at meals or hourly per day.
9. BROAD-SPECTRUM ANTIMICROBIALS
   Oral: Chloramphenicol, tetracycline, or oxytetracycline (0.25 gram), 1.0 gram per day in divided doses for 10 to 14 days; ampicillin (0.25 gram), 2.0 to 4.0 grams per day in divided doses; kanamycin (0.5 gram), 2.0 to 4.0 grams per day in divided doses; sulfisoxazole (0.5 gram), 1.0 to 2.0 grams daily in divided doses; lincomycin (0.25 gram), 1.0 to 2.0 grams daily. Repeated courses often necessary or administration for three to four days each week indefinitely.
10. HUMAN ALBUMIN, SALT POOR (0.25 gram/ml)
    Intravenous administration of 50 to 100 grams each day for three to seven days to elevate a severely depressed serum albumin level
11. GLOBULIN, IMMUNE SERUM (0.165 gram/ml)
    Intramuscular injection of 0.05 ml/kg each three to four weeks in patients with hypogammaglobulinemia and recurrent infection.
12. CORTICOTROPHIN AND ADRENOCORTICOSTEROIDS
    a. Corticotrophin, 30 to 40 units intravenously each day, 10 to 21 days or longer for severely ill patients.
    b. Prednisolone or prednisone, 30 to 60 mg orally each day as needed; 5.0 to 15.0 mg maintenance dose.
13. ANTIDIARRHEAL AGENTS
    Oral: Diphenoxylate hydrochloride (2.5 mg), 5.0 mg twice or three times daily. Deodorized tincture opium, 10 drops twice to three times per day. Propantheline (15.0 mg), 30 mg twice or three times daily.
14. CHOLESTYRAMINE, ORAL RESIN
    4.0 gram dose, three to six times daily, before feedings.
15. CALORIC SUPPLEMENTATION
    Oral: (a) Medium-chain triglyceride (MCT). "Home or Hospital Mix" (MCT: 45 per cent calories; caseinate, 15 per cent; dextrose, 40 per cent). Ingredients homogenized with H_2O to one liter (MCT: 75 mg; caseinate, 60 grams; dextrose 160 grams). Keep at 20°C for one year. Defrost day's formula each morning; give three ounces at meals; gradually increase between-meal feedings to six ounces. Portagen (MCT: 45.0 grams fat/quart; 30 cal/oz; 10 per cent carbohydrate). Formula mix. Prepare according to instructions. Give 16 oz every day.
    (b) Vivonex, 80 grams = 300 cal: 90.8% CHO; 0.7% fat; 8.5% amino acids, plus minerals and electrolytes. Dissolve in 100 ml water. Feed up to 480 grams q.d.
    Intravenous: Prepare solution of approx. 0.9 cal/ml: 20% dextrose and 5% fibrin hydrolysate (w/v). Give 1500–3000 ml q.d. Increase amounts cautiously. Solution contains electrolytes, including Po_4'''
16. DRUGS FOR PARASITES
    Oral: Thiabendazole (25 mg/kg/day). Strongyloidiasis, two to three days; *Capillaria philippensis,* 30 days. *A. duodenale, N. Americanus,* 25 mg/kg/day twice daily for two days.
    Oral: Metronidazole (0.25 gram), 0.25 gram three times daily for 7 days for *Giardia lamblia.*
    Oral: Bephenium (5 gram packet). *A. duodenale,* one packet twice for one day; *N. Americanus,* one packet twice daily for three days.

ture, by evidence of vitamin B deficiency and extreme malnutrition, or by chronic diarrhea. Diagnosis of the malabsorption syndrome as a cause for these symptoms and signs must first, however, be based upon demonstration of abnormal fat absorption.

As the patient with the malabsorption syndrome may have extreme weight loss, weakness, hypotension, and diffuse pigmentation, differentiation from *Addison's disease* must be made. Abnormalities of serum calcium, carotene, or plasma prothrombin and impaired absorption of fat and xylose indicate the presence of the malabsorption syndrome (Table 4). Addison's disease may be excluded by the responsiveness of the adrenal gland to an intravenous infusion of corticotrophin. However, it must be stressed that patients very severely, acutely, and chronically ill with malabsorption syndrome, particularly *celiac disease*, may have evidence of hypoadrenocorticism and that administration of steroids is an indicated component of initial therapy.

The principal distinctive features of the individual forms of the malabsorption syndrome are discussed according to the seven categories of Table 1.

As there are numerous conditions that can produce the malabsorption syndrome, its treatment must be individualized. In contrast to the often gratifying response to dietotherapy shown by patients with *adult celiac disease,* or to antimicrobials by patients with *Whipple's disease, diseases with bacterial overgrowth,* and *tropical sprue,* successful management of malabsorption resulting from various other diseases or alterations of the gastrointestinal tract is often difficult. Dosage schedules for agents used in the treatment of malabsorption syndrome are listed in Table 5.

Category 1: Defective Intraluminal Hydrolysis or Solubilization

Primary Pancreatic Insufficiency. Pancreatic insufficiency results from *chronic relapsing pancreatitis, carcinoma of the pancreas,* or *cystic fibrosis,* or *after extensive resection* of the gland. In the first three instances, it is due to extensive parenchymal destruction and/or obstruction of the major ductal system. In chronic pancreatitis with malabsorption (see Ch. 646), the patient is frequently diabetic, the gland is noted to be calcified on flat film of the abdomen, and frequently, but not always, there is a history of recurrent attacks of inflammation. Occasionally the dominant symptoms of *carcinoma of the pancreas* are those of malabsorption rather than pain, anorexia, or jaundice. *Cystic fibrosis* is most often clinically apparent in early childhood; increasingly, however, the diagnosis is being made in young adults.

Whatever the cause of pancreatic insufficiency, failure of lipolysis results in moderate to severe steatorrhea, depending to some degree on the amount of gland remaining. Patients with this disease may show evidence of deficiency of either vitamin B_{12} or fat-soluble vitamins. In contrast to adult celiac disease, d-xylose absorption is normal in pancreatic insufficiency except in the unusual instance of carcinoma of the pancreas that has invaded the small intestine. As noted earlier, the diagnosis of pancreatic insufficiency is facilitated by analysis of duodenal fluid after stimulation of the pancreas. When lipolysis is markedly depressed, hydroxy fatty acids are not produced, providing a possible way of distinguishing pancreatic steatorrhea from steatorrhea of bacterial

overgrowth and other nonpancreatogenous forms of malabsorption.

Secondary Pancreatic Insufficiency. Since pancreatic lipase is inactivated at an acid pH, conditions characterized by excessive gastric acid secretion, such as non-β islet cell tumor of the pancreas (Zollinger-Ellison syndrome) or massive small bowel resection, are associated with significant steatorrhea. As noted, defective lipolysis causes deficient formation of micelles. Although it is possible that a low pH in the upper small gut may also precipitate bile salts and cause mild histologic abnormalities, the importance of these factors as against inactivation of lipase remains to be determined.

Deficiency of Conjugated Bile Salts. Insufficient concentration of conjugated bile salt in the upper intestine, caused by severe liver disease or prolonged extrahepatic biliary tract obstruction, diminished bile salt pool, or significant reduction of conjugated bile salts resulting from bacterial overgrowth (see below), diminishes hydrolysis of neutral lipid and results in steatorrhea. The pathophysiologic mechanism is subnormal concentration (less than 2.5 mmoles per liter) of conjugated bile salts necessary for micelle formation.

Distal *ileectomy,* severely *diseased terminal ileum,* or *ileal bypass* (surgical or via cholecystocolonic fistula), by disrupting the enterohepatic circulation of conjugated bile salts, also causes steatorrhea, the degree proportional to the length of the resected, diseased, or bypassed segment (about 8 to 15 grams per 24 hours for distal 100 cm). Bile salt pool is diminished, the critical level of conjugated bile salts is not achieved in the jejunum, and micellar solubilization of lipid diminishes. Further, since bile salt absorption is subnormal, these substances make contact with colonic mucosa, inhibiting water and salt absorption, particularly in the ascending colon. Diarrhea—three to six loose to soft movements per day—results. When less than 100 cm of terminal ileum is involved, both the steatorrhea and diarrhea are mild. Patients with distal ileectomy generally lose from 15 to 30 grams of fat in stools per day. This large degree of steatorrhea may be due in small part to loss of absorptive function of the ileum, although it is likely that the diminished bile salt pool is responsible entirely.

Decreased conjugated bile salt pool is also notable in primary or *secondary biliary cirrhosis;* that the steatorrhea in these cases is due to liver disease is supported by disappearance of malabsorption with improvement of liver function. It is surprising, however, that the steatorrhea of complete obstruction is moderate, indicating other mechanisms for absorption in addition to proximal uptake of micellar lipid. Malabsorption of fat in *postnecrotic* (macronodular) or *portal* (micronodular) *cirrhosis* is usually mild unless *chronic pancreatitis* (usually caused by alcohol) is also present.

Bacterial Overgrowth (Increased Bile Salt Deconjugation). For many years, steatorrhea and vitamin B_{12} deficiency anemia have been clinically and experimentally associated with alterations in the anatomy of the small intestine, particularly surgically created "blind" loops; *enteroenteric, enterocolic,* or *gastrojejunocolic fistulas; afferent loop stasis* after subtotal gastrectomy and gastrojejunostomy; or *chronic obstruction* caused by adhesions or strictures, *jejunal diverticula,* or diseases with *motor abnormalities* such as scleroderma and pseudo-obstruction.

The common denominator in all conditions is bacterial overgrowth, which results from stasis in a segment of small bowel caused by anatomic factors, motor abnormalities, or contamination of small bowel by large bowel content. Concentration of anaerobic organisms greater than 10^7 per milliliter, particularly *bacteroides, clostridia,* and *lactobacilli,* is responsible for impairment of intraluminal solubilization of hydrolyzed lipid. Bacterial overgrowth may rarely play a role also in the malabsorption in *diabetes mellitus* with neuropathy (unclear), in *tropical sprue,* and after *subtotal gastrectomy* and Billroth II gastrojejunostomy. These patients may also have severe diarrhea as well as steatorrhea, possibly owing to impairment of Na^+ and water absorption by hydroxy fatty acids which result from bacterial action on unabsorbed fatty acids; also, short chain fatty acids, products of fermentation of sugars and amino acids, may cause diarrhea by increasing intraluminal osmolarity.

The mechanism of the malabsorption of vitamin B_{12} and fat caused by bacterial overgrowth is clear. Vitamin B_{12} is utilized by multiplying anaerobic organisms. Fat absorption is impaired by deconjugation of bile salts by bacterial enzymes. The decline in concentration of conjugated bile salts below a critical level (less than 2.5 mmoles per liter) impairs micelle formation, reducing uptake of lipid by the mucosa. Concentration of free bile acids is increased intraluminally; their absorption from the proximal small gut by passive diffusion is rapid, and their serum levels are elevated; these may also inhibit cellular resynthesis of triglycerides. Observations on patients with bacterial overgrowth indicate that less than 20 per cent of intraluminal fat is in a micellar phase 45 minutes after ingestion of a lipid meal (normal: more than 50 per cent). Since hydrolysis of fat is not impaired, steatorrhea is principally the result of impaired micelle formation.

Although the jejunal villi are not entirely normal in jejunal biopsy specimens of patients with bacterial overgrowth, demonstrating some infiltration of the lamina propria with lymphocytes, plasma cells, and occasionally polymorphonuclear cells, along with mild blunting, the appearance is strikingly different from the picture in adult celiac disease.

"Blind" Loops. A loop of intestine is "blind" either when it is disconnected from the main stream (rare) or when intestinal contents may gain access to it but not readily egress from it. An example would be a partly defunctionalized terminal ileal loop that has been partially excluded by either side-to-side or end-to-side ileotransverse colostomy (Fig. 2). Stasis and overgrowth of bacteria take place with subsequent invasion of the upper small intestine.

Multiple Strictures and Jejunal Diverticula. Strictures result from diffuse *granulomatous ileojejunitis, tuberculosis,* or *x-radiation* therapy. Frequently these patients have crampy abdominal pain, bloating, and other symptoms of progressive luminal narrowing, as well as other evidences of their underlying diseases. Most multiple jejunal diverticula are probably acquired. Stasis of intestinal content in these pockets of bowel leads to bacterial overgrowth.

Fistulas. Fistulas may complicate gastric or intestinal neoplasm or granulomatous enteritis, involving stomach, small gut and colon (gastrocolic), small gut and colon (enterocolic), or loops of small gut (enteroenteric). Malabsorption may also, of course, result from exclusion of significant lengths of absorbing surface from the main stream by large fistulas (gastroileostomy).

The diagnosis is greatly aided by a history of previous chronic enteric disease or of surgical procedure. Roentgenographic examination will often establish the diagnosis by the demonstration of one of these diseases or alterations. Frequently, however, the cause may not be demonstrated.

The megaloblastic anemia commonly associated with the "blind loop" syndrome will, unlike pernicious anemia, respond to the administration of broad-spectrum antimicrobial drugs. After 10 to 14 days of such therapy (tetracycline, 1.0 gram daily in divided dose), absorption of vitamin B_{12} is usually, but not always, restored to normal (Table 5). In contrast to those with pernicious anemia, these patients usually secrete hydrochloric acid.

Postgastrectomy. Afferent loop stasis after gastrectomy and gastrojejunostomy (Billroth II) is a cause for steatorrhea and malabsorption and may be due in part to bacterial contamination of the afferent loop (see Category 5).

Scleroderma and Pseudo-Obstruction. Although a disturbance of esophageal motor function is the most common gastrointestinal manifestation of scleroderma, severe involvement of the small bowel may cause malabsorption. Atrophy of the smooth muscle of the gut, submucosal fibrosis, and damage to the myenteric plexuses severely impair or abolish peristalsis. The resulting intermittent ileus may simulate closely the picture of complete intestinal obstruction. Severe involvement of the small intestine is usually associated with esophageal involvement, thickening of the skin, or other evidence of disseminated sclerosis, e.g., soft tissue calcification, telangiectasia, pulmonary diffusion defect, so that diagnosis is not difficult. Jejunal biopsy reveals normal villi, but there may be an increased number of inflammatory cells in the lamina propria.

Bacterial overgrowth is the principal factor in the steatorrhea and malabsorption of most patients with scleroderma involving the small intestine. As with the esophagus (see Ch. 634 and 635), small bowel smooth muscle is atrophic and is replaced with fibrous tissue. Motility is severely impaired; stasis and bacterial overgrowth result. Culture of small bowel content of such patients may yield a heavy growth of anaerobic organisms.

Pseudo-obstruction of the small and large intestine is a rare condition of unknown cause characterized by periodic episodes of prolonged ileus. It is chronic in some patients and may be associated with malabsorption resulting from bacterial overgrowth.

Treatment of Defective Intraluminal Hydrolysis

Primary Pancreatic Insufficiency. Replacement of digestive enzymes and insulin is important in the treatment of patients with primary pancreatic insufficiency. Among the available sources of enzymes are a commercial pancreatic extract, pancreatin, U.S.P.; a preparation containing whole raw pancreas, Viokase; and one containing hog pancreas extract, Cotazym. Doses of these preparations are listed in Table 5; occasionally, it may be necessary to increase the recommended amounts. Replacement therapy may be more effective when it is given in divided doses at regular intervals six times daily or even hourly during the day than when it is limited to mealtimes. Some patients with primary pancreatic insufficiency do not absorb vitamin B_{12} normally, a defect that may not be corrected by giving bicarbonate alone; pancreatic extracts, however, will increase absorption to normal. There is some indication that giving bicarbonate with pancreatic extracts may improve fat absorption, but this evidence is scanty.

Secondary Pancreatic Insufficiency. Hypersecretion of acid caused by *non-β islet cell tumor* is best treated by total gastrectomy (see Ch. 643); after *massive small bowel resection,* hypersecretion may appear and be relieved by vagotomy and pyloroplasty. In both conditions, large doses of anticholinergic drugs may be effective in reducing acidity.

Deficiency of Conjugated Bile Salts. Cases in which insufficient bile reaches the intestine pose a difficult problem in treatment. If possible, *cholecystocolonic fistulas* or chronic *obstruction* of the *biliary tree* should be corrected surgically. The keystone of medical management is a balanced diet without restriction of fat. For patients with chronic *cholestatic liver disease* it is important to provide calcium and fat-soluble vitamins A, K, and D in adequate amounts (Table 5). The demineralization of bone in patients with prolonged biliary obstruction results from osteoporosis and osteomalacia. Adequate supplements of vitamin D and calcium not only may prevent further osteomalacia but also may increase calcium deposition. The administration of a high protein diet and anabolic hormones, i.e., norethandrolone (Nilevar) or testosterone, and of estrogens intermittently, may help correct the osteoporosis. Because inactivity contributes to the skeletal demineralization, maximal ambulation must be encouraged.

Bacterial Overgrowth (Bile Salt Deconjugation). Absorption of vitamin B_{12} and of fat is impaired with *intestinal strictures, fistulas, blind loops,* and multiple *jejunal diverticula.* The surgical correction of the strictures, fistulas, or blind loops may effect a permanent cure and is therefore the therapy of choice.

In some patients with malabsorption syndrome associated with either *subtotal* (Billroth II) or *total gastrectomy* or *scleroderma,* long-term antimicrobial therapy should be undertaken. Tetracycline or oxytetracycline, 1.0 gram per day, or ampicillin, 2.0 to 4.0 grams per day, should be given for 10 to 14 days, and intermittently every other day for three days each week thereafter (Table 5). Chloramphenicol, also in a daily dosage of 1.0 gram, may be used in situations in which the risks of drug toxicity seem clearly to be outweighed by the potential dangers of the disease. Many of these patients, similar to those with bacterial overgrowth from other disorders, require continuous treatment. Rotation of antimicrobial drugs may be advisable in an effort to avoid the emergence of drug-resistant microbial populations. Aspiration of jejunal contents for cultures and periodic drug susceptibility determinations are necessary for therapeutic guidance. If organisms are not susceptible to the more usually employed drugs, courses of kanamycin (2.0 to 4.0 grams daily orally) may be given. All these drugs should be used in a rotational scheme. Occasionally, some patients with recurrent *regional enteritis* and strictures or fistulas, in whom the surgical approach is not feasible, will have to be managed in a similar fashion.

In addition to the assessment of clinical response, efficiency of antimicrobial therapy may be judged by the return of the bile salt breath test and urinary indican to normal or nearly normal levels.

Use of Medium-Chain Triglycerides (Table 5). Feeding preparations of medium-chain triglycerides, composed of fatty acids with six to ten carbons, appears to be valuable in a number of diseases that cause malabsorption, including those associated with defective intraluminal hydrolysis or solubilization of fat (see above).

Medium-chain triglycerides have been used in patients with defective intraluminal hydrolysis or solubilization and are most effective in those with pancreatic insufficiency who are also being given supplements of pancreatic enzymes (see above) and in patients with deficiency of conjugated bile salts (particularly biliary tract obstruction or bile fistulas).

Indication for medium-chain triglycerides is also strong in situations in which no specific therapy for malabsorption is available, such as after massive *small bowel resection* (short gut syndrome), *lymphatic obstruction,* and *biliary atresia.* Medium-chain triglycerides are a useful adjunct in malabsorption for which specific therapy is available (*celiac disease, bacterial overgrowth, Whipple's disease, parasitism,* and *tropical sprue*—all of which will be discussed in detail later in this section).

Category 2: Mucosal Cell Abnormality and Inadequate Surface

Primary Mucosal Cell Disorders

Disaccharidase Deficiency and Monosaccharide Malabsorption. Inability to split disaccharides because of disaccharidase deficiency (lactase or sucrase and isomaltase) may be primary or secondary. The primary type of *lactase deficiency* is either familial (very rare, fatal) or congenital with an autosomal dominant inheritance. Symptoms may appear during infancy, childhood, or adulthood. Primary lactase deficiency (as well as other primary disaccharidase deficiencies) is not associated with any discernible alteration of the villi or their brush borders which contain these enzymes. Bacterial fermentation of unsplit lactose produces lactic and other organic acids which increase osmotic load with water entering the lumen. Diarrhea, cramping abdominal pain, borborygmi, and flatulence result from ingestion of milk and milk products. Weight loss and steatorrhea are usually mild and appetite is good, although infants and children may not thrive well. This pathophysiologic concept applies equally to *sucrase deficiency.*

Lactase deficit is by far the most common, particularly in blacks, and is more common in Orientals than in whites. Dietary deficiency of lactose is not the cause. Adults diagnosed as having irritable colon syndrome (see Ch. 637) may be deficient in jejunal lactase. The reason for the clinical appearance of the disorder in adulthood is not clear; it is also occasionally unmasked after subtotal gastrectomy. Since no disease of the mucosal cells is evident, the deficiency is thought to be primary, but its clinical development is somehow acquired.

Diagnosis of lactase deficiency may be made by the measurement of blood glucose after the oral administration of lactose (Table 4). A rise of less than 20 mg per 100 ml is abnormal, and if the patient's blood glucose rises normally after he ingests a mixture of glucose-galactose of equal amount, lactase deficiency is extremely likely. Diagnosis may be confirmed only by the finding of low lactase activity in a jejunal biopsy specimen. Occasionally, these patients have lactosuria after administration of 50 grams of lactose during the lactose tolerance test.

Treatment of primary lactose deficiency is elimination of milk and milk products from the diet. It often dramatically relieves all symptoms. It may also be beneficial to patients with the secondary variety of deficiency.

Depression of lactase activity is also secondary to certain diseases affecting the brush borders of jejunal mucosal cells, such as *celiac disease*; but it is also found after *massive* small bowel *resection*, in *nonbacterial jejunitis, infectious diarrhea of childhood, Giardia lamblia infection, Whipple's disease, cystic fibrosis,* and *granulomatous* (regional) *enteritis.*

Deficiency of *sucrase* is rare; it is associated with deficiency of isomaltase. Recent studies indicate that it is a homozygotic deficiency affecting perhaps as many as 2 in 1000 individuals in the population. Symptoms include watery diarrhea and borborygmi, usually from infancy, and are caused by ingestion of sucrose and sucrose-containing foods. Secondary sucrase deficiency may often accompany secondary lactase deficiency.

Diagnosis of sucrase deficiency may be made by failure of blood glucose to rise at least 20 mg per 100 ml after ingestion of 100 grams of sucrose. Treatment may be either elimination or marked reduction of sucrose, dextrins, and starches from the diet.

Congenital *glucose-galactose malabsorption* is present from birth and is exacerbated by all sugars broken down to these hexoses. Diagnosis is made by failure of these children to absorb either of these substances. Treatment consists of feeding fructose or fructose precursor–containing foods.

Abetalipoproteinemia (Acanthocytosis). Abetalipoproteinemia is a disease characterized by a morphologic defect of erythrocytes, "spiny red cells," low to absent serum beta-lipoproteins, very low serum cholesterol, and, in some instances, mild steatorrhea, ataxia, nystagmus, motor incoordination, and retinitis pigmentosa. The cause of the disease is unknown, but it is related to an inability of the mucosal cells to invest lipid with a protein envelope necessary for entry to the lacteals. The severity varies – in milder cases, no steatorrhea or neurologic defects occur. Substitution of medium-chain triglycerides for ordinary triglycerides has led to weight gain in some patients, because the component fatty acids enter the portal, not the lacteal, system.

Vitamin B$_{12}$ Malabsorption. Very rarely, primary malabsorption of the vitamin B$_{12}$–intrinsic factor complex is noted, perhaps owing to absence of a specific but unidentified "receptor" in the ileal mucosa. These patients have been shown to have adequate intrinsic factor, normal ileal histology and calcium concentration, and alkaline pH. Treatment is monthly injections of vitamin B$_{12}$ intramuscularly (Table 5).

Cystinuria and Hartnup Disease. Rarely, patients may have genetic disorders of intestinal transport of amino acids. In *cystinuria* dibasic amino acids are involved – cystine, arginine, lysine, and ornithine; in *Hartnup disease,* neutral amino acids – e.g., phenylalanine and leucine. Tryptophan deficiency leads to nicotinamide deficiencies with rash, dementia, and ataxia. These patients are cured with adequate oral nicotinamide and protein, because they absorb small peptides normally.

Intraluminal Small Bowel Disease

These diseases include *adult celiac disease, Whipple's disease, nongranulomatous ileojejunitis, allergic* and *eosinophilic gastroenteritis, amyloidosis, small bowel ischemia,* and *Crohn's disease.*

Adult Celiac Disease. An important cause of chronic malabsorption in temperate climates is adult celiac disease (gluten enteropathy, celiac sprue, nontropical sprue). In some undemonstrated way, dietary gluten is related to this disease. Perhaps the intestinal mucosa of these patients is damaged by acidic peptides contained in the gliadin fraction of this substance, either because of a deficiency or absence of specific peptidases or by an immunologic reaction to them unrelated to enzyme activity. The process affects the mucosa principally with villous atrophy, columnar to cuboidal change of absorbing cells, and infiltration of the lamina propria with plasma cells and lymphocytes. Jejunum is more affected than ileum. The extent of this lesion may be roughly correlated with clinical severity.

Patients in this group have an abnormal incidence either of a history of childhood celiac disease or of evidence of the disease in relatives. The high incidence (80 per cent) of HLA-B in these patients suggests a genetic predisposition. Further, individuals with congenital IgA deficiency are predisposed to this disease.

Commonly, the symptoms of celiac disease disappear in later childhood and in adolescence, despite continued malabsorption. Although the clinical remission is sometimes permanent, the classic features of adult celiac disease may appear during the third to sixth decades. The patients then may present with a spectrum of disability, ranging from mild discomfort and diarrhea with perhaps some anemia to severe illness with an extreme degree of malabsorption, foul-smelling diarrheal stools, skeletal disorders, bleeding phenomena, and symptoms of hypocalcemia. There are no pathognomonic physical signs in this disease. There may be all degrees of malnutrition, as evidenced by muscle wasting and edema (Fig. 1). Hypotension and abdominal bloating are very common. Occasionally, there are clubbing of the fingers and pigmentation similar to that of Addison's disease. Signs and symptoms of celiac disease and their pathophysiologic bases are noted in Table 2.

Roentgenography of the small bowel gives findings that are characteristic but not specific. Frequently the only change is an altered pattern with some dilatation of proximal loops of small bowel and minimal coarsening of the jejunal folds. More severe impairment is manifested by marked dilatation of small bowel segments and clumping of the barium meal, with a waxy cast appearance of bowel segments (the *"moulage"* sign) (Fig. 3). As mentioned previously, the routine laboratory studies used in establishing the presence of the malabsorption syndrome are not specific.

Better techniques in diagnosis of adult celiac disease are measurement of d-xylose absorption and study of jejunal histology. Indeed, the diagnosis is untenable unless total or nearly total villous atrophy is found. Vitamin B$_{12}$ absorption is usually normal, but may be depressed if disease is extensive, involving the ileum. Other interesting findings, aside from those in Table 2, include frequent elevation of serum IgA and depression of IgM, along with reduced numbers of IgA-containing plasma cells in the biopsy.

A *trial of dietotherapy* may be important diagnostically in these patients. That the vast majority of adult celiac disease patients will respond favorably to an adequate gluten-free diet has been well established, and no other condition will respond so dramatically or so completely. Although clinical remission well within two months of institution of this therapy is the rule, nevertheless some patients may require six to twelve months or even longer.

Treatment of Celiac Disease. The basis for the use of the gluten-free diet in adult celiac disease lay in observations of its beneficial effects (in children initially) in celiac syndrome. Laboratory as well as clinical data strongly indicated that these patients cannot tolerate cereals with high gluten content. Thus when wheat, rye, oats, and barley are eliminated from the diet, diarrhea and steatorrhea cease, appetite improves, and rapid weight gain ensues. (Conversely, the introduction of gluten or gliadin into a histologically normal segment of small bowel causes mucosal inflammation with villous atrophy within 12 hours, associated with diarrhea and steatorrhea.)

The gluten-free diet excludes all cereal grains except rice and corn. To follow this diet, all labels must be carefully scrutinized to eliminate completely products that contain wheat, rye, barley, and oats as "fillers" (ice cream, salad dressings, canned foods, condiments, candy, etc.). As substitutes for the usual grains, rice, corn, and soy flours may be used. Recently, a wheat starch flour (Cellu Products Company) has become available. Beer and ale must be avoided, because they contain cereal residues; however, whiskies can be used, because the offending agent is not contained in the distillate. All other foods, except milk and milk products if they cause symptoms owing to lactase deficiency, are permitted, including fats. In general, the diet should be well balanced and high in protein. The complete diet is available in standard nutrition texts.

A substantial majority of the patients with adult celiac disease have responded to this diet, showing symptomatic improvement within a few days or a week, although a rare patient may require as long as 12 months. Weight gain has been so striking that patients have voluntarily restricted their caloric intake. The fact that a complete clinical remission with return to normal of pertinent blood components can be obtained in the majority of cases is significant, because previous treatment programs were usually only incompletely effective (Fig. 7). Follow-up biopsies demonstrate return to normal of mucosal histology in 50 per cent of patients who maintain that they adhere strictly to their diet, and marked improvement in most others. Complete restoration of villi and of the columnar epithelium in one patient is shown in Figure 4. Repeated biopsies in a minority of patients, however, reveal little or no improvement. It is difficult to ascertain whether they are ingesting some gluten; the physician should, however, also suspect other diseases which are associated with non-gluten-sensitive villous atrophy *(hypogammaglobulinemia,* particularly with *Giardia lamblia; lymphoma; dermatitis herpetiformis; collagenous sprue; Whipple's disease; and diffuse nongranulomatous ileojejunitis).* Absorption of d-xylose returns to normal, as does urinary excretion of 5-hydroxyindolacetic acid, within a few weeks of elimination of gluten. Steatorrhea diminishes remarkably in all instances, but fat absorption returns completely to normal only in those patients who carefully eliminate all gluten.

Corticosteroids have been shown to produce significant improvement in adult celiac disease without entirely correcting the steatorrhea or biochemical abnor-

Figure 7. Appearance of patient (M. S.) with adult celiac disease. *A,* Before treatment. Note wasting and edema. *B,* Six weeks after elimination of gluten from the diet.

malities. These agents should be used for long-term therapy only in cases refractory to the gluten-free diet, for impaired protein metabolism and osteoporosis are troublesome features in this chronic condition.

Occasionally, a patient with adult celiac disease is critically ill, with severe diarrhea, wasting and anorexia, and serious protein and electrolyte depletion. There may also be bleeding, tetany, and edema. This situation demands a rigorous therapeutic regimen, employing intravenous vitamin K and calcium as well as infusions of salt-poor albumin (Table 5). It is in this clinical situation that corticosteroids may be lifesaving by greatly stimulating the appetite and perhaps by increasing absorption. Initially, corticotrophin, 30 units, should be given intravenously over an eight-hour period daily. After 10 to 14 days, either prednisolone or prednisone, 60 mg a day, may be substituted. Simultaneously, a gluten-free diet should be offered, and, as the patient's condition improves, drug therapy should be discontinued by gradual reduction in dosage over three to four weeks. These patients should remain on such dietotherapy permanently. Supplements (vitamin D and K, calcium, iron, folic acid, B-soluble vitamins, and vitamin B_{12}) are gradually withdrawn as clinical and chemical improvement proceeds; the program is set by results of reported essential laboratory determinations and personal observations.

Special Considerations and Complications of Adult Celiac Disease.

LYMPHOMA AND CARCINOMA. The incidence of primary small bowel lymphoma and carcinoma in patients with adult celiac disease is high, about 13 per cent in a large collected series, with lymphoma contributing 10 per cent. Abdominal pain, weight loss, bleeding, obstruction, and perforation are the cardinal clinical features of this fatal complication. It is believed that lymphoma is more common in those not treated with a gluten-free diet. Relapse in those who have responded, associated with suggestive symptoms, should alert one to the possibility.

SMALL BOWEL ULCERATION. Nonmalignant ulcers of the jejunum and ileum may complicate celiac disease, and are manifested by exacerbation of severe diarrhea, abdominal pain, fever, and severe hypoproteinemia secondary to protein-losing enteropathy (see below). Perforation, bleeding, and/or obstruction are late manifestations.

NEUROLOGIC COMPLICATIONS. A syndrome similar to subacute combined degeneration of the spinal cord is noted early in celiac disease, despite remission with a gluten-free diet and no vitamin B_{12} deficiency (see Ch. 404 to 411 and Ch. 731).

CELIAC DISEASE AND THE SKIN. *Dermatitis herpetiformis* may be associated with patchy villous atrophy of the duodenum and upper jejunum; this abnormality does not extend beyond the proximal foot or so of the small gut, perhaps explaining why malabsorption in these patients is mild or even absent. Response to a gluten-free diet is poor, and instillation of gluten into the gut causes no inflammatory response as it does in gluten enteropathy. Partial and total villous atrophy have also been noted in *rosacea, atopic dermatitis,* and *psoriasis,* associated with varying degrees of steatorrhea and occasionally a dramatic response to a gluten-free diet. Conversely, a variety of skin disorders aside from hyperkeratosis have been reported in celiac disease, including *neurodermatitis* and *lichen planus.*

A rare patient with adult celiac disease who does not respond entirely to the diet may also have *pancreatic insufficiency* and will require oral pancreatic extract (Table 5).

COLLAGENOUS SPRUE. This disease resembles adult celiac disease in that it has the identical histologic picture, but it is not responsive to gluten elimination. Later, collagen is extensively deposited in the lamina propria beneath the epithelium.

HYPOSPLENISM. Recent studies indicate that an occasional patient will have splenic atrophy with hyposplenism and diminished immunologic response to antigens.

Whipple's Disease.

In Whipple's disease, or lipophagic intestinal granulomatosis (intestinal "lipodystrophy"), there is a heavy infiltration of the intestinal wall and lymphatics by macrophages filled with glycoprotein. It is a generalized disease with steatorrhea as its principal feature, and it occurs predominantly in males in the fourth to seventh decades.

It may be difficult to differentiate this entity from other serious to fatal causes of malabsorption, particularly *lymphoma* and *tuberculosis*. Several manifestations such as polyserositis and postprandial pain are seen in all three diseases. However, nondeforming arthritis is most characteristic of Whipple's disease and is frequently the initial complaint. When gastrointestinal symptoms occur, the disease usually progresses rapidly with marked diarrhea, weight loss, weakness, and symptoms of anemia and deficiencies of fat- and water-soluble vitamins. Physical findings that suggest this disorder include lymphadenopathy, found in 40 per cent of the patients, and the various manifestations of polyserositis. Fever may be noted in about one third of the patients. Indefinite plastic or doughy abdominal masses have been described in approximately one quarter of the patients. The most consistent findings in the routine laboratory studies are anemia and an increased sedimentation rate; eosinophilia is occasionally present. Classically, steatorrhea is severe, with d-xylose absorption depressed and thickened folds. The roentgenographic findings in the small bowel are nonspecific, usually showing a "sprue-like pattern."

The diagnosis of Whipple's disease can be verified either by peripheral lymph node biopsy or, when this is normal, by biopsy of a mesenteric lymph node at laparotomy. Diagnosis may be established by identification of macrophages containing periodic acid–Schiff positive material in jejunal biopsy specimens obtained perorally (Fig. 6). Patchy villous atrophy may also be noted; thus identification of the engorged macrophages is crucial. Electron microscopic studies have revealed bacilliform bodies in and near these macrophages that may be infectious agents. Recent studies suggest that a pleomorphic organism is involved. Infiltration of the lamina propria also causes enlargement of villi and thickening of the submucosa.

Treatment of Whipple's Disease.

Antimicrobial drugs by mouth are effective in treating Whipple's disease. Indeed, present information indicates that continuous treatment with penicillin G, 0.25 gram four times daily, or broad-spectrum antimicrobials, tetracycline or ampicillin, always brings about remission. The dose of tetracycline or ampicillin is 1.0 gram daily. The duration of therapy with antimicrobials is determined by the clinical response. Present data indicate that such treatment should be maintained indefinitely; otherwise, symptoms may return. Histologic as well as clinical improvement is noted after a period of weeks to months, with loss of diarrhea, reappearance of appetite, and tremendous gain of weight. The PAS-positive material slowly disappears from the mucosa, and the bacilliform bodies are no longer visible on electron microscopy. When remission has been sustained for nine months to one year, antimicrobial agents may be given intermittently, i.e., every other day or for three consecutive days each week (Table 5).

The symptoms of Whipple's disease may respond to corticosteroid therapy, as do those of other diseases characterized by arthritis and polyserositis, but the over-all result of such treatment is not satisfactory. Present evidence strongly indicates that only 40 per cent of patients achieve remission of the disease for two to six months while receiving corticotrophin or corticosteroids, and, in the majority, the disease relapses on cessation of such therapy. Many patients, particularly those whose illness is in a terminal phase, do not respond at all. The desperately ill patient should be given both corticotrophin intravenously, 40 units daily, *and* parenteral antimicrobial agents until the improvement of the patient permits withdrawal of the former agent.

Nongranulomatous Ileojejunitis. Steatorrhea and malabsorption may result not only from the complications of granulomatous enteritis (*strictures, fistulas,* or *massive resections*) (see Ch. 650), but also from nongranulomatous involvement of a large segment of the small intestine, particularly the jejunum. The small intestine is diffusely inflamed; mesenteric nodes are slightly enlarged, and serosal lymphatics are dilated. Although the mucosa is heavily infiltrated with inflammatory cells and has patchy ulcerations, the wall is not thickened as in Crohn's disease, nor are there strictures or fistulas.

The onset of this latter illness is abrupt, and signs and symptoms of malabsorption may predominate in a matter of one to two weeks. A daily remittent fever (39 to 40.5° C), abdominal cramping pain, usually periumbilical, and frequent watery stools are common complaints. Splenomegaly, occurring in 20 per cent of these patients with fever, may suggest an initial diagnosis of abdominal lymphoma. Usually, diffuse inflammatory changes are noted in roentgenograms of the small bowel. Stenotic segments and fistulas are not usually seen. The small bowel pattern may be indistinguishable from that of a wide variety of conditions associated with the malabsorption syndrome. One laboratory finding of help in the differential diagnosis is elevation of the leukocyte count, often with a substantial increase in the percentage of nonsegmented polymorphonuclear cells. Diagnosis may also be facilitated by a previous misdiagnosis of appendicitis. Often, however, diagnosis is made either by the response to treatment or by surgical exploration (see Ch. 650).

Treatment of Nongranulomatous Ileojejunitis. In diffuse ileojejunitis, corticosteroids may have a dramatic effect upon the clinical symptoms, including those that are due to malabsorption. Steatorrhea will diminish or cease; serum calcium, carotene, and plasma prothrombin concentration will return to normal. Serum albumin, often severely depressed to levels of 1.0 to 2.0 grams per 100 ml by "weeping" of serum protein into a large segment of inflamed gut, so-called protein-losing enteropathy (see below), likewise rises as the inflammation subsides. These improvements, as indicated by laboratory tests, accompany the disappearance of fever as well

as the increase in appetite, weight, and strength. Although such a therapeutic result is most salutary, it may not, unfortunately, be permanent. Recurrence is frequent, with progress of the disease in localized areas.

The consensus is that such patients, often acutely ill with fever and diarrhea, respond best to intravenous corticotrophin, 40 units daily, given over an eight-hour period for 10 to 14 days. The oral corticosteroid preparations are used after corticotrophin in the more serious cases and may be the principal therapeutic agents throughout the course of the less severe cases. The initial dose range in either instance is 40 to 60 mg of prednisone or prednisolone daily. The dose is gradually tapered over a week or longer to a maintenance level of 10 to 30 mg daily. The day-to-day clinical response best regulates the dose of drug at this stage of treatment. Broad-spectrum antimicrobials are not useful except in the presence of septic complications. Unfortunately, some of these patients have a relentless, refractory course and die of bowel perforation or intercurrent sepsis in two to three months, and the long-range outlook for permanent remission of this disease in those who initially respond is likewise not good.

Allergic and Eosinophilic Gastroenteritis. Increasingly, patients are seen with malabsorption, varying degrees of gastrointestinal bleeding, and protein-losing enteropathy; their small gut mucosa is infiltrated by eosinophils and is edematous but shows no vasculitis. The involvement in many instances is principally mucosal. In some patients, in whom the stomach is also involved, the deeper layers of the gut, including serosa, are infiltrated. In a minority of instances in adults, the disease is a response to a known allergen such as milk protein, meat, or even fruit. Even in the absence of an offending agent, these patients have histories of hay fever, eczema, and asthma, particularly in childhood, or other food idiosyncrasies.

The symptoms—cramping pain, diarrhea, weight loss, nausea, fever, and a degree of malabsorption—are related to the location and extent of the disease in the small bowel. Fat loss in stool is about 15 to 20 grams per day. If the stomach is also involved, epigastric pain, vomiting, and bleeding are common. Frequently, the patients have allergies, particularly hay fever and asthma, and many have urticaria as well as diarrhea after eating certain foods (milk, egg, cereal, meat). Marked eosinophilia is a constant finding and is greater than 20 per cent. The disease tends to be chronic with recurrent symptoms. Roentgenographic examination often reveals a nonspecific "malabsorption pattern" with coarsened folds of jejunum. Occasionally, narrowed segments may be seen. Hypoproteinemia caused by protein-losing enteropathy may be severe and may be associated with marked edema and ascites. Iron deficiency anemia resulting from occult gastrointestinal bleeding is common in children. Disease of the stomach, particularly antral, may cause hematemesis.

Another form of this disease is so-called *eosinophilic granuloma,* in which the process consists of localized nodular or pedunculated infiltrative eosinophilic lesions (involving the submucosa and muscle layer) without allergy or peripheral eosinophilia. *Eosinophilic gastroenteritis* may also involve the serosa of the bowel as well as peritoneum, with ascites the predominant manifestation.

Treatment of Eosinophilic Gastroenteritis. Effective therapy consists of withdrawal of offending foods, particularly milk for children. In more ill patients, prednisone, 20 to 40 mg daily orally with gradual tapering to a low maintenance dose, will bring remission of major symptoms and decrease of eosinophilia. With remission, edema and infiltrate of the jejunal mucosa also disappear in patients with no involvement of deeper layers. In patients with brisk bleeding from the stomach, surgery may have to be performed. Laparotomy, for severe pain or bleeding resulting from transmural small bowel disease, reveals thickened loops of jejunum, involved antrum, and enlarged mesenteric nodes. Biopsy differentiates this disease from granulomatous enteritis and tuberculosis. In the majority of patients the clinical picture, typical history, eosinophilia, obvious allergies, and response to treatment are sufficient to exclude *acute diffuse nongranulomatous ileojejunitis, lymphoma,* and *celiac disease.* Transoral jejunal biopsy will also be helpful.

Amyloidosis. Either the primary or the secondary form of the disorder may affect the gastrointestinal tract and cause malabsorption. Diffuse crampy pain and ileus are the most frequent abdominal symptoms. In the primary form of the disease, cardiac failure, macroglossia, and renal disease may be noted, but the Congo red test is negative. Roentgenographically, amyloidosis is characterized by dilated loops of bowel, occasionally with thickening of the jejuno-ileum and slow passage of the barium meal through the intestines. The diagnosis is made by tissue study. Gingival or tongue biopsies are frequently positive in *primary amyloidosis,* particularly when the disease is associated with myelomatosis; liver biopsy, although hazardous, may also establish the diagnosis. Biopsy of the liver or bowel at laparotomy may be necessary in some instances. Diagnosis may also be made from specimens of jejunal mucosa obtained by transoral suction biopsy.

In *secondary amyloidosis,* the presence of a chronic inflammatory illness and hepatosplenomegaly suggests the diagnosis. Congo red tests may show greater than 90 per cent retention of the injected material by the tissues.

Treatment is supportive, because the disease is too extensive for resection. If it is secondary to chronic infection or granulomatous disease, successful management of the underlying disorder may be helpful, although it is unlikely.

Small Bowel Ischemia. Chronic ischemia of the small bowel, caused by atherosclerosis of the celiac, superior, and inferior mesenteric arteries, may occasionally cause malabsorption, presumably because of impairment of mucosal cell function. No histologic damage, however, has been demonstrated in such instances (see Ch. 660).

The blood supply to the small intestine is occasionally severely compromised in patients with so-called collagen vascular disease, particularly *periarteritis nodosa* and *systemic lupus erythematosus.* Although malabsorption syndrome has been reported in these diseases, the documentation is unclear; *Degos' disease,* characterized by necrotic skin lesions and vasculitis of the small gut, may also cause malabsorption, although the far more serious and common clinical manifestation is infarction of the gut. A necrotizing type of arteriolitis leading to ulceration and perforation of the small gut is a serious form of vascular complication of the collagen vascular diseases.

Crohn's Disease. This important disease of the small bowel may cause malabsorption in a number of ways: by extensive damage to the mucosa; by multiple strictures (bacterial overgrowth); by fistulas between small bowel

and colon (bacterial overgrowth); or by necessitating ileectomy (defective solubilization and loss of absorptive surface) or massive resection (inadequate surface). Bacterial overgrowth and defective solubilization are discussed in Category 1 above; inadequate surface, a portion of Category 2, is discussed below. The clinical picture of diffuse Crohn's disease of the small intestine is discussed in Ch. 650. It is sufficient here to emphasize that an important part of this picture is the signs and symptoms of malabsorption, the range and severity of which are proportional to the extent (length of bowel involved), to severity (i.e., complications) of the disease, and to the type and extent of surgery which may have been performed.

Inadequate Surface

Most absorption takes place in the duodenum and first 90 cm of the jejunum. Clinical studies of patients who have had extensive resection of the small intestine indicate that survival is now reasonably certain with 90 to 120 cm of remaining normal small bowel, and is possible with shorter segments provided caloric intake is adequate. This length of jejunum is sufficient for normal carbohydrate absorption and, in most instances, for maintenance of positive nitrogen balance. The postoperative course is influenced by the site of resection—jejunum or ileum. Thus vitamin B_{12} absorption will be subnormal if a large length of ileum has been removed; conversely, sacrifice of a corresponding amount of jejunum will more seriously impair absorption of fat, calcium, and folic acid.

The three common causes for extensive resection of large segments of the small intestine are (1) *recurrent regional enteritis,* (2) *mesenteric vascular disease,* particularly thrombosis of the superior mesenteric artery, and (3) *malignant processes* involving the blood supply of the small bowel.

Treatment. Inadvertent surgical *jejunocolostomies* or *gastroileostomies,* which sidetrack large segments of small intestine, must be corrected surgically as soon as possible.

The patient who has had an *extensive resection of the small intestine,* nearly always right colon, ileum, and part of distal jejunum, requires continuous and meticulous medical care. For weeks or even for one or two months, nutrition may adequately be maintained by intravenous hyperalimentation which employs fluids containing adequate calories, protein, minerals, and vitamins. As little as 2 liters daily may satisfy nutritional requirements for an adult (Table 5). Certain complications may attend such therapy, and the physician must be aware of them. They are due to necessity for catheterizing the subclavian vein (sepsis, thrombosis, hemo- or pneumothorax). Hyperosmolar, hyperglycemic dehydration, or hypophosphatemia may also ensue. The patient's fluid and electrolyte balance must, of course, be meticulously monitored on a daily basis.

Oral feedings should be initiated as soon as possible, preferably containing substances which require minimal hydrolysis and are easily absorbed. Such preparations as Vivonex have been useful, because they contain simple sugars and amino acids; however, as with all hypertonic preparations, diarrhea may be aggravated.

For periods of up to 12 months postoperatively, the remaining segment of intestine will show progressive improvement in absorptive capacity, associated with elongation and dilatation. It is important to remember that, since the amount of fat absorbed is proportional to the amount presented to the absorbing surface, the maximal intake of fat that does not cause symptoms is desirable. Regardless of which segment or its part—ileum or jejunum—remains, the diet should be high in protein, and frequent feeding (six times daily) should be recommended and may consist in part of protein and amino acids (Table 5). Vitamins A, D, and K and the B-complex vitamins as well as calcium, iron, and magnesium may be given orally, except in those instances in which adequate replacement is possible only by the parenteral route (Table 5). In general, a high protein intake will adequately maintain the serum albumin; however, occasionally, infusions of salt-poor albumin must be given.

Supplementation of the diet by medium-chain triglycerides (see above; Table 5) has been of distinct benefit to patients with massive small bowel resection, diminishing diarrhea and helping to stabilize weight by improving fat absorption; however, it must be noted that weight gain attributable principally to medium-chain triglycerides in these patients is slight. Drugs that decrease intestinal motility, such as diphenoxylate hydrochloride (5.0 mg twice or three times daily), anticholinergics (propantheline, 15 to 30 mg twice to three times daily), and/or small doses of tincture of opium (10 drops twice to three times daily) may help reduce diarrhea (Table 5).

Category 3: Lymphatic Obstruction

Lymphoma. The malabsorption syndrome secondary to lymphoma of the small bowel and mesentery may be clinically and roentgenographically identical to the classic picture of adult celiac disease. Several features, however, suggest the correct diagnosis. The symptoms of this disease are likely to be of much shorter duration and to include crampy abdominal pain and fever. Lymphadenopathy and hepatosplenomegaly do not appear until late in the course. Although intramural small bowel masses may be present in some cases, the roentgenographic study of the intestine generally does not reveal them. Unexpectedly, the usual therapeutic measures, such as diet, fat-soluble vitamins, and vitamin B_{12}, may lead to a temporary clinical and laboratory remission. The incidence of malabsorption syndrome caused by small bowel lymphoma is difficult to ascertain. It appears that as many as 10 per cent of patients with adult celiac disease may develop lymphoma. Although lymphatic obstruction is important in the pathophysiology of steatorrhea in lymphoma, widespread disease of the intestine will also contribute significantly to the malabsorption.

The diagnosis is usually established by laparotomy necessitated by some complication of the underlying disease, such as bleeding, perforation, or obstruction. In some patients, the diagnosis may be made from jejunal tissue obtained by peroral biopsy. The average duration of this illness after onset of symptoms is 13 months, despite resection and roentgen therapy.

Primary intestinal lymphoma, with malabsorption, may be a chronic condition in certain parts of the world, particularly in the Middle East in young Arabs and Sephardic Jews, and in Mexico. The clinical picture strongly resembles adult celiac disease in terms of chronicity and jejunal villous atrophy; however, most of these patients do not respond to elimination of gluten,

and peroral biopsies will show evidence of lymphoma in the majority. In contrast to primary lymphoma of the small bowel with malabsorption in North America and Europe, which carries a prognosis of death one to two years after onset of symptoms (despite surgery, radiation, and chemotherapy), the young Middle Easterners may live with their disease for as long as ten years. Lymphoma also complicates *α-chain disease* in which heavy chains of IgA are produced excessively.

Treatment. Treatment of lymphoma of the small bowel and mesentery includes local resections as well as radiotherapy, and possibly therapy with chlorambucil and steroids or cyclophosphamide when the disease is disseminated. Despite this program, the course is frequently progressive, the average duration of life after onset of symptoms being one to two years. In these patients, continuous supportive therapy (high caloric diet, iron, vitamins, calcium, as needed) is frequently helpful and may result in successful maintenance of the patient's activity over a period of months. Indeed, these patients have also improved when given low-fat diets with vitamin and mineral supplementation.

Intestinal Tuberculosis and Tuberculous Lymphadenitis. Tuberculosis may result in a malabsorption syndrome through involvement of the mesenteric lymph nodes, although in some cases there may be associated disease of the intestinal wall. It is extremely rare in the United States, and it occurs almost always in persons with a history of severe pulmonary or lymph node tuberculosis.

Fever, palpable abdominal masses, a positive tuberculin skin test, evidence of old or recent disease on chest roentgenography, and calcification of mesenteric and pelvic lymph nodes on flat film all suggest the diagnosis, which may be confirmed by culture of sputum or gastric juice. Rarely, stool culture may be useful, but only if the other secretions are demonstrably free of tubercle bacilli. Roentgenographic studies, both barium enema and small bowel series, are particularly helpful when there is also deformity of the ileocecal segment resulting from hyperplastic lesions. Rarely, there may be diffuse small bowel abnormalities, such as coarsening of the folds, stricture formation, and edema, which suggest ileojejunitis. At times, exploratory laparotomy with node or bowel biopsy is necessary for diagnosis (see Ch. 234 and 240).

Treatment. Tuberculous involvement of the mesenteric lymph nodes should be treated by chemotherapy, as set forth in Ch. 240. A high caloric diet should be employed with calcium and vitamins as indicated. When there is an associated hyperplastic ileocecal tuberculosis with partial obstruction, appropriate local resection may be necessary.

Lymphangiectasia. In addition to the diseases just discussed, several other conditions may rarely cause the malabsorption syndrome by lymphatic blockade. These include *primary lymphangiectasia*, a genetically determined disease characterized by mild to moderate diarrhea, mild steatorrhea, and protein-losing enteropathy (see below), certain *protozoan diseases* (see Category 4), *the reticuloendothelioses, metastatic tumor* to the mesenteric nodes, and *neoplastic invasion of the main lymphatic channels* in the retroperitoneal tissues.

Category 4: Infection

Tropical Sprue. Tropical sprue can be differentiated from adult celiac disease. The disease occurs primarily in persons residing in certain areas of the Far East, India, and the Caribbean. Both nutritional deficiencies and bacterial contamination of the small gut appear to play causative roles. This disease responds to administration of broad-spectrum antimicrobial drugs, suggesting, but not proving, that infection is responsible. Histologic changes suggestive of tropical sprue may be noted in individuals newly arrived in the tropics; such changes may often be associated with an acute enteritis and a variable degree of malabsorption. Although the remarkable clinical improvement that follows folic acid therapy strongly suggests a vitamin deficiency, tropical sprue is not seen in some areas of the world where the population has a marginal or even inadequate diet; conversely, it has been noted in people with adequately "balanced" diets.

Clinically, three phases of the disease have been described. In the initial phase the patient complains only of fatigue, asthenia, and bulky stools. After weeks to months, the second phase of malnutrition is noted. Weight loss is prominent. Glossitis, stomatitis, cheilosis, and hyperkeratosis are observed in varying degrees. Moderate prothrombin depletion is present but is rarely associated with bleeding. Manifestations of impaired calcium absorption are not usually clinically apparent in patients with tropical sprue, in contrast to those with adult celiac disease. Iron deficiency anemia follows depletion of iron stores. Hypoalbuminemia with edema may be a late manifestation of this disease. Some laboratory criteria of impaired absorption are present (Table 4). The third stage is characterized by anemia and megaloblastosis and the symptoms of full-blown severe malabsorption described earlier in this section, although diarrhea may not be prominent. However, the clinical spectrum is wide—steatorrhea may be minimal, glossitis absent, and megaloblastosis inconstant. This inconsistent picture may indicate various causes.

Laboratory investigation reveals mainly steatorrhea and megaloblastic anemia. Small bowel roentgenographic findings and histologic changes of the jejunum are the same as those in adult celiac disease except that *total villous atrophy* is not as commonly encountered in tropical sprue. In many tropical areas, however, asymptomatic individuals often have histologic abnormalities suggestive of tropical sprue, making tissue diagnosis very difficult. Other routine laboratory studies, including d-xylose absorption, are also comparable in the two diseases. The gluten-free diet is ineffective.

Treatment for Tropical Sprue. The therapy for this disease is very effective. The similarity of tropical sprue to pernicious anemia, particularly in its hematologic aspects, prompted the use of liver extract, folic acid, and vitamin B_{12}, and remissions have also been noted with antimicrobial drugs, a low-fat, high-protein diet, and migration to a temperate climate. Administration of a broad-spectrum antimicrobial (tetracycline, 1.0 gram daily by mouth) along with 10 mg of folic acid daily is the best treatment and frequently brings remission, with disappearance of diarrhea and glossitis and gain in appetite and weight. However, response may be slow in some patients, and normal absorption and jejunal histology may not be noted for six months or longer. Parenteral vitamin B_{12} should be given for two months (Table 5). For those not responding completely within six months of treatment with antimicrobials and folic acid, therapy should be continued for as long as absorption continues to improve.

When remission has been achieved, 5.0 mg of folic acid daily is the maintenance therapy. In the presence of achlorhydria, addition of vitamin B_{12} to the regimen should be considered unless absorption of ^{60}Co B_{12} is normal (Table 5). If absorption of vitamin B_{12} remains subnormal after remission, monthly injections should be given.

Acute Infectious Enteritis. Bacterial and viral infections such as Salmonella, enteropathic *E. coli,* and a host of viruses may cause transient but severe malabsorption. Patients with this condition have steatorrhea and may have diminished xylose absorption. The serum calcium as well as the plasma prothrombin concentration may be depressed. Serum proteins may fall rapidly, largely owing to abnormal rate of loss into the inflamed gut. With recovery, absorption returns to normal.

Treatment. These patients may recover without specific antimicrobial therapy, provided that fluids and electrolytes have been rapidly and adequately replaced. Such infections are apt to attack patients who travel to tropical countries or are debilitated, or who have had abdominal surgery, particularly those also given broad-spectrum antimicrobials. Patients severely ill with salmonellosis (septicemia) may require treatment with broad-spectrum antimicrobials (see Ch. 213). The keystone of therapy for all infectious enteritis is rapid and complete replacement of fluid and electrolytes. Acidosis, hypokalemia, and hyponatremia are often severe (see Ch. 214).

Protozoan and Helminthic Diseases. Protozoan or helminthic diseases are a common cause of malabsorption in many tropical areas and are particularly associated with malnutrition. Because tropical sprue is also endemic in many of these countries, it is often difficult to assign a cause for malabsorption, especially in view of the histologic changes (blunting of villi, cellular infiltration of the lamina propria) which are present in many asymptomatic individuals who are malnourished with or without parasites. Some of these patients with mild to moderate steatorrhea (10 to 15 grams per 24 hours), however, have malabsorption syndrome caused by *hookworm, strongyloidiasis, Capillaria philippensis, coccidiosis,* and *giardiasis.* Parasites must be isolated and identified, and response to therapy, clinically, biochemically, and histologically, must be forthcoming before definite etiologic attribution of the malabsorption and malnutrition to parasitic infection can be made.

Patients with *Giardia lamblia* infection of the small bowel may suffer from malabsorption, particularly individuals with *subtotal gastrectomy; hypogammaglobulinemia* often associated with so-called "nodular lymphoid hyperplasia"; *tropical sprue;* or *severe malnutrition,* particularly in children. Thus the role played by the parasite is not completely clear despite demonstration of its invasion of the mucosa and report of some improvement in absorption after treatment with quinacrine (0.1 gram three times daily for one week). Recent evidence indicates that villous atrophy which is associated with the giardiasis of hypogammaglobulinemia is reversed with effective therapy for the parasite (see below, Category 6). In all doubtful cases it is wise to treat the patient (Table 5).

Category 5: Multiple Defects

Subtotal Gastrectomy. Steatorrhea and malabsorption after subtotal gastrectomy and gastrojejunostomy (Billroth II) or total gastrectomy are attributable to (1) loss of reservoir function with rapid emptying and dispersion of food through the small intestine, thereby diluting the normal output of pancreatic enzymes; or (2) stasis with bacterial contamination of the afferent loop of a Billroth II gastrojejunostomy. Deficiency of vitamin B_{12} will inevitably follow total gastrectomy, the lag period being determined by the liver store of the vitamin.

Treatment. Administration of ox bile extract is not helpful, probably because of its high content of unconjugated salts. As yet no preparation of pure conjugated bile salts is available for treatment. Pancreatic extracts may be tried in selected cases, although when given alone they have not produced consistent improvement. However, when pancreatic extract is combined with broad-spectrum antimicrobials (ampicillin or tetracycline, 1.0 gram per day in divided dosage, or lincomycin, 1.0 to 2.0 grams per day), in the treatment of patients after Billroth II operations, fat absorption may improve. These results indicate that in some patients bacterial contamination — probably originating in the afferent loop — plays an important etiologic role in the malabsorption syndrome that follows this procedure. Conversion of Billroth II to Billroth I has been reported to reduce steatorrhea in some patients.

Patients who have undergone Billroth II procedures should receive a high-calorie diet rich in protein, with frequent feedings containing as much fat as can be tolerated, in order to maintain good nutrition. After a total gastrectomy, 30 to 100 μg of vitamin B_{12} intramuscularly must be given monthly. Calcium, iron, and the fat-soluble vitamins may be added to this regimen as needed or when diarrhea or steatorrhea is so severe that deficient absorption of these substances may be anticipated (Table 5).

Distal Ileal Resection, Disease, or Bypass. As noted, resection, often required for granulomatous disease or vascular insufficiency, ileal bypass for obesity, or extensive ileal disease causes deficiencies of vitamin B_{12} and bile salts. Malabsorption is also in part due to loss of the reserve capacity of the ileum for absorbing fat, a function which would be carried on if proximal fat absorption were impaired by deficiency of bile salts.

Vitamin B_{12} should be replaced parenterally, as in pernicious anemia. If the megaloblastic anemia that appears does not respond entirely to vitamin B_{12}, folic acid should be added to the regimen (Table 5).

Treatment with cholestyramine, a bile salt–binding resin, is indicated and will often ameliorate the diarrhea caused by the effect of unabsorbed bile salts upon the colon. However, it may increase steatorrhea by further diminishing the bile salt pool. No replacement therapy for the bile salt deficiency is currently available clinically. Steatorrhea will be reduced, however, by feeding medium-chain triglycerides in place of dietary lipid (Table 5). Studies of the effect of potent pancreatic extracts and/or antimicrobials (broad-spectrum) are not available.

Radiation Enteritis. A few patients who receive high dosage x-ray therapy to the abdomen will develop a malabsorption syndrome on the basis of radiation injury to the bowel. It is difficult to assess how much of the defect in absorption is attributable to arterial damage, mucosal inflammation, or atrophy. Since the reaction to injury is slow, symptoms do not appear for weeks to months after exposure. In the usual patient, villous damage, mucosal and submucosal edema, and cellular infiltration are the main features and repair follows. However, larger doses cause ulceration of the mucosa and

endarteritis of submucosal vessels with transmural necrosis, followed by scarring with strictures and permanent loss of function. Thus malabsorption is principally due to disease of the small bowel wall; however, in some instances stasis caused by obstruction (bacterial overgrowth) contributes, and in others lymphatic obstruction (and perhaps ileal dysfunction) may contribute. Fibrosis and stricture are occasional sequelae of severe reaction, causing obstruction, usually chronic. Jejunal biopsy may reveal patchy villous atrophy.

Category 6: Unexplained

Hypogammaglobulinemia. The role of intraluminal immunoglobulins, particularly IgA, in maintaining the structure and function of the intestinal tract is not known, because their antibacterial activity as antibodies is minimal. Patients with hypogammaglobulinemia may, however, have steatorrhea and diminished d-xylose absorption, but the precise incidence is not known. Although the number of cases so documented is small, it is steadily growing. Evidence at hand indicates that most (if not all) of these patients have a deficiency of both plasma IgA and IgG and of intestinal IgA. Some patients have only plasma IgA ("selective") deficiency. IgM may be increased in serum and intestine in patients with selective IgA deficiency. The intestinal histology in diffuse hypogammaglobulinemia reveals normal histology or patchy villous atrophy, but *plasma cells are absent* and lymphocytes are reduced in all cases. Occasionally, it shows so-called "nodular lymphoid hyperplasia," and rarely it causes a granulomatous lesion. A high percentage of these patients with malabsorption will have *Giardia lamblia* infestation of their intestinal fluid, and in some the organism invades the mucosa. This infection is often associated with either villous atrophy or nodular lymphoid hyperplasia and appears to be present in a high percentage of these patients with steatorrhea. Although anaerobic bacteria may be present in the upper small bowel, their role in the pathogenesis of the steatorrhea is not proved. Other abnormalities include splenomegaly and gastric atrophy.

Treatment. Of those with villous atrophy, a rare patient will have a good to excellent response to the gluten-free diet. Antimicrobial drugs and injections of gamma globulin appear to be ineffective. The key to successful management appears to be eradication of giardiasis with atabrine or metronidazole (Table 5). Symptoms remit, absorption improves (including d-xylose), and villi regenerate. As noted above, patients with *celiac disease* have normal or elevated serum IgA, depressed IgM (one third), and normal IgG levels and have reduced IgA plasma cells and increased IgG and IgM plasma cells in the lamina propria.

Metastatic Malignant Carcinoid Syndrome. The presenting symptoms of this disease may be those of malabsorption. Steatorrhea may be caused by an increased production of 5-hydroxytryptamine (serotonin), which markedly increases gastrointestinal motility and thus impairs absorption. Other explanations for diarrhea and steatorrhea in this disease include lymphatic obstruction of the mesentery of the small bowel by tumor and ileal dysfunction. Treatment is that used for carcinoid syndrome in general. Methysergide (8.0 to 12.0 mg per day, orally) and cyproheptadine (80 mg per day in divided doses) have been reported to decrease diarrhea in this disease. Small doses of tincture of opium, however, seem most effective for the diarrhea. Parachlorphenylalanine, which inhibits hydroxylation of tryptophan to 5-HTP, has been effective in controlling diarrhea; however, side effects may preclude its general use. (see Ch. 869.)

Hypoparathyroidism and Pseudohypoparathyroidism. The association of steatorrhea and deficient parathyroid function has been recently confirmed. The mechanism by which parathormone is involved in fat absorption or transport is unknown. Symptoms of malabsorption may be the earliest manifestation of deficient parathyroid function. With vitamin D_2 therapy, diarrhea decreases, steatorrhea disappears, serum carotene and albumin levels rise, vitamin B_{12} absorption increases, and the roentgenographic appearance of the small bowel becomes normal. Diagnosis of hypoparathyroidism as a basis for malabsorption may be established by measuring hormone levels or by changes in urinary phosphate excretion after intravenous infusions of parathormone or calcium (see Ch. 839). Mild malabsorption (fecal fat about 10 grams per 24 hours) has been reported in pseudohypoparathyroidism. Parathormone in some way facilitates the effect of vitamin D upon calcium absorption by the intestinal tract. In pseudohypoparathyroidism the end organs, including the gut, are not responsive to parathormone. The effect of hypocalcemia per se upon intestinal absorption is not known.

Treatment. Administration of vitamin D and calcium will correct hypocalcemia and improve fat absorption as well as other manifestations of disease.

Diabetes Mellitus. Patients with longstanding diabetes mellitus may have severe diarrhea (see Ch. 637). Some with diarrhea will also have steatorrhea and malabsorption, and these patients are usually not well controlled by dietotherapy or insulin, or both, and a high percentage also have some evidence of neuropathy. In these patients, the intestinal difficulty may be due to involvement of the autonomic innervation of the small bowel, because they also have orthostatic hypotension, inability to perspire, and impotence. Possible changes in the microbial flora or mesenteric vascular insufficiency may also contribute to the malabsorptive state. Response to broad-spectrum antimicrobials supports the former hypothesis; however, careful bacteriologic studies of intestinal contents in a group of patients with diabetic neuropathy and diarrhea reveal that bacterial overgrowth is an uncommon cause for the steatorrhea of diabetic neuropathy. Although exocrine function is usually normal in diabetes, some patients have *pancreatic insufficiency* for which replacement therapy should also be given (Table 5) (see Ch. 646). Adrenal corticosteroids have been reported to benefit patients with this syndrome, but no satisfactory chemical documentation of such response has been presented. A disadvantage of such therapy would be the increased requirement for insulin. An increased incidence of *adult celiac disease* has also been reported in diabetics (see above).

Mastocytosis. Patients with overproduction of mast cells suffer not only from urticaria pigmentosa, but also from gastrointestinal symptoms. Perhaps the latter result from overproduction of histamine and perhaps of serotonin as well. Malabsorption is rare in these individuals. The lamina propria of the jejunal mucosa may or may not be infiltrated with mast cells; villi may be absent or stunted. Whether fat absorption is also impaired because of gastric hypersecretion or increased intestinal transit has not been determined.

Hyperthyroidism and Hypoadrenocorticism. Some patients with hyperthyroidism have steatorrhea. The pathogenesis is not understood. In one study of a group of patients with this disease, the possibility was raised that steatorrhea was due in part to excessive intake of fat in the diet (more than 120 grams per day). Successful therapy returns fat absorption to normal. Likewise, steatorrhea has been found in patients with Addison's disease in whom replacement therapy has corrected it.

Category 7: Drug-Induced Malabsorption

Some commonly used drugs may cause malabsorption. *Cholestyramine,* in doses of 12.0 or more grams per day, by binding bile salts renders them inactive in the process of fat solubilization and causes mild steatorrhea (7.0 to 15.0 grams of fat per day). *Colchicine* ingestion leads to mild malabsorption of fat (about 9.0 grams of fat per day), protein, and d-xylose by affecting epithelial cell replication and function. Certain *irritant laxatives,* presumably by markedly increasing transit, likewise may cause mild steatorrhea. *Neomycin,* frequently administered to patients with severe hepatic disease, causes steatorrhea, increased fecal loss of nitrogen, and impaired d-xylose absorption. The degree of malabsorption is dose related and may be noted with as little as 4.0 grams per day. It causes some blunting of villi and of their absorptive cells, reduces hydrolysis of fat, and precipitates bile salts. *Bacitracin, tetracycline, polymyxin,* and *kanamycin* may also cause malabsorption. Large doses (twice normal) of *p-aminosalicylic acid* lead to mild steatorrhea and decrease in absorption of d-xylose. *Phenindione,* an anticoagulant, may also cause steatorrhea. Anticonvulsants such as *diphenylhydantoin* in some way cause folic acid deficiency, as do *oral contraceptive* agents.

MALABSORPTION SYNDROME AND ENTERIC LOSS OF PROTEIN
(Protein-Losing Enteropathy)

Hypoalbuminemia without liver disease, inadequate protein intake, or albuminuria may be due to excessive loss of serum protein into the intestine. This loss has been noted in patients with mucosal ulceration of the stomach, small bowel, or colon; with mucosal disease without ulceration; or in lymphatic obstruction (Table 6). Intestinal lymphatic dilatation without obvious cause (lymphangiectasia, Fig. 8) is associated with abnormal enteric protein loss in some patients whose illness was previously termed "hypercatabolic hypoproteinemia." Many of these patients, regardless of the cause for plasma protein leakage, have some degree of malabsorption.

Edema or ascites, or both, secondary to hypoalbuminemia may overshadow enteric symptoms and, indeed, underlie presenting symptoms in patients with so-called *protein-losing enteropathy.* Most of these patients have specific diseases of the intestine. Thus the syndrome has been reported with gastric diseases such as *giant hypertrophic rugae* (Ménétrier's disease), *giant gastric ulcer, gastric cancer,* and *eosinophilic granuloma of the stomach.* A variety of inflammatory diseases of the small and large intestines are also associated with this syndrome: *granulomatous enteritis* and *enterocolitis; nongranulomatous ileojejunitis; acute infectious enteritis; ulcerative*

TABLE 6.   Classification and Therapy of Diseases
Associated with Enteric Loss of Plasma Protein

Disease	Therapy
A. Mucosal ulceration:	
Gastric carcinoma	
Gastric lymphoma	Surgical resection
Multiple gastric ulcers	
Colon cancer	
Granulomatous enteritis	
Diffuse nongranulomatous ileojejunitis	Corticosteroids
B. Mucosal disease without ulceration:	
Rugal hypertrophy (Menetrier's, etc.)	Resection, if local
Celiac disease	Gluten elimination
Tropical sprue	Antimicrobials; folic acid
Whipple's disease	Antimicrobials
Allergic gastroenteropathy	Elimination diet; steroids
Bacterial or parasitic enteritis	Antimicrobial drugs
Gastrocolic fistula	Resection
C. Lymphatic abnormalities:	
Capillaria philippensis	Thiabendazole
Primary lymphangiectasias	Low-fat diet or medium-chain triglycerides
Lymphenteric fistula	Resection
Lymphoma	Chemotherapy
Constrictive pericarditis	Pericardiectomy
Tricuspid valvular disease	Rx of heart failure

colitis; granuloma of the small bowel associated with *hypogammaglobulinemia, celiac disease, tropical sprue, lymphoma* of the small intestine, and *Whipple's disease;* and *lymphangiectasia* secondary to known causes such as *lymphoma* or *tuberculosis* or *Crohn's disease.*

Allergy to milk protein and, in rare cases, to cereals or even meat may underlie *protein-losing enteropathy* by affecting the small intestine. Biopsy is normal or shows mild infiltration of the lamina propria with eosinophils; the disorder usually begins in childhood; it is characterized by hypoproteinemia and edema; an iron deficiency anemia is common, as is diarrhea; eosinophilia is a permanent feature. This condition may well be a milder

Figure 8. Jejunal biopsy demonstrating dilated lacteals of lymphangiectasia associated with protein-losing enteropathy.

form of *eosinophilic gastroenteritis* in which both protein-losing enteropathy and malabsorption may be more serious (see above). Infestation with a roundworm, *Capillaria philippensis,* has been described in the Philippines; it causes diarrhea, protein-losing enteropathy, and malabsorption, and proves fatal in two to four months unless vigorously treated (Table 6) (see Ch. 303).

Clinical Picture.   As noted, the clinical picture may be dominated by signs and symptoms of hypoproteinemia. In most instances, the patient complains of some abdominal symptoms related to the underlying disease.

Diagnosis.   The diagnosis of protein-losing enteropathy should be suspected in any patient with low serum albumin who has normal liver function and does not have an abnormal amount of protein in the urine. The abnormal loss may be confirmed by abnormal fecal excretion of ^{51}Cr after intravenous injection of ^{51}Cr albumin or by a rapid decay curve after intravenous ^{51}Cr chloride or ^{131}I-albumin.

Treatment (Table 6).   Since therapy may be very successful, accurate diagnosis is extremely important. Resection of localized granuloma or ulcers of the stomach and bowel, or of localized giant gastric rugae, may lead to complete cessation of enteric protein loss. Patients with adult celiac disease and those with allergic gastroenteropathy who are sensitive to milk protein or other substances will respond to elimination of gluten or milk or other offending agents from the diet. Patients with intestinal lymphangiectasia of congenital origin respond to reduction of dietary fat to very low levels—5 grams or less—or to administration of medium-chain triglycerides in place of dietary fat. These regimens will usually reverse the abnormal protein loss in this disease, and may lessen it in any disease that obstructs lymphatics. Protein loss resulting from *acute, nongranulomatous ileojejunitis,* as well as *granulomatous enteritis* and *ulcerative colitis,* may disappear during therapy with corticosteroids, or, in the case of *viral enteritides,* with spontaneous recovery from the infection. *Acute bacterial enteritis* caused by Shigella or Salmonella, *Whipple's disease, enteric tuberculosis,* and instances of excessive protein loss associated with bacterial overgrowth in the small intestine *("blind loop syndrome")* all may respond to appropriate antimicrobial therapy. *Capillaria philippensis* is said to respond to thiabendazole, 25 mg per kilogram per day for 30 days (see Ch. 303). A similar effect has likewise been reported in enteric lymphoma after x-radiation and treatment with chlorambucil (Table 6).

Protein-losing enteropathy may be associated with *chronic constrictive pericarditis,* presumably caused by mediastinal lymphatic obstruction. Pericardiolysis or parietal pericardiectomy will alleviate or even completely reverse this enteric loss. Also, effective treatment of severe *right heart failure* may alleviate protein-losing enteropathy.

PROGNOSIS OF MALABSORPTION SYNDROME

The outlook for the patient with malabsorption syndrome depends upon both the nature of the underlying disease and the institution of appropriate therapy. (Proper treatment, of course, implies correct diagnosis.)

Specific therapy for patients with adult celiac disease (gluten-free diet) and effective agents for tropical sprue are available. Intelligent replacement therapy for those with deficient digestion (*gastrectomy, hepatobiliary dis-*

ease, *pancreatic insufficiency, massive resection* of the small intestine, or *ileectomy*) often alleviates the major symptoms (Table 5).

Whipple's disease now appears entirely manageable, and perhaps even reversible, with the use of broad-spectrum antimicrobial agents and adrenal steroids. The malabsorption of diffuse *nongranulomatous ileojejunitis*, involving large segments of the small intestine, may be completely abolished by administration of adrenal steroids or corticotrophin. Likewise, isoniazid and streptomycin are similarly effective in *tuberculosis enteritis.* Elimination of an offender in the diet and use of corticosteroids are an effective combination against *eosinophilic gastroenteritis.*

The correction of conditions in which intestinal microbes play an important role may be accomplished by appropriate surgery, such as resection of fistulas or strictures, or by administration of broad-spectrum antimicrobial drugs. In either case, a normal or nearly normal state of health may be achieved.

The prognosis for patients with malabsorption associated with endocrine disorders is good. The patient with intestinal *scleroderma* or with *diabetes mellitus* who has neuropathy and bacterial overgrowth may be helped by the intermittent administration of antimicrobial drugs. Vitamin D and calcium will restore absorption toward normal in cases of *hypoparathyroidism.* Appropriate management of *hyperthyroidism* will reverse abnormal fat absorption, as will replacement therapy for *Addison's disease.* Specific treatment for *Giardia lamblia* will likely cure the patient with *hypogammaglobulinemia.* Broad-spectrum antimicrobial drugs are effective in treating tropical sprue. Resection of a non-insulin-

secreting, *non-beta-cell tumor* of the pancreatic islets will diminish diarrhea and steatorrhea.

Because of the nature of the underlying disease, the outlook is bleak for a number of patients with malabsorption syndrome. These are the patients with advancing *biliary cirrhosis;* complicated *relapsing pancreatitis;* extensive *granulomatous enteritis* associated with recurrent fistulas, strictures, and mutilative surgery; progressive *scleroderma* of the intestine; *lymphoma* of the small bowel and mesenteric lymph nodes; and progressive *occlusive disease* of the *superior mesenteric artery.* Prognosis for those who have undergone *massive resection* of the small intestine—at once or in stages—is now vastly improved, however, because of intravenous hyperalimentation programs, improved feeding regimens of foods containing protein hydrolysates, and more potent antimicrobial drugs to treat infection. Therapy for *protein-losing enteropathy* is remarkably good if the correct diagnosis is made (Table 6).

On the whole, the prognosis for the malabsorption syndrome is optimistic, provided that the specific abnormality is identified and appropriate corrective measures are instituted.

Krone, C., and Sleisenger, M. H.: Studies on the pathogenesis of malabsorption: Lipid hydrolysis and micelle formation in the intestinal lumen. Medicine, 47:89, 1968.
Losowsky, M. S., Walker, B. E., and Kelleher, J.: Malabsorption in Clinical Practice. Edinburgh and London, Churchill, Livingstone, 1974.
Sleisenger, M. H., and Fordtran, J. S. (eds.): Gastrointestinal Disease. Philadelphia, W. B. Saunders Company, 1973, Chapters 4, 19–21, 66–67, 69–71, 73–76, 93, and 105.
Wilson, F. A., and Dietschy, J. M.: Differential diagnosis to clinical problems of malabsorption. Gastroenterology, 61:911, 1971.

Section Four. DISEASES OF THE PANCREAS

O. Dhodanand Kowlessar

645. ACUTE PANCREATITIS

GENERAL CONSIDERATIONS

During the past decade, rapid progress has been made in the understanding of basic pancreatic physiology and biochemistry. These advances have come from studies that have elucidated the factors controlling the secretion of pancreatic juice, the ultrastructure of the human pancreas by the use of the electron microscope, the sites of synthesis and discharge of pancreatic enzymes by the use of labeled amino acids and pulse chase radioautography, the precise electrolyte and enzyme contents of pancreatic juice, and the amino acid sequence and synthesis of potent pancreatic hormones. The information thus obtained, supplemented by contributions of clinicians, radiologists, and surgeons, has resulted in a better understanding of the pathogenesis of pancreatic inflammation, edema, and hemorrhage. It has further resulted in more exact and reliable diagnostic tests of pancreatic disease and, through utilization of therapeutic measures

directed against specific etiologic mechanisms, in more rational and efficacious treatment. A brief review of pancreatic function will be helpful in understanding the etiology and pathogenesis of acute pancreatitis.

PANCREATIC PHYSIOLOGY, BIOCHEMISTRY, AND ANATOMY

Each day the human pancreas secretes between 1000 and 2500 ml of a clear, colorless fluid, of low viscosity containing 5 to 8 grams of protein, with a pH of 7.5 to 8.5. Pancreatic juice consists mainly of water, electrolytes, and approximately 24 proteins, of which the vast majority are enzymes. The main ions are Na^+, K^+, HCO_3^-, and, in lesser concentrations, Cl^-, Ca^{++}, Zn^{++}, $HPO_4^=$, and $SO_4^=$. Hydrochloric acid stimulates the relase of *secretin,* which acts on the centroacinar cells to produce a watery secretion low in enzyme activity but high in bicarbonate. Secretin also acts in a feedback mechansim to inhibit *gastrin*-stimulated acid production and gastric motility. The augmentation of pancreatic secretion during digestion is the result of stimuli arising within the duodenum and a combination of integrated neurohumoral mechanisms acting on receptor sites on the acinar cells. Feeding stimulates vagal fibers originating in the hypothalamus to mediate the release of acetylcholine. Food distends the antrum, thereby releasing gastrin from "gastrin cells," and also causes the release of *cholecystokinin-pancreozymin* (CCK-PZ) from cells in the duodenal mucosa. Once released into the circulation, acetylcholine, gastrin, and CCK-PZ bind to receptor sites on the pancreatic acinar cell membrane where membrane-bound adenyl cyclase catalyzes the synthesis of cyclic 3-5′ AMP. A series of events is then activated which finally leads to the secretion of zymogen granules. At least two of the pancreatic proteins have been shown to be synthesized in attached ribosomes of the rough endoplasmic reticulum, whence they are transported into the intracisternal spaces to the Golgi complex for condensation, encapsulation, and formation of zymogen granules. The mature granules migrate toward the apex of the acinar cell, and under appropriate exogenous stimuli, a fusion of the zymogen granules and the external cell membrane occurs, allowing their contents to be ejected into the lumen by exocytosis.

Electrolytes are secreted by the human pancreas in a solution that is isotonic with the blood plasma. The concentrations of the cations Na^+, K^+, and Ca^{++} approximate the diffusible ionic content of the blood plasma. The Cl^- content varies inversely with the concentration of HCO_3^-, the latter increasing as the rate of secretion increases. The secretion of bicarbonate appears to be under the catalytic influence of carbonic anhydrase, which controls the formation of bicarbonate ion within the cell according to the following equation: $H_2O + CO_2 \rightleftharpoons H_2CO_3 \rightleftharpoons H^+ + HCO_3^-$. The main function of this balanced electrolyte pancreatic juice, apparently, is to adjust the duodenal contents to an optimal alkaline pH for the action of the pancreatic enzymes.

The proteolytic enzymes are synthesized and secreted as catalytically inert precursors or proenzymes and include trypsin(ogen), chymotrypsin(ogen) A and B, (pro)carboxypeptidases A and B, and (pro)elastase. (Pro)phospholipase A is also secreted in zymogen form. Enterokinase (secreted by the duodenal mucosa) in the presence of calcium catalyzes the transformation of trypsinogen to trypsin. In turn, trypsin catalyzes the formation of trypsinogen, chymotrypsinogen A and B, procarboxypeptidases A and B, proelastase, and prophospholipase A to their active forms.

The proteolytic enzymes hydrolyze dietary proteins to polypeptides of varying chain lengths and amino acids. The peptides undergo further hydrolysis by the brush border hydrolases followed by transport of the amino acids across the epithelial cell. α-Amylase splits starch to α-limit dextrins, maltose and maltotriose for further breakdown by brush border α-dextrinase and maltase. Lipase aided by conjugated bile salts acts on triglyceride to form monoglycerides and fatty acids. Once activated, phospholipase A in the presence of bile salts selectively removes the β-fatty acid from the lecithin molecule to form lysolecithin. The lysolecithin in human duodenal juice is an α-palmitoyl-lysolecithin.

ETIOLOGY OF ACUTE PANCREATITIS

A number of factors have been proposed for the etiology of pancreatitis. The three most important etiologic categories are gallstones, alcohol, and "idiopathic" processes, accounting for 90 to 95 per cent of all cases of acute pancreatitis; miscellaneous factors are implicated in the remaining 5 to 10 per cent of patients. The multiplicity of mechanisms for production of this disease demonstrates that this gland is capable of responding to a wide variety of stresses with a unitary reaction of varying degree.

Biliary Tract Disease. Biliary tract disease may be responsible for 10 to 95 per cent of various large series of pancreatitis. This wide range is related to the incidence of alcoholism in a given patient population.

The causative factors involved in the association of biliary tract disease and acute pancreatitis remain obscure. The importance of a mechanical factor in the pathogenesis of pancreatitis was stressed by Opie, who postulated his "common channel theory" from the observation of acute pancreatitis in a patient with a small stone impacted in the ampulla of Vater. This occurs in 8 per cent of the patients with gallstones and pancreatitis. In a recent study of patients with acute pancreatitis associated with gallbladder disease, there was a temporal relationship between an attack of pancreatitis and the appearance of gallstones in the feces, associated with transient jaundice and hyperamylasemia. Thus it would appear that the pancreatitis was due to an ephemeral mechanical blockage of the ampulla of Vater by migrating stones. It has also been suggested that duodenal contents, composed of unconjugated bile salts secondary to deconjugation of bile salts by microorganisms and lysolecithin secondary to the action of phospholipase A on bile lecithin, reflux into the pancreatic duct and initiate pancreatitis. It is equally possible that bacterial toxins derived from the biliary tree could reach the pancreas via anastomotic lymphatic channels, structurally altering the acinar cell membrane with release of pancreatic enzymes, which in turn initiates pancreatitis.

Alcohol. Alcoholism is responsible for 8 to 75 per cent of cases, depending upon the socioeconomic status of the patient population served by the hospital. The mechanisms whereby ethyl alcohol induces pancreatitis are not known. It is likely that after a large intake of alcohol, gastric acid secretion is stimulated by gastrin release and by direct stimulation of parietal cells. The acid in the duodenum promotes secretion of secretin and pancreozymin with an augmentation of pancreatic secretion by all three gastrointestinal hormones. Concomitantly, a direct effect of ethanol on the sphincter of Oddi would increase sphincteric resistance, with resultant increase in intrapancreatic ductal pressure. Another mechanism involves the reflux of bile into the pancreatic duct during vomiting and retching associated with heavy ethanol intake. Although the mechanical and reflux mechanisms appear cogent, it is possible, though not proved in man, that ethanol exerts a direct toxic effect on the pancreas. In long-term ethanol ingestion in rats, there are significant lipid droplets in the acinar cells, accompanied by mitochondrial swelling and reduction of their inner membranes, with associated degradation of acinar, centroacinar, and duct cells. There is also decreased protein synthesis in the pancreas, with inhibition of ^{32}P into pancreatic phospholipids. Although these experimental results are provocative, further work is needed to substantiate similar effects in man and to define the mechanism of the production of alcoholic pancreatitis.

Idiopathic Factors. Idiopathic factors consistently account for 20 to 50 per cent of large series and thus represent the third most common category; the precise etiology is unknown.

Miscellaneous Causes. A miscellaneous group of etiologic factors make up about 10 per cent of other causes of pancreatitis. Among these are the following: (1) *Metabolic-nutritional disturbances,* including hyperlipemia with genetically determined hyperlipoproteinemia (Types I and V), diabetic ketoacidosis, malnutrition (kwashiorkor), uremia, pregnancy (last trimester or early post partum), and *hypercalcemic states* (hyperparathyroidism, multiple myeloma, excessive doses of vitamin D, and sarcoidosis), which bring about excessive activation of trypsinogen by calcium ion, or by precipitation of calcium in an alkaline milieu in the ducts leading to obstruction. An increased incidence of parathyroid carcinoma causing hyperparathyroidism has been observed in those cases associated with severe pancreatitis. Of note also are the cases of severe pancreatitis occurring within the first 24 hours after the removal of a parathyroid adenoma. *Hereditary pancreatitis* appears to be transmitted as a non-sex-linked mendelian dominant trait modified by incomplete manifestation or sex-related expressivity. The attacks begin, in most cases, in childhood or early adult life, the average age of onset being 12 years, with approximately equal sex incidence. Cholelithiasis and alcoholism are infrequent concomitants. Pancreatic calcifications most often appear as discrete calculi in the larger pancreatic ducts. Aminoaciduria (increased lysine and cystine excretion and, to a lesser extent, arginine) has been observed in approximately 50 per cent of a small group of persons (with or without pancreatitis) so far studied in affected kindreds. However, aminoaciduria might be seen in some patients with nonfamilial pancreatitis. Carcinoma of the pancreas was a cause of death in a few members of kindreds with this entity. A particularly unique feature is the occurrence of portal vein thrombosis and splenic vein thrombosis complicating pancreatitis in a few cases. (2) *Infection* secondary to the reflux of infected material into the pancreatic duct, or from such systemic infections as scarlet fever, streptococcal food poisoning, typhoid fever, viral hepatitis, infectious mononucleosis, mumps, and coxsackievirus group B. (3) *Trauma:* Steering-wheel injuries, penetrating injuries from bullets or knife wounds, postoperative pancreatitis (after surgery in the area of the pancreas, as well as distant areas from the pancreas, e.g., transurethral resection), and electric shock. (4) *Vascular and autoimmune mechanisms:* Atheromatous embolization to intrapancreatic arteries, renal transplantation, extracorporeal circulation, polyarteritis nodosa, and systemic lupus erythematosus. (5) *Drugs:* Glucocorticoids, chlorothiazide, isoniazid, salicylates, sulfamethizole, indomethacin, salicylazosulfapyridine, L-asparaginase, immunosuppressive drugs (6-mercaptopurine and azathioprine), and oral contraceptives, especially in women who have Type 4 as well as Type 5 lipid patterns before therapy. (6) *Scorpion bite.* (7) *Pancreatic carcinoma.* (8) *Obstructive lesions* at the sphincter of Oddi secondary to benign polyps and regional enteritis of the duodenum.

PATHOGENESIS

The essential lesion in acute pancreatitis is necrosis of the acinar cells, and the clinical severity is determined by the extent of the damage to the exocrine pancreas. The underlying mechanism in the production of pancreatic inflammation is the escape of activated enzymes into the interstitial tissues, and the earliest responses to this chemical irritation are edema and vascular engorgement of the pancreas. Normally, the pancreatic proteases (trypsin, chymotrypsin, elastase, and carboxypeptidases) and phospholipase A are stored in the acinar cell as inactive precursors. The Golgi complex, ergastoplasm, zymogen granule, and the cell membrane segregate the exportable pancreatic enzymes in the acinar cell, as well as the lysosomal hydrolases. Two potent protease inhibitors which guard against intracellular activation of trypsinogen are also present in the exocrine cell. Theoretically, regardless of the etiology, a common denominator of the pathogenetic mechanism could be an increase in the permeability of the lipoprotein membranes which surround the exportable and lysosomal hydrolases with subsequent release of these enzymes with concomitant edema, coagulation necrosis, vascular injury, and hemorrhage.

Edema may occur anywhere in the gland, but is apt to be more severe in the head. The region affected becomes pale and indurated, with progressive engorgement of the blood vessels. In most instances the inflammatory edema subsides spontaneously, but in a small percentage of cases there is progression to hemorrhage, necrosis, and suppuration, or the inflammation becomes chronic. Progression of pancreatic edema to hemorrhagic necrosis is in part the result of enlargement of the pancreas within its capsule, which obstructs the pancreatic duct further and aggravates the vascular engorgement until ischemia supervenes. As elsewhere, ischemia superimposed on an inflammatory process results in infarction and hemorrhage. Activated elastase may bring about erosion of major blood vessels, with hemorrhage into the pancreas, the retroperitoneal tissues, and even the colon. Collections of blood, digested tissue, and pancreatic secretions may burrow along the tissue spaces into the gastrohepatic ligament and retroperitoneally into the lesser sac and flank, giving rise to the classic ascitic exudate of acute pancreatitis described as "beef broth," and to visible hemorrhagic areas in the costovertebral angle (Grey-Turner sign). The peritoneal effusion and peritoneal irritation during the early stages of acute pancreatitis are greatest in the lesser sac and at the base of the transverse mesocolon. This localized chemical peritonitis often results in a segmental paralytic ileus of the first jejunal loop, which has been described as a diagnostic sign, the "sentinel loop" of acute pancreatitis.

Thus the local pathology of pancreatitis at the inception is the result of edema, hemorrhage, and the onslaught of biochemical agents, i.e., the pancreatic enzymes. If the disease progresses without resolution, superimposed infection, especially by colonic bacteria, produces suppuration and results in pancreatic abscesses, as well as purulent collections in the various abdominal fossae, the lesser sac, the cul-de-sac, and the left subphrenic space.

Resolution may occur with fibrosis and calcification. The edema and other inflammatory changes subside during the first week of illness. Areas of necrosis are autolyzed and replaced by fibrous tissue. Cellular proliferation attempts to restore normal glandular architecture. By the end of the second week histologic repair may have proceeded to such a degree that the pancreas may appear normal. On the other hand, resolution is delayed in the more severe forms, with persistence of residual fibrosis, calcification, and acinar dysfunction.

DIAGNOSIS

Clinical Manifestations. *Pain* and *shock* are the outstanding symptoms of acute hemorrhagic pancreatitis; *pain* and *metabolic disturbances* dominate the clinical picture of acute edematous pancreatitis and chronic relapsing pancreatitis. However, all three—pain, shock, and metabolic disturbances—may be absent, as in painless pancreatitis.

The *pain* in acute pancreatitis results from distention of the pancreatic capsule, retroperitoneal extravasations, chemical peritonitis, and obstruction or spasm in the pancreatic ducts, extrahepatic biliary tract, and duodenum. Characteristically, the attack is sudden, and the pain is usually severe, constant, and widespread. It is frequently more intense when the patient is lying supine than when he is sitting or lying on the side with his spine flexed. Although usually originating in the epigastrium, the pain also may be experienced in other parts of the abdomen, and may radiate to the back, substernal area, and flanks. Physical examination discloses an acutely ill patient complaining of abdominal pain, with fever and tachycardia. The blood pressure may be slightly elevated in those in whom circulatory collapse has not supervened. *Cyanosis, cold* and *clammy skin, rapid* and *feeble pulse,* and *subnormal temperature* are present in the more severe attacks. The abdomen may be distended early as a result of paralytic ileus and the accumulation of peritoneal fluid. Peristalsis may be diminished or inaudible. *Tenderness* is invariably present in the epigastrium, and is associated with a moderate degree of muscular rigidity; it may be elicited elsewhere in the abdomen, depending on the sites of seepage of the pancreatic juice. Occasionally, a mass in the upper abdomen—an inflammatory *pseudocyst*—may be palpable. The systemic effects in acute pancreatitis are presumed to result from the absorption of activated pancreatic enzymes and the products of the activation of the bradykinin system.

Shock is the outstanding systemic phenomenon in *severe acute pancreatitis,* and may be so profound that death ensues within a few hours. The shock results from a combination of the following events: (1) presumed increase in serum proteolytic activity; (2) the release of the activated enzyme kallikrein, which in turn is responsible for the formation of kinins, whose main actions are stimulation of smooth muscle, dilatation of blood vessels, and lowering of blood pressure; (3) contraction of the blood volume, as great as 30 per cent, secondary to exudation of blood and plasma into the peritoneal cavity and possible protein leak; and (4) hyperlipasemia, which may then be related to hyperlipemia and to fat necrosis of the subcutaneous tissue and the bone marrow. Additional factors are (5) acute coronary insufficiency resulting from thrombosis and electrolyte disturbances (in turn, the lowered blood volume and shock contribute to the myocardial problem); (6) pulmonary embolus; (7) massive bleeding; and (8) intravascular coagulopathy.

In many cases, other metabolic disturbances can be uncovered. Serum calcium, potassium, and sodium are lowered. The depression of calcium is due partly to fixation by fatty acids in areas of fat necrosis and increased levels of circulating glucagon, which in turn stimulate the secretion of thyrocalcitonin with resultant inhibition of bone resorption. Glucagon can also directly inhibit bone resorption, induced either by parathyroid hormone or dibutyryl-3′-5′-adenosine monophosphate, indicating an additional glucagon action independent of thyrocalcitonin. Levels of calcium below 7 mg per 100 ml are usually accompanied by tetany.

Injury to the β-cells, as well as release of glucagon and glucocorticoids, secondary to pancreatic inflammation, are associated with *hyperglycemia, glycosuria,* and impaired glucose tolerance in about 50 per cent of the cases. These changes, although transient in the acute cases, may, with repeated attacks, progress to true "pancreatic" diabetes. *Coma* may be the presenting symptom of severe hemorrhagic pancreatitis; when associated with the commonly elevated blood sugar in acute pancreatitis, diabetic coma may be erroneously diagnosed. Likewise, confusion, restlessness, and disorientation have been observed during an acute attack ("pancreatic psychosis or encephalopathy").

Jaundice is seen in about 25 per cent of patients with acute pancreatitis, resulting primarily from obstruction of the terminal common duct as it traverses an edematous pancreas; in some patients, exacerbation of associated biliary tract disease may also be partly responsible. Intrahepatic cholestasis secondary to alcoholic liver disease may also contribute to the icterus.

Hyperlipemia with grossly opalescent serum has been observed in 3 to 8 per cent of patients with alcoholic pancreatitis and is due to a striking chylomicronemia or very low density lipoproteins. In follow-up studies of many of these patients, an underlying hyperlipidemia antedated the pancreatitis. Some authors have reported disseminated fat necrosis in the bone marrow and subcutaneous tissues. Acute and chronic bone lesions secondary to medullary necrosis have been described. *Pulmonary atelectasis, pneumonia,* and *pleural effusion,* particularly left-sided, are noted frequently. Significantly, pancreatic enzyme concentrations are higher in the pleural effusion than in simultaneously obtained serum. These enzymes are thought to reach the pleural fluid from the ascitic exudate by passage through the transdiaphragmatic lymphatic channels. Occasionally, *respiratory symptoms* may overshadow the abdominal complaints. Recently, mild to moderate degrees of respiratory insufficiency characterized by *arterial hypoxia* and *mild respiratory alkalosis* have been observed in a significant number of patients with acute pancreatitis.

The vascular phenomena in acute pancreatitis include peripheral *venous thromboses* and *thrombophlebitis* and mildly diffuse hemorrhage, widespread thrombosis, and disseminated intravascular coagulopathy.

Laboratory Diagnosis. *Serum Enzymes.* A diagnosis of acute pancreatitis may be made when an elevated serum amylase, usually greater than 300 Somogyi units, is found in a patient with acute, severe pain in the upper abdomen, tenderness, vomiting, fever, tachycardia, and leukocytosis. The serum amylase becomes elevated early in the course of the disease, usually within the first 24 to 48 hours. In most cases, values range from 300 to 800, but levels as high as 12,000 units have been reported. Apparently no constant relationship exists, however, between the severity of the disease and the height of the serum amylase values. Milder episodes may have considerable elevations. Conversely, in attacks with early fatality, the amylase values (as well as other enzyme levels) may be greatly decreased because of destruction of the pancreas. The serum *lipase* usually rises in parallel with the amylase activity, reaching its peak in 72 or 96 hours with a gradual fall; values greater than 2.0 ml of N/100 NaOH are significant. Elevations of the levels of glutamic oxaloacetic acid transaminase, alkaline phosphatase, and leucine aminopeptidase are usually secondary to obstruction of the common bile duct or associated liver disease.

A variety of diseases, intra-abdominal and extra-abdominal, may be accompanied by elevation of the serum enzymes, frequently posing a difficult diagnostic problem. Hyperamylasemia is encountered in *perforation of peptic ulcer, small bowel obstruction, salivary duct occlusion, parotitis,* and *uremia,* and after administration of opiates, notably codeine and morphine. Elevations of serum lipase have been reported in patients with *carcinoma of the pancreas; obstructive jaundice caused by stone, tumors,* and *cirrhosis of the liver; viral hepatitis; intestinal obstruction;* and *peritonitis.* It should be pointed out, however, that in these instances the serum enzyme elevations are not as high as in acute pancreatitis.

Urinary Amylase.   Elevation of urinary amylase concentration has been used to diagnose acute pancreatitis in the absence of renal failure. Levels of urinary amylase higher than 6000 units per 24 hours or 300 units per hour are usually seen in patients with acute attacks of pancreatitis. A more precise method of diagnosing and following patients with acute pancreatitis is to determine concomitant concentrations of amylase (units per milliliter) and creatinine (milligrams per milliliter) in serum and in a simultaneously voided urine specimen. Thus C_{Am}/C_{Cr} can be determined by the following formula:

$$C_{Am}/C_{Cr} (\%) = \frac{(Am)\ urine}{(Am)\ serum} \times \frac{(Cr)\ serum}{(Cr)\ urine} \times 100$$

In normal subjects this ratio is 2.3 ± 0.1 per cent, whereas in renal insufficiency the ratio is 2.1 ± 0.2 per cent. In acute pancreatitis there is a significant increase in the ratio of 6.6 ± 0.3 per cent, with gradual fall to normal levels in 9 to 15 days. Acute exacerbations during the clinical course of pancreatitis are characterized by an increase in the ratio. In contrast to pancreatitis, patients with macroamylasemia (amylases with molecular weights of at least 160,000) were consistently associated with a low ratio of 0.34 ± 0.13 per cent. This low ratio can serve as a simple screening test for macroamylasemia.

Other Laboratory Data.   Ancillary laboratory findings must be considered in making the diagnosis. The *leukocyte count* often ranges from 10,000 to 30,000 per cubic millimeter, with an increase in immature granulocytes. In mild cases, the leukocyte count may be normal. The hematocrit and erythrocyte count are usually not significantly lowered, except when there is hemorrhage into the gastrointestinal tract or peritoneal cavity. Elevation of *blood urea nitrogen* is not uncommon in the more severe cases, especially when shock and oliguria are present. *Glycosuria* appears in about 11 per cent of patients with acute pancreatitis, and disappears with resolution of the process. Transient *hyperglycemia* may be found more frequently than glycosuria. Bilirubin is usually slightly elevated – 2.0 to 4.0 mg per 100 ml; higher levels may indicate that common duct obstruction underlies the pancreatitis.

A slight depression of serum *calcium* occurs in most patients between the third and fifteenth days of the disease, the lowest level occurring about the sixth day. Serum calcium below 7.0 mg per 100 ml portends a poor although not invariably fatal prognosis. Diminished serum albumin lowers the total serum calcium, so that hypoalbuminemia should be evaluated in the assessment of serum calcium and in replacement therapy. An unexpectedly normal serum calcium level in severe pancreatitis may be the first indication of hyperparathyroidism. *Hypokalemia* may be observed, and is most likely related to alkalosis, intravenous administration of saline solution, and loss of gastric juice because of continuous nasogastric suction. In severe cases, in which there is considerable tissue destruction, *shock* with oliguria causes hyperkalemia.

Electrocardiography.   The electrocardiograms of some patients with acute pancreatitis may show depression of S-T segments in the limb leads and precordial leads as well as changes in the Q-T intervals. These changes may be due to the electrolyte imbalance or may be related to the shock in the more severe cases.

Roentgenographic Findings.   Although in no way pathognomonic of acute pancreatitis, certain roentgenographic abnormalities are encountered with sufficient frequency to suggest the diagnosis. A survey film of the abdomen may reveal a localized paralytic ileus of jejunum ("sentinel loop"), usually in the left midportion of the abdomen, or calcification in the region of the pancreas (see accompanying figure) or the "colon cut-off" sign. The latter consists of an isolated gaseous distention of the colon and hepatic flexure owing to partial obstruction caused by spread of the inflammatory process from the head of the pancreas. Barium swallow may demonstrate displacement of the stomach, enlargement of the duodenal loop, or collection and stasis of barium in the dependent parts of the duodenum caused by an enlarged head of the pancreas or an inflammatory *pseudocyst.* *Pancreatic ultrasonography* (echography) will show pseudocysts as smoothly rounded transonic spaces, often with a distinct wall. This technique reliably estimates the size of even small pseudocysts. Also there may be an

Left oblique roentgenogram of abdomen demonstrating pancreatic calcification.

enlarged edematous ampulla of Vater and irritability of the stomach and duodenum. In most instances the biliary tree may be adequately visualized by intravenous cholangiography, excluding bile duct obstruction as the precipitating event. Nonvisualization of the gallbladder after either oral or intravenous administration of dye, however, is a common finding during the acute episode, but does not necessarily indicate a disease of the gallbladder. Accordingly, the roentgenographic studies should be repeated several weeks after the attack has subsided, at which time, if the gallbladder is diseased, stones in the biliary tree and/or nonfilling of the gallbladder will be observed. The chest roentgenogram may show pleural effusion (usually on the left side), elevated left diaphragm, or linear focal atelectasis at the lung bases.

Other Diagnostic Procedures. Diagnostic tap of the peritoneum, performed under local anesthesia, in the left lower quadrant of the abdomen may reveal turbid yellow fluid in edematous pancreatitis or reddish-brown fluid in the hemorrhagic type. The peritoneal fluid amylase is considerably higher than serum amylase tested at the same time, and may remain elevated for two or three days after the serum amylase has fallen to normal levels. The determination of serum *methemalbumin* has been proposed as a diagnostic test for pancreatitis. Recent evidence suggests that elevated levels have occurred in other acute abdominal emergencies. However, if methemalbumin is detected within the first 24 hours in serum, pleural effusions, or ascitic fluid in a patient with clinical and biochemical evidence of pancreatitis, the diagnosis of necrotizing pancreatitis is justified.

Differential Diagnosis. The diagnosis of acute pancreatitis should be established as rapidly as clinical and laboratory facilities permit. However, the diagnosis is made difficult by the large number of abdominal catastrophes that may in many ways simulate this condition.

Perforated peptic ulcer, more than any other abdominal condition, may resemble acute pancreatitis. Usually a preceding history compatible with ulcer can be elicited, although occasionally perforation may be its first indication. Unlike pancreatitis, however, *boardlike rigidity of the abdomen* is the outstanding finding. A flat plate of the abdomen may show free air, usually under the right diaphragm. Hyperamylasemia, resulting from the escape of duodenal contents into the peritoneum or involvement of the pancreas in the process, may accompany perforation, but usually the values are not as high as in acute pancreatitis. (See Ch. 640 to 644.)

Biliary colic may resemble acute pancreatitis by virtue of pressure changes in the biliary tree and associated inflammation of the gallbladder. Pain, tenderness, and rigidity are frequently localized in the right upper quadrant of the abdomen. *Acute cholangitis,* caused by stones in the common bile duct, is usually associated with chills, fever, and jaundice. An elevated serum amylase is seen in about 20 per cent of cases of common duct stone, and differentiation may have to await the course of the disease.

The pain of *acute cholecystitis* is usually in the right upper quadrant and may radiate to the right scapula. Tenderness and guarding are present in the right upper quadrant. A striking feature is that, despite the pain, these patients do not usually look very ill, in contrast to patients with acute pancreatitis.

Acute *small bowel obstruction* may be a diagnostic problem in view of occasional associated hyperamylasemia. The history of vomiting and the cramplike periumbilical pain with abdominal distention and visible peristalsis are helpful. In mechanical ileus, auscultation will reveal high-pitched notes, succussion splashes, and peristaltic rushes. Acute appendicitis involving a retrocecal appendix in close contact with the gallbladder may require differentiation. The amylase is usually normal in this condition.

Mesenteric thrombosis may present as intestinal obstruction with a less acute onset. This may be associated with bloody diarrhea, which is rare in pancreatitis. Shock is more acute, and diffuse tenderness and rigidity are more common. A flat plate of the abdomen may show a large, dilated, fluid-filled loop of bowel, the site of infarction.

Dissecting aneurysm usually presents with severe pain, shock, absent pulsations in the femoral vessels, and lowered blood pressure in the legs. A pulsating mass may be felt.

Nephrolithiasis on the left side may simulate acute pancreatitis. Hematuria and a flat plate of the abdomen revealing a stone will help in the differentiation.

Acute coronary occlusion may present with left upper quadrant or epigastric pain, nausea, and vomiting. Electrocardiographic changes and elevation of the serum glutamic oxaloacetic transaminase occur in pancreatitis, but Q waves are not ordinarily present in pancreatitis. Also, the lack of elevation of serum enzymes of pancreatic origin will help exclude acute pancreatitis.

Acute intermittent porphyria is usually associated with a history of vomiting at intervals, severe and frequent episodes of abdominal pain, and chronic constipation. The demonstration of porphobilinogen in the urine by the Watson-Schwartz test is helpful in establishing the diagnosis.

Acute systemic lupus erythematosus and *periarteritis nodosa* may present with an abdominal picture requiring differentiation from pancreatitis. The situation is further confused by the fact that pancreatitis may be a complication of these diseases. The history, coupled with other common findings in these diseases, will help in the differential diagnosis.

TREATMENT

Acute pancreatitis varies greatly in the degree of its severity. The milder attacks are presumably due to edema of the pancreas, and in this situation therapy is directed primarily to the relief of pain. In the more severe form with hemorrhage and necrosis and their concomitant physiologic and biochemical disturbances discussed previously, treatment may conveniently be divided into several distinct phases.

Control of Pain. The pain is usually severe, and should be treated promptly with adequate doses of analgesics. Meperidine (Demerol), with its minimal effect on the tone of the sphincter of Oddi, is probably the drug of choice and should be given parenterally in doses of 75 to 100 mg every four to six hours to assure prompt and adequate relief. Morphine and codeine should be avoided because of their spasmogenic effects. Sympathetic nerve blocks and continuous or fractional epidural anesthesia can be used to supplement the effects of meperidine in patients whose pain is persistent.

Treatment of Shock. Circulatory collapse is often the most immediate and major problem of the severe form of pancreatitis. Whole blood is probably the most effective treatment and, in view of the diminution of blood volume to approximately 70 per cent in severe cases, should be given promptly. Large volumes of fluid are often required; constant monitoring of central venous pressure and careful measurement of fluid intake and urinary output are necessary. Albumin and plasma are adequate temporary substitutes. Low molecular weight dextran may be highly effective and should be tried. It can decrease blood viscosity, expand plasma volume, and improve peripheral blood flow, and has antithrombotic activity. Patients with severe, unresponsive disease may be given an infusion of 1:500,000 isoproterenol hydrochloride (Isuprel), commencing with a dose rate of 0.5 to 4.0 μg per minute with careful electrocardiographic monitoring.

Inhibition of Pancreatic Secretory Activity. An important principle in the management of acute pancreatitis is the "splinting of the injured pancreas" by suppression of pancreatic secretion. Achievement of this goal is accomplished by cessation of oral intake of food, continuous nasogastric suction to minimize release of secretin through stimulation by gastric acid, and administration of drugs to inhibit pancreatic secretion. Propantheline (Pro-Banthine) bromide, 30 mg, or methantheline (Banthine) bromide, 50 mg, given parenterally every six to eight hours, have enjoyed wide popularity, although their efficacy remains in doubt. Their pharmacologic effects include suppression of gastric acidity, relaxation of the sphincter, and partial inhibition of pancreatic enzyme production. However, in the presence of *paralytic ileus* and *shock,* these drugs may be harmful and should be avoided.

Recently, *glucagon* in an initial dose of 1 mg intravenously, followed by 1.0 to 1.5 mg in 5 per cent dextrose or normal saline every four hours, has been reported to result in clinical improvement and relief of pain associated with a fall of serum amylase. It has been suggested that the beneficial effect observed was due to the inhibition of pancreatic secretion, thus suppressing the activity of the acutely inflamed gland. The serum calcium should be monitored if this form of therapy is used.

Antimicrobials. The prophylactic use of antimicrobials for the prevention of infection in severe cases of acute pancreatitis is purely empirical and without controlled studies. It has been proposed that the protein-rich exudate in edematous, poorly perfused tissues is favorable for bacterial growth. Appropriate cultures of blood, urine, sputum, and effusions are taken. Antimicrobial drugs should be withheld unless there is reason to suspect infection, evidenced by sustained or high spiking fevers (higher than 39° C) strongly suggesting either pancreatic abscess or cholangitis. Intramuscular ampicillin, 500 mg, and kanamycin, 250 mg, every six hours must then be initiated. Abscesses must be drained or obstruction of the common bile duct relieved along with cholecystectomy and cholecystostomy with continued appropriate antimicrobial therapy. An important clue to underlying cholangitis is persisting jaundice with bilirubin levels above 4.0 mg per 100 ml.

Fluids and Electrolytes. The continued gastric suction and the abstinence from any oral intake make it necessary to replace body fluids and electrolytes carefully. The amount of normal saline with supplemental potassium chloride to be administered may vary between 3 and 6 liters daily and should be estimated by considering the insensible loss, the amount of sweating, the elevation of temperature, the volume of gastric suction, and the anticipated urinary output. Glucose must be administered cautiously, for it may aggravate a diabetic state that has been precipitated by acute pancreatitis. When hyperglycemia and glycosuria are marked and diabetic acidosis is imminent, small doses of insulin must be given.

Hypocalcemia is fairly frequent, and calcium gluconate solution may be given intravenously as needed. *Hypokalemia* is combated by cautious intravenous administration of potassium chloride. Blood potassium determinations and electrocardiograms should be done frequently to avoid potassium toxicity.

Miscellaneous Measures. Abdominal distention and ileus are usually adequately managed by gastric suction, but occasionally it may be necessary to insert a long intestinal tube to deflate the small intestine. The adynamic nature of this ileus makes the passage of such a tube rather difficult.

Many drugs have been used in the treatment of acute pancreatitis, but since the disease is self-limiting in most instances, it is difficult to assess their efficacy. In recent years, the use of corticotrophin and cortisone has been advocated in acute fulminant pancreatitis, particularly when an abdominal exploration has been performed without previous knowledge of the existence of the disease. However, evidence has accumulated that steroids, when used in other diseases, have brought about lesions similar to those seen in pancreatitis. Thus caution should be exercised, and these drugs should be reserved for those patients in whom shock has developed that is unresponsive to the usual measures.

Peritoneal dialysis should be attempted in those patients whose symptoms fail to improve after a period of conservative therapy and who appear to be dying of their disease. The dialysate recently used with some success consists of sodium, 141 mEq per liter, calcium, 3.5 mEq per liter, magnesium, 1.5 mEq per liter, chloride, 101 mEq per liter, and lactate, 4.5 mEq per liter, given via a standard peritoneal dialysis catheter. After a half hour of delay, the fluid is removed by straight drainage, and the procedure is repeated. Dramatic improvement in shock, oliguria, and correction of electrolyte imbalance has occurred in many patients.

Surgical Measures. It has become accepted generally that immediate operation for pancreatitis can do no good and that elective surgery should await the subsidence of the acute attack. In cases in which it is impossible to make the diagnosis and in which there is evidence of progressively serious pancreatitis that has failed to respond to medical management, laparotomy and surgery are justified. If hemorrhagic, suppurative, or necrotic pancreatitis is found, aggressive drainage of the pancreatic bed may improve the prognosis. A major indication for surgery is infection in the biliary tree, especially cholangitis. Even if pancreatitis appears fulminant, relief of obstruction and drainage are mandatory. Surgical consultation should be obtained in all cases of pancreatitis, particularly in patients with serum amylase greater than 1000, because it appears that these patients are more likely to have acute or chronic cholecystitis and cholelithiasis. Likewise, patients with *pancreatic abscesses* and those with *pseudocysts* which do not decompress are clearly surgical candidates.

Management after Acute Attack. Management should be directed toward the prevention of future attacks. Patients should be given a low fat diet and small, frequent meals to minimize pancreatic secretion; they should be told to avoid alcohol. Anticholinergic and analgesic drugs to minimize pancreatic secretion and pain are useful adjuncts. Overeating, obesity, and alcoholic abuse seem to be important precipitating factors and should be interdicted.

PROGNOSIS

Recovery is universal for patients with acute edematous pancreatitis; however, the fatality rate among those with hemorrhagic or necrotic disease is high, approximating 50 per cent. It is difficult to state the percentage of patients with acute pancreatitis who develop the chronic relapsing form of the disease. Suffice it to say that continued alcoholism or neglected biliary tract disease is often associated with recurrent attacks. Another important determining factor is the degree of ductal obstruction that is the residue of the initial bout of inflammation. Correction or control of an underlying cause, e.g., an endocrine disturbance such as hyperparathyroidism, or the withdrawal of a potentially noxious drug may help to prevent further attacks.

Condon, J. R., Knight, M., and Day, J. L.: Glucagon therapy in acute pancreatitis. Br. J. Surg., 60:509, 1973.

Creutzfeldt, W., and Schmidt, H.: Aetiology and pathogenesis of pancreatitis (current concepts). Scand. J. Gastroenterol. (Suppl.), 6:47, 1970.

Dreiling, D. A., Janowitz, H. D., and Perrier, C. V.: Pancreatic Inflammatory Disease: A Physiologic Approach. New York, Harper & Row, 1964.

Geokas, M. C.: Acute pancreatitis (medical progress). Calif. Med., 117:25, 1972.

Levitt, M. D., Rapport, M., and Cooperband, S. R.: The renal clearance of amylase in renal insufficiency, acute pancreatitis and macroamylasemia. Ann. Intern. Med., 71:919, 1969.

Ranson, J. H. C., Roses, D. F., and Fink, S. D.: Early respiratory insufficiency in acute pancreatitis. Ann. Surg., 178:75, 1973.

Webster, P. D., III.: Pancreatic acinar cells and their clinical significance. Viewpoints on Digestive Diseases, 4:No. 5, 1972.

646. CHRONIC PANCREATITIS AND CHRONIC RELAPSING PANCREATITIS

The most common clinical form of chronic pancreatitis is *chronic relapsing pancreatitis,* suggesting exacerbations of acute disease superimposed upon a previously injured gland. Acute pancreatitis may recur frequently and not progress to chronic pancreatitis, but such attacks invariably damage the pancreas. The parenchyma of the gland, subjected to cycles of fat necrosis, edema, and calcification, is gradually and extensively replaced by fibrotic tissue with disappearance of acinar and islet tissue. During the early stages of relapsing pancreatitis, the functional reserve of the gland and its capacity for protein synthesis and recovery are so great that enzyme deficiencies are only transiently demonstrable during the acute attacks. Since the disease process is frequently more severe in the region of the head of the gland, and the islets of Langerhans are concentrated in the body and tail, disturbed carbohydrate metabolism appears relatively late. Calcium is deposited in the obstructed

main duct and intralobular ducts as well as in areas of fat necrosis in the parenchyma (see figure in Ch. 645). In the later stages, with extensive destruction of the parenchyma and islet tissue (probably greater than 90 per cent of the pancreas), the biochemical abnormalities of altered carbohydrate metabolism (diabetes), increased excretion of stool fat (steatorrhea), and increased excretion of stool nitrogen (azotorrhea) will follow.

Etiology. Chronic relapsing pancreatitis may be caused by a wide variety of etiologic factors, but the principal one is the toxic effect of *chronic alcohol ingestion.* A second cause, although less frequent, is *untreated biliary tract disease* (gallstones). *Trauma* may also be an important cause, because the initial event may leave residual damage to the ductal system. Recently, because of the recurrent nature of the disease, the possibility of an autoimmune mechanism or a hypersensitivity state has been suggested. Indeed, the serum of patients with pancreatitis contains one or more precipitating antibodies that react with homologous pancreatic homogenate. The inability to create experimental pancreatitis by the injection of antiserum, coupled with the incomplete understanding of the mechanism of antibody formation, makes these observations only of experimental interest at this time.

Clinical Manifestations. Chronic pancreatitis begins most often in the third or fourth decade of life, but may begin in early childhood or old age. It is more common in men than in women and, unlike gallbladder disease, has no predilection for obese persons.

The clinical syndrome is readily divided into two stages. In the earlier stage the outstanding feature is recurrent attacks of severe abdominal pain (relapsing pancreatitis); the later stage is characterized by metabolic disturbances, e.g., *diabetes, steatorrhea,* and *azotorrhea,* with concomitant weight loss (chronic pancreatitis). Pseudocyst formation and pancreatic calcification are also common complications.

The abdominal pain in both stages is the same as that described in Ch. 645, and it may persist for days to weeks. Between attacks the patient may be asymptomatic except for occasional complaints of fullness, abdominal distention, and dull epigastric ache. As the disease progresses, the intervals between attacks become shorter, and the pain may eventually be continuous, requiring constant therapy with narcotics, which in some cases may lead to addiction. *Nausea, vomiting, chills, jaundice,* and *tachycardia* may be associated with these painful episodes.

Physical examination of the abdomen during an acute exacerbation may reveal the signs of acute pancreatitis. In addition, an epigastric mass may be found, representing either an inflamed pseudocyst of the pancreas or an enlarged fatty liver. With repeated attacks, the parenchymal disturbances become irreversible, and cause *steatorrhea* and *diabetes mellitus.* Loss of weight, despite a good appetite and a satisfactory caloric intake, results from faulty digestion and absorption of fat. The stools become bulky, frothy, glistening, and foul smelling, and they may increase in frequency (see Part XIV, Section Three). Sometimes, diabetes and/or steatorrhea first attracts attention to the existence of a destructive inflammatory process in the pancreas.

Course and Diagnosis. *Dysfunction of Acinar Cells.* The degree of disruption of acinar cells as reflected by serum levels of amylase and lipase depends on the stage of the disease. During an acute attack, levels of serum amylase and lipase are increased (see above). These enzyme values tend to rise early and return to normal after the acute attack. Elevations may persist when the attacks occur in rapid succession, when activity is prolonged, or in the presence of pancreatic ductal obstruction by stone or perisphincteric fibrosis. With repeated attacks, more and more of the gland is destroyed; thus late in the disease, even though active pancreatitis is present, serum levels of amylase and lipase do not rise. At this stage, abnormal fat excretion, usually greater than 7 grams of fat, and nitrogen excretion, greater than 2.5 grams of nitrogen daily, will be found.

Deficient secretion of pancreatic juice is consistently encountered in chronic pancreatitis. The characteristic changes in pancreatic juice are subnormal volume and bicarbonate concentration after the intravenous injection of 1 clinical unit of *secretin* per kilogram of body weight. The normal volume response is 2 ml or more per kilogram in 80 minutes, and the maximal bicarbonate concentration should reach 90 mEq per liter in any 20-minute specimen. Volume response as well as enzyme concentrations may be normal in the face of diminished bicarbonate except when the disease is advanced. It has not been established whether this dissociation indicates a differentiation of function between the acinar and intralobular cells or a differential loss of function of the secretory cells.

Disturbance of Function of Islet Cells. In the early stages of relapsing pancreatitis, acute attacks may demonstrate temporary islet cell dysfunction, characterized by *glycosuria, hyperglycemia,* and even abnormal glucose tolerance curves. However, with advanced disease, there is further destruction of islet tissue, and frank *diabetes mellitus* is encountered.

Roentgenographic demonstration of calcification in the region of the pancreas furnishes additional evidence of chronic pancreatitis (see figure in Ch. 645).

Forward and upward displacement of the stomach by inflammatory masses or pseudocysts with lifting of the antrum may be seen along with indenting or flattening of the duodenal sweep. Endoscopic pancreatocholangiograms may demonstrate strictures, stones, dilatation, narrowing, and tortuosity of the pancreatic ducts.

In the *differential diagnosis* of the acute painful episodes of chronic relapsing pancreatitis, the same causes of abdominal pain that were discussed in Ch. 645 must be considered. In the later stage, when steatorrhea and malabsorption are present, *adult celiac disease, carcinoma of the pancreas, and Whipple's disease* should be excluded (see Part XIV, Section Three). *Primary atrophy of the pancreas* should be excluded. This is a disease of unknown cause, appearing in both sexes after the fifth decade. The fully developed clinical picture of pancreatic atrophy is that of a deficiency syndrome characterized by steatorrhea, weight loss, normal or increased appetite, occasionally edema, anasarca, and diabetes mellitus. Abdominal pain, pancreatic calcification, and increase of serum enzymes are absent. By the time the disease is recognized clinically, the pancreas has undergone nearly complete atrophy. This observation underscores the great reserve capacity of this gland. The predominant chronic symptom, steatorrhea, usually begins insidiously and is generally mild. Edema and anasarca are frequently the initial signs in this disease. When there is an associated decrease of islet cells, diabetes mellitus of varying degrees develops. Exploratory laparotomy may be necessary for exact diagnosis.

Pathologically, this entity is characterized by almost complete disappearance of the acinar cells and, to a lesser extent, of the islets of Langerhans. Fatty replacement of the atrophic tissue may be an accompanying finding.

Painless Pancreatitis. Although clinically the hallmark of chronic pancreatitis is recurrent bouts of severe upper abdominal pain lasting for days or weeks and followed by epigastric tenderness for even longer periods, the disease may be painless. The diagnosis is to be suspected when one encounters a patient who, without having experienced abdominal pain, has the sequelae of chronic pancreatitis, i.e., pancreatic calcification, diabetes mellitus, and steatorrhea. All of these may coexist, or they may occur in various combinations. Infrequently, at operation, painless jaundice may be found to have resulted from obstruction of the common bile duct by a chronically inflamed pancreas. Recent evidence suggests that acute or subacute edematous forms of pancreatitis may occur without abdominal pain. In one review of 25 cases of chronic pancreatitis at necropsy in a 35-year period, the pathologist was unable to discover any clinical record that abdominal pain had occurred in 15 patients (60 per cent). Such observations suggest that acute edematous pancreatitis may occur more frequently than is suspected and that it may undergo progression either to irreversible change or to complete resolution without recognition by either physician or patient.

Treatment. Palliation of acute symptoms and efforts to terminate the acute exacerbation have been discussed in Ch. 645. Management comprises bed rest, limiting the oral intake of fluids, nasogastric suction, adequate sedation and narcotics, and appropriate fluids and electrolytes.

Nonsurgical Treatment. Medical means for preventing attacks of chronic relapsing pancreatitis and halting the progression of the disease are few and of limited value. Adherence to a bland, low-fat diet, avoidance of overeating, abstinence from alcohol, and the use of anticholinergics (propantheline bromide [Pro-Banthine], 15 to 30 mg, or methantheline bromide [Banthine], 50 to 100 mg, given one half hour before meals and at bedtime) are the principal measures. Management of pancreatic insufficiency secondary to progressive pancreatic destruction requires control of diabetes and of excessive losses of fat and nitrogen, with their associated abdominal distention, cramps, borborygmi, increased flatus, passage of large, malodorous and frequent stools, and loss of weight. The dietary intake of fat is usually restricted to 70 grams a day, and 120 grams of protein and up to 450 grams of carbohydrate are offered to compensate for the calories lost by restriction of fat intake.

Six to 9.0 grams of potent pancreatic extracts (Pancreatin, Viokase, or Pancrelipase, 0.3 gram) should be given in divided doses with meals, plus 0.6 gram with "snacks." Alternatively, 0.6 gram may be given while the patient is awake, a program which may especially benefit the patient with severe steatorrhea. In patients with high basal acid output, it may be helpful to give 30 ml of an antacid before each meal, or 0.5 gram of sodium bicarbonate when the hourly program is used. Sodium bicarbonate therapy should be avoided in older patients. With a greater degree of effective digestion, the insulin requirement may be increased. Nutritional replacement should include folic acid, vitamin B_{12}, calcium, vitamin D, and vitamin K, if these deficiencies are established (see Part XIV, Section Three). In rare patients vitamin B_{12} malabsorption is associated with pancreatic insufficiency and may be corrected by giving these extracts, or, very rarely, bicarbonate alone. Replacement of dietary triglyceride with medium-chain triglyceride (MCT) is effective in patients with pancreatic insufficiency. Although MCT can be given in appetizing form, its use is not very convenient. It may be important in the management of some patients, especially in the hospital, when early weight gain is a desirable goal.

Surgical Treatment. The large number of surgical procedures employed in the treatment of pancreatitis reflect the continued efforts to relieve pain and to prevent progression of the disease. Cholecystectomy, common duct exploration, sphincterotomy, sympathectomy, ablation of the celiac ganglia, and vagotomy with either a gastric drainage procedure or antrectomy and gastrojejunostomy, as well as a number of types of resective or drainage procedures on the pancreas, have been used with varying success. The best results seem to follow procedures which have been individualized to each patient, dependent on the gross findings of the pancreas at surgery and on operative and endoscopic pancreatography.

Surgical drainage of pancreatic pseudocysts has been relatively successful. Internal drainage of such cysts is preferable to external drainage because of the difficulties and unpleasantness of prolonged drainage of material rich in enzymes. Ninety-five per cent resection of the pancreas, leaving a thin rim of pancreas, with suturing of the main pancreatic duct close to the duodenal surface, appears to be effective. Bilateral thoracolumbar sympathectomy in selected cases for relief of pain is sometimes helpful, but the relief lasts for only two or three years.

It is clear that several variables complicate appraisal of the results of surgical therapy. Such variables include the number of spontaneous remissions, the presence or absence of disease of the biliary tract, the effect of previous operations, continued use of or abstinence from alcohol ingestion, the stage of destruction and the activity of the disease in the pancreas, the presence or absence of diabetes, calcification, and pseudocysts, and the degree of pancreatic insufficiency. Even though the results of different surgical procedures vary, it appears that surgery should be offered to patients with documented, well established but early phase chronic pancreatitis in an attempt to prevent or modify the inexorable sequelae of this disease process.

Prognosis. Replacement therapy has made the outlook good for those patients with chronic pancreatitis and pancreatic insufficiency whose painful attacks have ceased or become infrequent. Recurrent painful attacks will usually not be prevented simply by diet and antacid medication. The best hope lies in the surgical removal of a stone in the common bile duct, sphincteroplasty with unroofing or retrograde dilatation of the duct of Wirsung for fibrosis of the ampulla of Vater, or direct procedures of ductal drainage or pancreatic excision. In all other instances, especially if the patient partakes of alcohol, the prognosis for health and comfort is guarded.

Dixon, J. A., and Englert, E.: Growing role of early surgery in chronic pancreatitis: A practical clinical approach. Gastroenterology, 61:375, 1971.

Fitzgerald, O., Fitzgerald, P., Fennelly, J., McMullin, J. P., and Boland, S. J.: A clinical study of chronic pancreatitis. Gut, 4:193, 1963.

Littman, A., and Hanscom, D. H.: Current concepts: Pancreatic extracts. N. Engl. J. Med., 281:201, 1969.

647. CYSTIC FIBROSIS OF THE PANCREAS (Mucoviscidosis)

Cystic fibrosis of the pancreas is a generalized inheritable disease of unknown cause, associated with dysfunction of all exocrine glands, including those that are mucus producing. Although characteristically a disease of early childhood, cystic fibrosis is now recognized in adolescents and adults. The increased longevity has been attributed to earlier diagnosis, to increased use of antimicrobial drugs and other measures that control pulmonary infection, so frequently the cause of death, and to the effectiveness of potent pancreatic extracts and medium-chain triglycerides.

Etiology. The basic defect in cystic fibrosis is not known. The most commonly accepted theories for its pathogenesis are abnormal physicochemical secretions, autonomic dysfunction, humoral abnormality, and ion transport dysfunction. It appears that a humoral substance present in the body fluids of cystic fibrosis patients attaches to or acts upon the membrane surface of exocrine gland cells. This interaction results in a change in the metabolic activity within the cell with a concomitant alteration of cell membrane permeability with increased protein and mucopolysaccharide synthesis.

Whatever the nature of the basic defect in cystic fibrosis, it is an inherited disease expressed only in the homozygous state without X-linkage (autosomal recessive).

Incidence. The incidence of patients with the fully manifested disease (homozygotes) is estimated as 1 per 2000 live births, and that of heterozygotes as 2 to 5 per cent of the population. Approximately 5 per cent of all patients with cystic fibrosis survive past the age of 17, and the incidence in the white adult population is estimated to be 1 per 40,000. It affects equally all whites, is rare in blacks, and is very rare in Orientals.

Pathophysiology. The pancreas of patients with cystic fibrosis is characterized pathologically by obstruction of the large and small pancreatic ducts with amorphous eosinophilic concretions, followed by dilation of the acini, degeneration of the parenchyma, and fibrosis. The islets of Langerhans remain intact. The deficiency or absence of pancreatic enzymes, especially trypsin, lipase, and amylase, results in *steatorrhea* and *azotorrhea*. Carbohydrates are better utilized. *Diabetes mellitus* occurs in this disease, but ketosis is rare. The majority of these patients can tolerate protein better than fats, making a positive nitrogen balance possible with increased protein intake.

Generalized bronchial obstruction with secondary infection is a cardinal manifestation of the pulmonary involvement. The process leads to acute and chronic bronchitis, peribronchitis, patchy atelectasis, bronchiolectasis and bronchiectasis, poor alveolar aeration, hypoxia, hypercarbia, pulmonary hypertension, and cor pulmonale. In spite of their unusual susceptibility to respiratory infections, these patients are capable of developing good levels of circulating antibodies to many pathogenic bacteria to which they are exposed, and have adequate immunoglobulin responses to infections. Discovery of the constant presence of hemolytic *Staphylococcus aureus* and, more recently, of

Pseudomonas aeruginosa in their sputum and naso-pharynx suggests a metabolic basis for the striking association of these organisms and cystic fibrosis.

Sweat and Salivary Electrolytes. The eccrine sweat defect is characteristic of cystic fibrosis in the pediatric age group, and is rarely seen in other pediatric disease except adrenal cortical insufficiency. A striking increase in the levels of sodium, chloride, and to a lesser extent potassium is present in virtually all homozygote patients with cystic fibrosis. A similar but less striking elevation of sodium and chloride has been found in the saliva, hair, and nails of patients with cystic fibrosis (see below).

Biochemistry of Secretions. The abnormal secretions which occur in this disease have been recognized as the basic pathologic lesion which results in bronchial and pancreatic obstruction. The increased viscosity of these secretions has been attributed to an increased fucose and decreased sialic levels of the glycoproteins and to a complex formed by the glycoprotein and calcium. To date, there has been no delineation of the underlying biochemical defect.

Recent Observations. Recent observations which may have some bearing on the disease include the following: (1) The isolation of a heat-labile, nondialyzable factor in serum of patients with cystic fibrosis which chromatographs with the macroglobulin fraction. This substance disorganizes the ciliary rhythm in explants of respiratory epithelium. It has also been detected in parents of children with cystic fibrosis, but in a lower concentration. It is present in only 1 of 25 control sera, the expected incidence of heterozygotes in the population. (2) Easily recognizable cytoplasmic intravesicular metachromasia, found in skin-fibroblast cultures derived from children affected with cystic fibrosis of the pancreas. A similar cytoplasmic metachromasia was seen in 13 of the 14 parents, obligatory heterozygotes. The exact reason for the accumulation of the mucopolysaccharides within the fibroblasts is not known.

Clinical Manifestations. *Chronic pulmonary disease* is characterized by chronic cough, wheezing, thick tenacious sputum, and repeated respiratory tract infections, which are the hallmarks of the disease in both children and adults. With irreversible damage to the bronchi, the pulmonary disease becomes progressive and leads to the distressing picture of pulmonary insufficiency and eventually death through such complications as *lobar atelectasis, lung abscesses, cor pulmonale, pulmonary hypertension,* mediastinal and subcutaneous *emphysema, pneumothorax, hemoptysis,* and *asphyxia.* The chest is usually hyperresonant, with depressed diaphragms and increased anteroposterior diameter. Clubbing of the fingers may be present. *Pancreatic insufficiency,* characterized by abdominal distention, large, bulky, foul-smelling stools, diarrhea, and abdominal cramps, may appear alone or in combination with respiratory disease. Malnutrition may be severe despite an exorbitant appetite and an apparently adequate caloric intake. This may lead to shortened stature and delayed puberty if the disease is first discovered during adolescence.

Fecal masses that may be so persistent and tenacious as to produce acute mechanical intestinal obstruction occur frequently in older children and adults and are known as the *meconium ileus equivalent.*

Chronic involvement of the paranasal sinuses is a regular finding; with progressive pneumatization it leads to a nasal voice, postnasal drip, and formation of polyps that often require surgical removal. Enlargement of sub-maxillary salivary glands, hypertrophic osteoarthropathy, and ocular lesions (dilatation of the arteries and veins of the fundus with hemorrhage and papilledema) have been reported.

Diagnosis. The diagnosis of cystic fibrosis should be based on four criteria: (1) increase in electrolyte concentration in the sweat, (2) absence of pancreatic enzymes on assay of aspirated duodenal contents, (3) chronic lung disease, and (4) family history of the disorder. Usually two criteria are sufficient to establish the diagnosis.

An accurate *quantitative sweat test* performed by stimulation of the sweat glands by iontophoresis of a cholinergic substance (0.2 per cent pilocarpine nitrate) is mandatory. The sweat chlorides and sodium thus obtained will reveal mean values of 30 to 40 mEq and 60 mEq per liter, respectively, in normal children; in children with fibrocystic disease the means will be 105 to 125 mEq for chlorides and 120 mEq per liter for sodium, respectively. Values for sweat chloride greater than 60 mEq per liter and for sodium greater than 80 mEq per liter are considered diagnostic for children with cystic fibrosis.

Even though sweat tests have been used in the diagnosis of cystic fibrosis in adults, they are thought to be of limited value in this group. However, persistent elevated levels of sodium and chloride in the sweat of an adult or of an adolescent after strict salt deprivation constitute valid criteria for the diagnosis of cystic fibrosis of the pancreas. The clinical picture and duodenal aspiration appear to be more specific in the diagnosis of adult cystic fibrosis. A thick, viscid secretion with profound deficiency of amylase, lipase, and trypsin is obtained on duodenal drainage. Chest roentgenograms reveal generalized obstructive *emphysema* and *bilateral bronchopneumonia.* A family history of cystic fibrosis is of great diagnostic aid.

In patients with no lung involvement, but with symptoms and signs of *malabsorption,* the diagnosis of cystic fibrosis must be differentiated from that of *celiac disease,* with which it is most often confused, and from other causes of malabsorption. In celiac disease a jejunal biopsy will show virtual absence of villi, the d-xylose absorption test will be abnormal, urinary excretion of 5-hydroxyindolacetic acid will be elevated, and a clinical and biochemical response to a low gluten diet will be obtained (see Part XIV, Section Three).

Rectal biopsies in some patients with cystic fibrosis have shown widely dilated crypts packed with mucus, which can appear lamellated.

Treatment. Therapy of the chronic lung disease with various antimicrobials deserves major emphasis, because pulmonary involvement dominates the clinical picture and determines the fate of the patient. The choice of the antimicrobial regimen is the same as the treatment of chronic bronchitis and is discussed in Ch. 503.

Pulmonary physiotherapy in the form of postural drainage of each lobe three to four times daily often provides effective drainage of the involved lobe. In recent years, continuous nocturnal mist nebulization in a tent, with an appropriate small droplet nebulizer with a solution of 10 per cent propylene glycol, has been recommended. Agents such as deoxyribonuclease and N-acetyl cysteine have been recommended for daily nebulizations with the hope of diminishing the viscosity of pulmonary secretions. Pulmonary surgery is rarely indicated, because the pulmonary disease is usually bilateral and generalized.

The malabsorption seen in these patients can be ameliorated by a large intake of food with moderate restriction of fat intake and addition of pancreatic extracts to the diet. Concentrated pancreatic extract (Viokase or Pancrelipase) given hourly during the waking hours is satisfactory therapy (see Part XIV, Section Three). Medium-chain triglyceride preparations may aid in further decreasing steatorrhea and thereby help growth, development, and weight gain.

Prognosis. The prognosis in this disease is improving as early diagnosis and treatment become more effective. The pulmonary involvement usually determines the fate of the patient. Approximately 50 per cent of affected children die before the age of 10 years, more than 80 per cent before the age of 20 years, and most of the remaining survivors before 30 years of age.

Meconium ileus produces symptoms of intestinal obstruction shortly after birth and, unless surgically corrected, proves fatal. However, patients who survive the operation have essentially the same outlook as those without this complication.

Uncontrollable *gastrointestinal bleeding,* secondary to portal hypertension, and massive *salt depletion* in hot weather are additional hazards. In the older age group, *sinusitis* with its complications (notably polyps) has been a serious problem. Although pancreatic insufficiency is clearly present, digestive symptoms are minimal, and patients are able to tolerate an unrestricted diet. Sexual maturation proceeds normally, but with slight delay. A small number of women with this disease have given birth to healthy children. Only 2 to 3 per cent of males with cystic fibrosis who reach adulthood are fertile because of defective development of the wolffian duct derivatives.

Brusilow, S. W.: Cystic fibrosis in adults. Ann. Rev. Med., 21:99, 1970.
Danes, B. S., and Bearn, A. G.: A genetic marker in cystic fibrosis of the pancreas. Lancet, 1:106, 1968.
Lobeck, C. C.: Cystic fibrosis. *In* Stanbury, J. B., Wyngaarden, J. B., and Fredrickson, D. S. (eds.): The Metabolic Basis of Inherited Disease. New York, McGraw-Hill Book Company, 1972, pp. 1605–1626.
Spock, A.: Cystic Fibrosis. Current theories concerning pathogenesis. Minn. Med., 52:1429, 1969.

648. CARCINOMA OF THE PANCREAS

The diagnosis of malignant tumors of the pancreas and the periampullary region is a challenging and perplexing problem. The protean manifestations of this disease and retroperitoneal location of the gland make early diagnosis and treatment difficult. It is especially unfortunate that even the newer diagnostic techniques fail to establish an early diagnosis, because carcinoma of the pancreas is now the *fourth* leading cause of death among all sites of cancer in the United States.

Pancreatic carcinoma is predominantly a disease of males, with a sex ratio of 2 to 1. The mean age of onset of symptoms is 55 years. The most common tumors are adenocarcinomas, arising mostly from ductular epithelium. In two thirds of the cases, the head of the pancreas is the site; the body and tail contribute approximately 20 and 10 per cent, respectively. Extension of the tumor is by direct invasion of the remaining gland or duodenum and by adherence to adjacent structures. Extension via the perineural lymphatics and those accompanying the pancreaticoduodenal vessels is the rule. Metastases are most frequent to the regional lymph nodes and to the liver. Other sites of metastases, in their order of frequency, are lungs, intestines, adrenals, bone, and other organs.

Although not established, there are three frequently cited predisposing factors: chronic pancreatitis (especially calcific), heavy alcohol consumption, and diabetes mellitus.

Clinical Manifestations. *Symptoms.* Despite the still widely held opinion that carcinoma of the pancreas and ampulla of Vater is painless, *pain* is the most frequent first symptom. The pain is of three general types: (1) colicky, and frequently located in the right upper quadrant of the abdomen; (2) steady, dull, and midepigastric, radiating through to the low back; and (3) paroxysmal, near the umbilicus but felt over a wide area of the back, in the anterior chest, and over the abdomen. Other characteristic features of the pain are its severity, steady progression, and exacerbation at night, as well as its nonrelationship to normal events of the digestive cycle. This pain pattern may be due to the propensity of these tumors to infiltrate along nerve trunks and ducts with an accompanying desmoplastic response which tends to envelop and encase nerves, ducts, and blood vessels. The next most significant symptom is *jaundice,* which occurs in about 75 per cent of cases of carcinoma of the head of the pancreas, and is the symptom which causes most patients to seek therapy. It is almost always persistent and steadily progressive, and can become extremely deep, with accompanying pruritus. *Weight loss* occurs invariably and is usually extreme, frequently averaging more than 5 pounds per month. Gastrointestinal symptoms such as *anorexia, nausea,* and *vomiting,* although not specific for carcinoma of the pancreas, are very common complaints. An aversion for or complete rejection of food, rather than true anorexia, is considered distinctive of cancer of the pancreas. A feeling of *gastric fullness* and *flatulence* is common. Diarrhea, which may or may not be associated with steatorrhea, has been observed in 15 per cent of cases. *Constipation* is more common and may be related to the anorexia. *Bleeding* into the gastrointestinal tract, manifested by occult blood in the stool, is noted in about 50 per cent of cases, and is especially significant in lesions involving the stomach or duodenum and in carcinoma of the ampulla. *Thrombophlebitis* or phlebothrombosis, especially of the migrating type and resistant to anticoagulants, may be the first symptom in patients with carcinoma of the body and tail of the pancreas. *Emotional disturbances,* especially depression with crying spells, anxiety, intractable insomnia, and premonition of serious illness, are said to be unusually common with carcinoma of the pancreas, especially of the body and tail. Abnormal glucose tolerance or even frank *diabetes* is more common in carcinoma of the pancreas than in the general population. Uncommon manifestations of carcinoma of the pancreas include hypoglycemia, hypercalcemia, inappropriate antidiuretic hormone (ADH) secretion, excessive production of adrenocorticotrophic hormone (ACTH), and the carcinoid syndrome.

Physical Findings. Abnormal findings that may be noted on physical examination are evidence of weight loss, an enlarged, frequently hard liver, a distended gallbladder, jaundice, tenderness or resistance in the upper part of the abdomen, and a mass in the region of the pancreas. The gallbladder is visibly or palpably enlarged in about 50 per cent of patients with jaundice caused by carcinoma in contrast to patients with jaundice and chronic pancreatitis. Ascites and peripheral edema are noted in about 20 per cent of cases. Tumors arising in the tail of the pancreas may obstruct the splenic vein, leading to splenomegaly and hypersplenism; may obstruct the portal vein and produce esophageal varices; or may encase the splenic artery, resulting in an arterial bruit in the left upper quadrant. Subcutaneous fat necrosis, appearing as tender, subcutaneous nodules originating on the lower extremities and later involving other areas of the body, accompanied by polyarthralgia and eosinophilia, have been found only with the rarer *acinar cell carcinoma.* The high lipase content of these tumors may be responsible for this phenomenon.

Diagnosis. *Roentgenographic Findings.* Roentgenographic studies of the upper gastrointestinal tract may reveal a number of abnormalities owing to the tumor, such as changes in the mucosal pattern and rigidity of the duodenal wall, widening of the duodenal loop, "padding" of the gastric antrum, and disturbed motor activity of the small bowel. Occasionally, evidence of invasion of the duodenal wall—the "inverted 3" sign of Frostberg—will be noted. The ability to detect early changes is enhanced by *hypotonic duodenography,* performed with anticholinergic agents, glucagon or secretin. Spiculation (fine, sharply pointed serration along the inner aspect of the duodenal loop), flattening of folds, and nodular indentations along the inner aspect of the duodenal loop are the most reliable findings suggestive of pancreaticoduodenal cancer. Similar changes may occur in patients with chronic pancreatitis and collateral circulation secondary to portal hypertension. In the presence of obstructive jaundice, percutaneous transhepatic cholangiography will aid in the diagnosis of carcinoma of the head of the pancreas. These roentgenographic findings are invariably manifestations of progressive neoplastic change in the pancreas and surrounding structures.

Clinical Laboratory Findings. Early obstruction of the pancreatic duct will occasionally elevate the serum lipase and amylase. It is clear, however, that if the block has been prolonged, with resultant destruction of the acinar cells of the pancreas or replacement of the gland with tumor, these levels may be low. Unfortunately, significant change in either direction is infrequent. *Leucine aminopeptidase, nonspecific alkaline phosphatase,* and *5-nucleotidase* are elevated in carcinoma of the pancreas when there is an element of obstruction of the common bile duct or metastasis to the liver.

The *glucose tolerance test* is abnormal in 25 to 50 per cent of patients with carcinoma of the pancreas and is a more frequent abnormality than frank glycosuria or fasting hyperglycemia. Steatorrhea is found in approximately 10 per cent of the cases as judged by abnormal chemical fat excretion.

Pancreatic Drainage. Analysis of duodenal secretion after injection of *secretin* or *secretin followed by pancreozymin* is potentially of great diagnostic value. Precise localization of an obstructive lesion is possible. If both biliary and pancreatic secretions are absent, the obstruction must be in the head of the pancreas or in the ampulla of Vater. If the pancreatic and biliary flows are normal in volume, the lesion is not obstructive. If pancreatic secretions are ample despite absence of bile, the lesion must be in the extrahepatic biliary system, or duodenal obstruction is being bypassed by an anomalous pancreatic duct. With partial obstruction of the pancreatic duct, the quantity of bicarbonate and enzymes in the pancreatic secretion decreases, but the relative concentrations remain the same. Cytologic examination for malignant cells after secretin enhances the chance of positive diagnosis. The accompanying table presents a summary of the findings in carcinoma of the pancreas, chronic pancreatitis, and diseases of the biliary tract and liver after secretin stimulation. A significant rise in serum amylase or lipase, or both, after injection of secretin and pancreozymin strongly indicates pancreatic obstruction.

Radioactive Photoscanning. Radioactive photoscanning of the pancreas, utilizing ^{75}Se selenomethionine, results in decreased photoscan concentration in the area of tumors of the pancreas, as well as in pseudocysts. Uptake by the liver and inability to differentiate benign from malignant processes have limited the value of this technique.

Pancreatic Angiography. Pancreatic angiography, especially superselective angiography of vessels close to, or directly into, the pancreatic vessels, appears to help in establishing the diagnosis of carcinoma of the pancreas. The most reliable angiographic findings are irregular ar-

Significance of the Secretin* Test

	Total Volume Flow	Maximal HCO$_3^-$ Concentration	Total Enzyme Secretion	Biliary Pigment Response
Normal	2 ml or more/kg body weight/80 min	90 mEq/L in any 20-minute specimen	Normal	Normal
Pancreatic carcinoma				
Head	Greatly diminished	Normal to diminished	Normal to diminished	—
Body	Moderately diminished	Normal	Normal	—
Tail	Normal	Normal	Normal	—
With obstruction	Diminished	Normal to diminished	Normal to diminished	Obstructive (no bile)
Chronic pancreatitis				
Moderate	Normal	Diminished	Diminished to normal	Normal
Severe	Diminished	Diminished	Diminished	Normal
Biliary tract				
Common duct stone, stricture, or neoplasm	Normal	Normal	Normal	Obstructive (no bile)
Intrahepatic				
Hepatitis, cholangitis, and cancer	Normal	Normal	Normal	Normal (nonobstructive)
Cirrhosis and hemochromatosis	High	Normal	Normal	Normal

*With 1 clinical unit of secretin/kg of body weight.

terial or venous encasement, abrupt cut-off or occlusion of vessels, and occasional neovascular vessels. In the late phase of selective angiography the venous changes of occlusion or encasement of the splenic and superior mesenteric veins and their branches are best seen. Angiography also provides information regarding gall-bladder size, liver metastases, and enlarged intrahepatic bile ducts.

Retrograde Cholangiopancreatography. *Direct cannulation* of the ampulla of Vater via fiberoptic duodenoscopy and retrograde cholangiopancreatography is a new and useful approach in experienced hands in evaluating patients with suspected pancreatic carcinoma. The abnormal features observed by these techniques are strictures, obstruction, dilatations, displacements, and nonvisualization of the pancreatic ducts.

Carcinoembryonic Antigen. Preliminary studies have shown that the carcinoembryonic antigen is positive in 90 per cent of patients with proved pancreatic carcinoma and 30 to 70 per cent positive in other digestive tract tumors. The significance of this finding awaits further evaluation.

Carcinoma of the pancreas can usually be diagnosed either grossly or by biopsy at operation, although such biopsy of the pancreas frequently reveals only inflammation. This finding is usually due to the fact that pancreatic carcinoma is surrounded by inflammatory tissue.

Treatment and Prognosis. The natural course of disease, whether it is primarily in the head or in the body and tail of the pancreas, is one of swift progression to death after onset of symptoms, regardless of whether metastases or contiguous extensions are present, and is uninfluenced by any surgical procedure except radical extirpation in suitable cases. Unfortunately, the over-all resectability rate is less than 25 per cent for adenocarcinoma of the head of the pancreas, and is far less for tumors of the body and tail. Surgical exploration should be performed on patients with suspected localized pancreatic carcinoma to determine the size and spread of the tumor, because resection of periampullary tumors has a five-year survival rate of 40 per cent. Palliative surgery for relief of vomiting, jaundice, and pruritus can be accomplished by cholecystojejunostomy and provides an average survival of 12 months. Recent evidence suggests that a combination of 5-fluorouracil (as a single weekly intravenous injection of 10 mg per kilogram of body weight) with 50 mg of testolactose (Teslac) three or four times daily with meals resulted in a significant prolongation of life of over a year. Medical therapy is usually directed at maintenance of good nutrition, with insulin, pancreatic enzyme replacement, and medium-chain triglycerides. The pain invariably requires narcotics. With increasing severity of the pain, serious consideration should be given to nerve blocks, rhizotomy, or cordotomy to ensure the patient's comfort. Carcinoma of the body and tail is almost never resectable, and five-year cures are extremely rare.

Cotton, B.: Cannulation of the papilla of Vater by endoscopy and retrograde cholangiopancreatography (ERCP). Gut, 13:104, 1972.
Ferrucci, J. R., Jr., and Eaton, S. B.: Radiology of the pancreas (current concepts). N. Engl. J. Med., 288:506, 1973.
Gullick, H. D.: Carcinoma of the pancreas: A review and critical study of 100 cases. Medicine, 38:47, 1959.
Waddell, W. R.: Chemotherapy for carcinoma of the pancreas. Surgery, 74:420, 1973.
Watson, D. W.: Pancreatic carcinoma (clinical seminar). Am. J. Dig. Dis., 15:767, 1970.

Section Five. INFLAMMATORY DISEASES OF THE INTESTINE

CHRONIC INFLAMMATORY DISEASES OF THE INTESTINE

Henry D. Janowitz

649. INTRODUCTION

Chronic inflammatory bowel disease includes a group of disorders characterized by acute and chronic inflammatory changes in all portions of the small and large intestines. The best and oldest known is *ulcerative colitis,* an inflammatory disease confined to the colonic mucosa and submucosa. Almost as well characterized is *regional ileitis* or *regional enteritis,* an inflammatory disease involving the entire wall of a portion of small gut. A more confusing group of inflammatory diseases involve both colon and ileum *(ileocolitis).* Furthermore, some disease which involves the colon but not the small bowel never-theless exhibits all the distinguishing features of regional enteritis of the small bowel, and thus differs from ulcerative colitis. Therefore some have designated this latter disease as *regional enteritis of the colon,* whereas many physicians simply designate regional enteritis, ileocolitis, and regional enteritis of the colon as Crohn's disease (after the man who precisely described regional enteritis) to avoid confusion without commitment to any etiologic theory.

650. REGIONAL ENTERITIS (Crohn's Disease of Small Bowel)

Definition. Regional enteritis is a chronic inflammatory disorder of the intestinal tract of unknown origin which may appear at any site but characteristically involves the terminal ileum (hence its original name, "terminal ileitis"). Clinically, regional enteritis is a diarrheal disease often associated with fever, abdominal pain, weight loss, abdominal masses, and anal or perianal lesions. The disease is also characterized by the frequent formation of enteric fistulas or sinus tracts. Characteristically the regional enteritis produces linear ulcers and deep fissures in the gut; inflammation (characterized by aggregations of inflammatory cells and sarcoid-like granulomas) may extend through the full thickness of the bowel wall.

Etiology. Forty years after its original description (in 1932), regional enteritis remains a disease of unknown origin, although considerable search has been made for causes. No infectious agent has been isolated, although the resemblance of its histopathology to that of noncaseating tuberculosis was noted early. The psychosomatic approach to this disorder has evoked little interest and very little supportive research and documentation. The recent heavy emphasis has been on investigations of the immunologic reactivity of patients with Crohn's disease. No characteristic or significant alterations in serum immunoglobulins have been described. Impaired cutaneous responses to tuberculin, stressed in the earlier literature, are not supported by recent studies. We have noted an absolute lymphopenia in some patients. With a widely accepted test of delayed hypersensitivity, most patients are not sensitized to dinitrochlorobenzene. Further evidence of depressed lymphocyte immunologic competence has been obtained by several groups who have shown that the circulating lymphocytes have a diminished response in vitro to phytohemagglutinin, suggesting impairment of thymic derived lymphocytes. This depressed responsiveness was present in an equal number (40 per cent) of patients with ulcerative colitis as well. Controversy exists regarding immunologic cross-reactivity between sarcoidosis and Crohn's disease. The active international standard Siltzbach-Chase Kveim antigen does not give a positive skin reaction in patients with Crohn's disease. More important is the observation that tissue from Crohn's disease patients introduced into the footpad of the mouse produces a local granulomatous reaction. Confirmation is required, but this evidence suggests that Crohn's disease may be due to a transmissible agent, with a long latent period, in a susceptible population.

Incidence, Prevalence, and Epidemiology. Epidemiologic studies tend to lump all forms of Crohn's disease into one, regardless of the location of the disease, and have the added difficulty of separating Crohn's disease of the colon from ulcerative colitis. It has its highest incidence in the United States, is thought to be infrequent in Central Europe, and is recorded frequently in Britain and the Scandinavian countries. It appears to be seen only infrequently in Africa, Asia, and South America.

Variable *incidence rates* (rate of occurrence of the disease per 100,000 persons at risk per year) have been reported. In the Baltimore study of patients over 20 years of age which utilized hospital cases only, the incidence in males was 2.5 and in females 1.2, for an average of 1.8. In the Oxford study of Evans and Acheson (1967), the incidence for both men and women was approximately 1.0.

Evidence regarding *prevalence* (all the patients affected with this disease at any one moment per 100,000 persons at risk) is difficult to obtain. Based on 36 reports, Mendeloff has estimated the range of prevalence as between 20 and 40 per 100,000 population. Fragmentary evidence suggests that the incidence of Crohn's disease may be rising in the western world.

There is no significant difference in regard to sex. In contrast to ulcerative colitis, Crohn's disease under age

six appears to be extremely rare. The first incidence mode can be seen to occur between 15 and 20, with a second mode at age 55 to 60. In the United States, blacks and Indians are at low risk. Evidence has been accumulating that the incidence of inflammatory bowel disease in Jewish patients is strikingly higher than in the non-Jewish populations. In Baltimore, in Crohn's disease, the rate was six times higher for Jewish males and three times higher for Jewish females than the rates for non-Jews. Although these higher rates in Jews might be due to social, dietary, or genetic factors, current epidemiologic studies offer no explanation. There is a slight preponderance of urban over rural setting for Crohn's disease. Nevertheless, exhaustive study of socioeconomic status, for the United States, has demonstrated no significant difference for patient and control populations. Perhaps farmers are less vulnerable because of some occupational factor.

Genetics. Since the search for an exogenous (environmental) etiology in Crohn's disease has been fruitless, recent attention has been devoted to the problem of genetic susceptibility. No simple mendelian genetic mechanism has been forthcoming. A considerable number of family aggregations have been reported, the most frequent combination being two affected siblings, with parent (more often mother) and child combination a close second. This evidence may argue more for common environmental factors than for genetic influence. The literature contains no reference to a husband and wife both being affected, and studies on twins (concordance has been recorded in seven pairs of monozygotic twins) do not contribute to the solution of this problem. Family incidence of Crohn's disease is low; 1 in 15 to 1 in 50 patients have an affected first-degree relative. Although this incidence in first-degree relatives is higher than in the general population, lack of control data limits this interpretation. The association of Crohn's disease with other disorders of an inherited nature is pertinent. In one series eczema and hay fever were particularly common, possibly pointing to a genetically controlled immunologic mechanism. A stronger association exists with *ankylosing spondylitis,* which has some hereditary features, and which may appear before the clinical manifestations of the bowel disease. The association of Crohn's disease and ulcerative colitis within families is well recorded, but the uncertainties of this relationship do not advance our understanding. An interesting and curious feature in families with these diseases is that the index patient with Crohn's disease often has relatives with ulcerative colitis, whereas many series with families of ulcerative colitis patients have no relatives with Crohn's disease. One conclusion is that the genetic influence on etiology is likely to be polygenic, alleles at several different loci providing a genotype which determines susceptibility or resistance to environmental factors, although a virus-like maternal factor is a possibility.

Pathology. All areas of the gastrointestinal tract may be involved in regional enteritis, including rare lesions of the oral cavity and esophagus. Lesions of the stomach and duodenum occur more frequently, and the terminal ileum is the most common site of the disease. Although isolated regional jejunitis does occur, combined lesions of ileum and jejunum are more frequent. The lesion in the colon is discussed below (Crohn's disease of the colon). The *perirectal fistula* should be considered an integral part of Crohn's disease of the small bowel because of its frequency. All layers of the small intestine are involved, as are the regional lymph nodes. The bowel wall is remarkably thickened and rigid. Skip areas of disease are frequently seen with intervening normal bowel. Loops of affected small intestine may be adherent; frequently fistulas exist between these adherent loops. In addition, sinus tracts may extend into a thickened and inflamed mesentery, producing an inflammatory mass. Fistulas from the ileum to cecum and/or sigmoid are very common, but others may reach to the skin (often in old operative scars, occasionally to the navel), bladder, ureter, vagina, flank, and even the right hip joint. Frequently perianal inflammation arising in the crypts of Morgagni leads to anal and perirectal fistulas. An inflammatory mass may encase the ureter, producing ureteral obstruction and hydronephrosis. Superficial discrete ulcers which extend to form confluent linear ulcerations are characteristic of the macroscopic appearance of the intestinal mucosa, as are deep fissures which may extend through all coats and serve as the basis of fistulas. Microscopically, aggregations of inflammatory cells involving all layers predominate, with the sarcoid-granuloma most characteristic when present. Such granulomas are noncaseating collections of epithelioid cells (large mononuclear phagocytes) and multinucleated giant cells whose nuclei are arranged around the periphery or collected at the poles of the cell (Langerhans type) (Fig. 1). When a large number of sections are searched, granulomas have been found in the bowel wall in up to 75 to 85 per cent of patients.

The regional lymph nodes, often containing granulomas, are enlarged owing to nonspecific reactive changes. In one series, 38 per cent of lymph nodes contained granulomas, and in 63 per cent granulomas were present in the bowel wall. Further, 20 per cent of nodes may have this lesion without granulomas present in the bowel. Not all areas of the bowel and all regional nodes are equally affected in the same specimen.

A few available ultrastructural studies have not contributed to pathologic understanding or differential diagnosis but have confirmed the curious finding of neuronal hyperplasia in the mesenteric plexus.

Pathogenesis. An acute inflammatory reaction in the ileum has been well documented (albeit with little histologic confirmation), but most studies have demonstrated its disappearance without any of the sequelae of Crohn's disease, so that the transition from acute to chronic forms of regional enteritis is not recorded. Bacteriologic

and serologic evidence has associated some cases of acute ileitis with infection with the bacteria *Yersinia enterocolitica*, formerly known as *Pasteurella X*. (We need, however, to distinguish this situation from lymphoid hyperplasia of the ileum, frequently seen in the small bowel x-rays of youngsters studied for abdominal pain.)

Since all portions of the gastrointestinal tract from mouth to anus may participate in the pathologic process, an important question is the extent of dissemination. It is extremely rare to obtain characteristic pathologic changes in jejunal biopsies of patients with regional ileitis, and we have never had a positive rectal biopsy in patients with ileitis except when a local rectal or anal lesion was also present. Resected specimens show few lesions 6 cm beyond the edge. Although some scattered microscopic lesions have been noted in grossly normal colon adjacent to classic regional ileitis, in general the disease is localized and segmental rather than universal. Any scheme of pathogenesis must take into account other histologic features of this disease: hyperplastic reactive lymph nodes, the development of granulomas in regional nodes or in ectopic lymph follicles, inflammatory reactions in lymphatics and perilymphatics, ectasia of lymph channels, and the development of submucosal lymphedema secondary to obstructed lymphatics. Although the pathologic process may spread from ileum to adjacent large bowel by extension along sinus tracts with fistula formation, retrograde extension over any long segment does not occur in the absence of surgical intervention. Repeated surgical experience has demonstrated that in portions of the involved ileum excluded from the intestinal stream, completely diverting "bypass" operations lead quite regularly to subsidence of the inflammatory reaction and to recurrence of the pathologic process most frequently in the new "terminal ileum." One might postulate from this line of evidence that the exciting agent of the tissue reaction in Crohn's disease may be present in the intestinal stream, moving down and becoming more concentrated as it reaches the ileocecal area. Delay behind the ileocecal sphincter and above the anal sphincter favors its absorption and entry into submucosal lymphatics and lymphoid tissue with the characteristic tissue response in these loci.

Clinical Manifestations. The classic presentation of regional enteritis is that of a young person, in his or her late teens or early twenties, who has not been feeling well for an ill-defined time but whose indisposition has suddenly worsened. Whereas the past history may have included an occasional episode of cramps and diarrhea frequently ascribed to dietary indiscretions or "nerves," the patient now complains of more constant abdominal pain and more persistent diarrhea. The pain is most frequently cramping and periodic, and is often worse after eating; it is confined principally to the right lower quadrant; occasionally it radiates into the right upper thigh. At times it is more persistent, dull, and annoying. The stools become more frequent, small, loose to watery, often waking the patient at night as well, but are free of gross blood. Appetite clearly declines, and parents become alerted and alarmed by the obvious weight loss, which may be considerable. Often there is a low-grade fever, usually, however, not recorded at home. There may be a history of a recent appendectomy (performed for right lower quadrant pain and tenderness) or a slowly healing perirectal abscess.

Histories of some "allergic" phenomena, including pollen sensitivities and possibly intolerance to milk,

Figure 1.   Regional enteritis. Submucosa of ileum, showing noncaseating granulomas with multinucleated giant cells. Hematoxylin and eosin stain, × 150.

seem to be present more frequently than by chance, but no obvious association with other so-called "immune" diseases exists. There may be a history of recurrent crops of aphthous ulcers of the mouth which may not only plague the patient but may also herald an acute exacerbation. Less frequently, persistent fever, malaise, and anorexia may overshadow the abdominal complaints, and the patient may be labeled as having "fever of unknown origin" or rheumatic fever (especially in the younger child). Failure of sexual and somatic development may be the sole clinical feature.

Less frequent is the patient who presents with fecal fistula in the unhealed scar of an appendectomy, or persistent mucopurulent drainage from the wound. Equally striking are the extraintestinal clinical manifestations of regional enteritis. These include joint symptoms, ranging from fleeting *arthralgias* to obvious *arthritis* and tender, swollen, hot joints, particularly knees and ankles. Backaches may also precede intestinal symptoms, later found to be due to *ankylosing spondylitis.* Skin manifestations include *erythema multiforme,* and especially the painful *erythema nodosum* of shins and feet and the rarer *pyoderma gangrenosum.* An intense *conjunctivitis* (often phlyctenular in nature) and uveitis and iritis with eye pain and visual disturbances may also accompany an underlying chronic intestinal inflammatory disorder. Except for ocular involvements, these extraintestinal manifestations parallel the intensity of the bowel symptoms. Less frequent concomitants include biliary colic caused by *cholelithiasis,* and renal colic associated with either showers of uric acid crystals in the urine or the presence of mixed, especially oxalate, *kidney stones.*

Although the presentation thus far appears to stress the youth of patients, the symptoms may begin at any age; indeed, there seems to be a bimodal distribution, with a second peak in the forties and fifties. A frequent and distressing clinical manifestation is delayed reappearance of general and intestinal symptoms after surgical intervention. Such clinical behavior heralds the discovery of recurrent enteritis, readily confirmed radiographically.

Physical Examination. Physical examination often reveals a well-developed young adult, with some evidence of recent weight loss, moderate pallor, and lassitude. Clubbing of the phalanges is usually not present unless there is extensive involvement of jejunum and ileum, or of ileum and colon. A large number of patients have either a palpable loop of thickened inflamed ileum or a clear-cut mass in the right lower quadrant. Pedal edema may be present. The cutaneous, joint, and eye manifestation cited above may be present. Examination of the rectal area may disclose nothing abnormal or may reveal a perianal or perirectal abscess; evidence of the prior surgical attempts to treat perirectal abscesses and fistulas; or, in patients with colonic involvement, the curious florid indolent ulcers of the anus which often make rectal examination difficult. Proctoscopy demonstrates a normal mucosa except in those with Crohn's disease of the rectum and anus. In children, evidence of retarded growth and delayed secondary sexual characteristics may be striking.

Laboratory Studies. Laboratory findings may include evidence of a mild to moderate anemia; the white cell count is usually normal except in the presence of suppuration. Absolute lymphopenia may be present. Albuminuria is rare and may indicate renal amyloidosis. The

stools may reveal the existence of occult blood. The erythrocyte sedimentation rate, a crude but useful index of disease activity, is elevated. The serum albumin may be lowered, and often the gamma globulin fraction is elevated. Occasionally elevated blood uric acid levels in both females and males are present. Minor abnormalities in liver function tests may indicate the presence of fatty liver; more marked elevation in serum alkaline phosphatase or SGOT or SGPT determinations indicates the associated pericholangitis seen more frequently in ulcerative colitis and ileocolitis. Serum vitamin B_{12} levels and the Schilling test of vitamin B_{12} absorption may be abnormal, and variable amounts of unabsorbed fat can be detected by measuring fecal fat in a 72-hour collection (see Part XIV, Section Three); however, anorexia often precludes adequate fat intake, making this determination meaningless. The d-xylose test, a measure of carbohydrate absorption, is usually within normal limits.

Mechanisms of Disease Manifestations. The weight loss in regional enteritis is due in large part to failure of caloric intake, with a smaller contribution from failure of absorption. The reduced caloric intake derives mainly from loss of appetite but also from the generally restrictive diets that physicians recommend or patients adopt. The diarrhea of regional enteritis may arise from a multitude of causes: (1) failure of diseased ileum to resorb bile salts can result in excessive passage of bile salts into the colon where these products inhibit colonic fluid and electrolyte resorption; (2) loss of small bowel absorbing surface, as the result of disease or surgical resection, may produce general malabsorption with increased fecal output; (3) partial intestinal obstruction (caused by intestinal stenosis or mechanical obstruction from inflammatory masses or adherent loops of bowel) may produce diarrhea either as a result of excessive net secretion of fluid and electrolytes by dilated proximal bowel or as a result of intestinal stasis and bacterial overgrowth (see Part XIV, Section Three); and (4) lactase deficiency may be accentuated by the impaired nutritional status of these patients, because all brush border enzymes are decreased in the patients who are most ill (see below).

Absorptive Defects. Fat malabsorption is correlated with the length of inflamed or resected ileum, the incidence of steatorrhea increasing in those with more than 90 to 100 cm involved or resected. The mechanism is ascribed to the loss of bile salts (failure to be reabsorbed) in this portion of the gut, with resultant reduction of the bile salt pool and thus hepatic secretion of the bile salts needed for proper micelle formation and pancreatic lipase activity. Bacterial overgrowth in those with stenosis, stricture, fistulas, or surgically created blind loops may also contribute to steatorrhea. The bacterial overgrowth of colonic organisms is believed to deconjugate the bile salts needed for fat absorption. Carbohydrate absorption is usually quite normal (at least as measured by the d-xylose test) except in patients with jejunitis, or in those with stricture formation and consequent overgrowth of luminal bacteria which may metabolize this sugar. Lactose maldigestion secondary to intestinal lactase deficiency is seen in some patients, many of whom have themselves eliminated milk and milk products from their diets; the diarrhea of lactase deficiency in such patients arises from (1) the osmotic effects of unabsorbed lactose and (2) a lowered colonic pH (from bacterial breakdown products of lactose) which inhibits colonic water and electrolyte resorption. Vitamin

B_{12} malabsorption is related to the loss of normal ileal absorptive mechanism. When the length of involved or resected ileum exceeds 90 cm, the Schilling test is abnormal in all; thus malabsorption of vitamin B_{12} is correlated with fat malabsorption. The increased incidence of gallstones is ascribed to the alteration in bile salt pool and the secretion of "lithogenic" bile secondary to failure to reabsorb bile salts in the ileum (see Part XIV, Section Three).

Renal Calculi. Urinary uric acid crystals are more common in these patients. Several defects are believed responsible for this finding: (1) some patients have hyperuricemia, thought to result from increased catabolic rates; (2) the urine is more frequently acid, perhaps reflecting excessive loss of bicarbonate in the diarrheal stools; and (3) loss of excessive stool water results in the formation of a more concentrated urine. Some patients have in addition increased levels of blood uric acid, presumed to be associated with breakdown of tissue. Other types of renal calculi likewise appear to be correlated with fluid loss through the gut. The recognition of increased oxalate excretion in the urine and presence of oxalate stones has revealed a new metabolic complication. Ascribed at first to increased conversion of the glycine moiety of the deconjugated bile salts into the oxalate pathway, hyperoxaluria now appears to result from increased intestinal absorption of dietary oxalate.

Clinical Complications. Despite their frequency, certain manifestations of the disease are considered as complications. These include *local suppurative complications,* arising from extension of sinus tracts into the adjacent mesentery and giving rise to right lower quadrant abscess formation. These sinus tracts may also extend into the right psoas region, giving rise to a psoas syndrome of low backache, pain in the right upper thigh, and flexion deformity with limp. Healing takes place by a marked fibrotic reaction with narrowing of the intestinal lumen and *stricture formation,* accounting for the paradoxical increase in crampy abdominal pain with subsidence of systemic symptoms. The syndrome of incomplete intestinal obstruction rarely leads to complete obstruction unless there is a complicating local abscess or an impacted foreign body, usually of dietary origin (e.g., corn kernels, berries, peach pits). *Free perforation* of the ileum is reported with increasing frequency in recent years; usually, however, perforation of the bowel is confined by surrounding tissues and leads to sinus formation. *Massive hemorrhage* occurs in less than 5 per cent of patients with Crohn's disease of the small intestine, occasioned at times by stercorous ulceration proximal to a stenotic area. *Fistulization* may be considered an integral part of the basic disease; however, fistulas to the urinary bladder deserve some additional comment. Passage of frank feces through the urethra is quickly recognized by the patient. The passage of air or gas through the urethra, however, may require detailed specific inquiry by the physician. (This is also true of the passage of gas from the vagina.) Despite the frequently expressed fear of ascending urinary tract infections in the presence of an ileovesical fistula, patients tolerate this condition surprisingly well.

Renal Complications. Uric acid and *oxalate stones* have already been stressed. Right *hydronephrosis* and *hydroureter* from obstruction caused by a retroperitoneal inflammatory mass usually create few symptoms, and the urine is rarely infected. *Renal amyloidosis* is more common in Crohn's disease than in ulcerative colitis.

The writer has seen five instances in a series of 17 patients dying of ileitis in which the renal amyloid contributed to death.

Although *carcinoma* of the ileum or jejunum is rare, the 20 reported instances of adenocarcinoma in longstanding Crohn's disease of the small bowel, especially in excluded intestine, suggest that this is more than a matter of chance. Cancer in a "bypassed" loop is even more treacherous to diagnose, because these segments are almost always stenotic.

Neurologic Complications. Neurologic complications in the form of "startle reactions," tetany, and grand mal seizures, have been observed, usually on the basis of electrolyte and fluid disturbances, mainly hypocalcemia and hypomagnesemia. The clinical setting is one of a patient with profuse diarrhea, receiving steroids and intravenous fluids free of magnesium. We have seen a few patients with concurrent multiple sclerosis, one of whom had a diffuse vasculitis. Three of our younger patients suffered thrombosis of the middle cerebral artery without evidence of atherosclerosis.

Diagnosis. The history of malaise, anorexia with weight loss, and abdominal pain, especially in the right lower quadrant associated with increasing nonbloody diarrhea, together with the finding of thickened loops of intestine or a mass in the right lower quadrant, makes the diagnosis of Crohn's disease of the small bowel highly probable. The finding of an anal lesion or perirectal abscess or fistula or a cutaneous fistula increases the certainty of this diagnosis. Short of resection of bowel for histologic confirmation, characteristic x-ray findings in the small bowel (Fig. 2) confirm the diagnosis. Although the pathology of early regional enteritis may be insufficient to make the disease evident on barium contrast meal, patients with Crohn's disease should not be treated without x-ray confirmation. If the terminal ileum fails to visualize on barium enema examination because of failure of the barium to reflux from colon into ileum, an upper gastrointestinal series with small bowel follow-through is indicated. Failure to visualize ade-

Figure 2. Involvement of terminal ileum in regional enteritis. Note narrowing of lumen with hoselike configuration of ileal contours.

quately the terminal ileum with barium by mouth is the most frequent reason for the failure to find radiographic confirmation of a strong clinical impression. The characteristic x-ray finding is segmental involvement of the bowel, most frequently the terminal ileum; at times, several segments of the ileum may be separated by "skip areas" of normal intervening bowel. Thickened, edematous mucosa with a "cobblestone" appearance reflects the submucosal cellular aggregates. Narrowing of the lumen, the so-called "string sign," represents a functionally contracted irritable segment or, in a later stage of the disease, fibrotic stenosis. Progressive thickening of the bowel wall stiffens the loops, which may be widely separated because of the thickened swollen mesentery, agglutinated by serosal inflammatory changes, or draped over a right lower quadrant inflammatory mass. The presence of sinus tracts and fistulas to adjacent loops of small or large bowel, especially the cecum or sigmoid colon, are classic findings. With the development of stenosis, dilatation of proximal loops of gut appears, together with pseudodiverticula. In the less common ileojejunitis, similar changes are found throughout contiguous loops of jejunum and ileum.

Rectal biopsy is rarely of use except when amyloidosis is suspected or an obvious anal lesion is present. Biopsy of the perirectal fistula may reveal the characteristic granuloma.

Differential Diagnosis. The differential diagnosis includes *acute appendicitis, appendiceal abscess, cecal diverticulitis* with localized perforation, *ovarian carcinoma, carcinoma* of the *cecum* invading the ileum, *lymphosarcoma, Hodgkin's disease, lymphoid hyperplasia, ileocecal tuberculosis, ileal carcinoid,* and the *"backwash" ileitis* of ulcerative colitis. In diagnosis of regional jejunitis, *nodular lymphoid hyperplasia* with dysgammaglobulinemia, the *erosive jejunitis* of *Zollinger-Ellison syndrome,* nonspecific *erosive jejunitis,* and *metastatic melanocarcinoma* must be considered. The differential diagnosis for *regional ileojejunitis* includes *nodular lymphoid hyperplasia* with dysgammaglobulinemia, *lymphosarcoma,* the *diffuse nonerosive ileojejunitis* reported on occasion in patients with *sprue, diffuse nongranulomatous ileojejunitis,* and prior *severe ischemia* of *small intestines.*

Of this list only a few diseases present real problems. *Acute appendicitis* may be extremely difficult to separate from an acute episode of regional ileitis in the absence of an antecedent history of bowel problems. Exploration is the method of choice if any doubt exists; current experience justifies removal of the normal appendix to prevent confusion in the future if the cause of the patient's syndrome is Crohn's disease of the ileum; fecal fistulas arise mainly from unsatisfactory surgical technique in manipulating the ileum, not the appendiceal stump. Extremely rarely, Crohn's disease may be confined to the appendix. Patients with known Crohn's disease of the ileum only rarely develop acute appendicitis.

Appendiceal abscess frequently cannot be distinguished from regional enteritis with right lower quadrant mass, and the roentgenographic findings in the ileum may mimic ileitis. Occasionally the disappearance of the abscess and clearing of ileal x-ray changes under the influence of antimicrobial drugs may resolve this clinical dilemma.

Lymphosarcoma usually occupies longer segments than the ileum, often extending across the ileocecal valve; although the appearances are similar in some respects, roentgenograms usually show no luminal narrowing as noted in regional ileitis. Further, and most important, the clinical picture is quite different.

Ileocecal tuberculosis is a rare disease in the United States and therefore is rarely considered in the differential diagnosis in patients without pulmonary tuberculosis. However, this diagnosis is important to consider in patients with pulmonary tuberculosis and ileocecal disease, or in areas of the globe where tuberculosis—especially milk-borne tuberculosis—is very common. At times the differential diagnosis cannot be made except at laparotomy. A negative tuberculin test in a patient with ileal disease is more likely found with Crohn's disease than with tuberculous enteritis. Moreover, tuberculous enteritis most often involves ileum and cecum; thus patients with disease confined to the ileum most often have Crohn's disease, but since ileocecal disease is found both in granulomatous colitis and in tuberculous enteritis, the distribution of the lesions is rarely helpful in distinguishing these two diseases.

Carcinoid of the ileum usually presents no problem, except when it is invasive, and the x-ray appearance may resemble regional enteritis. The innocuous *lymphoid hyperplasia* of the ileum seen in young patients is easily distinguished from the acute inflammatory changes seen in regional enteritis. This is true also of the roentgenographic changes of *nodular lymphoid hyperplasia* with dysgammaglobulinemia.

Some special problems arise in patients with known regional enteritis. The problem of right lower quadrant suppuration and appendicitis has been discussed. The coexistence of ileitis and cancer of the right ovary and/or cecum has tripped the unwary. One must be alert for the development of *adenocarcinoma* of the *ileum* in the stenotic phase of ileitis, or in patients who have had "bypass" operations in the past.

"Backwash ileitis" is a poor but widely used term to describe the changes in a short segment of terminal ileitis associated with universal ulcerative colitis, and diagnosed by barium enema. It should be distinguished from regional enteritis and does not represent clinically significant disease. It probably represents a direct extension of the associated ulcerative colitis through a patulous ileocecal valve, and is confined to the mucosal surface. It is easily separated from classic regional ileitis, but its distinction from ileocolitis of the Crohn variety may be difficult.

Eosinophilic gastroenteritis is also important in the differential diagnosis, especially of ileojejunitis. This illness, usually associated with a significant blood and tissue eosinophilia representing a response in some to a dietary allergy, may present with diarrhea, malabsorption, and protein-losing enteropathy. The stomach, duodenum, and entire small bowel may be involved alone or in various combinations. Although it is superficially similar to Crohn's disease, the intestinal films do not present with the characteristic infiltrated thickened loops of the latter disease; further, strictures and fistula are not present.

Treatment. There is no known specific therapy for this disorder. Accordingly, treatment is essentially supportive. It is empirical; its efficiency is still undetermined; and it involves review of the patient's activity, dietary intake, life style, and personal habits. It also requires consideration of a number of drugs currently employed in the management of ileitis and imposes important decisions regarding the necessity of surgical intervention. It also requires an awareness of the mortality rate, ranging from 5 to 18 per cent.

Medical Management. All approaches to the medical management of the patient with regional enteritis begin with an awareness of the high rate of recurrence (up to 50 per cent in some series) after surgery. Accordingly, the current therapeutic stance of most experienced clinicians in this field is one of surgical conservatism unless the patient cannot be managed medically in the presence of a continuously unfavorable course or some of the more dramatic complications.

Although it has yet to be shown that prolonged rest favorably affects this illness, management of the patient must begin with an evaluation of the patient's energy balance. Caloric intake usually being suboptimal, some restriction of energy expenditure is clearly in order. This is an individual matter, but all patients must establish and accept some limitations of activity. Although the physician must avoid being arbitrary, he will have to be firm in some situations.

Efforts to improve the patient's nutritional status are necessary and difficult. The victim of this illness needs to be encouraged to take a well-balanced, high caloric, high protein diet. Care must be taken to discourage food faddism and avoid arbitrarily conceived medical dietary advice. The patient's ability to tolerate milk and milk-containing products should be the criterion for lactose intake rather than a lactose tolerance test. Most patients have already established their tolerance by the time they see the physician. In the presence of profuse diarrhea or stenotic lesions, some reduction of the noncaloric residue of the diet is prudent. For patients with marked reduction in absorptive mucosal surface, medium-chain triglycerides are a reasonable supplement; however, they are often of limited use because of patient reluctance to ingest the oil (free from any lactose fillers) owing to the induction of diarrhea. Vitamin supplementation is rational in view of the restricted food intake of many patients (see Table 5 in Part XIV, Section Three).

The anemia of enteritis is rarely due only to vitamin B_{12} deficiency and iron deficiency from bleeding but rather to the effects of the chronic illness on bone marrow synthesis. When there is significant loss of the ileum vitamin B_{12} replacement is required. Oral iron preparations seem to be tolerated poorly by these sick individuals, and a parenteral form such as Imferon is useful.

The symptomatic treatment of abdominal pain, cramps, and diarrhea is an integral part of management. Judicious and temporary use of analgesics, anticholinergics, and opiates is very frequently required. The overuse of deodorized tincture of opium or the diphenoxylate and atropine combination (Lomotil) may lead to dependence and addiction.

Antimicrobial Therapy. Antimicrobial drugs modify the symptoms and course of ileitis very little. Local suppurative complications involving gram-negative organisms of the bowel require the appropriate drug; ampicillin, in doses up to 4 grams daily by mouth or 4 to 6 grams intravenously, provides an acceptable regimen. When stenosis, stricture, or surgical bypass with blind loops or small bowel to colon anastomoses leads to intestinal overgrowth with colonic organisms, tetracycline (0.25 gram every four to six hours) may be helpful in treating the attendant vitamin B_{12} deficiency and/or steatorrhea (see Part XIV, Section Three). Its use should be closely supervised, however, because of the risk of staphylococcal enterocolitis.

For a long time the relatively poorly absorbed sulfonamide derivatives, succinylsulfathiazole and phthalylsulfathiazole in doses of 1.0 to 3.0 grams every six hours were commonly prescribed. More recently, salicylazosulfapyridine (Azulfidine) in doses of 1.0 to 2.0 grams every six hours is the drug more widely used. This sulfonamide whose metabolites are concentrated in the intestinal tissues is a relatively poor antimicrobial agent. The mechanism of its limited usefulness in ulcerative colitis is not known, and its value in Crohn's disease is yet to be deomonstrated. This fact, however, has not prevented its therapeutic popularity, which may reflect a measure of physician desperation. Adverse reactions to this drug, which include nausea, headache and vomiting, skin rashes, high fever, leukopenia and agranulocytosis, hemolysis, and occasional jaundice, may occur in up to 15 to 20 per cent of patients. Recent studies relate the majority of toxic reactions to the serum levels of sulfapyridine achieved in those taking 4 or more grams daily. Since sulfapyridine is acetylated after absorption and conjugated as a glucuronide in the liver before being excreted in the urine, the majority of patients with adverse effects phenotypically acetylate slowly.

Anti-inflammatory Agents: Corticotrophin (ACTH and Adrenal Corticosteroids. Because these anti-inflammatory agents appear to affect the course of ulcerative colitis favorably, and because ileitis and ulcerative colitis have certain nonintestinal manifestations (arthritis, uveitis, erythema nodosum), adrenocorticosteroids, especially prednisone, are now also widely used in these diseases. They improve the patient's sense of well-being and often stimulate his capricious and depressed appetite. It is doubtful, however, that they have been shown to influence the long-term course of the illness for the better, and they do not affect the histopathology of the disease. Indeed, their hazards impose serious limitations for their long-term use, and until the National Cooperative trial in Crohn's disease gives its definitive answer one would do well to avoid their use if possible. Occasionally, in some desperately ill patients, especially those with diffuse ileojejunitis or recurrent enteritis after multiple resections, the use of corticotrophin intravenously (25 units every eight hours continuously) may be more helpful than the conventional doses of prednisone, 40 to 60 mg daily or on alternate-day schedules. However, enthusiasm for corticosteroids must be tempered by the realization that in at least one good recent study a higher than expected mortality for Crohn's disease was related in part to prolonged corticosteroid therapy; however, the series included many patients who were extremely ill.

Immunosuppressive Therapy. Azathioprine (Imuran) was introduced for the therapy of Crohn's disease with fistulas in 1969. It has been used sporadically since then, but convincing evidence of its value is yet to be presented. In daily doses of 2 mg per kilogram, this writer has observed no catastrophes when the white blood count remained above 3500. Immunosuppression requires at least three weeks' therapy, and the long-term undesirable effects of this therapy are unknown. Although only patients with renal transplants have thus far been reported to develop lymphomas while being treated with azathioprine, the possible risks of therapy when balanced with therapeutic effects do not justify using this agent except as part of a controlled study or as a measure of desperation.

Surgical Therapy. The early expectation that surgical excision would lead to a permanent cure in regional ileitis was soon followed by an era of disillusion based upon increasing evidence of recurrence. Recognition of the limited value of steroid therapy, however, has refocused attention on the effects of surgical therapy. Current evidence indicates that many recurrences develop during the first two to three years after operation, followed by a period of three or four years with little increase in rate of recurrence, only to be followed by a period of more frequent recurrences. Two to three years after resection and ileocolostomy, perhaps 30 per cent of patients have a recurrence; 40 to 50 per cent have a recurrence at five years, and perhaps as many as 60 per cent at ten years. The recurrences are usually on the ileal side of the ileocolonic anastomosis; in some the recurrences are solely radiographic; in others clinical severity parallels the original disease. Since as many as half of the surgically treated patients are faring well at the end of five years, this form of treatment should not be deprecated, especially in the young person when growth and education are critical.

If surgery is elected, the operation of choice is resection of the diseased ileum with an ileoascending colostomy to preserve the right colon for water absorption. These patients may have some period of watery diarrhea after resection with removal of the ileocecal valve. This often responds to bile salt binding therapy with cholestyramine (Questran, 1 to 4 grams daily in divided doses). The mortality and morbidity of this procedure is no higher than that from the older bypass operation (side tracking of the involved ileum with exclusion), and eliminates the risk of the late development of neoplasm in the excluded loop. When a suppurative complication in the right lower quadrant makes resection hazardous, especially an abscess or inflammatory mass encroaching on the right ureter, a bypass operation is to be preferred. Few factors are known to influence recurrence rate after surgery. The rate is higher in patients whose symptoms first appeared below the age of 40, and is higher the more extensive the involvement of the small bowel.

The indications for surgery are the obvious ones of intestinal obstruction, massive hemorrhage, and fistulization to the bladder. An internal fistula between adjacent loops of bowel or an intra-abdominal mass per se does not necessarily indicate surgery. A cutaneous fistula, often after exploratory laparotomy and appendectomy, may on occasion close under treatment with sulfonamides but usually requires surgery. The more difficult clinical problem is the patient who fails to improve or deteriorates under our current supportive management. This patient can be remarkably helped, albeit often temporarily, by resection. On occasion, severe or nonhealing perirectal fistulas are an indication for resection of proximal ileal disease.

Prognosis. Regional enteritis is a disease of quite variable course. It has the interesting characteristic of not spreading in a retrograde fashion in the absence of surgery. Extension to sigmoid or cecum by fistulization, however, is common. Over-all, mortality ranges from 5 to 18 per cent; however, it is from 4 to 12 per cent when related to the ileitis itself. In view of current unsatisfactory medical therapy, it is not surprising that the majority of patients ultimately come to operation, many of whom have multiple procedures. Thus in one surgical center, of 332 patients with Crohn's disease (large as well as small bowel), 295 sooner or later were submitted to surgical treatment, with an operative mortality of 5.8 per cent.

651. ULCERATIVE COLITIS

Ulcerative colitis is an inflammatory disease of unknown cause which involves the mucosa of the colon. Confined in some patients to the rectum, involving the left colon in many, it may also involve the entire colon. Its onset may be acute and fulminant, and its course often continues chronically in an intermittent or continuous form. Diarrhea is a common symptom and bleeding is an almost constant concomitant symptom, because friability in the mucosa is an integral feature of the illness. Although ulcerative colitis is capable of the most startling resolution and reversal, the more typical course is one of unpredictable recurrences. Thus like the more recently defined regional enteritis, ulcerative colitis constitutes an enigmatic clinical entity.

Incidence, Prevalence, and Epidemiology. Estimating the incidence and prevalence of ulcerative colitis is difficult. Most estimates are based on studies of hospitalized patients. Some patients—particularly those with disease confined to the rectosigmoid colon (ulcerative proctitis)—have such mild symptoms that they are not commonly hospitalized and hence are not accounted for in such surveys. Also, physicians are reluctant to examine and investigate thoroughly patients with mild chronic diarrhea or children with diarrheal disorders; thus some of these patients may have undiagnosed ulcerative colitis. Finally, granulomatous colitis cannot always be distinguished on clinical grounds from ulcerative colitis.

Incidence Rates (rate of occurrence of the disease per 100,000 persons at risk per year). In a study of the Oxford area, the incidence was 7.3 for females and 5.2 for males for an average of 6.5. In a Baltimore study of hospitalized patients over 20 years of age, the corresponding figures were 5.2 and 3.9, for an average of 4.6. To these figures should be added the incidence of ulcerative proctitis, which may range from 3 to 6.

Prevalence (all the patients affected with this disease per 100,000 persons at risk). In the United Kingdom, the data suggest that for each patient admitted to a hospital for the first time with ulcerative colitis, there were 12 patients at large in the population with the same disease. The range of prevalence for this disease has been estimated for proctitis as 40 to 80, and for ulcerative colitis as 35 to 70.

Although inflammatory bowel disease as a whole is being increasingly recognized, there is no evidence to support impressions of increasing incidence. In the United States, between 200,000 and 400,000 persons have been estimated to suffer from the disease, with between 25,000 and 30,000 new cases each year. In almost all series there is a preponderance of females over males. The first peak of incidence occurs between the ages of 20 and 25, as in Crohn's disease. Again, almost all series show a second rise in incidence in the decade from age 50 to 60. Kirsner and co-workers have suggested that this second peak may be related to mesenteric vascular disease. In the Baltimore study the urban black population was one third as likely to have ulcerative colitis as the white population. Among veterans of World War II in England and the United States, the incidence of ulcerative colitis among Jewish patients was two to four times greater than might be expected. In the Baltimore study the frequency of ulcerative colitis among Jews was 3.5 times the rate for non-Jews. Although impressions exist that the ulcerative colitis population has a higher socio-economic and educational status than the general population, careful analysis does not confirm this.

Genetics. As with Crohn's disease, there is no simple mendelian genetic mechanism operative. Aggregation of families includes both ulcerative colitis and Crohn's disease; the incidence of familial disease is higher for Crohn's disease alone than for ulcerative colitis alone. In a recent study from Chicago, only 4 per cent of the control population had a family history of such bowel disease, whereas 11 per cent of those with chronic inflammatory disease had a family history of the same. Jews dominated this group and with onset at significantly lower age (less than age 20). Ulcerative colitis has been recorded in eight pairs of monozygotic twins with concordance in five. The association of *ankylosing spondylitis* with ulcerative colitis is similar to that of Crohn's disease. It may be that these two diseases have different environmental causes but occur in the same families because the genotypes determining susceptibility share genes in common.

Etiology. In the more than 100 years since Samuel Wilks separated nonspecific ulcerative colitis from epidemic forms of dysentery, many etiologic agents and concepts have been advanced. None has been convincingly demonstrated. No virus, bacterium, or protozoon has been shown to be specifically related to the disease. Occasionally after an epidemic of bacillary dysentery, a few individuals will be left with chronic ulcerative colitis, but this occurs in only a small minority. The disease occurring simultaneously in husband and wife is extremely rare, indicating that an environmental agent alone is not responsible. The relatively isolated dramatic response of the disease to withdrawal of milk from the diet has always raised the question of specific allergic factors.

Since all experienced clinicians have been impressed with exacerbation of ulcerative colitis in the setting of tensions, conflicts, and anxiety of their patients, much emphasis has been placed on the role of psychosomatic factors in initiating and perpetuating this disorder. George Engle, the most persuasive recent investigator of this aspect, has stressed the obsessive-compulsive immaturity of these patients and the dependency on parent or parent surrogate figures, and emphasized the "hopeless and helpless" reaction they experience at the loss of these figures by death, rejection, or removal. In similar approaches it is assumed that disturbances in secretory, vascular, and motor responses are mediated through the autonomic nervous system. Why only the colon should respond is obscure. More recently, these concepts have been both challenged and ignored by workers in the field. In the Baltimore study, in which the control population (patients with the irritable colon syndrome) and those with ulcerative colitis were meticulously interrogated for psychosomatic factors in their history, the results did not demonstrate that patients with inflammatory bowel disease had unusual health histories or significantly more of those factors which could be interpreted as evidence of life stresses and failure to adapt to them; indeed, there were more such factors in the patients with the irritable colon syndrome. Attention should also be paid to the failure of experienced clinicians to document the transition of the irritable colon syndrome into ulcerative colitis. However, the relatively crude investigative techniques used in these studies do not meet the criticism of more sophisticated psychiatrists. The inconclusive reports of the results of psychologic therapy cannot be interpreted in terms of etiology. Although the psychosomatic concept remains unproved, this does not gainsay the need to understand the emotional setting in which ulcerative colitis appears and exacerbates.

Immunologic mechanisms now occupy the forefront of investigations into the etiology, encouraged both by the concomitant presence of manifestations of hypersensitivity states such as *erythema nodosum, arthritis,* and *uveitis* and by the response to steroid therapy. More than 15 per cent of patients have high titers of circulating antibodies against colonic epithelial mucopolysaccharide antigens, and against certain cross-reacting bacterial lipopolysaccharide antigens, especially those of *E. coli* 014. These antibodies can bind to intestinal epithelial cells in vitro. But it has never been possible to demonstrate that these antibodies possess cytotoxic activity, or even that these antibodies are bound to colonic tissue in vivo. Anticolon antibodies also have been found in clinically healthy relatives of colitis patients, and classic ulcerative colitis has been reported in a patient with agammaglobulinemia. There is presently no evidence that anticolon or cross-reacting antibacterial antibodies in ulcerative colitis play any pathogenetic role in the disease. Individual patients with ulcerative colitis may have elevated serum levels of IgA and of secretory IgA in particular, in the presence of longstanding disease; but as a group, ulcerative colitis patients have no statistically different serum immunoglobulin levels or patterns from the general population, nor is there any consistent correlation between immunoglobulin patterns and disease severity. There is, however, some evidence to suggest that circulating immunoglobulins might be sequestered in diseased bowel, because a fall in concentration can be demonstrated across inferior mesenteric artery and vein during active disease. Moreover, serum IgM has been shown to rise acutely after bowel resection. Formation of antigen-antibody complexes in ulcerative colitis consumes the C1q component of complement. Pathologic processes might bind or catabolize immunoglobulins in diseased tissue in ulcerative colitis and initiate the formation of circulating immune complexes. Although no role has been identified for immunoglobulins in pathogenesis, circulating immune complexes could underlie such extracolonic manifestations as arthritis or erythema nodosum.

Lymphocytes from patients with ulcerative (and granulomatous) colitis are cytotoxic to intestinal epithelial cells in vivo and in vitro. There is also a cytophilic IgM antibody in the serum of patients with ulcerative colitis that confers this property upon normal lymphocytes. Neither lymphocyte cytotoxicity nor circulating cytophilic antibody reflects a basic underlying immune disorder in ulcerative colitis, because both disappear very rapidly when the inflamed colon is removed. The depressed responses of circulating lymphocytes to phytohemagglutinin in both Crohn's disease and ulcerative colitis in some patients appear also to be a secondary phenomenon.

Pathology and Pathogenesis. In contrast to the characteristic histopathologic features of Crohn's disease, the pathologic changes in ulcerative colitis are even more nonspecific. Throughout its course ulcerative colitis generally remains a disorder of the mucosa and submucosa of the colon. Under unusual circumstances the histopathologic process may extend through the muscular layer to reach the mucosa and may penetrate through the serosa.

The increasing use of rectal biopsy has made it possible to document the early pathologic features. The earliest lesion appears to involve the base of the crypts of Lieberkühn in the form of infiltration with polymorphonuclear leukocytes at the tip of the crypts with degenerative changes in the overlying epithelial cells. This is followed by the development of crypt abscesses with extension of the polymorphonuclear infiltrate into the crypts and necrosis of the crypt epithelium. A more heterogeneous cellular inflammatory reaction supervenes, involving lymphocytes, plasma cells, mast cells, and eosinophils, with vascular dilatation and engorgement. These so-called microabscesses of the crypts may next coalesce and separate the overlying mucosa from the lamina propria and its blood supply, producing ulceration of the mucosal surface and even its denudation. The extension of crypt abscess and ulceration results in the formation of residual islands of mucosa with undetermined edges. These fragments of epithelial tissue constitute the pathologic basis of *pseudopolyps.* Concurrent healing leads to some collagen deposition, but fibrosis is not prominent. Hypertrophy of the muscularis mucosae may also develop. Ineffective healing and regeneration lead to the presence of thin atrophic epithelium. These features are far from specific; similar changes have been described in a variety of infectious colitides, including *shigellosis* and *gonococcal infection,* and even in *amebic colitis.* However, the chronic recurrent nature of the changes, especially the crypt abscesses, and the development of either the atrophic mucosa or the multiple pseudopolypoid reactions are quite characteristic. Shortening of the bowel with narrowing of the lumen, loss of haustrations, and stricture formation in chronic cases appear to result infrequently from fixed fibrotic changes but more often from spasm and hypertrophy of the muscularis mucosae, which may account for their reversibility on occasion. Such reversals stand in marked contrast to the course of luminal narrowing in Crohn's disease.

In more severe forms the inflammatory necrotizing process may extend through all coats of the colon, leading to the clinical situation known as *toxic megacolon.* Here all elements are involved in the inflammatory reaction, and a vasculitis (swelling of the vascular endothelium, inflammatory changes in vessel walls, necrosis of blood vessels, and local thrombosis) is prominent. The inflammatory changes in the neural elements (especially ganglion cells) and musculature of the colon may account for the characteristic colonic dilatation in toxic megacolon. The extension of the pathologic process to the serosa, with deep ulceration through the muscular walls, together with loss of tone, sets the stage for free or walled-off perforations.

Grossly, the anatomic extent of the process differs widely. Perhaps as many as half the patients have the disease limited to the rectum alone, *ulcerative proctitis,* whose microscopic pathology in no way is different. Of the remainder, perhaps less than half involve the rectum and the left side of the colon from sigmoid to most of the descending colon. About one third of all patients have universal colitis. In about one fifth of the patients with involvement of the entire colon there is some superficial disease in the terminal ileum for a distance of 8 to 12 inches. The pathologic nature of "segmental colitis" involving portions of the right colon is more problematic; when significant ileal disease is present, patients are often found to suffer from Crohn's disease or regional (granulomatous) enterocolitis.

Clinical Manifestations. The wide diversity of clinical presentations is part of the highly variable course of this disease. Its onset may be most insidious or of catastrophic abruptness. In some patients (perhaps half) the initial symptoms of malaise, mild lower abdominal discomfort with slight increase in frequency, and softening of the stool with small amounts of blood are vaguely recalled. In another quarter of patients, the onset is more intense and more easily dated, often related by the patient to an upper respiratory infection, a "stomach virus," or a specific emotional trauma. More intense lower abdominal cramping pain, an increased number of loose to watery stools containing blood and often waking the patient at night, and mild systemic symptoms of easy fatigability and low-grade fever are characteristic of this moderately severe group. Perhaps in 15 per cent of patients there is an onset with profuse bloody diarrhea, high fever up to 39.5 to 40° C and severe abdominal diffuse pain. Such a sudden onset portends a grave illness.

Paralleling the diversity of the mode of presentation is the variability of the clinical course. A very small group will have but one attack and go into prolonged remission for years. The majority will have a chronic intermittent course with asymptomatic remissions between recurring attacks. The remainder (perhaps 5 to 15 per cent) will have a chronic, continuous, progressively relentless course. The outlook for survival after any episode is directly related to its severity. In an attack of mild disease the patient has few stools and lacks tachycardia, fever, and loss of appetite, whereas the patient with severe disease has severe bleeding, fever, anemia, and lowered serum albumin. Patients with mild disease rarely die, but as many as 35 per cent of those with severe attacks may die.

Those with mild colitis may also have vague lower abdominal distress, minor variations in the number and consistency of stools, and small amounts of rectal bleeding. This group of patients have few or no constitutional symptoms, except for perhaps a slight falling off of appetite. The patients usually continue their full activities, and if bleeding is not stressed, their symptoms may be interpreted as part of the irritable colon syndrome. Although in some the pathologic process is confined to the rectum or rectosigmoid, the mucosa of the entire colon may be involved. The group with the more limited distal disease, "ulcerative proctitis" or "idiopathic proctitis," may have all the attendant clinical features, both local and extraintestinal, as the more diffuse variants. Usually, however, the effects of illness are not striking, and reassuringly it tends to remain localized. Further, the immediate and long-term mortality in this variant is negligible and the risk of cancer is much reduced.

Intermediate in intensity, morbidity, and mortality between the "proctitis" variety and the severe form which may be fulminant and catastrophic is the group whose disease is moderate, about one quarter of patients. Diffuse lower abdominal pain, increasing number of stools both by day and—more troublesome—by night, tenesmus, more marked rectal bleeding than in the mild form, some anorexia, and low-grade fevers (37 to 37.5° C) are associated with disinclination to carry on usual activities.

The most dramatic and frightening presentation of ulcerative colitis is the severe disease which fulminates. Without any antecedent history, or in the first attack, or in the chronic course of mild and moderately severe ulcerative colitis, the illness begins explosively with high fever, profuse bleeding, marked diarrhea with profuse watery stools, associated with diffuse abdominal crampy pain, and prostration. With the extension of the pathologic process throughout all the coats of the colon, marked dilatation of the colon, "toxic dilatation," or "toxic megacolon," supervenes (Fig. 3). Death in an acute attack of ulcerative colitis is most frequent in this group.

In all forms of ulcerative colitis certain extracolonic manifestations may accompany the disease: they include *arthritis, uveitis,* and such skin manifestations as *erythema nodosum* and *pyoderma gangrenosum.* History-taking in the ulcerative colitis patient does not reveal any strikingly associated diseases except ankylosing spondylitis. In contrast to Crohn's disease, the extraintestinal manifestations (skin, eyes, joints) rarely precede the intestinal symptoms.

Physical Examination. In the mild forms, examination usually reveals no significant findings. In the more severe forms the physical examination reveals the ill, dehydrated, acutely or chronically sick and feverish patient. There may be diffuse abdominal tenderness, but except in patients with "toxic megacolon" or perforation, there is no evidence of peritonitis, localized or general. The spleen is rarely palpable. The skin, eye, and joint manifestations can at times all be present on physical examination. Clubbing of the fingers and toes is rare in the absence of concomitant small bowel involvement.

Laboratory Studies. Routine studies reveal a degree of blood loss which may be profound. Marked leukocytosis is usually present, as high, indeed, as 35,000 to 40,000. Remarkable increases in platelets may also be recorded in these same patients, and may play a role in thromboembolic phenomena. A hemolytic anemia may occur, usually in those receiving salicylazosulfapyridine (Azul-

fidine), but a Coombs-positive autoimmune hemolytic anemia may be present unrelated to sulfonamides. A prolonged prothrombin time may result from associated liver damage, or from the effects of antimicrobial drugs on intestinal bacterial synthesis of vitamin K. A reduction in platelets and fibrinogen levels may document disseminated intravascular coagulation. Fluid, electrolyte, and serum losses lead to marked reduction in levels of serum potassium and albumin. The flat film of the abdomen usually reveals some gas in the colon, and allows visualization of the thickened edematous colonic wall.

Mechanisms of Disease Manifestations. Rectal bleeding arises from friability of the colonic mucosa and deeper ulceration. The cause of this friability (manifested by the elicitation of bleeding when the surface is gently stroked at sigmoidoscopy with a cotton swab, a pathognomonic feature of the disease) is undetermined, although some evidence suggests increased local concentration of fibrinolysins. The anemia is secondary to blood loss, usually grossly visible; on occasion, however, occult bleeding may continue from the friable mucosa. Chronic colonic bleeding may give rise to *iron deficiency anemia.* Azulfidine-related and rare idiopathic hemolytic anemias also contribute to the anemia. Hypoalbuminemia ensues as the result of colonic loss of serum albumin from altered, more permeable mucosa, although diminished protein intake (caused by loss of appetite) and, rarely, liver disease contribute to a limited extent. The diarrhea, which may be profound, results from the inability of the damaged colonic mucosa to reabsorb water and sodium and from the increased secretion of potassium.

Disturbances in Colonic Motility. The colon is primarily a storage or reservoir organ, and the motility waves ordinarily recorded from it (designated types I, II, and III) are of low amplitude and are believed to have a segmenting, restraining, or mixing function. The "mass movement" activity of the colon which results in evacuation and defecation is associated with the normal, rarely occurring, large amplitude type IV wave, which may reach 80 to 100 cm of water pressure. Colonic pain and frequency of rectal evacuation in ulcerative colitis have been associated with a marked increase in type IV activity; there is also some increase in type I and lack of type III (increase in tone superimposed on type I or II). The net effect is a reduction in segmenting but an increase in propulsive motility.

Diagnosis. Ulcerative colitis is a syndrome—a constellation of clinical features—an abnormal, inflamed colonic mucosa (demonstrated by sigmoidoscopy and barium enema), and a characteristic histologic substrate (demonstrated by rectal biopsy). Since the disease by definition is mucosal in location, the sigmoidoscopic examination is the single most important diagnostic tool, and will establish the diagnosis in 95 to 98 per cent of cases, because the rectosigmoid is almost universally involved. On occasion the lesion is patchy, and the rectum may not be clearly involved (possibly as a result of local steroid therapy); in these few instances colonoscopy may be useful. On sigmoidoscopy the earliest changes are edema and hyperemia of the mucosa, which give the granular appearance. This is followed by the development of such fragility that gentle wiping with cotton, or the pressure of the instrument alone, leads to bleeding. This finding is the most characteristic. The colon bleeds spontaneously as well. Discrete ulcerations are not seen frequently on sigmoidoscopy, but the mucopurulent, slightly foul exudate is characteristic. Pseudopolyps are also hallmarks

Figure 3. Dilatation of the transverse colon in fulminating ulcerative colitis.

Figure 4. Diffuse ulcerative colitis with pseudopolyposis.

(Fig. 4). In most the diagnosis can be easily made by sigmoidoscopy; in some cases, however, the findings are extremely subtle, with friability the only positive finding. Here rectal biopsy may be helpful, with cellular infiltration, crypt abscesses, and atrophic epithelium (denudation of glands, evidence of previous mucosal ulceration). When the sigmoidoscopic examination is positive, there is little point in rectal biopsy except for serial study of the course of the patient; however, when the sigmoidoscopic lesion is equivocal, then biopsy may be helpful.

Radiologic Findings. Examination of the colon by barium enema is needed to determine the extent of disease beyond the sigmoidoscope, and to detect such complications as stricture, polyps, or cancer. Care must be used in the selection of patients for this examination. In the desperately ill patient, it is not only necessary but dangerous. The preparation of the colon for examination is also a serious concern. Cathartics and laxatives should not be used; rather, reliance is placed on several days of low-residue diet and gentle saline or tapwater enemas.

In the *acute stage* the roentgenographic findings are secondary to edema, ulceration, and alterations in motility. Spasm with narrowing and incomplete filling is associated with secretions within the lumen. Ulcerations are tiny and produce serrations along the contour of the filled bowel or small spicules in the film after evacuation. The bowel wall is fuzzy, and as ulceration proceeds "collar button"–like projections appear. In the *moderate* or *moderately severe stage,* the roentgenographic features are due to continued ulceration, beginning fibrosis, and epithelial regeneration, and pseudopolyps are the prominent features (Fig. 5). The results are shortening of the bowel, rigidity, and narrowing of the bowel lumen. The haustral markings, which are often missing in the normal left colon, disappear throughout. Some of the alterations in the shape of the colon are secondary to smooth muscle hypertrophy rather than collagen deposition. In this stage a patulous ileocecal valve allows visualization of the terminal ileum, which may (in 5 to 15 per cent of cases) have minimal involvement of the mucosa without narrowing of the lumen. In some patients early in the disease the barium enema may be entirely within normal limits. In others with "proctitis" the retrorectal space, which is increased owing to spasm and fibrosis of the rectal segment of the colon, may be the only evidence that this area has been involved in an inflammatory reaction.

Differential Diagnosis. Clinical presentation, the sigmoidoscopic findings, and the roentgenographic appearance usually establish the diagnosis with a high degree of accuracy. Yet certain other syndromes present real problems. Some acute *infectious colitides,* particularly shigellosis, may mimic the picture of acute fulminant colitis but usually are not chronic. The patient with the *irritable bowel syndrome* may have lower abdominal distress, intermittent cramps, and diarrhea. However, fever, the systemic symptoms, night stools, and bloody evacuations are absent, and a normal sigmoidoscopy establishes the difference authoritatively. *Amebic colitis* may be distinguished with some difficulty from acute ulcerative colitis, although the conventional teaching is that the ulcerations of amebic infection are larger and separated by islands of intact mucosa. If direct aspirates of the lesions fail to disclose the motile trophozoites, rectal biopsy may help by demonstrating them in the tissue. The patient with classic *ischemic colitis* is usually over 50 years of age, and has evidence of atherosclerotic vascular disease. However, *infarction of the colon* may be seen in young women taking oral contraceptive pills. The clinical picture of abrupt onset of lower abdominal pain, crampy in nature, fever, and rectal bleeding may mimic the acute onset of fulminant colitis, but the course with progression to gangrene or resolution with stricture formation helps to distinguish it. The typical x-ray features of intramural hemorrhage and edema with "thumbprinting" also help. But the occasional involvement of the rectosigmoid by ischemic colitis adds to the complexity of the differential diagnosis, because the proctoscopic features resemble nonspecific "proctitis." *Radiation colitis,* usually seen after radium treatment for carcinoma of the cervix, and occasionally seen in men after radiation and abdominal lymph node dissection for cancer of the testicle, presents with disturbances of bowel movements and bleeding at a variable time after the original exposure. Distinction from the other nonspe-

Figure 5. Evacuation film of colon of same patient as in Figure 4.

cific forms of colitis may be difficult, but the history is all important. *Acute proctitis* may occur after a large number of broad-spectrum antimicrobial agents; lincomycin has been especially stressed. *Gonococcal infection* of the rectum should also be considered. *Lymphogranuloma venereum* may simulate all the specific and nonspecific forms of proctitis. Positive Frei and complement fixation tests, together with presence or history of inguinal buboes, help to establish this diagnosis. *Cancer of the colon* and *diverticulitis of the sigmoid colon* may on occasion have a few clinical features in common with ulcerative colitis, but sigmoidoscopy and barium enema examination usually resolve the question. The interesting and important differential diagnosis of *ulcerative colitis* and *Crohn's disease of the colon* is discussed in Ch. 652.

Treatment. *Medical Therapy.* It must be recognized that ulcerative colitis is a disease with an extremely variable course and with no known specific therapy. The aim of therapy is therefore supportive: in the acute episode to reduce the still significant mortality (up to 35 per cent in severe cases), and in the chronic forms to induce and maintain remissions and reduce the number, severity, and duration of exacerbations. Therapy thus includes the establishment of a good relationship between patient and physician in view of the disturbing nature of this illness to recur, correction of nutritional deficits, the restoration of fluid and electrolyte equilibrium, replacement of blood loss, and symptomatic relief of pain and diarrhea.

General Symptomatic Therapy. In all but the mildest forms, a period of restricted energy expenditure with appropriate rest periods is useful, especially if accomplished in a stable supporting environment. The diet should be adequate in total calories, contain enough protein to replace the losses caused by colonic leak and offset the effects of fever, and be palatable enough to appeal to the capricious appetite of these sick patients. Granted that no convincing evidence exists regarding the widely prescribed unpalatable low residue diet, it seems rational during episodes of marked rectal frequency to limit the amount of calorically insignificant cellulose residue of the diet proffered to the already irritated, inflamed colon. There is much anecdotal and a little scientific evidence that some patients dramatically improve on a diet from which cow's milk is excluded. This can be related only in part to intestinal lactase deficiency, but the patient's prior experience should guide the decision to withdraw milk and its products. Massive blood loss requires adequate blood replacement. The anemia of chronically ill patients is in part due to iron deficiency of chronic bleeding, to hemolysis, and to bone marrow failure to incorporate iron. The intolerance of a considerable number of patients to oral iron preparations is genuine, and the use of parenteral iron in the form of dextrose iron complex (Imferon) is justified. Although some apprehension is justified regarding the use of anticholinergics and opiates for the control of pain and diarrhea, because they may play a role in precipitating toxic dilatation of the colon, the judicious use of these agents is valuable on the basis of clinical experience. Tincture of belladonna (15 drops), codeine (15 to 30 mg), deodorized tincture of opium (6 to 10 drops), paregoric (4 to 8 ml), or Lomotil (2.5 to 5 mg) before meals and at bedtime gives the patient considerable comfort.

Antimicrobial Therapy. Salicylazosulfapyridine (Azulfidine) has already been discussed in Ch. 650. This sulfonamide was introduced, however, for the treatment of ulcerative colitis, and in the opinion of most experienced clinicians it has a place in the management of milder forms of ulcerative colitis. The sulfonamide may be the sole drug used in treating patients who have mild disease and who are ambulatory. For those ill enough to be put to bed or hospitalized, however, it is inadequate. When used for those with mild disease, 2 to 8 grams in divided doses is prescribed; in view of the high percentage of patients developing nausea and anorexia or headache, it is wise to begin with smaller doses, or to add an antihistaminic to the regimen. Some clinicians are more comfortable with the use of other, non- or poorly absorbed sulfonamides in this group of patients.

In the sicker patients there is a place for maintenance therapy with the sulfonamide as well as for those who have gone into remission on corticosteroid therapy. In mild or moderately severe disease in remission, Azulfidine in doses of 2 grams per day is more effective in preventing relapses than are corticosteroids. Azulfidine has no place in the fulminatingly ill patient. Other antimicrobials also have no place in the management of ulcerative colitis except in the presence of toxic megacolon and suppurative complications.

Corticotrophin (ACTH) and Adrenocorticosteroids. Corticotrophin and corticosteroids were introduced into the therapy of ulcerative colitis on the assumption that their anti-inflammatory actions would be useful, especially because certain associated lesions of ulcerative colitis (*arthritis, uveitis,* and *erythema nodosum*) often responded to these compounds, and in the hope of reducing the colonic mucosal inflammatory reaction. Also, these agents stimulated appetite and elevated the patient's mood. Early studies revealed that a short course of cortisone induced an increased incidence of remission of this disease, but the effect was short lived and the long-term benefits have not been demonstrated. Yet the introduction of corticotrophin and steroid therapy with newer analogues of cortisone (prednisone or prednisolone) represents an advance in the management of the severe and the moderately severe attack.

In the mild forms, especially in those patients whose disease is confined to the rectosigmoid and distal colon, rectal instillations of steroids are of distinct use in inducing remissions, and their continued intermittent use may maintain remissions. Plastic disposable enema units containing 100 mg of hydrocortisone hemisuccinate or 20 to 40 mg of prednisolone phosphate are commercially available. This form of treatment may be used nightly as a retention enema until remission occurs, and maintained by instillation two to three times weekly. There is good evidence that these instillations may reach large sections of the colon (up to the hepatic flexure). The main effects are local, but some steroids are absorbed and the degree of adrenocortical suppression is minimal. In universal ulcerative colitis and in those sick enough to be hospitalized, rectal steroid therapy does not appear to be sufficient as the sole form of treatment.

In the moderately ill patient systemic oral steroids are the current drugs of choice. Forty to 60 mg of prednisone or its equivalent is a reasonable initial dose which should induce marked improvement and/or remission within two weeks, at which point it should be slowly tapered. In some patients the remission may be only partial and steroid therapy must be continued. Supplementation with Azulfidine at this point may be wise in the weaning period as well as for maintenance. Stepwise reduction in oral steroids should be continued while clinical well-being is maintained at a reasonably low dose. In view of the serious hazards of long-term corticosteroid therapy, which includes *profound suppression of endogenous adrenal activity, muscle weakness* and *wasting, osteoporosis* and *vertebral collapse, hypertension, diabetes, cosmetic deformities* with their attendant *psychologic disturbances, psychosis,* and *growth retardation* in children, doses above 15 to 20 mg should not be prescribed for longer than six to eight weeks. Although alternate-day therapy may minimize the incidence of undesirable side effects, the suppressive effect on symptoms is also lessened.

In the acutely ill patient with the fulminant presentation, intravenous therapy with corticotrophin or corticosteroids is the best current method of management. There is a general clinical impression that corticotrophin is superior to corticosteroids in this group; this judgment has, however, little supportive objective evidence. In these gravely ill patients corticotrophin should be given by continuous intravenous drip, 25 to 40 units per eight-hour period. If there is any question of adrenal responsiveness, intravenous hydrocortisone in doses of 100 mg given over each eight-hour period may be substituted. Fluid overload, sodium retention, and hypokalemia must be meticulously prevented. If a remission is to be achieved, it usually will be obvious within 7 to 10 days; it is hazardous to continue such therapy beyond 14 days. Failure of discernible response should lead to prompt colectomy at this point. If the expected clinical improvement occurs, the intravenous dose should be gradually reduced and supplemented by orally administered steroids. Dosage in turn is then gradually tapered until the patient can either be weaned or maintained on not more than 15 to 20 mg of prednisolone per day. The regimen may be supplemented in some by Azulfidine at this time.

Other complications of steroid therapy further limit the enthusiastic use of these compounds: *retinopathy, chemosis of lids, adrenocortical insufficiency* from too rapid withdrawal of the drug, or *inadequate adrenocortical reserve* which may persist for months after their use, and these agents may mask signs and symptoms of *sepsis* and *colonic perforation.* There is much discussion as to whether high-dose corticotrophin or prednisone therapy in the acutely ill patient increases the likelihood of perforation. Certainly in such circumstances the usual clinical signs and symptoms can be concealed. Demonstration of the preservation of liver dullness and measurement of abdominal girth should be part of the daily routine examination of this group of acutely ill patients. The activation of peptic ulcer and the precipitation of massive upper gastrointestinal hemorrhage are further reasons for close observation. Large doses of antacids, avoiding those containing magnesium which may aggravate the diarrhea, are widely and rationally used; their effectiveness in preventing ulceration and bleeding, however, is unproved. Cumulative experience supports the evidence that the mortality has been reduced considerably since the introduction of steroids, especially in the moderate to severe group in their acute attacks. It remains to be proved that the long-term outcome has been significantly altered. The earlier use of colectomy appears to be of major importance.

Immunosuppressive Therapy. Immunosuppressive therapy with azathioprine or 6-mercaptopurine has been used for a number of years for those patients not responsive to steroids or sulfonamides, or in an effort to reduce the dose of steroids needed to induce remission. There is little solid evidence to support this approach, although azathioprine (1.5 to 2.5 mg per kilogram of body weight daily) may be more effective than a placebo when given with steroids for exacerbations. Alertness for this drug's effect on the bone marrow as well as for possible intercurrent infections is essential. In view of its unproved nature and possible, albeit unknown, long-term effects, its use must be considered purely experimental and ethically should be confined to controlled clinical trials. This attitude is especially rational in view of the effectiveness of colectomy.

Psychotherapy. All who deal with patients with ulcerative colitis recognize the importance of the supportive role that the physician must play in this labile illness; indeed, most doctors act out their psychotherapeutic role intuitively. It is difficult to find convincing evidence that more formal psychotherapy by psychiatrists or lay analysts alters the long-term course of the illness. Despite this gap in knowledge, there is an obvious place for recommending psychotherapy for those patients and their families in whom personality problems and distorted interpersonal relationships exist. It is more difficult to decide whether all patients should have some exploration of possible psychic conflicts. If this is undertaken, the psychiatrist should be one who has experience with this illness and sensitivity to the often fragile psychic structures of these patients. There is little place for psychotherapy for the patient who is acutely ill. In general, psychotherapy should be reserved for the more quiescent interval phases of the disease.

Complications.   *Local Complications.*   These include the development of *anal fissures, rectal prolapse,* and *hemorrhoids* and are to be related to the intensity of the diarrhea. *Perianal abscess* and *fistulas* are rare in ulcerative colitis in contrast to Crohn's disease. *Rectovaginal fistulas,* however, may appear and do not heal with local surgical measures. The pseudopolyps carry with them no prognostic significance. They may disappear completely and have no relation to the development of cancer. *Massive hemorrhage* occurs in about 5 per cent of patients. Rapid replacement of blood and restoration of circulating blood volume are the initial factors in treatment. Hypoprothrombinemia should be corrected by ingestion of vitamin K. Although most patients will respond to medical management, an occasional patient may require colectomy, because the bleeding is from diffuse areas of the mucosa. At times inferior mesenteric arteriography may reveal a more discrete site of bleeding. The colectomy must be total to control bleeding; failure to remove the rectal stump usually requires further emergency surgery. *Strictures of the colon* occur in a little less than 10 per cent of patients, and are rarely of such magnitude as to compromise the intestinal lumen. They usually develop in the rectum or transverse colon, are of variable lengths, and may appear at any time in the course of the disease. They are not important symptomatically, because they only rarely cause abdominal cramping pain and obstipation. They require attention, because their differentiation from cancer is often difficult. *In fact, it is wise to consider every stricture in ulcerative colitis as carcinomatous until proved otherwise.* Exploratory laparotomy was the only method until recently, but colonoscopy and biopsy have been helpful when the strictured area can be thoroughly visualized and multiple biopsies taken.

Cancer of the Colon. The incidence of cancer of the colon is strikingly higher in patients with ulcerative colitis than in the control population, and contributes significantly to the colitis-related death rate. Current evidence relates this incidence to the duration of the colitis, rather than its activity, and to the extent of the colon involved. The risk of cancer rises regularly in all patients with the duration of the disease. After 20 years the cumulative risk of cancer in all patients is about 12 per cent, and at 25 years it is 25 per cent. In children it has been estimated that 3 per cent of those who develop the disease in childhood will have cancer of the colon after 10 years and 20 per cent per decade thereafter. The risk rises strikingly after the first decade of disease in children and after the second decade in adults.

The extent of colonic involvement with colitis plays an important role in determining the risk of subsequent cancer development. In proctitis it does not differ significantly from that in the control population. The incidence in left-sided colitis is much lower than in universal colitis. In this latter group the incidence may approach 13 per cent at 15 years, 25 per cent at 20 years, and 40 per cent at 25 years. Since childhood colitis is usually universal in type, this factor influences the high rate of malignancy. Most cancers of the colon are in the rectum, and this is true for ulcerative colitis, including universal colitis. Such cancers may, however, involve any segment of the colon, the transverse colon being the second most common location. The survival rate after surgery for cancer complicating ulcerative colitis is much lower than for cancer unrelated to ulcerative colitis. One reason is that cancer in ulcerative colitis is frequently multicentered (10 to 15 per cent). Clearly the population at greatest risk are those with universal colitis of more than 10 years' duration. Although prophylactic colectomy has been advocated for this group, no consensus exists at present on this point, although yearly sigmoidoscopy and barium enema examinations are widely proposed. The search for "precancerous" changes on biopsy may be more rewarding, particularly with the increasing use of colonoscopy as well as sigmoidoscopy. At present the value of serum carcinoembryonic antigen (CEA) levels in the diagnosis of malignancy in this disease remains to be established, because levels are elevated in 30 per cent of patients with inflammatory bowel disease.

Toxic Megacolon. At any time in the course of ulcerative colitis the patient may become gravely ill with the signs of systemic toxicity and marked dilatation of the colon. Although much ingenuity has been expended in establishing the criteria for defining this distention, usually the colon is more than 6 cm in width on the flat plate of the abdomen. This drastic episode coincides with extension of the previous mucosal inflammation through all coats of the colon, with evidence of involvement of neural and vascular components. Factors which decrease muscular tone or increase intraluminal pressure may be important in precipitating an episode of colonic dilatation: barium enema examination, injudicious use of opiates and anticholinergic drugs, or hypokalemia. In some patients no obvious triggering mechanism, except worsening of the pathologic process, can be found. Clinically, this is the most dramatic episode in all the variegated course of ulcerative colitis.

The patient is gravely ill, with high fever and rapid pulse, and dry. He complains of abdominal pain which may be continuous, and the abdomen is markedly distended. The previous diarrhea may cease abruptly. The abdomen is diffusely tender and ominously silent. Marked leukocytosis, hypokalemia, and a precipitous fall in serum albumin are usually present. The flat film reveals dilatation of all the colon or a segment, usually the transverse colon, and the edematous ragged colonic mucosa can be seen with the air contrast. If the colon has freely perforated, air may be seen under the diaphragm. Diffuse peritonitis and localized perforation are frequently overdiagnosed because of direct visceral tenderness elicited by pressure on the inflamed serosa of the dilated colon.

The diagnosis is made on the basis of the history of ulcerative colitis, acute worsening of the clinical picture, systemic toxicity, and dilatation of the colon on clinical and radiologic evidence. A few patients, however, will present initially with this condition. Barium enema examination should be avoided, and gentle proctoscopy in bed will make the diagnosis if the antecedent history of ulcerative colitis is not present.

Therapy of acute toxic dilatation of the colon should be intensive and meticulous. Correction of fluid and electrolyte deficits, especially of potassium, is needed. Anemia, hypoalbuminemia, and decreased circulatory blood volume require correction. Steroids are the therapy of choice, and if the patient has been on previous corticosteroids, corticotrophin or hydrocortisone in large doses is used as outlined above (25 to 40 units of corticotrophin or 100 mg of hydrocortisone, given over the course of each eight-hour period by intravenous drip). Since there is probably localized suppuration which has extended to the serosa, intravenous antimicrobial therapy is in order: ampicillin in doses of 8 to 12 grams daily intravenously is usually ordered. Daily flat film and physical examination two or three times a day are required. In view of the usual accompanying small bowel ileus, long-tube intubation should be promptly instituted along with cessation of feedings, anticholinergics, and opiates. The response to this vigorous form of therapy must be evaluated daily in terms of the patient's systemic improvement and regaining of colonic tone in terms of the distention of the colon clinically on flat film. The first 48 to 72 hours will usually indicate whether the hoped-for improvement is indeed beginning to take place. Failure to respond by the fourth or fifth day should lead to prompt subtotal colectomy (avoiding the trauma of the abdominoperineal resection in those desperately ill patients) and ileostomy. On occasion preliminary cecostomy or transverse colostomy has helped by decompressing the colon. The surgical difficulties in handling the thin, distended, often perforated colon should not be underestimated, even if performed by experienced surgeons, and the postoperative periods are often stormy, including localized or generalized peritonitis, walled-off abscesses, and the ominous iliofemoral thrombophlebitis. The mortality of toxic megacolon has been markedly reduced in recent years, in part because of steroid therapy and better systemic management, but probably in major part because of earlier surgical intervention. Of those who recover on current medical programs, the majority usually come to surgery during the next year because of persistent activity of the disease. An interesting clinical variant is the occasional patient who has a "subacute," perhaps a "chronic," megacolon, in contrast to the terribly sick "toxic" patient, and whose clinical course is more indolent, although similar.

Perforation of the Colon. Perforation of the colon is most likely to occur in the course of toxic dilatation, and is rare simply in the course of an acute attack. As noted, it is presumably the result of extension of the inflammatory ulcerative process through all layers of the bowel. Since the vast majority of these sick people are already receiving large doses of steroids, recognition is difficult, although sudden clinical worsening with increasing abdominal distention and tenderness of the colon may arouse suspicion. Obliteration of liver dullness must be sought for at all times, and the presence of free air under the diaphragm on x-ray examination makes the diagnosis. Surgical intervention is urgently required and colectomy indicated. Rarely, an episode of perforation may not be recognized and the patient survives; the perforation is documented later by an abdominal film showing free air in the peritoneal cavity.

Extracolonic Complications. As with Crohn's disease, a number of extracolonic complications or manifestations are part of the clinical syndrome. The *arthritis* may be severe, migratory, and accompanied by synovial swelling affecting knees, elbows, and ankles; however, the serologic factors of rheumatoid arthritis are missing, and there is no residual deformity. *Ankylosing spondylitis* and *sacroiliitis* occur with higher frequency than might be expected. *Iritis* and *uveitis,* unlike the arthritis, are not easily correlated with the degree of clinical colitis. Of the skin manifestations, *erythema nodosum* and *pyoderma gangrenosum* are the most common. The incidence of kidney stones is highest in those with ileostomies. The hepatic complications include *fatty infiltration, pericholangitis* and *chronic active hepatitis,* and, rarely, *sclerosing cholangitis* and its associated *carcinoma of the bile ducts.* It is not known at present whether colectomy improves liver function or structure. Massive peripheral or pelvic thrombophlebitis, especially *iliofemoral venous thrombosis,* is a grave complication, and may be related to marked thrombocytosis.

Surgical Therapy. Colectomy is curative in ulcerative colitis, at the cost of life with an ileostomy. The marked reduction in mortality from colectomy and the recent improvement in the quality of life with an ileostomy now makes colectomy an acceptable form of treatment for the patient with ulcerative colitis. Whether done in one or two stages, most experts agree that preservation of the rectum is not possible in this disease although ileoproctostomy (with or without active disease in the rectum) still has a few advocates. However, subsequent ileal dysfunction, intestinal obstruction, ileostomy prolapse or retraction, delayed healing of the perianal wound, and fear of psychogenic or neurogenic impotence present realistic limitations to the overenthusiastic use of surgery. The clearest indications for surgery are those complications for which no other therapy is available: massive uncontrollable hemorrhage, perforation of the colon, cancer of the colon, a stricture which cannot be distinguished from cancer, and medically unresponsive toxic dilatation. Close behind this group are the patients in a severe acute attack, which carries with it the highest mortality risk. This is the group which has until recently been usually treated with two to three weeks of intravenous steroids at high dosage plus massive antimicrobial therapy. Although continued disease activity, protein and electrolyte depletion, serious anemia, and localized suppuration make surgical intervention at this stage somewhat risky, it is the best choice. Some proponents of early surgery have advocated intervention after four to five days if the patient has not clinically shown remission in this period of time. Although this point of view

has yet to be unequivocably established, the trend of modern therapy is toward earlier intervention in the acutely ill patient. Moreover, there is probably little disagreement at present that the patient with intractable pyoderma gangrenosum and probably also persistent or serious uveitis should undergo colectomy. No solid evidence exists, however, that colectomy improves serious liver disease.

A decision for surgery in the patient with persistent symptomatic disease, sufficiently severe to prevent normal function, is indicated, especially for those who require unacceptably high levels of steroids (greater than 20 mg of prednisone daily) for suppression of symptoms. In others the decision for colectomy is more difficult, especially with childhood disease. These patients suffer a lower survival rate with or without malignancy, and growth and sexual maturation are retarded. Colectomy should be recommended for such children who are chronically ill, despite the reluctance and anxiety of both family and physician, but only after a period of medical trial, possibly not longer than two years.

The most difficult problem is the risk of cancer in the patient who has had the disease for ten years or more, either quiescent or with minimal medical therapy. Those with distal or only rectal involvement have little risk and can be followed with barium enema, proctosigmoidoscopy, and colonoscopy. It is those with universal colitis who raise the question of prophylactic colectomy. As indicated, no firm trend is visible at present. It should be pointed out that the development of the "continent" ileostomy of Kock of Sweden with its internal pouch and avoidance of an external mechanical appliance may simplify the decision in borderline patients.

652. CROHN'S DISEASE OF THE COLON
(Granulomatous Colitis)

Definition. Crohn's disease of the colon is a chronic inflammatory disease of the colon of unknown origin, characteristically of young adults, most frequently involving the proximal colon and its adjacent terminal ileum. Although any and all portions of the colon alone may be involved, it classically spares the rectum. A diarrheal disease of insidious onset and progressive course, it usually has little tendency to rectal bleeding, great tendency to fistulize both internally and externally, and, frequently, significant anal and perianal lesions. The characteristic pathology includes confluent linear ulceration, intramucosal fissuring, aggregates of mononuclear inflammatory cells, and epithelioid granulomas within the bowel wall or regional lymph nodes (hence the term granulomatous colitis). Because of similarities of clinical course, pathology, tendency to recur after resection, and coexistence with regional enteritis (Crohn's disease of the ileum), Crohn's disease of the colon is considered the same disease. The term "ileocolitis" is reserved for simultaneous involvement of the ileum and colon. The distinction from ulcerative colitis may be difficult on occasion, but this does not obliterate their differences and the therapeutic consequences of such differentiation.

Separation of Ulcerative Colitis and Crohn's Disease of the Colon. The year after the original description of regional enteritis, Colp described a patient with involvement of both ileum and cecum and demonstrated that the ileocecal valve is no barrier to the development of this process in the colon. Despite sporadic papers, it was not until 1960 that it became apparent that Crohn's disease could occur frequently in the colon as well as in the small bowel and could be differentiated from ulcerative colitis. The clinical and pathologic characters of Crohn's disease of the small bowel and ulcerative colitis have been presented in Ch. 650 and 651, respectively.

The features which distinguish ulcerative colitis and Crohn's disease of the colon should be emphasized: In Crohn's disease the small bowel is also involved in up to 80 per cent of cases; the lesion is segmental, sparing the rectum in perhaps more than half the patients; and fistulas are extremely frequent—all in marked contrast to ulcerative colitis. Clinically, in Crohn's disease rectal bleeding is a much less frequent occurrence, severe perianal and perirectal disease is often florid, free perforation and toxic dilatation are rarer, and, up to the present, development of cancer is extremely rare. In contrast to the mucosal pathology of ulcerative colitis, all coats are involved in Crohn's disease, with marked thickening and a high percentage of granulomas in the bowel wall and regional lymph nodes. Finally, in therapeutic contrast to ulcerative colitis, excision in Crohn's disease of the colon is often followed by recurrences in the small bowel. Our inability to differentiate these two entities even when adequate histologic material is present (in perhaps 15 per cent of cases) does not argue for their identity. The colon has a limited repertoire of disease, and other disorders are still to be separated from this group of inflammatory diseases, ischemic colitis being the most recently segregated entity.

Incidence and Distribution of Lesions. The available data regarding the incidence and prevalence of Crohn's disease have been cited in Ch. 650. Despite the increasing recognition of this entity, the impression that the incidence of Crohn's disease of the colon rivals that of ulcerative colitis appears erroneous. Of over 600 patients with inflammatory colonic disease sick enough to require ileostomy and colectomy in the writer's series, less than 10 per cent had Crohn's disease of the colon.

The colon may be involved in Crohn's disease in one of several ways. The least significant is by way of fistula formation from a contiguous loop of small bowel which is the site of regional enteritis. This is relatively trivial, because the disease does not appear to spread, and the colonic area heals when the small bowel is resected and the fistula closed. Second, the colon may become involved only after an anastomotic operation for regional ileitis, and almost always directly adjacent to the anastomosis. More important, the colon alone may exhibit the disease. Finally, the colon and small bowel are simultaneously the seat of the pathologic process, with continuity of disease in the colon, and occasionally normal segment intervenes. When the colon is involved, less than 20 per cent of patients have the lesion confined to that organ; 80 per cent have disease in the ileum. Over-all, about two thirds of Crohn's disease involves the small bowel alone. The anal involvement in Crohn's disease of the colon is noteworthy. It may be in the form of edematous anal tags, chronic fissuring, anorectal fistulas, and indolent undermining ulceration. About 75 per cent of patients with Crohn's disease of the colon and 25 per cent of those with Crohn's disease of the small bowel have an anal lesion at some time in the course of this illness.

Pathology. The pathology of Crohn's disease of the colon and rectum is fundamentally that of Crohn's disease of the small intestine. Because of the interest and difficulty at times of distinguishing colonic involvement from ulcerative colitis, some additional points should be mentioned. In contrast to ulcerative colitis, Crohn's disease is a discontinuous process, sparing the rectum generally in more than half the instances and involving the terminal ileum in a very high percentage of cases. Intense vascularity is characteristic of ulcerative colitis, not of Crohn's disease. Muscular shortening of the colon in ulcerative colitis contrasts with the fibrosis and stricturing of Crohn's disease. Pseudopolyp formation is characteristic of ulcerative colitis. External and internal fistulas are the hallmark of Crohn's disease, including such unusual sites as the stomach; the only fistula characteristic of ulcerative colitis is rectovaginal fistula.

The microscopic characteristics of both diseases have also been described under their respective categories. Ulcerative colitis is primarily a mucosal disease; Crohn's disease involves all layers. In Crohn's disease, in contrast to ulcerative colitis, fissuring is prominent, as well as aggregates of mononuclear inflammation and sarcoid granulomas in the bowel wall and regional lymph nodes. In biopsies of the rectum in Crohn's disease of the colon we have found about 10 per cent to have these granulomas when no gross lesion was visible on sigmoidoscopic or barium enema examination. Ultrastructural studies have disclosed no characteristic findings of these granulomas. Although crypt abscesses are not specific for ulcerative colitis, they are a prominent pattern in its histopathology, in contrast to Crohn's disease of the colon. The latter may also exist in a colon with sigmoid diverticular disease, and the clinical and radiographic features are as difficult to assign to each component as the pathologic findings.

Cancer as an important feature of the natural history of ulcerative colitis has already been emphasized; even in the small bowel in Crohn's disease, the incidence of adenocarcinoma is more frequent, especially in the bypassed ileum. Although some cancers have been observed in colons which are the seat of Crohn's disease, the data at present do not allow any firm statement regarding the risk of cancer development, for these patients have not been observed more than ten years, in part because the colons are usually removed before ten years of illness.

Clinical Manifestations. Crohn's disease of the colon, like Crohn's disease of the small bowel, begins in young adult life. About a third of the writer's patients had their first manifestations between 16 and 20 years of age. In comparison with ulcerative colitis, an acute fulminant presentation is rare, toxic dilatation is rarer, and free perforation, rarest. Onset is usually slow and insidious, with diarrhea as the principal symptom in the majority of patients. The stools are small, frequent, and soft but not necessarily watery; some patients may be constipated, especially if they have anal lesions. Over three quarters of the patients lose weight. Crampy abdominal pain of a diffuse nature is prominent. Gross bleeding is noted only in less than half the patients; indeed, important rectal bleeding is most unusual except in the presence of rectal involvement. The history of a perirectal abscess or fistula often precedes the obvious clinical onset by years. *Aphthous stomatitis, arthralgias* and *arthritis, uveitis, pyoderma gangrenosum* and *erythema nodosum,* and backache caused by *ankylosing spondylitis* and *sacroiliitis* are secondary manifestations, as in other variants of inflammatory bowel diseases.

Physical Examination. In contrast to regional ileitis, patients with Crohn's disease of the colon rarely have a palpable right lower quadrant mass, even when the ileum is involved. Clubbing of the fingers and curvature of the nails may be present. Edematous perianal skin tags and perirectal fistulas may be noted.

Diagnosis. Confirmation of the clinical suspicion of Crohn's disease of the colon depends upon sigmoidoscopy and barium enema examination, and, on occasion, upon the small bowel series. In half the cases, the sigmoidoscopic examination is negative; in the others it may reveal an edematous mucosa, mucoid secretions, or a cobblestoned surface. Rarely a few discrete ulcers may be seen. In contrast to ulcerative colitis, however, bleeding from a friable mucosa is not present. Rarely, diagnosis may be made by biopsy findings.

The roentgenologic features are the same as in regional enteritis of the small bowel, i.e., segmental involvement with normal skip areas, longitudinal ulcerations, fissures, eccentric involvement, pseudodiverticula, strictures, internal fistulas, and sinus tracts (Fig. 6). In early cases nodular defects or irregularity of the contour of a short segment of colon may be the only findings, and may be obscured on the filled films. At times the evacuation films or examination of the colon from above may be the only way of documenting these changes. Strictures, as in ulcerative colitis, are difficult to distinguish from cancer; when the entire colon is diffusely involved in a symmetrical fashion, and when the

Figure 6. Crohn's colitis. Note involvement of terminal ileum as well as right side of colon.

ileum is normal, it may be impossible to distinguish Crohn's disease of the colon from ulcerative colitis by x-ray examination.

Differential Diagnosis. The important conditions which must be differentiated from Crohn's disease of the colon include *ulcerative colitis, cancer* of the *colon, tuberculosis* of the *ileocecal area, amebiasis,* and, rarely, *radiation enteritis* and *colitis.* When a left-sided colonic segment is the site of disease, *ischemic colitis* and *sigmoid diverticulitis* are the disorders which must be distinguished. The intramural abscess of diverticulitis and the longitudinal submucosal ulceration of Crohn's disease are similar on barium enema, but the very long tracts are characteristic of Crohn's disease.

Therapy. Current approaches to therapy of Crohn's disease of the colon reflect the perspective of experience with Crohn's disease of the small bowel. The unpredictable course of the disease, the significant reduction in longevity, and the high rate of recurrence of surgically treated ileitis have engendered a cautious and somewhat pessimistic view of all therapies available at present for Crohn's disease of the colon. All the modalities of medical treatment for ileitis are used in Crohn's colitis: general supportive measures, nutritional supplements, sulfonamides (especially Azulfidine), steroids (corticotrophin and adrenocorticosteroids), and immunosuppressives (azathioprine [Imuran]). Even more than in regional ileitis, the therapeutic value of all these methods remains to be demonstrated in sound controlled clinical trials. When multiple enteric and cutaneous fistulas lead to marked malnutrition and malabsorption, hyperalimentation with a central venous catheter may be effective.

Surgical intervention is clearly indicated for those complications for which no medical therapy exists: perforation, cancer, obstruction resulting from stricture, massive hemorrhage, and fistulization into stomach, duodenum, and bladder. The more difficult decisions concern those patients who are not able to carry out their usual daily activities and those who require more than 20 mg of prednisolone daily to suppress their symptoms over a period of months. Almost 75 per cent of patients ultimately come to surgery. Since considerable controversy exists at present regarding the fate of patients with total extirpation of the colon for Crohn's disease, the decision is by no means easy in sick patients. Diversionary ileostomy in the hope of resting an inflamed colon and possibly even subsequently utilizing this organ has become discredited. When the disease is segmental and especially since the left colon and rectosigmoid are free in at least half the patients, resection and anastomosis with sigmoid or rectum is the operation of choice. The rate of recurrence in these localized extirpations clearly resembles the rate of recurrence of Crohn's disease of the ileum alone (approaching 50 per cent). In the writer's experience, of 67 patients with Crohn's colitis, 31, or 46 per cent, had significant recurrences in the ileum after ileostomy and colectomy, 8 required multiple operations, and 6 had severe nutritional deficits. This experience is not paralleled by all observers. In some series recurrences have been observed in none or only 3 per cent. A review of the experience at St. Mark's Hospital in London indicated four recurrences in 56 patients (7 per cent), but others have reported as many as 16 recurrences in 37 patients treated similarly. These differences may relate in part to the extent to which the ileum is involved; in our group almost all had the ileal involvement. Accordingly, some delay in deciding on colectomy seems warranted. Even the most vigorous proponents of ileostomy and total colectomy grant that the patients with Crohn's disease of the colon have a higher rate of stomal dysfunction and ileitis than patients with ulcerative colitis.

Regional Enteritis

Crohn, B. B., Ginzberg, L., and Oppenheimer, G. D.: Regional ileitis: A pathologic and clinical entity. J.A.M.A., 99:1323, 1932.

Gerson, C. D., Cohen, N., and Janowitz, H. D.: Small intestinal absorptive function in regional enteritis. Gastroenterology, 64:907, 1973.

Kayle, J.: Crohn's Disease. New York, Appleton-Century-Crofts, 1972.

Marshak, R. H., and Wolf, B. S.: Roentgen findings in regional enteritis. Am. J. Roentgenol. Radium Ther. Nucl. Med., 74:1000, 1955.

Monk, M., Mendeloff, A., Siegel, C., and Lilienfeld, A.: An epidemiological study of ulcerative colitis and regional enteritis among adults in Baltimore. I. Hospital incidence and prevalence, 1960 to 1963. Gastroenterology, 53:198, 1967. II. Social and demographic factors. Gastroenterology, 56:847, 1969.

Ulcerative Colitis

Edwards, F. C., and Truelove, S. C.: The course and prognosis of ulcerative colitis. I. Short term prognosis. Gut, 4:299, 1964. II. Long term prognosis. Gut, 4:309, 1964.

Engle, G. L.: Studies of ulcerative colitis. III. The nature of the psychological processes. Am. J. Med., 19:231, 1955.

Marshak, R. H., Korelitz, B. I., Klein, S. H., Wolf, B. S., and Janowitz, H. D.: Toxic dilatation of the colon in the course of ulcerative colitis. Gastroenterology, 38:165, 1960.

Sparberg, M., Genonessy, J., and Kirsner, J. B.: Ulcerative proctitis and mild ulcerative colitis: A study of 220 patients. Medicine, 45:391, 1966.

Wilks, S., and Moxon, W.: Lectures on Pathological Anatomy. London, Churchill, 1875.

Crohn's Disease of the Colon

Korelitz, B. I., Present, D. H., Alpert, L. I., Marshak, R. H., and Janowitz, H. D.: Recurrent regional ileitis after ileostomy and colectomy for granulomatous colitis. N. Engl. J. Med., 287:110, 1972.

Lindner, A. E., Marshak, R. H., Wolf, B. S., and Janowitz, H. D.: Granulomatous colitis, a clinical study. N. Engl. J. Med., 269:379, 1963.

Ritchie, J. K., and Lockhart-Mummery, H. E.: Nonrestorative surgery in the treatment of Crohn's disease of the large bowel. Gut, 14:263, 1973.

OTHER INFLAMMATORY DISEASES OF THE INTESTINE

Marvin H. Sleisenger

653. ACUTE APPENDICITIS (INCLUDING THE ACUTE ABDOMEN)

Definition. Appendicitis is acute inflammation of the vermiform appendix. It is rare before the age of two and reaches a peak incidence in the second and third decades. The vast majority of patients are between the ages of 5 and 30. Although incidence of the disease declines after the age of 40, the annual incidence is about 1.5 per thousand for males and 1.9 per thousand for females between the ages of 17 and 64. The disease is important because it is common and curable; it therefore constitutes the most important entity in the differential diagnosis of the acute abdomen.

Pathology. Usually, the appendix is swollen, hyperemic, warm, and covered with exudate. However, in the early stages it may appear only slightly discolored and, in the late stages, gangrenous with perforation. Microscopically, the picture ranges from some acute inflammatory cells in the lumen and mucosa to acute inflammatory changes transmurally with superficial mucosal ulcerations; in advanced stages, one or more perforations may be noted, particularly in patients over the age of 60.

Etiology and Pathogenesis. The initiating event in acute appendicitis appears to be obstruction, followed by increased intraluminal pressure, reduced venous drainage, thrombosis, hemorrhage, edema, and bacterial invasion of the wall. As the process proceeds, the appendiceal artery (an end artery) becomes occluded as a result of the inflammation, and venous stasis and perforation result.

Calculi are thought to be the most common cause of the initial obstruction. Indeed, about one third of inflamed appendices contain a radiologically demonstrable calculus, as compared with 2.7 per cent of normal ones. In turn, about a third of these are visible on plain films of the abdomen preoperatively, whereas they may be seen in only 1 per cent of a control population. The incidence of gangrene and perforation is significantly higher also in appendices which contain calculi. The nidus for these calculi is inspissated fecal material which is covered by a calcium phosphate–rich mucus; inorganic salts precipitate, hardening the calculus and increasing the likelihood for obstruction. It must be stressed, however, that two thirds to three quarters of patients with proved acute appendicitis do not have calculi. In these patients, obviously, an alternative pathogenetic mechanism must be responsible. Obstruction by parasites, lymphoid hyperplasia, and twisting of the appendix by adhesions have all been incriminated. An additional theory is malfunction of a valve system at the entrance of the appendix. Recently, mucosal ulceration has been considered by some to be the primary pathogenetic event rather than obstruction. Such ulceration may also result from viral infection.

Thus it is likely that the etiology of acute appendicitis is multiple. Regardless, increased intraluminal pressure, transmural swelling, and inflammation eventually compromise the appendiceal end artery and cause gangrene and perforation.

Clinical Picture and Diagnosis. The history of appendicitis is of short duration in the vast majority of cases—between 12 and 48 hours from onset to hospitalization. Over 95 per cent complain first of pain at onset, classically referred to the epigastric or periumbilical areas and later localizing in the right lower quadrant. This sequence, however, is found in only about half the patients. Further, a significant number will not localize clearly to the right lower quadrant, the pain being either diffuse or in the lower abdomen. When retrocecal, the pain may be referred to the thigh or right testicle and may even be felt as burning with urination.

Pain referred to the mid-epigastrium is due to stretching of the organ during early inflammation; later, when the process has reached the serosa and the peritoneum, it localizes over the site of disease. In some patients distress appears to be alleviated at the time of perforation; after perforation, localization of pain will depend on whether or not the process is quickly walled off locally. Thus if the spreading infection is not contained, generalized abdominal discomfort of variable severity will result. Anorexia and nausea (with or without vomiting) are the second and third most frequent symptoms. In almost all instances, pain precedes the appearance of these other complaints. About 10 per cent of patients will have constipation; diarrhea is relatively infrequent. Temperature usually ranges between 38 and 38.6° C; higher levels usually indicate perforation.

Physical Examination. The findings on physical examination differ widely and depend not only upon the stage of the inflammation but also upon the age of the patient. Tenderness to palpation is the most common and most reliable sign; indeed, without it, diagnosis is unlikely. It is usually confined to McBurney's point in the right lower quadrant, corresponding to the usual location of the organ. However, although rectal tenderness is present in about one third of patients, it may be so severe as to indicate pelvic peritonitis. On initial examination in a minority of patients, a mass may be felt in the right lower quadrant or in the pelvis or transrectally. Three quarters of patients will have unquestionable localized tenderness with localized rebound. Generalized rebound tenderness indicates diffuse peritonitis. Bowel sounds may be present or absent; absence associated with distention and generalized rebound tenderness is consistent with perforation and diffuse peritonitis.

On occasion, tenderness may be elicited in the case of retrocecal appendicitis by stretching the psoas by hip extension. Very rarely, because of the odd location of the appendix, tenderness may be in the right upper quadrant or even the left lower quadrant.

Laboratory studies consistently show a leukocytosis with an increase in polymorphonuclear cells—over 10,000 per cubic millimeter and greater than 75 per cent, respectively. Urinalysis is usually normal; however, about 15 per cent of patients have either a slight amount of protein or mild pyuria or hematuria. Presence of a calcified fecalith in the right lower quadrant on flat film of the abdomen is helpful, but its absence has no meaning in the diagnosis. Other findings on flat film include possible obliteration of the right psoas shadow, right lower quadrant sentinel loop ileus, and a right lower quadrant soft tissue mass with or without gas bubbles; with perforation and generalized peritonitis, fluid in the peritoneal cavity and obliteration of the peritoneal lines may be noted.

Differential Diagnosis of Appendicitis and of the Acute Abdomen. Appendicitis is first on the list of conditions causing acute abdominal pain which require surgery or immediate consultation with a surgeon. Here a few principles regarding the acute surgical abdomen in the setting of the differential diagnosis of acute appendicitis will be reviewed.

Pain Characteristics. Conditions associated with pain of sudden onset include perforated viscus or acute ischemia; occasionally, the onset of pain in acute small bowel obstruction is abrupt. The more gradual onset of pain usually indicates an inflammatory lesion, including appendicitis. However, the pain of diffuse inflammatory bowel disease is not localized as it is in appendicitis, except as a consequence of perforation or fistulization in granulomatous disease.

The type and radiation of the pain also help in differential diagnosis. For example, evidence of irritation of the diaphragm may be found on the right in *acute cholecystitis* and on the left in *acute pancreatitis;* sudden severe pain referred to the tips of the shoulders, associated with diffuse intra-abdominal pain and, later, distention, is more typical of perforated viscus, particularly

peptic ulcer. Ureteral obstruction causes pain which is frequently referred to the genitalia or groin. Steady continuous pain is more characteristic of inflammation, as in appendicitis; on the other hand, intermittent or crampy pain is more characteristic of *obstruction of a hollow viscus* such as the gallbladder or small bowel.

It is important again to stress that pain precedes nausea and vomiting in *appendicitis;* on the other hand, vomiting may be an earlier symptom of *acute cholecystitis* or *acute pancreatitis.* Bile-stained vomitus associated with acute cramping upper abdominal pain suggests *small bowel obstruction;* blood in the vomitus points toward a mucosal lesion proximal to the third portion of the duodenum. Relief of pain by vomiting suggests *gastric outlet obstruction.* Vomiting, of course, may accompany any intra-abdominal conditions, particularly if the patient has ileus or generalized peritonitis.

Physical Findings. Physical examination of the patient with an acute abdomen is of great importance, and the range of findings expected in acute appendicitis has been discussed. Localized tenderness and temperature elevation associated with continuing pain over a period of hours reflect either *localized peritonitis,* with or without perforation, or *vascular necrosis* of an ischemic organ. In such instances, the temperature is approximately 38.5 to 39.5° C. Higher temperatures are more often associated with urinary tract infections or bacterial pneumonias. A continuing rising pulse rate likewise indicates the possibility of gangrene or perforation of a viscus.

Careful examination of the abdomen is of extreme importance in differential diagnosis. *Diffuse peritonitis* is reflected by resistance of movement and change in position because of accentuation of pain; on the other hand, colic caused by *obstruction* of bile ducts, ureter, or small bowel early in its course is associated with restless movement. Later, in biliary tract and small bowel obstruction, infection and compromise of the blood supply may ensue and will cause the appearance of signs of localized tissue necrosis and peritonitis. The abdomen should be carefully examined for scars of previous surgery which may now underlie an *intestinal obstruction* caused by adhesions; hernias must be sought.

In examining the patient with an acute abdomen, the physician should palpate in that quadrant which is farthest removed from the site of distress. The important findings which indicate a surgical condition include persistent localized tenderness with unequivocal rebound, indicating localized peritonitis, and guarding. Guarding must be interpreted circumspectly, because it may be voluntary or involuntary. If it is the latter, underlying peritoneal irritation is likely. Generalized involuntary guarding is a classic finding for a perforated intra-abdominal viscus. The presence of an abdominal mass not previously noted, particularly when associated with other findings of inflammation, gangrene, or perforation, is very strong evidence for a surgical condition. Likewise, free air in the abdominal cavity, as evidenced by distention, absence of bowel sounds, and absence of liver dullness in the setting of acute abdominal pain, reflects a perforated viscus. Bowel sounds may be more active and high pitched in early obstruction or continuously active in diffuse acute inflammation (nonsurgical) of the small bowel. With increasing distention of small bowel loops, the sounds become less frequent and more high pitched. Bruits are an important finding, because they may reflect the presence of *arterial aneurysms*, the dissections of which may be the cause for the abdominal pain.

Rectal examination is crucial in differential diagnosis. Unequivocal tenderness indicates pelvic inflammation, and a mass usually reflects the presence of an abscess. As noted above, this examination often reveals positive findings in acute appendicitis. A glove specimen of stool must always be examined for occult blood. In females with acute abdominal pain, pelvic examination is essential to complement a careful gynecologic history.

Laboratory Aids in Diagnosis. The laboratory examination, consisting of urinalysis, complete blood count, serum electrolytes, BUN and creatinine, and x-ray examination of the abdomen and chest, is essential in differential diagnosis of the acute abdomen.

A *polymorphonuclear leukocytosis* strongly substantiates an acute intra-abdominal process with inflammation or necrosis; a low hematocrit reflects a disorder which is also capable of bleeding — *mucosal ulcerations, intestinal carcinoma,* or *ischemia* or *dissecting aneurysms.* An elevated hematocrit and BUN suggest dehydration, usually caused by vomiting and deficient fluid intake.

Urinalysis is vital in differential diagnosis, because the presence of pyuria, particularly white cell casts and bacteria on the smear of urinary sediment, is strong evidence for urinary tract infection and interdicts surgical exploration. Microscopic hematuria suggests stone or tumor of the genitourinary tract; red cell casts, on the other hand, suggest glomerulitis.

Important blood chemistries are *serum amylase,* elevation of which usually reflects acute pancreatitis; however, it may not be elevated in chronic relapsing pancreatitis, and it is elevated in other conditions such as *perforated peptic ulcer, strangulated obstruction* of the small bowel with perforation, and both *acute cholecystitis* and *acute common duct obstruction.*

Roentgenographic Studies in the Acute Abdomen. Roentgenologic examinations of importance include chest films, flat film of the abdomen, intravenous cholangiogram, and intravenous pyelogram. The flat and upright films of the abdomen may be specific for diagnosing free air in the peritoneal cavity, reflecting a perforation of a hollow viscus; in supporting the diagnosis of acute small bowel obstruction; in indicating the likelihood of calculus disease of either gallbladder or urogenital tract; of outlining a large obstructed stomach; and of revealing a variety of soft tissue masses which may reflect cysts or abscesses. Collections of extraintestinal gas often point to abscesses; occasionally, the biliary tree may be outlined by air, thus revealing a fistula to bowel. Diffuse calcification of the region of the pancreas indicates chronic pancreatitis. As noted, calculi in the right lower quadrant may help in the diagnosis of acute appendicitis. Flat film of the abdomen also may yield findings characteristic of acute pancreatitis, including "sentinel" loops and a "cut-off" of the colon. A routine chest x-ray is essential in order to reveal free intraperitoneal air under the diaphragm, to demonstrate pneumonia, or to show an elevated diaphragm on the left with or without pleural effusion and partial atelectasis as noted in acute pancreatitis, or on the right, reflecting subphrenic abscess.

The more special radiographic tests which may be of help in the differential diagnosis include an intravenous cholangiogram to evaluate the possibility of biliary tract obstruction and inflammation; cholangiographic demon-

stration of the gallbladder renders the diagnosis of acute cholecystitis highly unlikely. Intravenous pyelogram may establish the patency of the urinary tract or, conversely, establish ureteral obstruction or hydronephrosis unilaterally. Examination of the upper gastrointestinal tract with non-barium-containing radiopaque substances (Gastrografin) may help in the diagnosis of perforated ulcer.

Important in the differential diagnosis of acute appendicitis are those nonsurgical conditions which cause acute abdominal pain. These conditions may be excluded by appropriate attention to history, physical examination, and the laboratory studies enumerated in the preceding paragraphs. Chief among these are *pyelonephritis, pneumonia, pulmonary infarction, acute myocardial infarction,* and *pericarditis,* all of which may present with acute upper abdominal pain. Acute distention of the liver and its capsule resulting from acute right heart failure may simulate *acute cholecystitis; acute hepatitis,* viral or toxic (including alcohol), may closely simulate acute biliary tract disease. In these instances, however, an enlarged tender liver will be felt. Further, serum SGOT determinations will be markedly elevated (it is well to remember, however, that acute obstruction of the common duct with cholangitis may transiently raise SGOT to levels of a thousand units or more for 24 to 48 hours).

Systemic diseases, such as *sickle cell disease, acute intermittent porphyria, tabes dorsalis, heavy metal poisoning,* and *diabetic neuropathy,* all may present pictures simulating an acute surgical abdomen. Appropriate tests for sickling, for excretion of porphobilinogen (Watson-Schwartz test), for urinary lead, and for other evidences of syphilis or diabetes greatly aid in ruling out these conditions.

Acute pancreatitis, still considered a nonsurgical condition unless caused by common bile duct obstruction, usually presents with pain of many hours' to days' duration, associated with a history suggestive of biliary tract disease or indicative of acute and chronic alcoholism, and in its early stages abdominal tenderness is usually localized to the epigastrium. Markedly elevated plasma amylase (within 48 hours of onset) or urinary amylase (up to 5 days after onset) will help establish the diagnosis.

Special Considerations of Age in Differential Diagnosis of Acute Appendicitis. Great care must be extended to establish the diagnosis of this condition in the very young and very old. Children with diffuse abdominal pain which is preceded by anorexia, nausea, and vomiting and often associated with diarrhea are more likely to have *acute infectious gastroenteritis. Acute mesenteric adenitis,* presumably caused by viral illnesses and often associated with diffuse abdominal pain, is frequently confused with acute appendicitis in children. The difficulty is in those patients in whom there is some right lower quadrant tenderness and slight elevation of the white count. In such instances a diagnosis must be established at operation, because it is far safer to undertake a negative exploration than to neglect removal of an acutely inflamed appendix.

In young females diagnosis is confused by problems in the reproductive system, such as *ruptured graafian follicles, twisted ovarian cysts, ectopic pregnancies, dysmenorrhea, ruptured endometrioma,* and *acute pelvic inflammatory disease. Ruptured ectopic pregnancy* is usually of dramatic suddenness and is often associated with shock and massive blood loss; these findings in a pregnant woman make the diagnosis virtually certain. The *ruptured graafian follicle* is noted in midcycle; fever and leukocytosis are uncommon. Tenderness on moving of cervix on vaginal examination points toward a *twisted ovarian cyst*, the pain of which is out of proportion to the general well-being of the patient. *Gonococcal salpingitis* may be difficult to establish, because endocervical smears may be negative for the organism. Usually, however, the pain is more diffuse and tenderness not so well localized as in appendicitis. However, in questionable instances, exploration must be performed.

The differential diagnosis of appendicitis in the elderly may also be difficult. The classic picture is seldom noted, the history may be inadequate or misleading because of infirmity or the effects of medication, and the appendix perforates early. Findings on physical examination are usually not as dramatic, and, despite complications, fever may only be slightly elevated. Accuracy in diagnosis of patients over 60 years of age is below 70 per cent, and the incidence of perforation without a localized or generalized peritonitis at surgery is nearly 70 per cent—more than twice as high as all other age groups combined.

In elderly patients the principal problems in differential diagnosis are *cholecystitis, diverticulitis, mesenteric thrombosis, intestinal obstruction, incarcerated hernia,* and *perforated ulcer.* In these individuals it is well simply to recognize that one is dealing with a surgical abdomen, because, as stated, it is difficult to be clinically accurate in establishing acute appendicitis.

Right-sided acute diverticulitis may simulate acute appendicitis in every respect. In a few instances, *left-sided diverticulitis* may localize tenderness to the right lower quadrant, because the sigmoid is often more redundant in the elderly, and an excessively mobile loop may come to rest on the right side of the abdomen. In such instances, the patient also may have symptoms suggestive of diverticulitis, such as an episode of diarrhea associated with cramping or steady lower abdominal pain, slight temperature elevation, and, later, evidence of moderate to complete large bowel obstruction. When differential diagnosis is difficult, a cautious barium enema may help greatly in excluding acute diverticulitis as the cause of the problem.

Conversely, elderly patients must not be subjected to the risk of exploration falsely. Accordingly, all efforts should be extended to make certain that *acute myocardial* or *pulmonary infarction, pneumonia,* or other systemic disease or toxin is not responsible for acute abdominal pain simulating appendicitis.

Treatment.   Unless strongly contraindicated, the only therapy for acute appendicitis is surgical removal of the appendix. Since mortality correlates with perforation and, except in elderly patients, perforation correlates with duration of symptoms, early diagnosis and appendectomy are essential for the lowest acceptable morbidity and mortality for the disease. When surgery is performed early in the disease in an otherwise healthy individual, mortality is only slightly above that for general anesthesia. In view of these facts and since the diagnosis is often difficult to make early in the course of disease, some normal appendices will inevitably have to be removed. To avoid the catastrophe of unoperated-upon acute appendicitis, normal appendices may have to be removed in 20 to 25 per cent of patients.

In patients in whom complications have already occurred prior to surgery, necessary measures to correct dehydration and combat infection must be instituted. If perforation is very likely or suspected, continuous nasogastric suction should be instituted. Those patients with temperatures higher than 39° C and with findings indicative of localized abscess or generalized peritonitis should be given broad-spectrum antimicrobials, usually high-dose penicillin and gentamicin or high-dose ampicillin.

The surgical approach, i.e., whether the usual transabdominal or other, to institute drainage of an established abscess is a decision for the surgeon to make. In those patients with obvious acute appendicitis for whom no surgeon is available, the patients may be treated with head-up position of the bed, intravenous fluids, broad-spectrum antimicrobial drugs, and nasogastric suction. The chance for recovery in otherwise healthy individuals with this program is surprisingly good.

Morbidity and Mortality of Surgery.   Over-all, about 15 per cent of patients with acute appendicitis develop complications postoperatively; this figure is 35.6 per cent in those with perforation and localized peritonitis at the time of surgery and is 70 per cent in those with perforation and generalized peritonitis. The complications include *wound infection, intra-abdominal abscess,* mechanical *small bowel obstruction, fecal fistula,* and, much more rarely, *intraperitoneal hemorrhage. Pylephlebitis* is extremely rare (one in a thousand). In the elderly, of course, mortality is increased by the usual cardiovascular, pulmonary, renal, and cerebral complications.

The over-all mortality of acute appendicitis is now less than 1 per 100,000 population. It ranges from 0.18 to 1.6 per cent and is due principally to the interrelated factors of age and perforation. Indeed, mortality over the age of 60 ranges from 6.4 to 14 per cent. The cause of death in this group may be attributed equally to septic and nonseptic complications.

Special Considerations.   *Incidental Appendectomy.* In view of the decreasing risk of appendicitis with advancing age and the extremely low risk of developing acute appendicitis, it is difficult to advocate elective appendectomy during laparotomy (for example, at age 37 years the risk is 0.0431 for males and 0.369 for females). Nevertheless, if the procedure should be performed, the patient, as in any other operation, should be fully informed of what was done.

Prophylactic Appendectomy.   At present all data indicate that there is no place for prophylactic appendectomy. The one possible exception may be a move of indefinite duration to an area where neither adequate medical care nor surgical care is available on the part of an individual known to have a fecalith in the region of the appendix.

654.   DIVERTICULITIS

Definition.   Diverticulitis of the colon is a complication of diverticulosis defined as a micro- or macroperforation of a diverticulum. The etiology and pathogenesis of this complication are not clear; however, it is thought that increased segmental pressure causes a weakened area in the wall to perforate. There is no evidence for vascular occlusion or obstruction by stool as the cause.

Clinical Picture. The predominant clinical symptoms of diverticulitis are *pain* and *fever*. The pain is usually prominent and is frequently constant. Most commonly, it is localized in the left lower quadrant, because the sigmoid and descending colons are the sites of the largest number of diverticula. Occasionally, the patient will have a brief period of diarrhea or a few loose stools, and only rarely is rectal bleeding noted with diverticulitis. When the perforation and sepsis are of sufficient magnitude, the patient may also have chills with fever as high as 39 to 39.5° C. Usually, however, the fever is low grade, between 38 and 39° C.

Although the pain may be somewhat intermittent and even colicky at onset, it usually becomes steady and is of the same quality as noted in acute appendicitis. Indeed, acute diverticulitis has often been referred to as "left-sided appendicitis." The patient may present for examination after only a few hours or, when the situation is not so severe, after a few days of lingering but nagging left lower quadrant pain and low-grade fever.

Physical examination is extremely important in establishing the diagnosis. Since the process usually quickly involves the serosal surface and peritoneal cover, tenderness will be marked, and, as in acute appendicitis when the process has reached the peritoneal surface, will be both direct and rebound, though localized. Frequently, a tender mass may be discerned. When present for more than a few days, this mass may be astonishingly firm, even hard, and the distinction grossly from carcinoma is almost impossible. Rectal examination also will be painful, because inflamed bowel is often within reach of the finger; also, a mass may be palpable if a sizable abscess has formed.

In some instances the patient will present with complications of diverticulitis: *dysuria, pyuria,* and *pneumaturia,* all related to involvement of the urinary bladder. In extreme instances, the inflammatory process has perforated into the bladder; symptoms may be due to large collections of pus, not only adjacent to the colon, but also in the pelvis or under the diaphragm. Often the presenting symptom in these instances is simply septic fever. Rarely, the diverticulum perforates freely. In this instance the signs of free perforation are evident; that is, distention of the abdomen, generalized rebound tenderness, and absent bowel sounds.

Diagnosis. Diagnosis of diverticulitis should be suspected especially in patients with known diverticula who present with fever, leukocytosis, and signs of pericolic and peritoneal inflammation in the left lower quadrant. The diagnosis is even more likely if a mass is palpable. Fever between 38.5 and 39° C is also compatible with the diagnosis; when the process is more extensive and with formation of a *pericolic abscess* and its complications, the temperature is usually over 39° C, and the white count is proportionately higher. Urinalysis will reflect varying degrees of involvement of the urinary tract by this septic process; that is, with mild ureteral irritation a few red and white cells may be seen in the urinary sediment, but with direct involvement of the ureter or invasion of the ureter or the bladder by a pericolic abscess, the urine may be frankly septic and contain large numbers of red cells. Witnessing a patient pass gas on urination is also a sign, in the presence of other findings, that diverticulitis is the probable underlying diagnosis.

Some patients suffer much left flank pain owing to *hydronephrosis* resulting from obstruction of the ureter by a *pericolic abscess.* An intravenous pyelogram shows no function or an obstructed kidney on the left.

The use of x-rays is of crucial importance in the diagnosis, especially flat film of the abdomen. Evidence of pericolic perforation and abscess formation may be suspected from collections of air and fluid in the left lower quadrant; free air may be seen under the diaphragm in instances of free perforation, and with complete sigmoid obstruction the dilatation of the proximal colon down to the point of the obstruction affords important information.

Sigmoidoscopy should be carefully performed. Air insufflation should not be used, and the importance of the examination is to exclude other conditions (see below). Usually, diverticulitis per se produces no abnormalities on sigmoidoscopy except an undue amount of spasm at the rectosigmoid junction.

Clinicians debate the advisability of using a barium enema in the diagnosis of diverticulitis, particularly in its acute phase. The concern is that the increased intraluminal pressure may produce further complications. The history, physical examination, and laboratory information are sufficient to make the clinical diagnosis in the vast majority of instances, and barium enema should await some subsidence of the acute phase of the illness. The single exception to this dictum is in those instances in which the clinical picture does not permit distinguishing between *acute ischemic colitis* of the left colon and sigmoid diverticulitis.

The roentgenographic features characteristic of diverticulitis are the presence of barium outside a diverticulum, the delineation of a pericolic mass, or the demonstration of a fistula originating in the colon. In some instances the distinction between diverticulitis and carcinoma may be difficult. The presence of irregularity, thickening, or even a sawtooth appearance of the bowel is not sufficient to make the diagnosis of diverticulitis, because these are typical for diverticula without perforation.

After diagnosis of diverticulitis has been established, intravenous pyelography should be done to ascertain whether or not obstructive involvement of the urinary tract is present, particularly on the left side. In some instances, as noted above, urinary symptoms may be the predominant feature, and radiographic examination of the urinary tract may have to be performed early.

Differential Diagnosis. *Diverticulosis.* For many years symptoms of *diverticulosis* have been attributed incorrectly to diverticulitis. *Diverticulosis* may periodically be associated with marked local tenderness, a palpable sigmoid loop, and some degree of large bowel obstruction, and thus the picture suggests diverticulitis. However, such patients usually do not have fever, the localized tenderness gradually recedes, the white count is not elevated, and there is no evidence of involvement of contiguous organs. Barium enema will reveal an irregular luminal contour with a narrowed sigmoid, possibly even a so-called sawtooth appearance of the mucosa. Barium must be noted outside the diverticulum, a fistula seen, or evidences of a pericolic or intramural mass detected before the diagnosis of diverticulitis is definitely made.

Carcinoma of the colon must be distinguished from diverticulitis because of similarity of age during which both diverticulitis and cancer of the colon appear. The differential diagnosis is especially difficult, because diverticulitis also often causes luminal narrowing with partial or complete bowel obstruction, may be associated with mild rectal bleeding, and may appear rather insidiously. Chronic obstruction, more persistent rectal bleeding, and weight loss are more characteristic of *cancer,* whereas localized tenderness with rebound, leukocytosis, and fever support the diagnosis of diverticulitis. In some cases, however, it may be impossible to distinguish the two conditions, especially when the barium enema has features common to both; that is, a mass, luminal irregularities, and partial obstruction. The matter can only be settled at exploratory laparotomy. In those instances in which the signs and symptoms of obstruction rather rapidly recede, repeat barium enema will reveal marked improvement only in the patient with diverticulitis. In the event that a suspicious defect remains, exploration will have to be done.

Granulomatous colitis may be difficult to exclude in the face of marked luminal narrowing or multiloculated channels parallel to the bowel wall on x-ray. Clinically, although both may exhibit pain, partial obstruction and lower abdominal mass, some rectal bleeding, fever, and leukocytosis, the history preceding the inflammatory event is usually markedly different. The patient with granulomatous colitis usually will have had previous episodes of lower abdominal pain, fever, and diarrhea, and it is unusual for such patients to present for the first time with advanced localized colonic disease.

Sigmoidoscopy may be crucial in making the differential diagnosis if the rectum is involved with granulomatous disease. Also, evidence elsewhere in the bowel of granulomatous disease, such as cobblestoning, long intramucosal sinus tracts, and skip areas, will help in the differential diagnosis (see Ch. 652).

Ischemic colitis of the left colon in elderly patients may present with signs and symptoms of bowel necrosis and localized peritonitis which are difficult to distinguish from diverticulitis. In these instances, gross rectal bleeding is prominent, and a barium enema is of crucial importance, because so-called "thumb printing" will be found in ischemic colitis, especially in the area of the splenic flexure and descending colon (see Ch. 659).

Treatment of Diverticulitis. The patient is given nothing by mouth, and continuous nasogastric suction is instituted if signs of obstruction are present or if the patient is nauseated. Appropriate intravenous fluid is administered. Broad-spectrum antimicrobials should be given to cover gram-positive cocci and anaerobic bacteroides; e.g., high-dose penicillin or gentamicin or ampicillin and kanamycin. Tetracycline or chloramphenicol should be added if sepsis is severe. Some favor clindamycin (against *B. fragilis*) in the latter situation.

As noted above, an intravenous pyelogram should be performed early if the clinical picture suggests urinary tract infection or left ureteral obstruction. Surgical consultation must be obtained early in all cases in which a mass is palpable or when there is suspicion of peritonitis or involvement of a contiguous organ.

Most patients respond well to this type of therapy with abatement of the fever, tenderness, and evidence of partial obstruction. Long-term therapy becomes identical with that for diverticulosis (see Ch. 639).

Indications for Surgery. Surgical intervention is necessary for generalized peritonitis or for failure of medical therapy as evidenced by enlargement of a mass, appearance of a mass during therapy, persisting intestinal obstruction, or the development of a fistula. Elective surgery is indicated for recurrent attacks of diverticulitis and for the inability to exclude a carcinoma as the cause for persisting deformity after recovery from the acute phase.

655. RADIATION ENTEROCOLITIS

Damage to the small intestine and colon may result from radiation therapy for abdominal and pelvic malignancy.

Incidence. Incidence of radiation injury varies between 2.5 and 25 per cent of patients treated with radiotherapy for pelvic and intra-abdominal malignancy. It is noted most commonly after the total dosage exceeds 5000 rads. Transient histologic inflammatory change may, however, be found in the rectal mucosa of nearly 75 per cent of individuals receiving such therapeutic irradiation.

Pathogenesis and Pathology. Radiation damage results from interference with cell replication. Further, damage to the mesothelial cells of the small submucosal arterioles results in varying degrees of occlusion and mucosal transmural necrosis. Accordingly, hyperemia and ulceration of the mucosa are frequent. With extreme damage, diffuse edema is followed by extensive fibrosis with multiple strictures and irreversible damage.

The pathologic changes range from diminution of crypt cell mitosis, shortening of the villi of the small intestine to varying degrees of hyperemia, edema, and inflammatory cell infiltration of the mucosa. Progress of damage is marked by crypt abscesses, sloughing of epithelial cells, and, later, mucosal ulcerations, diffuse or localized, are found. Two to 12 months after radiotherapy, the damage to the blood vessels becomes prominent. In these instances, repair of acute damage does not ensue. The mucosa and submucosa become progressively ischemic and fibrotic. *Abscesses* and *fistulas* may form with sinus tracts between loops of intestine and between intestine and neighboring organs.

Clinical Picture. Symptoms may appear early, that is, during the first or second week of therapy, or late, that is, six months or more after completion of therapy. Early, diarrhea and mild rectal bleeding may appear, resembling ulcerative colitis. Sigmoidoscopy reveals an edematous mucosa which may be friable; in more extreme instances, the acute changes also reveal a patchy or diffusely necrotic mucosa.

Later, symptoms of radiation include gross rectal bleeding, decrease in stool caliber, and progressive difficulty in defecation with marked constipation, all indicating severe rectal involvement. Small intestinal symptoms result from either fibrosis and obstruction or fistulization and abscess formation. If the damage is especially diffuse, malabsorption may be noted, as described in Part XIV, Section Three.

Diagnosis. Diagnosis of radiation enteritis is suspected with any of the aforementioned symptoms in patients who have received significant radiation. Sigmoidoscopy shows a picture which ranges from variable degrees of edema to a markedly inflamed and necrotic mucosa. Multiple telangiectases are common, as is rectal stricture. Since most cases are fairly clear cut, biopsy is usually not indicated.

Barium studies of the intestine are not specific and range from changes of diffuse edema and spasm to diffuse fibrosis with strictures, fistulas, and ulceration in more severe cases. Thus the picture may resemble localized malignancy in the colon or diffuse granulomatous disease in the small intestine. Long strictured areas may also be noted, however, in the colon.

Differential diagnostic usefulness of small vessel angiography to the intestine in radiation enteritis remains to be confirmed.

Treatment. Improving methods for monitoring radiotherapy will probably reduce the incidence of this complication; however, the increasing incidence of malignancy and of the efficacy of radiotherapy will probably increase the total number of such patients.

Symptoms caused by early reaction consist of mild diarrhea and perhaps some minimal bleeding which can be managed with the judicious use of tranquilizers, anticholinergic drugs, local analgesics, and warm sitz baths. If rectal bleeding is prominent, treatment with steroid retention enemas should be initiated as in ulcerative colitis (see Ch. 651). If the bleeding is more significant, transfusions may be required and even, possibly, surgery. Rectal strictures may be dilated, providing that it is early in their course and they are not extensive. Lubricants and stool softeners are often helpful; however, the progress to symptomatic occlusion of the lumen may necessitate proximal colostomy. Fistulas should be resected and abscesses drained. Resection of bowel and anastomoses are hazardous in view of the impaired blood supply.

In patients with malabsorption, treatment is as outlined in Part XIV, Section Three.

Prognosis. Prognosis depends on the extent and degree of damage, the age of the patient, the course of the underlying malignancy, and whether or not the patient has systemic vascular disease. Unfortunately, extensive disease of the colon usually means significant disease in the small intestine. The prognosis is guarded in those with ulceration, fibrosis, or fistulas in whom repeated resections or other major surgical procedures must be carried out. In such cases, age and cardiovascular status are also crucial determining factors.

656. PSEUDOMEMBRANOUS ENTEROCOLITIS

Pseudomembranous enterocolitis is an inflammatory disease of the small and large bowel; occasionally it involves either the small bowel or the large bowel exclusively.

Etiology and Pathogenesis. The cause for this disease is not known; however, it is usually seen in patients with underlying serious illness, in the postoperative period, with intestinal obstruction, and in individuals receiving antimicrobial therapy for a variety of infections. In some instances it is associated with recovery of *Staphylococcus aureus* from intestinal contents, but the exact relationship of the organism to the disease is not clearly defined. Shock or ischemia of the intestine may also play a role in the pathogenesis of this entity.

Pathology. The involved bowel is covered with yellowish-green membranous plaques which may become confluent. The changes in the mucosa range from mild edema to marked friability and ulceration. The "membrane" is made up of fibrin, mucus, and a variety of mononuclear and polymorphonuclear cells; staphylococci may also be seen in clusters. Mucosal ulcerations may be scattered, and the submucosal tissue is edematous and congested. In its advanced stage, the intestine is completely covered with the membrane, and the underlying bowel exhibits extensive necrosis and ulceration.

Clinical Picture. As noted above, the disease appears in the setting of other illness or disability. Its onset is abrupt, with fever from 38 to 40° C, associated with watery diarrhea containing mucus, pus, and, on occasion, blood. The amount of fluid lost may be extreme, and dehydration and metabolic acidosis may be prominent.

Diagnosis. The disease should be suspected when the symptoms described appear in particular settings. Stool may reveal clusters of gram-positive cocci, suggesting *S. aureus*. Sigmoidoscopy may reveal hyperemia, some friability, and whitish exudate. In more severe instances, scattered ulcers may be noted with marked hyperemia and edema. Roentgenographic examinations with barium yield nondiagnostic findings, some of which resemble ulcerative colitis. Culture of the stool may reveal an overgrowth of *Staphylococcus aureus*.

Treatment. Attention must be first paid to dehydration and electrolyte imbalance which includes hyponatremia and hypokalemia. As in enterotoxic diarrhea, enormous amounts of fluid may be required—10 to 15 liters in 24 to 36 hours. Potassium must be replaced before bicarbonate may be given for acidosis.

Shock must be combated with intravenous fluids, pressor agents, and 100 mg of prednisolone per 24 hours intravenously. If staphylococci are seen on fecal smear, then appropriate antimicrobial agents such as methicillin or cephalothin should be given; if the patient is sensitive to penicillin, erythromycin, 2 to 4 grams intravenously per day, should be administered. After the initial 48 hours of therapy, attention must be paid to replacement of protein which has been lost into the intestine by administration of salt-free albumin (50 to 100 grams per 24 hours).

Prognosis. Unfortunately, the mortality is extremely high in pseudomembranous enterocolitis, 50 to 75 per cent. The reason is that this disease is superimposed upon an already serious clinical situation. If fluid and electrolyte balance is quickly restored and blood pressure returns to normal with increasing urinary output and cessation of diarrhea, the prognosis is good. Such signs are usually noted within 72 hours.

657. PRIMARY NONSPECIFIC ULCERATION OF THE SMALL INTESTINE

This inflammatory disease of unknown etiology is rare, although in a majority of instances it is attributable to ingestion of enteric-coated potassium chloride. Such ulceration may also be associated with *vascular disease, central nervous system disease, infection, trauma,* and *malnutrition.*

The clinical picture consists of symptoms of small bowel obstruction and, more rarely, perforation or bleeding. Earlier, the patient reveals periumbilical colicky pain and perhaps nausea and vomiting.

If the patient has small bowel obstruction, the findings associated with this condition would be noted. Distention, diffuse tympany, absence of liver dullness, and generalized tenderness with rebound may be found on examination if the ulcer has perforated.

Laboratory investigation is normal unless the patient has been bleeding or has had protracted vomiting; plain films of the abdomen are of great value if small bowel obstruction is present. Barium contrast studies in the uncomplicated cases are most often unrevealing, although in rare instances ulceration and narrowing in the jejunum may be noted.

Treatment for the disease is surgical with resection of the involved segment. Potassium supplements (if prescribed) in such patients should always be given in liquid form.

NONGRANULOMATOUS DIFFUSE ILEOJEJUNITIS AND EOSINOPHILIC GASTROENTERITIS

Diffuse nongranulomatous ileojejunitis and *eosinophilic gastroenteritis* are described in Part XIV, Section Three. *Tuberculous enteritis* and *enterocolitis* are discussed in Ch. 234.

Acute Appendicitis (Including the Acute Abdomen)

Babcock, J. R., and McKinley, W. M.: Acute appendicitis: An analysis of 1662 consecutive cases. Ann. Surg., 150:131, 1959.
Deal, R. D.: Acute appendicitis. *In* Sleisenger, M. H., and Fordtran, J. S. (eds.): Gastrointestinal Disease. Philadelphia, W. B. Saunders Company, 1973, p. 1494.
Kazarian, K. K., Roeder, W. J., and Mersheimer, W. L.: Decreasing mortality and increasing morbidity from acute appendicitis. Am. J. Surg., 119:681, 1970.
Stone, H. H., Sanders, S. L., and Martin, J. D.: Perforated appendicitis in children. Surgery, 69:673, 1971.

Diverticulitis

Loeb, P. M., and Sleisenger, M. H.: Diverticular disease of the colon. *In* Sleisenger, M. H., and Fordtran, J. S. (eds.): Gastrointestinal Disease. Philadelphia, W. B. Saunders Company, 1973, p. 1415.
Reid, D. R. K.: Acute diverticulitis of the caecum and ascending colon. Br. J. Surg., 39:76, 1957.
Rodkey, G. V., and Welch, C. E.: Diverticulitis of the colon. Evolution in concept and therapy. Surg. Clin. North Am., 45:1231, 1965.

Radiation Enterocolitis

DeCosse, J. J., Rhodes, R. S., Wentz, W. B., Reagan, J. W., Dwarken, H. J., and Holden, W. D.: The natural history and management of radiation-induced injury of the gastrointestinal tract. Ann. Surg., 170:369, 1969.
Earnest, D. L., and Trier, J. S.: Radiation enteritis and colitis. *In* Sleisenger, M. H., and Fordtran, J. S. (eds.): Gastrointestinal Disease. Philadelphia. W. B. Saunders Company, 1973, p. 1406.

Pseudomembranous Enterocolitis

Birnbaum, D., Laufer, A., and Freund, M.: Pseudomembranous enterocolitis, a clinicopathologic study. Gastroenterology, 41:345, 1961.
Curtis, K. J., and Sleisenger, M. H.: Infectious and parasitic diseases. *In* Sleisenger, M. H., and Fordtran, J. S. (eds.): Gastrointestinal Disease. Philadelphia, W. B. Saunders Company, 1973, p. 1369.
Jeffries, G. H., Steinberg, H., and Sleisenger, M. H.: Chronic ulcerative (non-granulomatous) jejunitis. Am. J. Med., 44:47, 1968.
Karz, S., Guth, P. H., and Plonsky, L.: Chronic ulcerative jejuno-ileitis. Am. J. Gastroenterol., 56:61, 1971.
Lawrason, F. D., Alpert, G., Mohr, F. L., and McMahon, F. G.: Obstructive-ulcerative lesions of the small intestine. J.A.M.A., 191:641, 1965.
Watson, M. R.: Primary nonspecific ulceration of the small bowel. Arch. Surg., 87:600, 1963.

Eosinophilic Gastroenteritis

Greenberger, N., and Gryboski, J.: Allergic disorders of the intestine and eosinophilic gastroenteritis. *In* Sleisenger, M. H., and Fordtran, J. S. (eds.): Gastrointestinal Disease. Philadelphia, W. B. Saunders Company, 1973, p. 1066.
Gryboski, J. D., Burkle, F., and Hillman, R.: Milk-induced colitis in an infant. Pediatrics, 38:299, 1966.
Heiner, D. C., Wilson, J. F., and Lahey, M. E.: Sensitivity to cow's milk. J.A.M.A., 189:563, 1964.
Klein, N. C., Hargrove, M. D., Sleisenger, M. H., and Jeffries, G. H.: Eosinophilic gastroenteritis. Medicine, 49:299, 1970.
Leinbach, G. E., and Rubin, C. E.: Eosinophilic gastroenteritis: A simple reaction to food allergens. Gastroenterology, 59:874, 1970.
Ureles, A. L., Alschibaja, T., Lodico, D., and Stabins, S. J.: Idiopathic eosinophilic infiltration of the gastrointestinal tract, diffuse and circumscribed. Am. J. Med., 30:899, 1961.

Section Six.   VASCULAR DISEASES OF THE INTESTINE

Robert K. Ockner

658. NORMAL ANATOMY AND PHYSIOLOGY OF THE SPLANCHNIC CIRCULATION

The supply of blood to the abdominal viscera depends upon three relatively large arteries which originate on the ventral aspect of the aorta. The most cephalad of these, the celiac axis, arises at the level of the twelfth thoracic or first lumbar vertebra, i.e., approximately at the insertion of the median arcuate ligament of the diaphragm (Fig. 1). Its subdivisions supply the liver and biliary structures (hepatic artery), spleen (splenic artery), and the stomach (left gastric and gastroepiploic, short gastrics, and branches of the gastroduodenal, including the right gastroepiploic). Important anastomotic connections between the hepatic branch of the celiac artery and the superior mesenteric artery (i.e., the pancreaticoduodenal arcades) are found in the region of the second portion of the duodenum, and branches of these also supply the pancreas and duodenum.

The second major splanchnic artery, the superior mesenteric, arises from the aorta just caudal to the celiac (Fig. 2). In addition to its pancreaticoduodenal anastomoses with the celiac arterial system, branches of the superior mesenteric artery supply those portions of the small and large intestines between the distal duodenum

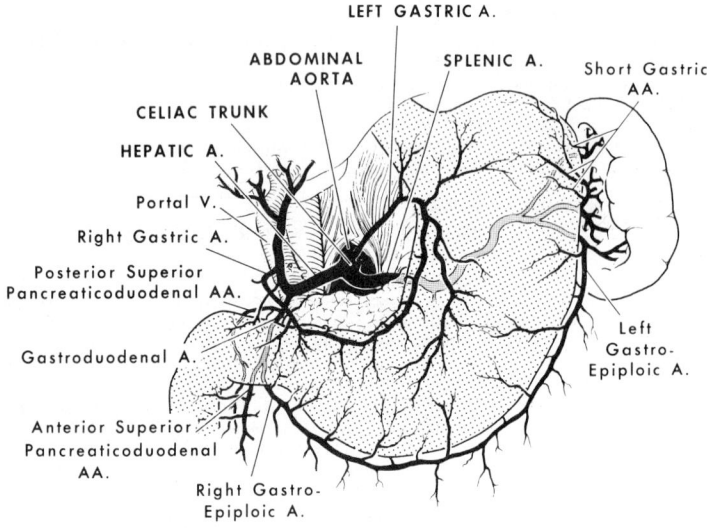

Figure 1. Arterial supply to the stomach and duodenum, showing major branches of the celiac axis and the superior portion of the pancreaticoduodenal arcades. (From Ockner, R. K., *In* Sleisenger, M. H., and Fordtran, J. S. [eds.]: Gastrointestinal Disease. Philadelphia, W. B. Saunders Company, 1973.)

and the distal transverse colon. The relatively large caliber of this vessel and its oblique take-off from the aorta render it particularly susceptible to entry by emboli originating in the heart and proximal aorta.

The third splanchnic arterial branch of the aorta is the inferior mesenteric. This vessel, the smallest of the three, arises at the level of the third lumbar vertebra and supplies the distal transverse and descending colon, sigmoid, and proximal rectum. Its branches connect with those of the superior mesenteric via the arc of Riolan ("meandering mesenteric artery") and the marginal artery (Fig. 2), and with the inferior and middle rectal branches of the hypogastric (internal iliac) arteries.

The system of abundant interconnections among the three major splanchnic arterial systems (i.e., the celiac, and the superior and inferior mesenterics) allows for the formation of collateral channels in the event that occlusive vascular disease develops. As a result, it is not uncommon for slowly developing complete or nearly complete occlusions of a single vessel to be associated with

little in the way of clinical sequelae. As with other systems, however, development of adequate collaterals requires time, and the sudden occlusion of even normal vessels (e.g., by emboli) usually results in infarction.

Blood flow in the splanchnic system depends not only on the patency of the large and medium-sized arteries described above, but also on systemic arterial pressure and the resistance at the arteriolar level. The latter is modulated not only in response to systemic arterial pressure itself (i.e., "autoregulation"), but also by a wide variety of other physiologic and pharmacologic factors. Thus resistance drops and flow increases during feeding and under certain neural and hormonal influences, including vagal stimulation, cholecystokinin, gastrin, secretin, and β-adrenergic stimulators, e.g., isoproterenol. Conversely, splanchnic vasoconstriction and decreased blood flow result from α-adrenergic stimuli, as occur in shock and other circumstances associated with endogenous catecholamine release. Digitalis glycosides also have been shown to cause splanchnic vasoconstriction. In the

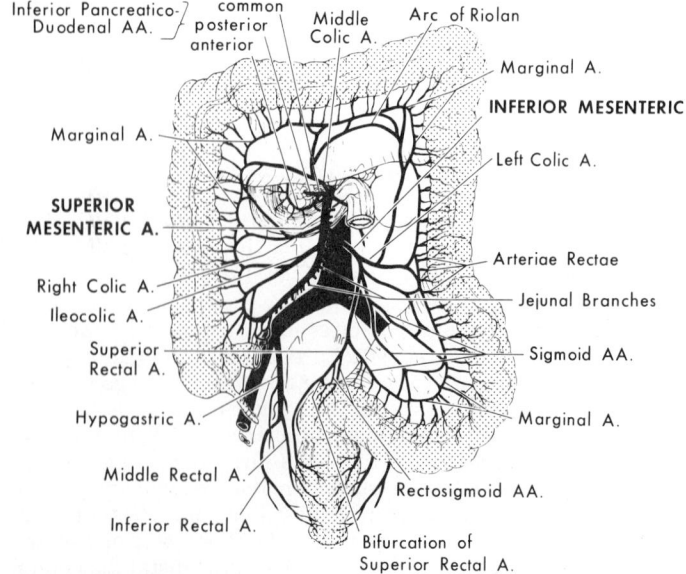

Figure 2. Arterial supply to the small and large intestines, showing the inferior portion of the pancreaticoduodenal arcades and the anastomoses between superior and inferior mesenteric arteries (arc of Riolan or "meandering mesenteric," and the marginal artery). (From Ockner, R. K., *In* Sleisenger, M. H., and Fordtran, J. S. [eds.]: Gastrointestinal Disease. Philadelphia, W. B. Saunders Company, 1973.)

final analysis, the adequacy of vascular perfusion is determined by the balance between tissue needs and local oxygen supply, and it is this balance, not merely the patency of any given vessel, that most often determines whether ischemia or infarction will occur.

659. ACUTE VISCERAL ISCHEMIC SYNDROMES

Acute Bowel Infarction: Mesenteric Artery Thrombosis. Thrombotic occlusion of the superior mesenteric artery may be asymptomatic if it evolves slowly enough to permit the formation of adequate collaterals, as noted above. More sudden occlusions, however, are associated with ischemic infarction of some or all of the supplied bowel. Most commonly, advanced atherosclerotic disease is responsible, but the syndrome may also occur in dissecting aneurysm, systemic vasculitis of all varieties, use of oral contraceptives, hypercoagulable states, and, rarely, without apparent explanation. Among causes of bowel infarction, the true incidence of arterial thrombosis is not certain, but it may be less common than previously thought in view of the increasingly recognized importance of *nonthrombotic* infarction (see below).

The clinical presentation of intestinal infarction (thrombotic or nonthrombotic) is often a misleading one. In its advanced stages, the associated abdominal pain, signs of intestinal obstruction, fever, leukocytosis, volume depletion, peritonitis with bloody abdominal fluid, hematemesis, and rectal bleeding are "classic" and render the diagnosis obvious. Earlier in the course, however, abdominal findings may be minimal, and the far less specific features of fever, leukocytosis, pain, and confusional state may dominate the clinical picture. Bowel sounds not only may be present, but may be hyperactive. The history is usually not helpful, but evidence of pre-existing "abdominal angina" (see below) or other conditions predisposing to thrombosis may aid in the evaluation of the problem.

The early diagnosis of bowel infarction depends upon a high index of suspicion, presumptive exclusion of other conditions likely to present as an acute abdomen, and, ultimately, surgical exploration. The demonstration of mesenteric vascular occlusion by abdominal angiography does not necessarily mean that the patient has an acute bowel infarction, because many patients with advanced occlusive disease are asymptomatic. On the other hand, the demonstration of *patent* vessels may serve to exclude *surgically correctable* vascular disease as a cause of bowel infarction (but will not exclude nonthrombotic infarction).

Initial therapeutic efforts should be supportive, i.e., correction of fluid and electrolyte imbalance (including administration of blood, plasma, or albumin as needed), cardiopulmonary support, and broad-spectrum antimicrobial drugs. Unoperated, acute bowel infarction carries essentially a 100 per cent mortality rate. Unfortunately, since many patients with this diagnosis are poor surgical risks because of age, advanced vascular disease affecting other vital organs, or poor general condition resulting from delay in diagnosis, surgery itself may contribute to a fatal outcome. As a rule, however, operation should be undertaken as soon as the patient is in optimal condition, because time is of the essence. At surgery, infarcted bowel should be resected and, if large vessel thrombi are present and the patient's condition permits, corrective vascular surgery (bypass or endarterectomy) may be attempted. Because it is often difficult to define accurately the limits of viable bowel, many surgeons have recommended a "second look" operation after 24 hours, in order to resect any additional nonviable intestine. It should be recognized, however, that even under the best of circumstances, massive bowel infarction carries a mortality rate of at least 60 to 70 per cent, except in those cases caused by emboli (see below), in which a somewhat more favorable prognosis may be expected.

Nonthrombotic Intestinal Infarction. This syndrome presents clinically in a manner quite similar to that of thrombotic infarction, but only more recently has its frequency been appreciated. Characteristically but not invariably, it occurs in a setting in which systemic anoxia, hypotension, congestive cardiac failure, or severe dehydration impairs the delivery of adequately oxygenated blood to the bowel, even though the splanchnic vessels themselves are patent. The mucosa, being most sensitive to oxygen deprivation, undergoes hemorrhagic necrosis first, but necrosis of the entire bowel wall usually supervenes. Although experience is accumulating with the potential usefulness of administration of vasodilator substances as a means of restoring intestinal vascular perfusion, treatment of this extremely grave condition is essentially the same as that of thrombotic infarction, i.e., supportive therapy and, as soon as feasible, surgical resection of infarcted bowel.

Mesenteric Embolic Disease. As noted, arterial emboli to the splanchnic viscera most commonly lodge in the superior mesenteric artery. They usually arise from endocardial mural thrombi or vegetations, or from atherosclerotic plaques in the proximal aorta. The condition is associated with diseases (e.g., mitral stenosis) which occur in a somewhat younger population than that at risk for thrombotic or nonthrombotic infarction, and because of this and the fact that its dramatic clinical presentation often leads to earlier diagnosis, embolic disease carries a somewhat more favorable prognosis. Classically, a patient with mitral stenosis will experience the sudden onset of severe periumbilical pain, followed by vomiting and diarrhea. Initially bleeding may be absent and bowel sounds present, but ultimately the picture progresses, if untreated, to one identical with that of advanced thrombotic infarction. Treatment consists of urgent exploration, with embolectomy and, if necessary, resection of infarcted bowel, followed by a "second look" procedure. It is important to note that there are well-documented examples of cases in which early embolectomy has obviated the need for bowel resection, although a transient malabsorption syndrome may result.

Ischemic Colitis. The large bowel is subject to most of the same problems associated with impaired blood supply which affect the small intestine, and many of the same pathophysiologic, diagnostic, and therapeutic principles apply. Thus outright infarction of the colon (thrombotic or nonthrombotic) may lead to perforation and peritonitis, and may require surgical intervention. The clinical presentation of ischemic colonic disease takes on a broader aspect, however, in that patients may present with a self-limited episode characterized by left-sided abdominal pain, fever, leukocytosis, and passage of bloody stools. The potential confusion resulting from this superficial resemblance to acute ulcerative colitis may be compounded by sigmoidoscopic findings which also suggest ulcerative colitis. Sigmoidoscopy, however, may disclose a normal mucosa, or one which shows discrete ulcers or blue-black hemorrhagic submucosal blebs or nodules. All or part of the colon may be involved, but the process usually affects the region of the splenic flexure or rectosigmoid. For those patients in whom surgery is not indicated, barium contrast studies performed after subsidence of the acute phase disclose mucosal edema and hemorrhage, as reflected by a sawtooth irregularity or by so-called "thumbprinting." Eventually, the healing process is often associated with scar and stricture formation, possibly necessitating surgery at a later date because of partial obstruction.

The true incidence of ischemic colitis is difficult to estimate, but its presence should be suspected in any patient over 50 who first presents with what clinically resembles acute ulcerative colitis. Although reconstructive surgery of the inferior mesenteric artery is generally not feasible, the recognition of this entity may avert the use of potentially harmful corticosteroid therapy.

660. CHRONIC VISCERAL ISCHEMIC SYNDROMES

Abdominal Angina.   This is an uncommon syndrome of postprandial epigastric or midabdominal pain resulting from relative bowel ischemia. It usually occurs 15 to 30 minutes after eating, i.e., at a time when intestinal blood flow and oxygen demand normally increase, and persists for one to two hours. The syndrome is almost invariably associated with extensive atherosclerosis affecting two or more of the major visceral arterial trunks. Clinically, in addition to the history of pain, patients exhibit marked weight loss. Although the over-all picture may suggest a diagnosis of advanced malignancy, careful questioning will usually elicit a fear of pain, which the patient has learned to associate with eating, resulting in diminished food intake. History and physical examination often provide evidence of atherosclerotic disease affecting other vessels, but the presence or absence of an abdominal bruit is of little help. Establishment of the diagnosis, which must be strongly suggested by the history, requires exclusion of other potentially confusing intra-abdominal pathology and the demonstration, by arteriography, of significant (i.e., more than 50 per cent) narrowing of at least two of the three major visceral arteries. If the occlusive lesions are close to their takeoff from the aorta, then surgical correction is possible in most patients, resulting in significant relief of symptoms.

Because a significant number of patients with bowel infarction give an antecedent history of abdominal angina, correct diagnosis and treatment of this disorder are essential. It must be emphasized, however, that in the absence of a convincing history, a positive arteriogram alone does not establish the diagnosis because of the relative frequency of advanced but asymptomatic occlusive disease. Furthermore, the long-term effect of surgery on the natural history of the disease has not been established conclusively.

Celiac Compression Syndrome.   This more recently described syndrome is characterized by vague, intermittent epigastric pain, occasionally associated with other nonspecific gastrointestinal symptomatology. There is no clear relation to meals, but, as with abdominal angina, it is believed to represent visceral ischemia caused in this instance by isolated narrowing of the celiac axis. Most cases have been ascribed to celiac compression by the adjacent median arcuate ligament of the diaphragm, but excess neurofibrous tissue of the celiac ganglion has also been incriminated. The patients are for the most part relatively young women, who are otherwise healthy, without evidence of atherosclerotic disease or other significant abdominal pathology. An epigastric bruit, failing to radiate inferiorly, has been an almost invariable finding. Celiac arteriography will successfully demonstrate the narrowing, and in many cases reconstructive or bypass surgery has been effective in relief of symptoms. Despite these favorable reports, however, the diagnosis should be made only with caution, because similar degrees of celiac axis narrowing have been found incidentally (autopsy or angiography) in asymptomatic subjects, and because of persisting uncertainty as to why this lesion should be associated with pain in the presence of an adequate collateral circulation. It has been suggested that the pain is not ischemic, but rather arises in the celiac ganglion itself.

661. MISCELLANEOUS DISORDERS

Intramural Intestinal Hemorrhage.   Bleeding into the wall of the intestine may occur as the result of spontaneous or iatrogenic hypocoagulable states (e.g., anticoagulant therapy), localized hemorrhagic infarction (e.g., vasculitis), or as the result of blunt abdominal trauma. Patients usually present with abdominal pain and exhibit variable findings suggestive of intestinal obstruction and bleeding. A significant obstructive picture is especially likely to be seen in those patients who sustain upper abdominal trauma, resulting in the formation of a large intramural hematoma in that portion of the duodenum which is fixed in position retroperitoneally. Barium studies show the "stacked coins" or "thumbprint" appearance typical of submucosal bleeding.

In most patients, intramural hemorrhage can be managed conservatively, including appropriate treatment of the underlying causative factors and nasogastric suction when indicated. In those patients with high-grade or unremitting intestinal obstruction, or in whom signs of peritonitis develop (suggesting perforation), surgery is necessary.

Abdominal Aortic Aneurysm.   Pathologic dilatation of the abdominal aorta is usually due to advanced atherosclerosis, and most commonly affects that segment distal to the origin of the renal arteries. Mild degrees of dilatation (i.e., 4 to 5 cm or less) are rarely symptomatic and are almost never associated with significant morbidity or mortality. Aneurysms larger than 6 to 7 cm, however, and those of any size which are observed to be increasing in caliber or to be causing symptoms (usually because of erosion of adjacent vertebrae) constitute serious threats to life. Such aneurysms may lead to a rapid exsanguination, by rupturing into either the bowel, the free peritoneal cavity, or the retroperitoneal space. Since the operative mortality under these urgent conditions is unacceptably high, such high-risk aneurysms should be resected electively.

Superior Mesenteric Artery Syndrome. In certain persons with an "asthenic" habitus, it has been suggested that the third portion of the duodenum may be compressed between the superior mesenteric artery and the uncinate process of the pancreas, causing symptoms of postprandial obstruction. Some of these patients obtain relief by assuming the knee-chest position. The validity of this syndrome as a cause of significant gastrointestinal symptoms is questionable, and surgery is rarely if ever indicated.

Vascular Malformations. Hemangiomas of the small intestine are very uncommon vascular tumors found throughout the bowel, particularly the jejunum. They assume clinical importance as one cause of gastrointestinal bleeding of undetermined source. These lesions are most reliably diagnosed by abdominal angiography. Telangiectasias may also be causes of gastrointestinal bleeding, and may be associated with mucocutaneous telangiectasias (Osler-Weber-Rendu disease) or Turner's syndrome.

Boley, S. J. (ed.): Vascular Disorders of the Intestine. New York, Appleton-Century-Crofts, 1971.

Bynum, T. E., and Jacobson, E. D.: Blood flow and gastrointestinal function. Gastroenterology, 60:325, 1971.

Fagin, R. R., and Kirsner, J. B.: Ischemic diseases of the colon. Ad. Intern. Med., 17:343, 1971.

Williams, L. F., Jr.: Vascular insufficiency of the intestine. Gastroenterology, 61:757, 1971.

Section Seven. DISEASES OF THE PERITONEUM, MESENTERY, AND OMENTUM

Robert K. Ockner

662. DISEASES OF THE PERITONEUM

Anatomy and Physiology. The abdominal cavity and viscera are lined by a continuous mesothelial membrane, the peritoneum. This structure forms a closed sac, except at the entry of the fimbriated ostia of the fallopian tubes, and consists of two anatomically distinct but contiguous portions. The *visceral* peritoneum encloses those organs which are entirely intraperitoneal, including the mesenteries by which they are suspended, whereas the *parietal* peritoneum lines the walls of the abdominal cavity (including the undersurface of the diaphragm and the pelvis) and the retroperitoneal organs (including the duodenum, ascending and descending colon, pancreas, kidneys, and adrenals). The two portions of the peritoneal membrane also differ in blood supply and innervation. The visceral peritoneum is supplied by the splanchnic arterial system, and its venous drainage enters the portal vein. In contrast, the parietal peritoneum receives branches of arteries which nourish the abdominal wall and diaphragm, and its venous drainage is by way of systemic veins. The visceral peritoneum does not contain pain receptors; afferent stimuli are transmitted via the visceral autonomics, whereas the parietal peritoneum is supplied by spinal nerves which also innervate the abdominal wall. As a result, irritation of the parietal peritoneum produces well-localized somatic pain (which may be referred to other sites in the same dermatome); in contrast, irritation of the visceral peritoneum produces a much less well-defined discomfort which is often poorly localized. The diaphragmatic portion of the peritoneum is supplied both by the phrenic nerve (spinal roots C3 to C5) and, in its more peripheral portions, by the intercostal nerves; as a result, pain resulting from diaphragmatic irritation may be referred either to the shoulder or to the thoracic or abdominal wall.

The peritoneal surface is a semipermeable membrane, and allows for the passive diffusion of water and solutes between the abdominal cavity and the subperitoneal vascular (blood and lymphatic) channels. In general, absorption of water and of solutes with a molecular weight of less than 2000 from the peritoneal cavity is accomplished via the blood vascular system; larger molecules and particulate substances enter the lymphatics. Movement of particles from the peritoneal cavity into the subdiaphragmatic lymphatics is facilitated by specialized areas of contact between the parietal peritoneum and the underlying lymphatics. In these areas, discontinuities exist between the peritoneal mesothelial cells and the lymphatic endothelial cells; basement membranes are scanty or absent. As a result, particles of substantial size (e.g., red blood cells) move freely from the abdominal cavity into the subdiaphragmatic lymphatics, a process which may be facilitated by respiratory motion of the diaphragm itself.

Water and electrolytes equilibrate rapidly (i.e., within two hours) between the blood vascular compartment and the free peritoneal cavity. *Net* fluid movement from the abdominal cavity into the plasma occurs at a maximal rate of approximately 30 to 35 ml per hour. This figure applies not only to the normal man, but also to patients with portal hypertension and ascites; this rate cannot be exceeded despite vigorous diuresis; rather, such diuresis only serves to remove fluid from other body compartments, and may cause hypovolemia.

Diagnosis. Because of their wide diversity, few generalizations can be made regarding history and physical examination in diseases of the peritoneum. Abdominal pain and ascites may be present, as may other less specific complaints of fever, nausea, and vomiting, depending on the nature and localization of the process. Diagnosis of known or suspected peritoneal disease is therefore greatly dependent upon special techniques, including radiology, abdominal paracentesis, peritoneal biopsy, peritoneoscopy, and exploratory laparotomy.

Radiographically, ascites may be manifest by haziness and separation of bowel loops on plain abdominal films. Otherwise, peritoneal disease reflects itself only indirectly. For example, an inflammatory process resulting in scar formation may cause angulation, separation, or narrowing of intestinal loops or evidence of mucosal edema (owing to mesenteric lymphatic or venous obstruction) on barium contrast studies. If ascites is present, abdominal paracentesis is essential in order to establish its cause (see below). Peritoneal biopsy, particularly with the Cope needle, is a relatively simple and safe bedside technique which may yield a positive diagnosis of neoplastic or infectious causes in 50 to 60 per cent of cases. Peritoneoscopy, performed under the proper circumstances by a physician experienced in this technique, can be accomplished with little morbidity or mortality. A successful examination may obviate the need for exploratory surgery and may permit biopsy under direct vision of involved portions of the peritoneum or liver. If a diagnosis cannot be made in a patient with obvious peritoneal disease by means of the aforementioned procedures, exploratory laparotomy may be necessary.

ASCITES

The accumulation of fluid within the peritoneal cavity may result from any or all of three different pathophysiologic mechanisms. These include (1) increases in the permeability of the peritoneal capillaries (e.g., in neoplastic and inflammatory diseases of the peritoneum) and (2) diminished plasma colloid osmotic pressure (e.g., severe hypoalbuminemia of any cause). An elevation in portal venous pressure alone (i.e., in the absence of hypoalbuminemia) is ordinarily not adequate cause for ascites formation, as evidenced by its relative rarity in portal vein thrombosis not associated with liver disease. A third important mechanism for ascites formation is elevation of the hydrostatic pressure within the hepatic sinusoids. This may result from any of the conditions associated with *postsinusoidal portal hypertension,* including *cirrhosis, hepatic vein,* or *inferior vena cava obstruction,* and advanced *congestive heart failure* or *constrictive pericarditis.* In these conditions, elevated sinusoidal pressure increases the movement of protein-rich plasma filtrate from the sinusoid into the space of Disse and the hepatic lymphatics. Although the fluid may ultimately enter the thoracic duct, hepatic lymph may be lost directly from the surface of the liver into the free peritoneal cavity. This mechanism undoubtedly accounts for the not infrequent finding that patients with postsinusoidal portal hypertension of any cause, including cirrhosis and congestive failure, may have ascites with an unexpectedly high protein concentration, despite the fact that its formation may be considered to represent "transudation" rather than "exudation" in the usual sense.

Ascites formation in the cirrhotic, and in other situations in which plasma volume or renal vascular perfusion is abnormal, may be aggravated by renal retention of sodium and water. It seems unlikely, however, that these latter factors alone are sufficient for the formation of ascites, because neither primary hyperaldosteronism nor increased antidiuretic hormone secretion is associated with ascites formation in the absence of other contributing factors.

Evaluation of Ascites Fluid. Although laboratory analysis of fluid removed from the abdominal cavity may not provide a specific etiologic diagnosis, no patient with ascites can be considered to have been properly evaluated without this examination. Fluids with protein concentrations exceeding 2.5 grams are usually regarded as "exudates," whereas those with lower concentrations are designated "transudates." Although this classification is useful, exceptions in both directions occur not infrequently. Thus cases of neoplasm or infection of the peritoneum in association with "transudative" fluids and of cirrhosis and congestive heart failure in association with "exudative" protein levels are numerous and well documented. For this reason, ascites fluid protein concentrations must be interpreted only in the context of all other clinical and laboratory findings. Other chemical determinations may be helpful, including amylase (markedly elevated in pancreatic ascites), glucose (often less than 60 mg per 100 ml in neoplastic ascites), and triglyceride (in excess of plasma concentrations in chylous ascites). Bloody ascites strongly suggests neoplasm, especially hepatoma. Elevated leukocyte counts (in excess of 250 per cubic millimeter) indicate peritoneal irritation, e.g., neoplasm or infection. The differential leukocyte count is of help in that a very high percentage of lymphocytes strongly suggests tuberculous peritonitis. Cytology is an essential part of the examination and may be expected to yield accurate results in more than half the cases. Ascites fluid should be cultured for routine pathogens, acid-fast bacilli, and fungi.

Differential Diagnosis of Ascites. Although a wide variety of disease processes may be associated with the

TABLE 1.   Causes of Ascites Not Associated with Peritoneal Disease*

I. Portal hypertension
   A. Cirrhosis
   B. Hepatic congestion
      1. Congestive heart failure
      2. Constrictive pericarditis
      3. Inferior vena cava obstruction
      4. Hepatic vein obstruction (Budd-Chiari syndrome)
   C. Portal vein occlusion
II. Hypoalbuminemia
   A. Nephrotic syndrome
   B. Protein-losing enteropathy
   C. Malnutrition
III. Miscellaneous
   A. Myxedema
   B. Ovarian disease
      1. Meigs' syndrome
      2. Struma ovarii
      3. Ovarian overstimulation syndrome
   C. Pancreatic ascites
   D. Bile ascites
   E. Chylous ascites

*From Bender, M. D., and Ockner, R. K., *In* Sleisenger, M. H., and Fordtran, J. S. (eds.): Gastrointestinal Disease. Philadelphia, W. B. Saunders Company, 1973.

TABLE 2. Diseases of the Peritoneum

I. Infections
  A. Acute peritonitis
  B. Tuberculous peritonitis
  C. Fungal and parasitic diseases
    1. Candidiasis
    2. Histoplasmosis
    3. Schistosomiasis
    4. Enterobiasis
II. Neoplasms
  A. Secondary malignancy
  B. Primary mesothelioma
  C. Pseudomyxoma peritonei
III. Miscellaneous
  A. Vasculitis
  B. Granulomatous peritonitis
    1. Sarcoidosis
    2. Crohn's disease
    3. Starch peritonitis
  C. Familial paroxysmal peritonitis
  D. Eosinophilic gastroenteritis
  E. Whipple's disease
  F. Gynecologic disease
    1. Endometriosis
    2. Deciduosis
  G. Peritoneal lymphangiectasia
  H. Peritoneal loose bodies
  I. Peritoneal encapsulation

presence of ascites, more than 90 per cent of patients with this complication are found to have cirrhosis, neoplasm, congestive heart failure, or tuberculosis. For purposes of classification, causes of ascites may be divided into diseases not involving the peritoneum on the one hand (Table 1) and diseases of the peritoneum on the other (Table 2). Of those cases not associated with peritoneal disease, *cirrhosis* is by far the most common; it is considered in Ch. 709. *Portal hypertension* caused by disease of the heart and great veins accounts for a substantial number of patients with ascites of obscure origin. Included in this group are patients with *congestive heart failure* (especially right-sided), *constrictive pericarditis,* and *inferior vena cava* and *hepatic vein obstruction (Budd-Chiari syndrome).* Clinically, patients with these conditions may not be readily distinguishable from those with hepatic cirrhosis; a high index of suspicion is necessary, and special diagnostic procedures may be required in order to establish or exclude the diagnosis. Hypoalbuminemia of any cause, including nephrotic syndrome and protein-losing enteropathy, may be associated with a classically "transudative" ascites.

Various endocrine conditions may be associated with ascites. These include *myxedema* and *diseases of the ovary,* among them *Meigs' syndrome,* in which transudative ascites is associated with ovarian fibroma or cystadenoma.

Ascites associated with pancreatic disease usually occurs in the presence of chronic *pancreatitis* and *pseudocyst.* The ascites fluid amylase concentration is elevated, often to very high levels, and drainage of the pseudocyst has usually been effective in managing this complication. Leakage of bile may be associated with the development of *bile ascites.* It is important to note that this situation is not necessarily associated with the fulminant clinical picture of fever, leukocytosis, and peritonitis which customarily is designated *bile peritonitis.* Rather, this latter, more ominous condition seems to occur primarily in those patients in whom the extravasated bile was infected originally.

Chylous ascites is due to the presence of lymph lipoproteins and chylomicrons in the peritoneal cavity. These lipid-rich particles impart a turbidity to the fluid which facilitates its diagnosis. It should be emphasized, however, that not all turbid abdominal fluids are "chylous." Establishment of the diagnosis requires direct evidence that the turbidity is indeed due to neutral lipid, a determination best made by analysis of the fluid for triglyceride concentration; alternatively, solvent extraction (ether or chloroform) which results in clearing of the fluid may be taken as presumptive evidence for the diagnosis. Other turbid abdominal fluids may be due to cellular debris, and are designated *"pseudochylous" ascites,* a condition occasionally associated with abdominal neoplasm or infection. The differential diagnosis of truly chylous ascites depends upon its chronicity and the age of the patient. *Chronic chylous ascites* in adults is caused in over 80 per cent of cases by abdominal neoplasm, usually *lymphoma,* with associated obstruction and disruption of the abdominal lymphatics resulting from extensive lymph node involvement. *Acute chylous ascites* ("chylous peritonitis") is associated with abrupt onset of abdominal pain. In some cases, this syndrome is due to *trauma, intestinal obstruction,* or *rupture* of a *chylous cyst,* but a specific etiologic diagnosis may not be possible even at laparotomy. In children, congenital malformations of the lymphatics, including intestinal *lymphangiectasia,* account for a higher proportion of the cases of chylous ascites.

INFECTIONS OF THE PERITONEUM

Acute Peritonitis

Although this syndrome may result from a chemical irritation or "burn" of the peritoneal surface (as in severe acute pancreatitis), most cases are due to *bacterial infection.* Most commonly, enteric organisms enter the peritoneal cavity through a necrotic defect in the wall of the intestine or other abdominal viscus resulting from *obstruction, infarction, neoplasm, foreign body,* or primary inflammatory disease such as *fulminant ulcerative colitis. Perforated peptic ulcer* and *ruptured appendix* are particularly frequent causes. If unchecked, bacterial contamination of the peritoneum results in a "spreading peritonitis," leading ultimately to marked exudation of protein-rich fluid into the abdominal cavity, paralytic ileus, and reflex spasm of the overlying abdominal musculature. The systemic consequences of this catastrophic event are predictable. Loss of fluid from the vascular compartment into both the free peritoneal cavity and the bowel lumen results in volume depletion and hemoconcentration; these factors, together with the possible systemic effects of the bacterial infection itself, may lead to shock and oliguria. The latter may progress to acute tubular necrosis.

Despite its often dramatic presentation, recognition of acute peritonitis may be difficult in those patients in whom the clinical manifestations are masked or suppressed. This applies particularly to the elderly and to those receiving corticosteroids, as, for example, in the treatment of acute ulcerative colitis. In these patients, a particularly high index of suspicion is necessary, and the only *early* manifestation may be a rise in pulse rate or unexplained hypotension. Diagnosis in such situations may depend upon the radiographic demonstration of free air in the peritoneal cavity and upon aspiration of abdominal contents to confirm the presence of polymorphonuclear leukocytes and bacteria. Fortunately, the peritoneum is often able to confine inflammatory processes of this type. As a result, acute peritonitis may be restricted to one portion of the abdomen and may not spread or become generalized.

Management of peritonitis includes restoration of fluid and electrolyte imbalance; the administration of fresh frozen plasma or albumin is often required. Antimicrobial therapy and nasogastric suction should be instituted. Analgesics are often necessary, but their premature use may hinder proper evaluation of the patient. The decision to operate must be individualized. In those patients who are seen early and who are good operative candidates, surgery should be undertaken as soon as feasible. However, in some patients (particularly those seen later in the course or who are poor operative risks), it may be desirable to attempt to control the process nonoperatively and to encourage its localization by means of antimicrobial drugs and other conservative measures. Localized abscesses so formed may be drained later, when circumstances are more favorable.

Subphrenic Abscess

Particularly challenging problems in diagnosis and treatment are posed by the collection of pus in one of the several more or less well-defined tissue spaces inferior to the diaphragm and adjacent to the liver, stomach, spleen, and lesser sac. Most often, subphrenic abscess develops secondary to other septic and inflammatory processes in the abdomen, especially *ruptured appendix* or *diverticulum, infected gallbladder, perforated ulcer* with bacterial contamination, *pancreatitis, penetrating abdominal wound,* or extension of an *intrahepatic abscess* beyond the liver capsule.

Clinically, the picture usually suggests a septic process, with malaise, fever, and leukocytosis. The subphrenic location is often not obvious, but may be suggested by a history of one of the aforementioned antecedent events, by direct clinical evidence such as pain, elevation, or impaired motion of the diaphragm, or by x-ray evidence of a pleural effusion associated with a subdiaphragmatic air-fluid level.

Antimicrobial therapy usually suppresses the process and helps to contain it, but may also obscure its recognition. Definitive therapy consists of surgical drainage.

Spontaneous ("Primary") Peritonitis

Bacterial peritonitis may also occur in the absence of an acute intra-abdominal precipitating factor. In this circumstance, the offending organism is often not enteric, and the syndrome is more likely to occur in patients who have pre-existing ascites, impaired immunologic defenses, or a cause for bacteremia such as localized infection elsewhere in the body or indwelling catheters. A well-recognized example of this circumstance is the child with nephrotic syndrome and ascites who develops *pneumococcal peritonitis* as a complication; the incidence of this entity has diminished considerably during recent decades because of the availability of antimicrobial drugs.

More common is spontaneous bacterial peritonitis in patients with advanced, decompensated *cirrhosis* and *as-cites.* This syndrome may occur in up to 10 per cent of such patients, and although enteric organisms (particularly *E. coli*) are most often cultured, pneumococci and streptococci are frequent offenders. The cause of the syndrome is not known; perforated viscus, pneumonia, biliary tract infection, and other local sites of bacterial infection cannot be implicated. Possibly, the cirrhotic liver with spontaneous portal-systemic shunting is less effective in clearing bacteria from the portal blood, but this would not explain the occurrence of nonenteric organisms. The syndrome may be recognized by the sudden onset of abdominal pain, fever, and leukocytosis, occurring in the setting of decompensated cirrhosis and ascites. Blood cultures are positive in 75 per cent of cases; abdominal fluid usually yields a positive culture and contains an elevated number of polymorphonuclear leukocytes. Although appropriate antimicrobial therapy may afford a satisfactory bacteriologic response in the majority of patients, the over-all mortality exceeds 90 per cent.

Other Infections

Tuberculous peritonitis is discussed in detail in Ch. 239. It should be emphasized, however, that this disorder may present in a variety of ways, ranging from an acute abdomen to an insidiously developing, otherwise unexplained ascites resembling (or associated with) cirrhosis. Accordingly, its presence should be suspected in all patients with ascites, with or without an apparently adequate cause. Tuberculosis skin testing and appropriate cultures of ascites fluid for tubercle bacilli should be regarded as routine in the evaluation of ascites. The diagnosis is strongly suggested by a high percentage of lymphocytes in the abdominal fluid, and may be confirmed by means of a positive culture, peritoneal biopsy, laparoscopy, or, if necessary, exploratory laparotomy. The very satisfactory response of this condition to appropriate chemotherapy adds to the importance of early diagnosis.

Fungal and parasitic diseases may be associated with peritoneal involvement and, occasionally, with ascites. These disorders, including *histoplasmosis, candidiasis,* and *schistosomiasis,* are quite uncommon, but deserve consideration in otherwise unexplained cases of peritoneal disease with or without ascites.

TUMORS OF THE PERITONEUM

Secondary malignancy is the most common form of neoplastic involvement of the peritoneum. More than 75 per cent of such tumors are *adenocarcinomas,* but peritoneal involvement by *sarcomas, lymphomas, leukemias, carcinoids,* and *multiple myeloma* has been described. It is assumed that in these patients there is increased permeability of the mesenteric and peritoneal capillary bed, accounting for the formation of "exudative" ascites. The clinical picture is usually that associated with advancing malignancy, including weakness and weight loss, and variable complaints referable to the abdomen such as pain, distention, nausea, or vomiting. On abdominal paracentesis, the fluid obtained usually has a high protein content (more than 2.5 grams per 100 ml); cellular composition is variable, and occasionally the fluid is grossly bloody. The diagnosis is reliably made in most patients by means of cytology or peritoneal biopsy, but peritoneoscopy or surgical exploration may be necessary at times.

Treatment of this condition involves the intraperitoneal administration of antitumor agents, including alkylators, antimetabolites, or radioactive isotopes. Unfortunately, the prognosis of patients in this advanced stage of malignancy is poor. Intra-abdominal quinacrine has occasionally been successful in producing a fibrous serositis, thereby obliterating the free peritoneal space and reducing further fluid exudation. The usefulness of this approach is limited, however, by the frequent occurrence of fever, nausea, vomiting, and abdominal pain.

Primary Mesothelioma

This uncommon primary tumor of the peritoneum is associated with the gradual onset of abdominal pain and distention, nausea, vomiting, weight loss, and development of ascites. Cytology or peritoneal biopsy reveals a variable histopathology in which epithelial and mesenchymal elements are combined and because of which differentiation from other malignancies may be difficult. It has been suggested on epidemiologic grounds that exposure to asbestos fibers may play an etiologic role in the development of this tumor. This conclusion is based on the association, in most patients, with environmental exposure to asbestos fibers and evidence of pulmonary asbestosis, including "asbestos bodies" in the lungs. Because of more recent evidence suggesting that these so-called "asbestos bodies" are nonspecific and occur in up to 50 per cent of the general population, the importance of asbestos in the etiology of this tumor is at present uncertain (see Ch. 526). A significant number of patients with peritoneal mesothelioma have a similar process affecting the pleura. The prognosis of the disease is exceedingly poor, averaging one to two years' survival after diagnosis. Chemotherapy and radiation therapy have generally been unsuccessful.

Pseudomyxoma Peritonei

Classification of this rare disorder as a tumor is a matter of some uncertainty, because in many cases it appears to arise as a complication of certain relatively benign processes, including mucocele of the appendix. On the other hand, its neoplastic nature is suggested by a high incidence of cellular atypia in carefully examined pathologic specimens, as well as by evidence for low-grade malignancy in a high percentage of those patients in whom the syndrome develops subsequent to *mucinous cystadenomas* of the *ovaries.* The syndrome is characterized by abdominal distention resulting from the accumulation of a mucinous, gelatinous, translucent material. Most cases seem to originate as an outgrowth of pre-existing mucinous cystadenomas and cystadinocarcinomas of the ovary and mucocele of the appendix, but other tumors of the genitourinary tract or gastrointestinal tract may be associated with the process.

The condition usually presents as an increase in abdominal girth, with little in the way of other clinical signs of disease. At surgery, the abdominal cavity is found to contain gelatinous material existing in a variety of states, including cystic masses, lying freely without apparent attachment, or anchored to the peritoneal surface.

If the tumor is indeed malignant, it appears to be of low grade and rarely metastasizes. As a result, the

course of the disease is prolonged and is characterized by recurrent episodes of intestinal obstruction and fistula formation. The most promising therapeutic approach at present appears to be one which combines surgical removal of the ovary, appendix, and as much mucin as possible, with intraperitoneal instillation of an alkylating agent.

Miscellaneous Diseases of the Peritoneum

The peritoneal membrane may be affected by a wide variety of systemic diseases, including *systemic lupus erythematosus* (see Ch. 81) and other "collagen vascular" diseases, *Whipple's disease* (see Part XIV, Section Three), and *sarcoidosis* (see Ch. 102).

Bender, M. D., and Ockner, R. K.: Diseases of the peritoneum, mesentery, and diaphragm. *In* Sleisenger, M. H., and Fordtran, J. S. (eds.): Gastrointestinal Disease. Philadelphia, W. B. Saunders Company, 1973, pp. 1578–1600.
Conn, H., and Fessel, M.: Spontaneous bacterial peritonitis in cirrhosis: Variations on a theme. Medicine, 50:161, 1971.
Levine, H.: Needle biopsy of the peritoneum in exudative ascites. Arch. Intern. Med., 120:542, 1967.

663. DISEASES OF THE MESENTERY AND OMENTUM

Mesenteric Inflammatory Disease. This syndrome includes a spectrum of conditions ranging from acute inflammation to a chronic fibrosing process associated with intestinal obstruction, ascites, and steatorrhea. Included are such conditions as *"mesenteric panniculitis"* and *"retractile mesenteritis."* The cause of this syndrome is not known, but it is believed to represent the sequel to some inciting event such as trauma, infection, or ischemia in the mesentery. Fat necrosis occurs, evoking an inflammatory reaction with subsequent scarring and granuloma formation.

Clinically, the acute syndrome ("mesenteric panniculitis") is characterized by recurrent abdominal pain, weight loss, nausea, vomiting, and fever. In most patients, a tender abdominal mass is palpable; leukocytosis may or may not be present. Radiographic examination is nonspecific, showing the effects of an abdominal mass and variable scarring, which include displacement and separation of intestinal loops, with angulation, stenosis, and extrinsic compression. In some patients the condition evolves into a more chronic process ("retractile mesenteritis"), characterized by continuing pain, fever, weight loss, and various signs of intestinal obstruction, ascites, and steatorrhea.

At surgery, the small bowel mesentery is found to be the principal site of involvement; it is thickened and fibrotic, particularly at the root. Microscopically in *mesenteric panniculitis,* there is infiltration of adipose tissue by foamy macrophages and lymphocytes, with fat necrosis, fibrosis, and calcification. In *retractile mesenteritis,* the thickening and fibrosis are more pronounced, and there is less evidence of acute necrosis and inflammation.

Although long-term experience with this syndrome is

limited, most patients seem to have a prolonged survival; many become asymptomatic after a period of months to years, whereas others exhibit the more chronic symptoms noted above. The role of corticosteroids is uncertain; although they may be effective in the management of those patients in whom acute symptoms predominate, there is no evidence that they affect the long-term prognosis or progression of the disease.

Mesenteric Cysts and Tumors. Mesenteric cysts usually develop as the result of anomalies in the mesenteric lymphatic system, but may also consist of enteric or urogenital epithelium or celomic mesothelium. They may spontaneously wax and wane in size, and usually do not present symptomatically in patients less than 10 years of age. Symptoms are related to the size and position of the cyst, which on physical examination is nontender, round, and mobile. Spontaneous rupture, hemorrhage, or infection may occur, but these complications are unusual. Treatment consists of surgical excision.

Mesenteric tumors are rare and usually arise from the cellular elements normally present in the mesentery. They include *fibromas, myxomas, lipomas,* and other less common neoplasms of mesenchymal or neural origin. Most are well differentiated, low-grade *fibrosarcomas* which produce symptoms such as pain, weight loss, abdominal mass, and compression of adjacent organs. They may be treated successfully by surgical excision. Others are more highly malignant and may metastasize distally. *Mesenteric lymphoid tumors* also occur, and certain of these have been associated with unexplained abnormalities in iron metabolism with hypochromic microcytic anemia.

Tumors of the omentum, unlike those of the mesentery, are chiefly muscular in origin (*leiomyomas, leiomyosarcomas*). About 40 per cent of these are malignant, and cause symptoms by virtue of local invasion and development of an abdominal mass; distant metastasis is unusual.

Bender, M. D., and Ockner, R. K.: Diseases of the peritoneum, mesentery, and diaphragm. *In* Sleisenger, M. H., and Fordtran, J. S. (eds.): Gastrointestinal Disease. Philadelphia, W. B. Saunders Company, 1973, pp. 1578–1600.

Section Eight.   NEOPLASTIC DISEASES OF THE ALIMENTARY TRACT

664.   INTRODUCTION

Lloyd L. Brandborg

Gastrointestinal cancer comprises 20 per cent of all cancers and accounts for 30 per cent of cancer deaths. In a single year in the United States there are about 133,000 new cancers and 97,000 deaths from cancers of the digestive organs. Cure rates of digestive organ cancer have remained constant for several decades. "Early" diagnosis and more effective treatment have not been achieved.

Striking geographic differences occur in the incidence of various gastrointestinal malignancies. There has been a marked decrease over the past several decades in carcinoma of the stomach in the United States. Carcinoma of the pancreas is increasing. Carcinoma of the colon has remained constant. Gastric carcinoma declines in migrants from countries with a high incidence to those with a low incidence, suggesting that environmental factors play a significant role in its causation. Carcinoma of the colon is virtually unknown in rural Africa, but the incidence in black people in the United States equals that in the white population. None of the factors identified in epidemiologic studies have been shown to cause any of the cancers of the gastrointestinal tract. Tantalizing clues are provided which require further intensive investigation.

Hereditary and genetic factors have been examined. There is an increase in gastric carcinoma in patients having blood group A, in pernicious anemia, and in patients having Lewis group specific substances, either Le[a] or Le[b] or both in saliva. Some families have been described with inordinately high incidences of carcinoma of the stomach or colon. Except for these patients and those with inherited multiple polyposis of the colon, gastrointestinal cancer does not have a familial distribution.

The symptoms of gastrointestinal cancer are not specific. Such phenomena as pain, bleeding, intestinal obstruction, weight loss, fever, or anemia should lead to a search for gastrointestinal malignancy. Most symptomatic gastrointestinal malignancies may be detected by roentgenographic, endoscopic, and cytologic techniques.

Specific chemical and serologic tests for gastrointestinal malignancy are not available. As the techniques become more sensitive, many of these tests become less specific. An example is the occurrence of carcinoembryonic antigen (CEA, see below) in many patients with nonmalignant disease.

Currently, surgery offers the main hope for cure of gastrointestinal cancer. It may also provide palliation. Preoperative irradiation therapy in gastrointestinal carcinomas may increase resectability and improve prognosis. Chemotherapy of gastrointestinal malignancy has been disappointing. Increased survival has not been shown. Occasional patients may enjoy striking remissions. Combination chemotherapy has not been widely studied in gastrointestinal malignancy. Hopefully, such an approach could improve survival as it has in leukemias, lymphomas, and other responsive cancers.

665.   NEOPLASMS OF THE ESOPHAGUS

Lloyd L. Brandborg

CARCINOMA OF THE ESOPHAGUS

Etiology.   Although the etiology of carcinoma of the esophagus is not known, a number of clinical conditions are associated with an increased incidence of the condition. Patients with *lye damage* of the esophagus have a

1000 times higher risk of developing carcinoma of the esophagus than the general population. Patients with *achalasia* have a reported incidence from 2 to up to 19 per cent. It is presumed that these lesions result from "irritation" caused by retention of esophageal contents. Whether successful brusk dilatation or myotomy, by virtue of eliminating stagnation, decreases the occurrence of carcinoma is not known. *Sideropenic dysphagia* is characterized by esophageal webs in the region of the cricopharyngeus, buccal mucosal atrophy, and a high incidence of carcinoma. This condition occurs most often in Scandinavia, particularly in northern Sweden, predominantly in elderly women. A strikingly high incidence of esophageal carcinoma occurs in some families with tylosis, an inherited disorder characterized by marked thickening of the skin of the hands and feet.

A statistical correlation exists between esophageal carcinoma and the use of cigarettes and alcohol. Atypical esophageal epithelium has been observed in the esophagus of smokers examined at autopsy. In view of the widespread use of cigarettes and alcohol, it is surprising that esophageal carcinoma is not more common.

Although it has been claimed that there is an association of esophageal carcinoma and hiatus hernia, prospective studies have failed to reveal such a relationship. Furthermore, most of the carcinomas associated with hiatus hernia are adenocarcinomas.

Incidence and Prevalence. The incidence of carcinoma of the esophagus is 5.8 per 100,000 in whites and 20.5 per 100,000 in nonwhites in the United States. Each year this amounts to 6800 new cases of esophageal cancer and 6400 deaths. Carcinoma of the esophagus is responsible for approximately 2 per cent of cancer deaths in the United States.

Epidemiology. The differences in geographic distribution of carcinoma of the esophagus are so striking throughout the world that it has been concluded that some environmental factors must have a role in etiology. The incidence in the United States in whites is 5.8 cases per 100,000 population per year, whereas in southern Rhodesia it is 157, in Transkei in South Africa it is 357, and in Kazakhstan in Asia it rises to 547 cases per 100,000 population. Statistical associations include long-term ingestion of very hot beverages, climate, vegetation, agriculture, trace metals in soils, and background irradiation. Genetic differences and chemicals in the diet may possibly contribute.

Pathology. Approximately one half of esophageal carcinomas occur at the level of the arch of the aorta, one third just above the esophagogastric junction, and the remainder in the hypopharynx and proximal esophagus.

If carcinomas arising in the cardia and fundus of the stomach are excluded, virtually all malignancies of the esophagus are squamous cell carcinomas. The gross appearance of carcinoma of the esophagus varies from hard, fibrotic infiltrative lesions to friable, exophytic papillary lesions. They are frequently ulcerated.

Esophageal carcinoma spreads by local invasion and lymphatic metastases. Microscopic lymphatic spread is common. These tumors frequently involve adjacent structures. The distal lesions invade the stomach and the left gastric and celiac lymph nodes. Extension into the diaphragm, vertebral bodies, pericardium, and heart is not rare. Lesions of the middle and upper third extend into the trachea and bronchi, and may involve the lungs and occasionally the recurrent laryngeal nerves.

Hematogenous metastases are less common than lymphatic extension and usually affect the liver, lungs, bones, and kidneys.

Clinical Manifestations. Carcinoma of the esophagus is unusual under the age of 40. The peak incidence occurs in the decade between the ages of 60 and 70. In most countries, males are afflicted approximately twice as often as females.

The most common symptom is progressive dysphagia. There is first difficulty in swallowing solid food, followed by inability to swallow semisolid foods and, finally, liquids. Occasionally, sudden esophageal obstruction occurs with a bolus of food that could have been easily swallowed a few days previously. Pain with swallowing, odynophagia, is due to extension of the tumor beyond the wall of the esophagus. It is located substernally, tends to be constant, is not always associated with swallowing, and is dull or burning. Occasionally, it may be felt in the back.

Other symptoms are due to chronic obstruction, extension of the tumor into adjacent organs, and hemorrhage. Brisk hemorrhage is uncommon (5 per cent of patients); however, occult bleeding is common.

Chronic obstruction leads to aspiration of secretions and undigested food, with severe coughing episodes and pneumonia; eating may become virtually intolerable. Food intake is reduced with ensuing weight loss. Regurgitation during the night, bad breath, bad taste, and thirst are frequent. Fever is common, usually because of pulmonary infection.

Symptoms of metastatic spread depend upon the organs involved. Involvement of the phrenic nerve or diaphragm may lead to unremitting hiccups. Extension into the trachea and bronchi produces coughing, infection, and tracheal or bronchoesophageal fistulas. Perforation into the mediastinum causes mediastinitis and empyema. Extension into the pericardium and heart causes pericardial effusions. A rare but dramatic symptom is exsanguinating hemorrhage caused by erosion into the aorta. Involvement of the recurrent laryngeal nerve will cause hoarseness. With distant metastases, patients may have jaundice, abdominal discomfort, ascites, cyanosis, dyspnea, and bone pain.

Diagnosis. *Every* patient with dysphagia should be investigated for carcinoma of the esophagus. The first procedure is a careful roentgenologic examination under fluoroscopic control (Fig. 1). Careful attention should be paid to the fundus of the stomach and cardia. Cineradiography is useful in detecting disordered motility. The most usual radiographic finding is a circumferential, irregular narrowing of the esophagus which is often ulcerated. There is slight or no dilatation proximal to the tumor. The mucosal folds are destroyed. In some smoothly tapering lesions, the differential diagnosis between benign stricture and carcinoma may be extraordinarily difficult.

Fiberoptic endoscopy permits direct visualization of the lesion. Directed biopsies give a diagnosis of malignancy in 50 to 75 per cent of patients. Directed cytology, either with lavage techniques or with the cytology brush, adds to the diagnostic accuracy. A benign biopsy cannot be relied upon, because in 25 to 50 per cent of patients biopsies taken out of obvious tumor reveal only "chronic inflammation."

Lavage cytology performed by skilled cytotechnicians and interpreted by skilled and interested physicians is

Figure 1. Extensive, sessile, ulcerated carcinoma of the esophagus.

Total obstruction is uncommon. The esophagus is dilated, often massively, and patients with achalasia may have symptoms of aspiration. The diagnosis may be made on a chest x-ray by finding a wide, mediastinal mass with a fluid level. The usual radiographic appearance is that of megaesophagus with a sharply tapering "beak" at the gastroesophageal junction. Test dilatation with a Hurst dilator has only a transient holdup at the cardioesophageal junction, whereas in malignancy the dilator usually cannot be passed. Manometric studies reveal absent peristaltic waves, a high pressure in the sphincter zone, and failure of the sphincter to relax in response to a swallow. The Mecholyl test is positive; however, a rare patient with carcinoma of the fundus or cardia which closely resembles achalasia radiographically may also have a positive Mecholyl test. Further, achalasia and carcinoma may coexist. (See Ch. 635.)

In *lye stricture,* the history of ingestion of caustic is usually clear; however, elderly patients may have ingested lye in childhood and not remember it. Because of the malignant potential of lye strictures, these patients should be followed periodically with roentgenologic examination, endoscopy, and exfoliative cytology.

Treatment and Prognosis. Treatment of esophageal carcinoma depends upon its location and whether it has spread. If distant metastases are absent, patients with distal esophageal carcinoma should have surgery. Lesions of the middle third are treated by either surgery or high voltage irradiation. Most patients with proximal esophageal carcinoma should receive irradiation therapy. Operative mortality for esophagectomy is between 15 and 20 per cent. Distal lesions are more favorable. Staged procedures, in selected patients, may improve the cure rate. A colon interposition, bypassing the cancer, is placed in the anterior mediastinum. The patient is then treated with therapeutic dosages of irradiation. Those patients surviving for six months then have an esophagectomy. Cure rates with irradiation alone or surgery alone are comparable and do not exceed 5 per cent.

Recent, uncontrolled observations suggest that preoperative irradiation in selected patients may improve resectability and perhaps even the incidence of cures. Irradiation, 4500 to 6000 rads tumor dose delivered to the entire esophagus, is followed in four to six weeks by resection. It is difficult to evaluate these observations, because only patients considered to be favorable candidates have received this treatment. However, a number of five-year cures have been reported.

Chemotherapy has not been shown to be of any value in esophageal carcinoma. Palliation is indicated in inoperable or incurable patients and consists of irradiation therapy, resectional surgery, or bypass surgery. Several prosthetic tubes are available which may be inserted through the tumor and which may relieve obstruction for some weeks or even months. Although nutrition may be improved, these devices may migrate through the tumor, erode into the mediastinum, or become occluded with tumor. Gastrostomy alone should not be done in patients with total obstruction caused by carcinoma of the esophagus, because this treatment only prolongs the patients' misery. They are unable to swallow their own secretions and suffer repeated pulmonary infections. If esophageal patency cannot be obtained with the aforementioned measures, these patients should be allowed to die with some dignity.

the most accurate means of diagnosing carcinoma when present and excluding it when suspected by other techniques. With an adequate test, carcinoma is diagnosed in 95 per cent or more of patients and false-positive diagnoses are exceedingly rare.

Differential Diagnosis. Only a few diseases may be confused with carcinoma of the esophagus. Most important is peptic *esophagitis* with *stricture* (see Ch. 635). Although most patients have a history of pyrosis, some have only a short history of dysphagia with little discomfort. The roentgenographic appearance may mimic malignant neoplasm. Eosphagoscopy with biopsy and cytology and lavage cytology will establish the benign nature of the stricture in virtually every patient.

The history of intermittent dysphagia in *achalasia* is much more characteristic than in carcinoma of the esophagus, which has a gradual increase in severity.

OTHER NEOPLASMS OF THE ESOPHAGUS

Carcinosarcomas

Carcinosarcomas are rare tumors of the esophagus. They tend to be polypoid and contain both carcinomatous and sarcomatous tissue. Exfoliative cytology may reveal both malignant sarcomatous and epithelial cells. Biopsy with histologic examination is probably more accurate. These tumors tend to be radiosensitive and should be treated with irradiation therapy if they are not resectable.

Malignant Lymphoma

Malignant lymphoma confined to the esophagus is extremely rare. The usual symptoms are either dysphagia or odynophagia. The roentgenographic appearance resembles monilial esophagitis. If the diagnosis can be established by exfoliative cytology or biopsy, irradiation therapy is the treatment of choice.

Leiomyomas

Leiomyomas are the most common benign neoplasms of the esophagus. Most often they cause no symptoms and are an incidental finding either at autopsy or surgery. They are usually less than 2 cm in diameter. They are intramural, extramucosal tumors and produce a smooth indentation in the esophagus on roentgenographic examination. Rarely, they may be "polyps" with a stalk. Even when they attain huge size, they may not produce symptoms. Rarely, patients have dysphagia and may even bleed. With large lesions, the diagnosis may be suspected by seeing a spherical mediastinal mass on chest x-ray. There is no evidence that leiomyomas undergo sarcomatous degeneration. The treatment of symptomatic esophageal leiomyomas is enucleation of the tumor. Resection is rarely necessary.

666. MALIGNANT NEOPLASMS OF THE STOMACH

Lloyd L. Brandborg

Ninety-five per cent of gastric neoplasms are malignant and 5 per cent benign. The most common benign neoplasm is the *leiomyoma,* which is usually an incidental finding at surgery or autopsy. The next most common is the *adenoma.* Other benign neoplasms of the stomach are exceedingly rare.

With the decreasing incidence of *adenocarcinoma* of the stomach in the United States and a constant incidence of gastric *lymphoma,* the proportion of malignant lymphomas has increased and possibly accounts for as many as 10 per cent of gastric malignancies. The other major malignant neoplasm of the stomach is the *leiomyosarcoma,* which accounts for about 1 per cent of gastric malignancies.

CARCINOMA OF THE STOMACH

Etiology. In spite of numerous experimental studies and epidemiologic investigations, a causative agent or agents responsible for carcinoma of the stomach remain elusive.

Genetic factors have been associated with an increased incidence of carcinoma of the stomach. Several families have been described with an unusually high occurrence. Studies of gastric carcinoma in twins have shown a higher frequency in monozygotic than in dizygotic twins. There is a 10 per cent increase in blood group A in gastric cancer patients when compared with suitable controls. Patients with pernicious anemia have been estimated to have a 10 per cent chance of developing gastric cancer. In these patients blood group A is also increased. Lewis group specific substances, either Le^a or Le^b or both, have been found in saliva in all patients with gastric carcinoma who have been examined. In the normal population 7 per cent of subjects are Lewis negative. These genetic factors are not etiologic, because the vast majority of subjects having them do not develop gastric carcinoma. They may be predisposing factors in response to other etiologic agents.

Adenomatous polyps have been considered to be "precancerous" in the past. Eight to 10 per cent of patients with adenocarcinoma of the stomach have one or more benign gastric polyps. However, many gastric adenomas observed over long periods of time have no growth, change in appearance, or malignant degeneration. Serial endoscopic observations have shown that some of these adenomatous polyps may even disappear. Benign adenomas may have small microscopic collections of cells that resemble carcinoma in situ. "Microinvasion" below the muscularis mucosae has been observed, but metastases have not been seen. Most often these cells have been found in proximity to areas of acute inflammation and granulation tissue and may not represent malignant change.

Atrophic gastritis, characterized by atrophy and intestinalization, is found in stomachs harboring carcinoma. In contrast to patients with adenomatous polyps, who are achlorhydric in 95 per cent of cases, 70 per cent of patients with gastric carcinoma secrete hydrochloric acid. It must be remembered also that decreased hydrochloric acid secretion is a feature of advancing age. Gastritis is probably not a predisposing factor, because histologic gastritis is very common in otherwise healthy individuals.

Patients with adult pernicious anemia have an increased incidence of gastric carcinoma. They are achlorhydric and achylic, and have intestinalization of their gastric mucosa and a high incidence of benign adenomas. Despite all these abnormalities, most of them do not develop carcinoma of the stomach.

Peptic ulcer of the stomach has been thought to be a precursor of carcinoma of the stomach. The finding of malignant cells in the margins of the ulcers has been offered as evidence. It is more likely, however, that ulcer in this circumstance develops as a result of peptic digestion of a small carcinoma. Further, virtually all such lesions have been described in patients secreting hydrochloric acid. Possibly neoplastic tissue is more susceptible to digestion than the surrounding mucosa. Although a benign gastric ulcer may degenerate into a malignant one, such an event must be extremely rare.

Previous surgery for benign peptic ulcer appears to be associated with an increase in carcinoma of the stomach. Several large reviews have shown that surgery for benign duodenal ulcer disease increases the risk of carcinoma in these patients. Carcinoma in association with duodenal ulcer is otherwise rare. The etiology and pathogenesis of gastric cancer in this situation are unknown. Possibly reflux of intestinal and pancreatic secretions into the gastric remnant may contribute. The interval between surgery for benign ulcer disease and the appearance of carcinoma of the stomach varies from 6 to up to 37 or more years. Any patient who develops gastric symptoms after several years of good health after surgery for benign peptic ulcer deserves a thorough investigation for malignancy.

Epidemiology. Striking geographic differences characterize the incidence and death rates from carcinoma of the stomach. The highest rates occur in Japan and Chile and the lowest in Egypt, Malaysia, and Nicaragua. Despite the marked differences, no environmental or dietary factor has been identified as being causative. Factors which have been found to be related to a high incidence include low socioeconomic status, urban dwelling, smoked fish in the diet, presence of carcinogens such as benzpyrene in barbecued meat or heated fats, background irradiation, trace metals in soil, types of soil, climate, and occupation.

Incidence and Prevalence. A striking and unexplained decrease in mortality from carcinoma of the stomach has occurred over the past four decades, from 33 per 100,000 population in 1930 to 7 to 8 per 100,000 population in the early 1970's. During the same interval, five-year cure rates have improved from 7 per cent to 9 per cent of all patients treated. These apparent small gains may be attributed to blood transfusion, better understanding of fluid and electrolyte therapy, better anesthesia, and the introduction of antimicrobial drugs.

Carcinoma of the stomach is twice as common in men as in women. This ratio tends to be maintained in all countries for which cancer statistics exist. In the United States the incidence in both men and women is approximately twice as high in blacks and Orientals as it is in whites. Carcinoma of the stomach has been observed in all age groups, but is most common in patients between the ages of 50 and 69.

Pathology. Carcinomas may be found at any site within the stomach. They may be divided into four gross classifications: polypoid, ulcerated noninfiltrating, ulcerated infiltrating, and the diffuse infiltrating varieties. (This classification corresponds to the Borrman classification.) The rare superficial spreading carcinoma is not included in the preceding classification. Most gastric carcinomas are adenocarcinomas of widely varying histology. The histology ranges from well-differentiated adenocarcinoma to mucoid carcinoma to undifferentiated carcinomas which may be difficult to differentiate from sarcomas.

Carcinoma of the stomach spreads by direct invasion and lymphatic channels. The pancreas, liver, and transverse colon are often invaded by tumor. Tumors in the proximal stomach often invade the esophagus for variable distances. The distensibility of the esophagus may be restricted. If the neural plexuses are invaded, these cancers may mimic achalasia. Extension across the pylorus from distal lesions is uncommon.

Probably lymph node metastases appear early. The local perigastric, preaortic, porta hepatis, and mediastinal nodes are frequently involved. Malignant deposits are frequently found in nodes in the hilum of the spleen and in the spleen itself. Occasionally metastases to the left supraclavicular space occur (Virchow's node), probably through the thoracic duct. Peritoneal implants are frequent, occurring in one third of patients coming to autopsy. In women the ovaries may have metastases, the so-called Krukenberg tumors.

Hematogenous metastases most often involve the liver, lungs, and bone. Pulmonary metastases may appear as a pneumonitis or as discrete masses, or may resemble miliary tuberculosis.

Clinical Manifestations. The mass survey studies in Japan have clearly shown that "early" gastric carcinoma confined to the mucosa does not produce symptoms. Most carcinomas of the stomach seen in the United States are already advanced. Symptoms are the result of ulceration, obstruction, necrosis, and disorders of gastric motility caused by tumor invasion.

Weight loss is the most common symptom and occurs in up to 96 per cent of patients. Approximately 70 per cent of patients have pain of variable intensity. Some patients have a mild and vague discomfort. Approximately 25 per cent of patients describe the pain as being similar to that of peptic ulcer. The pain may or may not be relieved by food or antacids. In a few patients it is of long duration. If the cancer has invaded the pancreas, pain may be referred to the back. The pain may be described as pressure sensations, fullness, aching, bloating, indigestion, dyspepsia, or gas pains. Some patients have pain immediately after eating. In others there is no apparent relationship to the ingestion of food.

Approximately 50 per cent of patients have vomiting. This usually implies pyloric obstruction, but occurs with carcinomas at any location within the stomach. Anorexia occurs in about 25 per cent of patients. The degree of weight loss often cannot be related to a reduction of food intake. Early satiety occurs in about 10 per cent of patients and is a fairly constant symptom in linitis plastica but may also occur with relatively small tumors.

Other gastrointestinal symptoms are changes in bowel habits such as constipation or diarrhea. Dysphagia is common with carcinoma of the fundus and cardia. A few patients may have odynophagia, and some have pyrosis. Gross hematemesis and melena are unusual, each occurring in 10 per cent of patients. Occult bleeding, on the other hand, is extremely common.

Other symptoms resulting from gastric carcinoma are unusual fatigability and symptoms of anemia such as dyspnea, dizziness and fainting, pallor, angina pectoris, and burning of the tongue. Some patients may have eructations, bad breath, and hiccups, and a few discover an abdominal mass. Peritoneal implants may cause ascites. Metastases in the liver or to the porta hepatis may produce jaundice. Bone pain may be the result of either pathologic fractures or invasion of the periosteum. Carcinomas may perforate and mimic perforated peptic ulcer.

Physical Examination. Only 45 to 50 per cent of patients with advanced gastric carcinoma have a palpable mass. Hepatomegaly is common but does not always indicate metastatic disease. Twenty per cent of patients will be emaciated or cachectic. Abdominal tenderness is noted in only 20 per cent of patients. Five per cent of patients have palpable peripheral lymph nodes caused by the metastases. Metastatic disease may also be manifest by hard nodular livers and palpable nodules on rectal examination. Rarely, a tumor nodule may be palpated or even seen in the umbilicus. Ascites is present in a few patients owing to hepatic or peritoneal metastases.

Jaundice may be seen with metastases to the porta hepatis or liver.

Differential Diagnosis. A number of other diseases may produce symptoms similar or identical to gastric carcinoma. The most important is benign *peptic ulcer. Cholelithiasis, pancreatitis, pancreatic neoplasm,* or *coronary artery disease* and other neoplasms of the stomach should be considered. Appropriate investigation will establish the correct diagnosis in most patients.

Laboratory Studies. The anemias of gastric carcinomas are of several varieties. Approximately two thirds of patients will have a hypochromic microcytic anemia. Macrocytic anemia caused by vitamin B_{12} or folate deficiency is not rare. A normochromic normocytic anemia may appear without bone marrow metastases. Occult blood is present in the stool in only about 45 per cent of patients on a single determination; when the stool is repeatedly tested, the percentage is much higher.

Gastric analysis is mandatory in every patient with a gastric ulcer. Ideally, the tube should be placed under fluoroscopic control with the tip in the middle of the antrum. If a fluoroscope is not readily available, the tube should be passed 55 to 60 cm from the nares. The secretagogue should be Histolog, 1.5 mg per kilogram subcutaneously or intramuscularly, or pentagastrin, 1 to 6 μg per kilogram intramuscularly. An ulcerating lesion in an achlorhydric patient is virtually pathognomonic of a malignant neoplasm. Presence of acid in no way excludes a diagnosis of cancer.

Roentgenologic Diagnosis. Roentgenologic examina-

Figure 2. Carcinoma of the stomach. The tumor has involved the entire antrum and produced a characteristic filling defect and mucosal destruction. An ulcer within the mass is indicated by the arrow.

tion will detect 95 per cent of gastric lesions. The radiologist must procure good mucosal detail to avoid overlooking small lesions. One of the more difficult differential diagnoses is between malignant and benign

Figure 3. Four gastric lesions photographed with the gastrocamera (reproduced from 5 mm color transparencies). *A,* Adenocarcinoma (arrow) seen on the posterior aspect of the stomach near the incisura angularis. *B,* Benign gastric ulcer (arrow) from a tangential view, showing the incisura angularis with the antral region to the left and fundus to the right. The edematous rolled margins of the ulcer surround the typical necrotic center; there is no evidence of neoplasia. *C,* This adenomatous polyp (arrow) in the gastric antrum had bled persistently, causing the patient to become severely anemic. The 5 to 6 mm lesion was seen in only one of several carefully performed upper gastrointestinal series. Its size, shape, and smooth contours are consistent with the subsequently proved diagnosis of adenoma. *D,* Leiomyoma (arrow) on the posterior wall of the body of the stomach lying above the incisura angularis. Note the obviously submucosal character of this lesion and its typical umbilication by an apical ulcer.

ulcers. In some ulcers, this distinction may be impossible. Some features which favor malignant ulcer are effacement of folds and abnormal mucosal folds, a niche in a notch (an ulcer within an ulcer), an ulcer with a flat wavy base, and a triangular-shaped wide-based ulcer. Linitis plastica is characterized by loss of distensibility of the stomach and absent or marked reduction of motility. Other malignant lesions are characterized by rigidity, mucosal distortion, irregular and enlarged mucosal folds, and fixed filling defects. An ulcer within a mass is characteristic of carcinoma of the stomach (Fig. 2). Some ulcers have features of both benignancy and malignancy.

Gastroscopy. Fiberoptic endoscopy permits a more complete examination of the stomach than was possible with the previous semiflexible instruments. Still and motion picture photography provide a permanent record (Fig. 3). These endoscopes have biopsy and directed cytology instruments. If six to ten biopsies and cytology specimens are taken from every lesion, a positive diagnosis is possible in 85 to 95 per cent of patients. In some lesions it may be technically impossible to place the biopsy forceps or the cytology instrument on the lesion. With the end-viewing instruments it may be impossible to biopsy the proximal edge of an ulcer. It is also not possible to sample the entire stomach to detect an otherwise unrecognized carcinoma.

Exfoliative Cytology. Skillfully collected and expertly interpreted, exfoliative cytology is one of the most sensitive techniques for either diagnosing or excluding cancer of the stomach. As with all other procedures, there are limitations. The technique cannot detect submucosal malignancies which do not penetrate into the lumen of the stomach. Leiomyosarcomas, even when ulcerated, do not exfoliate diagnostic cells. Some large, necrotic tumors may have fibrin or necrotic membranes overlying them, preventing exfoliation of diagnostic cells. The diagnosis in these lesions is usually apparent by radiographic and gastroscopic appearance.

Lavage cytology is superior to abrasive instruments. The highest accuracy has resulted from the utilization of chymotrypsin as a mucolytic enzyme. Lavage cytology provides a total mucosal "biopsy." In laboratories regularly performing gastric exfoliative cytology, accuracy ranges from 90 to 95 per cent in patients with proved malignancy, and cancer is falsely diagnosed in less than 1 per cent of patients with benign disease. The diagnosis rendered by the responsible physician should include only three possible categories: (1) malignant cells present with an interpretation of cell type, (2) no malignant cells present, and (3) unsatisfactory test which must be repeated after appropriate cleansing of the stomach.

Use of All Techniques. All available techniques should be used in gastric cancer suspects. Overconfidence in one method to the exclusion of others is to be avoided. The application of roentgenologic, gastroscopic, and cytologic methods affords the greatest benefit to the patient under consideration. If all these techniques indicate a benign lesion, the patient with gastric ulcer warrants a trial of medical therapy. However, it is mandatory that these patients be repeatedly examined to ensure ulcer healing.

Treatment. The only curative therapy for gastric carcinoma is surgical excision. The type and extent of the procedure must be left to the discretion of the surgeon. Polypoid carcinoma may be treated with a limited gastrectomy if no evidence of metastasis is present. Antral lesions may be treated by a subtotal gastrectomy, including the regional lymph nodes in the vicinity of the tumor. Patients with cancer of the cardia and fundus should have a proximal gastrectomy. Super-radical gastrectomy, in which all areas of *predicted* metastases are removed, was advocated in the past, but these procedures double surgical mortality and actually decrease cure rates. Total gastrectomy is almost never indicated for treatment of gastric carcinoma. Palliative resection is indicated for patients with incurable disease. Even though survival may not be improved, these patients may derive considerable benefit from relief of obstruction and hemorrhage and from improved nutrition.

Chemotherapy may provide palliation for some patients. 5-Fluorouracil (5-FU) produces an objective response in 20 per cent of patients and subjective improvement in 40 per cent. A recommended regimen is 5-FU, 15 mg per kilogram given once weekly either intravenously or orally. The drug should be administered by physicians skilled in its use.

Systematic studies of radiation therapy of gastric carcinoma are not available. Such therapy should be considered if the patient is inoperable but has tumor largely confined to the vicinity of the stomach. It is impossible to predict whether this form of treatment will be effective without attempting it. Irradiation therapy is of some use in selected patients in controlling hemorrhage.

Prognosis. Advanced carcinoma of the stomach has a dismal prognosis. Sixty-five per cent of patients subjected to surgery are found to be incurable. Fewer than 10 per cent of all patients with the disease can be cured. Factors which favor a more favorable prognosis are a long history as opposed to a brief history. The gross appearance of the tumor is related to prognosis. The polypoid tumors and the ulcerating but noninfiltrating tumors have the best prognosis, and the ulcerated, infiltrating, and diffuse infiltrating varieties have extremely low cure rates. Superficial spreading carcinoma, which is usually diagnosed cytologically, and carcinoma of the stomach confined to the mucosa have cure rates in the order of 90 to 95 per cent.

OTHER NEOPLASMS OF THE STOMACH

Lymphoma

Malignant lymphoma may be confined to the stomach. With the decreasing incidence of carcinoma, it assumes an increasingly important proportion of gastric cancers. *Reticulum cell sarcoma* and *lymphosarcoma* are the most common types. *Hodgkin's disease, giant follicular lymphoma,* and *plasmacytoma* may also involve the stomach primarily. The symptoms of malignant lymphoma are similar to carcinoma except that some patients have a history similar to that of peptic ulcer, sometimes for as long as several years. Men and women are equally affected. The peak incidence is between the ages of 40 and 60. Anemia, overt bleeding, and marked weight loss are somewhat less frequent than with carcinoma of the stomach.

There are no distinctive roentgenographic or gastroscopic appearances to permit differentiation from carcinoma. Exfoliative cytology is diagnostic in up to 90 per cent of patients. It is possible to differentiate reticulum cell sarcoma, lymphosarcoma, and Hodgkin's disease by cytologic criteria.

Treatment consists of resection of the tumor followed by irradiation therapy. The surgeon should attempt to excise as much tumor tissue as possible even if it cannot be resected in toto. Some patients who have been deemed inoperable and treated with radiation alone have had long survival. Cure rates, as judged by five-year survival, are 50 per cent in patients treated with surgery followed by irradiation therapy.

Leiomyosarcoma

The history of patients with leiomyosarcoma is similar to that of patients with carcinoma of the stomach; however, bleeding is more common, particularly massive hemorrhage, because these tumors are frequently ulcerated. Metastatic spread tends to be confined to the abdomen. Treatment is wide surgical excision. Five-year survival after surgery is 40 per cent and is dependent upon the degree of anaplasia of the tumor rather than its size.

667. BENIGN NEOPLASMS OF THE STOMACH

Lloyd L. Brandborg

ADENOMA

Adenomas of the stomach are generally seen in patients over the age of 50. Ninety-five per cent of patients with adenomas have achlorhydria, and they occur in 2 per cent of patients with achlorhydria. The incidence in pernicious anemia varies widely from series to series and may be as high as 20 per cent in these patients.

Probably most adenomas of the stomach are asymptomatic. The most common symptom is a nondescript upper abdominal pain. It is not related to food, is described as a dull ache and occasionally gnawing sensation, and is not relieved by antacids or food. Rarely, nausea and vomiting may be present. Overt hemorrhage is unusual, but the tumor may bleed occultly.

The physical examination is usually normal. In a few patients the signs of iron deficiency anemia are present. A palpable abdominal mass caused by adenoma is virtually never found.

The roentgenographic appearance of gastric adenoma is that of a spherical filling defect often on a stalk of variable length. Fiberoptic endoscopy is more sensitive than radiology in detecting small polypoid lesions. It also assists in differentiating the nature of these lesions and permits biopsy and cytologic examination. Endoscopy frequently detects several gastric polyps when one is identified on roentgenologic examination.

If it is highly likely that a patient's symptoms are due to gastric adenoma, therapy is local excision, including the stalk. Because of the low potential of malignancy, polyps less than 2 cm in diameter may be followed annually with cytologic examination and endoscopy. Polyps larger than 2 cm in diameter, particularly if they are sessile, have a higher probability of being malignant. If surgical contraindications are not present, these lesions should be locally excised.

LEIOMYOMA

Although leiomyomas are the most common benign tumors found in the stomach at autopsy, they are rarely responsible for clinical symptoms. Intramural, extramucosal tumors, they occur with equal frequency in men and women and are seen most often in subjects between the ages of 40 and 60. Most are between 1 and 2 cm in diameter, but they can attain huge size. Evidence of previous ulceration of the mucosa overlying the tumor is found in as many as 60 per cent of cases.

The most important symptom of gastric leiomyoma is bleeding. Usually it is occult and leads to iron deficiency anemia, but on occasion it may be massive. Some patients may also complain of epigastric burning or gnawing pain and anorexia.

The roentgenographic features are those of an intramucosal, usually spherical, intramural mass projecting into the lumen of the stomach. An ulceration may be detected within the mass. Gastroscopically, the tumor is covered by a normal but somewhat stretched mucosa with flattened rugae. The central ulcer is visible if present.

Symptomatic leiomyomas should be treated by local excision or limited gastrectomy. Prognosis is excellent.

See references after Ch. 669.

668. NEOPLASMS OF THE SMALL INTESTINE

Thomas F. O'Brien, Jr.

Primary neoplasms of the small intestine which are of clinical importance arise from the epithelial, muscular, vascular, and lymphatic components of the small intestine. Thus *adenomas, adenocarcinomas, leiomyomas, leiomyosarcomas, hemangiomas,* and *lymphomas* represent the most frequently observed tumors of the small intestine.

MALIGNANT NEOPLASMS

Types. *Adenocarcinomas, lymphomas,* and *leiomyosarcomas* are the three most common primary malignancies of the small intestine. Adenocarcinoma occurs with the greatest frequency and leiomyosarcoma with the least.

Etiology. Very little is known or hypothesized about the etiology of small intestinal malignancy. Dietary factors do not appear to play an important role in the development of adenocarcinoma, and no major differences in incidence have been observed among population groups. Chronic small bowel disease, however, may represent a predisposing factor, because *celiac sprue* and chronic *regional enteritis* appear to be associated with a disproportionate number of primary small bowel malignancies. An hereditary factor is suggested by the unusual frequency of *primary small bowel lymphoma* in the Middle East, particularly Israel and southern Iran.

Incidence. Primary small intestinal malignancies are rare. Excluding carcinoids, they represent only 1 to 2 per cent of all malignant gastrointestinal neoplasms.

Pathology. More than 90 per cent of the *adenocarcinomas* of the small intestine are located in the duodenum, and most lie within 20 cm of the ligament of Treitz. The lesions are usually annular in configuration and reveal a moderate degree of differentiation under the microscope. More than half the patients will show extension to or beyond regional lymph nodes at the time of initial diagnosis.

All varieties of lymphoma may arise primarily in the small intestine, although *reticulum cell sarcoma* is by far the most common. *Lymphomas* tend to involve the more distal portions of the jejunum and ileum and rarely arise in the duodenum.

Leiomyosarcomas of the small intestine may arise in any portion of the small intestine; however, the jejunum and ileum are the usual sites. They tend to be bulky tumors, exceeding 5 cm in diameter. Central necrosis is a common feature. Metastatic spread occurs primarily by the blood-borne route or by direct extension, rather than lymphatically.

Clinical Manifestations.   Malignant primary tumors of the small intestine are usually discovered in persons over 50 years of age. Lymphomas of the small intestine, however, tend to occur at a somewhat earlier age than adenocarcinomas or leiomyosarcomas. Men are afflicted with a frequency more than double that of women. Abdominal pain, malaise, anorexia, weight loss, and bleeding are common presenting symptoms. Although prodromal symptoms are usually present, sudden obstruction of the small intestine may be the first manifestation of a small bowel malignancy. A small bowel tumor, when palpable on physical examination, is almost invariably malignant. Free perforation is an important clinical manifestation of the sarcoma.

Diagnosis.   Most primary small intestinal malignancies are identified by radiographic examination of the small bowel. Certain roentgenologic features characterize the various histologic types. Annular lesions of short length are typically found with an *adenocarcinoma* (Fig. 1). Longer, ulcerating lesions producing so-called aneurysmal dilatation of the lumen favor lymphoma. Diffuse small bowel involvement suggesting a malabsorption syndrome is a less common manifestation of lymphoma. *Leiomyosarcomas* are bulky tumors which displace adjacent bowel loops.

Visceral angiography has become a valuable tool in identification of malignant small bowel tumors. The source of blood supply is an important clue in the differential diagnosis of benign and malignant lesions. Benign tumors are invariably fed by a branch of the gastroduodenal or superior mesenteric artery. Blood supply from a renal or lumbar artery (parasitic blood supply) is characteristic of a malignant lesion.

Treatment.   Surgery is required for the majority of patients with primary small bowel malignancies. Although in two thirds of the patients the disease will have spread at the time of surgical intervention, the procedure is usually indicated for relief of obstruction, control of hemorrhage, and alleviation of pain.

Radiation therapy, alkalating agents, and nitrogen mustard, together with corticosteroids, often prove effective for some patients with lymphoma. 5-Fluorouracil and its derivatives have not proved to be beneficial in most instances.

Prognosis.   Prognosis in primary bowel malignancy is dependent to some extent upon location, histology, and duration of disease. Under favorable circumstances five-year survivals of 20 per cent have been reported with adenocarcinoma, 60 per cent with lymphoma, and up to 50 per cent with leiomyosarcomas.

BENIGN NEOPLASMS

The small intestine may give rise to a variety of benign small bowel tumors. Among these are *adenomas, leiomyomas, lipomas, fibromas,* and *hemangiomas.* Of these, the *leiomyoma* is the most important of the group to the clinician. They may arise at any level of the small intestine but favor the jejunum. Central necrosis with ulceration, resulting in severe hemorrhage, is a characteristic feature of the leiomyoma.

Hemangiomas are much less frequently found than adenomas or leiomyomas. They, too, are clinically important because of their propensity to bleed.

Clinical Manifestations.   Benign small bowel tumors occur with equal frequency in men and women and are usually symptomatic in persons above 50 years of age. Colicky abdominal pain caused by luminal obstruction or intussusception is the predominant symptom. Massive gastrointestinal hemorrhage is suggestive of a leiomyoma. Benign small bowel tumors are rarely palpable.

Diagnosis.   Barium contrast studies of the small intestine and visceral angiography represent the principal diagnostic methods. A small bowel series occasionally demonstrates localized intussusception, an important clue that the lesion is benign.

Treatment and Prognosis.   Surgical excision is the treatment of choice for virtually all symptomatic primary benign small bowel tumors. Prognosis is excellent with resection.

669.   NEOPLASMS OF THE LARGE INTESTINE

Thomas F. O'Brien, Jr.

CARCINOMA OF THE LARGE INTESTINE

Incidence and Prevalence.   Colorectal cancer is the second most common malignancy of the adult population in the United States (excluding skin cancer). It is exceeded

Figure 1. Adenocarcinoma of the duodenum, close-up view. The characteristic features of a small bowel adenocarcinoma are demonstrated here. Note the "shelving" edges at the proximal portion of the tumor. The central lumen shows destruction of the normal mucosal pattern with ulceration (arrow). (From O'Brien, T. F., Jr., *In* Sleisenger, M. H., and Fordtran, J. S. [eds.]: Gastrointestinal Disease. Philadelphia, W. B. Saunders Company, 1973.)

only by lung cancer among males and breast cancer among females. Malignancies of the colon and rectum are responsible for approximately 15 per cent of all adult cancer deaths, resulting in an annual fatality rate of 16 to 18 patients per 100,000 population. A similar incidence has been noted in Great Britain, France, Germany, New Zealand, and a number of other countries which share an urbanized Western culture. In sharp contrast is a considerably reduced incidence in Japan, rural Africa, India, and a number of Latin American countries.

Etiology. The etiology of malignant tumors of the colon and rectum remains unknown. At least three factors must be considered in the development of large intestinal neoplasms, namely environmental factors, heredity, and pre-existing disease.

Environmental Factors. The contrasting prevalence of the disease among different cultures has led to increasing speculation that environmental factors, such as exposure to ingested carcinogens, play a primary role in pathogenesis. Considerable differences in dietary patterns exist between populations with high and low rates of large intestinal cancer. For example, those in cultures with a low incidence of large bowel cancer consume diets containing a large amount of plant fiber. Conversely, diets in areas where colon cancer is more prevalent tend to contain large amounts of highly refined carbohydrates and are generally low in fiber content. Perhaps related to these dissimilarities in diet are the significant differences in colonic bacterial flora which exist between the two groups. High fiber content diets produce bulky stools containing principally aerobic organisms (enterococci, streptococci), whereas the compact, small volume stools of low residue diets contain principally anaerobic organisms (bacteroides). Furthermore, it has been shown that some anaerobic organisms have the capacity metabolically to transform certain innocuous substances, such as bile acids, into potentially carcinogenic compounds. The latter phenomenon, together with the relatively prolonged colonic transit time of the small-volume stool, could lead to extended contact time between carcinogen and large bowel epithelium. Although unproved, this hypothesis is both popular and plausible.

In further support of the environmental theory is the observation that individuals from a "low-cancer" culture, such as native Japanese, develop large intestinal malignancies with an incidence similar to Americans when they establish residence in the United States and adopt Western dietary patterns.

Hereditary Factors. Genetic factors appear to play a primary role in several varieties of inherited colorectal neoplasms to be discussed.

FAMILIAL POLYPOSIS. Familial polyposis is inherited as an autosomal dominant trait. Multiple polypoid adenomas of the colon become apparent in patients between the ages of 10 and 15 years. In untreated cases, colorectal cancer will develop in 75 to 80 per cent of the patients. Unfortunately, some 40 per cent of index cases already have a malignancy at the time of original diagnosis. The identification of such an index case should prompt a thorough survey of all immediate family members with the usual diagnostic methods (see below). Subtotal colectomy with ileoproctectomy should be recommended to all asymptomatic patients in whom multiple polyps are present. The remaining rectal tissue, although subject to the development of polypoid adenomas and adenocarcin-

omas, can be inspected regularly with a proctoscope and suspicious lesions removed locally. The preservation of rectal function is desirable and more easily acceptable to asymptomatic patients.

GARDNER'S SYNDROME. Gardner's syndrome consists of multiple polyps of the small and large intestines associated with osteomas and soft tissue lesions. This disorder is also transmitted as an autosomal dominant trait. A variety of soft tissue lesions are seen, including sebaceous cysts, lipomas, fibromas, leiomyomas, and occasionally fibrosarcomas. These soft tissue tumors may occur in the skin, in subcutaneous tissues, or in a variety of mesenteric or retroperitoneal locations. Colorectal carcinoma occurs in these patients with a high frequency, similar to that observed in familial polyposis; however, the malignancies tend to develop at a later age in life. Prophylactic subtotal colectomy with ileorectal anastomosis is the treatment of choice.

FAMILY COLONIC CANCER WITHOUT POLYPS (THE CANCER FAMILY SYNDROME). Several kindreds have been described in which there is an unusual frequency of colonic cancer. The neoplasms tend to occur at an early age, and polyposis is *not* a feature. Pedigree studies suggest that the mode of inheritance is via an autosomal dominant trait.

PEUTZ-JEGHERS SYNDROME. Mucocutaneous pigmentation, primarily involving the buccal mucosa, perioral and periorbital skin, and distal extremities, characterizes this variety of gastrointestinal polyposis. The syndrome is transmitted by a single mendelian dominant trait responsible for both the melanin deposits and the polyps. Histologically, the latter are hamartomas rather than adenomas. In the great majority of cases the polyps are distributed primarily in the jejunum and ileum, although gastric polyps occur in approximately 25 per cent of cases, and colorectal polyps are seen in 30 to 50 per cent. The risk of associated gastrointestinal malignancy is small, of the order of 3 per cent of cases. In a recent review, it was reported that 15 of 125 female patients with Peutz-Jeghers syndrome had developed ovarian tumors. The wide distribution of the gastrointestinal polyps and the low incidence of associated malignancy make prophylactic bowel resection unrealistic.

TURCOT SYNDROME. This extremely rare condition features the association of malignant tumors of the central nervous system and familial polyposis. To date, only a single kindred has been described. No rational therapeutic management program has developed because of the insufficient case material.

CRONKHITE-CANADA SYNDROME. Diffuse gastrointestinal polyposis, alopecia, pigmentation, and onychotrophia characterize this syndrome. Diarrhea, hypoproteinemia, edema, and cachexia are important additional clinical manifestations. Patients with this syndrome have usually been in their fifth and sixth decades of life, and there is no predominant sex distribution. Although colorectal malignancy has not been associated with the polyposis, rapidly progressive cachexia and a fatal outcome are characteristic.

Predisposing Diseases. CANCER RISK AND POLYPOID ADENOMAS. Although formerly a subject of great controversy, there is general agreement that the polypoid adenoma of the colon is not a premalignant lesion. One or several such adenomas may be found in 15 per cent of the adult population (Fig. 2). One autopsy series in which meticulous inspection of the large bowel was

Figure 2. Adenomatous polyp, sigmoid colon (arrow).

carried out demonstrated adenomas in approximately three fourths of all those examined.

Most of the clinically detected polypoid adenomas are less than 1.5 cm in transverse diameter, and malignancy in lesions of this size is quite uncommon. Colorectal cancers, which assume a polypoid shape, are usually greater than 2.0 cm in transverse diameter at the time of discovery.

ULCERATIVE COLITIS. The development of colorectal carcinoma at a greatly increased rate in patients with chronic ulcerative colitis appears well established. Approximately 5 per cent of patients with prolonged disease develop this serious complication. At least three parameters appear important when considering the risk of malignancy in these patients: the duration of the disease, the age at initial onset of the disease, and the extent of colonic involvement with the disease. The majority of patients in whom ulcerative colitis is complicated by malignancy have usually had universal involvement of the colon by the inflammatory process, and their disease has been present in excess of 15 years on the average.

So-called childhood ulcerative colitis, with onset at less than 14 years of age, appears to have an unusual incidence of colonic carcinoma. An analysis of almost 400 cases from the Mayo Clinic places the cancer risk at 20 per cent for each 10 years of duration beyond the initial decade. This carcinogenic risk of longstanding ulcerative colitis makes duration of disease the most important single consideration in the decision for colectomy. To date there is insufficient evidence to establish a relationship between granulomatous-segmental colitis (Crohn's disease) and colorectal carcinoma.

Pathogenesis. *Normal and Abnormal Cellular Kinetics.* Radiothymidine-labeling studies of cellular proliferation in the colon have shown important differences between normal epithelium and areas of neoplasia. Mitosis of colonic epithelial cells is normally limited to a regeneration zone in the lower third of the base of the crypts of Lieberkühn. Newly formed epithelial cells then migrate to the mucosal surface over a period of approximately 72 hours, and are finally shed into the lumen in about 96 hours. No appreciable cellular division takes place once the cell has begun its journey out of the crypt. However, when surface epithelial cells of laboratory animals are exposed to chemical carcinogens, they begin to show considerable mitotic activity. Eventually polypoid adenomas develop which are histologically similar to those observed in humans. Parallel isotopic studies in humans with various hyperplastic colonic neoplasms have confirmed that increased cellular proliferation occurs within the superficial epithelium of such lesions. These studies support the theory that environmental carcinogens play an important role in colorectal neoplasms.

Pathology. The majority of rectal and colonic malignancies are adenocarcinomas. In a series of more than 50,000 cases of large intestinal malignancy, 86 per cent were adenocarcinoma in type. *Carcinoids, squamous cell carcinoma, leiomyosarcoma, adenoacanthoma,* and *lymphoma,* as a group, accounted for only 2 per cent of the total. The remainder were undifferentiated or poorly differentiated carcinomas. Multiple primary tumors within the colon are noted in approximately 5 per cent of patients at the time of initial diagnosis.

The distribution of large intestinal malignancies is similar in most large series. Approximately 15 per cent arise in the cecum and ascending colon, 10 per cent are distributed along the transverse colon, 5 per cent occur in the descending colon, 25 per cent occur in the sigmoid, and 45 per cent arise in the rectum. Metastatic spread may occur by direct invasion of surrounding tissues, by way of the regional lymphatics, or by multiple peritoneal implants. The liver is the principal site of major organ metastasis, with the lungs, brain, bones, and other viscera less frequently involved.

Microscopically, adenocarcinomas of the large intestine show a poorly formed acinar architecture, containing small amounts of mucus. A small number, perhaps 5 per cent, show considerable mucus production and have been assigned the term *mucoid adenocarcinoma.* Paradoxically, the well-differentiated mucoid carcinoma has a rather poor prognosis.

Clinical Manifestations. Carcinoma of the colon and rectum is primarily a disease of later life. Although sporadic cases may be observed in any age group, the disease occurs with increasing frequency above the age of 55 years and reaches its peak incidence beyond 65 years of age. Males and females develop tumors above the rectum with approximately equal frequency, whereas males predominate in rectal cancer.

The presenting clinical manifestations of colorectal cancer are primarily determined by the location of the tumor. Approximately 75 per cent of all large intestinal malignancies occur within, or distal to, the sigmoid colon. Characteristically, tumors in these locations grow circumferentially, producing some degree of bowel obstruction. For this reason a significant change in bowel pattern is reported by the majority of the patients. Common symptoms include increasing constipation or alternating constipation and diarrhea, usually accompanied by colicky lower abdominal pain.

Most tumors in this location have ulcerating surfaces, and because of their proximity to the rectum, visible blood is usually observed by the patient. When the tumors arise within or near the rectum, more severe obstipation, tenesmus, and visible blood are nearly always reported, and pencil-shaped stools are frequently observed.

In contrast, carcinomas arising in the cecum and ascending colon usually do not produce obstructive symptoms. Growths in this area often assume a polypoid configuration and may reach considerable size prior to discovery. Blood loss is typically occult, and is rarely observed by the patient. Frequently it is the symptoms of profound anemia which bring the patient to the physician. Quite often the tumor has metastasized to the liver at the time of initial examination, and jaundice, right upper quadrant pain, or a mass lesion may be noted.

Tumors arising in the middle third of the colon present with variable symptomatology. Vague discomfort, nonspecific dyspepsia, or colicky pain with gross or occult blood loss may be reported by the patient. Weight loss is variable, but when it exceeds 10 per cent or more of the patient's usual weight it usually indicates a poor prognosis.

Diagnosis. The diagnosis of a large intestinal malignancy is usually suggested by the patient's history. In addition, it must be strongly considered in all patients beyond the age of 45 years with unexplained anemia. A primary lesion in the large intestine must also be ruled out in those patients who present with evidence of metastatic liver disease such as jaundice and hepatic enlargement.

On physical examination, palpation of the abdomen may reveal a mass lesion, but this is highly variable and depends in large part upon the size of the tumor, degree of obesity, and location of the tumor in relationship to pelvic bony structures. Digital and proctoscopic examination of the rectosigmoid usually reveals two out of three lesions arising below the pelvic peritoneal reflection. The physician should be alert to those cutaneous manifestations suggestive of a familial syndrome asso-

ciated with colorectal cancer. Superficial forceps biopsy of the lesion can usually be obtained safely by an experienced physician and will lead to rapid histologic confirmation of the diagnosis. Reluctance toward biopsy on the grounds of tumor dissemination is not justified. Comparative five-year survival studies of patients with and without circulating malignant cells after surgical manipulation have demonstrated that their presence is without prognostic significance.

Lesions beyond the reach of the proctoscope are best revealed by barium contrast radiographic examination. Typical lesions in the sigmoid colon produce a sharply demarcated narrowing of the lumen usually not exceeding 8 to 10 cm in length. The "napkin ring" or "apple core" appearance with shelving edges is a most characteristic radiographic feature (Fig. 3). Tumors arising in the cecum often assume polypoid rather than annular configuration and may be obscured by excessive barium filling of the cecum. In suspicious cases, when an annular lesion is not demonstrated, an air contrast barium enema can be diagnostic. A carcinoma lying within an area of massed diverticula can easily be overlooked, and repeat studies with special emphasis to the area of interest should be performed in suspicious cases.

Fiberoptic colonoscopy offers considerable promise for the visual inspection and biopsy of lesions beyond the reach of standard proctoscopes. Perhaps the greatest utility for this technique lies in the examination of pedunculated or sessile growths whose benignity or malignancy cannot be established on radiographic grounds. Techniques are rapidly developing for the complete excision of these lesions at the time of colonoscopy, thereby avoiding the necessity of laparotomy. Such techniques, however, require considerable skill on the part of the endoscopist and should only be performed by those with adequate training.

Exfoliative cytology, although adovcated by Papanicolaou more than 20 years ago, has not gained wide acceptance in the diagnosis of colorectal cancer. Several series, however, have demonstrated a high degree of diagnostic accuracy for the method. A correct cytologic diagnosis is established in 80 to 95 per cent of patients with malignancy. The percentages of false-positive and false-negative reports are small in these series. Underutilization of the technique is probably accounted for by the belief that satisfactory specimens are difficult and unpleasant to obtain. In practice, however, quite satisfactory cytologic material may be obtained by a simple saline lavage of the colon preceded by several days of an elemental diet and a strong cathartic the night before the collection of the specimen.

Carcinoembryonic Antigen (CEA). A tumor-associated antigen, referred to as CEA, can be demonstrated in the serum of over 95 per cent of patients with disseminated colonic carcinoma and approximately 20 per cent of patients with localized disease. The CEA appears to be a glycoprotein with a molecular weight of approximately 200,000. In general, serum levels appear to be elevated in proportion to the mass of tumor tissue present. Serum levels of CEA below 2.5 ng per ml are clearly normal, whereas values which exceed 5.0 ng per ml are strongly suggestive of underlying disease (see below). Levels between 2.5 and 5.0 ng must be considered indeterminate, especially if underlying inflammatory disease is present.

The early promise of specific serologic diagnosis of large intestinal malignancy by means of the CEA has not been sustained.

Figure 3. Carcinoma of the colon. This annular lesion in the ascending colon has produced a typical appearance of mucosal destruction and overhanging margins.

Positive tests can be obtained in a significant percentage of other gastrointestinal diseases, both malignant (hepatoma and gastric, pancreatic, and small bowel carcinomas), and nonmalignant (alcoholic cirrhosis, pancreatitis, and ulcerative colitis). Positive CEA tests have also been reported in lung cancer, breast cancer, prostatic cancer, neuroblastoma, and osteogenic sarcoma. These findings cast much doubt on the utility of the CEA as a screening test for colorectal cancer. The test may be useful in postoperative cases, because elevated levels tend to fall with successful resection. A return to elevated values is indicative of recurrent or disseminated disease.

Differential Diagnosis.   Malignancies of the large intestine must be differentiated from other diseases which present with an abdominal mass, rectal bleeding, colicky abdominal pain, or a change in bowel habit. A number of diseases may produce these symptoms either singly or in combination. Included in the differential diagnosis are *diverticulosis coli,* with or without diverticulitis; inflammatory bowel diseases, including *ulcerative colitis* and *proctitis* and *ileocolitis* of the Crohn variety; and *benign tumors* (most frequently polypoid adenomas).

On rare occasions *pelvic endometriosis* may mimic a primary large bowel cancer. In this instance, usually the age, sex, and relationship of the rectal bleeding to menstrual flow are important differential diagnostic features in the history.

The finding of hemorrhoidal varices should not be accepted as sufficient explanation for rectal bleeding in any patient, especially in those over 45 years. Proctoscopy should be performed routinely in all patients with rectal bleeding, and radiographic studies should be obtained in most instances.

Treatment and Prognosis. *Surgical Resection.*   Most patients with colorectal carcinoma require surgical resection of the primary tumor. The operation may be either curative or palliative in intent. A palliative resection is justified when lower bowel obstruction is imminent, even though known metastases are present. In a series of over 1800 cases from the University of Minnesota, the overall five-year survival of patients with colorectal carcinoma was approximately 30 per cent. Patients with rectal carcinoma generally showed a poorer prognosis than those with tumors of other segments of the colon. Patients without lymph node involvement, whose surgery took place between 1958 and 1963, showed a five-year survival of 43.5 per cent for carcinoma of the rectum and 62.5 per cent for other colonic cancers. The operative mortality for rectal carcinoma was more than twice that for higher lesions.

Rectal Fulguration and Radiotherapy.   The higher operative mortality and poorer prognosis for rectal cancer has led to several innovations in therapy. Rectal fulguration and/or local radiation therapy have been successfully employed by some as an alternative mode of therapy for selected patients.

Chemotherapy.   There has been disappointingly little progress in the development of effective chemotherapeutic agents for colorectal carcinoma. 5-Fluorouracil (5-FU) remains the most widely used agent. Objective tumor regression occurs in approximately 20 per cent of the treated patients. The rather slow cellular doubling time of colorectal cancers has been offered as an explanation for the general unresponsiveness to chemotherapeutic agents.

Some are cautiously optimistic that immunotherapy may play a role in future treatment. The identification of tumor-specific antigens within human neoplastic colon cells justifies the hope that specific antibodies can be developed and directed against the neoplastic tissues.

VILLOUS ADENOMAS

The villous adenoma is a special form of colonic neoplasm with interesting gross anatomic, histologic, physiologic, and clinical features. Villous adenomas occur with much less frequency than polypoid adenomas, and are usually seen in patients in the seventh decade of life. Grossly, the tumors are broad based, usually measuring more than 4 cm in transverse diameter, and consist of numerous frond-like projections. The majority are in the rectum and rectosigmoid portion of the colon. Those which can be reached by digital examination are very soft to palpation and appear velvety on proctoscopy. The epithelial cells of these tumors are abundant in mucin, and patients with villous adenomas often note considerable mucoid content in their stools. In rare instances a villous adenoma will secrete considerable volumes of fluid, rich in potassium, leading to severe hypokalemia.

In the microscopic evaluation of these tumors a clear distinction between atypical focal hyperplasia and carcinoma in situ can be very difficult for the pathologist. Such foci of cellular atypia can be found in up to 50 per cent of all villous adenomas upon careful serial sectioning. It is very unlikely, however, that 50 per cent of the lesions advance to infiltrating adenocarcinoma. The unpredictable course, together with frequently distressing clinical symptoms, dictates complete surgical excision whenever possible.

Castleman, B., and Krickstein, H.: Current approach to the polyp-cancer controversy. Gastroenterology, 51:108, 1966.

Devroede, G. J., Taylor, W. F., Sauer, W. G., Jackman, R. J., and Stickler, G. B.: Cancer risk and life expectancy of children with ulcerative colitis. N. Engl. J. Med., 285:17, 1971.

Griffiths, J. D., McKinna, J. A., Rowbotham, H. D., Tsolakidis, P., and Salsbury, A. J.: Carcinoma of the colon and rectum: Circulating malignant cells and five-year survival. Cancer, 31:226, 1973.

Margulis, A. R., and Burhenne, H. J.: Alimentary Tract Radiology. St. Louis, C. V. Mosby Company, 1973.

Morrissey, J. F.: Gastrointestinal endoscopy. Gastroenterology, 62:1241, 1972.

Sherlock, P., Erlich, A. N., and Winawer, S. J.: Diagnosis of gastrointestinal cancer: Current status and recent progress. Gastroenterology, 63:672, 1972.

Sleisenger, M. H., and Fordtran, J. S. (eds.): Gastrointestinal Disease. Philadelphia, W. B. Saunders Company, 1973.

Section Nine. OTHER DISEASES OF THE COLON, RECTUM, AND ANUS

David L. Earnest

670. INTRODUCTION

Certain diseases of the colon are not conveniently classified with other vascular, motor, malignant, or inflammatory conditions. In general, these miscellaneous colonic diseases are uncommon, often of uncertain etiology, and frequently perplexing to diagnose and treat. Properly taken and processed rectal biopsy specimens can significantly contribute to their diagnosis. A pedunculated or sessile mucosal mass may be biopsied with either punch or cutting forceps. Biopsy of an ulcerating lesion should be taken at its margin and should include some normal tissue. A suction biopsy tube can be used when there is diffuse mucosal disease. This instrument is especially useful if the abnormality is located above the peritoneal reflection. The use of conventional biopsy forceps for small mucosal lesions 12 to 14 cm or more above the pectinate line always carries the potential hazard of bowel perforation. Tissue specimens should be mounted on a piece of monofilament mesh with the mucosal side up and then placed in a fixative solution. Proper orientation of the tissue on the mesh may facilitate diagnostic interpretation by making it easier to section the specimen perpendicular to the mucosa.

671. COLITIS CYSTICA SUPERFICIALIS AND PROFUNDA

There are two types of benign, cystic, mucus-filled lesions of the colonic mucosa: *colitis cystica superficialis* and *colitis cystica profunda*. The superficialis type occurs predominantly in patients with pellagra and may develop at a time when typical skin lesions are absent. It has also been described in a few cases of adult celiac disease. Diarrhea is frequently the presenting symptom. The condition is characterized by very small mucus-filled cysts which lie superficial to the muscularis mucosae of the colon. Grossly, the cysts appear as thousands of minute gray blebs on the mucosal surface from which mucus can be expressed. Treatment with niacin or tryptophan for the underlying pellagra is curative.

In colitis cystica profunda the cysts are located below the muscularis mucosae and occasionally appear to "invade" the muscularis propria. They are filled with basophilic mucoid material and are lined by colonic epithelium, showing varying degrees of pressure atrophy. Pathologically, colitis cystica profunda must be differentiated from mucus-producing adenocarcinoma. Misdiagnosis has resulted in extensive cancer surgery for this benign condition.

The pathogenesis of cyst formation is uncertain. Congenitally ectopic mucosa may be responsible. However, communications between the cyst and the bowel lumen have been demonstrated, suggesting a weakness in the muscularis mucosae which allows herniation of mucosal epithelium into the submucosa. Another possibility is downgrowth of colonic epithelium during the healing process into areas of inflammatory ulceration. The frequently obtained history of preceding severe diarrhea or dysentery supports an inflammatory origin.

Cramping lower abdominal pain, rectal tenesmus, and mild diarrhea associated with blood and mucus in the stool are the most consistent symptoms. If palpated on rectal examination, the cystic lesion usually has a rubbery firm consistency and is not adherent to surrounding tissue. It may be sessile or polypoid and have either normal or ulcerated overlying mucosa. A nodular irregularity in the bowel wall may be the only radiologic abnormality on barium enema and may stimulate a large differential diagnosis. Biopsy of one of the cystic nodules should settle the diagnostic dilemma. Treatment consists of local surgical excision. There are no reports of recurrence in uninvolved intestine.

672. PNEUMATOSIS CYSTOIDES INTESTINALIS

Pneumatosis cystoides intestinalis is characterized by multiple gas-filled cysts in the submucosa or subserosa of both the small intestine and the colon. The majority of cases with involvement of the small intestine are in patients between ages 25 and 50 years who have either chronic obstructive pulmonary disease or peptic ulcer with some degree of pyloric obstruction. The exact cause of the gas-filled cysts is unknown.

The composition of the gas is similar to that of atmospheric air. It is postulated that air, forced into tissue spaces around an ulcer or from rupture of a pulmonary bleb, dissects along facial planes into the retroperitoneal space and out along blood vessels in the mesentery to the intestinal subserosa. Patients with pneumatosis in the wall of the rectum and sigmoid colon usually have undergone previous sigmoidoscopy. Presumably air entered the rectosigmoid wall through a small mucosal tear. Scleroderma of the intestine and inflammatory or ischemic bowel disease have also been complicated by intestinal pneumatosis.

The gas-filled cysts may vary in size from a few millimeters to several centimeters and look like multiple lymphangiomas or even multiple sessile polyps. Microscopically, the gas cysts are lined by a layer of endothelial cells which have a tendency to coalesce to form giant cells. A progressive fibrotic reaction may develop and ultimately obliterate the cyst. Because the cysts do not communicate with the bowel lumen, cyst rupture does not result in peritonitis except in ischemic bowel disease when pneumatosis of the intestinal wall is produced by invading bacteria.

Pneumatosis cystoides intestinalis produces no specific symptoms. It is usually an incidental finding during radiologic examination of the abdomen or intestine. Nevertheless, lower abdominal cramping pain, recurrent diarrhea, rectal bleeding, tenesmus, and partial bowel obstruction have all been described in patients with colonic pneumatosis. In addition, pneumatosis should be considered in the patient who presents with vague abdominal discomfort and free air under the diaphragm on x-ray examination, and who has no other evidence for a perforated viscus.

The most useful way of establishing the diagnosis is by barium x-ray examination of the small bowel and colon. Pneumatosis involving the rectosigmoid area can be recognized during sigmoidoscopy as pale bluish soft masses which protrude into the lumen and often collapse when biopsied.

When pneumatosis involves the small bowel, often no specific treatment is necessary except for the underlying or primary disease. The value of correct diagnosis is mainly in preventing unnecessary surgery. In contrast, surgery may be required for colonic pneumatosis if there is severe tenesmus, bleeding, pain, or partial obstruction of the lumen with no other apparent cause. Unfortunately, pneumatosis may recur and become more extensive after resection. If surgery is performed, the rectum should be spared, because pneumatosis in the rectum usually regresses after resection of more proximally involved colon.

pains in the rectum and occasionally mild tenesmus. Endometriosis of the more proximal colon is usually asymptomatic. Implants on the small intestine are often discovered incidentally during abdominal surgery. Bowel obstruction may develop from endometriosis at any level of the intestinal tract owing to fibrous adhesions, stenosis from fibrosis, or volvulus.

Clinical diagnosis of intestinal endometriosis primarily requires a high index of suspicion. The first diagnostic maneuver should be a thorough pelvic examination with combined rectovaginal palpation. Tender nodules with irregular induration in the cul-de-sac are suggestive of rectosigmoid endometriosis. Repeated pelvic examination later in the menstrual cycle should demonstrate some variation in character of the lesion. When a mass is palpable in the free portion of the sigmoid colon and none in the cul-de-sac, the diagnosis of endometriosis is much less certain. Radiologic, sigmoidoscopic, and mucosal biopsy findings may not significantly contribute to the diagnosis. Persisting uncertainty about a constricting rectosigmoid lesion, especially in an older woman, should prompt needle biopsy or surgical exploration to exclude adenocarcinoma.

The therapy of symptomatic intestinal endometriosis lies between watchful waiting, hormonal therapy, surgical excision, and castration. Treatment must be individualized and flexible during the course of the disease. Progestin therapy occasionally produces regression and even disappearance of symptomatic colonic endometriosis. However, this result is inconstant, and unless symptoms are promptly alleviated, obstructing lesions should be excised.

673. ENDOMETRIOSIS

Endometriosis refers to the presence of extrauterine endometrial tissue and the clinical sequelae produced by its normal function in an abnormal site. It is a disease of the reproductive period, with peak incidence between the ages of 30 and 40 years. It is uncommon in the 20's and, rarely, may produce symptoms after menopause. Intestinal involvement with endometriosis is usually greatest in those parts of the bowel that are pelvic in location, especially the rectosigmoid colon.

It is uncertain exactly how the heterotopic endometrium reaches the subserosa of the bowel wall. Nevertheless, under hormonal influence there is maturation, slough of the surface endometrial epithelium, and bleeding as occurs in the uterine cavity. Debris generated from this process may produce pressure necrosis of adjacent tissue, resulting in progressive dissection of the endometriosis through both subserosa and muscularis of the bowel wall. The mucosa is seldom penetrated, a fact which explains why periodic intraluminal intestinal bleeding infrequently occurs from endometriosis. A large bulky intramural lesion can develop which contains areas of fibrosis and marked smooth muscle hyperplasia. This firm mass, known as an endometrioma, may produce luminal obstruction, especially in the sigmoid colon.

Symptoms of endometriosis include dysmenorrhea, menometrorrhagia, intermenstrual pelvic pain, sterility, dyspareunia, and low backache. Involvement of the rectosigmoid colon is usually signaled by cyclic cramping

674. MALACOPLAKIA

Malacoplakia is a rare granulomatous disease of unknown cause which usually affects the urinary tract but which has also been reported in the colon. It is characterized pathologically by the presence of histiocytes containing peculiar intracytoplasmic dark, round laminated inclusions called Michaelis-Gutman bodies. These inclusions are PAS positive, stain for both calcium and iron, and appear to be a cellular reaction to breakdown products of bacteria. Colonic malacoplakia is most often noted as an incidental finding in elderly debilitated patients and is usually histologically associated with coexisting malignancy such as adenocarcinoma of the colon. An abnormal delayed immune response has also been found in these patients. Fever, diarrhea, hematochezia, and even death have occurred in patients with only intestinal malacoplakia. When visualized at sigmoidoscopy, areas of malacoplakia may vary from soft grayish-tan nodular lesions with serpiginous borders to confluent superficial ulcerations. Correct diagnosis is made from biopsy tissue. Its known high association with colonic adenocarcinoma should prompt evaluation for this possibility.

There is no specific pharmacologic treatment for intestinal malacoplakia. In the urinary bladder the disease has been successfully treated with streptomycin, para-aminosalicylic acid, and isoniazid. Excision or fulguration may be tried for localized disease.

675. MELANOSIS COLI, CATHARTIC COLON, AND SOAP COLITIS

The use of "irritant" purgatives has been associated with at least three colonic abnormalities: *melanosis coli*, *cathartic colon*, and *soap colitis*.

MELANOSIS COLI

Melanosis coli is an abnormal black or brown discoloration of the colonic mucosa which has been compared in appearance to tiger or crocodile skin or cross-section of nutmeg. The discoloration is due to brownish-black pigment in large mononuclear cells or macrophages in the lamina propria of the mucosa. The pigment granules have histochemical staining characteristics of both melanin and lipofuscin. Its exact origin, however, is uncertain.

Melanosis coli appears to result from chronic use of anthracin cathartics in the presence of fecal stasis. The pigment has been noted as soon as four months after the onset of taking cascara preparations and may disappear after the laxative is discontinued.

By itself, melanosis coli produces no specific symptoms and has no known unfavorable long-term prognostic significance. However, a few patients with carcinoma of the colon have also had melanosis coli. It is uncertain how many of them actually took laxatives. Without an accompanying history of anthracin laxative abuse or fecal stasis, the presence of melanosis coli probably warrants radiologic evaluation for an occult colonic neoplasm.

CATHARTIC COLON

Cathartic colon occurs predominantly in women who have taken irritant laxatives (cascara segrada, senna, aloe, podophyllin, castor oil, phenolphthalein, calomel) for a period of at least 15 years. It is a radiologic diagnosis characterized by loss of haustral markings, with lengthy inconstant areas of constriction having long tapering margins. At fluoroscopy, the distensibility of the narrowed segments can be demonstrated, excluding a stricture. The terminal ileum and ascending colon are most commonly involved. The radiologic differential diagnosis includes chronic ulcerative colitis, granulomatous colitis, and amebic colitis. An adequate medical history and examination of the stools for amebae will help exclude these differential possibilities. There should be no history of recent fever, recurrent diarrhea, or the passage of mucus or blood in stool. Treatment is cessation of use of the offending laxative. Bulk-forming and emollient laxatives should be considered if persistent constipation requires treatment.

SOAP COLITIS

The use of cleansing "soapsuds" enemas may produce a spectrum of symptoms from slight discomfort to severe prostration. The colonic mucosal reaction also varies from mild irritation to frank necrosis. Severe reactions have usually occurred in cases in which a concentrated soap solution was administered. Symptoms, which begin within a few hours after the enema, may include severe abdominal cramps, abdominal distention, mucorrhea, and serosanguineous diarrhea. Hypovolemia and acute hemoconcentration can result from rapid exudation of fluid into the colon. Hypokalemia may develop when exudation of colonic mucus is massive. Most patients recover with treatment consisting of close observation, careful replacement of fluid and electrolytes, and possibly administration of broad-spectrum antimicrobial drugs.

676. FECAL IMPACTION AND STERCORAL ULCER

Incomplete evacuation of feces for an extended time may lead to formation of a large firm mass of stool in the rectum and distal colon known as fecal impaction. The large irregular mass of feces cannot be expelled from the dilated rectosigmoid through the disproportionately small anal canal. Fecal impactions most often occur in children who have undiagnosed megacolon or psychiatric problems, in elderly, debilitated, or sedentary persons, and in patients with painful anal disease.

A sensation of rectal fullness, lower abdominal discomfort, headache, mild anorexia with weight loss, and a general sense of ill-being are the most commonly reported symptoms. Liquid stool above the fecal mass can expand the already distended colon and pass around the impaction, thus preventing complete obstruction. Unfortunately, this watery stool is occasionally interpreted as diarrhea, and the patient is improperly treated with constipating agents. The true diagnosis could be easily made by rectal examination.

Small pieces of a large impaction in the rectum should be removed digitally. Thereafter, warm water or saline enemas may then be given as well as mineral oil orally. More proximal sigmoid impactions can be broken up by advancing a large bore rubber tube through a sigmoidoscope into the fecal mass and gently flushing small amounts of water through the tube. Warm oil enemas are unnecessary and may produce burns of the heat-insensitive colonic mucosa. Enemas containing a dilute (5 to 10 per cent) solution of hydrogen peroxide have been used, but this technique risks rupture of an already distended colon by the liberated gas. Dilatation of the anus under anesthesia to allow removal of the impaction is occasionally necessary.

Complications of fecal impaction include urinary tract obstruction, spontaneous perforation of the colon, and stercoral ulcer. Progressive enlargement of the rectosigmoid by the impaction can compress the ureters near the ureterovesical junction or elevate the bladder, producing marked angulation of the urethra. The resulting obstruction may present as symptomatic urinary tract infection.

Spontaneous perforation of the colon in patients with fecal impaction usually occurs during attempts by the patient to pass the fecal mass. Unfortunately, vague lower abdominal pain often precedes physical findings of a perforated viscus by only a few hours. Treatment requires surgical closure of the perforation.

Stercoral ulcers in the rectum and colon likely result from pressure necrosis produced by a large fecal mass. The ulceration has a dark yellow-gray to greenish-purple irregular outline. Microscopically, there is little acute inflammatory reaction around the necrotic center. The ulcer usually heals rapidly after removal of the fecal mass. Chronic stercoral ulcers occasionally can be asymptomatic. Complications are bleeding and perforation. Perforation, occurring either spontaneously or during disimpaction, can result in a localized abscess or suppurative peritonitis.

677. NONSPECIFIC OR SOLITARY ULCER OF THE COLON

Discrete, usually single, ulcerations of unknown cause may develop in any segment of the colon or rectum. The cecum, ascending colon, and rectosigmoid colon are the most frequent locations. Symptoms and clinical course of the ulceration vary, depending on the segment of colon involved. Nonspecific ulceration in the cecum or ascending colon frequently presents with right lower abdominal pain. A tender mass may develop. Gross bleeding is uncommon. The usual initial differential diagnosis includes *appendicitis, pelvic inflammatory disease, ovarian disease,* and *tuberculous* or *idiopathic regional enteritis.* Perforation of the cecum with peritonitis is a frequent complication.

The sigmoid colon is the second most common site of nonspecific ulceration. The diagnosis is seldom made prior to surgery. Chronic lower abdominal pain, recurrent rectal bleeding, and a high incidence of perforation characterize the ulcer in this location. Misdiagnosis of *diverticulitis* is common. An inflammatory mass may develop, and surgery may eventually be required to exclude *carcinoma.*

In contrast to the acute symptoms of nonspecific ulceration elsewhere in the colon, solitary ulcer of the rectum is a more chronic condition which tends to be resistant to therapy. Dull pain in the rectum or left iliac fossa, which is increased during defecation, and the passage of small amounts of bloody mucus with stool are typical symptoms. Massive bleeding is unusual. The shallow rectal ulceration frequently occurs 7 to 10 cm above the anal margin and is usually demarcated from normal mucosa by a narrow area of hyperemia. The lesion may be round, have an irregular outline, or even be linear. A symptomatic preulcer, hyperemic, or "granular" phase can antedate the actual crater.

Multiple biopsies of the ulcer margin will exclude malignancy. Almost all forms of local and systemic therapy have not affected the chronic course of the ulceration. The only certain cure is total excision. However, since perforation is uncommon, treatment with stool softener, local anesthetics, and periodic re-examination is indicated unless symptoms become severe. Spontaneous healing may occur even after many years.

678. NONSPECIFIC ULCERATIVE PROCTITIS

Patients may present with rectal bleeding, tenesmus, and occasionally a mucosanguineous anal discharge and are found to have inflammation of the rectal mucosa with a clearly demarcated upper border above which the mucosa is normal. Histologic changes in tissue from rectal biopsy are usually compatible with ulcerative colitis, but barium enema demonstrates no abnormality of the colon above the rectum. This disease, ulcerative proctitis, appears to be a localized milder form of generalized ulcerative colitis, but with a better prognosis (see Ch. 651). In general, the disease runs a relapsing course without complications, except rectal stricture. Less than 15 per cent of patients with this disease will progress to develop diffuse ulcerative colitis.

679. DISEASES OF THE ANUS

GENERAL CONSIDERATIONS

Functionally, the most important parts of the anus are the neural innervation and muscular elements comprising the internal and external anal sphincters which maintain rectal continence. Anal sphincter dysfunction without perianal disease, a history of prior anal surgery, or evidence of more generalized neurologic disease should prompt evaluation for rectal carcinoma. Although various reconstructive techniques appear to improve some patients with anal incontinence, surgery should be considered only after the cause of sphincter dysfunction has been thoroughly investigated. In general, anal and perianal diseases produce disproportionately great symptoms when compared with the extent of tissue involved. In this chapter, a number of anal diseases are discussed briefly to acquaint the reader with diagnostic possibilities.

HEMORRHOIDS

Hemorrhoids or piles are varicosities of the hemorrhoidal venous plexuses. External hemorrhoids occur below the anorectal line and are covered by pain-sensitive anal skin. Thrombosis or rupture of the vein leads to a small, very tender, tense, bluish lump which can be seen on the outside anal surface. Conservative treatment is usually effective and consists of hot sitz baths, stool softeners, a recumbent position if possible, and avoidance of straining or strenuous work. Small anal skin tags may be left after resolution of the acute process. If the pile ruptures, the clot should be removed or the area excised.

Internal hemorrhoids are varicosities of the superior hemorrhoidal vein above the anorectal line and are covered by relatively pain-insensitive mucosa. These hemorrhoids tend to prolapse during defecation and usually become symptomatic by bleeding. A mucoid anal discharge is common with chronic prolapse and may lead to irritation of the anal skin. Bleeding from hemorrhoids is often noted by the patient as streaks of blood on the outside of stool or on toilet tissue. It is usually intermittent. Prolonged or excessive bleeding can result in iron deficiency and anemia. Use of an astringent suppository and the conservative treatment outlined above are often adequate. Surgical therapy may be indicated for recurrent bleeding, protrusion, thrombosis, ulceration, infection, or coexistent severe pruritus ani. Surgery should be avoided in patients with only moderately symptomatic hemorrhoids who have portal hypertension, incurable cancer, intractable heart disease, or persistent hemorrhoidal symptoms for less than six months post partum. Rectal bleeding should not be attributed to hemorrhoids without complete anorectal examination.

ANORECTAL ABSCESS AND FISTULA IN ANO

Patients with a rapidly developing painful anal mass may have an abscess in the perianal and perirectal tissue. After diagnosis, proper treatment requires surgical drainage. *Perianal abscess* occurs superficially, adjacent to the anal opening and below the anorectal ring. Severe throbbing pain is the major symptom. An *ischiorectal fossa abscess* involves deeper tissue of the buttocks and presents with perirectal discomfort and fever. Digital examination of the lower part of the rectum will demonstrate a tender mass bulging into the lumen. A *submucous abscess* extends upward in the submucous space above the anal valves. It may cause fever and dull rectal pain with no visible perianal abnormality except occasionally a purulent rectal discharge. A *pelvirectal abscess* arises from a primary infection elsewhere in the pelvis and usually presents with systemic toxic symptoms. An *anorectal abscess* may develop as a complication of acute hemorrhoids, an anal fissure, or injections into the anorectal area. A *tuberculous anorectal abscess* often presents as a gradually enlarging perianal or ischiorectal mass with less pain than that caused by a similar acute infection.

After an acute infection in the anorectal area, a chronic suppurative process may develop and form a *fistula in ano.* This fistula is a tract of chronic granulation tissue which connects two epithelial surfaces, either cutaneous or mucosal, and may have several external openings. The main symptom is persistent or intermittent drainage which soils the patient's clothing and leads to soreness and pruritus in the perianal area. Treatment requires complete surgical excision of the fistulous tract.

ANAL FISSURE

An anal fissure is a painful, usually elliptical ulceration of unknown cause which is commonly located posteriorly in the midline of the anal orifice and may extend into the anal canal as far as the pectinate line. Early, the fissure appears as a simple slit in the anal skin, but secondary changes soon develop, the most striking of which is a swelling at the lower end of the fissure known as a sentinel pile. If untreated, the ulceration can "erode" down to the internal sphincter muscle. Chronic spasm of the sphincter and postinflammatory fibrosis can produce a fibrotic, tightly contracted anal opening. Pain, especially with defecation, is the main symptom. Bleeding is usually only modest, but can be severe.

Most fissures heal spontaneously. Dilatation of the spastic sphincter, hot sitz baths, local analgesics, and stool softeners give good results in most cases. When the ulceration is deep enough to expose the sphincter muscle fibers, surgical therapy is usually required.

PRURITUS ANI

Pruritus ani refers to perianal itching which is frequently intense. In early cases, the primary rugae of the anus may be edematous and red. The skin is often moist and macerated. Multiple excoriations are evidence of frequent scratching. Later the perianal skin may become thickened or lichenified and have increased pigmentation. Superficial ulcers may be present, and with extreme chronicity leukoplakia may develop.

In evaluating the cause of pruritus ani, dermatologic abnormalities such as *seborrheic dermatitis, atopic eczema, psoriasis, lichen planus, neurodermatitis,* and *contact dermatitis* must be excluded. Involvement of the perianal skin with fungal or yeast infection, or parasitic infestation such as scabies or pinworm, may produce intense pruritus. Pruritus ani may also complicate many of the so-called surgical diseases of the anus such as *prolapsed hemorrhoids, prolapse of the rectum, benign* or *malignant tumors of the rectum,* or *chronic anal fissure* or *fistula.* An increase in perianal moisture from chronic diarrhea or vaginal discharge may also play a causative role. Finally, many patients with idiopathic pruritus ani have been shown to have an abnormally alkaline anal discharge. This may produce a chemical dermatitis and alter perianal skin resistance to normal bacterial flora.

Treatment of pruritus ani should begin with an exclusion of correctable underlying causes. A large number of idiopathic cases are cured by strict anal hygiene. Anesthetic ointments, abrasive toilet tissue and clothing, constipation or diarrhea, and gas-producing foods should be avoided. The use of bland soap, dusting powders (zinc, starch, or boric acid), and hydrocortisone or betamethasone cream is often helpful. In cases of idiopathic pruritus ani, oral administration of capsules of *Lactobacillus acidophilus* or malt soup extract (Maltsupex) has been shown to normalize the alkaline anal discharge and lead to improvement in symptoms.

ANAL MALIGNANCY

The most common malignant tumor of the anus is *squamous cell carcinoma.* Treatment of this widely metastasizing lesion requires radical surgical excision. *Intraepithelial squamous cell* carcinoma or Bowen's disease may present as an irregular reddish plaque. Wide local excision is usually adequate therapy. *Basal cell carcinoma* of the anus produces a superficial ulcerating lesion. *Paget's disease* may involve the perianal dermal apocrine sweat glands and present as an anal mass. Since both of these tumors do not metastasize widely, excisional biopsy is usually adequate.

Malignant melanomas of the anus are highly lethal, but fortunately rare. Initially, a small melanoma may be interpreted as a hemorrhoid by both patient and physician. Later the tumor becomes more polypoid and tends to ulcerate. Wide excision biopsy of a suspect lesion should be done immediately when the diagnosis is considered. Radical surgery for an advanced melanoma does not seem to improve survival.

PROCTALGIA

There are several conditions in which the main symptom is anorectal pain and for which there is no obvious cause, even after full proctologic examination.

Coccygodynia refers to pain in the coccyx area. This is thought to be due to tonic spasm of the levator ani, coccygeal, and pyriform muscles and to result from trauma to the coccyx. Diagnosis is made by eliciting pain during palpation of these muscles and movement of the coccyx. Treatment consists of improved sitting posture, warm sitz baths, massage of the spastic muscles, and systemic analgesics or tranquilizers which have a muscle relaxant property such as diazepam.

Proctalgia fugax is a rectal pain syndrome which frequently awakens the patient at night and most commonly occurs in young men. Most patients describe the discomfort as a severe cramping rectal pain unassociated with straining efforts. The pain usually lasts 30 to 45 minutes. Spasms of a segment of the levator ani muscle may be the source of the pain, but the true cause is unknown. Various recommended treatments have included hot sitz baths or warm water enemas, passing flatus or stool, sublingual nitroglycerin, and firm pressure upward against the anus. In many patients the symptoms respond to no treatment but resolve spontaneously after a period of months or years.

The *puborectalis syndrome* is characterized by chronic constipation, rectal tenesmus, and pain during and after defecation. This is thought to result from hypertrophy and spasm of the puborectalis muscle sling. Diagnosis is made on rectal examination by finding a constricting tender muscular ring at the upper end of the anus. Conservative treatment includes anal dilatation prior to

defecation and the use of stool softeners. If this treatment is unsuccessful, surgical resection of a small segment of the puborectalis sling is usually curative without producing anal incontinence.

Tumors of the *cauda equina* of the spinal cord may also produce anal pain. Examination of the anus will demonstrate a weak sphincter and a small perianal area of diminished cutaneous sensation. Transient *sigmoidorectal intussusception* may also produce rectal pain which is difficult to diagnose.

Andrade, S., and Andrade, V. H.: Intestinal pneumatosis. Presentation of five cases. Am. J. Proctol., 19:39, 1968.
Epstein, S. E., Ascari, W. A., Ablow, R. C., Seaman, W. B., and Lattis, R.: Colitis cystica profunda. Am. J. Clin. Pathol., 5:186, 1966.
Folley, J. H.: Ulcerative proctitis. N. Engl. J. Med., 282:1362, 1970.
Gear, E. V., and Dobbins, W. O.: III. Rectal biopsy. A review of its diagnostic usefulness. Gastroenterology, 55:552, 1968.
Gray, L. A.: The management of endometriosis involving the bowel. Clin. Obstet. Gynecol., 9:309, 1966.
Lal, S., and Brown, G. N.: Some unusual complications of fecal impaction. Am. J. Proctol., 18:226, 1967.
Lewin, J., Harell, G. S., Lee, A. S., and Crowley, L. G.: Malacoplakia. An electron-microscopic study: Demonstration of bacilliform organisms in malacoplakic macrophages. Gastroenterology, 66:28, 1974.
Madigan, M. R., and Morson, B. C.: Solitary ulcer of the rectum. Gut, 10:871, 1969.
Nelson, S. W.: Extraluminal gas collections due to diseases of the gastrointestinal tract. Am. J. Roentgen., 115:225, 1972.
Pike, B. F., Phillippi, P. J., and Lawson, E. H.: Soap colitis. N. Engl. J. Med., 285:217, 1971.
Ziter, F. M.: Cathartic colon. New York State J. Med., 67:546, 1967.

Section Ten. DISEASES OF THE GALLBLADDER AND BILE DUCTS

Lawrence W. Way

680. INTRODUCTION

Biliary disease in adults includes congenital, metabolic, neoplastic, infectious, and parasitic conditions which cause considerable morbidity and pose challenging diagnostic problems to the clinician. Symptomatic cholelithiasis and its complications alone are responsible for over 300,000 operations in the United States annually, entailing great financial and emotional cost for the affected patients. Fortunately, improvements have recently been made in techniques of diagnosis and therapy, and preliminary findings suggest that even more dramatic advances may soon be made in the treatment of gallstone disease.

Physiology. Bile, an alkaline isotonic fluid (pH 7.8), is a mixture of the secretion of hepatocytes and the duct epithelial cells and has the composition given in Table 1. The volume of bile ranges from 500 to 1500 ml per day, depending on the amount and type of food ingested. The greatest fraction of the bile volume is produced by the hepatocytes and correlates directly with output of bile salts.

Bile salts are synthesized by hepatocytes from cholesterol by a process whose rate-limiting step involves the action of the enzyme 7α-hydroxylase. The two *primary bile salts*, cholate and chenodeoxycholate, are conjugated before secretion with either glycine or taurine to improve solubility. After entering the gut, bile salts aid in fat absorption, and then all but 5 per cent are reabsorbed in the ileum. Those that reach the colon are partially con-

verted by bacteria to the *secondary bile salts*, deoxycholate and lithocholate. Deoxycholate is absorbed and re-excreted in bile; lithocholate, being insoluble, is mostly excreted in the feces. The actual composition of bile is 40 per cent cholate, 40 per cent chenodeoxycholate, 18 per cent deoxycholate, and 2 per cent lithocholate, each conjugated with glycine or taurine in a ratio of 3:1. Other than bile salt, the major solids in bile are cholesterol and phospholipid (mainly lecithin). The close correlation between the output of lecithin and that of bile salt suggests that the former may be leeched from the canalicular membrane by the traversing bile salt molecules. Cholesterol output is largely independent of bile salt.

Normally, only 10 to 20 per cent of the daily hepatic secretion of bile salt consists of newly synthesized molecules, because efficient ileal reabsorption and hepatic re-excretion allow repeated recycling through the *enterohepatic* circulation. In this way the bile salt pool, normally 1.5 to 3.0 grams, passes through the liver and gut more than twice during each meal, producing 6 to 8 cycles daily (i.e., each day about 20 grams of bile salt enters the duodenum). During an average day involving three meals, the bile salt pool is in continuous motion until at night the stomach and bowel are empty and the gallblad-

TABLE 1. Average Composition of Human Gallbladder Bile (Gram/100 ml)

			% Total Solids
Lipids	Bile acids	12.00	
	Lecithin	3.00	91
	Cholesterol	0.50	
	Bilirubin	0.15	
	Protein	0.10	
	Potassium	0.05	9
	Calcium and magnesium	0.06	
	Chloride	0.08	
	Bicarbonate and phosphate	0.04	

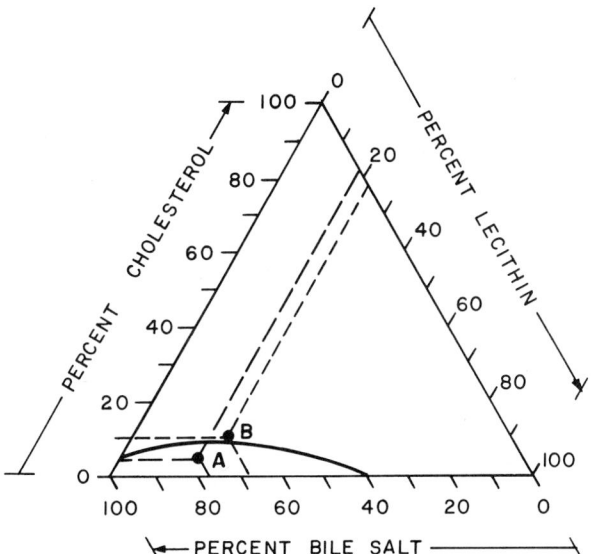

Figure 1. Phase diagram for plotting different mixtures of bile salt, lecithin, and cholesterol. The curved line represents the boundary of the micellar zone for aqueous solutions containing 4 to 10 per cent solids. Any mixture, such as A, falling within this area contains all its cholesterol in solution. Any mixture, such as B, falling outside this area has excess cholesterol as a precipitate or supersaturated solution. The points A and B actually depict the average composition of gallbladder bile obtained by Admirand and Small from normal persons and patients with cholesterol gallstones, respectively.

der fills. Reabsorption in the gut involves a mucosal active transport mechanism located in the terminal 100 cm of ileum. If the efficiency of the enterohepatic conservation is impaired by conditions such as a biliary fistula, Crohn's disease, or ileal resection, hepatic synthesis increases, but the maximal rate of 5 grams per day may be insufficient to restore intraluminal concentrations to normal if external losses exceed this amount.

The second component of bile, the ductular secretion, is generated by an active transport process which is stimulated by secretin, cholecystokinin, and gastrin, with vagal tone acting as a sensitizing influence. Ductular secretion results from active transport of Na^+ and HCO^- and seems to be useful in maintaining the alkalinity of bile.

Under basal conditions, tonic contraction of the sphincter diverts hepatic bile from the common duct into the gallbladder where it is concentrated by active absorption of Na^+, Cl^-, and HCO_3^- and passive return of H_3O. The absorptive mechanism is capable of concentrating gallbladder bile at a rate of 10 per cent of its volume per hour. Concentrations of bile salt may exceed 200 millimoles per liter, and since the gallbladder holds 40 ml, 8 millimoles (equivalent to 3 grams of cholic acid) or the entire bile salt pool can be sequestered here during prolonged fasting.

Cholecystokinin, released from the intestinal mucosa by fat, amino acids, and H^+, stimulates gallbladder contraction and simultaneous relaxation of the choledochal sphincter, emptying the gallbladder contents into the duodenum. Basal pressures in the biliary ducts and gallbladder are 10 to 15 cm H_2O. After eating, gallbladder pressure rises to 25 to 30 cm H_2O, slightly exceeding ductal pressure.

Bile salt molecules are amphophils possessing water-soluble and fat-soluble poles. In an aqueous medium, they are distributed randomly, until a critical concentration (about 2 millimolar) is reached, at which point spontaneous aggregation forms multimolecular structures called *micelles*. In micelles, the bile salt molecules line up with their hydrophilic portions facing the solvent (water) and their hydrophobic portions facing centrally. The hydrocarbon center of the micelle can incorporate biliary lecithin and cholesterol, and the entire aggregate remains water soluble. The addition of lecithin, a water-soluble compound, enhances the ability of bile salt micelles to incorporate other lipids. The ultimate cholesterol-carrying capacity of bile depends on the relative amounts of bile salt and lecithin (Fig. 1).

Pathogenesis of Cholesterol Gallstones. In Western cultures cholesterol is the principal ingredient (comprising over 50 per cent of total solids) of more than 90 per cent of gallstones, the remaining 10 per cent consisting mostly of bilirubin pigment stones in patients with hemolytic disease. In general terms an excess of cholesterol in bile seems to be a prerequisite, which in theory

could result either from diminished cholesterol holding capacity (bile salt and lecithin) or increased cholesterol concentrations.

Gallstones affect three times as many women as men, the differences beginning at puberty and declining somewhat in later years. This fact, combined with the higher incidence with multiparity and an apparently greater incidence in women who take birth control pills, suggests that female sex hormones may be partly responsible. In the United States the incidence in blacks, whites, and American Indians doubles in a stepwise fashion, so that at the upper extreme about 75 per cent of American Indian women over age 25 and 90 per cent of those over age 60 are affected.

Figure 1 is a phase diagram on which any aqueous mixture of bile salt, lecithin, and cholesterol can be represented by a point indicating the molar percentage each contributes to total solids. By in vitro testing, an area of the triangle (lower left) can be identified where cholesterol of the various combinations exists in stable micellar solution. Outside this area cholesterol forms a supersaturated solution or precipitates. The particular micellar zone depicted in Figure 1 pertains to solutions ranging from 4 to 10 per cent solids, which is comparable to bile.

Plotted on this diagram, bile from patients with gallstones tends to have relatively more cholesterol than that from normal persons, and simultaneous sampling from the gallbladder and hepatic ducts of patients with gallstones shows that bile is supersaturated as it emerges from the liver, implicating the hepatocytes rather than the gallbladder as the cause of the abnormality. Gallstone patients also have a total bile salt pool of 1.0 to 1.5 grams, about half the size of normal, and preliminary data indicate the presence of reduced amounts of the enzyme 7α-hydroxylase in their hepatocytes. These findings suggested the presence of diminished secretory rates of bile salts, but the few available measurements are conflicting; in one report, female American Indian patients had lower outputs, but in another (female whites) it was normal, presumably owing to more rapid recycling of the small pool.

The independence of cholesterol and bile salt output means that when bile salt secretion drops, the cholesterol:bile salt ratio climbs and the bile assumes greater lithogenicity. These observations appear to explain the shift in bile composition observed during fasting, a state that physiologically mimics interruption of the enterohepatic circulation. Instead of entering the gut, the bile salts during fasting become sequestered in the gallbladder, hepatic secretion drops, cholesterol secretion persists, and the bile becomes more lithogenic. Evidently supersaturation produced in this way is rather common in humans regardless of the presence of gallstones.

Therefore lowered micellar capacity caused by a scarcity of bile salt and lecithin has been demonstrated. One report on American Indian women also implicates abnormally high biliary cholesterol secretion, a consequence of obesity. So far neither men nor white women with gallstones, whether obese or not, seem to produce greater cholesterol than controls.

The aforementioned observations account for the production of lithogenic bile but do not explain why all persons with abnormal bile do not develop stones, why stone formation occurs mainly in the gallbladder, and why cholecystectomy is curative. Obviously, the gallbladder

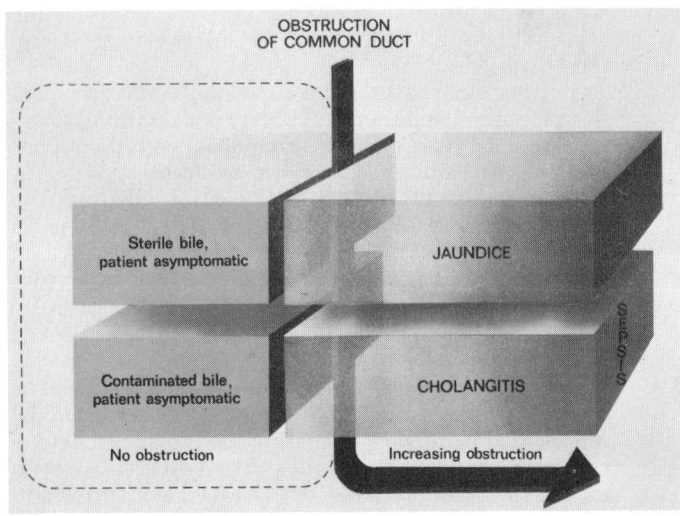

Figure 2. In the absence of obstruction there are no symptoms or active infection from bacterial contamination of bile. Obstruction, indicated by the arrow, produces either jaundice alone or cholangitis, depending on the original bacteriologic status of the duct.

possesses a critical role in the genesis of gallstones, possibly by supplying a nidus for crystallization (a small particle of bile pigment or mucoprotein can be found in the center of most stones), a mucoprotein lattice for further cholesterol deposition and stone growth, and an area of stasis to facilitate precipitation. Apparently the more supersaturated the bile, as in American Indian women, the more likely it is that gallstones will develop, but other initiating factors with quantitative importance must be postulated in any comprehensive theory on the pathogenesis of gallstones.

Dissolution of Gallstones by Chenodeoxycholic Acid. In preliminary experiments chenodeoxycholate given orally, 20 mg per kilogram per day, to patients with radiolucent gallbladder stones has partially or completely dissolved the stones within one to two years in a majority of cases. This treatment caused the bile to become unsaturated by lowering cholesterol output rather than by expanding the bile salt pool and increasing bile salt excretion (the expected mechanism). Other observations were that cholic acid had no beneficial effect, radiopaque gallstones were mostly resistant, and, after interruption of therapy gallstones returned in several patients. A nationwide clinical trial to determine the efficacy and safety of this treatment is in progress. Of concern is the possibility that lithocholate formed from chenodeoxycholate might damage the liver or that prolonged consumption of bile salts will interfere with endogenous cholesterol degradation. The potential impact of this or some analogous approach to curing cholesterol gallstones is certainly very great, but at this time treatment with chenodeoxycholic acid can only be justified within the framework of a clinical experiment.

Pathophysiology of Gallstone Disease. Obstruction caused by a stone is the primary cause of the manifestations of gallstone disease. By distending the gallbladder, blockage of the cystic duct produces biliary colic, and if the obstruction is unrelieved, acute cholecystitis may ensue. The intermediary steps leading from obstruction to acute inflammation are discussed later in more detail. The complications of empyema, perforation, and hydrops of the gallbladder develop, depending on whether a foothold is gained by secondarily invading bacteria. From the therapeutic standpoint, cholecystectomy cures cholecystitis, but it is important to appreciate that cholecys-

tostomy, which only relieves the obstruction, eliminates all the clinical manifestations of the disease.

An analogous situation holds for choledocholithiasis, in which obstruction is the key to all that follows. Pain, jaundice, pruritus, infection, and biliary cirrhosis are all dependent on the block to bile flow and, as with the gallbladder, surgical procedures which decompress the duct upstream from the stone allow acute symptoms to subside. The situation in the ductal system differs importantly from that in the gallbladder, because when ductal pressure exceeds about 25 cm per H_2O, bile is refluxed from the smallest ductules into hepatic venous blood. Pressures in this range and even higher are commonly produced by mechanical obstruction and are probably aggravated by infection. Regurgitation of ductal bacteria into the systemic circulation explains why the typical attack of cholangitis is accompanied by chills, positive blood cultures, and high fever. Fortunately, obstruction by calculus is rarely complete, because the combination of high-grade obstruction and infection (as in suppurative cholangitis) produces catastrophic sepsis (Fig. 2). It is also fortuitous that neoplasms, which uniformly give almost complete obstruction, occur most often in patients with sterile bile.

With unrelieved ductal obstruction, biliary cirrhosis gradually develops. About three months is the fastest that cirrhosis occurs; as might be expected, the earliest cases follow neoplastic (high-grade) obstruction. On the average, biliary cirrhosis from choledocholithiasis or biliary stricture takes five and seven years, respectively.

681. ROENTGENOLOGIC EXAMINATION

Because biliary disease usually results from obstructive lesions, radiologic techniques, if successful in outlining the system, are often diagnostic. Direct and indirect methods are available, and the diagnostic clinical strategy often revolves around the choice and timing of these procedures.

Plain roentgenograms can demonstrate the 10 to 15 per cent of gallstones which contain sufficient calcium to be radiopaque, but their relationship to the ductal system is not always obvious. Emphysematous cholecystitis, air in the bile ducts, and calcium in the wall of the gallbladder also have diagnostic appearances on plain films.

For *oral cholecystography,* the patient swallows tablets of iopanoic or tyropanoic acid, which are then absorbed from the gut, excreted in bile, and concentrated in the gallbladder. Films are exposed about 12 hours after the drug is taken. If the gallbladder is opacified, stones in its lumen are shown as radiolucent defects (Fig. 3). The gallbladder may not be visualized if the drug is not taken, if absorption by the gut or excretion by the liver is faulty, if the cystic duct is blocked, or if the diseased gallbladder mucosa cannot concentrate the bile. Oral cholecystography is the simplest and least expensive way of verifying gallstone disease in patients without acute symptoms. If hepatic and intestinal function are normal, nonvisualization is 95 per cent reliable in indicating gallbladder disease.

Intravenous cholangiography (IVC) relies on hepatic excretion of intravenously injected sodium or methylglucamine iodipamide in a concentration sufficient for ductal opacification. The procedure is used principally to identify common duct stones in patients who previously had a cholecystectomy and to verify acute cholecystitis when the findings of a normal duct and nonvisualized gallbladder are diagnostic. The disadvantage of intravenous cholangiography is that even with perfect liver function the concentration of contrast medium in bile is

Figure 4. Retrograde cholangiopancreatogram, showing a large gallstone in a dilated common duct and a normal pancreatic duct. (Courtesy of Dr. Jack Vennes.)

barely above the threshold level; tomography must be used routinely, and, even so, false negative results are common in the search for choledocholithiasis. When the bilirubin exceeds 3.0 mg per 100 ml, the study is rarely successful and, because of its high cost and the occasional allergic reaction, should usually be deferred.

Transhepatic cholangiography is obtained by direct percutaneous puncture of an intrahepatic duct by a needle inserted through the eighth or ninth right intercostal space into the center of the liver. An abnormal clotting mechanism, ascites, and severe cholangitis are contraindications. If a duct is entered, water-soluble contrast medium is injected through the needle, and roentgenograms are obtained. Transhepatic cholangiography has proved particularly valuable in diagnosing biliary stricture and neoplastic obstruction of the bile ducts. A technically successful study is correlated with the size of the ducts, and only rarely can useful films be obtained in a condition such as sclerosing cholangitis.

Retrograde endoscopic cholangiography, involving cannulation of the ampulla of Vater via the duodenoscope, is a recently developed technique which will probably supplant transhepatic cholangiography in most instances, because it obviates the potential for bleeding from the hepatic puncture site (Fig. 4). With experience, the duct can be entered successfully in 90 per cent of attempts. Concomitant pancreatography is often possible, and in fact pancreatitis is a complication to be avoided by controlling the pressure of injection.

682. ASYMPTOMATIC GALLSTONES

In the absence of a population survey to determine the prevalence of gallstones, the exact percentage of asymp-

Figure 3. Oral cholecystogram, showing gallstones. In this case the stones are considerably less distinct on the supine than on the upright film (inset), where they float as a layer.

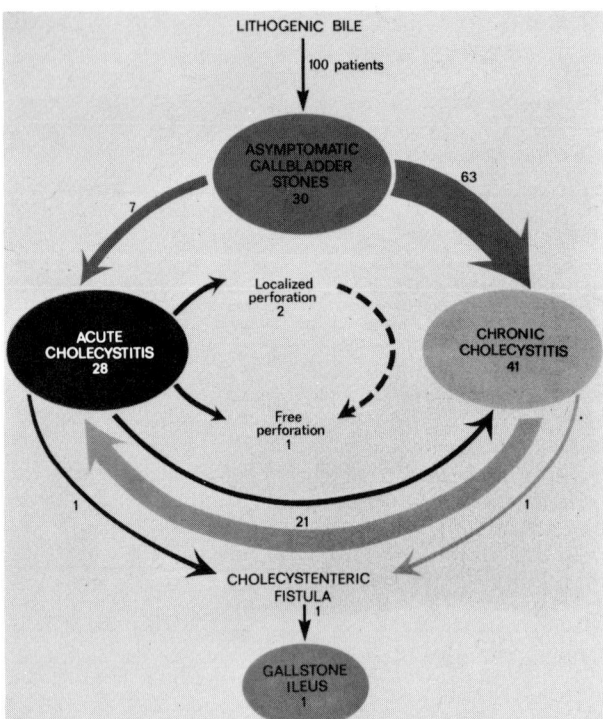

Figure 5. Natural history of cholecystolithiasis. The four ovals represent the major clinical syndromes, and the numbers represent the percentage of those operated on for each diagnosis. About 30 per cent remain asymptomatic.

tomatic stones, estimated now at 30 to 50 per cent of all cases, can only be guessed at (Fig. 5). Since the mortality of gallstone disease with the present plan of management, i.e., essentially treating only those patients with symptoms, is reasonably low, with a few exceptions asymptomatic patients should be followed expectantly and surgery advised only if symptoms develop. The asymptomatic patients for whom prophylactic cholecystectomy is recommended are (1) diabetics, because their mortality from acute cholecystitis is 10 to 15 per cent; (2) patients with nonfunctioning gallbladders or large (more than 2 cm diameter) stones, because their incidence of complications is considerably higher; and (3) patients with calcified gallbladders, because this change is so often associated with carcinoma of the gallbladder. Altogether these groups comprise less than half of the patients with asymptomatic gallstones. Confidence in the safety of expectant management is bolstered by knowing that at least three quarters of the asymptomatic patients who later develop symptoms will first experience episodes of biliary colic, and at that point cholecystectomy can still be performed electively.

683. CHRONIC CHOLECYSTITIS

The term chronic cholecystitis might be used to refer to any gallbladder, not acutely inflamed, which contains gallstones, or it might denote exclusively the presence of chronic inflammation. In actual practice,

chronic cholecystitis describes the *clinical* condition of symptomatic (nonacute) cholecystolithiasis. Chronic cholecystitis without gallstones is even less common than acute acalculous cholecystitis.

Two somewhat overlapping groups of patients are included in this category, depending on the occurrence of a previous attack of acute cholecystitis. In *primary chronic cholecystitis* the gallbladder appears grossly normal, the mucosa is slightly thinned, and the wall contains minor amounts of patchy scarring and cellular infiltration. Oral cholecystograms nearly always visualize the gallbladder and its stones. Symptoms tend to be vague, such as flatulence or food intolerance, and they sometimes persist after cholecystectomy.

In *secondary chronic cholecystitis* the gallbladder has been affected one or more times by acute cholecystitis. Signs of the resolved inflammatory disease consist of thickening of the wall by scar, adhesions to adjacent viscera, and patchy replacement of the mucosa by granulation tissue or collagen. In advanced cases the gallbladder may be so shrunken as to be almost unrecognizable. Nonvisualization is frequent on oral cholecystograms, biliary colic is the principal symptom, and relief is more predictable after cholecystectomy.

In about 5 per cent of patients with primary chronic cholecystitis, *cholesterolosis* gives the mucosal surface a streaked appearance, a condition which has been called "strawberry gallbladder." The changes are due to cholesterol located within clusters of large foamy macrophages in the submucosa. Cholesterolosis is seen occasionally without gallstones, but whether this situation gives symptoms is debated. That some patients become asymptomatic after removal of gallbladders which show only cholesterolosis is well documented, but it is also obvious that in most instances the condition is asymptomatic in the absence of gallstones.

Clinical Manifestations. The most specific symptom of chronic cholecystitis is biliary colic, a constant, severe, cramplike pain located in the epigastrium or right upper quadrant. It is caused by gallbladder contraction during obstruction of the cystic duct by a gallstone. Onset of pain takes only a few minutes; it quickly reaches a plateau in intensity and after an hour or two subsides more gradually. Even after the acute episode has resolved, a vague residual ache or soreness may remain. The absence of tenderness, muscular guarding, a palpable mass, fever, and leukocytosis distinguishes biliary colic from acute cholecystitis. Many patients have referred pain in the back at the level of the scapula. Vomiting may accompany the attack.

Considerably less reliable from the diagnostic standpoint are dyspepsia, fatty food intolerance, flatulence, and belching. Although these symptoms may be the result of chronic cholecystitis, they are often found in persons with normal gallbladders. The common occurrence of these complaints in the general population explains why cholecystectomy often fails to relieve them.

Hydrops, in which the lumen of the gallbladder contains mucus and gallstones, occasionally develops directly from chronic cholecystitis after cystic duct obstruction unaccompanied by acute inflammation. Hydrops produces constant discomfort in the right upper quadrant and a palapable mass without the clinical findings of acute cholecystitis.

Oral cholecystograms will demonstrate the gallstones in patients with primary chronic cholecystitis, but in secondary cholecystitis the gallbladder is often not visualized. In this case, a second examination should be performed; if nonvisualization persists and liver function and intestinal absorption are normal, significant gallbladder disease can be inferred. Because of the expense and risks of allergic reactions, an intravenous cholecystogram is not usually warranted for studying every patient with a nonvisualized gallbladder, but should be ordered selectively in puzzling cases.

Differential Diagnosis. The other common causes of chronic abdominal symptoms, such as *peptic ulcer* and *pancreatitis,* must be investigated in patients suspected of having chronic cholecystitis. Radicular pain from *spinal lesions* may mimic biliary colic, and vertebral films or, in some instances, myelograms of the T6-T8 segment may be indicated. *Angina pectoris* may cause pain thought to be abdominal, just as biliary colic may be felt in the precordial region. Postprandial pain or discomfort may result from the *irritable colon syndrome* or from *adenocarcinoma* of the *right colon.* Tragic delays in treatment have resulted from attributing pain from colonic carcinoma to gallstones.

Treatment. Dietary changes, anticholinergics, and antacids have no effect on the course of the disease but sometimes provide symptomatic relief for a while. Cholecystectomy is the treatment of choice. Cholecystolithotomy was tried at one time in patients whose gallbladders were normal in function and appearance, but gallstones recurred in most within a few years of surgery. At operation the common bile duct is inspected visually, operative cholangiograms are obtained, and the common duct is explored if there is evidence of choledocholithiasis.

Complications. *Choledocholithiasis* is the most common complication, affecting about 15 per cent of patients with cholecystolithiasis. The incidence of common duct stones increases with advancing age.

Mirizzi's syndrome results from gradual extrusion of a large gallstone from the gallbladder into the common duct. The cystic duct enlarges to accommodate the advancing stone, which eventually comes to reside in a common cavity comprising the residual gallbladder lumen, cystic duct, and common duct. Obstructive jaundice may develop.

About two thirds of patients with *acute cholecystitis* have previously had symptomatic chronic cholecystitis. The complication of acute cholecystitis is more common in the elderly and in patients with large gallstones.

Calcification of the *gallbladder,* relatively uncommon in acute and chronic cholecystitis, is of special significance because of its frequent association with carcinoma of the gallbladder. Whether it can be considered truly premalignant is not clear. The diagnosis is usually obvious when the abdominal x-ray shows an eggshell rim of calcium in the gallbladder wall.

Adenocarcinoma of the *gallbladder* is found mainly in elderly patients with cholelithiasis, most of whom have had biliary symptoms for many years. Since carcinoma of the gallbladder affects less than 1 per cent of patients with symptomatic cholelithiasis, it is hard to argue forcibly for early cholecystectomy just to prevent tumor.

Prognosis. Cholecystectomy predictably relieves biliary colic but is only 80 per cent successful in eradicating other types of preoperative complaints (e.g., dyspepsia or flatulence). Loss of the gallbladder does not impair gastrointestinal function.

The mortality of elective cholecystectomy is under 0.5 per cent, and most of the postoperative deaths follow cardiac and respiratory complications in elderly patients with pre-existing disease of these organs. The *postcholecystectomy syndrome* is discussed in Ch. 693.

684. ACUTE CHOLECYSTITIS

The patient with acute cholecystitis usually presents with acute right subcostal pain and tenderness. Obstruction of the cystic duct by a gallstone is usually the cause, and cholelithiasis is present in 95 per cent of patients. A variety of caustic agents produce cholecystitis when injected into gallbladders of animals, but the relation of this type of experiment to the human disease is obscure. More pertinent is the observation that when the gallbladder of dogs was filled with concentrated bile, obstruction of the cystic duct produced acute inflammation, presumably an effect of the bile salts. In control experiments, if the gallbladder was empty or distended with physiologic saline solution instead of bile, cystic duct obstruction was innocuous.

As in other biliary diseases, bacterial infection is secondary to the obstruction rather than a primary factor. Bacteria are present as contaminants in the gallbladders of about 25 per cent of patients with chronic cholecystitis. Early in acute cholecystitis the bile is positive in 50 per cent of the cases, but within a week after onset this figure reaches 90 per cent. Although infection is secondary, it is ultimately responsible for the most serious sequelae of acute cholecystitis—empyema and perforation.

Acalculous cholecystitis, accounting for 5 per cent of cases, is more common in men and in patients with unrelated sepsis. Many cases have been associated with prolonged fasting after major trauma, e.g., war injuries or surgical operations remote from the biliary system. At operation the bile is viscous and full of sludge. Perforation is more frequent, and the outcome is generally worse than in gallstone cholecystitis.

Primary gallbladder infection by *Salmonella typhosa* was responsible for cases of acalculous cholecystitis years ago when typhoid fever was more prevalent. *Polyarteritis nodosa* has occasionally been implicated.

Pathology. Subserosal edema, mucosal ulcerations, and submucosal hemorrhages are the earliest pathologic findings. The inflammatory process usually evolves slowly in contrast to that in appendicitis or diverticulitis, probably because the bacterial population within the gallbladder is relatively sparse at the moment of ductal obstruction. Cellular infiltration of the wall becomes prominent only after three to four days, reaching its greatest intensity at the end of the first week. During the second week, patchy mural gangrene and small intramural abscesses appear, the edema becomes organized, and the first signs of collagen deposition appear. Resolution of the acute changes takes another week or more.

The term *empyema* denotes a pus-filled gallbladder which clinically is characterized by a septic form of acute cholecystitis. On gross examination the condtion tends to be overdiagnosed, because gallbladder mucus containing precipitated calcium closely resembles pus. *Gangrene* and *perforation* are most common in the fundus where the blood supply is meager, or in the infundibulum where stones impact. With perforation, gallbladder contents may spill into the free abdominal cavity (bile peritonitis) or be confined by adhesions (pericholecystic abscess). Sometimes an adherent viscus is penetrated, making a *cholecystenteric fistula* through which the gallstones and pus may be discharged. If a large gallstone reaches the intestine and blocks its lumen, the presenting complaints are those of small bowel obstruction, i.e., *gallstone ileus*.

Chronic obstruction of the cystic duct causes *hydrops* (mucocele), a condition in which the gallbladder is distended with uninfected mucus (white bile). Hydrops may result either from resolved acute cholecystitis or from obstruction without inflammation.

Clinical Manifestations and Diagnosis. The attack begins with abdominal pain that mounts gradually in severity. The pain is usually located in the right subcostal region from the start, but sometimes begins in the epigastrium or left upper quadrant and then shifts to the region of the gallbladder as inflammation progresses. Two thirds or more of patients have had previous attacks of biliary colic. Early in the attack the patient may expect the symptoms to subside spontaneously as had happened before with similar pains, and medical aid is often not sought until 48 hours or more. Referred pain may be experienced in the back at the scapular level.

Anorexia, nausea, and vomiting are present in the average case, but the vomiting is rarely severe enough to be confused with bowel obstruction and is generally less than in acute pancreatitis. In the absence of complications, chills are rare; their presence should always suggest suppurative cholecystitis or associated cholangitis. Fever is also moderate, reaching an average temperature of 38° C in the absence of complications.

The right subcostal region is tender to palpation, and involuntary muscle spasm generally exists which limits the examination. If the patient takes a deep breath while the subhepatic area is being palpated, tenderness is suddenly worse and inspiratory arrest is produced *(Murphy's sign)*.

In somewhat more than a third of the patients, a distended, tender gallbladder can be felt as a distinct mass, usually located farther to the right than the normal gallbladder. The presence of the palpable gallbladder is an important finding which clinches the diagnosis in an otherwise typical case. The gallbladder cannot be felt in the rest of the patients because of obesity, rigidity of the abdominal wall, or a deep subhepatic location, or because it is small and shrunken from previous inflammation. Other related conditions characterized by a tender mass in the same area are *pericholecystic abscess*, acute cholecystitis complicating *carcinoma* of the *gallbladder, torsion* of the *gallbladder,* or the rare case of gallbladder distention in *obstructive cholangitis* (e.g., suppurative cholangitis or Oriental cholangiohepatitis).

About 20 per cent of patients with acute cholecystitis are slightly jaundiced. This is sometimes due only to edema of the nearby common duct; however, two thirds of jaundiced patients will have a mechanical cause such as *common duct stones* or, less often, a *biliary tumor*.

After hospitalization, improvement is usually noticeable within the first 12 to 24 hours, and the signs and symptoms gradually subside over five to seven days.

Oral feedings can usually be resumed after a few days. Persistent severe pain after hospitalization, a rise in temperature or leukocyte count, development of shaking chills, or the appearance of more severe local or generalized abdominal tenderness all indicate progression of the disease and suggest the need for emergency operation.

Empyema can produce systemic toxicity and may herald perforation. After empyema develops, if the infection is subsequently controlled with antimicrobial drugs, the large tender gallbladder may remain palpable for several weeks, and return of well-being is similarly prolonged. The leukocyte count is 10,000 to 15,000 per μl or even higher with complications. Mild rises in bilirubin, alkaline phosphatase, and SGOT are frequent.

Roentgenograms of the abdomen may show calcified gallstones or an enlarged gallbladder. Oral cholecystograms will not visualize during an acute attack and are diagnostically unreliable because of unpredictable absorption and excretion of the contrast agent. Except in patients who become asymptomatic rapidly, oral cholecystograms should not be scheduled until four to six weeks after the attack; the rate of nonvisualization remains high even then.

Intravenous cholangiograms (IVC) may give useful information and should be ordered when diagnostic uncertainty remains, liver function is good, and more information would be useful for clinical management. This situation usually occurs in a patient for whom early operation would be appropriate, but an enlarged gallbladder is not palpable on physical examination. If on IVC the gallbladder fills, the diagnosis of acute cholecystitis is essentially excluded; if the ductal system is demonstrated but the gallbladder does not opacify, the diagnosis is confirmed. More difficult to interpret is the situation in which neither gallbladder nor ducts are shown. If the bilirubin level is normal and the upper abdominal pain and tenderness are typical, most such patients will turn out to have acute cholecystitis exactly as suspected.

Differential Diagnosis. *Acute pancreatitis, acute appendicitis,* and *perforated peptic ulcer* are the conditions which most often cause major diagnostic problems. Diagnosis is complicated by the fact that in acute cholecystitis the serum amylase may rise to 1000 per 100 ml or more. Acute cholecystitis and acute pancreatitis may coexist, and intravenous cholangiography can be quite helpful in these situations, because visualization of the gallbladder is expected in acute pancreatitis.

In women, gonococcal perihepatitis *(Fitz-Hugh-Curtis syndrome)* may be mistaken for acute cholecystitis, but adnexal tenderness is usually present on pelvic examination, a cervical smear usually reveals gonococci, and the patients are younger, often have higher fever, and are in less distress than would be expected in cholecystitis. Shoulder pain and a friction rub over the liver, common in the Fitz-Hugh–Curtis syndrome, are not found in uncomplicated acute cholecystitis.

Acute hepatitis, either *viral* or *alcoholic,* sometimes produces marked right upper quadrant pain and tenderness. A history of recent binge drinking, high SGOT levels, and liver biopsy aid differentiation. *Pneumonitis, pyelonephritis,* and *cardiac disease* have all on occasion produced acute pain suggestive of cholecystitis.

Treatment. Most patients with acute cholecystitis will improve with either expectant treatment or cholecystectomy performed during the acute attack. In general, the decision regarding the type of treatment should include

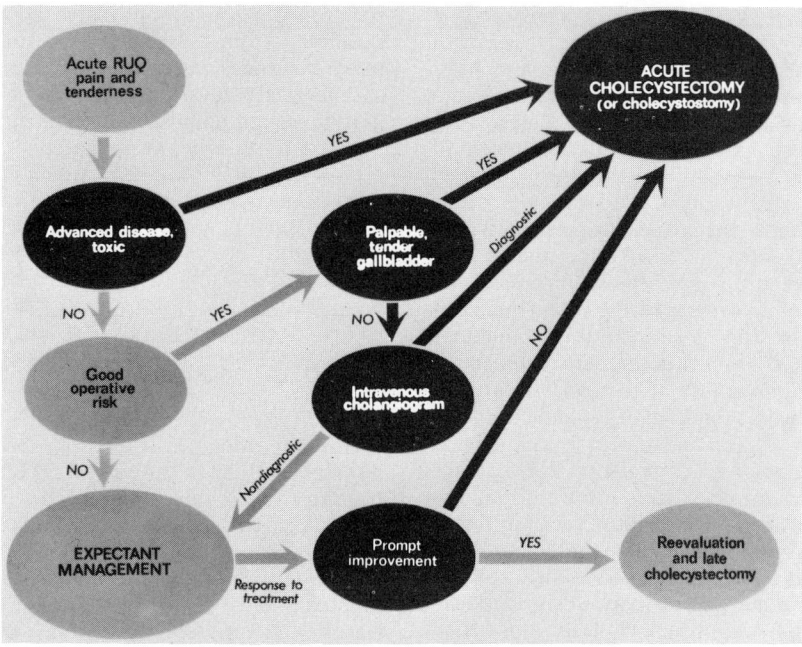

Figure 6. Algorithm for managing patients with acute right upper quadrant pain and tenderness, thought to have acute cholecystitis.

the following factors (Fig. 6): (1) whether the diagnosis is secure, (2) whether biliary complications have occurred or appear imminent, and (3) the over-all condition of the patient (operative risk).

Upon admission to the hospital, nasogastric suction should be started and fluid requirements given intravenously. Vomiting and fasting before hospitalization often cause dehydration which must be corrected. In many elderly patients, the acute biliary condition has aggravated pre-existing cardiac, pulmonary, or renal disease, and these systems must be evaluated and treated appropriately. Diabetes must be sought, because it is associated with a more ominous prognosis if surgery is delayed.

If the patient is first seen shortly after symptoms began, and if local signs and symptoms are mild, antimicrobial therapy need not be given. It is of more value later in the disease, especially for suppurative complications. Ampicillin, cephalosporin, or tetracycline is adequate, except in patients with empyema or perforation in whom cephalosporin plus gentamicin or kanamycin would be preferable.

Supported now by the results of controlled clinical trials, most experts advocate cholecystectomy during the acute attack, an approach which avoids the complications and prolonged morbidity of expectant treatment. This does not imply an emergency operation. The workup should proceed deliberately to confirm the diagnosis and to prepare the patient by procedures such as correcting fluid deficits. Cholecystectomy should then be scheduled for the next routine operating day.

In about 30 per cent of cases, the patient is a good surgical risk, the diagnosis is obvious within 12 to 24 hours, and cholecystectomy can be scheduled promptly. Another 30 per cent are good surgical candidates, but the gallbladder cannot be felt. In this situation the diagnosis should be regarded as tentative, because 10 to 15 per cent of patients whose only finding is tenderness will

have some other condition. An IVC should be performed preoperatively to verify the clinical impression.

Another third of patients will have serious coexistent cardiac, respiratory, or other disease whose treatment takes precedence. The cholecystitis should be treated expectantly while correcting the other problems. Progression of local abdominal findings requires continued reevaluation, balancing the risks of operation with the risks of continued delay.

About 10 per cent of patients require emergency surgery for complications present on admission or which appear later during observation and medical management. When emergency operation becomes necessary, *cholecystostomy* may be preferable to cholecystectomy in the seriously ill patient. In this procedure, the fundus is incised, stones and pus are removed from the lumen, and a catheter secured in the lumen is brought out through the abdominal wall and placed to gravity drainage. As in draining any abscess, this procedure allows the acute infection to resolve. Patients who recover should usually have a cholecystectomy six to eight weeks later. Those who continue to be poor surgical risks may be followed expectantly if postoperative cholecystography shows that the gallbladder and common duct contain no residual stones. If stones are present, surgery will be needed to avoid further acute attacks. In seriously ill patients, the cholecystostomy tube can be left in place indefinitely.

Recent experience suggests that postoperatively it is sometimes possible to extract residual gallbladder or common duct stones with flexible forceps or snares passed through the cholecystostomy fistula. The procedure is difficult to perform, and success is unpredictable.

After the cholecystostomy tube is removed from a patient whose biliary system contains no calculi, within the first year about 50 per cent of patients develop new stones and additional symptoms. Recurrent disease is less common after one year.

Complications. In *emphysematous cholecystitis,* a variant of acute cholecystitis, gas of bacterial origin can be seen in the gallbladder lumen and adjacent tissues. Clinically, emphysematous cholecystitis causes the same signs and symptoms as acute cholecystitis. Men are affected twice as frequently as women, about 30 per cent of patients have diabetes mellitus, and the gallbladder is acalculous in about half the cases. Gas does not occur until 24 to 48 hours after the attack begins, at which time a radiolucent halo outlines the lumen and an air-fluid level may be seen on upright films. Subserosal and then pericholecystic emphysema develop with time. Differential diagnosis of the x-ray findings includes *cholecystenteric fistula, appendiceal* or *subhepatic abscess,* and, rarely, *lipomatosis* of the *gallbladder.* In about half the cases the gas-forming organisms are clostridia, and the rest are *E. coli,* streptococci, and others. Treatment is the same as for acute cholecystitis in general, but the somewhat more aggressive nature of emphysematous cholecystitis and the association with diabetes mellitus mean that prompt surgery is usually required.

Empyema and *perforation* are usually manifested by greater sepsis and more marked abdominal signs. Perforation may take any of three forms: (1) free perforation into the abdominal cavity, (2) localized (contained) perforation with pericholecystic abscess, and (3) perforation into another viscus with fistula formation.

Free perforation, which has a 25 per cent mortality, is fortunately the least common type. It usually occurs early in the attack, often within the first three days, suggesting that when gangrene develops this quickly it cannot be walled off by adjacent viscera. Clinically, free perforation causes toxicity with high temperatures (greater than 39° C), leukocytosis over 15,000 per μl, and diffuse abdominal tenderness and rigidity. In more than half the cases, the correct diagnosis is unsuspected until laparotomy or autopsy, because a clear-cut history of preliminary right upper quadrant pain is often lacking. Treatment consists of intravenous antimicrobial therapy and emergency laparotomy with cholecystectomy.

Localized perforation most often appears in the second week of the attack at the peak of the inflammatory reaction. The diagnosis should be suspected with increasing local signs, especially when a mass suddenly appears. In most cases cholecystectomy can be performed; but in the severely ill patient, cholecystostomy and drainage of the abscess is the wiser procedure.

Fistula formation usually involves the nearby second portion of the duodenum or, less commonly, the colon, jejunum, stomach, or common bile duct. Rare fistulas have entered the renal pelvis or bronchus, or through the abdominal wall (empyema necessitatis). After intestinal fistulization the contents of the gallbladder are discharged into the gut, often aborting the acute attack. Clinically, the fistula itself may not be suspected, because it produces no unique findings; many are discovered incidentally during a later cholecystectomy. In the absence of biliary obstruction a cholecystenteric communication is not necessarily of pathophysiologic significance. Cholecystocolonic fistulas may cause malabsorption from diversion of bile, or from heavy bacterial contamination of the upper gut. If a particularly large gallstone enters through the fistula, it may obstruct the intestine, a condition called *gallstone ileus* (see Ch. 685).

Prognosis. The mortality of 5 to 10 per cent is almost confined to patients over 60 years of age with serious associated disease. Suppurative complications are more common in the elderly who can tolerate them least. In most instances, localized perforation can be managed satisfactorily at operation. Free perforation is considerably more ominous (25 per cent mortality), but is rare.

In patients who are treated expectantly, recurrent biliary symptoms are so common that an elective cholecystectomy should be planned in most cases. Another acute attack is not unusual during the month or two of waiting.

685. GALLSTONE ILEUS

Gallstone ileus is intestinal obstruction caused by a gallstone lodged in the intestinal lumen. The stone, passing through a cholecystenteric fistula, most often enters the gut in the duodenum, less commonly the jejunum, ileum, colon, or stomach. Although it is usually assumed that the initial event responsible for fistula formation is an attack of acute cholecystitis, only 30 per cent of patients with gallstone ileus give a history of recent right upper quadrant pain, and usually the clinical picture is that of bowel obstruction only.

After entering the gut, the gallstone moves downstream until is becomes too large for the intestinal lumen to accommodate. Obstruction is usually caused by gallstones over 2.5 cm in diameter, and because the lumen becomes progressively smaller aborally, the ileum is the final point of obturation in most cases. Typically, the patient's symptoms are intermittent at first as the stone transiently obstructs at various points and then dislodges, passing further along. This has been termed "tumbling obstruction," the brief periods of respite sometimes leading patient and physician to expect a spontaneous resolution of the symptoms. Eventually, however, vomiting, pain, and distention persist.

If the stone lodges in the duodenum, the diagnosis may be especially difficult in the absence of distention, hyperactive peristalsis, or x-ray findings of small bowel obstruction. Another uncommon variant is gallstone ileus of the large bowel. In these cases, the stone may have entered via a cholecystocolonic fistula or, less often, after traversing the entire small bowel. Obstruction of the colon, rare because its lumen is so wide, most often occurs when diverticulitis has narrowed the sigmoid.

Women are more often affected than men, and the average age is about 70 years. As a cause of intestinal obstruction, gallstone ileus is relatively uncommon but should always be high on the list in elderly patients, especially when incarceration in an external hernia is absent and there has been no previous laparotomy which might have produced adhesions.

On physical examination the findings are those of small bowel obstruction. Sometimes the large stone can be felt as a mass on abdominal, vaginal, or rectal examination, but it is rarely correctly identified as such.

Roentgenograms usually show air in the biliary tree if the films are carefully examined, and in some cases the radiopaque gallstone can be seen in its unusual location. Otherwise, the films are typical of bowel obstruction. Sometimes a gastrointestinal series is performed for the diagnosis of partial obstruction, revealing the cholecystoduodenal fistula.

Treatment consists of removing the obstructing gallstone through a small enterotomy and examining the proximal gut carefully to ensure that a second stone is not left which could produce an immediate recurrence. It is generally wise to leave the biliary disease undisturbed initially, because elderly patients tolerate long procedures poorly, and nothing much is gained by repairing the fistula primarily.

Postoperatively, if the patient has symptoms of biliary disease, an elective cholecystectomy may be scheduled several months later. Many patients become asymptomatic and the fistula closes spontaneously; for them, expectant management is best. About 50 per cent will require cholecystectomy.

The mortality rate, 15 to 20 per cent, remains high because of delay in diagnosis and the fragile state of cardiopulmonary function in elderly patients.

686. CHOLEDOCHOLITHIASIS AND CHOLANGITIS

In Western countries choledocholithiasis is usually the result of passage into the common duct of cholesterol gallstones formed in the gallbladder. Once there, they sometimes continue on into the duodenum, but the frequency of this event is not known and is rarely observed with certainty. The less common primary duct stone is usually associated with bile stasis caused by secondary dilatation of the duct from longstanding obstruction by stones, stricture, or ampullary stenosis. About 15 per cent of patients with gallbladder stones have concomitant choledocholithiasis. The incidence is even higher in elderly patients and in patients who seek medical care late. In rare instances choledocholithiasis is found in the absence of gallbladder stones; in such a case it is assumed that all the gallbladder stones escaped into the duct.

Clinical Manifestations. The natural history of choledocholithiasis is only vaguely known, because there is no solid information on the incidence and fate of asymptomatic patients. Available data suggest that 30 to 40 per cent of patients are asymptomatic at time of diagnosis, implying a relatively benign course in many cases. Obstruction by stones of the biliary or pancreatic ducts may produce any of the following syndromes: biliary colic, jaundice (without pain), cholangitis, pancreatitis, or a combination of these (Fig. 7). Secondary hepatic effects of persistent obstruction include biliary cirrhosis or hepatic abscesses.

Intermittent cholangitis, consisting of biliary colic, jaundice, and fever and chills *(Charcot's triad),* is the most common presenting symptom complex; in the absence of previous biliary surgery it is almost diagnostic in the Western Hemisphere of choledocholithiasis. Intermittency of symptoms is quite characteristic, a manifestation of intermittent partial obstruction. Whenever pain, chills with fever, and jaundice fluctuate together over a span of a few days or a week, cholangitis from biliary obstruction is almost certainly the cause. In a typical attack chills may precede the other symptoms, and dark urine from bilirubinuria may follow after a day or so. The pain, located in the epigastrium or right upper

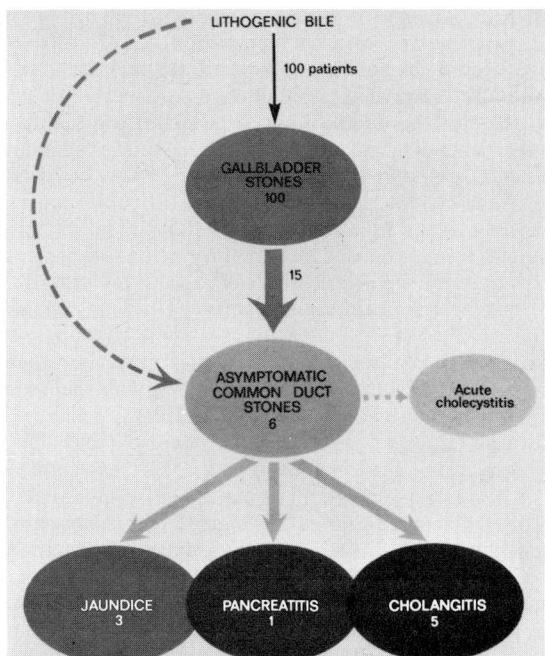

Figure 7. Natural history of choledocholithiasis, indicating that of 100 patients with gallbladder stones about 15 will develop this complication. Most acquire one of the syndromes in the bottom three ovals (with or without pain), but many probably remain asymptomatic.

quadrant, is indistinguishable from biliary colic caused by gallbladder stones and is steady, dull, and cramplike in quality. Pain may be referred to the upper back or even the precordium, occasionally suggesting coronary artery or esophageal disease.

The severity of the systemic reaction, i.e., fever and chills, varies widely from the usual mild transient illness to overwhelming sepsis with shock (see Suppurative Cholangitis, below). In the average case, the temperature rises to 38.5 to 40° C, preceded by chills and positive blood cultures. Localized tenderness in the subcostal region may be associated with extreme guarding and rigidity, but more often the local findings are minimal and are distinctly less severe than in acute cholecystitis. In most cases of common duct obstruction by stones, chronic inflammation and scarring of the gallbladder prevent it from becoming distended, as often occurs with periampullary malignancies. This serves as the basis for *Courvoisier's law:* a distended, nontender gallbladder in a jaundiced patient signifies neoplastic obstruction of the bile duct.

Laboratory Studies. In cholangitis the leukocyte count averages 15,000 μl but may go much higher in severe cases. Bilirubin values are usually in the range of 2 to 4 mg per 100 ml, and are uncommonly higher than 10 mg per 100 ml. Elevated serum alkaline phosphatase, leucine aminopeptidase, and 5'-nucleotidase levels indicate extrahepatic obstruction. The SGOT generally remains below 200 units, but values of 500 are not rare, and a few cases have been reported in which it has transiently exceeded 1000 units. In these instances the prompt drop within 48 hours and associated tenfold increase in LDH allows differentiation from serum hepatitis.

Differential Diagnosis. The same conditions considered for the patient with chronic cholecystitis must be excluded for biliary colic caused by ductal calculi. In patients who have had a cholecystectomy, differentiation between choledocholithiasis and biliary stricture as the cause of cholangitis usually depends on radiologic demonstration of the ducts. When the presenting syndrome is painless cholestatic jaundice, other causes, especially *periampullary* and *biliary neoplasms,* must be considered. With neoplastic obstruction the bilirubin averages about 18 mg per 100 ml and rarely fluctuates. Although jaundice from stones can certainly be as severe, the bilirubin is characteristically less than 10 mg per 100 ml and rises and falls episodically. The diagnosis of *intrahepatic cholestasis* from causes such as drugs, viral hepatitis, or pregnancy should in most cases be reached by exclusion only after visualization of normal bile ducts by direct or intravenous cholangiography.

Common duct stones may cause *acute pancreatitis* indistinguishable clinically from that resulting from alcohol or other causes and unaccompanied by specific signs of biliary disease. Pancreatitis caused by biliary calculi, despite numerous attacks, rarely progresses to pancreatic calcification, chronic pain, and pancreatic insufficiency, as so often occurs in the alcoholic variety. As a rule, gallstone disease should be searched for radiologically in every patient with acute pancreatitis, because further attacks can be avoided if the gallstones are removed.

Treatment. The potential seriousness of cholangitis warrants hospitalization for diagnosis and treatment in most cases. After blood cultures are drawn, antimicrobial drugs, chosen for their efficacy against enteric organisms, are given by the parenteral route. At present cephalosporin or ampicillin for mild attacks or either of these drugs plus gentamicin or kanamycin in severe infection has a good chance of controlling the infection. There is no strong rationale for choosing antimicrobial drugs based on their excretion in bile, because the block responsible for cholangitis also affects this process. Failure to obtain a rapid response may mean that the organisms were not susceptible to the initial drugs, justifying the addition of another drug or a shift from the initial regimen based upon the results of cultures and drug-susceptibility tests. The margin between mild and severe illness is small; antimicrobial therapy should be expected to control the acute attack within 48 to 72 hours, and if there is no improvement or worsening after this period, emergency surgery must be considered seriously.

Most acute cases respond satisfactorily to treatment and allow an orderly attempt at diagnosis. If oral cholecystography has already demonstrated gallbladder stones, laparotomy is indicated, and additional studies aimed at demonstrating the ductal pathology are usually not necessary. In patients with jaundice, acute pancreatitis, or upper abdominal pain who have had a cholecystectomy in the past, intravenous cholangiograms can be obtained if the bilirubin is below 3 or 4 mg per 100 ml, or direct opacification can be attempted by percutaneous transhepatic or, preferably, retrograde endoscopic cholangiography. Both these direct procedures are potentially hazardous in active cholangitis and should be postponed until infection is well controlled, proceeding then only under the protection of antimicrobial therapy.

Surgical exploration and choledochotomy should be scheduled after the diagnosis of choledocholithiasis has been made. If the gallbladder is present, cholecystectomy is done, and the common duct is opened and emptied of stones. A T tube is usually left in the duct to decompress biliary pressure in the postoperative period and to provide a route for additional cholangiograms a week or so later.

In patients with advanced disease, the common duct may be so packed with hundreds of stones that it is dilated to 3 cm or more in diameter. Rarely, the intrahepatic ducts become markedly dilated and contain innumerable stones, making complete extraction technically impossible. In either of these situations recurrent or persistent choledocholithiasis is almost certain unless a choledochoduodenostomy, sphincteroplasty, or Roux-en-Y choledochojejunostomy is performed to create a wide conduit between the duct and intestine through which residual stones can pass.

Retained Common Duct Stones. The methods for detecting duct stones at operation are about 95 per cent reliable, which means, unfortunately, that a few are overlooked only to be discovered on postoperative T tube cholangiograms. Two new approaches have recently made it possible to eliminate most residual stones without another laparotomy. One method depends on the ability of bile salt solutions to dissolve cholesterol gallstones. Several weeks after surgery a sterile solution of sodium cholate (100 mM) is infused into the T tube at 30 ml per hour continuously until the stone is gone. Oral cholestyramine must be given to prevent diarrhea from the large amount of bile salt delivered to the intestine. Disappearance of the retained stones occurs in about two thirds of patients within a two-week treatment period.

Instrumental extraction, an alternative technique, is somewhat simpler, faster, and about equally as successful. Under image intensification fluoroscopy the T tube is pulled out, a Dormia ureteral basket is passed into the duct, and the stone is grasped and withdrawn. If neither mechanical extraction nor chemical dissolution is successful, reoperation is usually necessary.

Prognosis. With accurate diagnosis and treatment, choledocholithiasis is cured by cholecystectomy and choledocholithotomy. Recurrent ductal stone formation is rare except as noted when the duct has become markedly dilated.

SUPPURATIVE CHOLANGITIS

The severest form of cholangitis, variously termed *suppurative* or *obstructive cholangitis,* involves the same causative factors as the "nonsuppurative" form but differs in that obstruction is complete, ductal contents become purulent, and clinically the manifestations of sepsis overshadow those of cholestasis. Hypotension and mental changes, such as lethargy or confusion, appear in addition to right upper quadrant pain, chills, fever, and jaundice. Because infection in the face of the high-grade obstruction progresses so rapidly, the serum bilirubin does not reach very high levels before the patient becomes moribund from sepsis. Costly delays in diagnosis are frequent, a consequence of failure to recognize the significance of mild icterus and abdominal pain in a patient with sepsis. All but a few cases are complications of choledocholithiasis, the others occurring with biliary stricture or neoplastic obstruction.

Laboratory tests reveal evidence of cholestasis with bilirubin values between 2 and 5 mg per 100 ml and elevated serum levels of alkaline phosphatase, 5'-nucleotidase, leucine aminopeptidase, and SGOT. The leukocyte count varies from normal to 40,000 per μl.

Tenderness is present to palpation in the right upper quadrant, but rigidity is rare. In some cases secondary cholecystitis develops, and an enlarged tender gallbladder may be found on abdominal examination.

There is no way to confirm the diagnosis by x-ray, because transhepatic or retrograde cholangiography would be extremely hazardous and intravenous cholangiograms are unsuccessful. Therefore diagnosis rests on recognizing the evidence of biliary obstruction and its relationship to the sepsis.

After initial resuscitation, consisting of intravenous infusions, antimicrobial drugs, and measures to restore cardiac, pulmonary, or renal function, emergency surgery offers the only hope of saving the patient. Hypoglycemia has been found in some patients whose depressed cerebral function seemed to improve with infusion of hypertonic glucose solutions.

At surgery when choledochotomy is performed, pus often squirts from the duct owing to the high pressure. If the patient's condition permits, thorough exploration can be performed to correct the obstruction by eliminating stones, repairing a stricture, or bypassing a tumor. Insertion of a T tube proximal to the obstruction is sufficient in patients who are unable to tolerate a longer operation, but sometime later it will be necessary to perform a second, more definitive procedure before the T tube can be removed.

The mortality is about 50 per cent, resulting from septic shock, renal failure, acute hepatic insufficiency, or a combination of these complications.

687. BILIARY STRICTURE

Biliary stricture, except in rare instances, results from surgical injury to the duct and usually follows cholecystectomy rather than procedures on the duct itself such as deliberate choledochotomy for common duct exploration. In some cases the surgeon may recognize the injury and attempt its repair. Often, however, it is not identified at the primary operation, and the first sign of trouble postoperatively might be excessive escape of bile along drains or the appearance of jaundice or cholangitis. A few noniatrogenic examples of biliary stricture stem from external trauma or scarring produced by choledocholithiasis.

Injury to the duct that is identified immediately or within a few days can sometimes be repaired without serious consequences. The patient who has signs of partial biliary obstruction and intermittent cholangitis weeks or months after cholecystectomy is the one who presents challenges for diagnosis and treatment. The symptoms closely resemble those of choledocholithiasis, the obvious clue being a history of previous cholecystectomy or attempt at repair of a stricture.

Leukocytosis and laboratory evidence of cholestasis parallel the clinical manifestations. The jaundice or cholangitis is generally mild and transient, and infection generally responds promptly to antimicrobial therapy.

Intravenous cholangiograms may be obtained if the bilirubin drops below 3 mg per 100 ml. Otherwise, transhepatic or retrograde cholangiograms will be necessary.

With persistent obstruction over several years, secondary biliary cirrhosis develops, and portal hypertension may give rise to bleeding esophageal varices, or hepatic failure may ensue gradually. In other cases, uncontrolled sepsis results in multiple intrahepatic abscesses and death.

Differential diagnosis must include all the various causes of obstructive jaundice and cholangitis, but in most cases the major consideration is *choledocholithiasis*. A useful differential feature is that the initial symptoms of stricture nearly always begin within two years of the cholecystectomy, whereas a symptom-free interval longer than this is common with residual or recurrent common duct stones.

In all but a few cases an attempt should be made to repair the stricture surgically by creating a new unobstructed conduit between normal duct on the hepatic side of the lesion and the proximal intestine. This can sometimes be accomplished by a direct end-to-end anastomosis of the duct after excising the lesion or more often by choledochoduodenostomy or choledochojejunostomy to a Roux-en-Y jejunal segment. Loss of the duodenal end of the duct and choledochal sphincter with the last two operations is of no physiologic significance. By diverting alkaline bile from the duodenum, choledochojejunostomy predisposes slightly to peptic ulcer disease, but the problem is not of sufficient magnitude to weigh heavily in the choice of procedure unless the patient already has a peptic ulcer.

The over-all success rate of these operations is about 75 per cent, but it is important to note that even when there has been one or more previous failures, the odds still favor a good result after another try. For this reason, it is rarely wise to keep a patient with a known stricture indefinitely on a regimen of intermittent antimicrobial drugs for symptoms. The obstruction invariably produces cirrhosis or uncontrollable infection, and the opportunity to obtain a real cure is lost.

The mortality of 10 per cent is from the complications mentioned above.

688. UNCOMMON CAUSES OF BILE DUCT OBSTRUCTION

The following inventory briefly covers several uncommon causes of common duct obstruction manifested clinically by jaundice, colic, cholangitis, or a combination of these. *Pancreatic* and *duodenal tumors* are covered in Ch. 648 and 668, respectively. Other causes rarely encountered are compression by *neoplastic* or *inflammatory paraductal lymph nodes* and *duodenal Crohn's disease.*

Choledochal cysts occasionally produce their initial clinical manifestations in adults, presenting with jaundice, cholangitis, and, in some, a right upper quadrant mass consisting of the dilated duct full of stones. Diagnosis may require transhepatic cholangiography or may not be obvious until operation. The most definitive surgical procedure is excision of the abnormal duct, followed by Roux-en-Y jejunal anastomosis to the stump of the hepatic duct. The simpler cystenteric anastomosis may be preferable in some situations.

Caroli's disease consists of saccular intrahepatic bile duct dilatation which in most cases becomes symptomatic in patients between the ages of 20 and 50 owing to intrahepatic stone formation and cholangitis. Two forms are recognized: one a disease of the ducts only, and the more common type which is associated with hepatic fibrosis and medullary sponge kidney. The latter patients often have complications of portal hypertension before cholangitis or obstructive jaundice appears. Antimicrobial therapy may control attacks of cholangitis, and surgical procedures to facilitate ductal emptying or to extract stones may help in some cases, but the intrahepatic anomaly cannot be definitively corrected. Rarely the left lobe alone is involved, and lobectomy is curative.

Hemobilia presents with the triad of biliary colic, obstructive jaundice, and occult or gross intestinal bleeding. Most cases are caused by hepatic injury with secondary bleeding into the ductal system, usually beginning several weeks after the trauma. Hemobilia is occasionally caused by *biliary* or *hepatic neoplasms*, ductal rupture of an *hepatic artery aneurysm, hepatic abscess,* or *biliary calculus.* Inflammatory hemobilia has been reported mostly from the Orient, where it accompanies *biliary parasitism (Ascaris lumbricoides)* or *cholangiohepatitis.* The diagnosis can be verified preoperatively by selective hepatic arteriography. Treatment may require hepatic artery ligation for hemobilia secondary to trauma, but for the other types direct surgical management of the lesion is usually necessary.

Pancreatitis can produce transient jaundice by obstruction of the distal common duct where it is encased by pancreatic tissue. Prolonged obstruction can result from pressure by a pseudocyst or entrapment in severe pancreatic scarring from chronic pancreatitis. Diagnosis may be difficult in alcoholic patients in whom elevated bilirubin values are usually attributed to hepatic parenchymal disease.

Most *duodenal diverticula* arise within 1 to 2 cm of the hepatobiliary ampulla, and in some patients the common duct empties directly into a diverticulum. Duodenal diverticula may obstruct the common duct by anatomic distortion of its duodenal entry, by diverticulitis, or by an enterolith (of bile acids) in the sac. Even in jaundiced patients most duodenal diverticula are only incidental findings, but when definite proof implicates them in ductal obstruction, either choledochoduodenostomy or Roux-en-Y choledochojejunostomy is simpler treatment than attempting to excise the diverticulum or surgically to enlarge its entry into the duodenum.

Echinococcosis, by rupture of an hepatic cyst into the ducts, can give rise to biliary colic, jaundice, and cholangitis. Treatment involves surgical removal of the obstructing hydatid debris and daughter cysts from the ducts and excision of the parent cyst from the liver after its contents are sterilized by sodium hypochlorite (0.05 per cent) or hypertonic saline (30 per cent) solution. The practice of injecting formalin into the hepatic cysts is fortunately no longer used, because in patients with a biliary communication serious damage to the bile ducts and even death have occurred.

Ascariasis may produce colic, jaundice, and cholangitis by worms which invade the bile ducts through the choledochal sphincter from the duodenum. The worm eventually dies, but in some cases not until after depositing ova. Air is sometimes seen in the ducts, presumably entering through the sphincter with the ascarid. Treatment entails antimicrobial drugs and then piperazine after the acute symptoms are controlled. If progressive cholangitis occurs despite antimicrobial therapy, common duct exploration and extraction of the parasites may be necessary. After the nonsurgical regimen, follow-up intravenous cholangiograms should be obtained to verify that no worms remain in the duct; if residual defects are present, they should be surgically removed.

Throughout coastal regions of the Orient, from Japan to Malaysia, many persons of low socioeconomic status are affected by *Oriental cholangiohepatitis,* a form of chronic recurrent cholangitis caused by calcium bilirubinate stones formed primarily within the bile ducts. Among the various etiologic possibilities are the effects of parasites in the ducts (especially *Clonorchis sinensis* and *Ascaris lumbricoides),* diet (low in fat and animal protein), and excessive bilirubin excretion. In some regions, ova or fragments of adult parasites have been demonstrated within the center of the stones, but the disease has also been reported in populations without heavy parasitic infestation. Within the ducts, Clornorchis is especially capable of inciting ductal inflammation and scarring. Whatever the initial event, there is good evidence that β-glucuronidase, produced in the bile by secondarily invading *E. coli,* hydrolyzes bilirubin diglucuronide which then precipitates as sludge and stones of calcium bilirubinate.

Acute cholangitis is the usual presenting syndrome. Subcostal abdominal tenderness is present, and the gallbladder, which contains stones in only 20 to 30 per cent, is usually palpable, or even visible on abdominal inspection. Strictures sometimes develop in the hepatic ducts, leading to further stasis and intrahepatic stone formation. In advanced cases, one (usually the left) or both lobar ducts may become honeycombed with cysts or abscesses, producing atrophy of the hepatic parenchyma. Laboratory abnormalities consist of leukocytosis, elevated serum bilirubin (2 to 10 mg per 100 ml), and elevated serum alkaline phosphatase. During symptomatic episodes neither plain films nor oral or intravenous cholangiograms will demonstrate the pathology.

Most acute cases can be controlled with antimicrobials, but severe toxicity, fever (39 to 40°C), or septic shock mandates emergency laparotomy in as many as 30 per cent. If nonsurgical management is initially successful, transhepatic cholangiograms can be used later to outline the ducts.

The common duct stones should be removed through a generous choledochotomy. If it is impossible to empty the intrahepatic ducts, transhepatic lithotomy or even lobectomy may be required if there is unilateral lobar atrophy or abscess formation. Recurrence of choledocholithiasis is almost certain unless the junction between duct and intestine is surgically enlarged by sphincteroplasty, choledochoduodenostomy, or Roux-en-Y choledochojejunostomy.

Sclerosing cholangitis, a rare condition of unknown etiology, consists of benign nonbacterial chronic inflammatory narrowing of the bile ducts. The entire ductal system may be involved, or, less commonly, the process may be confined to the extrahepatic or intrahepatic portion. Males predominate in a ratio of 3:1, and the peak incidence occurs in the third and fourth decades. About one third of the cases are associated with *retroperitoneal fibrosis, Riedel's thyroiditis, regional enteritis,* or especially *ulcerative colitis.* When both are present, the severity of sclerosing cholangitis and ulcerative colitis is not correlated, and colectomy has an uncertain effect on the biliary disease.

The initial complaint may be jaundice or pruritus, although both eventually appear in most cases. There may be mild upper abdominal pain and sometimes fever, but a clinical picture resembling bacterial cholangitis is uncommon in the absence of previous surgical exploration of the ducts. Hepatomegaly is the only abdominal finding until late when secondary cirrhosis produces ascites or splenomegaly.

Jaundice may be constant or fluctuating, and bilirubin values are usually in the range of 2 to 10 mg per 100 ml. The alkaline phosphatase is quite high and remains elevated despite variations in clinical manifestations. Antimitochondrial antibodies are absent. Other liver function tests are normal until late in the illness when hepatic failure develops.

Preoperative diagnosis is difficult to establish except by exclusion. Transhepatic cholangiography will demonstrate the pathology if the intrahepatic branches are not affected, but retrograde cholangiography via endoscopy may eventually be a more reliable technique. The x-rays show diffuse irregular ductal narrowing with only a tiny residual lumen in the most severely involved areas. When considering the differential diagnosis, a short stenosis (1 to 2 cm) of the duct more likely represents a neoplasm or traumatic stricture than sclerosing cholangitis. Other causes of persistent cholestatic jaundice must be considered, especially *primary biliary cirrhosis, drug cholestasis,* and *neoplastic ductal obstruction.*

At operation the lumen is identified, often a tedious process, and then dilated with progressively larger probes. An operative cholangiogram should be obtained to show the extent and severity of involvement, and as large a T tube as possible should be placed in the duct and left there for several months. Since differentiation from scirrhous biliary malignancy may be difficult even at operation, biopsy of the duct should be obtained in all cases, and even then the pathologist may have trouble distinguishing sclerosing cholangitis from neoplasm.

Many experts favor postoperative administration of systemic corticosteroids for 6 to 12 months; but in the absence of conclusive proof of their value, others argue that on balance corticosteroids are too dangerous, because they foster suppurative complications. After surgery which introduces a few bacteria and a foreign body, episodic mild cholangitis occurs in most patients, and short courses of antimicrobial therapy can be given to hasten their resolution. Cholestyramine may be useful for pruritus at any stage of the disease.

Significant palliation follows surgery in most cases, but unfortunately is not often permanent. A few patients seem to recover completely; however, most have episodic remissions and exacerbations over five to ten years during which time secondary biliary cirrhosis develops. Death may follow uncontrollable biliary sepsis with hepatic abscesses, liver failure, or bleeding from esophageal varices.

689. CARCINOMA OF THE GALLBLADDER

About 6000 people in the United States die each year from carcinoma of the gallbladder, a number equal to the mortality from benign disease of the biliary tract. Gallbladder cancer accounts for 1 per cent of all cancer deaths and 3 per cent of gastrointestinal malignancies. Women outnumber men by 3 to 1, and the average age is 70. Because 85 per cent of cases occur in patients with gallstones, cholelithiasis is thought to be etiologically important; somewhat less than 1 per cent of patients with cholelithiasis will develop gallbladder malignancy.

All but a few gallbladder carcinomas are adenocarcinoma, the remainder being squamous cell carcinoma. The earliest spread is usually to the liver by direct extension and metastasis. Nodal metastases in the liver hilum are somewhat less common, and distant metastases appear only late.

The patients present clinically in one of the following ways: (1) unremitting deep jaundice from common duct and hepatic involvement; (2) acute cholecystitis, usually with a palpable mass; (3) chronic cholecystitis with intermittent right upper quadrant pain; and (4) advanced carcinoma. The diagnosis is rarely considered preoperatively, but in some instances clinical clues are present. In about two thirds of the patients a mass can be felt, and in one third there is local tenderness. Gallbladder symptoms in patients 70 years or older are associated with carcinoma in about 10 per cent. In all but a few cases, the oral cholecystogram does not opacify, and even when the gallbladder is visualized, the tumor can rarely be demonstrated. Because the tumor becomes surgically incurable before it has grown very large, there is a strong correlation between presence of a palpable mass and incurability. More than half the patients have had chronic biliary symptoms for several years, and presumably earlier cholecystectomy in these would have avoided the development of carcinoma.

Surgery is indicated in most patients if for no more than diagnosis. Resection is rarely possible for cure, but in some cases palliative procedures will relieve jaundice. If it appears curative, cholecystectomy and resection of adjacent involved liver should be performed if the general health of the patient permits, but most elderly patients cannot tolerate an hepatic lobectomy. Most cures have resulted from excision of the gallbladder with a tumor so small that it was unsuspected by the surgeon. Only scattered reports of five-year survivors have appeared. Most patients live for only a few months after the diagnosis.

690. BENIGN TUMORS AND PSEUDOTUMORS OF THE GALLBLADDER

This is a heterogenous group of uncommon lesions with uncertain clinical significance. The roentgenographic appearance may be distinctive, especially for adenomyomatous hyperplasia, but often is not. A pathologic classification is presented in Table 2.

Adenomatous hyperplasia, consisting of mucosal thickening, may be focal or diffuse. Gallstones are present in some cases. The diagnosis cannot be made by x-ray.

Adenomyomatous hyperplasia, the most common lesion, has sometimes been called *adenomyomatosis, diverticulosis, cholecystitis glandularis proliferans,* or *cholecystitis cystica.* Focal, segmental, and diffuse forms

Benign pseudotumors:
1. Mucosal hyperplasia
    a. Adenomatous
    b. Adenomyomatous (adenomyoma)
2. Polyps
    a. Inflammatory
    b. Cholesterol
3. Mucosal heterotopia
4. Miscellaneous
    a. Fibroxanthogranulomatous inflammation
    b. Parasitic
    c. Other

Benign tumors:
1. Epithelial
    a. Adenoma, papillary
    b. Adenoma, nonpapillary
2. Supporting tissue
    a. Hemangioma
    b. Lipoma
    c. Leiomyoma
    d. Granular cell tumor

exist, but the first of these is by far the most common. Most pathologists agree that the lesion is not neoplastic; the absence of cases in children argues against a congenital origin. Located invariably in the fundus, the focal form consists of a thick button of smooth muscle invaded by cystic mucosal glands and punctuated by a central umbilication. Convincing cases have been reported in which patients were relieved of chronic abdominal complaints by cholecystectomy, but in most cases adenomyomatosis produces no symptoms.

Cholesterol polyps are a focal form of cholesterolosis consisting of submucosal histiocytes stuffed with cholesterol and located at a villous tip. Interestingly, diffuse cholesterolosis rarely gives rise to cholesterol polyps. The polyp is attached to the mucosa by a fragile stalk which can easily be broken. This has engendered speculation concerning a possible role for cholesterol polyps in the genesis of some cholesterol gallstones.

Papillary and *nonpapillary adenomas* are the only true benign neoplasms of the gallbladder seen with any frequency. Although the other lesions mentioned above clearly have no neoplastic potential, several cases of carcinoma have been reported in association with adenomas. It is doubtful, however, that many malignancies could arise in this way, because adenomas are rare compared with carcinoma of the gallbladder.

691. MALIGNANT BILE DUCT TUMORS

The main cause of early morbidity from tumors of the bile duct is biliary obstruction with gradual hepatocellular damage or secondary hepatobiliary infection. Except for a rare squamous cell tumor, bile duct malignancies consist of adenocarcinoma with either a scirrhous or a papillary pattern. Grossly, three types of pathologic presentations occur: focal stricture, diffuse thickening, and nodular mass. The first two varieties can easily be mistaken for a benign process, such as post-traumatic stricture or sclerosing cholangitis. To further complicate differentiation, some tumors are so marked by desmoplasia that tumor cells may be hard to find in the extensive collagen stroma. In many cases, spread is confined to local lymph node metastases or hepatic invasion for months or years before there is more widespread abdominal or systemic involvement. The common hepatic duct or common bile duct is the site of origin in about two thirds of the cases. By contrast with carcinoma of the gallbladder, cholelithiasis is found in only one third of patients, and men slightly outnumber women. The average age at diagnosis is 70 years. A number of cases have been reported in younger patients with ulcerative colitis, and since some of these had previously undergone colectomy, it is thought that elimination of the ulcerated colon is not protective. Exposure to the chemical carcinogens benzidine, 3,3-dichlorobenzidine, and M-toluene-diamine has been etiologically implicated in some cases. Japanese- and Mexican-Americans are more often affected than whites in the United States. In the Orient, infestation with *Clonorchis sinensis* probably contributes to the higher incidence of *intrahepatic cholangiocarcinoma*.

Clinical Manifestations.   The typical patient presents with unremitting deep jaundice, mild deep-seated upper abdominal pain, and weight loss. Pruritus is reported by many, usually after the jaundice, but preceding it in some cases. Diarrhea, presumably from steatorrhea, is reported by some. Pain, which affects over half the patients, is not of an intensity or character to be confused with biliary colic. In the absence of previous surgery, fever and chills are rarely present. Hepatomegaly without splenomegaly is found on abdominal examination. Tumors of the common duct sparing the cystic duct generally produce in addition to jaundice a distended nontender palpable gallbladder (*Courvoisier's law*). Otherwise, the abdomen is unremarkable, because palpation of the tumor itself is almost never possible. Most patients have occult blood in the stool.

The serum bilirubin exceeds 10 mg per 100 ml in most cases, with a mean value of around 18 mg per 100 ml. The alkaline phosphatase is raised and SGOT may be slightly elevated, although rarely higher than 200. Serum proteins are most often normal. The prothrombin time may be depressed but responds to parenteral vitamin K. Serum cholesterol averages about 400 mg per 100 ml.

Radiologic visualization of the biliary tree shows marked dilatation proximal to the obstruction. Excellent studies are usually obtained by transhepatic cholangiography, but retrograde cannulation of the duct, using fiberoptic endoscopy, may soon become the preferred technique. Only benign stricture of the duct is likely to create a similar radiographic picture, but if the patient has had no previous biliary surgery, benign stricture can be excluded.

Diagnostic confusion most often involves *primary biliary cirrhosis* and *jaundice* produced by *various drugs*. In neither of these does the bilirubin generally reach such high levels as with biliary tumors. Xanthelasma, found often with primary biliary cirrhosis, is only rarely seen with neoplastic obstruction. Antimitochondrial antibodies can be demonstrated in the serum of patients with primary biliary cirrhosis; how often they will be found with tumors is unclear, because the specificity of this test at present seems to vary between investigators, and there are reports of positive titers in some patients with longstanding extrahepatic obstruction.

Choledocholithiasis and *biliary stricture* are less likely to present with steady deep jaundice and weight loss. The clinical finding in these conditions is fluctuating, milder jaundice, usually associated with fever. Transhepatic cholangiograms can exclude calculous obstruction or stricture.

Treatment. Unfortunately, complete excision of the tumor is rarely possible, because unexpendable anatomic structures are involved early despite the slow growth of most biliary tumors. Nevertheless, a few cures can be expected when radical surgery is judiciously employed; and with new techniques for reestablishing bile flow, palliation is of increasing importance.

With proximal lesions, the findings at surgery consist of a collapsed gallbladder and small common duct, both grossly normal. That diagnostic pitfalls exist for the surgeon is underscored by the fact that many patients with tumors of the hepatic duct are subjected to at least one "negative" laparotomy before the problem is recognized. This could be largely obviated if operative cholangiograms that include the intrahepatic system were considered essential in diagnostic abdominal exploration for jaundice.

Distal lesions require radical pancreaticoduodenectomy (Whipple procedure) for complete removal. Because the operation has a 15 per cent mortality, it should rarely be performed if tumor would be left behind. Tumors of the supraduodenal duct are sometimes amenable to complete resection. Those of the left hepatic duct require a left hepatectomy, but secondary involvement of the right hepatic duct means this is rarely possible.

For most cases the goal is palliation. Distal tumors can be bypassed by cholecystojejunostomy or other types of biliary-enteric anastomosis. For proximal tumors a polyethylene tube is placed in the duct to maintain bile flow by spanning the tumor; the hepatic end is brought out directly through the liver substance, and the duodenal end is brought out through a choledochotomy. In this way the tube can be replaced later without reoperation when debris begins to plug the lumen, as usually happens after six months or so. Holes in the intraductal portion of the tube allow bile to reach the gut from the liver.

Prognosis. Cure is achieved in no more than 5 to 10 per cent, and survival is usually less than one year. If biliary drainage can be maintained, patients may survive for five to six years, even continuing their regular employment. Death eventually results from hepatic replacement with tumor or intrahepatic sepsis from recurrent ductal obstruction.

692. BENIGN TUMORS OF THE BILE DUCTS

The rare benign tumors of the bile ducts present with obstructive jaundice. *Papilloma,* the predominant morphologic type, is often multifocal and therefore difficult to cure. The next most common, *adenoma,* is more often localized. If the patient is an acceptable candidate, radical excision of the extrahepatic ducts is preferable to local curettement or limited resection.

693. POSTCHOLECYSTECTOMY SYNDROME

After cholecystectomy, a small percentage of patients continue to have significant abdominal symptoms. It was postulated by some that this postoperative disability resulted specifically from the absence of the gallbladder; hence the name postcholecystectomy syndrome. To avoid cholecystectomy, cholecystolithotomy was tried for chronic cholecystitis by several groups of surgeons, but an unacceptably high incidence of recurrent gallstones and persistent symptoms stimulated a return to cholecystectomy.

In many patients, the explanation for continued postoperative symptoms is that the gallstone disease was not the cause of their preoperative complaints. Patients with biliary colic, a symptom rather specific for chronic cholecystitis, are more often relieved than those with the vague symptoms of fatty food intolerance, dyspepsia, or flatulence. Success of cholecystectomy also correlates with the extent of pathologic change in the gallbladder wall; those with continued symptoms more often had minimal scarring and a functioning gallbladder.

In others, postcholecystectomy complaints can be attributed to overlooked organic disease, especially *choledocholithiasis, pancreatitis, peptic ulcer,* or *irritable colon syndrome.* These possibilities must be investigated by appropriate studies.

Last is a group of clinical entities whose clinical significance, incidence, or even existence in some instances remains in dispute. *Stenosis of the sphincter of Oddi, biliary dyskinesia, neuroma of the cystic duct stump,* and other cystic duct remnant lesions are the main examples. Perhaps it is fair to say that convincing evidence has been submitted to document the importance of each in specific cases, but as a group they are all quite rare. It should be appreciated in the management of patients with chronic abdominal pain that, in the absence of objective findings, exploratory laparotomy has a low rate of success for diagnosis and that surgical correction of minor variations in the gut anatomy usually fails to cure.

General

Kune, G. B.: Current Practice of Biliary Surgery. Boston, Little, Brown & Company, 1972.

Schein, C. J.: Acute Cholecystitis. New York, Harper & Row, 1972.

Sleisenger, M. H., and Fordtran, J. S. (eds.): Gastrointestinal Disease. Philadelphia, W. B. Saunders Company, 1973.

Specific

Adson, M. A.: Carcinoma of the gallbladder. Surg. Clin. North Am., 53:1203, 1973.

Dow, R. W., and Lindenauer, S. M.: Acute obstructive suppurative cholangitis. Ann. Surg., 169:272, 1969.

Dowling, R. H.: The enterohepatic circulation. Gastroenterology, 62:122, 1972.

Edlund, Y., and Olsson, O.: Acute cholecystitis: Its aetiology and course, with special reference to the timing of cholecystectomy. Acta Chir. Scand., 120:479, 1961.

Foulk, W. T.: Congenital malformations of the intrahepatic biliary tree in the adult. Gastroenterology, 58:253, 1970.

Grundy, S. M., Metzger, A. L., and Adler, R. D.: Mechanisms of lithogenic bile formation in American Indian women with cholesterol gallstones. J. Clin. Invest., 51:3026, 1972.

Longmire, W. P., Jr., McArthur, M. S., Bastounis, E. A., and Hiatt, J.: Carcinoma of the extrahepatic biliary tract. Ann. Surg., 178:333, 1973.

May, R. E., and Strong, R.: Acute emphysematous cholecystitis. Br. J. Surg., 58:454, 1971.

McSherry, C. K., and Glenn, F.: Biliary tract obstruction and duodenal diverticula. Surg. Gynecol. Obstet., 130:829, 1970.

Metzger, A. L., Adler, R., Heymsfield, S., and Grundy, S. M.: Diurnal variation in biliary lipid composition: Possible role in cholesterol gallstone formation. N. Engl. J. Med., 288:333, 1973.

Sandblom, P.: Hemobilia. Surg. Clin. North Am., 53:1191, 1973.

Schwartz, S. I.: Primary sclerosing cholangitis. Surg. Clin. North Am., 53:1161, 1973.

Small, D. M., and Rapo, S.: Source of abnormal bile in patients with cholesterol gallstones. N. Engl. J. Med., 283:53, 1970.

Thistle, J. L., and Hofmann, A. F.: Efficacy and specificity of chenodeoxycholic acid therapy for dissolving gallstones. N. Engl. J. Med., 289:655, 1973.

Thorpe, C. D., Olsen, W. H., Fischer, H., Doust, V. L., and Joseph, R. R.: Emergency intravenous cholangiography in patients with acute abdominal pain. Am. J. Surg., 125:46, 1973.

van der Linden, W., and Sunzel, H.: Early versus delayed operation for acute cholecystitis. Am. J. Surg., 120:7, 1970.

Way, L. W., Admirand, W. H., and Dunphy, J. E.: Management of choledocholithiasis. Ann. Surg., 176: 347, 1972.

Way, L. W., and Dunphy, J. E.: Biliary stricture. Am. J. Surg., 124:287, 1972.

Wenckert, A., and Robertson, B.: The natural course of gallstone disease. Gastroenterology, 50:376, 1966.

Section Eleven.   DISEASES OF THE LIVER

Graham H. Jeffries

694.   MECHANISMS OF HEPATIC DISEASE

An understanding of the pathophysiology of liver disease provides the basis for a rational clinical approach to the patient. The chapters that follow will review selective aspects of the biochemical and regulatory functions of the liver, the pathophysiology of clinical manifestations of liver disease, and the differential diagnosis and treatment of diseases of the liver.

JAUNDICE

Jaundice or *icterus* refers to a yellow discoloration of the skin or sclerae by bilirubin. Jaundice is usually apparent when the serum concentration of bilirubin exceeds 2 to 3 mg per 100 ml. Mucous membranes, colored by capillary blood, usually appear icteric only when serum bilirubin levels are considerably elevated. In patients with longstanding jaundice of the obstructive type, the skin may assume a greenish hue that is due in part to melanin pigmentation.

Bilirubin Metabolism

Production.   Bilirubin is a yellow tetrapyrrol pigment derived from heme-containing proteins. The hemoglobin of red blood cells is the major source of bilirubin (80 to 90 per cent). Normally, senescent red cells that have survived in the circulation for approximately 120 days are taken up by macrophages in the reticuloendothelial system (R-E system), and their hemoglobin is degraded to bilirubin. Biliverdin is an intermediate in the reactions that separate iron and protein (globin) from the molecule and open the tetrapyrrol ring at the α-methene bridge. The iron released from hemoglobin is stored in the R-E cells or is reutilized for heme synthesis.

When there is hemorrhage into tissues, the extravasated red cells are engulfed by macrophages which accumulate at the site of hemorrhage; the color changes of a subcutaneous hematoma reflect the conversion of hemoglobin to bilirubin.

Hemolytic disease states are usually accompanied by hyperplasia of the R-E system and an increased R-E cell production of bilirubin. When hemolysis is intravascular

and hemoglobin is released into the blood, the pigment may be cleared by hepatic parenchymal cells or alternatively excreted by the renal glomeruli and reabsorbed by renal tubule cells; these parenchymal cells also have the capacity to degrade hemoglobin to bilirubin.

Small amounts of bilirubin are derived from the breakdown of hemoproteins other than hemoglobin—e.g., myoglobin and cytochromes. In studies on the incorporation of N^{15}-labeled glycine into the fecal pigment *stercobilin* (urobilin) that is derived from bilirubin, a small fraction (10 to 20 per cent) of labeled bile pigment was excreted within a few days of isotope administration. This "early-labeled" bile pigment is derived from the degradation of cytochromes, particularly in the liver, and from hemoglobin which escapes incorporation into peripheral red blood cells.

Transport and Distribution.   Unconjugated bilirubin is a lipid-soluble molecule with minimal solubility in aqueous solution at the pH of plasma. The transport of bilirubin from the R-E cells and its subsequent distribution is determined by binding with plasma albumin; each albumin molecule has the capacity to bind two molecules of bilirubin. Unconjugated bilirubin, which is strongly albumin bound and thus nondialyzable, is not filtered by renal glomeruli and is not excreted in the urine. Conjugated bilirubin (see below) is water soluble and dialyzable from albumin solutions; in patients with obstructive jaundice and conjugated hyperbilirubinemia, the pigment is filtered and excreted in the urine. In patients with jaundice, bilirubin equlibrates between the intravascular and extravascular albumin pool. In the extravascular space, the pigment will distribute between tissue and plasma protein binding sites. Lipid-soluble, unconjugated bilirubin binds preferentially to albumin, and does not diffuse into cells other than the liver unless albumin binding sites are saturated (see Kernicterus in Ch. 696). The cerebrospinal and intraocular fluids do not become icteric in jaundiced patients.

Hepatic Uptake and Excretion.   The transfer of bilirubin from plasma to bile can be divided into four steps: (1) passage from sinusoidal blood across the liver cell membrane, (2) concentration in the liver cell, (3) conjugation to diglucuronide, and (4) secretion into the bile canaliculus. The passage of bilirubin from albumin-bilirubin complexes in plasma across the plasma membrane into the liver cell is facilitated by low molecular weight binding proteins, designated Y and Z, in the liver cell cytoplasm. These intracellular binding proteins also bind other organic anions. In the liver cell, bilirubin is conjugated to form bilirubin diglucuronide. Conjugation with glucuronic acid is catalyzed by a microsomal enzyme, *glucuronyl transferase,* in the presence of uridine diphospho-glucuronic acid, and converts nonpolar, lipid-soluble, unconjugated bilirubin to a polar, water-soluble compound, which is excreted in bile.

The secretion of conjugated bilirubin from the liver cell across the membrane lining the bile canaliculi is an active process which is probably carrier mediated. *Conjugation of the pigment is a prerequisite for its secretion into the bile.* In the absence of bilirubin glucuronyl transferase (see Crigler-Najjar syndrome in Ch. 696), the bile is colorless, and bile pigment is excreted by unidentified metabolic pathways.

Intestinal Degradation. Bacterial enzymes in the distal small intestine and colon convert conjugated bilirubin to colorless urobilinogens, which are excreted predominantly in the feces but are partly reabsorbed in the ileum and colon. Reabsorbed urobilinogen is either cleared by the liver and re-excreted in bile or excreted in the urine.

Pathophysiology of Jaundice

Hyperbilirubinemia with jaundice may be due to one or several mechanisms that include excessive pigment production, reduced hepatic uptake or conjugation of bilirubin, or decreased excretion of the conjugated pigment.

Excessive Bilirubin Production. *Hemolysis,* an excessive rate of red blood cell destruction, is the most common mechanism of excessive bilirubin production. In the normal subject, the low serum bilirubin concentration predominantly in the unconjugated fraction reflects the efficient hepatic clearance of the pigment. Hepatic bilirubin excretion may increase to maximal levels when pigment production is increased by hemolysis, but the serum concentration of bilirubin (predominantly unconjugated) rarely exceeds 3 to 5 mg per 100 ml unless hepatic excretion is impaired by reduced blood flow, impaired hepatocellular function, or ductal obstruction.

In some patients with unconjugated hyperbilirubinemia, bile pigment may be excreted in excess of the amount derived from peripheral red cell destruction. This is typical of thalassemia and pernicious anemia, but is sometimes unassociated with hemolytic disease. *Ineffective erythropoiesis* may account for excessive bilirubin production and jaundice in these patients. Although the "early-labeled" pigment excreted in bile is partly derived from the metabolism of heme enzymes (cytochromes) in the liver, there is currently no evidence that jaundice may result from increased hepatic metabolism of cytochromes.

Reduced Hepatic Uptake of Bilirubin. A defect in the transfer of plasma bilirubin to the liver cell may explain the unconjugated hyperbilirubinemia in *Gilbert's syndrome* (see Ch. 696), after recovery from acute *viral hepatitis,* in congestive heart failure and after portacaval shunt surgery. Certain drugs may also competitively interfere with bilirubin uptake (iodopanoic acid, novobiocin).

Reduced Hepatic Conjugation of Bilirubin. Bilirubin conjugation with glucuronic acid is essential for normal bilirubin excretion. A deficiency or inhibition of glucuronyl transferase activity causes unconjugated hyperbilirubinemia. *Neonatal jaundice* is commonly due to immaturity of the hepatic excretory system, particularly in premature infants. In the *Crigler-Najjar syndrome* (see Ch. 696), glucuronyl transferase activity is congenitally absent, the serum concentration of unconjugated bilirubin reaches high levels, and brain damage caused by deposition of pigment in the basal ganglia (kernicterus) is usual. Rare patients have survived to adulthood.

Inhibition of glucuronyl transferase activity by a steroid excreted in maternal milk is an unusual cause for neonatal jaundice.

Reduced Excretion of Conjugated Bilirubin. The excretion of conjugated bilirubin into the bile canaliculus is an active transport process which may be impaired by a variety of processes. In the *Dubin-Johnson* and *Rotor syndromes* there is a congenital defect in hepatic excretion of conjugated bilirubin and other organic anions including sulfobromophthalein (BSP); the normal excretion of conjugated bile salts in these patients suggests a separate transport pathway. Impaired excretion may result from hepatocellular injury as in *virus hepatitis,* or may be due to *drugs* that interfere with cell metabolism or increase the permeability of the biliary tree (methyl testosterone, estrogens), compete for excretion in bile, or damage bile ductules (chlorpromazine). Inflammatory, granulomatous, or neoplastic *infiltration* of the liver and extrahepatic *bile duct obstruction* by gallstone, stricture, or carcinoma commonly interfere with bile excretion. The mechanism by which water-soluble, conjugated bilirubin enters the plasma in patients with impaired hepatic excretion is uncertain. The pigment either may be transferred across the liver cell directly into sinusoidal blood or may diffuse from bile ductules or canaliculi when the permeability of the biliary system is modified by disease.

Classification of Jaundice

Patients with jaundice may be subdivided clinically into two groups in which the serum bilirubin is either predominantly unconjugated or conjugated. *Unconjugated hyperbilirubinemia* is due to excessive production, reduced uptake, or reduced conjugation of pigment, whereas *conjugated hyperbilirubinemia* may result from hepatocellular or biliary tract disease. The terms *hemolytic jaundice, hepatocellular jaundice,* and *obstructive jaundice* of intra- and extrahepatic types *(intra- and extrahepatic cholestasis)* are often used to describe these types of jaundice. *Cholestasis* refers to reduced bile flow and reduced excretion of bile constituents; pathologically, there is usually evidence of bile stasis with bile plugs in the canaliculi. Several of the mechanisms discussed previously may be responsible for jaundice in a particular patient. As an example, in acute viral hepatitis mild hemolysis may increase bilirubin production; parenchymal cell damage may impair uptake, conjugation, and excretion of pigment; and intrahepatic cholestasis resulting from disruption of bile canaliculi or inflammation may reduce bile excretion.

Fecal and Urinary Excretion of Bile Pigments

Unconjugated bilirubin, tightly bound to albumin and relatively nonpolar, cannot be dialyzed from plasma and does not pass the glomerular filter; jaundice with unconjugated hyperbilirubinemia is thus *acholuric.* Bilirubin diglucuronide, less avidly bound to plasma albumin, is partly dialyzable from plasma, and is excreted in the urine by glomerular filtration. In the presence of complete biliary obstruction, the urinary excretion of conjugated bilirubin will be equal to bilirubin production, and serum levels will stabilize at 15 to 25 mg per 100 ml.

The quantity of bile pigment excreted as urobilinogens in feces and urine is a reflection of the amount of bilirubin in the bile, the bacterial conversion of bilirubin to urobilinogens, and the capacity of the liver to excrete urobilinogen absorbed from the intestine. *Fecal urobilinogen* is increased by excessive bilirubin production, and is reduced when hepatobiliary disease impairs bilirubin excretion or when bacterial conversion of bilirubin to urobilinogens is inhibited by antimicrobial therapy. *Urinary urobilinogen* is increased when greater amounts of urobilinogen are absorbed from the intestine or when parenchymal liver disease impairs the hepatic excretion of this pigment. Reduced urinary levels suggest cholestasis or impaired renal function.

PHYSICAL CHANGES OF THE DISEASED LIVER

Liver enlargement is usually an indication of disease. A normal liver displaced by a depressed diaphragm or a Riedel lobe must be considered in the differential diagnosis. An increase in liver size may reflect changes in liver cells (infiltration with fat or glycogen, or an increase in the smooth endoplasmic reticulum), cholestasis (intrahepatic or extrahepatic), venous congestion, inflammation (hepatitis) or abscess formation, cellular infiltration (macrophages in Gaucher's disease, granuloma in sarcoidosis, hematopoietic cells in extramedullary hematopoiesis, tumor cells in primary or secondary neoplasms), or fibrosis with regeneration (cirrhosis in the alcoholic). A *small liver* is characteristic of acute and subacute hepatic necrosis and idiopathic cirrhosis. The *consistency* of the liver may indicate the nature of the underlying disease. Infiltration and fibrosis cause induration; palpable *nodules* may be neoplasm, cysts, abscesses, or regeneration nodules. *Tenderness* may be due to acute enlargement or inflammation, and may be elicited by direct palpation or by percussion over the right lower ribs. Expansile *pulsation* of the congested liver results from tricuspid regurgitation. Vascular *bruits* over the liver may be due to arteriovenous fistulas, vascular tumors, or pressure on the aorta by an enlarged liver. *Friction rubs* are usually associated with neoplastic infiltration of the liver capsule and peritoneum, but may be due to peritonitis.

PORTAL HYPERTENSION

The normal flow of blood through the liver approximates 1.5 liters per minute (25 per cent of the cardiac output); portal venous inflow from the splanchnic circulation contributes approximately 1 liter per minute, and the hepatic artery 0.5 liter per minute. Portal venous and hepatic arterial blood combine in the periphery of the hepatic sinusoids and flow centrally to the central vein and hepatic venous system. Hepatic blood flow is normally phasic with a pressure gradient between portal vein and inferior vena cava of 0 to 5 mm Hg.

Portal hypertension, an increased pressure gradient across the liver, may be due to an increased splanchnic blood flow, or to an increased resistance to blood flow through the liver.

An increase in splanchnic blood flow may be due to *arteriovenous fistulas,* either congenital or secondary to ruptured splenic or hepatic artery aneurysms. Massive *splenomegaly* in patients with *hematologic disorders* (polycythemia vera, agnogenic myeloid metaplasia, lymphoma, or leukemia) is sometimes associated with portal hypertension; both an increase in splenic blood flow and infiltration of hepatic sinusoids by hematopoietic cells or tumor cells contribute to the elevation of portal pressure. In patients with *tropical splenomegaly,* portal hypertension is also secondary to an increased splenic blood flow. *Cirrhosis of the liver* is often associated with an increased cardiac output and decreased peripheral vascular resistance. Spider angiomas and palmar erythema result from local arteriovenous shunts. It has been suggested that patients with cirrhosis and portal hypertension have a decreased splenic and splanchnic vascular resistance with increased blood flow that contributes to the portal hypertension. Splenic blood flow measured by injection of radioactive xenon into the splenic artery is increased in patients with cirrhosis, whereas portal blood flow measured after portacaval shunts was not increased. An increase in the vascular resistance within the liver is the major factor in the pathogenesis of portal hypertension in cirrhosis.

Portal hypertension secondary to an increase in vascular resistance across the liver is seen in patients with portal venous occlusion, in cirrhosis where blood flow from sinusoids is obstructed by fibrosis and nodular regeneration, and in patients with obstruction of the hepatic veins. *Presinusoidal obstruction* of the portal vein may be *intrahepatic* with occlusion of the distal branches of the portal system in portal triads as in *schistosomiasis* and *congenital hepatic fibrosis,* or may be *extrahepatic* when the portal vein is occluded by thrombosis or tumor. *Postsinusoidal obstruction* of the hepatic veins may be due to thrombus or tumor (Budd-Chiari syndrome). In *veno-occlusive disease* fibrosis around central veins and branches of the hepatic vein obstructs venous outflow. In patients with *acute alcoholic hepatitis,* acute sclerosing hyaline necrosis causes obstruction of central veins and adjacent sinusoids prior to the development of cirrhosis. With the progressive development of cirrhosis, scarring and nodular regeneration further obstruct blood flow. *Infiltrative disease* (secondary neoplasm or granuloma) sometimes leads to clinically significant portal hypertension.

Manifestations

The manifestations of portal hypertension are *splenomegaly,* the development of a *collateral circulation,* and *ascites.*

Splenomegaly. Splenic enlargement is commonly due to venous congestion, but may also result from lymphoid hyperplasia and cellular infiltration. The spleen is not always palpable in patients with portal hypertension, and, conversely, an enlarged spleen does not necessarily imply that a patient with liver disease has portal hypertension. Splenomegaly in cirrhotic patients is usually associated with an increased splenic artery blood flow.

Portal-Systemic Collateral Vessels. Collateral veins draining from the portal to the systemic venous system develop in response to an *increased pressure gradient* at sites of anastomosis between portal and systemic veins—in the esophagus and lower rectum, in the falciform ligament, in the retroperitoneal space, and in adhesions between the visceral and parietal peritoneum.

Esophageal collateral vessels between the left gastric and azygos veins develop as tortuous, dilated, thin-walled submucosal veins that may extend from the fundus of the stomach to the midesophagus *(esophageal* and *gastric varices).* Collateral vessels between the inferior mesenteric and internal iliac veins may form *hemorrhoids.* Collaterals from the left branch of the portal vein through patent umbilical or paraumbilical veins in the falciform ligament to the anterior abdominal wall may form a *caput medusae*—dilated, tortuous veins radiating from the umbilicus with centrifugal blood flow to epigastric, lateral thoracic, and saphenous vessels. A *venous hum* may be audible at the umbilicus (Cruveilhier-Baumgarten syndrome). These subcutaneous collaterals are most prominent when the patient is erect, and their origin from the portal system may be proved by showing that the glucose content of variceal blood exceeds that of peripheral venous blood during glucose absorption.

Acute upper gastrointestinal *bleeding from esophageal varices* is the major complication of portal hypertension.

Ascites. Ascites is an accumulation of lymph in the peritoneal cavity. Hepatic and intestinal lymph normally drains through the thoracic duct into the left subclavian vein. Ascitic fluid accumulates when hepatic and intestinal lymph is formed in amounts that exceed the capacity of the thoracic duct to drain lymph from the abdomen. Two factors, *portal hypertension* and a *lowered plasma colloidal osmotic pressure,* contribute to the increased transudation of fluid from hepatic sinusoids and splanchnic capillaries in patients with liver disease. A third factor, *increased plasma aldosterone* concentration, augments sodium and water retention by promoting distal renal tubular reabsorption of sodium.

Portal hypertension caused by hepatic venous outflow tract obstruction (hepatic vein occlusion or cirrhosis), with *increased hepatic sinusoidal pressure,* is the major factor that determines the *selective* accumulation of fluid in the peritoneal cavity of patients with liver disease. Large volumes of hepatic lymph drain from congested sinusoids through dilated hilar lymphatic vessels to the thoracic duct, or may leak from lymphatic vessels in the capsule and hilum of the liver into the peritoneal cavity. Ascites in patients with liver disease is not a stagnant pool. There is a rapid exchange of water and electrolytes between plasma and ascites across the visceral peritoneum, and an increased volume of lymph drains through the thoracic duct from the abdominal viscera and peritoneal cavity.

Portal hypertension without sinusoidal hypertension rarely causes ascites unless acute bleeding from esophageal varices precipitates hypoalbuminemia and stimulates aldosterone secretion. (See Hepatic Schistosomiasis in Ch. 702.)

Hypoalbuminemia with a lowered plasma colloidal osmotic pressure increases fluid transudation from hepatic sinusoids and splanchnic capillaries, and thus augments lymph flow from these congested vascular beds. Hypoalbuminemic patients without portal hypertension, however, develop ascites only as a manifestation of fluid accumulation in dependent parts, as in the nephrotic syndrome.

In cirrhotic patients with ascites there are increased urinary excretion and plasma concentration of *aldosterone,* owing in part to an *increased adrenal secretion* of aldosterone and in part to *reduced hepatic metabolism* of the hormone. Although it has been shown that inferior vena caval obstruction proximal to the hepatic veins in the dog stimulates aldosterone secretion, the exact mechanism of *secondary hyperaldosteronism* in patients with cirrhosis and portal hypertension has not been defined. A relative pooling of blood in the splanchnic bed with reduced renal blood flow may be the primary stimulus for the release of *renin* from the juxtaglomerular cells in the kidney and the subsequent secretion of salt-retaining hormone. Aldosterone secretion will be further augmented by hemorrhage, infection, and the administration of diuretic agents to these patients.

Ascites is sometimes precipitated by *peritonitis* (especially *tuberculous*) or *tumor* invasion of the peritoneal cavity. These complications must be considered in the differential diagnosis (see below).

The clinical manifestations of ascites are increasing *abdominal distention* with *weight gain* and an associated *decrease in urine output.* Distention of the abdominal wall may cause pain over the lower ribs at the insertion of the abdominal muscles, and may promote the formation of umbilical and inguinal hernias. On physical examination there may be *shifting dullness,* a *fluid wave,* and *elevation of the diaphragms.* Ascitic fluid may leak through the diaphragm to create a *pleural effusion;* this is more often seen on the right than on the left. The urinary excretion of sodium is considerably decreased and may be less than 1 mEq in 24 hours, whereas urinary potassium excretion is increased.

NEUROPSYCHIATRIC ABNORMALITIES ASSOCIATED WITH LIVER DISEASE

The neuropsychiatric manifestations of acute alcohol intoxication, prolonged excessive use of alcohol, alcohol withdrawal, vitamin deficiency in alcoholics, and head injury are often encountered in patients with cirrhosis. These are considered in Ch. 347. *Wilson's disease* (see Ch. 945) is important in the differential diagnosis of patients with juvenile cirrhosis.

Hepatic Coma and Precoma
(Hepatic Encephalopathy, Portal-Systemic Encephalopathy)

Patients with acute or chronic liver disease may develop a *metabolic encephalopathy* characterized by a variable disturbance of consciousness, psychiatric changes, a flapping tremor with hyperreflexia and increased muscle tone, hyperventilation with respiratory alkalosis, and a typical fetor.

Pathogenesis. Hepatic coma is associated either with severe impairment of liver function or with shunting of portal venous blood through collateral vessels into the peripheral circulation. There may be an accumulation of toxic substances which impair cerebral function or a lack of substances which are necessary for cerebral function. Of the several factors that may contribute to this metabolic encephalopathy, changes in *ammonium metabolism* have been studied most extensively. An increase in blood ammonium concentration parallels the severity of neuropsychiatric changes in cirrhotic patients with *chronic* encephalopathy after portacaval anastomosis. This increase in blood ammonium concentration resulting from enteric absorption of ammonia formed by bacterial deamination of amino acids or urea hydrolysis may be the major biochemical change that precipitates dysfunction of the central nervous system. In patients with *acute* hepatic coma, however, disturbances of ammonium metabolism may be of lesser importance, and blood ammonium levels may be normal.

Other agents which may impair central nervous system function in cirrhotic patients include *short chain fatty acids* (from the diet or from bacterial metabolism of carbohydrate) and bacterial metabolites of protein and amino acids, particularly biogenic amines which may function as false neurotransmitters.

The central nervous system of the patient with liver disease may be more susceptible to a variety of metabolic insults. Thus *hypoxia, electrolyte* and *acid-base imbalance, infection,* and *depressant drugs* may each contribute to metabolic encephalopathy in these patients. Although there may be changes in the serum concentration of electrolytes, elevation of blood ammonium concentration, and/or altered blood pH in patients with hepatic coma, these changes do not necessarily parallel electrolyte and pH changes and ammonium concentrations in the central nervous system. These changes *within the brain* are of primary importance in precipitating encephalopathy; alkalosis, which favors the diffusion of ammonia across the blood-brain barrier, increases ammonia toxicity. In patients with hepatic encephalopathy, there is a decrease in cerebral metabolism and oxygen utilization. There is some evidence that ammonia inhibits oxidative phosphorylation.

Clinical Features. The neuropsychiatric changes in hepatic encephalopathy are nonspecific. One of the more characteristic features of the metabolic encephalopathy associated with liver disease is its *rapid fluctuation. Disturbances of consciousness* may range from mild lethargy to deep coma. *Personality changes,* with depression or euphoria, irritability, anxiety, and paranoid features, together with a loss of concern for person or property, are evident. Intellectual function is variably impaired with *memory loss, inability to concentrate,* and a loss of the capacity for abstract thought. Speech may be slow and slurred, with a loss of modulation, and writing deteriorates; there may be dysphasia, perseveration, and apraxia. The common neurologic changes are asterixis, a "flapping" tremor of the outstretched hands, an increase in muscle tone, hyper-reflexia with clonus—often with flexor plantar responses—and ataxia. Hyperventilation causes repiratory alkalosis. The electroencephalogram shows the nonspecific changes of metabolic encephalopathy; high amplitude delta waves (2 to 3 per second) replace normal alpha waves.

Fetor hepaticus is a characteristic sweet, musty odor of the breath attributed to the excretion of mercaptans, particularly dimethylsulfide. Mercaptans produced by bacterial degradation of methionine escape hepatic detoxification and are excreted in excessive amounts in cirrhotic patients.

The *clinical course* of hepatic encephalopathy varies with its pathogenesis. In patients with *fulminant hepatitis* there is a rapid progression; mania and convulsions may precede the development of decerebrate rigidity and terminal deep coma. In patients with cirrhosis, encephalopathy may be acute or chronic and of varying severity.

Chronic encephalopathy usually improves with therapy (see below), but may progress to permanent neuropsychiatric syndromes (paraplegia, dementia) over a period of years.

CLINICAL MANIFESTATIONS RESULTING FROM IMPAIRED HEPATIC DETOXIFICATION

The liver cell is the major site of detoxification of many drugs and exogenous substances and of endogenous substances, including hormones. In general, by processes of oxidation, reduction, hydrolysis, or conjugation, mediated by enzymes in the smooth endoplasmic reticulum, relatively lipid-soluble substances are converted to water-soluble compounds that may be excreted in bile or urine.

Changes in Drug Metabolism. Several drugs (e.g., phenobarbital) stimulate the hepatic metabolism of drugs. Prolonged phenobarbital administration leads to hyperplasia of the smooth endoplasmic reticulum and an increase in the level of drug metabolizing enzymes. The concentration of hepatic binding proteins, Y and Z, which combine with drugs, also increases. The effects of alcohol (ethanol) on hepatic drug metabolism are of clinical importance. In the acutely intoxicated patient, drug metabolism is depressed; alcohol inhibits drug-metabolizing enzymes. The chronic alcoholic, withdrawn from alcohol, metabolizes drugs more rapidly than normal as a result of hyperplasia of the endoplasmic reticulum; this accelerated metabolism increases his tolerance to both alcohol and other drugs. When alcoholism causes alcoholic hepatitis or cirrhosis, drug metabolism is often depressed.

When hepatic detoxification is impaired in patients with liver disease, the pharmacologic action of some drugs may be augmented and prolonged as higher blood levels are maintained for longer periods of time than in normal subjects.

Endocrine Changes. The liver has a dual role in the metabolism of hormones. Several plasma proteins, alpha globulins, which bind hormones in the plasma, e.g., *thyroxin-binding protein, transcortin,* are synthesized by the liver; hormone activity may be influenced by protein binding in the plasma. Thyroxin and adrenal and gonadal steroid hormones are conjugated in the liver and partly excreted in bile. Conjugation forms polar, water-soluble molecules that have an enterohepatic circulation and are finally excreted in the urine.

Endocrine abnormalities in patients with liver disease may be due to malnutrition or chronic illness, to specific lesions of the endocrine glands (iron infiltration in hemochromatosis), or to altered hepatic metabolism, conjugation, and excretion of hormones by the diseased liver. Disturbances of gonadal function are particularly common in patients with cirrhosis. In males, there may be *hypogonadism,* with small testes, reduced libido and impotence, *gynecomastia,* and delayed development or regression of secondary sex characteristics. Depressed plasma levels of unbound 17β-hydroxy-androgens (particularly testosterone) with normal plasma levels of unbound estradiol have been documented in these patients with gynecomastia. In females there may be delayed menarche, oligomenorrhea, or amenorrhea with subnormal breast development. Normal cyclic hormonal activity is disturbed, and cessation of ovulation leads to sterility.

Cutaneous *striae, acne,* and *hirsutism* with truncal obesity and moon facies may suggest *Cushing's syndrome.* Although plasma cortisol levels may be slightly elevated in these patients, the urinary excretion of hydroxy- and ketosteroids is either normal or subnormal.

The appearance of some alcoholic patients with cirrhosis may suggest *hyperthyroidism.* There may be a tremor, peripheral vasodilatation with sweating, tachycardia, and a slight stare. Although the basal metabolic rate and the uptake and conversion of radioiodine by the thyroid may be increased (particularly if there is iodine deficiency), the serum protein-bound iodine concentration is normal.

NUTRITIONAL AND METABOLIC ABNORMALITIES IN LIVER DISEASE

Weight loss may be due to malabsorption, reduced caloric intake in patients with anorexia, or increased tissue catabolism in acutely ill febrile patients. The chronic alcoholic, deriving a major fraction of his calories from alcohol, consumes a diet that may be deficient in protein, folic acid, ascorbic acid, B vitamins, and minerals. Although body weight may be maintained by alcohol and carbohydrate, *muscle wasting* with progressive weakness is usual. *Hypokalemia,* magnesium deficiency, or alcoholic *myopathy* may accentuate muscle weakness in some patients.

Carbohydrate Metabolism. The liver has a central role in regulating blood sugar levels. During carbohydrate absorption, the monosaccharides glucose, fructose, and galactose are taken up from portal venous blood by liver cells, phosphorylated in the presence of specific hexokinases, and converted to glycogen or metabolized through pyruvate and Krebs cycle intermediates. During periods of fasting, or with secretion of epinephrine and glucagon, glycogenolysis or gluconeogenesis maintains or increases blood sugar levels.

Symptomatic *hypoglycemia* may occur in liver disease when hepatic glycogenolysis and gluconeogenesis are impaired. When liver glycogen stores are depleted by fasting, the ingestion of alcohol, which inhibits gluconeogenesis, may precipitate hypoglycemia *(alcoholic hypoglycemia).* Lowered blood sugar levels also result from massive hepatic necrosis (fulminant hepatitis) or a deficiency of enzymes necessary for glycogenolysis (glycogen storage diseases).

Diabetes mellitus in patients with cirrhosis is often due to associated pancreatic disease (chronic alcoholic pancreatitis, or hemochromatosis), or may be coincidental. Portal-systemic shunting is associated with a higher frequency of diabetes mellitus; plasma glucagon levels are significantly elevated in these patients. Cirrhotic patients often have an abnormal glucose tolerance curve owing to a reduced rate of glucose uptake and release from the diseased liver. Normal fasting blood sugar levels, with prolonged hyperglycemia and late hypoglycemia after a glucose load, are characteristic.

Triglyceride Metabolism. Postprandially, dietary triglyceride enters the circulation as a lipid emulsion (chyle) from the thoracic duct (fatty acids of chain length greater than C10), or passes directly as fatty acid into the portal venous blood (fatty acids of chain length less than C10). During periods of fasting, free fatty acid (FFA) is mobilized from peripheral fat depots and circulates as an albumin-FFA complex. Plasma FFA or triglyceride entering the liver cell is stored as triglyceride droplets, incorporated into plasma lipoproteins and thus transported to peripheral depots or catabolized to ketone bodies for peripheral utilization.

Triglyceride accumulates in the liver whenever there is excessive peripheral mobilization of fat or when liver cell injury prevents the normal metabolism of triglyceride. A fatty liver is commonly found in obese subjects, in diabetics, in normal subjects during starvation, and in alcoholics. The disturbances in triglyceride metabolism caused by acute and chronic alcohol ingestion are discussed in Ch. 709.

Cholesterol and Bile Acids. Cholesterol synthesized in the liver is either incorporated into plasma lipoproteins, excreted directly into bile, or converted to primary bile acids.

Plasma lipoproteins, containing varying amounts of cholesterol (both free and esterified), phospholipid, triglyceride, and specific proteins, are synthesized by the liver and intestinal epithelium. Cholestasis causes an increase in plasma cholesterol concentration; this is associated with an increase in high density lipoprotein with a high content of cholesterol and phospholipid. This does not cause a lipemic serum. Liver failure with impaired hepatic synthesis depresses serum concentrations of lipoprotein and cholesterol.

Cholesterol is excreted in bile as a micellar solution with conjugated bile salt and phospholipid. Changes in the concentration of these compounds may lead to the formation of gallstones (see Ch. 682 to 686).

The primary bile acids (cholic and chenodeoxycholic acids) are synthesized from cholesterol and are secreted in bile as their glycine and taurine conjugates (bile salts). These conjugated bile salts undergo an enterohepatic circulation with active reabsorption from the distal small intestine. Between 20 and 30 grams of conjugated bile salts are thus excreted in bile and reabsorbed daily; the daily fecal loss of bile acids (approximately 1 gram) is balanced by resynthesis from cholesterol.

The conjugated bile salts have important functions that depend on their detergent properties. In the bile they permit the formation of soluble micelles containing cholesterol; in the intestinal lumen they activate pancreatic lipase and form mixed micelles with monoglyceride and long-chain fatty acids, thus facilitating the absorption of fat and fat-soluble vitamins.

In patients with cirrhosis there is a greatly diminished total bile acid pool. This depressed bile acid pool does not lead to the formation of cholesterol gallstones, because decreased biliary bile acid secretion is accompanied by a parallel decrease in cholesterol excretion.

Liver disease may be complicated by *malabsorption* when biliary secretion of conjugated bile salts is insufficient to promote the formation of lipid micelles in the jejunum. The duration of malabsorption in patients with acute liver disease may be too short to cause deficiency states other than *hypoprothrombinemia* owing to malabsorption of vitamin K. In patients with chronic cholestasis (primary and secondary biliary cirrhosis, Ch. 709) steatorrhea may cause diarrhea and weight loss, whereas malabsorption of fat-soluble vitamins A, D, and K may lead to night blindness, bone demineralization, and hypoprothrombinemia.

Protein Metabolism. The liver cell contains enzyme systems that permit the synthesis of nonessential amino acids, synthesis of cellular and plasma proteins from amino acids, catabolism of plasma protein and amino acids, and conversion of ammonia to urea.

Amino acids derived from digested dietary proteins are absorbed in the upper small intestine, enter the portal venous blood, and are almost completely cleared by the liver to be catabolized or utilized in protein synthesis. During periods of fasting, amino acids are converted to pyruvate and phosphorylated hexose intermediates, which support gluconeogenesis and provide a source of glucose for brain metabolism.

Perfusion studies have shown that the liver is responsible for the synthesis of plasma proteins, with the exception of the immunoglobulins and antihemophiliac globulin (AHG). The factors which control protein synthesis are not well understood. Experimental studies suggest that the colloidal osmotic pressure of plasma has a regulatory function; albumin synthesis is depressed in laboratory animals or isolated liver preparations when the colloidal osmotic pressure of plasma is increased with dextran or gamma globulin. Adequate nutrition is essential for normal plasma protein synthesis; liver perfusion studies have shown that tryptophan exerts a specific role in activating albumin synthesis.

The sites of plasma protein degradation and the factors which regulate this are unknown. Studies with labeled albumin indicate that catabolism is in proportion to the total albumin pool. Catabolism by the liver, kidney, and gastrointestinal tract is well documented, but explains only a fraction of the total albumin catabolized daily.

Plasma proteins maintain the colloidal osmotic pressure of plasma, play a vital role in the transport of many substances (including iron, vitamin B_{12}, hormones, hemoglobin, bilirubin, and nonesterified fatty acids), and maintain normal blood clotting mechanisms.

Hepatic synthesis of plasma proteins may be impaired by hepatocellular failure. A reduced rate of plasma protein catabolism may partly compensate for reduced synthesis, which leads to *hypoproteinemia*. Severe *bleeding* may complicate a deficiency of blood-clotting factors. Excessive urinary excretion and elevated plasma levels of amino acids are manifestations of severe hepatocellular failure, particularly fulminant hepatitis. Although urea is synthesized by the liver, low blood urea levels are more often the result of dilution with fluid infused intravenously than of hepatocellular failure.

HEMATOLOGIC ABNORMALITIES

Anemia in patients with liver disease may be due to *blood loss* or *excessive destruction* and/or *reduced formation* of red cells. Changes in red cell morphology may reflect specific deficiency (iron or folic acid) or may result from changes in the lipid composition of the red cell membrane. Red blood cells from patients with cholestasis have an increased surface area related to the reversible accumulation of cholesterol from the plasma; these cells have a lowered osmotic fragility, and appear as target-cells on stained smears. Severe hemolysis in the alcoholic with liver disease may be associated with the appearance of poikilocytes (burr-cells) on peripheral smears.

Bleeding from the nose, upper gastrointestinal tract (esophageal varices, erosive gastritis, or peptic ulcer), or rectum (hemorrhoids) may precipitate acute anemia or chronic iron deficiency anemia. In the absence of blood loss, iron deficiency is uncommon in patients with liver disease; an increase in total body iron with hemosiderosis is more usual, particularly in alcoholic patients with pancreatic disease. The pathogenesis of this secondary hemosiderosis is not known.

Hemolysis is the most common cause of chronic anemia in patients with liver disease. Chronic, low-grade hemolysis in patients with splenomegaly is due to sequestration of red blood cells in the cortex of the congested spleen. Red cell production may fail to compensate for this increased destruction, particularly during periods of hepatic decompensation, so that the patient may exhibit a normochromic and sometimes macrocytic anemia with a normal reticulocyte count, reduced serum levels of haptoglobin, an increased serum level of unconjugated bilirubin, and a bone marrow showing cellular hyperplasia. Severe hemolytic anemia may be associated with hyperlipemia in alcoholic hepatitis *(Zieve's syndrome)* (see Ch. 709), but a causal relationship between the hyperlipemia and hemolysis has not been established. Acute viral hepatitis may precipitate hemolysis in patients with *glucose-6-phosphate dehydrogenase (G-6-PD) deficiency;* particularly high serum concentrations of bilirubin usually result.

A *deficiency of folic acid* may lead to a severe macrocytic anemia with *megaloblastic* bone marrow in alcoholic patients with liver disease. An inadequate vitamin intake, together with alcohol inhibition of folic acid utilization, contributes to the anemia. Treatment with a normal diet containing folic acid or with folic acid supplements corrects this deficiency. Rarely, a normochromic normocytic anemia may be due to *pyridoxine deficiency*.

Although *thrombocytopenia* (platelet counts less than 200,000 per cubic millimeter) and *granulocytopenia* (WBC counts < 4000 per cubic millimeter) may be associated with anemia in patients with liver disease and congestive splenomegaly, these abnormalities are rarely complicated by serious bleeding or infection. Severe thrombocytopenia and fatal aplastic anemia have been reported as complications of acute viral hepatitis.

Clotting abnormalities in patients with acute or chronic liver disease result from reduced synthesis of blood-clotting factors or their increased consumption. Many of the factors active in blood clotting—factors V, VII, IX, X, prothrombin, and fibrinogen—are synthesized by the liver. A lowered plasma concentration of these proteins, measured by blood-clotting tests (see Ch. 795), may be due to *malabsorption of vitamin K* which is required for the synthesis of prothrombin and factors VII, IX, and X, or may reflect *impaired hepatic protein synthesis*. Vitamin K malabsorption results from obstructive jaundice. Hepatic parenchymal disease, either acute or chronic, depresses the synthesis of clotting factors; the capacity of liver cells to produce fibrinogen appears to exceed that of other clotting factors, because fibrinogen levels are often maintained when other clotting factors are deficient. *Intravascular coagulation* with consumption of clotting factors, thrombocytopenia, and the appearance of fibrin split products in the plasma is a complication of fulminant hepatitis, decompensated cirrhosis, and metastatic cancer.

IMMUNE PHENOMENA IN LIVER DISEASE

Hypergammaglobulinemia is a common manifestation of *chronic active hepatitis, idiopathic cirrhosis,* and *primary biliary cirrhosis.* The gamma globulin increase is *polyclonal,* involving all classes of immunoglobulin (IgA, IgM, and IgG), although in primary biliary cirrhosis IgM may be increased selectively. Hypergammaglobulinemia is often associated with positive serologic tests for syphilis, heterophil antibody, antinuclear antibody, antimitochondrial antibody, and LE cell phenomena. Furthermore the titers of antibody against bacterial and viral antigens may be increased. An increase in circulating immunoglobulin in patients with liver disease usually reflects *infiltration of the liver* with plasma cells and lymphocytes, particularly in areas of parenchymal cell necrosis.

The role of *immunologic mechanisms* in the *pathogenesis* of chronic liver disease has not been established. The immune phenomena may be secondary to the release of antigens from damaged liver cells, or, alternatively, local immunologic processes may play an active role in destroying liver cells. The association between chronic liver disease, chronic thyroiditis, and Sjögren's syndrome suggests that autoimmune phenomena may indeed be important in pathogenesis (see Ch. 708 and 709). Depression of *serum complement* levels in patients with chronic liver disease cannot be correlated with immune phenomena, but appears to be related to impaired hepatic protein synthesis.

CARDIOVASCULAR CHANGES

Hepatocellular failure is often associated with an *increase* in *cardiac output* manifested by tachycardia, a precordial ejection systolic murmur, and peripheral vasodilatation. The cause for these circulatory changes is not known.

Some patients with cirrhosis exhibit central *cyanosis* with arterial oxygen unsaturation. In patients with portal hypertension, this may be due to portopulmonary venous shunts that bypass the pulmonary capillaries, or may result from pulmonary arteriovenous shunts or reduced aeration of basal lung segments in patients with tense ascites.

The plasma volume is usually normal or increased in cirrhotic patients prior to diuretic therapy. When patients with ascites are treated with diuretic agents, brisk diuresis is often accompanied by a fall in plasma volume which is particularly marked when fluid loss exceeds the volume of fluid mobilized from the ascitic pool. Hypovolemic shock may be a terminal complication of cirrhosis, precipitated by massive bleeding, by infection (especially gram-negative septicemia), or by paracentesis. Metabolic acidosis with hyperkalemia and hyponatremia are terminal events.

CHANGES IN RENAL FUNCTION

There are many causes for impairment of renal function in patients with liver disease. Many agents may cause acute cellular injury in both liver and kidneys; these include *hepatotoxins* (carbon tetrachloride,

Amanita phalloides), *infectious agents* (leptospirosis, infectious hepatitis virus; see below), and *hypoxia* (shock). *Metabolic diseases* may damage both organs; in Wilson's disease the deposition of copper in the tissues is associated with cirrhosis and impaired tubular reabsorptive function with glycosuria, aminoaciduria, and hypouricemia.

In patients with cirrhosis and ascites several factors modify renal function. There may be a physiologic response to secondary hyperaldosteronism with sodium retention and potassium excretion, reversed by aldosterone-blocking drugs (see below). Abnormal excretion of a water load usually accompanies cirrhosis with ascites.

Hepatorenal Syndrome. This term refers to the functional renal failure which is a common terminal event in patients with cirrhosis and ascites, and a less common complication of obstructive jaundice after surgery. Progressive azotemia with hyperkalemia and hyponatremia, a reduced creatinine clearance, and progressive oliguria with a concentrated urine free of protein and formed elements and low in sodium are usually observed. Spontaneous recovery is rare. At postmortem examination, no significant pathologic changes are present in the kidneys.

The functional renal failure in patients with cirrhosis and ascites has been attributed to a decrease in renal blood flow resulting from hypovolemia after vigorous diuresis, abdominal paracentesis, or massive bleeding. Alternatively, increased renal vein pressure caused by increased intra-abdominal pressure was suggested as a mechanism. Although hypovolemia will contribute to renal failure, these mechanisms do not explain this syndrome. Studies of renal blood flow by isotope scanning and by renal arteriography have demonstrated an intrarenal shunting of blood with reduced cortical perfusion in cirrhotic patients with ascites and reduced creatinine clearance. Vasoconstriction of cortical vessels reduces glomerular perfusion, although total renal blood flow may remain normal. The agents which cause cortical vasoconstriction have not been identified, but it is known that sympathetic blocking agents do not restore cortical flow.

When a cirrhotic patient with ascites develops the hepatorenal syndrome, increasing jaundice results from decreased bilirubin excretion in the urine, and azotemia with increased blood ammonia levels usually precipitates hepatic coma.

CUTANEOUS MANIFESTATIONS OF LIVER DISEASE

Pruritus. Patients with obstructive jaundice (both intrahepatic and extrahepatic cholestasis) may suffer from generalized itching. This is probably caused by retained *bile acids.* The intensity of pruritus parallels the serum concentration of bile acids, and the oral administration of the resin cholestyramine lowers serum bile acid levels and relieves itching by binding bile salts in the intestine and preventing their reabsorption. *Itching is not related to the intensity of jaundice;* anicteric patients may itch because of retained bile salts, whereas deeply jaundiced patients may be free of pruritus when cholesterol and bile acid synthesis is impaired by hepatocellular failure.

Pigmentation. An increase in *melanin pigmentation* of the skin is typical of chronic obstructive jaundice (biliary cirrhosis) and in hemochromatosis. The pathogenesis is not known.

Spider Angiomas (Vascular Spiders). These cutaneous lesions, found in areas drained by the superior vena cava, have a central pulsating arteriole from which small vessels radiate over an area 1 to 10 mm in diameter. Multiple lesions may appear and disappear during the course of both acute and chronic liver disease, but are most numerous when liver disease is chronic and progressive. Small arterial spiders are also seen in normal subjects, and often appear during pregnancy. Their pathogenesis is not known.

Palmar Erythema. Cutaneous erythema, maximal over the thenar and hypothenar eminences and the pulp of the fingers and less often seen on the soles of the feet, is due to local vasodilatation with increased blood flow. The cardiac output is usually increased in patients with prominent palmar erythema.

Other changes in the hands include *Dupuytren's contractures* in patients with cirrhosis associated with alcohol ingestion, *clubbing* of the nails in patients with biliary cirrhosis, and white, opaque nails with loss of lunules in hypoalbuminemic patients.

Xanthomas. Prolonged obstructive jaundice with elevation of serum lipoprotein may be associated with deposits of lipid, predominantly cholesterol, in macrophages in the dermis or subcutaneous tissue. Flat lesions *(xanthelasma)* are common on the eyelids, on the neck, and in the palm creases, as yellow, slightly raised, soft deposits. Tuberous lesions, more common over areas exposed to pressure, are firm, nodular, and slightly yellow. These lesions may appear when serum cholesterol levels exceed 450 mg per 100 ml for several months, and may disappear when serum cholesterol levels fall below that value.

NONSPECIFIC SYMPTOMS IN PATIENTS WITH LIVER DISEASE

Many symptoms in patients with liver disease are also common manifestations of nonhepatic disorders. It is often impossible to determine whether these symptoms are primarily due to liver disease or whether they result from extrahepatic effects of the primary noxious agent. The prodromal symptoms of acute viral hepatitis — malaise, weakness, unusual fatigability, anorexia, fever, myalgia, and headache — are good examples. Although these symptoms are nonspecific, they are often helpful in differential diagnosis.

Fever. Fever is common in patients with acute liver disease and is usually due to tissue necrosis, infection, or drug hypersensitivity. In patients with acute metabolic encephalopathy, fever may be due to dysfunction of central thermoregulatory mechanisms. This usually occurs in fulminant hepatitis and in the alcoholic with a severe withdrawal reaction (delirium tremens).

Abdominal Pain. Abdominal pain may be localized to the right upper quadrant and may result from inflammation or stretching of the pain-sensitive capsule of the liver. Epigastric or midabdominal pain may be due to associated peptic ulcer disease, acute gastritis, or pancreatitis. Stretching of the abdominal wall by tense ascites may cause pain over the lower costal margin.

695. DIAGNOSTIC PROCEDURES

TESTS OF LIVER FUNCTION

Many biochemical tests have been used to estimate liver function. In interpreting tests of liver function one must remember that no test is diagnostic of specific liver lesion, that many tests may be normal in the presence of liver disease, and that factors other than liver disease may cause abnormal tests.

Serum Bilirubin. Spectrophotometric measurement of the amount of diazo-pigment formed by the van den Bergh reaction after one minute in the absence of alcohol gives an estimate of the *direct-reacting* serum bilirubin concentration; this is approximately equal to the serum concentration of *conjugated bilirubin,* which is diazotized in the absence of alcohol. When alcohol is added in the van den Bergh reaction, unconjugated bilirubin is able to react with the diazo reagent, and the total concentration of bilirubin (direct plus indirect reacting) in the serum is estimated. Normal serum contains less than 0.2 mg of direct-reacting pigment and less than 0.8 mg of indirect-reacting pigment per 100 ml. Measurements of serum bilirubin (direct-reacting and total) are helpful in separating diseases associated with unconjugated bilirubinemia from those causing predominantly conjugated hyperbilirubinemia, but are of no value in differentiating jaundice resulting from hepatocellular disease from extrahepatic cholestasis. Serial determinations of serum bilirubin concentration provide a more accurate measure of the impairment of bilirubin excretion during the course of liver disease than can be gained by a clinical assessment of the degree of jaundice.

Tests for *bilirubin in the urine* are helpful in differentiating jaundice caused by unconjugated hyperbilirubinemia; only conjugated bilirubin is excreted in the urine. Bilirubin may be excreted in the urine when the elevation of serum bilirubin is insufficient to cause jaundice.

Urinary and Fecal Urobilinogen. Urinary excretion of urobilinogen increases when the amount of urobilinogen absorbed from the intestine is increased by excessive pigment production or when hepatic excretion of urobilinogen is impaired by liver disease. Normally, urobilinogen can be detected in urine diluted to 1 in 16. *An increase in urinary urobilinogen excretion in the absence of increased fecal excretion of pigment is a very sensitive indicator of liver disease.* A quantitative measurement of the 24-hour fecal excretion of urobilinogen is of diagnostic value in hemolytic states and in patients with biliary tract disease. An increased fecal excretion of urobilinogen confirms that there is excessive bilirubin production, and a total absence of urobilinogen in the stool indicates complete biliary tract obstruction owing to atresia or neoplasm.

Sulfobromophthalein Sodium (Bromsulphalein, BSP) Clearance. The measurement of the hepatic clearance of this organic, anionic dye is the most sensitive test of liver function. Injected BSP, bound by plasma proteins (albumin and alpha globulin), is cleared by the liver and excreted in bile. BSP excretion by the liver depends on the selective uptake and concentration of dye by Y and Z binding proteins in the liver cell and the rate-limiting active transport of both unconjugated and glutathione-conjugated BSP into the bile canaliculi. BSP clearance varies with bile salt excretion, and can be increased experimentally by intravenous infusion of bile salt which augments excretion by increasing canalicular bile flow.

In the standard liver function test, the amount of BSP retained in the plasma is measured 30 or 45 minutes after an intravenous injection of the dye (5 mg per kilogram of body weight). The normal subject excretes more than 90 and 96 per cent of the injected BSP in 30 and 45 minutes, respectively. A reduced plasma clearance of BSP (increased retention of dye in the plasma) may result from changes in hepatic blood flow as in congestive heart failure or portal vein thrombosis, from reduced ability of liver cells to concentrate or excrete the dye as in hepatocellular injury and metabolic abnormalities, or from obstruction to bile flow in intrahepatic and extrahepatic cholestasis. Thus abnormal BSP excretion does not indicate a specific hepatic lesion. The dye should be injected with care, because leakage outside the vein causes severe pain and tissue necrosis.

Although the standard BSP test is a sensitive measure of liver function, the maximal capacity of the liver to excrete the dye is not measured. The maximal capacity of the liver to concentrate and to excrete BSP may be estimated by measuring plasma clearance when infusions of the dye are given. Either of these maxima may be reduced when all other tests of liver function remain normal. In some patients with liver disease, the maximal excretion rate of the dye may be reduced when hepatic storage is normal or increased.

Albumin. Normal levels of plasma albumin are maintained by an equilibrium between hepatic synthesis and degradation or loss. When synthesis is reduced in liver disease, the serum albumin concentration and the total body albumin pool decrease until a new equilibrium is established between synthesis and degradation. In view of the slow rate of albumin degradation (the half-time of plasma albumin degradation varies between 12 and 18 days), the serum concentration of albumin does not immediately reflect rapid changes in liver function, but decreases slowly when synthesis is impaired. In patients with cirrhosis, a depressed level of serum albumin reflects reduced synthesis and/or distribution of the albumin pool in an expanded extravascular space (ascitic fluid).

Globulins. Changes in the concentration of the serum globulins can be assessed by salt fractionation or by electrophoresis of serum. *Alpha and beta globulin* concentrations increase in patients with infection or obstructive jaundice and decrease when hepatocellular failure impairs their synthesis. The serum concentration of the *immunoglobulins* increases when antibody production is stimulated by exogenous or tissue antigen. Although immunoglobulin synthesis is not a function of the liver, measurements of serum gamma globulin concentrations are helpful in diagnosis. Extreme hypergammaglobulinemia suggests a diagnosis of chronic active hepatitis, or cirrhosis. Positive tests for antinuclear and smooth muscle antibody and LE cell reaction are frequent in patients with chronic active hepatitis, whereas antimitochondrial antibody tests are usually positive in patients with primary biliary cirrhosis (see Ch. 708 and Primary Biliary Cirrhosis in Ch. 709).

The serum *flocculation tests* are nonspecific tests in which the plasma proteins are precipitated or flocculated by a variety of agents. Positive tests depend on relative changes in the concentration of several plasma proteins and are not specific for liver disease.

Blood-Clotting Tests. Tests of blood coagulation provide a sensitive measure of hepatic synthetic function. The relatively short half-life (two to four days) of several of the blood-clotting factors leads to a rapid change in the one-stage prothrombin time when synthesis is depressed by acute parenchymal liver disease. In acute hepatitis, the prothrombin time is a valuable guide to the severity of parenchymal damage; marked prolongation of the prothrombin time (greater than 20 seconds) is an early reflection of massive necrosis. Whenever clotting tests are used to measure liver function, possible deficiency of vitamin K should be first excluded by parenteral therapy.

Cholesterol. Changes in serum cholesterol concentrations reflect changes in serum lipoprotein. In cholestasis, when cholesterol and bile acid excretion is impaired but cholesterol synthesis is normal, serum lipoprotein and cholesterol concentrations increase. When hepatic lipoprotein synthesis is impaired by hepatocellular disease, serum cholesterol concentrations fall.

Serum Enzymes. A large number of enzymes normally concentrated in the liver (and other tissues) are also present at low activity in the plasma. The level of enzyme activity in the plasma is determined by the rate of release from cells and the rate of clearance from plasma, in addition to the presence of activators or inhibitors in the plasma. Three patterns of abnormal plasma enzyme activity which depend on differences in enzyme synthesis and release are seen in patients with liver disease.

1. *Increased enzyme activity due to release from damaged liver cells.* Enzymes present in high concentration in the liver cell are released with damage to parenchymal cells. These enzymes include the *transaminases* and *dehydrogenases* which are measured routinely in clinical laboratories. The wide tissue distribution of these enzymes limits their specificity in localizing the site of cell damage unless other diagnostic criteria are used concomitantly or unless the elevation of serum enzyme is of such degree that liver cell damage could be the only source. In *acute hepatitis,* serum transaminase levels are usually elevated to levels in excess of 500 iu, but the degree of enzyme elevation correlates poorly with the extent of liver cell necrosis seen on liver biopsy. In patients with fulminant hepatitis, progressive clinical deterioration is often accompanied by a fall in serum enzyme activity (see Ch. 698). In *chronic active hepatitis,* the level of serum transaminase reflects the activity of the disease process and is a useful guide to therapy with corticosteroids (see Ch. 708).

2. *Increased enzyme activity due to de novo synthesis by liver cells and/or bile ducts with release into plasma.* The serum levels of alkaline phosphatase, 5'-nucleotidase, and leucine aminopeptidase are increased in patients with cholestasis—either intrahepatic or extrahepatic. Experimental studies have shown that the increase in serum alkaline phosphatase activity after bile duct ligation is due to the release of enzyme that is newly synthesized in the liver. The level of serum alkaline phosphatase is of no value in the differential diagnosis of obstructive jaundice. When the origin of the serum alkaline phosphatase is uncertain (serum enzyme activity may be derived from bone, intestine, or liver), the hepatic origin of the enzyme can be confirmed by measurement of serum 5'-nucleotidase or leucine amino-

peptidase activity; these enzymes are more specific for liver disease. Alternatively, differences in the heat stability of enzymes of hepatic and bony origin suggest the site of origin. Hepatic alkaline phosphatase is more heat stable than bone alkaline phosphatase. In the *absence of jaundice,* an elevated alkaline phosphatase suggests early cholestasis or hepatic infiltration by tumor or granuloma. A normal alkaline phosphatase in a jaundiced patient is usually indicative of parenchymal cell disease.

3. *Decreased serum enzyme activity due to impaired hepatic synthesis.* The serum level of some enzymes may decrease in patients with impaired synthesis. These enzymes include *ceruloplasmin,* a copper-containing oxidase, and lecithin-cholesterol acyltransferase, an enzyme which normally esterifies plasma cholesterol. These enzymes are not routinely measured as tests of liver function.

NEEDLE BIOPSY OF THE LIVER

Percutaneous needle biopsy of the liver by an intercostal approach under local anesthesia is a simple, safe bedside procedure that provides a tissue diagnosis of liver disease without subjecting the patient to the greater risk of general anesthesia and laparotomy with open surgical biopsy.

Indications. Needle biopsy of the liver is of proved value in the following situations:

1. In the differential diagnosis of jaundice, hepatic enlargement, and splenomegaly.

2. In the differential diagnosis of unexplained fever. A liver biopsy may suggest or establish the diagnosis of *miliary tuberculosis,* sarcoidosis, brucellosis, or neoplasm.

3. To assess the degree of hepatic fibrosis in chronic hepatitis and cirrhosis, to evaluate the course of hepatitis and acute liver disease, and to estimate hepatic stores of iron in hemochromatosis.

Contraindications. Liver biopsy is contraindicated in the following circumstances:

1. In patients who are uncooperative or who cannot control movements of the diaphragm, e.g., with severe recurrent cough.

2. In patients with bleeding disorders, with clotting defects (prothrombin time elevations greater than two to three seconds over control), or with vascular tumors in the liver.

3. In patients with severe cardiopulmonary disease that would be a contraindication to surgery should a biopsy complication ensue.

4. In patients with prolonged jaundice, probably extrahepatic in origin.

Complications. Needle biopsy of the liver is usually painless, but is occasionally followed by right pleuritic chest pain referred to the shoulder; a transient pleural friction rub may be audible at the site of biopsy. Serious complications include *hemorrhage* from the biopsy site and leakage of bile from dilated intrahepatic bile ducts or gallbladder, with *bile peritonitis;* this is usually a complication of extrahepatic obstruction. The incidence of these major complications should be less than 0.1 per cent.

PROCEDURES USED TO DIAGNOSE BILIARY TRACT DISEASE

The *radiographic procedures* used to visualize the biliary tree depend on the hepatic excretion of radiopaque dye *(oral cholecystography* and *intravenous cholangiography)* or on the direct injection of contrast agents into the bile ducts either at operation *(operative cholangiography)* or after cannulation of the ampulla via the duodenoscope *(retrograde duodenoscopic cholangiography)* or by needle (at *peritoneoscopy,* or by *percutaneous transhepatic* and *transvenous* transhepatic approaches). These techniques, as well as examination of duodenal bile *(biliary drainage)* and the *secretin test,* are of value in the differential diagnosis of obstructive jaundice. They are discussed in detail in Ch. 681.

The hepatic excretion of the most commonly used oral cholecystographic agent, *iopanoic acid,* involves a sequence that is similar to the excretion of bilirubin. In the plasma, iopanoic acid is albumin bound. Excretion depends on diffusion across the liver cell membrane, concentration in the liver cell by binding to Y and Z proteins, conjugation with glucuronide to form a water-soluble complex, and active transport of the glucuronyl conjugate into the bile canaliculi. Impaired excretion of iopanoic acid should thus be expected in patients with parenchymal liver disease or cholestasis.

DIAGNOSTIC PROCEDURES IN PORTAL HYPERTENSION

Esophageal varices may be demonstrated roentgenographically by a *barium swallow,* although *esophagoscopy* is a more accurate method for their identification.

Portal venous pressure can be measured indirectly by inserting a needle into the splenic pulp or by wedging a catheter in a branch of the hepatic vein. Comparative studies have shown that portal vein pressures measured directly through a catheter in the umbilical vein correspond to pressures recorded from wedged hepatic vein catheters in patients with cirrhosis. Measurement of wedged hepatic vein catheter pressure has the advantage of providing baseline inferior vena cava pressures. Portal pressure measurements are of value in establishing the presence of portal hypertension when this is in doubt in patients with splenomegaly or ascites. An elevated pressure is consistent with the diagnosis of chronic liver disease rather than presinusoidal portal vein obstruction. Repeated pressure measurements provide evidence of changes in portal pressure which may be of prognostic value; with recovery from acute alcoholic hepatitis, a fall in portal pressure suggests a better prognosis than a stable or rising pressure which reflects progressive fibrosis. The degree of pressure elevation does not appear to indicate the risk of hemorrhage from esophageal varices or the prognosis after portacaval shunt surgery.

The portal circulation can be visualized roentgenographically by *selective celiac arteriography* or by injection of contrast material into the spleen *(transsplenic venography)* or directly through the catheterized umbilical vein. The portal vein and collateral circulation should be demonstrated before portacaval shunt surgery is performed.

LIVER SCANNING

When compounds that are concentrated in the liver (either by parenchymal or Kupffer cells) are labeled with gamma-emitting isotopes and injected intravenously, their uptake by the liver can be assessed by surface scanning. ^{131}I-labeled rose bengal, [198]Au colloidal gold, and [99]technetium have been used. Space-occupying lesions (cysts, abscesses, or tumors) appear as filling defects. In patients with cirrhosis, hepatic uptake is decreased and irregular and splenic uptake may be increased. A liver scan is of value in providing evidence of a space-occupying lesion when this was not evident clinically. A liver biopsy should be performed to confirm the pathologic diagnosis; the biopsy needle may be directed to the site of infiltration demonstrated by the scan. Serial liver scans may be of value in documenting the response of a patient with metastatic neoplasm to therapy.

696. METABOLIC DISORDERS

Inborn errors of metabolism may cause chronic liver disease. In some of these conditions specific enzyme defects have been demonstrated (glycogen storage diseases [see Ch. 809], galactosemia [see Ch. 808]), whereas in others the underlying metabolic abnormality has not yet been defined (idiopathic hemochromatosis [see Part XVI, Section Four], Wilson's disease [see Ch. 945], Gaucher's disease [see Ch. 776]).

Disorders of Bilirubin Metabolism. Knowledge of several metabolic disorders has contributed greatly to an understanding of bilirubin metabolism and excretion.

Unconjugated Hyperbilirubinemia. Acholuric jaundice with unconjugated hyperbilirubinemia in the absence of other signs of anemia or liver disease may be due to one of the following conditions:

1. *Compensated hemolysis* in which increased red cell production masks excessive red cell destruction. This abnormality may be suggested by lowered serum haptoglobin concentrations and increased fecal urobilinogen and reticulocyte counts, but can be confirmed only by direct measurement of red cell survival using tagged erythrocytes. An increase in bilirubin production alone is insufficient to account for the unconjugated hyperbilirubinemia in patients with compensated hemolysis. Studies of bilirubin clearance using labeled bilirubin indicate that these patients also have a delayed clearance of pigment; the excessive bilirubin load unmasks this excretory defect (see Gilbert's syndrome, below).

2. *Excessive bilirubin production without hemolysis* ("shunt hyperbilirubinemia"). This is a rare condition in which abnormal catabolism of hemoglobin in red cell precursors in the bone marrow results in excessive pigment production (early-labeled bilirubin) and increased fecal urobilinogen excretion; peripheral red cell survival is normal.

3. *Idiopathic unconjugated hyperbilirubinemia (Gilbert's syndrome).* Mild unconjugated hyperbilirubinemia (usually less than 3 mg per 100 ml) without hemolysis or excessive bilirubin production is commonly recognized in healthy young subjects. Jaundice may be intermittent with exacerbations during intercurrent illness and particularly during periods of fasting. The absence of physi-

cal abnormalities, normal liver function tests, and normal liver histology exclude a diagnosis of viral hepatitis. This syndrome appears to have an autosomal dominant inheritance; unconjugated hyperbilirubinemia was detected in 16.1 per cent of parents and 27.5 per cent of siblings of patients with this disorder.

A defect in the hepatic uptake of unconjugated bilirubin from plasma has been documented by a depressed plasma clearance of labeled unconjugated bilirubin in patients with Gilbert's syndrome. In some patients, excessive bilirubin production from compensated hemolysis accentuates the excretory defect. Whereas fasting increases serum bilirubin levels in patients with Gilbert's syndrome, the administration of drugs which induce microsomal enzyme systems (e.g., phenobarbital) lowers the serum bilirubin, presumably by increasing the efficiency of hepatic pigment excretion.

4. *Parenchymal liver disease* may be associated with unconjugated hyperbilirubinemia. This has been recognized in patients during recovery from viral hepatitis. Other abnormal tests of liver function (positive flocculation tests, mildly abnormal BSP), and histologic changes on liver biopsy suggest hepatitis in these patients. Unconjugated hyperbilirubinemia in patients with congestive heart failure, or after portacaval shunt surgery for portal hypertension, reflects reduced hepatic blood flow and bilirubin clearance.

5. *Impaired bilirubin conjugation.* A defect in bilirubin conjugation is usually manifest during the neonatal period, and may be due to immaturity of the liver, inhibition of glucuronyl transferase, or deficiency of this enzyme.

a. *The immature liver* of the premature infant exhibits a reduced level of glucuronyl transferase activity. It has not been established, however, that this is the primary cause for physiologic jaundice; there may be other defects in the excretory mechanism.

b. *Prolonged neonatal jaundice in breast-fed infants* may be due to inhibition of glucuronyl transferase activity by an abnormal steroid (pregnane-3α-20β-diol) excreted in the mother's milk. Jaundice is maximal during the second to third week, and subsides rapidly if breast feeding is discontinued, or over a four- to eight-week period with continued breast feeding.

Transient neonatal hyperbilirubinemia, described in successive infants of several mothers, has been related to the presence of an inhibitor of glucuronyl transferase in the maternal plasma during pregnancy. Several of these infants developed kernicterus.

c. *The Crigler-Najjar syndrome* (congenital, nonhemolytic, unconjugated hyperbilirubinemia with glucuronyl transferase deficiency). This syndrome, characterized by severe jaundice, usually from birth, is transmitted in some patients as an autosomal recessive defect, and in others as an autosomal dominant. Patients with the autosomal recessive defect are deeply jaundiced (mean bilirubin levels 25 to 31 mg per 100 ml) and develop kernicterus. Their bile is colorless, and phenobarbital administration does not lower the serum level of unconjugated bilirubin. The autosomal dominant defect may cause less severe hyperbilirubinemia so that some patients survive to adulthood without kernicterus. When phenobarbital is given to these patients, the serum bilirubin concentration falls dramatically; this effect may be due to induction of glucuronyl transferase activity.

The homozygous *Gunn rat,* deficient in glucuronyl

transferase, provides a laboratory model of the Crigler-Najjar syndrome.

Kernicterus (Bilirubin Encephalopathy). This neurologic complication of severe unconjugated hyperbilirubinemia usually develops in the jaundiced infant during the first week of life with the appearance of spasticity, leading to head retraction, opisthotonos, muscle twitching, or convulsions. The infant may die during the neonatal period, whereas survivors exhibit mental retardation and spastic paraplegia with athetosis.

Normally, the binding of unconjugated bilirubin by albumin restricts pigment diffusion into tissue cells. However, when the concentration of unconjugated bilirubin exceeds the albumin-binding capacity (approximately 20 mg of bilirubin per 100 ml of plasma in the normal infant), unconjugated bilirubin is free to diffuse into tissues; the lipid solubility of the pigment enhances its diffusion across cell membranes and the blood-brain barrier. Depression of the plasma albumin level, the administration of drugs which bind albumin and thus displace bilirubin (sulfonamides and salicylate), and metabolic acidosis all predispose to kernicterus. The biochemical mechanism for bilirubin encephalopathy has not been well defined.

Preventive therapy depends on the early recognition and treatment of conditions that may cause severe hemolysis in the newborn (ABO and Rh incompatibility or red cell enzyme defects). Infection and metabolic acidosis should be treated vigorously, and drugs which bind bilirubin should be avoided. Phototherapy (exposure to light of wavelength 440 mμ) may reduce the level of serum bilirubin by converting the tetrapyrrole pigment to colorless products with alternate pathways of excretion. Exchange transfusion is indicated when the serum bilirubin rises to dangerous levels; in sick premature infants with depressed albumin binding, serum bilirubin levels in excess of 10 mg per 100 ml plasma may be unsafe.

The Dubin-Johnson Syndrome. This is a familial metabolic disorder caused by impaired hepatic excretion of certain organic anions into the bile. Jaundice is associated with an increased serum level of conjugated bilirubin and bilirubinuria. The Dubin-Johnson syndrome is more common in females than in males, and often presents with jaundice during pregnancy when the hepatic excretory defect is accentuated by hormones. Jaundice is usually intermittent, and exacerbations are often associated with mild right upper quadrant abdominal pain. There is no hepatic enlargement. The excretion of oral cholecystographic agents is impaired so that the normal biliary system often cannot be visualized. Although BSP is concentrated and conjugated normally in the liver cell, biliary excretion of the dye is impaired, and large amounts of conjugated BSP passing back into the plasma may elevate the two-hour plasma BSP level above the 45-minute value. Patients with the Dubin-Johnson syndrome do not suffer from pruritus; there is no evidence for abnormal biliary secretion of the conjugated bile salts. In contrast to the retention of conjugated bilirubin and BSP, serum alkaline phosphatase levels are usually normal.

The diagnosis of the Dubin-Johnson syndrome is established by needle biopsy of the liver. Macroscopically the fresh liver tissue is black, and microscopically there are deposits of melanin-like pigment in the parenchymal cells, particularly in the centrilobular areas. The Kupffer cells do not contain pigment, the bile canaliculi

are normal, and the liver is free of fibrosis or inflammatory infiltrate. Recent studies on mutant Corriedale sheep with a similar defect in organic anion transport and liver pigmentation suggest that the pigment may be an oxidation product of metanephrine glucuronide, an epinephrine metabolite normally excreted in bile but poorly excreted by these animals and by patients with the Dubin-Johnson syndrome. The hepatic pigment accumulates with increasing age in both conditions. The *Rotor syndrome* is a variant of the Dubin-Johnson syndrome, differing only in the absence of hepatic pigment.

The more important considerations in managing patients with this disorder of bilirubin metabolism are the reassurance that the abnormality is benign and leads to no disability or reduction in life expectancy and the avoidance of unnecessary biliary tract surgery.

697. ACUTE VIRAL HEPATITIS

Acute viral hepatitis is a common acute inflammatory disease of the liver caused by at least two strains of hepatotropic virus. *Hepatitis A* or *short incubation hepatitis* (formerly called *infectious hepatitis*) is due to hepatitis virus (or viruses) A, and *hepatitis B* or *long incubation hepatitis* (formerly called *serum hepatitis*) is due to hepatitis viruses B.

Etiology. Early information relating to the viral etiology of human hepatitis was based on indirect evidence derived from studies of epidemic hepatitis and from human transmission experiments. Hepatitis A and B were both shown to be caused by filterable agents that were relatively resistant to heat and chemical disinfectants. Epidemiologic and clinical studies suggested differences in the biologic properties of the two viral agents. Infectious hepatitis was believed to be transmitted by the fecal-oral route in the majority of patients in both endemic and epidemic outbreaks. Experimental studies suggested a short incubation period of two to six weeks, with the appearance of the infective agent in both blood and feces during the prodromal and early icteric phases of illness. Infection conferred immunity against further attacks of infectious hepatitis, but did not protect against serum hepatitis infection. Serum hepatitis was considered to be transmitted only by parenteral inoculation of infected blood or blood products with a long incubation period of six weeks to six months. The infective agent was thought to be confined to the circulation and not excreted in feces. The transmission of disease by transfusion of blood from healthy donors indicated a prolonged carrier state.

Early attempts to isolate the viruses of human hepatitis, to propagate them in tissue culture, or to transmit them to laboratory animals were unsuccessful, and knowledge of these agents was thus limited. The identification of a virus-like antigen in the serum of patients with *hepatitis B* has advanced knowledge of the epidemiology of this infection. Hepatitis B virus antigen (HBAg) was first called *Australia antigen* after its identification immunologically in the serum of an Australian aborigine. HBAg (also called serum hepatitis antigen and hepatitis-related antigen) can be identified by immunodiffusion, immunoelectrophoretic, complement fixation, and radioimmunoassay techniques, using serum which contains *hepatitis B antibody* (anti-HB). Electron microscopic studies of HBAg positive sera have demonstrated the presence of free particles with virus-like structure; larger Dane particles (42 nm) have a central core and surface capsid, whereas smaller particles (20 nm spheres or filaments) lack the central core. Immunologic studies have identified both core and surface antigens, designated HB$_c$-Ag and HB$_s$-Ag, respectively; these antigens promote the formation of corresponding antibodies — anti-HB$_c$ and anti-HB$_s$. Two subtypes of HB$_s$Ag (designated D and Y) have been identified.

Recent experimental studies indicate that marmosets can be infected with human hepatitis A; the use of this animal model should provide further knowledge of this virus.

Epidemiology. *Hepatitis A (Short-Incubation, Infectious Hepatitis).* Transmission of the hepatitis A virus is usually by the fecal-oral route, although infusion of infected blood obtained from viremic donors may cause sporadic infection. The occurrence of both sporadic and epidemic hepatitis depends on the distribution of infected material and the susceptibility of the exposed population. Thus poor sanitation, overcrowding, and exposure of a nonimmune population will contribute to an epidemic situation with a high frequency of infection in the young. Adults without previous exposure to hepatitis A infection are particularly at risk when traveling in or moving to an area of high endemic infection with poor sanitation. Explosive epidemics have been described after fecal contamination of drinking water and milk, and the concentration of virus by shellfish in polluted sea water has been a recent cause of several epidemics in the eastern United States. The common epidemics in institutions that house small children — orphanages, schools, and homes for the mentally retarded — reflect the exposure of a nonimmune population to many cases of anicteric or preicteric infection. The frequency of viral hepatitis (HBAg negative) in persons handling primates suggests that these animals transmit hepatitis A.

Hepatitis B (Long-Incubation, Serum Hepatitis). Transmission of hepatitis B virus by the parenteral route is well documented. This is a hazard among recipients of transfused blood (particularly blood from paid donors), pooled plasma, fibrinogen, antihemophilic globulin (AHG), and vaccines contaminated with human serum (e.g., yellow fever vaccine during World War II). Inoculation with minute amounts of infected blood may transmit hepatitis B virus infection; inadequately sterilized syringes, hypodermic needles, dental and surgical instruments, tattoo needles, and razors have all been implicated in the transmission of infection. Hospital personnel, particularly operating room staff, dialysis unit staff, and laboratory personnel, have an increased risk of accidental parenteral exposure. A high frequency of parenteral drug abuse is a major cause for infection in the young adult population.

The development of immunologic methods for the detection of hepatitis B antigen (HBAg) and antibody (anti-HB) has led to major advances in the understanding of hepatitis B infection and provides a means for reducing infection, particularly among recipients of transfused blood. Tests for HBAg identify many carriers of the hepatitis B virus; between 1 and 2 per cent of paid donors were found to be HBAg positive, whereas volunteer blood donors have a hepatitis carrier rate of between 1 and 2 per 1000. A majority of patients transfused with HBAg positive blood either develop HBAg positive hepatitis (either anicteric or icteric) or exhibit a rise in the titer of anti-HB in their serum. The frequency of posttransfusion hepatitis B infection is significantly decreased when transfused blood is derived from volunteer rather than paid donors and when HBAg positive blood is discarded.

Studies on the infants of mothers who suffered from hepatitis B infection during the last trimester of pregnancy or during the immediate postpartum period have shown a high frequency of neonatal infection. Although HBAg is sometimes present in cord blood, the relative importance of transplacental, perinatal, or postnatal transmission remains uncertain.

In epidemiologic studies, Krugman and co-workers have proved that hepatitis B infection can be transmitted by nonparenteral (fecal-oral) as well as by parenteral routes. Thus the terms infectious hepatitis (IH) and serum hepatitis (SH), which implied differences in the mode of virus transmission, are no longer accurate. The increased frequency of hepatitis B (HBAg positive), together with a higher frequency of detectable anti-HB in the relatives of HBAg positive blood donors or chronic renal dialysis patients, is best explained by nonparenteral transmission of the infective agent.

It is of interest to consider the factors which determined the spread of hepatitis B infection among populations that do not have parenteral exposure to blood or blood products. Under conditions of poor sanitation, nonparenteral transmission may be of greater epidemiologic importance; this may explain the high HBAg carrier rate in tropical Africa. Alternatively, it has been suggested that an insect vector may be important in the transmission of infection; HBAg has been recovered from several arthropods, particularly mosquitoes, captured from human dwellings in tropical West Africa.

The significance of the HBAg subtypes, D and Y, with respect to the severity or chronicity of infection in man is currently under investigation. The D subtype has a higher frequency than the Y subtype among healthy carriers (volunteer blood donors) and patients with chronic liver disease. In patients with HBAg positive hepatitis, the D subtype appears to be more frequent in patients with sporadic hepatitis without parenteral exposure or association with drug users; the Y subtype is more common in patients with needle-associated hepatitis.

Pathology. The hepatic lesion in uncomplicated viral hepatitis (both hepatitis A and B, whether anicteric or icteric) is characterized by parenchymal cell degeneration and necrosis, proliferation of Kupffer's cells, inflammatory cell infiltration, and cell regeneration. Parenchymal cells throughout the lobule, and particularly in centrilobular areas, undergo rapid necrosis so that the cell cords are disrupted. Degenerating liver cells either show *ballooning* of their cytoplasm or hyalinize to form *acidophilic bodies* that may exhibit pyknotic nuclei. Cell necrosis is closely followed by cell regeneration; this may be recognized by the appearance of cells in mitosis and by large cells with multiple hyperchromatic nuclei. An increased number of macrophages containing a yellow, acid-fast pigment (lipofuscin) accumulate at sites of cell necrosis. Numerous lymphocytes, plasma cells, and polymorphonuclear cells, both neutrophil and eosinophil, also accumulate focally at sites of cell necrosis in the lobules and in the portal areas.

Although necrosis disrupts the normal cell cords, the reticulum framework surrounding the hepatic sinusoids is preserved, and cell regeneration restores normal lobules. During the recovery phase an increased number of fibroblasts with collagen may appear in the portal areas, together with proliferating bile ductules; these changes, together with the inflammatory cell infiltrate, disappear with full recovery.

Intrahepatic cholestasis — dilated bile canaliculi containing bile plugs — particularly in centrilobular areas, is often seen in viral hepatitis when there is prominent clinical evidence of cholestasis. This may be due to a disruption of bile canaliculi by parenchymal cell necrosis, or it may result from a change in the composition of bile due to cell injury.

Rarely, viral hepatitis may cause more extensive zones of parenchymal cell necrosis bridging adjacent portal triads and/or central veins with collapse of the normal reticulum framework. This lesion has been termed *subacute hepatic necrosis. Massive hepatic necrosis,* usually associated with fulminant hepatitis, is associated with widespread necrosis. The term *acute yellow atrophy* refers to the shrunken, bile-stained liver in which zones of collapsed reticulum and sinusoids lie between islands of surviving cells.

Although complete recovery can be anticipated in patients with typical focal necrosis, the prognosis of patients with massive necrosis or subacute hepatic necrosis with respect to full recovery is poor. Massive necrosis in patients with fulminant hepatitis is usually fatal. In patients who survive, liver cell regeneration may restore normal liver structure and function or may result in a macronodular cirrhosis. Subacute hepatic necrosis has a variable clinical course. Of 52 patients who exhibited this lesion on liver biopsy, 4 died with fulminant hepatitis, 6 died after a subacute illness of several weeks, and the remainder survived the acute illness; of the survivors, 7 exhibited the clinical and histologic features of chronic active hepatitis, 5 had residual abnormalities of liver function with cirrhosis documented by biopsy in 2, and 28 recovered with normal liver function but with biopsy evidence of inactive cirrhosis in 9 of 19 subjected to repeat liver biopsy.

There is evidence from HBAg studies that *chronic active hepatitis* (see Ch. 708) may complicate viral hepatitis. This condition usually has an insidious onset, but may also follow subacute hepatic necrosis.

Extrahepatic lesions in infectious hepatitis appear in the gastrointestinal mucosa and the kidney. The mucosae are edematous and infiltrated with mononuclear cells; renal biopsies reveal interstitial edema without inflammation.

Currently, the relationship between the various lesions (hepatic and extrahepatic) of viral hepatitis and the distribution of the viruses is unclear. HBAg has been localized by immunofluorescence in liver cells, but the source of HBAg in healthy carriers is not known, and the relative importance of persisting infection or host responses (e.g., immunologic reactions) in the pathogenesis of severe or chronic lesions must still be defined. There is evidence that skin and joint lesions occurring during the prodromal period may relate to the formation of complexes between HBAg and anti-HB.

Clinical Manifestations. Acute viral hepatitis is commonly a mild disease without jaundice, particularly in those with relative immunity from previous infection, or in infants and children. Infection may be followed by a mild illness without clinical evidence of hepatitis; a rise in viral antibody titer or transiently positive test for

HBAg may be the only evidence of infection. In many subjects exposed to either of the viral agents, there is evidence of hepatitis without jaundice — *anicteric hepatitis.* *Icteric hepatitis* is usually a short, uncomplicated illness, but sometimes has a prolonged course *(chronic persisting hepatitis).* Acute exacerbations may follow partial recovery, or *recurrent hepatitis* may follow complete recovery. When a clinical picture of cholestasis is the dominant abnormality, the term *cholestatic hepatitis* is used. In jaundiced patients with hepatitis A infection, the risk of *fulminant hepatitis* with massive necrosis is less than 1 per cent. The risk of massive or subacute hepatic necrosis in patients with hepatitis B infection is increased in elderly patients, in diabetics, and in patients with severe illness, particularly neoplasms, which have required surgery and transfusion.

The clinical features of each of these variants of viral hepatitis will be discussed below. *Fulminant hepatitis* and *chronic active liver* disease are discussed in Ch. 698 and 708, respectively.

Anicteric Hepatitis. The symptoms of anicteric hepatitis are similar to those of many other viral infections; the onset of disease may resemble the prodromal (pre-icteric) period of icteric hepatitis. The diagnosis is suspected only in epidemic situations, in patients exposed to known infection, or in those who develop tender enlargement of the liver. A diagnosis is confirmed by liver function tests and liver biopsy. There is often slight hyperbilirubinemia with an increase in urinary urobilinogen and bilirubin and BSP retention. The serum enzyme changes are most helpful in diagnosis; serum transaminase and dehydrogenase levels are elevated, and serum alkaline phosphatase and 5'-nucleotidase may be slightly increased. On liver biopsy, the hepatic lesion is indistinguishable from that of icteric hepatitis except for the absence of bile stasis.

Icteric Hepatitis. THE PREICTERIC PHASE. The preicteric phase of nonspecific constitutional and gastrointestinal symptoms varies in duration from a few days to several weeks. It is usually abrupt in onset in patients with hepatitis A and often of insidious onset with hepatitis B; these symptoms may mimic those of other viral infections of the respiratory or gastrointestinal tract. *Fever* is usually most pronounced at the onset, and may be accompanied by a shaking chill; it is unusual, however, for shaking chills to be recurrent, although fever may persist until the early icteric phase. *Anorexia, weakness, headache,* and *myalgia* are common symptoms; there may be a striking loss of taste for cigarettes. Right upper quadrant pain with local tenderness and muscle spasm may simulate an acute abdominal emergency. Joint pains or acute migratory arthritis and urticarial or erythematous maculopapular rashes are sometimes seen, particularly in patients with hepatitis B infection. During this preicteric phase, the liver may become enlarged and tender, and the urine may become discolored with bilirubin.

THE ICTERIC PHASE. Gastrointestinal symptoms — anorexia, nausea, and vomiting with right upper abdominal discomfort — usually increase during the early period of increasing jaundice, the liver becomes more enlarged and tender, and the spleen may be palpable. Fever usually subsides a few days after the onset of jaundice. Within a few days of hospitalization and bed rest, nausea subsides, and the appetite improves in most patients. Typically, the patient is maximally jaundiced within two weeks, and thereafter clinical jaundice and serum bilirubin levels gradually return to normal within six weeks. Hepatic enlargement may subside with symptomatic improvement, but often persists during the icteric period. The maximal changes in urinary and fecal bilirubin excretion coincide with maximal serum bilirubin levels.

In patients with *cholestatic hepatitis* jaundice is usually more severe and prolonged and accompanied by *pruritus* secondary to bile salt retention. Liver enlargement usually persists during the period of jaundice, whereas hepatic tenderness is usually observed early in the acute illness. *Diarrhea* may be due to the cathartic action of nonabsorbed fatty acids.

Some patients with otherwise typical acute viral hepatitis may remain icteric with hepatic enlargement and abnormalities of liver function for a period of several months. A liver biopsy is indicated in such patients to confirm a diagnosis of *chronic persisting hepatitis;* the histologic features of typical viral hepatitis in spite of the prolonged clinical course indicate an excellent prognosis for full recovery.

Occasionally there may be acute exacerbations with anorexia, nausea, recurrent liver enlargement, and tenderness and jaundice after partial recovery from the initial icteric illness. Such exacerbations are sometimes precipitated by vigorous physical activity, and usually resolve promptly without long-term complications.

THE CONVALESCENT PHASE. The convalescent phase, leading to complete recovery and resumption of normal activity, may last for several weeks or months. During this period variable tiredness and malaise with mild hepatic tenderness may persist. These symptoms may be quite troublesome to the patient. They are often precipitated by unaccustomed activity and may be accompanied by mild elevation of serum transaminase levels and minimal BSP retention.

Laboratory Features. The hemoglobin and hematocrit are usually normal early in the illness, but mild hemolysis and repeated venipuncture for laboratory tests may cause anemia later in the course of the acute disease. A normal or reduced white cell count, with atypical mononuclear cells (virocytes) on smear, is usual during the preicteric and early icteric periods. The erythrocyte sedimentation rate is slightly increased. Aplastic anemia is an unusual complication of acute viral hepatitis. Thrombocytopenic purpura is occasionally seen, as in other viral illnesses. Evidence of acute hemolysis, usually with deep jaundice, may be secondary to a red cell defect, particularly G-6-PD deficiency.

The urine contains an increased amount of both urobilinogen and bilirubin in the early icteric period; bilirubinemia increases with increasing jaundice, whereas urinary urobilinogen excretion decreases to minimal levels when jaundice is maximal. Minimal proteinuria with microscopic hematuria, pyuria, and granular casts during the early icteric period may reflect the renal abnormalities that have been demonstrated on renal biopsy.

During the icteric period both direct- and indirect-reacting bilirubin are almost equally elevated in the serum, but during the convalescent period indirect bilirubinemia may persist (see Gilbert's syndrome in Ch. 696). Serum transaminase (glutamic-oxaloacetic or glutamic-pyruvic) levels, maximally elevated in the late prodromal or early icteric periods, may exceed 500 to 1000 IU. These increased enzyme levels may be sustained during the icteric period but usually fall toward normal during the icteric period. Serum elevations of alkaline phosphatase, 5'-nucleotidase, and leucine aminopeptidase are usually minimal and return to normal during the late icteric period. In patients with *cholestatic hepatitis* the increases in serum alkaline phosphatase, 5'-nucleotidase, and conjugated bilirubin are usually more prominent than the rise in serum transaminase levels. Serum cholesterol levels will increase in these patients. The typical changes in plasma proteins include a slight decrease in albumin and a late increase in gamma globulin, and the flocculation tests may be abnormal late in the prodromal period and return to normal during convalescence. The increase in gamma globulin levels in patients with acute hepatitis or in patients with *chronic persisting hepatitis* is considerably less than that seen in patients with *chronic active hepatitis* (see below). BSP retention decreases to normal levels during the convalescent period.

Diagnosis. During the prodromal period, symptoms may suggest some other viral infection—*influenza* or *gastroenteritis*. Abdominal pain may mimic *acute cholecystitis, pneumonia,* or *acute appendicitis*. In the icteric patient, other causes for jaundice must be considered; *drug-induced or toxic hepatitis* is usually indicated by a history of drug exposure, but cannot be clearly differentiated by the preicteric symptoms from viral hepatitis. Choledocholithiasis with obstruction is suggested by a history of calculous disease, biliary colic, predominant cholestasis with pruritus, high alkaline phosphatase levels with only slight increases in transaminase, and signs of bacterial infection—shaking chills and polymorphonuclear leukocytosis. *Infectious mononucleosis* with hepatic involvement is distinguished by lymphadenopathy, pharyngitis, and a positive *heterophil* test. *Leptospirosis* is usually accompanied by headache and photophobia, signs of meningeal irritation with abnormal cerebrospinal fluid, persisting fever, leukocytosis, and proteinuria or renal insufficiency. It is important to exclude an exacerbation of chronic liver disease with jaundice; *acute alcoholic hepatitis* or *chronic aggressive hepatitis* may present with jaundice (see below).

A percutaneous liver biopsy is of diagnostic value whenever the clinical picture is atypical. Lesions of extrahepatic obstruction, subacute hepatic necrosis, chronic active hepatitis, acute alcoholic hepatitis, or active cirrhosis can be distinguished from the changes of acute viral hepatitis.

Tests for HBAg are of value early in the course of hepatitis, or in patients with prolonged illness. The HBAg test usually becomes positive during the preicteric phase of hepatitis B infection, and the antigen test usually becomes negative with the appearance of anti-HB within two to three weeks of the onset of jaundice. When HBAg persists in the serum for periods in excess of four weeks, chronic active hepatitis must be considered as a diagnostic possibility.

Management of Acute Viral Hepatitis. Hospitalization of patients with acute viral hepatitis is indicated during the early icteric phase when symptoms are severe (e.g., severe vomiting) or when there is clinical evidence at the time of diagnosis of serious illness, particularly manifestations of subacute or massive hepatic necrosis (see below). High risk patients—pregnant, diabetic, elderly, or those with complicating disease—should also be observed in hospital. Patients treated at home should be advised with respect to diet, alcohol intake, physical activity, and measures to reduce their infectivity. The routine precautions to reduce cross-infection in hospital are those applicable to enteric diseases, plus careful disposal of needles and syringes. During the early symptomatic period frequent careful clinical observation and assessment of liver function are necessary for early recognition and treatment of massive or subacute hepatic necrosis. Liver function tests should be performed as often as is necessary to assess the patient's progress; a daily estimation of the prothrombin time after parenteral vitamin K_1 (10 mg intramuscularly) is valuable in detecting a sudden deterioration in liver function. A daily measurement of caloric intake is also helpful in assessing the patient's progress.

A liver biopsy should be performed if the diagnosis is not firmly established on the basis of clinical and biochemical findings, or if an atypical course suggests subacute hepatic necrosis.

Rest. The value of rest in acute viral hepatitis is suggested by the remission and exacerbation of symptoms that follow bed rest and physical activity, respectively. Nevertheless, the only controlled study on the effect of rest and activity in infectious hepatitis indicated that enforced rest was of no value in therapy and that activity did not cause complications, lengthen the course of the disease, or lead to chronic residual abnormalities. This controlled study was carried out on military personnel who were young and fit and who, irrespective of therapy, suffered no mortality or long-term sequelae that could be attributed to the viral hepatitis. In a civilian population of varied age, with other disease states complicating viral hepatitis infection, there are significant morbidity and mortality from subacute and massive hepatic necrosis. *Complete bed rest during the acute phase of viral hepatitis may protect some of these patients from these complications.* Until there is further information relating to a civilian population, it is recommended that all icteric patients rest in bed during the early symptomatic period when it may be difficult to assess the severity of illness, and that limited activity during the icteric period be permitted only for young, otherwise healthy patients. Elderly patients and patients with complicating disease should be ambulated when the serum bilirubin has fallen below 2 mg per 100 ml. It is important that ambulation to normal physical activity should be gradual for patients who have been confined to bed for long periods.

Diet. During the preicteric and early icteric periods, a poor appetite and nausea or vomiting may limit food intake. The patient should be served and encouraged to eat those foods that appeal to him. For some patients, it is possible to increase the caloric content of the breakfast when they have difficulty in eating other meals. If a total intake of 2000 calories daily is not maintained, intravenous glucose supplements should be given.

Corticosteroids. Although glucocorticoids effect a dramatic remission of symptoms and biochemical improvement in patients with viral hepatitis, it has not been established by controlled studies that these agents shorten the course of the acute disease or reduce the complications. Thus in mild, uncomplicated hepatitis there is no indication for their use. Corticosteroids are recommended, however, for acutely ill patients whose symptoms are severe and persist for several days in spite of bed rest. A daily dose of 30 to 60 mg of prednisolone, or equivalent doses of other steroids, maintained for a week and tapered slowly over a period of several weeks is suggested.

Sedatives. Sedatives and other drugs should be used with caution in patients with viral hepatitis. Smaller doses may be necessary to achieve a therapeutic effect. In acutely ill patients their side effects may complicate the clinical assessment of the patient.

Surgery. All surgical procedures should be deferred to the postconvalescent period if possible. There is evidence that abdominal surgery under general anesthesia increases the risk of subacute or massive hepatic necrosis.

Management of the Hepatitis (HBAg) Carrier. The routine screening of blood donors and patients with liver disease for HBAg has raised special problems in the management and education of subjects who may be otherwise perfectly healthy. When a person is found to be HBAg positive, it should be confirmed that a chronic carrier state exists by repeated tests. If tests of liver function are abnormal, a liver biopsy is advised to define the nature of the associated liver disease. If there are no clinical manifestations of liver disease and liver function tests are normal, liver disease is very unlikely. The healthy HBAg carrier should be excluded from donating blood and should be advised to maintain careful personal hygiene.

Prophylaxis. A single dose of pooled gamma globulin (0.02 to 0.04 ml of 16 per cent solution per kilogram of body weight, intramuscularly) protects against, or modifies, hepatitis A infection in exposed subjects. Susceptible persons probably develop anicteric rather than icteric hepatitis. Susceptible travelers to zones of known poor sanitation should receive a larger dose, 0.06 to 0.12 ml per kilogram, to give protection for five to six months.

Commercially available pooled gamma globulin does not confer protection against post-transfusion hepatitis B infection; these preparations do not contain significant hepatitis B antibody. In preliminary studies, however, there is evidence that commercial gamma globulin and gamma globulin containing anti-HB may both protect children against hepatitis B infection caused by nonparenteral exposure; the gamma globulin may also reduce the frequency of the chronic HBAg carrier state.

Although experimental evidence indicates that active immunization with heat-inactivated HBAg is effective in reducing infection, the development of commercially available vaccines requires further characterization of the viral agents and their cultivation in the laboratory.

698.   FULMINANT HEPATITIS

Fulminant hepatitis resulting from massive hepatic necrosis may be due to *toxic liver injury* (e.g., carbon tetrachloride toxicity or acetaminophen overdosage), *hypersensitivity reactions* to therapeutic agents (e.g., halothane sensitivity), or *viral hepatitis.* In the case of toxic liver injury, the lesion is predictable and dose related; in the case of hypersensitivity reactions, the development of liver disease is unpredictable unless there has been a previous sensitivity reaction to the drug. Fulminant hepatitis may be caused by viruses A or B; predisposing factors have not been well documented, but the risk of infection during late pregnancy in malnourished patients is high.

Pathology. When a diagnosis of fulminant hepatitis is suspected by the clinical course, a percutaneous liver biopsy is usually precluded by the risk of bleeding caused by clotting abnormalities; the pathologic features are usually defined at postmortem examination. The liver is usually smaller than normal with a soft consistency and red-brown discoloration—thus the term *acute yellow atrophy.* Microscopically, there is confluent necrosis with disappearance of parenchymal cells, leaving a residual framework of collapsed reticulin, hepatic sinusoids, Kupffer cells, and inflammatory cells. Parenchymal cells surrounding portal tracts may be spared, or may exhibit evidence of degeneration or regeneration. The surviving Kupffer cells are usually hypertrophied and contain a yellow pigment—lipofuchsin. In portal areas, proliferation of bile ducts is commonly observed, and infiltration with inflammatory cells is usual. *Massive hepatic necrosis* usually leads to early death. *Subacute or submassive hepatic necrosis* represents a less extensive lesion in which areas of residual parenchyma are separated by zones of necrosis. Death may occur after a brief or protracted illness, or regeneration of parenchymal cells may permit survival. If the zones of parenchymal necrosis undergo fibrosis and surviving zones of parenchyma proliferate to form regeneration nodules, a macronodular cirrhosis will be the end result. Alternatively, prolonged survival may be accompanied by persisting piecemeal necrosis and the clinical picture of chronic active hepatitis (see below).

Pathologically, it is not possible to differentiate massive or submassive necrosis caused by toxic injury, drug hypersensitivity, or viral hepatitis.

Clinical Manifestations. In patients with fulminant hepatitis, the preicteric period is usually brief with severe symptoms, particularly abdominal pain, vomiting, and high fever. The clinical features which suggest a fulminant course are as follows: (1) High fever, severe abdominal pain, and vomiting which persist for several days after the initiation of bed rest. (2) A sudden decrease in the size of the liver. (3) Neuropsychiatric changes of early hepatic encephalopathy, including drowsiness, irritability, insomnia, and confusion. (4) Severe prolongation of the prothrombin time (more than 20 seconds with control of 12 seconds) with or without bleeding (uncorrected by parenteral vitamin K). (Serum bilirubin and transaminase levels do not reflect the severity of illness; patients may die in hepatic coma during the early icteric period, or may become deeply jaundiced, while serum transaminase levels often fall during the period of clinical deterioration.) (5) The appearance of ascites during the acute illness.

The complications of massive necrosis with acute liver failure include *hypoglycemia; bleeding* caused by deficient clotting factors; *disseminated intravascular coagulation,* which may accentuate liver cell necrosis; *acute hepatic encephalopathy* (described in Ch. 694) with terminal depression of medullary centers; *pneumonia* secondary to aspiration; *septicemia* with portals of entry at the sites of intravenous catheter lines, the gut, or urinary system; and terminal *renal failure* (hepatorenal syndrome).

Management. The patient with fulminant hepatitis requires intensive nursing care with monitoring and support of vital functions. In the comatose patient, a cuffed nasotracheal or tracheostomy tube should be inserted to ensure adequate ventilation, with respirator support if necessary, and to prevent aspiration. Continu-

ous intravenous infusion of glucose solution is required to prevent hypoglycemia in a patient who has no hepatic glycogen stores and has depressed glyconeogenesis. Fluid and electrolyte balance should be achieved by accurate measurement of intake and output. In the absence of hepatic plasma protein synthesis, plasma albumin levels can be maintained by intravenous infusion of solutions of salt-poor albumin. Deficiency of clotting factors can be partially corrected by infusion of fresh-frozen plasma. The agitated, hyperactive patient should be restrained to prevent injury and should be sedated with small doses of diazepam (5 mg by intravenous injection); heavy sedation will deepen coma. General measures to treat hepatic coma are indicated (see Hepatic Coma in Ch. 709).

High doses of *corticosteroids* are usually given by intravenous infusion—e.g., prednisolone, 100 to 500 mg daily; the benefit of this therapy has not been established by controlled clinical trials, but is based on clinical impressions. Although there is evidence for disseminated intravascular coagulation in patients with fulminant hepatitis, treatment with heparin has not been of benefit in limited clinical trials.

A variety of measures designed to support the patient in acute liver failure have been described. These include *exchange transfusion, plasmapheresis, cross-perfusion* with a human volunteer or primate, or *extracorporeal perfusion* through a mammalian liver. Although isolated case reports suggest that exchange transfusion or plasmapheresis may restore consciousness in some patients and thus prolong life, it has not been established that these support measures actually improve survival. In one prospective controlled study, exchange transfusion was of no benefit in decreasing mortality. Studies in experimental canine hepatitis showed that infusion of immune serum improved the survival of infected animals. Treatment of patients with fulminant viral hepatitis, type B, with plasma containing hepatitis B antibody has been suggested; controlled trials are needed to establish the value of this therapy.

Recovery from fulminant hepatitis depends on liver cell regeneration; currently there are no measures known to potentiate liver regeneration in these patients. The better prognosis for recovery in children probably relates to a greater regenerative capacity; any measures which prolong survival and increase the chance of liver cell regeneration should be used in treatment.

699. HEPATITIS DUE TO OTHER VIRUSES

The viruses of yellow fever, rubella, cytomegalic inclusion disease, and herpes simplex may cause hepatitis. Yellow fever is discussed in Ch. 154. Infection with *rubella, cytomegalic inclusion virus,* and *herpes simplex* may cause *neonatal hepatitis* with jaundice and hepatosplenomegaly. Rubella and cytomegalic inclusion viruses are transmitted transplacentally, whereas herpes virus infects the infant during delivery. Hepatitis resulting from these viral agents may be part of a generalized disease. Although there may be complete recovery, with normal liver function and structure, these infections may be important but previously unrecognized causes for juvenile cirrhosis.

Many viral illnesses may be accompanied by minor, nonspecific changes in liver function (positive flocculation tests and slight transaminase elevation). There may be hyperplasia of Kupffer's cells and infiltration with mononuclear cells in portal areas—nonspecific reactive hepatitis.

INFECTIOUS MONONUCLEOSIS

Infectious mononucleosis is a systemic disease which is commonly associated with liver disease (see Part XVI, Section Nine). Jaundice is unusual, although hepatic enlargement with mild tenderness is often seen. The disturbances of liver function are those associated with hepatic infiltration: an elevation of the serum alkaline phosphatase, 5'-nucleotidase and leucine aminopeptidase, and BSP retention. Serum transaminase levels may be slightly elevated. Histologically, there is mononuclear infiltration predominantly in the portal areas with minimal evidence of cell necrosis.

No case of chronic liver disease has been proved to result from an attack of infectious mononucleosis.

This disease must be considered in the differential diagnosis of acute viral hepatitis. An atypical mononuclear cell reaction is common to these diseases, but tests for heterophil antibody, Epstein-Barr virus, and cytomegaloviruses differentiate them.

700. LIVER DISEASE ASSOCIATED WITH BACTERIAL INFECTIONS

In bacterial infection, liver disease may result from the effect of bacterial toxins on cell metabolism, changes in liver blood flow caused by endotoxin, shock or fever, localization and multiplication of bacteria in the liver, or the effect of antimicrobial agents.

Severe infections, particularly intraperitoneal, may cause obstructive jaundice with conjugated bilirubinemia, increased alkaline phosphatase, and minimal elevation of serum transaminase. In the absence of demonstrable lesions of the extrahepatic biliary system and normal operative cholangiograms, the jaundice in these patients is due to intrahepatic cholestasis resulting from unknown toxic factors.

Gram-negative septicemia with shock may cause acute hypoxic necrosis of the liver with jaundice as a terminal manifestation. The liver may be enlarged and tender. In *typhoid fever* there is focal necrosis of liver cells with acute and chronic inflammatory cell infiltration. An elevation of serum transaminases reflects parenchymal cell injury. In *leptospirosis,* jaundice is usually disproportionally greater than other evidence of liver involvement; the associated renal disease may impair urinary excretion of conjugated bilirubin.

Although the mucocutaneous lesions are most prominent features of *secondary syphilis,* liver disease is well documented. Hepatic enlargement with mild jaundice and elevated levels of alkaline phosphatase and transaminase in the serum are associated with polymorphonuclear infiltration of the portal tracts. Hepatic *tuberculosis* is discussed in Ch. 235.

701. ACUTE LIVER ABSCESS

Amebic abscesses are discussed in Ch. 279.

Pyogenic organisms which cause liver abscess may reach the liver by the biliary system (cholangitis), the portal venous system (portal pyemia in patients with appendicitis or umbilical sepsis), or arterial blood (staphylococcal septicemia or bacteremia from distant foci); by direct spread from contiguous structures (empyema of gallbladder or subphrenic abscess); or by penetrating wounds. Infection complicating biliary tract disease—*suppurative (ascending) cholangitis*—is now the most common cause for liver abscesses; the early diagnosis and treatment of acute appendicitis and umbilical sepsis in the newborn has decreased the frequency of abscess caused by pylephlebitis. The responsible organism for liver abscess reflects the source of infection; cholangitis is usually due to enteric organisms, particularly *E. coli,* anaerobic streptococci and Bacteroides species. Abscesses formerly regarded as being sterile probably harbored anaerobic organisms which were not isolated because of inadequate anaerobic transport and culture techniques. Abscesses are more often multiple than solitary and involve the right lobe more frequently than the left. A decreasing frequency in the young and increasing frequency in the elderly reflect the decreasing morbidity after appendicitis and the greater relative frequency of abscesses caused by biliary tract disease.

The *clinical manifestations* of liver abscess are the result of sepsis and the presence of a space-occupying lesion(s) in the liver. *Paroxysmal fever* with *chills* and a *polymorphonuclear leukocytosis* are usual; a liver abscess should be considered in the differential diagnosis of persistent unexplained fever (FUO). Blood cultures are positive in approximately 50 per cent of patients. Gastrointestinal symptoms and abdominal signs are often nonspecific and include anorexia, nausea, epigastric or right upper quadrant pain, and liver enlargement with tenderness. Jaundice may not be an early clinical finding unless there is associated biliary tract obstruction.

Abnormalities of liver function reflect associated biliary tract disease and focal inflammatory disease in relation to the lesion. In the absence of biliary tract obstruction, serum alkaline phosphatase levels are usually only mildly elevated, and transaminase levels are often normal. A decrease in synthesis and an increased catabolism of albumin cause hypoproteinemia in the majority of patients. An enlarging liver abscess may elevate the diaphragm or may be associated with a pleural effusion.

Diagnosis. The diagnosis of liver abscess is made too frequently at postmortem examination in patients who did not have the benefit of treatment. When symptoms and signs suggest the possibility of a liver abscess, the presence of a space-occupying lesion must be confirmed by *liver scanning.* Selective *celiac arteriography* is of value in differentiating avascular (cysts and abscesses) and vascular (primary or metastatic neoplasms) space-occupying lesions in the liver. Amebic liver abscesses should be diagnosed by appropriate serologic tests (see Ch. 279); the clinical manifestations of pyogenic and amebic liver abscesses are similar.

Treatment. *Surgical drainage* of pyogenic liver abscess is usually recommended as the treatment of choice. Preoperative *antimicrobial therapy* to cover gram-negative and anaerobic organisms should be continued postoperatively until bacteriologic studies have identified the causal organism and specific drug therapy can be provided. There have been no clinical trials to determine whether antimicrobial therapy alone without surgical drainage is as effective as the surgical approach in treating liver abscesses; multiple small abscesses may be less accessible to the surgeon.

Complications. The major complications of liver abscess are septicemia and rupture of the abscess into the pleural space or peritoneum to produce an *empyema, subphrenic abscess,* or *generalized peritonitis.*

702. PROTOZOAN OR HELMINTHIC DISEASE OF THE LIVER

Parasites that commonly invade the liver include *amebae (E. histolytica* and malarial parasites*), schistosomes (S. mansoni), flukes (Clonorchis sinensis, Fasciola hepatica)* and *tapeworms (Echinococcus granulosus).* These diseases are discussed in Part IX.

Hepatic Schistosomiasis. Hepatic involvement in patients with *Schistosoma mansoni* results from portal seeding with ova that lodge in the portal areas and stimulate an inflammatory reaction with fibrosis. In acute schistosomiasis, the response to ova liberated two to eight weeks after infection is often associated with fever, diarrhea, hepatic and splenic enlargement, and intense eosinophilia. Transient abnormalities of liver function include increases in serum alkaline phosphatase and transaminase. In the later stage of hepatic parasitism, portal fibrosis interferes with hepatic blood flow and causes a presinusoidal portal hypertension, splenomegaly, and a collateral portal-systemic circulation. Bleeding from esophageal varices is a major complication. Liver function is usually good, so that patients may tolerate recurrent bleeding very well and do not usually develop ascites unless bleeding or malnutrition lowers serum albumin concentrations. Surgical decompression of the portal system by portacaval or splenorenal shunting is effective in preventing recurrent bleeding from esophageal varices, but it has not been established by prospectively controlled clinical trials that shunt surgery prolongs the life of these patients.

The diagnosis of hepatic schistosomiasis is established by demonstrating ova on liver biopsy; examination of "squash" preparations in glycerol is more helpful than routine histologic examination. The presence of ova in the stools or rectal biopsy of a patient with portal hypertension and splenomegaly suggests this diagnosis (see Ch. 296).

TOXIC AND DRUG-INDUCED LIVER DISEASE

703. TOXIC HEPATITIS

A *hepatotoxin* is defined as an agent that causes liver injury in both man and animals in a predictable manner.

Liver injury is dose related and is usually manifest after a relatively short latent period. Hepatotoxins may cause liver cell necrosis or biochemical changes with necrosis; these changes may be manifest by impaired formation of bile, disturbances of lipid metabolism with fat accumulation, or altered enzyme activity. Some hepatotoxins may exert their effect indirectly by interfering with hepatic blood flow (Senecio alkaloids in veno-occlusive disease).

With elimination of a number of industrial hazards, exposure to hepatotoxins other than alcohol (ethanol) is now usually accidental or suicidal. Hepatotoxic agents are not often used pharmacologically unless the therapeutic dose is considerably less than the toxic dose, or unless therapy despite toxic side effects may still benefit the patient. Immunosuppressive agents and certain agents used in the chemotherapy of cancer may be hepatotoxic.

Poisoning by several hepatotoxic agents is discussed in Part III.

CARBON TETRACHLORIDE LIVER INJURY

The hepatotoxicity of carbon tetrachloride is believed to be due to the formation of toxic metabolites which bind to microsomal proteins. The increase in carbon tetrachloride toxicity after alcohol ingestion in man and laboratory animals has been related to an increase in the activity of drug metabolizing enzymes with increased formation of toxic metabolites; phenobarbital also increases carbon tetrachloride toxicity in laboratory animals.

The clinical features of carbon tetrachloride liver injury are similar to those of acute viral hepatitis, but with a shorter symptomatic preicteric period and with more rapid recovery, unless massive necrosis causes early death or renal tubular necrosis leads to irreversible or fatal renal failure.

The symptoms that follow inhalation or ingestion of the agent are predominantly gastrointestinal, with *anorexia, nausea* and *vomiting,* and right upper quadrant *pain* with *tender hepatomegaly* preceding the onset of jaundice. In many patients there may be hepatic enlargement with acute elevation of serum transaminase levels without jaundice. Acute renal failure is often a more prominent manifestation of poisoning.

Pathologically, there is centrilobular necrosis without inflammation during the period of maximal liver injury, followed rapidly by regeneration of parenchymal cells and hyperplasia of Kupffer's cells. Complete restoration of structure and function follows recovery from a single exposure. There is some evidence, however, that repeated exposure may sometimes lead to cirrhosis of the liver.

LIVER INJURY DUE TO ALCOHOL

Experimental studies in man and animals have shown that alcohol (ethanol) is a direct hepatotoxin. All the lesions of alcoholic liver disease in man have been produced by feeding alcohol to baboons for periods up to four years; these lesions included fatty infiltration, alcoholic hepatitis, fibrosis, and cirrhosis. A nutritious diet did not protect these animals from developing liver disease.

The clinical and pathologic manifestations of alcoholic liver disease are discussed in detail in Ch. 709.

SEX HORMONES AND THE LIVER

Methyl testosterone and C-17 alkyl substituted steroids (norethandronone) may cause intrahepatic cholestasis with conjugated hyperbilirubinemia, reduced clearance of BSP (with normal hepatic uptake and conjugation), and increased serum alkaline phosphatase and 5'-nucleotidase activity. This effect is dose related in man, causes no permanent liver damage or acute parenchymal cell necrosis, and is reversible. This type of cholestasis may be due to a change in the permeability of the biliary tree to bile salts.

During the third trimester of normal pregnancy there may be increases in serum cholesterol, alkaline phosphatase, and 5'-nucleotidase with reduced clearance of BSP. Occasionally, impaired hepatic excretory function may cause jaundice that recurs in subsequent pregnancies—*recurrent jaundice of pregnancy*. Recent studies have shown that natural estrogens reduce hepatic BSP clearance. It is probable that the physiologic changes in liver function during the third trimester of pregnancy are due to hormone effects on the liver. These observations are of particular interest in view of the recent reports that hormones given to suppress ovulation may occasionally cause hepatic dysfunction.

ACETAMINOPHEN LIVER INJURY

Self-poisoning with excessive doses of acetaminophen is now recognized as a relatively common cause for centrilobular liver necrosis with severe hepatitis in Great Britain. Therapeutic doses of acetaminophen cause no liver injury, because potentially toxic metabolites are rapidly conjugated with glutathione to nontoxic compounds. Excessive doses of acetaminophen (particularly with blood levels in excess of 300 μg per milliliter four hours after drug administration) exhaust the available glutathione, and toxic metabolites which bind covalently to microsomal protein accumulate and cause liver cell necrosis. Preliminary studies in laboratory animals and patients suggest that the early intravenous administration of a glutathione percursor such as *cysteine* or the sulfhydryl compound *cysteamine* protects against liver injury after excessive acetaminophen ingestion.

704. LIVER DISEASE DUE TO HYPERSENSITIVITY DRUG REACTIONS

Liver injury after drug therapy is more often due to a *hypersensitivity reaction* than to a hepatotoxic effect. In contrast to hepatotoxic reactions, the hypersensitivity reaction is quite unpredictable unless a previous reaction has been recorded, is not dose related, follows a variable latent period after drug exposure, cannot be reproduced in experimental animals, and may be associated with other manifestations of hypersensitivity (skin rash, fever, eosinophilia).

Drug hypersensitivity reactions involving the liver may be minor local manifestations of a generalized reaction, e.g., minor changes in liver function in patients with exfoliative dermatitis, or may be the predominant manifestation of the reaction. The common hepatic le-

sions are *intrahepatic cholestasis* and *parenchymal cell necrosis*. The former is illustrated by reactions to *chlorpromazine,* and the latter by reactions to *halothane, isoniazid,* or *alpha-methyldopa.*

CHLORPROMAZINE JAUNDICE

Approximately 1 per cent of patients treated with this phenothiazine develop a hypersensitivity reaction with intrahepatic cholestasis and jaundice. A greater number of patients develop changes in excretory function without jaundice. Early symptoms, beginning acutely usually within one to four weeks of initial drug exposure, or within a few days of repeated challenge, include *nausea, vomiting,* and *epigastric pain* often associated with *fever, lymphadenopathy, skin eruptions,* and *arthralgias.* The liver becomes enlarged and variably tender. Jaundice is obstructive in type with severe pruritus, dark urine, and pale stools, and tests of liver function reflect predominant *cholestasis* with conjugated hyperbilirubinemia and increased serum alkaline phosphatase, 5'-nucleotidase, and cholesterol levels. The serum transaminase levels may be elevated in the range of 100 to 200 IU. The white blood count may be normal or slightly elevated, with peripheral eosinophilia.

On liver biopsy, intrahepatic cholestasis, with bile plugs in dilated bile canaliculi and bile staining of parenchymal cells, and variable periportal infiltration with mononuclear and eosinophil cells are the predominant findings. There may be minimal centrilobular necrosis of liver cells.

Jaundice usually subsides within a few days or weeks of onset, with complete recovery, but occasionally chronic intrahepatic cholestasis may develop in spite of cessation of drug therapy. The clinical features in these patients may be similar to those in primary biliary cirrhosis, but periportal fibrosis is less severe, and eventual recovery without cirrhosis is usual.

Treatment.   There is no specific therapy. The offending agent should be discontinued and avoided thereafter. Cholestyramine, 2 grams every four hours orally, may relieve pruritus by lowering serum bile acid levels. Vitamin K should be given parenterally if malabsorption causes an increase in prothrombin time. Corticosteroids are of little benefit either in relieving jaundice or in reducing pruritus.

HEPATITIS AFTER ANESTHESIA WITH FLUORINATED AGENTS

Acute liver disease, clinically and pathologically similar to viral hepatitis, is an uncommon complication of anesthesia with the fluorinated agents *halothane* and *methoxyflurane*. The mechanism of liver injury appears to be a *hypersensitivity reaction*. Liver disease is more common with repeated exposure to the anesthetic agent, and recurrent episodes have shorter latent periods between exposure and onset of symptoms; recurrent hepatitis has been well documented in several anesthetists after occupational exposure to halothane. Immunologic phenomena in patients with hepatitis after halothane exposure include peripheral eosinophilia, a transiently positive test for antimitochondrial antibodies in serum, and stimulation of cultured peripheral lymphocytes by halothane.

Several etiologic factors should be excluded before postoperative liver necrosis is attributed to an anesthetic agent; these include *hypoxia, hypotension, postoperative sepsis, biliary tract disease, viral hepatitis* (either coincidental or after transfusion), and *reactions to other drugs.* It is difficult to establish a diagnosis of hepatitis caused by anesthetic exposure with any degree of certainty unless there is a history of acute liver disease after previous exposure to the agent.

The treatment of patients with hepatitis caused by anesthetic agents is similar to that of acute viral hepatitis (see Ch. 697 and 698). When a patient has recovered from halothane or methoxyflurane hepatitis, further exposure to these anesthetic agents should be avoided.

ISONIAZID HEPATITIS

Severe hepatitis has been reported as a complication of *isoniazid* therapy for tuberculosis. Prospective studies in tuberculin-positive patients receiving isoniazid as a secondary chemoprophylactic agent have shown that approximately 10 per cent of patients exhibit transient elevation of serum transaminase levels (usually less than 100 IU). Overt hepatitis with jaundice is a rare complication which has usually been described during the first 12 weeks of treatment; jaundice is preceded by *fever, fatigue, weakness, myalgias* and *arthralgias,* and *anorexia.* Liver biopsies in jaundiced patients have shown focal necrosis, subacute necrosis (bridging), or multilobular necrosis with inflammation. Patients who continue drug therapy for longer periods after the onset of symptoms usually exhibit more severe liver lesions.

It is recommended that isoniazid therapy be discontinued in patients who develop symptoms associated with abnormal liver function tests; early cessation of therapy may prevent more serious and potentially fatal reactions.

705. FATTY LIVER

Fat accumulation in the liver (fatty liver) may be a physiologic response to an increase in lipid mobilization from peripheral fat, e.g., during early starvation, or may result from several disturbances of lipid transport and metabolism in a variety of disease states. Excessive lipid in parenchymal cells may arise from one or more of three sources: (1) the diet, (2) peripheral fat depots, and (3) hepatic synthesis. Lipid from any of these sources may accumulate when the supply is increased, or when a decrease in hepatic oxidation of fatty acids or reduced lipoprotein synthesis and release diminishes the clearance of lipid from the liver.

In *starvation,* free fatty acids are mobilized from adipose tissue, and are in part esterified in the liver to triglyceride. This physiologic response is probably the mechanism for the fatty infiltration of the liver observed in many patients after acute and chronic illnesses. In *protein malnutrition (kwashiorkor),* extreme fatty liver may be related in part to fat mobilization from depots (free fatty acid concentrations in serum are elevated), and in part to impaired lipoprotein synthesis. In *obese patients,* an excessive accumulation of fat in the liver may be a reflection of the general increase in the triglyceride stores. *Diabetic ketoacidosis,* with excessive mobil-

ization of depot fat, is usually accompanied by liver enlargement caused by fat. In each of these conditions the major clinical manifestation of fatty liver is hepatic enlargement; tenderness usually accompanies acute enlargement. *BSP retention* may be the only abnormality of liver function.

In several conditions fatty liver may be associated with severe derangement of liver function. This is particularly the case when fat accumulation is due to toxic injury causing decreased fatty acid oxidation or impaired lipoprotein synthesis. In *carbon tetrachloride* or *phosphorus* poisoning, fat accumulation is one manifestation of toxic liver injury. Large intravenous doses of *tetracycline* (usually more than 1 gram daily), particularly in pregnant women, have caused liver failure and death; a fine fatty vacuolization of the liver cells is the major pathologic change in the liver. In two syndromes, fatty liver is accompanied by severe encephalopathy with high mortality; the clinical picture is that of fulminant hepatitis. *Fatty liver of pregnancy* usually presents with vomiting, abdominal pain, and jaundice during the last month of pregnancy; bleeding, premature labor, renal failure, and coma with convulsions rapidly lead to death. The serum bilirubin and alkaline phosphatase elevations suggest severe cholestasis; disturbances of the clotting mechanism reflect impaired synthesis of clotting factors. *Reye's syndrome* is a rare disease described in children. Symptoms suggestive of an upper respiratory infection are followed by fever, progressive encephalopathy with delirium, convulsions, decerebrate posturing, coma, and death (see Ch. 397). Encephalopathy is associated with acute liver enlargement resulting from fatty infiltration; jaundice is unusual, probably because of the rapidly fatal outcome. Extremely high serum levels of transaminase, prolonged prothrombin time, and hypoglycemia indicate severe liver injury. The pathogenesis of this syndrome and the relationship between liver and brain injury are unknown; the suggestion that this syndrome may complicate viral infection has not been supported by virologic studies. *Small bowel bypass surgery* (particularly jejunocolic shunts) for the treatment of extreme obesity is often complicated by fatty infiltration of the liver with progressive impairment of liver function or the development of cirrhosis. Serial liver biopsies should be performed in these patients to monitor histologic changes.

The most common form of toxic liver injury leading to fatty infiltration of the liver is that due to *alcohol (ethanol) ingestion* (see Ch. 709).

Treatment of the underlying cause of fatty liver, e.g., correction or protein malnutrition, or withdrawal from alcohol, is usually effective in lowering the fat content of the liver. In patients with acute severe liver injury associated with encephalopathy, measures used in the management of patients with fulminant hepatitis have been applied with questionable success (see Ch. 698).

706. THE LIVER IN ACUTE HEART FAILURE AND SHOCK

Hypoxia secondary to reduced liver blood flow may cause centrilobular parenchymal cell necrosis. This often complicates *acute congestive heart failure* or *hypotension* of any cause. The liver may be enlarged and tender if the central venous pressure is raised. The predominant clinical manifestations are those of the underlying cardiovascular disease, which determines both therapy and prognosis. The biochemical changes in acute heart failure include slight hyperbilirubinemia with slight elevation of transaminases and alkaline phosphatase and BSP retention. In shock, the serum transaminase levels are sometimes markedly elevated but return quickly to normal levels with restoration of normal blood flow and parenchymal cell regeneration. Deep jaundice may be a terminal event in patients with prolonged shock.

707. HEPATIC VEIN OCCLUSION
(Budd-Chiari Syndrome)

Occlusion of the hepatic veins is a rare condition usually caused by *tumor infiltration* (hepatoma, metastatic tumor) or *thrombosis* of the vessels. This may be a local lesion, or may extend from the inferior vena cava. *Polycythemia vera* is one of the more common causes of thrombosis of these veins. The major clinical manifestations of this condition are *hepatic enlargement,* with *pain* and *tenderness,* and *ascites.* In the acute form, hepatic vein occlusion is characterized pathologically by centrilobular congestion and necrosis of the adjacent parenchyma. A needle biopsy of the liver should establish the diagnosis when hepatic congestion resulting from an increase in central venous pressure has been excluded. The obstruction may be subacute or chronic when ascites and portal hypertension are the major clinical problems. *Hepatic venography* by direct injection of contrast material into a hepatic catheter is the most valuable technique for establishing the diagnosis.

Patients with chronic hepatic vein occlusion usually respond to a diuretic program (see treatment of ascites). Polycythemia vera should also be treated vigorously (see Ch. 758).

CHRONIC LIVER DISEASE

708. CHRONIC ACTIVE (AGGRESSIVE) HEPATITIS

Chronic active hepatitis is characterized pathologically by a normal lobular architecture in which fibrous septa extend from enlarged portal tracts into the parenchyma, disrupting the liver cell plates adjacent to the portal zones and separating off rosettes of parenchymal cells. Piecemeal necrosis of liver cells adjacent to the expanding portal zones, infiltration of the portal areas with eosinophils, lymphocytes and plasma cells, and focal necrosis and inflammation within liver lobules are present in varying degrees and reflect the "activity" of the lesion. Progressive destruction of the normal lobular architecture with proliferation of fibroblasts in expanding portal areas and nodular regeneration of parenchymal cells may ultimately lead to cirrhosis in untreated patients.

Pathogenesis. It is now evident that the clinical and pathologic spectrum of *chronic active hepatitis* is a syndrome of diverse etiology. In a large percentage of patients the primary etiologic factor has not been identified. *Hepatitis B infection* is of importance in a significant number of patients; persistence of HBAg after acute hepatitis B is often associated with the development of chronic active hepatitis; chronic active hepatitis has been documented by liver biopsy in approximately 15 per cent of asymptomatic HBAg carriers without a past history of acute hepatitis; of patients diagnosed as suffering from chronic active hepatitis, between 10 and 30 per cent are HBAg positive. The clinical and pathologic features of chronic active hepatitis have been documented in patients with *drug-induced liver disease;* the laxative agent *oxyphenisatin* and *alphamethyldopa* cause hypersensitivity reactions with typical clinical, biochemical, immunologic, and pathologic changes of chronic active hepatitis. *Wilson's disease* may present with features of chronic active hepatitis.

The factors which determine the chronicity of the disease process are poorly understood. In some patients chronic active hepatitis may be a host response to persisting viral (hepatitis B) infection, and in others it may be a reaction to toxic liver injury. *Immunologic phenomena* are a common feature; hypergammaglobulinemia parallels disease activity, and the patients' serum may contain a variety of antibodies which lack organ specificity, including antimitochondrial, smooth muscle, and antinuclear antibodies. The hypothesis that immunologic mechanisms relate to the pathogenesis of chronic active hepatitis is supported indirectly by the increased frequency of other diseases considered to have an immunopathologic basis in both patients and relatives of patients with chronic active hepatitis; Sjögren's syndrome, thyroiditis or thyrotoxicosis, and fibrosing alveolitis with pulmonary diffusion defects are commonly associated diseases. Studies on serum complement levels in patients with chronic active hepatitis have revealed that depressed complement levels are related to impaired hepatic protein synthesis and do not reflect immunologic activity.

Clinical Manifestations. Chronic active hepatitis is a disease with a wide clinical spectrum and insidious onset; it may be clinically silent for long periods, as in patients who present as asymptomatic blood donors and are found to be HBAg positive with elevated SGOT levels; patients with more active disease may present with symptoms suggestive of acute hepatitis with malaise, arthralgias, anorexia, and low-grade fever. Amenorrhea commonly results from disturbances of endocrine function. On physical examination, the patient may exhibit signs of both acute and chronic liver disease; these include jaundice, spider angiomas, liver enlargement with variable tenderness, and splenomegaly. The presence of ascites or manifestations of portal hypertension suggests that cirrhosis is already established. The important laboratory features of chronic active hepatitis are changes in *serum transaminase* levels and *hypergammaglobulinemia,* because it has been shown that these tests reflect the activity of the disease—the extent of liver cell necrosis and the degree of associated round cell infiltration in the liver. Patients who present with clinical manifestations of acute hepatitis and subsequently exhibit elevated levels of serum transaminase and gamma globulin for periods in excess of ten weeks are likely to be suffering from chronic active hepatitis or subacute hepatic necrosis. The prognosis of patients with extreme hyperglobulinemia (gamma globulin levels greater than twice normal) and with five- to tenfold elevations of serum transaminase (SGOT) persisting without improvement over a ten-week period is extremely poor without therapy; more than a third of these patients die within a period of six months. When disease activity is minimal, patients may remain well for long periods. Increases in the level of serum bilirubin and alkaline phosphatase caused by intrahepatic cholestasis and depression of plasma albumin and clotting factor levels caused by impaired hepatic plasma protein synthesis are variable features of advanced disease.

Diagnosis. The diagnosis of chronic active hepatitis should be confirmed by percutaneous *liver biopsy* whenever there is clinical or laboratory evidence of this disease. It is important to differentiate chronic active hepatitis from other liver diseases, particularly *chronic persisting hepatitis* which has a favorable prognosis for full recovery without therapy. The degree of irreversible liver damage—cirrhosis—can be determined only by morphologic studies. In all patients with chronic active hepatitis, potential etiologic factors should be fully evaluated, i.e., exposure to drugs and the presence of circulating HBAg or anti-HB. Wilson's disease must be excluded by slit lamp examination of the eyes for Kayser-Fleischer rings, and by measurements of serum ceruloplasmin levels and urinary copper excretion.

Treatment. It has been established by controlled clinical studies that corticosteroids increase the survival of patients with chronic active hepatitis. In the Mayo Clinic study, patients with biochemical and histologic evidence of severe disease (SGOT levels five- to tenfold elevated, and gamma globulin more than twofold increased for periods of ten weeks) were treated with prednisone (20 mg daily), a combination of prednisone (10 mg daily) with azathioprine (50 mg daily), azathioprine (100 mg) alone, or placebo; treatment with prednisone or prednisone with azathioprine was significantly more effective than azathioprine alone or placebo in inducing clinical remission and prolonging survival. The current indications for corticosteroid therapy in patients with biopsy-proved chronic active hepatitis are (1) biochemical evidence of severe disease as cited above, and (2) clinical deterioration with development of ascites or evidence of progressing liver failure. Patients with clinical features of chronic active hepatitis and pathologic evidence of subacute hepatic necrosis on biopsy should also be treated in view of the evidence that their disease is progressive. Patients with relative contraindications to steroid therapy—e.g., with diabetes mellitus—and those who develop complications of steroid therapy may benefit from a combined regimen of low-dose prednisone (10 mg daily) with azathioprine (50 to 100 mg daily). The value of alternate-day corticosteroid therapy has not been assessed.

The duration of corticosteroid therapy should be determined by the clinical, biochemical, and histologic response. The goal of therapy is to induce remission of active hepatitis; the patient should be asymptomatic, with normal or minimally elevated SGOT (less than twice normal) and normal gamma globulin levels, and with resolution of inflammation and liver cell necrosis on

liver biopsy; this end result can be anticipated in approximately two thirds of patients treated for one to three years. When complete remission is established, corticosteroids can be slowly withdrawn and discontinued; subsequent relapses usually occur within six months and require further therapy.

The decision whether to treat a patient with chronic active hepatitis of low-grade activity, e.g., a patient with mild symptoms and minimal elevation of SGOT and gamma globulin, may be a difficult one. Guidelines derived from controlled clinical trials are not available, and the potential benefit from corticosteroid therapy may be exceeded by the risks of long-term therapy.

Prognosis. With adequate therapy, remission of active disease with restoration of normal liver morphology or with residual inactive cirrhosis is achieved in approximately two thirds of patients. Approximately 20 per cent of patients with severe chronic active hepatitis fail to respond to steroid therapy and die with liver failure caused by progressive cirrhosis within a period of one to three years. The long-term prognosis of patients with chronic active hepatitis of low-grade activity has not been defined.

709. CIRRHOSIS OF THE LIVER

Definition and Classification. The cirrhotic liver is one in which the normal lobular architecture is destroyed by bands of fibrous tissue which separate nodules of regenerated liver cells (regeneration nodules). Clinically, patients with cirrhosis usually present with symptoms that relate to the primary etiology (e.g., chronic active hepatitis or manifestations of excessive alcohol intake) or with complications of cirrhosis (e.g., ascites, bleeding from esophageal varices, or hepatic coma). At the time of diagnosis, major etiologic factors causing chronic liver disease may be evident (e.g., documented hepatitis progressing to *chronic active hepatitis, excessive alcohol intake,* or *chronic biliary tract obstruction),* but in many patients the etiology will never be determined. Macroscopic and/or microscopic examination of liver tissue is necessary to establish the diagnosis of cirrhosis, but the pathologic changes in the liver may be the end-stage of several alternative processes which are not always evident at the time of autopsy examination.

In this chapter an *etiologic* classification is used; alternative terminology for cirrhosis will be referred to in the text.

1. Posthepatitic and idiopathic cirrhosis.
2. Cirrhosis in the alcoholic.
3. Metabolic cirrhosis (hemochromatosis and Wilson's disease).
4. Biliary cirrhosis (primary and secondary).
5. Schistosomal fibrosis.
6. Cardiac cirrhosis.

Hemochromatosis is discussed in Part XVI, Section Four, Wilson's disease in Ch. 945, and schistosomal fibrosis in Ch. 296.

POSTHEPATITIC AND IDIOPATHIC CIRRHOSIS (POSTNECROTIC CIRRHOSIS)

Pathogenesis. It has been shown by serial liver biopsy studies that acute viral hepatitis (usually type B, either icteric or anicteric) or toxic hepatitis complicated by subacute hepatic necrosis or chronic active hepatitis may lead to a macronodular cirrhosis. In many nonalcoholic patients there is no history to suggest previous viral or toxic hepatitis; i.e., the cirrhosis is idiopathic (cryptogenic). Idiopathic cirrhosis is sometimes associated with chronic ulcerative colitis; it has been suggested but not proved that chronic pericholangitis resulting from portal bacteremia may cause cirrhosis in these patients.

The association of hypergammaglobulinemia, positive antinuclear reactions, positive LE cell phenomena, and other positive serologic reactions with idiopathic cirrhosis has led to a theory that cirrhosis may be caused by immunologic destruction of parenchymal cells; this has not been proved (see Ch. 708). An increased formation of immunoglobulins with hyperglobulinemia may be stimulated by antigens released from necrotic cells, and may have no primary etiologic significance.

Pathology. The liver in posthepatitic or idiopathic cirrhosis is typically shrunken, with irregular large regeneration nodules and broad zones of fibrous tissue. Pathologically, this is referred to as *macronodular (postnecrotic) cirrhosis.* During the phase of *progressive (active) cirrhosis* after subacute hepatic necrosis or chronic active hepatitis, there may be microscopic evidence of cell degeneration and regeneration, and mononuclear infiltration (both lymphocytes and plasma cells) is prominent in the zones of fibrosis. Intrahepatic cholestasis with bile plugs in dilated bile canaliculi varies with the degree of jaundice, and bile duct proliferation is usual.

Clinical Manifestations. The progressive cirrhosis that follows subacute hepatic necrosis and chronic active hepatitis is often associated with malaise, weakness, anorexia, and jaundice. The patient often has a low-grade fever, and multiple spider angiomas may be seen. The liver is sometimes enlarged and tender, but is more typically shrunken and associated with increased percussion resonance over the right lower costal margin; the spleen may be slightly or massively enlarged. Ascites or peripheral edema may complicate portal hypertension or hypoalbuminemia, and increased bruising may be due to hypoprothrombinemia. Manifestations of disturbed endocrine function—acne, striae, gynecomastia, and amenorrhea—are particularly common in juvenile patients with active cirrhosis. Hypergammaglobulinemia parallels the degree of lymphocytic and plasma cell infiltration in the liver, and may be accompanied by serologic abnormalities. Chronic intrahepatic cholestasis with jaundice, hypercholesterolemia, and high alkaline phosphatase levels sometimes mimics primary biliary cirrhosis. It is not unusual for the biochemical evidence of hepatocellular failure to exceed the clinical evidence of this condition.

The only clinical manifestations of compensated idiopathic cirrhosis may be the cutaneous stigmata of chronic liver disease and splenic enlargement. In these patients, ascites, hepatic coma, and bleeding from esophageal varices may be late complications.

Treatment. Patients with chronic active hepatitis or subacute hepatic necrosis should be treated with corticosteroids to induce clinical remission. When cirrhosis is already established in these patients (confirmed by liver biopsy), corticosteroids will not reverse the existing cirrhosis, but by suppressing continued destructive activity they may prevent progression of the liver disease (see Ch. 708). Corticosteroid therapy is not indicated in patients with inactive posthepatitic cirrhosis.

The management of the complications of cirrhosis is discussed later in this chapter under treatment of portal hypertension, ascites, and hepatic coma.

CIRRHOSIS IN THE ALCOHOLIC

Pathogenesis and Epidemiology. The incidence of cirrhosis in the United States parallels the consumption of alcohol. Little is known, however, of the factors that determine individual susceptibility to cirrhosis; these would explain why many persons with a chronic heavy intake of alcohol do not develop liver disease; both genetic and dietary factors may be of importance. Some insight into the problem of liver disease in the alcoholic has been gained from experimental studies on the effect of alcohol (ethanol) on liver metabolism.

The Effects of Alcohol (Ethanol) on the Liver. Both in man and in laboratory animals, alcohol ingestion is associated with two prominent morphologic changes: the accumulation of fat (triglyceride) in parenchymal cells and degeneration of cell organelles (visible as *alcoholic hyaline*–eosinophilic cytoplasmic inclusions). These changes may result from a direct *hepatotoxic effect of alcohol* rather than a deficiency of dietary factors; they are seen when alcohol is substituted for carbohydrate in an adequate diet.

The pathogenesis of cirrhosis in the alcoholic was not clarified by earlier studies in laboratory animals; in the rat, prolonged administration of alcohol caused fatty infiltration and parenchymal cell degeneration, but these lesions did not progress to cirrhosis. Recent studies in baboons fed alcohol for periods of nine months to four years have reproduced all the pathologic lesions of human alcoholic liver disease.

Pathology. The liver in *acute alcoholic hepatitis* is enlarged and firm, and on microscopic examination the parenchymal cells are distended with droplets of fat, and may contain eosinophilic cytoplasmic inclusions (alcoholic hyaline). Central veins and centrilobular areas may be replaced by zones of *hyaline sclerosis,* a lesion which undergoes subsequent fibrosis and may contribute to the development of portal hypertension. There is variable inflammatory cell infiltration in portal areas and throughout the parenchyma, and bile stasis occurs in jaundiced patients.

Cirrhosis in the alcoholic is usually of the *Laennec* or *micronodular type,* with small uniform regeneration nodules separated by fibrous bands containing mononuclear cells and proliferating bile ductules. The pathologic changes of acute alcoholic hepatitis—inflammation, cell degeneration, and infiltration with fat—are often seen in the cirrhotic liver. Occasionally the liver is of the *macronodular type,* with coarse, irregular regeneration nodules and broad intervening bands of fibrous tissue.

Clinical Manifestations. A patient with *acute alcoholic hepatitis* may seek medical help because of *abdominal pain* caused by acute hepatic enlargement, gastritis, or pancreatitis; *vomiting,* with or without *hematemesis,* caused by gastritis, ulcer, or sometimes esophageal varices; *jaundice; abdominal swelling* with ascites; or because of symptoms caused by head injury, alcohol withdrawal, or thiamin deficiency.

On admission to hospital, the patient is usually *febrile*

and *dehydrated* and has an alcoholic fetor. An *enlarged, firm, tender liver,* abdominal distention with *ascites* and *jaundice,* with prominent spider angiomas and palmar erythema, are typically present. The early hospital course is often complicated by *delirium tremens.* Intense jaundice with *pruritus* in febrile patients may simulate extrahepatic biliary tract obstruction.

Liver function tests reveal conjugated hyperbilirubinemia, elevated serum transaminase levels (50 to 300 units), variable increases in alkaline phosphatase activity, and normal or depressed levels of albumin and clotting factors. The serum cholesterol concentration may be increased, normal, or depressed. *Hypokalemia* often results from increased urinary excretion of potassium. *Hyperuricemia* resulting from depressed urinary excretion of uric acid parallels lactic acidosis. Anemia may be due to bleeding or *hemolysis;* acute severe hemolysis is sometimes associated with *hyperlipemia* (Zieve's syndrome).

Cirrhosis in the alcoholic may present insidiously with anorexia, fatigue, and weakness, and a gradual onset of jaundice and ascites, or may present acutely with one or several major complications: acute upper gastrointestinal *bleeding,* sudden onset of *ascites,* liver failure with *jaundice* or *coma,* or symptoms of hepatic *carcinoma.* When the cirrhotic patient shows manifestations of acute alcoholic hepatitis, the term *florid cirrhosis* is often used. In the absence of these complications the only stigmata of cirrhosis may be a firm, enlarged, nontender liver with or without splenomegaly, and the cutaneous manifestations of chronic liver disease.

In *compensated cirrhosis* the only abnormalities of liver function may be mild BSP retention and an increased urinary excretion of urobilinogen. With progressive decompensation, serum protein concentrations fall, and hyperbilirubinemia and BSP retention increase. Serum enzyme levels are usually only slightly elevated.

Differential Diagnosis. In the differential diagnosis of acute alcoholic hepatitis other causes for acute jaundice must be considered, i.e., *viral hepatitis, extrahepatic obstruction,* and *drug reactions.* Infection should be considered in the febrile patient, although fever may be due to cell necrosis. In the compensated cirrhotic, an enlarged, firm liver may be suggestive of infiltrative disease. A needle biopsy of the liver usually resolves these differential diagnostic problems.

When cirrhosis is complicated by bleeding, ascites, or coma, other causes for these complications must be excluded. In cirrhotic patients, acute upper gastrointestinal *bleeding* may come from esophageal varices; but acute gastric erosions, peptic ulcer, and neoplasm must also be considered. Esophagoscopy, gastroscopy, and roentgenologic evaluation of the esophagus, stomach, and duodenum are necessary to establish the site of bleeding (see Ch. 644). Although *ascites* is usually due to portal hypertension with hypoalbuminemia, *constrictive pericarditis, bacterial peritonitis* (especially *tuberculous*), and *intra-abdominal neoplasm* must also be considered. Measurement of the venous pressure and a diagnostic paracentesis with analysis for protein, enzymes, bacteria, and cells are of value in differential diagnosis. In tuberculous peritonitis the protein concentration of ascitic fluid may exceed 2.5 grams per 100 ml and the ascitic fluid white cell count usually exceeds 250 per cubic millimeter, with lymphocytes predominant. Malignant effusions are often hemorrhagic, with a protein content greater than 2.5 grams per 100 ml and elevated lactic

dehydrogenase activity; malignant cells may be found on cytologic examination.

Treatment. Long-term abstinence from alcohol is the single major factor that may modify the course of liver disease in the alcoholic. With abstinence, liver function may return to normal after an episode of acute alcoholic hepatitis, and minimal hepatic fibrosis may persist without progression. When cirrhosis is well established and portal hypertension with esophageal varices complicates the liver disease, abstinence from alcohol may not prolong the patient's survival.

Patients with *acute alcoholic hepatitis* should be treated with bed rest, alcohol withdrawal, and a diet containing adequate proteins, vitamins, minerals, and calories. Intravenous infusions of 5 per cent glucose, with potassium, magnesium and vitamin supplements, may be needed by the febrile, dehydrated patient. Oral supplements of ferrous sulfate (0.3 gram three times a day) or folic acid (5 mg daily) should be given to correct anemia caused by iron or folic acid deficiency. Salt intake should be restricted to 1 gram per 24 hours in patients with ascites, and fluid intake and output should be monitored with daily weights. On this regimen clinical and biochemical improvement is usual within two to three weeks, and is accompanied by a spontaneous diuresis and disappearance of ascites unless portal hypertension is already established by fibrosis.

Although corticosteroid therapy has been recommended for the treatment of severely ill patients, a recent controlled study indicated that prednisone was of no benefit.

TREATMENT OF THE COMPLICATIONS OF CIRRHOSIS

Portal Hypertension with Upper Gastrointestinal Bleeding. In the early management of bleeding, treatment is directed toward restoring blood volume and controlling the bleeding at the same time that diagnostic efforts are made to determine the site of bleeding. The alcoholic patient may bleed from *acute gastric erosions, peptic ulcer,* or *esophageal varices;* appropriate therapy depends on the site of bleeding. The several measures that may be used to control bleeding in cirrhotic patients include gastric lavage with ice water, local gastric hypothermia using an esophagogastric balloon, intravenous infusions of Pitressin, esophageal tamponade with an inflated balloon, or direct surgical procedures. *Lavage* with ice water is unlikely to control esophageal bleeding, but may be effective when bleeding is from gastric erosions. Infusions of Pitressin (20 units intravenously in 10 minutes) constrict the splanchnic arterioles, reduce splanchnic blood flow, and lower portal venous pressure. Bleeding from varices may thus be temporarily controlled. Similar results may be achieved without systemic side effects by continuous infusion of vasoconstrictor drugs into the superior mesenteric artery, selectively catheterized. *Esophageal tamponade* (with a Sengstaken esophageal tube) may be the only nonoperative procedure that will control massive bleeding from esophageal varices. The disadvantage of this procedure is the many complications that result from tamponade: asphyxia resulting from upward displacement of the balloon, aspiration, and esophageal erosion by pressure necrosis. These complications, however, will be minimized by using an additional smooth bore tube attached to the Sengstaken tube for aspiration of secretions proximal to the balloon and by tracheal intubation with a cuffed endotracheal tube.

Several surgical procedures have been recommended to control bleeding from esophageal varices. These include direct ligation of varices, transection of the esophagus with division of varices, esophagogastric resection, splenectomy, and splenorenal or portacaval anastomosis. Each procedure carries a high risk in the poor-risk patient with hepatic decompensation. The surgical procedure of choice is a *portacaval anastomosis,* which controls bleeding by lowering portal pressure; with the subsequent disappearance of esophageal varices, recurrent bleeding is unusual.

A portacaval anastomosis is recommended for the good-risk patient with documented bleeding from esophageal varices, unless bleeding has been precipitated by acute alcoholic hepatitis. In the latter instance, portal pressure may return to normal, and varices may disappear upon recovery from acute hepatic decompensation and resolution of hepatic inflammation and fatty infiltration. When esophageal bleeding complicates hepatocellular failure, surgery is contraindicated even when medical therapy is ineffective in controlling hemorrhage. There is no evidence that a prophylactic portacaval shunt is of value in prolonging the life of a patient with portal hypertension and esophageal varices that have not bled. Although prophylactic shunt surgery reduces the risk of subsequent variceal hemorrhage, the complications of surgery—hepatic encephalopathy and hepatic failure—result in considerable morbidity.

Ascites. When ascites complicates acute alcoholic hepatitis, therapy aimed at improving liver function usually leads to a spontaneous diuresis as the portal pressure falls toward normal and serum albumin levels rise. Sodium intake should be restricted to 1 gram daily, and diuretics should be used with caution.

When ascites is of longer duration and is associated with sustained portal hypertension and hypoalbuminemia, diuretic agents together with a restricted intake of sodium may be necessary to control sodium and water retention. Water intake may need to be restricted to a volume that equals insensible losses plus urine output in patients who fail to excrete a fluid load. The sole use of diuretic agents that act principally on the proximal tubule (mercurials and chlorothiazides) is contraindicated. These agents do not counteract the effect of aldosterone on the distal tubule; not only are they ineffective diuretics in cirrhotic patients with secondary hyperaldosteronism, but they also augment potassium loss and may precipitate *hypokalemic alkalosis* with hepatic coma in spite of oral potassium supplements.

To promote an *effective* and *safe* diuresis, an *aldosterone blocking agent* should be given in combination with one of the aforementioned diuretic agents. Spironolactone (50 to 200 mg daily) with hydrochlorothiazide (50 to 100 mg daily) is recommended. Oral potassium supplements (KCl in cherry syrup, 1 gram three times a day) may be necessary during the initial two to four days of combined drug therapy to prevent hypokalemia. Whereas edema fluid can be mobilized rapidly during diuresis, the maximal rate at which ascitic fluid can be removed by diuresis in the cirrhotic is approximately 900 ml per 24 hours. In patients free of peripheral edema, the rate of diuresis should not produce a daily

weight loss in excess of 0.5 kg; if diuresis is more rapid, there will be a fall in plasma volume.

The complications of diuretic therapy include the following: (1) *Hyperkalemia* often results from the use of aldosterone-blocking drugs in patients with impaired renal function. (2) *Hyponatremia* may be associated with an abnormal distribution of sodium between the intracellular and extracellular fluid pools in patients with an increased total body sodium, with disproportionate water retention, or with sodium depletion after prolonged diuresis. (3) *Azotemia* may be due to contraction of the extracellular fluid pool or a decrease in glomerular blood flow owing to intrarenal shunting of blood. (4) *Hepatic encephalopathy* may follow rapid diuresis or disturbances of pH and electrolyte balance. These complications will be reduced if serum electrolyte concentrations and urinary electrolyte excretion are measured frequently during therapy. Diuretics should be discontinued when neuropsychiatric symptoms complicate rapid diuresis or electrolyte imbalance, and no attempt should be made to mobilize all ascitic fluid by prolonged therapy that increases the risk of complication without benefit to the patient. When long-term diuretic therapy is necessary to control ascites, diuretics should be given intermittently rather than continuously.

When ascites is associated with severe hypoalbuminemia, intravenous infusions of salt-poor albumin (50 to 100 grams daily) may potentiate a diuresis, but pulmonary edema caused by an expanded plasma volume must be avoided.

Paracentesis with removal of less than 1000 ml of ascitic fluid should be performed for diagnostic purposes, but is now rarely indicated for therapy of ascites except when impaired renal function prevents safe or effective diuretic therapy. Ascitic fluid should then be removed slowly through a small plastic catheter, and salt-poor human albumin (50 to 200 grams) should be infused intravenously over a period of 12 to 24 hours to prevent hypovolemia and shock that may result from a shift of fluid from the intravascular compartment into the peritoneal cavity.

Hepatic Coma. When a cirrhotic patient develops hepatic encephalopathy it is important to identify the precipitating cause. It may be due to gastrointestinal bleeding; fluid and electrolyte imbalances and pH disturbances, particularly during diuretic therapy; the administration of depressant drugs, both analgesic and sedative; intercurrent infection with fever; or increased dietary intake of protein. In the treatment of hepatic coma, gastrointestinal bleeding and infection must be controlled, depressant drugs withheld, and disturbances of fluid, electrolyte, and acid-base balance corrected. In all patients, measures that lower blood ammonium concentration by reducing enteric bacterial breakdown of amino acids and urea should be instituted. These measures include dietary *protein restriction* (complete in the comatose patient, or partial—20 to 40 grams—in patients with mild encephalopathy), *cathartics* (magnesium citrate, 240 ml twice daily), *enemas* to clear the intestine of its nitrogenous content, and *neomycin* (4 to 6 grams daily by mouth or by nasogastric tube) to reduce the bacterial flora.

Patients with chronic hepatic encephalopathy, who usually have extensive portal-systemic shunts, may be helped by long-term restriction of protein intake to 40 grams and the administration of neomycin, 2 to 3 grams daily. Lactulose, a disaccharide that is not absorbed but is metabolized by intestinal bacteria to organic acids, is effective in lowering the blood ammonia levels of patients with chronic encephalopathy; the unabsorbed sugar produces an osmotic diarrhea, and ammonia is retained in the fecal content at the acid pH.

A surgical approach to the management of the patient with chronic hepatic encephalopathy is excision or exclusion of the colon; the complications of surgery in chronically ill patients usually balance the potential benefit of removing a bacteria-laden gut.

BILIARY CIRRHOSIS

Primary biliary cirrhosis (chronic nonsuppurative destructive cholangitis) is a disease of unknown etiology. *Chronic intrahepatic cholestasis* is associated with progressive periportal fibrosis and chronic inflammation. Cirrhosis with nodular regeneration is a late pathologic finding. Although hypersensitivity reactions to drugs sometimes cause prolonged intrahepatic cholestasis, there is no evidence that acute intrahepatic cholestasis leads to primary biliary cirrhosis. It has been suggested that the primary lesion may be an injury to small bile ducts; these are often absent in liver biopsy specimens taken early in the course of the disease, but regenerate in the cirrhotic liver. Patients with primary biliary cirrhosis may exhibit hypergammaglobulinemia with circulating antibodies reactive against mitochondria (antimitochondrial antibody), but the significance of immunologic phenomena has not been established.

In *secondary biliary cirrhosis,* bile duct obstruction with or without infection causes periportal inflammation with progressive fibrosis, parenchymal cell destruction, and nodular regeneration.

Clinical Features. Primary biliary cirrhosis is most often diagnosed in women aged 40 to 60. The earliest symptom may be generalized *pruritus.* Jaundice with dark urine and pale stools and cutaneous xanthomas appear later with increasing intrahepatic cholestasis. At the time of onset of symptoms, the liver is usually firm and enlarged, and the spleen is palpable. Liver function tests at this time reflect cholestasis with good hepatocellular function; alkaline phosphatase, 5′-nucleotidase, and cholesterol levels may be markedly elevated, whereas serum albumin levels remain normal. During the period of maximal cholestasis the manifestations of malabsorption may become evident: *weight loss, diarrhea* with pale bulky stools, *bleeding* resulting from hypoprothrombinemia, and collapse of vertebrae and *pathologic fractures* with bone demineralization caused by malabsorption of vitamin D and calcium. *Xanthomas* usually appear when the serum cholesterol level exceeds 450 mg per 100 ml. Acute upper gastrointestinal bleeding is more often from a duodenal ulcer than from esophageal varices; a reduced flow of alkaline bile with normal gastric acid secretion may contribute to peptic ulcer.

The terminal stage of biliary cirrhosis is one of hepatocellular failure with rising serum bilirubin levels, a decrease in serum albumin and cholesterol with disappearance of xanthomas, and the onset of ascites.

Differential Diagnosis. The diagnosis of primary biliary cirrhosis must always be confirmed by exploratory laparotomy, with liver biopsy and operative cholangiography. Stenosing cholangitis, extrahepatic bile duct obstruction resulting from stone or stricture, and carcinoma involving the major extrahepatic or intrahepatic bile ducts should be excluded. The presence of antimitochondrial antibody is of diagnostic importance – patients with acute extrahepatic biliary obstruction do not exhibit this antibody.

Treatment. Supplements of fat-soluble vitamins should be given to prevent or correct deficiency caused by malabsorption. Vitamin K_1, 5 to 10 mg, and vitamins A and D, 10,000 units, should be given by mouth daily, together with calcium lactate or gluconate, 6 to 12 grams. *Pruritus* may be relieved by methyltestosterone or norethandrolone, 10 mg twice or three times daily, but these agents increase the jaundice. The bile acid sequestrant resin, *cholestyramine,* 8 to 12 grams daily in divided doses, is effective in relieving pruritus, lowering serum cholesterol levels, and reducing xanthomas when cholestasis is incomplete. Patients with duodenal ulcer or with complications of cirrhosis should be treated appropriately as outlined elsewhere.

Prognosis. The average life expectancy in primary biliary cirrhosis from the time of onset of symptoms is approximately five years. With supportive therapy the patient will be more comfortable and will suffer fewer complications during this period.

CARDIAC CIRRHOSIS

Chronic congestive heart failure with valvular heart disease and tricuspid incompetence or constrictive pericarditis may cause progressive fibrosis extending peripherally from centrilobular to portal areas. Regeneration nodules are not prominent. Fat may accumulate in hypoxic cells.

The liver is usually firm, with tenderness and an increase in size during more severe episodes of heart failure. Hepatic pulsation may be detected with tricuspid insufficiency. The changes in liver function are those of acute hepatic congestion, but hypoalbuminemia may be more severe when there is excessive enteric leakage of plasma protein. (See Part XIV, Section Three.) Although chronic congestive heart failure may raise the portal venous pressure, a portal-systemic collateral circulation, e.g., esophageal varices, does not develop in the absence of an increased pressure gradient between these systems.

710. CONGENITAL HEPATIC FIBROSIS

Congenital hepatic fibrosis is a variant of polycystic disease. Broad bands of fibrous tissue containing bile ducts surround the liver lobules and obstruct portal blood flow. Splenomegaly, portal hypertension, and bleeding from esophageal varices are the usual presenting manifestations in childhood or adolescence. With normal liver function these children usually tolerate recurrent bleeding and portacaval shunt surgery better than patients with cirrhosis. In adults, *polycystic disease of the liver* may cause massive liver enlargement without interfering with liver function. The complications include hemorrhage into a cyst with abdominal pain and bleeding from esophageal varices.

711. INFILTRATIVE DISEASE OF THE LIVER

less effective than biopsy through a peritoneoscopy in establishing the presence of liver involvement.

HEPATIC GRANULOMAS

Hepatic granulomas are most commonly due to *sarcoidosis* and *tuberculosis,* but also occur in beryllium poisoning, brucellosis, fungal and parasitic infections, and Hodgkin's disease.

In sarcoidosis there are noncaseating granulomas, with mononuclear, epithelioid, and giant cells, and variable fibrosis. In patients with pulmonary tuberculosis or miliary tuberculosis, hepatic granulomas are particularly common. Small lesions may exhibit no caseation, and no organisms may be demonstrated; but larger lesions may have a central area of caseation.

Granulomatous disease of the liver may be associated with enlargement of the liver and BSP retention with elevation of alkaline phosphatase and 5'-nucleotidase without jaundice. A needle biopsy of the liver should be performed to establish the diagnosis of granulomatous disease. This is particularly helpful in the diagnosis of miliary tuberculosis in an ill, febrile patient without typical radiologic changes in the chest.

SECONDARY CARCINOMA OF THE LIVER

Primary carcinomas of the lung, gastrointestinal tract, and breast are the most common neoplasms that metastasize to the liver. Abdominal swelling or pain and jaundice are the presenting symptoms, but the liver is usually massively enlarged with multiple nodules before jaundice develops. The earlier biochemical manifestations of hepatic metastases are BSP retention and elevations of serum alkaline phosphatase and 5'-nucleotidase. Needle biopsy of the liver is helpful in providing a tissue diagnosis of secondary carcinoma, and may save the patient from the discomfort of an exploratory laparotomy. External radioisotopic scanning of the liver after the intravenous injection of a gamma-emitting radioisotope that is concentrated in the liver may be helpful in localizing large metastases that appear as "cold" areas in the surface scan. The presence of hepatic metastases from carcinomas of the colon and pancreas is usually associated with positive tests for carcinoembryonic antigen (CEA) in the serum; false positive tests have been reported in patients with decompensated alcoholic liver disease.

SARCOMAS OF THE LIVER

Hepatic infiltration with lymphoma, lymphosarcoma, or Hodgkin's disease is usually a manifestation of disseminated disease. Firm liver enlargement and biochemical evidence of intrahepatic cholestasis suggest, but are not necessarily diagnostic of, hepatic infiltration. Jaundice is more often the result of hepatic infiltration than invasion of the extrahepatic bile ducts by tumor; jaundice caused by intrahepatic cholestasis may develop, however, in the absence of liver infiltration. Splenomegaly is commonly associated with hepatic involvement in Hodgkin's disease. Percutaneous liver biopsy is

PRIMARY CARCINOMAS OF THE LIVER (HEPATOMA)

Hepatic carcinoma usually complicates cirrhosis of the liver; it has a higher incidence in postnecrotic cirrhosis and hemochromatosis than in Laennec's cirrhosis. This lesion should be suspected whenever a cirrhotic patient exhibits unexplained clinical deterioration with enlarging liver, right upper quadrant pain, or sudden onset of ascites. A vascular bruit may be heard over these tumors. Hypoglycemia is sometimes a prominent clinical manifestation. Changes in liver function include a rising alkaline phosphatase and elevated lactic dehydrogenase. A laboratory manifestation of hepatoma is the appearance of a fetal plasma protein, alpha-fetoprotein, in the plasma; sensitive radioimmunoassay techniques have recently detected this protein in the plasma of patients recovering from hepatitis. Hepatomas localized to one lobe of the liver have been excised successfully on several occasions, but usually cirrhosis and invasion of hepatic veins or local spread prevent surgical therapy.

Hepatoma can be produced with a high degree of regularity in several species of laboratory animals by injection of minute doses of the microtoxin known as *aflatoxin.* This substance is produced by Aspergillus growing on peanut (groundnut) meal that has been stored in appropriately hot, humid conditions. The incidence of hepatoma in man has long been known to show a marked geographic variation, and there is a correlation between the localities where hepatoma is the most frequently occurring carcinoma and the particular complex of circumstances that favors the production of aflatoxin. Obviously, it cannot be stated as yet that hepatoma in man is caused by aflatoxin, but this possibility that hepatoma is thus environmentally induced is being actively pursued in epidemiologic, clinical, and laboratory studies.

General

Davidson, C. S.: Liver pathophysiology. Its Relevance to Disease. Boston, Little, Brown & Company, 1970.
Scheuer, P. J.: Liver Biopsy Interpretation. London, Balliere, Tindall and Cassell, Ltd., 1968.
Schiff, L.: Diseases of the Liver. 3rd ed. Philadelphia, J. B. Lippincott Company, 1969.
Sherlock, S.: Diseases of the Liver. 4th ed. Oxford, Blackwell Scientific Publications, 1968.

Manifestations of Liver Disease

Berk, P. D., Bloomer, J. R., Howe, R. B., and Berlin, N. I.: Constitutional hepatic dysfunction (Gilbert's syndrome). A new definition based on kinetic studies with unconjugated radiobilirubin. Am. J. Med., 49:296, 1970.
Kaplan, M. M.: Alkaline phosphatase. N. Engl. J. Med., 286:200, 1972.
Reynolds, T. B., Ito, S., and Iwatsuki, S.: Measurement of portal pressure and its clinical application. Am. J. Med., 49:649, 1970.
Rothschild, M. A., Oratz, M., and Schreiber, S. S.: Albumin metabolism. Gastroenterology, 64:324, 1973.
Scheuer, P. J.: Liver biopsy in the diagnosis of cirrhosis. Gut, 11:275, 1970.
Schmid, R.: Bilirubin metabolism in man. N. Engl. J. Med., 287:703, 1972.

Acute Liver Disease

Chalmers, T. C., Eckhardt, R. D., Reynolds, W. E., Cigarroa, J. G., Jr., Deane, N., Reifenstein, R. W., Smith, C. W., and Davidson, C. S.: The treatment of acute infectious hepatitis. Controlled studies of the effect of diet, rest, and physical reconditioning on the acute course of the disease and on the incidence of relapses and residual abnormalities. J. Clin. Invest., 34:1136, 1955.
Chalmers, T. C., and Alter, H. J.: Management of the asymptomatic carrier

of the hepatitis-associated (Australia) antigen. N. Engl. J. Med., 285:613, 1971.

Klatskin, G., and Kimberg, D. V.: Recurrent hepatitis attributable to halothane sensitization in an anesthetist. N. Engl. J. Med., 280:515, 1969.

Krugman, S., Giles, J. P., and Hammond, J.: Infectious hepatitis. Evidence for two distinctive clinical, epidemiological and immunological types of infection. J.A.M.A., 200:365, 1967.

Maddrey, W. C., and Boitnott, J. K.: Isoniazid hepatitis. Ann. Intern. Med., 79:1, 1973.

Redeker, A. G., and Yamahiro, H. S.: Controlled trial of exchange-transfusion therapy in fulminant hepatitis. Lancet, 1:3, 1973.

Sabbaj, J., Sutter, V. L., and Finegold, S. M.: Anaerobic pyogenic liver abscess. Ann. Intern. Med., 77:629, 1972.

Schweitzer, I. L., Dunn, A. E. G., Peters, R. L., and Spears, R. L.: Viral hepatitis B in neonates and infants. Am. J. Med., 55:762, 1973.

Sherlock, S.: Halothane hepatitis. Gut, 12:324, 1971.

Sherlock, S.: The course of long incubation (virus B) hepatitis. Br. Med. Bull., 28:109, 1972.

Shulman, N. R.: Hepatitis-associated antigen. Am. J. Med., 49:669, 1970.

Vittal, S. B. V., Thomas, W., Jr., and Clowdus, B. F.: Acute viral hepatitis. Course and incidence of progression to chronic hepatitis. Am. J. Med., 55:757, 1973.

Williams, R.: Problems of fulminant hepatic failure. Br. Med. Bull., 28:114, 1972.

Chronic Liver Disease

Boyer, J. L., and Klatskin, G.: Patterns of necrosis in acute viral hepatitis.

Prognostic value of bridging (subacute hepatic necrosis). N. Engl. J. Med., 283:1063, 1970.

Campra, J. L., Hamlin, E. M., Kirshbaum, R. L., Olivier, M., Redeker, A. G., and Reynolds, T. B.: Prednisone therapy in acute alcoholic hepatitis. Report of a controlled trial. Ann. Intern. Med., 79:625, 1973.

Conn, H. O.: A rational approach to the hepatorenal syndrome. Gastroenterology, 65:321, 1973.

Conn, H. O., Lindenmuth, W. W., May, C. J., and Ramsby, G. R.: Prophylactic portacaval anastomosis. Medicine, 51:27, 1972.

Gabuzda, G. J.: Cirrhosis, ascites and edema. Clinical course related to management. Gastroenterology, 58:546, 1970.

Golding, P. L., Smith, M., and Williams, R.: Multisystem involvement in chronic liver disease. Studies on the incidence and pathogenesis. Am. J. Med., 55:772, 1973.

Lieber, C. S.: Hepatic and metabolic effects of alcohol. Gastroenterology, 65:821, 1973.

Rubin, E., and Lieber, C. S.: Fatty liver, alcoholic hepatitis and cirrhosis produced by alcohol in primates. N. Engl. J. Med., 290:128, 1974.

Schenker, S., Breen, K. J., and Hoyumpa, A. M.: Hepatic encephalopathy; current status. Gastroenterology, 66:121, 1974.

Sherlock, S., and Scheuer, P. J.: The presentation and diagnosis of 100 patients with primary biliary cirrhosis. N. Engl. J. Med., 289:674, 1973.

Soloway, R. D., Summerskill, W. H. J., Baggenstoss, A. H., Geall, M. G., Gitnick, G. L., Elveback, L. R., and Schoenfield, L. J.: Clinical, biochemical and histological remission of severe chronic active liver disease. A controlled study of treatments and early prognosis. Gastroenterology, 63:820, 1972.

Soterakis, J., Resnick, R. H., and Iber, F. L.: Effect of alcohol abstinence on survival in cirrhotic portal hypertension. Lancet, 2:65, 1973.

Part XV
DISEASES OF NUTRITION

712. NUTRIENT REQUIREMENTS

Nevin S. Scrimshaw

GENERAL CONSIDERATIONS

The nutrient intakes recommended by most national and international organizations are defined as the amounts sufficient for the physiologic needs of virtually all healthy persons in a population. Conceptually, they are intended to cover the mean plus two standard deviations, although the data for actually calculating a standard deviation are rarely available. It is important for the physician to recognize that existing recommended dietary allowances for nutrients do not cover the additional needs that arise from microbial disease, trauma, advanced malignancies, disorders of the gastrointestinal tract, or metabolic diseases and abnormalities. Moreover, the intake recommended for any one nutrient presupposes that the requirements for energy and for all other nutrients are fully met.

Persons receiving less than the recommended allowance are not necessarily malnourished; it depends on their individual requirements, on the margin of safety inherent in the recommendation, and on whether other deficiencies are more limiting. On the other hand, persons consuming the recommended allowance are not necessarily adequately nourished. The presence of disease may interfere with absorption, increase utilization, or accelerate loss of an essential nutrient. This should be taken into account in prescribing diets for persons with acute or chronic disease. Moreover, imbalance among nutrients can render inadequate an intake which would otherwise be ample.

The 1974 Recommended Dietary Allowances of the Food and Nutrition Board (FNB) of the National Academy of Sciences are given in Table 1. They differ from those of the United Kingdom and FAO/WHO in their higher recommendations for calcium and ascorbic acid and slightly lower recommendations for calories.

The following nutrients have been established as necessary dietary constituents for man under physiologic or pathologic conditions, or both.

NECESSARY NUTRIENTS

Calories. The body requires a source of energy to maintain the normal processes of life and to meet the demands of activity and growth. Calorie requirements depend mainly on body size, basal metabolic rate, activity, age, sex, and environmental temperature. Clinical diseases associated with calorie deficiency are marasmus in children and cachexia in adults. A 70-kg male requires approximately 70 calories per hour under basal conditions and up to 600 calories per hour for very heavy muscular work, so that activity levels largely determine gain or loss of weight on a given diet. Carbohydrate and protein furnish about 4 calories per gram, alcohol about 7, and fat about 9. The report of the FAO Expert Committee on Calorie Requirements provides more detailed information.

Protein. Proteins in the diet vary in their usefulness, depending on the extent to which they contain those eight essential amino acids that cannot be synthesized within the body in the proportions needed for making new tissue. When protein is severely deficient relative to calories, kwashiorkor develops.

Protein requirements have two components: sufficient amounts and proportions of the essential amino acids, and adequate additional nitrogen from any utilizable source. The latter comes from both the dietarily dispensable amino acids and those essential amino acids present in excess of requirements. If the diet does not supply adequate calories, dietary protein will be utilized to meet energy needs at the expense of fulfilling requirements for protein. Protein requirements are greatly increased by microbial disease, trauma, and most other pathologic states.

Protein requirements are expressed in terms of reference protein which, in theory, is 100 per cent absorbed and utilized. Since only egg and milk approach this ideal, recommended dietary allowances for protein must be expressed in terms of the quality of the protein of the actual diet. In industrialized countries it can be assumed that the protein of the ordinary mixed diet is about 70 per cent utilized, but for cereal-based diets in most developing countries a figure of 60 per cent or less is more appropriate. Proteins of animal origin are generally the best utilized, followed by those from legumes, oilseeds, rice, oats, and Opaque-2 corn. Most other cereal proteins are of relatively poor quality.

Carbohydrates and Fats. Carbohydrates supply dietary energy and are necessary constituents of a balanced and palatable diet. There is no fixed requirement for carbohydrates, however, since they can be completely replaced as energy sources in the diet by protein and fats. Fats supply more than twice the energy of carbohydrate and protein per gram, and thus contribute a concentrated source of calories as well as palatability in the diet. The actual requirement for fat, however, is limited to a minute quantity of linoleic, linolenic, or arachidonic acid – all polyunsaturated fatty acids. Deficiency of these in young children leads to defective growth and scaly skin.

Fat-Soluble Vitamins

Vitamin A. Vitamin A (retinol) is essential for integrity of mucosal surfaces and is required in the form of its aldehyde for vision, particularly in dim light. Avitaminosis A results in skin and eye lesions and reduced resistance to infection (see Ch. 717), and hypervitaminosis A is equally serious (see Ch. 722).

Vitamin A is found preformed in animal tissue, and the beta-carotene of green and yellow vegetables is converted in the body to vitamin A with an efficiency of about 50 per cent. There are several other forms of carotene that have some activity but are still less efficiently

TABLE 1. Food and Nutrition Board, National Academy of Sciences–National Research Council
Recommended Daily Dietary Allowances,* Revised 1974
Designed for the Maintenance of Good Nutrition of Practically All Healthy People in the U.S.A.

	Age (years) From–Up to	Weight (kg)	Weight (lbs)	Height (cm)	Height (in)	Energy (kcal)†	Protein (grams)	Vitamin A Activity (RE)‡	Vitamin A Activity (IU)	Vitamin D (IU)	Vitamin E Activity¶ (IU)	Ascorbic Acid (mg)	Folacin (µg)	Niacin†† (mg)	Riboflavin (mg)	Thiamin (mg)	Vitamin B_6 (mg)	Vitamin B_{12} (µg)	Calcium (mg)	Phosphorus (mg)	Iodine (µg)	Iron (mg)	Magnesium (mg)	Zinc (mg)
Infants	0.0–0.5	6	14	60	24	kg × 117	kg × 2.2	420§	1400	400	4	35	50	5	0.4	0.3	0.3	0.3	360	240	35	10	60	3
	0.5–1.0	9	20	71	28	kg × 108	kg × 2.0	400	2000	400	5	35	50	8	0.6	0.5	0.4	0.3	540	400	45	15	70	5
Children	1–3	13	28	86	34	1300	23	400	2000	400	7	40	100	9	0.8	0.7	0.6	1.0	800	800	60	15	150	10
	4–6	20	44	110	44	1800	30	500	2500	400	9	40	200	12	1.1	0.9	0.9	1.5	800	800	80	10	200	10
	7–10	30	66	135	54	2400	36	700	3300	400	10	40	300	16	1.2	1.2	1.2	2.0	800	800	110	10	250	10
Males	11–14	44	97	158	63	2800	44	1000	5000	400	12	45	400	18	1.5	1.4	1.6	3.0	1200	1200	130	18	350	15
	15–18	61	134	172	69	3000	54	1000	5000	400	15	45	400	20	1.8	1.5	2.0	3.0	1200	1200	150	18	400	15
	19–22	67	147	172	69	3000	54	1000	5000	400	15	45	400	20	1.8	1.5	2.0	3.0	800	800	140	10	350	15
	23–50	70	154	172	69	2700	56	1000	5000		15	45	400	18	1.6	1.4	2.0	3.0	800	800	130	10	350	15
	51+	70	154	172	69	2400	56	1000	5000		15	45	400	16	1.5	1.2	2.0	3.0	800	800	110	10	350	15
Females	11–14	44	97	155	62	2400	44	800	4000	400	12	45	400	16	1.3	1.2	1.6	3.0	1200	1200	115	18	300	15
	15–18	54	119	162	65	2100	48	800	4000	400	12	45	400	14	1.4	1.1	2.0	3.0	1200	1200	115	18	300	15
	19–22	58	128	162	65	2100	46	800	4000	400	12	45	400	14	1.4	1.1	2.0	3.0	800	800	100	18	300	15
	23–50	58	128	162	65	2000	46	800	4000		12	45	400	13	1.2	1.0	2.0	3.0	800	800	100	18	300	15
	51+	58	128	162	65	1800	46	800	4000		12	45	400	12	1.1	1.0	2.0	3.0	800	800	80	10	300	15
Pregnant						+300	+30	1000	5000	400	15	60	800	+2	+0.3	+0.3	2.5	4.0	1200	1200	125	18‡‡	450	20
Lactating						+500	+20	1200	6000	400	15	80	600	+4	+0.5	+0.3	2.5	4.0	1200	1200	150	18	450	25

*Reprinted from Recommended Dietary Allowances. 8th revised edition. Washington, D.C., National Academy of Sciences, 1973. The allowances are intended to provide for individual variations among most normal persons as they live in the United States under usual environmental stresses. Diets should be based on a variety of common foods in order to provide other nutrients for which human requirements have been less well defined. See text for more detailed discussion of allowances and of nutrients not tabulated.

†Kilojoules (KJ) = 4.2 × kcal.

‡Retinol equivalents.

§Assumed to be all as retinol in milk during the first six months of life. All subsequent intakes are assumed to be one half as retinol and one half as β-carotene when calculated from international units. As retinol equivalents, three fourths are as retinol and one fourth as β-carotene.

¶Total vitamin E activity, estimated to be 80 per cent as α-tocopherol and 20 per cent other tocopherols. See text for variation in allowances.

**The folacin allowances refer to dietary sources as determined by Lactobacillus casei assay. Pure forms of folacin may be effective in doses less than one fourth of the RDA.

††Although allowances are expressed as niacin, it is recognized that on the average 1 mg of niacin is derived from each 60 mg of dietary tryptophan.

‡‡This increased requirement cannot be met by ordinary diets; therefore the use of supplemental iron is recommended.

utilized. One international unit (IU) is equivalent to 0.3 μg of retinol, or 6 μg of beta-carotene.

Vitamin D. Vitamin D is essential at all ages for maintenance of calcium homeostasis and skeletal integrity. It can be acquired by ingestion of vitamin D_2 (ergocalciferol) or D_3 (cholecalciferol) and by exposure to certain ultraviolet wavelengths of light that convert 7-dehydro-cholesterol in the skin to vitamin D_3.

One IU of vitamin D is 0.025 μg of pure vitamin D_3. Excessive amounts of vitamin D (of the order of 1000 to 3000 IU per kilogram per day) are potentially dangerous and may lead to hypercalcemia and attendant complications.

Most foods of animal origin have some vitamin D activity, and 1 quart of vitamin D–fortified milk supplies the daily requirement.

Vitamin E. The earliest evidence of vitamin E deficiency differs with the species, but eventually the hematopoietic, muscular, vascular, and central nervous systems are affected. The normal resistance of red blood cells to rupture by oxidizing agents is also markedly reduced in vitamin E deficiency. One IU of vitamin E is 1 mg of synthetic dl-alpha-tocopherol acetate. Recommendations are based on the formula, IU = 1.25 $\times$ body weight in kg.[0.75]

Abundant vitamin E is supplied by salad oils, shortening, margarine, fruits and vegetables, and whole-grain products. However, high intakes of polyunsaturated fatty acids may increase requirements sufficiently to induce a deficiency of this vitamin.

Vitamin K. The K family of vitamins occurs throughout nature and is required in microgram amounts by man and certain animals to maintain prothrombin and other clotting factors. The average diet apparently contains adequate amounts of vitamin K, and additional amounts are supplied by the gastrointestinal flora. Thus few malnourished human beings have presented findings indicating inadequate dietary vitamin K. Because of the lack of reliable information, a daily allowance for this vitamin has not been established. A group of older adults experimentally depleted of vitamin K were found to require slightly more than 0.03 mg per kilogram of body weight intravenously to obtain normal blood clotting.

(For the clinically important states in which deficiency of vitamin K develops, see Ch. 799.)

Water-Soluble Vitamins

Ascorbic Acid (Vitamin C). Ascorbic acid has many biochemical functions in the body and is essential for normal wound healing and resistance to infection. Man, higher apes, and the guinea pig lack the metabolic pathway to synthesize adequate amounts of ascorbic acid, and in these species a lack of sufficient dietary ascorbic acid leads to scurvy. The minimal daily intake of ascorbic acid to prevent scurvy in the adult is about 10 mg, but this does not allow tissue saturation. Ascorbic acid is furnished by fruits, particularly citrus fruits, as well as by most fresh vegetables. (For more information on ascorbic acid deficiency, see Ch. 721.)

Biotin. Biotin is essential for the activity of many enzyme systems in bacteria, animals, and, presumably, man. Biotin deficiency does not occur naturally in man because the vitamin is so widely distributed in all common foods. Experimental biotin deficiency in man, induced by feeding the metabolic antagonist avidin found in egg white, results in the development of serious clinical and pathologic changes. These include scaly dermatitis, pallor, extreme lassitude, anorexia, muscle pains, insomnia, precordial pain, and slight anemia.

Choline. Choline serves as a source of labile methyl groups in the body, and in addition is a constituent of several compounds necessary for nerve function and lipid metabolism. Choline is generally considered to be an essential nutrient in the diet, although human choline deficiency has not been demonstrated. The average mixed diet consumed by persons in industrialized countries has been estimated to contain 500 to 900 mg per day of choline, mostly from egg yolk, vegetables, and milk. Beef liver contains about 0.6 per cent choline.

Folacin. Folacin coenzymes function in the transfer of single carbon units in a number of intracellular metabolic processes, particularly in the synthesis of purine and pyrimidine ribotides and deoxyribotides and in amino acid interconversions. A folacin deficiency may arise from inadequate dietary intake, impaired absorption, excessive demands by tissues of the body, and metabolic derangements. Megaloblastic anemias resulting from folacin deficiency have been recognized with increasing frequency (see Ch. 731). The intake of food folacins depends on the highly variable amount destroyed by cooking. Folic acid (phenylmonoglutamic acid) and folacin (tetrahydropteroyl glutamic acid) occur in a wide variety of foods of animal and vegetable origin, particularly in glandular meats, yeasts, and green leafy vegetables.

Niacin. The term "niacin" is generic for both nicotinic acid and nicotinamide. Nicotinamide functions in the body as a component of two important coenzymes that are primarily concerned with glycolysis, tissue respiration, and fat synthesis. Tryptophan is a precursor of niacin in man, and the efficiency of conversion is such that an average of 60 mg of dietary tryptophan is equivalent to 1 mg of niacin. Good dietary sources of niacin are liver, other meats, fish, whole-grain cereals and enriched breads, dried peas, nuts, and peanut butter.

Pantothenic Acid. Pantothenic acid is of biologic importance because of its incorporation into CoA, on which acylation and acetylation and other interactions depend. Pantothenic acid deficiency induced in human volunteers by feeding the metabolic antagonist, omega-methylpantothenic acid, together with a deficient diet, resulted in serious clinical signs and symptoms within a few months. An important feature of the syndrome produced by pantothenic acid deficiency was reduced antibody formation. Neuropathy associated with low serum pantothenic acid has been observed in alcoholic patients habitually consuming extremely poor diets. A daily intake of 5 to 10 mg is probably adequate for children and adults. Ordinary cooking does not cause excessive losses of pantothenic acid, and the vitamin is so widely distributed in plant and animal tissues that deficiency does not occur spontaneously in human populations.

Food sources include organ meats, egg yolk, peanuts, plants of the cabbage family, and whole grains. Other meats, vegetables, milk, and fruits also contain moderate amounts of pantothenic acid.

Riboflavin. Riboflavin functions as a coenzyme or active prosthetic group of flavoproteins concerned with the oxidative processes. The requirement for riboflavin is related to body size, metabolic rate, and rate of growth. Deficiency of riboflavin produces lesions in mucous membranes, most easily seen in the tongue, lips, and cornea (see Ch. 718).

Riboflavin is soluble in water. It is widely distributed in all leafy vegetables, in the flesh of animals and fish, and in milk, but may be destroyed when food is exposed to sunlight or cooked.

Thiamin. Thiamin functions in carbohydrate metabolism as a coenzyme in the decarboxylation of alpha-keto acids and in the utilization of pentose in the hexose monophosphate shunt. Thiamin deficency leads to beriberi, still seen among populations subsisting primarily on rice; but in the industrialized countries, signs of thiamin deficiency are limited almost entirely to chronic alcoholics (see Ch. 720).

Thiamin is widely distributed in foods and readily available. It is soluble in water, sensitive to oxidation, and destroyed rapidly by heat in neutral or alkaline solutions. Roasting and stewing of meat may reduce the thiamin content by 30 to 50 per cent, and vegetables may lose 25 to 40 per cent in cooking.

It has been generally assumed that thiamin need is related to caloric intake, particularly to those calories derived from carbohydrate. Although dietary fat does "spare" thiamin to some extent, the reduction in requirement appears to be small. Because it is possible that older persons use thiamin less efficiently, it is deemed advisable to recommend that a thiamin intake of 1 mg per day be maintained by older adults, even when they are consuming less than 2000 calories daily.

Vitamin B$_6$. Vitamin B$_6$ in the form pyridoxal phosphate or pyridoxamine phosphate has been shown to function in carbohydrate, fat, and protein metabolism. Vitamin B$_6$ is a collective term for a group of naturally occurring pyridines that are metabolically and functionally interrelated; namely, pyridoxine, pyridoxal, and pyridoxamine. The vitamin appears to be part of the molecular configuration of glycogen phosphorylase. Pyridoxine deficiency has occurred in children fed a proprietary formula in which the B$_6$ content was largely destroyed as a result of changes in the sterilization process. Symptoms were restlessness and irritability, and some developed convulsions. Pyridoxine deficiency may be responsible for anemia in adults.

Good dietary sources are liver, other meats, whole-grain cereals, soybeans, peanuts, corn, and many vegetables.

Vitamin B$_{12}$. Vitamin B$_{12}$ is essential for the normal functioning of all cells, but particularly those of the bone marrow, nervous system, and gastrointestinal tract, because it facilitates reduction reactions and participates in the transfer of methyl groups. Its chief importance seems to be in nucleic and folic acid metabolism. Deficiency of vitamin B$_{12}$ results in the development of megaloblastic anemia and signs of degeneration of the long tracts of the spinal cord. Sore tongue, paresthesias, and amenorrhea may also be present (see Ch. 411 and 731).

Cyanocobalamin is the principal one of several compounds with vitamin B$_{12}$ activity. As little as 1.0 μg daily will cure most cases of megaloblastic anemia resulting from deficiency of this vitamin, but will not replenish liver stores. In a dose of 0.5 μg more than 70 per cent is absorbed, but as the dosage of vitamin B$_{12}$ increases, absorption gradually decreases to 30 per cent in a dose of 5 μg. Vitamin B$_{12}$ occurs predominantly in foods of animal origin, with very little present in vegetables. Nevertheless, except in vegetarians, deficiency states are likely to arise only as a result of superimposed infections, malabsorption, or lack of intrinsic factor (pernicious anemia).

Mineral Elements

Calcium. Calcium is a major mineral constituent of the body and makes up about 1.5 to 2.0 per cent of the body weight of the mature human, more than 99 per cent of it in bones and teeth. Active processes of bone formation and resorption constantly exchange calcium with body fluids. The small proportion of calcium distributed in body fluids and tissues contributes importantly to other functions, such as blood coagulation, neuromuscular irritability, muscle contractility, and myocardial function. Calcium is incompletely absorbed, and phytate, oxalate, and fatty acids of the diet form nonionized or poorly soluble calcium complexes, further interfering with intestinal absorption. Calcium requirements are increased during periods of growth, and in pregnancy and lactation, but intestinal absorption is more efficient as need increases.

Good sources of calcium include milk and most other dairy products, shellfish, egg yolk, canned sardines and salmon (with bones), soy beans, and many green vegetables. Adequate vitamin D is required for efficient absorption of calcium.

Copper. Copper-containing proteins in the body include ceruloplasmin, erythrocuprein, hepatocuprein, cerebrocuprein, cytochrome-C oxidase, tyrosinase, and monoamine oxidase. Copper depletion of a degree severe enough to cause hypocupremia has been observed in a few patients with iron deficiency anemia and edema, kwashiorkor, sprue, and the nephrotic syndrome. Anemia, neutropenia, and bone changes caused by copper depletion have been reported in Peruvian children.

A copper intake of 2 mg per day appears to maintain balance in adults, and an intake of 0.08 mg per kilogram per day is recommended.

Copper is widely distributed in foodstuffs, and a diet of even mediocre quality contains more than the recommended amount. The richest sources are liver, kidney, shellfish, nuts, raisins, and dried legumes. Milk is poor in both copper and iron.

Fluorine. Fluoride is incorporated into the structure of teeth and bone, and is necessary for maximal resistance to dental caries. In areas where natural water supplies do not contain this amount, the addition of fluoride to bring the concentration to 1 part per million has proved to be a safe, economical, and efficient way to reduce the incidence of dental decay. In communities where fluoridation has been introduced, the incidence of tooth decay in children has been decreased up to 50 per cent or more. The range of safety in fluoride intake is wide enough for safe accommodation to normal fluctuations in the fluoride content of foods among populations with fluoridated water supplies, without risk of inducing the first indication of an excess — slight mottling of the enamel. Some natural water supplies contain sufficient fluoride to induce mottling of the enamel, but no other associated adverse effects have been found (see Ch. 892).

Iodine. Iodine is an integral part of the thyroid hormones thyroxine and triiodothyronine, which have important metabolic roles. Dietary iodine deficiency leads to thyroid enlargement (goiter) as a result of increase in size and number of the epithelial cells in the gland (see Ch. 841).

Balance studies in adults indicate a daily requirement of 50 to 75 μg of iodine, approximately 1 μg per kilogram. Sources of iodine are food and water, but in large sections of the world, the amount of iodine in the water supply and locally produced foods is too low to meet human needs without hypertrophy and hyperplasia of the thyroid gland. Although today's wide diversification in the origin of foodstuffs has reduced the problem in many countries, iodization of salt is a desirable and effective measure of ensuring an adequate iodine intake for all segments of the population.

Iron.   Iron is an essential constituent of hemoglobin and a variety of enzymes. An absolute deficiency owing to a low dietary intake, or a relative deficiency owing to high body losses of iron, results in the development of microcytic anemia and other clinical signs (see Ch. 737).

Iron is widely distributed in both animal and vegetable foods, but intake estimates based on food iron values in food composition tables are of limited value. Foods lose iron during preparation, gain iron from cooking vessels or from other contamination, or have much of the iron in poorly utilized bound forms.

Magnesium.   Magnesium appears to activate the enzymes that catalyze the transfer of phosphate from ATP to a phosphate receptor, or from a phosphorylated compound to ADP. It appears to be associated with thermoregulation, neuromuscular contraction, and protein synthesis. Magnesium deficiency disease in man is similar to hypocalcemic tetany, and is reversed by administration of magnesium sulfate. Low serum magnesium levels have been observed in a variety of clinical conditions, including alcoholism, diabetes, malabsorption syndromes, kwashiorkor, neuromuscular conditions associated with parathyroid disease or without parathyroid disease, in surgical patients on restricted dietary regimens or parenteral feeding, and in patients receiving diuretic therapy.

Magnesium is widely distributed in ordinary foods. For example, cocoa, nuts and soy flour, barley, lima beans, corn, whole wheat flour, and oatmeal all contain over 100 mg per 100-gram edible portion.

Chromium, Cobalt, Manganese, Molybdenum, Selenium, and Zinc.   Direct evidence for the essentiality of these trace or microelements in human nutrition is often difficult to obtain. Clear evidence that an element is required by mammals has provided a reliable index of a human requirement. Identification of elements in normal human enzyme systems has also afforded substantial evidence of a nutritional requirement.

There is evidence that *chromium* is a required nutrient. Continuing investigations of the relationship of this element to carbohydrate metabolism suggest its possible role in human nutrition.

Cobalt is an integral part of vitamin B_{12}. It is found in most common foods, and is readily absorbed from the gastrointestinal tract. Cobalt deficiency in man is unknown.

Manganese is an essential element, needed for normal bone structure, and is a part of enzyme systems that occur in man. A human deficiency has not been demonstrated, nor a recommended dietary allowance established.

Molybdenum and selenium have been shown to be essential in laboratory animals, and may also function nutritionally in man. There are insufficient data to establish a recommended dietary allowance. The close parallel of the functions of selenium and vitamin E in laboratory animals suggests a need for an evaluation of selenium in man.

Zinc has been recognized as an essential element in the nutrition of animals and humans, and there is some evidence for the occurrence of zinc deficiency in man under some circumstances. Patients exhibiting anemia, hepatosplenomegaly, short stature, hypogonadism, and geophagia have responded to zinc therapy when tissue levels of zinc and zinc intakes were low.

A mixed diet may be expected to supply adequate amounts of these microelements, and the risk of a deficiency in the United States is slight. Green leafy foods, fruit, whole grains, organ meats, and lean meats usually serve as generous sources of these elements.

At high levels of intake, all the elements are known to cause injury and to interfere with the utilization of other elements. Supplements should be used with caution and only with clear evidence of deficiency.

Beaton, G. H., and McHenry, E. W. (eds.): Nutrition: A Comprehensive Treatise, Vol. II: Vitamins, Nutrient Requirements, and Food Selection. New York, Academic Press, Inc., 1964.

Canadian Bulletin on Nutrition, Vol. 6, No. 1, Dietary Standard for Canada. Ottawa, Department of Public Printing and Stationery, March, 1964.

Department of Health and Social Security: Recommended Intakes of Nutrients for the United Kingdom (Report of the Panel on Recommended Allowances of Nutrients). Department of Health and Social Security Reports on Public Health and Medical Subjects No. 120. London, Her Majesty's Stationery Office, 1969.

Food and Agriculture Organization of the United Nations: Calorie Requirements: Report of the Second Committee on Calorie Requirements. FAO Nutritional Studies, No. 15. Rome, Italy, FAO, 1957. (Third printing, 1965.)

Food and Agriculture Organization of the United Nations/World Health Organization: Report of an FAO/WHO Expert Group, Rome, Italy, 23 to 30 May, 1961. Published jointly by FAO and WHO, FAO Nutrition Meetings Report Series No. 30 and World Health Organization Technical Report Series No. 230. Rome, FAO, 1962.

Food and Agriculture Organization of the United Nations/World Health Organization: Requirements of Vitamin A, Thiamin, Riboflavin and Niacin; Report of a Joint FAO/WHO Expert Group, Rome, Italy, 6–17 September, 1965. FAO Nutrition Meetings Report Series No. 41, World Health Organization Technical Report Series No. 362. Rome, FAO, 1967.

Food and Nutrition Board, National Research Council: Recommended Dietary Allowances, eighth revised edition, 1974. Publication 2216. National Academy of Sciences, 1974. Washington, D.C., Printing and Publishing Office, National Academy of Sciences.

World Health Organization: Energy and Protein Requirements. Report of a Joint FAO/WHO ad hoc Expert Committee. Rome, 22 March–2 April, 1971. WHO Technical Report Series No. 522 and FAO Nutrition Meetings Report Series No. 52. Geneva, World Health Organization, 1973.

713.   ASSESSMENT OF NUTRITIONAL STATUS

Nevin S. Scrimshaw

The physician should always look for the clinical signs suggestive of nutritional disease in his patients. Inspection of those body areas in which signs of deficiency are most likely to be detected—the hair, eyes, lips, mouth, and skin of the face, neck, and arms—can be part of any examination, no matter how cursory, because neither formal examination facilities nor disrobing is essential. Suspicions aroused by clinical examination can then be verified by medical and dietary history and appropriate biochemical tests.

A manual of procedures developed primarily to guide

surveys of the assessment of nutritional status in populations has been developed by the U.S. Interdepartmental Committee on Nutrition for National Development (ICNND, 1963); a more concise document was prepared by a committee of experts convened in 1962 by the World Health Organization (WHO, 1963).

Clinical Examination: Inspection and Measurement. The over-all nutritional appearance of each patient should be appraised before examination of specific areas. This will indicate whether a person has excessive pallor, generalized skin lesions, or other indications of unsatisfactory health, possibly related to diet. Although simple inspection also reveals obvious overweight and underweight in individuals, weight for height is a more reliable means of discrimination. Similarly, a gross subjective estimate of subcutaneous fat can be obtained by pinching a double fold of skin over the outer surface of the upper arm (midtriceps region), but skin calipers provide a more precise estimate.

Hair. Protein malnutrition causes the hair to change color and become fine, dry, and brittle. Characteristically, the hair of persons with severe protein deficiency can be pulled out of the scalp without discomfort; whole tufts of hair come out readily by the roots. Since the hair is brittle, the tips also break off easily. In whites, Indians, and Orientals who normally have brown or black hair, the change to a lighter color is readily detected, but without knowledge of prior hair color it might be thought to be genetic. The hair of blacks tends to become reddish in cases of protein deficiency before becoming lighter. In persons with naturally light and fine hair, the change is more difficult to detect.

Eyes. Both vitamin A and riboflavin deficiencies are known to affect the eyes. The xerophthalmia caused by avitaminosis A begins with a dryness of the bulbar conjunctiva, loss of the light reflex, lack of luster, and decreased lacrimation. It may proceed to keratomalacia, which is a softening of the cornea, and lead to ulceration, perforation, rupture, and destruction of the cornea. The final result is a scarred, opaque cornea and a sightless eye.

Bitot spots are often associated with vitamin A deficiency, although they cannot be regarded as specific to it. They appear as frothy, irregular, white or light yellow spots from one to several millimeters in diameter, most often on the conjunctiva lateral to the cornea. They look as if they could be wiped away, but are beneath the conjunctival epithelium. A small Bitot spot may consist of only a few tiny bubbles visible in the triangles, especially the outer ones. Both photophobia and the inability to see in dim light may be due to vitamin A deficiency.

The circumcorneal injection seen in riboflavin deficiency consists of penetration of the corneal limbus by the subconjunctival arterioles that normally terminate within 0.5 mm of the limbus. However, proliferation and congestion of the blood vessels in the sclerae and their extension into the clear corneal tissue is by no means pathognomonic of riboflavin deficiency. Excessive exposure to sunlight, smoke, dust, and other irritants is a recognized factor. Ariboflavinosis may also produce a moist, red lesion of the external angles of both eyes.

Skin. The areas of the skin most affected by nutritional deficiency usually are those most exposed to the environment. The skin of the face, neck, arms, and legs, and over pressure points such as the elbows, knees, and ankles is most likely to show positive findings in nutritional deficiencies.

Dyssebacea refers to a series of disturbances of the sebaceous glands characterized by increased oiliness, dermatitis, fissuring, and exfoliation. For positive identification, the lesion must be red and moist. In riboflavin deficiency, it occurs at the external angles of the eye, the nasolabial fold, and behind the ears, and may appear in other skin folds of the body. The nasolabial lesions should not be confused with acne in adolescents or with the irritation from nasal discharge in small children.

Xerosis, or generalized dryness of the skin, is thought to be characteristic of vitamin A deficiency, but difficult to evaluate in the individual because the appearance of the skin is influenced so much by bathing habits and exposure to dust and sunlight. The follicular hyperkeratosis widely ascribed to vitamin A deficiency consists of a "goose flesh" appearance which is not altered by temperature or brisk rubbing, and is most prominent on the skin of the outer forearm and thigh. Fully developed lesions consist of symmetrically distributed, rough, horny papules formed by keratotic plugs projecting from hypertrophied hair follicles; they make the skin look and feel like coarse sandpaper. Several well conducted therapeutic trials have failed to demonstrate any relationship between this hyperkeratosis and vitamin A deficiency, even when dietary fat is sufficient, and its specific etiology is not yet understood.

It is important to differentiate follicular hyperkeratosis from the perifolliculitis of ascorbic acid deficiency. The latter consists of perifollicular congestion, swelling, and, eventually, hypertrophy of the follicles. Only in this late stage is the skin rough to the touch. Other skin changes observed in severe ascorbic acid deficiency include petechiae, purpura, and hematomas. Because of increased capillary fragility, they are readily caused by a blood pressure cuff, shoes, or accidental bruising. Obviously, other factors increasing capillary fragility or interfering with blood clotting could cause these phenomena.

The cutaneous lesions of pellagra vary because of differences in the degree of deficiency, natural skin color, and conditioning factors, but they are sufficiently characteristic to be diagnostic in many instances. The most common chronic form is thickening, inelastic, fissured, and deeply pigmented areas of skin where exposed to sunlight or covering pressure points. Eventually, the skin in affected areas becomes dry, scaly, and atrophic. Erythema upon exposure to sunlight is an acute manifestation, with subsequent vascularization, crusting, and desquamation out of proportion to the precipitating exposure. In intertriginous areas a common, acute, but highly nonspecific reaction is redness, maceration, abrasion, and superimposed infection. Heat friction and poor personal hygiene contribute importantly to these signs. The symmetrical distribution of pellagrous lesions over skin exposed to sunlight and over pressure points is the most characteristic feature. Casal's necklace is a virtually diagnostic distribution of pellagrous dermatitis which sharply follows the neckline when a low-necked dress or an open shirt collar is habitually worn outdoors by persons on a niacin-tryptophan – deficient diet.

In severe protein deficiency, the skin of the legs, arms, and thighs shows marked pitting edema (which is a *sine qua non* of the diagnosis), and a dermatosis characterized by hyperkeratosis, hyperpigmentation, and desquamation. Although often similar in appearance to the lesions of pellagra, they are not limited to the exposed areas, and often extend to the thighs and lower trunk.

Neck. Endemic goiter resulting from a deficiency of iodine available to the thyroid gland usually can be detected by inspection and palpation (see Ch. 841).

Mouth. The mouth is one of the areas most sensitive to nutritional deficiencies, but the changes are nonspecific, confusing, and difficult to evaluate. Pallor of the lips and mucous membranes, like pallor of the skin and fingernails, may be a consequence of anemia, but its clinical appraisal is so subjective as to be of little value unless the anemia is severe. The stomatitis which may be a consequence of riboflavin deficiency has already been mentioned. Angular scars may be the result of past episodes of acute ariboflavinosis, but may also be wholly non-nutritional in origin. Poorly fitting dentures are a common cause.

The gums may reflect any of a variety of nutritional deficiencies, but the changes are difficult to differentiate from those resulting from local irritants and poor hygiene. This is especially true because neglect of both diet and oral hygiene are likely in the same individual. Marginal gingivitis and periodontal disease are reported to be common in persons whose diets are deficient in ascorbic acid, but attempts to prove such a relationship by ascorbic acid therapy have been failures. On the other hand, engorged, dark red, and bleeding gums are characteristic of scurvy.

Marginal and generalized gingivitis may also be found associated with deficiencies of vitamin A, niacin, and riboflavin. The problem is that many factors may play a causal role simultaneously so that the experimental correction of a single factor, even if contributory, does not necessarily effect a cure. General improvement of both diet and oral hygiene is usually required.

Marked hypertrophy of the filiform and fungiform papillae of the tongue is more frequently seen in populations in which vitamin B deficiencies, particularly of thiamin and riboflavin, are present. Papillary atrophy is also sometimes related to niacin or iron deficiency. Both nutritional megaloblastic anemia and the microcytic anemia of iron deficiency result in a smooth tongue. A markedly furrowed, so-called scrotal tongue is a possible manifestation of vitamin A deficiency.

Impression of the teeth on the borders of the tongue may be due to the edema resulting from protein deficiency as well as to defective dentures and a variety of other causes. When protein deficiency is the cause, evidence is likely to be present in the extremities as well.

Nutritional deficiencies may also cause changes in the color of the tongue, although they are usually difficult to evaluate. Reddening, either generalized or limited mainly to the distal third, may be associated with sprue. It affects first the tip and lateral margins, but may

TABLE 2.   Suggested Guide for Interpretation of Clinical Signs*

Dietary Obesity	Sensory loss and motor weakness
Excessive weight	Calf-muscle tenderness
Excessive skin folds	Cardiovascular dysfunction
Excessive abdominal girth	Edema
Undernutrition	*Niacin Deficiency*
Lethargy, mental and physical	Pellagrous dermatosis
Low weight in relation to height	Scarlet and raw tongue
Diminished skin folds	Tongue fissuring
Exaggerated skeletal prominences	Atrophic lingual papillae
Loss of elasticity of skin	Malar and supraorbital pigmentation
Protein-Calorie Deficiency Disease	*Vitamin D Deficiency*
Edema	Spongy and bleeding gums
Muscle wasting	Folliculosis
Low body weight	Petechiae
Pyschomotor change	Ecchymoses
Dyspigmentation of the hair	Intramuscular or subperiosteal hematoma
Thin, sparse hair	Epiphyseal enlargement (painful)
Moon face	
Flaky paint dermatosis	*Vitamin D Deficiency*
Areas of hyperpigmentation	1. *Active rickets* (in children)
	Epiphyseal enlargement (over 6 months of age), painless
Vitamin A Deficiency	Beading of ribs
Xerosis of skin	Craniotabes (under 1 year of age)
Follicular hyperkeratosis	Muscular hypotonia
Xerosis conjunctivae	2. *Healed rickets* (in children or adults)
Keratomalacia	Frontal and parietal bossing
Bitot's spots	Knock-knees or bow legs
	Deformities of thorax
Riboflavin Deficiency	3. *Osteomalacia* (in adults)
Angular stomatitis	Local or generalized skeletal deformities
Cheilosis	
Magenta tongue	*Iron Deficiency*
Central atrophy of lingual papillae	Pallor of mucous membranes
Nasolabial dyssebacea	Koilonychia
Angular palpebritis	Atrophic lingual papillae
Scrotal and vulval dermatosis	
Corneal vascularization	*Iodine Deficiency*
	Enlargement of the thyroid
Thiamin Deficiency	
Loss of ankle jerks	*Excess of Fluorine (Fluorosis)*
	Mottled dental enamel

*Adapted from World Health Organization Technical Report Series No. 258, Expert Committee on Medical Assessment of Nutritional Status. Geneva, WHO, 1963, pp. 59–61.

progress to include not only the entire tongue but all of the oral mucous membranes as well. A beefy red glossitis resembling raw beefsteak most frequently represents a deficiency of niacin, but other B vitamin deficiencies may be involved. Riboflavin deficiency is probably most often responsible for the purplish discoloration known as magenta tongue. Patchy areas of paler discoloration give rise to the name "geographic" tongue, which has no nutritional significance.

Teeth. The frequency and severity of dental caries is increased by a diet relatively high in soluble carbohydrates and decreased by adequate fluoride and phosphate intake. Any severe dietary deficiency in infancy and early childhood will delay tooth eruption and contribute to malposition of teeth. Malposition resulting from retarded mandibular development is a common sequela of early protein deficiency.

In children of many underdeveloped countries, a so-called hypoplastic line across the upper primary incisors has been described, in which a yellow or brown pigment becomes deposited. This is followed by the development of caries on the labial surface of the teeth. Subsequently, the teeth may break off along this line. A nutritional or febrile insult in the neonatal period is a probable cause.

Fluorosis, occurring in regions where the fluoride content of the water supplies is above about 2 to 6 parts per million of fluoride in drinking water, is characterized by mottled enamel and chalky white patches distributed over the surface of the teeth. In some cases, the entire tooth surface may be dull white and lusterless. Although cosmetically undesirable, the lesion is harmless, and such teeth are usually resistant to caries.

Edema. Edema of the lower extremities is characteristic of protein deficiency, and may also be seen in acute beriberi. In severe cases it becomes generalized.

Evaluation of Signs. The signs suggesting nutritional deficiency are easier to evaluate and more specific in children than in adults. In adults, lesions from other causes, such as aging and repeated trauma, and confusing signs such as pinguecula, pterygium, and geographic tongue, are more likely to be present. The clinical signs that suggest more or less strongly the possibility of a nutritional deficiency are summarized in Table 2.

It must be emphasized again that the aforementioned signs are largely nonspecific. Moreover, they are more reliable in the assessment of nutritional status of population groups than of single individuals. Excellent color illustrations will be found in several of the references listed at the end of this chapter.

It should be clear from the foregoing that clinical examination alone will rarely be sufficient to establish a definite diagnosis. Many of the signs are so nonspecific that they cannot be relied upon in a given individual even when appropriate for population surveys. A medical history and confirmatory dietary and biochemical data are required when clinical examination raises the question of nutritional deficiency in the individual.

Physical Methods Complementary to Clinical Examination. Although routine roentgenographic studies are rarely possible, or indeed required, it is valuable to carry out roentgenographic examinations if physical signs and other circumstances suggest that rickets, osteomalacia, infantile scurvy, beriberi, fluorosis, or protein-calorie malnutrition is present.

The test of dark adaptation is sometimes used as a measure of vitamin A deficiency. It is, however, difficult to perform, and is influenced by factors other than vitamin A. The same appears to be true of electroretinography.

Biochemical Tests. A single biochemical determination, if accurate, may decisively confirm or deny the nutritional origin of an uncertain complex of clinical signs. Here again, biochemical measures vary in their reliability and specificity. Serum levels of vitamin A and ascor-

TABLE 3. Tentative Guide to the Interpretation of Selected Biochemical Data Useful in the Appraisal of Nutritional Status of Adults*

	Deficient (High Risk)	Low (Medium Risk)	Acceptable (Low Risk)
Serum protein: gram/100 ml	<6.0	6.0–6.4	>6.5
Serum albumin (electrophoretic method): gram/100 ml	<2.8	2.8–3.4	>3.5
Nonessential/essential amino acid ratio (NE/E)†	<3.0	3.0–2.0	>2.0
Urea/creatinine ratio‡	<6.0	6.0–12.0	>12.0
Hemoglobin: gram/100 ml sea level			
Men	<12.0	12.0–13.9	>14.0
Women§	<10.0	10.0–11.9	>12.0
Hematocrit % (sea level)			
Men	<37	37–43	>44
Women§	<31	31–37	>38
Serum ascorbic acid: mg/100 ml	<0.20	0.20–0.29	>0.30
Plasma retinol: μg/100 ml	<10	10–19	>20
Thiamin, urinary excretion μg/gram creatinine	<27	27–65	>66–129
Riboflavin, urinary excretion μg/gram creatinine	<27	27–79	>80
N-methylnicotinamide, urinary excretion mg/gram creatinine	<0.5	0.5–1.59	>1.6–4.29
Pyridoxine, urinary excretion μg/gram creatinine	<20	—	>20
Serum folacin ng (mμg)/ml¶	<3.0	3.0–5.9	>6.0
Red cell folacin¶	<140	140–159	>160
Serum vitamin B_{12} pg ($\mu\mu$g)/ml	<150	150–200	>200
Serum vitamin E (α-tocopherol) level, mg/100 ml (levels will vary according to method of analysis)	<0.50	0.50–0.70	>0.70

*Adapted from Sauberlich, H. E., Dowdy, R. P., and Skala, J. H.: Crit. Rev. Lab. Clin. Sci., 4:215, 1973.
†Value depends upon the analytical method employed and the procedure used to calculate the ratio.
‡These values are considered exceedingly tentative in view of the effect of age and the wide range of values reported in the literature.
§Nonpregnant, nonlactating.
¶Guidelines should be regarded as tentative and must be considered in terms of the microbiologic assay procedure employed. Values are based on the use of *Lactobacillus casei* as the test organism.

bic acid are quite useful, although very low levels may be present for some time before lesions appear.

For the B vitamins, blood serum levels are relatively insensitive, and measurement of thiamin, riboflavin, and niacin excretion in 24-hour urine samples is recommended.

Total serum protein and serum albumin are decreased markedly in protein deficiency, but only when the deficiency has progressed to the point at which it is beginning to be clinically evident. The ratio of urea to creatinine has been recommended recently as a measure of the loss of lean body mass in protein-calorie malnutrition. Anemia is also a laboratory-based diagnosis. A tentative guide to the interpretation of selected biochemical data is given in Table 3. It should be noted that most biochemical measures show only the current state of the patient, so that chronic nutritional lesions are possible even in those with normal serum levels of various nutrients.

Beaton, G. H., and McHenry, E. W. (eds.): Nutrition: A Comprehensive Treatise. Vol. III. New York, Academic Press, Inc., 1966.
Davidson, S., Passmore, R., and Brock, J. F.: Human Nutrition and Dietetics. 5th ed. Edinburgh, Churchill Livingstone, 1972.
Jelliffe, D. B.: The Assessment of the Nutritional Status of the Community. World Health Organization Monograph Series No. 53. Geneva, World Health Organization, 1966.
Jolliffe, N.: Clinical Nutrition. 2nd ed. New York, Hoeber Medical Book, Harper & Brothers, 1962.
Sauberlich, H. E., Dowdy, R. P., and Skala, J. H.: Laboratory tests for assessment of nutritional status. Crit. Rev. Lab. Clin. Sci., 4:215, 1973.
World Health Organization Technical Report Series No. 258: Expert Committee on Medical Assessment of Nutritional Status. Geneva, World Health Organization, 1963.

714. NUTRITION AND INFECTION

Nevin S. Scrimshaw

Malnutrition in man is inseparable from the occurrence and effects of microbial disease. Infection precipitates nutritional disease in the malnourished, and malnutrition worsens the consequences of infection. The interaction between the two is synergistic. Both are major health problems wherever poverty and ignorance result in poor dietary habits, as well as inferior environmental sanitation and personal hygiene. The World Health Organization monograph, *Interactions of Nutrition and Infection,* provides extensive documentation for the statements and conclusions of this chapter.

EFFECT OF INFECTION ON NUTRITIONAL STATUS

General.   One of the earliest and most constant consequences of infection is loss of appetite and a decrease in the amount of food tolerated. Another is the almost universal tendency to change the diet to one that is more liquid and higher in carbohydrates at the expense of foods that are good sources of protein and other essential nutrients. This is a particularly common practice in the feeding of young children in less developed areas. Often milk as well as solid food is removed from the diet in favor of starchy gruels and cooking water from cereal grains or plant leaves when a child has diarrheal disease or other acute infections. In addition, therapeutic agents such as purgatives may reduce intestinal absorption, or antimicrobial drugs may interfere with intestinal synthesis of some nutrients. The direct influence of fever in increasing both basal metabolism and the loss of nutrients in sweat must also be taken into account. Sweat losses may amount to as much as 4 grams of nitrogen per day, together with significant quantities of electrolytes and iron.

Protein.   Acute infections cause a stress response qualitatively the same as that observed in states of pain, anxiety, fear, and other psychologic stress. The stress reaction, mediated by cortisone and insulin, mobilizes amino acids from skeletal muscle and other tissues from which they can be spared for gluconeogenesis in the liver. This is necessary because in man the contribution of liver glycogen to maintain blood glucose is relatively limited. The stress reaction undoubtedly arose to enable individuals to fight, flee from sudden danger, or recover from wounds and infections, regardless of the timing of meals. However, it necessarily depletes the body of protein because the amino acids thus mobilized are deaminated to provide the carbons of glucose, and the nitrogen is excreted in the urine, largely as urea.

Nitrogen losses during severe infectious diseases have long been recognized and can be equivalent to the nitrogen of 2 or 3 kg of muscle during the acute phase of the illness. It is now clear that even such mild infections as vaccination against smallpox and immunization with the 17-D strain of yellow fever vaccine, as well as tonsillitis, otitis media, bronchitis, and localized abscesses, will also provoke this stress reaction.

The duration of the metabolic effect of stress depends upon the nature and extent of the precipitating cause. If the stress is of short duration, it may be balanced by an increase in nitrogen retention during the succeeding 24 hours. The catabolic period associated with an infectious disease episode, however, is likely to last for several days, and the anabolic period of increased nitrogen retention is generally at least twice as long. After the acute stress is over, dietary amino acids are returned to the depleted tissues; hence protein intakes above maintenance levels are required at this time. In individuals already depleted by low levels of protein intake, the urinary loss of nitrogen measured during stress is less than that observed in those who are well nourished. Nevertheless, increases in urinary loss of nitrogen during minor infections have been found even in experimental subjects receiving a nitrogen-free diet.

In infections associated with diarrhea, reduced absorption of nitrogen and other nutrients adds to the nutritional consequences. However, even in severe diarrheal disease the drop in nitrogen absorption may be only 10 to 15 per cent, and seldom exceeds 50 per cent. *Thus it is worthwhile to continue feeding persons with diarrhea even though stool volume may be increased.*

With so many factors adversely affecting protein nutritional status during infectious disease, it is not surprising that in underdeveloped countries the protein deficiency disease, kwashiorkor, is commonly precipitated by diarrheal disease, measles, or other infections in children who are already in a precarious nutritional state. Similarly, infections, especially of a chronic nature, are responsible for much of the protein deficiency seen in adults.

Vitamins. Blood levels of vitamin A are reduced in acute infections. Diarrheal and other infectious diseases, particularly measles, are frequently responsible for precipitating xerophthalmia and keratomalacia in children receiving diets deficient in vitamin A. It is probable that most clinical cases of avitaminosis A follow an acute infection. The absorption of vitamin A has been found to be reduced by severe *Giardia lamblia* infections. It is probable that other intestinal infections have this effect when sufficiently severe.

As was observed among prisoners of war of the Japanese during World War II, clinical beriberi is frequently precipitated in thiamin-deficient individuals by an infectious episode. The synthesis of thiamin and other B vitamins by intestinal bacterial flora may also be affected by both intestinal infections and chemotherapy.

Spontaneous respiratory infections have been found to induce megaloblastic anemia in monkeys maintained on a diet low in folic acid. Also, the dietary intake of hemopoietic B vitamins is not low enough to account for the megaloblastic anemia seen in many patients with complicating infections.

Well confirmed is the appetite of the fish tapeworm, *Diphyllobothrium latum,* for vitamin B_{12}. These tapeworms are a significant cause of anemia in people infected from eating raw fresh-water fish, a common custom in Scandinavia and among persons of Scandinavian descent in the United States.

The role of infections in lowering serum ascorbic acid and increasing urinary excretion of this vitamin has been demonstrated by many experimental studies in guinea pigs. In poorly nourished children, otitis media, pneumonia, pyelonephritis, and other infections have long been recognized as precipitators of scurvy. Malaria, typhoid fever, influenza, measles, tuberculosis, and vaccination against smallpox are among other specific infections reported responsible for the appearance of scurvy in vulnerable children.

Minerals. Early in an infectious episode there is a sharp decrease in blood levels of iron and zinc. It is well recognized that hookworm infection, if sufficiently severe, causes enough loss of blood to produce microcytic-hypochromic anemia even when dietary intakes of iron appear adequate. This may also occur with *Schistosoma haematobium* infections. Increased losses of calcium and phosphorus have been reported for tuberculosis in both guinea pigs and man. Losses of sodium, chloride, potassium, and phosphorus, which are sometimes severe enough to cause death, occur in diarrhea of infectious origin.

EFFECT OF MALNUTRITION ON INFECTION

There are large numbers of laboratory, clinical, and field observations which demonstrate that the severity and outcome of infection are frequently worsened by malnutrition. The prevalence of diarrheal disease, both upper and lower respiratory infections, and some other types of microbial disease is also influenced by malnutrition. Moreover, much of the high infant and preschool mortality in developing countries attributed to microbial disease would not occur in well nourished children. The relative influence of the various potential mechanisms whereby nutritional deficiencies influence resistance to infectious disease under field conditions is not really known. The following must be considered.

Antibody Formation. Although other mechanisms may be equally important in defense against infections, formation of antibodies specific for infectious agents or their toxins has received the most attention. This is because there are excellent techniques for detecting the presence of antibodies, and protective immunizations have been developed against many infections. Severe deficiencies of protein, vitamin A, ascorbic acid, riboflavin, thiamin, pantothenic acid, biotin, and niacin-tryptophan in laboratory animals are known to interfere with antibody formation. A number of studies confirm that protein deficiency in man can interfere with formation of antibodies. There have been several reports of false-negative tuberculin reactions in malnourished patients with tuberculosis. In human volunteers, antibody formation has been suppressed by inducing metabolic deficiencies of pantothenic acid or pyridoxine by feeding the corresponding antimetabolites, desoxypyridoxine and omega-methylpyridoxine. The same effect has been observed in cases of severe pellagra and moderately severe deficiency of several of the B vitamins.

Phagocytic Activity. The macrophages and microphages of the reticuloendothelial system are important protectors of the body against microbial diseases, particularly those caused by bacteria. Nutritional deficiency can reduce both the number and the phagocytic capacity of these cells. Children with kwashiorkor have little or no leukocyte response to superimposed infections. Macrophage activity is decreased in the presence of vitamin A, ascorbic acid, thiamin, and riboflavin deficiency in laboratory animals. Both animal studies and clinical observations of folic acid deficiency have shown production of phagocytes in mammalian bone marrow to be depressed to the extent of nullifying the effect of protective antibodies. Recently, relatively mild iron deficiency has been shown to reduce the killing power of leukocytes. Reduced cell-mediated immunity, as measured by delayed hypersensitivity skin tests, DNCB sensitivity, and lymphocyte transformation by PHA, has been demonstrated in children with protein-calorie malnutrition.

Tissue Integrity. The integrity of the skin, mucous membranes, and other epithelial tissues helps to prevent entry of the infectious agent. Various pathologic changes occur in tissues, depending on the type and severity of the nutritional deficiency. Mucous secretions may be reduced or absent, mucosal surfaces may become easily permeable, changes may take place in intercellular substance, or there may be epithelial metaplasia, edema in underlying tissues, and accumulation of cellular debris to form a favorable culture medium for the infectious agent. Deficiencies in vitamin A, ascorbic acid, thiamin, riboflavin, niacin, and protein are especially likely to cause tissue changes that lower resistance.

Wound Healing and Collagen Formation. How long an infection will be disabling depends on how rapidly it can be localized and contained. Nutritional deficiencies affect not only tissue integrity, but also wound healing, fibroblastic response to trauma, walling off of abscesses, and collagen formation. In protein-deficient rats, the walls of induced sterile subcutaneous abscesses were much thinner than those of spontaneous or induced abscesses in well nourished animals. The fibroblastic response in the deficient rats was markedly reduced, and as a result fatal septicemia frequently developed.

Ascorbic acid intake must be adequate for synthesis of the amino acids from which collagen is formed, particularly hydroxyproline and hydroxylysine, which are almost unique to collagen. The skin at the edges of wounds in scorbutic guinea pigs showed almost no hydroxyproline. Restoration of ascorbic acid to the diet induced rapid production of hydroxyproline and the onset of wound healing.

Nonspecific Resistance Factors. It is hard to assess the importance of various nonspecific mechanisms of resistance to infection such as those requiring properdin, interferon, or lysozymes. All would appear vulnerable to nutritional deficiencies, but there is no evidence of this occurring.

Destruction of Bacterial Toxins. Most of the destruction of bacterial toxins or resistance to them in the animal host occurs as the result of the toxins combining with specific antibodies. There is some evidence that other mechanisms may exist as well. For example, rats suffering from deficiencies of B vitamins or vitamin A are more susceptible than controls to diphtheria toxin, even though antitoxin titers and rate of disappearance of injected toxin are similar in the two groups. Probably because of the ethical difficulties of investigating the problem directly in man, there are no clinical observations of this phenomenon.

Intestinal Flora. There is evidence that changes in the intestinal flora induced by diet can influence susceptibility to some intestinal pathogens. In kwashiorkor, there is a tendency for the bacteria of the lower intestinal tract to appear at a higher level. In milder degrees of protein malnutrition it seems likely that intestinal organisms that are not normally pathogenic to the well nourished host may cause diarrhea. Not only is no known pathogen identified in most diarrheal episodes in malnourished children, but also the frequency and severity of these episodes are decreased when dietary supplements are provided. Changes in gastrointestinal motility secondary to malnutrition may also play a role in the severity of protozoal and helminthic infections.

Endocrine Balance. Prolonged adrenocorticotrophic hormone (ACTH) or cortisone therapy increases the spread of many infections, presumably by inhibiting local inflammatory reactions at the site of bacterial proliferation. These observations may have a bearing on the question of how malnutrition influences resistance to infection, since protein deficiency, caloric deprivation, and a number of other nutritional deficiencies influence endocrine balance.

Chung, A., and Visčorová, B.: The effect of early oral feeding versus early oral starvation on the course of infantile diarrhea. J. Pediatr., 33:14, 1948.

Gallin, J. I., Kaye, D., and O'Leary, W. M.: Serum lipids in infection. N. Engl. J. Med., 281:1081, 1969.

Law, D. K., Dudrick, S. J., and Abdou, N. I.: Immunocompetence of patients with protein-calorie malnutrition. Ann. Intern. Med., 79:545, 1973.

Scrimshaw, N. S.: Protein deficiency and infective disease, In Munro, H. N., and Allison, J. B., (eds.): Mammalian Protein Metabolism, Vol. II. New York, Academic Press, Inc., 1964, chap. 23, p. 569.

Scrimshaw, N. S., Taylor, C. E., and Gordon, J. E.: Interactions of Nutrition and Infection, World Health Organization Monograph Series No. 57. Geneva, World Health Organization, 1968.

Smythe, P. M., Brereton-Stiles, G. G., Grace, H. J., Mafoyane, A., Schonland, M., Coovadia, H. M., Loening, W. E. K., Parent, M. A., and Vos, G. H.: Thymolymphatic deficiency and depression of cell-mediated immunity in protein-calorie malnutrition. Lancet, 2:939, 1971.

Taylor, P. E., Tejada, C., and Sánchez, M.: The effect of malnutrition on the inflammatory response as exhibited by the granuloma pouch of the rat. J. Exp. Med., 126:539, 1967.

715. KWASHIORKOR, MARASMUS, AND INTERMEDIATE FORMS OF PROTEIN-CALORIE MALNUTRITION

Nevin S. Scrimshaw

Definition. The clinical spectrum of protein-calorie deficiency ranges from forms characterized only by growth retardation to the extremes of kwashiorkor and marasmus. Kwashiorkor results from a deficiency of protein relative to calories, is found in children whose caloric intake is adequate and even excessive, or may be superimposed on varying degrees of protein-calorie deficiency. When protein and calories are limited to about the same degree, the clinical condition that develops is marasmus.

Pathogenesis. The various forms of protein-calorie malnutrition are of major public health significance in most underdeveloped countries. They result from diets that are quantitatively and qualitatively inadequate in individuals with superimposed stress, usually episodes of infectious disease. A deficient diet results in turn from varying combinations of low food production, inadequate preservation and distribution of foods, restricted purchasing power, poor food habits, and deficient knowledge of the relation between diet and health. The excessive incidence of infectious disease is a consequence of poor environmental conditions, inadequate knowledge of epidemiologic factors, poor personal hygiene, and insufficient health services.

The clinical result depends on the severity and duration of the nutritional deficiencies of protein and calories, on the relative importance of the deficiency of protein to that of calories, on the nature and severity of other associated nutritional deficiencies, on the age of the person affected, and on the presence of other complications. The mild and moderate forms in children, frequently unrecognized or misinterpreted, are primarily characterized by inadequate growth and development. In adults they reduce work performance and resistance to infection.

Mild to Moderate Protein-Calorie Malnutrition in Children. Retarded growth is greatest in the first two years of life, when dietary inadequacy and frequency of infections are most pronounced. Insufficient or improper supplementation of breast feeding is usually a factor. After weaning, the usual diet is cereal grains, starchy roots, overdiluted milk, or even cornstarch. Often such a regimen not only fails to provide the needed calories but also is deficient in many essential nutrients, particularly proteins of high biologic value.

Not until the third to fifth year of life is the usual child in underdeveloped countries permitted an adult type of diet. The period of greatest dietary inadequacy coincides in general with increased exposure to an unsanitary environment and a greater frequency of diarrheal and parasitic diseases, measles, whooping cough, and other diseases of childhood. By the time children enter school this critical period of high morbidity from infection is largely past because of an acquired immunity and better nutrition.

The assumption that reduced growth of children in underdeveloped countries is due more to environmental than to genetic factors is supported by observations of children of different races living under similar adverse conditions. Conversely, well nourished children of the same genetic origins usually follow the growth pattern of well fed North American or European children in a healthy environment.

The shorter limb-to-trunk ratio often observed in poorly nourished populations is caused mainly by primary or secondary malnutrition during the period when growth, particularly of the long bones, is normally rapid in the young child. There is also x-ray evidence that such children have retarded ossification of centers in their wrists and hands. Children with early growth retardation experience a parallel impairment of psychomotor development that persists at least through the school years, although the latter stems partly from social deprivation.

Mild to Moderate Protein-Calorie Malnutrition in Adults. The consequences of the mild to moderate chronic protein-calorie malnutrition common among adult populations has been little studied. Adaptation to insufficient calories includes low weight for height and reduced caloric expenditure. Accordingly, it is probable that it seriously reduces work capacity and thereby contributes to the low social and economic development in these areas. The effects of such malnutrition on resistance to stress, particularly that resulting from infectious disease, also needs further attention. Pregnant and lactating women are a particularly vulnerable segment of adult populations of underdeveloped countries. Many women do not gain a normal amount of weight during pregnancy, and average weights of their children at birth are generally at least 200 to 300 grams lighter than those of well nourished mothers. Associated with this lower birth weight is higher neonatal and perinatal mortality as well as higher morbidity and poorer growth in infancy. The consequences of repeated pregnancy and lactation on poorly nourished mothers have received too little attention. It is noteworthy that such women look older than their chronologic age.

MARASMUS

The extremely low calorie diets responsible for the syndrome of marasmus are obviously also deficient in proteins and many other essential nutrients. Because calories are so inadequate, the child utilizes amino acids from the skeletal muscles and other less essential tissues for gluconeogenesis in addition to energy from fat deposits. Growth stops, but the amino acids and other nutrients liberated from the child's tissues permit a continuing synthesis of serum albumin, enzymes, and other essential metabolites, and no serious metabolic disturbances are observed.

The child with marasmus is emaciated owing to a loss of subcutaneous fat, extreme muscle wasting, and atrophy of most organs. Although the liver and other essential organs are much reduced in size, histologic changes are minimal. Despite the apt description of being reduced to "skin and bones," the child remains clinically alert, and maintains an appetite.

KWASHIORKOR

Clinical Characteristics. Clinically, the syndrome of kwashiorkor presents a pitting edema varying from a mild form localized in feet and ankles to severe, generalized edema, with eyelids swollen shut. Movement of the extremities may be limited, and fluid accumulates in the peritoneal cavity. Patients are usually extremely apathetic, with a weak, monotonous cry if disturbed. Anorexia is frequently severe; diarrhea is an almost constant finding. The characteristic alterations of the skin resemble the dermatosis of pellagra, with which they have been mistakenly identified. The lesions are pigmented, dry, hyperkeratotic, and sometimes desquamating, and vary in size from punctiform to large, confluent areas. They are most numerous where subject to irritation, especially in the perineal region. They frequently occur on the extremities and face, and may extend to the trunk.

Normally curly hair becomes dry, fine, brittle, and straight. It is easily pulled out or may even fall out. It may become reddish, yellowish, or even white. These pigmentation changes are often observed in stripes, indicating successive periods of normal and abnormal hair growth. The extremities are frequently cold and cyanotic. The abdomen may be distended owing to flaccid abdominal muscles and ascites. Hepatomegaly is sometimes found.

Biochemical Alterations. *Protein.* Low total serum protein is a diagnostic characteristic. It is due almost entirely to a low level of albumin, and is sometimes partially obscured by a relatively high level of gamma globulin resulting from a concurrent infectious process. There is a tendency for the beta globulin fraction to be both relatively and absolutely decreased; a relative increase in the alpha$_2$ globulin has also been found. Studies with I^{127}-labeled albumin indicate that the lowering of this fraction is due to a decrease in rate of synthesis and not to abnormal catabolism.

Total α-amino nitrogen in plasma is abnormally low because most amino acids are present in decreased amount. The greatest reductions are in tryptophan, cystine, valine, tyrosine, and methionine. Low levels of urea in both blood and urine indicate decreased protein metabolism. The synthesis of antibodies is also inhibited. A very marked increase in the proportion of urinary nitrogen excreted as purine derivatives has been taken as evidence of cellular breakdown in kwashiorkor. Other abnormal substances in the urine indicating impairment of important metabolic pathways are β-aminoisobutyric acid and ethanolamine.

Although the liver protein concentration in kwashiorkor is greatly reduced by fat, it is not decreased in absolute amount in relation to body size. However, a lowered ratio of nitrogen to deoxyribonucleic acid has been reported, suggesting a true loss of protoplasmic nitrogen. In any case, the level of nitrogen in the liver of children with kwashiorkor is markedly decreased over that for normal children of the same age. There is also a marked loss of muscle nitrogen in kwashiorkor, the degree depending largely upon the severity of pre-existing marasmus.

Lipids and Carbohydrates. All the lipid fractions that have been determined in the blood of children with kwashiorkor, including neutral fat, fatty acids, phospholipids, and cholesterol, have been found to be low, and levels of these substances rise rapidly in the course of treatment. An increase in fat content of the liver, found by gross and microscopic examination, is another diagnostic criterion. In true marasmus, on the other hand, the amount of liver fat is decreased. Blood glucose levels

Figure 1.　Edema and skin lesions in child with kwashiorkor. (Courtesy of Institute of Nutrition of Central America and Panama.)

are generally low. Although glucose tolerance is sometimes reduced, and a diabetic type of glucose tolerance curve is observed, this is not an invariable feature of the disease.

Enzymes.　In acute kwashiorkor, lipase, trypsin, and amylase activities in the duodenal secretion are lowered almost to zero, and marked reductions in serum pseudocholinesterase, amylase, carbonic anhydrase, and alkaline phosphatase are recognized characteristics. The activity of these enzymes returns rapidly to normal with the administration of an adequate diet. Alkaline phosphatase levels, however, show a slight further drop before rising with therapy.

The activity of a number of enzymes has also been measured in liver obtained by needle biopsy from children with kwashiorkor. The outstanding finding is a decrease in xanthine oxidase activity per unit of protein, although cholinesterase and D-amino acid oxidase activity are also definitely lowered. Alkaline phosphatase activity in the liver is generally increased. These findings suggest that, although the activity of many key enzymes is maintained even in the presence of extreme protein deficiency, some are sufficiently affected to initiate the train of events culminating in death.

Vitamins.　Levels of vitamin A and carotene in the serum of children with kwashiorkor are extremely low. It was assumed that this was due to low intake of vitamin A, until studies demonstrated that children with acute kwashiorkor upon admission to the hospital did not have an increase in serum vitamin A after a 75-mg oral dose of vitamin A palmitate. After three to five days of intensive protein therapy, however, a similar dose gave the same sharp increase in serum vitamin A that is found in normal children. It was also found that, in most cases, serum vitamin A levels rose with protein therapy, even when the diet contained no carotene or vitamin A. Analysis of liver biopsy material demonstrated that this

phenomenon occurred whenever there were adequate stores of vitamin A in the liver, and that in those few cases in which there was gross depletion of vitamin A, administration of protein alone produced no serum response. From this and similar studies, it appears probable that the *transport* of vitamin A and possibly of vitamin E, which also occurs in abnormally low amounts in blood plasma of children with kwashiorkor, is inadequate because of the lack of a protein carrier.

Blood levels of thiamin and riboflavin are within normal limits. Even though the pigmented skin lesions superficially resemble those of pellagra, there is no evidence of niacin deficiency. The urinary excretion of N-methylnicotinamide, in cases in Central America at least, is within normal limits. Levels of serum ascorbic acid are relatively low, but are not in the range commonly associated with clinical deficiency. No significant alterations of levels of vitamin B_{12} in the blood have been found.

Electrolytes and Other Minerals.　Potassium depletion is a major biochemical characteristic of kwashiorkor, and is a direct consequence of the protein deficiency. Other electrolyte changes are secondary to diarrhea (a symptom almost always present in kwashiorkor) or vomiting. Interpretation and correction of electrolyte changes in kwashiorkor are complicated by the abnormal distribution of water and the severe degree of potassium depletion. Magnesium deficiency may occur and lead to tetany.

Endocrine Function.　On the basis of observed normal adrenal cortex function in marasmus and decreased glucocorticoid production in kwashiorkor, the hypothesis has been proposed that the severe restriction of calories in children in whom marasmus develops results in increased production of ACTH by the anterior pituitary gland which in turn stimulates the adrenal cortex to produce more corticosteroids. These hormones assure catabolism of muscle and other labile proteins sufficient to furnish amino acids to the liver for gluconeogenesis and likewise provide the liver with amino acids for synthesis of essential proteins. This mechanism does not operate when the child receives a diet with enough calories to meet minimal energy needs even though it is extremely deficient in proteins. Under these circumstances, children do not mobilize amino acids from their muscles, and instead present the serious metabolic disturbances of protein deficiency without further muscle wasting. The result is kwashiorkor.

Other Physiologic Changes. In the marasmic type of kwashiorkor seen in Central America, a relatively small heart, which rapidly increases in size with treatment, is found upon radiologic examination. Electrocardiographic findings have consisted of low voltage and minor abnormalities, including alterations in the T wave and changes in rhythm. To judge by the volume of feces excreted by children with kwashiorkor, these children suffer from a malabsorption syndrome which is not completely corrected even after some weeks of treatment. Good digestion and absorption of proteins still take place during the acute state, but fat is poorly handled at first. Although fat absorption improves very rapidly as the child recovers, some degree of steatorrhea persists even into late recovery. Despite the marked histologic alterations in the liver, the common tests for liver function have been found to give results within normal limits, with the possible exception of sulfobromophthalein retention, which is frequently high.

Electroencephalographic studies have shown diminished voltage and excessively slow rhythmic activity. Some authors have also reported abnormal focal activity and other alterations. These abnormalities tend to disappear as recovery progresses.

Pathology. The main pathologic alterations in kwashiorkor include fatty changes in the liver, of the large droplet type, beginning in periportal areas of the lobule and extending progressively to the central vein. The pancreas and other endocrine glands become atrophic, along with marked atrophy of the intestinal mucosa, to give changes like those in primary malabsorption. The skin shows atrophy of the epidermis, with varying degrees of hyperkeratosis and parakeratosis.

Coexisting Deficiencies. The clinical manifestations of protein-calorie malnutrition are further complicated by the presence of other nutritional deficiencies. Vitamin A deficiency with severe ocular lesions is frequent in both marasmus and kwashiorkor. Concurrent deficiencies of components of B vitamins, particularly riboflavin, are also common. The mild normocytic, normochromic anemia attributable to protein deficiency is often complicated and becomes much more severe because of simultaneous deficiencies of iron, vitamin E, folic acid, and other hematopoietic factors of the B vitamins. A recent report suggests that vitamin E deficiency is sometimes responsible. Dehydration and serious electrolyte imbalance are usual because of the coexisting diarrhea.

Treatment. The correction of dehydration and associated electrolyte imbalance and the treatment of infections are the immediate demands in management of protein-calorie malnutrition. The basic requirement, however, is a diet providing all essential nutrients. Three to 4 grams of protein of high biologic value and 100 to 140 calories per kilogram of body weight are useful in children with kwashiorkor, and up to 200 calories per kilogram in those with marasmus.

Prevention. The prevention of protein-calorie malnutrition depends upon teaching mothers the importance of feeding their young children properly. Efforts should be made to increase the availability of low-cost protein foods suitable for feeding to infants and young children, ensuring that the mother can obtain them through either commercial channels or welfare programs. There must also be effective public health measures for reducing the burden of microbial disease in vulnerable populations.

Béhar, M., Viteri, F., and Scrimshaw, N. S.: Treatment of severe protein deficiency in children (kwashiorkor). Am. J. Clin. Nutr., 5:506, 1957.

National Academy of Sciences–National Research Council: Pre-School Child Malnutrition: Primary Deterrent to Human Progress. An International Conference on Prevention of Malnutrition in the Pre-School Child, Washington, D.C., December 7-11, 1964. NAS–NRC Publication No. 1282, 1966.

Scrimshaw, N. S., and Béhar, M.: Protein malnutrition in young children. Science, 133:2039, 1961.

Scrimshaw, N. S., and Béhar, M.: Malnutrition in underdeveloped countries. N. Engl. J. Med., 272:137, 193, 1965.

Viteri, F., Béhar, M., Arroyave, G., and Scrimshaw, N. S.: Clinical aspects of protein malnutrition. *In* Munro, H. N., and Allison, J. B. (eds.): Mammalian Protein Metabolism. Vol. II. New York, Academic Press, 1964, Chap. 22, p. 523.

Waterlow, J. C., and Alleyne, G. A. O.: Protein malnutrition in children: Advances in knowledge in the last ten years. Adv. Protein Chem. 25:117, 1971.

Waterlow, J. C., Cravioto, J., and Stephen, J. M. L.: Protein malnutrition in man. Adv. Protein Chem., 15:131, 1960.

716. UNDERNUTRITION, STARVATION, AND HUNGER EDEMA

Nevin S. Scrimshaw

When a person's caloric intake is far below his daily energy expenditure, he must either bring the two into balance by reduced activity or draw upon his own tissues for energy. Initially, tissue fat is a major energy source, but protein is also required as a source of amino acids for gluconeogenesis. Cahill has shown that after several weeks of fasting, dependence on endogenous amino acids decreases, because even the central nervous system can then utilize fatty acids.

Once adipose tissue has been exhausted, lassitude, loss of ambition, hypotension, collapse, and death follow if the caloric intake deficit continues. The late stages of this syndrome are also observed in anorexia nervosa, terminal carcinoma, and other wasting diseases.

Keys provides the most comprehensive review of the world literature on starvation, and adds important experimental observations of his own. Others have described severe malnutrition in the prisons and concentration camps of World War II and famines in many parts of the world.

Dependent edema often accompanies severe, prolonged undernutrition (starvation). The edema is soft and pitting, and usually disappears when the person is recumbent for some time, as during sleep. The causes of the edema are not entirely clear. Hypoproteinemia (specifically hypoalbuminemia, thus lowering the colloid osmotic pressure) is frequent but by no means invariable. Loss of fat and muscle, leaving a "loose sack" of skin with fluid filling the empty spaces, has been thought of as a contributing phenomenon. Diminished renal blood flow and glomerular filtration resulting from diminished cardiac output would presumably lead to sodium retention and edema.

Treatment of starvation demands caution. *In all forms of severe undernutrition, refeeding must be instituted slowly.* Overeating was a cause of shock and death of concentration camp victims at the end of World War II. The same is true for nutritional treatment of patients severely undernourished because of non-nutritional disease, e.g., esophageal carcinoma. Sudden flooding of the intestine with rich food through a feeding jejunostomy or gastrostomy may produce shock and death.

Benedict, F. G.: A Study of Prolonged Fasting. Carnegie Institute of Washington, Publication No. 203, 1915.
Keys, A.: The Biology of Human Starvation. Minneapolis, University of Minnesota Press, 1950.
Mollison, P. L.: Observations on cases of starvation at Belsen. Br. Med. J., 1:4, 1946.
Owen, O. E., Morgan, A. P., Kemp, H. G., Sullivan, J. M., Herrera, M. G., and Cahill, G. F., Jr.: Brain metabolism during fasting. J. Clin. Invest., 46:1589, 1967.
Young, V. R., and Scrimshaw, N. S.: The physiology of starvation. Sci. Am., 225:14, 1971.

DEFICIENCIES OF INDIVIDUAL NUTRIENTS: VITAMIN DISEASES

Nevin S. Scrimshaw

717. HYPOVITAMINOSIS A (INCLUDING XEROPHTHALMIA AND KERATOMALACIA)

Etiology and Distribution. The term vitamin A is used to include all compounds having vitamin A activity, but requirements are now expressed by the Food and Agriculture Organization and World Health Organization in terms of crystalline vitamin A_1 alcohol (retinol). The international unit, still used in many countries, is equivalent to 0.3 μg of retinol (or 0.344 μg of retinyl acetate) or to 0.6 μg of the provitamin beta-carotene. The recommended intake for adult males is 1000 μg of retinol per day, and for adult females, 800 μg, increasing to 1000 μg during pregnancy. During lactation 1200 μg of retinol per day is recommended. For children the recommendations are estimated from expected body weight for age, ranging from 420 μg per day at three to five months of age to the adult levels. Requirements are not influenced by physical activity or climate, but any pathologic condition that interferes with fat absorption is likely to impede vitamin A absorption, and infections can increase vitamin A needs.

Signs and symptoms of hypovitaminosis A are particularly common in Indonesia and most other countries of Southeast Asia and the Indian subcontinent, but are seen at least occasionally in nearly all economically underdeveloped countries. They are most often precipitated by infectious disease in infants and young children who already suffer from chronic malnutrition. Sporadic cases occur among particularly underprivileged infants in most of the industrialized areas of the world.

Clinical Manifestations; Pathology and Pathologic Physiology. The best known and generally the earliest physiologic effect of hypovitaminosis A is the loss of night vision (nyctalopia). The retinal rods responsible for vision in dim light contain a light-sensitive pigment, rhodopsin, an aldehyde of vitamin A that breaks down to retinene when light strikes a rod. In vitamin A deficiency rhodopsin regeneration fails.

Xerophthalmia is a dryness of the only transparent epithelial structures of the body that are exposed to air and light. The conjunctiva is affected earlier and more constantly than the cornea. Typical is a fatty dryness, most pronounced at the thickened wrinkles of the corners; the eye loses its porcelain aspect and looks muddy-greasy, like oil paint.

Bitot spots are often present, ranging in severity from a few tiny air bubbles visible on the exposed conjunctiva between the corneal rim and limbus, to a frothy white coating that overflows onto the cornea. The meibomian glands sometimes enlarge to look like a string of beads along the margin of the eyelids. The cornea is more resistant, but becomes hazy, rough, and dry and insensitive to touch. Punctate superficial infiltrations or small erosions may be seen on the surface. As the disease progresses to *keratomalacia*, one of these erosions may enlarge rapidly, with protrusion and eventually prolapse of the iris and loss of the lens. Sometimes there is a rather sudden spongy swelling and melting down of the cornea, a colliquative necrosis, with subsequent shrinkage of the eyeball (Fig. 2).

The skin becomes dry as the sebaceous glands become covered with keratin, so that secretions are diminished. *Phrynoderma*, an elevated papular lesion caused by plugging of the mouth of the hair follicles with a dense keratotic mass together with hyperplasia of the epithelium lining the plugged follicles, has been mistakenly listed as a sign of vitamin A deficiency. This condition is not necessarily associated with low serum levels of vitamin A, and does not respond to prolonged vitamin A therapy. Moreover, it is different from the follicular lesion of vitamin A deficiency in laboratory animals, in which the upper third of the hair follicles contains loose keratin and becomes dilated.

The small intestine is the main site of the conversion of active forms of carotene to vitamin A and its absorption. Therefore, when the intestine is affected by diseases such as sprue, fibrocystic disease of the pancreas, lymphomas, or lipodystrophy (Whipple's disease), hypovitaminosis A is likely to result. The liver contains 90 per cent of vitamin A stores, but these may be markedly reduced in some hepatic diseases.

Lowered dietary intake of preformed vitamin A or of an active carotene precursor is the most obvious and common factor in hypovitaminosis A, but any condition interfering with the intestinal absorption and conversion of carotene to vitamin A and its transport to the liver will contribute to deficiency of this vitamin. Surgical removal of sections of the small bowel and excessive consumption of mineral oil are in this category. So are

Figure 2. *A*, Keratomalacia in four year old boy. *Left eye:* Perforation of cornea, through which lens has escaped, with drop of vitreous substance visible on lower lid. *Right eye:* Necrosis of cornea with small ulcer. *B*, Bitot spot on transparent conjunctiva, nine year old child. *C*, Xerosis conjunctivae, showing Bitot spot and dryness of mucosal folds, four year old boy. *D*, Xerophthalmia with subtotal leukoma, after measles with perforating xerosis of cornea, in three year old child. (Courtesy of Dr. H. A. P. C. Oomen.)

massive intestinal infections with *Giardia lamblia* and probably also ascaris and hookworm. Severe protein deficiency (kwashiorkor) decreases the availability of transport protein. Dried skim milk fed to protein-deficient children in Indonesia increased the frequency of xerophthalmia, presumably by removing the limitation of protein and calories on growth and thereby increasing the need for vitamin A which the milk did not contain.

Treatment. Treatment consists of administration of therapeutic amounts of vitamin A, correction of the pattern of dietary intake, and, in cases of secondary deficiency, therapy of the underlying disease. In young children without serious eye involvement, the daily oral administration of 3000 µg of retinol is recommended. When there is reason to suspect that dietary fat, including the fat-soluble vitamin A, is not properly absorbed, the new water-miscible vitamin A preparations are indicated rather than fish liver oil. If no response is observed, or signs of keratomalacia are present, daily doses of 15,000 to 25,000 µg of retinol should be given intramuscularly for the first week in an attempt to prevent permanent impairment of vision. Improvement may be seen within a week, but maximal healing may take many weeks. If the lens is intact, residual corneal scarring can sometimes be treated by transplant.

When hypovitaminosis A is associated with protein deficiency, dietary protein alone will bring a prompt increase in serum vitamin A levels if the stores in the liver are adequate. Conversely, if protein deficiency is present, hypovitaminosis A will not respond to treat-ment with the vitamin alone owing to the lack of transport protein.

Prevention. Primary prevention depends upon assuring a diet with adequate vitamin A activity to meet all body needs and to maintain good stores of vitamin A in the liver. Foods of animal origin such as dairy products containing butter fat, egg yolk, liver, and fish liver oils are excellent sources. Sufficient quantities of the provitamin beta-carotene and other active carotenoids are also found in many vegetables and fruits. For populations in tropical and less developed countries, most of the vitamin A activity in the diet can come from fruits such as the mango and papaya. African palm oil, used in cooking in many parts of the world, is rich in vitamin A activity.

When processing has reduced the vitamin A activity of a food or when substitute foods of lower vitamin A content are introduced, fortification may be indicated. For example, margarine is routinely fortified with 10,000 IU of vitamin A per pound because it replaces butter, a good source of this vitamin. Similarly, skim milk for human consumption should be fortified with water-miscible vitamin A, because all vitamin A activity has been removed with the cream. Synthetic breakfast drinks replacing natural fruit juices can be made good sources of vitamin A.

Prevention of deficiency secondary to other disease requires measures to control the primary cause. Most important will be environmental sanitation and other public health measures to reduce the prevalence of infections.

Federation of American Societies for Experimental Biology: Nutritional Disease, Proceedings of a Conference on Beriberi, Endemic Goiter and Hypovitaminosis A, held at Princeton, New Jersey, June 1–5, 1958. Fed. Proc. 17:Part II, Supplement No. 2, 1958, pp. 103–143.

McLaren, D. S.: Malnutrition and the Eye. New York, Academic Press, Inc., 1963.

Scrimshaw, N. S., Taylor, C. E., and Gordon, J. E.: Interactions of Nutrition and Infection. World Health Organization, Monograph Series No. 57. Geneva, World Health Organization, 1968.

RICKETS AND OSTEOMALACIA

See Ch. 885 to 890.

ENDEMIC GOITER

See Ch. 841.

718. ARIBOFLAVINOSIS

Etiology and Distribution. The intake of riboflavin must be low for many months before symptoms become evident. Among persons whose diets contain limited riboflavin, the disease often appears during periods of physiologic stress such as pregnancy and lactation, and during the rapid growth of childhood. Ariboflavinosis is so commonly associated with diets deficient in niacin and protein that for years it was considered part of the pellagra syndrome.

Characteristic deficiency signs appear in persons on deficient diets for three to eight months, depending upon the exact level of riboflavin and individual variation.

Low urinary riboflavin excretion levels and mild clinical signs of ariboflavinosis are common among the low-income populations of developing countries. Moderate to severe ariboflavinosis is usually seen only in association with other deficiency diseases such as pellagra and kwashiorkor. In the industrialized countries it is likely to be one of the deficiencies seen in alcoholics and persons with long-standing infections, malignancies, and other chronic debilitating diseases.

Clinical Signs. Early symptoms of ariboflavinosis are soreness and burning of the lips, mouth, and tongue, and photophobia, lacrimation, burning, and itching of the eyes. The lesions of the lips may progress so that fissures extend from the angles of the mouth for a centimeter or more, and the lips themselves may appear dry and chapped. Shallow ulcerations and crusting sometimes develop. Neither the cheilosis nor the angular stomatitis is pathognomonic of riboflavin deficiency, because similar lesions may result from deficiency of niacin, iron, or pyridoxine.

The seborrheic type of dermatitis has a scaly, greasy appearance and is associated with erythema. Hard sebaceous plugs or fine filiform comedones may be seen over the bridge of the nose and on the malar prominences and chin. Dermatitis of the scrotum and vulva may also appear. In some instances, the redness, scaling, and desquamation of the skin of the scrotum extend to adjacent areas of the thigh which become raw and weeping.

The tongue in ariboflavinosis is characteristically purplish red or magenta and often has deep fissures. The papillae may be swollen, flattened, or mushroom-shaped, giving a pebbled appearance. In chronic deficiency the papillae may become atrophic. The glossitis of riboflavin deficiency cannot be clearly differentiated from that caused by lack of niacin, folic acid, or vitamin B_{12}.

Eye signs responding to administration of riboflavin include diffuse inflammation of the conjunctivae, and red, swollen eyelids with a sticky exudate. Photophobia may be intense. Injection and proliferation of the capillaries of the limbic plexus may develop.

Biochemical Function. Riboflavin functions as a coenzyme of the active prosthetic group of flavoproteins concerned with oxidative processes. Among these are cytochrome-c reductase, D- and L-amino oxidases, succinic dehydrogenase, diaphorase, and xanthine and aldehyde oxidases.

The concentrations of free riboflavin, flavin mononucleotide, and flavin dinucleotide in plasma can be readily measured, but are not reliable indicators of deficiency, nor are white or red blood cell levels of riboflavin any more specific. Either 24-hour urinary excretion of riboflavin or the excretion four hours after subcutaneous administration of 1.0 mg will be found reduced in those whose diets have been deficient in riboflavin for an extended period. Less than 50 mg in 24 hours or 20 μg in the four hours after the test dose indicate that prior intake has been inadequate.

Prevention and Treatment. Prevention requires a diet that includes foods that are rich sources of riboflavin such as milk, liver, other meats, eggs, and many green and yellow vegetables. For treatment, an adequate diet should be prescribed, and 5 mg of riboflavin given orally twice a day. Symptoms disappear in a few days, and the lesions clear up in a few weeks. In general, it is better to give a multivitamin preparation in treating ariboflavinosis because of the frequency of simultaneous deficiency of other B vitamins. When signs suggestive of such deficiencies are present, therapeutic doses of the appropriate vitamins should also be given.

Goldsmith, G. A.: The B vitamins: Thiamine, riboflavin, niacin. In Beaton, G. H., and McHenry, E. W. (eds.): Nutrition: A Comprehensive Treatise. Vol. II. New York. Academic Press, Inc., 1964, chap. 2, p. 145.

719. PELLAGRA

Etiology and Distribution. Although pellagra is caused by a primary dietary deficiency of niacin, the adequacy of dietary niacin is influenced by the quantity and quality of dietary protein, and particularly by the availability of tryptophan, which is a metabolic precursor of niacin. The term "niacin" is generic for both nicotinic acid and nicotinamide. One niacin equivalent is defined as 1 mg of niacin or 60 mg of tryptophan. The minimum required to prevent pellagra is 4.4 niacin equivalents per 1000 kcal per day, and a recommended allowance of 6.6 niacin equivalents per 1000 calories per day allows for individual variation.

Pellagra is traditionally associated with maize (corn) diets because this cereal grain has a low tryptophan as well as niacin content. It does not occur, however, where maize diets are supplemented with sufficient legume protein, as they are in Central America. It is still seen in the Yucatan peninsula of Mexico where the raising of henequen, maguey, hemp, or sisal takes most of the land, and in corn-eating populations of several Middle Eastern and African countries, notably in Egypt and Lesotho. In the 1930's it was still common in the southern United

States among low-income groups whose diets consisted mainly of pork fat and hominy grits made from degerminated corn, but the disease has now disappeared from the United States except in alcoholics. Until recently it was still seen among corn-eating populations of rural Yugoslavia, Rumania, and Greece.

The pellagra common in Indian populations subsisting on a diet of jowar (millet, *Sorghum vulgare*) is reported to be influenced by the relative excess of leucine as well as the low tryptophan and niacin of this cereal. Diets containing protein of animal origin or vegetable proteins of good quality contain enough tryptophan to prevent pellagra even when niacin intakes are low.

Experimental niacin-tryptophan deficiency in human subjects duplicates most but not all of the features of pellagra as it occurs in populations, because in the latter there are nearly always other complicating diseases and deficiencies. Pellagra in the industrialized countries at present is generally a result of the vitamin- and protein-deficient diets of chronic alcoholics.

Deficiency of folic acid probably accounts for the frequency of megaloblastic anemia in pellagra. The cheilosis, angular stomatitis, proctitis, scrotal dermatitis, and vaginitis may be more related to concomitant deficiency of riboflavin (vitamin B_2) or vitamin B_6 than to that of niacin. The neurologic and mental symptoms, especially the cord degeneration sometimes found, could possibly be caused by poor vitamin B_{12} absorption. Reversible achlorhydria often occurs. The peripheral neuropathy and occasional mental changes, suggesting Korsakoff's psychosis, are possibly due to concomitant deficiency of thiamin or pyridoxine. Because fatty liver may be present, deficiency of protein and especially of choline and methionine must also be considered.

Pellagra is encountered in patients with cirrhosis of the liver, chronic diarrheal disease, diabetes mellitus, and neoplasia. Prolonged infectious diseases, such as tuberculosis, or thyrotoxicosis may lead to deficiency owing to an increase in niacin requirement. Pellagrous dermatitis has also been reported in patients with malignant carcinoid, a rare tumor which may convert as much as 60 per cent of the body's tryptophan to serotonin in-

stead of the usual 1 per cent. Decreased food intake and diarrhea presumably contribute to the development of pellagra in this condition.

Clinical Manifestations. The early signs of pellagra are nonspecific and include lassitude, anorexia, weakness, digestive disturbances, and often anxiety, irritability, and depression. As the deficiency progresses, soreness of the tongue gives way to severe inflammation of mucous membranes manifested by glossitis, stomatitis, esophagitis, diarrhea, urethritis, proctitis, and vaginitis. The mouth may be so painful that it is difficult to take even liquids, and the mucous membranes become bright red. The tongue is scarlet and swollen, with atrophy of the papillae. Not surprisingly, severe weight loss ensues.

The chronic dermatitis of pellagra may be difficult to distinguish from extensive exposure to dust and sunlight. It varies with the acuteness and severity of the deficiency state. At the earlier, acute stages it resembles sunburn. In chronic pellagra, which has developed more slowly, skin changes include thickening, scaling, hyperkeratinization, and pigmentation. Either type will usually be found on areas of skin exposed to sunlight—the backs of the hands and forearms, the anterior surfaces of the feet and lower legs, and the face and neck. Lesions following the sharp neckline of a dress or an open shirt are known as Casal's necklace. Other areas which may be involved are the axillae, groin, perineum, genitalia, elbows, knees, and skin under the breasts.

The early nonspecific psychic and emotional changes of early pellagra may, with increasing severity, progress to disorientation, delirium, and hallucination. The dementia may be hyperactive and manic or apathetic, lethargic, and stuporous. Other sensory and neurologic abnormalities and acute encephalopathy have been described in some cases. Anemia from associated deficiencies is common.

Biochemistry and Pathology. Nicotinamide functions in the body as the component of two important coenzymes, DPN (diphosphopyridine nucleotide) and TPN (triphosphopyridine nucleotide), which are functional groups in intracellular oxidation-reduction enzyme systems necessary for tissue respiration, glycolysis, and fat

Figure 3.   Modern pellagra. Egypt and the Balkans. (Courtesy of Dr. William J. Darby.)

synthesis. In endemic pellagra the combined excretion of the niacin metabolites, N^1-methylnicotinamide and pyridone, seldom exceeds 2 grams daily.

The skin lesions are hyperkeratotic, often with vesicles containing erythrocytes, fibrin, and melanin pigment. Microscopic examination reveals atrophy of the sebaceous glands and hair follicles and degeneration of the peripheral nerves of the skin. Pathologic changes have also been reported in the brain, spinal cord, and peripheral nerves. Mucous membranes show inflammation and atrophy.

Treatment and Prevention. The treatment of pellagra is a diet adequate in niacin and tryptophan and the administration of therapeutic doses of the vitamin. The best food sources of niacin are yeast, liver, lean meat, poultry, peanuts, and legumes. Potatoes, other vegetables, and whole wheat cereal and bread are fair sources. Most of these are also good sources of tryptophan as well. Although milk and eggs contain little niacin, they are also protective against pellagra because of their high tryptophan content. Enrichment of cereal flours with niacin and other B vitamins is a simple and inexpensive way of ensuring an ample intake of these nutrients.

In severe deficiency, niacinamide may be given in divided doses of 50 to 100 mg to a total of 300 to 500 mg for the first few days and then decreased to 150 mg daily. When circumstances make oral administration difficult, niacinamide can also be given intramuscularly in a dose of 100 mg three times daily. In advanced pellagra, bed rest is essential, and calorie intakes up to 3500 per day may be required. Acute symptoms improve within a few days, but several weeks of therapy may be required for complete recovery. Because concurrent deficiencies of other B vitamins are generally present, a multivitamin tablet containing 5.0 mg each of thiamin, riboflavin, and pyridoxine, should be given daily in the treatment of pellagra. Associated anemia may require either folic acid or iron therapy.

Goldsmith, G. A.: The B vitamins: Thiamine, riboflavin, niacin. *In* Beaton, G. H., and McHenry, E. W. (eds.): Nutrition: A Comprehensive Treatise. Vol. II. New York, Academic Press, Inc., 1964, chap. 2, p. 161.

Goldsmith, G. A., Sarett, H. P., Register, U. D., and Gibbens, J.: Studies of niacin requirements in man. I. Experimental pellagra in subjects on corn diets low in niacin and tryptophan. J. Clin. Invest., 31:533, 1952.

Spies, T. D.: Niacinamide malnutrition and pellagra. *In* Jolliffe, N. (ed.): Clinical Nutrition. 2nd ed. New York, Hoeber Medical Book, Harper & Brothers, 1962, chap. 18, p. 622.

Spies, T. D., Aring, C. D., Gelperin, J., and Bean, W. B.: The mental symptoms of pellagra. Their relief with nicotinic acid. Am. J. Med. Sci., 196:461, 1938.

720. BERIBERI

Etiology and Distribution. Beriberi occurs mainly in countries where polished rice provides a diet low in thiamin and high in carbohydrate. Among prisoners subsisting largely on polished rice in Japanese prison camps during World War II, beriberi developed when the thiamin supply was less than 0.3 mg per 1000 nonfat calories, with the acute episode usually precipitated by dysentery or other infectious disease. Deficiency signs may be anticipated when dietary intakes are less than 0.2 mg per 1000 calories, and intakes of 0.5 mg or more per 1000 calories are recommended. Because it is possible that older persons utilize thiamin less efficiently, they should maintain an intake of 1.0 mg per day, even when they are consuming less than 2000 kcal daily. The allowance of 0.5 mg per 1000 calories also applies to pregnant and lactating women and to children.

Beriberi is still seen occasionally in the rice-eating populations of Southeast Asia and the Indian subcontinent, and infantile beriberi has actually increased in some villages where newly introduced gasoline mills more completely separate the germ from the endosperm than does traditional hand-pounding. It has been described in some populations of Brazil and Africa among persons consuming cassava as the primary source of calories. It may also occur in association with pathologic states that interfere with the ingestion or absorption of food, and it is the most important of the B vitamin deficiencies common to alcoholism. Wernicke's syndrome is often associated with beriberi. Korsakoff's psychosis found among alcoholics is closely related to it (see Ch. 406).

Clinical Characteristics. The great majority of cases of beriberi are of the mild, subacute form, in which paresthesias and altered reflexes are the most characteristic findings. The muscle groups involved seem related to the length of the nerve controlling them, the amount of work they do, and possibly their blood supply. Laborers complain of disturbances of the lower legs, women more often of sensations in the fingers; other distributions can be related to the occupational use of muscle groups. Fullness or tightening of the muscles and fatigue pains resembling those of muscle ischemia are prominent, and, especially at night, muscle cramps occur.

In well developed cases, tachycardia is present, and the heart is enlarged. The edema may be generalized and massive or minimal without clear relation to the severity of the other symptoms. The most common characteristics of acute beriberi in prisoners of the Japanese in World War II were persistent tachycardia, symmetrical foot and wrist drop associated with muscle tenderness, mild disturbances of sensation over the outer aspects of the legs and thighs, and in patches over the abdomen, chest, and forearms. Most of these signs and symptoms have been reproduced experimentally in 30 to 120 days in adult subjects on thiamin intakes from 0.075 to 0.2 mg per 1000 calories.

The acute fulminating form of beriberi has been called Shoshin; it is dominated by circulatory insufficiency. The milder forms may develop into this often fatal type, but more often it is of sudden onset. When nerve lesions develop early, the heart is saved from extreme insufficiency because the patient is forced to rest. In terminal cases, severe dyspnea and violent palpitations of the heart allow the patient no rest, and precordial pain may be intense. The patient tosses and turns about violently and complains of heaviness, constriction, oppression, and sometimes actual pain over the epigastrium. The moans and shrieks of the patient are distorted by the coincident hoarseness and sometimes aphonia. Pupils are dilated, and respirations are frequent and superficial. The liver and heart are enlarged and the heart action tumultuous. Cyanosis is obvious, and the pulse is weak but regular.

The chronic, dry, atrophic type—with wrist drop and foot drop—is generally found only in older adults. They no longer show the biochemical changes characteristic of acute beriberi, nor do they respond satisfactorily to therapy.

The beriberi seen in *infants*, particularly from one to four months of age, is associated with poor thiamin content of, and possibly abnormal metabolites in, the breast milk of mothers subsisting on a rice diet. It begins with vomiting, restlessness, pallor, anorexia, and insomnia, and evolves variously. In acute infantile beriberi, the infant develops cyanosis, dyspnea, and running pulse with cardiac crises which are often fatal. If the process is more chronic, the symptoms are vomiting, inanition, anorexia, aphonia, opisthotonos, edema, oliguria, constipation, and meteorism. A subacute form that may evolve into either the acute or chronic type is also described. The infant develops puffiness, vomiting, oliguria, abdominal pain, dysphagia, aphonia, and even convulsions. These forms are not really distinct, and the signs and symptoms may be present in almost any combination. Case fatality is very high unless treatment is given.

Biochemistry and Pathology. Pyruvic acid tends to accumulate in the tissues in severe thiamin deficiency. Because thiamin pyrophosphate is a coenzyme in the reaction, reduced transketolase activity can be detected in the red blood cells of persons consuming diets low in thiamin. Urinary excretion of thiamin of 0 to 14 μg in 24 hours has been reported in beriberi, and early signs have been observed with excretions of less than 40 μg in 24 hours.

The pathology of thiamin-deficient states ranges from maximal disturbance of function with minimal histologic abnormalities in acute, severe deficiency to minimal biochemical changes and well defined peripheral nerve lesions in chronic deficiency. In fatal cases, hypertrophy of the heart is a constant finding.

Degeneration is found not only in peripheral, but also in cerebrospinal nerves, in terminal branches of the vagus and phrenic nerves, and sometimes in the spinal cord and fibers of the posterior root. In Wernicke's encephalopathy, histologic changes are found chiefly in the mamillary bodies, the related walls of the third ventricle, and the aqueduct and tegmentum of the medulla.

Treatment and Prevention. The treatment of beriberi consists of a balanced diet plus the administration of 5.0 to 10.0 mg of thiamin three times daily. In severe beriberi the thiamin should be given parenterally for the first few days, but oral administration is satisfactory for the treatment of most cases. Delay in the treatment of Wernicke's syndrome may result in cardiac death or in permanent cerebral damage with signs of Korsakoff's syndrome. Because other B vitamin deficiencies are often present in beriberi, a multivitamin preparation is also advisable.

The biochemical lesions are rapidly reversed, but structural defects require long recovery periods. Signs of heart failure disappear within a few days; within a few weeks the heart returns to normal size, and electrocardiographic abnormalities disappear. In longstanding cases of advanced neuropathy, complete restoration to normal may be impossible, although improvement may continue for many months.

Prevention requires an increase in the intake of thiamin for persons consuming rice diets. Parboiling causes the thiamin to pass into the grain so that it is not removed in the milling process. In practice, efforts to encourage parboiling or the use of home-pounded and undermilled rice have not been successful. Enrichment of rice at the mill with thiamin, riboflavin, and niacin has not been adopted by those countries needing it most. A generally improved diet, containing foods which are good sources of thiamin, and extensive distribution of synthetic thiamin are the measures that have been most effective in Asia.

Federation of American Societies for Experimental Biology: Nutritional Disease, Proceedings of a Conference on Beriberi, Endemic Goiter and Hypovitaminosis A, held at Princeton, New Jersey, June 1–5, 1958. Fed. Proc., 17: Part II, Supplement No. 2, September, 1958, pp. 3–56.

Goldsmith, G. A.: The B Vitamins: Thiamine, riboflavin, niacin, In Beaton, G. H., and McHenry, E. W. (eds.): A Comprehensive Treatise, Vol. II. New York, Academic Press, 1964, chap. 2, p. 109.

Spillane, J. D.: Nutritional Disorders of the Nervous System. Baltimore, Williams and Wilkins Company, 1947.

Weiss, S., and Wilkins, R. W.: The nature of the cardiovascular disturbances in nutritional deficiency states (beriberi). Ann. Intern. Med., 11:104, 1937.

721. SCURVY

Etiology and Distribution. Most mammals are able to synthesize ascorbic acid from glucose by way of glucuronic acid. Man, the primates, and the guinea pig lack the enzyme required for conversion of gluconate to ascorbate. If dietary intake of ascorbic acid ceases for several months, clinical scurvy develops. Scurvy has most commonly occurred in the spring in temperate climates or at the end of the dry season in tropical ones, because of the relative lack of fresh fruit and vegetables during the preceding months and because several months are required for the disease to become manifest. Although now rare, the disease is still seen in exceptional circumstances, and the treatment is specific and effective. The minimal daily requirement for ascorbic acid is controversial. A group of British volunteers remained in good health and had normal wound healing on a daily intake of 10 mg for almost a year, although plasma and leukocyte ascorbic acid contents were very low. In a notable human experiment by Crandon, under controlled conditions with complete deficiency of the vitamin, the plasma level of ascorbic acid fell to zero by the forty-first day, but abnormal hair and hair follicles appeared only after four months. Perifollicular hemorrhages were not evident until after five months on the experimental diet. Subjective symptoms of a less specific nature—fatigability and anorexia—preceded the appearance of objective signs.

Biochemistry and Pathology. The effect of ascorbic acid on enzymes depends on its properties as either a strong reducing agent or the source of peroxide from its oxidation with air. It is a reactant in such well defined enzyme systems as hydroxylation to form norepinephrine, 5-hydroxylation of tryptophan, tyrosine oxidase, and a number of others. In the oxidation of p-hydroxyphenylpyruvic acid, it protects the enzyme involved from inhibition by its substrate, a necessary function when large amounts of tyrosine are being metabolized. It is also a specific reductant of the ferric ion in its transfer from plasma transferrin to liver ferritin.

It is needed also for the conversion of proline to hydroxyproline and the synthesis of chondroitin sulfate in the ground substance of collagen; hydroxyproline is an amino acid found only in collagen. Ascorbic acid is a necessary component of the mucopolysaccharides of ground substance. In the vitamin's absence, defective ground substance is formed, and can be seen by electron microscopy to have lost its characteristic periodicity. At any rate, scar tissue does not form. Ascorbic acid is involved in the preservation of folinic acid, the reduced form of folic acid. Perhaps this contributes to the occasional macrocytic anemia seen in scurvy by diminishing the amount of folinic acid available. There is no good evidence that ascorbic acid is itself required for erythropoiesis.

The pathologic changes in scurvy are predominantly in the mesenchymal tissues of the body, especially in collagen, growing bones, teeth, and blood vessels. In growing bones the histopathology of scurvy is distinctive: a suppression of the orderly growth process and of the normal calcification of the cartilage matrix. In addition, hemorrhages may be found in the interior of the bone at the cartilage-shaft junction, together with fractures of the minute columns of cartilage matrix and, at times, dislocation, separation, or impaction of the epiphyses.

Subperiosteal hemorrhages are relatively uncommon in the adult but frequent in infantile scurvy. Loosening of the periosteal attachment leads to capillary bleeding, which may dissect the periosteum free over a large area. Most frequently these subperiosteal hemorrhages are found at the lower end of the femur, the upper end of the humerus, both ends of the tibia, and the costochondral junctions of the middle ribs.

Capillaries in the skin become fragile, and petechiae, ecchymoses, and hematomas result. Hemorrhages into the gums lead to swelling, tissue friability, and even gangrene.

The teeth become loose because of resorption of alveolar bone. In children the teeth also show abnormalities of development, with poorly formed matrix and porous dentine.

The laboratory detection of this deficiency or confirmation of the clinical diagnosis of scurvy requires measurement of the plasma or leukocyte concentration of ascorbic acid, or the urinary excretion of the vitamin with or without a "loading" test. With low levels of dietary ascorbic acid intake, plasma ascorbic acid levels fall sharply, but even levels below 0.2 mg may be associated with a wide range of tissue saturations, from 0 to approximately 50 per cent. At this level of nutriture, the white blood cell–platelet ascorbic acid level is most useful. It will average 20 to 30 mg per 100 ml in a well nourished subject, and on an ascorbic acid-free diet will decrease to 0 to 2 mg per 100 ml in three to five months. Clinical scurvy usually appears shortly thereafter.

Clinical Manifestations. Malaise, weakness, and lassitude are early and constant symptoms. Shortness of breath and aching in the bones and joints follow. The most distinctive physical sign and one of the earliest is perifollicular hemorrhage, usually in hyperkeratotic hair follicles, appearing particularly on the posterior thighs, anterior forearms, and abdomen. The hairs become fragmented, coiled, and buried in the follicles.

Petechiae are characteristic features of fully developed scurvy, and are usually most prominent in the same hair-bearing areas and in dependent parts of the body. Scorbutic petechiae are usually larger and more purplish than those in other forms of purpura, for example, in thrombocytopenia. Similarly, a tourniquet produces petechiae that are typically large and dark in color, appearing mostly on the hair-bearing areas of the forearm rather than on the flexor surface usually examined.

As scurvy becomes more advanced, ecchymoses appear, first at areas of irritation, pressure, or trauma. The "saddle area" and posterior thighs are the most frequent locations. Larger hemorrhages occur later in subcutaneous tissue, muscles, or joints, but are uncommon in the viscera, heart, or brain. Gums become swollen, inflamed, and "spongy," bleed easily, and are usually infected. Gum changes are less pronounced in edentulous subjects.

In untreated disease of long duration, postural hypotension and syncope are common. They may be part of the preterminal state in which vomiting and frank hypotension occur, resembling an Addisonian crisis.

Anemia, normocytic or macrocytic, with resultant pallor, is frequent. Two major causes of anemia must be considered. First, and most important, is the blood loss into the skin and deeper tissues or, uncommonly, into the gastrointestinal tract. Second is the possibility that dietary intake of folic acid may also be deficient. Many foods are important sources of both folic acid and ascorbic acid, and the two deficiencies may potentiate one another.

Most cases of scurvy seen in infancy *(Barlow's disease)* develop 6 to 12 months after the institution of artificial feeding. A few examples have been reported in infants considerably younger, but in these instances the mothers habitually subsisted on a diet inadequate in ascorbic acid. The concentration of ascorbic acid in human milk, invariably higher than that in maternal plasma, closely reflects the mother's intake.

Loss of appetite, listlessness, and irritability are early and insidious signs of infantile scurvy. The bony lesions and subperiosteal hemorrhages lead to tenderness, swelling, and evidence of pain on movement. Bleeding into the costochondral junctions of the ribs is noted externally as swellings—the "scorbutic rosary." Purpura and gum changes are similar to those in the adult except that pre-existing gum infection is less common.

Significance of Ascorbic Acid in Clinical Medicine. Although scurvy is now a rare disease, in several important clinical situations the state of ascorbic acid nutrition is a significant consideration. Resistance to infection is reduced in ascorbic acid deficiency, and microbial diseases have long been recognized to precipitate scurvy in individuals on borderline intakes of this vitamin.

Healing of wounds is defective in scurvy because of poor collagen formation. Experimentally deficient subjects fail to form new collagen in experimental wounds until the vitamin is administered. Delayed healing of wounds, postoperative breakdown of incisions, and delayed union of fractures may sometimes be at least partly the result of unrecognized but severe ascorbic acid deficiency. It is also known that extensive trauma and infectious diseases lower the plasma concentration of the vitamin. Ascorbic acid appears to be transported to wounds soon after injury, its concentration rising there as the plasma concentration falls, perhaps because the vitamin is needed for new ground substance and collagen formation.

Patients with thermal burns may develop ascorbic

Figure 4. Ecchymoses, petechiae, and perifollicular hemorrhages on legs of patient with scurvy.

acid deficiency, especially when the burns are extensive and deep. Large doses of the vitamin may be necessary to maintain even low-normal plasma concentrations. Such deficiency leads to delayed healing of burns and impaired skin graft "takes."

Attention to nutrient intake, including that of ascorbic acid, is an essential part of the medical care of many illnesses. For example, the diet prescribed for peptic ulcer may be almost free of ascorbic acid, a situation which favors bleeding rather than healing.

Treatment and Prevention. Small amounts of ascorbic acid will promptly reverse the florid clinical manifestations of scurvy. Even in severe scurvy, 100 mg per day for several days, accompanied by a normal diet, usually produces rapid cure. Because retention is high in the deficient state, this is also sufficient to restore the normal 4- to 5-gram body content of the vitamin in a few weeks.

Prevention requires a diet containing adequate ascorbic acid. The vitamin is present in most fresh fruits and vegetables, and in liver. Citrus fruits are particularly good sources. Synthetic ascorbic acid is chemically identical, and is very cheap.

Attention must be paid to the prevention of infantile scurvy, for the disease continues to occur sporadically in the United States in spite of our knowledge of prevention. At least 2 ounces of orange juice or its ascorbic acid equivalent should be given to all infants after the first month.

When extensive wounds, fractures, or chronic infections are treated, supplementary ascorbic acid should be given if any reasonable doubt exists regarding previous nutrition with this vitamin. Patients with deep and extensive burns may require large amounts of ascorbic acid (200 to 500 mg daily) to maintain measurable blood concentrations.

Crandon, J. H., Lund, C. C., and Dill, D. B.: Experimental human scurvy. N. Engl. J. Med., 223:253, 1940.
Gupta, S. D., Chaudhuri, C. R., and Chatterjee, I. B.: Incapability of L-ascorbic acid synthesis by insects. Arch. Biochem. Biophys., 152:889, 1972.
Levenson, S. M., Green, R. W., Taylor, F. H. L., Robinson, P., Page, R. C., Johnson, R. E., and Lund, C. C.: Ascorbic acid, riboflavin, thiamin, and nicotinic acid in relation to severe injury, hemorrhage and infection in the human. Ann. Surg., 124:840, 1946.
Sebrell, W. H., Jr., and Harris, R. S. (eds.): The Vitamins: Chemistry, Physiology, Pathology, Methods. New York, Academic Press, Inc., 1967. (See Chapter 2, Ascorbic Acid, p. 305.)
Woodruff, C. W.: Ascorbic Acid, *In* Beaton, G. H., and McHenry, E. W. (eds.): Nutrition, a Comprehensive Treatise. Vol. 2. New York, Academic Press, Inc., 1964, p. 265.

722. HYPERVITAMINOSIS A AND D

Vitamin A is not normally excreted except during disease states. Therefore, massive doses may lead to increased storage in the liver and hepatomegaly. Toxicity from hypervitaminosis A brought on by eating polar bear liver has been reported since 1596 by Arctic explorers. A 500-gram polar bear liver may contain over nine million IU of vitamin A, more than twenty times the total normal liver reserves in man. Toxic symptoms are drowsiness, irritability, severe headache, and vomiting within a few hours after ingestion. Acute hypervitaminosis A was reported in an infant given a single dose

of 300,000 IU. Drowsiness, hydrocephalus with protrusion of the fontanel, and vomiting ensued 12 hours after administration. Hepatosplenomegaly, hypoplastic anemia, leukopenia, precocious skeletal development, clubbing of the fingers, and coarse, sparse hair have been reported from long-continued high doses in children. Most symptoms, but not the hepatomegaly and abnormal bone growth, clear with discontinuation of the vitamin.

Overdosage of any form of vitamin D is dangerous. The syndrome of hypervitaminosis D is characterized by hypercalcemia and by generalized calcinosis (deposition of calcium phosphate in a matrix of mucoproteins) affecting joints, synovial membranes, kidneys, myocardium, pulmonary alveoli, parathyroid glands, pancreas, skin, lymph glands, arteries, conjunctivae and cornea of the eyes, and the acid-secreting portion of the stomach. In advanced stages, demineralization of the bones occurs.

The exact borderline between tolerable and noxious doses is not known. Certainly the continuous ingestion of 150,000 IU per day may result in symptoms. It is possible that some infants may show hypercalcemia on relatively small doses of 2500 to 4000 IU per day. Retardation of linear growth in children has been reported with 1800 IU per day. Complete recovery usually occurs when vitamin D is temporarily withdrawn. Treatment should include lowering of the calcium intake and a generous fluid intake.

Dam, H., and Søndergaard, E.: Fat-soluble vitamins. *In* Beaton, G. H., and McHenry, E. W. (eds.): Nutrition, A Comprehensive Treatise. Vol. II. New York, Academic Press, 1964, pp. 34–35.
Sebrell, W. H., Jr., and Harris, R. S. (eds.): The Vitamins: Chemistry, Physiology, Pathology, Methods. Vol. I. 2nd ed. New York and London, Academic Press, 1967.
Stimson, W. H.: Vitamin A intoxication in adults. Report of a case with summary of the literature. N. Engl. J. Med., 265:369, 1961.

723. OBESITY

Margaret J. Albrink

The differentiation of adipose tissue was a triumph of evolution. Phylogenetically the ability to store fat in true adipose tissue appeared first in the arthropods and became fully developed in birds and mammals; it was very likely an important factor in the liberation of life from the sea with its constant source of food. However, the ability to store fat in compact form, of great survival value when food was scarce, has become a handicap in affluent societies where overnutrition and underactivity have upset the ancient balance between caloric supply and demand. The consequence is obesity of epidemic proportions and the associated diseases of atherosclerosis, hypertension, and diabetes.

Definition. Obesity may be defined as excess adipose tissue. The dividing point between normal and excessive may be determined esthetically as fatness beyond the socially acceptable norms, or medically as adipose tissue in excess of that consistent with good health of mind and body. The latter definition includes the mild to moderate obesity characteristic of a large segment of our population, of paramount public health significance because of the associated toll of cardiovascular and other diseases.

Incidence. The exact incidence is uncertain because of difficulty in measuring degree of obesity. When compared to their desirable weight, 30 per cent of men and 40 per cent of women are 20 pounds or more overweight.

Etiology. Obesity results from the relative excess of caloric intake over caloric expenditure. Most cases of obesity seen in common clinical practice are due to the interaction of cultural forces that encourage excess intake with genetic factors that, other things being equal, favor the synthesis of fat.

Cultural Factors. First the agricultural, then the industrial, and finally the computer revolution have all served to make food increasingly available and life livable with a minimum of physical exertion. An important cause of widespread moderate obesity in the United States is the plethora of purified foods of high caloric content but low nutrient value.

Genetic Factors. Obesity, especially in its extreme form, tends to be familial. Obesity in children is much more common when both parents are obese than when neither parent is obese. Anabolic forces appear to be in operation from birth in very heavy people. (See below: Central Nervous System Regulation.) Heavy children usually become heavy adults, and differ constitutionally from lean persons in being statistically of shorter stature and greater breadth of trunk and in having small hands and feet. The localization of extreme deposits of fat, such as the massive adipose tissue over the buttocks of certain Bushmen, the so-called "Hottentot bustle," is an instance of genetically determined localized adiposity. This extreme example suggests that the number of adipose cells may be in part genetically determined and that the number and location of such cells or their precursors will determine in part the magnitude as well as the location of obesity.

Endocrine Factors. Many endocrine and metabolic abnormalities have been reported in very obese persons. Most are probably secondary to obesity (see below: Complications).

Sex. Women have a greater amount of subcutaneous fat than men. The relationship between parity and obesity and the frequent menopausal gain in weight, although difficult to document, suggest a possible role of female sex hormones in the regulation of fat metabolism. Administration of estrogens in rather high doses such as are present in birth control pills may cause obesity. The obesity of eunuchs suggests further that absence of male sex hormones also promotes adiposity. The hypogonad obesity that occurs in children just prior to adolescence disappears with puberty, at which time the adult fat distribution of each sex takes place. The effect of sex hormones could be explained by emotional factors and physical activity rather than by a direct effect on fat metabolism.

Age. The tendency to gain weight with advancing age is associated with increased mortality from cardiovascular and other diseases, and cannot be considered normal.

Central Nervous System Regulation of Food Intake. The role of the central nervous system in controlling food intake resides chiefly in the hypothalamus. A satiety center in the ventral medial hypothalamus exerts an inhibitory influence on a neighboring feeding center. Destruction of the inhibitory center releases the feeding center, with resultant massive overeating and hypothalamic obesity. Brain injury in man on occasion causes obesity, but the extent to which variation in the balance between these centers contributes to ordinary obesity is unknown. Very early overfeeding may "set" the regulatory centers in such a manner that obesity, manifest by

an irreversibly increased number of adipose cells, persists in later life.

Behavioral and Emotional Aspects. Decreased activity rather than increased food intake is recognized in many obese persons, particularly obese women. Associated depression is a frequent concomitant of inactivity, and may be exaggerated by weight loss. The very obese person has a characteristic eating pattern in which the major caloric intake occurs at the evening meal or later.

Some distinctive behavioral traits have been described in obese persons, although whether they are causes or effects is uncertain. Unlike slender persons, the obese seem to depend on external rather than internal cues to initiate feeding. They eat in response to clock time, to the attractiveness and availability of food, and to other external cues rather than to internal signals of hunger and satiety. Correspondingly there is an inability to recognize and cope with inner needs and feelings. Behavior such as eating that should be dictated from inner needs is attached, rather, to external cues. Such lack of self-direction could result from lack of early life experiences which normally encourage development of ego identity. Another interpretation of dependence on external cues is that the obese are inwardly always hungry but outwardly always trying to exhibit socially acceptable behavior.

Like most of man's ills at one time or another, obesity has been blamed on the world's domineering mothers. The role of mothers in causing obesity in children can as well be attributed to their enforcement in early life of patterns of overeating as to the psychologic effects of overprotection.

Pathology. Two general types of distribution of obesity are described. Obesity in the male is most pronounced in the upper trunk and spares the extremities. In the female, distribution is predominantly in the lower trunk and involves also the extremities, particularly the lower extremities.

Excess adipose tissue is found subcutaneously, interspersed in muscle and about all organs. Extremely obese persons have generally enlarged organs; cardiac enlargement is mainly left ventricular, and may be due to the increased circulating blood volume and/or hypertension commonly present. The kidney, liver, and, indeed, the entire splanchnic area are of greater size than normal. Large fatty livers are frequently found in extreme obesity.

Cellularity. Hirsch, Salans, and Knittle and their colleagues, using a new method for estimating adipose cell size and number from adipose tissue sampled by needle biopsy, have studied the cellularity of adipose tissue. In man and in several other species the number of adipose cells increases until the onset of adult life. Thereafter the adipose mass is expanded only by increasing the size of existing cells. In man, probably no new adipose cells are laid down after age 20, although methodologic variability prevents exclusion of possible later addition of cells. Two periods of rapid adipose cell number expansion have been identified: very early in the first few years, and again between ages 9 and 13.

Two groups of obese persons can be identified: those with normal numbers of cells but increased cell size (hyperplastic) and those with increased numbers of cells which might or might not also be enlarged (hypercellular). The two types can best be separated by age of onset. Obesity of onset early in life is associated with increased numbers of adipose cells, whereas adult onset obesity is associated with normal cell number but increased size of cell. Extreme obesity is usually of the juvenile onset hypercellular type.

Sims and colleagues confirmed the hyperplastic nature of obesity of the adult onset type. Lean volunteers who purposely gain weight expand their existing adipose cells but do not add any new adipose cells. By the same token, weight loss in the obese is accomplished by shrinkage of existing adipose cells, not by loss of cells. Once laid down, the number of cells is immutable.

Hirsch et al. found behavioral differences between "adult onset" and "juvenile onset" diabetes. The lifelong hypercellular obese experience depression, fatigue, anxiety, and distortion in timing perception and body image during weight reduction. On both theoretic and practical grounds, therefore, weight reduction might seem more practical in adult onset obesity, where weight reduction and cell shrinkage should restore normal adipose cell size and number, than in the hypercellular obese, in whom no amount of dieting will reduce the number of adipose cells.

The cellularity of adipose tissue varies greatly from site to site so that information obtained by biopsy is of more statistical than diagnostic value in a single individual. There is some evidence that hypercellular obesity is distributed both on the trunk and on the extremities, whereas acquired hypertrophic obesity is more confined to the trunk. The finding of an obese trunk with thin arms and legs would thus suggest acquired obesity.

Pathogenesis. The balance between fat synthesis and fat mobilization depends on several key reactions in the adipose cell and the influence of various hormones, as well as state of nutrition, on these reactions. A shift in the adipose cell toward increased synthesis of fat or decreased mobilization of fat would operate to cause obesity.

Synthesis of Triglyceride. Triglycerides are synthesized within the adipose cell from one alpha-glycerol-phosphate molecule and three fatty acid molecules. The latter may be synthesized within the adipose cell from glucose, a reaction favored by reduced nicotinamide adenine dinucleotide phosphate (NADPH) (reduced triphosphopyridine nucleotide), or may be derived from circulating fatty acids of dietary or endogenous origin. By contrast, the alpha-glycerol-phosphate must be derived from glucose metabolized within the adipose cell. The glycerol liberated from triglyceride breakdown cannot serve this purpose since adipose tissue lacks appreciable glycerol kinase, the enzyme necessary for converting glycerol into alpha-glycerol-phosphate. The availability of glucose thus determines the availability of alpha-glycerol-phosphate, which in turn is obligatory for triglyceride synthesis in adipose tissue.

Circulating triglycerides such as those present in chylomicrons are evidently available to the adipose cell only if they are first broken down into glycerol and free fatty acids, a reaction taking place at or near the adipose cell wall under the influence of the enzyme lipoprotein lipase. This enzyme is increased in the carbohydrate-fed state, decreased in starvation. Since the enzyme appears in the circulation after heparin injection, it is also called post-heparin lipoprotein lipase. The free fatty acids liberated by the action of lipoprotein lipase enter the adipose cell, where they are re-esterified into triglyceride, provided alpha-glycerol-phosphate is present.

The latter must be derived from carbohydrate combustion. Carbohydrate combustion has the additional effect of generating NADPH via the pentose phosphate shunt, and NADPH favors the synthesis of fat from two-carbon precursors.

Insulin occupies a central role in the regulation of adipose cell metabolism. High insulin concentration inhibits lipolysis and favors fat synthesis. When insulin concentration is low, fat synthesis ceases and lipolysis proceeds. Insulin acts by stimulating the lipogenic actions of glucose metabolism noted above. In addition, insulin directly inhibits lipolysis.

In man and certain other species, the liver is an important site for new triglyceride synthesis. The triglycerides are packaged as very low density lipoproteins (VLDL) and secreted into the bloodstream. The VLDL triglyceride, just as with chylomicron triglyceride, is taken up by adipose tissue for storage under the influence of lipoprotein lipase when metabolic factors favor fat synthesis, that is, when carbohydrate metabolism is active and insulin is available.

Fat Mobilization. Fat is mobilized entirely in the form of free fatty acids. The release of fat from the adipose cell is accomplished by activation of an intracellular lipolytic system different from lipoprotein lipase. The activation is dependent upon generation of cyclic adenosine monophosphate (cyclic AMP). This system splits triglycerides into free fatty acids and glycerol. The liberated free fatty acids are either re-esterified into triglyceride, provided conditions favor fat synthesis, or are transported into the circulation bound to albumin as free fatty acids, either to be utilized by tissue or transported to the liver for re-esterification into triglyceride. A rise in concentration of circulating free fatty acids is evidence of fat mobilization.

Fat mobilization is favored by various hormones that activate the lytic system, of which epinephrine, norepinephrine, and growth hormone are probably of the greatest physiologic significance. Factors that stimulate epinephrine secretion such as exercise and trauma thus activate mobilization of fat. The absence of carbohydrate combustion as in starvation or diabetic acidosis also results in fat mobilization. Low concentration of circulating insulin characterizes both situations. The removal of the suppressing effect of insulin on lipolysis permits lipolysis to proceed. Alpha-glycerol-phosphate ceases to be synthesized from glucose in amounts sufficient for re-esterification of all the liberated fatty acids, and net loss of triglyceride from adipose tissue takes place. Through these systems the deposition or mobilization of fat is regulated by the presence or absence of food, especially carbohydrate, and by the presence or absence of emergencies that require fat as fuel for sudden bursts of energy.

Adipose Cell Metabolism in Obesity. Certain aspects of adipose tissue metabolism of obese persons are referable to the increased cell size of adult onset obesity. Hirsch and Salans and their colleagues have reported that the well known insulin resistance of obese persons is related to the oversized adipocytes and that normal insulin responsiveness is restored by weight loss and resulting cell size reduction. The large adipocyte is characterized by insensitivity to the stimulating effect of insulin on glucose oxidation and on synthesis of fatty acids from glucose and by increased basal and epinephrine-stimulated lipolysis. Similar abnormalities are found in the expanded adipocytes of lean individuals who have undergone forced weight gain. The abnormal findings are reversed by weight loss.

The decreased antilipolytic and lipogenic effect of insulin in large adipose cells has been proposed as a possible cause for the insulin resistance of the obese. Several theories have been advanced to account for the lack of insulin responsiveness. A lack of insulin binding sites on adipose cells or a defect in some aspect of intracellular glucose metabolism has been proposed, but no specific metabolic locus has been identified with certainty.

Prior diet exerts an important influence on adipose cell metabolism. The insulin insensitivity of both spontaneous and forced obesity can be overcome if sufficient carbohydrate is fed prior to biopsy. The large adipose cell thus appears to require more carbohydrate calories to maintain triglyceride storage than does the small adipose cell.

Several arguments can be made against the existence of a primary deficit in insulin responsiveness specific to large adipose cells. Similar insulin resistance is demonstrable in many, perhaps all, tissues of obese persons. The insulin resistance can be induced by forced weight gain and can be reversed by weight loss, and is therefore secondary. The resistance may, rather, be caused by a general lipolytic state which can be overcome by sufficient carbohydrate calories. The lipolytic state, in turn, perhaps through the known anti-insulin effects of increased intracellular free fatty acids, could be responsible for the insulin resistance at the tissue level. That increased lipolytic tendency and obesity coexist must mean that the weight-stable or weight-gaining obese person eats more than enough to overcome the lipolytic state.

Lipolysis is an adrenergic function. Its regulation and its modulation by nutrient intake may be controlled by the central nervous system, probably through certain hypothalamic centers. Such centers may also control the level of nutrient intake necessary to reverse the lipolytic state and may control the feeding behavior needed to ensure such intake. The observed lipolytic tendency of large adipocytes may merely reflect recent caloric deprivation relative to the requirements of the hypothalamic "set" for that individual. The nature of such a "set" if it exists, the signals to which it responds, and its potential for change are uncertain.

Manifestations and Complications. The sheer mechanical trauma of excessive body weight either aggravates or causes such troublesome ailments as osteoarthritis and flat feet, intertriginous dermatitis, varicose veins, and ventral and diaphragmatic hernias. Cholelithiasis and cholecystitis are more common in the obese than in the lean.

Obesity-Hypoventilation Syndrome. Dickens' graphic description of Fat Joe, a character in *Pickwick Papers* who fell asleep at the most inopportune moments, led to the eponym *pickwickian syndrome.* This condition, which appears in some very obese persons, is characterized by hypoventilation, somnolence, and carbon dioxide retention (Pco_2 values consistently elevated above 48 mm of mercury). Decreased compliance of the thoracic wall and consequent increased work of respiration are thus evidently penalties of extreme obesity. Failure to make the necessary increased respiratory effort to move the ponderous thoracic wall initiates the syndrome. Ventilation-perfusion disturbances also occur. Possible underlying pulmonary disease may be a factor in some patients. Hypoxia, pulmonary hypertension, secondary polycythemia, and, eventually, cardiopulmonary failure ensue. All symptoms are improved by weight loss.

Hemodynamic Complications. Very obese persons have a greater than normal total circulating blood volume and increased cardiac output, stroke volume, and cardiac work, probably because of the additional vascular bed of the excess adipose tissue. The blood volume per unit weight of adipose tissue, however, is less than that for lean tissue, with the result that the circulating blood volume per kilogram of body weight is less than for a lean person.

Hypertension. Studies around the world show a correlation between blood pressure and obesity. To a large extent the increased death rate of obese persons is due to hypertension. Increased stroke volume, a consequence of the increased cardiac output in the presence usually of a normal heart rate, may be in part responsible for the hypertension and left ventricular hypertrophy in obese persons. Peripheral resistance is normal or low. The hypertension and hemodynamic abnormalities are improved by weight loss.

Endocrine Complications. Sims and his colleagues, in studies of experimental obesity in man, have compared the metabolic abnormalities found in spontaneous obesity with those induced in normal subjects by forced overeating. Most of the abnormalities found in spontaneous obesity could be induced in the volunteers, and were reversed by weight loss in both spontaneous obesity and induced obesity. The abnormalities are therefore probably the result rather than the cause of the obesity. The picture in intact obese man, as in the large adipose cell, is that of decreased sensitivity to insulin. Increased concentrations of plasma glucose, amino acids, and insulin are the result. Since the induced obesity was achieved entirely by increasing cell size rather than number, the metabolic abnormalities were associated with adipose cell hypertrophy. The only metabolic difference between spontaneous and induced obesity was the greater number of calories required to maintain weight in induced obesity. The plasma free fatty acid concentration in induced obesity was found to be low, secondary to the high carbohydrate diet needed for weight gain. Free fatty acid concentration is elevated in spontaneous obesity only when there is associated diabetes, free fatty acids being normal in nondiabetic obese.

HYPERINSULINEMIA. Elevation of plasma insulin is a striking feature of obese nondiabetics. Fasting plasma insulin concentrations of 30 μU per milliliter or higher and postcibal concentrations in excess of 300 μU per milliliter are not uncommon in nondiabetic obese. In contrast, fasting and postcibal values for lean persons are usually well below 20 μU per milliliter and 150 μU per milliliter, respectively.

The insulin increase after a glucose challenge in the obese, when expressed relative to the basal insulin concentration, is appropriate for the degree of hyperglycemia. The basal insulin, however, is inappropriately high for the degree of fasting glycemia in obese persons. The increase in fasting insulin is thus the critical difference between thin and obese persons.

According to Felig and colleagues, the explanation for the elevated basal insulin may be the high fasting concentrations of those amino acids which stimulate the release of insulin and which are decreased in response to insulin. Insensitivity of the tissue to insulin accounts for the increase in insulin-sensitive substrates, such as certain amino acids as well as glucose and probably others. The fact of insulin insensitivity is communicated to the pancreas by increased concentrations of such substrates, but the resulting increased insulin concentration is less effective in restoring substrate levels to normal than is a similar concentration of insulin in slender persons. The reason for the insulin insensitivity of the obese is not known. In the case of obese adipose tissue, insulin insensitivity is related to increased cell size (see above). With weight reduction cell size returns to normal, and insulin sensitivity is restored.

THYROID FUNCTION IN OBESITY. Although the usual parameters of thyroid function are normal in obesity, Bray has reported an abnormality in the adipose tissue of obese persons which is corrected by administration of triiodothyronine. The defect is a deficiency in the mitochondrial oxidation of glycerol phosphate. Since this reaction may favor energy wastage and thus prevent weight gain in overfed persons, such a deficiency might cause obesity. However, in later studies similar deficiency was induced by forced weight gain in normal volunteers. Bray has also found an increase in the concentration of circulating triiodothyronine. The increase is probably secondary to tissue resistance to the action of triiodothyronine. Thus the demonstrated abnormalities in thyroid metabolism are the result of obesity, not the cause.

GROWTH HORMONE IN OBESITY. Several hormones of the anterior pituitary cause mobilization of fat from adipose tissue. The most important is growth hormone, which promotes mobilization and utilization of fat and conservation of protein and carbohydrate during caloric restriction. Growth hormone is secreted in response to hypoglycemia, hyperaminoacidemia, exercise, and other stimuli, and is spontaneously secreted during deep sleep. In both spontaneous and induced obesity the growth hormone response to hypoglycemia and to arginine infusion is reduced, as is the nocturnal rise. The normal increase in growth hormone in response to starvation is less marked in obese than in nonobese subjects. Obese persons respond to prolonged fasting with a less than normal rise in free fatty acids, a phenomenon probably reflecting the decreased secretion of growth hormone. The growth hormone hyposecretion is secondary to the obesity and is corrected by weight loss.

ADRENOCORTICAL FUNCTION IN OBESITY. Increased plasma cortisol concentration may occur in obesity. Increased cortisol secretory rate reported in spontaneous and induced obesity is related merely to increased body mass. The abnormalities are secondary to the obesity.

Diabetes. Diabetes is four times more common in obese than in lean adults, and with its toll of vascular disease accounts for some of the risk of obesity. The hyperinsulinemia of the obese may be a contributing factor to their increased susceptibility to diabetes. Over many years such increased insulin production may lead to pancreatic exhaustion and diabetes, accounting for the association between obesity and diabetes. When diabetes coincides with obesity, the rise of plasma insulin relative to plasma glucose after glucose ingestion is blunted, as in nonobese diabetics. The insulin increments, being superimposed on the increased basal levels, result in higher insulin values for each degree of glucose tolerance in the obese than in the nonobese. Weight loss greatly relieves the burden on the pancreas by decreasing both the basal and postcibal needs for insulin, with the result that glucose tolerance may become normal.

Atherosclerosis. The influence of obesity on atherosclerotic vascular disease and on serum lipids is discussed later in this chapter.

Diagnosis. Simple precise methods for measuring degree of obesity are lacking. The amount of body fat can be estimated from whole-body specific gravity or from the thickness of subcutaneous fat measured by skin-fold calipers or roentgenographically. The contribution of lean body mass to the total body mass can also be determined from whole-body radioactive potassium and the fat body mass indirectly calculated. The discussion of assessment of nutritional status (see Ch. 713) contains further information on methods for evaluating nutritional state.

The most commonly used method, however, remains the height-weight tables. In Table 1 may be seen the ranges of desirable weight, i.e., weight associated with lowest mortality according to insurance company data obtained from large numbers of policyholders. Desirable weight approximates that at age 25; this stresses the fact that weight gain during adult life is associated with increased mortality.

If a person weighs more than the upper limit of his ideal weight for his frame, he may be considered overweight, and if he is 20 pounds in excess of his ideal weight he is generally considered obese. Degree of obesity is often denoted as relative weight, the actual weight expressed as a percentage of desirable weight.

TABLE 1. Desirable Weights for Men and Women According to Height and Frame, Ages 25 and Over*

Height (in Shoes)†	Weight in Pounds (in Indoor Clothing)		
	Small Frame	Medium Frame	Large Frame
Men			
5 ft 2 in	112–120	118–129	126–141
5 ft 3 in	115–123	121–133	129–144
5 ft 4 in	118–126	124–136	132–148
5 ft 5 in	121–129	127–139	135–152
5 ft 6 in	124–133	130–143	138–156
5 ft 7 in	128–137	134–147	142–161
5 ft 8 in	132–141	138–152	147–166
5 ft 9 in	136–145	142–156	151–170
5 ft 10 in	140–150	146–160	155–174
5 ft 11 in	144–154	150–165	159–179
6 ft 0 in	148–158	154–170	164–184
6 ft 1 in	152–162	158–175	168–189
6 ft 2 in	156–167	162–180	173–194
6 ft 3 in	160–171	167–185	177–199
6 ft 4 in	164–175	172–190	182–204
Women			
4 ft 10 in	92–98	96–107	104–119
4 ft 11 in	94–101	98–110	106–122
5 ft 0 in	96–104	101–113	109–124
5 ft 1 in	99–107	104–116	112–128
5 ft 2 in	102–110	107–119	115–131
5 ft 3 in	105–113	110–122	118–134
5 ft 4 in	108–116	113–126	121–138
5 ft 5 in	111–119	116–130	125–142
5 ft 6 in	114–123	120–135	129–146
5 ft 7 in	118–127	124–139	133–150
5 ft 8 in	122–131	128–143	137–154
5 ft 9 in	126–135	132–147	141–158
5 ft 10 in	130–140	136–151	145–163
5 ft 11 in	134–144	140–155	149–168
6 ft 0 in	138–148	144–159	153–174

*Prepared by the Metropolitan Life Insurance Company. Derived primarily from data of the Build and Blood Pressure Study, 1959.
†1 inch heels for men and 2 inch heels for women.

Several height-weight indices are commonly used to express obesity, but, like other measures based on height and weight, actually measure body bulk rather than obesity. Of these indices the ponderal index, height/$\sqrt[3]{weight}$, and the body mass index, weight/height² × 100, are best, the latter being most independent of height.

The chief drawback of height-weight indices is their failure to take into account the variable contributions of lean and fat body mass to total body weight. The measurement of subcutaneous fat with skin-fold calipers avoids this difficulty. Skin-fold thickness, preferably measured at several sites, correlates rather well with total body fat estimated from specific gravity, and has the advantage of ease and simplicity of measurement. Special calipers have been designed for the purpose. The results of the community-wide study of Tecumseh, Michigan, although not necessarily representative of the world, provide guide lines for comparison of individual readings (Table 2). Ideal standards for skin-fold thickness are not yet available. As with weight, mean subscapular skin-fold thickness at age 25 (12.4 mm.) might be considered desirable.

Differential Diagnosis. *Hypothyroidism.* The weight gain in hypothyroidism is usually only moderate, and is due in part to accumulation of myxedematous fluid as well as to adipose tissue. The reduction in caloric expenditure contributes to the obesity. The usual measurements of thyroid function such as serum thyroxine concentration and I^{131} uptake are normal in ordinary obesity, and thus can be used to exclude hypothyroidism as a contributing cause of obesity. Hypothyroidism is rarely the cause of obesity.

TABLE 2.   Subscapular and Triceps Skinfold by Age and Sex (Values in Millimeters)*

	Age (Yr)	Male Subjects, Percentiles			Female Subjects, Percentiles		
		20	50	80	20	50	80
Subscapular	20–24	8.0	12.1	19.2	8.6	13.2	21.7
	25–29	8.8	12.4	20.9	9.1	13.2	20.4
	30–34	9.1	15.1	24.3	9.0	13.6	21.2
	35–39	8.9	14.7	21.4	9.7	16.9	24.8
	40–44	10.9	16.3	23.5	11.4	17.6	28.2
	45–49	11.0	17.3	25.9	13.0	20.8	29.1
	50–54	9.9	17.3	24.6	13.4	21.0	33.2
	55–59	11.8	18.8	30.7	13.5	22.3	32.0
	60–64	9.3	16.8	24.8	15.5	22.4	33.6
	65–69	8.0	12.5	17.4	13.0	20.9	30.0
	70–74	8.7	14.3	23.1	14.0	22.6	29.9
	75–79	9.9	14.8	20.8	10.0	21.6	31.2
Triceps	20–24	7.2	11.0	17.8	12.5	17.5	23.4
	25–29	7.1	10.4	16.7	12.1	17.5	23.8
	30–34	7.9	12.3	17.8	13.0	18.1	25.0
	35–39	7.4	11.8	17.3	14.1	20.0	26.0
	40–44	8.0	12.4	17.6	15.2	20.7	27.3
	45–49	8.6	12.5	17.3	16.3	22.1	27.7
	50–54	8.7	12.0	18.7	18.1	22.7	26.9
	55–59	9.9	14.0	18.7	17.3	22.9	28.8
	60–64	8.6	11.7	17.8	18.3	24.7	31.5
	65–69	7.1	10.9	15.4	17.2	21.8	26.6
	70–74	8.1	11.8	15.3	16.0	21.2	26.0
	75–79	7.4	13.5	17.2	12.2	20.0	26.0

*From Montoye, H. J., Epstein, F. H., and Kjelsberg, M. O.: Am. J. Clin. Nutr., 16:417, 1965.

Cushing's Disease. Hyperadrenocorticism causes moderate obesity that chiefly involves the face, causing the typical moon facies, the thorax, and abdomen, but spares the buttocks and extremities. The fat pad over the last cervical vertebra, the so-called buffalo hump, is characteristic, but may also occur in ordinary obesity, for example, the "dowager's hump" of the postmenopausal woman.

The presence of purple striae of the skin of the abdomen and elsewhere suggests Cushing's disease. However, striae are common in persons who gain weight rapidly. Obese adolescents frequently have striae of the upper arms, breasts, abdomen, hips, and thighs, although adrenal function is normal.

The differentiation of obesity with and without Cushing's disease may present difficulties because of the frequency with which the results of tests used to diagnose Cushing's disease are slightly abnormal in obesity. Elevated urinary 17-ketosteroids and 17-hydroxycorticosteroids as well as increased rate of cortisol secretion are common in obesity. The two most helpful tests for excluding Cushing's disease in obese patients are the diurnal variation in plasma cortisol conentration (usually lost in Cushing's disease but preserved in obesity) and the dexamethasone suppression test. Suppression is normal in the obese but impaired in Cushing's disease.

Stein-Leventhal Syndrome. In a woman, obesity, hirsutism, and infertility suggest this syndrome. The finding of large cystic ovaries on physical examination is confirmatory, although surgical exploration may be necessary for verification. Tests of adrenal cortical function are normal as a rule.

Insulinoma, Hyperinsulinism. The carbohydrate feeding necessary to counteract frequent hypoglycemic attacks may lead to obesity.

Treatment of Obesity. *General Considerations.* Reduction of excess weight in obese persons is associated with improvement in hypertension, in the hemodynamic abnormalities, and in diabetes, as well as with amelioration of the mechanical effects of the adipose mass. Weight reduction is highly desirable for a large segment of our population yet it is singularly difficult to achieve.

There is no satisfactory treatment for obesity. Once established, it is remarkably self-sustaining. Even if weight is temporarily lost, the former weight is regained with astonishing regularity—within months as a rule, within five years almost certainly. A patient who has successfully lost weight must be prepared for a lifetime of vigilance if he is to maintain his success. Nonetheless, the benefits to be expected from weight loss justify the utmost effort on the part of both physician and patient to bring about and maintain optimal weight. If successful, such measures correct or improve the hypertension, the diabetes, and the abnormal serum lipids associated with excess calories, and relieve the mechanical injuries resulting from the increased adipose mass.

Of the three main approaches to obesity—drugs, diet, and exercise—diet is the mainstay of treatment. An understanding of the physiologic changes that accompany caloric restriction is essential if the patient's progress is to be understood. Under dietary treatment, the outlook for the extremely obese patient who has as much as a hundred pounds or more to lose is dismal. Perhaps the most hopeful outlook can be expected for the slightly obese patient who has only a few pounds to lose. Because such patients account for the great majority of cardiovascular disease victims in this country, every effort should be made to reach them and to achieve weight reduction.

Diet. EFFECT OF CALORIC RESTRICTION. The seemingly simple and logical limitation of calories below caloric expenditure is often made difficult by the metabolic changes that occur in response to caloric restriction. After initial satisfactory weight loss of one to two or more pounds a week, a plateau is reached. The patient claims continued adherence to the diet, yet no further weight is lost. He finally yields to discouragement, abandons the diet altogether, and gains back all of the lost weight or even more.

One reason for this failure is that too much is expected of caloric restriction. Of the tissue lost, fat and protein tissue differ in their caloric density. Pure fat yields 9 calories per gram. Adipose tissue, consisting mainly of fat with little water, contains about 8 calories per gram of tissue. Protein, on the other hand, gives 4 calories per gram of protein, and carries with it about three or four times its weight in intracellular water. Protein tissue thus gives only about 0.8 calorie per gram, one tenth that of adipose tissue on a weight basis. If, for instance, a caloric deficit of 500 calories were derived only from protein tissue, it could be calculated that 620 grams of protein and water or more than a pound a day would be lost. If only fat tissue were lost, a mere 62-gram tissue loss a day, chiefly fat, would account for the 500 calories.

Actually a mixture of protein and fat tissue is lost. Some nitrogen loss is acceptable since the excess tissue of obese persons contains 10 to 30 grams of nitrogen per kilogram of excess weight. The tendency for negative nitrogen balance in the early days of caloric restriction favors loss largely of protein tissue and thus large weight loss. However, particularly in the very obese, with continued caloric restriction the body reacts by defense of its nitrogen reserves, and the nitrogen balance becomes less negative. If nitrogen balance is established, weight loss then results only from loss of adipose tissue, and occurs very slowly. The nitrogen-conserving defense is so great that positive nitrogen balance can occur on the same diet that initially caused nitrogen loss. Conceivably, protein synthesis taking place concomitantly with loss of calories from adipose tissue could create new protein-rich tissue that would more than equal in weight the adipose tissue lost, with resulting net weight gain despite continued caloric deficit. How long this state of affairs could last is not known, but the tendency toward positive nitrogen balance when undernourished persons are refed full diets may last for months.

The adaptation to caloric restriction includes a strong anabolic tendency that may be manifest not only as nitrogen retention but also as increased synthesis of fat from available carbohydrate. Adaptive hyperlipogenesis in laboratory animals is the greatly augmented synthesis of fat from carbohydrate on refeeding after a period of starvation. If this phenomenon occurs in humans, it would account further for the tendency to regain lost weight.

Not only do the logistics of weight loss from protein and fat tissue favor plateau and even weight gain in obese persons undergoing caloric restriction, but the tendency of such patients to retain sodium and extracellular water is further reason for weight gain. The resultant edema may be refractory to thiazide diuretics or salt restriction. The likelihood of depression, decreased activity, hunger, decreased metabolic rate, and weakness all operate against the successful continuation of a calorically restricted diet.

SPECIFIC DIETS. Conservative nutritionists recommend a balanced diet, including 1 gram of protein per kilogram of ideal body weight and fat roughly equal in weight to the protein, the remainder of the calories to be made up from carbohydrate. From 800 to 1800 calories are commonly recommended, depending on activity, size, and desired speed of weight loss. However, the few available long-term studies show discouraging results on all diets. There is no basis for recommending any one diet over any other.

UNBALANCED DIETS. A variety of unbalanced diets have been proposed. Because they stimulate the patient's imagination, so-called "fad" diets, though the despair of dietitians, may elicit greater patient cooperation than conservative diets.

Two possibilities which might justify the various unbalanced diets are better patient acceptance or greater caloric loss for a given level of caloric intake. Some experimental evidence exists for both possibilities. Dietary imbalance of nutrients such as amino acids fed to laboratory animals may be recognized by the central nervous system and may lead to spontaneous decrease in food intake. Similar mechanisms interpreted as unpalatability or anorexia may limit intake of unbalanced diet in man and might facilitate adherence.

The second rationale, that certain foodstuffs are less efficiently used than others, has received some support from experiments in man and animals. The old concept of "luxuskonsumption," or the ability to maintain stable weight despite varying caloric intake, has been the subject of renewed interest and has been reviewed by Sims et al. Implicit in the concept is the assumption that calories fed in excess of those needed are less efficiently utilized and are in part lost as heat, with the result that less weight is gained than expected. The energy wastage of excess calories is explained in part by the greater number of energy-requiring metabolic steps required when fuel must first be converted to its storage forms than when it is utilized directly. The energy wastage of a high protein diet is well known and is attributed in part to the energy required for conversion of excess nitrogen to urea and its subsequent excretion by the kidneys. In hypocaloric diets the efficiency of protein, fat, and carbohydrate utilization is increased. This, together with a well-known decrease in metabolic rate with caloric deprivation, tends to minimize weight loss on weight reduction diets. Whether any particular hypocaloric diet will cause more rapid weight loss has not been demonstrated.

LOW PROTEIN DIET. On the assumption that a certain amount of excess tissue is nitrogen, and that the tendency of obese patients to retain nitrogen may defeat efforts at weight loss, some argument may be made for a low protein diet. The dangers of severe protein deficiency, especially liver disease, must be remembered. The classic concept that 1 gram of nitrogen per kilogram per day is needed for nitrogen balance has been revised downward by the World Health Organization to about 0.5 gram of nitrogen per kilogram per day.

LOW CARBOHYDRATE DIET. On theoretical grounds a low carbohydrate diet should be effective by discouraging lipogenesis and preventing reactive hypoglycemia with its attendant hunger. As noted under pathogenesis, dietary carbohydrate favors lipogenesis at several steps. It is also required for the manifestation of salt and water retention so commonly encountered during weight reduction. Limitation of carbohydrate to 50 or 60 grams a day but with *ad libitum* intake of protein and fat causes initial rapid weight loss (largely water), mild ketosis, and absence of hunger, and is usually well tolerated. Total calories are voluntarily limited to 1300 or so because of reduced palatability of fat without carbohydrate. More extreme, nearly total carbohydrate restriction may cause hypercholesterolemia. The safety of associated prolonged ketonemia and ketonuria has not been established. The complications of total carbohydrate restriction are similar to those of total starvation noted below.

STARVATION. The treatment of obesity by total starvation is usually well tolerated for repeated periods of 10 to 15 days each, sometimes much longer, and causes an average weight loss of a pound a day. Marked persistent ketosis occurs, but less than 100 calories a day are lost as ketones. Complications include decreased uric acid excretion, and hyperuricemia, sometimes manifested as clinical gout. Postural hypotension, anemia, and cardiac irregularities may also occur. Upon refeeding, excess excretion of uric acid may cause uric acid nephropathy. Intense retention of sodium and water causes edema and weight gain. Both the uric acid excretion and sodium retention are dependent on dietary carbohydrate, as little as 40 grams a day being sufficient. Unless dietary supervision is continued, the lost weight is readily regained. Starvation is best reserved for hospitalized patients in whom rapid weight loss is mandatory, for some reason such as planned surgery.

FORMULA DIETS. Prepared liquid diets of high satiety value have the advantage of simplicity but the drawback of monotony. Long-term studies indicate no greater success with these than with any other diets.

Drugs. Appetite-suppressant drugs are effective for only a few weeks, whereas treatment of obesity is lifelong. Dependence on the stimulatory effect of the amphetamine group makes withdrawal a problem. Such drugs have no demonstrated role in the long-term management of obesity. Although thyroid hormone is occasionally prescribed for obesity, weight loss occurs only with toxic doses. Negative nitrogen balance may occur. Such treatment makes evaluation of thyroid function difficult because of suppression of endogenous thyroid secretion.

Exercise. The notoriously poor state of physical fitness of Americans undoubtedly contributes to their problem of obesity. Exercise, in addition to its obvious effect of expending calories, engenders a state of physical fitness with an accompanying sense of well-being. A program of gradually increasing exercise is an important part of the treatment of obesity. The caloric expenditure also varies with occupation (Table 3).

Jejunoileal Shunt. Bypass of all the small intestine except for a few inches of proximal jejunum and terminal ileum causes weight loss because of malabsorption. Severe nutritional cirrhosis and serious loss of water and electrolytes may occur unless patients are meticulously managed. The long-term results are not known.

Prevention. Prevention of weight gain after maturity is clearly more desirable than treatment of existing obesity. Once established, obesity seems to be self-perpetuating; the five-year cure rate is almost zero. Prevention means even further education of our already diet-conscious civilization. Such education might properly start with mothers who are responsible for establishing in their children life-long dietary patterns. Institutions, such as the army, that are responsible for feeding large segments of the population have an opportunity not only to establish restrained eating habits but to prevent weight gain in men during their tour of duty. Most important of all, and perhaps least achievable, would be the restraint by the food industry of its promotion of foodstuffs of high caloric but low nutritive value. The excess calories which contribute to mass obesity in the western world are derived mainly from products which the food industry has made too readily available. Purified fats and carbohydrates, either alone or combined in the form of rich pastries and other delicacies, are the worst offenders. Since an almost invariable result of food processing is the concentration of calories with loss of minerals and vitamins, a simple rule to apply would be to reduce the consumption of foodstuffs which require manufacturing at some stage of their preparation. The adoption in American homes of such simple diets with reservation of

TABLE 3.   Illustrations of How the Energy Expenditure May Be Distributed over 24 Hours and the Effect of Occupation*

| | Reference Man (65 kg, Age 20 to 39) | | | |
	Light Activity	Moderately Active	Very Active	Exceptionally Active
In bed (8 hours)	500	500	500	500
At work (8 hours)	1100	1400	1900	2400
Nonoccupational activities (8 hours)	700–1500	700–1500	700–1500	700–1500
Range of energy expenditure (24 hours)	2300–3100	2600–3400	3100–3900	3600–4400
Mean (24 hours)	2700	3000	3500	4000
	Reference Woman (55 kg, Age 20 to 39)			
	Light Activity	Moderately Active	Very Active	Exceptionally Active
In bed (8 hours)	420	420	420	420
At work (8 hours)	800	1000	1400	1800
Nonoccupational activities (8 hours)	580–980	580–980	580–980	580–980
Range of energy expenditure (24 hours)	1800–2200	2000–2400	2400–2700	2800–3200
Mean (24 hours)	2000	2200	2600	3000

*Adapted from "Energy and Protein Requirements." Report of a Joint FAO/WHO Ad Hoc Expert Committee. World Health Organization Technical Report Series, No. 522, Geneva, 1973, p. 29.

rich treats for special occasions would enhance appreciation of the special occasions and do much to eliminate obesity and its toll of vascular disease.

ATHEROSCLEROSIS AND OBESITY

The urgency of the problem of obesity is its role in the etiology of atherosclerosis and its most common lethal manifestation, ischemic heart disease.

Definition. Atherosclerosis is a type of arteriosclerosis in which the primary lesion is a thickening of the intimal layer of the aorta and large and medium-sized arteries.

Incidence. Most epidemiologic studies of atherosclerosis are concerned with coronary artery disease, which appears to have been increasing alarmingly in the United States during the current century. The annual incidence estimated from the Framingham study increased with age in males from less than 3.8 per 1000 at age 30 to 16 or more at age 55. Half of all deaths in men aged 50 are caused by ischemic heart disease. The incidence is much lower in females, but ten years postmenopausally approaches that of men. The annual death rate from atherosclerosis and degenerative heart disease in the United States for men aged 50 to 59 is the highest in the world. Sixty per cent or more of deaths from coronary artery disease are sudden deaths.

Etiology. Atherosclerosis is a multifactorial disease. Factors which have been most clearly implicated are serum cholesterol, smoking, and hypertension. Other important predisposing factors are serum triglycerides, diabetes, and obesity. Increased concentration of circulating serum insulin has been implicated by several studies. Although most epidemiologic studies have been concerned with ischemic heart disease, the same risk factors apply to other manifestations of atherosclerosis.

Obesity. Epidemiologic data show that members of ethnic groups with low incidence of ischemic heart disease, with a few unexplained exceptions, are leaner than Americans and do not gain significant weight after maturity. Among Americans, the prevalence of coronary artery disease is lowest in persons below normal weight, and increases proportionally with degree of overweight.

Considerable evidence suggests that adult onset obesity of mild degree, the type associated with increased size of adipose cells, is more closely related to atherosclerosis than is the juvenile onset hypercellular type. The Framingham study showed that certain manifestations of coronary heart disease, i.e., angina pectoris, preinfarction angina, and sudden death, were best predicted from subscapular skin-fold thickness. Triceps thickness, which when taken alone had no prognostic value, when taken in conjunction with other measurements was actually negatively associated with these manifestations. Unpublished studies by the author show, moreover, that skin-fold thickness is better correlated with serum triglycerides, glucose, and insulin concentrations when measured at the subscapular than at the triceps site, and that when adjustment is made for the former relationship, the correlations with triceps skin-fold are negative. There is no simple way to determine cell number and size in epidemiologic studies, but obesity which involves the trunk relatively more than the limbs is thought to be an indication of adult onset obesity and therefore of large adipose cells. The finding suggests that acquired obesity predisposes to electrical

abnormalities of the heart or to thromboembolic phenomena.

A large share of the effect of obesity on the atherosclerotic plaque may be explained by the fact that in the United States obesity is the single most important influence on virtually all other risk factors. The role of obesity in the etiology of hypertension, diabetes, and hyperinsulinemia has already been discussed. Obesity also has an influence on what could be the most important risk factor, the serum lipids. The status of glucose tolerance and serum lipids can best be ascertained after an overnight fast of 12 to 24 hours when the subject has been living and eating normally at least three months after an acute illness.

Serum Lipids. Two main groups of hyperlipoproteinemia are associated with increased incidence of atherosclerosis: hyperbetalipoproteinemia, in which lower density lipoproteins (LDL) are increased (Fredrickson Types IIA and IIB), and hyperprebetalipoproteinemia, in which very low density lipoproteins (VLDL) or endogenous triglycerides are increased (Type IV will constitute most of this group) (see Ch. 819). The predominant lipid in the first group is cholesterol; in the second, triglycerides. A classification based on lipid concentration is empirically useful: pure hypercholesterolemia (Type IIA) and hypertriglyceridemia. The latter in turn can be divided into mixed lipemia (cholesterol also elevated, Type IIB and some Type IV's) or pure hypertriglyceridemia (cholesterol normal, Type IV). Pure hypercholesterolemia may carry the greatest risk of coronary artery disease, but mixed lipemia and pure hypertriglyceridemia are more prevalent. Hypercholesterolemia and hypertriglyceridemia probably contribute about equally to the population of patients with ischemic heart disease. Recent investigations have shown that VLDL is the probable precursor of LDL. An increase in concentration of circulating VLDL as well as of LDL could be responsible for the LDL seen in the atherosclerotic plaque (see below).

HYPERCHOLESTEROLEMIA. According to the Framingham study, the incidence of coronary heart disease increases as serum cholesterol concentration increases. Between the ages of 45 and 54 the annual incidence of coronary artery disease is about six per 1000 among men with cholesterol concentrations below 200 mg per 100 ml; this increases to about 15 per 1000 among men with cholesterol over 260 mg per milliliter. There is no low concentration below which absence of myocardial infarction can be guaranteed and no upper limit above which it is inevitable. The overlap is great between normal persons and those with coronary artery disease; however, a cholesterol below 200 mg per 100 ml may be considered desirable and one above 260 undesirable. For laboratories which measure the cholesterol by an automated technique, which gives values a little higher than the true values, the aforementioned levels should be modified according to the criteria for the laboratory.

Comparison of different ethnic and geographic groups suggests that hypercholesterolemia is caused by the combined effects of obesity and of high intake of saturated fat and of cholesterol, acting on a genetic predisposition. Saturated fat intake constitutes nearly 20 per cent of calories in countries characterized by highest serum cholesterol concentrations.

The amount of cholesterol in the diet has an influence on serum cholesterol concentration which is most marked in the range between no intake and intake of 300 mg per day. Further increase in dietary cholesterol has only a small effect, if any, on serum cholesterol. The average dietary cholesterol intake of most Americans exceeds this and may be over 1000 mg per day. Weight gain and relative weight were the only factors measured in the Framingham study which were related to cholesterol concentration. Variations in diet had no discernible effect, probably because the intake of saturated fat and cholesterol was above the range in which a hypocholesterolemic effect of low intake of these components can be demonstrated. Obviously other as yet unidentified factors contribute to variation in serum cholesterol in the United States. Other dietary constituents such as pectins and cereal fiber may have a cholesterol-lowering effect.

HYPERTRIGLYCERIDEMIA. Epidemiologic data concerning the risk of elevated triglycerides are still rather meager but suggest that, as with cholesterol, the risk increases continuously throughout the range. The upper limit of normal is considered to be about 150 mg per 100 ml. Peripheral vascular disease may be a more common manifestation than in pure hypercholesterolemia. Endogenous hypertriglyceridemia is frequently associated with obesity of the adult onset type, and with impaired glucose tolerance, insulin resistance, and high basal insulin concentrations. In nondiabetics the postcibal rise in insulin, being superimposed on an elevated fasting level, may be high. In diabetics the insulin response is blunted. As in obesity, the high insulin output may eventually lead to pancreatic exhaustion and low insulin-output diabetes, thus accounting for the frequency of impaired glucose tolerance. Also as in obesity, the insulin-resistant state may be a fundamental aspect of endogenous lipemia.

The causal sequences among obesity, hypertriglyceridemia, hyperinsulinism, insulin resistance, impaired glucose tolerance, and ultimately atherosclerosis are not known.

Although it is not certain whether endogenous hypertriglyceridemia is caused by increased synthesis or impaired removal, it is exaggerated by factors which increase fat synthesis such as weight gain and very high carbohydrate diet. The latter causes so-called carbohydrate-induced lipemia, probably by increasing VLDL synthesis. Weight reduction or a low carbohydrate diet improves the lipemia. The amount of carbohydrate necessary to induce the lipemia is subject to marked individual variation. The triglyceride-lowering effect of a low calorie diet overrides the triglyceride-raising effect of a high carbohydrate diet.

Pathogenesis of Atherosclerosis. Of the three layers of an artery, atherosclerosis is a disease only of the intima. The characteristic lesion is the subendothelial atherosclerotic plaque. The earliest lesion is the "fatty streak," a subendothelial accumulation of fat which occurs in early childhood. This lesion is universal and is reversible. Its importance lies in the fact that during the third decade it progresses to the second stage, the raised subendothelial fibrous plaque in which fibrous connective tissue, collagen, and mucopolysaccharide appear and cause the lesion to encroach on the vessel lumen. Ischemia or necrosis of the organ supplied is the end result. The lesion progresses to ulceration, necrosis, calcification, and hemorrhage, the so-called complicated lesion. With each stage reversibility is lessened.

Progression of the universal innocuous fatty streak to the fibrous plaque is not inevitable but depends on dietary and other environmental factors. The single most important factor determining whether the fatty streak progresses to the atherosclerotic plaque is the lipid, particularly cholesterol, content of the lesion.

Study of the lipid components of the plaque show that cholesterol and triglycerides are probably derived from plasma, whereas phospholipids may be synthesized by the vessel wall. Little is known of the mechanism whereby lipids are transported across the endothelial barrier into the vessel wall. High density lipoproteins (HDL), low density lipoproteins (LDL), and possibly smaller very low density lipoproteins (VLDL) are small enough to enter by diffusion. The identification of LDL apoprotein within the plaque suggests that entire lipoproteins do enter the vessel wall from the serum. A certain amount of lipid exchange between intima and plasma is normal. The triglyceride can be metabolized by the vessel wall, and the remaining cholesterol-rich LDL disposed of in a manner unknown. Only when the rate of entry of LDL becomes greater than the rate of disposal does abnormal accumulation occur.

The localization of atherosclerotic plaques at sites of injury and at points of bifurcation of arteries and the greater incidence of atherosclerosis in hypertensive persons demonstrate that local injury and pressure relationships are important factors in plaque formation. Atherosclerosis is rare in pulmonary arteries unless pulmonary hypertension is present.

Recent work has focused on proliferation of the smooth muscle cell in the intima as the key event in the pathogenesis of the atherosclerotic plaque. The smooth muscle cells may proliferate from a few pre-existing intimal cells or may migrate from the media, the usual location of smooth muscle cells. Early in the atherosclerotic process the intimal smooth muscle cell accumulates LDL, thus becoming the well-known lipid-laden foam cell. Smooth muscle cells grown in tissue culture react to LDL accumulation by proliferation and by secretion of other constituents of the plaque: elastic fiber protein, collagen, and mucopolysaccharides. They later may secrete lipids into the extracellular space.

In summary, factors which increase endothelial permeability to lipoproteins, such as injury to the vessel wall, and factors which increase lipid concentration presented to the vessel wall in the circulation, would act to promote intimal smooth muscle cell proliferation which in turn leads to the atherosclerotic plaque.

An alternative theory attributes plaque formation to the intravascular coagulation initiated by increased platelet stickiness and platelet agglomeration or by a shift in the balance between fibrin formation and fibrinolysis in the direction of fibrin deposition, with secondary enmeshment of circulating lipids. Increased coagulability, superimposed on underlying atherosclerotic disease, may be of importance in the 50 per cent of myocardial infarctions in which thrombosis is a prominent part of the pathologic change.

Although atherosclerosis is a generalized disease, coronary artery disease may occur without atherosclerotic involvement elsewhere. Such isolated coronary artery disease is a common cause of morbidity and mortality among younger men and is associated, more than is generalized atherosclerosis, with overnutrition. Cerebral atherosclerosis occurs in taller, thinner persons about 20 years later than coronary atherosclerosis.

Treatment of Atherosclerosis. Specific treatment is directed toward individual organs. General treatment consists of identifying and correcting all the known risk factors (see above). The most important aspects of treatment are weight reduction, correction of hyperlipidemias, correction of hypertension, and cessation of smoking.

The general principles of weight reduction have been discussed above. Special attention to the diet is necessary when hyperlipidemias are not corrected by simple weight reduction. Whether such dietary intervention will reverse the atherosclerotic process is unknown, but optimism seems permissible on the basis of available knowledge.

Dietary Treatment of Hypercholesterolemia. In spite of lack of correlation between prevailing diet and serum cholesterol in the Framingham study, dietary *change* will have a small but definite effect on serum cholesterol concentration.

The National Diet Heart Study showed that reduction of total fat intake from 40 to 30 per cent of calories, reduction of saturated fat from 18 to 9 per cent of calories, reduction of dietary cholesterol intake from 700 to 400 mg per day, and an increase in the polyunsaturated to saturated fat (P/S) ratio from 0.4 to 1.5 effected an 8 per cent reduction of serum cholesterol in weight-stable persons. The effect was nearly doubled by weight loss, and weight loss in the control group caused a 5 per cent reduction. A further decrease of dietary cholesterol to 100 mg will be more effective, but such a diet is difficult to follow. The addition of polyunsaturated oils will have a cholesterol lowering effect which is about half the cholesterol raising effect of saturated fats. The safety of large amounts of unsaturated dietary fat is not certain. Most authorities now recommend only enough polyunsaturated fat to raise the P/S ratio to 1.0. Dietary cholesterol is derived entirely from animal sources. The important dietary sources of cholesterol may be seen in Table 4. Because one problem of cholesterol restriction is the maintenance of adequate protein intake, the protein values are also shown.

The elimination of eggs from the diet will do much to lower the cholesterol intake. Further reduction can readily be achieved by eliminating butter, organ meat, shrimp, and crab, and by substituting skimmed milk for whole milk. Recent studies have shown lower cholesterol in shellfish than previously thought. Protein can be supplied either by lean meat or by cheese, as preferred, as well as by vegetable sources. Although even lean meat contains substantial amounts of cholesterol, meat is the mainstay of the American diet, and its elimination will jeopardize patient cooperation. If meat is the only significant source of cholesterol in the diet, as much as 8 ounces a day can be permitted without exceeding 200 mg of dietary cholesterol.

The carbohydrate content of a very low fat diet may be sufficiently high to cause hypertriglyceridemia in susceptible persons (see below). In the average person moderate increases in dietary carbohydrate have little influence on triglycerides.

Treatment of Hypertriglyceridemia. The first step in the treatment of hypertriglyceridemia is weight reduction to or toward ideal weight (Table 1), or to weight at age 25. If simple weight loss does not lower serum triglycerides, restriction of carbohydrate to 40 or even 30 per cent of calories or more may be necessary. A decrease in serum triglyceride by as much as 50 per cent may be achieved.

Some evidence exists for the possibility that carbohydrate-induced lipemia is a response more to highly purified carbohydrates such as sucrose than to carbohydrate in general. For this reason it would be wise to eliminate sugar as such from the diet of obese or atherosclerotic patients, particularly if the triglycerides are elevated. Alcohol ingestion may raise the triglycerides and should be used only sparingly.

Prevention of Atherosclerosis. Preventive measures are the same as therapeutic measures except that they are directed toward patients of high risk who do not yet have atherosclerosis. Opinion is divided as to the advisability of drastic changes in the diet for children and young

TABLE 4. Approximate Cholesterol Content of Foods*

Item	Size Serving, Edible Portion as Purchased	Amount of Cholesterol (mg)	Amount of Protein (Grams)
Milk, whole	One glass (200 ml)	22	7
Milk, skim	One glass (200 ml)	6	7
Whole milk cheeses, as American, Cheddar, and cream	100 grams	85–100	21–36
Cheese, cottage	100 grams	15	13
Butter	1 tablespoon (15 grams)	38	0
Animal fat (lard)	1 tablespoon (15 grams)	14	0
Egg yolk	1 egg	300	3
Egg white	1 egg	0	5
Lean cuts of any poultry, meat except organs, fish except shrimp and crab	100 grams of meat only	30–90	16–32
Shrimp and crab	100 grams of meat only	100–150	16–24
Caviar	100 grams	>300	26–34
Organ meats	100 grams	150–375	16–26
Brain	100 grams	>2000	12

*Estimated from values listed in U.S. Department of Agriculture Handbook No. 8, Composition of Foods, 1963, and Feeley, R. M., Criner, P. E., and Watt, B. K.: J. Am. Dietet. Assoc., 61:134, 1972.

adults, not because of any doubt that prevention is desirable, but because of uncertainty regarding the best methods of prevention. Certain preventive measures can be recommended for the entire population: avoidance of cigarette smoking, of high intake of foods of high caloric density but low nutritive value such as sugar and fats, and of weight gain after maturity.

Albrink, M. J.: Overnutrition and the fat cell. *In* Bondy, P. K., and Rosenberg, L. (eds.): Duncan's Diseases of Metabolism. 7th ed. Philadelphia, W. B. Saunders Company, 1974.

Alexander, J. K., and Peterson, K. L.: Cardiovascular effects of weight reduction. Circulation, 45:310, 1972.

Bray, G. (ed.): Fogarty International Center Conference on Obesity. U. S. Government Printing Office, in press.

Damon, A., Damon, S. T., Harpending, H. C., and Kannel, W. B.: Predicting coronary heart disease from body measurements of Framingham males. J. Chronic Dis., 21:781, 1969.

Grinker, J., and Hirsch, J.: Metabolic and behavioral correlates of obesity. *In* Physiology of Emotion and Psychosomatic Illness. Ciba Foundation Symposium 8 (new series). Amsterdam, Elsevier Publishing Company, 1972.

Hatch, F. T.: Interactions between nutrition and heredity in coronary heart disease. Am. J. Clin. Nutr., 27:80, 1974.

Keys, A., Aravanis, C., Blackburn, H., Van Buchem, F., Buzina, R., Djordjevic, B. S., Fidanza, F., Karvonen, M. J., Menotti, A., Puddu, V., and Taylor, H.: Coronary heart disease: Overweight and obesity as risk factors. Ann. Intern. Med., 77:15, 1972.

Ross, R., and Glomset, J. A.: Atherosclerosis and the arterial smooth muscle cell. Science, 180:1332, 1973.

Sims, E. A. H., Danforth, E., Jr., Horton, E. S., Bray, G. A., Glennon, J. S., and Salans, L. B.: Endocrine and metabolic effects of experimental obesity in man. Recent Prog. Horm. Res., 29:457, 1973.

724. ANOREXIA NERVOSA

G. F. M. Russell

Definition. Anorexia nervosa is a chronic illness principally affecting young girls after puberty. It is characterized by severe weight loss which is self-induced, amenorrhea, and a specific psychopathology.

Historical Note. Sir William Gull described anorexia nervosa in 1868 and 1874 and concluded that "the want of appetite is due to a morbid mental state." This he attributed to the wiles of young women whom he considered "specially obnoxious to mental perversity." He advised that "the patients should be fed at regular intervals, and surrounded by persons who would have more control over them, relations and friends being generally the worst attendants." For a long time, confusion resulted from the concept of "Simmonds' cachexia," which embodied the mistaken view that panhypopituitarism usually caused loss of weight and wasting. Thus much needless effort was spent on the differential diagnosis of these two disorders which do not resemble each other.

Etiology. The cause of anorexia nervosa is unknown. Little is known about genetic aspects: morbidity is higher among sisters of patients (6.6 per cent), and concordance for the illness has been described in identical twins, but these observations are also explicable by the similarity of the home environment. Anorexia nervosa used to be considered a rare illness. However, a fivefold increase in incidence was reported in Malmö, Sweden, by Theander when he compared the 1950's with the 1930's. Similar observations in Britain have led to the hypothesis that culturally determined attitudes might lead to the illness. In recent years the upper social class bias for

anorexia nervosa has tended to disappear. The incidence of new cases ranges from 0.6 to 1.6 per 100,000 of the whole population, but the prevalence among schoolgirls around puberty may be as high as one in a hundred. The usual age of onset is 14 to 17 years, but it can be earlier (10 to 13 years) or later (up to 40 years). The illness is at least ten times more frequent in girls than in boys.

Psychopathology and Pathogenesis. Anorexia nervosa is usually thought to be a disorder of psychologic origin, especially from conflicts engendered by the experience of puberty and adolescence. The illness can also be viewed from a predominantly somatic perspective as a disorder of the feeding and endocrine functions normally controlled by the hypothalamus.

The psychologic basis of anorexia nervosa is supported by the observation that food refusal is often purposive. Psychodynamic formulations (not equivalent to causal explanations) emphasize the ambivalent emotional ties between the patient and her mother, conflicts caused by the advent of puberty, and the uncertainties that surround the search for a personal identity during adolescence. Psychologic explanations postulate an abnormal reaction to puberty (Thomä) or a disturbance of "body image" (Bruch). Some support has been given to the last hypothesis (Slade and Russell). Patients with anorexia nervosa have been shown to be abnormally responsive to their impressions of body size and weight. They eat less whenever they feel that their body is too large, instead of relying on the physiologic signals of hunger. Moreover, they tend to overestimate the width of their own body. They therefore see themselves as wider and fatter than normal girls, and further starvation ensues.

It has also been proposed that the pathogenesis of anorexia nervosa involves a disorder of hypothalamic function on the ground that destruction of the "feeding centers" in animals causes refusal of food and water. However, studies in anorexia nervosa have not revealed any primary disorder in the control of food intake, and there is often no true loss of appetite, so that the term "anorexia" is a misnomer. Emaciation has been described as a consequence of hypothalamic lesions in humans, but in such cases the clinical picture does not otherwise resemble anorexia nervosa.

The strongest evidence of a hypothalamic disorder in anorexia nervosa is specific failure in the function of the hypothalamic–anterior pituitary–gonadal axis: gonadotrophins are not released from the anterior pituitary, the ovarian production of estrogens drops, and ovulation fails to occur. These abnormalities often persist long after the malnutrition is corrected; gonadotrophins and estrogens rise again in the blood and urine, but cyclical variations in their levels and ovulation do not return for several months. These findings, together with the early onset of amenorrhea which may precede weight loss, indicate that the endocrine disorder is not simply the sequel of the malnutrition. The precise nature of the hypothalamic disorder is unknown. In male patients there is a corresponding endocrine disorder with reduction in gonadotrophin and testosterone levels in the blood and urine. There is also evidence of disordered thermoregulation in anorexia nervosa, but this can be corrected by restoring body weight to normal and is therefore probably secondary to malnutrition.

Clinical Manifestations. The illness usually begins in a girl aged 14 to 17 years. Her previous personality may have been normal. In some patients, however, there may be a preceding history of food fads or difficulty in making friendships; other signs of maladjustment are excessive tidiness or fears of meeting strangers or of taking school examinations. Loss of weight may be the first feature noticed by the parents, who draw the patient's attention to it. She is likely to explain the weight loss as the result of dieting for the purpose of improving her figure. Menstruation will have ceased by the time there has been a significant loss of weight, or this may happen as the first feature of the illness. There is often a change in the girl's temperament, consisting of impatience, irritability, and depression. She may become preoccupied with schoolwork or indulge in solitary exercises, thus withdrawing from her customary social life. The loss of weight can be very rapid, with a fall from 55 kg (121 pounds) to 35 kg (77 pounds) within two to three months. This is achieved mainly by avoiding carbohydrate-containing foods, but self-induced vomiting, the abuse of purgatives, and excessive exercising, in various combinations, may accelerate the loss of weight. The patient's life becomes unhappy and constricted. If she had a boyfriend, she loses interest in him and avoids any sexual contact. Relations with members of the family become strained. Parents may react to their daughter's food refusal by alternately pleading with her and trying to force her to eat. Food refusal leads to malnutrition which may persist for months or even years. The patient subsists on a diet of vegetables, fruit, and cheese, and avoids bread, potatoes, cakes, sugar, and other carbohydrate-containing foods. On some days she may take only black coffee. Sometimes, food avoidance alternates with orgiastic bouts of overeating, especially at night when the patient can no longer resist her cravings for food. These bouts are followed by vomiting. In severe cases the patient presents a pitiable sight of emaciation, apathy, weakness, and severe depression. There is a risk of death from suicide or complications of malnutrition – infections, potassium depletion, or hypothermia.

In spite of progressive malnutrition, the patient may reject her parents' entreaties to see a doctor, and she minimizes the extent of her dieting. When she does agree to seek help, she is likely to deny that she is unwell or admit only to insomnia, constipation, sensitivity to cold, or some depression of mood.

Mental Examination. Examination of the patient's mental state may reveal a variety of disturbances. There may be depression and agitation; compulsive features may be prominent, such as elaborate feeding rituals and the counting of calories eaten daily; hysterical mechanisms may account for her assertion that she is eating well, whereas at the same time she hides food surreptitiously or vomits in secret. In addition, however, more specific psychologic abnormalities will be present. Their central theme is the patient's fear of becoming fat as a result of "losing control over eating." To play safe she resolves to remain thin and sets herself a sharply defined weight threshold above which she is unwilling to rise, defending her chosen weight as "right" for her. She may betray an abnormal sensitivity about the shape and size of her body, saying that fat would go to her stomach (hips, thighs, or some other part of the body). She may overestimate her weight and maintain, with all sincerity, that she eats large amounts of food. In an extreme case she may deny that she is thin, or even state that she is fat in spite of obvious emaciation. The patient's distorted awareness of her size can be measured by getting her to estimate the width of her body at various levels

(e.g., face, bust, waist, and hips) by means of an apparatus which permits the separation of two lights until it corresponds to the selected body dimension. The patient's estimate is liable to exceed her actual measurements by as much as 50 per cent. Patients may offer a variety of other reasons for their reluctance to return to a normal weight, or they may conceal their abnormal attitudes which nonetheless become explicit by their behavior when they are under observation in hospital.

Physical Examination. Physical examination will reveal the signs of severe malnutrition in a young girl who has developed secondary sex characteristics. The malnutrition is of a calorie-deficiency type. The disappearance of subcutaneous fat leads to gaunt, hollow facial features; bony prominences stand out sharply, the limbs are reduced to sticks, the belly is flat, the breasts shrunken, and the buttocks wasted. The hands and feet remain cold and blue, even when the room temperature is warm. The central body temperature may be reduced by 1° C. The blood pressure is low (e.g., 90/60), and the heart rate is slow (50 to 60). The skin is dry, and there is an excessive growth of dry, downy hair over the nape of the neck and the cheeks, forearms, and legs (lanugo hair), changes attributed to a follicular keratosis. In older patients purpuric patches resembling senile purpura may appear over the dorsum of the hands, the forearms, and the legs after minor knocks.

In patients who vomit, dehydration ensues, together with a marked reduction in the levels of serum potassium (e.g., to 1.4 mEq per liter), which may lead to muscular weakness, tetany, and electrocardiographic abnormalities. There may also be a moderate fall in serum sodium and hypochloremic alkalosis. Serum cholesterol levels may be raised, especially in patients who overeat intermittently. Carotenemia may follow a high intake of carrots or spinach, and causes a yellow pigmentation of the palms and soles. Vitamin deficiencies occur only rarely.

Endocrine Changes. Patients who are wasted show a fall in the urinary output of gonadotrophins and estrogens; blood levels of luteinizing hormone (LH) are low. A course of clomiphene fails to raise the low serum LH levels. Specific measures of thyroid function fall within the normal range. Plasma levels of growth hormone and cortisol are normal or elevated, and can be raised further by the administration of insulin. Most of the physical abnormalities disappear when the malnutrition is corrected, and the patient's mental state is also likely to improve. An exception to this recovery is the disorder of gonadotrophin activity, as described above.

Side Effects of Refeeding. Peripheral edema may occur, especially when the diet has a high content of salt, water, and carbohydrates which cause water retention. A moderate normochromic normocytic anemia may result from hemodilution, or a more severe anemia may result from temporary hypoplasia of the bone marrow; occasionally, moderate iron deficiency anemia may occur. Acute dilatation of the stomach is a rare complication of too rapid refeeding.

Anorexia Nervosa in the Male. The illness in the male is rare, but resembles closely that in the female. The onset occurs around the time of puberty. The young boy rapidly loses weight as a result of avoiding carbohydrate-containing foods. Like the female, he expresses a fear of becoming fat, and resorts to a similar abnormal behavior of food refusal, possibly with vomiting, purgation, or exercising to excess. Because of the later age of physical maturation in the male, there is a greater risk of malnutrition causing retardation of growth and delayed puberty. The malnutrition is more likely to be of a type combining a deficiency of calories and proteins. The endocrine disorder in the male is analogous to that in the female. Urinary gonadotrophins and blood LH levels are low; the urinary output of testosterone is reduced. Questioning will elicit loss of recently acquired sexual interest and potency. As in the female, these hormonal abnormalities can be slowly reversed by treatment resulting in weight gain.

Treatment.   There is no specific treatment; nevertheless the general management of patients can be rewarding. The approach is essentially empirical; the treatments used are those which have been found to be effective in practice. The immediate aim is to treat the patient's malnutrition, which can become severe and dangerous. Even during the early stages of treatment it is desirable to try altering abnormal attitudes, for the course of the illness is much affected by the psychologic state. Thus treatment is best administered in a psychiatric unit, but it is essential that there should be good nursing facilities. The long-term aim of treatment is to reduce the duration of the illness and prevent relapses.

Short-Term Treatment.   SECURING THE PATIENT'S CO-OPERATION.   The first need is to obtain as much cooperation from the patient as possible, notwithstanding her denial of illness. By the time there has been severe loss of weight, admission to hospital is the only certain way of restoring her nutrition to normal. The doctor's skills must therefore be focused on persuading the patient to come into hospital. Compulsory admission is best avoided whenever possible, because the patient's continued cooperation is essential throughout the course of the illness, which may last for a few years.

NURSING TREATMENT.   The refeeding of the patient is best achieved by skilled nurses. After having assessed the severity of the feeding disorder, the nurse should try to establish a good relationship with her patient, one based on trust but not dependent on giving way to the patient's abnormal wishes to avoid food and weight gain. This is best achieved by the nurse asking the patient to look upon her as a person whom she can trust to decide on the amount of food to be eaten each day, and who will not allow her to become fat. The patient is told frankly that because of her illness she will be tempted to be deceitful about eating, vomiting, or taking purgatives. The nurse thus explains that close supervision will be necessary at first to reduce the strength of these temptations. The patient must be observed throughout every meal, and the nurse will cajole her into finishing all the food put on her plate. The avoidance of self-induced vomiting can be difficult. It requires round-the-clock nursing supervision, limiting the fluid intake to 1.5 liters daily, preventing access to the toilet for at least two hours after meals, and removal of vomit-bowls. The use of purgatives should also be stopped. As soon as the patient gains weight, she is complimented on her improved looks and is encouraged to use cosmetics and buy new clothes suitable for a person of normal weight.

The techniques of nursing are also important, but they will only succeed within the context of a good relationship with the patient. They consist of a close supervision and a positive encouragement to eat. Complete bed rest is seldom necessary for more than a few days, but it may facilitate a close watch being kept.

The nurse will decide on a judicious balance between restrictions and privileges, in collaboration with the doctor and psychologist. The balance is gradually altered in favor of added privileges which will be viewed by the patient as rewards for continuing progress. Thus the general management can also be fitted within a model of behavior therapy.

DIET.   No special diets are needed. The patient is given her own choice of food so long as she does not exclude carbohydrate-containing foods. To begin with, the food intake should be 1500 calories daily; within seven to ten days she should be persuaded to accept full meals totaling 3000 to 5000 calories daily. Concentrated foods may be used to achieve this high intake (e.g., Complan, Metrecal, or Carnation breakfast food) by adding them to milk. Potassium supplements do not remedy the hypokalemia unless vomiting is controlled, and then they become unnecessary.

ADDITIONAL MEASURES.   The nursing care described should be viewed as a form of *psychologic treatment* embodying the principles of psychotherapy and behavior therapy. Formal psychotherapy has only a limited place during the early stages of treatment.

Large doses of chlorpromazine are sometimes advocated to reduce the patient's resistance to eating, but they can be dangerous in undernourished patients, and are seldom necessary. In very agitated patients the nursing task can be facilitated by administering moderate, divided doses of chlorpromazine up to a total of 300 mg daily. There is no place for tube feeding. It is doubtful whether a modified leukotomy is ever justified. Weight gain can be achieved by conservative treatment, and the risk of suicide is increased after leukotomy.

ASSESSMENT OF PROGRESS.   The patient is weighed daily before breakfast, and this provides the best check on her progress. A weight gain of up to 28 pounds (12.7 kg) in eight weeks should be possible. The patient should be seen to maintain a healthy weight for about two weeks before being discharged from hospital.

Long-Term Treatment.   There is less known about the efficacy of long-term treatments. After discharge from hospital, it is necessary to provide outpatient supervision. Psychotherapy should be directed to whatever emotional problems have been identified in the patient and her family. Even when a normal weight is maintained, amenorrhea may persist for months or years. When the patient is eager to resume normal menstruation, one or two courses of clomiphene (50 to 100 mg daily for seven days) may be effective, but only when body weight has been restored to a normal level. In the event of a serious relapse, readmission to hospital will be necessary.

Prognosis.   The short-term prognosis is usually excellent. Treatment should lead to a return to a normal weight; at the same time, the majority of patients show a marked improvement in their mental state. Deaths from malnutrition should not occur.

The long-term prognosis is more problematical. Relapses requiring readmissions occur in about half the patients. The illness often lasts two to three years or even longer. In a follow-up of severely ill patients who had been treated at least four years previously, 40 per cent had recovered, 27 per cent had menstrual irregularity or a moderately low body weight, 29 per cent had serious weight loss with amenorrhea, and 5 per cent had died. Poor prognostic signs are a later age of onset (early twenties as opposed to early teens), or an illness which has lasted more than five years. Even in these patients, however, good results can still be obtained from energetic treatment. In many patients the prognosis is good – their health returns to normal and they may marry and can bear children.

Bruch, H.: Eating Disorders: Obesity, Anorexia Nervosa and the Person Within. New York, Basic Books, 1972.

Gull, W. W.: Anorexia nervosa (apepsia hysterica, anorexia hysterica). Trans. Clin. Soc. London, 7:22, 1874.

Mecklenburg, R. S., Loriaux, D. L. Thompson, R. H., Andersen, A. E., and Lipsett, M. B.: Hypothalmic dysfunction in patients with anorexia nervosa. Medicine, 53:147, 1974.

Russell, G. F. M.: Anorexia nervosa: Its identity as an illness and its treatment. *In* Price, J. H. (ed.): Modern Trends in Psychological Medicine. 2d ed. London, Butterworth & Co. (Publishers) Ltd., 1970.

Russell, G. F. M.: The management of anorexia nervosa. *In* Robertson, R. F. (ed.): Symposium – Anorexia Nervosa and Obesity. Edinburgh, The Royal College of Physicians, 1973.

Slade, P. D., and Russell, G. F. M.: Awareness of body dimensions in anorexia nervosa: Cross-sectional and longitudinal studies. Psychol. Med., 3:188, 1973.

Theander, S.: Anorexia nervosa. A psychiatric investigation of 94 female patients. Acta Psychiatr. Scand., Supplement 211, 1970.

Thomä, H.: Anorexia Nervosa. Translated by G. Brydone. New York, International Universities Press, 1967.

NUTRITIONAL MAINTENANCE AND DIET THERAPY IN ACUTE AND CHRONIC DISEASE

Philip Felig

725. INTRODUCTION

Diseases resulting from deficiencies of specific nutrients in the diet are well recognized and have been covered in detail elsewhere (see Ch. 717 to 722). Except in underdeveloped areas of the world, problems of nutritional homeostasis in hospitalized patients are generally a secondary consequence rather than a cause of disease processes. The normal intake of nutrients may be interfered with in a variety of inflammatory, septic, or malignant disorders as a result of anorexia or vomiting, in association with primary disturbances of the gastrointestinal tract, and in the postoperative state. Nutritional maintenance also poses a problem in patients placed on therapeutic diets designed to limit the intake of calories, carbohydrate, protein, sodium, or potassium. Generally attention is focused on correcting the primary disorder, and little concern is attached to over-all nutritional requirements, since most patients are expected to tolerate limited periods of subnutrition without difficulty. Considerations of nutritional factors are often limited to providing vitamin supplements, with little attention to caloric and nitrogen balance. It is noteworthy, however, that sepsis secondary to debilitation, in the form of terminal bronchopneumonia, is a major cause of death in hospitalized patients. The sequence of events in

such patients is often as follows: primary disease (e.g., uremia, malignancy, ulcerative colitis) → poor nutrition and protein catabolism → depletion of body protein reserves (i.e., muscle) → weakness of respiratory muscles → atelectasis → pneumonia → death. In less severe circumstances, failure of adequate nutrition may prolong convalescence, predispose to infection, and interfere with wound healing.

An important goal in the medical management of disease is thus the maintenance of normal body composition in the face of reduced intake, increased metabolic requirements, or disordered metabolic machinery. From a practical standpoint nutritional considerations become an integral aspect of the therapeutic decision process in patients requiring short-term or long-term parenteral feeding, particularly when an anabolic response is necessary, and in patients on restrictive diets. To understand the principles underlying such nutritional interventions, it is first necessary to consider body composition in healthy subjects prior to the onset of illness, the metabolic response to nutritional deprivation in normal man, and the accelerated catabolism observed in disease states.

726. FUEL HOMEOSTASIS IN HEALTH AND DISEASE

Body Composition. Normal man may be considered not only in terms of his constituent organ systems, but also with respect to his underlying fuel reserves. The energy resources available in a 70-kg man are shown in Table 1. Body fat, comprising 15 to 25 per cent of body weight, constitutes the primary fuel depot, each gram providing 9 kcal. Smaller amounts of calories are available in the form of protein (4 kcal per gram), whereas carbohydrate stores (4 kcal per gram) are calorically insignificant. The enormity of fat stores relative to other nutrients is readily apparent. Furthermore, an increase in body weight, such as occurs in obesity, involves little change in the quantity of protein or carbohydrate but is associated primarily with an increase in fat. Thus a 25 per cent gain in weight is accompanied by a doubling in body fat. In contrast, weight loss, as observed in chronic debilitated states, involves a substantial reduction in body protein as well as fat. The ability to withstand a debilitating illness is accordingly reduced in the already wasted patient.

Short-Term Starvation. In individuals of normal weight or in those who are obese, even under circumstances of heavy exercise or the increased demands engendered by severe injury (Table 2), the magnitude of

TABLE 1. Body Composition and Fuel Reserves in a Normal 70-kg Man

Fuel	Tissue	kg	% Body Weight	Energy Value (kcal)
Fat	Adipose tissue	11–17	15–25	100,000–150,000
Protein	Primarily muscle	8–12	12–17	32,000– 48,000
Carbohydrate	Liver glycogen	0.070	<1	280
	Muscle glycogen	0.200	<1	800
	Blood glucose	0.020	<1	80

body fat stores is such that they might be expected to meet the total energy needs during periods of total starvation extending at least two months. However, it is not the depletion of fat which is the limiting factor in survival during food restriction. Death caused by starvation is a consequence of protein loss and generally occurs when one third to one half of total protein stores has been depleted. The continuous, obligate utilization of protein in the face of more plentiful fat reserves is a consequence of three factors: (1) protein constitutes the sole source of noncarbohydrate precursors which can be converted to glucose, inasmuch as net glucose synthesis from fatty acids does not occur in mammalian tissue; (2) certain tissues are obligate consumers of glucose; and (3) carbohydrate reserves (particularly liver glycogen) are extremely limited (Table 1) and are dissipated in less than 24 hours of starvation.

During short-term starvation the brain is the major site of glucose utilization. Glucose is consumed by the brain at a rate of 100 to 150 grams per day and undergoes terminal oxidation to CO_2 and water. Smaller amounts of glucose (50 to 75 grams) are converted to lactic acid by the formed elements of the blood, the renal medulla, and muscle tissue. The bulk of the energy requirements of muscle, heart, and visceral tissues are not dependent on glucose utilization (in either the fed state or starvation), but are met by the oxidation of free fatty acids mobilized from adipose tissue, and ketone acids formed in the liver in association with fat oxidation.

Since, as noted above, liver glycogen stores are limited to less than 100 grams, hepatic glycogenolysis can sustain brain glucose requirements for less than 24 hours. Synthesis of glucose from noncarbohydrate precursors (gluconeogenesis) consequently begins in the immediate postabsorptive state (10- to 12-hour fast). Amino acids, particularly large amounts of alanine, are released from muscle tissue and are taken up by the liver where they are converted to glucose. The rate of protein breakdown is approximately 60 to 75 grams per day, resulting in the appearance of 10 to 12 grams of nitrogen in the urine (6.25 grams N/gram of protein). Since muscle tissue is about 75 to 80 per cent water, this rate of protein catabolism results in a loss of approximately one half pound (200 to 300 grams) of lean body mass per day. A more rapid rate of weight loss reflects either a loss of body fluids (diuresis) or a catabolic state (see below).

The primary hormonal modulators of the gluconeogenic and ketogenic response to short-term starvation are insulin and glucagon. Fasting evokes a prompt decrease in serum insulin and a rise in circulating levels of glucagon. These hormonal changes, particularly the fall in insulin, provide the signal which stimulates lipolysis in adipose tissue and augmented gluconeogenesis by the liver. Insulin does not disappear entirely from the circulation; the small amounts remaining probably serve to prevent the massive ketogenesis and gluconeogenesis observed in diabetic ketoacidosis.

The catabolic processes precipitated by starvation may be dramatically altered by providing minimal amounts of carbohydrate. Administration of 100 grams of carbohydrate (400 calories) in the absence of other foodstuffs results in a marked diminution in urinary nitrogen losses to as little as 2 to 3 grams per day. This protein-sparing effect of calorically insignificant amounts of carbohydrate is of prime consideration in determining the composition of fluids administered to patients in whom food intake must be withheld for short periods (see below). Two points deserve emphasis regarding carbohydrate intake in otherwise fasted individuals: (1) increasing the carbohydrate content above 100 grams does not increase the protein-sparing effect; (2) positive nitrogen balance (anabolism) cannot be achieved unless an exogenous source of protein is provided as well.

Long-Term Starvation. As fasting continues beyond several days, a series of adaptations occurs designed to limit the rate and magnitude of protein breakdown. Total glucose utilization decreases as the brain consumes ketone bodies as an alternative oxidative fuel. Since less glucose is required, gluconeogenic processes are curtailed, and the outflow of alanine and other amino acids from muscle is greatly reduced. Urinary nitrogen excretion falls to as little as 3 grams per day, reflecting the catabolism of no more than 20 grams of protein and depletion of less than 100 grams of lean body mass. The expendable nature of fat as compared to protein is indicated by the fact that 95 per cent of caloric needs are met by combustion of free fatty acids and ketone bodies. The patient in this circumstance is on an "endogenous high-fat diet" in which protein breakdown continues, but at a greatly reduced rate. The precise signal (? hormonal) triggering this decrease in protein catabolism has not been identified.

Catabolic States: Inflammation, Sepsis, Trauma. The orderly adaptive processes directed at minimizing protein losses in prolonged or short-term starvation are predicated upon the absence of significant underlying disease. In association with acute or chronic inflammation, sepsis, or trauma (burns, injuries, or surgery), the response to nutritional deprivation is characterized by an accelerated rate of protein catabolism. The magnitude of the catabolic response is related in part to increases in energy expenditure. Oxygen consumption is increased by fever at a rate of 7 per cent per degree Fahrenheit. Thus a fever of 103° F results in a 25 to 30 per cent elevation in energy requirements (Table 2). In addition to the effects of fever, the nature of the underlying disease or injury will influence caloric expenditure. The trauma associated with elective surgery causes no increase in basal oxygen consumption. In contrast, compound fractures or severe infections (e.g., peritonitis) are associated with an increase of 50 per cent, whereas extensive body burns are followed by elevations of 100 per cent above normal (Table 2). These increased demands for energy are met by an accelerated rate of protein dissolution. Urinary nitrogen losses in the poorly fed patient with an extensive inflammatory process may amount to 25

TABLE 2.   Caloric Expenditure in Normal and Disease States

Normal Activity	Calories/kg Body Weight/Day	Disease States
Bed rest	25	Bed rest
Light exercise (light housework, office work)	30–35	Fever of 103° F
Moderate exercise (industrial work, heavy housework)	35–40	Peritonitis, sepsis
Heavy exercise (construction work, farm work)	40–45	Extensive burns

grams per day (more than twice the rate observed in uncomplicated starvation), reflecting the breakdown of over 150 grams of protein and resulting in a loss of more than 1 pound per day of lean body mass. The origin of the protein loss is primarily muscle, inasmuch as the integrity of visceral tissues (e.g., liver) is maintained. Although the fate of the amino acids mobilized from muscle has not been precisely defined, recent studies by Kinney suggest that this rapid loss of protein is coupled with an accelerated rate of gluconeogenesis. This increased production of glucose may serve to meet the needs of reparative tissues such as fibroblasts and phagocytes.

The over-all metabolic picture thus contrasts markedly with that which occurs in prolonged starvation in normal subjects. Oxygen consumption, protein dissolution, and gluconeogenesis are all accelerated. Even more striking is the dissimilarity in the response to glucose administration. In contrast to the protein-sparing effects of minimal amounts of carbohydrate in starvation, administration of 100 to 400 grams of glucose fails to influence substantially the course of protein breakdown. Positive nitrogen balance or even a substantial reduction in net nitrogen losses is achieved only by providing an exogenous source of amino acids as well as sufficient calories (in the form of carbohydrate and/or fat) to meet the increased energy demands of catabolic states.

Accelerated Starvation: Alcoholic Ketoacidosis and Alcohol-Induced Hypoglycemia. The response to nutritional deprivation in normal man not only is directed at minimizing protein losses but also involves a limitation of ketone acid (beta-hydroxybutyrate and acetoacetate) production so as to avoid metabolic acidosis. In addition, continuous production of glucose assures the maintenance of blood glucose concentrations above the hypoglycemic range. During periods of total starvation extending for several days to weeks in healthy subjects, ketone acid accumulation in blood does not exceed 8 mM per liter, serum bicarbonate remains above 14 mEq per liter, and blood glucose concentration remains above 50 mg per 100 ml. In contrast, in alcoholic patients, particularly after binge drinking and protracted vomiting, starvation-induced metabolic acidosis (caused by excessive ketone acid accumulation) and/or hypoglycemia may be observed. Clinically, patients with alcoholic ketoacidosis present in a comatose state or are alert but appear acutely ill and have rapid, deep respirations. Arterial pH is reduced to less than 7.2, and an increased anion gap is observed. In about 25 per cent of cases the blood glucose level is less than 50 mg per 100 ml. The nature of the metabolic acidosis is often not recognized or is mistakenly attributed to lactate, since the semiquantitative nitroprusside reaction for ketones (Acetest, Ketostix, Ames Co.) is often only faintly positive. The failure to detect the extent of ketonemia is due to the high ratio of betahydroxybutyrate (which is not detected in the nitroprusside test) to acetoacetate. The mechanism whereby alcohol accelerates the ketotic response to starvation involves augmented lipolysis and altered intramitochondrial oxidative pathways. In most instances a prompt clinical response follows the administration of parenteral fluids containing glucose.

Alcohol-induced hypoglycemia is observed in circumstances in which liver glycogen stores have been depleted by a period of one or more days of food abstinence or vomiting. Alcohol interferes with glucose homeostasis by inhibiting hepatic gluconeogenesis from lactate, pyruvate, and amino acids. This effect is mediated by changes in cytoplasmic redox (i.e., an increase in hepatic NADH) that accompany the metabolic degradation of alcohol. The hypoglycemic action of alcohol therefore does not become apparent until glycogen stores have been exhausted, and maintenance of the glucose supply to the brain is solely dependent on gluconeogenic processes. Consequently, this disorder is most likely to be encountered in the chronic alcoholic who has been eating poorly or has had protracted vomiting. In addition to the usual signs and symptoms of hypoglycemia, alcohol hypoglycemia is frequently accompanied by hypothermia. In contrast to insulin-induced hypoglycemia, glucagon is ineffective in raising the blood sugar level since glycogen reserves have already been depleted. As in the case of ketoacidosis, patients promptly respond to infusion of glucose.

727. PARENTERAL NUTRITION

The problem of assuring nutritional maintenance or minimizing losses in body composition in association with acute or chronic disease is particularly challenging in patients in whom feeding via the gastrointestinal route is precluded. Until recently the primary focus in parenteral nutrition has been mainly on water and electrolyte replacement with little emphasis on meeting total caloric and protein requirements. The development of new techniques involving the infusion of markedly hypertonic solutions containing glucose and amino acids (parenteral hyperalimentation) has revolutionized the field of parenteral nutrition. Weight gain and positive nitrogen balance are now attainable goals in patients fed intravenously. However, total parenteral nutrition is not without morbidity (as noted below, a variety of infectious and metabolic complications have been described), and consequently is not indicated for all patients in whom oral or tube feeding cannot be maintained. The factors determining the composition, tonicity, and volume of fluid to be administered will depend in large part on whether feeding via the intravenous route must be sustained for a relatively brief period of up to a week or whether one is dealing with a prolonged period of parenteral alimentation. In the former instance the goal is primarily to minimize losses in body composition, whereas in the long-term situation the objective is positive caloric and protein balance to facilitate repair and healing of inflamed or traumatized tissue and to hasten convalescence.

Short-Term Intravenous Nutrition. In the patient requiring intravenous feeding for a period of several days, treatment is directed at providing sufficient carbohydrate to meet cerebral glucose requirements without depleting liver glycogen stores. In this manner, the need for gluconeogenesis and its attendant dissolution of body protein is minimized. Simultaneously, the glucose infusion prevents the fall in serum insulin levels which would otherwise occur in a nonfed individual, thereby inhibiting the development of starvation ketosis. These protein-sparing and antiketogenic effects are achieved with as little as 100 grams of carbohydrate, which may be infused over 24 hours as 2 liters of a 5 per cent dextrose solution. The net effect of the conventional glucose infusion is not one of stimulation of glucose uptake by muscle or fat tissue, but inhibition of hepatic glycogenolysis and replacement of the liver (by the infusion) as the source of glucose for brain oxidative requirements. Such an infusion doubles circulating insulin levels (as compared to the five- to tenfold increase observed after a carbohydrate meal) and elevates blood glucose by 15 to 30 mg per 100 ml. Increasing the amount of glucose infused above 100 grams per day will not further reduce the small degree of protein catabolism which persists in nonfed patients, unless one achieves caloric balance by administering markedly hypertonic solutions (see below).

An alternative form of carbohydrate available in commercial parenteral fluids is fructose. There is no evidence, however, that fructose has any advantage over glucose. Furthermore, rapid administration of large amounts of fructose (0.5 gram per kilogram per hour) can result in the development of lactic acidosis.

In addition to meeting nutritional needs, the major goal in short-term intravenous therapy is the maintenance of fluid and electrolyte balance. Basal fluid requirements may be estimated at 2000 ml per day, which consists of (1) 800 ml to provide for insensible losses via the lungs and skin and sensible losses as sweat, and (2) 1200 ml to maintain a reasonable urine output. The electrolyte requirements are in the form of sodium and potassium. Although the urine will become free of sodium after five to eight days of total sodium restriction, negative sodium balance (and the possibility of plasma volume contraction) will prevail during this interval if exogenous sodium is not provided. The usual intake of sodium in the diet is 4 to 6 grams (174 to 261 mEq), which is ingested as 10 to 12 grams of NaCl. Sodium depletion can be readily prevented in normal man by infusing 500 ml of isotonic (0.9 per cent) sodium chloride containing 77 mEq of NaCl. Potassium supplementation is also necessary, because there is an obligatory daily loss of about 40 mEq per day.

The total carbohydrate, fluid, and electrolyte requirements during short-term intravenous therapy may thus be met with the following daily infusion regimen: 1500 ml of 5 per cent dextrose in water containing 40 mEq KCl; and 500 ml of 5 per cent dextrose in isotonic (0.9 per cent) saline.

It should be noted that this regimen is designed to meet basal fluid and electrolyte requirements in patients without cardiac or renal failure and does not take into account pre-existing deficits or abnormal losses. For the modifications necessary to meet problems of hydration and electrolyte imbalance, see Ch. 805.

Long-Term Intravenous Nutrition (Total Parenteral Nutrition, Parenteral Hyperalimentation). In circumstances requiring long-term intravenous nutrition, particularly in debilitated patients, the optimal goal is positive nitrogen balance and weight gain. The infusion program outlined above for short-term therapy is obviously nutritionally inadequate in that it provides only 400 calories and no amino acids. Although protein hydrolysates have been available for over 30 years, a major problem has been the provision by parenteral means of an adequate amount of calories (2500 or more calories per day) to promote anabolism. Fat emulsions providing 9 calories per gram are potentially the most efficient energy source; however, none are currently approved for clinical use in the United States. Ethyl alcohol (7 calories per gram) is also a relatively efficient source of calories, but the toxic effects associated with infusion of alcohol limit its usefulness. The achievement of caloric balance by infusion of carbohydrate (4 calories per gram) necessitates

the infusion of massive amounts of isotonic or moderately hypertonic fluid (6 liters of a 10 per cent solution), or, alternatively, the infusion of hypertonic solutions (20 to 25 per cent or four to five times the tonicity of plasma). The former regimen results in problems of fluid overload, whereas the latter approach leads to thrombosis of peripheral veins. These difficulties in providing adequate calories were solved by Dudrick and his colleagues with their introduction of parenteral hyperalimentation, a technique involving placement of a catheter in the superior vena cava followed by infusion of a hypertonic glucose–amino acid mixture.

Indications. Although total parenteral nutrition has been applied in a variety of clinical conditions, its usefulness has been documented in specific circumstances only. Furthermore, this technique involves a serious risk (in view of the complications enumerated below), and should be restricted to patients in whom a definite indication exists. The following disorders are likely to benefit from this form of therapy: (1) Gastrointestinal disorders, particularly chronic inflammatory bowel disease (regional enteritis, ulcerative colitis) complicated by fistula formation; the "short bowel syndrome" after extensive intestinal resection; and congenital lesions of the gastrointestinal tract amenable to surgical repair. (2) Extensive body burns and traumatic injuries in which caloric requirements are markedly increased. In such cases parenteral nutrition may be used as a supplement to oral feeding. (3) Acute renal failure. Over-all mortality and duration of azotemia have been demonstrated to decrease in patients with acute renal failure treated with a mixture of glucose and 1.8 per cent essential amino acids.

It should be emphasized that neither the presence of an acute focal, septic condition nor the requirement to "put the alimentary tract at rest" is a sufficient indication for this form of treatment.

Composition of Solutions. A variety of hypertonic glucose and amino acid mixtures are currently available in commercial form. The solution to be administered is generally prepared by mixing 500 to 600 ml of the commercial protein hydrolysate or synthetic amino acid mixture with 400 to 500 ml of 50 per cent dextrose. The resulting solution should provide 900 to 1200 calories per liter. The recommended concentrations of nutrients and electrolytes in the infusate are shown in Table 3. Inasmuch as commercial preparations vary markedly in their content of sodium, potassium, and phosphate, supplemental electrolytes may have to be added to the infusate to achieve desired concentrations. Particular attention should be focused on administration of adequate phosphate, inasmuch as the phosphate requirement in parenterally alimented patients may exceed the 40 mEq per day recommended in patients fed via the oral route. The concentrations of nutrients shown in Table 3 do not apply to patients in renal failure or with congestive heart failure. In the former circumstance, a sodium-free solution containing only essential amino acids (1.8 per cent) is employed. In cardiac failure the sodium content of the infusate is reduced to 20 mEq per liter or less.

Solution Administration and Patient Management. Because of the hypertonicity of the infusate, rapid dilution of the infusion mixture by high blood flow is necessary to prevent phlebitis or thrombosis. Consequently total parenteral nutrition necessitates administration of nutrient solutions through a catheter in the superior vena cava. The latter may be cannulated via an infra-

TABLE 3.   Nutrient Concentration in Hypertonic
Solutions Used in Total Parenteral Nutrition*

Glucose	200–250 grams
Protein hydrolyzate or synthetic amino acids	30–50 grams
Calories	920–1200 kcal
Sodium	40–50 mEq
Potassium	30–40 mEq
Calcium	5–10 mEq
Magnesium	4–8 mEq
Phosphate	15–20 mEq
Multivitamin concentrate†	2 ml

*Expressed per liter of infusate.
†Vitamin K and folic acid which are not present in the multivitamin
concentrate are administered by intramuscular injection.

clavicular percutaneous subclavian vein puncture.
Alternatively, a surgical cutdown may be performed
with exposure of a peripheral vein through which the
catheter is threaded to the superior vena cava. Strict
asepsis must be used in inserting and maintaining
catheters. The dressing over the puncture site should
be changed every two to three days and an antibiotic
ointment reapplied.

The solution is initially administered at a rate of 2
liters per day, and thereafter is gradually increased to 3
liters per day. In dealing with a markedly catabolic
state, 4 to 5 liters may be administered. The solution
should be infused at a constant rate over the entire 24-
hour period.

While the patient is receiving total parenteral nutrition, a number of laboratory parameters should be followed so as to prevent or minimize metabolic complications. Fluid intake and output, body weight, and
fractional urine glucose concentrations should be recorded daily. Blood sugar, blood urea nitrogen, electrolytes, and calcium and phosphate concentration should
be determined at two- to three-day intervals. The importance of such monitoring is obvious from the complications reported in patients infused with hypertonic solutions.

Complications. Total parenteral nutrition is not
without risk to the patient. The reported complications
relate to either infection or metabolic disorders.

SEPSIS.   This is the most frequently observed complication; it may occur in 25 per cent or more of patients.
Fungemia caused by *Candida albicans* accounts for half
the cases, with the remainder attributable to
Staphylococcus aureus and *Klebsiella aerobacter.* In most
instances the organism can be cultured from the catheter
tip, implicating the catheter as the source of sepsis. Factors which may predispose to sepsis are prior antimicrobial use, the nutrient content of the infusate (which may
serve as growth medium), and possible adverse effects of
hypertonicity on phagocytic function. The incidence of
septicemia may be reduced by placing an on-line membrane filter of 0.22 μ pore size in the infusion apparatus,
frequent changing of the catheter, and meticulous care of
the skin puncture site.

HYPERGLYCEMIA.   In patients with normal pancreatic
islet cell function, the dextrose-rich infusate invokes a
hyperinsulinemic response which permits disposal of the
administered glucose load without the development of
hyperglycemia in excess of 200 mg per 100 ml. In pa-

tients with a predisposition to diabetes, the islet cell
response is inadequate and hyperglycemia and glycosuria develop. In some instances this may take the form
of *hyperglycemic nonketotic hyperosmolar coma* in which
the blood glucose reaches levels of 1000 mg per 100 ml
and is accompanied by dehydration, azotemia, obtundation, and occasionally seizures. Such patients should be
treated with rapid-acting insulin intravenously and
large volumes of water containing 2.5 per cent glucose.
The development of a severe hyperosmolar state can generally be prevented by frequent monitoring of the urine
and blood glucose levels and by administering insulin in
doses of 10 to 20 units to patients with persistent hyperglycemia (above 200 mg per 100 ml) and glycosuria.

POSTINFUSION HYPOGLYCEMIA.   If the intravenous infusion is suddenly dislodged or discontinued, a rapid fall
in blood glucose occurs which may reach hypoglycemic
levels. Presumably this is due to persistence of hyperinsulinemia and suppression of counter-regulatory hormones (glucagon, epinephrine, growth hormone, cortisol). This complication may be avoided by maintaining a
constant infusion rate and by switching to a solution containing 5 per cent glucose several hours before terminating the infusion.

HYPOPHOSPHATEMIA.   A decline in serum phosphate
concentration to levels less than 1 mg per 100 ml is almost uniformly observed after hyperalimentation with
phosphate-free solutions for periods of seven to ten days.
Accompanying the hypophosphatemia is a decline in red
cell levels of 2,3-diphosphoglycerate and an increase in
red cell oxygen affinity as indicated by a left-shift in the
oxygen dissociation curve. The clinical picture consists of
circumoral paresthesias, obtundation, hyperventilation,
and, in severe cases, seizures and coma. The hypophosphatemia is not due to urinary losses but is probably a
consequence of shifts in body phosphate. Insulin-
mediated glucose uptake in muscle and liver brought
about by the hypertonic glucose infusion is accompanied
by phosphate deposition in these tissues. This redistribution apparently occurs at the expense of plasma and red
cell phosphate reserves. The syndrome may be prevented
by adding phosphate supplements to the nutrient solution; in debilitated patients the requirement may be as
high as 20 to 25 mEq per liter.

HYPERCHLOREMIC ACIDOSIS.   In patients receiving synthetic amino acid mixtures rather than protein hydrolysates, the concentration of cationic amino acids (histidine, arginine, lysine) is substantially greater than that
of metabolizable anions as reflected in a large cation gap.
These cationic amino acids contribute hydrogen ions
(thereby lowering blood pH) and chloride to body fluids
upon conversion to urea or incorporation into peptide
chains. The resulting effect is hyperchloremic metabolic
acidosis. This syndrome may be prevented by adding a
portion of the sodium supplements to the infusate in the
form of bicarbonate rather than chloride when using
synthetic amino acid mixtures.

HYPERAMMONEMIA.   Abnormally elevated concentrations of blood ammonia have been reported in premature
infants and in adults with liver disease receiving infusions containing casein or fibrin hydrolysates. It is
probably due to an inability to metabolize preformed ammonia which may account for as much as 8 to 10 per cent
of the total nitrogen content in protein hydrolysate solutions. This complication can be prevented or minimized
by utilizing synthetic amino acid mixtures in patients
with liver disease and in premature infants.

728. DIET THERAPY

Diets are employed in the care of the sick for the following purposes: (1) to regulate (either decrease or increase) the total caloric intake; (2) to restrict (or less frequently augment) the content of specific nutrients, such as protein, fat, sodium, or potassium; (3) to provide foods which are bland in flavor, as in patients with peptic ulcer disease; (4) to reduce fiber content, as in disorders characterized by chronic diarrhea; (5) to eliminate specific foods, as in allergic conditions; and (6) to modify the consistency of foods, as in "soft" or "liquid" diets. Here we will consider specific conditions (diabetes, obesity) and diets in which the treatment program is restrictive in total calories and/or specific nutrients (protein, carbohydrate, sodium, potassium). The use of bland or fiber-restricted diets is discussed in Ch. 637. The dietary treatment of hyperlipidemias is described in Ch. 723.

In prescribing a diet it is important to recognize not only the therapeutic goals but also the likelihood of patient acceptance. The patient's likes and dislikes as well as cultural, sociologic, and economic factors must all be considered. For example, the high protein, low carbohydrate diet advocated by some in the treatment of obesity has been referred to as a "rich man's diet," since the cost of a diet made up primarily of foods high in protein content (meat, fish) may be prohibitively expensive. On the other hand, diet treatment based on an extremely restrictive protein content (20 grams) may fail because the basic unpalatability and limited food selection result in noncompliance.

A second factor to be considered in the make-up of a diet is the influence of restriction of one nutrient on the availability of other dietary components. A diet which is extremely low in sodium (250 mg) requires restriction in protein intake inasmuch as unlimited ingestion of milk or meat will increase the sodium content of the diet. The use of such a diet for the patient with chronic congestive heart failure may contribute to mobilization of edema fluid, but at the expense of a depletion in lean body mass. Similarly, a diet low in protein (20 to 40 grams) as used in cirrhotic patients with portal-systemic shunting and in renal disease will generally be calorically inadequate. Caloric balance can only be achieved by means of a very high intake of carbohydrate in the form of concentrated sweets, which may cause difficulty if there is an associated diabetic tendency. Deficiencies in vitamins are also likely to occur on severely restrictive diets but are more readily corrected by giving a single multivitamin tablet daily.

A third principle requiring emphasis is the requirement for precision in nomenclature and the need for close communication between the physician and dietician. The term "diabetic diet" has no meaning as such. However, a prescription for a 1900-calorie, 200-gram carbohydrate, 80-gram protein, and 90-gram fat diet is readily interpretable. Similarly, a "low salt diet" does not specify the precise level of sodium restriction as indicated by a "500-mg sodium diet." Few physicians have adequate knowledge of nutrition to construct a palatable and effective diet. On the other hand, the dietician, even when given a precise diet order, may not be aware of the therapeutic priorities for a particular patient. Communication between the physician and dietician will permit the minor modifications which may transform an unpalatable regimen into an acceptable program. For example, in the case of the patient in chronic renal failure on a restricted protein, sodium, and potassium intake, it is important for the dietician to know which nutrient may be most safely liberalized so as to improve patient acceptance without imposing serious difficulties in overall management.

The Normal Diet. In prescribing a therapeutic diet it is useful to begin by considering the normal diet. In an individual with a stable body weight and no marked shifts in body fluid, caloric intake equals caloric expenditure. As indicated in Table 2, the caloric requirements in a 70-kg man engaged in moderate activity are approximately 2500 to 2800 calories per day. In the "average" diet consumed in the United States, 15 per cent of these calories are derived from protein, 45 to 50 per cent are in the form of carbohydrate, and the remaining 35 to 40 per cent are derived from fat.

The normal diet can also be defined in terms of the relative contributions of six basic food groups (Table 4). Each of these basic food groups has a specific content of calories, protein, fat, and carbohydrate. In addition, for each of these groups an "exchange list" may be prepared, in which all of the specific food items of approximately equal carbohydrate, protein, and fat value are grouped. In this manner it becomes relatively simple to determine which foods are to be eliminated or reduced when intake of a specific nutrient is restricted. For example, it is clear that a diet low in protein entails a restriction in milk and meat. It is also obvious that a reduction in total calories can be achieved by substituting nonfat milk for whole milk and by restricting fat intake, while increasing vegetables (group A) as desired. It should be noted that certain vegetables such as potatoes, beans, peas, and corn are placed in the "bread group" because of their relatively high content of carbohydrate. The use of exchange lists, which is the fundamental tactic employed by the dietician in constructing a specific diet, is also extremely helpful to the patient in that it allows variety in food choices while maintaining specific nutritional guidelines.

Diabetes Mellitus. The fundamental role of diet in the management of diabetes is well recognized. Nevertheless, the specific principles involved in diet therapy have been poorly understood. The generally held notion is that carbohydrate is bad for people with diabetes and that a "diabetic diet" is a carbohydrate-restricted diet. In fact, the major emphasis in diet treatment in the diabetic should be directed at the following points in decreasing order of priority:

1. Regulation of total caloric intake so as to achieve an ideal body weight. For the maturity-onset diabetic in whom the incidence of obesity is 60 per cent or more, this generally entails a reduction in caloric intake. The importance of weight reduction in these patients is based upon the fact that obesity results in resistance to endogenous insulin; this is reversed by a return to ideal weight. With restoration to normal weight, the demand for endogenous insulin is reduced and an improvement in glucose tolerance will ensue. In contrast to the obese, maturity-onset diabetic, a hypercaloric intake is indicated in the thin, wasted insulin-dependent diabetic, particularly in childhood. Such patients require an increase in calories to restore body fat and protein and to permit normal growth.

2. The total carbohydrate content of the diet should not be disproportionately restricted, but the intake of concentrated sweets (candies, table sugar, pastries)

TABLE 4. Nutritive Values for Food Groups*

Food Group	Serving	Weight (grams)	Calories	Carbo-hydrate (grams)	Fat (grams)	Protein (grams)	Sodium (mg)	Potassium (mg)
1. Milk								
Whole milk	1 cup	240	170	12	10	8	120	335
Nonfat milk	1 cup	240	80	12	–	8	120	335
Low-sodium milk	1 cup	240	170	12	10	8	7	600
2. Meat								
Lean meat or fish	3 oz	90	219	–	15	21	75	300
Egg	1	50	73	–	5	7	60	65
3. Vegetables								
Group A†	½ cup	100	2–8	–	–	0.5–2.0	9	100–250
Group B‡	½ cup	100	35	7	–	2	9	100–200
4. Fruits	½ cup	100	40	10	–	0–1.0	2	75–250
5. Bread§								
Regular	1 slice	30	68	15	–	2	160	30
Low-sodium	1 slice	30	68	15	–	2	5	30
Low protein and low electrolyte	1 slice	30	68	17	–	0.1	9	3
Potatoes	1 small	100	68	15	–	2	4	407
Spaghetti	½ cup	100	68	15	–	2	1	61
6. Fat								
Butter, unsalted	1 tsp	5	45	–	5	–	–	–
Butter, salted	1 tsp	5	45	–	5	–	50	–

*Based on the Manual of Diets, Departments of Dietetics, Hospital of St. Raphael, Veterans Administration Hospital, and Yale–New Haven Hospital, New Haven, Connecticut, 1972.

†Includes all vegetables not listed in Group B or classified in "bread" group.

‡Beets, carrots, onions, green peas, turnips, squash.

§Includes high carbohydrate vegetables (potatoes, beans, and corn), cereals, and noodle products.

should be limited. There is no compelling evidence that isocaloric reduction in the carbohydrate content to 30 per cent results in improvement of the diabetic state. Such an approach may be deleterious in the long run, because the calories not taken as carbohydrate are generally made up in the form of a high fat intake which may have an adverse effect in accelerating atherosclerosis. Once the appropriate caloric intake has been determined, approximately 45 per cent of the calories should be provided in the form of carbohydrate. An exception is the diabetic with a carbohydrate-inducible (Type III or Type IV) form of hyperlipidemia, in whom a low carbohydrate, high fat intake is indicated (see Ch. 723). To avoid marked swings in the blood glucose concentration, particularly in insulin-dependent diabetics, simple sugars in the form of concentrated sweets should be avoided. Instead the carbohydrate in the diet should be primarily in the form of complex carbohydrates or starches (such as potatoes, beans, bread, and noodle products), because the glucose derived from these foods is released more slowly into the bloodstream.

3. Day-to-day regularity of food intake with respect to total consumption of calories and carbohydrates and with regard to the timing of meals is of importance in insulin-dependent diabetics so as to prevent insulin-induced hypoglycemia. An increase in the number and frequency of feedings in the form of a mid-morning, afternoon, and bedtime snack is also helpful in this regard. The regularity and frequency of feedings are predicated on the fact that, in contrast to the normal subject in whom insulin secretion is dictated by food ingestion, the insulin-dependent diabetic must match his food intake to the continuing action of injected insulin. The consistency in the pattern of food ingestion does not apply on those days in which there is a marked increase in caloric expenditure as a consequence of moderate to severe exercise. In normal subjects exercise causes an inhibition in beta cell secretion, resulting in a fall in endogenous insulin levels which permits an increase in hepatic glucose output. In the diabetic subject receiving insulin injections such homeostatic changes in circulating insulin levels will not occur in response to exercise. Here, extra food should be taken so as to meet the needs of contracting muscles and to prevent hypoglycemia.

Dietary management in diabetes must be related to the two primary types of the disease. In the obese, adult-onset diabetic the primary goal is a hypocaloric intake and weight reduction. In the insulin-dependent diabetic the major dietary objective is regularity of food ingestion so as to prevent hypoglycemia. Despite the simplicity of these principles, less than 50 per cent of the diabetic population adheres to the recommended dietary regimen. Poor understanding on the part of the patient as well as the physician with respect to dietary goals and tactics is frequently responsible for failure. Often the basic prescription is clearly in error and unsuitable for the specific patient. For example, to many physicians a "diabetic diet" almost by definition means an 1800-calorie intake. Such a diet in a vigorous, nonobese 160 pound insulin-dependent diabetic is obviously too restrictive and is likely to have adverse consequences: (1) the patient will not follow the diet and will supplement his intake, generally with concentrated sweets, resulting in marked swings in the blood glucose; or (2) he may stick to the diet but will develop hypoglycemic episodes and/or lose weight. An 1800-calorie diet is equally inappropriate in the 180 pound, 5 foot 2 inch, 50-year-old, sedentary, noninsulin-dependent diabetic woman, in whom the major objective should be weight reduction by means of a more limited caloric intake.

Diet treatment is also useful in the prevention of diabetes. The most important nutritional factor contributing to the development of diabetes is obesity, irrespective of the ratio of individual foodstuffs in the diet. The notion that an increased intake of concentrated carbohydrate is in itself a major causative factor in diabetes has not been substantiated. Thus in patients with a predisposition to diabetes (e.g., strong family history; mothers with a history of large babies), the emphasis should be on *total caloric regulation* so as to prevent obesity rather than on disproportionate restriction in carbohydrate intake.

Obesity. The situation in which diets are most commonly used in the general population is in obesity (see Ch. 723). A wide variety of "fad" diets have been heralded in the lay press (water diet, grapefruit diet, the low carbohydrate "diet revolution," etc.). Unfortunately none of these provides more rapid weight loss or a greater likelihood for long-term success than is achieved by more conventional caloric restriction. To be particularly condemned is the practice of restricting carbohydrate intake to virtually zero while permitting unlimited ingestion of fat. Such a diet will cause ketosis and hyperuricemia and will result in weight loss only so long as total calories as well as carbohydrate are restricted. On the other hand, if fat intake is increased to high levels, weight loss will not occur, and the tendency toward hyperlipidemia may be exaggerated.

Generally, the most appropriate dietary approach to obesity is to restrict total caloric intake to 1000 to 1400 calories per day, while maintaining the protein contribution at 20 per cent or more. In this manner the amount of bulk in the diet is increased, thereby prolonging the amount of time spent on eating and providing the patient with more oral gratification.

A major cause for the failure of diet treatment in obesity is the patient's loss of motivation because of his expectation of totally unrealistic results (e.g., continued weight reduction at a rate of 4 pounds or more per week). It is therefore imperative that the following points be stressed to the patient: (1) Weight loss is most rapid in the first one to two weeks as a consequence of an initial (hypocaloric-induced) diuresis. (2) Subsequent weight loss will be dictated by the caloric value of the tissue lost (adipose tissue) and the extent of negative caloric balance. (3) Adipose tissue has a caloric value of 3500 calories per pound. (4) It is unlikely that on a long-term basis intake can be adequately restricted and/or activity substantially increased to achieve a negative caloric balance of greater than 500 calories per day. (5) The expected rate of weight loss should therefore be no greater than approximately 1 pound per week.

Protein-Restricted Diets. Protein, as noted above, contributes approximately 15 per cent of the total calories consumed in the American diet. The daily intake of protein by healthy adults in the United States varies between 70 and 125 grams, averaging about 100 grams. Diets in which protein content is restricted to 60 grams or less are frequently used in the treatment of chronic renal failure (see Ch. 603) and to a lesser extent in the management of patients with cirrhosis of the liver complicated by portal hypertension. In these conditions the concomitant requirement to limit the intake of sodium and (in patients with renal disease) restrict the ingestion of potassium complicates the over-all nutritional approach.

Since it has long been recognized that dietary protein contributes to the endogenous pool of urea, diets low in protein have been advocated in the treatment of acute or chronic renal disease for over 50 years. The nutritional management of renal disease gained impetus, however, after the classic observations by Giordano and Giovannetti in the early 1960's that patients with chronic renal failure achieved symptomatic relief, a decrease in blood urea nitrogen, and positive nitrogen balance when essential amino acid requirements were met by providing no more than 20 grams of dietary protein. This limited intake of nitrogen could be either in the form of natural foods containing proteins of high biologic value or as a synthetic mixture of essential amino acids. The principle is that with adequate calories and minimal requirements for essential amino acids, retained nitrogen, principally in the form of urea, can be used for the synthesis of nonessential amino acids which are then incorporated into tissue proteins. In this manner the accumulation of urea is reduced, and, to the extent that breakdown products of nitrogen metabolism contribute to the symptoms of uremia (nausea, vomiting, anorexia), clinical improvement is obtained. The extrarenal metabolism of urea and its incorporation into protein have subsequently been confirmed by a variety of techniques. In fact, recent data indicate that urea utilization can be further stimulated and dietary nitrogen requirements can be further reduced by feeding patients the alpha-keto analogues of the essential amino acids.

Despite its rational basis and initially enthusiastic reception, the over-all usefulness and frequency of implementation of the Giordano-Giovannetti diet are currently rather limited. It was early recognized that dietary manipulation provided symptomatic relief but in no way improved underlying renal function. Second, the increasing use of dialysis and renal transplantation programs lessened the need for purely symptomatic maneuvers. Third, implementation of the diet has proved to be extremely difficult with respect to food preparation and patient acceptance.

In addition to restricting total protein intake, the success of the Giordano-Giovannetti diet depends on two additional constraints: (1) the protein ingested must be of high biologic value; and (2) the caloric intake must be maintained at 2000 to 3000 calories per day. The biologic value or quality of food proteins is an index of the efficiency with which these foodstuffs can be used for anabolic processes and is dependent on the amounts and ratios of the constituent essential amino acids. Proteins such as eggs, meat, fish, and milk are of high biologic value since they can meet the essential amino acid requirements when supplied in minimal quantities. In contrast, bread, cereals, fruits, and vegetables contain significant amounts of protein (Table 4), but are lacking in one or more essential amino acids and consequently are of low biologic value. Formulation of a 20-gram protein diet thus involves the administration of one egg (or 1 ounce of meat, cheese, or fish) plus three fourths of a cup of milk (to provide 14 grams of high quality protein) plus one serving each of a fruit and vegetable. To provide the patient with an adequate amount of calories without increasing protein content, it is necessary to add to the diet low-protein bread, biscuits, and noodle products which are specially prepared from wheat starch (rather than wheat flour). A major problem is the lack of palatability and difficulty in preparation of such a diet. The result is poor compliance and often an angry, frustrated patient with a limited caloric intake and progressive wasting of lean body mass.

To meet the twin goals of symptomatic improvement plus maintenance of body protein reserves in chronic renal disease, a more moderate degree of protein restriction than that in the 20-gram protein diet is generally recommended. In *symptomatic* patients (i.e., patients with nausea, anorexia, or vomiting) in whom glomerular filtration rate (GFR) is between 5 and 10 ml per minute, dietary management consists of a 40-gram protein intake, composed primarily of high quality protein. In patients with a GFR below 5 ml per minute who fail to achieve relief with a 40-gram intake, the 20-gram protein diet is used while awaiting initiation of dialysis treatment or transplantation. The 20-gram protein diet should be used on a long-term basis only in circumstances in which dialysis is unavailable or impracticable. Institution of chronic dialysis treatment should not be delayed solely because a symptomatic response has been obtained while the patient is on a 20-gram protein intake. In patients on dialysis treatment, the recommendations regarding dietary protein content vary from 40 to 80 grams per day. The general trend at present is toward more liberalized protein intake so as to ensure adequate caloric ingestion and avoidance of wastage of lean body tissue.

In addition to reducing protein ingestion, a restriction in sodium (see below) and potassium content of the diet is generally necessary in patients with renal failure. The average intake of potassium in the normal diet is 3000 mg per day. In renal failure potassium ingestion is generally reduced to levels of 1000 to 2000 mg. Because potassium is so widely distributed in foods (Table 4), restriction in potassium becomes an important factor limiting the palatability and choice of foods. Since fruits and vegetables are quite variable with respect to their potassium content, diet planning is facilitated by grouping these foods on the basis of their potassium content (Table 5). It should be noted that the number of permissible foods can be increased by extracting their potassium content during preparation. For example, the potassium content of potatoes is 407 mg per serving when prepared in the usual manner, but is greatly reduced by cutting the potatoes into small pieces and boiling in a large volume of water. The caloric value of the protein-potassium restricted diet may be increased with such carbohydrate-rich foods as hard candies, honey, jams, jellies, and granulated sugar. However, chocolate candies should be avoided because of their potassium content.

Sodium Restriction. The intake of sodium in the normal diet ranges between 4 and 6 grams (174 to 261 mEq) per day, ingested primarily in the form of sodium chloride. The sources of sodium in the diet include naturally occurring sodium in foods (Table 4) and sodium added to foods. Among the foods rich in natural sodium are the milk, egg, and meat groups, particularly organ meats and shellfish. Bread is another important source of sodium (160 mg per slice) because of the baking soda and baking powder used in its preparation. Sodium is also added in the canning and freezing of vegetables, as a preservative in the form of sodium benzoate, and as a seasoning in the form of monosodium glutamate. An additional important source of sodium is table salt used at the time of cooking or eating. Each teaspoonful of table salt provides 2000 mg of sodium.

A restricted sodium intake is employed in the management of edematous states such as congestive heart failure, cirrhosis, and renal disease (nephrotic syndrome and oliguric renal failure), and in the treatment of hypertension. Since it is the sodium ion rather than chloride which must be limited in these conditions, and inasmuch as sodium may be present in the diet in a variety of forms (e.g., bicarbonate, glutamate, benzoate, propionate, or chloride), it is inappropriate to characterize diets in terms of *salt* intake. Instead the diet prescription should designate the precise number of *milligrams of sodium* to be provided each day. In general one of four categories of sodium restriction is employed: 2000 to 4000 mg, 1000 mg, 500 mg, and 250 mg.

The 2000 to 4000 mg (87 to 174 mEq) sodium diet represents a mild degree of sodium restriction which is attained by (1) elimination of table salt and sodium-rich seasonings added at meal times and (2) avoidance of salted foods such as pretzels, potato chips, processed meats (bacon, sausages, etc.), and salty fish (anchovies, sardines). Small amounts of salt may be used in cooking with this diet. This level of sodium restriction is useful as a maintenance diet in subjects in whom a diuresis has already been achieved.

A reduction in sodium intake to 1000 mg (43 mEq) requires, in addition to the measures outlined above, the elimination of salt in cooking and the avoidance of canned or frozen fruits and vegetables, unless specially

TABLE 5. Potassium Content of Fruits and Vegetables*

Fruits	Vegetables

Group I (less than 100 mg; average 75 mg)
  Applesauce, cranberries, pears (canned), pineapple (canned),
  blueberries (canned)
	Group I (100–150 mg)
	  Lettuce, cucumber, onions, cabbage, carrots (canned), corn (canned)

Group II (100–150 mg)
  Apples (raw or juice), grapefruit, cherries, tangerine, watermelon,
  pineapple juice, grape juice, peaches (canned)
	Group II (150–200 mg)
	  Carrots (raw or cooked), celery, beets, turnips, asparagus (canned),
	  mushrooms (canned)

Group III (150–200 mg)
  Oranges (raw or juice), grapes, grapefruit juice, fruit cocktail
	Group III (200–250)
	  Tomatoes (fresh, canned, or juice), asparagus (fresh or frozen),
	  broccoli, cauliflower, lima beans, spinach

Group IV (greater than 200 mg)†
  Apricots (canned), bananas, cantaloupe, dates, honeydew melon,
  prunes (raw or juice), raisins
	Group IV (over 250 mg)†
	  Potatoes, artichokes, Brussels sprouts

*Potassium content is given per serving (1/2 cup or small size for raw fruits such as apples, oranges and pears) and is based on the Manual of Diets, Department of Dietetics, Hospital of St. Raphael, Veterans Administration Hospital, and Yale–New Haven Hospital, New Haven, Connecticut, 1972.
†Fruits and vegetables in Group IV are generally omitted in potassium restricted diets.

processed as low-sodium dietetic foods. The ingestion of foods containing significant amounts of sodium such as regular bread and milk must be limited, generally to three slices and 1 pint per day, respectively. This level of sodium intake is often used when therapy is initiated in edematous patients.

In patients with severe refractory edema, it may be necessary to reduce the level of sodium intake to 500 mg (22 mEq) or less to effect a diuresis. This degree of restriction in sodium (500 mg) requires avoidance of all the foods omitted in the 1000 mg diet, substitution of low sodium bread for regular bread, and strict limitation in the intake of allowable foods (particularly meat, fish, eggs, and milk) to carefully measured amounts. A further reduction in sodium intake to 250 mg (11 mEq) is achieved by substituting low-sodium milk for regular milk. Because of the restriction in choices and amounts of food involved in such diets, it is difficult to maintain an adequate caloric or protein intake or to provide sufficient palatability to assure patient compliance. Con-

sequently, severe sodium restriction (250 or 500 mg diets), particularly on a long-term basis, should be employed only for patients who are clearly refractory to more moderate degrees of sodium restriction.

Cahill, G. F., Jr.: Starvation in man. N. Engl. J. Med., 282:668, 1970.

Cowan, G. S., and Scheetz, W. L.: Intravenous Hyperalimentation. Philadelphia, Lea & Febiger, 1972.

Dudrick, S. J., Macfadyen, B. V., Jr., Van Buren, C. T., Ruberg, R. L., and Maynard, A. T.: Parenteral hyperalimentation. Metabolic problems and solutions. Ann. Surg., 176:259, 1972.

Felig, P., Marliss, E., Owen, O. E., and Cahill, G. F., Jr.: Blood glucose and gluconeogenesis in fasting man. Arch. Intern. Med., 123:293, 1969.

Hyne, B. E. B., Fowell, E., and Lee, H. A.: The effect of caloric intake on nitrogen balance in chronic renal failure. Clin. Sci., 43:679, 1972.

Levy, L. J., Duga, J., Girgis, M., and Gordon, E. E.: Ketoacidosis associated with alcoholism in nondiabetic subjects. Ann. Intern. Med., 78:213, 1973.

Long, C. L., Spencer, J. L., Kinney, J. M., and Geiger, J. W.: Carbohydrate metabolism in man: Effect of elective operations and major surgery. J. Appl. Physiol., 31:110, 1971.

West, K. M.: Diet therapy of diabetes: An analysis of failure. Ann. Intern. Med., 79:425, 1973.

Part XVI
HEMATOLOGIC AND HEMATOPOIETIC DISEASES

729. INTRODUCTION

Ralph L. Nachman

This edition includes a number of new and exciting advances in the area of clinical hematology. Much of this new knowledge, which bears directly on the diagnosis and care of patients with hematologic disease, results from the direct application of the principles of molecular biology to clinical hematologic disorders. This is particularly appropriate since modern molecular biology stems in a real sense from the original observations made over a quarter of a century ago by Pauling on sickle cell hemoglobin. With this growing complexity and sophistication it has become obvious that many of the several areas within hematology have rapidly become the province of superspecialists such as red cell enzymologists, hemoglobinopathy experts, chemotherapists, and clotters. Despite this fragmentation, it is important to note that, although many primary hematologic disorders are relatively rare, hematologic symptoms, signs, and laboratory abnormalities are frequent secondary components of many common clinical disorders. A good history and physical examination still remain the essential prerequisites for adequate evaluation of a hematologic problem. It is true that many clinical hematologic disorders require complicated laboratory procedures before the final diagnosis is verified; it is clear, however, that these studies must be performed as part of an evaluation of the whole patient and not as a fragmented dissection of an isolated organ system.

In the chapters which follow, new information will be presented relating to several different areas which will have a long-range impact on the diagnosis and therapy of hematologic disease. Some of the most important new advances are noted here.

Red cell 2,3-diphosphoglycerate (DPG) plays an important role in the regulation of oxygen dissociation. DPG binds to the beta chains of deoxyhemoglobin and decreases oxygen affinity. As DPG rises, more oxygen is released to the tissue without a change in the tissue oxygen tension. Intraerythrocytic DPG levels thus play an important role in the physiologic adaptation to anoxia and anemia. Patients with severe chronic anemia tolerate very low hemoglobin levels owing to the elevated levels of red cell DPG.

Chronic granulomatous disease of childhood results from an inability of neutrophils to kill certain species of bacteria. The study of this disorder and similar related illnesses has greatly increased our knowledge of intracellular bactericidal mechanisms. Neutrophils generate H_2O_2 which in the presence of halide and the lysosomal enzyme myeloperoxidase kills phagocytized bacteria. Several new clinical disorders have been observed in which other qualitative defects in neutrophil function have been defined.

Viruses continue to play important roles in various hematologic disorders. Epstein-Barr (EB) virus causes infectious mononucleosis in man. The etiologic role of this virus in other lymphoproliferative states such as Burkitt's lymphoma remains to be determined. Considerable information has been accumulated concerning the etiologic role of RNA tumor viruses in a variety of animal cancers. Reverse transcriptase is a well-defined biochemical attribute of these tumor viruses. White cells from leukemic patients have been demonstrated to contain reverse transcriptase, which in the test tube synthesizes DNA homologous to certain tumor virus RNA. The story is inconclusive, but the evidence suggests that in the future viruses may be shown to be the causative agent of some forms of human leukemia.

Chemotherapy of leukemia and the lymphomas has made major strides in recent years. Combination chemotherapy and newer concepts of induction, consolidation, and maintenance have led to significant prolongation of survival in acute lymphocytic leukemia in childhood and in Hodgkin's disease in adults.

Some progress has been made in our understanding of hemorrhagic diseases. The role of the platelet as a first line of defense in hemostasis has been greatly clarified. It seems that this cell also significantly contributes to pathologic processes associated with arterial intimal disease. Much has been learned about the blood coagulation proteins and some of the control mechanisms which regulate the enzymatic conversion of fibrinogen to fibrin. Much interest and work have geen generated by clinical and molecular studies of the factor VIII diseases—hemophilia A and von Willebrand's disease.

These are only a few of the major advances which may well transform the face of clinical hematology in the coming years. It is certain that this is an area of medicine which is bound to substantially change in the next decade.

Section One.   THE ANEMIAS

730. INTRODUCTION

M. C. Brain

The function of the red blood cell is the transport of oxygen from the capillaries in the lungs to the systemic capillaries of the tissues and the facilitation of carbon dioxide transport from the tissues to the lungs. In physiologic terms, anemia can be regarded as a reduction in oxygen transporting capacity of the blood. The normal response to increased demand by the tissues for oxygen is met by an increase in cardiac output, and the symptoms of anemia first become apparent on exercise. Since oxygen is transported by the red blood cell in combination with hemoglobin, the principal protein constituent of the cell, anemia can be most simply and practically defined as a lowering of the hemoglobin concentration of the blood below the normal range for a population of comparable age and sex. However, the definition of anemia solely in terms of whole blood hemoglobin concentration makes several assumptions. First, the whole blood hemoglobin concentration does not take into account the influence of changes in plasma volume, nor does it provide information on the concentration of hemoglobin within the red blood cells, although the latter can be determined from knowledge of the cell count and the packed red cell volume or hematocrit. Second, and physiologically of greater importance, the definition of anemia in terms of hemoglobin concentration might be thought to imply that the hemoglobin concentration is the sole determinant of oxygen delivery by the red blood cells. Recent work on the regulation of the affinity of hemoglobin for oxygen has shown this not to be true. A number of factors are known to influence hemoglobin-oxygen affinity and hence both the amount and rate at which oxygen is released from red blood cells at the lowered partial pressure of oxygen in the systemic capillaries. These factors include blood pH, temperature, the concentration of hemoglobin within the red blood cell (the mean corpuscular hemoglobin concentration [MCHC]), the red blood cell concentration of organic phosphates (principally 2,3-diphosphoglycerate [DPG] and, to a lesser extent, adenosine triphosphate [ATP]) which are products of red cell metabolism, and the presence of genetically determined substitutions in key positions in the polypeptide chains of the hemoglobin molecule. All these factors may either increase or reduce hemoglobin-oxygen affinity and thereby enhance or diminish the amount and rate of oxygen release. Thus the physiologic consequences of anemia must reflect the hemoglobin concentration of the blood and the hemoglobin-oxygen affinity of red blood cells in the circulation. Whereas the hemoglobin concentration of the blood can be readily and rapidly determined, the measurement of hemoglobin-oxygen affinity is less simple. However, changes in hemoglobin-oxygen affinity caused by variations in pH and the MCHC can be readily calculated, as can the effects of DPG and ATP if the concentrations of these compounds in the red blood cell are known. Although changes in hemoglobin-oxygen affinity are rare and are therefore of less clinical importance than changes in hemoglobin concentration, it is important to be aware that they exist, because they may modify the physiologic effects of anemia.

An understanding of the pathologic and physiologic factors which give rise to anemia and its consequences requires an appreciation of the following: (1) the structure and function of the normal red blood cell, (2) the formation of red blood cells in the bone marrow and the factors which regulate erythropoiesis, (3) the disorders which influence the quantity and/or the normal constitution of red blood cells produced by the bone marrow, (4) the factors which influence the distribution and/or survival of red blood cells within the circulation, and (5) the disorders which result in loss of erythrocytes from the circulation.

The mammalian red blood cell is remarkable in that it carries out its function after loss of the nucleus which determined and controlled the synthesis of its constituents. The nucleus is normally extruded from the cell as it enters the circulation by passing into the venous sinuses of the bone marrow. For the first few days after entering the circulation the red blood cell retains cytoplasmic organelles, including mitochondria and ribosomes, and ribonucleic acids, and can be identified with supravital dyes which stain these constituents. The filamentous or reticulin-like pattern of the stained structures gave rise to the term *reticulocyte* for these cells. Once the mitochondria and ribosomes are lost, the cell's capability to synthesize proteins ceases. Thereafter the mature red blood cell has only a limited capacity to reconstitute membrane lipid and other nonlipid cytoplasmic constituents. As a consequence it has a finite life span of approximately 120 days. The maintenance of normal numbers of red blood cells in the circulation is thus dependent on continuous production from precursor cells in the bone marrow. In anemia the number of circulating red blood cells depends upon the capacity of the bone marrow to increase the number produced to compensate for the loss from the circulation—a response which may be ultimately restricted by the limitations imposed by the bony skeleton upon the expansion of the bone marrow within it.

The mature red blood cell is a highly deformable cell which in the resting state assumes the shape of a biconcave disc with an average diameter of 8.4 μ. The biconcave shape is primarily determined by the inherent physical strains within the membrane in relation to the ratio of membrane surface area to volume of the cell. The remarkable deformability of the red blood cell accounts for the low viscosity of blood at high flow rates despite the high proportion of red blood cells present in blood. Furthermore, the deformability enables the cell to pass repeatedly through the capillaries of the microcirculation, some of which have a diameter of 3 μ or less. Reduction in deformability resulting from a change in shape, or from a change in solubility or stability of hemoglobin with the formation of intracellular inclusions, predisposes the red blood cell to selective sequestration in the microcirculation, especially in the spleen, and can lead to shortened survival in the circulation.

Hemoglobin comprises approximately 95 per cent of the dry weight of the red blood cell and on average 34 per cent of the wet weight, the remainder being made up of water, anions, cations (principally potassium), glucose, phosphorylated glycolytic intermediates (principally 2,3-diphosphoglycerate which is present in the same molar concentration as hemoglobin), glutathione, adenosine and pyridine nucleotides, and the enzymes responsible for the metabolism of glucose to lactic acid. Glucose is metabolized by two linked metabolic pathways. The principal function of the Embden-Meyerhof pathway is the formation of ATP which is utilized in maintenance of the normal cation content of the red blood cells through ATP-dependent transport mechanisms, in maintenance of membrane lipid composition, and in cell shape. The hexose monophosphate shunt, the subsidiary pathway of glucose metabolism, is responsible for maintaining glutathione in a reduced state and thereby in protecting the cellular constituents (notably hemoglobin) from oxidative denaturation.

The hemoglobin within the red blood cell is formed of spheroidal molecules of a molecular weight of 64,458. Ninety-seven per cent of the molecule consists of the polypeptide chains of globin, and 3 per cent of the heme groups. Each molecule is formed from four subunits, comprising two pairs of identical polypeptide chains, to each of which is attached a heme group partially buried in the outer aspect of the molecule. In the red blood cells of adults, 97 per cent of the hemoglobin is made up of two α and two β chains and is designated *hemoglobin A*. *Hemoglobin A_2*, consisting of two α and two δ chains, forms 2 per cent, and *hemoglobin F*, formed from two α and two λ chains, provides the remaining 1 per cent. Hemoglobin F is the principal hemoglobin in the red blood cells of the fetus, and is gradually replaced by hemoglobin A with the onset of β chain synthesis in the last trimester of pregnancy. Hemoglobin F levels fall from birth and reach adult levels by the end of the first year of life. For the red blood cell to contain a normal concentration of hemoglobin requires balanced synthesis of both the α and β chains and of the heme groups by the erythroblasts in the bone marrow. Disorders of hemoglobin constitution and/or concentration within the red blood cell can arise through abnormalities of synthesis either of the globin (polypeptide chain) or of heme groups. Disorders of the constitution of the globin chains are not usually associated with major reductions in the amount of hemoglobin synthesized. Although many genetic variations in the primary amino acid structure of hemoglobin molecule have been recognized, they only become clinically important when such substitutions are at critical sites in the molecule, thereby influencing the function, solubility, or stability of the molecule. Deficient hemoglobin synthesis within the erythroblast can result from failure or imbalance of the synthesis of the polypeptide chains (the thalassemia syndrome), or through disturbances of heme synthesis, commonly caused by lack of iron, and more rarely caused by disorders in the porphyrin synthetic pathway.

The red blood cell formed in the bone marrow is the final stage in a sequence of cell divisions arising from a common multipotential hematopoietic stem cell. This common hematopoietic stem cell gives rise to a number of committed stem cells from which develop the erythroid, granulocyte, and megakaryocyte cell lines. The committed stem cells form a self-regenerating stem cell pool, as well as giving rise to differentiated erythroblasts which undergo three mitotic divisions during the course of maturation to the late normoblast and finally through extrusion of the nucleus to the reticulocyte. The time taken between an erythropoietic stimulus and the outpouring of reticulocytes from the bone marrow is approximately five days. It has long been recognized that anemia or hypoxia stimulates increased erythropoiesis. The response is mediated through the action of a specific erythropoiesis-stimulating hormone, *erythropoietin.* Erythropoietin is a relatively heat-stable glycoprotein with a molecular weight of between 40,000 and 70,000. It has been shown experimentally that erythropoietin stimulates the erythroid stem cell to undergo mitosis and accelerates the rate of cell division of the developing erythroblasts. Raised levels of erythropoietin have been demonstrated in the serum and urine of anemic patients. The primary stimulus to its release into the circulation has been shown to be hypoxia. There is much evidence to suggest that the kidneys are the principal site of erythropoietin formation or release. Destruction or removal of the kidneys is associated with diminished erythropoiesis; yet other organs and tissues must be responsible for erythropoietin formation, because erythropoiesis continues in anephric patients and erythropoietin has been detected in their serum. Although hypoxia is the principal stimulus to erythropoietin release, clinical evidence indicates a greater erythropoietic response to hemolytic anemia than to comparable anemia resulting from blood loss. Thus the products of red blood cell destruction may provide an additional stimulus to erythropoietin release.

The continuous formation of red blood cells from precursor cells within bone marrow is dependent upon both normal bone marrow function and the stimulus of erythropoietin. Disorders of red blood cell formation can arise from diminution of the number of pluripotent hematopoietic stem cells, as in aplastic or hypoplastic anemias, or from disturbances in maturation of the committed erythropoietic stem cell, as in isolated red cell aplasias. In acute and chronic leukemias the disorder of stem cell differentiation will adversely affect erythropoiesis. Similarly, infiltration of the bone marrow by malignant cells arising from other organs or the progressive sclerosis of the bone marrow in myelosclerosis will reduce erythropoiesis. In the latter circumstance, hematopoiesis, including erythropoiesis, may be undertaken at *extramedullary sites* in the body such as the liver and spleen. Erythropoiesis is quantitatively reduced in acute and chronic infections, by chronic inflammatory disorders such as rheumatoid arthritis, and by renal failure. It is influenced by the nutritional status of the individual, being particularly affected by deficiencies of vitamin B_{12}, folic acid, iron, and protein. Vitamin B_{12} and folic acid are essential cofactors in the synthesis of DNA. Deficiency of either one results in impairment of cell division with formation of megaloblasts, macroerythroblasts with defective nuclear maturation, and production of large red blood cells (*macrocytes*). Conversely, deficiency of iron through the impairment of hemoglobin synthesis results in the production of *hypochromic microcytic* (small) red blood cells. Defective hemoglobinization of the red blood cell is also a feature of the defective hemoglobin synthesis resulting from imbalanced globin synthesis of the thalassemia syndromes. Disorders of red blood cell maturation within the bone marrow, whether caused by disorders of cell division as in the megaloblastic anemias or by defective hemoglobin synthesis, are associated with *ineffective erythropoiesis,* a considerable proportion of the abnormal erythroblasts undergoing phagocytic destruction within the bone marrow and therefore failing to gain entry to the circulation. The extent of ineffective erythropoiesis can be assessed by measurement of the rate of clearance of radioactive iron from the plasma and of the proportion of the radioactive iron entering the circulation in labeled hemoglobin. In ineffective erythropoiesis there is rapid clearance of radioactive iron from the plasma, but only 20 to 40 per cent of the iron enters the blood compared with the 70 to 90 per cent in normal subjects. Ineffective erythropoiesis can also be assessed by the early excretion of C^{14}-carbon monoxide and C^{14}-stercobilin derived from the catabolism of newly synthesized heme after the administration of C^{14}-glycine. This latter method has shown that even in normal subjects a small proportion of the newly synthesized heme is catabolized to bilirubin, which may reflect the rapid turnover of nonhemoglobin heme proteins in the liver. In ineffective erythropoiesis the proportion of newly synthesized heme which is catabolized and the products excreted are greatly increased.

Red blood cells entering the circulation are normally uniformly distributed within the circulation, and the hematocrit of the venous blood corresponds closely to the whole-body hematocrit derived from simultaneous measurements of the red blood cell and plasma volumes. The distribution of red blood cells within the circulation is influenced by the spleen. Reticulocytes, until they mature, are preferentially sequestered within the spleen. In conditions which cause massive enlargement of the spleen, such as the congestive splenomegaly of portal hypertension, the proportion of red blood cells sequestered may be greatly increased. The sequestration of red blood cells in the spleen together with the associated increase in plasma volume can result in a lowering of the red blood cell count and hematocrit in the venous blood to produce an apparent anemia, although the red blood cell mass may be normal or only slightly below normal.

Red blood cells normally survive in the circulation for 120 days. The degree of anemia caused by shortened red blood cell survival is governed by the rate of the hemolysis and the ability of the bone marrow to compensate. Hemolytic anemia can usually be recognized by the association of an anemia, in the absence of evidence of blood loss, with an increase in the catabolism of hemoglobin as reflected by hyperbilirubinemia, and by reticulocytosis. Minor degrees of hemolysis accompany many disorders associated with ineffective erythropoiesis. Shortened red blood cell survival may be due to abnormalities inherent to the cell, such as congenital or familial disorders of the membrane, metabolism, or hemoglobin, or may be brought about by the action of extrinsic or environmental factors in the circulation. The latter include the effects of plasma factors (antibodies), the action of drugs or toxins, or changes in the vascular environment through which the red blood cells circulate. The extrinsic factors influencing red blood cell survival in general tend to be acquired rather than congenital or familial in etiology. But this distinction is not always valid, because congenital disorders of metabolism or of hemoglobin may predispose the cell to deleterious action of extrinsic agents such as oxidative drugs.

Loss of red blood cells from the circulation through frank or occult hemorrhage is a common cause of acute or chronic anemia, the degree of anemia reflecting the magnitude and duration of the blood loss and the reduction in body iron stores through loss of hemoglobin from the body. Thus chronic blood loss rapidly produces iron deficiency, with consequent impairment of erythropoiesis by the bone marrow.

The normal range of red blood cell values in adults is shown in Table 1.

The values of the red blood cell count, hemoglobin concentration, and packed cell volume in children between the ages of three months and puberty are approximately 10 to 20 per cent lower than the adult values, the difference being more marked in younger children. The differences between the sexes become apparent only at puberty. The lower values in children probably reflect the diminished affinity of hemoglobin for oxygen in children. Thus the lower red blood cell count and hemoglobin concentration meet the normal physiologic needs for oxygen transport.

CLASSIFICATION

Anemias can be classified according to the etiology of the disorder giving rise to anemia (Table 2) or in relation to the morphologic appearance and quantitative abnormality of red blood cell size (mean corpuscular volume [MCV]), hemoglobin content (MCH), and hemoglobin concentration (MCHC). Any attempt at classification is at best somewhat arbitrary, because in many disorders the degree of anemia and the morphologic appearance of the red blood cell are consequences of the effects of both the primary cause and the erythropoietic response by the bone marrow. Furthermore, it is difficult to combine a

TABLE 2.   Anemias: Etiologic Classification

I. Principally caused by impaired production
  A. Disturbances of the proliferation and differentiation of stem cells
    1. Aplastic anemia: idiopathic; due to physical or chemical injury (radiation, benzol, lead, or cytotoxic and other drugs such as chloramphenicol, phenylbutazone, etc.)
    2. Pure red blood cell aplasia
    3. Anemia of chronic renal failure
    4. Endocrine deficiency (pituitary, thyroid, adrenal, or testicular hormones)
  B. Disturbances of proliferation and maturation of differentiated erythroblasts
    1. Defective DNA synthesis (vitamin B_{12}, folic acid, and metabolic defects in purine and pyrimidine metabolism)
    2. Defective hemoglobin synthesis
      a. Deficient globin synthesis (thalassemia)
      b. Deficient heme synthesis (iron deficiency)
      c. Sideroblastic anemia
    3. Protein malnutrition
    4. Anemia of chronic infections or inflammatory or neoplastic disease
    5. Myelophthisic anemias due to bone marrow infiltration or replacement (leukemias, myelofibrosis, Hodgkin's disease, multiple myeloma, metastatic carcinoma, etc.)
II. Principally caused by shortened red blood cell survival (increased rate of destruction)
  A. Intrinsic or red blood cell abnormalities
    1. Membrane disorders
      a. Inherited disorders of cell shape; spherocytosis, elliptocytosis, stomatocytosis
      b. Inherited disorders of membrane lipid synthesis
      c. Paroxysmal nocturnal hemoglobinuria
    2. Disorders of red blood cell metabolism
    3. Congenital or inherited enzyme deficiencies
    4. Disorders of hemoglobin (globin) structure, solubility, and stability (sickle cell anemia, hemoglobin C disease, unstable hemoglobins, etc.)
  B. Extrinsic or extraerythrocytic abnormalities
    1. Plasma factors
      a. Antibody mediated destruction
      b. Disturbance of cholesterol or plasma lipids (abetalipoproteinemia, liver disease)
    2. Physical factors (cardiac, microangiopathic, burns)
    3. Chemical or toxic agents (copper, lead, oxidative drugs: dapsone, phenacetin)
    4. Bacterial or other organisms: (Cl. welchii, malaria)
    5. Reticuloendothelial sequestration (splenomegaly)
III. Anemia of blood loss (acute or chronic)

TABLE 1.   Red Cell Values in Adults: Normal Range

	Men	Women
Red blood cells	5.11 ± 0.38	$4.51 \pm 0.36 \times 10^6$ μl blood
Hemoglobin	15.5 ± 1.1	13.7 ± 1.0 gram/100 ml blood
Packed cell volume	46.0 ± 3.1	40.9 ± 3.0 ml/100 ml blood
Mean corpuscular volume	90.0 ± 4.8	90.4 ± 4.8 μm^3/red blood cell
Mean corpuscular hemoglobin	30.2 ± 1.8	30.2 ± 1.9 pg/red blood cell
Mean corpuscular hemoglobin concentration	33.9 ± 1.2	33.6 ± 1.1 grams/100 ml red blood cells
Reticulocytes	0.2 to 2.0	0.2 to 2.0 per 100 red blood cells

logical pathophysiologic classification with the expected frequency with which the various etiologies may be encountered, the latter being influenced by the age, racial background, socioeconomic factors, and geographic location of the population encountered.

A classification of anemia on the basis of red blood cell morphology, as seen in the peripheral blood smear and supported by the quantitative measurements of cell size (MCV) and hemoglobin content and concentration (MCH and MCHC), can provide a valuable indication as to the possible etiologic mechanisms (Table 3). The introduction of automatic equipment for the rapid and accurate enumeration of red blood cells and determination of the MCV, MCH, and MCHC has greatly enhanced the diagnostic value of these measurements.

The classification shown in Table 3 fails to include much additional information which can be obtained from examination of stained blood smears. Quantitative data with the emphasis on mean values cannot reflect variations in cell shape, size, or hemoglobin content or cell staining, such as the polychromasia indicative of reticulocytosis. Only examination of the stained smear can lead to the recognition of intracellular inclusions such as *Howell-Jolly bodies* (nuclear remnants indicative of splenectomy or splenic dysfunction), *Pappenheimer bodies* (granules of hemosiderin), *punctate basophilia* (a feature of disorders of hemoglobin synthesis often seen in lead poisoning and in thalassemia), and malarial parasites. Disturbances of cell size *(anisocytosis),* shape *(poikilocytosis),* and staining can lead to the recognition of congenital or acquired causes of spherocytosis, of elliptocytosis, or of stomatocytosis. Poikilocytosis is a frequent accompaniment of disordered erythropoiesis, and is associated with disorders of hemoglobin synthesis as in iron deficiency or thalassemia. The abnormal shape of the *sickle cell* was recognized long before the molecular pathology of the sickle cell anemia was understood. Likewise, *target cells* in the absence of macrocytosis may suggest the presence of hemoglobin C. The presence of *red blood cell fragments* in the presence of hemolysis suggests a cardiac or microangiopathic mechanical hemolysis. Variation in hemoglobinization of erythrocytes can suggest partial response to iron therapy, be compatible with recent blood transfusion, or be a feature of the sideroblastic anemias. The recognition of megaloblastic anemia when associated with iron deficiency may not be accompanied by macrocytosis; however, the presence of multilobed polymorphonuclear leukocytes may provide the clue to an underlying vitamin B_{12} or folate deficiency. Likewise, knowledge of the differential white cell count and platelet count can lead to the recognition of hypoplastic anemias, myelophthisic anemias, and leuke-

mic disorders. Further information may be derived from examination of the reticulocyte preparation in the detection of *Heinz bodies* (precipitated denatured hemoglobin) and *hemoglobin H bodies* (β_4 inclusions). It may be helpful to examine a diluted wet preparation of blood in determining the nature of shape changes which can arise from the drying of conventional stained smears. Finally, the presence of intense rouleaux formation may indicate the presence of a paraprotein, whereas frank agglutination can point to the presence of cold-agglutinating antibodies.

Although knowledge of the red blood cell count, hemoglobin concentration, and MCV, MCH, and MCHC provides valuable information as to whether an anemia is macrocytic, normocytic, or microcytic, examination of the blood film can often give a more specific indication of the etiology of the disorder. This in turn can lead to further diagnostic investigations of erythropoiesis, such as a bone marrow biopsy, or of disorders of red blood cell membrane, metabolism, or hemoglobin, including the detection of antibodies on the membrane surface, or to evidence of frank or occult blood loss by appropriate inquiry or investigation.

PRINCIPLES OF THERAPY

As in all conditions, the principles of the treatment of anemia are primarily dependent on recognition of the cause of an anemia and, when possible, the correction of the cause with appropriate treatment. Consideration of the classification of the etiology of anemia provides a useful framework on which to base the principles of treatment. When a cause for aplastic or hypoplastic anemia can be identified, exposure to the agent or agents should cease and an incriminated drug should never again be given to the patient. Heavy metals may be excreted in response to appropriate chelating agents. In general the principal measures are supportive with blood transfusions. Erythropoiesis may be improved by androgenic steroids. Renal failure and endocrine deficiency states should be treated appropriately.

The cause of megaloblastic anemia should be sought and appropriate replacement therapy with either vitamin B_{12} or folic acid given. Neither of these vitamins should be prescribed without clear-cut indications. Among these indications is the folate deficiency associated with increased requirement for this vitamin in pregnancy and in the erythropoietic response to hemolytic anemia. Iron therapy should be given when anemia is recognized as being due to iron deficiency resulting either from inadequate intake or increased demand, as in pregnancy, or from blood loss. Patients with sideroblastic anemia may respond to treatment with pyridoxine. Iron therapy should be avoided in patients with anemia of other causes such as thalassemia or sideroblastic anemia, in both of which the hypochromic anemia may be mistaken for iron deficiency; nor should iron be given to patients with chronic hemolytic anemia. In all these disorders iron therapy can lead to tissue damage through iron overload. In the secondary anemias caused by infective or inflammatory disorders, the anemia only responds to the treatment of the underlying disease. The same is true for the myelophthisic anemias caused by marrow infiltrations. In hemolytic anemias treatment with corticosteroids may be indicated, depending upon the nature of the hemolysis, and splenectomy may be in-

---

TABLE 3. Anemias: Morphologic Classification

1. Macrocytic (MCV 93 cu mm)
   a. Megaloblastic erythropoiesis (deficiency of vitamin B_{12} or folic acid)
   b. Liver disease and obstructive jaundice
   c. Reticulocytosis
2. Normocytic
   a. Acute blood loss before reticulocytosis
   b. Hemolytic anemia when not associated with spherocytosis
   c. Anemia of chronic disease
3. Microcytic and hypochromic
   a. Iron deficiency
   b. Thalassemia
   c. Sideroblastic anemia

dicated when there is evidence that the spleen is playing a major role in red blood cell destruction. Anemia caused by acute blood loss and the anemias which fail to or cannot be expected to respond to specific hematinics may require blood transfusions. It must be recognized that blood transfusions are not without the risk of serious and sometimes fatal reactions, and that multiple transfusions increase the risk of both serum hepatitis and iron overload. Except for replacement of acute blood loss, the risk of circulatory overload and of transfusion reactions can be reduced by transfusing red blood cell concentrates from which the plasma has been removed. There is little cause to give blood transfusions if the hemoglobin is greater than 10 grams per 100 ml or to endeavor to maintain the hemoglobin above that level. Blood transfusions should be given after a full cross-match, including an indirect Coombs test, has established that the blood to be transfused is compatible. However, in patients with life-threatening autoimmune hemolytic anemia, the most compatible blood should be given despite the presence of a positive indirect Coombs test, because the survival of the transfused cells is likely to be no shorter than that of the patient's own red blood cells, and death from anemia can be prevented until more specific treatment with corticosteroids and/or splenectomy becomes effective.

Finch, C. A., and Lenfant, C.: Oxygen transport in man. N. Engl. J. Med., 286:407, 1972.
Gordon, A. S.: Regulation of Hematopoiesis. Vol. 1, Red Cell Production. New York, Appleton-Century-Crofts, 1970.
Harris, J. W., and Kellermyer, R. W.: The Red Cell Production, Metabolism, Destruction: Normal and Abnormal. 2nd ed. Cambridge, Mass., Harvard University Press, 1970.
Williams, W. J., Beutler, E., Erslev, A. J., and Rundles, R. W. (eds.): Hematology. New York, McGraw-Hill Book Company, 1972.

731. MEGALOBLASTIC ANEMIAS

Victor Herbert

Definition. The megaloblastic (Greek: megas=large + blaste=germ) anemias are characterized by a common morphology of giantism of every proliferating cell and an underlying common biochemical defect of slowed DNA synthesis. Classically, the diagnosis of megaloblastic anemia is made when the first-visit evaluation of a new patient reveals anemia, often with pancytopenia, and the peripheral blood smear reveals the progeny of a megaloblastic bone marrow, namely, macro-ovalocytic red cells, granulocytes whose nuclei are hypersegmented ("hypersegmented polys"), and giant platelets. Although megaloblastic anemia is a single *morphologic* entity, the underlying slowed DNA synthesis may result from any of a wide variety of causes. Thus the *diagnosis* of megaloblastic anemia is usually very easy, but the *differential diagnosis* of underlying cause and therefore *proper therapy* rest on determination of the precise etiologic classification into which the patient fits.

Pernicious anemia is *not* a synonym for megaloblastic anemia. It is that etiologic subcategory of megaloblastic anemia which is due to inadequate intrinsic factor secretion of uncertain etiology (Table 1).

Etiologic Classification and Pathogenesis. In about 95 per cent of cases, megaloblastic anemia proves to be a nutritional anemia (or, more broadly, a nutritional pancytopenia) caused by deficiency of vitamin B_{12}, folic acid, or, in some cases, both. Classification therefore usually falls in one of the six etiologic categories common to all nutritional deficiencies: inadequate ingestion, absorption, or utilization, and/or increased requirement, excretion, or destruction. Table 1 presents an etiologic classification of the causes of slowed DNA synthesis and therefore of the megaloblastic anemias, and Figures 1 and 2 present the flow charts of vitamin B_{12} and folate metabolism which provide the nutritional, physiologic, and biochemical underpinnings on which much of the etiologic classification rests.

As indicated in Figure 1, food vitamin B_{12} is liberated from its bonds by gastric acid and gastric and intestinal enzymes. The freed B_{12} (of which there is less when there is no gastric acid) attaches to the intrinsic factor (IF), a glycoprotein of molecular weight about 50,000 secreted by gastric parietal cells, and the B_{12}-IF complex dimerizes and passes into the ileum, where it is plastered onto specific brush border receptors for the IF-B_{12} complex in the presence of ionic calcium and a pH of more than 6. In the presence of trypsin and appropriate but unknown biochemical circumstances ("releasing factor"), the vitamin is absorbed and transported in the bloodstream, attached to the B_{12}-delivery protein, transcobalamin II (TC II, B_{12}-binding beta globulin), to be rapidly delivered to the liver, hematopoietic system, and other proliferative cells. Some B_{12} attaches in an apparently permanent fashion to granulocyte-related serum B_{12}-binding glycoproteins (TC I, a B_{12}-binding alpha globulin, and TC III, a B_{12}-binding globulin which moves with approximately the speed of transferrin on electrophoresis at pH 8.6). Normally, when a sample of blood is drawn, plasma B_{12}-binding protein is found to be approximately one third saturated with B_{12}, almost none of which is on TC II. Of the unsaturated B_{12}-binding protein, approximately 90 per cent is TC II. TC II delivers B_{12} to cells in an ionic calcium- and pH-dependent manner similar to the delivery of B_{12} to the brush border of the ileal cell by IF. The liver is the main storage organ for B_{12} in man, normally containing about 1 μg B_{12} per gram of liver, and there is a large enterohepatic circulation of the vitamin. It is this which explains why vitamin B_{12} deficiency occurs so slowly in vegetarians (whose enterohepatic circulation of B_{12} is usually intact) and relatively rapidly when B_{12} absorption (and therefore reabsorption) is shut off.

As indicated in Figure 2, food folates are predominantly in polyglutamate form. Prior to absorption, the excess glutamates must be split off by conjugases (gamma-glutamyl carboxypeptidases) present in bile and intestine; this process is variably inhibited by inappropriate pH (optimal pH for conjugase action is 4.6) and by conjugase inhibitors in beans, yeast, and some other foods. Once deconjugated, folate is absorbed primarily across the upper third of the small bowel, mainly as reduced monoglutamate, but partly as pteroylglutamic acid (PGA). The absorption of 5-methyl tetrahydrofolate (5-methyl THF) may be B_{12} dependent. Dilantin and certain other drugs inhibit folate absorption at step 2 in Figure 2. After absorption, folate is transported, mainly as 5-methyl THF, probably by a carrier protein, to cellular sites of utilization. Vitamin B_{12} appears necessary to get 5-methyl THF across cell walls (step 5 in Fig. 2), and this vitamin B_{12}-dependent cell uptake of folate helps explain why patients with uncomplicated vitamin B_{12} deficiency have a "pile-up" of folate in serum, resulting in a high serum folate and a low red cell folate. The "folate trap" in vitamin B_{12} deficiency consists in this folate "pile-up" compounded by inability to convert body folate stores (which are mainly methyl THF) to metabolically usable tetrahydrofolate (THF) because this conversion (step 6 in Fig. 2) is vitamin B_{12} dependent. Normal total body folate stores are in the range of 5 to 10 mg, about half of which is in the liver. There is an enterohepatic circulation of about 100 μg folate daily.

The defective DNA synthesis is due to inadequate thymidylate synthesis (step 11 in Fig. 2). Folate deficiency directly reduces the amount of 5,10-methylene THF available for thymidylate synthesis, and vitamin B_{12} deficiency reduces production of 5,10-methylene THF by blocking utilization of 5-methyl THF (at step 6 in Fig. 2) and possibly by directly reducing synthesis of thymidylate synthetase.

Incidence and Prevalence. Dietary vitamin B_{12} deficiency megaloblastic anemia is common among vegetarians because animal protein is the sole source of the vitamin. Conversely, it rarely occurs among meat eaters because the vitamin is almost indestructible by cooking or other processing. On the other hand, dietary folate deficiency megaloblastic anemia occurs in about one third of all the pregnant women in the world ("megaloblastic anemia of pregnancy") despite the fact that folate is found in nearly all natural foods, because folate is heat labile and is rapidly destroyed by extensive cooking, especially of finely divided foods such as beans and rice. Any pregnant women whose daily diet contains neither a fresh uncooked fruit nor a fresh lightly cooked vegetable, and all of whose food is heated at 100° C for periods in excess of 15 minutes, can be assumed to have folate deficiency until proved otherwise. Dietary folate deficiency is also present in over 90 per cent of hard-liquor alcoholics, a majority of wine and beer alcoholics, and about half of narcotic addicts, because these groups waste little money on solid food.

Pernicious anemia (megaloblastic anemia caused by inadequate secretion of gastric intrinsic factor) is age related, with an approximate incidence of 1 per million persons at ages 6 months to 1 year, 1 per 10,000 at ages 1 to 10, 1 per 5000 at ages 30 to 40, and a progressive increase in frequency thereafter so that the incidence is approximately 1 per 200 persons at ages 60 to 70. When statistics are corrected for age, there appears to be no specific sex or race predilection, and only a predilection for following by some years the incidence of gastric atrophy with its consequent histamine-refractory achlorhydria, which is present in about 15 per cent of people between ages 40 and 60, 25 per cent between ages 60 and 70, and 30 per cent over the age of 70.

Megaloblastosis caused by subnormal intestinal absorption of vitamin B_{12} (often with associated folate deficiency) is almost always present in active tropical sprue, which is endemic in the Caribbean and Southeast Asia, and has been most studied in Puerto Ricans, Haitians, Vietnamese, Pakistanis, and Indians, but is also found in other nationals from these two geographic regions. For unknown reasons, a person born in an endemic sprue region who gets sprue may have remissions and exacerbations of the disease throughout life; recurrences are seen in such persons even after they have been in a temperate zone and apparently symptom free for up to 20 years. For this reason, when a person born in Puerto Rico develops megaloblastic anemia in the continental United States, he should be considered to have tropical sprue until proved otherwise. Subnormal absorption of vitamin B_{12} is also present in the majority of patients with regional enteritis, and is also present in a majority with chronic pancreatic disease.

Hematologic and Other Pathology. The pathology of megaloblastic anemia is generated by slowed DNA synthesis per unit time, and this is observed in all proliferating cells. Normally, cells capable of reproducing themselves are in the resting state (i.e., 1 unit of DNA) most of the time. When they reproduce, they do so by rapidly doubling their DNA, dividing, and returning to the resting state. Thus at any instant 100 such normal cells may contain 101 units of DNA (99 cells with 1 unit each plus 1 cell which is about to divide and has rapidly doubled its DNA to do so). Unlike such normal cells, at any given instant few megaloblastic cells are resting, because nearly all are engaged in a slowed attempt to complete doubling their DNA, with frequent arrest in the S (synthesis) phase and lesser arrest in other phases. Thus the amount of DNA observed per cell may be almost 2 units, so that instead of the hypothetical 101 units of DNA per 100 normoblastic cells, there may be close to 200 units of DNA per 100 megaloblastic cells. This largely explains the apparent anomaly that megaloblastic cells are seen under the microscope to have larger than normal nuclei with *increased DNA* content and yet they have biochemically *defective DNA synthesis.* Megaloblasts have an even larger cytoplasm than nucleus, as compared with normal cells, because, although their synthesis of DNA is impaired, their ability to synthesize RNA is usually relatively unimpeded. This disparity or nuclear-cytoplasmic dissociation or asynchrony, as it is variously termed, is reflected in the finely particulate nuclear chromatin ("young nucleus," or nucleus with retarded maturation) of the erythroid megaloblasts at all stages of their development, even when hemoglobin is clearly visible in the cytoplasm ("old cytoplasm"), easily differentiating them from normoblasts with their coarsely clumped "old" nuclear chromatin.

Another striking feature of megaloblastic hematopoiesis is the megaloblastic myelopoiesis, manifested most dramatically by the presence of many giant metamyelocytes, whose increased DNA is eventually packaged in an increased number of mature neutrophil lobes.

The evolutionary biochemical and hematologic sequence in development of folate deficiency is indicated in Figure 3; the sequence in development of vitamin B_{12} deficiency is similar, but is measured in years rather than months.

When there is concomitant iron deficiency, as is often the case in pregnancy, various malabsorption syndromes, and alcoholism, and in about a third of cases of pernicious anemia, the erythroid megaloblastosis and macrocytic "overcolored" erythrocytes may be masked by the countervailing tendency of iron deficiency to produce microblasts and hypochromic microcytic erythrocytes. The result may be "intermediate megaloblasts" (cells halfway between megaloblasts and normoblasts) in the bone marrow, and in the peripheral blood both red cell forms may be present ("dimorphic anemia"), or one may dominate. The myeloid megaloblastosis in the bone marrow and the hypersegmented polymorphonuclear leukocytes ("hypersegmented polys") in the peripheral blood are not masked by iron deficiency, and they provide the

TABLE 1. Etiologic Classification of Megaloblastic Anemias; A Tabular Lexicon

I. Vitamin B_{12} Deficiency (normal B_{12} body stores last 3 to 6 years after cessation of B_{12} absorption, but 20 to 30 years after cessation of only B_{12} ingestion, because of continuation of reabsorption of the 3 to 6 μg of B_{12} excreted daily in bile):

A. Inadequate ingestion
  1. Poor diet (lacking microorganisms and animal foods, which are the sole B_{12} sources)
    a. Strict vegetarianism (eating no meat, fowl, seafood, eggs, milk, or any products thereof)
    b. Chronic alcoholism (no B_{12} or folate in hard liquor) (folate deficiency occurs first, and is more common, partly because body stores of B_{12} last much longer than those of folate)
    c. Poverty, religious tenets (Hinduism, Seventh-Day Adventism, certain Catholic orders), dietary faddism
B. Inadequate absorption
  1. Gastric disorder, producing inadequate or absent secretion by gastric parietal cells of intrinsic factor
    a. Addisonian pernicious anemia (PA) (PA is that form of B_{12} deficiency disease due to inadequate intrinsic factor secretion of uncertain etiology)
      (1) Hereditary absence of normal intrinsic factor secretion; absent secretion at birth (circulating antibody to intrinsic factor never present) (supports theory that antibody only occurs when antigenic stimulus is produced by intrinsic factor which enters bloodstream from damaged parietal cells and is recognized as foreign by the immunologic surveillance system); rare
      (2) Congenital production of defective intrinsic factor molecule (one published case)
      (3) Autoimmunity-associated gastric atrophy. These patients almost always have nondiagnostic-for-PA circulating parietal cell antibody, which is index only of past or present gastric damage and *not* of amount of intrinsic factor secretion (circulating diagnostic-for-PA antibody to intrinsic factor is always present under age 21; there is a gradual decrease in measurable antibody, so that by age 65 only two thirds of cases present with measurable circulating antibody to intrinsic factor)
        (a) Juvenile pernicious anemia (usually presents between ages 3 and 14)
        (b) Hereditarily determined degenerative gastric atrophy (gradually progressing with increasing age) (almost half of all adult PA cases fall in this category)
        (c) Acquired gastric atrophy as the end result of superficial inflammatory gastritis; superficial gastritis with atrophy (almost half of all adult PA cases fall in this category, which includes acquired gastric damage related to iron deficiency, alcohol, etc.)
        (d) Endocrine disorders (hypothyroidism, polyendocrinopathy, etc.) associated with gastric damage
    b. Gastrectomy
      (1) Total
      (2) Subtotal (approximately 20% develop PA within ten years after surgery, associated with atrophy of remaining parietal cells)
        (a) Proximal
        (b) Distal
    c. Lesions which destroy the gastric mucosa (ingested corrosives, linitis plastica, etc.)
    d. Intrinsic factor inhibitor in gastric secretion
      (1) Antibody to intrinsic factor (in saliva or gastric juice)
        (a) "Blocking" antibody (attaches to intrinsic factor so as to block ability of intrinsic factor to take up B_{12})
        (b) "Binding" antibody (attaches to intrinsic factor at site distal to site of B_{12} attachment)
  2. Small intestinal disorder (affecting ileum, which is the main site of B_{12} absorption)
    a. Gluten-induced enteropathy (childhood and adult celiac disease); idiopathic steatorrhea; nontropical sprue
    b. Tropical sprue (B_{12} is often the first nutrient to be subnormally absorbed and the last to return to normal absorption)
    c. Regional enteritis
    d. Strictures or anastomoses of the small bowel
    e. Intestinal resection

  f. Malignancies and granulomatous lesions involving the small intestine
  g. Other conditions characterized by chronically disturbed intestinal function
  h. Drugs damaging B_{12} absorption
    (1) Para-aminosalicylic acid (PAS) (therapy of tuberculosis)
    (2) Colchicine (therapy of gout)
    (3) Neomycin (antimicrobial)
    (4) Ethanol (societal)
    (5) Metformin (and other biguanide oral antidiabetic agents?)
    (6) Oral contraceptive agents?
  i. Specific malabsorption for vitamin B_{12}
    (1) Due to long-term ingestion of calcium-chelating agents (ionic calcium required for B_{12} absorption)
    (2) Due to inadequately alkaline pH in ileum (Zollinger-Ellison syndrome, pancreatic disease, etc.) (pH > 6 required for B_{12} absorption)
    (3) Unknown causes (absence of intestinal receptors for B_{12}-intrinsic factor complex? absence of "releasing factor"?)
      (a) Congenital (Imerslund-Gräsbeck syndrome) (receptors probably functioning)
      (b) Acquired (forme fruste of sprue?) (receptors absent or nonfunctioning)
  3. Competition for vitamin B_{12} by intestinal parasites or bacteria
    a. Fish tapeworm (*Diphyllobothrium latum*) (decreasing in Finland because of pollution of fresh water killing the host fish)
    b. Bacteria: The blind loop syndrome (B_{12} adsorbing bacteria)
  4. Pancreatic disease (normal pancreatic exocrine secretion of trypsin and bicarbonate required for normal B_{12} absorption)
C. Inadequate utilization
  1. Vitamin B_{12} antagonists
    a. Substituted B_{12} amides and anilides (experimental agents)
    b. Cobaloximes (experimental agents)
  2. Congenital or acquired enzyme deficiency or deletion
    a. Methylmalonyl-CoA mutase
    b. Methyltetrahydrofolate-homocysteine methyltransferase
    c. B_{12a} reductase
    d. B_{12r} reductase
    e. Deoxyadenosyltransferase
    f. Other enzyme reduction or deletion
  3. Abnormal B_{12}-binding protein in serum, irreversibly binding B_{12} and making it unavailable to tissues
    a. Increased TC I and/or TC III glycoprotein (myeloproliferative disorders) ("granulocyte-related" B_{12} binders)
    b. Increased TC II protein (liver disease) ("liver-related" B_{12} binders)
    c. Other abnormal B_{12} binding (a glycoprotein in some hepatoma cases, etc.)
  4. Inadequate serum B_{12}-binding protein (congenital or acquired)
    a. TC II protein (lack produces megaloblastic anemia) (it delivers B_{12} to blood cells, as transferrin delivers iron)
    b. TC I glycoprotein (lack not known to produce megaloblastic anemia) (it is mainly a storage protein for B_{12}, somewhat akin to ceruloplasmin for copper)
    c. TC III (lack not yet clearly established) (large amounts produced in vitro by granulocytes)
  5. Protein malnutrition?
  6. Malignancy?
  7. Liver disease?
  8. Renal disease?
  9. Thiocyanate intoxication?
D. Increased requirement (normal adult daily requirement from exogenous sources is 0.1 μg)
  1. Hyperthyroidism
  2. Increased hematopoiesis?
  3. Infancy (increased requirement for growth)
  4. Parasitization
    a. By fetus
    b. By malignant tissue?
E. Increased excretion
  1. Inadequate B_{12}-binding protein in serum (inadequate TC II particularly?)
  2. Liver disease (inadequate storage capacity for B_{12})
  3. Renal disease?

F. Increased destruction
   1. By pharmacologic doses of ascorbic acid
II. Folic acid deficiency (normal folate body stores will last only 3 to 6 months after cessation of folate ingestion or absorption):
  A. Inadequate ingestion
    1. Poor diet (lacking unprocessed fresh, uncooked, or slightly cooked food) (or fruit juices) (folates are heat labile)
     a. Nutritional megaloblastic anemia
      (1) Tropical
      (2) Nontropical
      (3) Scurvy (diets poor in vitamin C are also poor in folate)
     b. Chronic alcoholism with or without cirrhosis
  B. Inadequate absorption (affecting upper third of small intestine which is the main site of folate absorption) (since most food folates are in polyglutamate forms, biliary and intestinal gamma glutamyl conjugases are necessary to split off excess glutamates to make folates absorbable)
    1. Malabsorption syndromes
     a. Gluten-induced enteropathy (childhood and adult celiac disease) (idiopathic steatorrhea, nontropical sprue) (coincident B_{12} malabsorption rare)
     b. Any other chronic functional or structural disorder involving the upper small intestine
      (1) Tropical sprue (coincident B_{12} malabsorption almost invariably present)
      (2) Associated with herpetic and other skin disorders
     c. Drugs
      (1) Diphenylhydantoin (Dilantin) (anticonvulsant)
      (2) Primidone (anticonvulsant)
      (3) Barbiturates
      (4) Oral contraceptive agents (?)
      (5) Cycloserine (tuberculosis)
      (6) Ethanol (societal)
      (7) Metformin (diabetes therapy)
      (8) Dietary amino acid excess of glycine and/or methionine
      (9) Nitrofurantoin? (antimicrobial)
      (10) Glutethimide? (sedative)
    2. Specific malabsorption for folate
     a. Congenital nonconjugase defects (four cases published)
     b. Acquired nonconjugase defects
     c. Inadequate biliary or intestinal conjugase
     d. Conjugase inhibitors (such as are contained in some beans)
    3. Blind loop syndrome (folate-greedy bacteria) (more commonly, bacteria make folate and actually raise serum folate level of host)
  C. Inadequate utilization (metabolic block)
    1. Folic acid antagonists (dihydrofolate reductase inhibitors)
     a. 4-amino-4-deoxyfolates (Chemotherapy, immunosuppression, psoriasis) (i.e., methotrexate)
     b. 2,4-Diaminopyrimidine (Malaria, toxoplasmosis) (i.e., pyrimethamine)
     c. Triamterene (Diuretic)
     d. Diamidine compounds (*Pneumocystis carinii*, protozoacidal) (i.e., pentamidine isethionate)
     e. Trimethoprim (Antibacterial)
    2. Diphenylhydantoin and possibly other anticonvulsants (possibly block cell uptake or use of folate)
    3. Enzyme deficiency
     a. Congenital
      (1) Formiminotransferase
      (2) Dihydrofolate reductase
      (3) Methyltetrahydrofolate transmethylase
      (4) Other enzymes
     b. Acquired
      (1) Liver disease
       (a) Formiminotransferase
       (b) Other enzymes
    4. Vitamin B_{12} deficiency (reduces methylfolate uptake by cells)
    5. Alcohol (both specific and nonspecific damage to folate metabolism)
    6. Ascorbic acid deficiency (increased hematopoiesis associated with bleeding reduces folate stores) (may also decrease ability of body to retain folates in their metabolically active reduced state)
    7. Dietary amino acid excess (glycine, methionine)
  D. Increased requirement (normal adult daily requirement from exogenous sources is 50 μg)

    1. Parasitization
     a. By fetus (especially in multiple and twin pregnancies)
     b. By malignant tissue (especially lymphoproliferative disorders, myeloproliferative disorders to a lesser extent, extensive carcinomatosis, etc.)
    2. Infancy (increased requirement for growth)
    3. Increased hematopoiesis (hemolytic anemias; chronic blood loss [including scurvy])
    4. Increased metabolic activity (hyperthyroidism, chronic temperature elevations)
  E. Increased excretion
    1. Vitamin B_{12} deficiency? (? of obligatory excretion of folate in urine and bile) (possible inability to reabsorb methylfolate excreted in bile, because B_{12} required for it)
    2. Liver disease?
    3. Kidney dialysis
    4. Chronic exfoliative dermatitis
  F. Increased destruction
    1. Oxidant in diet?
III. Interference with purine ring synthesis and interconversion of purine bases:
  A. Purine antagonists
    1. 6-Mercaptopurine (6-MP)   Chemotherapy, immunosuppression
    2. Thioguanine   Chemotherapy, immunosuppression
    3. Azathioprine   Immunosuppression
  B. Enzymatic defects in ability to make purine nucleotide from preformed bases
    1. Lesch-Nyhan syndrome (there is an associated increased requirement for folate, which is needed at two steps in the increased de novo biosynthesis of purine)
IV. Interference with pyrimidine synthesis:
  A. Pyrimidine antagonists
    1. 5-Fluorouracil (5-FU)   Chemotherapy (blocks thymidylate synthetase)
    2. 6-Azauridine   Chemotherapy, psoriasis
  B. Enzymatic defects in ability to make pyrimidine
    1. Hereditary oroticaciduria (not responsive to therapy with vitamin B_{12} or folic acid, but responsive to yeast extract or its active ingredients, uridine or the pyrimidine nucleotides, cytidylic and uridylic acids)
V. Inhibition of ribonucleotide reductase (cytidylic to deoxycytidylic acid):
  A. Cytosine arabinoside (inhibits DNA polymerase also)   Chemotherapy, antiviral
  B. Hydroxyurea   Chemotherapy, psoriasis
  C. Iron deficiency: iron is required for ribonucleotide reductase, but it is not yet established that lack of iron can produce megaloblastosis; some workers have reported hypersegmented polys in iron deficiency which disappear with iron therapy, but coincident folate deficiency has not yet been excluded fully
  D. Procarbazine (depolymerizes DNA)
VI. Inhibition of protein synthesis:
  A. L-Asparaginase   Chemotherapy
VII. Mechanism unknown:
  A. Benzene   Solvent
  B. Azulfidine   Ulcerative colitis
  C. Arsenic   Poison
  D. Pyridoxine-responsive megaloblastic anemia (only about 10% of patients with pyridoxine-responsive sideroblastic anemia have megaloblastic morphology)
  E. Thiamine-responsive megaloblastic anemia (one case reported)
  F. Megaloblastoid anemias (differentiated from megaloblastic anemias by bizarre morphology, including marked polyploidy and few to no orthochromatic megaloblasts)
    1. Di Guglielmo's syndrome (erythremic myelosis) (a myeloproliferative disorder usually presenting as refractory anemia and eventuating in death from "erythroleukemia" or myelogenous leukemia); preleukemia
    2. Occasional cases of polycythemia vera and other myeloproliferative disorders
    3. Occasional cases of aplastic anemia (which cases may subsequently develop myeloproliferative disorders)
    4. Occasional cases of miliary tuberculosis (in such cases, the megaloblastoid marrow is often accompanied by monocytosis and leukopenia or leukocytosis)

*MDR = Adult minimum daily requirement from exogenous sources to sustain normality

Figure 1. Flow chart of vitamin B_{12} metabolism.

morphologic key to the existence of vitamin B_{12} or folate deficiency even in the presence of severe iron deficiency.

"Hypersegmented polys" are sought by either the simple "Rule of Fives" (i.e., if more than five of 100 neutrophils have five or more lobes, hypersegmentation is present) or the more elaborate "lobe average" (i.e., count the number of lobes in 100 "polys" and divide by 100; the normal lobe average is 3.17 ± 0.25; hypersegmentation is present if the lobe average is greater than 3.5; normally 20 to 40 per cent of "polys" have two lobes, 40 to 50 per cent have three lobes, and 15 to 25 per cent have four lobes; a substantial increase in percentage with four or more lobes means megaloblastosis, congenital hypersegmentation, or chronic renal disease). As Figure 3 indicates, in incipient megaloblastic anemia, hypersegmentation is present prior to the appearance of an obviously megaloblastic bone marrow or anemia. When the peripheral blood smears of all new patients are screened on a routine basis for hypersegmentation, one third of those found to have it are subsequently proved to have early vitamin B_{12} or folate deficiency, with low serum vitamin level but no anemia and no clinical suspicion of the diagnosis. The "Twenty Per Cent Rule" (i.e., if less than 20 per cent of 100 neutrophils have two or less lobes, hypersegmentation is present) is particularly useful when there are few or no "polys" with more than five lobes.

The megaloblastic anemias are due to ineffective erythropoiesis, and as such they have both a hemolytic component and an iron overload pathologic picture. The increased intramedullary "fetal" death rate of the erythroid cells is dramatically illustrated by the frequent finding of up to 25 per cent reticulocytes among

the bone marrow erythrons but 1 per cent or less in the peripheral blood, the high serum lactate dehydrogenase, and the modestly elevated serum bilirubin. Ineffective utilization of iron results in increased saturation of the iron-binding capacity and increased iron stores; this is so prominent that when a patient presents with megaloblastic anemia and normal rather than elevated serum and bone marrow iron, one should suspect iron deficiency, and should repeat the measurements of serum and bone marrow iron after vitamin therapy to determine whether overt iron deficiency has now been unmasked. Since megaloblastic anemia is usually associated with low normal total iron binding capacity, an elevated iron binding capacity is a clue to occult iron deficiency.

Megaloblastosis with underlying defective DNA synthesis is present in all proliferating cells; this is almost as striking in epithelial cells, particularly those of the alimentary tract and vagina, as in hematopoietic cells. Thus defective DNA synthesis results in a variable degree of secondary atrophy in epithelial cells of the tongue, stomach, and small intestine. It is this atrophy which produces secondary failure of gastric intrinsic factor secretion in one third of patients with tropical sprue, secondary failure of intestinal absorption of vitamin B_{12} in about half of patients with primary failure of intrinsic factor secretion, and the variety of other vicious cycles whereby vitamin B_{12} deficiency results in secondary decreased absorption of folate (and B_{12}) and folate deficiency results in secondary decreased absorption of vitamin B_{12} (and folate). These secondary malabsorption phenomena disappear after a variable period of vitamin therapy.

In addition to the defective DNA synthesis common to all megaloblastic anemias, a primary defect of unknown cause in ability to synthesize myelin is present only in vitamin B_{12} deficiency. This results in the insidious development of demyelinating vitamin B_{12} deficiency neuropathy, often beginning in peripheral nerves and progressing to involve the posterior and lateral columns of the spinal cord (variously called subacute combined degeneration, combined system disease, posterolateral sclerosis, and funicular degeneration) and the cerebrum ("megaloblastic madness"). (See Ch. 411.)

Clinical Manifestations.   Infrequently, the patient with megaloblastic anemia presents with bleeding caused by the thrombocytopenia, or infection caused by the leukopenia, but usually the presentation is with one or more of the symptoms of a gradually developing and slowly progressive anemia: easy fatigability, weakness, tiredness, shortness of breath, occasional faintness (particularly on suddenly arising from a recumbent or sitting position), headache, palpitations, and syncope. Before such symptoms are brushed off as "neurotic" (which they frequently prove to be), laboratory testing for anemia should be carried out, consisting at the least of determination of hematocrit (and/or hemoglobin) and examination of peripheral blood smear morphology.

If the patient has vitamin B_{12} deficiency and a good diet supplying adequate folate to substantially mask the hematologic picture, he may have no anemia and only slight morphologic evidence of megaloblastosis, and may present as a neurologic or neuropsychiatric problem, with paresthesias (especially numbness and tingling in the hands and feet) and diminished vibration and/or

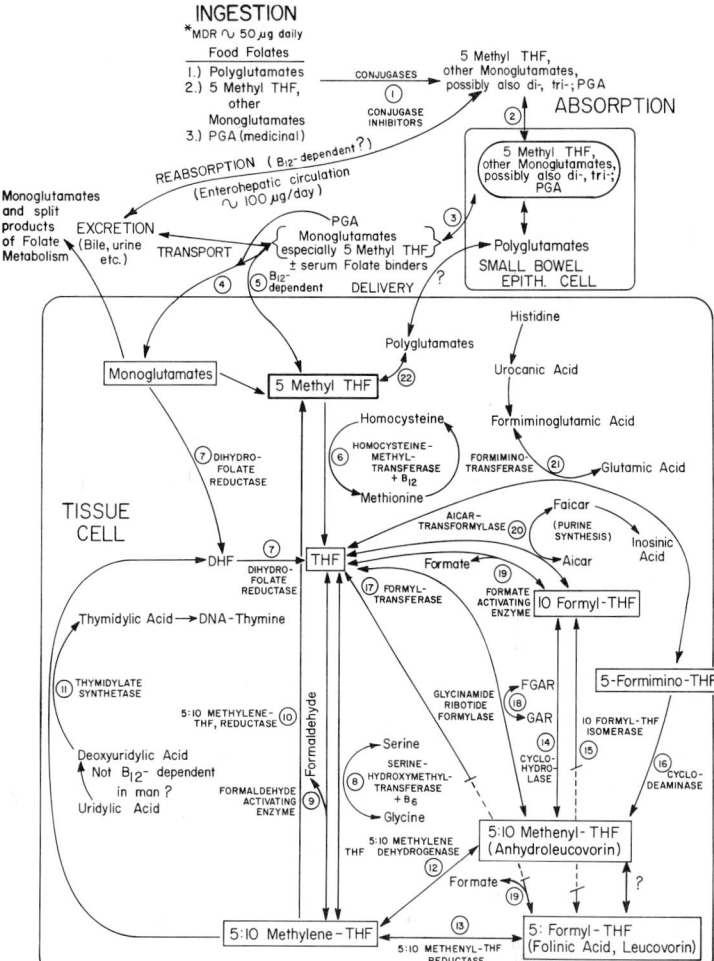

Figure 2. Flow chart of folate metabolism.

position sense (with loss of perception of 256 vps preceding by many months loss of perception of 128 vps, and loss of position sense in the index toes preceding by many months loss of position sense in the great toes). Examination with a "256" tuning fork may reveal complete loss

Figure 3. Biochemical and hematologic sequence of events in folate deficiency.

of vibration sense from toes to iliac crest bilaterally before any loss of perception of vibration of a "128" tuning fork.

The classic neurologic disorder associated with vitamin B_{12} deficiency is combined system disease (subacute combined degeneration). Usually slow and insidious in onset, it is characterized by degeneration of the dorsal and lateral columns of the spinal cord, with paresthesias of the hands and feet, ataxia of the legs with variable spasticity and weakness, and eventual paraplegia. The classic symptoms are symmetrical paresthesias (numbness, tingling, burning) in feet and/or hands, followed by unsteadiness of gait associated with loss of position sense, manifested by inability to detect passive movements of the great toes. Prior to the appearance of deficits in the great toes, there may be inability to detect passive movements of the index toes. Knee and ankle jerks may be diminished or lost, or the knee jerks increased; extensor plantar responses, indicating damage to the spinal cord, commonly occur. Mental changes are variable, may include paranoid ideation and depression, and may be sufficiently severe to mimic paranoid schizophrenia or senility. (British workers have referred to this phenomenon as "megaloblastic madness"). Ataxic paraplegia similar to that resulting from vitamin B_{12} deficiency results from any kind of damage to the dorsal or lateral columns of the spinal cord, as may occur with multiple sclerosis or chronic meningeal syphilis.

Subjective neurologic dysfunction, such as irritability, forgetfulness, and sleeplessness, occurs not only with vitamin B_{12} deficiency but even more frequently with folate deficiency. Such subjective stigmata are of limited differential diagnostic value in separating the two vitamin deficiency states; when caused by folate deficiency, these stigmata disappear dramatically within 24 hours of the start of folate therapy.

Occasionally, a chronic alcoholic with megaloblastic anemia caused by folate deficiency is erroneously diagnosed as having vitamin B_{12} deficiency because he has neurologic damage, including impaired position and vibration sense. However, associated thiamin deficiency in the alcoholic produces peripheral neuropathy mimicking that caused by vitamin B_{12} deficiency. Confusion may also arise in patients with folate deficiency and diabetes mellitus, because diabetic neuropathy may also mimic the neuropathy resulting from vitamin B_{12} deficiency.

The skin may have a lemon-yellow cast owing to the combination of pallor from anemia and low-grade icterus from the hemolytic component of the disorder. The "classic" pernicious anemia patient still appears as described by Addison in 1855:

> The countenance gets pale, the whites of the eyes become pearly, *the general frame flabby rather than wasted;* the pulse perhaps large but remarkably soft and compressible, and occasionally with a slight jerk, especially under the slightest excitement. There is an increasing indisposition to exertion with an uncomfortable feeling of faintness or breathlessness on attempting it; the heart is readily made to palpitate; the whole surface presents a blanched, smooth and waxy appearance; the lips, gums and tongue seem bloodless; *the flabbiness of the solids increases;* the appetite fails, extreme languor and faintness supervene, breathlessness and palpitation being produced by the most trifling exertion or emotion; some slight edema is probably perceived about the ankles. The debility becomes extreme; the patient can no longer arise from his bed; *the mind occasionally wanders;* he falls into a prostrate and half torpid state, and at length expires. *Nevertheless, to the very last, and after a sickness of perhaps several months' duration, the bulkiness of the general frame and the obesity often present a most striking contrast to the failure and exhaustion observable in every other respect.*

The parts of Addison's classic description which do not fit folic acid deficiency states as generally as those caused by vitamin B_{12} deficiency have been italicized. In folate deficiency, emaciation is more common than flabbiness, and diarrhea is more common than the constipation often seen in vitamin B_{12} deficiency.

About one third of patients with megaloblastic anemia have splenomegaly, but this may be observable only on abdominal radiography, because the spleen exceeds two to three times normal size in less than 10 per cent of cases. Moderate hepatomegaly may also be present.

A smooth or sore tongue is frequent, owing to megaloblastosis of the cells of the papillary surface. Almost 10 per cent of patients have hyperpigmentation, often most marked in the palmar creases, but occasionally in bizarre patterns such as occur with Addison's disease, sometimes with vitiligo. Occasionally low-grade fever is present.

Laboratory Findings and Differential Diagnosis. *Primary* laboratory findings include macro-ovalocytic anemia, leukopenia (with "hypersegmented polys"), thrombocytopenia (with giant platelets), and megaloblastic bone marrow. Reticulocyte count below 1 per cent is common with vitamin B_{12} deficiency, and that of 1.5 to 8 per cent is common with folate deficiency. *Secondary* findings include reduced haptoglobin, hyperbilirubinemia, increased fecal stercobilin, elevated serum lactate dehy-

TABLE 2.   Separating Vitamin B_{12} Deficiency from Folate Deficiency: Laboratory Differential Diagnosis

Before therapy only:
1. Serum vitamin B_{12} (microbiologic: *Euglena gracilis, Ochromonas malhamensis; Escherichia coli, Lactobacillus leichmannii,* etc.) (radioassay using coated charcoal); normal: 200–900 pg/ml
2. Serum folate (*Lactobacillus casei*) (radioassay using coated charcoal); normal: 7–16 ng/ml
3. Erythrocyte vitamin B_{12}; normal: >100 pg/ml
4. Erythrocyte folate; normal: >150 ng/ml
5. Methylmalonate in urine; ↑ usually means B_{12} deficiency
6. Formiminoglutamate (FIGLU) (FGA) and urocanate in urine after oral histidine load; ↑ in B_{12} deficiency, folate deficiency, liver disease
7. "dU suppression" test (i.e., in vitro therapeutic trial)

Before or after therapy:
8. Gastric analysis: acid, pepsin, quality, quantity, intrinsic factor (IF) content
9. Tests of radio-B_{12} absorption (radioactivity in stool, plasma, liver, whole body, or urine) after physiologic dose (0.5–2 μg) of radio-B_{12} orally
   a. Urine (Schilling test)
      Stage 1: Radio-B_{12} orally + 1000 μg "cold" B_{12} IM, followed by 24-hour urine collection, another 1000 μg "cold" B_{12} IM, another 24-hour urine collection (normal result: >5% in 48-hour urine) (2 μg dose)
      Stage 2: Repeat Stage 1, but this time mix IF with radio-B_{12} before administering to patient (normal result: >5% in 48-hour urine) (2 μg dose)
      Stage 3: See text
10. Circulating antibody to human IF; normally absent

drogenase, formiminoglutamic aciduria (found not only in primary folate deficiency but also in primary vitamin B_{12} deficiency and primary liver disease), high serum iron and high saturation of transferrin, loss of gastric acid and abnormal liver function, and intestinal absorption tests. Megaloblasts are usually present in the buffy coat of centrifuged peripheral blood.

A serum B_{12} level below 100 pg per milliliter is essentially diagnostic for primary vitamin B_{12} deficiency and *both* a serum folate of less than 3 ng per milliliter and a red cell folate below 150 ng per milliliter are diagnostic for primary folate deficiency. (Low serum folate alone may occur long before tissue folate depletion, and low red cell folate occurs also in primary vitamin B_{12} deficiency, because B_{12} is necessary to get methylfolate into red cells). One caveat: when the serum levels of both vitamins are low, the primary deficiency may be of just one, with resultant intestinal megaloblastosis producing malabsorption and therefore secondary deficiency of the other. For example, in megaloblastic anemia of pregnancy, both vitamin levels may be low, but treatment with only folic acid results in gradual rise to normal of the serum B_{12} level.

Methylmalonic aciduria occurs only in vitamin B_{12} deficiency and not in folate deficiency.

Absence of intrinsic factor in the gastric juice on in vitro assay is essentially diagnostic for pernicious anemia. One caveat: primary intestinal malabsorption of B_{12} or folate deficiency may produce secondary loss of intrinsic factor secretion; this will return to normal after vitamin therapy.

In vivo tests for detection of vitamin B_{12} malabsorption involve feeding 0.5 to 2 μg of the vitamin, labeled with ^{56}Co (half-life, 77 days), ^{57}Co (half-life, 270 days), ^{58}Co (half-life, 71 days), or ^{60}Co (half-life, 5.26 years), and measuring the amount absorbed by the amount of radioactivity in either stool, urine, blood, liver, or whole body. The test is divided into three stages: (1) Feed radio-B_{12} alone. Subnormal absorption means gastric or ileal dysfunction. It need not be done if in vitro radioassay for intrinsic factor is carried out. (2) Feed radio-B_{12} plus intrinsic factor concentrate. Subnormal absorption means ileal dysfunction, but does not rule out concomitant gastric dysfunction. (3) Only done if second stage is subnormal: Feed antimicrobial (or anthelmintic) for appropriate period, then feed radio-B_{12}. A normal result means that the patient had blind loop syndrome (or fish tapeworm). When pancreatic dysfunction is suspected, the third stage consists in feeding the radio-B_{12} with added bicarbonate or pancreatin, or both. When drug-induced B_{12} malabsorption is suspected, the third-stage test is carried out after withdrawal of the offending agent.

Every patient in whom tests reveal gastric or intestinal malabsorption of B_{12} that is not of a clear single cause should have the tests repeated after therapy with B_{12} (or after therapy with folic acid, if deficiency of folic acid is present). Vitamin B_{12} deficiency is a vicious-cycle disease (as is folic acid deficiency); severe deficiency of either B_{12} or folic acid may produce a variable degree of gastric and/or intestinal damage, and therefore may itself produce a variable degree of secondary reduction of gastric secretion of intrinsic factor and/or ileal ability to absorb B_{12} (and/or intestinal ability to absorb folate). This secondary malabsorption of B_{12} or folate is corrected by therapy.

Repetition of tests after therapy will establish which damage was secondary (i.e., a result of deficiency of B_{12} or folic acid) and which was primary (i.e., a lesion not produced by deficiency of B_{12} or folate). The B_{12} deficiency of a patient with regional enteritis may produce secondary gastric damage which may reduce intrinsic factor secretion; this secondary gastric damage may be corrected by B_{12} therapy. Conversely, the B_{12} deficiency of a patient with pernicious anemia may produce secondary ileal damage and resultant malabsorption of a test dose of B_{12} fed with intrinsic factor; this secondary ileal damage may be corrected by B_{12} therapy. Additionally, the B_{12} deficiency of either patient may make the malabsorption worse owing to his primary lesion.

Circulating antibody to intrinsic factor is present in two thirds of patients with pernicious anemia and, when found, is essentially diagnostic. Less than 10 per cent saturation of serum vitamin B_{12} binding capacity is also essentially diagnostic.

The dU suppression test on bone marrow cells aspirated from the patient is diagnostic for folate deficiency if a deficit in deoxyuridine suppression of radioactive iododeoxyuridine incorporation into DNA is found, and is corrected in vitro by pteroylglutamic acid (PGA) and methylfolate; it is diagnostic for vitamin B_{12} deficiency if corrected by B_{12} but not by methylfolate. This "therapeutic trial in the test tube" is the laboratory equivalent of the classic clinical trial discussed below.

Therapy. *Therapeutic trial* is diagnostic for vitamin B_{12} or folate deficiency. Such trial is carried out by giving the patient a diet devoid of foods high in vitamin B_{12} and folate, i.e., devoid of all fresh uncooked fruits and vegetables, fruit juices, nuts or other uncooked natural foods, and liver. After ten days on such a diet, and while continuing the diet, the patient is then treated with 1 μg of vitamin B_{12} parenterally daily if vitamin B_{12} deficiency is suspected, and with 50 to 100 μg of folic acid parenterally daily if folic acid deficiency is suspected. Unless

hematopoiesis is suppressed by infection, uremia, chloramphenicol, alcohol, or some other chronic systemic disease or drug, approximately three days after the start of therapy reticulocytosis will appear and will reach a peak at approximately seven days (range: five to twelve days) after the start of the daily vitamin therapy. The lower the initial red count, the higher the reticulocyte peak. The hemoglobin will gradually rise, and by approximately seven days after the start of therapy the white cell and platelet counts will rise to normal. The platelet count will usually, and the white count will in 10 per cent of cases, exceed normal before falling back into the normal range. It is important that the therapeutic trial vitamin dose not be larger than the aforementioned, to avoid "nonspecific" response (Fig. 4).

Immediate therapy is advisable in patients with megaloblastosis accompanied by anemia so severe as to be associated with dyspnea, congestive failure, and occasionally angina. Such symptoms, when found, usually occur in association with a hematocrit below 15 per cent. Rapid and dramatic relief of these symptoms may be obtained by administration of packed cells into one arm, accompanied by withdrawal of a slightly lesser quantity of whole blood from the contralateral arm. Venous pressure should be monitored, and only that amount of whole blood removed which is necessary to prevent elevation of the venous pressure. Packed cells may be given at the rate of 1 unit per five minutes by interposing a three-way stopcock and a 50-ml syringe between the bottle or bag of packed cells and the vein, drawing the packed cells from source into the syringe and then injecting into the vein. Using the three-way stopcock, venous pressure can be monitored and whole blood drawn off as required. In this procedure, packed cells with a hematocrit of approximately 80 are going into one arm while whole blood with a hematocrit of less than 15 is coming out the same or the other arm; there is therefore no dangerous sudden rise in circulating blood volume to induce the irreversi-

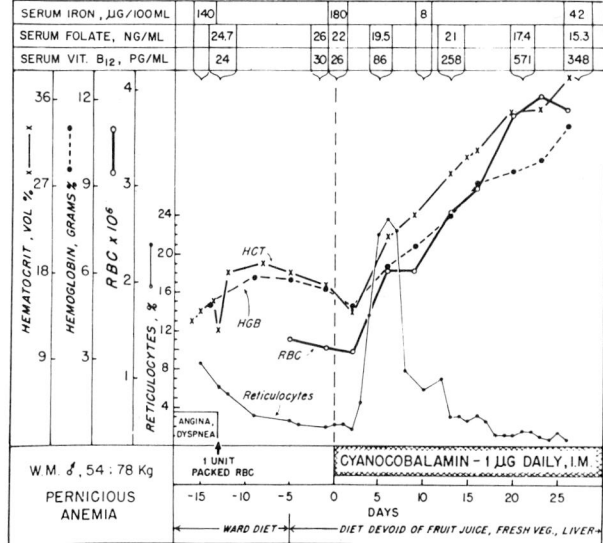

Figure 4. Therapeutic trial with 1μg of vitamin B_{12} daily. Note the "spontaneous" reticulocytosis present on admission (more frequent in folate deficiency), the termination of angina and dyspnea by a single unit of packed red blood cells (RBC), the initial high serum iron and folate, and their fall on vitamin B_{12} therapy.

ble congestive failure so dreaded when chronically ane-mic patients are given packed cells or whole blood in the conventional manner.

Immediate therapy with vitamin B_{12} and/or folate is advisable in patients with severe megaloblastic anemia and bleeding associated with platelet levels below 50,000 per cubic millimeter of blood or associated with infec-tion accompanied by leukopenia with a white cell count below 2000 per cubic millimeter of blood. Immediate therapy with vitamin B_{12} and/or folate is also advisable in patients with severe infection, coma, severe disorien-tation, marked neurologic damage, severe liver disease, uremia, or other markedly debilitating illness complicat-ing the deficiency of vitamin B_{12} and/or folate. When one of these reasons makes necessary immediate vitamin therapy before establishing the etiologic diagnosis, such therapy should be given intramuscularly with a mini-mum of 30 μg (1 ml) of vitamin B_{12} (cyanocobalamin) and 1 mg (1 ml) of folic (pteroylglutamic) acid, followed by 1 tablet (1 mg) of folic acid by mouth daily for a week and a minimum of 30 μg of vitamin B_{12} by intramuscular injec-tion daily for a week. Some have recommended that po-tassium chloride be given at the onset of immediate vi-tamin B_{12} therapy to avoid the potential hazard of hypokalemia with subsequent arrhythmias.

After a week of therapy to carry the patient from the critical state to a state of well-being, all vitamin therapy should be stopped if necessary to make an etiologic diag-nosis. However, with a combination of foresight and laboratory facilities, blood will have been obtained from the patient immediately on admission and prior to treat-ment, and diagnosis of vitamin B_{12} and/or folate defi-ciency will have been made from determination of the serum and erythrocyte levels of these vitamins, supple-mented by the various tests which may be performed even when the patient is in a treated state. Initial ther-apy for inadequate absorption of vitamin B_{12} is 30 μg (or more) of cyanocobalamin daily for a week, or every other day for a total of five doses, to help replenish the body stores, followed by a minimum of 30 μg monthly. This quantity is not adequate to sustain complete normality and allows morphologic damage of moderate degree to persist; therefore a monthly injection of 100 μg of cyano-cobalamin is preferable, because it will sustain in com-plete remission all patients with uncomplicated vitamin B_{12} deficiency.

Monthly maintenance therapy must be carried out for life in the patient whose inadequate absorption of B_{12} is due to lack of intrinsic factor secretion or to a noncorrect-able structural or functional lesion of the ileum. Al-though there is no evidence that greater or more frequent therapy has any value, it has become general practice to give patients with neurologic damage 250 μg or more of vitamin B_{12} once or twice weekly for several months, followed by similar doses once or twice monthly for another year. Neurologic damage resulting from vi-tamin B_{12} deficiency, when of behavioral nature such as paranoia, may improve very rapidly (even within 24 hours) after the start of therapy. Objectively ascertaina-ble neurologic damage, such as loss of position and/or vibration sense, improves more slowly, and there may be return of ability to perceive 128 vps before return of abil-ity to perceive 256 vps, as well as return of ability to per-ceive passive motion of the great toes before return of ability to perceive passive motion of index toes. *Any neu-rologic damage which has not been corrected at the end of approximately 1 to 1 1/2 years may be considered to*

be irreversible. Neurologic damage caused by vitamin B_{12} deficiency begins as inability to make myelin, followed by gradual deterioration of the axon, followed by deterio-ration of the nerve head. This process occurs very slowly and is reversible until the nerve head deteriorates.

Oral therapy with large doses of vitamin B_{12} (500 to 1000 μg daily) should only be used when the patient with B_{12} malabsorption refuses parenteral therapy. Although there is usually sufficient diffusion-absorption from such doses to maintain patients in remission, this is not always reliable.

Oral therapy with vitamin B_{12}-intrinsic factor com-plexes should not be used, because such preparations are valueless to patients with structural or functional dis-orders of the small bowel and produce unreliable absorp-tion of B_{12} in patients with pernicious anemia, many of whom become refractory owing to development in the gut wall of local antibody to intrinsic factor.

"Shotgun" antianemia preparations may actually harm the patient, because they may obscure the real na-ture of the anemia. For example, response to folic acid in a patient with megaloblastic anemia secondary to gas-tric carcinoma may obscure and delay the correct diag-nosis.

The only recommended use of low (5 μg) daily dose oral B_{12} maintenance therapy is in the management of vege-tarians who refuse to eat any animal matter.

Satisfactory clinical and hematologic remission may be obtained in any patient with uncomplicated vitamin B_{12} deficiency disease by daily parenteral administration of only 1 μg of vitamin B_{12} for ten days. Larger doses sim-ply allow more rapid repletion of body stores. Initial therapy with doses of cyanocobalamin greater than 1 μg daily is desirable only when the vitamin B_{12} deficiency is complicated by other debilitating illness. Parenteral amounts of vitamin B_{12} greater than 30 μg daily have no proved therapeutic advantage, although it is possible that larger daily doses may result in slightly more rapid repletion of body stores. However, the percentage of the injected dose of vitamin B_{12} excreted in the urine rises logarithmically as the quantity of cyanocobalamin in-jected rises above 30 μg daily.

The most frequent complications of vitamin B_{12} deficiency, especially that caused by pernicious anemia, are infections, especially of the genitourinary tract, and variable degrees of congestive failure. These should be managed appropriately. Since the incidence of carcin-oma of the stomach in patients with pernicious anemia is approximately threefold higher than chance, this entity should be looked for at yearly intervals.

In patients with chronic pancreatic disease, the intrin-sic factor mechanism may not be operative and may be enhanced by feeding sodium bicarbonate, pancreatin, or trypsin.

Initial therapy with larger doses of pteroylglutamic acid than 0.1 mg daily is desirable when the folate deficiency state is complicated by conditions which may suppress hematopoiesis (infection, uremia, tumor; active inflammatory lesions such as rheumatoid arthritis, ul-cerative colitis, or hepatitis; chloramphenicol or alcohol administration), or conditions which increase folate requirements (pregnancy; hypermetabolic states; states of increased hematopoiesis such as occur with hemolytic anemia or protracted blood loss). Therapy should then be 0.5 to 1 mg of pteroylglutamic acid daily.

There is no evidence that doses greater than 1 mg daily have greater efficacy than does 1 mg. Additionally, loss of folate in the urine becomes roughly logarithmic as quantities of administered pteroylglutamic acid exceed 1 mg. It is possible that the use of larger daily doses, especially if given in several spaced doses each day, may more rapidly replete the body folate stores, but the value of such rapid replenishment is uncertain.

When folate deficiency is due to malabsorption rather than inadequate ingestion, parenteral therapy is preferable initially, and maintenance therapy is preferably with 500 to 1000 μg (0.5 to 1.0 mg) of PGA daily rather than 100 μg (at least until further studies support the current impression that PGA is well absorbed even when the patient is only poorly capable of absorbing other nutrients [such as food folates]).

The best maintenance therapy for dietary folate deficiency is correction of the diet rather than permanent supplementation. Such correction often simply requires less prolonged cooking of the same foods the patient has always eaten, because prolonged cooking destroys folates. In other instances, such correction involves switching from canned to fresh fruits and vegetables, because the canning process may destroy 50 to 95 per cent of food folate.

Summary of Response to Therapy. Objective and subjective improvement occurs within a few days and a sense of well-being often within a day of the start of therapy with the lacking vitamin. Within 48 hours, the bone marrow returns sharply toward normoblastic. Reticulocytosis begins within two to five days after therapy is started and usually reaches its peak on about the fifth to twelfth day. The shape and height of the reticulocyte curve depend on the dose of vitamin B_{12} or folic acid, the route of its administration, and the severity of the anemia. At approximately the time the reticulocytes reach their peak, the leukocytes and platelets will have risen to normal levels. Serum iron is usually elevated in untreated patients and falls abruptly within one to two days after starting therapy. This sequence of events should be followed by obtaining a blood count just prior to the start of therapy and a reticulocyte count at least once every two days from then until the reticulocyte peak has passed, plus a hemoglobin or hematocrit determination at weekly intervals for the first month and then every two weeks for the next month or two. If hematologic recovery does not follow the outlined response pattern, then either the diagnosis is wrong or complications suppressing hematopoiesis are present.

Arnstein, H. R. V., and Wrighton, R. J. (eds.): The Cobalamins. Edinburgh and London, Churchill Livingstone, 1971.

Beck, W. S.: Erythrocyte disorders—anemias related to disturbance of DNA synthesis (megaloblastic anemias). *In* Williams, W. J., Beutler, E., Erslev, A., and Rundles, R. W. (eds.): Hematology. New York, McGraw-Hill Book Company, 1972, pp. 249, 256; 278, 297.

Chanarin, I.: The Megaloblastic Anemias. Oxford, Blackwell; Philadelphia, F. A. Davis Company, 1969.

Herbert, V. (ed.): Symposium on vitamin B_{12} and folate. Am. J. Med., 48:539, 541, 549, 555, 562, 570, 584, 594, 599, 602, 1970.

Herbert, V.: Detection of malabsorption of vitamin B_{12} due to gastric or intestinal dysfunction. Semin. Nucl. Med., 2:220, 1972.

Herbert, V.: Drugs effective in megaloblastic anemias. *In* Goodman, L. S., and Gilman, A. (eds.): The Pharmacological Basis of Therapeutics, 5th ed. New York, Macmillan, 1975.

Herbert, V.: Folic acid and vitamin B_{12}. *In* Goodhart, R. S., and Shils, M. E. (eds.): Modern Nutrition in Health and Disease. Philadelphia, Lea & Febiger, 1973, p. 221.

Herbert, V., and Tisman, G.: Effects of deficiencies of folic acid and vitamin B_{12} on central nervous system function and development. *In* Gaull, G. (ed.): Biology of Brain Dysfunction, Vol. 1. New York & London, Plenum Press, 1973, p. 373.

Herbert, V., Tisman, G., Go, L. T., and Brenner, L.: The dU suppression test using ^{125}I-UdR to define biochemical megaloblastosis. Br. J. Haematol., 24:713, 1973.

Jerzy Glass, G. B.: Gastric Intrinsic Factor and Other Vitamin B_{12} Binders. Biochemistry, Physiology, Pathology and Relation to Vitamin B_{12} Metabolism. Stuttgart and New York, Thieme Verlag and Intercontinental Medical Book Corporation, 1974.

Stebbins, R., Scott, J., and Herbert, V.: Drug-induced megaloblastic anemias. Semin. Hematol., 10:235, 1973.

Sullivan, L. W.: The megaloblastic anemias. *In* Mengel, C. E., Frei, E., and Nachman, R. (eds.): Hematology, Principles and Practice. Chicago, Year Book Medical Publishers, 1972.

Wellcome Trust Collaborative Study: Tropical Sprue and Megaloblastic Anemia. Edinburgh and London, Churchill Livingstone, 1971.

NORMOCHROMIC NORMOCYTIC ANEMIAS

732. ACUTE HEMORRHAGIC ANEMIA

Elmer B. Brown

Definition. Acute hemorrhagic anemia caused by loss of a large volume of blood may result from trauma, ulcerative lesions, abnormal blood vessels, or coagulation defects; it may occur from a severed blood vessel, from the gastrointestinal, respiratory, or genitourinary tracts, into a large muscle mass, or into various body cavities such as cysts or the pleural, peritoneal and retroperitoneal spaces. The hemorrhage is grossly evident except when blood is lost into the gastrointestinal tract, body cavities, or tissues. Clinical manifestations vary with the size, rate, and site of the hemorrhage, with the lesion responsible for the bleeding, and with the state of consciousness of the patient.

Clinical Manifestations. The manifestations of acute severe hemorrhage are remarkably consistent regardless of the underlying cause, because they depend on the volume of blood lost. As outlined in the accompanying table, the loss of as much as 500 ml of blood in five minutes usually produces only trivial effects on the circulation without changes in blood pressure or pulse rate. Withdrawal of a liter of blood often produces no fall in blood pressure in the recumbent subject, although if

Clinical Manifestations of Acute Blood Loss

Volume of Blood Lost		Clinical Manifestations
% of Blood Volume	*ml**	
10	500	Usually none; rarely vasovagal syncope
20	1000	Few changes supine; upright or with exercise, tachycardia and mild hypotension are often present
30–40	1500–2000	Marked postural hypotension and tachycardia; central venous pressure, cardiac output, and arterial blood pressure are reduced; pulse is thready; skin is cold and clammy; thirst, air hunger, headache, and syncope are frequent
50	2500	Severe shock, often leading to death

*Based on 5000 ml blood volume.

he sits up or attempts to walk, tachycardia occurs, the blood pressure often falls, and consciousness may be lost. When apprehension is added to the loss of even small amounts of blood, syncope caused by a vasovagal reaction may occur. Loss of 1500 to 2000 ml of blood leads to a fall in right atrial pressure, diminished cardiac output, hypotension, and a rapid, thready pulse. Additional symptoms are prostration, restlessness, thirst, tachypnea and air hunger, pallor with cold clammy skin, sweating, pounding headache, and frequent syncope. Rapid blood loss of greater than 40 per cent of the patient's blood volume leads to shock, the risk of renal tubular necrosis, myocardial infarction, and a high risk of death unless immediate replacement therapy is initiated. However, a previously healthy person may survive the gradual loss of as much as 50 per cent of his blood volume over a period of 24 hours. Hemorrhage into pleural, peritoneal, or retroperitoneal spaces usually causes pain, fever, and signs of serosal inflammation; bleeding into muscles may also produce marked limitation of motion.

Diagnosis. Initial assessment of the degree of hemorrhage may be difficult. When associated with multiple trauma, the amount of swelling surrounding the area of a wound correlates roughly with the amount of blood lost. Wounds of the thigh involving large muscles may be associated with a blood loss of 2500 ml or more. With gross disruption of tissues, as in gunshot or automobile injuries, the size of the wound correlates fairly well with the degree of blood loss — for an area of tissue damage the size of the patient's hand, loss of approximately 10 per cent of the patient's blood volume should be assumed. Upper gastrointestinal bleeding can be roughly quantitated by the fact that frank hematemesis indicates a large hemorrhage (usually more than 25 per cent of the blood volume), whereas melena alone indicates a much smaller blood loss. Generalizations of this type are important, because the initial hematocrit does not adequately reflect the size of the hemorrhage. Blood vessels of the skin and muscles constrict in an attempt to compensate for the decreased blood volume and to provide blood flow and adequate oxygen supply for vital organs. Replacement of plasma from endogenous sources is slow. The initial changes in blood counts after hemorrhage reflect the mobilization of platelets and leukocytes from marginated storage pools. Thrombocytosis to levels approaching 1 million per cubic millimeter may occur within an hour; a polymorphonuclear leukocytosis with white cell counts as high as 20,000 to 30,000 occurs within two to three hours. Metamyelocytes, myelocytes, and nucleated red blood cells often appear in the peripheral blood after severe hemorrhage. Replacement of plasma volume by fluid from the extravascular space is a relatively slow process, with the limiting factor being the rate at which albumin and other proteins are mobilized. After loss of 10 per cent of the blood volume, about half of the lost red cells and plasma are replaced by plasma alone after 24 hours. Loss of about 20 per cent of the blood volume requires 24 to 60 hours for restoration of the normal blood volume as reflected by a decreasing hematocrit for two or three days. Loss of red blood cell mass causes decreased tissue oxygenation only partially compensated for by adjustments in cardiovascular dynamics. Tissue hypoxia by a still unknown mechanism triggers erythropoietin production with measurable increases in plasma levels of this hormone within six hours. Increased levels of 2,3-diphosphoglycerate in circulating erythrocytes contribute to a shift of the hemoglobin oxygen dissociation curve for more efficient tissue oxygenation. Erythropoietin-stimulated erythropoiesis causes a fall of the plasma iron during the two to five days required for marrow stem cells to proliferate and mature into circulating reticulocytes to expand the red cell mass. Some reticulocytes are released prematurely from the marrow in response to hemorrhage, and their numbers increase to peak levels of 10 to 15 per cent after seven to ten days. Since reticulocytes are larger than mature erythrocytes, the mean corpuscular volume (MCV) rises (approximately 1 fl for each per cent of increase in reticulocyte count) and polychromatophilic macrocytes are seen in Wright-stained blood films. Depending on the size of the hemorrhage and the adequacy of iron stores, the red cell volume and hematocrit are restored to normal in about five or six weeks. Elevated platelet counts and leukocytosis have usually returned to the normal range within three to five days. Bleeding into the gastrointestinal tract produces an elevation of the blood urea nitrogen which may be accentuated if renal function is impaired. Resorption of blood from body cavities or tissues results in increased production of unconjugated bilirubin and may be associated with mild jaundice; iron released from hemoglobin bled into tissues is reutilized for new erythropoiesis.

Treatment. Treatment should be directed at stopping the hemorrhage, combating shock, and restoring blood volume. The patient should be kept warm and quiet; sedation and analgesics may be required. It is essential to begin an infusion through a needle or catheter of adequate bore to permit rapid fluid replacement, and this will sometimes require a surgical cutdown to find collapsed veins. The choice of solutions for initial replacement therapy depends on how critical the patient's condition is and what solutions are available. Most quickly available for rapid expansion of plasma volume are noncolloid electrolyte solutions (e.g., isotonic saline and Ringer's lactate) or dextran solutions, either a 10 per cent solution of low molecular weight dextran in isotonic saline (dextran 40, with an average molecular weight of 40,000) or a 6 per cent solution of high molecular weight dextran (dextran 70, with an average molecular weight of 70,000). Dextran 40 has the advantage of increasing the plasma volume by one to two times the amount infused, but is more rapidly cleared in the urine. Its effect is rapidly dissipated during the succeeding 12 hours, and in a few patients it may precipitate acute renal failure. Dextran 70 is cleared more slowly and sustains the plasma volume expansion for 24 to 48 hours. Both may produce circulatory overload, which can usually be avoided by administering the first 500 ml rapidly and the remainder more slowly with frequent monitoring of central venous pressure. When volumes of dextran solution in excess of 1000 ml are used, interference with platelet adhesiveness and coagulation mechanisms may accentuate bleeding. Plasma protein solutions and 5 per cent albumin in saline have the advantage of predictable volume expansion with physiologic materials, but carry the disadvantages of relatively high cost, slower time for reconstitution, and, with plasma solutions, the risk of hepatitis. Noncolloid electrolyte solutions such as isotonic saline or Ringer's lactate may be given quickly in acute emergencies for support of blood volume, but since they are rapidly distributed throughout the intravascular and extravascular compartments they must be supplemented with blood or colloid solutions. Use of fresh whole blood, packed erythrocytes, or saline-resuspended, concentrated red blood cells requires typing and cross-matching that cause too great a delay for routine use in the initial treatment of life-threatening hemorrhage. Use of uncross-matched universal donor blood cannot be condoned except in extreme emergencies. Rarely is red cell depletion so severe that blood transfusions cannot wait for careful cross-matching. Blood transfusions supplement initial volume expansion with dextran or other colloidal solutions and are the mainstay of the definitive treatment of acute hemorrhage. When bleeding is due to absence of platelets or coagulation factors, transfusion of fresh whole blood or concentrates of blood components is essential and may be lifesaving. With prolonged bleeding requiring replacement of more than 5000 ml of stored blood within 48 hours, thrombocytopenia caused by transfusion of nonviable platelets may cause bleeding. Anticipation of this complication as well as the risks of severe uncontrolled bleeding may favor early surgical attempts to identify and correct the cause of bleeding from gastrointestinal or other obscure sites. After the emergency is over, provision of a high protein diet and iron by mouth are indicated to replace the stores depleted by blood loss; no other supplements are needed.

Adamson, J., and Hillman, R. S.: Blood volume and plasma protein replacement following acute blood loss in normal man. J.A.M.A., 205:609, 1968.

Collins, J. A., and Ballinger, W. F.: The treatment of shock. *In* Ballinger, W. F., Rutherford, R. B., and Zuidema, G. D. (eds.): The Management of Trauma. Philadelphia, W. B. Saunders Company, 1973, Chapter 3.

Harris, J. W., and Kellermeyer, R. W.: The Red Cell. Production, Metabolism, Destruction: Normal and Abnormal, Revised ed. Cambridge, Harvard University Press, 1970, Chapter 4.

Mollison, P. L.: Blood Transfusion in Clinical Medicine. 5th ed. Oxford, Blackwell Scientific Publications, 1972.

733. ANEMIA ASSOCIATED WITH INFECTION AND CHRONIC SYSTEMIC DISEASES
(Simple Chronic Anemia, Anemia of Chronic Disorders)

Elmer B. Brown

Definition. The anemia of infection and many chronic disorders is usually mild and nonprogressive in severity. It develops over a period of one to two months, is usually normochromic normocytic, and is characterized by decreased plasma iron, decreased transferrin iron-binding capacity, decreased bone marrow sideroblasts, increased reticuloendothelial iron deposits, mild hemolysis, and relative bone marrow failure. The occurrence of anemia in association with chronic disease of multiple etiologies makes the selection of an appropriate descriptive name difficult. The term "anemia of chronic disorders" may be the least restrictive for the anemia underlying cancer, lymphomas, connective tissue disorders, hepatic, renal and endocrine disorders, fractures and tissue injury, and chronic viral and suppurative infections. Other types of anemia, such as those related to blood loss, iron or vitamin deficiency, or hemolysis, may accentuate and complicate the underlying anemia of a chronic disorder. By its widespread association with many chronic diseases this anemia is the most common form seen in hos-

pital populations, and it is frequent in the population at large.

Etiology and Pathogenesis. The mechanism can generally be framed in terms of three basic abnormalities: (1) moderate shortening of erythrocyte life span; (2) failure of the bone marrow to increase erythropoiesis sufficiently to compensate for the mild hemolytic anemia; and (3) an unexplained impairment of iron release from reticuloendothelial cells throughout the body. Examination of the interaction of these three basic abnormalities is essential before special features of anemias associated with specific diseases can be defined.

Decreased erythrocyte life span is of moderate degree and requires measurements with special erythrocyte labeling techniques; half-time survival of ^{51}Cr-tagged cells is reduced from a normal range of 30 ± 3 days to about 20 to 25 days. In absolute terms, erythrocyte survival is about 80 days instead of the normal 120 days. Cross-transfusion experiments have shown normal survival of red cells from anemic patients transfused into normal recipients, whereas cells from normal subjects transfused into the patient show decreased survival indicative of an extracorpuscular factor responsible for the decreased erythrocyte life span. Whether this unidentified factor acts in the plasma or adversely influences other portions of the erythrocyte's environment has never been defined.

Ordinarily, this mild degree of hemolysis would be compensated for by greater erythropoietic activity of the bone marrow which can increase red cell production six to eight times the normal rate. However, erythropoiesis in patients with chronic disorders rarely increases more than twofold; as a result, production of red cells falls behind destruction until a new balance is reached at mildly anemic levels. Normally the body responds to tissue hypoxia of anemia by increasing the output of erythropoietin which stimulates the differentiation of marrow stem cells into erythroblasts and speeds their maturation to circulating erythrocytes. One might suppose, under conditions of chronic disease, that either the stimulation of erythropoietin production is defective or the marrow is incapable of responding to this hormone. Experimental evidence indicates that erythropoietin levels are low and that the marrow is quite capable of responding to erythropoietin when injected in pure form or when stimulated by external hypoxia or cobalt administration. Thus the block to an appropriate erythropoietic response seems to be an insensitive "thermostat," failing to stimulate erythropoietin release in response to slowly developing anemia. The precise mechanism of this defect is unknown.

The third basic abnormality common to the anemias of chronic disorders is the impairment of iron release from reticuloendothelial cells. Normally, senescent erythrocytes are removed from the circulation by reticuloendothelial cells which digest hemoglobin, free its iron from the heme ring, and release it to plasma transferrin for transport to the marrow and reutilization in erythropoiesis. Within hours after infection or injury a block occurs to the normal release of iron by the reticuloendothelial cells, as evidenced by a precipitous fall in plasma iron concentrations. Further experimental evidence for this block was obtained by injecting ^{59}Fe-labeled, heat-damaged red cells that are rapidly cleared by reticuloendothelial cells and measuring the release and reutilization of ^{59}Fe into newly formed erythrocytes. Normal subjects reutilize 55 to 70 per cent of the ^{59}Fe for hemoglobin synthesis, whereas patients with the anemia of chronic disorders utilize less than 40 per cent. As a result of this block to normal iron flow, there is a buildup of ferritin and hemosiderin in reticuloendothelial cells in the bone marrow and throughout the body. The paucity or iron available for erythropoietic cells in turn leads to decreased numbers of marrow sideroblasts and other evidence of iron-deficient erythropoiesis. The three basic abnormalities are balanced so that the resultant anemia is mild and self-limiting. However, if blood loss, red cell fragmentation, or immune hemolysis increases the rate of red cell loss, if folate or vitamin B_{12} deficiency further decreases erythropoietic response, or if iron deficiency accentuates the block to iron flow, the anemia may be much more severe.

Various diseases have additional specific etiologic factors that might profitably be examined separately from the basic abnormalities that characterize the anemia of chronic disorders.

Renal failure is usually accompanied by anemia which may be quite severe. Anemia correlates roughly with the elevation of blood urea nitrogen, although a more nearly linear relationship exists between elevated BUN and decreased red cell life span. The factor or factors in uremic plasma that damage erythrocytes and cause anemia have not been identified, although many substances have been suggested. In some patients mechanical trauma and increased fragmentation of red cells lead to severe hemolytic anemia when renal failure is associated with malignant hypertension or various types of hemolytic-uremic syndrome. Other patients with renal failure have hemorrhagic tendencies caused by decreased numbers and function of platelets.

Deficiency of folate and iron aggravates the *anemia of patients undergoing dialysis;* folate is dialyzable and is lost into the dialysis bath, whereas iron is lost with blood in the dialysis coil. Since approximately 90 per cent of erythropoietin originates in the kidney, either directly or through a renal activating system, progressive renal disease leads to decreased erythropoietin production. In addition, the presence of uremia may blunt the bone marrow's response to the reduced amounts of erythropoietin released by damaged kidneys; dialysis may salvage some of the effectiveness of the available erythropoietin and cause amelioration of the anemia.

Rheumatoid arthritis in the active phase is frequently accompanied by the anemia of chronic disorders. A unique feature is the microscopic bleeding into the inflamed joints that leads to massive accumulation of iron in the hyperplastic synovial tissue. Sequestration of several hundred milligrams of iron in hypertrophied synovium may contribute to an iron deficiency state superimposed on the anemia of inflammation. Bleeding induced by the gastrointestinal irritation of aspirin, corticosteroids, and other anti-inflammatory therapeutic agents may further accentuate the iron deficiency.

Cancer in its later stages is almost always accompanied by the anemia of chronic disorders. Frequently there is no correlation between the degree of anemia and the extent of the tumor. Bone marrow invasion by cancer is often associated with the release of immature leukocytes and nucleated erythrocytes, but the extent of marrow metastases correlates poorly with the degree of anemia. Substances released from necrotic cancer cells and the red cell fragmentation from fibrin strands in vessels narrowed by tumor invasion have been postulated to explain the hemolytic anemia in cancer. Bleeding from tumors of the alimentary or genitourinary tracts or from vascular lesions of the skin causes hemorrhagic or iron deficiency anemia, and the inanition leading to calorie, protein, and vitamin deficiency accentuates the underlying simple chronic anemia.

Liver disease is associated with various complications in addition to the underlying anemia of chronic disorders. The increased plasma volume of cirrhosis may give an exaggerated impression of anemia when the concentration of erythrocytes is measured by hematocrit and hemoglobin determinations. Bleeding related to peptic ulcers, varices, and deficient coagulation factors may produce rapid blood loss anemia or slowly developing iron deficiency. Alcohol depresses erythropoiesis acutely and leads to folate deficiency anemia because of inadequate intake and defective absorption of the vitamin. Erythrocyte abnormalities—thin macrocytic target cells or burr cells—may contribute to the decreased red cell survival. Hypersplenism frequently associated with portal hypertension of liver disease also accentuates the hemolytic anemia of chronic disorders.

Endocrine disorders, including thyroid, pituitary, and adrenal insufficiency, are associated with a normochromic normocytic anemia most severe in hypothyroidism. Presumably these endocrine deficiencies lead to decreased erythropoietin production. In the case of *hypothyroidism* the diminished need of the tissues for oxygen leads to an adaptive partial atrophy of the erythron. Frequently, coexistent iron, folate, and especially vitamin B_{12} deficiencies are present with the anemia of hypothyroidism.

Clinical Manifestations. The symptoms are primarily those of the underlying disease. As the anemia is mild and develops slowly, the patient can adjust to it with minimal accentuation of fatigue, dyspnea, and palpitations. When bleeding or hemolysis complicates the underlying anemia of chronic disorders in patients with leukemia, lymphoma, or chronic renal failure, symptoms of anemia may be disabling and lead to coronary insufficiency and congestive failure. Pallor, tachycardia, cardiac dilatation, and low-grade sustained fever are nonspecific signs common to many types of chronic anemia.

Diagnosis. The anemia of chronic disorders is usually normocytic normochromic (MCV 87 to 103 fl and MCHC 32 to 36 grams per deciliter), but may be normocytic hypochromic or even microcytic hypochromic. When microcytosis or hypochromia is present, it is usually milder than that seen in well-developed iron deficiency anemia. The hematocrit usually remains constant in a range between 25 and 39 per cent at full development of the anemia after six to eight weeks. Erythrocyte morphology is unremarkable except for burr cells of uremia and some types of cancer and the thin, flat macrocyte of chronic liver disease. Reticulocytosis or polychromasia indicative of increased erythropoiesis is rare. Leukocytes and platelets are normal unless they reflect changes related to the underlying disease. Bone marrow morphology on Wright-stained specimens shows no specific abnormality; changes related to the underlying disease may include increased numbers of plasma cells in cirrhosis or rheumatoid arthritis and leukemic or tumor cell infiltration. Prussian blue stains for iron in bone marrow disclose decreased numbers of erythroid precursors with iron granules (sideroblasts), whereas reticuloendothelial cells show increased hemosiderin deposits. Plasma iron and total iron-binding capacity are both reduced; the per cent saturation of transferrin is normal or low. Differentiation from the plasma iron changes of iron deficiency anemia may be difficult; the major difference is a tendency toward increased transferrin concentration and absence of stainable marrow iron in iron deficiency. When iron deficiency and the anemia of chronic disorders occur together, the rise in transferrin usually seen in iron deficiency is blunted; absent marrow hemosiderin is the key diagnostic observation. Despite the underlying hemolysis, the serum bilirubin is usually normal unless there is associated liver dysfunction. Hemolysis is usually detectable only by special red cell survival measurements.

Treatment. The only effective therapy is that directed toward correction of the underlying disease. Since the anemia typically is mild and nonprogressive, no attempt at correction may be necessary. When symptoms of underlying heart disease are triggered by anemia, transfusions with packed erythrocytes to a hematocrit of 30 to 35 per cent may be temporarily beneficial. Attempts to stimulate erythropoiesis by administration of cobalt have been abandoned, because undesirable side effects outweigh the modest improvement of the anemia. Androgenic steroids may be effective in some patients with cancer or chronic renal disease. Purified erythropoietin is not yet available in sufficient amounts for adequate clinical trials. Corticosteroids frequently ameliorate the anemia of rheumatoid arthritis and other connective tissue diseases; they may also be beneficial in treatment of complicating immune hemolysis. No means has been found to bypass the block to iron flow in the anemia of chronic disorders. Since colloidal iron preparations given parenterally must be processed by the reticuloendothelial cells before iron is made available to transferrin, the colloidal iron is blocked as effectively as that from senescent erythrocytes. When bleeding causes superimposed iron deficiency, giving iron by mouth or parenterally will restore hemoglobin levels to those of the underlying chronic disorder, but not back to normal. Similarly, folate deficiency of alcoholic cirrhosis will respond to folate therapy by partial correction of anemia.

Cartwright, G. E.: The anemia of chronic disorders. Semin. Hematol., 3:351, 1966.

Harris, J. W., and Kellermeyer, R. W.: The Red Cell. Production, Metabolism, Destruction: Normal and Abnormal. Cambridge, Mass., Harvard University Press, 1970.

Kimber, C., Deller, D. J., Ibbotson, R. N., and Lander, H.: The mechanism of anaemia in chronic liver disease. Quart. J. Med., 34:33, 1965.

Strandberg, O.: Anemia in rheumatoid arthritis. Acta Med. Scand. [Suppl.], 454:1, 1966.

Williams, W. J., Beutler, E., Erslev, A. J., and Rundles, R. W. (eds.): Hematology. New York, McGraw-Hill Book Company, 1972.

734. APLASTIC ANEMIA

M. C. Brain

Definition. Aplastic or hypoplastic anemia is the term applied to a group of disorders characterized by reduction in all the cellular elements of the blood (pancytopenia), and associated with hypocellularity of the bone marrow. The degree of panctyopenia reflects the severity of the disorder and may vary during the course of the illness. Less marked reduction in cell counts may be encountered in hypoplastic anemia than in aplasia of the bone marrow. The bone marrow aspiration or biopsy may

on rare occasions yield a hypercellular or normocellular specimen. Such a finding probably reflects the chance sampling of a residual focus of marrow showing normal or increased cellularity. The distribution of active marrow by isotopic scanning techniques and the findings at necropsy usually reveal a diffusely hypocellular fatty marrow throughout the normally hematopoietic skeleton, although residual foci of hematopoietic marrow may be present. Reduced erythropoiesis may be confirmed by ferrokinetic studies with impaired clearance of iron from the plasma and greatly diminished, often negligible, incorporation of iron into red blood cells. Although the exact etiology of aplastic anemia is frequently unknown, the generalized failure of hematopoiesis, including erythropoiesis, granulopoiesis, and megakaryopoiesis, suggests that the primary defect is due to an absolute reduction in the numbers of pluripotent hematopoietic stem cells.

Although the term aplastic anemia is descriptive, it appears reasonable in the light of present knowledge to draw a distinction between the failure of bone marrow function associated with a hypoplastic or aplastic marrow and the failure of hematopoiesis that may be associated with hypercellular marrow, ineffective hematopoiesis. However, it must be recognized that certain bone marrow toxins which are known to produce aplastic anemia, such as benzol, may also give rise to pancytopenia with a hypercellular marrow exhibiting ineffective hematopoiesis. Furthermore, it seems reasonable to draw a distinction between the pancytopenia associated with aplastic anemia and the isolated reductions in red blood cells, granulocytes, or platelets through failure of formation of the differentiated cell lines. Disorders of formation of isolated cell lines probably reflect the action of toxic agents or the influence of immune mechanisms on the differentiation of committed rather than the pluripotent stem cell precursors in the bone marrow. Lack of fundamental knowledge of the precise etiologic mechanisms which can result in either aplastic anemia or isolated failures of formation of one of the hematopoietic cell lines may make the distinction between the disorders somewhat arbitrary. However, recent knowledge regarding the association of pure red cell aplasia with immunologic disorders and thymic tumors does suggest that different mechanisms may be operative and therefore validate the distinction. Aplastic anemia may develop without an apparent or recognized cause, or may follow exposure to ionizing radiation or a variety of chemical agents, including drugs, either known to be potentially toxic to hematopoiesis or recognized to only occasionally have this effect, or it may be familial or constitutional in etiology, becoming manifest in childhood or early adult life. The clinical course is influenced by the severity of the pancytopenia and especially by the degree of leukopenia or thrombocytopenia. If severe infective and hemorrhagic complications do not take place, or can be prevented, the patient may survive for a number of years, and occasionally complete or partial remissions may take place.

Etiology. A general classification of the etiology of aplastic anemia is given in Table 1. The exact cause of aplastic anemia is often obscure. In a considerable proportion of the cases no etiologic agent can be incriminated with certainty, and these are described as idiopathic. A small proportion of the idiopathic group occur in childhood or in early adult life, and when associated with other congenital abnormalities and a history of

TABLE 1.   Etiologic Classification of Aplastic Anemia

Idiopathic
    Familial or constitutional (Fanconi's anemia)
    Acquired
Secondary
    Physical or chemical agents
        Ionizing radiation
        Drugs (cytotoxic; normally noncytotoxic)
        Nonpharmacological chemicals
    Infections
        Viral hepatitis
        Bacterial: miliary tuberculosis
    Metabolic
        Pancreatitis
        Pregnancy
    Immunologic
        Antibody mediated
        Graft versus host reaction
    Neoplastic
        Myelophthisic
        Paroxysmal nocturnal hemoglobinuria

aplastic anemia in other members of the family their separate designation as the constitutional type of aplastic anemia *(Fanconi's anemia)* is warranted. The majority of idiopathic cases are presumed to be acquired, and although no etiologic agent may be incriminated, this designation does not preclude exposure to some unrecalled or unrecognized environmental or ingested agent. In the secondary aplastic anemias in which a history can be obtained of exposure to chemical or physical agents, or when the onset was preceded by an event known to be associated with aplastic anemia, the exact causal relationship between the implicated agent or agents and the fundamental disturbance of hematopoiesis often remains obscure.

The agents which may give rise to aplastic anemia can be divided into two categories. First come agents that regularly produce bone marrow damage if the magnitude or the duration of the exposure is sufficient to produce cytotoxicity. These include exposure to ionizing radiations from x-rays, radioactive elements, or nuclear explosions; chemical agents such as benzol; and a variety of cytotoxic drugs used in the treatment of malignant disease, including nitrogen mustard, cytoxan, busulfan, the vinca alkaloids, and antimetabolites such as 6-mercaptopurine and methotrexate. The second category contains agents which have been recognized as being associated with aplastic anemia in only a small proportion of the population exposed to them. The incidence of aplastic anemia in this second category is so low that considerable periods of time have elapsed before the adverse reaction has been sufficiently widely recognized and reported for it to be appreciated as being a statistically significant risk. Drugs are the most common group in this second category. Chloramphenicol is now widely recognized as a potential cause of aplastic anemia. Inquiry as to exposure to drugs must include both drugs prescribed by physicians and drugs that can be purchased without prescription, including analgesics, hypnotics, and antihistamines. Inquiries should be made and evidence sought for the possibility of self-administration or abuse of mood-changing drugs, or the inhalation of organic solvents for the same purpose. When no history of drug ingestion can be established, the incrimination of possible etiologic agents may be exceedingly difficult, because many chemical compounds in common

daily use contain benzene derivatives or allied compounds which must be regarded with suspicion. Many such chemicals are used as solvents in common household cleaning agents, in dyes and paints, and in insecticides and fertilizers, and have been identified in animal feed supplements in which the manufacturing processes have resulted in toxic products derived from relatively nontoxic precursors. Thus the risks of exposure to potentially toxic compounds are well-nigh limitless. Despite frequent difficulty in establishing a definite etiologic agent, it is important that a full and detailed inquiry be made of the patient and relatives as to the possible exposure at work or in the home to potentially toxic chemicals, through a detailed history of daily activities and hobbies.

Since its introduction in 1948, *chloramphenicol* became recognized as the drug most commonly associated with aplastic anemia. It achieved rapid and widespread popularity with physicians by virtue of the range of its antimicrobial activity and the ease with which it could be administered. In 1952 a number of reports were published associating chloramphenicol with aplastic anemia, an association which was directly responsible for the establishment of a registry of drugs giving rise to aplastic anemia and other adverse hematologic drug reactions. The reports published in 1965 and 1967 by the Registry on Adverse Reactions showed that of 771 cases of pancytopenia 338 (44 per cent) followed the use of chloramphenicol, and that in 154 (23 per cent) chloramphenicol was the only drug taken in the preceding six months. Although the risk of developing pancytopenia and aplastic anemia after chloramphenicol is approximately 1 in 20,000 to 30,000, this is about 13 times greater than the risk of idiopathic aplastic anemia in the population as a whole. Awareness of the risk has resulted in a considerable and commendable reduction in the prescribing of chloramphenicol, partly through the increasing availability of other broad-spectrum antimicrobials of comparable activity and ease of administration. It is now generally accepted that chloramphenicol should only be prescribed in specific and serious infections in which it can be shown to be the *only* antimicrobial agent suitable on the basis of sensitivity testing. However, the awareness of the hazards of this serious complication of chloramphenicol differs in different countries, and there are still countries where it is widely prescribed or may, indeed, be obtained without prescription. The higher incidence of aplastic anemia in clinical practice in certain countries may reflect relative lack of control over the availability of this drug. Thus with increasing air travel the risks of exposure to chloramphenicol may persist despite the adverse publicity and the application of more stringent indications for its prescriptions in many nations.

It is now recognized that there are two independent types of bone marrow toxicity produced by chloramphenicol. It is well established that this drug induces a dose-related reversible bone marrow lesion characterized by maturation arrest and vacuolization in early erythroid cells, reticulocytopenia, and ferrokinetic changes indicative of suppressed erythropoiesis. This reversible effect of the drug results from inhibition of mitochondrial protein synthesis and consequent mitochondrial injury. It appears to be quite distinct from the much rarer and devastating complications of aplastic anemia, which may not be dose dependent or even directly temporally related to exposure to the drug. There is some evidence that the bone marrow aplasia may occur on the basis of a genetically determined biochemical predisposition to toxicity involving the DNA synthetic pathway. Although knowledge as to the mechanism of the reversible pharmacologic toxicity of chloramphenicol in the bone marrow may ultimately throw light onto the mechanism of marrow aplasia, it must be emphasized that currently these two mechanisms appear to be distinct and that the onset of aplasia cannot be predicted nor is it readily reversible. Thus the only way to avoid the calamitous consequence of aplastic anemia is to not expose the patient to chloramphenicol in any form.

Although the association of aplastic anemia with drugs other than chloramphenicol is well recognized, the low incidence of this complication and the fact that, as mentioned already, it is common for patients with aplastic anemia to give a history of exposure to a number of potentially toxic agents makes it difficult to calculate with any accuracy the possible risk of this complication. However, phenylbutazone was the second most frequently recorded drug in the A.M.A. Registry, having been administered alone or concomitantly with an apparently innocuous agent to 27 patients and having been associated with other potentially toxic agents in a total of 52 patients (6.3 per cent). Other drugs, including the hydantoin analogues used in treating epilepsy, sulfonamides, sulfonylureas, gold compounds, organic arsenicals, potassium perchlorate, and quinacrine, are known to be associated with aplastic anemia. At least 50 other drugs have been implicated, and many of them are chemically related to drugs established as being associated with aplastic anemia. Among those obtainable without prescription are a wide variety of antihistamine preparations. In addition, salicylamide, widely available as a sedative without prescription, has been reported in three patients as being associated with aplastic anemia.

Benzol and a wide variety of *aromatic hydrocarbons* derived from the refining of petroleum and coal products are included in many cleaning solvents and form the basis of many compounds used in the petrochemical and plastic industries. Aplastic anemia has been reported as following exposure to aromatic hydrocarbons by siphoning gasoline from gas tanks. The widespread use of these compounds in dyes, solvents, insecticides, cements, glues, and fingernail polish, and as diluents to paints, varnishes, and lacquers as thinners and paint removers, makes the risk of exposure of the general population very considerable. Furthermore, in many instances the relative purity of organic solvents is unknown and significant amounts of benzene may be present. Aplastic anemia is recognized to follow the ingestion of benzene trinitrotoluene or exposure to Stoddard solvent, widely used in the automobile industry as a cleaning agent.

Aplastic anemia is a recognized complication of "glue-sniffing," and many of the glues and cements may contain benzene or benzene derivatives.

Insecticides such as gamma benzene hexachloride (Lindane), chlordane, and chlorophenothane (DDT) have been associated with aplastic anemia, and have been reported in the A.M.A. Registry. Many of these organic insecticides are used suspended in petroleum solvents which may contain benzene.

Aplastic anemia has occasionally been reported after exposure to hair dyes, tints, rinses, and sprays, but in view of the widespread use of these agents it appears that they represent a negligible risk.

Aplastic anemia has been associated with *hepatitis* in more than 50 patients. The onset of aplastic anemia is usually within two to six months after the hepatitis has resolved. The nature of the etiologic relationship between hepatitis and aplastic anemia is unclear. Viral etiology of the hepatitis has seldom been established. Furthermore, it is well recognized that many agents capable of producing aplastic anemia are also hepatotoxic; thus both the hepatitis and the aplastic anemia may have a common etiology. Even when the viral nature of the hepatitis is established, the possibility remains that hepatic dysfunction itself may increase the risk of aplastic anemia because of impaired or abnormal handling of potentially marrow-toxic agents.

The etiology of *pure red cell aplasia* can, like that of aplastic anemia, be divided into constitutional and acquired forms. More than 100 cases of chronic erythroid hypoplasia and aplasia have been described in childhood. The onset may be at birth but is more commonly recognized within the first two years of life. The occasional occurrence of the disorder in a sibling has suggested a genetic or inherited abnormality, although detailed family studies have not provided evidence to support this. A metabolic defect in the handling of tryptophan has been described in some of the affected children. The children may go into remission either spontaneously or in response to adrenal steroid administration. Acquired red cell aplasia may occur as an acute transient episode, particularly in children with congenital hemolytic anemia. This disorder, most frequently reported in hereditary spherocytosis, is thought to be due to suppression of erythropoiesis in association with viral illnesses and may reflect a direct action of viruses on erythropoiesis or be a consequence of an immunologic response to a viral infection. The recognition of this disorder in association with chronic hemolytic anemia probably reflects the dramatic onset of anemia caused by cessation of erythropoiesis and an increased rate of hemolysis, and may indicate increased susceptibility of an actively erythropoietic bone marrow to a variety of toxic factors. Pure red cell aplasia in the adult is associated with thymic tumors in about 30 to 50 per cent of patients. The presence of a thymoma and the response of these patients to either thymectomy or adrenal steroid or immunosuppressive treatment have suggested that the selective disturbance of erythropoiesis is due to an immunologic mechanism. Support for this has come from demonstration of antibodies in the patient's serum which react against erythroid precursor cells and from the selective suppression of erythropoiesis in laboratory animals given gamma globulin prepared from the patient's serum. Although anti-erythropoietin antibodies have also been demonstrated, the presence of high levels of erythropoietin in the serum of these patients makes it unlikely that this is the primary mode of action.

Incidence. Idiopathic aplastic anemia is rare and occurs predominantly in children and young adults of either sex. The incidence of secondary aplastic anemia will be directly related to the size of the population exposed to the causal agents. Increasing use of atomic energy and of radioactive isotopes and x-rays in both industry and medicine has increased the risks of exposure to ionizing irradiation. However, the widespread recognition of the hazard makes it unlikely that aplastic anemia will increase through this cause except by accidents or negligence. Nevertheless, numerous cases of aplastic anemia resulted from the two atomic bombs exploded over Japan in 1945, and the risk of aplastic anemia through atomic warfare and, indeed, other chemical agents under such conditions is ever present. The incidence of secondary aplastic anemia caused by drugs and other toxic chemical agents is difficult to estimate with accuracy. It has been calculated that 1 of every 20,000 to 30,000 patients receiving chloramphenicol develops pancytopenia. The incidence of secondary aplastic anemia will be dependent on the population exposed to known toxic agents. The increasing use of cytotoxic drugs in malignant disease, in order to produce suppression of immune system in a wide variety of disorders, and the use of methotrexate in the treatment of psoriasis have greatly increased the risk of the development of hypoplastic or aplastic anemia as a complication of treatment. In patients exposed to phenylbutazone, the incidence rises with age and reflects the relative preponderance of women receiving this and other related agents in the treatment of rheumatoid arthritis. The incidence of pure red cell aplasia depends on whether the disorder is constitutional or acquired. Both the constitutional and the acute acquired red cell aplasia seen in congenital hemolytic anemia are most commonly seen in childhood. Acquired pure red cell aplasia in the adult is mainly seen in middle age. There is a significant preponderance of females over males when pure red cell aplasia is associated with thymoma, whereas males exceed females in those patients in whom a thymoma cannot be demonstrated either radiologically or on exploration of the anterior mediastinum.

Pathology and Pathogenesis. The peripheral blood count reveals a reduction in all cellular elements, with lowering of the red cell count, packed red cell volume, and hemoglobin concentration, and reduction in the total circulating white cells, particularly those of the granulocyte series, although absolute monocytopenia is usually present. The platelet count is invariably reduced and may be very low. The anemia is usually normochromic but may be slightly macrocytic with red blood cells showing some slight changes in size and shape. The reticulocyte count varies from 0 to 5 per cent, but the absolute reticulocyte count is usually subnormal. The reticulocytes may be large and immature, possibly reflecting a response of the remaining erythroid cells to increased erythropoietin stimulation with a short bone marrow transit time. The presence of nucleated red blood cells in the peripheral blood is unusual and implies some other disorder of hematopoiesis. Absolute granulocytopenia is an invariable feature and is of importance in relation to the immediate prognosis, because an absolute granulocyte count of less than 200 per cubic millimeter puts a patient at great risk from infectious complications. The absolute monocyte count is usually reduced, and an absolute lymphocytopenia is a common finding. It is unusual to find immature cells of the granulocytic or lymphocytic cell lines in the peripheral blood.

These peripheral blood findings reflect the disordered hematopoiesis in the bone marrow. The specimens of bone marrow are usually aspirated without difficulty or pain and usually yield fragments which consist of fat spaces with few cellular elements. Occasionally bone marrow aspiration reveals a normocellular or hypercellular specimen, which may reflect the chance aspiration of a sample of bone marrow with residual normal activity, in which case aspiration should be carried out at other sites if the diagnosis is to be confirmed. Further information regarding over-all cellularity of the bone marrow can be obtained from the histology of needle or trephine biopsies. The relative proportions of the different cellular elements in the bone marrow seen on aspiration or on biopsy can vary from patient to patient. Both the degree of cellularity and the relative involvement of the different cell lines may reflect the nature and severity of the action of the toxic agent inducing disordered hematopoiesis. Although increases in precursor cells may be present, suggesting a "maturation arrest," or may be accompanied by changes in the chromatin pattern of the erythroid precursors with some megaloblastic-like features, an absolute increase in blast cells is uncommon. The presence of an increase in granulocyte precursors and a reduction in cytoplasmic granules within the maturing cells may make the distinction between aplastic anemia and subleukemic myelocytic leukemia difficult. However, the absence of blast cells in the peripheral blood and the presence of a hypoplastic or aplastic marrow at other sites usually distinguish between aplastic anemia and subleukemic leukemia. When the patient has received multiple blood transfusions, hemosiderosis of the bone marrow may be present and in due course will involve other organs, notably the liver, spleen, and heart. Enlargement of the liver and spleen may be due to hemosiderosis, because extramedullary hematopoiesis is uncommon. Other pathologic changes are related to infectious and hemorrhagic complications which are frequently encountered during the course of the illness and are the usual causes of death.

The mechanism by which exposure to irradiation or chemical agents induces the cellular damage which results in aplastic anemia is incompletely understood. Ionizing radiations and radiomimetic drugs are thought to inhibit mitosis, probably by causing disturbances of DNA replication or synthesis. The antimetabolites used in treatment of malignant disease either interfere with the formation of purines or nucleic acids or, in the case of the vinca alkaloids, inhibit chromatin separation through interaction with spindle proteins. Although exposure to radiation or cytotoxic drugs characteristically produces a transient depression of hematopoiesis, the persistent disorder of hematopoiesis characterizing aplastic anemia implies a more fundamental defect in stem cell proliferation and differentiation. A similar distinction must be drawn between the transient, reversible, and dose-related disturbance of hematopoiesis that follows ingestion of chloramphenicol and the more fundamental and probably unrelated disturbance of hematopoiesis characterizing aplastic anemia caused by this agent. Although the transient disorder of hematopoiesis caused by chloramphenicol can be regarded as a direct or metabolic effect on cell maturation, aplastic anemia would appear to imply some more fundamental derangement of the genetic information necessary for stem cell proliferation and differentiation. A variety of evidence supports the latter view.

Exposure to irradiation may be followed by persistent disorders of the chromosomal structure of lymphocytes which may be detected months or years after the radiation exposure. In aplastic anemia from any cause, the level of fetal hemoglobin in the erythrocytes produced by the bone marrow may be increased, suggesting some persistent derangement of the control of globin chain synthesis. Although initial results suggested that a high hemoglobin F might be a good prognostic sign, this interpretation has been questioned. In Fanconi's anemia, in which some as yet unknown inherited influence can result in the appearance of aplastic anemia in childhood or early adult life, chromatin breaks and other disturbances of the karyotype have been described. Furthermore, abnormalities of the red cell enzymes have also been described. The common association of Fanconi's anemia with developmental abnormalities affecting the structure or position of the kidneys and radiologic evidence of abnormalities of the bony skeleton suggests the presence of some fundamental derangement of genetic factors influencing development, although the causal relationship between these abnormalities and the subsequent development of aplastic anemia is as yet unexplained.

Still further support for the view that a fundamental disturbance of stem cell structure and function is the basis for aplastic anemia comes from the association between aplastic anemia and *paroxysmal nocturnal hemoglobinuria.* Hypoplastic or aplastic anemia may develop as a complication of paroxysmal nocturnal hemoglobinuria (PNH), or a small proportion of the red blood cells in aplastic anemia may show the increased susceptibility to complement lysis characteristic of PNH. The PNH red blood cells may be found at the onset or during recovery from aplastic anemia and be associated with frank hemolytic anemia. Since the membrane disorder characterizing PNH can be shown to be present in red blood cells, granulocytes, and platelets, it is probable that the lesion is due to proliferation of a modified stem cell line. In pure red cell aplasia there is an isolated failure of differentiation of the erythroid cell line which may reflect different susceptibilities of the various hematopoietic cell lines to agents capable of inducing aplastic anemia. A variety of drugs may induce transient erythroid hypoplasia and, in the case of chloramphenicol, be associated with morphologic changes in the erythroid precursors; however, the relationship of this response to pure red cell aplasia is ill understood and appears to be a fundamentally different reaction. As mentioned under Etiology, the association of pure red cell aplasia in adults with thymoma points strongly to an immunologic mechanism specifically directed against erythroid precursor cells.

Clinical Manifestations. The patient's symptoms are related to the rapidity of onset and the extent to which the different hematopoietic cell lines are affected. Acute aplasia induced by ionizing radiation or by cytotoxic drugs can develop rapidly, and in such circumstances the symptoms are predominantly due to the infective or hemorrhagic complications of severe granulocytopenia or thrombocytopenia. Anemia, unless it is due to some underlying disease, develops more insidiously, although gastrointestinal hemorrhage or increase in menstrual blood loss or uterine bleeding can rapidly exacerbate it. When the granulocyte and platelet counts are at levels which provide some protection against infection and spontaneous hemorrhage, the presenting symptoms are usually those of anemia: pallor, fatigue, dyspnea and tachycardia on exertion, and headache. Severe granulocytopenia may be accompanied by infections of the skin and oral and rectal mucosa, with the development of painful ulceration at these sites which may cause difficulties in swallowing and defecation, or by urinary tract infections. Thrombocytopenia is usually associated with bleeding into the skin from mucous membranes and spontaneous bleeding from the gums, nose, vagina, and rectum. Occasionally patients appear to tolerate severe thrombocytopenia without serious bleeding except at sites subjected to minor degrees of trauma. Intracerebral

or subarachnoid hemorrhage may take place and is one of the causes of death. However, it is often remarkable how long patients survive with an increased hemorrhagic tendency caused by thrombocytopenia before this serious complication occurs.

The principal features on physical examination relate to the changes that result from anemia, the infective or hemorrhagic complications. At the onset of the illness physical examination may be unremarkable apart from petechiae of the skin at sites exposed to undue pressure and on the lower limbs. Larger bruises may be present at sites subjected to trauma, including venipuncture. Examination of the optic fundi often reveals flame-shaped hemorrhages and occasional Roth spots. The extent of the retinal changes is frequently related to the degree of anemia as well as to the severity of the thrombocytopenia. It is unusual for the spleen to be enlarged in the early stages of the disease; indeed, the finding of splenic enlargement usually suggests the presence of some other disorder causing pancytopenia. Severe anemia is accompanied by tachycardia, cardiac enlargement, a systolic hemic murmur, and signs of congestive cardiac failure. In the later stages of the disease, particularly when multiple transfusions have been given, increased pigmentation of the skin and enlargement of the liver and spleen may indicate development of hemosiderosis. Infective complications can be accompanied by chronic ulceration of the oral and rectal mucosa, and can give rise to fever. Hectic fever and rigors are usually due to widespread infections, which in the absence of a granulocyte response may be accompanied with few localizing symptoms or signs. Neurologic signs may be present when hemorrhagic or infective complications involve the brain, spinal cord, or peripheral nerves.

Diagnosis. Pancytopenia is a cardinal feature of aplastic anemia, and although the blood count may vary, it is unwise to make the diagnosis unless there is severe depression of all cellular elements at some stage in the disease.

The degree of anemia may vary, depending on when the patient is seen and the relationship of the blood count to previous blood transfusions. The morphology of the red blood cells in peripheral blood smears is usually normal, but slight macrocytosis and anisocytosis may be present. There is usually an absolute reticulocytopenia, although because of the degree of anemia the percentage of reticulocytes may be increased, and an absolute reticulocyte count should be calculated, because it is usually subnormal. The presence of an increased reticulocyte count should lead one to suspect the possibility of the development of paroxysmal nocturnal hemoglobinuria. It is unusual for nucleated red cells to be present in the peripheral blood, and, when found, some other disorder of hematopoiesis should be considered. The total white cell count is usually low, and an absolute granulocytopenia is a feature. The severity of the granulocytopenia is of considerable immediate prognostic significance, because a count of 200 per cubic millimeter or less suggests that the patient is in imminent danger of infective complications. The neutrophil granulocytes may be deficient in granules. Metamyelocytes, myelocytes, and blast cells are rarely found, and, if present, suggest the presence of leukemia rather than aplastic anemia. The absolute monocyte and lymphocyte counts are often depressed in severe cases. Thrombocytopenia is frequently present and may be severe. Large and bizarre-shaped platelets may be present in the blood smear. Severe thrombocytopenia is associated with prolonged bleeding time and positive tests for capillary fragility. Neither of these tests is of diagnostic value, and they do not warrant the discomfort they may produce for the patient. Coagulation tests are usually normal except for those dependent upon normal numbers of platelets. *Bone marrow* aspiration should be carried out and may be performed safely if attention is paid to aseptic techniques and to the prevention of subsequent hemorrhage by applying firm pressure to the site of aspiration for 15 to 20 minutes. Aspiration is achieved with little pain. The specimen often contains an adequate number of bone marrow fragments, although diluted with blood. A needle or trephine biopsy of the bone marrow may be helpful in the assessment of cellularity. Smears from the bone marrow aspirate usually reveal marked hypocellularity of the marrow fragments with a predominance of reticulum cells, mast cells, lymphocytoid cells, and plasma cells. Cells of the myeloid series are often grossly reduced in numbers, and those that are present are usually at the promyelocyte and myelocyte stages of maturation. Megakaryocytes may be absent or very infrequent. Erythroid precursors may be more numerous than those of the myeloid series and, although usually normoblastic, may show abnormal nuclear maturation with some megaloblastic features. Iron can usually be demonstrated in the reticulum cells and may be greatly increased if the patient has received blood transfusions. In view of the selective involvement of the bone marrow, a hypercellular specimen may be obtained, in which case aspiration at another site is advisable and a needle biopsy may be helpful.

The serum iron level is usually elevated, and the total iron binding capacity of the serum is reduced. Ferrokinetic studies may reveal a normal rate of plasma iron clearance and turnover but marked diminution of iron utilization. External scanning of the iron distribution into organs has shown that most of the iron is taken up by the liver rather than the bone marrow. The ferrokinetic studies are of little diagnostic value. The levels of erythropoietin in plasma and excreted in the urine are high and often exceed values found in patients with comparable degrees of anemia. The levels of fetal hemoglobin (hemoglobin F) may be increased. Except for the association with paroxysmal nocturnal hemoglobinuria, evidence for shortened red blood cell survival caused by hemolysis is usually absent and of little value in the presence of frank or occult hemorrhage.

The diseases most likely to be confused with aplastic or hypoplastic anemia are those which lead to pancytopenia by other mechanisms. They include subacute leukemia or preleukemia and other forms of myelophthisic anemia.

The greatest difficulty may be encountered in distinguishing between a hypoplastic anemia and subacute or subleukemic myelocytic leukemia. The presence of an increased number of blast cells and myelocytic precursors in the bone marrow can usually enable the distinction to be made, as can the finding of blast cells and other immature cells in the peripheral blood. The distinction usually becomes apparent during the course of the illness when a more obviously leukemic blood picture may develop. The distinction between a preleukemic state and a true aplastic anemia is sometimes rendered difficult by the development of acute myelocytic leukemia in a patient who has had aplastic anemia for many months or years. It is possible that the agent or agents

provoking aplasia, such as irradiation, are also leukemogenic. The finding of enlargement of the spleen or lymph nodes, generalized bone tenderness, or radiologic evidence of bone destruction should lead one to doubt the diagnosis. It is unusual for the level of immunoglobulins to be raised, and the finding of a monoclonal protein in the serum should arouse suspicion. Infiltration of the bone marrow by metastatic malignancy, metastasis, plasma cells, Hodgkin's disease, lymphosarcoma, or myelofibrosis, all of which can cause a myelophthisic anemia, can usually be recognized by the cellular infiltration seen in smears and histologic sections of biopsies.

Treatment. The principles underlying treatment are to recognize and, wherever possible, to prevent further exposure to any recognized or implicated causative agent, and then to endeavor to prevent hemorrhagic and infective complications, while correcting anemia by blood transfusion in the hope that the patient may go into spontaneous remission.

Whenever possible, all drug therapy should be discontinued unless specifically indicated, in which case drugs thought to have the least risk of marrow toxicity should be used. Only in the case of heavy metals, such as gold, are measures directed toward increasing excretion of the toxic agent from the body likely to be helpful. The patient should be advised against coming into contact with organic solvents in any form, and should only take those drugs specifically prescribed.

The general supportive measures required are determined by the severity of the pancytopenia. An ambulatory patient will often tolerate an anemia of 8 grams per 100 ml, and therefore a blood transfusion is only indicated when the anemia is more severe than this or when hemorrhage or intercurrent infections result in a fall in the hemoglobin concentration below this level. Blood should be given as packed cells which have been stored for less than seven days, and care should be taken in the cross-matching procedure, because it is not uncommon for the patient to develop group-specific antibodies after receiving multiple transfusions. The transfusion of platelet concentrates is indicated to control hemorrhagic complications when the platelet count falls to 10,000 to 20,000 per cubic millimeter. The platelets transfused should be blood group compatible and can be shown to have improved survival if they are drawn from an HL-A-compatible donor if this is feasible. The use of platelet transfusions is probably best reserved for the control of serious thrombocytopenic bleeding, because the development of antibodies to transfused platelets often limits their effectiveness when given on a regular or prophylactic basis. When severe granulocytopenia is accompanied by blood-borne bacterial infections, the transfusion of granulocytes prepared by using a cell separator or by filtration techniques may enable an infection which is not responding to appropriate antimicrobial therapy to be brought under control. The granulocytes so prepared have a very short survival and therefore can only be used to combat serious infective complications.

Apart from these specific measures, meticulous care should be given to the acutely ill pancytopenic patient with regard to the prevention of infection by scrupulous attention to aseptic techniques in setting up intravenous infusions, regular oral hygiene, and protection of the skin, particularly at pressure points. At no time should intramuscular injections be given, because the hematoma at the site of injection impedes the absorption of a drug and greatly increases the risk of infection at the injection site. The principal benefit of isolation procedures may be to constantly remind those looking after the patient of the risks of inappropriate procedures. Microbial cultures should be obtained on all infected lesions, and blood cultures should be performed whenever the patient's condition suggests systemic infection. Antimicrobial therapy should be given after cultures have been taken and should be modified in the light of the sensitivities of the organisms cultured. It is not uncommon for patients with granulocytopenia to have serious infections with bacteria which in other circumstances would not be regarded as pathogens. The prophylactic administration of antimicrobial drugs is of doubtful benefit and may predispose to infection with resistant organisms.

There is little evidence that adrenal steroids influence the degree of pancytopenia or the prognosis. Transient remissions have been documented, but these may reflect the natural history of the disease. Steroids may lessen the bleeding caused by thrombocytopenia and may occasionally reduce the fever in patients unresponsive to antimicrobial therapy. In view of the uncertainty as to the beneficial effects of adrenal steroids, it may be warranted to give prednisone or prednisolone in a dose of 20 mg per day for a trial period of one or two months. The possible benefits of adrenal steroid administration have to be weighed against the known side effects and the greater risk of bacterial infections. Likewise, there is no substantive evidence that splenectomy is beneficial; it should be considered only after multiple blood transfusions are associated with enlargement of the spleen and evidence that the survival of the transfused blood is significantly reduced. The immediate risks of hemorrhage at splenectomy have been reduced with the increasing availability of platelet transfusions, but any benefit must be balanced against the risk of increased susceptibility to bacterial infections that have followed splenectomy, particularly when associated with persistent hematopoietic disorders.

A variety of drugs have been used to enhance the hematopoietic activity of the bone marrow. There is no evidence that administration of vitamin B_{12} is of benefit; indeed, the fact that this has to be given as an intramuscular injection is a valid contraindication. Occasionally patients may become deficient in folic acid, but this is unlikely to take place if the patient is able to tolerate an adequate diet. Treatment with iron is contraindicated, because it will further add to the iron overload induced by multiple blood transfusions. There is evidence in childhood that the combined use of androgens and steroids in patients with constitutional aplastic anemia (Fanconi's anemia) or acquired aplastic anemia may be accompanied by partial or complete remission of the anemia, although the response of the granulocytes or platelets tends to be less satisfactory. Nevertheless, the reduction in blood transfusion requirements may be considerable and thereby both reduce symptoms and reduce the risks of iron overload and other complications of multiple transfusions. The experience of adult aplastic anemia with androgens has been far less encouraging, and although the anemia may improve, the over-all survival curve of adults with aplastic anemia has not been significantly influenced. Nevertheless, it is reasonable to try androgen therapy for a period of three to six months in the hope that a partial remission may be induced or that transfusion requirements may be reduced. The oral synthetic testosterone, oxymetholone (2 to 4 mg per kilo-

gram per day), is the drug of choice, because it has fewer side effects than intramuscular injections of testosterone enanthate (3 to 10 mg per kilogram once a week) or oral administration of testosterone propionate (0.25 mg per kilogram per day). Liver function tests should be performed regularly on all patients receiving androgen therapy, because cholestatic hepatitis may develop as a toxic manifestation of the treatment. In the absence of a remission in two to three months the drug should be discontinued, because the side effects of hepatotoxicity, fluid retention, and hirsutism, particularly in women, do not justify their continued use.

Bone marrow transplantation has been used successfully in a number of patients. This procedure should only be carried out in centers which have the ability to HL-A type the patient and potential donors, and must be accompanied by use of immunosuppressive drugs to prevent both graft rejection and the development of graft versus host disease. Although this approach is being actively explored in a number of centers and has been accompanied by dramatic success with recovery of hematopoiesis when the graft has taken, it is too early to assess its relative benefits and cost-effectiveness as against careful supportive therapy with the ultimate development of a spontaneous remission. It seems unlikely at present that this treatment will be applicable to more than a few highly selected patients for whom HL-A-compatible donors are readily available.

In patients with pure red cell aplasia and radiologic evidence of a thymoma, surgical excision of the thymic tumor has been associated with remission in approximately half the cases. These patients may benefit from use of adrenal steroids, although the dose required can maintain a sustained remission but may be too high to be tolerated by the patient without producing serious side effects. The evidence that pure red cell aplasia may have an autoimmune basis has led to the use of immunosuppressive drugs such as cyclophosphamide and 6-mercaptopurine, and a few patients seem to have successfully responded to such treatment. It is thus worthwhile giving a course of treatment with these drugs at a dosage which does not induce severe depression of the granulocyte or platelet counts. There is no evidence that splenectomy is of benefit in patients with pure red cell aplasia.

Prognosis. The immediate prognosis is related to the severity of pancytopenia and the degree of bone marrow aplasia. The initial prognosis of the severely pancytopenic patient is grave; approximately 30 per cent of them die within the first year. The initial survival may improve with the increased availability of platelet transfusions and of antimicrobial drugs in overcoming bacterial infections. Patients with less severe pancytopenia survive for a number of years despite persistent anemia, granulocytopenia, and thrombocytopenia. Spontaneous or drug-induced remissions may take place and are most likely to be seen in patients with mild pancytopenia and moderate hypocellularity of the bone marrow. Death usually results from infective or hemorrhagic complications. Hemosiderosis of the heart and liver may be a late sequel of patients requiring repeated blood transfusions.

Allen, D. M., Fine, M. H., Nechles, T. F., and Dameshek, W.: Oxymetha-lone therapy in aplastic anemia. Blood, 32:83, 1968.
Buckner, C. D., Clift, R. A., Fefer, A., Neiman, P., Storb, R., and Thomas, E. D.: Human marrow transplantation—current status. In Brown, E. B. (ed.): Progress in Hematology, Vol. 8. New York, Grune & Stratton, 1973, p. 299.

Dacie, J. V., and Lewis, S. M.: Paroxysmal nocturnal haemoglobinuria: Clinical manifestations, haematology and nature of the disease. Ser. Haematol., 3:3, 1972.

Dameshek, W., Brown, S. M., and Rubin, A. D.: "Pure" red cell anemia (erythroblastic hypoplasia) and thymoma. Semin. Hematol., 4:222, 1967.

Erslev, A. J.: Aplastic anemia. In Williams, W. J., Beutler, E., Erslev, A. J., and Rundles, R. W. (eds.): Hematology. New York, McGraw-Hill Book Company, 1972, p. 207.

Erslev, A. J.: Pure red cell aplasia. In Williams, W. J., Beutler, E., Erslev, A. J., and Rundles, R. W. (eds.): Hematology. New York, McGraw-Hill Book Company, 1972, p. 227.

Harris, J. W., and Kellermyer, R. W.: The Red Cell. Production, Metabolism, Destruction: Normal and Abnormal. 2nd ed. Cambridge, Mass., Harvard University Press, 1970.

Krantz, S. B., and Kao, V.: Studies on red cell aplasia. II. Report of a second patient with an antibody to erythroblast nuclei and a remission after immunosuppressive therapy. Blood, 34:1, 1969.

Registry on Adverse Drug Reactions, Panel on Hematology. Council on Drugs, American Medical Association. April-May 1965, June 1, 1967.

Sanchez-Medal, L., Gormez-Leal, A., Duarte, L., and Guadalupe, M. G.: Anabolic androgenic steroids in the treatment of acquired aplastic anemia. Blood, 34:283, 1969.

Williams, D. M., Lynch, R. E., and Cartwright, G. E.: Drug-induced aplastic anemia. Semin. Hematol., 10:195, 1973.

Yunis, A. A.: Chloramphenicol-induced bone marrow suppression. Semin. Hematol., 10:225, 1973.

735. SIDEROBLASTIC ANEMIA

M. C. Brain

The sideroblastic anemias are a heterogeneous group of disorders in which a normocytic or slightly macrocytic anemia is accompanied by ineffective erythropoiesis and defective hemoglobin synthesis, manifested by hypochromasia of a proportion of red cells in the peripheral blood, with the finding of *ringed sideroblasts* in the bone marrow. Ringed sideroblasts are nucleated red blood cell precursors, often showing defective hemoglobinization, which can be shown on iron staining to have a perinuclear ring distribution of iron-staining granules. The perinuclear distribution of the iron distinguishes this disorder from the increase in iron-staining granules which may be seen in megaloblastic anemias and in thalassemia. Electron microscopic studies have shown that the nonheme iron is located between the cristae of the perinuclear mitochondria, and may also be present as ferritin and ferritin aggregates in the cytoplasm. The presence of ringed sideroblasts may be suspected when basophilic granules are observed in hypochromic

TABLE 2.   Sideroblastic Anemias: Classification

1. Primary
   a. Acquired sideroblastic anemia in adults (synonyms: chronic refractory anemia with sideroblastic bone marrow, refractory normoblastic anemia, sideroachrestic anemia, refractory sideroblastic anemia)
   b. Hereditary (sex-linked) sideroblastic anemia
2. Pyridoxine-responsive sideroblastic anemia
3. Secondary
   a. Sideroblastic anemia associated with rheumatoid arthritis, polyarthritis, carcinoma, myelofibrosis, leukemia, multiple myeloma, hereditary and acquired hemolytic anemias, malabsorption syndromes, or chronic alcoholism
   b. Drug-induced: isoniazid, cycloserine, and other antituberculous drugs
   c. Lead poisoning

erythroblasts in Romanovsky-stained preparations. Studies of heme and globin synthesis have demonstrated that the defective hemoglobin synthesis is due to failure of incorporation of iron into protoporphyrin to form heme. Increased levels of erythrocyte protoporphyrin may be found, and the defective hemoglobin synthesis observed in vitro can be corrected by the provision of heme. The sideroblastic anemias may be classified as in Table 2.

Primary acquired sideroblastic anemia of adults is thought to be due to acquired disorder of the heme synthetic pathway. It has been thought by some to be a variant of erythroleukemia, and a proportion of patients subsequently develop either erythroleukemia or a chronic subacute myeloid leukemia. This type of sideroblastic anemia occurs most frequently in men and women late in life, and has no distinguishing clinical features. *Hereditary sex-linked* sideroblastic anemia is rare, but appears to be transmitted as a sex-linked recessive abnormality. The precise metabolic defect is still incompletely understood, and may involve different enzymatic steps in the protoporphyrin synthetic pathway in different subjects. Anemia occurs in early childhood and presents problems analogous to the chronic anemia caused by defective globin chain synthesis which characterizes thalassemic syndromes. However, it requires blood transfusions less commonly but, as in thalassemia, the chronic anemia and enhanced dietary iron absorption can lead to development of hemosiderosis of the liver and myocardium.

Pyridoxal phosphate functions as a coenzyme in the synthesis of delta amino levulinic acid, the product of the first synthetic step in porphyrin synthesis. Pyridoxal-responsive sideroblastic anemias may thus arise as an unexplained primary disorder; in alcoholism, in which the formation of pyridoxal phosphate from pyridoxine may be impaired; or as a consequence of isoniazid therapy, a drug which is a metabolic antagonist of pyridoxine. Sideroblastic anemia may also be due to pyridoxine deficiency as a complication of severe malabsorption syndromes. In patients in whom there is pyridoxal phosphate deficiency caused by ethanol ingestion, malabsorption, or drug antagonism, the anemia responds to the administration of physiologic concentrations of pyridoxal phosphate. Patients with acquired pyridoxine-responsive anemia not apparently caused by isoniazid ingestion or ethanol occasionally respond to pharmacologic doses of pyridoxine. The biochemical explanation for this is as yet unclear. Still other patients have been described who appear to respond to crude liver extract and may have a fundamental disorder of tryptophan metabolism. The sideroblastic anemia that results from lead poisoning is due to inhibition of delta levulinic acid dehydrase and ferrochetalase (heme synthetase), important steps in heme synthesis.

The degree of anemia may vary but is usually in the range of 7 to 8 grams of hemoglobin, with a lowered mean cell hemoglobin concentration. The red cells may show a varying degree of hypochromasia, and not uncommonly there may be a dimorphic blood picture with a varying proportion of normochromic normocytic cells with hypochromic microcytic red cells. Macrocytosis and a moderate degree of poikilocytosis may be present. The red cells may contain Pappenheimer bodies, demonstrable as iron-containing siderocytes on iron staining. Basophilic stippling is a feature of lead poisoning. The absolute reticulocyte count is usually reduced. The leukocyte and platelet counts are usually normal. The plasma iron and transferrin saturation are either normal or high. As mentioned earlier, the diagnosis is made on examination of the bone marrow which shows erythroid hyperplasia, defective hemoglobinization, and increased iron both in the marrow fragments and in the developing erythroblasts. The erythroblasts may show megaloblastic features and the associated defective maturation of white cell precursors. These changes are usually indicative of an accompanying folate deficiency, which can be confirmed by finding a low serum folate level. Myelopoiesis is usually normal, although an increase in blast cells and early precursor cells of the myeloid series may point to an associated subacute myeloid leukemia.

It is not uncommon for acquired sideroblastic anemia in the adult to be confused with iron deficiency anemia, although the high serum iron and the presence of iron in the bone marrow preclude this diagnosis.

Treatment should be directed toward correcting a folate deficiency when it is present and vitamin B_{12} deficiency has been excluded. A trial of pyridoxine of 50 mg a day for two to four weeks is indicated. A variable response may take place to either folate and/or pyridoxine treatment. Patients have been reported who only respond to pyridoxal phosphate given parenterally. Blood transfusions may be required when the hemoglobin level falls to below 8 grams per 100 ml and when symptoms or complications caused by anemia are present. The blood transfusion requirements may increase and will tend to exacerbate iron overload. Iron treatment by any route is absolutely contraindicated. When sideroblastic anemia is due to a drug, removal of the agent or treatment with pyridoxine can result in complete recovery. Except in those patients in whom the anemia is associated with a subacute leukemia, the prognosis in terms of survival is good, although chronic anemia usually persists.

Hines, J. D., and Cowan, D. H.: Studies on the pathogenesis of alcohol-induced sideroblastic bone marrow abnormalities. N. Engl. J. Med., 283:441, 1970.

Hines, J. D., and Grasso, J. A.: The sideroblastic anemias. Semin. Hematol., 7:86, 1970.

Moore, C. V.: Sideroblastic anemia. *In* Williams, W. J., Beutler, E., Erslev, A. J., and Rundles, R. W. (eds.): Hematology. New York, McGraw-Hill Book Company, 1972, p. 349.

736. MYELOPHTHISIC ANEMIA

M. C. Brain

The term myelophthisic anemia is applied to those anemias accompanied by the presence of nucleated red cell precursors and immature white cells in the peripheral blood resulting from a disturbance in the microarchitecture of the bone marrow brought about by infiltration of the bone marrow by abnormal cells or progressive fibrosis of the bone marrow, as in myelosclerosis. The disorder occurs when the bone marrow is extensively invaded or replaced with leukemic cells, the plasma cells of multiple myeloma, metastatic carcinoma or sarcoma, Hodgkin's disease and other malignant lymphomas, infectious or noninfectious granulomas, or lipid storage cells. Carcinomas of the breast, lung, prostate, stomach, kidney, and thyroid and neuroblastomas are most frequently associated with metastatic infiltration of the bone marrow. Extramedullary hematopoiesis can often be demonstrated at necropsy and can give rise to massive enlargement of the spleen and liver in a patient with a chronic myelophthisic anemia such as myelosclerosis.

The anemia may be moderate to severe; the white blood cell count may be elevated or depressed; and the platelet count may be normal or increased, but is more commonly reduced. A degree of anemia is often unrelated to the extent of bone marrow infiltration, suggesting that there is a more fundamental disturbance of hematopoiesis than can be accounted for by the extent of bone marrow infiltration. Survival of red cells may be reduced.

The clinical manifestations are usually those of the underlying disease, although not infrequently a myelophthisic anemia may be the presenting feature in a patient with widespread metastasis from a small primary tumor which may itself have given rise to few symptoms or signs. Bone pain may be severe, and may be either generalized or localized to the site of pathologic fractures. Symptoms may arise from the severity of the anemia, and bleeding may be associated with the thrombocytopenia. In patients with widespread metastatic adenocarcinoma, activation of coagulation within the blood can contribute to the thrombocytopenia and may rarely be associated with a microangiopathic hemolytic anemia. Enlargement of lymph nodes and the liver may be a manifestation of the underlying malignant disease; enlargement of spleen usually reflects the duration of the anemia and the extent of extramedullary hematopoiesis.

Myelophthisic anemia should be suspected whenever nucleated red blood cell precursors are found in the peripheral blood in association with a normocytic anemia and in the absence of other obvious disorders of hematopoiesis. In patients with known malignant diseases, the appearance of nucleated red cells in the blood is highly suggestive of bone marrow infiltration. In patients with moderate anemia the red blood cells show few morphologic changes. The presence of teardrop cells is suggestive of myelofibrosis, and when anemia is marked there may be greater degrees of poikilocytosis, polychromasia, and basophilic stippling. The blood picture may be complicated by a concomitant hypochromic anemia resulting from iron deficiency, by gastrointestinal blood loss, or by macrocytosis caused by folate deficiency in myelofibrosis. The reticulocyte count may be normal or increased. The total leukocyte count is often elevated, and usually exhibits a left shift with the presence of myelocytes and metamyelocytes. The platelet count will vary with the extent of the disease; large and bizarre platelets and occasionally megakaryocytic nuclei may be seen. The diagnosis of myelophthisic anemia is made by the finding of abnormal cells in the bone marrow. Aspiration of this may be difficult or, indeed, unsuccessful, or at best may yield a specimen containing few if any fragments diluted with blood. Owing to the focal nature of the infiltration, a normal actively hematopoietic bone marrow may be obtained. Nevertheless, all the slides should be surveyed extensively for presence of malignant cells; not infrequently these are found in small groups. A needle or trephined biopsy of the bone marrow is very helpful in the assessment of hematopoiesis, the recognition of bone marrow infiltration, and the demonstration of an increase in reticulin and fibrosis by silver stains characteristic of myelofibrosis. Bone marrow aspiration and biopsy may have to be carried out at more than one site before the diagnosis can be made with certainty. The diagnosis of the cause of myelophthisic anemia depends upon the identification of the underlying disease.

Treatment and prognosis depend on the cause of the disorder, and blood transfusions may be required to overcome the anemia.

Beutler, E.: Anemias associated with marrow infiltration. In Williams, W. J., Beutler, E., Erslev, A. J., and Rundles, R. W. (eds.): Hematology, New York, McGraw-Hill Book Company, 1972.

HYPOCHROMIC ANEMIAS

Elmer B. Brown

737. IRON DEFICIENCY ANEMIA

Definition. Iron deficiency anemia occurs when the supply of iron is inadequate to support optimal erythropoiesis. In its fully developed form it is characterized by hypochromia and microcytosis of the circulating erythrocytes, low plasma iron, low transferrin saturation, and marked depletion of bone marrow and other body iron stores.

Prevalence. Throughout the world iron deficiency is almost certainly the most common cause of anemia. In parts of Africa and Asia, where marginal dietary intake and excessive iron loss owing to intestinal parasites occur together, more than 50 per cent of the population may suffer from iron deficiency anemia. Variable figures of the incidence of iron deficiency have been reported from surveys in temperate countries. Reasons for variation include the criteria used for detecting borderline iron deficiency as well as the nature of the population sampled in terms of age, sex, economic status, and local environmental factors. Fewer than 3 per cent of men are affected in most population surveys; 10 to 30 per cent of all women may show signs of iron deficiency; and 10 to 60 per cent of pregnant women and infants in the first year of life have iron deficiency anemia. Much more information is needed to define precisely the prevalence of iron deficiency in representative geographic and socioeconomic cross sections of the United States.

Iron Metabolism. Iron is essential to human life because of its central role in the heme molecule that permits oxygen and electron transport. Every cell in the body contains some iron.

Distribution. The body's iron can be divided into two main compartments: (1) an essential, functional component composed of hemoglobin, myoglobin, enzyme and cofactor iron, and plasma transport iron, and (2) a nonessential storage component made up predominantly of ferritin and hemosiderin, not required for health but providing a reserve of iron readily mobilizable into the essential functional compartment in time of need.

In the normal adult man there is about 50 mg of iron per kilogram of body weight, approximately 80 per cent of which is in the functional compartment and 20 per cent in a storage form. Women, with a reduction in red cell mass and hemoglobin concentration as well as

smaller iron stores, have a body iron concentration of about 40 mg per kilogram. Total body iron ranges between extremes of 2 and 6 grams in small women and large men. These differences are reflected in the amount and percentage distribution of iron in the body (Table 1). Approximately 85 per cent of the functional iron in the body is present in the red blood cells as hemoglobin, which contains 0.34 per cent iron by weight. Divalent iron in each of the four disc-shaped heme groups carefully positioned in the pocket of coiled globin chains binds oxygen reversibly for transport to all tissues. Oxidation of the iron to the ferric state (as in methemoglobin) causes hemoglobin to lose its capacity to carry oxygen. Myoglobin, one fourth the size of hemoglobin and with one iron atom per molecule, accounts for about 15 per cent of the functional iron. It is present in concentrations of 0.9 to 2.2 grams dry weight of human muscle; cardiac muscle contains consistently less myoglobin than skeletal muscle. Myoglobin functions as a reservoir of oxygen for muscle metabolism. A small but extremely important component of body iron is that bound to transferrin. Approximately half of the transferrin iron is in extravascular tissue fluids while a more easily measured fraction is circulating in the plasma in transit from sites of hemoglobin destruction, iron absorption, or storage depots to the bone marrow and other areas of utilization. Lactoferrin, an iron-binding protein of milk, mucosal tissues, and leukocytes, is similar to transferrin structurally but appears to function in the body's defense against bacterial infection by binding iron essential to bacterial growth. Iron present as an integral part of various enzymes or as a cofactor constitutes a small but important part of the functional iron compartment. Iron enzymes may be classified as heme-proteins (cytochromes a, b, c, c_1, a_3, cytochrome c oxidase, catalase, peroxidases, tryptophan pyrrolase, lipoxidase, and homogentisic oxidase) and iron-flavoproteins (cytochrome c reductase, NADH dehydrogenase, xanthine oxidase, succinate dehydrogenase, and acyl CoA dehydrogenase). Iron as an essential cofactor is required by aconitase and succinic dehydrogenase. Most of these enzymes function as reversible donors or acceptors of electrons and are critical to the metabolism of every cell in the body.

Nonessential storage compounds that account for the remaining body iron are ferritin and hemosiderin. Ferri-

TABLE 1. Distribution of Iron in the Body

Compartment	Iron Content (grams)		Fraction of Total Body Fe (%)	
	Men	*Women*	*Men*	*Women*
Functional				
Hemoglobin	3.050	1.700	71.8	73.5
Myoglobin	0.430	0.300	10.1	13.0
Enzymes	(?) 0.010	0.010	0.2	0.4
Transferrin	0.008	0.006	0.2	0.2
Subtotal	3.498	2.016	82.3	87.1
Storage				
Ferritin-hemosiderin	0.750	0.300	17.7	12.9
Total	4.248	2.316	100.0	100.0

Values are based on data from various sources. Assumptions include a body weight for men of 80 kg, blood volume of 70 ml/kg, and Hgb of 16 grams/dl; for women the values used were a weight of 55 kg, blood volume of 65 ml/kg, and Hgb of 14 grams/dl.

tin, composed of a large, water-soluble, crystalline protein surrounding micelles of iron (up to 20 per cent by weight), is a ubiquitous compound found in many tissues of the body but predominantly in liver parenchymal cells and reticuloendothelial cells of the liver, spleen, and bone marrow. Hemosiderin is a water-insoluble protein with higher concentrations of iron (up to 35 per cent by weight) that is readily identified by Prussian blue staining of tissues. Since the iron in these compounds is readily mobilizable for use by the essential functional iron compounds, there is wide variation in their amounts and percentage of total body iron.

Absorption. Iron absorption assumes great importance in human iron metabolism, because iron balance is regulated by controlled absorption rather than by excretion. Despite intensive investigation, many facets of the mechanism and control of iron absorption remain unexplained or controversial. Current information suggests that iron entering the stomach in various organic compounds of food is digested to soluble ferric salts that may be either reduced to ferrous ions or chelated in either the ferrous or ferric valence state to maintain stability and promote absorption. The presence of hydrochloric acid in the stomach is not essential for iron absorption, although an acid milieu prevents the formation of insoluble complexes of ionized iron. Other unidentified iron-stabilizing substances in gastric secretions — possibly mucoproteins — promote iron absorption. Entry of iron at the brush border of mucosal cells appears to be mainly by passive diffusion; exit from the cells to the plasma transferrin probably requires metabolic energy for active transport. Most of the iron destined to enter the bloodstream traverses the mucosal cell rapidly in the form of small molecules. Attempts to identify specific mucosal iron carrier substances have been unsuccessful. Likewise, efforts to identify subcellular fractions in the sequence of iron transfer across the mucosal cell have added little to our understanding of the precise process of iron absorption. Older theories implicating mucosal ferritin as a carrier of iron and the key to regulation of iron absorption through a "mucosal block" mechanism have been abandoned. The small quantities of ferritin in intestinal mucosal cells appear to function as a storage compound to accept a proportion of iron in excess of the rapid transport capacity. The ferritin is then lost when the cells are desquamated at the end of their three- to five-day life span. Luminal factors modifying the form in which iron is presented to the mucosal cell play an important role in the amount of iron that can be absorbed. Sugar, sorbitol, cysteine and other amino acids, ascorbic and succinic acids, mucoproteins, and various other components of the dietary constituents or intestinal secretions tend to stabilize iron in a soluble form and to promote iron absorption. Phytates, phosphates, carbonate, oxalate, pancreatic bicarbonate, and gastroferrin bind iron as relatively insoluble complexes and decrease iron absorption. The means by which the body's need for increased or decreased iron absorption is transmitted to the mucosal cell have not been completely defined. Multiple signals, including mucosal cell iron concentration, local hypoxia, tissue iron stores, rate of erythropoiesis, plasma transferrin saturation, plasma iron turnover, and humoral factors, have been suggested, but without compelling evidence for any precise mechanism.

Measurement of iron absorption has progressed from the tedious and cumbersome dietary iron balance studies to the use of radioactive iron with determination of unabsorbed iron in the feces, absorbed radioactivity in the circulating red blood cells, or total body radioiron using sensitive whole body counters. Studies of iron absorption can be divided conveniently into two groups: (1) those using simple iron salts such as ferrous sulfate or ferric chloride which give information applicable to the behavior of iron given therapeutically; and (2) those measuring the absorption of iron from foods.

Ferrous salts are better absorbed than ferric compounds, and various agents such as ascorbic and succinic acids and sorbitol enhance iron absorption. Other substances such as phytates, phosphates, and various antacid preparations bind iron and diminish its absorption. Maximal absorption occurs in the duodenum and upper jejunum where the villous surface is maximal and in which the luminal contents are acid or neutral; there is progressively less absorption distally from a more alkaline environment, although the potentiality for some iron absorption exists throughout the length of the gut from the stomach to the rectum. Iron absorption from mucosal cells is via intestinal capillaries with little lymphatic participation, and is virtually complete within several hours after ingestion. Uptake of iron is unidirectional without any back-flux except for iron lost into the gut lumen by desquamation of mucosal cells. There is no enterohepatic circulation. Small doses of iron are absorbed from the duodenum by an active process; with large doses of iron, passive diffusion occurs. Increasing the ingestion of simple iron salts results in increasing absorption of iron until toxicity becomes the limiting factor. Conditions associated with increased iron absorption include iron deficiency, hemolytic and sideroblastic anemias, hypoxia, cobalt and erythropoietin administration, hemochromatosis, cirrhosis and portacaval shunts, some types of pancreatic insufficiency, and the later stages of pregnancy. Decreased iron absorption is present in patients with iron overload, erythroid hypoplasia, generalized malabsorption states, malignant, infectious, and inflammatory diseases, and achlorhydria.

Less information is available about the absorption of food iron. Attempts have been made to classify the "availability" of iron in various foods by its release after incubation in digestion mixtures or by its ability to increase hemoglobin formation in anemic animals or human subjects. These efforts have been relatively unsuccessful. Radioactive iron biosynthetically incorporated into various foods or added as a simple salt to dietary food mixtures has allowed comparison of dietary iron absorption with that of simple iron salts. From these studies it was learned that heme iron is absorbed differently from various nonheme iron compounds in the diet. Heme is taken up by the mucosal cell where the porphyrin ring is split open to make iron available to the body. Heme iron absorption is not influenced by dietary composition (ascorbic acid, phytates, or phosphates) as is the case with nonheme iron compounds. Furthermore, the nonheme iron compounds of food behave as a single pool in their absorption characteristics and can be labeled with a single radioiron salt. ^{55}Fe labeling of heme (intrinsic tag) and ^{59}FeCl$_3$ for labeling of nonheme vegetable components (extrinsic tag) have allowed the precise measurement of the absorption of complex dietary iron mixtures. Results of this type of study indicate that iron in meat (primarily heme) is better absorbed (12 to 20 per cent) than iron from vegetable sources (primarily nonheme). Iron from vegetable sources is absorbed to a variable extent — about 1 to 7 per cent of usual doses in a meal—with substances such as phytates accounting for the diminished absorption. Rice and spinach are at the lower end of the absorption scale, whereas wheat and soybean iron are better absorbed. When mixtures of foods approximating those of usual diets are given, the percentage of iron absorption of the total mixture is similar to that of the least well-absorbed vegetable source, except for the heme component whose absorption is uninfluenced by other dietary components. Of importance in the consideration of food iron supplementation to prevent iron deficiency is the finding that diets containing foods with little heme (meat) and with a predominance of poorly absorbed vegetable iron sources, such as rice, impart their poor iron absorbability to the supplementary iron salt irrespective of the compound used.

Transport. Iron is transported in plasma bound to a specific carrier protein, transferrin. This β-globulin of about 75,000 molecular weight is synthesized in the liver and has an eight- to ten-day half-time in plasma; the 7 to 15 grams present in the body is almost equally distributed in the extravascular and intravascular spaces, with plasma concentrations varying from 215 to 350 mg per deciliter. At least 19 genetic variants have been described, but all that have been studied appear to be identical in their iron-binding properties. Transferrin can bind two atoms of ferric iron per molecule in the presence of bicarbonate. Binding of iron to transferrin receptor sites is a random process in vitro, and there is no exchange of iron from one molecule to another. Recent evidence suggests that release of iron to tissue receptor sites is a selective process, with one transferrin iron site being erythroblast oriented and the other site oriented toward receptors on liver parenchymal cells. If these functional differences in selective iron delivery are confirmed, the concept of transferrin as a passive plasma carrier of homogeneous iron atoms will be changed to one of actively controlling the distribution of iron in the body. Measurement of functional iron-binding capacity rather than direct determination of transferrin is employed clinically. Iron is present in equal amounts in plasma and serum; normal values range from 60 to 160 μg per deciliter, with a mean of 120 for men and 110 for women. Plasma transferrin is normally about one third saturated and the total plasma iron-binding capacity is 280

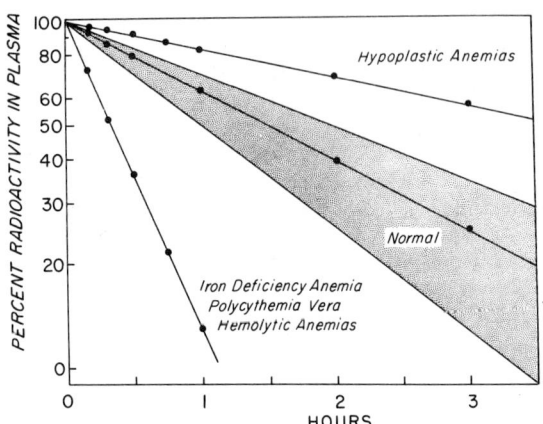

Figure 2. Plasma radioiron disappearance curves for normal subjects and for patients with increased and decreased erythropoiesis.

to 400 μg per deciliter. Plasma iron shows a diurnal variation, with morning values about 30 per cent higher than those in the evening. Menses, exercise, or normal meals have no appreciable effect on plasma iron concentrations. Highest concentrations are seen during reproductive years in both sexes, with a modest decline in old age. Variations in plasma iron and iron-binding capacity are seen in a variety of disorders, as illustrated in Figure 1.

Ferrokinetics. Since the pioneering studies of the kinetics of iron transfer were published by Huff and co-workers in 1950, there have been many refinements in technique that have added much to the precision of measurement and the complexity of mathematical analysis, but little to the clinical interpretation of ferrokinetic data. Measurement of plasma radioiron clearance and erythrocyte utilization are simple, useful tests available to any clinician with access to radioisotope facilities. If more sophisticated interpretation of deranged iron metabolism in a variety of diseases is desired, computer evaluation of prolonged plasma iron disappearance curves and external monitoring over liver, spleen, and sacrum are needed. By this type of analysis a number of compartments with various rates of iron interchange can be identified with analyses too complex for routine use. However, useful basic information is obtained by measuring the rate of disappearance of radioactive iron bound to plasma transferrin after intravenous injection and its subsequent incorporation into circulating erythrocytes 7 to 14 days later (Figs. 2 and 3). Plasma radioiron disappearance, measured at 10- to 15-minute intervals and plotted semilogarithmically, is linear with a half-time rate of disappearance normally between 60 and 120 minutes. More rapid disappearance rates (shorter half-time values) are found in iron deficiency and conditions with increased erythropoiesis such as polycythemia vera and hemolytic anemias. Slow rates of radioiron disappearance indicate erythroid hypoplasia from various causes. By extrapolating the plasma iron disappearance line back to zero time, one may obtain a close estimate of plasma volume by dividing the total count rate of the injected radioiron by the count rate at time zero. Calculation of the plasma iron turnover rate (PITR) requires only the additional measurement of plasma iron concentration. The formula for this calcula-

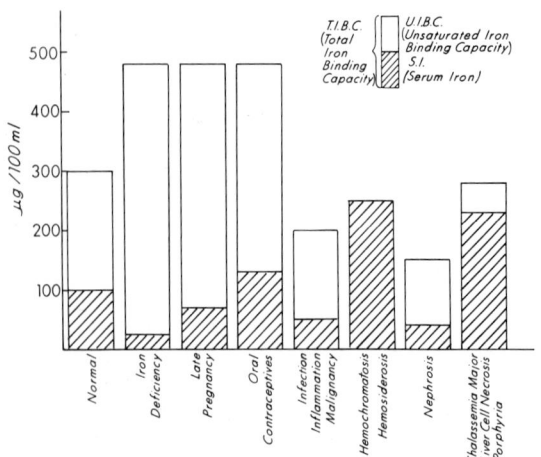

Figure 1. Representative serum iron and iron-binding capacity values in a variety of conditions.

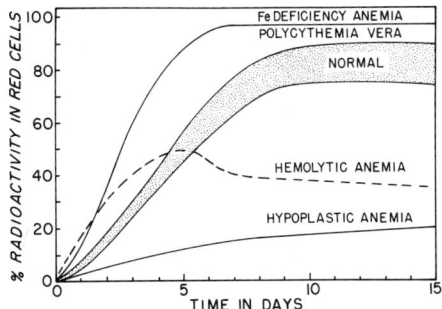

Figure 3. Patterns of radioiron utilization in peripheral erythrocytes for normal subjects and for patients with various disorders with increased or decreased erythropoiesis.

tion is shown at the bottom of this page. The PITR reflects changes in two variables, the size of the plasma iron pool and the rate of disappearance of ^{59}Fe from plasma. Normal values of PITR range from 25 to 40 mg per day. Increased PITR is observed in patients whose plasma radioiron disappearance is rapid and whose plasma iron values are normal or increased, e.g., hemolytic states and ineffective erythropoiesis with values four to ten times normal. Decreased PITR is seen in some patients with hypoplastic anemias, infection, or uremia or after irradiation when slow plasma radioiron disappearance rates are combined with normal or low plasma iron values. In iron deficiency anemia, in which there is rapid radioiron disappearance and low plasma iron values, the PITR is usually normal.

Measurement of the utilization of radioiron incorporated into hemoglobin of red cells during the one to two weeks after a plasma radioiron clearance study provides valuable information about the effective production of erythrocytes compared to total erythropoiesis reflected by the PITR. Iron utilization is calculated from the radioactivity in 1 ml of packed red cells multiplied by the red cell volume (calculated from the previously determined plasma volume and the hematocrit) divided by the count rate of injected radioiron, and is expressed in percentage terms. Normally 70 to 90 per cent of the injected radioiron can be accounted for in circulating cells two weeks after injection. Decreased radioiron utilization reflects decreased erythropoiesis with extreme reductions in aplastic anemia. Radioiron utilization to levels slightly above the normal range occurs sooner in iron deficiency or polycythemia. Complex intermediate curves reflecting rapid red cell production and destruction may be seen in various hemolytic anemias.

Storage. Iron in excess of the needs for hemoglobin, myoglobin, and essential intracellular enzymes is stored as ferritin and hemosiderin. Major sites of storage iron are hepatic parenchymal cells, reticuloendothelial cells of the bone marrow, liver, and spleen, and a poorly defined store in skeletal muscle. The immediate source of most reticuloendothelial iron stores is hemoglobin iron conserved from the breakdown of red cells at the end of

their life span. Hepatic parenchymal iron comes from plasma transferrin. Accurate measurement of diffusely distributed iron stores is difficult. Qualitative estimates are usually based on histochemical appraisal of bone marrow or liver hemosiderin deposits. More quantitative estimates can be obtained from measurement of iron excreted into the urine after injections of deferoxamine or other chelating agents; chelate iron mobilization correlates closely with the amount of iron mobilized by phlebotomy before iron deficiency anemia supervenes. Minute amounts of ferritin circulating in plasma are related to the amount of iron stores, and plasma ferritin measurement provides another means of determining body iron stores. Estimates of storage iron in normal adults have decreased in recent years to an average in men of 750 mg (range 200 to 1400 mg) and an average in women of 300 mg (range 60 to 500 mg). Approximately 65 per cent of storage iron is normally in the form of ferritin; the remainder is hemosiderin. In disorders of iron overload the proportion of hemosiderin increases progressively. Both storage forms are readily mobilized in response to need such as bleeding. Regulatory mechanisms controlling the buildup and mobilization of iron stores are poorly understood. Mobilization is frequently interfered with by infection, inflammation, and malignancy.

Excretion. The body has a limited capacity to excrete iron except by means of hemorrhage. Normally, excretion balances absorption, because most of the iron released from hemoglobin of senescent red blood cells is conserved and reutilized. Total daily excretion amounts to slightly less than 1 mg for men and postmenopausal women. Of this amount approximately 0.1 mg is excreted in the urine, and about 0.6 mg in the feces from mucosal cell desquamation, bile, and small amounts of blood loss; the remainder is lost from skin as desquamated cells and in sweat. Approximately 0.5 mg of iron is present per milliliter of blood. With normal menstrual blood losses of 25 to 60 ml monthly, this normal bleeding accounts for an additional 12 to 30 mg of iron lost monthly, or 0.4 to 1.0 mg per day, in women during their reproductive years. Iron loss occurs in pregnancy and delivery in amounts totaling more than 500 mg. Obligatory daily iron losses are about 50 per cent less than normal in patients with iron deficiency anemia.

Requirements. Since iron absorption must balance excretion for the body's iron stores to stay in balance, one may construct a table of iron requirements for different physiologic states (Table 2). In addition to the exceptional stresses on iron balance imposed by menstrual losses and pregnancy, one must also add the needs related to growth. These needs of iron to build hemoglobin, myoglobin, and other intracellular iron compounds are greatest at growth spurts of infancy and adolescence. An increment of 0.5 mg per day is an acceptable estimate in the absence of precise measurements.

These requirements of iron to meet special circumstances can be translated into terms of nutritional iron intake to prevent a negative balance from occurring. Assuming that absorption of iron from food mixtures nor-

$$\text{PITR (mg/day)} = \frac{0.693}{^{59}\text{Fe T/2 (hrs)}} \times \text{mg Fe/ml plasma} \times \text{plasma vol (ml)} \times 24 \text{ hrs}$$

TABLE 2. Estimated Dietary Iron Requirements

	Absorbed Iron Requirement, mg/Day	Daily Food Iron Requirement,* mg/Day
Normal men and nonmenstruating women	0.5–1.0	5–10
Menstruating women	0.7–2.0	7–20
Pregnant women	2.0–4.8	20–48†
Adolescents	1.0–2.0	10–20
Children	0.4–1.0	4–10
Infants	0.5–1.5	1.5 mg per kg‡

*Assuming 10 per cent absorption.

†This amount of iron cannot be derived from diet and should be met by iron supplementation in the latter half of pregnancy.

‡To a maximum of 15 mg.

mally averages about 10 per cent, the figures for dietary iron intake can be derived (Table 2). Iron concentrations of foods in most Western diets are related to calories, with about 6 mg of iron per 1000 calories. Although iron absorption may increase to about 20 per cent with the onset of iron deficiency, it is obvious that pregnant women can hardly eat enough food to provide for their markedly increased iron needs and that they, with many menstruating women and adolescent girls, are likely to fall behind in meeting dietary iron needs.

Pathogenesis. Iron deficiency develops because of one or a combination of the following factors: inadequate dietary iron intake, malabsorption, blood loss, or repeated pregnancies. Since excretion of iron is limited, assigning the cause of iron deficiency in adults to inadequate intake or malabsorption implies chronicity measured in years. More important are iron losses which occur most often from the gastrointestinal tract of men and from abnormal menstrual bleeding in women. A convenient way to consider these causes of iron deficiency is to divide them into two categories—low intake and high output.

Low Intake. Restrictions of dietary iron because of economic, religious, or cultural considerations lead to iron deficiency in many parts of the world. Economic and religious factors weigh heaviest in underdeveloped nations, whereas in the United States one might cite the inadequate meals of weight-conscious young women and mothers caught up in the harried pace of rearing children. In old age, absent or ill-fitting dentures combined with apathy, inactivity, and financial restrictions reduce the intake of foods with high iron nutritive value. Continual refinement and cleanliness of our food supplies combined with the use of noniron cooking vessels may have the undesired effect of reducing our iron intake. Assimilation of iron is often reduced owing to interaction of phytates from cereals, phosphates, and other substances in the foods we eat. Malabsorption of iron rarely if ever occurs as an isolated absorptive defect, but is present in sprue syndromes and is associated with iron deficiency. (Surprisingly, the steatorrhea of pancreatic insufficiency allows normal or even increased iron absorption.) Abnormal gastrointestinal motility secondary to gastrectomy or to a variety of causes for diarrhea is usually associated with decreased iron absorption. Patients with achlorhydria have inefficient absorption of food iron, and cannot increase iron uptake effectively when they become iron deficient.

High Output. Identification of the site of blood loss responsible for high output iron deficiency may be quite difficult. One reason for this difficulty is that increased menstrual blood loss, the single most common cause of iron deficiency in temperate countries, is often not recognized, and is difficult to quantitate. The best estimates of the frequency and extent of menorrhagia in randomly selected women indicate that the normal menstrual flow (25 to 60 ml) is exceeded in about 20 per cent of women, with occasional blood losses as high as 500 ml per month. Unfortunately, predictions of menstrual loss by the patient's account of the number and saturation of sanitary napkins and the number of days of flow are only partially successful. Contraceptive pills of the combined estrogen-progesterone type reduce menstrual blood loss by 50 to 60 per cent, whereas intrauterine devices tend to increase menstrual blood loss. Iron loss associated with pregnancy is easier to estimate and totals about 500 mg. Unless iron supplementation is provided, repeated pregnancies are almost invariably accompanied by iron deficiency.

Blood loss from the alimentary tract is frequently occult and intermittent, and may elude careful search with a battery of sophisticated techniques. In a recent study no demonstrable source of blood loss could be found in 16 per cent of patients with gastrointestinal bleeding. In those whose bleeding could be explained, the cause was hemorrhoidal bleeding in 10 per cent, salicylate ingestion in 8 per cent, peptic ulceration and hiatus hernia in 7 per cent each, diverticulosis in 4 per cent, neoplasm in 2 per cent, and a sprinkling of additional cases of esophageal varices, hemorrhagic gastritis, regional enteritis, ulcerative colitis, hemorrhagic telangiectasia, and intestinal polyps. Hookworm and other intestinal parasites are important causes of blood loss and iron deficiency in many countries. Blood donation—which must be specifically inquired about—doubles the amount of iron that must be absorbed when only three pints are removed per year. Blood removed for diagnostic studies from patients undergoing prolonged or repeated hospitalization is a cause for iron deficiency that can easily be overlooked. Rare causes of excess iron loss include the hemosiderinuria from chronic intravascular hemolysis of paroxysmal nocturnal hemoglobinuria and cardiac prostheses, and the iron that is trapped in the lungs of patients with pulmonary hemosiderosis. One cannot overemphasize the dictum that iron deficiency anemia in the adult man and the postmenopausal woman is due to blood loss until proved otherwise.

The sequence of changes in slowly developing iron deficiency is fairly predictable. Initially iron stores in reticuloendothelial and parenchymal cells are mobilized to provide the metal for functional iron needs. When demands for functional iron cannot be met from the stores, a signal of some sort is transmitted to the intestine to increase iron absorption. Transferrin concentration increases while the plasma iron concentration falls as demands of the bone marrow exceed the supply of iron released from senescent erythrocytes and intestinal absorption. Anemia appears when the supply of iron restricts erythropoiesis. Distorted cells reflecting skipped divisions and hypochromic cells reflecting insufficient iron for heme synthesis gradually replace the normal cells of the circulating blood. Later, increased cell division or more severe maturation defects lead to microcytosis and dyserythropoiesis of the fully developed iron deficiency anemia. The extent of the depletion of cell enzyme iron is variable in different tissues sampled in man, and little is known of the rate of these changes.

Clinical Manifestations. Iron deficiency anemia is accompanied by a wide diversity of symptoms. Some patients have no awareness of ill health despite marked anemia which may be recognized by chance examinations. Symptoms usually appear insidiously, and their onset is difficult to date. The gradual development of iron deficiency often allows remarkable adaptation, and may permit strenuous work with few symptoms. At the other extreme, marked tiredness, easy fatigability, dyspnea on exertion, palpitations, headache, irritability, paresthesias, lightheadedness, and other vague symptoms may trouble patients with borderline or mild anemia.

Examination usually discloses pallor, although on casual observation this finding may not be noticed. A peculiar greenish appearance of the skin of young girls, vividly described by careful observers before 1900 and termed chlorosis, has mysteriously disappeared. Vitiligo is a rare skin change in blacks. Angular stomatitis—most marked in edentulous patients—frequent papillary atrophy, and varying degrees of glossitis comprise the oral lesions associated with iron deficiency. Dysphagia resulting from postcricoid esophageal webs or strictures, associated with hypochromic anemia and achlorhydria, and most frequently seen in middle-aged women—the Paterson-Kelly or Plummer-Vinson syndrome—is rare in the United States, but is fairly common in the British Isles and Scandinavia. Whether this syndrome is due to iron deficiency or some associated disorder is not known. Multiple gastrointestinal complaints, such as anorexia, pyrosis, flatulence, nausea, eructation, and constipation, are common in association with iron deficiency. Occasionally bizarre cravings for cornstarch, ice, clay, and other substances may appear. These forms of pica are especially common in iron-deficient black women, but probably have a world-wide distribution. Gastritis, which is reversible after iron therapy, and permanent gastric atrophy have been described in numerous gastroscopic investigations of iron-deficient patients. Whether these gastric lesions are cause or effect of iron deficiency is debatable. Spoon nail (koilonychia) is the most advanced abnormality of the nails and is becoming very rare. Often, milder nail changes such as thinning, brittleness, lusterless appearance, longitudinal ridging, and flattening accompany prolonged iron deficiency, and are associated with depletion of cysteine in the nails. The frequent suggestion that these epithelial changes are related to the severity or chronicity of iron deficiency anemia may be questioned because of their virtual absence in patients with severe, lifelong iron deficiency owing to hookworm infestation. An attractive but unproved hypothesis is that the epithelial changes may reflect a chronically depressed intake of iron (and possibly other substances) rather than chronically increased loss of iron from bleeding.

Severe anemia often leads to cardiac dilatation, the occurrence of hemic murmurs, and, in older patients, the development of congestive heart failure. Enlargement of the spleen to slightly below the costal margin is observed in about 10 per cent of patients, and recedes after treatment. Claims of aggravation of menorrhagia by iron deficiency anemia and improvement after treatment are difficult to substantiate. Numbness and tingling without objective neurologic abnormalities are reported by about 25 per cent of patients. Extremely rare are the papilledema and increased pressure of cerebrospinal fluid that may be confused with intracranial tumors. Infants often show marked irritability and present difficulties in feeding.

Laboratory Findings. A number of laboratory procedures facilitate the identification of iron deficiency anemia. A well-stained blood film shows small erythrocytes (microcytosis) poorly filled with hemoglobin (hypochromia) with marked variation in size (anisocytosis) and shape (poikilocytosis). Mean corpuscular volume is less than 80 fl and mean corpuscular hemoglobin concentration is less than 30 per cent. Since the introduction of the Model S Coulter electronic counter into many hematology laboratories, the mean corpuscular hemoglobin concentration in iron deficiency anemia has been observed to be in the low normal range. The explanation for this seems to be that the volume of the erythrocytes, calculated from their number and degree of interference with the electrical field across the aperture through which they pass, is different from that measured by packing in a high speed centrifuge. Erroneous estimates of packed cell volume occur because of increased plasma trapping between distorted iron-deficient cells. Thus to identify iron deficiency, the key measurement to note in the printout of the Model S Coulter Counter is the mean cell volume. Plasma iron concentration is usually less than 80 μg per deciliter, associated with a total plasma iron-binding capacity of more than 400 μg per deciliter. Transferrin saturation (the product of plasma iron divided by total iron-binding capacity multiplied by 100) is 15 per cent or less. Examination of bone marrow particles shows normoblastic erythroid hyperplasia; sideroblasts and hemosiderin in macrophages are absent when the marrow particles are stained for iron. Defective heme synthesis is associated with elevated erythrocyte protoporphyrin concentration and decreased plasma bilirubin. Reticulocytes are present in normal numbers except for elevations secondary to recent hemorrhage. Erythrocyte osmotic fragility is decreased, reflecting the diminished hemoglobin concentration. The life span of erythrocytes is usually normal, although shortened survival has been reported. Thrombocytosis in the range of one million platelets per cubic millimeter, or, less often, thrombocytopenia, both of which return to normal after iron therapy, may be observed. Abnormalities of the leukocytes are rare and are usually confined to slight leukopenia and occasional hypersegmented neutrophils. Unfortunately there is no practical laboratory test to measure depletion of tissue enzyme iron.

Treatment. The two objects of treatment of iron deficiency anemia are (1) to replace the blood and tissue iron deficits, and (2) to recognize and, if possible, correct the underlying cause. Despite the vast array of therapeutic preparations containing iron, simple ferrous salts (ferrous sulfate, ferrous gluconate, and ferrous fumarate) given by mouth remain the mainstay of treatment for iron deficiency anemia. Large doses of ascorbic or succinic acid will increase iron absorption but only to a small extent that hardly warrants the extra expense. The addition of other substances found in "shotgun" mixtures such as copper, cobalt, molybdenum, intrinsic factor, and various B vitamins is of no benefit. The use of these shotgun hematinics must be condemned, because they may obscure the correct diagnosis as indicated by a response to iron alone; further, they encourage sloppiness in diagnosis, and they are unnecessarily expensive.

Enteric-coated and delayed-release iron preparations are poorly designed to exploit the fact of maximal absorption in the upper gastrointestinal tract. All too often their delay in iron release serves to dump the metal in the lower intestine, in which absorption is greatly diminished. When iron medication is prescribed in tablet form, the physician should warn the patient to keep the tablets out of reach of small children to reduce the danger of severe iron intoxication. Suitable warnings on the label and the use of child-proof containers will further reduce this risk.

A total daily dose of iron in the range of 180 to 240 mg provides for maximal rates of hemoglobin regeneration in adults. Three or four tablets of ferrous sulfate (60 mg of elemental iron) or ferrous fumarate (66 mg of iron) provide the requisite daily dose. Ferrous gluconate, with only 36 mg of elemental iron per tablet, requires a dosage of six tablets per day. These iron preparations are given in equal doses with or after meals and with a snack at bedtime. The advantage of increased absorption of iron salts taken on an empty stomach is often overweighed by the undesirable side effects of gastrointestinal irritation.

Approximately one patient in ten will experience unpleasant side effects such as nausea, epigastric pain, abdominal cramps, diarrhea, or vomiting of sufficient severity to require discontinuation of treatment. No effective iron preparation is free from causing gastric or intestinal irritation. Gastric symptomatology is dose dependent, and may be minimized by a gradual buildup of the iron dose during the first three days of treatment. A few patients are completely unable or unwilling to take iron by mouth; patience and understanding on the part of the physician can keep this group small. Treatment with iron should be continued for four to six months and even longer in the face of recurrent bleeding. Restoration of iron stores to provide a buffer against recurrent iron deficiency is a slow process.

Infants and toddlers are best treated with liquid iron preparations. Infants should receive a total of 60 to 90 mg of iron daily in water or fruit juices. Ferrous sulfate is available in concentrated drops containing 15 mg of iron per 0.6 ml, as a syrup with 30 mg of iron per 5 ml, or as an elixir with 44 mg of iron per 5 ml. Transient staining of the teeth by liquid iron preparations can be prevented by using a dropper or a straw. Most children weighing 35 to 75 pounds can satisfactorily take iron tablets in half the adult dosage; larger children usually receive adult doses of iron.

Response to adequate doses of iron given to a patient with iron deficiency anemia is quite predictable (Fig. 4). An initial sense of well-being is often observed within 48 hours. This improvement appears to be more than a psychologic effect from taking medications, as infants often lose their irritability and begin to eat better. Because this response occurs before any change in blood values is measurable, it has been attributed, without any real evidence, to replenishment of some vital cellular iron compound. The height of the reticulocyte peak and the rate of hemoglobin regeneration are proportional to the severity of the anemia; maximal daily rates of hemoglobin regeneration are 0.3 gram per deciliter.

Failure to respond to iron given by mouth should call forth the following considerations: (1) the patient failed to take the iron as prescribed; (2) the patient did not have iron deficiency anemia, and re-evaluation of the diagnosis is necessary; (3) blood loss exceeded new blood formation; (4) intercurrent infection, inflammation, or malignancy interfered with the response to iron; (5) the patient was unable to absorb the iron; and (6) an ineffective iron preparation was administered.

Parenteral administration of iron should be reserved for the following indications: (1) patients with malabsorption syndromes; (2) the relatively small group of patients who are unable or unwilling to take iron by mouth, including some people with ulcerative colitis, regional enteritis, and colostomies; (3) selected patients who prove unreliable in taking their prescribed iron; and (4) some patients with chronic uncorrectable bleeding with iron loss in excess of that which can be replaced by the oral route. Two satisfactory preparations are available for parenteral use. Both iron dextran (Imferon) and iron sorbitex (Jectofer) contain 50 mg of iron per milliliter. Iron sorbitex should be administered only by intramuscular injection, but iron dextran can be given by either the intramuscular or the intravenous route. The technique of deep intramuscular injections is important. The skin at the injection site (preferably the buttock) should first be displaced laterally before the needle is inserted into the muscle, so that reflux of the dark brown iron solution along the injection path, causing skin staining, can be prevented. After a test dose of 0.5 ml, 2 to 5 ml doses are given daily into alternate extremities until a calculated total dose is administered. Intravenous injection of iron dextran is reserved for patients in whom insufficient muscle mass or the discomfort of massive and prolonged intramuscular therapy precludes the intramuscular route. Usually iron dextran is injected undiluted in a dose of 2 to 5 ml per day, although the total dose may be diluted in 250 to 1000 ml of isotonic saline and infused during a two-hour period without untoward reactions. Dosage is calculated by the following formula: Normal Hgb (grams per deciliter) − patient's Hgb × 0.255 = iron dose in grams. This formula provides sufficient iron to replace the circulating hemoglobin deficit plus a 50 per cent excess for creation of tissue stores. Side effects such as local pain, lymphadenitis, headache, dizziness, fever, urticaria, arthralgias, myalgias, and hypotension occur in about 5 per cent of patients; rare fatal anaphylactic reactions have been reported. Urine that turns black on standing and urinary irritation may occur after injections of iron sorbitex, because one third of the dose is excreted into the urine, a fact that should be considered in total dose calculations.

Preventive iron therapy for groups prone to develop iron deficiency (infants, pregnant women, and blood donors) requires special consideration. Fortification of foods with iron salts seems a reasonable and fairly effective way to improve the iron intake of infants. Iron enrichment of bread remains a hotly debated subject both in terms of its efficacy in preventing iron deficiency of groups at special risk and in terms of risks of eventual iron overload in other groups. Pregnant women should be given iron during the last half of pregnancy, after the early period of "morning sickness" that might erroneously be attributed to the iron tablets and influence the patient's subsequent willingness to take this medication. One tablet of ferrous sulfate (60 mg of iron daily) is sufficient to provide for the extra iron needs of pregnancy. For repeated blood donors the dose of iron will depend on the rate of donation—one to three tablets daily may be required.

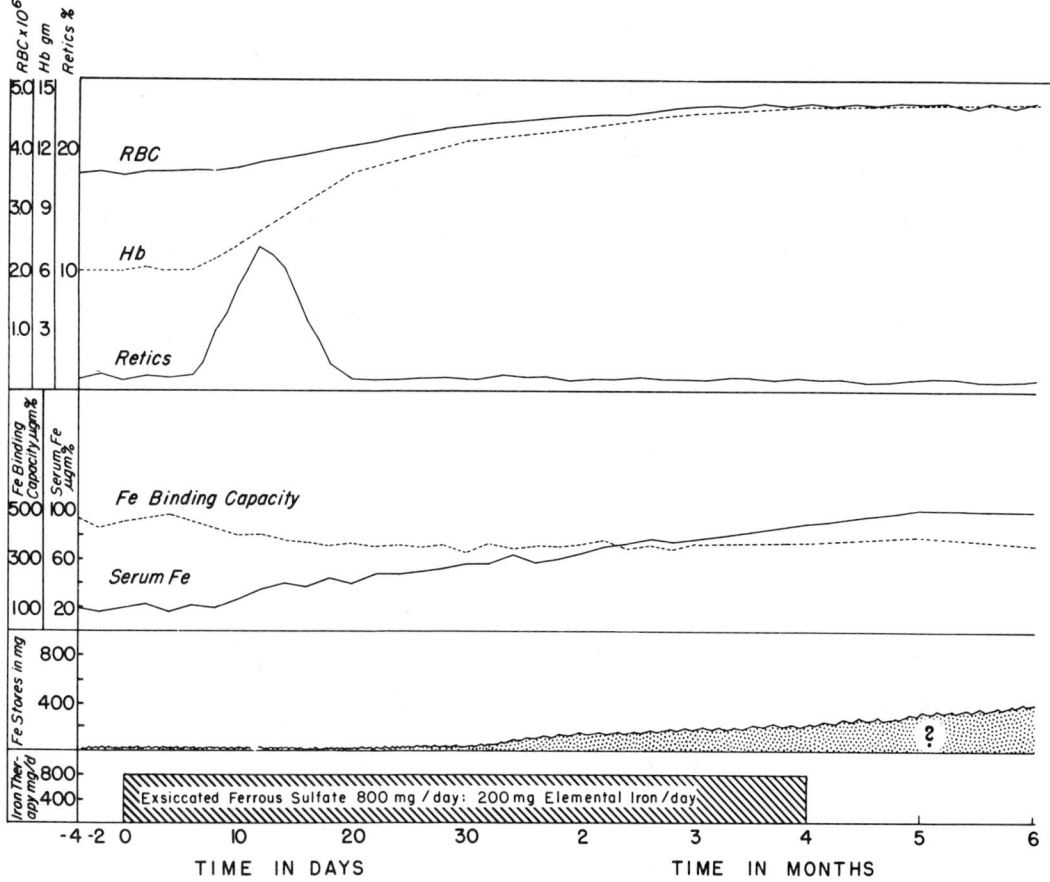

Figure 4. Schematized response to iron therapy. Reticulocytes begin to rise about the fifth to seventh day after iron therapy is started, reach a peak between the tenth and fourteenth days, and then fall to normal levels. Hemoglobin level begins to increase on about the seventh to tenth day. From four to eight weeks are required before normal values are attained. No accurate data are available to describe the reappearance of storage iron; its reaccumulation may be slower than shown; hence the question mark.

Prognosis. Prognosis in iron deficiency can only be applied to the underlying disorder causing the anemia. A vastly different prognosis is expected in a patient with a bleeding carcinoma of the alimentary tract and another with hemorrhoids. Patients rarely die of iron deficiency anemia itself, but they often die of the underlying cause. Recurrence of iron deficiency anemia after treatment is common; one third of women and one fourth of men have a recurrence in extended follow-up studies. These recurrence rates emphasize the importance of identifying and correcting the cause of iron deficiency.

Bothwell, T. H., and Finch, C. A.: Iron Metabolism. Boston, Little, Brown & Company, 1962.

Committee on Iron Deficiency: Iron deficiency in the United States. J.A.M.A., 203:407, 1968.

Fairbanks, V. F., Fahey, J. L., and Beutler, E.: Clinical Disorders of Iron Metabolism. New York, Grune & Stratton, 1971.

Gross, F. (ed.): Iron Metabolism—An International Symposium. Berlin, Springer-Verlag OHG, 1964.

Hallberg, L., Harwerth, H.-G., and Vanotti, A. (eds.): Iron Deficiency. Pathogenesis, Clinical Aspects, Therapy. New York, Academic Press, 1970.

Harris, J. W., and Kellermeyer, R. W.: The Red Cell. Production, Metabolism, Destruction: Normal and Abnormal. Cambridge, Mass., Harvard University Press, 1970.

Moore, C. V.: Iron nutrition and requirements. Scand. J. Haematol. (Series Haematologica), 6:1, 1965.

Williams, W. J., Beutler, E., Erslev, A. J., and Rundles, R. W. (eds.): Hematology. New York, McGraw-Hill Book Company, 1972.

Wintrobe, M. M.: Clinical Hematology. 6th ed. Philadelphia, Lea & Febiger, 1967.

738. HYPOCHROMIC ANEMIAS NOT CAUSED BY IRON DEFICIENCY

Hypochromic anemia occurs predominantly when hemoglobin synthesis is interfered with out of proportion to defects in erythrocyte proliferation. Biosynthetic abnormalities have been identified at one or more stages of protoporphyrin synthesis, iron incorporation into the heme ring—the prime defect in iron deficiency anemia—or globin synthesis. Compared to iron deficiency anemia, these disorders of hemoglobin synthesis are rare. As a group they can be differentiated from iron deficiency anemia by increased body iron stores with increased hemosiderin in marrow particles, the presence of sideroblasts and siderocytes, and increased plasma iron and transferrin saturation. Special distinguishing features are included with the following list of these disorders. (1) By far the most common of the hypochromic anemias not caused by iron deficiency are thalassemia and its variants resulting from interaction with abnormal hemoglobins. The basic defect is in the synthesis of globin chains. Thalassemia and its variants can be distinguished from iron deficiency by hemoglobin electrophoresis and detection of elevated levels of hemoglobins A_2 and F. (2) Homozygous Hgb-C disease and Hgb-

S-D are hypochromic anemias readily identified by appropriate hemoglobin electrophoresis. (3) Sideroblastic anemias can be subdivided into congenital, acquired, and pyridoxine-responsive categories. They share the common features of disordered heme synthesis with prominent ringed sideroblasts observable on iron staining of bone marrow particles. Electron microscopy discloses the siderotic granules to be diffuse iron aggregates in the intercristal spaces of mitochondria surrounding the nucleus of an erythrocyte precursor. Abnormalities in tryptophan metabolism and partial improvement of the anemia after pyridoxine or crude liver extract administration, as well as a high rate of leukemic transformation, have been reported in this group of disorders. (4) Chronic lead intoxication produces a hypochromic anemia resulting from defective hemoglobin synthesis. Stippling of erythrocytes and abnormal urinary excretion of coproporphyrin and aminolevulinic acid distinguish this disorder from iron deficiency, although in young children whose lead poisoning is due to pica of lead-based paint the two disorders may coexist. (5) Inadequate delivery of iron from plentiful stores to the marrow for hemoglobin synthesis has been observed in rare instances, such as in a child with congenital absence of transferrin, in pulmonary hemosiderosis, and in older people with an unexplained block in the release of iron from reticuloendothelial sites of hemoglobin catabolism.

Williams, W. J., Beutler, E., Erslev, A. J., and Rundles, R. W. (eds.): Hematology. New York, McGraw-Hill Book Company, 1972.
Wintrobe, M. M.: Clinical Hematology. 6th ed. Philadelphia, Lea & Febiger, 1967.

Section Two.   HEMOLYTIC DISORDERS

739.   INTRODUCTION

Lawrence E. Young

Definition. The essential feature of a hemolytic disorder is shortening of the life span of the red blood cells. The patient may have a compensated hemolytic state without anemia if the bone marrow responds adequately. As the marrow of adult man appears to be capable of increasing red blood cell production about eightfold, and as the normal life span of human red cells is about 120 days, anemia may not develop in some cases even if the average life span of the red cells is reduced to 15 to 20 days. The reserve capacity of the liver to excrete an increased quantity of bilirubin resulting from hemolysis may likewise result in maintenance of a normal concentration of bilirubin in the blood plasma. In a large proportion of the hemolytic states recognized clinically, however, patients are either anemic or mildly icteric, or both, so that the terms *hemolytic anemia* and *hemolytic icterus* are applicable.

Clinical Manifestations. In addition to pallor and mild icterus, the patient with a hemolytic disorder may present with fever, dyspnea, or shock if hemolysis is severe and anemia develops rapidly. The spleen is frequently enlarged but is by no means always palpable. In some instances, notably in hereditary spherocytosis, splenomegaly may be associated with accumulation of red cells in the splenic pulp; in others, enlargement may be due chiefly to proliferation of one or more cellular elements. The liver is also enlarged in many cases. Other clinical findings are related chiefly to the severity of the anemia and to the condition responsible for the hemolytic process. Chronic ulceration of the skin over or proximal to the malleoli may develop in sickle cell anemia, and rarely in hereditary spherocytosis and other chronic hemolytic disorders.

Gallstones containing chiefly bile pigment develop frequently in patients with chronic hemolytic disorders. Obstructive jaundice associated with choledocholithiasis or with cholestasis may develop rapidly and with extremely high concentrations of serum bilirubin because of the combination of excessive pigment production and biliary obstruction. Another major complication of chronic hemolytic disorders is rather sudden depression of erythropoiesis and fall in reticulocyte count, most often associated with acute infection. In such cases, the bone marrow may show hypoplasia or arrested maturation of erythroid cells. Folate deficiency may be demonstrable in some patients with chronic hemolytic anemia and may at times be associated with a megaloblastic marrow. Many of the "crises" in chronic hemolytic states are due chiefly to decrease in erythropoiesis for one reason or another. Anemia may suddenly become severe under these circumstances without significant increase in hemolysis above the patient's usual rate. Such episodes are often referred to as "hyporegenerative crises." Because folate requirement may be increased by persistent hemolysis, administration of 1 mg of folic acid by mouth daily may be justified in chronic hemolytic states of any type to prevent deficiency of this vitamin.

Diagnosis. Persistent reticulocytosis, with or without nucleated red blood cells in the peripheral blood, in the absence of blood loss should arouse suspicion of hemolysis. Large, diffusely basophilic red cells, which appear on supravital staining as prematurely released reticulocytes, are especially indicative of heightened bone marrow response. Estimates of compensatory increase in rate of erythropoiesis by use of reticulocyte counts require calculation of the number per cubic millimeter (normal is about 60,000) and recognition of the fact that maturation time of reticulocytes in the circulation may increase two- to threefold as anemia becomes severe. The rate of red cell destruction can be estimated most conveniently by measuring the survival time of the patient's cells after tagging with radioactive chromium (^{51}Cr). Rapid disappearance of similarly labeled normal donor cells from the patient's circulation points to an extracorpuscular hemolytic mechanism. Measurement of fecal urobilinogen excretion, usually in four-day collections of stool, also provides an estimate of the rate of red cell destruction, but such estimates may be falsely low in some cases. Fecal urobilinogen determinations have been made much less frequently in most centers since isotopic tagging of red cells became available. Since the amount

Classification of Hemolytic Disorders

I. Intracorpuscular abnormalities (sometimes combined with extrinsic challenge):
  A. Membrane defects
     Spherocytosis
     Elliptocytosis
     Stomatocytosis
     Chronic hemolytic anemia with paroxysmal nocturnal hemoglobinuria
  B. Enzyme deficiencies
     Defect in Embden-Meyerhof pathway of glycolysis
     Hexokinase
     Glucose phosphate isomerase
     Phosphofructokinase
     Fructosediphosphate aldolase
     Triosephosphate isomerase
     Diphosphoglyceromutase
     Phosphoglyerate kinase
     Pyruvate kinase
     Deficiency in enzyme activity related to the hexose monophosphate shunt pathway
     Glucose-6-phosphate dehydrogenase
     Phosphogluconate dehydrogenase
     Glutathione reductase
     γ-Glutamyl-cysteine synthetase
     Glutathione synthetase
     Glutathione peroxidase
  C. Hemoglobinopathies—qualitative defect in alpha or beta chains of globin
     Aggregating hemoglobins (S, C, D, I)
     Unstable hemoglobins (Zürich, Köln, etc.) with Heinz body formation
  D. Thalassemias—quantitative deficiency in synthesis of alpha or beta chains (may be combined with qualitative defect)
  E. Other types
     Low ATP concentration
     High ATP concentration
     ATPase deficiency
     Erythropoietic porphyria
     Increased red cell lecithin

II. Extracorpuscular causes (sometimes acting upon defective red cells):
  A. Immune mechanisms
     Warm-reacting antibodies
       Isoimmune
         Transfusion reactions
         Hemolytic disease of newborn
       Autoimmune
     Cold-reacting antibodies
       Cold agglutinin syndrome
       Paroxysmal cold hemoglobinuria
     Paroxysmal nocturnal hemoglobinuria (discussed in Ch. 740)
  B. Intravascular fragmentation
     Microangiopathic—intravascular clotting hemolysis
     Cardiac valvular hemolysis
     March hemoglobinuria
  C. Acquired membrane alterations
     Chemicals
       Drugs
         Nonimmune
         Immune
       Poisons
         Animal—spider bites, snake venoms
         Vegetable—castor beans, mushrooms
         Mineral—Cu^{++}
     Accumulated metabolites
       Due to kidney failure
       Due to liver failure
     Infectious agents
       Direct infestation
         Malaria
         Bartonella
       Indirect alteration
         Immunologically
         Nonimmunologically
  D. Hemolysis due to abnormal sequestration of normal red cells by the reticuloendothelial system
     Hypersplenism
     Eosinophilic granuloma syndromes (histiocytic reticuloendothelioses)

of urobilinogen excreted in the urine is affected by liver function, measurements of urinary urobilinogen are unreliable as indicators of the rate of red cell destruction. In the presence of modest hemolysis, urinary urobilinogen excretion may be normal if liver function is well preserved, or it may be greatly increased if liver function is impaired.

The concentration of bilirubin (predominantly unconjugated) seldom exceeds 8.0 mg per 100 ml of plasma. Hemolytic icterus has been recognized for many years as "acholuric"; little or no bilirubin is excreted in the urine unless liver function is impaired or the biliary tract becomes obstructed.

Since hemoglobinemia is largely the result of rapid intravascular hemolysis outside the microcirculation of the spleen, liver, and/or bone marrow, it is absent or minimal in many hemolytic states. The renal threshold for hemoglobin depends on the capacity of plasma haptoglobins to bind hemoglobin (normally 100 to 150 mg of hemoglobin per 100 ml of plasma) and on the ability of renal tubular cells to remove hemoglobin from glomerular filtrate. The haptoglobins, which are alpha-2 globulins with remarkable capacity to bind hemoglobin, are markedly reduced in the plasma in most of the clinically recognized hemolytic states, acute and chronic, including those with little or no hemoglobinemia. Reduction in haptoglobin concentration is due to rapid clearing of the hemoglobin-haptoglobin complex by the recticuloendothelial system.

Morphologic abnormalities of the red blood cells are best discussed in connection with the individual hemolytic disorders. In some examples of hemolytic disease, no abnormality of size or shape of the red cells is apparent. Fragmentation, best observed with phase microscopy or scanning electron microscopy, but also evident in customary examination of stained blood smears, is recognized increasingly as a final common pathway in many hemolytic states. Platelets and granulocytes are usually present in normal or increased numbers, but either or both may be decreased in some instances. The bone marrow typically shows normoblastic hyperplasia in response to hemolysis except during hyporegenerative periods which are most commonly associated with infection.

Splenectomy. Since the estimated benefits and hazards of splenectomy must be weighed in the management of many patients with hemolytic disorders, certain general considerations can be presented to advantage at this point. Often decision can be reached easily on the basis of precise diagnosis and abundant documentation in the literature of favorable or unfavorable results with a given disorder. In some of the disorders to be described, decision regarding splenectomy may be influenced by measurements of radioactivity over the body surface above the spleen in comparison with counts above the liver after transfusion of autogenous or normal donated red cells tagged with ^{51}Cr. Such measurements help to reveal the relative importance of the spleen in the hemolytic process. There are well-documented examples, however, of patients benefiting from splenectomy despite the fact that excessive splenic localization was not found in this type of preoperative study.

Immediate operative mortality from splenectomy performed primarily to relieve hemolytic disease is very low in the hands of experienced surgeons. Two possible sequelae of splenectomy deserve emphasis. The risk of sepsis with sudden onset and high mortality rate must be recognized in all asplenic persons regardless of the reason for splenectomy. The risk is greatest during infancy but persists throughout adulthood, especially with blood-borne inocula of pneumococcus, Meningococcus, *E. coli*, and *H. influenzae*. Splenectomized patients and their families as well as responsible nurses and physicians should be aware of the need for prompt diagnosis and treatment of infection in the absence of defense mechanisms normally provided by the spleen.

Another consequence of splenectomy is thromboembolism in patients with persistent thrombocytosis. Such patients are usually those who continue to have anemia and reticulocytosis as well as thrombocytosis for many years. The patient whose hemolytic anemia is not significantly relieved by splenectomy thus incurs the added risk of thrombophlebitis and embolic complications.

Classification. The classification in the accompanying table is based chiefly upon current concepts of pathogenic mechanisms. The disorders listed with intracorpuscular abnormalities of the red cell are hereditary except for that associated with nocturnal hemoglobinuria. Intrinsically defective red cells with shortened life span may be produced in patients with myeloid metaplasia, chronic myelocytic leukemia, deficiency of vitamin B_{12} folate, or iron, and in patients with lead intoxication. These conditions will not be discussed here because other features of the respective illnesses are usually more important than the hemolytic component of the anemia.

740. INTRACORPUSCU-LAR ABNORMALITIES

Lawrence E. Young

Erythrocytes from patients with certain types of intracorpuscular abnormality have been found to disappear rapidly from the circulation after transfusion to normal recipients. Normal donor cells, on the other hand, survive normally in the circulation of such patients unless there are complicating hemolytic mechanisms such as hypersplenism or the development of immune isoantibodies as a result of previous transfusions. Although there are unmistakable abnormalities of the red blood cells in this group of patients, hemolysis may be dependent upon or heightened by the presence of environmental factors that provide a critical challenge to the defective cells. The sequence of events by which most recognized types of abnormal red cells are destroyed in vivo becomes clearer each year. This group of disorders provides excellent material for studies in cellular biology.

MEMBRANE DEFECTS

Hereditary Spherocytosis (HS)

Definition. This condition is inherited as an autosomal dominant disorder and is characterized by the presence of spherocytes or abnormally thick red blood cells in the circulation. It has been found in many populations, but appears to be most common in northern European stocks. In such populations, the incidence has been estimated at from 200 to 300 per million.

Clinical Manifestations. Diagnosis may be made at birth if the condition is suspected, but in mild cases diagnosis may not be made until late in life. Moderate splenomegaly develops in nearly all cases. Leg ulcers are encountered infrequently. Roentgenographic examination reveals striation and thickening of the frontal and parietal bones in some cases. Anemia is rarely severe in the absence of hyporegenerative crises or other complications such as infection or hemorrhage.

Diagnosis. Spherocytosis is usually evident in blood smears or in wet preparations which show bizarre rouleau formation. The increase in osmotic fragility provides a reliable measure of the degree of spherocytosis. Mechanical fragility of the red cells is also increased. Both types of fragility are increased by sterile incubation of the blood at body temperature for 24 hours, a procedure that may cause changes in red cells similar to those produced during sequestration within the spleen. Autohemolysis, or spontaneous lysis of red cells in defibrinated blood incubated at body temperature, is best measured at 48 hours and is markedly increased in most cases of HS. The percentage of lysis after incubation is computed by measuring the concentration of hemoglobin in the serum in relation to the hemoglobin content of the blood sample prior to incubation. Autohemolysis is strikingly inhibited by addition of glucose or by slight acidification of the blood from HS patients. Such inhibition of autohemolysis is less evident in other types of chronic spherocytosis, and is sometimes not demonstrable in HS until after splenectomy. In order to establish the diagnosis, similar abnormalities should be sought in relatives of patients with spherocytosis, even when there is no history of anemia, jaundice, or splenomegaly. In some cases only the measurements of fragility with incubated red cells are clearly abnormal. In instances of suspected low gene manifestation or gene mutation, both parents of patients with suspected HS may be hematologically normal by all available criteria.

Pathogenesis. Spherocytes are readily trapped, probably for variable periods of time, within the splenic pulp. When washed from that site after splenectomy, they show much greater osmotic fragility than do spherocytes in the peripheral blood, although normal donor cells in the splenic pulp show little increase in fragility. Transfused spherocytes are readily trapped and destroyed in the spleen of hematologically normal recipients but survive normally in splenectomized normal recipients.

The red cell membrane in this disease is less deformable and more permeable to sodium than the membrane of normal red cells. Trapping of HS red cells within the cords of Billroth of the spleen is probably related to cellular rigidity, which depends both on the decreased surface area to volume ratio and on increased intrinsic rigidity of the cell membrane. Abnormality of contractile protein in the membrane is under continuing study. The relatively low pH and oxygen tension within the splenic pulp render ATP bound to deoxyhemoglobin less available than needed to maintain integrity of the red cell membrane. Hereditary spherocytosis cells lose lipid and protein from the membrane surface as they make their way through the cords, with the result that they become more nearly spherical and still more rigid. Eventually the cells are unable to escape through the small openings into the venous sinusoids. Fragmentation of the rigid cells to the point of ultimate destruction has been observed by phase microscopy and electron microscopy in the spleens of mice afflicted with a comparable disorder. Hemoglobinemia is not encountered in HS patients, but plasma haptoglobin concentration is consistently low.

Treatment. Splenectomy is invariably effective in lengthening the life span of the red cells to a nearly normal range. In most cases anemia is fully corrected and there is a decrease to normal in reticulocytes and serum bilirubin concentration. Spherocytosis and other demonstrable abnormalities of the red cells persist after splenectomy, but are of little or no consequence once the splenic trap is removed. Splenectomy can be recommended in most cases, even when well compensated, because of the threats of cholelithiasis and of severe anemia during periods of suppressed erythropoiesis. Splenectomy may prevent development of hemochromatosis, a recently reported complication in older patients. Operation is usually deferred to about age five to make minimal the risk of sepsis explained previously. Transfusion of normal red blood cells is seldom indicated except during the periods of severe anemia associated with hyporegenerative bone marrow.

Hereditary Elliptocytosis

Hereditary elliptocytosis is similar to hereditary spherocytosis in many respects. It has been found in many populations, and may be encountered more frequently than spherocytosis in some localities. It is inherited as an autosomal dominant abnormality with wide variations in gene manifestation both within and between families. In some families there is evidence for location of the gene or genes determining elliptocytosis on the chromosome bearing genes for the Rh blood group system. The degree of elliptocytosis varies from person to person and also among the red cells of any affected person. Many of the cells are usually abnormal in shape, some are greatly elongated, and others are slightly oval. There is no apparent relationship between the degree of elliptocytosis and the life span of the red cells. In the presence of active hemolysis, microspherocytes may be found in small numbers. Some affected persons have red cells with normal life span; others have a compensated hemolytic state; and a minority have overt hemolytic anemia. The very rare homozygous state is associated with severe hemolysis. Factors determining chronic hemolysis in the heterozygotes are unknown. Coexistence of elliptocytosis with hemoglobin S or hemoglobin C trait or with erythrocyte glyoxalase II deficiency does not appear to cause an additive, deleterious effect on the red cells. Coexistence of elliptocytosis with heterozygous beta thalassemia, on the other hand, may be associated with hemolysis.

Splenomegaly is common, and sequestration of red cells in the spleen is evident. Most patients splenectomized because of hemolysis associated with elliptocytosis have been benefited.

Stomatocytosis

Stomatocytosis is characterized by red cells with the appearance of a linear, mouthlike area of central pallor on stained films and with the appearance of bowls in wet preparations. There is marked increase in osmotic fragility, and in one form there is high concentration of calcium and sodium and low concentration of potassium with increased energy requirement for active cation transport. Reports to date suggest that this is an autosomal dominant character. Response to splenectomy is variable. Stomatocytosis may be produced in vitro by a variety of chemical agents, many of which are cationic detergent-like molecules.

Chronic Hemolytic Anemia with Paroxysmal Nocturnal Hemoglobinuria*

Definition. This rare disorder has been encountered in many parts of the world. It occurs in both sexes, with onset most common during the third or fourth decade. There is no report of familial incidence.

Clinical Manifestations. The disease is characterized by chronic hemolysis of a highly variable degree, with hemoglobinemia and usually, but not always, hemoglobinuria. Hemolysis is usually increased during sleep, regardless of the time when the patient sleeps. Episodes of increased hemolysis, sometimes lasting several days, occur irregularly, particularly after infections. During the period of hemolysis sufficient to cause hemoglobinuria, the urine passed on arising is usually brown or reddish brown. In severely affected patients, hemoglobinuria may be continuous, with further darkening of the urine after sleep. Hemosiderinuria, a regular feature of the disease, results in considerable loss of iron from the body. Renal function is usually unimpaired, but there may be complications such as pyelonephritis. Hemosiderin is not found in any significant quantity in the body outside the cells of the convoluted tubules and ascending loops of Henle in the kidney, unless the patient has had frequent transfusions. The liver and spleen may be slightly enlarged. No characteristic abnormality of the red cell is evident in blood smears or in tests of osmotic or mechanical fragility. Neutropenia and thrombocytopenia are commonly found. Alkaline phosphatase activity in the neutrophils is markedly decreased. Although erythroid hyperplasia of the bone marrow is usually present, marked hypoplasia of all elements is being found increasingly before or, rarely, after the hemolytic disorder becomes apparent. It has been suggested that in some cases the abnormal red cells may be derived from a mutant clone of precursors originating during a period of marrow aplasia, even when the aplasia seems related to drug usage. The recently recognized development of stem cell or acute myelocytic leukemia in patients with antecedent nocturnal hemoglobinuria has led to the suggestion that this hemolytic disorder may represent a somatic mutation which, at times, involves the stem cells. Thrombotic complications, particularly involving hepatic and cerebral veins, are frequently associated with greatly accelerated hemolysis. Dysphagia caused by increased esophageal pressure waves may occur, particularly during hemolytic crises. Severe abdominal pain of uncertain cause is also seen with such episodes.

Pathogenesis. The disease is characterized by the presence of a proportion of red cells which are more susceptible to the lytic action of complement than normal

---

*The author thanks Dr. Wendell F. Rosse for advice in the wording of this article.

cells. The proportion of abnormal cells may vary from 1 to over 90 per cent, and the severity of the disease roughly parallels this proportion. The activation of complement by unknown mechanisms results in the intravascular lysis of these abnormal cells, particularly during sleep. The nature of the membrane defect leading to increased lysis by complement is not known, but it appears to result in an increased binding of the later components (C3 and beyond) and an increased effectiveness of these components. Membrane-bound acetylcholinesterase is deficient on these cells, but the relationship of this to the increased lysis by complement is problematic.

Because of the membrane defect, the cells are lysed, no matter how the complement sequence is activated. In vitro activation by antibody is useful in demonstrating the presence of the lesion, but activation by the so-called alternate, or properdin, pathway which bypasses the initial steps of the classic antibody pathway in activating C3 is probably more important in initiating hemolysis in vivo.

The diagnosis is made by demonstrating increased lysis by complement in any of several systems. In the Ham test (acidified serum lysis test), complement is activated through the alternate pathway by the mild acidification of normal serum. It may be rendered more sensitive by augmentation of the magnesium concentration to 0.005 M. This test is specific for PNH if suitably controlled, including demonstration that the patient's serum lyses his own cells. The red cells of some patients with congenital dyserythropoietic anemia may be hemolyzed in normal serum because of the occurrence of naturally occurring antibodies against membrane antigens; these cells are not lysed by the patient's own serum nor by normal serum in any of the tests listed below.

Complement may also be activated by reduced ionic strength in an osmotic solution of sucrose. This provides a convenient method for diagnosis, but the test must be carefully performed. Lysis of PNH cells may also be induced by a factor from cobra venom and inulin, both of which activate the alternate pathway.

Treatment.   Transfusion of washed, normal red blood cells is needed during periods of severe anemia. Transfusion of whole blood should be avoided in most cases, because constituents of normal plasma as well as leukocytes may accelerate hemolysis. Use of coumarin derivatives may be indicated in patients who have developed thrombosis, but it is difficult to justify for prevention of thrombosis. Their inhibitory effect on hemolysis is transient with tolerable doses. Use of heparin is controversial. Intravenous administration of 1000 ml of 6 per cent dextran daily or at longer intervals may inhibit hemolysis during critical periods of the disease but is not recommended for sustained use. All operative procedures, including splenectomy, are to be avoided if possible. Administration of iron, preferably by mouth, may be beneficial for patients who are not transfused and who develop evidence of iron deficiency. Administration of androgens, such as fluoxymesterone, 20 to 30 mg daily by mouth, may be beneficial by stimulating erythropoiesis and perhaps by reducing hemolysis. Prednisone, 20 to 30 mg every other day, may be useful in control of hemolysis in severely affected patients. Folic acid, 1 mg daily by mouth, is indicated to meet increased folate requirement.

Prognosis.   This is a chronic disorder that terminates fatally in many cases. The patients may lead active lives between complicating episodes if suitably managed. In some instances, the abnormality of the red cells eventually disappears. A few women with this disease have borne normal children, but usually with complications during pregnancy or the puerperium.

ENZYME DEFICIENCIES

The accompanying figure shows the pathways of glycolysis in the mature human erythrocyte, with lines drawn under the names of enzymes thus far demonstrated to be deficient in certain individuals with hemolytic states. Although the hemolytic mechanisms are only partially understood, the relationship between enzyme deficiency and hemolysis is well documented in most instances. Under normal conditions about 90 per cent of glucose is metabolized anaerobically through the Embden-Meyerhof pathway with net increase in high energy adenosine triphosphate (ATP) serving multiple purposes. Another product of glycolysis is 2,3-diphosphoglycerate (2,3-DPG) which exerts major influence on the binding of oxygen to hemoglobin (see Ch. 730).

Defects in Embden-Meyerhof Pathway of Glycolysis

Hemolytic states associated with deficiencies of eight enzymes involved in the anaerobic pathway of glycolysis

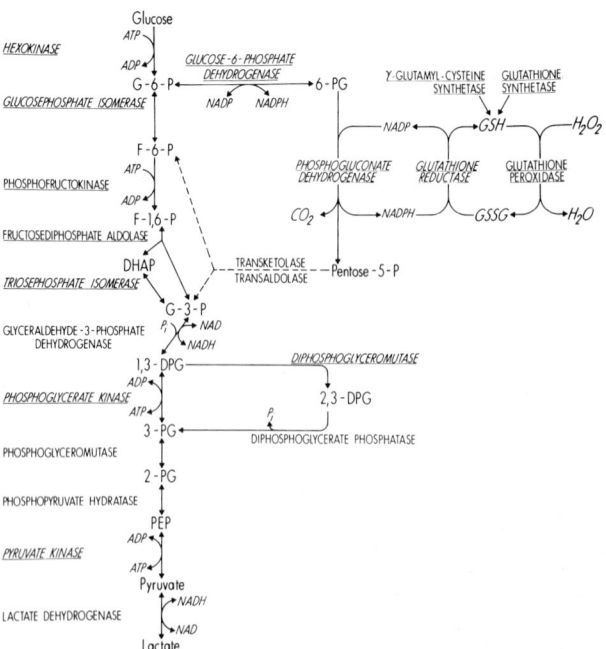

Pathways of glycolysis in mature human red cell (modified from Valentine).

Abbreviations: ATP = adenosine triphosphate; ADP = adenosine diphosphate; NADP = nicotinamide-adenine dinucleotide phosphate (TPN); NADPH = reduced nicotinamide-adenine dinucleotide phosphate (TPNH); G-6-P = glucose-6-phosphate; 6-PG = 6-phospho-3-ketogluconate; Pentose-5-P = pentose-5-phosphate; GSH = reduced glutathione; GSSG = oxidized glutathione; F-6-P = fructose-6-phosphate; F-1,6-P = fructose-1,6-phosphate; DHAP = dihydroxyacetonephosphate; G-3-P = glyceraldehyde-3-phosphate; P_i = inorganic phosphorus; 1,3-DPG = 1,3-diphosphoglycerate; 2,3-DPG = 2,3-diphosphoglycerate; 3-PG = 3-phosphoglycerate; 2-PG = 2-phosphoglycerate; PEP = phosphoenol pyruvate.

in red cells have been identified since 1962. Pyruvate kinase (PK) deficiency is the most frequently encountered example of this uncommon group of disorders and was the first to be described. The pattern of inheritance is autosomal recessive, except for phosphoglycerate kinase deficiency which is X-linked.

In PK deficiency, the prototype of this group, heterozygotes are phenotypically normal, but have measurable deficiency of enzyme activity in the red cells. Homozygotes have a lifelong hemolytic state of variable severity with splenomegaly and only partial relief from hemolysis after splenectomy. Spherocytosis is not prominent, but may be noted on close inspection of blood smears and wet preparations. Crenated red cells are frequently noted and are probably crenated spherocytes or irregularly contracted cells. Finding crenated spherocytes on the blood smear of a patient with splenomegaly and with a history suggesting hemolytic anemia since early childhood should stimulate the clinician to obtain enzyme assays on the patient's red cells.

Genetically determined heterogeneity of erythrocyte PK has been demonstrated, including evidence of kinetic abnormality of the enzyme. Most patients with PK deficiency develop anemia and jaundice in the neonatal period. Anemia is usually more severe than in hereditary spherocytosis. Osmotic fragility of the red cells is normal with fresh blood but is abnormally increased after the blood has been incubated for 24 hours at 37° C. Autohemolysis is moderately increased except in patients with a presumed variant of PK deficiency and usually is not diminished when glucose is added to the blood. In some cases of PK deficiency, however, glucose may inhibit autohemolysis. Use of the autohemolysis test for differential diagnosis must take into account these exceptional cases of PK deficiency along with the exceptional cases of hereditary spherocytosis in which glucose fails to inhibit autohemolysis until after splenectomy.

Hemolysis in PK deficiency generally is attributed to impaired glycolysis and consequent reduction in ATP generation, but further studies of the hemolytic mechanism are needed. PK-deficient reticulocytes may be spared to some extent from destruction in the general circulation, because their mitochondria provide ATP from aerobic metabolism. The PK-deficient reticulocytes, like normal reticulocytes, tend to be sequestered within the spleen. Within the hypoxic environment of the splenic pulp, aerobic metabolism, upon which the PK-deficient reticulocytes are dependent, is inhibited with consequent decrease in ATP content, increase in cellular rigidity, and irreversible sequestration of the reticulocytes. The partial relief of anemia and frequent reduction in transfusion requirement in this disorder after splenectomy may be attributable to removal of the hypoxic trap. Reticulocyte counts are frequently higher after splenectomy despite amelioration of anemia, thus reflecting the survival of reticulocytes which previously had been eliminated from the circulation by the spleen. Although splenectomy is much less effective than in hereditary spherocytosis, it can be recommended after infancy for patients requiring transfusions to maintain acceptable concentrations of hemoglobin.

In triosephosphate isomerase deficiency, enzyme activity is also low in leukocytes, muscle, and cerebrospinal fluid. A severe, progressive neurologic disorder develops in addition to hemolytic anemia. The hematologic picture is similar to that of PK deficiency except that

autohemolysis is inhibited more constantly by glucose.

Glucosephosphate isomerase deficiency may be second in incidence to PK deficiency among the enzymes involved in the anaerobic pathway. Other examples of enzyme deficiency in the red cell related to anaerobic glycolysis are rare. In general, the clinical findings and course are similar to those of PK deficiency. Severe deficiency of lactate dehydrogenase, transmitted as an autosomal recessive trait, is not associated with overt hemolysis.

Deficiency in Enzyme Activity Related to the Hexose Monophosphate (HMP) Shunt Pathway

Glucose-6-Phosphate Dehydrogenase (G-6-PD)

The enzyme G-6-PD is involved at the beginning of the oxidative HMP shunt pathway, which under usual conditions accounts for about 10 per cent of glucose metabolism of the red cell. In normal red cells the proportion of total glucose metabolized through the shunt pathway may be increased many-fold if the cells are subjected to oxidants such as those derived from certain drugs. The resulting increase in generation of the reduced form of nicotinamide adenine dinucleotide phosphate (NADPH) and consequently of reduced glutathione (GSH) helps to resist oxidant stresses. Otherwise, these stresses may inactivate essential thiol (SH) groups on membrane proteins, and within the cell may cause formation of methemoglobin and degradation of hemoglobin to form Heinz bodies. Drugs such as phenylhydrazine may overwhelm this protective mechanism, especially in older red cells because there is a decline in G-6-PD activity with aging of red cells in the circulation. Red cells with a genetically determined deficiency of G-6-PD are unable to withstand lesser oxidative stresses. The outcome in any given red cell presumably is determined by the amount of stress and the severity of enzyme deficiency, but predictions based on estimates of enzyme activity by the usual methods may nevertheless be inaccurate.

Studies on hemolytic disorders related to the HMP shunt pathway constitute one of the most fascinating and clinically significant chapters in the history of hematology. G-6-PD deficiency in red cells has been shown to be due to a wide range of genetic variants, each of which is X-linked. The defect is fully expressed in male hemizygotes and female homozygotes. It is variably manifest in female heterozygotes because two populations of red cells are present, deficient cells and normal cells, in varying proportions. It is not known whether the heterogeneity in G-6-PD formation is produced by different mutations at a single locus on the X chromosome or whether mutations at different loci affect the production and function of the enzyme. There are two common types of G-6-PD. Type A, moving rapidly on starch-gel electrophoresis, is found in about 30 per cent of American blacks, including most of those who are enzyme deficient. Type B, moving more slowly on electrophoresis, is found in about 70 per cent of blacks and in nearly all Caucasians.

Manifestations in Blacks. The most common type of G-6-PD deficiency is found in blacks: about 10 per cent of American blacks, 8 to 20 per cent of blacks in West Africa, but only 2 per cent of South African Bantus. Activity of this enzyme in the red cells is reduced to 5 to 15 per cent of normal in hemizygous males and homozygous females. Enzyme activity in heterozygous females ranges from normal to figures nearly as low as those obtained from homozygotes. Red cell life span is only slightly reduced in G-6-PD-deficient blacks unless the cells are subjected to stress imposed by derivatives of certain drugs or by infection or possibly by diabetic ketoacidosis. More than 40 drugs have been found to produce hemolysis in G-6-PD-deficient persons. These include the antimalarial drugs primaquine and quinine (the latter also used in popular beverages), the antipyretics and analgesics acetylsalicylic acid and phenacetin in large doses, the nitrofurans, sulfones, many sulfonamides, para-aminosalicylic acid, probenecid, quinidine, phenylhydrazine, and water-soluble analogues of vitamin K. Naphthalene, of which moth balls are composed, is often ingested by children with effects similar to those of the drugs listed. Blacks whose G-6-PD-deficient red cells are challenged develop hemolytic anemia of varying severity, depending upon the dose and oxidative capacity of the derivatives of the chemical agent involved; in female heterozygotes the degree of enzyme deficiency appears also to influence the extent of hemolysis. Patients suffering from infection, acidosis, or impaired liver or kidney function, with consequent delay in drug excretion, may be more subject to hemolysis with a given dose of a potentially oxidant drug. Moreover, infection or acidosis may provoke hemolysis in the absence of an offending drug, and they may in fact be the most common precipitants of hemolytic anemia in these individuals. Infection may lead to hemolysis through increased production of hydrogen peroxide by leukocytes engaged in phagocytosis of organisms.

Hemoglobinemia and hemoglobinuria are usually of only moderate degree and short duration, and may not be observed. Plasma haptoglobin is usually reduced even in the cases of little or no hemoglobinemia. Many of the red cells may contain Heinz bodies during the first few days of hemolysis, but in typical cases most of the red cells containing Heinz bodies have been eliminated by the time the hematocrit reaches its lowest point. The red cells show fragmentation of widely varying degree from case to case prior to onset of the recovery phase. The cells may appear as though a portion had been torn away, but they do not as a rule show crenation or appear as irregularly contracted spherocytes. Careful inspection of the blood smear together with consideration of the patient's history and ethnic group helps to differentiate this type of hemolytic anemia from that caused by a defect in the Embden-Meyerhof pathway within the red cell. Typically hemolysis is limited in duration because of the more nearly normal G-6-PD activity in younger red cells which become more abundant in the circulation in response to hemolysis. Consequently, the erythrocyte level may return to normal even though administration of the offending drug is continued. Diagnosis by estimates of enzyme activity in the red cells may be difficult at the time of acute hemolysis and reticulocytosis. Confirmation of the clinical diagnosis by enzyme assay often must await the return to normal of the red cell age distribution unless special methods are used.

Manifestations in Other Populations. G-6-PD deficiency in populations other than blacks is usually more severe, with red cell enzyme activity in most cases in the range of 0 to 5 per cent of normal and with reduced G-6-PD activity in leukocytes and platelets as well as in red cells. At least 100 different forms of G-6-PD have been demonstrated among Caucasian and Oriental populations on the basis of biochemical characteristics of the enzyme. Among Caucasian populations G-6-PD Mediterranean is by far the most common variant enzyme, with a gene frequency of less than 0.1 per cent in Northern Europeans and of about 50 per cent among male Kurdish Jews. The frequency in Greeks is 2 to 9 per cent, in Italians 0.5 to 1.0 per cent, and in Sardinians 3 to 35 per cent. The distribution of variant enzyme types in other populations is less clearly determined; the incidence of G-6-PD deficiency is about 2 to 4 per cent in Chinese, 12 per cent in Thais, and 1 to 5 per cent in Indians.

Studies of Caucasians with G-6-PD activity in the range of 0 to 18 per cent of normal have shown that about 20 per cent of the circulating red cells are destroyed after ingestion of a single standard prophylactic antimalarial dose of primaquine (45 mg). The degree of hemolysis under these circumstances is not related to the estimated level of enzyme activity. G-6-PD-deficient Caucasians are generally more subject than are blacks to hemolysis after use of potentially oxidant drugs or as a complication of infection or of diabetic ketoacidosis.

Chronic hemolytic anemia in the absence of drugs or other extrinsic challenge is encountered in Caucasian and occasionally in Oriental males with marked deficiency of G-6-PD activity. Hemolysis appears to be continuous from infancy, but may be accelerated by the same types of challenges causing acute hemolysis in the much more common, nonanemic G-6-PD-deficient Caucasian or black. Most of the G-6-PD variants associated with a chronic hemolytic state are abnormally labile at temperatures of 40 to 46° C. Osmotic fragility of the red cells in the chronic state is normal or nearly so. Autohemolysis is increased only slightly and usually is inhibited by glucose. Ovalocytes are noted in some cases, but spherocytes are seen rarely. Data on spleen size and results of splenectomy are meager. Splenomegaly is not a regular feature as it is in hereditary spherocytosis and in PK deficiency. Studies with ^{51}Cr-tagged red cells show no unusual concentration of radioactivity over the spleen.

Favism is an acute hemolytic anemia occurring after ingestion of fava beans or after inhalation of pollen from the plant *Vicia faba* by persons with G-6-PD-deficient red cells. Several other plants may have a similar effect. Favism has been observed only in Caucasians and is most common among certain groups of Kurdish Jews, Sardinians, Greeks, and Italians. Since many Caucasians with G-6-PD deficiency suffer no hemolysis after challenge by bean or plant, an additional mechanism is suspected. Studies on isolated populations with high incidence of favism suggest that the additional determinant may be inherited. Anemia may be very severe and accompanied by hemoglobinemia. During the early phase of an attack the hemoglobin appears to be concentrated on one side of some of the red cells, leaving the cell envelope visible on the opposite side. Heinz bodies and spherocytes may be seen, and osmotic fragility may be increased transiently. There is marked leukocytosis, often with transient eosinophilia.

Neonatal Jaundice. Neonatal jaundice with development of kernicterus is a hazard for infants, especially males, with some types of G-6-PD deficiency. Hemolysis and hyperbilirubinemia can be induced in the newborn, particularly if premature, by use of drugs such as water-soluble, synthetic vitamin K preparations or by drugs given to the mother before delivery. Caucasian and Oriental infants may develop jaundice without exposure to drugs. In Hong Kong, for example, G-6-PD deficiency is claimed to be the most common cause of neonatal jaundice and kernicterus. Even in the presence of normal G-6-PD activity in the red cells, glutathione is unstable during the first few days of life. Since this instability can be corrected in vitro by addition of glucose, it is believed that hypoglycemia in the newborn may increase the risk of neonatal jaundice.

Use of Screening Tests. It is estimated from population surveys that at least 100 million persons in the world have red cells deficient in G-6-PD. Wide use of a simple screening test for this deficiency, such as that based on reduction of methemoglobin, is indicated as a part of comprehensive health care for populations known to be at relatively high risk. Tests done when the patient is well serve to forewarn both patient and physician. Tests performed during or immediately after a period of hemolysis are unreliable because some genetic variants, chiefly in blacks, have a high activity of G-6-PD in reticulocytes; i.e., the tests may yield "false negative" results.

Drug-Induced Hemolysis of Older Normal Red Cells. Since G-6-PD activity declines with aging of red cells in the circulation, even red cells with normal enzyme activity initially may become susceptible to hemolysis if challenged by large doses of a drug such as the commonly used phenacetin or by modest doses of a drug such as phenylhydrazine with high oxidizing potential. It seems likely that this type of drug-induced hemolysis of normal aging red cells would be accentuated in the presence of infection or of diabetic acidosis. This potential hazard should be kept in mind by the physician as he estimates the risk of contemplated therapy in many clinical situations.

Other Deficiencies Related to the HMP Pathway

Deficiency of 6-phosphogluconate dehydrogenase has been the subject of recent studies revealing genetic polymorphism with respect to this enzyme; relationship to hemolysis is not yet clear.

Glutathione reductase deficiency, inherited as an autosomal dominant trait, is found in leukocytes and platelets as well as in red cells, and is associated with hemolytic anemia, thrombocytopenia, and, in some cases, with leukopenia. A neurologic disorder characterized by spasticity may develop in these patients. Use of oxidant drugs may cause severe pancytopenia. The enzyme deficiency may be corrected by oral administration of 5 mg of riboflavin daily, at least in some cases.

Deficiency of red cell glutathione with an associated chronic hemolytic state may be caused by deficiency in either of the two enzymes involved in synthesis of glutathione, γ-glutamyl-cysteine synthetase or glutathione synthetase. Both types of enzyme deficiency probably are inherited as autosomal recessive traits. Use of potentially oxidant drugs causes acceleration of hemolysis in persons with deficiency of red cell glutathione synthetase; comparable observations are not yet reported in persons having deficiency of red cell γ-glutamyl-cysteine synthetase. Deficiency of the latter enzyme is associated with chronic neurologic disease in the cases reported, but relationship between the degenerative neurologic disorder and the enzyme deficiency is not established.

Deficiency of red cell glutathione peroxidase is associated with relatively mild hemolytic states. Since this enzyme normally helps to prevent peroxidative injury, increased susceptibility to hemolysis after use of oxidant drugs is anticipated and has been demonstrated in one presumably homozygously deficient patient. Available data suggest that this deficiency is most likely an autosomal recessive trait.

OTHER INTRACORPUSCULAR ABNORMALITIES

The hemoglobinopathies and thalassemias, some of which are associated with a hemolytic state, are considered in Ch. 746 to 751. It is noteworthy that the Heinz body anemias associated with unstable hemoglobins usually are detectable by the simple procedure of heating hemolysates at 50° C for one to two hours. The resulting turbidity owing to precipitation of unstable hemoglobin is not observed in the Heinz body anemias associated with deficiency in enzyme activity related to the HMP shunt pathway.

Patients have been described with hemolytic anemia associated with low ATP concentration in the red cells and very high glycolytic rate. The cause of increased ATP utilization by the cells is unknown. Several different types of red cells have been described with high ATP concentration but without an associated hemolytic state. In one patient with high ATP concentration and deficiency of ribosephosphate pyrophosphokinase, chronic hemolysis was documented. Examples of hemolytic anemia have been reported in association with ATPase deficiency in the red cells, probably as an autosomal dominant trait.

A large share of patients with erythropoietic porphyria have hemolytic anemia which is relieved to varying degree by splenectomy. Improvement both in the hemolytic state and in photosensitivity after splenectomy may be marked.

Other types of hereditary abnormalities of the red cell associated with hemolysis are not easily classified. An example is the hemolytic anemia associated with increased red cell content of lecithin (phosphatidyl choline) probably inherited by an autosomal dominant pattern.

General

Dacie, J. V.: The Haemolytic Anaemias: Congenital and Acquired. 2nd ed. Parts 1, 2, 3, and 4. London and New York, J. & A. Churchill, Ltd., and Grune & Stratton, 1960–1967.
Harris, J. W., and Kellermeyer, R. W.: The Red Cell. Production, Metabolism, Destruction: Normal and Abnormal. Revised ed. Cambridge, Mass., Harvard University Press, 1970, pp. 517–593.
Singer, D. B.: Postsplenectomy sepsis. *In* Rosenbert, H. S., and Bolande, R. P. (eds.): Perspectives in Pediatric Pathology. Chicago, Year Book Medical Publishers, 1973, 1:285, 1973.
Weed, R. I. (ed.): Hematology for Internists. Boston, Little, Brown & Company, 1971, pp. 49–127.
Williams, W. J., Beutler, E., Erslev, A. J., and Rundles, R. W. (eds.): Hematology. New York, McGraw-Hill Book Company, 1972. pp. 381–409, 460–474.

Specific Hemolytic States

Beutler, E.: Abnormalities of the hexose monophosphate shunt. Semin. Hematol., 8:311, 1971.
Konrad, P. N., Richards, F., II, Valentine, W. N., and Paglia, E. D.: γ-Glutamyl-cysteine synthetase deficiency: A cause of hereditary hemolytic anemias. N. Engl. J. Med., 286:557, 1972.
Rosse, W. F.: Variations in the red cells in paroxysmal nocturnal haemoglobinuria. Br. J. Haematol., 24:327, 1973.
Valentine, W. N.: Hereditary enzymatic deficiencies of erythrocytes. Introduction. Deficiencies associated with Embden-Meyerhof pathway and other metabolic pathways. Semin. Hematol., 8:307, 348, 1971.

EXTRACORPUSCULAR MECHANISMS

Wendell F. Rosse

741. INTRODUCTION

Hemolysis not resulting from intrinsic defects of the red cell itself may be caused by a variety of abnormalities. In some instances, this is the only manifestation of disease; more frequently it is secondary to some other pathologic process which adversely affects the ability of the red cell to survive. The general manifestations of the hemolytic anemia resulting from extracorporeal causes do not differ from those for hemolysis resulting from intracorpuscular lesions, which are discussed in Ch. 740.

742. HEMOLYSIS DUE TO IMMUNE MECHANISMS

Alteration of the red cell membrane by immunologic reactions is one of the more common mechanisms by which the life span of the red cell may be shortened. These immune processes are usually initiated by IgG or IgM immunoglobulins; the diagnosis often depends upon demonstration of an antibody on the cells or in the serum of the patient.

Antibodies may sometimes be demonstrated by ability to agglutinate the cells. This is effected by the fixation of one antigen binding site of the antibody molecule on one cell and the other on another cell. When several cells are thus bound together, an agglutinate forms. IgM molecules are able to do this readily, because they are large enough to bridge the distance imposed by forces responsible for mutual repulsion of the red cells (the "zeta potential"). Many IgG antibodies cannot directly agglutinate, because they are not able to bridge this distance. Their presence on the red cell surface is often detected by the addition of antibodies directed against antigens present on the antibody molecules (*antiglobulin reaction; Coombs' reaction*). These heterologous antibodies are able to react with IgG antibodies on two red cells, thus linking the cells and forming the agglutinate. This reaction has immeasurably increased our ability to define immunologic reactions involving red cells.

The mechanisms by which immune reactions effect hemolysis depend upon the nature of the antibody, its interaction with antigen, and its ability to fix complement. When most IgG antibodies interact with red cell antigens, an area changes in the heavy chain portion of the molecule which permits it to interact with receptor sites on phagocytic cells, neutrophils, and macrophages (monocytes). The red cell may thus be held in place, and the whole cell or a portion of the membrane may be ingested; the remaining membrane may reseal across the defect, and the resulting cell fragment is capable of escaping from the phagocyte. Since it has lost more membrane than contents, the red cell must assume the shape of a spherocyte.

The spleen plays an important role in hemolysis by this mechanism. Because of peculiarities of its circulation and the rich layer of phagocytic cells lining the sinusoids, it is the chief site of interaction between macrophages and red cells with IgG antibody on the surface. In addition, those spherocytes which survive the initial interaction are rigid and on subsequent circulation through the spleen may be trapped and destroyed in the fine interstices. However, even when the spleen is removed, if sufficient antibody is present, the cells may be destroyed in other parts of the reticuloendothelial system.

Red cells may be destroyed because of fixation of complement. The complement sequence is initiated when two IgG antibody molecules or one IgM antibody molecule react with two antigen sites in close proximity to one another. This fixes a molecule of the first component of complement (C1), which acts upon the fourth component (C4) which may be then firmly affixed to the red cell surface. The second component, also activated by C1, is affixed to the fourth component, and this combination is able to activate a third component (C3) which is also fixed to the membrane. The fixed, active C3 molecule may interact with membrane receptors on phagocytic cells different from those interacting with IgG. This allows the phagocytic cell to ingest either a portion of the membrane or, more commonly, the entire cell. Such phagocytosis may be prevented by an enzyme which cleaves the C3 molecule, leaving an inactive portion of the molecule on the red cell membrane; it is this fragment which is usually detected by anti-C3 antiserum in an antiglobulin (Coombs) reaction like that used to detect IgG antibodies.

The active C3 molecule on the red cell membrane is able to propagate the complement sequence; if the sequence is successfully completed, disruption of the membrane occurs and intravascular hemolysis follows. For reasons not clearly understood, the completion of the complement sequence is singularly inefficient on normal human red cells, and therefore intravascular hemolysis is uncommon in immune hemolytic anemia, except under unusual circumstances.

The hematologic manifestations and the mechanism of destruction depend in large part upon the nature of the antibody initiating the immune reaction. Although many classifications could be constructed according to the various properties of the antibodies, it has been found most convenient to classify the syndromes by whether the antibody is able to react with the cell at body temperature (*warm-reacting antibodies*) or only at reduced temperatures (*cold-reacting antibodies*).

Antibodies may also be classified as isoimmune and autoimmune. The former arise in response to antigens not present on the red cells of the patient. Autoimmune antibodies react with antigens of the patient's own red cells. This distinction is usually relatively simple to make in the untransfused patient, because the direct antiglobulin test will be negative if the antibodies are isoimmune and positive if the antibodies are autoimmune. In complex clinical situations in which transfusion has taken place, this distinction may be more difficult.

HEMOLYSIS DUE TO WARM-REACTING ANTIBODIES

Warm-reacting antibodies are those capable of reacting with the red cell antigens at 37° C. They may or may not fix complement, depending upon the spacing of the antigen sites with which they interact and the immunoglobulin subclass of the antibody. In some instances, the antibody is not readily detectable on the red cell membrane by the antiglobulin test, but fixed complement components indicate that the immune reaction has taken place.

Hemolysis Due to Isoimmune Antibodies

Transfusion Reactions

See Part XVI, Section Three.

Hemolytic Disease of the Newborn

Hemolytic disease of the newborn is due to the transplacental infusion of isoimmune antibodies from the mother to the infant when the infant's red cells contain an antigen against which they may react. The antibody is, in most instances, formed in the mother in response to the prior transplacental transfer of "incompatible" red cells from that infant or previous infants, with the resultant production of isoimmune antibodies; occasionally, prior transfusion may be the cause of maternal sensitization. Hemolytic anemia in the infant results from the interaction of the maternal antibody and the infant's red cells.

Clinical Manifestations. The clinical manifestations are dependent in part upon the degree of sensitization of the mother, the immunoglobulin class of the antibody, and the antigen with which the antibody is reacting. In its most severe manifestations, the infant is born with anasarca, marked anemia, and hepatosplenomegaly; such infants rarely survive. In other instances, marked hemolytic anemia with jaundice may result. The anemia may persist for days to weeks. If appropriate treatment is instituted quickly, the resultant outcome is usually good; in some instances of marked sensitization, the infant is delivered prematurely in order to institute treatment. Where there is lesser sensitization, the extent of hemolytic anemia may be minimal.

Diagnosis. Hemolytic disease of the newborn is usually diagnosed by finding a positive direct antiglobulin test on the cells of the infant. The antibody may be eluted and its specificity determined. Occurrence of the illness may be anticipated by demonstration of an isoantibody in the mother's serum before birth where a rising titer may be assumed to indicate increasing sensitization and therefore increased chance of severe hemolysis. In some instances, prenatal hemolytic anemia is diagnosed by examination of the amniotic fluid for bilirubin-like catabolic products.

Prevention and Treatment. The chief complications of hemolytic disease of the newborn are anemia and excessive bilirubinemia, leading to kernicterus. The standard treatment is exchange transfusion. More recently, exposure of the infant to ultraviolet light has been shown to lower the bilirubin level and reduce the number of exchange transfusions needed.

Since most of the transplacental infusion of fetal cells into the mother occurs at birth, it has been found possible to prevent sensitization of the Rh_0 (D) negative mother to the Rh_0 (D) antigen by injection of a large quantity of anti Rh_0 (anti-D) antibody shortly after parturition. Any cells that have leaked from the fetus to the mother are destroyed by the injected antibody, and sensitization of the mother does not occur. Clearly, this preventive treatment does not work if the mother has been previously sensitized by other pregnancies or by transfusion.

Hemolysis Due to Autoimmune Antibodies

When the antibody is directed against an antigen on the red cells of the host (autoimmune hemolytic anemia), the warm-reacting antibodies are usually IgG; although IgM and IgA antibodies have been described, their pathogenetic role is unclear. In approximately two thirds of the instances, the IgG antibodies will fix complement; when complement is not fixed, the antibody usually has specificity for the Rh locus of one of its antigens.

The hemolytic anemia which results may vary greatly in intensity. Usually the amount of hemolysis is related to the amount of antibody detectable on the red cell surface, but this is not clearly the case in some instances. In approximately one instance in fifty, immunoglobulin may not be detected on the red cell surface (*Coombs-negative immune hemolytic anemia*). In general, an antibody fixing complement probably causes a greater degree of hemolysis than one which does not.

Approximately one third of the time, there may be no other manifestation of disease, except perhaps for immune thrombocytopenia. In the remaining half to two thirds of the instances, an underlying disease may be defined at the time of the initial diagnosis or during the clinical course. The most common diseases associated with immune hemolytic anemia of the warm antibody type are *chronic lymphocytic leukemia* and *lymphoma* or *systemic lupus erythematosus.* It may be seen with other immune system diseases such as the *Wiskott-Aldrich syndrome, agammaglobulinemia,* and *malignant thymoma,* as well as a variety of other syndromes such as *rheumatoid arthritis, systemic sclerosis,* or *ulcerative colitis.*

Clinical Manifestations. The degree of hemolysis varies from patient to patient. In its classic presentation, immune hemolytic anemia is rapid in onset; well-documented instances of the development of severe anemia within a few days have been seen. The anemia can be so severe as to be fatal if not competently treated. The spleen is frequently enlarged and may vary in size according to the degree of hemolysis. The liver is less commonly enlarged. Jaundice and pallor may be present. The peripheral blood frequently shows spherocytosis and marked reticulocytosis; however, considerable hemolysis can take place in the absence of spherocytes. The white blood count may be elevated slightly. Hemoglobinemia may be chemically detectable, but hemoglobinuria is rare. There are few other manifestations associated with the anemia itself, although, if it is secondary to some underlying disease, symptoms of that disease may be manifest.

Diagnosis. The diagnosis usually depends upon the demonstration of immunoglobulins or components of complement on the red cells of the patient. This is usually done with specific antisera containing only antibodies against IgG or the inactive fragment of the third component of complement (C3). Tests with these reagents may reveal the presence of either or both on the surface. When complement alone is found, further efforts must be made to demonstrate the antibody. Cooling the cells to 4° C may reveal an IgG antibody on the surface (*cold-detectable antibody*) capable of reacting with the cell at 37° C but detectable only at reduced temperature. An antibody of low affinity may be detected in the serum, using papainized normal cells to increase the interaction of the antigen and antibody. The antibody may rarely be IgM or IgA, and specific anti-IgM or anti-IgA antisera may be needed to reveal its presence. The antibody may be cold reactive or drug related, and appropriate steps will be needed to reveal its presence, as described later in this chapter (Diagnosis) and in Ch. 744.

Treatment. The initial treatment of autoimmune hemolytic anemia caused by IgG warm-reacting antibodies is prednisone. In general, 1 mg per kilogram per day in divided doses is sufficient for initial therapy. If response to this dose of the drug is seen in elevation of the hematocrit, the amount of prednisone being administered can be rapidly tapered to approximately 0.3 mg per kilogram per day. Thereafter the dose may be tapered more slowly, at about the rate of 5 mg per day each month. In many instances of immune hemolytic anemia in childhood, remission occurs and prednisone may be omitted entirely; however, in adults, this is unusual, and great caution must be used in discontinuing prednisone completely. Many patients will maintain total remission on 2.5 to 10 mg per day; alternate-day dosage appears to be as good as daily dosage and may be attended by less severe side effects.

The mode of action of prednisone is not clear but appears to be multiple. Evidence has been adduced that it causes the removal of antibody from the red cell membrane when given in high doses. This effect appears to account for many of the instances of rapid remission obtained with the drug. In addition, it appears to suppress the production of antibody in two to three weeks in those patients achieving remission which can be maintained on small doses. Finally, it is thought that prednisone can interfere with sequestration of cells by the reticuloendothelial system. The basic mechanism of any of these actions is not known.

If prednisone is unsuccessful in initial therapy or if the dose of prednisone required to maintain remission is too high, other measures must be sought. In general, these consist of *immunosuppression* by other drugs (azathioprine, 100 to 150 mg per day; cyclophosphamide, 50 to 100 mg per day) or splenectomy. *Splenectomy* is generally preferred in younger patients, whereas in older patients immunosuppression may be wiser. If one of these treatments fails to bring about an adequate remission, the other method may be required. Seldom is a patient resistant to a combination of prednisone, immunosuppression, and splenectomy.

Transfusion may be necessary during the acute hemolytic phase of the disease. This is often attended by difficulty because of problems in obtaining an adequate cross-match; however, if it is clinically indicated, a transfusion that is not appropriately cross-matched is preferable to having the patient succumb to the anemia. The best chance of a proper cross-match is obtained if the antibody is isolated, either from eluates or from the serum, to determine whether specificity exists and, if it does, in selecting units of blood which are compatible. If the specificity cannot be identified, the blood bank is often obliged to test the patient's serum against all units of blood available of the appropriate type to determine which are optimal. When this procedure is carefully performed, few transfusion reactions will occur; however, one must be cautious about the simultaneous presence of isoantibody in addition to the autoimmune antibody.

HEMOLYSIS DUE TO COLD-REACTING ANTIBODIES

The term *"cold-reacting antibodies"* is probably a misnomer, because it has recently been shown that when the antigens against which these antibodies interact are isolated in vitro, interaction between antigen and antibody can occur at any temperature, including 37° C. Antigens against which these antibodies interact are located on a species of glycoprotein on the red cell surface; the placement of the antigen is probably temperature dependent such that in the warm, it is not available for interaction.

The fact that these antibodies are unable to interact with the red cell at 37° C means that the mode of destruction cannot be mediated by antibody (see above); since these antibodies are able to fix complement, complement is responsible for the hemolysis.

Cold Agglutinin Syndrome

The cold agglutinin syndrome is due to antibodies, usually IgM, which are able to act at reduced temperature and cause agglutination of the red cells. The presence of the antibody is readily demonstrable in the serum of the patient; the serum may on occasion be diluted several thousand fold and still be able to agglutinate red cells.

The antigens with which these antibodies interact are of three general sorts, called "I", "i," and "Pr." The *"I" antigens* are those which are most strongly expressed on adult cells; the *"i" antigens* are most strongly expressed on cells of newborn infants and of rare adults; the *"Pr" antigens* are equally well expressed on both cells and are destroyed by neuraminidase. The antigens are polysaccharide in nature, and some of them appear to be related to the polysaccharides of the ABH and Lewis groups.

The maximal temperature at which the antibody interacts with the red cell is variable. Since the interaction in vivo of antigen and antibody depends upon lowering the temperature of the blood below 37° C in the peripheral areas (arms, legs, and appendages), those antibodies which are able to interact at higher temperatures will, in general, have a greater opportunity to cause hemolysis than those which react only at lower temperatures.

Clinical Manifestations. The clinical manifestations of the cold agglutinin syndrome are due to two phenomena: (1) intravascular agglutination, which occurs when blood is cooled in peripheral parts of the body, and (2) hemolytic anemia, which occurs consequent upon the fixation of complement. Upon exposure to cold, patients with cold agglutinin syndrome may note that the hands, ears, nose, or feet may turn purple and become painful; this process is rapidly reversed upon rewarming and is distinguished from Raynaud's phenomenon in that there is no blanching phase and little evidence of hyperemia. If the symptoms of agglutination are sufficiently severe, pain may result upon breathing cold air or eating cold food, or from so small a stimulus as holding a glass of ice water.

The hemolytic anemia which accompanies cold agglutinin syndrome is rarely severe. Usually the patient has moderate hemolytic anemia which is exacerbated during the winter. The spleen may or may not be enlarged. Spherocytosis is usually absent. If the patient is exposed to severe chilling, he may have a sudden bout of hemolysis with consequent hemoglobinemia and hemoglobinuria. In some whose antibody has a high thermal amplitude, the anemia may be severe even when the patient is carefully protected from the cold; these people may require transfusion.

Cold agglutinin syndrome is seen in two major clinical settings: (1) *chronic cold agglutinin disease* of the elderly and (2) *postinfectious cold agglutinin syndrome*. Chronic cold agglutinin disease of the elderly is characterized by a gradual onset of symptoms and a chronic course. The antibody seen is usually monoclonal and is nearly always of the κ light chain type. Some patients with this syndrome have been found to have lymphoma; this is particularly true when the antibody is anti-i.

Postinfectious cold agglutinin syndrome usually follows infection with *Mycoplasma pneumoniae* (in which case the antibody is anti-I) or *infectious mononucleosis* (in which case the antibody is anti-i). Antibodies in these instances are not monoclonal, as in the chronic idiopathic type, but may be restricted in their molecular variation. The antibodies in infectious mononucleosis are highly variable; some may even be IgG. Although most patients with either Mycoplasma infection or mononucleosis may have a rise in the titer of the cold agglutinins in their serum, reaching a peak two to three weeks after onset of the illness, clinically manifest hemolytic anemia is uncommon, usually only when the amount of antibody is very great. The course of the illness is self-limited, and all manifestations usually disappear within two to three months.

Diagnosis. The presence of cold agglutinins is often suspected by casual observation of an anticoagulated sample of blood at room temperature. The sample may appear to be coagulated or show marked clumping, which disappears when warmed to 37° C. This is more rigorously tested by diluting the serum and testing it against normal adult and newborn cells; in some instances dilutions as high as 1 in 100,000 may cause agglutination.

The patient's cells invariably have on them relatively large amounts of the inactive fragment of the third component of complement which is detectable with antiglobulin reagents containing anti-C3. The reaction with anti-IgG is negative. The hemolytic ability of the antibody may also be tested by appropriate in vitro reactions.

Treatment. The treatment of chronic cold agglutinin disease is usually simplified if the patient is able to avoid cold exposure during the winter months. This may require near-incarceration in heated rooms and wearing heavy, warm clothes. Sometimes it may require traveling to warmer climates. If this is insufficient or not possible, treatment with chlorambucil (2 mg per day) has been suggested. In general, little benefit results from treatment with prednisone or splenectomy.

Paroxysmal Cold Hemoglobinuria

Paroxysmal cold hemoglobinuria was the first hemolytic disease to be specifically defined. It formerly was encountered in patients with syphilis; it now more commonly occurs as an autoimmune or postviral disease. The antibody is IgG in type and reacts with the P blood group antigen which is possessed by nearly all red cells. For reasons not clearly understood, the antibody is able to effect marked lysis by complement. This is detectable clinically by episodes of hemoglobinemia and hemoglobinuria after exposure to cold and is detected in vitro by the *Donath-Landsteiner test,* by which the syndrome is frequently diagnosed. In some instances, the syndrome may be so severe as to threaten life; this usually occurs after viral infection in children. Paroxysmal cold hemoglobinuria is treated by protection from exposure to cold, by prednisone, and by cyclophosphamide, just as any other IgG antibody syndrome.

743. FRAGMENTATION HEMOLYTIC ANEMIA

The membrane of the normal red cell is readily deformable but with limits to its elasticity. When sufficient shear stress is placed upon the cell, it undergoes progressive deformation and, eventually, membrane rupture. The amount of shear stress required has been estimated at about 3000 dynes per square centimeter. Such stresses do not occur in the normal circulation, because the vessels of the circulatory system are designed to allow the smooth passage of the blood, and the turbulence of the blood passing through the normal heart does not generate forces of this magnitude. However, such shear stress forces may be generated when abnormalities occur in the circulatory system, and fragmentation of the red cells may result. The characteristic red cell fragments resulting from this phenomenon are called *schistocytes;* these usually have sharp points and have been called *"helmet" cells, "triangle" cells,* and other similar names.

Fragmentation within the circulation occurs in two general clinical situations: (1) when intravascular fibrinous coagulation or abnormalities of the vessel walls in small arterioles cause irregularities upon which red cells may be fragmented, much as cells may be fragmented by being pushed through a fine wire screen, and (2) when alterations in the heart and major vessels occur such that turbulence and other factors yield shear stress forces sufficient to fragment the red cells.

HEMOLYSIS DUE TO ABNORMALITIES OF THE MICROCIRCULATION
(Microangiopathic Hemolytic Anemia)

The first clear-cut description of fragmentation hemolytic anemia in patients in whom abnormalities of the arterioles could be demonstrated was in 1963 by Brain, Dacie, and Hourihane. They named the syndrome "microangiopathic hemolytic anemia." The mechanism of this hemolysis was elucidated by members of the same group, using an artificial circulatory system. They demonstrated that if blood were pumped through a bed of fibers of sufficiently small diameter so that the red cells could be looped over the fibers like clothes hung on a clothesline (without clothespins) and if sufficient force were applied as pressure, the cells would be severed by the strand much as a wire cheese knife cuts cheese. Since the opposite sides of the membrane were brought into apposition, they were sometimes able to reseal and the fragment was able to float away.

Fragmentation in vivo results when threads of sufficiently small size (usually fibrin) occur in the arteriolar side of the circulation where the blood pressure provides sufficient force to fragment the cells. The accompanying table lists some of the clinical states in which this occurs.

In many instances, there is a greater or lesser degree of intravascular coagulation. When the primary defect appears to be arteriolar damage, the amount of intravascular coagulation demonstrable by a diminution in procoagulants may be small or even absent. On the other hand, when intravascular coagulation is the major event and occurs on both the arteriolar and venous sides, marked diminution in procoagulants may be present with only minor amounts of fragmentation hemolysis.

Clinical Manifestations. The degree of hemolysis may vary, depending upon the underlying process. Fragmentation hemolysis occurs in malignant hypertension, usually only when renal failure and papilledema are present; pathologically the kidneys usually show fibrinoid necrosis. The fragmentation hemolysis in carcinoma is usually seen only in adenocarcinoma and then only when widely metastatic; the degree of hemolysis may be considerable. The hemolysis in vasculitic lesions (e.g., Rocky Mountain spotted fever, periarteritis nodosa, Wegener's granulomatosis) is generally relatively minor, and the major manifestations are those of the underlying disease.

Diagnosis. The diagnosis of fragmentation hemolysis is made by the demonstration of schistocytic forms in the peripheral blood. Evidences of intravascular hemolysis (increased plasma hemoglobin and lactic acid dehydrogenase, urine hemosiderin, and, perhaps, urine hemoglobin) are usually present. Ancillary evidence may include evidence of disseminated intravascular coagulation (see Ch. 801).

Treatment. Treatment of fragmentation hemolysis depends in large part on the management of the underlying lesion. Reduction in blood pressure in malignant hypertension will reduce the rate of fragmentation hemolysis. Resolution of the septic shock or the Rocky Mountain spotted fever will also end the hemolytic episode. Irradiation or removal of vascular abnormalities (giant hemangioma, traumatic arteriovenous fistula) will usually end the hemolytic process. In those instances in which intravascular coagulation plays a major role, treatment with heparin may be of value. Heparin does not appear to be of value in widely metastatic carcinoma.

HEMOLYSIS DUE TO ABNORMALITY OF THE HEART AND GREAT VESSELS
(Traumatic Cardiac Hemolytic Anemia)

Abnormalities of the heart and great vessels may lead to such degrees of turbulence that fragmentation may occur. The resultant hemolytic anemia is in general mild. Instances of fragmentation hemolysis have been described in aortic stenosis, ruptured sinus of Valsalva, congenital stenosis of the aorta, traumatic arteriovenous fistula, marked aortic regurgitation, and marked tachycardia. In general, only lesions of the left side of the heart and general circulation lead to traumatic fragmentation hemolysis, because only on that side are the shear stress forces of sufficient strength.

When prosthetic devices are inserted into the heart or great vessels, fragmentation hemolysis is frequent. In one large series, 60 to 80 per cent of all patients with prosthetic aortic or mitral valves demonstrated clinically significant hemolysis. Patients with both aortic and mitral prostheses are more likely to have hemolysis than are those with only one.

Causes of "Microangiopathic" Fragmentation Hemolysis

Vascular abnormality predominant:
1. Thrombotic thrombocytopenic purpura (hemolytic-uremic syndrome)
2. Renal lesions
   a. Malignant hypertension
   b. Glomerulonephritis
   c. Transplant rejection
   d. Preeclampsia
3. Vasculitis
   a. Polyarteritis nodosa
   b. Rocky Mountain spotted fever
   c. Wegener's granulomatosis
4. Vascular anomalies
   a. Giant cavernous hemangioma (Kasabach-Merritt syndrome)
   b. Arteriovenous fistula

Intravascular coagulation predominant:
1. Septicemia with shock
2. Abruptio placentae

A frequent cause of severe hemolysis is regurgitation around the outside of the valve owing to poor seating; this is particularly common in prosthetic aortic valves. The material of which the valve is composed is of some importance; cloth-covered valves tend to give more hemolysis than others, and those with steel balls show less hemolysis than those with Silastic balls. When variance of the Silastic ball occurs, increased hemolysis may result. In general, increased hemolysis occurs in situations of increased turbulence, as when large quantities of blood are forced through small apertures by high pressure.

Fragmentation hemolysis may also occur after surgery for correction of the ostium primum defect with a patch. In certain instances, the defect in the mitral valve is insufficiently closed, and blood regurgitates forcefully against the patch. When this occurs, epithelialization of the patch may be prevented, and since the surface is relatively rougher than the endothelium, the forceful jet of blood may create forces sufficient to fragment the cells.

Clinical Manifestations. The degree of hemolysis is variable from patient to patient, depending upon the underlying abnormality. In a given patient the amount of hemolysis tends to vary with the cardiac output. Hence patients tend to have more hemolysis during the daytime when active than at night. If the patient becomes markedly anemic, in compensation the cardiac output is raised and the degree of hemolysis may increase. This may be manifest to the patient as increasing hemoglobinuria.

As in all chronic intravascular hemolysis, considerable iron is lost into the urine as hemosiderin and hemoglobin. Hence the patients may become iron deficient, thus suppressing erythropoiesis. This will lead to more severe anemia which will lead to an increase in cardiac output and thus more severe hemolysis.

Treatment. All patients with evidences of fragmentation hemolysis ought to be given iron supplementation (ferrous sulfate, 300 mg three times a day). When the degree of hemolysis is severe, parenteral iron therapy with iron-dextran may be needed. Transfusion may be required. However, if chronic transfusion is necessary, some consideration should be given to replacement of the valve if, as is usually the case, some defect in the valve placement is present. When hemolysis is due to a patch on an ostium primum defect, it may be necessary to replace the patch and further to replace the mitral valve so that regurgitation against the patch does not occur.

In those instances of traumatic fragmentation hemolysis in which no prosthesis has been inserted, the hemolysis is usually not severe enough to require treatment.

MARCH HEMOGLOBINURIA

March hemoglobinuria was first described in 1881 in an infantryman in the Prussian army who, after long marches, noted passage of dark urine. Since that time, many instances of hemoglobinuria occurring after running or after repeated trauma to some part of the body have been described. *Marathon runners* commonly demonstrate this syndrome, especially those with a stomping gait or those who run barefoot or in poorly cushioned shoes. *Karate experts* who practice their art by repeatedly striking their hand against hard surfaces, *pelota players, bongo drummers,* and *patients who strike their heads* repeatedly against the wall have all been found to have hemolysis as a result of their particular activity.

The red cells do not appear to be abnormal. The hemolysis apparently occurs because the red cells are forceably smashed within the microcirculation when the body part is struck against a hard surface or object. The cells may be popped like a balloon, and schistocytes are rarely if ever seen. The syndrome can be stopped by altering the activity so that forceable striking of a body part does not occur; e.g., marathon runners may be advised to use cushioned shoes or to alter their gait.

Clinical Manifestations. The patient commonly notes dark urine immediately after the activity; it generally clears by the second or third voiding. Anemia seldom occurs, and no other serious side effects, save for the fright of seeing dark urine, have been noted.

744. HEMOLYSIS DUE TO ALTERATIONS OF THE RED CELLS BY EXOGENOUS MATERIALS

During the normal circulation of red cells, the red cell membrane is not appreciably altered in such a way as to effect hemolysis until 120 days are reached. However, certain alterations in the environment have been defined which can alter the red cell membrane and shorten the life span of the red cells.

DRUGS

Drugs and other chemicals may diminish the life span of the red cell in several ways: (1) they may interact directly with the membrane of the normal cell, resulting in abnormalities which lead to hemolysis; (2) they may stimulate the formation of antibodies which then lead to the destruction of the red cell; or (3) they may effect certain reactions which are not usually toxic for the normal red cell but are injurious to red cells deficient in detoxifying mechanisms, usually related to deficiencies of the hexose monophosphate shunt. Since these deficiencies are usually on a congenital basis (e.g., glucose-6-phosphate dehydrogenase deficiency), this form of hemolysis is considered elsewhere (see Ch. 740).

Drugs which cause hemolysis directly are few in number, because this effect is readily detected and the drugs are not used. *Amphotericin* may do so by its ability to interact with lipids of the membrane. Certain lipid solvents may interact with the membrane and bring about its dissolution. This form of hemolysis is probably rare.

Immune hemolysis initiated by drugs is more common. There are basically two types: (1) "autoimmune" hemolytic anemia, in which the drug induces an antibody which reacts with antigens normally present in the red cell, and (2) "immune" hemolytic anemia, in which the antibody formed is directed against the drug and the red cell is lysed as a consequence of the interaction between antibody and drug. In this latter group, the drug may be firmly fixed to the red cell membrane *(haptene-like reaction)* or only loosely attached to the membrane *("innocent bystander" reaction).*

"Autoimmune" drug-induced hemolysis is almost exclusively due to a single drug, α-*methyldopa (Aldomet),* although L-dopa and mefanemic acid have been implicated as well. After taking the drug for at least two to three months, about 5 to 10 per cent of all patients will have a positive indirect antiglobulin (Coombs) test caused by the presence of IgG antibody directed against components of the Rh complex locus; complement is almost never fixed. Antibody may be detected in the serum without addition of the drug to the test. In most patients, little if any hemolysis will result, but in a small proportion of patients taking the drug, significant hemolysis occurs. The syndrome produced is that of warm-reacting IgG antibody with spherocytosis, splenomegaly, and response to prednisone therapy, if its use becomes necessary. When the drug is stopped, the antibody usually disappears within two to three months, and the direct antiglobulin test reverts to negative. The reason a drug should stimulate production of an antibody capable of reacting with autologous red cell antigens is not clear.

Many drugs serving as haptens apparently stimulate the production of antibodies. These antibodies may be capable of destroying red cells as a result of their reaction with the drug. In some cases, the drug may be firmly attached to the red cell, as in the case of penicillin; in those instances, the IgG antibody will also be detectable on the red cell surface in the direct antiglobulin test. Since relatively small amounts of antibody are attached, complement is usually not fixed. In other instances, the drug is not firmly attached to the red cell. However, the interaction of drug and antibody results in the activation of complement at the red cell surface. If sufficient complement is fixed, hemolysis results, as outlined above. Since the initial steps of the immune reaction are not firmly associated with the red cell, antibody will not be detected on the direct antiglobulin test. In these reactions, the red cell has been called an "innocent bystander"; some doubt has been raised as to its complete innocence in this reaction.

Numerous drugs have been implicated in an "innocent bystander" reaction: *Fuadin* (an antischistosomal agent), *sulfonamides, quinidine, chlorpropamide,* and *thorazine,* to name a few. When the "innocent bystander" reaction is responsible for hemolysis, only complement will be present on the patients' cells (antibody having been washed away during the preparation of the cells for the test), and the indirect antiglobulin test will be positive only when the responsible drug is present in the reaction mixture.

MEMBRANE ALTERATION BY TOXIC SUBSTANCES

Toxins and Poisons

Toxic substances ("poisons") may bring about hemolysis by alteration of the membrane. These substances may be of animal origin, as in the case of hemolysis after snake bites or spider bites (see Ch. 57 and 59). In the former, phospholipases are thought to release the lipids of the membrane and destroy its integrity. Hemolysis, if present at all, is only a minor part of the complex clinical syndrome.

Some vegetable poisons such as *castor beans* and certain *mushrooms* may cause hemolysis. The mechanism of this has not been delineated. Certain minerals may also cause hemolysis, the best known of which is *copper.* This is thought to be the cause of the hemolysis which occasionally occurs in Wilson's disease. Its role has been very clearly demonstrated in patients undergoing dialysis in which the medium became so alkaline that copper salts were dissolved from the machine. The precise mechanism of its action is not clear; it may have to do with the fact that the copper ion is able to bind to the membrane sulfhydryl groups. Patients with *arsenical* intoxication sometimes have hemolytic anemia. Again, interference with the membrane structure is probably the cause, although the details have not been ascertained.

Failure of an Excretory Organ

The milieu in which the red cells circulate may be altered by failure of one of the excretory organs. When this occurs, some of the accumulated abnormal metabolites may alter the red cell membrane and result in hemolysis. With *liver failure,* commonly secondary to cirrhosis or alcoholic hepatitis, the red cells may become markedly overloaded with cholesterol. This at first leads to a spreading of the membrane, resulting in target cells which have a normal life span. However, if the process is further exaggerated and if the ratio of cholesterol to phospholipids is further altered, the membrane may become markedly abnormal, and a *spur cell,* a contracted, irregular cell fancifully resembling a spur for horses, may result. When this occurs, marked intravascular hemolysis may result.

Some patients with renal failure also exhibit hemolysis. The precise nature of the accumulated metabolite which is responsible for this phenomenon has not been demonstrated. In some instances, the defect may be demonstrated by an abnormal autohemolysis (sterile incubation) test.

Infectious Agents

Hemolysis is a frequent accompaniment of infections. This may be due to the fact that the infectious agent invades the red cell and directly effects its lysis. This most commonly occurs in malaria, particularly by *Plasmodium falciparum.* The sudden release of merozoites may result in sufficient hemolysis to cause hemoglobinuria *(blackwater fever).* The bacterial organism *Bartonella* may also invade the red cells and cause hemolysis.

Red cells may be altered indirectly by infections. In some instances, reactions may occur as the result of the infection which may result in immunologic damage to the cell. This is particularly true in cold agglutinin syndrome secondary to Mycoplasma or Epstein-Barr virus infections, but may also be found in bacterial and other viral infections as well. In these instances, the direct antiglobulin test will be positive.

Several infections with clostridial organisms causing gas gangrene may result in marked hemolysis; instances of hemolysis of all circulating red cells have been recorded. This is thought to be due to alteration of the membrane phospholipids by enzymes elaborated by the organisms, but this has not been proved. The red cells show marked spherocytosis, and readily apparent evidences of intravascular hemolysis are present. The occurrence of this complication usually indicates a very poor prognosis, although instances of recovery have been reported when the infection is adequately treated.

In other instances of infection of various sorts (e.g., *Salmonella, Neisseria, E. coli, D. pneumoniae*), hemolysis of a less dramatic degree may occur in the absence of evidence of immunologic reaction on the red cell membrane. This has been thought, as in the case of the clostridial infection, to be due to alteration of the membrane by the organism or some product elaborated by it; this theory remains to be proved.

745. HEMOLYSIS DUE TO OVERACTIVITY OF THE RETICULOENDOTHELIAL SYSTEM

Red cells are presumably destroyed normally in the reticuloendothelial system, although the causes and the details of this destruction are not known. In certain instances, overactivity of the reticuloendothelial system, resulting from either anatomic alteration or malignancy of its cells, has been thought to cause premature destruction of normal cells.

HYPERSPLENISM

See Ch. 788.

EOSINOPHILIC GRANULOMA SYNDROMES

See Part XVI, Section Ten.

Immune Hemolytic Anemia

Mollison, P. J.: Transfusion in Clinical Practice. 5th ed. Oxford, Blackwell Scientific Publications, 1973.
Pirofsky, S. M.: Autoimmunization and the Autoimmune Hemolytic Anemias. Baltimore, Williams & Wilkins Company, 1960.
Rosse, W. F., and Dacie, J. V.: Immune lysis of normal human and paroxysmal nocturnal hemoglobinuria (PNH) red blood cells. II. The role of complement components in the increased sensitivity of PNH red cells to immune lysis. J. Clin. Invest., 45:749, 1966.
Worlledge, S. M.: Immune drug-induced haemolytic anaemias. Semin. Hematol., 6:181, 1969.

Fragmentation Hemolysis

Brain, M. J.: Microangiopathic hemolytic anemia. Ann. Rev. Med., 21:133, 1970.
Bull, B. S., Rubenberg, M. L., Dacie, J. V., and Brain, M. C.: Microangiopathic haemolytic anaemia: Mechanisms of red-cell fragmentation. Br. J. Haematol., 14:643, 1968.
Davidson, R. J. L.: March or exertional hemoglobinuria. Semin. Hematol., 6:150, 1969.
Marsh, G. W., and Lewis, S. M.: Cardiac hemolytic anemia. Semin. Hematol., 6:133, 1969.

HEMOGLOBIN, THE HEMOGLOBINOPATHIES, AND THE THALASSEMIAS

C. Lockard Conley

746. INTRODUCTION

The primary role of the red cells is transport of oxygen, a function made possible by the hemoglobin within the erythrocytes. The amount of oxygen delivered by fully oxygenated blood is dependent not only on the hemoglobin content and rate of flow, but also on the affinity of the hemoglobin for oxygen at existing oxygen tensions. The effectiveness of hemoglobin in oxygen transport is the result of its variable oxygen affinity, a unique property dependent upon the tetrameric structure of the hemoglobin molecule.

The major hemoglobin component of the normal adult (Hb A) contains four polypeptide chains, two alpha chains each with 141 amino acid residues, and two beta chains each with 146 residues; it is designated $\alpha_2\beta_2$. A heme group containing an iron atom is affixed to each chain. A minor component comprising 2 to 3 per cent of the hemoglobin is designated Hb A_2, consisting of alpha and delta chains ($\alpha_2\delta_2$). The predominant hemoglobin of the fetus and newborn (Hb F) contains pairs of alpha and gamma chains ($\alpha_2\gamma_2$). There are multiple differences in amino acid sequences of beta, delta, and gamma chains, but the physiologic properties of the hemoglobins are similar. The fashion in which the globin chains and their heme groups are bonded together provides the iron atoms with precisely the environment necessary for reversible combination with oxygen. As oxygen is bound successively to each of the four iron atoms, stereochemical changes occur in the hemoglobin molecule that cause an increased affinity of the remaining iron atoms for oxygen. The sigmoid oxygen dissociation curve is the graphic representation of these relationships. Because of these allosteric effects, hemoglobin is fully oxygenated in the lungs even if the alveolar oxygen tension is appreciably less than normal; as oxygen is unloaded in the tissues, progressive reduction in the oxygen affinity of the hemoglobin provides for maximal delivery of oxygen with little change in oxygen tension.

OXYGEN AFFINITY OF THE RED CELLS

Pure hemoglobin has too high an affinity for oxygen to release appreciable amounts at normal tissue oxygen tensions. Within the red cell the oxygen affinity of the hemoglobin is modified by several mechanisms. Hydrogen ions stabilize the deoxy-state of hemoglobin, lessening oxygen affinity (Bohr effect). Carbon dioxide binds to hemoglobin and decreases its affinity for oxygen. Both these reactions facilitate release of oxygen in the tissue capillaries. Hemoglobin concentration in the erythrocyte influences oxygen affinity, with high values of the mean corpuscular hemoglobin concentration as-

sociated with lowered oxygen affinity. Certain phosphate compounds within the red cells significantly reduce the oxygen affinity of hemoglobin. Of these, 2,3-diphosphoglycerate (DPG) occurs in highest concentration (almost 1 mol per mol of hemoglobin), and is most important in regulation of oxygen dissociation. The deoxy-conformation of hemoglobin facilitates DPG binding to the beta chains, stabilizing this conformation and lessening oxygen affinity. Fetal hemoglobin binds less DPG than Hb A; therefore the oxygen affinity of red cells containing Hb F is higher than that of normal adult red cells, even though the oxygen dissociation curves of purified Hb A and Hb F are similar. The position of the oxygen dissociation curve is expressed as the P_{50}, the oxygen tension required to half-saturate the hemoglobin with oxygen. Because of its high concentration of Hb F, the blood of the fetus has a higher oxygen affinity than that of adult blood; the P_{50} is reduced and the oxygen dissociation curve is shifted to the left.

Each red cell produces its own DPG, an intermediate in glycolytic metabolism. The concentration of DPG within the red cell is markedly influenced by the environment of the erythrocyte. Anemia or anoxia causes the concentration of DPG within normal erythrocytes to rise. When normal red cells are transfused to anemic patients, the DPG level of the transfused red cells increases, demonstrating that the effect is initiated by extracellular mechanisms. In addition, alterations of DPG concentration may result from intrinsic disorders of the metabolism of the red cell; for example, in erythrocyte pyruvate kinase deficiency, DPG is usually elevated. The presence of DPG is largely responsible for reducing the oxygen affinity of the hemoglobin within normal red cells to a value appropriate for release of oxygen at tissue oxygen tensions. When the concentration of DPG rises, oxygen affinity is lessened, so that more oxygen is released in the tissues without a change in the tissue oxygen tension. This phenomenon is significant in adaptation to anoxia and anemia. In persons acclimatized to low oxygen tensions, as at high altitude, values for DPG are high, assuring that relatively large amounts of oxygen are released at tissue tensions even though the arterial blood is not fully saturated. The remarkable ability of patients with chronic severe anemia to tolerate extremely low concentrations of hemoglobin in the blood is largely attributable to the high values of DPG in the erythrocytes, permitting release of greatly increased amounts of oxygen per red cell at normal tissue oxygen tensions. These adaptive changes are promptly and effectively regulated, the oxygen affinity of red cells changing within hours after the onset of anemia or anoxia.

DEFINITIONS AND GENETIC CONSIDERATIONS

A *hemoglobinopathy* is an abnormality of hemoglobin synthesis manifested by the production of globin in which there is a structural abnormality. More than 180 genetically determined abnormalities of hemoglobin have been discovered. A separate gene determines the amino acid sequences of each of the globin chains. A single amino acid substitution in one type of polypeptide chain is accounted for by replacement of one nucleotide in an RNA codon. Thus the abnormality of sickle hemoglobin can be attributed to a change in a single purine base in the codon which specifies the sixth amino acid of the beta chain, with the result that glutamic acid is replaced by valine. Such a point mutation accounts for most of the inherited abnormalities of hemoglobin. Rarely two amino acid substitutions occur within a single polypeptide chain, as in Hb C Harlem. In certain abnormal hemoglobins, including Hb Gun Hill and Hb Freiburg, amino acid residues are missing from a globin chain, an abnormality that can be accounted for by loss of a segment of DNA ("deletion" of part of a gene) during nonhomologous crossing-over of genes. The hemoglobins Lepore contain the amino-terminal portion of the delta chain and the carboxy-terminal portion of the beta chain, an abnormal structure that can be explained by loss of DNA from portions of closely linked genes, with formation of a "fusion" gene. Hb Kenya contains the amino-terminal sequence of the gamma chain and the carboxy-terminal segment of the beta chain. Hb Constant Spring contains elongated alpha chains, an abnormality that may be explained by a mutation affecting a terminator codon. *Thalassemia* is an inherited impairment of hemoglobin synthesis caused by retarded production of a specific type of globin chain, not associated with a primary structural abnormality. The mechanism is not clearly understood, but is related to insufficiency of messenger RNA. *Hereditary persistence of fetal hemoglobin* is an anomaly occurring in several forms. In the type occurring in blacks, beta and delta chains are not produced at all, perhaps because of deletion of closely linked genes. Complete compensation for the deficit is achieved by synthesis of gamma chains, and the homozygous carrier has exclusively Hb F but no anemia or other clinical manifestations.

The hemoglobinopathies are inherited as autosomal codominant traits; heterozygous carriers have both the normal and the abnormal hemoglobin in each red cell. The normal component almost always constitutes the larger fraction. The genes that determine the structure of one class of globin chains are alleles; thus a person heterozygous for Hb S and Hb C, both of which contain abnormalities of the beta chain, has no Hb A and transmits one or the other but never both of the abnormal hemoglobins to each child. Thalassemia is inherited as if closely linked to the structural gene for the same chain. The beta and delta chain genes are closely linked, but the alpha chain gene segregates independently; accordingly a person heterozygous for both Hb G Philadelphia (an

Clinical Disorders Associated with Some Abnormal Hemoglobins

Disorder	Abnormal Hb	Structural Change		Electro-phoretic Mobility, Starch Alkaline pH*	Comments
Hemolytic anemia	S	beta 6	glu → val	−	Forms molecular aggregates when deoxygenated, producing sickle cell anemia in homozygotes
	C	beta 6	glu → lys	−	Low solubility lessens plasticity of red cells, causing hemolytic anemia in homozygotes
	D Punjab	beta 121	glu → gln	−	Mechanism unknown
	E	beta 26	glu → lys	−	
	Zürich	beta 63	his → arg	−	Unstable hemoglobin is precipitated by certain drugs, producing hemolytic anemia in heterozygotes
	Torino	alpha 43	phe → val	0	
	L Ferrarra	alpha 47	asp → gly	−	
	Hasharon	alpha 47	asp → his	−	
	Ann Arbor	alpha 80	leu → arg	−	
	Bibba	alpha 136	leu → pro	−	
	Leiden	beta 6 or 7	glu deleted	−	
	Savannah	beta 24	gly → val	−	
	Riverdale-Bronx	beta 24	gly → arg	−	
	Genova	beta 28	leu → pro	0	
	Abraham Lincoln	beta 32	leu → pro	0	
	Philly	beta 35	tyr → phe	0	
	Hammersmith	beta 42	phe → ser	0	
	Louisville	beta 42	phe → leu	0	Unstable hemoglobin causes chronic hemolytic anemia in heterozygotes; precipitated hemoglobin tends to form inclusion bodies within red cells, under certain conditions
	Toulouse	beta 66	lys → glu	−	
	Bristol	beta 67	val → asp	0	
	Sydney	beta 67	val → ala	−	
	Seattle	beta 70	ala → asp	0	
	Shepherd's Bush	beta 74	gly → asp	+	
	Santa Ana	beta 88	leu → pro	−	
	Borås	beta 88	leu → arg	−	
	Sabine	beta 91	leu → pro	−	
	Gun Hill	beta deletion of 5 residues between 91 and 97		−	
	Istanbul	beta 92	his → gln	−	
	Köln	beta 98	val → met	−	
	Casper	beta 106	leu → pro	0	

alpha chain variant) and Hb S (a beta chain variant) may transmit either, both, or neither of the abnormal hemoglobins to a child. The gamma chain gene appears to be duplicated, i.e., there are two gamma chain genes on one chromosome. The alpha chain gene also may be duplicated, at least in some individuals.

Hemoglobinopathies and thalassemias occur as a result of genetic mutations. Very high gene frequencies for harmful mutants are maintained in some areas of the world, presumably by strong selection pressures. Heterozygosity for Hb S appears to protect infants against the lethal effects of falciparum malaria, accounting for the maintenance of a high frequency of this deleterious abnormality in Africa. What selective advantage is conferred by Hb C in Africa, by Hb E in Southeast Asia, and by thalassemia in several parts of the world is unknown. New mutations account for a surprising number of the unstable hemoglobins; in these cases the abnormal hemoglobin is not detected in other members of the family.

Not all variations in hemoglobin are genetically determined. Increased levels of Hb F may occur in several acquired conditions, including pregnancy, aplastic anemia, leukemia, myeloproliferative disorders, and hemo-

lytic anemias. Hemoglobin A$_2$ may be increased in pernicious anemia and decreased in iron deficiency and aplastic anemia. Hemoglobins with abnormal electrophoretic mobility have been encountered in lead poisoning and diabetes, presumably as a result of chemical alterations in Hb A induced by the metabolic disturbance.

CLINICAL SYNDROMES ASSOCIATED WITH HEMOGLOBINOPATHIES

Substitutions of amino acids in the globin chains do not necessarily cause untoward effects, and most of the known abnormal hemoglobins are not associated with disease. Two types of clinically important abnormalities have been identified: (1) Replacements on the surface of the molecule may cause abnormal *intermolecular* reactions, phenomena which explain the pathologic effects of Hb S and Hb C. Individual molecules function satisfactorily, and the peculiar interactions between molecules tend to occur only with the high intraerythrocytic concentrations of the abnormal hemoglobin found in homozygotes. Therefore the disease appears to be

Clinical Disorders Associated with Some Abnormal Hemoglobins (*Continued*)

Disorder	Abnormal Hb	Structural Change		Electrophoretic Mobility, Starch Alkaline pH*	Comments
	Peterborough	beta 111	val → phe	0	
	Wien	beta 130	tyr → asp	0	
	Olmstead	beta 141	leu → arg	−	
	H	alpha$_2$beta$_2$ → beta$_4$		+	Unstable hemoglobin occurring in some forms of alpha thalassemia; precipitation of hemoglobin and hemolysis are accelerated by certain drugs
Cyanosis due to methemoglobinemia	M Boston	alpha 58	his → tyr	0	Methemoglobin causes cyanosis in heterozygotes; some also have evidence of hemolytic anemia
	M Iwate	alpha 87	his → tyr	0	
	M Milwaukee	beta 67	val → glu	0	
	M Saskatoon	beta 63	his → tyr	0	
	M Hyde Park	beta 92	his → tyr	−	
	Freiburg	beta 23	val deleted	−	
Cyanosis due to increased deoxyhemoglobin	Kansas	beta 102	asn → thr	−	Decreased oxygen affinity of hemoglobin causes cyanosis in heterozygotes
Erythrocytosis (polycythemia)	Chesapeake	alpha 92	arg → leu	+	Increased oxygen affinity of hemoglobin hinders release of oxygen to tissues, causing compensatory erythrocytosis in heterozygotes
	J Cape Town	alpha 92	arg → gln	+	
	Olympia	beta 20	val → met	0	
	Malmö	beta 97	his → gln	0	
	Yakima	beta 99	asp → his	−	
	Kempsey	beta 99	asp → asn	−	
	Ypsi	beta 99	asp → tyr	−	
	Brigham	beta 100	pro → leu	0	
	San Diego	beta 109	val → met	0	
	Little Rock	beta 143	his → glu	0	
	Rainier	beta 145	tyr → cys	0	
	Bethesda	beta 145	tyr → his	0	
	Hiroshima	beta 146	his → asp	+	
Hydrops fetalis	Bart's	alpha$_2$gamma$_2$ → gamma$_4$		+	Unstable hemoglobin with high oxygen affinity occurring in high concentration in stillborn fetuses with homozygous alpha thalassemia

*Symbols indicate relative mobility as compared with Hb A, less rapid (−), more rapid (+).

recessively inherited. When a red cell contains two major hemoglobin components (for example, Hb S and Hb C), interactions may occur that importantly influence the pathologic effects. (2) Replacements in critical areas of the molecule may lead to *intramolecular* abnormalities with resultant alteration in oxygen binding or in molecular stability. These effects are manifested in heterozygotes, and in some the homozygous state presumably would be lethal.

Amino acid substitutions are likely to impair molecular function or stability when they occur in the area in which the heme group is attached, when they distort the conformation of the molecule, or when they occur at points of interaction between the polypeptide chains. The net result may be formation of methemoglobin, alteration of oxygen affinity, denaturation of the hemoglobin, or a combination of these effects.

Most of the known variant hemoglobins were discovered because of abnormal electrophoretic mobility under usual conditions of measurement. The electrophoretic method continues to be useful, but many amino acid substitutions do not alter net charge on the molecule and may be electrophoretically neutral. A number of abnormal hemoglobins have the same electrophoretic pattern. The method therefore has important limitations in the detection as well as in the recognition of mutant hemoglobins. Other types of investigation, including detailed analysis of the functional properties of the hemoglobin, may be required for identification.

747. SICKLING DISORDERS

The single amino acid substitution in the beta chain in Hb S, located on the surface of the molecule, has no significant effect on oxygen affinity or molecular stability. It causes a unique *intermolecular* reaction in which molecules of deoxygenated Hb S align in spirally arranged polymers, forming insoluble fiber-like structures which distort the erythrocyte, increase its rigidity, and thereby cause the sickling deformation. The attractive forces between molecules operate only at short distances, so that the sickling phenomenon is markedly influenced by the concentration of deoxygenated Hb S in the red cell. Conditions influencing the intracellular concentration of deoxyhemoglobin, in particular oxygen tension and pH, are critical determinants of the degree of sickling. Sickling may be enhanced by the low oxygen affinity of the red cells of patients with sickle cell anemia; the low affinity is attributable in part to elevated values of 2,3-DPG and in part to the high concentration of hemoglobin in irreversibly sickled cells. Sickling is not instantaneous when hemoglobin is deoxygenated, so that duration of exposure of red cells to low oxygen tension is also a conditioning factor. Whether intravascular sickling occurs depends on local conditions of blood flow, oxygen tension, and pH; on the concentration of Hb S in the red cell; and on the presence in the erythrocyte of another hemoglobin which may interact with Hb S to lessen or enhance sickling. Except for irreversibly sickled cells, the number of which seems to be correlated with severity of disease, erythrocytes quickly resume their normal shape when the hemoglobin is reoxygenated.

Manifestations of disease attributable to Hb S are caused by intravascular sickling of partially deoxygenated erythrocytes. The rigid sickle cells tend to be tangled, trapped, and fragmented in small vascular channels; in addition, the cell membrane may be damaged by the sickling distortion. Both factors shorten red cell survival with predominant destruction of erythrocytes within the RE system. The unyielding elongate and crescentic cells increase the viscosity of the blood, retard flow, occlude small blood vessels, and produce infarcts and other lesions as a result of local anoxia.

SICKLE CELL ANEMIA

Definition. Sickle cell anemia, the clinical expression of homozygosity for Hb S, is a serious disease characterized by unrelenting hemolytic anemia, recurrent episodes of pain and fever, and pathologic involvement of many organs. Affected persons are predominantly blacks who have obtained the mutant gene from both parents. Since sickle cell trait occurs in about 8 per cent of American blacks, about 16 per 10,000 are expected to be homozygous at the time of conception; the actual incidence of sickle cell anemia is lower because of its high mortality. First described by J. B. Herrick in 1910, the disease is of unique historic significance. Study of the sickling phenomenon led Hahn and Gillespie in 1927 to discover that the distortion of the red cells is related to the state of oxygenation of the hemoglobin. Pauling and his associates in 1949 demonstrated the existence of an abnormal hemoglobin and developed the concept of "molecular" disease. Subsequently the investigations of Ingram and others showed that the abnormality in Hb S is limited to a single amino acid substitution within a polypeptide chain of globin. These discoveries initiated an unprecedented era of scientific advancement, with rapid evolution of knowledge pertaining to molecular biology, genetics, and pathophysiology.

Clinical Manifestations. Manifestations of the disease appear after the newborn period, when Hb F is replaced by Hb S. Persistent hemolytic anemia, although usually severe, is remarkably well tolerated and is not often the cause of the presenting symptoms. Many patients lead reasonably normal lives, at least for long intervals, and may be capable of a surprising amount of physical exertion. Much of the havoc of the disease is related to the periodic occurrence of disabling "crises," acute self-limited episodes of pain and fever, usually incapacitating but often not associated with increase in the degree of anemia. Precipitating factors may not be apparent; but attacks tend to occur at night, on exposure to cold, or during infections, times at which erythrostasis may be enhanced. Pain frequently is experienced in the bones and large joints of the extremities and in the back. Agonizing pain of great severity may be localized to a single area, involve multiple sites, or have a migratory character. Episodes tend to subside within a few days, but some patients have more persistent grumbling discomfort. Dramatic episodes of severe abdominal pain and fever simulate acute appendicitis and other urgent intraabdominal disorders.

Most patients have a characteristic asthenic habitus with disproportionately long extremities and "spider" fingers, probably as a result of delayed closure of epiphyses. Sexual maturation tends to be delayed, and fertility is reduced. Pregnancies often are concluded successfully, although fetal loss and maternal morbidity and mortality are increased. Susceptibility to infection is enhanced. Pneumococcal infections, including meningitis, occur with increased frequency, probably because of decreased serum opsinizing activity related to an abnormality of the properdin pathway. A unique predisposition to salmonella osteomyelitis is a remarkable feature of the disease. Chronic ulcers of the legs, overlying the malleoli, tend to occur at puberty or later. Multisystemic involvement is caused principally by ischemia resulting from anemia, erythrostasis, and vascular occlusions. Segmentation of blood flow can be seen in conjunctival vessels, and the retinal vessels may be tortuous, sometimes with peripheral vascular occlusions. Many symptoms are referable to infarction of bones and bone marrow. In infancy the earliest manifestation may be the "hand-foot" syndrome, a painful swelling of the hands or feet, associated with appearance on roentgenograms of rectangular deformities of metacarpals, metatarsals, and phalanges. Later avascular necrosis of the femoral or humeral heads may cause permanent disability. Bone involvement is readily seen in dental films, which show radiolucency, abnormal trabeculation, and infarcts. Similar changes, with widening of marrow cavities and elevation of the periosteum, may be seen in other bones. Osteoporosis of the spine may be associated with a "fish" deformity of the vertebrae.

Repeated episodes of pneumonia tend to occur, sometimes in conjunction with painful crises. Infarction of the lung is responsible for many pneumonia-like illnesses. Pulmonary vessels are occluded by masses of sickled erythrocytes or by emboli arising in veins or in infarcted marrow. Rarely, repeated emboli lead to cor pulmonale. The heart is enlarged, and the dilated chambers and accelerated circulation give rise to impressive murmurs. These are most often systolic; they simulate the murmurs of valvular heart disease. Electrocardiographic abnormalities are not unusual. Congestive heart failure, uncommon in childhood, becomes more frequent as age advances. Vascular lesions in the nervous system may produce focal or multifocal neurologic manifestations, sometimes with convulsions. Hemolytic jaundice is persistent, and the chronic overproduction of bilirubin predisposes to formation of gallstones, cholecystitis, and obstruction of the biliary tract. The liver is usually enlarged. Erythrostasis in hepatic sinusoids may cause necrosis of liver cells, leading to episodes of marked jaundice with high levels of conjugated bilirubin and aberrations of liver function tests, suggesting both hepatocellular damage and intrahepatic biliary obstruction. Damage to the liver may cause chronic hepatic dysfunction, and the end result may be a peculiar form of cirrhosis. In addition to these disorders hepatitis may be acquired through blood transfusions. The spleen is enlarged in infancy, but infarctions lead to its shrinkage to a fibrous remnant, and splenomegaly is rare in adults. Even when enlarged the spleen does not function normally, probably a factor in the increased susceptibility to infection. Hyposthenuria is the most common evidence of renal dysfunction. Infarcts of the kidney or papillary necrosis may cause hematuria, and recurrent infarction may lead to progressive renal insufficiency. The nephrotic syndrome occurs more often than would be expected by chance and is sometimes associated with renal vein thrombosis. Priapism may lead to permanent deformity and impotence.

Anemia is normocytic, with hemoglobin concentrations ranging between 5 and 10 grams per 100 ml. The reticulocyte count persistently exceeds 10 per cent, and polychromatophilia, stippling, and target cells are usual;

siderocytes and Howell-Jolly bodies may be seen. Sickled erythrocytes may not be numerous in the blood smear, but in blood deoxygenated with sodium metabisulfite virtually all the red cells are sickled. Hemolytic jaundice is associated with a slight increase in the plasma hemoglobin. Thrombocytosis and leukocytosis tend to persist and increase during crises, when leukocyte counts of more than 20,000 per cubic millimeter are common. The bone marrow is hyperplastic with a predominance of erythroid precursors. At times necrotic marrow can be aspirated from areas of acute bone pain. Profound anemia may be the result of "aplastic crises," transient episodes of retarded erythropoiesis associated with reticulocytopenia; these occur most often in association with infections. Folate deficiency, attributable in part to the high folate requirement of chronic hemolytic anemia, may lead to a superimposed megaloblastic anemia.

Diagnosis. In typical cases the diagnosis is readily established by the demonstration of hemolytic anemia, positive sickling preparation with sodium metabisulfite, and the abnormal mobility of the hemoglobin on electrophoresis. Anemia may be overlooked in blacks, and the dramatic nonhematologic manifestations can be misleading. Recurrent joint pain and striking cardiac abnormalities often suggest rheumatic fever. Differentiation between the painful abdominal crises and other intra-abdominal disorders may be extremely difficult. Differential diagnosis of marked jaundice in patients with sickle cell anemia may require meticulous evaluation, including liver biopsy in appropriate cases. Limitations of the electrophoretic method should be recognized. Sickle cell anemia is clearly distinguished from sickle cell trait by this procedure in untreated patients, but after transfusions the patterns may be similar. The electrophoretic pattern of hemoglobin in untreated sickle cell anemia may be indistinguishable from that of other disorders, including sickle cell–thalassemia, sickle cell–hemoglobin D disease, sickle cell–hereditary persistence of fetal hemoglobin, and homozygous sickle cell anemia with heterozygosity for hemoglobin Memphis or alpha thalassemia, disorders which tend to be less severe. Accordingly, proof of diagnosis may require family studies and additional analysis of the hemoglobin. Special investigations are warranted when the clinical disorder is atypical, for example, when splenomegaly persists into adult life, when anemia is mild or absent, or when the disease is unusually benign.

Prognosis. The disease in the past has had a high mortality rate in early childhood, few patients reaching adult life. Recent decades have seen progressively increasing longevity, and increasing numbers of patients survive beyond the age of 50. This improvement in outlook is not attributable to advances in specific therapy, but is largely the result of better nutrition and more adequate prevention and treatment of infections. Infection remains the most common cause of death. Aplastic crises are a serious threat to life if not treated promptly. Death may result from renal or hepatic insufficiency, cardiac failure, or vascular occlusions in the nervous system. Widespread intravascular sickling is found in some patients dying suddenly or during a painful crisis. The clinical spectrum of the disease is broad, and mild cases of sickle cell anemia are increasingly recognized. Some older patients have chronic anemia but have not had the characteristic symptoms associated with the disease.

Treatment. Specific therapy is not available. The

painful episodes are self-limited; accordingly they appear to respond to a variety of therapeutic measures, but convincing evidence of efficacy is lacking. None of the drugs or agents reported to shorten a crisis has stood the test of a properly conducted controlled trial. A recent wave of enthusiasm for the therapeutic use of urea appears to be unjustified, and careful clinical trials have not demonstrated a beneficial effect of this drug. The lesions underlying the painful crisis are related to ischemia and infarction, and there is no proof that unsickling the red cells will relieve pain after the crisis has occurred. A more promising approach to treatment of sickle cell disease is the long-term use of an agent that modifies the hemoglobin molecule in such a way as to lessen the tendency to sickling. Sodium cyanate preferentially carbamylates the N-terminal residues of the hemoglobin polypeptides, increasing oxygen affinity and thereby lessening the tendency of the red cells to sickle. Clinical trials are in progress to determine whether therapeutic benefits of cyanate can be achieved at doses that are not excessively toxic; the preliminary results are not very encouraging, because neurotoxic and other untoward effects have occurred with doses of cyanate too low to improve anemia. Severe pain justifies the use of narcotics, with care to avoid respiratory depression. Narcotic addiction attributable to appropriate therapy is rare, because the painful episodes are too short to induce dependence. Hydration should be maintained by use of intravenous fluids as needed during the crisis. Careful attention should be given to oxygenation of the blood in patients with pulmonary lesions. Patients with sickle cell anemia should continuously receive supplemental folic acid (0.5 mg per day). Infections should be treated promptly. Transfusions may be lifesaving in aplastic crises and in the shock of abdominal crises, but their use in other situations should be carefully considered. Administration of usual volumes of blood raises the hematocrit value without markedly diluting the sickle cells, increasing the viscosity of deoxygenated blood and potentially enhancing the production of vascular occlusions. Partial exchange transfusions are effective in preventing crises when about 50 per cent of the red cells are replaced by normal erythrocytes. This procedure is particularly useful in preparing patients for surgical operations, and may be used in other critical situations. Leg ulcers tend to heal with conservative measures, particularly when anemia is corrected by transfusions and during bed rest; however, they often recur even after grafting procedures. When anesthesia is administered, good ventilation and high oxygen tensions in the inspired gas mixture should be maintained. Surgical procedures can be safely performed in patients in good general condition; nevertheless, major elective procedures such as removal of asymptomatic gallstones appear to be unjustified.

SICKLE CELL TRAIT

Persons heterozygous for hemoglobin S are said to have sickle cell trait, with rare exceptions innocuous and not associated with anemia. It occurs in Africa, the Mediterranean area, Arabia, and India. About 8 per cent of American blacks are affected. Each erythrocyte contains both Hb S and Hb A, and all the red cells sickle when deoxygenated; but the concentration of Hb S in the red cells is sufficiently low that intravascular sickling does not occur at physiologic oxygen tensions. Clinical mani-

festations may appear when unusual circumstances foster intravascular sickling. Hemolytic anemia simulating sickle cell anemia has been encountered in heterozygous carriers of Hb S with anoxemia owing to congenital heart disease. Infarction of the spleen has occurred during travel in unpressurized aircraft. Very rarely sudden death has been attributed to sicklemia, but documentation of the role of the sickle cells is not adequate. Hyposthenuria is relatively common. Unilateral renal hematuria may appear without demonstrable cause and may persist for weeks; it usually ceases without relation to therapeutic efforts, none of which are clearly effective. Recurrent gross bleeding from either kidney may occur, and nephrectomy is contraindicated. Infection of the urinary tract in pregnancy is reported to be increased in frequency in women with sickle cell trait. Diagnosis requires demonstration of the sickling phenomenon in addition to the electrophoretic abnormality of the hemoglobin.

OTHER HETEROZYGOUS SICKLING DISORDERS

Persons heterozygous for hemoglobin S and for another abnormality of either the alpha or beta chain may have no evidence of disease. Thus persons heterozygous for Hb S and J (an innocuous beta chain variant) have no Hb A in their red cell hemolysates, yet appear perfectly well. In certain other heterozygous states intravascular sickling of red cells is enhanced by the additional genetic abnormality.

Sickle cell–thalassemia resembles sickle cell anemia but is generally less severe, with atypical features including relatively mild anemia and persistent splenomegaly. It occurs predominantly in persons of black or Mediterranean ancestry. The beta thalassemia gene lessens production of Hb A, which occurs in low proportion. Electrophoresis of hemoglobin shows that the predominant hemoglobin is Hb S, with smaller fractions of Hb A and Hb F; sometimes Hb A cannot be detected and family studies are required to differentiate the disorder from sickle cell anemia.

Sickle cell–hemoglobin C disease occurs in American blacks with about one fourth the frequency of sickle cell anemia. Anemia tends to be mild, and some patients are asymptomatic. Splenomegaly is usual and may persist to old age; but atrophy of the spleen attributable to infarction occurs in some cases. The disease has special importance because of its predominantly nonhematologic manifestations. Symptoms may be referable to the eye, where peripheral vascular occlusions in the retina cause retinal avascularity and neovascular proliferations; these tend to bleed, producing vitreous hemorrhages with subsequent fibrosis and retinal detachment. Pain and dysfunction of the hip or shoulder are caused by avascular necrosis of capital epiphyses, especially the femoral head. Acute abdominal pain after anesthesia or during flight in unpressurized aircraft is the result of infarction of the spleen. Gross unilateral renal hematuria is not uncommon. Pregnancy may be complicated by severe anemia, infarcts of bone, and pulmonary emboli; but in many instances pregnancy is uncomplicated. Diagnosis is suggested by examination of the blood smear in which almost all the red cells are target forms. Electrophoresis of hemoglobin shows two major components, Hb S and Hb C; Hb A is absent.

Sickle cell–hemoglobin D Punjab disease has many of the features of sickle cell anemia and may be incapacitating because of vascular occlusive lesions, although anemia tends to be less severe. The rarity of the disease, its predominant occurrence in white persons, and the nonhematologic presenting manifestations obscure the diagnosis. Standard electrophoretic methods yield a pattern indistinguishable from that of sickle cell anemia, but Hb D separates from Hb S on agar gel at low pH.

748. DISORDERS ASSOCIATED WITH HEMOGLOBINS C, D, AND E

Homozygous hemoglobin C disease is an uncommon disorder occurring in blacks. Affected persons usually have few symptoms, but the spleen is enlarged. Chronic hemolytic anemia is rarely severe and is often discovered incidentally. Hb C is relatively insoluble, causing increased rigidity of the red cells with fragmentation and accelerated destruction. The blood film contains populations of target cells and microspherocytes, the latter representing older fragmented cells. *Hemoglobin C–thalassemia* causes a similar disorder. Heterozygosity for Hb C, *hemoglobin C trait,* occurs with high frequency in some areas of East Africa and in 2 to 3 per cent of American blacks. Some target cells are seen in the blood smear without anemia or other evidence of disease.

Homozygous hemoglobin D Punjab disease is a rare disorder causing mild or moderately severe anemia with numerous target cells in the blood smear. Hb D Punjab occurs in India but also in many other parts of the world, and several instances of the disease have been encountered in white families. Hemoglobin D–thalassemia resembles the homozygous disorder but can be differentiated by family studies. Persons heterozygous for Hb D alone have no hematologic abnormalities.

Homozygous hemoglobin E disease is manifested by mild microcytic and normochromic anemia, usually without splenomegaly. Large numbers of target cells are seen in the blood smear. The disease has been encountered with considerable frequency in Orientals. Persons heterozygous for Hb E and beta thalassemia have a more severe anemia, and the spleen is usually enlarged. The high frequency of the genes for Hb E and various types of thalassemia in Southeast Asia has led to the appearance of some complex genetic disorders, for example, hemoglobin E–alpha thalassemia disease, in which affected persons appear to have the characteristics of hemoglobin H disease in addition to hemoglobin E. Heterogeneity of the hemoglobin E diseases is related in part to the diversity of genetic factors.

749. HEMOLYTIC ANEMIAS CAUSED BY UNSTABLE HEMOGLOBINS

Congenital hemolytic disorders attributable to unstable hemoglobin molecules have been discovered in a few widely scattered cases. The patients present with ane-

mia of varying severity, jaundice, and often splenomegaly. Affected persons are the heterozygous carriers of the abnormal hemoglobin, and homozygotes are unknown. Persons with *Hb Zürich* have a compensated mild hemolytic disorder without anemia except after administration of sulfonamides or during infections, when fulminant hemolytic anemia may occur. Drug-induced hemolytic episodes have been described in carriers of *Hb Torino* and *Hb Shepherd's Bush. Hb Köln* causes chronic hemolytic anemia, with recurring bouts of more severe anemia, jaundice, and dark urine; splenectomy has sometimes appeared to have a beneficial effect. Other unstable hemoglobins are not associated with distinguishing clinical features. Mild methemoglobinemia accompanies the hemolytic process in some instances, and the variant hemoglobin may have abnormal oxygen affinity. Increased oxygen affinity in Hb Zürich appears to have no clinical importance; reduced oxygen affinity in *Hb Seattle* is thought to increase anemia by lessening the stimulus for compensatory erythropoiesis. Diagnosis is suggested by demonstration of precipitates of denatured hemoglobin (Heinz bodies) in the red cells. In patients with Hb Zürich these may appear during hemolytic episodes as large globular inclusions. Heinz bodies are seen in many of the red cells of patients with Hb Köln after splenectomy. They can be demonstrated in other cases by incubating red cells with brilliant cresyl blue, a redox dye. The abnormal hemoglobin tends to precipitate when hemolysates are heated at 50° C. The dark urine contains a dipyrrole pigment thought to originate from heme groups dislodged from unstable hemoglobin molecules.

750. DISORDERS CAUSED BY HEMOGLOBINS WITH ABNORMAL OXYGEN AFFINITY

Cyanosis is caused by methemoglobinemia in the heterozygous carriers of the hemoglobins M and *Hb Freiburg.* The concentration of methemoglobin is not sufficiently high to cause major symptoms. In some instances there is an associated hemolytic disorder. Carriers of *Hb Kansas* also display cyanosis, in this instance caused by an increased concentration of deoxyhemoglobin in the blood in capillaries and venules. Hb Kansas has a low affinity for oxygen which facilitates the unloading of oxygen in the tissues, a phenomenon without apparent harmful effects.

Erythrocytosis (polycythemia) is the clinical expression of several abnormal hemoglobins with increased oxygen affinity. These variants have been discovered in scattered cases, and it is noteworthy that they cause one form of familial polycythemia without leukocytosis, thrombocytosis, or splenomegaly. Hematocrit values of heterozygotes have not exceeded 65 per cent, and homozygotes are unknown. Impaired release of oxygen activates the erythropoietin mechanism, producing the compensatory erythrocytosis. These hemoglobins should be sought by direct measurement of oxygen affinity in cases of unexplained erythrocytosis; electrophoretic mobility of the variant hemoglobin is not always abnormal. (See Ch. 754 to 758.)

751. THE THALASSEMIA SYNDROMES

The thalassemia syndromes are a heterogeneous group of inherited disorders manifested in the homozygote by profound anemia or death in utero, and in the heterozygote by red cell abnormalities of relatively trivial significance. Two major categories are recognized: *alpha thalassemia,* caused by retarded production of alpha chains of globin, and *beta thalassemia,* caused by retarded production of beta chains. Delta thalassemia has been described but is of no clinical significance. Impaired hemoglobin synthesis causes anemia and microcytosis. In addition, unbalanced production of globin chains leads secondarily to accumulation of uncombined alpha chains in beta thalassemia and to formation of the abnormal molecules γ_4 (Hb Bart's) and β_4 (Hb H) in alpha thalassemia; these tend to precipitate within red cells, hastening their destruction. In rare instances a thalassemic disorder is associated with one of the Lepore hemoglobins or Hb Constant Spring.

HOMOZYGOUS BETA THALASSEMIA

Definition. Homozygous beta thalassemia is the inherited disorder described by Cooley and Lee in 1925 and subsequently known as Cooley's anemia, Mediterranean anemia, target cell anemia, or thalassemia major. Occurring primarily in persons of Mediterranean ancestry, the disease is characterized by profound anemia, marked hepatosplenomegaly, and, typically, death in childhood.

Clinical Manifestations. Anemia appears after the newborn period and thereafter is severe, with marked pallor and mild to moderate hemolytic jaundice. The spleen and liver become tremendously enlarged. Deformation of the bones, particularly those of the head, contributes to the characteristic "Mongoloid" facies, and distorts the mouth and disturbs the alignment of the teeth. Roentgenograms show a "hair-on-end" appearance of the skull, enlargement of other marrow cavities with thinning of cortical bone, and abnormalities of trabeculation related to the marked hyperplasia of marrow. Cardiac enlargement and failure are explained by the anemia and by the deposition of large amounts of iron in the myocardium. Hemosiderosis is largely the result of the many transfusions required to maintain life. The hypochromic microcytic red cells are flattened, usually with numerous target and stippled forms and variable numbers of nucleated erythrocytes, polychromatic cells, and reticulocytes. Inclusion bodies can be demonstrated in many normoblasts and reticulocytes when stained with methyl violet. Leukocytosis may be marked and persistent. Much of the hemolytic activity appears to be intramedullary with resulting ineffective erythropoiesis. Serum iron is elevated with increased saturation of iron-binding protein. The proportion of Hb F is usually between 20 and 60 per cent, but values as high as 90 per cent may occur. Hemoglobin A_2 is not increased.

Treatment and Prognosis. With frequent transfusions and appropriate prevention and treatment of infections, life may be improved and prolonged. Massive deposition of iron is often the cause of cardiac failure and death. In selected cases splenectomy is beneficial when the spleen is actively sequestering red cells, but susceptibility to infection may be enhanced. Supplemental folic acid (0.5 mg per day) provides for the increased requirement. Chelating agents such as desferrioxamine have been used in an effort to reduce iron stores.

HETEROZYGOUS BETA THALASSEMIA

Heterozygous beta thalassemia (thalassemia minor) is manifested by mild anemia, usually with microcytosis, hypochromia, stippling, and target cells. Most frequent in Mediterranean populations, it is widely distributed throughout the world, occurring not rarely in blacks and less often in white persons from northern Europe. Symptoms are unusual, but some persons have anemia of moderate severity associated with jaundice and splenomegaly. Red cell abnormalities, which are variable and sometimes hardly detectable, are associated with resistance to osmotic lysis. Genetic heterogeneity is suggested not only by the clinical variability but also by differences in proportions of hemoglobins in hemolysates. Typically Hb A_2 is increased to about 5 per cent, sometimes with a slight increase in Hb F. But in some cases Hb F tends to be more elevated; in others Hb A_2 is reduced ($\delta\beta$ thalassemia). "Thalassemia intermedia," a term applied to instances of thalassemia which on clinical grounds appears to be intermediate between the typical heterozygous and homozygous disorders, has no specific meaning. Thalassemia minor is most often discovered during routine blood examination of blood smears or by detection of a low MCV using an electronic cell counter. It is often mistaken for iron deficiency anemia. Lead poisoning may be suggested by the numerous stippled cells, or other iron-refractory microcytic anemias may be considered. Diagnosis is suggested by demonstration of the same blood abnormality in other members of the family. An elevated level of Hb A_2 is confirmatory.

ALPHA THALASSEMIA

Homozygous alpha thalassemia is thought to be incompatible with life, and in a number of instances has appeared to be the cause of fetal death at about the thirtieth week. Most cases have been described in Orientals. The stillborn infant displays severe hydrops fetalis. Red cell hemolysates contain about 80 per cent Hb Bart's, a functionally inadequate hemoglobin with high oxygen affinity.

Heterozygous alpha thalassemia is manifested by very slight thalassemic abnormalities of the red cells with little or no anemia and by increased proportions of Hb Bart's (5 to 20 per cent) in cord blood. Identification is virtually impossible after the newborn period, although minor abnormalities of erythrocytes persist. It is widely distributed, occurring most frequently in Asiatic, African, and Mediterranean populations, and has been detected in almost 2 per cent of American blacks at birth. Rarely, heterozygous alpha thalassemia has occurred in persons who also had an alpha chain structural abnormality. Hemoglobin Q–alpha thalassemia, described in Orientals, is manifested by severe anemia. Hemoglobin I–alpha thalassemia was encountered in a black with mild anemia.

Hemoglobin H disease is a chronic hemolytic anemia associated with splenomegaly and intermediate levels of Hb H in erythrocytes. It has been found in persons of various ethnic backgrounds, including persons of apparently Northern European origin. Hemolytic episodes may be precipitated by sulfonamides. Red cells are hypochromic and microcytic. Intracellular inclusions of Hb H appear in erythrocytes after splenectomy, and may be induced before splenectomy by incubating blood with brilliant cresyl blue. The disease is thought to occur in persons heterozygous for alpha thalassemia and for a different alpha thalassemia gene with milder effects. The resulting deficiency of alpha chains is not so severe as in homozygous alpha thalassemia, and the disease is compatible with long life.

Charache, S., Weatherall, D. J., and Clegg, J. B.: Polycythemia associated with a hemoglobinopathy. J. Clin. Invest., 45:813, 1966.
Diggs, L. W.: Sickle cell crises. Am. J. Clin. Pathol., 44:1, 1965.
Herrick, J. B.: Peculiar elongated and sickle-shaped red corpuscles in a case of severe anemia. Arch. Intern. Med., 6:517, 1910.
Pauling, L.: Abnormality of hemoglobin molecules in hereditary hemolytic anemias. Harvey Lecture, 1953–1954, p. 216.
Weatherall, D. J. (ed.): The haemoglobinopathies. Clin. Haematol., 3:No. 1, 1974.
Weatherall, D. J., and Clegg, J. B.: The Thalassaemia Syndromes. 2nd ed. Oxford, Blackwell Scientific Publications, 1972.
White, J. M., and Dacie, J. V.: The unstable hemoglobins—molecular and clinical features. Prog. Hematol., 7:69, 1971.

752. METHEMOGLOBINEMIA AND SULFHEMOGLOBINEMIA

Ernst R. Jaffé

METHEMOGLOBINEMIA

Definition. Methemoglobinemia occurs when the concentration of methemoglobin within circulating erythrocytes is increased above the normal level of about 1 per cent. Since the abnormal pigment is intracellular, methemoglobinemia is perhaps a misnomer, but methemoglobincythemia and methemoglobinia are too clumsy, and convention dictates the use of the former term. Methemoglobin (ferrihemoglobin, hem*i*globin, ferric protoporphyrin IX-globin) is defined as an oxidation product of hemoglobin in which the sixth coordination position of ferric heme is bound to a water molecule (acid form) or to a hydroxyl group (alkaline form), each with its characteristic optical spectrum. Because of the additional positive charge, the sixth coordination position of iron is no longer available to bind molecular oxygen reversibly.

Etiology and Pathogenesis. The intracellular environment of hemoglobin is such that some oxidation of heme iron might be expected. Although the intrinsic structure of hemoglobin shields the iron against oxidation, metabolic processes are also normally active to protect hemoglobin against oxidation or irreversible denaturation and to reduce any methemoglobin which is formed to hemoglobin. An increase in the concentration of methemoglobin above the normal level can result from (1) the presence of a hemoglobin with an abnormal structure that makes it more susceptible to oxidation and/or unsuitable for reduction, (2) deficiency in the ability to reduce methemoglobin, and (3) exposure to drugs or chemicals which increase the rate of oxidation beyond the protective and reductive capacities of the cell. Whereas the first two mechanisms are associated with inherited disorders, the latter occurs in toxic or acquired methemoglobinemia.

Hereditary Methemoglobinemia Due to an Abnormal Hemoglobin (Hemoglobin M) (see Ch. 746 to 751). Substitution of tyrosine for histidine occurs at or across from the heme-binding site in the α chains of hemoglobin M Iwate and M Boston and in the β chains of hemoglobin M Hyde Park and M Saskatoon. Glutamic acid replaces valine in the β chain of hemoglobin M Milwaukee-1 one helical turn away from, but still facing, the heme iron. These alterations in the primary structure of hemoglobin increase the tendency of the heme iron to be oxidized and/or stabilize the methemoglobin form so that the normal mechanism for the reduction of methemoglobin is ineffective. Thus the methemoglobinemia does not respond significantly to conventional therapy (see below). As with other abnormal hemoglobins, hemoglobin M is transmitted as a codominant characteristic. Only heterozygotes for hemoglobin M have been identified, presumably because the homozygous state would be incompatible with life. Because only one pair of chains (either α or β) of a hemogloblin M is affected, and in the oxidized state, the concentration of methemoglobin does not exceed 25 to 30 per cent. Since α chains are already present in large amounts at birth, M hemoglobins with α chain substitutions are usually apparent immediately, whereas β chain abnormalities are often not manifest until later.

Hereditary Methemoglobinemia Due to a Deficiency in the Ability to Reduce Methemoglobin. The reduction of methemoglobin in human erythrocytes depends, primarily, on the activity of a reduced nicotinamide adenine dinucleotide (NADH or DPNH)-dependent methemoglobin reductase system. This system utilizes NADH generated by glyceraldehyde-3-phosphate dehydrogenase in the Embden-Meyerhof pathway of glycolysis to reduce methemoglobin to hemoglobin. Three other pathways capable of reducing methemoglobin are present in human erythrocytes, but are much less important: nonenzymatic reduction by ascorbic acid or reduced glutathione (GSH) and a reduced nicotinamide adenine dinucleotide phosphate (NADPH or TPNH)-methemoglobin reductase system, which requires an artificial electron carrier, such as methylene blue, to become effective in reducing methemoglobin. Significant methemoglobinemia is not observed in scurvy, glucose-6-phosphate dehydrogenase deficiency, marked GSH deficiency, or NADPH–methemoglobin reductase deficiency. Although other defects in the metabolic pathways of erythrocytes theoretically might lead to methemoglobinemia, they have not been identified.

The limited ability of erythrocytes from patients with hereditary methemoglobinemia not due to an abnormal hemoglobin to reduce methemoglobin in vitro has been demonstrated in numerous investigations. In most cases, this handicap has been traced to decreased activity of the NADH–methemoglobin reductase system. Methemoglobinemia as high as 40 to 50 per cent results from the accumulation of spontaneously formed methemoglobin in the absence of the normal mechanism for reduction. Data from family and biochemical studies are consistent with an autosomal codominant mode of inheritance. Marked deficiency in activity is seen in erythrocytes of affected homozygous patients, whereas approximately half normal activity is usually evident in cells from acyanotic, asymptomatic heterozygous subjects. At least eight different electrophoretic variants of NADH–methemoglobin reductase have been demonstrated. One variant is associated with only a slight decrease in activity. Thus, as is true for hemoglobin, glucose-6-phosphate dehydrogenase and other enzymes, multiple aberrations in the NADH–methemoglobin reductase system apparently exist, some with and some without functional consequences.

Toxic (Acquired) Methemoglobinemia. Methemoglobinemia occurs when oxidative stress overwhelms the protective capacities of erythrocytes and exceeds the ability of the cells to reduce methemoglobin. The heme iron may be oxidized directly by ferricyanide, ferric tartrate, bivalent copper, chromate, chlorate, certain quinones, alloxans, and some dyes with a high oxidation-reduction potential. Nitrite, a powerful reducing agent and one of the most common methemoglobin-forming compounds, produces methemoglobinemia by a reaction that is not completely understood, although the generation of hydrogen peroxide has been suggested. Nitrates, upon conversion to nitrites, especially in the gastrointestinal tract of infants, can lead to toxic methemoglobinemia. Erythrocytes of newborns also are less able than adults' cells to protect hemoglobin against oxidation and to reduce methemoglobin, owing to decreased activities of NADH–methemoglobin reductase and other enzymes. More complex reactions are postulated to explain the methemoglobin-forming properties of aromatic amino and nitro compounds (acetanilid, phenacetin, nitrosobenzene, phenazopyridine, primaquine, sulfonamides, prilocaine, benzocaine) and of aniline dyes in laundry marks and wax crayons. These compounds may be converted to metabolites which either act as direct oxidants or participate in a coupled oxidation with oxyhemoglobin. In the latter reaction, generation of hydrogen peroxide, peroxyhemoglobin, or free radicals is thought to cause the formation of methemoglobin. In addition to producing methemoglobinemia, some of these agents also can induce alterations which lead to hemolysis, especially in erythrocytes deficient in glucose-6-phosphate dehydrogenase activity.

Incidence and Prevalence. Although hereditary methemoglobinemia is rare, over 450 probable cases have been recorded. It is impossible to determine accurately how many are the result of a deficiency in NADH–methemoglobin reductase activity and how many are due to hemoglobin M. Patients in whom complete biochemical studies have not been performed, but whose chronic methemoglobinemia responds to therapy, presumably have had an abnormality in erythrocyte metabolism. Most of these patients probably have a deficiency in NADH-methemoglobin reductase activity; about 250 examples can be cited. The abnormality has a worldwide distribution, and is particularly prevalent in inbred populations.

The M hemoglobins also have a worldwide distribution with about 200 examples. Although many patients are of Northern European origin, a number have been reported from Japan, and the patient with hemoglobin M Hyde Park was a 77-year-old black man.

There have probably been thousands of instances of acquired methemoglobinemia, but most have been transient and either clinically insignificant or coincidental complications of another disease. The chronic methemoglobinemia ("enterogenous cyanosis") which is be-lieved to result from the absorption of nitrites produced in a gastrointestinal (or urinary) tract persistently infected with nitrite-producing bacteria is extremely rare. More than 700 cases of toxic methemoglobinemia have been reported in infants fed formulas prepared with well-water containing high concentrations of nitrate; the mortality has been as high as 10 per cent. The anticipated increase in susceptibility to toxic methemoglobinemia of individuals heterozygous for NADH-methemoglobin reductase deficiency is seen in such subjects while receiving primaquine, chloroquine, or diaminodiphenylsulfone as malarial chemoprophylaxis.

Clinical Manifestations. The characteristic clinical picture of hereditary methemoglobinemia is presented by a patient with diffuse, persistent slate-gray cyanosis, often present from birth and not associated with clubbing of the fingers or evidence of cardiopulmonary disease. Concentrations of methemoglobin of 10 to 25 per cent are tolerated without apparent ill effect, but levels of 30 to 40 per cent may be associated with mild exertional dyspnea and headaches. These patients are really more blue than sick.

Toxic methemoglobinemia, especially if it develops rapidly, will produce symptoms of anoxia. Levels of 20 to 30 per cent methemoglobin are accompanied by dyspnea, tachycardia, headache, fatigue, fainting, nausea, anorexia, and vomiting. Some of these symptoms may reflect direct toxic effects of the causative agent. Lethargy and stupor may appear with methemoglobin concentrations above 55 or 60 per cent. The lethal concentration probably is greater than 70 per cent.

The decreased oxygen-carrying capacity resulting from untreated hereditary methemoglobinemia is sometimes associated with a mild compensatory erythrocytosis. This is often not as great as expected and is not observed with M hemoglobins. Segregation of methemoglobin in a population of older erythrocytes in NADH–methemoglobin reductase deficiency has been invoked to explain, in part, the absence of erythrocytosis. The heme groups of the normal hemoglobin chains in the M hemoglobins retain their capacity to bind oxygen, and normal oxygen affinities are observed with hemoglobin M Saskatoon and Hyde Park. The oxygen affinity, however, is decreased in hemoglobin M Boston, Iwate, and Milwaukee-1. This looser binding of oxygen may facilitate delivery to the tissues and may make an erythrocytosis unnecessary. In toxic methemoglobinemia, the methemoglobin not only decreases the available oxygen-carrying pigment, but also increases the affinity of the unaltered hemoglobin for oxygen, thereby further impairing the delivery of oxygen and enhancing symptoms.

Systemic effects usually do not occur in hereditary methemoglobinemia. The association of severe mental retardation has been noted in 21 children from 12 different families with NADH–methemoglobin reductase deficiency, perhaps caused by a generalized disorder not limited to the erythrocytes. Toxic methemoglobinemia may be associated with hemolysis, central nervous system depression, hepatic damage, or renal dysfunction, depending upon the causative agent or associated disease.

Diagnosis. Methemoglobinemia should be considered, even if only briefly, in the differential diagnosis of cyanosis. About 5 grams of deoxyhemoglobin per 100 ml of blood are required to produce visible cyanosis, but a comparable discoloration is produced by 1.5 to 2 grams per 100 ml of methemoglobin and by about 0.5 gram per 100 ml of sulfhemoglobin (see below). The greater visible effect of these abnormal pigments is due to the alterations in the absorption spectra. Blood which contains more than about 10 per cent methemoglobin (or sulfhemoglobin) appears unusually dark red or even brown, and does not change color upon vigorous shaking with air. Addition and mixing of a few drops of 10 per cent NaCN or KCN results in the rapid formation of bright red cyanmethemoglobin, but has no effect on the color of sulfhemoglobin.

Determination of the absorption spectrum is required to define the nature of the abnormal pigment. Acid methemoglobin has a characteristic spectrum with peaks at 502 and 632 mμ that disappear upon the addition of cyanide. Sulfhemoglobin has a peak at 620 mμ that is not altered by cyanide. The absorption spectra of methemoglobin M variants differ from those of normal methemoglobin with displacement of the peaks at 502 and 632 mμ toward lower wavelengths. Sulfhemoglobin, however, may be difficult to differentiate from methemoglobin M. The rate of formation of a complex with cyanide, the resulting absorption spectrum, and the electrophoretic migration of the methemoglobin form of hemoglobin M variants often differ from those of normal methemoglobin and help to establish the diagnosis.

NADH–methemoglobin reductase deficiency can be detected by a simple spot test, but confirmation of the diagnosis requires assay of this enzyme system in a hemolysate.

A careful history should provide clues to possible toxic methemoglobinemia. Parent-to-child transmission of congenital cyanosis should suggest the possibility of a hemoglobin M, whereas unexplained cyanosis in siblings but not in parents or offspring is more consistent with NADH–methemoglobin reductase deficiency.

Treatment. With toxic methemoglobinemia, concentrations of 20 to 30 per cent will disappear spontaneously in 24 to 72 hours after exposure to the offending agent terminates. More vigorous therapy is indicated if unconsciousness, stupor, or methemoglobinemia greater than 40 per cent supervenes. Oxygen administration and hemodialysis or exchange transfusion to remove the toxic agent may be helpful. Methylene blue, 1 to 2 mg per kilogram given intravenously during five minutes, will often correct the methemoglobinemia within 30 to 60 minutes. Repeated doses may be needed. Toxicity from methylene blue is uncommon, but doses over 15 mg per kilogram may cause hemolysis in infants. Individuals with glucose-6-phosphate dehydrogenase deficiency may respond suboptimally, and may develop hemolysis. Since neither methemoglobin M nor sulfhemoglobin will respond to methylene blue administration, failure to observe a significant change in color should alert the physician to the possibility of these abnormal pigments. Ascorbic acid has no place in the management of toxic methemoglobinemia because the rate at which it reduces methemoglobin is so much slower than that of the normal intrinsic mechanism.

Hereditary methemoglobinemia resulting from NADH–methemoglobin reductase deficiency usually does not require treatment except for cosmetic reasons. Intravenous methylene blue will reduce the methemoglobinemia rapidly, and daily oral administration of 100 to 300 mg will maintain the concentration below 10 per cent. Somewhat less effective is oral administration of ascorbic acid, 500 mg daily, to maintain the concentration of methemoglobin between 5 and 13 per cent. De-

spite good control of methemoglobinemia, therapy does not influence the mental retardation suffered by some patients.

Since the causal abnormality in the M hemoglobins resides in the structure of the hemoglobin, no effective form of therapy has been discovered.

Prognosis and Prevention. Methemoglobinemia, as an isolated alteration, does not have an adverse effect on the life expectancy of the patient or on the life span of the erythrocyte. The prognosis in toxic methemoglobinemia, once the acute episode is over, depends upon the precipitating circumstances. Toxic methemoglobinemia can be avoided by careful supervision of potential methemoglobin-producing drugs and chemicals, including thorough laundering of diapers to remove excess aniline dyes.

SULFHEMOGLOBINEMIA

Sulfhemoglobin, an incompletely characterized pigment not normally present, arises from the interaction of hemoglobin with soluble sulfides, especially hydrogen sulfide, in the presence of an oxidizing agent, usually hydrogen peroxide. Sulfhemoglobinemia is caused by the same aromatic amino drugs (acetanilid, phenacetin) that are associated with toxic methemoglobinemia. Why some patients develop methemoglobinemia and others have sulfhemoglobinemia is unknown. The concentration of GSH in the erythrocytes of some of the latter patients is elevated. Sulfhemoglobinemia may occur in patients with "enterogenous cyanosis," and has been attributed to the absorption of H_2S from the diseased gastrointestinal tract. The effect of sulfhemoglobin on the life span of human erythrocytes is uncertain, but many patients with sulfhemoglobinemia also have hemolysis. Since sulfhemoglobin cannot bind oxygen, the clinical effects are similar to those of methemoglobin. Sulfhemoglobin cannot be converted to hemoglobin, and there is no effective treatment. The pigment disappears when the erythrocytes containing sulfhemoglobin leave the circulation.

Cumming, R. L. C., and Pollock, A.: Drug-induced sulphaemoglobinaemia and Heinz body anaemia in pregnancy with involvement of the foetus. Scott. Med. J., 12:320, 1967.

Hsieh, H.-S., and Jaffé, E. R.: The metabolism of methemoglobin in human erythrocytes. *In* Surgenor, D. MacN. (ed.): The Red Blood Cell. 2nd ed. New York, Academic Press, 1975.

Jaffé, E. R., and Hsieh, H.-S.: DPNH-methemoglobin reductase deficiency and hereditary methemoglobinemia. Semin. Hematol., 8:417, 1971.

Kiese, M.: The biochemical production of ferrihemoglobin-forming derivatives from aromatic amines, and mechanisms of ferrihemoglobin formation. Pharmacol. Rev., 18:1091, 1966.

753. HEMOGLOBINURIA

Hugh Chaplin, Jr.

Definition and Mechanism. Hemoglobinuria (the presence of free hemoglobin in the urine) is a sign of variety of pathologic states and not a disease entity in itself. Hemoglobin generally finds its way into the urine by filtration from the plasma; uncommonly, it may be released from red cells which lyse within the kidney or urinary outflow tract. Normal human plasma contains an alpha$_2$ globulin, haptoglobin, present in amounts sufficient to bind 75 to 175 mg of hemoglobin per 100 ml of plasma. The tightly bound hemoglobin-haptoglobin complex, which has a molecular weight above 280,000, is not filtered by the normal glomerulus but is metabolized independent of the kidney at a linear rate of approximately 10 mg per 100 ml of plasma per hour. The total plasma hemoglobin binding capacity of the average normal adult, e.g., 3 liter plasma volume, is $125 \times 30 = 3750$ mg of hemoglobin, the amount contained in 11 ml of red blood cells. When hemoglobin entering the total plasma pool exceeds this relatively modest amount, the pigment exists free in the plasma, and is either metabolized or filtered into the urine and excreted. During metabolism of free plasma hemoglobin, some of the heme moiety is split from the parent molecule and binds to albumin, forming methemalbumin, which is readily distinguishable chemically and spectroscopically from free hemoglobin and hemoglobin-haptoglobin complex, and which is relatively slowly metabolized over 24 to 48 hours. Normal plasma also contains a beta globulin, hemopexin (50 to 100 mg per 100 ml), which selectively binds free heme in equimolar amounts.

It has been puzzling that free hemoglobin (molecular weight 66,000) should pass so readily into the glomerular filtrate when albumin (molecular weight 60,000) is filtered so poorly. It is known that under physiologic conditions oxyhemoglobin in dilute solution partially and reversibly dissociates into two alpha beta dimers each with a molecular weight of about 32,000. Recent studies by Bunn et al. suggest that it is this phenomenon occurring in the glomerulus that is responsible for the increased filtration of hemoglobin into the urine. The kidney has a limited capacity for tubular reabsorption of filtered hemoglobin; free hemoglobin will be excreted in the urine when the plasma free hemoglobin concentration exceeds 15 to 25 mg per 100 ml.

Occurrence. *Hemoglobinuria Following Intravascular Hemolysis.* Lysis of red cells within the circulation may occur under a variety of circumstances. The plasma will appear pink or red (free and haptoglobin-bound hemoglobin) or brown (methemalbumin). Isoimmune hemolysis occurs in relation to transfusion when the patient's plasma contains antibodies to donor red cell antigens. Hemolytic transfusion reactions usually involve incompatibility within the ABO system, but may occur within the other blood group systems, especially when complement-binding antibodies are involved, e.g., anti-Jk^a. Repeated transfusion of group A, B, or AB recipients with group O "universal donor" blood may result in isoimmune hemolysis of the recipient's red cells owing to the cumulative effect of donor isoantibodies. Autoimmune hemolysis, particularly when complement components are part of the erythrocyte-autoantibody complex, may result in massive hemoglobinemia (as in "cold" autoimmune hemolytic anemia and in the rare condition of paroxysmal cold hemoglobinuria). It should be emphasized here that hemoglobinemia is not an inevitable accompaniment of severe iso- and autohemolysis; when red cell destruction occurs primarily extravascularly, i.e., by phagocytosis within the reticuloendothelial system (especially in the spleen), plasma hemoglobin levels will be low, and haptoglobin levels may be only minimally depressed. Severe hemoglobinemia has also occurred in relation to certain drug-antibody-erythrocyte complexes, as in patients sensitized to Fua-

din and quinidine. A number of intrinsic red cell defects may result in massive intravascular hemolysis under appropriate conditions. The most striking example is the poorly understood cell membrane defect in patients with paroxysmal nocturnal hemoglobinuria (PNH); also important are the enzyme-deficient cells, e.g., cells deficient in G-6-PD, which may lyse massively when exposed to sufficient concentrations of oxidant drugs or to components of the fava bean. Rarely, mechanical damage to red cells, as in severe microangiopathic hemolytic states or after extensive body surface burns, may cause gross hemoglobinemia; physical damage also accounts for the hemoglobinemia that accompanies many extracorporeal perfusion procedures. A number of snake and spider venoms contain enzymes that provoke rapid red cell lysis (lecithinase in the venom of the brown recluse spider, reported mainly in the south central United States). Massive destruction of red cells may result from direct erythrocyte parasitism in falciparum malaria. Hypotonic red cell lysis follows the intravenous infusion of distilled water, and may occur inadvertently when water is used to irrigate the bladder during exposure of the vascular prostatic bed in the course of transurethral resection procedures. A rare but interesting condition, "march (or exertional) hemoglobinuria," has been described, wherein hemoglobinuria follows prolonged exercise (usually, running) in susceptible individuals. Because of the variety of conditions under which this poorly understood phenomenon has been reported, it is likely that multiple factors may be responsible for its occurrence. The condition is clearly distinguishable from myoglobinuria.

Hemoglobinuria Originating in the Urinary Tract. Hemoglobinuria may accompany infarction of the kidney. Presumably, red cells lyse in the infarcted tissue, and the liberated hemoglobin "leaks" into the urinary outflow tract directly; cystoscopy reveals the unilateral origin of the pigmenturia. Rarely, when hematuria occurs coincident with a very dilute urine (specific gravity less than 1.006), hypotonic lysis of the cells occurs within the collecting system. In neither of the aforementioned conditions is hemoglobinemia found, and plasma haptoglobin levels are normal.

Clinical Manifestations and Implications. Hemoglobinemia and hemoglobinuria, when induced by the experimental infusion of hemoglobin, when occurring from nonimmune causes, and when unaccompanied by shock or dehydration, are generally asymptomatic and benign phenomena. Stroma-free hemoglobin administered intravenously has no demonstrable effect on renal function. Red cell stroma is known to have coagulant properties; signs of mild disseminated intravascular coagulation and mild transient impairment of inulin and creatinine clearances have been observed in monkeys receiving large amounts of hemoglobin-free autologous stroma intravenously. Nonetheless, massive hemoglobinuria occurring in patients with PNH and in human subjects mistakenly given distilled water intravenously has not been associated with renal impairment. Thus any symptoms occurring in association with hemoglobinuria are likely to be related to the cause of the hemolysis and not to the hemoglobinuria per se.

By contrast, hemoglobinuria can contribute importantly to severe renal damage when it occurs in association with a major antigen-antibody reaction, e.g., incompatible blood transfusion, and/or in association with markedly reduced renal blood flow, as in shock or severe dehydration. That hemoglobinuria per se is not necessarily the cause of renal shutdown after transfusion reaction has been demonstrated by Schmidt et al., who observed renal failure after the infusion of hemoglobin-free incompatible red cell stroma. Since hemoglobin and its breakdown products are relatively insoluble when in high concentration and at acid pH, the precipitation of hemoglobin products in the renal tubules will be favored by any condition that results in reduced urine volume and acid urine pH.

Diagnosis. Investigation of suspected hemoglobinuria should include studies of the plasma as well as of the urine. Plasma obtained at the time of active intravascular hemolysis will be pink or red; free hemoglobin and haptoglobin-bound hemoglobin (in acute hemolysis) will be demonstrable by electrophoretic, spectrophotometric, and gel filtration methods. If a blood sample is not obtained until 18 to 48 hours after intravascular hemolysis has ceased, the plasma will have a brown discoloration, and the only heme-containing pigment present will be methemalbumin, demonstrable spectroscopically by Schumm's test (appearance of a sharply defined band at 558 mμ after treatment with one tenth volume of concentrated ammonium sulfide).

During acute hemoglobinuria, the freshly voided urine will be pink, red, or deep port wine in color, depending on the hemoglobin concentration. Over a period of hours (whether in the bladder or during storage after voiding) the color turns brownish red or almost black owing to the formation of reduced hemoglobin, methemoglobin, acid hematin, and other breakdown products. Differential diagnosis should include hematuria, myoglobinuria, porphyrinuria, bilirubinuria, melanuria, betaninuria (beet pigment sometimes excreted in urine), and alcaptonuria (darkens only after storage and at alkaline pH). Hematuria can be quickly ruled out by centrifugation of the specimen. Several techniques employing benzidine reagents (which react with the iron-containing heme portion of the molecule) will help to rule out porphyrinuria, bilirubinuria, melanuria, and alcaptonuria, each of which can be separately identified by appropriate laboratory tests. Benzidine reagents will not, however, make the important distinction between hemoglobinuria and myoglobinuria, because they react with the heme groups of both molecules. The excretion of myoglobin in the urine should be suspected on clinical grounds when pigmenturia follows extreme excessive exercise (especially in the untrained individual who complains of severe postexercise muscle pain and weakness) and infarction of, or trauma to, a large muscle mass (crush syndrome). Although there are minor spectroscopic differences between hemoglobin and myoglobin, differentiation of these pigments is made easier by two physicochemical properties of myoglobin. Myoglobin does not bind to haptoglobin, and, because of its small molecular size (molecular weight 17,500), is rapidly excreted in the urine. Therefore during acute myoglobinuria, the plasma will be only slightly discolored or normal in appearance, and plasma haptoglobin levels will be normal. Second, hemoglobin is essentially insoluble at 80 per cent saturation with ammonium sulfate, whereas myoglobin remains in solution under these conditions. Thus the addition of 2.8 grams of ammonium sulfate to 5 ml of benzidine-positive red-brown urine will result in precipitation of the abnormal pigment if hemoglobinuria is present. Rarely, both pigments may occur together in the urine and may be identified by a variety of immunologic, electrophoretic, or gel filtration techniques.

Chronic hemoglobinuria, even at levels too low to discolor the urine, is always accompanied by *hemosiderin granules* in the urinary sediment. The hemosiderin is formed within tubular cells after reabsorption of hemoglobin, and is either released from the cells or appears within cells sloughed into the outflow tract. The brown granules are readily identified by the Prussian blue reaction with potassium ferrocyanide. Hemosiderinuria is a common accompaniment of many chronic hemolytic states, and is occasionally seen in patients with hemochromatosis. When hemolysis is sufficiently prolonged and severe (as in PNH), the cumulative loss of hemoglobin and hemosiderin in the urine may lead to frank iron deficiency.

Treatment. Therapy must be directed to the primary cause of the red cell lysis that is ultimately responsible for the hemoglobinuria. Assurance of adequate urine volume (by maintenance of adequate systolic blood pressure and good hydration) is essential. Special measures (including the use of mannitol and alkali) of importance in treating acute hemoglobinuria of isoimmune origin or under any circumstances, e.g., shock, in which acute renal shutdown is threatened are described in detail in Part XVI, Section Three.

Allison, A. C., and Rees, W.: The binding of hemoglobin by plasma proteins (haptoglobins). Br. Med. J., 2:1137, 1957.

Birndorf, N. I., Lopas, H., and Robboy, S. J.: Disseminated intravascular coagulation and renal failure. Production in the monkey with autologous red cell stroma. Lab. Invest., 25:314, 1971.

Blondheim, S. H., Margoliash, E., and Shafrir, E.: A simple test for myohaemoglobinuria (myoglobinuria). J.A.M.A., 167:453, 1957.

Bunn, H. F., Esham, W. T., and Bull, R. W.: The renal handling of hemoglobin. I. Glomerular filtration. J. Exp. Med., 129:909, 1969.

Ham, T. H.: Hemoglobinuria. Am. J. Med., 18:990, 1955.

Rabiner, S. F., Helbert, J. R., Lopas, H., and Friedman, L. H.: Evaluation of a stroma-free hemoglobin solution for use as a plasma expander. J. Exp. Med., 126:1127, 1967.

Schmidt, P. J., and Holland, P. V.: Pathogenesis of the acute renal failure associated with incompatible transfusions. Lancet, 2:1169, 1967.

Section Three. TRANSFUSION REACTIONS

Hugh Chaplin, Jr.

GENERAL CONSIDERATIONS

The true frequency of untoward reactions to transfusions of whole human blood is unknown. Incidences varying from 10 per cent to less than 0.2 per cent have been reported; the wide variation reflects principally the care with which the observer followed the recipients and the strictness of the criteria employed for defining reactions. A conservative estimate would be that 2 per cent of all transfusions are accompanied by some sort of unfavorable response. Thus with approximately 8 million units of whole blood administered annually in the United States, at least 160,000 recognizable reactions can be expected.

Caution must be exercised against erroneous diagnoses of transfusion reactions. Most of the symptoms of transfusion reactions are nonspecific (see accompanying table). Patients who receive transfusions are often seriously ill with disorders which themselves may be responsible for the acute onset of chills, fever, shock, or jaundice. The temporal association of the transfusion with the onset of symptoms certainly constitutes presumptive evidence of cause and effect, but important errors in patient care may result if wisdom and restraint are not exercised to assure a comprehensive consideration of possible causes other than transfusion.

Several complications of transfusions do not strictly qualify as transfusion "reactions," and thus are not included in the table. Among these are the development of *transfusion hemosiderosis* in the chronically anemic patient who receives a great many transfusions (usually more than 50) over a period of months or years, and the possible prejudicial effect of *sensitization to blood donor histocompatibility antigens* with respect to subsequent homograft survival. Another complication is the *transmission of diseases* such as syphilis, malaria, and hepatitis. The value of gamma globulin as prophylaxis against transmission of serum hepatitis has been controversial; a comprehensive evaluation of available evidence by the Public Health Service Advisory Committee on Immunization Practices has provided no justification for the prophylactic administration of conventional immune serum globulin. The possible value of hepatitis hyperimmune serum globulin for high-risk transfusion recipients is under investigation. An additional recognized complication of transfusion is the *"post-pump syndrome,"* an infectious mononucleosis–like illness occurring in 5 to 10 per cent of patients approximately one month after open-heart surgery. Possible causes include transmission of infectious mononucleosis or cytomegalovirus organisms via the transfusions, or transient host versus graft or graft versus host reactions involving recipient and donor leukocytes (principally lymphocytes).

There are several *complications of massive transfusion* (usually more than 3000 ml to an adult recipient within 12 hours). Citrate toxicity may occur, particularly during rapid intra-arterial transfusion or in patients with hepatic insufficiency or shunt bypass of the portal venous circulation. At citrate concentrations higher than 100 mg per 100 ml, skeletal muscle tremors may occur, along with prolongation of the QT segment of the electrocardiogram. Cardiac arrest may result if the citrate concentrations rise even higher. The manifestations of citrate intoxication can be prevented or eliminated by the simultaneous administration of calcium gluconate into another vein. Two other complications of massive transfusion are related to changes that take place in blood during storage in the blood bank. A hemorrhagic diathesis may develop, caused principally by the absence of viable donor platelets in blood stored more than 24 to 48 hours, even under ideal blood bank conditions. Depletion of the patient's own platelets by preceding massive blood loss is thus not compensated by the transfusion of viable donor platelets, and thrombocytopenia develops. Other

Categories of Transfusion Reactions

Cause of Reaction	Common Symptoms	Frequency	Shock	Prognosis
Contaminated blood	Chills, fever, headache, backache, delirium, bloody vomitus, and diarrhea	Rare	Yes ("red shock")	Serious
Bacterial pyrogens	Chills, fever, headache, malaise	Rare	No*	Good
Circulatory overload	Dyspnea, cough, hemoptysis, tachycardia	Rare	Rare*	Good
Air embolism	Sudden onset of cough, cyanosis, syncope, convulsions	Rare	Yes	Serious
Allergy	Itching, urticaria, fever, angioneurotic edema, bronchospasm	Common	No*	Good
Red cell incompatibility: intravascular hemolysis, extravascular hemolysis	Chills, fever, headache, backache, hemoglobinemia, hemoglobinuria, oliguria, jaundice	Moderate	Yes	Serious
Sensitivity to:				
Donor leukocytes	Chills, fever, headache, malaise, confusion	Common	Rare*	Good
Donor platelets	Chills, fever, headache, malaise, confusion	Rare	Rare*	Good
Donor plasma (IgA)	Anaphylaxis, collapse, chest pain	Rare	Yes	Serious
Unexplained (febrile)	Chills, fever, headache, malaise	Common	No*	Good

*Although shock is absent or rare as a general feature of these types of reactions, in the seriously ill or injured patient shock may be precipitated by the added stress of the transfusion reaction.

causes for hemorrhagic tendency are deficiencies of labile plasma coagulation factors in stored donor blood. Abnormal bleeding may occur on this basis in an adult who receives more than 8 to 10 successive units of stored blood in less than 24 hours; the complication can be largely prevented if every fourth unit of blood given within a 12- to 18-hour period is a "fresh" unit, i.e., drawn within three to four hours of administration. A unit of fresh-frozen plasma may be substituted at the same intervals if the patient's platelet count is adequate. A less frequent complication of massive transfusion of stored blood is the occurrence of clinically significant hyperkalemia in the recipient. During storage in ACD preservative solution at 4° C, donor red blood cells continuously lose potassium ion; thus the concentration of potassium in the suspending donor plasma will average 15 to 20 mEq per liter after two weeks of storage and 25 to 30 mEq per liter after three weeks. The danger of hyperkalemia is increased in the presence of impaired renal function. When renal insufficiency is known to exist, transfusion should employ blood stored less than five to seven days, and packed red cells should be used, whenever possible.

MECHANISMS OF REACTIONS

Contaminated Blood. The transfusion of banked blood contaminated by endotoxin-producing bacteria (usually gram-negative rods that grow well at refrigerator temperature) may give rise to extremely serious reactions in the recipient, with a fatal outcome likely in more than 50 per cent of the patients. Death usually results from profound and persistent vascular collapse. In addition to the symptoms listed in the table, a characteristic feature is the occurrence of "red shock"; i.e., unlike the more common hypovolemic shock in which peripheral vasoconstriction results in cold, gray, clammy skin, endotoxin shock may be accompanied by marked peripheral vasodilatation so that the skin is dry, warm, and pink. Thus it is essential that blood pressure be measured frequently in patients suspected of having reactions to contaminated blood, because dangerous hypotension may coexist with an outward appearance that belies the severity of the circulatory collapse.

Fortunately, with current blood banking procedures, contamination of stored blood rarely occurs. It is also fortunate that the diagnosis of significant bacterial contamination can be established within ten minutes. A small sample of residual donor blood from the container or tubing used for administration is centrifuged lightly (500 rpm for two to three minutes); a drop of the supernatant plasma is smeared, fixed by heating, and Gram stained. Unless most oil immersion fields contain several clearly definable organisms, contamination can be disregarded as the primary cause of the reaction. If the blood is cultured to confirm the diagnosis, incubation should be carried out at 30° C as well as at 37° C, because some contaminants will not grow at temperatures as high as 37° C.

Because of the extreme gravity of reactions owing to contaminated blood, rapid institution of comprehensive supportive therapy is essential. Intravenous therapy should include sufficient vasopressor drug to maintain the systolic pressure above 100 mm of mercury, corticosteroids (100 to 150 mg of hydrocortisone), broad-spectrum antimicrobials in high dosage, and additional

whole blood if the estimated blood loss has not been corrected. Special measures to mitigate renal complications are discussed later.

Pyrogenic Reactions. The term "pyrogenic reactions" should be reserved for reactions related to the presence of demonstrable bacterial pyrogens (endotoxins) in the infused blood or in the transfusion equipment. Now that commercially manufactured pyrogen-tested disposable transfusion equipment is widely employed, the frequency of pyrogenic transfusion reactions has diminished strikingly. When parenteral therapy equipment does contain pyrogens, febrile reactions are "epidemic" among patients receiving intravenous infusions, and the aid of a specialized laboratory qualified to demonstrate the presence of bacterial pyrogens should be sought. Treatment is symptomatic.

Circulatory Overload. The onset of acute left-sided heart failure during transfusion may reflect actual hypervolemia caused by administration of excessive amounts of blood to a patient whose volume deficit has been seriously overestimated. Even in the absence of hypervolemia, pulmonary edema may be precipitated by the too rapid administration of blood to a patient who is profoundly anemic (hemoglobin concentration less than 4 to 5 grams per 100 ml) or in cardiac failure. A further cause for the symptoms of circulatory overload may be the presence of mechanical circulatory obstruction, e.g., mitral or aortic valve disease. Whatever the cause, treatment consists of slowing the rate of transfusion (cessation if necessary), changing to packed red blood cells, and digitalization. Rarely, a small phlebotomy is required. When there is reason to be concerned about possible circulatory overload in an elderly or severely anemic patient, or in one suffering from either cardiac or renal insufficiency, venous pressure should be monitored at frequent intervals during transfusion.

Air Embolism. Air embolism is rarely encountered as a life-threatening cause of transfusion reaction except when blood is being administered under air pressure after massive exsanguination. The accident occurs when all the blood in the container into which air has been pumped has been delivered and air is allowed to flow into the patient. This complication has been largely eliminated with the increasing use of plastic blood containers to which external pressure can be safely applied without the possibility of air infusion (provided that air has not inadvertently got into the bag, e.g., during prior component preparation). When air embolism has occurred, the administration tubing should be immediately clamped and the patient turned on his left side in the head-down, feet-up position so that air in the right ventricle floats away from the pulmonary outflow tract.

Allergy. Allergic reactions are relatively common and are generally mild (hives, bronchial wheezing, and congestion of mucous membranes). Treatment is symptomatic (antipyretics, antihistaminics). The drugs should be administered directly to the patient; under no circumstances should they be added to the container of blood. Marked angioneurotic edema or anaphylaxis may require prompt parenteral administration of epinephrine, vasopressor drugs, and corticosteroids.

Red Blood Cell Incompatibility. Incompatibility within the ABO system, with the resultant destruction of donor cells by alloantibodies in the recipient's circulation, is the most common cause of life-threatening reactions in contemporary transfusion practice. These preventable transfusion accidents almost always occur because of technical or logistic errors—the use of faulty techniques of blood typing and improper identification of blood samples, donor bottles, and patients. When the recipient's blood contains potent allohemolysins, acute intravascular hemolysis of the donor cells occurs. When the plasma hemoglobin concentration exceeds the hemoglobin binding capacity of the recipient's plasma (normally 75 to 175 mg of hemoglobin per 100 ml of plasma), *hemoglobinuria* occurs. Whereas many patients tolerate severe hemoglobinuria, e.g., paroxysmal nocturnal hemoglobinuria, without serious impairment of renal function, intravascular hemolytic reactions are potentially dangerous, especially when accompanied by shock, because of the possible development of oliguria, anuria, and uremia.

When donor red blood cell destruction occurs predominantly extravascularly, as for example in the presence of Rh antibodies demonstrable only by the indirect antiglobulin (Coombs) reaction, hemoglobinemia is generally much less severe, and jaundice is a more prominent feature, reflecting reticuloendothelial cell destruction of antibody-coated donor erythrocytes sequestered from the circulation predominantly in the spleen and/or liver.

Although the occurrence of an acute hemolytic transfusion reaction can generally be suspected on the basis of the symptoms and signs shown in the table, a special problem is presented by *anesthetized patients,* in whom the only sign of serious hemolytic reaction may be oozing of blood at the operative site. The bleeding tendency, which is often accompanied by severe transient thrombocytopenia, is generally thought to be the consequence of disseminated intravascular coagulation in response to thromboplastic substances liberated from the hemolyzing cells.

To determine quickly whether acute intravascular hemolysis has occurred, a blood sample is drawn from the patient into a clean, dry syringe or a syringe rinsed with physiologic saline. The blood is mixed with an anticoagulant by repeated gentle inversion (with care to avoid foaming, which causes in vitro hemolysis) and immediately centrifuged. If the plasma is obtained within two to eight hours of massive intravascular lysis, it will appear frankly pink or red. Plasma examined 12 to 48 hours after intravascular lysis is more apt to be brown, reflecting the presence of methemalbumin, which can be demonstrated spectroscopically by Schumm's test (appearance of a sharply defined band at 558 mμ after treatment with one tenth volume of concentrated ammonium sulfide). When donor red blood cell destruction has been largely extravascular, the plasma will show increased indirect-reacting (unconjugated) bilirubin; peak levels generally occur four to six hours after the transfusion.

To ascertain the basis for incompatibility, blood freshly drawn from the recipient should be sent immediately to the blood bank along with the donor blood container so that a thorough serologic review can be carried out. Along with the conventional retesting of the recipient's serum for the presence of antibodies against donor erythrocytes, such a review should include search for antibodies in the donor plasma that might cause destruction of the patient's cells, or cells of the other donors in the case of multiple transfusions.

In addition to general supportive measures, therapy of acute hemolytic transfusion reactions should be especially directed to minimizing possible renal complications (see below).

Delayed hemolysis of donor cells may occur (usually three to ten days after the transfusion) as a result of post-transfusion sensitization of the recipient. Red blood cell destruction generally occurs by an extravascular mechanism, and is manifested principally by jaundice and progressive anemia. The latter, if severe, may be treated safely by further transfusion, provided that serologic investigation has clarified the cause of the erythrocyte destruction so that repetition may be avoided.

Dangerous Universal Donor. A special instance of hemolytic transfusion reaction is the destruction of the group A, B, or AB patient's cells by high-titer alloantibodies in the plasma of a group O donor blood. In modern practice, every effort is made to screen group O donor bloods so as to detect those with dangerously high titers of alloantibodies. Except under emergency conditions, group O blood should be given to A, B, or AB recipients only if screening tests have defined the blood as "low titer." When a "dangerous universal donor" reaction does occur, its severity is usually tempered by the dilution effect of the recipient's plasma volume, the neutralizing effect of soluble group-specific A or B substance (or both) in the recipient plasma, and the large recipient red cell mass. Nonetheless, hypotension, hemoglobinemia, hemoglobinuria, and renal shutdown may result. Clinical management is similar to that described above for hemolytic reactions resulting from destruction of donor cells.

When an A, B, or AB recipient must be transfused with multiple units (4 or more) of low-titer group O whole blood, a cumulative effect of donor alloantibodies may result in relatively slow extravascular destruction of the patient's red blood cells. Jaundice and progressive anemia are the chief signs. If the patient requires further transfusion, it is advisable to continue with low-titer O blood and to resume type-specific blood only after two weeks have elapsed from the time of multiple Group O transfusions.

A special category of "dangerous donors" consists of those whose plasma contains alloantibodies (which may be of any blood group specificity) as a result of multiple prior transfusions or incompatible pregnancies, the latter usually associated with evidence of hemolytic disease of the newborn. In many blood banks, donor alloantibodies against red cells will be detected by routine screening of all donor sera against commercially available cells containing all the clinically important erythrocyte antigens. Even when such screening has not been performed, the donor alloantibodies will be detected if a sensitive technique is employed for the minor cross-match.

Sensitivity to Donor Leukocytes, Platelets, or Plasma. Transfusion reactions in this category are observed in patients who have had multiple previous exposures to the homologous antigens either by repeated transfusions or by pregnancies. The aid of an experienced serologic laboratory should be sought to demonstrate the presence in the patient's plasma of antibodies to donor leukocytes, platelets, and plasma proteins. The majority of such reactions are caused by recipient sensitization to donor *leukocytes;* symptoms appear within 30 to 90 minutes from the start of transfusion and subside over the succeeding four to eight hours. Treatment is symptomatic. The reactions can be prevented by several effective procedures for removing leukocytes from the blood prior to transfusion. In addition, there have been increasingly frequent reports that *donor* plasma containing antileukocyte antibodies active against recipient white cells may cause an anaphylaxis-like reaction with hypotension, tachycardia, prolonged fever (up to 48 hours), tachypnea, cyanosis, and x-ray findings of "allergic pneumonia." Eosinophilia is sometimes observed. Treatment is symptomatic. Although antibodies to donor *platelets* are commonly demonstrable in multitransfused recipients, symptomatic reactions to the platelets in a single unit of transfused blood rarely if ever occur. Reactions may be observed when a sensitized recipient receives multiple platelet concentrates in a single infusion. Shulman has described a rare form of delayed post-transfusion thrombocytopenia representing a complex immune response to incompatible donor platelets. The patients are generally multiparous women; profound thrombocytopenia develops five to seven days after transfusion and may persist for up to six weeks thereafter. Steroid therapy has been ineffective, but there are two reports of prompt termination of thrombocytopenia after exchange transfusions. An additional complication of platelet transfusion has been observed in severely leukopenic sensitized recipients; immediately after transfusion of multiple HLA-incompatible platelet concentrates, leukopenia becomes more profound and may not recover to pretransfusion values for 48 to 72 hours. Finally, dangerous acute post-transfusion thrombocytopenia may result when the plasma from multitransfused donors contains antibodies to recipient platelets. Rare but extremely serious anaphylactic reactions have been observed in recipients whose sera contain antibodies to donor *IgA globulin*. The patient's own serum lacks IgA globulin, and precipitating anti-IgA antibodies are demonstrable by agar immunodiffusion. Marked anxiety, collapse, and unconsciousness may occur immediately upon receipt of as little as 2 to 5 ml of donor plasma; measures to combat anaphylaxis must be undertaken immediately. Because the reactions may be provoked by such small amounts of IgA globulin, prevention requires extensive washing of donor red cells to accomplish virtual elimination of residual donor plasma.

Unexplained Febrile Reactions. These continue to make up a large proportion of the febrile reactions observed on a busy hospital service. Incompatibility between recipient's plasma and donor's red cells, white cells, platelets, and plasma cannot be demonstrated, nor can pyrogens be detected. There have been several well documented reports of symptomatic reactions associated with rapid destruction of donor red cells in the absence of any evidence of incompatibility by an elaborate battery of in vitro serologic tests. Therefore transfusion reactions that remain unexplained should not be comfortably dismissed as "idiopathic" but should stimulate persistent diagnostic investigation. Until the cause is found, the patient remains prey to recurring reactions with all subsequent transfusions.

MANAGEMENT OF RENAL COMPLICATIONS

A patient who has experienced severe hemorrhage with actual or impending hypovolemic shock, or who is suffering from bacteremia, may be precipitated into more severe circulatory collapse by any of the transfusion reactions described above. Under these circumstances the hazard of oliguric renal failure is ever present. The hazard is greatly increased when the reaction is of the acute hemolytic variety, in which the free hemoglobin that enters the urine may precipitate in the renal tubules.

The following recommendations for treatment of threatened or actual renal failure complicating transfusion reactions are based on a program developed by Barry and Crosby at the Walter Reed Medical Center. Urine flow, as a reliable indicator of renal function, is an important guide to management, and such measures as may be necessary should be taken to assure accurate measurement of urine volume at hourly intervals. The objective of treatment is to maintain a urine flow of at least 100 ml per hour until the effects of the reaction have subsided. Systolic blood pressure should be maintained at a sufficient level (above 100 mm of mercury) to assure adequate renal perfusion. Excessive elevation of blood pressure is to be avoided because of accompanying renal vasoconstriction. As soon as the reaction has occurred, 20 grams of mannitol as a 20 per cent aqueous solution should be infused intravenously during a five-minute interval. This dose should initiate diuresis in the patient capable of responding to mannitol. In the event of an acute hemolytic reaction, the infusion of 45 mEq of sodium bicarbonate subsequent to the test dose of mannitol may be indicated. Because some of the urine obtained at the end of the first hour may have been in the bladder before the reaction, an additional one-hour collection should be obtained to enable reliable evaluation of the patient's response to mannitol. If the urine flow is greater than 40 ml per hour, intravenous fluid containing approximately 50 mEq of sodium per liter as chloride or bicarbonate, e.g., 300 ml normal saline plus 700 ml 5 per cent dextrose in water, should be administered in sufficient volume to match the desired urine flow (100 to 150 ml per hour) until the possibility of renal injury is past and the patient is able to take oral fluids in sufficient volume to maintain satisfactory urine flow. The original dose of mannitol may be repeated whenever urine flow drops below 100 ml per hour for any two-hour period, but not more than 150 grams of mannitol should be administered in any 24-hour period.

If the patient does not respond to the aforementioned measures and renal shutdown has become established, Barry and Crosby recommend the following:

1. Restriction of fluid intake to 500 ml plus visible output per 24 hours.

2. Provision of 100 grams of carbohydrate per day at a constant rate to avoid periods of hypoglycemia and to decrease catabolism.

3. Control of hyperkalemia by the administration of 15 to 30 grams of sodium polystyrene sulfonate resin every six hours by mouth or by rectum.

4. Transfer of the patient within the first few days of oliguria to a renal center. Prior to transport, any EKG abnormality associated with hyperkalemia should be corrected by the infusion of 25 per cent glucose in distilled water containing 25 units of regular insulin and 200 ml of 10 per cent calcium gluconate per liter. An infusion rate of 3 ml per minute or more may be required during the first 30 minutes to return the electrocardiogram to normal. Thereafter, during transportation, rates of 0.25 to 1 ml per minute will usually protect the patient from cardiac arrest.

SUBSEQUENT TRANSFUSION OF THE REAC-TION-PRONE PATIENT

There is always an increased hazard in transfusing a recipient who has had a previous transfusion reaction. Therefore the indications for subsequent transfusions in these patients should be subjected to especially critical scrutiny, and transfusion should be avoided whenever possible. On the other hand, the added hazard should not engender indecision and delay, to the detriment of the patient. Informed of the possible causes for transfusion reactions, supported by the results of thorough investigation of previous reactions in the patient, and possessing a variety of sensitive cross-matching procedures as well as methods for separating donor blood to provide only the components actually needed by the patient, the physician can proceed with confidence to meet such a patient's transfusion needs. The transfusion should be administered slowly, and the patient should be watched especially carefully to detect the earliest signs of recurrent reaction so that the procedure can be discontinued if serious symptoms develop.

Barry, K. G., and Crosby, W. H.: The prevention and treatment of renal failure following transfusion reactions. Transfusion, 3:34, 1963.

Bjerrum, O. J., and Jersild, C.: Class-specific anti-IgA associated with severe anaphylactic transfusion reactions in a patient with pernicious anemia. Vox Sang., 21:411, 1971.

Cassell, M., Phillips, D. R., and Chaplin, H., Jr.: Transfusion of buffy coat-poor red cell suspensions prepared by dextran sedimentation. Transfusion, 2:216, 1962.

Chaplin, H., Jr., and Cassell, M.: The occasional fallibility of in vitro compatibility tests. Transfusion, 2:375, 1962.

Greenwalt, T. J., Finch, C. A., Pennell, R. B., et al.: General Principles of Blood Transfusion. 2nd ed. Chicago, American Medical Association, 1970.

Public Health Service Advisory Committee on Immunization Practices: Immune serum globulin for protection against viral hepatitis. Ann. Intern. Med., 77:427, 1972.

Shulman, N. R., Marder, V. S., Hiller, M. C., et al.: Platelet and leukocyte isoantigens and their antibodies: Serologic, physiologic and clinical studies. Prog. Hematol., 4:222, 1964.

Ward, H. N.: Pulmonary infiltrates associated with leukoagglutinin transfusion reactions. Ann. Intern. Med., 73:689, 1970.

Section Four. HEMOCHROMATOSIS

(IRON STORAGE DISEASE)

Thomas H. Bothwell

Definition. The term hemochromatosis implies the presence of massive, generalized iron deposits in parenchymal tissues together with evidence of fibrotic changes and functional impairment in the most severely affected organs.

Pathogenesis. The amounts of iron normally absorbed and excreted daily are small, being between 0.5 and 1.0 mg in men and twice this figure in women. Any variations in absorption that do occur are directed toward maintaining a normal body iron content. There are three basic ways in which excessive amounts of iron can accumulate in the body.

First, there are conditions in which mucosal behavior is abnormal and amounts of iron are absorbed that are inappropriate to body needs. This occurs in idiopathic hemochromatosis, in which a daily absorptive rate of no more than 3 to 5 mg extending over half a lifetime leads eventually to massive iron overload with its attendant pathologic sequelae. The tendency to absorb iron excessively in the condition is inherited, being transmitted by a dominant or partially dominant autosomal gene. Inappropriate absorption of iron has also been noted in certain anemias, being a feature of thalassemia major and of other refractory anemias. The common denominator in such "iron-loading" anemias appears to be increased but ineffective erythropoietic activity. Excess iron absorption has also been noted sometimes in liver disease and in porphyria cutanea tarda, but why this should be so is not known.

A second cause of iron overload is too much iron in the diet. When large amounts of absorbable iron reach the lumen of the upper small intestine, the mucosal mechanism for excluding unwanted iron is overwhelmed, and excessive quantities are absorbed. This occurs most commonly in South African blacks who brew fermented drinks in iron containers. As a result, iron overload of varying degrees is found in the majority of adult men, and a small proportion exhibit fully developed hemochromatosis. Other potential sources of excessive iron in the diet are medicinal tonics and red wine.

Finally, there are situations in which iron is introduced into the body by another route. Multiple transfusions are used in the mangement of hypoplastic and other forms of refractory anemia. Each unit of blood contains approximately 200 mg of iron, and massive quantities of the metal can be introduced by this means. Since the body's capacity to excrete iron is very limited, subjects on regular transfusion therapy accumulate large amounts.

The eventual outcome in an individual patient can be modified by several factors. Caloric intake and hence iron intake tend to be greater in males, whereas menstruation and pregnancies increase iron losses in females. As a result, clinical manifestations of idiopathic hemochromatosis are four times more common in males than in females and occur at a younger age. Approximately a third of patients presenting clinically with the disease give a history of an excessive intake of alcohol. There are several reasons for the association. As mentioned previously, some alcoholic beverages, such as red wines, contain appreciable amounts of iron. Alcohol also stimulates iron absorption. Finally, the hepatoxicity of alcohol and iron are almost certainly additive. A similar interplay between genetic and environmental factors is seen in the hemochromatosis that occurs as a complication in thalassemia major. Such subjects have an inherent tendency to absorb increased amounts of iron. In addition, they receive multiple blood transfusions and are often subjected to misguided therapy with oral iron.

Pathology. Approximately one quarter of the 3 to 4

grams of iron normally present in the body is stored in the liver and reticuloendothelial system as a soluble complex, ferritin, and as a closely related but insoluble golden-brown compound, hemosiderin. In hemochromatosis the total body iron content is increased to between 20 and 40 grams, most of the extra iron being deposited as hemosiderin. Concentrations are greatest in the parenchymal cells of the liver and pancreas, but significant deposits are also present in other endocrine organs and in the heart. Varying degrees of fibrosis occur in affected organs, and in the liver cirrhosis is almost invariably present. Deposits in the reticuloendothelial system are relatively scanty in the genetic disorder idiopathic hemochromatosis, but are often heavy after multiple transfusions and are also prominent in the dietary iron overload that occurs in South African blacks. The degree to which the iron from transfused blood is redistributed from reticuloendothelial cells depends on the activity of the erythroid marrow and the plasma iron level. Redistribution, with offloading onto parenchymal cells, is particularly liable to occur when there is a hyperplastic marrow and when the transferrin of plasma is saturated with iron. Why reticuloendothelial deposits are so prominent in the dietary iron overload occurring in South African blacks is not known. A similar distribution has, however, been noted in animals given large amounts of oral iron. The cellular localization of the iron is important, because parenchymal deposits are noxious to tissues, whereas iron in reticuloendothelial cells seems to be harmless.

Clinical Features. Idiopathic hemochromatosis is usually regarded as a model of the effects of the slow accumulation of large amounts of iron in parenchymal tissues. Symptoms usually develop between the ages of 40 and 60 years, and presenting clinical features relate to one or more of a number of organs. The most prominent are skin pigmentation, diabetes mellitus, hepatomegaly with symptoms of hepatic dysfunction, cardiac failure, and evidence of panhypopituitarism.

In half the patients the skin is bronzed owing to the presence of excess quantities of melanin; hemosiderin is also present in the remaining half, and the skin has a slate-gray appearance. Pigmentation is most prominent on the exposed parts. Although a firm hepatomegaly is almost invariably present, liver function in the absence of associated alcoholism is often surprisingly good. Hepatic failure with coma can, however, be precipitated by intercurrent infections and other acute insults. The spleen is enlarged in about 50 per cent of patients, but complications as a result of portal hypertension are not common. Hepatoma may occur as a complication in older patients.

Diabetes occurs in the majority of subjects and may be mild or severe; insulin, occasionally in large doses, is usually needed for its control. Complications, such as nephropathy, neuropathy, and peripheral vascular disease, occur in about 20 per cent of patients. It has been customary to ascribe the diabetes to inadequate islet function as a result of iron deposits in the pancreas. There is, however, evidence that insulin levels are often normal. In addition, it has been shown that the incidence is high in the relatives of affected individuals, and that this is not related to the presence of iron overload.

Arrhythmias and refractory cardiac failure occur in a proportion of affected persons and are particularly troublesome in younger patients. Sexual impotence, testicular atrophy, and sparsity of body hair are commonly present. Although these are usually secondary to the liver dysfunction, the pituitary and other endocrine glands are sometimes directly affected. Recently, attention has been drawn to an arthropathy in some patients, affecting both small and large joints. It seems to result from chondrocalcinosis and iron deposits in the joints.

The symptom complex that is such a characteristic feature of idiopathic hemochromatosis is sometimes found in other forms of iron overload. For example, cirrhosis and diabetes have been reported both in South African blacks and in subjects who have had many transfusions; cardiac failure is also common in the hemochromatosis that occurs in thalassemia major. Other complications of excessive iron deposits have been recognized in South African blacks. Ascorbic acid deficiency and osteoporosis are both common in affected individuals, and there is some evidence that the iron overload is a causal factor in their occurrence.

Diagnosis. The diagnosis is not difficult when the classic tetrad of skin pigmentation, liver disease, diabetes, and heart failure is present. In fact, the combination of any two of these should alert the physician. Laboratory tests are required to confirm the diagnosis. The best screening test is the measurement of the plasma iron concentration and the plasma iron–binding capacity. In the absence of intercurrent infection or complicating hepatoma, the plasma iron is usually greater than 200 μg per 100 ml, and the transferrin is virtually completely saturated. It must be emphasized that this test does not define the degree of iron overload. The plasma is often saturated with iron both in affected relatives at a time prior to the development of significant stores and in patients with anemias resulting from ineffective erythropoiesis. Insight into the amount of parenchymal iron present can be gained in several ways. Injecting chelating agents such as deferoxamine (Desferal) and measuring the quantity of iron passed in the urine is helpful, because it has been established that this is positively correlated with the size of the iron stores. With an intramuscular dose of deferoxamine of 10 mg per kilogram, a normal person excretes less than 2 mg of iron over the next 24 hours, whereas subjects with idiopathic hemochromatosis usually excrete more than 10 mg. The test is particularly useful in distinguishing between idiopathic hemochromatosis and alcoholic cirrhosis with only moderate iron overload. Liver biopsy provides the final proof, with evidence of heavy parenchymal iron deposits together with a fibrous reaction. The amount of connective tissue varies from a fine portal-tract fibrosis to frank macronodular cirrhosis. Further useful information can be obtained by chemical estimation of the concentration of iron present in a needle biopsy specimen. In passing, it is important to emphasize that the physician's role extends beyond the diagnosis and treatment of affected patients. With up to one half of siblings showing a predisposition to develop the disease, it is important that they be defined and treated prior to the accumulation of massive quantities of iron.

Treatment and Prognosis. Apart from the management along conventional lines of complications, such as diabetes and heart failure, the specific treatment is to remove the iron as rapidly as possible. This objective is normally achieved by repeated phlebotomies. The 200 to 250 mg of iron removed in each pint of blood creates a deficit that leads to the mobilization of a similar quantity of iron from the body's stores. Weekly phlebotomies are tolerated well by most patients, and hemoglobin levels greater than 11.0 grams per 100 ml are often maintained with venesection programs that are even more vigorous. Once the stores are exhausted, venesections are continued at less frequent intervals to prevent reaccumulation of the iron. Successful removal of all the iron deposits, which is heralded by a drop in the plasma iron concentration, may occur only after weekly venesections have been carried out for two years or more. Provided the patient is eating a well balanced diet, no specific supplementation is required. When venesections are not feasible (e.g., in thalassemia), deferoxamine can be given on a daily basis. The amounts of iron excreted are, however, usually not more than 10 to 20 mg, and this method of treatment has not been widely applied.

Without therapy, idiopathic hemochromatosis is a fatal disease. Death usually results from cardiac failure in younger patients and from liver disease or its complications in older ones. Some subjects succumb to an acute abdominal crisis followed by shock. Although the cause has not been definitely established, it may result from gram-negative bacteremic shock. In one recent study only 33 per cent of untreated patients were alive at five years. In contrast, 89 per cent of those treated by repeated venesections survived. Such therapy is associated with a gain in weight, an increased sense of well-being, regression of skin pigmentation, and an improvement in hepatic and cardiac function; insulin requirements are also often reduced. Hepatoma can, however, still occur as a late complication.

Bothwell, T. H., and Finch, C. A.: Iron Metabolism. Boston, Little, Brown & Company, 1962.
Charlton, R. W., Bothwell, T. H., and Seftel, H. C.: Dietary iron overload, Clin. Haematol., 2:383, 1973.
Fairbanks, V. F., Fahey, J. I., and Beutler, E.: Clinical Disorders of Iron Metabolism. 2nd ed. New York, Grune & Stratton, 1971.

Section Five.   POLYCYTHEMIA

Edward H. Reinhard

754.   INTRODUCTION

Definition and Classification. Polycythemia is better defined as a sustained abnormal increase in red blood cell volume than as an increase in the number of red blood cells per cubic milliliter of blood; an abnormal increase in hemoglobin is invariably accompanied by an increase in erythrocytes, but the converse is not always so. Some writers apply the term *erythrocytosis* to polycythemias secondary to recognized causes, and the term *erythremia* to the idiopathic disorder otherwise known as *polycythemia (rubra) vera*. Polycythemic syndromes include polycythemia rubra vera, *"benign polycythemia,"* *familial polycythemia,* and *polycythemia secondary to a variety of causes;* although relative polycythemia does not fit our definition of polycythemia in that there is no absolute increase in red blood cell mass, it will be discussed in Ch. 755, because this condition must always be considered in the differential diagnosis.

The polycythemic syndromes can be classified under the following headings: (1) *Relative polycythemia* includes polycythemia caused by fluid loss, fluid deprivation, or extravascular shift of fluid, and at least some cases of so-called benign or "stress" polycythemia. (2) *Familial polycythemia* is usually due to an inherited hemoglobinopathy (which will be discussed under secondary polycythemias), but there are rare reports of what appears to be familial polycythemia vera. (3) *Secondary polycythemias* can be divided into those that are due to an appropriate (or physiologic) increase in erythropoietin production, and those due to an inappropriate (or nonphysiologic) increase in erythropoietin production. (4) *Polycythemia vera* ("primary" polycythemia).

755.   RELATIVE POLYCYTHEMIA

Relative polycythemia occurs when there is a decrease of plasma without comparable decrease of red blood cells so that the erythrocytes become more concentrated. Restricted fluid intake alone may lead within a few days to lowered plasma volume. More common mechanisms are increased loss of water and electrolytes because of diabetic acidosis, the postoperative state, diuretic therapy of congestive heart failure, vomiting, diarrhea, abnormal sweating, hyposthenuria, adrenal insufficiency, or excessive plasma loss owing to extensive burns or traumatic shock. The hemoconcentration accompanying dehydration rarely gives rise to more than a 25 per cent increase in hematocrit, but the leukocyte level may rise considerably more owing to mobilization from marrow and marginal leukocyte pools or stimulation of leukopoiesis by the disorder producing the dehydration. Restoration of fluid balance with appropriate amounts of water and electrolytes promptly abolishes the relative polycythemia. Release of erythrocytes from storage in the spleen in normal man is never sufficient to produce significant polycythemia.

GAISBÖCK'S SYNDROME, STRESS POLYCYTHEMIA, AND BENIGN POLYCYTHEMIA

Gaisböck in 1905 described 18 patients with hypertension associated with an elevated red blood cell count but without splenomegaly; subsequently this combination of findings became known as Gaisböck's syndrome. This term gradually fell into disuse, and some authors believed that these were patients in whom mild erythrocytosis and hypertension coexisted by coincidence.

In 1952 Lawrence and Berlin reported 18 patients with erythrocytosis in whom blood volume determinations revealed normal red blood cell mass and decreased plasma volume. It was thus apparent that these patients had relative polycythemia. Half of them had hypertension. The authors were so impressed by the anxiety-tension state of these patients that they attributed the relative polycythemia to "stress." Similar cases were described by other authors, and the diagnosis of "stress polycythemia" became popular. In 1964 Russell and Conley studied 25 patients with polycythemia who did not have the associated symptoms, the splenomegaly, the leukocytosis, and the thrombocytosis characteristic of polycythemia vera and in whom dehydration and arterial oxygen unsaturation were excluded. These patients formed a strikingly homogeneous group. They were predominantly white males with a mean age of 45 years, somewhat younger than that for patients with polycythemia vera. They tended to be moderately overweight and of stocky habitus. Slight plethora and suffusion of the eyes were common. Many of the patients were tense and nervous. Almost all smoked cigarettes. Twelve of the 25 had persistent hypertension. None of them had congenital heart disease, pulmonary disease, vascular shunts, clubbing of the fingers, or palpable spleen. The highest documented hematocrit values for the group ranged between 54.5 and 65 per cent. Blood volume determinations were done on ten of the patients. Some had a mild absolute polycythemia, whereas others had only relative polycythemia. Seven of these 25 patients had had significant vascular disease (myocardial infarction, intermittent claudication, cerebrovascular accident, Leriche syndrome, or thrombophlebitis). Russell and Conley believed that the recurring pattern of manifestations justified the concept of a unique syndrome that they called benign polycythemia. They emphasized that this is the same syndrome described by earlier authors under the designation Gaisböck's syndrome or stress polycythemia. They doubted, however, that stress played any part in the etiology of the erythrocytosis, and were of the opinion that multiple features of the syndrome are of constitutional pathogenesis and, at times, of familial occurrence. Some patients with high hematocrit values are undoubtedly normal persons whose hematocrit and red blood cell counts fall rather far from the mean on the normal curves of distribution. Patients with the Gaisböck or benign polycythemia syndrome do not require any specific treatment.

756. FAMILIAL POLYCYTHEMIA

It now appears clear that most instances of what were reported in the past as examples of familial polycythemia were, in fact, cases of genetically transmitted hemoglobin abnormalities, in which inheritance follows an autosomal dominant pattern. However, the incidence of polycythemia vera appears to be higher among American Jews and lower among American blacks even after correction for all biases which might lead to lower detection among blacks and higher detection among Jews. This different prevalence according to ethnic groups living in a somewhat similar environment suggests the influence of genetic factors. Furthermore, rare examples of what appear to be familial incidence of polycythemia vera have been reported in the literature. These findings, if valid, are best explained by polygenic inheritance (the operation of several genes often transmitted from both parents). There is an increased incidence of aneuploidy in polycythemia vera, but the chromosomal abnormalities are nonspecific and have been attributed by some authors to the abnormal and increased cellular proliferation of the marrow.

757. SECONDARY POLYCYTHEMIAS

SECONDARY POLYCYTHEMIAS ASSOCIATED WITH AN APPROPRIATE (PHYSIOLOGIC) INCREASE IN ERYTHROPOIETIN PRODUCTION

A variety of conditions associated with *tissue* hypoxia may lead to the development of this type of secondary polycythemia.

Pathologic Physiology. When there is prolonged lowering of the oxygen *tension* of the arterial blood despite a normal or elevated hemoglobin content, sustained secondary polycythemia often results. In this situation, the oxygen tension of the arterial blood is less than normal in spite of the increased oxygen carrying capacity. This, together with increased viscosity of the blood and the underlying circulatory burden imposed by the primary cardiac or pulmonary disease, results in decreased delivery of oxygen to the tissues. The plasma of hypoxic animals and of man has been shown to produce accelerated erythropoiesis in recipient animals. The mechanism by which erythropoietin-producing cells detect tissue hypoxia is not known, but the oxygen tension of arterial blood passing through the renal parenchyma somehow initiates a sequence of events in which the kidneys produce a *renal erythropoietic factor* (REF) which, in turn, may combine with or cleave an alpha-2 globulin in the plasma to form *erythropoietin*. This, when carried to the marrow, initiates the differentiation of erythroblast precursors into erythroid cells. Experimentally, erythropoietin also shortens the transit time of radioactive iron through the marrow compartment, which suggests that the maturation of the erythroid cells is speeded up. As the red blood cell mass is increased, the oxygen supply to the kidneys increases and the production of REF is reduced or shut off completely, thus slowing or stopping red cell production.

Some patients with significant arterial oxygen unsaturation caused by chronic obstructive pulmonary disease do not have erythrocytosis, or they may have considerably less erythrocytosis than comparable degrees of hypoxia resulting from high altitude or cyanotic heart disease would produce. The reason is not always clear. However, in some cases the red blood cell volume may actually be increased, but the hemoglobin and hematocrit values remain normal owing to a comparable increase in the plasma volume. Furthermore, acidosis makes more oxygen available to the tissues than would be predicted for a given degree of oxygen saturation (the *Bohr effect)*, and many patients with chronic lung disease have respiratory acidosis. Lastly, the concentration of 2,3-DPG in the red cells influences the availability of oxygen to the tissues, and this may be increased in chronic lung disease. Thus many factors other than the arterial oxygen saturation may influence the P_{O_2} in and around the cells in the kidneys responsible for erythropoietin production.

Situations and Disorders Causing Secondary Polycythemia Associated with an Appropriate Increase in Erythropoietin Production

Polycythemia secondary to *cardiac or pulmonary disease* occurs when there is less than normal oxygen saturation of the blood entering the aorta because of short-circuiting of the pulmonary capillary bed by passage of part of the venous blood from the right directly into the left side of the heart or into the aorta, e.g., patent atrial or ventricular septum, dextroposition of the aorta, or pulmonary arteriovenous fistula; when the alveolar ventilation is restricted because of chronic pulmonary disease, e.g., emphysema or silicosis; or when there is thickening of the alveolar membranes, e.g., in mitral stenosis, or diffuse pulmonary fibrosis preventing normal transfer of oxygen from the alveoli to the blood. Tremendous obesity (pickwickian syndrome), massive abdominal tumor, or ascites may decrease pulmonary ventilation and thus contribute to the development of secondary polycythemia. Healthy persons living at high altitudes have polycythemia proportional to the diminution in oxygen tensions of the inspired air (and hence in the arterial blood).

Another important cause of secondary polycythemia associated with an appropriate increase in erythropoietin production is the presence in the red blood cells of an *abnormal hemoglobin* with an increased affinity for oxygen (approximately 50 per cent of the total hemoglobin). These patients are heterozygotes with mutant hemoglobin and normal hemoglobin. The abnormality is transmitted as an autosomal dominant. The first such report involved an 81-year-old man and 15 members of his family covering three generations, in all of whom a hemoglobin variant designated as hemoglobin Chesapeake comprised about 30 per cent of the total hemoglobin. Since the initial report, familial polycythemia has been found to be caused by many other hemoglobin variants, including J. Capetown, Yakima, Kempsey, Ypsilanti, Hiroshima, Rainier, Bethesda, and Malmö (see Ch. 746 to 751). In all these familial polycythemias, the affected members of the families have had hematocrits in the range of 45 to 58 per cent, with a proportionate elevation of the erythrocyte count and hemoglobin levels; none have had leukocytosis, thrombocytosis, or splenomegaly. There has been no significant associated disability.

All the hemoglobin variants associated with erythrocytosis have amino acid substitutions located at one of the structural sites involved in subunit rearrangement during oxygenation. These substitutions usually involve amino acids which play a direct part in chain-chain interactions, as a result of which the mutant hemoglobin has an abnormal or abolished interaction between subunits resulting in an increased affinity for oxygen. The affinity of hemoglobin for oxygen may be expressed as the partial pressure of oxygen at which hemoglobin is half saturated (P_{50}). At $37°$ C and pH 7.4, the P_{50} of normal blood is 26.5 mm Hg. All these hemoglobins associated with erythrocytosis have an increased affinity for oxygen, and the oxygen dissociation curve is shifted to the left. The P_{50} value for the blood of patients with Hb Chesapeake is 18 to 20 mm Hg, and for the blood of patients with Hb Rainier, Yakima, and Kempsey it is 12 to 14 mm Hg. This left shift of the oxygen dissociation curve has little effect on the uptake of oxygen in the lungs, but is associated with a significant decrease in oxygen release to the tissues, so that tissue oxygen tension is decreased at a normal hematocrit with resultant stimulation of erythropoietin production. Hence red blood cell production increases until tissue oxygen tension is restored to normal. Many abnormal hemoglobins have normal electrical charges and cannot be detected by electrophoretic mobility studies. In addition to screening hemoglobin electrophoresis, laboratory confirmation of the diagnosis is based on study of the oxygen dissociation curves of the whole blood and of dialyzed hemolysates from which 2,3-DPG has been removed.

A mild compensatory erythrocytosis may occur in patients with longstanding *methemoglobinemia* or *sulfhemoglobinemia*, particularly when the pigment abnormality is secondary to certain chemicals such as analine dyes or gum shellac. Methemoglobinemia associated with hemoglobin M is only rarely associated with erythrocytosis. Cobalt is thought to produce secondary polycythemia by indirect stimulation of erythropoietin production.

Polycythemia occurs in association with primary aldosteronism, and may be induced by the administration of large doses of androgens or vasopressin. Relative polycythemia is common in Cushing's syndrome, but a true polycythemia may occur if both corticosteroid and androgen production are increased.

Clinical Manifestations. The clinical symptoms associated with these secondary polycythemias vary widely. In contrast to the disabling acute symptoms that appear in normal individuals on ascent to an altitude of 10,000 feet or more, most permanent residents at such elevations make a satisfactory adjustment and are asymptomatic. By virtue of the increased oxygen-carrying power of the blood and an increase in erythrocyte 2,3-diphosphoglycerate, sufficient compensation for its lowered oxygen tension is achieved so that these people are able to carry on muscular work with comparative ease. However, Monge has described *chronic mountain sickness* in occasional persons living at such altitudes who presumably have chronic pulmonary disease as a superimposed additional cause of arterial anoxia. Recurrent bronchitis and laryngitis over a long period of time develop into an incapacitating illness characterized by headache, tinnitus, dyspnea, anorexia, vomiting, and lethargy. These symptoms are greatly aggravated by slight exertion. The chest is emphysematous, and the vital capacity is reduced. Cyanosis, clubbing of the digits, and congestion of the scleral capillaries are prominent. Examination of the blood reveals polycythemia greater than that of other residents at the same altitude. The blood volume is increased, and reticulocytosis, moderately increased bilirubinemia, and sometimes leukocytosis are found. Return to sea level promptly relieves the symptoms, and the polycythemia gradually subsides. *Brisket disease,* affecting 1 to 5 per cent of cattle grazing in certain areas at high altitudes in Utah and Colorado, is an interesting counterpart of chronic mountain sickness in man. Brisket disease affects young calves mainly and, unlike *Monge's disease,* is characterized by pulmonary hypertension followed by right heart failure. The animals do not have sustained arterial oxygen desaturation, and they do not develop significant polycythemia. All animals that have been studied show a thick muscular coat around the small pulmonary arteries; it has been postulated that excessive development of this muscular coat as well as excessive fluid and salt intake caused by grazing on marshy ground are factors that contribute to the pulmonary hypertension and cor pulmonale in the affected animals.

Polycythemias secondary to cardiac or pulmonary disease are accompanied by symptoms and signs characteristic of the primary disease. The patients are invariably cyanotic and often have clubbing of the digits. Cardiac failure is common. Slight splenomegaly may be due to congestive failure or chronic pulmonary infection. *Ayerza's syndrome* is a condition characterized by slowly developing symptoms of pulmonary insufficiency, cyanosis, and polycythemia owing to primary disease of the pulmonary artery and its branches (arterial and arteriolar sclerosis, syphilis, or congenital hypoplasia of the pulmonary artery), aggravated, in some cases, by emphysema and pulmonary fibrosis. In this condition right-sided heart failure eventually develops (see Ch. 546 to 550).

In some secondary forms of polycythemia the erythrocyte level may reach 8 million and occasionally 10 million cells per cubic millimeter, usually with somewhat less than corresponding hemoglobin and hematocrit values. Reticulocytosis and slight hyperbilirubinemia are characteristic. Leukocytosis is absent except when there is associated infection, which also seems in some cases to restrict the polycythemic response to the arterial unsaturation. The essential diagnostic criterion of secondary polycythemia of this type is decreased oxygen saturation of the blood, almost always less than 90 per cent. The arterial oxygen saturation should always be determined at rest and after standard exercise; under the latter circumstances the arterial oxygen saturation remains approximately 95 per cent in normal persons and in most patients with polycythemia vera, whereas in patients with polycythemia secondary to anoxemia the arterial oxygen saturation after exercise always falls to less than 80 per cent and usually to much less than this (occasionally as low as 30 per cent).

Treatment. The treatment of polycythemia secondary to heart or lung disease is chiefly that of the underlying cardiac or pulmonary disorder. Elimination of the offending drug or toxic exposure relieves the polycythemia caused by methemoglobinemia, sulfhemoglobinemia, or carboxyhemoglobinemia. In acute episodes of cyanosis, oxygen administration may be helpful. The polycythemia with resultant increased oxygen-carrying capacity of the blood is a useful compensatory physiologic response. However, if the hematocrit value rises to levels above 65 or 70 per cent, phlebotomies may result in temporary relief of symptoms, perhaps because the bleeding lowers blood volume and viscosity. When hematocrit values are plotted against blood viscosity, blood viscosity rises slowly with increasing hematocrit until the level exceeds 60 per cent, when the slope of the curve increases more rapidly.

SECONDARY POLYCYTHEMIAS ASSOCIATED WITH AN INAPPROPRIATE (NONPHYSIOLOGIC) INCREASE IN ERYTHROPOIETIN PRODUCTION

In all the types of secondary polycythemia discussed above, the increased production of erythropoietin appears to be appropriate in that normal animals or man exposed to similar hypoxia, cobalt, or androgens would respond in a similar fashion. However, there is another group of secondary polycythemias in which the mechanism for the elaboration of erythropoietin is nonphysiologic, because there is no hypoxia and only a small proportion of individuals with each of these disorders develop increased erythropoietin levels. Secondary polycythemia of this type has been reported in association with many types of *cancer* and a few *benign tumors*. The

tumors which produce secondary polycythemia most frequently are malignant renal tumors and brain tumors; the brain tumors have usually been vascular tumors most commonly located in the posterior fossa. Papilledema was present in most of them. In one series of 37 cases of brain tumor (usually hemangioblastoma) with associated polycythemia, the hemoglobin returned to normal after removal of the tumor in 21 instances. Polycythemia has also been observed in association with carcinomas of the liver, prostate, lung, rectum, and breast, as well as with melanosarcomas, multiple myeloma, and pheochromocytoma. Secondary polycythemia also occurs in association with many types of *renal disease* other than tumors, including medullary cystic disease, renal tuberculosis, hydronephrosis, and renal artery stenosis, as well as after renal transplantation. There is evidence that many tumors and even some benign cysts of the kidney elaborate a substance having erythropoietin-like activity that is responsible for the excessive erythropoiesis.

758. PRIMARY POLYCYTHEMIA
(Polycythemia Vera, Erythremia)

Primary polycythemia is a chronic disease of unknown cause characterized by hyperplasia of all the cellular elements of the bone marrow, nucleated red blood cells being most prominently involved, with resultant sustained elevation of the erythrocyte count and hemoglobin and usually, to a lesser extent, leukocytosis and thrombocytosis. It has been regarded by many persons as a malignant neoplastic disease of the erythropoietic tissue analogous to leukemia. The relationship of these two diseases is emphasized by the fact that in primary polycythemia the leukocytosis is sometimes so pronounced as to suggest a diagnosis of chronic granulocytic leukemia, and some patients with well-established polycythemia eventually have developed blood and bone marrow findings, and even pathologic changes at autopsy, suggestive of leukemia even when no radiation therapy has been given. Conversely, several patients with typical granulocytic leukemia have been observed to develop polycythemia. In patients with primary polycythemia treated with radioactive phosphorus, the incidence of acute leukemia as a late manifestation has varied in different series of cases from 0 to greater than 20 per cent.

Aneuploidy and several other nonspecific chromosomal aberrations have been reported in untreated patients with polycythemia vera. In P^{32}-treated patients, the frequency of these aberrations is somewhat higher. According to one study, the finding most typical of P^{32}-treated patients is dicentric chromosomes, and a dose response curve to the last P^{32} dose was demonstrated. A Philadelphia-like chromosome was observed in two patients with polycythemia vera and in one with benign erythrocytosis, all after P^{32} therapy. The authors speculated whether the development of leukemia complicating P^{32}-treated polycythemia might be dependent on the type and location of radiation-induced chromosomal damage, with subsequent establishment of a clone of cells with a selective developmental advantage. There is no evidence that tissue anoxia or excessive production of any known endocrine or humoral factor, including erythropoietin, constitutes the stimulus to excessive blood cell production in primary polycythemia. When marrow from patients with polycythemia vera is incubated in vitro with erythropoietin, the rate of heme synthesis increases over that of controls by only one tenth. Marrows from polycythemia vera patients in remission respond normally to erythropoietin. These data suggest that the disease is due to an abnormal cell line whose intrinsic stem cell defect does not allow normal control of erythrocytic production by the usual regulatory substance, erythropoietin. There is now considerable evidence for the existence of two different lines of primitive cells in the marrow of patients with polycythemia vera: an abnormal cell line which differentiates at an increased rate and is not responsive to erythropoietin, and a normal cell line which lies relatively dormant so long as the differentiated products of the abnormal cells are present in sufficient numbers to suppress erythropoietin production.

It is now well established that many types of fowl and animal leukemia are due to viruses. Likewise, it has been observed that a "polycythemic virus" (a variant of Friend virus, or a passenger virus present in spleen filtrate prepared originally from mice infected with Friend virus) when injected into normal mice results in polycythemia and splenomegaly. Furthermore, this virus can initiate erythropoiesis in hypertransfused-polycythemic mice. The only other substance known to initiate erythropoiesis in a hypertransfused-polycythemic state is erythropoietin. The fact that this polycythemia-inducing virus causes an increase in proerythroblasts, erythroblasts, and reticulocytes and an increase in Fe^{59} uptake in the bone marrow and spleen without detectable erythropoietin activity in the plasma and urine suggests that the virus acts directly on erythropoietic stem cells and not through the mediation of erythropoietin. It is not presently known whether these animal data are relevant to human polycythemia vera.

In untreated polycythemia vera, the erythropoietic cells in the bone marrow do not respond normally to erythropoietin. The erythropoietin activity of plasma and urine is not increased. However, when the hematocrits of patients with polycythemia vera are reduced to normal or anemic levels by bleeding, measurable amounts of erythropoietin appear in the urine. Patients with hypoxia-induced erythrocytosis usually have increased levels of urinary erythropoietin, but an occasional patient with polycythemia of this type may have a normal level of urinary erythropoietin. If this situation is suspected, it is helpful to measure urinary erythropoietin content before and after phlebotomy. In polycythemia vera, phlebotomy results in little or no increase in erythropoietin excretion, but in patients with polycythemia secondary to tissue hypoxia with normal urine erythropoietin content, phlebotomy results in a marked increase in erythropoietin excretion.

The *incidence* of polycythemia vera is high among Jews and low among blacks. Men are more commonly affected than women. The usual age of onset is in middle or later life, although, rarely, young adults or children are affected. Familial polycythemia has been reported, and in these families onset of the disease in childhood is more common; as previously stated, at least some familial polycythemias are due to inherited hemoglobin variants.

Pathologic Physiology. In uncomplicated primary polycythemia the cardiac output and work are normal, but the velocity of blood flow is slowed. Pulmonary functions

are normal or nearly so. The arterial saturation of the blood is normal in most instances. Hypoxia has been demonstrated in some patients with polycythemia vera, but in such cases it has usually been attributed to unrelated coexisting cardiorespiratory disease. However, one study of 26 patients with polycythemia vera who had no evident heart or lung disease revealed that, although all of them had normal ventilatory function, 9 patients had an arterial oxygen saturation of less than 92 per cent, and 11 patients had a mean arterial oxygen tension that was significantly lowered (that is, less than 80 mm Hg). The diffusing capacity for carbon monoxide was significantly lower than normal in 10 of these patients, and the defect in diffusing capacity appeared to correlate well with the level of hypoxia. It was suggested that these abnormalities might be due to widespread thrombosis in small pulmonary arteries. Whether this is the correct explanation or not, it is important to emphasize that many studies have confirmed the fact that mild hypoxemia is not uncommon in patients with well established polycythemia vera, and the arterial oxygen saturation is of little value in distinguishing between primary and secondary polycythemia unless it is less than 88 per cent.

Many of the clinical manifestations, as well as intravascular thrombosis, the most common complication of untreated primary polycythemia, can be attributed directly or indirectly to three factors: (1) increased total blood volume, (2) increased viscosity of the blood, and (3) thrombocytosis. The feeling of fullness and aching in the head and the fatigability characteristic of this disease can be relieved by phlebotomies so promptly and consistently that the increased blood volume seems a major factor in their genesis. Some patients with this disease continue to have mild symptoms when the red blood cell level and hematocrit are in the upper normal range, and yet are completely asymptomatic when these values are reduced to the lower normal range. The extent to which the increased viscosity of the blood contributes to these symptoms and to the high incidence of intravascular thrombosis is not entirely clear, but the circulation time may be greatly prolonged with resultant visceral stasis; increased blood viscosity is at least an important contributory factor. As the hematocrit level rises above normal, there is a progressively more rapid increase in the blood viscosity; the higher the hematocrit rises above 60 per cent, the more imperative becomes the need to lower the hematocrit, and hence the viscosity, in order to relieve symptoms and minimize the danger of intravascular thrombosis. Paradoxically, when the hematocrit is greatly elevated, there is a tendency to bleed excessively from minor injuries; this may be caused, in part, by the distention of the capillaries and veins required to accommodate the huge blood volume. However, abnormal platelet function has been reported in patients with polycythemia vera who have thrombocytosis. The thrombocytosis may be pronounced, and undoubtedly contributes to the production of intravascular thromboses, because the incidence of thromboses is low in secondary polycythemia (high viscosity, normal platelet level).

In untreated polycythemia vera, the marrow iron stores are often depleted, and hypoferremia is not uncommon. Furthermore, as would be expected under these circumstances, the plasma iron disappearance time (T 1/2) is often markedly shortened. After repletion of iron stores by parenteral iron dextran administration, the plasma iron disappearance time approaches normal. In uncomplicated secondary polycythemia, the marrow iron stores are normal or increased, and the plasma iron disappearance time is more nearly normal than in polycythemia vera.

In polycythemia vera, there is very poor correlation between the hemoglobin value and the packed red blood cell volume on the one hand and the *total* red blood cell mass on the other. This is because the plasma volume in polycythemia vera may be normal, decreased, or increased.

The basal metabolic rate is frequently elevated. The increased production of blood cells results in an increased destruction of blood cells, and this increased cell turnover increases the metabolic rate. Since an end product of nucleic acid degradation is uric acid, it is not surprising that hyperuricemia or increased urate excretion occurs in 75 per cent of cases of untreated polycythemia vera and that at least 5 per cent of patients develop clinical gout.

Clinical Manifestations.   Symptoms vary from none to so many that psychoneurosis is suspected. Common presenting complaints include headache or a feeling of fullness in the head, itching that is aggravated by a hot bath, paresthesias, dizziness, weakness, fatigability, dyspnea, and visual disturbances. A ruddy complexion usually of considerable duration, skin or mucous membrane hemorrhages, or awareness of a heavy sensation or fullness in the left side of the abdomen owing to enlargement of the spleen may be initial manifestations. The plethora is especially noticeable in the face, mouth, neck, hands, and feet. The veins of the scleras and retinas are distended and dark. Elevation of the systolic pressure occurs in more than half the cases, but diastolic hypertension is no more common than in the general population. Hepatomegaly occurs in about half the cases and splenomegaly in over three fourths.

The red blood cells frequently number from 7 to 10 million or more per cubic millimeter when patients are first seen. The erythrocytes usually appear normal, but the hemoglobin value may be increased less, in proportion, than the erythrocyte level because of a low mean corpuscular volume and mean corpuscular hemoglobin. Sometimes there is hypochromia (low mean corpuscular hemoglobin concentration) in addition to microcytosis, especially after large hemorrhages or repeated phlebotomies. The reticulocyte percentage is usually normal, but the absolute number is increased. Reticulocytosis occurs, and normoblasts may appear in the blood, especially after hemorrhage. The leukocyte count is greater than 10,000 per cubic millimeter in more than half the patients; it is frequently over 25,000, and rarely as high as 50,000. Metamyelocytes and occasional myelocytes are seen in the blood. The platelets are usually increased in number, and counts as high as 3 million and even 6 million have been reported (counts above 3 million are now rarely encountered when modern "direct" platelet counting techniques are employed). The serum bilirubin levels, urine urobilinogen, and stool urobilin values are commonly slightly increased. The bone marrow in polycythemia vera classically shows hyperplasia involving all the cellular elements, orderly maturation, and decreased or absent stainable iron. By contrast, in secondary polycythemia the marrow hyperplasia involves only the erythroid cells, and iron stores tend to be normal. There are many exceptions to these classic concepts and, in actual practice, bone marrow examination is of lim-

ited differential diagnostic value. Determination of the *absolute red blood cell volume* is the single most important procedure in establishing the diagnosis. Unless the red blood cell volume is greater than 38 ml per kilogram for males and 36 ml per kilogram for females, the diagnosis of polycythemia vera cannot be considered established. The serum uric acid concentration may be greatly elevated in either primary or secondary polycythemia.

Among the common complications of the disease are the vascular thromboses already referred to; the incidence of such thromboses can be greatly reduced by adequate therapy. Cirrhosis of the liver and occlusion of the hepatic veins *(Budd-Chiari syndrome)* have been observed. Hemorrhage from varices in the esophagus, stomach, bowel, or rectum may be massive, as may be bleeding from duodenal ulcers, which occurs in 8 to 16 per cent of cases. Many patients with polycythemia vera, after an extremely variable interval ranging from a few years to over 20 years, develop compensated myeloid metaplasia. During this phase they usually have severe splenomegaly and occasionally considerable leukocytosis with the appearance of increasing numbers of immature granulocytic leukocytes in the blood. The red blood cell count and hematocrit may remain perfectly normal without therapy. This phase may last from six months to several years, and is usually followed by the development of myelofibrosis, progressive myeloid metaplasia, often with a leukemoid blood picture, and progressive anemia.

Treatment.   The treatment of primary polycythemia is directed toward maintenance of a reasonably normal blood volume, viscosity, and thrombocyte level. When the hematocrit rises above 55 per cent, blood should be withdrawn. Myelosuppressive therapy should be employed (1) whenever, in order to keep the hematocrit below 55 per cent, it is necessary to withdraw blood so frequently that iron deficiency of sufficient degree to produce symptoms develops, or (2) when the platelet count rises significantly above normal.

Radioactive phosphorus therapy is a very effective means of suppressing excessive hematopoiesis; 3.5 to 5 mc intravenously (or 4.5 to 6.5 mc by mouth) is a reasonable dose. If too much radioactive phosphorus is given, leukopenia, thrombocytopenia, anemia, or any combination of these may develop. Further treatment should not be given for at least two or three months, for this length of time is required before the red blood cell counts stabilize. An additional, somewhat smaller dose of P^{32} may then be necessary. Once the blood has been restored to normal by such treatment, it is desirable not to give further radiation therapy for at least one year and preferably several years, occasional phlebotomies being resorted to in the meantime as necessary. It seems likely that such conservative therapy will minimize the danger of a radiation-induced acute leukemia. Control of the manifestations of polycythemia vera by radioactive phosphorus is so smooth that patients so treated have a greater number of symptom-free days than from any other form of treatment available.

Nitrogen mustard, triethylene melamine, busulfan, chlorambucil, cyclophosphamide, phenylalanine mustard, procarbazine, cytosine arabinoside, and hydroxyurea have all been used successfully to reduce excessive hematopoiesis in this disease; the first two drugs are seldom employed for this purpose any longer, and there are only limited data concerning the long-term effectiveness of the last three drugs. If chemotherapy is being employed as the only form of therapy, busulfan should probably be avoided, because it produces the most persistent and prolonged platelet depression. However, if the red blood cell level is being controlled by phlebotomies and the only indication for drug treatment is control of marked thrombocytosis, busulfan may be the drug of choice. Any of these drugs may also be used as an adjunct to P^{32} therapy in the occasional patient who develops severe thrombocytosis or progressive leukocytosis refractory to P^{32}. During therapy with any alkylating agent, much closer supervision of the patient is necessary than when P^{32} is used.

It is apparent that at present there are many different ways of treating this disease. The author believes that phlebotomy should be used as the primary method of control of the hematocrit; busulfan, chlorambucil, cyclophosphamide, or phenylalanine mustard should be used as an adjunct to phlebotomies when needed to control a markedly elevated platelet count; and P^{32} should be reserved for treatment of elderly patients, patients who cannot be seen by the physician at frequent intervals, and those rare patients who are refractory to other forms of treatment. Irradiation of the spleen, if it becomes uncomfortably large, may relieve the discomfort. Splenec-

tomy is contraindicated, because an increase in the platelet level with resultant fatal thrombosis may result. Elective surgery of any sort should never be done until the platelet and hematocrit levels have been restored to normal. If emergency major surgery is unavoidable in a polycythemic patient with very high hematocrit and platelet levels, an immediate phlebotomy and P^{32} administration can be done within half an hour; rapid ambulation of the patient after surgery is imperative. Allopurinol should be given to control hyperuricemia.

It is paradoxic that after blood has been withdrawn repeatedly over a period of many years, in the late stages of the disease transfusions are often necessary, because myelofibrosis develops.

Adamson, J. W., and Finch, C. A.: Erythropoietin in the polycythemias. Ann. N. Y. Acad. Sci., 149:560, 1968.
Jepson, J. H.: Polycythemia: Diagnosis, pathophysiology and therapy. Can. Med. Assoc. J., 100:271, 1969.
Klein, H.: Polycythemia—Theory and Management. Springfield, Ill., Charles C Thomas, 1973.
Lertzman, M., Frome, B. M., and Israels, L. G.: Hypoxia in polycythemia vera. Ann. Intern. Med., 60:409, 1964.
Modan, B., and Lilienfeld, A. M.: Polycythemia vera and leukemia—the role of radiation treatment. Medicine, 44:305, 1965.
Reinhard, E. H., and Hahneman, B.: The treatment of polycythemia vera. J. Chronic Dis., 6:332, 1958.

Section Six.   DISEASES OF THE WHITE BLOOD CELLS

759.   NEUTROPHIL FUNCTION

S. J. Klebanoff

The primary function of the neutrophilic polymorphonuclear leukocyte is the phagocytosis and destruction of microorganisms, and this functional specialization is reflected in its unique morphologic and biochemical characteristics. The neutrophil develops in the bone marrow in a continuous process, beginning with the pluripotential stem cell and continuing through the committed stem cell, myeloblast, promyelocyte, myelocyte, metamyelocyte, and band cell to the fully segmented mature cell. The most important morphologic feature of the mature neutrophil is the abundance of membrane-bound cytoplasmic granules. At least two granule populations exist. Dense, relatively large granules which stain reddish purple with azure dyes (azurophil or primary granules) develop in the promyelocyte. These granules, which contain myeloperoxidase, basic proteins, acid mucopolysaccharides, and a number of acid hydrolases, are primary lysosomes. During the myelocyte stage smaller, less dense granules are formed which contain alkaline phosphatase, lactoferrin, collagenase, and lysozyme. These specific or secondary granules are free of acid hydrolases and thus are not lysosomes in the strict sense of the term. No further granule formation occurs beyond the myelocyte stage. Approximately three fourths of the granules of the mature neutrophil are of the specific (secondary) variety, and the remainder are azurophil (primary) granules. Subpopulations with more limited enzyme composition

have been described. The mature neutrophil has a relatively short life span. It disappears from the circulation at an exponential rate with a mean half-life of 6.5 hours. Its extravascular life span is a day or two. Some of the cells which leave the circulation are removed by the fixed macrophages of the liver and spleen. The remainder pass into the tissues or migrate to areas of direct contact with the environment (oral cavity, bronchotracheal tree, cervical canal).

The neutrophil response to microbial invasion can be divided into several stages: (1) chemotaxis, (2) phagocytosis, (3) intracellular killing, and (4) digestion (Fig. 1). Neutrophils are discharged from the bone marrow in large numbers, producing a leukocytosis. The total blood granulocyte pool (TBGP) normally consists of a circulating granulocyte pool (CGP) of actively circulating cells and a marginated granulocyte pool (MGP) of cells which are sequestered or marginated along the walls of small blood vessels. This latter process is accentuated in areas of inflammation. The neutrophil extends pseudopods between the endothelial cells of small venules, opening up a passageway through which it passes. The channel immediately closes behind it, and the neutrophil migrates by ameboid movement along an increasing concentration gradient of a specific chemotactic agent or agents. Chemotactic agents are formed in a number of ways: (1) Bacteria elaborate low molecular weight (approximately 1000) factors which are directly chemotactic for neutrophils. (2) The components of the complement (C) system are activated sequentially with the release of chemotactic factors. Bacterial antigens combine with specific antibody to form complexes which activate complement either by the "classic" pathway involving the first three functional complement components, C1, 4, and 2, or by

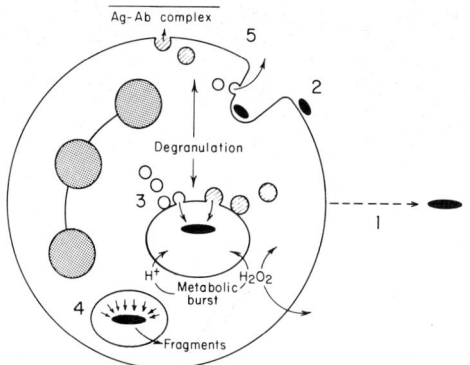

Figure 1. Schematic representation of the neutrophil response: (1) chemotaxis; (2) phagocytosis; (3) intracellular killing; (4) digestion; (5) extracellular enzyme release.

the "alternate" or properidin pathway which bypasses the early complement components. Activation by the "alternate" pathway also occurs when complement reacts with the endotoxic lipopolysaccharides of gram-negative bacteria. Three complement-derived components, C3a, C5a, and the trimolecular complex C567, have chemotactic activity. C5a is the predominant chemotactic factor in activated serum. (3) Proteinases released by bacteria, leukocytes, or damaged tissue act directly on complement components without activation of the entire complement sequence. C5 and C3 are cleaved to form the neutrophil chemotactic factors C5a and C3a. (4) Initiation of the kinin-generating and fibrinolytic pathways by Hageman factor activation results in the formation of kallikrein and plasminogen activator, respectively, which are chemotactic.

The chemotactic stimulus brings the neutrophil into direct contact with the microorganism, and phagocytosis rapidly follows. Cellular pseudopods surround the organism and isolate it from the extracellular environment in a vacuole lined by the invaginated cell membrane. A number of virulent organisms resist phagocytosis by virtue of the nature of their capsular material. These organisms are ingested when they can be trapped against a surface by the leukocyte (surface phagocytosis) or when the antiphagocytic nature of the capsular material is neutralized. Substances which react with particles to render them more susceptible to phagocytosis are termed opsonins. They may be heat stable or heat labile. Specific antibodies to surface antigens function as heat-stable opsonins. They attach to the bacterium through the antibody combining site on the $F(ab')_2$ portion and to the phagocyte through the Fc portion of the antibody molecule. The heat-labile opsonins are derived largely from complement, particularly C3. They are polyspecific and are not dependent on previous exposure to the organism. C3 when activated (C3b) attaches both to the bacterial cell wall and to receptor sites on the surface of the phagocyte. In general, antibody and complement combine to prepare the particle for ingestion, antibody serving both to identify the invading organism and to initiate adjacent complement activation.

Phagocytosis initiates a sequence of morphologic and biochemical events which result in the death of most ingested organisms. The granules adjacent to the phagocytic vacuole fuse with the vacuole, the common membrane ruptures, and the granular contents are discharged into the vacuolar space. All granular types

participate in the degranulation process. The metabolic machinery of the neutrophil is geared primarily to the production of energy (ATP) for chemotaxis and phagocytosis and to the production of H_2O_2 for microbicidal activity (Fig. 2). Energy production is dependent on glycolysis; it occurs in the absence of oxygen. H_2O_2 production, on the other hand, is dependent on the burst of metabolic activity which is associated with phagocytosis. There is an increase in glucose oxidation, particularly by the hexosemonophosphate (HMP) shunt. This is measured by the conversion of glucose carbon 1 to CO_2. There is a lesser increase in the conversion of glucose carbon 6 to CO_2 which measures the oxidation of glucose via the glycolytic pathway and Krebs cycle. Glycogen, which is present in large amounts in the neutrophil as particulate deposits, is broken down at an accelerated rate. Oxygen consumption is increased many fold and H_2O_2 is formed, possibly through a superoxide anion intermediate. Formate oxidation serves as a measure of H_2O_2 formation. Lactic acid production and phospholipid turnover also are increased.

Studies of the enzymic mechanisms responsible for the metabolic burst have focused on the oxidase responsible for the increased oxygen consumption and H_2O_2 production and on the link between this oxidase and the activation of the HMP shunt. The first two enzymes of the HMP shunt, glucose-6-phosphate dehydrogenase (G-6-PD) and 6-phosphogluconate dehydrogenase, reduce NADP to NADPH, and the continued activity of the shunt is dependent upon the reoxidation of NADPH. There are two prevalent views: (1) Oxygen is converted to H_2O_2 by NADH oxidase, a soluble enzyme which utilizes the NADH formed in the glycolytic pathway, and the H_2O_2 so formed activates the HMP shunt by a sequence of reactions, the oxidation of GSH by glutathione peroxidase and the reduction of GSSG by glutathione reductase, which result in the reoxidation of NADPH. (2) A granular NADPH oxidase is activated which meets the total requirements of the metabolic burst—increased oxygen consumption, H_2O_2 formation, and NADPH oxidation. The H_2O_2 formed by these or other mechanisms reacts with myeloperoxidase in the vacuolar space to form a microbicidal system (see below), whereas cytoplasmic components are protected from excess H_2O_2 by the glutathione system and by catalase.

A number of granular components released into the

Figure 2. Leukocyte metabolism: (1) glucose-6-phosphate dehydrogenase and 6-phosphogluconate dehydrogenase; (2) NADPH oxidase; (3) glutathione reductase; (4) glutathione peroxidase; (5) NADH oxidase.

phagocytic vacuole during the degranulation process have antimicrobial properties. These include cationic proteins, lactoferrin, lysozyme, and myeloperoxidase. The pH in the vacuole falls, and H_2O_2 accumulates. Myeloperoxidase combines with H_2O_2 and a halide such as iodide or chloride to form a potent antimicrobial system which is effective against bacteria, fungi, viruses, and mycoplasma. Chloride ions are present in the leukocyte in excess, and small amounts of iodide are absorbed from the extracellular fluid or are released by the deiodination of the thyroid hormones. When iodide is the halide employed, iodination of the microorganisms occurs, and the extent of the iodination in intact leukocytes is a measure of the activity of this system in situ. H_2O_2 or other products of oxidative metabolism have some antimicrobial activity in the absence of myeloperoxidase. The ingested organisms vary in their sensitivity to the intravacuolar microbicidal systems. Some organisms (e.g., pneumococci) are susceptible to acid, whereas others (e.g., lactobacilli) are acidophilic; some are readily lysed by lysozyme, whereas most organisms resist the action of this enzyme; some organisms (e.g., streptococci, pneumococci) secrete H_2O_2 or acid into the vacuolar space, and this contributes to their own destruction, whereas others contain catalase and thus resist H_2O_2-dependent systems. The level and variety of the antimicrobial systems endow the neutrophil with an overkill capacity which allows it to function adequately despite a decrease in the activity of one of the systems. The death of the ingested organisms is followed by their digestion to low molecular weight fragments by acid hydrolases.

Although the neutrophil primarily serves a protective function, tissue damage may result from the release of granule components into the extracellular fluid because of cell disintegration, leakage during phagocytosis, or secretion when leukocytes are in contact with antigen-antibody complexes on a nonphagocytizable surface (Fig. 1). Neutrophil-mediated injury is seen in the Arthus and Shwartzman reactions and in experimental immune complex disease. In man, it may contribute to the tissue damage in acute glomerulonephritis, polyarteritis nodosa, rheumatoid or gouty arthritis, and transplantation rejection.

Karnovsky, M. L.: Chronic granulomatous disease—pieces of a cellular and molecular puzzle. Fed. Proc., 32:1527, 1973.
Klebanoff, S. J., and Hamon, C. B.: Role of myeloperoxidase-mediated antimicrobial systems in intact leukocytes. J. Reticuloendothel. Soc., 12:170, 1972.
Mayer, M. M.: The complement system. Sci. Am., November 1973, p. 54.
Stossel, T. P.: Phagocytosis. N. Engl. J. Med., 290, 717, 774, 833, 1974.
Ward, P. A.: Leukotactic factors in health and disease. Am. J. Pathol., 64:521, 1971.

760. NEUTROPHIL DYSFUNCTION SYNDROMES

S. J. Klebanoff

Metchnikoff over 70 years ago proposed that the destruction of microorganisms by "microphages" is essential to the host defense, and the increased incidence of infection in severe neutropenia or agranulocytosis fully

Neutrophil Dysfunction Syndromes

Defects of chemotaxis
Defects of phagocytosis
Defects of microbicidal activity
    H_2O_2 deficiency
        Hereditary
            Chronic granulomatous disease (CGD)
                X-linked
                Autosomal
            Familial lipochrome histiocytosis
            Severe leukocytic G-6-PD deficiency
        Acquired
    Myeloperoxidase deficiency
        Hereditary
        Acquired
Mixed defects
    Granule dysfunction
        Hereditary
            Chédiak-Higashi syndrome
        Acquired
            Toxic granulation

supports this thesis. What has become apparent within the past decade is that neutrophils may be present in adequate numbers in the bloodstream, yet still be unable to perform their function adequately. Defects have been described involving several aspects of the neutrophil response, namely, chemotaxis, phagocytosis, and microbicidal activity (see accompanying table).

DEFECTS OF CHEMOTAXIS

Decreased chemotaxis may result from a cellular defect in which the leukocytes are incapable of responding appropriately to a chemotactic factor, from a serum defect in which formation of chemotactic factors in the patient's serum is decreased, or from the presence of an inhibitor of chemotaxis in serum. A combined cellular and serum defect may exist. Chemotaxis is evaluated in vivo by the skin window technique and in vitro by the Boyden chamber technique. In the *skin window technique,* coverslips, applied to areas of abraded skin, are replaced at intervals, and the cells which have adhered to their undersurface are stained and counted. The cells which enter the lesion during the first six hours are predominantly neutrophils, after which mononuclear cells predominate. The *Boyden chamber* consists of two compartments separated by a membrane filter. The leukocytes present in one compartment migrate through pores in the filter under the influence of a chemotactic agent and are counted.

A cellular defect in chemotaxis has been described in the lazy leukocyte syndrome, congenital ichthyosis, the Chédiak-Higashi syndrome, newborn infants, diabetes mellitus, rheumatoid arthritis, some patients with acute infection, particularly those with toxic granulation, and in other isolated cases. A serum defect in the generation of chemotactic factors is seen in newborn infants, hereditary C2 deficiency, C3 hypercatabolism, C5 dysfunction, systemic lupus erythematosus, and diabetes mellitus. An inhibitor of chemotaxis is found in the serum of patients with cirrhosis and in the serum of isolated patients with multiple infections. Normal serum contains a chemotactic factor inactivator which is decreased in $\alpha 1$ antitrypsin deficiency.

The *lazy leukocyte syndrome* is characterized by low-grade fever, neutropenia, and recurrent gingivitis, stomatitis, and otitis media. The response of the patient's neutrophils to a chemotactic stimulus is decreased, as are random mobility (i.e., mobility in the absence of a specific chemotactic stimulus) and the release of granulocytes from the bone marrow. The formation of chemotactic factors in the patient's serum, however, is normal.

Job's syndrome is characterized by recurrent "cold" superficial staphylococcal abscesses, eczematous dermatitis, hyperkeratotic nails, and high IgE levels. Extensive neutrophil function studies failed to reveal a metabolic or microbicidal defect, suggesting that Job's syndrome should not be included as a variant of chronic granulomatous disease. A cellular defect in chemotaxis has recently been found in this condition as well as in some other patients with high IgE levels.

DEFECTS OF PHAGOCYTOSIS

Decreased phagocytosis may be due to a cellular defect or to a deficiency or dysfunction of either immunoglobulin or complement resulting in decreased opsonic activity. A cellular defect in phagocytosis has been described in some patients with diabetes mellitus, systemic lupus erythematosus, chronic myelocytic leukemia, myelofibrosis, and megaloblastic anemia. The sera of patients with hypo- or agammaglobulinemia have decreased levels of heat-stable opsonins resulting in an increased susceptibility to infection by encapsulated bacteria.

The opsonic activity of complement is dependent largely on C3. *C3 deficiency* with decreased opsonic activity is seen in systemic lupus erythematosus and progressive glomerulonephritis. Newborn infants, particularly with low birth weight, have decreased serum opsonic activity related either to C3 deficiency or to lack of transplacental transfer of IgM. Hereditary defects involving C3 include homozygous C3 deficiency and essential hypercatabolism of C3. The latter has been subdivided into Type I associated with a deficiency in the C3 inactivator KAF (conglutinogen activating factor), and Type II caused by the enhanced activity of a C3 inactivating enzyme. The patient's serum was deficient in a number of complement-mediated functions, namely, bactericidal activity and opsonic activity, and in the generation of chemotactic factors, resulting in an increased susceptibility to infection with pyogenic bacteria. The administration of normal serum or, in some instances, purified C3 produced a temporary increase in C3 levels with restoration of the complement-mediated functions. *C5 dysfunction* is found in infants with a syndrome consisting of generalized seborrheic dermatitis, intractable severe diarrhea, recurrent local and systemic infections, usually with gram-negative organisms, and marked wasting and dystrophy *(Leiner's syndrome)*. Total hemolytic complement activity is normal, as is the level of the individual complement components. However, dysfunction of C5 is indicated by inability of the serum to opsonize particles dependent on C5 for optimal opsonization and reversal of this defect with purified C5. The generation of chemotactic factors in serum is defective in some patients.

The serum in *sickle cell disease* is deficient in heat-labile opsonins for pneumococci. It has normal levels of immunoglobulin, total complement, and the opsonic components of complement (C3, C5). A 5–6S pseudoglobulin of normal serum restores the opsonic activity of sickle cell serum. Decreased splenic clearance resulting from functional splenectomy also contributes to the decreased resistance to the pneumococcus in sickle cell disease.

CHRONIC GRANULOMATOUS DISEASE

Definition. Chronic granulomatous disease (CGD) is characterized by repeated and severe infection affecting lymph nodes, skin, lung, liver, bone, and many other tissues. *Staphylococcus aureus* and certain low-grade gram-negative organisms are the predominant pathogens. Tissue examination reveals multiple abscesses and granulomas and characteristic lipid-filled macrophages. The neutrophils (and monocytes) of these patients fail to kill certain ingested bacteria or fungi normally, and this is correlated with impaired leukocyte metabolic activity.

Incidence. CGD is a rare disease seen predominantly in males. Although generally found in infants and children, it is also seen in young adults.

Pathology. Miliary abscesses, varying in size from a few millimeters to several centimeters in diameter with occasional large abscesses, are seen on gross examination. Although any tissue may be involved, liver, spleen, lung, and lymph nodes are particularly susceptible. Patchy areas of hemorrhage and necrosis are common. Microscopic examination reveals evidence of an acute and a chronic inflammatory response; indeed, their coexistence is suggestive of CGD. An influx of polymorphonuclear leukocytes with abscess formation is seen, particularly in early lesions. Granulomas are a prominent feature, with areas of central necrosis surrounded by numerous plasma cells, lymphocytes, macrophages, and a few multinuclear giant cells. Tissue macrophages may be large with a foamy or vacuolated cytoplasm containing a characteristic yellow-brown lipid material. In some patients, the lipid-laden macrophages dominate the histologic picture, whereas, in others, only an occasional cell is seen. The organisms most commonly found in the lesions are staphylococci, enteric bacilli (Klebsiella-Aerobacter organisms, *Escherichia coli, Serratia marcescens,* Pseudomonas, Proteus, Salmonella, and Paracolon bacilli), and certain fungi (Candida, Aspergillus). Conspicuous by their rarity or absence from the lesions are β-hemolytic streptococci, pneumococci, and *Hemophilus influenzae.*

Pathogenesis. CGD is characterized by impaired host defense against certain microorganisms. Immunoglobulin levels are normal or elevated, and delayed hypersensitivity is unimpaired. Leukocytosis, with a high proportion of neutrophils, is characteristic of CGD as it is of infection in the general population. The peripheral neutrophils are morphologically indistinguishable from normal cells, although toxic granulation may be seen with longstanding infection. Chemotaxis and phagocytosis are unimpaired; however, the neutrophils do not kill normally those microorganisms generally found in the lesions. Other organisms (e.g. streptococci, lactobacilli, pneumococci) are readily killed by the patient's cells. This microbicidal defect is associated with a marked decrease in the phagocytosis-induced metabolic burst. The role of H_2O_2 deficiency in the microbicidal defect is emphasized by the improvement in microbicidal activity in vitro on the introduction of an H_2O_2-generating system into the cell. Indeed, those organisms which are killed well by CGD leukocytes generate H_2O_2, and their susceptibility to the intracellular microbicidal systems is due partly to the replacement of a defective leukocytic H_2O_2-generating system with H_2O_2 of microbial origin. The variability in the clinical course and in the mode of transmission suggests that different intraleukocytic molecular lesions can result in decreased H_2O_2 production and microbicidal activity. Several have been described. Leukocyte NADH oxidase activity was decreased in some patients, and two female patients were deficient in leukocyte glutathione peroxidase. Neutrophil dysfunction is also associated with a severe leukocytic deficiency of glucose-6-phosphate dehydrogenase, which is discussed later in this chapter.

A decrease in the intraleukocytic microbicidal activity results in the prolonged intracellular survival of ingested organisms. These sequestered organisms are protected from certain antimicrobials and from extracellular microbicidal systems, and multiplication and dissemination occurs. The organisms spread via the lymphatics and the bloodstream to the second line of defense, the fixed cells of the mononuclear phagocyte system. Lymphadenopathy and hepatosplenomegaly result. It is not known whether a defect exists in the fixed macrophage; however, its precursor, the blood monocyte, has decreased microbicidal activity. The fixed macrophages are unable to control the spread of infection, and miliary abscesses result.

Clinical Manifestations.   CGD is characterized by repeated, severe, and widespread infections with staphylococci and certain gram-negative pathogens. Chronic suppurative lymphadenitis is the most common feature, with cervical lymphadenitis often its first manifestation. Enlargement of the inguinal, axillary, mesenteric, and mediastinal nodes also occurs regularly. The initial and most striking feature in some patients is a refractory eczematoid dermatitis, particularly around the eyes, nose, mouth, and other body orifices. Stomatitis, conjunctivitis, and persistent rhinitis occur with regularity. Wounds often are infected. Pneumonitis is seen in most patients, although it may be a late manifestation. The lesion progresses from a patchy bronchopneumonia with hilar node enlargement to massive consolidation, involving the entire lobe or lung. Lung abscesses are common, and pleural effusion and empyema may occur. A distinctive roentgenologic finding in some patients is discrete, usually round, homogeneous areas of consolidation ("encapsulating" pneumonia). The pulmonary lesions run a protracted course, leading in some instances to progressively increasing pulmonary insufficiency and death. Hepatosplenomegaly is a consistent feature of the disease. Liver scans may reveal focal lesions, either abscesses or sterile granulomas. Chronic subphrenic abscesses occur frequently. Osteomyelitis, often at multiple sites, is common. The metacarpal and metatarsal bones are particularly susceptible; however, the large bones may also be involved. A feature of the osteomyelitis of CGD is absence of sclerosis. Complete healing occurs with long-term antimicrobial therapy. Gastrointestinal manifestations include persistent, often bloody diarrhea, nausea, anorexia, and abdominal pain. Perianal and perineal abscesses with fistula formation occur frequently. Pigmented lipid histiocytes and granulomas with giant cells are seen in rectal biopsies. Pericarditis may occur, and anemia, either hypochromic microcytic or normochromic normocytic, is found in almost all patients.

Diagnosis.   Any patient with severe staphylococcal or gram-negative infections since childhood who has normal or elevated immunoglobulin and WBC levels and normal delayed hypersensitivity should be suspected of having CGD. The diagnosis can be made with confidence by neutrophil function tests. A simple and commonly employed procedure is the nitroblue tetrazolium (NBT) reduction test. NBT is reduced to a blue-black substance (blue formazan) with low solubility by neutrophils activated by phagocytosis or exposure to endotoxin. Precipitation of formazan can be visualized microscopically or the dye extracted and measured spectrophotometrically (quantitative NBT reduction test). NBT is not reduced by CGD leukocytes. The leukocytes of many non-CGD patients with bacterial infection have increased spontaneous NBT reduction, i.e., NBT reduction in the absence of phagocytosis. A false negative result in this test should suggest the possibility of CGD. The diagnosis of CGD is confirmed by a decrease in leukocytic microbicidal activity, oxygen consumption, glucose C1 oxidation, formate oxidation, or iodination. The microorganism employed in the measurement of microbicidal activity is important, because the defect is selective, affecting staphylococci, gram-negative pathogens, and certain fungi.

Genetic Transmission.   The most common form of CGD exhibits *X-linked* transmission. The affected children are males, and the mother and approximately 50 per cent of female siblings are carriers. The female carrier of the abnormal X chromosome has two populations of granulocytes, one with normal metabolic and microbicidal activity and a second with the same defect as affected children (Lyon hypothesis). When the leukocytes of carriers are treated as a single population, intermediate activity in the neutrophil function tests is observed. Two populations of cells are seen in procedures (slide NBT test, radioautographic iodination test) which measure the activity of individual cells. The presence of a variant or variants of CGD with *autosomal* inheritance is indicated by female patients, particularly female siblings with clinical and laboratory findings similar to those of the X-linked variety.

Clinical Manifestations in Female Carriers of X-Linked CGD.   Unequal X inactivation may result in a preponderance of defective cells and in an increased incidence of infection. This, however, is rare in proved carriers, who are generally healthy. A chronic lupus-like illness, sometimes limited to the skin lesions of discoid lupus but on other occasions characterized by a more systemic disease, with arthralgia, cutaneous manifestations of lupus erythematosus, photosensitivity, fever, Raynaud's phenomenon, and recurrent stomatitis, has been noted in several CGD carriers. Tests for antinuclear antibodies are negative.

Therapy.   The treatment of CGD remains the vigorous treatment of infection, namely antimicrobial administration and surgical drainage or excision. Both should be instituted promptly and antimicrobial administration maintained until healing is complete. Surgical excision of circumscribed suppurative lesions, e.g., lymph nodes, is preferable to incisional drainage, because the latter heals slowly with seeding at other sites. There are two considerations in the choice of antimicrobial agent: (1) sensitivity of the microorganism and (2) ability of the antimicrobial to reach and destroy the intracellular organisms. Viable microorganisms sequestered within intact leukocytes are protected from the lethal effects of many antimicrobials. The preferred antimicrobial based on sensitivity should be used despite poor penetrance, to combat extracellular organisms. Rifampin, which readily penetrates into leukocytes, is effective against sensitive intracellular staphylococci in vitro and in animal models, but has not yet been proved effective in man. It should be used in conjunction with other antimicrobials to minimize the development of resistance. Continuous antimicrobial therapy during periods of remission may be beneficial. Granulocyte transfusion has been advocated for life-threatening infections.

Whole blood transfusions may be required when the anemia is severe. The coexistence of CGD and the very rare Kell phenotypes, Kell null (K₀) or McLeod, has been observed in five patients, suggesting an association between the two genetic loci. Such patients are sensitized by transfusions with blood containing Kell antigens, making subsequent transfusions difficult. The Kell phenotype of patients with CGD should be determined, and those with either K₀ or McLeod phenotypes should not be transfused unless a compatible blood is available or the clinical situation warrants the risk of sensitization. Most patients with CGD have normal Kell antigens.

Prognosis. In some patients, the disease is apparent within the first year of life and progresses relentlessly, with remissions measured in weeks or months to death within the first decade. In others, there is a relatively late onset and long periods of remission measured in years.

Variants of Chronic Granulomatous Disease

Variants of CGD have been described which can be separated from "classic" CGD by clinical and/or laboratory findings but which have in common a leukocytic microbicidal defect caused by decreased oxidative metabolism.

Familial Lipochrome Histiocytosis. Three female siblings have been described with splenomegaly, pulmonary infiltration, hypergammaglobulinemia, arthritis, and an increased susceptibility to infection. The most striking histologic feature was the presence of numerous large, pigmented lipid-filled histiocytes. As in CGD, the patients' leukocytes were defective in microbicidal activity and in phagocytosis-induced oxygen consumption, glucose C1 oxidation, formate oxidation, NBT reduction, and iodination. This condition differed from "classic" CGD, not only in sex affected but also in the late onset of symptoms, absence of a chronic granulomatous response, and occurrence of arthritis.

Severe Leukocytic Glucose-6-Phosphate Dehydrogenase Deficiency. Patients with glucose-6-phosphate dehydrogenase (G-6-PD) levels which are 20 per cent of normal or greater do not have an increased incidence of infection and have leukocytes with normal metabolic and microbicidal activity. This includes all patients with the common African Gd A⁻ variant of G-6-PD who have normal leukocyte G-6-PD activity and most patients with the Mediterranean Gd B⁻ variant who have a partial deficiency of leukocyte G-6-PD. Patients with leukocyte G-6-PD levels of 5 per cent of normal or below, however, have neutrophil dysfunction and increased susceptibility to infection. The leukocyte abnormality differs from the more common variants of CGD in that the decrease in hexosemonophosphate shunt activity is not reversed by methylene blue. Further, the metabolic and microbicidal defect is not as severe, which correlates well with the milder clinical course. All the patients described have chronic nonspherocytic hemolytic anemia.

MYELOPEROXIDASE DEFICIENCY

Neutrophils in a normal human blood smear contain an abundance of peroxidase-positive granules. Myeloperoxidase (MPO) deficiency is indicated by a decrease in this peroxidase reaction. It may be hereditary or acquired.

Hereditary MPO Deficiency. Six patients from four families with a complete absence of MPO from neutrophils and monocytes have been described. The eosinophil peroxidase is present in normal amounts. The leukocytes are otherwise morphologically indistinguishable from normal cells. Genetic studies suggest autosomal recessive inheritance. Of these patients, four were reported to be in good health, the clinical history of one was not described, and one had severe disseminated candidiasis which began in adulthood and responded well to amphotericin B therapy. MPO-deficient leukocytes have decreased fungicidal and bactericidal activity despite normal phagocytosis, although the defect is not as severe as in CGD. Iodination also is impaired; however, in contrast to CGD, there is not a decrease in phagocytosis-induced NBT reduction, oxygen consumption, glucose C1 oxidation, or formate oxidation.

Acquired MPO Deficiency. Acquired MPO deficiency may involve all or a portion of the neutrophils; myeloperoxidase may be undetectable or decreased in amount, and the deficiency may be permanent or temporary. It has been observed in some patients with severe untreated bacterial infection, in acute encephalitis lethargica Economo, in a few patients with refractory megaloblastic anemia, and in some patients with acute myelogenous leukemia, chronic myelogenous leukemia with blast-cell transformation, or myelomonocytic leukemia. When tested, the microbicidal defect in the isolated leukocytes was comparable with that found in hereditary MPO deficiency.

THE CHÉDIAK-HIGASHI SYNDROME

The Chédiak-Higashi syndrome is a rare autosomal recessive disease characterized by the presence of giant lysosome-like granules in all granule-containing cells. It is seen in man, mink, cattle, and mice. Less than 100 cases have been described in man, with a roughly equal proportion of males and females. Its main clinical features are (1) partial oculocutaneous albinism with photophobia, rotatory nystagmus, and hair with a characteristic silken sheen when exposed to light; (2) repeated febrile episodes resulting chiefly from staphylococcal infections of the skin, lungs, and upper respiratory tract; and (3) a lymphoma-like "accelerated phase," with widespread tissue infiltration by lymphoid and histiocytic elements, characterized by lymphadenopathy, hepatosplenomegaly, neutropenia, hypogammaglobulinemia, hemolytic anemia, a bleeding tendency caused by thrombocytopenia and coagulation factor deficiencies, and peripheral neuropathy.

The diagnosis of the Chédiak-Higashi syndrome is made by demonstration of giant granules in circulating leukocytes. In the bone marrow, abnormally large, pleomorphic, azurophil (primary) granules are seen in promyelocytes which undergo a series of fusions to form giant granules containing myeloperoxidase and acid phosphatase. The specific (secondary) granules develop normally. The bone marrow neutrophil reserve is low, and neutropenia is common, particularly in the accelerated phase when lymphocytic infiltration of the bone marrow is apparent. The presence of giant granules in mature neutrophils is associated with some impairment in function. Chemotaxis, as measured by migration into a skin window in vivo or by the response to a preformed chemotactic agent in vitro, is decreased. Phagocytosis and the related metabolic burst are unimpaired; indeed, an increase in the initial rate of phagocytosis has been reported. However, degranulation with the release of the contents of the giant granules into the phagocytic vacuole is delayed or absent, and a delay in the killing of some bacterial species has been described. These abnormalities in neutrophil function combine to increase the susceptibility of the patients to pyogenic infections. The partial albinism is a consequence of the abnormal distribution of melanin in giant melanosomes, and the neurologic manifestations are associated with a lympho-histiocyte infiltration in the region of the degenerated peripheral nerves. Giant lysosomes are seen in both peripheral and central nervous system elements.

Treatment. The infections generally respond to conventional antimicrobial therapy, and the anemia and hemorrhagic tendency to multiple blood or platelet transfusions. The low serum folic acid levels and megaloblastic bone marrow changes can be corrected by folic acid therapy. Treatment of the accelerated phase with combined vincristine and prednisone administration has been advocated. Death usually occurs within the first two decades owing to infection but less commonly to hemorrhage or to the extensive lymphocytic infiltration of the accelerated phase.

Baehner, R. L.: Disorders of leukocytes leading to recurrent infection. Pediatr. Clin. North Am., 19:935, 1972.

Blume, R. S., and Wolff, S. M.: The Chédiak-Higashi syndrome: Studies in four patients and a review of the literature. Medicine, 51:247, 1972.

Dossett, J. H.: Microbial defenses of the child and man. Pediatr. Clin. North Am., 19:355, 1972.

Good, R. A., Quie, P. G., Windhorst, D. B., Page, A. R., Rodey, G. E., White, J., Wolfson, J. J., and Holmes, B. H.: Fatal (chronic) granulomatous disease of childhood: A hereditary defect of leukocyte function. Semin. Hematol., 5:215, 1968.

Johnston, R. B., Jr., Lawton, A. R., III, and Cooper, M. D.: Disorders of host defense against infection. Pathophysiologic and diagnostic considerations. Med. Clin. North Am., 57:421, 1973.

Klebanoff, S. J.: Intraleukocytic microbicidal defects. Ann. Rev. Med., 22:39, 1971.

Lehrer, R. I.: The role of phagocyte function in resistance to infection. Calif. Med., 114:17, 1971.

Nathan, D. G., and Baehner, R. L.: Disorders of phagocytic cell function. Prog. Hematol., 7:235, 1971.

Quie, P. G.: Infections due to neutrophil malfunction. Medicine, 52:411, 1973.

761. THE LEUKOPENIC STATE AND AGRANULOCYTOSIS

William N. Valentine

Leukopenia exists when a reduction below about 4000 per cubic millimeter occurs in the total blood leukocytes. Although the differential count may remain essentially normal, much more frequently the neutrophils are disproportionately low and the terms *neutropenia* or *granulocytopenia* are more accurately descriptive. *Lymphopenia* exists when the lymphocytes number below about 1400 per cubic millimeter in children or 1000 per cubic millimeter in adults. Although severe leukopenia merges into *agranulocytosis* with its frequently fulminant clinical manifestations, the more moderate and usual degrees of leukopenia are often well tolerated. No hard and fast rule exists, and host factors as well as the numbers of monocytes influence the incidence and severity of infections. In general, subjects with absolute granulocyte counts of 500 to 1000 per cubic millimeter have moderately increased risks, whereas below this the invasion of mucous membranes, skin, and blood by microorganisms becomes increasingly frequent and severe. With absolute counts below 200 per cubic millimeter, severe infectious complications become the rule.

Etiology and Pathogenesis. The kinetics of leukopoiesis have been more difficult to approach experimentally than those of erythropoiesis. In granulocytic leukopoiesis three compartments exist: the marrow, the circulating blood, and the body tissues in general. The marrow consists of a mitotic compartment containing cells capable of division and a postmitotic compartment composed of a reservoir of mature, nondividing cells in numbers perhaps 15 to 20 times as great as those present in the peripheral blood. This "ready reserve" can be rapidly mobilized, and its availability provides a source of additional granulocytes while granulopoiesis is increasing in response to sustained increases in demand. The total intravascular granulocytes are thought to be normally about twice those calculated from leukocyte counts and blood volume. Some are margined along vessel walls, but are in rapid equilibrium with actively circulating cells. The normal granulocyte circulating half-time in man appears to be about six to seven hours, and once granulocytes exit into the tissues there is little evidence of return to the intravascular compartment. The extravascular life span of leukocytes is difficult to ascertain, but in the steady state it has been estimated that there may be some 20 times as many tissue granulocytes as intravascular granulocytes. The numbers of circulating leukocytes are a result of their rate of production, rate of exodus from the blood to extravascular tissue, and rate of destruction. In the long term, supply and demand must be equal if normal balance is to be maintained; in the short term, excesses of demand may temporarily be met by drawing on the marrow reserve pool of mature granulocytes. The feedback mechanisms by which control is modulated are not fully understood. However, the techniques for in vitro culture of marrow in soft media have demonstrated that the formation of distinct colonies containing granulocytic and monocytic cells requires the presence of a "colony stimulation factor" (CSF). Variations in CSF presumably affect net granulopoiesis and may constitute one mechanism of control. However, there are probably multiple stimulatory and inhibitory controls modulating production rate, maturation, and release of granulocytes into the blood. At present, assessment of granulocytopenia depends upon evaluation of marrow cellularity, the marrow myeloid to erythroid cell ratios, the distribution of marrow granulocytes of different stages of maturation, the response of marrow cultures to various levels of CSF and to graded doses of bacterial endotoxin, and sophisticated granulocyte labeling procedures necessary in assessing leukocyte life span outside the marrow. The difficult availability and partial inadequacy of these procedures often render the peripheral leukocyte total and differential count the principal modality for evaluating granulocytopenia.

The granulocytopenic state may result, then, from (1) interference with normal marrow production of leukocytes and their delivery to the periphery, (2) increased utilization and destruction of granulocytes in the circulating blood and tissues other than marrow, or (3) combinations of the above. In addition, redistribution of leukocytes among the various body pools may result in relative or pseudogranulocytopenia when peripheral white cell counts form the basis of the evaluation.

Those disorders *interfering with normal granulopoiesis* can be subclassified. The marrow may be aplastic or hypoplastic on an idiopathic basis. There may be a similar lack of granulocyte precursors owing to exposure to ionizing radiation or certain drugs which predictably have cytolytic effects and interfere with marrow function on a dose-related basis. Such drugs include many of the chemotherapeutic agents used in the treatment of neoplasia or in producing immunosuppression: the alkylating agents such as nitrogen mustard, cyclophosphamide (Cytoxan), chlorambucil (Leukeran), and their congeners, busulfan (Myeleran), procarbazine which interferes with deoxyribonucleic acid (DNA) polymerization, and the mitosis inhibitors such as vinblastine and vincristine sulfate (Velban and Oncovin). Chemotherapeutic agents which act as antimetabolites have similar effects. Among these are purine and pyrimidine antagonists such as cytosine arabinoside (Ara-C), 6-mercaptopurine, azathioprine (Imuran), thioguanine and 5-fluorouracil, and the folic acid antimetabolites such as methotrexate. The commonly employed phenothiazines have been intensively investigated, and appear to produce marrow aplasia or hypoplasia through inhibition of DNA synthesis, with resulting prolongation of marrow granulocyte generation time and reduction in cell division. Although adverse reactions are related to dose, there is considerable variation in host susceptibility. Mepazine and promazine have been relatively more frequently implicated than chlorpromazine. Other drugs whose administration carries a relatively or moderately high risk of causing either acute or chronic granulocytopenia and diminished granulopoiesis include the antithyroid drugs such as thiouracil, and to a lesser extent propylthiouracil and methimazole (Tapazole); the antimicrobials chloramphenicol, sulfonamides, and arsenobenzols; the anti-inflammatory agent phenylbutazone; and such therapeutic agents as gold preparations. Although adverse reactions to sulfonamides and the antithyroid drugs have some relationship to dose and duration of therapy, there are again wide variations in host susceptibility. For most of the other agents mentioned, idiosyncratic reactions appear to provoke granulocytopenia in certain sensitive individuals without much obvious relationship to dosage. This is particularly true of the severe aplasia produced by chloramphenicol, which, although rare, is chronic and often irreversible. This contrasts with the much more frequent occurrence of reversible and usually inconsequential leukopenia in many subjects receiving the drug. Other drugs at times producing granulocytopenia include the antidepressant dibenzazepine compounds such as imipramine; the antidiabetic drugs tolbutamide, chlorpropamide, and carbutamide; and the chinchona alkaloids such as quinidine. More rarely reported apparent offenders are procainamide, quinacrine (Atabrine), tripelennamine (Pyribenzamine), ethacrynic acid, thiazides, allopurinol, and various antimicrobial drugs. The list of offending or possibly offending agents is large and expanding. Exposure to environmental agents such as benzol, other solvents, insecticides, and sprays likewise carries the risk of quantitative granulopoietic depression. The hazards of exposure to benzol are particularly well documented.

In some disorders, *granulopoiesis is ineffective,* and there is increased intramarrow leukocyte death and inadequate delivery of granulocytes to the circulating blood despite normal or even increased cellularity of myeloid precursors. Ineffective granulopoiesis and granulocytopenia may be present at times in subjects with refractory anemia, leukemia, and other myeloproliferative disorders. They are classically present in folate and vitamin B$_{12}$ deficiency states, and may be induced by drugs which impair absorption (diphenylhydantoin) or interfere with the metabolism (methotrexate) of substances such as folic acid. Certain other antimetabolites in large doses produce an aplasia and, in smaller doses, a hypercellular marrow characterized by a variety of morphologic abnormalities and degenerative changes. Alcohol ingestion in large amounts may at times produce a similar picture.

Granulocytopenia and/or agranulocytosis may also result from *replacement of normal marrow elements* by fibrous tissue, by leukemic blasts, by plasma cells in multiple myeloma, by lymphocytes in lymphosarcoma, and, more rarely, by carcinoma cells in large numbers.

Finally, there are certain *hereditary or familial disorders* characterized by impaired production of granulocytes. In *infantile genetic agranulocytosis,* there is a usually severe granulocytopenia, although the marrow contains abundant myeloid precursors. Late myeloid forms are conspicuously absent or severely reduced, however. Neutrophil survival has been reported as normal. *Familial benign chronic leukopenia* is a rare condition with little increased susceptibility to infection. Marrows are cellular, but late granulocytic precursor cells (bands and segmented forms) are reduced. *Cyclic neutropenia* is characterized by periodic, recurring episodes of severe granulocytopenia with intervening intervals of complete normality. Its familial nature has been sometimes demonstrable and sometimes not. Its cause is unclear. It has been suggested that there is mild marrow failure with the periodicity regulated by feedback mechanisms. During periods of granulocytopenia, the myeloid marrow elements are hypoplastic, and mature forms beyond the myelocyte are markedly reduced in number. In certain heritable conditions, granulocytopenia has coexisted with other abnormalities. In *pancreatic insufficiency with neutropenia,* a hyperplastic marrow, neutropenia, and deficient exocrine pancreatic secretion coexist. The disorder is not X chromosome linked. *Neutropenia with immunoglobulin abnormalities* is probably familial, and is associated with hypogammaglobulinemia and a cellular marrow. *Myelokathexis* is an unusual syndrome in which a high proportion of myeloid precursors in marrow have severe degenerative changes. The ineffective granulopoiesis and evidence of increased intramarrow death of granulocytes are also accompanied by shortened peripheral life span of granulocytes. In some cases of the *Chédiak-Higashi syndrome,* a disorder characterized by defective lysosomal membranes, ineffective granulopoiesis also appears to be present.

In contrast to defective production, granulocytopenia may also result from *increased utilization and destruction* of leukocytes, even in the presence of normal marrow function. *Infections* are common causes: bacterial (typhoid and paratyphoid fever, brucellosis, tuberculosis, and overwhelming infections even with microorganisms characteristically producing leukocytosis); viral (influenza, measles, infectious mononucleosis, infectious hepatitis, rubella); rickettsial, at times; protozoal (malaria, relapsing fever, kala-azar). *Splenic dysfunction* and almost any condition associated with splenomegaly may result in leukopenia alone or in combination with anemia or thrombocytopenia, or both. Thus leukopenia is frequently found in congestive splenomegaly caused by portal vein hypertension, in certain collagen vascular disorders such as lupus erythcmatosus and Felty's syndrome (rheumatoid arthritis, splenomegaly, and leukopenia), in Gaucher's disease, and in granulomatous disorders and lymphomas with splenic involvement. A nonhereditary, splenomegalic disorder of unknown cause, *primary splenic neutropenia,* has also been reported to be due to increased peripheral destruction of leukocytes. *Neonatal immunization neutropenia* is a somewhat controversial entity, thought by some to be secondary to fetomaternal leukocyte incompatibility and transplacental passage of a specific leukoagglutinin from mother to fetus. Others question its existence as an established entity.

Certain drugs (amidopyrine is the prime example, but sulfonamides, phenylbutazone, and gold have been implicated in rare instances) act as haptens and elicit antibodies leading to neutrophil destruction and severe agranulocytosis *(agranulocytic angina).* The initial administration of the drug does not cause agranulocytosis for at least 7 to 14 days, and sensitization may not develop for weeks or months. The experiments of Moeschlin convincingly support an immune mechanism of this type in the pathogenesis of amidopyrine-induced agranulocytosis. Blood from a sensitized subject receiving this drug and administered to a normal recipient promptly produced severe neutropenia in the latter. Further, agglutination of both homologous and heterologous leukocytes occurred when they were exposed to plasma from a sensitive subject receiving amidopyrine. The serum of a sensitized donor is totally inactive in the absence of the sensitizing drug. It is postulated that the agglutinated leukocytes are destroyed and lysed, perhaps mainly in the lungs. Although the explosive production of agranulocytosis by other drugs has often been attributed to a similar mechanism, this often is not the case, and the phenomenon is probably considerably rarer than originally believed. In this reaction to amidopyrine, not only is there profound destruction of granulocytes in the periphery, but granulocytic precursors in marrow are also temporarily eliminated.

Often the etiology of granulocytopenia is multifactorial. Thus infections may suppress marrow function by toxicity, by interference with metabolism of substances such as folic acid, and by causing accelerated leukocyte destruction. Nutritional deficiencies may interfere with leukocyte production and simultaneously result in production of defective cells with shortened life span. Antibodies may damage both marrow precursors and circulating granulocytes. Lymphomatous involvement of marrow and spleen may lead to the coexistence of diminished granulopoiesis and accelerated peripheral destruction of white cells.

Although the clinician most commonly equates the term leukopenia with granulocyte deficiency, certain lymphopenic states are also associated with profound susceptibility to infections. Thus lymphopenia is observed in hereditary thymic aplasia (hereditary lymphopenia or Swiss type of agammaglobulinemia) commonly in conjunction with agammaglobulinemia. Affected children are liable to progressive viral infections and susceptibility to generalized vaccinia after vaccination; death usually occurs before the age of two years. Less severe or episodic lymphopenia has also been documented in other hereditary defects involving the thymus-dependent lymphocyte. These include the Wiskott-Aldrich syndrome, ataxia telangiectasia, and certain patients with "immunologic amnesia" in whom a complement-dependent lymphocytotoxic factor could be demonstrated in the serum during episodes of lymphopenia. In these situations, the lymphopenia is related to an underlying defect in the cellular immune mechanism which renders the patient extremely susceptible to bacterial, viral, protozoan, or fungal infections. In certain forms of Hodgkin's disease lymphopenia may be severe and anergy present.

Incidence. Agranulocytosis has become increasingly common with the proliferation of marrow-damaging chemotherapeutic agents utilized in the treatment of neoplasia and in immunosuppressive therapy, and by the more aggressive use of multi-drug therapy in malignancy. Indeed, with many protocols employed in the treatment of leukemia as one example, a period of agranulocytosis is accepted as the expected event to be endured prior to any evidence of remission. With other types of medication, agranulocytosis occurs in only a small number of patients exposed even to those drugs that cause the greatest number of cases. The gravity of complication rather than its frequency accounts for its great importance. Estimates of frequency have varied widely, but a recent estimate of phenothiazine-induced agranulocytosis has been 1 case in 1200 treated. Similarly, antithyroid drugs have been reported to cause this complication in about 4 of 1000, and chloramphenicol in as few as 0.01 per 1000 cases treated. The absolute frequency of agranulocytosis caused by each agent is a function of its rate of occurrence in those at risk and the frequency of its use in the general population. Although agranulocytosis occurs with a worldwide distribution, its induction by drugs or environmental factors parallels that of exposure of the population to offending agents.

Pathology. In granulocytopenias caused by underlying disease, the pathology of bone marrow and extramedullary tissues is that secondary to the disorder. Marrow may be replaced by fibrous tissue or by foreign or abnormal cells, or may be hypoplastic or aplastic. On the other hand, a hyperplastic but dysplastic marrow may accompany ineffective agranulopoiesis in certain leukemias, refractory anemias, and other myeloproliferative disorders. The myeloid precursors may exhibit vacuolization, asynchronous cytoplasmic-nuclear maturation, and other morphologic abnormalities. In vitamin B_{12} and folate deficiency, the marrow is hypercellular, and megaloblastic erythropoiesis is present, together with abnormal granulocytes such as giant metamyelocytes. In granulocytopenias in which peripheral leukocyte destruction is the predominant mechanism, the marrow granulocytes are most commonly increased, though with a paucity of mature forms owing to exhaustion of the marrow postmitotic reserve pool. In drug-induced agranulocytosis of the amidopyrine type, the marrow changes vary with the stage of the disease. Megakaryocytes and erythroid precursors are present in normal abundance. At the height of severe agranulocytosis, granulocytic elements, including myelocytes and metamyelocytes, are greatly reduced or absent. The prevalence of blast forms may erroneously arouse the suspicion of leukemia. In later stages, or in milder cases, there may be normal or hyperplastic granulocytopoiesis with a preponderance of less mature precursor cells. The marrow picture in agranulocytosis induced by the phenothiazines in its severe form is one of extreme aplasia. In the rare but exceedingly serious disorder sometimes induced by chloramphenicol, the chronic aplasia involves all cell series. In severe agranulocytosis, ulcerative lesions in the mouth, rectum, skin, and elsewhere are necrotic and contain large numbers of bacteria, but granulocytes are conspicuously absent. If death occurs as the granulocytic elements are returning to the blood, abscesses may make their appearance at affected sites. The localization of tissue reactions to invading microorganisms determines the remaining pathologic changes.

Clinical Manifestations.   In leukopenia without infectious complications, the clinical manifestations either are nonexistent or are those of an underlying disorder. In acute, drug-induced agranulocytosis of the amidopyrine type (agranulocytic angina), the onset of the disease is sudden, usually with chills, high fever, and prostration. This pattern was initially regarded as being due to bacterial invasion, but since symptoms may follow within an hour of drug administration, the initial manifestations of this type of drug-hapten-antibody reaction are probably due to the period of rapid granulocyte lysis. Similar pyrogenic reactions occur in the absence of infection in patients developing antibodies and reactions against homologous leukocytes as a result of repeated transfusions. These prodromal symptoms, either mild or severe, are often followed by a brief but variable period in which fatigue, prostration, and neutropenia persist, but no new symptoms develop. This second stage is followed by return of fever, chills, and headache, frequently with ulceration of the oral pharynx and sometimes of the rectum and vagina, and manifestations of sepsis. This third stage is concomitant with bacterial invasion of the tissues, the most frequent lesions occurring at the sites where bacterial flora normally flourish in the absence of infection. In agranulocytosis not associated with an immunologic mechanism of the amidopyrine type, initial symptoms may represent invasive infection per se. In severe agranulocytosis of any etiology, fever is often as high as 40 or 40.5° C and prostration is extreme. In the absence of treatment or of spontaneous recovery, mental confusion, stupor, and death frequently supervene within the next few days. The ulcerated lesions are covered with a dirty gray membrane, but gross pus and abscesses are absent. Bacilluria may occur in the absence of pyuria. Regional lymph nodes become enlarged, pneumonitis may develop, and hypotension and hyperventilation may be prominent. Death is usually due to massive infection, often with gram-negative bacilli. The peripheral blood has few if any granulocytes, and these few, when present, usually show pyknotic nuclei, vacuolization, and toxic granulation. In acute, self-limited forms of agranulocytosis such as those often induced by amidopyrine, antithyroid drugs, phenothiazines, and sulfonamides, erythrocytes and platelets are usually normal. When hematopoiesis is widely depressed, other cytopenias coexist with lack of granulocytes. In amidopyrine-induced *agranulocytic angina* as well as in many other drug-caused agranulocytoses, if the offending agent is withdrawn, the granulocytopenia usually persists for five to ten days. Immature granulocyte precursors reappear in the marrow before return of mature

cells to the peripheral blood and tissues. A transient monocytosis and appearance of a few myelocytes often herald the beginning of recovery, the percentage of myelocytes sometimes being as high as 10 to 15 per cent. In a few days the white blood cell count rises rapidly to normal levels, or substantial leukocytosis may supplant the leukopenia.

In other circumstances in which severe neutropenia or agranulocytosis is slightly less severe, develops more slowly, or continues on a chronic basis, the onset of symptoms may be less explosive, and the course more indolent or fluctuating. In *cyclic neutropenia* the usual history is that at intervals of 15 to 35 days but most frequently at about 21 days, the patient experiences a few days of fever, oral ulceration, or skin infection corresponding with the development of profound neutropenia. The neutropenia usually lasts three to four days, during which time granulocytes may disappear from the blood. A compensatory monocytosis is sometimes present. Between the cyclic attacks, which most often develop in infancy or childhood, but which may have a later onset, affected subjects are completely well. Some of the hereditary disorders such as *infantile genetic agranulocytosis*, transmitted as an autosomal-recessive disorder, are very severe, with early onset, frequent infections, and usually early death. In some, such as *familial benign chronic leukopenia,* there is little increased susceptibility to infection and neutropenia is modest.

Differential Diagnosis.   In the differential diagnosis of granulocytopenia and agranulocytosis, the history, physical examination, and marrow examination are crucial. Acute aleukemic leukemia and aplastic anemia are associated with characteristic marrow changes and usually with pancytopenia. Underlying disease in the form of neoplasia, collagen-vascular disorders, infections, and the presence of hepatosplenomegaly is defined by the history and physical examination and by laboratory studies. The history of drug ingestion or exposure to hazardous environmental agents is obviously of great importance. The familial or cyclic nature of certain granulocytopenias may also afford clues pointing to the correct diagnosis.

Prognosis.   Prognosis depends upon the nature and severity of the underlying disorder and the granulocytopenia itself, upon the self-limited duration or chronic peristence of granulocytopenia, upon the initiation of proper antimicrobial and other therapy, upon the presence or absence of associated erythrocyte and platelet depression, and upon the potential reversibility of the lack of granulocytes. Before the advent of antimicrobial drugs, mortality in severe agranulocytosis, such as that associated with certain coal tar derivative drugs in Germany and the United States in the 1920's and early 1930's, was 50 to 90 per cent. This approached 100 per cent in patients over 60 years of age or with less than 1000 leukocytes per cubic millimeter. At present, with early and proper antimicrobial management most patients recover. Another factor clearly influencing prognosis is the recognition of offending drugs or environmental agents and their complete, immediate withdrawal.

Treatment.   Patients with mild neutropenia without infection require only observation. Patients with sustained neutropenia are often managed on an ambulatory basis, sometimes with intermittent hospitalization for acute episodes of infection or for treatment of underlying disease. All patients with significant neutropenia should be carefully instructed on avoidance of crowds or undue exposure to infection in any form, on reporting promptly any untoward symptoms or febrility, and on the proper hygiene of skin, nails, and mucous membranes. Skin tests should be performed to provide information as to the patient's ability to express cellular immunity, and immunoglobulin levels of serum should be measured.

When agranulocytosis is detected, the patient should be hospitalized immediately even in the absence of signs of infection, because the earliest possible institution of antimicrobial therapy with the first indication of infection is important for survival. If infection or ulcerative mucous membrane lesions develop, early cultures of the lesions, the blood, the urine, and, if indicated, the cerebrospinal fluid are desirable, and should be repeated as indicated by the clinical course. Antimicrobial therapy should be directed toward broad coverage, and should not be withheld until the cultural results are known. However, therapy may require modification when the predominating organisms have been identified. It is, of course, important that all organisms cultured be tested for antimicrobial susceptibility. In many instances, the infecting organisms are those constituting "normal flora" rendered invasive by the presence of agranulocytosis in the patient. However, any microorganisms may be offending, and the possibility of sepsis with gram-negative organisms such as Pseudomonas and Proteus or with penicillin-resistant staphylococci must be recognized by the treatment regimen. For sepsis of unidentified type a satisfactory regimen includes gentamicin, 1.5 mg per kilogram of body weight every eight hours intravenously if the kidneys are functioning normally. The dosage should be reduced in subjects with uremia, but the drug may still be used with careful observation of renal function. In addition, 2 grams of cephalothin every four hours or 450 mg of 7-chlorolincomycin phosphate every six hours, both intravenously, should be administered. In patients with fulminant sepsis, 2 to 4 grams of carbenicillin every three hours intravenously may be used as a third drug. In many forms of acute agranulocytosis caused by drugs, the clinician can take some comfort that *if the offending agent is withdrawn,* agranulocytosis, and hence antimicrobial therapy, will be self-limited. In cases of doubtful etiology, *all* even remotely etiologic drugs should be withdrawn. The patient with agranulocytosis should be hospitalized in a single room, nurses or physicians with respiratory or other infections excluded, and visitors rigidly limited or excluded temporarily. The necessity for total "reverse isolation" with cap, gown, and mask precautions is advocated by some; but in the opinion of the writer, it is of doubtful efficacy if the regimen recommended above is employed. Nevertheless, in studies conducted in special facilities and dealing with severely neutropenic patients over prolonged periods (chiefly those being treated with extended chemotherapy), more stringent measures, employing "life islands" or laminar airflow rooms, vigorous measures to reduce skin and intestinal flora, and even sterilization of food, have probably further reduced intercurrent infections. Such facilities exist in only a few centers.

In patients in whom marrow function can be reasonably expected to return after agranulocytosis induced by therapy, every effort is required to support the patient during the critical period when granulocytes are absent. Neutrophil replacement by transfusion has proved to have some efficacy, but replacement of functional neutrophils in beneficial numbers is not feasible presently in most hospitals. However, in a few centers an increasing number of continuous-flow centrifuges designed to harvest leukocytes and platelets from large amounts of blood of compatible donors are being employed. Such harvesting techniques are becoming increasingly available, and may be a practical factor in the management of more cases of agranulocytosis in the not-too-distant future. The same can be said for currently experimental procedures such as marrow transplantation in subjects with leukemia and aplastic anemia. There is also increasing interest and, hopefully, potential for practical usefulness in techniques designed to bank or store patient's marrow for future use when it is expected that marrow function will be depressed or ablated by chemotherapy or radiation. These technical advancements, not yet available for most hospitals, are being increasingly evaluated for practicality and efficacy. In the meantime, transfusion of whole blood and separated platelets are of benefit when concomitant anemia and severe thrombocytopenia are present.

Granulocytopenia resulting from arsenic and gold may be treated by administration of BAL (British antilewisite; 2,3-dimercaptopropanol) in dosage of 1.5 ml of a 10 per cent solution in oil intramuscularly every four hours for two days, followed by similar dosage at 12-hour intervals for an additional eight to ten days. Of considerable importance in the treatment of agranulocytosis are attention to proper mouth care with frequent cleansing washes, avoidance of constipation and attendant anal abrasions by means of gentle enemas, and the maintenance of proper fluid balance by parenteral fluid administration when indicated. When the disorder is of short duration, maintenance of nutrition is usually not a major problem. Of great importance is the detection of an offending agent and its absolute prohibition at any future time.

Boggs, D. R.: The kinetics of neutrophilic leukocytes in health and disease. Semin. Hematol., 4:359, 1967.

Crosby, W. H.: How many "polys" are enough? Arch. Intern. Med., 123:722, 1969.

Finch, S. C.: Granulocyte disorders — benign, quantitative abnormalities of granulocytes. *In* Williams, W. J., Beutler, E., and Erslev, A. J. (eds.): Hematology. New York, McGraw-Hill Book Company, 1972, pp. 628–654.

Kostman, R.: Infantile genetic agranulocytosis. Acta Paediatr. Scand., 45 (Suppl. 105):6, 1956.

Kretschmer, R., August, C. S., Rosen, F. S., and Janeway, C. A.: Recurrent infections, episodic lymphopenia, and impaired cellular immunity. N. Engl. J. Med., 281:285, 1969.

Moeschlin, S.: Immunological granulocytopenia and agranulocytosis (clinical aspects). Sang, 26:32, 1955.

Morley, A. A., Carew, J. P., and Baikie, A. G.: Familial cyclical neutropenia. Br. J. Haematol., 13:719, 1967.

Pisciotta, A. V.: Immune and toxic mechanisms in drug-induced agranulocytosis. Semin. Hematol., 10:279, 1973.

Wiseman, B. K., and Doan, C. A.: Primary splenic neutropenia: A newly recognized syndrome, closely related to congenital hemolytic icterus and essential thrombocytopenic purpura. Ann. Intern. Med., 16:1097, 1942.

762. LEUKEMOID REACTIONS

Richard T. Silver

A leukemoid reaction is defined as a clinical syndrome in which changes are found in the peripheral blood suggesting leukemia. Usually, the white blood cell count is elevated, but a picture resembling leukemia may develop even when the white blood cell count is normal or reduced.

The most important distinction between a leukemoid reaction and leukemia is that the former is not an unregulated proliferation of leukocytes but an expression of a bone marrow response to some underlying cause. Thus the peripheral blood and bone marrow abnormalities return to normal when the cause has disappeared. Leukemoid reactions involve any of the white blood cells and can occur in a variety of diseases caused by bacterial and viral infections, allergy, poisonings, and malignancy, as well as in acute conditions such as hemolytic anemia, in hemorrhage, and after burns. It is unclear why certain leukemoid reactions are seen in some patients and some diseases and not in others. Leukocyte stimulatory and maturation factors and leukocyte kinetics are not well defined. Different types of leukemoid reactions occur with the same frequency as those cells which appear in the peripheral blood. Thus neutrophilic leukemoid reactions are most frequent; lymphocyte and then eosinophilic leukemoid reactions are next most common; and monocytic leukemoid reactions are relatively infrequent.

Neutrophilic leukemoid reactions are associated with neutrophilic granulocytic hyperplasia in the marrow. Such increases in neutrophilic leukocytes are seen, for example, in certain types of acute bacterial infections, acute hemolytic anemias, and metastatic disease of the bone marrow. Often, there is shift toward immaturity in both the marrow and the peripheral blood, for increased numbers of metamyelocytes and myelocytes are observed. Vacuoles and heavy, coarse granules may be seen in the cytoplasm of the granulocytes. Differentiation of a neutrophilic leukemoid reaction from chronic granulocytic leukemia is difficult if based only upon microscopic examination of the peripheral blood and bone marrow. Abnormalities suggestive but not diagnostic of chronic granulocytic leukemia include an increased platelet count (and correspondingly increased megakaryocytes in the marrow), increased numbers of circulating basophils and eosinophils, slight marrow fibrosis, and complete obliteration of marrow fat spaces. Anemia is less helpful in differentiating a benign from a malignant elevation of the white blood cell count, because it may be related either to the leukemia or to the disease causing the leukemoid reaction. Much more useful is the leukocyte alkaline phosphatase (LAP) score of the mature neutrophils in the peripheral blood. It is difficult to attribute an elevated white blood cell count to a leukemoid reaction unless there is a significant increase in the LAP score, whereas in the typical case of chronic granulocytic leukemia, the LAP score is low. Striking elevations of serum B_{12} and its binding proteins which are found in chronic granulocytic leukemia are rarely seen in neutrophilic leukemoid reactions, and this test can be helpful in differential diagnosis.

Leukemoid reactions should be readily distinguishable from acute granulocytic leukemia, even though in the latter disease the LAP score may also be increased. In a leukemoid reaction, the marrow shows relatively good preservation of erythropoiesis and granulocytes in all stages of maturation. There is no diffuse replacement of normal cellular elements by abnormal, immature cells as occurs in acute leukemia. *Auer rods*, usually considered strong morphologic evidence for acute granulocytic leukemia, have been seen in leukemoid reactions associated with disseminated tuberculosis.

Eosinophilic leukemoid reactions are often seen in parasitic and collagen-vascular diseases and in drug reactions. They are accompanied by eosinophilic proliferation in the marrow with a shift toward immaturity, and eosinophilic myelocytes and metamyelocytes may be observed. Eosinophilic (granulocytic) leukemia is indeed a rare clinical entity. Thus when a patient is observed with a high white blood cell count and a predominance of eosinophils, the condition is far more likely to represent a benign proliferation. It is noteworthy that eosinophils do not have alkaline phosphatase activity. Hence, in contrast to neutrophilic cells, eosinophilic leukemoid reactions and chronic eosinophilic leukemia cannot be distinguished by using the LAP determination.

Leukemoid reactions involving lymphocytes are seen, for example, in whooping cough, chickenpox, and infectious mononucleosis. In these conditions, the peripheral blood contains an increased number of lymphocytes, many of which are atypical and are known as "virocytes." There is considerable morphologic heterogeneity in contrast to the singular lymphocyte type seen in acute lymphocytic leukemia. The cytoplasm is vacuolated, and the cell border is serrated and wavy. Nuclear configuration and staining characteristics range from dark, clumped chromatin to lighter and more open or vesicular patterns. Most often, the bone marrow does not show a marked increase in lymphocytes or suppression of erythropoiesis or thrombopoiesis. Therefore marrow examination may be quite useful in excluding acute lymphocytic leukemia. Helpful distinction in diseases such as infectious mononucleosis, for example, may be made by utilizing serologic tests such as the heterophil reaction.

Striking increase in number of peripheral blood monocytes occurs infrequently, and rarely should cause difficulty in distinction from myelomonocytic or monocytic leukemia. Monocytosis has been seen in disseminated tuberculosis, in brucellosis, in other granulomatous diseases, and during marrow recovery after the vigorous use of chemotherapeutic drugs.

No therapy is required for a leukemoid reaction per se, although obviously the underlying condition should be appropriately treated. In those few but difficult instances in which it is initially impossible to distinguish a leukemoid reaction from leukemia, specific treatment must be deferred until the situation has clarified. The premature use of potent drugs in a patient without a primary hematologic malignancy is far more hazardous than deferring the onset of chemotherapy in a patient who subsequently proves to have leukemia.

763. THE ACUTE LEUKEMIAS

James F. Holland

Definition. The acute leukemias are a group of neoplasms which are manifest in the bone marrow. They are characterized by cells analogous to, and often individually indistinguishable by light microscopy from, normal immature hematopoietic cells. In the untreated state, acute leukemic cells enter the blood, where they usually become the predominant leukocyte, and invade other organs. The untreated disease leads to death after a brief and stormy illness, rarely lasting more than a year. Therapy has markedly altered prognosis, however, and the name "acute" as distinguished from "chronic" leukemia is no longer wholly descriptive.

Acute myelocytic leukemia arises from the marrow hematopoietic stem cell or its progeny; the term subsumes several subtypes of leukemia: *myeloblastic leukemia, promyelocytic leukemia, myelomonocytic leukemia, acute myelocytic leukemia* that is none of the foregoing, and *erythroleukemia*. Special forms of acute myelocytic leukemia often occur as the terminal events of chronic myelocytic leukemia, polycythemia vera, and myelofibrosis. Acute "pure" *monocytic leukemia* (Schilling) is characterized by monoblastic proliferation which can be distinguished cytochemically. Acute lekemias apparently derived from eosinophilic, megakaryoblastic, plasmablastic, and mast cells, although uncommon, display unique characteristics as well as some features in common with the other acute leukemias of marrow origin.

Acute lymphocytic leukemia arises in lymphoid tissue and is ordinarily first manifest by its presence in marrow. In some instances thymic infiltration precedes overt marrow disease, but it is not known whether the initial leukemogenic event in man is usually extramedullary. Many instances of lymphocytic lymphosarcoma and histiocytic lymphoma culminate in an acute leukemic phase which bears some resemblance to acute lymphocytic leukemia.

Acute leukemias and related lymphoreticular neoplasms occur throughout the vertebrate animals; examples are even known in some invertebrates. In the mouse, the species most extensively studied, a single transplanted leukemic cell can give rise to the full-blown disease. Removal of lymphoid target organs, such as thymus and spleen, causes a much higher frequency of acute myelocytic leukemia after leukemogenic viral infection than ordinarily would be the case. This indicates that host factors may in large part determine the type of leukemia which evolves.

Etiology. The etiology of human leukemia has not been established. It is known that leukemias and related sarcomas of chicken, mouse, rat, hamster, guinea pig, cat, dog, cow, baboon, monkey, and gibbon are caused by RNA virus infection. In inbred laboratory mice the infection is not spread horizontally by contact, but transmission may occur through the germ line. Some selectively inbred strains such as AKR eventually develop leukemia in nearly every mouse. Mice may harbor and transmit the incorporated leukemic virus without manifestations of leukemia, allowing it to become apparent in progeny as if sui generis. In chickens, hamsters, and cats, horizontal leukemia or sarcoma *viral transmission* has been conclusively proved. The risk of neoplasm in healthy cats after known viral infection has been shown to be several hundredfold higher than in the general cat population.

When analyses are made of all cases of human acute leukemia, clusters in space and time cannot be shown. When analyses have been limited to children less than six years of age, however, significant clustering has been found in different parts of the world. Rare anecdotal instances of contact transmission are also provocative. Leukemic families have been reported in which several offspring have been affected. In one such family, fibroblasts from surviving members showed increased suscep-

tibility to transformation in vitro by SV 40 virus, a suggestive analogy to ease of induction of the neoplastic state in vivo.

Radiation leukemogenesis in man is well known. Radiologists sustained nearly tenfold the death rate from leukemia of other physicians before the widespread use of protective measures. Survivors of atomic bombings, patients who formerly were x-irradiated for spondylitis, and those who received therapeutic doses of ^{131}I for thyroid cancer all showed increased incidence of acute myelocytic leukemia. Patients with multiple myeloma, Hodgkin's disease, or other cancers, who were previously treated with alkylating agents, with or without x-irradiation, have increased frequency of acute myelocytic or acute histiocytic leukemia.

Chronic benzene exposure is leukemogenic in mice and can cause human acute myelocytic leukemia. Anecdotal data on other aromatic solvents suggest their possible human leukemogenicity, but less widespread use. Acute myelocytic leukemia has been reported after marrow aplasia induced by chloramphenicol and by phenylbutazone.

A few *constitutional diseases* lead to disproportionate frequency of acute leukemia. In trisomy 21 *(Down's syndrome)* both acute lymphocytic and acute myelocytic leukemia are increased. *Bloom's syndrome* characterized by chromosomal fragility and rearrangements, the pancytopenia of *Fanconi's syndrome*, and *idiopathic aplastic anemia* are sometimes followed by acute myelocytic leukemia. *Paroxysmal nocturnal hemoglobinuria* may represent a clonal stem cell disorder, first manifest by production of abnormal erythrocytes, culminating occasionally in acute myelocytic leukemia.

None of these data on family clusters, radiologic initiation, chemical induction, or constitutional predisposition are inconsistent with the possibility of underlying viral leukemogenesis in man. Available molecular biologic data from human experiments are essentially congruent with observations made in the known viral leukemias of mice. The discovery of an RNA-instructed DNA polymerase (reverse transcriptase) in the avian sarcoma and murine leukemia viruses was a monumental step. This enzymatic activity provides an explanation for the mechanism of transcribing oncogenic information from the RNA of an infecting virus into DNA polymers. Such heteropolymers can be incorporated into the host cell DNA, thereby introducing a heritable template for transcription in daughter cells. This provides information to maintain the neoplastic state and, under proper circumstances, to make new virus. The enzyme has been found in high concentration in every RNA oncogenic virus studied.

An RNA-instructed DNA polymerase has also been found in virtually every instance of fresh human acute leukemic cells. A DNA transcript prepared from the RNA of a murine leukemia virus underwent partial hybridization with RNA from human leukemic cells. This suggests that the human RNA had itself been transcribed from a DNA codon similar to the nucleic acid sequences of mouse leukemia.

An antibody to the purified reverse transcriptase of a known primate sarcoma virus cross-reacted with and inactivated the human enzyme, suggesting their near identity. In extracts of human acute leukemic cells, a virus-like particulate is found on centrifugation in a sucrose gradient, corresponding to the known density of murine leukemogenic viruses. On rupture of this particulate, reverse transcriptase activity is released. In the presence of labeled deoxynucleotide triphosphates, and using the RNA of the particulate as template, a DNA transcript is synthesized similar to the DNA transcribed from known primate sarcoma virus. In other experiments, the labeled transcribed DNA specifically hybridized with segments of DNA in human leukemic cells, but not in normal cells. This implies that nucleic acid sequences in the particular RNA template had been transcribed from sequences uniquely found in the DNA of the leukemic cell.

In two pairs of identical twins, each with one normal and one leukemic member, the patients' DNA's contained segments that hybridized with DNA transcribed from the 70s RNA recovered from particulates in the leukemic leukocytes. The normal twins had no such particle-related sequences in the DNA of their leukocytes. These data support the concept that the leukemia-associated DNA sequences were inserted after twinning, and not through the germ line.

These data, taken together, provide strong molecular biologic support for the viral etiology of human leukemia. Infectivity of the isolated particulate remains to be demonstrated. Since there is no proof of utility of laboratory animals or in vitro systems for this purpose, reservations must still be held until this investigative impasse is surmounted.

Pathogenesis. The recognizable leukemogenic event may precede clinical disease by many years. The time of appearance of the first leukemic cell and the interim behavior of the population of leukemic cells can only be inferred from data in man obtained during evident leukemia, or from animal models. Under the conditions of marrow crowding inherent in the fully developed leukemic state, the thymidine labeling index is substantially lower for leukemic blasts than for normal myeloblasts. This indicates that a large proportion of cells are not entering the DNA synthetic phase during the availability of labeled thymidine. It is clear evidence that many leukemic blasts are dividing slowly if at all. The largest leukemic myeloblasts or lymphoblasts are the cells which have the highest frequency of labeling. These large blasts mature, partially, to smaller blasts.

In some experimental murine leukemias, the doubling time progressively lengthens as the population density of cells becomes greater, thus deviating from exponential growth. This could be a result of lengthening of the cell cycle, cell death, and an increasing number of cells that do not divide. Some nondividing cells are sterile, whereas others may again be recruited into the mitotic cycle. Early in the pathogenesis of the human acute leukemic process, cells might divide more rapidly than normal cells, but this is usually not true when the disease has become advanced enough to measure.

Acute leukemic cells generally lack the appropriate metabolic programming for the physiologic aging that dictates leukocyte death or loss from the body across membrane surfaces. Such cells therefore accumulate, and, relatively insensitive to whatever humoral mechanisms control normal hematopoietic cell population size, they become an ever-increasing tumor that "spills over" into the blood. Normal immature hematopoietic cells are ordinarily excluded from the blood, perhaps because their nondeformability precludes traversing the interstices of the marrow sinusoids. Leukemia, in its literal sense, occurs late in the disease. The reason why imma-

ture acute leukemic cells eventually appear in the blood is not known; it probably depends on complex interactions with or invasion of the sinusoidal wall.

Myeloblasts demonstrate positive staining reactions for peroxidase and Sudan black which are negative in *lymphoblasts* and *monoblasts*. Myeloblasts do not stain, or at most have diffuse cytoplasmic periodic acid–Schiff (PAS) staining, whereas lymphoblasts often show large, coarse granules with this stain. Fluoride inhibits esterase activity of monoblasts for naphthol AS-D acetate, but not that of myeloblasts. Electron microscopic studies often show dissociation in nuclear and cytoplasmic age and other ultrastructural characteristics which distinguish leukemic blasts from other types of hematopoietic cells.

On direct preparations made from bone marrow, about half the patients with acute leukemia have a normal *karyotype*. This establishes that grossly visible chromosomal abnormalities are not essential in the pathogenesis. The half of patients with acute lymphocytic leukemia and half of those with acute myelocytic leukemia who have abnormal karyotypes (hyperdiploid for acute lymphocytic leukemia, hypo-, pseudo-, and hyperdiploid for acute myelocytic leukemia) are of great significance in studying pathogenesis. Indeed, in both major forms of acute leukemia, the aneuploid modal chromosome pattern disappears when a complete remission of the disease is achieved and is replaced by a normal karyotype. On relapse of the disease, the original leukemic karyotype reappears, almost without exception. This indicates that the acute leukemias are clones of abnormal cells, rather than abnormally functioning normal cells. This distinction has great importance when devising a therapeutic strategy.

The fact that cells are fundamentally abnormal does not preclude their demonstrating many normal characteristics, including maturation, albeit impaired. Leukemic cells form much smaller colonies of granulocytes and macrophages in agar cultures than do normal marrow cells, and then only in the presence of a glycoprotein colony-stimulating factor. Since the colony-stimulating factor(s) also enhance normal colony growth and are found in abundant quantity in the urine of some patients with acute myelocytic leukemia, a possible role of this bioregulatory substance in the evolution and pathogenesis of the leukemic state has been postulated.

The maturing granulocytes in acute myelocytic leukemia may have abnormal size and distribution of specific granules, sometimes appearing as a regional haze of eosinophilic dust. *Auer bodies* are highly refractile cytoplasmic rods derived from coalescence of azurophilic granules. They are seen in some of the myeloblasts or promyelocytes of about one third of patients with acute myelocytic leukemia. Rarely, these nearly pathognomonic markers are also seen in mature polymorphonuclear neutrophilic granulocytes of acute myelocytic leukemia, demonstrating that some maturation has occurred. The granulocytes of acute myelocytic leukemia show diminished migration across capillary membranes; this test also returns to normal during remission when granulocytes derive from the euploid stem cells.

In *acute lymphocytic leukemia,* it is commonplace to see different stages of lymphoid maturation in the marrow, up to and including lymphocytes morphologically indistinguishable from normal. The degree of immaturity of the predominant acute lymphocytic leukemic cell in the marrow is of prognostic importance. Patients with large primitive lymphoblasts do not respond so well as patients whose cells appear more mature.

The proliferation of acute leukemic cells in the marrow impairs normal hematopoiesis, even at population densities of leukemic cells when mechanical crowding alone cannot be responsible. One explanation relates this to inhibition of normal hematopoiesis by a hypothetical biochemical product of the leukemic cells. Alternatively, the affected cell in acute myelocytic leukemia may in fact be the early progenitor cell whose progeny are the stem cells for myeloblasts, erythroblasts, megakaryoblasts, and monoblasts. Leukemic proliferation of one cell might be associated with concomitant abnormalities of the other progeny, including hypoplasia. This interpretation would help explain the abnormalities in erythrocyte maturation commonly seen in acute myelocytic leukemia, which in the extreme are called *erythroleukemia*. In its end stages the natural evolution of erythroleukemia is for a clonal selection to myeloblastic proliferation. Megakaryocytes in acute myelocytic leukemia are also often bizarre in appearance and maturation, and their derived platelets may be abnormal.

Leukemic cells invade tissues; infiltration with enlargement of spleen, liver, and lymph nodes is common in all types of acute leukemia. Central nervous system leukemia, characterized by infiltration of the pia and arachnoid, occurs in about half the patients with acute lymphocytic leukemia and less frequently in acute myelocytic leukemia. It ordinarily becomes clinically manifest only in patients whose early death from hematologic manifestations of disease has been prevented by therapy. Leukostasis, infiltration of vascular walls, invasion into surrounding tissues, and hemorrhage occur particularly at high myeloblast counts, and may account for rapid death when the vessel is in the brain substance. Infiltrates of skin, testes, serosal membranes, and bone may be prominent. Enlargement of liver and kidney may also occur without infiltration by leukemic cells.

Acute myelocytic leukemic cells, particularly in promyelocytic leukemia, may secrete a vitamin B_{12}–binding protein in large quantity, accounting for high serum levels of B_{12}. Acute myelocytic leukemic cells, particularly those with monocytoid characteristics, may secrete *muramidase*. This low molecular weight lysosomal enzyme, also known as lysozyme, may appear in the urine, leading to tubular damage and renal insufficiency. In promyelocytic leukemia, and rarely in other types of acute myelocytic leukemia, secretion of thromboplastic substances accounts for the frequent (but not invariable) syndrome of disseminated intravascular coagulation, fibrinolysis, and major hemorrhage.

Epidemiology. The annual incidence per million of acute myelocytic leukemia is quite constant from birth throughout the first 10 years at about 10 cases. A slight peak in late adolescence occurs, and the incidence remains at a nearly constant 15 per million until age 55, after which the incidence progressively rises to 50 at age 75. This suggests some ubiquitous agent and cumulative injury.

The incidence of acute lymphocytic leukemia is sharply different. There is a peak incidence from 2 to 4 years reaching 50 per million annually, falling to 20 or less by age 8 until puberty, when the rate declines to about 10. The incidence remains below 10 until age 65, when it again climbs to about 15 per million at age 75.

These data are not inconsistent with an infectious disease with greatest susceptibility in childhood.

Numerous clusters of leukemia have been reported, although it has not been persuasively demonstrated that they occur more frequently than by chance. In three separate series, however, coincidences in time (within 60 to 75 days) and space (within 1 kilometer or 1 mile) have been seen in a total of 15 pairs of children less than six years old, sufficiently frequently to make their occurrence by chance highly improbable ($P<<0.01$). Of the 30 children involved, 27 were under four years. These occurrences, taken in conjunction with the virologic data aforementioned, are compatible with a contagious infectious origin of acute lymphocytic leukemia of young childhood. Further information about induction periods and periods of infectivity might provide additional clues that would bear on the appearance of leukemia in older patients.

Clinically, approximately 80 to 90 per cent of children with acute leukemia have acute lymphocytic leukemia, and 80 to 90 per cent of adults with acute leukemia have the acute myelocytic varieties.

Clinical Manifestations. The symptoms and signs of acute leukemia relate to decrease or disordered function of normal hematopoietic cells, and to tumefaction by leukemic cells.

Anemia. Asthenia, pallor, headache, tinnitus, dyspnea, angina, edema, and congestive heart failure may all indicate anemia. The anemia may result in part from diminished erythropoiesis; excessive hemolysis and blood loss are also often contributory. Evidence of specific antibody mediated hemolysis (positive Coombs test) is uncommon. Erythrocytes may show considerable variation in size and shape. Normoblasts and erythroblasts are common in the peripheral blood in erythroleukemia, but occasional nucleated red cells can also be seen in other types of acute leukemia.

Hemorrhage. Oozing gums, epistaxis, petechiae, ecchymosis, menorrhagia, melena, and excessive bleeding after tooth extraction are common initial manifestations of coagulation disorder in acute leukemia. Retinal hemorrhages, subarachnoid bleeding, and gross hematuria are rare initial manifestations, but may occur later. In nearly all instances the abnormal hemostasis can be correlated with decrease in circulating thrombocytes. Hemorrhagic manifestations are uncommon when circulating levels are above 50,000 per cubic millimeter; below this level, hemorrhage is inversely related to platelet count. Most thrombocytopenic bleeding occurs when platelets are 20,000 per cubic millimeter or less. Increased intravascular pressure (venous occlusion or dependency) augments the appearance of petechiae. Sepsis markedly accentuates thrombocytopenic bleeding, not only locally as in hemorrhagic pneumonia, but also systemically.

In promyelocytic leukemia, thromboplastic substances released from the cells can initiate disseminated intravascular coagulation which leads to activation of normal fibrinolytic systems and the appearance of fibrin split products in the blood. Massive ecchymosis and exsanguinating hemorrhage can occur if not promptly treated.

Infection. Acute leukemia is often first recognized by the occurrence of a respiratory infection from which the patient never fully recovers. Other bacterial infections are frequent before therapeutic control is attained: dental infections, sinusitis, bronchitis, pneumonia, perirectal abscess, urinary tract infections, paronychiae, and skin infections. Infections appear to be attributable to absolute granulocytopenia and, to some extent in acute myelocytic leukemia, to impaired function of the granulocytes present. Fever without recognizable infection is also common in acute leukemia, but this is always a diagnosis by exclusion. Every new fever in an acute leukemic patient could be the beginning of a bacterial infection with potential life-threatening consequences. Early, diligent, and repeated search is required before accepting an interpretation of "leukemic fever."

Infiltration. Lymphadenopathy, particularly of the cervical nodes in children, may be the first sign of the disease. It is often generalized. Splenomegaly is present in most patients with acute lymphocytic leukemia, and in about half of those with acute myelocytic leukemia. Hepatomegaly is usually present. Bulging interdental papillae are highly characteristic of acute monocytic or myelomonocytic leukemia. Tumefaction in bone may lead to bone or joint pain and tenderness. These are common in children, and the disease may present as a limp or protective restriction of motion. Confusion of acute leukemia with acute rheumatic fever was once common. Subepiphyseal decalcification in children and small areas of osteolysis may be recognized on x-ray films.

A diagnosis can be long delayed by failure to obtain a blood count. Pancytopenia without recognizably abnormal leukocytes is found in a small proportion of patients, the so-called aleukemic leukemia. Granulocytopenia with a normal number of circulating lymphocytes may occur in any kind of acute leukemia. Ordinarily, however, the peripheral blood contains immature myelocytic or lymphocytic cells, and the leukocyte count is elevated owing to the abnormal cells, sometimes in excess of 100,000 per cubic millimeter.

A suspicion or presumption of acute leukemia necessitates an examination of the bone marrow, because a diagnosis ordinarily cannot be established with certainty on peripheral blood findings alone. If cells are not obtained in adequate quantity (a circumstance that occurs from entrapment in reticulin fibers or cellular "packing"), a needle biopsy is also required. Other causes of hematologic disorders which mimic acute leukemia must be excluded. Among these are toxic cytopenias, isolated or multiple, and conditions such as infections, neoplasms, or marrow infiltrations that may lead to leukocytosis and to immature cells in the peripheral blood. The most commonly confused disorders are infectious mononucleosis, hematogenous tuberculosis, and drug-induced myelotoxicity. Drug-induced marrow aplasia may be succeeded by a marrow filled with myeloblasts. This normal cohort of repopulating cells matures in a few days, thus establishing the differential diagnosis.

Preleukemia is a term which has been applied to patients with symptoms and findings suggesting acute myelocytic leukemia but whose diagnosis cannot be established on the basis of the evidence then available. The marrow may be hypo-, normo-, or hypercellular. The change of marrow differential to a younger cell type, ordinarily with peripheral leukocytosis, may come suddenly after years of desultory mild illness. Adequate studies have not been performed to establish if karyotypic or other characteristics of neoplasia are present from the beginning.

Therapy. The treatment of acute leukemia is aimed at eradication or at least at marked destruction of the tumor, and at supporting the patient through manifestations of the disease per se, its complicating disorders, and the effects of therapy. The strategy of antileukemic treatment is conveniently divided into remission induction, sustaining or maintaining the remission, reinforcement of the remission, treatment of central nervous system disease, and, on an investigational basis, immunotherapy. Conversion of leukemic to normal or nonleukemic cells has not been achieved in vivo.

The possibility of cure of acute lymphocytic leukemia has become realistic. Although not yet at this level of accomplishment, chemotherapy of acute myelocytic leukemia is much better than a few years ago, and several long-term survivors without evident disease are known. Before undertaking the induction treatment of patients with acute leukemia, the conscientious physician should establish that he has the most current information, drugs, and professional resources available. Since the therapy has been progressively improving, much important information is embodied in current research undertakings. Several drugs of great usefulness have not yet been released from investigational status. Many supportive services are not available except in large centers participating in leukemia research. For these reasons, care of an acute leukemia patient should be carried out by a physician in cooperation with the closest leukemia center. Strategy can be planned and induction accomplished there, and the patient can be managed by his own physician during remission. This participation in ongoing research is also critical to continued progress toward universally curative therapy.

Single drug treatments of acute leukemia have largely given way to combinations of therapeutic procedures tailored to different body burdens of leukemic cells. Induction treatments are effective in abruptly lowering the leukemic population but are less effective in prolonging remissions. Drugs of value in maintaining remissions are somewhat less active in inducing them. Experimentally, immunotherapy is known to be ineffectual when leukemic populations are sizable.

Classification of Response. After therapeutic reduction of leukemic infiltration of the marrow, restitution of normal elements occurs. Clinical improvement and survival correlate well with disappearance or decrease of detectable leukemic infiltration and return of normal hematopoiesis. For convenience, codification systems have been devised for marrow (M), peripheral hematologic data (H), physical status (P), and symptomatic status (S).

In the best remission, the marrow is classified as M_0, indicating no recognizable abnormality in any constituent. When the blast cells are less than 5 per cent by Wright's stain, it is difficult if not impossible to be certain a blast cell is a leukemic blast and not a normal myeloblast. M_1 allows up to 5 per cent blasts and M_2 up to 25 per cent blasts; M_3 and M_4 are more abnormal. In similar fashion, the hematologic values in the peripheral blood can be classified as H_0, indicating no abnormalities whatever in erythrocytes, leukocytes, or platelets; H_1, for minor abnormalities within the range of normal; and H_2, H_3, and H_4, for more pronounced departures from normal. Similar rating scales exist for physical abnormalities (P) and symptomatic manifestations (S). These allow classification of individuals for clinical purposes into those with complete remission (M_1, H_1, P_1, S_1, or better), partial remission (all values 2 or better), improvement, no change, and progression.

Acute Lymphocytic Leukemia. Induction of remission is successfully accomplished in 85 per cent of children with vincristine and prednisone. The use of daunorubicin, methotrexate, 6-mercaptopurine, or asparaginase during this induction period has not significantly increased the induction frequency. The sequence of events includes a rapid fall in leukemic cells in the peripheral blood, often beginning within 48 hours. Leukopenia usually ensues, which is not ordinarily a cause for alteration in dose during vincristine and prednisone administration. In 7 or 14 days the population of leukemic cells in the bone marrow is noticeably decreased and the marrow cellularity is less. By 28 days half of children have less than 5 per cent leukemic cells remaining in their marrow, and a brisk erythroid hyperplasia is often present. Repopulation of the marrow with normal hematopoietic cells follows. The appearance of increasing platelet counts and granulocyte counts in the blood precedes return of marrow entirely to normal and is a favorable prognostic sign of an oncoming remission.

Administration of *E. coli* asparaginase immediately after the vincristine and prednisone administration significantly lengthens the subsequent remission duration without serious addition to the toxicity which simultaneous administration entails.

MAINTENANCE. Combined use of 6-mercaptopurine and methotrexate delays the emergence of resistant clones of cells. The probability of a single cell being or becoming refractory to both drugs simultaneously is much less than for a single drug, thereby accounting for some of the benefits which accrue to combination chemotherapy. Although immunosuppression exists during this drug regimen, attempts to change the dose and schedule of the combination, allowing for periods of immunologic recovery during the intermittency, have not yet proved superior to the uninterrupted administration of both drugs.

REINFORCEMENT. During remission maintenance, reinforcement with one or two doses of vincristine plus prednisone for one or two weeks has been applied every four to 12 weeks. Reinforcement has been proved of value when contrasted to maintenance chemotherapy alone.

CENTRAL NERVOUS SYSTEM TREATMENT. Central nervous system leukemia is rare early in the disease. CNS leukemia became clinically frequent only after systemic manifestations of the disease yielded to control, precluding early death. Without specific treatment to the central nervous system, nearly half of affected children develop infiltration of the meninges and brain substance, often as the first manifestation of relapse, giving rise to headaches, irritability, vomiting, personality change, meningismus, papilledema, cranial nerve palsies, and, in young children, separation of the cranial sutures. The failure of systemic treatment to control the central nervous system manifestations probably results from sanctuary of the leukemic cells beyond the blood-brain barrier where drug concentrations are substantially lower. Because of the high frequency of CNS manifestations, regional treatment for central nervous system leukemia with intrathecal methotrexate has been applied effectively before the clinical syndrome emerges. This therapy decreases the central nervous system manifestations and improves the duration of the hematologic remission as well.

The early administration of cranial radiation (2400 rads in 12 treatment days) to include the entire brain,

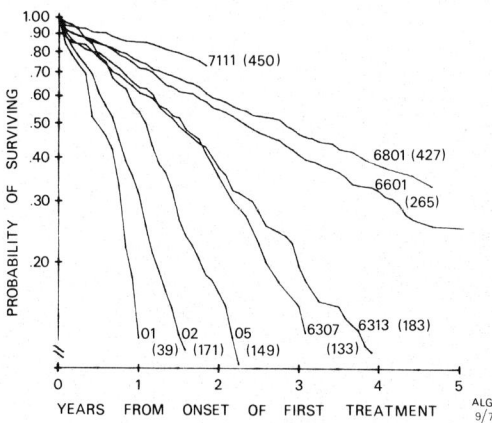

STUDIES IN ACUTE LYMPHOCYTIC LEUKEMIA (UNDER 20 YEARS OLD)

Successive improvement of survival in studies of Acute Leukemia Group B. Studies 01, 02, and 05 were begun between 1956 and 1962. The year when later studies began is given in the first two digits of subsequent numbers. The number of patients in each study is shown in parentheses. Each protocol contained several alternative therapeutic choices allocated at random.

retinas, and upper cervical cord has further reduced the appearance of CNS leukemia in patients treated with systemic chemotherapy at standard doses plus intrathecal methotrexate.

TREATMENT DURATION. The optimal duration of treatment for patients with acute lymphocytic leukemia is not well established. Some patients have sustained long-term remissions on particular regimens. Relapses in patients on these same regimens have almost always occurred within three years. Some investigators thus terminate chemotherapy after three years of treatment, whereas others are engaged in study programs which allocate patients at random to continue or terminate treatment after five years. Premature termination might, of course, lead to relapse, whereas adverse effects of unnecessary continuation would be cumulative toxicity and immunosuppression, leading to opportunistic infections or possibly to reinduction of leukemia through a repetition of the leukemogenic stimulus. Apparent freedom from disease has been produced in 50 per cent or more in recent protocols of at least four research centers.

Immunotherapy, using allogeneic leukemic myeloblasts and the BCG strain of tubercle bacilli, has been successful in reports by Mathe and colleagues. Seven of 20 patients repetitively treated with these immunologic stimuli after a short chemotherapeutic course have remained in remission for three to seven or more years. Unfortunately, this experience has not been duplicated elsewhere. This appears related in part to failure to reproduce the exact experimental design and in part to the progressive success of chemotherapy, which has preempted investigators' attention.

In children who fail to remain disease free, relapse of the leukemia can be detected in the marrow weeks or months before it is apparent in the peripheral blood. Reinduction into remission with vincristine and prednisone is ordinarily successful, but sustaining the remission with the drugs from which the child has just relapsed, or with new drugs, becomes progressively more difficult, and after a shorter remission florid leukemia reappears. Death usually comes during the florid uncontrolled leukemic state, although a small percentage of children die of intercurrent infection while in remission.

Acute Myelocytic Leukemia in Adults. The chemotherapy of acute myelocytic leukemia is more difficult than that of acute lymphocytic leukemia. Drugs known to affect the leukemic myeloblast also affect the normal myeloblast. Selective toxicity is heavily dependent on differences in kinetics of the leukemic and normal populations. Indeed, at the outset in florid leukemia, the population of normal myeloblasts is diminished if not absent; normal hematopoietic stem cells, through unknown mechanisms, are apparently in prolonged G_1 or in G_0 cell cycle status. The leukemic population is primarily in cell cycle, however. Because of this kinetic difference, maximal therapeutic advantage appears to derive from treatment programs of relatively short duration, five to ten days, which seriously injure the cycling leukemic population before substantial numbers of normal stem cells enter into the cycle. In the hiatus before a second course of treatment is administered, two to four weeks after the initiation of the first course, recovery of antibody synthesis and cellular immunologic functions is recognizable. It is presumed that the normal hematopoietic stem cell pool is similarly replenished, thus explaining the avoidance of irreversible marrow aplasia. Failure of remission induction or eventual relapse is ascribable to cells in the leukemic population which are, or become, relatively insusceptible to the drugs which can be given within the tolerance of nonlethal toxicity.

Age is a significant determinant of successful induction frequency in acute myelocytic leukemia; patients over 60 fare worse in virtually every study. This is not inherently a difference in the susceptibility of leukemic cells, but is rather due to a lesser recovery of normal stem cell functions and decreased resiliency in withstanding the nearly invariable complications of the induction phase.

Cytosine arabinoside, a highly specific inhibitor of the "S" or DNA synthetic phase of the cell cycle, can cause 20 to 35 per cent complete remissions of acute myelocytic leukemia. Given in combinations with other active antileukemic drugs, the remission rates reach 50 to 80 per cent. Cytosine arabinoside must be given frequently daily or by continuous infusion, to ensure that drug is present at some time during the S phase of each leukemic cell in cycle. Effective combinations of cytosine arabinoside with thioguanine, cyclophosphamide, CCNU, and, most successfully, the anthracycline antimicrobial drugs daunorubicin or adriamycin have been reported. Some investigators also add vincristine and prednisone. After induction, which can be accomplished in the majority of patients under 60 years of age with a single course of seven days of cytosine arabinoside and three days of daunorubicin (other regimens often require two or three repeated courses), efforts to sustain the remission are necessary.

The continuous drug administration regimens so useful in maintaining remission in acute lymphocytic leukemia of childhood are without equivalent impact in acute myelocytic leukemia of adults. Remissions can be sustained by intermittent courses resembling the induction treatment, or by rotating cycles of active agents in combinations. Median remission duration is 10 to 15 months on different programs, with second remissions, if they occur, of short duration. Central nervous system leukemia is substantially less common than in acute lymphocytic leukemia, in part because of earlier demise from systemic disease. Intrathecal methotrexate or intrathecal cytosine arabinoside given in combination with cranial irradiation is temporarily effective in controlling central nervous system manifestations. Efforts to prevent clinical emergence of central nervous system leukemia will become more appropriate as increasing numbers of longer remissions are achieved.

The majority of patients with acute myelocytic leukemia show blastogenesis when their lymphocytes are incubated in vitro with their autologous leukemic cells. This is a manifestation of immune cellular recognition. Competence of the efferent immunologic arm is demonstrable by delayed skin hypersensitivity to leukemic cell membranes. Complete immunologic responses are detectable in animal leukemias, and are subject to augmentation with immunotherapy. First attempts to immunize patients with acute myelocytic leukemia in remission, using repeated BCG and allogeneic leukemic cell inoculations, have appreciably prolonged remission duration.

Less Common Acute Leukemias. Acute lymphocytic leukemia in adults can be effectively treated with nearly as good induction results as in children, using the programs for this disease outlined previously. Vincristine and prednisone induction, asparaginase intensification, 6-mercaptopurine and methotrexate maintenance with vincristine and prednisone reinforcement, and intrathecal methotrexate therapy with cranial irradiation have produced 70 per cent remission rates lasting two years in 40 per cent. Investigators whose programs for acute myelocytic leukemia of adults include vincristine and prednisone have treated adults with acute lymphocytic leukemia similarly, and have reported equally good induction results.

Acute myelocytic leukemia in children is even more responsive than the adult disease to the identical treatments.

The subvarieties of acute myelocytic leukemia have rates of response which are not importantly different from unclassified acute myelocytic leukemia, except for promyelocytic leukemia, which is particularly sensitive to daunorubicin. No in vitro or in vivo tests are sufficiently developed to predict reliably which drugs will be best for which tumor.

Supportive Measures. Massive leukemic cellular destruction releases a sudden load of purines to be oxidized to urate. This can lead to hyperuricemia and to urate nephropathy with uremia. If this possibility appears likely, short-term prophylaxis with a xanthine oxidase inhibitor such as allopurinol is appropriate.

Anemia is common and erythrocyte replacement is necessary to keep levels of hemoglobin above the threshold of physiologic dysfunction, at least above 7 grams per 100 ml. Thrombocytopenic bleeding should be prevented. The value of prophylactic platelet administration to preclude hemorrhage has been clearly demonstrated. Optimal platelet survival occurs when the genetic mismatch between donor and recipient is minimal. A sibling, particularly one who is HLA identical, is the best repetitive donor. Random donors are also of value, however, and enough platelets should be administered to protect against hemorrhage during the critical hypoplastic phase before remission ensues if the platelet count is less than 30,000 per microliter. Platelets which have been separated by flotation centrifugation suvive longer and are required less frequently than those which are precipitated and resuspended.

Prevention of infection is of great significance. Barrier

isolation with sterile filtered air circulating in a laminar flow pattern essentially eliminates exposure to exogenous airborne infection, and the likelihood of serious and fatal infections should thereby be decreased. Although most investigators have combined this isolation with oral nonabsorbable or systemic antimicrobial administration, equivalent effects have also been reported in patients isolated without prophylactic antimicrobial administration.

The nature of many serious infections depends upon the prevalence of particular organisms selected by the prior use of antimicrobial drugs in the hospital environment. In hospitals where extensive use has been made of antimicrobial drugs, Pseudomonas and Enterobacter infections outnumber infections caused by staphylococci and *E. coli,* the ordinary organisms in hospitals where extensive antimicrobial use has not been practiced. Opportunistic infections from fungi, *Pneumocystis carinii,* or cytomegalovirus may occur in granulocytopenic or immunodepressed patients who are protected against bacterial infection by early use of antibacterial drugs.

In the presence of granulocytopenia, new symptoms, signs, or unexplained fever require vigorous and immediate action. If infection is suspected, appropriate. cultures and other diagnostic tests should be made and treatment started before results are returned. Evolving insusceptibilities in hospital organisms dictate the antimicrobials to be used which provide broad and effective coverage for gram-positive organisms and the likely spectrum of gram-negatives. Cephalothin or clindamycin has largely superseded ampicillin or methicillin, and Gentamicin has largely superseded kanamycin or polymyxin. Carbenicillin may be added if the suspicion of Pseudomonas is particularly strong. The antimicrobial regimen can be discontinued or changed early, if the initial clinical impression proves incorrect.

When visceral infection occurs in the presence of granulocytopenia, mortality is high despite treatment with antimicrobials, unless marrow recovery occurs nearly simultaneously, with the consequent return of granulocytes. Transfusion of allogeneic normal donor granulocytes, collected by differential centrifugation or by filtration leukophoresis on nylon filters, with subsequent elution, has proved a component of major effectiveness in the treatment of sepsis during granulocytopenia. Recovery of transfused granulocytes is best when donated by histocompatible sibling donors, but even granulocytes from random donors in adequate quantity, more than 10^{10} daily for several days, can cause significant improvement in survival from serious infections.

Baxt, J., et al.: Leukemic-specific DNA sequences in leukocytes of the leukemic member of identical twins. Proc. Natl. Acad. Sci. U.S.A., 70:2629, 1973.

Clarkson, B. D.: Acute myelocytic leukemia in adults. Cancer, 30:1572, 1972.

Cronkite, E. P.: Kinetics of leukemic cell proliferation. *In* Dameshek, W., and Dutcher, R. (eds.): Perspectives in Leukemia. New York, Grune & Stratton, pp. 158–186.

Doll, R.: The Epidemiology of Leukemia. Seventh Annual Guest Lecture, Leukemia Research Fund, 61 Great Ormond Street, London, WC1N3JJ.

Ellison, R. R.: Acute myelocytic leukemia. *In* Holland, J. F., and Frei, E., III (eds.): Cancer Medicine. Philadelphia, Lea & Febiger, 1973, pp. 1199–1234.

Henderson, E.: Acute lymphoblastic leukemia. *In* Holland, J. F., and Frei, E., III (eds.): Cancer Medicine. Philadelphia, Lea & Febiger, 1973, pp. 1173–1199.

Holland, J. F., and Glidewell, O.: Chemotherapy of acute lymphocytic leukemia of childhood. Cancer, 26:1480, 1972.

Holland, J. F., and Glidewell, O.: Survival expectancy in acute lymphocytic leukemia. N. Engl. J. Med., 287:769, 1972.

Todaro, G. J., and Gallo, R. C.: Immunological relationship of DNA polymerase from human acute leukaemia cells and primate and mouse leukaemia virus reverse transcriptase. Nature, 244:206, 1973.

Yates, J. W., and Holland, J. F.: A controlled study of isolation and endogenous microbial suppression in acute myelocytic leukemia patients. Cancer, 32:1490, 1973.

Yates, J. W., Wallace, H. J., Jr., Ellison, R. R., and Holland, J. F.: Cytosine arabinoside and daunorubicin therapy in acute myelocytic leukemia. Cancer Chemother. Rep., 57:485, 1973.

THE CHRONIC LEUKEMIAS

Charles M. Huguley, Jr.

764. CHRONIC GRANULOCYTIC LEUKEMIA
(Chronic Myelocytic Leukemia [CML], Chronic Myeloid Leukemia, Chronic Myelogenous Leukemia)

Definition. Chronic granulocytic leukemia (CGL) is characterized by abnormal proliferation of immature granulocytes—neutrophils, eosinophils, and basophils—in the bone marrow, the spleen, the liver, and sometimes other tissues.

Etiology. Except in a small percentage of patients, the etiology of chronic granulocytic leukemia remains obscure. Epidemiologic studies have been essentially negative with the exception of two well-established factors: exposure to ionizing radiation and chronic exposure to benzene. Evidence for a viral etiology has not been forthcoming. Genetic factors have seldom seemed to play a role.

The relationship to ionizing radiation was first demonstrated through the increased incidence of chronic granulocytic leukemia among radiologists who practiced in the era when careful shielding was not generally used. Later an increased frequency of the disease was found in patients with ankylosing spondylitis treated by radiation to the entire spine and in the Japanese population exposed to a single massive dose of radiation from atomic bomb explosions. There is also a clearly demonstrated increase in CGL among workers with chronic occupational exposure to benzene, mostly among those who had acute hematologic damage from the chemical. A relationship to other chemicals and drugs such as chloramphenicol and phenylbutazone is not established. There is no association with other cancer.

Incidence and Prevalence. Chronic granulocytic leukemia accounts for 15 to 20 per cent of all leukemia and has an over-all incidence of about 12 cases per million population per year. The disease is unusual below age 35 and thereafter increases steadily. It is slightly more common in males than in females.

Pathology. The essential feature of chronic granulocytic leukemia is accumulation of granulocytic precursors in the marrow, spleen, and blood. The marrow is usually devoid of fat, and 80 to 90 per cent of the cells are granulocytes. The distribution of granulocytes shows only a slight shift toward immaturity. In the early stages megakaryocytes are nearly always strikingly increased. Needle biopsy of the marrow will reveal some degree of fibrosis with positive stain for reticulin in about 25 per cent of cases. This fibrosis tends to become progressively more severe, and many patients end with a marrow picture similar to that of myelofibrosis. The spleen is usually very much enlarged. Its normal architecture is replaced by extramedullary myelopoiesis, including not only granulocytes but also erythroblasts and megakaryocytes. Infarcts are common. The liver is usually enlarged, although not massively. There are infiltrations with myeloid cells but usually not much damage to the liver cells. Other tissues are usually not involved early.

Although the numbers of granulocytes in the marrow, blood, and spleen are greatly increased, the mitotic index is usually lower than normal, because the mean generation time of immature cells is longer. There is an exchange of cells between the blood, the spleen, and the marrow.

About 90 per cent of patients with chronic granulocytic leukemia exhibit an abnormal chromosome called the Philadelphia chromosome (Ph¹). This abnormality results from the deletion of a short arm from a chromosome of group 22. When present the Ph¹ chromosome is found in virtually all metaphases observed in the marrow, including erythroid precursors and megakaryocytes as well as granulocytes. It is not found in lymphocytes, skin, or connective tissue, indicating that the Ph¹ chromosome is an acquired abnormality of a common stem cell for granulocytes, red cells, and megakaryocytes. Since it nearly always persists despite vigorous treatment, there has been pessimism as to the possibility of ridding the body of the abnormal cell in order to permit repopulation by normal cells. Recently it has been possible, after vigorous therapy, to replace Philadelphia chromosome cells with normal cells. Whether this will alter the course of the disease remains to be seen, but it offers a basis for optimism.

Eventually 60 to 80 per cent of patients will develop a transformation into a pattern virtually indistinguishable from acute granulocytic leukemia. This change is called the *"blast crisis."* The pathologic manifestations are those of acute granulocytic leukemia. Occasionally a blast transformation will occur in extramedullary sites, particularly in lymph nodes, producing a histologic pattern resembling sarcoma. The demonstration that such cellular infiltrations contain the Ph¹ chromosome proves that the cells are immature granulocytes rather than other cells. Such tumors have been called *chloromas* or *granulocytic sarcomas*.

Patients who do not have the Ph¹ chromosome generally pursue an atypical course; e.g., the response to therapy is less predictable than it is in a typical patient with the Ph¹ chromosome, and prognosis is poorer.

Clinical Manifestations. Sometimes the disease may be diagnosed at an early stage by an incidental blood count. More commonly the patient experiences insidious onset of fatigue, sometimes accompanied by anorexia and weight loss. There may be fullness or heaviness in the left upper quadrant, or the discovery of a mass may bring the patient to the doctor. More rarely, the physician is consulted because of the manifestations of anemia, pain in the splenic region secondary to a splenic infarct, hemorrhagic or thrombotic manifestations, or an attack of gout.

The spleen is palpable in nearly all patients at the time of diagnosis and is usually quite large, frequently extending beyond the umbilicus. If there has been a recent splenic infarct, the organ may be tender and a rub may be heard over the area of infarction. The liver is also palpable. Less commonly it is possible to elicit sternal tenderness. Lymphadenopathy is rare. In short, the typical patient has relatively minor symptoms, and the usual physical finding is splenomegaly.

The essential laboratory abnormality is leukocytosis. The patient who presents with symptoms will characteristically have more than 75,000 WBC per cubic millimeter, and the count may exceed 500,000. The differential white cell count shows a spectrum of immature granulocytes similar to that seen in normal bone marrow. Myeloblasts rarely exceed 5 per cent of the count. Eosinophils and basophils are increased in percentage, which means a striking absolute increase. Monocytes may also be increased.

Anemia of varying degree may be present, but usually not until the white cell count exceeds 50,000 per cubic millimeter. About half of all patients at the time of diagnosis will have thrombocytosis which may be associated with bleeding as well as thrombotic manifestations. Some patients present initially with thrombocytopenia, and as the disease progresses thrombocytopenia becomes increasingly frequent.

The bone marrow is as described under Pathology.

Alkaline phosphatase activity in the mature neutrophils is strikingly decreased. Uric acid is elevated. The serum vitamin B_{12} level is high, as is the B_{12} binding protein transcobalamin I. The level of serum lactate dehydrogenase is considerably elevated in CGL.

Diagnosis. Leukocytosis with the characteristic shift to immaturity of the granulocytes and the increase in eosinophils and basophils suggests the diagnosis of chronic granulocytic leukemia. The presence of splenomegaly in most cases will serve to distinguish CGL from leukemoid reactions, although not from other myeloproliferative syndromes. The cellular marrow with granulocytic and megakaryocytic hyperplasia is characteristic. A bone marrow biopsy should be done to help distinguish CGL from myelofibrosis and also to search for some degree of fibrosis which is commonly present.

A cytogenetic study should be made on the marrow to establish the presence of the Ph¹ chromosome. If present, this abnormality corroborates the diagnosis of chronic granulocytic leukemia and indicates the probability of a rather typical course. Determination of leukocyte alkaline phosphatase activity of mature neutrophils in the peripheral blood, which is very low in chronic granulocytic leukemia and high in leukemoid reactions and in the other myeloproliferative syndromes, is an important test.

In the unusual case identified by a routine blood count, the diagnosis may at first be difficult. Sometimes patients are seen who have a persistent leukocytosis of 15 to 20,000 WBC per cubic millimeter with a mild shift toward immature forms. At this point the neutrophil alkaline phosphatase may not be much reduced. Many months may elapse before the more characteristic findings of the disease appear. In such cases the demonstration of the Philadelphia chromosome is especially helpful.

Treatment. Chronic granulocytic leukemia is remarkably easy to control until complications develop. Benzene was first used a century ago. Later, arsenic in the form of Fowler's solution was found to be effective. With the advent of radiotherapy, it was shown that the disease was readily responsive to radiotherapy directed to the spleen or to the whole body. Later radiophosphorus ^{32}P also proved effective. More recently it has been demonstrated that extracorporeal irradiation of the blood will control the disease.

With the advent of chemotherapy it was readily shown that most of the agents which produce leukopenia and are effective against any tumor are also effective against CGL. Busulfan has been found to be the drug which combines effectiveness with ease of use and is the standby of treatment. More recently dibromomannitol has proved equally effective.

Standard treatment consists of oral administration of busulfan (Myleran). It is available in 2 mg tablets, and the dose is 6 mg daily. The blood count must be monitored at weekly intervals and the dose adjusted as indicated. The fall in the white count is usually exponential after about two weeks. A safe rule is to reduce the dose of busulfan by half as the white count is reduced by half. However, if the white count falls more gradually and smoothly, the original dose may be maintained until the count is in the neighborhood of 15,000 per cubic millimeter. In any event therapy should cease when the count reaches this level, because there is a tendency for the decline to continue for a week or two after the busulfan is discontinued. Once the white cell count plateaus, it is advisable to resume busulfan in a reduced dose (2 to 4 mg daily) in order to bring the count down somewhat below 10,000 per cubic millimeter. The dose will then have to be titrated, ordinarily between 2 mg every other day and 4 mg daily and maintained until the spleen is no longer palpable and the platelet count has been reduced to normal. Both of these usually take longer than the return of the leukocyte count to normal. Control of the leukocyte count is achievable in over 90 per cent of patients. In perhaps 60 to 70 per cent it is possible to eradicate splenomegaly and have the platelet count, the hemoglobin, and the white cell differential return to normal, thus eradicating diagnostic features of the disease. At this point the leukocyte alkaline phosphatase may return to normal but the Ph^1 chromosome will persist.

Once control has been established, it is possible to continue treatment with a small dose of busulfan. Experienced hematologists, more commonly, will discontinue treatment and observe the patient. Relapse may occur within a few weeks or may require many months. In the latter case, the ordinary approach is to reinduce a remission and again stop treatment just as with the initial episode. Successive remissions become increasingly more difficult to achieve, and their duration will be shorter. If relapse occurs promptly after discontinuing busulfan, it will be easier to maintain the patient on regular dosage once a second remission has been obtained. Maintenance requires careful monitoring not only of the leukocytes but also of the platelets at intervals not to exceed two weeks because of the sometimes unexpected appearance of hematologic toxicity.

Other manifestations of busulfan toxicity usually occur with prolonged treatment and include the development of amenorrhea in females or aspermia in males and a dark pigmentation of the skin. These patients may develop a rare syndrome resembling Addison's disease but not accompanied by evidence of adrenal insufficiency. In addition, the so-called "busulfan lung," a fibrosing process, is only partially relieved by steroid therapy.

Complications. Anemia, when present, is attributable primarily to crowding of the marrow and responds to control of the leukemia. Thrombocytosis may be accompanied by thrombotic complications. Bleeding may be associated with either thrombocytosis or thrombocytopenia which may be due to disease or to treatment. The mature neutrophils of CGL have been shown to be effective in control of infection when transfused into granulocytopenic recipients. Infection is not a usual complication of CGL. The patient in remission ordinarily leads a normal life until the resultant phase of the disease develops. Sixty to 80 per cent of patients will develop the "blast crisis," which occurs fairly suddenly and presents the picture of acute granulocytic leukemia. It is treated with various chemotherapeutic agents effective against acute granulocytic leukemia but less successfully. Remissions seldom last long.

About 25 per cent of patients with CGL will have some degree of fibrosis of the marrow at the time of diagnosis. This tends to progress and occasionally develops into a picture indistinguishable from myelofibrosis. At this point the hypocellularity of the marrow makes continued chemotherapy difficult, and the prognosis is poor. Another unusual outcome is development of a refractory state to chemotherapy. It becomes no longer possible to control the white cell count without producing unacceptable degrees of thrombocytopenia. Hydroxyurea or 6-mercaptopurine may be somewhat more effective than busulfan at this stage.

The untreated patient, or one in florid relapse with high leukocyte count and large spleen, has an elevated uric acid and greatly elevated uric acid excretion. This will be exaggerated by the destruction of leukocytes after treatment, which occasionally causes precipitation of uric acid in the renal tubules and anuria. Therefore it is advisable to administer allopurinol, 100 mg three times a day, during the initial weeks of treatment.

Prognosis. Recent reports of survival of patients with chronic granulocytic leukemia do not indicate an improved survival over the series of untreated patients reported by Minot in the 1920's. The median survival is between 2 1/2 and 3 1/2 years, and the range is ordinarily between one and ten years. It is somewhat paradoxical that the most easily controlled of all malignant conditions treated with chemotherapy has been so refractory to efforts at improving survival. Nevertheless, the quality of life is strikingly improved by treatment and is approximately normal until the appearance of the blast crisis. No means of preventing this complication is yet known. There is no clear evidence that any treatment accelerates or delays its onset. This failure has cast a pall of pessimism over all attempts at controlling chronic granulocytic leukemia. However, a recent clinical study has succeeded in eliminating the Ph^1 chromosome and repopulating the marrow with normal cells. The demonstration that there is indeed a clone of normal cells in the marrow suggests the possibility that the abnormal clone can indeed be destroyed and that some cases of chronic granulocytic leukemia may be curable.

The blast crisis often appears suddenly and is marked

by more than 30 per cent myeloblasts and promyelocytes in the peripheral blood and/or marrow. Some cases develop more insidiously and may be preceded by a rise in white count on a dose of busulfan which formerly controlled the white count, or by anemia, or thrombocytopenia or sustained unexplained fever. Another bad prognostic sign is rising percentage of basophils. Once the blast crisis develops, the duration of life is in weeks or months.

The immediate outlook for patients with chronic granulocytic leukemia is excellent. The major manifestations of the disease can be controlled in nearly all patients, and in the majority the blood counts and splenomegaly can be reverted to normal. However, within one to ten years, usually two to four years, complications will develop as described which lead to death within a few months.

Dowling, M., Jr., Haghbin, M., Gee, T. J., Wakonig-Vaar Tara, T., and Clarkson, B.: Attempt to induce true remissions in chronic myelocytic leukemia (CML). Am. Soc. Clin. Oncol., April 1973 (Abst. No. 50).

Ezdinli, E. Z., Sokal, J. E., Crosswhite, L., and Sandberg, A. A.: Philadelphia-chromosome-positive and -negative chronic myeloid leukemia. Ann. Intern. Med., 7:175, 1970.

Galton, D. A. G.: Chemotherapy of chronic myelocytic leukemia. Semin. Hematol., 6:323, 1969.

Gralnick, H. R., Harbor, J., and Vogel, C.: Myelofibrosis in chronic granulocytic leukemia. Blood, 37:152, 1971.

Haut, A., Abbott, W. S., Wintrobe, M. M., and Cartwright, G. E.: Busulfan in the treatment of chronic myelocytic leukemia. The effect of long-term intermittent therapy. Blood, 37:152, 1971.

Medical Research Council's Working Party for Therapeutic Trials in Leukaemia: Chronic granulocytic leukaemia: Comparison of radiotherapy and busulfan therapy. Br. Med. J., 1:201, 1968.

Tjio, J. H., Carbone, P. P., Whang, J., and Frei, E., III: The Philadelphia chromosome and chronic myelogenous leukemia. J. Natl. Cancer Inst., 36:567, 1966.

765. CHRONIC LYMPHOCYTIC LEUKEMIA

(Chronic Lymphatic Leukemia)

Definition. Chronic lymphocytic leukemia (CLL) is characterized by accumulation in the lymphoid organs, bone marrow, and blood of long-lived cells with uniform appearance similar to that of the small lymphocyte. There is mild to severe immunologic deficiency characterized by hypogammaglobulinemia. Conversely, phenomena such as autoimmune hemolytic anemia and increased delayed hypersensitivity reaction to stimuli such as insect bites are common.

At present the whole subject of the lymphoproliferative diseases, including chronic lymphocytic leukemia, is in process of re-evaluation, stimulated by two developments: (1) our increasing sophistication in the morphologic separation of the various lymphoproliferative disorders and (2) the recognition of the important differences between T lymphocytes and B lymphocytes (see Ch. 60). The cells in nearly all cases of CLL tested have had the features of B cells.

Etiology. Epidemiologic studies have given very little insight into the etiology of chronic lymphocytic leukemia. It is clear that exposure to ionizing radiation is not a factor. It is also clear that genetic factors play some role, as evidenced by the appearance of multiple cases of CLL in some families. CLL is comparatively rare in Japanese, even among Japanese living in the United States. There has been no evidence of a relationship to any chemical carcinogen or to oncogenic viruses.

Incidence and Prevalence. Chronic lymphocytic leukemia is the most common type of leukemia and represents about 30 per cent of all cases. The annual incidence has been given as 15 per million. It is predominantly a disease of older people, being unusual below the age of 40. It is more common in males, in a ratio of about 3:2.

Pathology. Chronic lymphocytic leukemia must be considered as a leukemic form of well-differentiated lymphocytic lymphoma. It is not possible to distinguish between the lymph node pathology in the two diseases. The normal architecture is replaced by a sea of small lymphocytes. Lymph nodes are characteristically enlarged. The spleen is also nearly always enlarged but usually not to a conspicuous degree. Infarction is uncommon. Its architecture is similarly replaced by monotonous infiltration of small lymphocytes. The liver is often enlarged and demonstrates a lymphocytic infiltration which may be minimal or may consist of nodular masses. The bone marrow is involved. In early cases this may be patchy, and a bone marrow aspirate may be hypocellular without a particularly large number of lymphocytes, whereas a biopsy will show nodules of lymphocytes interspersed in normal marrow. Later the marrow becomes almost completely replaced with lymphocytes to the detriment of granulocytes, erythrocytes, and megakaryocytes, yielding a so-called "packed marrow" syndrome. Other organs may be involved, in particular the gastrointestinal tract and the skin.

Clinical Manifestations. In at least a quarter of patients with CLL, symptoms are absent and the diagnosis is suggested by a blood count obtained as part of a routine examination or for the diagnosis of some other illness. In other patients there is insidious onset of noncharacteristic symptoms, and in some the first sign of the disease is a complicating infection. There may be a vague feeling of malaise with easy fatigability. Sometimes there is loss of appetite and weight or a low-grade unexplained fever associated with night sweats. In an appreciable percentage of patients, with or without other symptoms, the physician will be consulted because enlarged lymph nodes or spleen have been observed by the patient. More rarely, bleeding manifestations bring the patient to the physician. Although generalized leukemia cutis may occur, it is rare. Nevertheless, skin manifestations are common. They may take the form of nonspecific leukemids represented by scattered papular or vesicular lesions, often intensely pruritic. These must be distinguished from hyperreactivity to insect bites or a generalized herpes simplex infection. Herpes zoster occurs frequently and may become generalized. Smallpox vaccination may produce a very severe local lesion, and it may go on to generalized vaccinia. The expanding lesions in the marrow encroach upon the bone, leading to demineralization and sometimes to collapse of vertebrae. (The use of steroids in treatment will aggravate demineralization.)

The blood picture is characterized by an absolute lymphocytosis composed mostly of uniform, small, mature-appearing lymphocytes. There will be some large lymphocytes, perhaps with a cleaved nucleus or nucleoli. Smudge cells are common. Early in the disease the absolute number of granulocytes is normal. There is often no thrombocytopenia or anemia at the time of diagnosis. The total white count is usually more than 20,000 but not usually more than 100,000. An occasional patient will have a normal or low white cell count consisting of the same type of abnormal lymphocytes. Most authorities would include such patients within the group of CLL. Examination of the marrow reveals an infiltration with small lymphocytes similar to those in the blood. The marrow may be difficult to aspirate, and a needle biopsy will demonstrate the infiltration of lymphocytes which may be patchy, In more advanced disease, the marrow will be packed with lymphocytes at the expense of the normal myeloid cells. At this point there will be neutropenia, thrombocytopenia, and anemia.

In chronic lymphocytic leukemia there is an accumulation of long-lived lymphocytes; the rate of cell production appears to be little if any above normal. These cells, predominantly of the B cell type, are characterized by an immunoglobulin coating of a monoclonal type. The percentage of T cells which react to antigen or phytohemagglutinin stimulation is reduced, and their absolute number is reduced. T cells may return to normal with treatment.

B cells are necessary for antibody formation. In CLL they appear to be abnormal so that the antibody response to antigens is diminished. Hypogammaglobulinemia is characteristic of the disease, and it increases in severity as the disease progresses. This leads to an increased susceptibility to infection which is the major cause of morbidity in patients with CLL. In advanced disease all patients will have hypogammaglobulinemia with a reduction in normal immunoglobulins. A monoclonal spike may be present, usually of IgM type. There is often a positive Coombs test, which may be accompanied by autoimmune hemolytic anemia. However, excessive hemolysis may occur in the absence of a positive Coombs test, and, in addition, anemia is caused by marrow replacement.

Although the serum uric acid concentration is usually normal, it may be elevated in rapidly progressive cases or after treatment.

Diagnosis.   The diagnosis of CLL depends upon examination of the blood and marrow, as described under Pathology. Lymph node biopsy will show a diffuse, well-differentiated lymphocytic lymphoma. Lymphadenopathy and splenomegaly are usually present. Either may be massive but usually is not. Studies at the time of diagnosis should include careful history with an attempt to identify the earliest manifestations of the disease. There should be special examination of the skin, lymph nodes, liver, and spleen. The patient must have a complete blood count, including reticulocytes and platelet count, and a bone marrow examination. A needle biopsy of the marrow as well as the aspirate is desirable.

Other studies should include chest film, bilirubin, direct Coombs test, and studies of liver and kidney function. Determination of total protein and serum electrophoresis is important, and it is helpful to monitor the immunoglobulins. An abnormal electrophoretic pattern should be studied by immunoelectrophoresis to identify a monoclonal peak.

Treatment.   Many forms of treatment have been effective, but in the past all have been of somewhat limited value, and there is therefore a considerable opinion that only the symptomatic patient should be treated.

As discussed under Clinical Manifestations, many patients (up to half) have the diagnosis of CLL made incidental to examinations carried out for other reasons. These patients may exhibit no morbidity from the disease and may show no progression for many years. Patients with "active" disease, by contrast, may be defined as those who have one or more of the following: unexplained weight loss, unexplained fever of more than two weeks' duration, rapidly enlarging or painful lymph nodes or spleen, anemia, thrombocytopenia, or such complications as hemolytic anemia, recurrent infections, or skin involvement.

Present experience suggests that the asymptomatic patient has little to gain from treatment and may be harmed. Active disease is an indication for treatment.

Radiation therapy can reduce the size of the spleen and lymph nodes. Whole body radiation has been particularly effective in controlling all manifestations of the disease. Of the various chemotherapeutic agents available, chlorambucil has been the most effective. It is usually administered daily, beginning with an oral dose of 12 mg and reducing the dose as the white cell count comes under control. More general improvement will be observed if treatment is maintained after the white cell count has been brought to normal for at least 12 weeks. Administered in this way, chlorambucil will lead to some improvement in all measurable parameters of disease in about two thirds of patients. About 10 per cent will obtain a return to normal status, including a normal blood differential and a reduction in marrow lymphocytes below 30 per cent, qualifying for a rating of "complete remission."

Since the abnormal lymphocytes of CLL proliferate slowly, they will not replenish themselves after treatment as rapidly as the normal cells of the marrow. Therefore it is logical to use chlorambucil in a single dose every two weeks, thus permitting time for recovery of normal cells between doses. This schedule has about the same effectiveness as daily chlorambucil, although response is slower, but with much less toxicity to the granulocytes and platelets. The dose is 0.8 mg per kilogram given at bedtime once every two weeks (this differs from the manufacturer's recommendations).

The addition of prednisone to chlorambucil has been shown to be associated with a much higher percentage of complete remissions. It has usually been given in a dose of 20 to 30 mg daily, but is also effective if given in a dose of 60 to 80 mg for four to five days every two weeks. The intermittent schedule may possibly protect the patient against some of the side effects of steroid therapy. Prednisone is mandatory for the treatment of autoimmune hemolytic anemia and other autoimmune phenomena. It is particularly effective in reducing the size of lymph nodes and may be helpful for thrombocytopenia.

Treatment should be maintained in an individualized dose for at least three months and certainly until maximal effect appears to have been achieved. This may require as long as a year. During this time careful monitoring of blood counts for hematopoietic toxicity will necessitate counts weekly until stability is achieved and then every two weeks. Treatment can then be stopped until the evidences of active disease return. A majority of patients will require constant treatment. It has not been shown that continued regularly spaced titrated therapy is more effective than the regimen described.

Complications. Most complications have already been mentioned. About 20 per cent of patients will develop an autoimmune hemolytic anemia which is usually responsive to prednisone. Not infrequently hemolysis may be precipitated by treatment. If the disease is controlled with chlorambucil, the hemolytic anemia may not recur. The anemia and sometimes the thrombocytopenia and neutropenia of advanced disease may be helped by the administration of an androgen on a daily basis. Fluoxymesterone in a dose of 10 mg three times daily has often been quite effective.

Infections require specific and vigorous treatment. The regular administration of gamma globulin has not been shown to be effective in preventing infections.

Monoclonal immunoglobulinopathy is present in 5 per cent or more of patients. It is usually of the IgM type and may be associated with a hyperviscosity syndrome.

Prognosis. Extensive tumor registry data indicate that patients diagnosed since 1955 have fared better than those diagnosed previously in the same hospitals. Although these data correspond to the introduction of chlorambucil, it may be that longer survival should be attributed to wider availability of blood banks, introduction of better antimicrobial drugs, and use of prednisone for treatment of hemolytic anemia and thrombocytopenia. Series reported from centers particularly interested in the care of patients with chronic lymphocytic leukemia seem to show a much better median survival (on the order of five to six years) than do series of patients derived from tumor registry data which indicate a median survival of less than four years. The difference may be artifactual in that referral centers tend to attract patients whose disease was discovered in the indolent phase because of routine yearly examinations, whereas district hospitals may handle a higher proportion of patients who have only sought help when symptoms had interfered with ability to work.

Have we been too impressed with the long, "benign" course of some patients? Has our pessimism about the past failure to prolong survival by treatment led us to be too conservative and nihilistic in our approach? Although many patients do survive for ten years or more before any treatment is deemed necessary, and some have lived longer than 25 years, we must not lose sight of the poor survival of the average patient. Patients with "indolent" disease have a median survival of only about two years longer than patients with "active" disease.

A number of "complete remissions" have been reported. A review indicates that such remissions have usually lasted many months and that the survival of such patients is considerably lengthened. Recent reports indicate a frequency of 10 to 50 per cent "complete remissions" after use of chlorambucil, chlorambucil plus prednisone, whole body irradiation, and a combination of cytosine arabinoside and cyclophosphamide. These reports should give us hope that a more aggressive attack upon the disease may lead to better survival than we have achieved in the past. Remissions have corrected all complications, and in some of those tested the normal immunoglobulins have returned to normal.

Boggs, D. R., Sofferman, S. A., Wintrobe, M. M., and Cartwright, G. E.: Factors influencing the duration of survival of patients with chronic lymphocytic leukemia. Am. J. Med., 40:243, 1966.
Cutler, S. J., Axtell, L., and Heise, H.: Ten thousand cases of leukemia: 1940–62. J. Natl. Cancer Inst., 39:993, 1967.
Han, T., Ezdinli, E. Z., Shimaoka, K., and Desai, D. V.: Chlorambucil vs. combined chlorambucil-corticosteroid therapy in chronic lymphocytic leukemia. Cancer, 31:502, 1973.
Huguley, C. M., Jr.: Survey of current therapy and problems in chronic leukemia. In Leukemia-Lymphoma, A Collection of Papers Presented at the 14th Annual Clinical Conference on Cancer, 1969, at The University of Texas M.D. Anderson Hospital and Tumor Institute at Houston. Chicago, Year Book Medical Publishers, 1970.
Johnson, R. E., Kagan, A. R., Gralnick, H. R., and Foss, L.: Radiation-induced remissions in chronic lymphocytic leukemia. Cancer, 20:1382, 1967.
Silver, R. T.: The treatment of chronic lymphocytic leukemia. Semin. Hematol., 6:344, 1969.
Zimmerman, T. S., Godwin, H. A., and Perry, S.: Studies of leukocyte kinetics in chronic lymphocytic leukemia. Blood, 31:277, 1968.

MYELOPROLIFERATIVE DISORDERS

Richard T. Silver

766. INTRODUCTION

The bone marrow, an organ diffusely spread throughout the bones of the body, consists of several different cell types that are strikingly different with regard to their physiologic roles. Depending upon the stimulus, a normal marrow response is unique and selective, occurring, for example, with an elevated white blood cell count after a pyogenic infection or with an elevated platelet count after hemorrhage. These reactions are self-limited, for the marrow reverts to its normal status once the provocative stimulus subsides. The myeloproliferative disorders refer to certain diseases in which the marrow proliferates more or less en masse. This proliferation is self-perpetuating, thus resembling a neoplastic disease, and results in common clinical, hematologic, biochemical, and morphologic characteristics. The concept of the myeloproliferative syndrome as a spectrum of disease with transitions from one form to another has achieved a certain popularity. There is a wide difference of opinion, however, as to which diseases should be included in the "myeloproliferative disorders," and a few hematologists find the term neither precise nor productive. Most would include in this group of diseases chronic granulocytic leukemia, polycythemia vera, myelofibrosis with myeloid metaplasia, and essential (idiopathic) thrombocythemia. At the onset of these illnesses, despite predominant proliferation of one cell type, there is evidence that the marrow *is* reacting en masse. Thus, for example, patients with chronic granulocytic leukemia initially may have an increased platelet count or even an increased red cell count in addition to an elevated white blood cell count. When first diagnosed, patients with polycythemia usually have, in addition to an increased red cell mass, elevations of white blood cell and platelet counts. Most patients with chronic myeloproliferative disorders have increased reticulin fibers in the bone marrow, presumably reflecting mesenchymal cell proliferation which reaches its greatest expression in the disease myelofibrosis with myeloid metaplasia (agnogenic myeloid metaplasia). All these illnesses involve the spleen as well as marrow. In some cases at diagnosis the bone marrow biopsy in the four conditions may be indistinguishable. Alterations are also seen in the levels of serum uric acid, vitamin B_{12} and its binding proteins, and leukocyte alkaline phosphatase activity. The terminal episode in many of these patients is often a disease resembling acute granulocytic leukemia.

The caveat regarding the myeloproliferative concept clearly relates to causation. The *Philadelphia chromosome,* the hallmark of about 90 per cent of the cases of chronic granulocytic leukemia, has not been found in the other diseases of the myeloproliferative group. Moreover, there is no current reason to indicate a common cause for these diseases. Although myelofibrosis may be seen in end-stage patients with polycythemia vera and chronic granulocytic leukemia, it is unlikely that this is the same disease as the idiopathic form. The similarities seen in these disorders may be explained on the basis of the limited manner in which the marrow can express itself in different disease states. Finally, transitions of chronic granulocytic leukemia and agnogenic myeloid metaplasia to polycythemia vera or idiopathic thrombocythemia are difficult to document.

In summary, whereas the term "myeloproliferative disorder" in a restricted sense is useful to refer to certain chronic proliferative diseases of the marrow which share certain characteristics, it should not embrace all the malignant hematologic disorders known to man.

Dameshek, W.: Some speculations on the myeloproliferative syndrome. Blood, 6:372, 1951.

Glasser, R. M., and Walker, R. I.: Transitions among the myeloproliferative disorders. Ann. Intern. Med., 71:284, 1969.

Myeloproliferative Disorders of Animals and Man. Proceedings of the Eighth Annual Hanford Biology Symposium at Richland, Washington, May 20–23, 1968, edited by W. J. Clarke, E. B. Howard, and P. L. Hackett. U.S. Atomic Energy Commission, published June 1970.

767. AGNOGENIC MYELOID METAPLASIA

Definition and Pathogenesis. The degree of confusion and controversy regarding the etiology, pathogenesis, and treatment of agnogenic myeloid metaplasia *(myelofibrosis with myeloid metaplasia* or *myelofibrosis with extramedullary hematopoiesis)* has been proportional to its polysyllabic length. No wonder this entity has been described in the hematologic literature under at least 35 additional names, ranging from *leukoerythroblastic anemia* to *pseudoleukemic-pseudoerythremic myelosis.* In order to understand this disease it is helpful to review the meaning of some terms constituting the name of this disorder. *Agnogenic* is derived from the Greek *agnostos* meaning unknown. *Myeloid,* as a general hematologic term, refers either to myeloid (or granulocytic) cells or to the marrow as a whole. In this sense it should be interpreted as referring to the marrow. *Metaplasia* is characterized by the proliferation of cells which are not usually histologically or functionally important in an organ or tissue. Therefore the term agnogenic myeloid metaplasia can be redefined as the causally unknown proliferation of cells which normally arise from the bone marrow in organs and tissues which are not usually involved in blood cell formation. What is *extramedullary hematopoiesis?* In the early developmental stages of the human embryo, hematopoiesis is a function of embryonic connective tissue or mesenchyme. Erythrocytes are first formed in the blood islands of the yolk sac, followed by active hematopoiesis in the liver, spleen, and lymph nodes. Intramedullary blood formation within the bone marrow cavity has its onset at about the fifth month of gestation, and by the eighth month the marrow is the principal site of hematopoiesis as extramedullary (outside the marrow) hematopoiesis gradually subsides. At birth, significant extramedullary blood cell formation no longer exists. Nevertheless, the mesenchymal cells originally responsible for hematopoiesis persist throughout life. Normally inactive, they nevertheless retain their embryonic potential, and under a variety of stimuli they are capable of resuming active hematopoiesis. When the mesenchymal cells of the spleen and liver resume blood formation, once again there is extramedullary hematopoiesis (or myeloid metaplasia), for now there is production of marrow cells by organs not usually concerned with hematopoiesis. Such formation of blood outside the marrow cavity may occur secondary to a variety of clinical conditions, including, for example, severe hemolytic anemias, Hodgkin's disease, metastatic neoplasms to the marrow, irradiation, and infections such as tuberculosis, or may occur after poisoning of the bone marrow by fluorine, phosphorus, benzol, or strontium. In some patients with chronic granulocytic leukemia or polycythemia vera, myeloid metaplasia or extramedullary hematopoiesis occurs in association with fibrosis of the marrow during the course of the illness and/or as a consequence of therapy. In a certain number of patients the cause of the myeloid metaplasia is unknown; thus the term *agnogenic myeloid metaplasia.* This occurrence is most commonly (but not always) associated with fibrosis of the marrow; thus the term *myelofibrosis.*

Clinical Manifestations. Agnogenic myeloid metaplasia (AMM) occurs primarily in the older age groups. Nearly two thirds of the cases occur between the ages of 50 and 70 years, about equally in men and women. Symptoms may be of several years' duration, are usually insidious in onset, and are referable to anemia or to abdominal discomfort owing to splenic enlargement. Deafness caused by otosclerosis has been reported in 10 per cent of cases. Less often, migratory bone pain and symptoms of gouty arthritis may occur. The spleen is almost always enlarged when the patient is first seen, and without this physical finding the diagnosis on clinical grounds must be held suspect. On the other hand, the liver is palpable in only one third of the cases, and this finding may be associated with mild liver function test abnormalities. Hepatomegaly without splenomegaly does not occur in AMM. When an enlarged liver without splenomegaly is found in a patient with proved extramedullary hematopoiesis, a diagnosis of *secondary* myeloid metaplasia is almost certain.

Laboratory Findings. Severe degrees of anemia are uncommon when the patient is first seen. Usually the hemoglobin ranges between 9 and 13 grams per 100 ml. The white blood cell count is elevated in about half the patients, normal in one third, and low in the remainder. The leukocyte alkaline phosphatase score is variable, but usually it is normal or increased. The Philadelphia chromosome, the hallmark for the typical case of chronic granulocytic leukemia, is absent. Karyotypic abnormalities have occasionally been reported in AMM, although the majority of studies have been negative. A peripheral blood smear shows striking changes; typically there is a shift toward granulocyte immaturity, even with the appearance of a few myeloblasts and progranulocytes. The presence of these immature cells does not imply a shortened survival time. Marked changes in the red cells include variations in size and shape and teardrop forms. Polychromatophilia and nucleated red cells are characteristic. The reticulocyte count is usually elevated and reflects either dyspoiesis or hemolysis. The platelets may appear large and bizarre and may be increased, normal, or low in number. Megakaryocyte fragments may be seen. Normal or slightly elevated serum levels of vitamin B_{12} and its binding proteins have been reported in AMM, but a clear separation between the extremely high values in chronic granulocytic leukemia (CGL) and AMM is usually apparent. Radioactive iron studies reflect ineffective erythropoiesis and decreased red cell formation in medullary and extramedullary sites. Radioactive chromium-51 studies demonstrate shortened red cell survival in the majority of cases. Most likely this is due to hypersplenism, because the Coombs test is rarely positive and tests for red cell enzyme deficiencies are inconclusive.

The frequency of radiographic evidence of *osteosclerosis* in patients with AMM has ranged from 30 to 70 per cent and may be severe enough to be recognized on a routine chest x-ray in about one third of the cases. The distribution of osteosclerosis is primarily in the axial skeleton where changes are most apparent in the vertebrae, ribs, clavicles, pelvis, scapulae, and metaphyseal ends of the femur and humerus. Bones distal to the elbow and knee are rarely involved. Osteosclerosis of the skull may occur. The most frequent radiographic finding is a "ground-glass appearance" of the bones with loss of definition of individual trabeculae.

In almost every case (even when the marrow is very cellular) the bone marrow aspiration yields a "dry tap," but this finding must not be used as sole evidence for diagnosis. A closed needle biopsy can be readily obtained from the posterior iliac crest. If not, then an open surgical biopsy should be performed. In more than 90 per cent of the cases, the marrow shows fibrosis, and in some, osteosclerosis which is marked by the formation of broad irregular bone lamellae. Islands and clumps of megakaryocytes may remain. In a small but significant percentage of cases, the marrow at the time of diagnosis may be hypercellular, although the architecture in these instances is disorganized. When panhyperplasia occurs, the marrow findings may not be distinguishable from the histologic changes seen in polycythemia vera. Granulocytic hyperplasia is never found to the degree that occurs in chronic granulocytic leukemia. Striking increase in the amount of reticulin fibers is demonstrated by silver impregnation stain and may be found even before the classic increase in collagenous tissue is observed. Although the sine qua non for the diagnosis rests on the demonstration of myeloid metaplasia in the liver or spleen, the risks involved in biopsying these organs are rarely justified.

Course. As the disease progresses, the spleen gradually enlarges, and so may the liver. Anemia becomes more severe in degree and may be complicated by iron deficiency owing to blood loss or to folic acid deficiency. Bacterial infections occur more frequently and can be a major contributing factor leading to death. Of particular importance is the association of tuberculosis with myelofibrosis, and particular efforts should be made to exclude this infectious disease. Nearly all patients have elevated levels of serum uric acid, and attacks of gouty arthritis may develop. Within the past decade, the association of portal hypertension and ascites has been reported in a significant percentage of patients with AMM. Thrombosis of the hepatic vein and the development of the Budd-Chiari syndrome have been recognized. It has been suggested that portal hypertension is a manifestation of both high portal blood flow and a relative obstruction of portal flow at the hepatic sinusoidal level.

Treatment and Prognosis. No treatment affects the basic fibrosis of the marrow, and no form of therapy has been shown to prolong life. Survival time in AMM is difficult to state with assurance because of the problem of accurately determining the onset of the illness. Suggested estimated median survival times are approximately ten years from onset of disease and five years from diagnosis, although there is considerable heterogeneity with both shorter- and longer-lived survivors. Insofar as AMM can thus be a disease of long duration, presently no specific treatment should be undertaken unless the patient becomes symptomatic. All patients should receive at least 200 to 400 mg of *allopurinol* daily in order to avoid the complications of elevated serum uric acid levels. If a patient becomes symptomatic from anemia, *androgens* may be employed, although the high doses used to stimulate erythropoiesis lead to excess fluid accumulation and to masculinizing effects in women. Doses of testosterone enanthate, 600 mg weekly intramuscularly, or oxymetholone, 50 to 100 mg daily by mouth, can be used. Treatment must be continued for 6 to 12 weeks to evaluate its efficacy. It seems most effective in women whose spleen had been removed prior to the onset of therapy or in whom it had not been massively enlarged. Treatment becomes less impressive in patients with more advanced disease. The hemolytic anemia which is most often due to hypersplenism rarely responds to *corticosteroids*. In those patients who initially present with markedly elevated platelet counts, *busulfan* in a dose of 4 mg per day, followed by lower doses as the platelet count falls, may be instituted. In most cases, busulfan cannot be used for definitive reduction in spleen size, because prohibitive degrees of suppression of erythropoiesis and thrombopoiesis result. *Radiation therapy* to the spleen rarely produces meaningful reduction in spleen size, and the dose required often causes severe leukopenia, anemia, and thrombocytopenia. Although *splenectomy* is not automatically interdicted in patients with AMM, it should be reserved for those individuals with severe hemolytic anemia, thrombocytopenia and clinical bleeding, portal hypertension, or mechanical symptoms secondary to splenomegaly. Nevertheless, the postoperative morbidity of splenectomy is significant. Striking thrombocythemia after splenectomy, with thrombosis and hemorrhage, may develop. Often there is further gradual enlargement of the liver, and recurrent hemolysis and thrombocytopenia may occur owing to sequestration by the liver.

In summary, one cannot be categorical about the therapy of AMM, and each treatment modality has its significant attendant risks. On the other hand, future studies may show that earlier treatment, including splenectomy, of the relatively asymptomatic patient may alter the heretofore slow but nevertheless inexorable course of the illness.

Gardner, F., and Nathan, D.: Androgens and erythropoiesis. Further evaluation of testosterone treatment of myelofibrosis. N. Engl. J. Med., 274:420, 1966.

Silver, R. T., Jenkins, D., and Engle, R. L.: Use of testosterone and busulfan in the treatment of myelofibrosis with myeloid metaplasia. Blood, 23:341, 1964.
Silverstein, W. M., Gomes, M. R., ReMine, W. H., and Elveback, L. R.: Agnogenic myeloid metaplasia: Natural history and treatment. Arch. Intern. Med., 120:546, 1967.
Ward, H. P., and Block, M. H.: The natural history of agnogenic myeloid metaplasia (AMM) and a critical evaluation of its relationship with the myeloproliferative syndrome. Medicine, 50:357, 1971.

Section Seven.   LYMPHORETICULAR NEOPLASMS

768.   INTRODUCTION

Paul P. Carbone

Neoplasms of the reticuloendothelial system are characterized as myeloproliferative or lymphoreticular. The myeloproliferative disorders include erythroid, myeloid, and megakaryocytic neoplasms that start in the bone marrow and only secondarily invade other tissues of the reticuloendothelial system (lymph nodes, spleen). Lymphoreticular neoplasms arise in lymphocytic cells, reticulum cells, or primitive precursor cells. The lymphocytic cells, primarily involved in immune reactions, are either T cells (thymus derived) or B cells (bone marrow derived). Malignant diseases of lymphoid cells, referred to as lymphoproliferative disorders, may be associated with immune disturbances or monoclonal gammopathies. Reticulum cells, referred to as histiocytic or macrophage cells, form the background population of all lymphoreticular tissues. The lymphoreticular cells are located primarily in lymph nodes, thymus, spleen, and liver, but components of the lymphoreticular system are also found in the submucosal areas of the respiratory and gastrointestinal tracts as well as in the marrow.

Lymphoreticular tumors may become clinically apparent as single or multiple tumors in the lymph nodes, spleen, or gastrointestinal tract and may or may not involve the bone marrow. Since lymphocytes and macrophages also normally occur in the peripheral blood, lymphoreticular tumor cells may circulate. Much confusion can be avoided by understanding these concepts. The term malignant lymphoma commonly refers to patients who present predominantly with solid tumors and must be further classified as to cell type, i.e., histiocytic, lymphocytic, or Hodgkin's. Since the tumor cells may exhibit different degrees of differentiation, i.e., well differentiated or poorly differentiated, that affect prognosis and response to therapy, subclassification for differentiation also is important. Occasional patients have such primitive cells that the terms stem cell and Burkitt's tumor are applied to indicate less differentiated populations. In the lymph node or tissue section, two populations of malignant cells may occur simultaneously with neoplastic lymphocytic and histiocytic components, and the term mixed lymphomas is used. When the marrow and peripheral blood manifestations are prominent, as contrasted to tumor or nodal enlargement, the term leukemia or leukemic phase is applied. Thus in patients with lymphoreticular neoplasms, one sees a complete spectrum from localized tumors only to multiple tumors, leukemia, and mixtures. The presentation at the time of diagnosis reflects only a point in time, and the natural progression—untreated or after ineffective therapy—is toward dissemination.

Two other points deserve mention in understanding these disease processes. First, the cell type and disease progression may change with time to a less differentiated state. Patients with relatively well differentiated tumors may have subsequent biopsies that indicate less differentiation and even a stem cell–like picture. Clinically, this is important to appreciate, because therapy may need to be changed drastically in form or intensity. A second point relates to the identification of the pattern of lymph node involvement. The term giant follicle lymphoma, originally proposed by Brill and Symmers, referred to a *benign* form of involvement. Subsequent investigators recognized the fact that these patients did indeed die of cancer and that nodular involvement (follicular) occurred in patients with Hodgkin's disease, lymphocytic lymphoma, and, rarely, histiocytic lymphoma. Data from several centers indicate that the involvement pattern of follicular or diffuse can be applied to most histologic subtypes except Burkitt's tumor. In general, the prognoses of nodular forms are better than those of corresponding histologic varieties with diffuse patterns.

The current approach to classification of lymphoreticular neoplasms, as well as the previously applied terms, is shown in Table 1. The use of this classification and the appreciation of chronologic changes in cell type should clear up many of the previous difficulties with confusing names that encompassed grossly different prognostic categories.

The diagnosis of lymphoreticular neoplasms must always be based on an adequate tissue biopsy. Occasionally, multiple biopsies may be needed before the decision as to pathologic classification can be definitively made. Imprint preparations as well as cytochemical studies will help clarify the specific cell type and degree of differentiation. More recently, specific markers of the cell surface such as immunoglobulin receptors, complement receptors, immunoglobulin fluorescence, or rosette cell formation have classified cell variants that heretofore were difficult or impossible to categorize. Current histologic variants may in fact be lymphocytic cells but with cytologic variations. Electron microscopy studies may also be helpful in identifying the nature of the cell involved in the malignant process.

Besides insisting on adequate tissue for diagnosis, the physician responsible for the patient's care must work

TABLE 1. Classification of
Lymphoreticular Neoplasms*

Proposed Name	Old Name
Lymphoma, lymphocytic type, well differentiated	Lymphosarcoma
Lymphoma, lymphocytic type, poorly differentiated	
Lymphoma, histiocytic type	Reticulum cell sarcoma
Lymphoma, mixed lymphocytic-histiocytic type	Mixed lymphoma
Lymphoma, undifferentiated pleomorphic type	Stem cell lymphoma
Lymphoma, undifferentiated Burkitt type	Stem cell lymphoma

*From Berard, 1972. All varieties except Burkitt's may be classified
as nodular or diffuse.

in concert with the clinical pathologist, nuclear medicine specialist, radiologist, and surgeon to establish the extent of disease. This process is known as staging. The complete extent of staging procedures has not been determined. One must do a careful history and physical examination, asking for symptoms, examining all nodal areas, determining liver and spleen involvement, and searching for abdominal or testicular masses. Careful examination of the oropharynx is a necessity, because much lymphoid tissue is located in those regions. In addition to routine laboratory studies, radioisotope scans (particularly bone and ⁶⁷Ga studies), bone marrow biopsy, x-rays of chest and abdomen, intravenous pyelogram, and lymphograms are all helpful in evaluating the extent of disease. Further emphasis on evaluating liver involvement has shown that liver function tests and even closed hepatic biopsies can be misleading. To achieve a greater degree of accuracy, laparoscopy with several direct biopsies of the liver and laparotomy have been used. Diagnostic laparotomy has been adopted by many centers because of the opportunity to do biopsies of other suspicious abdominal areas and to perform a splenectomy. In patients with Hodgkin's disease and non-Hodgkin's lymphoma, the spleen if involved seems to predict liver spread. The more extended procedures also aid in the shaping of radiotherapy fields to fit the specific pattern of involvement. Moreover, Kaplan and his colleagues have utilized these extended staging procedures to map out the natural history and pattern of spread so useful to modern approaches to treatment. Since patients with lymphoreticular disorders tend to be older than patients with Hodgkin's disease and generalized disease is more common, these additional staging procedures must be justified on the basis of risk and morbidity in relation to possible therapeutic benefit. The therapeutic benefit should be realized as leading to significant changes in approach or intensity of treatment.

769. LYMPHOCYTIC AND HISTIOCYTIC LYMPHOMAS

Paul P. Carbone

The non-Hodgkin's lymphomas include lymphocytic, histiocytic, mixed lymphocytic and histiocytic, pleomorphic (or stem cell type), and Burkitt's tumor. (Burkitt's

tumor is described in Ch. 769a.) As described in Ch. 768, each of the major cell types of lymphocytic and histiocytic lymphomas can be further classified by the degree of differentiation of the cell and by the presence or absence of a nodular histologic pattern. The pathologist identifies the cell type, but the designation of leukemia or lymphoma (solid tumors) must be integrated by the physician from all the information learned by physical examination, laboratory study, and further biopsies.

Epidemiology. Many animal lymphoid tumors have been associated with viruses, radiation, and genetic factors. Although virus-like particles have been reported in tissues from patients, no direct causal agent has been identified with certainty. Some animal viruses infect human tissues, but no increased incidence of lymphoid tumors has been seen in owners of sick animals. Using biochemical markers of viral information such as reverse transcriptase, tissue from patients has yielded positive results. An increased incidence of lymphocytic lymphoma and Hodgkin's disease has been reported in survivors of the atomic bomb explosions in Japan. Genetic and acquired immune deficiency disorders predispose to the development of lymphoid malignancies. Patients with ataxia telangiectasia, Wiskott-Aldrich syndrome, congenital sex-linked agammaglobulinemia, and Chédiak-Higashi syndrome all have associated increased risks of developing lymphoid tumors presumably related to immune deficiencies. Patients with acquired hypogammaglobulinemia, autoimmune disorders, and Sjögren's disease likewise seem to have increased risks of developing malignant lymphomas. Patients with kidney grafts and those on long-term immunosuppression have an increased incidence of secondary malignancies. More than half of such malignancies are primary lymphomas, particularly involving the central nervous system, an unlikely site for spontaneous occurrences.

Pathology. Misinterpretations as to histologic type as well as differentiating benign from malignant disorders are common problems. The lymph node biopsy result must be related to bone marrow, peripheral blood, and ancillary laboratory studies, particularly serum or urine immunoelectrophoresis. The classification of non-Hodgkin's lymphoma and the characteristic histopathologic sections are shown in Table 1 and the accompanying figure.

Lymphocytic, Well Differentiated Type. The pattern of lymph node involvement is usually diffuse, replaced by small, normal-appearing lymphocytes. The cytoplasm cannot be seen in most of the cells. The bone marrow is usually involved focally or diffusely. The disease most often occurs in elderly individuals, may be asymptomatic, and may present with small scattered lymph nodes. Bulky lymph node enlargement and splenomegaly also occur. Examination of the peripheral blood may reveal lymphocytosis, and with marrow invasion the diagnosis of chronic lymphocytic leukemia can be made. In young persons, the diagnosis of reactive hyperplasia or Hodgkin's disease, lymphocyte predominant type, should be entertained in the differential diagnosis. Occasionally admixtures of plasma cells occur that are associated with immunoglobulin paraproteins, particularly IgM, in the serum or urine.

Lymphocytic, Poorly Differentiated. The range of lymphocyte size and differentiation seen in the node is more heterogeneous. In children, mediastinal or abdominal tumors with a progression to leukemia are commonly seen with this pattern. This is called "convoluted cell" lymphocytic leukemia by Lukes (1973). Adults are more likely to show peripheral node enlargement and less often manifest frank leukemia. In the node, the cells are variable in size and often have clefted nuclei. Sometimes these abnormal cells in adults enter the peripheral blood and have been characterized as lymphosarcoma cell leukemia. Nodular varieties rearely occur in children.

Histiocytic Type. A wide spectrum of cell sizes and morphology occur, indicating various degrees of differentiation. Some cells may be multinucleate and confused with Reed-Sternberg cells. Phagocytosis and fibroblastic differentiation with marked sclerosis may be seen. The term malignant histiocytosis refers to a relatively benign-looking proliferation of histiocytes that exhibit phagocytosis. Erythrophagocytosis and progressive pancytopenia may be seen that lead to the patient's death. Other variants include leukemic reticuloendotheliosis and histiocytic medullary reticulosis. The former is relatively benign, with "hair cells" in the peripheral blood. The latter is a more fulminant disease, with fever, erythrophagocytosis, jaundice, pancytopenia, and hepatosplenomegaly.

Mixed Histiocytic-Lymphocytic Type. The pattern of involvement is usually nodular, but characteristically malignant histiocytic and lymphocytic cells occur. The histologic pattern of the disease may progress to a more malignant histiocytic type with time. Newer approaches to histologic identification by immunoglobulin markers have recognized the two populations as variants of B lymphocytes.

Undifferentiated or Pleomorphic Type. These tumors usually lack histiocytic or lymphocytic differentiation. The cells are pleomorphic and include bizarre giant forms. Subsequent evidence of cytologic differentiation to lymphocytic or histiocytic forms may occur. Unlike Burkitt's lymphoma, in which uniformity of cell size occurs, these tumors show striking variation on touch preparations.

Clinical Manifestations. The major clinical manifestation of lymphoreticular neoplasms is painless enlargement of one or more peripheral lymph nodes. The glands characteristically are firm and symmetrical, and tend to enlarge progressively. Systemic manifestations of fever, night sweats, or weight loss usually are not prominent features, occurring in only 20 per cent of the patients. In about 20 per cent, lymphoid structures of the oropharynx, nasopharynx, or tonsils are involved. Palpable *splenomegaly* occurs in about 20 per cent of the patients and is more common in the lymphocytic than in the histiocytic varieties. *Gastrointestinal signs and symptoms* include obstruction, and malabsorption syndromes as a consequence of involvement of the intestinal tract occur in 15 per cent of patients. Diffuse patterns are more often associated with gastrointestinal involvement than nodular forms. The stomach and small intestine are the common gastrointestinal sites of disease. Primary lymphomas of the stomach may be confused with gastric cancer. Large mediastinal nodes are seen in about 20 per cent of the patients with non-Hodgkin's lymphomas as compared with 50 to 70 per cent of patients with Hodgkin's disease. Secondary findings related to intrathoracic tumor include superior vena caval obstruction and pleural effusions. Primary lymphomas of the lung are rare, whereas secondary spread to the lungs occurs commonly.

Hepatic enlargement and jaundice are relatively rare findings, but percutaneous biopsy evidence of liver involvement occurs in about 20 per cent. Further diagnostic procedures to evaluate the liver, including laparotomy, laparoscopy, and open biopsies, increase the yield of positives to about 50 per cent. The histologic subtypes of nodular or diffuse poorly differentiated lymphocytic forms are most likely to have liver spread.

Abnormalities in renal function may be secondary to parenchymal infiltration, obstruction of the outflow system, uric acid precipitation, anomalous protein excretion, or amyloid. Primary lymphomas of the *bone,* particularly histiocytic tumors, have been reported. The most frequent sites are the femur, pelvis, tibia, scapula, and humerus. They present as lytic lesions. Secondary lesions of the bone can be seen in advanced stages.

Primary lymphoreticular tumors of the *nervous system* are rare, but secondary compressions of the spinal cord or nerves may occur when large tumors impinge upon or invade the vertebral axis. The occurrence of free-floating cells or meningeal disease seems to be a late manifestation. Small cell glioblastoma (probably a lymphocytic tumor) with monoclonal gammopathy and primary histiocytic central nervous system tumors are seen.

Skin tumors, described as nodular infiltrations, dusky or blue colored, may be seen in few or many areas. The tumors occasionally ulcerate and become painful. Diffuse skin infiltration and exfoliative lesions may be a dramatic clinical presentation described as the "red

A, Normal lymph node (×11). Nodal architecture clearly shows nodules, germinal centers, and sinuses, particularly under capsule.

B, Diffuse lymphoma (×7). The normal nodal architecture is completely obliterated by a diffuse infiltrate of lymphoid malignant cells. The capsule, although intact here, can be disrupted with tumor cells extending outside the lymph node.

C, Nodular lymphoma (×7). The nodal structure is replaced by large nodules of malignant cells. The subcapsular area reveals fibrosis characteristic of an inguinal lymph node.

D, Well-differentiated lymphocytic lymphoma (×600). The malignant cells are small and uniform, with minimal cytoplasm, compact nuclear chromatin, and absence of mitoses.

E, Poorly differentiated lymphocytic lymphoma (×600). The cell size varies, particularly nuclear size with occasional mitoses. The nuclei are often irregular in shape. The nuclear chromatin is finely dispersed.

F, Mixed lymphocytic-histiocytic lymphoma (×600). Two morphologic populations of cells are clearly seen, small irregular lymphoid cells and large histiocytic cells with prominent nuclei.

G, Histiocytic lymphoma (×600). The cells are large and irregular, with clearly evident cytoplasm and large nucleoli.

H, Undifferentiated, non-Burkitt (×600). The pleomorphic cells are large and lack clear histologic differentiation with primitive nuclear pattern. A large multinucleate cell is also seen.

(Illustrations were kindly supplied by Dr. Costan Berard, Head, Hematopathology Section, Laboratory of Pathology, National Cancer Institute.)

See opposite page for legend.

man's syndrome." Patients with B cell variant of *Sézary's syndrome* may have peripheral blood involvement without much marrow invasion.

In 10 per cent of the patients *anemia* may be present at the onset, but it occurs more often as the disease progresses. A brisk or chromic hemolytic anemia, often Coombs positive, may complicate the onset of more aggressive disease. Peripheral white blood counts are usually normal, but lymphocytosis occurs particularly in association with the well differentiated lymphocytic variety of lymphoma. Immature circulating cells occur in most children with poorly differentiated or stem cell lymphomas at some time during the clinical course. Leukemic transformation approaches 50 to 70 per cent during the first 12 months even if the initial bone marrow is not involved. Poorly differentiated lymphocytic cells occasionally invade the peripheral blood, appearing as moderate to large lymphocytes with notched nuclei. This manifestation has been called *"lymphosarcoma cell leukemia."*

Initial involvement of the marrow is seen in about 20 per cent of the patients with non-Hodgkin's lymphoma; however, the incidence is much higher, 40 per cent, in lymphocytic varieties as compared to histiocytic types. The finding of bone marrow involvement is usually associated with clinical Stage III disease (90 per cent) and rarely with Stage I disease.

Differential Diagnosis. The major considerations in the differential diagnosis of lymph node enlargement include infections, reactive lymphadenopathy, and other neoplastic illnesses. Principal among the infectious causes are diseases such as infectious mononucleosis, tuberculosis, syphilis, toxoplasmosis, cytomegalovirus infection, and many pediatric viral illnesses. Reactive hyperplasias of the lymph nodes may accompany acute or chronic infections of the extremities or throat, particularly after vaccinations. Lymphadenopathy has also been associated with diphenylhydantoin administration. Nonlymphoreticular neoplasms characteristically spread to local lymph nodes only. A careful search of the oropharynx and mucosal surfaces may reveal a primary cancer that should be biopsied rather than the neck nodes. Breast cancer may present as lymph node enlargement in the axilla with a small primary tumor in the breast that may escape initial evaluation. Occasionally, diffuse adenopathy with histologic features of a lymphoma can be seen in association with immunoglobulin abnormalities characteristic of Waldenström's macroglobulinemia. Differentiation between a primary macroglobulinemia and a lymphoma with paraproteinemia may be difficult. Immunoglobulin M paraproteinemia with lymphoma occurs in the diffuse varieties more often than in the nodular forms. Examination of the marrow may reveal the characteristic lymphoid plasma cell along with the hyperviscosity, purpura, and bleeding tendency in patients with macroglobulinemia.

Staging. After establishing the diagnosis, evaluating the extent of disease is the most important responsibility of the attending physician. The staging procedures currently recommended are shown in Table 2. More recent data with ^{67}Ga scan indicate that this is an important adjunct in finding disease sites for further evaluation, because inflammatory lesions and other tumors also take up ^{67}Ga. The staging originally applied to Hodgkin's disease appears to be most widely used

TABLE 2.   Staging Procedures

1. History and physical examinations
2. Chest x-rays and tomograms as indicated
3. Complete blood counts
4. Liver function tests, serum electrophoresis, BUN, and creatinine
5. Bone marrow biopsy
6. Lower extremity lymphograms
7. Intravenous pyelogram
8. Bone and liver scans
9. Laparoscopy
10. Laparotomy when indicated

(Table 3). In it, extranodal sites are designated E. A clinical stage is based on the initial biopsy evidence of lymphoma and on the history, physical examination, and radiographic studies. A pathologic stage as a result of information derived from further special surgical procedures, such as liver biopsy or laparotomy, is included in the definition. The pathologic staging evaluation tends to result in an advance in the clinical stage in about 50 per cent. In one large series the distribution by stage for nodular and diffuse lymphomas is shown in Table 4.

A major tool in the evaluation of patients with lymphoreticular neoplasms is the *retroperitoneal lymphogram*. A radiopaque dye is injected into the small lymphatics of the foot under pressure. The dye is taken up by the abdominal lymph nodes and can be seen on the abdominal x-ray. In two thirds of patients with neck node enlargement, despite clinical evidence of localized disease, the lymphograms are abnormal. Since the dye persists in the nodes, the lymphogram findings may be used to follow the results of treatment. Repeat studies can be used to confirm disease activity.

The role of *laparotomy and laparoscopy* in the staging of patients with non-Hodgkin's lymphoma has become increasingly important, particularly in determining evidence of liver and extranodal involvement. The usual plan of staging is to do closed liver biopsies and bone marrow biopsy first in all patients. If the biopsy does not indicate disease in liver or marrow and the clinical evaluation of the patients does not reveal other evidence of Stage IV disease, then laparoscopy or laparotomy is indicated. The laparoscopic examination increases the yield of liver positives, precluding further exploration. Some institutions prefer to go directly to the laparotomy for wedge and needle biopsies of the liver, splenectomy, and thorough examination of abdominal lymph nodes and extranodal sites. Laparotomy

TABLE 3.   Ann Arbor Staging Classification

Stage   I: Involvement of a single lymph node region (I) or a single extralymphatic site (IE)

Stage II: Involvement of two or more lymph node regions on the same side of the diaphragm (II) or a solitary extralymphatic site and one or more of lymph node areas on the same side of the diaphragm (IIE)

Stage III: Involvement of lymph node regions on both sides of the diaphragm (III), accompanied by spleen involvement (IIIS), or by solitary involvement of an extralymphatic organ or site (IIIE) or both (IIISE)

Stage IV: Diffuse involvement of extralymphatic sites with or without lymph node enlargement

Clinical stage and pathologic stage defined for each patient; extranodal sites are designated by specific denominators; presence or absence of symptoms is designated B or A, respectively

TABLE 4. Distribution of Stage and Histology*

Clinical Stage	Histiocytic		Mixed		Lymphocytic, Poorly Differentiated		Lymphocytic, Well Differentiated		Pleomorphic		Total
	D†	N†	D	N	D	N	D	N	D	N	
I	9	3	5	5	6	9	3	1	3	—	44
IE	4	—	1	1	—	—	—	—	—	—	6
II	20	8	4	15	7	9	—	1	2	—	66
IIE	18	1	5	2	4	3	1	—	—	—	34
III	18	6	8	29	8	20	1	2	—	—	92
IIIE	2	1	1	1	—	1	—	—	—	—	6
IV	45	10	19	21	19	27	5	2	9	—	157
Total	116	29	43	74	44	69	10	6	14	0	405

*Modified from Jones, S. E., et al.: Cancer, 31:806, 1973.
†D = Diffuse.　N = Nodular.

has indicated evidence of liver involvement in at least 25 per cent of patients with prior negative percutaneous and laparoscopy biopsies. Mesenteric nodes are often found to be involved and must be considered in shaping radiation fields. The complications of laparotomy include occasional mortality, left side pleural effusions, infarction, pulmonary emboli, pancreatitis, gastrointestinal bleeding, and increased liability to subsequent infection. Because of these risks the indication for laparotomy must take into account the associated medical illnesses and the treatment program. If the treatment planned will not be influenced by laparotomy regardless of the result, the surgical exploration is not justified.

Treatment. The major modalities are irradiation, antineoplastic chemotherapeutic agents, and surgery. Historically, surgery was used for diagnosis, but also to remove obvious localized disease. This approach rarely resulted in long-term control unless the diagnosis was wrong or the histology extremely favorable (well differentiated lymphocytic, nodular). Therefore radiotherapy and/or chemotherapy form the basis of modern treatment.

Radiotherapy was recognized more than 30 years ago as an effective modality if administered in sufficiently high doses to forestall recurrences in the irradiated site. The usual dose for curative intent is 3500 to 4500 rads in patients with lymphoreticular neoplasms, administered at a rate of 1000 rads per week. The problem remains to define how much of the lymphoreticular system to radiate. In general, adequate radiotherapy should be administered to all involved sites in Stages I and II. Since more than half the patients have noncontiguous sites of involvement, more recent clinical trials have proposed extended radiotherapy to include all nodal areas and the spleen. With use of megavoltage equipment, total nodal irradiation appears to be well tolerated and capable of sterilizing disease. At some centers, experimental approaches to irradiate the entire body, the liver, and/or the lung are being tried, but the total dose administered has to be cut considerably. Radiotherapy may be used in combination with chemotherapy. Since we know that local disease may be controlled directly by radiotherapy, chemotherapy is used to treat occult disease in other sites.

Two additional points about radiotherapy must be emphasized. Since the abdomen is a major site of extranodal disease and mesenteric nodes are frequently involved, therapy techniques are available to permit total abdominal radiation. This includes spray radiation of the entire abdomen, with shielding of the liver and kidneys as the dose exceeds 1500 to 2000 rads. Another approach is the strip technique, in which the abdomen is radiated in a piecemeal fashion. The other use of radiotherapy is for special clinical problems. Obstruction of ureters, biliary system, bowel, and the respiratory airway, as well as compression of the nervous system, are medical emergencies. Radiotherapy to specific sites is very effective in relieving severe symptoms and signs quickly to prevent irreversible damage. Radiotherapy of the cranium combined with intrathecal chemotherapy is an accepted approach to meningeal disease.

The use of *chemotherapeutic* agents in the treatment of lymphoreticular neoplasms began in the 1940's, and their clinical usefulness spawned the search for many other new agents. Several have been used to treat patients with non-Hodgkin's lymphoma. The major categories of drugs and toxicities are shown in Table 5. The early trials indicated a relatively high proportion of responses as measured by tumor shrinkage in 30 to 50 per cent of patients using single drugs, but these responses were short-lived and clinical resistance followed. Following the lead of successful drug treatment programs in patients with acute leukemia, effective combination chemotherapy regimens were developed whereby tumor regressions were regularly achieved in most patients with non-Hodgkin's lymphoma. Most importantly, complete disappearances of tumor occurred in 50 per cent of the patients. Drugs with independent effectiveness and nonoverlapping toxicities were able to be combined at almost full doses, and the resultant effect against the tumor was additive or even synergistic. Most of the combinations employ an alkylating agent, a vinca alkaloid (usually vincristine) and a corticosteroid, and procarbazine. Some of the more common combinations are shown in Table 6.

The management of any patient should take into account the histologic type, the pattern of node involvement, the stage of the disease, and the associated medical condition of the patient. The initial approach should include a planned intent to achieve curative therapy or palliation. The decision must be firmly supported by what can be done under optimal circumstances with the best therapeutic modalities. For example, the physician must decide whether the x-ray equipment, expertise in treating with drugs, or management of complications is within the scope of his abilities and facilities. Respectable cure rates can be achieved by modern therapy. After frank discussion with the patient, the physician must advise on optimal therapy and where it

TABLE 5.   Doses and Toxicities of Drugs Used in Non-Hodgkin's Lymphoma

Drug	Dose and Schedule	Limiting Toxicities
1. Nitrogen mustard	0.4 mg/kg IV repeated q 3–4 weeks	Bone marrow suppression; nausea and vomiting
2. Cyclophosphamide	40 mg/kg q 3 weeks IV 15 mg/kg weekly IV 1–4 mg/kg/day PO	Bone marrow suppression; nausea and vomiting; cystitis; alopecia
3. Vincristine	0.025 mg/kg weekly IV	Neuromuscular; alopecia
4. Prednisone	1 mg/kg/day PO	Osteoporosis; diabetes
5. Asparaginase	200 units/kg/day IV	Allergic reactions; pancreatitis; renal failure
6. Bleomycin	5 to 30 mg twice a week or weekly IV (limited to 300 mg total)	Pulmonary fibrosis; skin ulcerations
7. Adriamycin	60 mg/m² q 3 weeks IV (maximum dose 500 mg/m²)	Cardiac toxicity; bone marrow suppression; alopecia
8. Bis-chloroethyl nitrosourea	3.4 mg/kg q 6–8 weeks IV	Bone marrow depression

should be given, either locally or by referral to special treatment centers. These decisions are often difficult, but they must be considered carefully before embarking on a therapeutic course. Since the answers to many questions are not yet settled or merely reflect personal opinion rather than scientific fact, the physician must be well informed or ask for help.

Although the therapy of patients with lymphoreticular neoplasms is changing rapidly, certain general statements appear valid. For patients with localized disease Stage I or II, the optimal therapy involves radiotherapy to the tumor-bearing areas, including the adjacent normal lymph nodes. The dose to be administered should be at least 4000 rads given over four weeks. Since disease extent is hard to determine with certainty, many oncologists are extending the treatment fields to include all lymph node areas and the splenic area, or bed, if splenectomy has been performed. The upper half of the body is treated en bloc, followed by a short rest and then treatment of the lower half. The anatomic sequence varies if disease exists only below the diaphragm. For patients with localized Stage IE or IIE in the abdomen, consideration should be given to the special abdominal radiation approaches mentioned above. Since the volume of tissue and potential damage to the normal tissues such as marrow, lung, and kidney are great, care must be taken to have well calibrated machines and expertly shaped fields. Therapists prefer megavoltage (linear accelerator) machines

that markedly restrict the amount of scatter to adjacent normal tissues. The ill effects of therapy of this intensity have been pulmonary or cardiac fibrosis, myelitis, pericarditis, bowel ulcerations, and marrow insufficiency.

The approach to patients with Stage III disease is not agreed upon by experts in the field. Even with the most aggressive total nodal radiotherapy, x-ray only produces median survivals of less than three years. Investigators tend to use a combination of chemotherapy and x-ray. The approach may be with chemotherapy first, followed by radiotherapy, or the alternate sequence.

For patients with Stage IV disease, which represents about 40 to 50 per cent of patients, most oncologists prefer combination chemotherapy programs attempting to achieve complete tumor regressions. The one possible exception relates to nodular or diffuse well differentiated lymphocytic lymphomas, in which less aggressive and even single agent chemotherapy may prove to be highly effective. Here one can choose one of several alkylating agents and add corticosteroids for certain clinical indications such as thrombocytopenia and hemolytic anemia. These patients often have marrow involvement and peripheral blood abnormal cells characteristic of chronic lymphocytic leukemia and immunoglobulin deficiencies of immunoglobulin G.

The characteristic effect of combination chemotherapy is rapid resolution of tumor with any of several combinations, but varying proportions will show re-

TABLE 6.   Combination Chemotherapies*

Hoogstraten (1969)	Cyclophosphamide Vincristine Prednisone	15 mg/kg weekly IV × 6 0.025 mg/kg weekly IV × 6 1.0 mg/kg daily PO × 42 days
Luce (1971)	Cyclophosphamide Vincristine Prednisone	800 mg/M² day 1 2.0 mg/M² day 1 60 mg/M² daily × 5 } repeat q 15–21 days
Bagley (1972)	Cyclophosphamide Vincristine Prednisone	400 mg/M² daily × 5 1.4 mg/M² day 1 100 mg/M² days 1–5 } repeat q 21 days
Lowenbraun (1970)	Cyclophosphamide Vincristine Procarbazine Prednisone	600 mg/M² day 1 + 8 IV 1.4 mg/M² day 1 + 8 IV 100 mg/M² days 1–10 PO 40 mg/M² days 1–14 } repeat q 28 days
Bonadonna (1973)	Adriamycin Bleomycin Prednisone	75 mg/M² day 1 15 mg/M² day 1 + 8 100 mg/M² daily × 5 } repeat q 21 days

*From Carbone, P. P.: Cancer, 30:1511, 1972, and Bonadonna, personal communication.

bound tumor growth during rest periods or after cessation of therapy. To avoid this, other combinations are being evaluated and the use of maintenance treatment added. No single regimen has been agreed on for any single disease category. Moreover, some of the drugs still in the stage of investigation require special permission to use as part of an exploratory approach.

The *complications of chemotherapy* reflect the fact that the drugs injure all rapidly dividing cells, including the normal marrow and gastrointestinal tract, with resultant increased risks of infection, hemorrhage, and ulcerations. *Alopecia* appears common to many of the drugs, because the hair follicle is also dividing its germinal cells rapidly. It is usually reversible, as are most of the other side effects. Modification of the dose may be necessary to make the toxicity manageable.

Some of the newer agents have other toxicities, such as *pulmonary fibrosis* and *cardiac myopathy,* that restrict total dosages. Consideration must be given to the fact that drugs interact with each other or even synergize the effect of x-ray therapy. This is particularly true of adriamycin, a new agent. Some long-term toxicities have been uncovered, including hemorrhagic cystitis, azoospermia or anovulation, cytologic dysplasia, and even pulmonary or hepatic fibrosis; these must be explained carefully to the patient and his family. More recently, information is accumulating that, as patients do better and treatment becomes prolonged, *second cancers* develop, substantiating the effects seen in animals of the carcinogenic potential of x-ray and antineoplastic drugs. However, despite these hazards and risks, under optimal conditions more effective therapies are being devised, and patients are doing better for extended periods of time.

Several *special therapy problems* should be mentioned. First, the rapid turnover of tumor cells results in the production of excessive amounts of uric acid. Treatment itself may result in marked destruction of tumor, and *hyperuricemia* may ensue. Allopurinol, a metabolic inhibitor of xanthine oxidase, should be administered routinely at the start of therapy as a prophylactic measure, along with fluids to ensure adequate urinary output to prevent precipitation of uric acid in the renal tubules. *Hypercalcemia,* an uncommon complication of bone marrow involvement or the production of parathormone-like activity, can be managed with corticosteroids, oral phosphates, or mithramycin, a new antimicrobial that affects bone resorption. *Immune disturbances,* induced by the disease or occurring after treatment, result in an increased *risk of infections,* sometimes with exotic organisms. Accurate diagnosis must be attempted to institute effective therapy. These include fungus infections, viral illnesses, toxoplasmosis, and pneumocystis, whose treatment demands accurate elucidation. Platelet and white cell transfusions, particularly the former, should be available to treat acute problems that arise during the therapy. Pleural effusions and ascites caused by tumor cells on the parietal surfaces can be treated by using a variety of sclerosing agents or chemotherapeutic drugs.

Prognosis.   Over-all survival figures for lymphoreticular neoplasms are meaningless, because survival is dependent on histologic subtype, presence or absence of nodularity, stage, sex, age, and treatment program. Such uncorrelated information is available from the End Results Studies of the National Cancer Institute.

Median survivals for localized lymphocytic and histiocytic lymphomas were three and six years, respectively. In disseminated disease the corresponding figures are twelve and six months, respectively. Few investigators report data based on the breakdown mentioned above. The best prognosis is associated with well differentiated lymphocytic lymphoma group, with median survivals of five or more years. In other cell types, nodular varieties do better than corresponding histiocytic forms. Nodular lymphocytic poorly differentiated and nodular mixed lymphomas have the next best prognosis (approximately four to five years). The diffuse poorly differentiated lymphocytic, diffuse histiocytic, and pleomorphic groups fare poorly, with median survivals in the order of one to two years. In most categories, females fare better than males. Age does not consistently affect survival but varies with subtypes. Unlike Hodgkin's disease, symptoms or absence of symptoms does not seem to affect the survival figures corrected for stages.

Data on survival by stage indicate that again histologic pattern influences the outcome. In Stage I patient survivals of five years or more range from 50 to 100 per cent, probably related to histologic differences between series. Stage II and III patients with nodular lymphocytic poorly differentiated and mixed lymphomas have a median survival of three to five years, whereas survival in the diffuse forms ranges from three to four years. Patients with the Stage II and III histiocytic lymphomas, rarely nodular, have a median survival of one to two years. For Stage IV patients, those with the nodular mixed and poorly differentiated variety have an estimated survival of three to four years. Patients with the same cell types and stage but diffuse forms have a median survival of one to two years. Poorest end results are reported in patients with histiocytic Stage IV disease, in which the median survival is six to twelve months. The figures quoted are to be reinterpreted as estimates based on retrospective reviews and analysis when therapy was not systematically controlled. More recent data with more aggressive radiotherapy and chemotherapy indicate that survivals may become considerably better as more attention is paid to staging evaluation and intensive treatment programs are applied.

Berard, C. W.: Lymphoreticular disorders; malignant proliferative responses; lymphoma: Histopathology of the lymphomas. *In* Williams, W. J. (ed.): Hematology. New York, McGraw-Hill Book Company, 1972, p. 901.

Carbone, P. P.: Non-Hodgkin's lymphoma: Recent observations on natural history and intensive treatment. Cancer, 30:1511, 1972.

Carbone, P. P., and DeVita, V. T.: Malignant lymphoma. *In* Holland, J. F., and Frei, E., III (eds.): Cancer Medicine. Philadelphia, Lea & Febiger, 1973, p. 1302.

Carbone, P. P., and Spurr, C.: Management of patients with malignant lymphoma: A comparative study with cyclophosphamide and vinca alkaloids. Cancer Res., 28:811, 1968.

Jones, S. E., Fuks, Z., Bull, M., Kadin, M. E., Dorfman, R. F., Kaplan, H., Rosenberg, S. A., and Kim, H.: Non-Hodgkin's lymphomas. IV. Clinicopathologic correlation in 405 cases. Cancer, 31:806, 1973.

769a.   BURKITT'S LYMPHOMA

Paul P. Carbone

Burkitt's lymphoma has attracted a great deal of interest because of its unique geographical distribution, response to treatment, and epidemiologic features highly suggestive of an infectious origin. The clinical and pathologic features were originally described by Dennis Burkitt, a British surgeon, in East Africa in 1958. Burkitt's lymphoma also occurs in the United States, South America, and New Guinea. In Africa, Burkitt's lymphoma accounts for over 50 per cent of all childhood tumors; the incidence in the United States is not known, but more than 100 cases have been reported. The features of the disease and response to treatment are quite similar in Africa and in the United States.

Etiology and Pathogenesis. Burkitt's observations suggested that there were climatic restrictions for expression of this disease in Africa. These were weather and terrain conditions conducive to malaria, i.e., adequate rainfall and lack of freezing temperatures. Epidemiologic studies have confirmed these initial observations as well as time-space clustering of cases, further suggesting a viral etiology. Serologic and virologic studies have indicated that the Epstein-Barr virus (EBV) was associated with many cases. More recently, EBV has been proposed as the cause of infectious mononucleosis and possibly as a passenger virus in Burkitt's lymphoma. Malaria has also been associated with Burkitt's lymphoma, because those places that have eliminated malaria do not have a high incidence of this tumor. Malaria has been implicated as a possible co-carcinogen, i.e., priming the reticuloendothelial system, or as an immunosuppressive agent. Recently reverse transcriptase (RNA-dependent DNA polymerase) and Rauscher virus material have been found in some tumors. Despite all these associations, the cause of Burkitt's lymphoma and the causes of its peculiar distribution have not been uncovered.

Pathology. Burkitt's lymphoma, histologically, contains undifferentiated lymphoid cells of uniform size. The nuclei are round and vesicular with prominent nucleoli. The cytoplasm is basophilic with small vacuoles shown to contain fat by special stains. Large histiocytes ingesting tumor debris are scattered throughout the section. The cells can be differentiated from other lymphomas by their characteristic large size and lack of differentiation.

Clinical Features. The tumor affects primarily children (median age 7, range 3 to 60). Males are slightly more prone to develop the disease than are females. The clinical history of illness is short. In Africa, the most common presenting features relate to facial tumors (60 per cent). Abdominal masses occur in 30 per cent, usually as a result of ovarian, mesenteric, or retroperitoneal tumors. Peripheral adenopathy, splenomegaly, and/or hepatomegaly are rarely the main presenting features. Neurologic manifestations, such as paraplegia, cranial nerve paresis, and/or meningeal involvement, occur less frequently (10 per cent). In American patients abdominal manifestations predominate (75 per cent), and less than 25 per cent present with primary localized involvement elsewhere. Hematologic manifestations, such as marrow involvement and/or frank leukemia, are rare in contrast to other childhood lymphomas.

Because these tumors grow rapidly and because they involve the kidneys or obstruct the ureters, hyperuricemia and azotemia are common. The serum LDH may be extremely elevated and is of prognostic value; generally, high abnormal values that do not fall are associated with the poorest results. Metabolically, the tumor produces large amounts of lactic acid, and lactic acidosis may be an added complication. After chemotherapy, tumor lysis may be so rapid that hyperkalemia may be fatal unless treated prophylactically by maintaining high fluid volumes and frequent serum K^+ determinations.

Diagnosis. The diagnosis can be established only by biopsy, because many of the clinical features, even in endemic areas, can be mimicked by other lymphomas, acute granulocytic leukemia (chloromas), and pediatric solid tumors such as Wilms' tumor, retinoblastomas, embryonal rhabdomyosarcomas, and neuroblastoma. Cytologic material should be prepared by touching a freshly cut surface of the tumor to the glass slides and then staining with standard hematologic techniques.

In the absence of the classic jaw tumor, Burkitt's lymphoma may not be suspected. The surgeon may first encounter the disease in the abdomen at laparotomy because of an expanding mass or intestinal obstruction. Attempts should be made to debulk the tumor as much as possible, because this may improve the over-all prognosis. Additional staging procedures include intravenous pyelogram, bone survey, bone marrow biopsy, lumbar puncture, lymphograms, and [67]gallium scans. It must be emphasized, however, that the tumor grows so fast that undue delay may be deleterious to the patient's eventual prognosis. Clinical staging schemes have generally acknowledged the good prognosis of facial tumors and limited abdominal disease. Conversely, central nervous system and bone marrow involvement convey a poor prognosis.

Management and Prognosis. Even in the localized cases, chemotherapy plays a major role in management. Cyclophosphamide, 40 mg per kilogram every three weeks intravenously for two to six courses, is the major therapeutic regimen. Patients who suffer a relapse quickly or fail to respond may receive vincristine, 1.4 mg per square meter, on day 1 and methotrexate, 15 mg per square meter, on days 1 to 4, alternating with cytosine arabinoside, 250 mg per square meter per day given in six-hour doses for three days.

When complete remission has been achieved, maintenance treatment has not been shown to be of value. X-ray therapy has not been a major modality in this disease except for treatment of obstructive symptoms. Ninety per cent of all patients achieve complete disappearance of tumor. About 30 per cent of these patients never relapse. The disease in one third of the remaining patients recurs early or produces central nervous system manifestations. These patients have a poor prognosis and will die usually in six months. The remainder have late recurrence (after six months) after a complete response. Characteristically, they respond to the same initial treatment. As mentioned above, care must be taken to prevent or manage the metabolic complications, particularly hyperuricemia, lactic acidosis, and hyperkalemia.

The long-term survival with Burkitt's lymphoma both in the United States and in Africa is extremely good, about 50 to 60 per cent. Best results are obtained in those patients with localized disease. Extensive abdominal disease or liver, central nervous system, or bone marrow involvement carries the poorest prognosis. Despite the strong evidence for tumor-associated antigens and spontaneous regressions in some patients, immunotherapy with BCG and/or allogenic tumor cells has not been shown to be better than chemotherapy alone.

Burkitt, D., and O'Conor, G. T.: Malignant lymphoma in African children: Clinical syndrome. Cancer, 14:256, 1966.

Cohen, M. H., et al.: Burkitt's tumor in the United States. Cancer, 23:1259, 1969.

Ziegler, J. L., et al.: Intensive chemotherapy in patients with Burkitt's lymphoma. Int. J. Cancer, 10:254, 1972.

Ziegler, J. L., and Magrath, I. T.: Burkitt's lymphoma. Pathobiology Annual 129. New York, Appleton-Century-Crofts, 1974.

770. HODGKIN'S DISEASE

Saul A. Rosenberg

Definition and History. Hodgkin's disease can be defined as a malignant disease, usually arising in the lymph nodes, with a histopathologic appearance which includes characteristic giant cells in an appropriate cellular background. The affliction has challenged clinicians and investigators because of its unknown etiology, its clinical and histopathologic features suggesting a granulomatous infection as well as neoplasia, the extreme variability of its microscopic and clinical picture, its peculiar associated immunologic abnormalities, and its frequent responsiveness to modern therapeutic approaches, which can result in cure of the disease.

In the absence of a known etiology or satisfactory animal model, it is being increasingly challenged that the characteristic giant cell of Hodgkin's disease, the so-called Reed-Sternberg cell, identifies a single disease entity. Nonetheless, considerable information and literature have supported the clinical value of considering Hodgkin's disease as a disease which can be variable yet reasonably predictable in its expression.

Thomas Hodgkin's name has been immortalized for his description, in 1832, of seven patients with a fatal illness in a report entitled *On Some Morbid Appearances of the Absorbent Glands and Spleen.* On later histopathologic review, Fox confirmed only two of Hodgkin's cases, and on clinical grounds suggested that a third patient of the original seven belonged to the entity now bearing Hodgkin's name.

Although numerous names have been given to this disease, such as *lymphogranuloma, lymphogranulomatosis, lymphadenoma,* and *malignant granuloma,* the name of Hodgkin's disease, initially suggested by Sir Samuel Wilks, has now received international recognition. Many pathologists have contributed to the characterization of this disease, but Dorothy Reed and Carl Sternberg are given credit for the clearest description of the virtually pathognomonic giant cell which bears their names.

Etiology and Pathogenesis. The cause of Hodgkin's disease is unknown. Although various etiologic agents, including bacteria, protozoa, and viruses, have been proposed, none have withstood the tests of time and confirmation. The problem of secondary invaders in the infection-susceptible patient with late-stage Hodgkin's disease has plagued the efforts of investigators for almost a century. The very nature of Hodgkin's disease, whether infectious in the usual sense or neoplastic, has long been a controversy and remains unsettled. The finding of aneuploidy and marker chromsomes in cells from Hodgkin's disease tissue is preliminary evidence that Hodgkin's disease is a true neoplasm. Whether this holds for all clinical and histologic types of Hodgkin's disease remains to be determined.

Any view of the cause of Hodgkin's disease must take into account the wide variety of histopathologic and clinical pictures, the usual rarity of neoplastic-appearing giant cells, the signs of an inflammatory reaction, the frequent infection-like symptoms, its anatomic predilections, its characteristic immunologic deficiencies, and its peculiar epidemiologic characteristics.

Epidemiology. In the United States the annual incidence of Hodgkin's disease is 35 per million for white males and 26 per million for white females, with an annual death rate of 23 per million and 13 per million, respectively. Nonwhites have a somewhat lower reported incidence than whites in all age groups, although the rates approach each other in the age range between 35 and 59 years. Hodgkin's disease has an unusual bimodal age-specific incidence curve, with one mode at ages 15 to 34 and another after the age of 50. The disease is distributed throughout the world, but the incidence peaks differ somewhat for various regions, e.g., absence of the first age mode in Japan.

Approximately 60 to 65 per cent of reported patients are male; 85 per cent of children with disease at age ten or younger are male, but between ages 15 and 35 the sex incidence is about the same.

Occurrence of the disease in two or more members of the same family has been documented in numerous reports and studies. Although the data are inadequate, it is likely that close relatives of patients with Hodgkin's disease experience a slightly increased risk of developing the disease. Observations suggesting a higher incidence of Hodgkin's disease among close unrelated contacts of those with the disease have been made recently. These provocative reports require confirmation and are difficult to establish statistically.

Pathology. The minimal requirement for the pathologic diagnosis of Hodgkin's disease is the presence of characteristic giant cells of the Reed-Sternberg type in an appropriate histologic setting. The morphologic findings, however, can be very diverse.

The most reliable characteristics of the Reed-Sternberg cell are the large inclusion-like nucleoli and the double or multiple nuclei of large size. Mononuclear forms are also found in typical lesions of Hodgkin's disease, but cannot be considered as reliably diagnostic. The Reed-Sternberg cells may vary considerably in appearance, depending on the type of histologic response and category. The distinctive multinucleated giant cells associated with the nodular sclerosis variety are presumed to be variants of the Reed-Sternberg cell, with abundant pale eosinophilic cytoplasm, well-defined cellular borders in lacuna-like spaces (in formalin-fixed tissue) with small to medium-sized nucleoli, and an unusual hyperlobation.

Recent reports have emphasized that cells indistinguishable from, or closely resembling, Reed-Sternberg cells may be found in conditions other than Hodgkin's disease. The appropriate cellular and architectural environment for these cells is required to permit the diagnosis of Hodgkin's disease.

There have been two major histopathologic classifications for Hodgkin's disease: that proposed by Jackson and Parker, and the Rye classification proposed in 1965. The relative frequency of the subgroups of these clas-

TABLE 1.   Histopathologic Classification
of Hodgkin's Disease

Relative Frequency (%)	Jackson and Parker	Rye, 1965	Relative Frequency (%)
5–10	Paragranuloma ——→	Lymphocyte predominance	10–15
80–90	Granuloma ——→	Nodular sclerosis	30–70
		Mixed cellularity	20–40
5–10	Sarcoma ——→	Lymphocyte depletion	5–15

sifications is shown in Table 1. The major advantage of the Rye classification lies in recognition of the important subgroup of nodular sclerosis described by Lukes and his colleagues.

Clinical Manifestations. The presenting and subsequent clinical manifestations of patients with Hodgkin's disease can be extremely varied and considerably influenced by therapy.

A typical onset is in the observation, usually by the patient, of a painless, enlarging mass, most commonly in the neck, but occasionally in the axilla or inguinal-femoral region. Upon examination this is found to be a discrete, rubbery, painless lymphadenopathy, frequently with surrounding enlarged lymph nodes. In other instances, a chest roentgenogram, taken for a routine purpose, demonstrates mediastinal node enlargement; examination may then disclose lower cervical lymphadenopathy, which had not been noticed by the patient. Although these typical presentations may occur at any age with any histopathologic type, these patients are usually between 15 and 35 years of age and have the histologic variety of nodular sclerosis.

As the typical asymptomatic patient is evaluated more thoroughly with available diagnostic methods, the anatomic extent of disease is usually more widespread than was apparent on physical examination. In particular, mediastinal enlargement is found on routine or detailed radiologic examination, para-aortic involvement is noted on lower extremity lymphography, or splenic involvement is found at exploratory laparotomy in significant numbers of such patients.

Occasionally the lymphadenopathy makes itself known to the patient or his physician by producing local symptoms of pain, lymphatic or venous obstruction of an extremity, vena caval obstruction, or airway narrowing. The duration of lymphadenopathy prior to diagnosis is extremely variable. Some patients report that a particular mass had been present for several years, even waxing and waning in size. Typically several weeks to several months elapse between the time of the patient's first observation and the diagnostic biopsy.

Another group of patients with Hodgkin's disease have unexplained and persistent fever and/or night sweats as initial symptoms. Fatigue and weight loss may be associated complaints as these symptoms become more severe and prolonged. These patients tend to be in the older age group, are more often male than female, and, when evaluated, are found to have more widespread disease than the typical patient presenting without symptoms. Occasionally, in older patients, usually past the age of 40, the systemic symptoms are severe, often with associated anemia, but the lymphadenopathy is minimal. Extensive diagnostic efforts may be required to uncover the cause of the symptoms, including lymphography, bone marrow and liver biopsies, or even exploratory laparotomy. In rare cases, the diagnosis is not made before a postmortem examination. These older patients, with predominant systemic symptoms at the onset, usually show the histologic varieties of mixed cellularity or lymphocyte depletion.

Occasional patients with Hodgkin's disease have intermittent evening fever lasting several days, alternating with afebrile periods lasting days or weeks. Usually, the fever gradually becomes more severe and more continuous. This *cyclic fever* has been labeled as the *Pel-Ebstein* or *Murchison* type and is rarely a presenting manifestation of the disease.

Pruritus, usually generalized and severe, is another characteristic systemic symptom of Hodgkin's disease. It may appear as a mild localized symptom, but, if caused by Hodgkin's disease, it usually progresses and becomes generalized. The pruritus may be the only systemic symptom in the otherwise typical presentation of a young person, especially in women. Generalized severe pruritus may occur in patients with lymphoma other than Hodgkin's disease and in other medical and dermatologic conditions, but its presence should always suggest Hodgkin's disease. Its cause is unknown.

Rarely, patients complain of *pain* in the region of enlarged lymph nodes within a few minutes *after drinking alcoholic beverages.* Although this is suggestive of Hodgkin's disease, it is not diagnostic. Its mechanism is not known.

A wide variety of other symptoms may initially call the attention of the patient and his physician to the disease. These same problems occur more commonly as the course of the disease progresses.

The *clinical course* of the disease can be extremely variable. In addition, almost all patients receive treatment that may profoundly affect the course, sometimes resulting in apparent cure, and in many instances resulting in complications that become difficult to separate from the disease itself.

In the typical young patient with Hodgkin's disease, the disease progresses at a variable rate, over a period of months or years, to involve lymph nodes adjacent to those initially involved. In time, if not adequately controlled, typical extensions beyond the lymph nodes occur. There may be intrathoracic problems with compression of the airway or great veins, involvement of the pleura and/or pericardium with resultant effusions, increasing pulmonary parenchymal involvement, or local osseous involvement of sternum, clavicle, ribs, or vertebrae.

It is not uncommon for patients with early disease, apparently localized to the neck, to develop disease in the lymph nodes in the upper para-aortic region and/or spleen. Later, even the young patient with an initially favorable prognosis may develop widespread problems, as if there has been a loss of defense mechanisms. At this stage the *bone marrow* may become focally and then diffusely involved, with eventual marrow failure. Multiple *osseous lesions* may occur, usually of an osteoblastic or mixed osteoblastic and osteolytic radiologic appearance. These often produce pain, but rarely fractures. The *liver* may become progressively involved, diffuse infiltration of the portal spaces causing serious and even fatal hepatic dysfunction and laboratory features of intrahepatic biliary obstruction. Liver involvement in Hodgkin's disease has been noted to be closely, if not uniformly, associated with involvement of the spleen. Peripheral *neuropathies* as a direct result of tumor growth and epidural cord compression are seen increasingly as the disease progresses.

In time, virtually all patients with Hodgkin's disease develop increasingly severe systemic symptoms as their disease progresses beyond control. High continuous fever, drenching night sweats, malaise, fatigue, anorexia, and weight loss are all characteristic of the terminal picture of patients with Hodgkin's disease. Generalized pruritus is seen in a proportion of patients during their course but is not uniform in its appearance. Selected aspects of some of the clinical problems of patients with Hodgkin's disease require emphasis.

Hematologic Abnormalities. It is especially difficult to separate the effects of therapy for Hodgkin's disease from the effects of the disease itself on hematologic parameters. Anemia of a moderate degree may be found in patients who present with widespread disease, often associated with systemic symptoms. This is usually with normal indices, normal or low reticulocyte count, and a negative Coombs test. When analyzed in detail, there may be shortened red blood cell survival with inadequate marrow response, as is also seen in patients with advanced cancer or chronic infection. Excluding effects of therapy, which can greatly aggravate the situation, some patients develop profound anemia occasionally at the onset, but more commonly during the course of the disease. This may be due to extensive bone marrow involvement with the disease, hypersplenism, or, rarely, a Coombs-positive hemolytic picture. Often, combinations of these factors are responsible for the most severe anemias.

Bone marrow involvement by Hodgkin's disease can only rarely be demonstrated by the usual marrow aspirate technique and examination of marrow smears. The involvement is focal, is often associated with fibrosis, and can be discovered more readily by a marrow biopsy performed with a large-bore needle or open surgical technique.

The erythrocyte sedimentation is commonly elevated in patients with active disease, and sometimes it may be the only evidence that the disease has been inadequately treated or that clinical recurrence is imminent. Numerous other laboratory abnormalities have been reported to be correlated with disease activity. These include elevations of serum alpha-2-globulin, fibrinogen, haptoglobin, copper, zinc, and ceruloplasmin; depression of serum iron and iron-binding capacity; elevation of leukocyte alkaline phosphatase; and increase in urinary hydroxyproline and muramidase.

In the untreated patient, or if therapy has been minimal, moderate to marked neutrophilic leukocytosis and thrombocytosis are characteristic of active, symptomatic Hodgkin's disease. Occasionally, the granulocytosis may be so marked as to suggest chronic granulocytic leukemia. More careful study, however, usually demonstrates that this is a "leukemoid" reaction. Eosinophilia of a mild degree is not uncommon, but occasionally it is moderate or marked, tending to occur in patients with severe and longstanding pruritus. Absolute lymphopenia, even in untreated patients, is seen in a small percentage of cases and, when present, is a poor

prognostic sign. Absolute lymphocytosis rarely if ever is seen in Hodgkin's disease and should always suggest an error in diagnosis. Reed-Sternberg cells have been described in the peripheral blood in studies employing special techniques, but they are seldom seen with usual hematologic techniques. Rarely, leukemia of the acute myelomonocytic type occurs in patients with longstanding Hodgkin's disease.

Immunologic Abnormalities. The observation that patients with Hodgkin's disease frequently fail to develop a delayed type of skin reaction to tuberculin, even in the presence of active tuberculosis, has stimulated considerable study and speculation. Patients with Hodgkin's disease, even when apparently well, have a higher frequency of cutaneous anergy than does a control population.

Numerous studies have confirmed that patients with Hodgkin's disease have a defect in delayed hypersensitivity. In general, the more widespread and advanced the clinical extent of the Hodgkin's disease, the more complete is the loss of this immunologic reaction. The therapy used for Hodgkin's disease almost certainly contributes to the immunologic deficiencies observed. However, despite the immunosuppressive effects of therapy, recovery of parameters of delayed hypersensitivity has been observed as disease activity has been controlled.

It remains to be determined whether the defect in cellular immunity is uniformly observed in Hodgkin's disease, and thus may be of etiologic importance, or is a result of the disease and its therapy. Techniques of measuring cellular immunity are not yet sufficiently precise to be certain. It appears that the more sensitive the test, the more frequently it is abnormal, even in limited disease and prior to therapy.

The relatively well patient with Hodgkin's disease cannot be shown to be more susceptible to infections of any kind, even though he may be anergic to the usual skin tests. As the disease progresses with greater use of radiotherapy, chemotherapy, corticosteroids, and antimicrobials, bacterial, viral, and mycotic infections become more frequent. However, this is not substantially different from other hematologic and immunologic diseases in the late stages.

Selected Clinical Problems. *Epidural tumors* occur in Hodgkin's disease and other lymphomas. These may be seen in patients with otherwise favorable prognosis and must be recognized and managed as a medical emergency. Any patient who complains of back or neck pain, numbness, tingling or weakness of an extremity, or bladder or bowel dysfunction should be carefully examined for a transverse *spinal cord* or *cauda equina lesion.* This will require the cooperative efforts of neurologic, neurosurgical, radiologic, and radiotherapeutic consultants.

The problem of the *pulmonary infiltrate* in Hodgkin's disease is especially challenging. Involvement of the lungs is common, but its appearance is variable and must be distinguished from radiation effects, partial lung collapse, drug reactions, and especially the wide variety of pulmonary infections which occur in these patients. In some situations the therapeutic significance of these lesions is so great that a diagnostic thoracotomy is justified.

Virtually all patients with uncontrolled Hodgkin's disease who succumb to their disease will have episodes of serious infections. These occur most frequently during the later stages of the disease and are associated with the more intensive use of therapy, especially of myelosuppressive drugs and corticosteroids.

At the turn of the century, tuberculosis was so prevalent in patients with Hodgkin's disease that a causal relationship was proposed. Since tuberculosis has come under relative control in the United States and elsewhere, this infection is only rarely observed to coexist with Hodgkin's disease and is only rarely a cause of death in these patients. Although bacterial infections are commonly identified and respond to the modern use of antimicrobials, other infections complicate the later clinical course.

Fungal infections, especially of the lungs and meninges, with almost any species but especially Cryptococcus, are encountered in most series of patients with hematologic neoplasms, especially when corticosteroids are employed. *Pneumocystis carinii* and toxoplasmosis are being recognized with increasing frequency and must be sought, because effective therapy is now available. Viral infections, especially herpes zoster and cytomegalovirus infection, have frequently been described.

Diagnostic Evaluation. The progress being made in the treatment of Hodgkin's disease has paralleled the improvement in techniques for identifying the extent of the disease in the untreated patient. In view of the current choices of therapy, it is essential that all patients with Hodgkin's disease be evaluated completely by physicians experienced with the disease before therapeutic decisions are made.

A careful history and physical examination are essential to uncover characteristic systemic symptoms and to describe all the lymph node areas of the body. Not all palpable lymph nodes are pathologic in the sense that they contain Hodgkin's disease. However, if there are suspicious lymph nodes which, if involved, would change the therapeutic approach, biopsy should be done for confirmation. The lymphoid tissues in the oropharynx and nasopharynx should be evaluated by a skillful examiner. The size of the liver and spleen must be determined as carefully as possible. The bones should be examined for areas of tenderness.

Radiologic examinations should include routine chest films and whole lung tomography to identify mediastinal and hilar lymphadenopathy and pulmonary involvement. Lower extremity lymphography is essential in all patients, unless pulmonary function is seriously limited or bone marrow or other disseminated extralymphatic involvement has been documented. A skeletal survey complemented by bone scans is desirable to detect osseous lesions, most often first seen in the vertebrae and pelvis. Routine blood cell counts and determination of sedimentation rate, serum alkaline phosphatase, and urinalysis and evaluation of renal function are the minimal laboratory studies required for evaluation. Bone marrow biopsy, using a needle or an open technique, should be performed in all patients with advanced lymph node involvement.

In recent years, exploratory laparotomy and splenectomy have been employed to identify and confirm the presence of Hodgkin's disease in the abdomen and pelvis. Studies have demonstrated that approximately half the patients with clinical enlargement of the spleen do not have histologic involvement of that organ; conversely, in approximately one patient in four, spleens of normal size have demonstrable foci of Hodgkin's disease. The identification of involvement of the liver by Hodgkin's disease is especially difficult. It is unusual for marked and obvious liver involvement to occur early in the course of the disease. Abnormalities of liver function tests, including the Bromsulphalein excretion, serum alkaline phosphatase, and other enzymes, modest hepatomegaly, and nonspecific hepatic scan abnormalities may all be misleading. These abnormalities may occur nonspecifically, especially in patients with systemic symptoms, and histologic verification of hepatic involvement should be sought. Conversely, liver involvement can be demonstrated, although rarely, at laparotomy, with no laboratory abnormalities thought to be characteristic of that condition.

The advances in diagnostic ability and the results of detailed study of patients early in their course provide strong evidence that Hodgkin's disease presents in relatively orderly patterns of involvement, suggesting a unifocal origin. Before the distribution of disease has been altered by treatment, the lymph node involvement is not a random affair, but nodal disease occurs in contiguous regions (or those directly connected by lymphatic channels, such as the low neck and upper para-aortic lymph nodes) in 90 per cent or more of the cases when a second node group is involved.

Staging in Hodgkin's Disease. There have been several attempts to classify the extent of the disease, in previously untreated patients, to provide useful prognostic and therapeutic indicators. All the proposals acknowledge the poor prognostic significance of widespread disease and of systemic symptoms. The importance of an accepted staging classification in any disease is to facilitate the selection of appropriate treatment programs, to give an estimate of prognosis, and to permit a valid comparison among medical centers for evaluation of their therapeutic results and investigative programs. The disease stage of classification in current use is shown in Table 3 of Ch. 769.

Treatment. The treatment of Hodgkin's disease has undergone radical changes since 1940. These have resulted from advances in the availability and techniques of supervoltage radiotherapy, effectiveness of chemotherapeutic agents, and the realization that patients can be cured.

The advances and enthusiasm for aggressive treatment since 1960 have appeared and evolved rapidly. It is not yet possible to make an accurate assessment of the true curative potential of modern treatment. Nonetheless, there can be no doubt that considerable improvement in over-all survival rates is being observed, and a significant number of patients are being cured by appropriate evaluation and staging and the application of concepts of tolerable aggressive therapy.

Radiotherapy. The basic concepts of modern radiotherapy for Hodgkin's disease were enunciated years ago by the Swiss radiotherapist René Gilbert and were effectively put into practice during the kilovoltage era by Vera Peters, utilizing megavoltage apparatus by Kaplan, Johnson, and others.

The major considerations which determine the success of radiation therapy are the radiation dose per field, the extent of the fields employed, and the beam energy. It is inappropriate to employ kilovoltage x-rays in a curative attempt for a patient with Hodgkin's disease. Doses of 3500 to 4500 rads are required to relatively large fields to effect permanent eradication of any given site. Because of the limitations of present diagnostic methods in determining the true extent of the disease, lymphoid regions adjacent to known disease or contiguous via lymphatic channels are usually treated to full dose to achieve the best results. Modern equipment and methods permit the treatment of most of the commonly involved lymphoid tissues in two or three large single fields, the "mantle" or supradiaphragmatic field and the "inverted-Y" below the diaphragm.

Data are accumulating which support this philosophy of therapy for all carefully studied patients with Stage I, II, and III disease in providing relapse-free survival and probably increased cure rates as well. Extended field, so-called total lymphoid or total nodal radiotherapy should not be attempted by radiologists who do not devote their entire time to radiation therapy.

Chemotherapy. Chemotherapy has developed significantly since the initial experience with nitrogen mustard during World War II. Successful palliation now can be obtained in the majority of patients. Not infrequently, treatment with one agent will eliminate all evidence of Hodgkin's disease, but inevitably the disease recurs. No documented instance of apparent cure by single drug chemotherapy is on record. It is therefore not justifiable to utilize chemotherapy as initial treatment for patients with localized disease who have a chance for cure by intensive radiotherapy.

The alkylating agents vinblastine and procarbazine are valuable drugs for palliation of patients with Hodgkin's disease. In addition, vincristine and the corticosteroids are utilized in intensive combination approaches.

The principal alkylating agents are mechlorethamine (nitrogen mustard, HN-2), chlorambucil (Leukeran), cyclophosphamide (Cytoxan), and thiotriethylenephosphoramide (thio-tepa). *Nitrogen mustard* has the advantage of rapid action, but it must be given intravenously and causes brief but occasionally severe nausea and vomiting. The average duration of benefit is two to three months after a single dose. The advantage of *chlorambucil* is that it may be given orally, and its effect may be titrated more readily against both tumor and bone marrow response.

Cyclophosphamide is a good drug for Hodgkin's disease. Its gastrointestinal toxicity is mild, and it may be used intravenously or orally. An advantage is its lesser toxicity for blood platelet formation. However, it causes alopecia in many patients in whom administration of the drug is carried to the point of marrow toxicity, and hemorrhagic cystitis occurs in 10 to 20 per cent of patients with long-term administration.

Vinblastine provides significant objective improvement for the majority of patients with Hodgkin's disease. Although oral preparations have been tested, the clinically available form of the drug must be given intravenously. It is well tolerated, granulocytopenia being its major toxic effect. There is little or no depression of the platelet count when usual doses are used. The drug is usually given at weekly intervals. Although pronounced leukopenia may develop, rapid recovery is the rule. In some patients, injections may be spaced at two- to four-week intervals after the initial response is obtained. With maintenance therapy, the disease may be kept in remission for many months, occasionally for several years.

Procarbazine represents another class of drug which has definite activity against Hodgkin's disease. A high proportion of patients experience objective benefit for at least a short time. Its bone marrow toxicity is similar to that of nitrogen mustard, affecting all the formed elements. When used as the third sequential drug for Hodgkin's disease, the responses have been relatively short in duration, averaging two or three months, and marrow suppression may be prolonged.

There is no doubt that objective regression of Hodgkin's disease is observed in some patients treated with *corticosteroids*. However, the general experience is that the responses are brief in duration and overshadowed by the serious toxic effects of steroids, which are particularly distressing in leukopenic patients. The corticosteroids have been employed in combination drug programs, because they are not myelosuppressive.

Combination Chemotherapy. In recent years there has been great interest in the use of combinations of chemotherapeutic agents. It is possible to achieve greater cell destruction when drugs that do not have overlapping toxicity can be combined at relatively full dosage. The most successful and widely tested combination has been developed at the National Cancer Institute and consists of six two-week cycles of therapy with nitrogen mustard, vincristine, procarbazine, and prednisone — the so-called MOPP program. Since two-week rest periods intervene between successive cycles, the entire course requires six months. Although this is a prolonged and occasionally difficult therapeutic program, complete suppression of evidence of Hodgkin's disease can be obtained in 70 to 80 per cent of previously untreated patients. The value of this approach has been the high percentage of complete regression of disease and of long disease-free intervals without maintenance therapy.

In some series, the median duration of remissions is two to three years, with some patients in their first continuous unmaintained remissions approaching ten years in duration. This raises the realistic possibility that clinical cure of Hodgkin's disease can be achieved with combination chemotherapy, a result which had not been observed with effective but only palliative single-drug therapy.

Combination Radiotherapy and Chemotherapy. There have been numerous attempts to improve the results of radiotherapy by combining chemotherapy with it. To date, however, there are no convincing reports that such combined therapy has been beneficial. Moreover, the routine supplementation of radiotherapy with concurrent single-drug chemotherapy in localized Hodgkin's disease seems distinctly unwise, because the drug, by depressing hematopoiesis, may jeopardize completion of a potentially curative course of radiotherapy.

Recently there have been studies of the possibility of administering the MOPP cyclic combination chemotherapy after total lymphoid radiotherapy. This is an area of active clinical investigation at this time. Carefully controlled therapeutic trials will be required to prove if there is an advantage in terms of prolonged high quality survival of programs which of necessity are associated with greater morbidity and prolonged inconvenience to the patient.

TABLE 2.   The Treatment of Hodgkin's Disease (November 1973)

Ann Arbor Pathologic Stage	Recommended Therapy	Estimated Five-Year Disease-Free Survival (%)	Experimental Therapy
IA, IEA, IIA, IIEA	Total lymphoid radiotherapy	90	Limited radiotherapy ± combination chemotherapy
IB, IEB, IIB, IIEB	Total lymphoid radiotherapy	75	Total lymphoid radiotherapy + combination chemotherapy
IIIA, IIIEA, IIISA	Total lymphoid radiotherapy	60	Combination chemotherapy ± total lymphoid radiotherapy
IIIB, IIIEB, IIISB	Total lymphoid radiotherapy or combination chemotherapy	40	Total lymphoid radiotherapy + combination chemotherapy
IVA, IVB	Combination chemotherapy	25	Total lymphoid radiotherapy + combination chemotherapy

Recommended Therapy.   The recommended therapy for a patient with Hodgkin's disease must be individualized. Considerations of age, extent of disease, prior therapy, and availability of modern skills in radiotherapy and chemotherapy are important in making therapeutic decisions. However, the improving results of aggressive therapy after accurate clinical evaluation and staging in the untreated patient must be acknowledged. Although the value of some therapeutic regimens remains to be established, in terms of survival the recommended therapeutic approaches for the previously untreated patient with various stages of Hodgkin's disease are listed in Table 2. Estimated results are expressed as the percentage of patients likely to achieve a disease-free interval of five years. Careful evaluation and observation of a high proportion of patients, perhaps 90 or 95 per cent, who have survived disease-free for five years show them to be clinically cured of their disease. Trials are being conducted to further improve these results or to reduce the morbidity of their therapy. These newer approaches are also listed in Table 2.

Prognosis.   Hodgkin's disease can no longer be accepted as a uniformly fatal disease. The advances in histopathologic classification and diagnostic evaluation and the selection of appropriate aggressive therapy are resulting in a continuous improvement in over-all survival.

Survival figures and prognostic factors which were accepted twenty or even ten years ago are not acceptable today. This is dramatically demonstrated by comparing over-all survival figures for all patients seen, not only from individual institutions, but from Public Health reports. The five-year survival rate has increased from approximately 25 to 50 per cent over the past twenty years. In some institutions the five-year survival rate is exceeding 75 per cent for all patients seen with the disease.

Even prognostic variables are being obscured by modern aggressive therapy. Such important factors as histology, stage of the disease, and presence of systemic symptoms, for example, are becoming less significant as the therapy has become more successful.

Within the context of the foregoing considerations, certain prognostic indicators can be re-emphasized. In general, the more widespread the disease, the poorer the prognosis. Patients with systemic symptoms as defined by the Ann Arbor Conference have a poorer prognosis than those without symptoms, independent of the extent of disease. Patients with the histologic varieties of mixed cellularity and lymphocyte depletion have a much shorter survival, on the average, than those with lymphocyte predominance and nodular sclerosis. All series show that female patients survive longer than males. Patients over the age of 40 have a poorer prognosis than children and younger adults. An important observation is that limited involvement of nonlymphoid structures does not indicate a poor prognosis.

The prognostic variables described above are not completely independent of each other. For example, systemic symptoms are correlated with the extent of disease, and the histologic type is correlated with the sex of the patient. Nonetheless, these prognostic variables are of practical value in considering the management of each patient and in evaluating the relative success of various therapeutic approaches.

Table 2 presents a reasonable estimate of prognosis, recommended therapy, and current appropriate investigative approaches for the various stages of Hodgkin's disease, as of November 1973. That such estimates and recommendations must be dated is testimony to the fact that the understanding and management of patients with Hodgkin's disease are dynamic and gratifying endeavors.

DeVita, V. T., Serpick, A., and Carbone, P. P.: Combination chemotherapy in the treatment of advanced Hodgkin's disease. Ann. Intern. Med., 73:881, 1970.

Easson, E. C., and Russell, M. H.: The cure of Hodgkin's disease. Br. Med. J., 1:1704, 1963.

International Symposium on Hodgkin's Disease, N.C.I. Monograph No. 36, May, 1973.

Jackson, H., Jr., and Parker, F. Jr.: Hodgkin's Disease and Allied Disorders. New York, Oxford University Press, 1947, p. 177.

Kaplan, H. S.: Hodgkin's Disease. Cambridge, Mass., Harvard University Press, 1972.

Rosenberg, S. A., and Kaplan, H. S.: Hodgkin's disease and other malignant lymphomas. Calif. Med., 113:23, 1970.

Symposium: Obstacles to the Control of Hodgkin's Disease, Rye, N.Y. Cancer Res., 26, 1966.

Symposium: Staging in Hodgkin's Disease, Ann Arbor, Mich. Cancer Res., 31, 1971.

Section Eight. CYTOTOXIC AND IMMUNOSUPPRESSIVE AGENTS

Paul Calabresi

771. INTRODUCTION

Although all active drugs exert a certain degree of toxicity on some cells in the body, the term *cytotoxic agents* usually denotes those compounds that affect the proliferative capacity of cells by their inhibitory action on DNA, RNA, or protein biosynthesis. Accordingly, they are sometimes also called *antiproliferative agents.* The desired result is selective cell death, with destruction of malignant·neoplastic cells and relative sparing of viability and function of normal cells. From the large number of compounds studied in experimental systems, only a few have demonstrated sufficient clinical antineoplastic activity, at acceptable levels of toxicity, to deserve the designation of *chemotherapeutic agents.*

Because these drugs inhibit biochemical sites that are not unique to cancer cells, they have also proved valuable in the management of several non-neoplastic disorders. Among these are certain conditions characterized by altered immune reactivity, including those observed in recipients of organ transplantations and in patients afflicted with connective tissue or autoimmune diseases. The term *immunosuppressive agents* has been used properly to describe drugs capable of suppressing measurable immune responses. It is an oversimplification, however, to attribute all beneficial effects of these drugs to suppression of the immune responses, because this does not take into consideration their anti-inflammatory action or selective enhancement and alterations of complex cellular and humoral immunologic interactions that are probably involved in these disorders.

Other non-neoplastic conditions that have been markedly improved by drugs originally developed for *cancer chemotherapy* include metabolic disorders, such as hyperuricemia and gout, dermatologic diseases, such as psoriasis, and infections caused by DNA viruses and other microorganisms. For these reasons, antiproliferative agents are attracting increasing interest, and their practical importance has expanded beyond the treatment of neoplastic disorders into many other areas of medicine.

772. PRINCIPLES OF CHEMOTHERAPY AND RATIONALE

THE CHEMOTHERAPEUTIC TRIANGLE

When using cytotoxic agents, the physician should always keep in mind the three principal entities involved in the chemotherapeutic triangle: (1) the host, (2) the drug, and (3) the tumor (see accompanying figure).

A series of primary effects and secondary responses involving these factors are illustrated in the figure. The relative preponderance or effectiveness of these interactions determines the final outcome for patients receiving chemotherapy. The effect of the tumor on the host is recognized as the "disease." The effects of the drug on the tumor are called "therapy," and those on the host are designated as "toxicity." The tumor may escape from the effects of the drug by one or more mechanisms of resistance. Although the mechanisms for natural and acquired resistance to drugs are not completely established, increased levels of target enzyme, deficiency of enzymes required for "lethal synthesis" of the active agent, impaired transport into cells, and increased catabolism of the drug have all been implicated. These and other mechanisms are usually exerted through selection by the drug of resistant cells, as a result of elimination of the susceptible population. The host responds to the toxic effects of the drug by metabolizing and eliminating the compound from the body. It is necessary therefore to be familiar with the mechanisms of detoxification and route of elimination of the drugs administered, as well as with the functional status of the organs involved. This is particularly true for cytotoxic agents, because the therapeutic:toxic ratio is small and the margin for error is slight.

Least understood are the defenses of the host against the tumor, although some degree of natural resistance and considerable variation between different individuals and types of tumors have been recognized for a long time. Recently, specific immunologic mechanisms have received considerable attention, and the importance of

The chemotherapeutic triangle.

cell-mediated immunity through the lymphocyte has been clearly established. The role of humoral antibodies, on the other hand, may be beneficial to the host, when "cytotoxic antibodies" are present, or protective for the tumor when "blocking factors" are involved. Even more nebulous are nonspecific host defense mechanisms, including interferon, local inflammatory responses, phagocytic activity, reticuloendothelial system function, and others yet to be explored. Administration of cytotoxic agents to the host may have profound effects on host defenses, thereby altering a delicate balance that may exist between host and tumor. It is important to remember that these relationships also apply to other parasitic infestations in the body, including viruses, fungi, and bacterial microorganisms. Accordingly, suppression of host defenses may not only facilitate tumor growth, but may render the host more susceptible to infectious complications by pathogenic bacteria or opportunistic organisms.

CONCEPT OF TOTAL CELL-KILL

In order to achieve complete cure of a neoplastic process, every last clonogenic cell, i.e., one capable of giving rise to malignant proliferating daughter cells, must be eradicated. This may be attained surgically when the entire cancer can be excised or it may be accomplished by x-irradiation if sufficient mean lethal doses can be delivered without irreversible damage to normal tissues, so that less than one tumor cell remains. Although the same principles are applicable to chemotherapy, the result has been more difficult to achieve. This is both due to the limitations of currently available cytotoxic agents and because medical oncologists are usually asked to treat patients when the neoplastic process is large, widely disseminated, and not amenable to surgery or radiotherapy.

A number of fundamental principles established by Skipper and his colleagues, using the experimental leukemia L1210 model, offer an excellent basis for understanding the problems involved, and appear to have valid clinical implications. Briefly condensed, they are as follows: (1) A single clonogenic leukemia cell is capable, through its progeny, of producing enough cells eventually to kill the host; (2) the life span of the host is inversely related to either the number of leukemia cells inoculated or the number remaining at the end of therapy; (3) first-order kinetics obtain with respect to leukemic cell-kill by chemotherapy, i.e., a given dose of a given drug kills a constant percentage of cells, not a constant number, regardless of the cell numbers present at the time of therapy (fractional kill hypothesis); (4) it is possible to calculate the chances of killing the last cell in populations that are homogeneous with respect to drug sensitivity; and (5) host immune defenses can be augmented, but are detectable only when small numbers of leukemic cells remain.

It is clear that a reliable assay for determining surviving tumor cells would be a highly desirable guide for effective chemotherapy. Unfortunately, this has been available only for trophoblastic tumors of women. In patients with choriocarcinoma and related disorders, it is possible to measure quantitatively chorionic gonadotrophins in the urine. This enables assessment of the amount of tumor remaining after each course of treatment and continuation of chemotherapy until the assay indicates that all tumor cells have been killed. In certain leukemias and lymphomas, rough approximations of cell-kill can be made by counting the number of abnormal cells in the peripheral blood and the marrow or measuring changes in size of visible tumors. These neoplasms have responded most successfully to chemotherapy, not only because we are able to monitor the presence of residual tumor cells, but more important, because they are characterized by rapid growth and are more susceptible to cytotoxic drugs. In order to begin to understand the reasons underlying the results obtained with cytotoxic agents, it is essential to have a basic knowledge of cell-cycle kinetics.

CELL-CYCLE KINETICS

The percentage of cells in a tumor or a normal organ undergoing division at any given time represents the *growth fraction* or *proliferating pool*. The larger the growth fraction, the more rapid the growth. Since our most effective cytotoxic agents kill cells that are undergoing DNA synthesis and mitosis, the tumors with larger growth fractions are more susceptible to currently available drugs. These include choriocarcinoma in women, acute lymphocytic leukemia, lymphocytic lymphosarcoma, Burkitt's lymphoma, reticulum cell sarcoma (histiocytic lymphoma), Hodgkin's disease, testicular neoplasms, Wilms' tumor and Ewing's sarcoma. Other tumors characterized by a small growth fraction, including carcinoma of the lung and various types of adenocarcinomas, are less responsive to, or not inhibited by, cytotoxic drugs. Several normal rapidly proliferating tissues, particularly the bone marrow, the epidermal appendages (hair follicles and nails), and the epithelium of the alimentary tract, are extremely sensitive to cytotoxic drugs, and often constitute the limiting factor to the amount of chemotherapy that can be administered.

The intermitotic time of proliferating cells, i.e., the average time from one mitosis to the next, can be determined by using ^{3}H-thymidine. This interval can be divided into three phases: (1) the presynthetic phase (G_1), (2) the phase of DNA synthesis (S) and (3) the postsynthetic phase (G_2). At this point in the cycle, mitosis (M) transforms one G_2-cell into two G_1-cells, and the cycle may begin again. Implicit in the discussion of growth fraction is the concept that some cells in a tumor, or a normal organ, may be resting and nonproliferating. Some may be permanently incapable of reproduction, and others may be recruited into the proliferating compartment upon receiving an appropriate, but as yet unidentified, stimulus. These recruitable cells are considered to be in a fourth phase, designated as G_0.

Cells that are in cycle are the most vulnerable to cytotoxic drugs, particularly those that are S-phase specific, such as arabinosylcytosine (ara-C) and hydroxyurea. Other drugs, including methotrexate (MTX), 5-fluorouracil (FU), and 6-mercaptopurine (6-MP), exert their major effects during S-phase but, because of their inhibitory effects on RNA and protein synthesis, are self-limiting because they also produce delay of entry into S-phase. The vinca alkaloids are considered cell-cycle specific agents because they interfere with the process of mitosis.

Cells that are not in cycle (G_0) are almost completely insensitive to S-phase specific drugs but may still be affected by cycle-phase nonspecific agents. Alkylating agents, such as cyclophosphamide and 1,3-bis(2-chloroethyl)-1-nitrosourea (BCNU), are called cycle-phase nonspecific, because they react with DNA during any phase of the cell cycle, leading directly to the cell death or to a delayed lethal effect at mitosis. Actinomycin D and the anthracycline antibiotics, daunorubicin and adriamycin, bind to DNA and interfere with transcription, and are also cycle-phase nonspecific.

Normal tissues with large growth fractions, such as the bone marrow, may have fewer resting cells in G_0 than a slow-growing tumor with a small growth fraction. In this situation, chemotherapy with inhibitors of DNA biosynthesis (S-phase specific drugs) probably would be ineffective, because life-threatening marrow suppression would occur before significant antineoplastic effects. By contrast, the tumors that have responded best to our present generation of cytotoxic agents probably have a larger growth fraction of clonogenic cells than the marrow stem cells of the host. In these patients, judicious administration and scheduling of selected cytotoxic agents can progressively destroy the neoplastic cells while sparing significant numbers of marrow stem cells in G_0, which subsequently could reconstitute the host hematologically.

773. CLASSIFICATION OF DRUGS

ALKYLATING AGENTS

Alkylating agents were studied extensively during World War II in programs concerned with chemical warfare research. They became generally available in 1946, when secrecy restrictions were removed. Hundreds of biologically active compounds have been synthesized, using modifications of the basic chemical structure. A number of substances occurring naturally, including certain antimicrobial drugs with antineoplas-

tic activity, such as mitomycin C, porfiromycin, and streptozotocin, probably function as alkylating agents.

Five major types of alkylating agents have established clinical usefulness: (1) the nitrogen mustards, (2) the ethylenimines, (3) the alkyl sulfonates, (4) the nitrosoureas, and (5) the triazenes. The mechanism of cytotoxic action is thought to be similar for most of the agents in this class.

Mechanism of Cytotoxic Action

Most alkylating agents, except busulfan, generate highly reactive electrophilic carbonium ions that alkylate, by forming convalent linkages, with various nucleophilic substances. Although many biologically important groups may be targets for the reaction, it is thought that one of the most significant sites is the strongly nucleophilic 7 nitrogen of the purine base, guanine. This could lead to miscoding errors or depurination and, in the case of bifunctional alkylating agents, to cross-linking of adjacent macromolecules, which would interfere with normal mitosis by preventing separation of the strands of DNA. Polyfunctional alkylating agents are more cytotoxic than monofunctional alkylators, although the latter may cause mutagenic and carcinogenic damage that is not lethal to the cell and can therefore be reproduced indefinitely as an inherited mutation. Cells are most susceptible to cytotoxic action of nitrogen mustards or alkyl sulfonates when they are in G_1 or in mitosis (M). Progression from G_1 and S phases to mitosis is impaired after exposure to nitrosoureas, nitrogen mustards, and ethylenimine derivatives. Inhibition of mitosis with double complement of DNA and continuing synthesis of RNA and protein can lead to unbalanced growth, giant cells, and lethal cytotoxicity. Nonproliferating cells in G_0 can also be destroyed by alkylating agents. Cell death may occur during interphase, when many sites, including RNA and protein, are damaged, or may be delayed until mitosis when only cross-linking of DNA has occurred. Lymphocytes appear to be most sensitive to rapid cellular disintegration and lysis by highly reactive nitrogen mustards, whereas busulfan is more toxic to granulocytes. Suppression of the immune response may be pronounced, and depression of erythropoiesis and of platelet production also occur. The intestinal mucosa, the hair follicles, and the reproductive system can be damaged to varying degrees by different drugs in this class.

Nitrogen Mustards. *Mechlorethamine (Mustargen, HN_2).* The first of the nitrogen mustards to be used clinically, this compound is often abbreviated as HN_2, its chemical warfare code name. Mechlorethamine is a highly reactive agent and a powerful vesicant. For this reason, it is usually administered intravenously (0.4 mg per kilogram)* into the tubing of a rapidly flowing intravenous infusion. Since thrombosis and thrombophlebitis may occur when relatively high concentrations of the drug are in prolonged and direct contact with the intima of the injected vein, its administration into areas of elevated venous pressure, such as superior vena caval obstruction resulting from mediastinal tumors, must be avoided. The use of surgical gloves is advised to protect

Cytotoxic and Immunosuppressive Agents

I. Alkylating agents:	II. Antimetabolites:	III. Natural products:
Nitrogen mustards	Folic acid analogue	Vinca alkaloids
Mechlorethamine	Methotrexate	Vinblastine
Cyclophosphamide		Vincristine
Melphalan	Pyrimidine analogues	
Uracil mustard	Fluorouracil	Enzyme
Chlorambucil	Fluorodeoxyuridine	Asparaginase
	Fluorocytosine	
Ethylenimine	Trifluorothymidine	Antibiotics
derivatives	Cytaribine	Dactinomycin
TEM	Azaribine	Daunorubicin
Thiotepa	Idoxuridine	Adriamycin
		Mithramycin
		Bleomycin
Alkyl sulfonate	Purine analogues	IV. Miscellaneous
Busulfan	Mercaptopurine	agents:
	Azathioprine	Hydroxyurea
Nitrosoureas	Thioguanine	Procarbazine
BCNU	Adenine	Mitotane
Streptozotocin	arabinoside	Dacarbazine

---

*For conversion of milligrams per kilogram of body weight to milligrams per square meter of body surface, a ratio of 1:30 may be used. The conversion factor varies between 1:20 and 1:40, depending on age and body build.

the hands of the physician preparing and administering the solution. The drug must be dissolved and administered in a few minutes, because it decomposes on standing. Within a few minutes after administration, the drug is no longer detectable in active form and is bound to proteins or intracellular macromolecules. Less than 0.01 per cent is excreted in the urine. HN_2 has been administered intra-arterially, using techniques involving isolation and perfusion of a tumor-bearing area. The intracavitary use of mechlorethamine (0.2 to 0.4 mg per kilogram) after drainage of malignant pleural effusions can be an effective palliative measure. Intraperitoneal administration is often accompanied by severe gastrointestinal toxicity and is not recommended. Very dilute solutions (0.25 per cent) can be painted on the skin of patients with generalized mycosis fungoides with good results.

The major indications for HN_2 are in the treatment of generalized (Stage III and IV) Hodgkin's disease and other lymphomas, alone or in combination with other agents. The usual dose is 0.4 mg per kilogram administered as a single intravenous dose, because divided consecutive daily doses merely prolong the duration of nausea and vomiting, a direct central nervous system side effect which regularly follows administration of the drug. Premedication with a short-acting barbiturate and an antiemetic is recommended. When extensive neoplastic infiltration of the marrow is suspected, as in malignant lymphoma, lymphocytic type, a reduced dose of 0.2 or 0.3 mg per kilogram is recommended. Beneficial palliative results have also been observed in carcinomas of the lung, breast, and ovary and, occasionally, in less common tumors.

The most serious toxic effect of nitrogen mustard is bone marrow depression, with resulting leukopenia and thrombocytopenia. After four weeks, recovery is usually adequate to permit administration of another course. Dermatologic complications include an idiosyncratic nonrecurring maculopapular skin eruption, overt clinical manifestations of herpes zoster, and local reactions caused by extravasation and vesicant action. The last-named complication may produce a painful, tender, brawny induration, which, in severe cases, may slough. If accidental extravasation occurs, the area should be promptly infiltrated with a sterile isotonic solution of sodium thiosulfate (1/6 molar), or normal saline if this is not immediately available, and an ice compress should be applied intermittently for six to twelve hours.

Cyclophosphamide (Cytoxan, Endoxan). Originally devised as a carrier or transport form of nitrogen mustard, cyclophosphamide is activated by enzymatic cleavage of the phosphorus-nitrogen linkage within the molecule. Although levels of phosphatases and phosphamidases capable of accomplishing this cleavage may be relatively high in some tumors, no evidence for this type of selective activity has been observed and the drug is mainly activated in the liver. Since this occurs through the drug-metabolizing microsomal oxidase system, it is subject to the influence of other compounds that affect these systems. Barbiturates stimulate these enzymes and would increase the activation and toxicity of cyclophosphamide, whereas corticosteroid and sex hormones appear to inhibit the effect. Since cyclophosphamide is frequently used in patients also receiving corticosteroid therapy, special caution is necessary, because a reduction in steroid dosage may increase the toxicity of a previously well-tolerated dose of the alkylating agent. After oral administration, maximal plasma levels are achieved in approximately one hour. Disappearance from the plasma is rapid, with a half-life of about four hours; urinary recovery of unchanged drug is less than 14 per cent.

The major advantage of cyclophosphamide is its versatility which permits a wide, intermediate range of activity, extending from that of the highly reactive intravenous mechlorethamine to that of the slow-acting oral chlorambucil. It can be administered intravenously at usual initial loading doses of 40 to 50 mg per kilogram, given at the rate of 10 to 20 mg per kilogram over two to five days. In patients with compromised bone marrow function, a reduction of one third to one half is recommended. Oral doses usually range between 1 and 5 mg per kilogram daily. The drug can also be administered intramuscularly or into body cavities, and is not associated with vesicant action. A good objective guide for prolonged regulation of maintenance therapy is the total leukocyte count, which should be kept between 2500 and 4000 cells per cubic millimeter.

The major clinical indications for cyclophosphamide are in the lymphoproliferative and myeloproliferative disorders. It is highly effective and has produced cures in Burkitt's lymphoma and is very beneficial in acute lymphoblastic leukemia of childhood, Hodgkin's disease, and other lymphomas. It is active in multiple myeloma, chronic lymphocytic leukemia, ovarian carcinoma, neuroblastoma, and retinoblastoma. Temporary beneficial results have also been observed in carcinoma of the breast, bronchogenic carcinoma, and other neoplasms. Because of its potent immunosuppressive action, it has been used clinically in Wegener's granulomatosis, rheumatoid arthritis, nephrotic syndrome in children, and other conditions associated with altered immune reactivity.

The most important toxic effects are on the bone marrow, but severe thrombocytopenia is probably less common than with other nitrogen mustards. By contrast, alopecia is more frequent and often more severe, though usually reversible. Nausea and vomiting are common, and mucosal ulcerations, hepatic toxicity, increased skin pigmentation, and interstitial pulmonary fibrosis have been reported. Sterile hemorrhagic cystitis, probably caused by accumulation of active metabolites in concentrated urine, has been reported in about 5 per cent of cases. Ample fluid intake and frequent voiding are helpful measures in the prevention of this complication. Because gonadal suppression resulting in sterility has been observed and the mutagenic and carcinogenic potential is high, the use of the drug in patients with reproductive capacity should be carefully considered with respect to possible benefits and risks.

Melphalan (Alkeran). This compound is a phenylalanine derivative of nitrogen mustard. It has the general pharmacologic properties of an alkylating agent of intermediate strength, demonstrating activity in the blood for about six hours. The drug can be administered orally, usually in daily divided doses of 6 mg for two to three weeks; then, after interrupting therapy for four weeks, a daily maintenance dose of 2 to 4 mg is instituted. It is particularly useful in multiple myeloma, alone or in combination with other agents. As with other alkylating agents, the clinical toxicity is mainly hematologic. Nausea and vomiting are infrequent, and alopecia does not occur.

Uracil Mustard. Although synthesized in an attempt to obtain more specificity for the alkylating moiety in pyrimidine biosynthesis, this agent behaves like other nitrogen mustards of intermediate activity. Plasma disappearance is rapid, with no detectable drug after two hours, and less than 1 per cent is recovered intact in the urine. The usual oral daily dose is 1 to 2 mg for three weeks or 3 to 5 mg for one week, with maintenance doses of 1 mg daily. The spectrum of clinical activity is similar to that of other nitrogen mustards. Bone marrow depression is the major toxic manifestation; nausea, vomiting, diarrhea, and dermatitis have been reported, but frank alopecia has not been observed.

Chlorambucil (Leukeran). An aromatic derivative of mechlorethamine, chlorambucil is the slowest-acting and least toxic nitrogen mustard in clinical use. Absorption after oral administration is good, but information on biologic persistence and elimination is inadequate. The usual oral dose is 0.1 to 0.2 mg per kilogram daily for at least three to six weeks. The total daily dose, usually 4 to 10 mg, is given at one time. The dosage is adjusted according to the clinical response, and when maintenance therapy is required, 2 mg daily is recommended. Chlorambucil is the treatment of choice in chronic lymphocytic leukemia. It is effective in Hodgkin's disease, malignant lymphoma, lymphocytic type, polycythemia vera, multiple myeloma, and, particularly, primary macroglobulinemia. It is useful in carcinoma of the ovary, breast, and testes, usually in combination with other agents. Good responses have been reported in the treatment of vasculitis as a complication of rheumatoid arthritis, and in autoimmune hemolytic anemias associated with cold agglutinins. Toxicity to the bone marrow is usually moderate, gradual, and readily reversible. Gastrointestinal and dermatologic toxicity are seldom encountered.

Ethylenimines. Triethylenemelamine (TEM) and triethylenethiophosphoramide (thiotepa) have been largely replaced by the nitrogen mustards, and have similar clinical indications and toxic manifestations.

Alkyl Sulfonate. ***Busulfan (Myleran).*** The cytotoxic action of this drug is quite selective, affecting primarily granulocyte production, and, to some extent, platelets. More than 90 per cent disappears from the blood within three minutes and is almost entirely excreted in the urine as methanesulfonic acid and other metabolites. The initial oral dose is 4 to 12 mg daily, and maintenance doses of 1 to 3 mg daily are recommended. It is the treatment of choice in chronic granulocytic leukemia and may be useful in polycythemia vera and myelofibrosis with myeloid metaplasia. It is of no value in acute leukemia or in the "blastic crisis" of chronic granulocytic leukemia. Gastrointestinal toxicity is rare. Occasionally, unusual complications have been reported, including generalized hyperpigmentation of the skin, gynecomastia, cheilosis, glossitis, anhidrosis, and pulmonary fibrosis, but their relation to the drug is poorly understood.

Nitrosoureas. ***BCNU.*** This abbreviation is used for 1,3-bis(2-chloroethyl)-1-nitrosourea; a related cyclohexyl compound is called CCNU. Disappearance of BCNU from the plasma occurs within five minutes. The

usual intravenous dose is 1 to 2 mg per kilogram monthly. Bone marrow depression is the principal toxicity, with delayed onset and the nadir occurring after four or five weeks. Although useful in Hodgkin's disease and occasionally in malignant melanomas, the unique property of the nitrosoureas is that they cross the blood-brain barrier, probably because they are lipid soluble, and have demonstrated some promise in the treatment of primary and metastatic brain tumors.

Streptozotocin. This naturally occurring glucosamine nitrosourea is diabetogenic in animals and has been effective in patients with islet cell carcinoma of the pancreas and malignant carcinoid tumors. The usual dose is 1 gram per square meter intravenously for four weeks. Bone marrow toxicity is not significant, but nephrotoxicity may be severe.

ANTIMETABOLITES

Antimetabolites of nucleic acid biosynthesis are structural analogues of normally occurring substances, metabolites. They interfere with normal biosynthesis by competing with purines, pyrimidines, and their precursors for important enzymatic reactions. They may also be incorporated into nucleic acids in place of the corresponding normal nucleotides. Although the site of action for most of them has been defined, the mechanisms of cell death are incompletely understood. Cytotoxicity may be related to unbalanced growth of cells capable of synthesizing RNA and protein, but not DNA, or to coding, transcription, or translation errors after incorporation of the analogue into DNA or RNA.

The agents with recognized clinical value may be classified as follows: (1) folic acid analogues, (2) pyrimidine analogues, and (3) purine analogues.

Folic Acid Analogues. ***Methotrexate (Amethopterin).*** The folic acid analogues, aminopterin and subsequently methotrexate, were the first class of antimetabolites to demonstrate effective antineoplastic activity. Other "small-molecule" folate antagonists, pyrimethamine and cycloguanil, have been effective against malaria, and more recently trimethoprim has been useful in bacterial infections of the urinary and respiratory tracts. The primary site of action of methotrexate is the enzyme dihydrofolate reductase which catalyzes the reduction of folate and dihydrofolate to tetrahydrofolate. The kinetics of this inhibition are often referred to as "pseudo-irreversible," because the binding of the inhibitor to the enzyme is tight. This interferes with the transfer of single carbon fragments and blocks the conversion of deoxyuridylate to thymidylate, blocking DNA synthesis. Although RNA and protein synthesis are also inhibited by lack of tetrahydrofolate coenzymes, the thymidylate block is considered to be the most important site of cytotoxic action leading to "thymineless death."

Methotrexate is readily absorbed after oral administration. The mean plasma half-life is approximately two hours, and about 50 per cent of the drug is bound to plasma proteins. Transport across the blood-brain barrier is very poor, and intrathecal administration (0.2. to 0.4 mg per kilogram) is necessary to obtain high concentrations in the cerebrospinal fluid. The major route of elimination is through the kidney, with 50 to 90 per cent of the drug excreted unchanged in the urine, usually within eight hours. Impaired renal function can produce marked increase in toxicity.

The usual daily oral dose is 2.5 to 10.0 mg. Intravenous doses of 25 to 50 mg can be given once or twice weekly. Constant daily infusions of much higher doses have been administered but only when using the technique of leucovorin "rescue."

Methotrexate has produced cures in women with choriocarcinoma and related trophoblastic tumors in approximately 75 per cent of the cases. It is capable of inducing complete remissions in acute lymphoblastic leukemia of childhood, but is of more value for maintenance therapy. It can be useful in Burkitt's lymphoma, mycosis fungoides, and carcinomas of the breast, testes, and oropharynx. It is also effective in severe, recalcitrant psoriasis and as an immunosuppressive agent. In addition to bone marrow depression, it causes ulcerative stomatitis and gastrointestinal toxicity. These adverse reactions can reach serious proportions and even cause death, particularly in the presence of pre-existing folate deficiency or renal insufficiency. Other complications include dermatitis, alopecia, and hepatic dysfunction, sometimes leading to cirrhosis.

Pyrimidine Analogues. *Fluorouracil (FU) and Fluorodeoxyuridine (FUdR).* Both the fluorinated pyrimidine base (5-FU) and its corresponding nucleoside (FUdR) are converted in vivo to 5-fluoro-2'-deoxyuridine-5'-phosphate (F-dUMP). This fraudulent nucleotide has great affinity for thymidylate synthetase, the enzyme involved in transfer of a methyl group from N^5,N^{10}-methylenetetrahydrofolic acid to deoxyuridylic acid (dUMP) in the synthesis of thymidylate. This site of action is responsible for the major cytotoxic effects by blocking DNA synthesis. Inhibition of RNA synthesis and incorporation into RNA also occur and may explain why these compounds are cycle-specific but not phase-specific agents.

These drugs are usually administered intravenously; three hours after injection, no FU can be detected in the plasma. Metabolic degradation occurs primarily in the liver, and special caution must be observed in patients with impaired liver function or extensive hepatic metastases. Approximately 15 per cent of an injected dose of FU appears intact in the urine, most of it within one hour.

The recommended dosage schedule of FU is 12 mg per kilogram intravenously daily for four days and, after toxicity has subsided, 12 mg per kilogram weekly (not to exceed 1 gram) as a single intravenous weekly maintenance dose. FUdR can be administered either at twice the daily dose of FU intravenously or by continuous intra-arterial infusion at doses of 0.1 to 0.4 mg per kilogram daily.

FU and FUdR have been most useful in the palliative treatment of carcinomas of the breast, colon, and rectum. Occasional responses have been noted in carcinomas of the stomach, pancreas, ovary, urinary bladder, and oropharynx. Topical FU (Efudex) as a 2 or 5 per cent solution of propylene glycol or in a hydrophilic cream base has been successful in eradicating premalignant actinic keratoses, as well as superficial basal cell carcinomas.

The major toxic manifestations are bone marrow depression and ulceration of the epithelium of the alimentary tract, with stomatitis, esophagopharyngitis, nausea, vomiting, and diarrhea. The nadir of the leukopenia is between 9 and 14 days. Dermatitis, hyperpigmentation of the skin, hair loss, and nail changes have been observed.

Other Fluorinated Pyrimidines. 5-Fluorocytosine (FC) is converted to the deoxyribonucleoside (FCdR), an active antimetabolite, by fungi such as *Candida albicans.* It is administered in oral doses of 50 to 150 mg per kilogram daily for one to three months, and is useful in fungal and cryptococcal infections.

Trifluorothymidine (F_3TdR) is beneficial as an antiviral agent when applied topically to the eyes of patients with herpes simplex keratitis. It is active also against vaccinia, another DNA virus.

Cytarabine (Cytosine Arabinoside, Ara-C, Cytosar). This analogue of 2'-deoxycytidine has a structural alteration in the sugar moiety instead of the base. Although the most important site of action has not been completely established, inhibition of DNA polymerase appears to be a primary locus, a concept supported by its cytotoxic effects as an S-phase specific inhibitor. The drug is also incorporated into DNA and RNA, and blocks ribonucleotide reductase. The drug is rapidly deaminated in the blood to an inactive metabolite, uracil arabinoside, which accounts for about 90 per cent of the material in the urine. Ara-C disappears from the blood in approximately 20 minutes, but after intrathecal injection may persist for several hours because of low levels of deaminase in the CSF. The drug is administered intravenously daily for 10 to 20 days, either by rapid injection, 2 to 4 mg per kilogram, or by continuous infusion, 0.1 to 1.0 mg per kilogram. Ara-C is a potent immunosuppressive agent and, depending on the dosage schedules used, can suppress either humoral or cellular responses, or both. It is effective against DNA viruses and has been used topically with beneficial results in patients with herpes simplex keratitis. In contrast to IUdR, systemic ara-C may have greater immunosuppressive than antiviral action, with detrimental effects in disseminated herpes zoster. Although it has not proved successful against solid tumors, it is the most active drug available in acute myelogenous leukemia, and is particularly effective in combination with thioguanine. Myelosuppressive toxicity can be severe, with leukopenia, thrombocytopenia, and anemia characterized by striking megaloblastic changes. Gastrointestinal disturbances, stomatitis, thrombophlebitis, hepatic dysfunction, dermatitis, and fever have been reported.

Azaribine (Triacetyl-6-Azauridine, Triazur). This triacetyl derivative of 6-azauridine blocks orotidylate decarboxylase and, thereby, the de novo synthesis of uridylate. Azaribine is well absorbed after oral administration, and provides good levels of 6-azauridine in the blood for approximately six to eight hours, almost 100 per cent of which is recovered intact in the urine. Occasionally, further metabolism to 6-azauracil, probably by gastrointestinal microorganisms, may produce reversible neurologic disturbances. The recommended oral dose is 125 mg per kilogram daily. It is extremely effective in the treatment of psoriasis and psoriatic arthritis. Recent evidence indicates that increased occurrence of thromboembolic disease in psoriasis is reduced by azaribine therapy. Relative absence of toxic manifestations makes it a safe and desirable agent, although at higher doses (270 mg per kilogram daily), it can produce reversible suppression of erythropoiesis. In this dosage it has been beneficial in patients with polycythemia vera and mycosis fungoides.

Idoxuridine (5-Iododeoxyuridine, IUdR, IDU, Stoxil, Herplex, Dendrid). Because the iodine atom in the 5-position of the pyrimidine ring is larger than hydrogen or fluorine and of similar size to the methyl group of thymine, IUdR behaves as an analogue of thymidylate, competitively inhibiting its utilization, and even replacing it in DNA. After parenteral administration, it disappears from the blood within two hours and is metabolized to, and excreted in, the urine as 5-iodouracil, uracil, and iodide. Topical therapy of herpes simplex keratitis is highly effective. Intravenous eight-hour infusions of 60 to 100 mg per kilogram daily for five days are used for systemic DNA virus infections. Beneficial results have been observed in patients with disseminated herpes zoster, vaccinia gangrenosum, and herpes simplex encephalitis. Immunosuppression has not been detected. Major toxic manifestations include bone marrow depression, stomatitis, and alopecia. Gastrointestinal toxicity is less frequent than with FU or FUdR. Transverse ridging of the nails and sensitivity to iodine are sometimes encountered.

Purine Analogues. *Mercaptopurine (6-MP, Purinethol).* This antimetabolite, after formation of the 5'-phosphate ribonucleotide, blocks by "pseudo-feedback inhibition" the formation of ribosylamine-5-phosphate catalyzed by PRPP-amidotransferase, the first committed step in the de novo pathway of purine biosynthesis. It can also block the synthesis of adenylate and guanylate from the "bridgehead" nucleotide, inosinate. The drug is well absorbed after oral ingestion, and about 50 per cent of the dose is recovered in the urine in 24 hours, largely metabolized to 6-thiouric acid and inorganic sulfate. Attempts to inhibit this degradation led to the development of allopurinol (Zyloprim), a xanthine oxidase inhibitor capable of blocking the catabolism of 6-MP, as well as the formation of uric acid from hypoxanthine and xanthine. Allopurinol has become an important agent in the management of hyperuricemia and gout. The usual oral daily dose of 6-MP is 2.5 per kilogram, but *this must be reduced to 25 per cent when allopurinol is being administered concomitantly* at doses of 200 to 600 mg daily to reduce or prevent hyperuricemia. The major clinical indication for 6-MP is acute lymphoblastic leukemia in children. It may be useful in adults with acute leukemia or in chronic granulocytic leukemia. It is not effective in chronic lymphocytic leukemia, Hodgkin's disease, malignant lymphoma, lymphocytic type, or solid tumors. Although active as an immunosuppressive agent, 6-MP has been superseded by its imidazolyl derivative, azathioprine (Imuran). The primary toxic effect is bone marrow depression. Stomatitis and gastrointestinal symptoms are uncommon. Cholestatic jaundice has been reported in as many as one third of adult patients; this is usually reversible upon discontinuation of therapy.

Azathioprine (Imuran). This imidazolyl derivative of 6-MP is probably the most widely used immunosuppressive agent in organ transplantation and disorders with altered immune reactivity. It is cleaved slowly to 6-MP and has similar actions, catabolism, and toxicity. The usual oral dose is 3 to 5 mg per kilogram daily, but this must also be reduced to 25 per cent if allopurinol is administered simultaneously.

Thioguanine (TG, Tabloid). In addition to being a potent "pseudofeedback inhibitor" and blocking interconversion of purines in a manner analogous to 6-MP, it is more significantly incorporated into DNA and RNA. After oral administration, peak blood levels are reached in six to eight hours, and approximately 40 per cent of the dose is excreted in the urine in 24 hours, mainly as inorganic sulfate and 2-amino-6-methylthiopurine, instead of 6-thiouric acid. Because of this, unlike 6-MP and azathioprine, no reduction in dose of TG is necessary when used together with allopurinol. The usual daily oral dose is 2 mg per kilogram. Clinically, it has a spectrum of antileukemic and immunosuppressive activity similar to that of 6-MP, and similar toxicity. It is particularly useful, together with ara-C, in acute myelogenous leukemia.

Adenine Arabinoside (Ara-A). This investigational compound appears to inhibit DNA polymerase and perhaps ribonucleotide reductase, with little effect on RNA or protein. It has demonstrated activity against several DNA viruses.

NATURAL PRODUCTS

An increasing number of naturally occurring substances have attracted attention because of their cytotoxic action. Some are derived from plants that were known for their toxic manifestations many centuries ago, such as the colchicine derivatives of the autumn crocus (*Colchicum autumnale*), and some are of more recent vintage, including the vinca alkaloids from the periwinkle (*Vinca rosea*). The enzyme asparaginase represents an interesting and unique approach to antineoplastic therapy. Finally, countless antimicrobial drugs have been isolated and tested for antitumor activity. Of these, only a few with special clinical pertinence will be discussed.

Vinca Alkaloids. The mechanism of action of these compounds is not clearly defined. Inhibition of the cell cycle occurs at metaphase as a result of spindle protein damage. Despite their structural similarity, remarkable differences in cytotoxic action and lack of cross-resistance have been noted among these agents. Oral absorption is unpredictable. Extravasation during intravenous injection may cause considerable irritation and should be treated with local injection of hyaluronidase and heat. The compounds are cleared in less than one hour from the blood and are excreted primarily through the biliary system. Increased toxicity may be encountered in obstructive jaundice. The drugs penetrate the blood-brain barrier poorly.

Vinblastine (Velban, VLB). This drug is administered at weekly intervals, intravenously. The initial recommended dose is 0.1 mg per kilogram, increased by weekly increments of 0.05 mg per kilogram until either moderate leukopenia or the desired beneficial effects are attained, up to a maximum of 0.5 mg per kilogram. Vinblastine is effective in the treatment of lymphomas, particularly Hodgkin's disease. Objective responses have been observed in neuroblastomas, Letterer-Siwe disease, choriocarcinoma, and carcinomas of the breast and testes. The major toxicity is bone marrow depression, usually leukopenia. Gastrointestinal manifestations may be encountered. Neurologic toxicity and alopecia occur less frequently than with vincristine.

Vincristine (Oncovin, VCR). This agent is administered intravenously, at weekly intervals. The initial recommended dose is 0.05 mg per kilogram, increased by weekly increments of 0.025 mg per kilogram to a maximum of 0.15 mg per kilogram, or until the desired response or toxicity is encountered. Vincristine is particularly effective in the induction of remission in children with acute lymphoblastic leukemia. Vincristine (2 mg per square meter) used together with prednisone (40 to 150 mg per square meter) daily can induce complete remissions in 90 per cent of cases, and with a third drug, such as daunorubicin (25 mg per square meter), this rate approaches 100 per cent. It is also very effective in Hodgkin's disease, malignant lymphoma, lymphocytic type, Wilms' tumor, and rhabdomyosarcoma. Responses have been described in choriocarcinoma and carcinomas of the breast, prostate, cervix, and kidney. In contrast to vinblastine, it does not produce bone marrow depression, which makes it particularly useful in combination with other myelosuppressive agents. The combination of nitrogen mustard, Oncovin, procarbazine, and prednisone, the so-called MOPP regimen, is considered the treatment of choice in advanced Hodgkin's disease. The dose-limiting toxicity is neurologic, with paresthesias, loss of deep-tendon reflexes, paresis manifested by footdrop, hoarseness, ptosis, and double vision. Neurogenic constipation may be severe and should be anticipated with an appropriate prophylactic regimen. Alopecia occurs in about 20 per cent of patients. The syndrome of inappropriate antidiuretic hormone (ADH) secretion has been observed in patients treated with vincristine.

Asparaginase. This enzyme, naturally present in guinea pig serum and currently prepared from *E. coli* as an investigational agent, catalyzes the hydrolysis of plasma asparagine to aspartic acid and ammonia. Because, in contrast to normal cells, certain neoplastic cells lack asparagine synthetase and are dependent on exogenous asparagine, a selective nutritional deficiency is produced. The resulting antineoplastic effect has stimulated considerable hope that exploitable biochemical differences may exist between normal and neoplastic cells. Unfortunately, this expectation has been somewhat tempered by the briefness of the remissions, by rapid development of resistance, and by allergic reactions after repeated administrations of foreign protein. Recommended intravenous doses range from 200 IU per kilogram daily for 28 days to 1000 IU per kilogram for periods not exceeding ten days. Asparaginase can produce complete remissions in up to 60 per cent of children with acute lymphoblastic leukemia; it is sometimes beneficial in other leukemias and lymphomas, and occasionally in malignant melanoma. Despite its notable immunosuppressive properties, hypersensitivity reactions occur in 5 to 20 per cent of patients, ranging from urticaria to anaphylactic shock. Inhibition of protein synthesis often results in mild impairment of hepatic, renal, pancreatic, central nervous, or clotting functions. Although usually expressed only as reversible aberrations of laboratory values, toxicity may occasionally be more severe.

Antibiotics. Antitumor antibiotics may (1) inhibit DNA synthesis, (2) impair RNA synthesis, or (3) block protein synthesis. Most of those with established clinical usefulness appear to belong to the second category and, after binding with DNA, inhibit DNA-dependent RNA biosynthesis. Bleomycin, however, inhibits DNA synthesis and reacts with DNA, causing strand scission. Most of these agents are rapidly cleared from the blood and are excreted mainly in the bile. They do not penetrate the blood-brain barrier significantly.

Dactinomycin (Actinomycin D, Cosmegen). This agent is administered intravenously in doses of 0.015 mg per kilogram daily for five days, to be repeated after two to four weeks if no toxicity persists. Dactinomycin is highly effective in gestational trophoblastic tumors and, in combination with radiotherapy and surgery, in Wilms' tumor. It is active in testicular tumors and rhabdomyosarcomas. It has an immunosuppressive effect and has been used in renal transplantation. Toxicity includes primarily bone marrow depression, stomatitis, and gastrointestinal reactions. Dermatologic manifestations include alopecia, as well as erythema, desquamation, and hyperpigmentation in areas subjected to radiotherapy. Extravasation can produce severe local injury.

Daunorubicin (Daunomycin, Rubidomycin, Daunoblastin). This anthracycline antibiotic is administered intravenously at doses of 0.8 to 1.0 mg per kilogram daily for three to six days. It is particularly effective in induction of remissions in children with acute lymphoblastic leukemia, usually in combination with vincristine and prednisone, and has some activity in lymphomas. The drug frequently causes bone marrow depression, stomatitis, alopecia, and gastrointestinal disturbances. A peculiar cardiac toxicity has been observed with arrhythmias and congestive failure, not relieved by digitalis. Vesicant action can occur if extravasated.

Adriamycin (Doxorubicin, Adriablastina). This 14-hydroxy-derivative of daunorubicin is also effective in acute leukemias but differs markedly in its strong activity in solid tumors. The currently recommended dose is 60 to 75 mg per square meter administered intravenously every three weeks. Vesicant action can occur if extravasated. Adriamycin is effective in the treatment of osteogenic, Ewing's, and soft tissue sarcomas. It is particularly beneficial in carcinomas of the thyroid and breast, and is active against neuroblastoma, lymphomas, and carcinomas of the bronchus and genitourinary systems in males and females. Myelotoxicity is a major complication, and alopecia, stomatitis, and gastrointestinal manifestations are common. Cardiomyopathy frequently occurs at total doses above 550 mg per square meter, and this level should generally not be exceeded. The structural similarities of the anthracycline antibiotics to the cardiac glycosides and their avid binding to cardiac DNA have been invoked as possible explanations for the arrhythmias and rapidly progressive congestive heart failure, unresponsive to digitalis. Since the drug is metabolized and excreted primarily by the liver, reduced dosages must be administered in the presence of impaired hepatic function.

Mithramycin (Mithracin). The usual daily dose is 0.025 mg per kilogram, administered during four to six hours intravenously for eight to ten days, as indicated for the treatment of patients with testicular tumors. The drug has an interesting and unique capacity for lowering the serum calcium level, possibly by interfering with calcium resorption from bone. Prompt reversal of dangerous hypercalcemia and hypercalciuria associated with metastatic disease has been observed with daily intravenous doses of 0.025 mg per kilogram for three to four days. The major toxic manifestation is a dangerous hemorrhagic diathesis, usually beginning with epistaxis. This is probably due to a combination of thrombocytopenia, abnormalities in multiple clotting factors, and capillary damage. Other myelosuppressive effects, gastrointestinal disturbances, and hepatic and renal abnormalities also occur.

Bleomycin (Blenoxane). The recommended dose is 10 to 20 mg per square meter, administered intravenously or intramuscularly once or twice weekly to a total dose of 400 mg. Preferential localization of drug occurs in the skin and the lung; other tissues inactivate the compound by removing 1 mole of ammonia. This probably accounts for the selectivity of therapeutic and toxic effects. It is of palliative value in patients with squamous cell carcinoma of the head, neck, and skin, lymphomas, and testicular tumors. Bleomycin alone does not produce bone marrow depression. The most serious toxicity is pulmonary. This begins with a picture indistinguishable from pneumonitis and may, in 2 to 15 per cent of cases, progress to pulmonary fibrosis, which has been fatal in about 1 per cent of patients. Stomatitis, alopecia, and marked dermatologic manifestations frequently occur, including hyperkeratosis, ulceration, and hyperpigmentation. Because anaphylactic reactions have been observed in patients with lymphomas, administration of a 1 mg test dose, followed by a 24-hour observation period, is recommended.

MISCELLANEOUS AGENTS

There are several substances, active as antineoplastic or immunosuppressive agents, that cannot be conveniently categorized under the aforementioned classification of cytotoxic drugs. Some of these are discussed elsewhere, including the steroid hormones—androgens, estrogens, progestins, and adrenocorticosteroids—and radioactive isotopes. Four other clinically useful compounds are listed below.

Hydroxyurea (Hydrea). This structurally simple compound inhibits DNA synthesis, probably by interfering with the enzymatic reduction of ribonucleotides to deoxyribonucleotides. It is an S-phase specific agent and does not block RNA or protein synthesis. It is well absorbed orally, peak plasma concentrations are reached in two hours, and it is undetectable in the blood within 24 hours. About 80 per cent is recovered in the urine; the rest is probably metabolized in the liver. The usual oral dose is 20 to 30 mg per kilogram daily, or 80 mg per kilogram every third day. Hydroxyurea is useful in patients with chronic granulocytic leukemia, who are refractory to busulfan and mercaptopurine. It has produced temporary remissions in malignant melanoma and is beneficial in psoriasis. Toxicity includes bone marrow depression, stomatitis, gastrointestinal disturbances, and, more rarely, alopecia, dermatitis, and neurologic manifestations.

Procarbazine (Matulane). The mechanism of action of this methyl hydrazine derivative is unknown, but it is capable of inhibiting DNA, RNA, and protein synthesis. It is rapidly absorbed from the gastrointestinal tract and readily equilibrates between the plasma and cerebrospinal fluid. Because of rapid metabolism, its half-life in the blood is approximately seven minutes, and in 24 hours 25 to 40 per cent is excreted as a metabolite in the urine. The recommended oral daily dose is 50 to 300 mg. It is effective in Hodgkin's disease, particularly in combination with nitrogen mustard, Oncovin, and

prednisone (the so-called MOPP regimen), and apparently lacks cross-resistance to other agents. Notable immunosuppressive activity has been reported. Major toxicity includes bone marrow depression and gastrointestinal manifestations. Neurologic, psychic, and dermatologic disturbances have been noted. Augmentation of sedative effects may accompany the concomitant use of CNS depressants. Ethyl alcohol may cause a reaction resembling the acetaldehyde syndrome produced by disulfiram (Antabuse). Because it is a weak monoamine oxidase inhibitor, sympathomimetics, tricyclic antidepressants, and other drugs or foods with high tyramine contents, such as bananas and ripe cheese, should be avoided.

Mitotane (o,p′-DDD, Lysodren). This derivative of the insecticides DDD and DDT causes selective destruction of normal or neoplastic adrenocortical cells. It also modifies the peripheral metabolism of corticosteroids. Approximately 40 per cent of the drug is absorbed after oral administration, and about 10 to 25 per cent is recovered as a metabolite in the urine. Blood levels are measurable for six to nine weeks after cessation of therapy. The drug is distributed in all tissues, fat being the primary site of storage. The initial daily dose is 8 to 10 grams, usually given in three or four portions. Maximal tolerated doses vary from 2 to 16 grams per day. Treatment should be continued for at least three months. Beneficial effects have been observed in 35 to 40 per cent of patients with unresectable adrenocortical carcinoma. Gastrointestinal disturbances are common. Somnolence, lethargy, vertigo, and dermatitis also occur. Adverse reactions are usually reversible with reduction in dosage, and do not contraindicate continuation of therapy. Discontinuation of drug and administration of exogenous corticosteroids are indicated if shock or severe trauma supervenes.

Dacarbazine (Dimethyltriazeno-imidazole Carboxamide, DTIC). The mechanism of action of this drug is uncertain. Originally considered an antimetabolite, it has demonstrated alkylating activity. It is not cell-cycle phase specific. After intravenous injection, plasma half-life is about 35 minutes, with 43 per cent excreted intact in the urine in six hours. Elevated urinary levels of 5-aminoimidazole-4-carboxamide (AIC) result from catabolism of DTIC and not inhibition of de novo purine biosynthesis. Intravenous daily doses of 4.5 mg per kilogram for five days every month are recommended. It is currently the most popular drug in disseminated malignant melanoma, used alone or in combination. Bone marrow depression and gastrointestinal manifestations are the major toxic effects. Fever, myalgias, malaise, alopecia, facial flushing, and paresthesias have been reported.

774. SELECTION OF PATIENTS

Proper use of cytotoxic agents requires more than a knowledge of their pharmacology. The physician must be thoroughly familiar with the natural history and pathophysiology of the disease before undertaking therapy. Most important is a careful evaluation of each patient in order to determine the benefit : risk ratio. Special attention must be directed toward factors that may potentiate acute toxicity. Among these, the presence of overt or occult infections, bleeding dyscrasias, poor nutritional status, and severe metabolic disturbances are important considerations. The functional condition of the major organs involved in metabolism and elimination of drugs, usually the liver and kidneys, must be determined. Of cardinal importance is the status of the bone marrow, which may be compromised by the disease process, earlier chemotherapy, or previous irradiation, particularly to the spine or pelvis. Cytotoxic agents have a potential risk for teratogenesis, mutagenesis, and carcinogenesis. Their use during pregnancy or during the reproductive years should be undertaken only after thoughtful consideration and appropriate precautions. Predictive tests for tumor sensitivity or selective immunosuppression are still research endeavors, but rational selection of patients for chemotherapy is feasible with the judicious application of available clinical and pharmacologic information.

775. SUPPORTIVE CARE

Notwithstanding careful precautions, moderate or severe toxicity may be encountered. The physician must be prepared to provide vigorous supportive therapy. Component blood therapy is often required, particularly platelet transfusions. Granulocyte transfusions are more difficult to obtain, unless access to a continuous flow cell separator is available. Accordingly, infectious complications in leukopenic and immunosuppressed patients are common. Although fever may be a manifestation of neoplastic disease, it generally indicates infection. Specific antimicrobial therapy requires prompt

identification of the responsible organism. Bacterial pathogens and opportunistic fungal, viral, or protozoal organisms may be causative agents. Some of these respond to the newer drugs described in Ch. 773. Cytotoxic drugs may produce metabolic complications. Hyperuricemia can be prevented by allopurinol; hypercalcemia can be controlled by corticosteroids and mithramycin; and inappropriate ADH secretion can be corrected by fluid deprivation. Other specific measures are discussed above in reference to individual agents. Finally, the importance of psychologic support cannot be overemphasized. Frank discussion of expected but unpleasant complications, such as gastrointestinal disturbances, paresthesias, and alopecia, should include appropriate reassurance of their reversibility. Because palliation is more frequent than cure, the physician's attitude is most important and should combine honesty with compassion.

Brodsky, I., Kahn, S. B., and Moyer, J. H.: Cancer Chemotherapy II. New York, Grune & Stratton, 1972.

Calabresi, P., and Parks, R. E., Jr.: Chemotherapy of neoplastic disease. *In* Goodman, L. S., and Gilman, A. (eds.): The Pharmacological Basis of Therapeutics. 5th ed. New York, Macmillan, 1975, in press.

DeVita, V. T., and Schein, P. A.: The use of drugs in combination for the treatment of cancer. N. Engl. J. Med., 288:998, 1973.

Greenwald, E. S.: Cancer Chemotherapy. Flushing, N.Y., Medical Examination Publishing Company, 1973.

Holland, J. F., and Frei, E.: Cancer Medicine. Philadelphia, Lea & Febiger, 1973.

Kaplan, S. R., and Calabresi, P.: Immunosuppressive agents. N. Engl. J. Med., 289:952, 1234, 1973.

Krakoff, I. H. (ed.): Medical Aspects of Cancer. Med. Clin. North Am., May 1971.

Proceedings of the National Conference on Cancer Chemotherapy. Cancer, 30:1473, 1972.

Sartorelli, A. C., and Johns, D. G.: Antineoplastic and Immunosuppressive Agents. Berlin–Heidelberg–New York, Springer-Verlag, 1974.

Skinner, M. D., and Schwartz, R. S.: Immunosuppressive therapy. N. Engl. J. Med., 287:221, 281, 1972.

Steinberg, A. D., Plotz, P. H., Wolff, S. M., Wong, V. G., Agus, S. G., and Decker, J. L.: Cytotoxic drugs in treatment of nonmalignant disease. Ann. Intern. Med., 76:619, 1972.

Young, C. W., and Burchenal, J. H.: Cancer chemotherapy. Ann. Rev. Pharmacol., 11:369, 1971.

Section Nine.   INFECTIOUS MONONUCLEOSIS

William N. Valentine

Definition. Infectious mononucleosis is characterized typically by irregular fever, pharyngitis, lymph node enlargement, splenomegaly, absolute lymphocytosis with variably numerous morphologically atypical lymphocytes, the development in the patient's serum of heterophil antibodies against sheep, horse, and ox erythrocytes, and the development of antibodies to the herpes-like Epstein-Barr virus (EBV) present in certain Burkitt-lymphoma cell lines. It appears probable that EBV is the causative agent.

History. Although the first account of the disease is generally credited to Emil Pfeiffer, who in 1889 described an epidemic in children that he termed "glandular fever," substantial clinical differences from the typical syndrome and absence of serologic or hematologic

data render this assumption highly doubtful. Sprunt and Evans in 1920 first applied the name "infectious mononucleosis" to the disorder recognized as such today, and directed attention to the abnormal blood leukocytes. The latter were described in detail in 1923 by Downey and McKinlay. Paul and Bunnell in 1932 discovered the unusual concentrations of sheep cell agglutinins in the serum of subjects with the disease. In 1968, Gertrude and Werner Henle reported that patients with infectious mononucleosis acquired antibodies to EBV.

Etiology. The evidence supporting EBV as the etiologic agent of infectious mononucleosis is increasingly strong. Seroepidemiologic data have indicated that students entering college whose sera contains antibodies to

EBV subsequently fail to develop infectious mononucleosis. In contrast, the attack rate in EBV antibody-negative individuals ranges up to 15 per cent during the college years. EBV antibodies are regularly demonstrated in typical, heterophil-antibody-positive mononucleosis. Anti-EBV antibody has been shown to be absent in preillness sera, and to appear and rise in titer during the course of the disease. Unlike the transiently present heterophil antibodies, those directed against EBV persist for years. EBV has the capacity to "transform" lymphoid cells of subjects lacking antibody to it or lymphoid cells derived from umbilical cord blood or fetal lymphoid organs into lymphoblasts capable of long-term survival in tissue culture. Such transformation of cord blood lymphocytes by a factor convincingly identified as EBV has now been demonstrated when filtered throat washings from patients with classic mononucleosis (but not washings from healthy donors) are added to cultures. Moreover, the initial antibodies developing against EBV during acute mononucleosis have now been shown to be IgM in type. These are initially present in high titer, but subsequently become unmeasurable and are succeeded by IgG antibodies. This is precisely the expected course of events if EBV is the causative immunogen and the disease follows initial exposure to it. Nonetheless, there are some reservations, and it has been suggested that EBV could be a "fellow traveler" or latent virus emerging during the lymphoproliferative events of infectious mononucleosis. EBV has also been implicated in such diverse conditions as Burkitt's lymphoma, sarcoidosis, and viral hepatitis, and lymphoblastic cell lines containing EBV have been derived from other lymphoproliferative disorders and even on occasion from normal persons. Although the evidence for an etiologic relationship of EBV to infectious mononucleosis is very compelling, the transmission of EBV to a susceptible host with resultant unequivocal development of the disease is required if the last of Koch's postulates is to be fulfilled.

Incidence and Prevalence. Infectious mononucleosis is widely distributed, having been recognized in Europe, Asia, Australia, America, and elsewhere. Sporadic cases occur mainly, but not exclusively, between the ages of 15 and 30 years, with a slightly greater incidence in males. Epidemics have been reported chiefly in younger children, although in World War II a number of epidemics were observed in young adults. Unfortunately, in many reported epidemics clinical data fail to preclude other diagnoses, and hematologic and serologic data are inadequate or not convincingly confirmatory. Infectious mononucleosis has a low order of contagiousness, is rare in the endemic form among children, and most probably is largely, if not entirely, a sporadic disease. Large series of sporadic cases have been reported from college health dispensaries. Although earlier experience suggested the comparative rarity of the disease in blacks, it is now clear that it is not uncommon in this race. A high incidence has been found among hospital personnel, nurses, and medical students, but it must be recognized that hematologic studies are more frequent with mild illnesses in this group. In Connecticut from 1948 to 1967, the reported incidence of the disease increased some 25-fold. Although the increase was in part undoubtedly related to better recognition and reporting, similar upward trends in various parts of the world suggest that a true increase in incidence may

have occurred. At Yale University, about 75 per cent of entering students lacked EBV antibodies, and the annual student attack rate from 1962 to 1967 was 1.3 to 2.2 per cent.

Epidemiology. In the sporadic form of the disease, cases seldom appear in roommates, families, or other close contacts of patients with the disease. Evidence suggests that kissing may be one important mode of transmission. In epidemics reported before the development of the heterophil antibody test in 1932, serologic confirmation was unattainable, and those before about 1920 (and often later) were not substantiated by adequate hematologic studies. Variability in hematologic and serologic criteria for diagnosis in different reports, an unusual prevalence of atypical and subclinical cases in certain epidemics, and the handicap of the inability to demonstrate a specific etiologic agent combine to cast doubt upon whether reported epidemic and sporadic cases are necessarily the same disorder.

Pathology. The wide variety of clinical manifestations in infectious mononucleosis reflects the diffuse distribution of tissue lesions observed histologically. However, gross changes are confined almost exclusively to lymphoid tissues. Hyperplasia of nasopharyngeal lymphoid tissue is constant, and lymph node enlargement is present in varying degree. Histologically, lymph node reactions vary from a predominantly follicular hyperplasia to a blurred pattern, owing to proliferation of lymphocytic and reticuloendothelial elements in the medullary cords, and resemble malignant lymphoma in some instances. In properly prepared sections, the abnormal lymphocytes seen in the blood are also observed in nodal tissue. The spleen may be tense and swollen, the capsule and trabeculae being thinned and sometimes dissolved by lymphocytic infiltration. The normal splenic histologic pattern is usually partially effaced, with widely spaced follicles and with accumulations of normal and abnormal lymphocytes about the intratrabecular arteries, beneath the intima of veins, and in the blood sinuses. The changes in the spleen render it susceptible to rupture.

Other gross changes include hepatic enlargement and, occasionally, icterus and a skin rash. However, histologic lesions may be observed in virtually every body tissue, varying in distribution from case to case. These generalized lesions consist predominantly of perivascular aggregates of normal and abnormal lymphocytes, and resemble those of certain known viral diseases. Focal lesions are described in the myocardium, kidneys, lungs, skin, central nervous system, and elsewhere. The liver usually contains periportal lymphoid collars, and these occasionally attain the proportions seen in leukemia. Changes similar to those noted in the spleen are found in the capsule of the liver. Meningoencephalitis of mild to severe degree may be observed. In patients with severe nervous system involvement the meninges may be congested and edematous, and may contain increased numbers of mononuclear cells; perivascular cuffing with round cells may be found in brain tissue. Swelling and disruption of myelin sheaths and cellular infiltration of anterior nerve roots have been observed in patients with the Guillain-Barré syndrome associated with infectious mononucleosis. Custer and Smith are of the opinion that the widespread "infiltrates" of connective tissue and the cells composing the perivascular collars arise in situ from cells of the reticuloendothelial system rather than as cell migrations from distant locations. Particle sections of bone marrow fail to show lymphocytic infiltration, although smears of aspirates may contain increased mononuclear elements owing to dilution with peripheral blood. Granulomatous lesions have been described in particle sections on occasion.

Clinical Manifestations. The incubation period is uncertain, but in young adults it is usually in the range of 30 to 50 days. Initial symptoms are nonspecific; malaise followed by fever, sore throat, and headache frequently appears with increasing intensity during the first five or more days of illness. Nearly all patients seeking medical advice experience fever, most commonly from 37.5 to 39.5° C, although sometimes higher. A variably severe pharyngitis is commonly present in the first week of illness, but onset may be delayed to the second week or very occasionally later. Fusospirochetal organisms and hemolytic streptococci are frequently secondary invaders. In some patients (with the so-called "typhoidal" type of the disease) sore throat is absent, although pharyngeal injection and lymphoid hyperplasia are almost invariably present. The throat may be diffusely injected, or membranous pharyngitis may be observed. A palatal enanthem consisting of sharply circumscribed red spots, probably petechial, appearing in crops of usually 6 to 20 lesions, is commonly seen between the fifth and twelfth days of illness.

Lymph node enlargement is present in virtually all cases, but it may be relatively transient in some. The cervical lymph nodes are almost always involved, and posterior cervical nodal enlargement is of value in differentiation from other forms of pharyngitis. Cervical adenopathy is generally moderate but may be massive, and there is little correlation with the severity of pharyngitis. Axillary and inguinal adenopathy are common but not invariable, and enlarged mediastinal nodes may be detected roentgenographically in rare instances. There is no correlation between degree of lymph node enlargement and severity of illness. The enlarged nodes are normally discrete, nontender or slightly tender (unless they drain a secondarily infected area), firm, elastic, and nonsuppurating. Local heat and redness are not present. The spleen is variably enlarged in about 75 per cent of cases. Most commonly the enlarged spleen extends 2 to 3 cm below the costal margin, but more severe enlargement has been recorded.

The liver is palpable less frequently, but jaundice with or without hepatomegaly may occur, most commonly between the fourth and fourteenth days of illness. It is usually mild to moderate and is associated with bilirubinemia, but only rarely with acholic stools. Anicteric hepatitis occurs in most cases.

Although this constellation of signs and symptoms usually predominates in varying degree, giving rise to classification into pharyngeal, typhoidal, and icteric types, involvement by the offending agent is diffuse, and may result in symptoms involving almost every body system. Skin rashes—most commonly transient maculopapular or faintly erythematous eruptions—have been described in different proportions of cases in different series. Their incidence and importance as a physical finding are in dispute, and evaluation is complicated by possible confusion of infectious mononucleosis with other diseases producing exanthems. The most frequently observed lesions are small (2 to 5 mm),

usually pinkish or pinkish-brown, and involve mainly the trunk and upper arms. In Hoagland's extensive experience, skin rashes attributable to infectious mononucleosis itself occurred at the most in 3 to 4 per cent of cases. Neurologic manifestations indicative of involvement of the central and peripheral nervous systems may occur. Headache is common and frequently severe. Instances of isolated cranial and peripheral nerve palsies, nystagmus, papilledema, ataxia, skin hyperesthesia, paresis of an extremity, and toxic psychoses are recorded. Death from the Guillain-Barré syndrome, with ascending paralysis, involvement of multiple peripheral nerves, and high cerebrospinal fluid protein, has occurred.

Electrocardiographic and pathologic evidence of focal cardiac or pericardial involvement may be noted, but clinically significant cardiac involvement or permanent cardiac damage appears to be very rare. Likewise, pulmonary symptoms in the form of cough, sputum, and parenchymal infiltrates demonstrable by roentgenographic examination are uncommon, but have been described. Clinically significant renal disease does not ordinarily occur, but red blood cells, leukocytes, and albumin are sometimes found in the urine. In this regard, however, it must be remembered that hemolytic streptococcal infections are common complications of the pharyngitis. In somewhat less than half the cases, edema of the eyelids and a consequently narrowed ocular aperture are present. It should be emphasized, in addition, that, as with many illnesses, asymptomatic or subclinical cases occur and that the severity of the illness is extremely variable.

The characteristic "mononucleosis" most commonly appears by the fourth or fifth day of illness and persists two to eight weeks, occasionally for several months. Normal small lymphocytes and monocytes are found in abundance. A common, abnormal lymphocyte (Type I of Downey) has an oval, kidney-shaped, or lobulated nucleus with vacuolated, foamy, and usually nongranular cytoplasm. Others are larger with less condensation of nuclear chromatin and a nonvacuolated, more homogeneous cytoplasm (Type II of Downey), or may possess a finer chromatin pattern and one or two nucleoli, and may resemble lymphoblasts (Type III of Downey). Other forms of abnormal lymphocytes are also noted; the "Downey" cells individually are not specific for the disease. Their abundance in typical cases is characteristic, however. In the first two weeks of the disease, isotopic labeling evidence suggests that a high proportion of circulating lymphocytes are synthesizing DNA. The atypical lymphocyte in infectious mononucleosis is not only capable of in vivo proliferation, but has an increased potential for long-term in vitro proliferation as well. Thus long-term cultures derived from peripheral blood may be established, whereas in normal persons such cultures usually fail to thrive. Although cytochemical studies indicate some differences from normal lymphocytes or monocytes, differences observed by electron microscopy are insufficient to classify three types of "Downey" cells by this modality. The total leukocyte count is usually 10,000 to 20,000 per cubic millimeter at some point in the disease, but may be normal or appreciably higher. In the fully developed disease, mononuclear cells usually comprise 60 per cent or more of the leukocytes, and values of more than 90 per cent have been reported. At the outset, counts in the normal or leukopenic range without lymphocytosis are often present. Anemia and clinically significant thrombocytopenia are normally absent, although both acute hemolytic anemia and thrombocytopenic purpura are observed in rare instances; in the former the Coombs test may or may not be positive.

Heterophil antibodies agglutinating sheep and horse cells and hemolyzing ox cells almost always appear in the first two weeks of illness, and persist from four to eight weeks up to several months. Highest titers are usually observed in the second and third weeks of illness. The characteristic heterophil agglutinins are absorbed by beef erythrocyte antigen, but not completely by guinea pig kidney. Differential absorption studies are imperative in atypical cases, and serve in most instances to differentiate infectious mononucleosis from other conditions in which occasionally increased heterophil antibodies are observed. In most of the latter the antibody present is of the Forssman type, and is absorbable by guinea pig kidney. In serum sickness, the heterophil agglutinins are absorbed by both guinea pig kidney and beef antigen. However, a positive test for properly absorbed heterophil antibodies requires the presence also of appropriate clinical and hematologic manifestations if acute infectious mononucleosis is to be diagnosed. Purely serologic evidence may indicate persisting antibodies from a recent attack of the disease, or, rarely, a nonspecific anamnestic resurgence of heterophil antibodies during an unrelated illness.

In addition to heterophil antibodies, several other antibodies obviously not directed specifically at the original immunogen may be noted. Most common of these is a cold-reacting antibody against the human erythrocyte antigen i, most abundantly present in fetal red cells. When this is of sufficient titer and has a wide thermal range, hemolytic anemia in rare instances is the result. Sera from subjects with infectious mononucleosis may also react against Rhesus monkey erythrocytes, may possess cryoglobulins, and may have low titers of antinuclear antibodies. Early reports of frequent occurrence of a false positive VDRL test for syphilis now appear probably to be in error, and this serologic manifestation is probably rare. Its true incidence is currently controversial. In view of the rich serology, it is not surprising that immunoglobulin levels are elevated, usually returning to normal within three months. Although both heterophil and cold agglutinin antibodies are of the IgM class, their absorption from even high-titered sera removes less than 5 per cent of the increase in IgM.

Hepatitis with or without icterus occurs in most patients. Transaminase, alkaline phosphatase, and sulfobromophthalein retention tests for liver function are abnormal in a high proportion of cases. Elevations in SGOT and SGPT enzyme levels have been reported to be the most consistent abnormality. In one study the levels of both enzymes usually increased in the first week of illness, peaked in the second week, and returned to normal in about five weeks. Electrocardiographic changes such as abnormal T waves and prolonged P-R intervals are not uncommon. The cerebrospinal fluid may exhibit pleocytosis up to several hundred cells (chiefly lymphocytes). Moderate elevations in cerebrospinal fluid pressure have been observed.

Diagnosis. Diagnosis until recently rested on the triad of (1) clinical features of fever, pharyngotonsillitis, lymph node enlargement, and splenomegaly; (2) absolute lymphocytosis persisting over a period of several days or longer and characterized by the presence of atypical lymphocytes, usually constituting 20 per cent or more of the leukocytes at some time during the acute stages; and (3) a positive heterophil agglutination test, with specific absorption studies when indicated. The time-consuming titrations and absorptions characterizing earlier serologic tests have largely been supplanted by a reliable, simple, quite specific and rapid screening slide test. This incorporates absorption with the classic combination of guinea pig kidney and boiled ox erythrocytes. It requires only a drop of serum, and sensitivity has been increased by substituting horse for sheep erythrocytes. Since antibody to EBV can be demonstrated with great consistency in infectious mononucleosis, the immunofluorescence, complement fixation, and membrane fluorescence tests for its presence may be extremely valuable, particularly in atypical or heterophil antibody negative cases. Antibodies to EBV are lacking in preillness serum where this is available; are present, often in high titer, early in the illness; and in any event develop within two to three weeks after the onset of symptoms. However, no single titer is diagnostic, because high titers may be present in other disorders. Although the absence of antibody would preclude the diagnosis, the usefulness of its presence is unfortunately limited by its lack of specificity, by the fact that high titers are often present when the patient is first seen and hence a rise may be difficult to demonstrate, and by inability to obtain anti-EBV titers except in comparatively few laboratories.

Typical cases are readily recognized. Atypical cases present substantial diagnostic problems. It must be remembered that transient lymphocytosis with a few atypical lymphocytes occurs in a number of febrile illnesses. A persisting negative heterophil antibody test does not exclude the diagnosis completely, but a firm diagnosis in its absence throughout the entire course of the disease is dangerous and unconvincing. However, heterophil antibody-negative cases, otherwise typical, have been shown to develop EBV antibody during the course of illness. Conversely, for reasons previously discussed, a positive slide test is not grounds for diagnosis in the absence of "mononucleosis" and appropriate clinical features. In the past, reliance on incomplete criteria for diagnosis or, indeed, at times on a single criterion has resulted in diagnostic confusion and frequent inclusion of questionable illnesses as instances of the disease.

Differential   Diagnosis.   Infectious   mononucleosis may be confused with a variety of febrile illnesses, particularly viral, accompanied by some degree of lymphocytosis and atypical cells. The prominent *pharyngotonsillitis* requires differentiation from streptococcal infections, Vincent's angina, diphtheria, aphthous stomatitis, and other causes of acute sore throat. Generalized infections may be considered in the differential diagnosis in some cases. Constitutional symptoms associated with a skin rash may suggest a variety of exanthems. Adult *toxoplasmosis* may mimic the clinical syndrome of infectious mononucleosis, including the findings of pharyngitis, cervical lymphadenopathy, splenomegaly, fever, and lymphocytosis with atypical lymphocytes. No cross-reaction has been found, however, between heterophil and Toxoplasma dye test antibodies. A syndrome resembling infectious mononucleosis may accompany infection with cytomegalovirus. CMV mononucleosis and infectious mononucleosis both may be characterized by indistinguishable hematologic abnormalities, protracted fever, hepatitis and abnormal liver function tests, splenomegaly, and a variety of non-specific immunologic aberrations. CMV mononucleosis occurs occasionally in healthy individuals, or some 21 to 34 days after massive transfusion therapy for nonsurgical conditions, or after open-heart surgery with extracorporeal circulation. In CMV mononucleosis the heterophil test is negative, pharyngitis is ordinarily absent, and lymphadenopathy is often not present. With special studies the virus may sometimes be isolated and specific CMV antibodies demonstrated. Syndromes simulating infectious mononucleosis in many respects have also been reported in infection with adenovirus. The hepatitis of infectious mononucleosis may simulate *infectious hepatitis* or homologous serum jaundice, and, indeed, lymphocytosis may also be observed in these disorders. Prominent neurologic features may simulate *encephalitis, poliomyelitis, Guillain-Barré syndrome,* or *lymphocytic choriomeningitis.* The abnormal blood picture may raise the question of *leukemia* or *infectious lymphocytosis.* The latter disorder is not accompanied by splenomegaly or lymph node enlargement, nor are the characteristic atypical lymphocytes or serologic features of infectious mononucleosis present. Hemolytic anemia and thrombocytopenia, when present, must be differentiated from similar findings in a variety of disorders.

Treatment. No specific therapy is available. Secondary bacterial invasion with streptococcal pharyngitis or Vincent's angina should be sought and treated with appropriate antimicrobial drugs and perborate mouth washes. In view of the peculiar liability of patients with infectious mononucleosis to allergic reactions to ampicillin, that antimicrobial should be avoided. Symptomatic treatment of the fever and pharyngitis with salicylates and sedation for pain is indicated when necessary. Splenic rupture occasionally occurs and may be heralded by abdominal pain and shock. This complication calls for prompt surgical intervention. Corticotrophin and 17-hydroxycorticosteroids have been reported to produce dramatic clinical improvements, but do not specifically influence the disease. They are not indicated, except possibly for very ill patients in extreme degrees of pharyngeal lymphoid hyperplasia or edema of the glottis threatening occlusion of the respiratory tract, and in rare instances of acute hemolytic anemia and thrombocytopenic purpura. They may be given to adults as a six-day course: prednisone, 80 mg the first day, and 40 mg a day for three additional days, followed by gradual reduction over the final two days of therapy. Although chloroquine has been advocated, there is little evidence of any significant effect on the basic disease. Very rarely, tracheostomy has been required for edema of the glottis or tracheal occlusion. The hepatitis is usually mild, and permanent sequelae are rare. However, it is probably wise to treat severely icteric patients with bed rest and close observation of liver function tests, as in other forms of hepatitis. Adequate rest and avoidance of activities in which splenic rupture may occur are important in the acute and convalescent period. The friability of the spleen is such that repeated or heavy-handed attempts at splenic palpation are to be avoided. The low order of contagiousness in sporadic cases precludes the necessity for strict isolation.

Prognosis. Infectious mononucleosis is essentially a benign disorder, although rare fatalities have occurred because of rupture of the spleen or severe neurologic involvement, particularly ascending paralysis with the Guillain-Barré syndrome. Very rarely myocarditis has been reported as a cause of death; also very rarely, edema of the glottis or secondary sepsis may be life threatening.

In terms of morbidity, the prognosis is extremely variable. As with other disorders, some patients have clinically inapparent disease or mild, transient illnesses that may or may not be diagnosed. In the more severely ill patients, the febrile period is usually of one to three weeks' duration, and there is a variable but definite period of postconvalescent asthenia. Brief recrudescences are sometimes seen. Serologic and hematologic abnormalities can persist for some time after convalescence. Although longstanding "chronic" infectious mononucleosis has been reported, most observers are of the opinion that a true chronic form of the disease has not been definitely recognized. Clinically significant sequelae of hepatic or cardiac involvement are ordinarily not observed. Occasional focal neurologic residuals are reported, but complete recovery is the general rule.

Carter, R. L., and Penman, H. G. (eds.): Infectious Mononucleosis. Oxford and Edinburgh, Blackwell Scientific Publications, 1969.

Evans, A. S., Niederman, J. C., and McCollum, R. W.: Sero-epidemiologic studies of infectious mononucleosis with EB virus. N. Engl. J. Med., 279:1121, 1968.

Henle, G., Henle, W., and Diehl, V.: Relation of Burkitt's tumor-associated herpes-type virus to infectious mononucleosis. Proc. Natl. Acad. Sci. USA, 59:94, 1968.

Klemola, E., von Essen, R., Wager, O., Haltia, K., Koivuniemi, A., and Salmi, I.: Cytomegalovirus mononucleosis in previously healthy individuals. Ann. Intern. Med., 71:11, 1969.

Remington, J. S., Barnett, C. G., Meikel, M., and Lunde, M. N.: Toxoplasmosis and infectious mononucleosis. Arch. Intern. Med., 110:744, 1962.

Stites, D. P., and Leikola, J.: Infectious mononucleosis. Semin. Hematol., 8:243, 1971.

Section Ten. EOSINOPHILIC GRANULOMA AND RELATED SYNDROMES

Philip H. Lieberman

Eosinophilic granuloma is a benign disorder characterized by infiltrates of eosinophils and mononuclear cells which have been considered to be histiocytes. This disease is complicated by a complex terminology which has its origin in the empiricism of yesteryear. "Histiocytosis X" is an old concept which refers to a spectrum of disease encompassing both the benign disorder eosinophilic granuloma and malignant lymphomatous diseases. The concept of "histiocytosis X" has been challenged recently on both historical and clinical grounds. The "Hand-Schüller-Christian syndrome" has been redefined over the years and is probably synonymous with the more exact designation "multifocal eosinophilic granuloma."

EOSINOPHILIC GRANULOMA

Eosinophilic granuloma occurs most frequently in children and young adults but is occasionally seen in the sixth and seventh decades of life. Approximately twice as many males as females are affected. Of particular importance is whether it is *unifocal* or *multifocal,* for if dissemination is present, one must expect a chronic disease state with generalized manifestations. If a unifocal bone lesion is found (verified by skeletal x-ray survey) and no secondary lesions develop within six months, one can be reasonably certain that the process is limited and that no further defects will develop. Unifocal bone lesions are found in long or flat bones, frequently in the calvarium or femur in children and not infrequently in ribs in adults. Multifocal lesions may involve any site, but are less frequent in the hands and feet. Bone pain and swelling are common presenting complaints, and pathologic fractures may occur.

In addition to orthopedic problems, patients with multifocal lesions frequently manifest fever, malaise, irritability, anorexia, pallor, and malnutrition. Many of the patients have recurrent bouts of otitis media, mastoiditis, and gum ulcerations and infiltrates. Careful history often reveals an allergic background. The periodicity of disease with attacks of hepatosplenomegaly, adenopathy, and debility is impressive. The patient may have transient or permanent diabetes insipidus at the onset of the disease, or it may develop at a later date. Despite the chronicity of the disease with periodic bouts of frequently severe illness, these patients almost all recover; some will have residual orthopedic defects or persistent diabetes insipidus. Much has been written about skin lesions in this disorder, with attempts to classify benign versus malignant forms on the basis of skin or mucous membrane histology. In general, skin biopsies are not helpful. Many patients develop dermatologic lesions which clinically and morphologically can best be described as seborrheic dermatitis. Laboratory studies have been disappointing. The blood counts are generally within normal range, except for occasional slight normochromic normocytic anemia in very ill patients or a slight shift to the left in differential counts when the patient develops secondary infections. Eosinophilia is not uncommon. Serum lipid and cholesterol studies have not been helpful. Immunoglobulin levels and tests of cellular immunity (dinitrochlorobenzene and tuberculin skin tests) have been within normal limits. Almost invariably studies of stools for ova and parasites have not been helpful. Occasional cases of infection by uncommon mycobacteria have been reported, but these are most unusual.

The basic lesion of eosinophilic granuloma of bone consists of aggregates of mature eosinophils and mononuclear cells; the latter have been considered to be benign histiocytes. Varying degrees of necrosis are encountered as well as the multinucleated giant cells common in many bone lesions. In areas of suppuration, foamy histiocytes can be seen. There may be some fibrosis, especially when the lesion is healing. Serial biopsies do *not* show a progression of the typical eosinophilic and histiocytic mixtures to a lipid phase followed by healing fibrosis, as was originally thought. More commonly, the lesion heals by direct fibrosis. Aside from skin there have been very few tissue studies of nonosseous lesions, presumably because of the benign course. However, lymph node biopsies are sometimes performed which show either nonspecific hyperplastic changes or large collections of eosinophils and benign histiocytes. The term "eosinophilic granuloma" has been used for apparently unrelated disorders such as diffuse or polypoid eosinophilic enteritis or cystitis. Nevertheless, it is believed that soft tissue lesions may also be present in the classic cases. Many of the children with multifocal eosinophilic granuloma have had episodes of pneumonitis, documented by roentgenograms, some of which may show diffuse pulmonary infiltration. Some of these attacks of pneumonitis probably represent secondary bacterial infections, for they respond to appropriate antimicrobial therapy. Occasionally typical morphologic lesions of eosinophilic granuloma may involve the mandible, maxilla, or orbital bones. Such patients present with ulcerative lesions of gums or classic proptosis. Although the classic triad of the Hand-Schüller-Christian syndrome, namely unilateral or bilateral exophthalmos, diabetes insipidus, and unifocal or multifocal areas of bone destruction, may be found in multifocal eosinophilic granuloma, they are also seen in other disorders such as malignant lymphoma or carcinoma.

Recent observations have indicated that the mononuclear cells involved in eosinophilic granuloma have an unusual type of membrane configuration similar to that seen in the Langerhans cell of the skin. These mononuclear cells thus may not be conventional histiocytes.

Electron micrograph showing a mononuclear cell characteristically found in eosinophilic granuloma. Arrows indicate two of the numerous Langerhans-type granules found in these cells. ($\times$ 10,800.) Inset: Langerhans granule. ($\times$ 128,000.)

The membranous "bodies" found in these cells result from an inversion of the plasmalemma. The pathogenesis of the peculiar membrane structures and the role the eosinophil plays, if any, in these changes is as yet unknown, but the suggestion that eosinophilic granuloma is an immunologic reaction is intriguing. Recent studies have shed much light upon the mechanisms of eosinophilia and its suppression by agents known to modify immune responses. Some of these latter agents have proved very effective in the clinical management of multifocal eosinophilic granuloma.

LETTERER-SIWE SYNDROME

The Letterer-Siwe syndrome, as formally defined by Abt and Denenholz, consists of (1) marked splenomegaly with moderate to considerable enlargement of the liver; (2) hemorrhagic diathesis; (3) lymphadenopathy; (4) localized tumefactions over bones (may be diagnosed radiologically); (5) secondary anemia with normal or somewhat diminished leukocyte count, normal differential count, and unremarkable platelet count; (6) splenic aspirates, containing increased numbers of nonlipid-containing macrophages; (7) no familial or hereditary disposition; (8) occurrence exclusively in infants; (9) acute onset unrelated to infection;

downhill course with duration from a few weeks to several years; (10) unknown etiology; and (11) generalized hyperplasia of nonlipid-storing macrophages in various organs. These criteria have been variously altered by authors throughout the years, but they are *nonspecific* and have included both benign and malignant disorders, causing much confusion. After eliminating various infectious diseases and nonspecific case reports, one is left with a group of malignant neoplasms principally characterized by the presence of histiocytic elements. On purely morphologic grounds, these disorders probably represent unusual forms of malignant lymphoma. It is probable that the Letterer-Siwe syndrome or disease and eosinophilic granuloma are independent entities. If it is true that eosinophilic granuloma may represent an immunologic response to an unknown etiologic agent, one would expect that rare overlapping of disease entities might take place and that the picture of eosinophilic granuloma might occur not only in rare lymphomatous disorders but also in other disorders, as, indeed, has been the case.

FURTHER NOTES ON TERMINOLOGY

It should be pointed out that, in addition to the inadvisability of using expressions such as "Hand-Schüller-

Christian syndrome," "histiocytosis X," and the "histiocytoses," the terms "reticuloendotheliosis" and "reticulosis" likewise do not belong in the lexicon of the modern clinician. The term "reticuloendotheliosis" was intended to describe proliferation of reticuloendothelial cells giving rise to circulating monocytes, thus being analogous to the terms "myelosis" and "lymphadenosis" used to describe disorders of the bone marrow and lymph nodes, respectively. The term "reticulosis" was introduced by Letterer as a synonym for reticuloendotheliosis. The use of these terms has caused confusion. "Reticulosis" has unfortunately become synonymous with malignant lymphoma in some parts of the world, and "reticuloendotheliosis" (and later "histiocytosis") has been used to describe not only the disorders under discussion in this section but also various lipid storage diseases and infectious granulomas.

TREATMENT

Management of Unifocal (Solitary) Eosinophilic Granuloma of Bone

1. Open biopsy for exact diagnosis.
2. Curettage (with or without bone chip packing).
3. Supervoltage radiation therapy to local "hazardous" sites such as cervical vertebrae or weight-bearing bones (300 to 600 r TD fractionated). Such noncancericidal dosages arrest progression of lesions and stimulate repair. High dosage radiotherapy can lead to tissue damage with resultant poor healing.
4. Supportive therapy, e.g., bed rest as indicated, a brace or cast to protect collapsed vertebra. (See below for diabetes insipidus.)
5. Surgery: (a) to relieve cord compression; (b) partial mastoidectomy if indicated; (c) skin grafts if necessary.
6. Observe for development of other lesions, which usually occur within the first six months after diagnosis. Incidence of solitary bone lesions increases with age. Patients with lesions in the mandible, mastoid, or facial or orbital bones are more likely to develop further disease. (a) Monthly history and physical examination. (b) Skeletal survey six months after biopsy if indicated. If necessary, repeat surveys every six months for one to two years.

Management of Multifocal Eosinophilic Granuloma of Bone

1. Open biopsy for exact diagnosis.
2. Curettage (with or without bone chip packing).
3. Chemotherapy is essential in management in order to prevent prolonged disease and to lessen morbidity and permanent deformity. This probably non-neoplastic disorder can best be treated with drugs used

in cancer chemotherapy. Bone marrow depression is *not* necessary to achieve desired effect. Vinblastine, prednisone, and methotrexate used judiciously by experienced physicians can lead to marked suppression of the disease process. *Acute phase* (repeat every 4 to 6 months if new lesions develop): (a) Vinblastine, 0.1 mg per kilogram intravenously every week for three to five weeks. (b) Prednisone, 2 mg per kilogram by mouth three days each week for three to five weeks, with each cycle starting on days vinblastine is given. Total dosage should never exceed 80 mg per day. *Maintenance phase:* Methotrexate, 0.025 to 2.5 mg by mouth for three days, then without medication for 4 days.
4. Supervoltage radiation therapy to local "hazardous" sites, 300 to 600 r TD fractionated. There should be a prompt response, especially if radiation is administered after vinblastine-prednisone therapy is initiated.
5. Antimicrobial agents – used to treat otitis externa, mastoiditis, and sinusitis.
6. Surgery – for cord decompression, to relieve mastoid problems, and to excise calvarial lesions eroding through skin.
7. Supportive therapy: (a) maintain good nutrition; (b) whole blood transfusion when indicated; (c) bed rest, casts, braces, as indicated; (d) physical therapy as indicated; (e) *Reassurance* that the process is not neoplastic and that the patient will be able to regain normal life.
8. Diabetes insipidus: Pitressin tannate in oil and/or Diapid insufflation in conventional dosages (see Ch. 834).

Management of the Letterer-Siwe Syndrome (When Presenting as Histiocytic Lymphoma)

See Ch. 769.

Abt, A. F., and Denenholz, E. J.: Letterer-Siwe's disease. Splenohepatomegaly associated with widespread hyperplasia of nonlipoid-storing macrophages; discussion of the so-called reticuloendothelioses. Am. J. Dis. Child., 51:499, 1936.
Boyer, M. H. Basten, A., and Beeson, P. B.: Mechanism of eosinophilia. III. Suppression of eosinophilia by agents known to modify immune responses. Blood, 36:458, 1970.
Jones, C. R., and Lieberman, P. H.: Unpublished data.
Lichtenstein, L.: Histiocytosis X. Integration of eosinophilic granuloma of bone, "Letterer-Siwe disease," and "Schüller-Christian disease" as related manifestations of a single nosologic entity. Arch. Pathol., 56:84, 1953.
Lieberman, P. H., Jones, C. R., Dargeon, H. W. K., and Begg, C. F.: A reappraisal of eosinophilic granuloma of bone, Hand-Schüller-Christian syndrome and Letterer-Siwe syndrome. Medicine, 48:375, 1969.
Nyholm, K.: Eosinophilic xanthomatous granulomatosis and Letterer-Siwe's disease. Acta Pathol. Microbiol. Scand., Supp. 216, 1971.
Symmers, W. St. C.: The lymphoreticular system. In Wright, G. P., and Symmers, W. St. C. (eds.): Systemic Pathology, Vol. 1. London, Longmans, Green & Co., 1966, Chapter 5.
Tusques, J., and Pradal, G.: Analyse tridimensionnelle des inclusions rencontrées dans les histiocytes de l'histiocytose "X," en microscopie électronique. Comparaison avec les inclusions des cellules de Langerhans. J. Microscopie, 8:113, 1969.

Section Eleven.   LIPID STORAGE DISORDERS

Donald S. Fredrickson

776. GAUCHER'S DISEASE

Definition.   Gaucher's disease is a relatively common familial disorder characterized by abnormal accumulation of glucocerebrosides in reticuloendothelial (RE) cells; the accumulation occurs because an enzyme necessary for the degradation of these glycolipids is deficient. The increasing mass of the storage cells accounts for most of the clinical manifestations of the disease, including hepatosplenomegaly, lymph node enlargement, and bone lesions owing to expansion of the involved marrow. At least three syndromes have been recognized: (1) a chronic non-neuronopathic or "adult" form, which is by far the most common, becoming evident at any age and associated with hypersplenism, bone lesions, skin pigmentation and pingueculae, and preponderance among Ashkenazic Jews; (2) an acute neuronopathic form, which is manifest in infancy, is associated with severe neurologic abnormalities, and is usually fatal by three years of age; and (3) a "juvenile" form, which may begin at any time in childhood, combining the features of the chronic form with slowly progressive neurologic dysfunction. At least three different mutations are represented by the different forms of Gaucher's disease. No specific treatment is available.

Pathologic Physiology and Pathogenesis.   Cerebrosides are compounds that contain equimolar amounts of sphingosine, fatty acid, and hexose. In the brain the hexose component is galactose, and the galactocerebrosides form an essential part of the myelin in the white matter. In tissues outside the brain, except for the kidney, practically all the small amounts of cerebroside present contain only glucose. These glucocerebrosides arise mainly from the degradation of more complex sphingoglycolipids, the most important source probably being the normal breakdown of both white and red blood cells. In Gaucher's disease there is a specific deficiency in the activity of glucosylceramide-β-glucosidase (glucocerebrosidase), one of the acid hydrolases found in the lysosomes. Glucocerebroside, a *relatively* insoluble compound, then accumulates in RE cells.

The morphologic hallmark of Gaucher's disease is the *Gaucher cell*, a round or polyhedral pale reticulum cell 20 to 80 μ in diameter, with a small eccentrically placed nucleus and a wrinkled ("crumpled silk") cytoplasm that contains an irregular network of fibrils. With electron microscopy the fibrils are shown to represent tubules or strands of glucocerebroside contained within secondary lysosomes having a single limiting membrane. Evidence of active phagocytosis or pinocytosis is present at the cell border, and fragments of erythrocytes are often visible. A few cells may have two or more nuclei. The cytoplasm does not stain with fat stains, but numerous wavy fibrillae are stained deeply with the periodic acid–Schiff reaction or with Mallory's

trichrome connective tissue stain. The cytoplasm also demonstrates strong acid phosphatase activity. Examination of unstained smears of aspirated bone marrow by phase microscopy affords the best visualization of the cells (see accompanying figure, part A).

Proliferation and expansion of the Gaucher cells are responsible for the enlargement of spleen, liver, and intrathoracic and intra-abdominal lymph nodes. The concentration of glucocerebrosides may be increased 50 to 100 times normal in these organs. The spleen may become tremendous in size. Hemosiderin may be increased in the skin and other organs. Gaucher cells are also scattered diffusely throughout the marrow, and in some areas form tumor-like accumulations that may expand, erode the cortex, and lead to pathologic fractures. Infiltration of the lungs, kidneys, thymus, tonsils, thyroid, adrenals, and lymphatic tissue of the intestinal tract also occurs. Functional impairment of these

Appearance of the typical Gaucher cell (*A*) and a foam cell seen in Niemann-Pick disease (*B*). Both are viewed under phase microscopy in unstained smears of aspirated bone marrow. Magnification can be estimated from adjacent red cells.

organs is unusual, except for the lungs. Serious pulmonary infections are common in children, and pulmonary hypertension may occur in adults. Pathologic changes in the brains of adults are restricted to the presence of perivascular adventitial cells swollen in the typical Gaucher configuration. In children with the acute neuronopathic type of disease, such "perivascular cuffing" is accompanied by acute nerve cell degeneration with active phagocytosis of the cellular remains by histiocytes and microglia, and cytoplasmic storage of periodic acid–Schiff positive lipid in either neurons or glial cells. These changes are distributed focally in the cerebrum, cerebellum, brainstem, and spinal cord. In the juvenile form the ballooning of neurons is accentuated. An accumulation of both glucocerebrosides and gangliosides has been reported in the brains of infants with the acute neuronopathic type. It is not known why the severity of the effect on the brain is so different in the several forms of the disease.

Acid phosphatase activity, not inhibited by L-tartrate (in contrast to the prostatic enzyme), is characteristically elevated in plasma and has diagnostic value. The enzyme is apparently spilled into plasma from the Gaucher cells. Plasma cerebroside concentrations are elevated after splenectomy.

Clinical Manifestations. *Chronic Non-neuronopathic Type.* The disease affects both sexes equally. It has been reported in Caucasians, Negroes, and Orientals; but a very high proportion of cases occurs among Ashkenazic Jews. Manifestations may appear at any age; the diagnosis has been made in the first month of life and past the age of 80 years. The course is extremely variable and tends to be more severe in affected children. Often, particularly in adults, the patient has no symptoms for a long time except awareness of a progressively enlarging mass in the left upper abdomen. The spleen may become very large; the liver is usually palpable. The second most common presenting abnormality is related to bone lesions. From 50 to 75 per cent of patients have roentgenographic changes, mostly asymptomatic. A common change is expansion of the cortex of the lower end of the femur, producing a characteristic radiolucent area with the configuration of an Erlenmeyer flask. The phalanges, long bones, vertebrae, ribs, and pelvis are more commonly involved than the skull. Bone pain or aching and pathologic fractures may appear at sites of skeletal lesions. With destruction of the head and neck of the femur, walking may become progressively more difficult. The hip abnormalities are sometimes confused with Legg-Perthes disease. In younger patients episodic attacks of bone pain simulating acute osteomyelitis are common. The long bones are usually affected; fever, joint tenderness, and redness occur, and draining sinus tracts may form. The cause is believed to be interference with the blood supply of the highly vascular metaphysis. Attacks usually last several weeks and no longer recur when growth is complete.

A high percentage of patients with Gaucher's disease develop hematologic changes of hypersplenism at some time during the course of their disease: hemolytic anemia, leukopenia, thrombocytopenia, or any combination of the three. The peripheral cytopenia is accompanied by a normal or increased number of the progenitors of the involved formed element in the bone marrow. Chronic Gaucher's disease usually involves only a single generation, but it has been observed in two generations. Otherwise normal parents, siblings, and other close relatives of patients sometimes have slight splenomegaly or small Gaucher cells in the marrow. Although the disease sometimes appears to behave like a dominant trait, most patients probably are homozygous for an autosomal recessive allele or alleles.

Acute Neuronopathic Type. This "infantile" form of the disease is usually evident by three months of age but may become so any time between birth and 18 months. Among the earliest signs are splenomegaly, chronic cough, and psychomotor retardation. Other neurologic signs indicative of brainstem and cranial nerve involvement usually appear by the age of six months. The children have a stereotyped appearance: hepatosplenomegaly, strabismus, head retroflexed, lips retracted, and often spastic extremities held in flexion. The disease is fatal within three years; the average life span is about one year, respiratory infection and distress being the principal cause of death. Sex distribution is about equal. If one child in a family is afflicted, all other affected sibs will have the same form of disease. The disease appears to be transmitted as an autosomal recessive gene and is expressed only in the homozygote. The mutant gene is present in low frequency in many ethnic groups. Four of about 70 reported cases have occurred in Jews.

Juvenile Type. About 25 examples of subacute neuronopathic Gaucher's disease have been described. Hepatosplenomegaly, hypersplenism, bone lesions, and other features of the chronic type appear from infancy onward. These are combined with mental retardation, behavioral problems, seizures, choreoathetoid movements, and sometimes strabismus, trismus, and other evidence of brainstem involvement. In several related Swedish families, glucocerebrosidase deficiency was demonstrated. Glycolipids other than glucocerebrosides may be stored in the spleen and liver, and a clear-cut phenotype has not been established.

Diagnosis. Gaucher's disease should be ruled out in any patient with unexplained splenomegaly, especially with elevated plasma acid phosphatase activity (not inhibited by L-tartrate). A presumptive diagnosis is made from detection of Gaucher cells, usually in marrow aspirates. Diagnosis should be confirmed by demonstration of absence or severe deficiency in activity of glucosylceramide β-glucosidase. The enzyme activity can be measured most accurately in fibroblasts cultured from skin, bone marrow, or amniotic fluid (for prenatal diagnosis). Circulating white cells have also been used for this purpose. If there is any doubt, liver biopsy will permit confirmation of both specific enzyme deficiency and accumulation of glucocerebrosides, provided that the tissue is stored in the absence of fixatives.

Treatment and Prognosis. No specific therapy exists. X-ray therapy to bone lesions may alleviate pain, but usually does not arrest the destructive process. Bone pain may also respond well to corticosteroid therapy. Splenectomy corrects the manifestations of hypersplenism but does not otherwise influence the course of the disease. Because of the possibility that bone involvement may be accelerated by splenectomy, the indication for the procedure should be clear cut. The course is protracted, often extending over many years. Most older patients die of intercurrent diseases rather than Gaucher's disease per se.

Brady, R. O., and King, F.: Gaucher's disease. *In* Hers, H. G., and Van Hoof, F. (eds.): Lysosomes and Storage Diseases. New York, Academic Press, 1973, pp. 381–394.

Fredrickson, D. S., and Sloan, H. R.: Glucosylceramide lipidoses: Gaucher's disease. *In* Stanbury, J. B., Wyngaarden, J. B., and Fredrickson, D. S. (eds.): The Metabolic Basis of Inherited Disease. 3rd ed. New York, McGraw-Hill Book Company, 1972, pp. 730–759.

Reich, C., Seife, M., and Kessler, B. J.: Gaucher's disease: A review and discussion of twenty cases. Medicine, 30:1, 1951.

Schettler, G., and Kahlke, W.: Gaucher's disease. *In* Schettler, G. (ed.): Lipids and Lipidoses. New York, Springer-Verlag, 1967, pp. 260–287.

777.   NIEMANN-PICK DISEASE

Definition.   The eponym Niemann-Pick disease refers to several rare disorders characterized by extensive tissue storage of sphingomyelin. All patients have hepatosplenomegaly and large macrophages filled with lipid droplets in the bone marrow (see figure in Ch. 776, part B); some also have severe neurologic abnormalities. The "sphingomyelin lipidoses" fall into two major groups. In the first, there is clear-cut inheritable deficiency of activity of sphingomyelinase, a lysosomal enzyme that catalyzes the hydrolysis of phosphorylcholine from sphingomyelin. Sphingomyelin concentrations in tissues are 10 to 100 times normal. The second includes a heterogeneous group of disorders with clinical manifestations similar to the first. The tissue activity of sphingomyelinase is normal or only slightly deficient, however, and increases in sphingomyelin concentrations of liver or spleen are relatively small.

The sphingomyelinase-deficient disorders usually occur in either an acute neuronopathic form (type A) or a chronic, non-neuronopathic form (type B). All affected members of the same family are phenotypically the same, and the two disorders are presumably "allelic," i.e., they represent different mutations at or near the same locus governing the activity of sphingomyelinase.

Clinical Manifestations. *Type A.* Type A is usually manifested by six months of age by abdominal enlargement and evidence of physical and mental retardation. Hepatosplenomegaly and roentgenographic evidence of diffuse pulmonary infiltration may be present as early as one month of age. Throughout the nervous system the neurons and glial cells are ballooned with lipid, the nuclei are pushed to one side, and Nissl substance disappears. Neuronal loss, gliosis, and demyelination are severe. Retinal degeneration in the macular area usually causes a cherry-red spot to appear. The disease progresses to a vegetative state, and death nearly always occurs by the fourth year of life. There are a few exceptional patients, perhaps representing different mutations, who early have retinal changes and other central nervous system signs and who have a much more prolonged course. Both sexes are affected. The disease occurs in all races; it is disproportionately frequent in Ashkenazic Jews.

Type B.   Children with type B may develop evidence of visceral involvement as severe and as early as those with type A, but the central nervous system apparently is spared, and mental development is normal. Chronic pulmonary infections and hypersplenism are sometimes life-threatening, but a reasonably normal life span may be possible. Types A and B are inherited as autosomal recessives.

Diagnosis.   The typical presentation of Niemann-Pick disease is a very young child with hepatosplenomegaly in whose bone marrow foam cells (see figure in Ch. 776, part B) are present. From the appearance of the cells Gaucher's disease can be excluded but the diagnosis of Niemann-Pick disease cannot be made. Indistinguishable foam cells occur with severe hyperglyceridemia and many other lysosomal enzyme deficiencies. The next diagnostic step should be the culture of skin or marrow fibroblasts for assay of sphingomyelinase. When the assay is appropriately controlled, sphingomyelinase activity between 0 and 20 per cent of normal permits a presumptive diagnosis. Distinction between type A and type B rests on frequent observation for development of neurologic abnormalities. Niemann-Pick disease is also detectable prenatally by enzyme assays of fetal cells grown from amniotic fluid. Separation of types A and B in utero can only be presumed from phenotype of a previously affected sib. No certain test exists for diagnosis of the heterozygotes.

Indeterminate Forms of Sphingomyelin Storage. When the patient has unexplained hepatosplenomegaly and marrow foam cells and the tissue assay for sphingomyelinase is normal or slightly deficient, open liver biopsy is advisable. Tissue must be kept frozen without fixatives for chemical and enzymatic analyses. Careful morphologic examination is also advisable, but neither light nor electron microscopy is capable of distinguishing between most of the lipid storage diseases. Exhaustive analyses of the concentrations of phospholipids, neutral lipids, and glycolipids, in combination with assay of various lysosomal hydrolases and other appropriate enzymes, must be carried out.

In a number of patients an increase of only one- to twofold in sphingomyelin and cholesterol has been detected. These are usually children who have appeared normal for one or more years before moderate hepatosplenomegaly is noted. Later neurologic abnormalities appear; these may include seizures, behavioral disorders, and mental retardation. Frequently such abnormalities are familial and have been referred to as chronic neuronopathic forms of Niemann-Pick disease. If the sphingomyelinase activity is modestly decreased, such patients have been referred to as Niemann-Pick disease, Type C, or as Type D for a similar disorder occurring in related patients of Nova Scotian ancestry. They may possibly represent other mutations affecting sphingomyelinase, but probably they and other similar phenotypes in which the enzyme activity is unequivocally normal represent other undetermined lysosomal enzyme deficiencies in which sphingomyelin metabolism is only incidentally affected.

Treatment.   There is no specific treatment for any of the sphingomyelin storage disorders. Chronic administration of sphingomyelinase has not been attempted. Because phospholipid storage leads to excessive lipid peroxidation and ceroid pigment deposition in tissues, long-term administration of an antioxidant, such as vitamin E, has been empirically recommended.

Brady, R. O., and King, F.: Niemann-Pick Disease. *In* Hers, H. G., and Van Hoof, F. (eds.): Lysosomes and Storage Diseases. New York, Academic Press, 1973, pp. 439–452.

Crocker, A. C., and Farber, S.: Niemann-Pick disease: A review of 18 patients. Medicine, 37:1, 1958.

Fredrickson, D. S., and Sloan, H. R.: Phosphorylcholine ceramidoses: Niemann-Pick disease. *In* Stanbury, J. B., Wyngaarden, J. B., and Fredrickson, D. S. (eds.): The Metabolic Basis of Inherited Disease. 3rd ed. New York, McGraw-Hill Book Company, 1972, pp. 783–807.

Section Twelve. PLASMA CELL DYSCRASIAS

Elliott F. Osserman

778. INTRODUCTION

Definition and Terminology. The term "plasma cell dyscrasia" is employed to encompass the wide range of pathologic conditions and biochemical abnormalities considered to represent unbalanced proliferative disorders of the cells that normally synthesize gamma (immuno-) globulins. The extent of the proliferative abnormality in the various plasma cell dyscrasias ranges from apparently autonomous, malignant proliferation (neoplasia) in typical multiple myeloma to apparently benign and stable dyscrasias manifested principally by their associated gamma globulin abnormalities. The plasma cell dyscrasias are characterized by (1) the proliferation of plasma cells in the absence of an identifiable antigenic stimulus; (2) elaboration of electrophoretically and structurally homogeneous, monoclonal, "M-type" (myeloma, macroglobulinemia) gamma globulins and/or excessive quantities of comparably homogeneous polypeptide subunits of these proteins, i.e., Bence Jones proteins, H-chains; and (3) commonly, an associated deficiency in the synthesis of normal immunoglobulins.

The major clinical patterns associated with plasma cell dyscrasia are listed in Table 1. Certain of these categories, such as myeloma, macroglobulinemia, amyloidosis, and heavy chain diseases, have sufficiently well defined clinical patterns to permit precise diagnostic classification. With increasing use of electrophoresis, however, many cases of M-type gamma globulin abnormalities are being found that apparently do not represent typical plasma cell myeloma or primary Waldenström's macroglobulinemia at the time of initial study. The fact that some of these patients ultimately develop

TABLE 1. Plasma Cell Dyscrasias

Clinically overt forms, with distinctive clinical and pathologic features:
  Plasma cell myeloma (multiple myeloma, myelomatosis, "solitary" and multiple plasmocytomas, plasma cell leukemia)
  Waldenström's (primary) macroglobulinemia
  γ Heavy chain (Franklin's) disease
  α Heavy chain (Seligmann's) disease (abdominal "lymphoma")
  μ Heavy chain disease
  Amyloidosis (Pattern I and Mixed Pattern I and II amyloidosis)
  Lichen myxedematosus (papular mucinosis, lichen amyloidosus)

Clinically occult (asymptomatic or presymptomatic) forms
  Plasma cell dyscrasia of unknown significance (PCDUS)
    Associated with chronic inflammatory and infectious processes, e.g., osteomyelitis, tuberculosis, chronic biliary tract disease, pyelonephritis, rheumatoid arthritis, chronic pyoderma, etc.
    Associated with nonreticular neoplasms, particularly cancers of the bowel, biliary tract and breast
    Associated with lipodystrophies, particularly Gaucher's disease, familial hypercholesteremia, and xanthomatosis
  Transient plasma cell dyscrasias
    Associated with drug hypersensitivity, sulfonamides
    Associated with (presumed) viral infections
    Associated with cardiac surgery: valve prosthesis

clinically typical myeloma or macroglobulinemia is well documented, but there are many cases (of the order of 20 to 30 per cent of patients with M-type gamma globulin abnormalities) that almost certainly do not belong in the diagnostic categories of myeloma or primary macroglobulinemia. Various designations have been given to these cases, including premyeloma, essential hyperglobulinemia, essential benign hyperglobulinemia, essential macroglobulinemia, idiopathic or essential cryoglobulinemia, the dysgammaglobulinemic syndromes, idiopathic or essential monoclonal gammopathy, paraimmunonoglobulinopathy, and others. The probable inaccuracies of all these terms are evident.

It is recommended that the inclusive term "plasma cell dyscrasia" be used, modified by the clinical pattern, e.g., myeloma, Waldenström's macroglobulinemia, or amyloidosis, when this is overt and evident. When no recognizable clinical pattern is associated with the finding of an M-type protein, the condition is classified as a plasma cell dyscrasia of unknown significance, because the ultimate course is not presently predictable. However, many, if not all, of the diagnostic categories listed in Table 1 overlap. Thus either amyloidosis can be the predominant feature of a plasma cell dyscrasia, in which case the diagnosis of "primary amyloidosis" is commonly, although inappropriately, applied, or the amyloid infiltrates can occur in association with otherwise typical myeloma. Also, a given case can progress from an asymptomatic status, i.e., plasma cell dyscrasia of unknown significance, to symptomatic myeloma, macroglobulinemia, amyloidosis, and so forth. Accordingly, the categories listed in Table 1 are tentative and somewhat indefinite diagnostic groupings in many instances.

In a significant percentage of cases the finding of an M-type protein abnormality is associated with another chronic disease such as recurrent cholecystitis and cholelithiasis, a chronic infection (particularly tuberculosis), or a nonreticular neoplasm (particularly rectosigmoid and biliary carcinoma). *These associations may not be coincidental,* but may represent plasma cell dyscrasias related to and possibly induced by these diverse chronic reticuloendothelial stimuli. For this reason, it is considered useful to document the associations by designations such as "plasma cell dyscrasia associated with chronic biliary tract disease" or "plasma cell dyscrasia associated with adenocarcinoma of the rectosigmoid."

Pathogenesis of Plasma Cell Dyscrasias. Although the etiologic factors responsible for production of plasma cell dyscrasias in man are still unknown, it is possible that some clues may have been provided by studies of experimental plasma cell tumors in mice. These studies have established the importance of genetic factors with the demonstration of the particular susceptibility of the inbred C_3H mouse strain and the F^1 hybrids of CBA $\times$ DBA/2 mice to develop plasma cell tumors spontaneously. In an effort to document genetic factors, chromosome studies have been carried out in several of these murine tumors as well as in human myeloma and macroglobulinemia, but thus far no consistent karyo-typic abnormalities have been documented.

The *interdependence of genetic and carcinogenic mechanisms* is apparent in the interesting group of experimental *plasma cell tumors* that have been induced in BALB/c strain mice. A variety of plasma cell neoplasms can be induced in this strain by the intraperitoneal implantation of plastics, mineral oil–adjuvant mixtures, and mineral oil alone. The importance of genetic mechanisms is evident from the particular susceptibility of the BALB/c strain to develop plasma cell tumors in response to these forms of chronic peritoneal (reticuloendothelial) irritation. Significantly, strain C₃H mice, which develop spontaneous plasma cell tumors, are *not susceptible* to the induction of these tumors by intraperitoneal adjuvants and the like. With many other experimental tumors the intimate interaction of genetic factors, oncogenic viruses, and chemical and physical carcinogens has been established.

Cytology. The synthesis of specific proteins is the principal and probably the sole function of plasma cells. The abundant cytoplasmic RNA is responsible for the characteristic basophilia and pyroninophilia of plasma cells, and the highly developed Golgi apparatus is responsible for the typical paranuclear "halo" or clear zone. Electron microscopy of plasma cells has shown that the cytoplasmic RNA is organized in the form of granules (ribosomes) attached to a highly developed network of endoplasmic reticulum. All these structural features have now been related to the complex functions of protein synthesis and secretion. The nucleus of the plasma cell with its characteristically clumped chromatin (DNA) contains the genetic information that determines the structure of the protein to be synthesized. The synthesis of ribosomal RNA is carried out on DNA localized in the nucleolus. Messenger RNA's, which determine the structure of the specific proteins to be synthesized on these ribosomes, are derived from the nonnucleolar DNA's.

The different classes of immunoglobulins are probably synthesized by different cells. The possibility that a single cell may under certain conditions synthesize two types of immunoglobulins (e.g., IgG and IgM) either simultaneously or sequentially has not been excluded, but most studies have indicated the synthesis of only one type of immunoglobulin by a single cell. Immunohistochemical studies, using fluorescein-labeled antisera specific for each of the immunoglobulin groups, have generally shown IgG globulin synthesis in typical, mature, Marshalko-type plasma cells. IgA globulin has been localized in cells with relatively more abundant and vacuolated cytoplasm but still having the major features of plasma cells; IgM synthesis has been related to a population of somewhat smaller cells with proportionately less cytoplasm. These cells have been variously classified as lymphocytoid-plasma cells, plasmacytoid-lymphocytes, atypical plasma cells, and atypical lymphocytes.

Typical, ovoid plasma cells with eccentric nuclei, clumped chromatin, prominent nucleoli, paranuclear halo, and basophilic cytoplasm are widely distributed in lymph nodes, spleen, marrow, intestinal wall, and other tissues and organs. They constitute less than 5 per cent of the normal bone marrow population but increase significantly in association with infection, sensitivity reactions (particularly serum sickness), collagen diseases,

cirrhosis, parasitism, and certain neoplasms. In these conditions, the increase in plasma cells includes both "typical" and "atypical" forms (including multinucleated cells and cells with prominent nucleoli), and there are *no reliable morphologic criteria to distinguish these reactive plasmacytic populations from the cells that are found in the plasma cell dyscrasias.*

Normal Immunoglobulins and the Paraproteins of the Plasma Cell Dyscrasias. Figure 1 is a schematic summary of the present working hypothesis relating the synthesis of individual gamma globulin molecules (1, 2, 3, 4 . . . n) to specific plasmacytic clones. The normally broad, polydispersed serum gamma globulin peak represents the balanced synthesis of small quantities of a very large and presently indeterminate number (n) of individual and specific gamma globulin molecules by specific plasma cell populations. Normally, most of the proteins synthesized by these cells are complete immunoglobulin molecules, and there is only a small quantity of incomplete polypeptide subunits elaborated. These incomplete proteins, designated "gamma-u," are low molecular weight constituents (M.W. 20,000 to 25,000) and closely resemble Bence Jones proteins. Because of their small molecular size, gamma-u polypeptides are rapidly excreted by the kidney. Normally, 20 to 40 mg of gamma-u is excreted per 24 hours.

A plasma cell dyscrasia is considered to represent the excessive proliferation of a single clone of plasma cells, resulting in the synthesis of large quantities of a single protein related to one of the major classes of immunoglobulins and/or the synthesis of excessive quantities of a constituent polypeptide subunit of one of these proteins, usually of the Bence Jones type.

The proteins elaborated in the plasma cell dyscrasias have been shown to be very closely related and structurally similar to the normal immunoglobulins. As large quantities of these single proteins are synthesized in the plasma cell dyscrasias, they are more suitable for structural studies than the heterogeneous and polydispersed normal immunoglobulins. Significantly, much of our present knowledge regarding the structure and properties of normal immunoglobulins has been obtained from studies of the M-type paraproteins.

The biochemical and physiologic properties of the presently recognized immunoglobulins, IgG, IgA, IgD, IgE and IgM globulins, are presented in Ch. 60. In typical multiple myeloma, approximately 70 per cent of the serum "spikes" are IgG, 28 per cent are IgA, and 2 per cent are IgD. There have been only three cases of IgE myeloma reported to date. Bence Jones proteins, which represent free light chains, are elaborated in large quantities and excreted in the urine in approximately 50 per cent of cases of myeloma. Bence Jones proteins have molecular weights in the range of 20,000 to 25,000 but are commonly excreted as disulfide-bonded dimers. In any given case of plasma cell dyscrasia with Bence Jones proteinuria, the Bence Jones protein is *either* Type κ *or* Type λ, in contrast to excretion of small quantities of *both* Type κ and Type λ constituents in normal urine. In those cases of plasma cell dyscrasia in which there is a synthesis of both an M-type serum paraprotein and a Bence Jones–type protein, the Bence Jones protein is apparently identical to the constituent light chains of the corresponding serum paraprotein. This evidence is interpreted as indicating that a portion of the abnormal cells has retained the capacity to elaborate

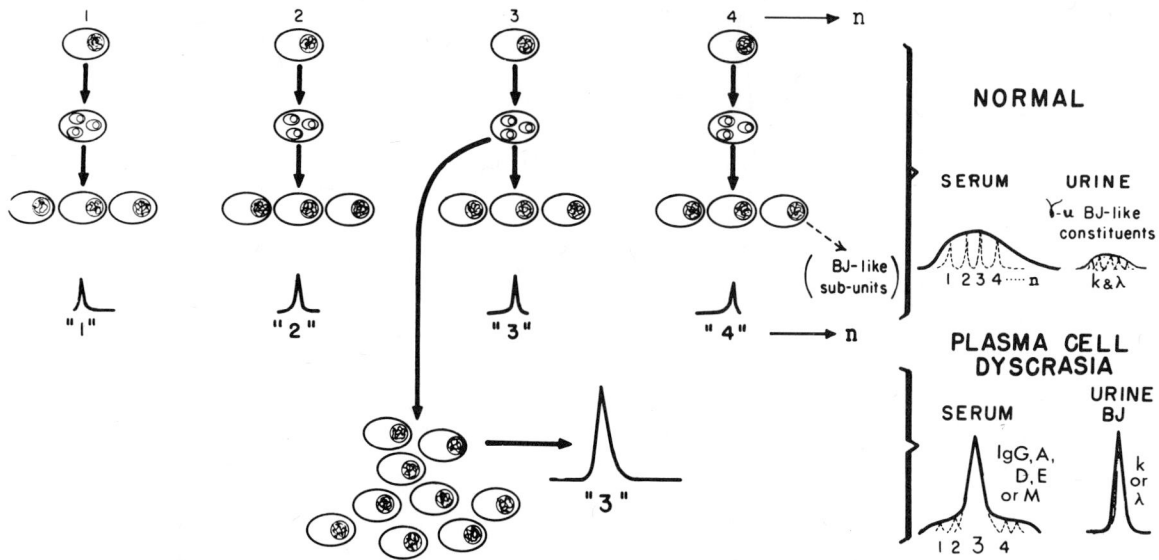

Figure 1. Schematic representation of the clonal hypothesis of immunoglobulin synthesis and the derangements in protein synthesis associated with plasma cell dyscrasias.

complete molecules with light and heavy chains, whereas others are capable of synthesizing only one of the constituent polypeptide subunits, i.e., light chains.

A fundamental question that remains unanswered is whether the proteins elaborated in the plasma cell dyscrasias are truly abnormal or whether they are, in fact, functional antibodies elaborated in great quantitative excess as a consequence of the proliferative abnormality. An increasing body of evidence obtained in recent years lends support to the latter hypothesis. Thus many human and mouse myeloma proteins and macroglobulins have been found to interact with a variety of synthetic haptens, polysaccharides, lipids, and bacterial antigens. The present consensus is that some of these reactions are probably cross-reactions between these proteins and antigens which are structurally related but not identical to the true antigens. Investigations are presently underway to identify the true antigens to which the myeloma proteins are directed, and this will unquestionably shed light on the pathogenic mechanisms responsible for plasma cell dyscrasias in man.

Electrophoretic Patterns of Serum and Urinary Proteins in the Plasma Cell Dyscrasias. As a result of the more general use of electrophoresis, increasing numbers of cases of plasma cell dyscrasia are being documented by the electrophoretic demonstration of M-type serum or urinary protein abnormalities, or both. These M-type abnormalities (see Figs. 3 and 4) are best appreciated by comparison with the patterns of normal serum and urine and the serum in certain disease states affecting the reticuloendothelial system generally (Fig. 2). The electrophoretic analyses illustrated were performed by the Spinco cellulose acetate method, which has certain advantages over filter paper techniques. For diagnostic purposes, the *contours of electrophoretic patterns are more significant* than the precise quantitation of individual peaks. A careful appraisal of the contours of each peak, particularly distinguishing a diffuse gamma elevation from an M-type spike, in conjunction with a rough

quantitative comparison of the patient's serum albumin, alpha-1, alpha-2, beta, and gamma globulins with a normal serum pattern will yield most of the clinically important information offered by this method.

In Figure 2, the normal serum pattern shows the characteristically broad contour of the major slow gamma peak, sometimes referred to as gamma-2, and a small secondary peak in the fast gamma region (between gamma and beta), which at times is designated gamma-1. The gamma-1 peak is detectable by cellulose acetate electrophoresis in most but not all normal sera. It is not resolved as a distinct peak by filter paper electrophoresis. The gamma-1 peak has been related to the faster migrating IgA and IgM globulins.

The electrophoretic pattern of the normal urinary proteins in Figure 2 shows albumin to be the major constituent, with lesser quantities of alpha, beta, and gamma globulins. Because of the extremely low concentration of protein in normal urine, the sample must be concentrated 50- to 100-fold by dialysis against 25 per cent dextran or polyvinylpyrollidone (PVP) prior to electrophoresis. As in the case of serum proteins, the clinically important abnormal urinary proteins are detected as changes in the contours of the pattern and the relative concentrations of albumin and proteins of alpha, beta, and gamma mobility. Serial quantitation of 24-hour urinary protein excretion is useful for evaluating therapy but is not of particular importance diagnostically.

As illustrated in the lower patterns in Figure 2, the general suppression of plasmacytic function associated with the congenital and acquired forms of hypogammaglobulinemia is reflected in a *broad decrease* in gamma globulin, and, conversely, the generalized hyperactivity of the reticulendothelial system associated with certain chronic infections, cirrhosis, collagen diseases, etc., is reflected in a *broad elevation* of gamma globulin. The pattern illustrating a diffuse hypergammaglobulinemia shows an elevation of the slow, major gamma (gamma-2) peak owing to an increase in IgG

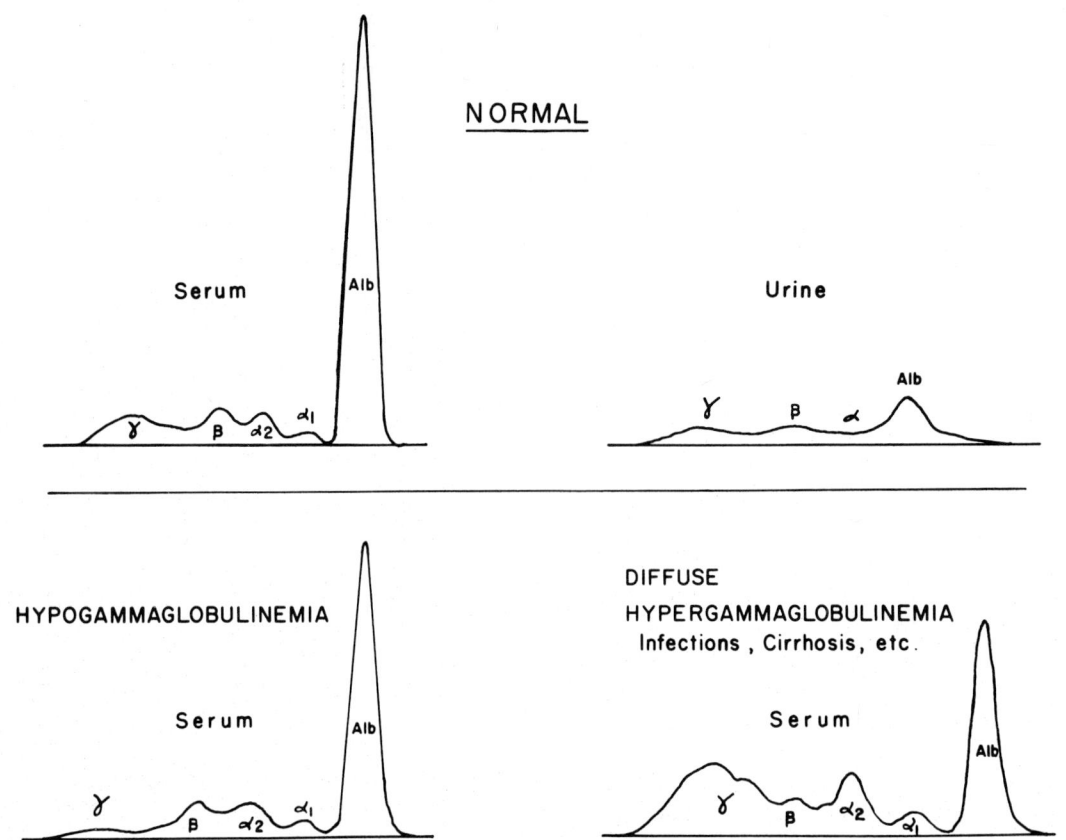

Figure 2.   Representative electrophoretic patterns (Spinco, cellulose acetate system). *Top,* Normal serum and normal urinary proteins (concentrated 50×). *Bottom left,* Hypogammaglobulinemia (adult, idiopathic). *Bottom right,* Diffuse hypergammaglobulinemia.

globulins, and also an increase in the fast gamma (gamma-1) peak, reflecting an increase in IgA and IgM globulins.

The M-type serum and urinary protein abnormalities observed in myeloma, macroglobulinemia, and the other plasma cell dyscrasias are illustrated in Figures 3 and 4. In Figure 3, three sets of serum and urinary patterns from three cases of myeloma illustrate different combinations of abnormalities. Bence Jones proteinuria was present in all three cases of myeloma and was confirmed by the classic heat precipitation and re-solution at 90 to 100° C. Because of their small molecular size, the Bence Jones proteins are rapidly excreted, and their serum concentration is usually too low to be detected by conventional electrophoretic methods. Urine electrophoresis, however, demonstrates the Bence Jones proteins to have the same relative homogeneity as the myeloma serum globulins and electrophoretic mobilities, ranging from slow gamma through beta and into the alpha-2 mobility range. Urine electrophoresis is a more reliable method for the detection of Bence Jones proteins than the usual heat-precipitation procedure. *The finding in the urine of an electrophoretically homogeneous M-type component of gamma, beta, or alpha-2 mobility present in a concentration exceeding that of albumin indicates that the protein has a molecular size smaller than albumin (M.W. 70,000).* This is strong evidence in favor of Bence Jones proteinuria and can generally be confirmed by precipitation at 55 to 60° C and re-solution at 90 to 100° C *if the pH is carefully ad-*

justed to 4.5 to 5.0. False negative reactions will be obtained if inadequate attention is given to pH adjustment.

In the case of myeloma illustrated in Figure 3A the serum pattern shows a large, electrophoretically homogeneous peak of slow gamma mobility, and the urine pattern shows a large, abnormal M-type peak with a somewhat faster (more anodally positioned) mobility than the serum M-type peak. The lack of correspondence in mobilities of the serum and urinary proteins establishes their *nonidentity.* Immunoelectrophoretically, the serum protein was identified as an IgG globulin and the urinary protein as a Type κ Bence Jones constituent.

In Figure *3B,* the serum shows a small abnormal peak of slow gamma mobility and an obvious decrease in normal gamma globulin. The urine shows a very large abnormal peak of slow gamma mobility and a minimal amount of albumin. The serum and urinary proteins were both identified immunoelectrophoretically as Type λ Bence Jones protein. Bence Jones protein*emia* is usually not detectable by conventional electrophoresis, although it is almost always demonstrable by the more sensitive technique of immunoelectrophoresis when Bence Jones proteinuria is present.

In Figure 3C, the serum pattern shows two overlapping abnormal peaks of fast gamma (gamma-1) and beta mobility. The urine pattern has an abnormal beta peak along with significant quantities of albumin. In occasional cases of myeloma and other plasma cell dyscrasias, double peaks are found in serum patterns. Most frequently these have been shown to be due to an unusually high concentration of Bence Jones protein in the serum along with an M-type IgG or IgA globulin. Rarely, two distinct globulins or an IgG *and* an IgA or IgM globulin are found in the serum of a patient with a plasma cell dyscrasia. It is presumed that these double peaks indicate the simultaneous proliferation of more than one plasmacytic clone. In Figure 3C, the two serum peaks were immunoelectrophoretically identified, respectively, as IgA globulin and a Type λ Bence Jones protein. The abnormal urinary protein was identified as the same Type λ Bence Jones constituent present in the serum. There was no detectable IgA globulin in the urine.

In Figure 3D the serum and urinary patterns from a case of primary (Waldenström's) macroglobulinemia are illustrated. The serum has an M-type peak of slow gamma mobility indistinguishable from the IgG abnor-

mality illustrated in Figure 3A. Definitive identification of the abnormal protein as an IgM globulin in this as in all cases of macroglobulinemia was accomplished only by immunoelectrophoretic and ultracentrifugal analyses. The urinary protein pattern revealed nonspecific proteinuria with albumin as the predominant constituent. The virtual absence of the IgM globulin from the urine is noteworthy. Bence Jones proteinuria occurs in a smaller percentage (10 to 20 per cent) of cases of macroglobulinemia than of myeloma (50 to 60 per cent).

Serum and urinary electrophoretic patterns from plasma cell dyscrasias other than typical myeloma and macroglobulinemia are illustrated in Figure 4. The patterns in Figure 4A are from a case of generalized amyloidosis with predominant involvement of the tongue, heart, and gastrointestinal tract, classified as "Pattern I amyloidosis." There were no detectable skeletal lesions, but plasma cell dyscrasia was indicated by the finding of Bence Jones proteinuria,

Figure 3. Serum and urinary protein patterns in three cases of multiple myeloma (*A*, *B*, and *C*), each with an M-type protein abnormality in the serum and Bence Jones proteinuria. *D*, Macroglobulinemia with nonspecific proteinuria.

Figure 4. Representative electrophoretic patterns in plasma cell dyscrasias. *A*, Plasma cell dyscrasia and amyloidosis of "Pattern I" distribution with a characteristic Bence Jones–type abnormality in the urine pattern. *B*, γ Heavy chain (Fc fragment) disease with corresponding serum and urinary M-type peaks of β mobility. *C* and *D*, Asymptomatic plasma cell dyscrasias with a small (*C*) and a large (*D*) M-type serum peak. *E*, Plasma cell dyscrasia associated with an adenocarcinoma of the rectosigmoid colon. *F*, Plasma cell dyscrasia associated with chronic and recurrent cholecystitis and cholelithiasis.

and was confirmed by the finding on marrow aspiration of abnormal numbers of plasma cells. The abnormal urinary protein was immunoelectrophoretically identified as a Type λ Bence Jones constituent. The serum pattern shows an elevated alpha-2 globulin and a decreased gamma globulin, without an M-type peak.

In Figure 4*B*, the serum and urinary proteins from a case of γ heavy chain (Fc fragment) disease are shown. The protein elaborated in this conditon has been characterized as representing the major portion (Fc fragment) of the IgG H-chain with a molecular weight in the range of 50,000 to 55,000. Because these proteins are relatively larger than Bence Jones proteins, their renal clearance rate is relatively lower, and they are retained in the serum in sufficiently high concentrations to be detectable by conventional electrophoretic analysis. The abnormal serum and urinary protein peaks are of identical mobility and electrophoretically somewhat more polydispersed than the abnormal peaks in the

other plasma cell dyscrasias. The urinary protein pattern, however, is indistinguishable from the patterns observed with Bence Jones proteinuria, and identification of the abnormal protein as related to the IgG heavy chain and unrelated to Bence Jones proteins and light chains must be accomplished by appropriate immunochemical and physicochemical studies.

The serum electrophoretic patterns illustrated in Figures 4*C* and 4*D* are from two cases in which M-type protein abnormalities were discovered in the absence of overt signs or symptoms of myeloma, macroglobulinemia, or any other recognizable disease. These cases are classified as "plasma cell dyscrasia of unknown significance." As will be noted subsequently, the clinical and pathologic significance of protein abnormalities of this type are presently still obscure. In some cases, progression to overt forms of plasma cell dyscrasia, such as myeloma, has been documented, but in many cases the protein abonormality has been found to persist for as long as 20 years without the development of clinically recognizable disease. Rarely, protein abnormalities of this type have been found on subsequent analyses to have disappeared—i.e., transient paraproteinemias—and these almost certainly represent examples of the synthesis of excessively large quantities of functional antibodies.

The M-type gamma globulin abnormalities illustrated in Figures 4E and 4F were found in association with clinical conditions that may have been related to the development of plasma cell dyscrasias, notably an adenocarcinoma of the rectosigmoid with an intense plasmacytic infiltration surrounding the tumor and in the resected nodes (Fig. 4E), and chronic and recurrent cholecystitis and cholelithiasis with extensive plasmacytosis in the gallbladder wall and along the biliary tract (Fig. 4F). Until a direct relationship is established between these conditions and the plasma cell dyscrasias, their association must be considered coincidental, but the relative frequency of these associations warrants the search for an occult neoplasm or biliary tract disease in patients found to have asymptomatic M-type gamma globulin abnormalities.

Edelman, G. M.: The antibody problem. Ann. Rev. Biochem., 38:415, 1969.

Metzger, H. M.: Editorial. Myeloma proteins and antibodies. Am. J. Med., 47:837, 1969.

Osserman, E. F., and Takatsuki, K.: Considerations regarding the pathogenesis of the plasmacytic dyscrasias. Scand. J. Haemat., 4 (Suppl.): 28, 1964.

Potter, M.: Antigen binding M-components in man and mouse. In Azar, H. A., and Potter, M. (eds.): Multiple Myeloma and Related Disorders. Vol. I. Hagerstown, Md., Harper & Row, 1973, p. 195.

Potter, M.: The developmental history of the neoplastic plasma cells in mice. Semin. Hematol., 10:19, 1973.

Putnam, F. W.: Immunoglobulin structure: Variability and homology. Science, 163:633, 1969.

Seligmann, M., and Brouet, J. C.: Antibody activity of human myeloma globulins. Semin. Hematol., 10:163, 1973.

Solomon, A., and McLaughlin, C. O.: Immunoglobulin structure determined from products of plasma cell neoplasms. Semin. Hematol., 10:3, 1973.

CLINICAL PATTERNS OF THE PLASMA CELL DYSCRASIAS

779. MULTIPLE MYELOMA
(Plasma Cell Myeloma, Myelomatosis)

Multiple myeloma is generally defined as a neoplasm of plasma cells manifested primarily by widespread skeletal destruction and frequently associated with anemia, hypercalcemia, renal functional impairment, and increased susceptibility to infections. Amyloidosis, coagulation defects, and symptoms and signs related to cryoglobulins or increased serum viscosity are less commonly associated manifestations. Diagnosis depends upon the roentgenographic demonstration of diffuse osteolytic lesions and/or osteoporosis, documentation of increased numbers of plasma cells in the marrow, and the finding of M-type serum or urinary proteins.

The frequency of myeloma has apparently increased in recent years and now is comparable to that of Hodgkin's disease in many large clinics. Improved diagnostic techniques are unquestionably partly responsible for the apparent increase. Males and females are approximately equally affected. The age of onset of symptoms ranges from young adulthood to advanced years, the peak incidence being in the mid-fifties.

The symptomatic stage of myeloma is preceded by a significant asymptomatic or presymptomatic period in most, and perhaps all, cases. In this presymptomatic period, M-type serum and/or urinary proteins are demonstrable and are usually first suggested by the finding on routine examination of an increased erythrocyte sedimentation rate or unexplained and persistent proteinuria. Because intravenous pyelography may precipitate renal shutdown in the presence of Bence Jones proteinuria, the increased hazard of the procedure should be considered in planning the investigation of a case with unexplained proteinuria. The duration of the presymptomatic period in myeloma is impossible to define, but apparently can range up to 20 years. Repeated bacterial infections, particularly pneumonias, can occur during this period, presumably as a consequence of impaired immunologic mechanisms.

When myeloma becomes symptomatic, skeletal pains are the presenting and predominant manifestations in most cases. These may at first be mild and transient, or their onset may be sudden with severe back, rib, or extremity pain after an abrupt movement or effort. The abrupt onset of pain frequently indicates a pathologic fracture. With progression of the disease, more and more areas of bone destruction develop, frequently resulting in marked skeletal deformities, particularly of the sternum and rib cage, and shortening of the spine with as much as 5 or more inches decrease in stature. With earlier diagnosis and more effective chemotherapy and general management, these extreme degrees of skeletal deformity have become less common.

In most cases, multiple osteolytic ("punched-out") lesions are apparent on initial roentgenographic examination (Fig. 5). The skull, spine, ribs, clavicles, sternum, pelvis, and proximal long bones exhibit the greatest destruction, but any part of the skeleton, including the phalanges, may be involved.

In many cases, the initial roentgenographic appearance of the skeleton is that of diffuse osteoporosis without discrete osteolytic lesions. Histologic studies demonstrate a diffuse infiltration of the marrow spaces by myeloma cells, with generalized thinning of trabeculae not detectable by standard roentgenographic techniques. Virtually all patients with this initial pattern of diffuse osteoporosis eventually develop osteolytic lesions as the disease progresses. Possibly the rarest finding in myeloma is an osteoblastic reaction in the absence of a pathologic fracture; there are now several reported examples of this.

In occasional cases, myeloma presents as an *apparently single* skeletal lesion. Although these lesions are commonly designated as solitary plasmacytomas, most patients ultimately develop disseminated disease even if the original lesion is radically excised or irradiated. In cases of apparently solitary plasmacytomas, M-type protein abnormalities are almost invariably demonstrable.

Figure 5.   Characteristic x-ray abnormalities in multiple myeloma. Skull (left) shows multiple osteolytic ("punched-out") lesions. Thoracic spine (right) shows extensive osteoporosis and partial collapse of several vertebral bodies.

Skeletal destruction results in the release of bone salts, negative calcium balance, and hypercalciuria in virtually all cases. This is generally well tolerated if adequate hydration is maintained. Hypercalcemia ensues, however, if the renal excretory capacity for calcium is exceeded, usually as a consequence of inadequate hydration and diminished urine output. All too frequently, there develops a menacing sequence of hypercalciuria → osmotic diuresis + impairment of renal tubular reabsorption → dehydration → diminished urine output → hypercalcemia + azotemia → anorexia, nausea, vomiting, and further dehydration. This set of circumstances constitutes a major threat requiring prompt therapeutic intervention with rehydration as the primary goal. Prednisone is a useful adjunct in the management of hypercalcemia, but other chemotherapy is contraindicated until hydration is accomplished and renal function restored.

In occasional cases, particularly those of diffuse osteoporosis rather than local skeletal destruction, the initial symptoms are the nonspecific gastrointestinal complaints related to hypercalcemia and the polyuria and polydipsia secondary to hypercalciuria.

Anemia of variable severity is present in virtually all cases, either at the time of diagnosis or developing subsequently as the disease progresses. It may remain moderate (hemoglobin in the range of 7 to 10 grams) and be well tolerated or become severe enough to require repeated transfusions. The anemia is usually normocytic and normochromic, but may be macrocytic. It is characteristically refractory to iron, vitamin B_{12}, folic acid, and liver therapy. In occasional cases a hypochromic anemia may be related to blood loss from the gastrointestinal tract, to a defect in coagulation, or to plasmacytic or amyloid infiltrates of the intestinal wall. Several factors participate in the production of anemia in myeloma, including marrow replacement, accelerated erythrocyte destruction, blood loss, renal insufficiency, the effects of radiotherapy and chemotherapy, associated infections, and nutritional factors.

Erythrocyte rouleau formation is observed in peripheral blood and marrow films, and in vivo erythrocyte aggregation ("sludged blood") is often demonstrable. This aggregation is probably due to erythrocyte coating by M-type proteins and may contribute to shortened red cell life span. Coombs reactions, however, are usually negative.

Leukocyte and platelet counts are usually within normal limits prior to cytotoxic therapy. Occasionally, however, moderate to severe leukopenia or thrombocytopenia may be observed prior to treatment and, indeed, with therapy, the white cell and platelet counts may rise toward normal. Thrombocytopenia may contribute to a bleeding diathesis and leukopenia to an increased susceptibility to infection. The precise mechanisms responsible for leukopenia and thrombocytopenia in the plasma cell dyscrasias are unknown. The differential white cell count frequently reveals a relative lymphocytosis (40 to 55 per cent) with a variable proportion of immature lymphocytic and plasmacytic forms. Plasma cells in the peripheral blood have been reported in up to 70 per cent of cases. An outpouring of plasma cells into the peripheral blood is occasionally seen in the later stages of disease, and is considered to represent a displacement phenomenon.

A clinical pattern consistent with a diagnosis of plasma cell leukemia, with hepatosplenomegaly and white cell counts in excess of 15,000 and over 50 per cent plasma cells, is occasionally observed, with weakness, anemia, and bleeding manifestations. In the peripheral blood the cells range from typical plasmacytes to immature and atypical forms. Bence Jones proteinuria and abnormal serum globulins occur with the same frequency as in myeloma. The majority of these cases pursue an acute or subacute clinical course. It is of interest that two known cases of IgE myeloma exhibited the clinical pattern of plasma cell leukemia.

Eosinophilia, with eosinophil counts as high as 15 to 25 per cent, is observed in occasional cases of myeloma and somewhat more commonly in macroglobulinemia and γ heavy chain disease. The significance of eosinophilia in these diseases is unknown.

Marked elevation of the erythrocyte sedimentation rate (ESR) is found in most cases of myeloma. When the M-type serum proteins are cold precipitable (cryoglobulins), the ESR may be markedly temperature dependent, i.e., slower at room temperature or in the cold and accelerated when performed at 37° C.

Pathologic Effects of M-type Serum Globulins and Bence Jones Proteins. Each M-type protein must be recognized to be individually specific and to possess specific physiochemical properties, such as solubility, intrinsic viscosity, thermostability, and reactivity with other proteins. Certain of these properties can be correlated with specific clinical and pathologic manifestations. Thus coagulation defects are related in certain cases to the interaction (protein:protein complexing) of specific M-type IgG or IgA globulins with specific coagulation factors, including fibrinogen, factors V, VII, prothrombin, and the antihemophilic globulin. Another group of protein-related symptoms are those produced by M-type IgG globulins which are cold precipitable, i.e., cryoglobulins. These include a Raynaud-type phenomenon, circulatory impairment, and, at times, occlusion and gangrene after relatively mild exposure to cold. Circulatory impairment, particularly in the central nervous system and retina, can also be related in certain cases to IgA and IgG globulins with a high intrinsic viscosity.

An association between Bence Jones proteinuria and renal functional impairment has long been implied, and is generally ascribed to the tubular precipitation of these proteins and blockage owing to cast formation. More recently, it has been found that Bence Jones proteinuria is occasionally associated with specific defects in renal tubular reabsorption mechanisms, including the adult Fanconi syndrome, indicating that certain Bence Jones proteins have the capacity to interfere with specific tubular transport mechanisms through direct (protein:protein) interaction with tubular cytoplasmic constituents. There is no evident correlation between the antigenic type of a Bence Jones protein and its nephrotoxic potential. The fact that a nephrotoxic potential is *not* common to *all* Bence Jones proteins is indicated by the persistence of apparently normal renal function in many cases with protracted and profound Bence Jones proteinuria. This is further evidence that several factors in addition to Bence Jones proteinuria, particularly hypercalciuria and dehydration, contribute to renal dysfunction in myeloma.

Bence Jones proteins have also been implicated in the pathogenesis of amyloidosis. It is postulated that Bence Jones proteins traverse capillary beds because of their small molecular size and polymerize and/or coprecipitate with as yet unidentified tissue proteins or polysaccharides to yield the complex proteinaceous tissue infiltrates designated amyloid (see Ch. 781).

Additional Clinical Manifestations. Hyperuricemia and hyperuricosuria are observed in most cases as a result of increased turnover of nucleic acids in the proliferating cell population. Hyperuricosuria is not infrequently associated with renal functional impairment resulting from precipitation of urate crystals or stone formation, or both. The danger of increased urate excretion is particularly great in the initial stages of cytotoxic chemotherapy, and warrants special attention to the maintenance of adequate hydration and possibly therapy with allopurinol. Gouty arthropathy is a rare complication.

Neurologic manifestations may develop from direct pressure on the spinal cord, nerve roots, or cranial or peripheral nerves, or as a result of a pathologic fracture of a vertebral body or long bone. Spinal cord compression leading to weakness and ultimately paraplegia is an especially serious complication because the osteoporosis and negative calcium balance produced by the myeloma are compounded by the osteoporosis of immobilization. Again, this complication of myeloma has become less common with improved therapeutic management.

Infiltration of peripheral nerves and nerve roots by amyloid can cause peripheral neuropathies or root symptoms that are usually symmetrical and are associated with other evidence of amyloidosis such as macroglossia, cardiac manifestations, and the carpal tunnel syndrome. Rarely, polyneuropathies develop in myeloma and the other plasma cell dyscrasias without demonstrable tumor or amyloid infiltration. The pattern of these polyneuropathies is nonspecific; apparently they are similar to the polyneuropathies of obscure origin occasionally associated with other neoplastic diseases.

Myopathies involving principally proximal muscle groups are also rarely associated with myeloma and other plasma cell dyscrasias and, again, the pathogenic mechanisms are completely unknown.

An apparent increase in the incidence of nonreticular neoplasms, particularly of bowel, breast, and biliary tract carcinomas, has been noted in association with myeloma in one comprehensive postmortem study (19 per cent) and in the author's series (22 per cent).

Immunologic Deficiency. Increased susceptibility to bacterial infections, particularly pneumococcal pneumonia, exists in many cases of myeloma and is at least partially the result of an impaired capacity for antibody formation. This is generally reflected in a decrease in the serum concentration of normal IgG, IgA, and IgM immunoglobulins irrespective of the type of M-protein elaborated. The basis for these deficiencies is presently unknown, but available studies indicate that diminished production is a more significant factor than increased catabolism or loss. Herpes zoster and generalized varicella infections occur with increased frequency in myeloma and other plasma cell dyscrasias, but apparently no more so than in Hodgkin's disease and lymphosarcoma. Susceptibility to other viral infections apparently is not increased. Studies of the homograft rejection reaction have demonstrated a significant prolongation of rejection time, indicating that the immunologic deficiencies in myeloma may include cell-mediated immune mechanisms.

Treatment. Both the comfort and useful life of patients with myeloma can unquestionably be extended by proper management. The importance of *ambulation and adequate hydration* cannot be overemphasized. The constant threats of hypercalcemia, hypercalciuria, and hyperuricemia necessitate continual attention to these cardinal aspects of general care. Many patients are immobilized and bedridden with pain when first seen. In these circumstances, all effort should be made to achieve ambulation by a combination of analgesics, orthopedic supports (particularly Taylor spine bracing), and local radiotherapy, as indicated. Plasma cell tumors are characteristically radiosensitive, and x-ray therapy is of established value in the control of localized symptomatic lesions. The field of irradiation and the dosage should be limited in order to spare the marrow as much as possible. A total dose of 1200 to 1500 roentgens is usually adequate for symptomatic control and for the facilitation of ambulation. Pain relief is frequently noted after as little as 200 to 400 r. Salicylates and codeine are usually more effective analgesics for the pain of myeloma than meperidine (Demerol) or propoxyphene (Darvon). Prednisone, as previously indicated, is a useful agent in the management of hypercalcemia, but hydration sufficient to achieve a 24-hour urine output of over 1500 ml is the principal need. Unless mobilization and hydration are accomplished by these measures, it is usually impossible to maintain a patient for the time required to accomplish a remission with chemotherapy.

Of the chemotherapeutic agents presently available, melphalan (1-phenylalanine mustard, Alkeran) and cytoxan (cyclophosphamide) are the two drugs most useful in the long-term management of myeloma. When properly administered, both agents can achieve significant objective and subjective remissions in approximately 80 per cent of cases. Although both melphalan and cytoxan are alkylating agents, their precise mechanisms of action must be different, because sensitivity or resistance to one agent does not necessarily imply the corresponding sensitivity or resistance to the other. Thus the two agents can be used sequentially with an increased possibility of achieving a remission. As yet it is not known whether there is a preferential order, but melphalan is generally the first agent employed in the author's clinic. Therapy is usually initiated with an eight- to ten-day course of 8 to 10 mg per day, i.e., an initial course of 64 to 100 mg, depending upon the patient's size, hematologic status, and general condition. After this initial course, continuous maintenance therapy at a dose of 2 mg a day is instituted. It is no longer considered necessary to interrupt therapy between the initial loading dose and institution of maintenance therapy. With this dosage regimen, it may be anticipated that the peripheral leukocyte count will fall to the range of 3000 to 4000 and be maintained in this range with continued therapy. This degree of marrow suppression is tolerated without complications and provides an index of the adequacy of dosage. In some cases, a decrease in white count below 3000 necessitates reducing the maintenance dose to 1 mg per day. With cytoxan, therapy is initiated at a dosage level of 200 mg a day for seven to ten days, after which the dose is reduced to 100 mg a day for maintenance. Again, in some cases it is necessary to reduce the maintenance dose to 50 mg a day because of leukopenia or thrombocytopenia, or both. With both melphalan and cytoxan, present evidence indicates that continuous drug administration is preferable to interrupted therapy.

With chemotherapy, the objective signs of improvement include a decrease in the concentration of abnormal M-type serum globulins, decreased Bence Jones proteinuria, hematologic improvement, cessation of further skeletal destruction, and occasionally recalcification of osteolytic lesions. In some cases, it has also been found that the concentrations of normal immunoglobulins increase, and this is associated with improved resistance to bacterial infections. It should be recognized, however, that several weeks may elapse between the institution of therapy and the first signs of improvement. Because of the rapid turnover of Bence Jones proteins, a decrease in Bence Jones proteinuria is the earliest objective sign of chemotherapeutic effect, and this has been noted within one week of initiating chemotherapy. A decrease in myeloma serum globulins is usually not observed until the fourth or fifth week. The duration of the remissions which can be achieved with chemotherapy has steadily increased in the past several years; there are now many patients who have been maintained in excellent clinical and functional remission for periods of six years or more. Thus the prognosis in myeloma has greatly improved in the past several years with the introduction of these agents.

An attempt to increase skeletal density by inducing fluorosis with sodium fluoride has been made in some cases with generally equivocal results. At present, this therapy is not recommended. The maintenance of ambulation and the encouragement of exercise are equally as important in the long-term management of myeloma as in the initial phase of therapy. Patients should be encouraged to walk, swim, or engage in other forms of exercise to the extent of their ability, avoiding only those activities which involve excessive lifting and straining.

Azar, H. A., and Potter, M.: Multiple Myeloma and Related Disorders. Vol. I. Hagerstown, Md., Harper & Row, 1973.

Farhangi, M., and Osserman, E. F.: The treatment of multiple myeloma. Semin. Hematol., 10:149, 1973.

Korst, D. R., Clifford, G. O., Fowler, W. M., Louis, J., Will, J., and Wilson, H. E.: Multiple myeloma. II. Analysis of cyclophosphamide therapy in 165 patients. J.A.M.A., 189:758, 1964.

Osserman, E. F.: Plasma-cell myeloma: II. Clinical aspects. N. Engl. J. Med., 261:952, 1006, 1959.

Snapper, I., and Kahn, A.: Myelomatosis: Fundamental and Clinical Features. Basel, S. Karger, 1971.

Waldenström, J.: Diagnosis and Treatment of Multiple Myeloma. New York, Grune & Stratton, 1970.

780. MACROGLOBULINEMIA
(Primary or Waldenström's Macroglobulinemia)

Macroglobulinemia is presently classified as a plasma cell dyscrasia involving those cell populations normally responsible for the synthesis of IgM globulins. The excessive proliferation of these cells results in the elaboration of large quantities of electrophoretically homogeneous (M-type) IgM globulins and a variable clinical pattern with anemia, bleeding manifestations, and symptoms related to the serum macroglobulins as the predominant features. Males and females are approximately equally affected. Symptoms generally begin in the fifth or sixth decade. As the disease slowly evolves, lymphadenopathy, splenomegaly, and hepatomegaly develop in a variable percentage of cases, producing a clinical pattern resembling a malignant lymphoma or lymphatic leukemia. Skeletal lesions of the type seen in myeloma are exceptionally rare.

Histologic studies of lymph nodes demonstrate a proliferation of lymphocytic-plasmacytic forms often arranged in a pattern of follicular hyperplasia. Immunofluorescent studies have confirmed the synthesis of IgM globulin in these cells, as well as in the corresponding lymphocytic-plasmacytic forms demonstrable in peripheral blood and bone marrow preparations. It is generally impossible to ascertain whether the cellular proliferations observed in macroglobulinemia represent reactive responses or autonomous neoplasia. The possibility that initially benign and reactive proliferations may undergo transformation to neoplastic proliferations is suggested in many cases of macroglobulinemia as in other forms of plasma cell dyscrasia.

When macroglobulinemia becomes symptomatic, anemia is the most common presenting manifestation, and is frequently profound, with hemoglobin levels in the range of 4 to 6 grams per 100 ml. Usually the anemia is due to a combination of factors, including accelerated red cell destruction, blood loss, and decreased erythropoiesis. Coating of erythrocytes with IgM globulin is apparently responsible for the marked rouleaux formation, positive Coombs reactions, and cross-matching difficulties encountered in many cases.

As previously noted, a large percentage of IgM globulins have specific physicochemical properties that are responsible for specific symptom patterns in certain cases. These properties include cold-insolubility (cryoglobulins), high intrinsic viscosity, and the capacity to form complexes with coagulation factors and other plasma proteins. *Cryoglobulin-related symptoms* include Raynaud's phenomenon, cold sensitivity, cold urticaria, and vascular occlusion with gangrene after exposure to cold. *Viscosity-related manifestations* are most evident in the retinal vasculature, in which a pattern of patchy venous bulging and localized narrowing ("sausage-effect" or "fundus paraproteinemicus") develops, frequently associated with hemorrhages, exudates, and visual impairment. Circulatory impairment in the central nervous system caused by increased plasma viscosity produces changing patterns of neurologic signs and symptoms, e.g., transient paresis, reflex abnormalities, deafness, impairment of consciousness ("coma paraproteinemicum"), frequently terminating with cerebral vascular hemorrhage. Cardiac decompensation and pulmonary symptoms may also develop secondary to increased viscosity in the systemic and pulmonary vascular beds. *Protein:protein interactions* with formation of complexes between IgM globulins and coagulation factors (fibrinogen, prothrombin, factors V, VII, etc.) are an important contributing factor to the bleeding diatheses (particularly epistaxes, oral mucosal bleeding, and purpura) exhibited in many cases. Interference with platelet function (platelet agglutination) and capillary damage secondary to increased serum viscosity are additional factors contributing to bleeding manifestations. It must be recognized that all these symptom patterns are also observed in occasional cases of myeloma with M-type IgG and IgA globulins possessing similar physicochemical properties.

Bence Jones proteinuria is present in approximately 10 per cent of cases of macroglobulinemia, but renal functional impairment is much less common than in myeloma, presumably because of the absence of the con-

tributing factors of hypercalcemia and hypercalciuria. Amyloidosis has been observed in only a few cases of macroglobulinemia, and in all of these, the liver, spleen, and parenchymal organs have been the major areas of involvement (Pattern II) in contrast to the primary, atypical mesenchymal distribution (Pattern I) of amyloid usually observed in myeloma.

Peripheral neuropathies *(Bing-Neel syndrome)* and myelopathy may be progressive and incapacitating. Circulatory impairment in vasa nervorum is a postulated but still unsubstantiated mechanism. Myopathies and rheumatoid-like arthropathies have also been observed.

In the author's series of 57 cases, 15 had clinical or postmortem evidence of an associated nonreticular neoplasm, and an additional 12 had a background of long-standing infection, particularly tuberculosis.

Many of the laboratory findings in macroglobulinemia have already been considered. The presymptomatic cases are usually detected initially as a result of finding an unexplained elevation of erythrocyte sedimentation rate on routine examination, followed by electrophoretic demonstration of an M-type serum protein (Fig. 3) and, finally, its characterization as an IgM globulin by ultracentrifugation or immunoelectrophoresis, or both. The majority of IgM globulins are euglobulins and give a positive Sia water-dilution reaction, but this is not specific for macroglobulins because certain IgG globulins are also Sia-positive euglobulins. Approximately one third of IgM globulins are cryoglobulins, yielding a white precipitate or a thick clear gel on cooling. The temperature and duration of cooling needed for precipitation varies with individual cryoglobulins. With some cryoglobulins, precipitation or gel-formation occurs almost immediately after venipuncture, and a prewarmed syringe is necessary for blood sampling. Others require several hours at 10° C for precipitation. Similarly, the increased viscosity of serum containing a viscous M-type macroglobulin may be readily apparent when a tube of serum at room temperature is inverted, or viscosimetric determinations at different temperatures may be required.

Hematologic abnormalities, in addition to anemia, include an absolute lymphocytosis with "atypical, immature, and plasmacytic" forms in many cases, occasionally reaching leukemic proportions. Polymorphonuclear leukopenia, thrombopenia, and eosinophilia are also observed. Bone marrow aspirations characteristically reveal an increase in lymphocytic-plasmacytic forms, accompanied by eosinophils and mast cells in many cases. The small lymphocyte, with a dense pyknotic nucleus, which has been considered most typical for macroglobulinemia, probably represents a degenerating cell undergoing cytoplasmic shedding (so-called "clasmatosis").

Additional laboratory abnormalities in certain cases of macroglobulinemia include positive flocculation reactions, false positive serologic reactions, and positive rheumatoid factors. The latter are occasionally associated with rheumatic symptoms and arthropathy.

Treatment. The principal indications for therapy in macroglobulinemia are anemia, bleeding manifestations, and symptoms related to increased plasma viscosity. When the latter symptoms are severe and threaten central nervous system function and vision, plasmapheresis is indicated as a temporary measure. Sufficient plasma should be removed to effect a lowering of viscosity, and the red cells should be returned. In certain cases, a prompt and dramatic improvement in clinical status follows the removal of as little as 500 ml of plasma. Repeated plasmapheresis for a period of several weeks may be required until effective chemotherapy can be instituted.

Chlorambucil (Leukeran) is presently regarded as the chemotherapeutic agent of choice in macroglobulinemia. This should be administered continuously at a dosage level of 8 to 10 mg daily. Although this dosage level is significantly higher than the average employed in most cases of lymphatic leukemia or lymphosarcoma, it is usually well tolerated in macroglobulinemia. A large number of patients have been maintained in objective and subjective remission for periods up to nine years with continuous chlorambucil therapy. More limited studies with melphalan indicate it to be less effective in macroglobulinemia than chlorambucil. Prednisone may be of some value in the control of capillary bleeding.

MacKenzie, M. R., and Fudenberg, H. H.: Macroglobulinemia: An analysis of 40 patients. Blood, 39:874, 1972.
McCallister, B. D., Bayrd, E. D., Harrison, E. G., Jr., and McGuckin, W. F.: Primary macroglobulinemia. Review with a report on 31 cases and notes on the value of continuous chlorambucil therapy. Am. J. Med., 43:394, 1967.
Waldenström, J.: Studies on conditions associated with disturbed gamma globulin formation (gammopathies). Harvey Lect., Series 56:211, 1961.

781. AMYLOIDOSIS

Amyloidosis is a term applied to a variety of conditions associated with tissue infiltrates comprised of insoluble proteins and/or protein-polysaccharide complexes. With the relatively recent development of methods for the isolation and chemical and immunologic analysis of amyloids, it has become evident that there are *at least* two chemical types of amyloid. In one (Ig-type), immunoglobulin light chains appear to be the principal protein component; in the other (protein A-type), an apparently nonimmunoglobulin constituent (protein A) is the major protein. It must be stressed that other chemical types of amyloid will probably be defined by further studies, but the Ig-type and protein A-type probably comprise the majority of amyloidosis cases encountered clinically. In both types, the tissue infiltrates apparently represent noncovalently bonded polymers of the basic protein subunit, either alone or in combination with other proteins or polysaccharides. The polymers are sufficiently large to yield a characteristic fibrillar structure which can be visualized by electron microscopy and a distinctive green-yellow dichroic birefringence seen by polarization microscopy after Congo red staining.

As outlined in Table 2, there is some correlation between the chemical type of amyloid and the clinical pattern of amyloid distribution. Thus IgG-type amyloid has been mainly found in cases with either occult plasma cell dyscrasia or overt multiple myeloma. The pattern of distribution of amyloid in these cases is most frequently that previously referred to as primary-type, i.e., principal involvement of the tongue, heart, gastrointestinal tract, skeletal and smooth muscles, carpal ligaments, nerves, and skin. This distribution pattern, referred to as Pattern I, was manifested in 50 per cent of the cases in the author's series.

Protein A-type amyloid has thus far been mainly found in cases of amyloidosis associated with chronic infections (e.g., tuberculosis), rheumatoid arthritis, Hodgkin's disease, and familial Mediterranean fever. The pattern of distribution of amyloid in these cases most frequently is that previously referred to as secondary-type, i.e., principal involvement of the liver, spleen, kidneys, and adrenals. This distribution pattern, now designated Pattern II, was displayed by 17 per cent of the author's cases.

In a significant proportion of cases (30 per cent of the author's series), amyloid involves both Pattern I and II sites to varying degrees, and these cases are now referred to as Mixed Pattern I and II. Monoclonal IgG, A, D, and M globulins, indicative of associated plasma cell dyscrasias, are demonstrable in the majority (82 per cent) of Mixed Pattern I and II cases, but the specific role of these proteins in the amyloid deposits has not been determined. In a small percentage of cases (3 per cent in the author's series) amyloid is apparently localized to one tissue or organ. In all our cases of localized amyloidosis, abnormal collections of plasma cells were found in immediate juxtaposition to the amyloid deposits, and monoclonal immunoglobulins were also demonstrated in all three cases.

Ideally, disease classifications should be based on etiologic factors, and this should eventually be possible

TABLE 2. Patterns of Amyloidosis

	Previous Designations	Distribution	Associated Conditions	Type of Amyloid Protein
Pattern I	Primary-type, atypical, para-amyloid, pericollagen, mesenchymal	Tongue, heart, GI tract, muscles, ligaments, skin	Plasma cell dyscrasia, usually with Bence Jones only; overt myeloma	Ig-light chain
Pattern II	Secondary-type, typical, perireticular, parenchymal	Liver, spleen, kidney, adrenal	Chronic infections, rheumatoid arthritis, familial Mediterranean fever	Protein A
Mixed Pattern I and II	—	Various combinations of I and II sites	Plasma cell dyscrasia with complete IgG, A, D, and M globulins	Not known
Localized	Tumor-forming	Lung, GI tract, bladder, eye	Plasma cell dyscrasia	Not known

Figure 6. Lichen myxedematosus (papular mucinosis). A form of amyloidosis with extensive involvement of the dermis.

with amyloidosis. Until this is achieved, however, the presently suggested classification based on the predominant clinical patterns of amyloid distribution is considered preferable to previously employed designations such as primary, secondary, typical, and atypical. The terms primary and secondary have been particularly confusing, because in usage they have referred either to *presumed* etiologic factors or to particular patterns of amyloid distribution. Because of the prevalence of chronic infections and suppuration in the preantibiotic era, Pattern II amyloid was relatively more common and "typical" than Pattern I ("atypical"). In more recent series, however, Pattern I cases predominate.

The clinical manifestations of amyloidosis are variable and depend on the distribution and extent of the tissue infiltrates. In Pattern I amyloidosis the clinical manifestations may be any one or a combination of the following: cardiac involvement with decompensation (low output failure) characteristically refractory to digitalis and associated with decreased pulse pressure, low EKG voltage, conduction defects, and arrhythmias; tongue and salivary gland involvement with progressive macroglossia, change in taste sensation, xerostomia, and dysphagia; gastrointestinal manifestations, particularly anorexia, alternating diarrhea and constipation, abdominal cramps, borborygmi, spruelike manifestations with malabsorption, and gastrointestinal bleeding; carpal tunnel syndrome with median nerve involvement and arterial insufficiency caused by infiltration of the carpal ligaments; joint and muscle stiffness and limitation of motion, usually not painful or tender and readily distinguishable from rheumatoid arthritis; neuropathies and radiculopathies with varying sensory and motor deficits; or skin and subcutaneous tissue involvement evidenced by subcutaneous hemorrhages and purpura after minimal trauma, particularly in the eyelids and periorbital tissues. Monoclonal immunoglobulins, particularly Bence Jones proteins, and abnormal marrow plasmacytosis can be demonstrated in virtually all Pattern I cases, and overt skeletal lesions consistent with multiple myeloma develop in approximately 50 per cent of these cases.

In Pattern II amyloidosis, the process is usually man-

ifested by the insidious onset of hepatosplenomegaly and progressive hepatic failure, proteinuria, and renal functional impairment, culminating in the nephrotic syndrome. Peripheral edema and anasarca frequently develop as a consequence of the combined effects of hypoalbuminemia (decreased albumin synthesis caused by hepatic dysfunction plus urinary loss) and abnormal arteriolar capillary permeability secondary to amyloid infiltration.

As would be expected, the clinical manifestations in Mixed Pattern I and II amyloidosis also reflect the extent of involvement of specific tissues and organs. Six of 30 cases of Mixed Pattern I and II amyloidosis in our series were associated with overt myeloma.

Lichen myxedematosus (lichen amyloidosus, papular mucinosis) is a rare form of amyloidosis or tissue proteinosis characterized by the progressive deposition of amyloid in the dermis of the face, trunk, and extremities (Fig. 6). Recent studies have established that this form of amyloidosis is apparently consistently associated with the elaboration of unusually basic (cationic) M-type IgG globulins. It has further been demonstrated in one case that the amyloid infiltrates of the skin were comprised, at least in part, by this specific protein, presumably deposited in combination with the mucopolysaccharides of the dermis. The possibility that lichen myxedematosus may be an autoimmune disease in which a monoclonal antibody is directed against antigenic constituents of the dermis has been suggested.

Diagnosis. The diagnosis of amyloidosis depends on biopsy documentation. If possible, an accessible site with apparent involvement should be biopsied (e.g., skin, muscle), but tongue biopsy should be avoided because of pain and the risk of infection. Liver and kidney biopsy are possibly associated with a risk of bleeding, but this has not been a significant problem in most series. Because amyloidosis of Pattern I and Pattern II frequently involves the arterioles of the rectal submucosa, rectal biopsy is a relatively safe and useful diagnostic procedure. All biopsy material should be stained with Congo red and examined by polarization microscopy. This technique not infrequently discloses amyloid deposits not revealed by the usual staining procedures.

In all cases of amyloidosis, detailed examination of the serum and urinary proteins by electrophoresis and immunoelectrophoresis is indicated, along with bone marrow studies, to document a plasma cell dyscrasia. In a case of amyloidosis with proteinuria, the finding of a negative Bence Jones reaction on heat-testing does not exclude the presence of an abnormal constituent of the Bence Jones type, because albumin and other serum proteins in the urine may mask a Bence Jones reaction.

Treatment. There is no known method to reverse the deposition of amyloid infiltrates except the identification and control of associated conditions, particularly osteomyelitis, pulmonary abscess, and tuberculosis. Several cases have been reported in which effective antimicrobial therapy or surgery or both for a chronic suppurative process have resulted in cessation of amyloid deposition and reabsorption of existing infiltrates. Unfortunately, this is rare; in most cases the amyloidosis continues despite apparently effective control of associated conditions.

Experience with melphalan therapy in cases of amyloidosis with overt myeloma or occult plasma cell dyscrasia is limited, but results have been generally discouraging. Most patients have continued to pursue a downhill course, succumbing to cardiac decompensation or complications related to tongue and gastrointestinal involvement. Corticosteroids occasionally provide slight symptomatic benefit. In cases of macroglossia, careful attention to oral hygiene is important to avoid irritation and ulceration of the tongue.

Cohen, A. S.: Amyloidosis. N. Engl. J. Med., 277:522, 574, 628, 1967.

Franklin, E. C., and Zucker-Franklin, D.: Current concepts of amyloid. *In* Dixon, F. J., and Kunkel, H. G. (eds.): Advances in Immunology. Vol. 15. New York, Academic Press, 1972, p. 249.

Glenner, G. G., Terry, W. D., and Isersky, C.: Amyloidosis: Its nature and pathogenesis. Semin. Hematol., 10:65, 1973.

Isobe, T., and Osserman, E. F.: Patterns of amyloidosis and their associations with plasma cell dyscrasia, monoclonal immunoglobulins and Bence Jones proteins. N. Engl. J. Med., 290:473, 1974.

Osserman, E. F., Takatsuki, K., and Talal, N.: The pathogenesis of "amyloidosis." Studies on the role of abnormal gamma globulins and gamma globulin fragments of the Bence Jones (L-polypeptide) type in the pathogenesis of "primary" and "secondary amyloidosis," and the "amyloidosis" associated wilh plasma cell myeloma. Semin. Hematol., 1:3, 1964.

782. γ HEAVY CHAIN DISEASE

γ heavy chain disease is a relatively rare form of plasma cell dyscrasia characterized by the elaboration of excessive quantities of polypeptide related to the heavy chains and, more specifically, to the Fc fragment of IgG globulin. The clinical pattern resembles a lymphoma with lymphadenopathy, splenomegaly, and hepatomegaly as the predominant manifestations associated with the nonspecific symptoms of weakness, fever, weight loss, and marked susceptibility to bacterial infections. Several patients have exhibited transient palatal erythema and edema resembling that of infectious mononucleosis, and in some there was transient spontaneous regression of the lymphadenopathy after an initially rapid onset. None have had clinical or roentgenographic evidence of skeletal destruction. Most have shown anemia, leukopenia, and thrombopenia, presumably owing to hypersplenism, and moderate to marked eosinophilia. Bone marrow aspirations and lymph node biopsies demonstrated proliferation of plasmacytic and lymphocytic forms along with eosinophils and large reticulum or reticuloendothelial cells.

Persistent proteinuria (4 to 15 grams per 24 hours) was generally the initial indication of an abnormality of protein metabolism. The characteristic serum and urinary protein electrophoretic patterns are illustrated in Figure 4*B* and have been described in Ch. 778. Total serum protein concentrations were generally within normal limits. The serum concentration of the abnormal protein ranged from 2 to 4 grams per 100 ml associated with marked decrease in the concentration of normal gamma globulin. Identification of the abnormal protein as related to the γ heavy chain (Fc fragment) and unrelated to Bence Jones and light chain polypeptides must be accomplished by immunochemical and physicochemical analyses.

In contrast to myeloma, erythrocyte sedimentation rates have been normal or only slightly elevated. Additional laboratory findings have included hyperuricemia with normal or only slightly elevated blood urea nitrogen levels and no other evidence of renal functional impairment.

Survival from the time of onset of symptoms has ranged from four months to over five years. Bacterial pneumonia and sepsis caused death in all cases.

Splenic radiation has produced temporary remissions with hematologic improvement. Limited trials of cyclophosphamide, melphalan, and steroids gave little or no benefit.

783. IgA HEAVY CHAIN (α-CHAIN) DISEASE

IgA heavy chain (α-chain) disease is the most recently identified plasma cell dyscrasia. As defined by Seligmann and his associates, the clinical pattern is that previously referred to as "Mediterranean-type abdominal lymphoma." The predominant features are a diffuse lymphoma-like proliferation in the small intestine and mesentery, chronic diarrhea, and malabsorption unresponsive to gluten withdrawal. Although all of Seligmann's cases were either non-Ashkenazi Jews or Israeli Arabs, we have recently documented the syndrome, with the specific α-chain abnormality, in a South American (Colombia) male of Spanish and Indian (Mestizo) descent. Thus, although genetic factors were considered to be of major importance, the disease is not exclusively restricted to the Mediterranean population.

Chronic diarrhea, malabsorption, and progressive wasting are the major clinical features. Small intestinal biopsies demonstrate a profound infiltration of the lamina propria with abnormal plasma cells. Intestinal absorption studies demonstrate impaired absorption of vitamin B_{12}, glucose, lactose, and fat. Roentgenograms of the small intestines show thickened mucosal folds, segmentation, and dilated intestinal loops. Bone marrow aspiration reveals moderate increases in plasma cells, and skeletal roentgenograms show moderate diffuse osteoporosis but no destructive lesions.

On electrophoretic analysis of serum, the distinctive increase in IgA heavy chains (α chains) has been evidenced by a markedly elevated, broad peak traversing the beta and alpha-2 mobility range. The electrophoretic polydispersity has been shown to be due to polymeric heterogeneity of the alpha chains. This tendency to polymerize also explains the relatively low concentration of alpha chains in the urine as compared with the excretion of gamma chains in IgG heavy chain disease. Confirmation of the identity of the abnormal serum protein as free α-chains is accomplished by demonstrating the absence of associated light chains by appropriate immunologic and chemical analyses.

The association of this particular form of plasma cell dyscrasia with the small intestine is of particular interest in view of the known preponderance of IgA-producing plasma cells in the intestinal tract. The possible role of antecedent chronic infection or irritation of the intestines in the pathogenesis of IgA heavy chain disease cannot be presently defined.

Frangione, B., and Franklin, E. C.: Heavy chain diseases: Clinical features and molecular significance of the disordered immunoglobulin structure. Semin. Hematol., 10:53, 1973.

Franklin, E. C., Lowenstein, J., Bigelow, B., and Meltzer, M.: Heavy chain disease. A new disorder of serum γ-globulins. Am. J. Med., 37:332, 1964.

Osserman, E. F., and Takatsuki, K.: Clinical and immunochemical studies of four cases of heavy (Hγ2) chain disease. Am. J. Med., 37:351, 1964.

Seligmann, M., Danon, F., Hurez, D., Mihesco, E., and Preud'homme, J. L.: Alpha-chain disease: A new immunoglobulin abnormality. Science, 162:1396, 1968.

784. PLASMA CELL DYSCRASIA OF UNKNOWN SIGNIFICANCE AND PLASMA CELL DYSCRASIA ASSOCIATED WITH CHRONIC INFECTIONS, BILIARY DISEASE, AND NONRETICULAR NEOPLASMS

Use of serum electrophoresis as a routine clinical laboratory procedure has resulted in the detection of M-type protein abnormalities, such as are illustrated in Figure 4C and D, in otherwise asymptomatic persons. As previously noted, certain of these later develop signs and symptoms of myeloma, macroglobulinemia, or amyloidosis after many months or years. A fundamental question is whether M-type protein abnormalities are invariably manifestations of plasma cell dyscrasia that will produce clinical symptoms if the patient survives "long enough" (possibly several decades), or whether certain M-type abnormalities are truly benign and "essential." Since this question is presently unanswerable, the term "plasma cell dyscrasia of unknown significance" is considered preferable to "premyeloma" or "essential or benign monoclonal gammopathy."

In general, asymptomatic M-type protein abnormalities are more commonly observed in older subjects. In many cases there is a background of tuberculosis, syphilis or other chronic infection, chronic biliary tract disease, or a nonreticular neoplasm, particularly large bowel, breast, oropharyngeal, and biliary tract carcinomas. Although a coincidental association cannot be excluded, particularly in older subjects, there is increasing evidence that certain plasma cell dyscrasias in man may be induced by diverse forms of protracted reticuloendothelial stimuli comparable to those described in

mice. Because of the frequency of these associations, a careful search for an occult infection or neoplasm should be periodically carried out in all patients with asymptomatic M-type protein abnormalities, with particular attention to the bowel and biliary tracts.

To date, chemotherapy with melphalan or any other agent has not been deemed warranted in asymptomatic subjects, despite the knowledge that a certain percentage of them will later develop overt myeloma. Although there are obvious theoretical advantages to earlier chemotherapy, the unpredictability of the course in any one case and the significant toxicities of presently available agents are strong arguments against the institution of chemotherapy before a distinct clinical pattern is evident.

785. ASSOCIATION BETWEEN PLASMACYTIC AND MONOCYTIC DYSCRASIAS

A close functional relationship is known to exist between the monocyte-histiocyte-macrophage system and plasma cells in the processing of antigens and the synthesis of antibodies. As an apparently related phenomenon, there is a significant association between plasmacytic and monocytic dyscrasias in man. Thus monocytic leukemia develops late in the course of a small but significant number of cases of longstanding plasma cell myeloma, generally after several years of effective chemotherapeutic control of the myeloma. In all cases, the monocytic leukemia is associated with markedly elevated serum and urine lysozyme levels. The onset of monocytic leukemia is usually abrupt, although in some cases transient episodes of peripheral monocytosis and fever precede the development of the terminal leukemic phase.

Additional evidence linking monocytic and plasmacytic dyscrasias has been the finding of M-type gamma globulin abnormalities or diffuse hypergammaglobulinemia, or both, in several cases of monocytic leukemia not associated with overt myeloma. Significantly, many of these latter patients have had protracted chronic illnesses, particularly chronic pulmonary infections, tuberculosis, and osteomyelitis, similar to those associated with plasma cell dyscrasia. Thus comparable pathogenic mechanisms may be operative, and may constitute a proliferative stimulus to both plasma cells and monocytes, either simultaneously or sequentially.

Hallen, J.: Discrete gamma globulin (M−) components in serum. Clinical study of 150 subjects without myelomatosis. Acta Med. Scand. (suppl.) 462, 127 pp., 1966.

Isobe, T., and Osserman, E. F.: Pathologic conditions associated with plasma cell dyscrasia: A study of 806 cases. Ann. N. Y. Acad. Sci., 190:507, 1971.

Osserman, E. F.: Clinical and biochemical studies of plasmacytic and monocytic dyscrasias and their interrelationships. Trans. Studies, Coll. Physicians, Phila., 36:134, 1969.

Osserman, E. F., and Lawlor, D. P.: Serum and urinary lysozyme (muramidase) in monocytic and mono-myelocytic leukemia. J. Exp. Med., 124:921, 1966.

Waldenström, J. G.: Benign monoclonal gammapathies. In Azar, H. A., and Potter, M. (eds.): Multiple Myeloma and Related Disorders. Vol. I. Hagerstown, Md., Harper & Row, 1973, p. 247.

Young, V. H.: Transient paraproteins. Proc. R. Soc. Med., 62:778, 1969.

Zawadzki, Z. A., and Edwards, G. A.: Dysimmunoglobulinemia associated with hepatobiliary disorders. Am. J. Med., 48:196, 1970.

Section Thirteen.   DISEASES OF THE SPLEEN

Robert I. Weed

786.   INTRODUCTION

Aristotle may have been one of the first to suggest that the spleen was not necessary for the maintenance of life. In fact, there are references in ancient writings to removal of the spleen, in the belief that it would improve the wind of runners (perhaps, especially in runners who might have had splenomegaly because of malaria or another parasitic disease). Although today we are beginning to understand the functions of the normal spleen, it is an impressive fact that normal individuals can tolerate splenectomy, e.g., after trauma, with little evident ill effect. Indeed, we know far more about pathologic function than we do about normal function of the spleen, although much remains to be learned about the pathophysiology in disease states. The discussion in this section will include mention of splenic hypofunction as well as splenic diseases. Splenic diseases can be divided into primary hypersplenism, in which the abnormality appears confined to the spleen with no apparent associated systemic illness; secondary hypersplenism associated with a systemic disease, either malignant or nonmalignant; and a third group of miscellaneous disorders associated with splenomegaly, with or without hypersplenism.

Anatomy and Normal Functions.   There is considerable variation in ultrastructure as well as function of the spleen from one species to another, e.g., the spleens of sheep, cats, and dogs appear to act as erythrocyte reservoirs, whereas the human spleen normally contains only 20 to 30 ml of red cells. As illustrated in the accompanying figure, the spleen can be considered to contain three regions, structurally and functionally distinct, along the course of each branch of the splenic artery. The entire organ is encased in a capsule with supporting trabeculae, which extend into the splenic pulp. The splenic artery divides into trabecular branches which first enter the white pulp (on right in figure). This is made up primarily of periarterial collections of lymphocytes with germinal centers that contain variable numbers of monocytes, macrophages, and plasma cells. The location of the white pulp along branches of the artery proximal to the red pulp may be related to the relative rigidity of lymphoid cells compared to erythrocytes. Thus, as terminal arterioles branch out within the white pulp, the efficient filtering mechanism of the spleen may remove the lymphoid cells that arrive via the general circulation, permitting the erythrocytes to pass on into the red pulp.

Encircling the white pulp and interposed between it and the red pulp is a marginal zone that communicates with the periphery of the lymphoid follicles and contains lymphatic vessels that represent the efferent limb of the lymphatic circulation through the spleen. The arterioles that traverse the white pulp may terminate directly in splenic sinuses, or the terminal arterioles may simply end within the red pulp (on left in figure).

The red pulp consists of cords made up of fixed macrophages, a finger-like network of reticulin extending throughout the cords, and a basement membrane separating the cords from sinuses, with overlying endothelial cells lining the interior of the sinuses. Normally, less than 5 per cent of the blood passing through the spleen traverses the splenic cords in the red pulp, the rest being shunted directly through the sinuses without traversing the cords. However, for those cells that do traverse the cords, the challenge is formidable. Those that pass must be deformable and able to squeeze between the high endothelial cells at the terminal end of

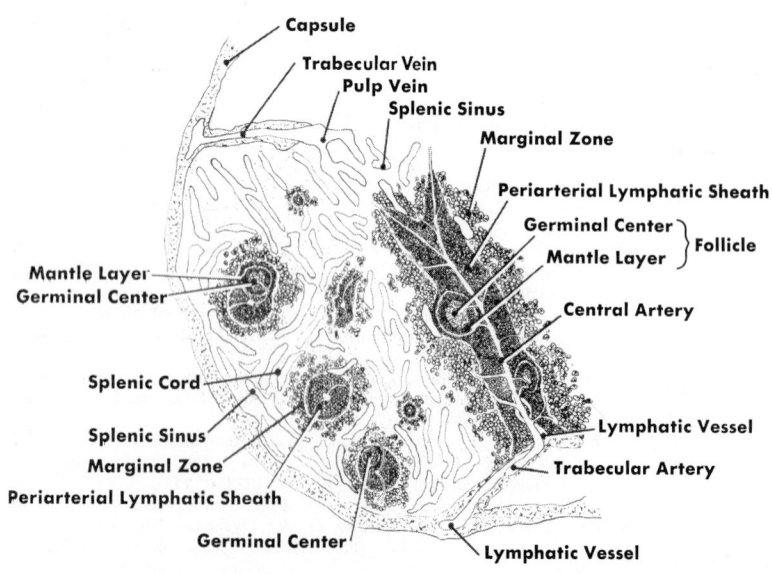

Diagrammatic representation of the structure of the spleen. (From Weiss, L.: Semin. Hematol., October 1970, p. 373.)

the arteriole, then between the macrophages lining the potential spaces which represent the normal circulatory pathways through the cords, and then to pass through 0.5 to 3 μ diameter slitlike openings or potential openings in the basement membrane which separates the cords from sinuses. After re-entering the sinuses, the cells then pass back into trabecular veins and into the general circulation. Under normal circumstances, erythrocytes make approximately 500 passages through the splenic circulation each day.

787. HYPOSPLENISM

Definition. As mentioned in Ch. 786, absence of the spleen is generally tolerated without evidence of clinical illness. There are, however, certain clinical and laboratory features which characterize "hyposplenism," whether it follows splenectomy or is associated with agenesis of the spleen or splenic atrophy secondary to multiple infarction.

Mechanisms. One of the functions of the normal spleen is to remove various inclusions from erythrocytes. Consequently, functional or genuine absence of the spleen is invariably associated with the persistence of such inclusions as *Howell-Jolly bodies.* The presence of Howell-Jolly bodies after splenectomy, or their disappearance at some interval after splenectomy, is an excellent illustration of how the peripheral blood may be used to evaluate splenic function (see next paragraph).

Diagnosis. Absence of splenic function is invariably associated with the appearance and persistence of these inclusions, and their subsequent disappearance after splenectomy may be taken as an indication of hypertrophy of an accessory spleen or spleens. Additional changes seen in erythrocytes after splenectomy include the appearance of target cells and acanthocytes (irregularly spiculated cells). Acanthocytes are noted regularly in the blood of all postsplenectomy patients, and after splenectomy their number often reaches a steady level between 10 and 20 per cent, although in some cases, up to 90 per cent of the cells may be acanthocytes. After splenectomy, *nucleated red cells* are found in the peripheral blood, especially when the spleen is removed for the treatment of hemolytic disease and also when the stimulus for increased erythroid production and release from the marrow persists after splenectomy. When the spleen is present and functioning normally, *siderocytes* (cells with iron-containing inclusions that are normally present in the bone marrow) are not seen in the peripheral blood, because the siderosomes are "culled" from the cells. After splenectomy, however, siderocytes are present in abundance in the peripheral blood, although it is necessary to use Prussian blue (PB) stain to identify them.

In *Heinz body anemias,* presplenectomy blood smears may show no evidence of the Heinz bodies, because the Heinz bodies have been pitted from the pathologic red cells. However, postsplenectomy, there is often an abundance of Heinz body–containing cells in the peripheral blood.

Leukocytosis, up to 20,000 per cubic millimeter or higher, if the patient is being treated with corticosteroids, and *thrombocythemia* to values of 500,000 to 800,000 per cubic millimeter are features that regularly characterize the peripheral blood of patients who have had their spleens removed. In evaluating leukocytosis in these individuals, it is important to recognize the predisposition of the splenectomized patient to develop leukocytosis. Potentially more important, however, is the thrombocytosis which normally rises to a maximum between the fourth and thirteenth postoperative day, and usually disappears within a month after surgery.

Treatment. If the platelet count exceeds values of 1,000,000 per cubic millimeter, there may be danger of thrombosis, including such serious complications as thrombosis of the portal vein. If the platelet count does rise above 1,000,000 per cubic millimeter, anticoagulation is indicated. Current investigations may establish that postoperative administration of aspirin interferes with platelet function sufficiently to justify the administration of aspirin in order to tide a patient over a period of thrombocytosis.

Prognosis. Potentially, the most significant consequence of absence of the spleen relates to the predisposition to develop serious infections, particularly those produced by *Diplococcus pneumoniae* and *Hemophilus influenzae,* although this is a controversial subject. There is general agreement regarding the increased risk of infection in children who undergo splenectomy under the age of four years. In older children and adults with hematologic disorders that require splenectomy, the increased incidence of infection associated with the diseases themselves makes it difficult to assess whether this risk is enhanced by splenectomy. There is no clear evidence that splenectomy in normal adults, e.g., after trauma, predisposes to infectious complications. Nevertheless, this potential complication of splenectomy, which is perhaps related to the role of the spleen as a large lymph node responsible for filtering and processing foreign antigenic material, as well as removal of foreign matter or injured cells by phagocytosis, requires further investigation to determine whether there is a significant predisposition of adults to infection after splenectomy.

788. HYPERSPLENISM

Definition. Hypersplenism, as a descriptive term, was first used by Chauffard in the last century to describe the role of the spleen in hereditary spherocytosis. The concept of hypersplenism which is generally accepted, however, was probably best defined by Dameshek during the period beween 1941 and 1955. This definition includes (1) splenomegaly, (2) pathologically low levels of one or more of the formed elements in the peripheral blood, (3) hypercellularity of the marrow precursors of those elements which are low in the peripheral blood, and (4) correction of the cytopenia by splenectomy. This definition of hypersplenism covers a variety of disorders, although it may exclude certain hematologic disorders that are improved by splenomegaly. Idiopathic thrombocytopenic purpura is an example, and even hereditary spherocytosis may satisfy all the criteria except for cytopenia, because in some cases there may be a compensated hemolysis without anemia.

Disorders which satisfy all the criteria of hypersplenism may be divided into primary disorders that have no apparent underlying cause and those states in which hypersplenism is clearly secondary to an underlying systemic illness.

PRIMARY HYPERSPLENISM

As with many disorders, the term primary or idiopathic represents a confession of ignorance, although ultimately an underlying diagnosis of lymphoma or collagen disease may become apparent months to years later. Nontropical splenomegaly has been suggested as a designation to describe this syndrome if one cannot establish a specific diagnosis based on pathologic findings or other distinctive clinical features. Nontropical splenomegaly, however, should be distinguished from the tropical splenomegaly syndrome (see below).

Pathogenesis. By definition, the pathogenesis remains poorly understood, and although it has been suggested that the splenic enlargement may represent an unusual or exaggerated response to an exogenous infection or insult, there is no conclusive evidence for this suggestion.

Pathology. Commonly, there is a wide separation of the fibrous trabeculae, although this is a feature common to all enlarged spleens. In some patients, lymphoid tissue constitutes an increased percentage of the total splenic tissue. In some cases, the sinuses in the red pulp are dilated and the hemosiderin within macrophages may be increased. Even in patients who may later prove to have an underlying lymphoma, the splenic histology is often nondiagnostic.

Clinical Manifestations. The clinical manifestations are those that one might anticipate with the classic picture of hypersplenism, and their extent depends on the degree of anemia, granulocytopenia, and/or thrombocytopenia.

Diagnosis. Evaluation of splenic size and abnormal function has become simpler in recent years by virtue of radioisotope techniques. In addition to careful palpation for splenic enlargement as part of the physical examination and examination of a roentgenogram of the abdomen for the size of the splenic shadow, more precise estimation can be obtained by a splenic scan after injection of damaged erythrocytes tagged with ^{197}Hg-labeled mercurihydroxypropane or ^{99}technetium, or ^{113}indium-tagged colloids. Removal of these labeled particles from the circulation by the spleen permits visualization and estimation of its size. Splenic scan may also identify defects suggestive of tumors or abscesses, although precise evaluation of tumors may require angiography. Evaluation of the destructive role of the spleen depends on the specific labeling of red cells or platelets with subsequent characterization of splenic radioactivity, compared to hepatic and precordial counts. In general, evaluation of splenic function in a hemolytic state may be helpful in predicting the possible benefit of splenectomy. Contribution of the spleen to hemolysis can be appraised by labeling of red cells with ^{51}Cr sodium chromate, reinjection, and following the cell survival, in conjunction with surface counting over the liver and spleen. In patients with hereditary or acquired anemias and enlarged spleens, the patients' own cells should be used. In other patients with splenomegaly who seem to be destroying transfused cells at an increased rate,

fresh cells from a normal donor should be used to evaluate whether splenectomy may decrease the transfusion requirement. Although there is considerable variation in the techniques employed and evidence of sequestration will not invariably predict benefit from splenectomy, an increasing splenic count in relation to the liver at the half-time (T/2) for red cell survival is evidence of significant splenic sequestration which supports a decision for splenectomy. Finally, it should be emphasized that "hypersplenic anemia" may represent (1) hemolysis, (2) splenic pooling, or (3) compensatory increase in plasma volume. These possibilities should be evaluated in each case.

Platelet sequestration can also be characterized with ^{51}Cr sodium chromate–labeled platelets. Studies of platelet survival are technically difficult and therefore are best done by those with experience in the technique. Careful studies of platelet distribution and survival have demonstrated that even in a normal-sized spleen, approximately one third of the total platelet mass in the peripheral circulation is sequestered there, and in splenomegaly the proportion of the total platelet mass may be even greater in the spleen. Studies of splenic platelet sequestration must therefore be evaluated in the light of this splenic pool both in normal and in pathologic spleens.

Treatment. Although by definition a preoperative diagnosis cannot be established in any patient with splenic enlargement, the condition is indicated by hypercellularity of normal bone marrow elements and peripheral blood cytopenia in one or more cell lines. Splenectomy is advisable when the hypersplenic syndrome becomes life-threatening as indicated by platelet counts of less than 20,000 per cubic millimeter or granulocyte counts less than 500 per cubic millimeter. Platelet counts of between 20,000 and 50,000 per cubic millimeter and/or granulocyte counts between 500 and 1000 per cubic millimeter constitute relative indications for splenectomy which may otherwise be called for because of mechanical or pressure symptoms.

Prognosis. The outcome of splenectomy in primary hypersplenism is generally satisfactory, provided that the criteria, as defined above, are satisfied. The long-term prognosis, however, depends upon the underlying disease, and, in fact, the establishment of idiopathic hypersplenism as the diagnosis is based on exclusion of specific causes of hypersplenism as demonstrated by splenic pathology, portal hypertension, or demonstration of systemic disease elsewhere.

HYPERSPLENISM SECONDARY TO AN UNDERLYING SYSTEMIC DISORDER

The accompanying table lists a wide variety of disorders which may be associated with hypersplenism. The reader is referred to specific chapters elsewhere within the book for discussion of the individual disorders. Nevertheless, it is important to recognize that the hypersplenic syndrome, including splenomegaly, hypercellular marrow, and cytopenia of one or more of the formed elements of the peripheral blood, may all be associated with a wide variety of underlying disease states that can be benefited by splenectomy.

Collagen Diseases. *Lupus erythematosus* is commonly associated with splenomegaly, and thrombocytopenia is

Secondary Hypersplenism

Collagen diseases:
  Lupus erythematosus, Felty's syndrome
Hematologic diseases:
  Hemolytic anemias: hereditary spherocytosis, hereditary ellipto-
  cytosis, thalassemia, sickle cell disease (in children), S-C, S-T dis-
  ease at all ages, autoimmune hemolytic anemia, unstable hemo-
  globin syndromes, pyruvate kinase deficiency, hereditary stomato-
  cytosis
  Myeloproliferative disorders: myeloid metaplasia, chronic granulo-
  cytic leukemia
  Lymphomas: Hodgkin's disease, non-Hodgkin's lymphomas (histio-
  cytic and lymphocytic)
Infections:
  Subacute bacterial endocarditis, malaria (tropical splenomegaly),
  kala-azar
Portal hypertension:
  Cirrhosis of the liver, portal vein thrombosis, myeloid metaplasia
Miscellaneous:
  Aneurysm of splenic artery, cavernous hemangioma

a clinical feature in approximately 15 per cent of patients with this disease. Leukopenia characterized by
both granulocytopenia and lymphopenia is also a
frequent clinical feature. Ten to 15 per cent of lupus patients have a hemolytic anemia, often with a positive
antiglobulin test. Thrombocytopenia may also be associated (see Ch. 81).

Felty's syndrome is a form of hypersplenism which
may occur in association with rheumatoid arthritis (see
Ch. 88). In Felty's syndrome, leukopenia may occasionally be severe enough to be life-threatening, and in
these cases splenectomy may be genuinely beneficial.

Hematologic Diseases. Several hematologic diseases
are associated with some type of hypersplenism. These
include congenital hemolytic anemia such as hereditary
spherocytosis and hereditary elliptocytosis, in which
splenectomy is clinically curative. In other congenital
hemolytic anemias such as thalassemia, sickle cell disease, unstable hemoglobin syndromes, pyruvate kinase
deficiency, and hereditary stomatocytosis, splenectomy
ameliorates the severity of the disorder. In autoimmune
hemolytic anemia, splenectomy may be clinically curative in some cases, and in other cases may fail to alter
the course of the disease. Patients who respond to
steroid therapy generally are benefited by splenectomy,
but some may benefit even though steroids are not effective.

In myeloproliferative disorders, particularly myeloid
metaplasia, splenomegaly is common. Although hematopoiesis can be demonstrated within the spleen, it is
not clear whether these marrow precursor cells have
arisen de novo within the spleen itself, or may represent marrow precursors that escaped from a pathologic
marrow, are trapped in the spleen, and continue to mature. Frequently, the enlarged spleen is a site for increased destruction of erythrocytes and platelets, so that
consideration of splenectomy becomes a major clinical
problem. In myeloid metaplasia, in particular, splenectomy should not be undertaken unless bone marrow
biopsy reveals an active bone marrow. Otherwise, although splenectomy may decrease transfusion requirements, no significant long-term benefit can be anticipated. The same applies to malignant lymphomas
associated with splenomegaly. Pancytopenia associated
with splenomegaly in malignant lymphoma should not
be interpreted as hypersplenism unless careful examination of the bone marrow reveals the latter to be active.

Infectious Etiologies. The hypersplenic syndrome is a
common feature of subacute bacterial endocarditis.
Splenomegaly is also a common accompaniment of malaria and of kala-azar. It may also be a feature of
tuberculosis and histoplasmosis.

Some patients who live in malarial areas develop a
syndrome that is characterized by marked splenomegaly and elevated levels of macroglobulin (IgM). This
has been called the *tropical splenomegaly syndrome*. An
important feature is that one finds normal transformation of the lymphocytes from affected individuals after
stimulation with phytohemagglutinin (PHA). These patients may have moderate lymphocytosis in the peripheral blood and lymphocytosis in the hepatic sinusoids as
well. Although the etiology is not clearly established,
patients with the tropical splenomegaly syndrome come
from malarial zones, many have positive trypanosomal
agglutination tests, and one of the hallmarks of the
disorder is a clinical response to antimalarial therapy
with proguanil. Thus it appears likely that this is a
complication of malaria associated with an exaggerated
response on the part of the lymphatic system, particularly the spleen. The red cell destruction is often characterized by splenic fragmentation of erythrocytes with
resultant spherocytosis but a negative antiglobulin test.

Portal Hypertension. Portal hypertension secondary to
cirrhosis of the liver, portal vein thrombosis, or disorders such as myeloid metaplasia in which there may
be major arteriovenous shunting occurring within the
pathologic spleen itself often leads to clinical hypersplenism. It is clear, however, that in many such patients the size of the spleen correlates rather poorly
with the severity of the cytopenias observed.

Miscellaneous. A variety of vascular anomalies, including aneurysm of the splenic artery or cavernous
hemangioma of the spleen, may be associated with
hypersplenism. In splenic artery aneurysm, the syndrome may exist for a long time and may even represent a lifelong disease state. In these vascular anomalies, in addition to splenomegaly, there may be
thrombocytopenia and also evidence of chronic intravascular coagulation with or without red cell fragmentation and destruction in the spleen. Physical examination may reveal a bruit over the splenic bed.

Diagnosis and Treatment. In all disorders in which
the hypersplenic syndrome is secondary to another
disease, attention must be paid to establishing the nature of the systemic illness, and primary treatment
should be directed toward that illness. However, if the
cytopenia(s) is severe enough and constitutes a clinical
problem, and if the bone marrow is demonstrated to be
hyperactive, splenectomy should be considered.
Frequently, the diagnostic work-up should include
liver biopsy except when thrombocytopenia is present,
and at the time of surgery portal vein pressures should
be measured. If elevated, a portacaval or a splenorenal
shunt should be considered at that time. Removal of a
large spleen in which there was significant shunting
may cause decrease in portal hypertension.

MISCELLANEOUS SPLENIC DISEASES WHICH MAY OR MAY NOT BE ASSOCIATED WITH HYPERSPLENISM

Splenic Abscess. Splenic abscesses are uncommon.
Most are secondary to metastatic spread of infection

from some remote site. About 10 per cent result from extension of contiguous infections, e.g., a perforated peptic ulcer, and 15 per cent develop secondary to some other splenic disorder or trauma, such as a hematoma. When small, they may be difficult to recognize. They may or may not cause left upper quadrant pain, but commonly cause fever, and, if large enough, splenomegaly. Rupture of a splenic abscess may lead to subdiaphragmatic abscess and, ultimately, pain in the left chest. A difficult diagnostic problem arises when the abscess is small and splenic enlargement is nil or minimal and the clinical problem is of septic fever without evidence of localization.

Splenic Infarcts. Splenic infarcts are encountered principally in hematologic disorders associated with vascular occlusive phenomena as in sickle cell disease or in disorders with marked and/or rapid hypertrophy, such as myeloid metaplasia. In sickle cell disease, the repeated infarctions ultimately result in splenic atrophy and "autosplenectomy." Sharp pain, splinting of the left diaphragm, and referred pain to the left shoulder, with or without friction rub, are the diagnostic features of a splenic infarct. Splenic infarction is generally managed conservatively, and the treatment should be based primarily on the underlying disorder.

Splenic Cysts. Splenic cysts are rare causes for splenomegaly. These may be divided into *true cysts,* which are formed from embryonal rests and lined with flattened cuboidal or squamous epithelium. Dermoids and mesenchymal inclusion cysts are included in this category. *False cysts* are more common, and usually result from trauma to the left upper abdomen. Histologically, they lack a true lining, although portions of the wall may consist of flattened cuboidal or squamous epithelium. The third type of cyst that may be encountered in the spleen is the *parasitic cyst,* usually caused by Echinococcus, which is often associated with calcification of the wall and eosinophilia in the peripheral blood.

Splenic cysts may give rise to a sense of fullness in the left upper quadrant and early satiety after ingesting food because of compression of the stomach. Angiography may help distinguish splenic cysts from splenic tumors.

Splenic Tumors. The most frequent tumors of the spleen are lymphocytic, lymphoblastic, or histiocytic lymphomas. Even though initial clinical examination may reveal no evidence of lymphoma elsewhere, the very nature of these disorders necessitates caution in designating splenic involvement by these generally systemic diseases as primary splenic tumors. Much less common are tumors of the vascular endothelium such as hemangiomas, lymphangiomas, and endothelial sarcomas. Rare primary splenic tumors include fibrosarcomas, leiomyosarcomas, or myomas involving the cap-

sule or trabecular framework; extremely rarely, one may encounter embryonic inclusions within the spleen. Again, angiography may be helpful in establishing the diagnosis.

Rupture of the Spleen. Trauma to the upper abdomen, such as an automobile accident, may cause the normal spleen to rupture. Less obvious reasons for splenic rupture may include spontaneous or postpalpation rupture of spleens enlarged because of infectious mononucleosis, sepsis (acute splenic tumor), abscess, or, rarely, leukemia. The hallmarks of splenic rupture include evidence of acute abdominal disease with sharp pain and muscle wall rigidity in the left upper quadrant, hemorrhage with shock, ånd pain which is commonly referred to the left shoulder and associated with splinting of the left diaphragm. This is a surgical emergency which should be dealt with immediately.

Aster, R. H.: Pooling of platelets in the spleen: Role in the pathogenesis of "hypersplenic thrombocytopenia." J. Clin. Invest., 45:645, 1966.

Battaxe, H. A., Watson, R. C., and Levin, D. C.: The angiographic appearance of splenic masses. Angiology, 23:316, 1972.

Boiger, L. E., Edhog, O., and Forsgren, L.: Splenectomy — indications and results. Acta Med. Scand., 192:213, 1972.

Christensen, B. E.: Pathophysiology of "hypersplenism syndrome." Scand. J. Haematol., 11:5, 1973.

Cormia, F. E., and Campos, L. T.: Infection after splenectomy. Ann. Intern. Med., 78:149, 1973.

Crosby, W. H.: Hypersplenism. Ann. Rev. Med., 13:127, 1962.

Crosby, W. H.: Hyposplenism: An inquiry into normal function of the spleen. Ann. Rev. Med., 14:349, 1963.

Dacie, J. V., Brain, M. C., Harrison, C. V., Lewis, S. M., and Worlledge, S. M.: Non-tropical idiopathic splenomegaly (primary hypersplenism): A review of the cases and their relationship to malignant lymphomas. Br. J. Haematol., 17:317, 1969.

Dameshek, W.: Hypersplenism. Bull. N.Y. Acad. Med., 31:113, 1955.

Das Gupta, T., Coombes, B., and Brashfield, R. D.: Primary malignant neoplasms of the spleen. Surg. Gynecol. Obstet., 120:947, 1965.

Eraklis, A. J., Kevy, S. V., Diamond, L. K., and Grass, R. E.: Hazard of overwhelming infection after splenomegaly in childhood. N. Engl. J. Med., 276:1225, 1967.

McIntyre, P. A., and Wagner, H. N., Jr.: Newer technics in hematology. In Progress in Hematology, Vol. 6. New York, Grune & Stratton, 1969.

Mitchell, J.: Lymphocyte circulation in the spleen. Marginal zone bridging channels and their possible role in cell traffic. Immunology, 24:93, 1973.

Nightingale, D., Prankerd, T. H. J., Richards, J. D. M., and Thompson, D.: Splenectomy in anaemia. Quart. J. Med., 41:261, 1972.

Sagoe, A. S.: Tropical splenomegaly syndrome. Long-term proguanil therapy correlated with spleen size, serum IgM, and lymphocyte transformation. Br. Med. J., 3:378, 1970.

Schwartz, S. I., Adams, J. T., and Bauman, A. W.: Splenectomy for hematologic disorders. In Current Problems in Surgery, May 1971.

Szur, L., Marsh, G. W., and Pettit, J. E.: Studies of splenic function by means of radioisotope-labeled red cells. Br. J. Haematol., 23:183, 1972.

Weed, R. I., and Weiss, L.: The relationship of red cell fragmentation occurring within the spleen to cell destruction. Trans. Assoc. Am. Physicians, 79:426, 1966.

Weiss, L.: The Spleen. In Histology. Third Edition. New York, McGraw-Hill Book Company, 1973, p. 445.

Section Fourteen.   HEMORRHAGIC DISORDERS: DISORDERS OF PRIMARY HEMOSTASIS

Ralph L. Nachman

789.   INTRODUCTION

The major hemorrhagic disorders are associated with malfunction of three physiologic systems either separately or in combination: (1) abnormalities of platelets, (2) abnormalities of blood vessels, and (3) abnormalities of plasma coagulation factors. Clinical disorders associated with qualitative or quantitative platelet defects and/or abnormalities of the blood vessel wall have been referred to as diseases of primary hemostasis or "purpuric syndromes." There are several important clinical and laboratory features which help differentiate this spectrum of diseases from those associated with disorders of coagulation factors (Table 1). Purpuric syndromes are characterized by capillary hemorrhages occurring chiefly in the skin and mucous membranes. Occasionally excessive bleeding may follow trauma; however, the usual lesions encountered are spontaneous petechiae and ecchymoses which result from a breakdown in the anatomic and physiologic integrity of small blood vessel walls. Gastrointestinal and genitourinary bleeding may occur spontaneously with either abnormalities of platelets or coagulation factors. Deep hematomas and hemarthroses are more frequently associated with a coagulation factor abnormality. It is important to note the relationship of excessive bleeding to antecedent trauma or surgery, such as circumcision, tonsillectomy, or tooth extraction. Recurrent bleeding for two to three days or more usually indicates an underlying coagulation disorder. In general, bleeding caused by platelet or blood vessel defects is immediate and responds to direct pressure. A strong familial history of a serious bleeding problem should clearly raise the possibility of a coagulation disorder; however, it is important to note that as many as one third of all hemophilic patients have a negative family history. Several simple bedside procedures are useful for the initial evaluation of a hemorrhagic disorder. The Rumpel-Leede vascular fragility test is usually positive in patients with a purpuric syndrome; however, the procedure is superfluous in patients with spontaneous diffuse petechiae and ecchymoses The Duke bleeding time is also a valuable bedside test which can help differentiate patients with purpuric disorders from those with underlying coagulation abnormalities. The rebleeding phenomenon should not be confused with the prolonged primary bleeding time. Patients with hemophilia may rebleed one to two hours after an essentially normal Duke or Ivy bleeding time. This results from the formation of a poorly formed friable clot owing to the deficiency of a coagulation factor.

An understanding of the physiology of primary hemostatic mechanisms is important for the interpretation of diagnostic laboratory tests and for the subsequent management of patients with purpuric disorders. The formation of a hemostatic platelet plug can be divided into several separate but interrelated stages. The initial event in the development of the primary plug occurs with great rapidity and involves the adhesion of circulating platelets to exposed subendothelial collagen fibers, microfibrils, or basement membrane at the site of vessel wall injury. The adhesion reaction is mediated by specific chemical and physical determinants on the collagen molecule and possibly by a platelet membrane enzyme system. ADP which is stored in platelet granules is released by a process analogous to endocrine gland secretion and leads to platelet aggregation (cohesion). A chain reaction of aggregating platelets releasing intracellular ADP which in turn recruits more platelets characterizes the growing plug. Platelet factor 3, a surface lipoprotein complex, and endothelial cell tissue factor become available at the site of the vessel injury probably owing to conformational changes of platelet and endothelial cell membranes. This soon results in the evolution of thrombin by activation of the intrinsic and extrinsic coagulation pathways. These biochemical events lead to consolidation and contraction of the platelet plug with eventual sealing of the injured vessel wall. The thrombin generated at the local site polymerizes fibrinogen, and the resulting fibrin reinforces the platelet mass at the periphery of the plug.

TABLE 1.   Differentiation of Purpuric and Coagulation Disorders

Features	Purpuric Syndromes	Coagulation Disorders
Family history	Generally negative	Usually positive
Sex	More common in females	More common in males
Type of bleeding	Skin and mucosal surfaces	Visceral and intramuscular
	Petechiae and ecchymoses	Deep hematomas
	Spontaneous	Usually traumatic
Hemarthroses	Very rare	Frequent
Duration	Recent in onset	Usually lifelong
Bleeding time	Generally prolonged	Normal
Capillary fragility (tourniquet test)	Positive	Negative

QUANTITATIVE PLATELET ABNORMALITIES

790. THROMBOCYTOPENIA

Thrombocytopenia is the most common cause of hemorrhagic disease. Thus the peripheral blood of every patient who bleeds should be carefully examined. With experience, it is possible to approximate the platelet count by careful evaluation of a peripheral blood smear. Depending on the individual observer, the microscope, and the technique used in making the smear, there should be approximately three to ten platelets per oil immersion field. Smears prepared from "finger stick" blood samples show platelets which are less evenly distributed than smears from anticoagulated blood. Fewer than 50 platelets per 50 oil immersion fields usually suggests moderate to severe thrombocytopenia. With modern automated counting devices, the average normal platelet count varies from 200,000 to 400,000 per cubic millimeter.

The relationship of the platelet count and clinical bleeding is sometimes obscure. Some patients with severe thrombocytopenia may have little bleeding, but others with only a moderate decrease in platelet number present with a marked hemorrhagic diathesis. It is obvious that a number of contributing variables influence the integrity of the blood vessel wall. Sudden precipitous drops in platelet count, fever, and anemia appear to contribute significantly to petechial hemorrhage. Hormonal influences also can affect vascular integrity, as demonstrated by the beneficial effects of steroids in some patients in the absence of improvement in the platelet count. At very low levels, such as 10,000

platelets per cubic millimeter, major hemorrhagic manifestations such as central nervous system bleeding or massive gastrointestinal hemorrhage are more frequent. It is useful to categorize the many causes of thrombocytopenia in the framework of decreased production, decreased survival or excessive utilization, sequestration, and intravascular dilution (Table 2).

DECREASED PRODUCTION OF PLATELETS

Multiple anatomic as well as biochemical alterations may alter megakaryocyte number and function in the marrow. In such conditions, the erythroid and myeloid cellular elements may also be involved to varying degrees. Megakaryocyte depression from bone marrow infiltration may occur in leukemia, myeloma, carcinoma, lymphoma, granuloma, or myelofibrosis. Drugs, in particular the thiazide derivatives, ionizing radiation, and various toxins may cause major injury and megakaryocytic depletion. Familial aplastic anemia (Fanconi's anemia) with thrombocytopenia is a rare fatal childhood illness associated with multiple congenital and skeletal anomalies. A rare syndrome of infancy, congenital amegakaryocytic thrombocytopenia, is associated with bilateral absence of the radii. In congenital rubella, megakaryocytes are decreased in number with an associated decreased platelet production. In this disease the megakaryocyte may provide a preferred site for viral replication.

Impaired platelet production may also result from ineffective thrombopoiesis. Under these circumstances, adequate to increased numbers of megakaryocytes are present in the marrow; however, thrombocytopenia results from interference with the functional integrity of the marrow. This is seen in megaloblastic anemias, in paroxysmal nocturnal hemoglobinuria, and in various hereditary thrombocytopenias, including the Wiskott-Aldrich syndrome and the May-Hegglin anomaly.

DECREASED PLATELET SURVIVAL—INCREASED DESTRUCTION

Drug Purpura

Drugs must be considered a possible cause in every adult with thrombocytopenic purpura. Patients with drug purpura may develop hemorrhagic symptoms after weeks or even years of symptom-free use of an agent. Thrombocytopenia may develop within minutes to hours after administration of a drug to a sensitized patient. The bleeding at first is characterized by petechiae, purpura, occasionally hemorrhagic bullae of the oral mucosa, and not infrequently gastrointestinal and/or genitourinary hemorrhage. The petechiae do not itch, are not tender, and are not associated with wheals. In general the skin lesions are distributed over the lower extremities; they are not found on the soles or palms. In the majority of cases, the thrombocytopenic purpura will clear within a few days after removal of the offending drug. Purpura which persists for more than two to three weeks after drug exposure has been terminated should no longer be considered drug induced, and other conditions should be suspected. However, the duration of the purpura may be variable and

TABLE 2. Thrombocytopenia

I. Decreased production
  A. Reduced marrow megakaryocytes
    Marrow infiltration
    Marrow hypoplasia—radiation, toxins, chemicals, drugs, idiopathic
    Fanconi's anemia
    Congenital amegakaryocytic thrombocytopenia
    Infection—congenital rubella
  B. Normal or increased marrow megakaryocytes
    Megaloblastic anemia
    Paroxysmal nocturnal hemoglobinuria
    Hereditary thrombocytopenia
      Wiskott-Aldrich syndrome
      May-Hegglin anomaly
II. Decreased platelet survival
  A. Increased destruction
    Drug-induced purpura
    Idiopathic thrombocytopenic purpura
    Post-transfusion purpura
    Neonatal purpura
    Secondary immunologic purpura
  B. Increased consumption
    Disseminated intravascular coagulation
    Hemangioma
    Thrombotic thrombocytopenic purpura
    Hemolytic-uremic syndrome
    Acute infections
III. Sequestration (splenomegalic states)
IV. Dilutional

depends to a large extent on the metabolic fate of the drug. Thus certain toxic agents such as gold remain in the body for long periods of time after the last injection. Many patients forget that they have been chronically ingesting various common remedies such as aspirin, sedatives, and/or various tranquilizers, which can cause thrombocytopenia.

Etiology and Pathogenesis. Many agents have been implicated as causes of thrombocytopenia (Table 3). These agents can produce thrombocytopenia by several different mechanisms. Thiazide derivatives, estrogens,

TABLE 3. Drugs Associated with Thrombocytopenic Purpura

I. Marrow suppression
  Thiazides, alcohol, estrogens
II. Direct cytotoxic effect
  Ristocetin
III. Immunologic mechanisms – peripheral destruction
  A. Etiologic relationship established
    Acetazolamide
    Allyl-isopropyl carbamide (Sedormid)
    Arsenical antiluetic drugs
    Carbamazepine
    Chlorothiazide
    Digitoxin
    Diphenylhydantoin sodium
    Hydrochlorothiazide
    Hydroxychloroquine
    Methyl dopa
    Novobiocin
    Para-aminosalicylic acid
    Quinidine
    Quinine
    Stibophen
    Sulfathiazole
  B. Etiologic relationship suspected but not confirmed
    Acetaminophen
    Aminopyrine
    Aspirin
    Butabarbitone
    Carbabutamide
    Chloramphenicol
    Chlorpheniramine maleate
    Chlorpromazine
    Chlorpropamide
    Codeine
    Desipramine
    Dextroamphetamine
    Digitalis
    Digoxin
    Disulfiram
    Erythromycin
    Ethyl-allyl-acetylurea
    Gold
    Iopanoic acid
    Isonicotinic acid hydrazide
    Meperidine
    Meprobamate
    Mercurial diuretics
    Penicillin
    Phenacetin
    Phenylbutazone
    Prednisone
    Prochlorperazine
    Promethazine
    Propylthiouracil
    Reserpine
    Streptomycin
    Sulfadiazine
    Sulfadimidine
    Sulfamethoxypyridazine
    Sulfamerizine
    Sulfisoxazole
    Tetracycline
    Thiouracil
    Tolbutamide

and alcohol may interfere with bone marrow megakaryocyte number and function. The antibiotic ristocetin may directly damage platelets in vivo. Among the drugs listed in Table 3, *particularly frequent offenders include quinidine, quinine, sulfonamides, and the thiazides.* One should have a high level of suspicion of drug sensitivity when thrombocytopenic purpura develops in a patient receiving any of these drugs. Widely used drugs such as aspirin, penicillin, and phenobarbital have also been reported as offenders. In effect, any drug taken by a patient is a possible cause of purpura.

The most common mechanism implicated in drug purpura is immunologic platelet destruction. In recent years, a convincing body of experimental and clinical evidence has been accumulated that clearly demonstrates the participation of the platelet in immunologic reactions. The external platelet surface is capable of nonspecifically adsorbing certain antibody drug complexes which then lead to platelet damage by an "innocent bystander" effect. According to this theory, the administered drug as hapten binds to a plasma protein or "carrier" to form an antigen. Antibodies stimulated by the immunogen bind to the drug, and these immune complexes secondarily interact with the platelet membrane, leading to cellular damage. Recent evidence also suggests that specific metabolic products of certain drugs rather than the primary agent may act as the offending immunogen.

Diagnosis. A careful history of drug ingestion is an absolute necessity in any patient with thrombocytopenia. In addition to the usual medications, specific questioning is necessary regarding intake of beverages which contain quinine. In general the purpuric lesions with thrombocytopenia develop within hours after exposure to the agent by a sensitized patient. There may be an increased percentage of circulating large young platelets in the peripheral blood which is indicative of increased platelet turnover. A number of laboratory tests have been utilized to demonstrate drug, platelet, and antibody interactions as evidence of drug prupura. Tests involving complement fixation and platelet factor 3 release have proved to be relatively sensitive. Inhibition of clot retraction in the presence of the suspected offending agent is the simplest to perform but only detects high titer antibody. These in vitro tests are based on the premise that the underlying mechanism of the drug purpura is platelet adsorption of immune complexes consisting of drug and antibody with subsequent secondary cell damage. Direct challenge of the patient by a test dose of suspected drug in vivo is potentially hazardous. No single test is capable of detecting all cases of drug purpura. The most sensitive tests are difficult to perform and require expert laboratory assistance.

Treatment. All drugs should be discontinued. Medications which are indisputably needed should be replaced with pharmacologically equivalent but chemically different preparations. Adrenal corticosteroids should be given for their beneficial effect on vascular integrity. Platelet transfusions should be used only for life-threatening hemorrhage.

Idiopathic Thrombocytopenic Purpura

Definition. *Acute.* Acute idiopathic thrombocytopenic purpura (ITP) is essentially a disease of young children, affecting both sexes equally. It is characterized by sudden onset of severe thrombocytopenic purpura in an otherwise healthy child, frequently occurring one to two weeks after a sore throat or ordinary cold. Acute ITP is seen most frequently between the ages of two and six years. The manifestations are extensive petechial hemorrhages and purpura with gingival, gastrointestinal, and genitourinary bleeding. There is frequently severe thrombocytopenia (platelet counts below 20,000 per cubic millimeter) with marked hyperplasia of bone marrow megakaryocytes. The spleen is usually not palpable. In over 80 per cent of the patients the disorder is self-limited, clearing spontaneously within two weeks. Patients should be treated with prednisone, 1 to 2 mg per kilogram of body weight, during the period of maximal thrombocytopenia. In some cases the thrombocytopenia may persist for two to six months. Approximately 10 to 15 per cent of affected children will develop chronic ITP, which eventually requires splenectomy.

Chronic.   Chronic ITP is predominately a disease of young adults, affecting females three to four times as often as males. The disorder is characterized by insidious onset with a relatively long history of easy bruising and menorrhagia. Many patients give a history of mild to moderate bleeding after trauma or minor surgery such as dental extractions. The platelet count is usually in the range of 50,000 to 100,000 per cubic millimeter. Bone marrow examination reveals megakaryocytic hyperplasia with predominance of early young forms.

In a typical patient the physical findings are minimal except for petechiae and ecchymoses. There is no characteristic pattern of ditribution of the hemorrhagic lesions. The patient is afebrile, and in most cases the spleen is not palpable. The presence of an easily palpable spleen should direct attention away from the diagnosis of ITP. The disease may be present for a number of months to years and may be characterized by remissions and relapses. In most cases, the hemorrhagic complications are not life threatening; however, a rare individual may show central nervous system signs with intracerebral bleeding. In some patients the disorder appears to have cyclical characteristics, with striking exacerbations of systemic hemorrhagic symptoms with menstruation. These patients generally feel quite well except for complaints relating to the four or five days of hemorrhage per month.

Etiology and Pathogenesis.   In approximately 85 per cent of cases, ITP is a disorder produced by a platelet autoantibody that develops in a patient with no evidence of underlying disease or significant exposure to drugs. For this reason, some authors now prefer to define this disease as *autoimmune thrombocytopenic purpura* (ATP).

Although platelet autoantibodies are difficult to demonstrate, a significant body of clinical and experimental evidence has suggested their presence. Thus pregnant women with ITP frequently give birth to thrombocytopenic infants, a situation strongly suggesting the transplacental transfer of antiplatelet antibody. Plasma from patients with ITP produces severe thrombocytopenia when infused into normal individuals. This plasma also produces thrombocytopenia in the donor individual when reinfused at a time of remission. The activity causing thrombocytopenia upon transfusion of ITP plasma has been identified as a 7S gamma globulin which is absorbed by incubation with autologous and homologous platelets.

A number of in vitro test systems have been devised to demonstrate platelet antibodies in ITP. These include platelet agglutination, complement fixation, platelet factor 3 release, anti-gamma globulin consumption tests, and inhibition of labeled serotonin uptake. These tests are generally difficult to perform and are not yet part of routine laboratory studies. With sensitive in vitro systems it has been demonstrated that approximately 85 per cent of chronic ITP patients have antiplatelet antibodies. It is of interest that antibody production has been demonstrated in surgically removed spleens.

Diagnosis.   The diagnosis of chronic ITP is in large part an exercise in clinical exclusion. This is because the in vitro tests used to demonstrate circulating antiplatelet antibodies are difficult to perform and are generally not available in most clinical centers. Thus the diagnosis is made by a consideration of the major clinical and laboratory hallmarks as outlined above, paucity of physical findings, absence of underlying systemic disorders, exclusion of other primary immunologic thrombocytopenic conditions, and, finally, response to therapy. In most patients, perhaps the most significant diagnostic differential involves the exclusion of primary drug purpura. It is useful initially to remove or replace all drugs for at least two to three weeks. Thrombocytopenia which persists beyond this period is only rarely associated with previous drug administration, with the possible exception of a gold preparation.

Therapy and Prognosis.   Adrenal corticosteroids in a fairly high dose range, e.g., 60 mg of prednisone daily, are employed initially in an attempt to promote a significant rise in the platelet count and decrease bleeding. With steroid therapy, reduction in capillary fragility and decreased bleeding are often observed before an appreciable rise in the platelet count occurs. Most patients (approximately 70 per cent) with chronic ITP will respond to this therapy within two to three weeks. Unfortunately most of them will relapse within weeks to months after discontinuation of the steroids. Less than 15 per cent of adults with ITP will make a complete permanent recovery after an initial course of steroid therapy. In general, if significant clinical improvement does not occur within four to eight weeks or can be maintained only with toxic levels of steroids, splenectomy should be considered. For those patients who respond initially to steroids, the drug should be decreased gradually over several weeks so as to maintain the platelet count above 50,000 per cubic millimeter. In practical terms, most patients will require long-term doses of steroids which eventually lead to undesirable side effects. Thus unless the patient represents an unusual surgical risk, splenectomy should be performed.

Approximately 70 per cent of patients will achieve long-term and even permanent remissions after splenectomy. This is due to (1) removal of a major site of platelet destruction and (2) elimination of a major source of synthesis of platelet antibody. Most patients who enter remission after splenectomy show significant rises in the platelet count, often well above normal levels, within a few days. After surgery, up to 10 per cent of patients may require weeks or even months before a significant remission develops. Recent studies suggest that the effectiveness of splenectomy correlates with the response to prior corticosteroid therapy. A good or excellent response to splenectomy may be expected in a high percentage of patients who have shown a significant rise in the platelet count while on steroids.

Postsplenectomy failure with significant bleeding may respond to high-dose steroids even if the patient previously was refractory to the steroid effect. Immunosuppressive agents such as azathioprine and cyclophosphamide have proved useful in the treatment of these patients. These agents should also be considered for use in patients with symptomatic chronic ITP in whom splenectomy cannot be performed. As noted previously, a small group of women with ITP who do not respond to splenectomy may develop exacerbations of the hemorrhagic symptoms during the menses. Some of these patients show striking improvement in clinical manifestations after suppression of ovarian function with hormonal agents.

Platelet transfusions should be reserved for life-threatening hemorrhage in chronic ITP. Platelets should not be given prophylactically, because they will be rapidly destroyed by the circulating platelet antibodies.

Post-Transfusion Purpura

Post-transfusion purpura is a rare form of immunologic purpura which must be distinguished from ITP and drug purpura. The disease is characterized by sudden explosive onset of thrombocytopenic purpura about five to eight days after transfusion of whole blood. The disease develops because of the mismatching of an inherited platelet antigen with the subsequent development of a complement-fixing antiplatelet isoantibody. The antigen PL^{A1} is found in 98 per cent of the normal population and is absent from the platelets of the patient who develops the disorder. The process is self-limited; however, purpura may last up to six weeks. Conclusive diagnosis rests on the serologic demonstration of platelet antigen mismatching. Post-transfusion purpura should be suspected in any patient who develops sudden purpura in the absence of an overt underlying cause shortly after a blood transfusion. Owing to the danger of intracranial hemorrhage, the therapy consists of exchange transfusion and steroids in high dosage.

Neonatal Purpura

Neonatal thrombocytopenia may develop because of isoimmunization of the mother against fetal platelets with subsequent transplacental transfer of maternal antibody. The disease is the platelet analogue of erythroblastosis fetalis, with platelets rather than red cells serving as the antigenic stimulus. The infant shows generalized purpura at delivery, and platelet counts are usually below 30,000 per cubic millimeter. Intracranial hemorrhage has occurred in approximately 10 per cent of cases.

At least four well-defined platelet antigen systems have been elucidated and appear to be involved in the development of maternal-fetal incompatibility. These include the PL^{A1}, PL Gc Ly^{B1}, PL Gc Ly^{C1}, and PL^{E2} antigens. These antigens, which are distinct from erythrocyte antigens, are inherited as dominant characteristics. The B1 and C1 platelet antigens are shared by granulocytes and lymphocytes. Adrenal corticosteroids, transfusion with maternal platelets, and exchange transfusion have been tried in severe cases.

Secondary Immunologic Purpura

Idiopathic thrombocytopenic purpura may be associated with *autoimmune hemolytic anemia (Evans' syndrome)*. Patients with this disorder present with clinical and laboratory features of Coombs-positive hemolytic anemia and marked to moderate thrombocytopenia.

Autoimmune thrombocytopenia presenting in a manner identical to that of classic ITP occurs in approximately 10 per cent of patients with *systemic lupus erythematosus*. This entity may present as the only significant clinical feature of early lupus. For this reason, immunologic tests for lupus erythematosus should be performed on all patients who present with ITP.

A chronic ITP syndrome can be observed during the course of *chronic lymphocytic leukemia* and *malignant lymphoma*. It should be emphasized that the great majority of cases of thrombocytopenia associated with these diseases are secondary to marrow involvement. The pathogenesis in these rare cases appears to be the same as that described in the idiopathic (autoimmune) disorder. Certain postinfectious thrombocytopenic states, such as those occasionally seen with *rubella* or *infectious mononucleosis,* result from a temporary stimulation of circulating antibody to platelets. The antibody in some cases of infectious mononucleosis is a cold agglutinin with "i" specificity which coats platelets upon exposure to cold. The antibody-coated cells are sequestered in the spleen.

DECREASED PLATELET SURVIVAL—INCREASED CONSUMPTION

Disseminated Intravascular Coagulation

This group of disorders, which is discussed in Ch. 801, is generally associated with significant thrombocytopenia. The platelets are consumed throughout the vascular tree secondary to the generation of excessive amounts of thrombin in the circulation.

Cavernous Hemangioma (Kasabach-Merritt Syndrome)

Giant cavernous hemangioma of infancy is generally detected at birth. Thrombocytopenia, which may be severe, results from excessive consumption of circulating platelets on the damaged subendothelial surface of the neoplasm. Intravascular coagulation takes place within the tumor. Occasionally the tumors are located in visceral sites. In many of these the thrombocytopenia is the most prominent feature of the generalized coagulation disorder. Surgical excision of the tumor if possible and radiation have been used successfully in therapy.

Thrombotic Thrombocytopenic Purpura

Thrombotic thrombocytopenic purpura (TTP) is an acute disease which presents a clinical spectrum, including thrombocytopenic purpura, microangiopathic hemolytic anemia, transient fluctuating neurologic symptoms, kidney disease, and fever. Approximately 80 per cent of patients die within one month of onset of the illness. The most frequently observed symptoms are related to the fluctuating and, at times, bizarre central nervous manifestations and the severe hemorrhagic complications. The anemia is usually brisk, with hematocrits often below 20 per cent on initial examination. An important diagnostic feature is the striking microangiopathic peripheral blood picture; the blood smear shows an increased number of schistocytes, burr cells, and helmet-shaped red cell fragments. Careful evaluation of the coagulation parameters early in the illness does not support the premise that disseminated intravascular coagulation (DIC) has a primary role in this disorder. Later, as the illness becomes more severe and hepatic failure and sepsis occur, secondary DIC may be seen. Diagnostic confirmation of TTP requires histologic demonstration of a characteristic pathologic lesion: the deposition of hyaline thrombi within the lumina of arterioles and capillaries in the absence of vasculitis. These lesions are probably composed of aggregates of degenerating platelets and fibrin. The relationship of the platelet to the primary process in this disease remains unclear. Fibrin has been demonstrated in the thrombotic lesions of TTP by immunofluorescence techniques. Since fibrinogen constitutes approximately 10 per cent of the platelet proteins, focal platelet deposition on blood vessel walls would produce positive immunofluorescence reactions for fibrin. Radioisotope labeling studies have demonstrated decreased platelet survival but normal fibrinogen survival in patients with TTP.

The cause of TTP is unknown. The disorder should be considered a syndrome with multiple etiologic factors producing microcirculatory pathology resulting from the consumption of circulating platelets throughout the microvasculature at sites of vascular damage. In some cases, the primary lesion may reside in small blood vessels. Electron microscopic studies of capillaries have revealed subendothelial prethrombotic fibrin and accumulations of platelets. TTP has occurred in association with systemic lupus erythematosus and other collagen vascular disorders, supporting the possibility of an immune cause in some cases. Bartonella-like bacteria have been isolated from the blood of several patients with TTP. It is possible that other bacterial agents as well as viruses may act as intravascular platelet aggregating agents. Platelet aggregates which are formed in the circulation have been demonstrated to cause microvascular damage by deposition in small vessels and release of vasotoxic factors. Thus under some circumstances, the lesions of TTP could result from insults which primarily affect normal circulating platelets. Whether platelet aggregation is primary or secondary to vessel wall damage, platelet consumption is important in the disease process.

Acute TTP is a medical emergency. Therapy to date has been relatively ineffective, and the current approach is to some extent empirical. Steroids (60 to 100 mg of prednisone daily) and antiplatelet aggregating agents should be started as soon as the diagnosis is made. An effective antiplatelet aggregating combination includes combined dipyridamole and aspirin. If the clinical situation deteriorates, splenectomy should be performed. Anticoagulant therapy in general has not proved beneficial in this disorder.

Hemolytic-Uremic Syndrome

The hemolytic-uremic syndrome (*Gasser's syndrome*) is a disease of early childhood characterized by acute microangiopathic hemolytic anemia, thrombocytopenia, and renal failure. The explosive onset may follow a minor febrile illness or even prophylactic immunization. Neurologic symptoms are rarely seen, and the patients frequently have hemorrhagic diarrhea. The lesions are usually limited to the kidney and are characteristically focal thromboses of glomerular arterioles and capillaries with renal cortical necrosis. The pathogenesis of the hemolytic-uremic syndrome is unknown. Disseminated intravascular coagulation resulting from circulating immune complexes with deposition of circulating fibrin in the renal microvasculature has been considered as the most likely pathogenetic mechanism. Therapy has been primarily directed at management of the acute renal failure. Corticosteroids are probably not helpful. Heparin has appeared to be beneficial in some cases.

The hemolytic-uremic syndrome may also be seen in pregnant or postpartum women. The explosive onset of microangiopathic hemolytic anemia, thrombocytopenia, and acute renal failure may develop in the setting of premature separation of the placenta or toxemia of pregnancy. The pathologic lesions are identical to those seen in young children.

Acute Infections

Thrombocytopenia may occasionally develop during an acute viral or bacterial infection. Direct platelet damage caused by platelet-bacterium or platelet-virus interaction probably contributes significantly to thrombocytopenia. Extracellular toxins from both staphylococci and streptococci as well as endotoxins from gram-negative organisms lead to platelet damage and aggregation. In cases of severe sepsis, thrombocytopenia may in fact reflect consumption of circulating platelets in association with DIC. In contrast, the thrombocytopenia of some viral infections may be caused by suppression of megakaryocytic function, as is seen in congenital rubella.

SEQUESTRATION THROMBOCYTOPENIA

Thrombocytopenia may occur in any disorder associated with an enlarged spleen. The characteristic clinical picture is prominent splenomegaly with moderate thrombocytopenia (50,000 to 100,000 platelets per cubic millimeter). This entity has also been referred to as *hypersplenic thrombocytopenia*. Under normal circumstances, approximately one third of the total body platelet mass is in the spleen and the splenic platelet pool exchanges with the freely circulating platelets. In splenomegaly of any cause, the splenic platelet pool may be greatly expanded and up to 90 per cent of the platelets can be trapped at any one time. Thus a redistribution of platelets can occur, resulting in thrombocytopenia despite normal platelet production and normal platelet survival. In addition, young platelets tend to accumulate in the spleen to a greater extent than old platelets. The clinical picture will reflect the underlying etiology of the splenomegaly, e.g., cirrhosis with portal hypertension, myelofibrosis, or infiltrative disease such as Gaucher's disease or malignant lymphoma. The thrombocytopenia secondary to splenomegaly is rarely severe enough to produce hemorrhagic disease. Splenectomy, however, will generally restore a normal or even elevated platelet count.

DILUTIONAL THROMBOCYTOPENIA

Massive blood transfusions, extracorporeal circulation, and exchange transfusion may result in moderate thrombocytopenia because of blood volume replacement with platelet-poor banked blood. The severity of the thrombocytopenia is directly related to the number of transfusions.

791. THROMBOCYTOSIS

Thrombocytosis refers to clinical situations in which the platelet count is significantly elevated. Benign or secondary thrombocytosis usually occurs as a temporary event in the setting of another condition such as splenectomy, acute or chronic inflammatory disease, hemolytic anemia, acute hemorrhage, or iron deficiency, or as a response to exercise. Asymptomatic secondary thrombocytosis with platelet counts in the range of 700,000 to 1,000,000 per cubic millimeter has been reported in a number of patients with carcinoma, Hodgkin's disease, and other malignant lymphomas. The nature of the reactive thrombocytosis in these conditions is unknown, but it may represent a nonspecific megakaryocytic proliferative response to tissue necrosis. It is of interest that thrombocytosis has been noted after the use of drugs such as vincristine, which interferes with microtubules.

Essential thrombocythemia is characterized by spontaneous bleeding, at times alternating or coinciding with thrombotic episodes accompanied by a sustained elevation in the platelet count. The process may be considered one of the myeloproliferative diseases and can accompany or develop into chronic myelogenous leukemia, polycythemia vera, or myelofibrosis. The platelet count is usually in the range of 1,000,000 per cubic millimeter, and giant irregular forms and aggregates of platelets are seen on the peripheral smear. Platelet function studies such as the bleeding time, platelet factor 3 release, and platelet aggregation in response to epinephrine are frequently abnormal. The platelets are probably qualitatively defective; however, the precise mechanisms underlying the thrombotic and hemorrhagic symptoms are unknown. In some patients essential thrombocythemia has been unmasked after splenectomy for unrelated conditions. *Pseudohyperkalemia* is an interesting laboratory artifact seen in some of these patients. Serum potassium levels may be strikingly elevated in the absence of electrocardiographic evidence of hyperkalemia. In this circumstance the plasma potassium levels are normal, and the elevated serum levels are caused by release of potassium from platelets

during blood clotting. Clinically the hemorrhagic and thrombotic symptoms improve as the platelet count is lowered. Busulfan and other myelosuppressive agents have proved useful in the long-term management of these patients. Antiplatelet aggregating agents, such as aspirin and dipyridamole, may prove useful in preventing thrombotic complications.

792. QUALITATIVE PLATELET ABNORMALITIES

Several hemorrhagic disorders have been attributed to abnormalities in platelet function occurring in the presence of adequate numbers of circulating platelets. The abnormalities may result from (1) defects in the primary hemostatic process involving adhesion or cohesion, leading to ineffective platelet plug formation, and/or (2) defects in the procoagulant activity of platelets associated with abnormal platelet factor 3 availability. The bleeding time is probably the most useful in vivo test for rapid evaluation of platelet function. In addition, a number of in vitro test systems to monitor platelet aggregation and to measure the platelet adhesiveness to glass bead columns have helped to clarify these different defects. The presence of a qualitative platelet abnormality in a patient is established by the following criteria: (1) hemorrhagic history in the absence of a disorder of the coagulation factors, (2) normal platelet count, and (3) abnormal platelet function.

A large group of qualitative platelet disorders have not yet been satisfactorily characterized. Some exceedingly rare congenital disorders have been reported, including the *Bernard-Soulier syndrome*, a potentially fatal hemorrhagic condition with circulating giant lymphocytoid platelets. Both morphologic and functional platelet abnormalities have been observed in patients with certain inherited disorders of connective tissue, including *Ehlers-Danlos syndrome, osteogenesis imperfecta*, and *pseudoxanthoma elasticum*. Abnormal platelet function has been reported in the *Wiskott-Aldrich syndrome*. The more important diseases of abnormal platelet function are discussed below.

THROMBASTHENIA
(Glanzmann's Disease)

Thrombasthenia is a rare congenital hemorrhagic disease in which there is a profound aberration of the primary hemostatic process. The patients characteristically present with severe bleeding from mucous membranes, usually beginning in childhood. However, some suffer only a minor hemorrhagic problem. There is an autosomal recessive inheritance pattern. The bleeding time is markedly prolonged, and clot retraction is greatly reduced or absent. Platelets from these patients do not aggregate with ADP or thrombin. Although the precise nature of the platelet abnormality is unknown, defects in cellular size and shape as well as various enzyme abnormalities have been reported. Markedly diminished content of platelet fibrinogen in the presence of normal levels of plasma fibrinogen is a characteristic feature in most patients. The platelets also fail to provide surface platelet factor 3 activity after exposure to activating agents. If clinically significant bleeding occurs, they usually respond to therapy with platelet transfusions.

THROMBOPATHIA—DEFECTIVE ADP RELEASE

This is a relatively mild common platelet disorder. Patients present with easy bruising and mild to moderate postoperative bleeding, and the bleeding time may be moderately prolonged. Their platelets when studied in vitro respond normally to high ADP levels but show decreased aggregation with collagen and impaired aggregation with epinephrine. There are probably several types of abnormality within this group. For example, some patients appear to have decreased intracellular pools of ADP, whereas others have normal storage pools of ADP but are unable to release the nucleotide. The latter category resembles the defect seen after aspirin ingestion by normal subjects.

DRUG-INDUCED PLATELET ABNORMALITIES

Aspirin ingestion results in abnormal platelet function because of inhibition of the release of intrinsic platelet ADP. The bleeding time may be slightly prolonged, and platelet aggregation induced by collagen or epinephrine is abnormal. The mechanism by which aspirin inhibits ADP release is not known; however, acetylation of a platelet membrane protein may be an important component of the process. It is of interest that the effect of a single dose of aspirin may last for several days. In some individuals administration of small amounts of aspirin may prolong the bleeding time and lead to a significant hemorrhagic disorder, particularly if the patient is subjected to a surgical stress. This exaggerated aspirin response may reflect the unmasking of an underlying platelet functional abnormality. Patients with thrombocytopenia or blood coagulation disorders should avoid aspirin.

Other agents also can interfere with normal platelet function. Plasma expanders such as *dextran* and *hydroxyethyl starch* prolong the bleeding time, presumably by interrupting the normal process of adhesion. Numerous other agents currently used in clinical medicine adversely affect normal hemostasis. Included in this group are the anti-inflammatory agents *Butazolidin, sulfinpyrazone,* and *Indocin,* some *antihistamines,* various *local anesthetics, clofibrate,* and *dipyridamole.* Some of these pharmacologic agents or structural analogues may be useful as agents to counteract platelet aggregation in thrombotic disorders.

ACQUIRED PLATELET FUNCTIONAL ABNORMALITIES—SYSTEMIC DISEASE

Uremia. The bleeding time in uremic patients is frequently prolonged out of proportion to that caused by the moderate thrombocytopenia which is commonly present. The most consistent laboratory abnormalities include decreased platelet adhesiveness to glass bead columns and impaired release of the coagulant activity, platelet factor 3. Normal platelets in uremic plasma function abnormally, and the defect in uremia improves significantly after dialysis. It is therefore probable that the platelet functional aberration in uremia results from the accumulation of small molecular weight metabolic waste products.

Dysglobulinemia. Abnormal platelet function has been observed in patients with macroglobulinemia as well as in multiple myeloma. Macroglobulin probably coats the platelet surface and sterically interferes with the normal hemostatic reactions. Improvement has been noted in patients after plasmapheresis.

Defects in platelet aggregation with prolonged bleeding times have been seen in a number of systemic conditions such as *cirrhosis, systemic lupus erythematosus,* and *pernicious anemia.* The hemorrhagic symptoms in these conditions may be related to the associated qualitative platelet abnormalities.

793. VASCULAR PURPURA

A varied group of clinical syndromes are characterized by intrinsic abnormalities of the blood vessel wall which result in mucosal and skin hemorrhages in the absence of overt defects in platelet function and number or plasma clotting factor defects. These syndromes are listed in Table 4.

Among the most common examples is *purpura simplex.* This is seen in otherwise healthy females who present with frequent but relatively harmless purpuric lesions. The disorder is lifelong, and there is occasionally a positive family history. It is disturbing cosmetically, and there is no effective treatment. It is significant only that this benign condition should be distinguished from the more serious purpuric states.

Senile Purpura. This is a relatively harmless, common condition primarily affecting the elderly. Purpuric lesions are mainly localized over the back of the hands and the extensor surfaces of the forearms. Large superficial ecchymotic areas may develop after mild trauma. The lesions occur in thin parchment-like atrophic skin and are presumably related to the degeneration of sub-

TABLE 4. Causes of Vascular Purpura

Senile purpura
Dysproteinemia
 Macroglobulinemia
 Multiple myeloma
 Cryoglobulinemia
 Benign hyperglobulinemic purpura
Nonthrombocytopenic drug purpura
Henoch-Schönlein purpura
Hereditary connective tissue disorders
 Ehlers-Danlos syndrome
 Pseudoxanthoma elasticum
 Marfan's syndrome
 Osteogenesis imperfecta
Cushing's syndrome
Scurvy
Autoerythrocyte sensitivity

cutaneous elastic tissue. They are of little clinical significance.

Dysproteinemia. Vascular purpura may be seen in *macroglobulinemia, myeloma,* and *cryoglobulinemia.* As noted previously, the nonthrombocytopenic purpura may develop because of protein coating of the platelet surface as well as coating of endothelial vascular surfaces, leading to impairment in blood vessel integrity. Epistaxis is a common symptom in these patients. It is probable that platelet dysfunction as well as coagulation factor abnormalities contributes to the bleeding diatheses in patients with myeloma, particularly those of the IgA type. Hyperviscosity with sludging of red cells also contributes to capillary anoxia. In cryoglobulinemia, purpuric lesions appear after exposure to cold and are more frequent during the winter months.

Benign hyperglobulinemic purpura primarily affects middle-aged females who present with successive crops of petechiae on the legs occurring at variable intervals, leading to pigmentary changes in the skin. Occasionally local itching or urticaria precedes the petechial eruptions. In half the cases other conditions such as Sjögren's syndrome, disseminated lupus erythematosus, or rheumatoid arthritis are also present. The hypergammaglobulinemia is due to the presence of high titer IgG antiglobulins.

Nonthrombocytopenic Drug Purpura. Some of the agents listed in Table 3 (Ch. 790) may lead to purpura in the absence of thrombocytopenia. The chlorothiazides and chemically related compounds are probably the most common offenders. In these situations, it is probable that the vascular endothelium rather than the circulating platelet serves as a target tissue. Whether this is a true immunologic reaction remains to be determined. The bleeding disorder is usually mild, and the only necessary therapy is removal of the suspected offending agent.

Henoch-Schönlein Purpura. This allergic vasculitis occurs most frequently in children after a streptococcal infection or, occasionally, after ingestion of a sensitizing food or drug. The skin is invariably involved, usually with extensive elevated purpuric or ecchymotic lesions scattered over the extensor surfaces of the extremities. Initially, the skin lesion is urticarial in nature and gradually becomes hemorrhagic. The rash typically occurs in recurrent crops and may involve the face. Other systems frequently affected include the joints, especially knees and ankles, gastrointestinal tract, and kidneys. Intestinal complications include intramural hematomas and gross mucosal hemorrhage, both of which may be accompanied by severe colicky pain, hematemesis, and melena. Renal involvement with hematuria is seen in approximately 50 per cent of the patients. Chronic nephritis with uremia may also develop (see Ch. 611). In the younger patients, the disease is usually self-limited. Steroids have been used, particularly in the more severely ill patients with visceral involvement.

Hereditary Connective Tissue Disorders. Vascular purpura may be seen in certain inherited disorders of connective tissue, including the *Ehlers-Danlos syndrome, pseudoxanthoma elasticum, osteogenesis imperfecta,* and *Marfan's syndrome.* In some of these disorders abnormal platelet function has also been reported.

Cushing's Syndrome. Nonthrombocytopenic purpura predominantly distributed over the trunk and lower extremities is seen after prolonged administration of exogenous steroids as well as in patients with Cushing's syndrome. The nature of the vascular lesion is unknown; however, some observers believe that chronic exposure of the vasculature to steroids produces a catabolic effect which interferes with vascular integrity.

Scurvy. Chronic vitamin C deficiency is primarily a disease of extremes of age—the very young and the very old. Epistaxis, hematuria, and gastrointestinal bleeding are seen in infants. In adults, deep intramuscular hematomas are frequently encountered. In addition to the vessel wall defect, qualitative platelet defects may also contribute to the bleeding.

Autoerythrocyte Sensitivity. This unusual condition is seen only in women and is characterized by the spontaneous appearance of painful ecchymoses. The lesions occur over the anterior aspects of the upper and lower extremities and spread superficially. Many patients give a history of trauma preceding the onset of the ecchymoses. In general, the lesions appear over areas which are liable to superficial trauma. The etiology of the illness is not known; however, some evidence suggests that certain of these women are sensitive to their own red cells. Many of the patients have significant emotional difficulties, and the lesions at times may be self-inflicted.

794. HEREDITARY HEMORRHAGIC TELANGIECTASIA
(Osler-Weber-Rendu Disease)

Hereditary hemorrhagic telangiectasia is an inherited disorder associated with intermittent bleeding from vascular abnormalities scattered throughout the body, particularly on mucosal surfaces. Skin lesions appear as small, flattened telangiectases or dilated, raised small vascular nodules which blanch with pressure. The lesions are common on the face and in the mucous membranes of the tongue, lips, and nose. They are also found in the scalp, fingertips, conjunctival surfaces, vagina, and rectum. Visceral lesions are most common in the gastrointestinal tract, but the respiratory and genitourinary systems may also be involved. Approximately 20 per cent of the patients have pulmonary arteriovenous fistulas. Recurrent spontaneous epistaxis is the most common symptom. Severe gastrointestinal bleeding may also be a major clinical problem. The patients invariably have iron deficiency anemia which is sometimes severe. The pathologic lesions involving arterioles, venules, and capillaries are characterized by marked thinning of the vessel wall with ballooning and aneurysm formation. Management consists of symptomatic care of recurrent bleeding. Various plastic surgical procedures have been utilized to diminish the particularly troublesome recurrent episodes of epistaxis. Local pressure with packing is helpful. Systemic estrogen therapy has not proved particularly beneficial. All patients should be maintained on long-term iron administration.

Aster, R. H.: Thrombocytopenia due to enhanced platelet destruction. *In* Williams, W., Beutler, E., Erslev, H., and Rundles, R. (eds.): Hematology. New York, McGraw-Hill Book Company, 1972, Chap. 139, p. 1131.

Aster, R. H., and Keene, W. R.: Sites of platelet destruction in idiopathic thrombocytopenic purpura. Br. J. Haematol., 16:61, 1969.

Capra, D. J., Winchester, R. J., and Kunkel, H. G.: Hyperglobulinemic purpura. Studies on the unusual anti-γ globulins characteristic of the sera of these patients. Medicine, 50:125, 1971.

Horowitz, H. I., and Nachman, R. L.: Drug purpura. Semin. Hematol., 2:287, 1965.

Jaffé, E., Nachman, R., and Merskey, C.: Thrombotic thrombocytopenic purpura. Coagulation parameters in twelve patients. Blood, 42:499, 1973.

Karpatkin, S., and Siskind, G.: In vitro detection of platelet antibody in patients with idiopathic thrombocytopenic purpura and systemic lupus erythematosus. Blood, 33:795, 1969.

Marcus, A. J.: Platelet function. N. Engl. J. Med., 280:1213, 1278, 1330, 1969.

Nachman, R. L.: Disorders of primary hemostasis. *In* Mengel, C., Frei, T., and Nachman, R. L. (eds.): Hematology. Chicago, Year Book Medical Publishers, 1972, p. 600.

Shulman, N. R.: A mechanism of cell destruction in individuals sensitized to foreign antigens and its implications in autoimmunity. Ann. Intern. Med., 60:506, 1964.

Section Fifteen.   HEMORRHAGIC DISORDERS: COAGULATION DEFECTS

Oscar D. Ratnoff

795.   INTRODUCTION

A hemorrhagic disorder often appears when blood coagulation is impaired. Defective hemostasis may be caused by (1) inadequate production of one or more of the procoagulant substances of blood, (2) depletion of components required for clotting as a result of increased utilization, (3) the presence in blood of inhibitors of coagulation, or (4) activation of proteolytic mechanisms of plasma. Blood normally contains a relative abundance of each clotting factor, and hemorrhage is rarely the result of deficiency of one of these substances unless its concentration has been reduced to less than 50 per cent of the normal value. Abnormal bleeding may result from lack of each of the known clotting factors, with three exceptions. Hageman factor (factor XII) and Fletcher factor (plasma prekallikrein), proteins concerned with the initiation of blood clotting upon contact with foreign surfaces, are apparently not required for normal hemostasis. Depletion of calcium is not a cause of abnormal bleeding, because the cardiovascular and neuromuscular effects of profound hypocalcemia are incompatible with life. Deficiency of a single clotting factor is usually the result of an inherited disorder. Acquired coagulation defects are more likely to involve multiple components of the clotting system. In some clinical situations several mechanisms operate to impair hemostasis, and the extent to which each contributes may be difficult to analyze.

A knowledge of the physiology of blood clotting is essential in interpreting the results of laboratory tests useful in the diagnosis of hemostatic defects. Blood clots when fibrinogen (factor I) is converted to fibrin through the action of a proteolytic enzyme, thrombin (Fig. 1). Fibrinogen is a dimer, each half consisting of three subunits, Aα, Bβ and γ chains. Thrombin splits off from each half of fibrinogen fibrinopeptides A and B, from the Aα and Bβ chains, respectively. What remains, fibrin monomer, then polymerizes to form insoluble strands of fibrin. The polymerization of fibrin is accelerated by calcium ions at physiologic concentrations, and probably by a heat-labile accelerator in normal plasma.

Under physiologic conditions, the molecules of fibrin are chemically bonded to each other by a second enzyme, fibrin-stabilizing factor (factor XIII), a transamidase which provides mechanical strength to the fibrin strands. Thrombin does not exist in detectable amounts in normal blood. When blood is shed, thrombin evolves through one or both of two convergent sequences of chemical reactions, the extrinsic and intrinsic pathways. Presumably, similar mechanisms operate to induce clotting in vivo. Thrombin formation via the extrinsic pathway is initiated by components of tissue known as tissue thromboplastin which interact with several plasma agents, factor VII, Stuart factor (factor X), proaccelerin (factor V), and calcium ions, to bring about the formation of a prothrombin-converting principle (Fig. 2). Blood also clots without the participation of tissue thromboplastin upon contact with certain negatively charged surfaces such as glass; in vivo, collagen and sebum may serve this function. This intrinsic pathway requires the successive participation of Hageman factor (factor XII), Fletcher factor, plasma thromboplastin antecedent (PTA, factor XI), Christmas factor (PTC, factor IX), antihemophilic factor (factor VIII), Stuart factor, and proaccelerin (Fig. 2). Some or all of these factors are "activated" during the clotting process. A prothrombin-converting principle, probably identical with that developed through the extrinsic pathway, evolves when calcium ions and phospholipids are available, the latter supplied by platelets and the plasma it-

Figure 1.   The formation of fibrin in human plasma. The site of action of the plasma accelerator, if this exists, is not known.

THE INTRINSIC CLOTTING MECHANISM

Figure 2. The intrinsic and extrinsic pathways for the formation of thrombin. Omitted from the diagram are inhibitors of the various steps. The phospholipid portion of tissue thromboplastin may function in the formation and action of the prothrombin-converting principle. The phospholipid for the intrinsic pathway is furnished by platelets and by the plasma itself. A proposed action of kallikrein on factor VII is not depicted.

self. Once the prothrombin-converting principle has formed, it liberates thrombin from its precursor, prothrombin (factor II), by an enzymatic process. In addition to its action on fibrinogen, thrombin promotes clotting in several ways, liberating phospholipid from platelets, activating fibrin-stabilizing factor from an inert precursor, and altering antihemophilic factor and proaccelerin so as to heighten their activity. Plasma contains potent inhibitors of the clotting process, of which those inhibiting thrombin, tissue thromboplastin, and the activated forms of Hageman factor, PTA, and Stuart factor are most clearly defined. It also contains the precursor of plasmin, a powerful proteolytic enzyme which can digest fibrinogen, fibrin, and other clotting factors as well as certain other substrates. The sole or principal site of synthesis of several clotting factors—namely, fibrinogen, prothrombin, factor VII, proaccelerin, Stuart factor, and Christmas factor—is the hepatic parenchymal cell. Vascular endothelium has been implicated in the synthesis of antihemophilic factor; the locus of synthesis of other factors is not certain.

The laboratory procedures used to differentiate disorders of blood clotting are based upon these physiologic considerations. Thus defects in the extrinsic pathway of coagulation are readily detected by measuring the one-stage prothrombin time, in which tissue thromboplastin and calcium ions are added to decalcified plasma, and the interval of time elapsing until clotting takes place is measured. Defects in the intrinsic pathway are reflected in the test tube by delayed clotting of whole blood, retarded "thromboplastin generation" (a misnomer for the evolution of the prothrombin-converting principle), deficient conversion of prothrombin to thrombin, i.e., prothrombin consumption, and a prolonged partial thromboplastin time, i.e., the clotting time of recalcified plasma in the presence of phospholipid to which an activator of Hageman factor, such as kaolin, is often added. The one-stage prothrombin time is normal in persons whose defect is restricted to the early part of the intrinsic pathway, before the participation of Stuart factor, but is prolonged if defects of the later parts of the

pathway are present. Defects in the conversion of fibrinogen to fibrin are measured by testing the effect of preformed thrombin on the clotting time of plasma, i.e., the thrombin time, whereas a deficiency of fibrin-stabilizing factor is detected by noting the solubility of fibrin in 5 molar urea or 1 per cent monochloroacetic acid, which cannot dissolve fibrin bonded by this factor.

The laboratory procedures available for investigation of defects of coagulation are often crude, nonspecific, and influenced by variations in technique. Accordingly, care is required in selection and performance of the tests and in interpretation of results. Assays are available for each of the known clotting factors. Final identification of a specific deficiency requires mixing of the patient's plasma with that of a patient with a known coagulation defect to determine whether correction occurs. Only fibrinogen can be measured in gravimetric terms, by its conversion to fibrin and by determination of the protein content of the clot.

Biggs, R. (ed.): Human Blood Coagulation, Hemostasis and Thrombosis. Oxford, Blackwell Scientific Publications, 1972.

Harker, L. A. (ed.): The Hemostasis Manual. 2nd ed. Philadelphia, F. A. Davis Company, 1974.

Poller, L. (ed.): Recent Advances in Blood Coagulation. London, J. & A. Churchill, Ltd., 1969.

Ratnoff, O. D. (ed.) Treatment of Hemorrhagic Disorders. New York, Harper & Row, 1968.

HERITABLE DISORDERS OF BLOOD COAGULATION

796.   INTRODUCTION

The familial occurrence of a deficiency of each of the organic clotting factors is well established. The cause is either deficient synthesis or the synthesis of functionally defective factors. Transmission of the defect is genetically determined. In most instances, severe function deficiency of a single clotting factor is encountered in homozygotes in autosomal recessive traits and in male hemizygotes and female homozygotes in X-linked recessive disorders. In some cases, heterozygous carriers can be shown to have a reduced plasma level of the procoagulant, but, except in von Willebrand's disease, the deficiency is rarely sufficient to impair hemostasis. In one anomaly, dysfibrinogenemia, an autosomal dominant gene appears to be responsible for synthesis of a protein that may be normal in quantity but abnormal in structure and function. Rarely, familial deficiency of more than one clotting factor has been encountered. The genetic basis for multiple hemostatic defects is not understood.

797. CLASSIC HEMOPHILIA

Classic hemophilia, the best known of the familial disorders of blood coagulation, is the result of functional deficiency of antihemophilic factor (factor VIII). The plasma does not lack antihemophilic factor. Rather, it appears to contain a nonfunctional variant of this clotting factor. The abnormality is attributable to an X-linked recessive gene so that the disorder occurs almost exclusively in males. The sons of a male hemophiliac are unaffected and do not transmit the disease, although all his daughters are carriers. Heterozygous females do not bleed, but half their sons have hemophilia and half their daughters are carriers. Homozygous females, very rarely encountered, have the typical disease. The clinical manifestations vary from family to family, correlating with the intensity of the functional deficiency of antihemophilic factor, but within a family the degree of the bleeding tendency among affected members is about the same. A positive family history is obtained in only about two thirds of cases.

Clinical Manifestations. In severe hemophilia, in which virtually no functional antihemophilic factor is detectable in plasma, serious or lethal hemorrhage may occur in the neonatal period after circumcision, but bleeding from the umbilicus is unusual. In infancy, the bleeding tendency is frequently manifested by the appearance of cutaneous ecchymoses or hematomas in soft tissues, often after injuries so trivial as to be unnoted. Bleeding from the mouth, in particular from the frenum of the upper lip, is sometimes encountered in young children. After the early years of life, hemorrhages into the joints are characteristic. Increasing deformity, limitation of motion, and destruction of joints result from repeated hemarthroses, commonly the most disabling manifestation of the disease. The ankles, knees, and elbows are particularly likely to be involved, whereas the hands are usually spared. Bleeding is limited by the tension of the joint capsule, and ceases when the synovial space becomes distended. Hemorrhages into soft tissues are not similarly restricted, and may extend widely, dissecting through subcutaneous tissue, along fascial planes, or into muscles. Even enormous hematomas are usually reabsorbed, but sometimes they persist, leaving firm masses that calcify. Pseudotumors can produce symptoms by pressure on other structures, or

may erode bone and simulate neoplasms. Hemorrhages into the muscles sometimes cause contractures and deformities such as a claw hand. Bleeding into the lax tissues beneath the tongue, in the pharynx, or in the neck is particularly dangerous, because it may interfere with swallowing or may occlude the respiratory passage. Retroperitoneal hemorrhage can produce symptoms simulating those of appendicitis, or can give rise to other manifestations such as obstructive jaundice owing to occlusion of the common bile duct or fulminant hypertension from compression of the kidneys. Hemorrhage into the mesentery can cause abdominal pain, digestive symptoms, or even avascular necrosis of the bowel. Episodes of hematuria, often accompanied by ureteral colic, are common and tend to persist for weeks if untreated. Hemorrhage into the gastrointestinal tract may occur. Excessive bleeding is the rule after dental extraction or minor surgery, and tonsillectomy or major operative procedures may lead to fatal hemorrhage. Subdural hematomas and other hemorrhages into the central nervous system, although uncommon, are an important cause of disability or death, and may result from relatively trivial injury. Hematomas encroaching on nerve trunks may cause sensory loss or paralysis.

Only about half of hemophiliacs present this grim picture. Such individuals have little or no functional antihemophilic factor in their plasma. In others, in whom the concentration of this factor may be as high as 30 per cent of normal, the symptoms are proportionately milder, and bleeding may occur only after such challenges as injury, operative procedures, or dental extractions.

Diagnosis. Specific diagnosis can be established only by laboratory tests of blood coagulation, although the character of the bleeding and the family history provide important clues. Tests that detect abnormalities in the intrinsic pathway of coagulation usually give abnormal results, but the clotting time of whole blood may be normal in mildly affected patients. The prothrombin time, thrombin time, and bleeding time are normal. Proof of diagnosis requires the use of appropriate tests to demonstrate the functional deficiency of antihemophilic factor, preferably including an assay using the plasma of a known hemophiliac. A normal bleeding time helps to differentiate mild cases from von Willebrand's disease; careful analysis of the pattern of inheritance and tests of other relatives may be necessary. Further support for the diagnosis in doubtful cases can be obtained by demonstrating the presence of normal or elevated antigenic material related to antihemophilic factor in the plasma, typical of classic hemophilia, using antiserum raised in rabbits. All patients deficient in antihemophilic factor must be tested for the presence of circulating anticoagulants directed against this substance.

Treatment. Patients with hereditary hemorrhagic disease often have difficulty adjusting to the problems inherent in a disorder that poses unexpected threats to normal behavior and to life itself. As soon as the diagnosis is made, the patient or his parents should be instructed concerning the care, prognostic implications, and hereditary nature of his disorder. The parents should be encouraged to rear their afflicted children in as normal a way as is consistent with safety, for emotional crippling is as devastating as that resulting from hemorrhage. While the patient is too young to guard himself, the parents should arrange his environment so that it is as danger-free as possible, in order to lessen the need to restrain his behavior. As he grows older, the patient should be advised to indulge in such sports as swimming, running, tennis, and golf, and to avoid those involving body contact or predisposing to injury. The hemophiliac should prepare for a vocation which is not inherently dangerous; he and his parents should be reminded that hemophilia does not preclude a useful life in business or the professions. The object of therapy is to allow the patient to become a self-supporting adult, capable of caring for himself and living as full a life as possible.

The mainstay of therapy for episodes of bleeding is the transfusion of normal plasma or fractions of plasma rich in antihemophilic factor to correct temporarily the specific defect. The use of whole blood is restricted to the maintenance of blood volume after severe blood loss. Enough plasma or its fractions must be administered to raise the blood level of antihemophilic factor sufficiently to permit normal hemostasis. Once transfused, antihemophilic factor disappears rapidly from the circulation, only about half remaining after 10 to 12 hours, so that repeated transfusions must be given until bleeding has been controlled. Therapy with plasma or its fractions carries with it risks of transmitting hepatitis and of inducing the formation of circulating anticoagulants that specifically inhibit antihemophilic factor.

In the event of major injury or in preparation for surgical procedures, the plasma level of antihemophilic factor must be raised to at least 30 or 40 per cent that of a normal individual; lesser amounts may be adequate to control bleeding into joints or minor soft tissue hemorrhage. When only fresh or fresh-frozen plasma was available as a source of antihemophilic factor, adequate plasma levels of this substance were difficult to achieve without danger of circulatory overload except by exchange transfusion. Fortunately, during the last few years concentrates of antihemophilic factor that can be administered in a small volume have become generally available. One preparation in wide use is *cryoprecipitated antihemophilic factor,* separated during the cold thawing of fresh-frozen plasma. Plasma levels sufficient for adequate hemostasis can be achieved with the administration of the cryoprecipitate of 1 unit of plasma for each 4 kg of body weight, sustaining the plasma level of antihemophilic factor by administering half this amount every 12 hours. Larger doses may be needed if surgical procedures are undertaken. Another useful preparation is *lyophilized antihemophilic factor,* separated from plasma either by cryoprecipitation or by addition of glycine or other protein precipitants. Such material can be used under conditions in which frozen cryoprecipitated antihemophilic factor is not available. No rule of thumb can be provided as to how long therapy should be continued. In general, after surgery, dental extraction, or severe bleeding, concentrated antihemophilic factor is administered in the manner described for at least two days after all signs of bleeding have ceased, and the dose is then gradually decreased over the succeeding three or four days. Shorter courses of therapy are used when the danger of renewed bleeding is less threatening, as in most instances of hemarthrosis.

The availability of concentrates of antihemophilic factor has made it possible to abort hemorrhage more readily than was formerly possible without circulatory embarrassment. It has reduced the risk of surgical procedures and dental extractions in hemophiliacs. Indeed, in many patients, elective surgical procedures may be carried out, although surgery should be performed only in hospitals equipped to deal with this special problem.

This optimistic picture must be tempered by the fact that in as many as 20 per cent of severe hemophiliacs a circulating anticoagulant appears in plasma that specifically inactivates antihemophilic factor. The presence of this agent, which is an antibody directed against antihemophilic factor, vitiates the beneficial results of transfusion. Patients in whom this complication is present should under no conditions be subjected to surgery. Experimentally, immunosuppressive therapy has been attempted, but the results are usually disappointing.

If the bleeding site is accessible, *hemostasis* may be most effectively achieved by local measures. By appropriate use of local hemostatic agents such as bovine thrombin and the application of cold and gentle pressure, bleeding may often be controlled. These measures must be sustained, for recurrent bleeding is likely over a period of days. Dental extractions in particular require meticulous local measures. Extractions should be carried out only in the hospital and by dental surgeons with special training in the care of hemophiliacs. Except in patients with mild hemophilia, hemostasis should be enhanced by the transfusion of concentrates of antihemophilic factor. The administration of *epsilon-aminocaproic acid* (4 grams every four hours for ten days in adults) may reduce the need for transfusion therapy.

The transfusion of concentrated antihemophilic factor is also useful in aborting *bleeding into joints.* A single dose of cryoprecipitated antihemophilic factor, one bag for every 2 2/3 kg of body weight, combined with a short course of prednisone, 1 mg per kilogram daily for three days, with a maximum of 80 mg per day, followed by 0.5 mg per kilogram for two days, with a maximum of 40 mg per day, has been useful. Acutely swollen joints should be immobilized. Local chilling and application of elastic bandages may be beneficial, but the application of a constricting bandage is contraindicated. Aspiration of the joint is occasionally advantageous, and should be performed only after adequate transfusion therapy. Active motion without weight-bearing is essential after bleeding has stopped in order to prevent persistent limitation of motion. Careful use of physiotherapy, traction, and splints may be helpful in preventing and correcting deformities. Surgical correction of certain deformities has been successfully accomplished, but should be attempted only by experts and under the supervision of someone skilled in the transfusion therapy of hemophiliacs. Increased mobility of joints has sometimes been achieved by synovectomy.

Other forms of bleeding require special types of care. Particularly hazardous is bleeding into the soft tissues of the neck, in which tracheostomy, performed under the cover of transfusion therapy, may be needed. Hemophiliacs should not be given intramuscular injections, but venipunctures are not hazardous if performed with care. Immunization against tetanus is important, because bleeders are particularly prone to infection with this organism, but this is wisely delayed in severe hemophiliacs until the first course of replacement therapy. Immunization may be carried out without such preparation in mildly affected patients. Regular prophylactic care of the teeth should be provided. Bleeders should avoid the use of aspirin, because this agent may impair hemostasis. Acetaminophen, 0.65 gram every four hours in adults, and proportionately less in children, is a useful substitute.

Prognosis. The outlook for the hemophiliac has been greatly improved by modern methods of treatment. Those with moderately severe or mild hemophilia may seem so little affected that they live virtually normal lives, but even these patients may have exsanguinating hemorrhage after dental extraction, injury, or surgery. Those in whom the defect is more pronounced may require frequent admission to the hospital, and may be crippled by joint deformities. Some meet the challenge and are reasonably productive individuals, although others seem foredoomed to chronic invalidism. The life expectancy of hemophiliacs has lengthened with the availability of transfusion therapy, but death as the result of the complications of hemorrhage still occurs with disturbing frequency.

Detection of Carriers. Certain women in hemophilia families are necessarily carriers—the daughters of affected men, the mothers of more than one hemophiliac, and the mother of one hemophiliac who has other affected relatives. The carrier state in other women can be detected with a high degree of certainty by simultaneous measurement of functional antihemophilic factor and antigens related to this agent. In normal women, these two modalities vary from individual to individual, but in proportion. In contrast, in carriers, relative excess of antigenic material is nearly always present. Because of variation of functional antihemophilic factor titers both in normal women and in known carriers, this procedure alone successfully detects only a small proportion of carriers.

Biggs, R. (ed.): Human Blood Coagulation, Hemostasis and Thrombosis. Oxford, Blackwell Scientific Publications, 1972.

Biggs, R., and Macfarlane, R. G.: Treatment of Hemophilia and Other Coagulation Disorders. Oxford, Blackwell Scientific Publications, 1966.

Douglas, A. S. (ed.): Blood coagulation and fibrinolysis in clinical practice. Clinics in Haematology, Vol. 2, No. 1. London, W. B. Saunders, Ltd., 1973.

Hardisty, R. M., and Ingram, G. I. C.: Bleeding Disorders. Investigation and Management. Philadelphia, F. A. Davis Company, 1965.

Ratnoff, O. D. (ed.): Treatment of Hemorrhagic Disorders. New York, Harper & Row, 1968.

Rossi, E. D. (ed.): Symposium on Hemorrhagic Disorders. Medical Clinics of North America, Vol. 56, No. 1. Philadelphia, W. B. Saunders Company, 1972.

Spaet, T. H. (ed.): Progress in Hemostasis and Thrombosis. Vol. 1. New York, Grune & Stratton, 1972.

798. OTHER HERITABLE DISORDERS OF BLOOD COAGULATION

Von Willebrand's disease (vascular hemophilia) is a hemorrhagic disorder characterized by a long bleeding time and deficiency of antihemophilic factor (factor VIII). Both functional antihemophilic factor and antigens in plasma related to antihemophilic factor are reduced, and in proportion. The disease is transmitted by a dominant autosomal mutant gene, but has been detected more often in women than in men. The severity of symptoms varies considerably among affected members of the same family, some of whom may be asymptomatic. Menorrhagia and postpartum bleeding are common. The patient may experience epistaxes and gingival bleeding in severe cases; cutaneous ecchymoses or hematomas may occur. Hemorrhage follows injury or surgical procedures. Hemarthroses are relatively uncommon, but visceral bleeding or severe and even lethal hemorrhage into the gastrointestinal tract has been observed. Occasionally, petechiae may be found.

A unique feature of von Willebrand's disease is the prolonged bleeding time, an abnormality not usually associated with other hemophilia-like diseases. The coagulation defect can be corrected in vitro by normal but not by hemophilic plasma. In contrast, transfusion of hemophilic as well as of normal plasma or serum is followed by a delayed but pronounced and protracted rise in the patient's plasma level of functional antihemophilic factor. A single unit of normal plasma may lead to the elevation of the antihemophilic activity of the patient's plasma to normal levels for many hours. Paradoxically, no corresponding rise in antigens related to antihemophilic factor occurs. These interesting observations are unexplained, although they suggest that the synthesis of antihemophilic factor takes place in at least two steps, the first of which is defective in von Willebrand's disease and the second in classic hemophilia. Whether the abnormality in bleeding time is due to a second plasma defect is disputed; the administration of plasma, but not of purified antihemophilic factor, is reported to shorten the bleeding time. Diagnosis is readily made when a markedly long bleeding time is encountered in a patient with functional deficiency of antihemophilic factor. Additionally, adhesion of platelets to glass beads is often impaired, although the specificity of this test is doubtful. Aggregation of platelets by the antimicrobial ristocetin, which occurs in normal or hemophilic platelet-rich plasma, is impeded in von Willebrand's disease. Sometimes, within a given family, affected individuals may be found in whom the bleeding time may be prolonged without significant deficiency of antihemophilic factor, or vice versa. Careful study of the patient's relatives may help to differentiate mild classic hemophilia from von Willebrand's disease. When the bleeding time is not significantly prolonged, recognition of the disease is facilitated by demonstration of a concomitant deficiency of antigens related to antihemophilic factor. Treatment of bleeding episodes consists of measures for local control of hemostasis and the administration of fresh blood, plasma, or cryoprecipitates of plasma, all of which contain the agent that induces synthesis of antihemophilic factor in von Willebrand's disease. Menorrhagia may be terminated by suppression of menstrual bleeding with hormonal preparations such as norethynodrel. During pregnancy, the titer of antihemophilic factor may rise to levels which would be normal in nonpregnant women, and parturition may occur without hemorrhage, although the bleeding time remains long.

Christmas disease is attributable to functional deficiency of Christmas factor (factor IX, plasma thromboplastin component), an abnormality transmitted by an X chromosome–linked gene. In most cases, patients seem unable to synthesize Christmas factor, whereas in a minority nonfunctional Christmas factor is demonstrable in plasma. The disorder typically occurs in males, and is less common than hemophilia, from which it is clinically indistinguishable. All the clinical manifestations of hemophilia are encountered in patients with Christmas disease. The disorder varies in severity from family to family, manifestations roughly paralleling the degree of the deficiency of Christmas factor measured in the laboratory. Heterozygous female carriers may have a partial deficiency of Christmas factor, and some have a mild bleeding tendency. A positive family history is obtained in only about two thirds of cases. Diagnosis is established by laboratory tests that demonstrate a defect in the early steps of the intrinsic pathway of thrombin formation, and by specific assay for Christmas factor, using a substrate plasma from a patient with known Christmas disease. Treatment is basically the same as for hemophilia, but cryoprecipitates of plasma lack Christmas factor. Christmas factor is relatively stable, so that the patient can be treated effectively with blood that has been stored under usual conditions in a blood bank. Large volumes of plasma are required to raise the level of Christmas factor sufficiently to provide normal hemostasis; thereafter smaller amounts will sustain the titer of this substance, because half the transfused Christmas factor is still present in the circulation after 20 or more hours. Concentrates of the vitamin K–dependent clotting factors, including Christmas factor, are now available, and can be used to provide large amounts of the missing factor without dangerous expansion of the circulating blood volume. These fractions, however, are often contaminated with hepatitis virus. In a few cases, the beneficial effects of transfusion are vitiated by the presence in the patient's plasma of a circulating anticoagulant, presumably an antibody directed against Christmas factor.

Plasma thromboplastin antecedent deficiency, a rare familial hemorrhagic disorder encountered in both sexes, is attributable to deficiency of PTA (factor XI). The disorder is inherited in an autosomal recessive manner; in most reported cases, the patients have been Jewish. Bleeding episodes often follow trauma or surgical procedures, but spontaneous bleeding occasionally occurs. Hemorrhage is usually less severe than in hemophilia, and hemarthrosis is rare. Sometimes the disorder is asymptomatic. Laboratory tests demonstrate a defect in the early steps of the intrinsic pathway of clotting, but the specific diagnosis is often difficult to establish even with appropriate tests, and requires careful confirmation, including matching the plasma with that of a patient known to have PTA deficiency. Transfusion of blood or plasma is used in the treatment of bleeding episodes. Since half of the infused PTA is still present in the circulation 60 hours after transfusion, correction of the defect is relatively simple.

Hageman trait is the hereditary deficiency of Hageman factor (factor XII). It occurs in both sexes, and is in most instances inherited as an autosomal recessive defect. Hageman trait is usually asymptomatic, although minor bleeding has occasionally been encountered. The diagnosis may be suspected when the clotting time is prolonged and a defect in the early steps of the intrinsic pathway is detected, but it can be established only by comparison with plasma of patients known to have this disorder. No treatment has been needed in reported cases, but in the event of hemorrhage normal plasma should be efficacious.

Fletcher trait is a rare, asymptomatic disorder of blood coagulation in which the intrinsic pathway of

clotting is defective as demonstrated by prolongation of the partial thromboplastin time. The defect is due to a deficiency of Fletcher factor, apparently identical with a plasma prekallikrein, needed for the optimal action of Hageman factor upon PTA. No therapy is needed.

Parahemophilia, a familial bleeding disorder affecting both sexes, is caused by a functional deficiency of proaccelerin (factor V); in some cases, the plasma is said to contain normal amounts of a nonfunctional agent immunologically related to proaccelerin. The disease is inherited in an autosomal recessive manner. Spontaneous bleeding may occur at numerous sites, but the joints are rarely involved. Menorrhagia and postoperative bleeding may occur, but in some patients the disease is mild or latent. The clue to diagnosis is provided by a prolonged prothrombin time which is not shortened by plasma deficient in proaccelerin. A presumptive diagnosis can be made by demonstrating that the prothrombin time is shortened by addition of plasma from which the vitamin K–dependent clotting factors have been removed, but this test does not rule out a deficiency of fibrinogen. During surgical procedures or when abnormal bleeding is sufficiently severe to justify transfusion, fresh blood or plasma should be given in amounts adequate to maintain the plasma level of proaccelerin at about 25 per cent of normal; half the amount of proaccelerin infused disappears from the circulation in 12 to 36 hours.

Congenital deficiency of factor VII is transmitted in an autosomal recessive manner. Homozygous individuals of both sexes display a bleeding tendency of varying severity correlating with the severity of the deficiency. In some patients the plasma contains no material recognizable as nonfunctional factor VII, whereas in others a nonfunctional variant of the protein is present. Numerous hemorrhagic manifestations have been encountered, including umbilical bleeding in the neonatal period, epistaxis, ecchymoses, hemarthroses, menorrhagia, and hemorrhages into the gastrointestinal tract and central nervous system. The one-stage prothrombin time is prolonged, an abnormality that is not affected by plasma or serum from patients known to have factor VII deficiency. Factor VII is stable so that stored plasma is of therapeutic value. Large volumes of plasma, infused repeatedly, are required for effective hemostasis because of the rapid disappearance of factor VII from the circulation, half the amount infused being removed in only one or two hours; concentrates of the vitamin K–dependent clotting factors may also be used. Menorrhagia may be controlled by the administration of oral contraceptive agents.

Stuart factor deficiency, a rare congenital disorder of blood coagulation, is characterized by deficiency of Stuart factor (factor X), and is attributable to an autosomal mutant gene. Only homozygotes have a bleeding tendency, which is similar to that of congenital deficiency of factor VII. In some instances a functionally defective form of Stuart factor is demonstrable in plasma, whereas in others a true deficiency of this agent is apparently present. The prothrombin time is prolonged and is not shortened by plasma from patients with known Stuart factor deficiency. The clotting time of recalcified plasma is not shortened to a normal degree by the addition of Russell's viper venom, which requires Stuart factor for its procoagulant effect. Treatment is the same as that for factor VII deficiency, but transfusions have a much more prolonged action, half of the Stuart factor remaining in the blood after two or three days, so that transfusions need not be repeated as frequently.

Prothrombin deficiency, an extremely rare autosomal recessive trait, is clinically similar to factor VII and Stuart factor deficiencies. Two varieties have been discerned, a true deficiency of prothrombin and a condition in which nonfunctional prothrombin is detectable in plasma. The prothrombin time is prolonged and is not shortened by the addition of normal serum or of plasma from which the vitamin K–dependent clotting factors have been removed. The treatment of bleeding is the same as that for factor VII deficiency; about half of infused prothrombin disappears from the circulation in nine hours.

A rare anomaly has been described in which individuals have unusual *resistance to coumarin-like drugs.* As much as 20 times the usual dose is required to achieve a therapeutic effect. The disorder is inherited in an autosomal dominant manner. The mechanism underlying the defect is unknown, but in an analogous disease of rats, the microsomal membranes lack the normal capacity to bind warfarin.

Congenital deficiency of fibrinogen, a rare disorder occurring in both sexes, is apparently transmitted as an autosomal recessive trait. Clinical manifestations may begin at birth with hemorrhage from the umbilicus. In general, bleeding is hemophilia-like, except that permanent joint damage from hemarthroses is uncommon. Some patients have remarkably little bleeding, and even menstrual blood loss may not be excessive, but others have severe hemorrhages that can be fatal in early life. The blood does not clot even after the addition of thrombin, and little or no fibrinogen can be detected in plasma by physical, chemical, or immunologic methods. Bleeding episodes can be satisfactorily treated by intravenous administration of fibrinogen, either in the form of Cohn fraction I or of cryoprecipitates of plasma, in amounts sufficient to maintain a plasma fibrinogen level in excess of 100 mg per 100 ml. Several instances in which therapy has been impeded by the development of antibodies against fibrinogen have been reported. Strangely, death from obstruction of the pulmonary circulation by "thrombi" composed of platelets has been described.

Congenital dysfibrinogenemia is a recently described group of familial disorders in which fibrinogen is usually present in normal amounts, but is abnormal in structure and coagulability. The abnormality has occurred in both sexes and in consecutive generations, suggesting autosomal dominant inheritance. The anomaly appears to be different in different families. In some the release of fibrinopeptides is impeded; in others aggregation of fibrin monomers is defective; in one family chemical bonding by fibrin-stabilizing factor is impaired. The disorder is usually recognized because the prothrombin time is prolonged, reflecting the presence of the anomalous fibrinogen. The bleeding tendency is usually mild, although severe bleeding has been reported. In some patients wounds have dehisced, whereas in others a paradoxical thrombotic tendency has occurred. Clots are small and friable and form slowly upon the addition of thrombin to plasma, but fibrinogen concentration as measured immunologically is usually normal. In one family, in which recurrent thrombotic episodes were prevalent, the abnormal fibrinogen clot-

ted unusually rapidly upon the addition of thrombin.

Congenital deficiency of fibrin-stabilizing factor (factor XIII) is a rare disorder in which affected individuals have repeated episodes of serious bleeding after injury. Bleeding from the umbilicus is common. Hematomas, hemarthroses, hematuria, and habitual abortion have been described, and intracranial bleeding is a common cause of death. Sometimes wounds appear to heal slowly, occasionally breaking down repeatedly. The plasma of affected persons usually contains nonfunctional material antigenically similar to fibrin-stabilizing factor. The mode of inheritance of fibrin-stabilizing factor deficiency is not certain. In some families, the disorder is attributable to autosomal recessive mutant genes, whereas in others the syndrome seems limited to males. Diagnosis is established by demonstrating that clots of the patient's plasma are soluble in 5 molar urea or 1 per cent monochloroacetic acid, in contrast to normal clots which are insoluble. More sophisticated tests of the transamidation function of fibrin-stabilizing factor have been used. Transfusion of normal blood or plasma transiently corrects the hemorrhagic tendency and facilitates the healing of wounds.

Simultaneous congenital deficiency of several clotting factors has been repeatedly described. Only the *coexistent deficiencies of antihemophilic factor and proaccelerin* appear well established. The defect is probably inherited as an autosomal recessive trait. The bleeding tendency is usually mild, but should treatment of hemorrhage be needed, fresh-frozen plasma should be effective.

Biggs, R. (ed.): Human Blood Coagulation, Hemostasis and Thrombosis. Oxford, Blackwell Scientific Publications, 1972.

Biggs, R., and Macfarlane, R. G.: Treatment of Hemophilia and Other Coagulation Disorders. Oxford, Blackwell Scientific Publications, 1966.

Jackson, D. P., Beck, E. A., and Charache, P.: Congenital disorders of fibrinogen. Fed. Proc., 24:816, 1965.

Ratnoff, O. D. (ed.): Treatment of Hemorrhagic Disorders. New York, Harper & Row, 1968.

Rossi, E. D. (ed.): Symposium on Hemorrhagic Disorders. Medical Clinics of North America. Vol. 56, No. 1. Philadelphia, W. B. Saunders Company, 1972.

Spaet, T. H. (ed.): Progress in Hemostasis and Thrombosis. Vol 1. New York, Grune & Stratton, 1972.

ACQUIRED DISORDERS OF BLOOD COAGULATION

799. VITAMIN K DEFICIENCY

Vitamin K is required for the synthesis of prothrombin, factor VII, Stuart factor, and Christmas factor. If a defiency of vitamin K is present, polypeptides are formed and, indeed, released into the plasma, but they lack clot-promoting properties. The role of vitamin K appears to be to transform these polypeptide chains to functional clotting factors.

If vitamin K is not available in adequate amounts, the plasma levels of these procoagulant substances fall and a hemorrhagic disorder ensues. The normal diet contains an abundance of vitamin K; deficiency rarely if ever can be attributed to inadequate diet alone. The bacteria of the intestinal tract synthesize relatively large amounts of the vitamin, which may contribute to the body's supply. Prolonged *oral administration of antibacterial agents* has been associated with depletion of vitamin K and a hemorrhagic disorder responsive to treatment with this vitamin. This syndrome is most likely to occur in patients undergoing parenteral feeding to whom no vitamin K is provided.

The infant at birth may be deficient in vitamin K and as a result may have *hemorrhagic disease of the newborn.* Melena is common, but bleeding may occur from numerous sites. In some cases transfusion is required, and hemorrhage may be fatal. The disorder is self-limited within a few days, because the minute amounts of vitamin K needed by the infant are provided in milk; cow's milk contains more vitamin K than human milk. The establishment of intestinal flora may contribute to the supply, and the administration of antimicrobial drugs to infants requiring correction of congenital gastrointestinal lesions may precipitate hemorrhagic disease of the newborn. The frequency of this disease can be lessened by administration of small amounts of vitamin K to the mother before delivery or to the infant at birth.

Naturally occurring compounds with vitamin K activity are fat soluble and are poorly absorbed from the intestine in the absence of bile salts. Bleeding that accompanies obstructive jaundice or biliary fistula is usually the result of impaired absorption of vitamin K and is promptly responsive to the parenteral injection of the vitamin. Vitamin K should always be given preoperatively in cases of biliary obstruction, for the first evidence of a hemorrhagic disorder often does not appear until the surgical procedure is performed. Deficiency of the vitamin of a degree sufficient to cause bleeding is encountered in *malabsorption syndromes* such as *sprue* or *celiac disease,* and is readily prevented by parenteral administration of vitamin K.

Derivatives of *coumarin* and *indandione* behave as antagonists of vitamin K. These substances, commonly employed in therapy of thromboembolic disease, impair synthesis of prothrombin and other vitamin K–dependent clotting factors. *Salicylates,* related in chemical structure to coumarin, may produce the same effect when given in large amounts; possibly *propylthiouracil* may have this action in rare instances. Hemorrhage associated with the administration of vitamin K antagonists is usually a complication of therapy. The possibility that hemorrhage complicating anticoagulant therapy is due to potentiation of vitamin K antagonists by other drugs—for example, phenylbutazone, allopurinol, chloral hydrate, salicylates, sulfonamides, glucagon, indomethacin, quinidine, clofibrate, or anabolic steroids—must be kept in mind. Some patients with an obscure hemorrhagic disorder have been discovered to have taken coumarin compounds surreptitiously or because these agents were dispensed in error. A characteristic of the coagulation defects produced by vitamin K antagonists is failure to respond rapidly to injection of large amounts of menadione, a synthetic derivative of naphthoquinone, which ordinarily has potent vitamin K activity; in contrast, vitamin K_1 (phytonadione) is promptly effective. Psychiatric treatment of patients suspected of ingesting coumarin compounds surreptitiously is imperative, because this bizarre behavior may be a manifestation of depression, and the patient may seek more effective means of committing suicide.

Bleeding associated with deficiency of prothrombin and related clotting factors is similar to that occurring with other coagulation defects. Cutaneous ecchymoses, epistaxes, hematuria, gastrointestinal bleeding, and postoperative hemorrhage are common, and intracranial hemorrhage may occur. The hemorrhagic disorder may be fatal.

Diagnosis of vitamin K deficiency is established by the demonstration of a significantly prolonged prothrombin time that is shortened within a few hours after administration of vitamin K.

Treatment consists of oral or parenteral administration of a preparation of the vitamin. For most deficiency states, including those associated with biliary obstruction and malabsorption syndromes, water-soluble derivatives of menadione (menadiol sodium diphosphate or menadione sodium bisulfite) are rapidly and completely effective in correcting the abnormalities of coagulation. An injection of 10 mg of the menadione preparation is adequate, but should be repeated at weekly intervals for patients with a persistent absorption defect. Menadione in moderate amounts can produce serious hemolytic anemia and kernicterus in the newborn, even if given to the mother before delivery. Vitamin K_1 (phytonadione) is preferable, and a single dose of 1 mg, given intramuscularly to the infant at the time of birth, is adequate to prevent hemorrhagic disease of the newborn. To overcome the effects of coumarin derivatives and related drugs, only vitamin K_1 is effective. It is given orally or intramuscularly in doses of 5 to 20 mg. Vitamin K_1 may be administered by slow intravenous injection, but this route should be avoided except in an urgent situation because of the possibility of untoward reactions. Immediate but transient correction of multiple deficiencies of the vitamin K–dependent clotting factors may be provided in life-threatening situations by transfusion of plasma or of concentrates of these factors.

Girdwood, R. H. (ed.): Blood Disorders Due to Drugs and Other Agents. Amsterdam, Excerpta Medica, 1973.

Rossi, E. D. (ed.): Symposium on Hemorrhagic Disorders. Medical Clinics of North America, Vol. 56, No. 1. Philadelphia, W. B. Saunders Company, 1972.

800. LIVER DISEASE

Diffuse hepatic disease often produces a hemorrhagic disorder. Ecchymoses and pretibial petechiae are common, and hemorrhage may occur from many sites; bleeding from surgical wounds is frequent. The bleeding tendency may have multiple causes, including vascular abnormalities, thrombocytopenia, and impairment of blood coagulation. Hypoprothrombinemia and deficiencies of the other vitamin K–dependent clotting factors are common; deficiencies of proaccelerin and PTA may contribute to the hemostatic defect. The catabolism of fibrinogen is often accelerated, and rarely, when parenchymal disease is severe, the concentration of plasma fibrinogen may be decreased. In some patients with advanced liver disease, depletion of plasma clotting factors and platelets may reflect diffuse intravascular coagulation. Another rarely encountered disturbance in chronic hepatic disease, particularly primary hepatoma, is the synthesis of a qualitatively abnormal form of fibrinogen which is converted to fibrin by thrombin at an abnormally slow rate. In cirrhosis of the liver, clots prepared from plasma or its euglobulin fraction dissolve abnormally rapidly, but evidence that this test tube phenomenon correlates with a bleeding tendency is insecure. Although the prothrombin time is usually prolonged in patients with hepatic disease who exhibit a bleeding tendency, the administration of vitamin K usually has little or no corrective effect. Transfusion of fresh blood or fresh-frozen plasma may provide transitory correction of the coagulative defect, but is usually not satisfactory in maintaining hemostasis. The use of currently available concentrates of the vitamin K–dependent clotting factors should be avoided, because fibrinolytic reactions have been described.

Ratnoff, O. D.: Disordered hemostasis in hepatic disease. *In* Schiff, L. (ed.): Diseases of the Liver, 3rd ed. Philadelphia, J. B. Lippincott Company, 1969, p. 147.

801. ACQUIRED HYPOFIBRINOGENEMIA AND SYNDROMES OF INTRAVASCULAR COAGULATION AND FIBRINOLYSIS

Deficiency of fibrinogen of a degree sufficient to cause abnormal bleeding is encountered in a number of different clinical syndromes. It occurs only rarely because of retarded production of fibrinogen and more often as a result of rapid utilization. A bleeding tendency encountered in some patients with *cyanotic congenital heart disease* is attributable in part to the very high hematocrit; the fibrinogen concentration of whole blood is so low that an adequate clot cannot form. Although fibrinogen is synthesized in the liver, *hepatic disease* is seldom the cause of profound deficiency.

Normal plasma contains, on the average, about 300 mg of fibrinogen per 100 ml, although individual variation is wide. During pregnancy, infection, inflammation, myocardial infarction, and other stresses, the concentration of fibrinogen in plasma may be much higher, an alteration principally responsible for the elevated erythrocyte sedimentation rate in these conditions. The biologic half-life of fibrinogen is about three days, but the nature of its normal catabolism is unknown. Neither consumption by intravascular coagulation, nor deposition at extravascular sites of inflammation, nor fibrinolysis by the proteolytic enzyme, plasmin, seems adequate to explain its continual destruction.

Plasmin is present in circulating plasma in the form of a protein precursor, plasminogen. In the test tube, this proenzyme can be converted to plasmin in many ways, including addition of streptokinase (a product of certain beta-hemolytic streptococci), urokinase (a proteolytic enzyme in normal urine), or a plasminogen activator found in many tissues, most impressively in the endothelium of venules and veins. Under certain conditions, the clotting process itself appears to initiate formation of plasmin, an effect mediated by activated Hageman factor via one or more intermediate agents. The long-recognized activation of plasminogen by incubation of plasma or its euglobulin fraction (that is, the fraction insoluble at low ionic strength and low pH) with chloroform is apparently brought about through this Hageman factor–determined mechanism.

Plasmin can digest a wide variety of substrates, including fibrinogen, fibrin, antihemophilic factor, proaccelerin, gamma globulin, and corticotrophin (ACTH). It converts the first component of complement, C1, to its esterolytic form, C$\bar{1}$, and separates biologically active kinins, such as bradykinin, from their precursor in plasma, kininogen. Additionally, plasmin digests casein, gelatin, and certain synthetic esters of arginine and lysine, all of which have been used for in vitro assay of plasmin.

Plasma also contains several potent inhibitors of plasmin, notably α1-antitrypsin, α2-macroglobulin, and C$\bar{1}$ inactivator, a protein which also inhibits C$\bar{1}$, activated Hageman factor, activated PTA, and plasma kallikrein. Platelets, too, possess plasmin-inhibitory properties. Recent evidence also suggests that plasma may inhibit the activation of plasminogen.

Although purified fibrinogen and fibrin appear to be digested by plasmin at comparable rates, this is apparently not true in plasma. For example, fibrin formed in the presence of streptokinase dissolves rapidly, whereas the digestion of fibrinogen in an unclotted mixture of plasma and streptokinase proceeds more slowly. One likely explanation is that plasminogen, adsorbed to fibrin, can be converted to plasmin in situ and then induce fibrinolysis. Presumably, fibrinolysis takes place because the plasmin is physically separated from inhibitors of the activation of plasminogen and of plasmin itself. In unclotted plasma, these inhibitors protect fibrinogen from hydrolysis by plasmin. This phenomenon is of major importance in attempts at therapeutic dissolution of thrombi by the administration of plasminogen activators, with minimal digestion of circulating plasma proteins.

The digestion of fibrinogen by plasmin takes place by steps. The first cleavage of fibrinogen, whose molecular weight is about 340,000 D, splits this molecule into a fragment with a molecular weight of about 240,000 D (fragment X), which can still be clotted by thrombin, and several small fragments. Further digestion of fragment X leads ultimately to the formation of three incoagulable fragments, two with a molecular weight of about 83,000 D each (fragments D), and one with a molecular weight of about 50,000 D (fragment E). Similar fragments appear during the digestion of fibrin, but in this case fragment X is incoagulable. Fragments X and E are powerful anticoagulants, interfering primarily with polymerization of fibrin, apparently by forming complexes with monomeric units of fibrin, formed by the action of thrombin on fibrinogen. Clots formed in the presence of digestion products of fibrinogen and fibrin are structurally defective. The *degradation products of fibrinogen and fibrin (FDP)* also interfere with earlier stages of clotting, and perhaps with platelet aggregation, but the physiologic significance of these actions is unclear.

EXPERIMENTAL INTRAVASCULAR COAGULATION

When a massive amount of tissue thromboplastin or thrombin is injected intravenously into an animal, its blood clots, presumably because the extrinsic pathway of coagulation has been activated. Death ensues from circulatory obstruction. When, instead, the clot-promoting agent is injected slowly, the animal survives but its blood becomes incoagulable. The slower rate at which thrombin forms under these conditions results in slower, and perhaps incomplete, formation of fibrin, so that plasma may contain intermediates of fibrin formation, such as fibrin monomer, soluble fibrin polymers, or complexes of fibrin monomer and fibrinogen. These products are rapidly removed from the circulation by the reticuloendothelial system, whose cells then contain material recognizable immunologically as related to fibrinogen, whereas the circulating blood is depleted of this protein. Usually thrombi cannot be detected by microscopic examination, although occasionally the smallest blood vessels of the kidneys, adrenals, and other organs contain thrombi. Concomitant with the evolution of afibrinogenemia, the concentration of other clotting factors decreases, particularly prothrombin (presumably utilized in the formation of thrombin), proaccelerin, and antihemophilic factor (the latter two, perhaps, inactivated by thrombin). The platelet count falls, possibly because these cells are clumped by thrombin and removed from the circulation. Animals which have undergone experimental defibrination may undergo hemolysis, and their red blood cells may appear to have been fragmented, as if ruptured by intravascular strands of fibrin. Inconstantly, evidences of intravascular fibrinolysis may be detected, either by demonstration of products of digestion of fibrinogen or fibrin in the animal's serum, or by depletion of plasminogen, the precursor of the fibrinolytic enzyme, plasmin; direct evidence for the presence of fibrinolytic activity in the animal's plasma is more difficult to demonstrate. Nonetheless, fibrinolysis has been invoked as one cause for failure to find thrombi in animals injected with tissue thromboplastin; the plasma often acquires clot-inhibitory properties attributed to the presence either of degradation products of fibrin formed through the action of plasmin, or of complexes of these degradation products, fibrinogen, and dissolved fibrin monomers and polymers, in various combinations.

LABORATORY DIAGNOSIS OF INTRAVASCULAR COAGULATION

When intravascular coagulation has been extensive enough to induce hypofibrinogenemia or afibrinogenemia, rapid diagnosis may be made by observing the appearance of coagulating blood in a test tube. A simple qualitative test for hypofibrinogenemia is the addition of 1 ml of blood to 0.1 ml of bovine thrombin solution containing 1000 NIH units per milliliter. Unless virtually no fibrinogen is present, the blood clots quickly. The size of the clot can then be estimated by tapping the tube and observing the degree to which the clot retracts. The retracted clot may be so small that it is difficult to find among the extruded red blood cells and serum, leading to the misinterpretation that fibrinolysis has occurred. The existence of hypofibrinogenemia is confirmed by additional tests, including quantitative measurement of fibrinogen concentration.

In patients thought to have undergone intravascular coagulation, the thrombin time (that is, the time elapsing until a mixture of plasma and thrombin clots),

Disorders Accompanied by Intravascular Coagulation*

A. Hypofibrinogenemic or afibrinogenemic states:
 1. Secondary to the introduction of extrinsic clot-promoting agents
   Amniotic fluid embolism
   Envenomation by snakebite
   Premature separation of the placenta
 2. Secondary to intravascular elaboration of clot-promoting agents
   Acute hemolytic processes (e.g., mismatched blood transfusion)
   Extracorporeal circulation
   Massive arterial or venous thrombosis; pulmonary embolism
   Near drowning
 3. Secondary to vascular injury, exposing clot-promoting tissues
   Purpura fulminans
   Sepsis with gram-positive or -negative organisms; septic abortion; Waterhouse-Friderichsen syndrome
   Infectious disease (e.g., generalized herpes simplex, dengue, cytomegalic inclusion disease, scrub typhus, Rocky Mountain spotted fever, miliary tuberculosis, subacute bacterial endocarditis, trypanosomiasis)
   Heat stroke
   Aortic aneurysm
   Traumatic shock; burns; head injury; surgical procedures
   Thrombotic thrombocytopenic purpura; hemolytic-uremic syndrome
 4. Secondary to vascular stasis
   Giant hemangioma
   Hemangioendotheliosarcoma
   Cavernomatous transformation of veins
 5. Pathogenesis uncertain (introduction of clot-promoting agents?)
   Malignancy (e.g., carcinoma of prostate, pancreas, etc., neuroblastoma, leukemia)
   Administration of L-asparaginase
   Acute pancreatitis
   Hydatidiform mole
B. Conditions in which intravascular coagulation has been implicated in the absence of hypofibrinogenemia:
 1. Secondary to intravascular elaboration of clot-promoting agents
   Hemolytic processes (e.g., paroxysmal nocturnal hemoglobinuria)
   Rejection of organ transplants
 2. Secondary to vascular injury
   Purpura fulminans
   Sepsis with gram-positive or -negative organisms
   Infectious diseases (e.g., exanthematous diseases, viral hemorrhagic fevers, influenza, rickettsial or mycotic disorders, falciparum malaria, bubonic plague, subacute bacterial endocarditis)
   Thrombotic thrombocytopenic purpura, hemolytic uremic syndrome, eclampsia
   Chronic glomerulonephritis, renal cortical necrosis, lupus erythematosus with renal disease, polyarteritis nodosum, nephrotic syndrome with proliferative glomerulonephritis
   Traumatic and anaphylactic shock, burns, surgical procedures
 3. Secondary to vascular stasis
   Malignant hemangioendothelioma
 4. Pathogenesis uncertain
   Malignancy (e.g., metastatic carcinoma of stomach, lung, breast, etc., especially mucin-producing tumors; Wilms' tumor)
   Idiopathic respiratory distress syndrome; hyaline membrane disease
   Cirrhosis of the liver
   Amyloidosis
   Fat embolism
   Poisoning with *Amanita phalloides,* mercuric oxide, alkyl phosphates, dichlorethane
   Cyanotic congenital heart disease
   Cardiogenic shock

*This tabulation is not all-inclusive; the classification is tentative, and the evidence supporting the existence of intravascular coagulation as an important component of the disease state varies in its cogency.

prothrombin time, and partial thromboplastin time may all be prolonged, both because necessary reactants have been depleted and because of the presence of clot-inhibitory agents. In some cases, intravascular coagulation may be suspected because the concentration of fibrinogen, although within the range found in normal individuals, is decreased below the level anticipated in the light of the patient's clinical condition. In parallel to the changes observed in laboratory animals, the platelet count may be reduced, and deficiencies of prothrombin, proaccelerin, and antihemophilic factor may be observed. Inconstantly, too, rapid dissolution of clots formed from plasma or its euglobulin fraction may suggest that *secondary fibrinolysis* has taken place. More frequently, the concentration of plasminogen may be diminished, as if this proenzyme had been converted to plasmin and then inactivated by its inhibitors in plasma, and the plasma may acquire inhibitory properties directed against the clotting process.

Direct evidence that intravascular coagulation has taken place has been provided in several ways. Thus free fibrinopeptide A, separated from fibrinogen through the action of thrombin, can be detected immunologically in the plasma of patients thought to be undergoing intravascular coagulation. Further, the incorporation of radioactive glycine methyl ester into a fraction of plasma rich in fibrinogen has been thought to reflect the presence of dissolved fibrin monomers or polymers; this ester is incorporated into fibrin, but not fibrinogen, through the action of fibrin-stabilizing factor. High molecular weight complexes, seemingly of fibrinogen and fibrin monomer, have been separated from plasma by physical means. And the half-disappearance time of intravenously injected radioactive fibrinogen is dramatically shortened in patients in whom intravascular coagulation is believed to be taking place. These four techniques are not yet firmly established, nor translated into practical methodology.

Indirect support for the existence of intravascular coagulation can be obtained by demonstrating that the patient's serum, normally devoid of fibrinogen, contains antigenic material related to this protein. Many techniques have been used to demonstrate these fibrinogen-related antigens (FRA), often called by the more restrictive term, fibrinogen degradation products (FDP), which implies that the materials identified are the product of the action of plasmin. Immunodiffusion, immunoelectrophoresis, tanned red blood cell hemagglutination inhibition, and agglutination of latex particles coated with heterologous antifibrin antiserum have all been used to detect fibrinogen-related antigens. Less reliably, gelation of plasma by addition of ethanol or protamine sulfate, or aggregation of certain strains of *Staphylococcus aureus* by the patient's serum may reflect the presence of dissolved polymers, particularly of fibrin monomer and fibrinogen but also, perhaps, of fibrin monomer and degradation products of the action of plasmin on fibrinogen or fibrin. Similarly, chilling plasma may induce precipitation of "cryofibrinogen," composed of complexes of fibrinogen and fibrin monomers. And in some patients evidences of intravascular damage to erythrocytes, similar to those seen in experimental animals undergoing defibrination, may be found.

The laboratory abnormalities described have been detected in the blood of patients undergoing disseminated intravascular coagulation. Similar changes, however, are observed in some patients with extensive localized thrombosis, for example, pulmonary embolism or aortic aneurysm.

HYPOFIBRINOGENEMIC SYNDROMES ASSOCIATED WITH LOCALIZED THROMBOSIS

Rarely, after massive arterial or venous thrombosis or pulmonary embolism, the blood is incoagulable, and marked thrombocytopenia is present. Presumably, the fibrinogen, platelets, and other clotting factors are depleted in the formation of thrombi. A similar coagulation defect may be encountered in *purpura fulminans*, a disease in which acute necrosis of superficial and peripheral parts of the body is associated with thrombosis at the sites of vasculitis in small blood vessels in the affected areas. This rare disorder, which is most prevalent in children and often follows shortly after an apparently banal infection, is usually self-limited, but its course may be aborted by administration of heparin, which inhibits further thrombin formation. Perhaps the rare instances of patchy *cutaneous necrosis during therapy with coumarin-like anticoagulants* have a similar pathogenesis, although hypofibrinogenemia has not been described in this situation. The lesions are most likely to appear at sites rich in fatty tissue, such as the breast and buttocks. The necrotic lesions are preceded by an evanescent, painful erythematous patch, and treatment with vitamin K_1 may abort the episode.

Unusually, hypofibrinogenemia has also been observed with *thrombotic thrombocytopenic purpura,* in which noninflammatory thrombosis of small blood vessels is associated with fever, acute hemolytic anemia, neurologic symptoms, thrombocytopenia, and acute renal failure (see Ch. 790); in this disorder, the administration of heparin is usually without benefit. Hypofibrinogenemia may occur in patients with *giant cavernous hemangioma, hemangioepithelioma,* or *cavernomatous transformation of veins,* particularly of the portal system; in these disorders, fibrin thrombi form in the relatively static blood within the vascular lesions. Other syndromes in which widespread thrombosis of relatively large vessels is commonplace, such as *paroxysmal nocturnal hemoglobinuria, sickle cell disease,* and *homocystinuria,* have not been associated with hypofibrinogenemia.

HYPOFIBRINOGENEMIC SYNDROMES ASSOCIATED WITH DIFFUSE INTRAVASCULAR CLOTTING

Hypofibrinogenemia or afibrinogenemia may be encountered in other disorders in which thrombosis may be difficult or impossible to demonstrate. In such cases, procoagulant substances are thought to be introduced into the bloodstream sufficiently slowly that massive thrombosis does not ensue. The fate of the fibrin that forms intravascularly is not clear. Perhaps, as is true in laboratory animals, fibrin is removed from the circulating blood by the reticuloendothelial system. Alternatively, soluble fibrin monomers or polymers, perhaps complexed with fibrinogen, are cleared from the bloodstream before insoluble fibrin strands can form, or fibrin is dissolved by plasmin, and the fibrin degradation products, some of which may be complexed with fibrinogen or fibrin monomer, are removed by the reticuloendothelial cells.

The clearest examples of defibrination by these mechanisms are *amniotic fluid embolism,* in which amniotic fluid and its contaminants enter the maternal bloodstream during parturition, *envenomation* by the bite of snakes whose venom contains procoagulant agents, and the administration of several hundred milliliters of *incompatible blood.* In this last circumstance, the products of lysis of the transfused cells may initiate intravascular coagulation and defibrinate the recipient's blood. Envenomation by the bite of the Malayan pit viper, *Agkistrodon rhodostoma,* has been extensively studied; the venom has a thrombin-like action upon fibrinogen, resulting in afibrinogenemia without any of the depletion of other clotting factors or platelets seen in other cases of intravascular clotting. These properties have led to its experimental use in the treatment of thromboembolic disorders.

Similar mechanisms have been evoked to explain hypofibrinogenemia in other disorders, although the evidence is more inferential. For example, hypofibrinogenemia has been encountered in patients with severe *sepsis,* particularly *septic abortion,* and *Waterhouse-Friderichsen syndrome.* In these syndromes, vascular damage may expose the circulating blood to subendothelial tissues which may induce thrombosis through activation of Hageman factor or localized aggregation of platelets. A wide variety of both gram-positive and gram-negative organisms have been implicated. The possibility that in some cases intravascular coagulation is part of the human counterpart of the generalized Shwartzman reaction has been advocated. Hypofibrinogenemia has been reported with peculiar frequency in individuals with *pneumococcal sepsis* who have asplenia, usually as the result of splenectomy, or splenic atrophy, such as occurs in sickle cell disease. Vascular damage may also be important in initiating disseminated intravascular coagulation in patients with *viral hemorrhagic fevers* or certain other infectious diseases.

Some cases of *premature separation of the placenta* may be complicated by hypofibrinogenemia; although the introduction of highly thromboplastic placental tissue into the maternal bloodstream has been invoked as an explanation, other mechanisms, such as the formation of a massive retroplacental clot, may be operative. The pathogenesis of hypofibrinogenemia in *prolonged retention of a dead fetus* or *neoplastic diseases* is less clear, although in such cases intravascular coagulation induced by procoagulants derived from the pathologic tissue has been surmised. *Metastatic carcinoma of the prostate* is the most frequent of the many neoplasms that may produce hypofibrinogenemia; this defect has also been encountered in patients with carcinoma of the breast, stomach, gallbladder, pancreas, lung, and colon, disseminated rhabdomyosarcoma, leukemia, most often of the acute promyelocytic type, and other tumors as well.

Hypofibrinogenemia, thrombocytopenia, and other coagulation defects have been encountered during various types of *extracorporeal circulation.* The apparatus may defibrinate the blood if insufficient heparin is employed. *Abnormal bleeding during cardiovascular surgical procedures* may have multiple causes, including the use of too much or too little heparin, as well as the operative procedure itself. Hypofibrinogenemia has also been observed during other surgical procedures, most frequently during pulmonary resection, although this is a rare complication. Hypofibrinogenemia may accompany *aneurysm of the aorta,* particularly *dissecting aneurysm,* presumably because the exposed subendothelial tissue is clot promoting. Widespread vascular damage may also explain the occurrence of hypofibrinogenemia in patients with *shock* of different origins and *heat stroke.*

Bleeding associated with the defibrinating syndromes is often severe, but the character of the bleeding, as well as the prognosis, is influenced by the nature of the underlying disease. Often, the first indication that defibrination is taking place is bleeding at the sites of arterial or venous puncture. In women with *premature separation of the placenta* or *amniotic fluid embolism,* major hemorrhage is usually from the uterus, although a generalized bleeding tendency may be evident. In patients with more chronic forms of hypofibrinogenemia, ecchymoses, hematoma formation, and bleeding from the gastrointestinal tract may be prominent. Patients with syndromes of diffuse intravascular coagulation may also have symptoms consequent upon the obstruction of the circulation by small thrombi; renal tubular and cortical necrosis caused by thrombosis in the smallest blood vessels are of the greatest moment.

Primary treatment of hypofibrinogenemia or afibrinogenemia caused by intravascular coagulation is that of the basic disease; if this can be eradicated or ameliorated, the coagulation defects are rapidly corrected. Thus the hypofibrinogenemia associated with *amniotic fluid embolism* is self-limited, whereas in patients with *premature separation of the placenta* or *retention of a dead fetus,* recovery follows shortly after the uterus is emptied. Severe bleeding associated with *carcinoma of the prostate* may subside, and the coagulation abnormalities may disappear within days of the institution of estrogen therapy. Transfusion of fresh blood is often required. Although administration of fibrinogen may be of temporary value and tide the patient over an acute episode of bleeding, if the basic pathologic process continues, the transfused fibrinogen is rapidly removed from the circulation and may participate in the formation of new disseminated thrombi. Moreover, the use of human fibrinogen preparations is all too often followed by serum hepatitis. In cases in which the primary disease cannot be treated, intravenous injection of heparin may impede intravascular defibrination by inhibiting the clotting process and raise the levels of depleted clotting factors. A typical course of therapy includes an initial dose of 50 to 100 units of heparin per kilogram of body weight, followed by 10 to 15 units per kilogram per hour, administered by intravenous infusion; more may be needed, and smaller doses may be appropriate if severe thrombocytopenia is present. This seemingly paradoxical approach to treatment is most effective when the disease is self-limited, as in the case of *extensive arterial or venous thrombosis* or *purpura fulminans,* or in cases of chronic defibrination, as in instances of *metastatic disease.* The risks of bleeding from operative wounds or the placental site limit the usefulness of heparin therapy in acute forms of hypofibrinogenemia.

DISSEMINATED INTRAVASCULAR COAGULATION WITHOUT HYPOFIBRINOGENEMIA

A widely held view is that many pathologic states may induce widespread intravascular coagulation, perhaps insufficient to cause significant hypofibrinogenemia, but adequate to bring about ischemic damage. Under such conditions, the thrombin time, prothrombin time, and partial thromboplastin time may be prolonged; serum may contain agents immunologically resembling fibrinogen; plasma may undergo coagulation upon addition of ethanol or protamine sulfate, and the platelet count may be depressed. In some patients, intravascular hemolysis may be detected, and the erythrocytes may have the morphologic characteristics of those of animals undergoing experimental defibrination, appearing fragmented and often triangular in shape. Such cells, often called *schistocytes*, are characteristic of *microangiopathic hemolytic anemia*, a state seen pre-eminently in *thrombotic thrombocytopenic purpura* and the *hemolytic-uremic syndrome*. In some cases, too, accelerated turnover of fibrinogen and platelets suggests that intravascular coagulation has occurred even though the blood levels of these substances may not be decreased because other compensating mechanisms are operative.

Application of these criteria has led to the assumption that myriad clinical disorders are accompanied by intravascular coagulation. Besides thrombotic thrombocytopenic purpura and the hemolytic-uremic syndrome, these diseases include fulminant *eclampsia* with hemolytic anemia and thrombocytopenia, *malignant hypertension, chronic glomerulonephritis, nephrotic syndrome* with proliferative glomerulonephritis, *renal cortical necrosis, cirrhosis of the liver, hyaline membrane disease, sepsis*, especially *meningococcemia* and *rickettsial* and *viral* disorders, *metastatic carcinoma, systemic lupus erythematosus, polyarteritis nodosum*, and *shock* of diverse origins. Intravascular coagulation has also been thought to be important in rejection of *organ grafts*, and may complicate *therapeutic abortion*. This by no means exhausts the disorders in which intravascular coagulation, disseminated or localized to specific organs, is thought to be an important feature (see accompanying table).

Evidences for the role of intravascular coagulation in the pathogenesis of these various disease states varies in degree of conviction. Particular criticism has been leveled at diagnostic reliance upon hemolysis or changes in red blood cell morphology, because these may occur in the absence of other changes associated with intravascular coagulation, and hemolysis may be the cause rather than the result of defibrination.

The beneficial effects of heparin in some cases of hypofibrinogenemia have led to its use in individuals in whom disseminated intravascular coagulation is suspected in the absence of hypofibrinogenemia. In some cases, a trial of heparin therapy, as outlined for patients with hypofibrinogenemic states, may be justified, and may be followed by clinical and laboratory improvement. In most instances, unfortunately, the results have been disappointing, and skepticism concerning the importance of disseminated intravascular coagulation in pathogenesis seems appropriate.

McKay, D. G.: Disseminated Intravascular Coagulation. An Intermediary Mechanism of Disease. New York, Hoeber Medical Division, Harper & Row, 1965.

Minna, J. D., Robboy, S. J., and Coleman, R. W. (eds.): Disseminated Intravascular Coagulation in Man. Springfield, Ill., Charles C Thomas, 1974.

Poller, I. (ed.): Recent Advances in Blood Coagulation. London, J. & A. Churchill, Ltd., 1969.

Rossi, E. D. (ed.): Symposium on Hemorrhagic Disorders. Medical Clinics of North America, Vol. 56, No. 1. Philadelphia, W. B. Saunders Company, 1972.

802. FIBRINOLYTIC STATES

An attractive hypothesis envisions that minor degrees of fibrinolytic activity operate under normal conditions to maintain the fluidity of blood by dissolving thrombi in the microcirculation. Evidence in support of this view is, however, equivocal. As measured in vitro, the fibrinolytic activity of blood or its euglobulin fraction is exaggerated in chronic hepatic disease, under such conditions of stress as traumatic shock, anxiety, electroconvulsive therapy or anoxia, and after the injection of certain vasoactive substances, for example, epinephrine or nicotinic acid. The enhanced fibrinolytic activity is thought to be due to the presence in plasma of circulating activators of plasminogen, perhaps derived from venous endothelium and, in the case of chronic hepatic disease, inadequately removed from the bloodstream by the liver. The clinical significance of these in vitro observations is uncertain, because the enhanced fibrinolytic activity is not ordinarily reflected in clinical symptomatology, and in vivo the array of inactivators of plasmin in plasma may limit the evolution of significant proteolytic activity. Moreover, demonstration of increased fibrinolytic activity in vitro usually requires the formation or presence of a fibrin clot, to which plasminogen and its activators may be adsorbed. Under these conditions, plasmin may form, physically separated from its inhibitors in plasma, allowing fibrinolysis to take place. In vivo, on the other hand, the array of inactivators of plasmin may limit the evolution of significant proteolytic activity.

Under the stress of intravascular coagulation, local fibrinolysis appears to be an important mechanism in dissolution of small thrombi. Here, as in vitro, plasmin may be capable of digesting clots without reaching effective levels in circulating plasma. Under these conditions, products of fibrinolysis may be found in circulating plasma, where they may inhibit the coagulation process and interfere with the polymerization of fibrin. Usually, direct evidence that fibrinolysis is taking place is meager, but fibrinolysis has been inferred from a fall in the concentration of plasminogen in plasma. The concentrations of antihemophilic factor and proaccelerin may also be decreased, and the patient's serum may contain antigenic material related to fibrinogen, possibly products of fibrinolysis but, as has been noted earlier, sometimes the result of incomplete clotting of fibrin. In some patients undergoing intravascular coagulation, fibrinolysis may be so extensive that clotted blood undergoes spontaneous dissolution within minutes or a few hours. This *secondary fibrinolytic state* is most often found in patients in whom defibrination is particularly severe, such as those with *amniotic fluid embolism, premature separation of the placenta, profound hemorrhagic shock,* or *neoplasms*, such as *metastatic carcinoma of the prostate* or *acute leukemia*. In some cases, despite the demonstration of potent fibrinolytic activity in vitro, the concentration of fibrinogen does not fall dramatically, recalling the observation noted earlier that fibrinolysis occurs more readily than fibrinogenolysis.

A few patients have been described who, under severe stress, have developed a fulminant hemorrhagic syndrome attributable to excessive fibrinolytic activity. Thus during laparotomy, blood may seem to ooze from every cut tissue; fibrinolysis may be so rapid that whole blood appears to be incoagulable, whereas the patient's plasma can be clotted by thrombin, only to redissolve within minutes. Although this rare syndrome has been ascribed to a *primary fibrinolytic state,* it is uncertain whether in fact the disorder does not reflect an episode of diffuse intravascular clotting in which fibrinolysis rather than thrombosis dominates the clinical picture. In contrast to the usual case of disseminated intravascular clotting, the platelet count may be normal; but other laboratory features, including prolongation of the thrombin time, prothrombin time, and partial thromboplastin time, depletion of clotting factors, and the demonstration of fibrinogen-related antigens in serum, do not distinguish the disorder from diffuse intravascular coagulation. If the diagnosis seems certain, the administration of large amounts of *epsilon-aminocaproic acid,* a drug which inhibits the activation of plasminogen, may be helpful. A typical regimen in an adult is 4 grams every four hours for two or three days. Unfortunately, this agent is strongly contraindicated in individuals undergoing intravascular coagulation, for it may stabilize thrombi which would otherwise dissolve. Thus great circumspection must be used in treating patients with suspected primary fibrinolysis with this agent.

A more certain primary fibrinolytic state may be induced during therapeutic attempts at dissolution of thrombi by administration of streptokinase or urokinase, activators of plasminogen. In such cases, more plasmin forms within the bloodstream than can be effectively neutralized by plasma inhibitors of this enzyme, and fibrinogen and other clotting factors may be depleted, without a concomitant fall in the platelet count. Hemorrhagic symptoms, apparently induced by excessive fibrinolytic activity, are a relatively common complication of experimental fibrinolytic therapy. If bleeding symptoms are alarming, therapy with epsilon-aminocaproic acid in the manner described for primary fibrinolytic states may be indicated, but caution must be exercised in its use, lest the thrombotic state for which therapy was initiated be worsened.

Local fibrinolysis after prostatectomy may lead to protracted and sometimes severe hematuria. The pathogenesis of bleeding under these conditions is uncertain; clots in the operative bed may be dissolved by plasmin, formed through the action either of urinary urokinase or of tissue activators in exposed prostatic tissue. Therapy with epsilon-aminocaproic acid is effective, and is not attended by the dangers inherent in the treatment of thrombotic states.

Douglas, A. S. (ed.): Blood coagulation and fibrinolysis in clinical practice. Clinics in Haematology, Vol. 2, No. 1. London, W. B. Saunders, Ltd., 1973.
Rossi, E. D. (ed.): Symposium on Hemorrhagic Disorders. Medical Clinics of North America, Vol. 56, No. 1. Philadelphia, W. B. Saunders Company, 1972.

803. ANTICOAGULANTS

The presence of an anticoagulant in the circulating blood causes a bleeding tendency that may be severe. This occurrence may follow parenteral administration of heparin, a substance that interferes with generation of the prothrombin converting principle as well as with the conversion of fibrinogen to fibrin. Heparin rapidly disappears from the circulation so that the hemorrhagic disorder subsides within an hour or two after intravenous injection is terminated. Rarely, inadvertent administration of heparin may be responsible for sudden, unexpected bleeding. A tentative diagnosis can be made by demonstrating that the patient's plasma clots abnormally slowly upon addition of thrombin (whose action is antagonized by heparin) but at a normal rate upon addition of Reptilase, i.e., the venom of *Bothrops atrox* (whose clotting action upon plasma fibrinogen is not blocked by heparin). A number of hemorrhagic disorders have been attributed to the production of heparin in vivo, but there are few if any cases in which this claim is supported by convincing evidence. Antiheparin agents, including protamine sulfate and toluidine blue, effectively counteract the action of heparin when given intravenously in precisely calculated amounts. Bishydroxycoumarin (Dicumarol) and related compounds are often referred to as anticoagulants, but they interfere with the synthesis of clotting factors and do not retard coagulation directly.

Endogenously produced anticoagulants are encountered under several circumstances and may produce a hemophilia-like disease. These circulating anticoagulants appear to be IgG antibodies, and they most often interfere with the early stages of coagulation. One frequently demonstrable in the plasma of patients with hemophilia specifically inactivates antihemophilic factor and is an antibody against this agent. An anticoagulant of similar nature and specificity sometimes occurs in the plasma of women after pregnancy, producing a hemophilia-like disorder. Hemorrhagic disease attributable to an apparently identical anticoagulant has appeared without obvious cause in persons who were previously healthy or who have a chronic disease. Comparable substances, specifically inactivating other clotting factors, have been encountered in patients with congenital deficiency of the clotting factor in question. A circulating anticoagulant occurring in the plasma of some patients with systemic lupus erythematosus is unusual, because it interferes with the conversion of prothrombin to thrombin; less commonly, patients with this disease have circulating anticoagulants against antihemophilic factor.

The presence of an anticoagulant is detected by demonstrating the retarding action of small proportions of the patient's plasma on the coagulation of normal blood or recalcified plasma. Circulating anticoagulants may disappear spontaneously, sometimes after a period of many months or years, but therapy is difficult. Because of the anticoagulant effect of the patient's plasma, transfusions do not correct the clotting defect. When bleeding is life threatening, exchange transfusion and the injection of massive amounts of the missing factor may be tried. The use of steroids or immunosuppressive agents has been disappointing. Patients with myeloma and with other diseases causing dysproteinemia may display impairment of blood coagulation attributable to the presence of the abnormal protein. The bleeding manifestations frequently associated with dysproteinemia are not, however, clearly related to retarded clotting.

Spaet, T. H. (ed.): Progress in Hemostasis and Thrombosis. Vol. 1. New York, Grune & Stratton, 1972.

Part XVII
DISEASES OF METABOLISM

804. INTRODUCTION

Nicholas P. Christy

The term "metabolism" used to be defined as the sum of the processes concerned in the building up and breaking down of living protoplasm, and as the chemical changes in living cells by which energy is provided for cellular work and for cellular repair. Such a definition depicts metabolism as a kind of cellular nutrition. Nowadays, the term is broadened to stand for "the sum of the processes by which a particular substance is handled...in the living body," i.e., the processes that are essential for survival, growth, maturation, and reproduction. Defined in this more general way, almost any disease is a "disease of metabolism" (from the Greek, μεταβολή, change; "metabolic" from μεταβολικός, changeable). After *trauma*, e.g., fracture of a hip, calcium may be lost from bone during prolonged immobilization, with accompanying hypercalcemia. An *infectious disease*, chronic pyelonephritis, may lead to renal insufficiency, uremia, and the familiar renal mismanagement of H^+, phosphate, and other ions; cholera is associated with tremendous gastrointestinal losses of sodium and water. *Hereditary diseases* of several systems are characterized by disordered "handling" of particular substances: in congenital adrenal hyperplasia, deficiency of one or another adrenal cortical enzyme results in reduced synthesis of cortisol, excessive secretion of androgens, and precocious virilism; the disordered synthesis of hemoglobin in sickle cell anemia, the classic "molecular disease," results in the specific amino acid difference in the beta chain that underlies the misshapen erythrocytes, the hemolysis, and the microinfarctions. A major clinical manifestation of a disease of *unknown etiology,* chronic pancreatitis, is steatorrhea with diarrhea, largely owing to deficiency of pancreatic exocrine secretion and the failure to hydrolyze triglycerides in the gut. Thus diseases of all systems and of diverse etiologies are metabolic diseases, in the sense that they show some change in the way the body deals with (metabolizes) a particular chemical substance.

Metabolism itself must be changeable; the internal environment is only relatively constant. In his famous and much quoted generalization, Claude Bernard said: "All the vital mechanisms, varied as they are, have only one object: that of preserving constant the conditions of life in the *milieu intérieur.*" But, as the American physiologist L. J. Henderson wrote in 1926, "This should not be thought of as absolute constancy, and it should be understood that variations in the properties of the internal environment may be both cyclical and adaptive, that is, functional...." Normal metabolism thus operates to keep the cellular environment in a state appropriate to constantly changing conditions, e.g., growth, reproduction, and aging; changes in body temperature, hydration, and nutrition. It is a mistake to think of the constancy of the *milieu intérieur* as simply a ceaseless struggle of the cells to return to some fixed and immutable baseline. The baseline is continually changing. Abnormal metabolism (or disease), as defined by Bernard, can be viewed as a "perturbation or dislocation" of the mechanisms that make possible appropriate adjustments to change.

Part XVII contains an account of hereditary and acquired diseases characterized by derangement of the internal environment, diseases which have in common *disordered production or fate of a well-defined, specific chemical substance.** Consequences of these disorders are an excess or deficiency of that substance or a substance closely related to it. The excess or deficiency gives rise to a well-defined, specific clinical syndrome which involves either predominantly one or in some cases several organs or systems.

In Part XVII are placed most of the clinical conditions in which there is a demonstrated abnormality of a specific protein, either a "deficiency in a specific enzymatic activity...[or] a normal amount of a structurally abnormal protein" (see Ch. 7). Thus the various forms of glycogen deposition disease, galactosemia, pentosuria, Type I hyperlipoproteinemia, alcaptonuria, and xanthinuria are examples of the operation of the "one-gene, one-enzyme" hypothesis (Beadle and Tatum).

In addition, Part XVII includes examples of disorders of more than one gene (in association with envoronmental influences). The inheritance of gout may be polygenic. The endogenous hyperlipemias (Types IIb and IV hyperlipoproteinemia) represent several genotypes. There is heterogeneity of the mutations that lead to the enzyme deficiency present in the Lesch-Nyhan syndrome. The reader will observe that many of the diseases of metabolism are rare (not diabetes mellitus, with a prevalence in the United States of about 5 per cent, but, for example, primary hyperoxaluria, of which there are fewer than 200 reported cases) or of no clinical importance (fructosuria, pentosuria). If apologies are needed, one might offer these: (1) study of rare diseases has very often made possible a better understanding of normal metabolic processes (certain aminoacidurias); (2) discovery of some of these rare conditions early enough in life may lead to prevention of clinical disease simply by adjustment of the diet (galactosemia, phenylketonuria; (3) precise identification of a rare enzyme deficiency may lead to methods for replacement therapy with that enzyme (Fabry's disease); and (4) no disease is rare to the patient who has it.

Bernard, C.: An Introduction to the Study of Experimental Medicine (translated by H. L. Green). New York, Dover Publications, 1957, p. viii.

Bondy, P. K., and Rosenberg, L. E. (eds.): Duncan's Diseases of Metabolism. 7th ed. Philadelphia, W. B. Saunders Company, 1974.

Brady, R. O., Tallman, J. F., Johnson, W. G., Gal, A. E., Leahy, W. R., Quirk, J. M., and Dekaban, A. S.: Replacement therapy for inherited enzyme deficiency. Use of purified ceramidetrihexosidase in Fabry's disease. N. Engl. J. Med., 289:9, 1973.

Frimpter, G. W.: Aminoacidurias due to inherited disorders of metabolism. N. Engl. J. Med., 289:835, 895, 1973.

Garrod, A. E.: Inborn errors of metabolism (Croonian Lectures). Lancet, 2:1, 73, 142, 214, 1908.

---

*Part XXI includes conditions which are difficult to classify under standard categories and in which the biochemical defect is in most instances not completely understood (e.g., Marfan's syndrome, dysautonomia).

Seegmiller, J. E.: New prospects for understanding and control of genetic diseases. Arch. Intern. Med., 130:181, 1972.

Smith, L. H.: Pyrimidine metabolism in man. N. Engl. J. Med., 288:764, 1973.

Stanbury, J. B., Wyngaarden, J. B., and Fredrickson, D. S. (eds.): The Metabolic Basis of Inherited Disease. 3rd ed. New York, McGraw-Hill Book Company, 1972.

Tatum, E. L.: A case history in biological research. Science, 129:1711, 1959.

805. DISORDERS OF FLUID, ELECTROLYTE, AND ACID-BASE BALANCE

William B. Schwartz

Fluid and electrolyte disturbances usually occur as complications of an underlying illness, and the disorders to be considered in this chapter must therefore be viewed not as isolated entities but in the context of the specific clinical settings in which they appear.

As general background to the following discussion, it should be recalled that the water content of the body (approximately 50 to 60 per cent of body weight) is distributed between the intracellular and the extracellular compartments. Approximately two thirds of the water is within cells, and the remaining third is divided between the interstitial space and plasma, which together comprise the extracellular compartment. Water moves freely across cell boundaries, and for this reason changes in tonicity in one compartment induce a transfer of fluid that continues until a new steady state of osmotic equilibrium is established. By contrast, electrolytes are distributed in an asymmetric pattern, most of the ions in the extracellular fluid consisting of sodium, chloride, and bicarbonate and those in the intracellular fluid of potassium and organic anions. Except for the slight deviations attributable to the Donnan effect of the plasma proteins, the electrolyte compositions of plasma and interstitial fluid are virtually identical. Thus for clinical purposes plasma composition can be taken as representative of the entire extracellular compartment.

Ch. 601 and 602 summarize the renal regulation of electrolyte and acid-base equilibrium. In the present chapter relevant physiology will be presented entirely within the context of the clinical disorder under consideration.

DEPLETION OF VOLUME

The most common disturbance of fluid and electrolyte equilibrium is volume depletion. Loss of volume may occur from simple dehydration, but is seen more frequently in association with a combined loss of water and electrolytes.

Clinical Manifestations. The symptoms of volume depletion are few and nonspecific. The patient may complain of thirst, especially if the body fluids are hypertonic, but nausea, light-headedness, and weakness are perhaps the most frequent and troublesome manifesta-

tions. The major effects of volume depletion are on the circulation and on renal function. As plasma volume is diminished, blood pressure falls, heart rate rises, and a decrease in renal perfusion leads to oliguria and azotemia. When volume depletion is severe, profound shock becomes an immediate and serious threat to survival. The management of these clinical problems will be discussed after the individual causes of volume depletion have been considered.

Pathogenesis. The specific clinical circumstances in which volume depletion is encountered are listed in Table 1. These are discussed in the succeeding paragraphs.

Simple Dehydration (Loss of Water Without Electrolyte). The fluid requirement of the body is determined by the insensible losses through skin and lungs and by the amount of water that is required to excrete the daily solute load. Ordinarily the minimal intake that will serve to maintain water balance is 700 to 1000 ml per day. Thirst ordinarily serves to maintain water intake well above this basal level; but if weakness or disability sharply curtails fluid intake, dehydration will develop. The magnitude of the fluid deficit will be aggravated when insensible losses are increased by factors such as fever and hyperventilation or when urinary losses are abnormally large—for example, in uncontrolled diabetes insipidus.

Whenever water is lost in excess of electrolyte, hypertonicity and elevation of the serum sodium concentration accompany the depletion of volume. The clinical features and consequences of hypernatremia are discussed later in this chapter.

Combined Depletion of Water and Sodium. Severe volume deficits occur most commonly in patients who have suffered a combined loss of water and sodium, usually from the gastrointestinal tract, the kidneys, or the skin.

GASTROINTESTINAL LOSSES. Volume depletion may occur as the result of losses from any portion of the gastrointestinal tract. Gastrointestinal secretions normally amount to some 8 to 10 liters per day, and, if the body is deprived of a significant fraction of this total, severe volume depletion will result. Depletion is most commonly the consequence of vomiting, gastric drainage, or diarrhea. It also is seen with small-bowel drainage, ileostomy, colostomy, and pancreatic or biliary fistulas.

TABLE 1. Causes of Volume Depletion

Simple dehydration
  (Loss of water without electrolyte)

Combined depletion of water and sodium
  Gastrointestinal losses
    Vomiting
    Gastric or small bowel drainage
    Diarrhea
    Bowel fistulas (colostomy, ileostomy, etc.)
  Renal losses
    Chronic renal failure
    Diuretic phase of acute tubular necrosis
    Postobstructive nephropathy
    Adrenal insufficiency
    Osmotic diuresis
    Diuretics
  Skin losses
    Sweating
    Burns
  Paracentesis

Most gastrointestinal secretions are either isotonic or slightly hypotonic and, for this reason, enteric losses per se should not produce a striking change in serum sodium concentration. However, because serum sodium concentration is ultimately determined by over-all water balance (as influenced by fluid intake, skin losses, etc.), either hyponatremia or hypernatremia may be encountered.

RENAL LOSSES. Patients with *chronic renal failure* commonly have a reduced ability to conserve sodium, but the sodium-wasting tendency is seldom severe enough to become apparent if dietary intake of salt is normal. If salt intake is restricted, however, continued excretion of sodium and the associated loss of water may produce severe depletion of extracellular volume. Contraction of volume, in turn, causes a further reduction in glomerular filtration rate, and may even precipitate frank uremia. Sodium intake in the azotemic patient should not be curtailed, therefore, without careful sequential observations of body weight and sodium excretion.

An occasional patient wastes sodium even while ingesting a normal quantity of salt; most of these appear to have *medullary cystic disease* as their underlying renal lesion. In such cases of severe salt-wasting, the diet must be supplemented with sodium chloride if volume depletion is to be avoided. It is important to remember that in the patient with renal disease volume depletion should always be considered as a possible explanation for a sudden, otherwise unexplained increase in azotemia.

During the *diuretic phase of acute tubular necrosis* a defect in the ability of the damaged tubules to reabsorb sodium may lead to a considerable loss of sodium and water. Sodium wasting does not usually persist for more than several days, and is not likely to become clinically significant if the patient is taking a diet of normal salt content. At times it may be difficult to distinguish between an abnormal diuresis and the physiologic diuresis that will occur if an excessive quantity of fluid and electrolyte has been administered during the oliguric phase of the disease. If one is uncertain about the cause, treatment can ordinarily be delayed for a day or two until the issue is resolved either by the cessation of the diuresis or by the appearance of early signs of volume depletion. In this way an unnecessary and prolonged cycle of saline loading and saline loss can be avoided. A similar period of uncontrolled sodium and fluid loss by the kidney may be observed during *acute rejection episodes* after renal transplantation.

Postobstructive nephropathy occasionally produces severe sodium and volume depletion in patients in whom complete or nearly complete obstruction has been present for a prolonged period. The defect in sodium reabsorption results from tubular damage, and becomes manifest promptly after the relief of obstruction permits the filtered load of sodium to increase. Loss of salt may lead to an obligatory diuresis of as much as 5 or 10 liters per day and, thus, to an acute contraction of extracellular and plasma volume. Just as with the diuretic phase of acute tubular necrosis, the disorder is usually self-limiting, because the tubules generally recover their capacity to transport sodium within a few days.

Volume depletion consequent to excessive renal losses of fluid and electrolyte may also occur in the absence of structural renal disease. In patients with *adrenal insufficiency* (Addison's disease) a deficiency of salt-retaining steroids reduces the activity of renal transport mechanisms, and may allow large quantities of sodium and water to escape into the urine. Continued administration of *diuretics* to the patient who has been but is no longer edematous will also sometimes produce volume depletion.

Abnormal losses of sodium and water are also induced by the obligatory excretion of a large solute load. Such an osmotic diuresis is seen most frequently in association with the glycosuria of *diabetic ketoacidosis* (see Ch. 806) and of *nonketotic hyperosmolar coma*. This latter disorder typically occurs in middle-aged or elderly mild diabetics and is characterized by hyperglycemia, hyperosmolality, and profound dehydration. Blood sugar is often in the range of 1000 mg per 100 ml, but the disorder is readily distinguished from diabetic coma by the absence of ketoacidosis. Salt and water depletion caused by osmotic diuresis also sometimes occurs with administration of *tube feedings containing large quantities of protein*. Repeated infusions of *mannitol* may have the same effects.

SKIN LOSSES. Large losses of water and electrolyte from the skin may result either from excessive sweating or from burns. *Sweat* is a hypotonic solution normally containing no more than 50 mEq of sodium per liter, and for this reason sweating will produce a relatively larger deficit of water than of sodium. *Burns* can lead to two types of deficits: isotonic extracellular fluid may be lost by transudation; and water may be lost without electrolyte as the result of increased evaporation through damaged epithelium. An additional factor contributing to a severe depletion of circulating volume is the capillary damage that results in the interstitial accumulation of fluid, particularly during the first days after the burn has occurred. Such fluid loss, because it takes place internally, can readily be overlooked.

PARACENTESIS. An occasional patient with cirrhosis and ascites has been noted to develop circulatory collapse after *paracentesis*. Reduction of pressure within the peritoneal cavity may allow transudation of a large quantity of fluid with consequent contraction of plasma volume. Clinically significant contraction is not likely to occur in patients who have a substantial amount of peripheral edema, apparently because plasma volume can be readily replenished by transfer of fluid from the expanded interstitial space.

Diagnosis. The *history* is frequently of great value in an appraisal of the origin and magnitude of a volume deficit. The patient should be questioned closely about fluid intake and about losses of fluid that may have resulted from vomiting, diarrhea, sweating, polyuria, or other disturbances. In many cases, particularly when a reliable history is not available, *physical examination* is the single most valuable diagnostic tool. Reduction in turgor of the skin, particularly over the arms, legs, and face, is the most characteristic finding, and is usually accompanied by postural hypotension. The facies are usually pinched, and the tongue is dry. Lowered tension of the eyeballs, a rapid resting pulse, and hypotension in the recumbent position may be observed when dehydration is severe.

Laboratory findings are likely to be of less value. The serum sodium concentration reflects only the ratio of sodium to water and, whether low, normal, or high, gives

(2) normal tissue turgor and normal blood pressure; (3) normal blood urea nitrogen and creatinine concentrations; (4) normal adrenal function; and (5) specific gravity of the urine inappropriately high for a hypotonic subject, that is, in excess of 1.002 or 1.003. Edema is not a usual feature, because water retention does not ordinarily exceed 3 or 4 liters and because a large fraction of the retained fluid probably moves into cells.

It should be noted that although sodium loss is a classic feature of SIADH, the presence of a significant quantity of sodium in the urine is not a prerequisite for the diagnosis of the syndrome. As serum sodium concentration falls, a new balance is struck between the reduced filtered load of sodium and the reduced renal capacity for sodium reabsorption. Thus when a new steady state of serum sodium concentration has been achieved, the urine will become virtually sodium free if sodium intake is extremely low. The salt-wasting abnormality can, however, be readily unmasked by the administration of salt either by mouth or by vein.

When serum sodium concentration is so low that it produces signs of severe water intoxication (such as coma or convulsions), hypertonic sodium chloride solution should immediately be infused to raise plasma osmotic pressure. Since administered salt will rapidly be excreted if expansion of extracellular volume persists, one should also promptly undertake correction of the state of overhydration. Diuretic therapy with an agent such as furosemide is an effective means of producing such volume contraction and, when combined with hypertonic salt infusion, will produce a rapid and sustained elevation of serum sodium concentration.

If severe manifestations of water intoxication are not present, appropriate treatment consists simply of restricting fluid intake and allowing insensible and urinary losses of water to contract the volume of extracellular fluid. This program of management not only will restore the capacity for normal renal conservation of sodium but will also correct that component of hyponatremia which has developed as a consequence of dilution. Correction of that element of the hyponatremia caused by renal sodium loss does, of course, require provision of salt either by mouth or by vein. It should be emphasized that fluid restriction will not be effective unless it is stringent enough to produce a loss of several kilograms in weight. An intake of 400 to 500 ml per day over three to five days will usually accomplish this goal.

If the patient fails to conserve sodium subsequent to a large loss of weight, the diagnosis of SIADH must be called into serious question, and other disorders, in particular Addison's disease, must be considered. Addison's disease, it should be noted, can easily be overlooked unless one recognizes that sodium depletion in adrenal insufficiency need not be accompanied by volume depletion; in some patients the deficiency of cortisol causes an impairment of water excretion of such magnitude that, despite the loss of sodium, hydration remains normal. In such patients the clinical picture can closely mimic SIADH. For this reason, it is always advisable to carry out studies of adrenal function before concluding that the hyponatremia is due to inappropriate secretion of antidiuretic hormone.

In a disorder such as meningitis or pneumonitis, the water-excreting defect disappears as recovery from the underlying illness takes place. With permanent brain damage, or with carcinoma of the lung, the defect can persist indefinitely, and a moderate degree of water restriction may be necessary to prevent recurrence of severe hyponatremia and salt wasting.

Whether the transient water retention and hyponatremia frequently encountered in the postoperative state are the result of an inappropriate secretion of antidiuretic hormone remains to be determined.

Renal Disease with Defective Excretion of Water. During the oliguric phase of *acute renal failure* dilutional hyponatremia will regularly occur if fluid intake is not adequately restricted. The net loss of water from skin and lungs is normally about 400 to 500 ml per day, and if severe oliguria or anuria is present, administration of significantly more than this quantity (for example, 1000 to 1200 ml) will produce overhydration within a relatively short time.

Water intoxication is occasionally seen in *chronic renal failure,* and occurs primarily in patients who have been urged to ingest large quantities of fluid in an effort to increase urine volume and thus to promote urea excretion. Such attempts to force a diuresis not only may be hazardous, but also appear to have little beneficial effect on the clinical course, even when they produce a slight reduction in blood urea concentration.

Idiopathic Hyponatremia. Hyponatremia frequently appears without warning in the edematous patient entering the late stages of *congestive heart failure* or *cirrhosis of the liver.* In this setting it is an ominous prognostic sign that appears to be the reflection (rather than the cause) of the underlying clinical deterioration.

The factors responsible for this electrolyte disturbance have not been clearly defined. Salt depletion induced by diuretic therapy cannot be held accountable, because the edematous patient has a larger than normal quantity of sodium in his extracellular space and, in theory, could readily restore plasma sodium concentration to normal simply by excreting surplus water. Furthermore, the disorder has been observed in patients who have not received diuretics or in whom diuretics have failed to promote salt excretion. In some cases it can be demonstrated that retention of water is responsible for the hyponatremic state, but in others measurements of body weight give no evidence that fluid was retained during the period that sodium concentration fell. In the latter circumstance it has been proposed that a primary reduction in intracellular osmolality allows water to shift into the extracellular space and that the lowered osmotic pressure of the plasma is simply a passive reflection of the change in cellular tonicity. According to this thesis, failure to increase the excretion of water is explained by the absence of an osmotic gradient between plasma and the osmoreceptors of the hypothalamus.

In some patients with congestive heart failure or cirrhosis, the development of hyponatremia is apparently an indirect consequence of enhanced proximal reabsorption of sodium and water; the delivery of an abnormally small volume of glomerular filtrate from the proximal tubule to the distal nephron prevents the elaboration of a hypotonic urine and leads to pathologic water retention. Inappropriate secretion of antidiuretic hormone has also been invoked as a factor in the genesis of the hyponatremia, but clear support for this hypothesis has yet to be obtained.

As noted above, the appearance of hyponatremia in

the edematous patient is usually a grave prognostic sign. Even if the patient does not appear to be critically ill, prolonged survival is uncommon unless treatment directed toward improvement of the underlying cardiac or liver disease is successful. Elevation of the serum sodium concentration by either water restriction or the administration of hypertonic sodium chloride usually has no beneficial effect. Water restriction usually induces severe thirst before osmolality is restored to normal, and if the patient is then permitted to increase his fluid intake, he quickly re-establishes the hyponatremic state. The administration of hypertonic saline not only seems to be of little clinical value, but appears, in many instances, to hasten rather than retard the downward clinical course.

Hyponatremia of unknown cause is sometimes seen in seriously ill patients with a debilitating disease such as metastatic carcinoma or leukemia. Neither dehydration nor edema is present, and there is no evidence of extrarenal or urinary loss of sodium. The explanation for this disturbance is obscure.

Excessive Water Intake in the Presence of Normal Renal Function (Psychogenic Polydipsia). A syndrome virtually identical to that already described for inappropriate secretion of antidiuretic hormone may be produced by the ingestion of more water than the normal kidney can excrete; that is, more than 1000 or 1200 ml per hour. Intakes in excess of these amounts are unusual, but are occasionally seen in patients who have a severe psychiatric illness. In such cases the expansion of extracellular volume induced by the positive water balance leads to both hyponatremia and renal wasting of sodium. Characteristically, the urine is maximally dilute (specific gravity of 1.001), and it is this finding that unequivocally demonstrates that the syndrome is the result of excessive ingestion of water rather than of inappropriate secretion of antidiuretic hormone.

If signs of water intoxication are present, hypertonic saline solution should be given intravenously, but in most cases reduction of water intake and increased ingestion of salt will be the only treatment required.

Hyponatremia Without Disturbance in Water Balance. ACCUMULATION OF SOLUTE IN THE EXTRACELLULAR FLUID. Solutes such as glucose and mannitol, which do not distribute freely throughout body water, can accumulate in the extracellular space and create an osmotic gradient between cells and interstitial fluid. As a result, water shifts from the intracellular compartment, and the serum sodium concentration falls. Hyponatremia resulting from such a redistribution of fluid is a characteristic feature of the severe hyperglycemia seen in patients with uncontrolled diabetes mellitus; each 100 mg per 100 ml increment in blood sugar concentration above normal respresents the addition of slightly more than 5 milliosmoles of solute per kilogram to the extracellular compartment, and leads to a reduction in serum sodium concentration of approximately 1.5 mEq per liter. A blood sugar concentration of 1000 mg per 100 ml can thus be expected to lower sodium concentration from 140 to 126 mEq per liter. Failure to consider the role of hyperglycemia in the genesis of hyponatremia in the diabetic can lead to the administration of an excessive amount of sodium during the treatment of ketoacidosis.

The accumulation of mannitol in the extracellular fluid can also cause a shift of water sufficient to reduce serum sodium concentration. This problem is most likely to be encountered in the patient with acute renal failure in whom an unsuccessful attempt has been made to increase urine volume by repeated mannitol infusions.

Hyperosmolality will *not* produce hyponatremia if the solute distributes freely across cell membranes, and thus increases the osmolality of cells and interstitial fluid to a proportional degree. In uremia, for example, serum sodium concentration is unaffected by the hypertonicity induced by urea accumulation because urea penetrates cells readily, and its concentration is elevated throughout body water.

PSEUDOHYPONATREMIA. Pseudohyponatremia refers to a spurious reduction in sodium concentration resulting from a displacement of some fraction of plasma water by an abnormal accumulation of lipid or protein. Although plasma sodium concentration is usually measured as milliequivalents per liter of plasma, the physiologically significant measurement is the sodium concentration expressed as milliequivalents per kilogram of plasma water. Thus a sodium concentration of 140 mEq per liter, as measured on whole plasma, reflects an actual concentration of 150 mEq per kilogram of water in normal plasma containing 93 per cent water. Since the percentage of plasma that is water does not vary appreciably under most circumstances, reductions in plasma sodium concentration can generally be taken as reflecting a decrease in the sodium concentration per unit of plasma water and in the tonicity of extracellular fluid. On the other hand, if severe hyperlipemia (or hyperproteinemia) is present, the fraction of plasma that is water will be lower than normal, and a striking reduction in the sodium concentration per unit volume of plasma will be observed despite the absence of a significant change in the electrolyte concentration per kilogram of plasma water.

Hyperlipemia of sufficient magnitude to produce pseudohyponatremia occurs in a number of diseases, including diabetes mellitus, nephrotic syndrome, and biliary cirrhosis. In nearly all cases in which sodium concentration is reduced by lipidemia the plasma is frankly lactescent, and lactescence will thus often be the first finding that points to the correct diagnosis. *Hyperproteinemia* severe enough to cause pseudohyponatremia is a rare occurrence, and has been seen only in multiple myeloma. In this disease the plasma sodium concentration may be lowered to a value of 125 or 130 mEq per liter.

The contribution of an increased concentration of lipid or protein to a reduced plasma sodium concentration can be readily assessed by determination of plasma osmotic pressure (estimated from freezing-point depression). If osmotic pressure is normal despite the hyponatremia, it will be evident that the concentration of sodium in the aqueous phase of plasma is normal.

Aviram, A., Pfau, A., Czaczkes, J. W., and Ullmann, T. D.: Hyperosmolality with hyponatremia, caused by inappropriate administration of mannitol. Am. J. Med., 42:648, 1967.
Bartter, F., and Schwartz, W. B.: The syndrome of inappropriate secretion of antidiuretic hormone. Am. J. Med., 42:790, 1967.
Harrington, J. T., and Cohen, J. J.: Clinical disorders of urine concentration and dilution. Arch. Intern. Med., 131:810, 1973.
Langgard, H., and Smith, W. O.: Self-induced water intoxication without predisposing illness. N. Engl. J. Med., 266:378, 1962.
Leaf, A.: The clinical and physiologic significance of the serum sodium concentration. N. Engl. J. Med., 267:24, 1962.
Tarail, R., Buchwald, K. W., Holland, J. F., and Selawry, O. S.: Misleading reductions of serum sodium and chloride associated with hyperproteinemia in patients with multiple myeloma. Proc. Soc. Exp. Biol. Med., 110:145, 1962.

HYPERNATREMIA

Virtually all cases of hypernatremia result from a loss of water that produces a relative excess of sodium in the body fluids. Any hypotonic loss, such as that occurring with sweating or vomiting, will cause a modest degree of hypernatremia which will persist if adequate fluid replacement is not provided. Extreme elevations of plasma sodium concentrations (160 mEq per liter or above) are uncommon and are usually encountered in only one of three clinical settings: decreased or absent fluid intake, diabetes insipidus, or osmotic diuresis. Such extreme increases in tonicity of the extracellular fluid, when they occur, lead to marked cellular dehydration.

The most common cause of hypernatremia is a fluid intake that is inadequate to replace urinary losses and insensible losses of water from skin and lungs. This problem is most frequently encountered in the patient who is stuporous or who has some other disability that prevents him from drinking normally. In the comatose patient in whom *diabetes insipidus* develops after a head injury or a neurosurgical procedure, a large negative water balance is likely to appear with unusual speed. In most cases of diabetes insipidus, polyuria will quickly draw attention to the nature of the problem, but if solute intake is low, the diagnosis can readily be overlooked, because urine volume may not exceed 2 or 3 liters per day.

Osmotic loading can also produce severe hypernatremia. During osmotic diuresis water is lost in excess of sodium, and with sustained or repeated diuresis the serum sodium concentration sometimes rises to values greater than 175 mEq per liter. This sequence of events is often observed in comatose patients who are confronted with a massive urea load as the result of being given tube feedings containing large amounts of protein. In such patients maintenance of a normal urine volume by continued solute loading may sometimes obscure the fact that dehydration and hypertonicity are present. Under such circumstances, the progressive loss of weight, the physical signs of volume depletion, and the development of hypernatremia should draw attention to the correct diagnosis.

The specific signs and symptoms produced by a marked elevation of serum sodium concentration have not been clearly defined; most patients with hypernatremia are already seriously ill and the role of the hypertonicity, as distinguished from that of the underlying disease, is frequently difficult to evaluate. Clinical experience suggests, however, that when hypernatremia is encountered water should be administered (either orally or as 5 per cent glucose intravenously) in quantities sufficient to restore serum sodium concentration to normal. The quantity of water required must be calculated with an appreciation that hypertonicity is present not only in the extracellular fluid but throughout total body water. Thus a 70-kg man with a plasma sodium concentration of 170 mEq per liter will require a 20 per cent expansion of body water, that is, 8 liters of fluid, to restore serum sodium concentration to a normal value of 140 mEq per liter. Observations during the treatment of hypernatremia indicate that full correction should not be carried out rapidly, i.e., over a few hours, because a rapid reduction in tonicity may produce signs of water intoxication.

Gault, M. H., Dixon, E. E., Doyle, M., and Cohen, W. M.: Hypernatremia, azotemia, and dehydration due to high-protein tube feeding. Ann. Intern. Med., 68:778, 1968.
Leaf, A.: The clinical and physiologic significance of the serum sodium concentration. N. Engl. J. Med., 267:24, 1962.
Ross, E. J., and Christie, S. B. M.: Hypernatremia. Medicine, 48:441, 1969.
Weiner, M., and Epstein, F. H.: Signs and symptoms of electrolyte disorders. Yale J. Biol. Med., 43:76, 1970.

DISTURBANCES OF POTASSIUM EQUILIBRIUM

Potassium, the major intracellular cation, plays a significant part in control of osmotic pressure, and also serves as an essential activator in a number of enzymatic reactions. In addition, the potassium concentration of body fluids has an important influence on the excitability of both skeletal and cardiac muscle and on the structure and function of the kidneys. Disturbances in potassium equilibrium may therefore produce a wide range of clinical disorders.

The potassium concentration in extracellular fluid is normally 3.8 to 5 mEq per liter and in intracellular fluid approximately 150 mEq per liter. Since about 20 per cent of body weight is extracellular fluid, it can readily be calculated that only a small fraction of the 2500 to 3000 mEq of potassium within the body is contained in the extracellular space. On the other hand, changes in plasma potassium concentration often mirror changes in cellular potassium content, and plasma concentration thus usually provides a useful clinical guide to disturbances in potassium balance. Furthermore, relatively small absolute changes in extracellular concentration, by producing large differences in the ratio of intracellular to extracellular potassium, may have important effects on neuromuscular activity.

Despite the usual wide variations in dietary intake of potassium (40 to 120 mEq per day), plasma potassium concentration is normally stabilized within the narrow range of 4 to 5 mEq per liter by virtue of close renal regulation of potassium balance. As discussed earlier, renal potassium excretion is accomplished largely, if not exclusively, by a process of potassium secretion in the distal portion of the nephron; it has been demonstrated that essentially all filtered potassium is reabsorbed in the proximal tubule and that the potassium that appears in the urine is added to the filtrate by a distal process of sodium-cation exchange. Fecal excretion of potassium normally amounts to only a few milliequivalents per day and does not play a significant role in potassium homeostasis.

If a large potassium load is suddenly administered, renal mechanisms do not respond quickly enough to prevent a rise in serum potassium concentration to abnormal levels. Under such circumstances, sequestration of potassium within cells helps to prevent a dangerous degree of hyperkalemia. If renal function is normal, the elevation of serum potassium concentration usually persists only briefly.

The clinical aspects of disturbances in potassium metabolism will be considered under two headings, *potassium deficiency* and *potassium intoxication*.

Hypokalemia and Potassium Deficiency

Potassium deficiency may occur as the result of either *renal* or *extrarenal losses*. Typically, serum potassium concentration is reduced to a level of 2.5 to 3.5 mEq per liter, but with severe potassium depletion it may fall below 2 mEq per liter. In some circumstances, the reduction in potassium concentration is minimized or prevented by the concomitant presence of acidosis. Acidosis shifts the equilibrium between cells and extracellular fluid, tending to make serum potassium concentration high in relation to total body stores.

Hypokalemia can also occur without a loss of potassium from the body in the uncommon disorder known as *hypokalemic familial periodic paralysis*. This disorder is discussed in Ch. 480.

Pathogenesis and Diagnosis. Table 3 lists the common causes of potassium deficiency grouped according to whether the losses are of renal or extrarenal origin. As is evident from the table, a large variety of factors, including adrenal steroids, diuretics, and renal tubular disease, may promote abnormal renal excretion. Nearly all appear to increase sodium-potassium exchange in some fashion. *Adrenal steroids*, whether produced in excessive quantities by the body or given therapeutically, directly stimulate the sodium-cation exchange mechanism and thereby induce a urinary potassium loss. An excess of adrenal steroids resulting from overproduction is seen in *primary aldosteronism*, Cushing's syndrome, and various forms of *secondary aldosteronism* (see Ch. 850 to 852).

One uncommon cause of secondary aldosteronism and hypokalemia is *Bartter's syndrome*. This disease is characterized by juxtaglomerular hyperplasia, hypersecretion of renin, and metabolic alkalosis. Neither hypertension nor edema is present, and there is a subnormal pressor response to the administration of angiotensin. Renal salt wasting and accompanying hyponatremia are frequently striking features of the clinical picture.

Bartter's syndrome occurs most commonly in children and in some instances is familial in nature. The clinical manifestations of the disorder appear to result from an abnormal activation of the renin-angiotensin mechanism; nearly all the findings are accounted for by hyperplasia of the juxtaglomerular apparatus with a consequent excessive rate of renin production and of aldosterone secretion. The factors responsible for the juxtaglomerular hyperplasia have not been clearly defined, but several mechanisms have been proposed. It has been suggested, for example, that the stimulus to hyperplasia arises from a decreased responsiveness of

blood vessels to angiotensin and a consequent chronic state of subclinical hypotension. Another postulate is that renal sodium wasting, with resulting chronic hypovolemia, produces the abnormal stimulus to the juxtaglomerular cells.

A disorder closely mimicking Bartter's syndrome has recently been observed in states of chronic volume depletion induced by vomiting, diarrhea, or diuretics. Juxtaglomerular hyperplasia, high rates of renin and aldosterone secretion, hypokalemic alkalosis, and a normal blood pressure are present, just as in the classic form of Bartter's syndrome. It thus appears that juxtaglomerular hyperplasia can be produced by a variety of stimuli and that a number of types of Bartter's syndrome will eventually be delineated.

Hypokalemia has also been observed as a cardinal feature of another disorder involving the juxtaglomerular apparatus, namely *juxtaglomerular cell tumor*. This tumor, as might be expected, produces excessive renin and thereby causes secondary aldosteronism and hypokalemic alkalosis. In striking contrast to Bartter's syndrome, however, blood pressure is markedly elevated rather than normal.

Studies of renal venous renin in the patient with a juxtaglomerular cell tumor will quickly identify one kidney as the source of the excessive renin production. Selective renal angiography will usually demonstrate the tumor, but in an occasional instance the lesion may be so small that it is overlooked; under such circumstances a decision regarding surgery must be made on the basis of the other clinical features. Blood pressure and electrolyte abnormalities usually return to normal shortly after the tumor is removed.

Renal potassium wasting and hypokalemia also occur as the result of *therapy with diuretics* such as thiazides, ethacrynic acid, and furosemide. These agents exert their effect on potassium balance by increasing the delivery of sodium to sodium-avid distal exchange sites and by thus accelerating the rate of sodium-potassium exchange. Diuretics which act through inhibition of carbonic anhydrase also cause potassium loss but exert their influence directly on the distal exchange mechanism; inhibition of carbonic anhydrase reduces the availability of hydrogen for exchange and thus enhances the exchange of sodium for potassium.

The derangements in function responsible for potassium wasting and hypokalemia in renal tubular diseases such as *renal tubular acidosis* are discussed in Ch. 619 to 624.

The only significant *extrarenal* route of potassium depletion is through the loss of gastrointestinal secretions. Gastric juice contains potassium in a concentration somewhat higher than plasma, and diarrheal fluid may have a potassium content as high as 50 to 60 mEq per liter. Thus prolonged vomiting, drainage of the upper gastrointestinal tract, or diarrhea typically produces a considerable deficit of potassium. If intake of potassium is poor, the severity of potassium deficiency will be further aggravated by renal losses; inefficient renal conservation allows considerable quantities of potassium to escape into the urine for as long as ten days or two weeks after potassium intake is lowered sharply. As much as 150 or 200 mEq can be lost before excretion is reduced to a level of less than 10 mEq per day.

In *hypokalemia of unknown origin* the quantity of potassium in the urine frequently provides the clue to the

TABLE 3. Causes of Potassium Deficiency

A. Renal
  1. Adrenal steroids
    Primary aldosteronism
    Secondary aldosteronism (including Bartter's syndrome and juxtaglomerular cell tumor)
    Cushing's syndrome
    Adrenal steroid therapy
  2. Diuretics
    Mercurials
    Ethacrynic acid
    Thiazides
    Furosemide
    Carbonic anhydrase inhibitors
  3. Renal tubular diseases
B. Extrarenal
  1. Vomiting
  2. Gastric drainage
  3. Diarrhea

correct diagnosis. If a patient with persistent hypokalemia is excreting considerable quantities of potassium in the urine (30 mEq or more per day), the deficit is clearly of renal origin, and attention can therefore immediately be focused on those disorders listed under Section A of Table 3. Ordinarily the history and other clinical findings will clarify the etiology of such renal losses. There are several exceptions to this statement, however. A common problem, for example, is the evaluation of hypokalemia in the hypertensive patient who has received an agent such as a thiazide as part of his antihypertensive regimen. In such a patient it may be difficult to decide whether potassium deficiency is the result of diuretic therapy or is caused by primary aldosteronism. This question can usually be resolved by observation of the serum potassium level for at least several weeks after the drug has been discontinued.

In the patient with hypokalemia in whom potassium excretion is low (less than 15 mEq per day), the depletion is usually of extrarenal origin (Section B of Table 3). In nearly all such instances a history or other evidence pointing to gastrointestinal losses will easily be obtained, but sometimes the diagnostic problem is more difficult. Occasionally, a patient with *laxative-induced diarrhea* will deny both laxative ingestion and diarrhea, and it will then be necessary to obtain the relevant history from members of the family. Similarly, some patients with *psychogenic* or *self-induced vomiting* do not admit to their difficulties. Patients with *villous adenomas of the rectum* may also pose a diagnostic problem, because they usually have normally formed stools and, unless asked specifically, may neglect to mention the nearly continuous rectal leakage of mucus-like material which is characteristic of their illness. Accordingly, whenever unexplained chronic hypokalemia is associated with a low urinary potassium excretion, each of these uncommon disorders should be sought carefully.

Clinical Manifestations. The clinical effects of potassium deficiency may be manifested in one or more organ systems, including skeletal muscle, heart, kidneys, and the gastrointestinal tract. Perhaps the most serious disturbances are those affecting the neuromuscular system. At serum potassium concentrations in the range of 2 to 2.5 mEq per liter, muscular weakness is likely to occur, and with more severe hypokalemia the patient may develop areflexic paralysis. In this latter state respiratory insufficiency is an immediate threat to survival. The severity of the neuromuscular disturbance tends to be proportional to the speed with which the potassium level has declined. In an occasional instance, *myoglobinuria* has been noted in association with marked hypokalemia.

Finally, it should be noted that the patient who has developed potassium depletion as the result of diuretic therapy will sometimes demonstrate a low renal excretion of potassium even though the potassium loss was of renal origin. If diuretics are no longer being administered and if metabolic alkalosis is not present, the kidney will promptly begin to conserve potassium, and urinary excretion will remain low until the deficit is fully repaired.

Abnormalities in the electrocardiogram that commonly occur in hypokalemia are a sagging of the S-T segment, depression of the T wave, and elevation of the U wave (Fig. 1). With marked reductions in serum concentration, the T wave becomes progressively smaller,

Figure 1. Typical electrocardiographic abnormalities induced by hypokalemia. (Serum potassium concentration 2.8 mEq per liter.) Note in lead II how the merger of the T and U waves might lead to the erroneous interpretation that the Q-T interval is prolonged.

whereas the U waves show increasing amplitude. In some cases the merging of a flat or positive T with a positive U wave may erroneously be interpreted as a prolonged Q-T interval. Ordinarily, there are no serious clinical consequences from the abnormalities in cardiac excitation, but in digitalized patients the sudden development of hypokalemia may precipitate serious arrhythmias.

Longstanding potassium depletion is apt to produce renal tubular damage—so-called *hypokalemic nephropathy.* This disorder is discussed in detail in Ch. 619. Potassium deficiency is believed to cause dysfunction of the smooth muscle of the gastrointestinal tract and in some patients has been held responsible for the development of *paralytic ileus.*

Potassium deficiency is also a regular concomitant of *metabolic alkalosis.* The role of potassium in the genesis and maintenance of alkalosis is considered later in this chapter.

Treatment. Under many circumstances potassium deficiency can be corrected by oral administration of potassium salts. The oral route should be used whenever feasible, because the relatively slow absorption from the gastrointestinal tract prevents a sudden large increase in serum potassium concentration of the sort that can occur during the injudicious administration of potassium intravenously. In this connection, it should be appreciated that correction of a typical deficit of 200 to 500 mEq requires the transfer through the extracellular compartment of a quantity of potassium that has the potential of raising serum concentration to well above lethal levels. For this reason, when potassium is administered intravenously, it should ordinarily be given at a rate not exceeding 15 to 20 mEq per hour and at a concentration no higher than 40 to 60 mEq per liter. It is also generally prudent to limit the supplement to 100 or 150 mEq per day and to use the serum potassium concentration as a guide to the need for further replacement. If acidosis is present, the serum potassium may be higher than is appropriate to the degree of potassium deficiency, and this discrepancy must be taken into account when treatment is planned. As acidosis is corrected, a more accurate appraisal of further potassium requirements will be possible. Unfortunately, there is no way of directly calculating the quantity of potassium that will be required for full replacement.

The *electrocardiogram* does not provide a reliable guide to the need for replacement therapy, but is extremely useful as a convenient and rapid means for determining whether an excessive quantity of potassium has been given. The electrocardiogram in hyperkalemia and potassium intoxication is discussed later.

The chloride salt of potassium is used almost exclusively for intravenous therapy, but it has fallen into some disfavor for purposes of oral administration because it often produces annoying upper gastrointestinal symptoms. Such symptoms can be avoided if potassium chloride is used in the enteric-coated form, but this mode of administration occasionally creates other problems. Dissolution of the enteric coating in the small intestine, and the resulting high local concentration of potassium on the mucosa, may produce ulceration, obstruction, or bleeding. For this reason, organic potassium salts, which are more palatable than potassium chloride and which can be given without an enteric coating (and without untoward local effects on the intestine), have come into widespread use. Potassium gluconate and potassium "triplex" (citrate, acetate, and bicarbonate) are among the agents frequently employed and are effective in patients who are not depleted of chloride. They are, however, relatively ineffective in repairing potassium deficiency when the patient is hypochloremic, alkalotic, and on a low-salt (low-chloride) intake. The explanation for this can be summarized as follows: In hypochloremic alkalosis a smaller than normal fraction of filtered sodium is reabsorbed with chloride and an increased fraction is reabsorbed by exchange with potassium and hydrogen. As long as hypochloremia and avidity for sodium persist, the accelerated rate of sodium-cation exchange forces a continued high rate of potassium excretion. For this reason, full repair of potassium deficiency cannot be achieved by administration of an organic potassium salt. Potassium must instead be provided as the chloride salt, or chloride must be made available in some other form, such as ammonium chloride or sodium chloride.

Hyperkalemia and Potassium Intoxication

Pathogenesis. Hyperkalemia is most often due to defective renal excretion of potassium. It may arise as the result of primary renal disease, deficiency of adrenal steroids, or the use of aldosterone antagonists (spironolactones) or other agents that inhibit sodium-potassium exchange by the tubule. Excessively rapid intravenous administration of potassium may also elevate plasma concentration to dangerous levels, as has been mentioned earlier in connection with the treatment of potassium deficiency. Potassium given by mouth rarely causes severe hyperkalemia unless renal function is severely impaired.

Hyperkalemia secondary to renal damage occurs frequently in *acute tubular necrosis* or in any other form of acute renal failure that is characterized by oliguria or anuria. In *chronic renal failure* potassium intoxication is usually encountered only in the terminal stages of the disease, but is sometimes seen earlier as a sequel to the inadvertent administration of potassium supplements. A deficiency of mineralocorticoid, caused either by *Addison's disease* or by *primary hypoaldosteronism,* a rare disorder, also impairs potassium secretion and may produce hyperkalemia.

The *spironolactones,* agents which are used in diuretic therapy for the purpose of antagonizing the sodium-retaining effects of aldosterone, do not usually cause sig-

nificant elevation in serum potassium concentration. They do, however, impair the ability of the kidney to respond to a potassium load, and should not be given in conjunction with potassium supplements. The same caution concerning administration of potassium applies to patients receiving diuretic agents such as *triamterene* and *amiloride,* which also impair the exchange of sodium for potassium by the tubule.

Hyperkalemia also occurs in an uncommon and puzzling disorder known as *familial hyperkalemic periodic paralysis.* In individuals with this disorder, attacks can be induced by the ingestion of potassium. This disease is discussed in detail in Ch. 480.

Pseudohyperkalemia has been observed in a few patients with thrombocytosis secondary to a myeloproliferative disorder. The spurious elevation of serum concentration results from release of potassium from platelets during the coagulation process. Concentrations as high as 9 mEq per liter can be found in the serum at a time when plasma (platelet-free) has a normal potassium level. Similar spurious elevations in serum potassium concentration resulting from the release of potassium from white blood cells have also been reported in a few patients with chronic myelogenous leukemia. The possibility that one is dealing with pseudohyperkalemia should be considered whenever an elevated serum potassium concentration cannot otherwise be explained.

Clinical Manifestations. The clinical manifestations of potassium intoxication are related primarily to the heart and the neuromuscular system. *Electrocardiographic abnormalities* are the earliest and most frequent sign of disturbed membrane excitability, and are characterized by the development of tall, "tent-shaped" T waves, by decreased amplitude of the P waves, and later by atrial asystole (Fig. 2). Intraventricular block, with widening of the QRS complex, may lead to the development of a sine wave pattern and ultimately to ventricular standstill. Changes in the electrocardiogram usually appear when the serum potassium concentration reaches 7 to 8 mEq per liter, and cardiac standstill is likely to occur at a concentration of 9 to 10 mEq per liter. *Weakness* and *flaccid paralysis* appear only in association with severe hyperkalemia, but are not always present even at plasma levels sufficiently high to produce serious deterioration in the electrocardiogram. Indeed, death from cardiac arrest may occur even before muscular weakness is evident. For this reason the electrocardiogram is the single most important guide in appraising the threat posed by hyperkalemia and in determining how aggressive a therapeutic approach is necessary.

Figure 2. Typical electrocardiographic abnormalities induced by a moderate degree of hyperkalemia. (Serum potassium concentration 6.5 mEq per liter.) Note the typical "tent-shaped" T waves.

Treatment. The first goal in the treatment of severe potassium intoxication should be to promote the rapid transfer of potassium into cells in order to lower serum potassium concentration and prevent cardiac arrest. Two approaches to this goal are likely to prove effective. Infusion of glucose and insulin induces the cellular deposition of glycogen and at the same time brings about a shift of potassium to the intracellular space; 1 liter of a 10 per cent glucose solution with 30 to 40 units of insulin is generally employed for this purpose. In the acidotic patient further redistribution of potassium can be achieved by the administration of sodium bicarbonate (150 to 300 mEq). In many cases these measures will induce a striking reduction in plasma potassium concentration and prompt improvement in the electrocardiogram. In some instances the administration of calcium (as 2 grams of calcium lactate) is also useful, because calcium, though it has no effect on the plasma potassium concentration, opposes the cardiotoxic effects of potassium. It should be noted, incidentally, that calcium cannot be given in the same solution with sodium bicarbonate, because precipitation of the calcium ion will result.

Because the techniques described above do not remove potassium from the body and may be only temporarily effective, longer-term efforts should be directed toward promoting gastrointestinal losses of potassium. A cation-exchange resin in the sodium cycle, such as Kayexelate, will usually achieve this purpose if administered by mouth in a dose of 20 to 30 grams every six hours. Each gram of resin binds approximately 1 mEq of potassium, and within 24 hours a significant effect on plasma potassium concentration should be achieved. To enhance potassium loss and assure the rapid movement of the resin through the gastrointestinal tract, sorbitol, a nonabsorbable polyhydric alcohol, should be given in quantities sufficient to induce a soft or semiliquid bowel movement every few hours. The usual dose for this purpose is 20 ml of a 70 per cent solution three or four times a day. If the patient is unable to take medication by mouth, the resin can be administered by rectum as a retention enema of 100 grams in several hundred milliliters of water.

Hemodialysis is an efficient alternative means of removing excess potassium, but usually will not be required if the program outlined above can be implemented.

Cannon, P. J., Leeming, J. M., Sommers, S. C., Winters, R. W., and Laragh, J. H.: Juxtaglomerular cell hyperplasia and secondary hyperaldosteronism (Bartter's syndrome): a reevaluation of the pathophysiology. Medicine, 47:107, 1968.
Conn, J. W., et al.: Primary reninism. Arch. Intern. Med., 130:682, 1972.
Fleischer, N., Brown, H., Graham, D. Y., and Delena, S.: Chronic laxative-induced hyperaldosteronism and hypokalemia simulating Bartter's syndrome. Ann. Intern. Med., 70:791, 1969.
Ingram, R. H., and Seki, M.: Pseudohyperkalemia with thombocytosis. N. Engl. J. Med., 267:895, 1962.
Schwartz, W. B., and Relman, A. S.: Effects of electrolyte disorders on renal structure and function. N. Engl. J. Med., 276:383, 1967.
Welt, L. G., Hollander, W., and Blythe, W. B.: The consequences of potassium depletion. J. Chronic Dis., 11:213, 1960.

DISTURBANCES OF ACID-BASE EQUILIBRIUM

The pH of extracellular fluid normally ranges between 7.35 and 7.45, and is stabilized within these limits despite wide variations in the dietary load of acid or alkali. A large number of body functions are importantly influenced by the pH of body fluids, disturbances in acid-base regulation often having serious effects on metabolic activity, on the circulation, and on the central nervous system.

As background to a discussion of acid-base disturbances, it is instructive to consider briefly the way in which the body deals with the *normal daily acid load* and thus maintains a steady state of acid-base equilibrium. As food is oxidized, both carbon dioxide (carbonic acid) and nonvolatile acids such as sulfuric and phosphoric acids are added to the extracellular fluid. Immediate buffering within the interstitial fluid, plasma, and red blood cells minimizes the change in pH and permits large quantities of acid to be transferred to the lungs and kidneys for excretion. *Carbon dioxide* is excreted almost entirely by the lungs, and for this reason alveolar carbon dioxide tension is the prime determinant of P_{CO_2} in body fluids. With usual rates of carbon dioxide production, alveolar ventilation maintains the P_{CO_2} of blood at approximately 40 mm of mercury, that is, 1.2 millimoles of dissolved carbon dioxide per liter of plasma.

Nonvolatile acids are excreted solely by the kidney. The process by which this is accomplished is complex, because no significant fraction of the daily hydrogen ion load (some 50 to 100 mEq) can be excreted in an unbuffered form at the minimal urinary pH of 4.0 that the kidney can establish. Virtually all hydrogen must thus be removed as either *titratable acid* or *ammonium*. Acidification of the glomerular filtrate by a process of sodium-hydrogen exchange titrates buffers such as phosphate and also favors the diffusion of ammonia (NH_3) from the tubular cells to the lumen, where it reacts with hydrogen ions to form ammonium (NH_4^+). Bicarbonate generated in tubular cells as the result of acid excretion moves into peritubular blood and replenishes the bicarbonate stores that previously were depleted by the buffering of dietary acid. From all these considerations it is evident that derangements in either pulmonary or renal function, or the imposition of stresses that overwhelm normal regulatory mechanisms, can be expected to produce disturbances of acid-base equilibrium.

Because the carbonic acid–bicarbonate buffer pair is the major buffer system in the extracellular fluid, its parameters provide a meaningful and convenient expression of the acid-base status of the organism. The relation between pH and the bicarbonate and carbonic acid concentrations can be expressed in a general fashion according to the familiar Henderson-Hasselbalch equation,

$$pH = pK + \log \frac{HCO_3^-}{H_2CO_3} \qquad (1)$$

where pK is the dissociation constant of carbonic acid. In the normal subject this expression will be

$$7.4 = 6.1 + \log \frac{24 \text{ mM/L}}{1.2 \text{ mM/L}} \qquad (2)$$

Traditionally, disturbances in acid-balance equilibrium are considered in terms of a change in the ratio of bicarbonate to carbonic acid, but this approach, in the opinion of some, does not always provide the immediate and intuitive insight that can be derived from the following expression:

$$
\begin{array}{c}
40 \text{ mm Hg} \\
\text{Pco}_2 \\
\searrow\ \searrow \\
H_2CO_3 \ \rightleftarrows \ H^+ \ + \ HCO_3^- \\
1.2 \text{ mM/L} \quad \text{pH } 7.4 \quad 24 \text{ mM/L}
\end{array} \qquad (3)
$$

This equation allows ready visualization of the directional changes that can be anticipated in both metabolic and respiratory disturbances of acid-base equilibrium. It is apparent, for example, that a primary reduction in bicarbonate concentration (*metabolic acidosis*) will cause the reaction to shift to the right, thus increasing hydrogen ion concentration, whereas a primary elevation in bicarbonate concentration (*metabolic alkalosis*) will cause the reaction to shift to the left, thus decreasing hydrogen ion concentration. Respiratory disorders can be analyzed in the same fashion. A rise in Pco_2 increases the hydrogen ion concentration by shifting the reaction to the right (*respiratory acidosis*), and a fall has the reverse effect (*respiratory alkalosis*). In both metabolic and respiratory acid-base disturbances, the widest range of pH values compatible with life is approximately 6.8 to 7.8.

Metabolic Acidosis

Metabolic acidosis results whenever acid is added to the body, alkali is lost from the body, or impaired renal function prevents the excretion of the normal endogenous acid load. In each case the reduction in bicarbonate concentration is accompanied by a rise in hydrogen ion concentration, that is, a decrease in pH.

Physiologic Considerations. The normal organism confronted with a large acid load has a remarkable ability to maintain hydrogen ion concentration within tolerable limits until augmented excretion of acid (and concomitant regeneration of buffer stores) allows restoration of a normal plasma bicarbonate concentration. This resiliency is explained by the magnitude of the total body buffer capacity and the prompt respiratory adjustment of Pco_2.

Body buffers provide a large reservoir of hydrogen ion acceptors distributed through both the extracellular and intracellular compartments. In the extracellular space bicarbonate provides the bulk of the buffer capacity; hemoglobin and plasma proteins, though they make a significant contribution to the buffering ability of *blood*, are of little quantitative importance when viewed in terms of the entire extracellular compartment. Intracellular buffers, which consist largely of protein and organic anions, provide an additional buffer reserve that is responsible for sequestering half or more of an acid load and that thus serves the important function of protecting against lethal reductions in extracellular pH.

As the price for maintaining electroneutrality during cellular accumulation of hydrogen, both potassium and sodium are forced out of cells. If renal function is normal, the displaced potassium is ultimately lost in the urine. On the other hand, if renal function is impaired or if dehydration has reduced urine volume to oliguric levels, potassium will be retained and potentially dangerous elevations of serum potassium concentration may occur.

Respiratory compensation takes place promptly after the development of metabolic acidosis, an increase in both depth and rate of respiration lowering alveolar and arterial Pco_2. The magnitude of the fall in Pco_2 becomes larger as the reduction in bicarbonate concentration becomes greater, but respiratory defense is never sufficient to restore pH to normal.

Even with the most severe metabolic acidosis, Pco_2 does not fall below 10 mm of mercury because the physical effort required to produce a further increase in alveolar ventilation increases carbon dioxide production more rapidly than it does pulmonary gas exchange. Thus if bicarbonate concentration is very low and maximal reductions in Pco_2 have already been achieved, a slight further fall in bicarbonate concentration will produce a large decrement in pH.

The foregoing comments on respiratory defense have been based, of course, on the assumption that there will be a normal ventilatory response when metabolic acidosis occurs. Indeed, the clinical significance of a given reduction in plasma bicarbonate concentration is judged almost automatically (in the absence of pH measurements) on the basis of experience with the usual degree of respiratory compensation. In some circumstances, however, Pco_2 does not fall in the anticipated manner, and the increase in hydrogen ion concentration will therefore be far greater than is customary. This difficulty will be encountered if the respiratory center has been depressed by sedatives or other medications. It is also seen in the patient with pulmonary disease who, though able to maintain a normal Pco_2 under usual conditions, cannot increase alveolar ventilation to a significant degree under stress. In the patient with a plasma bicarbonate concentration of 10 mEq per liter, for example, normal respiratory compensation will usually reduce the Pco_2 to approximately 25 mm of mercury and keep the pH in the range of 7.20 to 7.25, whereas without a reduction in Pco_2 the pH would be 7.00. The measurement of pH or Pco_2 therefore is often important even in circumstances in which the diagnosis of metabolic acidosis is not in question.

Renal compensation is the final step in the defense against metabolic acidosis, but takes place slowly and does not contribute to the immediate protection of pH. Several days are required before excretion of ammonium and titratable acid rises sufficiently to regenerate bicarbonate and restore plasma concentration to normal. If renal function is impaired, or if underlying renal tubular disease is present, an even longer period may be required for correction to take place.

Pathogenesis (Table 4). *Large Acid Loads as a Cause of Acidosis.* Probably the most frequent cause of metabolic acidosis is the addition of a large acid load to the body fluids. *Diabetic ketoacidosis* is a familiar example of such a disturbance. In diabetic acidosis there is an imbalance between the production and utilization of

TABLE 4. Causes of Metabolic Acidosis

With Increase in Unmeasured Anions	Without Increase in Unmeasured Anions
Diabetic ketoacidosis	Diarrhea
Alcoholic ketoacidosis	Drainage of pancreatic juice
Salicylate poisoning	Ureterosigmoidostomy
Ethylene glycol poisoning	Carbonic anhydrase inhibitors
Methyl alcohol poisoning	Ammonium chloride
Paraldehyde (rarely)	Renal tubular acidosis
Lactic acidosis	
Renal failure	

beta-hydroxybutyric and acetoacetic acids, with the result that both accumulate in the extracellular fluid. Because these acids are almost completely dissociated at the pH of body fluids, nearly 1 millimole of bicarbonate is dissipated by the addition of each millimole of ketoacid.

Severe *ketoacidosis associated with alcoholism* has also been noted in nondiabetic patients. This disorder is seen in patients with chronic alcoholism who have been drinking heavily and who have eaten little or no food over several days. Typically such patients also have a history of protracted vomiting. Blood sugar is usually normal or mildly elevated. The acidosis, which is often severe, results from the accumulation of β-hydroxybutyric and acetoacetic acids (and sometimes lactic acid as well), but the severe ketosis can readily be overlooked because the ratio of β-hydroxybutyrate to acetoacetate in the plasma is unusually high; as a result, the nitroprusside test, which detects only acetoacetate, may be negative or only slightly positive. However, the characteristic history and the findings of a large "anion gap" should point strongly to the correct diagnosis.

Accumulation of lactic acid is now recognized as a relatively frequent cause of metabolic acidosis. *Lactic acidosis* is most often encountered in patients with circulatory failure caused by dehydration, hemorrhage, or endotoxic or cardiogenic shock. In these conditions the failure to supply sufficient oxygen to the tissues induces a shift from aerobic metabolism to anaerobic glycolysis and produces a lactic acidosis analogous to that occurring with severe exercise. Lactic acidosis may also occur in the absence of any obvious predisposing cause such as hypotension or hypoxemia. The onset is usually abrupt and without warning, and the acidosis is often of great severity. This syndrome of *spontaneous lactic acidosis* is seen in association with a variety of major illnesses, including diabetes mellitus, hepatic failure, subacute bacterial endocarditis, and leukemia. The etiology remains obscure. Lactic acid may also accumulate in significant quantities during *total fasting in the presence of obesity* and in *glycogen-storage disease.* Severe lactic acidosis has also been seen in association with *phenformin therapy* in diabetics and in association with the ingestion of huge doses of *isoniazid* (15 to 20 grams) taken by accident or in a suicide attempt.

Poisoning caused by the ingestion of *salicylates, methyl alcohol, ethylene glycol,* or (occasionally) *paraldehyde* leads to the accumulation of relatively strong and highly dissociated organic acids in the body fluids and to marked reductions in plasma bicarbonate concentration. The specific organic acids responsible for the acidosis in these disorders have not been adequately identified.

Metabolic acidosis can also result from the ingestion of mineral acid such as *ammonium chloride.* The release of hydrogen, as ammonium is converted by the liver to urea, makes the administration of ammonium chloride analogous to the administration of an equivalent quantity of hydrochloric acid. *Lysine hydrochloride* and *arginine hydrochloride* have the same effect on acid-base equilibrium, because they too deliver hydrochloric acid to the body fluids. Acidosis resulting from administration of acidifying salts is uncommon, however, because these agents are ordinarily administered only in conjunction with diuretic agents that tend to produce metabolic alkalosis.

Loss of Alkali as a Cause of Acidosis. Severe *diarrhea* frequently produces metabolic acidosis, because liquid stools usually contain bicarbonate in concentrations considerably higher than those in extracellular fluid. Loss of *pancreatic juice,* another highly alkaline solution, also leads to a reduction in plasma bicarbonate concentration. Acidosis of this latter origin is encountered almost exclusively in patients who have undergone prolonged drainage of a pancreatic fistula or of the upper portion of the small bowel.

Transplantation of the ureters into the sigmoid colon for the purpose of urinary diversion *(ureterosigmoidostomy)* leads to pooling of urine in the bowel, and sets into motion two physiologic events that tend to produce metabolic acidosis: movement of bicarbonate from plasma to urine in exchange for chloride directly depletes bicarbonate stores; and absorption of urinary ammonium from the bowel, with the consequent addition of hydrogen ions to the body fluids, further reduces plasma bicarbonate concentration. The more prolonged the period during which urine is in contact with the colonic mucosa, the larger will be these exchanges and the greater the compensatory increase in acid excretion that will be required. If kidney function is normal, this recycling can often be accomplished without serious disturbance in acid-base equilibrium. With impairment of kidney function, a common complication of ureterosigmoidostomy, severe acidosis is likely to occur. Acidosis can usually be avoided or minimized if the rectum is frequently emptied of urine, either voluntarily or by the use of a rectal tube.

Renal Dysfunction as a Cause of Acidosis. Inability of the diseased kidney to deal with the normal dietary load of nonvolatile acid will result in a positive acid balance and consequently in a reduction in plasma bicarbonate concentration. In *acute renal failure* the acid-base disturbance is usually transient and mild. In *chronic renal failure* metabolic acidosis is commonly present over an extended period and can be severe. In most patients with chronic renal failure the problem in acid excretion does not arise from any serious difficulty in acidifying the urine or in forming titratable acid, but is primarily the result of an inability to excrete normal quantities of ammonium. Defective renal reabsorption of bicarbonate is sometimes an additional contributory factor. Despite these abnormalities, plasma bicarbonate is usually stabilized at a level of 15 to 20 mEq per liter. This new steady state is achieved in part by the enhanced excretion of acid that accompanies the fall in plasma pH and in part by buffering of some portion of the acid load, probably by alkaline bone salts. The equilibrium is precarious, however, and any factor that increases either the intake or the production of acid (or induces a loss of alkali) is likely to precipitate a dangerous degree of metabolic acidosis.

In the foregoing discussion of renal acidosis, no mention has been made of the traditional view that retention of "acid anions" such as sulfate and phosphate is responsible for the reduction in plasma bicarbonate concentration. Such a view is inconsistent with modern concepts of physical chemistry that define an acid as any substance that donates hydrogen ions and a base as any substance that accepts hydrogen ions. In these terms substances such as sulfate and dibasic phosphate are actually weak bases rather than acids, and accumulation of these ions could not be expected to have a significant influence on either plasma bicarbonate concentration or pH. The tendency in many patients for bicarbonate to vary more or less reciprocally with the concentration of accumulated anions appears to be the fortuitous consequence of a parallel progression of glomerular and tubular damage, the reduction in filtration rate causing sulfate and phosphate retention, and the damage to tubules impairing acid excretion. It should also be realized that such a parallel change is not inevitable. In some patients, particularly those with chronic pyelonephritis, tubular capacity for acid excretion may be impaired at a time when glomerular filtration rate is only slightly reduced; under these circumstances the fall in plasma bicarbonate concentration is accompanied by an increase in chloride reabsorption that produces a state of so-called hyperchloremic acidosis.

Hyperchloremic acidosis is also seen in an uncommon form of renal dysfunction known as *renal tubular acidosis.* It is also observed in *Fanconi's syndrome,* a rare disease characterized by a multiplicity of tubular defects. These disorders are discussed in detail in Ch. 621 and 820, respectively.

Metabolic acidosis accompanied by hyperchloremia also follows the administration of *carbonic anhydrase inhibitors* such as acetazolamide. Carbonic anhydrase has an essential role in making hydrogen available for secretion by renal tubular cells, and inhibition of this enzyme impairs the cation-exchange process and reduces both sodium reabsorption and acid excretion. Carbonic anhydrase inhibitors, because of their ability to increase sodium excretion, were at one time widely used as diuretics. They proved, however, to be of relatively limited value because the modest diuresis which they produce is short lived; the prompt development of metabolic acidosis quickly impairs the effectiveness of these agents, and a rest period of several days must then be allowed to permit regeneration of bicarbonate and restoration of a normal plasma bicarbonate concentration.

Diagnosis. Hyperventilation is the only clinical finding characteristic of metabolic acidosis, and even this sign is sometimes difficult to detect. For example, patients with acidosis of long duration often appear to be breathing nearly normally at a time when measurements of Pco_2 demonstrate a striking increase in alveolar ventilation. Other clinical disturbances such as lethargy and coma are frequently seen in the patient with severe acidosis, but it is frequently difficult to decide whether these abnormalities are a manifestation of the acidosis per se or of the underlying disease, for example, diabetic acidosis or uremia.

In most cases, the history, in conjunction with the low plasma bicarbonate concentration and other routine chemical studies, will provide the basis for a tentative diagnosis of metabolic acidosis. However, since plasma bicarbonate concentration can also be reduced by primary hyperventilation (see below), a measurement of pH will be necessary in order to distinguish with certainty between respiratory alkalosis and metabolic acidosis. Subsequent measurements of pH will also serve the important function of providing a guide to effective clinical management.

Once the presence of metabolic acidosis has been documented, it is important to determine the exact cause. In many cases the cause is obvious, but in other

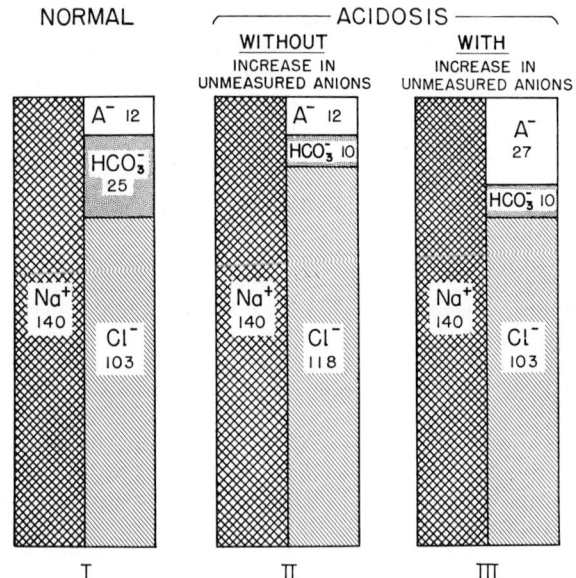

Figure 3. Composition of plasma in various forms of metabolic acidosis, with special reference to the concentration of unmeasured anions ("anion gap"). Column I shows that anions other than chloride and bicarbonate normally make up approximately 12 mEq per liter of the total anion content of plasma. Columns II and III indicate that acidosis can develop with or without an associated increase in concentration of unmeasured anions. The various causes of acidosis that will produce these patterns are listed in Table 4, and the way in which the "anion gap" can be used in differential diagnosis is discussed in the text.

instances it is obscure, and some rapid and systematic approach to differential diagnosis is invaluable. Particularly helpful is the calculation of the so-called "anion gap," or concentration of unmeasured anions, in plasma. This value, which is estimated by subtraction of the sum of chloride and bicarbonate concentrations from that of sodium, is normally about 10 to 12 mEq per liter (Fig. 3, column I), and represents negative charges contributed to plasma by ions other than chloride and bicarbonate (chiefly phosphate, sulfate, organic anions, and the anionic groups of plasma proteins).

In the patient with metabolic acidosis the reduction in bicarbonate concentration may or may not be accompanied by an increase in the "anion gap"; this distinction, which can be made on the basis of routine electrolyte measurements, immediately narrows the range of diagnostic possibilities (Table 4). If the concentration of unmeasured anions is increased (Fig. 3, column III), it can be concluded that hydrogen has been added to the body fluids with some anion other than chloride. This finding suggests a diagnosis of diabetic ketoacidosis, drug poisoning, renal failure, or lactic acidosis, and gives direction to further studies designed to identify the specific cause of the acid-base disturbance. Lactic acidosis is likely to pose the only special diagnostic problem, because in many hospitals lactate determinations are not yet routinely available. In nearly all cases, however, a tentative diagnosis of lactic acidosis can be made by exclusion of the other disorders characterized by an increased concentration of undetermined anions.

If, on the other hand, the "anion gap" is not increased (Fig. 3, column II), the reduction in bicarbonate concentration can clearly be attributed either to the accumulation of hydrogen with chloride or to a loss of bicarbonate. With the spectrum thus narrowed, it should again be relatively easy to identify the underlying disorder. A history of diarrhea, or of the ingestion of an acidifying agent such as ammonium chloride or acetazolamide, will often clarify the problem. The finding of a relatively alkaline urine and of nephrocalcinosis on roentgenographic examination of the abdomen will strongly suggest the diagnosis of renal tubular acidosis.

In some patients, of course, several causes of metabolic acidosis may be present simultaneously, and this possibility should not be overlooked. If, for example, the disappearance of ketonemia during the treatment of diabetic acidosis is not accompanied by restoration of a normal plasma bicarbonate concentration, the presence of a coexistent disorder such as lactic acidosis should be suspected.

Treatment. *General Principles.* Treatment should ordinarily be directed toward any reversible abnormality, such as ketosis or shock, which may be responsible for the acidosis. However, if the underlying disturbance is not amenable to treatment, or if acidosis is life threatening, alkali therapy will be necessary. Calculation of the amount of alkali to be administered must take into account not only the depletion of extracellular bicarbonate stores but also the magnitude of the intracellular acidosis. As mentioned earlier, a large fraction of an acid load is sequestered in cells, and restoration of normal acid-base equilibrium therefore involves repair of total body buffer stores. Estimates of alkali requirements should thus assume "distribution" of bicarbonate through a volume equivalent to 50 per cent of body weight. The calculation for full repair can be summarized by the following expression:

$$\text{(25 mEq per liter} - \text{observed plasma HCO}_3 \text{ conc.)} \times 0.5 \text{ body weight (kg)} = \text{mEq of alkali}$$

The figure of 50 per cent for the distribution of bicarbonate is only approximate, but clinical experience has demonstrated that therapy based on this assumption usually induces a rise in plasma bicarbonate concentration close to the predicted level.

In most patients with severe acidosis immediate correction of the entire alkali deficit is unnecessary; if bicarbonate concentration is increased to 15 or 20 mEq per liter, plasma pH will be returned to a safe level, and renal adjustments (or continued treatment of the underlying metabolic abnormality) can be relied upon to complete the corrective process. More rapid correction may, in fact, be undesirable. If bicarbonate concentration is quickly restored to normal or nearly normal levels, blood pH may become frankly alkaline. This apparently paradoxical behavior is the consequence of persistent hyperventilation which often maintains a state of hypocapnia for as long as one or two days after bicarbonate stores have been replenished.

During the correction of metabolic acidosis, the movement of potassium into cells in exchange for hydrogen tends to lower serum potassium concentration. In the patient with hyperkalemia and potassium intoxication this serves a useful therapeutic purpose, as discussed earlier. If, however, serum potassium concentration is normal initially, the transfer of potassium from the extracellular fluid may produce hypokalemia and signs of potassium deficiency. This sequence of events has been noted with particular frequency during the correction of diabetic ketoacidosis, but it may also occur during the

repair of other acidotic states. For this reason careful clinical observation and occasional measurements of serum potassium concentration should be carried out in the course of treatment to determine the need for replacement of potassium deficits.

Special Problems in Management. Some of the disorders that cause metabolic acidosis present particular problems in management. This discussion considers such problems as they occur in lactic acidosis, diabetic ketoacidosis, and renal acidosis; salicylate poisoning and methyl alcohol poisoning are dealt with in detail in Ch. 26.

In metabolic acidosis resulting from the accumulation of either ketoacids or lactic acid there is the potential for prompt and full correction of the bicarbonate deficit without administration of exogenous alkali. In both diabetic and lactic acidosis, the anion that has accumulated in the body fluids, if fully oxidized, will regenerate an equivalent quantity of bicarbonate, and will restore plasma bicarbonate concentration to normal. A familiar physiologic example of this behavior is seen with the lactic acidosis of exercise; after exertion is discontinued, acidosis is rapidly corrected according to the following reaction:

$$Na^+ + CH_3CH(OH)COO^- + HOH + 3O_2$$

$$\rightarrow \underbrace{Na^+ + OH^-} + \underbrace{3CO_2} + 3H_2O \qquad (4)$$

$$Na^-HCO_3^- + 2CO_2$$

In *diabetic ketoacidosis* full and rapid oxidation of the organic anion occurs promptly after the administration of adequate quantities of insulin and glucose, and it is for this reason that most patients with ketoacidosis do not require alkali therapy. On the other hand, it is reasonable to administer small quantities of alkali if, at the time of admission, the patient is found to have acidosis of life-threatening severity. Such treatment will have an important influence on pH at a time before insulin can exert a significant effect, and will lead to only an inconsequential degree of alkalosis after ketosis has been fully corrected.

In the *ketoacidosis associated with alcoholism,* the only treatment necessary is administration of glucose and isotonic saline solution. Insulin is not required, but small amounts of bicarbonate should probably be given in the early phase of treatment if the metabolic acidosis is of life-threatening proportions.

The ease with which *lactic acidosis* can be corrected depends on the cause of the metabolic abnormality. If shock is responsible for the shift to anaerobic glycolysis, transfusions or other means of restoring blood volume and blood pressure will usually correct the acid-base disturbance. Lactic acidosis of unknown cause *(spontaneous lactic acidosis)* poses a completely different problem. Specific means for remedying the defect in lactate metabolism are not available, and one must therefore rely solely on alkali therapy. Treatment is often further complicated by the unpredictable response to administration of alkali; in some cases there is little or no rise in bicarbonate concentration despite administration of an amount of bicarbonate that, by usual estimates, would be more than sufficient to restore the plasma level to normal. The explanation for this "resistance" to therapy presumably lies in continued addition of lactic acid to the body fluids during the period of treatment.

In an occasional patient, the rate of addition of lactic acid to the body fluids may be so great that as much as 400 to 500 mEq of sodium bicarbonate must be administered over a period of a few hours in order to prevent the development of lethal acidosis.

On the other hand, bicarbonate concentration will sometimes rise spontaneously as a sudden increase in the oxidation of lactate regenerates large quantities of bicarbonate. In the patient who has previously been given alkali, frank metabolic alkalosis may be the result. For these reasons the acid-base status must be monitored closely during the course of therapy.

It should be emphasized that even when the acid-base disorder is well controlled, the majority of patients with spontaneous lactic acidosis do not survive. Any therapeutic approach directed toward the acid-base disturbance alone will obviously be far from satisfactory, because it deals with effect rather than cause. In this connection it should be noted that problems analogous to those seen in spontaneous lactic acidosis were encountered in the management of diabetic acidosis during the preinsulin era; resistance to alkali therapy was common, and death frequently occurred even after plasma bicarbonate concentration was restored to normal.

Chronic *renal acidosis* poses still a different problem. There is no accumulation of organic anion from which bicarbonate can be regenerated, and irreversible renal damage ordinarily precludes correction of the underlying tubular abnormality responsible for the acid-base disturbance. For this reason, reliance must be placed on alkali therapy alone. Fortunately, in most patients with renal insufficiency the degree of metabolic acidosis is not sufficiently great to demand treatment; reductions in bicarbonate concentration to 16 to 18 mEq per liter, which occur commonly, do not appear to cause symptoms or to aggravate the uremic syndrome. If, however, acidosis becomes severe, either sodium bicarbonate or sodium citrate should be given by mouth in doses of several grams per day; plasma bicarbonate concentration need not and, in fact, probably should not be raised to normal because of the risk of precipitating tetany if hypocalcemia is present. Sometimes the ingestion of alkali precipitates nausea or vomiting, and under these circumstances it may be necessary to discontinue treatment. Sodium bicarbonate is more likely than sodium citrate to produce gastrointestinal symptoms.

If the patient has a sodium-retaining state such as congestive heart failure, it is wise to defer administration of alkali as long as possible and, if treatment must be given, to restrict dietary sodium intake sharply.

The management of *renal tubular acidosis* and that of *Fanconi's syndrome* are discussed in Ch. 621 and 820, respectively.

Choice of an Alkalinizing Agent. Two agents, *sodium bicarbonate* and *sodium lactate,* have been widely employed in patients requiring the intravenous administration of alkali. Sodium lactate is usually an effective and satisfactory means of treatment, but has the disadvantage that it depends on the intervention of oxidative processes to make bicarbonate available (Equation 4). Thus if there is a defect in lactate metabolism, as in lactic acidosis, the prompt and quantitative conversion of lactate to bicarbonate cannot be relied upon. Bicarbonate, on the other hand, is ideally suited to the treatment of metabolic acidosis, because it directly replenishes

depleted buffer stores. There thus appears no basis for the continued use of lactate in the treatment of acidotic states.

Bicarbonate can also be provided by the administration of *THAM* (tris-[hydroxymethyl]aminomethane), an organic buffer with a pK of 7.8, which reacts with carbonic acid according to the following equation:

$$THAM + H_2CO_3 \leftrightarrows THAMH^+ + HCO_3^- \quad (5)$$

It is not clear, however, that any advantage accrues from the administration of bicarbonate with, in effect, cationic THAM rather than sodium. THAM, or tris buffer, is toxic when given in large doses and furthermore may produce serious injury to tissue at the site of infusion because it must be administered as an intensely alkaline solution (pH 10). Parenthetically, it should be noted that the slight and transient reduction in carbon dioxide tension that follows an infusion of THAM is of no clinical significance in the patient with metabolic acidosis. The possible role of THAM in the treatment of *respiratory acidosis* will be discussed later in this chapter.

Metabolic Alkalosis

Metabolic alkalosis results from either an abnormal loss of acid or an excessive retention of alkali. In each case the rise in bicarbonate concentration induces a fall in hydrogen ion concentration, that is, an increase in pH.

Physiologic Considerations. As in metabolic acidosis, pH is defended to a significant extent by *tissue buffering.* In response to alkalinization of the extracellular fluid, hydrogen ions migrate from cells to extracellular space (in exchange for sodium and potassium), and thus mitigate the severity of the acid-base disturbance.

Respiratory compensation may serve as an additional mitigating factor. Diminished ventilation and a resulting rise in Pco_2 tends to restore a more normal ratio between the concentrations of carbonic acid and bicarbonate. Even with severe metabolic alkalosis, Pco_2 does not usually rise above 50 mm Hg, but values between 50 and 60 mm Hg are not rare, and in a very occasional patient Pco_2 may even reach a level of 65 mm Hg. In contrast to metabolic acidosis, however, the magnitude of the respiratory compensation is usually small, and becomes significant only when plasma bicarbonate concentration rises to 35 or 40 mEq per liter.

Renal excretion is the route for removal of excess alkali, and is thus ultimately responsible for the correction of metabolic alkalosis. Normally, the kidneys reabsorb approximately 25 mEq of bicarbonate per liter of glomerular filtrate, and when plasma concentration is elevated above this level by ingestion or infusion of alkali, the excess bicarbonate is rapidly and quantitatively excreted. Thus even a large alkali load induces only a transient alkalosis. The following theoretical example will serve to illustrate this point. If plasma bicarbonate is raised from 25 mEq per liter to 35 mEq per liter by alkali administration, approximately 10 mEq of bicarbonate will be excreted each time a liter of glomerular filtrate is formed. With a glomerular filtration rate of 180 liters per day, daily excretion would thus be 1800 mEq. Maintenance of the metabolic alkalosis would therefore require either the daily administration of 150 grams of sodium bicarbonate or the loss per day of 18 liters of gastric juice containing 0.1N HCl. Although such circumstances are rarely if ever encountered clinically, sustained elevations of plasma bicarbonate concentration do occur with considerable frequency. Indeed, plasma concentrations of 40 to 50 mEq per liter are seen even in patients who are neither receiving bicarbonate nor losing gastric juice. This finding clearly indicates that renal reabsorption of bicarbonate must be abnormally large, a conclusion borne out by the fact that the urine of the alkalotic patient typically has a pH in the acid range and contains virtually no bicarbonate. The problem confronting the physician therefore is the identification and correction of the cause of the defect in bicarbonate excretion.

Before the causes of metabolic alkalosis are considered, it seems desirable to review briefly the mechanism of bicarbonate reabsorption. Reabsorption of bicarbonate takes place by an indirect process involving the transport of sodium from the glomerular filtrate and the secretion of hydrogen into the lumen in its place. The addition of hydrogen to the filtrate converts bicarbonate to carbonic acid, but at the same time generates an equivalent quantity of bicarbonate in the renal tubular cells; the subsequent diffusion of this bicarbonate into the peritubular blood serves as the mode of bicarbonate "reabsorption." It is evident that any stimulus that increases the rate of sodium-hydrogen exchange will also increase bicarbonate reabsorption, and will sustain a metabolic alkalosis.

Pathogenesis (Table 5). A variety of clinical disturbances can produce metabolic alkalosis, but most of these can be grouped under the general headings of *losses from the upper gastrointestinal tract, diuretic therapy,* or *hyperadrenocorticism*. In each instance, as mentioned earlier, the urine is virtually free of bicarbonate, indicating that the rate of sodium-hydrogen exchange is increased. The nature of the mechanisms responsible for the enhanced bicarbonate reabsorption can perhaps best be understood by considering the renal adjustments that occur during vomiting or as the result of gastric drainage. As hydrochloric acid is lost from the stomach, bicarbonate is generated and plasma bicarbonate concentration rises, with the result that sodium formerly filtered with chloride is now filtered with bicarbonate. Because bicarbonate is not as readily reabsorbable as chloride, sodium reabsorption in the proximal tubule cannot proceed normally, and much of the newly generated bicarbonate is therefore delivered with sodium to distal exchange sites. Since the distal exchange sites, even when stimulated by a low sodium diet, cannot fully conserve this additional sodium, some sodium is initially lost into the urine with bicarbonate. A loss of potassium also occurs because a portion of the

sodium which is conserved by the distal nephron is exchanged with potassium.

As sodium loss and contraction of the extracellular volume stimulate sodium reabsorption, and as the depletion of tubular potassium stores reduces the availability of this cation for exchange, sodium-hydrogen exchange is accelerated. As a result, all further sodium and bicarbonate that escapes proximal reabsorption is conserved and there is a sustained elevation of plasma bicarbonate concentration.

These same basic mechanisms account for the metabolic alkalosis seen with diuretic therapy in the edematous patient. Diuretic agents such as mercurials, furosemide, and ethacrynic acid block sodium chloride reabsorption and deliver sodium and chloride to sodium-avid exchange sites where some fraction of the sodium is exchanged with hydrogen and potassium. Hydrogen is therefore lost into the urine with chloride, and an equivalent quantity of bicarbonate is generated. As with gastric alkalosis, two conditions are required for maintenance of the high rate of sodium-hydrogen exchange and of the state of metabolic alkalosis. First, there must be a continued intense stimulus to sodium reabsorption; second, there must be a persistent deficiency of chloride which maintains the abnormally high ratio of bicarbonate to chloride in the glomerular filtrate.

The exact sequence of events leading to the rise in bicarbonate concentration in both *primary aldosteronism* and *Cushing's syndrome* remains to be determined, but the fundamental renal mechanisms at play are almost certainly the same as those responsible for the alkalosis seen with gastrointestinal losses or diuretic therapy. The syndrome of *posthypercapneic alkalosis* is discussed later in this chapter under Respiratory Acidosis.

Diagnosis. There are no signs or symptoms specific for metabolic alkalosis. The diagnosis is usually suspected because there is a history of vomiting, because therapy with diuretics or adrenal steroids has been given, or because the patient has undergone prolonged gastric drainage. Occasionally, an elevation of bicarbonate concentration is discovered accidentally in the course of routine measurements of serum electrolyte values. An unequivocal diagnosis of metabolic alkalosis can be made only after pH is shown to be increased, but, as a practical matter, an elevated bicarbonate concentration in a patient without significant pulmonary disease can be taken as virtually diagnostic.

The finding of unexplained metabolic alkalosis will sometimes lead to the diagnosis of *Cushing's syndrome* even when there are few, if any, clinical signs of the disease. This sequence of events is most likely to occur with adrenal hyperfunction associated with extra-adrenal neoplasms. The tumor most likely to produce this syndrome is bronchogenic carcinoma.

Treatment. The treatment of metabolic alkalosis (other than that caused by an excess of adrenal steroids) consists of correction of dehydration and of the various ionic deficits. It will be recalled from the discussion of the etiology of metabolic alkalosis that the combination of chloride deficiency and increased avidity for sodium is responsible for the abnormally high rate of bicarbonate reabsorption. Correction can therefore usually be accomplished promptly by administration of sodium chloride and water. Potassium chloride is also effective in the treatment of metabolic alkalosis and is particu-

---

TABLE 5. Causes of Metabolic Alkalosis

Vomiting or gastric drainage
Diuretic therapy
   Mercurials
   Ethacrynic acid
   Thiazides
   Furosemide
Cushing's syndrome
Primary aldosteronism
Bartter's syndrome
Adrenal steroid therapy
Relief of chronic hypercapnia

larly useful in edematous states because sodium administration is usually contraindicated. Organic potassium salts, for example, "triplex" and gluconate, will not correct either alkalosis or potassium deficiency unless adequate amounts of chloride are available in the diet.

In cases of metabolic alkalosis of mild or moderate severity, the speed of correction of the acid-base disorder is not a critical factor. Slow correction over several days, achieved by the renal response to repair of the fluid and electrolyte deficit, usually represents optimal management. On occasion, however, an extreme degree of metabolic alkalosis may necessitate a more direct and intensive approach to therapy. In the Zollinger-Ellison syndrome, for example, continuous and massive losses of hydrochloric acid may elevate the plasma bicarbonate concentration to 60 mEq per liter or above. Under such circumstances, direct titration of the excess bicarbonate by the intravenous administration of hydrochloric acid, as ammonium chloride or arginine hydrochloride, may be imperative.

If ammonium chloride is used, it must be given slowly and under close observation, because if the rate of infusion exceeds the capacity of the liver to convert ammonium to urea, lethal ammonium intoxication may occur. This risk will be greatly increased if there is any element of underlying hepatic disease. Arginine hydrochloride has come into widespread favor as an alternative and safer means of providing hydrochloric acid intravenously.

In treating patients who are receiving diuretics that tend to produce metabolic alkalosis, it may at times be desirable to administer an acidifying salt by mouth. Ammonium chloride is the agent most commonly used for this purpose, and can be given without hazard if liver disease is not present. It is usually administered as an enteric-coated form, because it otherwise gives rise to unpleasant gastric symptoms. An amino acid salt such as lysine monohydrochloride is another useful vehicle for the oral provision of acid.

The management of alkalosis in the patient with hyperadrenocorticism *(Cushing's syndrome, primary aldosteronism)* poses a problem different from that encountered in more common clinical states. First, both the elevated plasma bicarbonate concentration and the hypokalemia persist despite a normal dietary intake of potassium, sodium, and chloride. Furthermore, even a large sodium chloride supplement does not correct the electrolyte abnormalities. Correction of both the alkalosis and potassium deficiency can, however, readily be accomplished over several days by administration of potassium chloride either by mouth or by vein. The explanation of this phenomenon remains obscure. Definitive treatment of the electrolyte disturbances associated with hyperadrenalism consists, of course, in the surgical removal of the offending adrenal tissue.

The alkalosis and potassium deficiency encountered in the syndrome of juxtaglomerular hyperplasia with secondary aldosteronism *(Bartter's syndrome)* has the characteristic of often being quite resistant to correction by potassium chloride. Daily supplements of several hundred milliequivalents of potassium may be necessary to hold the plasma bicarbonate concentration at normal or near-normal levels. In such instances spironolactone administration may be a useful adjunct to therapy.

Respiratory Acidosis

Respiratory acidosis results from any disturbance in ventilation that increases arterial Pco_2. An elevation of Pco_2 shifts the normal equilibrium of the bicarbonate–carbonic acid buffer system and increases the plasma hydrogen ion concentration (that is, it decreases pH). This effect on pH is mitigated, however, by a secondary *increase* in plasma bicarbonate concentration that is dependent on two mechanisms. During acute hypercapnia bicarbonate is generated by the titration of body buffers. With more prolonged elevation of Pco_2, additional bicarbonate is added to the extracellular fluid as the result of augmented renal acid excretion. A concomitant rise in the renal capacity for bicarbonate reabsorption permits conservation of the new bicarbonate and allows plasma concentration to be stabilized at an elevated level (Fig. 4). Experimental studies indicate that the complete process of renal adaptation requires several days or longer. It is apparent from these considerations that the extent of physiologic adjustment to a given degree of hypercapnia varies as a function of time and that intelligent appraisal of the acid-base changes in respiratory acidosis requires a knowledge of the duration of the ventilatory disturbance.

Pathogenesis. *Acute respiratory acidosis* occurs in a variety of clinical settings. Airway obstruction or hypoventilation resulting from central nervous system depression, neuromuscular disorders, or chest wall injuries are perhaps the most frequent causes. Acute hypercapnia may also occur as a result of decreased alveolar ventilation in disorders such as bacterial and viral pneumonias, aspiration pneumonitis, and pulmonary edema. Extreme respiratory acidosis is also often encountered in cardiopulmonary arrest.

Chronic respiratory acidosis is seen with progressive lung diseases such as emphysema or chronic bronchitis. The disturbance in gas exchange results from ventilation-perfusion mismatching and decreased effective alveolar ventilation. Pulmonary diseases characterized primarily by restrictive changes, such as pulmonary

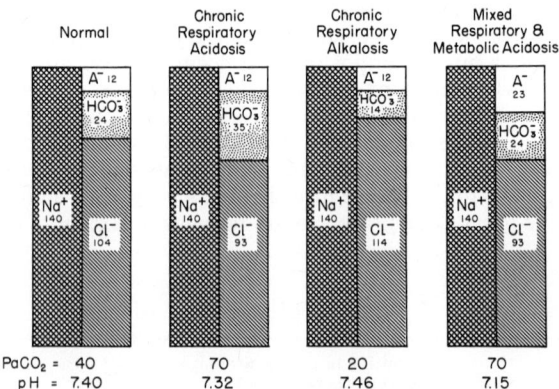

Figure 4. Composition of plasma in representative instances of chronic respiratory acid-base disorders. Note that in *chronic respiratory acidosis* plasma bicarbonate concentration is elevated, whereas in *chronic respiratory alkalosis* it is depressed; in each instance the change in bicarbonate concentration serves to minimize the effect on plasma pH of the abnormality in carbon dioxide tension. The column to the far right depicts a representative example of a *mixed respiratory and metabolic acidosis* in which the "anion gap" is elevated as the result of a disorder such as diabetic ketoacidosis or lactic acid acidosis.

Figure 5. Schematic diagram of pathways followed by the acid-base disturbances that may complicate chronic respiratory acidosis. The *solid* lines represent the bicarbonate concentrations observed during acute hypercapnia in man, and the *dashed* lines the bicarbonate concentrations seen during chronic hypercapnia in the dog. The origin of each vector has been placed arbitrarily at a point depicting physiologically complete adaption to a Pco_2 of 65 mm of mercury. Each panel is discussed in detail in the text. (Reproduced by permission of the American Journal of Medicine.)

fibrosis, do not cause hypercapnia until late in the course of the illness.

Diagnosis. The tentative diagnosis of *acute respiratory acidosis* can often be made on clinical grounds alone if there is obvious impairment of ventilation. The definitive diagnosis depends, however, on demonstration that Pco_2 is elevated and that plasma pH is reduced. These measurements are of particular importance when clinical observation cannot be relied upon to reveal an impairment of gas exchange, as, for example, in the patient who is being artificially ventilated or who is suffering from intoxication with barbiturates or other central nervous system depressants.

Chronic respiratory acidosis should be suspected in any patient with the symptoms and physical findings of severe lung disease. Classically, the diagnosis rests on the finding of an elevated Pco_2 accompanied by a low pH. However, it is now recognized that in some patients with chronic pulmonary disease hypercapnia may occur in conjunction with a normal or even a high pH. Such values of pH have sometimes been interpreted as indicating full compensation or even "overcompensation" for the respiratory acidosis, but they are, in fact, almost always attributable to a complicating metabolic alkalosis (see below). This problem in interpretation illustrates the difficulty the physician faces in deciding whether a patient with chronic pulmonary insufficiency is suffering from respiratory acidosis alone or from a mixed disorder in which metabolic components are also present.

Hypercapnia and Mixed Acid-Base Disorders. Just as a variety of illnesses, e.g., vomiting, lactic acidosis, or diabetic ketoacidosis, may produce a metabolic acid-base disturbance in the normal subject, they can do the same in the patient with hypercapnia (Fig. 4). To recognize and quantitate the magnitude of a complicating metabolic disturbance in pulmonary insufficiency, *one must have prior knowledge of the pH and bicarbonate concentration appropriate to the given degree of uncomplicated hypercapnia.* Recent observations on changes in plasma composition during exposure of normal subjects

to various degrees of acute hypercapnia have provided a background for the appraisal of the acid-base status in *acute* respiratory acidosis. As shown in Figure 5, over a range of carbon dioxide tension up to 90 mm of mercury there is only a slight rise in plasma bicarbonate concentration. From this response curve and other available information, it appears that in uncomplicated acute hypercapnia of mild or moderate severity the bicarbonate concentration should lie between 25 and 30 mEq per liter. Concentrations above 30 mEq per liter indicate the presence of a complicating metabolic alkalosis, and those below 25 mEq per liter, the presence of a complicating metabolic acidosis.

Unfortunately, physiologic observations on the response to *chronic* hypercapnia are available only in the dog, but data on patients with chronic lung disease suggest that the pattern of response which has been defined experimentally is closely similar to that which occurs clinically. Figure 5 illustrates schematically how data on the adaptation to chronic hypercapnia can be utilized in the analysis of complex acid-base disorders. This figure contains four schematic diagrams depicting, by vectors, the ways in which the acid-base status in pre-existing chronic respiratory acidosis can be deranged. For purposes of discussion, the initial Pco_2 is assumed to be 65 mm of mercury.

Figure 5a contains the vector for a superimposed metabolic alkalosis. The bicarbonate concentration lies above the level appropriate for chronic adaptation to a Pco_2 of 65 mm of mercury, and indicates that there has been a pathologic loss of acid or retention of alkali. Such deviations of bicarbonate in the alkaline direction, occurring as a result of diuretics, steroid therapy, or vomiting, could have important clinical consequences, because an inappropriately high pH may diminish respiratory drive and aggravate the pre-existing degree of hypoxemia.

Figure 5b shows the pathway of a superimposed metabolic acidosis. A mild degree of metabolic acidosis, as indicated by the solid portion of the vector, will produce bicarbonate concentrations in the zone lying between the acute and chronic response curves. With a more severe metabolic disturbance, as shown by the dotted extension of the vector, the bicarbonate concentration will be depressed to a level below even the acute response curve.

Figure 5c demonstrates the sequence that will ensue when an acute increase in P_{CO_2} is superimposed on chronic hypercapnia. This disturbance occurs in association with such common complications as pneumonia, heart failure, and excessive sedation, all of which may further compromise alveolar ventilation. As an element of *acute* hypercapnia develops, body buffers can be expected to generate only a small additional amount of bicarbonate, and, as indicated by the vector, plasma bicarbonate concentration should follow a course roughly parallel to the acute titration curve. For a period of several days—that is, until there is renal compensation appropriate to the new level of hypercapnia—the bicarbonate concentration will remain at a point below the chronic response curve. It should be noted in Figure 5 that when either mild metabolic acidosis (Fig. 5b) or acute hypercapnia (Fig. 5c) is superimposed on chronic respiratory acidosis, the bicarbonate values will lie between the acute and chronic response curves. Obviously, the acid-base parameters per se cannot be used to differentiate these two complications, and additional clinical information will be required.

Figure 5d contains the vector resulting from a recent improvement in alveolar ventilation. A sudden fall in P_{CO_2} will titrate body buffers toward normal and induce a fall in bicarbonate concentration. This titration cannot be expected, however, immediately to erase the renal component of the initial increment in extracellular bicarbonate stores. Plasma bicarbonate concentration therefore will be high in relation to the P_{CO_2}, a condition that has been termed "*posthypercapneic alkalosis*." If the diet contains sodium chloride or if the patient is given potassium chloride, the kidney will excrete the excess bicarbonate and the condition will disappear within several days. However, if chloride intake is low, metabolic alkalosis is likely to persist indefinitely. The physiologic mechanisms responsible for this behavior are the same as have already been discussed in connection with the metabolic alkalosis that results from vomiting or from diuretic therapy.

Treatment. The treatment of *acute respiratory acidosis* should be directed toward the underlying cause of the impaired ventilation. The measures required obviously will depend on the nature of the clinical problem. If, for example, alveolar gas exchange is impeded by bronchospasm, bronchodilators should be used. If inadequate ventilation is the result of a neuromuscular disturbance, artificial ventilation may be necessary.

The treatment of *chronic respiratory acidosis* should also be directed primarily toward improving alveolar ventilation, not toward the restoration of a normal pH. Bronchodilators, adrenal steroids, antimicrobials, postural drainage, and artificial ventilation all have a valuable place in therapy at one time or another in the course of the illness. The management of pulmonary insufficiency is dealt with in detail in Ch. 507, but a word of caution should be repeated here concerning the possible hazards of oxygen therapy in worsening chronic respiratory acidosis. In severe hypercapnia the sensitivity of the respiratory center to carbon dioxide may be diminished and, if this occurs, hypoxemia becomes the major stimulus to respiratory activity. If hypoxemia is then partially or totally corrected, ventilation often undergoes further serious impairment, hypercapnia becomes increasingly severe, and the patient can lapse into coma and die. Thus during oxygen therapy the patient must be watched closely to ensure that improvement in the degree of hypoxemia does not depress ventilation.

The use of an organic buffer such as THAM for the purpose of lowering P_{CO_2} (Equation 5) has little or nothing to recommend it; the rise in pH that follows the reaction of THAM with carbonic acid usually reduces minute ventilation and thus aggravates the pre-existing hypoxemia. This problem can be circumvented if the patient is given artificial ventilation, but even under such circumstances, THAM has little practical value; control of hypercapnia for more than one or two hours would require amounts of THAM far in excess of what can safely be administered.

Respiratory Alkalosis

Respiratory alkalosis results from any disturbance in ventilation that lowers arterial carbon dioxide tension. A reduction in P_{CO_2} shifts the normal equilibrium of the bicarbonate–carbonic acid buffer system and decreases the plasma hydrogen ion concentration (that is, it increases pH). This effect on pH is mitigated, however, by a secondary *decrease* in plasma bicarbonate concentration. During acute hypocapnia bicarbonate is removed from the extracellular fluid by a process of buffering in both blood and tissues, renal excretion of alkali playing only a minor role. During chronic hypocapnia there is a further reduction in bicarbonate concentration which is mediated largely if not entirely by the kidneys. If hyperventilation is sufficiently prolonged (as in persons living at high altitude), these adjustments are sufficient to restore plasma pH to normal or nearly normal levels (Fig. 4).

Pathogenesis. Probably the most common cause of respiratory alkalosis is the hyperventilation resulting from extreme anxiety. Other causes are central nervous system injury involving the respiratory center, artificial ventilation, fever, hepatic coma, and salicylate intoxication. Hypocapnia is also encountered in the early phase of pulmonary disease if a disturbance in the relation between ventilation and perfusion has produced hypoxemia and hyperventilation.

Finally, as discussed earlier, the persistence of respiratory compensation after the correction of metabolic acidosis may produce a picture indistinguishable chemically from a primary respiratory alkalosis.

Diagnosis. The presence of hyperventilation in a patient suffering from any one of the disorders considered under Pathogenesis should suggest the diagnosis of respiratory alkalosis. In many cases characteristic signs and symptoms provide evidence that one is dealing with primary hyperventilation rather than respiratory compensation for metabolic acidosis. Respiratory alkalosis produces a typical clinical syndrome in which the cardinal features are lightheadedness, numbness, tingling of the extremities, and circumoral paresthesia. In some patients, frank carpopedal spasm occurs.

The finding of an abnormally low plasma bicarbonate concentation and P_{CO_2} does not in itself distinguish between metabolic acidosis and respiratory alkalosis; the measurement of plasma pH is often vital to the differentiation. The problem of diagnosis sometimes is further complicated by the presence of a mixed acid-base disorder—that is, one with both respiratory and metabolic components. This combination occurs very often in salicylate poisoning.

Treatment. The treatment of respiratory alkalosis should be directed toward correction of the underlying disturbance responsible for the hyperventilation. In the patient with salicylism the goal is to promote removal of the offending drug. One can accomplish this purpose either by augmenting the renal excretion of salicylate (by means of urinary alkalinization and the administration of osmotic diuretics) or by hemodialysis. With injury to the central nervous system or with liver failure, the ability to correct respiratory alkalosis will be determined by the effectiveness of therapy directed toward the underlying pathologic process. The hyperventilation syndrome resulting from anxiety can often be effectively controlled if the patient rebreathes into a paper bag. If this fails, sedation will usually put an end to the acute episode. Recurrences can sometimes be prevented by reassurance and by explanation of the nature of the disorder to the patient, but if these techniques fail, psychotherapy may be indicated.

Arbus, G. S., Hebert, L. A., Levesque, P. R., Etsten, B. E., and Schwartz, W. B.: Characterization and clinical application of the "significance band" for acute respiratory alkalosis. N. Engl. J. Med., 280:117, 1969.

Brackett, N. C., Jr., Wingo, C. F., Muren, O., and Solano, J. T.: Acid-base response to chronic hypercapnia in man. N. Engl. J. Med., 280:124, 1969.

Levy, L. J., Duga, J., Girgis, M., and Gordon, E. E.: Ketoacidosis associated with alcoholism in nondiabetic subjects. Ann. Intern. Med., 78:213, 1973.

Oliva, P. B.: Lactic acidosis. Am. J. Med., 48:209, 1970.

Relman, A. S.: The acidosis of renal disease. Am. J. Med., 44:706, 1968.

Schwartz, W. B., van Ypersele de Strihou, C., and Kassirer, J. P.: Role of anions in metabolic alkalosis and potassium deficiency. N. Engl. J. Med., 279:630, 1968.

Seldin, D. W., and Rector, F. C.: The generation and maintenance of metabolic alkalosis. Kidney Int., 1:306, 1972.

DISORDERS OF CARBOHYDRATE METABOLISM

806. DIABETES MELLITUS

George F. Cahill, Jr.

General Considerations. *Diabetes mellitus* is a diagnostic term applied to a constellation of anatomic and biochemical abnormalities which share in common, as part of a syndrome, a disturbance in glucose homeostasis, which is secondary to a deficiency in the beta cells of the endocrine pancreas. This bulky and vague definition cannot be made more specific owing to the marked variability in the disorder. As was once said of syphilis, knowledge of diabetes and its sequelae touches on all areas of medicine.

The syndrome can be completely asymptomatic, or it can appear as an isolated disorder of any organ or system. Fulminant ketoacidosis, fatal unless immediately treated, may be the first sign. Often it is manifested by one of the long-term complications, such as foot ulcer, retinopathy, or proteinuria. Other pathologic states noted to be more frequent in diabetics as compared to the general population may be the clue. For example, the presenting event may be of a myocardial infarction in a young man, an unexpectedly large newborn or pruritus vulvae in the female, recurrent skin infections, or many other phenomena which at first glance appear unrelated. Diabetes mellitus is protean in its manifestations, and this variability is central to its diagnosis and treatment.

History. Descriptions of the disease were made 3000 years ago in Egypt. About 400 B.C., Charak and Susrut in India noted not only the sweetness of the urine but also the correlation between obesity and diabetes, the tendency of the disease to be passed from one generation to another through the "seed," and even two types of disease, one associated with emaciation, dehydration, polyuria, and lassitude, and the other characterized by "stout build, gluttony, obesity, and sleepiness." Near the beginning of the Christian era, the Romans Areteus and Celsus described the disease and gave it the name diabetes (= siphon) mellitus (melli = honey or sweet). Its correlation with gangrene was mentioned by the Arab, Avicenna, 1000 A.D. The sweetness of the urine was again described by Thomas Willis (1675). Dodson, 100 years later, demonstrated that the sweetness was due to sugar and suggested it was not formed de novo by the kidney, but rather that the kidney removed it from the body, a fact scientifically confirmed by the great French physiologist, Claude Bernard, in the mid-1800's.

In 1889 Von Mering and Minkowski first produced experimental diabetes by removing the dog's pancreas. Subsequently Opie (1901) noted changes in the islets of cells in the pancreas (the islets having been described by Langerhans in 1869) in humans dying with the disease. This led to attempts by many to prepare pancreatic extracts which would correct the deficiency. Active fractions were obtained by some, but not until 1921 did Banting and Best in Toronto achieve continuous success, and their discovery was rapidly applied to clinical therapy within six months of their first report. Until then, only a careful semistarvation diet with elimination of excess carbohydrate was even partially effective in prolonging life in the more insulin-deficient juvenile form of the disease, or in ameliorating the symptoms in many patients with the milder maturity-onset variety.

The Banting-Best era changed the outlook of the juvenile diabetic from certain death within two to three years to a nearly normal, albeit shortened, life expectancy. In 1936 the use of long-acting insulin was introduced, simplifying the management of the insulin-requiring diabetic. It became apparent at that time, however, that although insulin therapy prevented many of the acute metabolic problems such as ketoacidosis or those closely correlated with the hyperglycemia, e.g., pruritus vulvae or furunculosis, other sequelae such as retinitis, diabetic neuropathy, or renal glomerulosclerosis appeared in most patients with the juvenile form of the disease for two or more decades in spite of insulin therapy. These complications had been noted prior to the advent of insulin but were relatively unusual, because death from ketoacidosis or infection shortened the life of the patient before these could become manifest. Thus insulin, although a tremendous step forward, did not provide the total solution for the diabetic and his problem. Another development, although less significant than that of insulin, stemmed from the German observation during World War War II that certain sulfonamide derivatives lowered blood glucose, and subsequently Loubatières initiated trials in France which established their clinical efficacy. In 1955, oral sulfonylureas began to be generally used as hypoglycemic therapy in diabetics with the milder maturity-onset type of the disease.

Pathophysiology. Before discussing the etiology, epidemiology, pathology, and clinical aspects of diabetes, the metabolic effects of insulin in normal and abnormal states must be described. Simply, insulin is the animal's "fed" signal. After a large meal, the high circulating levels of insulin tell the body's tissues to take up and store fuel not required for immediate metabolic needs. An intermediate level of insulin resulting from a smaller intake signals the tissues to take up and store fuel less avidly. In contrast, a low level of insulin such as occurs during fasting tells the body that no fuel is entering, and the body's depots should therefore release

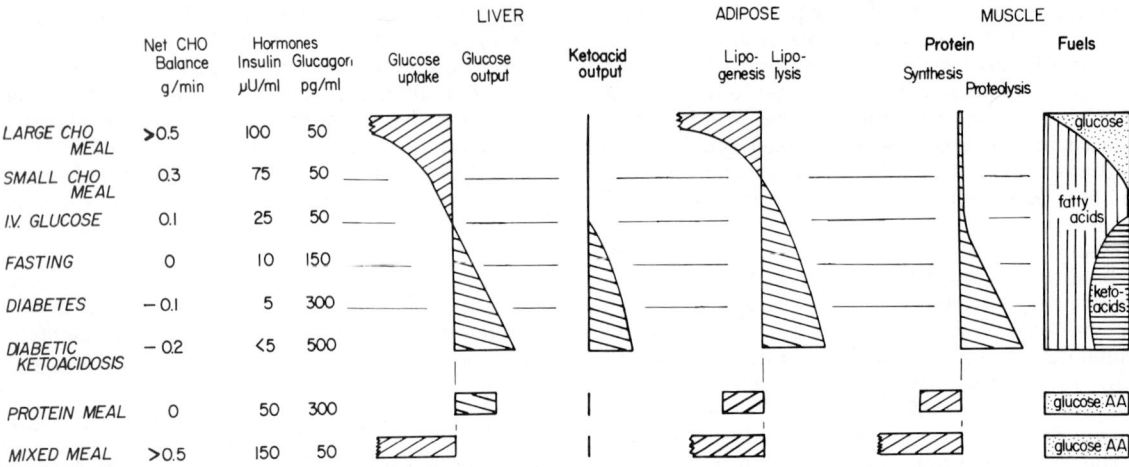

Figure 1.   Insulin and glucagon levels and varying rates of organ metabolism as a function of net carbohydrate (CHO) balance in man. The progression from a large positive carbohydrate balance after a large CHO meal to a negative balance as in ketoacidosis forms a continuum of decreasing insulin levels and increasing glucagon levels. Relative metabolic fluxes after protein and mixed meals are also shown. Since the relative contributions of glucose or amino acids (AA) to muscle fuel are not known, these are not differentiated in the scheme.

their stored nutrients back into the blood. Insulin and its normal and abnormal metabolic effects form a continuum of metabolic events (Fig. 1), ranging from those seen when there is a total or near-total lack of insulin's metabolic effects (diabetic ketoacidosis) to those which occur when there are very high levels of insulin (after a large orally ingested mixed meal in a normal individual possessing adequate pancreatic beta cell reserve).

Body Fuels.   As shown in Table 1 of Ch. 726, average man is about one fifth fat, which stores approximately a two- to three-month supply of calories. Carbohydrate reserves, in contrast, are minimal, about 70 grams (280 kcal) as liver glycogen and 200 grams (800 kcal) in muscle glycogen. Glucose in body fluids is even less, about 15 to 20 grams. Slightly more than 1 kcal per minute is required for basal metabolic needs in a normal resting adult; thus total available carbohydrate in the entire body provides less than one day's supply of fuel. Unlike carbohydrate and fat, there is no depot of protein purely for storage. All is being used for structure, for enzymes, or for other essential purposes. These points emphasize the role of fat as the primary energy storage depot in man and the minimal role of carbohydrate.

Tissue Fuel Utilization.   In contrast to storage, in which fat predominates, fuel utilization by brain and, to a lesser degree, by certain other tissues requires a constant supply of glucose. Thus glucose concentration in normal man is confined to a zone between 50 and 150 mg per 100 ml, concentrations above the minimum required by brain and below that saturating the renal reabsorption capacity. Insulin plays the dominant role in maintaining glucose in this range. All other tissues are capable of using glucose and do so when ample amounts are present in the diet, but only if insulin levels are increased. Most of these, particularly fat and muscle, do not utilize glucose when insulin levels are low, and consume instead fat in the form of free fatty acids released from adipose tissue. The capacity of the endocrine pancreas to respond rapidly and adequately to the nutritional state by its rate of insulin release is thus critical to fuel homeostasis.

FED STATE.   After eating a mixed meal, gastrointestinal digestion hydrolyzes proteins to single amino acids and carbohydrates to simple sugars, and these enter the portal blood. The liver is easily permeable to all simple sugars and related molecules, and possesses specific enzymes for the phosphorylation and subsequent metabolism of these, particularly of galactose and fructose (see Ch. 808 and 811). Glucose is phosphorylated and incorporated into glycogen or metabolized by the liver both for its own energy needs and for fat synthesis. These processes require increased insulin levels. After a large carbohydrate-containing meal, much glucose also passes through to the periphery, and the increased insulin levels accelerate the transport of glucose across the muscle and adipose cell wall (Fig. 1).

In muscle, as in liver, glucose is rapidly phosphorylated and used for glycogen synthesis. It is also metabolized to lactate or pyruvate in the cell's cytosol and then, in the presence of adequate oxygen, to carbon dioxide by the cell's mitochondria to provide the bulk of the cell's ATP and, thereby, the muscle's energy needs. In adipose tissue, the augmented glucose uptake in the presence of high insulin levels is metabolized to pyruvate, but instead of the acetyl CoA from the pyruvate being oxidized to CO_2 for energy as in muscle, most is returned to the cytosol and long chain fatty acids are synthesized. In simple terms, the original potential energy available in glucose is converted into potential energy as fatty acid, and the fatty acids are then included, three at a time esterified to glycerol, as triglyceride, into the oil vacuole in the center of the fat cell. The net effect is transformation of a poor economy type of fuel expressed per unit weight as stored in tissues (carbohydrate) into a much more efficient form (fat).

The amino acids absorbed with the meal are removed by many tissues, particularly by muscle. It has been shown that insulin augments the transfer of certain amino acids across muscle cell membrane. Insulin also, when exposed to intact muscle, increases the protein-synthetic machinery inside the cell, and the net effect is to increase muscle protein. Thus, as was shown 50 years ago, insulin is anabolic, expanding the body's protein mass.

The third component of the diet, the ingested fat or triglyceride, is partly hydrolyzed in the gut lumen, absorbed by the mucosa where the triglyceride is resynthesized, and incorporated in association with several lipoproteins into a particle, or chylomicron, which is secreted into the lymphatics between the intestinal cells and then, via the thoracic duct, carried into the general circulation. A major part of these chylomicrons is removed in adipose tissue by an enzyme located at or near the fat-cell membrane, lipoprotein lipase, and this enzyme hydrolyzes the triglyceride to yield three free fatty acids, which, in turn, enter into the fat cell, and, like the fatty acid synthesized de novo from glucose, are esterified and incorporated as triglyceride into the central oil droplet. The acceptor for the intracellular re-esterification for fatty acids is glycerol phosphate derived from glucose metabolism. A high insulin level is necessary for the activity of lipoprotein lipase as well as to provide adequate glycerol phosphate for the intracellular esterification of the fatty acids.

In summary, in the "fed" state, a high insulin level is necessary for incorporation of glucose into liver and muscle glycogen, for muscle to consume glucose for energy needs, for both liver and adipose tissue to make fatty acid from glucose, for amino acids to be incorporated into muscle protein, for circulating chylomicrons to discharge their fatty acids into adipose tissue, and for these, in turn, to be re-esterified and incorporated into the triglyceride storage droplet in the middle of the cell.

INTRAVENOUS D AND W. Between the "fed" state, described above, and the fasted state is one in which small amounts of carbohydrate are ingested or administered. This is termed intravenous dextrose and water (IV D and W), because it is frequently employed during partial starvation in patients who cannot or should not be fed by mouth. Glucose, at 100 mg per minute, closely approximates the energy needs of the brain, about one fourth to one fifth the basal caloric need of the body, and thus its administration obviates the need for hepatic glycogenolysis or gluconeogenesis. The body achieves this by the beta cells slightly increasing insulin secretion as a response to the small increase in glucose concentration. This causes circulating insulin levels to rise sufficiently to decrease the release of amino acid from muscle and to prevent hepatic glycogenolysis and gluconeogenesis. It does not increase insulin concentration enough to open up muscle cell and adipose cell membranes to glucose utilization. Thus glucose is yet excluded from most tissues and spared for brain, and, most important, the breakdown of protein to provide precursor for glucose synthesis is no longer necessary. This is the basis for the well-known "nitrogen-sparing effect of carbohydrate." It must again be emphasized that this is achieved via levels of insulin slightly above those in simple fasting, and it is the beta cell which increases the insulin level, thanks to its exquisite sensitivity to the minimal but significant increase in blood glucose concentration.

FASTED STATE. As described above, man has minimal carbohydrate reserves, and these are rapidly depleted even during overnight fast. Between meals, glucose levels can be maintained by glycogenolysis, but during more prolonged periods of caloric deprivation, hepatic gluconeogenesis must be initiated to maintain adequate glucose concentrations. This is achieved by a reduction in beta cell release of insulin as glucose falls and thereby in reduced insulin levels, the low levels initiating (1) net muscle proteolysis, (2) the release of amino acids to the liver via the circulation, and (3) gluconeogenesis from these. Subsequently the glucose so produced is consumed by brain. Other tissues, such as renal medulla, red blood cells, peripheral nerve, and, to a limited degree, skeletal muscle, also utilize glucose, but mainly to pyruvate and lactate, and these are returned to the liver for resynthesis to glucose—the so-called Cori cycle. Some of the pyruvate is transaminated to alanine, which also participates in the cycle analogous to lactate and pyruvate. Thus brain is the major tissue metabolizing glucose completely to carbon dioxide and water and requiring gluconeogenesis from amino acids.

For a better understanding of fasting, and particularly of diabetes, more detail is necessary. As insulin level falls, muscle proteolysis outweighs synthesis, certain amino acids are metabolized in the muscle, and those which are glucogenic such as alanine are released. Liver, owing to low insulin and normal or high glucagon levels, is enzymatically poised in the direction of glucose synthesis, and the alanine and other glucogenic amino acids are made into glucose. This process requires both energy and hydrogen (reducing equivalent), and these are met by fat oxidation in the liver. The long-chain fatty acids, originally derived from adipose tissue, are partially oxidized to molecules of acetyl CoA, but few of these gain access for terminal combustion via the citric acid cycle to carbon dioxide for reasons not biochemically clarified. Instead they are condensed and exported from the liver, two at a time, as the *ketone bodies, acetoacetate* and *β-hydroxybutyrate.* Thus during fasting, coupled with gluconeogenesis is the production of ketoacids (ketone bodies).

Acetoacetate and β-hydroxybutyrate are readily utilized by muscle as fuel, and their rate of production by liver in simple fasting closely approximates their utilization, with little "spilling over" into the urine. However, after more than several days of fasting, peripheral tissues diminish their utilization of ketoacids, and their total level in blood rises to approximately 6 to 8 mM. In parallel with this increase is a gradual increase in cerebrospinal fluid ketoacids, sufficient in concentration to provide the major proportion of the brain's energy needs, displacing glucose utilization accordingly. This permits less gluconeogenesis and less mobilization of muscle protein as glucogenic precursor, and survival, thanks to this sparing of body nitrogen, is dramatically prolonged. All these are a result of a continuously low level of insulin, but it must be emphasized that insulin is still playing the central feedback role in the relationship between fuel utilization and mobilization.

Diabetes. With the metabolic states briefly described, it is apparent that abnormalities in insulin secretion must result in altered fuel homeostasis. If insulin secretion cannot be rapidly increased after ingestion of a meal, the rate of intestinal absorption (an insulin-independent process for carbohydrate, amino acid, and fat) will greatly surpass the peripheral uptake of all fuels, resulting in alimentary hyperglycemia, hyperaminoacidemia, and hyperlipemia. This is most easily tested by a simple glucose meal (glucose tolerance), whereby the blood level of glucose given orally or intravenously is followed over time. If insulin release is inadequate, the glucose level is high and remains higher for a longer time owing to failure of the body to receive an adequate "fed" signal. If the insulin deficiency is more marked and is insufficient to facilitate glucose ingress into muscle and adipose cells or glucose incorporation into liver glycogen, but yet enough to depress hepatic ketogenesis and gluconeogenesis, the glucose load will stay in the circulation. Glucose concentration then surpasses the renal threshold and spills into the urine, and dehydration, hypovolemia, and severe hyperglycemia ensue, possibly leading to hyperosmolar coma.

If the insulin deficiency is severe, irrespective of glucose concentration, peripheral amino acid release from muscle protein will provide the liver with more and more glucogenic substrate, and gluconeogenesis and ketogenesis will be rapidly increased. As in prolonged starvation, there is also a decreased peripheral ketoacid utilization, levels of β-hydroxybutyrate and acetoacetate rise quickly in the body, and life-threatening ketoacidosis occurs in addition to the marked hyperglycemia, dehydration, and volume deficiency.

Endocrine Pancreas. The entire carbohydrate, fat, protein, and lipid disorder, as seen in diabetic ketoacidosis, is precisely mimicked by acute pancreatectomy, by chemical destruction of the beta cells with agents such as alloxan or streptozotocin, or by administration of antibody to insulin. Subtotal destruction or removal of beta cells results in less severe degrees of diabetes. Likewise, postmortem examination of human pancreas has shown either total absence of beta cells in juvenile diabetics after several years of the disease or minimal reductions in number with variable nonspecific morphologic changes in the older, maturity-onset type of diabetic.

Little is known of the natural history of the beta cell. It appears early in the human embryo and continues to divide slowly through life. In states in which there is resistance to insulin's effects, beta cell hyperplasia may be noted. Why the diabetic cannot generate more beta cells to replace his deficiency is unknown, and this deficiency as well as a temporal delay in insulin release by the remaining cells may possibly be the primary underlying defect.

The beta cell responds both to the ambient concentration of *glucose* and to changes in glucose concentration by insulin release. This appears to be in two phases, one occurring almost immediately after the increase in glucose concentration and peaking in five to ten minutes, and a later phase occurring 15 to 30 minutes later and persisting as long as the glucose concentration remains elevated. Glucose taken by mouth elicits a greater insulin release than glucose infused parenterally; this is due to a hormonal effect in the gut during carbohydrate absorption which sensitizes the beta cells to release even more insulin in response to changes in glucose concentration. This gut hormone(s) has yet to be identified, but is probably similar to secretin; it also cross-reacts with some nonspecific antibodies to glucagon.

Amino acids also can provoke insulin release. Of particular interest are leucine and arginine, the former being an essential branched-chain amino acid which, in certain children, can induce excessive insulin release, causing symptomatic hypoglycemia (see Ch. 807). Arginine, as well as several other amino acids, also induces insulin release, and its administration has been used as one of a battery of research tests for assessing beta cell function. Eating a protein meal results in an apparently greater insulin release than one might expect from the constituent amino acids. This has been explained by the capacity of CCK-pancreozymin, the gut hormone released after protein ingestion to stimulate excessive pancreatic secretion, to affect also the endocrine pancreas by promoting insulin release from the beta cells (as well as glucagon from the alpha cells).

Other factors known to stimulate insulin release are the *sulfonylurea class of oral antidiabetic agents,* stimulation of parasympathetic nerves leading to the pancreas, and, to a lesser degree, elevated concentrations of fatty acids, ketoacids, and the potassium ion. The relative importance of innervation and these last-named factors appears to be less than that of glucose and amino acids in man. In other animals, such as the ruminants, ketoacids and related compounds are very active insulin secretagogues.

INSULIN.   Insulin is synthesized inside the beta cell as a single chain proinsulin of 86 amino acids which then folds back on itself; closure of sulfur bridges then follows (Fig. 2). As shown by Steiner in the mid-1960's, the "connecting peptide" is then split out, leaving two amino acid chains of 31 and 20 amino acids connected

Figure 2.   Probable sequence of human proinsulin, containing 86 amino acids in a single chain folded back on itself, with closure of 2 sulfhydryl bridges between the beginning and end as well as a bridge between amino acids 71 and 76. When the C-peptide (connecting peptide) is split out in the beta cell as the insulin is being collected into storage granules, the A and B chains are left connected by the sulfhydryl bridges. The eventual human A chain has 21 amino acids and the B chain 30 amino acids. The A-B chain insulin differs from pig insulin by a threonine (Thr) instead of an alanine at the end of the B chain. Many more differences exist in the connecting peptides between species; hence the higher antigenicity of the impure insulins. (Illustration courtesy of Dr. D. Steiner.)

by sulfur bridges. The insulin and connecting peptide are packaged together into granules; when the beta cell is stimulated to release insulin, the granules are brought to the surface of the cell, and insulin is discharged with the metabolically inert connecting peptide into the adjacent capillary. Normally a small amount of proinsulin is also released, but this hormone is either inactive or much less active than insulin itself. In abnormal states such as islet cell tumor or in diabetes, the proportion of proinsulin may be increased, a circumstance which has been helpful in diagnosis.

Insulin in blood is unbound. Approximately half is removed as it passes through liver, and most of the remainder is removed by the kidney, being small enough (5734 daltons) to be filtered and catabolized by the tubules on resorption. Thus insulin has a short half-life, approximately ten minutes. All data suggest that changes in its concentration are regulated by alterations in beta cell secretion, not by alterations in removal rates.

Insulin, like other peptide hormones, binds to specific receptors on cell membranes and elicits the release of one or more second messengers, which in turn alter enzyme levels and activities inside the cell. In muscle and adipose tissue, there is also a rapid acceleration of glucose transport across the cell wall after exposure to insulin, as well as augmented transport of certain amino acids and potassium into the cell and change in the membrane electrical potential. Which of these are primary insulin effects and which are secondary to one or more intracellular messengers remain to be established. In certain tissues, levels of cyclic AMP are reduced by insulin, but the numerous intracellular effects cannot be explained solely by the reduced level of cyclic AMP.

GLUCAGON. Glucagon is composed of a single strand of 29 amino acids and is secreted by the alpha cells in the islets. Its primary effect is to increase the activity of adenylcyclase in liver by reacting with sites on the liver cell membrane, and thereby to increase hepatic cyclic AMP. This in turn initiates activation of glycogen breakdown, by increasing the activity of the glycogen phosphorylase system and by decreasing the activity of the glycogen synthetase system (see Ch. 809). It also increases gluconeogenesis in the liver, again probably because of its effect on adenyl cyclase activity. The precise role of glucagon in man is as yet unclear, but it is probably important in the disposition of the amino acids in a pure protein meal. Its release is prompted by certain amino acids such as arginine and alanine and also by enteric hormones such as CCK-pancreozymin. Its level also increases in many states of stress, such as trauma, hypoglycemia, infection, exercise, and starvation. Unger has shown that at a given glucose concentration it is increased in diabetics as compared to nondiabetics, suggesting either a direct effect of insulin on the alpha cell or a primary alpha cell abnormality. Since destruction of the total pancreas or of beta cells specifically or removal of circulating insulin by administration of antibody in laboratory animals can produce the full-blown diabetic state, the role of glucagon, if any, may be minimal and secondary to that of insulin. In milder degrees of diabetes, its relatively increased level as compared to that of normals may play a role, but this has yet to be characterized.

Etiology. As known to the Hindis centuries ago, dia-

betes is familial. Environment also plays a large role, particularly overnutrition, as evidenced by the marked decrease in incidence of the disease in Europe during World War II. The geneticist's best tool, a comparison of identical versus fraternal twins, has been used several times, and a much higher concordance rate has been noted in identical twins, indicating an important genetic component. As mentioned before, the disease is a continuum ranging from a total or near total absence of insulin, resulting in death in two or three days in diabetic ketoacidosis, to a slightly elevated glucose level after a glucose load as compared to the disposition of a similar glucose load in a "normal" population. Terms used for either end of the spectrum include "*juvenile-onset*" or "*ketosis-prone*" for the markedly insulin-deficient, and *maturity-onset* "*mild*" or "*late-onset*" for the individual whose insulin release after a challenge is insufficient to effect normal glucose tolerance. Although most children exhibit the "juvenile-onset" form of diabetes, they can develop a very mild or "maturity-onset" type of the disease, and this latter predisposition, often associated with obesity, appears to be marked in certain families. Likewise, four fifths or more of all diabetics develop the "maturity-onset" type of the disease in later life and usually are overweight at diagnosis. Ketoacidosis is infrequent in this older-age-onset group, but does occur. Nonhereditary diabetes, such as that secondary to pancreatitis, should be considered when ketoacidosis develops early in diabetes in this older age group. Curiously, subjects in the eighth or ninth decade of life may also develop the juvenile type of diabetes, but this is infrequent.

Paradoxically, concordance for diabetes is much greater in identical twins developing the disease in middle or later life, approaching 90 to 100 per cent when tested by glucose tolerance. In the juvenile-onset type of diabetes, concordance, which occurs in approximately half of twin pairs, is within one or two years of the diagnosis in the first twin. If the second twin does not develop it within a few years, he frequently never will, suggesting juvenile-type diabetes to be less familial than the adult-onset type and possibly more influenced by environment—exactly the reverse of other inherited diseases, in which the more severe form appears to be more transmissible through heredity. Another strong possibility is that there are different forms of diabetes with a different genetic basis.

It has been suggested that juvenile diabetes may be due to viral destruction of beta cells, and British studies have shown juvenile diabetes to occur in clusters associated with certain common viral epidemics (e.g., group B, coxsackievirus). One still must note the greater prevalence of both types of diabetes in a given kindred as compared to the population as a whole, and this might be explained by a lesser capacity for beta cells to divide within the diabetic kindred. Although a single autosomal recessive was suggested at one time, a double dose being necessary for phenotypic expression, the inheritance is certainly polygenic. No difference in sex that cannot be attributed to the tendency of middle-aged females to be more obese in certain cultures has been consistently observed.

Siperstein has questioned whether a beta cell abnormality is the primary etiologic event, and his studies have shown offspring of two diabetic parents to possess significant thickening of the capillary basement membrane as shown by electron microscopic examination of tissues obtained by biopsy of the quadriceps muscle. Also it has been noted that fibroblasts of diabetic subjects grow less well in tissue culture, suggesting a more ubiquitous lesion in cell replication. Williamson has attributed Siperstein's observations simply to a progressive age-related thickening of the basement membrane. The subject remains controversial, but the high association with degenerative vascular disease suggests some underlying generalized tissue abnormality.

The high incidence of diabetes noted in many other hereditary diseases, such as Turner's and Werner's syndromes, and in various muscular disorders, such as amyotrophic lateral sclerosis, suggests the beta cell to be uniquely sensitive to inherent defects in metabolism, again possibly because of defective replication. Surprisingly, the body's most rapidly replicating cells, those in the gut mucosa and the hematopoietic cells, do not appear to be affected by such a replicative lesion in diabetic kindreds as would be true if this were fundamental in the diabetic pathogenesis. However, certain hematologic disorders such as Fanconi's anemia have a very high prevalence of diabetes both in affected subjects and in relatives. In certain multiple endocrine deficiencies an autoimmune process has been involved, but for other forms of diabetes, autoimmunity has not been adequately demonstrated.

Diagnosis.   The sine qua non for diagnosis is demonstration of the inability of a given subject to dispose appropriately of a glucose load, as evidence of a relative or absolute decrease in insulin release and circulating concentration. This legalistic description is, however, markedly qualified. Anxiety, prior carbohydrate deprivation, old age, acute illness, infection, delayed gastric emptying, certain pharmacologic agents,

hypokalemia, and many other factors can all result in abnormal glucose tolerance. A normal unstressed subject, having had adequate amounts of dietary carbohydrate (over 200 grams per day for several days), on ingesting 75 or 100 grams of glucose should have a venous whole blood glucose level below 110 mg per 100 ml before glucose ingestion, under 160 mg per 100 ml at one hour, and below 120 mg per 100 ml at two hours (Fig. 3). Capillary levels (mainly arterial) and levels in plasma (caused by the volume occupied by hemoglobin and red cell stroma) will be proportionally higher, and appropriate corrections should be made. The glucose is given as either pure glucose or commercially available flavored dextrins (i.e., Glucola), which are rapidly hydrolyzed to free glucose in the gut and then absorbed. The glucose may also be given intravenously, 0.5 gram per kilogram, and blood levels determined at several ten-minute intervals up to one hour after its rapid infusion. The per cent disappearance, calculated from half-life ($t^{1/2}$) of blood glucose (e.g., the minutes elapsed when glucose levels decrease from 300 to 150 mg per 100 ml, as plotted semilogarithmically) is defined as:

$$K \left(\frac{\text{per cent disappearance}}{\text{minute}} \right) = \frac{0.69}{t^{1/2} \text{ minutes}} \times 100$$

and should normally be greater than unity. This test has been utilized mainly as a research tool, because it bypasses the gut factor effect elicited by oral glucose. It has been found, however, to be clinically less discriminant than the oral glucose tolerance test.

Rarely, one is presented with a patient with classic diabetic retinopathy or nephropathy but a normal fasting glucose level, and even more rarely the same patient might have a normal glucose tolerance. Is this a diabetic? Probably yes, so the strict adherence to the legalistic glucose tolerance as being pathognomonic is not warranted. It is highly probable that this subject had had glucose intolerance at one time. This introduces a problem shared by most other diseases of the endocrine system, namely their fluctuating nature and capacity to remit and relapse without known cause.

Natural History and Definitions.   The disease may present as fulminant diabetic ketoacidosis at any age, but most frequently in childhood or adolescence. It is common for the disease then to remit, little or no insulin being required for several weeks to months, and then to recur as the remission ends. Glucose tolerance through the remission is usually abnormal, but occasionally it may even be normal. Also, the remission may last as long as one or two years, and very rarely the diabetes may not recur. Once the diabetes has recurred in the young individual, it may be relatively easy to manage with a simple morning injection of intermediate-duration insulin, but after several years the glucose levels become more difficult to manage, suggesting termination of all endogenous insulin release. Rubenstein and Steiner have shown connecting peptide (Fig. 2) to be present in plasma, suggesting that some endogenous insulin synthesis and secretion do persist through the early phases of the disease. The diabetes then becomes labile or "brittle" after endogenous insulin secretion ceases and requires more careful matching of diet and insulin, the latter usually necessary twice ("split-dose") instead of once a day.

In the maturity-onset type of diabetic, the insulin

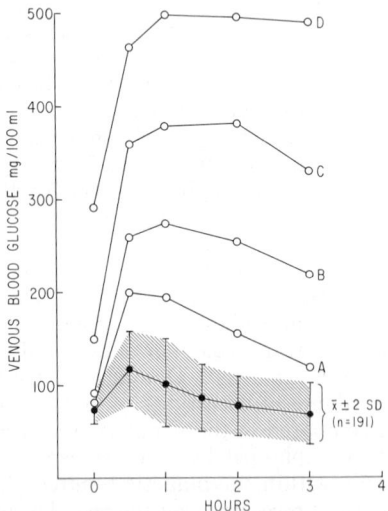

Figure 3. Glucose tolerance tests in four diabetics (A-D) and range of values in 191 healthy controls. Shaded area shows range of two standard deviations in the normal population. Diabetics A and B have sufficient insulin for fasting glucose homeostasis, but an inability to increase insulin release appropriately. Diabetic C has fasting hyperglycemia and marked glucose intolerance. The late fall-off at the end of the curve may be due mainly to glucose loss in urine. Subject D, in whom the tolerance test was clinically unnecessary, is probably almost totally lacking in insulin, and, with this degree of fasting hyperglycemia, is a candidate for the development of ketoacidosis. In such a subject, glucose in the urine may even surpass the load given for the tolerance itself. (Unpublished data of R. Gleason and J. S. Soeldner.)

Figure 4. Glucose and insulin levels in five groups of subjects during 16 hours of the day. The glucose levels are lumped together into nondiabetics and diabetics. The diabetics were specifically selected to be those with a significant degree of fasting hyperglycemia. The obese diabetics show the marked hyperinsulinemia necessary to overcome their generalized resistance to insulin. The estimated peripheral insulin secretion rate in the obese diabetic is calculated as 114 units per day, almost four times that of the normal nonobese.

The obese diabetic has also a greater insulin secretion than does the normal, 46 units per day. The thin adult diabetic does less well than the normal, and the juvenile diabetic shows an almost total failure to increase the very meager insulin level after changes in fuel loads. (Data of S. Genuth.)

deficiency is less severe and may be evidenced only by glucose intolerance of varying degrees. Obesity, for as yet unexplained reasons, requires a higher insulin concentration and therefore a greater rate of insulin release for insulin to exert its metabolic effects (Fig. 4). Binding of insulin to various cells taken from experimentally obese animals has been shown to be decreased, as have the metabolic effects of insulin. Thus obesity unmasks diabetes (as do pregnancy and other endocrine disturbances associated with peripheral resistance to insulin). If the patient loses weight and normal glucose tolerance ensues, the patient is spoken of as a latent diabetic. This same term is applied to a mother with normal glucose tolerance post partum but a diabetic tolerance when pregnant. A "chemical diabetic" is one who is also asymptomatic at the time but has abnormal glucose tolerance or even an elevated fasting blood glucose value.

The maturity-onset type of diabetic, as just mentioned, may lose the glucose abnormality with weight loss, or, occasionally, may even lose it without weight loss by dietary therapy alone, meaning carbohydrate restriction. Conversely, the glucose intolerance may progress, with initial worsening of the glucose tolerance itself, followed by insufficient insulin to maintain normal fasting glucose concentrations, with exogenous insulin required to prevent ketoacidosis. Generally, however, the diabetes tends to remain at the severity at which the original diagnosis was made.

Incidence and Prevalence. Surveys in the United States have shown 1 to 2 per cent of the population to have documented diabetes and a similar number to have abnormal glucose tolerance without having been previously diagnosed. The "softness" of this statistic is grossly apparent in view of the "softness" of the criteria for diagnosis. In Michigan, 1 in 600 school children requires insulin; this is probably a good statistic for juvenile diabetes, but there are probably additional children with milder maturity-onset diabetes undiagnosed. In the total diabetic population, the juvenile type of diabetes comprises approximately 10 per cent, but again this is not a firm statistic, because many patients

who have insulin-requiring diabetes do not go into ketoacidosis without insulin but stabilize at a high glucose concentration, thanks to deficient yet significant endogenous insulin production. Thus the disease is a continuum between total insulin lack and the normal, and the characterization of the normal is made arbitrarily. With advanced age, a greater proportion of the population, as high as 40 to 60 per cent in the ninth decade, has abnormal glucose tolerance; so again the definition is arbitrary.

There are diverse cultural and racial differences in incidence and prevalence. Diabetes is rare in the Eskimo; in certain American Indians such as the Pima in Arizona, up to 50 per cent of the population develop diabetes. Similar high rates are observed in Asian Indians who have moved to South Africa and adopted a sedentary, high-caloric style of life. Ketoacidosis is less frequent to absent in these and in blacks in Africa or in the Oriental races, particularly homeland Japanese. The extent to which these differences are genetic on the one hand or environmental or nutritional on the other is under study.

Clinical Manifestations. The classic juvenile diabetic is a child with one or two weeks or longer of progressive polydipsia and polyuria, weight loss, lassitude, blurred vision, leg cramps, inattentiveness at school, irritability, and frequently a craving for sweet beverages. Such a child, if diabetes is undiagnosed, develops mild and then severe nausea, followed by vomiting, dehydration, stupor, coma, and finally death. The progression may be more rapid, particularly in infants or small children, or it may continue as the three "polys," polydipsia, polyuria, and polyphagia, for from weeks to months, with marked weight loss even to the point of emaciation. These latter subjects apparently still have some endogenous insulin production. Thus the initial presentation of the juvenile diabetic may be due to (1) ketoacidosis; (2) marked hyperglycemia, dehydration, and collapse without ketoacidosis, namely hyperosmolar coma; or (3) an intermediate between these two. Diabetic ketoacidosis always has some degree of hyperosmolarity.

If the insulin deficiency is less marked but fasting hyperglycemia and glucosuria are present, the patient may not be aware of the insidious onset of polydipsia and polyuria and may be brought to the physician's attention by superimposed infection. Females with glycosuria are particularly susceptible to bacterial and fungal infections of the vulva and vagina, with marked pruritus, excoriation, and bad odor. The hyperglycemia may predispose the subject to other soft tissue infection such as cellulitis, furunculosis, gingival abscess, otitis media, or paronychia. There is also a predisposition to other internal infective processes, such as appendicitis and cholecystitis, and particularly to pulmonary tuberculosis or systemic mycotic infections.

The patient with the milder, maturity-onset type of disease may be asymptomatic, and the diagnosis may be made by finding glycosuria or hyperglycemia or by glucose intolerance. The predisposition of diabetes to premature atherosclerosis frequently provokes medical attention, and the diabetes is then recognized. Myocardial infarction in a young man or, particularly, a woman in the reproductive age, premature peripheral vascular insufficiency, or occasionally diabetic neuropathy or nephropathy may be the first manifestation.

Eye. The ocular manifestations of diabetes are numerous. Hyperglycemia increases glucose concentration in the lens and optic humors, resulting in blurring of vision, weakness of accommodation, and myopia. Very rarely the lens itself may become opacified (the metabolic or *"snowflake" cataract*) presumably owing to sorbitol formation and accumulation; this may disappear after correction of the hyperglycemia. Another manifestation of acute or subacute diabetes is *lipemia retinalis,* the retinal arteries and veins appearing as if they contain cream of tomato soup rather than demonstrating their usual dark red color. Treatment of these conditions is directed to correction of the hyperglycemia (and hyperlipidemia) with appropriate therapy, namely insulin and diet, and other specific agents according to the type of hyperlipidemia.

More serious and much more prevalent are the *microvascular complications* of the chronic diabetic state. For example, about one sixth of all cases of acquired blindness are due to *diabetic retinopathy.* Approximately two thirds of diabetics with disease for 15 years and over 90 per cent of those with disease for three or four decades have evidence of retinopathy. It most often appears after ten years of known diabetes as an increased tortuosity and widening of the vessels, with scattered, barely visible dots caused by microaneurysms, usually about the macula or about the periphery of the temporal area. Later, small punctate hemorrhages may appear with "waxy" exudates which may either persist or disappear after months to years, leaving a small whitish scar, but with loss of visual elements in that area. Increased capillary permeability leads to extravasation of protein seen as fluffy "cotton-wool" exudates, which also are variable, appearing and disappearing with time.

In the next phase, small new vessels may appear over the disc and along the nerves, and these may then grow into the vitreous. More ominous, they frequently rupture with large hemorrhages and, depending on whether the macular area is involved, with either loss of areas of vision or transient total blindness (Fig. 5). They usually undergo moderate to marked resorption with return of some vision until the next hemorrhage. However, these newly formed vessels, part of the syndrome of retinitis proliferans, usually portend an ominous prognosis unless treated. If there is hemorrhage anteriorly into the vitreous, resorption may be associated with contraction and tearing and detachment of the retina. However, the retinitis may arrest or even regress at any stage without known cause. More commonly, however, proliferating vessels usually lead to legal blindness in the affected eye within four to six years.

The microvascular disease is not limited to the retinal vessels but may also occur in the ciliary body and iris (*rubeosis iridis*), leading to occlusion of the outflow tract, resulting in open-angle neovascular glaucoma, or to hemorrhagic glaucoma after rupture of a vessel.

The pathogenesis of the retinal microangiopathy, as described by Kuwabara and Cogan, is a loss of the pericytes (mural cells) about the capillaries, followed by thickening and weakening of the wall forming the microaneurysm which, in turn, may rupture to cause the visible punctate hemorrhage. In addition shunt vessels surrounded by areas of capillary closure appear, and it is in these that microaneurysms frequently appear. Another theory postulates small capillary thromboses, vessel distention, rupture, and hemorrhage.

The Joslin Clinic staff and many other specialists have stressed the better visual prognosis in patients who control their diabetes with optimal insulin-carbohydrate homeostasis than in patients taking poorer care of their disease, especially for the first ten years of the disease. Rigid prospective studies on this point are not available, but the rapid acceleration of retinopathy noted in the diabetic decompensation with pregnancy or with infection supports the hypothesis. It is rare to see a patient with normal fundi who has had

---

Figure 5.   *A,* Vitreous and preretinal hemorrhage from the disc area secondary to disc neovascularization.

B, Fibrous band resulting from going into a quiescent stage of retinopathy one year after slide *A* was taken. Patient maintained quiescent stage for eight years until he died a cardiac death.

C, Preretinal hemorrhages in region of macula which also has exudates and superficial hemorrhages. Note boat-shaped dependency type of hemorrhage.

D, Preretinal hemorrhage at site of frond of neovascularization. Note the new vessel fan underneath the boat-shaped preretinal hemorrhage. It is these new vessels which rupture spontaneously or with minimal stress.

E, Extensive fan of new vessels with fibrous network elevated forward into vitreous. Feeding vessels come from multiple arteries and veins at the retinal level, the entire process being analogous to an angioma.

F, Characteristic waxy exudates in macular zone accounting for decrease in vision, apparently due to incompetent capillaries and leaking from central areas of rings of waxy exudates where the red blotches are noted.

G, Fluorescein angiography in a diabetic, showing some very fine microaneurysms and some tiny areas of capillary closure but with good parafoveal network of vessels and 20/20 vision. These are early changes of diabetic retinopathy probably not seen on ophthalmoscopy. (Courtesy of Dr. L. Aiello.)

Figure 5.   *See opposite page for legend.*

several episodes of ketoacidosis after 15 to 20 years of the disease; those with normal fundi after many years of the disease usually, but again not always, tend to be the "better controlled."

Treatment of the microangiopathy, if we adhere to the "control" hypothesis, calls for optimal treatment of the diabetes itself through adjustment of insulin and diet from the earliest recognition of the disease. Since many conscientious patients, even with the best effort, still develop retinopathy, numerous therapies, including various vitamins, dietary alterations, and hormones, have been used without effect.

An observation that a patient with diabetic retinopathy underwent remission after spontaneous pituitary necrosis prompted a wave of *pituitary ablative procedures* in the 1960's, including total surgical hypophysectomy, surgical section of the pituitary stalk, proton bombardment of the pituitary, transsphenoidal implantation of yttrium-90, freezing of the pituitary, and others, and a significant delay of the retinopathy or even improvement was observed in many. Many patients with hormonal evidence of total pituitary destruction nevertheless progressed, and a few others, in whom the pituitary was not destroyed, improved. The procedure has since been all but abandoned. It is still not clear why the procedure provided some benefit to the average patient; most authorities attribute its effect to reduction or removal of growth hormone.

Direct therapy of the fundus, using photocoagulation, has been a major advance. Patients with unilateral retinitis pigmentosa and diabetes were observed to have less diabetic retinopathy in the eye with the previous retinitis. This has prompted Aiello and Beetham and others to use the ruby laser to apply numerous scattered destructive lesions to the retina as the light is absorbed by the pigment layer, heating and coagulating the adjacent elements. These scattered lesions result in no field defect, and patients with early diabetic neovascularization have had progression of the disease halted or delayed, probably secondary to a diminished vascular need because of diminished tissue in the area treated. Similar results were previously obtained by Wetzig and others, using the polychromatic light of the xenon arc lamp. More recently a green source, the argon laser, has been used to specifically coagulate lesions in the vessels themselves, such as bleeding points, microaneurysms, or the newly forming vessels near or overlying the optic disc; optimal therapy involves treatment of both the specific lesions and the scattered destructive lesions described above.

The eye is occasionally the site of nerve lesions, most frequently the third, resulting in diplopia and strabismus. This disturbing lesion, probably caused by a small vascular infarction, may be preceded by severe pain; it usually reverses itself within several months. The pupil reaction, however, is maintained, because the infarct is usually with the nutrient vessels of the nerve, whereas the pupillary fibers on the outside of the nerve remain nourished by adjacent vessels. Finally, diabetics appear to be more susceptible to the common senile cataract, which appears at an earlier chronologic age and matures more rapidly than usual, and, as mentioned elsewhere, to infections of the eye. Corneal lesions are more pernicious than similar injuries in nondiabetics.

Kidney. The kidney is also a focal point for diabetes and its complications. The predisposition to infection makes pyelonephritis fairly frequent and serious, and the more severe renal infections may lead to papillary necrosis or perinephric abscess, grave conditions almost unique to the diabetic. For this reason urinary tract instrumentation such as catheterization should be avoided in a diabetic unless absolutely necessary, because subsequent infection is so often observed.

The main problem, however, is the *microangiopathy*. Proteinuria appears in two thirds of patients with diabetes for 20 years and portends progressive renal involvement, with uremia developing in the average patient in five years. Forty per cent of juvenile-type diabetics die from renal failure. Biopsies of kidneys in newly discovered diabetics by Lundbaek's group in Denmark have shown no demonstrable lesion, but after several years there is increased thickness of the capillary basement membrane and accumulation of material in the mesangial area as seen by the electron microscope, which then may become visible by standard light microscopy after 10 to 15 years. In some unfortunate patients, the nephropathy may be more rapid, occasionally leading to renal failure after only nine to ten years of diabetes. In a very fortunate few, and these appear to be those patients in whom the diabetes has been best controlled by insulin and diet, the signs or symptoms of nephropathy may not develop even after 50 years of the disease. With the progressive thickening and folding of the vascular basement membrane, composed of glycoprotein, as well as the mesangial accumulation of similar material, the lesion is seen as (1) a *nodular glomerulosclerosis* as described by Kimmelstiel and Wilson over 30 years ago, (2) a diffuse accumulation of glycoprotein in all areas of the glomerulus, or (3) a mixture of the two. Paradoxically, the thickened basement membrane is more permeable to macromolecules; hence the proteinuria. As the lesion progresses, entire glomeruli may become occluded, with loss of renal function, uremia, and death. Added to these microvascular lesions are the accelerated atherosclerosis and high frequency of hypertension and arteriolar nephrosclerosis in diabetics with nephropathy.

Beisswenger and Spiro have shown the accumulated material to be a specific complex glycoprotein and to contain an excess of hydroxylysine to which is attached a glucose-galactose disaccharide. Insulin-deficient laboratory animals show an increased activity in the enzymes involved in formation of this material, but the precise biochemical correlation between it and the diabetes awaits clarification. Transplantation of normal kidneys in experimentally diabetic animals has shown similar lesions to appear and to disappear with retransplantation back into nondiabetic animals.

As with retinopathy, treatment of diabetic nephropathy is directed to the treatment of the diabetes itself. Infection in the genitourinary system in particular, as well as any infection elsewhere with diabetic decompensation, tends to accelerate the nephropathy as well as the retinopathy. With renal failure, chronic dialysis and/or transplantation are the only direct forms of therapy; however, the generalized atherosclerosis makes vascular shunts difficult to create and maintain, and the diabetic's susceptibility to infection creates an even greater problem. Added to this, immunosuppression for transplantation poses such a risk that only subjects with advanced renal failure but otherwise in good condition should be considered as candidates. Basically, therefore, the treatment of diabetic nephropathy is no different from that of renal failure resulting from chronic glomerulonephritis, polycystic kidneys, or other causes; such treatment involves judicious use of diuretics and antihypertensives, a restricted protein diet, and careful adjustment of electrolyte intake.

Nervous System. Diabetes affects the nervous system in many ways as it does other organs and tissues. The marked predilection of the diabetic to atherosclerosis, particularly of medium-sized and small arteries, predisposes him to infarction. If the artery is to the spinal cord, *paraplegia* may result, a very infrequent but disastrous event. Rarely the occlusion may be to a nerve root, resulting in a radiculopathy confined to a dermatome. More frequently, a single peripheral nerve is involved, with sudden loss of sensory and motor function and pain. This may involve the ulnar or peroneal nerve or, more frequently, one of the oculomotor nerves, resulting in acute ophthalmoplegia of the facial nerve, producing Bell's palsy. Fortunately collateral circulation corrects most or all of the deficit and the mononeuropathy disappears in weeks or months.

By far the most frequent neurologic problem in diabetics is the *peripheral neuropathy* (see Ch. 465). This occurs in over 90 per cent of diabetics who have had the disease for one or more decades. The typical case presents after eight to twelve years of overt diabetes with a grossly symmetrical stocking-type of anesthesia, mainly of the lower extremities, producing decreased vibratory and fine-touch sensation and occasionally progressing after months to years to near-total or total anesthesia. Paradoxically, there may be marked hyperesthesia and pain, frequently nocturnal and occasionally excruciating in character. Fortunately for the patient, the progressive nature of the neuropathy provides relief of the pain after several months or occasionally a year or longer, resulting in hypesthesia to total anesthesia of the area, probably owing to total loss of sensory nerve function. Deep tendon reflexes in the lower extremity are almost always decreased to absent in these subjects. Many elderly subjects may exhibit similar changes; whether these are due to the diabetic syndrome associated with the mild glucose intolerance of the aged can be argued.

Histologic examination reveals segmental demyelinization. Experimental diabetes in animals is associated with an accumulation of sorbitol and fructose in peripheral nerves, probably in the Schwann cells, as well as delayed nerve conduction velocity. Whether this pathogenic sequence explains most instances of diabetic neuropathy is debatable, because the neuropathy occurs with almost equal frequency in diabetics without fasting hyperglycemia, particularly in older people; hence the biochemical basis remains conjectural. The similar findings in elderly subjects without diabetes suggest that the peripheral neuropathy is part of the accelerated senescence of the diabetic as manifested in the nervous system. Occasionally patients with marked hyperglycemia, peripheral pain, and delayed nerve conduction lose their symptoms and signs with reduction of glucose concentration, and this acute diabetic "neuropathy" is more probably related to the direct metabolic disorder of sorbitol and fructose accumulation.

The diabetic neuropathy may progress to total sensory anesthesia, and, as occurs to the hip and knee in syphilis with tabes, the safeguards of the normal foot to protect its structure by afferent signals is lost, and

chronic trauma to the joints leads to destruction, the so-called "*Charcot joint.*" Loss of position sense also leads to *ataxia,* the *pseudotabes of diabetes.* Likewise a callus may act as a foreign body, repeatedly injuring the anesthetized foot, leading to ulcer and infection, the "*neuropathic*" ulcer. Worse yet, the anesthesia of the foot prevents the patient from recognizing not only the aforementioned problem but also true foreign bodies such as thumb tacks. Daily inspection of the foot, careful and professional management of calluses and bunions, and properly fitted shoes are mandatory to prevent infection, ulcer, and subsequent amputation.

A peculiar syndrome, *diabetic amyotrophy,* usually occurring in middle-aged or older males, involves the anterior thigh muscles, frequently with pain; this may be due to some metabolic aberration at the nerve terminal. Like other mononeuropathy, it may persist without remission, but usually clears in 12 to 24 months.

The *autonomic nervous system* is also affected in the neurologic sequelae, involving both sympathetic and parasympathetic pathways. In the circulatory system this may be manifested as *orthostatic hypotension* caused by involvement of the afferent and efferent autonomic nerves. Decreased angiotensin production resulting from involvement of renal renin production may also contribute to the problem. *Decreased sweating* is also a common observation, although rarely *hyperhidrosis* may occur. *Impotence* in diabetic males is extremely frequent, again resulting from autonomic involvement; retrograde ejaculation is not uncommon. The gastrointestinal system is frequently affected, as evidenced by *delayed gastric emptying* (diabetic gastropathy), with nausea, anorexia, vomiting, and marked weight loss, not unlike that seen in a patient with mental depression or with gastrointestinal malignancy. The bowel itself, both small and large, may be involved, the former leading to a *malabsorption*-like syndrome and the latter to a distressing *diarrhea,* usually nocturnal, or, conversely, to *constipation* and occasionally *megacolon.* Also involved in the autonomic neuropathy is the *bladder,* leading to asymptomatic distention, occasionally with several liters of residual urine. This can be detected by enlargement of the lower abdomen and around-the-clock urination of small overflow volumes. Obviously, the predilection to urinary tract infection is marked in these subjects. Catheterization, unless essential, is contraindicated.

The treatment of all these disorders is depressingly nonspecific, namely better control of the diabetes. Paradoxically, many patients with peripheral neuropathy who are then placed into better carbohydrate-insulin homeostasis have a worsening of the neuropathy, possibly owing to transient improvement in the afferent nerves. In the specific problems, treatment is at best supportive. The patient with bladder involvement may need chronic catheterization or else genitourinary surgery to revise the outflow tract for better bladder decompression. Various cholinergic agents may be of help to the bladder dysfunction and also for the gastropathy. Occasionally antimicrobial drugs as well as anticholinergics may be palliative to the bowel disorder when diarrhea is severe.

The predisposition of the diabetic to *central nervous system vascular accident,* owing to the accelerated atherosclerosis, has already been mentioned. Of much interest, however, and not correlated with the vascular disease but purportedly associated with peripheral neuropathy is the frequent elevation of cerebrospinal fluid protein, occasionally to levels of 200 to 400 mg per 100 ml. In some patients the protein may be elevated without the neuropathy, and in others neuropathy may be present without the protein. Cellular elements, however, are low to absent, ruling out an infectious or other inflammatory process.

Skin. Dermatologic manifestations of diabetes result from the microvascular and macrovascular abnormalities, from the diabetic's predisposition to infection, and from the secondary lipid disorders in blood.

Necrobiosis lipoidica diabeticorum is a rare but dramatic skin condition, found more frequently in females than in males, which may even antedate the other clinical signs and symptoms of diabetes. Although usually in the pretibial area, it may appear elsewhere, particularly on the dorsum of the foot. The mature lesion is a clearly demarcated painless area of atrophic skin, usually deeply pigmented with small telangiectases about the border. Frequently it follows trauma to the area, but many times its appearance is unprovoked. The lesions, which start as red raised papules that coalesce and expand, may remain stationary or even regress without relation to other problems the patient may have. Many diabetics, particularly those of long standing, have a waxy hue of the skin, and small freckle-like brown spots are frequently seen over the lower extremities. Both these and the necrobiosis are probably due to a microangiopathy similar to that in the renal glomerulus and retinal capillary.

Macrovascular disease, or atherosclerosis, often involves the skin in the form of *gangrene* secondary to ischemia. Most commonly one or more toes are affected, but occasionally the entire foot or lower limb may be involved. Rarely the fingers or localized areas of skin anywhere on the body may be affected, probably secondary to occlusion of a small artery, the collaterals having been previously compromised by the same process.

Skin infections are extremely frequent, particularly if the patient is in poor control. The usual staphylococcal and streptococcal infections occur much more frequently than in nondiabetics and may lead to rapid and massive destruction unless antimicrobials are administered and the diabetes is brought under better control. Rectal abscesses, furunculosis, hidradenitis, cellulitis, and intertriginous infections caused by fungi such as dermatophytosis of the feet are all more frequent in the diabetic. Obviously, ischemic areas, especially the feet, are exquisitely susceptible to infection.

Xanthoma diabeticorum (eruptive xanthomatosis): A small percentage of uncontrolled diabetics have a marked elevation in circulating lipids. When triglycerides are chronically elevated, they accumulate not only in macrophages in liver and spleen but also as collections in the skin; these appear as clusters of raised papules, usually on a red base with a pale yellow center, and are referred to as eruptive xanthoma. Most often they are found over the buttocks and extremities, but they may appear anywhere. Diagnosis is made by finding the lipemia in the retinal vessels or by the turbidity or frank creaminess of the serum, and classification is made by electrophoresis into Type I (hyperchylomicronemia), IIb (mixed hypercholesterolemia and hyperchylomicronemia), IV (endogenous hypertriglyceridemia), or V (hyperchylomicronemia and endogenous hypertriglyceridemia) hyperlipidemias. If the diabetes is secondary to Type IV, standard diabetic treatment is indicated with restriction of dietary carbohydrates and, most important if the patient is overweight, a hypocaloric diet. Types IIb, IV, and V are also frequently associated with diabetes, and the hyperlipidemia and diabetes are treated according to the type and severity of each.

Atherosclerosis. Diabetes in all ages is associated with accelerated atherosclerosis. *Coronary insufficiency* in the premenopausal female is twenty times more common than that in the nondiabetic female. A *myocardial infarction* in a male under 40 is almost always associated with either diabetes or a familial lipid disorder. Fifty per cent of all diabetics die prematurely of myocardial infarction. In a diabetic with a myocardial infarction, five-year survival is limited to 30 per cent, whereas 60 per cent of a nondiabetic population would survive this period. *Peripheral arteries* are more severely affected, and gangrene of the feet caused by ischemia is 70-fold more frequent in diabetics. Many explanations have been offered for this accelerated atherosclerosis; one of these implicates defective lipoprotein metabolism. Approximately one fifth of all diabetics have an elevated circulating triglyceride level, mainly in the pre-beta region (endogenous hypertriglyceridemia), and these are diagnosed as Type IV hyperlipoproteinemics. Conversely, over 90 per cent of subjects with Type IV hyperlipoproteinemia have overt diabetes or glucose intolerance. Other lipid disorders, particularly Types IIb, III, and V, have an increased prevalence of diabetes (see Ch. 819). However, for the minimal or absent demonstrable circulating lipid abnormality present in most diabetics, their premature atherosclerosis is far out of proportion. Direct cholesterol synthesis in the vessels has been indicted, as has the basement membrane defect, leading to a microangiopathy of the vasa vasorum and then to atherosclerosis. As in the nondiabetic population, the pathogenic sequence is not clear.

Treatment poses a quandary, because most diabetic diets are restricted in carbohydrate, calling for a high fat intake which may contribute to the atherosclerosis. A compromise is usually suggested with a diet containing one half the calories as fat, but polyunsaturated in nature. For the specific dyslipidemias, clofibrate or nicotinic acid is used, as is cholestyramine. Interestingly, the waxy exudates in the retinal fundus have been significantly decreased with clofibrate therapy, but visual improvement has not been documented. Most important, the synergistic effect of smoking in augmenting vascular disorders with the diabetic predisposition makes *smoking abstinence* a most important part of therapy in any diabetic. Finally, although there is evidence that optimal diabetic control may mitigate the microvascular complications of diabetes, there is little evidence of any effect of control on the accelerated atherosclerosis, suggesting that this predisposition may be an inherent abnormality closely related to the inheritance of the diabetes itself but independent of the abnormality in insulin-glucose homeostasis.

Infection. At any stage of diabetes, infection is both a diagnostic indicator and a major threat. The reasons are manifold, including a decrease in macrophage mobility, a decrease in the potential of macrophages to phagocytose infectious particles, and the relative substrate richness of hyperglycemia itself for microorganisms. Added to these factors is decreased vascularity, particularly in the lower extremity, which makes infection an even greater threat. Noninvasive organisms, such as various fungi, find the diabetic a unique organism in which to flourish, similar to the patient with immunodeficiency caused by hereditary or acquired disorders. The diabetic is predisposed not only to soft tissue infection such as furunculosis, gingival abscess, or perinephric abscess, but also to meningitis, osteomyelitis, and many others. *Mucormycosis* occurs almost uniquely in the uncontrolled or ketoacidotic diabetic and is evidenced by a rapid invasive and destructive infection of the orbit or nasal sinuses eroding directly into major vessels, into the eye itself, and even into brain substance.

Lipoatrophic Diabetes. Patients with this relatively rare syndrome have a peculiar form of diabetes with minimal to absent ketoacidosis, marked resistance to insulin, hypermetabolism, and either congenital or acquired absence of grossly demonstrable adipose tissue. Other prominent features may include marked hyperlipidemia and hepatomegaly, leading to cirrhosis and occasionally to esophageal varices. There are frequently increased musculature, acanthosis nigricans, phlebomegaly, curly hair, thickened skin, and other peculiar anomalies such as cystic angiomatous lesions in bones, genital enlargement, and polycystic ovaries. How these diverse features (Lawrence's syndrome or the *Lawrence-Seip syndrome)* are genetically or metabolically interconnected is obscure. Treatment is symptomatic, and the marked insulin resistance usually makes insulin therapy ineffectual; however, most patients adapt to their marked polydipsia, polyuria, and glucosuria. Histologic examination may demonstrate a diminished number of scattered small adipose cells with minimal lipid. In the congenital variety the paucity of adipose tissue is evident at birth or soon thereafter, but the diabetes and other sequelae may not appear until several years later. In the later or acquired form, the adipose tissue may gradually atrophy through childhood, and again the diabetes occurs several years later. Both forms appear to be inherited as autosomal recessive traits. Hypotheses for this peculiar disorder include a lack of cellular receptors for insulin, a lack of intracellular effects of the insulin response itself, or possibly one or more factors produced in excess by the hypothalamus or pituitary which inhibit insulin's metabolic effects. (See Ch. 931.)

Secondary Diabetes. *Hemochromatosis.* Hemochromatosis is a hereditary disease resulting from iron deposition in various tissues such as liver, skin, and pituitary, and includes the endocrine pancreas (see Part XVI, Section Four). Treatment is directed to the hemochromatosis by iron depletion through phlebotomy and to the diabetes by standard insulin replacement and diet therapy, depending on the severity of the diabetes. Many patients require more insulin than might be expected from simple destruction of beta cells, and this relative insulin resistance may result from the accompanying liver disease.

Pancreatitis. The endocrine pancreas is also involved in the destruction and scarring that occur with acute and chronic pancreatitis. Thus diabetes occurring with episodic abdominal pain, periumbilical and boring through to the back, particularly in the alcoholic, and associated with elevations of circulating or urinary amylase, makes pancreatitis probable. Treatment of the diabetes is again as indicated by the severity of the disturbed carbohydrate homeostasis; with extensive destruction of the pancreas, total insulin replacement with split doses (two doses daily) of intermediate (with or without rapid-acting insulin) is indicated. The malabsorption resulting from exocrine deficiency may require oral pancreatic enzyme therapy. In patients with surgical removal of the pancreas because of tumor or, occasionally, pancreatic replacement by tumor or infection, therapy is similar to that for the patient pancreatectomized because of pancreatitis. Many patients in acute diabetic ketoacidosis may have transient elevations of amylase, possibly caused by mild pancreatitis associated with the acute metabolic decompensation, but residual pancreatic exocrine insufficiency is not observed.

Stress Diabetes. During severe stress, sufficient to increase circulating catecholamines and to activate sympathetic innervation of the endocrine pancreas, insulin release is suppressed and glucagon release provoked. The stress-induced hyperglycemia resulting from hepatic glycogenolysis serves to provide emergency fuel for anaerobic metabolism in muscle or in reparative tissue after trauma, without insulin promoting glycogen or fat synthesis from the glucose. Thus there is a true functional diabetes in severe trauma, septicemia, peritonitis, pneumonia, burns, stroke, and myocardial infarction, to name a few. Of course, if the patient had been a mild diabetic previously, the carbohydrate abnormality would be more marked or more easily unmasked. If parenteral glucose is administered, the hyperglycemia resulting from the absolute or relative lack of insulin may become extreme and the patient may progress into hyperglycemic hyperosmolar coma. These patients may have no evidence of diabetes before or after this episode. Should the hyperglycemia be greater than 400 mg per 100 ml, transient insulin therapy is advisable to prevent excess osmolarity. With lesser degrees of injury, or even with the physical incapacity associated with milder diseases, less severe depression of insulin release may occur, resulting in diabetic glucose tolerance; hence, for diabetes the diagnostic tolerance tests should not be performed until the patient is in good health with adequate nutrition and physical activity.

Acromegaly. Growth hormone administration provokes insulin resistance, and, likewise, excess endogenous growth hormone secretion requires a high concentration of insulin to maintain glucose homeostasis. In some series, 20 to 50 per cent of patients with acromegaly have been found to have either frank diabetes or glucose intolerance. In all patients there is a decreased sensitivity to administered insulin, as evidenced by a markedly decreased hypoglycemic effect of 0.1 unit of insulin per kilogram of body weight given intravenously. Before growth hormone immunoassays became available, diagnosis was made on clinical grounds and on the findings of enlargement of the sella turcica, elevated serum phosphate, and insulin resistance. Now any patient with suggestive acromegaloid features or evidence of postpubertal growth of extremities and jaw, thickening and coarsening of facial features and of skin, particularly fingers, increased sweating, and the many other signs or symptoms of excess growth hormone should be tested for diabetes and treated accordingly in addition to treatment for the acromegaly (see Ch. 832).

Cushing's Syndrome. Excess glucocorticoid, whether administered exogenously or secreted endogenously, may produce either glucose intolerance or frank clinical diabetes in one of five adults. Although there is a slight resistance to the metabolic effects of insulin, the glucose intolerance appears also to be related to increased gluconeogenesis and perhaps to a decrease in beta cell capacity to release insulin. Fajans and Conn have administered small doses of glucocorticoid followed by a glucose tolerance test the next morning as a test for latent diabetes, especially in subjects with strong family histories of diabetes.

Any diabetic, particularly one with early features suggestive of the rounded moon facies, buffalo hump, and truncal obesity, with abdominal striae, osteoporosis, hypertension, or psychosis, must be studied for adrenal hyperactivity. But the clinical challenge is in the less overt or earlier form of the syndrome, and this possibly should always be considered in any newly diagnosed diabetic (see Ch. 850). Again, the diabetes is treated according to its signs and symptoms, until the primary cause of the excess glucocorticoid is corrected. It is believed that most of these patients who require insulin have independent diabetes mellitus that has been aggravated by the excess glucocorticoid.

Other Endocrine and Metabolic Disorders. *Pheochromocytoma* is frequently associated with diabetes mellitus because of the suppression of insulin release from beta cells as well as the capacity for adrenal catechols to provoke hepatic glycogen breakdown and peripheral inhibition of glucose uptake. As in patients with major trauma and high levels of catecholamines, this type of diabetes probably may occur in an individual without inherent diabetes, never to return after removal of the tumor. *Thyrotoxicosis,* on the other hand, appears to be able to unmask latent diabetes mellitus, but its direct effect on carbohydrate metabolism is minimal and is possibly related to the relative starvation of the hypermetabolic patient. Also, accelerated gastric emptying and absorption may cause marked hyperglycemia early in an oral glucose tolerance test, similar to that seen in an individual with gastric resection. Other endocrinopathies that are diabetogenic include pregnancy (to be discussed) and the simulated pregnancy found in patients receiving exogenous estrogen. Many latent diabetics can be made overt if given *oral contraceptive agents,* and the estrogen moiety appears more diabetogenic than the progestin. The hypokalemia of *hyperaldosteronism* or during *diuretic therapy* diminishes insulin release from the pancreas and may contribute to diabetes or carbohydrate intolerance. Another factor leading to glucose intolerance is hyperlipidemia, but again many of these patients probably have independent diabetes, and the pathophysiologic relationship is obscure.

Finally, a large number of metabolic and endocrine disorders are associated with a higher incidence of diabetes than one might expect from the general population. These include the Prader-Willi syndrome, sexual ateliotic dwarfism, Schmidt's syndrome, Werner's syndrome, Refsum's syndrome, Friedreich's ataxia, optic atrophy and nerve deafness, Turner's syndrome, and many others. One wonders why the incidence of diabetes is so high in almost all chromosomal aberrations and inborn errors of metabolism. No clear answer is apparent.

Treatment. The specific treatment of diabetes depends upon the signs and symptoms of the individual

patient presenting with the disease and can be subdivided accordingly. Since the spectrum has at one end fulminant ketoacidosis, which can result in death in coma within several days in the previously well-controlled subject omitting insulin (or in 24 to 48 hours in the child), and at the other end only a slightly abnormal glucose tolerance, the therapy is likewise varied. There is really no fixed regimen for any single patient, even one in ketoacidosis, so only general guidelines will be discussed.

In the terminal ketoacidotic patient in coma, the thready pulse, decreasing blood pressure, rapidly falling arterial pH, and rising Pco_2 (signifying inability to achieve compensation of the acidosis by hyperventilation) portend irreversible shock and death, and rapid heroic treatment is mandatory to reverse the fatal outcome. On the other hand, many patients will walk in with mild ketoacidosis, feeling poorly, without nausea or vomiting, but with a glucose level of 500 mg per 100 ml or higher and a total HCO_3 of 4 to 16 mEq per liter. A liter or two of saline plus 20 to 30 units of crystalline insulin intravenously or intramuscularly may be all that is necessary, as evidenced by correction of the metabolic disorder. This may be followed by the standard insulin dose eight to twelve hours later or, if these patients were not previously on insulin, by a small dose of intermediate-acting insulin (about 20 units) in order to initiate their standard replacement regimen.

The less severe type of diabetic, presenting with polydipsia and polyuria or with any of the sequelae, such as pruritus vulvae, may be handled by diet alone, particularly if over 30 to 40 years of age and overweight. By diet is meant a low calorie, carbohydrate-restricted regimen distributed between meals to avoid excessively large meals at any one time. Should this regimen not be effective in controlling hyperglycemia after one to two months' trial, insulin or one of the oral antidiabetic medications may be indicated in addition to the diet. If insulin is used, it is usually given as a single dose of one of the intermediate types, either NPH or lente, one half hour before breakfast, in order to supplement the endogenously produced insulin. The philosophy, of course, is the reciprocal of the normal physiology wherein the beta cells release insulin proportional to the composition and size of the ingested meal; in the diabetic, the meals are proportioned to match the rate of absorption of the injected intermediate-acting insulin (e.g., a smaller breakfast, a moderate-sized lunch, a mid-afternoon snack, a moderate-sized supper, and a small bedtime snack). Should a larger breakfast be desired, some crystalline insulin may be mixed with the intermediate insulin.

Since ketoacidosis is the most dramatic and life-threatening event, its treatment will be discussed first in greater detail.

Diabetic Ketoacidosis. As in most acute, life-threatening crises, the primary concern is lack of effective circulating volume. The marked hyperglycemia leads to marked glycosuria and an osmotic "washout" of water and electrolyte, mainly sodium and chloride. In addition, as a result of the elevated circulating levels of ketoacids, which are relatively poorly reabsorbed by the renal tubule from the glomerular filtrate, these relatively strong organic acids with pK's below 4 appear in the urine and are coupled with excretion of sodium, potassium, and ammonium, leading to further volume depletion. The ketoacidosis also leads to systemic acidosis, which, in itself, depresses cardiac contractility as well as the capacity of arterioles to respond to catecholamines, both the circulating epinephrine and the norepinephrine released locally from sympathetic nerve endings. Thus the thready pulse, hypotension, and poor organ perfusion reflect both hypovolemia and poor physiologic compensation to the decreased volume, the two processes enhancing each other's threat to survival.

Therapy first involves correct diagnosis; the history of polydipsia and polyuria in a patient with marked hyperglycemia and glycosuria together with the demonstration of excess ketoacid in plasma establishes the diagnosis. Usually the patient has omitted insulin because of intercurrent illness, with the mistaken thought that insulin is unnecessary if food is not eaten. Other explanations include the insulin resistance associated with infection or the first trimester of pregnancy, or even emotional stress. In the previously undiagnosed diabetic, the typical history may also include severe abdominal pain, frequently with a rigid, tender abdomen. The marked leukocytosis with immature granulocytes in the blood smear may make an acute surgical abdomen a reasonable diagnosis until the hyperglycemia, glycosuria, ketonemia, and ketonuria provide the correct cause.

In simplest terms, a large indwelling needle is inserted in a vein of the suspect patient, blood is drawn and checked for hyperglycemia by either an approximate bedside procedure (Testape or Reflectometer) or rapid automatic glucose determination, using glucose oxidose, and plasma or serum ketosis is assessed by a drop placed on one of several commercial preparations (e.g., Acetest, Ketotest, Ketostix). If hyperglycemia and marked ketosis are present, the diagnosis is immediately confirmed and therapy initiated.

The original needle inserted is obviously left in place after drawing the blood, and isotonic saline is run in at a rapid pace, because volume deficit is usually severe. If the patient is critically ill with marked hypotension and barely detectable peripheral pulse, plasma expanders such as plasma itself, albumin, or synthetic colloids can be given in order to improve the circulating hypovolemia. In this case, drawing of arterial gases and pH is mandatory; if the pH is below 7.1, sodium bicarbonate, 1 ampule (44 mEq), should be added to each liter of isotonic saline to help correct myocardial contractility as well as to improve vascular tone. With documentation of the hyperglycemia and the marked increase in ketone bodies, insulin should be given. The precise amount varies between clinics, but usually about five times the daily dose is given; for the average diabetic therefore approximately 200 units is given, half intravenously and half subcutaneously. Recently, some clinics have reported what they regard as improved results by giving 5 to 10 units per hour by continuous intravenous infusion or by giving 10 to 20 units hourly intramuscularly during the first hours of treatment. For the present the writer prefers to follow the philosophy that early vigorous reversal of the pathogenic sequence is indicated to spare life, and, once the progression of the metabolic lesion has been reversed, to proceed more slowly in making the final corrections in volume deficit and electrolytes. Of importance is the urinary loss of potassium during the development of ketoacidosis, owing partly to the osmotic diuresis and partly to loss of potassium from cells. With volume deficit, aldosterone is also called into play, and distal tubular exchange of potassium for sodium results in an even more marked deficit in body potassium. With the metabolic acidosis there is usually hyperkalemia, approximately 5 to 6.5 mEq per liter in spite of the total body deficit. An initial serum potassium of 4 to 5 mEq per liter or, more striking, of less than 4 mEq per liter signifies severe potassium deficiency. Therefore potassium, as the phosphate or chloride (preferably the phosphate), should be added to the infusion (40 mEq per liter), particularly after the insulin is injected, because that will accelerate potassium movement into cells, and life-threatening hypokalemia can ensue. Usually potassium administration can be withheld until glucose levels are shown to fall. If bicarbonate is administered because of severe acidosis and hypotension, the fall in potassium may be accentuated and replacement should be more vigorous.

Three or 4 liters of isotonic saline, with bicarbonate in the severely acidotic patient or with potassium in the patient predisposed to hypokalemia, may be given in the first two or three hours of therapy. If there is gastric atony with emesis of a black and frequently benzidine-positive fluid, gastric aspiration helps to return gastric compensation as well as lessening the risk of aspiration pneumonia. These patients may have a demonstrable succussion splash before decompression.

Except in very severe cases, when one may wish to monitor renal perfusion, urinary catheterization is contraindicated. The hyperosmolarity induced by the hyperglycemia exerts a protective effect on the kidney, and acute tubular necrosis after severe diabetic ketoacidosis is extremely rare. Electrocardiographic tracings help to monitor the physiologic effects of the potassium levels.

Of prime importance is close observation of the patient, together with the compilation of a detailed bedside flowsheet of all events: insulin administered, chemistries, pulse, blood pressure, and so forth. If blood glucose levels do not fall after the initial insulin injection, the infrequent but serious problem of insulin resistance may be present, requiring intravenous or subcutaneous injection of hundreds to thousands of units. This need to follow the glucose levels is one of the contraindications to giving exogenous glucose in the initial intravenous therapy until a significant insulin effect is observed, as evidenced by a definite fall in glucose concentration.

Although it appears more logical initially to administer hypotonic saline, since the patient has lost more water than electrolyte, isotonic saline provides a better defense for the maintenance of extracellular fluid volume. As glucose levels fall, thanks to insulin exerting its physiologic effects, the extracellular osmolarity falls and fluid tends to move into cells, decreasing, thereby, extracellular fluid volume; hence the preference for giving isotonic instead of hypotonic solutions initially. Also, the shift of water from the extracellular fluid into cells is shared by the central nervous system, leading tragically, but fortunately rarely, to cerebral edema and death. Hence, again, the principle in the treatment of diabetic ketoacidosis is to initiate treatment rapidly, in order to reverse the process and to correct circulatory fluid volume. Once the patient has begun to improve, the management can proceed more conservatively.

Should bicarbonate and potassium salts be added to

the infusate, 0.45 per cent sodium chloride can be used in the basic fluid in order to avoid overly hypertonic solutions.

As blood glucose levels fall, if potassium was not administered initially, it should be added subsequently, 1 ampule per liter (40 mEq) of solution, preferably as the phosphate salt. When the blood glucose level approaches the renal threshold of 180 to 200 mg per 100 ml, glucose as 5 per cent D/W or 5 per cent D/S can be infused in order to prevent hypoglycemia. The patient is returned to long-acting insulin therapy once the threat of hypoglycemia has passed.

Should the initial insulin therapy be ineffective as evidenced by a failure to reduce blood glucose levels in the first or second hour, a second injection must be given, and this is usually twice the first, unless the patient's condition has deteriorated markedly, in which case much larger doses should be given as well as alkali, volume expanders, and all other maneuvers used in the treatment of the patient in shock. If, however, the glucose level is decreased, for example, falling from 600 to 300 mg per 100 ml, a second insulin injection need not be given unless the progressive fall later ceases or glucose levels begin to increase, in which case a small second injection of insulin can be given, perhaps one quarter to one half the initial dose. Thus continuous monitoring and charting of blood glucose concentrations, first at hourly intervals and later at two-hour intervals, are essential. The availability of rapid bedside glucose techniques such as the glucose-oxidase analyzer has greatly simplified this task.

The precipitating event leading to ketoacidosis should always be kept in mind. Usually it is lack of understanding owing to poor education, the patient having omitted insulin when slightly ill from an upper respiratory infection or a gastrointestinal disturbance, believing that the decreased food intake obviated the need for daily insulin. Frequently, an unrecognized infection may provoke sufficient insulin resistance to tip the patient into ketoacidosis. Thus appendicitis, pyelonephritis, meningitis, and other disorders should be considered. The marked leukocytosis with immature forms associated with diabetic ketoacidosis makes exclusion of infection all the more difficult.

Alcohol is metabolized in liver to acetate which is then released for further metabolism by peripheral tissues. Thus alcohol compounds the rate of hepatic acetate production during fasting, particularly in the insulin-deficient diabetic, and severe ketoacidosis may occur with varying degrees of hyperglycemia. In the previously fasting nondiabetic, an alcoholic debauch may even provoke severe ketoacidosis with normal or low blood glucose levels. Thus a careful history is indicated, and in such a subject with severe ketoacidosis, glucose as well as electrolyte may be indicated in the initial therapy.

Hyperosmolar Coma. Coma, usually occurring in an elderly patient, with hyperglycemia caused by dehydration, prerenal azotemia, and marked but not total insulin deficiency, can mimic that of the subject in ketoacidosis. However, the Kussmaul respirations of severe acidosis and the smell of acetone are lacking owing to the low or absent ketonemia. On the other hand, if there are hyperventilation, a low pH, and low bicarbonate without demonstrable ketoacidosis, *lactic acidosis* is a probable diagnosis. The patient in hyperosmolar coma is treated like the patient in diabetic ketoacidosis with an indwelling large needle in a peripheral vein through which isotonic saline is administered rapidly. The usual insulin resistance of ketoacidosis may be absent; if the hyperglycemia is in the range of 500 to 1000 mg per 100 ml or even higher, only 10 to 25 units of insulin need be first given intravenously. In these subjects, the requirement for isotonic as opposed to hypotonic fluid replacement is even more strongly indicated, because reduction of glucose levels markedly decreases extracellular osmoles and fluid entry into tissues will markedly compromise extracellular fluid volume as well as producing intracellular fluid overload, especially in the brain. Hence *hypotonic solutions should not be administered* until the patient's circulatory volume is stabilized, and then only slowly and judiciously. Also, as in ketoacidosis, the primary reason for the decompensation should be considered. Bronchopneumonia, myocardial infarction, and local or generalized infections are all included in the differential diagnosis. Again, with the decrease in glucose levels as treatment continues, potassium moves into cells and parenteral potassium replacement may be required. The needed amounts are usually far less than in ketoacidosis, but the same precaution, close observation with frequent monitoring such as precordial electrocardiographic tracings and serum electrolyte levels, is indicated.

Nonketotic or Nonhyperosmolar Patient. In the diabetic with marked fasting and postprandial hyperglycemia, the urgency of the aforementioned two syndromes is not present. In the young individual, particularly under age 20, with polyuria, thirst, and fasting hyperglycemia, insulin therapy is indicated, because deficiency of the hormone, although not as severe as in the patient with ketoacidosis, will eventually be complete or nearly complete. In an adolescent, 20 units of intermediate-duration insulin (lente or NPH) given each morning is a good start, followed by the adjustment of diet and insulin treatment based on urine and blood glucose levels. Since endogenous insulin secretion is moderately compromised, the diet is made to match the rate of insulin absorption within some structure as dictated by social convenience. Thus total calories might be distributed with two sevenths at breakfast, two sevenths at lunch, two sevenths at supper, and the other one seventh split between mid-afternoon and bedtime snacks. Many manuals and texts published by the American Diabetes Association and various hospitals and clinics describe this in further detail and should be

TABLE 1. Insulin in Clinical Usage*

	Peak Effect (Hours)	Duration of Effect (Hours)
Regular or crystalline	2–3	6–8
Semilente	3–6	10–14
NPH	6–10	16–24
Lente	6–10	16–24
Ultralente	10–16	36+
PZI (protamine zinc insulin)	10–16	36+

*Insulin preparations in the United States and their duration of action. They are available in 40, 80 and 100 units per milliliter, termed U40, U80 and U100 respectively. Standard and disposable syringes calibrated accordingly are available. The use of the two lower doses is being phased out in view of the simplicity of use of U100. Also available are U500 and U5000 for the rare patient with marked insulin resistance.

consulted for specifics. The patient is taught to test urine for glucose levels and to alter insulin and diet accordingly. If a larger breakfast is desired, or if the present insulin regimen does not cover the breakfast, regular or clear insulin can be added to the intermediate-duration insulin. Likewise, if there is glycosuria at bedtime, a short-acting insulin can be given before supper. Since the peak action of intermediate insulin is in the mid-afternoon, hypoglycemia at that time necessitates reduction of the dose (making sure the patient is not omitting the mid-afternoon snack). Conversely, late afternoon hyperglycemia necessitates increasing the morning dose of intermediate-duration insulin. Careful daily records should be kept by the patient of his urine sugar tests as well as hypoglycemic reactions, even if minimal.

If the patient does well through the day but has early morning hyperglycemia and glycosuria, a small injection of intermediate insulin may be necessary before supper or bedtime to carry through the night. This is usually not necessary in the juvenile diabetic in the first years of the disease, thanks to the small endogenous production of insulin. However, after about five years of disease all beta cell function has usually ceased, and the "split" dose of insulin, one in the morning and the other before supper, becomes the rule. In many juvenile-type patients, even the "split" dose with a most careful adherence to diet cannot adequately control the diabetes, and mild hyperglycemia is the compromise to prevent excessive hypoglycemic reactions. In these, occasional collection of a 24-hour urine with quantification of glucose may give an index of over-all control, with the hope that excretion is less than 5 to 10 per cent of dietary carbohydrate intake.

In the patient over 20 with marked fasting hyperglycemia, if not overweight but with minimal or mild ketosis, insulin therapy will also probably be necessary. If the patient is overweight, however, the insulin resistance of obesity calls for a trial of rigid dietary restriction and weight reduction, keeping close observation that he does not go into ketoacidosis. Rarely, a fat child without ketosis may fall in this group. Not infrequently, with weight loss, endogenous insulin becomes sufficient to maintain glucose homeostasis for at least several years, occasionally permanently. Too often, unfortunately, weight loss may be minimal because of failure to adhere to a calorically restricted diet; insulin or sulfonylurea therapy is then indicated. The insulin is usually given as a single injection of intermediate acting (NPH or lente) one half hour before breakfast and regulated according to urine and blood tests. Because urine glucose may represent hyperglycemia many hours previously, patients are usually advised to empty the bladder one half hour before the anticipated time of testing, to drink water, and then to void again—the "double-voided" urine specimen.

Oral Hypoglycemic Agents. Although weight reduction by caloric restriction is the ideal approach to the middle-aged overweight diabetic subject, it is almost universally unsuccessful. Thus in these patients, as well as in nonoverweight subjects with maturity-onset type diabetes, addition of the oral hypoglycemic agents is indicated should hyperglycemia persist, although, as discussed below, some controversy exists between experts in the field as to their value and contraindications.

TABLE 2. Oral Agents

Sulfonylureas	Dosage	Duration of Effect (Hours)
Tolbutamide (Orinase)	0.5–3 grams/day	6–12
Acetohexamide (Dymelor)	0.25–1.5 grams/day	12–24
Chlorpropamide (Diabinese)	0.1–0.5 gram/day	24–48
Tolazamide (Tolinase)	0.1–0.75 gram/day	12–24
Glyburide (Micronase, Diabeta)	5–35 mg/day	12–24

Biguanides	Dosage	Duration of Effect (Hours)
Phenformin (Meltrol, DBI)	25–200 mg/day	4–6
Phenformin (Meltrol-50, DBI-TD)	50–200 mg/day	8–14

Table 2 lists the oral agents available in the United States. Those of the sulfonylurea type acutely increase insulin release from beta cells in man and in experimental preparations, and their chronic effect is allegedly through this same mechanism, but non-beta-cell effects have also been described, such as inhibition of hepatic glucose output. They differ from each other by their potencies, duration of action, and mechanism of elimination. Tolbutamide, the drug most commonly used, has a relatively shorter duration of action, and its lesser potency requires larger doses to be given as indicated in Table 2. Usually the patient is started on 1 to 2 grams per day, half in the morning and the other half in the evening. Tolbutamide is primarily metabolized to inert products by the liver and then excreted. Should its action not be reflected in lowered glucose levels, a larger dose (3 grams) can be given or else one of the other more potent and longer-acting agents. Acetohexamide is also metabolized by the liver, but its principal product retains hypoglycemic activity. Chlorpropamide, on the other hand, is excreted unchanged by the kidneys and is obviously contraindicated in renal insufficiency. Extremely infrequently these drugs cause skin rashes or other allergic manifestations; an even more rare but serious problem has been protracted hypoglycemia, particularly in elderly individuals, usually from the more potent, long-acting sulfonylureas. Other pharmacologic agents, such as anticoagulants and salicylates, compete with hepatic removal of the sulfonylurea (except chlorpropamide) and drug-drug interactions must always be considered when they are used. If the patient's abnormal glucose tolerance is successfully corrected toward normal or—more easily determined—a one- or two-hour postprandial glucose is less than 160 or 120 mg per 100 ml, respectively, the drug may be continued and later reduced in dosage or perhaps, after a year or so, terminated with the patient observed at quarterly or so intervals to see if glucose intolerance returns.

In a large multicenter study, the University Group Diabetes Project, sponsored by the National Institutes of Health and performed through the 1960's, it was demonstrated that middle-aged subjects on a fixed dose of one of the sulfonylureas, tolbutamide, although showing a small but significant lowering of blood glucose levels, had an increased incidence of sudden death, presumably resulting from myocardial infarction or arrhythmia. This study has limited the indiscriminate use of sulfonylureas, and has placed further emphasis on diet as the primary approach to the maturity-onset type of diabetic. Many experienced students of the disease question the significance of the study and continue to use the agents. Nevertheless, if one adheres to the hypothesis that hyperglycemia is deleterious, in that it leads to the microvascular complications, then the sulfonylureas may be indicated if their benefit outweighs the possible risk of increased myocardial instability. Certainly, in the elderly female with glycosuria, the correction of her discomfort associated with the glycosuria may far outweigh the theoretical increased risk of sudden death as found in the UGDP study. One is obviously hesitant to start older, debilitated individuals on insulin injections unless absolutely necessary, and in these the sulfonylureas may play an important role.

The biguanides, of which, at the time of this writing, only phenformin is available in the United States, apparently work independently of beta cell insulin release and thus can be used independently of or supplementary to the sulfonylureas. Their mode of action is not yet known, although many experimental metabolic effects have been demonstrated, such as delayed glucose absorption in the gut, augmented peripheral glucose uptake, and inhibition of gluconeogenesis. A predilection to lactic acidosis in patients receiving biguanides, has been described, and these agents are thereby contraindicated in elderly individuals with congestive failure or similar debilitated states. Their major use has been as an adjunct to the sulfonylureas when the latter have failed to reduce blood glucose levels sufficiently. A slight anorexigenic effect has also been attributed to the biguanides, with the suggestion that they might be all the more indicated in the obese diabetic. Thus persistent hyperglycemia and glycosuria in an individual on a full dose of one of the more potent sulfonylureas can be treated with one to two capsules of the longer-acting biguanide preparation, and a satisfactory hypoglycemic effect is frequently observed. This combined therapy is particularly useful in patients, such as those with visual problems, who are physically or emotionally unable to inject insulin. Unfortunately, a "metallic" taste in the mouth or even persistent nausea and, occasionally, vomiting may limit full usage of biguanide, and it is therefore logical to start with but a single capsule daily, increasing the dosage either until the desired metabolic effect is achieved or just before the gastrointestinal side effects are observed. In the same University Group Diabetes Project discussed above for tolbutamide, patients placed on phenformin given singly without sulfonylurea developed more hypertension and tachycardia than a placebo-treated control, and a significant increase in death from cardiovascular causes was recorded. These patients, however, were asymptomatic middle-aged diabetics, in whom dietary treatment should be the primary mode of therapy.

With both the sulfonylureas and biguanides, many patients may become refractory to their hypoglycemic effects after several years, and these "secondary failure" patients must be started on insulin therapy.

In the milder diabetic with normal fasting glucose and only intermittent or absent glucose in the urine, diet may be all that is necessary. This diet involves reduction or elimination of the easily and rapidly absorbed free sugars; hence no candy, preserves, cookies, or cakes may be eaten, and calories must be distributed throughout the day. Thus a typical diabetic diet of 2200 calories may be composed of 200 to 250 grams of carbo-

hydrate, 100 grams of protein, and the remainder as fat. Again, the standard diabetic texts and handbooks should be used for details such as caloric contents and types of foods as well as exchanges of similar types of foods to provide palatable variability in the diet.

Insulin Problems. The most frequent complication of insulin therapy is hypoglycemia, which can generally be prevented by readjustment of insulin type or dose and of diet. A well-controlled juvenile diabetic may experience occasional mild autonomic symptoms indicating a low glucose and respond by eating some carbohydrate, and this is not felt to be deleterious. In fact it may be helpful to demonstrate that ambient glucose levels are in the physiologic range. However, unconsciousness or convulsions are strongly contraindicated, and the insulin therapy is made less stringent in order to prevent these episodes. In many juvenile diabetics, hyperglycemia, as indicated by slightly positive urine tests, may be the compromise to prevent the physiologic and certainly the social consequences of hypoglycemia.

Allergy. Since insulin is a foreign protein, most patients experience slight reddening, discomfort, and occasionally itchiness at the site of injection after the first two or three weeks. These usually disappear in several weeks or months. In rare patients, the insulin may cause generalized hives and itching, requiring antihistamines, or, if more severe, desensitization to insulin according to schedules delineated in the standard diabetes texts. When allergy to insulin occurs, the patient is re-evaluated as to whether insulin per se is mandatory, because a more restricted diet with or without sulfonylureas or biguanides may suffice. In a juvenile, "ketotic type" diabetic, insulin is mandatory and desensitization must be performed. Also, as discussed under Insulin Resistance, the insulin preparation containing factors least foreign to man should be used.

Insulin Resistance. ANTIBODY-RELATED. Until 1972–73, commercially available insulin preparations contained small amounts of proinsulin and insulin with connecting peptide (C-peptide) still attached to the A or B chains, in addition to other contaminants such as insulin dimers. Thus all patients on daily insulin therapy for several weeks developed antibodies to insulin and these foreign proteins, since beef insulin and pig insulin differ from human insulin by 4 and 1 amino acids respectively. This antibody production, however, did not compromise the effectiveness of insulin except in about 1 in 1000 patients, in whom increasing amounts of insulin were necessary to saturate antibody binding sites in order to permit enough insulin to be physiologically active. By definition, patients receiving 200 units of insulin for two or more days were said to be insulin resistant. Many of these had been on and off insulin therapy on several occasions, an excellent antibody-inducing regimen. Treatment entailed use of the insulin closest in structure to man, pig insulin or pig insulin with the terminal beta-chain alanine removed, making it identical to human insulin minus the terminal beta-chain threonine. In some this decreased the daily insulin dosage, but in others with "resistance" little difference was observed.

In the early 1970's, insulin preparations without contaminants were prepared and found to be much less antigenic than those used formerly. This "single peak" insulin has induced less antibody formation, and the over-all incidence of insulin resistance on this preparation is much less, although its precise rate has yet to be determined. Thus patients with increasing insulin requirement should be started on "single peak" insulin (or "single component," an electrophoretically pure insulin) and, if available, with the amino acid sequence closest to that of man, namely pig.

Formerly, in those patients with insulin resistance, the insulin doses required for effective therapy frequently fluctuated. The patient might need several thousand units daily for several weeks; then because of unexplained alterations in insulin-antibody interrelationships, he might have frequent hypoglycemic reactions, with daily insulin needs being reduced to 100 or fewer units per day. This instability in management occasionally necessitated treatment with glucocorticoids to reduce antibody formation; indeed, even immunosuppressive therapy with antimetabolites was used in certain difficult cases in which management became extremely difficult.

ANTIBODY-UNRELATED. A non-antibody-related insulin resistance is seen in many metabolic states and these have been discussed under Secondary Diabetes. Rarely, a patient without prior immunization to insulin may require 100,000 units or more of insulin to correct the metabolic disorder. These patients are usually young females, and the precise metabolic defect is as yet unknown. It is for these rare patients that the physician must remember that preparations of U500 and U5000 are commercially available and may be lifesaving.

OBESITY. In both laboratory animals and man, obesity is associated with a decreased metabolic response to exogenous and endogenous insulin. Decreased binding sites for insulin have been demonstrated on cell membranes from obese animals and man; Ogilvie, many years ago, found obese man to have true pancreatic hyperplasia at autopsy unless diabetes was present.

The hyperinsulinemia, both basal and postprandial, in obese man is shown in Figure 4. Since insulin degradation rates are equal in normal subjects and in the obese, the pancreas in the latter must secrete five to ten times more insulin to achieve fuel homeostasis. It is thus obvious that a deficient beta cell population is unmasked by obesity, and that, in any diabetic, obesity is a major problem. As discussed previously, the primary therapy in the obese diabetic is the hypocaloric weight-reducing diet. Many middle-aged obese diabetics may require 50 to 100 units of insulin daily, but with weight loss they may not require insulin, or possibly may not even need supplementary oral hypoglycemic agents. Only with weight loss in a given patient can the endogenous insulin secretory reserve be assessed.

SOMOGYI EFFECT. After a hypoglycemic reaction, counterregulatory processes such as increased sympathetic nerve activity and increased circulating catecholamines, glucagon, and cortisol and growth hormone (although the metabolic effects of these latter two are less than those of the first two) all induce peripheral insulin resistance as well as increasing hepatic glucose production from both glycolysis and gluconeogenesis. In addition, overzealous correction by oral intake of carbohydrate adds to the hyperglycemia. Thus as in starvation and diabetic ketoacidosis, the trend is toward hyperglycemia, and a larger than usual dose of insulin is necessary to correct the rebound. Occasionally another hypoglycemic reaction can follow and the sequence be repeated, resulting in marked metabolic swings of hyper- and hypoglycemia. This pattern has been em-

phasized by Somogyi, and his name is frequently applied to this diabetic instability. Therapy is to reduce the dose of the principal insulin injection and, unless already in use, to administer a second, smaller dose of intermediate-acting insulin before supper in order to "smooth out" the patient's metabolic state. In fact, a true "brittle" diabetic, one in whom glucose levels are highly unstable and unpredictable, is best treated by the "split" or double dose of insulin and occasionally might even do better on a third or, rarely, a fourth injection, judged according to premeal urine tests, the experience of the previous day or two, and anticipated meal size.

Lipoatrophy and Hypertrophy. Not infrequently, and most often in girls in their late teens, lipoatrophy is seen at sites of insulin injection. This disfiguring event, occurring in up to one third of all patients, is treated by rotating insulin injections to different sites; however, the new, purer insulin preparations have presumably decreased the incidence of this problem. In many cases, injection of the single peak or single component insulins has even reversed the lesion when injected into the same site.

The hypertrophy that occurs at the site of insulin injection of many diabetics, more often in males than in females, is a direct result of insulin's lipogenic action on fat cells. This can also be disfiguring and usually results from repetitive injections into the same site. Treatment is rotation of injection sites, using thighs, buttocks, abdominal wall, and triceps areas as loci, so that no one site is used more than once a week, even in a patient taking two injections daily.

Hypoglycemia. Any patient on insulin and occasional patients on oral hypoglycemic agents are subject to episodes of hypoglycemia. This is usually evident first as a disturbance in cerebration, such as inability to perform addition or subtraction, or mood changes, followed by parasympathetic signs and symptoms, salivation, hunger, and increased gastric motility. There may then be sympathetic hyperactivity, with sweating, tachycardia, piloerection, and anxiety. The pattern in a given patient may vary, and between patients it varies markedly. Bizarre behavior may arouse suspicion of alcohol or drug intoxication. As hypoglycemia becomes more severe, unconsciousness and convulsions occur which, if prolonged, may lead to severe organic deficit and possibly to an irreversible decorticate or decerebrate state or death. Patient education is most important. Deliberately causing a mild hypoglycemic reaction in a newly discovered and treated diabetic may be advisable so that he is aware of the symptoms and signs. Treatment is by administration of carbohydrate as candy or as a sweetened beverage; however, if the patient is stuporous, oral therapy of any sort must not be given because of danger of aspiration. Instead, glucagon, 1 mg given subcutaneously or intramuscularly by a trained family member or friend, or intravenously by a physician, causes sufficient glycogenolysis to elevate glucose transiently to awaken the patient, so further carbohydrate can be given by mouth. Thus glucagon should be in every diabetic kit. Of course, if the hypoglycemia occurs in a hospital or office setting, drawing a blood sample for glucose analysis can be done to document the diagnosis, and glucose (10 to 25 grams) can be given immediately intravenously, usually as a 50 per cent solution.

Symptoms and signs of hypoglycemia may occur literally within minutes and may rapidly progress to total unconsciousness. Thus any diabetic behaving in a bizarre fashion or, particularly, unconscious should be treated as if hypoglycemic until proved otherwise. Ketoacidosis, on the other hand, takes many hours to days to develop; in contrast to hypoglycemia, the patient appears and behaves chronically ill.

Patients on sulfonylureas, particularly the longer-acting agents, may also develop a severe and prolonged hypoglycemia requiring continuous intravenous glucose therapy for as long as two or three days. These are usually elderly patients with mild diabetes or with compromised renal function. As with insulin-induced hypoglycemia, the unconsciousness may be associated with a variable neurologic examination, including unilateral or bilateral Babinski reflexes and hyperactive or hypoactive deep tendon reflexes, and may mimic a cerebrovascular accident. A superimposed diabetic neuropathy may make the event all the more confusing, particularly because the deep tendon reflexes in the lower extremity may be decreased to absent.

If a patient taking insulin is found to need a progressive reduction in insulin dosage because of recurrent hypoglycemic episodes, particularly if the daily insulin requirement is less than 15 to 20 units, reasons other than simple fluctuations in insulin responsiveness should be considered. An islet cell tumor, partial hypopituitarism, adrenal insufficiency, hypothyroidism, and pregnancy are all possibilities, particularly pituitary disease, thanks to the diabetic's predilection for vascular infarction secondary to generalized atherosclerosis.

Pregnancy and Delivery. In the first trimester of pregnancy, a juvenile diabetic receiving insulin frequently needs a reduction in daily dosage owing to recurrent hypoglycemic episodes. In the second trimester, the diabetes tends to become more labile, and more insulin is needed. Ketoacidosis occurs more readily and, if severe, usually results in death of the fetus. Compounded with this lability, particularly in the third trimester, is the increased renal glomerular filtration rate, lowering the threshold and making urine tests less indicative of blood levels. Immediately after delivery there is a dramatic reduction in insulin need, literally within hours, but after one or two weeks the insulin requirement returns to the prepregnancy level.

The pregnant diabetic has a greater tendency to retain sodium and chloride, making her more susceptible to toxemia and to the development of hydramnios. The latter, caused by increased volume, may result in premature labor and delivery before maturation of the infant. Salt restriction and diuretics are indicated. Mothers with juvenile diabetes for less than ten years or with a milder maturity-onset type of diabetes have large babies, which may cause obstetrical difficulties. In a longstanding juvenile diabetic, particularly with microangiopathic complications or atherosclerosis as evidenced by calcified pelvic vessels, placental function may be decreased and the infant inadequately nourished and "small-for-dates." In both the hypermature or dysmature pregnancy there is a likelihood of sudden intrauterine death, and delivery prior to this catastrophic event is advised. However, the infant is also particularly subject to respiratory distress, and too early delivery is accordingly contraindicated. The thirty-seventh week is usually approximately optimal, but fetal movements, maternal hormone excretion (estrogen and estrogen metabolites, placental lactogen),

and amniotic fluid concentrations of pulmonary surfactants are all evaluated to select the best time for delivery.

The newborn possesses markedly hyperplastic pancreatic islets and is placed on intravenous dextrose and water to prevent prolonged and severe hypoglycemia. More important, the predisposition to the respiratory distress syndrome makes close supervision mandatory.

A successful obstetrical outcome results mainly from frequent observation of the pregnant patient and optimal insulin control of her diabetes, with weekly or twice-weekly visits and hospitalization for the last two to three weeks. Because diabetic complications such as retinopathy are frequently aggravated by pregnancy, delivery of one or certainly of two viable infants in a juvenile diabetic should raise consideration of measures to prevent further pregnancies.

General Principles in Diabetic Management. Since diabetes is a lifelong event, the patient must learn to become his own physician. This is accomplished through extensive education. If he is taking insulin, urine testing, with results recorded before each meal and at bedtime, is mandatory, and the insulin dose should be adjusted according to the previous one or two days' records. He is instructed to reduce insulin or take extra food before strenuous physical activity, or to increase insulin dosage in times of stress, whether it be physical or, occasionally, emotional, particularly as dictated by previous experience. Also if treated with insulin, he should be taught about insulin hypoglycemia and should always be in contact with someone who knows of his disease and the therapy of hypoglycemia. If he is traveling, identification bracelets or cards in the purse or wallet are mandatory. He should also be instructed in foot care, particularly if elderly and with peripheral vascular disease or neuropathy. For educating the young insulin-dependent diabetic, summer camps have been of great help; they have the additional advantage of exposing the child to others with the disease in order to minimize his inferiority as being "singled out." Finally, he should be especially warned of the threat of infection and of wounds, particularly of the lower extremities. The large number of juvenile and maturity-onset diabetics who have achieved major successes in all walks of life, including athletics, attests to the minimal impact of the disease in many. Unfortunately in many others, particularly with the juvenile-onset form of the disease occurring in childhood, inadequate or improper emotional support and guidance frequently result in gross maladjustment; these patients can become a burden to society as well as a major threat to their own well-being by neglect of their therapy.

Alberti, K. G. M. M., Hockaday, T. D. R., and Turner, R. C.: Small doses of intramuscular insulin in the treatment of diabetic coma. Lancet, 3:515, 1973.

Beisswenger, P. J., and Spiro, R. G.: Studies on the human glomerular basement membrane. Diabetes, 22:180, 1973.

Ellenberg, M., and Rifkin, H.: Diabetes Mellitus: Theory and Practice. New York, McGraw-Hill Book Company, 1970.

Fajans, S. S., and Sussman, K. E.: Diabetes Mellitus: Diagnosis and Treatment. Vol. III. New York, American Diabetes Association, 1971.

Gabbay, K. H.: The sorbitol pathway and the complications of diabetes. N. Engl. J. Med., 288:831, 1973.

Gamble, D. R., and Taylor, K. W.: Seasonal incidence of diabetes mellitus. Br. Med. J., 2:631, 1969.

Genuth, S. M.: Plasma insulin and glucose profiles in normal, obese, and diabetic persons. Ann. Intern. Med., 79:812, 1973.

Kilo, C., Vogler, N., and Williamson, J. R.: Muscle capillary basement membrane changes related to aging and to diabetes mellitus. Diabetes, 21:881, 1972.

Lundbaek, K.: Recent contributions to the study of diabetic angiopathy and neuropathy. Adv. Metab. Disord., 6:99, 1972.

Marble, A., White, P., Bradley, R. D., and Krall, L. P.: Joslin's Diabetes Mellitus. 11th ed. Philadelphia, Lea & Febiger, 1971.

Rimoin, D. L., and Schimke, R. W.: Genetic Disorders of the Endocrine Glands. St. Louis, C. V. Mosby Company, 1971.

Siperstein, M. D., Unger, R. H., and Madison, L. L.: Studies of muscle capillary basement membranes in normal subjects, diabetic and pre-diabetic patients. J. Clin. Invest., 47:1973, 1968.

Stanbury, J. B., Wyngaarden, J. B., and Fredrickson, D. S.: The Metabolic Basis of Inherited Disease. 3rd ed. New York, McGraw-Hill Book Company, 1972.

Steiner, D. G., and Freinkel, M. (eds.): Handbook of Physiology, Section 7, Endocrinology. Vol. I, Endocrine Pancreas. Washington, D.C., American Physiological Society, 1972.

Tattersall, R. B., and Pyke, D. A.: Diabetes in identical twins. Lancet, 2:1120, 1972.

Vracko, R.: Basal lamina layering in diabetes mellitus. Diabetes, 23:94, 1974.

807. HYPOGLYCEMIC DISORDERS

Norbert Freinkel

Homeostatic mechanisms are geared to preserve blood sugar within a narrow range. Fall of blood sugar to a concentration which elicits symptoms caused by glucose deprivation in the central nervous system constitutes hypoglycemia. It is a manifestation of homeostatic failure and can be caused by a variety of diseases. By arbitrary definition, hypoglycemia in adults has been equated with values for blood sugar below 40 mg per 100 ml (or plasma or serum glucose below 45 to 50 mg per 100 ml).

Because of intermittent eating, all human intermediary metabolism can be subdivided into two categories: the fed state and the fasted state. The fed state begins whenever we eat, and regulation at this time is designed to provide *synchronized* storage and anabolism from the ingested nutrients. When levels of circulating fuels have returned to pre-eating values, the fasting state is initiated. Regulatory processes are then geared to recall the various foodstuffs from stores in an integrated fashion that is parsimonious and yet appropriate to the prevailing needs for fuel in the central nervous system and periphery.

The pathophysiology of hypoglycemia and its attendant symptoms are substantially different in the fed state and in the fasting state. The distinctions justify classification of the hypoglycemic disorders on the basis of their relation to meals (see accompanying table).

HYPOGLYCEMIA IN THE FED STATE

Pathophysiology. Increased amounts of insulin can be demonstrated in the peripheral circulation within a few minutes after eating. Concentration of plasma insulin parallels the rise and fall of blood sugar. However, the decrement of insulin lags somewhat behind that of glucose so that normoglycemia is restored before circulating insulin returns to pre-eating levels.

Because of the anatomic location of the pancreas, insulin reaches the liver sooner and in greater amounts

---

Pathophysiologic Classification of Hypoglycemic Disorders

I. Hypoglycemia in the fed state ("overutilization" during the disposition of meals; reactive hypoglycemia)
  A. Relative excess of insulin
    1. Alimentary hyperinsulinism
    2. Reactive hypoglycemia of mild maturity-onset diabetes mellitus
    3. Leucine hypersensitivity of infancy and childhood
  B. Accumulation of metabolites which inhibit resumption of hepatic glucose output
    1. Fructose-1-phosphate aldolase deficiency (hereditary fructose intolerance)
    2. Galactose-1-phosphate uridyl transferase deficiency (galactosemia)
    3. Familial fructose and galactose intolerance
  C. Mechanism unknown
    1. Functional hypoglycemia

II. Hypoglycemia in the fasting state ("underproduction" during the metabolism of endogenous fuels; spontaneous hypoglycemia)
  A. Absolute production failure (intrinsic limitations in the hepatic capacity for glucose output)
    1. Diffuse hepatoparenchymal disease
    2. Defects in liver enzymes for
      a. Final common pathway
        (1) Glucose-6-phosphatase deficiency (glycogen storage disease, Type I)
      b. Glycogen turnover
        (1) Amylo-1,6-glucosidase deficiency (glycogen storage disease, Type III)
        (2) Defects in the phosphorylase enzyme system (glycogen storage diseases, Types VI and VIII)
        (3) Glycogen synthetase deficiency (aglycogenosis)
      c. Gluconeogenic formation of glucose-6-phosphate from smaller fragments
        (1) Pyruvate carboxylase deficiency
        (2) Fructose-1,6-diphosphatase deficiency
  B. Relative production failure (insufficient glucose output from intrinsically normal hepatocytes)
    1. Insulin excess
      a. Functioning pancreatic islet cell tumors
      b. Pancreatic islet cell hyperplasia
      c. Multiple endocrine adenomatosis (MEA I syndrome)
      d. Epithelioid tumors from foregut anlage
      e. Neonatal hypoglycemia in infants of diabetic mothers
      f. Neonatal hypoglycemia in erythroblastosis fetalis
    2. Deficiency of contrainsulin hormones
      a. Panhypopituitarism
      b. Primary hypoadrenocorticism
      c. Isolated deficiency of growth hormone
      d. Isolated deficiency of ACTH
      e. Hypothyroidism
    3. Limitations in the availability of gluconeogenic substrates
      a. Ketotic hypoglycemia of childhood
      b. Fasting hypoglycemia of late pregnancy
    4. Insulin-independent, supranormal removal of glucose
      a. Severe exercise
      b. Renal glycosuria
    5. Mechanism unknown
      a. Massive nonpancreatic tumors associated with hypoglycemia
      b. Neonatal hypoglycemia in low birth weight infants
      c. "Idiopathic hypoglycemia" of infancy and childhood

III. Hypoglycemia induced in the fasting state (pharmacological interruption of gluconeogenesis, fatty acid oxidation, or both)
  A. Induced insulin excess
    1. Administration of insulin
    2. Administration of oral hypoglycemic agents
  B. Direct inhibition, independent of insulin
    1. Alcohol hypoglycemia
    2. Ingestion of unripe ackee fruit ("Jamaican vomiting sickness"; hypoglycin intoxication)
  C. Mechanism unknown
    1. Salicylates

than any other structure. During an acute insulin secretory response to eating, net hepatic production of glucose is "turned off" almost immediately. It is "turned on" again when blood sugar returns to normal. However, even in normal subjects, there may be some lag resulting in a transitory hypoglycemic overshoot. The lag is exaggerated in those regulatory disturbances of the fed state which manifest themselves by symptomatic hypoglycemia during the disposition of meals. Such disorders reflect sluggish or thwarted resumption of hepatic glucose output with consequent prolongation of the period of net utilization of alimentary glucose (i.e., "overutilization").

Classification. In pediatric practice, hypoglycemia in reaction to eating may be caused by dietary components which produce excessive release of insulin (e.g., leucine sensitivity of infancy or childhood) or inhibitory metabolites which accumulate owing to inherited enzyme defects (e.g., galactose-1-phosphate in galactosemia; fructose-1-phosphate in hereditary fructose intolerance). However, in adults the hypoglycemias in the fed state are usually caused by one of the following three patterns of disturbed interactions between glucose and insulin during alimentation.

When prior *gastrectomy or surgical bypass of the pylorus* enables ingested glucose to have more rapid access to absorptive sites in the small bowel, the prompt rise in blood sugar may elicit secretion of insulin that is greater than normal, although appropriate to the hyperglycemia. Rapid utilization of glucose follows as blood sugar falls to pre-eating levels, and the "extra" insulin is not buffered by continuing absorption from a reservoir of carbohydrate within the gastrointestinal tract. This has been designated as "alimentary hyperinsulinism." An analogous situation can occur in normal persons when prolonged infusions of glucose sufficient to sustain hyperglycemia are abruptly terminated, or in patients undergoing hemodialysis when dialysates containing large amounts of glucose are withdrawn suddenly.

When *glucose absorption is normal and releases of insulin are sluggish,* attenuation of hepatic glucose output and net deposition of glycogen may be retarded, so that blood sugar rises more than normally. This can occur in mild, early maturity-onset diabetes mellitus and lead to another type of reactive hypoglycemia. The continuing stimulus to insulin secretion produces plasma levels of insulin that are high but perhaps subnormal in relation to the blood sugar. In such a setting of laggard islet cell response, relative hyperinsulinism may prevail once the utilization of glucose exceeds the rate of influx from the intestine.

More than two thirds of the hypoglycemias that occur in the fed state in adults remain unexplained and have been designated as *"functional hypoglycemia."* Herein, normal or exaggerated "hypoglycemic rebounds" with profound attendant symptoms may occur with seemingly normal rates of glucose absorption, disposition, and insulin release. Functional hypoglycemia is particularly frequent in thin, tense, hyperkinetic young women and tends to occur in subjects with vagotonia and compulsive, conscientious, and intense personality patterns. It may also be encountered in patients with peptic ulcer.

Signs and Symptoms. Signs and symptoms of the hypoglycemias in the fed state can be readily understood when viewed as "overutilization" during *non-steady-state conditions.* They are characterized by precipitous onset and by features of acute epinephrine release, e.g., tachycardia, tremulousness, sweating, weakness, anxiety, nervousness, and hunger. Although the hyperepinephrinemia is triggered by glucose deprivation in the central nervous system, the duration of hypoglycemia is usually too brief to elicit additional signs of central glucopenia other than faintness, inability to concentrate, and sometimes mental confusion or visual disturbance. Consciousness is almost always preserved. The hypoglycemia is evanescent and self-limited, because the extra insulin released in response to alimentation has a finite persistence and glycogen is deposited in the liver during the induction of the hypoglycemia. Thus as soon as sufficient counter-regulation is activated (the hyperepinephrinemia is one expression), glycogenolysis corrects the hypoglycemia.

However, such a benign course is not invariable. Hypoglycemic coma can occur in subjects with reactive hypoglycemia, especially when they are receiving therapy with autonomic blocking agents such as propranolol. Thus beta receptor blockade can impair the activated lipolysis and muscle glycogenolysis by which resistance to insulin may be induced and alternate fuels and gluconeogenic precursors mobilized during hypoglycemic rebound. Similarly, in subjects with compromised cardiovascular function, even evanescent hypoglycemia and hyperepinephrinemia may provoke angina, ectopic cardiac rhythms, pulmonary edema, and episodes of transient cerebral ischemia.

Diagnosis. Since *fasting* blood sugar is never abnormally low in the aforementioned disorders, diagnosis depends upon eliciting the hypoglycemia during reproduction of the fed state with oral tests of glucose tolerance. The time at which hypoglycemia becomes manifest depends on the factors that determine the hypoglycemic rebound. Thus in alimentary hyperinsulinism, hypoglycemia usually occurs one to three hours after glucose administration; in maturity-onset diabetes, the characteristic diabetic oral glucose tolerance curve is followed by transitory hypoglycemia during the fourth or fifth hour; and functional hypoglycemia is seen during the third or fourth hour. To maximize the diagnostic value of the test, blood samples are obtained at least every 30 minutes for five hours. The signs and symptoms ascribed to hypoglycemia should coincide with nadir values for blood sugar. Professional personnel should be in attendance throughout so that vital signs may be monitored regularly and blood sampled as soon as symptoms occur. The evanescent nadir may be missed by adherence to a fixed schedule of blood sampling even with intervals as short as 30 minutes. Increments in plasma cortisol should also be demonstrable 30 to 60 minutes after the symptomatic event and may be used as further evidence that the hypoglycemia threatens homeostasis. Rigid diagnostic criteria are imperative because neurasthenic symptoms unrelated to blood sugar, such as the hyperepinephrinemia of anxiety attacks, are easily confused with true reactive hypoglycemia. Particularly in functional hypoglycemia, oral glucose tolerance may be normal when tested in the hospital under conditions divorced from daily stresses, and abnormal only in a "real-life" outpatient setting. Hence a single negative glucose tolerance test need not exclude the diagnosis of hypoglycemia in the fed state; more frequent monitoring of blood sugars during symptomatic episodes may be required.

Treatment. General objectives are to dampen the elevations in blood sugar which elicit the subsequent excessive hypoglycemic rebounds. Multiple small feedings have constituted one approach. However, regular meal-eating with diets high in protein (120 to 140 grams), low in carbohydrate (75 to 100 grams), and sufficient in fat to maintain caloric adequacy have been more efficacious. Although long experience has corroborated that high protein, low carbohydrate diets diminish the frequency of all the hypoglycemias in the fed state, their mechanism of action remains unexplained.

Certain more specific therapies may be useful. Phenformin, a drug that slows absorption of glucose from the gastrointestinal tract, has been reported to help in alimentary hyperinsulinism. The postprandial hypoglycemia of early maturity-onset diabetes mellitus may be ameliorated by improving insulin-glucose interrelationships with weight reduction or oral hypoglycemic agents. However, the entity may also disappear spontaneously as the diabetes worsens and lesser absolute amounts of insulin are released in response to dietary stimulation. Reassurance and judicious use of mild sedatives or tranquilizers may be beneficial in functional hypoglycemia. In the light of existing knowledge, adrenocortical steroids have no place in the treatment of these hypoglycemic disorders.

SPONTANEOUS HYPOGLYCEMIA IN THE FASTING STATE

Pathophysiology. By the time of waking from overnight sleep, all energy requirements of the body are fulfilled from endogenous resources. Prevailing blood sugar then reflects a balance between the continuing utilization of endogenously derived glucose and the production of additional glucose via gluconeogenesis from smaller fragments to replace the glucose lost. The reliance of the brain on glucose for its oxidative demands determines the major metabolic objective of the fasted state, that is, to produce sufficient glucose for normoglycemia to be preserved. Since net production of glucose requires catabolism of structural protein, the second objective is to restrict utilization of glucose to a minimum. The following adaptations facilitate these objectives: (1) glucose utilization is restrained in most extracerebral tissues, and the more expendable fatty acids are substituted as oxidative fuels; (2) hepatic gluconeogenesis effects essentially complete recovery of lactic acid so that tissues which rely upon glycolysis for energy (e.g., red blood cells, renal medulla) can function without a *net* expenditure of glucose; and (3) hepatic ketogenesis generates lipid products which can cross the blood-brain barrier and replace glucose for *some* of the oxidative needs of the brain once *sufficient ketonemia becomes established.*

The net rate of glucose removal is the physiologic pacesetter for the equilibrium between glucose utilization and production by which normoglycemia is maintained in the fasted state. Hypoglycemia occurs when the liver is unable to "keep up" with rates of glucose removal.

As detailed elsewhere in this text, recent studies permit the relationships in adults to be formulated in quantitative terms. Splanchnic glucose output in normal man after overnight fast approximates 180 grams

per day; 80 per cent of that is oxidized completely to carbon dioxide by nervous tissue, chiefly the brain, whereas the remainder undergoes only glycolysis with the formation of lactate which is recycled to glucose. Since postprandial hepatic glycogen averages only 70 to 75 grams, some de novo formation of glucose is mandatory even after overnight fast. The precursors for the net formation of new glucose have been estimated as originating approximately 50 per cent from amino acids (of which alanine accounts for more than half) and 10 per cent from glycerol derived during lipolysis.

Data are not available concerning the maximal capacity for gluconeogenesis in normal human liver. However, extrapolations from in vitro studies and infusions of gluconeogenic precursors suggest that the biosynthetic ceiling is several-fold greater than the aforementioned values. Thus normal regulation may be delimited largely by the factors which influence the extrahepatic generation of substrates for gluconeogenesis.

Classification. Spontaneous hypoglycemias in the fasting state represent "underproduction" of hepatic glucose and may be classified as "absolute" or "relative" (see table).

The "absolute" production failures are uncommon and arise when intrinsic anatomic or enzymic abnormalities in the liver compromise its capacity to elaborate enough glucose to offset normal rates of glucose utilization in the periphery. Limitations resulting from enzyme deletions are usually confined to pediatric practice. In adults, it used to be held that fasting hypoglycemia via "absolute" production failure occurs only with fulminant hepatic necrosis, very extensive destruction of parenchyma, or severe hepatic congestion secondary to heart failure. However, the recent finding of asymptomatic low blood sugars after overnight fast in patients with viral hepatitis suggests that less severe hepatic disease can cause hypoglycemia.

"Relative" production failures are far more common. They occur when normal hepatocytes cannot "keep up" with normal or supranormal rates of glucose utilization owing to functional restraints to hepatic glucose output, inadequate generation of endogenous substrates for gluconeogenesis, or both. In most instances, additive factors are operative. For example, direct inhibition of glucose release and ketogenesis in the liver may be combined with restrained lipolysis and protein catabolism and enhanced peripheral glucose utilization to effect the fasting hypoglycemia of insulin excess (see table).

Signs and Symptoms. The fasting hypoglycemias develop slowly, so that manifestations of acute epinephrine discharge are usually not observed. Instead, the clinical picture is dominated by signs and symptoms of more prolonged and severe glucose deprivation in the brain. These may range from confusion, disorientation, and memory lapses to psychotic behavior, paresthesias, transient paralysis, convulsions, and coma. Sclerotic cerebral vessels with selectively compromised blood supply may account for focal abnormalities such as hemiplegias and monoplegias. Vulnerability of different parts of the brain to glucopenia is in reverse order of phylogenetic development. Hence the cerebral cortex is affected first. However, no single constellation of nervous system involvement is diagnostic. Fasting hypoglycemia should be suspected whenever a neuropsychiatric or neurologic complex occurs repeatedly, especially *before breakfast* or after "skipped meals," and is ameliorated almost immediately by food. In these states, reactive hypoglycemia can also occur, presumably because the factors impairing glucose production during fasting may equally restrain resumption of hepatic glucose output during the postprandial hypoglycemic rebound.

Diagnosis. Diagnosis of fasting hypoglycemia presupposes that inadequate delivery of glucose to the brain can be duplicated by simply withholding all food. In normal subjects, normoglycemia and mental acuity are preserved even with prolonged fasting, although blood sugar stabilizes at somewhat lower plateaus from the second or third day onward. Sex differences become manifest after 24 hours; nadirs for plasma glucose averaging 66 mg per 100 ml in normal men compared with 48 mg per 100 ml in normal women have been observed during the second or third day of fasting. Hence criteria for "fasting hypoglycemia" based solely on arbitrary lower limits for normal blood sugar may require modification.

Certain findings may occur in all the fasting hypoglycemias without regard to etiology. For example, Whipple's triad of (1) symptomatic hypoglycemia, (2) low blood sugar, and (3) alleviation by glucose ingestion is not pathognomonic for any single entity. Similarly, exercise may precipitate symptomatic hypoglycemia in any of these disorders, because it promotes glucose utilization independent of insulin action and thereby overtaxes marginal glucose production. Procedures should be designed to differentiate between hypoglycemia resulting from insulin excess, lack of contrainsulin factors, or compromise of other factors which preserve the normal equilibrium between glucose production and utilization in the fasting state (see table).

For optimal interpretability, safety, and rigorous exclusion of pharmacologic lowerings of blood sugar by drugs or other *exogenous* agents, diagnostic evaluation should be conducted in the hospital.

FUNCTIONING ISLET CELL TUMORS

Functioning adenomas of the beta cells of the pancreatic islets are the most common cause of fasting hypoglycemia. They are usually single, although multiple adenomas have been reported in 4 to 10 per cent of the cases. Approximately 10 per cent are malignant and 0.5 to 1 per cent are ectopic, usually within the splenic hilum, pancreatic bed, or duodenal wall. A family history of diabetes mellitus is present in approximately 25 per cent of the cases. Peak incidence is encountered between ages 40 and 60; however, cases have been seen in all age groups, although with extreme rarity in infancy and early childhood. Single adenomas are distributed with equal frequency in the head, body, and tail of the pancreas. The incidence of benign adenomas shows no sex difference, whereas malignant functioning islet tumors may be more common in males. In certain instances, functioning islet cell tumors are associated with other endocrine adenomas, particularly in the pituitary, parathyroid, and adrenal (multiple endocrine adenomatosis, Type 1), so that search for multiple endocrinopathy should be instituted whenever disorders of any of these glands occur, especially on a familial basis. Peptic ulcer disease also deserves investigation, because it has been reported in 10 per cent of all islet cell tumor patients, and many believe that the Zollinger-Ellison

syndrome (see Ch. 640 to 644) and multiple endocrine adenomatosis may represent phenotypic variants of the same mutant gene.

Diagnosis. Specific diagnosis of functioning islet cell tumors requires demonstration of (1) inappropriately elevated insulin levels during hypoglycemia when food is withheld, and (2) excessive insulin release in response to certain islet secretagogues.

Levels of plasma total immunoreactive insulin above the upper limits of normal (25 μU per milliliter) in association with subnormal blood sugar occur in approximately two thirds of patients when blood samples are obtained after overnight fast on at least three separate days. Recognition that meaningful quantities of circulating insulin should no longer be demonstrable at plasma glucose levels of 30 mg per 100 ml has expanded the diagnostic potential of insulin measurements. In this context, "normal" insulin levels may be abnormal when associated with fasting hypoglycemia. Such inappropriate relationships between insulin and glucose may be unmasked by prolonging the period of dietary deprivation (and sampling blood repeatedly at six-hour intervals) whenever normoglycemia still prevails after overnight fast. The recent demonstration that proinsulin can account for a greater than normal proportion of fasting plasma total immunoreactive insulin (i.e., greater than 20 per cent) in some, but not all, patients with islet cell tumors may provide yet another diagnostically useful characterization. It should be emphasized that modest elevations of basal insulin per se can be encountered in a variety of states associated with insulin resistance, such as obesity or acromegaly. However, these are never associated with fasting hypoglycemia.

For provocative challenge with islet secretagogues, oral or intravenous glucose has proved unrewarding, and no characteristic patterns have emerged. On the other hand, the insulin secretory response to intravenous tolbutamide (1 gram dissolved in 20 ml of saline and given intravenously over two minutes) is supranormal (i.e., increments greater than 120 μU per milliliter above baseline) in approximately 80 per cent of patients with functioning islet cell tumors; leucine (0.2 gram per kilogram orally or intravenously) elicits greater than normal increases of plasma insulin (i.e., in excess of 30 μU per milliliter) in approximately 70 per cent; and the stimulated release of insulin that follows 1 mg of intravenous glucagon exceeds the peak normal response (i.e., greater than 130 μU per milliliter) in somewhat more than 50 per cent. Since maximal insulin responses occur early, within 3 to 30 minutes after administration of the secretagogue, diagnostic evaluation can be terminated before serious hypoglycemia supervenes. Although equally exuberant releases of insulin may follow tolbutamide or glucagon administration in obesity, acromegaly, pregnancy, and other states associated with heightened basal insulin secretion, the subsequent hypoglycemia is not commensurate with the hyperinsulinemia under such circumstances. Therefore both blood sugar and insulin values should be monitored during provocative tests for insulinoma.

Treatment. *Surgery* constitutes the treatment of choice. Preoperative attenuation of hypoglycemia may be achieved with 100 to 200 mg hydrocortisone per day and appropriate dietary supplementation. The nondiuretic benzothiadiazine, diazoxide, in doses of 200 to 800 mg per day has proved more effective, by inhibiting insulin secretion directly as well as by exerting peripheral actions. Because of its sodium-retaining properties, diazoxide should be combined with a natriuretic thiazide such as trichlormethiazide (2 to 4 mg per day). These medications should be discontinued two days preoperatively.

At surgery, the pancreas should be mobilized and explored carefully for single or multiple lesions that can be "shelled out." Preoperative localization by selective pancreatic arteriography has been successful in approximately 40 per cent of the limited number of instances in which it has been tried. Quite frequently, however, all efforts at visualization and palpation of the tumor fail. Under such circumstances, the tail and then the body of the pancreas should be excised sequentially, because this will remove a significant proportion of the insulinomas. Failure to find tumor on serial sectioning justifies subsequent excision of most of the head of the pancreas but avoiding duodenal and bile duct resection. Such surgical aggressiveness requires unequivocal preoperative diagnostic confidence—a circumstance that insulin immunoassays have made possible today. Monitoring of blood samples during surgery may also be helpful; a sharp rise in blood sugar within 30 minutes after excision of tumor affords presumptive evidence against residual functioning tumor in situ or additional tumors elsewhere.

Successful extirpation of tumor (or tumors) effects complete and prompt cure. However, nonresectable islet cell carcinomas may be functional and accompanied by hypoglycemia. Long-term symptomatic palliation with diazoxide and trichlormethiazide or hormones such as glucocorticoids, long-acting glucagon, or growth hormone has been tried. *Streptozotocin,* a broad-spectrum antimicrobial with relatively selective cytotoxicity for pancreatic beta cells, has proved more rewarding. In 52 patients with metastatic pancreatic islet cell carcinoma treated with streptozotocin, measurable response has been observed in 50 and 63 per cent of those with functional and nonfunctional tumors, respectively. Response included tumor regression, rectification of hyperinsulinism, and more than threefold improvement in survival. The renal and hepatic toxicities of streptozotocin, although appreciable, usually have been reversible.

EXTRAPANCREATIC NEOPLASMS ASSOCIATED WITH HYPOGLYCEMIA

Over 200 instances of massive extrapancreatic neoplasms (ranging from 1.5 to 20 pounds) associated with fasting hypoglycemia have been reported. Four major tumor groups have been involved. Approximately half have been mesothelial tumors (most commonly classified as fibromas, fibrosarcomas, spindle cell sarcomas, and leiomyosarcomas); 20 per cent have been malignant hepatomas; gastrointestinal carcinomas (particularly of the stomach, colon, and bile ducts) and adrenocortical carcinomas have each accounted for about another 10 per cent. The rest have been miscellaneous tumors. About 80 per cent of the tumors have been intra-abdominal.

Although the pathophysiology of this hypoglycemia is not fully understood, it has been associated in a number of cases with heightened glucose utilization by the tumor and restrained hepatic glucose output. Increased plasma immunoreactive insulin has not yet been demonstrated unequivocally with any of these neoplasms.

In this they differ from the smaller epithelioid tumors which are embryologically derived from the same foregut anlage as the islets. The latter on rare occasions have insulin secretory potential, and one bronchial carcinoid tumor has been described in which increased immunoreactive insulin was demonstrated in plasma as well as in primary and metastatic tumor tissue.

Massive extrapancreatic tumors associated with fasting hypoglycemia can be readily distinguished from insulinomas. Plasma immunoreactive insulin is low and usually appropriate to the prevailing hypoglycemia. Responses to tolbutamide and leucine are usually subnormal in terms of glucose as well as insulin, most likely because islet function has been dampened by the antecedent hypoglycemia.

Therapy should be directed toward total surgical excision, or as much tumoricidal ablation as possible. When such therapy is successful, the hypoglycemia has usually disappeared. Glucocorticoids, glucagon, growth hormone, and dietary manipulations have been helpful in managing the hypoglycemia during preparation for surgery and, occasionally, when tumor therapy has been unsuccessful. Diazoxide has been tried also; efficacy has been somewhat less than in other fasting hypoglycemias, perhaps because of the smaller role played by pancreatic insulin.

HYPOGLYCEMIA INDUCED IN THE FASTING STATE

Pathophysiology. The hypoglycemias which arise *spontaneously* in the fasting state must be differentiated from another group of disorders, the hypoglycemias *induced* in the fasting state. Here, an *exogenous* agent has been introduced which can block the endogenous realignments by which normoglycemia is preserved when food is withheld. The resulting hypoglycemia may persist for the duration of the biologic effectiveness of the exogenous agent and engender considerable diagnostic confusion in the unwary.

Classification and Manifestations. Two broad groups can be delineated: the hypoglycemias caused by *induced* insulin excess and those caused by drugs which directly impair homeostatic mechanisms, independent of insulin action (see table).

Induced insulin excess should always be suspected when hypoglycemic episodes have no well-defined, recurring pattern and when they involve individuals with ready access to hypoglycemic medications such as diabetics, relatives of diabetics, or medical and paramedical workers. The clinical picture in instances of *surreptitious or accidental administration of insulin* depends on the nature of the insulin involved. Short-acting preparations may elicit the hyperepinephrinemia and the clinical features characteristic of the hypoglycemias in the fed state. Contrariwise, long- or intermediate-acting preparations of insulin may effect a picture indistinguishable from the spontaneous hypoglycemias of the fasting state.

All the *sulfonylureas* have also been associated with life-threatening hypoglycemic comas, presumably owing to stimulation of excessive insulin release (see table). Vulnerability to this exaggeration of their action is greatest in the elderly, in newborns of diabetic mothers who have received sulfonylureas, and in subjects with reduced hepatic or renal capacities for metabolizing or excreting the drugs. Chlorpropamide has posed the greatest problem. As the longest-acting sulfonylurea, it has been implicated in 120 of the 220 known cases of coma caused by sulfonylurea drugs when used alone. The clinical hypoglycemic syndromes with all these agents have consisted of slowly evolving cerebral dysfunction progressing to coma.

Perhaps the most frequent cause of the hypoglycemias induced in the fasting state in adults is *ethanol* (see table). Although other factors may participate, the principal mechanism is by direct inhibition of gluconeogenesis resulting from the metabolism of alcohol in the cytoplasm of the liver. As each mole of ethanol is oxidized to acetaldehyde and then to acetate (or acetyl CoA) via alcohol and aldehyde dehydrogenase, respectively, two moles of NAD^+ are reduced. The ratio of $NADH/NAD^+$ thereby increases, a reductive environment supervenes, and NAD^+ is diverted from other reactions in the liver. Thus the citric acid cycle is restrained, and there is attenuation of the flux of precursors such as glycerol, lactate, and amino acids which enter the gluconeogenic sequence via NAD^+-dependent reactions. The duration of prior fasting required to lower blood sugar under such circumstances and the latency between imbibition and hypoglycemia depend upon (1) how much glycogen is present for sustaining hepatic glucose output while gluconeogenic renewal is blocked, and (2) how rapidly circulating glucose is being removed in the periphery. In normal adults, more than 24 hours of fasting are usually necessary; infants and children are far more vulnerable, and hypoglycemia may occur shortly after exposure to ethanol and after only minimal dietary deprivation.

The clinical signs differ little from other types of hypoglycemia occurring in the fasting state. However, the early mental changes are often mistaken for alcoholic inebriation so that help is not usually sought until patients become comatose. Even then, the transition from alcoholic stupor to hypoglycemic coma may be unsuspected. Hypothermia is common; trismus may be present; and convulsions are particularly prominent in infants and children. The relationship to prior ethanol ingestion need not be obvious. Alcohol oxidation is a linear function so that a relatively constant amount is oxidized per unit time. Therefore, depending upon initial intake, the generation of reducing equivalents within the liver may persist for many hours and at low blood alcohol levels. If there has been no intake of food, hypoglycemia can thus occur 6 to 20 hours after imbibition, and without any clinical signs of alcoholism.

The situation may be particularly complex and dangerous when several agents interact concurrently. For example, irreversible brain damage and even death have occurred from alcohol hypoglycemia in diabetic alcoholics who have received insulin during periods of spree drinking and dietary dereliction.

Salicylates warrant inclusion, because they account for most of the drug-induced hypoglycemias during the first two years of life. Because of the age group involved, salicylates have been associated with the greatest mortality of any hypoglycemic drug (33 per cent in 15 reported cases). The mechanism of hypoglycemic action remains unsettled (see table).

Diagnosis and Treatment. Recognition of hypoglycemia in these comatose patients is imperative. Failure to do so, and to treat accordingly, accounted for fatal ter-

minations in 25 per cent of the children and 11 per cent of the adults with alcohol hypoglycemia reported before 1962. As in all hypoglycemic comas, a high index of suspicion improves prognosis, and response to glucose is usually dramatic unless brain damage has been sustained. However, in the induced hypoglycemias, especially when caused by sulfonylureas, the effect of the drug may be prolonged, and continued administration of glucose, with frequent monitoring of blood sugar, may be necessary for several days. After the patient has been stabilized, it must be established whether the hypoglycemia in the fasting state was *spontaneous* or *induced*. This can only be done in a hospital, because rigorous supervision may be required to exclude *exogenous* agents (as in factitious hyperinsulinism). After the cause of induced hypoglycemia has been established, no definitive therapy may be required save for dietary instruction, psychiatric help when necessary, and other attempts to modify exposure to the offending agent. However, it must be appreciated that vulnerability to the hypoglycemic potential of drugs like alcohol is far greater in individuals in whom endogenous capacities for gluconeogenesis or lipolysis are already marginal. Therefore diagnostic work-up of the functions that influence blood sugar homeostasis in the fasting state is also indicated. Such evaluations have unmasked occult diseases (e.g., hypopituitarism, hypoadrenocorticism) in several instances.

Broder, L. E., and Carter, S. K.: Pancreatic islet cell carcinoma. Ann. Intern. Med., 79:101, 108, 1973.
Cahill, G. F., Jr.: Starvation in man. N. Engl. J. Med., 282:668, 1970.
Conn, J. W., and Pek, S.: Current concepts: On spontaneous hypoglycemia. Scope Monograph. Kalamazoo, Michigan, The Upjohn Company, 1970, pp. 1–33.
Felig, P., Brown, W. V., Levine, R. A., and Klatskin, G.: Glucose homeostasis in viral hepatitis. N. Engl. J. Med., 282:1436, 1970.
Freinkel, N., and Bleicher, S. J.: The physiologic basis for evaluation of "fasting hypoglycemias." Am. J. Surg., 105:730, 1963.
Freinkel, N., Cohen, A. K., Sandler, R., and Arky, R. A.: Alcohol hypoglycemia: A prototype of the hypoglycemias induced in the fasting state. In Proceedings of the VIth Congress of the International Diabetes Federation, Stockholm, July 30–August 4, 1967. Amsterdam, Exerpta Medica International Congress Series No. 172, 1969, pp. 873–886.
Freinkel, N., and Metzger, B. E.: Oral glucose tolerance curve and hypoglycemias in the fed state. N. Engl. J. Med., 280:820, 1969.
Merimee, T. J., and Fineberg, S. E.: Homeostasis during fasting. II. Hormone substrate differences between men and women. J. Clin. Endocrinol. Metab., 37:698, 1973.
Pagliara, A. S., Karl, I. E., Haymond, M., and Kipnis, D. M.: Hypoglycemia in infancy and childhood, Parts I and II. J. Pediatr., 82:365, 558, 1973.
Seltzer, H. S.: Drug-induced hypoglycemia. Diabetes, 21:955, 1972.
Sherman, B. M., Pek, S., Fajans, S. S., Floyd, J. C., Jr., and Conn, J. W.: Plasma proinsulin in patients with functioning pancreatic islet cell tumors. J. Clin. Endocrinol. Metab., 35:271, 1972.
Smith, H. M. (ed.): Diazoxide and the treatment of hypoglycemia. Ann. N.Y. Acad. Sci., 150:191, 1968.
Unger, R. H.: The riddle of tumor hypoglycemia. Am. J. Med., 40:325, 1966.
Yalow, R. S., and Berson, S. A.: Dynamics of insulin secretion in hypoglycemia. Diabetes, 14:341, 1965.

808. GALACTOSEMIA

Ernest Beutler

The galactosemias are disorders characterized by inability to metabolize galactose normally. When individuals with galactosemia ingest galactose, either in its free form or as the galactose-containing disaccharide, lactose, galactose and some of the products of its incomplete metabolism accumulate in the blood, tissues, and usually the urine. Two types of galactosemia may be distinguished: "classic" or *transferase deficiency galactosemia* caused by a lack of galactose-1-phosphate uridyl transferase activity, and *galactokinase deficiency galactosemia.*

CLASSIC GALACTOSEMIA

Etiology. "Classic galactosemia" is due to a marked deficiency of the enzyme galactose-1-phosphate uridyl transferase. This deficiency is inherited as an autosomal recessive disorder.

Incidence. The incidence of classic galactosemia is approximately 1 per 80,000 births in the white population. The incidence may be somewhat higher in the black population.

Pathogenesis. The galactose molecule is identical to the glucose molecule except for the relative position of the hydroxyl and hydrogen groups attached to the fourth carbon. However, the body is unable to utilize this sugar until it has been converted to glucose. Only one pathway for the metabolism of galactose has been clearly established. First, galactose is phosphorylated in the 1-position by ATP through the mediation of the enzyme galactokinase:

$$\text{Galactose} + \text{ATP} \xrightarrow{\text{galactokinase}} \text{galactose-1-P}$$

Next, the galactose-1-P formed exchanges with the glucose-1-P moiety attached to a uridine disphosphate carrier. This reaction is catalyzed by galactose-1-phosphate uridyl transferase (transferase):

$$\text{Galactose-1-P} + \text{UDPG} \xleftrightarrow{\text{transferase}} \text{glucose-1-P} + \text{UDPGal}$$

Finally, the uridine diphosphogalactose (UDPGal) formed may be converted to uridine diphosphoglucose (UDPG) through the action of epimerase:

$$\text{UDPGal} \xleftrightarrow{\text{epimerase}} \text{UDPG}$$

In classic galactosemia the absence of galactose-1-phosphate uridyl transferase activity results in accumulation of both galactose and galactose-1-P. Galactose may serve as a substrate for aldose reductase and for L-hexonate dehydrogenase. These enzymes oxidize NADPH, reducing galactose to its polyol derivative, dulcitol, to which cell membranes are relatively impermeable. In the lens of the eye, this creates an unbalanced osmotic force, resulting in excessive hydration. At the same time, it may deplete the lens of its supply of NADPH. The result of these changes is the irreversible precipitation of the lens protein with the formation of cataracts.

In addition, cirrhosis of the liver and mental retardation are characteristics of classic galactosemia. Since these changes do not occur in galactokinase deficiency (see below), it may be presumed that they are the result of galactose-1-phosphate accumulation.

Clinical Manifestations. Occasionally galactosemic infants may have cataracts at birth. More typically the symptoms of galactosemia begin within a few days or weeks of birth. The infant takes feedings poorly, vomits frequently, and may have diarrhea. Many galactosemic infants die in the first few weeks of life. The abdomen may enlarge owing to progressive hepatomegaly and ascites. Jaundice usually appears quite early, and the disorder has at times been mistaken for hemolytic disease of the newborn. Proteinuria and generalized aminoaciduria are constant findings. If they are not present at birth, cataracts may develop within a few weeks or, in some instances, not for many months. Mental retardation becomes evident as the infant matures. Administration of large galactose loads, as in the performance of galactose tolerance tests, may produce dangerous hypoglycemia.

Diagnosis. Classic galactosemia is diagnosed by demonstrating that galactose-1-P uridyl transferase activity is absent from the erythrocytes.

Treatment. The treatment of galactosemia consists of institution of a diet with a very low galactose content as soon as the diagnosis is established. Because milk contains a high concentration of lactose, a disaccharide of glucose and galactose, a milk substitute such as Nutramigen must be fed during infancy. Although the effectiveness of the low-galactose diet is established in infants, no data are available regarding the necessity for maintaining strict dietary control after the first few years of life. It is likely that the ingestion of small amounts of galactose is relatively harmless after the fifth or sixth year of life. However, until further evidence is available regarding the possible harmful effects of galactose when fed to older galactosemic children and adults, it is probably wise to continue a moderate degree of dietary restriction throughout life.

Prognosis. Untreated infants with classic galactosemia rarely survive more than a few months, and may succumb within a few days. A few cases first diagnosed in later childhood or early adult life are known. With the prompt institution of a low-galactose diet, the development of galactosemic children appears to be normal or nearly so. If treatment is delayed, however, some degree of permanent mental retardation and irreversible cataracts is often present. Signs of liver failure and growth retardation appear to respond promptly to therapy in most instances, however, and treated galactosemics generally survive into adult life.

Prevention. Galactosemia itself can only be prevented through genetic counseling. Heterozygotes for classic galactosemia have one half normal galactose-1-P uridyl transferase activity in their red cells. However, not all persons with this level of enzyme activity are carriers of galactosemia. Persons homozygous for another gene, that for the Duarte variant, also have one half of normal transferase activity, but may be differentiated from those heterozygous for galactosemia on the basis of the electrophoretic properties of the red cell enzyme.

Prevention of the clinical sequelae of galactosemia by early diagnosis and prompt institution of treatment is the most practical means of control. Microbiologic and enzymatic methods for the detection of galactose in the blood or in the urine have been developed and will detect most cases of classic galactosemia in the neonatal period. However, some false positive results are encountered, and false negative results will be found in infants who are so ill as to refuse their feedings. A fluorescent screening test which depends directly upon galactose-1-P uridyl transferase activity will reliably detect classic galactosemia even from cord blood. Prenatal diagnosis can be achieved by assaying cultured amniotic cells for galactose-1-P uridyl transferase.

Segal, S.: Disorders of galactose metabolism. *In* Stanbury, J. B., Wyngaarden, J. B., and Fredrickson, D. S. (eds.): The Metabolic Basis of Inherited Disease. 3rd ed. New York, McGraw-Hill Book Company, 1972, pp. 174–195.

Beutler, E., Matsumoto, F., Kuhl, W., Krill, A., Levy, N., Sparkes, R., and Degnan, M.: Galactokinase deficiency as a cause of cataracts. N. Engl. J. Med., 288:1203, 1973.
Kalckar, H. M., Kinoshita, J. H., and Donnell, G. N.: Galactosemia: Biochemistry, genetics, patho-physiology, and developmental aspects. Biol. Brain Dysfunct., 1:31, 1972.

GALACTOKINASE DEFICIENCY

Etiology. Galactokinase deficiency is a genetically determined disorder caused by an autosomally inherited enzyme deficiency.

Incidence. Only about 20 families with galactokinase deficiency have been described. However, the true incidence of the disorder is probably larger than this very small number of cases would suggest, because the disorder was first described only in 1965. Limited data suggest that the incidence may be of the order of 1 in 500,000 births, and that as many as 1 in 100 patients developing cataracts of unknown origin during the first year of life may have this defect.

Pathogenesis. Galactokinase catalyzes the first step of galactose metabolism (see above). In galactokinase deficiency, galactose accumulates in the body and produces cataracts through the same mechanism outlined under Classic Galactosemia.

It is uncertain whether only individuals with virtually total absence of galactokinase develop cataracts from galactokinase deficiency. Since galactose is the limiting enzyme in galactose metabolism, it is possible that repeated large galactose loads may result in lenticular damage even in individuals heterozygous for galactokinase deficiency who have one half normal galactokinase activity. An increased incidence of cataracts has been noted among heterozygotes in some families of galactokinase-deficient persons. However, most individuals heterozygous for galactokinase deficiency do not develop cataracts, and the link between partial galactokinase deficiency and cataracts cannot be considered to be firmly established.

Clinical Manifestations. The only clinical manifestation of galactokinase deficiency is the development of cataracts. After ingestion of galactose, elevated blood galactose levels and galactosuria may be found.

Diagnosis. The diagnosis of galactokinase deficiency should be considered in any person developing cataracts of unknown cause during childhood. The diagnosis is established by assaying the galactokinase activity of the red blood cells.

Treatment. The treatment of galactokinase deficiency consists of institution of a low-galactose diet (see above).

Prognosis. If a low-galactose diet is initiated at the time of birth or shortly thereafter, cataract formation is prevented. When cataracts are already present, some improvement may occur on institution of galactose restriction, particularly in the very young.

Prevention. The effects of galactokinase deficiency can be prevented by early detection and institution of a low-galactose diet. Detection of heterozygotes can be accomplished by measuring galactokinase activity in red cells. Genetic counseling can therefore be carried out with families in which a case of galactokinase deficiency has been found. Screening of the blood of neonates by methods which detect increased blood galactose level makes possible early detection so that treatment can be instituted promptly.

809. GLYCOGEN STORAGE DISEASE

J. B. Sidbury, Jr.

Definition. The glycogenoses are a group of heritable disorders of altered glycogen metabolism. Excluded are conditions associated with secondary glycogen accumulation such as Mauriac's syndrome and steroid therapy. A glycogen storage disease was the first inborn error of metabolism to be enzymatically defined. Cori's original classification into four types has been extended progressively to 13. Additions to the original classification have been made in the chronology of the enzymatic definition, except for Type 0 which is so designated because it is characterized by a deficiency of glycogen. Subtypes are designated to reflect different clinical presentation of the same enzymatic defect or when differences in the enzyme can be discerned without a distinguishing phenotypic pattern.

Etiology. The evidence available is compatible with autosomal recessive transmission except in Type IX which is sex linked. The symptoms associated with Types 0, I, III, IV, IX, XI, and XII can be ascribed to the inadequacy of liver glycogen availability, and the severity of symptoms is related to the degree of impediment in glycogen conversion to blood glucose. In Type IV the symptoms evolve from the resultant cirrhosis. The muscle glycogenoses, Types V, VII, VIII, and X, have symptoms resulting from the inadequacy of glycolysis in the muscle which is usually evident only with vigorous exercise.

Clinical Manifestations. The enzymatic deficiency of Type 0 results in inadequate rate of glycogen synthesis, and since the rate of degradation is normal, the inadequate glycogen stores are rapidly depleted and hypoglycemia results. Gluconeogenesis alone is inadequate in the infant to sustain the blood glucose. Symptoms are often not manifest until the frequency of feedings is decreased. The other *liver forms* of glycogenosis (see accompanying table) may have symptoms so similar as to be clinically indistinguishable, and the symptoms vary from difficult, symptomatic hypoglycemia and ketoacidosis to essentially asymptomatic hepatomegaly. Types I and III are more likely to be symptomatic, and the associated findings seen are susceptibility to infections, bleeding tendency, short stature, mild cushingoid features, excessive sweating, and eruptive xanthoma. Gout is unique to Type I, and it is not generally symptomatic until after puberty despite an elevation of uric acid throughout the course. The clinical management of the more symptomatic individuals is most difficult in the first five years of life. As a rule all symptoms and the hepatomegaly resolve with puberty or before in all the classic hepatic types except Type I. In patients with Type IV defect, death almost invariably supervenes as a result of the cirrhosis and portal hypertension before puberty. This is the only glycogen storage disease with splenomegaly.

The Enzymatically Defined Glycogenoses

Type	Defect	
0	UDPG-glycogen transferase	(L)
Ia	Glucose-6-phosphatase	(L)
Ib	Glucose-6-phosphatase, functionally	(L)
IIa,b	Lysosomal α-1,4-glucosidase	(M)
IIIa,	Amylo-1,6-glucosidase and/or	
b,c,d	oligo-1,4→1,4-glucantransferase*	(L)
IV	Amylo-1,4→1,6-transglucosylase*	(L)
V	Muscle phosphorylase	(M)
VI	Liver phosphorylase	(L)
VII	Phosphofructokinase	(M)
VIII	Phosphohexosisomerase	(M)
IX	Phosphorylase kinase	(L)
X	Phosphorylase kinase	(M)
XI	Phosphoglucomutase	(L)
XII	Cyclic 3′,5′-AMP dependent kinase	(L)

*Glycogen structure abnormal.
(L) Symptoms related to liver.
(M) Symptoms related to muscles.

The *muscle types* of glycogenosis, V, VII, VIII, and X, involve striated muscle. The symptoms may be first noted in early childhood (V, VII, and X) or not until the mature years (VIII). The day-to-day symptoms are unimpressive as are the physical findings, and these individuals are often labeled psychoneurotic for several years before the diagnosis is made. Vigorous exercise is associated with weakness, muscle cramps, and occasionally myoglobinuria. Symptoms tend to be slowly progressive. Seizures associated with myoglobinuria have been reported in individuals with the phosphorylase defect.

Type IIa designates classic *Pompe's disease* or generalized glycogenosis which is seen in infants who appear to be normal for the first two or three months of life and progress to flaccidity, absent reflexes, gross cardiomegaly, and death by one year of age. Patients with Type IIb, with apparently the same enzyme defect, do not have the heart involvement and present simulating relatively severe muscular dystrophy in the first few years of life or as a progressive myopathy in the teen years or later.

Diagnosis. The definitive diagnosis of glycogen storage disease is made by enzymatic assay of liver and/or muscle obtained by biopsy. The glycogen is characterized and the content determined. Enzymatic assays of leukocytes can be useful in Types III, IV, VI, and IX. Skin fibroblasts grown in culture have been shown to be useful in diagnosis and in the determination of heterozygosity in Types II and IV, and antenatal diagnosis is possible using these techniques. An antibody to glucose-6-phosphatase has been prepared which will detect the enzyme in the serum of normal individuals and gives no precipitin lines with the sera of patients with Type I glycogenosis. The response of blood glucose and lactate to the glucagon tolerance test is useful in that the blood glucose usually does not respond in Types I, III, and VI, and in Type I the lactate is high in the fasting state with a further increase in response to the glucagon. The red cell glycogen may be elevated markedly in Type III.

Types V, VII, VIII, and X are characterized by absence of rise in blood lactate consequent to anoxic exercise. This is performed by having the subject exercise the hand with the blood pressure cuff above the elbow inflated above systolic pressure and by obtaining blood from the antecubital vein at intervals for several minutes. The normal individual will have a two- to fourfold rise, whereas the muscle glycogen patients will have none. Type II glycogenosis patients show no abnormality of carbohydrate metabolism that can be approached through blood sampling. Electromyography can be helpful. In the muscle glycogenoses of impaired glycolysis, the signal becomes isoelectric after a period of vigorous exercise. The "dive bomber" effect is characteristically found in Type IIb glycogen storage. Type IIa muscle does not demonstrate a characteristic finding.

Treatment. Types I, II, III, and IV are the most likely to be management problems. Individuals with the Type I defect are at risk of severe ketoacidosis in association with infection in the early years. This complication, like the symptomatic hypoglycemia which is frequently seen, is best managed by frequent high carbohydrate feedings. Portacaval shunt has been found to relieve many of the biochemical aberrations, and preoperative intravenous hyperalimentation for two to three weeks reduces the operative risk. This approach should be considered only for the more severely ill patients. Patients with Type III glycogenosis and the occasional patient with the other forms of hepatic glycogenoses who are symptomatic will respond to a high protein diet with additional carbohydrates when symptomatic. Patients with Type IV glycogenosis are treated symptomatically as one would treat any other child with cirrhosis and portal hypertension. The infant with Type II glycogenosis is managed symptomatically. Digitalis is used for heart failure, but there is little evidence of its efficacy. Patients with glycogen myopathies associated with impaired glycolysis are symptomatic when engaged in vigorous exercise. They must be taught to modulate their activity and seek employment appropriate to their physical capacities. It is reported that fructose administration will help patients with Type VIII glycogen storage disease.

Cori, G. T.: Glycogen structure and enzyme deficiencies in glycogen storage disease. Harvey Lectures, 48:145, 1953.

Moses, S. W., and Gutman, A.: Inborn errors of glycogen metabolism. *In* Schulman, I. (ed.): Adv. Pediatr., 19:95, 1972.

810. PENTOSURIA
(Essential Pentosuria)
J. B. Sidbury, Jr.

Pentosuria is a clinically asymptomatic, rare, heritable abnormality of carbohydrate metabolism limited almost exclusively to Jews. It is transmitted as an autosomal recessive condition, with estimated incidence of 1:2000 to 1:5000 of the population at risk. Loading of the glucuronic acid cycle by oral administration of glucuronolactone will cause an increase in urinary 1-xylulose excretion in the homozygote and a lesser response in the heterozygote. Assay of the erythrocytes of affected individuals has demonstrated a deficiency of the specific NADP-linked xylitol dehydrogenase which converts 1-xylulose to xylitol and has further shown that the affinity of the mutant enzyme for NADP is significantly less than that from normal individuals. As a consequence of the enzyme reduction in the liver, affected individuals excrete 1 to 4 grams of 1-xylulose in the urine daily. The sugar can easily be distinguished from others by paper or thin-layer chromatography.

Glucose oxidase, which is the reagent in the dip-stick type of urine test, will not react with this sugar, whereas the reducing methods will. The practical importance of proper identification is in preventing the individual from being labeled a diabetic for treatment and insurance purposes.

Hiatt, H. H.: Pentosuria. *In* Stanbury, J. B., Wyngaarden, J. B., and Fredrickson, D. S. (eds.): The Metabolic Basis of Inherited Disease. 3rd ed. New York, McGraw-Hill Book Company, 1972, p. 119.
Wang, Y. M., and VanEys, J.: The enzymatic defect in essential pentosuria. N. Engl. J. Med., 282:892, 1970.

811. FRUCTOSURIA AND HEREDITARY FRUCTOSE INTOLERANCE

J. B. Sidbury, Jr.

Fructosuria (Essential Fructosuria). Fructosuria is an asymptomatic, rare, autosomal recessive condition resulting from a deficiency of fructokinase, which is the first reaction in the major pathway of fructose metabolism. The incidence of the condition is estimated to be 1:130,000. Fructokinase is normally found only in the liver, kidney, and intestinal mucosa. The diagnosis can be surmised by performing a fructose loading test determining the fructose rise in the blood by difference between total reducing substance and glucose and by identifying the fructose excreted in the urine by chromatography. Normally, under loading conditions the blood fructose will peak at one hour and not exceed 25 mg per 100 ml. No significant fructosuria occurs. Fructose will not react with glucose oxidase but will reduce copper sulfate, even at 80° C. The proper diagnosis is important to the patient in order to prevent his being labeled or treated as a diabetic.

Hereditary Fructose Intolerance. This is an autosomal recessive condition associated with a structural alteration of phosphofructoaldolase B. The adult will commonly note dyspepsia and anxiety with fructose ingestion but usually will have learned to avoid offending foods through personal observation. The untreated infant will have vomiting, failure to grow, hypotonia, jaundice, hepatosplenomegaly, ascites, bleeding disorder, hypoglycemia, hypophosphatemia, abnormal liver function tests, aminoacidemia, acidosis, uric acid elevation, proteinuria, mellituria (fructose and sometimes galactose and glucose also), and aminoaciduria. The clinical presentation and findings often make the differential diagnosis between this condition, tyrosinosis, and galactosemia very difficult indeed. Liver biopsy reveals portal and interlobar fibrosis without cellular infiltrate, steatosis, bile retention, and rosette formation. The reported pathology in the kidney is variable. The brain may show diminished neurons. The mechanism of the symptomatology is unclear when the defect is defined in terms of the inability to cleave fructose-1-phosphate to the corresponding trioses. That the symptoms might be similar to those of galactosemia is not surprising, because galactose-1-phosphate accumulates in the cells in galactosemia. In fructose intolerance fructose-1-phosphate accumulates in the liver and kidney, the two primary organs in which fructose is metabolized. Thus symptoms are secondary or tertiary phenomena. The hypoglycemia results from a marked decrease in glucose production by the liver very shortly after fructose loading in these individuals. In spite of the recurrent hypoglycemia in infancy, the affected adults evaluated have had normal intelligence.

The defective enzyme, phosphofructoaldolase B or liver aldolase, has been shown to be decreased in total activity but more specifically to function in a manner analogous to aldolase A or muscle aldolase in that aldolase B normally demonstrates a 1:1 ratio of activity for fructose-1-phosphate and fructose-1,6-diphosphate, whereas aldolase A normally has a ratio of activity for these substrates of approximately 0.1 to 0.2. Kinetic studies of the mutant enzyme have shown a markedly reduced affinity for fructose-1-phosphate. Immunologically the mutant enzyme cross-reacts with the normal and quantitatively correlates with the activity for fructose diphosphate. The enzyme in the liver of parents showed no abnormality.

A presumptive *diagnosis* can be made in an individual whose symptoms are suggestive by an oral or intravenous loading test. Serious hypoglycemia can be induced; hence modified loading doses are recommended, e.g., 0.5 gram per kilogram of body weight orally or 0.25 gram per kilogram intravenously, or 3 grams per square meter of body surface area in children. Demonstrating resultant hypoglycemia, fructosemia, hypophosphatemia, and fructosuria constitutes presumptive evidence for the diagnosis. *Management*, once the diagnosis is made, is simply avoidance of fruits and foods with sucrose.

Froesch, E. R.: Essential Fructosuria and Hereditary Fructose Intolerance. *In* Stanbury, J. B., Wyngaarden, J. B., and Fredrickson, D. S. (eds.): The Metabolic Basis of Inherited Disease. 3rd ed. New York, McGraw-Hill Book Company, 1972, p. 131.
Nordmann, Y., and Schapira, F.: Intolérance au fructose. Biochimie, 54:741, 1972.
Odievre, M., Gantier, M., and Rieu, D.: Intolérance héréditaire au fructose du nourrisson. Arch. Franç. Péd., 26:433, 1969.

812. PRIMARY HYPEROXALURIA

Lloyd H. Smith, Jr.

Primary hyperoxaluria is a general term for two rare genetic disorders of glyoxylate metabolism productive of excessive synthesis and urinary excretion of oxalic acid. Both disorders are transmitted as autosomal recessive traits. The diseases are characterized by the onset in childhood of recurrent calcium oxalate nephrolithiasis or nephrocalcinosis, or both, usually leading to early death secondary to renal failure. At postmortem examination calcium oxalate may be found widely deposited in extrarenal sites, a condition known as oxalosis. More rarely, milder forms of the disease may be found in adults. Athough oxalate is an important constituent in approximately two thirds of all kidney stones, most adult patients with calcium oxalate nephrolithiasis excrete normal amounts of urinary oxalate.

Primary hyperoxaluria Type I (glycolic aciduria) represents a genetic defect in the soluble enzyme α-ketoglutarate: glyoxylate carboligase. The resulting accumulation of glyoxylate leads to its excessive oxidation to oxalate and its reduction to glycolate, both of which are excreted in increased amounts in the urine (more than 60 mg per 1.73 square meters per 24 hours each).

In *primary hyperoxaluria Type II* (L-glyceric aciduria) there is a defect in the enzyme D-glyceric dehydrogenase. Hydroxypyruvate accumulates and is reduced by lactic dehydrogenase (LDH) to L-glyceric acid, a compound which is undetectable in normal urine. The reduction of hydroxypyruvate to L-glycerate is probably coupled to the oxidation of glyoxylate to oxalate, both catalyzed by LDH. Each disease can be diagnosed by the characteristic pattern of metabolites in urine: Type I, oxalate and glycolate; Type II, oxalate and L-glycerate. Pyridoxine deficiency in laboratory animals and man also leads to hyperoxaluria and even oxalosis with a urinary pattern similar to that of the genetic disease Type I. With the onset of renal failure the clearance of oxalate is reduced (normally about 1.2 times the creatinine clearance) so that its urinary excretion may return to normal. The diagnosis may then be difficult to establish because of the unreliability of current methods for measuring serum oxalate.

No specific methods of treatment are now available. Efforts are directed toward reducing the amount of oxalate excreted and increasing its solubility. Large amounts of pyridoxine (200 to 400 mg per 24 hours) may decrease oxalate excretion in the Type I disease. Dilute urine should be maintained by forcing fluids, and a phosphate supplement seems to offer partial protection against stone formation. Attempts at renal homotransplantation have been disappointing because of rapid deposition of calcium oxalate in the transplanted kidney. A search for a more effective inhibitor of oxalate synthesis is being conducted.

An important cause of secondary hyperoxaluria has recently been found. Increased urinary excretion of oxalate and stone diathesis (in the absence of glycolic aciduria or L-glyceric aciduria) occurs in many patients who have small bowel disease and malabsorption. This form of acquired hyperoxaluria results from excessive absorption of dietary oxalate. It can be controlled by a low oxalate diet.

Boquist, L., Lindquist, B., Östberg, Y., and Steen, L.: Primary oxalosis. Am. J. Med., 54:673, 1973.
Chadwick, V. S., Modka, K., and Dowling, R. H.: Mechanism of hyperoxaluria in patients with ileal dysfunction. N. Engl. J. Med., 289:172, 1973.
Hockaday, T. D. R., Clayton, J. E., Frederick, E. W., and Smith, L. H., Jr.: Primary hyperoxaluria. Medicine, 43:315, 1964.
Williams, H. E., and Smith, L. H., Jr.: Disorders of oxalate metabolism. Am. J. Med., 45:715, 1968.
Williams, H. E., and Smith, L. H., Jr.: Primary hyperoxaluria. In Stanbury, J. B., Wyngaarden, J. B., and Fredrickson, D. S. (eds.): The Metabolic Basis of Inherited Disease. 3rd ed. New York, McGraw-Hill Book Company, 1972, p. 196.

DISORDERS OF LIPID METABOLISM

Richard J. Havel

813. INTRODUCTION

Changes in the concentration of lipids in blood plasma occur in a variety of disease states or as a result of inborn errors. In the former, they may provide a clue to diagnosis of the underlying condition. More important, deleterious consequences may occur in both, in-

cluding premature atherosclerotic vascular disease and recurrent pancreatitis. Taken together, the inborn hyperlipidemias are among the most common metabolic diseases. It is important to recognize them, because reasonably effective treatment is available which may prevent disability and delay death.

814. TRANSPORT OF LIPIDS IN THE BLOOD

Because of their insolubility in aqueous environment, essentially all lipids in blood plasma are in complexes (lipoproteins) containing amphiphilic substances which permit the dispersal of the lipids into small particles. The major lipids transported are fatty acids and cholesterol. Fatty acids exist as such in a complex with albumin and as esters of which the main transport form is triglyceride. The former are called free fatty acids (FFA) to indicate that their carboxyl groups are not in ester linkage. Cholesterol is also transported in the "free" state (alcohol group not in ester linkage) or esterified with fatty acids. The amphiphilic substances which coat the surface of microdroplets of the neutral lipids or form soluble complexes with them are mainly phospholipids and specific proteins.

Exogenous Fat (Triglyceride) Transport. Dietary fat, after hydrolysis to form partial glycerides and fatty acids, is absorbed from micelles containing conjugated bile acids. From these products, triglycerides are resynthesized in the mucosal cells of the small intestine, appear in particulate form in the Golgi region, and are secreted into the intestinal lacteals. In the lymph, they appear as chylomicrons and are delivered into the blood through the thoracic duct. Normally, chylomicrons are present only during active absorption of fat, because their life span in the blood is only a few minutes. Triglycerides in chylomicrons are removed primarily in tissues other than the liver which contain on the endothelial surface of their capillaries an enzyme, lipoprotein lipase, which hydrolyzes the triglycerides to FFA and glycerol. These products readily diffuse across the capillary and other cell membranes where they are stored or oxidized.

Endogenous Fat Transport. Triglycerides, derived from fat transported in the blood or synthesized from nonlipid precursors, are stored mainly in adipose tissue. Normally, these triglycerides are hydrolyzed to FFA and glycerol at a variable rate controlled by the action of hormones and the adrenergic innervation of the tissue on a "hormone-sensitive" lipase. Catecholamines and growth hormone increase lipase activity, whereas insulin reduces it. The FFA, as albumin complexes, are rapidly transported to various tissues to be oxidized or stored temporarily as lipid esters. They are also the major precursors of endogenous plasma triglycerides, secreted continuously by the liver in particles similar to, but smaller than, chylomicrons (very low density, pre-beta lipoproteins, VLDL; Fig. 1). In the postprandial state, these triglycerides may be derived from dietary fatty acids or from fatty acids synthesized de novo in the liver; in the fasting state, they are derived mainly from plasma FFA. This pathway appears to provide a mechanism for exporting excess fatty acids to sites of storage or oxidation. The metabolism of VLDL-

PROPERTIES OF PLASMA LIPOPROTEINS

CLASS	HDL	LDL	VLDL			CHYLOMICRONS		
	100	200	300	500	800	800	2000	5000
• DIAMETER (Å)	○	○						
• DENSITY	1.06–1.21	1.006–1.063	0.95 – 1.006			0.94		
• ELECTROPHORETIC MOBILITY	α_1	β	PRE-β			ORIGIN		
PER CENT COMPOSITION								
• PROTEIN	50	20	15	7	4	4	2	1
• PHOSPHOLIPIDS	25	25	25	18	13	13	8	3
• CHOLESTEROL (FREE + ESTERS)	20	50	45	22	13	13	8	3
• TRIGLYCERIDES	5	5	15	53	70	70	82	93

Figure 1.   Properties of plasma lipoproteins. (From Havel, R. J.: Adv. Intern. Med., 15:117, 1969.)

triglycerides resembles that of chylomicrons, but their disposal is less efficient, and they remain in the blood for a considerably longer period.

Transport of Cholesterol.   Cholesterol (both free and esterified) is also transported in chylomicrons. The esterified cholesterol remaining in chylomicrons, "remnants," which are formed when triglycerides are taken up in various extrahepatic tissues, is removed in the liver. The free cholesterol may also be removed in the liver; alternatively, it may be transferred to high density lipoproteins (HDL), where it receives a fatty acid residue from lecithin in a transesterification catalyzed by the enzyme lecithin–cholesterol acyl transferase. Eventually, these esters are also taken up in the liver. The transferase may also promote the transport of cholesterol transferred to HDL from various tissues.

Role of Apolipoproteins.   Three major groups of apoproteins (termed A, B, and C apoproteins) have essential roles in lipid transport. The C apoproteins are transferred from HDL to newly secreted triglyceride-rich lipoproteins. One of them facilitates the hydrolysis of triglycerides by lipoprotein lipase. One of the A apoproteins has a similar role in the action of lecithin–cholesterol acyl transferase in HDL. The B apoprotein is essential for the formation of VLDL and chylomicrons. In the process of metabolism of triglycerides and cholesterol in chylomicrons and VLDL, this apoprotein appears in low density, beta lipoproteins (LDL). Normally, LDL contain most of the cholesterol and cholesteryl esters present in blood plasma; the latter presumably are transferred to LDL from HDL after they are

synthesized through the action of lecithin-cholesterol acyl transferase.

Fredrickson, D. S., Levy, R. I., and Lees, R. S.: Medical progress. Fat transport in lipoproteins—an integrated approach to mechanisms and disorders. N. Engl. J. Med., 276:34, 1967.

Glomset, J. A., and Norum, L. R.: The metabolic role of lecithin–cholesterol acyltransferase: Perspectives from pathology. *In* Advances in Lipid Research, Vol. 11. New York, Academic Press, 1973, p. 1.

Havel, R. J.: Mechanisms of hyperlipoproteinemia. *In* Holmes, W. F., Paoletti, R., and Kritchevsky, D. (eds.): Pharmacological Control of Lipid Metabolism. New York, Plenum Press, 1972, p. 57.

815. CLASSIFICATION AND ANALYSIS OF PLASMA LIPOPROTEINS

Plasma lipoproteins can be separated by electrophoresis or in the ultracentrifuge into the four main classes shown in Figure 1. In most disorders involving plasma lipoproteins, these classes do not differ substantially from normal in gross chemical and physical properties so that they are classified as hyper- or hypolipoproteinemias. In some states, lipoproteins differing from those normally comprising the bulk of a given class may accumulate; these are classified as dyslipoproteinemias.

For most clinical purposes, relatively simple methods will characterize these states. Two approaches are now

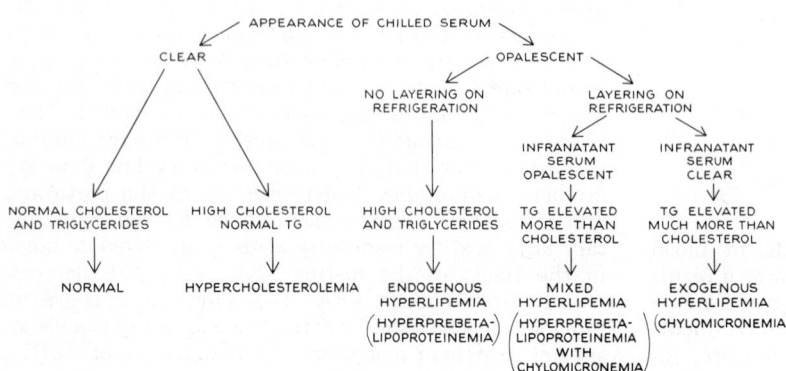

Figure 2.   Evaluation of hyperlipoproteinemias with simple techniques. (From Havel, R. J.: Adv. Intern. Med., 15:117, 1969.)

generally used. In both, the concentration of cholesterol and triglycerides is measured in fasting serum or plasma. From the actual and relative values of these constituents, certain inferences can be made concerning the lipoprotein class or classes involved. For better subclassification of the hyperlipemias (increased concentration of triglycerides), it is necessary to establish whether their source is *exogenous* (chylomicrons), *endogenous* (VLDL), or *mixed* (chylomicrons plus VLDL). This can usually be achieved by evaluating lactescence of serum chilled overnight in a refrigerator, because chylomicrons tend to form a creamy layer spontaneously, whereas VLDL do not (Fig. 2). Additional studies that can be used include electrophoresis on a supporting medium, such as paper, agarose gel or cellulose acetate, or measurement of light scattering before and after passing diluted serum through a microporous filter. The last-named method has the advantage of simultaneously providing a quantitative estimate of triglyceride concentration. In some instances, particularly in certain dyslipoproteinemias, classification may be uncertain so that additional methods are needed. However, combined information gained from examination of the patient and from the simple laboratory tests will permit classification in almost all cases.

Beaumont, J. L., Carlson, L. A., Cooper, G. R., Fejfar, Z., Fredrickson, D. S., and Strasser, T.: Classification of hyperlipidaemias and hyperlipoproteinaemias. Bull. WHO, 43:891, 1970.
Havel, R. J.: Hyperlipidemia: The significance and management. Modern Medicine, January 24, 1972.

816. NORMAL REGULATION OF PLASMA LIPOPROTEIN CONCENTRATION

Apart from chylomicrons, all lipoprotein classes are present in blood plasma at all times. Among these, the concentration of VLDL, the carrier of endogenous triglycerides, is most variable and is a function rate of hepatic triglyceride synthesis. This rate, in turn, depends upon rate of uptake of FFA from the blood or synthesis of fatty acids from glucose, and also upon the extent to which the fatty acids are oxidized or converted to triglycerides. Ingestion of glucose initially causes a rapid fall in level of VLDL, presumably related to the accompanying decrease in mobilization of fat from adipose tissue. After one to three days on a high carbohydrate, low fat diet, VLDL level tends to rise. The extent to which this reflects increased hepatic triglyceride synthesis or impaired removal of triglycerides in extrahepatic tissues is uncertain. Ingestion of foodstuffs in excess of need is accompanied by rapid increase in level of VLDL. In addition, in stable obesity, VLDL levels are increased. This has been equated with associated insulin resistance and hyperinsulinism, but the precise mechanism is not clear (see Ch. 723). Increased triglyceride and VLDL levels accompany several other states in which insulin resistance and hyperinsulinism are present.

Plasma levels of LDL and HDL tend to fall as VLDL levels rise, presumably because some components of these lipoprotein species also are constituent parts of VLDL. The concentration of HDL is regulated by sex hormones and hence is sex dependent; increases are

produced by estrogens and a fall by androgens. The level of LDL is also moderately sensitive to caloric intake, but is influenced more by specific dietary factors. In particular, fats containing saturated fatty acids and cholesterol increase the level of this cholesterol-rich lipoprotein. Substantial differences in lipoprotein levels occur in various population groups throughout the world. The major cause of these differences, which occur predominantly in cholesterol-rich LDL, appears to be dietary (see also Ch. 723).

Conner, W. E., Stone, D. B., and Hodges, R. E.: The interrelated effects of dietary cholesterol and fat upon human serum lipid levels. J. Clin. Invest., 43:1691, 1964.
Havel, R. J.: Caloric homeostasis and disorders of fuel transport. N. Engl. J. Med., 287:1186, 1972.

817. INBORN ERRORS OF LIPOPROTEIN METABOLISM

HYPERLIPOPROTEINEMIAS

Whereas characterization of the lipoprotein class or classes responsible for hyperlipoproteinemia in a patient is generally straightforward, establishment of a definitive diagnosis in inherited forms of hyperlipoproteinemia frequently is difficult and may not be possible. There are two major reasons for this. First, lipoprotein concentrations vary with time in an affected individual as well as among affected family members. Second, a given abnormality may represent more than one disorder and pattern of inheritance. Thus both monogenic and polygenic disorders may lead to the same phenotype. The most widely used system of classification, introduced by Fredrickson, defines six patterns or phenotypes: I, elevated chylomicrons; IIa, elevated LDL; IIb, elevated LDL and VLDL; III, elevated beta-migrating VLDL with increased content of cholesterol; IV, elevated VLDL; and V, elevated VLDL and chylomicrons. In the three most common types, IIa, IIb, and IV, classification by this system frequently fails to identify a specific disorder. Thus an obese individual, initially classified as Type IV, may, with sufficient loss of weight, be classified as Type IIa. Further, individuals classified as Type IV may belong to kindreds in which IIa, IIb, and IV all occur commonly; in other kindreds all affected individuals belong to Type IV. Fortunately, treatment of such individuals may be determined simply from quantitative estimation of serum cholesterol and triglycerides, as described earlier, after exclusion of the acquired disorders described below.

Familial Hyperbetalipoproteinemia
(Hypercholesterolemia, Type IIa Hyperlipoproteinemia)

Familial hyperbetalipoproteinemia, inherited as a mendelian dominant trait, is characterized by increased concentration of LDL of normal composition. Xanthomas in the tendons, particularly the Achilles, plantar, patellar, and digital extensors of the hands, as well as tuberous xanthomas, xanthelasmas, and early onset of corneal arcus, are frequently encountered. In adults, serum cholesterol concentration usually exceeds 350 mg per 100 ml. Its prevalence is not established, but it may occur in up to 1 per cent of the American population.

Etiology and Pathogenesis. The specific molecular or enzymatic defect responsible for the increased concentration of LDL is unknown, but recent studies suggest the presence of a cellular defect in the regulation of 3-hydroxy-3-methylglutaryl reductase, the enzyme controlling the rate-limiting step in cholesterol biosynthesis.

Clinical Manifestations. The hyperlipoproteinemia is present from birth or shortly thereafter, and is generally detected as hypercholesterolemia with little or no increase in triglycerides; the xanthomas usually do not appear until after puberty. The patient may not be aware of the presence of large xanthomas in the Achilles or plantar tendons, and the latter may be missed by the physician unless the tendon is put under tension by having the patient extend his toes. Small xanthomas of the extensor tendons of the hands are best detected by observing the tendon while the patient flexes and extends the finger, and small xanthomas in the Achilles tendon are detected by palpation of irregular contour, usually in the central region. Xanthelasmas (raised, yellow plaques about the eyelids near the inner canthus) and corneal arcus are not diagnostic, because they may also be seen in individuals with no discernible abnormality of plasma lipoproteins. The incidence of premature coronary heart disease is several times that of control populations in countries with a "western" culture, and the incidence of peripheral atherosclerotic occlusive disease is also increased. In the homozygous states, the disease is much more severe, with large xanthomas occurring in childhood, together with "malignant" atherosclerotic disease, including calcific aortic stenosis. A possible variant of the disease is seen in the Near East in which early occurrence of large xanthomas is common.

Diagnosis. Hypercholesterolemia without hypertriglyceridemia in the absence of known cause, such as hypothyroidism, is not sufficient basis for making a diagnosis unless the cholesterol level exceeds 400 mg per 100 ml. Presence of characteristic xanthomas is diagnostic, and demonstration of familial occurrence (at least one parent should have hyperbetalipoproteinemia) provides strong presumptive evidence. Some individuals or families may have moderate hypertriglyceridemia (Type IIb). This must be distinguished from familial dysbetalipoproteinemia, described below. Most normotriglyceridemic individuals whose cholesterol level is 275 to 325 mg per 100 ml (also classified as Type II hyperlipoproteinemia) have a different disorder, which may be polygenic (see Ch. 819).

Treatment. No simple method has been devised to reduce lipoprotein levels to normal. Some reduction can be achieved by a diet restricted in saturated fats and cholesterol, with sufficient polyunsaturated fats to provide a total fat intake of 30 to 35 per cent of calories. Nonabsorbable bile acid–binding substances, such as cholestyramine (15 to 30 grams daily in divided doses with meals), are more effective. Large doses of nicotinic acid (5 to 12 grams daily in divided doses) may also be effective. These drugs may in some cases reduce lipoprotein levels to normal. Surgical bypass of the terminal 150 cm of the ileum, which also prevents absorption of bile acids, generally gives good results. Frequent, loose stools are generally produced by this operation. In post-

menopausal women, estrogens may provide some improvement. Thyroxine and its analogues, especially d-thyroxine (4 to 8 mg daily) and the ethyl ester of p-chlorophenoxyisobutyrate, occasionally give good results. Xanthomatous lesions regress slowly; tendinous lesions seldom disappear. It is reasonable to begin treatment in childhood, although it has not been established that reducing the lipoprotein level will prevent or delay onset of ischemic vascular disease.

Familial Dysbetalipoproteinemia
(Broad-Beta Disease, Type III Hyperlipoproteinemia)

Definition. Familial dysbetalipoproteinemia is characterized by accumulation of abnormal beta lipoproteins, which resemble normal pre-beta migrating VLDL in size and flotation characteristics, but differ from them in composition. Planar xanthomas, particularly in the palmar and digital creases, are peculiar to this form of primary hyperlipoproteinemia, but tuberous, tuberoeruptive, and tendinous lesions also occur. It is much rarer than familial hyperbetalipoproteinemia; in the older literature, it was frequently called *xanthoma tuberosum*. The mode of inheritance is uncertain.

Etiology and Pathogenesis. The abnormal lipoprotein contains predominantly the B apoprotein together with a basic protein, unusually rich in arginine, in particles with more cholesteryl ester and less triglyceride than normal VLDL. Its electrophoretic mobility is also abnormal, encompassing the beta and extending toward the pre-beta region ("broad beta"). This lipoprotein is thought to represent remnant-VLDL which accumulate because of abnormality in the mechanism responsible for uptake of cholesteryl esters in the liver.

Clinical Manifestations. The disorder is seldom discovered before early adult life and is usually manifested by appearance of xanthomas when the patient gains weight. The patient may be unaware of the characteristic planar xanthomas which are yellow to orange and tend to fill the palmar and digital creases; they may also appear over the dorsal surfaces of the hands. The tuberous xanthomas tend to be smaller and more numerous than in hyperbetalipoproteinemia and are often confluent and surrounded by an erythematous halo ("tuberoeruptive"). They occur most commonly over the knees and elbows and on the buttocks. Tendinous lesions are usually in the extensors of the hands. Premature coronary and peripheral atherosclerotic vascular disease are quite common. Overt diabetes mellitus is seldom seen, but slight degrees of glucose intolerance usually can be detected, as in the other forms of endogenous hypertriglyceridemia described below.

Diagnosis. Combined hypercholesterolemia and hypertriglyceridemia are always present. The levels of these two lipids are often similar, and they change rapidly with alterations in diet. Most patients have the characteristic planar xanthomas which, in the absence of obstructive biliary tract disease, are pathognomonic. The serum is usually lactescent. Lipoprotein electrophoresis shows a "broad-beta" pattern with normal or reduced content of alpha lipoproteins. Slight chylomicronemia is often present when hyperlipoproteinemia is severe. Spurious "broad-beta" bands may be seen in other states, particularly in some of the secondary hyperlipemias. Definitive laboratory diagnosis requires additional tests, such as ultracentrifugation of serum at its own density to demonstrate "floating-beta" lipoproteins.

Treatment. The mainstay of treatment is diet. In obese subjects, caloric restriction is almost always very effective. The diet should be restricted in simple sugars and in cholesterol but not in fat, which should provide 40 to 50 per cent of calories. Concentration of cholesterol and triglycerides will usually fall almost to normal. For patients who will not adhere to a dietary program and for the few who respond inadequately, the ethyl ester of p-chlorophenoxyisobutyric acid, 500 mg four times daily, will almost always produce a good response. Xanthomas invariably regress or disappear with effective reduction in lipid levels. There is some evidence that atheromatous lesions also regress (see Ch. 819). This disorder is greatly aggravated by hypothyroidism, in which a similar lipoprotein may accumulate. For this reason, thyroid function should always be carefully evaluated.

Primary Hyperlipemias

Exogenous Hyperlipemia
(Bürger-Grütz Syndrome, Type I Hyperlipoproteinemia)

Definition. This rare disease, inherited as a recessive trait, is characterized by accumulation of chylomicrons proportional to intake of dietary fat and manifested by recurrent acute pancreatitis, usually beginning in childhood.

Etiology and Pathogenesis. This disorder is caused by deficient activity of lipoprotein lipase with resultant defective removal of triglycerides from the blood. Hydrolytic activity with the characteristic properties of this enzyme on lipoprotein-bound triglycerides is almost absent in blood plasma obtained a few minutes after intravenous injection of heparin, although another lipase, thought to be derived from the liver, is present. In one family, no lipoprotein lipase activity could be demonstrated in adipose tissue.

Clinical Manifestations. Chylomicronemia develops as soon as fat is ingested, and the disorder has been diagnosed during the first week of life. Pancreatitis is very common, and many patients diagnosed in adult life have a history of bouts of abdominal pain in childhood. Abdominal pain, not definable as pancreatitis, has been reported frequently, but causes other than pancreatitis have not been established. Other complications, described rarely, include melena and pretibial ulcers. Like the pancreatitis, they may result from ischemia related to agglomeration of chylomicrons in capillaries. Hepatosplenomegaly, presumably the result of phagocytosis of chylomicrons by reticuloendothelial cells, is common, and hypersplenism has been described. Foam cells may be found in the bone marrow. The endogenous hyperlipemia occurring normally during pregnancy is greatly magnified and may lead to repeated attacks of pancreatitis. In infants and children especially, eruptive xanthomas—small yellow papules in the skin, surrounded by an erythematous halo—may occur when lipemia is severe. Lipemia retinalis—whitish reflection from retinal arterioles and venules—can usually be detected when triglyceride levels in plasma exceed 3000 mg per 100 ml and becomes florid with levels above 5000 mg

per 100 ml. Other xanthomas do not occur, and premature atherosclerotic vascular disease has not been described. Carbohydrate metabolism is normal.

Diagnosis. Markedly lactescent blood plasma in a young patient with severe midabdominal pain and no history of alcoholism is presumptive evidence for this disorder or one of the other primary hyperlipemias. In exogenous hyperlipemia, the chylomicrons rise to form a creamy layer when the serum is allowed to stand overnight in the refrigerator and the infranatant serum is usually limpid. Triglyceride concentration is increased far more than that of cholesterol, and the chylomicron band predominates on electrophoresis. Triglyceride levels fall dramatically when intake of dietary fat is severely restricted for two to three days. Lipolytic activity, measured in blood plasma obtained ten minutes after intravenous injection of 0.2 mg of heparin per kilogram of body weight, is reduced, and activity sensitive to inhibition by 0.5 M NaCl (a characteristic of lipoprotein lipase) is virtually undetectable.

Treatment. The only established measure is restriction of dietary fat ("saturated" and "polyunsaturated" fats are equivalent) sufficient to reduce fasting triglyceride levels to 500 mg per 100 ml or less. This usually requires an intake of no more than 30 grams per day by adults. On this regimen, xanthomas disappear and pancreatitis is uniformly prevented. Pretibial ulcers have also healed, and hypersplenism has subsided on this regimen. Once pancreatitis occurs, recurrence is very common when large amounts of fat are ingested and may happen within hours. During pregnancy, complete elimination of fat from the diet may be necessary to control hyperlipemia and minimize the possibility of pancreatitis.

Endogenous Hyperlipemia
(Types IIb and IV Hyperlipoproteinemia)

Definition. The term endogenous hyperlipemia encompasses a group of disorders, frequently shown to be familial, which are common in middle life. These disorders are characterized by accumulation of VLDL of normal composition and electrophoretic mobility and by insulin resistance. In some kindreds, the trait appears to be an autosomal dominant. The concentration of VLDL depends upon several environmental factors, and the true prevalence is unknown.

Etiology and Pathogenesis. Secretion of hepatogenous triglycerides in VLDL varies with quantity and quality of food intake, including ethanol, and with neural and hormonal responses to stress. These responses are generally magnified in endogenous hyperlipemia, in which there is evidence for impaired catabolism of VLDL-triglycerides as well as increased hepatic secretion, but the nature of these abnormalities is not known. Evidence that severity of the hypertriglyceridemia is related to hyperinsulinism and insulin resistance, together with the fact that gain in weight, which increases insulin resistance, almost uniformly increases the hyperlipemia, indicates a close relationship with disordered carbohydrate metabolism. The concentration of LDL may be low, normal, or elevated. In the latter case, the disorder is usually called combined hyperlipidemia (Type IIb). As indicated earlier, in some kindreds hyperlipoproteinemic individuals may have elevated LDL, elevated VLDL, or both, whereas in others all those affected have only elevated VLDL. The en-

XVII. DISEASES OF METABOLISM

dogenous hyperlipemias evidently represent several genotypes which condition the responses of VLDL and LDL to common environmental influences.

Clinical Manifestations.   Most commonly, the disorder is detected when patients with ischemic vascular disease are screened for metabolic abnormalities. Although endogenous hyperlipemia is commonly found in individuals who develop such disease prematurely, the incidence of vascular complications has not been established. The great majority of patients are at least moderately obese when hyperlipemia is found, but only a few have fasting hyperglycemia. With severe hyperlipemia, eruptive xanthomas and pancreatitis may occur, as in exogenous hyperlipemia.

Diagnosis.   The disorder should be suspected in obese subjects with premature vascular disease. It is diagnosed presumptively when fasting serum is lactescent with no layering on standing. When serum cholesterol is normal or is less than half the concentration of triglycerides, VLDL alone are generally increased. When serum cholesterol is elevated and equal to or greater than the triglyceride level, both LDL and VLDL are increased. Numerous other causes of endogenous hyperlipemia must be excluded (see Ch. 818).

Treatment.   Effective measures are available to reduce the level of VLDL, but it has not been shown that atherosclerotic lesions regress or that the progress of ischemic vascular disease is slowed. For obese patients, caloric restriction alone usually produces rapid reduction of serum triglycerides, often almost to normal. The diet should also be restricted in simple sugars as described for familial dysbetalipoproteinemia. If cholesterol remains elevated, dietary measures used to reduce LDL should also be employed. Ethyl ester of p-chlorophenoxyisobutyrate may be used for individuals with inadequate dietary response, as in familial dysbetalipoproteinemia. When added after the patient has responded partially to a dietary program, it usually reduces triglycerides further, but cholesterol levels often remain unchanged, indicating an increase in level of LDL at the expense of VLDL. Since there is no evidence that such a change is beneficial, treatment with the drug should be discontinued in such patients. Drugs used to reduce the level of LDL in familal hyperbetalipoproteinemia, such as cholestyramine, nicotinic acid, and d-thyroxine, may then be employed.

Mixed Hyperlipemia
(Type V Hyperlipoproteinemia)

Definition.   This is a rare disorder of adolescence and adult life, in which VLDL and chylomicrons of normal composition accumulate in the blood on ordinary diets. It is usually accompanied by overt, insulin-independent diabetes mellitus and often by eruptive xanthomas and recurrent acute pancreatitis.

Etiology and Pathogenesis.   The metabolic abnormalities in this disorder partake of both endogenous and exogenous hyperlipemia. In familial cases, insulin resistance is usually accompanied by fasting hyperglycemia, and postheparin lipolytic activity in plasma is often somewhat reduced. Possibly, multiple genetic defects are present which combine insulin resistance with defective activity of lipoprotein lipase. Some patients with endogenous hyperlipemia may accumulate chylomicrons when their lipemia is severe, particularly with ingestion of substantial quantities of ethanol; in these cases, the chylomicronemia may represent an "overload" phenomenon. In others, the distinction between endogenous and mixed hyperlipemia is blurred.

Clinical Manifestations.   The disorder usually presents in adolescence or early adult life with recurrent attacks of obscure abdominal pain, sometimes definable as acute pancreatitis. At onset of pain, lipemia is usually severe. Eruptive xanthomas are often present and frequently are confluent. As in exogenous hyperlipemia, hepatosplenomegaly and lipemia retinalis are often found. Overt hyperglycemia is only occasionally severe enough to produce symptoms of diabetes, and evidences of microangiopathy are usually absent. Hyperuricemia is also common. Obesity is frequent but by no means universal. In some patients, evidences of premature atherosclerotic vascular disease may be found, but incidence is not known to be increased.

Diagnosis.   Markedly lactescent serum, which separates into a creamy layer with persistent lactescence in the infranatant serum, provides presumptive evidence for mixed hyperlipemia. This can be confirmed by nephelometry or electrophoresis. Alcoholic hyperlipemia must be considered, particularly in patients presenting with abdominal pain, and diabetic hyperlipemia must be ruled out when hyperglycemia is severe and accompanied by ketoacidosis. Differentiation from exogenous hyperlipemia usually presents no problem and depends on the accompanying severe endogenous hyperlipemia, hyperglycemia, and normal or slightly reduced lipolytic activity in postheparin plasma.

Treatment.   For obese patients, restriction of caloric intake and ethanol usually reduces levels of both chylomicrons and VLDL effectively. For patients of normal body weight, avoidance of intermittent excesses of sugars, fat, or ethanol generally provides some improvement. The hyperglycemia usually responds to the caloric restriction or to addition of sulfonylurea drugs. Neither the sulfonylureas nor insulin, however, have a specific effect on the hyperlipemia. The ethyl ester of p-chlorophenoxyisobutyrate, given as described for familial dyslipoproteinemia, may be effective in some patients not responding to diet. Nicotinic acid, in doses of 1 to 2 grams three times daily, is frequently useful. As in exogenous hyperlipemia, recurrent pancreatitis is prevented by effective reduction of lipoprotein levels, and eruptive xanthomas disappear.

Fredrickson, D. S., and Levy, R. I.: Familial hyperlipoproteinemia. *In* Stanbury, J. B., Wyngaarden, J. B., and Fredrickson, D. S. (eds.): The Metabolic Basis of Inherited Disease. 3rd ed. New York, McGraw-Hill Book Company, 1972, p. 531.

Goldstein, J. L., and Brown, M. S.: Familial hypercholesterolemia: Identification of a defect in the regulation of 3-hydroxy-3-methylglutaryl coenzyme A reductase activity associated with overproduction of cholesterol. Proc. Natl. Acad. Sci. USA, 70:2804, 1973.

Havel, R. J., and Kane, J. P.: Drugs and lipid metabolism. *In* Elliott, H. W. (ed.): Annual Review of Pharmacology. Vol. 13. Palo Alto, Calif., Annual Review, Inc., 1973, p. 287.

Havel, R. J., and Kane, J. P.: Primary dysbetalipoproteinemia: Predominance of a specific apoprotein species in triglyceride-rich lipoproteins. Proc. Natl. Acad. Sci. USA, 70:2015, 1973.

Levy, R. I., et al.: Dietary and drug treatment of primary hyperlipoproteinemia. Ann. Intern. Med., 77:267, 1972.

Slack, J., and Nevin, N. D.: Hyperlipidaemic xanthomatosis: I. Increased risk of death from ischaemic heart disease in first degree relatives of 53 patients with essential hyperlipidaemia and xanthomatosis. II. Mode of inheritance in 55 families with essential hyperlipidaemia and xanthomatosis. J. Med. Genet., 5:4, 8, 1968.

Strisower, E. H., Adamson, G., and Strisower, B.: Treatment of hyperlipidemias. Am. J. Med., 45:488, 1968.

Thompson, G. R., and Gotto, A. M.: Ileal bypass in the treatment of hyperlipoproteinemia. Lancet, 2:35, 1973.

HYPOLIPOPROTEINEMIAS

These conditions are exceedingly rare, but they have considerable importance for the light that they shed on normal functions of plasma lipoproteins.

Abetalipoproteinemia
(Bassen-Kornzweig Syndrome)

This disease, inherited as an autosomal recessive, is characterized by complete absence of LDL, VLDL, and chylomicrons. The absence of the B protein appears to be accompanied by virtually complete loss of ability to transport triglycerides in the blood. It is manifested by severe malabsorption, beginning in early childhood, followed by progressive ataxia, nystagmus, distal sensory loss, weakness, and visual impairment with scotomas. These are related, respectively, to inability to deliver triglycerides into the intestinal lymph; demyelination of spinocerebellar tracts, posterior columns, and, occasionally, peripheral nerves; and pigmentary retinal degeneration ("atypical retinitis pigmentosa"). Other findings include peculiar thorny or spiny red cells (acanthocytes) and fatty liver (resulting from failure to export triglycerides in very low density lipoproteins). This disorder is also discussed in Ch. 438 and in Part XIV, Section Three.

Diagnosis is established by finding very low cholesterol concentration (about 50 mg per 100 ml) and almost no triglycerides in blood plasma in an individual with one or more of the characteristic symptoms. The disorder should be considered in any patient with hereditary ataxia. On paper electrophoresis only alpha lipoproteins are present, and blood smears or wet preparations show the characteristic acanthocytes. Treatment is limited to restriction of ordinary fat and supplementation with fat-soluble vitamins. Medium-chain triglycerides are well tolerated. Such measures have not been shown to alter the progressive and disabling course of the disease.

Hypobetalipoproteinemia

A few families have been described with low concentrations of beta lipoproteins. Some patients have had acanthocytes and late onset of neuromuscular difficulties.

Tangier Disease
(Alpha-Lipoprotein Deficiency)

This disorder, in the homozygous state, leads in childhood to diffuse deposition of cholesterol esters in reticuloendothelial tissues, with enlargement of liver, spleen, and lymph nodes, and especially to grossly enlarged tonsils with a characteristic orange color. Foam cells may be found in the bone marrow. In adults, flocculent corneal infiltrates may occur. Usually, the disorder does not affect growth, nutrition, or general health. Electrophoretic or ultracentrifugal examination shows almost no alpha lipoproteins or HDL, and one of the A proteins is reduced to about 1 per cent of the normal level. Heterozygotes have low concentrations of HDL but no other detectable abnormalities. In homozygotes, levels of LDL tend to be reduced, although

those of triglycerides and VLDL are high. No treatment is available. There is limited evidence that premature vascular disease may develop.

Lecithin–Cholesterol Acyltransferase Deficiency

This disorder has been found only in a few individuals in Scandinavia. Affected subjects have proteinuria, anemia, and corneal deposits of lipids. HDL are almost absent, levels of VLDL and chylomicrons are variably increased, and abnormal lipoproteins bearing some resemblance to those found in cholestasis are present (see Biliary Obstruction in Ch. 818). Cholesteryl esters comprise less than 10 per cent of total cholesterol in plasma (normal value about 72 per cent) and are found almost entirely in the triglyceride-rich lipoproteins. Their fatty acids are much more saturated than those produced normally by the plasma enzyme lecithin–cholesterol acyltransferase, and this enzyme cannot be detected. Other findings include foam cells in the bone marrow and renal glomeruli and increased concentration of cholesterol and lecithin in the red blood cells. The relationship between the enzyme deficiency and the various clinical and chemical abnormalities is uncertain.

Fredrickson, D. S., Gotto, A. M., and Levy, R. I.: Familial lipoprotein deficiency. *In* Stanbury, J. B., Wyngaarden, J. B., and Fredrickson, D. S. (eds.): Metabolic Basis of Inherited Disease. 3rd ed. New York, McGraw-Hill Book Company, 1972, p. 493.

Gjone, E., and Norum, K. R.: Familial serum cholesterol ester deficiency. Acta Med. Scand., 183:107, 1968.

818. ACQUIRED DISORDERS OF LIPOPROTEIN METABOLISM

HYPERLIPOPROTEINEMIAS

These conditions are important as clues to diagnosis or because they may be associated with premature atherosclerotic vascular disease.

Hyperbetalipoproteinemia

Hypothyroidism. Hyperbetalipoproteinemia is a characteristic finding in myxedema; hypothyroidism must be considered in all patients with this abnormality. All forms of hyperbetalipoproteinemia are accompanied by hypercarotenemia, but this is particularly striking in myxedema because of the additional defect in conversion of carotene to vitamin A. Occasionally, increased levels of VLDL are also present.

Dietary. Moderate degrees of hypercholesterolemia may occur in subjects ingesting large amounts of cholesterol, usually in eggs and dairy products.

Nephrotic Syndrome. Hyperbetalipoproteinemia is frequently observed in nephrotic states when serum albumin concentration falls below 3 grams per 100 ml. As the level of albumin falls below 1.5 grams per 100 ml, concentration of VLDL rises to produce the characteristic nephrotic hyperlipemia. Treatment is that of the underlying disorder.

Resolving Lipemias. As levels of chylomicrons or VLDL are reduced in various hyperlipemic states, the concentration of LDL usually rises, presumably reflecting the removal of triglyceride with liberation of constituent B protein and associated lipids. Such hyperbetalipoproteinemia may persist for days to weeks and can lead to confusion if the sequence is not appreciated.

Hyperadrenocorticism. Hyperbetalipoproteinemia of moderate degree is commonly seen in Cushing's syndrome and subsides with appropriate treatment.

Endogenous and Mixed Hyperlipemias

Diabetic Hyperlipemia. Mixed hyperlipemia is characteristic of prolonged insulin deficiency with ketosis. It is generally accompanied by fatty liver and by weight loss and other evidences of a catabolic state. It is not ordinarily seen with acute diabetic ketoacidosis. Defective removal of triglycerides and reduced lipolytic activity in postheparin plasma can be demonstrated. Eruptive xanthomas and lipemia retinalis are commonly seen. With administration of adequate insulin, triglyceride levels fall rapidly and cholesterol levels more slowly. Diabetic hyperlipemia must be differentiated from primary endogenous hyperlipemia and especially mixed hyperlipemia with its frequent associated hyperglycemia. These states are not accompanied by ketosis or wasting and do not respond to insulin.

Alcoholic Hyperlipemia. This lipemia, usually mixed, is seen in chronic alcoholics with fatty liver and good hepatic function. Diversion of fatty acids entering the liver to triglyceride synthesis accompanies oxidation of ethanol to acetate and appears to be the most important abnormality, but decreased activity of lipoprotein lipase has also been implicated. Some of these patients have underlying primary hyperlipemias, and ingestion of ethanol is an important factor aggravating primary endogenous and mixed hyperlipemias. The association of jaundice and hemolytic anemia with hyperlipemia has been described in patients with alcoholism (Zieve's syndrome), but it has not been shown that the features of this triad are causally interrelated. Pancreatitis and hyperlipemia may also coexist. It is unlikely that pancreatitis causes the hyperlipemia, because the association is confined almost entirely to alcoholics in whom these complications can occur separately. This situation must be clearly distinguished from occurrence of pancreatitis as a complication of one of the primary (usually exogenous or mixed) hyperlipemias.

Hyperlipemia in Glycogen Storage Disease Type I. Endogenous or mixed hyperlipemia is consistently found in children and adults. It is related both to increased hepatic secretion of triglycerides in VLDL and decreased activity of lipoprotein lipase. Measures decreasing delivery of absorbed carbohydrate to the liver may be helpful.

Hyperlipemia in Lipodystrophy. Hyperlipemia is consistently observed in generalized as well as in partial forms of lipodystrophy. The mechanism is not understood, especially in partial lipodystrophy; but, as in primary endogenous hyperlipemia, insulin resistance and hyperinsulinism are associated phenomena.

Stress Hyperlipemia. In a variety of situations, increased secretion of catecholamines, together with growth hormone and ACTH, can lead to hyperlipemia by increasing mobilization of fatty acids from adipose tissue to liver with resultant increased secretion of triglycerides in VLDL. Such hyperlipemia, appearing soon after myocardial infarction, can lead to confusion with primary endogenous hyperlipemia.

Administration of Contraceptive Steroids. Mild endogenous hyperlipemia is commonly produced by the estrogenic component of estrogen-progestogen mixtures and is associated with insulin resistance, hyperinsulinism, and decreased lipolytic activity in postheparin plasma.

Other Causes. Endogenous hyperlipemia has been described in uremia, after renal homotransplantation, and in hypopituitarism, Niemann-Pick disease, Gaucher's disease, Werner's syndrome, and hepatoma. The prevalence of hyperlipemia is increased in gout.

Dyslipoproteinemias

Biliary Obstruction. A low-density lipoprotein which has not been detected in health appears in the plasma of patients with extrahepatic or intrahepatic biliary obstruction. It is a spherical vesicle about 400 Å in diameter, the wall of which is a lipid bilayer composed of a 1:1 molar mixture of cholesterol and phospholipids, together with a small amount of C apoproteins. This "cholestasis lipoprotein" or "LP-X" can be detected in virtually all patients with biliary obstruction, but very high levels are most characteristic of the early stages of primary biliary cirrhosis and are frequently accompanied by eruptive and planar xanthomas and xanthelasmas. Bile acid-binding agents, such as cholestyramine, may reduce the concentration of the lipoprotein. Spontaneous subsidence of the hyperlipoproteinemia and disappearance of xanthomas usually signify failing hepatic parenchymal cell function in primary biliary cirrhosis.

Paraproteinemias. The abnormal globulins in patients with multiple myeloma and macroglobulinemia may be associated with lipid. In some cases, lipoprotein-globulin complexes have been demonstrated with accompanying hyperlipemia and various xanthomas.

HYPOLIPOPROTEINEMIAS

The secondary states are characterized chiefly by hypobetalipoproteinemia and are the result of malnutrition, malabsorption, or parenchymal liver disease. Presumably they reflect decreased transport of exogenous and endogenous triglycerides, so that formation of LDL is decreased. Reduced concentrations of LDL also occur in healthy individuals when intake of calories and saturated fats is habitually low.

Bagdade, J. D., Porte, D., and Bierman, E. L.: Diabetic lipemia. A form of acquired fat-induced lipemia. N. Engl. J. Med., 276:427, 1967.

Beck, P.: Contraceptive steroids: Modifications of carbohydrate and lipid metabolism. Metabolism, 22:841, 1973.

Earley, L. E., Havel, R. J., Hopper, J., Jr., and Grausz, H.: Nephrotic syndrome. Calif. Med., 115:23, 1971.

Glueck, C. J., Kaplan, A. P., Levy, R. I., Greten, H., Gralnick, H., and Fredrickson, D. S.: A new mechanism of exogenous hyperglyceridemia. Ann. Intern. Med., 71:1051, 1969.

Hamilton, R. L., Havel, R. J., Kane, J. P., Blaurock, A., and Sata, T.: Cholestasis: Lamellar structure of the abnormal human serum lipoprotein. Science, 172:475, 1971.

Havel, R. J., Balasse, E. O., Kane, J. P., and Segel, N.: Splanchnic metabolism in von Gierke's disease (glycogenosis type I). Trans. Assoc. Am. Physicians, 82:305, 1969.

Piscatelli, R. L., Vieweg, W. V. R., and Havel, R. J.: Partial lipodystrophy: Metabolic studies in three patients. Ann. Intern. Med., 73:963, 1970.

819. HYPERLIPOPROTEINEMIA IN ATHEROSCLEROTIC VASCULAR DISEASE

Although atherosclerosis develops under the influence of a variety of factors, the role of plasma lipoproteins may be decisive in the muscular arteries supplying the heart and lower extremities. Plasma levels of LDL, VLDL, or both, tend to be elevated in patients with occlusive atherosclerotic disease in these vessels, particularly before the sixth decade. The level of cholesterol, which closely reflects that of LDL in large population groups, is a powerful predictor of the incidence of, and mortality from, coronary artery disease in middle-aged men. Retrospective studies indicate that the level of triglycerides, which closely reflects the level of VLDL, is also associated with premature ischemic vascular disease, but prospective studies suggest that solitary elevation of triglycerides is a less powerful predictor than elevation of serum cholesterol alone.

The level of serum cholesterol is subject to strong familial influence even in the absence of a major gene effect, such as that operating in familial hyperbetalipoproteinemia. The influence could be environmental, but genetic data suggest that multifactorial inheritance is mainly operative. However, the level of serum cholesterol (and that of LDL) is also influenced by content of cholesterol and saturated fats in the diet. In industrialized countries, where intake of these nutrients is large, cholesterol levels are substantially higher than in underdeveloped countries where habitual intake of animal fat is low. The much lower incidence of coronary artery disease in underdeveloped countries is consistent with the putative role of LDL-cholesterol in the early development of the atherosclerotic plaque.

In the absence of the major gene effects described in Ch. 817, the level of serum triglycerides is less subject to familial influence. The substantial effects of caloric intake and ethanol on serum triglyceride concentration accord with this fact and suggest that sporadic cases of mild to moderate hypertriglyceridemia largely reflect alterations in lipid transport produced by nutritional or other environmental influences.

Recent studies of survivors of myocardial infarction indicate that hyperlipoproteinemia occurs in about half of those under the age of 50. More than half of the hyperlipoproteinemic survivors, in turn, appear to carry major gene defects. Familial hyperbetalipoproteinemia accounts for only about one fifth of these; the remainder have endogenous hyperlipemia, usually with associated elevation of LDL cholesterol (combined hyperlipidemia). Families in whom most affected individuals have combined hyperlipidemia are more common than families characterized by elevation of VLDL alone; however, many affected individuals in families with combined hyperlipidemia have solitary elevation of VLDL, and some may have only elevated LDL. These variations presumably reflect the influence of obesity, diet, and other factors on lipid transport as described in Ch. 816. In addition, polygenic hypercholesterolemia and sporadic cases of hypertriglyceridemia are also common among survivors of myocardial infarction, so that a genetic diagnosis is seldom possible without extensive studies of the patient's family. The major exception to this situation is the patient with severe hyperbetalipoproteinemia (cholesterol exceeding 350 mg per 100 ml); such individuals frequently have tendinous xanthomas. In them, the diagnosis of familial hyperbetalipoproteinemia can generally be made with confidence and with the knowledge that dietary measures alone will be of limited benefit. In all other situations, diets designed to reduce the level of VLDL or LDL may be recommended as described earlier, with drug therapy reserved for those individuals who do not respond adequately.

The important question of whether reduction of lipoprotein levels will prevent progression or cause regression of atherosclerotic lesions has not been answered convincingly. Regression of experimentally induced atherosclerosis occurs in animals under some circumstances, and recent studies suggest that reduction of dietary cholesterol and saturated fats may delay death from ischemic vascular disease in survivors of myocardial infarction and in elderly men. In patients with primary dysbetalipoproteinemia, more direct evidence of regression of occlusive lesions in muscular arteries of the leg has recently been obtained in subjects treated with diet and clofibrate. Thus specific dietary or pharmacologic treatment of hyperlipoproteinemia is probably indicated in established coronary artery disease and peripheral atherosclerotic vascular disease as well as for prophylaxis.

Since the risk of developing coronary artery disease is a graded function of the concentration of LDL-cholesterol, the presence of normal levels of cholesterol and triglycerides in survivors of myocardial infarction cannot be taken to exclude a major influence of plasma lipoproteins in the pathogenesis of their disease. Statistical normality of LDL-cholesterol level in industrialized countries should therefore not be confused with the level consistent with maintenance of health. Rather, levels in the range of 90 to 130 mg per 100 ml serum (equivalent to total cholesterol level of 140 to 180 mg per 100 ml) may be normal in this context. The relative immunity of premenopausal women to complications of atherosclerosis may result from their lower levels of LDL. This is not reflected in the level of total serum cholesterol, because the level of HDL-cholesterol is higher in premenopausal women than in men. These differences presumably result from actions of sex hormones and disappear after the menopause.

Immediately after myocardial infarction, the concentration of VLDL tends to rise as a result of increased fat mobilization produced by secretion of "stress" hormones and increased sympathetic nervous activity. At the same time, the level of LDL-cholesterol may fall as a result of reduced caloric and fat intake. Therefore evaluation of the nature and magnitude of associated hyperlipoproteinemia should be postponed for two to three months after the acute episode.

Carlson, L. A.: Serum lipids in men with myocardial infarction. Acta Med. Scand., 167:399, 1960.

Goldstein, J. L., Hazzard, W. R., Schrott, H. G., Bierman, E. L., and Motulsky, A. G.: Hyperlipidemia in coronary heart disease: I. Lipid levels in 500 survivors of myocardial infarction. II. Genetic analysis of lipid levels in 176 families and delineation of a new inherited disorder, combined hyperlipidemia. III. Evaluation of lipoprotein phenotypes of 156 genetically defined survivors of myocardial infarction. J. Clin. Invest., 52:1533, 1544, 1569, 1973.

Kannel, W. B., Garcia, M. J., McNamara, P. M., and Pearson, G.: Serum lipid precursors of coronary heart disease. Human Pathol., 2:129, 1971.

Turpeinen, O.: Control of atherosclerosis: Pr gress in primary diet trials. In Jones, R. J. (ed.): Atherosclerosis. Proceedings, Second International Symposium. New York, Springer-Verlag, 1970, p. 572.

Zelis, R., Mason, D. T., Braunwald, E., and Levy, R. I.: Effects of hyperlipoproteinemias and their treatment of the peripheral circulation. J. Clin. Invest., 49:1007, 1970.

820. INBORN ERRORS OF AMINO ACID METABOLISM

Charles R. Scriver

HYPERAMINOACIDURIA

General Comments. A certain amount of L-aminoaciduria, representing less than 2 to 3 per cent of the total urinary nitrogen, is a normal phenomenon. A small fraction, usually less than 5 per cent, of the filtered load of the amino acids in plasma is not absorbed completely by the proximal portion of the renal tubule and is excreted in the urine. In the healthy person, the efficiency of renal tubular transport for the individual amino acids is related to their chemical and steric structure, the amount in the glomerular filtrate, and the sex, age, and physiologic state of the subject. Data for normal range and mean values of endogenous renal clearance rates, plasma levels, and urinary excretion rates of approximately 20 L-amino acids are now available for infants, children, and adults, both male and female, in fasting and nonfasting states. Advances in the knowledge of aminoaciduria have come primarily from the development of chromatographic methods, which allow rapid qualitative screening and reliable quantitative estimation of the complex amino acid composition of physiologic fluids.

Renal tubular absorption of amino acids is mediated by reactive sites which are believed to be membrane proteins, and whose catalytic relationships to the individual amino acids observe Michaelis-Menten kinetics. This means that the transport mechanism is saturable (equivalent to the T_m) and is susceptible to competitive and noncompetitive inhibition. The specificity of the site (protein) is genetically controlled.

Flux of the site–amino acid complex transfers the amino acid across the membrane (a directional process) by a mechanism which either is coupled to metabolic reactions which produce energy (nondirectional reactions) or elicits coupled fluxes in the same or opposite direction of other solutes.

Abnormal aminoaciduria will result when there is an acquired or hereditary disturbance of cellular metabolism or transport of amino acids. The known hyperaminoacidurias (Table 1) can be classified according to four basic mechanisms:

1. *Saturation:* Substrate is at elevated concentration and approaches or exceeds the capacity of the system ("overflow" aminoaciduria).

2. *Competition:* One substrate itself at elevated concentration competes with other members for access to the system ("combined" aminoaciduria).

3. *Modification of reactive site(s):* Substrate(s) not transported efficiently because access to the system is modified ("renal" aminoaciduria).

4. *Inhibition of substrate transfer:* Impaired energy-dependent processes, coupled to the transfer of substrates across membrane ("renal" aminoaciduria).

In some diseases, e.g., in Group III of Table 1, gene mutation affects amino acid transport in both the renal tubule and the intestine. Furthermore, it appears that the individual mechanisms required for transport of each amino acid can be grouped into at least five major gene-controlled and nonoverlapping systems, each having a particular *preference for a group of amino acids* normally found in plasma and usually elucidated in a particular aminoacidopathy. Another series of reactive sites *recognizes individual amino acids,* one site for each of the protein amino acids. Yet *another series permits transepithelial absorption of oligopeptides* in the intestine, with hydrolysis following uptake of the peptides. The *group-specific sites* used by free amino acids, and particularly evident through the inborn errors of amino acid metabolism, are classified as follows:

1. *The β-amino system:* β-alanine, β-aminoisobutyric acid, and taurine (viz., hyper-β-alaninemia).

2. *The α-amino systems:*

a. "Basic" system: lysine, arginine, ornithine (and cystine, although not as a "basic" amino acid, viz., cystinuria).

b. "Acidic" system: aspartic, glutamic.

c. Neutral-I system: prolone, hydroxyproline, and glycine (viz., hyperprolinemia and renal iminoglycinuria).

d. Neutral-II system: the remaining neutral α-amino acids (viz., Hartnup disease).

It is usually possible to classify the aminoaciduria by analyzing the amino acid content of plasma and urine collected conjointly (Table 1). Chromatographic techniques will reveal the details of hyperaminoaciduria more accurately than any other method. The recognition of a specific aminoaciduria can provide an accurate clinical diagnosis for which there may be appropriate therapy.

Scriver, C. R., and Rosenberg, L. E.: Amino Acid Metabolism and Its Disorders. Philadelphia, W. B. Saunders Company, 1973.

THE HYPERPHENYLALANINEMIAS

Mass screening of newborn infants in recent years has shown that all that is hyperphenylalaninemia is not necessarily phenylketonuria. Hence this section has been broadened to include mention of several hyperphenylalaninemic phenotypes evident in the human race. As position papers of their time, the conference reports edited by Anderson and Swaiman (1968) and by Bickel et al. (1971) should be read to supplement this brief discussion.

Metabolism of Phenylalanine. L-Phenylalanine is an essential amino acid for man. In infancy half or more of its dietary intake is used for protein synthesis, and the remainder is oxidized to tyrosine by hydroxylation in the liver. As body size increases, the phenylalanine intake increases from $1/2$ gram per day at birth to as much as 4 grams daily in the older child and adult; at the same time that the rate of growth slows, a larger fraction of phenylalanine is catabolized to tyrosine, and the amount required for anabolism decreases proportionately. Any impairment of oxidation, without change in the other parameters, will cause the phenylalanine free pool to enlarge and its plasma concentration to rise above the normal maximum (1.2 mg per 100 ml). When this happens, other minor pathways of phenylalanine catabolism are called upon, and increased amounts of normal minor metabolites will appear in body fluids.

The key step in L-phenylalanine catabolism, namely, hydroxylation to tyrosine, has received much attention. This complex reaction involves several genes which control various components. Not surprisingly, several types of hyperphenylalaninemias are known; further variants will undoubtedly be discovered in the future.

Classic Phenylketonuria

Definition. The disease was first described by Følling in 1934. In its fully expressed form, there is persistent hyperphenylalaninemia in excess of 1 mMolar (16.5 mg per 100 ml), mental retardation (in most cases), and excessive urinary excretion of phenylpyruvic acid and other phenylalanine derivatives. The condition is autosomal recessive, being the result of complete absence of phenylalanine hydroxylase activity. If mass screening of newborn infants for this trait and genetic counseling are to be effective, the patient with classic untreated phenylketonuria should become an oddity, often mentioned but rarely seen in modern medical practice.

Prevalence. The homozygote occurs once in about 12,000 live births in Caucasians, with significant variation in frequency among ethnic groups. The disease is rare in the black and in the Ashkenazic Jew; in the latter cases, the mutation may not be allelic with the gene causing Caucasian phenylketonuria.

Clinical Manifestations. The most important and consistent feature is mental retardation. This becomes evident at six months of age, and in later childhood 98 per cent of untreated patients have an I.Q. below 70. Phenylketonuric patients are clinically normal at birth, distinguishable only by hyperphenylalaninemia, which is established in the first postnatal week. Other manifestations, such as seizures (often with the hypsarrhythmic EEG pattern), psychotic behavior, eczema, dermatographia, "mousy" odor (owing to excretion of phenylacetic acid), and pigment dilution, are found in untreated patients. None of these are seen in patients who benefit from early diagnosis and proper treatment.

The Metabolic Error. Homozygotes are almost completely lacking in phenylalanine hydroxylase activity; heterozygotes have partial activity, sufficient to maintain normal phenylalanine metabolism under ordinary circumstances.

Phenylalanine accumulates when the catabolic pathway is blocked, and is found in excessive amounts in blood, urine, and cerebrospinal fluid. Minor pathways are then overutilized, and, characteristically, phenylpyruvic acid is formed and excreted in urine. Additional compounds such as the lactic and acetic derivatives and the glutamine conjugate are also formed and excreted. Orthohydroxylation can occur and the corresponding ortho series of metabolites may be present.

Excessive amounts of phenylalanine and its derivatives can inhibit other enzymes. As a result disturbances of tyrosine and tryptophan metabolism occur. Diminished formation of catecholamines, melanin, and serotonin is observed in untreated phenylketonuria.

The cause of mental retardation in phenylketonuria is still unknown. It is probably due to many chemical abnormalities which occur as a consequence of the disturbed chemical environment during the critical early postnatal stage of brain development.

Diagnosis. Recognition of the trait should result from early postnatal detection of hyperphenylalaninemia. Subsequent studies to assess the degree of hyperphenylalaninemia, the dietary phenylalanine tolerance, and the persistence of the trait will help to distinguish it

from other genetic variants affecting phenylalanine metabolism. Testing of the urine and ferric chloride (a few drops of 5 per cent solution in 0.1N HC1 added to 1 to 2 ml urine) is not recommended for diagnosis in the newborn, because this test requires the excretion of phenylpyruvic acid, whose formation is dependent on transamination of phenylalanine; the latter function may not mature for at least three weeks after birth, even in full-term babies. All current newborn screening programs employ a specific microbiologic assay, fluorometric assay, or partition chromatography to detect excess phenylalanine in a few microliters of capillary blood collected from the heel of the infant.

Treatment. Replacement or induction of phenylalanine hydroxylase is not feasible. Partial liver transplantation from a normal homozygote or heterozygote would give the patient a stable source of enzyme, and perhaps this mode of treatment will be possible in the future. At present dietary restriction of phenylalanine is the only practical therapy. By means of semisynthetic diets containing a low-phenylalanine hydrolysate, it is possible to restrict L-phenylalanine intake to about 250 to 500 mg daily while providing the recommended amounts of other essential amino acids and of calories and other nutritional factors. Close supervision of this treatment is important, and is best performed at centers experienced with such regimens.

Reduction of hyperphenylalaninemia to about 4 to 12 mg per 100 ml (relaxed regimen), when begun within 60 days of birth, will allow normal physical and mental development. Delayed or inadequate treatment impairs normal mental development. There is no agreement whether dietary treatment should be continued after the fifth year of life when human brain growth is complete. Female homozygous phenylketonurics should be treated during pregnancy to prevent harm to the fetus from intrauterine hyperphenylalaninemia.

Hyperphenylalaninemic Variants

The following phenotypes behave as independent autosomal recessive traits. Their recognition is important in order to avoid confusion with classic phenylketonuria and subsequent inappropriate treatment and counseling.

Atypical Phenylketonuria (Mild Variant). This variant is characterized by its high dietary tolerance for phenylalanine, which allows the patient to ingest between 700 and 2000 mg of the amino acid in the diet. Phenylalanine hydroxylase deficiency in the liver is probably incomplete; impaired intestinal absorption or excessive renal or fecal loss of phenylalanine does not account for the different phenotype.

Transient Phenylketonuria. Several sibships are known in which disappearance of the phenylketonuric phenotype and restoration of normal or nearly normal dietary phenylalanine tolerance occur spontaneously during infancy or childhood. The precise enzymatic basis for the phenotype has not been established.

Benign Persistent Hyperphenylalaninemia. This trait was first observed in families of Mediterranean origin but now also in other ethnic groups, including Jews. The concentration of phenylalanine in plasma of homozygotes consuming normal diets is usually less than 1 mMolar (16.5 mg per 100 ml). Mental and physical development is normal without treatment in these subjects.

TABLE 1. Hereditary and Acquired Aminoacidopathies:* Classified According to Mechanism and Preferred Fluid for Detection

Group IA: Primary defect in catabolism
Low renal clearance of amino acid
Hyperaminoaciduria by saturation of transport system
Detection preferable in plasma

Condition or Disease	Amino Acids Affected	Abnormal Enzyme	Comment
I.A.1 *Common perinatal (adaptive) traits*			
Neonatal hyperphenyl-alaninemia*	Phenylalanine	Phenylalanine hydroxylating system (?)	Benign; may respond to folic acid; often occurs with tyrosinemia
Neonatal tyrosinemia†	Tyrosine	p-Hydroxy-phenyl pyruvic acid hydroxylase (EC 1.14.2.2)	Benign; responds to ascorbic acid and reduced protein intake
Hypermethioninemia†	Methionine	ATP: 1-methionine S-adenosyl transferase (?) (EC 2.5.1.6)	Benign; usually found with high protein intake
Hyperhistidinemia†	Histidine	L-Histidine ammonia lyase (?) (EC 4.3.1.3)	Benign; related to high protein intake
I.A.2 *Inherited aminoacidopathies*			
1. The hyperphenylalaninemias			
(i) "Classic" phenylketonuria	Phenylalanine	L-Phenylalanine tetrahydropteridine; oxygen oxidoreductase (4-hydroxylating) (EC 1.14.3.1) (residual activity <1%)	(i) Plasma phenylalanine >16 mg/100 ml; causes mental retardation; when treated, L-phenylalanine tolerance in diet is 250–500 mg phe/day
(ii) "Atypical" phenylketonuria†	Phenylalanine	L-Phenylalanine tetrahydropteridine: oxygen oxido-reductase (4-hydroxylating) (EC 1.14.3.1) (residual activity >1%)	(ii) Plasma phenylalanine >16 mg/100 ml; similar to (i), but dietary tolerance for L-phenylalanine is >500 mg/day
(iii) "Transient" phenylketonuria†	Phenylalanine	L-Phenylalanine tetrahydropteridine: oxygen oxido-reductase (4-hydroxylating) (EC 1.14.13.1)	(iii) Plasma phenylalanine >16 mg/100 ml; change in status to (iv), or normal, several months or years after birth
(iv) "Benign" hyper-phenylalaninemia†	Phenylalanine	L-Phenylalanine tetrahydropteridine: oxygen oxido-reductase (4-hydroxylating) (EC 1.14.3.1)	(iv) Plasma phenylalanine <16 mg/100 ml; on normal diet; benign trait
2. The hypertyrosinemias			
(i) Tyrosinosis (Medes)	Tyrosine	L-tyrosine: α-ketoglutarate amino transferase (?) (EC 2.6.1.20)	One case known; myasthenia gravis, probably incidental finding
(ii) Hypertyrosinemia†	Tyrosine	Soluble (cytosol) tyrosine aminotransferase	One case; associated developmental retardation
(iii) Hereditary tyrosinemia†	Tyrosine (and methionine)	p-HPPA hydroxylase (EC 1.14.2.2) Primary or secondary defect?	Hepatic cirrhosis, and renal tubular failure, eventually fatal; responds to tyrosine restriction
3. The hyperhistidinemias			
(i) "Classic" form†	Histidine (alanine in some cases)	L-Histidine ammonia lyase (EC 4.3.1.3.) (liver and skin)	Usually associated with mental retardation and speech defect
(ii) Variant form	Histidine	L-Histidine ammonia lyase (EC 4.3.1.3) (liver only)	As above
4. The branched-chain hyper-aminoacidemias			
(i) "Classic maple syrup urine disease"†	Leucine isoleucine, valine, allo-isoleucine	Branched-chain α-keto acid; lipoate oxidoreductase (acceptor acylating) (EC 1.2.4.-) (<2 per cent of normal)	Postnatal collapse, mental retardation in survivors; early diet therapy effective
(ii) Intermittent form	Same	Same (2–15 per cent of normal)	Intermittent symptoms; development may be otherwise normal
(iii) Mild form	Same	Same	Unremittent; milder than (i)
(iv) Thiamin-responsive	Same	Same	Mild form; B₁-responsive (10–20 mg/day)
(v) Hypervalinemia	Valine	Valine amino-transferase (EC 2.6.1.-)	Retarded development and vomiting; responds to diet
(vi) Hyperleucinemia	Leucine/isoleucine	Leucine-isoleucine transferase (EC 2.6.1.-)	Retarded development
(vii) Others§			

TABLE 1.   Hereditary and Acquired Aminoacidopathies:* Classified According to Mechanism and Preferred Fluid for Detection (*Continued*)

Group IA: Primary defect in catabolism
Low renal clearance of amino acid
Hyperaminoaciduria by saturation of transport system
Detection preferable in plasma

Condition or Disease	Amino Acids Affected	Abnormal Enzyme	Comment
5. Sulfuraminoacidemias			
(i) Homocystinuria‡	Methionine and homocystine	L-Serine hydrolase (deaminating); ("cystathionine synthetase") (EC 4.2.1.13)	Usually associated with thromboembolic disease, mental retardation, ectopia-lentis, and Marfan phenotype; some cases respond to Vitamin B₆
(ii) Cystathioninuria‡	Cystathionine	L-Homoserine hydrolyase (deaminating) (EC 4.2.1.15)	Probably benign trait; vitamin B₆ corrects biochemical trait in most patients
6. The hyperglycinemias			
(i) Ketotic form†	Glycine and other glucogenic acids	Propionyl-CoA; carbon dioxide ligase (ADP) (EC 6.4.1.3)	Ketosis, neutropenia, mental retardation; often fatal
(ii) Nonketotic form†	Glycine	"Glycine decarboxylase" (?)	Different trait; poor prognosis
7. Sarcosinemia‡	Sarcosine (ethanolamine)	Sarcosine: oxygen oxidoreductase (demethylating) (EC 1.5.3.1)	Benign trait (probably)
8. The hyperprolinemias			
(i) Type I†	Proline	L-Proline: NAD(P) 5-oxido-reductase, ("proline oxidase") (EC 1.5.1.2) (partial defect)	Benign trait, which is sometimes associated with hereditary nephritis
(ii) Type II	Proline	"Δ¹-pyrroline-5-carboxylate dehydrogenase"? or more complete deficiency of oxidase?	Benign trait, sometimes associated with CNS disease; ΔPC excreted in urine; proline concentration greater than Type I
9. Hydroxyprolinemia	Hydroxyproline	"Hydroxyproline oxidase"	Two cases, associated with CNS disease; others normal
10. The hyperlysinemias			
(i) Type I	Lysine (and glutamine)	Lysine: α-ketoglutarate: triphosphopyridine nucleotide (TPNH), oxidoreductase (ε-N-[L-glutaryl 1-2]-L-lysine forming)	Associated with mental retardation and hypotonia
(ii) Type II	Lysine, arginine (NH₃)	(Partial defect of above [10, i]) or different enzyme?	Hyperammonemia symptoms, related to protein intake
(iii) Saccharopinuria‡	Lysine, saccharopine, citrulline	"Saccharopinase"(?)	First case associated with mental retardation and short stature
11. Pipecolicacidemia‡	Pipecolic acid	"Pipecolate oxidase" (?)	Hepatomegaly and mental retardation
12. The hyperammonemias			
(i) Type I	Glycine, glutamine	ATP: carbamate phosphotransferase (EC 2.7.2.2)	
(ii) Type II†	Glutamine (and orotic acid)	Carbamoylphosphate: L-ornithine carbamoyl-transferase (EC 2.1.3.3.)	Type II is X-linked; it and the autosomal recessive diseases show ammonia intoxication, protein intolerance, hepatomegaly, vomiting, etc.; ASAuria also has trichlorrhexis nodosa
(iii) Hyperornithinemia	Ornithine	Unknown	
(iv) Citrullinemia†	Citrulline	L-Citrulline: L-aspartase ligase (AMP) (EC 6.3.4.5)	
(v) Argininosuccinicaciduria‡	ASA	L-Argininosuccinate argininelyase (EC 4.3.2.1)	
(vi) Argininemia	Arginine	"Arginase": L-Arginineamidino hydrolase (EC 3.5.3.1)	
(See also 10, Type II)			
13. Glutamicacidemia	Glutamate	Unknown	X-linked mental retardation; possibly the same as Menkes' (kinky hair) syndrome
14. The hyperalaninemias	Alanine	(i) Pyruvate dehydrogenase (EC 4.1.1.1) decarboxylase (EC 1.2.4.1) deficiency	Lactic acidosis, intermittent ataxia, mental retardation

(Table continued on following pages)

TABLE 1. Hereditary and Acquired Aminoacidopathies:* Classified According to Mechanism and Preferred Fluid for Detection (*Continued*)

Group IA: Primary defect in catabolism
Low renal clearance of amino acid
Hyperaminoaciduria by saturation of transport system
Detection preferable in plasma

Condition or Disease	Amino Acids Affected	Abnormal Enzyme	Comment
		(ii) Pyruvate carboxylase deficiency (EC 6.4.1.1)	Intermittent lactic acidosis, intermittent hypoglycemia
15. Aspartylglucosaminuria	Glucoasparagines	2-acetamido-1-(β^1-L-aspartamido)-1,2-dideoxyglucoseamido hydrolase	Lysosomal disease? mental retardation
16. "Glutathionemia"	Glutathione or related peptide	γ-Glutamyl-transpeptidase deficiency	Mental retardation associated with finding

1.A.3 *Nutritional and other diseases which may affect amino acids in plasma*

Protein-calorie malnutrition	Tryptophan/leucine / isoleucine/valine ↓ ; tyrosine/glycine/ proline ↑		Severity of change related to severity of malnutrition
Prolonged fasting	Alanine ↓ ; threonine; glycine ↑		Early fasting does not show same pattern
Obesity	Leucine/isoleucine/ valine/phenylalanine/ tyrosine ↑ ; Glycine ↓		Reflects insulin insensitivity
Hepatitis	Methionine/tryosine ↑		Reflects severity of liver disease

Group IB: Primary defect in catabolism
High renal clearance of amino acid
Hyperaminoaciduria by saturation
Detection preferable in urine

Condition or Disease	Amino Acids Affected	Abnormal Enzyme	Comment
1. (a) Hypophosphatasia	Phosphoethanolamine	? Deficiency of o-phosphoryl-ethanolamine phospho-lyase (EC 4.2.99.-)	"Rickets" unresponsive to vitamin D; craniosynostosis; hypercalcemia
(b) Pseudohypophosphatasia	Phosphoethanolamine	"Alkaline phosphatase" activity present but altered (Km mutant)	(Same as 1a)
2. β-Aminoisobutyricaciduria	βAIB	?	Benign polymorphic trait
3. Hyper-β-alaninemia	β-Alanine	β-Alanine transaminase?	Seizures; somnolence; mental retardation
4. Carnosinemia	Carnosine	Carnosinase	Seizures and mental retardation
5. Pyroglutamicaciduria	5-oxo-L-proline (pyr-rolidone-2-carboxylic acid)	Overproduction secondary to defective glutathione synthesis?	5-O-P in urine; origin in kidney ?

See also homocystinuria (I.A.2.5.i), cystathioninuria (I.A.2.5.ii), and argininosuccinicaciduria (I.A.2.12.v)

Group II: Primary defect in catabolism; secondary defect in transport
Hyperaminoaciduria of combined origin (saturation and competition)
Detection possible in plasma and urine

Disease	Amino Acids Affected in Plasma	Amino Acids Present in Urine	Comment
1. Hyperprolinemia Types I and II	Proline	Proline plus hydroxyproline and glycine	See I.A.2.8; competition occurs on iminoglycine transport system (see III, 2)
2. Hyper-β-alaninemia	β-Alanine	β-Alanine plus βAIB and taurine	See I.B.3; competition occurs on β-amino transport system
3. Hyperlysinemia	Lysine	Lysine plus ornithine and arginine	See I.A.2.10; competition occurs on "di-basic" transport system (see III, 1)

TABLE 1. Hereditary and Acquired Aminoacidopathies:* Classified According to Mechanism and Preferred Fluid for Detection (*Continued*)

Group III: Primary defect in membrane transport site
High renal clearance of amino acid
Detection possible only in urine

Disease or Trait	Amino Acids Affected	Abnormal Transport System	Comment
III.A *Common perinatal (adaptive) traits*			
1. Neonatal iminoglycinuria	Proline, hydroxyproline, and glycine	Low capacity system for proline; same for glycine	Iminoaciduria persists about 3 months; glycinuria persists 5–6 months
III. B. *Hereditary traits*			
1. Cystinuria†	Dibasics and cystine	High capacity, diaminomonocarboxylic (involving cysteine during efflux only)	
a. Type I	In homozygote, not in heterozygote	Kidney plus gut	Cystine stone formation in urinary tract is major hazard
b. Type II	In homozygote and heterozygote	Kidney plus gut	
c. Type III	In homozygote and heterozygote	Kidney (plus gut, partial or normal)	
2. Hypercystinuria	Cystine only	Substrate-specific system for cystine	
3. Renal iminoglycinuria†	Proline, hydroxyproline, and glycine	High capacity system for imino acids and glycine	
a. Type I		Kidney and gut	Benign trait
b. Type II		Kidney alone	
4. Hartnup disease†	Neutral mono-amino acids and monocarboxylic acids (except imino acids and glycine)	High capacity system shared by neutral amino acids	Pellagra-like symptoms under condition of marginal protein nutrition
a. Type I		Kidney and gut	
b. Type II		Kidney only	
5. Blue diaper syndrome	Tryptophan	Low capacity system for specific amino acid (in the intestine)	Hypercalcemia
6. Methionine malabsorption	Methionine		Mental retardation

Group IV: Generalized inhibition of transport processes
High renal clearance of substrates
Detection best in urine

Primary Abnormality	Aminoaciduria and Other Findings	Comment
1. Acquired		
e.g., Degraded tetracyclines, salicylates, heavy metals, vitamin D deficiency, scurvy, etc.	Generalized aminoaciduria, plus combinations of glucosuria, hyperphosphaturia, etc. (Fanconi's syndrome)	Early removal of toxin or correction of deficiency usually followed by recovery of normal transport function
2. Hereditary		
Galactosemia	Generalized + galactosuria	Can be induced by galactose feeding and treated by removal of galactose
Oculocerebro-renal syndrome	Generalized + phosphaturia and renal tubular acidosis	X-linked glaucoma, hypotonia, and mental retardation; defect in ammonia synthesis?
Other Fanconi syndromes, related to:	Generalized + loss of glucose, phosphate, K, bicarbonate, water, etc.	Symptoms related to functional defect (Po_4 and K loss, etc.) plus primary disease
a. Cystinosis		a. Cystine storage; recessive gene
b. Idiopathic (infants)		b. No cystine storage; sporadic cases
c. Idiopathic (adults)		c. Recessive inheritance; no cystinosis
d. Luder-Sheldon variety		d. Onset in late childhood
e. Secondary to Wilson's disease		e. Onset in late childhood
f. Secondary to tyrosinemia (Baber's syndrome)		f. Onset usually in late infancy
g. Others, including fructosemia (aldolase deficiency)		g. Differentiate from f

*Table refers only to those conditions associated with perturbation of the normal content of ninhydrin-reactive metabolites in plasma or urine.
†These conditions have been detected by screening methods applied in the newborn period of life.
‡Urine screening is probably preferable in these conditions.
§A number of disorders of branched-chain amino acid catabolism cause accumulation of substances which are ninhydrin-negative. These compounds can usually be detected by gas-liquid chromatographic methods.
EC=Enzyme classification number.

Recognition of the trait is important, for it must not be confused with phenylketonuria.

Anderson, J. A., and Swaiman, K. F. (eds.): Proceedings of a Conference on Phenylketonuria and Allied Disorders. U.S. Department of Health, Education, and Welfare, Social and Rehabilitation Service, Children's Bureau. U.S. Government Printing Office, 1967–0–282–371.

Bickel, H., Hudson, F. P., and Woolf, L. I. (eds.): Phenylketonuria and Some Other Inborn Errors of Amino Acid Metabolism. Biochemistry, Genetics, Diagnosis, Therapy. Stuttgart, Georg Thieme Verlag, 1971.

Justice, P., O'Flynn, M. E., and Hsia, D. Y.: Phenylalanine-hydroxylase activity in hyperphenylalaninaemia. Lancet, 1:928, 1967.

BRANCHED-CHAIN AMINOACIDURIA

Maple Syrup Urine Disease. The colloquial term describes a characteristic odor of patients with *branched-chain ketoaciduria, and aminoacidopathy.* The disease is autosomal recessive, and its apparent rarity may reflect, in part, missed diagnoses in patients dying in infancy. Severe hypotonia, apnea, feeding difficulty, and hypoglycemia appear in the first week of life, progressing to seizures, decorticate rigidity, severe mental retardation, and death. At least three variants with episodic illness or mild mental retardation presenting in later infancy have been reported.

The primary enzymatic defect is a block in decarboxylation of branched-chain α-keto acids; consequently leucine, isoleucine, alloisoleucine, and valine and their equivalent α-keto acids and α-hydroxyacids accumulate after birth; symptoms are primarily related to abnormal leucine metabolism. The aminoacidopathy can be detected in blood and urine within the first week of life; the enzyme defect can be assayed in leukocytes and in cultured skin fibroblasts.

The disease responds to dietary control of leucine, isoleucine, and valine intake, the best results following the earliest possible treatment. One variant is responsive to thiamin at ten times the normal daily intake.

Hypervalinemia. Symptoms of vomiting, blindness, and retardation of physical and mental development in a single Japanese infant were reported, which improved abruptly with a valine-restricted diet. Valine transaminase is the defective enzyme; hence only valine accumulates in body fluids.

HYPERHISTIDINEMIA

Many cases of this rare and apparently autosomal recessively inherited disease are now known. Inactivity of the enzyme histidase, which nonoxidatively deaminates histidine to uraconic acid, can be detected in skin biopsy material. Accumulation of histidine (and sometimes of alanine) above normal levels and depressed serotonin levels are found in blood; increased excretion of imidazolepyruvic acid and a positive ferric chloride test are found in urine. The risk of mild mental retardation and/or short auditory memory span, reflected as delayed speech development, is apparently about 1 in 2. Low-histidine therapy is feasible and, in view of the risk of delayed mental development, is probably indicated.

THE HYPERPROLINEMIAS AND HYDROXYPROLINEMIA
(Iminoacidopathies)

Hyperprolinemias. *Type I* (L-proline oxidase deficiency) is a recessively inherited condition. Proline is the only amino acid elevated in plasma, but a "combined" aminoaciduria involving proline, hydroxyproline, and glycine is found. In *Type II* hyperprolinemia the block is apparently at the second step in proline degradation (Δ-pyrroline-5-carboxylate dehydrogenase); the pyrroline derivative is also excreted in urine. Type I hyperprolinemia is sometimes associated with familial hematuric nephropathy, but pedigree studies show that prolinemia and nephropathy are not the consequences of a single gene effect; seizures also occur in both types of hyperprolinemia.

Hydroxyprolinemia. Mental retardation was the principal finding in the first patient described. The enzymes for free hydroxy-L-proline catabolism are distinct from those for L-proline, and the deficient enzyme is a hydroxyproline-specific "oxidase." Subsequent patients have been free of clinical symptoms.

DISEASES OF THE UREA CYCLE

A number of enzymes are involved in the incorporation of ammonia and its delivery as urea. Differences in their relative activity (Table 2) and their location in the cell may account for some of the differences in clinical severity of the inborn errors of the urea cycle. In addition to the catalytic steps, two transport steps across the mitochrondrial membranes are involved, one of which delivers citrulline to the cytoplasm from the mitochondria, the other returning ornithine to the mitochondrion. *Carbamyl phosphate synthetase deficiency* is an intramitochondrial disease with severe hyperammonemia and a rapidly fatal course after birth; inheritance is probably autosomal recessive. *Ornithine transcarbamylase deficiency* is an X-linked disease, with males severely, even fatally, affected and females exhibiting a variable range of clinical symptoms as expected in an X-linked trait. *Citrullinemia* and *argininosuccinicaciduria* are each autosomal recessive, their names identifying the substrate which accumulates in the presence of their respective enzyme deficiencies. *Argininemia* is an autosomal recessive disorder of the last step of the cycle. *Ornithinemia* is yet another apparently autosomal recessive disease of the cycle in which the defective catalytic reaction (perhaps the transport step) has not yet been identified.

Each disease of the urea cycle is accompanied by a set of similar findings which include hyperammonemia, metabolic alkalosis, failure to thrive, convulsions, hepatomegaly, and mental retardation. A fatal outcome is common.

The severity of symptoms and biochemical imbalance varies with the site of the defect and with its completeness. It is interesting that most patients maintain normal or nearly normal urea synthesis, presumably

TABLE 2.   Enzymes in Urea Cycle and Relative Activities*

Carbamyl phosphate synthetase	4.5
Ornithine transcarbamylase	163.0
Argininosuccinic acid synthetase	1.0
Argininosuccinic acid lyase	3.3
Arginase	149.0

*From Scriver, C. R., and Rosenberg, L. E.: Amino Acid Metabolism and its Disorders. Philadelphia, W. B. Saunders Company, 1973.

reflecting a partial block only in the urea cycle compensated for by marked substrate accumulation. Symptomatic treatment with low protein diet and prevention of ammonia intoxication is sometimes feasible. Careful genetic counseling, coupled with the option for prenatal diagnosis in some of the diseases, is recommended.

DISORDERS OF METHIONINE DEGRADATION

Homocystinuria. The full spectrum of clinical features of this autosomal recessive disease is diagnostic: ectopia lentis, downward and forward, mental retardation, lax ligaments, lengthened extremities, malar flush, and fine sparse hair; death from thromboembolic phenomena is frequent. Late-surviving patients have ocular, skeletal, and vascular changes likened to those of Marfan's syndrome (see Ch. 933). Cystathionine synthetase is deficient; its substrate, homocysteine, and the precursor, methionine, accumulate; the product, cystathionine, is deficient in brain. Homocysteine is oxidized and excreted in urine as homocystine, where it can be detected by the cyanide-nitroprusside test. Early dietary therapy with methionine restriction (and cystine supplementation) has apparent benefit. Some patients respond to large doses of pyridoxine (vitamin B_6).

Cystathioninuria. This condition is transmitted in autosomal recessive fashion. It appears to be a benign and not uncommon condition often found in patients with other diseases that attract attention first. Acquired cystathioninuria also occurs secondary to hepatic failure and neuroblastoma. In the hereditary form, the presumed heterozygote exhibits modest elevation, and the homozygote has marked elevation of cystathionine levels in body fluids related to a deficiency of cystathionine-cleaving enzyme activity. Biochemical improvement with pyridoxine therapy demonstrates that the cleaving enzyme is present in the patient's tissues, but is inactive until an excess of pyridoxal-5-phosphate is available, indicating a specific defect in co-factor binding by the apoenzyme.

β-AMINOISOBUTYRICACIDURIA

β-Aminoisobutyric acid (β AIB) is a derivative of thymine and valine metabolism. High urinary excretion (more than 100 μM per gram total N) occurs in some humans who are probably homozygous for a gene controlling β AIB metabolism. In these subjects, plasma levels of β AIB are elevated; the renal clearance rate of the natural isomer, D-(-), β AIB, exceeds that for inulin, indicating net renal "secretion" of β AIB; probenecid can suppress excretion. Hyperexcretors are common in the Mongolian race but infrequent (approximately 5 per cent) in Caucasians; the adaptive significance for the mutation is unknown. Increased β AIB excretion can also be acquired under catabolic stress.

RENAL HYPERAMINOACIDURIAS

Certain hyperaminoacidurias reflect impairment of specific transport systems; the transport lesion is frequently demonstrable in the gut as well as in the kidney. The renal clearance rates of affected amino acids are high, and their plasma levels are low or normal, rather than elevated.

Cystinuria. Three homozygous cystinuric phenotypes are now recognized; in all, there is elevated urinary excretion of cystine, lysine, ornithine, and arginine. In Type I, gut transport of the four amino acids is also abnormal; the heterozygote has normal aminoaciduria (complete recessive). Type II has defective gut transport of the basic amino acids but not of cystine; the heterozygote has elevated urinary lysine and cystine (incomplete recessive). Type III has normal gut transport; the heterozygote phenotype is "incomplete." The exact mechanism of the hyperaminoaciduria is unclear; net tubular "secretion" of the affected amino acids in patients may indicate exaggerated back-flux from cell into urine.

Genetic classification of patients now extends to include "genetic compounds," that is, individuals who resemble homozygotes in their findings but who have inherited two *different* mutant alleles (e.g., I-III, I-II, or II-III).

Urinary cystine calculi are the predominant clinical problem, related to the poor aqueous solubility of cystine in acid urine. Prevention of calculi formation and attendant complications can be attained with copious free water excretion throughout day and night and the use of sodium bicarbonate (10 to 30 grams per day). Rapid solubilization of cystine by formation of a mixed disulfide with D(-) penicillamine (0.5 to 1.0 gram every six hours) may be useful in some patients. Cystinuric patients also have modest growth retardation, perhaps related to fecal and urinary loss of lysine. In a few children severe growth failure and generalized intestinal malabsorption occur with cystinuria as a particular syndrome.

Hartnup Disease. Episodic clinical features include pellagra-like symptoms with photosensitive dermatitis, cerebellar ataxia, and psychosis. Biochemical findings include reduced blood levels of tryptophan metabolites, e.g., nicotinic acid and serotonin, and a fluctuant increase in urinary excretion of indolic acids and derivatives. A constant transport defect for certain neutral α-amino acids is demonstrable in kidney and intestine. The abnormal "indoluria" is dependent on intestinal flora degrading unabsorbed L-tryptophan, with absorption and renal excretion of the products. Defective intracellular transport of tryptophan may account for the deficiency of its endogenous metabolites. Good protein nutrition, normal general intestinal health, and nicotinamide supplements (40 to 200 mg per day) can maintain good general health of the patient.

Proline-Hydroxyproline-Glycinuria (Iminoglycinuria). This finding is normal in early infancy. Failure of the group-specific transport system to develop has been observed as a frequent, benign autosomal recessive trait. Presence or absence of an associated intestinal transport defect indicates at least two mutant genotypes.

FANCONI'S SYNDROME

The term "Fanconi's syndrome" describes a disturbance of proximal renal tubular function of multiple causation and comprising generalized hyperaminoaciduria, renal glucosuria, and hyperphosphaturia, as well as renal loss of potassium, bicarbonate and water, and other substances conserved by the proximal tubule. Fanconi's syndrome should be considered as the final result of any one of many possible primary insults to proximal tubular function (see Group IV aminoacidurias, Table 1). The patient's symptoms reflect the disturbance of tubular function, in addition to the primary cause of the syndrome. Osteomalacia is a particularly prominent clinical finding primarily reflecting phosphate wasting. Acidosis accompanies the bicarbonate loss, whereas muscular weakness may be a prominent manifestation of hypokalemia.

Fanconi's syndrome may be inherited or acquired. The various hereditary forms are predominantly recessive, different alleles being responsible for the different diseases causing the syndrome. For example, cystinosis is a recessive, inherited disease, with cystine accumulation occurring in tissues and accompanied by the syndrome that first appears about six months after birth. The idiopathic Fanconi syndrome in adults is a recessively inherited disorder of early middle age. Acquired causes are numerous; deteriorated tetracycline (epianhydrotetracycline) is an interesting example of a toxic cause of the syndrome.

The syndrome appears to follow inhibition of cellular mechanisms sustaining transport function in the proximal tubule. As a result, the tubular capacity for transport is impaired. In severe cases, morphologic changes also occur, with reduction in cell organelles and cell mass of the proximal portion of the proximal convoluted tubule (swan-neck lesion). There is considerable experimental evidence that solutes enter urine in excess not only because of impaired absorption but also by backflux from renal cells after entry into kidney tissue from peritubular capillaries.

The disturbance of proximal tubular function results in the alterations in urine and plasma composition referred to above. The final levels of expression of the syndrome are more peripheral, and are related to both the disturbances in renal physiology and the primary causes of the syndrome. Pitressin-resistant diabetes insipidus is sometimes diagnosed in children before the syndrome is recognized. There may also be evidence for the primary cause of the syndrome, e.g., cystine crystals in the cornea, Kayser-Fleischer rings of Wilson's disease, a history of exposure to antimicrobial drugs or toxins, or other affected family members.

Treatment. Attempt to eliminate the primary cause, e.g., removal of exogenous toxic agents or deficiency states. Other primary conditions may be ameliorated, e.g., removal of milk in galactosemia or removal of copper in Wilson's disease.

Offset the disturbance in tubular physiology. Osteomalacia is readily treated, and prevented, with oral phosphate supplements (1.0 to 2.0 grams phosphorus per day, equivalent to 20 grams of "neutral" phosphate salt); supplemental vitamin D_2 may also be required in doses adjusted to the patient's need. Shohl's solution, 30 ml three times daily for adults, usually controls the acidemia. Hypokalemia may be corrected with potassium salts (as phosphate or citrate). Adequate fluid intake is indicated to prevent dehydration.

Efron, M. L.: Aminoaciduria. N. Engl. J. Med., 272:1058, 1107, 1965.

Nyhan, W. L. (ed.): Amino Acid Metabolism and Genetic Variation. New York, McGraw-Hill Book Company, 1967.

Scriver, C. R., and Rosenberg, L. E.: Amino Acid Metabolism and Its Disorders. Philadelphia, W. B. Saunders Company, 1973.

THE HYPERGLYCINURIAS

Six forms of isolated hyperglycinuria are known:

1. Hyperglycinemia with "overflow" hyperglycinuria.

a. Type I (ketotic): Vomiting, acetonuria, neutropenia, thrombocytopenia, and leucine intolerance occur in the neonatal period; retardation of growth and mental development follow if the infant survives. The findings to a lesser or greater degree are found in propionicacidemia (propionyl CoA carboxylase deficiency), methylmalonicacidemia (methylmalonyl CoA mutase deficiency), and a disorder of isoleucine catabolism (β-ketothiolase deficiency). Restriction of dietary protein intake may be helpful.

b. Type II (nonketotic): There is severe developmental and mental retardation. Conversion of glycine to carbon dioxide, methylenetetrahydrofolate, and ammonia is apparently impaired.

2. Renal glycinurias.

a. Impaired renal conservation of glycine occurs as the heterozygous phenotype in one form of familial iminoglycinuria.

b. Resistant rickets and renal hyperglycinuria occur in association with (i) hyperphosphaturia, (ii) hyperphosphaturia and glucosuria (both renal).

c. Dominantly inherited, asymptomatic renal glycinuria with renal glucosuria has been reported from Switzerland.

ALCAPTONURIA AND OCHRONOSIS

Definition. Alcaptonuria (homogentisicaciduria) is a disorder of tyrosine metabolism which results from deficiency of the enzyme homogentisic acid oxidase. Alcaptonuria is the predecessor of ochronosis, the condition which results from chronic deposition of an oxidized brown-black pigment of homogentisic acid in connective tissue, causing spondylosis and arthropathy. Alcaptonuria is one of the inborn errors of metabolism originally described by Garrod, and the first disease for which autosomal recessive inheritance was proposed.

Pathogenesis. Homogentisic acid (2,5-dihydroxyphenylacetic acid) is normally oxidized in liver and kidney to maleylacetoacetic acid. In the absence of this reaction, homogentisic acid accumulates in tissues, and is secreted into urine by alcaptonuric subjects. There is no significant homogentisicacidemia, because the compound is rapidly secreted by kidney, its renal clearance greatly exceeding the glomerular filtration rate. The damage to connective tissue characteristic of ochronosis results from prolonged exposure to homogentisic acid. Its oxidized pigment, benzoquinoneacetic acid, is believed to polymerize to form a melanin-like pigment, which binds irreversibly with collagen. It has been suggested that such binding cross-links collagen, thus altering its physicochemical properties, which in turn leads to the degenerative changes observed in ochronosis. Although alcaptonuria may be detected in the newborn period, changes in connective tissue do not appear until adulthood, perhaps because the enhanced remodeling of connective tissue during childhood and adolescence removes the chemically modified collagen.

Diagnosis. Homogentisicaciduria is present from birth onward, and its intensity is proportional to the dietary intake and catabolism of phenylalanine and tyrosine. With modern sanitation patients may not know for many years that their urine can darken on standing. Thus the diagnosis usually rests on clinical suspicion, a family history, and chemical tests.

Urine. Freshly voided urine is normal in appearance; darkening occurs slowly from the exposed surface downward on standing in air, and rapidly when made alkaline. Homogentisic acid reduces Benedict's reagent to a brown-orange color, and produces a purple-black reaction with ferric chloride reagent. Large amounts of ascorbic acid may give false positive reactions with these chemical tests, and it will prevent spontaneous darkening. Coloration of urine caused by bile, porphyrins, myoglobin, and hemoglobin should be distinguished. Homogentisic acid can be confirmed by chromatography and a specific enzymatic method.

Ochronosis

Deposition of brown-black pigment in connective tissue is the legacy of prolonged exposure to homogentisic acid. It can occur in dermis and sweat glands, conjunctiva and cornea, sclera, pinna, tympanic membrane, and ossicles of the middle ear, laryngeal and tracheal cartilages, heart valves, genitourinary tract, tendons, large diarthrodial joints, and spine. Pigment granules occur as both intracellular and extracellular deposits. Characteristically the pinnae are stiff and opaque to transillumination; the corneas are black; conduction hearing loss may accompany involvement of tympanum and ossicles. Renal stones and prostatic calculi occur but usually do not cause renal disease, although prostatitis may be caused by alcaptonuria. Heart disease is not more frequent in alcaptonuria despite pigmentation of the endocardium and intima of the aorta.

Ochronotic Arthropathy. The most serious complication of ochronosis is arthropathy. Unlike rheumatoid disease, it spares the small joints of hands and feet. Onset of arthropathy is earlier and more severe in males, and the knee is the most frequently and severely affected peripheral joint. Spondylosis, which is very often present, appears slowly with pain and stiffness, usually in the low back. Ultimately involvement of the lumbar and thoracic spine results in loss of motion and disappearance of the normal lumbar lordosis. Herniation or calcification of the intervertebral discs is also characteristic. As a consequence of ochronotic arthropathy, the typical patient assumes a wide-based stance with forward stoop, rigid spine, and flexed hips and knees.

Roentgenographic examination reveals narrowing of the intervertebral spaces, disc calcification, and gradual fusion of vertebral bodies. However, the annular ossification ("bamboo spine") of ankylosing spondylitis is not seen. In the peripheral joints there may be evidence of synovial effusion and osteochondral bodies in the knee joint; the osteophytes and periarticular cystic changes of osteoarthritis are not prominent. With time, degenerative changes occur, with narrowing of the joint space, eburnation, sclerosis, and calcification of adjacent tendons.

Prognosis. Life expectancy is normal. Alcaptonuria and ochronotic pigmentation are symptomless manifestations of homogentisic acid accumulation. Patients with the disease usually marry noncarriers, and will transmit the trait, with a 1 in 2 probability, to their offspring.

Treatment. There is no specific treatment for alcaptonuria. Limitation of phenylalanine and tyrosine intake would be of theoretical value to prevent homogentisic acid accumulation, but such lifelong dietary treatment is not feasible. The reducing agent, vitamin C, impedes oxidation and polymerization of homogentisic acid and large amounts in the diet might delay ochronotic changes. Occupations which stress the spine and large joints should be avoided. Families expressing this autosomal recessive trait should be given appropriate genetic counseling.

Garrod, A. E.: The incidence of alkaptonuria. A study in chemical individuality. Lancet, 2:1616, 1902.

LaDu, B. N.: Alcaptonuria. *In* Stanbury, J. B., Wyngaarden, J. B., and Fredrickson, D. S. (eds.): The Metabolic Basis of Inherited Disease. 3rd ed. New York, McGraw-Hill Book Company, 1973, pp. 308–325.

LaDu, B. N., Zannoni, V. G., Laster, L., and Seegmiller, J. E.: The nature of the defect in tyrosine metabolism in alcaptonuria. J. Biol. Chem., 230:251, 1958.

O'Brien, W. M., LaDu, B. N., and Bunim, J. J.: Biochemical, pathologic and clinical aspects of alcaptonuria, ochronosis and ochronotic arthropathy. Am. J. Med., 34:813, 1963.

Stoner, R., and Blivaiss, B. B.: Reaction of quinone of homogentisic acid with biological amines. Arthritis Rheum., 10:53, 1967.

DISORDERS OF PURINE METABOLISM

Lloyd H. Smith, Jr.

821. GOUT

Definition. Gout represents a group of *genetic* diseases of purine metabolism or excretion ordinarily identifiable by *hyperuricemia*. When clinically manifest, gout presents as an acute inflammatory *arthritis,* the accumulation of sodium urate deposits as *tophi, uric acid nephrolithiasis,* or *renal failure.* These manifestations can occur in any combination. This definition, which must remain arbitrary until the pathogenesis of each gouty syndrome has been more firmly established, has several points of emphasis which will be discussed more fully later in this chapter. First, it emphasizes the genetic or familial origin of gout. This attribute has long been recognized. Galen attributed gout to "debauchery, intemperance, and an hereditary trait," and Sydenham emphasized its early occurrence in patients "when they have received the ill seeds of this disease from their parents by inheritance." Second, gout is defined here in terms of its chemical derangement, essentially hyperuricemia. This is analogous to the diagnosis of diabetes mellitus as essential hyperglucosemia. The clinical manifestations are complications of hyperuricemia (or hyperuricaciduria) which may or may not occur in the individual patient. It has been estimated that these complications in some combination occur in only 10 to 20 per cent of individuals with hyperuricemia, the incidence increasing in rough proportion to the level of serum uric acid. Finally, the definition emphasizes the heterogeneity of gout. Several different diseases lead to the common feature of persistent hyperuricemia (see Pathogenesis and Table 1).

In a sense all of us have inappropriate hyperuricemia

because of two errors in evolution. Uricase catalyzes the conversion of relatively insoluble urate to soluble allantoin, which would be a much more appropriate end product for the mammalian kidney. The evolutionary retention of this enzyme would have obviated both gout and uric acid nephrolithiasis. A second error compounds the first. The mechanism by which the human kidney excretes uric acid is complex, including glomerular filtration, tubular reabsorption, and tubular secretion. The net result is renal retention of more than 90 per cent of that filtered. At equilibrium, the same amount of uric acid is presumably excreted but at the cost of relative hyperuricemia. Renal tubular reabsorption of filtered uric acid is not present in other primates, which therefore have serum uric acid levels of less than 0.05 mg per 100 ml. The suggestion has been made that renal retention might help to modulate bursts of uric acid excretion owing to purine ingestion, and also might shunt more urate into the gut for bacterial destruction. Whether this is true or not, it seems clear that gout represents an exaggeration of a genetic legacy of hyperuricemia common to all.

History. Gout has figured largely in history, perhaps rivaled only by pandemics of infectious diseases and mental illness. Its classic manifestations were noted in classical times, and the occurrence of osseous tophi and uric acid stones has allowed archeologic diagnoses to be made with confidence. Hippocrates, who recognized and described podagra, devoted three of his aphorisms to the disease, saying in effect: 28, Eunuchs do not take the gout, nor become bald; 29, Women do not take the gout until their menses be stopped; 30, Young men do not take the gout until they indulge in coition. Galen described tophaceous gout and commented upon the familial occurrence of the disease. The term gout, derived from the Latin word *gutta*, came into usage during the Middle Ages to reflect a theory of pathogenesis that this form of arthritis resulted from the "dropping" of a poisonous *"noxa"* into the joint. It is interesting to see the recent confirmation of this theory and the identification of sodium urate microcrystals as the *noxa*. In the seventeenth century, Thomas Sydenham (1683), sometimes called the Shakespeare of gout, wrote clinical descriptions of the disease which have yet to be improved on. He wrote with an authority based on intense personal experience with gouty arthritis and stones. Uric acid was first discovered as a component of stones by Scheele in 1776 (designated lithic acid), followed two decades later by its identification in tophi by Wollaston (1797). In the middle of the nineteenth century the elder (A. B.) Garrod developed a crude but ingenious method for estimating uric acid in serum (crystallization on a linen fiber), and found it to be elevated in patients with gout, demonstrating for the first time the chemical hallmark of the disease. His postulate that acute gouty arthritis was due to deposits of sodium urate was convincingly supported by the work of Freudweiler (1899), who demonstrated the inflammatory potential of sodium urate microcrystals and leukocytic phagocytosis of such crystals in acute gout. This contribution was lost in the sediment of subsequent investigations, the phenomenon of *microcrystalline synovitis* being independently rediscovered within the past few years. In 1931, the younger (A. E.) Garrod proposed that gout should be classified as one of the inborn errors of metabolism. Over the past two decades studies in many laboratories, notably those of Buchanan, Greenberg, Seegmiller, and Wyngaarden, have elucidated the pathways of purine biosynthesis and degradation and the controlling mechanisms for modulating the appropriate rate of control of purine metabolism. It is against this background that current studies of pathogenesis, to be reviewed below, are being conducted.

The history of gout has been intermingled with sociologic and cultural variables as well as the march of medical and biochemical progress. From earliest observations the disease has been associated with dissipation and venery. Even gouty Sydenham wrote, "the gout generally attacks those aged persons who have spent most of their lives in ease, voluptuousness, high living, and too free use of wine and other spirituous liquors." It gradually became a disease in caricature in the eighteenth and nineteenth centuries, used by novelist, satirist, and political cartoonist alike as symbolic of medical retribution for excessive indulgence of natural appetites. Ambrose Bierce defined gout as "a physician's name for the rheumatism of a rich patient." The disease gradually won grudging respect ("disease of kings and king of diseases") because of its remarkable association with men of genius and exceptional achievement. An incomplete list of those alleged to have suffered from the gout includes Alexander the Great, Louis XIV, Isaac Newton, William Harvey, Martin Luther, John Calvin, Leonardo da Vinci, Samuel Johnson, and Benjamin Franklin. It is an amusing sequel that several recent studies have confirmed positive statistical correlations of serum uric acid levels and intelligence or social status. In this context it is unkind to recall, with Hippocrates, that gout is rare in the premenopausal female.

Genetics of Gout. Family aggregation of clinical gout has been observed since the first clinical descriptions of the disease in antiquity. Gout has appeared in an irregular pattern both in successive generations and in sibships. A positive family history for clinical gout is found in about 10 to 20 per cent of patients with the primary disorder. Attempts have been made to use hyperuricemia as a more precise marker for the presence of the gouty trait. Within the restrictions imposed by the statistical uncertainties of the boundary between normal and abnormal serum urate levels (Fig. 1), hyperuricemia has been found in 15 to 25 per cent of close relatives of patients with clinical gout. It is sometimes stated that primary gout is transmitted as an autosomal dominant with incomplete penetrance. The pattern of inheritance of hyperuricemia has varied so widely that it may be polygenic in origin. Many variables affect the phenotypic expression of the gouty trait: age, sex, diet, and renal function. It is noteworthy that in the form of gout in which a specific enzyme defect of purine metabolism has been most clearly established, the syndrome of hypoxanthine–guanine phosphoribosyltransferase deficiency, the genetic transmission has been established as that of a sex-linked recessive trait. Glycogen storage disease Type I, which is associated with a specific form of secondary renal gout, is transmitted as an autosomal recessive trait. It seems probable that the mode of inheritance of other forms of gout will not be clearly established until genetic markers more specific than hyperuricemia are available. This must await clarification of the pathogenesis of the various gouty syndromes in more specific phenotypic terms.

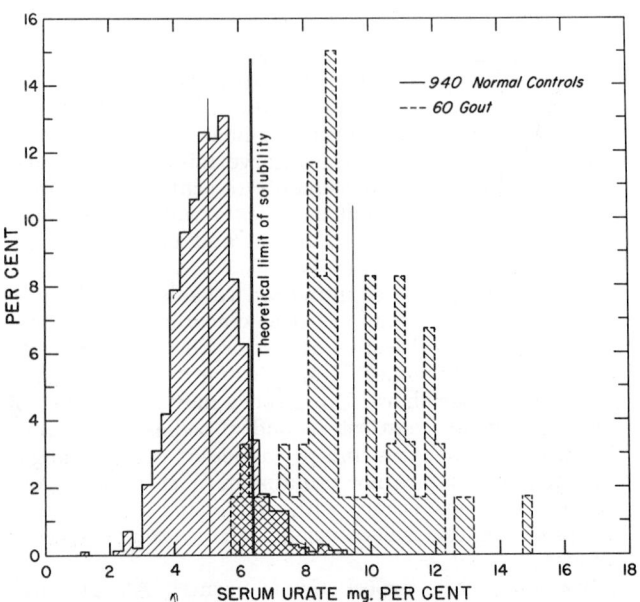

Figure 1. Distribution of serum urate concentrations in normal and gouty male subjects and calculated limit of solubility of sodium urate in serum. (From Seegmiller, J. E.: Diseases of purine and pyrimidine metabolism. *In* Bondy, P. K., and Rosenberg, L. E. [eds.]: Duncan's Diseases of Metabolism. 7th ed. Philadelphia, W. B. Saunders Company, 1974.)

ALLOPURINOL   ALLO-XANTHINE

INHIBITION

XANTHINE OXIDASE

HYPOXANTHINE   XANTHINE   URIC ACID

Figure 2. Pathway of uric acid synthesis catalyzed by xanthine oxidase and the site of action of allopurinol.

Pathogenesis. It has been established for over 100 years (A. B. Garrod) that the hallmark of gout is hyperuricemia. All of the clinical manifestations of gout, with the single exception of uric acid nephrolithiasis, derive from the cystallization of sodium urate from extracellular fluids where it has accumulated in a supersaturated concentration. No one has shown that sodium urate in solution is toxic. There are several questions which relate to the pathogenesis of gout: What leads to the accumulation of urate in extracellular fluid? What are the variables in its precipitation? How do sodium urate crystals lead to inflammatory arthritis?

The Cause of Hyperuricemia. The accumulation of any metabolite in excess must result from one (or a combination) of four variables: increased absorption, decreased metabolism, decreased excretion, or increased biosynthesis. There is no evidence that gouty patients habitually ingest excessive purines or have an increased avidity for purine absorption. Elimination of purine ingestion usually results in a reduction of serum urate of about 0.6 mg per 100 ml in normal subjects and about 1.0 mg per 100 ml in gouty patients. Under experimental conditions, ingestion of a diet very high in nucleic acids may lead to hyperuricemia in normal subjects comparable to gouty levels. In summary, absorption of preformed purines from dietary sources may

modify extracellular urate levels, but does not represent a primary cause of gout.

Uric acid is the end product of purine metabolism, most of it being excreted as free urinary urate. Recent studies have indicated at least two mechanisms by which it is partially destroyed in man. Leukocytes contain verdoperoxidases capable of degrading uric acid to allantoin and carbon dioxide. Of much greater importance quantitatively, uric acid is secreted into the gut where uricolysis is carried out by bacterial enzymes. Approximately one quarter of that synthesized daily is degraded through these mechanisms. Studies in gout have not supported decreased uricolysis as a mechanism for hyperuricemia. In fact, with high urate concentrations, especially after the onset of renal insufficiency, excretion into the gut, and uricolysis there, may be enhanced as an important second line of defense. Particular attention has therefore been directed toward increased synthesis or decreased excretion as primary mechanisms for hyperuricemia in gout.

Uric acid is synthesized from xanthine and from hypoxanthine (via xanthine), these successive oxidations being catalyzed by xanthine oxidase (Fig. 2). The free purine bases bear complex metabolic relationships to various pools of purine nucleotides. In part the free bases are reutilized to form functioning nucleotides; in part they are converted to uric acid for excretion. Be-

Figure 3. De novo pathway of purine nucleotide biosynthesis and the feedback control mechanisms (— — — →). E_1, Glutamine 5-phosphoribosylpyrophosphate amidotransferase; E_2, inosine 5′-phosphate dehydrogenase; E_3, adenylsuccinic acid (AMP-S) synthetase; XMP, xanthosine 5′-phosphate.

PP—RIBOSE—P + GLUTAMINE

E_1

5-PHOSPHORIBOSYLAMINE

GLYCINE   GLUTAMINE

FORMATE   ASPARTATE

CO_2 ATP

GUANYLIC ACID ← XMP ←E_2← INOSINIC ACID →E_3→ AMP-S → ADENYLIC ACID
GMP   IMP   AMP

cause of this reutilization, sometimes called "salvage synthesis," uric acid synthesis, as reflected in urinary excretion and intestinal destruction, represents only a part of the purine nucleotide turnover rate. At equilibrium, however, that part should approximate the de novo synthetic rate of purine nucleotides. Small amounts of hypoxanthine, xanthine, and other trace purines are normally excreted in the urine as well. Several methods have been widely applied in an attempt to determine whether there is excessive purine synthesis in gout: measurement of urate excreted on a low purine diet, use of isotopic urate to determine its pool size and turnover rate, and study of the time course of incorporation of a purine precursor, usually glycine, into urate (Fig. 3). Each of these methods is subject to limitations which cannot be detailed here. The following information has emerged from such studies. In normal man the daily rate of production of uric acid on a low purine diet averages about 750 mg. The miscible pool of uric acid is about 1.0 to 1.3 grams, so that two thirds to three fourths of the body pool turns over daily. Urinary excretion of urate varies widely even during dietary regulation, averaging in men 426 ± 81 mg per 24 hours. The difference between the estimated production rate of urate and that excreted in the urine represents uricolysis, mostly by bacterial action in the gut.

By use of these methods, evidence for excessive synthesis of uric acid has been obtained in about two thirds of patients with primary gout. Overproduction is readily understood in patients with diseases resulting in increased tissue breakdown, e.g., myeloid metaplasia, polycythemia vera, and leukemia. The hypoxanthine–guanine phosphoribosyltransferase deficiency syndrome will be discussed later in this chapter as the biochemical basis for excessive purine synthesis in one form of gout. The first step unique to purine nucleotide biosynthesis and the major site of metabolic regulation is that of the synthesis of phosphoribosylamine, catalyzed by the enzyme glutamine 5-phosphoribosyl-pyrophosphate (PRPP) amidotransferase:

$$\text{Glutamine} + \text{PRPP} + H_2O \xrightarrow{Mg^{++}} \text{glutamic acid} +$$
$$\text{5-phosphoribosylamine} + \text{pyrophosphate}$$

There are several possibilities for loss of normal rate control at this regulatory site; these include excessive concentrations of the substrate glutamine, PRRP, or both, a genetic alteration in the enzyme rendering it less sensitive to normal feedback control by purine nucleotides, or a partial deficiency of one of the nucleotides (adenylic, guanylic, and inosinic acids) which, in concert, exert allosteric modulation of the enzyme (Fig. 3). Recent work from two laboratories has demonstrated increased activity of PRPP synthetase in a few patients with gout, presumably driving purine synthesis by excessive availability of PRPP. Glutamate but not glutamine is raised in the plasma of a number of gouty patients. It can be anticipated that future studies will document further heterogeneity in the mechanisms by which purine synthesis is enhanced in various types of overproduction gout.

In about one third of patients with gout there is no evidence for overproduction of uric acid by any of the methods now available. Evidence suggests that these patients have an inherited disorder (or group of dis-

orders) of the renal tubule resulting in decreased urate clearance as the cause of hyperuricemia. Renal clearance of urate is a complex function of filtration, tubular reabsorption, and tubular secretion. There is partial binding of urate to plasma proteins, but this does not seem to represent a significant fraction under physiologic conditions at 37° C. Using the assumption that urate is completely filterable at the glomerulus, there is net tubular reabsorption of 90 to 95 per cent. Urate which is excreted is in part and perhaps in toto that secreted by the tubule. Patients with "renal gout" exhibit reduced clearances of urate, the differences being most evident when compared to normal controls with dietary induction of comparable plasma levels of uric acid. The differences have not always been striking, and in some cases may be difficult to interpret because of early impairment of renal function by gout. In renal gout reduced net clearance of urate probably results from a defect in its tubular secretion, although enhanced tubular reabsorption of urate has not been excluded. In theory, an increase in the bound fraction of urate would also reduce clearance by reducing that filtered. An impaired tubular secretion of urate might be an intrinsic defect of the transport mechanism, which has not yet been clarified biochemically. It might also result from a genetic or acquired metabolic disorder in some other pathway which leads to the accumulation of a metabolite which secondarily interferes with tubular urate secretion. An example of this latter mechanism is the hyperuricemia associated with the lactic acidosis of Type I glycogen storage disease (see Ch. 809). Idiopathic renal gout might similarly result from the accumulation of other uric acid transport inhibitors not yet identified. When over-all reduction of renal function occurs, as happens not infrequently in gout, hyperuricemia is further exacerbated, and an increased percentage of urate is excreted into the gut for uricolysis.

In summary, the important causes of persistent hyperuricemia are those of excessive synthesis and decreased renal clearance. This allows for a rational classification of gout as shown in Table 1. Such a classification reflects only a progress report. Although hypoxanthine–guanine phosphoribosyltransferase deficiency and PRPP synthetase excess represent the only types of metabolic gout for which specific enzymatic defects have been established, new defects in the rate control mechanisms will almost certainly be established shortly, possibly as abnormalities of phosphoribosyl-

TABLE 1.   Classification of Hyperuricemia and Gout

I. Metabolic gout—excessive synthesis
  A. Genetic
    1. Hypoxanthine–guanine phosphoribosyltransferase deficiency —Lesch-Nyhan syndrome or incomplete forms
    2. Excessive activity of 5-phosphoribosylpyrophosphate synthetase
    3. Other defects of rate control
  B. Acquired—excessive tissue turnover
II. Renal gout—reduced clearance
  A. Genetic— ↓ renal tubular secretion?
    1. Idiopathic
    2. Lactic acidosis—glycogen storage disease Type I
  B. Acquired
    1. Inhibition of urate transport—drugs, metabolites (lactic acid, β-hydroxybutyric acid)
    2. Renal failure

pyrophosphate amidotransferase. Similarly, the genetic types of renal gout will probably prove to be more heterogeneous in future studies. A variety of drugs (notably the chlorothiazide diuretics) and metabolites (lactate, β-hydroxybutyrate) diminish urate clearance in the normal kidney, and may precipitate clinical gout.

Precipitation of Urate. Uric acid is not toxic to man in its soluble state. Although hyperuricemia has been associated epidemiologically with a number of conditions, e.g., coronary artery heart disease and hypertension, there is no evidence that it has any pathogenic relationship to those disorders. Uric acid seems to produce disease "physically" rather than "chemically" when precipitated as sodium urate at pH 7.40, or as uric acid in acidic urine. Its precipitation as amorphous sodium urate, which may occur in virtually any tissue in the body except for the central nervous system, results in tophi with tissue disruption and destruction but with minimal inflammatory response. Its precipitation as microcrystals of critical size in certain tissues, especially in synovial tissues and spaces, leads to an acute inflammatory reaction to be described below. Its precipitation in the renal distal collecting tubules as uric acid may rarely lead to acute renal failure. The precipitation of uric acid in a protein matrix in the renal pelvis, or more rarely in the ureter or bladder, leads to uric acid nephrolithiasis.

Sodium urate is soluble in human plasma to a concentration of only about 7 mg of urate per 100 ml. Values above this denote supersaturated solutions, although sodium urate may remain in supersaturated solution with considerable stability. Why do some patients with serum uric acid levels of 9 mg per 100 ml have severe tophaceous gout or acute gouty arthritis or both, whereas others may maintain similar levels for years or even for life with no evidence of precipitation, i.e., of clinical gout? The reasons for these differences in threshold of precipitation are not known. One recently described variable is that of protein binding of urate in plasma to a specific α_1-α_2 globulin (Alvsaker) and to albumin. The report that some patients with tophaceous gout have reduced protein-binding of urate is provocative but has not been confirmed. Furthermore, the importance of protein-binding of urate remains to be established.

The solubility of urate in urine decreases with increasing acidity because of the shift to free uric acid. The titration curve is such that the undissociated uric acid increases to 85 per cent at pH 5.0. At this pH only 6 to 8 mg of urate is soluble per 100 ml of urine so that supersaturation is required to excrete an average uric acid load in a normal urine volume. The solubility increases 20-fold at pH 7.0 over that at pH 5.0. Three factors are therefore important in the urinary precipitation of uric acid: urine volume, the amount of urate excreted per 24 hours, and urine pH. It is possible that the availability of stone matrix and the level of stabilizing substances in urine may also play important roles.

Cause of Acute Gouty Arthritis. The four clinical manifestations of gout are those of tophaceous deposits, acute gouty arthritis, uric acid nephrolithiasis, and gouty kidney with various degrees of impairment of renal function. Of these clinical manifestations or complications associated with hyperuricemia, acute inflammatory arthritis is that which has been most obscure in its pathogenesis. Garrod the elder, in the second of his

ten propositions on "the true nature or essence of gout" (1859), wrote: "Investigations recently made in the morbid anatomy of gout prove incontestably that true gouty inflammation is always accompanied with a deposition of urate of soda in the inflamed part." This proposition was strongly supported by the experimental work of Freudweiler (1899), who was able to produce inflammation with sodium urate crystals and observe their subsequent presence in leukocytes. For many years, however, this work was ignored because of evidence which seemed to indicate that retention of uric acid, the seemingly obvious basis of tophi, was unrelated to the sudden acute attacks of inflammatory arthritis. Several pieces of evidence supported that view. The onset of acute attacks bore no relation to changes in serum urate levels. Joints severely involved with tophaceous deposits were often free from acute attacks. Despite its almost specific therapeutic effectiveness, colchicine had no demonstrable effect on urate metabolism. During reductions of serum urate levels with uricosuric drugs, attacks of acute gouty arthritis were fairly often exacerbated. Because of these and other observations, major attention was directed toward alternative explanations, such as abnormalities in the metabolism of trace purines.

Within the past few years gouty arthritis has been clearly shown to be an inflammatory reaction to microcrystals of sodium urate, mediated by a series of chemical changes accompanying phagocytosis of the crystals by leukocytes. The presence of sodium urate microcrystals in synovial fluid from gouty joints during acute inflammation, both free and in leukocytes, is so con-

Figure 4. Sodium urate monohydrate crystals phagocytized by leukocytes in synovial fluid from acute gouty arthritis examined by polarized light. (Reproduced with permission of Dr. Daniel J. McCarty, Jr.)

stant as to be of diagnostic value (Fig. 4). This was the key observation that led to the experiments supporting the early Garrod-Freudweiler concept. The injection of sodium urate microcrystals into joints of normal controls or gouty patients produces typical gout responsive to colchicine. Aspiration of these joints demonstrates phagocytosis of some of the injected crystals. In fact, no experimental gouty arthritis can be produced in laboratory animals in the absence of leukocytes. The inflammatory reaction of microcrystalline synovitis is a nonspecific one, being produced by injection of other crystals of appropriate size and shape, such as sodium orotate or calcium pyrophosphate.

The exact mechanism by which sodium urate crystals initiate inflammation has not been established. The crystals can activate Hageman factor, and in this way initiate the chain of events resulting in bradykinin synthesis. Bradykinin levels are raised in synovial fluid from gouty joints, but injection of carboxypeptidase B, which destroys bradykinin, does not prevent experimental gout. The requirement for leukocyte-crystal interaction was noted above. Uric acid has been found to be leukotactic. Phagocytosis of the crystals leads to increased metabolic activity of the leukocyte, release of lysosomal enzymes, and increased lactic acid production. Interesting studies on the molecular basis of crystal-induced inflammation have been carried out recently (Weissmann, McCarty). Phagocytosis of sodium urate crystals leads to rapid destruction of the phagolysosome membrane, releasing its hydrolytic enzymes into the cell cytoplasm. This results in cell lysis. The original crystal, the hydrolytic enzymes, and the cytoplasmic enzymes from the destroyed leukocyte are released into the surrounding tissue. This crystal-membrane interaction, which can be simulated with artificial lipid membranes ("liposomes") as well, is thought to result from hydrogen bonding between the rigid crystal and elements in the lipid membrane surface, leading to breaks in its continuity. The attack of the leukocyte on the sodium urate crystal is therefore both suicidal and counterproductive, setting in motion an inappropriate inflammatory response which is injurious to the host.

Although the biochemical events of inflammation are poorly understood, the establishment of the general mechanism of microcrystalline synovitis has allowed a rational explanation of acute gouty arthritis. Still unexplained are the mechanisms by which the acute attack is initiated, i.e., what leads to the presumed burst of microcrystallization at a given time. How are the known precipitating events of acute gouty arthritis, which may be roughly grouped together as stresses, translated into microcrystallization?

The model of leukocyte-crystal interaction may offer an explanation for the action of colchicine. As stated, in the therapeutic range colchicine has no effect on net purine metabolism as reflected in levels of extracellular uric acid or in its excretion. On the other hand, colchicine diminishes leukocyte migration and modifies many of the metabolic concomitants of phagocytosis in the leukocyte. The use of such an in vitro model may allow the rational development of other therapeutic agents in the future.

Clinical Manifestations. As previously stated, the clinical manifestations of gout can be arbitrarily divided into four categories: acute gouty arthritis, tophaceous gout, uric acid nephrolithiasis, and gouty kidney. Although the basic metabolic abnormalities of genetic gout must be presumed to have been present since conception, clinical gout is extraordinarily rare before the rise in extracellular uric acid levels which accompany puberty in the male. Exceptions to this are seen in the juvenile gout of the Lesch-Nyhan syndrome and in glycogen storage disease Type I. Clinical gout usually makes its appearance in middle life in men, although the majority of patients with hyperuricemia never exhibit these complications. As observed by Hippocrates, clinical gout in women rarely occurs before the menopause, at which time there is a further rise in uric acid levels. In most series, gout in women accounts for only 5 to 10 per cent of cases.

The epidemiology of gout and hyperuricemia has received increasing attention beyond the genetic studies of families. The positive statistical correlation of uric acid levels with education, intelligence, and social status was pointed out above. Exceptionally high frequencies of hyperuricemia have been found in Filipinos (in the United States but not in the Philippines), in Maoris, and in the natives of the Marianas Islands. The over-all incidence of clinical gout in the United States has been estimated as 3 patients per 1000 population. As a generality it has been stated that gout makes up about 5 per cent of arthritis.

Acute Gouty Arthritis. Acute gouty arthritis is the most frequent first clinical manifestation of the disease. It has been eloquently described by many who have endured it, but by none more effectively than Sydenham, who wrote, "it [the affected part] is not able to bear the weight of the cloths upon it, nor hard walking in the chamber." He further alluded to the pain as being "like the gnawing of a dog." Acute gouty arthritis often follows a precipitating event: surgery, injury, alcohol ingestion, dietary excess, emotional stress, or even the minor stress of excessive walking. In view of the current concept of the pathogenesis as that of microcrystalline synovitis, such stress must somehow be translated into localized sodium urate crystallization, or must alter the tissue reaction to such crystals. Since sodium urate usually exists in a supersaturated solution in the gouty patient, the initiating event need introduce only a single crystal focus for seeding a cascade of precipitation. Some of the precipitating events, such as starvation and alcohol ingestion, increase urate levels by inhibition of renal urate excretion through the accompanying ketosis and lactic acidosis, respectively. The particular association of gout with spirituous liquors, legendary in medieval history ("in the young wine goes to the head; in the aged it goes to the feet"), therefore finds some scientific basis at the level of the renal tubule. A particularly puzzling and important kind of exacerbation of acute gouty arthritis is that which frequently occurs during early stages of treatment designed to lower extracellular urate levels. This may complicate the use of uricosuric agents or of allopurinol, to the great distress of both patient and physician. It has been difficult to explain the exacerbation of gout in the face of a falling urate concentration. It is possible that mobilization of amorphous tophaceous deposits may allow for local precipitation of the microcrystals conducive to inflammation. The frequent occurrence of this complication may occasionally obviate or delay effective treatment.

Gout usually presents as a sudden, exquisitely painful arthritis. After a few premonitory twinges the onset of inflammation may occur within minutes with severe arthritis within a few hours. Typically a patient may retire for the night in good health, yet be awakened a few hours later with excruciating pain in the affected joint. He may develop podagra (gouty arthritis of the first metatarsophalangeal joint) with such rapidity that he is unable to remove his shoe in time. More rarely the warning signals of impending arthritis develop into a crescendo pattern ending in the acute attack.

Gouty arthritis exhibits a marked predilection for the larger joints, particularly in the feet and ankles. Hippocrates described podagra, which still represents the most frequent site of involvement (Fig. 5). This may reflect the trauma of weight-bearing which in the normal foot produces the greatest force per unit area (pressure) there. Other frequent sites of early attacks are the ankle, the instep, or occasionally the knee. Less frequently the elbow, wrist, or metacarpophalangeal joints are the sites of gouty arthritis. The hips, shoulders, and spine are very rarely the sites of microcrystalline synovitis, and almost never the sites of initial involvement. Gouty arthritis is usually monoarticular, especially in the earliest attacks. Some patients may have marked tophaceous gout with bone and articular destruction and few if any attacks of acute gout. Involvement of a joint by tophi does not seem to predispose that area to acute attacks, and some clinicians have even suggested that tophaceous areas enjoy relative immunity from acute inflammation.

Acute gouty arthritis is characterized by severe inflammation, not only in the joint itself but typically in the periarticular tissues and skin. The presence of heat, marked swelling, exquisite tenderness, and rubor extending well beyond the immediate vicinity of the joint capsule has often led to the erroneous diagnosis of septic arthritis or cellulitis. Occasionally lymphangitis may be evident. The skin over the area of inflammation is usually tense and shiny, and after subsidence of the attack undergoes superficial desquamation as is seen in erysipelas. Systemic signs of inflammation may include fever, leukocytosis, and elevation of the sedimentation rate which may further suggest an infectious etiology. The severity of the associated pain has been referred to above, and commands respect and attention rather than the traditional jocularity. When untreated, an attack of acute gouty arthritis usually subsides gradually over a period of one to two weeks. Generally there are no residual signs or symptoms; more rarely, stiffness persists, or a second flareup supervenes before there is complete recovery.

As stated, only about one of six patients with hyperuricemia will eventually have one or more of the complications of clinical gout. Moreover, the clinical course of gout after an initial attack of acute arthritis is highly variable. Some patients have only a single attack of monoarticular arthritis and then remain free of symptoms despite the persistence of hyperuricemia. More often, after a symptom-free interval, but usually within the first year, there is recurrence of an attack. In Gutman's series, 62 per cent have had recurrences within the first year, 16 per cent in one to two years, 11 per cent in two to five years, 4 per cent in ten years, and 7 per cent, no recurrence as yet during prolonged follow-up. In the usual pattern, subsequent attacks come with increasing frequency over the years unless prophylactic measures are taken, with gradual reduction in the duration of the symptom-free intervals (sometimes called intercritical gout). In about one third of patients, the number of attacks occurring each year has remained constant, and, rarely, there has been a spontaneous decline in frequency with increasing age of the patient. When attacks become more frequent they also tend to become more severe, both in the extent and duration of the inflammation and in the number of joints affected. The patient may reach a state at which he is rarely free of gouty inflammation, and at which even with subsidence of an acute attack there is enough residual swelling, stiffness, and pain in the involved joints to give permanent disability not responsive to the measures usually effective in acute attacks.

Tophaceous Gout. Sodium urate may accumulate in virtually any tissue in the body with the exception of the central nervous system, where the concentration is reduced by the blood-brain barrier. Tophi occur most

Figure 5. Acute gouty arthritis of great toe.

often in and around joints in cartilage, bone, bursae, and subcutaneous tissue. As foreign bodies, these deposits elicit a low-grade chronic inflammatory process with disruption of tissues and fibrosis. Destruction of tissue is particularly evident in cartilage and bone, leading to radiolucent "punched-out" lesions of bone and gross deformities of joints (Figs. 6 and 7). Deposits of sodium urate may be massive, particularly in the hands and feet and around the olecranon bursa. Subcutaneous deposits may be easily visible as yellowish-white excrescences, which on occasion may erode through the skin and discharge a pale paste composed largely of crystalline needles of sodium urate. In advanced cases, deposits of several hundred grams may lead to grotesquely deformed extremities. Rarely, involvement of the heart has been observed with tophi causing conduction disturbances. A frequent site of tophaceous deposits is the external ear, especially in the helix and antihelix. The local factors that control the sites of crystallization are not known. Massive tophi may be found in the hands, feet, and elbows with none of the typical auricular deposits. Conversely, the external ear may be the only site of visible tophi over many years of gouty diathesis. As stated above, recent work suggesting that patients most susceptible to tophi may have reduced protein binding of urate has not been confirmed.

About one half of all patients with clinical gout have visible tophi at some stage of their disease. Other patients may have more diffuse deposition of sodium urate without local nodules or infiltrates demonstrable by physical or radiologic examination. The destruction and gross distortion of articular structures (cartilage, bone, capsule, synovial membranes) by tophi leads to a form of chronic gouty arthritis which compounds the stiffness, pain, and fibrosis that may follow repeated attacks of acute gouty arthritis. Although symptomatic and objective improvement may occur with proper therapy, this late stage of destructive gout cannot be completely reversed. One of the objectives of modern management is to prevent the excessive accumulation of urate that results in tophaceous destruction and connective tissue reaction.

Uric Acid Nephrolithiasis. Kidney stones are very common. It has been estimated that 1 in every 1000 inhabitants of the United States is hospitalized annually because of a kidney stone. This figure does not include those whose stones remain in situ or are passed without hospitalization. In large series it has been found that 5 to 10 per cent of all kidney stones in adults are composed mainly of uric acid deposits within a protein matrix. Uric acid may serve as the nidus for a stone of mixed composition, in particular in association with calcium oxalate. Pure uric acid stones are radiolucent, being demonstrable only by the use of contrast media. Other radiolucent stones, so-called matrix stones which are predominantly proteinaceous and xanthine stones, are extremely rare.

Most patients with uric acid stones do not have clinical gout. On the other hand, patients with gout are much more likely to have stones. The frequency of stones in primary or genetic gout has been estimated at 15 to 20 per cent, and in secondary overproduction gout (e.g., myeloid metaplasia, polycythemia vera) at 35 to 40 per cent. Stone formation may occur at any stage in the disease, as the first manifestation of gout or as a late complication in the course of crippling arthritis. Stones may be infrequent or, rarely, they may be the main problem, with almost constant uric acid gravel and superimposed episodes of acute renal colic from passage of larger stones.

As noted earlier, the absolute amount of uric acid excreted per 24 hours is only one of the factors conducive to stone formation. A concentrated acidic urine increases the likelihood of stones at any level of uricaciduria. Some investigators have reported that patients with gout, and certain other patients with uric acid stone diathesis, habitually excrete more acid urine. It is postulated that this reflects a shift toward increased titratable acidity rather than ammonia excretion because of a relative defect in renal ammonia production. These data have been both confirmed and denied, perhaps an indication in part of the difficulty in choosing proper controls.

Gouty Renal Disease. A selective defect in urate

Figure 6. Chronic gouty arthritis with tophaceous destruction of bone and joints.

Figure 7. Advanced tophaceous gout, with ulcerations.

excretion may be the basic defect in possibly one third of all patients with gout. Extracellular urate rises non-specifically in all patients with renal insufficiency, uric acid representing one component of nonprotein nitrogen. The onset of renal failure in gout tends to exacerbate the disease, especially the frequency and severity of tophaceous deposits. More generally, renal tubular reabsorption of urate in man, as opposed to other primates, leads to inappropriate urate retention without which there would be no gout. The kidney therefore plays a significant role in the pathogenesis and progression of gout.

Conversely, gout may impair renal function and lead to death in uremia. The so-called gouty kidney represents a variable mixture of factors. Sodium urate may crystallize in the renal interstitial tissue, especially in the pyramids, with tissue destruction and distortion and a low-grade inflammatory reaction leading to fibrosis. In addition to this primary lesion, uric acid stones lead to obstruction with hydronephrosis and increased susceptibility to chronic pyelonephritis, a complication quite often found in late-stage gouty kidney. Finally, gout, or at least hyperuricemia, carries a statistical association with accelerated vascular disease and hypertension, so that nephrosclerosis may contribute in some measure to impairment of renal function. There are no characteristic clinical or laboratory find-

ings to distinguish gouty kidney from chronic glomerulonephritis except for the association of the former with clinical gout. The question whether gout (i.e., hyperuricemia) ever leads to renal failure in the absence of the other three manifestations of the disease, i.e., arthritis, tophi, and stones, is pertinent to the prophylactic treatment of patients discovered to have essential hyperuricemia (considered here to be gout without complications). Gouty kidney in the absence of these manifestations of clinical gout is extraordinarily rare, and even then the entity may be open to question because of variable interpretations of renal pathology. One unusual family has been described in which this syndrome occurred.

A particular form of uric acid nephropathy may be found in the absence of clinical gout. With sudden exceptionally high levels of uric acid excretion, seen almost exclusively after chemotherapeutic or radiation therapy of certain malignant myeloproliferative disorders, crystals may occlude the distal collecting tubules, leading to acute renal failure. These intraluminal crystals are uric acid rather than sodium urate, precipitate in the distal tubule in which maximal concentration and acidification occur, and lead to intranephronic hydronephrosis. This complication is easy to prevent with fluids, alkalinization of the urine, and allopurinol inhibition of urate synthesis. Oliguria, once established, usually follows a course similar to that seen with acute renal failure secondary to shock or to an incompatible blood transfusion.

Diseases Associated with Gout (Table 2). Several diseases have been described in association with gout. In some cases, the relationship seems to be clear pathogenically, as outlined in the classification of gout in Table 1. Some associations have not yet been so explained. Many diseases which lead to continued tissue synthesis and breakdown may produce hyperuricemia and clinical gout because of the resulting increased turnover of nucleic acids and functional nucleotides. This form of secondary or acquired metabolic gout is that seen with polycythemia vera, myeloid metaplasia, chronic leukemia, mast cell disease, extensive psoriasis, and sarcoidosis. The triad of sarcoidosis-psoriasis-gout has been described in a small number of patients, although this may represent the fortuitous coincidence of two quite common diseases, both of which may be productive of secondary gout. Severe gout may be a major complication in surviving patients with glycogen storage disease Type I because of the constant lactic acidosis which inhibits renal tubular urate secretion. Studies with isotopic glycine also suggest excessive synthesis of urate in this disease. It has been suggested that this may result from excessive synthesis of PRPP, one of the substrates for the rate-limiting initial step in purine synthesis catalyzed by glutamine 5-phosphoribosylpyrophosphate amidotransferase. The hyperuricemia of starvation has a similar mechanism in that β-hydroxybutyrate, as one of the ketone bodies, also inhibits renal urate excretion. The association of gout and diabetes mellitus is not a strong one. Three to 5 per cent of patients with gout have diabetes, but this figure is not far from that of the incidence of diabetes in the general population when adjusted for age. Some diabetic patients considered to have atypical gout in the past in fact have pseudogout, as described in Ch. 97. Over the last decade several clinics have documented a high incidence of hyperuricemia and clinical gout in patients with primary hyperparathyroidism even in the absence of renal failure. This relationship is obscure, because the hyperuricemia has not always responded to successful surgical treatment of the hyperfunctioning parathyroid glands. Hyperuricemia may also be found in hypothyroidism. Renal insufficiency is a common cause of hyperuricemia. It is surprising how rarely this results in clinical gout in view of the high concentrations of uric acid which may be found. It may be that hyperuricemia in uremia does not have sufficient duration, i.e., time at risk, to result in a high incidence of sodium urate precipitation. Uremia may also interfere in some way with the crystallization potential of sodium urate, as it does for bone salts in osteoid, or diminish

the inflammatory response to such crystals when they occur. Garrod commented upon the association of lead poisoning and gout in his treatise of 1876, and this has been repeatedly confirmed in subsequent reports. Saturnine gout, as it has been called, occurs late in the course of chronic plumbism. The mechanism has not been established but it has been supposed that enhanced breakdown of tissue, including the erythropoietic series, is the origin of excessive urate synthesis in lead poisoning. Hyperuricemia has also been described in Down's syndrome and in nephrogenic diabetes insipidus.

Pseudogout. The syndrome of pseudogout, also called *chondrocalcinosis articularis,* is considered as a separate entity in Ch. 97.

Hypoxanthine–Guanine Phosphoribosyltransferase (HG-PRT) Deficiency. The X-linked genetic disease HG-PRT deficiency is a form of gout associated with overproduction of urate in which a specific enzymatic defect has been clearly established. It is important beyond its relative infrequency, because (1) the enzymatic defect can be demonstrated as a cause of excessive purine synthesis; (2) the mechanism of genetic transmission is known, in contrast to other forms of gout except for glycogen storage disease Type I; and (3) in its complete form it produces a distinct clinical picture with neurologic abnormalities: the Lesch-Nyhan syndrome.

In 1964, Lesch and Nyhan described a distinctive syndrome characterized by mental retardation, choreoathetosis, spasticity, weakness, and compulsive self-mutilation. Patients with this syndrome generally appear normal at birth but show evidence of neurologic deficits and retarded mental development within the first few months of life. Bizarre self-mutilation of extremities, lips, and other oral structures may require constant restraint of the patient, despite the evident pain which accompanies this uncontrollable self-destructive process. These patients often develop uric acid stones and gouty nephropathy which may lead to death in uremia. In contrast, gouty arthritis rarely occurs despite very high levels of extracellular urate. The severity of the neurologic damage usually leads to institutionalization, and most patients with the Lesch-Nyhan syndrome die in childhood, although a few survive to early adult life. Some of the patients have had a megaloblastic anemia resistant to the usual hematinic agents. The enzyme HG-PRT is coded on the X chromosome and the disease is transmitted as an X-linked recessive with no clinical phenotypic expression in hemizygous females. As predicted in the Lyon hypothesis, mothers of children with the Lesch-Nyhan syndrome can be shown by tissue culture of their fibroblasts to exhibit mosaicism, with one cell population deficient in HG-PRT and one in which there is normal enzymatic activity.

The Lesch-Nyhan syndrome as defined above represents one end of the clinical spectrum associated with HG-PRT deficiency. There are some patients who have some incomplete deficiency of HG-PRT with severe clinical gout, marked by excessive synthesis of urate, but without the characteristic mental and neurologic derangements. A minority of these patients have exhibited some neurologic abnormalities: mild spastic quadriplegia, cerebellar ataxia, dysarthria, and seizures. This group of patients, like those with the Lesch-Nyhan syndrome, have been particularly susceptible to uric acid stones as a consequence of the excessive uricaciduria. As might be anticipated, genetic transmission of partial HG-PRT deficiency resembles that of the Lesch-Nyhan syndrome, with relative constancy of phenotypic expression within a given family.

In the catabolism of purine nucleotides, free bases are released as adenine, guanine, and hypoxanthine. In part these undergo deamination and further oxidation to uric acid via hypoxanthine and xanthine, these oxidations being catalyzed by xanthine oxidase. In part, the free bases are reutilized, being coupled with PRPP to form purine nucleotides, a process sometimes described as "salvage synthesis" to distinguish it from de novo synthesis from simple precursors (Fig. 8). To the extent that salvage synthesis preserves the purine bases, the requirement for de novo synthesis is reduced, and at equilibrium urate synthesis and excretion are correspondingly reduced. One enzyme, HG-PRT, catalyzes the salvage synthesis of inosine-5'-phosphate and guanosine-5'-phosphate from hypoxanthine and guanine, respectively. A separate enzyme, A-PRT, catalyzes the synthesis of adenosine-5'-phosphate from adenine (and PRPP). The Lesch-Nyhan syndrome is secondary to a selective, almost complete deficiency of HG-PRT, the activity of adenine PRT being normal, or, more often, significantly increased. By immunologic techniques HG-PRT protein has been found to be present in normal amounts in the Lesch-Nyhan syndrome, indicating that the decrease in enzyme activity is secondary to a structural mutation. The defect, most conveniently shown in hemolysates of erythrocytes, has also been found in fibroblasts and brain. The enzyme activity is normally found in highest concentration in the basal ganglia, a major site of neurologic deficit in the Lesch-Nyhan syndrome. In HG-PRT deficiency, tissue levels of PRPP are increased. Uric acid synthesis is massively increased, with urinary excretion in the range of 50 mg per kilogram per 24 hours (normal being about 6). Patients with partial deficiency of HG-PRT also have severe overproduction gout, with levels of uric acid excretion intermediate in amount between the normal range and those found in the Lesch-Nyhan syndrome (about 20 to 25 mg per kilogram per 24 hours). This excessive purine synthesis probably results from inadequate allosteric inhibition of phosphoribosylamidotransferase, the rate-limiting first step in the biosynthetic sequence, because of reduced tissue levels of guanosine-5'-phosphate and inosine-5'-phosphate. The mechanism of neurologic injury has not been established. It may represent localized purine starvation owing to the inability of de novo synthesis to keep pace with the demands generated by failure of salvage synthesis. It is also possible that the resulting high levels of oxypurines (hypoxanthine and xanthine) in the central nervous system are injurious.

The diagnosis of the Lesch-Nyhan syndrome offers no difficulties when the typical neurologic and mental deficits are combined in a male with marked hyperuricemia, and in particular with grossly abnormal uricaciduria. Partial HG-PRT deficiency may be suspected in a male patient with severe gout, possibly with minor neurologic abnormalities, who excretes uric acid in an amount greater than 0.75 times that of creatinine. The final diagnosis can best be made by enzymatic assay of a hemolysate preparation, preferably sent to one of the laboratories engaged in research on purine metabolism. Therapy is ineffective in preventing or reversing neurologic damage, but may reduce the complications directly related to urate accumulation and excretion, as described below.

Diagnosis. The diagnosis of acute gouty arthritis rarely offers difficulties when there is sudden onset of typical inflammatory involvement of a susceptible joint in a patient with hyperuricemia. Rarely, the serum uric acid concentration may be within the upper range of normal at the time of measurement (Fig. 1), or the arthritis may be atypical in its location or persistence. Rapid response of the pain and inflammation after administration of colchicine is so characteristic as to be of diagnostic usefulness. Some response of rheumatoid arthritis or sarcoid arthritis has been described with colchicine, but the effects are not so dramatic as those in gout. Demonstration of the typical needle-shaped birefringent crystals of sodium urate in leukocytes of synovial fluid is diagnostic of gout. With proper technique, intraleukocytic sodium urate crystals are found in over 95 per cent of aspirates from joints affected by acute gout (Fig. 4). Although use of a polarizing microscope is preferable, sodium urate crystals can also be demonstrated in centrifuged, heparinized joint fluid by examining the sediment with an ordinary microscope. Positive identification of the crystals may be achieved by incubation of the synovial fluid preparation with uricase. The particular characteristics of pseudogout or *chondrocalcinosis articularis* are described in Ch. 97. Occasionally, gout may simulate infectious arthritis or be confused with monarticular rheumatoid arthritis. Examination of the joint fluid, measurement of serum uric acid, and response to colchicine should suffice to establish the diagnosis.

Figure 8. Pathways for salvage synthesis of purine nucleotides from free purine bases in normal subjects (left) and in the metabolic abnormality of hypoxanthine-guanine phosphoribosyltransferase (HG-PRT) deficiency (right). APRT, Adenine phosphoribosyltransferase.

A classification of types of gout according to pathogenesis has been outlined in Table 1. It is clearly important to determine whether gout is secondary to a myeloproliferative disorder, renal failure, or drug or metabolite interference with renal tubular secretion or urate. In the study of the average patient with idiopathic gout, in the absence of the aforementioned disorders, it is not necessary to establish whether the disease is metabolic (overproduction) gout or renal (underexcretion) gout in order to institute proper treatment. In the absence of clear-cut hyperuricaciduria on a low purine diet, this further classification is still a laborious procedure requiring isotopic studies.

Treatment. Genetic gout cannot be cured, but its phenotypic expression can usually be modified and progression of its clinical complications controlled or reversed. The therapeutic program differs according to the complications present. Generally, in the majority of patients, the treatment of gout is now quite adequate with the introduction of potent uricosuric drugs and allopurinol, and more skilled use of colchicine as a prophylactic agent. The purpose of every therapeutic program is to prevent the complications of gout or, failing complete prophylaxis, to treat each complication specifically when it occurs.

Acute Gouty Arthritis. Although acute gouty arthritis is self-limited in duration, the severity of the pain and the persistence of the untreated inflammatory process over one to two weeks call for early intervention. The earlier the onset of treatment, the more likely a rapid response. The affected joint should be placed at rest. Usually the degree of pain will demand this, and on occasion specific medication, i.e., a narcotic, for pain may be required. Four types of drugs have been utilized with repeated success in the treatment of acute gout: colchicine; phenylbutazone, indomethacin, and glucocorticoids (or ACTH).

Colchicine is still widely used and is a relatively specific agent for the treatment of acute gout. A number of regimens can be used. It is recommended that an initial dose of 1.0 mg be given orally, followed by 0.5 mg every hour until the relief of pain or the onset of diarrhea. These responses often occur more or less spontaneously. No more than 6.0 mg of colchicine should be given for an acute attack; no more than that should be given over a 72-hour period. Colchicine may also be given intravenously (2.0 mg given in 20 ml of saline over a ten-minute period) instead of orally, with less gastrointestinal reaction, and repeated if necessary after an interval of four to six hours. Not more than 5.0 mg should be administered intravenously within a 24-hour period. Diarrhea is the most frequent complication of colchicine therapy and often requires treatment, e.g., paregoric, for rapid relief. Colchicine is excreted by the kidney and should be used cautiously in uremia. Large amounts of colchicine may cause transient leukopenia. The probable mechanism of action of colchicine has been discussed earlier. Because of the frequent occurrence of gastrointestinal symptoms during its use, colchicine has been replaced by the anti-inflammatory agent phenylbutazone as the first drug of choice in the treatment of acute gouty arthritis in many if not most clinics.

Phenylbutazone (Butazolidin) or *oxyphenbutazone* (Tandearil) is given in a dose of 200 mg four times a day for two days, with rapid tapering to discontinuation over the following two days. With such brief therapeutic periods, toxicity is minimized. *Indomethacin* (Indocin) may be given in amounts of 50 mg three times daily with early resolution of an acute attack, but it may produce more side effects. Glucocorticoid (or ACTH) therapy is not recommended for routine use in acute gouty arthritis because of variability in response and the high incidence of rebound arthritis after its discontinuation. ACTH has proved to be useful in postoperative gout when parenteral therapy is mandatory. Here it may be given as 40 units by slow intravenous drip on the first day, combined with 40 units of ACTH gel intramuscularly on each of the first three days.

When effective treatment has been given, improvement in symptoms usually begins within 6 to 12 hours, with virtually complete remission within 24 to 48 hours. In about 5 to 10 per cent of patients, no rapid relief is obtained, especially if treatment is begun late in the course, and the resolution of the inflammatory arthritis is more gradual. The use of uricosuric agents is not indicated in the management of acute gout.

One of the purposes of therapy is to prevent acute attacks of arthritis. By experience, patients may become aware of stressful experiences or dietary or alcoholic excesses which precipitate attacks, and in this way be able to avoid them. The proper use of uricosuric agents or allopurinol will lower urate levels below the saturation concentration over time, and in this way help to prevent the crystallization which precedes attacks. The short-term effect of such treatment, however, usually leads to exacerbation of gouty arthritis during periods of mobilization of urate deposits. Gutman has established the usefulness of daily colchicine (0.5 mg once or twice a day) as a simple measure to prevent acute attacks in patients subject to recurrent arthritis. Colchicine prophylaxis is not recommended for patients with a single attack (which may never recur) but should be instituted for all patients with frequent attacks of arthritis. Finally, the importance of aborting acute attacks by the use of colchicine or phenylbutazone during the earliest premonitory symptoms should be stressed. This will be the responsibility of the patient himself.

Tophaceous Gout. There are two ways to remove or reduce the size of tophi: surgical removal or redissolving sodium urate crystals. In extracellular fluid, sodium urate crystals can be dissolved only by lowering urate below the saturation level (approximately 7 mg per 100 ml, assuming normal protein binding). The rate of redissolving sodium urate bears a direct relationship to the degree of unsaturation achieved, although it may be modified by blood supply, fibrosis, and the area of crystal surface exposed. Two methods are in general use to lower urate levels: the use of uricosuric drugs to increase renal clearance, and the use of allopurinol to inhibit urate synthesis. Dietary restriction may help to reduce urate synthesis from preformed purines, but with the advent of the aforementioned methods of treatment it has become less important. In theory, an ideal approach to treatment would be to increase urate excretion into the gut (normally one fourth to one third of that synthesized) for bacterial uricolysis. No agent has yet been found which selectively increases gut excretion of urate.

Two uricosuric agents are most often employed, *probenecid* (Benemid) or *sulfinpyrazone* (Anturan). Either of these drugs should be started in small amounts with forced fluids and mild alkalinization of the urine (if no contraindications exist), in order to prevent uric acid stone formation. If the patient has been subject to acute arthritis, prophylactic colchicine should be administered simultaneously to anticipate the exacerbation of gouty arthritis during the early phases of uricosuric therapy. Probenecid should be started at a dose of 0.25 gram twice daily, gradually increasing over a two-week period to a maintenance dose of 0.5 gram two or three times daily. A few patients, particularly those with reduction in renal function, may require 2.5 to 3.0 grams daily in order to reduce serum urate to satisfactory levels, preferably lower than 6.0 mg per 100 ml. Sulfinpyrazone may be used as an alternate in beginning doses of 50 mg twice daily, gradually increasing to a maintenance dose of 100 mg three to four times daily. Exceptionally, sulfinpyrazone may be required in doses of 200 mg four times daily for effective uricosuria. In general, both drugs are well tolerated. The most frequently reported reactions are those of gastrointestinal intolerance and drug-induced dermatitis. Very rarely, marrow suppression and hepatic necrosis have been reported. Although uricosuric in large doses, salicylates should not be used in the treatment of gout. At usual therapeutic levels they may primarily inhibit renal tubular secretion of urate and therefore be uricoretentive.

The availability of *allopurinol* (Zyloprim) has introduced a new approach to the treatment of gout. This analogue of hypoxanthine and its oxidation product allo-xanthine competitively inhibit xanthine oxidase, and in this way reduce the oxidation of hypoxanthine to xanthine and of xanthine to uric acid (Fig. 2). The human kidney clears hypoxanthine and xanthine much more efficiently than uric acid, so that their extracellular fluid concentrations do not rise commensurately with the fall in urate. The total amount of purine bases excreted is generally somewhat reduced, owing probably to increased reutilization of the oxypurines for salvage synthesis of nucleotides. Furthermore, the more equitable distribution of purines excreted among the three metabolites reduces the tendency toward urinary saturation by either xanthine or uric acid (hypoxanthine being highly soluble). Allopurinol is usually given in divided doses of 300 to 600 mg per day. As in the case of uricosuric drugs, its use may initially increase the number of acute attacks of gouty arthritis unless colchicine prophylaxis is used. The pharmacologic production of xanthinuria, an analogue of the genetic disorder, has rarely resulted in difficulties from xanthine stone formation, notably in two patients with the Lesch-Nyhan syndrome and in a few patients being treated with antineoplastic agents. The nucleotide of allopurinol is formed in vivo, and inhibits the enzyme orotidylic decarboxylase with secondary orotic aciduria and orotidinuria. This partial inhibition of pyrimidine synthesis has not been shown to be adverse, and no incorporation of allopurinol nucleotide into nucleic acid as a possible mutagenic agent has been found. Toxic effects of allopurinol are rare (3 to 5 per cent of patients), and consist of dermatitis, fever, headache, diarrhea, transitory leukopenia, and elevation of serum transaminase enzymes of hepatic origin. Intramuscular crystals of xanthine and oxipurinol have been described in patients receiving allopurinol. The significance of this observation in terms of ultimate toxicity is not clear.

The availability of two general methods of treatment allows choice in the management of tophaceous gout or marked hyperuricemia productive of acute gout. It is recommended that uricosuric agents be given an initial trial in treatment, allopurinol being withheld for more specific indications. Probenecid has been widely used for over 20 years, whereas the use of allopurinol, although the known toxic effects are few and rarely severe, represents the introduction of a foreign purine base and nucleotide with which there has been extensive experience for only eight or nine years. This expression of some therapeutic restraint in the use of allopurinol is a conservative position, for there is a definite trend toward using this agent in the initial treatment of hyperuricemia. Allopurinol is definitely indicated for certain patients: when uricosuric treatment proves ineffective in lowering the extracellular urate level sufficiently (to less than 6 mg per 100 ml); when there are toxic reactions to uricosuric drugs; when tophaceous gout is particularly severe (which often accompanies some degree of renal functional impairment and poor response to uricosuric agents); or when there have been recurrent uric acid stones. In general, the allopurinol regimen is more effective in rapidly lowering urate levels without the added hazard of passing extra uric acid through the kidney and urinary tract. Although a uricosuric drug may be used in conjunction with allopurinol, this is not usually wise, because probenecid may increase urinary excretion of allopurinol and alloxanthine, making it less effective, and may also decrease the excretion of the oxypurines. Combined treatment has been used successfully for patients with severe tophaceous gout with good renal function when neither drug alone has sufficed to lower urate levels adequately.

With prolonged treatment, remarkable reversal of tophaceous gout may be obtained. Treatment should then be continued for life to prevent recurrence of hyperuricemia and its complications.

Gouty Kidney. There is no specific way to treat gouty kidney when renal failure has occurred. There is rarely any evidence of improvement in renal function when urate values are reduced enough to mobilize tophaceous deposits. Treatment is limited to control of pyelonephritis if it exists, prevention of further stone formation, lowering extracellular urate levels by the methods previously described in order to prevent further injury, treatment of hypertension to modify the progress of nephrosclerosis, and the general metabolic measures used to treat any patient with diminished renal function. With early diagnosis and treatment, renal failure is becoming a much rarer complication of gout. With uremia, the dose of allopurinol used should be lower.

A particular form of gouty kidney, acute tubular blockade by uric acid with oliguria or anuria, can be prevented in patients being treated with cytotoxic agents by the use of fluids, alkalinization of the urine, and, in particular, full doses of allopurinol *before* the treatment of the myeloproliferative disorder. If anuria occurs, the usual measures for the treatment of acute renal failure should be instituted in anticipation of tubular regeneration over a 10- to 14-day period.

Uric Acid Stones. As previously described, the tendency to form uric acid stones is a function of the concentration of free uric acid, as opposed to sodium urate, in urine. Preventive measures attempt to reduce uric acid concentration by increasing urine volume (forcing of fluids, particularly at night), increasing urine pH (administration of sodium citrate or bicarbonate to maintain urine pH greater than 6), or reducing urate excretion (allopurinol). In most patients, fluids and mild alkalinization suffice to prevent uric acid stones. When uricaciduria is marked, when excess sodium is contraindicated, or when these measures are not successful, the use of allopurinol offers a specific method for the prevention of uric acid stones. As stated, the theoretical possibility of substituting xanthine stones for uric acid stones exists, but this complication has so far occurred only in the Lesch-Nyhan syndrome.

Essential Hyperuricemia.   In this chapter, essential hyperuricemia is considered to be gout without complications. The incidental discovery of elevated serum urate values in the absence of any of the clinical manifestations of gout has increased with the broader use of screening laboratory determinations. One of the most vexing problems facing the physician is whether asymptomatic hyperuricemia should be treated. There are few firm data on which to base a decision. Although hyperuricemia is associated epidemiologically with hyperlipidemia, hypertension, obesity, glucose intolerance, and accelerated vascular disease, there is no evidence that it is primary in any of these derangements, or that lowering uric acid levels affects their course. Similarly, gout may lead to renal failure, but documentation of gouty kidney in the absence of other clinical manifestations is exceedingly rare. Finally, only a minority of patients develop complications of gout despite a lifetime of hyperuricemia in the postpubertal period, although the incidence of complications is roughly proportional to the degree of sodium urate supersaturation in extracellular fluid. Because of these uncertainties, it does not seem justified to start therapy for life in essential hyperuricemia. On the other hand, when serum uric acid values are consistently above 9.0 mg per 100 ml, the degree of supersaturation is such that the incidence of complications is perhaps 90 per cent. It would seem reasonable to treat such patients with uricosuric agents, or allopurinol, in order to maintain safer uric acid levels.

Garrod, A. B.: A Treatise on Gout and Rheumatic Gout. 3rd ed. London, Longmans, Green & Co., Ltd., 1876.

Gutman, A. B., and Yü T.-F.: Uric acid nephrolithiasis. Am. J. Med., 45:756, 1968.

McCarty, D. J., Jr.: Mechanisms of the crystal deposition diseases—gout and pseudogout. Ann. Intern. Med., 78:767, 1973.

Rieselbach, R. E., and Steele, T. H.: Influence of the kidney upon urate homeostasis in health and disease. Am. J. Med., 57:665, 1974.

Seegmiller, J. E. (ed.): Symposium on clinical and biochemical features of X-linked uricaciduria. Arch. Intern. Med., 130:181, 1972.

Seegmiller, J. E.: Diseases of purine and pyrimidine metabolism. *In* Bondy, P. K., and Rosenberg, L. E. (eds.): Duncan's Diseases of Metabolism. 7th ed. Philadelphia, W. B. Saunders Company, 1974, p. 655.

Smyth, C. J., and Percy, J. S.: Comparison of indomethacin and phenylbutazone in acute gout. Ann. Rheum. Dis., 32:351, 1973.

Steele, T. H.: Control of uric acid excretion. N. Engl. J. Med., 284:1193, 1971.

Watts, R. W. E., Scott, J. T., Chalmers, R. A., Bitensky, L., and Chayen, J.: Microscopic studies on skeletal muscle in gout patients treated with allopurinol. Quart J. Med., 40:1, 1971.

Weissman, G.: Crystals, lysosomes, and gout. Adv. Intern. Med., 19:239, 1974.

Weissman, G., and Rita, G.: Molecular basis of gouty inflammation: Interaction of monosodium urate crystals with lysosomes and liposomes. Nature (New Biol.), 240:167, 1972.

Wyngaarden, J. B.: The metabolic defects of primary hyperuricemia and gout. Am. J. Med., 56:651, 1974.

Wyngaarden, J. B., and Kelley, W. N.: Gout. *In* Stanbury, J. B., Wyngaar-

den, J. B., and Fredrickson, D. S. (eds.): The Metabolic Basis of Inherited Disease. 3rd ed. New York, McGraw-Hill Book Company, 1972, p. 889.

Yü, T.-F.: Milestones in the treatment of gout. Am. J. Med., 56:676, 1974.

822. XANTHINURIA

Xanthinuria is a rare genetic disorder secondary to deficiency of xanthine oxidase. Approximately a dozen cases have been described, and some of these have not been fully investigated. It is probably transmitted as an autosomal recessive trait, although this has not been firmly established and there is no method now available for detection of heterozygotes. Deficient activity of xanthine oxidase has been demonstrated in liver and gut mucosa in xanthinuria. The normal function of this enzyme is to catalyze the oxidation of hypoxanthine to xanthine and of xanthine to uric acid.

Most patients with xanthinuria have been asymptomatic, being discovered in the investigation of hypouricemia (serum urate less than 1 mg per 100 ml). Three patients had xanthine kidney stones, which resemble uric acid stones in their radiolucency. Two of the patients had muscle cramps, made worse by exercise, and were found on muscle biopsy to have intracellular crystals of xanthine and hypoxanthine. Although one patient with xanthinuria had hemochromatosis, no other patients have shown abnormal avidity for iron absorption.

The diagnosis is established by the demonstration of hypouricemia and hypouricaciduria with increased excretion of hypoxanthine and xanthine. In xanthinuria these oxypurines are usually excreted in amounts somewhat less than the normal value for uric acid. Hypoxanthine is partially reutilized to form inosine-5′-phosphate, a reaction catalyzed by hypoxanthine guanine phosphoribosyltransferase, the enzyme which is deficient in the Lesch-Nyhan syndrome. Xanthinuria is simulated pharmacologically by the use of allopurinol which is a competitive inhibitor of, as well as a substrate for, xanthine oxidase. (See Ch. 821.) Hypouricemia may also occur in proximal renal tubular disease (Fanconi's syndrome, Wilson's disease) and during treatment with uricosuric agents. Uricosuric agents include aspirin, x-ray contrast agents, and glyceryl guaiacolate. Hypouricemia has been described repeatedly in association with neoplastic diseases. It has also been described in several healthy individuals who had an isolated defect in renal tubular reabsorption of urate (clearance of urate 1.3 times creatinine clearance), similar to that found in the Dalmatian coach hound and in primates other than man. Probably a few patients have had xanthine stones or mixed stones containing xanthine as one component in the absence of the genetic disease. The solubility of hypoxanthine prevents its precipitation in the urinary tract.

Treatment is usually not required. A program for the prevention of xanthine stones would be similar to that for uric acid stones, i.e., forcing fluids, alkalinization of the urine (although the enhancement of solubility of xanthine by alkalinization is not as great as that of urate), and possibly a low purine diet if the above does not suffice. Despite the very low levels of xanthine oxidase, studies on a single patient suggest that allopurinol might increase the amount of oxypurine excreted as the more soluble hypoxanthine.

Engelman, K., Watts, R. W. E., Klinenberg, J. R., Sjoerdsma, A., and Seegmiller, J. E.: Clinical, physiological and biochemical studies of a patient with xanthinuria and pheochromocytoma. Am. J. Med., 37:839, 1964.

Seegmiller, J. E.: Xanthine stone formation. Am. J. Med., 45:780, 1968.

Seegmiller, J. E.: Hereditary xanthinuria. In Bondy, P. K., and Rosenberg, L. E.(eds.): Duncan's Disease of Metabolism. 7th ed. Philadelphia, W. B. Saunders Company, 1974, p. 739.

Wyngaarden, J. B.: Xanthinuria. In Stanbury, J. B., Wyngaarden, J. B., and Fredrickson, D. S. (eds.): The Metabolic Basis of Inherited Disease. 3rd ed. New York, McGraw-Hill Book Company, 1972, p. 992.

823. DISORDERS OF PYRIMIDINE METABOLISM

Lloyd H. Smith, Jr.

Pyrimidine nucleotides share equally with purine nucleotides the chemical chore of transmitting genetic information for reproduction or for phenotypic expression within the cell. They also function in the intermediary metabolism of lipids and carbohydrates. Only a few disorders of pyrimidine metabolism have been recognized.

Hereditary orotic aciduria is a rare genetic disorder of pyrimidine metabolism characterized by megaloblastic anemia resistant to the usual hematinic agents, leukopenia, failure of normal growth and development, and the continued excessive urinary excretion of orotic acid. Orotic acid is highly insoluble and often forms a heavy sediment of urinary crystals which may on occasion result in ureteral or urethral obstruction. The disorder, which is transmitted as an autosomal recessive trait, is usually characterized by reduced activities of two consecutive enzymes in pyrimidine biosynthesis, orotate phosphoribosyltransferase (OPRT) and orotidine 5'-phosphate decarboxylase (ODC). A single patient has been described with isolated deficiency of ODC. There is a prompt and sustained hematologic and general clinical response to oral uridine (2 to 4 grams per day), which must be continued indefinitely as replacement therapy. The disease has attracted special attention because it represents a block in the de novo pathway of pyrimidine synthesis, is an example of a double enzyme defect, and produces a requirement for replacement of a normal metabolic intermediate, uridine.

Orotic aciduria, without the characteristic hematologic abnormalities, also occurs in *ornithine transcarbamylase deficiency*. It is presumed that this results from the overflow of carbamyl phosphate from urea synthesis (partially blocked in this disease) to pyrimidine synthesis.

Excessive urinary excretion of orotic acid and orotidine occurs during treatment with *allopurinol* or *6-azauridine*. Metabolic products of both compounds inhibit orotidine 5'-decarboxylase activity.

Beta-aminoisobutyric aciduria is a benign hereditary disorder of thymine catabolism which occurs in 5 to 10 per cent of Caucasians and in a much higher percentage of Asians. The defect presumably lies in the transamination of beta-aminoisobutyric acid to methylmalonic acid semialdehyde. The aminoaciduria which results, representing the only known disorder of pyrimidine catabolism, has no known biologic disadvantage.

Smith, L. H., Jr.: Pyrimidine metabolism in man. N. Engl. J. Med., 288:764, 1973.

Smith, L. H., Jr., Huguley, C. M., Jr., and Bain, J. A.: Hereditary orotic aciduria. In Stanbury, J. B., Wyngaarden, J. B., and Fredrickson, D. S. (eds.): The Metabolic Basis of Inherited Disease. 3rd ed. New York, McGraw-Hill Book Company, 1972, p. 196.

Weissman, S. M.: Human pyrimidine metabolism. J.A.M.A., 195:27, 1966.

Part XVIII
DISEASES OF THE ENDOCRINE SYSTEM

824. INTRODUCTION

Nicholas P. Christy

FUNCTIONS OF THE ENDOCRINE SYSTEM

Like the nervous system, the endocrine system provides mechanisms by which the mammalian organism adapts itself to a constantly changing environment. Parts of the endocrine system may indeed be regarded as extensions of the nervous system: the adrenal medulla, which secretes epinephrine in response to environmental change, is of ectodermal origin, arising from the neural crest; many environmental stimuli cause cells in the hypothalamus to secrete neurohumoral peptides which are carried in the hypothalamic-hypophysial portal venous system to cells in the anterior pituitary, which then secrete growth hormone, adrenocorticotrophin, or gonadotrophins (see Ch. 826). These two glands, the adrenal medulla and the anterior pituitary, are particularly clear examples of endocrine organs whose secretions mediate between the external and internal environments. Less dramatic but no less important examples are the neurohypophysial response to changes in hydration and the fluctuations of adrenocortical secretion of aldosterone with changes in dietary Na+. These and the other endocrine glands, by steady or by waxing and waning secretion of hormones, wield an important *regulatory* influence on cellular metabolism (see Ch. 806).

Again like the nervous system, the endocrine system has both *vegetative* and *adaptive* functions. The essential roles of pituitary growth hormone and thyroxine on normal growth and the effects of the sex steroids, testosterone and estradiol, on the gradual and orderly maturation of the secondary sex characters are examples of *vegetative* activity. Rapid *adaptive* functions are numerous: insulin secretion in response to hyperglycemia; epinephrine secretion during profound hypoglycemia; antidiuretic hormone secretion in the presence of increased osmolarity of the plasma; and the instantaneous hypersecretion of pituitary adrenocorticotrophic hormone (ACTH) in response to many noxious stimuli, of growth hormone to severe muscular exercise, and of aldosterone to hemorrhage-induced hypovolemia. It is apparent that both the vegetative and adaptive, that is, the slowly acting and rapidly acting functions are in effect homeostatic (see Ch. 804). However, it is probably a mistake to think of the endocrine system as a system in a rigid sense. It is true that the endocrine organs are all by definition ductless glands which secrete hormones that have many actions at sites remote from those glands. It is also true that several hormones may conspire to affect single, well-defined functions or substances. For instance, it can be shown that all the following hormones have the capacity to influence the concentration of blood glucose: pituitary growth hormone, ACTH, thyroxine, cortisol, epinephrine, insulin, and glucagon. Pituitary growth hormone, ACTH, cortisol, aldosterone, and antidiuretic hormone all influence serum Na+ concentration. But in any of these groupings, it is difficult to know in a given set of circumstances which hormone is quantitatively the most important and to calculate accurately how the several hormones, with their complementary, supplementary, synergistic, or opposing actions, operate together to regulate the serum concentration of glucose or Na+. Further, it is hard to see, for example, how epinephrine secretion by the adrenal medulla relates to the secretion of parathyroid hormone, how growth hormone secretion bears on thyroxine secretion, and how aldosterone and gonadotrophins inter-relate. There are at least as many examples of independent as of interdependent functions among the endocrine glands. Therefore it seems most reasonable not to regard the endocrine glands as such a tightly integrated system as the anatomically distinct nervous system, but rather as a loose group of secretory organs, arising from different embryologic sources, having made their appearance at different stages in evolution, and possessing a broad range of functions, some separate and distinct and some interdigitated. These regulatory functions are exerted by circulating chemical substances upon biochemical processes of all cells and tissues.

The *disorders of the endocrine glands* become clinically apparent through excessive, deficient, or untimely secretion of a hormone, owing either to primary disease of the endocrine gland or to an abnormal secretion by that gland in response to disease of some other organ (see Categories of Endocrine Disease, below). All endocrine diseases have this property in common: the secretion of the hormone is not regulated or is improperly regulated by the control mechanisms that operate under normal conditions; that is, the production of the hormone is *autonomous, anarchic,* or *inappropriate,* a state of affairs that leads to disordered homeostasis.

BIOCHEMISTRY AND MODE OF ACTION OF HORMONES

The *chemical nature* of human hormones is now well known. The substances are amines (epinephrine), amino acids (thyroxine), peptides (vasopressin or antidiuretic hormone), proteins (pituitary growth hormone, parathyroid hormone), and steroids (aldosterone). Many hormones have been chemically synthesized, e.g., epinephrine, thyroxine, most of the steroids, and even some of the peptides and proteins, as vasopressin, oxytocin, thyrotrophin-releasing hormone (TRH), and ACTH. For some of the hormones of high molecular weight, e.g., growth hormone, amino acid sequences have been worked out; knowledge of the structures of thyrotrophin and the gonadotrophins is still not complete. Methods have now been developed for accurate measurement of nearly all the important human hormones. These chemical techniques, although difficult and time consuming, are enormously superior to the indirect or biologic assay methods investigators and clinicians used to rely on. The chemical methods, including the revolutionary radioimmunoassay techniques introduced by Berson and Yalow, have now made it possible to quantify the plasma or urinary concentrations of virtually all the known hormones. These advances have put endocrine diagnosis on a firm footing, and have enabled workers in the field not only to measure blood levels but also to determine secretory rates or production rates of several classes of hormones. Thus it is now possible to measure accurately the daily secretion rate of steroid hormones, e.g., aldosterone and cortisol, and even to estimate the daily turnover rate of such protein hormones as growth hormone and ACTH.

Despite intensive study by many workers, the mode of action of hormones is still not completely understood. There is a good deal of information about the *structural determinants of hormonal activity,* e.g., the number, sequence, and identity of the amino acids that determine the immunologic reactivity and the biologic potency of the ACTH molecule (see Ch. 828). Small changes in the molecular structure of hormones profoundly affect their biologic activity and metabolism, both qualitatively and quantitatively; for example, among the steroid hormones, cortisone, with a ketone group at the carbon-11 position of the steroid nucleus, is quite inactive in vitro, whereas cortisol, the principal adrenocortical glucocorticoid of man, which differs structurally from cortisone only by having a hydroxyl (-OH) instead of a ketone group (-O) at carbon-11, is highly active; among the thyroid hormones, L-thyroxine has a half-time in plasma twice that of its stereoisomer, D-thyroxine, and ten times its calorigenic potency. What is not yet definitely known is the exact chemical form of any hormone that is active at the cellular level; it remains to be shown how the known alterations of any hormone molecule brought about by peripheral metabolism are necessary steps in hormone action.

The significance of the *physical state* of a given hormone in the *plasma* is also not clear. The conventional view is that only the portion of a hormone that is *not* bound to a plasma protein is "active" in the sense that only the unbound, "free" form is available to cells. There is some evidence to support this view. Under various conditions—e.g., rare hereditary abnormalities in the serum concentration of certain α-globulins, pregnancy, estrogen therapy, nephrotic syndrome, severe hepatic disease, and several acute illnesses—there are definite changes in the plasma levels of thyroxine-binding globulin or of corticosteroid-binding globulin. Yet, although these changes give rise to easily measurable changes in *total* serum concentration of thyroxine or cortisol, there is no clinical evidence of an altered thyroid or adrenal state, presumably because the "free" thyroxine and "free" cortisol levels are not significantly abnormal.

The biochemical mode of action of hormones at the cellular level is discussed in detail in Ch. 825.

UBIQUITY OF HORMONAL EFFECTS

Since all hormones circulate in the blood, their actions are to be found everywhere. The effects of disordered endocrine function impinge upon most organs and systems. Some examples are the characteristic changes in the skin, central nervous system, muscles, gastrointestinal tract, heart, and blood vessels (increased susceptibility to atherosclerosis) in severe *hypothyroidism;* the changes in the psyche, the eyes, the regulation of blood glucose (hypoglycemia), the blood pressure, water metabolism, and the structure and function of the sexual apparatus in fully developed *pituitary insufficiency;* and the changes in the psyche, central nervous system (lethargy, coma), muscles, gastrointestinal tract (constipation, ileus), kidneys (stones), and skeleton that are characteristic of *hyperparathyroidism.*

Many acute and chronic diseases impinge on the endocrine glands. Examples are such changes as increased adrenocortical and adrenal medullary secretion of cortisol and epinephrine during *acute myocardial infarction,* increased aldosterone secretion in the accelerated phase of *hypertension,* decreased pituitary gonadotrophin secretion with hypogonadism accompanying the inanition and emotional disorder of *anorexia nervosa* (see Ch. 724), and the secondary hyperparathyroidism of *renal insufficiency* (see Ch. 890).

Looking at endocrine disease from another point of view, many common symptoms and signs may be parts of endocrine syndromes. *Hypertension* is common in acromegaly and *Cushing's syndrome;* not all patients with these diseases can be diagnosed on inspection. Fixed hypertension is also present in *pheochromocytoma, aldosteronism, renal artery stenosis,* and in some patients with *congenital adrenal hyperplasia.* In the differential diagnosis of *coma,* one must consider the hypercalcemia of *hyperparathyroidism,* the hypoglycemia associated with *islet cell tumors* or *panhypopituitarism,* and the severe water intoxication sometimes associated with the syndrome of *inappropriate secretion of antidiuretic hormone.* Serious *psychologic disturbance,* including psychosis, may be an important feature of *pituitary insufficiency, hypothyroidism, hyperthyroidism, hyperparathyroidism,* any of the *hypoglycemias, Addison's disease,* and *Cushing's syndrome.*

The aim here is to sensitize the reader to the systemic but less obvious signs of endocrine disease; he does not need to be reminded that the patient with clear signs of thyrotoxicosis may have disease of an endocrine gland.

CATEGORIES OF ENDOCRINE DISEASE

In the light of the discoveries made during the past two decades, it is no longer enough to think of endocrine disease simply as too much or too little hormone. For clinical purposes, the following may be a helpful classification:

Primary Hyperfunction of Endocrine Glands. Most diseases in this group are due to *benign tumors* of endocrine glands, such as the pituitary adenoma of acromegaly, the "toxic adenoma" which produces hyperthyroidism, the parathyroid adenoma of hyperparathyroidism, the insulin-secreting islet cell adenoma of the pancreas, benign pheochromocytoma, and the adrenal cortical adenoma of Cushing's syndrome.

Malignant hormone-secreting tumors of the anterior

pituitary and thyroid are extremely rare, but cancers of the parathyroids, islet cells, adrenal medulla, and adrenal cortex are occasional causes of severe and intractable endocrine disease. No more is known about the etiology of these endocrine cancers than about that of any other cancer.

There are hyperfunctional states *not associated with endocrine tumors.* An example is Graves' disease or toxic diffuse goiter, which was formerly believed to be due to pituitary oversecretion of TSH. It is not; plasma TSH concentrations are low (see Ch. 837).

Secondary Hyperfunction of Endocrine Glands. This term defines overactivity of a "target" gland owing to *hyperfunction of the anterior pituitary.* Cushing's syndrome not associated with adrenal tumor is caused by excessive and unremitting ACTH secretion; there are very rare instances of hyperthyroidism associated with TSH overproduction by pituitary tumors.

Primary Hypofunction of Endocrine Glands. Primary glandular failure is the usual cause of endocrine deficiency syndromes. The etiology is often obscure. Fibrosis or even absence of the anterior pituitary has been discovered at autopsy *without anatomic evidence of any cause.* Destruction of a gland by formation of *autoantibodies* to that gland has been postulated as a cause of the hypothyroidism of Hashimoto's thyroiditis, and also as a cause of hypoparathyroidism and of "idiopathic" Addison's disease. Autoantibodies to thyroid, parathyroid, and adrenals have indeed been demonstrated in many patients with these disorders, but it is not clear whether the antibodies are the primary cause of the glandular destruction or are secondary consequences, arising from damage to the glands by unknown agents. There has been recent interest in the possibility that delayed or cellular hypersensitivity related to abnormal "lymphoid recognition" may play a part, especially in cases of polyglandular insufficiency. *Tumors* may destroy a gland. Breast cancer and lymphomas may metastasize or spread to invade the neurohypophysis or supraoptic nuclei, giving rise to diabetes insipidus; chromophobe adenoma is the most common cause of anterior pituitary insufficiency. Several cancers, especially lung cancer, very often metastasize to the adrenals, but rarely cause enough destruction to produce adrenocortical insufficiency. *Infections* are not very common causes of glandular failure: tuberculosis and syphilitic gummas used to be occasional causes of pituitary destruction, but are now museum pieces; tuberculosis, histoplasmosis, and blastomycosis may destroy the adrenals with ensuing Addison's disease. *Chromosomal disorders,* such as Klinefelter's syndrome and gonadal dysgenesis (Turner's syndrome), are not rare as causes of primary gonadal deficiency in phenotypic males and females (see Ch. 859 and 867).

Secondary and Tertiary Failure of Endocrine Glands. This term means failure of the gonads, thyroid, or adrenals owing to *pituitary insufficiency.* Although it is true that the growth hormone–secreting and gonadotrophic functions of the pituitary are usually the first to drop out during the course of destructive pituitary disease, and, as a corollary, if only one function is affected, it is likely to be either growth (hypopituitary dwarfism) or gonadal function, the other functions, i.e., thyrotrophic or adrenocorticotrophic, may fail singly or in any combination (see Ch. 831). The key to diagnosis is to study the patient carefully for the presence of pituitary disease in every instance of growth failure, hypogonadism,

hypothyroidism, or hypoadrenocorticism. There may be good clinical evidence to implicate or rule out pituitary involvement, but, if not, assessment of thyroid or adrenal response to TSH or ACTH or direct measurement by radioimmunoassay of the trophic hormones in plasma or urine will clarify the diagnosis. When the anterior pituitary insufficiency is the result of hypothalamic disease, the target gland failure is defined as "tertiary," e.g., "tertiary hypothyroidism" (see Ch. 826).

"Functional" Disorders of the Endocrine Glands. The response of endocrine glands to certain disease states may be clinically important or clinically trivial. Important endocrine responses are the secondary hyperparathyroidism of renal failure, leading to renal osteodystrophy; and the secondary aldosteronism of portal cirrhosis and of the nephrotic syndrome with ascites and edema – aldosterone is an important contributing factor in edema formation. Responses which are either trivial or not yet of proved clinical significance are altered metabolism of thyroxine in liver disease and in patients acutely ill from a variety of causes; the altered metabolism of cortisol in portal cirrhosis; the altered metabolic disposition of androgens in thyroid disease and acute intermittent porphyria; and many others.

Failure of an End-Organ to Respond to a Hormone. There are several examples of this in human medicine. One is *nephrogenic diabetes insipidus,* a heritable defect in which the kidney fails to respond to vasopressin in the face of adequate secretion of vasopressin by the supraoptic nuclei. Another is *pseudohypoparathyroidism,* a hereditary disease characterized by renal and osseous resistance to measurable effects of parathyroid hormone (PTH), which is secreted in normal or greater than normal amounts by normal or hyperplastic parathyroids. In both these diseases, the respective hormones, vasopressin and PTH, fail to activate the adenylate cyclase system of the appropriate renal tubular cells; there is no rise in cyclic AMP and no metabolic effect of the hormone. Still another type of failure of end-organ response, the so-called *pseudohypoparathyroidism type II,* is characterized by adequate cyclic AMP response to PTH but absence of phosphaturia or rise in serum calcium concentration. The inference is that there is a failure to receive the intracellular cyclic AMP "message." A third example is the syndrome of *testicular feminization,* a developmental defect in which "target tissues" are unresponsive to endogenous or administered androgen. In this entity the mechanism of end-organ failure has not been worked out.

Production by an Endocrine Gland of an Abnormal or Unusual Hormone. Such lesions are characteristic of the inborn errors of metabolism. In *congenital adrenocortical hyperplasia,* deficiencies of C-21 and C-11 hydroxylases cause metabolic blocks in the synthesis of cortisol, with the additional result that several cortisol precursors, e.g., pregnanetriol and 17α-hydroxyprogesterone, normally present in very small amounts, are secreted in amounts much greater than normal, as are C_{19} androgens. In *goitrous cretinism* enzymic blocks in the synthesis of thyroxine give rise to thyroidal secretion into the bloodstream of large quantities of mono- and diiodotyrosines. In "T_3 *thyrotoxicosis*" hyperthyroidism is present and serum PBI and thyroxine concentrations are normal; for unknown reasons the goiter or thyroid nodule apparently synthesizes excessive quantities of the normally less abundant hormone, triiodothyronine

(T_3). A form of hypoparathyroidism *("pseudoidiopathic hypoparathyroidism")* has been described in which the glands secrete a biologically ineffective PTH, possibly because of a defect in conversion of proparathyroid hormone to an active form.

Production of a Hormone by a Nonendocrine Organ. Cancers of many organs (lung, thymus, pancreas) may produce substances that cannot be chemically or immunologically distinguished from normal endocrine products, usually proteins, such as ACTH, MSH, gonadotrophins, erythropoietin, and others. The clinical features and hypotheses concerning the mechanisms by which these "hormones" are secreted are discussed in Ch. 870.

Prostaglandins. The status of *prostaglandins* is not yet clear. These 20-carbon, unsaturated, cyclic fatty acids were originally found in seminal fluid, but are now known to be present in most tissues and biologic fluids. At least 16 prostaglandins have been isolated and described. Their effects are widespread and varied. In addition to many actions on the central nervous, cardiovascular, and gastrointestinal systems and the kidney, the prostaglandins have many effects upon the endocrine organs. Prostaglandins have been shown to affect the hypothalamus–anterior pituitary "axis," to augment pituitary growth hormone release in vitro, to mediate the effect of luteinizing hormone on the ovary, to exert a lytic effect on the corpus luteum, to alter thyroidal response to TSH, and to affect adrenal cortical steroidogenesis. Prostaglandins have been shown to mimic the "hormonal" effects of cyclic AMP and, under certain conditions, to attenuate cyclic AMP effects. The *physiologic* importance of the prostaglandins in regulating endocrine function remains to be worked out. Although their actions often appear to be "hormonal," there is still no agreement as to whether they should be considered hormones.

Iatrogenic Endocrine Disease. By far the most common of these is iatrogenic Cushing's syndrome caused by administration of ACTH or cortisol and its derivatives in pharmacologic doses for many allergic, inflammatory, and neoplastic diseases. In the United States, there are hundreds of thousands of patients receiving long-term steroid therapy. An unknown number of these are getting very large doses (more than 50 mg per day of cortisol, or equivalent), and an unknown proportion of them have overt hyperadrenocorticism. The features of this entity are the physical signs of spontaneously occurring Cushing's syndrome, but with a lesser incidence in the iatrogenic form of diabetes, hypertension, and psychosis, and a higher incidence of peptic ulcer and certain rarer untoward effects, e.g., pseudotumor cerebri, glaucoma, pancreatitis, and "aseptic necrosis" of the hip joint. In addition, an unpredictable and probably small number have enough suppression of pituitary-adrenal function to be important in times of intercurrent acute illness or surgical emergency. The writer has developed elsewhere the idea that these patients are addicted to corticosteroids (see References; also Ch. 849). The point is that one should be as ungenerous as possible in the dosage of corticosteroids.

Prescription of sex hormones and thyroid hormone to patients without gonadal or thyroidal deficiency rarely produces iatrogenic disease, but there have been instances of surreptitious thyroxine ingestion leading to thyrotoxicosis. Overenthusiastic use of estrogen may induce endometrial hyperplasia and breakthrough bleeding; some patients are apparently hypersensitive to methyl testosterone, which may cause cholestatic jaundice. The abnormalities in glucose tolerance, serum triglycerides, and liver function tests and the increased incidence of thromboembolic disease associated with administration of oral contraceptives have become familiar.

The protein hormones are sometimes troublesome. There are more than 80 reported instances of anaphylaxis owing to ACTH. For further details about the toxicity of hormonal products, the reader is referred to textbooks of pharmacology. The keys to successful hormone therapy are accurate diagnosis and great restraint in dosage.

HORMONES AS MEDICINES

Hormones are legitimately given to patients in three sets of circumstances: (1) for replacement of lost functions, (2) as tests of endocrine function, and (3) to achieve a pharmacologic purpose.

Replacement Therapy. This is probably the most gratifying use of hormones to both patient and physician, and is the easiest to defend. So long as an endocrine deficiency is clearly and definitely demonstrated, in most instances a realistic goal owing to the availability of good chemical tests for most hormonal diseases, the physician can achieve brilliant clinical results with small doses of hormones. Cortisol for adrenal insufficiency, thyroid hormone USP or thyroxine for hypothyroidism, and human growth hormone for hypopituitary dwarfism are all given in amounts very close to the estimated daily production rates of the respective hormones. It is common practice to give too much cortisone to patients with primary or secondary adrenal insufficiency, i.e., enough to induce signs of mild Cushing's syndrome; daily doses of not more than 10 to 25 mg per day are usually quite sufficient. With thyroid hormone replacement, restraint is also necessary, especially in older people with coronary artery disease, in whom the maintenance dose should be attained gradually. The writer believes that triiodothyronine is never indicated for treatment of longstanding myxedema; too many older patients with atherosclerosis have had bouts of severe coronary insufficiency or even myocardial infarction when this rapidly acting hormone is given. Triiodothyronine may have a place in the treatment of myxedema coma (see Ch. 839).

Replacement dosages of sex hormones have been arrived at by "clinical experience." In the writer's experience, treatment to develop deficient secondary sex characters is best given just before or at the expected time of puberty. If replacement therapy with estrogen or testosterone is delayed until late in the second or well into the third decade, the induced sexual development is suboptimal. This puts a premium on early diagnosis as the basis for early treatment.

Few protein hormones are used routinely in treatment. Although it would be theoretically most correct, say in hypopituitarism, to replace absent trophic hormones by giving gonadotrophins, TSH or ACTH, this is not practical, owing to antibody formation, short supply, and the need for parenteral administration. Gonadotrophins are given only in short courses to induce ovulation in women (see Ch. 867); to stimulate ovarian or testicular function over a long period of time is cumbersome, so sex hormones, which can be administered orally, are used instead. Treatment of secondary hypothyroidism and hypoadrenalism is much more easily done with thyroid hormone and cortisone; allergic reactions to ACTH have been alluded to above. Parathyroid hormone from human sources is not available; vitamin D and calcium salts are simpler to give. The only protein hormone other than insulin that is generally used as replacement therapy is human growth hormone, because there is still no satisfactory substitute for it.

Testing. TSH and ACTH are useful for assessing thyroidal and adrenal response in differentiating between primary and secondary deficiencies of these glands, and the triiodothyronine suppression test of thyroidal ^{131}I uptake is a useful adjunct in diagnosis of some patients with hyperthyroidism. These testing procedures entail the direct chemical or physical measurement of a hormone or of a glandular function. Such methods have largely superseded indirect methods of estimating endocrine activity (e.g., the BMR and the eosinophil count). Some of the older techniques, being provocative tests, were potentially dangerous, e.g., the water-loading and salt withdrawal tests for Addison's disease. These should now be abandoned.

By testing, the writer does not mean the administration of a hormone as a *therapeutic trial,* that is, to determine by the patient's response whether he has or does not have an endocrine deficiency. This approach may be tolerable in an emergency, as for a patient in acute shock when there seems to be some possibility of adrenocortical insufficiency and there is no time for careful chemical study. Under any other conditions, failure to establish a diagnosis is an inexcusable basis for giving hormonal therapy.

Hormones Given to Achieve a Pharmacologic End. Hormones customarily are given to patients in high doses to achieve some pharmacologic, not physiologic, goal in three sets of circumstances: treatment of diseases in which large doses of hormones are *often beneficial;* treatment of diseases for which large doses of hormones are *possibly* or *sometimes beneficial;* and treatment of diseases for which large doses of hormones are *never beneficial* or of very doubtful value.

Beneficial Uses. The obvious examples are of course ACTH and cortisol and its congeners. Although ACTH is usually associated with fewer serious untoward effects and with less danger of a "withdrawal syndrome" when treatment is stopped, the corticosteroids are preferred because of the convenience of the oral route of administration, more flexibility in spacing of doses, shorter action, the larger doses attainable, and the absence of serious allergic reactions. The ideal use of high-dosage corticosteroids is in acute, self-limited diseases such as serum sickness owing to penicillin allergy or bouts of status asthmaticus. In serious inflammatory diseases such as pemphigus, ulcerative colitis, acute rheumatic fever, and lupus erythematosus, in hematologic disorders such as acute lymphoblastic leukemia of childhood, and in bronchial asthma of allergic origin, among other conditions, there is good evidence that corticosteroids often alter the course of the disease in a favorable direction. As in giving any other medicinal agent, the physician has to balance the probability of benefit from corticosteroid therapy against the disability or danger incurred by giving the patient corticosteroids, with the attendant risk of iatrogenic Cushing's syndrome. To make this semiquantitative judgment,

the doctor has to have the fullest possible knowledge of the *natural history* of what he proposes to treat, that is, the natural course of the disease untreated (Feinstein).

Possibly or Sometimes Beneficial Uses. The efficacy of corticosteroids in such disorders as scleroderma and endotoxin shock remains arguable. The same statement applies to the use of testosterone or estrogen, or both, in the treatment of postmenopausal osteoporosis (q.v.); the use of vasopressin or mineralocorticoids in the management of idiopathic postural hypotension; administration of small doses of corticosteroids to women with "acquired adrenal virilism," an entity which may or may not exist; and many others. In this group of diseases, further work is needed toward an understanding of pathogenesis; only this will provide a rational basis for giving or withholding treatment.

Uses That Are Never Beneficial. These uses are derived by the trial and error method, with emphasis on the latter. Examples are numerous; outstanding ones are the widespread administration of thyroid hormone for obesity, for fatigability, and for infertility and menstrual disturbances, the use of estrogens to treat frigidity in the female, and the use of testosterone for impotence in the male. The major objection to such therapies is that they are ineffective. Further, they are often expensive and raise false hopes. The physician must resist the temptation to keep trying one hormonal remedy after another in the hope that something will work. "The empiricist," said Claude Bernard, "is never at a loss." It is the patient who loses.

HORMONES AND MAGIC

By now, it is apparent to the reader that endocrinology is inseparable from the rest of internal medicine. Until the 1920's, endocrinology was entirely an empirical branch, not quite respectable, not quite accepted as professional, lurking on the outskirts of medicine. The endocrinologist dealt with patients who were too fat, too thin, too short, too tall, too tired, too hairy, or not hairy enough. With the discovery of insulin in 1922, with the elucidation of the structures of thyroxine and the steroid hormones in the next decade, and with good studies of hormone metabolism in the period from 1950 to the present, there began to be a firm scientific basis for the practice of endocrinology. But three factors have contributed to the persistence of empiricism. One was the isolation and synthesis of cortisone and cortisol and their derivatives; it is easier to list the diseases for which these compounds have not been given than those for which they have been at least tried. Second is the dramatic and gratifying clinical response that follows administration of a hormone in a deficiency state, or the surgical removal of a hyperfunctioning gland. The physician is sometimes irresistibly tempted to achieve such magical results even when the diagnosis of endocrine deficiency or excess is not firmly established. The third factor, a corollary of the second, is that endocrine diagnostic procedures are time consuming, technically difficult, and sometimes not available locally, and that the data produced are not always easy to interpret. The physician grows impatient. Enough has been said previously about the need for accurate diagnosis as an essential basis for endocrine replacement therapy. Accuracy is equally essential for establishing a diagnosis of glandular hyperfunction; since most of the treatments for such conditions are ablative, the physician should be on solid ground before consigning the patient to such major surgical procedures as thyroidectomy, parathyroidectomy, partial pancreatectomy, or adrenalectomy. Fortified by accurate diagnosis, the endocrinologist no longer has any excuse to treat blindly or to practice magic.

Bloodworth, J. M. B. (ed.): Endocrine Pathology. Baltimore, Williams & Wilkins Company, 1968.

Christy, N. P. (ed.): The Human Adrenal Cortex. New York, Harper & Row, 1971.

Cope, C. L.: Adrenal Steroids and Disease. 2nd ed. Philadelphia, J. B. Lippincott Company, 1972.

Deane, H. W., and Rubin, B. L. (eds.): The Adrenocortical Hormones. Part 3. Handbook of Experimental Pharmacology, Vol. XIV/3. Berlin, Springer-Verlag, 1968.

Drezner, M., Neelon, F. A., and Lebovitz, H. E.: Pseudohypoparathyroidism, Type II: A possible defect in the reception of the cyclic AMP signal. N. Engl. J. Med., 289:1056, 1973.

Edmonds, M., Lamki, L., Killinger, D. W., and Volpé, R.: Autoimmune thyroiditis, adrenalitis and oophoritis. Am. J. Med., 54:782, 1973.

Ezrin, C., Godden, J. O., Volpé, R., and Wilson, R. (eds.): Systematic Endocrinology. Hagerstown, Md., Harper & Row, 1973.

Gardner, L. I. (ed.): Endocrine and Genetic Diseases of Childhood. Philadelphia, W. B. Saunders Company, 1969.

Labhart, A. (ed.): Klinik der inneren Sekretion. 2nd ed. Berlin, Springer-Verlag, 1971.

Nusynowitz, M. L., and Klein, M. H.: Pseudoidiopathic hypoparathyroidism. Hypoparathyroidism with ineffective parathyroid hormone. Am. J. Med., 55:677, 1973.

Rimoin, D. L., and Schimke, R. N.: Genetic Disorders of the Endocrine Glands. St. Louis, C. V. Mosby Company, 1971.

Schwartz, T. B., Ryan, W. G., and Becker, F. O. (eds.): The Year Book of Endocrinology. Chicago, Year Book Medical Publishers, 1973.

Sterling, K., Refetoff, S., and Selenkow, H. A.: T_3 thyrotoxicosis. Thyrotoxicosis due to elevated serum triiodothyronine levels. J.A.M.A., 213:571, 1970.

Sutherland, E. W.: Studies on the mechanism of hormone action. Science, 177:401, 1972.

Werner, S. C., and Ingbar, S. H. (eds.): The Thyroid. 3rd ed. New York, Harper & Row, 1971.

Wilkins, L.: The Diagnosis and Treatment of Endocrine Disorders in Childhood and Adolescence. 3rd ed. Springfield, Ill., Charles C Thomas, 1965.

Williams, R. H. (ed.): Textbook of Endocrinology. 5th ed. Philadelphia, W. B. Saunders Company, 1974.

Wilson, D. E. (ed.): Symposium on prostaglandins. Arch. Intern. Med., 133:29, 1974.

Wurtman, R. J. (ed.): Symposium: Biogenic amines and endocrine functions. Fed. Proc., 32:1769, 1973.

825. MODE OF ACTION OF HORMONES

John N. Loeb

The physiologic effects of the endocrine secretions have long been recognized as among the most dramatic in clinical medicine. The conspicuous consequences of castration in the male have been known since ancient times, and by the mid-nineteenth century the results of ablation of various other endocrine tissues had begun to be appreciated. By the end of the first quarter of the present century most of the currently recognized syndromes of endocrine hypersecretion had been described as well, and at the present time it is recognized that an enormous diversity of metabolic processes, exerting profound effects on growth and differentiation, are under endocrine control.

In recent years there has been a concerted effort to understand the biochemical mechanisms by which these processes are regulated, and in particular to account, in molecular terms, for the diverse and dramatic effects of the endocrine secretions on structure and function. The development of sensitive biochemical techniques has permitted a shift in focus from simple observations of hormonal effects to efforts at defining mechanisms by which such effects are mediated. It is becoming increasingly clear that, despite the variety of their physiological effects, the fundamental modes of action of many hormones are similar. This chapter outlines some of the patterns which are beginning to emerge and discusses some of their implications.

PROPERTIES COMMON TO ALL HORMONES

As non-neuronal carriers of information between different organs, hormones must interact specifically and reversibly with target cells, and this interaction must have the capacity to result in widespread cellular effects. The fact that hormones are normally present in extraordinarily low concentrations (e.g., 10^{-11} to 10^{-8} molar) moreover requires that target tissues be sensitive to even minute changes in hormone concentration. It follows that hormone–target cell interactions must have at least two characteristics: *specificity,* and the capacity for *amplification* of an initial hormone signal in terms of subsequent biochemical events. These two characteristics will be discussed in some detail below for different classes of hormones.

STEROID HORMONES

A general model for the mode of action of a steroid hormone is shown in Table 1. After secretion, the hormone, either alone or complexed to a specific plasma-binding protein, circulates to its target cell. The free hormone then diffuses into the cytoplasm, where it becomes attached to another specific binding protein called a "receptor" protein. This attachment results in a steroid-receptor complex which has a high affinity for a specific region of the nuclear chromatin (DNA–histone protein complex). The steroid-receptor complex then enters the nucleus, becomes attached to this region of the chromatin, and, through mechanisms still unknown, interacts with the chromatin to bring about an increased rate of transcription (synthesis) of specific messenger RNA (mRNA). The resulting mRNA molecules leave the nucleus and enter the cytoplasm where they are "translated" into molecules of corresponding specific protein (see Part IV). These latter proteins, at least some of which are enzymes, then influence specific intracellular biochemical pathways and account for the ultimate "biologic effects" of the hormone. In recent years a number of steroid hormones have been studied, and in all instances their mechanism of action, insofar as it has been elucidated, appears to conform to this model.

CATECHOLAMINE, POLYPEPTIDE, AND PROTEIN HORMONES

In contrast to the steroid hormones, which must reach the cell *nucleus* before influencing cellular events, many other hormones exert their biochemical effects by

TABLE 1.   Outline of Modes of Action of Some Different Classes of Hormones

Hormone Class	Location of Receptor	Primary Result of Interaction with Receptor	Consequences	
Steroids ? Thyroid hormones	Target cell cytoplasm	Steroid-receptor complexes in cytoplasm migrate to nucleus, bind to specific region(s) of chromatin, and result in increased rate of synthesis ("transcription") of specific mRNA molecules	mRNA molecules migrate to cytoplasm, where they are "translated" into molecules of protein (e.g., specific enzymes) →	Changes in enzyme concentrations, which can then influence the rates of specific biochemical events within the cell
Catecholamines Polypeptides Most proteins	Target cell outer membrane	1. Modification of adenyl cyclase activity: a. Stimulation of cAMP synthesis (e.g., catecholamines, majority of polypeptide and protein hormones — see Table 2)	Increased intracellular concentration of cAMP →	Changes in enzyme activities, changes in cell permeability, etc. (effects of cAMP dependent upon nature of particular target cell — see Table 2)
		b. ? Inhibition of cAMP synthesis (e.g., to account for known effects of insulin on liver and fat cell cAMP levels)	Decreased intracellular concentration of cAMP →	Increased rate of liver glycogen synthesis; decreased rate of gluconeogenesis, glycogenolysis, and lipolysis
		2. ? Direct effect on membrane transport processes (e.g., effects of insulin on glucose uptake by adipose tissue and skeletal muscle)	Increased rate of glucose entry →	Increased rate of glucose utilization and glycogen synthesis

interacting directly with the external cell surface. These latter hormones include many polypeptide and protein hormones as well as the catecholamines, and in these instances the hormone receptors, instead of being located in the cytoplasm of the target cell, appear to be located in the external cell membrane ("plasma membrane") itself. As shown in Table 1, the result of the interaction of one of these hormones with its receptor in the cell membrane depends upon the nature of the hormone. As first shown by the brilliant work of Sutherland, a large number of membrane-active hormones exert their effects by interacting specifically with the enveloping cell membrane to activate *adenyl cyclase*, an enzyme present in the membranes of a great variety of cells. Activation of adenyl cyclase causes an increased rate of synthesis of 3′,5′-cyclic adenosine monophosphate ("cAMP") from ATP. This mechanism leads to an increase in the intracellular concentration of cAMP and accounts for the action of the catecholamines and of most polypeptide and protein hormones for which mechanisms are currently known. An increase in cAMP concentration in a target organ can have diverse and important biochemical consequences which depend upon the cell type and which account for the physiologic effects of the hormone on its target tissue. The diversity of these effects is illustrated in Table 2. In contrast to the steroid hormones, the effects of which require new RNA and protein synthesis (see above), the catecholamine and most of the polypeptide hormones act directly to influence the activity of pre-existing enzyme systems. Many of their physiologic effects can thus be observed almost instantaneously (e.g., those of epinephrine), in contrast to those of the steroid hormones which often require many minutes or longer to become clinically apparent (e.g., the effects of hydrocortisone).

Insulin, in contrast to the hormones discussed in the preceding paragraph, is known to produce a *decrease* in the cyclic AMP content of several tissues. Although it is possible that a fall in intracellular cAMP accounts for many of the effects of insulin on the liver and adipose tissue, it is by no means clear that it explains *all* the biologic effects of the hormone. Other important effects of insulin, such as the stimulation of glucose uptake by

skeletal muscle, appear thus far to take place in the absence of any demonstrable change in adenyl cyclase activity or total intracellular cAMP concentration and may instead reflect direct and independent effects of the hormone on membrane transport processes. Two other examples of protein hormones whose mechanism of action remains unclear are growth hormone and calcitonin.

TABLE 2.   Some Hormonal Responses Dependent Upon an Activation of Adenyl Cyclase

Hormone	Target Tissue	Response
Catecholamines	Liver	Activation of phosphorylase Inactivation of glycogen synthetase
	Skeletal muscle	Activation of phosphorylase Inactivation of glycogen synthetase
	Heart	Activation of phosphorylase Positive inotropic response
	Adipose tissue	Lipolysis
	Salivary gland	Amylase secretion
	Kidney	Renin production
	Pineal gland	Melatonin synthesis
Glucagon	Liver	Activation of phosphorylase
	Pancreatic beta cell	Insulin release
	Adipose tissue	Lipolysis
ACTH*	Adrenal cortex	Steroidogenesis
	Adipose tissue	Lipolysis
LH (ICSH)*	Corpus luteum	Steroidogenesis
	Testis	Steroidogenesis
Angiotensin	Zona glomerulosa	Steroidogenesis
Vasopressin	Renal collecting tubule	Increase in permeability to water
TRH*	Anterior pituitary	TSH release
TSH*	Thyroid	Thyroid hormone release
Gastrin	Gastric parietal cell	Production of HCl
Parathormone	Renal tubule	Excretion of phosphate
	Bone	Calcium mobilization

*ACTH, adrenocorticotrophic hormone; LH (ICSH), luteinizing hormone (interstitial cell–stimulating hormone); TRH, thyrotrophin-releasing hormone; TSH, thyroid-stimulating hormone (thyrotrophin). (Modified after Sutherland, E. W., et al.: Circulation, 37:279, 1968.)

SPECIFICITY OF HORMONAL EFFECTS; "AMPLIFICATION" OF HORMONAL SIGNALS

Two characteristics of hormonal effects have already been mentioned: their *specificity* and the fact that hormones exert their biochemical effects at extremely low molecular concentrations. Both characteristics will be considered briefly as they apply to the two different models for hormone action presented above. In the first model, that for *steroid hormone* action, specificity resides in the affinity of the steroid hormone for its appropriate receptor protein in the cytoplasm of the target tissue. Thus tissues which are estrogen sensitive contain an estrogen-binding receptor protein in their cytoplasm, whereas those which are unresponsive to estrogen do not. "Amplification" of the initial steroid signal can occur at several subsequent steps: interaction of the steroid-receptor complex with the nuclear chromatin can bring about the transcription of more than one molecule of mRNA from a given DNA gene; each of these can then be translated into many enzyme molecules, each of which in turn can catalyze the transformation of many molecules of intracellular substrate into product.

The model presented for *those hormones which operate through cAMP* provides a similar opportunity for both specificity of hormone effect and amplification of the hormonal signal. The mechanisms, however, are different. In the case of the polypeptide and catecholamine hormones, specificity is determined not only by the presence or absence of specific hormone receptors in a cell membrane, but also by the response of that cell to an increased level of cAMP once adenyl cyclase has been activated (see, e.g., Table 2 and References). Mechanisms by which the adenyl cyclase system can amplify an initial hormonal signal are described under the following heading.

CYCLIC AMP

Biologic Effects. The effects of changes in the intracellular concentration of cAMP depend upon the nature of the cell in which these changes occur. Thus in various cells an increase in intracellular cAMP may affect enzyme activities (for example, that of phosphorylase in liver or muscle), may affect permeability of the external cell membrane (as in the renal collecting tubule), may influence gene transcription, or, in certain tissues, may actually stimulate the production or release of certain hormones (see Table 2). The generation of cAMP in response to a hormonal signal at the surface of the cell permits the conversion of an external hormonal signal into a new kind of *(intracellular)* signal, referred to by Sutherland as a "second messenger," and can greatly amplify the original hormonal signal; by stimulating adenyl cyclase activity, a single hormone molecule can potentially cause the synthesis of many molecules of cAMP, which in turn can produce a whole cascade of events within the cell. Both the complexity of these events and their extraordinary rapidity, despite this complexity, are illustrated by the familiar example of hepatic glycogenolysis in response to epinephrine. The steps involved are illustrated in Figure 1; the many steps which intervene between the binding of epinephrine to receptor sites in liver cell membranes and the clinical "result" (an elevation of the blood sugar) are evident.

Figure 1. Steps required in the activation of liver phosphorylase by epinephrine resulting in glycogenolysis and hyperglycemia. The activation of phosphorylase is only one of the consequences of an increased level of cAMP in the liver, and the precise mechanism by which cAMP produces a shift in the balance between inactive and active phosphorylase in favor of the active form is still somewhat conjectural for this tissue. ($P \sim P$, pyrophosphate; P_i, inorganic phosphate; enzymes are indicated in small type.)

Regulation of Intracellular Cyclic AMP Concentration. The intracellular concentration of cAMP is controlled both by regulation of its rate of synthesis and by regulation of its rate of degradation. Degradation of cAMP occurs via a phosphodiesterase which rapidly hydrolyzes cAMP (3',5'-cyclic AMP) to the noncyclic monoester 5'-AMP. It has been found that many substances not conventionally considered hormones are capable of affecting intracellular cAMP levels and hence of mimicking the effects of certain hormones (Fig. 2). Epinephrine and theophylline, for example, have very different primary biochemical actions, yet through entirely different mechanisms they both cause an in-

Figure 2. Influence of various physiologic and pharmacologic substances on the formation and degradation of cyclic AMP. → ⊕ implies stimulation; → ⊖ implies inhibition. Prostaglandins may also affect adenyl cyclase activity, but whether they result in an increase or a decrease in the level of cyclic AMP depends upon target cell type. (Modified after Sutherland, E. W., et al.: Circulation, 37:279, 1968.)

creased concentration of cAMP in many cells. In view of this "final common path" it is not surprising that many of the familiar physiologic effects of theophylline and epinephrine (e.g., tachycardia, positive inotropic effect, dilatation of the coronary arteries, bronchodilatation, nervousness, sweating, glycogenolysis, lipolysis) are so similar.

OTHER HORMONES

The modes of action of certain other hormones remain obscure. Perhaps the most conspicuous example is that of the thyroid hormones, thyroxine and triiodothyronine, which, despite the relative simplicity of their chemical structures, exert their biologic effects by mechanisms still unclear. Although early effects of thyroid hormones include both stimulation of nuclear RNA synthesis and stimulation of mitochondrial protein synthesis and oxygen consumption, and although some of the latter effects can be mimicked by the addition of thyroid hormones to isolated mitochondria in vitro, recent reports of specific nuclear hormone-binding sites suggest the nucleus as a primary site of action. There is evidence that the calorigenic effect of these hormones may be mediated by an increased utilization of ATP in the process of intracellular sodium extrusion, but this phenomenon, in contrast to effects on nuclei and mitochondria, is a relatively late consequence of thyroid hormone administration. (See References for further discussion of some current hypotheses about thyroid hormone action.)

HORMONE STRUCTURE AND SPECIFICITY

The relation between hormone structure and specificity is imperfectly understood, but studies of the relation between molecular structure and function in simpler systems suggest concepts that may apply to hormones and their target-cell receptors. In most of the systems studied so far it appears that the number of indispensable functional groups per molecule is small. For steroid hormones, for example, it is probable that the steroid nucleus itself functions little more than as a rigid spacer to hold essential functional groups in fixed relation to each other. Thus the stilbestrol molecule, a potent but nonsteroidal synthetic estrogen, bears only superficial resemblance to estradiol except in the relative (and fixed) positions of its phenolic hydroxy groups.

In the more complex polypeptide hormones it is possible that one portion of the molecule is responsible for specific binding to a membrane receptor, while another portion interacts with adenyl cyclase to stimulate the synthesis of cAMP. Thyroid-stimulating hormone (TSH) and luteinizing hormone (LH), for example, both exert their biologic effects by stimulating adenyl cyclase in their respective target tissues. Both hormone molecules consist of subunits made up of two different proteins, and one of these two subunits is identical in both hormones. It is tempting to speculate that the subunit which is shared in common contains the site that interacts with adenyl cyclase, whereas the other subunit, which is different in the two hormones, contains the determinants for their tissue specificity.

It now seems likely that those hormone molecules which act by influencing cAMP synthesis and which have tissue specificity contain not only functional groups capable of interacting with adenyl cyclase, but also functional groups which confer an affinity for specific receptors in their target cell membranes. An ingenious and attractive, though still unproved, hypothesis has recently been advanced by Beers and Reich. They have suggested that certain essential tyrosinyl, histadyl, and tryptophanyl residues in the polypeptide hormones may represent the evolutionary descendents of three "primeval" adenyl cyclase–stimulating amines, epinephrine, histamine, and serotonin, and that these amino acids may play an analogous role in the stimulation of adenyl cyclase in target tissues. The rest of the polypeptide molecule is regarded as an elaborate appendage which has been acquired in the course of evolution to confer necessary tissue specificity and to maintain the amino acid at the adenyl cyclase–active site in an appropriate three-dimensional orientation. Epinephrine, for example, is a simple amine and stimulates adenyl cyclase in a great variety of target cells (see, e.g., Table 2); in contrast, the specificity of a substance like parathormone may, by this hypothesis, be attributed to the acquisition of a portion of the molecule which is capable of binding to a more restricted range of target tissues, and which may in fact be at some distance from the site which interacts with adenyl cyclase.

"PHYSIOLOGIC" VS. "PHARMACOLOGIC" EFFECTS

The diversity of the human hormones and their striking tissue specificity are apparent. With the ready availability of many of these hormones in pure form, and with the present ability of the biochemist to detect even subtle effects, an ever-increasing number of hormonal "effects" are being described. One must be cautious in interpreting some of these observations, particularly those made at hormone concentrations which greatly exceed those present in the normal organism. At high concentrations of hormone it is possible that certain exquisite end-organ specificities are simply overcome; under such conditions occasional "anomalous effects" on "surprising" target organs may have little *physiologic* significance.

Buchanan, J., and Tapley, D. F.: Thyroid hormones: Subcellular effects. *In* Werner, S. C., and Ingbar, S. H. (eds.): The Thyroid: A Fundamental and Clinical Text. New York, Harper & Row, 1971, p. 90.

Cahill, G. F., Jr.: Glucagon (editorial). N. Engl. J. Med., 288:157, 1973.

Ismail-Beigi, F., and Edelman, I. S.: The mechanism of the calorigenic action of thyroid hormone: Stimulation of Na$^+$ + K$^+$-activated adenosine triphosphatase activity. J. Gen. Physiol., 57:710, 1971.

Jesen, E. V., and DeSombre, E. R.: Estrogen-receptor interaction. Science, 182:126, 1973.

Lefkowitz, R. J.: Isolated hormone receptors: Physiologic and clinical implications. N. Engl. J. Med., 288:1061, 1973.

Levine, R.: Action of insulin: An attempt at a summary. Diabetes, 21 (suppl.): 454, 1972.

Loeb, J. N.: Models for hormone action. *In* Christy, N. P. (ed.): The Human Adrenal Cortex. New York, Harper & Row, 1971, p. 191.

Maddaiah, V. T.: A model for hormone specific activation of adenyl cyclase. J. Theor. Biol., 25:495, 1969.

O'Malley, B. W.: Mechanisms of action of steroid hormones. N. Engl. J. Med., 284:370, 1971.

Oppenheimer, J. H., Koerner, D., Schwartz, H. L., and Surks, M. I.: Specific nuclear triiodothyronine binding sites in rat liver and kidney. J. Clin. Endocrinol. Metab., 35:330, 1972.

Pitot, H. C., and Yatvin, M. B.: Interrelationships of mammalian hormones and enzyme levels in vivo. Physiol. Rev., 53:228, 1973.

Robison, G. A., Butcher, R. W., and Sutherland, E. W.: Cyclic AMP. New York, Academic Press, 1971.

Roth, J.: Peptide hormone binding to receptors: A review of direct studies in vitro. Metabolism, 22:1059, 1973.

Samuels, H. H., and Tsai, J. S.: Thyroid hormone action in cell culture: Demonstration of nuclear receptors in intact cells and isolated nuclei. Proc. Natl. Acad. Sci. (USA), 70:3488, 1973.

Sutherland, E. W.: Studies on the mechanism of hormone action. Science, 177:401, 1972.

Sutherland, E. W., Robison, G. A., and Butcher, R. W.: Some aspects of the biological role of adenosine 3',5'-monophosphate (cyclic AMP). Circulation, 37:279, 1968.

Thompson, E. B., and Lippman, M. E.: Mechanism of action of glucocorticoids. Metabolism, 23:159, 1974.

Tomkins, G. M., Gelehrter, T. D., Granner, D., Martin, D. W., Samuels, H. H., and Thompson, E. B.: Control of specific gene expression in higher organisms. Science, 166:1474, 1969.

826. THE CONTROL OF ANTERIOR PITUITARY SECRETION

Seymour Reichlin

Although the anterior pituitary gland lacks a direct nerve supply, the secretion of each of its hormones is under the control of the central nervous system. Through specialized secretory neurons localized in the ventral hypothalamus, the function of the pituitary and, in turn, of its target glands becomes responsive to changes in the external and internal environment. In addition, the neurohumoral connections of the anterior pituitary are important in the "feedback" regulation of a number of hormones such as cortisol, the gonadal steroids, thyroxine, and prolactin, and serve as part of the integrated mechanism by which behavioral and metabolic adaptation to the external environment is accomplished.

During the last few years, as the importance of neural factors in the control of pituitary secretion has become increasingly apparent, a division of study of endocrinology has developed which is termed *neuroendocrinology*. This area deals mainly with the interaction of neural and hormonal factors in endocrine and metabolic control systems.

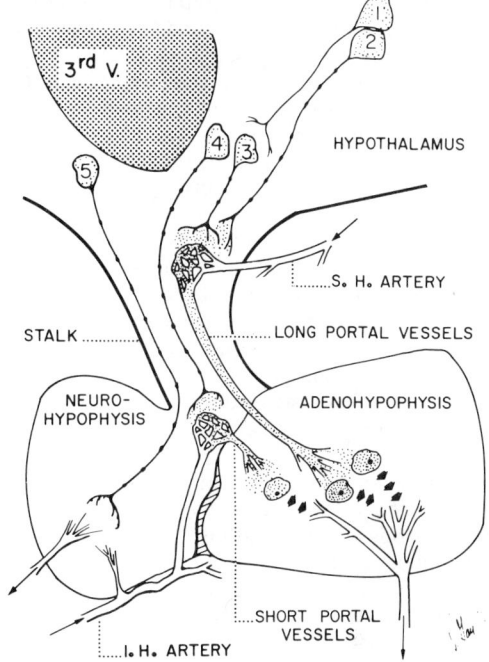

Figure 1. The functional elements of control of the hypothalamic-pituitary unit. Two general types of neurons are involved in anterior pituitary regulation. One type, the peptidergic neuron, forms the releasing hormones (shown here as No. 3, ending in the median eminence, and No. 4, ending in the pituitary stalk), both in relation to the capillary plexus of the hypophysial-portal vessels. These neurons (corresponding to the designation "tuberohypophysial" neurons) are neurosecretory. That is, they combine the function of excitable electrical tissue and secretory function and serve as "neuroendocrine transducers" (Wurtman, 1971) to convert neural information to hormonal information. Their function is analogous to the function of the classic supraoptico-hypophysial neuron (No. 5), the structure responsible for secretion of vasopressin. The second type of neuron is the link between the rest of the brain and the peptidergic neuron. These are largely monaminergic and are believed to end on the cell body of the peptidergic neuron in a conventional manner (No. 1), or to end on the axon terminus of the peptidergic neuron (No. 2) in a manner termed by Schneider and McCann "axo-axonic." Abbreviations: S.H., superior hypophysial; I.H., inferior hypophysial; 3rd V., third ventricle. (From Gay, V.: Fertility and Sterility, 23:50, 1972.)

HYPOTHALAMIC NEUROSECRETION: HYPOPHYSIOTROPHIC NEURONS

The pituitary gland and hypothalamus are closely related anatomically, as may be seen in Figure 1. This relationship has both embryologic and functional significance. The neural lobe develops as a downgrowth of axons from the diencephalon, whose cells of origin are located in the paraventricular and supraoptic nuclei of the hypothalamus. These nerve fibers pass as unmyelinated axons through the neural stalk and terminate in the neural lobe. Like neurons elsewhere, supraopticohypophysial and paraventriculohypophysial neurons are electrically excitable, conduct action potentials, and are responsive to neurotransmitters. Unlike most other neurons, these cells are neurosecretory, that is, they synthesize hormonal substances which are released into blood vessels for action at a remote site rather than locally at synapses, as is characteristic of most neurons. Hormones of the neurohypophysis are synthesized

mainly in cell bodies located in the hypothalamus and pass in granule form (associated with a protein carrier substance) to the nerve endings in the neural lobe, where they are stored. Neurosecretory neurons thus manifest the properties of both nerve and gland. These cells, of which the neurohypophysial neurons are the classic example, have been termed by Wurtman *"neuroendocrine transducers."* Cells of this type are the major effector links between the nervous system and the endocrine gland. Although the neural lobe lies close to the anterior lobe of the pituitary and neurohypophysial secretory products are identifiable in blood reaching the pituitary, the secretions of the neurohypophysis (oxytocin, vasopressin, neurophysin) have no established regulatory action in the anterior lobe but are released into the systemic circulation to affect remote tissues such as the kidney, breast, and uterus.

The phylogenetically more primitive neuroendocrine "transducer" for anterior pituitary control is located within the median eminence of the hypothalamus.

Nerve endings here contain "hypophysiotrophic" hormones; these substances, also called *"releasing factors,"* reach the anterior pituitary through a specialized system of capillaries and veins, the hypophysial-portal circulation. The cells of origin of the median eminence neurons are clustered around the medial-basal hypothalamus in the so-called hypophysiotrophic area. They resemble neurohypophysial neurons in being electrically active, pharmacologically excitable, and responsive to a wide variety of nerve impulses arising from other sites in the brain and to feedback hormonal stimuli. Neuron endings of the stalk–median eminence region (tuberohypophysial neurons) and the associated blood vessels have been likened to the posterior lobe and can be looked upon as a "median eminence gland"; taken together, these structures constitute the "final common pathway" for neural control of the anterior pituitary gland.

This outline of anterior pituitary regulation is the *portal vessel chemotransmitter hypothesis.* According to this view, lesions of the hypothalamus (and of the portal vessel complex of the stalk) reduce most anterior pituitary functions by causing a deficiency of releasing factors. Direct electrical stimulation of the tuberohypophysial neurons, or reflex activation of these neurons, caused, for example, by emotional stress, activates the anterior pituitary by the release of hypophysiotrophic hormones.

Initially based on indirect physiologic experiments, this hypothesis has been established by demonstration of hypothalamic substances which selectively affect each of the known pituitary hormones. These are CRF (corticotrophin-releasing factor), TRF (TRH) (thyrotrophin-releasing factor), GHRF (growth hormone–releasing factor), LRF (LRH) (luteinizing hormone–releasing factor), FSHRF (follicle-stimulating hormone-releasing factor), and PRF (prolactin-releasing factor). Because the existence of these substances seems so well established, it has been proposed that they be called releasing hormones. Inhibitory hypophysiotrophic hormones have also been identified. These are PIF (prolactin inhibitory factor) and GHRIF (growth hormone release inhibitory factor [somatostatin]). MSH secretion by intermediate lobe cells (which do not form a definite anatomic subdivision in the human subject) appears to be regulated by both excitatory (MSHRF) and inhibitory factors (MSHIF).

The chemical nature of TRF, now termed thyrotrophic-releasing hormone (TRH), was identified in 1969 as a tripeptide amide, pyroglutamyl histidyl prolineamide (Fig. 2). The chemical nature of LRF (LRH) was identified in 1971 as a decapeptide (Fig. 2), the amino terminal of which (like TRH) is pyroglutamic acid and the carboxyl terminal an amide. A substance with powerful growth hormone release inhibitory activity, chemically identified in 1973 as a linear peptide composed of 14 amino acids (Fig. 2), was named by its discoverers *somatostatin.* The chemical nature of the MSH-regulating peptides is still somewhat uncertain, but fractions of oxytocin (the terminal tripeptide, and the five-membered ring tocinoic acid) have been reported to have powerful effects on MSH secretion in various test situations. Although the primary activity of the aforementioned chemically identified releasing hormones is related to the original bioassay properties used in purification and identification, it is now apparent that there are certain

pyroGlu-His-Pro Amide

TRH, Thyrotrophin-releasing hormone

pyroGlu-His-Trp-Ser-Tyr-Gly-Leu-Arg-Pro-Gly Amide

LRH, Luteinizing hormone–releasing hormone, gonadotrophin-releasing hormone, GnRH

H-Ala-Gly-Cys-Lys-Asn-Phe-Phe-Trp-Lys-Thr-Phe-Thr-Ser-Cys OH

GHRF-IF, Somatostatin

Figure 2.   Structural formulas of the established hypophysiotrophic hormones.

crossover effects of these hormones. Thus TRH is a potent releaser of prolactin in man and certain other species and releases GH in some acromegalics. LRH releases FSH as well as LH and may therefore be the only gonadotrophin-releasing hormone (GnRH) for regulation of both of these gonadotrophins. Somatostatin inhibits TSH secretion as well as somatotrophic hormone secretion and, when given in "pharmacologic" doses, inhibits pancreatic secretion of glucagon and insulin. The chemical nature of CRF and GHRF has not been identified.

In the human subject, TRH and LRH have been widely used for physiologic and diagnostic studies of pituitary function.

One of the important consequences of these discoveries is that means have now been provided for selective manipulation of the secretion of TSH, LH-FSH, prolactin, and GH.

BIOGENIC AMINE CONTROL OF HYPOPHYSIOTROPHIC FUNCTIONS

The hypophysiotrophic neurons are in turn innervated by specialized monaminergic neurotransmitter neurons (Fig. 1), the principal ones of which secrete dopamine, norepinephrine, and serotonin. It appears probable, though not completely established, that norepinephrine stimulates the secretion of LRH, TRH, and GHRF, and that dopamine stimulates the secretion of PIF. There is evidence that serotonin may inhibit the secretion of PIF and of TRF. A noradrenergic link in the regulation of CRF appears to be inhibitory. Since the central nervous biogenic amine network is also involved in the regulation of affective states (such as depression), many drugs commonly used as psychopharmacologic agents, e.g., reserpine and phenothiazines, may alter anterior pituitary function. Clinical examples of such effects are irregular menstrual cycles or anovulation in women (owing to blockade of the cyclic discharge of LRH), galactorrhea (owing to inhibition of PIF release), and inhibition of reflex somatotrophin release (owing to inhibition of GHRF). Certain of the drug effects have been used to test hormonal secretion. For example, chlorpromazine and other phenothiazines stimulate prolactin release and have been used as a means of testing prolactin secretory reserve. Chlorpromazine has been used to treat acromegaly, because it lowers GH levels in some cases, presumably through changes in secretion of GHRF. L-Dopa, a drug used in the treatment of Parkinson's disease, which increases central nervous system concentration of dopamine, brings about the release of GH and the inhibition of prolactin secretion. In acromegalics L-dopa may paradoxically inhibit growth hormone secretion.

Hormonal feedback effects are also involved in the control of the hypophysiotrophic neurons. The relative importance of hypothalamic and pituitary feedback appears to differ to some degree from one system to another. The pituitary-thyroid axis is the best worked out of these control systems. Thyroid hormone regulates TSH secretion through a direct inhibitory effect on the anterior pituitary. These inhibitory effects are opposed by the stimulatory effect of hypothalamic drive brought about by TRH secretion. TRH secretion, a neurogenic function, is responsive to a variety of neural signals, including those involved in temperature regulation. It has been proposed that the secretion of TRH may also be stimulated by thyroid hormone as a *positive* feedback effect, although the opposite effect of thyroid hormone has also been reported to occur.

Gonadotrophic hormone secretion is regulated by a complex interaction of ovarian or testicular hormone feedback on both the pituitary and hypothalamus. Evidence has been adduced in man which shows that LRH secretion may be stimulated by the positive feedback effects of estrogen on the hypothalamus. Estrogenic hormones inhibit pituitary responsiveness to LRH, but can also transiently *sensitize* the pituitary to releasing hormone, depending upon the effects of time and dose. In addition to this hormonal interaction, gonadotrophin secretion is subject to "open-loop" effects such as emotional stress (which in the human can inhibit ovulation), and in animals such as the rabbit copulation can trigger reflex ovulation.

Growth hormone secretion is almost exclusively controlled by the central nervous system. Estrogenic hormones appear to sensitize the pituitary to the growth hormone–releasing factor, and metabolic (as well as stress-related) events are mediated at the level of the hypothalamus. An important aspect of GH regulation is so-called short-loop feedback control. Plasma GH itself is capable of inhibiting the secretion of GHRF.

Prolactin secretion, like GH secretion, is largely regulated by the nervous system; there is a short-loop feedback control, and estrogen also appears to sensitize the pituitary to the effects of PRF.

Cortisol feedback inhibition of the pituitary-adrenal axis appears to act primarily on the median eminence of the hypothalamus, but there is an important negative feedback effect on the pituitary, and cortisol may also act on suprahypothalamic neural structures. Some workers believe that all feedback control is directed at the pituitary and that results of experiments in which intrahypothalamic injection of cortisol was effective in inhibiting ACTH were due to transport of the cortisol via the median eminence to the pituitary.

An important recent insight is that pituitary secretion of growth hormone, prolactin, and ACTH is regulated by intrinsic brain rhythms related to the sleep-wake cycle or to changes in lighting, rather than by specific homeostatic requirements. Nocturnal GH secretion (largely related to early deep sleep) accounts for more than half of total daily GH secretion, values at night approaching the levels found in acromegaly. Nocturnal prolactin secretion begins about the same time that GH secretion does but appears to last longer. The

secretion of ACTH with a peak in the early morning hours is linked to the day-night lighting cycle. Nocturnal rhythms for TSH and (under certain circumstances) gonadotrophins have also been shown. Disturbances in sleep-related hormonal secretion may be the earliest indication of incipient or mild hypothalamic-pituitary disturbance. Proper evaluation of total endocrine function under physiologic or pathologic states must take into account these diurnal rhythms.

NEUROENDOCRINE DISEASES OF THE PITUITARY GLAND

It is apparent that any consideration of the neuroendocrine diseases of the pituitary overlaps the descriptions of diseases of the pituitary itself (see Ch. 830 to 832). The following paragraphs emphasize, primarily, neuroendocrine disorders of the anterior pituitary.

In the context of the foregoing description of the hypothalamic-pituitary unit, disorders of pituitary se-

TABLE 1.   Endocrine Syndromes of Hypothalamic Origin

Hypophysiotrophic hormone deficiency:
  Surgical pituitary stalk section
  Basilar meningitis and granuloma, sarcoidosis, tuberculosis,
    sphenoid osteomyelitis, eosinophilic granuloma
  Craniopharyngioma
  Hypothalamic tumor
    Infundibuloma
    Teratoma (ectopic pinealoma)
    Neuroglial tumors, particularly astrocytoma
  Maternal deprivation syndrome
  Isolated GHRF deficiency
  Hypothalamic hypothyroidism
  Panhypophysiotrophic failure

Disorders of regulation of LRH and FRH:
  Female
    Precocious puberty
    Delayed puberty
    Neurogenic amenorrhea
      Pseudocyesis
      Anorexia nervosa
      "Functional amenorrhea"
      "Functional oligomenorrhea"
      Drug-induced amenorrhea
  Male
    Precocious puberty
    Fröhlich's syndrome
    Olfactory-genital dysplasia (Kallmann's syndrome)

Disorders of regulation of prolactin-inhibiting hormone (nonpuerperal galactorrhea):
  Tumor
  Sarcoid
  Drug-induced
  Reflex
    Herpes zoster of chest wall
    Post-thoracotomy
    Nipple manipulation
    Spinal cord tumor
  "Psychogenic"
  Chiari-Frommel syndrome
  Hypothyroidism
  CO_2 narcosis

Disorders of regulation of CRF:
  Paroxysmal ACTH discharge (Wolff's syndrome)
  Loss of circadian variation
  Cushing's disease?

Hypersecretion of GHRF:
  Acromegaly?

cretion can be viewed as occurring at many "levels" of function. Defects may arise resulting from destruction of the pituitary itself (as by a tumor), or from genetically determined deficiency of a particular type of pituitary cell. At a higher level, disorders may arise through disruption of the stalk–median eminence neurons or of their essential vascular channels to the anterior pituitary gland. Such destruction of the "final common path" of anterior pituitary regulation occurs after surgical stalk section, in tumors of the stalk region, e.g., craniopharyngioma, infundibuloma, or teratomas, and in such inflammations as sarcoidosis. In precocious puberty, the tonically active inhibitory system which determines the time at which the hypophysiotrophic neurons will become active may be destroyed or inactivated too soon. Disease may also arise from abnormal stimulation of the hypophysiotrophic neurons. In Table 1 the major endocrine diseases of hypothalamic origin are listed.

Hypophysiotrophic Hormone Deficiency

Introduction of TRH and LRH into clinical medicine has made it possible to identify several syndromes of hypophysiotrophic neuron failure. Isolated TSH deficiency secondary to isolated TRH deficiency has been identified as a rare cause of thyroid failure. This disorder has been termed "hypothalamic hypothyroidism" or "tertiary" hypothyroidism. Isolated LRH deficiency accounts for the endocrine deficiency in many patients with isolated gonadotrophin deficiency, as in Kallmann's syndrome (hypogonadotrophic hypogonadism with hyposmia). Isolated GHRF deficiency appears to underlie the growth hormone secretory failure in the bulk of patients with idiopathic dwarfism. There also appears to be a disorder of "panhypophysiotrophic failure" in which all pituitary functions are lost. Most children with idiopathic panhypopituitarism fall into this category.

Hypophysiotrophic deficiency can be induced by destruction of the hypophysiotrophic area of the hypothalamus, of the stalk, or of the vascular supply to the anterior pituitary. The association of hypophysiotrophic deficiency with abnormal EEG's, and a history of birth trauma in some cases, or its occurrence as a congenital loss of hypophysiotrophic secretion, suggests an analogy with other forms of birth injury.

Under most circumstances, acquired hypophysiotrophic deficiency (as in surgical stalk section) results in a moderate to severe degree of pituitary failure, but the extent of endocrine deficit is not as extreme as that seen after hypophysectomy. This residuum of function (which is readily duplicated in laboratory animals) has been thought in the past to represent the "autonomous" capacity of the pituitary to function independent of the hypothalamus. With the identification of syndromes of hypophysiotrophic failure, as in "hypothalamic hypothyroidism" and panhypophysiotrophic failure, has come the recognition that pituitary deficiency as severe as that observed after hypophysectomy can at times follow loss of hypothalamic function. It is probable that most of the so-called pituitary autonomy after stalk section is the result of residual hypothalamic hypophysiotrophic function.

The main endocrine manifestations of hypothalamic failure are variable loss of TSH secretion, abolition of gonadotrophin secretion, loss of normal GH secretory responses to hypoglycemia and other stimuli, and loss of normal sleep pattern. Circadian and tonic baseline corticotrophin secretion is abolished, as is feedback control by circulating cortisol levels, but the response to certain kinds of stress, such as pyrogens, may be retained, suggesting that there are extrahypothalamic sites of formation of CRF. In sharp contrast to the hypophysectomized patient, individuals with hypothalamic disease usually have high circulating levels of prolactin owing to loss of PIF influence. Galactorrhea develops in about one fourth of women after section of the pituitary stalk, although all have elevated prolactin levels in plasma. The most sensitive signs of hypothalamic damage appear to be loss of diurnal GH rhythms, loss of GH secretory responses to stress, and the capacity to have an ovulatory surge of LH secretion.

Disorders of Regulation of GHRF

In addition to idiopathic hypophysiotrophic failure and specific damage to the hypothalamus or stalk, growth hormone deficiency may arise on a psychogenic basis in the so-called maternal deprivation syndrome (MDS). Such patients, generally children from grossly disturbed homes, may fail to grow despite adequate food intake. When they are brought into the hospital and given a degree of tender, loving care, growth rate returns to normal. GH secretion is impaired or absent in such children, and they do not respond to the usual stimuli such as hypoglycemia or arginine infusion. Since this disturbance is reversible after psychologic management, it has been concluded that a functional inhibition of the hypophysiotrophic GH-regulating neurons has taken place in these children. Deprivation in infants can cause severe marasmus.

In adults a somewhat analogous situation is seen in severe "monopolar" depression. Failure to release GH in response to hypoglycemia or to L-dopa administration suggests that in such patients there is an abnormality in central hypophysiotrophic function. In the light of modern ideas about the role of biogenic amines in determination of affective states, it is believed that the GH unresponsiveness in depression may be a reflection of abnormalities in central noradrenergic pathways in the hypothalamus.

In addition to GH unresponsiveness, some children with MDS may have unresponsive pituitary-adrenal function with loss of the circadian rhythm and of the response to the metyrapone test of ACTH reserve.

Excessive GHRF secretion has been proposed to be the cause of some cases of acromegaly.

Disorders of Regulation of GnRH

The concept of "levels" of neurogenic disruption of pituitary control is best illustrated in abnormalities of secretion of the gonadotrophins. Deficiency of both LH and FSH occurs after destruction of the hypophysiotrophic neurons. But disturbances also occur if the hypophysiotrophic neurons are themselves abnormally stimulated. The characteristic pattern of male gonadotrophin regulation is one of tonic low-level secretion of LH and FSH which leads to growth, development, and maturation of the spermatozoa, a process taking place over a 70-day period. The characteristic pattern of human female regulation is that of the recurring menstrual cycle, dependent upon a recurring surge of LH secretion which is in turn dependent upon cyclic secretion of estrogens by the ovary. In certain forms of hypothalamic disease, the characteristic normally recurring cyclic pattern of LH secretion may be lost. Because this often occurs transiently in a setting of severe psychologic stress, as after incarceration in concentration camps, in bombing attacks, or after minor stress such as going away to school, and develops in the absence of evident structural disease of the pituitary or hypothalamus, it is probable that loss of LH cycling may be an acquired psychologic disorder. The terms "functional amenorrhea," "functional oligomenorrhea," and "hypothalamic amenorrhea" have been applied to such cases. These probably represent a neural inhibition of normal estrogen-induced LRH secretion. A similar correlation appears likely in pseudocyesis, most often a manifestation of hysteria, and in anorexia nervosa. In about half the cases of anorexia nervosa, amenorrhea begins coincident with the disturbance in eating, and for this reason must be regarded as a concomitant rather than a consequence of inanition. Resumption of menstrual cycling does not occur until the patient has returned to a "critical weight," thus supporting the role of nutritional factors in this disease.

Besides these more obvious psychogenic changes in menstrual function, many women with "secondary" amenorrhea are encountered who have no apparent psychologic distress, but in whom the pattern of menstrual irregularity, amenorrhea, and oligomenorrhea is similar to that seen in the neurogenic syndromes. In one series, fully one fourth of the women in this category who were placed into a research study after one year or more of anovulation developed normal cycles within a month of their entry into the research project.

Next to pregnancy, "functional" amenorrhea is the most common cause of a secondary failure to menstruate. A clear-cut differential diagnosis between functional amenorrhea and disease of the anterior pituitary or hypothalamus can now be made. The patient with pituitary or hypothalamic disease most often has more than one trophic hormone deficiency, may have evidence of local pituitary damage, e.g., enlarged sella by x-ray, visual field defects, and behavioral or other neurologic abnormalities of the hypothalamus. Sixty to 80 per cent of patients with "functional" amenorrhea release luteinizing hormone after treatment with the drug clomiphene. Synthetic LRH stimulates LH and FSH release in patients whose disease is due to hypothalamic and not pituitary disorder. In patients with longstanding LRH deficiency, the pituitary may become relatively resistant to LRH. Repeated injections are required to restore normal responsivity. This finding indicates that LRH stimulates either the synthesis of LH or the secretory machinery for LH, or both, a conclusion supported by laboratory studies.

Drug-induced anovulation should be borne in mind as a cause of amenorrhea. Reserpine and the phenothiazines are particularly common causes. Patients who fail to resume normal menses after discontinuance of contraceptive pills ("post-pill amenorrhea") usually have underlying functional abnormalities of the pituitary-gonad axis evident before taking the pill. Such patients release LH in response to LRH. Excessive prolactin secretion (as in certain chromophobe adenomas) has recently been recognized as a cause of amenorrhea. Prolactin is thought to inhibit hypothalamic secretion of LRH. The tumor may not be detectable by usual neuroradiologic diagnostic methods, and cures have been achieved by removal of very small adenomas by microsurgical techniques.

Gonadotrophin regulatory difficulties may arise from loss of hypophysiotrophic function, from failure of the intrinsic cycling mechanism, and, at a higher functional level, from precocious or delayed development of sexual maturation. The timing of the onset of puberty is a neural function, and involves a patterned development of brain analogous to the patterns of development of other brain functions such as crawling, sitting, or walking and the development of abstract ability. Both delayed and accelerated puberty can be observed. When sexual function is normal in other respects, the term *precocious puberty* is applied, in contradistinction to the condition arising from primary secretory abnormalities of the gonads, properly termed *pseudoprecocious puberty*. All true precocious puberty is neurogenic in origin. In males, more than half the cases are due to brain lesions which directly or indirectly impinge upon the hypothalamus. In girls, fewer than 10 per cent have demonstrable lesions, although a high proportion have EEG abnormalities and may be regarded as suffering from mild degrees of brain damage.

In the male, primary isolated gonadotrophin failure is a well recognized cause of delayed puberty. In one type, there is an association with failure to develop rhinencephalic brain structures, manifested clinically by hyposmia. Such cases have been termed olfactory-genital dysplasia (Kallmann's syndrome), and appear to be due to failure to develop hypophysiotrophic function, because the patients usually respond to injections of LRH, albeit sluggishly. Cases of isolated gonadotrophic failure resulting from intrinsic pituitary disease have also been identified.

Disorders of Regulation of PIF

Many conditions cause lactation unrelated to pregnancy (nonpuerperal galactorrhea). Certain chromophobe pituitary tumors may secrete prolactin (Forbes-Albright syndrome) and induce lactation. Hypothalamic disturbance or "psychogenic" factors are important causes of galactorrhea. Causes listed in Table 1 have in common a presumed deficiency of prolactin inhibitory hormone, whether caused by irritation of the neural pathways involved in normal suckling reflexes (herpes zoster, nipple stimulation, post-thoracotomy) or by drugs, encephalopathy, hypothyroidism, or direct damage to the hypothalamus or stalk. Still uncertain is the relative frequency of small chromophobe adenomas as a cause of prolactin hypersecretion. Improved criteria for making the diagnosis of chromophobe adenoma are being developed. Values for prolactin over 150 ng per millimeter are very suspicious for tumor.

USE OF THE HYPOTHALAMIC HORMONES IN DIAGNOSIS OF ANTERIOR PITUITARY DISEASE

Synthetic TRH and LRH have been widely used for diagnostic purposes. The intravenous injection of TRH (15 to 800 μg; usual dose, 400 μg) is followed within five minutes by a rise in TSH which peaks between 15 and 45 minutes (Fig. 3). Changes in TSH secretion lead to a detectable increase in T_3 and a slight and less consist-

RESPONSE   TO   I.V.   TRH   800 µg   IN   HUMANS

Figure 3.   Effect of TRH on plasma TSH and prolactin in the human. (Data replotted from Bowers, C. Y., Friesen, H. G., Hwang, P., Guyda, H. J., and Folkers, K.: Biochem. Biophys. Res. Comm., 45:1033, 1970.) This figure illustrates the response of plasma TSH to injection of TRH in normal men and women and in patients with thyrotoxicosis. Note that the response is greater in women than in men, and is abolished by the thyrotoxic state. The latter effect is due to thyroxine- and triiodothyronine-induced inhibition of response at the pituitary level. TRH also acts as a prolactin-releasing hormone, and, like the TSH response, it is blocked by the administration of thyroxine, or the spontaneous occurrence of thyroid hormone excess.

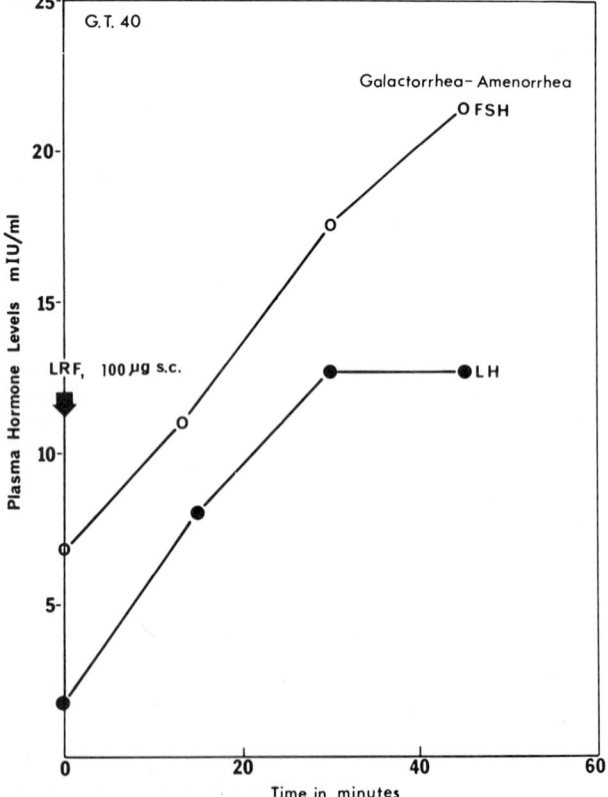

Figure 4.   Changes in plasma LH and FSH after injection of LRH. This patient with a chromophobe adenoma of the pituitary had been amenorrheic for 15 years. Plasma prolactin levels (not shown) were 365 ng per ml. The prompt and striking response to LRH indicates that the amenorrhea was secondary to hypophysiotrophic failure, in this case owing to prolactin-induced inhibition of LRH secretion.

TABLE 2.*   Changes in Plasma LH and FSH After Intravenous Injection of a Standard Test Dose of 100 µg of LRH

	LH (µIU/ml)	FSH (µIU/ml)
Males	83.9 ± 42.7	9.3 ± 4.4
Females		
Adult premenopausal	61.8 ± 26.2	5.2 ± 2.2
Menopausal	154.4 ± 46.9	49.1 ± 19.3

*From Hashimoto, T., Miyai, K., Izumi, K., and Kumahara, Y.: J. Clin. Endocrinol. Metab., 37:910, 1973.

ent increase in T_4. Mean responses in normal men are slightly less than in normal women, presumably owing to the estrogen sensitization of the anterior pituitary. In one series of normal subjects, mean maximal increment ±S.D. after 400 µg was 16.0 µU per ml ±2.5; in another, mean response to 500 µg was 25 µU ±10 of TSH. In normal people, prolactin levels also rise (Fig. 3), and in many acromegalics (unlike the normal) GH levels may also rise. Pituitary failure causes a loss of the response to TRH or a reduction in response, and in patients with TRH hypophysiotrophic failure the response may be slightly delayed in onset, but may rise higher, presumably owing to the associated hypothyroidism. This test thus permits the differentiation between pituitary and hypothalamic forms of secondary hypothyroidism. Because of the fact that thyroid hormone inhibits the pituitary, the response to TRH is also abolished in patients being treated with thyroid hormone, or in individuals with hyperthyroidism which may be so mild as to be barely detectable (Fig. 3). This response, in fact, is a very sensitive test for mild degrees of hyperthyroidism. Recovery of TSH responsiveness may be very much delayed (as long as six weeks) after a course of thyroxine treatment.

The administration of 20 to 500 µg of LRH (usual dose 100 µg subcutaneously or intravenously) is followed by a prompt rise in LH and a somewhat less marked and much more delayed rise in FSH (Fig. 4). Many patients will show only the LH response to the lower doses. There may be a shift in these responses according to prior hormonal state. In one well-studied series of patients, normal values ± S.D., as shown in Table 2, were obtained for peak increment in plasma gonadotrophins after intravenous injection of 100 µg of LRH.

Responses are abolished in patients with pituitary failure, and they may be excessive if the patient is in a state of increased gonadotrophic secretion, e.g., in menopausal or certain hypogonadal states. Individuals with hypothalamic failure may have reduced LH secretory responses to LRH, but these values return toward normal after repeated injections of the releasing hormones. The administration of estrogen in usual therapeutic doses usually causes a transient increase in the sensitivity of the pituitary to LRH in women, and a decrease in men.

Side effects after TRH include mild nausea and a sense of urinary urgency. "Allergic" symptoms have occasionally been observed, but no serious reactions have been reported, and even these mild symptoms are prevented if the material is injected over a two-minute period instead of as a single rapid "bolus." No side effects have been observed after LRH injection.

TREATMENT

Treatment of granulomatous disease of the hypothalamic region consists of treating the specific disease, e.g., adrenal corticosteroids for sarcoidosis; these have been effective in some cases. Surgery for tumors of this region may entail a high risk. Decision about the best therapeutic method depends upon the nature of the tumor (cyst, craniopharyngioma, infundibuloma) as best one can interpret it clinically and radiographically, the precise location of the tumor, and the presence or absence of encroachment on important nearby structures, e.g., the optic chiasm. (For the treatment of pituitary tumors that rise up out of the pituitary fossa and impinge upon the hypothalamus, see Ch. 830).

Bardin, C. W., Ross, G. T., Rifkind, A. B., Cargille, C. M., and Lipsett, M. B.: Studies of the pituitary–Leydig cell axis in young men with hypogonadotropic hypogonadism and hyposmia: Comparison with normal men, prepubertal boys, and hypopituitary patients. J. Clin. Invest., 48:2046, 1969.

Bowers, C. Y., Schally, A. V., Hawley, W. D., Gual, C., and Parlow, A.: Effect of thyrotropin-releasing factor in man. J. Clin. Endocrinol. Metab., 28:978, 1968.

Frohman, L. A.: Clinical neuropharmacology of hypothalamic releasing factors. N. Engl. J. Med., 286:1391, 1972.

Gual, C.: Clinical effects and uses of hypothalamic releasing and inhibiting factors. In Ganong, W. F., and Martini, L. (eds.): Frontiers in Neuroendocrinology. New York, Oxford University Press, 1973, pp. 89–131.

Guillemin, R.: Hypothalamic hormones: Releasing and inhibiting factors. Hosp. Prac., 8:111, 1973.

Kastin, A. J., Schally, A. V., Gual, C., Midgley, A. R., Jr., Bowers, C. Y., and Diaz-Infante, A., Jr.: Stimulation of LH release in men and women by LH-releasing hormone purified from porcine hypothalami. J. Clin. Endocrinol. Metab., 29:1046, 1969.

Martin, J. B.: Neural regulation of growth hormone secretion. N. Engl. J. Med., 288:1384, 1973.

Martini, L., and Ganong, W. F. (eds.): Neuroendocrinology. New York, Academic Press, Vol. 1, 1966; Vol. 2, 1967.

Martini, L., and Ganong, W. F. (eds.): Frontiers in Neuroendocrinology. New York, Oxford University Press, Vol. 1, 1969; Vol. 2, 1971; Vol. 3, 1973.

McCann, S. M., and Porter, J. C.: Hypothalamic pituitary-stimulating and -inhibiting hormones. Physiol. Rev., 49:240, 1969.

Reichlin, S.: Hypothalamic-hypophysial function. In Scow, R. (ed.): Proceedings of the Fourth International Congress of Endocrinology. Amsterdam, Excerpta Medica, 1973.

Sawyer, C. H., and Gorski, R.: Steroid Hormones and Brain Function. The UCLA Forum in Medical Sciences, Nuber 15. University of California Press, 1971.

Siler, T. N., VandenBerg, G., and Yen, S. S. C.: Inhibition of growth hormone release in humans by somatostatin. J. Clin. Endocrinol. Metab., 37:632, 1973.

THE ANTERIOR PITUITARY
(Adenohypophysis)

Nicholas P. Christy

827. INTRODUCTION

Diseases of the anterior pituitary manifest themselves in two ways: mechanically, when space-occupying pituitary tumors impinge upon adjacent structures; and functionally, when there is deficient or excessive secretion of some or all of the several hormones secreted by the gland.

History. The pituitary gland was first described by Vesalius in 1543. The earliest known artistic representation of pituitary disease is found in a sculptured figure on the Rheims Cathedral (thirteenth century): one of the gargoyles has distinctly acromegalic features. Good clinical and pathologic descriptions of acromegaly were provided by Verga (1864) and Fritzsche and Klebs (1884). Pierre Marie (1886) named the disease "acromegaly" because of the hypertrophy of the extremities. The pituitary tumor was recognized by Minkowski (1887) and by Broca (1888). In 1900, Benda ascribed the disorder to eosinophilic adenoma of the hypophysis.

Hypofunction of the pituitary was suspected by Lorain (1871), who associated dwarfism with pituitary destruction in man. Simmonds (1914) described the necropsy findings in an emaciated woman who proved to have extreme atrophy of the anterior pituitary and ovarian fibrosis and splanchnomicria. He correctly attributed the clinical picture to pituitary destruction, which he later showed could also result from tuberculosis or tumor (1916). Many later authors described clinical features now interpreted as those of pituitary insufficiency in patients with tumors of the infundibulum and chromophobe adenomas of the anterior lobe (Honlinger, Cushing and others, 1923–1938). The association of pituitary destruction with the puerperium was definitely established by H. L. Sheehan (1937–1949). He demonstrated acute pituitary necrosis in women dying shortly after difficult labor. He also traced the syndrome of chronic hypopituitarism and pituitary atrophy to episodes of postpartum hemorrhage, and showed that cachexia is not an essential feature of the syndrome.

Experimental elucidation of the functions of the pituitary began with Aschner's demonstration (1909) that hypophysectomy caused arrest of growth in young dogs. Splanchnomicria was found in hypophysectomized animals (Livon and Peyron, 1912), and P. E. Smith observed failure of growth after hypophysectomy in the frog and the rat (1916–1926). In 1921, Evans and Long made the important observation that administration of pituitary extracts restored normal growth in the hypophysectomized animal and that large amounts of such growth-promoting extracts produced gigantism in the rat. Smith (1927–1930) described the repair by hypophysial extracts of the gonadal, thyroidal, and adrenocortical atrophy that follows hypophysectomy. He also showed the distinctive effects of destruction of the pituitary (hypopituitarism) as opposed to the hypothalamus (obesity).

The last four decades have witnessed rapid progress in knowledge of the physiologic and biochemical effects of ablation of the pituitary in animals and man. The work of many investigators has led to methods for the extraction of progressively purer pituitary hormones for physiologic study and clinical use, to knowledge of the chemical structure of several, to the total synthesis of at least two (ACTH, MSH) and to the measurement of all in plasma by radioimmunoassay (Berson and Yalow). Current experimental and clinical interest centers around the central nervous system control of anterior pituitary function (Harris and others), especially the role of the hypothalamic "releasing hormones" (see Ch. 826).

Anatomy. The adult pituitary gland weighs 0.4 to 0.9 gram, averaging about 0.6 gram. It enlarges during pregnancy, and after repeated pregnancies may attain a weight of 1.0 to 1.5 grams; the weight tends to decrease in old age. The gland rests in the bony sella turcica and is bounded superiorly by the tough diaphragma sellae, a lamina of the dura mater. The pituitary stalk perforates the diaphragma and connects the pituitary to the hypothalamus; it contains the neurosecretory fibers, which pass from the supraoptic and paraventricular nuclei to the posterior pituitary (neurohypophysis) and the complex arterial and hypothalamic-hypophysial portal venous system, which serves as the functional connection between the nuclei of the hypothalamus and the anterior pituitary. For clinical purposes, the *gross anatomy* of the pituitary is the anatomy of the sella turcica; roentgenographic changes in that structure provide evidence of pituitary enlargement in the form of increase in the linear measurements of the sella and erosion, demineralization, or displacement of its bony borders. The normal sella can be oval, round, or flat. In normal adults, the anteroposterior diameter (sagittal plane) should not exceed 17 mm, the vertical diameter should not be greater than 14 mm, and the normal width (frontal projection) is about 19 mm. Measured roentgenographically, the calculated area of the normal adult pituitary fossa (sagittal plane) does not exceed 130 sq mm; the volume is about 1100 cu mm. Even when sellar measurements are normal, pituitary tumor is suspected if there is suprasellar calcification (Fig. 1), elevation or

Figure 1. Craniopharyngioma in a 69-year-old woman. The lateral (sagittal) film of the skull shows suprasellar calcification and a normal-sized sella with depression of the sellar floor and some flattening of the dorsum sellae.

destruction of the anterior or posterior clinoids, demineralization or depression of the floor of the sella (Fig. 1), or "ballooning" of the fossa.

The pituitary fossa is enlarged in many but not all instances of intrasellar tumor; intrasellar calcification may be present. The fossa is also large in some suprasellar tumors with intrasellar extension, e.g., craniopharyngioma, metastases to the sella (as from carcinoma of the breast or prostate), longstanding increase of intracranial pressure from any cause, the so-called "empty sella syndrome," and hypothyroidism (see Ch. 830). The fossa is often small in patients with postpartum pituitary necrosis (Sheehan's syndrome), hypopituitary dwarfism without pituitary tumor, and myotonic muscular dystrophy. Rarely observed in presumably normal people, the significance of the small sella is not clear. Roentgenographic changes in the base of the skull may involve the sella in several disorders, e.g., osteoporosis, Paget's disease, Hand-Schüller-Christian disease, and Hurler's syndrome.

When pituitary tumors extend upward through the diaphragma sellae they encroach upon the optic chiasm to produce the familial bitemporal hemianopia. When such tumors impinge on the pituitary stalk or the diencephalon there may be symptoms of hypothalamic involvement (diabetes insipidus, galactorrhea). Such upward extensions can often be seen roentgenographically with the use of pneumoencephalography or carotid artery angiography.

The *microscopic anatomy* of the anterior pituitary is complex. The classic concept of secretory acidophilic (eosinophilic) and basophilic cells and functionless chromophobes has to be modified in the light of recent data. There appear to be five or six distinct kinds of cells; it is probable that each pituitary hormone is secreted by one of the distinct cell types. Somatotrophic cells are acidophils which secrete growth hormone. The pituitary

tumors associated with acromegaly (excessive secretion of growth hormone) are usually composed of acidophils; sometimes the tumors consist of acidophils mixed with chromophobes, chromophobes alone, or cells which have features of both types of cell ("amphophils"). Another kind of acidophil has been identified in the primate and human pituitary. This larger acidophil (known as "lactotrophic" or "mammotrophic") can be distinguished from the growth hormone–secreting acidophil by special stains. Increased numbers of these cells, now accepted as *prolactin*-secreting, are found in the pituitaries of pregnant and lactating women and patients with galactorrhea. A recognizable type of basophil secretes gonadotrophins; there is some evidence that two distinct subtypes of basophils are associated with FSH and LH secretion. Gonadotrophin-secreting basophils are few or absent in childhood, but increase in number at puberty; there are subtle changes during the menstrual cycle; marked changes are observed after castration and menopause. The thyrotrophin-secreting cell is another identifiable type of basophil. The number of these cells increases, and the morphology changes with thyroprivic states. The corticotrophin- (ACTH-) secreting basophil, known as the (R) basophil, probably also secretes MSH in man; the human pituitary lacks a definite intermediate lobe, the source of MSH secretion in lower animals. The pituitary tumors described by Cushing in hyperadrenocorticism are basophilic. In the absence of pituitary tumor, the most notable feature of pituitary cytology in patients with Cushing's syndrome is in the basophils; the cytoplasm becomes hyalinized ("Crooke's change"), a change also found in patients whose hyperadrenocorticism is due to very large doses of administered adrenocortical steroids. In the rather aggressive pituitary tumors that occur after bilateral adrenalectomy in 10 to 15 per cent of patients with Cushing's syndrome associated with bilateral adrenal cortical hyperfunction (owing to oversecretion of ACTH by the pituitary), the cell type is a distinctive kind of chromophobe which often has the capacity to secrete MSH as well as ACTH (see Ch. 850).

Adams, J. H., Daniel, P. M., and Prichard, M. M. L.: Observations on the portal circulation of the pituitary gland. Neuroendocrinology, 1:193, 1965/66.

Bergland, R. M., Ray, B. S., and Torack, R. M.: Anatomical variations in the pituitary gland and adjacent structures in 225 human autopsy cases. J. Neurosurg., 28:93, 1968.

Daughaday, W. H.: The adenohypophysis. *In* Williams, R. H. (ed.): Textbook of Endocrinology. 5th ed. Philadelphia, W. B. Saunders Company, 1974, p. 31.

Harris, G. W., and Donovan, B. T. (eds.): The Pituitary Gland, 3 vols. Berkeley, University of California Press, 1966.

Meador, C. K., and Worrell, J. L.: The sella turcica in postpartum pituitary necrosis (Sheehan's syndrome). Ann. Intern. Med., 65:259, 1966.

New, P. F. J.: The sella turcica as a mirror of disease. Radiol. Clin. North Am., 4:75, 1966.

Ney, R. L.: The Anterior Pituitary Gland. *In* Bondy, P. K., and Rosenberg, L. E. (eds.): Duncan's Diseases of Metabolism. 7th ed. Philadelphia, W. B. Saunders Company, 1974, p. 961.

Russfield, A. B.: Adenohypophysis. *In* Bloodworth, J. M. B. (ed.): Endocrine Pathology. Baltimore, Williams & Wilkins Company, 1968, p. 75.

828. THE HORMONES OF THE ANTERIOR PITUITARY

Seven *protein* or *peptide hormones* have been isolated from human pituitary tissue: growth hormone, prolactin, follicle-stimulating hormone, luteinizing hormone, thyrotrophin, adrenocorticotrophin and melanocyte-stimulating hormone. Each is regulated by the *releasing hormones of the hypothalamus* which stimulate the secretion of pituitary peptides; it is not yet certain that the releasing factors act to increase the synthesis of pituitary hormones. *Hypothalamic inhibitory factors* also exert an important regulatory influence. The tonic control of prolactin secretion is exerted by prolactin-inhibiting factor (PIF), and there are inhibitory peptides for growth hormone ("somatostatin") and MSH.

Pituitary hormones act directly (prolactin) or through "second messengers." The growth-promoting activity of growth hormone is probably via an intermediary protein, "somatomedin" (see below); the gonadotrophins, TSH and ACTH, stimulate hormone synthesis in their corresponding target glands via cyclic AMP.

Largely controlled by the central nervous system (see Ch. 824 and 826), the anterior pituitary hormones profoundly affect growth, maturation, and metabolism. The paragraphs immediately following deal with the chemistry, physiology, and regulation of these hormones under normal conditions; pathologic states are discussed in Ch. 829.

Brazeau, P., Vale, W., Burgus, R., Ling, N., Butcher, M., Rivier, J., and Guillemin, R.: Hypothalamic peptide that inhibits the secretion of immunoreactive growth hormone. Science, 179:77, 1973.

Frohman, L. A.: Clinical neuropharmacology of hypothalamic releasing factors. N. Engl. J. Med., 286:1391, 1972.

GROWTH HORMONE
(Somatotrophin)

Pituitary growth hormone is the substance that, secreted or given in excessive amounts, induces gigantism and acromegaly in animals and man; its absence results in failure to grow. The hormone exerts a major influence on somatic growth in man from an early stage of infancy. It also has widespread metabolic effects in both young and adult subjects.

Chemically, human growth hormone (HGH) is a single-chain peptide containing 190 amino acids whose sequence is now known; the molecular weight is 21,500.

Within the substance of the gland and in the plasma, HGH is heterogeneous, existing in at least two forms. "Orthodox" HGH (the 21,500 peptide) has in common with prolactin and placental lactogen several segments of identical amino acid sequence; all three hormones may be phylogenetically descended from a single primordial peptide. The daily production rate is about 500 μg per day.

The physiologic effects of HGH are many. The salient action is anabolic. In the hypophysectomized, dwarfed animal, GH administration induces symmetrical growth of the skeleton (chondrogenesis and osteogenesis), the musculature, and viscera. Several effects of HGH on cartilage appear to operate through the obligatory intermediate, *"sulfation factor"* or *"somatomedin,"* a protein of molecular weight 8000 whose site of origin is the liver. Somatomedin is thought to play a vital role in HGH-induced skeletal growth. Optimal growth response also requires the presence of thyroid hormone and insulin. HGH causes both cellular hypertrophy and hyperplasia; there is an increased rate of cellular mitosis, as well as an increase in tissue and organ weight. The hormone induces accelerated transport of specific amino acids into cells, stimulates synthesis of messenger and ribosomal RNA, and influences the activity of several enzymes.

HGH augments protein anabolism in hypophysectomized or hypopituitary human subjects. Nitrogen retention occurs within 24 to 48 hours; BUN concentration falls even earlier, within 12 to 24 hours. Nitrogen storage is great (3 to 4 grams per day) for the first several days of treatment, then falls to an amount compatible with growth requirements, about 0.3 gram of nitrogen retained per day in children 9 to 13 years of age. Linear growth can be induced in hypopituitary dwarfs (see Pituitary Insufficiency in Childhood, in Ch. 831).

HGH brings about changes in electrolyte and water metabolism. Tissue protein and water are increased. Phosphorus and potassium are stored, the latter in amounts larger than can be accounted for by the estimated quantity of new tissue formed. Moderate sodium retention occurs. Hypercalciuria is the rule, but most studies of calcium metabolism indicate an over-all positive calcium balance.

The increase in tissue mass induced by administration of HGH is not accompanied by fat deposition. The hormone is in fact adipokinetic. Although many other pituitary hormones have fat-mobilizing properties, e.g., prolactin, thyrotrophin, corticotrophin, MSH, and several other peptides, HGH appears to be the major adipokinetic principle of the human anterior pituitary. Administration of this hormone to hypophysectomized man rapidly stimulates the release of fat from adipose tissue, with a rise in plasma free fatty acids. This HGH effect on fat metabolism may operate in the anabolic response by ensuring a supply of calories, yet sparing protein breakdown through gluconeogenesis. In acromegalic patients, fat deposition is notably absent; obesity is extremely rare.

HGH also affects carbohydrate metabolism. The hormone is well known to be diabetogenic; many acromegalics have diabetes. The diabetic state is characterized by fasting hyperglycemia, impaired glucose tolerance, insulin resistance, lipemia, and ketosis. HGH given to normal subjects produces only minor changes; in diabetics the diabetes is often substantially exacerbated. Nondiabetic and diabetic subjects are much more sensitive to this effect of growth hormone after hypophysectomy.

The closely interrelated effects of HGH on fat and carbohydrate metabolism may be of great importance in concert with insulin, not only in promoting growth but also in maintaining homeostasis during feast or famine.

Most important observations have followed the recent development of accurate methods for the measurement of HGH in serum by radioimmunoassay (see Ch. 829). The findings have provided new insights into the role of the hormone in the growth of children. Basal serum concentrations and secretion rates are slightly higher in young children and adolescents than in older children or adults. It is now clear that HGH is required for the normal growth rate of infants but not of the fetus; growth hormone–deficient mothers bear children of normal birth weight.

The serum concentration of HGH in *adults* is extremely labile, responding to a variety of stimuli, and being spontaneously secreted in periodic bursts, probably under the influence of the CNS. Serum values rise at the onset of deep sleep. Rapid rises in the serum levels of HGH are induced by hypoglycemia, fasting, and exercise; in some obese subjects these responses are blunted. HGH response to hypoglycemia is inhibited by corticosteroids. Hypoglycemia-induced rises in HGH level are quickly suppressed when glucose is given. Ambulation raises the serum levels of HGH in women, not in men; estrogen administration reproduces this increase. Increases in ambulatory (not basal) serum levels of growth hormone occur during the luteal phase of the menstrual cycle. Growth hormone also participates in the response to *stress,* e.g., surgery, but the pattern of response differs from that of ACTH; this suggests that the neural pathways influencing the two hormones are different. Infusion of amino acids, ACTH, glucagon, and large amounts of catecholamines and oral administration of L-dopa also stimulate HGH secretion. The production rate of HGH is subnormal in hypothyroidism, raised in hyperthyroidism.

Apart from the obvious value of measuring serum levels of HGH for the diagnosis of hypopituitarism and acromegaly, the aforementioned findings have clearly shown that HGH is not secreted at a uniform rate in adults. The lability of response to many metabolic events indicates that the hormone is not functionless in adults, as formerly thought, but participates in the day-to-day regulation of organic metabolism.

The use of the hormone in treatment of HGH deficiency is discussed in Ch. 831 under Pituitary Insufficiency in Childhood.

Berson, S. A., and Yalow, R. S.: Radioimmunoassay of peptide hormones in plasma. N. Engl. J. Med., 277:640, 1967.
Catt, K. J.: Growth hormone. Lancet, 1:933, 1970.
Daughaday, W. H.: Sulfation factor regulation of skeletal growth: A stable mechanism dependent on intermittent growth hormone secretion. Am. J. Med., 50:277, 1972.
Glick, S. M., Roth, J., Yalow, R. S., and Berson, S. A.: The regulation of growth hormone secretion. Rec. Prog. Hormone Res., 21:241, 1965.
Li, C. H.: Hormones of the adenohypophysis. Proc. Am. Philosoph. Soc., 116:365, 1972.
Martin, J. B.: Neural regulation of growth hormone secretion. N. Engl. J. Med., 288:1384, 1973.
Yalow, R. S., Varsano-Aharon, N., and Berson, S. A.: HGH and ACTH secretory responses to stress. Horm. Metab. Res., 1:3, 1969.

PROLACTIN
(Lactogenic Hormone)

Because of many chemical and biologic similarities to HGH, prolactin was not recognized as a separate hormone in man until recently. Human prolactin is now definitely established as a distinct hormone, distinguishable from HGH. The evidence is this: the human pituitary during pregnancy and lactation and in galactorrhea contains many acidophils that are unlike HGH-secreting acidophils; patients with galactorrhea do not have high plasma HGH concentrations; plasma HGH is not raised in lactating women; normal postpartum lactation occurs in mothers with isolated HGH deficiency; pituitary tumors from women with galactorrhea have been shown to contain large amounts of prolactin activity not neutralizable with anti-HGH antiserum; bioassay experiments have indicated high prolactin activity in the presence of low immunoassayable HGH in normal and pathologic lactation; and prolactin has been found to be immunologically distinct from HGH.

In women, prolactin governs growth, development, and milk formation in the breast. These effects require the presence of estrogens, progestogens, adrenocortical steroids, insulin, and perhaps HGH. The physiologic role of prolactin in men is not yet clear.

The hormone is a single polypeptide chain (molecular weight about 23,000) containing 198 amino acids; its chemical similarity to HGH and human placental lactogen (HPL) has been described above.

Prolactin has more than 20 physiologic actions in animals and man, most of them related to reproduction. Apart from its effect on the primate breast, prolactin controls cutaneous "milk" secretion in certain teleost fish, the renal osmoregulatory adaptation of salmon migrating to fresh water, hormone secretion by the corpus luteum in some rodents, and broodpatch formation in birds. In man, prolactin has growth-promoting (and nitrogen-retaining) effects similar to but much weaker than those of HGH; the hormone may also induce renal sodium, potassium, and water retention. The role of prolactin in human breast cancer is now under intense study.

Prolactin is secreted throughout the day in *periodic bursts* unrelated to those of HGH. Plasma levels are lowest during the waking hours, rising 60 to 90 minutes after the onset of sleep and reaching highest concentrations at 5 to 7 A.M. Plasma levels do not vary from day to day throughout the normal *menstrual cycle,* but rise progressively during *pregnancy;* there are sharp rises during *breast feeding.*

Many *physiologic stimuli* elicit increased secretion of prolactin. These include suckling in postpartum women, stimulation of the nonlactating breast (women show a greater response than men), strenuous physical exercise, sexual intercourse in women (most striking when orgasm occurs), profound hypoglycemia, and surgical stress; plasma prolactin values fall with prolonged fasting. Several *pharmacologic agents* alter plasma prolactin levels. Rises follow the administration of TRH, estrogens (but not progesterone), arginine, phenothiazines and other tranquilizing drugs (which sometimes cause galactorrhea), and reserpine. L-Dopa, nicotine, and ergot alkaloids induce falls in plasma prolactin concentration. Chlorpromazine and L-dopa appear to exert their effects by respectively inhibiting and stimulating the hypothalamic secretion of PIF.

Frantz, A. G.: The regulation of prolactin secretion in humans. *In* Ganong, W. F., and Martini, L. (eds.): Frontiers in Neuroendocrinology. New York, Oxford University Press, 1973, p. 337.
Friesen, H. G.: Prolactin: Its physiologic role and therapeutic potential. Hosp. Pract., 7:123, 1972.
Friesen, H. G., Guyda, H., Hwang, P., Tyson, J. E., and Barbeau, A.: Functional evaluation of prolactin secretion: A guide to therapy. J. Clin. Invest., 51:706, 1972.
Hwang, P., Guyda, H., and Friesen, H. G.: A radioimmunoassay for human prolactin. Proc. Nat. Acad. Sci. U.S.A., 68:902, 1971.
Kleinberg, D. L., and Frantz, A. G.: Human prolactin: Measurement by in vitro bioassay. J. Clin. Invest., 50:1557, 1971.
Schwartz, T. B.: Prolactin. *In* Schwartz, T. B. (ed.): The Year Book of Endocrinology. Chicago, Year Book Medical Publishers, 1973, p. 7.
Tyson, J. E., Friesen, H. G., and Anderson, M. S.: Human lactational and ovarian response to endogenous prolactin release. Science, 177:897, 1972.

FOLLICLE-STIMULATING HORMONE
(FSH)

Follicle-stimulating hormone is the pituitary hormone essential for the normal cyclic growth of the ovarian follicle and for restoration of follicular growth in the hypophysectomized female; it stimulates spermatogenesis in the male without significant influence on the androgen-secreting interstitial cells of the testis. For optimal effect upon both ovary and testis, FSH seems to require the presence of luteinizing hormone (LH).

The molecular weight of human FSH is not finally established; estimates vary between 24,000 and 35,000. It is a glycoprotein, containing 7 per cent carbohydrate. Sialic acid is an integral part of the molecule; biologic activity is lost on exposure to neuraminidase. The purest preparations contain slight LH activity. FSH comprises two subunits: an α subunit which resembles the α subunits of LH and human chorionic gonadotrophin (HCG), and a unique β subunit in which the specific biologic activity of FSH probably resides.

Administration of purified human FSH to amenorrheic women elicits increased secretion of estrogens and may stimulate the ovary to polycystic enlargement; given together with HGC, FSH sometimes provokes spermatogenesis. Discussion of the use of human gonadotrophins in the treatment of infertility in men and women is found in Ch. 859 and 867.

Gonadotrophin concentrations are low in the pituitaries and in the plasma and urine of infants and young children. The hormones rise to reach detectable levels well before puberty. In adult women, the values are about the same as those for men during the preovulatory (follicular) and postovulatory (luteal) phases of the menstrual cycle. In adult men, FSH and LH are secreted in arrhythmic, pulsatile bursts (like ACTH [q.v.]), during sleep, but without relation to the phasic peaks of HGH and prolactin secretion.

Secretion of Gonadotrophins During the Normal Menstrual Cycle. Hypothalamic control of FSH and LH secretion by one or more hypothalamic releasing factors is discussed in Ch. 825, and the role of positive and negative feedback control of gonadotrophin release by estrogens and progesterone is dealt with in Ch. 866. This chapter sets out the pattern of hormone secretion during the normal menstrual cycle. Figure 2 shows the cyclic secretion of FSH, LH, estradiol, and progesterone. During the early *follicular phase,* plasma FSH rises from its nadir during menstruation, and then, while estrogen secretion is rising, falls toward mid-cycle. In this phase, plasma LH progressively rises toward mid-cycle. Just after the peak level of estrogen, now thought to stimulate gonadotrophin (LH) release, both FSH and LH reach their maximal secretion rate (day 0 in Fig. 2); the average daily production rates of FSH and LH are 15 and 30 μg per day, respectively, increasing 10- to 15-fold at *mid-cycle,* when *ovulation* occurs. Values for plasma FSH and LH then decline through the *luteal phase* (FSH being lowest when progesterone levels are high), LH rising slightly as estrogen and progesterone values fall just before menses.

Unopposed by the negative feedback action of gonadal hormones, plasma and urinary FSH values are high, as in ovariectomized and postmenopausal women. In females, the negative feedback is in part due to estrogen inhibition of hypothalamic gonadotrophin-releasing hormone; in the male, the inhibiting testicular hormone may be elaborated by the seminiferous tubule, testosterone being a weak suppressor of FSH secretion.

SECRETION OF PITUITARY AND OVARIAN HORMONES IN THE NORMAL MENSTRUAL CYCLE

Figure 2. Notice the fall of plasma estradiol values on the day before the midcycle peak of FSH and LH. Plasma estradiol and progesterone concentrations both rise during the luteal phase after the midcycle "surge" of gonadotrophin. The luteal rise in progesterone is reflected by a rise in basal body temperature (BBT) and increased urinary excretion of pregnanediol. The black bar denotes menses. (Adapted from Yen, S. C. C., Vela, P., Rankin, J., and Littell, A. S.: J.A.M.A., 211:1513, 1970; and Catt, K. J.: Lancet, 1:1097, 1970.)

Albert, A.: Bioassay and radioimmunoassay of human gonadotrophins. J. Clin. Endocrinol. Metab., 28:1683, 1968.

Baghdassarian, A., Guyda, H., Johnson, A., Migeon, C. J., and Blizzard, R. M.: Urinary excretion of radioimmunoassayable luteinizing hormone (LH) in normal male children and adults, according to age and stage of sexual development. J. Clin. Endocrinol. Metab., 31:428, 1970.

Catt, K. J.: Reproductive endocrinology. Lancet, 1:1097, 1970.

Rifkind, A. B., Kulin, H. E., and Ross, G. T.: Follicle stimulating hormone (FSH) and luteinizing hormone in the urine of prepubertal children. J. Clin. Invest., 46:1925, 1967.

Ross, G. T., Cargille, C. M., Lipsett, M. B., Rayford, P. L., Marshall, J. R., Strott, C. A., and Rodbard, D.: Pituitary and gonadal hormones in women during spontaneous and induced ovulatory cycles. Recent Prog. Horm. Res., 26:1, 1970.

Rubin, R. T., Kales, A., Adler, R., Fagan, T., and Odell, W.: Gonadotropin secretion during normal sleep in normal adult men. Science, 175:196, 1972.

Schally, A. V., Nair, R. M. G., Redding, T. W., and Arimura, A.: Isolation of the luteinizing and follicle-stimulating hormone-releasing hormone from porcine hypothalami. J. Biol. Chem., 246:7230, 1971.

Vande Wiele, R. L., Bogumil, J., Dyrenfurth, I., Ferin, M., Jewelewicz, R., Warren, M., Rizkallah, T., and Mikhail, G.: Mechanisms regulating the menstrual cycle in women. Recent Prog. Horm. Res., 26:63, 1970.

LUTEINIZING HORMONE OR INTERSTITIAL CELL–STIMULATING HORMONE
(LH or ICSH)

Luteinizing hormone is essential for ovulation, for the formation of the corpus luteum, and for stimulation of steroid hormone secretion by that structure. Acting alone, it does not produce follicular growth; to be effective, LH requires the prior action of FSH on the follicle. Human LH is assumed to be the luteotrophic hormone; there is evidence that the corpus luteum has an intrinsic life span that is not much influenced by pituitary hormones. LH also stimulates the growth and secretory activity of the testicular interstitial cells. This interstitial cell–stimulating activity is sufficient to correct the testicular endocrine defect of hypophysectomy, producing androgen secretion and maintenance of the secondary sex organs. The steroidogenic action of LH on the corpus luteum and the Leydig cells is mediated by cyclic AMP. Spermatogenesis in man requires the synergism of FSH.

Like FSH, LH is a glycoprotein. Human LH (ICSH) has a molecular weight estimated at about 28,000. It is composed of two subunits, designated α and β; the α subunit is chemically similar to that of FSH and TSH, so that the hormonal specificity of LH probably resides in the β subunit. The hormone has been little used therapeutically; the more readily available human chorionic gonadotrophin (HCG), which also contains an α subunit similar to that of human LH, has predominantly LH properties and is used instead.

The circadian and cyclic secretion of LH is described above (see FSH). Partly through their action on the elaboration of hypothalamic FSH/LH-releasing hormone, testosterone, estrogen, and progestogens inhibit the secretion of LH. In men testosterone lowers plasma LH levels; in women estrogen-progestin combinations (as in antiovulatory drugs) suppress the mid-cycle "surge" of LH and reduce LH secretion in the postmenopausal state. Conversely, LH values are high in castrate men and postmenopausal women. It appears that the concentration of circulating estrogen in the follicular phase of the menstrual cycle *stimulates* LH release.

Lipsett, M. B., Cargille, C. M., and Ross, G. T.: Reproductive endocrinology: Methodologic advances and clinical studies. Ann. Intern. Med., 72:933, 1970.
Marsh, J. M., Butcher, R. W., Savard, K., and Sutherland, E. W.: The stimulating effect of luteinizing hormone on adenosine-3',5'-monophosphate accumulation in corpus luteum slices. J. Biol. Chem., 241:5436, 1966.
Rathnam, P., and Saxena, B. B.: Subunits of luteinizing hormone from human pituitary glands. J. Biol. Chem., 246:7087, 1971.
Schalch, D. S., Parlow, A. F., Boon, R. C., and Reichlin, S.: Measurement of human luteinizing hormone in plasma by radioimmunoassay. J. Clin. Invest., 47:665, 1968.

THYROTROPHIN
(Thyrotrophic or Thyroid-Stimulating Hormone, TSH)

Throtrophin repairs the atrophy of the thyroid gland that follows hypophysectomy. The hormone also restores the ability of the thyroid to synthesize and secrete thyroxine and triiodothyronine. If given in large doses to normal or hypophysectomized animals or man, thyrotrophin evokes the morphologic and secretory changes of hyperthyroidism. TSH elicits a rapid release of thyroxine and triiodothyronine from the gland; the content of colloid is reduced, and the quantity of organic iodine is decreased.

Thyrotrophin is a glycoprotein, containing hexose and glucosamine. The molecular weight is about 28,000; there are two subunits, the α subunit being essentially identical to the α subunit of LH and similar to those of FSH and HCG, and the β subunit comprising the hormone-specific properties. The linear amino acid sequences of the two subunits are known. There is evidence that the TSH molecule is heterogeneous. The hormone stimulates many metabolic processes in the thyroid, e.g., the uptake and oxidation of glucose, the production of TPNH, and many others. The rapid discharge of thyroxine from the thyroid follicles is in part due to the action of TSH upon a proteolytic enzyme that accelerates the release of the hormone from the intrafollicular protein thyroglobulin. Within 24 hours after the administration of TSH, hypertrophy and hyperplasia of the thyroid epithelium occur. The weight of the thyroid increases. TSH augments the capacity of the thyroid to take up iodide, to convert iodide to organic iodine, and to synthesize thyroxine. These effects can be reproduced by cyclic AMP; this and other evidence indicates that the nucleotide is an important mediator of TSH action on the thyroid.

Hypothalamic TRH appears to be the most important regulator of TSH secretion; the daily production rate of TSH is about 100 μU. Circadian rhythm of plasma TSH levels in man is slight, and, in contrast to other anterior pituitary hormones, TSH secretion remains remarkably constant in the face of many kinds of stimuli. Except for a transitory increase in early neonatal life, there is no age-related change in plasma TSH values; they are the same in both sexes and do not change in response to exercise, the stress of surgery, or the administration of vasopressin, glucagon, arginine, or, surprisingly, antithyroid drugs. Corticosteroids suppress TSH secretion, and prolonged exposure to cold slightly increases it. Thyroxine and triiodothyronine also exert important effects on the hypothalamic and pituitary control of TSH secretion; values are high in primary hypothyroidism and low in naturally occurring and iatrogenic hyperthyroidism (see Ch. 837).

Bovine thyrotrophin and synthetic TRH are available for medical use; diagnostic tests of thyroid function are discussed in Ch. 829.

Anderson, M. S., Bowers, C. Y., Kastin, A. J., Schalch, D. S., Schally, A. V., Snyder, P. J., Utiger, R. D., Wilber, J. F., and Wise, A. J.: Synthetic thyrotropin-releasing hormone. N. Engl. J. Med., 285:1279, 1971.
Hershman, J. M., and Pittman, J. A.: Control of thyrotropin secretion in man. N. Engl. J. Med., 285:997, 1971.
Pierce, J. G., Liao, T., Howard, S. M., Shome, B., and Cornell, J. S.: Studies on the structure of thyrotropin: Its relationship to luteinizing hormone. Recent Prog. Horm. Res., 27:165, 1971.
Shenkman, L., Mitsuma, T., and Hollander, C. S.: Modulation of pituitary responsiveness to thyrotropin-releasing hormones by triiodothyronine. J. Clin. Invest., 52:205, 1973.
Utiger, R. D.: Radioimmunoassay of human plasma thyrotropin. J. Clin. Invest., 44:1277, 1965.

ADRENOCORTICOTROPHIN
(ACTH, Corticotrophin)

Adrenocorticotrophin repairs the adrenocortical atrophy and failure to synthesize steroid hormones that follow hypophysectomy. In most species, ACTH administration causes hypertrophy and hyperplasia of the adrenal. The main effect appears to be upon the fascicular and reticular zones. The hormone stimulates the synthesis and release of cortisol, corticosterone, and androgens; it also elicits a moderate increase in the secretory rate of aldosterone, but this increase is not sustained. Large amounts of exogenous corticotrophin cause enlargement and hyperemia of the adrenal, and hemorrhagic infarction has occurred rarely.

The chemical nature of adrenocorticotrophin is known. It is a single polypeptide made up of 39 amino acids. Smaller fragments of the ACTH peptide, e.g., that containing amino acids 1 to 20, have full biologic potency. The complete hormone has been synthesized; its molecular weight is 4567, its potency 100 to 140 units per milligram. ACTH exists in two forms in the pituitary; "big ACTH" may serve as a precursor, whereas "little" ACTH (molecular weight 4500) is the circulating, biologically active hormone. One international unit, equal to 1 USP unit, is the biologic activity of 1 mg of international standard. The daily production rate of ACTH in man is small, about 10 μg per day.

The action of the hormone upon the adrenal cortex is complex. It stimulates increased mitotic activity. The increase in steroidogenesis is the result of an increase in the rate of steroid biosynthesis, not simply of accelerated release of steroid into the bloodstream. The precise point in the biosynthetic pathway at which corticotrophin acts is debatable; the increased steroid production may be mediated by ACTH stimulation of a particular messenger RNA. An important mechanism by which ACTH induces increased steroid synthesis is its capacity to stimulate the synthesis of active adrenocortical phosphorylase by raising the concentration of cyclic AMP in the gland. The increased phosphorylase activity makes available more glucose-6-phosphate from the hexose monophosphate shunt, thus providing larger quantities of NADH (TPNH), a compound essential for the synthesis and hydroxylation of steroids.

Corticotrophin has extra-adrenal actions. It stimulates the release of free fatty acids from adipose tissue; the importance of this effect is unknown. In large doses it causes darkening of the skin.

In man, the short-term administration of adrenocorticotrophin causes a rapid increase in the secretion of cortisol, reflected by an abrupt rise in plasma cortisol concentration. This effect has proved useful in the diagnostic assessment of adrenocortical response, as has the biologic and immunologic assay of ACTH in human serum. Radioimmunoassay measurements of plasma ACTH concentration have confirmed earlier ideas about the extraordinary lability of this hormone in response to physiologic and pathologic stimuli. Plasma ACTH undergoes a free-running circadian cycle under CNS (hypothalamic CRF) influence. The hormone is secreted in episodic bursts, with highest levels tending to be in the early morning; a nadir is reached by late evening. Plasma cortisol levels roughly reflect this circadian rhythm. Hospitalized patients not acutely ill often have ACTH concentrations higher than normal, and severely ill patients occasionally show extremely elevated levels. Plasma ACTH rises in addisonian and adrenalectomized patients and in response to metyrapone, and falls when suppressive doses of adrenocortical steroids, e.g., dexamethasone, are given (see Ch. 845). Stressful stimuli, such as surgery under general anesthesia, electro-

shock, and hypoglycemia, and the administration of histamine and vasopressin are usually followed by raised plasma ACTH concentrations.

The long-term effects of adrenocorticotrophin in human subjects are the same as those produced by cortisone, cortisol, and their synthetic analogues. In contrast to the adrenocortical steroids, corticotrophin evokes sensitivity reactions, but antihormone formation does not occur. Corticotrophin brings about a greater degree of sodium and water retention, more androgenicity, and a more constant elevation in serum cholesterol than do steroids. Large doses elicit the stigmata of Cushing's syndrome (e.g., osteoporosis, hyperglycemia, psychosis). The unpleasant symptoms associated with abrupt withdrawal of steroid therapy are said to occur rarely after a course of ACTH therapy.

Adrenocorticotrophin regulates the growth, structural integrity, and steroid secretion of the adrenal cortex. This constantly changing regulatory influence is exerted by central nervous system control of the anterior pituitary and by a reciprocal relation between the amounts of circulating cortisol and ACTH. In man, noxious stimuli such as acute illness or severe and prolonged emotional disturbance provoke an increased or abnormally regulated output of adrenocortical steroids, mediated via an increased rate of endogenous corticotrophin release.

ACTH is available for diagnostic purposes in lyophilized and repository (with gelatin or zinc) forms. Two synthetic ACTH preparations are also available in unmodified and repository forms: α^{1-24} ACTH (Synacthen, Cortrosyn), and α^{1-18} ACTH (see Ch. 829 and 846). ACTH has also been used *therapeutically*, but most clinicians think that the diseases which respond to hyperadrenal therapy are more simply managed with corticosteroids than with ACTH.

Berson, S. A., and Yalow, R. S.: Radioimmunoassay of ACTH in plasma. J. Clin. Invest., 47:2725, 1968.
Grahame-Smith, D. G., Butcher, R. W., Ney, R. L., and Sutherland, E. W.: Adenosine-3',5'-monophosphate as the intracellular mediator of the action of adrenocorticotrophic hormone in the adrenal cortex. J. Biol. Chem., 242:5535, 1967.
Weitzman, E. D., Fukushima, D., Nogiere, C. Roffwarg, H., Gallagher, T. F., and Hellman, L.: Twenty-four hour pattern of the episodic secretion of cortisol in normal subjects. J. Clin. Endocrinol. Metab., 33:14, 1971.

MELANOCYTE-STIMULATING HORMONE
(MSH)

MSH produces darkening (addisonian pigmentation) in human skin. Two MSH peptides have been identified in pituitary tissue. The smaller and more potent molecule, α-MSH, is made up of 13 amino acids and has a molecular weight of 1823; it is found in the pituitaries of pigs, cows, and monkeys, and may be present in the neurohypophysis of man. The characteristic human peptide, β-MSH, contains 22 amino acids and has a molecular weight of 2734. α-MSH has a common 13-amino acid sequence with ACTH; β-MSH a 7-amino acid sequence. These partial identities of structure may account for common physiologic properties among the three molecules: ACTH has a slight pigmentary effect on skin; both MSH molecules and ACTH are adipokinetic; both MSH's have weak adrenal-stimulating activity. Studies of plasma β-MSH concentration in man have shown that the hormone undergoes a circadian rhythm in normal subjects and that its secretion is regulated by the same factors that control ACTH. Metyrapone raises and adrenocortical steroids depress plasma β-MSH levels.

The functional significance of human β-MSH is unknown. Plasma values are the same in pigmented and nonpigmented races, and are normal in albinism and in several diseases characterized by increased dermal pigmentation.

Abe, K., Nicholson, W. E., Liddle, G. W., Orth, D. N., and Island, D. P.: Normal and abnormal regulation of β-MSH in man. J. Clin. Invest., 48:1580, 1969.
Lerner, A. B., and McGuire, J. S.: Effect of alpha- and beta-melanocyte stimulating hormones on skin colour of man. Nature (London), 189:176, 1971.

829. ASSESSMENT OF ANTERIOR PITUITARY FUNCTION

Clinical Detection of Pituitary Disease. Clinical suspicion of hypopituitarism must be entertained in patients with short stature, delayed puberty, primary and secondary amenorrhea, sterility, and hypothyroidism. Typical ocular findings or the incidental discovery of an enlarged pituitary fossa (as in a skull film taken for head injury) also require diagnostic study of pituitary function (see below).

Functional Detection of Pituitary Disease. This is based on measurement of hormones in plasma or urine. In addition to detection of abnormally high or low levels of pituitary hormones, such measurements permit an evaluation of abnormal *regulation* of pituitary hormone secretion (see Ch. 824). *Direct* measurement of pituitary hormones is made when possible, as for growth hormone and gonadotrophins; *indirect* evaluation of TSH and ACTH is usually done by measuring the hormones of glands that are under their trophic control, because the methods are more generally available, e.g., thyroidal response to TSH, adrenocortical response to ACTH (see below).

GROWTH HORMONE

Radioimmunoassay of plasma growth hormones is becoming a routine procedure, and can be done at many medical centers and commercial laboratories. This is the most direct method for detecting hypopituitary states and acromegaly. In *hypopituitary dwarfism,* radioimmunoassay for growth hormone has superseded the crude indirect indices that clinicians have had to rely on, e.g., measurements of body proportions, chromosomal analysis, roentgenographic estimate of bone age, and laborious exclusion of all other causes of short stature. In pituitary dwarfism, basal plasma HGH values of less than 1.0 ng per milliliter may be found; these low values are not diagnostic, because the normal range is 0 to 5 ng per milliliter. One must demonstrate failure of growth hormone to respond to a stimulus, e.g., hypoglycemia. When suspicion is strong, the starting dose of insulin should be 0.05 unit per kilogram, given intravenously; if the hypoglycemia is inadequate, the dose can be increased to 0.1 or even 0.15 unit per kilogram, given under careful supervision to avoid prolonged hypoglycemia. Adequate stimulus requires a lowering

of blood glucose to one half the basal value or to 40 mg per 100 ml for at least ten minutes; if this condition is satisfied, patients without growth hormone deficiency show a rise in HGH value of at least 7 ng per milliliter above the basal level 60 minutes after injection. *Failure of growth hormone response to hypoglycemia is the most common laboratory abnormality in adult hypopituitarism, and is characteristic only of the dwarfism associated with growth hormone deficiency.* Certain amino acids also have the property of inducing growth hormone release; intravenous administration of neutralized arginine hydrochloride, 0.5 gram per kilogram, is preferred by some workers, because one avoids possibly dangerous hypoglycemia. The rise in growth hormone value is again 7 ng per milliliter above the resting levels.

In *acromegaly* also, HGH radioimmunoassay has begun to replace the highly unsatisfactory indirect methods clinicians have struggled with for years: histologic changes in the cartilage of the costochondral junction, measurement of serum phosphorus, PBI, urinary calcium, hydroxyproline excretion, and so forth. Basal plasma HGH may be in the range of 50 to more than 100 ng per milliliter. Many patients with untreated acromegaly fail to show a sharp drop in plasma HGH concentration, as do normal people, after administration of glucose (given as for a standard glucose tolerance test, blood samples being taken for glucose and growth hormone determinations at 30-minute intervals for at least three hours). It will require protracted follow-up studies of acromegalic patients before and after treatment and careful correlation with clinical findings, e.g., acral growth, to assess the usefulness of this nonresponse to hyperglycemia as an index of "acromegalic activity." In some acromegalics, plasma HGH paradoxically *rises* in response to glucose.

Glucagon and L-*dopa* have been recently introduced as provocative tests of HGH adequacy. Both have the virtue of simplicity. One mg of glucagon is given subcutaneously or intramuscularly; in normal subjects plasma HGH rises to 8 ng per milliliter or more within two to three hours. L-Dopa, 0.5 gram, is given orally; normal subjects raise HGH levels more than 5 ng per milliliter with a peak rise at 90 minutes. Response is said to be subnormal or absent in pituitary disease. These two maneuvers are promising but require further trial.

Eddy, R. L., Gilliland, P. F., Ibarra, J. D., Jr., McMurry, J. F., Jr., and Thompson, J. Q.: Human growth hormone release: Comparison of provocative test procedures. Am. J. Med., 56:179, 1974.
Fraser, R.: Human pituitary disease. Br. Med. J., 2:449, 1970.
Mitchell, M. L., Byrne, M. J., Sanchez, Y., and Sawin, C. T.: Detection of growth hormone deficiency: The glucagon stimulation test. N. Engl. J. Med., 282:539, 1970.
Nelson, J. C., Kollar, D. J., and Lewis, J. E.: Growth hormone secretion in pituitary disease. Arch. Intern. Med., 133:459, 1974.
Rabkin, M. T., and Frantz, A. G.: Hypopituitarism: A study of growth hormone and other endocrine functions. Ann. Intern. Med., 64:1197, 1966.

PROLACTIN

The development of sensitive bioassay and radioimmunoassay measurements for plasma prolactin has introduced a new and useful method for evaluating pituitary disease and *galactorrheic states.* Normal values are the same for adult men and women, usually less than 15 ng per milliliter, with an extreme upper limit of 25 ng per milliliter. Plasma prolactin is usually elevated in patients who have had *pituitary stalk section,* owing to interference with the action of hypothalamic PIF (see Ch. 826). A finding of major importance is detection of high plasma prolactin levels in patients with various kinds of *pituitary tumors,* often in the absence of galactorrhea and when all other pituitary hormones are low and there is clinical panhypopituitarism. The mechanism is either mechanical interference with PIF action or actual oversecretion of prolactin by the pituitary tumor. Plasma prolactin measurement may turn out to be valuable as an early hormonal sign of "nonfunctional" chromophobe adenoma. Raised prolactin levels are usually but not always found in patients with *galactorrhea:* e.g., in the *Chiari-Frommel syndrome* (postpartum amenorrhea and low gonadotrophin levels), *Del Castillo's syndrome* (amenorrhea and low gonadotrophin levels but not in relation to parturition), the *Forbes-Albright syndrome* (the same but associated with chromophobe adenoma), and the *"oversuppression" syndrome* (the same after cessation of anti-ovulatory medication), occasionally in *acromegaly,* and rarely in *primary hypothyroidism* (especially when the pituitary is enlarged) and injury to the chest wall. Prolactin levels are often high in renal failure but are usually normal in gynecomastia.

Provocative tests have been devised to distinguish between hypothalamic and pituitary disorders of prolactin secretion: stimulation with TRH and chlorpromazine and suppression with L-dopa. Panhypopituitary patients have low plasma prolactin levels which fail to respond to all three tests; patients with hypothalamic involvement respond abnormally to one or more of the three agents. Details of protocols and interpretation are given by Tolis et al.

Besser, G. M.: Galactorrhea. Br. Med. J., 1:280, 1972.

Forsyth, I. A., Besser, G. M., Edwards, C. R. W., Francis, L., and Myres, R. P.: Plasma prolactin activity in inappropriate lactation. Brit. Med. J., 2:225, 1971.

Frantz, A. G., Kleinberg, D. L., and Noel, G. L.: Studies on prolactin in man. Recent Prog. Horm. Res., 28:527, 1972.

L'Hermite, P., Copinschi, G., Golstein, J., Vanhaelst, L., Leclercq, R., Bruno, O. D., and Robyn, C.: Prolactin release after injection of thyrotropin-releasing hormone in man. Lancet, 1:763, 1972.

Tolis, G., Goldstein, M., and Friesen, H. G.: Functional evaluation of prolactin secretion in patients with hypothalamic-pituitary disorders. J. Clin. Invest., 52:783, 1972.

GONADOTROPHINS
(FSH and LH)

Biologic assay of urinary gonadotrophin is useful in distinguishing primary from secondary gonadal failure after the expected age of puberty. In the former, urinary gonadotrophin titers are elevated; in the latter (resulting from pituitary deficiency), levels are not detectable. Results of urinary gonadotrophin (human pituitary gonadotrophin) assays, done by the mouse uterine weight or rat ovarian weight method, are expressed in mouse uterine units (muu) or rat units (RU). In the mouse assay, a reported value of "positive at 20 muu" means that one twentieth of the extract of a 24-hour urine just produced a definite response in the injected mice. If one twentieth of a 24-hour urinary extract produces a definite response in the rat assay, results are reported as "20 RU per 24 hours." The rat assay is the more sensitive; normal people occasionally have undetectable values in the mouse assay. There is no official reference

TABLE 1.   Plasma Gonadotrophin Values as Measured by Radioimmunoassay in Normal People (with the "2nd IRP–Human Menopausal Gonadotrophin" as Standard)

	FSH, mIU/ml	LH, mIU/ml
Children	3–19	5–15
Adult males	3–42	3–32
Adult females		
Follicular phase	10–18	7–27
Mid-cycle	20–30	70–100
Luteal phase	6–18	7–22
Postmenopausal	35–215	0–90

standard for this bioassay. Representative mean values for the rat assay are as follows: adult men, 10; women in the follicular and luteal phases, 7; women at mid-cycle, 15; postmenopausal women, 75 – all values being expressed in RU per 24 hours. Corresponding figures for the mouse assay are 35, 20, 55, and 200 – all expressed in muu per 24 hours. In pituitary insufficiency, urinary gonadotrophins are usually undetectable; this abnormality is one of the earliest laboratory signs to appear in the course of the disease.

The highly sensitive radioimmunoassays for plasma FSH and LH are becoming available for routine clinical use, and they may very well supplant the bioassay methods in time. As expected, values are low or undetectable in pituitary insufficiency and high in primary gonadal failure. The normal ranges for various stages of the reproductive cycle are set out in Table 1.

Use of FSH and LH radioimmunoassay measurements has permitted sharper diagnostic accuracy in *delayed puberty* and the identification of patients with *hypogonadotrophic hypogonadism,* e.g., isolated FSH deficiency and gonadotrophin deficiency associated with *anosmia* or *hyposmia (Kallmann's syndrome),* in some of whom the defect may be in the synthesis or release of gonadotrophin-releasing factor (FSH-LH/RF). *Provocative tests* which entail administration of FSH-LH/RF or clomiphene have been used in attempts to distinguish hypothalamic from pituitary hypogonadotrophism. Clomiphene may be therapeutically effective in some patients with gonadotrophin deficiency. (For detailed protocols, see references.)

Hamiliton, C. R., Henkin, R. I., Weir, G., and Kliman, B.: Olfactory status and response to clomiphene in male gonadotrophin deficiency. Ann. Intern. Med., 78:47, 1973.

Marshall, J. C., Harsoulis, P., Anderson, D. C., McNeilly, A. S., Besser, G. M., and Hall, R.: Isolated pituitary gonadotrophin deficiency: Gonadotropin secretion after synthetic luteinizing hormone and follicle stimulating hormone–releasing hormone in man. Br. Med. J., 2:643, 1972.

Newton, J., Ramsay, I., and Marsden, P.: Clomiphene as a test of pituitary function. Lancet, 2:190, 1971.

Rabin, D., Spitz, I., Bercovici, B., Bell, J., Laufer, A., Benveniste, R., and Polishuk, W.: Isolated deficiency of follicle-stimulating hormone: Clinical and laboratory features. N. Engl. J. Med., 287:1313, 1972.

Saxena, B. B., Beling, C. G., and Gandy, H. M. (eds.): Gonadotropins. New York, John Wiley & Sons, 1972.

THYROTROPHIN
(TSH)

Radioimmunoassay for serum thyrotrophin is becoming available for general clinical use; normal values are

0.5 to 11.5 μU per milliliter. The values in primary myxedema, as expected, are high, falling to normal when thyroid hormone is given, and are undetectable in Graves' disease (see Ch. 837). A *provocative test*, in which 200 to 500 μg of TRH is given intravenously and plasma TSH rise is measured 30 to 60 minutes later, has permitted differentiation between "hypothalamic" and pituitary hypothyroidism. TSH rise may be normal in the former and absent in the latter. In intrinsic pituitary disease, the basal TSH level is low; if this measurement cannot be obtained, an acceptable method for distinguishing primary myxedema from secondary thyroid deficiency is the thyrotrophin stimulation test. The most reliable technique seems to be measurement of 24-hour ^{131}I uptake by the thyroid before and after intramuscular administration of bovine TSH, 10 USP units per day intramuscularly for three days. In primary myxedema, there is no response; normal subjects respond briskly; patients with myxedema secondary to pituitary failure respond, but subnormally. Exceptions are some patients with Sheehan's disease of long duration, who may be unresponsive.

Burke, G.: The thyrotrophin stimulation test. Ann. Intern. Med., 69:1127, 1968.

Costom, B. H., Grumbach, M. M., and Kaplan, S. L.: Effect of thyrotropin-releasing factor on serum thyroid-stimulating hormone. J. Clin. Invest., 50:2219, 1971.

Foley, T. P., Jr., Owings, J., Hayford, J. T., and Blizzard, R. M.: Serum thyrotropin responses to synthetic thyrotropin-releasing hormone in normal children and hypopituitary patients. J. Clin. Invest., 51:431, 1972.

Nelson, J. C., Johnson, D. E., and Odell, W. D.: Serum TSH levels and the thyroidal response to TSH stimulation in patients with thyroid disease. Ann. Intern. Med., 76:47, 1972.

Pittman, J. A., Haigler, E. D., Hershman, J. M., and Pittman, C. S.: Hypothalamic hypothyroidism. N. Engl. J. Med., 285:844, 1971.

Shenkman, L., Mitsuma, T., Suphavai, A., and Hollander, C. S.: Triiodothyronine and thyroid-stimulating hormone response to thyrotropin-releasing hormone. Lancet, 1:111, 1972.

ADRENOCORTICOTROPHIN
(ACTH)

Measurement of the ACTH secretion of the pituitary is usually done *indirectly* by testing adrenocortical response. A safe and specific method is intravenous administration of 25 units of lyophilized ACTH in 500 ml of 0.9 per cent saline over a four-hour period. Five per cent glucose in water should not be used as a diluent, because it may aggravate pre-existing hyponatremia. In primary adrenocortical failure (Addison's disease) there is no response of plasma corticosteroids; in pituitary deficiency with secondary adrenal failure, response is present but subnormal. Equally useful is intravenous infusion of ACTH over several days with measurement of urinary steroid excretion; some workers think this is a more certain method for differentiating primary and secondary adrenal insufficiency. It is prudent to give 0.5 to 1.0 mg of dexamethasone orally to obviate untoward reactions to ACTH. Use of the synthetic corticotrophins avoids these reactions, but results are not yet standardized. The nonspecific methods, insulin tolerance test and water loading, can be dangerous and are not recommended.

Four other methods have been used to assess pituitary ACTH release; like the ACTH-response test described above, the index is rise or failure to rise of plasma or urinary corticosteroid values. Three of the methods entail stimulation of ACTH release by giving a more or less noxious stimulus: insulin-induced hypoglycemia, vasopressin, and bacterial pyrogen. Although it is true that patients with hypopituitarism show absent or subnormal rises in plasma cortisol concentration after all three of these, there is no agreement about which is the most discriminating or the most sensitive. The insulin, vasopressin, and pyrogen tests have not found favor as clinical methods in this country. The fourth method, the metyrapone test, a measure of pituitary ACTH reserve, is described in Ch. 845 and 848. To make certain that the adrenal has the capacity to respond to ACTH, a standard ACTH response test should be done before metyrapone is given. In a few patients with severe hypopituitarism, metyrapone blockade of adrenocortical biosynthesis coupled with poor or absent ACTH reserve has resulted in clinically significant adrenal insufficiency. In patients with possibly advanced hypopituitarism, "coverage" with 0.5 to 1.0 mg of dexamethasone is therefore a reasonable safeguard during a metyrapone test.

Biologic assay and radioimmunoassay of plasma ACTH, although not yet available for clinical purposes, are *direct* techniques which have yielded valuable information about the fluctuations of this hormone. Normal values are a mean of about 0.3 mU per 100 ml by bioassay and a mean of 22 pg per milliliter by radioimmunoassay (normal range, 12 to 80 pg per milliliter). Values are occasionally ten times higher than those in severely ill patients; as expected, levels are low or not detected in hypopituitarism. The changes in plasma ACTH concentration that occur in the various forms of Cushing's syndrome are discussed in Ch. 850.

Christy, N. P., Wallace, E. Z., and Jailer, J. W.: The effect of intravenously administered ACTH on plasma 17,21-dihydroxy-20-ketosteroids in normal individuals and in patients with disorders of the adrenal cortex. J. Clin. Invest., 34:899, 1955.

Staub, J. J., Jenkins, J. S., Ratcliffe, J. G., and Landon, J.: Comparison of corticotrophin and corticosteroid response to lysine vasopressin, insulin, and pyrogen in man. Br. Med. J., 1:267, 1973.

Wood, J. B., Frankland, A. W., James, V. H. T., and Landon, J.: A rapid test of adrenocortical function. Lancet, 1:243, 1965.

MELANOCYTE-STIMULATING HORMONE
(MSH)

A radioimmunoassay for plasma β-MSH has been developed but is not used for clinical purposes. Normal levels are 20 to 110 pg per milliliter. The values are raised in untreated Addison's disease and congenital adrenal hyperplasia, and fall during corticosteroid administration. Plasma β-MSH is slightly elevated, as is plasma ACTH, in the "pituitary" form of Cushing's syndrome (see Ch. 850), and is very much elevated in patients who develop pituitary tumors and dermal hyperpigmentation after bilateral adrenalectomy for this disease. Elevations of plasma β-MSH tend to parallel those of plasma ACTH, and large amounts of each peptide have been found in extracts of hormone-secreting tumors (see Ch. 870). A new finding of great interest is the detection of raised plasma β-MSH levels in patients with parkinsonism; this raises the possibility that β-MSH functions as a neuroregulatory hormone.

Abe, K., Nicholson, W. E., Liddle, G. W., Island, D. P., and Orth, D. N.: Radioimmunoassay of β-MSH in human plasma and tissues. J. Clin. Invest., 46:1609, 1967.

Shuster, S., Thody, A. J., Goolamali, S. K., Burton, J. L., Plummer, N., and Bates, D.: Melanocyte-stimulating hormone and parkinsonism. Lancet, 1:463. 1973.

830. DIAGNOSIS AND TREATMENT OF PITUITARY TUMORS

Epidemiologic studies indicate that there are 2500 newly diagnosed pituitary tumors per year in the United States. Tumors of the pituitary may be *asymptomatic*. In an autopsy study of 1000 "normal" pituitaries, adenomas were found in nearly 25 per cent, over half being chromophobic, more than a quarter basophilic, and the rest (7.5 per cent) acidophilic. Although some pathologists believe, on the basis of special stains, that most pituitary tumors are chromophilic and contain stainable, possibly hormone-secreting granules, the majority of tumors are chromophobic by conventional light microscopy, whatever implication this may have for their secretory capacities. Thus in a recent collection of nearly 1000 cases of known pituitary adenoma, 98 per cent were chromophobic, the remaining 2 per cent being acidophilic. Malignant chromophobe adenomas are rare. Extrasellar and suprasellar cysts and tumors, especially gliomas of the optic chiasm and craniopharyngiomas, are less common tumors that may involve the pituitary, either by direct extension into the pituitary fossa or by impingement upon the adjacent hypothalamus or pituitary stalk.

Patients with pituitary tumor are more likely to seek medical aid because of visual or neurologic symptoms than for complaints of endocrine dysfunction. In a recent series, about three quarters of the patients had headaches (not by themselves sufficiently typical to be diagnostic); two thirds had impairment of visual fields, and the same proportion had impairment of visual activity; about 40 per cent complained of decreased libido, and one third had diplopia, decrease in potency, dizziness (postural hypotension), change in distribution of sexual hair, or intolerance to cold. By far the most common visual field defect is *bitemporal hemianopia*, occurring in 70 to 80 per cent of patients; it is noteworthy that about 15 per cent of patients with this defect are unaware of it. Paralysis of cranial nerves III, IV, and VI usually denotes a large tumor extending outside the sella turcica. Among *endocrine symptoms*, about 90 per cent of patients give a history of some degree of gonadal insufficiency on careful questioning, about 80 per cent have symptoms of thyroid failure, and perhaps half give evidence of adrenocortical deficiency. Even when pituitary tumors rise up out of the sella turcica and exert pressure on the diencephalon, they rarely cause *hypothalamic symptoms;* diabetes insipidus and disorders of sleep or temperature regulation are rare and do not occur unless the diencephalon is grossly damaged. About one eighth of patients may have symptoms caused by *"pituitary apoplexy"* (abrupt hemorrhage into the tumor).

Physical findings in pituitary tumor are also more

Figure 3. Chromophobe adenoma in a 36-year-old man. Roentgenogram of the skull shows moderate enlargement of the sella (24 mm in the anterior-posterior diameter, 16 mm in depth on the original film). The sellar floor shows a double contour, indicating uneven downward growth of the tumor, which depresses one side of the sella more than the other. The dorsum sellae is thin; the posterior clinoids are intact. The texture and appearance of the skull and facial bones are normal (cf. acromegaly, Fig. 4).

Figure 4. Skull roentgenogram typical of acromegaly; 66-year-old woman with acromegaly of 43 years' duration. Radiotherapy to sella within five years of onset. Intermittent increases in the acral parts. No symptoms of endocrine deficiency (serum protein-bound iodine normal, normal blood glucose two hours after a meal). The film shows thickening and hyperostosis of the cranial vault and occipital protuberance, and overdevelopment of the frontal sinuses. As is not uncommonly true in acromegaly, the sella is only slightly enlarged (18 mm. in the sagittal plane). The dorsum sellae is pneumatized. Prognathism is indicated by the overlapping lower teeth.

Figure 5. X-ray of the hands in acromegaly. There is tufting of the distal phalanges, but the most characteristic finding is increase in soft tissue mass.

commonly related to the eyes than to the endocrine system. In addition to bitemporal hemianopia, up to 85 per cent of patients can be shown to have reduced visual acuity, more than half have optic atrophy, and one third have cranial nerve palsies. About two fifths of patients are found to have loss of body hair, and a third or fewer have changes in the skin or genital atrophy.

Roentgenographic detection (see Anatomy in Ch. 827) should be based on frontal as well as sagittal views of the skull and sella. In addition to changes in the length and depth of the pituitary fossa, the examiner looks for erosion or destruction of the anterior and posterior clinoids and of the tuberculum sellae, suprasellar calcification (chromophobe adenoma, craniopharyngioma), and "double floor" of the sella, seen when a tumor extends downward unevenly (Fig. 3). Laminagraphy may show intrasellar calcification or extension of a tumor into the sphenoid sinus. Carotid artery angiography and particularly pneumoencephalography may show quite accurately the degree of upward extension of an intrasellar tumor; these procedures, at least the latter, should always be done before craniotomy for pituitary tumor, and are also necessary guides in the design of a radiotherapeutic program. In *acromegaly,* plain films of the skull show not only enlargement of the sella turcica in 80 to 90 per cent of patients, but also thickening of the calvarium, enlargement of the paranasal sinuses, and widening of the mandibular angle with prognathism (Fig. 4). Films of the hands disclose gross increase in the mass of soft tissue, a more characteristic finding than tufting of the distal phalanges (Fig. 5). Spinal films may reveal anterior lipping of vertebral bodies; lateral films of the os calcis often show thickening of the heel pad.

Chromophobe Adenoma. *Natural History.* These tumors may occur in adolescence but are most common between the ages of 30 and 60, with equal distribution between men and women. They are the largest of pituitary tumors, having a tendency to extend upward for a considerable distance. The clinical picture is variable. The tumors may be asymptomatic; the symptoms may be predominantly ocular or neurologic; or *endocrine symptoms* and signs may predominate, the most common being secondary gonadal failure (amenorrhea, decreased frequency of shaving, impotence), with evidence of secondary thyroidal and adrenocortical failure being less common and occurring later in the course. *Galactorrhea* may be the only endocrine symptom (Forbes-Albright syndrome) or may coexist with elements of hypopituitarism. Recent studies have called attention to the possibility that longstanding *primary hypogonadism* or *hypothyroidism* may give rise to pituitary enlargement, owing to chromophobe adenoma in most cases (Bower; Lawrence et al.). In contrast, there are rare instances of *oversecretion* of a *pituitary* hormone, e.g., TSH, by a chromophobe adenoma.

Treatment. It is now clear that chromophobe adenoma must be treated; it is not safe to manage "expectantly" a patient suspected to have this lesion. A recent study has shown that of 16 such patients left untreated, 14 eventually required treatment, and during the observation period (6 months to 15 years) growth of the adenoma produced further and irreversible damage in 8. The best treatment appears to be *surgery,* followed by *conventional radiotherapy* (4000 to 5000 rads over five to six weeks); this method yields a control rate of about 75 per cent. Surgery (mortality rate 5 to 7 per cent) is

mandatory if there is evidence of recent or rapid growth of the adenoma or if there is a major threat to vision. Since surgery alone is followed by an appreciable recurrence rate, radiotherapy should be added. In selected cases, radiotherapy alone may suffice. Preliminary results suggest that treatment with *heavy particles* (protons, α-particles) may be as effective as conventional radiotherapy for this tumor; the method is available only at those few centers that have cyclotrons.

Treatment of *galactorrhea* is either *surgical* or *pharmacologic.* If the tumor is large and threatens vision, surgery must be done. Hardy has had considerable success with *transsphenoidal* removal of laterally located prolactin-secreting microadenomas without producing hypopituitarism (Kohler and Ross). With or without pituitary tumor, treatment of galactorrhea with L-*dopa* and *ergot alkaloids* has shown promise, eliciting falls in plasma prolactin levels and, after several weeks, suppressing the inappropriate lactation.

Acidophilic Adenoma with Acromegaly. *Natural History and Pathogenesis.* There is some evidence that acidophilic tumors may arise through an abnormality in HGHRF secretion by the hypothalamus. The course and prognosis of this lesion are more unfavorable than used to be thought. Life expectancy is reduced; in one series half the patients were dead before age 50 and nearly 90 per cent by age 60; among 194 patients followed for up to 30 years in London, the death rate was almost twice that in a matched group of patients without acromegaly (see Ch. 832). Treatment is therefore mandatory, even in "mild" cases without ocular or neurologic symptoms.

Treatment. Several modes of therapy are available; each is more or less effective and more or less hazardous. As Gorden and Roth have put it (Kohler and Ross): "At the present time patients are treated largely on the basis of regional expertise or preference. No single mode of therapy has emerged as ideal or clearly preferable. All therapeutic modalities to date leave some patients with distinctly elevated growth hormone concentrations." *Conventional pituitary radiation* (4000 to 5000 rads over five weeks) probably controls tumor growth in over 70 per cent of patients; if one is willing to wait, plasma HGH values will fall somewhat by one to two years after radiation and will be reduced by nearly 80 per cent after 3 to 6 years, with some values in the normal range; untoward effects are not common. Treatment with *heavy particles* (4500 to 6500 rads over 11 days) sometimes produces dramatic results; there are more untoward effects than with conventional external radiation. The method works best when there is no major extrasellar extension of the tumor. Plasma HGH falls to levels below 10 ng per milliliter within two years after radiation in about three fourths of patients; at these levels metabolic improvement is almost always seen.

More in Europe than in the United States, *transsphenoidal implantation of radioactive isotopes* (^{90}Y, ^{198}Au) into the pituitary has found favor. There are many reports of beneficial effect, with resolution of soft tissue and osseous abnormalities and reduction of plasma HGH levels, but there is an appreciable rate of complications (meningitis, CSF rhinorrhea), and a still higher rate may be expected during the developmental phase at a given institution.

Many *surgical approaches* have been tried. *Transfrontal hypophysectomy* is effective and has a mortality rate of well under 5 per cent in experienced hands; the difficulty is in achieving total removal of the tumor, for short of that plasma HGH values remain elevated. *Transsphenoidal* removal, especially of small adenomas, may be highly successful in skilled hands; in a recent series of 40 patients, 25 had clinical "cure" with return of plasma HGH to normal levels, and 10 showed improvement with substantial falls of plasma HGH; there was one late postoperative death. Both *stereotaxic* and *transsphenoidal cryohypophysectomy* have also been used in small numbers of patients.

A number of *pharmacologic agents* have been tried: *estrogens, chlorpromazine, progestins,* and *somatostatin* (HGH-inhibiting hormone). These drugs may prove to be suitable in selected "mild" cases; further trials over long periods will be required for full evaluation of efficacy.

Basophilic Adenoma with Cushing's Syndrome. *Natural History.* These tumors are *small,* being rarely visible radiographically. If the sella is enlarged, it is most likely owing to a chromophobe adenoma; those occurring after bilateral total adrenalectomy for Cushing's syndrome have chromophilic granulations, are aggressive, and may secrete ACTH and β-MSH with dermal pigmentation (Nelson's syndrome).

Treatment. Conventional external pituitary radiation (up to 4000 rads) in Cushing's syndrome may yield results better than the 30 to 40 per cent of incomplete or temporary remissions that could be achieved in the past (Orth and Liddle). In *Nelson's syndrome,* tumors may be aggressive or malignant, and require more radiation; with *heavy particles,* doses of 12,000 to 16,000 rads have been given with control of most tumors. In the faster-growing adenomas, particularly those with large extrasellar extension, *surgery* is required.

Transsphenoidal surgery for removal of these tumors, especially when small (microadenomas), has corrected the ACTH and β-MSH oversecretion and controlled the tumor without producing hypopituitarism. When there is a large suprasellar component, the *transfrontal* approach is preferable.

Craniopharyngioma (Rathke's Pouch Tumor, Adamantinoma). Although they may first appear in adult life, most of these tumors become manifest in childhood. Signs of increased intracranial pressure, changes in visual fields and acuity, and slowing or cessation of growth in late childhood are typical; because of the suprasellar location of the major portion of the tumor mass, *hypothalamic symptoms,* especially *diabetes insipidus,* occur occasionally. About 80 per cent of craniopharyngiomas display suprasellar calcification on x-ray (Fig. 1); the sella may be normal, eroded, or enlarged. Since these tumors are cystic (lined with squamous or columnar epithelium not resembling pituitary cells), they are not very radiosensitive; *transfrontal surgery* is usually indicated.

Multiple Endocrine Adenomatosis. *Clinical Characteristics.* Acidophilic or chromophobic adenomas of the pituitary are occasionally accompanied by functioning islet cell tumors of the pancreas and adenomas of the parathyroids and adrenal cortex. Intractable peptic ulcer (hypergastrinemia, Zollinger-Ellison syndrome; q.v.) is often associated. The disorder is familial in many instances. Presenting symptoms may be those of pituitary tumor (ocular, neurologic, acromegaly), hypoglycemia, hyperparathyroidism (e.g., renal colic), or gastrointestinal hemorrhage. Acromegaly with hypertension has been associated with surgically proved, primary *aldosterone-secreting adrenal adenoma.* It is probably more correct to regard multiple endocrine adenomatosis as a complex of separate genetic abnormalities than as a series of consequences of a single primary disease. This syndrome (known as multiple endocrine adenomatosis Type I or MEA I) should not be confused with MEA Type II: medullary carcinoma of the thyroid, pheochromocytoma, and parathyroid hyperplasia (also known as Sipple's syndrome) which is transmitted as an autosomal dominant trait with a high degree of penetrance (see Ch. 837 and 843).

Treatment. This syndrome may present the physician with a nice problem in deciding which tumor to treat first. Generally, the pituitary tumors are not so

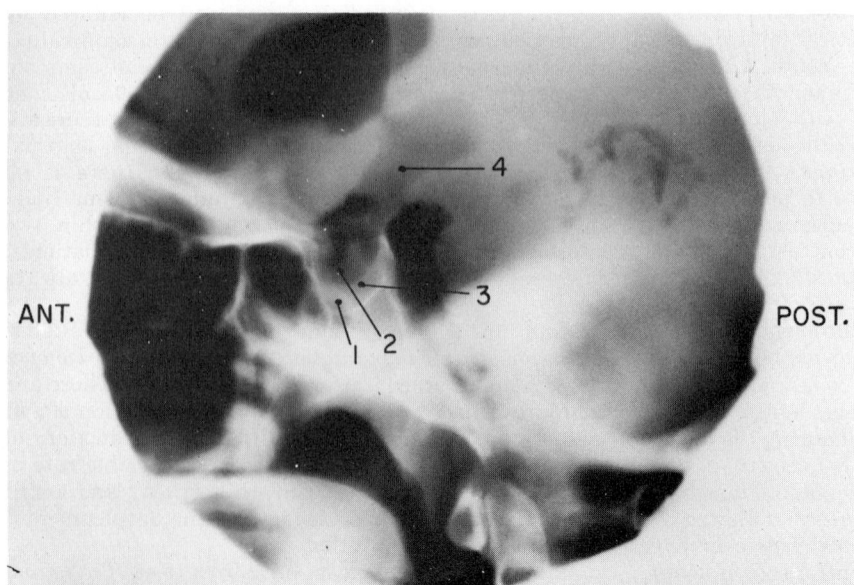

Figure 6. "Empty sella" in a 56-year-old woman. Pneumoencephalogram, lateral (sagittal) view of the sella which shows depression of the sellar floor (1). The striking abnormality is downward extension of air (2) into the sella; the pituitary is flattened downward and posteriorly (3). Normally, no air should enter the sella. If an intrasellar tumor were present, one would expect it to elevate the air column above the sella and encroach upward upon the third ventricle (4).

threatening as the others; unless there is a major or rapidly progressive impairment of vision, treatment of the pituitary adenoma or of acromegaly can wait. Obviously, the gastrointestinal problem, the hypoglycemia, or the hypercalcemia will have to be attacked first, depending upon which is the most acute or the most incapacitating.

The "Empty Sella" Syndrome. *Pathogenesis and Clinical Characteristics.* In an unknown proportion of cases, enlargement of the pituitary fossa as seen on lateral x-rays of the skull is not due to pituitary tumor. In a recent study, nearly a third of enlarged sellae were found on pneumoencephalography to contain not too much but too little pituitary tissue (Fig. 6). One autopsy series has revealed a 5.5 per cent incidence of this lesion in nearly 800 presumably normal people, the space above the pituitary remnant being replaced by a subarachnoid sac filled with cerebrospinal fluid. "Empty sella" may occur as a consequence of Sheehan's syndrome or of necrosis of a pituitary adenoma, either spontaneous or after x-irradiation. The sella may be radiologically enlarged or normal. The pathogenesis is debated. Possible mechanisms include a defective diaphragma sellae through which an outpouching of subarachnoid membrane may descend, and medial kinking of the internal carotids compressing the "waist" of the dorsum sellae, with consequent expansion ("ballooning") of the pituitary. The *clinical picture* may show *no endocrine abnormality* or *frank hypopituitarism.* Usually symptoms of pituitary deficiency are not prominent, but one or more defects in anterior pituitary hormone secretion can be shown by test. There seems to be a curious predisposition to "empty sella" in obese middle-aged women who have had many children.

Diagnosis and Treatment. This lesion emphasizes the need for *pneumonencephalography* in all cases of enlarged sella (Fig. 6) in which radiotherapy is contemplated; such treatment, directed to an unsuspected empty sella, is likely to produce a permanent CSF fistula. If an empty sella is found, the only therapy required is replacement of lost hormonal functions if any are shown to exist.

Ballard, H. S., Frame, B., and Hartsock, R. J.: Familial mulitple endocrine adenoma–peptic ulcer complex. Medicine, 43:481, 1964.

Besser, G. M., Parke, L., Edwards, C. R. W., Forsyth, I. A., and McNeilly, A. S.: Galactorrhea: Successful treatment with reduction of plasma prolactin levels by brom-ergocryptine. Br. Med. J., 2:669, 1972.

Bower, B. F.: Pituitary enlargement secondary to untreated primary hypogonadism. Ann. Intern. Med., 69:107, 1968.

Brisman, R., Hughes, J. E. O., and Holub, D. A.: Endocrine function in nineteen patients with empty sella syndrome. J. Clin. Endocrinol. Metab., 34:570, 1972.

Craven, D. E., Goodman, D., and Carter, J. H.: Familial multiple endocrine adenomatosis: Multiple endocrine neoplasia, type I. Arch. Intern. Med., 129:567, 1972.

Fürst, E.: On chromophobe pituitary adenoma. Acta Med. Scand. (Suppl. 452), 1966.

Hall, R., Schally, A. V., Evered, D., Kastin, A. J., Mortimer, C. H., Tunbridge, W. M. G., Besser, G. M., Coy, D. H., Goldie, D. J., McNeilly, A. S., Phenekos, C., and Weightman, D.: Action of growth-hormone-release inhibitory hormone in healthy men and in acromegaly. Lancet, 2:581, 1973.

Hamilton, C. R., Jr., Adams, L. C., and Maloof, F.: Hyperthyroidism due to thyrotropin-producing pituitary chromophobe adenoma. N. Engl. J. Med., 283:1077, 1970.

Keiser, H. R., Beaven, M. A., Doppman, J., Wells, S., Jr., and Buja, L. M.: Sipple's syndrome: Medullary thyroid carcinoma, pheochromocytoma, and parathyroid disease. Ann. Intern. Med., 78:561, 1973.

Kohler, P. O., and Ross, G. T. (eds.): Diagnosis and Treatment of Pituitary Tumors. New York, American Elsevier Publishing Company, 1973.

Kolodny, H. D., Sherman, L., Singh, A., Kim, S., and Benjamin, F.: Acromegaly treated with chlorpromazine: A case study. N. Engl. J. Med., 284:819, 1971.

Lawrence, A. M., and Kirsteins, L.: Progestins in the medical management of active acromegaly. J. Clin. Endocrinol. Metab., 30:646, 1970.

Lawrence, A. M., Wilber, J. F., and Hagen, T. C.: The pituitary and primary hypothyroidism: Enlargement and unusual growth hormone secretory responses. Arch. Intern. Med., 132:327, 1973.

Lawrence, A. M., Pinsky, S. M., and Goldfine, I. D.: Conventional radiation therapy in acromegaly: A review and reassessment. Arch. Intern. Med., 128:369, 1971.

Lawrence, J. H., Tobias, C. A., Linfoot, J. A., Born, J. L., Lyman, J. T., Chang, C. Y., Manougian, E., and Wei, W. C.: Successful treatment of acromegaly: Metabolic and clinical studies in 145 patients. J. Clin. Endocrinol. Metab., 31:180, 1970.

LeMay, M.: The radiologic diagnosis of pituitary disease. Radiol. Clin. North Am., 5:303, 1967.

Neelon, F. A., Goree, J. A., and Lebovitz, H. E.: The primary empty sella: Clinical and radiographic characteristics and endocrine function. Medicine, 52:73, 1973.

Orth, D. N., and Liddle, G. W.: Results of treatment in 108 patients with Cushing's syndrome. N. Engl. J. Med., 285:243, 1971.

Roth, J., Gorden, P., and Brace, K.: Efficacy of conventional pituitary irradiation in acromegaly. N. Engl. J. Med., 282:1385, 1970.

Snyder, N., III, Scurry, M. T., and Deiss, W. P.: Five families with multiple endocrine adenomatosis. Ann. Intern. Med., 76:53, 1972.

831. HYPOPITUITARISM

PITUITARY INSUFFICIENCY IN THE ADULT

Definitions. Hypopituitarism is the clinical condition resulting from destruction of the anterior pituitary; it is accompanied by secondary atrophy of the gonads, thyroid, and adrenal cortex. The term *panhypopituitarism* has been used to designate total absence of all the known pituitary secretions. *Simmonds' disease* is used synonymously. The term *Sheehan's disease* describes hypopituitarism resulting from postpartum necrosis of the gland. The designation *pituitary insufficiency* is inclusive.

Etiology, Pathology, and Pathogenesis. The most common cause of pituitary insufficiency in adult life is *pituitary tumor,* particularly chromophobe adenoma; the most common cause of *very severe* adult hypopituitarism is probably postpartum necrosis of the gland. The pathogenesis is debated. The common denominator is obstetric accident. According to Sheehan, peripheral vascular collapse is followed by spasm of local vessels, then thrombosis, and then infarction. McKay holds that the primary event is not arteriolar spasm but thrombosis of pituitary vessels as part of generalized intravascular coagulation. Neither view accounts for the peculiar susceptibility of the pituitary to damage in the postpartum period. The well-demarcated infarctions are small or nearly total. Sheehan and Summers have shown that pituitary insufficiency does not occur unless the lesion is very large. The late lesion is fibrosis with residual small nests of normal chromophils.

Lesions other than tumors (see Ch. 830) are fibrosis of unknown cause, granulomas, which may be nonspecific, syphilitic, or tuberculous, and aneurysms of the *internal carotid artery.* Ischemic necrosis has occasionally followed acute infection (usually associated with diabetes mellitus), meningitis, basal skull fracture, and septic cavernous sinus thrombosis. In some patients the primary defect may be in the hypothalamus (e.g., sarcoidosis, metastatic cancer, idiopathic).

General pathologic findings in pituitary insufficiency include widespread *splanchnomicria* with particularly striking atrophy of the gonads, thyroid, and adrenal cortex.

Clinical Manifestations and Natural History.   The speed of onset of pituitary insufficiency depends upon the nature and size of the lesion. When *postpartum necrosis* of the pituitary is extensive and severe, acute symptoms such as *diabetes insipidus* and *hypoglycemia* occur during the puerperium and may be only transitory; the patient may suddenly die within weeks, probably as a consequence of acute adrenocortical insufficiency. More commonly, the onset after obstetric accident is slow, occurring over months to years. The first symptom is usually failure to lactate; pubic and axillary hair fails to grow; menses do not return owing to gonadal failure, or the periods are scanty and transitory; amenorrhea follows. Libido is lost. Symptoms of *thyroid and adrenocortical failure* occur later as a rule than do those of ovarian deficiency, but *there is no set pattern.* General

Fig. 7   Fig. 8

Figure 7.   A patient with documented hypopituitarism 21 years after postpartum necrosis of the pituitary. Pubic and axillary hair is gone. Notice the absence of cachexia. Compare with Figure 8. (Reproduced by permission from Sheehan, H. L., and Summers, V. K.: Quart J. Med., 42:319, 1949.)

Figure 8.   The patient is a 30-year-old unmarried woman with anorexia nervosa who had lost 55 pounds (compare with the good nutritional state of the patient with hypopituitarism, Fig. 7). Pubic hair was present and menses continued but were scanty and irregular. (Reproduced by permission from Bliss, E. L., and Branch, C. H. H.: Anorexia Nervosa. New York, Paul B. Hoeber, Inc., 1960.)

deterioration ensues. Patients become weak, easily fatigued, indifferent to their surroundings, slothful, and negligent of household duties. *Personality changes* range from mild idiosyncrasies to frank psychosis. Intolerance of cold, as in primary hypothyroidism, may be extreme. *Hypopituitary coma* with hypotension and hypothermia, probably in most instances resulting from *hypoglycemia,* may have its onset gradually with no apparent cause, or rapidly in response to minor illness. At times collapse is preceded by clinical manifestations of *adrenal crisis* with nausea, vomiting, high fever, and hypotension. Although *anorexia* is a prominent feature in some patients, cachexia is uncommon and is a terminal event in the neglected patient. Pre-existing diabetes is on rare occasions ameliorated abruptly, with sudden lowering of the insulin requirement, after pituitary destruction ("Houssay phenomenon").

The *physical examination* discloses a fair state of nutrition as a rule (Fig. 7). The skin is thin, smooth, cool and pale, with fine wrinkling about the eyes (geroderma). The dry, scaly skin and puffy face of primary myxedema are unusual but occur on occasion. Pubic and axillary hair is absent or sparse. The pulse is slow and thin, the blood pressure low. Symptomatic hypotension on orthostasis is common. The breasts may appear well preserved, but genital atrophy is the rule.

General *laboratory examination* shows a moderate normochromic anemia that is less striking than the pallid appearance suggests. Roentgenogram of the skull is normal (there is no expanding intrasellar lesion). Blood glucose concentration is often low. The serum sodium concentration may be 120 mEq per liter or lower without symptoms of adrenal insufficiency. Hyponatremia is probably related to hemodilution owing to inadequate excretion of water, which in turn is due to deficient cortisol secretion. Episodic hyponatremia in patients with pituitary insufficiency is correlated with measurable water retention (increased total body water), not with sodium depletion. The level of serum potassium is normal. As in the hypophysectomized animal or man, the aldosterone function of the adrenal cortex is fairly well preserved; the hypopituitary patient responds to salt withdrawal by a slow but adequate increase in aldosterone secretion and consequent retention of sodium. In very severe hypopituitarism with complete adrenal destruction, this capacity may be lost. The urinary 17-ketosteroids and corticosteroids are decreased. The basal metabolic rate is low, and serum protein-bound iodine is depressed; but thyroidal uptake of ^{131}I is often inexplicably normal even when the patient is clinically hypothyroid.

The typical clinical picture becomes obvious as late as 15 to 20 years after the obstetric accident. Acute adrenocortical failure with or without superimposed infection is the chief cause of death in untreated patients.

Expanding intrasellar tumors—e.g., chromophobe adenoma—may have a similar insidious onset. The clinical picture and natural history are discussed in Ch. 830. In patients with intrasellar tumor, both the chief complaint and the ultimate cause of death are more commonly mechanical results of the adenoma than of pituitary failure.

Diagnosis.   A history of postpartum hemorrhage, symptoms and signs of an intracranial tumor with chiasmal pressure, or evidence of multiple glandular deficiencies should raise the question of hypopituitarism. Diagnosis is difficult early in the course of the disease, before symptoms and signs of deficiency of more than one target gland are definite. Hypopituitarism should be suspected in patients with onset of gonadal failure in adult life. Amenorrhea occurring in a fertile woman before the expected age of menopause requires inquiry about obstetric hemorrhage in the past. Loss of axillary and pubic hair and atrophy of the external genitalia make hypopituitarism likely in a relatively young woman with amenorrhea. In men, loss of previously normal libido and potency and loss of body hair with or without genital atrophy are suggestive; roentgenogram of the skull shows sagittal stretching or ballooning of the sella if a pituitary tumor is present. Reduced visual acuity, optic atrophy, and bitemporal hemianopia provide evidence of suprasellar expansion of an intrasellar mass (see Ch. 830). Failure of sexual development late in the second decade raises the question of hypopituitarism in either sex.

In the *differential diagnosis,* primary gonadal failure and primary hypothyroidism must be considered. *Primary gonadal failure,* in the *male* especially, may resemble pituitary insufficiency. The degree of eunuchoidism (disproportionately long arms and legs owing to late closure of the epiphyses of the long bones) depends on the age of onset of hypoleydigism, being extreme if early, absent if late. Many males with gonadal failure have the fine, pale, wrinkled skin of hypopituitarism, but thyroid and adrenal function is normal. *Anorexia nervosa* is not difficult to differentiate, because only gonadotrophic deficiency is present and the degree of emaciation is extreme (Fig. 8; see Ch. 724).

Levels of urinary gonadotrophin are elevated in testicular deficiency, undetectable in pituitary failure. Klinefelter's syndrome (seminiferous tubule dysgenesis) is easily distinguished. In the female the same principles apply: The level of urinary gonadotrophin is undetectable in hypopituitarism, high in natural menopause. *Primary myxedema* is generally characterized by more noticeable dryness and puffiness of the skin, and the serum cholesterol tends to be higher. In hypothyroidism resulting from pituitary failure, other glandular deficiencies are often present and should be sought. Measurement of thyroidal response to thyrotrophin may be helpful (see Ch. 829). *Primary adrenocortical failure* (Addison's disease) is not hard to differentiate. The skin is darkly tanned (MSH) rather than pale, gonadal function is often normal, and thyroidal function is unimpaired, unless Hashimoto's thyroiditis is associated (Schmidt's syndrome). Diagnosis of this entity is discussed in Ch. 846. Primary adrenal failure is ruled out, and subtle adrenal insufficiency caused by pituitary failure is diagnosed by measuring the response of plasma or urinary corticosteroids to intravenous corticotrophin. This constitutes more specific evidence of adrenal deficiency than do low urinary steroid values, which are reduced in a great variety of chronic, debilitating diseases.

Treatment. *Long-term medical management* of the patient with hypopituitarism consists of careful replacement of lost functions. (Management of intrasellar mass lesions is discussed in Ch. 830.) Trophic hormones are not used because of expense and the bother of daily injections. By far the most important defect is that of the *adrenal cortex;* acute adrenal crisis may come on abruptly and without warning, and may lead to death. Under ordinary conditions, cortisone or hydrocortisone (10 to 25 mg per day in two divided doses, by mouth)

provides a sense of well-being and adequate protection against hypotension, hypoglycemia, and water and electrolyte imbalance. Small doses are preferred, because patients with hypopituitarism have a peculiar susceptibility to the effects of larger doses of corticosteroids (peptic ulcer, facial rounding, psychosis) possibly because of coexisting secondary hypothyroidism in which metabolism of corticosteroids is much delayed. Added salt and a mineralocorticoid are only occasionally required. In the female, diethylstilbestrol, 0.5 to 1.0 mg per day for 20 days of each month, provides good maintenance of developed secondary sex characters and, in time, leads to an artificial menstrual cycle. Induction of ovulation in women with hypopituitarism is discussed in Ch. 867. In the male, a fair degree of libido and potency can be conferred by androgens (methyltestosterone, 20 to 30 mg per day orally; testosterone propionate, 25 to 100 mg two to three times per week by intramuscular injection; or a long-acting ester once per month intramuscularly). Thyroid replacement should be started with small doses (8 to 15 mg per day of USP thyroid orally), which are gradually increased over a period of several weeks; for optimal effect a dose as large as 0.180 gram may be needed. Roughly equivalent doses of L-thyroxine are 0.1 to 0.2 mg per day. It is probably wise to begin corticosteroid therapy first, because adrenal crisis has allegedly been precipitated by vigorous treatment with thyroid hormone.

Treatment of an acute illness or management during a surgical procedure, e.g., craniotomy for intrasellar tumor, is essentially that of adrenal crisis. Thyroid hormone is not necessary. *Corticotrophin should never be relied upon,* because the degree of endogenous adrenal response is unpredictable. Correct treatment is hydrocortisone (100 to 300 mg per day of a water-soluble ester in isotonic saline intravenously). It is better to err on the side of *moderately* excessive doses, because untoward reactions are not likely to occur during the few days of vigorous treatment generally required; the dose should be reduced as quickly as possible to the maintenance level. If in an emergency there is doubt concerning the presence of secondary hypoadrenalism, one should assume that it exists rather than attempt a time-consuming laboratory evaluation of adrenal status. If *diabetes insipidus* occurs postoperatively, treatment is as set out in Ch. 834.

Keller, P. J.: Induction of ovulation by synthetic luteinizing-hormone releasing factor in infertile women. Lancet, 2:570, 1972.

Martin, L. G., Martul, P., Connor, T. B., and Wiswell, J. G.: Hypothalamic origin of idiopathic hypopituitarism. Metabolism, 21:143, 1972.

McKay, D. G.: Pituitary. Disseminated Intravascular Coagulation. New York, Hoeber Medical Division, Harper & Row, 1965, pp. 405, 460.

Sheehan, H. L., and Davis, J. C.: Pituitary necrosis. Br. Med. Bull., 24:59, 1968.

Sheehan, H. L., and Summers, V. K.: The syndrome of hypopituitarism. Quart. J. Med., 42:319, 1949.

Sherman, B. M., Gorden, P., and diChiro, G.: Postmeningitic selective hypopituitarism with suprasellar calcification. Arch. Intern. Med., 128:600, 1971.

Stocks, A. E., and Powell, L. W.: Pituitary function in idiopathic haemochromomatosis and cirrhosis of the liver. Lancet, 2:298, 1972.

Warren, M. P., and Vande Wiele, R. L.: Clinical and metabolic features of anorexia nervosa. Am. J. Obstet. Gynecol., 117:435, 1973.

DEFICIENCY OF SINGLE ANTERIOR PITUITARY HORMONES

It is hard to determine in an individual case whether there is isolated deficiency of a pituitary hormone or whether one is observing an early stage of what will ultimately be panhypopituitarism. Whereas some *pituitary dwarfs* are panhypopituitary, others have *isolated HGH deficiency,* either of pituitary or hypothalamic origin. Patients who have Hand-Schüller-Christian disease with short stature have also been shown to have isolated HGH deficiency. It is not yet known whether women who have failure of postpartum lactation are deficient in *prolactin* secretion. Idiopathic isolated gonadotrophin failure exists in several forms, with or without anosmia, in men and women (see Ch. 867). *Isolated deficiencies of TSH and ACTH* have been reported; in one instance of the latter, pituitary basophils were virtually absent. Isolated corticotrophin deficiency has been found as part of the hypothalamic disorder of acute intermittent porphyria.

The most common form of isolated ACTH deficiency occurs in patients receiving *long-term corticosteroid therapy,* which is discussed in Ch. 849. Prolonged treatment with thyroid hormone and antiovulatory drugs usually induces *self-limited* TSH and gonadotrophin deficiency; rarely, the latter persists ("oversuppression syndrome"; see Ch. 867).

Treatment. Thyrotrophin and adrenocorticotrophin deficiencies are usually treated with thyroid hormone (or thyroxine) and corticosteroids, respectively. Administration of purified human FSH and HCG is effective in the induction of ovulation in hypopituitary women and, sometimes, spermatogenesis in men (see Ch. 857 and 867).

Braunstein, G. D., and Kohler, P. O.: Pituitary function in Hand-Schüller-Christian disease: Evidence for deficient growth-hormone release in patients with short stature. N. Engl. J. Med., 286:1225, 1972.

Christy, N. P.: Iatrogenic Cushing's syndrome. *In* Christy, N. P. (ed.): The Human Adrenal Cortex, New York, Harper & Row, 1971, p. 395.

Males, J. L., Townsend, J. L., and Schneider, R. A.: Hypogonadotropic hypogonadism with anosmia—Kallmann's syndrome. Arch. Intern. Med., 131:501, 1973.

Miyai, K., Azukizawa, M., and Kumahara, Y.: Familial isolated thyrotropin deficiency with cretinism. N. Engl. J. Med., 285:1043, 1971.

Spitz, I. M., Diamant, Y., Rosne, E., Bell, J., David, M. B., Polishuk, W., and Rabinowitz, D.: Isolated gonadotropin deficiency: A heterogenous syndrome. N. Engl. J. Med., 290:10, 1974.

Tagatz, G., Fialkow, P. J., Smith, D., and Spadoni, L.: Hypogonadotropic hypogonadism associated with anosmia in the female. N. Engl. J. Med., 283:1326, 1970.

Waxman, A. D., Berk, P. D., Schalch, D., and Tschudy, D. P.: Isolated adrenocorticotropic hormone deficiency in acute intermittent porphyria. Ann. Intern. Med., 70:317, 1969.

HYPOPHYSECTOMY-INDUCED HYPOPITUITARISM

Since 1952, pituitary ablation has been used as a palliative treatment for metastatic cancer and for diabetic retinopathy.

The metabolic consequences of hypophysectomy in man are familiar. They are repaired by hormonal replacement therapy. If diabetes insipidus is present, it is treated with vasopressin as set forth in Ch. 834. Loss of gonadotrophic function, observed as disappearance of detectable urinary gonadotrophin, occurs within a week after hypophysectomy. Gonadal steroids are not given, especially to patients with cancer, because hypogonadism may be an important part of the palliative therapy. Loss of thyrotrophic function is apparent from fall of serum PBI values to myxedematous levels at one week and of thyroidal uptake of ^{131}I at two weeks after pitu-

itary ablation. If hypophysectomy is incomplete, these indices decline, only to return to normal within a month after surgery. Loss of adrenocorticotrophic function is notable only if hypophysectomy has been virtually total. Some investigators believe that the metyrapone test and measurement of plasma prolactin concentration are the most sensitive indices of completeness of hypophysectomy.

Conventional medical treatment consists of thyroid USP in daily doses of 0.120 gram and cortisone acetate, 25 mg or less, both given by mouth.

Methods for pituitary ablation are numerous: transfrontal and transsphenoidal hypophysectomy, cryosurgery, stereotaxic radiofrequency surgery, pituitary stalk section, implantation of radioactive gold or yttrium (^{198}Au, ^{90}Y), and external delivery of heavy particles (proton beam) from the cyclotron. It is not yet possible to decide which of these techniques is the safest or the most effective. It is also not clear why pituitary ablation is effective at all; there is evidence that adequate palliation may not be closely or uniquely related to the degree of reduction in growth hormone or prolactin secretion.

The present position can be summarized in this way. Carefully selected patients with advanced, widespread metastases from cancer of the breast have objective remissions in bony, cutaneous, and pulmonary metastases in about 50 per cent of cases treated with surgical hypophysectomy. In metastatic prostatic cancer, remissions occur in fewer than half the patients. The methods which bring about less complete ablation of the pituitary tend to be associated with lower remission rates (see Ch. 877).

In patients with diabetic retinopathy, surgical hypophysectomy is rarely done now (see Ch. 806). It is ineffective in proliferative retinopathy, and in several series the remission rate of hemorrhages and exudates is about the same in hypophysectomized as in untreated groups of patients.

Juret, P.: Endocrine Surgery in Human Cancers. 2nd ed. Springfield, Ill., Charles C Thomas, 1966.

Krieger, D. T., Sirota, D. K., and Lieberman, T.: Cryohypophysectomy for diabetic retinopathy: Ophthalmological and endocrine correlation. Ann. Intern. Med., 72:309, 1970.

Ray, B. S.: Hypophysectomy as palliative treatment. J.A.M.A., 200:974, 1967.

PITUITARY INSUFFICIENCY IN CHILDHOOD

Lesions involving the pituitary in childhood cause *dwarfism;* like that of gonadotrophin, secretion of HGH appears to be more sensitive to impairment than the thyrotrophic or adrenocorticotrophic functions of the pituitary. Pituitary insufficiency is an uncommon cause of short stature, accounting for fewer than 10 per cent of instances. About two thirds of pituitary dwarfs have no evidence of pituitary tumor; usually there is no evidence of an anatomic lesion. The lesion may in some cases be hypothalamic. Idiopathic hypophysial *fibrosis* has been occasionally observed. Of the tumors, *craniopharyngioma* (adamantinoma) is the most common. This neoplasm arises from fragments of oral epithelium remaining from the embryologic invagination (see Ch. 830). Other causes are *suprasellar cysts* and *Hand-Schüller-Christian disease.* Reversible isolated HGH deficiency has been documented in children with the maternal deprivation syndrome.

Diagnosis of pituitary dwarfism is often difficult early in life. The infant's size may be normal at birth. Growth does not stop entirely, but is obviously retarded in early infancy. Evidence of thyroid and adrenocortical insufficiency, e.g., hypoglycemic attacks, is strongly suggestive, but may be subtle or absent. If, however, the patient reaches the early years of the second decade with continued retardation of growth and complete failure of sexual development, suspicion of pituitary dwarfism is raised. The physical examination discloses relatively normal proportions. The facies is childish, but the skin may become wrinkled early, imparting an incongruous aspect of aging. Laboratory study shows absence of urinary gonadotrophin, reduced concentration of serum protein-bound iodine, and subnormal response of plasma corticosteroids to intravenous adrenocorticotrophin. Idiopathic hypopituitary dwarfism may occur either as an isolated, recessively inherited deficiency of growth hormone, or sporadically. When sporadic, the deficiency may involve growth hormone alone or several pituitary hormones.

The *differential diagnosis* of pituitary dwarfism includes constitutional retardation of growth and delay in the onset of puberty (see Ch. 857); in the latter condition, the family history is often positive, evidence of thyroidal and adrenocortical insufficiency is lacking, and in time normal growth and maturation take place. *Systemic and other endocrine diseases* may cause dwarfism; among these are chondrodystrophy, rickets, Hurler's syndrome, intestinal malabsorption, chronic renal disease, hypoxia associated with congenital cardiac malformations, hypothyroidism, and sexual precocity with premature fusion of the epiphyses. These conditions are distinguished by the inappropriately short extremities, osseous deformities, overt malnutrition and evidence of fat intolerance, gross proteinuria and nitrogen retention, cyanosis and heart murmur, mental deficiency and other stigmata of cretinism, or precocious development of the genitalia. D. W. Smith has presented a list of 52 conditions associated with short stature, some of which are recognized at a glance by seasoned pediatricians; Smith also lists the very numerous systemic diseases in which growth retardation is observed.

One of the most difficult disorders to distinguish from pituitary dwarfism before puberty is *primordial dwarfism.* The patients, also known as sexual ateliotic (incomplete) dwarfs, become miniature adults, often capable of producing normal offspring. McKusick and his co-workers have shown that in some of these patients the failure to grow in association with normal gonadal and secondary sexual development and normal thyroid and adrenal function is due to a deficiency of end-organ response to growth hormone. With radioimmunoassay measurements of serum growth hormone, it is possible to define four subgroups of ateliotic dwarfs, some of whom fail to raise sulfation factor (somatomedin) activity when HGH is administered. It is interesting that the African pygmy also has subresponsiveness to administered growth hormone, whereas endogenous growth hormone release is apparently normal (Table 2). The differentiation of pituitary dwarfism in the female and *gonadal dysgenesis (Turner's syndrome)* may be difficult before puberty; patients with this disorder are phenotypic females who often have associated congenital anomalies (webbed neck, coarctation of the aorta) and short stat-

TABLE 2. Classification of Pituitary Dwarfism*

I. *HGH undetectable:*
A. Idiopathic hypopituitarism (primary disorder of pituitary or secondary to deficiency of hypothalamic HGHRF)
1. Panhypopituitarism
2. Isolated HGH deficiency (may be familial)
B. Organic hypopituitarism
1. Tumors
2. Trauma
3. Infection
4. Hand-Schüller-Christian disease
C. HGH unreactive immunologically, partially active biologically (Merimee's Type II ateliotic dwarf)
1. Absent HGH response to provocative tests
2. Evidence that endogenous HGH has some activity
3. Resistance to exogenous HGH (including no rise in somatomedin)
4. Autosomal dominant inheritance in some cases

II. *HGH detectable but ineffective:*
A. Laron dwarf
1. Normal plasma HGH response to provocative tests
2. Plasma HGH normal or high
3. Deficient generation of somatomedin when HGH is given
B. African pygmy
1. Normal plasma HGH response to provocative tests
2. Plasma HGH normal
3. Somatomedin low and showing no rise when HGH is given

*Compiled from many sources by Dr. C. A. L. Abrams of the Pediatric Service, The Roosevelt Hospital, and the Department of Pediatrics, The College of Physicians and Surgeons, Columbia University. See references to the text (Merimee, Najjar).

ure; the distinguishing features are less immature facies, less delay in epiphysial closure, slight but definite growth of pubic hair at puberty, a frequently negative (male) chromatin pattern on buccal smear, and, after the age of 9 to 13, an elevated rather than absent titer of urinary gonadotrophin (see Ch. 867). Recognition of *progeria* is easy; this rare idiopathic condition is characterized by retardation of growth, baldness, loss of subcutaneous fat, premature fusion of epiphyses, and atherosclerosis or arterial calcification, all occurring within the first few years of life. The life span is short; there is no evidence of endocrine disease.

As indicated in Ch. 829, the best way to detect growth hormone deficiency is to test the response of serum growth hormone values to insulin-induced hypoglycemia. If a metabolic ward is available, demonstration of a sharp increase in nitrogen retention in response to administered growth hormone is diagnostic of classic idiopathic HGH deficiency (see also Table 2). Analysis of the growth curve determines whether or not to subject the patient to elaborate testing procedures.

As to *treatment,* a moderate degree of linear growth can be achieved in pituitary dwarfs through the administration of thyroid hormone in combination with gonadal steroids. Impressive skeletal growth can be induced with the administration of purified human growth hormone. The optimal dose is about 20 to 45 mg per month (see Tanner et al.). This therapy is limited by the short supply of the hormone; if it is used, gonadal steroids should not be given until maximal linear growth is attained so that epiphysial closure will not occur; thyroid hormone augments the somatotrophic effects. Crawford and his colleagues have set out detailed criteria for diagnosis and treatment of pituitary dwarfism and have described the response to growth hormone. The hormone causes only minimal if any increase in linear growth rate in children whose short stature is not due to deficiency of HGH. Since growth hormone should therefore be reserved for patients with growth hormone deficiency, a high premium is placed upon accurate diagnosis.

Goodman, H. C., Grumbach, M. M., and Kaplan, S. L.: Growth and growth hormone: II. A comparison of isolated growth hormone deficiency and multiple pituitary hormone deficiencies in 35 patients with idiopathic hypopituitary dwarfism. N. Engl. J. Med., 278:57, 1968.

Grumbach, M. M., and Kaplan, S. L.: The pathogenesis of growth hormone deficiency. Proceedings of the XIII International Congress of Pediatrics, 15:10, 1971.

Lacey, K. A., and Parkin, J. M.: Causes of short stature: A community study of children in Newcastle upon Tyne. Lancet, 1:42, 1974.

Laron, Z., Pertzelan, A., Karp, M., Kowaldo-Silbergeld, A., and Daughaday, W. H.: Administration of growth hormone to patients with familial dwarfism with high plasma immunoreactive growth hormone: Measurement of sulfation factor, metabolic and linear growth responses. J. Clin. Endocrinol. Metab., 33:332, 1971.

Merimee, T. J., et al.: An unusual variety of endocrine dwarfism: Subresponsiveness to growth hormone in a sexually mature dwarf. Lancet, 2:191, 1968.

Merimee, T. J., Hall, J. D., Rimoin, D. L., and McKusick, V. A.: A metabolic and hormonal basis for classifying ateliotic dwarfs. Lancet, 1:963, 1969.

Merimee, T. J., Rimoin, D. L., and Cavalli-Sforza, L. L.: Metabolic studies in the African pygmy. J. Clin. Invest., 51:395, 1972.

Najjar, S. S., Khachadurian, A. K., Ilbawi, M. N., and Blizzard, R. M.: Dwarfism with elevated levels of plasma growth hormone. N. Engl. J. Med., 284:809, 1971.

Root, A. W., Rosenfield, R. L., Bongiovanni, A. M., and Eberlein, W. R.: The plasma growth hormone response to insulin-induced hypoglycemia in children with retardation of growth. Pediatrics, 39:844, 1967.

Silver, H. K., and Finkelstein, M.: Deprivation dwarfism. J. Pediatr. 70:317, 1967.

Smith, D. W.: Compendium on shortness of stature. J. Pediatr., 70:463, 1967.

Tanner, J. M., Whitehouse, R. H., Hughes, P. C. R., and Vince, F. P.: Effect of human growth hormone treatment of 1 to 7 years on growth of 100 children with growth hormone deficiency, low birthweight, inherited smallness, Turner's syndrome, and other complaints. Arch. Dis. Child., 46:745, 1971.

832. HYPERPITUITARISM

ACROMEGALY

Definition. Acromegaly is a chronic disease of middle life characterized by overgrowth of bone, connective tissue, and viscera in response to prolonged and excessive secretion of adenohypophysial growth hormone. The term "acromegaly" denotes the typical enlargement of acral or distal parts of the body—the hands, feet, face, and head.

Etiology. The increased secretion of growth hormone results from overactivity of the acidophil cells of the pituitary. The evidence for excessive growth hormone is that (1) similar pathologic changes are produced in animals by administration of the hormone, and (2) increased concentrations of growth hormone have been detected in plasma of patients with acromegaly. Hyperactivity of the anterior pituitary is deduced from (1) the almost invariable necropsy finding of pituitary enlargement, (2) histologic observation of overgrowth of the acidophilic cells, and (3) the clinical improvement that frequently follows destruction of the gland.

Incidence and Prevalence. Acromegaly is a rare disorder with about 300 new cases per year being discovered in the United States. The sexes are affected equally often. Acromegaly starts most commonly in the third and fourth decades; a few patients trace the start

of acromegaly to adolescence. Some 30 acromegalic children have been reported.

Pathology and Pathogenesis. Acidophilic or mixed acidophilic and chromophobe adenoma is found in 75 per cent or more of autopsied patients with acromegaly. Rarely, acidophil cell hyperplasia is observed, malignancy almost never. The growth of the tumor may obliterate normal cells. The assumption is that if hypopituitarism occurs, it is a result of atrophy of normal pituitary tissue owing to the pressure of the tumor. Over 90 per cent of adenomas cause sufficient enlargement of the sella turcica to be visible in roentgenograms of the skull. Sellar enlargement may be minimal or gross. Upward extension rarely produces clinical evidence of hypothalamic involvement, e.g., diabetes insipidus, but invasion of the optic tracts of chiasm is of clinical significance (visual field changes, optic atrophy) in about 60 per cent of patients.

The excessive secretion of growth hormone affects virtually all organs and tissues. The response of cartilage and bone is obvious and distinctive. The histologic appearance of chondrogenesis and osteogenesis is somewhat disorderly. The cartilaginous and bony response occurs at points of special sensitivity, e.g., mandible, zygoma, ribs, and clavicles. The uneven growth is thought to be due to the effect of pressure or of muscular traction. Increased *chondrogenesis* is most obvious in hypertrophy of the costal cartilages, which contributes to the increased circumference of the thorax. *Acromegalic arthritis,* affecting chiefly the large joints and the spine, resembles osteoarthritis and results from proliferation of deep layers of joint cartilage with thinning of articular cartilages. Hypertrophy of nasal and aural cartilage accounts for part of the enlargement of nose and ears. *Osteogenesis* from the thickened periosteum is accelerated; absorption of bone is also rapid; late in the disease *osteoporosis* may be striking. There is overgrowth of the supraorbital ridge. The anterior temporal ridge advances with forward growth of the lateral portions of the orbit, expansion of the frontal sinuses, and forward displacement of the zygoma. Overgrowth of the maxilla lengthens the face, and the teeth are separated by heaping up of alveolar bone. The ramus of the mandible grows longer; the angle between ramus and body opens out to produce mandibular prognathism. The ribs and clavicles widen and reach a length 2 to 3 inches greater than normal. The *long bones* thicken and become massive. The humerus and femur may be lengthened, and the latter may be deformed by bowing. The vertebral bodies are increased in the anteroposterior diameter; the greatest changes occur in the thoracic spine with deposit of new bone upon diaphyses, particularly anteriorly; this change makes forward flexion of the spine difficult.

The visible *enlargement of distal parts* is chiefly due to proliferation of soft tissue, not bone. Subcutaneous connective tissue is grossly increased, giving the characteristic thick and fleshy appearance of the *hands* and *feet,* enlargement of the *lips,* and *accentuation of skin folds.* The skin itself is greatly thickened; there are increased sweating and seborrhea; hirsutism occurs in a few female patients. The *tongue* may be so large as to protrude from the mouth.

Widespread splanchnomegaly is the rule. The heart, lungs, liver, spleen, and intestines are variously enlarged two- to fivefold. The kidneys are enlarged by the growth of individual nephrons; studies of renal function indicate increased glomerular filtration rate and proximal tubular activity. The endocrine glands participate in the splanchnomegaly. A possible role of accompanying oversecretion of trophic hormones is not proved. The gonads, although often functioning subnormally and showing histologic evidence of failure, may be large. The *adrenal cortex* is hyptertrophied, and nodules are often found. The *thyroid* may be eight to nine times the normal size; goiters are diffuse or nodular. True hyperthyroidism is uncommon. The *parathyroids* are usually enlarged, and adenomas occur. Although there is generalized enlargement of tissues and organs and a considerable gain in weight, obesity is almost unknown, possibly because of the adipokinetic effect of growth hormone. The muscles enlarge somewhat but without conspicuous hypertrophy; edema and deposition of mucopolysaccharide in muscle have been reported; atrophy is a late finding.

Clinical Manifestations and Natural History. The onset of acromegaly is usually so insidious and so subtle that it escapes detection by the patient and his intimate associates. The gradualness and subtlety of onset are such that a third of the patients seek medical help for unrelated diseases, being unaware of their acromegaly. In Davidoff's series of 100 patients, the mean age of onset was estimated as 27 years, but the mean age at which the patients presented themselves was over 40; this average lapse of 13 or 14 years implies chronicity and a generally slow course. Careful analysis of the history reveals that early symptoms are related to peripheral effects of growth hormone or, much less commonly, to the mechanical pressure of the intrasellar tumor. Even before the obvious changes in appearance are noticed patients may complain of excessive sweating, paresthesias of the hands and feet, and pain and stiffness of the slowly expanding fingers and toes. Arthralgias are common. Accounts of hypersexuality and greatly increased muscular strength early in the course of the disease are rare. Complaints of hypogonadism (amenorrhea, loss of libido) are common. Headache may be extremely severe; the mechanism is not clear, because, in many instances, there is little clinically detectable enlargement of the pituitary tumor. Impairment of visual acuity or symptomatic encroachment upon visual fields occurs in over 60 per cent of patients at one time or another.

The *clinical picture* of advanced acromegaly is easily recognized on physical examination, but the changes are occasionally subtle. The typical acromegalic is large and burly; in late stages the forward carriage of the head, prognathism, kyphosis, bowing of the legs, and rolling gait are distinctive. The features are blunt and coarse, the nose and ears large; the brow is prominent and the jaw prognathous; the facial wrinkles are exaggerated; the lips are full. The skin is thick and hairy, the voice husky and cavernous. The hands and feet are enlarged; shaking hands with an acromegalic patient gives the startling impression of losing one's hand in a mass of dough. The superficial veins of the extremities are thick and prominent. The thoracic cage is widened and deepened and thoracic kyphosis is present. Galactorrhea is an occasional finding in both men and women.

Most routine *laboratory data* are within normal limits. The basal metabolic rate is elevated in more than half the patients, but other evidence of hyperthyroidism (increased thyroidal uptake of ^{131}I or level of serum PBI) is usually lacking even when the thyroid is palpably enlarged. Appraisal of adrenocortical function reveals normal plasma cortisol values, normal response to ACTH, occasionally increased excretion of urinary 17-ketosteroids or corticosteroids, and sometimes raised cortisol secretory rate and a degree of adrenal refractoriness to suppression by dexamethasone. Urinary gonadotrophin titer is normal or reduced; semen analysis generally shows oligospermia. Despite the reported increased insulin activity of acromegalic plasma, glycosuria or glucose intolerance is found in about a third of acromegalic subjects and frank diabetes in about one fifth. The diabetes is usually mild and somewhat resistant to insulin, but management of the diabetes presents no unusually difficult problems, and ketoacidosis is rare. Hypercalciuria is a common finding, and hypercalcemia occurs in a few patients; in some this abnormality is apparently due to hypersecretion of growth hormone, because it disappears with successful treatment of the acromegaly. However, in others the hypercalcemia persists and can be shown to be due to associated hyperparathyroidism as part of the syndrome of *multiple endocrine adenomatosis*.

As the disease progresses, muscular weakness (predominantly of proximal muscle groups) supervenes; kyphosis increases, partly because of osteoporosis. Visual impairment may become aggravated to the point of blindness. Partial or total pituitary insufficiency may ensue. The course is extremely variable; it is hard to know with accuracy the natural history, because the onset is usually so insidious and because most patients have received some sort of treatment. Life expectancy is reduced (see Ch. 830). The course may be fulminant, resulting in death within three years (usually because of tumor growth in younger patients), or benign and intermittent, lasting 50 years or longer. Death comes from the tumor (expansion, hemorrhage into its substance, "pituitary apoplexy"), cardiac failure (owing to "acromegalic heart disease"), or the effects of hypertension (found in 20 to 50 per cent of patients) or degenerative vascular disease. The causes of death in years past were diabetes and hypopituitarism; these are now rarely lethal because of the availability of adequate treatment.

Diagnosis. The typical acromegalic is recognized at a glance. *The great need is a means of early diagnosis.* If acromegaly is suspected, a history of increasing size of gloves and shoes and of increasingly poor fit of dentures provides useful clues. Tightness of old rings is suggestive; comparison of the patient's features with old photographs is helpful. Roentgenogram of the skull and tests of the visual fields usually give confirmatory evidence.

The differential diagnosis rarely presents difficulties. The large tongue, hoarse voice, and periorbital edema may suggest myxedema, but the other physical and laboratory abnormalities of hypothyroidism are absent. Patients with pachydermoperiostosis, some of whom look quite acromegalic, do not have involvement of the pituitary, and plasma HGH values are normal. Some patients receiving anticonvulsants for long periods may develop "acromegaloid" coarsening of the features. The articular pains of acromegaly are usually distinguishable from those associated with other forms of arthritis by the typical acromegalic aspect.

There is no generally satisfactory method for the *indi-*

rect assessment of the *secretory activity* of the adenoma. History of recent acral enlargement is the best evidence of active secretion, and some clinicians believe that excessive sweating and seborrhea are good guides. Laboratory data are disappointing. Elevation of serum phosphorus follows administration of human growth hormone, but is an unreliable index of "activity" of the disease in acromegaly. The same may be said of the glucose tolerance test and basal metabolic rate. Some investigators consider the insulin tolerance test useful. Biopsy of costal cartilage may show active endochondral bone formation. Urinary excretion of hydroxyproline is increased. None of these laboratory indices has been conclusively proved to correlate closely with the clinical course of the disease. If plasma growth hormone measurements cannot be made, one must rely on a synthesis of historical, physical, and laboratory findings. Without documentary evidence of recent acral growth, judgment of secretory activity is highly subjective.

The use of *radioimmunoassay of plasma growth hormone* is the method of choice for *direct* assessment of the secretory activity of the acidophilic tumor. It is known that most untreated acromegalics have high concentrations. After hypophysectomy these fall, often to normal, but sometimes they remain elevated, presumably when hypophysectomy is not complete. After pituitary radiation, levels often do not fall. Not enough data are yet available to allow a complete appraisal of growth hormone response to physiologic stimuli (hypoglycemia, glucose administration) as a measure of "activity" in acromegaly. What is needed is careful correlation (over a period of years) of plasma growth hormone levels with objective studies of acral growth. Such studies will reveal the value of plasma growth hormone measurements as indices of secretory activity. At the moment, it appears that sharp falls in basal plasma growth hormone value, or recovery of growth hormone responsiveness to administered glucose, are closely related to clinically arrested disease.

Treatment. Treatment is discussed in detail in Ch. 830. No single method has been shown to be ideal (Fig. 9).

Figure 9. Evolution of acromegaly. *A*, Age 38, within a year after onset of the disease. *B*, Age 55, after two courses of radiation therapy to sella; disease has progressed with moderate coarsening of features: thickening of lips, enlargement of nose and ears. *C, D,* Age 64, 26 years after onset, after a third series of x-ray treatments to sella (total dose of radiation to the pituitary, 10,000 rads); nose and ears have enlarged further, supraorbital ridge and zygoma have become more prominent, and jaw is more prognathous; frontal view shows deepening of skin wrinkles (temporal atrophy is a result of x-irradiation). *E, F,* Age 64, volar and dorsal aspects of hand, showing broadened fingers and characteristically "meaty" appearance owing to gross increase in soft tissue, not bone (compare Fig. 5). The patient died 12 years later at age 76 of cardiac and respiratory failure. By that time diabetes mellitus and hypopituitarism (thyroid and adrenocortical deficiency) had developed and were treated, but the last plasma HGH measurement, six years before death, was still elevated, 27 ng per ml.

Clinicopathological Conference: A case of acromegalic heart disease. Br. Med. J., 1:718, 1973.

Davidoff, L. M.: Studies in acromegaly: III. The anamnesis and symptomatology in one hundred cases. Endocrinology, 10:461, 1926.

Falconer, M. A., and Davidson, S.: Coarse features in epilepsy as a consequence of anticonvulsant therapy: Report of cases in two pairs of identical twins. Lancet, 2:1112, 1973.

Goldfine, D., and Lawrence, A. M.: Hypopituitarism in acromegaly. Arch. Intern. Med., 130:720, 1973.

Gordon, D. A., Hill, F. M., and Ezrin, C.: Acromegaly: A review of 100 cases. Can. Med. Assoc. J., 87:1106, 1962.

Mastaglia, F. L., Barwick, D. D., and Hall, R.: Myopathy in acromegaly. Lancet, 2:907, 1970.

Strauch, G., Vallotton, M. B., Touitou, Y., and Bricaire, H.: The renin-angiotensin-aldosterone system in normotensive and hypertensive patients with acromegaly. N. Engl. J. Med., 287:795, 1972.

GIGANTISM

Gigantism is arbitrarily defined as height exceeding 78 to 80 inches or, in children, exceeding a height three standard deviations above the mean for age. This rare disorder has been conventionally regarded as the childhood counterpart of acromegaly, i.e., as oversecretion of growth hormone by a pituitary adenoma in a growing organism *before closure of the epiphyses*. However, acromegaly occurs in young children. It is reasonable to doubt a pituitary cause when (1) there is no evidence of acromegaly, (2) the sella is not enlarged, or (3) there is a strong familial history of unusually tall stature suggesting constitutional gigantism. A form of "cerebral gigantism" is described in children; associated features are macrocrania, large extremities, large hands and feet, evidence of cerebral dysfunction, and normal values and normal response of plasma growth hormone. An additional cause of tall stature is hypogonadism or late puberty, resulting in prolongation of the period of linear growth because of delayed epiphysial closure. In such patients, the bodily proportions are eunuchoidal, with a lower segment greater than the upper segment and arm span greater than height.

In those giants who are acromegalic (about 50 per cent), management is that of acromegaly. Treatment of the pituitary adenoma must be vigorous. The radioimmunoassay for growth hormone provides more accurate assignment of cause in gigantism and a more objective criterion as a guide to management

Baumann, G., Cain, J. P., and Dingman, J. F.: Gigantism with hypopituitarism: A re-evaluation. Am. J. Med., 53:805, 1972.

Haigler, E. D., Jr., Hershman, J. M., and Meador, C. K.: Pituitary gigantism: A case report and review. Arch. Intern. Med., 132:589, 1973.

Hook, E. B., and Reynolds, J. W.: Cerebral gigantism: Endocrinological and clinical observations of six patients, including a congenital giant, concordant monozygotic twins, and a child who achieved adult gigantic size. J. Pediatr., 70:900, 1967.

Ludwig, G. D., Chaykin, L. B., and Escueta, A. V.: Cerebral gigantism with intermittent fractional hypopituitarism and normal sella turcica. Ann. Intern. Med., 67:123, 1967.

POSTERIOR PITUITARY

Alexander Leaf

833. ANTIDIURETIC HORMONE

Normal Physiology. Antidiuretic hormone is produced in nuclei of the anterior hypothalamus. The major source of this hormone is the supraoptic nuclei, but contributions from the paraventricular and filiform nuclei are thought to be added. The hormone produced in these neural centers is transported by a process of neural secretion down the supraopticohypophysial tract to the neurohypophysis or posterior pituitary where the hormone is stored until released into the blood according to the state of hydration of the subject.

The antidiuretic hormone in man was identified by du Vigneaud as the octapeptide arginine vasopressin. The hormone is released normally in response to osmotic stimuli; a rise in concentration of solute, largely the salts of sodium, in the plasma or extracellular fluid, serves as the stimulus for release of vasopressin from the neurohypophysis. The hormone circulates to the kidney where its major action is on the epithelium lining the collecting ducts. In the presence of vasopressin this epithelium becomes more permeable to water so that water is transported from the tubular lumen to the more concentrated peritubular fluids. This serves to reduce urine volume and increase its concentration, thereby conserving body water. Dilution of plasma or extracellular fluids, as occurs after water ingestion, inhibits release of antidiuretic hormone. The dilute luminal fluid entering the distal convoluted tubule is excreted with little modification in concentration, with the result that a copious flow of dilute urine characterizes the absence of antidiuretic hormone. This rids the body of any excess of water.

The thirst center is functionally and anatomically closely related to the antidiuretic mechanism. Andersson has shown that osmotic or electrical stimulation of the anterior portion of the supraoptic nuclei creates a sensation of thirst; dilution of plasma inhibits thirst. The integrated activity of thirst and antidiuretic mechanism serves to regulate the concentration of body fluids as follows:

This double negative feedback system works with remarkable effectiveness to preserve the concentration of sodium in the serum between some 136 and 143 mEq per liter. Since intracellular fluids are in osmotic equilibrium with the extracellular fluids, this mechanism regulates the tonicity of the body fluid compartments.

In addition to the usual osmotic stimuli regulating release of vasopressin, other factors may affect this process. Pain and emotional states have been associated with antidiuresis, as have a number of pharmacologic agents which act to release the hormone. These include cinchoninic acid, acetylcholine, nicotine, morphine, barbiturates, ferritin, and bradykinin. Alcohol may inhibit release of antidiuretic hormone, but the effect is weak and is often obscured. Physiologically, reduction in the effective plasma volume appears to be a stimulus for secretion of antidiuretic hormone; at least this has been documented after acute large blood loss.

It is now appreciated that in a considerable number of clinical conditions there is an apparent inappropriate secretion of substances possessing antidiuretic activity. The adjective "inappropriate" is used to indicate that neither osmotic nor circulatory (volume) stimuli are responsible for the excessive persistent antidiuretic activity. Furthermore, the antidiuretic substances may not arise in all instances from the neurohypophysis but may be secretory products of the tumors or inflammatory tissue which give rise to the syndrome of inappropriate antidiuretic hormone secretion (see Ch. 805).

Andersson, B.: Polydipsia, antidiuresis and milk ejection caused by hypothalamic stimulation. In Heller, H. (ed.): The Neurohypophysis. London, Butterworth Scientific Publications, 1957.
Bartter, F. C., and Schwartz, W. B.: The syndrome of inappropriate secretion of antidiuretic hormone. Am. J. Med., 42:790, 1967.
du Vigneaud, V.: Hormones of the posterior pituitary gland: oxytocin and vasopressin. In The Harvey Lectures 1954–1955. New York, Academic Press, 1956.
Leaf, A.: The clinical and physiologic significance of the serum sodium concentration. N. Engl. J. Med., 267:24, 77, 1962.
Leaf, A., Bartter, F. C., Santos, R. F., and Wrong, O.: Evidence in man that urinary electrolyte loss induced by pitressin is a function of water retention. J. Clin. Invest., 32:868, 1953.
Schwartz, W. B., Bennett, W., Curelop, S., and Bartter, F. C.: A syndrome of renal sodium loss and hyponatremia, probably resulting from inappropriate secretion of antidiuretic hormone. Am. J. Med., 23:529, 1957.
Verney, E. B.: The absorption and excretion of water: The antidiuretic hormone. Lancet, 2:739, 781, 1946.

834. DIABETES INSIPIDUS

Etiology. Diabetes insipidus is an uncommon disturbance resulting from any condition which damages the neurohypophysial system. Idiopathic cases constitute the major group, comprising approximately 45 per cent. The idiopathic condition may become manifest at any age and affect either sex. It is unusual in infancy, but may commence in early childhood. Familial diabetes insipidus is very uncommon, but may occur in infancy or childhood and affect either sex. The condition has been noted in seven generations of one family. Familial diabetes insipidus is to be distinguished from nephrogenic diabetes insipidus, which is a renal tubular defect, inherited largely by males, in whom the affected tubules are unresponsive to antidiuretic hormone.

Head trauma (accidental or neurosurgical) and neoplasms (primary or metastatic) are the major causes of acquired diabetes insipidus. Of the metastatic tumors, breast cancer seems to have a special predilection for the hypothalamic area. Other rarer etiologic factors include sarcoidosis, birth injuries, eosinophilic granuloma, and a variety of local infections. Even with lesions directly in the hypothalamus, diabetes insipidus is rare, because a small fraction of normal tissue suffices to protect against manifest dysfunction. Since the posterior and anterior pituitary have separate blood supplies, infarction of the latter need not be associated with failure of the former; a space-occupying lesion is suspect when insufficiency of both occurs.

Clinical Manifestations. The polyuria and polydipsia can be so dramatic that adult patients may remember an exact date or even hour when symptoms started. The fluid exchanges may reach the distressing proportions of 5 to 10 liters or more per 24 hours. The specific gravity of the urine is usually 1.001 to 1.005; corresponding concentrations will be about 100 to 200 mOsm per liter. With restriction of fluid intake the specific gravity may reach 1.010, or even slightly higher with severe water lack, and urine concentration may increase to 300 mOsm per liter. Urine slightly hypertonic to serum has been produced experimentally in the complete absence of antidiuretic hormone by greatly reducing the glomerular filtration rate. The elaboration of a hypertonic urine by a patient with diabetes insipidus during severe dehydration or with acute reduction of the glomerular filtration rate from any cause need not therefore indicate the presence of residual neurohypophysial function.

Other than the annoyance of polyuria and polydypsia, there may be no evidence of ill health or of other physiologic disturbance associated with the condition, unless the patient suffers from the underlying local or systemic disease which has destroyed the neurohypophysial system. The assumption that patients with diabetes insipidus suffer from severe dehydration is not supported by measurements of serum sodium or total solute concentrations. A slight elevation of sodium and total solute concentrations of serum has been demonstrated statistically, but the overlap in individual cases is such as to make these determinations of little assistance diagnostically: 297 ± 12 mOsm per liter (S.D.) for diabetes insipidus and 285 ± 4 mOsm per liter (S.D.) for normal persons. As long as the patient's thirst center remains intact, the total solute concentration of the body fluids will be preserved close to normal values, but at the expense of polydipsia and the large fluid exchange characteristic of the condition. After a period of water restriction, these differences may be accentuated and have greater diagnostic value.

With unconsciousness resulting from trauma or anesthesia, the inability of the patient to demand water may be fatal. This situation may occur at the onset of diabetes insipidus secondary to head injury or intracranial surgery, and is one of the causes of hypernatremia after trauma to the head. A careful record of urine volumes and urine and serum concentrations in patients with acute head trauma and coma will prevent the occurrence of severe dehydration.

Differential Diagnosis. A patient with persistent polyuria and urine of low concentration may have one or more of three basic disturbances: (1) inability of the kidney to elaborate a concentrated urine despite adequate vasopressin, (2) deficient vasopressin, or (3) persistent excessive water intake. Any condition which disturbs the renal concentrating mechanism, rendering it unresponsive to vasopressin, may produce polyuria. Hypercalcemia, potassium depletion, or renal failure (both chronic and acute) may impair maximal concentrating ability, but none of these conditions cause the urine to be persistently hypotonic, and in only a few patients does the resulting polyuria suggest diabetes insipidus. These conditions are readily excluded in establishing the diagnosis of diabetes insipidus. The rare nephrogenic diabetes insipidus results from a failure of the renal tubule to respond to vasopressin. Patients with uncontrolled diabetes mellitus may exhibit extreme polyuria and polydipsia, but the specific gravity of the urine is high, although its osmolality may not be over 300 mOsm per liter; the large contribution which glucose makes to the specific gravity accounts for this seeming discrepancy.

Although it is evident that polyuria in diabetes insipidus is primary to polydipsia, compulsive water drinking may give rise to a condition which closely mimics diabetes insipidus. Chronic ingestion of large volumes of water impairs the renal concentrating mechanism, making it sometimes quite difficult to distinguish this psychogenic disturbance from true diabetes insipidus.

Several special procedures have been devised to assist in establishing the diagnosis of diabetes insipidus in patients with polyuria and polydipsia. They all test ability to respond to osmotic stimuli by elaboration of a concentrated urine, whether failure to do so is the consequence of a lack of endogenous vasopressin or of an inability of the renal tubules to respond to the hormone.

Water restriction with observation of urine volume and concentration constitutes the simplest test. Weight should be followed to avoid the hazards of incurring loss of more than 3 to 5 per cent of body weight. Small children and infants are especially liable to serious circulatory disturbances if dehydration is allowed beyond this limit. A normal subject may be expected to reduce urine flow to less than 0.5 ml per minute and increase urine concentration to greater than 800 mOsm per liter (corresponding to a specific gravity of 1.020 or above). In patients with diabetes insipidus, urine volumes well above this limit persist, and urine concentration remains below 200 mOsm per liter (specific gravities of 1.001 to 1.005) until advanced states of dehydration are present. Unfortunately, the differences are often not so clear, and patients with neurohypophysial insufficiency may concentrate their urine to 300 to 400 mOsm per liter (specific gravities of 1.008 to 1.014) with marked dehydration.

Another means of increasing plasma osmolarity to test the release of antidiuretic hormone is by the infusion of hypertonic solutions. After an initial hydrated state is established, 2.5 per cent sodium chloride is infused intravenously at a rate of 0.25 ml per minute per kilogram of body weight for 45 minutes. Urine flow is measured at 15-minute intervals. If neurohypophysial and renal functions are normal, urine flow will drop promptly to 25 per cent or less of control.

If either the water deprivation test or the infusion of hypertonic saline fails to reduce urine flow or to increase urine concentration, as expected, the ability of the patients' kidneys to respond to exogenous vasopressin must be demonstrated, in order to separate nephrogenic causes from hormone deficiency. For this purpose 5mU per minute of aqueous vasopressin (vasopressin injection, USP) may be administered intravenously for at least one hour by a slow drip, or 5 units of the long-acting vasopressin tannate in oil may be administered intramuscularly. An injection of the latter material in the evening, with urine samples collected on arising the following morning and hourly for three successive hours thereafter, should induce maximal concentration.

These simple measures will readily distinguish diabetes insipidus from nephrogenic causes of diminished response to vasopressin. To distinguish true diabetes insipidus from compulsive water drinking may be more difficult, because continued polydipsia lowers the max-

imal urinary concentrations achievable after dehydration, infusions of hypertonic saline, or exogenous vasopressin. Barlow and de Wardener have pointed out that a normal subject with intact neurohypophysis will achieve a higher urinary concentration after water deprivation than after administration of vasopressin without water restriction. The patient with diabetes insipidus has just the opposite response, i.e., higher urine concentration after vasopressin than after water restriction. Patients with psychogenic polydipsia respond in this regard normally; whatever the absolute value of urine concentration they achieve, concentrations during dehydration will exceed those attained after injections of vasopressin. In addition to the laboratory studies it should be remembered that compulsive water drinking to a degree which is confused with diabetes insipidus constitutes a severe psychogenic disorder. Clinical evaluation is usually rewarding in revealing other neurotic symptoms supporting the suspicion of a serious personality or behavioral disturbance.

Treatment.   If symptoms are mild, no therapy may be warranted, although a thorough search for underlying causative factors should be conducted. When symptoms interfere with sleep or interrupt work, treatment is indicated. Replacement therapy intramuscularly with long-acting vasopressin in oil (1.0 ml ampule contains 5 units per milliliter; 0.5 to 1.0 ml injected every 24 to 72 hours, as necessary to control polyuria) is generally reserved for the more severe cases, whereas an aqueous nasal spray, self-administered as necessary every two to six hours, may suffice to alleviate symptoms. The oral hypoglycemic agent chlorpropamide has been found to enhance the antidiuretic activity of residual endogenous antidiuretic hormone; 100 to 500 mg once daily will usually relieve polyuria and polydipsia in patients with incomplete neurohypophysial failure. Thiazide diuretics – 250 mg of chlorothiazide two or three times daily – presumably by sustaining a condition of persistent mild salt depletion, will blunt a water diuresis, and in patients with diabetes insipidus may reduce urine flow by some 50 per cent. In patients with nephrogenic diabetes insipidus this form of antidiuretic agent is also effective.

Barlow, E. D., and de Wardener, H. E.: Compulsive water drinking. Quart. J. Med., 28:235, 1959.
Coggins, C. H., and Leaf, A.: Diabetes insipidus. Am. J. Med., 42:807, 1967.
Dashe, A. M., Cramm, R. E., Crist, C. A., Habener, J. F., and Solomon, D. H.: A water deprivation test for the differential diagnosis of polyuria. J.A.M.A., 185:71, 1963.
Leaf, A.: Diabetes insipidus. In Astwood, E. B. (ed.): Clinical Endocrinology, I. New York, Grune & Stratton, 1960.
Williams, R. H., and Henry, C.: Nephrogenic diabetes insipidus: Transmitted by females and appearing during infancy in males. Ann. Intern. Med., 27:84, 1947.

835.   THE PINEAL

Seymour Reichlin

The pineal gland was discovered more than 20 centuries ago, and its function has long been a matter of scientific and philosophic speculation. Arising embryologically from ependyma lining the roof of the third ventricle, the pineal consists of parenchymal cells supported by a meshwork of neuroglia. In the adult, the gland weighs between 100 and 180 mg and is a cone-shaped organ lying in the groove formed by the superior colliculi. Although connected to the epithalamus by a peduncle, the pineal does not receive a direct nerve supply from this source. Instead, it is innervated by postganglionic nerve fibers which arise in the cervical sympathetic ganglia and travel along the great vein of Galen. A number of humorally active substances have been isolated from the pineal. In addition to norepinephrine, serotonin, histamine, and melatonin are found. Melatonin is formed by a series of enzymatic steps from tryptophan (Fig. 1). One of the intermediates is serotonin, which in turn is converted to N-acetylserotonin by the enzyme N-acetyl transferase; the conversion of N-acetylserotonin to melatonin is accomplished by the enzyme hydroxy-o-methyl transferase (HIOMT). Measurement of the activities of these enzymes has been used to study the factors controlling melatonin synthesis and, by inference, melatonin secretion. Both enzyme activities are influenced by alterations in the light-dark cycle (in rats and other laboratory forms), a change mediated by a special retinal-hypothalamic neural pathway (the inferior accessory optic tract) which does not involve the visual cortex. It was initially believed that the HIOMT enzyme was the rate-limiting step for melatonin synthesis. More recent work indicates that the acetyltransferase system is more important, but both enzymes may be involved in final control of pineal secretion. Enzymic activity of the pineal gland and its secretory function are regulated by noradrenergic nerve endings on pinealocytes (Fig. 2). Beta norepinephrine receptors activate adenyl cyclase with the formation of cyclic AMP through the classic second messenger mechanism. The activated ATP-protein kinase is believed to promote the formation of the melatonin-synthesizing enzymes. Norepinephrine also stimulates pineal uptake of the precursor tryptophan (Fig. 2). Although melatonin is a potent hormone in lower animals (it causes contraction of granules dispersed in melanocytes) and inhibits gonadotrophic and possibly thyrotrophic function through actions at the hypothalamic level, it has no known action in man. Lacking a method for measurement of melatonin in peripheral blood, there is no clear evidence for changes in pineal secretion of melatonin in the human

subject under any of the conditions in which the activity of the pineal is altered in the laboratory animal. Recent development of a radioimmunoassay for melatonin may change this situation. Recently, three of the hypothalamic releasing factors have also been demonstrated. These are TRH, LRH, and somatostatin. The functional significance of these findings is unknown.

The pineal gland has no known function in man but becomes of clinical significance because of the occurrence of calcification and of tumor formation. Calcific nodules termed *acervuli* form in a matrix of ground substance secreted by pinealocytes. This process begins in early childhood and becomes increasingly evident by roentgenography beginning in the second decade of life. Calcification has no known effect on pineal function, as inferred from the fact that the characteristic enzymes of the pineal (HIOMT, monoamine transferase, and histamine N-methyl transferase) maintain normal concentrations throughout life.

Pineal tumors are rare, and their classification and nature are still disputed by pathologists, some of whom believe that the pineal cell in situ or situated in ectopic regions of the brain (chiefly the infundibular area) can give rise to neoplasms. The most common pineal cell tumor is the parenchymal tumor, classified as a pineoblastoma or pineocytoma according to the degree of differentiation. Convincing evidence that at least certain of these tumors are truly of pineal origin comes from the finding by Wurtman and collaborators that tissue from a parenchymal and from an ectopic pinealoma contained the marker enzyme HIOMT. Pineal cell tumors may also resemble seminomas of the testis (seminomatous pinealomas); the relationship of these tumors to teratomas is not well understood. The pineal also gives rise to teratomas of dermoid type and to tumors of the supporting structures such as gliomas, astrocytomas, and endothelial tumors.

Pinealomas occur mainly in young males. The symptoms and signs of the tumor reflect both local effects on the brain and, in a minority of cases, more remote changes in sexual maturation. Enlargement of a mass in the pineal region compresses the aqueduct of Sylvius and distorts the quadrigeminal plate. Internal hydrocephalus gives rise to characteristic manifestations of

Tryptophan

5-Hydroxytryptophan

Serotonin

N-Acetylserotonin

Melatonin

Figure 1. Biosynthesis of melatonin from tryptophan in the pineal gland. Step 1 is catalyzed by tryptophan hydroxylase; Step 2 by L-aromatic amino acid decarboxylase; Step 3 by N-acetylating enzyme; and Step 4 by HIOMT. (From Wurtman, R. J., Axelrod, J., and Kelly, D.: The Pineal. New York, Academic Press, 1968, p. 60.)

Figure 2. The effect of norepinephrine on tryptophan metabolism in the pineal. 5-HIAA = 5-hydroxyindole acetic acid. (From Shein, H. M.: *In* Wolstenholme, G., and Knight, J. (eds.): The Pineal Gland. London, Churchill Livingstone, 1971.)

increased intracranial pressure such as headache, vomiting, papilledema, and disturbance of sensorium. Pressure on the superior colliculi causes conjugate paralysis of upward gaze (Parinaud's syndrome). Disturbances of gait, resulting from either hydrocephalus or possibly cerebellar damage, are also observed.

Pineal tumors arising in male children may, in about one third of cases, cause precocious puberty; over-all, however, pineal tumors are exceedingly rare and are therefore a relatively rare cause of sexual precocity. The mechanism of effect of the tumor on gonadotrophic function is controversial. It has been suggested that the pineal secretes a hormone which tonically inhibits onset of sexual maturation; destruction of the pineal permits the earlier development of puberty. In support of this hypothesis is the finding in laboratory animals that melatonin injections delay puberty, that tumors destroying the pineal are three times as likely to cause precocious puberty as are parenchymal tumors, and that some cases of precocious puberty occur in the absence of local brain damage.

On the other hand, there is impressive evidence that pineal tumors, like certain other types of hypothalamic tumors, cause precocious puberty by direct physical damage to the gonadotrophin-regulating areas of the brain. For example, Bing and co-workers found that whenever precocious puberty was caused by a pineal tumor, neuroanatomic evidence indicated extension beyond the pineal region with internal hydrocephalus or invasion of the third ventricle or hypothalamus. Clinical evidence of hypothalamic involvement, e.g., diabetes insipidus, polyphagia, somnolence, obesity, or behavioral disturbance, was observed in 71 per cent of cases. These clinicopathologic correlations strongly support the view that neoplasms of the pineal gland produce sexual precocity indirectly through involvement of the hypothalamus. In a few cases, precocity or infantilism (also reported to occur) may prove to be due to altered pineal hormone secretion, but convincing evidence of this occurrence has not yet been adduced.

A special type of pinealoma is sufficiently distinctive to be noted here. "Ectopic" pinealomas arising from pineal rests in midline areas most commonly occur in the region of the infundibulum and produce diabetes insipidus, compression of the optic chiasm, and hypopituitarism. Precocious puberty may also occur in such patients.

Treatment of pineal tumors is generally unsatisfactory. Because of their critical location in the epithalamic region above the midbrain, or in the infundibulum, surgical removal is hazardous and usually impossible. Most of them are radiosensitive, and respond at least partially to deep x-ray therapy. A few apparent radiotherapeutic cures have been reported, but the long-range prognosis is poor.

Wolstenholme, G. E. W., and Knight, J. (eds.): The Pineal Gland. Ciba Foundation Symposium. Edinburgh and London, Churchill Livingstone, 1971.

Wurtman, R. J., Axelrod, J., and Kelly, D. E.: The Pineal. New York, Academic Press, 1968.

THE THYROID

Leslie J. DeGroot

836.   INTRODUCTION

Thyroid hormone serves as a metabolic thermostat, regulating the level of biochemical activity of most tissues. In general, malfunction of the thyroid gland leads to two sets of symptoms: those related to the local effects of a mass in the neck, and the generalized effects of an excess or deficiency of hormone. Illnesses involving this gland are relatively common medical disorders and, excluding diabetes, account for nearly four fifths of endocrine disease.

DEVELOPMENT AND ANATOMY

The embryonic thyroid gland develops from segments of the fourth pharyngeal pouches, joined by a midline anlage from the base of the tongue. During the first three months of growth, the thyroid gland is unable to synthesize and release thyroid hormone. Accordingly, if hormone is needed in this period, the fetus must depend upon the maternal supply of thyroid hormone. By the end of the first trimester, the gland has assumed its

adult shape and position, concentrates iodide, synthesizes thyroglobulin, and functions under the control of
the fetal pituitary. During the remainder of intrauterine life, the gland produces the hormone required for
the developing fetus. If necessary because of malfunction of the fetal gland, the fetus derives some hormone
from the maternal circulation, but it is not established
whether an adequate supply reaches the fetus when
maternal hormone levels are in the normal range for
pregnancy. During the first 18 or 20 years after birth,
the gland doubles in size three to four times to attain a
weight of 15 to 20 grams. In the absence of disease or
changes in iodine supply, the size and function of the
gland remain relatively constant throughout life until
advanced age, when hormone production gradually diminishes.

The normal thyroid gland is butterfly shaped, firm,
smooth, and red-brown. It consists of two elongated
lobes on either side of the trachea connected by a thin
isthmus of tissue at or below the level of the cricoid
cartilage. (Often, a remnant of the lingual anlage, the
pyramidal lobe, extends superiorly from one side of the
isthmus. Under normal circumstances, this is too small
to be detected by external palpation.) The fine structure
consists of numerous follicles, each approximately 300 μ
in diameter and made up of clusters of cells surrounding a colloid-filled luminal space. The colloid is a mixture of proteins, of which thyroglobulin comprises about
80 per cent.

The thyroid cells are 15 μ high; the borders facing the
lumen have microvilli, thought to be involved in secretory and resorptive activities. In hyperplastic glands
the cells are taller, and colloid space is reduced. Certain
cells do not contact the luminal surface and have
slightly different staining properties; these perifollicular or "C-cells" secrete the hormone calcitonin
and are involved in regulation of calcium metabolism.
The parathyroid glands occur as two pairs, one posterior
to the upper poles of the thyroid and the other below or
embedded in the substance of the lower poles. The recurrent laryngeal nerves pass immediately beneath the
lower poles of the thyroid, or are sometimes embedded
in the substance of the thyroid gland. Occasionally bits
of normal-appearing thyroid tissue are present adjacent
to the gland.

PHYSIOLOGY OF THE THYROID

It is best to view the thyroid gland as part of a system
designed to provide a constant supply of hormone to
somatic cells. Thyroid hormone is transported from
blood to the peripheral tissues, where it produces its
characteristic metabolic stimulation, and is in turn
degraded. The thyroid gland replenishes this supply by
secreting about 75 μg of tetraiodothyronine (thyroxine,
T_4) and 25 μg of triiodothyronine (T_3) daily. If the hormone supply to tissue is depleted, the change is sensed
by the pituitary (and possibly the hypothalamus), which
increases the secretion of thyroid-stimulating hormone
(TSH). TSH increases secretion of hormone by the
thyroid gland in a feedback control system until the
circulating level of hormone returns to the original
level and suppresses TSH to its control level.

Iodide Metabolism (Fig. 1).   Iodine bears a unique
relation to thyroid physiology, because the element is a
major and characteristic constituent of the hormones.

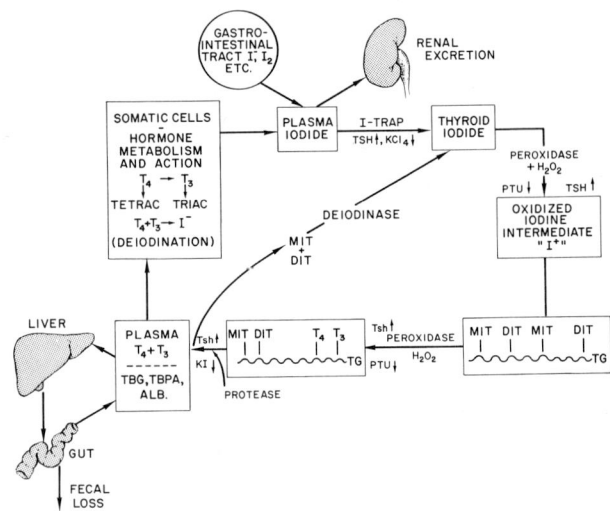

Figure 1.   The iodide cycle and thyroid hormone metabolism. The
pathway includes iodide absorption, thyroid trapping, oxidation by
peroxidase, iodination of tyrosine and intramolecular coupling, proteolysis, plasma hormone transport, and finally hormone action and
metabolism with recirculation of iodide.

The average daily American diet contains 150 to 600 μg
of iodide, depending in part on the consumption of certain varieties of bread, which may contain much iodate,
and milk, which may contain considerable iodide. Another major source is iodized salt. Most forms of ingested
iodine are reduced to iodide in the gastrointestinal tract
before absorption. Absorption is usually complete in one
hour. Iodide is cleared from plasma by the salivary
glands and gastric parietal cells into their secretions,
but normally this iodide is recycled to plasma. Iodide is
cleared unidirectionally by the kidney from plasma at a
rate of about 30 ml per minute. The normal thyroid
clears plasma iodide at a rate of 4 to 12 ml per minute.
The TSH feedback control system regulates the clearance rate to provide the gland with enough iodide for
hormone production, and this control point is probably
the prime determinant of thyroid hormone production.
If iodide intake is low and thyroid uptake of iodide is
diminished, thyroxine production is reduced and the
level of hormone in plasma falls. TSH secretion is then
increased and augments iodide clearance by the thyroid
gland. Under the influence of TSH or in thyroid hyperactivity of thyrotoxicosis, clearance may be elevated
5 to 20 times the normal range. With augmented levels
of iodide ion in the body, e.g., during therapy with
Lugol's solution, thyroid clearance falls to a fraction of
a milliliter per minute. The thyroid cells actively transport iodide and maintain a concentration gradient of 20
to 1 over the level in plasma. The iodide concentration
process is blocked competitively by perchlorate or thiocyanate ions. These drugs can thus interfere with formation of thyroid hormone. They are also used to establish the presence of elevated amounts of free iodide
in the gland (see below).

Hormonogenesis.   As rapidly as iodide is transported
into the normal thyroid cell it is oxidized by a peroxidase and bound to tyrosine residues present in thyroglobulin. This iodination process takes place near the
apical cell border, either in secretory vesicles before liberation of thyroglobulin to colloid or inside the colloid

space. The iodine acceptor protein, thyroglobulin, is a huge glycoprotein of 670,000 molecular weight. Each thyroglobulin molecule contains about 120 tyrosine residues and, after iodination, 26 atoms of iodine. The iodination of the tyrosyl residues in thyroglobulin leads to the production of monoiodotyrosine (MIT) and diiodotyrosine (DIT) in the peptide chain. Then two iodotyrosyl groups couple to form an iodothyronine (T_3 or T_4), still within the peptide chain of thyroglobulin. In the iodine-replete gland, each thyroglobulin molecule contains about one iodothyronine molecule (T_3 or T_4). The ratio of T_4 to T_3 molecules is about 4 to 1.

Hormone Secretion. As thyroglobulin is iodinated and coupling of iodotyrosines occurs, some molecules are hydrolyzed to release hormone and others are stored in the colloid for days or weeks. Resorption from colloid occurs by pinocytosis; microvilli or pseudopods on the surface of the thyroid cell surround a small fragment of colloid, and a droplet is thus formed within the cell. The colloid droplet then fuses with a lysosome, producing a phagosome within which thyroid protease hydrolyzes thyroglobulin to its component amino acids. MIT and DIT are released and deiodinated by a dehalogenase present in the microsomal fraction of the cell; the liberated iodide is reincorporated into new MIT and DIT in thyroglobulin. The thyroxine and triiodothyronine released from thyroglobulin are secreted into blood, along with some unhydrolyzed thyroglobulin, small amounts of iodotyrosines, and small amounts of iodide. The thyroid also iodinates other proteins, including a protein very similar to serum albumin, and secretes this iodinated protein into the circulation. Other particulate and soluble iodoproteins are formed in the gland, but their metabolic role is unknown. Some T_4 may be mono-deiodinated to form T_3 within the thyroid cell.

Hormone Transport. The T_4 and T_3 secreted by the gland are transported in plasma largely bound by non-covalent bonds to plasma proteins. Of these, the main and most specific hormone-binding protein is thyroxine-binding inter-alpha-globulin, or TBG. Approximately 70 per cent of T_4 in the blood is carried by this protein. Perhaps 15 per cent of thyroxine is bound to thyroxine-binding prealbumin (TBPA), and the remainder is bound to albumin. Triiodothyronine is less tightly bound to TBG, and insignificant amounts bind to TBPA. T_4 binds firmly to the proteins; only 0.04 per cent of the hormone exists free in solution at any one time. The plasma protein–hormone interaction is reversible. The binding proteins control distribution of hormone between serum and cells, serve as a reservoir constantly replenishing free hormone, and also prevent the iodinated thyronines from being excreted in urine. Free hormone gains access to cells and appears to be the metabolically important fraction. The level of TBG is raised by estrogen treatment and lowered by testosterone. TBG is rarely absent or present in excess on a congenital basis, and its formation is depressed in serious malnutrition or liver disease. In these conditions there may be wide variations in the total thyroid hormone content of plasma, but since the absolute level of free hormone remains constant, the patients remain metabolically normal (Fig. 2).

Free hormone penetrates cells and controls the feedback mechanism in the hypothalamus and pituitary. Approximately one third of the extrathyroidal hormone is loosely bound in the liver. The hormone slowly pene-

Figure 2. Variations in plasma hormone level. Plasma T_4 (and T_3) is largely bound to protein, whose capacity for holding the hormone is partially saturated. The small fraction of free hormone regulates metabolism. Variations in total hormone primarily reflect the protein bound fraction, and must be combined with analysis of the fraction that is free in order to assess properly that hormone which is active on body tissues.

trates most other tissues, reaching an equilibrium within tissue (e.g., muscle) in two or three days.

T_4 leaves the blood with a disappearance half-time of about six days, and T_3 with a half-life of approximately one day. The usual ratio of T_4 to T_3 secreted by the thyroid is 4 to 1. Because of the difference in T_4 and T_3 binding to plasma proteins and metabolism, the ratio of T_4 to T_3 in plasma is about 40 to 1. About 30 per cent of T_4 is converted to T_3 by monodeiodination in peripheral tissues. A significant fraction of this T_3 returns to plasma. T_4 may be considered to be a plasma hormone, or pro-hormone, and T_3 the main tissue hormone. T_3 is less firmly bound to plasma proteins, and enters the cells much more rapidly. T_3 is somewhat selectively taken up and bound by receptor molecules in the cell nuclei. Because of extensive conversion of T_4 to T_3, and the threefold greater metabolic potency of T_3 in comparison to T_4, a large proportion of the metabolic stimulation caused by the hormones may be due to T_3.

Metabolic Action. The exact metabolic action of the hormone is unclear. In animals made hypothyroid by ablation of the gland, administration of thyroid hormone is followed by stimulation of liver nucleic acid synthesis in about 12 hours, increased protein synthesis in 24 hours, and increased mitochondrial oxidative phosphorylation, reaching a peak within two to seven days. Coincident with this increased synthetic and oxidative activity in the cell, the activity of many enzymes, including alpha-ketoglutarate dehydrogenase and isocitrate dehydrogenase, is stimulated.

Usually several hours elapse before any action of the

hormone is observed after administration to animals or man. After a single dose, peak action is seen within two to five days, and gradually decays over a period of two to three weeks. T_3 has a slightly more rapid onset of action than T_4, and its action is more rapidly dissipated. It is of interest that some tissues (brain, spleen, and testes) do not appear to respond to thyroxine.

Treatment of animals with large doses of thyroid hormone or addition of thyroid hormone in vitro induces uncoupling of mitochondrial oxidative phosphorylation. For years one theory of the primary action of thyroid hormone action has centered around this phenomenon. There are two objections to this theory. (1) The change from the sluggish metabolic activity of the hypothyroid state to the normal or mildly hyperactive state induced by administration of physiologic doses of thyroid hormone to animals is accompanied by an increased rate of oxidative phosphorylation *without* loss of efficiency. (2) Studies of mitochondria taken by biopsy from patients with severe hyperthyroidism have shown increased metabolic activity but normally coupled oxidative phosphorylation.

Many other actions of thyroid hormone have been observed, including stimulation of protein synthesis in isolated mitochondria and microsomes, inhibition of pyridine nucleotide-linked dehydrogenases, and swelling of mitochondria.

Recent studies indicate that T_3 and, to a lesser extent, T_4 are accumulated rapidly in the nuclei of responsive tissues and are found tightly but noncovalently linked to a protein associated with chromatin. Although no specific effects of this T_3-protein complex are known, it is postulated that the complex may modulate nuclear RNA synthesis, leading to subsequent increases in protein synthesis and enzyme actions.

Thyroid hormone seems to differ in its mechanism of action from the peptide hormones which act on the adenyl cyclase system at the cell membrane, or the steroid hormones which cause an almost immediate stimulation of nuclear RNA synthesis.

Thyroid Hormone Metabolism. A major portion of T_4 is metabolized by monodeiodination in peripheral tissues to form T_3. In fact T_4 is considered by some as only a pro-hormone, but evidence indicates that T_4 can independently affect tissue metabolism. In any event, T_4 to T_3 conversion must be considered a very important aspect of normal hormone metabolism. In a few instances (in the fetus, in severe illness), low serum and tissue T_3 levels occur in the absence of clinical hypothyroidism. The significance of these findings is not clear.

T_4 and T_3 are metabolized to form butanol-insoluble iodoprotein, some of which may be covalently bound hormone. This material is formed in the microsomal fraction of cells, and some in plasma. Most likely it is a degradative product of thyroid hormone. The alanine side chain of the molecule is metabolized to the acetic acid and pyruvic acid derivatives, analogues which are significantly less active than the parent compound. The hormone is also metabolized extensively by deiodination without rupture of the ether linkage. In some tissues the ether linkage is broken with formation of a hydroquinone and protein-bound DIT. As a final result of metabolism, the hormone is deiodinated and the iodide is returned to plasma to follow the same fate as newly absorbed dietary iodine.

Approximately 10 to 20 per cent of hormone is lost in the feces after secretion by the liver as glucuronide and in other conjugates. A small amount of hormone derived from free T_4 and T_3 in plasma is cleared by the kidneys to urine.

Feedback Control. Each day the thyroid releases approximately 60 to 100 μg of hormonal iodide, of which three fourths is thyroxine and one fourth triiodothyronine. If production falls because of inefficiency in the gland or diminished iodide supply, the level of free hormone in blood decreases, and this alteration is detected by the pituicytes which synthesize increased TSH. The signal recognized by the pituicyte requires RNA and protein synthesis. It is presumed that T_3 and T_4 exert the same sort of metabolic activity on the tissues involved in feedback control as they do in other cells and that this metabolic process constitutes the feedback signal.

In turn, the feedback control of T_4 on the pituitary is modulated by the hypothalamus. Neural centers in the hypothalamus synthesize and secrete the tripeptide pyro-glutamyl-histidyl-proline amide known as thyrotrophin-releasing hormone (TRH). This hormone travels down the hypophysial-portal vessels and stimulates TSH release. There is a delicate balance between the TRH stimulation and T_3-T_4 feedback inhibition of the pituicyte; excess of either can overcome the effect of the other.

TRH is needed for normal tonic control of TSH secretion, as evidenced by the hypothyroidism occurring when the hypothalamus is damaged and TRH is no longer formed. However, the physiologic control of TRH is unclear. Secretion may be altered in response to neural stimuli or cold, but there is no evidence that an excess or deficiency of thyroid hormone alters secretion of TRH. TRH is also a potent stimulant of pituitary prolactin release, but its exact role in the physiologic control of prolactin synthesis and secretion is unknown.

TSH Action on the Thyroid. TSH released by the pituitary binds to a receptor on the thyroid cell membrane and initiates a sequence of reactions, including stimulation of adenyl cyclase and formation of increased intracellular cyclic adenosine monophosphate (cAMP). It is believed that this cAMP "second messenger" somehow mediates all the metabolic stimulatory actions of TSH, including increased uptake and binding of iodide, increased thyroglobulin synthesis, increased colloid resorption, proteolysis, and hormone release.

Other Controls of Thyroid Function. As described above, pituitary TSH is the main regulator of thyroid function. The adrenal gland exerts some control; excess cortisol depresses pituitary production of TSH, possibly by blunting the pituitary sensitivity to TRH. Cortisol also directly depresses the level of TBG in plasma, and augments urinary excretion of iodide. Pregnancy, associated with its increased estrogen production, augments the level of circulating TBG, and increases the concentration of circulating T_4 and T_3. However, the turnover rate of the hormone in blood is proportionately decelerated, so that net hormone utilization remains unchanged. Androgens have a converse effect. Severe illness and stress appear to accelerate thyroid hormone disappearance from plasma. Thyroid hormone utilization is also accelerated in animals by exposure to cold and in man by conditioning to strenuous exercise.

In a very real sense, the average daily intake of iodide controls thyroid function. The feedback control system is designed to maintain a constant level of serum T_4 and T_3. To achieve this the gland must accumulate a constant amount of iodide each day. Thus variations in iodide intake are countered by reciprocal changes in thyroid activity (uptake and binding of iodide, for example) which achieve homeostasis.

THYROID FUNCTION TESTS

In examining a patient with thyroid disease, one seeks to determine the level of tissue metabolic activity and the nature of the thyroid disease. The most direct measure of metabolic activity is the basal metabolic rate (BMR), but the wide range of normal values and the changes in the BMR caused by nonthyroidal factors make the determination of limited diagnostic value. There is no other good approach to assaying the peripheral action of thyroid hormone, although numerous measurements can be made. The serum cholesterol is elevated in hypothyroidism and depressed in hyperthyroidism. The relaxation half-time of the deep tendon reflexes is sometimes shortened below 240 msec in hyperthyroidism, and characteristically prolonged beyond 360 msec in hypothyroidism. Plasma tyrosine levels are elevated in hyperthyroidism, urinary hydroxyproline excretion is depressed in hypothyroidism, and CPK, SGOT, and LDH are elevated in hypothyroidism. None of these tests are useful for definitive diagnosis, because they are nonspecific and similar alterations can be caused by other disease processes.

Protein-Bound Iodine. Lacking a good measure of hormone action in the tissues, most physicians turn to a measure of thyroid hormone in blood. The standard determination for years was the serum protein-bound iodine (PBI) or butanol-extractable iodine (BEI). In the past decade, direct measurements of serum T_4 and T_3 by competitive displacement (T_4D and T_3D) or radioimmunoassay (T_3-RIA and T_4-RIA) have been developed and have replaced PBI and BEI because of their unique specificity. When combined with a measure of saturation of TBG by hormone, such as thyroxine dialyzable fraction (per cent DT_4) or resin uptake (T_3RU), a measure of serum-free thyroxine (FT_4) or triiodothyronine (FT_3) is obtained. The latter values are the most precise measures of thyroid hormone supply to tissues that are currently available.

The PBI measures all iodine in serum precipitable by protein-denaturing agents. Ordinarily this consists mainly of thyroid hormone, but if large quantities of iodide are present, or if any of the roentgenographic contrast medium used for gallbladder examinations, intravenous pyelograms, or arteriograms is present in plasma, the level is falsely elevated. Iodoproteins, formed by the thyroid in augmented amounts in some conditions, e.g., thyroiditis, are also precipitated. Nevertheless, the test is useful as a screening examination and is still widely available. The normal range is 4 to 8 μg of iodine per 100 ml. It is wise to determine total plasma iodine as well; if the level is no more than 2 or 3 μg per 100 ml above the PBI, it can be assumed that contamination with excess quantities of free iodide is not present. The butanol-extractable iodine (BEI) procedure is technically more sophisticated and is more specific for thyroid hormone because it excludes iodopro-

teins. If the PBI exceeds the BEI by more than 20 per cent, abnormal amounts of iodoprotein are present. Neither of these tests is widely used for diagnosis at present.

Serum Thyroxine and Triiodothyronine. A competitive protein-binding assay for thyroxine, similar in principle to the radioimmunoassay of peptide hormones, is widely available. The technique is in practice like the resin uptake test. T_4 is extracted from a serum sample. The T_4 of the plasma sample is then mixed with isotope-labeled T_4 in a standard TBG-containing solution, and its capacity to displace some of the radioactive-labeled hormone from the TBG to a resin is quantitated, by comparison to a standard curve made with known amounts of T_4. The test is technically demanding, but is extremely useful because it is specific for tetraiodothyronine and triiodothyronine. In practice it measures mainly T_4, because so little T_3 is present in plasma. Serum T_4 by displacement analysis (T_4D) is usually 4 to 10 μg per 100 ml, expressed as quantity of thyroxine, not iodide. Serum T_3 can also be measured specifically by this technique if the T_3 is first extracted from serum and separated chromatographically from T_4.

Specific antibodies to T_4 and T_3 have been generated, allowing radioimmunoassay of T_4 (T_4-RIA) and T_3 (T_3-RIA). These techniques are gradually becoming available in most medical centers and commercial laboratories. T_4 (RIA) results are similar to $T_4(D)$. The levels of T_3 reported from various laboratories have varied widely, but most results suggest that normal T_3 (RIA) is about 140 (100 to 200) ng per 100 ml. Usually T_4 and T_3 vary concordantly. Under some circumstances (limited availability of iodine, diminished peroxidase, thyroid hyperplasia), excess T_3 may be produced relative to T_4. Thus measurement of T_3 (RIA) may ultimately replace T_4 (D) or T_4 (RIA) as the standard measure of serum hormone.

Variation in total T_4 or T_3 in serum may occur because of excess or diminution of hormone supply, or because of increase or decrease in serum TBG. Changes in hormone supply represent chemical thyrotoxicosis or hypothyroidism. Increased TBG resulting from pregnancy, estrogen administration, or heredity, or decreased TBG or TBPA resulting from liver disease, severe malnutrition, severe illness, steroids, or testosterone is accompanied by concordant alterations in T_4 and T_3 but reciprocal alterations in per cent free T_4 and T_3, resulting in normal quantities of FT_4 and FT_3. To differentiate between these two possible causes of high or low serum thyroid hormones, one must make an independent assessment of the level of TBG, or measure per cent DT_4 (Fig. 2).

T_3 Resin Uptake (T_3RU). Serum is incubated with a trace amount of labeled T_3 and a resin. Uptake of the tracer by the resin varies directly with total serum T_4 and T_3 and per cent FT_4 if TBG levels are normal, and inversely with serum TBG if it is altered. Resin uptake is *inversely* proportional to, and can be used as an estimate of, unoccupied TBG and varies *directly* with free hormone fraction.

Per Cent FT_4. Serum plus a labeled T_4 tracer is dialyzed to equilibrium against a buffer. The dialyzable fraction, normally ± 0.04 per cent of the total T_4, represents the free hormone fraction.

Free Thyroid Hormone. Multiplication of the total serum $T_4 \times$ per cent FT_4 yields FT_4, the actual concentration of free—non-protein-bound—T_4. The usual range is 1.5 to 3.5 ng per 100 ml. The same measure can be derived for T_3 (FT_3) if T_3 concentration and per cent FT_3 are available.

In most laboratories advantage is taken of the relationship of the resin uptake to per cent FT_4 in order to calculate an "index," as first suggested by Clark and Horn. Total $T_4 \times \dfrac{\text{Patient's } T_3 \text{ RU}}{\text{Standard } T_3 \text{ RU}}$ equals the free thyroxine index (FTI), which is a very good approximation of free T_4 and correlates exactly with FT_4.

FT_4 or FTI constitutes the best available contemporary measure of hormone supply to tissues, is independent of variations in plasma thyroid hormone binding proteins, and is not affected by excess iodide or iodide-containing compounds.

Two problems must be remembered when performing function tests. Excess iodine in any form may elevate the PBI and BEI and depress the radioactive iodide uptake test. Roentgenographic contrast dyes may for a short time depress the radioactive uptake test, and for periods of weeks or months falsely elevate the PBI and BEI. Alterations in binding proteins caused by heredity, hormones, illness, liver disease, or malnutrition can cause increases or decreases in the PBI, BEI, serum thyroxine, and T_3 values without altering the level of free thyroid hormone.

Radioactive Iodine Uptake. Another commonly used measure of thyroid activity is the thyroidal radioactive iodide uptake (RAIU). The patient is given a trace dose of radioactive iodide, and the fraction accumulated in the gland is determined at 2, 6, or 24 hours, the last of these being the most widely used end-point. The normal uptake is inversely dependent upon available iodide supply. In areas where the iodide intake is 150 to 200 μg per day, it ranges from 20 to 50 per cent. In most of the United States, an increase in iodide in the diet up to 400 to 600 μg per day has reduced the normal range to 10 to 25 per cent. This procedure measures the activity of the thyroid trapping and binding process, which can be augmented owing to excess TSH stimulation or because of inherent thyroid hyperactivity. The RAIU is characteristically elevated in areas of iodide deficiency.

Perchlorate Discharge Test. The presence of trapped but unbound iodide in the thyroid gland can be ascertained by administering 1 gram of $KClO_4$ orally two hours after a ^{131}I tracer. Discharge of more than 10 per cent is characteristic of thyroid organification defects of congenital (e.g., Pendred's syndrome) or acquired (e.g., Hashimoto's thyroiditis) types (Fig. 3).

Serum TSH Assay. Measurement of serum TSH by RIA is now a standard and useful determination. Normal TSH varies from undetectable to 8 μU per milliliter. TSH is characteristically suppressed by exogenous or endogenous excess of thyroid hormone. Elevations of 20 to 400 μU per milliliter occur in primary thyroid failure of any cause. Mild elevations (10 to 20 μU) are of less certain significance and may represent mild hypothyroidism or euthyroidism (compensated hypothyroidism) achieved by the elevated TSH. Undetectable or normal TSH levels are found in pituitary hypothyroidism, hypothalamic damage, and in almost all patients with thyrotoxicosis.

Tests for Specific Conditions. The nature of the disease process affecting the thyroid can be evaluated by a number of other procedures.

Figure 3. $KClO_4$ discharge test. In the usual test thyroid RAIU is measured sequentially over two to three hours after a tracer dose of ^{131}I. One gram of $KClO_4$ is given orally, and thyroid uptake determinations are continued. In this patient with organification defect resulting from complete lack of peroxidase, $KClO_4$ caused nearly complete release of accumulated iodide, indicating that the tracer existed in the gland as iodide and had not been bound in the normal manner to thyroglobulin.

T_3 Suppression Test. A high thyroid ^{131}I uptake caused by endogenous TSH can be reduced in most circumstances to or below the normal range by administration of 100 μg of triiodothyronine daily for one week. Serum T_4 will also be lowered, and its determination is useful when administration of radioiodine is contraindicated (e.g., pregnancy). Thyroid activity is not suppressible in most patients with active Graves' disease (see Ch. 837). This response is seen whether the basal RAIU is elevated or normal and is accepted as the most characteristic abnormality in this illness. However, nonsuppressibility also occurs in the closely related syndrome of Hashimoto's thyroiditis and if autonomous functioning thyroid nodules are present.

TSH Stimulation Test. The presence of functioning thyroid tissue can be evaluated by administration of 5 units of TSH subcutaneously daily for three days, with a radioactive iodine uptake test (and sometimes a scan) before and after. TSH should raise the radioactive

Figure 4. TSH responses to intravenous TRH. The normal rapid elevation of plasma TSH after TRH is obliterated in thyrotoxicosis, by thyroid hormone administration, or in pituitary destruction. An excessive response occurs in primary thyroid failure.

NORMAL   THYROIDITIS

Figure 5. Fluorescent thyroid scan. Fluorescence induced by [241]Americium indicates distribution and concentration of stable [127]I in the normal gland. By contrast, the gland affected by Hashimoto's thyroiditis is nearly devoid of iodine.

iodide uptake to a normal level or at least double it in a patient whose basal function is low because of deficient TSH. The test is also useful for demonstrating normal tissue which has been suppressed by a functioning "hot" nodule.

TRH Test (Fig. 4). The ability of the pituitary to secrete TSH can be elevated by administration of 400 μg of TRH intravenously and measuring serum TSH during the subsequent 90 minutes. Hypothalamic hypothyroidism is associated with normal basal TSH, responding normally to the administration of exogenous TRH. Primary thyroid failure is associated with a high basal level of TSH hyper-responsive to TRH. Hypothyroidism resulting from pituitary failure causes low serum TSH and absent TRH response. Administration of replacement doses of T_4 or T_3 or excess endogenous or exogenous T_4 or T_3 obliterates the response to TRH.

Antibodies and LATS. Autoimmunity against thyroid antigens can be demonstrated by measuring antithyroglobulin antibodies by the tanned red cell agglutination procedure, or antithyroid microsomal antibodies by the immunofluorescent, complement fixation, or tanned red cell agglutination methods. Positive tests are found in Hashimoto's thyroiditis, primary thyroid failure, and Graves' disease.

Long-acting thyroid stimulator (LATS), measured by a bioassay described in Ch. 837, is characteristic of Graves' disease.

Thyroid Scans. A scintiscan performed after administration of [199]Te or radioactive iodine provides anatomic localization of functioning thyroid tissue. Adenomas may appear inactive ("cold") or hyperactive ("hot"). Graves' disease and Hashimoto's thyroiditis show diffuse uptake, whereas multinodular goiter gives a mottled picture. Uptake outside the thyroid identifies aberrant thyroid tissue, metastatic thyroid cancer, and struma ovarii.

Recently, fluorescent scanning with a [241]Am source has been developed. This technique identifies concentration and distribution of the stable [127]I present in the

gland (Fig. 5). It is a useful technique when radioisotopes should be avoided (children, pregnant women, lactation). In addition, it provides another independent index of thyroid function. The Hashimoto's gland is characteristically and diagnostically found to be devoid of stored iodine. Also, the thyroid can be shown to have a normal appearance and iodine content in pituitary hypothyroidism and when uptake of a tracer is suppressed by administration of exogenous hormone or iodide.

Needle Biopsy. Needle biopsy of the thyroid is a useful procedure in properly selected cases and can provide a histologic diagnosis when all other techniques fail.

Initial Selection of Function Tests. In most thyroid diseases careful history and physical examination lead to the diagnosis, and laboratory procedures serve to confirm the clinical impression. In the initial evaluation of most patients, it is useful to measure the serum thyroxine, the free thyroxine index, and occasionally the radioactive iodine uptake. A scan can be done at the same time if there is a question of nonuniformity of gland function raised by history or examination of the neck. The TSH level should be checked if hypothyroidism is suggested. The test for antithyroglobulin antibodies is also useful in the initial evaluation of many patients. To follow the progress of therapy, the most useful procedures are serial determinations of serum thyroxine. Frequent measurement of the patient's weight also constitutes an excellent measure of whole body metabolism.

Further tests are dictated by the progress of the evaluation. Many specialized assays are available if needed to define unusual congenital or acquired diseases.

Davis, P. J.: Factors affecting the determination of the serum protein bound iodine. Am. J. Med., 40:918, 1956.

DeGroot, L. J.: Kinetic analysis of iodine metabolism. J. Clin. Endocrinol. Metab., 26:149, 1966.

Dowling, J. T., Appleton, W. G., and Nicoloff, J. T.: Thyroxine turnover during human pregnancy. J. Clin. Endocrinol. Metab., 27:1749, 1967.

Dumont, J. E.: The action of thyrotropin on thyroid metabolism. Vitam. Horm., 29:287, 1971.

Hershman, J. M., and Pittman, J. A.: Utility of the radioimmunoassay of serum thyrotrophin in man. Ann. Intern. Med., 74:481, 1971.

Hoffer, P. B., Gottschalk, A., and Refetoff, S.: Thyroid scanning techniques: The old and the new. Curr. Prob. Radiol., 2:5, 1972.

Kaplan, S. L., Grumbach, M. M., Friesen, H. G., and Costom, B. H.: Thryotropin-releasing factor (TRF) effect on secretion of human pituitary prolactin and thyrotropin in children and in idiopathic hypopituitary dwarfism. J. Clin. Endocrinol. Metab., 35:825, 1972.

Lieblick, J., and Utiger, R. D.: Triiodothyronine radioimmunoassay. J. Clin. Invest., 51:157, 1972.

Oppenheimer, J. H.: Role of plasma proteins in the binding, distribution and metabolism of the thyroid hormones. N. Engl. J. Med., 278:1153, 1968.

Ormston, B. J., Garry, R., Coyer, R. J., Besser, G. M., and Hall, R.: Thyrotrophin releasing hormone as a thyroid function test. Lancet, 2:10, 1971.

Rapoport, B., and DeGroot, L. J.: Current concepts of thyroid physiology. Semin. Nucl. Med., 1:265, 1971.

Robin, N. I., Hagen, S. R., Collaco, F., Refetoff, S., and Selenkow, H. A.: Serum tests for measurement of thyroid function. Hormones, 2:266, 1971.

Roitt, I. M., and Doniach, D.: Thyroid autoimmunity. Br. Med. Bull., 16:152, 1960.

Sterling, K., and Brenner, M. A.: Free thyroxine in human serum. Simplified measurement with the aid of magnesium precipitation. J. Clin. Invest., 45:153, 1966.

Taunton, O. D., McDaniel, H. G., and Pittman, J. A.: Standardization of TSH testing. J. Clin. Endocrinol. Metab., 25:266, 1965.

Vale, W., Burgus, R., and Guillemin, R.: On the mechanism of action of TRF: Effects of cycloheximide and actinomycin on the release of TSH stimulated in vitro by TRF and its inhibition by thyroxine. Neuroendocrinology, 3:34, 1968.

Wolff, J.: Transport of iodide and other anions in the thyroid gland. Physiol. Rev., 44:45, 1964.

837. GRAVES' DISEASE AND HYPERTHYROIDISM

Hyperthyroidism refers to a state of heightened thyroid gland activity associated with the production of excess quantities of thyroid hormone. The clinical state is also referred to as *thyrotoxicosis*. Most commonly hyperthyroidism is part of a syndrome which may include goiter, exophthalmos, and pretibial myxedema, known as *Graves' disease* or *Basedow's disease*. Thyrotoxicosis can also be caused by excessive production of hormone by a *single "toxic" nodule*, by a *toxic multinodular goiter*, by occasional *functioning thyroid carcinomas*, or by *medication*. Rarely, it is caused by a TSH-secreting pituitary adenoma, is associated with acromegaly, occurs because of production of TSH-like material in trophoblastic tumors or embryonal-cell carcinomas, or is due to hyperfunctioning teratoma (struma ovarii).

Incidence. Hyperthyroidism is not a reportable condition, so exact data on incidence are unavailable. Incidence is probably in excess of 3 per 10,000 adults per year. It is largely a disease of adult women, with a sex ratio of approximately 5 to 1. Peak incidence is between 30 and 50 years of age.

Etiology and Pathogenesis. The manifestations of Graves' disease fall into two categories: (1) the primary disease involving the thyroid (plus eyes and skin), and (2) the circulatory, neurologic, and metabolic abnormalities, described below, which are secondarily caused by excess thyroid hormone produced by the thyroid gland impinging on tissues.

There are two recurring themes in discussions of the etiology of Graves' disease: (1) It may be the result of

emotional trauma, or (2) it may be an "autoimmune" disease. The previous impression that the thyroid in Graves' disease was responding to excess TSH is erroneous, because TSH in plasma of patients with this disorder is characteristically reduced or absent, apparently suppressed by increased circulating thyroid hormone.

For decades it has been suggested that Graves' disease is induced by emotional stress, because of the frequency with which physicians obtain a history of emotional trauma occurring before the onset of hyperthyroidism. Characteristically the event is a marital problem or death of a loved one. Although such testimonials are frequent, the meager factual data available are inconclusive. Psychiatric evaluations indicate that there is nothing special about the individual who becomes a victim of Graves' disease, and that the incidence of emotional stress in these patients is comparable to that in a control population. Perhaps, in the individuals who report a stressful circumstance, Graves' disease was already present and made the emotional reaction more dramatic. Also, the patient suffering from Graves' disease has anxiety and tremulousness as a result of the illness; these symptoms may be misinterpreted as causal.

Autoimmunity directed against thyroid antigens is currently thought to be the most probable cause. Antibodies directed against endogenous thyroid antigens were detected in patients with Hashimoto's thyroiditis in 1956, and several thyroid antibody-antigen systems have since been found in patients with thyroiditis, idiopathic myxedema, and Graves' disease (see Ch. 838). Sixty to 80 per cent of patients with Graves' disease have antibodies directed against thyroglobulin or against thyroid microsomes. In addition, Adams and Purves described in 1956 a factor (long-acting thyroid stimulator, LATS), present in the serum of about half the patients with Graves' disease, which stimulated the release of hormone from the prelabeled thyroid of a test animal. LATS is now known to be a polyclonal gamma globulin, probably an autoantibody directed against a component of the thyroid cell membrane. LATS can be neutralized by reacting with antibodies prepared against 7S human IgG. LATS adsorbs to thyroid microsomes, but the reaction is not entirely specific and does not require complement. In addition to causing release of hormone, LATS stimulates increased synthesis of nucleic acids and proteins, increases incorporation of phosphate into phospholipids, stimulates glucose metabolism, and causes thyroid growth. A contemporary interpretation is that LATS is an autoantibody which mimics the action of TSH and stimulates the synthesis and release of thyroid hormone. In patients whose thyroids are capable of responding to such a trophic stimulus, LATS may be the mediator of hyperthyroxinemia. LATS crosses the placenta and is the cause of transient hyperthyroidism in some neonates born to mothers who have high circulating levels of the antibody.

LATS is, however, found in at most 80 per cent of patients with Graves' disease, and its presence or level does not correlate uniformly with thyroid hyperactivity. Recent data suggest that there may be other "thyrotrophic" antibody systems present which can be detected in different assays. One of these is the "human thyroid stimulator" (HTS) of Onaya et al.; another possible factor is the "LATS protector" of Adams.

In addition to circulating antibodies (humoral immune response), there is much evidence for cell-mediated immunity (CMI) in Graves' disease, as well as in Hashimoto's thyroiditis and primary myxedema. The CMI is probably involved in a cell-destructive response. Our theory is that Graves' disease is due to autoimmunity, and that its manifestations represent a balance between the stimulatory or blocking effect of circulating antibodies such as LATS and HTS and the cell-destructive effects of CMI.

Exophthalmos has also been related to autoimmunity. In serum of patients with exophthalmos, a factor causing experimental exophthalmos in animals is found. Various reports also indicate an abnormality in binding of gamma globulin from exophthalmic patients to orbital antigens, and two studies indicate that patients with exophthalmos have CMI against these antigens.

Why the body should develop a humoral antibody and CMI response active against its own tissues remains unknown. There is no evidence for an abnormal antigen in these conditions, or for an abnormal sequestration or release of antigen. Because of the association of thyroid autoimmunity with immunity against several other organs of the body, it seems possible that Graves' disease is basically a manifestation of deranged immune homeostasis.

Much evidence indicates that *a strong hereditary factor is involved in Graves' disease, Hashimoto's thyroiditis, and myxedema,* and that the three diseases are intimately related. Patients with Graves' disease and thyroiditis usually have a family history positive for the same condition. Thyroid autoantibodies, including LATS, are found in relatives of patients with these diseases. The incidence of any one of the other two diseases is increased in relatives of patients who have one of the three. Some patients appear to have a combination of thyroiditis and Graves' disease that has been called "Hashitoxicosis."

Another intriguing bit of circumstantial evidence related to etiology is the occasionally reported occurrence of Graves' disease after consumption of desiccated thyroid for weight reduction. It is as if the ingestion of thyroid hormone somehow conditioned the body to a high level of the substance and "demanded" continued thyroid hyperfunction after the exogenous hormone was withdrawn.

Iodine administration occasionally induces hyperthyroidism. This Jod-Basedow phenomenon typically occurs in areas of endemic goiter when iodinization of salt is introduced, but can occur after administration of iodine to patients in nonendemic areas. Apparently the thyroid was functioning autonomously at a hyperactive level before the introduction of iodine, but was unable to manifest hyperthyroidism owing to the limitation of hormone synthesis imposed by the low iodide intake.

Little is known about other causes of hyperthyroidism. The etiology of the toxic nodular goiter, the toxic solitary nodule, or the hyperfunctioning thyroid carcinoma is related to the problem of tumor formation. Hyperthyroidism found in association with acromegaly may be due to increased TSH production, although this has not been established. Hyperthyroidism associated with trophoblastic tumors is due to the production of a trophic substance by the tumor. Placental thyrotrophin is a normal placental product; a slightly different protein is formed in excess in patients with hydatidiform mole and in choriocarcinoma. It is immunologically related to bovine thyrotrophin, but does not cross-react with antibodies to human thyrotrophin.

Pathology. The main pathologic abnormality in Graves' disease is evident in the size of the thyroid cells. The cells are tall, and the size of the average follicle is reduced. Small amounts of colloid are present in the lumen. The picture is analogous to a gland under intense TSH stimulation. In addition there is characteristically an infiltration of mononuclear cells, mainly small lymphocytes and some plasma cells, and lymphoid germinal centers may be apparent. Sometimes the process shades into a picture characteristic of Hashimoto's thyroiditis. There is generalized lymph node hyperplasia, the thymus is enlarged, and the proportion of active thymic tissue is increased. Active germinal centers are also found in the thymus, and the histology is similar to that of myasthenia gravis or lupus erythematosus. The muscles are usually microscopically normal, but occasionally the cells are atrophic, multiple nuclei are present, striations are indistinct, and a lymphocyte infiltrate is apparent. Hepatic changes include cellular edema, focal necrosis, and lymphocyte infiltrates. The epidermis and dermis are thinned. Bones may show osteoporosis or osteomalacia. Pathology of the eye and "localized myxedema" are described below.

Clinical Manifestations. In many patients the changes are so obvious as to be inescapable; in others the subtlety of the disease defies anything except a laboratory diagnosis. The patient may notice weakness, increased fatigue, insomnia, weight loss, or tremulousness. The skin becomes fine and moist, and there is excess perspiration. The hair thins, and the nails become thin and brittle. Increased tolerance to cold or decreased tolerance to moderate heat is noted. Friends observe that the eyes are prominent, and the patient appears to be staring. Double vision, blurred vision, burning, tearing, and decreased visual acuity may occur. Often the patient finds a mass in the neck, although this produces few local symptoms. A hyperactive heart, palpitations, dyspnea on exertion, and ankle edema may be evident, usually in the absence of congestive failure. Weight loss occurs despite increase in appetite. There may occasionally be abdominal pain reminiscent of an ulcer and frequent loose bowel movements. Subdeltoid bursitis may occur. Menstrual periods become scanty, the cycle is shortened, some periods may be missed, and fertility is reduced. Usually libido is not altered. Thirst and polyuria are sometimes noted. Weakness of the muscles is prominent; it may be the primary symptom in older persons who have had chronic low-grade thyroid hyperfunction for months or years. Such patients report that they cannot climb stairs or get up easily from a chair. Pruritus is frequently noticed, and occasionally hives occur.

On examination the patient appears anxious, tremulous, and restless, and is typically quick to cooperate. The hair is fine and thin, and females may show some temporal recession of the hairline. The skin feels moist, hot, thin, or even silky, and pigmentation may be increased. Vitiligo, especially of the hands and feet, is present in about 7 per cent of cases. The nails are thin, and the hyponychium is often seen to have receded, forming an irregular concave erosion under the distal portion of the nail. This change (onycholysis or Plummer's nails) is most typically found bilaterally on the fourth digit. The elbows are sometimes red, as are the palms.

The eyes may appear prominent, and the sclera is visible above the iris on upward or downward gaze (lid lag). The lids may be grossly puffy. Proptosis (forward displacement of the globes in the orbits) may be evident, and if severe the lids may not close adequately. Edema of the scleral conjunctiva may form loose pockets filled with clear liquid (chemosis). Extraocular muscle function may be diminished, often first with a loss of upward gaze, and later with a fixed strabismus caused by contracture of a damaged muscle. In severe cases total loss of ocular motility and convergence are present. With proptosis the edge of the lacrimal gland may be felt bulging below the supraorbital ridge. The beefy red insertion of the lateral rectus can sometimes be seen. Depending on the severity of the process, there may be papilledema or hemorrhages and exudates in the retina. Visual acuity may be severely reduced.

The thyroid typically is enlarged, usually three to four times the normal size, although rarely the gland may be of normal dimensions. Usually the gland is symmetrically involved and may be lobulated. It characteristically feels rather firm and beefy, and often the pyramidal lobe is palpable. Lymph nodes are often present in the supraclavicular fossae and may be tender. A systolic bruit may be heard over the thyroid or palpated ("thrill") in very vascular glands.

The precordium is hyperactive, and the heart sounds are intensified. A systolic murmur is usually audible, and sometimes a scratching systolic sound (Lerman's sound) is heard in the second or third left intercostal space. Murmurs present before the onset of thyroid disease are louder. Occasionally murmurs suggestive of mitral insufficiency or stenosis are audible; they disappear after hyperthyroidism is controlled. Tachycardia is usually present, and there is an increased propensity to atrial fibrillation. Axillary lymph nodes are frequently palpable; on examination of the abdomen, the spleen or liver or both may be minimally enlarged. Muscle strength and bulk may be reduced. Reflexes are exaggerated in speed and strength.

Rarely, typical attacks of hypokalemic periodic paralysis occur during severe hyperthyroidism, especially in young men of Oriental extraction.

Occasionally patients develop severe hyperthyroidism but present few classic manifestations. In this picture, termed *masked hyperthyroidism,* to which older people are most prone, the tremor, anxiety, and hyperkinesis may be lacking. Instead, the patient is apathetic, sometimes mentally confused, or obtunded. There may be extreme weakness and muscle atrophy. The skin may not be thinned, and the sweating and eye signs may also be lacking. Usually, however, tachycardia, goiter, and low-grade fever are present. A coincidental atrial fibrillation and weight loss should suggest this diagnosis.

Diagnosis.   The flagrant case with all the characteristic manifestations is usually recognized by laymen who refer the patient to the physician for therapy. Other patients do not present with more than a few of the signs and symptoms of Graves' disease, and in these patients laboratory studies become critical. Diagnosis begins with the history and physical examination. Serial weights should be recorded, because progressive loss of weight is a strong clue to the diagnosis. To prove the diagnosis, the serum thyroxine (or better, the free thyroxine index) and RAIU are probably the most useful tests. The BMR, cholesterol, T_3RU, and reflex time may occasionally be helpful. The antithyroglobulin or antimicrosomal antibody tests are useful, because a positive test indicates that the patient has some variety of thyroid autoimmune disease. Often patients develop a normochromic and normocytic anemia with 9 to 11 grams of hemoglobin per 100 ml. Alkaline phosphatase may be elevated because of increased rate of bone turnover, and serum calcium, urinary calcium, and hydroxyproline excretion may be increased. Bilirubin is occasionally elevated. Roentgenograms of the skull and views of the orbits should be obtained if there is a question of an intracerebral or orbital space-occupying lesion, especially if unilateral exophthalmos occurs before the onset of hyperthyroidism. All the tests must be carefully evaluated in the light of the patient's known iodide intake, exposure to radiographic contrast media, and medications. If there is doubt about the diagnosis, a T_3 suppression test may be useful. *Nonsuppressibility of the thyroid is considered the most characteristic feature of Graves' disease.*

T_3 Toxicosis.   In some patients who have clinical symptoms suggestive of hyperthyroidism, but in whom the radioactive iodide uptake and serum thyroxine are normal, measurement of elevated plasma triiodothyronine may confirm the condition known as "T_3 toxicosis." This condition can be the presenting feature of Graves' disease, but is more frequently found in patients with an autonomous nodule or residual tissue after radioiodide (RAI) or surgical therapy, or in areas of iodine deficiency. Some reports indicate that as many as one tenth of patients have T_3 toxicosis without elevated T_4 levels. This has not been the author's experience. Although it is imperative to remember that T_3 toxicosis can explain the unusual case, the great majority of patients present with both high T_4 and high T_3, and cause no difficulty in diagnosis by the more commonly available serum T_4 measurement.

It is especially important to consider this diagnosis in elderly patients who have atrial fibrillation or congestive heart failure. Other diagnostic hints are unexplained diarrhea, severe muscle weakness, bursitis, and vitiligo of the hands and feet.

Severe pulmonary disease, anxiety, carcinoma, malabsorption, cirrhosis, and myasthenia can have features similar to thyrotoxicosis, and must be considered in the differential diagnosis.

In this age of dependence upon chemistry, it is not rare to be faced with a patient who has negligible signs and symptoms but in whom an elevated T_4 or T_3 has been detected by chance. In such patients it is wise to establish as carefully as possible the presence or absence of disease by RAIU, T_3 suppression test, and FT_4 or FT_3 levels, and then to observe events for a period of time. The process may subside, show evidence of damage to cardiac, hepatic, or osseous tissues, indicating need for treatment, show no change, or progress gradually into overt thyrotoxicosis.

In fact, major reliance is placed on the laboratory tests. A significant elevation of FT_4 or FT_3 can alone be the determining feature of Graves' disease and demand therapy.

The RAIU, formerly a very useful test, is now of less value because elevated intake of iodide has depressed the normal and thyrotoxic values and confused the area of overlap between them. It is not necessarily required for diagnosis, but is useful when planning RAI therapy and with a scan when defining autonomous thyroid function caused by an adenoma or multinodular goiter.

Differentiation from Other Mitochondrial Diseases. The symptoms and signs of thyrotoxicosis are due to hypermetabolism, and theoretically could be mimicked by any cause of uncontrolled mitochondrial function. In fact few conditions have been reported in which mitochondrial oxidative phosphorylation is disturbed, and only one syndrome has caused confusion in diagnosis. A unique illness suggestive of thyrotoxicosis was reported by Luft. Weakness, excessive perspiration, marked hypermetabolism, and weight loss led to thyroidectomy, but induction of overt hypothyroidism failed to control the illness. Muscle mitochondria from this patient were unusually abundant and large, and had excessive crista formation. Respiration was not controlled as in normal tissues, and uncoupled oxidative phosphorylation was demonstrated. The cause of this illness is unknown.

Other cases that less clearly represent mitochondrial disease have been described, but none resemble thyrotoxicosis. Distorted mitochondria in hepatocytes and a defect in electron transport between dehydrogenases and the cytochromes have been observed in the fatal congenital "cerebro-hepato-renal syndrome." Abnormal increased, diminished, and absent muscle mitochrondria have been detected in various idiopathic myopathies, in steroid-induced myopathy, and in cardiac muscle in experimental left ventricular failure. Experimental iron deficiency can lower tissue cytochrome content, and copper deficiency may be associated with diminished cytochrome oxidase. The clinical correlates of these observations are unknown. Considering the importance of mitochondria in cell homeostasis, they so far appear to be remarkably immune from disease-related pathology.

Therapy. The choice of therapy for hyperthyroidism resulting from Graves' disease has been debated for decades, and final resolution is not yet in sight. During the period from 1950 to 1970, sentiment gradually swung to the use of RAI in most adults because of its simplicity and absence of surgical complications or hospitalization. When hypothyroidism was observed to occur in 40 to 70 per cent of patients in the 5- to 10-year period after treatment with "conventional" doses of RAI, many clinics adopted a "low dose" [131]I treatment program. This clearly reduced the incidence of early hypothyroidism, but is associated with a need for multiple doses and continued treatment of many patients with various other agents over one to five years. Dissatisfaction with ^{131}I has swung the pendulum, to some extent, back toward surgery. In fact this treatment is now the author's first choice for most young adults through age 40. Although the three common treatments for hyperthyroidism are excellent, each has its built-in disadvantages and none of the therapies can be considered ideal.

Radioactive Iodide. For adults older than 25, administration of radioactive iodide appears to be a satisfactory form of treatment. So far there is no evidence that this therapy causes an increased incidence of leukemia or significant somatic damage. Hypothyroidism, attributable to an "overeffective" treatment, is a disadvantage and will be discussed below. The radiation dose delivered to the gonads during treatment is similar to that given during an intravenous pyelogram or barium enema and is probably inconsequential. Patients have now been treated with this agent for nearly three

decades, and there is still no evidence of ^{131}I-induced tumor formation. Evidence on this point must continually be accumulated, but for the moment it does not appear that radiation of the adult thyroid with ^{131}I leads to subsequent thyroid malignancy.

A major difficulty with radioactive iodine treatment has been the onset of hypothyroidism, either immediately or long after the treatment. The incidence of hypothyroidism may approach 40 to 70 per cent after ten years. Most patients are now treated with a dose of radioactive iodide approximately half that used five or ten years ago, in an effort to diminish the incidence of hypothyroidism.

Therapy is planned to deliver a retained dose of 40 to 100 μC per estimated gram of weight at 24 hours, the dose per gram increasing with thyroid size from 20 to 100 grams. With this dose, many patients do not achieve immediate euthyroidism, and require ancillary therapy such as administration of potassium iodide solution or an antithyroid drug if hyperthyroidism is not controlled within two or three months. These agents should be continued for 6 to 12 months, because the full effect of radiation is not obtained until then. At the end of 6 or 12 months, the potassium iodide or the antithyroid drug or both are discontinued, and if hyperthyroidism recurs, a second treatment of radioactive iodide is given. Thirty to 50 per cent of the patients need a second treatment, and occasionally a third dose is required (Fig. 6). In selected individuals, in whom it is imperative that hyperthyroidism be rapidly controlled, a two- to threefold larger dose is administered, and re-treatment is given at three months if required. If prompt control is necessary, antithyroid drug and then KI can be instituted within one day of administration of the therapeutic ^{131}I dose, with loss of about one fifth of the radiation effect. Control of the disease with this combined treatment is usually achieved in one to four weeks.

All women in the reproductive age who are to receive

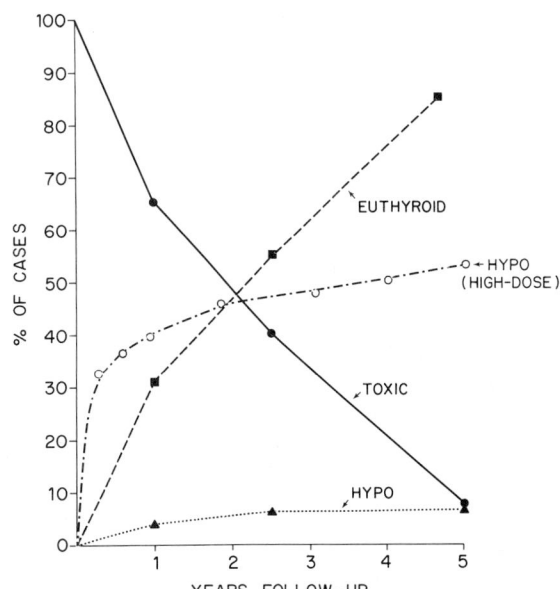

Figure 6. Graphic representation of current therapeutic results achieved with "low-dose" [131]I therapy of thyrotoxicosis. Although hypothyroidism is infrequent in the first five years, many patients remain toxic for a prolonged period after initial therapy. The high and progressively increasing incidence of hypothyroidism after "high-dose" therapy is also indicated.

radioactive iodide must be questioned for possible pregnancy or lactation, which are contraindications to this treatment. It is best to give the radioactive iodide shortly after a menstrual period. Women should be advised to avoid pregnancy for a period of at least one year, because the possible need for re-treatment will not be eliminated before this time has elapsed.

There was a recent wave of interest in the use of ^{125}I for therapy, on the basis that it would be less likely to produce hypothyroidism. The few reported trials do not establish any improved efficacy of ^{125}I over ^{131}I.

Antithyroid Drugs. Children and young adults are best treated initially by a long-term course of antithyroid drug. Patients with small goiters, recent onset of disease, and mild symptoms respond most frequently to this therapy and are thus the preferred candidates. Usually propylthiouracil, 100 mg every eight hours, or methimazole, 10 mg every eight hours, is given orally. If this is not effective within two to four weeks, the dose may be doubled. Rarely, 1 gram of propylthiouracil or 100 mg of methimazole will be needed daily. It is imperative that the patient be instructed to take the medication at the scheduled times. Antithyroid drugs have a short duration of action, and one of the main causes of treatment failure is that patients do not adhere to a rigorous time schedule. As a response is obtained, the dose is progressively lowered to 50 or 100 mg of propylthiouracil every 12 hours, or a comparable dose of methimazole. Many patients can be maintained on a single daily dose of medication. Some physicians prefer to maintain a higher dose of the antithyroid drug and to add replacement doses of thyroid hormone in order to avoid hypothyroidism. Overtreatment with antithyroid drugs will of course block formation of thyroid hormone, lower the T_4, and cause a TSH response. This is usually evident in rapid enlargement of the thyroid.

Symptoms of thyrotoxicosis usually abate within two to six weeks, and the patient should be metabolically normal after this period of time. The thyroid gland, in the absence of induced hypothyroidism, either remains at the original size or gets smaller. The latter is a favorable prognostic sign. Another favorable prognostic sign is return of thyroid suppressibility after administration of T_3 (T_3 suppression test), which has been documented to occur in some patients as early as eight weeks after the start of antithyroid drug treatment. The medication is continued for one to two years and then is gradually discontinued. Half the treated patients will enter a prolonged remission. Others will relapse within 1 to 12 months, and are either re-treated with the same drug or given an alternative form of therapy. The incidence of remission is higher after the first year of therapy, and decreases among patients who have failed to remit with each subsequent year of treatment.

During antithyroid drug administration, patients must be carefully monitored for occurrence of side effects such as pruritus, rash, and epigastric pain, and for the more serious but less frequent occurrence of neutropenia or even agranulocytosis. A mild skin rash may disappear spontaneously. Pruritus can be treated by the addition of an antihistaminic drug. A severe rash calls for discontinuation of the antithyroid drug. It is often useful to institute therapy with an alternative antithyroid medication, because cross-reactions do not always occur. The leukocyte count should be checked at each visit during administration of antithyroid drugs. Occa-

sionally, a count as low as 3500 cells per cubic millimeter may be observed spontaneously in patients with thyrotoxicosis. If, however, the blood count falls from a normal range down to a level of 3500 or lower during therapy, the antithyroid drug should be discontinued. Occasionally agranulocytosis develops, requiring intensive care in a hospital, but is usually reversible.

Surgery. Subtotal thyroidectomy performed by a skilled surgeon is also very effective. It is the preferred therapy in children who fail to respond to antithyroid drugs or have had adverse reaction to the drug, in young adults who do not wish to pursue a prolonged course of treatment, in patients who are apprehensive about the possible adverse effects of radioactive iodide, in patients who have huge thyroids, and in patients whose glands are believed to harbor a carcinoma. As the initial mode of treatment for adults of 20 to 40 years, it usually offers the most prompt return to normal function. Although no hard data can be offered, it also seems preferable to RAI therapy in patients with marked exophthalmos. The procedure is accompanied by a mortality rate of less than 1 in 1000, an incidence of permanent hypothyroidism in from 5 to 40 per cent, recurrence of thyrotoxicosis in 5 per cent or more (depending on the extent of the initial resection), occasional instances of damage to the recurrent laryngeal nerves and parathyroids, need for hospitalization, and considerable expense. Patients should be rendered euthyroid with an antithyroid drug in preparation for surgery, and should be given potassium iodide (saturated solution of potassium iodide, 2 drops twice daily) or Lugol's solution (ten drops twice daily) for a period of one to two weeks before the operation. Iodide decreases vascularity of the gland and makes the surgical procedure less difficult. Induction of euthyroidism before surgery is imperative, because cardiac arrhythmias during surgery are frequent in patients with thyrotoxicosis.

Iodine. Iodine was introduced for control of hyperthyroidism 50 years ago but is rarely used today as the sole treatment. When given in doses of greater than 6 mg per day, iodide blocks further formation of iodotyrosines (Wolff-Chaikoff effect), and diminishes release of thyroid hormone by inhibiting proteolysis of thyroglobulin. Most patients are benefited initially by iodide, although some respond only partially, and some have an exacerbation of their illness despite continuation of iodine. Iodine treatment may induce hypothyroidism, especially in patients who have previously been treated with surgery or radioactive iodide. Addition of iodine to the regimen of patients who are already receiving antithyroid drugs has been known to induce a severe exacerbation of hyperthyroidism. At present the three more certain and well defined modes of treatment described above seem preferable to the use of potassium iodide, but it is probable that further study of this treatment will be forthcoming in future years, especially in treatment of mild hyperthyroidism.

Potassium perchlorate is rarely used at present for control of hyperthyroidism because of its reported association with fatal aplastic anemia.

Cortisone and immunosuppressive treatments have been tried experimentally, but no data indicate that they are appropriate for routine use.

Ancillary Treatments. Most patients benefit from a period of rest, a good diet, and added vitamins and calcium. The response to a few days in a hospital bed is often remarkable even before specific therapy is instituted. Phenobarbital, diazepam, and reserpine are useful for sedation.

Much recent interest has been given to propranolol as a specific therapy because of its ability to counteract the alleged beta-adrenergic mediated features of thyrotoxicosis. Although the mechanism may be uncertain, in doses of 10 to 40 mg by mouth four times daily, propranolol will reduce tachycardia and provide a beneficial calming effect in some patients. The author believes it is a useful drug, but does not find it to be more than an adjunct to usual therapy.

Therapy in Pregnancy. The choice of therapy in pregnancy is between antithyroid drug and surgery during the middle trimester. At present most patients are probably treated by administration of antithyroid drugs, although there is no certain superiority of one method. It is advisable to use the smallest dose necessary to bring the FTI into the high normal range, that is, between 9 and 13, if this coincides with a remission of symptoms. This precaution is taken because induction of fetal hypothyroidism by the antithyroid drug could result in mental damage. Therapy is followed by measurement of the FTI, or FT_4. These tests avoid the problem of interpreting the effect of pregnancy on T_4 and T_3 (high TBG). An alternative (although not preferred) program is to continue the antithyroid drug and to institute coincident therapy with thyroid hormone. Since this method exposes the fetus to a higher level of antithyroid drug than is needed in the absence of added hormone, and since there is no evidence that the added hormone has any protective effect, it is not recommended.

Therapy in Children. Thyrotoxicosis in children is usually less severe than in adults. Restlessness, inability to concentrate, weight gain or loss, emotional lability, and poor performance at school may be the presenting signs. Exophthalmos is rarely severe, and pretibial myxedema does not occur.

After surgery, there is a pronounced tendency for the disease to recur, unless an extensive subtotal resection is done; this increases the likelihood of postoperative hypothyroidism. RAI is avoided in individuals under the age of 25, if possible, because of the belief that children are most susceptible to induction of tumors. Thus individuals under age 25 are typically given a one- to two-year trial of antithyroid drugs before considering an alternative approach. Sometimes the drugs are continued for four to seven years if a remission does not occur after one year, in an attempt to delay a more drastic form of therapy until the child is older. Subtotal resection is an appropriate alternative therapy if a one- to two-year trial of drug treatment fails to induce remission or if the child is unable for some reason to maintain a drug regimen satisfactorily over the required months or years. RAI has been used only rarely, when some problem such as a severe reaction to both propylthiouracil and methimazole occurred, preventing adequate preparation for surgery and making the radiation hazard the least of the several evils.

Prognosis. Untreated hyperthyroidism can result in death from inanition, congestive heart failure, and other causes. All three major forms of therapy should result in prompt control of hyperthyroidism, and most patients subsequently lead a normal life. It is interest-ing to observe that none of the treatments are directed toward the cause of the illness. There is a tendency for a patient who responds to antithyroid drugs (less so to surgery) to have recurrence of the illness years later. This rarely if ever occurs in patients who have been adequately treated with radioactive iodide. *Delayed onset of hypothyroidism must always be watched for,* and therefore patients who have been treated with surgery, RAI, or antithyroid drugs should be followed indefinitely at yearly intervals. The prognosis for the ophthalmologic and dermatologic complications of Graves' disease is not so sanguine. Often these complications persist for years or even decades and may be incapacitating. As set out below, their course seems to be little influenced by the course of hyperthyroidism.

COMPLICATIONS OF GRAVES' DISEASE

Ophthalmopathy. Mild lid retraction and stare are probably effects of hyperthyroxinemia and in themselves are inconsequential. The remaining abnormalities of Graves' ophthalmopathy (described previously) appear to be due to infiltration of the retro-orbital tissues, extraocular muscles, and lacrimal gland by lymphocytes, plasma cells, and polymorphonuclear leukocytes, as well as an increase in tissue water, mucopolysaccharides, and mucoproteins. The extraocular muscles are often swollen to five or ten times their normal diameter, and the muscle fibers may be largely destroyed, leading in time to contractures. The lacrimal gland may likewise be severely swollen and damaged, although keratitis sicca does not appear. The initial presentation is as a cosmetic defect owing to proptosis and lid edema, often with tearing, burning, or retrobulbar pain. As the condition increases, the patient's difficulties include diplopia, susceptibility to infection, and the more severe complications such as loss of visual acuity, corneal ulceration, and panophthalmitis. Occasionally the process presents essentially as retrobulbar neuritis with loss of vision and few other signs. Infiltrative ophthalmopathy may occur at any time in relationship to the hyperthyroidism of Graves' disease. Most typically it develops with the onset of hyperthyroidism and subsides coincident with therapy. Changes of infiltrative ophthalmopathy are present in 10 to 20 per cent of patients with Graves' disease, and severe progressive ("malignant") exophthalmos occurs in 2 to 3 per cent.

The cause of this complication is unknown. Plasma of patients with progressive exophthalmos has been found to contain a factor which stimulates exophthalmos in certain test animals; the material is known as exophthalmos-producing substance (EPS). Some data suggest that EPS may be a fragment of TSH. Although LATS is present more frequently in patients with exophthalmos and typically in higher titers than in the average patient with Graves' disease, there is no evidence that LATS itself causes exophthalmos. No localization of gamma globulin in orbital tissue has been recognized, and retro-orbital tissue does not bind and neutralize LATS. Gamma globulin from exophthalmic patients is reported to bind to retrobulbar antigens in what may be a pseudoimmunologic reaction. These patients also have CMI against orbital antigens. Thus the belief exists that exophthalmos is an autoimmune phenomenon, but the cause and nature of the antigen are unknown. Although there is usually little diagnostic confusion, some degree of exophthalmos may occur in Cushing's syndrome, Turner's syndrome, and cirrhosis. Orbital tumor, sphenoid ridge meningioma, and thrombosis of the cavernous sinus must also be considered in reaching a diagnosis, especially when the exophthalmos is unilateral, and differentiation from other causes of optic neuritis must be considered.

Treatment. Patients with any degree of exophthalmos should be reassured that the process is almost invariably self-limiting. The eyes usually return to an essentially normal condition, although some degree of proptosis may persist. Useful local measures include shielding the eyes from excessive light and dust, avoidance of smoke and other irritants, and instillation of 10 per cent methylcellulose. Patients may find it useful to sleep with the head of the bed elevated, and to cover the eyes at night with cold saline compresses. If proptosis is severe, the lids may be taped together with cellophane tape which holds a piece of wet gauze and Saran Wrap over the eyelids. Diuresis (chlorothiazide, 500 mg every day) may be useful. Diplopia can be alleviated in part by covering one eye with a patch or obscuring one lens of the patient's glasses. Any sign of infection should be treated by appropriate antimicrobial ointments or, if necessary, by parenteral administration of antimicrobial drugs. If proptosis is severe, muscle function is progressively lost; if vision deteriorates, glucocorticoids may be helpful. Most patients who have active exophthalmos respond, whereas those who have stable changes do not. A common starting dose is 20 to 40 mg of prednisone daily in divided doses, although occasionally, and especially in patients with retrobulbar neuritis, doses up to 120 mg daily may be required. This medication induces Cushing's syndrome. It should be given for a few weeks, after which an attempt should be made to reduce the dose gradually. Sometimes improvement can be maintained with 10 to 20 mg of prednisone daily or every other day The response is variable, ranging fron none at all to a complete remission of muscle paresis, papilledema, improvement in visual acuity, and recession of exophthalmos.

In patients resistant to steroids but requiring therapy, a Kronlein lateral decompression may be useful. In some clinics, other operative procedures such as the Naffziger supraorbital decompression or decompression into the antrum and ethmoids may be performed. The results are unpredictable, but often improvement is gained, and a few patients respond dramatically. In more chronic cases, operations on the muscles may restore binocular vision, and recession of the levator palpebrae superioris can help alleviate a disturbing stare. Muscle surgery, however, should not be done during the stage of progression but should be reserved for a time when fibrosis has occurred and diplopia is stable.

Lateral tarsorrhaphy is useful in patients whose eyes become damaged because the lids do not close during sleep. It provides some protection against corneal abrasions and infection and, sometimes, cosmetic benefits but has little effect on the basic process.

When these procedures have been exhausted, one sometimes resorts to methods whose basis is speculative. Some patients have been treated with azathioprine. Total surgical ablation of the thyroid followed by radioactive iodide has been proposed as being univer-

sally effective, but reports from several clinics indicate that it has no predictable effect on exophthalmos. Hypophysectomy, hypophysial stalk section, x-ray treatment of the pituitary, and x-ray treatment to the posterior aspects of the orbits have all been espoused, but none is of consistent value. The latter procedure, used extensively in earlier years, has been resuscitated recently by several thyroidologists who report sufficiently frequent successes to make it a possible first-line therapy, useful before steroids.

The *course and prognosis* of this illness are difficult to predict. In general, patients whose thyroid disease is successfully controlled will in time do well, although they may go through a period of severe discomfort. Typically, in 6 to 18 months, the activity of the process appears to abate, and there is subsequent slow but progressive evolution toward normality. Rarely sight is severely impaired or even lost, despite the administration of steroids and use of local x-ray and decompressive surgery. In general it is best to treat coincident hyperthyroidism by the most logical means irrespective of the ophthalmologic complication, and to maintain the patient in a *euthyroid* state after the initial control of the thyrotoxicosis. It is possible that RAI therapy, perhaps by inducing release of antigens and an augmented immune response, may exacerbate exophthalmos. With considerable reservation about the scientific basis for the recommendation, surgery or antithyroid drug therapy is preferred over RAI by the author for patients who have evidence of possibly dangerous exophthalmos.

Pretibial Myxedema (Fig. 7). In the simplest form, pretibial or localized myxedema presents as a firm bulging over the lateral aspect of the lower leg, just above the lateral malleolus. Often the skin is shiny and has an orange-peel appearance. The deposits may extend from an area of a few centimeters to involve multiple areas or even the entire anterior leg and foot. Occasionally, similar deposits can be found on the abdomen, hands, or face. Histologically there is an infiltration of mucopolysaccharide and mucoprotein material in the dermis, an increase in fluid, fraying of connective tissue fibers, and increase in collagen. The pattern is very similar to that observed in thyroid hormone deficiency, although there is no evidence that local thyroid hormone deficiency is present. There is a characteristic increase in hyaluronic acid in the lesions and also in uninvolved skin. The process almost invariably occurs in patients who have exophthalmos. It typically is first noted during the onset of hyperthyroidism, but may occur without associated hyperthyroidism and even in some patients whose thyroid appears to have been destroyed by thyroiditis and who are euthyroid or hypothyroid. Usually the process is not incapacitating, and except for its cosmetic disadvantage it requires no therapy. Topical application of triamcinolone ointment under Saran Wrap may be temporarily useful. It is striking that patients with this lesion characteristically have high and sometimes remarkable levels of serum LATS. If LATS disappears, so does the pretibial myxedema. Nevertheless, no etiologic relationship with LATS or other autoimmunity has been shown.

Thyroid Storm. Sudden severe exacerbation of hyperthyroidism may occur as a feature of the basic disease process or because of coincident infection, trauma, or surgery. Without treatment, and even with

Figure 7. A, An example of severe "localized myxedema" involving the entire legs, feet, and hands, and coincident exophthalmos. B, Deposits of localized myxedema on the dorsum of the second, third and fourth digits, which are unusual manifestations of this condition.

therapy, the illness carries a *high mortality*. The patients develop severe hyperkinesis, tachycardia, hyperpyrexia, vomiting, and shock, and may drift into coma. Dehydration may be prominent.

If the diagnosis seems reasonable, treatment of the hyperthyroidism should begin at once, pending laboratory confirmation. Oral or parenteral blocking doses of an antithyroid drug should be given, followed in one hour with potassium iodide. The latter agent should cause a rapid remission in the symptoms of hyperthyroidism, and it is active in the presence of a methimazole block. The prior introduction of an antithyroid drug block ensures that the gland will not be flooded with iodide and guards against a subsequent flare of the illness. If the patient is not obtunded, sedatives such as phenobarbital (60 mg intramuscularly every four to six hours) or reserpine (1 to 3 mg every eight hours) should be given. Propranolol, 10 to 40 mg every six hours orally, or 2 to 10 mg every four hours intravenously, has recently been introduced for therapy of this condition and probably is useful, although experience is limited. This drug should be given with caution in the presence of congestive heart failure. Dehydration should be treated by appropriate fluid supplementation. Cultures should be taken to exclude infection, and antimicrobial therapy given as indicated. Adrenocortical steroids (50 to 100 mg of hydrocortisone intramuscularly every six hours) are given empirically. Occasionally plasma, blood, or norepinephrine is required to support the circulation. Hyperthermia can be treated by cooling. Digitalization may be needed to control congestive heart failure.

Treatment in the Presence of Heart Disease. Usually this complication occurs in older patients who would typically receive RAI. The FTI usually decreases progressively after RAI therapy, and no exacerbation of the heart disease (angina, congestive heart failure, myocardial infarction, arrhythmia) is seen. But if there is concern about therapy because of the gravity of the heart disease, several not very certain approaches can be suggested. RAI, followed in 24 hours by methimazole and then Lugol's solution, is probably safe and effective. Multiple low doses of RAI can be used, but therapeutic response is delayed.

Buhler, U. K., and DeGroot, L. J.: Effect of stable iodine on thyroid iodine release. J. Clin. Endocrinol. Metab., 29:1546, 1969.

Das, G., and Krieger, M.: Treatment of thyrotoxic storm with intravenous administration of propranolol. Ann. Intern. Med., 70:985, 1969.

Goldfischer, S., Moore, C. L., Johnson, A. B., Spiro, A. J., Valsamis, M. P., Wisniewski, H. K., Ritch, R. H., Norton, W. T., Rapin, I., and Gartner, L. M.: Peroxisomal and mitochondrial defects in the cerebro-hepato-renal syndrome. Science, 182:62, 1973.

Graves' Disease – 1972. Second F. Raymond Keating, Jr., Memorial Symposium, April 14 and 15, 1972. Mayo Clinic Proceedings, November and December, 1972, pp. 803–995.

Lamki, L., Row, V. V., and Volpe, R.: Cell-mediated immunity in Graves' disease and in Hashimoto's thyroiditis as shown by the demonstration of migration inhibition factor (MIF). J. Clin. Endocrinol. Metab., 36:358, 1973.

Luft, R., Ikkos, D., Palmieri, G., Ernster, L., and Afzelius, B.: A case of severe hypermetabolism of non-thyroidal origin with a defect in the maintenance of mitochondrial respiratory control: A correlated clinical, biochemical, and morphological study. J. Clin. Invest., 41:1776, 1962.

McKenzie, J. M.: Humoral factors in the pathogenesis of Graves' disease. Physiol. Rev., 48:252, 1968.

Munro, R. E., Lamki, L., Row, V. V., and Volpe, R.: Cell-mediated immunity in the exophthalmos of Graves' disease as demonstrated by the migration inhibition factor (MIF) assay. J. Clin. Endocrinol. Metab., 37:286, 1973.

Nofal, M. M., Beierwaltes, W. H., and Patno, M. E.: Treatment of hyperthyroidism with sodium iodide I131. J.A.M.A., 197:605, 1966.

Rapoport, B., Caplan, R., and DeGroot, L. J.: Low dose sodium iodide I131 therapy in Graves' disease. J.A.M.A., 224:1610, 1973.

Sterling, K., Refetoff, S., and Selenkow, H. A.: T3 toxicosis – thyrotoxicosis due to elevated serum triiodothyronine levels. J.A.M.A., 213:571, 1970.

Wilson, W. R., Theilen, E. O., Hege, J. H., and Valenca, M. R.: Effects of beta-adrenergic receptor blockade in normal subjects before, during, and after triiodothyronine-induced hyperthyroidism. J. Clin. Invest., 45:1159, 1966.

838. THYROIDITIS

Three types of thyroiditis are recognized: chronic, acute, and subacute. Chronic thyroiditis is not an infection nor, in the usual sense, an inflammation, and therefore the name may be inappropriate. Two varieties are defined by pathologists: lymphocytic thyroiditis and Riedel's struma. In lymphocytic thyroiditis (Hashimoto's thyroiditis, struma lymphomatosa), the thyroid is replaced to a varying degree by lymphocytes forming germinal centers and fibrous tissue, leading to goiter, parenchymal destruction, and thyroid hormone insufficiency. Riedel's thyroiditis (ligneous thyroiditis) is a possibly related, slowly progressive fibrosis of the thyroid, of great rarity. These two processes will be considered separately, with the main emphasis on Hashimoto's thyroiditis.

HASHIMOTO'S THYROIDITIS

Etiology and Pathogenesis. Hashimoto's thyroiditis is thought to be an autoimmune disease. In 1956, Doniach and Roitt, and Witebsky, coincidentally discovered antibodies to thyroid antigens in patients with this illness. The thyroid antigen-antibody systems that are now known include (1) antibodies reacting with thyroglobulin, usually detected by the tanned red cell agglutination test; (2) antibodies reacting with a component of thyroid cytoplasm, detected by the immunofluorescent technique, by a complement-fixing reaction with thyroid microsomes, or by a variation of the tanned red cell technique; and (3) antibodies reacting with a colloidal antigen which is distinct from thyroglobulin. When antibodies against thyroglobulin and thyroid cell cytoplasm are both measured, about 95 per cent of patients with Hashimoto's thyroiditis have a positive titer in one or both tests, and frequently the titers are very high.

Thyroiditis with a similar histologic pattern can be induced by immunization of animals with thyroid tissue. The experimentally induced disease cannot be transferred from animal to animal by serum, but can be transferred in inbred guinea pigs by transfer of lymphocytes. This observation, as well as the poor correlation of circulating antibody titers with the course of the disease, suggested that *cell-mediated immunity* (CMI) was important in the destruction of thyroid cells. This has been abundantly confirmed in the past few years by studies demonstrating CMI by in vitro techniques such as leukocyte migration inhibition assay and lymphotoxin assay. Patients with thyroiditis, primary thyroid failure, and Graves' disease are found to have lymphocytes presensitized to thyroid antigens. The antigens are associated with particulate fragments of the cell. CMI is most obvious in patients with primary myxedema, and is less intense in patients with thyroiditis or Graves' disease.

Why individuals should produce antibodies against thyroid antigens remains a mystery. It might be supposed that an abnormal antigen exists in the cells, but none has been found. It has been suggested that thyroglobulin or other thyroid antigens are normally hidden from the organism during fetal life when immune tolerance is established, and that subsequent escape of the thyroglobulin from the thyroid follicle could induce immunity in the adult. This seems unlikely, because thyroglobulin normally circulates in the blood. Possibly viral infection or other injury could alter thyroid tissue and produce neoantigens. There is a strong hereditary pattern for the illness, and the propensity to produce antibodies is transmitted as a dominant trait. Further, thyroiditis is associated with a number of other possibly autoimmune diseases, including pernicious anemia, idiopathic adrenal insufficiency, rheumatoid arthritis, Sjögren's syndrome, ulcerative colitis, lupoid hepatitis, disseminated lupus erythematosus, and hemolytic anemia. The relationship to pernicious anemia is especially prominent. Fifty per cent of patients with pernicious anemia have antibodies against thyroid tissue antigens, and the converse is also true. There is also an associated increased incidence of antibodies against parathyroid tissue, and possibly of antibodies against the pancreas and ovary. These observations suggest that some ill-understood hereditarily defined abnormality in immune homeostasis occurs in these patients, predisposing them to develop reactivity to self-antigens.

In the author's view, Graves' disease, Hashimoto's thyroiditis, and myxedema are variants of a common process. Among the relatives of patients with one of these three diseases, it is typical to find examples of the other two. The histology of Graves' disease shades into that of Hashimoto's thyroiditis, and the histology of idiopathic thyroid failure is interpreted by some as the end-stage of lymphocytic and fibrotic replacement of the thyroid. Antibody titers against thyroid cell antigens are high in each condition. It is as if an abnormality in immune homeostasis were at the root of each illness, possibly triggered by some environmental factor. Perhaps with the development of antithyroglobulin and anticytoplasmic antibodies, plus a cell-mediated response, Hashimoto's thyroiditis occurs. If the destructive cell-mediated response is severe, the process may go on to thyroid failure. If, in addition to or in the absence of the other antibodies, LATS or other thyroid-stimulating antibodies are formed, and if the thyroid is capable of responding, thyroid hyperplasia and hypersecretion occur with the picture of Graves' disease. Although this formulation is by no means universally accepted, it embodies the thinking of many workers in the field.

Pathology (Fig. 8). On gross inspection the thyroid appears pale yellow-tan and has a lumpy surface. The normal thyroid structure is replaced with dense infiltration by lymphocytes, and lymphoid germinal centers are evident. The remaining thyroid tissue often shows hyperplasia, with small empty follicles. The cells frequently are enlarged and eosinophilic. In many specimens, fibrosis is prominent. The thymus is characteristically enlarged, and germinal centers are seen. There may be lymph nodes showing reactive hyperplasia in the area surrounding the thyroid.

Clinical Manifestations. This illness occurs with an incidence roughly similar to that of Graves' disease. There is good evidence that it has tripled in frequency in the past three decades. Hashimoto's thyroiditis may present with thyroid enlargement or symptoms of hypothyroidism. The disease is 20 times as frequent in women as in men. It can occur even in young children, but is most common between ages 30 and 50. In children the process is occasionally seen to subside spontaneously. In other instances, extensive destruction of the gland can lead to thyroid failure and growth retardation (Fig. 8). Most characteristic is the thyroid enlargement, which varies from two to five times normal, averaging 30 to 50 grams. The gland may be soft, normal, or firm, and there is no thrill or bruit. The surface may feel lobulated, but distinct nodules are usually not found. Their presence suggests that a mass of lymph nodes is present or that a thyroid adenoma or malignancy is present. Typically the pyramidal lobe is palpable. Sometimes patients complain of choking or difficulty in swallowing or of a sensation of local pressure, but usually the goiter is asymptomatic. Rarely, the illness proceeds more rapidly, and there are pain and tenderness in the thyroid gland. The trachea is charac-

Figure 8. *A,* Identical twins, age 12, both of whom developed Hashimoto's thyroiditis. One boy ceased growing at age 8 and was hypothyroid. *B,* Biopsy specimen from one twin, showing small hyperplastic residual follicles, fibrosis, and lymphocytic infiltration. (Photographs provided by Dr. Frank Milgram.)

teristically in the midline. The remainder of the physical examination is unremarkable unless there are signs of hypothyroidism.

The presence of an asymptomatic diffuse thyroid enlargement (with a palpable pyramidal lobe) in a middle-aged woman who appears to be euthyroid is indicative of Hashimoto's thyroiditis. The serum thyroxine may be normal or depressed, depending on the stage of development of the process. The PBI may be low, normal, or elevated owing to butanol-insoluble iodinated albumin in plasma. This can be detected by simultaneous determination of the PBI and BEI, or the PBI and serum T_4. The RAIU test may be elevated, normal, or low, but usually is normal unless the patient has developed hypothyroidism. Other tests of thyroid function reflect the ability of the thyroid to produce hormone. Characteristically, the scintiscan shows an enlarged thyroid with a smooth outline and diffuse distribution of the isotope. Fluorescent scans show a diminution or virtual absence of thyroid-stable iodine. The diagnosis can be made if the tanned red cell (TRC) agglutination titer is positive at a greater than 1:2560 dilution or if there is a very strongly positive test for anticytoplasmic antibodies. However, only 60 per cent of the patients have a positive TRC, and only 95 per cent are positive if both tests are performed. If it seems imperative that the diagnosis be established and the antibody response is not in the diagnostic range, needle biopsy is both safe and effective. A diagnostic piece of tissue will be obtained in perhaps 80 per cent of the biopsies. Failure of

radioactive iodide uptake to rise after administration of TSH is also suggestive, indicating the syndrome of low thyroid reserve. Further, some patients will show a positive perchlorate discharge test. Occasionally there are striking elevations of the serum gamma globulin.

Therapy. In patients with thyroid deficiency, therapy with thyroid hormone is indicated. It is also useful to give replacement therapy to euthyroid individuals who have developed a goiter causing a cosmetic defect or local symptoms, or to prevent further thyroid enlargement. In young patients, treatment results in disappearance of the goiter, but in older persons whose thyroid enlargement has been present for a prolonged period, it may have little effect. When the thyroid is minimally enlarged, it is debatable whether therapy is indicated. Serial biopsies have shown that the histologic picture may not change over a decade. Further, there is no evidence that the process tends to spread to other organs.

Usually therapy is with thyroid hormone, although there are reports of other approaches. In children steroid therapy causes diminution of goiter and suppresses antibody titers, but the entire process recurs when therapy is withdrawn. This approach does not appear to have merit.

Prognosis. There is a tendency for the involved thyroid to enlarge slowly and for hypothyroidism to develop. Spontaneous thyroid atrophy may occur, and it is hypothesized that this sequence may be the cause of "idiopathic" myxedema.

RIEDEL'S THYROIDITIS

In Riedel's thyroiditis, a very uncommon condition, the gland is replaced by a mass of dense, infiltrative fibrotic tissue which extends into the capsule of the thyroid, the trachea, and the surrounding strap muscles. Patients seek attention because of local symptoms such as choking or difficult swallowing, because a small goiter is observed, or because of hypothyroidism. The disease is more frequent in women than in men and characteristically occurs after age 40. Some circumstantial evidence suggests that it is a variant of Hashimoto's thyroiditis. Patients have been observed who first had typical lymphocytic thyroiditis but later had the histology of Riedel's struma. On examination, the thyroid is found to be of normal size, reduced in bulk, or moderately enlarged, and is unusually firm and densely adherent to the trachea. Thyroid function tests reveal normal function or hypothyroidism. There is no specific diagnostic test, and antibody titers to thyroid antigen are not elevated in this condition as in Hashimoto's thyroiditis.

Diagnosis is usually made at operation, when the surgeon finds fibrotic thyroid tissue bound to the trachea. Often the process suggests a sclerosing carcinoma, and the diagnosis is made on frozen sections. The only known therapy is surgery if pressure symptoms are sufficient to warrant this approach. The gland may be resected or the isthmus may be exposed and divided, allowing the two halves of the gland to fall laterally, thus avoiding tracheal constriction. Since resection may cause loss of the parathyroids or recurrent laryngeal nerve, simple division of the isthmus and mobilization of the lateral lobes is the preferred approach. Thyroid hormone therapy may be required.

An association has been suggested between this process and sclerosing cholangitis, mediastinal fibrosis, and periureteral fibrosis (see Ch. 107). Since some of these processes may respond to steroid administration, it is possible that this would be a useful therapy in Riedel's thyroiditis; information on this therapeutic approach is not available.

ACUTE THYROIDITIS

Acute and subacute thyroiditis are etiologically unrelated. Both are transient inflammatory reactions involving the thyroid, and they are clinically distinct from chronic thyroiditis. "Acute thyroiditis" (acute infectious thyroiditis, suppurative thyroiditis) means an uncommon condition in which the thyroid gland is invaded by pathogenic bacteria. This occurs as part of a cellulitis in the neck or because of infection of a cyst in a multinodular goiter. Usually the patient presents with fever, pain in the neck, and a mass involving the thyroid area. The area is erythematous and tender to palpation. Often only one portion of the thyroid is involved, and contiguous infection is evident. The leukocyte count is elevated. The serum thyroxine is normal. On scintiscan there may be some depression of radioiodine uptake in a portion of the thyroid, but RAIU is usually normal.

Cultures should be taken and appropriate antimicrobials administered. With suitable therapy, the process subsides rapidly. Occasionally resection of a portion of the thyroid is indicated.

SUBACUTE THYROIDITIS

Subacute thyroiditis (granulomatous thyroiditis, acute thyroiditis, De Quervain's thyroiditis) is an inflammatory condition of the thyroid causing painful enlargement, lasting over a period of weeks or months, with a prominent tendency to relapse. Its incidence is not known, but it appears to be about one tenth as common as Graves' disease.

Etiology. Subacute thyroiditis frequently occurs two to three weeks after viral upper respiratory infection. This association suggests that the thyroiditis represents an immunologic response to the viral infection. Other data imply that direct viral invasion of the thyroid may be the cause. Thyroiditis has occurred in outbreaks of mumps, and the mumps virus has been cultured from the thyroid. Numerous other attempts at viral culture have been negative. Volpe finds that most patients have antiviral antibody titers which are high at the time of diagnosis, and tend to fall progressively over subsequent weeks. Antibodies are frequently found against common pathogens such as echovirus, coxsackievirus, and adenovirus, and often one finds significant changes in titers against two or even three viral antigens. The reported occurrence with mumps virus or in mumps epidemics may represent one possible etiology, but is not the most common. The causation remains obscure.

Pathology. The thyroid may be enlarged with dense infiltration by polymorphonuclear cells, lymphocytes, and plasma cells. Fibrosis is prominent. Many pyknotic thyroid follicular cells are apparent. The follicular structure is often destroyed, and in its place are found small granulomas with giant cells. There is poor correlation between the histologic abnormalities, which may be extreme, and the clinical picture.

Clinical Manifestations. Subacute thyroiditis may be painful and disabling, but it does not last long. The patient usually notices gradual onset of severe pain and tenderness involving one or both sides of the lower neck, sometimes localized to the thyroid. The process may begin in one lobe and travel over several days to the other. There may be fullness and the sensation of pressure. Pain typically radiates up the lateral aspects of the neck and into the jaw and ear. Swallowing may be uncomfortable, causing the patient to choke over saliva. There are often mild fever, sore throat, malaise, and fatigue. Sometimes the process is entirely asymptomatic.

On examination the thyroid is enlarged and often extremely tender. The process may be restricted to one portion of a lobe or may involve the entire gland. Lymph nodes are usually not enlarged. Sometimes the patient develops symptoms and signs of mild hyperthyroidism, but usually the clinical status is that of euthyroidism or rarely hypothyroidism. The disease tends to remit spontaneously or because of therapy, only to recur after a period of two to three weeks, and this cycle may recur several times. Over the course of one to twelve months the process finally subsides.

Diagnosis. The typical history of pain and the tender enlargement of the thyroid are highly suggestive of subacute thyroiditis. The leukocyte count may be elevated to 15,000 to 20,000, or may be normal. The sedimentation rate is characteristically high, and may reach 100 mm per hour (Westergren). Anemia is said to accompany the illness, although the cause is unknown.

On scan, RAIU is suppressed in the involved portion of the gland, which may be one lobe or the entire thyroid, and the RAIU is often zero. Fluorescent scanning shows the involved thyroid tissue to have lost all iodine stores. The PBI, T_4, and FTI may be elevated because of iodoprotein or excess thyroid hormone released during the acute phase of the illness, making the patient thyrotoxic. During recovery, the TSH and RAIU may be transiently elevated while T_4 is depressed, and then over a period of two to three months all tests return to normal. Antibody titers against thyroid antigens may be transiently demonstrable, but they rarely if ever reach the levels found in Hashimoto's thyroiditis, and the responses are not sustained.

This process can usually be differentiated from acute thyroiditis because of the localization to the thyroid, absence of signs of infection, characteristically high sedimentation rate, and depressed radioactive iodide uptake. Occasionally, aspiration biopsy may be necessary to prove the diagnosis. Rarely, Hashimoto's thyroiditis presents with a rather acute and painful onset, and it may be difficult to make the distinction short of biopsy. Sometimes the diagnosis of Graves' disease is suggested by a painless goiter and thyrotoxicosis, but in these cases the patient fails to have the appropriate history or physical evidence of long-term thyrotoxicosis. Exogenous iodine can depress RAIU in Graves' disease to near zero, offering another source of confusion. Serial observations over a few weeks will identify the proper diagnosis.

Therapy. In mild cases the inflammatory process subsides spontaneously, and all that is needed is mild analgesia. Aspirin, up to 6 grams daily, is useful in suppressing the pain. It is probably advantageous to give desiccated thyroid if the disease has gone on for more than a few days, because TSH stimulation may exacerbate the process. If the illness does not subside with these simple measures, corticosteroids are useful; 20 to 40 mg of prednisone is given daily for a period of one to four weeks, with progressive diminution of the dose as symptoms are controlled. Often withdrawal of steroids is followed by exacerbation of the process, and such a cycle may recur several times before the illness eventually subsides. Rarely, a chronic, tender enlargement of the thyroid persists despite therapy and requires surgical resection.

Prognosis. In the author's experience, all patients with subacute thyroiditis, with the exception of one who required surgery, have eventually returned to normal thyroid function and become asymptomatic. It is reported that up to 10 per cent of the patients develop permanent hypothyroidism.

Bastenie, P. A.: Contribution à l'étiologie du myxoedème spontane de l'adulte. Bull. Acad. R. Med. Belg., 9:179, 1944.
Calder, E. A., McLeman, D., Barnes, E. W., and Irvine, W. J.: The effect of thyroid antigens on the in vitro migration of leukocytes from patients with Hashimoto's thyroiditis. Clin. Exp. Immunol., 12:429, 1972.
DeGroot, L. J., Hall, R., McDermott, W. V., and Davis, A. M.: Hashimoto's thyroiditis, a genetically conditioned disease. N. Engl. J. Med., 267:267, 1962.
Greene, J. N.: Subacute thyroiditis. Am. J. Med., 51:97, 1971.
Ling, S. M., Kaplan, S. A., Weitzman, J. V., Reed, G. B., Costin, G., and Larding, B. H.: Euthyroid goiter in children: Correlation of needle biopsy with other clinical and laboratory findings in chronic lymphocytic thyroiditis and simple goiter. Pediatrics, 44:695, 1969.
McConahey, W. M., Keating, F. R., Jr., Beahrs, O. H., and Woolner, L. B.: On the increasing occurrence of Hashimoto's thyroiditis. J. Clin. Endocrinol. Metab., 22:542, 1962.
McMaster, P. R. B., and Lerner, E. M.: The transfer of allergic thyroiditis in histocompatible guinea pigs by lymph node cells. J. Immunol., 99:208, 1967.
Rapoport, B., Block, M. B., Hoffer, P. B., and DeGroot, L. J.: Depletion of thyroid iodine during subacute thyroiditis. J. Clin. Endocrinol. Metab., 36:610, 1973.
Roitt, I. M., and Doniach, D.: Thyroid autoimmunity. Br. Med. Bull., 16:152, 1960.

839. HYPOTHYROIDISM AND MYXEDEMA

Hypothyroidism (Gull's disease) refers to the morbid state characterized by progressive slowing of all bodily activities owing to deficiency in thyroid hormone. The severest form is known as myxedema because of the characteristic infiltration of the skin by nonpitting, mucinous edema.

Etiology. Probably most cases of "idiopathic" hypothyroidism and myxedema develop as the end-stage of Hashimoto's thyroiditis. The histologic pattern confirms this suggestion; antithyroglobulin and anticytoplasmic antibody are frequently present in high titers, and progress from Hashimoto's thyroiditis to hypothyroidism can be observed. More commonly, thyroid failure occurs because of administration of RAI to control the thyrotoxicosis in Graves' disease or after subtotal thyroidectomy for Graves' disease, multinodular goiter, or Hashimoto's thyroiditis. Hypothyroidism sometimes occurs as part of the presentation of Graves' syndrome, with coincident exophthalmos and pretibial myxedema. Less frequently, hypothyroidism occurs as the only feature of hypopituitarism because of isolated failure of the pituitary to produce TSH or because of damage in the hypothalamus inhibiting TRH secretion. Hypothyroidism is reported to occur in 10 per cent of patients who have had subacute thyroiditis (see Ch. 838). Some patients with multinodular goiter are hypothyroid. Hypothyroidism is also found in patients with congenital metabolic defects of thyroid hormone synthesis, is sometimes caused by severe iodine deficiency in areas of endemic goiter, and can be induced by medications such as the antithyroid drugs, resorcinol, or para-aminosalicylic acid. In some individuals, administration of iodine (more than 6 mg per day) induces inhibition of thyroid hormone synthesis and release, with the development of goiter and hypothyroidism.

Pathogenesis and Pathology. Whatever the cause of thyroid hormone deprivation, the effects are similar. Over a period of months and years, there is progressive infiltration of the skin by mucoprotein and mucopolysaccharides, giving a puffy appearance. Similar deposits of mucopolysaccharide are reported to occur under the sarcolemma of striated muscle. Muscle fibers become frayed, and the cells may become necrotic. Effusion can occur in any serosal space. Thickening of joint capsules and joint effusion also occur. There is a generalized decreased rate of nucleic acid and protein synthesis, and almost all enzyme systems are reported to be underactive.

In idiopathic myxedema the thyroid is replaced by scar tissue containing a few scattered thyroid cells and many lymphocytes. In secondary hypothyroidism resulting from pituitary failure, the thyroid is small, with flattened, cuboidal epithelium and acini filled with colloid. In other conditions the pathology is that of the primary process. In goiter resulting from metabolic defects in hormone formation or the action of thyroid blocking drugs or iodide, the characteristic picture is extreme hyperplasia, which may look much like papillary adenocarcinoma.

Clinical Manifestations. Quite typically the patient has no complaints. He or, more commonly, she may be brought to the doctor because someone else recognized unusual sluggishness, weight gain, or sleepiness. Sometimes the presenting symptom is edema or menorrhagia. We have seen several women whose menorrhagia, caused by myxedema, was treated first by hysterectomy and only later by thyroid hormone. The symptoms and signs are in proportion to the severity and duration of the illness. In advanced cases the diagnosis is obvious. The patient notices fatigue and somnolence, often falling asleep at inopportune times. There is marked increase in sensitivity to cold. Hearing may be diminished. The eyes are puffy or watery. The hair is brittle, sparse, and coarse; curl tends to be lost. The eyebrows are sparse, and the outer third may be missing. The skin is thickened and dry, and sweating rarely occurs. There is generalized thickening and puffiness of the face and extremities; pitting is not characteristic, but may occur in the presence of fluid retention or congestive heart failure. True obesity is not characteristic. The patients have a jocular air about them, their answers to questions often being delayed and seemingly humorous but inappropriate. As a group they tend to be uncomplaining and hardly recognize the marked change that may have occurred in their appearance and behavior. The tongue is thick, and papillae may be atrophic, especially if there is coincident pernicious anemia, which occurs in 12 per cent of patients with idiopathic thyroid failure. The thyroid may be absent or palpable, depending on the etiology. The heart is quiet, the pulse is slow, and diastolic blood pressure may be elevated. Although pericardial effusion is frequently present, physical signs of tamponade are rarely if ever found. Pleural effusion may occur, and the abdomen may be distended by ascites. These fluids may have a high specific gravity. The patient complains of severe constipation, and ileus and megacolon have been reported. Irregular menstrual pattern and severe menorrhagia frequently occur in younger women. Deep tendon reflex relaxation time is markedly prolonged. Other neurologic signs include diminished hearing, paresthesias, vertigo, and ataxia with lateral column signs. Often the skin shows perifollicular keratoses. The nails may be thickended. Joint stiffness, thickening of the joint capsules, joint effusion, arthritis, and bursitis are occasionally seen.

Overt *psychosis* may develop as a manifestation of prolonged and severe myxedema. Hallucinations, disorientation, paranoia, and attempted suicide have been reported. With substitution therapy, the psychosis usually clears, although some patients never regain sanity. Occasionally patients develop overt psychosis as therapy is introduced. The name "myxedema madness" has been applied to these conditions.

The degree of abnormality is by no means always as great as that described. In mild hypothyroidism it may be impossible to make a clinical distinction from the normal state.

Diagnosis. In the classic case the diagnosis can be confirmed at the bedside by evaluation of the slow relaxation time of the Achilles tendon reflexes. Other tendon jerks are less reliable. The PBI and serum T_4 are characteristically low, as is the RAIU, except in individuals who have a block in thyroid hormone formation as a cause of their thyroprivia. Both the T_4 and the RAIU tend to be less severely depressed in patients with hypothyroidism of pituitary origin, and in these subjects the values tend to overlap the normal range. The RAIU is not a very useful test now, because normal values (down to 10 per cent) overlap the values found in hypothyroid patients. The BMR is depressed, the serum cholesterol and carotene are elevated, and there may be marked elevation of the enzymes GOT, LDH, and CPK. Uric acid is sometimes elevated. The EKG shows slow rate and low voltage. Most patients have anemia. This may be due to menorrhagia causing iron deficiency or to coincident pernicious anemia, or may be normocytic or macrocytic and be related solely to hypothyroidism. Pernicious anemia, nephritis, uremia, and mongolism are occasional causes for confusion in differential diagnosis.

After the conclusion is reached that the patient is hypothyroid, it is imperative that the cause be evaluated. It there is atrophy of thyroid tissue, the presence of thyroiditis may be ascertained by tests for antithyroglobulin and anticytoplasmic antibodies. Goiter and a positive $KClO_4$ discharge test may be found in hypothyroidism caused by congenital metabolic defects, including Pendred's syndrome and Hashimoto's thyroiditis. Pituitary dysfunction should be considered unless there is strong evidence incriminating primary thyroid failure. In primary thyroid failure, the sella turcica is usually normal, but it may be enlarged in cretins and in some adults with longstanding myxedema. Plasma cortisol is normal, although ketosteroid and hydroxycorticoid excretion is depressed, and the adrenal response to metyrapone may be delayed and low. Follicle-stimulating hormone is characteristically elevated in postmenopausal women with primary thyroid failure, but is occasionally low, returning to an elevated level after therapy with thyroid hormone has been started. Growth hormone should be present in primary thyroid failure, but the response to insulin hypoglycemia is often depressed. TSH is characteristically very high in primary thyroid failure, often 20 to 1000 μU per milliliter. Absent or normal TSH and a failure to respond to exogenous TRH indicate pituitary damage. Hypothyroidism and a normal TSH which responds to exogenous TRH identify "hypothalamic hypothyroidism." This condition may be the cause of most instances of secondary hypothyroidism in children, and can be acquired by trauma or neoplastic lesions.

Therapy. Treatment with desiccated thyroid is a remarkably satisfactory therapeutic maneuver. Usually it is advantageous to initiate treatment with a low dose of hormone, such as 15 or 30 mg of USP desiccated thyroid daily or the equivalent dose of one of the synthetic mixtures of T_4 and T_3 (liotrix). Subsequent increments of 15 or 30 mg are made at intervals of 7 to 14 days, until a full replacement dosage is reached in two to three months. Marked improvement should be seen with 30 mg. The usual replacement dosage is 90 to 120 mg of desiccated thyroid daily given in one dose, although a range of 60 to 200 mg per day is found, with some dependence upon patient's size. Equivalent doses of L-thyroxine (100 μg = 60 mg USP desiccated thyroid) or L-triiodothyronine (37.5 μg = 60 mg USP desiccated thyroid), may be used for replacement therapy. If desiccated thyroid or liotrix is used to achieve replacement therapy, the FTI should be in the normal range when the patient is optimally replaced. Using thyroxine alone, the T_4 or FTI will be in the upper range of normal or slightly elevated. When T_3 is given, the T_4 or FTI will be near zero even when replacement is quite adequate.

In patients who have congestive heart failure, previous myocardial infarction, or angina pectoris, it is best to initiate therapy very gradually. Often such conditions are exacerbated by therapy, although some patients cease to have angina pectoris on replacement of the hormone. Triiodothyronine is theoretically useful because of the more rapid disappearance of its effect should toxicity be encountered, but in most patients, replacement with desiccated thyroid or liotrix is preferred, because with these medications the T_4 is within the normal range during adequate therapy and is a useful guide.

The best guide to treatment is the patient's and the physician's progressive re-evaluation of the clinical status. There should be a return to a normal and steady weight, a disappearance of all symptoms, and a feeling of well-being. Severe myalgias and arthralgias may occur during therapy, but disappear gradually if therapy is continued. It is sometimes useful to increase the dose until symptoms of thyroid hormone excess appear and then return to a slightly lower dose, in order to be certain that sufficient medication is administered. Once the dosage is established, the patient may take exogenous hormone for years or decades without change. Patients must be cautioned to continue taking the medication indefinitely, for some will feel that treatment is no longer needed once well-being has been restored. It is especially important that women be urged to continue the medication without interruption and at the same dosage level throughout pregnancy. Dosage need not be changed in preparation for or during surgery.

Prognosis. The prognosis for treatment of hypothyroidism in the ambulatory patient is excellent; usually there is a complete return to normal health.

SPECIAL PROBLEMS IN HYPOTHYROIDISM

Myxedema Coma. As myxedema worsens, the affected individual becomes more and more lethargic, and episodes of apparent sleep may become frequent, culminating in severe obtundation or even coma from which the paient cannot be aroused. In other instances coma develops abruptly during an intercurrent illness such as pyelonephritis, pneumonia, or cellulitis. Patients with severe myxedema may develop sepsis with minimal symptoms, no fever, and little leukocytosis.

Typically, if a history is available, it is that the patient had previous surgery or radioactive iodine therapy for hyperthyroidism, did well for a number of years afterward, but then over five or ten years gradually lapsed into hypothyroidism, finally developing coma. Often such people have received replacement therapy with thyroid hormone, but have for some reason discontinued it.

The mechanism of myxedema coma is unknown.

Blood flow to the brain is diminished, but oxygen consumption is allegedly not diminished. Altered cortical activity is apparent in sluggish mentation and slowing of the alpha rhythm of the EEG. The pathologic correlates of these changes are not well known. Progressive hypothermia, hypoglycemia, and carbon dioxide retention may be specific causes of coma in some patients.

The clinical manifestations are fundamentally those of severe myxedema, as described before. Localizing neurologic signs are characteristically absent. The reflexes are symmetrical and depressed, and the relaxation time is delayed. Babinski reflex may be evident. Often the patients are severely obtunded rather than comatose, and they are typically disoriented. It may be possible to arouse the patient from his stupor, only to have him immediately slip back into a depressed state. The temperature should be carefully recorded, and may be as low as 29.5 to 30.5° C.

The diagnosis is usually suggested by physical examination which reveals signs of advanced hypothyroidism and cutaneous myxedema. The scar of a thyroidectomy, a history of previous thyroid surgery or radioactive iodide treatment, and a history of thyroid therapy are important diagnostic clues. The thyroid is impalpable or replaced by fibrous tissue. Careful search should be made for precipitating causes such as infection of the lungs or urinary tract, as well as other causes of coma, e.g., cerebrovascular accidents, renal and hepatic failure, and drug ingestion. The last-named cause is important, because hypothyroid patients are excessively sensitive to the usual doses of barbiturates and opiates. Diagnosis rests on finding abnormally low blood levels of thyroid hormone, but usually these tests are not immediately available. Clinical judgment is called for in the interim; this can sometimes be supplemented by measurement of the deep tendon reflex relaxation time. Severe hyponatremia and hypoglycemia may occur as a manifestation of primary or secondary thyroid failure. The usual measures needed for differential diagnosis of primary and secondary thyroid failure, including FTI, antibody tests, TSH levels, measurement of plasma cortisol, skull films, and measurement of plasma LH and FSH, should be carried out. Carbon dioxide retention should be excluded, if necessary, by arterial gas determination, because hypoventilation may induce coma in some patients. If the diagnosis seems probable but cannot be established at the time the patient is admitted, it is best to institute treatment without a diagnosis because of the urgency of the condition.

The appropriate treatment remains a matter of debate. Failure has consistently been reported in patients treated with very slow supplementation of thyroid hormone, and an impressive series of successes has been reported in patients given a massive intravenous dose of T_4 or T_3 in an attempt to return the circulating thyroid hormone to normal levels without delay. Approximately 300 μg of thyroxine is administered intravenously and 100 to 200 μg is given daily thereafter with monitoring of the plasma thyroid hormone blood levels. Hypothermia is best treated by covering the patient with warm blankets and allowing endogenous body heat to bring up the temperature gradually. Rapid warming by means of electrical blankets or hot baths has resulted in shock and death. Appropriate antimicrobial therapy should be given if there is evidence of infection. If there is carbon dioxide retention, the patient should be placed on a respirator to provide an adequate ventilatory exchange. If there is any suggestion of pituitary failure, shock, or hyponatremia suggestive of adrenal steroid insufficiency, the patient should be given 100 to 200 mg of hydrocortisone intravenously. Occasionally blood pressure must be supported by transfusions or by use of norepinephrine. Fluid and electrolyte therapy should be given with caution; since cutaneous and respiratory losses are extremely small, 600 to 1000 ml of fluid per day, of which one third to one half is a balanced electrolyte solution, is sufficient. Overhydration is the major problem in therapy and often leads to congestive failure, cerebral edema, and death. Hyponatremia should be treated preferably by fluid restriction rather than by administration of hypertonic saline, because with thyroid hormone therapy excess stored salt in myxedema tissue is mobilized and may precipitate congestive failure.

If the patient survives the critical first few days and is able to take medication orally, replacement therapy can be switched to any standard preparation of thyroid hormone. The blood thyroxine level should be checked to assay adequacy of replacement.

Despite some advances in understanding of the precipitating causes of this illness, therapy remains unsatisfactory, and mortality rates of 50 to 90 per cent are reported.

Myxedema Heart. Cardiomegaly and congestive failure often accompany myxedema. The EKG shows low voltage, flattened T waves, and occasionally first degree AV block. Is there a specific variety of heart disease associated with thyroid hormone deficiency? Obviously patients who develop myxedema may be in the older age groups expected to have a high incidence of hypertension and coronary artery disease. The coexistence of mild hypertension, which may be alleviated by therapy with thyroid hormone, has previously been noted. Another and probably more common cause of presumptive cardiomegaly is the frequent pericardial effusion found in this illness. The pericardial effusion is usually functionally insignificant, but rare instances of cardiac tamponade have been reported.

Atherosclerosis was for many years thought not to be accelerated by hypothyroidism, but present evidence indicates that there is an association between these two conditions.

In addition, it appears that severe myxedema can be associated with a specific cardiac lesion, evident pathologically as an edema of the myocardium, deposition of mucopolysaccharides and mucoproteins between the cells, fraying of cardiac myofibrils, and death and necrosis of cells. Probably this represents a very advanced stage of myxedema, and these changes are not found in most patients dying of myxedema coma.

Although the effusion, decreased cardiac output, and EKG changes are manifestations of hypothyroidism per se, most instances of heart failure associated with myxedema are probably due to coexistent organic heart disease. Occasionally the problem may not be overt before institution of therapy because of the lesser cardiac output required in the hypothyroid patient. With therapy increased demands are put upon the heart, and congestive failure, angina, and even myocardial infarction may occur.

Begg, T. B., and Hall, R.: Iodide goiter and hypothyroidism. Quart. J. Med., 32:351, 1963.

Bland, J. H., and Frymoyer, J. W.: Rheumatic syndromes of myxedema. N. Engl. J. Med., 282:1171, 1970.
Holvey, D. N., Goodner, C. J., Nicoloff, J. T., and Dowling, J. T.: Treatment of myxedema coma with intravenous thyroxine. Arch. Intern. Med., 113:89, 1964.
Sanders, V.: Neurologic manifestations of myxedema. N. Engl. J. Med., 266:547, 1962.

840.　MULTINODULAR GOITER

Multinodular goiter refers to an enlargement of the thyroid associated with more than one identifiable nodule. In fact the condition more specifically refers to a replacement of the normal homogeneous cytostructure of the thyroid by a collection of nodules of variegated histologic pattern, ranging from colloid-filled cysts and colloid adenomas to follicular and fetal adenomas. There may be some residue of histologically normal thyroid between the lumps, but more typically the structure between the more discrete adenomatous nodules consists of follicles with distended colloid-filled lumina. Often there is considerable associated fibrosis, sometimes there is calcification in the fibrous tissue or in the nodules, and hemorrhage into the nodules may be evident. Sometimes there is lymphocytic infiltration.

Etiology. The causation of this condition is not known with certainty, but there is evidence that mild deficiency in thyroid hormone production with consequent long-term stimulation of the gland (by TSH?) is one etiology. In areas of iodide deficiency, children under age 10 typically have diffuse enlargement of the thyroid, which on histologic examination shows a pattern of follicles distended with colloid and low cuboidal epithelium. Between ages 10 and 20, there is a gradual transformation of the process into the multinodular structure. Alternate periods of iodide deficiency with thyroid hyperplasia, and iodide sufficiency with involution, may lead first to colloid goiter and later to the typical multinodular goiter. Experimental proof of this theory in man is lacking. Presumably the hypertrophy of the thyroid in the iodide-deficient areas is due to TSH stimulation, but why this should lead to a colloid goiter rather than to hyperplasia is uncertain. For some reason the iodide-deficient gland forms excessive poorly iodinated thyroglobulin which is resistant to hydrolysis by intrathyroidal proteases, and thus accumulates.

Another possible cause is an inherited partial defect in hormone synthesis. Some patients with typical multinodular goiter secrete a large proportion of the iodide from the thyroid in a butanol-insoluble form, apparently an iodinated protein. These patients are usually euthyroid. Multinodular goiter tends to occur with high incidence in some kindreds. It has been generalized from this evidence that mild forms of metabolic defects in hormone synthesis, or perhaps the heterozygous carrier state for such a defect, may lead to the development of sporadic multinodular goiter.

Prevalence. The prevalence of multinodular goiter is related to geography, age, and heredity, among other factors. In iodide-deficient areas, multinodular goiter may occur in most individuals. In the United States a conservative estimate of the prevalence of palpable multinodular goiter among adults is 2 per cent, but this is probably low. Identical pathologic changes in the thyroid which do not produce gross enlargement of the gland are present in a much higher proportion of individuals at autopsy.

Clinical Presentation. Most commonly the condition exists throughout life and is not detected. In some patients enlargement and nodularity of the thyroid are found on routine physical examination. Since the incidence is 10 to 20 times as great in women as in men, and since it develops and progressively increases in size during life, it is often found in females of 50 to 70. Usually the condition is asymptomatic, but with progressive growth there may be a visible enlargement in the neck; tracheal compression, producing a sensation of choking or coughing; and occasionally pressure on the recurrent laryngeal nerve or edema, causing hoarseness. Sometimes there is hemorrhage into a cyst, producing sudden enlargement and tenderness in one area of the goiter. The problems of thyrotoxicosis and malignancy are discussed below.

Diagnosis. The diagnosis of multinodular goiter is usually made on the basis of physical examination. In its most typical form, the goiter feels like a bunch of grapes. The nodules vary in size from 0.5 to several centimeters in diameter and are of variable consistency. The patients are usually euthyroid on clinical examination, and this is confirmed by measuring the serum T_4 or FTI and the RAIU. Single nodules and Hashimoto's thyroiditis are the most common sources of confusion with multinodular goiter. Extensive development of one portion of the gland may lead to the impression of a single nodule; up to half of all thyroid enlargements thought to be single nodules turn out at operation to be multinodular goiters. The gland of Hashimoto's thyroiditis may have a lobulated texture, making it impossible to distinguish from multinodular goiter. Thyroid scintiscan may be useful if it shows a mottled distribution of radioisotope in the gland. Fluorescent thyroid scans show the same mottled distribution of stable iodine, in contrast to the uniform and diminished stable iodine in the gland of thyroiditis. Roentgenographic examination of the neck may give evidence of broad septate calcification or ringlike calcification in nodules. Often the trachea is deviated because of pressure by the goiter; this is rare in Hashimoto's thyroiditis. If diagnosis is imperative and cannot be made on the basis of the examinations already mentioned, needle biopsy is useful.

Therapy. Small nodular goiters in euthyroid subjects require no therapy. However, the natural history is progressive enlargement, and therefore it is appropriate to place patients on permanent therapy with desiccated thyroid in the hope that this will suppress TSH and prevent further enlargement of the gland. This should be done with careful observation, because some of the glands become autonomous, and the additional metabolic effect of exogenous hormone occasionally causes thyrotoxicosis. If the gland is grossly enlarged and causes a cosmetic defect or tracheal compression, resection may be indicated. Subsequently such patients should be placed on replacement therapy, because there is a pronounced tendency for regrowth. Sudden swelling and pain in the gland owing to hemorrhage into a cyst usually subside spontaneously over several weeks, and can be treated with analgesics. Nodular goiters that have progressively enlarged and have become displaced below the clavicles (substernal goiter) may cause tra-

cheal compression and should be resected. Such lesions can usually be removed through a cervical incision. Long-term pressure on the trachea occasionally produces tracheomalacia. The cartilaginous rings of the trachea are destroyed with a loss of normal rigidity. In such patients it is imperative that the function of the trachea be examined during inspiration and expiration at operation. Occasionally it is necessary that a tracheostomy be performed. The tracheostomy tube is left in place for 10 to 14 days to induce a fibrous reaction in the trachea and give it some rigidity.

Prognosis. The prognosis in untreated multinodular goiter is for slow enlargement of the gland. Administration of thyroid hormone may prevent progressive growth. It is also typical for longstanding multinodular goiter to develop autonomy and produce clinical hyperthyroidism.

COMPLICATIONS OF MULTINODULAR GOITER

Toxic Nodular Goiter. Many years ago Plummer observed that after nodular goiters had been present for an average of 17 years, thyrotoxicosis tended to develop. This may be due to the coincident occurrence of Graves' disease in the normal tissue between the nodules, but more often it is due to the uncontrolled hyperfunction of one or more nodules in the multinodular gland. In areas of endemic goiter this is the most common cause of hyperthyroidism, especially when iodine supplementation is first introduced into a previously deficient area. It is presumed that nodules developing because of TSH stimulation eventually become autonomous. Also, some autonomously functioning nodules in which hormone production has been limited by restricted iodine supplies are, in the presence of iodide supplementation, able to augment greatly the production of thyroid hormone. Patients with toxic nodular goiter are typically elderly, and symptoms are often minimal. Although the pathophysiology does not differ from that of other forms of thyrotoxicosis, congestive heart failure, atrial fibrillation, and muscle weakness tend to be prominent. The diagnosis should be suspected in any individual with a multinodular goiter and symptoms suggestive of hyperthyroidism, especially if heart failure or atrial fibrillation is present. The RAIU and serum T_4 may be in the high normal range or elevated. The diagnosis is further substantiated by a thyroid scan which localizes radioactivity to one or more of the nodules of the gland. In some of these patients it has been shown that there is a preferential secretion of T_3, leading to an increased ratio of T_3 to T_4 in blood. If the thyrotoxicosis is caused primarily by the excess T_3, the serum T_4 level may be normal. This diagnosis can be partially corroborated by observing failure of suppressibility of the gland, but must be confirmed by direct measurement of T_3.

Toxic multinodular goiter may be treated either by thyroidectomy after appropriate preparation with antithyroid drugs and potassium iodide or by administration of larger doses of radioiodine than are used in the treatment of Graves' disease, typically 10 to 15 mCi. Hypothyroidism is rarely produced because the isotope is distributed unevenly throughout the gland, and some portions are spared from radiation. The gland usually shrinks, but does not disappear. If the patient has significant heart disease, it is best to pretreat with antithyroid drugs before giving RAI, or to use multiple small doses of isotope (5 mCi every two to three months) until euthyroidism is achieved. Release of stored hormone after vigorous RAI therapy can otherwise precipitate congestive failure or infarction.

Administration of small doses of iodine (1 to 4 mg per day) occasionally induces thyrotoxicosis in previously euthyroid individuals with multinodular goiter. The thyrotoxicosis may be transient or may require treatment.

The Cancer Problem. Although the vast proportion of patients with multinodular goiter are never referred for evaluation or for surgery, the occurrence of sudden growth of one area of a multinodular gland, the palpation of an unusually firm area, or the development of hoarseness may raise the question of malignancy. Patients who come to surgery are obviously highly selected because they have developed symptoms that brought them to a physician and that were considered significant enough for referral to a surgeon. Among those who are operated upon, the incidence of verified carcinoma, usually papillary adenocarcinoma, varies from 2 to 20 per cent. Because of this frequency, some physicians view the presence of multinodular goiter as sufficient indication for thyroidectomy. The gross illogic of this reasoning can be seen by some simple calculations. If 2 per cent of the population have multinodular goiter and 10 per cent of these have thyroid malignancy, at least 400,000 papillary cancers would be present in the United States. In fact it is known that the prevalence of multinodular goiter is much greater than the figure used. In contrast, only 5000 thyroid cancers are detected annually, and the majority of these are found in patients whose thyroids are normal except for the malignancy. Because of this, it seems more logical to accept multinodular goiter as a measure of assurance that malignancy is not present. Multinodular goiter should not be resected because of a general fear of malignancy, but thyroidectomy is logical in the presence of signs that in themselves are suggestive of malignant change. In contrast, glands harboring a single nodule carry a real increase in risk of thyroid carcinoma.

Mortensen, J. C., Woolner, L. D., and Bennett, W. A.: Gross and microscopic findings in clinically normal thyroid glands. J. Clin. Endocrinol. Metab., 15:1270, 1955.

Sokal, J. E.: The incidence of thyroid cancer and the problem of malignancy in nodular goiter. *In* Astwood, E. B. (ed.): Clinical Endocrinology. New York, Grune & Stratton, 1960, Vol. 1, pp. 168–178.

Vagenakis, A. G., Wang, C. A., Burger, A., Maloof, F., Braverman, L. E., and Ingbar, S. H.: Iodide-induced thryotoxicosis in Boston. N. Engl. J. Med., 287:523, 1973.

Vander, J. B., Gaston, E. A., and Dawber, T. R.: The significance of nontoxic thyroid nodules. Ann. Intern. Med., 69:537, 1968.

Veith, F. J., Brooks, J. R., Grigsby, W. P., and Selenkow, H. A.: The nodular thyroid gland and cancer. A practical approach to the problem. N. Engl. J. Med., 270:431, 1964.

841.   ENDEMIC GOITER

In the United States the average iodide intake is 200 to 600 μg or more per day, and detectable thyroid enlargement occurs in 2 to 4 per cent of adults. In contrast, in areas where iodide deficiency is present, as evidenced by urinary iodine excretion below 50 μg per day, the incidence of palpable enlargement of the thyroid increases in inverse relation to the average urinary iodide excretion. Endemic goiter exists in many mountainous areas of the world, including the Andes, central New Guinea, and Switzerland, as well as in many lowland areas such as the Baltic Plains and Zaïre. In almost all well-studied endemics, the cause is deficient iodide in the soil and water, leading to deficient iodide intake. Presumably, iodide privation leads to diminished production of thyroid hormone, which is sensed by the pituitary, resulting in augmented secretion of TSH, and thus to increased thyroidal clearance of plasma iodide. With this there is also growth (both hyperplasia and hypertrophy) of the thyroid. The thyroid strives to gain the necessary 60 to 100 μg of iodide needed daily for hormonogenesis, and does so by accumulating almost all the iodide ion entering the vascular compartment, either from the diet or from degradation of hormone within the body. The uptake of a radioactive tracer is 90 to 98 per cent in some endemic areas. Initially the gland is diffusely enlarged, and the histologic picture in adolescence is a "colloid goiter" with large follicles and flat cuboidal epithelium. In time the picture changes into the multinodular goiter described previously; the histology is identical with that of sporadic multinodular goiter found in other regions. Usually diffuse goiter predominates in youth, and multinodular goiter in older persons. The incidence is higher in women than in men unless the endemic is unusually severe. In some areas, practically all adults have thyroid enlargement.

Pathogenesis. The biochemical abnormalities that lead to the formation of multinodular goiters in response to iodide deficiency are not known. Alternate periods of iodide deficiency and repletion may lead to hyperplasia and involution and produce the picture of endemic goiter. TSH is elevated in some severe endemics, but in Argentina adults have been found to have endemic goiter in the presence of normal levels of plasma TSH. Possibly these people had elevated TSH levels earlier in their lives, or perhaps owing to iodide deficiency the gland is more sensitive to TSH. The thyroglobulin of endemic goiters is iodine poor and characteristically has an excess of MIT over DIT, and the content of T_4 and T_3 tends to be low. Possibly these alterations of iodide content or distribution in the amino acids of thyroglobulin lead to abnormalities in degradation of thyroglobulin and produce the picture of a colloid-filled goiter.

Goitrogens. In a few instances factors other than iodide deficiency operate to cause endemic goiter. Thus a factor present in water appears to be associated with an endemic in Colombia. Thiocyanates are derived from some plants, e.g., cassava eaten in Central Africa. Potent goitrogens related in action to the thioureas are found in some plant species and are transmitted through cow's milk to humans in Tasmania and Finland. As fascinating as these examples are, they account for only a minute fraction of endemic goiter, a condition that involves many millions of people throughout the world.

Clinical Manifestations. Patients with goiter in endemic zones present with thyroid enlargements that may be diffuse or nodular and that vary in size from barely detectable to as large as the head (Fig. 9). In some places monstrous enlargement of the thyroid is accepted as normal. Usually such individuals, when adult, are euthyroid, and thus appear to have adapted to iodide deficiency by growth of the goiter. All the problems related to thyroid enlargement, such as dysphagia, respiratory difficulty, tracheal deviation and compression, and cosmetic problems may of course be associated with the thyroid enlargement. Occasionally, in severe endemics, some people are hypothyroid clinically and by laboratory examination. In contrast to the condition known as endemic cretinism, described below, patients with endemic goiter do not have neurologic signs or gross mental retardation. Aside from what might be considered by foreigners a cosmetic blemish, endemic goiter itself is inconsequential to most adults with this condition. However, there is evidence, discussed below, that the neural complications of iodide privation may be important.

Diagnosis. The diagnosis of endemic goiter is best made by study of a population group. The characteristic feature is reduced excretion of iodide in the urine. Iodide excretion is often 30 to 50 μg per day, although values as low as 5 μg per day have been recorded. RAIU values are elevated to the 70 to 95 per cent range.

Figure 9. A young woman from the Nepalese village of Wapsa which has severe iodine deficiency and a high incidence of endemic goiter. (Photograph kindly provided by Professor Kaye Ibbertson of the University of Auckland, Private Bag, New Zealand.)

Thyroid hormone in blood, as measured by the PBI or T_4, is normal, or rarely is depressed, and the patients are hypothyroid. The T_4 may be low in the presence of euthyroidism; these patients maintain normal metabolism by producing relatively more T_3. The findings of diminished urinary iodide, augmented thyroid uptake, and high incidence of goiter are sufficient to incriminate iodide as the cause of the endemic. If iodide intake is sufficient, i.e., above 100 μg per day in the presence of endemic goiter, some other cause must be sought, such as a goitrogenic agent in foodstuffs.

Treatment. The best treatment for endemic goiter is iodine prophylaxis applied to the entire population group. The most convenient approach is salt iodinization, adding about 50 μg of iodide per gram of salt as iodate or as potassium iodide. Another approach is to inject population groups with iodinated poppyseed oil. This provides a depot of 1 to 2 grams of potential iodide, and is sufficient to supply iodide for one to four years. Treatment with desiccated thyroid should prevent further enlargement of the goiters and suppress diffuse goiters in children. It usually has little effect on the multinodular goiters of adults. Local symptoms caused by massive enlargement of the thyroid may require thyroidectomy.

Thyrotoxicosis is rarely seen in areas of severe endemic goiter, apparently because the limitation of iodide supply prevents its development. Occasionally it does occur, and may be difficult to recognize because RAIU values are elevated even in "normal" subjects. The PBI or serum T_4 may be elevated, or may be normal if the patient secretes an excess of T_3. After administration of iodine in salt or by injection, some patients develop thyrotoxicosis. Sometimes this process (Jod-Basedow) is self-limiting, but therapy with antithyroid drugs, radioactive iodide, or surgery may be required.

There is no convincing evidence that carcinoma occurs with increased frequency in areas of endemic goiter, but there is a strong suggestion that a higher proportion of the tumors that do occur are poorly differentiated or sarcomatous.

ENDEMIC CRETINISM

This term refers to defective individuals having a typical constellation of signs and symptoms found with increased frequency in areas of severe endemic goiter. If recognized shortly after birth and if the children are hypothyroid, there is a typical appearance with increased hair, low forehead, puffy features, umbilical hernia, enlarged tongue, and sluggish behavior. Other abnormalities may be detected: deaf-mutism, mental retardation, and evidence of spastic paraplegia. These may occur with or without overt hypothyroidism, or as individual entities. If there is continued hypothyroidism, retarded growth and retarded bone age and epiphysial stippling occur. The individual may be goitrous, or no thyroid tissue may be present. In childhood, most endemic cretins achieve a euthyroid metabolic state, but stunted growth, deaf-mutism, mental subnormality, and diplegia give evidence of the syndrome. Endemic cretinism is probably caused by severe iodide deficiency leading to hypothyroidism in both mother and child during fetal development. Athyrotic individuals born to normal mothers in nonendemic zones rarely if ever develop the full-blown syndrome, apparently because significant quantities of thyroid hormone are transported from the mother to the fetus across the placenta. When investigated during childhood or adult life, endemic cretins may be hypothyroid or euthyroid. Treatment of euthyroid adult cretins with thyroid hormone has had no beneficial effect on mental function, deafness, or neurologic damage. The only known therapy is iodine prophylaxis, as described above for endemic goiter. Studies by Fierro in Ecuador suggest that in severe endemics associated with cretinism, mental subnormality may afflict a much larger portion of the population. Thus the effects of endemic iodide deficiency, goiter, and cretinism appear to be even more devastating than was previously known, making iodine prophylaxis of crucial importance in these areas.

Butterfield, I. H., Black, M. L., Hoffmann, M. J., Mason, E. K., and Hetzel, B. S.: Correction of iodine deficiency in New Guinea natives by iodized oil injection. Lancet, 2:767, 1965.
Dumont, J. E., Ermans, A. M., and Bastenie, P. A.: Thyroidal function in a goiter endemic. IV. Hypothyroidism and endemic cretinism. J. Clin. Endocrinol. Metab., 23:325, 1963.
Ermans, A. M., Bastenie, P. A., Galperin, H., Beckers, C., Van Den Schrieck, H. G., and DeVisscher, M.: Endemic goiter in the Uele region. II. Synthesis and secretion of thyroid hormones. J. Clin. Endocrinol. Metab., 21:996, 1961.
Fierro-Benitez, R., Penafiel, W., DeGroot, L. J., and Ramirez, I.: Endemic goiter and endemic cretinism in the Andean region. N. Engl. J. Med., 280:296, 1969.
Stanbury, J. B. (ed.): Endemic Goiter. Scientific Publication No. 193. Washington, D.C., Pan American Health Organization, 1969, p. 447.
Stanbury, J. B., and Kroc, R. L. (eds.): Human Development and the Thyroid Gland. Relation to Endemic Cretinism. New York, Plenum Press, 1972.

842. METABOLIC DEFECTS IN THYROID HORMONE FORMATION, TRANSPORT, AND ACTION

CONGENITAL METABOLIC DEFECTS IN THYROID HORMONE FORMATION
(Sporadic Goitrous Hypothyroidism or Goitrous Cretinism)

The biosynthesis of thyroid hormone proceeds via transport of iodide into the thyroid, binding of iodide to tyrosine in thyroglobulin, coupling of iodotyrosines, subsequent proteolysis of thyroglobulin with release of iodotyrosines and thyronines, intrathyroidal deiodination of iodotyrosines and reutilization of their iodide, and release of thyroid hormone to the blood. Specific enzymatic defects causing diminished efficiency in the formation of thyroid hormone have been identified as several of these steps. The various genotypes usually produce a common phenotype, characterized by the presence of a hyperplastic thyroid plus hypothyroidism or euthyroidism.

Defect in Iodide Trapping. A few patients have been recognized with hyperplastic thyroid glands and congenital hypothyroidism associated with inability to transport iodide into the thyroid and thyroidal uptake of tracer isotope near zero. Thyroid tissue from such patients, studied in vitro, is unable to establish an iodide

concentration gradient. The patients also fail to transport iodide into saliva and gastric juice; this observation forms the basis of a simple test for the defect. The concentration of iodide in saliva is compared with that in plasma two hours after administration of a radioactive iodide tracer. In affected individuals the ratio is 1, whereas in normal individuals and in presumed heterozygotes it is from 10 to 100. Thyroid tissue of these patients contains the other enzymes needed for hormone synthesis. It should be remembered that the usual cause for failure of iodide uptake during a tracer test is that the gland is saturated by exogenous iodine, rather than a faulty iodide-concentrating mechanism.

Iodide Organification Defect. The most common defect in hormone synthesis is at the iododide-binding step. The patients are able to transport and concentrate iodide in the thyroid, but the iodide is not bound to tyrosine in thyroglobulin. Iodide in the thyroid remains in equilibrium with that in plasma, and as iodide in plasma is cleared to the urine, the free thyroidal iodide gradually returns to plasma. Such patients have an elevated thyroid uptake shortly after administration of a tracer and a low uptake at 24 hours. The iodide content of the gland is greatly reduced. Reduced amounts of iodinated compounds are formed or released to plasma. T_4 is low.

A defect in binding can be identified by administration of potassium perchlorate two hours after administration of a radioactive iodide tracer. The potassium perchlorate will effectively block the iodide transport mechanism. If there is a large pool of free intrathyroidal iodide, potassium perchlorate will cause a release of this material to plasma, with a dramatic drop in the thyroid iodide content. A release of 10 per cent or more of the iodide present at two hours is considered a positive test.

A variant of this condition is found in association with congenital nerve deafness (Pendred's syndrome). This condition is transmitted as a mendelian dominant, but is expressed to varying degrees. Deafness ranges from complete through nearly normal hearing, and hypothyroidism may be severe or thyroid function may be normal.

The biochemical basis of the organification defect syndromes has been identified in patients studied in the author's laboratory. Some patients have diminished or absent peroxidase. Others have an abnormal peroxidase apo-protein which fails to bind the hematin prosthetic group firmly; thus the enzyme is not fully active. In other patients, an abnormality of thyroglobulin synthesis results in a diminished quantity of iodide acceptor. Other proteins are iodinated, but apparently inefficiently, resulting in a buildup of free intrathyroidal iodide and failure to produce iodothyronines.

"Coupling" Defect. Some individuals with congenital goiter have large, hyperactive thyroids and low thyroid hormone in plasma. Large amounts of MIT and DIT are found in their thyroglobulin. An abnormality of the coupling process is implied by these observations, but it is by no means certain what this abnormality is. It could, for example, be an abnormality in energy supply, an abnormality in the structure of the thyroglobulin, or perhaps lack of peroxidase enzyme related to the coupling process. It is currently believed that there is no "coupling enzyme," rather that peroxidase mediates this process as well as initial iodination of thyroglobu-

lin. Although patients with congenital thyroid disease, hypothyroidism, low plasma T_4, and plentiful iodotyrosines in the thyroid must have a defect of the coupling process, a more exact definition will require new information about the normal synthetic process.

Iodotyrosine Dehalogenase Defect. Thyroglobulin is degraded in the thyroid by a combination of protease and peptidases, and each amino acid of the thyroglobulin peptide chain is thus separated. Normally the iodotyrosines are deiodinated by a dehalogenase present in the microsomes. The liberated iodide is reutilized for the iodination of tyrosine to form more MIT and DIT. Each day about four times as much iodide goes through this cycle as enters the thyroid from the blood. Some patients have a specific defect of the dehalogenase. In the most carefully studied cases, the enyzme defect also exists in other tissues. Because of the defect in the thyroid, iodotyrosine is liberated from the gland into the blood. Because of lack of the enzyme in other tissues, iodotyrosines are not deiodinated, but are excreted in the urine. This iodide loss causes marked hypothyroidism and thyroid enlargement. The disease can be diagnosed by the identification of labeled iodotyrosines in plasma or urine after administration of a radioactive iodide tracer. Also, infused iodotyrosine is not deiodinated, but is excreted unchanged in the urine. Parents of affected individuals, who are presumed to be heterozygous, often show a minor abnormality in their ability to deiodinate iodotyrosine.

Butanol-Insoluble Iodide Defect. Many patients with congenital or familial thyroid enlargement and hypothyroidism have in their plasma iodine insoluble in acidified butanol, and thus not T_4 or T_3. This material is formed in the thyroid, and is of heterogeneous nature. Some glands secrete large amounts of iodinated albumin, prealbumin, or both. Others seem to secrete iodinated proteins that do not react with antihuman albumin serum, and do react in part with antithyroglobulin antibodies. Possibly these are abnormal subunits or fragments of thyroglobulin. The iodoproteins usually contain mainly MIT and DIT and no T_4 or T_3.

This inefficient utilization of glandular iodide restricts the formation of T_4 and causes thyroid hyperplasia. The basic abnormality is poorly understood. There may be inadequate production of normal thyroglobulin. Other proteins may then gain access to the gland and be iodinated. Another possibility is an abnormality in the proteolytic enzymes of the thyroid so that iodinated subunits of thyroglobulin are released to plasma. Attempts to identify defective protease activity have been inconclusive.

Epidemiology. The metabolic defects in hormone synthesis occur sporadically or in family groupings. Affected siblings may be identifiable, and occasionally parents are found to have a minor metabolic abnormality. Typically there is inbreeding in the family. The metabolic defects usually represent the expression of a homozygous recessive genetic abnormality. The exception to this is in Pendred's syndrome, which is inherited as a mendelian dominant.

Pathology. Typically there is marked hyperplasia of the thyroid. The gland is beefy, the cells are columnar, there is little or no colloid, and hypervascularity is marked. The extreme hyperplasia may take on the appearance of a papillary carcinoma. In other instances the longstanding thyrotrophin stimulation to the gland results in change into a carcinoma, metastases, and death. Disease, other than in the thyroid, depends upon the degree of hypothyroidism. In Pendred's syndrome there is in addition nerve deafness, but information on the nature of the lesion is lacking.

Clinical Presentation. Patients present a common phenotype. Usually the illness is not suspected at birth but becomes apparent within the first few months or, more frequently, during childhood. If the illness is severe, the child will develop evidence of hypothyroidism. There is symmetrical enlargement of the thyroid from two to ten times normal size. The gland is usually very vascular, and typically a bruit and thrill are present. The signs and symptoms of hypothyroidism are those described previously. The presence of metastases, including pulmonary infiltrates, indicates malignant change in the goiter.

Diagnosis. The diagnosis is suggested by observation of a hyperplastic thyroid in an individual who is apparently euthyroid or hypothyroid. The iodide-trapping defect can be demonstrated by the inability of the gland to accumulate iodide during a tracer uptake study. A corroborative finding is lack of concentration of iodide in the saliva. An iodide organification defect can be shown by a positive perchlorate discharge test and hypothyroxinemia. The iodotyrosine dehalogenase defect can be identified by chromatography revealing iodotyrosine in plasma and urine after administration of a tracer. The butanol-insoluble iodoprotein defect is detected by an abnormal difference between the PBI and BEI or between the PBI and serum T_4 iodine. Normally the difference is no more than 20 per cent. In patients with the syndrome, the BEI or T_4 iodine may be only 30 to 40 per cent of the PBI. Identification of the labeled protein can be made by electrophoresis of plasma or thyroid proteins obtained at biopsy after administration of a radioiodide tracer.

Therapy. Since the patients have a goitrogenic response to TSH caused by deficiency of thyroid hormone, the obvious therapy is to replace thyroid hormone. This corrects existing hypothyroidism and in children usually results in complete regression of the goiter. In older people in whom multinodular goiter has developed, there may be little change in size. In patients with the iodide trapping or dehalogenase defects, administration of a few drops of Lugol's solution daily will compensate for the defect. Development of thyrotoxicosis during iodide therapy for dehalogenase defect has been reported.

Prognosis. It is imperative that individuals with these syndromes be treated with suppressive doses of thyroid hormone or potassium iodide, as indicated, for the duration of their lives. Inadequate therapy will allow continued TSH stimulation of the gland, and malignant degeneration may occur. In general the patients and parents can be reassured that if the defect has been detected early so that there is no neurologic abnormality, treatment will result in normal health and longevity. Further, it is highly unlikely that progeny will be affected if there is no inbreeding.

DEFECTS IN HORMONE TRANSPORT

Occasionally patients have a great elevation or depression of blood thyroid hormone in the absence of corresponding clinical symptoms, owing to the presence of abnormal quantities of thyroxine-binding globulin (TBG). In well-studied kinships, the abnormalities have been shown to be transmitted as X-linked traits. Thus the affected or "carrier" females are typically heterozygous, and affected males are homozygous. In families with hypo-TBG-nemia, the males have extremely low or undetectable levels of TBG, with PBI or T_4 values in the range of 1 to 2 μg per 100 ml. Affected females usually have about half-normal TBG and PBI or serum T_4 values. The abnormality is the altered production of a normal protein, because no protein immunologically related to TBG is found in the serum of TBG-deficient subjects and turnover of labeled normal TBG injected into these subjects is similar to turnover in unaffected individuals. The decrease in total bound hormone in the plasma of such patients is counterbalanced by an increased fraction of free hormone. The absolute free hormone concentration is therefore normal, and the patients are eumetabolic. Aside from the confusion caused in the interpretation of laboratory tests, there is no known physiologic abnormality associated with this defect.

A few individuals have been reported with elevations of TBG to approximately two times normal and gross elevation of serum T_4. Again this appears to be genetically X-linked, with affected males exhibiting TBG elevation about twice that of affected (carrier) females. The patients are euthyroid, and no change in the availability of thyroid hormone to tissues can be shown.

The possibility of genetically induced decreased or (rarely) increased TBG should always be kept in mind when a thyroid hormone test reveals a level that appears to be discordant with the observed clinical state and no hormonal or disease-related cause exists. Measurement of absolute free T_4 content, or of the FTI, will indicate that the amount of functioning thyroid hormone in the plasma is normal. Another way to show the nature of the condition is by measurement of the T_4 carrying capacity of TBG. Evaluation of other members of the family will help verify the diagnosis.

HEREDITARY RESISTANCE TO THE ACTION OF THYROID HORMONE

Three of eight children in one reported sibship have apparent resistance to the action of thyroid hormone. The children have a characteristic facial appearance, retarded growth, delayed bone age, stippled epiphyses, deaf-mutism, and elevated thyroid hormone concentration in blood. The hormone in blood is T_3 and T_4, and there is no abnormality of binding proteins. Their thyroids produce about five times the normal amount of hormone daily, and this quantity is likewise degraded in the peripheral tissues. They appear to be euthyroid. A large body of laboratory data supports the conclusion that these children are resistant to the action of thyroid hormone. In compensation, an increased quantity of hormone is made available to the peripheral tissues. Even with this, some organs (e.g., the ears and bones) receive an insufficient supply of hormone. It is hypothesized that the hypothalamus shares in the decreased sensitivity. Studies designed to identify the basic enzymatic defect have not been revealing, and no therapy

has been devised. Conceivably, treatment of the mothers of such individuals with large doses of thyroid hormone during early pregnancy would be advantageous to the neurologic development of the fetus.

DeGroot, L. J., and Stanbury, J. B.: The syndrome of congenital goiter with butanol insoluble serum iodine. Am. J. Med., 27:586, 1959.

Lissitzky, S., Bismuth, J., Codaccioni, J. L., and Cartouzou, G.: Congenital goiter with iodoalbumin replacing thyroglobulin and defect of deiodination of iodotyrosines. Serum origin of the thyroid iodoalbumin. J. Clin. Endocrinol. Metab., 28:1797, 1968.

Niepomniszcze, H., Castells, S., DeGroot, L. J., Refetoff, S., Kim, O. S., Rapoport, B., and Hati, R.: Peroxidase defect in congenital goiter with complete organification block. J. Clin. Endocrinol. Metab., 36:347, 1973.

Niepomniszcze, H., DeGroot, L. J., and Hagen, G. A.: Abnormal thyroid peroxidase causing iodide organification defect. J. Clin. Endocrinol. Metab., 34:607, 1972.

Refetoff, S., DeGroot, L. J., Benard, B., and DeWind, L. T.: Studies of a sibship with apparent hereditary resistance to the intracellular action of thyroid hormone. Metabolism, 21:723, 1972.

Refetoff, S., Robin, N. I., and Alper, C. A.: Study of four new kindreds with inherited thyroxine binding globulin abnormalities. Possible mutations of a single gene locus. J. Clin. Invest., 51:848, 1972.

Stanbury, J. B., and Chapman, E. M.: Congenital hypothyroidism with goiter. Absence of an iodide-concentrating mechanism. Lancet, 1:1162, 1960.

Stanbury, J. B., Kassenaar, A. A. H., Meijer, J. W. A., and Terpstra, J.: The occurrence of mono- and di-iodotyrosine in the blood of a patient with congenital goiter. J. Clin. Endocrinol. Metab., 15:1216, 1955.

843. THYROID NEOPLASMS

Thyroid neoplasms are adenomas and malignant tumors. Pathologically, adenomas are classified into fetal, follicular, Hürthle cell, and papillary forms. Carcinomas are usually grouped into papillary, follicular, mixed, Hürthle cell, medullary, and anaplastic varieties. Lymphoma and lymphosarcoma are also found in the thyroid.

Etiology. As in all other neoplasms, the exact etiology is unknown. In the case of thyroid cells, it is certain that both radiation and TSH stimulation may be in some way involved. After the original observation by Duffy and Fitzgerald, a relation between x-ray to the pharyngeal or thymic area in early childhood and subsequent development of thyroid carcinoma (usually papillary) was well documented. In children who develop thyroid carcinoma under the age of 20, this association is characteristically present. Although the tumors are presumed to occur because of x-ray damage to the thyroid, it is possible that the pathogenesis involves damage to the immunologic surveillance system of the thymus, or that the response is fundamentally due to x-ray damage to the thyroid with subsequent TSH hypersecretion. Another known relationship is between chronic TSH stimulation and the formation of invasive thyroid carcinoma, best identified in patients with congenital metabolic defects. A third relationship is to a variety of the multiple endocrine adenomatosis syndrome (Type 2), involving pheochromocytoma and medullary thyroid carcinoma, which is transmitted as a dominant genetic trait. Multiple cutaneous neuromas are also seen in association with this syndrome, and occasionally parathyroid adenomas. Many thyroid tumors are known to be TSH dependent, in that administration of suppressive doses of thyroid hormone leads to decrease in or regression of the malignancy. The exact relation of x-ray or TSH to induction of autonomous growth is unclear, although it is presumed to involve a mutational change with deletion of genes that restrict growth of the thyroid cells.

Little is known about the development of thyroid adenomas, although it may be presumed that the same sort of change that causes thyroid carcinoma is involved in the pathogenesis of adenomas. Thyroid adenomas, or at least nodularity, are present with increased frequency in patients who have received x-ray therapy to the thymus, and adenomas are produced in laboratory animals subjected to long-term TSH stimulation. Multiple follicular adenomas are occasionally found in family groups. Although adenomas may develop into thyroid carcinomas, this is not a common process.

A high incidence of thyroid carcinoma has been found in patients coming to surgery with multinodular goiter. The reasons for this have been discussed in Ch. 840. It has been stated for years that the incidence of thyroid cancer in Graves' disease is diminished, but this is not certain. In a recently reported large series, 0.5 per cent of patients undergoing thyroidectomy for Graves' disease were found to have papillary thyroid carcinoma.

THYROID ADENOMAS

Pathology. Adenomas are new growths of thyroid tissue having a homogeneous histologic pattern, surrounded by a capsule composed of fibrous tissue or compressed normal cells. They may present as single structures in otherwise normal glands or, less frequently, as two or three discrete adenomas, or they may be a feature of the multinodular goiter. The most common variety is the follicular adenoma, composed of large colloid-filled follicles with flattened cuboidal epithelium. A common variety of this growth has large colloid-filled follicles and an ill-defined capsule, leading to its designation as a "colloid nodule." Whether or not these are true adenomas is debated. Occasionally there may be degeneration, and the adenoma is then cystic and filled with a gelatinous material. Evidence of old or recent hemorrhage into a degenerating adenoma is common. Some adenomas have the histologic appearance of normal thyroid tissue. Adenomas with smaller follicles and more cellularity are termed fetal or embryonal and are occasionally transitional forms between adenomatous and carcinomatous growths. In the Hürthle cell adenoma the cells are eosinophilic and have the appearance of liver cells. All of these are variants of the follicular adenoma. Papillary "adenomas" have characteristic fronds of cells projecting into a sparsely filled lumen; these may in fact be carcinomas.

Clinical Presentation. *The clinical problem most often presented by the thyroid adenoma is management of a solitary thyroid nodule.* This may be asymptomatic, or, less commonly, may be brought to attention because of hoarseness, pain, or difficulty in swallowing. Single nodules may be present in 2 per cent of the adult population. They are much less frequent in men than in women. It is certain that most remain without significant danger for long periods of time.

The problem is in differentiation of such lesions from thyroid cancer. In the vast majority of persons, the clinical finding is limited to a nodule in an otherwise normal gland. On clinical and laboratory examination,

most patients are euthyroid, although some are clinically toxic. RAIU and scanning studies may show that the nodule is "cold" (most commonly), that it is equal in uptake of radioactive iodide to that of the normal tissue, or that it concentrates radioactive iodide selectively. Some of the "hot" nodules produce excessive hormone and suppress the normal gland, or produce clinical thyrotoxicosis. Nodules may be "cold" because they are biochemically unable to transport radioactive iodide into the thyroid or are unable to bind it, but most frequently they are "cold" because they are cystic. If the nodule is "cold," is unusually firm, is fixed to the trachea or surrounding structures, is irregular in contour, or is known to have recently grown, or if cervical nodes are felt, the likelihood of malignancy is increased. However, it is certain that clinical examination and isotope scanning cannot segregate carcinomas from benign adenomas. Carcinoma may occur in nodules that are clinically "hot" on scanning; from 3 to 10 per cent of carcinomas are warm or hot by this technique. Solitary nodules in the thyroids of children and men are particularly dangerous. It cannot be taken for granted that a nodule known to have been present for a few years is benign. Further, it is probably not advantageous to treat such lesions for a long time with desiccated thyroid in an attempt to suppress their growth, because this rarely causes disappearance of the nodule. Short-term therapy before surgery may be of value since it makes the lesion more discrete and facilitates a localized resection. Positive diagnosis of cancer can be made in the infrequent medullary carcinomas by detection of elevated thyrocalcitonin levels, if this assay is available.

Since clinical differentiation between benign and malignant lesions is very difficult, and since most physicians are reluctant to perform a needle biopsy for diagnosis of possible neoplasm, *a logical approach is to resect most single nodules unless there is a clear contraindication to surgery.* The operative procedure is usually subtotal lobectomy if the lesion appears to be benign and if there are no observable lymph nodes. Frozen sections are made; if the diagnosis of adenoma is confirmed, no further procedure is done. If the lesion is malignant, a more extensive procedure is carried out, as discussed below. Patients who have a subtotal resection for a benign adenoma should be placed on permanent thyroid hormone replacement therapy. *Up to half the "single nodules" subjected to surgery are found to be multinodular goiters, and from 10 to 20 per cent are diagnosed by the surgical pathologist as thyroid carcinoma.*

A significant fraction of thyroid nodules, perhaps one third, are largely cystic. This differentiation can sometimes be made by palpation, and by echograms. Some surgeons are currently treating lesions thought to be cystic by aspiration, and early results indicate that this may effectively reduce the nodule. Other physicians are performing diagnostic needle biopsy to select lesions for surgery. Both these approaches carry the possible objections of spreading tumor or of false negative diagnosis. However, the techniques now being employed on a trial basis may prove beneficial; if so, they will greatly alter the indications for surgery noted above.

THYROID CARCINOMAS

Papillary Carcinoma. Nearly 80 per cent of thyroid carcinomas are papillary tumors, and there is debate over whether a benign papillary adenoma actually exists. The tumors have fronds of cellular tissue projecting into slitlike lumina containing scant or no colloid. Other portions of the lesion may show differentiation into a relatively normal follicular structure. The lesions are frequently very small and often are found as incidentally observed microscopic tumors in glands removed for some other lesion. Papillary tumors tend to metastasize early to lymph nodes in the neck, often when the primary tumor cannot be detected by physician examination or by scanning. The tumor remains confined to cervical lymph nodes for a long time, but may invade locally into strap muscles and the larynx, and metastasize to lungs. The histologic patterns of the primary and metastatic disease may be quite different, with follicular elements in either area. Growth tends to be partially dependent on TSH. The disease is less aggressive in individuals under age 40. Ten-year survival with various forms of therapy is 80 to 90 per cent.

Up to two thirds of the thyroid tumors in the differentiated papillary group cannot be categorized as either purely papillary or follicular, but are mixed. These tumors behave more or less like pure papillary lesions. It is impossible to tell which element has metastasized, and there may be major discrepancies in architecture and function between the primary and the metastatic deposits.

Follicular Carcinoma. Follicular thyroid carcinoma varies in appearance from relatively normal-looking thyroid tissue, to microfollicular structures, large follicles, or areas of solid, rather anaplastic-appearing tumor. Often some areas have Hürthle cell changes. These tumors metastasize early via the bloodstream to lung and bones. The tumors are TSH responsive and tend to pick up and metabolize iodide and to form thyroid hormone. Occasionally the unchecked biosynthetic activity of the tumor results in clinical thyrotoxicosis. The ten-year survival in patients with this illness is approximately 50 per cent.

Hürthle cell carcinoma tends to invade and metastasize locally in the neck. It has a morbidity approximately like that of follicular carcinoma.

Medullary Carcinoma. Medullary cell carcinoma is derived from the "C" cells, or calcitonin-secreting parafollicular cells of the thyroid. These tumors form sheets of cells with large nuclei. There is usually extensive deposition of amyloid and considerable fibrosis; lymphocyte infiltration may also be prominent. The tumors tend to metastasize locally to the neck and finally to the lungs and soft tissues. Their course is like that of follicular carcinoma, despite their undifferentiated "solid tumor" appearance. The tumors are associated with pheochromocytoma and a variety of other endocrine syndromes. It is clear that they produce calcitonin and rarely cause hypocalcemia. In response to this they may induce parathyroid adenomas. The tumors may also secrete "hormonal" polypeptides and, through this mechanism, may cause Cushing's syndrome and may produce excess serotonin. A history of familial cancer, pheochromocytoma, or hypocalcemia should suggest this diagnosis, and assay for calcitonin should be done.

Anaplastic Carcinomas. Anaplastic thyroid cancer ranges from small cell tumors through carcinosarcomas, giant cell tumors, and epidermoid tumors. These tend to invade locally and behave much as malignant neoplasms in any other portion of the body. Survival is usually less than 10 to 20 per cent after one year.

Lymphoma and lymphosarcoma may also involve the thyroid. It is doubtful that this is related to the occurrence of Hashimoto's thyroiditis. The mortality rate depends upon the histologic nature of the lesion.

Treatment of Thyroid Cancer. The selection of patients for operation has been discussed above. Patients with a neck mass thought to be due to thyroid cancer, or those with a thyroid mass plus cervical nodes, should have *thyroidectomy* unless some contraindication to surgery is present. At surgery diagnosis is made on the basis of examination of the primary lesion by the physician, resection of lymph nodes, and examination of frozen sections. If the lesion is differentiated (papillary or follicular cancer) and is confined to the thyroid, a total lobectomy is done on the involved side, resection of the lymph nodes in the tracheoesophageal groove is carried out, and a subtotal resection is performed on the opposite side. If there is evidence of multicentricity, a more radical resection is performed. If the lesion involves the thyroid and has metastasized to the neck, a total thyroidectomy is done, with preservation of the parathyroids by careful dissection or transplantation, and a homolateral limited neck dissection is performed. Occasionally patients will present with metastatic disease. If there is proved thyroid cancer with a solitary metastasis, it may be profitable to extract both the thyroid and the metastasis, because some patients will survive for a long time. In preparation for surgery and after surgery, patients with thyroid cancer should be on hyperphysiologic doses of thyroid hormone in order to suppress endogenous TSH. Many tumors are TSH dependent, and this therapy will prevent growth or actually cause tumor involution over years or decades.

If there is definite evidence of lymph node involvement or metastases, the patients are given one or more doses of 50 mCi ^{131}I to ablate residual thyroid tissue. If uptake in the metastasis can be demonstrated by scanning techniques after stimulation by endogenous or exogenous TSH, then patients are given courses of approximately 150 mCi of radioactive iodide-131 at intervals of three months (Fig. 10). Except when receiving ^{131}I therapy, all should receive thyroid hormone in doses sufficient to induce mild clinical hyperthyroidism. Some spectacular cures of metastatic thyroid cancer are obtained by ^{131}I, but all too frequently tumor uptake is low or declines with treatment, and there is a gradual overgrowth of tumor which does not concentrate isotope.

Medullary thyroid cancer is treated by surgery followed by x-ray therapy to the neck, because this tumor rarely concentrates radioactive iodide.

Anaplastic thyroid cancer is treated by local dissection to the extent possible. A radioactive iodide scan should be performed, but it is most unlikely that these tumors will concentrate radioactive iodide. Roentgen therapy is useful. After surgery, patients are placed on suppressive doses of thyroid hormone. Patients with lymphoma or lymphosarcoma are usually treated by surgery combined with postsurgical radiotherapy. The long-term survival is excellent in the lymphomas, and is perhaps 50 per cent at ten years in lymphosarcoma.

Recent reports indicate that the antitumor agents bleomycin and adriamycin may be useful in treating

Figure 10. *A,* Chest roentgenogram demonstrating pulmonary and mediastinal deposits of functioning follicular thyroid cancer in a 43-year-old woman. *B,* Two years and 450 mC ^{131}I later, the original nodules are invisible. However, nonfunctioning osseous metastasis has destroyed the body of D2 requiring a steel brace to alleviate spinal cord compression.

thyroid cancer unresponsive to surgery, ^{131}I, or x-ray therapy.

Black, B., Yadeau, R., and Woolner, L.: Surgical treatment of thyroidal carcinomas. Arch. Surg., 88:610, 1964.

Buckwalter, J.: Surgical treatment of thyroid carcinoma. Arch. Surg., 98:597, 1969.

DeGroot, L. J., and Paloyan, E.: Thyroid carcinoma and radiation. J.A.M.A., 225:487, 1973.

Duffy, B. J., Jr., and Fitzgerald, P. J.: Cancer of the thyroid in children: A report of twenty-eight cases. J. Clin. Endocrinol. Metab., 10:1296, 1950.

Leeper, R. D.: The effect of ^{131}I therapy on survival of patients with metastatic papillary or follicular thyroid carcinoma. J. Clin. Endocrinol. Metab., 36:1143, 1973.

Melvin, K. E. W., Miller, H. H., and Tashjian, A. H.: Early diagnosis of medullary carcinoma of the thyroid gland by means of calcitonin assay. N. Engl. J. Med., 285:1115, 1971.

ADRENAL CORTEX

Grant W. Liddle

844. THE ADRENAL STEROIDS AND THEIR FUNCTIONS

The function of the adrenal cortex is to secrete hormonal steroids, and the major disorders of the adrenal cortex arise from deficiencies or excesses of one or another of the adrenal steroids.

Table 1 lists the major adrenal steroids, their most abundant metabolites, their functions, and the clinical consequences of steroid deficiencies or excesses.

It has been known since the publication of Thomas Addison's classic monograph in 1855 that the adrenal cortex is essential for life. The two essential hormones are cortisol and aldosterone. The former provides resistance to a variety of stresses and maintains the activity of a number of enzyme systems; the latter enables the organism to withstand salt deprivation. In the quantities normally secreted, all the other adrenal steroids may be regarded as relatively weak or inactive precursors, metabolites, or by-products of cortisol and aldosterone. Cortisol and aldosterone are, indirectly, self-regulating, because each one is capable of initiating a series of physiologic events that result in the suppression of their respective stimulators.

Although cortisol and aldosterone are essential for life, when secreted in excessive quantities they can be life threatening. Beyond the scope of this chapter is the fact that supraphysiologic doses of cortisol and certain of its synthetic analogues can be used to modify the courses of a wide variety of nonendocrinologic disorders, particularly inflammatory and allergic processes.

Cortisol is the most important product of the human adrenal cortex in the sense that it is the one steroid that corrects most of the pathophysiologic effects of adrenalectomy when given in doses comparable to the amounts normally secreted. Cortisol is synonymous with hydrocortisone (the official pharmaceutical term) and, chemically, is 11β,17α,21-trihydroxy-pregn-4-ene-3,20-dione. It is closely related to *cortisone,* the glucocorticoid first produced synthetically on a large enough scale for widespread use as a therapeutic agent. Chemically, cortisone differs from cortisol in only one small detail: it has an 11-keto group instead of an 11β-hydroxyl group. This small chemical difference is extremely important biologically, however, for cortisone itself is lacking in biologic activity. It becomes effective in the body only because it can be converted to cortisol.

Cortisol is secreted by the zona fasciculata in response to adrenocorticotrophic hormone (ACTH). A specific biosynthetic step that is catalyzed by ACTH is the conversion of cholesterol to pregnenolone (3β-hydroxy-pregn-5-ene-20-one). Pregnenolone is then transformed by a series of adrenal enzymes to progesterone → 17α-hydroxyprogesterone → 11-deoxycortisol → cortisol. An inborn error in one of these enzymes or pharmacologic inhibition of one of them diminishes the efficiency of cortisol production and results in hypersecretion of the precursor occurring immediately before the inhibited step.

Upon entering the circulation, cortisol is reversibly bound to an α₂-globulin, transcortin. The major process of metabolic inactivation is carried out in the liver and involves reduction of ring A: Cortisol → dihydrocortisol → tetrahydrocortisol → tetrahydrocortisol glucuronide. The glucuronide is rapidly excreted by the kidneys. Some of the cortisol is oxidized to cortisone and then reduced and excreted as tetrahydrocortisone glucuronide. Tetrahydrocortisol and tetrahydrocortisone are the two most abundant end-products of cortisol metabolism; together, they account for almost 50 per cent of the total disposition of cortisol.

A widely used method for measuring cortisol in biologic fluids is the Porter-Silber reaction, utilizing the chromogenicity of the product resulting from the combination of phenylhydrazine with steroids having 17,21-dihydroxy-20-keto side chains (17-hydroxycorticosteroids, 17-OHCS). Normally, cortisol is the only major 17-OHCS in plasma, and tetrahydrocortisol and tetrahydrocortisone are the only major 17-OHCS in urine.

Another simple method for estimating plasma cortisol is based on the fact that it fluoresces; the fluorogenic steroid method is not applicable to the measurement of tetrahydrosteroids. Urinary tetrahydrocortisol and tetrahydrocortisone can be oxidized to 17-ketosteroids by bismuthate and are, therefore, 17-keto*genic* steroids

TABLE 1.   Properties of the Major Adrenal Steroids

Steroid	Regulated by	Major Metabolites*	Methods of Measurement	Major Actions	Clinical Consequences of Deficiency	Clinical Consequences of Excess
Cortisol	ACTH	Tetrahydro-cortisol Tetrahydro-cortisone	17-OHCS (Porter-Silber) Fluorogenic 17-KGS	Suppression of ACTH and MSH Protein catabolism Impairs glucose utilization Stabilizes lysosomes Suppresses inflammation Na retention K excretion	Hyperpigmentation (high ACTH, MSH) Fasting hypoglycemia Anorexia and vomiting Weight loss Apathy Impaired water excretion	Impaired glucose tolerance Thinning of skin Ecchymoses Poor wound healing Osteoporosis Weakness Hypertension Impaired growth Central obesity
Aldosterone	Angiotensin K,Na ACTH Volume	Tetrahydro-aldosterone Aldosterone-18-glucuronide	Isotopic	Na retention K excretion	Hypotension Hyponatremia Hyperkalemia	Hypertension Hypokalemia
Deoxycorticosterone (DOC)	ACTH	Tetrahydro-DOC	Isotopic	Na retention K excretion		Hypertension Hypokalemia
Dehydroisoandrosterone	ACTH	Androsterone Etiocholanolone	17-KS	Weakly androgenic and anabolic	Lack of axillary hair in women	Virilization of women and children
Unidentified androgens	ACTH			Androgenic	Lack of axillary hair in women	Virilization of women and children
Unidentified estrogens	ACTH			Estrogenic		Feminization in men and children
Substance S	ACTH	Tetrahydro-S	17-OHCS 17-KGS			
17α-OH-progesterone	ACTH	Pregnanetriol	17-KGS			
Corticosterone	ACTH	Tetrahydro-corticosterone	Isotopic			

*Methods such as 17-OHCS, 17-KS, and 17-KGS are not specific; isotopic and chromatographic methods are used in specific identification of individual steroids.

(17-KGS). This method is somewhat less specific than the Porter-Silber reaction; nevertheless, it is widely used for estimating cortisol metabolites.

Cortisol is ubiquitous as a physiologic regulator; hardly a tissue in the body is unaffected by this hormone. Cortisol influences the level of activity of certain enzymes. It restrains the secretion of ACTH and melanocyte-stimulating hormone (MSH) by the pituitary. It accelerates the catabolism of protein and the hepatic metabolism of amino acids. It increases the appetite and promotes the deposition of fat in the facial, cervical, and truncal portions of the body. It retards the uptake of glucose by muscle cells and promotes hepatic gluconeogenesis from amino acids, pyruvate, lactate, and bicarbonate. It stabilizes lysosomes and suppresses a variety of inflammatory processes. It stimulates a number of electrolyte transport systems. As will become apparent in the discussions of Addison's disease and Cushing's syndrome, most of the manifestations of these clinical disorders can be understood in terms of inadequacies or exaggerations of the physiologic actions of cortisol.

Aldosterone is secreted by the zona glomerulosa in response to angiotensin, potassium, and ACTH. Like cortisol, it is metabolized by the liver to an inactive tetrahydro derivative; but, in addition, about 10 per cent is conjugated by the liver and kidneys to aldosterone-18-glucuronide. This is an acid hydrolyzable conjugate which recovers its identity as biologically active aldosterone when exposed to acid, a fact which has been exploited in the measurement of urinary aldosterone. Aldosterone is extremely potent, and the concentrations encountered in clinical situations are so low that they can be measured precisely only with highly sophisticated isotopic methods.

The physiologic effects of aldosterone stem from its property of stimulating transport of electrolytes by epithelial cells of the sweat glands, gastrointestinal tract, and, of greatest importance, the nephron. In response to aldosterone all these tissues tend to conserve sodium and lose potassium. Aldosterone deficiency leads to sodium depletion, loss of extracellular fluid, hypovolemia, and hypotension. An excess of aldosterone leads to sodium retention, expansion of extracellular volume, and hypertension.

11-Deoxycorticosterone (DOC) is normally secreted at about the same rate as aldosterone (of the order of 0.1 mg per day), but since it has only about one thirtieth the mineralocorticoid potency of aldosterone it is usually of little physiologic importance. DOC normally occurs in the biosynthetic pathway as a precursor of corticosterone and aldosterone, but in certain varieties of congenital adrenal hyperplasia it may be secreted in quantities sufficient to cause hypertension. It is metabolized to tetrahydro-DOC, but the quantities of either DOC or its metabolite that appear in biologic fluids are so small that isotopic techniques are usually required to measure them.

Dehydroisoandrosterone, a weakly androgenic 17-ketosteroid, is the most abundant steroid secreted in response to ACTH. A small portion is excreted as such; some is excreted in the form of androsterone and etiocholanolone; a minute portion is converted to testosterone. Dehydroisoandrosterone is the major precursor of the urinary 17-ketosteroids. Except in states in which it is secreted in grossly excessive quantities, such as

virilizing congenital adrenal hyperplasia, it is of little physiologic importance.

11-Deoxycortisol (Reichstein's substance S) is the immediate precursor of cortisol and is, therefore, produced in response to ACTH. Normally, it is retained by the adrenal long enough to undergo 11β-hydroxylation, resulting in formation of cortisol. Inefficiency of 11β-hydroxylase can occur as an inborn error of metabolism (hypertensive congenital adrenal hyperplasia), in carcinomatous adrenals, and as a consequence of treatment with an 11β-hydroxylase inhibitor (metyrapone). It has little biologic activity. Like cortisol it has a 17,21-dihydroxy-20-ketone side chain and is, therefore, measurable either as a 17-OHCS or as a 17-KGS.

17α-Hydroxyprogesterone is the cortisol precursor preceding the formation of 11-deoxycortisol and is under the regulatory control of ACTH. It has little biologic activity, and probably has no important role in the clinical manifestations of virilizing congenital adrenal hyperplasia. It is normally secreted in trivial quantities, but in the most common variety of congenital adrenal hyperplasia (21-hydroxylase deficiency) it is secreted in large amounts. This steroid is metabolized to a tetrahydro derivative, pregnanetriol, which is excreted in the urine and is of diagnostic value: a large excess of urinary pregnanetriol is practically pathognomonic of virilizing congenital adrenal hyperplasia owing to 21-hydroxylase deficiency. Although pregnanetriol is not a 17-OHCS by the Porter-Silber reaction, it is a 17-KGS and thus contributes to the nonspecificity of the latter as an index of cortisol production.

845. REGULATION OF ADRENAL STEROID SECRETION

The adrenal cortex may be regarded as two related but distinct organs. The inner portion of the cortex (zona fasciculata and zona reticularis) is under the control of ACTH and secretes all the adrenal steroids except aldosterone. The outer portion of the cortex (zona glomerulosa) secretes aldosterone in response to angiotensin, potassium, and ACTH.

ACTH activates adrenal adenyl cyclase, stimulating the formation of adenosine-3',5'-monophosphate (cyclic AMP). Cyclic AMP is thought to activate an enzyme system that catalyzes the conversion of cholesterol to 20α-hydroxy-cholesterol, which in turn is converted to pregnenolone. The latter serves as a precursor for all hormonal steroids. The pattern of steroids secreted depends upon the enzymatic makeup of the adrenal cortex. Under normal circumstances the most abundant secretory products of the human adrenal cortex are cortisol and dehydroisoandrosterone, but a deficiency of one of the enzymes involved in the conversion of pregnenolone to its normal derivatives results in increased secretion of the biosynthetic intermediates occurring before the impaired step. Such distortions of adrenal secretory patterns are observed in congenital adrenal hyperplasia, in certain adrenal neoplasms, and during treatment with pharmacologic inhibitors of adrenal enzymes.

Since the secretory activity of the adrenal cortex is directly controlled by ACTH, many questions concerning the regulation of adrenal steroid secretion can be transformed into questions of what controls the secretion of ACTH. In brief, there are three major determinants of ACTH secretion in man. The *first* of these is the level of cortisol. Of all the products of the human adrenal cortex, only cortisol has significant ACTH-regulating potency. The higher the cortisol level, the greater is its restraining influence on ACTH secretion; the lower the cortisol level, the less the restraint on ACTH secretion. A *second* factor governing the secretion of ACTH is the sleep schedule. In people in the habit of sleeping at night, plasma ACTH (and cortisol secretion) begins to rise at about 2 A.M. It crests at about the time of awakening; then during the day it falls irregularly to low values during the evening. Thus there is a "diurnal rhythm" in the secretion of ACTH. The *third* factor governing the secretion of ACTH has been referred to as stress. Such experiences as pyrogenic reactions, acute hypoglycemia, electroconvulsive treatments, and major surgical operations bring about increases in ACTH secretion. Whether various stresses influence ACTH secretion through a common mechanism or separate mechanisms is unknown.

For practical purposes, in people with normal adrenal responsiveness, the plasma cortisol concentration can be used as an indirect index of ACTH secretion. Within the physiologic range of ACTH concentrations the adrenal response is directly proportional to the amount of ACTH reaching it. The cortisol secretory response to ACTH begins within minutes and continues as long as the plasma ACTH concentration is maintained. Once ACTH secretion has ceased, the plasma ACTH concentration falls with a half-time of about ten minutes; and once cortisol secretion has ceased, the plasma cortisol concentration falls with a half-time of one to two hours.

The secretion of aldosterone is only partially under the control of ACTH. Large amounts of ACTH induce increases in aldosterone transiently; but if ACTH is administered for more than two or three days, aldosterone secretion diminishes to pretreatment levels. Aldosterone is also influenced by potassium; depletion of bodily potassium diminishes aldosterone secretion. Impressive increases in aldosterone secretion can be brought about simply by depletion of bodily sodium, thus inducing hypovolemia. Hypovolemia of any cause induces renal production of renin, which catalyzes the generation of angiotensin; and angiotensin stimulates adrenocortical secretion of aldosterone. It is currently thought that the renin-angiotensin system is the principal regulator of aldosterone secretion in most of the conditions grouped under the heading Secondary Aldosteronism (see Ch. 852).

846.   ADDISON'S DISEASE
(Primary Adrenal Cortical Insufficiency)

Incidence and Etiology.   Addison's disease has been estimated to occur with an incidence of 1 case per 100,000 population. It is usually caused by granulomatous destruction or idiopathic atrophy of the adrenal cortex. Clinical adrenal insufficiency usually does not occur unless at least 90 per cent of the adrenal cortex has been destroyed. The most common granulomatous disease destroying the adrenal cortex is tuberculosis, but, in certain regions, disseminated fungal infections are almost equally common. Idiopathic atrophy of the adrenal cortex is thought by some to be a consequence of an autoimmune process. All other causes of Addison's disease are decidedly rare. They include amyloidosis, adrenal apoplexy, and destruction of the adrenal cortex by metastatic tumor.

Pathogenesis.   From the foregoing comments, it should be apparent that Addison's disease commonly arises in association with other significant disease processes. Thus the patient with Addison's disease resulting from granulomatous destruction of his adrenal glands should be considered to have had hematogenous spread of a tuberculous or fungal infection, and should be carefully surveyed for evidence of an active infection of other organs, particularly the genitourinary and respiratory systems. Patients with "autoimmune" atrophy of their adrenals have an increased probability of having other diseases such as diabetes mellitus, hypothyroidism, and hypoparathyroidism. Patients with Addison's disease preceded by the nephrotic syndrome should be suspected of having amyloidosis.

The pathology of the granulomatous adrenal was described in masterful detail in a monograph written in 1931 by Rowntree and Snell. Of interest to physiologists in later years was the fact that the few remaining adrenal cells were often "arranged in adenoma-like nodules . . . suggesting . . . compensatory hypertrophy." All the pathophysiologic consequences of Addison's disease can now be understood in terms of deficiencies of cortisol, aldosterone, and adrenal androgen.

Cortisol deficiency results in increased pituitary secretion of ACTH and melanocyte-stimulating hormone (MSH), and these pituitary hormones are responsible for the mucocutaneous accumulation of melanin in classic Addison's disease. Cortisol deficiency also results in loss of appetite, loss of vigor, inability to maintain adequate blood glucose levels during prolonged fasting, inability to excrete a load of free water with normal rapidity, and inability to withstand severe or even rather minor stresses without going into shock.

Aldosterone deficiency renders the distal convoluted tubule of the nephron unable to carry out cation exchange at a normal rate. Consequently, there is failure to conserve sodium and excrete potassium normally. As a result of sodium wastage, there is depletion of extracellular fluid volume, blood volume decreases, blood pressure falls, cardiac output falls, and heart size diminishes. This process may culminate in peripheral vascular collapse, and is a prominent feature of addisonian crisis. Hyponatremia results from failure to conserve sodium and, as noted before, impaired ability to excrete a water load. Impaired ability to excrete potassium causes serum potassium concentrations to rise. If serum potassium concentrations exceed about 7 mEq per liter, disturbances of cardiac electrophysiology occur, manifested by sharp peaking of the T waves of the electrocardiogram and cardiac standstill in diastole.

Adrenal androgen deficiency is of no consequence in the male, because testicular androgen production suffices to induce adequate virilization. In women, however, the adrenal is responsible for a major portion of the total production of androgen, and loss of adrenal function results in a decreased growth of axillary and pubic hair.

The clinical manifestations of Addison's disease are usually insidious, and often exist in mild form for several weeks or months before correct diagnosis leads to proper treatment. Throughout this time, however, the patient with severely compromised adrenal function is in jeopardy of fatal addisonian crisis, either through progression of the chronic abnormalities or through superimposition of some acute stress such as fasting (vomiting), injury (surgical operation), or infection.

The mechanisms of death are peripheral vascular collapse (shock) and hyperkalemic cardiac standstill; perhaps hypoglycemia plays a role in some cases.

Clinical Manifestations. One can hardly do better than to quote or paraphrase the clinical descriptions in the monographs by Addison and by Rowntree and Snell, written before synthetic steroids became available to alter the natural course of Addison's disease. Addison wrote:

> The patient, in most of the cases I have seen, has been observed gradually to fall off in general health; he becomes languid and weak, indisposed to either bodily or mental exertion; the appetite is impaired or entirely lost; ...the pulse small and feeble...excessively soft and compressible; the body wastes...slight pain or uneasiness is from time to time referred to the region of the stomach, and there is occasionally actual vomiting...it is by no means uncommon for the patient to manifest indications of disturbed cerebral circulation. . . . We discover a most remarkable, and, so far as I know, characteristic discoloration taking place in the skin,—sufficiently marked indeed as generally to have attracted the attention of the patient himself, or of the patient's friends. . . . It may be said to present a dingy or smoky appearance, or various tints or shades of deep amber or chestnut-brown. . . . The body wastes . . . the pulse becomes smaller and weaker, and . . . the patient at length gradually sinks and expires.

In their experience with 108 cases of Addison's disease, Rowntree and Snell noted that asthenia, weight loss, gastrointestinal symptoms (anorexia, nausea, vomiting, and abdominal pain), and hypotension were almost always part of the syndrome. Hyperpigmentation was present in most cases and was described in such terms as "a suntan which does not wear off . . . tinged somewhat with blue or gray . . . dirty in appearance." The exposed portions of the body (hands, face, neck, and arms), points of pressure and friction, nipples, freckles, recently formed scars, genitalia, and creases of the palms often showed exaggerated pigmentation. Brown, blue, or gray spots on the lips and buccal mucous membranes were common.

Nowadays, earlier diagnosis and specific therapy make it possible to correct the compensatory hypersecretion of ACTH and MSH before development of prominent mucocutaneous hyperpigmentation, so that this manifestation may disappear in the patient who has been treated for a long time. Hyperpigmentation is not present in all untreated patients, so one should not take the position that the absence of characteristic hyperpigmentation rules out the diagnosis of Addison's disease.

The mental state of the untreated addisonian patient was frequently characterized as "asthenia, languor, exhaustion, or disinclination to physical or mental effort." Less frequently, irritability, confusion, and delusions were noted. Almost invariably the patients lacked the vigor to carry on productive lives.

Fever was not found in "uncomplicated" cases of Addison's disease. When it did occur it was attributable to coexisting infection.

It is of historical interest that the laboratory abnormalities of Addison's disease as listed by Rowntree and Snell were limited to such items as gastric achlorhydria, elevated serum urea, and delayed excretion of phenolsulfonphthalein and water. It was only later that hyponatremia and hyperkalemia were recognized as being commonplace abnormalities in the chemical profile of Addison's disease.

It is important to remember that Addison's disease often occurs in association with other diseases. Since the clinical manifestations of Addison's disease are shared by many other debilitating disorders, it is easy to overlook the possible presence of Addison's disease while attributing all the manifestations to some coexisting condition. Fortunately, it is now possible to establish with certainty whether a patient has Addison's disease with a specific test for adrenocortical reserve, and this should be carefully performed without hesitation whenever the possibility of Addison's disease seems realistic, for example, in any patient with a syndrome of hypotension, weakness, anorexia, and weight loss.

Diagnosis and Differential Diagnosis. To establish the diagnosis of Addison's disease one should measure the steroid secretory response to a standard dose of ACTH. A standard test, which has a number of modifications, all valid in experienced hands, is to give 50 units of ACTH as a constant intravenous infusion for eight hours and measure the resulting rise in plasma cortisol. Individuals with normal adrenal glands should respond with increases in plasma cortisol to at least 30 μg per 100 ml. Addisonian patients show little or no increase in plasma cortisol, which is usually less than 15 μg per 100 ml both before and during the infusion of ACTH. Intermediate (subnormal) responses are observed in patients with adrenocortical insufficiency secondary to hypopituitarism or prolonged corticosteroid therapy; these conditions can be distinguished from Addison's disease by demonstrating that repetitive treatment with ACTH, over several successive days, induces a stepwise increase in adrenal steroids until normal values are attained. Among the acceptable modifications of this standard test are procedures employing intramuscular injection of a good quality of depot ACTH and measurement of urinary 17-OHCS, 17-KGS, or 17-ketosteroids. The crucial point is that the patient with Addison's disease has little or no adrenocortical capacity to respond to ACTH (Fig. 1).

Treatment. The most important principles to observe in the management of Addison's disease are (1) that only two adrenal hormones, cortisol and aldosterone, are vitally important; (2) that the physiologic requirements for these two hormones fluctuate; (3) that cortisol substitution therapy should never be totally withdrawn unless it can first be demonstrated that the diagnosis of Addison's disease was erroneous, and (4) that sodium chloride must be administered in liberal quantities in order to correct extracellular fluid depletion.

Treatment of Addisonian Crisis. The patient in addisonian crisis is in immediate danger of losing his life because of glucocorticoid deficiency, extracellular fluid depletion, and hyperkalemia. Without delay, he should be treated with an intravenous infusion of physiologic sodium chloride; the infusion should be given rapidly, on the assumption that the patient probably has a deficit of at least 20 per cent of his extracellular volume (at least 3 liters in the adult). A water-soluble glucocor-

Figure 1. Urinary 17-OHCS:(1) during a control day and (2) during a day on which 50 units of ACTH was administered intravenously over a period of eight hours. In contrast to normal subjects and patients with Cushing's disease, patients with Addison's disease have low steroid values on both days.

ticoid such as hydrocortisone phosphate, 100 mg, should be added to the infusion. Within a few hours, if the electrolyte imbalance is corrected, the endocrinologic crisis may be considered to be over, and therapy should be adapted to meet the patient's current needs; if there is no stressful complication, the dose of glucocorticoid may be reduced to the physiologic range of approximately 20 mg of hydrocortisone daily; but if the patient is stressed, larger doses will be required. An attempt should be made to determine whether the crisis might have been precipitated by some stress such as an infection, and if so, this should be treated specifically.

If the diagnosis of Addison's disease has not previously been established and the patient's illness is suggestive of addisonian crisis, one should without delay initiate therapy and, at the same time, carry out a definitive diagnostic test for Addison's disease. Physiologic sodium chloride solution should be administered as outlined above. Instead of adding hydrocortisone phosphate to the saline infusion, one should add the potent water-soluble glucocorticoid dexamethasone phosphate, 4 mg. This will be equivalent to 100 mg of hydrocortisone in biologic potency, but will not obscure the adrenal response to an infusion of ACTH. To the intravenous infusion one may add ACTH in a dose sufficient to assure that the patient receives at least 5 units each hour for eight hours. Plasma cortisol should be measured prior to the addition of ACTH and again toward the end of the ACTH infusion. An adequate rise in plasma cortisol in response to ACTH excludes the diagnosis of Addison's disease; a negligible adrenal response confirms the diagnosis.

Chronic Treatment of Intercritical Addison's Disease. Therapeutic strategy in Addison's disease aims at simulating normal rates of secretion of cortisol and mineralocorticoid. Normal adults secrete about 20 mg of cortisol per day, and adults with Addison's disease usually require approximately 20 mg of cortisol (hydrocortisone) daily in the form of medication; it may be administered orally or parenterally in single or divided doses. Various synthetic glucocorticoids may be substi-

tuted for hydrocortisone, providing that proper adjustment is made for their differences in biologic potency.

Normal adults receiving unrestricted diets usually consume 100 to 300 mEq of sodium daily, and while on such diets they secrete approximately 0.1 mg of aldosterone daily. Aldosterone is not available for therapeutic use, but a synthetic mineralocorticoid, fludrocortisone (9α-fluorohydrocortisone), is available, and a tablet containing 0.1 mg taken once daily usually suffices as an aldosterone substitute. Another useful preparation is *desoxycorticosterone pivalate,* a slowly absorbed suspension given intramuscularly in doses of about 50 mg (2 ml) per month. A patient who has a history of hypertension prior to the onset of Addison's disease may not require mineralocorticoid replacement therapy as long as he receives glucocorticoids and ordinary amounts of dietary sodium. No addisonian patient will do well, however, without an ample intake of sodium chloride.

Children with Addison's disease require smaller doses of steroids than adults. The daily cortisol dose should be about 12 mg per square meter of body surface. If the child's linear growth does not proceed normally, it should be assumed that the dose of cortisol might be excessive, and the dose should be adjusted downward. The dose of mineralocorticoid should be adjusted as necessary to maintain normal blood pressure.

Treatment During Stresses. The maximal response of the normal pituitary-adrenal system to extreme stress results in the secretion of 200 to 500 mg of cortisol per day. This is the dosage range of hydrocortisone phosphate to be administered parenterally to patients undergoing bilateral adrenalectomy or to addisonian patients undergoing extensive surgical procedures. Hydrocortisone phosphate administered parenterally in doses of 100 mg every four to six hours should suffice as glucocorticoid replacement therapy in any severely stressed addisonian patient. As the stress subsides, the dose of hydrocortisone should be diminished accordingly. For example, after a major surgical operation, the daily dose of hydrocortisone can usually be decreased by decrements of 50 per cent each day until the usual dosage employed in chronic substitution therapy is reached.

For one reason or another, severely stressed patients usually do not consume adequate diets. It is important that addisonian patients be given at least 1 liter of physiologic sodium chloride solution daily until they resume their normal diets; a particularly hazardous period in convalescence is that during which orders are ordinarily given for the patient to take a "soft diet" or "surgical liquids." During this period the patient often does not even take all that is offered and may become depleted of extracellular fluid.

Mild stresses such as minor surgical operations and injuries require only minor increases in corticosteroid therapy. Usually a two- to fourfold increase in glucocorticoid treatment on the day of the stress will suffice. Oral medications may be used if they can be retained. Again, it is important that the addisonian patient who is fasting or vomiting be given parenteral sodium chloride solution.

Treatment in the Presence of Infection. In the presence of infection, it is particularly important that glucocorticoid dosage should simulate the cortisol secretion rate of the similarly infected but endocrinologically normal person. Overtreatment might impair the patient's mechanisms for defending against invading microorganisms, whereas undertreatment might predispose the infection-stressed patient to addisonian crisis. As a rule, an endocrinologically normal person secretes no more than 20 to 100 mg of cortisol per day in response to infection. This then is the hydrocortisone dosage range that is appropriate for the addisonian with an intercurrent infectious illness. A practical rule is to be guided by the patient's body temperature. If it is in excess of 39° C, the dose of hydrocortisone should be increased to whatever amount is needed to reduce the temperature to less than this level. If the temperature is normal, the hydrocortisone dosage should be lowered until maintenance doses are reached. If the temperature is between 38 and 39° C, it may be assumed that the dose of hydrocortisone is appropriate (presumably between 20 and 100 mg per day). It is of utmost importance that infections be specifically diagnosed and specifically treated as quickly as possible.

Mineralocorticoid vs. Sodium Chloride Therapy. Mineralocorticoids are used in treating intercritical adrenal insufficiency in order to assist the well-fed patient in maintaining adequate sodium stores without taking supplemental sodium chloride. Ordinary doses of mineralocorticoids do not adequately protect the addisonian patient from sodium and extracellular fluid depletion during periods of fasting or vomiting. Once sodium depletion has occurred, it must be corrected by the administration of sodium chloride; if adequate attention is given to this matter, upward adjustment of mineralocorticoid dosage (simulating the normal aldosterone secretory response to sodium depletion) will be unnecessary. Patients who sustain losses of sodium chloride but who are still capable of retaining oral medication, e.g., patients who sweat excessively, may be given supplemental sodium chloride tablets in doses of 2 grams two to four times daily.

Identification Bracelet and Injectable Hydrocortisone. The patient with Addison's disease should wear an identification bracelet stating his name, nearest kin's name and telephone number, and physician's name and telephone number. It should also state: "I have adrenal insufficiency. In any emergency involving injury, vomiting, or loss of consciousness, the hydrocortisone in my possession should be injected under my skin, and my physician should be notified." The patient should carry a small, clearly labeled kit containing 100 mg of hydrocortisone phosphate solution in a sterile syringe ready for injection. Even if never used, the bracelet and kit are of educational value to the addisonian patient who must understand that his survival depends upon the timely use of steroids.

Prognosis. With the advent of synthetic corticosteroids the prognosis of Addison's disease became radically altered from one of almost certain fatal termination within months (rarely years) to one of normal activity and life expectancy. The well-treated addisonian patient should have essentially normal steroid and electrolyte values under all circumstances; therefore he should not be incapacitated or have his life expectancy shortened by the fact that he has Addison's disease. All of the author's addisonian patients are productively employed unless they suffer from some additional disorder which is in some way incapacitating. Addisonians must, however, face the perils of emergencies in which they are incapable of caring for themselves and in

which they might depend upon the assistance of others to assure that the essential steroids and electrolytes are administered. Their prognosis might also be limited by other diseases sometimes associated with Addison's disease, such as tuberculosis, histoplasmosis, diabetes mellitus, or amyloidosis. Most of the addisonian patients who have been discovered since synthetic cortisone became generally available are still living, and there are no accurate data to indicate whether Addison's disease per se, when adequately treated, alters life expectancy.

ADRENAL INSUFFICIENCY SECONDARY TO BILATERAL ADRENALECTOMY

Adrenal insufficiency secondary to bilateral adrenalectomy is one variant of Addison's disease which should never present any diagnostic difficulty inasmuch as it is iatrogenic. Treatment is the same as that outlined under Addison's Disease.

847. ADRENAL APOPLEXY

Hemorrhagic infarction of the adrenal glands can occur in the course of meningococcal septicemia (Waterhouse-Friderichsen syndrome) or as a complication of anticoagulant therapy. The occurrence of hypotension in either of these clinical settings should alert the physician to the possibility of adrenal apoplexy, and treatment similar to that outlined under the heading Treatment During Stresses (Ch. 846) should be undertaken on an emergency basis. Specific treatment for the underlying disorder (meningococcemia or coagulation defects) should also be carried out without delay. If the patient survives, he may at some later date undergo a standard test for adrenocortical reserve in order to determine whether steroid replacement therapy can be withdrawn safely.

Although the adrenal glands are hemorrhagic in the Waterhouse-Friderichsen syndrome, hypotension, shock, and death in this condition are usually not attributable to adrenal insufficiency. Cortisol should be given in large doses, because it is impossible to rule out adrenal insufficiency within the time that is available to initiate decisive therapy; the patient who might have true adrenal insufficiency in association with adrenal apoplexy should not be denied the benefits of adequate cortisol therapy.

848. ADRENAL INSUFFICIENCY SECONDARY TO HYPOPITUITARISM

Definition and Incidence. Since normal adrenal function is dependent upon the stimulatory action of ACTH secreted by the pituitary, it follows that any disorder in which the pituitary is damaged in such a way as to reduce ACTH secretion to subnormal values leads to secondary adrenocortical hypofunction. This situation is encountered in approximately 1 of 1000 patients admitted to hospitals. (See Ch. 831.)

Pathogenesis. Whether associated with tumor, infarction, infection, histiocytosis, surgical resection, or intensive irradiation, loss of pituitary function is attributable to loss of pituitary tissue or to interruption of the connections between the hypothalamus and the pituitary. The degree of hypopituitarism is variable from patient to patient, ranging from such profound deficiencies as to be incompatible with survival to such mild deficiencies that special tests of pituitary reserve are required to demonstrate an abnormality.

Absence of ACTH results in decreased secretion of cortisol and adrenal androgen, but aldosterone secretion remains relatively intact. Cortisol deficiency results in loss of appetite, loss of vigor, inability to maintain adequate blood glucose levels during prolonged fasting, inability to excrete free water with normal rapidity, and inability to withstand severe stresses without going into shock. Hyponatremia is commonly encountered in patients with hypopituitarism who have been given liberal amounts of fluid, and it is directly attributable to the difficulty these individuals have in excreting free water. If they are given glucocorticoid so that they can excrete water adequately, they can be shown to have the capacity to adapt to simple sodium chloride deprivation by increasing their aldosterone secretion sufficiently to enable them to excrete urine that is virtually sodium free.

Absence of adrenal androgen is itself of little consequence; but when adrenal insufficiency is secondary to hypopituitarism, it is usually accompanied by a deficiency of gonadotrophins with secondary hypogonadism and a consequent decrease in testicular secretion of testosterone. Therefore, in contrast to Addison's disease, in which only the adult female shows evidence of androgen deficiency, in hypopituitarism patients of either sex are likely to exhibit manifestations of androgen deficiency.

Clinical Manifestations. There are several similarities and a few important differences between hypopituitarism and Addison's disease with regard to their clinical manifestations. Like the addisonian, the patient with hypopituitarism "falls off in general health; he becomes languid and weak, indisposed to either bodily or mental exertion; the appetite is impaired...and there is occasionally actual vomiting." Fasting may lead to hypoglycemia, and hypoglycemic symptoms (including loss of consciousness) are probably more common in untreated hypopituitarism than in Addison's disease. A liberal intake of water may lead to severe hyponatremia and manifestations of water intoxication such as confusion, incoordination, stupor, and convulsions. Severe stress may precipitate peripheral vascular collapse.

In contrast to the addisonian, the patient with hypopituitarism does not show mucocutaneous hyperpigmentation (this abnormality, in Addison's disease, is a consequence of *excessive* secretion of the pituitary hormones ACTH and MSH). Unlike the addisonian, the patient with hypopituitarism can tolerate simple sodium deprivation without developing shock or hyponatremia. In addition to the manifestations of adrenal insufficiency, the patient with hypopituitarism usually exhibits manifestations of hypogonadism and hypothyroid-

ism, and may show other evidence of pituitary or intracranial disease, e.g., erosion of the sella turcica and temporal visual field defects.

Diagnosis and Differential Diagnosis. The diagnosis of secondary adrenal insufficiency is established by the demonstration that cortisol levels in blood and cortisol metabolite levels in urine are subnormal and that they can be induced to rise to normal or above normal by repetitive treatment with ACTH over a period of one to three days. Urinary 17-ketosteroids are also subnormal, but rise in response to ACTH.

Primary adrenal insufficiency (Addison's disease) is easily differentiated from secondary adrenal insufficiency by the failure of steroids to rise substantially regardless of the dosage or duration of treatment with ACTH.

It is advisable to measure both plasma and urinary steroids in order to avoid pitfalls in differentiating secondary adrenal insufficiency from certain disorders of cortisol metabolism in which a normal relationship between plasma and urinary corticosteroids is lacking. Thus in primary hypothyroidism, hepatic insufficiency, and severe renal insufficiency, and during treatment with drugs that alter the extra-adrenal metabolism of cortisol (diphenylhydantoin, aminoglutethimide, amphotericin, o,p'-DDD, triparanol), the urinary 17-OHCS do not adequately reflect cortisol secretion rates and are falsely low in relation to plasma cortisol levels. In these situations, plasma cortisol concentrations accurately reflect cortisol secretion under basal conditions and in response to ACTH, whereas urinary 17-OHCS might falsely suggest the presence of secondary adrenal insufficiency. In contrast, there is a familial disorder in which plasma transcortin concentrations are subnormal, even though cortisol secretion rates, plasma free cortisol concentrations, and urinary 17-OHCS are all normal. In this situation, plasma cortisol concentrations alone might erroneously suggest the presence of secondary adrenal insufficiency.

Various clinical clues are also helpful in arriving at a correct diagnosis of secondary adrenal insufficiency, e.g., hypothyroidism with normal responsiveness to thyrotrophin, hypogonadism with subnormal gonadotrophin levels in plasma or urine, or growth failure with consistently negligible levels of growth hormone in serum (even after provocative maneuvers such as arginine infusion or insulin-induced hypoglycemia). Other evidence of pituitary disease, such as erosion of the sella turcica or a history of postpartum hemorrhage, should also alert the physician to the possibility that the patient might have hypopituitarism, subnormal ACTH production, and secondary adrenocortical deficiency.

A mild degree of ACTH deficiency can exist with normal or slightly subnormal plasma and urinary corticosteroids and normal or slightly subnormal responses to ACTH. Such mild degrees of ACTH deficiency are referred to as limited pituitary reserve, and are characterized by failure of the pituitary to secrete normal quantities of ACTH (and therefore a failure of the adrenal glands to secrete normal quantities of corticosteroids) in response to stress or to standard test doses of metyrapone.

Treatment. Secondary adrenocortical insufficiency requires cortisol replacement therapy in the same doses and under the same conditions as outlined for Addison's disease (see Ch. 846). Mineralocorticoid therapy is unnecessary. An identification card and hydrocortisone phosphate for emergency use should be employed as in Addison's disease.

If the patient suffers from hypogonadism, hypothyroidism, or diabetes insipidus, these conditions should be treated with androgens or estrogens, thyroid, or pitressin, as outlined in Ch. 859, 839, and 834, respectively.

Prognosis. As in the case of Addison's disease, the prognosis in secondary adrenal insufficiency is excellent if intelligent use is made of hormones for replacement therapy and if the primary basis for the hypopituitarism is not otherwise incapacitating or life threatening (see Ch. 831).

849. ADRENAL INSUFFICIENCY SECONDARY TO PITUITARY-ADRENAL SUPPRESSION BY CORTICOSTEROIDS

Prolonged administration of glucocorticoids or prolonged secretion of cortisol by an adrenal tumor in quantities sufficient to cause Cushing's syndrome consistently causes suppression of ACTH secretion and consequent adrenocortical atrophy. Withdrawal of steroid therapy or removal of the adrenal tumor results in adrenal insufficiency. Diagnosis should not be difficult in view of the physician's or surgeon's role in bringing about the condition. If the hypercortisolism has been severe and has existed continuously for at least one year, the course of pituitary-adrenal recovery may be slow, requiring several months for completion. Early in the course the basal corticosteroid levels, the adrenal response to ACTH, and the pituitary-adrenal response to metyrapone are all subnormal, simulating adrenal insufficiency secondary to hypopituitarism. Treatment consists of giving a physiologic dose of hydrocortisone, 20 mg once daily, to prevent symptoms of adrenal insufficiency. Over a period of months this dose can gradually be reduced to 5 mg daily and finally withdrawn altogether as pituitary-adrenal function gradually returns to normal. Until pituitary-adrenal recovery is complete, one should treat the patient as if he had hypopituitarism during periods of stress or infection (see Ch. 831).

850. CUSHING'S SYNDROME

Definition. Cushing's syndrome is the clinical and metabolic disorder resulting from a chronic excess of glucocorticoids. *Cushing's syndrome medicamentosus* is a common iatrogenic disorder caused by any of several synthetic glucocorticoids. Spontaneous Cushing's syndrome, on the other hand, is caused solely by cortisol, the only glucocorticoid produced in significant quantities by the human adrenal cortex.

Etiology. Normally, cortisol is not secreted except in response to ACTH, and ACTH is not secreted in the presence of supraphysiologic levels of cortisol. Therefore the very occurrence of Cushing's syndrome implies a

disorder in the regulation of cortisol or ACTH secretion: either the adrenal gland has acquired the capability of secreting cortisol in the absence of ACTH, or ACTH secretion is not normally suppressible by cortisol. There are three well-established causes of Cushing's syndrome. *First,* adrenocortical tumors can secrete cortisol autonomously, that is to say, in the virtual absence of ACTH. The tumors may be carcinomas, solitary adenomas, or (rarely) multiple adenomas. *Second,* certain nonpituitary neoplasms secrete ACTH, which stimulates the adrenal cortices to secrete supraphysiologic quantities of cortisol. This clinical entity is sometimes referred to as the ectopic ACTH syndrome (see Ch. 870). *Third,* pituitary function can become disordered so that ACTH is secreted in excessive quantities, thus stimulating excessive secretion of cortisol by the adrenals. This condition is referred to by the specific term Cushing's disease. The pituitary can be normal in appearance, contain a small basophil adenoma, or contain a large chromophobe adenoma; regardless of the morphologic appearance of the pituitary, virtually all patients with excessive pituitary ACTH show similar patterns of ACTH secretion. There is loss of normal diurnal rhythmicity, relative but not absolute resistance to suppression by glucocorticoids, and increased secretion of ACTH in response to a reduction of cortisol levels to normal.

Incidence. Cushing's syndrome resulting from adrenal tumor occurs in approximately 1 of every 10,000 hospital admissions. Cushing's disease occurs in approximately 1 of every 4000 admissions. The incidence of the ectopic ACTH syndrome is difficult to estimate, because it is frequently overlooked. There is evidence that ectopic ACTH might be produced by as many as 8 per cent of visceral carcinomas. Careful screening of patients with nonpituitary tumors might reveal the production of ectopic ACTH to be the most common cause of hypercortisolism.

Pathogenesis. The major features of Cushing's syndrome are understandable in terms of the known actions of cortisol. When present in excessive quantities, this hormone accelerates the catabolism of protein and stimulates the hepatic uptake and deamination of amino acids. It also inhibits the transport of amino acids into extrahepatic tissues. As a consequence of these actions, prolonged high concentrations of cortisol cause clinical manifestations of protein wasting. Children show retardation of linear growth. Wasting of the integument and increasing capillary fragility result in ecchymoses. Cutaneous striae form in areas where the skin is stretched by an accumulation of adipose tissue. In extreme cases, wasting of muscle results in pronounced weakness. Wasting of bone matrix results in osteoporosis.

Abnormally high levels of cortisol alter the body's responses to injury and infection. Cortisol stabilizes lysosomal membranes, thus diminishing the tendency of injured tissues to perpetuate their own damage. It suppresses the sticking of leukocytes to endothelial surfaces, and diminishes the accumulation of leukocytes at sites of tissue injury. It inhibits the diapedesis of white blood cells and impairs their migration through tissues. In high concentrations over long periods of time, cortisol impairs antibody production and inhibits the proliferation of lymphocytes. Thus almost every aspect of the normal cellular response to injury or infection is suppressed by high concentrations of cortisol, leaving the patient with impaired capacity to limit the spread of invading organisms.

Cortisol promotes potassium excretion and sodium retention by stimulating cation exchange by the distal convoluted tubules. A severe excess of cortisol can result in depletion of bodily potassium to such a degree that hypokalemia, electrocardiographic abnormalities, muscular weakness, and impairment of renal concentrating capacity develop. Retention of sodium and elevated blood pressure occur. Steroid hypertension, like other varieties of hypertension, leads to left ventricular hypertrophy and predisposes the patient to congestive heart failure and strokes. Even without frank congestive heart failure, some patients experience expansion of their extracellular fluid volumes to the point of edema.

In addition to stimulating the formation of new glucose from amino acids, lactate, pyruvate, and bicarbonate, cortisol impairs the action of insulin in transporting glucose across cell membranes. Consequently, abnormally high amounts of cortisol tend to raise the level of blood glucose; this is most readily apparent in the prolongation of hyperglycemia after a glucose load; a minority of patients with hypercortisolism have abnormally high fasting blood glucose levels (see Ch. 806).

Adrenal carcinomas that secrete cortisol usually secrete significant quantities of adrenal androgen as well. In men this is of no clinical consequence, but in women and children it gives rise to virilism. Benign adenomas that cause Cushing's syndrome are somewhat less likely to produce excessive quantities of androgen. Mild virilism, usually amounting to nothing more than acne, thinning of scalp hair, and some degree of facial hirsutism, is common in women with Cushing's disease or the ectopic ACTH syndrome. In these disorders the increased levels of ACTH result in increased production of adrenal androgens as well as cortisol.

Although Cushing's syndrome is due entirely to an excess of corticosteroids, one must realize that the clinical illness of the patient may be affected by other factors as well. This is readily apparent in the ectopic ACTH syndrome when the clinical picture is usually dominated by other effects of the ACTH-secreting tumor. These patients often have a degree of weakness out of proportion to the severity of their hypercortisolism, and they often lose weight, in contrast to patients with classic features of Cushing's syndrome.

Clinical Manifestations. The clinical manifestations of Cushing's syndrome are familiar to every physician who has seen a patient treated with large doses of a cortisol-like steroid for several weeks or longer. In addition to the picture of cortisol excess, there will, in some patients, be features of virilism and mineralocorticoid excess as well. The frequencies of various clinical manifestations in Cushing's syndrome are listed in Table 2.

General Appearance and Physiognomy. The typical patient with Cushing's syndrome has central obesity, with rounding of the face, thickening of the fat pads in the supraclavicular fossae, and thickening of the thoracicoabdominal panniculus (Fig. 2). In longstanding cases, the abdominal obesity can progress to grotesque proportions while the extremities remain remarkably slender. People with pre-existing obesity from other causes can, of course, develop Cushing's syndrome; under such circumstances it is difficult to decide on clinical grounds

TABLE 2.   Frequency of Clinical Manifestations in Cushing's Syndrome

	Per Cent
Impaired glucose tolerance	94
Central obesity	88
Hypertension	82
Oligomenorrhea	72
Osteoporosis	58
Purpura and striae	42
Muscle atrophy	36
Hirsutism	30
Edema	20
Hypokalemia (unprovoked)	18
Kidney stones	12
Psychotic mentation	6

alone whether the patient has Cushing's syndrome and, if so, to what extent his obesity is attributable to the steroid excess. Patients with malignant tumors often show little or no obesity, even though their steroid levels are high and other features of Cushing's syndrome are fully expressed.

Cutaneous Manifestations. The face and neck often have a ruddy hyperemic appearance. Trivial trauma often results in ecchymosis. In advanced cases, the skin

Figure 2. The appearance of a patient with Cushing's syndrome (*A*) before and (*B*) one year after removal of an adrenal adenoma. (*C*) Profile, before treatment.

over the forearms and legs becomes thin, having the appearance of parchment. Slight injury to the skin can result in purpuric extravasation of blood; the sites of venipunctures sometimes show extensive subcutaneous hemorrhage. Removal of adhesive tape sometimes denudes the delicate skin of the patient with the advanced protein-wasting of Cushing's syndrome. Wounds heal slowly and often become the sites of indolent infections. In areas where the weakened skin is stretched by the underlying accumulation of fat (particularly the abdomen, shoulders, and hips), wide purplish striae may form.

The reaction to infection is attenuated in Cushing's syndrome. Superficial fungal infections, e.g., tinea versicolor, occur in about 20 per cent of cases. In more severe cases, bacterial infections are not well confined in the form of discrete abscesses of short duration, but are more likely to be chronic and to give rise to cellulitis and bacteremia. This is a dangerous situation which may escape notice, because the patient with Cushing's syndrome often has less discomfort and experiences less of a febrile reaction than would ordinarily be expected with a given degree of infection.

Largely as a function of an associated excess of androgens, acne and hirsutism commonly occur in patients with Cushing's syndrome. The hirsutism is usually slight, downy, and distributed over the cheeks and shoulders, but coarse hairs may appear in the beard area and on the chest and abdomen. In men, of course, this aspect of hyperadrenocorticism is unnoticed.

Reproductive Functions. Most women with Cushing's syndrome have oligomenorrhea. Although it is difficult to evaluate with certainty, many of them may have diminished fertility; however, this is by no means uniform. Men with Cushing's syndrome are sometimes said to be troubled with impotence; this is certainly not always so, and might not be related to the hyperadrenocorticism when it does occur. Infertility is probably not a feature of Cushing's syndrome in men.

Musculoskeletal Manifestations. Children with Cushing's syndrome experience arrest of linear growth. If obesity in a child is associated with growth arrest, the possibility of Cushing's syndrome should receive strong consideration; continued normal linear growth is strong evidence that the child's obesity is not due to Cushing's syndrome. Insidious atrophy of the skeleton results in mild hypercalciuria and, in time, in frank osteoporosis. Severe osteoporosis of the vertebral bodies may result in bulging of intervertebral discs, giving the appearance of codfish vertebrae in lateral roentgenographic views. Compression fractures with anterior wedging of the vertebral bodies result in kyphosis and loss of height. Pathologic fractures of ribs and hips occasionally occur.

In severe Cushing's syndrome, muscular atrophy may progress to such an extent that the patient is too weak to rise from a squatting position without assistance. Muscular weakness is usually not noticeable in milder cases.

Cardiovascular and Renal Manifestations. Most patients with Cushing's syndrome have hypertension, the course and complications of which are similar to those of essential hypertension. Edema can occur as a manifestation of congestive heart failure, but in 10 to 20 per cent of cases, mild edema occurs in the absence of congestive failure.

Hypokalemia with hypochloremic alkalosis occurs spontaneously in about 10 to 20 per cent of the cases (usually those with the most severe excesses of steroid secretion), and may occur in others as a complication of diuretic therapy.

Renal lithiasis can occur in chronic cases of Cushing's syndrome.

Hematologic Features. Some patients with Cushing's syndrome have erythrocytosis, granulocytosis, lymphopenia, and eosinopenia.

Carbohydrate Tolerance. Impaired carbohydrate tolerance occurs in more than 90 per cent of cases of Cushing's syndrome. In the majority it is manifested merely by a failure of the blood glucose to return to normal fasting levels during the first three hours after a glucose load. In about 20 per cent it is manifested as clinical diabetes mellitus.

Psychologic Abnormalities. Alterations of mood are common in Cushing's syndrome. Many patients feel irritable and weep with little provocation. A few experience psychotic mentation with delusional content. A few patients are depressed, and some attempt suicide. Manic and hypomanic behavior may also occur.

Diagnosis and Differential Diagnosis. It is important for the physician to know when to suspect Cushing's syndrome and then how to prove or disprove the diagnosis, keeping in mind the need for economy and precision. Taken singly, the various clinical manifestations of Cushing's syndrome are not very specific. Thus only a minute percentage of all hypertensive patients have Cushing's syndrome; only a minute percentage of diabetic patients have Cushing's syndrome; only a minute percentage of patients with renal lithiasis have Cushing's syndrome, and so forth. The coexistence of multiple clinical manifestations greatly increases the probability that a given patient might have hypercortisolism. If one encounters a patient with a single manifestation of Cushing's syndrome, he should always ask himself if hypercortisolism could be present; but if no other symptoms or signs of the syndrome can be found in the course of a complete medical evaluation, it will usually be unrewarding to pursue this line of investigation. Here we are discussing only probabilities, and should recognize that rare examples of hypercortisolism have been unequivocally diagnosed in the virtual absence of clinical manifestations.

Under certain conditions, one can make a clinical diagnosis quite confidently. For example, a patient with protein wasting (osteoporosis, easily denuded skin) and centripetal obesity probably has hypercortisolism. A child who simultaneously develops central obesity and experiences arrest of linear growth probably has Cushing's syndrome. Osteoporosis occurs commonly in patients beyond the age of 50 and is of limited value in diagnosis in this group; but osteoporosis in children and young adults should make one alert to the possibility of Cushing's syndrome. Although impaired glucose tolerance, taken by itself, is not especially suggestive of Cushing's syndrome, *normal* glucose tolerance is rare in Cushing's syndrome (about 10 per cent) and is therefore useful in discounting the probability of hypercortisolism. Patients with tumors of any organ and unprovoked hypokalemia should be suspected of having hypercortisolism, regardless of lack of obesity or signs of protein wasting.

Whenever the suspicion of Cushing's syndrome cannot be dismissed confidently, one should proceed with assays of plasma cortisol or urinary 17-hydroxycortico-steroids under basal conditions and during treatment with standard small doses of dexamethasone. At this point, a reliable laboratory with well-established ranges of normal values is indispensable. Equally important is close supervision of the patient so that specimens are collected properly, so that stresses or medications which might lead to high steroid values are avoided, and so that the physician knows that the dexamethasone is taken as prescribed.

Normal subjects have plasma cortisol concentrations of 8 to 25 μg per 100 ml in the morning and less than 8 μg per 100 ml in the evening. Patients with untreated Cushing's syndrome almost always have plasma cortisol concentrations in excess of 15 μg per 100 ml at all times. Normal subjects have urinary 17-OHCS of 3 to 7 mg per gram of urinary creatinine. Patients with untreated Cushing's syndrome almost always have urinary 17-OHCS in excess of 10 mg per gram of creatinine.

In response to small doses of dexamethasone (0.5 mg every six hours for two days), normal subjects show decreases in plasma cortisol to less than 5 μg per 100 ml and excrete less than 2 mg of 17-OHCS per gram of creatinine. Under similar conditions, patients with Cushing's syndrome almost always maintain plasma cortisol concentrations above 8 μg per 100 ml and excrete more than 3 mg of 17-OHCS per gram of creatinine.

Having established the fact that a patient has hypercortisolism, the physician must then determine whether it is caused by autonomous adrenal function, ectopic secretion of ACTH, or inappropriate secretion of pituitary ACTH. There are many useful guides in making this differential diagnosis, but the most reliable approach is to perform a large-dose dexamethasone suppression test and then, if pituitary-adrenal suppressibility cannot be demonstrated, to perform an assay for plasma ACTH if this measurement is available. The purpose of the large dose of dexamethasone is to determine whether adrenal function is under pituitary control. In almost all cases of Cushing's syndrome caused by inappropriate secretion of ACTH by the pituitary, it is possible to suppress adrenal function distinctly and reproducibly (though not necessarily profoundly) by administering dexamethasone in doses of 2 mg every six hours for two days. If a distinct, reproducible decrease in adrenal function does not occur, one should assume that adrenal function is autonomous or that it is under the control of ectopic ACTH. The distinction between these two disorders can be made by assaying plasma ACTH. In patients with autononous adrenal function, plasma ACTH concentrations should be subnormal; but in patients with the ectopic ACTH syndrome plasma ACTH is high-normal or distinctly elevated (Fig. 3). The reason for emphasizing the importance of reproducibility in the large-dose dexamethasone suppression test is to avoid diagnostic errors that might result if spontaneous decreases in tumor activity should occur or if inadequate urine collections happen to be made at the same time as the administration of dexamethasone. Such coincidences should not be reproducible, but suppression of pituitary ACTH secretion should be. Frequently it is unnecessary to carry out the large-dose dexamethasone test, because all the information one requires can be derived from an analysis of the results

Figure 3. Diagnostic flow sheet for Cushing's syndrome.

of the small-dose test. Many patients with an excess of pituitary ACTH show partial suppression of their steroid output in response to 0.5 mg of dexamethasone every six hours. Definite, reproducible suppression of adrenal function with any dose of dexamethasone implies that adrenal function is under the control of the pituitary.

Blind reliance upon a single set of laboratory values is not to be recommended; for example, high levels of estrogen, such as those encountered in pregnancy or during treatment with oral contraceptives, lead to elevations of plasma cortisol by raising the concentration of cortisol-binding globulin, but there is no increase in cortisol secretion rate or in urinary 17-OHCS. Hyperthyroidism can lead to accelerated removal of cortisol from the circulation and a compensatory increase in cortisol secretion rate, accompanied by an increase in urinary 17-OHCS, but plasma 17-OHCS values are not elevated. Awareness of the total clinical condition and use of more than one dimension in evaluating adrenal function should protect one from making diagnostic errors.

Although the approach described above is the most economical and reliable method of establishing a definitive diagnosis of Cushing's syndrome, the following points may often offer additional help (Fig. 4):

1. Patients with Cushing's disease almost invariably respond to metyrapone with increased secretion of ACTH and total 17-OHCS (the increase in 17-OHCS is attributable to a large increase in 11-deoxycortisol). Patients with Cushing's syndrome caused by adrenal tumor do not respond to metyrapone with increased 17-OHCS production. Patients with the ectopic ACTH syndrome vary in their responses; some show increases in 17-OHCS and others do not.

2. In patients with hypercortisolism, a grossly disproportionate elevation of urinary 17-ketosteroids is highly suggestive of adrenal carcinoma. The same may be said if more than 30 per cent of the urinary 17-OHCS are made up of 11-deoxy-cortisol and its tetrahydrometabolite.

3. Virtually all patients with Cushing's disease respond to exogenous ACTH with large increases in cortisol secretion; this is also true of patients with the ectopic ACTH syndrome unless their basal levels of cortisol are very high. Patients with Cushing's syndrome resulting from adrenal carcinoma almost never

	NORMAL	ADRENAL TUMOR	"CUSHING'S DISEASE"	ECTOPIC ACTH SYNDROME
PLASMA CORTISOL	10-25µg% RHYTHMIC	HIGH, NO RHYTHM	HIGH, NO RHYTHM	HIGH, NO RHYTHM
PLASMA ACTH	0.1 - 0.4 mU%	LOW	HIGH	HIGH
17-OHCS RESPONSE TO ACTH	3-5 FOLD RISE	+,0	+	+,0
RESPONSE TO METYRAPONE	2-4 FOLD RISE	0	+	+,0
RESPONSE TO DEXAMETHASONE	0-3mg/d	NO FALL	PARTIAL FALL	NO FALL
PLASMA ACTH AFTER ADRENALECTOMY, ON NORMAL CORTISOL	NORMAL	LOW	HIGH	HIGH

Figure 4. Typical cortisol, ACTH, and urinary 17-OHCS values in normal subjects and in the hypercortisolism associated with (a) adrenal tumor, (b) Cushing's disease (pituitary ACTH excess), and (c) the ectopic ACTH syndrome. (From Liddle, G. W.: Am. J. Med., 53:638, 1972. By permission.)

respond to brief infusions of ACTH. Patients with cortisol-secreting adenomas vary in their responses; about half of them respond and half do not.

4. Adrenal carcinomas are usually so inefficient in producing steroids that they do not cause Cushing's syndrome until they have become large enough to be readily demonstrated by intravenous urography or arteriography; some are so large that they can be palpated through the anterior abdominal wall by the time the patient exhibits Cushing's syndrome.

Treatment. The prime therapeutic objectives in Cushing's syndrome are to reduce cortisol levels to normal and to eradicate any associated tumors. Secondary objectives are to avoid producing hormonal deficiencies and to avoid making the patient chronically dependent upon medication. All these objectives can be achieved in some patients in each of the three categories of Cushing's syndrome. In many cases, however, compromises must be made. Sound therapeutic strategy begins with precision in diagnosis.

In Cushing's disease, ideal therapeutic results can be achieved in about 25 per cent of cases by irradiation of the pituitary with about 4500 R. Although this mode of therapy was abandoned in many medical centers when the availability of cortisone substitution therapy made it feasible to perform bilateral adrenalectomy, it remains the only form of therapy that offers the patient a chance of achieving all the therapeutic objectives listed above. The author has 24 patients who have been in remission from 1 to 17 years after pituitary irradiation. None of the patients appear to have developed deficiencies of any pituitary hormones as a consequence of therapy. There are only three drawbacks to this therapeutic approach. First, one must be certain that his diagnosis is correct; pituitary irradiation is clearly inappropriate for patients with adrenal tumors or for patients with the ectopic ACTH syndrome. Second, many patients do not respond, and ultimately require other therapy. Third, the results of pituitary irradiation are not apparent for one to four months; and the patient with fulminant hypertension, rapidly progressive osteoporosis, or psychosis not well controlled by psychoactive drugs should be treated more aggressively.

A technical advance in pituitary irradiation has been achieved recently through careful use of a cyclotron to deliver intensive irradiation to a sharply localized region. Through this means, it is possible to deliver 10,000 R to the pituitary gland with little risk of injury to neighboring structures. Information thus far available indicates that this form of therapy might cure at least two thirds of the patients with Cushing's disease; however, there is at least a small risk of producing hypopituitarism, a problem that did not arise in connection with conventional irradiation with less than 5000 R.

Only three other modes of therapy have been consistently effective in Cushing's disease. With each of them, normalization of cortisol is usually achieved, but the patient incurs life-threatening hormonal deficiencies which require lifelong substitution therapy. Bilateral adrenalectomy is most widely practiced. Substitution therapy with a glucocorticoid (and usually a mineralocorticoid) must begin at the time of adrenalectomy and continue for the duration of the patient's life. The principles of substitution therapy are outlined in Ch. 846. Subtotal adrenalectomy is not to be recommended because of the likelihood of recurrence of hyperadrenocorticism and the frequent impossibility of finding and removing all the regenerative remnant from a scarred mass of perinephric fat at a second operation.

Hypophysectomy and subtotal ablation of the pituitary by means of transsphenoidal microdissection, cryosurgery, or the implantation of radioactive gold or yttrium have been mastered in several medical centers. These forms of therapy carry the risk of producing hypopituitarism and are therefore not be be recommended for the young patient to whom reproductive capacity and normal growth are, obviously, important matters.

Selective destruction of the zona fasciculata and zona reticularis without the induction of aldosterone deficiency can be achieved with prolonged administration of the adrenocorticolytic drug mitotane (o,p'-DDD). This mode of therapy is attended by at least minor gastrointestinal side effects and entails the risk of producing virtually complete loss of glucocorticoid secretory capacity unless the physician is able to follow the patient closely enough to adjust the dose of o,p'-DDD so that plasma cortisol concentrations remain within the optimal range. The advantage of this form of treatment, apart from the avoidance of operative risks, is the preservation of the aldosterone secretory mechanism so that the patient is not so vulnerable to sodium depletion as is the totally adrenalectomized patient.

In the ectopic ACTH syndrome, ideal therapeutic results can be achieved only if the ACTH-secreting tumor can be completely removed. Thus far this has been possible in only a score of cases. In those cases in which the ACTH-secreting tumor cannot be removed, it is still possible to curtail the hypercortisolism by treatment with metyrapone. This drug inhibits the final step in cortisol synthesis and leads to secretion of the biologically weak precursor, 11-deoxycortisol. One can start with small doses of 250 mg every eight hours and increase them if necessary to achieve the desired reduction of cortisol production (under these circumstances the simplest way to estimate cortisol levels is to measure plasma fluorogenic steroids). Doses in excess of 500 mg every six hours are rarely required. Bilateral adrenalectomy or o,p'-DDD therapy might be employed in selected patients in whom the hypercortisolism offers a more immediate threat to life than does the ACTH-secreting tumor. It should be borne in mind that o,p'-

DDD so alters the extra-adrenal metabolism of cortisol that the measurement of urinary 17-OHCS is unreliable in evaluating cortisol secretion; the patient's progress should be followed by measurements of plasma cortisol.

The only completely satisfactory treatment of Cushing's syndrome resulting from adrenal tumor is the surgical removal of the tumor. Most tumors are benign and unilateral, and removal of the tumor-bearing gland is curative. It is essential that the patient be supported with glucocorticoids during and for several days after the operation, because chronic suppression of ACTH production will have resulted in atrophy of the non-tumorous adrenal. A regimen similar to that employed during bilateral adrenalectomy is appropriate. Post-operatively, glucocorticoid therapy should be progressively reduced so that within a week or so the patient receives only 20 to 30 mg of cortisol per day. This supportive therapy should be withdrawn gradually over the ensuing year. It is possible during this period to give the entire daily steroid supplement as a single dose in the morning, thus permitting the pituitary-adrenal system to escape from the suppressive influence of cortisol for a portion of each day. On this schedule the daily dose of cortisol can gradually be reduced from 30 mg to 5 mg and then discontinued altogether. Throughout this first year the physician and patient should be alert to the possible need for increased cortisol dosage in the event of an acute stress. The principles of therapy in this situation are the same as those described for patients with adrenal insufficiency. After steroids have been withdrawn for a time, the patient's recovery of normal pituitary-adrenal function can be verified by a metyrapone test. A normal response should indicate that the patient no longer needs to be concerned about pituitary-adrenal insufficiency.

Approximately 5 to 10 per cent of patients with Cushing's syndrome resulting from benign adrenal adenomas have bilateral tumors. These patients require bilateral adrenalectomy followed by lifelong treatment, as for Addison's disease.

Although adrenal surgery is curative in some patients with adrenal carcinoma, a majority have either apparent or occult metastases by the time they seek medical attention. In about two thirds of these patients, the adrenocorticolytic drug o,p'-DDD will induce a temporary remission of hyperadrenocorticism, and about one half of these experience regression of tumor mass for several months to a few years. The dose ranges from 3 to 10 grams per day, depending upon the severity of gastrointestinal side effects. If measures to control growth of the tumor are unsuccessful, it is still possible to control hypercortisolism with metyrapone given in divided doses totaling 1 to 2 grams daily. In patients with adrenal tumors, overtreatment with adrenal inhibitors can result in adrenal insufficiency; this can be avoided by erring on the side of undertreatment or by giving 0.5 mg of dexamethasone daily as a supportive measure.

Significance of Virilism in Association with Cushing's Syndrome. Clinical and chemical evidences of androgen hypersecretion are not uncommon in Cushing's syndrome. Although not a highly reliable rule, it is usually true that when a patient with Cushing's syndrome exhibits marked evidence of androgen excess, the cause is likely to be adrenocortical carcinoma. In other varieties of Cushing's syndrome, virilism is usually mild or inapparent.

The most important question to be settled early in the evaluation of any patient with virilism is whether or not this is associated with hypercortisolism, for virilism associated with hypercortisolism should be managed according to the principles outlined above for Cushing's syndrome, but virilism without hypercortisolism represents an entirely different group of disorders requiring drastically different treatment (see Ch. 853, 854, 858, and 867).

851. PRIMARY ALDOSTERONISM

Definition, Etiology, and Incidence. Narrowly defined, "primary aldosteronism" is the constellation of chemical and clinical abnormalities resulting from the "autonomous" hypersecretion of aldosterone. The words "primary" and "autonomous" are employed to set this condition apart from "secondary aldosteronism," which refers to hypersecretion of aldosterone in response to a known stimulus such as angiotensin. Usually primary aldosteronism is due to an aldosterone-secreting adenoma (Conn's syndrome), but occasionally it is associated with adrenal hyperplasia or with morphologically normal adrenals (idiopathic hyperaldosteronism).

The incidence of primary aldosteronism is a subject of controversy. Conn has suggested that it might be present in 7 per cent of patients who otherwise appear to have essential hypertension. Others believe it to be less common, perhaps occurring in 1 per cent of the hypertensive population. It has been reported in about twice as many females as males.

Pathogenesis. Virtually all the features of primary aldosteronism are attributable to the fact that aldosterone promotes the conservation of sodium and the excretion of potassium.

Excessive conservation of sodium leads to expansion of extracellular volume, elevation of the blood pressure, and suppression of renin production. In the absence of circulatory insufficiency, modest expansion of extracellular volume leads to physiologic adjustments which enable the excretory system to come into equilibrium with the sodium intake; progressive expansion of extracellular volume is thus avoided, and overt edema is absent or only slight. (These adjustments are sometimes referred to as the "escape phenomenon.")

Excessive excretion of potassium can result in potassium depletion, hypokalemic alkalosis, muscular weakness, areflexia, tetany, paresthesias, electrocardiographic abnormalities (S-T depression, flattening of T waves, and appearance of U waves), idioventricular arrhythmias, and kaliopenic nephropathy, with impaired renal concentrating capacity that cannot be corrected by vasopressin. Despite the hypokalemia, urinary potassium excretion usually exceeds 30 mEq per day. Since potassium secretion in the distal convoluted tubule is, in part, a function of the quantity of sodium reaching that portion of the nephron, a high sodium intake tends to exaggerate the potassium-wasting process, and a low sodium intake tends to mask it.

The action of aldosterone in promoting the conservation of sodium and the rejection of potassium is observable not only in the kidney but in all epithelialized organ systems which carry on cation exchange. Thus in hyperaldosteronism one can often demonstrate depression of the sodium:potassium ratio in sweat, saliva, and gastrointestinal secretions.

Apart from the relatively rare patients who develop alarming ventricular arrhythmias or incapacitating muscular weakness as a result of potassium depletion, the great dangers of primary aldosteronism are the common complications of hypertensive cardiovascular disease: cardiac hypertrophy, congestive heart failure, strokes, and progressive impairment of renal function. Although uncommon, malignant hypertension can occur as a complication of primary aldosteronism and can be associated with either elevated or suppressed plasma renin activity.

Clinical Manifestations. All patients who have been proved to have primary aldosteronism have had hypertension. This is somewhat tautologic because physicians do not usually consider the diagnosis in the absence of hypertension. Nevertheless, the clinical importance of primary aldosteronism is in the main related to hypertension and its sequelae. There are no characteristics of the hypertension of primary aldosteronism that are helpful in distinguishing it from "essential" hypertension.

The coexistence of hypertension and *unprovoked* hypokalemia is highly suggestive of primary aldosteronism. Indeed, in some studies as many as 50 per cent of patients with this combination of abnormalities have ultimately been shown to have primary aldosteronism. In a large percentage of patients the hypokalemia is asymptomatic. In an uncertain but probably small percentage it is not demonstrable at all. The clinical manifestations of potassium depletion have been summarized under Pathogenesis. Another possible consequence of potassium depletion in primary aldosteronism is impairment of carbohydrate tolerance.

Diagnosis and Differential Diagnosis. In practice, the diagnosis of primary aldosteronism usually begins with the recognition that the patient has hypertension. Serum potassium should be determined on several occasions while the patient is on a liberal sodium intake and is not receiving kaliuretic drugs (diuretics) or experiencing diarrhea or vomiting. The finding of unprovoked hypokalemia in association with hypertension calls for measurements of aldosterone and renin. If the aldosterone secretion rate is elevated, it may be assumed that the patient has either primary or secondary aldosteronism. If plasma renin activity is suppressed, one may assume that the patient has primary rather than secondary aldosteronism. Anecdotal evidence indicates that some patients have coexistent primary and secondary aldosteronism, but it is impossible to diagnose primary aldosteronism with certainty until the secondary aldosteronism has been corrected and it can be demonstrated that the hypersecretion of aldosterone persists in spite of subnormal plasma renin activity.

Hypokalemia is not an essential feature of primary aldosteronism, but the diagnosis is not easy to establish in its absence, when total reliance must be placed on the aldosterone and renin determinations. There is no substitute for a sophisticated and reliable laboratory if one is to practice competently in this area of medicine.

Conditions that can lead to concomitant hypertension and hypokalemia include malignant hypertension, Cushing's syndrome (especially the ectopic ACTH syndrome), congenital adrenal hyperplasia caused by 17-hydroxylase deficiency or 11-hydroxylase deficiency (see below), ingestion of large quantities of licorice, and a familial renal disorder simulating primary aldosteronism but with negligible aldosterone secretion (Liddle, Bledsoe, and Coppage). Except for the last condition, all these disorders should be recognizable in the course of a routine evaluation, which includes a determination of 17-OHCS.

Once the diagnosis of primary aldosteronism has been established by demonstrating that, under carefully standardized conditions, the patient has an abnormally high aldosterone secretion rate and abnormally low plasma renin activity, one would like to know whether the hypersecretion of aldosterone is unilateral or bilateral. If the source of aldosterone is a unilateral adenoma, the condition can usually be cured by unilateral adrenalectomy with the expectation that the contralateral adrenal gland will then function normally. If the source of aldosterone is bilateral (with or without adenomas), the disorder usually cannot be surgically corrected short of bilateral adrenalectomy, and this is too high a price to pay in view of the fact that medical therapy with the mineralocorticoid antagonist spironolactone will generally correct both the hypokalemia and the hypertension of primary aldosteronism.

Unfortunately, the art of distinguishing between unilateral and bilateral hypersecretion of aldosterone is not highly developed. Kahn and Melby have found it possible to determine which of the two adrenal glands contains an aldosterone-secreting adenoma by catheterizing the adrenal veins (via a femoral vein) and measuring aldosterone concentrations in the adrenal effluents before and after brief injection of angiotensin. This procedure is not generally useful owing to the extraordinary expertise that is required in placing the adrenal venous catheters properly. Adrenal venography has been used to demonstrate the location of aldosterone-secreting tumors, but this procedure carries the danger of rupturing the adrenal vein. Scanning of adrenals with radioactive iodocholesterol has been used to demonstrate the location of a small number of adenomas, but this procedure is not highly reliable and is still limited to a few centers where active investigative programs are in progress. Robertson has developed a computer program for distinguishing between unilateral adenoma and bilateral hypersecretion, combining a large variety of clinical and laboratory data, but the applicability of the program to patients in other medical centers does not yield distinctions having the reliability that Robertson found in his original study in Scotland, presumably because other medical centers employ somewhat different standard conditions for collecting and reporting their data. In summary, most medical centers still find it necessary to explore both adrenals surgically in order to determine whether primary aldosteronism is attributable to unilateral or bilateral hypersecretion of aldosterone.

Treatment. Unless the patient is a poor surgical risk, the treatment of choice in primary aldosteronism is surgical excision of an adenomatous adrenal gland. During the weeks prior to operation the patient's hypertension and potassium depletion should be corrected by treatment with the aldosterone antagonist spironolactone in doses of 200 to 400 mg daily. Both glands are exposed, inspected, and palpated before a decision is made as to what should be resected. If one gland is found to contain an adenoma, it should be removed, and the contralateral gland should be left intact. If no adenoma can be found, one gland may be removed and sectioned carefully in search of a small tumor; if one is found, nothing further is required. If a tumor is not found in the first gland to be removed, half of the second gland may be resected in search of an adenoma. Even if an adenoma is not encountered, the operation should be terminated at this point rather than risk permanent adrenal insufficiency.

Patients who are poor surgical risks, those who are unwilling to undergo adrenal exploration, and those whose hyperaldosteronism persists after subtotal adrenalectomy should be treated chronically with spironolactone in doses of 100 to 400 mg daily.

Prognosis. Without treatment, patients with primary aldosteronism will sooner or later have the disabling and fatal complications common to hypertensive cardiovascular disease in general; they have been known to die of strokes, congestive heart failure, and renal insufficiency. Within several days to several months after the successful removal of an aldosterone-secreting tumor, 70 per cent of the patients become normotensive, 25 per cent exhibit significant lowering of blood pressure but not to normal levels, and only 5 per cent are unimproved. Correction of the electrolyte disturbance is uniformly observed after correction of the aldosterone excess. Adequate treatment with spironolactone is almost equally effective in correcting the hypertension and potassium depletion of primary aldosteronism, but not infrequently it leads to gynecomastia, impotence, or menstrual irregularity.

852. SECONDARY ALDOSTERONISM

The normal response of the adrenal cortex to increased stimulation by the renin-angiotensin system is to secrete increasing quantities of aldosterone. The aldosterone, in turn, promotes sodium conservation and potassium excretion. The retention of sodium results in expansion of extracellular volume and tends to restrain further production of renin. In many circumstances the renin–angiotensin–aldosterone–sodium-volume sequence can be viewed teleologically as a compensatory mechanism designed to support the blood flow to the kidney by expanding extracellular volume. Thus severe dehydration, sodium depletion, hemorrhage, hypoalbuminemic states, renal arterial constriction, and sequestration of blood on the venous side of the circulation are all conditions in which blood flow to the kidney is diminished, calling forth increased production of renin and aldosterone. Secondary aldosteronism, then, is not a disease but, rather, is a response of the normal adrenal to physiologic demands arising in the course of a variety of disease processes, notably the nephrotic syndrome and hepatic cirrhosis.

853. CONGENITAL ADRENAL HYPERPLASIA

General Considerations, Definition, Etiology. Steroidal hormones are derived from cholesterol through a long series of enzymatically controlled steps. Each enzyme system carries the biosynthetic process one step along the pathway from ultimate precursor through an orderly series of intermediates to the final, biologically potent derivative. Many of these enzyme systems are common to both the zona fasciculata and zona glomerulosa, and some are important in the biosynthesis of gonadal androgens and estrogens as well as corticosteroids.

An inborn error in an adrenal enzyme system which impairs the efficiency of any step in the biosynthesis of cortisol or aldosterone can lead to congenital adrenal hyperplasia. Impairment of cortisol synthesis leads to a compensatory increase in ACTH secretion by the pituitary, and impairment of aldosterone synthesis leads to a compensatory increase in the production of renin and angiotensin. These trophic hormones stimulate the production of cortisol and aldosterone precursors and induce hyperplasia of the adrenal cortex. If the block in cortisol or aldosterone biosynthesis is not complete, and if the compensatory increase in ACTH or renin secretion is adequate, the resultant production of cortisol and aldosterone may be within the normal range. However, the chemical hallmark of an intra-adrenal enzyme deficiency would still be evident: a distortion of steroid secretory pattern with conspicuous overproduction of the intermediates that occur in the biosynthetic pathway immediately prior to the blocked step. The clinical manifestations of congenital adrenal hyperplasia are determined in part by the biologic properties of the biosynthetic intermediates which are excessively secreted and in part by the degree of deficiency of cortisol, aldosterone, or gonadal steroids.

Beyond the fact that the enzymatic defects that lead to congenital adrenal hyperplasia are genetically determined, little is known about their etiology. The pattern of familial occurrence is usually consistent with the view that congenital adrenal hyperplasia is inherited as a recessive trait. Within any one family, the same enzyme appears to be defective in all affected members.

Varieties of Congenital Adrenal Hyperplasia. Thus far, six varieties of congenital adrenal hyperplasia have been described, each resulting from impaired function of a different enzyme (Fig. 5).

Deficiency of 20α-Hydroxylase. The first step in the conversion of cholesterol into hormonal steroids is 20α-hydroxylation. Impairment of this process results in clinical adrenal insufficiency and, in the male fetus, incomplete differentiation of the external genitalia. The adrenal glands are hyperplastic and contain high concentrations of cholesterol. This is an extremely rare disorder.

Deficiency of 3β-Hydroxysteroid Dehydrogenase. This too is a rare disorder; it is characterized by genital ambiguity in infants of either sex. The explanation for this is that these patients have impaired capacity to transform Δ^5 steroids into Δ^4 steroids. Cortisol, aldosterone, and the potent androgens are all Δ^4 compounds; therefore these hormones are subnormal in this disorder, and affected patients have clinical adrenal insufficiency. Males have inadequate genital differentiation owing to lack of testicular androgen during fetal life. In response to increased levels of ACTH, both males and females secrete superabundant amounts of the Δ^5 steroids, pregnenolone and dehydroisoandrosterone. Although the latter is not a very strong androgen, it is secreted in large enough quantities to cause partial masculinization of the external genitalia of the female fetus. Both males and females therefore have adrenal

GLAND	ENZYME	ENZYME DEFICIENCY RESULTS IN:	
		UNDERPRODUCTION OF:	OVERPRODUCTION OF:
Adrenal and Gonad	20-Hydroxylase	Cortisol, Aldosterone, 17-KS, Testosterone, Estrogen	Cholesterol
Adrenal and Gonad	3-OH-Dehydrogenase	Cortisol, Aldosterone, Testosterone, Estrogen	Pregnenolones, 17-KS
Adrenal and Gonad	17-Hydroxylase	Cortisol, 17-KS, Testosterone, Estrogen	DOC and Corticosterone
Adrenal	21-Hydroxylase	Cortisol, Aldosterone	17-OH-Progesterone, 17-KS
Adrenal	11-Hydroxylase	Cortisol, Aldosterone	DOC, Substance S, 17-KS
Adrenal	18-Hydroxylase	Aldosterone	Corticosterone

Figure 5. Summary of the enzymatically regulated reactions through which cholesterol is converted to hormonal steroids. A deficiency of each enzyme results in underproduction of certain important adrenal or gonadal hormones and overproduction of their precursors and by-products.

insufficiency, ambiguous genitalia, and elevated urinary 17-ketosteroids (derived from dehydroisoandrosterone).

Deficiency of 17 α-Hydroxylase. Congenital adrenal hyperplasia resulting from a deficiency of 17α-hydroxylase has only recently been described; it is undoubtedly a very rare disorder but is nevertheless important because it represents a curable cause of hypertension. Cortisol synthesis is impaired at the step where progesterone is converted to 17α-hydroxyprogesterone. Androgen and estrogen synthesis, whether by the adrenal, ovary, or testis, also depend upon hydroxylation at the 17α-position prior to cleavage of the 17-20 carbon-carbon bond. Thus impairment of 17α-hydroxylation leads to a deficiency of estrogen and androgen. The patient with 17-hydroxylase deficiency has subnormal cortisol production, a compensatory increase in ACTH, and a consequent increase in the secretion of 17-deoxycorticosteroids, the most prominent of which are DOC and corticosterone. The excessive mineralocorticoid results in hypertension and suppression of renin production; aldosterone production is subnormal. Estrogen and androgen deficiencies result in sexual infantilism and compensatory increases in gonadotrophin secretion.

Deficiency of 21-Hydroxylase. The most common variety of congenital adrenal hyperplasia is attributable to a deficiency of 21-hydroxylase activity. This condition affects approximately one person in 10,000 of our general population. Cortisol synthesis is impaired at the step at which 17-hydroxyprogesterone should be converted to 11-deoxycortisol, and aldosterone synthesis is impaired at the step where progesterone is normally converted to 11-deoxycorticosterone. If the defect is severe, the patient during the first weeks of life may show signs of adrenocortical insufficiency such as salt-wasting, dehydration, hypotension, shock, prerenal azotemia, hyponatremia, hyperkalemia, vomiting, hypoglycemia, and poor tolerance to stress. Plasma ACTH and renin levels are high. Plasma concentrations of melanocyte-stimulating hormone (β-MSH) are also raised, and occasionally the patient may exhibit mucocutaneous hyperpigmentation. Hypersecretion of 17-hydroxyprogesterone is of no clinical consequence, but it results in the excretion of a diagnostically specific urinary metabolite, *pregnanetriol.*

Adrenal androgens do not require 21-hydroxylation for their synthesis, and as part of the adrenal response to high levels of ACTH they are produced in excessive quantities. Chemically, this is reflected in excessive levels of urinary 17-ketosteroids. The clinical consequence is virilization. The precise clinical manifestations of virilism depend upon the sex of the patient, the age at which the androgen excess occurs, and the severity of the androgen excess. In the male fetus, testicular production of androgen is sufficient to bring about completely masculine differentiation of the genitalia, and even a large excess of adrenal androgen has no obvious effect on genital differentiation or growth. The female fetus, though lacking gonadal androgen, is nevertheless very sensitive to androgens. In females with virilizing congenital adrenal hyperplasia, an excess of adrenal androgen results in partial masculinization of those portions of the genitourinary system that are the last to undergo differentiation. The abnormalities include the development of a urogenital sinus, fusion of labioscrotal folds, and hypertrophy of the clitoris. In extreme cases the external genitalia may be so ambiguous that on superficial examination the patient appears to be a male with hypospadias and bilateral cryptorchidism. In general, female infants with the most profound deficiencies of cortisol and aldosterone (the so-called salt-wasters) are likely to have conspicuous genital abnormalities, and the diagnosis should be suspected at birth, well in advance of any clinical difficulty from adrenal insufficiency. Salt-wasting males, on the other hand, lacking abnormalities of genital differentiation, are unlikely to attract special attention until they are in trouble with vomiting, dehydration, and other consequences of adrenal insufficiency. A positive family history, however, sometimes assists the pediatrician in considering the diagnosis before clinical complications arise.

Unless he or she succumbs or is treated, the patient with 21-hydroxylase deficiency grows rapidly and becomes quite muscular; at some time between two and ten years of age, pubic and axillary hair appear; this is followed by facial hirsutism and deepening of the voice. Investigation at this time reveals that the bone age is advanced beyond the height age, which, in turn, is advanced beyond the chronologic age. Early epiphysial closure foredooms the patient to short stature during adult life.

Clinically, the male patient may appear normal except for precocious puberty. The untreated female patient, however, does not undergo true pubertal changes but simply shows slowly progressive virilization; she lacks the feminization, mammary development, uterine development, and menstrual cycles that are a part of true puberty in the female.

The definitive diagnosis of 21-hydroxylase deficiency is based upon the demonstration of excessive quantities of pregnanetriol in the urine together with *easy* suppressibility of pregnanetriol and 17-ketosteroids by administration of glucocorticoids. This maneuver aids in distinguishing patients with congenital adrenal hyperplasia from those with Cushing's syndrome and those with adrenal tumors.

Deficiency of 11β-Hydroxylase. The second most common variety of congenital adrenal hyperplasia is attributable to a deficiency of 11β-hydroxylase. Fewer than 100 cases have been recognized thus far. The final step in cortisol synthesis is impaired so that cortisol secretion is subnormal, ACTH secretion is excessive, and the biologically inactive precursor of cortisol, *11-deoxycortisol,* is secreted in large quantities. Normally, corticosterone is secreted by the zona fasciculata in quantities of the order of 2 mg daily, but in patients with 11β-hydroxylase deficiency the final step in corticosterone synthesis is impaired, and large quantities of *11-deoxycorticosterone (DOC)* are secreted. DOC is a mineralocorticoid having about one thirtieth the potency of aldosterone. When secreted in quantities of several milligrams daily, DOC induces hypertension. Renin and aldosterone levels are low.

Adrenal androgens do not require 11β-hydroxylation for synthesis, and they are produced in excessive quantities as part of the adrenal response to high levels of ACTH. The consequent virilization is similar in its pathogenesis to that observed in patients with 21-hydroxylase deficiency.

The clinical manifestations of 11β-hydroxylase deficiency are simply those of hypertension and virilism. Plasma and urinary 17-OHCS are elevated because 11-deoxycortisol and its tetrahydro derivative behave like cortisol and its tetrahydro derivatives in chemical tests based on the presence of the 17,21-dihydroxy-20-keto configuration. Despite the elevation of 17-OHCS, this condition should not be confused with Cushing's syndrome, because plasma fluorogenic steroids should be normal or low in 11β-hydroxylase deficiency, the elevated steroids should be *readily* suppressible by the administration of glucocorticoids, and the clinical features of central obesity, protein wasting, and impaired carbohydrate tolerance are absent. The history of lifelong abnormalities together with *easy* suppressibility of the high steroid levels should distinguish 11β-hydroxylase deficiency from an adrenal tumor.

Deficiency of 18-Hydroxysteroid Dehydrogenase. This rare disorder results in a selective impairment of the final step in aldosterone biosynthesis. As a consequence the patient suffers excessive sodium loss, dehydration, and hypotension; there is a compensatory increase in formation of the aldosterone precursor 18-hydroxycorticosterone.

Treatment of Congenital Adrenal Hyperplasia. The major abnormalities in congenital adrenal hyperplasia stem from deficiencies of cortisol or aldosterone or both. Compensatory increases in secretion of ACTH or renin or both then stimulate overproduction of the precursors or by-products of these important steroids. The rationale of therapy is to provide physiologic quantities of glucocorticoid and mineralocorticoid, thus correcting the deficiency state, suppressing the trophic hormones, and curtailing the secretion of steroid precursors and by-products.

The technique of treatment is similar to that employed in adrenal insufficiency. For the first several days it is advisable to employ slightly greater than physiologic doses of glucocorticoid in order to hasten the involution of the hyperplastic, very responsive adrenal cortex. Thereafter only physiologic doses are required, and overtreatment must be assiduously avoided so that growth will not be inhibited.

In those varieties of congenital adrenal hyperplasia that are characterized by the excessive excretion of 17-ketosteroids, glucocorticoid dosage should be adjusted from time to time so as to bring daily 17-ketosteroid excretion to approximately 1 mg for each year of chronologic age, up to 12 years. More profound suppression of 17-ketosteroids is not necessary to prevent progression of virilism, but would be indicative of excessive glucocorticoid dosage. During intercurrent stressful illnesses, corticosteroid doses should be adjusted upward in the same manner and for the same reason as in treating adrenal insufficiency.

Several steroid preparations are available, and with proper consideration of relative potencies, effective routes of administration, and duration of effect, one can substitute one glucocorticoid for another and one mineralocorticoid for another at will. Many patients do well on approximately 12 mg of hydrocortisone and 0.06 mg of 9α-fluorohydrocortisone per square meter of body surface per day. In any case, the dosage must be adjusted to suit individual requirements; the objectives of therapy are to avoid adrenal insufficiency, to normalize 17-ketosteroid excretion, and to maintain normal blood pressure.

Certain therapeutic considerations are peculiar to the specific varieties of congenital adrenal hyperplasia. Mineralocorticoid therapy is required only for patients with salt-wasting varieties of congenital adrenal hyperplasia and not for those with the hypertensive varieties. Glucocorticoid therapy is not required in treating 18-hydroxysteroid dehydrogenase deficiency. Estrogen and androgen therapy may be needed to induce secondary sex characteristics in patients with 17α-hydroxylase deficiency, those with 20α-hydroxylase deficiency, or those with 3β-hydroxysteroid dehydrogenase deficiency.

Plastic surgery to correct gross abnormalities of the external genitalia should be carried out before the age of two years, by which time the child's psychosexual identity should be unambiguously established.

Prognosis. Without treatment, patients with various salt-wasting forms of congenital adrenal hyperplasia are unlikely to survive infancy. Patients with the hypertensive varieties also have decreased life expectancy. Many experience psychosexual problems arising from pseudohermaphroditism in the females and precocious puberty in the males.

If recognized early and treated properly, patients with any variety of congenital adrenal hyperplasia should theoretically be able to live normal lives. This is true for the patients with 21-hydroxylase and 11β-hydroxylase deficiency, except that they have usually not attained normal height. It appears that reproductive functions will be normal if proper treatment is started before adulthood. It is of interest that a child whose bone age has advanced beyond about 13 years before suppressive treatment with glucocorticoids is instituted will exhibit adult pituitary-gonadal relationships (females will undergo breast development and establish their menstrual cycles) when glucocorticoid treatment is finally begun; this is true even if the chronologic age is only seven or eight years.

The other varieties of congenital adrenal hyperplasia have less favorable prognoses. In 17α-hydroxylase deficiency, reproduction will probably not be possible even though the hypertension can be controlled and all other clinical manifestations of steroid deficiency corrected. The survival of patients with deficiencies of 20α-hydroxylase or 3β-hydroxysteroid dehydrogenase has been unaccountably poor up to the present time.

854. VIRILIZING TUMORS

Adrenal tumors that produce a clinically significant excess of androgen along with cortisol have been discussed in Ch. 850. Somewhat less common are adrenal tumors that secrete androgen without significant quantities of cortisol. Most of these tumors are malignant, and the majority are large and have metastasized by the time they are clinically apparent. The clinical hallmark of such tumors is virilization; this manifestation, of course, is limited to children and women; adult males usually recognize no increased virilization as a result of even large excesses of the relatively weak adrenal androgens. The common chemical hallmark of a purely virilizing tumor is the excessive excretion of 17-ketosteroids. This is a remarkably uniform characteristic of adrenal carcinomas. Several adrenal carcinomas have, probably erroneously, been reported as being nonfunctioning simply because they did not give rise to clinical virilization. Evidence was inadequate to support this conclusion, however, whenever 17-ketosteroid excretion was not measured.

It is not sufficient just to measure urinary 17-keto-steroids; under basal conditions one should also carry out dexamethasone suppression tests and demonstrate that urinary 17-ketosteroids can reproducibly be reduced to less than 6 mg per day within three days before concluding that an adrenocortical carcinoma is nonfunctioning.

Suprarenal "masses" that are discovered accidentally during roentgenographic examinations almost never prove to be adrenal cortical tumors if basal 17-OHCS and 17-ketosteroids are normal and normally suppressible, and they almost never prove to be adrenal medullary tumors if catecholamines are consistently normal.

Virilizing adrenal tumor must be differentiated from congenital adrenal hyperplasia, Cushing's syndrome with virilism, ovarian tumor, idiopathic hirsutism, and precocious puberty. This can be accomplished by a history of late onset of first clinical manifestations, absence of Cushing's syndrome, presence of a palpable abdominal mass, abnormal resistance to suppression of 17-ketosteroids with dexamethasone, absence of ovarian mass, and presence of an adrenal mass on urography or arteriography.

Treatment is with surgical resection and with o,p'-DDD. A sizable minority responds favorably to each mode of therapy, at least temporarily.

855. FEMINIZING ADRENAL TUMORS

Feminization as a clinical manifestation of adrenal tumor is exceedingly rare. The most common sign is gynecomastia, and this is one of the least common causes of gynecomastia. The diagnosis is made by the observation of other signs of adrenal overactivity, e.g., hypertension, demonstration of excessive estrogen in the urine, and demonstration of a suprarenal mass by intravenous urography or arteriography. If positively diagnosed, the tumor may be treated by surgical resection, and, if this fails, with o,p'-DDD. Experience is too limited to support a generalization as to prognosis.

Addison, T.: On the constitutional and local effects of diseases of the suprarenal capsules. London Med. Gaz., 43:517, 1849, 1855.

Bartter, F. C., Albright, F., Forbes, A. P., Leaf, A., Dempsey, E., and Carroll, E.: The effects of adrenocorticotropic hormone and cortisone in adrenogenital syndrome associated with congenital adrenal hyperplasia: An attempt to explain and correct its disordered hormonal pattern. J. Clin. Invest., 30:237, 1951.

Baulieu, E. E., and Robel, P. (eds.): Aldosterone: Prague Symposium. Oxford, Blackwell Scientific Publications, 1964.

Blizzard, R. M., and Kyle, M.: Studies of the adrenal antigens and antibodies in Addison's disease. J. Clin. Invest., 42:1653, 1963.

Bongiovanni, A. M., Eberlein, W. R., Goldman, A. S., and New, M.: Disorders of adrenal steroid biogenesis. Recent Prog. Horm. Res., 23:375, 1967.

Christy, N. P. (ed.): The Human Adrenal Cortex. New York, Harper & Row, 1971.

Conn, J. W., Knopf, R. F., and Nesbit, R. M.: Clinical characteristics of primary aldosteronism from an analysis of 145 cases. Am. J. Surg., 107:159, 1964.

Cope, C. L.: Adrenal Steroids in Disease. 2nd ed. Philadelphia, J. B. Lippincott Company, 1972.

Cushing, H.: The basophil adenomas of the pituitary body and their clinical manifestations (pituitary basophilism). Bull. Johns Hopkins Hosp., 50:137, 1932.

Eisenstein, A. B. (ed.): The Adrenal Cortex. London, J. & A. Churchill, Ltd., 1967.

Gabrilove, J. L., Sharma, D. C., Wotiz, H. H., and Dorfman, R. I.: Feminizing adrenocortical tumors in the male: A review of 52 cases including a case report. Medicine, 44:37, 1965.

Glaz, E., and Vecsei, P.: Aldosterone: International Series of Monographs in Pure and Applied Biology. New York, Pergamon Press, 1971.

Graber, A. L., Ney, R. L., Nicholson, W. E., Island, D. P., and Liddle, G. W.: Natural history of pituitary-adrenal recovery following long-term suppression with corticosteroids. J. Clin. Endocrinol. Metab., 25:11, 1965.

Liddle, G. W.: Tests of pituitary-adrenal suppressibility in the diagnosis of Cushing's syndrome. J. Clin. Endocrinol. Metab., 20:1539, 1960.

Liddle, G. W., Bledsoe, T., and Coppage, W. S., Jr.: A familial renal disorder simulating primary aldosteronism but with negligible aldosterone secretion. Trans. Assoc. Am. Physicians, 76:199, 1963.

Liddle, G. W., Island, D., and Meador, C. K.: Normal and abnormal regulation of corticotropin secretion in man. Recent Prog. Horm. Res., 18:125, 1962.

Orth, D. N., and Liddle, G. W.: Results of treatment in 108 patients with Cushing's syndrome. N. Engl. J. Med., 285:243, 1971.

Rowntree, L. G., and Snell, A. M.: A Clinical Study of Addison's Disease. Mayo Clinic Monographs. Philadelphia, W. B. Saunders Company, 1931.

Temple, T. E., and Liddle, G. W.: Inhibitors of adrenal steroid biosynthesis. Ann. Rev. Pharmacol., 10:199, 1970.

Thorn, G. E. (ed.): Symposium on the adrenal cortex. Am. J. Med., 53:No. 5, 1972.

THE TESTIS*

Mortimer B. Lipsett

856. INTRODUCTION

FETAL DEVELOPMENT

The primordial gonad arises in the urogenital ridge from intermediate mesoderm during the fifth week of gestation. Early in its development, the bipotential primitive gonad (Fig. 1) is composed of two unipotential mesodermal primordia, each with a distinct physiologic as well as morphologic capacity: (1) a cortical component, consisting of the germinal epithelium; and (2) a medullary component, made up of the primary sex cords derived from the germinal epithelium, and mesonephric and blastemal elements. A third constituent, the primordial germ cell, which appears to be bipotential, arises in an extragonadal site and migrates to the gonads. The cortical component can differentiate only as an ovary, and the medullary component only as a testis (Fig. 1); normally, the dominant element follows the genetic sex of the zygote, and the recessive element retrogresses.

When the gonad destined to become a testis begins to differentiate in a male direction during the seventh to eighth week of embryonic life, the cortical component involutes. Within the medulla, seminiferous tubules form from the primary sex cords and anastomose with the rete testis and testicular ducts, and Leydig cells develop. Leydig cells proliferate predominantly during the first half of gestation, but then gradually involute, persisting until shortly after birth. With morphologic differentiation, the Leydig cells acquire the capacity to synthesize testosterone, and this steroid hormone has been found in the fetal testis.

*In the four previous editions this chapter was written by Dr. Melvin M. Grumbach, who has kindly given me permission to include portions of this material. M.B.L.

ACCESSORY SEX STRUCTURES

Fetal castration experiments in placental mammals have clarified the regulation of development of the accessory sex structures. Jost and others demonstrated that castration of male fetuses at an early critical period prevented the differentiation of male structures and led to entirely female development of ducts, urogenital sinus, and external genitalia. These studies, in the light of recent observations of anomalies of sex in man, support the notion that a fetal testicular morphogenetic substance causes regression of the müllerian (female) duct system and that testosterone, which does not have this property, brings about masculinization of the urogenital sinus and external genitalia.

Intrinsic or extrinsic factors that adversely affect any stage of the mechanisms of sex determination and sex differentiation can lead to sexual anomalies. Most disorders of sexual differentiation can be understood by reference to the separate action of each of these fetal testicular substances. These disorders will be discussed in Ch. 859 and 860.

CHEMISTRY AND PHYSIOLOGY OF THE TESTICULAR HORMONES

The testicular hormone *testosterone,* secreted from the Leydig cell, has the primary role in the development and maintenance of the male accessory sex organs, prostate, and seminal vesicles, in the elaboration of semen, and in the development of masculine secondary sexual characteristics. These properties define a class of substances, the androgens; the important androgen secreted by the testis is testosterone. Recent evidence suggests that the 5α reduced derivative of testosterone, 5α-dihydrotestosterone, may be the active form of the hormone at the nuclear receptor within the male accessory sex structures, and is responsible for inducing growth of these organs.

The adrenal cortex secretes little testosterone. The weak androgenic potency of adrenocortical steroids such as androstenedione and dehydroepiandrosterone can be attributed to their conversion to testosterone in small yield.

The contention that testosterone is the principal testicular androgen has been confirmed by the measurement of this steroid in human spermatic vein blood. Healthy young men secrete about 7 mg of testosterone per day. From animal experiments in which the seminiferous tubules were destroyed without affecting the Leydig cells, it has been concluded that testosterone originates in the Leydig cells, although the seminiferous tubule has a weak capacity for testosterone synthesis. Clinical signs of androgen deficiency are absent in certain testicular disorders in man associated with defective seminiferous tubules but with intact Leydig cells.

Pathways for the biosynthesis of testosterone by the Leydig cell resemble those in other steroid-synthesizing glands. Precursors such as acetate and cholesterol are converted enzymatically to testosterone via 17-hydroxypregnenolone and 17-hydroxyprogesterone. The testis can also aromatize testosterone to estradiol. In adult man 15 to 20 μg of estradiol is secreted daily; an additional 25 to 30 μg is produced peripherally by aroma-

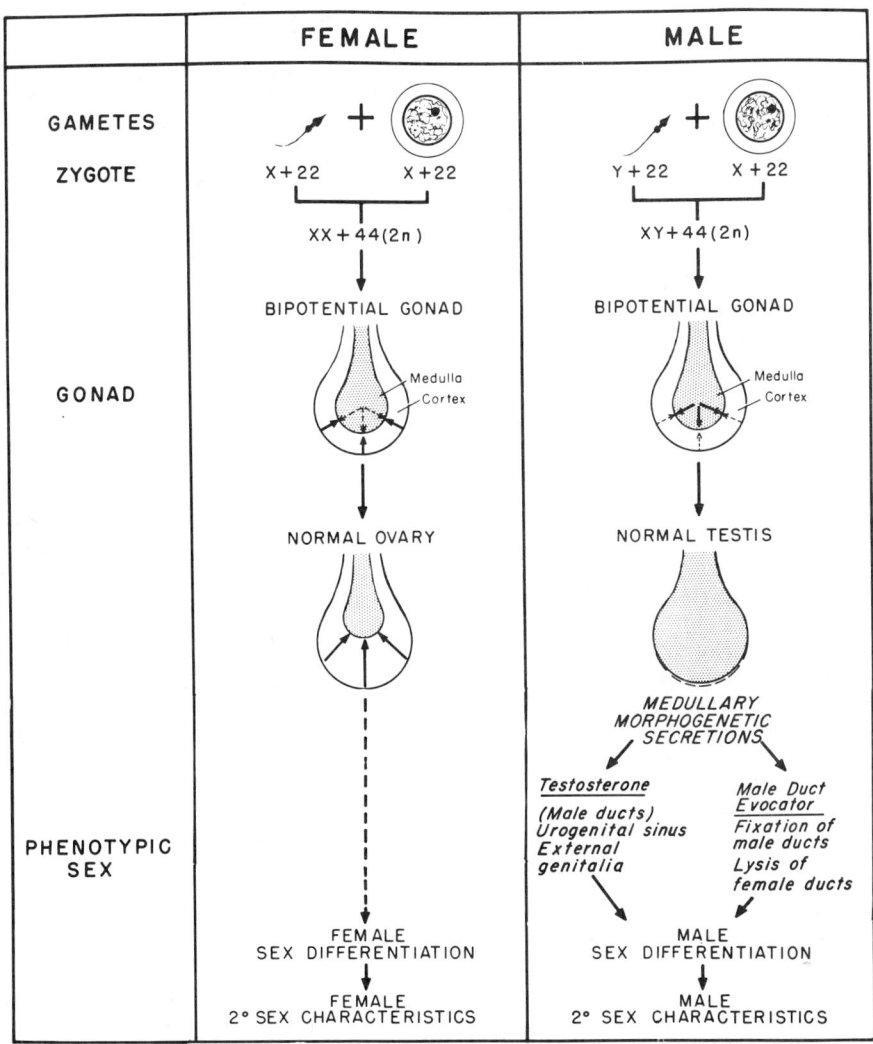

Figure 1. Diagrammatic scheme of human sex determination and differentiation. (Modified from Grumbach, M. M.: *In* Astwood, E. B. (ed.): Clinical Endocrinology I. New York, Grune & Stratton, Inc., 1960.)

tization of blood testosterone in other tissues. Estrone, however, is predominantly a product of adrenal cortical secretions.

The liver is the main site of catabolism of testosterone and of the conjugation of its known metabolites with glucuronic or sulfuric acid; other tissues play a less important role in its metabolism. The major identifiable urinary metabolites are the 17-ketosteroids androsterone and etiocholanolone, which are excreted principally as glucuronides and account for 20 to 40 per cent of the testosterone secreted. A small amount of testosterone (0.2 to 2 per cent) is excreted as testosterone glucuronide.

The two functions of the testis, the synthesis of testosterone and sperm production, are under the control of the hypothalamic-pituitary unit. Luteinizing hormone (LH) acts on the Leydig cell to induce testosterone synthesis, although FSH may synergize to a limited extent. FSH is necessary to initiate spermatogenesis, but it is uncertain whether it has any other role in the process.

The seminiferous tubule is a target tissue for androgen, and there are many data showing that the high concentration of testosterone in the fluid bathing the tubule is functionally important. In hypophysectomized man or monkey it has been shown that spermatogenesis continues if intratesticular testosterone concentration is maintained by human chorionic gonadotrophin (HCG) administration or testosterone implants, respectively. The identification of a tubular androgen-binding protein regulated by FSH may be the link that connects FSH, androgen, and spermatogenesis.

Testosterone exerts a negative feedback on LH secretion, although it is not clear whether the steroid combining at the hypothalamic receptor sites is testosterone or one of its metabolites, dihydrotestosterone or estradiol. The hypothalamus has the capacity to metabolize testosterone to dihydrotestosterone and estradiol. Plasma FSH is also suppressed by testosterone, but an additional factor, derived probably from the Sertoli cell, also modulates FSH secretion. Thus plasma FSH and LH are high in the absence of Leydig cell secretions, but FSH alone is increased when there is severe seminiferous tubule disease. These relationships are shown diagrammatically in Figure 2.

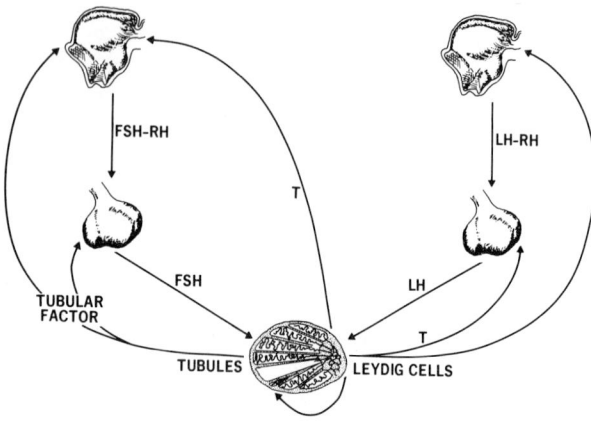

Figure 2. Diagram of hypothalamic-pituitary-testis interactions. (From Lipsett, M. B., and Sherins, R. J.: The testis. *In* Bondy, P. K., and Rosenberg, L. E. [eds.]: Duncan's Diseases of Metabolism. 7th ed. Philadelphia, W. B. Saunders Company, 1974.)

EVALUATION OF TESTICULAR FUNCTION

Clinical Assessment. A clinical estimate of the adequacy of androgen production may be obtained by ascertaining the degree of development of the penis and scrotum, size of the prostate, general maturity and status of male secondary sex characteristics, habitus and skeletal proportions, muscular development, and sexual potency. This assessment has limitations in the mature adult, however, because regression of secondary sexual characteristics is slow even after complete loss of Leydig cell function. Furthermore, distribution of facial and body hair can be highly variable owing to differences in responsiveness of these skin appendages to hormonal stimulation. In this regard, the American Indian, the black African, and some Orientals have sparse or absent facial and body hair despite normal testicular function and plasma testosterone concentration.

Urinary 17-Ketosteroids. About 80 per cent of the urinary 17-ketosteroids (17-KS) is derived from adrenocortical steroids that have little intrinsic androgenic activity. Less than 3 mg daily is derived from Leydig cell secretions. Androsterone and etiocholanolone, the principal urinary metabolites of testosterone, are also metabolites of adrenocortical 11-deoxysteroids. Thus, since urinary 17-KS are an index chiefly of adrenal cortical function, they cannot be used to assess testicular function. Testosterone, which has a hydroxyl group at carbon atom 17, is not a 17-ketosteroid.

The normal range of 17-KS excretion in men is 8 to 25 mg per day (mean, 15 mg). Before puberty only small amounts are detectable in urine. In adult men and women after the third decade, urinary 17-KS decrease gradually owing to lessening adrenal secretion of dehydroepiandrosterone. The excretion of 17-KS may be reduced in eunuchoidism, although the values obtained in such patients are often within the normal range. In panhypopituitarism the function of both the testis and the adrenal cortex is impaired, and the excretion of urinary 17-KS is greatly decreased. Low values are also frequently found in chronic debilitating disease and renal insufficiency. Measurement of urinary 17-KS has little clinical value in disease of the testis or adrenal cortex except as a screening test for congenital adrenal hyperplasia and adrenal tumors (see Ch. 853 to 855).

Urinary Estrogens. It was suggested by Maddock and Nelson that the increase in urinary estrogen after the administration of chorionic gonadotrophin (a placental gonadotrophin with LH-like activity) could be a useful index of Leydig cell function. It has been shown recently that the Leydig cell is the source of almost all of the plasma estradiol in men. Nevertheless, neither measurement of plasma estradiol concentration or that of urinary estrogen excretion is a practical index of Leydig cell function.

Plasma and Urinary Testosterone. The measurement of plasma and urinary testosterone, the latter as the glucuronide conjugate, provides reliable indices of Leydig cell function. The production rate of testosterone can be estimated, but the method is too cumbersome for routine use. Young adult males excrete 40 to 100 μg per day of testosterone glucuronide; women excrete less than 6 μg, and boys before puberty less than 0.5 μg. The concentration of testosterone in plasma of young adult men ranges from 0.3 to 1.2 μg per 100 ml (mean 0.65 μg per 100 ml), and the concentration in women varies from 0.034 to 0.06 μg per 100 ml (mean, 0.054 μg per 100 ml). More than 95 per cent of testosterone in plasma is bound to a specific β-globulin, and thus only 1 to 2 per cent is available for diffusion into cells. The administration of HCG to adult men induces a rise in plasma and urinary testosterone; this procedure has been used to assess the responsiveness of the Leydig cell and to distinguish between primary and secondary testicular disease.

Plasma and Urinary Gonadotrophins. Only a small proportion of the FSH and LH secreted daily appears in the urine in a biologically active form. The normal range of gonadotrophin excretion by the mouse uterine weight method is 10 to 100 mouse uterine units per day, and by the rat ovarian weight method 5 to 20 rats units per day. The common bioassays of urinary gonadotrophins measure the combined excretion of LH and FSH and cannot therefore give meaningful information about variations in individual hormones. Further, the imprecision of the measurements is such that only successive determinations will permit a statement about low or normal levels. Gonadotrophins are detectable by bioassay in 15 per cent of samples obtained randomly from prepubertal children and are diminished or absent in hypogonadism secondary to pituitary or hypothalamic disturbances and frequently in chronic debilitating disease, malnutrition, and starvation. The excretion of gonadotrophin is increased in many but not all primary testicular disorders. In general, elevated levels appear to be related to the degree of damage to the seminiferous tubules, reflecting increased urinary FSH.

The advent of radioimmunoassay procedures has led to the development of sensitive, accurate, practical methods for measurement of these glycoproteins in serum and urine. Determination of plasma or urinary FSH and LH is a useful diagnostic procedure replacing urinary gonadotrophin bioassay. The values obtained by immunoassay are expressed in terms of International Units of the Second International Reference Preparation (2nd IRP) of human menopausal gonadotrophin or in ng of a human pituitary FSH and LH standard. The mean plasma FSH concentration in adult men is 11.7 mIU per milliliter (range 4 to 27 mIU per milliliter) and the mean plasma LH concentration is 9.1 mIU per milliliter (range 4 to 18.9 mIU per milliliter) in terms of the 2nd IRP-HMP (see Ch. 828 and 829).

Plasma FSH levels remain fairly constant throughout the day; nonsystematic pulsatile fluctuations of LH are commonly noted. It has been estimated that 200 to 300 IU of each hormone is secreted daily; of this only 5 to 20 IU is excreted in the urine.

Assessment of Hypothalamic-Pituitary Gonadotrophin Release. Clomiphene citrate, an analogue of the nonsteroidal estrogen chlorotrianisene, is an estrogen antagonist and competes with both androgen and estrogen at hypothalamic receptor sites. When administered to normal men by mouth, 100 to 200 mg per day for five to seven days, it evokes a mean increase in the concentration of plasma FSH of 130 per cent and of plasma LH of 160 per cent. It also induces a rise in urinary FSH and LH and of plasma testosterone. Little or no increase in FSH or LH secretion is elicited in men with pituitary disease.

The recent identification and synthesis of a hypothalamic decapeptide with predominantly LH-releasing activity has enabled the physician to establish pituitary responsiveness directly (see Ch. 829). It may prove valuable in distinguishing between normal and decreased pituitary synthesis of gonadotrophins.

Testicular Biopsy. This procedure can be of great value in the diagnosis and prognosis of testicular disorders. It provides information concerning primarily the gametogenic function of the testis—the status of the seminiferous tubules and the stages of spermatogenesis. Biopsy examination of the testis is of use in diagnosis of tubular disease, in assessing processes of sperm maturation, and in distinguishing azoospermia resulting from obstruction to the passage of sperm from azoospermia of other causes.

Examination of Semen. Specimens of semen for analysis are usually obtained two to three days after the last ejaculation. The volume of the specimen, the total number of sperm, and the motility and morphology of the sperm are determined. The minimal number of sperm necessary for normal fertility is unknown, but a total sperm count of 60 million may be considered normal. Less than this in general means decreased fertility. Because of the wide variations in sperm count among several specimens from the same patient, evaluation of therapy requires long control periods. Assessment of motility and morphology may require examination of many specimens to establish an accurate baseline.

Sex Chromatin Pattern. The number of X chromosomes in the sex chromosome complex can be assessed indirectly by cytologic methods because of sexual dimorphism in the nuclear structure of somatic cells. Preparations suitable for examination can be obtained from smears of buccal mucosa, skin biopsy specimens, or blood (see Ch. 13). This test is widely used in the investigation of abnormalities of sex differentiation, particularly of males with defective testes and azoospermia or severe oligospermia. When a chromatin-positive (female-type) nuclear sex chromatin pattern is detected in a phenotypic male with bilateral testes, it suggests that an associated congenital primary testicular disorder may be present (see Ch. 859).

Instances have been described in which some of the nuclei from phenotypic males or females contained two or more sex chromatin bodies. The maximal number of sex chromatin bodies in somatic nuclei is equivalent to one less than the number of X chromosomes in the sex chromosome complex. For example, XO and XY individuals have chromatin-negative (male-type) somatic nuclei (no chromatin bodies), whereas a high proportion of diploid nuclei in individuals with XX or XXY sex chromosome constitution contain a maximum of one sex chromatin body. Similarly, in XXX females and XXXY males a maximum of two bodies is found in somatic nuclei.

It has been found that quinacrine hydrochloride, an acridine derivative, when utilized as a stain, produces intense fluorescence of the Y chromosome in interphase nuclei, in metaphase preparations, and in sperm. This discovery makes it possible to detect XYY, XXYY, and other double Y syndromes by the simple buccal smear technique.

857. PUBERTAL DEVELOPMENT IN THE MALE

There are wide variations in the age of onset, duration, and sequence of events that characterize the biologic pattern of male puberty. In normal boys signs of puberty may appear at any age between 10 and 17 years; the average age of onset is 12 to 13 years. Once initiated, the major changes are usually completed or well advanced in three to four years; in a small percentage of normal persons, maturity is not attained until the age of 21, and rarely thereafter.

A substantial body of evidence suggests that the stimulus for release of pituitary gonadotrophin at puberty originates in the hypothalamus and is mediated by a neurohormonal secretion, LH-releasing hormone (LHRH). It seems likely that a certain level of physiologic maturation, presumably including the central nervous system, is necessary before this complex and incompletely understood mechanism is activated. This level of development can be best correlated with the degree of osseous and epiphyseal development (bone age) rather than with the chronologic age. Of interest is the observation that small amounts of FSH and LH are secreted by prepubertal children. There is good evidence in animals as well as some data in man showing that the hypothalamic-pituitary-testicular negative feedback mechanism is operative and set at a low level before pubescence.

The sequence of events that marks the pubertal period starts with an acceleration in the growth of the testes and scrotum. The initial increase in testicular size is largely attributable to changes in the seminiferous tubules, which occupy about 90 per cent of the volume of the testis. After initial acceleration of testicular growth, there is an increase in the size of the penis, the appearance of pubic hair, which has at first a transverse growth, and gradual enlargement of the prostate and other accessory organs and glands. It should be noted that the increase in testis size precedes the first appearance of pubic hair by approximately two years and peak height velocity by three years, and is an important clinical feature in ascertaining onset of early puberty. With pubescence, pulsatile and increased release of LH is observed, first at night and then throughout the 24 hours.

Concomitantly, usually between the ages of 13 and 15, an acceleration of growth takes place. This adolescent growth spurt is completed in about three years and, in boys, accounts for an average increment in height of about 8 inches (4 to 12 inches) and a gain in weight of about 40 pounds.

It is necessary that the physician be cognizant of the wide range of normality of the pubertal process in time of onset, intensity, and duration, and also of normal variations in the degree of development of the secondary sex characteristics. In normal men, the pitch of the voice, the size of the external genitalia, the amount of body hair, and the body habitus vary from individual to individual, and are largely attributable to genetic factors and not to differences in the secretion of testosterone.

Delayed Adolescence. Commonly, failure to undergo sexual maturation by the average age is ascribable to the normal variation in pubertal development. Delayed adolescence, although inherently a benign condition, is often a severe psychologic handicap to the patient and a cause of parental anxiety. Many of these boys are short, and a delay of several years in osseous development is not uncommon. Frequently there is a history of late onset of puberty in other members of the family. Retardation of puberty may also be due to inadequate dietary intake or to chronic illness, because these may be associated with diminished secretion of pituitary gonadotrophin.

Pubertal failure or arrest in pubertal development secondary to pituitary-hypothalamic dysfunction or gonadal disease must be excluded in cases of delayed puberty. To exclude pituitary tumor, roentgenographic examination of the skull and careful examination of the fundi and visual fields are required, as well as search for other signs of neurologic involvement in boys who are significantly delayed in their sexual development, particularly when this is accompanied by stunting of growth. It is advisable to assess other pituitary functions (see Ch. 829), especially if the delayed maturation is accompanied by short stature or a decreased rate of growth. In addition, a buccal smear for sex chromatin and determination of urinary or plasma gonadotrophins may clarify the clinical situation. The response to clomiphene will not differentiate between delayed puberty and hypogonadotrophic hypogonadism, because both groups are clomiphene unresponsive. LHRH usually causes LH release in both groups so that the response to this agent also is not diagnostic.

Treatment. Treatment should be directed toward correction of the basic disturbance, e.g., measures to improve nutrition or surgical removal or irradiation of a pituitary neoplasm. Substitution therapy with male sex hormone should be started at about 13 or 14 years of age so that the onset of the patient's maturation coincides with that of his contemporaries. The use of this regimen does not preclude subsequent induction of spermatogenesis with FSH in those individuals with hypogonadotrophic hypogonadism.

Less well defined is the treatment of boys in whom no apparent etiologic factor is found. Many will mature spontaneously before 17 years of age and merely represent an extreme of the normal range. Indiscriminate use of hormonal treatment in this group is unwise, and a conservative approach is indicated. Nonetheless, at times, sociopsychologic considerations may make it expedient to treat such boys. A therapeutic trial with human chorionic gonadotropin, 500 to 1000 IU three times weekly injected intramuscularly, or with a testosterone preparation for three to six months will cause

virilization, and often maturation will progress after treatment is discontinued.

858. SEXUAL PRECOCITY

Isosexual precocity in boys is defined as the occurrence of signs of masculinization before the age of ten years. Skeletal maturation is accelerated and the epiphyses fuse at a premature age, leading to short stature in adult life. On the other hand, mental and dental development are not precocious. Sexual precocity occurs about three times more frequently in girls than in boys. There are four main causes of isosexual precocity in boys: *cerebral, adrenocortical, testicular,* and *extra-endocrine tumors secreting HCG.*

The cerebral causes of sexual precocity may be functional or organic. They are associated with premature activation of the hypothalamic-pituitary mechanism and the release of pituitary gonadotrophic hormones. This form, designated true precocious puberty or complete isosexual precocity, is manifested by maturation of the Leydig cells and spermatogenesis.

True precocious puberty may be caused by organic lesions of the brain either directly or indirectly involving the posterior hypothalamus, such as hypothalamic and pineal tumors, hamartoma of the tuber cinereum, craniopharyngioma, hydrocephalus, postencephalitic lesions, congenital defects, tuberous sclerosis, and neurofibromatosis. The *McCune-Albright syndrome* of sexual precocity, polyostotic fibrous dysplasia, and pigmented areas of skin is rare in boys. The mechanism whereby such lesions activate the hypothalamic-pituitary secretion of gonadotrophins is unknown. Cerebral lesions, particularly tumors, accompanied by precocious puberty may affect other hypothalamic functions, causing diabetes insipidus, bulimia, obesity, somnolence, emotional lability, or disturbances in temperature regulation. Diabetes insipidus in association with precocious puberty is a syndrome that tends to occur in the presence of an aberrant pinealoma. Involvement of the optic nerves or visual pathways causes visual disturbances. In some instances signs of puberty precede the onset of detectable neurologic involvement, and a prolonged period of observation with repeated careful neurologic examinations, roentgenograms of the skull, and determinations of the visual fields is necessary before it is possible to exclude cerebral neoplasm. When no organic cause is found, the condition is described as *idiopathic precocious puberty;* in some instances, it is transmitted as a sex-limited autosomal dominant trait. In the idiopathic cases, seizure disorders and abnormal electroencephalographic patterns are appreciably more frequent than in normal children.

In all varieties of true precocious puberty, the excretion of urinary 17-ketosteroids rises slowly to normal adolescent values; initially, levels are between 2.5 and 4.0 mg per day. Plasma and urinary testosterone values are increased, because Leydig cell secretion is stimulated. In contrast to precocious pseudopuberty, pituitary gonadotrophin is excreted in the urine; frequently, however, this is not detectable early except by the more sensitive radioimmunoassay procedures for FSH and LH. The pulsatile secretion of LH that normally occurs with pubescence has been noted in precocious puberty. Medroxyprogesterone acetate, a synthetic long-acting progestin, administered intramuscularly, is occasionally of value in the management of patients with idiopathic precocious puberty by virtue of its capacity to inhibit pituitary LH secretion. Rarely, extrapituitary neoplasms, such as hepatoma, that secrete a HCG-like gonadotrophin cause isosexual precocity.

In other forms of isosexual precocity not related to intracranial causes, the testes remain immature, in contrast to the enlarged phallus, and true puberty does not occur. Accordingly, this type has been called *incomplete sexual precocity* or *precocious pseudopuberty*.

The most common cause of incomplete sexual precocity in boys is adrenocortical hyperfunction resulting from congenital virilizing adrenal hyperplasia or a virilizing adrenocortical tumor. With few exceptions the testes remain prepubertal in size despite enlargement of the penis and scrotum and development of other secondary sexual characteristics. An ectopic nodule of hyperplastic adrenal tissue is occasionally palpable in the testis, sometimes bilaterally, and may be confused with Leydig cell tumor, especially in rare instances in which striking enlargement of the testis is found. The excretion of 17-KS is increased in relation to chronologic age, and urinary pregnanetriol is high (see Ch. 853).

Interstitial cell tumor of the testis is a rare cause of isosexual precocity. In almost all reported cases the tumor has been unilateral, and the contralateral testis is immature. Gynecomastia is occasionally present. The excretion of 17-KS varies from 3 to 64 mg per day. Plasma testosterone concentration has generally been in the normal male range, although an occasional high value has been reported. Spermatogenesis has been observed in the tubules surrounding the tumor only, thereby confirming the importance of high intratesticular androgen concentrations for spermatogenesis.

Iatrogenic sexual precocity has been produced by the administration of male sex hormone, but is seen most frequently in boys who have been treated with large doses of HCG for cryptorchidism.

859. HYPOGONADISM

Hypogonadism may refer to a decrease in either the endocrine or the gametogenic function of the testis or to both. Hypogonadism is most commonly classified as primary or secondary, depending on the site of the defect. Primary hypogonadism is due to testicular disease, whereas secondary hypogonadism is a result of hypothalamic-pituitary disease. The excretion or blood level of gonadotrophins is normal or high in primary hypogonadism, and is decreased in secondary hypogonadism. Of common occurrence are primary lesions of the testis involving only spermatogenesis, resulting in infertility. On the other hand, when testosterone secretion is deficient, spermatogenesis is impaired.

Androgen Deficiency. The clinical signs of androgen deficiency depend upon the age of onset and upon severity and duration of the deficiency. Total loss of testicular androgenic function, usually secondary to surgical castration or congenital defects of the testes, before or during early puberty results in eunuchoidism in adulthood. Eunuchoidism causes disproportionate growth of the long bones owing to delay in epiphysial closure. The span exceeds the height by several inches, and the distance between the symphysis pubis and the sole (lower segment) measures more than 55 per cent of the height. Tall stature is common, but not invariable. (The characteristic skeletal proportions of the eunuch are not pathognomonic and may be found in otherwise normal men.) The shoulders tend to be narrow and, although the habitus may be lean or obese, excessive fat deposition often occurs about the pectoral region, hips, thighs, and lower abdomen. Muscular development is poor. Except for the appearance of sparse pubic hair, secondary sex characteristics fail to appear, and the voice remains juvenile. Gynecomastia occurs in association with Klinefelter's syndrome and with male pseudohermaphroditism. Acne and baldness do not occur. Sex drive and potentia are absent or greatly reduced. The hematocrit and hemoglobin levels are characteristic of those for women and increase with administration of androgen.

The effects on somatic and sexual development of partial loss of testicular androgenic function are less striking and vary greatly in degree. Characteristic of the milder forms of eunuchoidism are the scant growth of facial hair and a female distribution of pubic hair. In men who have attained sexual maturity, castration does not result in complete regression of secondary sexual characteristics, and the signs of androgen deficiency are less conspicuous. The most common signs are reduction in prostatic size, diminished rate of growth of the beard and body hair, the appearance of fine wrinkles around the eyes, and a pasty, sallow complexion. Semen volume is reduced. Potentia and libido, although usually diminished, occasionally persist. There may be vasomotor phenomena, including hot flushes.

The most useful substances for the treatment of androgen deficiency are the preparations of testosterone that are available in forms suitable for intramuscular, oral, and buccal or sublingual administration. The mode of administration depends, for the most part, on the preference of the patient and the cost.

Esterification of testosterone with organic acids potentiates its activity when injected as an oily solution. Testosterone propionate in doses of 25 to 50 mg by intramuscular injection two or three times weekly is usually adequate for replacement therapy. However, longer-acting esters are available that can be administered less frequently. One dose of 200 to 400 mg of testosterone cyclopentylpropionate or testosterone enanthate is highly effective when injected at two- to four-week intervals.

Methyltestosterone is an effective preparation for oral and buccal or sublingual use. It is usually administered in doses of 50 mg (30 to 75 mg) orally or about 25 mg per day by sublingual absorption. It is not metabolized to 17-KS as is testosterone. No potent protein anabolic steroid lacking androgenic properties in man is available at present, although intensive efforts have been made to obtain one.

Undesirable effects of androgens include edema caused by retention of extracellular electrolyte (an uncommon effect except with use of large doses or in elderly persons with diminished cardiac reserve), polycythemia, acne, gynecomastia, depression of spermatogenesis in some fertile men when administered in large doses, and premature closure of the epiphyses. Rarely, methyltestosterone causes intrahepatic cholestatic jaundice. Androgen therapy may be contraindicated in patients with carcinoma of the prostate.

PRIMARY HYPOGONADISM
(Primary Failure of the Testis)

The problem of classification of primary hypogonadism has not been entirely resolved, because the etiology of many of the disorders in this group is uncertain. Primary hypogonadism may result from genetic and developmental defects, such as seminiferous tubule dysgenesis and Laurence-Moon-Biedl syndrome, or from other causes: trauma, destruction of spermatogonia after orchitis, exposure to ionizing radiation, chemotherapy, and surgical castration. Disorders in this group may or may not be accompanied by androgen deficiency, although in some eunuchoidism is a constant or frequent feature. Disorders of spermatogenesis characterized only by oligospermia and infertility are likewise examples of primary hypogonadism. The excretion of gonadotrophin is normal or increased, depending, apparently, upon the integrity of some component of the seminiferous tubules. Increase of plasma FSH signifies severe tubular damage.

Klinefelter's Syndrome; Seminiferous Tubule Dysgenesis

This syndrome was described in 1942 by Klinefelter, Reifenstein, and Albright and is characterized classically by small, firm testes, azoospermia, gynecomastia, and elevated urinary gonadotrophins. The features become apparent during early puberty, and also include eunuchoidism. Histologically there are atrophy and hyalinization of the seminiferous tubules; Leydig cells tend to occur in large clumps and are apparently increased in number, but total Leydig cell volume is probably normal. The tubules are lined by Sertoli cells; rarely, germ cells are present in isolated tubules. The cause of the syndrome is a developmental defect of the gonad associated with and probably resulting from a sex chromosome abnormality. More recently Klinefelter's syndrome and its variants have been defined by the single constant finding of an increase in the number of X chromosomes in at least one cell line.

The discovery in 1956 that most persons with the classic features of Klinefelter's syndrome are chromatin positive, followed by the detection of sex chromosome abnormalities, served to identify an especially well-defined disorder caused by a nonfamilial, genetically determined gonadal defect. In accordance with this observation and the histopathologic characteristics of the testicular lesion, the term "seminiferous tubule dysgenesis" has been suggested. This disorder, which occurs sporadically, is an important cause of male infertility and a common type of sexual anomaly. The results of several large surveys of newborns in nurseries indicate that the frequency of chromatin-positive seminiferous tubule dysgenesis is of the order of 1 in 500 newborn males.

The most frequent clinical feature of Klinefelter's

Figure 3. A and B, Typical 19-year-old phenotypic male with chromatin-positive seminiferous tubule dysgenesis (Klinefelter's syndrome). This patient had a positive sex chromatin pattern and an XXY karyotype. His 17-ketosteroid excretion was 11.2 mg per 24 hours, and his urinary gonadotrophin excretion was more than 100 mu. These patients vary widely in their habitus and degree of virilization. This patient is well virilized, but had long extremities with eunuchoidal proportions and exhibited gynecomastia. The testes measured 1.8 × 0.9 cm and were small and firm. Testicular biopsy, C, revealed a severe degree of hyalinization of his seminiferous tubules and Leydig cell hyperplasia. D, Forty-eight-year-old man with chromatin-positive Klinefelter's syndrome who came to medical attention only because his severe leg varicosities were thought to reveal a "female trait." (From Van Wyk, J. J., and Grumbach, M. M.: Disorders of sex differentiation. In Williams, R. H. (ed.): Textbook of Endocrinology. 4th ed. Philadelphia, W. B. Saunders Company, 1968.)

syndrome is the small size of the testes, the long diameter usually being less than 2 cm. The testes are firmer than normal owing to hyalinization of the tubules. Gynecomastia is present in fewer than 50 per cent of cases, and eunuchoidism is variable. Patients with this disorder are often tall, and the skeletal proportions frequently are eunuchoid as a consequence of the disproportionately long lower extremities, even though epiphysial fusion is not delayed and skeletal maturation usually follows the normal male pattern (Fig. 3). Cryptorchidism and hypospadias are infrequent. Mental retardation and psychopathic behavior are not uncommon, and there is often evidence of poor social adaptation. This disorder has been reported in association with mongolism and with leukemia. It has been suggested that chronic pulmonary disease and varicose veins are more prevalent in affected adults. The frequency of impaired glucose tolerance and of mild diabetes is increased.

The excretion of urinary gonadotrophin is almost invariably increased, and plasma FSH is always increased as a result of the extensive tubular disease. Plasma LH may be either high or normal, depending perhaps on whether Leydig cell function is normal. In general, urinary 17-KS are within the normal range. The plasma concentration of testosterone is often low, and may increase only slowly with the daily administration of human chorionic gonadotrophin for four to five days.

The abnormality of the sex chromosomes in chromatin-positive Klinefelter's syndrome, characterized by an XXY sex chromosome constitution and a chromosome number of 47, was first demonstrated in 1959 by Jacobs and Strong and by Ford and his associates. Subsequently, less common types of sex chromosome abnormalties have been reported in this disorder. These include phenotypic males with the genotypes 48,-XXYY; 48,XXXY; or 49,XXXXY, which have been found so far only in mentally retarded persons. Unusually tall stature has been found in the XXYY group, along with a tendency to more aggressive and delinquent behavior. The 48,XXXY sex chromosome complex is associated with two sex chromatin bodies in a proportion of diploid somatic nuclei, and the 49,-XXXXY constitution with three sex chromatin bodies. In addition to mental retardation, the XXXXY men have had severe congenital malformations, including very small, usually undescended testes, hypoplastic external genitalia, minor skeletal deformities, including radioulnar synostosis, and other congenital anomalies. It seems that with increasing numbers of X chromosomes, the severity of the abnormalities increases.

Instances of sex chromosome mosaicism have also been described in which at least two populations of cells with different cell chromosome complexes were found in the same individual, e.g., XY/XXY (one cell line with an XY sex chromosome complex and another with an XXY sex chromosome complex), XY/XXXY, XX/XXY, and XXXY/XXXXY. Sex chromosome mosaics arise from a mitotic error in an early division after fertilization in a zygote that originally had either a normal or an abnormal sex chromosome constitution. The detection of a chromatin-positive sex chromatin pattern on buccal smear should not by itself be used as incontrovertible evidence of sterility. Active spermatogenesis was found in the testes of an XY/XXXY mosaic, and additional examples of potential fertility may be found in chromatin-

positive males with other forms of sex chromosome mosaicism, especially XY/XXY. In several carefully studied men with Klinefelter's syndrome, only an XX sex chromosome constitution was found. The maternal origin of the two X chromosomes suggests that a Y chromosome was present early in ontogeny and was lost or more likely translocated to an X chromosome or autosome, or that these men were mosaics and the Y-bearing cell line has escaped detection.

The typical XXY sex chromosome constitution of seminiferous tubule dysgenesis may arise from an abnormality of meiosis during gametogenesis or from a mitotic error in the fertilized zygote (see Ch. 13 to 16). The positive association of this disorder with advanced maternal age and the results of surveys of color blindness (a sex-linked recessive trait) and of the Xg blood group suggest a maternal origin with nodisjunction occurring during oogenesis. Using X-linked markers, a paternal origin of one X has been established in several informative pedigrees, nondisjunction during spermatogenesis giving rise to an XY-bearing sperm and fertilization yielding an XXY zygote. More complex sex chromosome anomalies may arise from meiotic or mitotic errors, or from a combination of both.

The gonadal defect is a consequence of the abnormal sex chromosome constitution. The single Y chromosome is a sufficiently powerful male determiner to suppress the cortical component (ovarian anlage) of the primordial gonad despite the presence of two (or even four) X chromosomes. The fetal testes that develop may have either an adequate number or a deficiency of germ cells, but bring about normal male differentiation of the genital tract. At puberty, if the function of the Leydig cells is adequate, male secondary sexual characteristics develop, but the seminiferous tubules lack or are severely deficient in germ cells. Tubular hyalinization usually does not begin until the later prepubertal period. It seems likely that the characteristic appearance of the testes in adolescent and adult cases depends on the direct or indirect action of pituitary gonadotrophins from the onet of puberty on an inherently defective testis, which, before this time, shows only subtle signs of an abnormal histologic structure.

Treatment. If there is evidence of androgen deficiency, testosterone replacement is indicated. Mastectomy may be necessary in some patients, primarily for cosmetic reasons. It should be noted that testosterone treatment may produce transient increase in gynecomastia and nipple tenderness.

Chromatin-Negative Klinefelter's Syndrome

This term is a misnomer and was bestowed before the fundamental distinction was made on the basis of karyotype. The small testes and azoospermia suggest the Klinefelter phenotype. The testicular lesion resembles that of Klinefelter's syndrome, but it should be remembered that the testis can react to injury in only a limited number of ways. The patients have none of the associated anomalies seen in Klinefelter's syndrome, but hypogonadism is sometimes present. It is probable that so-called chromatin-negative Klinefelter's syndrome is the end-stage of several different disease processes, the final result being hyalinization of the tubules with loss of spermatogonia. Some of these patients may be unrecognized mosaics with one cell line bearing an XXY karyotype and would thus be classified as

Klinefelter's syndrome. Plasma testosterone levels have varied from normal to low.

XYY Syndrome

Although the XYY syndrome is discussed under the topic of primary hypogonadism, in fact primary hypogonadism is unusual in XYY subjects. The XYY syndrome is characterized by a chromosome complement of 47 with an extra Y chromosome and a sex chromatin–negative buccal smear that contains nuclei with two small fluorescent Y chromatin masses, and is estimated to occur in 1 per 500 to 1 per 1000 male births. Newborn males and young boys with this syndrome have a normal phenotype. A number of associated characteristics have been reported in the adolescent and adult XYY male. These include tall stature (often over 6 feet), severe acne, and skeletal abnormalities, e.g., radioulnar synostosis. In studies of criminals with a history of aggessive crimes, an increased frequency of the XYY genotype has been noted. On the other hand, some adult XYY males are physically and mentally normal.

Although the extra Y apparently confers the potential for increased stature, Leydig cell function and plasma and urinary testosterone concentrations have been normal.

Germinal Aplasia
(Sertoli-Cell-Only Syndrome)

This condition is characterized by seminiferous tubules lined with Sertoli cells, little or no tubular fibrosis, and absent germinal cells. The patients are first seen by the physician because of sterility. Leydig cell function is normal. Azoospermia is an invariable finding. The testes are normal or moderately reduced in size. Urinary gonadotrophins are usually increased owing to increased FSH excretion, and plasma FSH is increased four- to fivefold, whereas LH levels are within normal limits. The sex chromosome constitution is XY. Germinal aplasia probably is a developmental defect; but the lesion has also been described after exposure of the testes to ionizing radiation and after extensive chemotherapy with cytotoxic agents. There is no treatment for the spontaneous form, but the lesion after damage to the spermatogenic epithelium may be reversible.

Myotonic Muscular Dystrophy

Testicular atrophy, occurring in middle age, is found in about 80 per cent of affected men with myotonic dystrophy. This syndrome is characterized by myotonia, muscle wasting, frontal baldness, and lenticular opacities. In the series of Drucker et al., signs of androgen deficiency occurred in 18 per cent of the patients and gynecomastia in 12 per cent. The excretion of urinary gonadotrophins was usually normal. The histology of the testis shows tubular fibrosis, hyalinization, and disordered spermatogenesis. There are other metabolic abnormalities which, in association with the testicular findings, have been described as accelerated aging.

Anorchia

Absence of both testes in phenotypic males has been described but is exceedingly rare. Careful surgical exploration is required to establish the diagnosis. Unilateral anorchia is more common, and may result from testicular atrophy after herniorrhaphy, from attempted orchiopexy, or from a developmental disturbance, in which case there may be associated anomalies of the genitourinary tract. Arrest at an early stage of pubescence has been described in association with anorchia. In a few cases, catheterization of the spermatic vein revealed a testosterone gradient, suggesting that a nidus of Leydig cells in the expected position of the testis remained functional.

Infertility

In many testicular lesions, the defect involves only spermatogenic function and results in infertility. Endocrine manifestations are absent. Either the semen lacks sperm or the number or quality of sperm is impaired. Testicular biopsy has a major role in differentiating the various disturbances in spermatogenic activity and in determining prognosis. Azoospermia is usually associated with severe tubular fibrosis, germinal aplasia, or spermatogenic arrest, and oligospermia with germinal cell desquamation, hypospermatogenesis, incomplete spermatogenic arrest, and less severe forms of tubular fibrosis. In general, only azoospermia or severe oligospermia is associated with increased plasma FSH concentrations. In most cases the cause is unknown. Azoospermia may also result from obstruction in the afferent ducts secondary to gonorrhea, tuberculosis, or a nonspecific infection. Absence or atresia of the vas deferens and a rudimentary epididymis are common bilateral lesions in boys with cystic fibrosis, but may occur spontaneously. Hypospermatogenesis is of unknown cause and is not accompanied by other measurable abnormalities.

Sterility is a common sequel of bilateral cryptorchidism and may occur in association with unilateral cryptorchidism. Sterility may follow orchitis caused by mumps, gonorrhea, brucellosis, leprosy, or occasionally other systemic infection; it may result from radiation of the testes or treatment with chemotherapeutic agents; it may be of developmental origin, as in seminiferous tubule dysgenesis. Even relatively minor illnesses may cause profound depression in sperm count. Starvation and chronic debilitating diseases associated with inanition adversely affect spermatic function. Estrogen and androgen administration also inhibit spermatogenesis by suppression of gonadotrophins with concomitant decrease in intratesticular testosterone concentration.

Treatment of Infertility in the Male. Although important advances have been made in the evaluation of spermatogenic function, treatment of infertility caused by primary testicular disease is unsatisfactory. The results of therapy of hormonally normal men with testicular defects of spermatogenesis by the use of large doses of androgenic steroids, gonadotrophins, pregnenolone, thyroid hormone, clomiphene, and vitamin preparations have been unsuccessful. Claims of success in the treatment of oligospermia with human gonadotrophins usually stem from a lack of appreciation of the variability of the sperm count. In published reports the dose of FSH has been about 75 IU three times a week. Since subjects with oligospermia have normal plasma FSH concentrations, their daily FSH production rates are 200 to 300 IU. Thus the "treatment" does not increase FSH "production rate" to a significant extent.

The intermittent use of large doses of testosterone to take advantage of the "rebound effect" on spermatogenesis has not been established as efficacious.

SECONDARY HYPOGONADISM

Secondary hypogonadism is due to decreased secretion of gonadotrophins, and may result from neoplastic, inflammatory, traumatic, vascular, and degenerative lesions involving the pituitary or hypothalamus. These lesions include such entities as pituitary adenoma, craniopharyngioma, astrocytoma, infarction, carotid aneurysm, granulomas such as tuberculosis, histiocytosis X, and hemochromatosis. In many instances, the nature of the underlying lesion is not known. A functional and reversible depression of gonadotrophin secretion occurs in malnutrition, in chronic disease states associated with inanition and nutritional deficiencies, and in some patients with myxedema. High concentrations of androgen and estrogen, as in the adrenogenital syndrome, may cause secondary hypogonadism by suppression of gonadotrophin secretion. Excessive estrogen, either from ingestion or endogenous, as from a feminizing adrenal tumor, depresses the secretion of pituitary gonadotrophin. The testicular atrophy and gynecomastia that occur in some patients with severe liver disease have been ascribed by some to increased levels of estrogen. Decreased gonadotrophin secretion may also result from the nutritional and metabolic disturbances accompanying hepatic cirrhosis.

Decreased secretion of pituitary gonadotrophins occurs either as an isolated defect, *hypogonadotrophic hypogonadism,* or, more commonly, in association with a deficiency of growth hormone and other anterior pituitary hormones. On the other hand, hypoadrenocorticism or hypothyroidism secondary to pituitary failure is rarely found without concurrent involvement of gonadotrophic function and secondary hypogonadism. Although only LH secretion may be impaired, usually secondary hypogonadism is characterized clinically by both inadequate androgenic function and, with rare exceptions (see below), absent or deficient spermatogenesis.

The clinical manifestations vary with age of onset, degree of the deficiency, and whether there is coexistent deficiency of other anterior pituitary hormones. Hypopituitarism occurring during childhood, commonly designated "pituitary dwarfism," results in proportionate dwarfism and complete sexual infantilism. The characteristic features of prepubertal or pubertal gonadotrophic failure are eunuchoid habitus, small testes, lack of development of secondary sexual characteristics, an increased frequency of anosmia or hyposmia, low or absent gonadotrophins, low 17-ketosteroid excretion, low plasma testosterone concentration, and failure of response to clomiphene. Kindreds have been described in which the pattern of inheritance was consistent with either an X-linked or sex-linked dominant trait or as an autosomal recessive trait. The absence of gynecomastia, regarded by some as a salient feature, is of no clinical value in differentiating primary from secondary hypogonadism. It is important to detect organic disease of the pituitary region. Such evaluation should include study of the visual fields, roentgenography of the sella turcica, and, when indicated, such procedures as tomography of the sella, pneumoencephalography, and carotid and venous angiography.

A familial form of isolated hypogonadotrophic hypogonadism limited to males occurs in association with anosmia or hyposmia *(Kallmann's syndrome)* and is transmitted as either an X-linked or a sex-linked dominant trait. Aplasia of the olfactory lobes has been found in autopsied cases. Leydig cell responsiveness to HCG in some of these patients may be decreased. Both familial and sporadic forms of isolated FSH and LH deficiency are known, and these may be associated with a variety of somatic anomalies and neurologic defects. Although the response to LHRH has been variable, the data suggest that hypothalamic synthesis or release of LHRH is impaired in some of these patients.

The testis in patients with hypogonadotrophic hypogonadism remains infantile, the tubular diameter being the same as that of the fetal testis. When the pituitary function is decreased in adult life, tubular collapse, fibrosis, and hyalinization occur at variable times after the onset of gonadotrophic failure.

Isolated LH Deficiency. Pasqualini and Bur described a group of eunuchoidal men with relatively normal-sized testes and some spermatogenic function. Later, McCullagh applied the term "fertile eunuch" to patients with this syndrome. The patients are not fertile, however, because spermatogenesis is decreased, and libido and potentia are absent. Leydig cells are absent or hypoplastic, and androgen deficiency is always present. The excretion of urinary gonadotrophin is usually normal. However, the concentration of plasma LH and the excretion of urinary LH are low or undetectable, whereas the secretion of FSH is normal. Chorionic gonadotrophin stimulates Leydig cell function and ameliorates the androgen deficiency. These patients have an isolated deficiency of LH, which may arise from an abnormality in the hypothalamus (and the synthesis or release of LHRH) or in the pituitary gland. A kindred with two affected brothers has been reported. Rarely, a pituitary tumor or idiopathic delayed adolescence may manifest itself as isolated LH deficiency.

The pathogenesis of the testicular atrophy that follows injury to the spinal cord is uncertain. Both primary and secondary hypogonadism have been described in the Laurence-Moon-Biedl syndrome.

Treatment. A physiologic approach to the treatment of secondary hypogonadism characterized by decreased spermatogenesis requires the use of gonadotrophins. Unfortunately, FSH preparations derived from animal sources are not consistently effective and, when injected repeatedly, stimulate antibody formation that reduces the effect of the hormones. Although human pituitary FSH is not available commercially, gonadotrophin prepared from menopausal urine has been used successfully in combination with chorionic gonadotrophin to induce spermatogenesis in patients with hypogonadotrophic hypogonadism. Here, 75 IU of FSH three times a week has induced normal spermatogenesis. Testosterone cannot be used in place of HCG, because intratesticular testosterone concentrations do not reach the levels attained when the Leydig cells are stimulated. HCG stimulates the Leydig cells to secrete androgen, but must be administered at frequent intervals (three to four times a week). It does not have a direct effect on the seminiferous tubules, although in a few instances of partial gonadotrophic failure spermatogenic as well as Leydig cell function improved after its use. HCG has been effective in maintaining spermatogenesis after hypophysectomy for diabetic retinopathy. When only androgen substitution therapy is needed, one of the long-acting testosterone preparations is preferred.

860. MALE PSEUDOHERMAPHRODITISM

Male pseudohermaphroditism may be considered a form of fetal hypogonadism, because those fetal structures normally responsive to androgen develop incompletely or not at all. Depending on the degree of androgen deficiency, the adult phenotype may range from almost normal female to male with minimal abnormalities. Male pseudohermaphroditism is most often familial and is transmitted either as a sex-linked autosomal dominant or as a sex-limited recessive trait manifest in the male.

SYNDROME OF TESTICULAR FEMINIZATION

This form of familial male pseudohermaphroditism deserves detailed consideration because the pathophysiology illuminates areas of hormone action and fetal regulation. The patients have primary amenorrhea, absent or sparse axillary and pubic hair, female external genitalia, a short blind vaginal pouch, absence of uterus and usually of the male genital ducts, and undescended or labial testes. The phenotypic women are usually tall, have good breast development, and show cornification of the vaginal mucosa. The karyotype is 46 XY.

The cause of the syndrome is a congenital resistance to androgens. Exogenous androgens have been shown to be ineffective in causing axillary or pubic hair growth, virilization, or nitrogen retention. From studies of rat and mouse models of this syndrome, it is probable that the androgen resistance is due to absence of the cytosol androgen-binding protein receptor present in androgen-responsive tissues. This receptor is also present normally in the male gonaducts. In its absence, the male fetus receives no effective androgenic stimulus, resulting in failure of fusion of the genital folds and swellings to form penis and scrotum, respectively, and a lack of posterior migration of the labioscrotal folds. The fetal testicular inducer of müllerian duct regression is not an androgen and continues to be secreted by the fetal testis in this syndrome. Thus, since the upper third of the vagina is a müllerian duct derivative, it regresses and the vagina remains short. Wolffian duct derivatives such as the vas deferens, however, are induced by androgen and therefore are usually absent in this syndrome.

The hormonal relationships in the adult are likewise of interest. Plasma testosterone concentrations are within the normal range for men. Plasma LH is increased, presumably because of end-organ resistance of hypothalamic receptors. Plasma FSH is normal, however, suggesting that feedback is normal owing to a combination of normal estradiol concentration and "tubular factor."

The testes in these patients have tubules containing only Sertoli cells and showing considerable peritubular fibrosis. Spermatogenesis is rare. The Leydig cells appear hyperplastic.

Treatment consists of orchiectomy, because the risk of cancer in these gonads is several times that of gonads in the normal individual. The patients should receive replacement doses of an estrogen such as 0.5 mg of diethylstilbestrol or 0.05 mg of ethinyl estradiol daily to prevent the vasomotor instability characteristic of castration and to maintain normal female secondary sexual characteristics.

OTHER FORMS OF MALE PSEUDOHERMAPHRODITISM

When androgen secretion or effect is decreased during fetal development, the male infant shows varying degrees of ambiguity of the external genitalia. The most extreme example of this would be testicular feminization. The family reported by Lubs et al. has a lesser degree of abnormality because the children were raised as girls but the genitalia were ambiguous. In *Reifenstein's syndrome* and the patients reported by Gilbert-Dreyfus, the phenotype was male. The former syndrome is characterized by severe hypospadias, incomplete fusion of the labioscrotal folds, and gynecomastia. In the latter syndrome, the abnormalities were similar but less marked. Virilization at pubescence in these patients was slow or incomplete, and spermatogenesis was quantitatively decreased. The pathologic physiology of these syndromes has been clarified by Wilson, who showed that decreased 5α-reductase activity with resultant decreased dihydrotestosterone formation would selectively alter the external genitalia.

There have been a few reports of patients with hypospadias and gynecomastia. These may be examples of the least severe form of the syndrome.

861. CRYPTORCHIDISM

The terms "cryptorchidism" and "undescended testes" are used synonymously to designate testes that have never descended into the scrotum. Unilateral cryptorchidism is approximately four times as common as bilaterally undescended testes. A cryptorchid testis may be situated in the abdomen, within the inguinal canal, or in an ectopic position outside the scrotum and the normal pathway of descent. The majority of undescended testes are inguinal. To avoid needless treatment, it is essential to distinguish this condition from retractile testes, which lie in the lower or upper scrotum and are withdrawn into the inguinal region and occasionally into the abdomen by slight stimulus.

The testes usually descend into the scrotum about the eighth fetal month; but occasionally descent is delayed until shortly after birth. Incomplete descent is common in premature male infants. Scorer found undescended testes at birth in 3.4 per cent of 1500 full-term male infants; during the first month of life 50 per cent of the undescended testes reached the scrotum. In a prospective study of the incidence of congenital anomalies by McIntosh and associates, only 0.5 per cent of 2793 liveborn male infants had undescended testes at 12 months of age. The incidence of unilateral and bilateral cryptorchidism in large series of adult males has been variously estimated at 0.2 to 0.4 per cent. Spontaneous descent occurs frequently during the first year of life and is less common after this age.

The etiology is not understood. Not infrequently a normal testis resides in the superficial inguinal pouch, its descent arrested by Scarpa's fascia. However, the cryptorchid testis is often dysgenetic. In rare instances, unilateral or bilateral cryptorchidism is the only overt anatomic abnormality of the external genitalia in individuals with fetal testicular dysfunction.

Diagnosis. The most difficult aspect of diagnosis is distinguishing the true undescended testis from the more common retractile testis of childhood; repeated examinations may be necessary, especially in obese boys. It is important to ascertain by careful inquiry whether the testes have at any time been observed in the scrotum. In cryptorchidism the ipsilateral side of the scrotum is empty and poorly developed. The patient should be carefully examined while standing, squatting, and in a recumbent position, in a warm room and with warm hands. Bimanual examination and palpation while the patient performs a Valsalva maneuver or while the examiner applies pressure to the lower abdomen are also useful procedures. In boys with retractile testes, elicitation of the cremasteric reflex often results in a localized puckering of the scrotal skin. If the testis is palpated in the normal pathway of descent, gentle manipulation should be used in an attempt to displace it into the scrotum. Such mobile testes do not require therapy and will remain in the scrotum with the advent of puberty. Failure to palpate a testis on multiple occasions suggests that the testis is intra-abdominal, atrophic, or absent.

Treatment. The treatment of undescended testes is a vexing and controversial subject; experienced observers differ in their approach to the problem. Major considerations are (1) the potential fertility of the undescended testis, (2) the likelihood of spontaneous descent, and (3) the propensity of the undescended testis to undergo malignant change.

It is well established that during or after puberty the undescended testis shows degenerative changes that eventually proceed to atrophy. With good reason these changes have been ascribed to the deleterious effect of the higher temperature of an extrascrotal environment on the testes, especially on the germinal epithelium. The tubules gradually undergo progressive fibrosis and loss of germinal elements, although androgenic function may persist for many years. These degenerative changes may also be manifestations of a dysgenetic testis. This distinction is important, because the risk of cancer in the dysgenetic gonad is considerably greater than in the normal gonad.

Men with bilateral undescended testes are sterile. However, general agreement is lacking as to the age at which the fertility potential of the cryptorchid testis is impaired. A lag in development of the seminiferous tubules and, in some instances, a mild degree of fibrosis in testes retained after the age of six to ten years have been observed. The significance of these changes is uncertain, but after puberty irreversible degenerative changes frequently occur.

The incidence of cancer in undescended testes is considerably greater than in scrotal testes, and more so in abdominal than in inguinal testes. Although precise statistics are not available, the over-all risk appears to be small, with the exception of the dysgenetic, frequently undescended gonads of intersexes, which are especially prone to malignant degeneration.

The most important problem in the treatment of patients with cryptorchidism is the age at which it is advisable to attempt correction. Treatment consists of orchiopexy or of the administration of HCG followed by orchiopexy when necessary. It is generally agreed that therapy must be started before pubescence if irreparable testicular damage is to be prevented, but opinions differ about the optimal age for treatment. In the more common unilateral cryptorchid, the scrotal testis, if normal, is adequate for fertility. Treatment is recommended for cosmetic reasons, to facilitate examination for neoplasm, and as additional insurance against infertility in the event that the scrotal testis is defective or impaired at a later age.

In bilateral cryptorchidism preservation of fertility is the major consideration. Here the risk of damage to the testis by orchiopexy, which even in experienced hands is not negligible, must be weighed against the possibility of infertility if surgical treatment is delayed too long. When bilateral orchiopexy is followed by atrophy of the testes, the patient will be eunuchoid as well as sterile. Since many undescended testes descend before puberty, it is justifiable to delay treatment until nine years of age unless the testis is ectopic or associated with a hernia.

In some cases hormonal therapy is effective and orchiopexy is unnecessary. It is the opinion of most that testes that descend with such therapy would have descended spontaneously at puberty under the stimulus of endogenous gonadotrophin. To minimize a theoretical risk of damage to the tubule, short intensive courses of 4000 units of HCG administered intramuscularly daily for three days or 4000 units three times a week for three weeks may be used. Hormonal treatment is contraindicated when the testis lies outside the normal pathway of descent.

If the undescended testis is atrophic and biopsy examination at the time of surgery shows irreversible changes, it is generally advisable to perform orchiectomy, provided that the contralateral testis is in the scrotum. This also applies to a testis that, despite all attempts at mobilization, cannot be brought into the scrotum.

862. IMPOTENCE

Impotence is a complicated problem that may be either relative or complete and may involve any phase of the sexual act. Although it is a symptom of androgen deficiency and of genitourinary or neurologic disease, in most instances it is psychic in origin. Multiple sclerosis, tabes dorsalis, and diabetic neuropathy are commonly associated with impotence. Impotence without apparent impairment of libido has been described in patients with temporal lobe lesions. Ganglionic blocking agents, used in the therapy of hypertension, are also a notable cause of impotence. When impotence is the principal complaint of a patient, it is usually the result of an emotional disturbance, and androgen therapy is valueless and at times may add to the psychic trauma. Several recent studies show clearly that, in men as well as in women, stress can decrease gonadotrophic secretion and thereby affect androgen secretion and spermatogenesis (see Ch. 867).

863. "MALE CLIMACTERIC"

The spontaneous occurrence of a male climacteric is still controversial. Although in women during the fifth or sixth decade ovarian failure with a compensatory rise in gonadotrophin excretion is an anticipated and physiologic accompaniment of the aging process, spontaneous testicular deficiency of sufficient degree to produce symptoms is an exceedingly rare occurrence. Many of the symptoms ascribed to this syndrome are common in psychoneurotic syndromes in middle-aged and elderly men. The diagnosis should be documented by finding an increased excretion of gonadotrophin and a low concentration of plasma testosterone, and should be confirmed by obtaining a therapeutic response to androgen therapy, but not to placebos. Plasma testosterone concentrations show little change until after 70 years of age. However, increasing concentrations of testosterone-binding globulin (TeBG) are associated with the gradually decreasing concentration of plasma-free testosterone that has been noted after the age of 50. A progressive increase in plasma LH levels after age 50 has been described.

864. ORCHITIS

Acute orchitis, a common complication of mumps, is a rare occurrence in the course of other specific infectious diseases (see Ch. 125).

Chronic orchitis is associated with painless, hard, sometimes nodular enlargement of the testis. *Syphilis,* the most common cause, may produce an interstitial orchitis in which the testis is characteristically smooth and wooden in consistency ("billiard ball" testis); involvement is frequently bilateral. Other causes include *tuberculosis, leprosy, brucellosis, glanders,* and certain parasitic infections such as *filariasis* and *bilharziasis.* In these diseases, Leydig cell function almost always remains intact, but severe tubular destruction may result.

865. TUMORS OF THE TESTIS

Tumors of the testis are uncommon, comprising about 0.7 per cent of all forms of cancer in the male, occur in about 0.002 per cent of men, and frequently are malignant. The greatest incidence occurs in the third and fourth decades. Testicular tumors may arise from any of the cellular components of the testis or their embryonal precursors.

Considerable uncertainty applies to classification, especially of those neoplasms whose origin has been ascribed to the totipotent germ cell. Melicow has suggested the classification shown in the accompanying table.

GERMINAL TUMORS

Most common are germinal tumors, and, of these, seminoma exceeds in frequency all other testicular tumors. *Seminoma,* although usually fairly uniform in

Tumors of Testis: Classification

I. Primary tumors
  A. Germinal
    1. Seminoma
    2. Embryonal tumors
      a. Embryoma
      b. Choriocarcinoma
      c. Embryonal carcinoma
      d. Teratocarcinoma
      e. Adult teratoma
    3. Combinations of seminoma and embryonal tumor and of the various types of embryonal tumors
    4. Gonadal tumors in intersexes (gonadoblastomas)
  B. Nongerminal tumors
    1. Interstitial cell tumor
    2. Sertoli cell tumor
    3. Tumors of testicular stroma: fibroma, lipoma, etc.
II. Secondary tumors
  A. Lymphoma, plasmacytoma, leukemia, etc.
  B. Metastatic carcinoma

cellular architecture, may contain embryonal elements such as chorionic syncytium in the primary growth or in metastatic lesions. In contrast to the embryonal tumors, which tend to invade the spermatic cord and to metastasize early, especially to lung, seminomas in general are relatively slow growing and commonly invade the iliac and periaortic lymph nodes before generalized dissemination is demonstrable. In addition, seminomas are frequently highly radiosensitive, whereas embryonal tumors are usually resistant to radiotherapy. The significantly increased incidence of germinal tumors, particularly seminoma, in undescended testes and in the dysgenetic gonads of intersexes has been discussed above.

Many patients with germinal tumors excrete increased amounts of chorionic gonadotrophin. This may almost always be attributed to the presence of trophoblastic elements in the tumor. Response to therapy or evidence of recurrence may be monitored by measurement of plasma HCG levels.

INTERSTITIAL CELL TUMORS

Tumors of this type are rare, occur at any age, and are usually but not invariably benign. The tumors are small and often difficult to palpate. In boys interstitial cell tumors cause sexual precocity but not true puberty, because spermatogenesis is absent in the contralateral testis. The only recognizable endocrine manifestation in the adult is gynecomastia, which has been observed in about 10 per cent of cases. Malignant interstitial cell tumors that retain their steroid-synthesizing capacities have been reported.

Bardin, C. W., Ross, G. T., and Lipsett, M. B.: Site of action of clomiphene citrate in men: A study of the pituitary–Leydig cell axis. J. Clin. Endocrinol. Metab., 27:1558, 1967.

Bardin, C. W., Ross, G. T., Rifkind, A. B., Cargille, C. M., and Lipsett, M. B.: Studies of the pituitary–Leydig cell axis in young men with hypogonadotropic hypogonadism and hyposmia: Comparison with normal men, prepubertal boys, and hypopituitary patients. J. Clin. Invest., 48:2046, 1969.

Bergada, C., Cleveland, W. W., Jones, W. H., and Wilkins, L.: Variants of embryonic testicular dysgenesis. Bilateral anorchia and the syndrome of rudimentary testes. Acta Endocrinol., 40:521, 1962.

Bowen, P., Lee, S. N. C., Migeon, C. J., Kaplan, N. M., Whalley, P. J., McKusick, V. A., and Reifenstein, E. C., Jr.: Hereditary male pseudohermaphroditism with hypogonadism, hypospadias, and gynecomastia. Ann. Intern. Med., 62:252, 1965.

Brasel, J. A., Wright, J. C., Wilkins, L., and Blizzard, R. M.: An evaluation of seventy-five patients with hypopituitarism beginning in childhood. Am. J. Med., 38:484, 1965.

Clermont, Y.: Kinetics of spermatogenesis in mammals: Seminiferous epithelium cycle and spermatogonial renewal. Physiol. Rev., 52:198, 1972.

Court Brown, W. M.: Males with an XYY sex chromosome complement. J. Med. Genet., 5:341, 1968.

Davidson, J. M.: Neuroendocrine mechanisms in the control of spermatogenesis. J. Reprod. Fertil., 2:103, 1967.

Dorfman, R. I., and Shipley, R. A.: Androgens: Biochemistry, Physiology, and Clinical Significance. New York, John Wiley & Sons, 1956.

Drucker, W. D., Blanc, W. A., Rowland, L. P., Grumbach, M. M., and Christy, N. P.: The testis in myotonic muscular dystrophy: A clinical and pathologic study with a comparison with the Klinefelter syndrome. J. Clin. Endocrinol. Metab., 23:59, 1963.

Faiman, C., Hoffman, D. L., Ryan, R. J., and Albert, A.: The "fertile eunuch" syndrome: Demonstration of isolated luteinizing hormone deficiency by radioimmunoassay technique. Mayo Clin. Proc., 43:661, 1968.

Faiman, C., and Ryan, R. J.: Radioimmunoassay for human follicle stimulating hormone. J. Clin. Endocrinol. Metab., 27:444, 1967.

Federman, D. D.: Abnormal Sexual Development. Philadelphia, W. B. Saunders Company, 1967.

Foss, G. L., and Lewis, F. J. W.: A study of four cases with Klinefelter's syndrome, showing motile spermatozoa in their ejaculates. J. Reprod. Fertil., 25:401, 1971.

French, F. S., Baggett, B., Van Wyk, J. J., Talbert, J. M., Hubbard, W. R., Johnston, F. R., and Weaver, R. P.: Testicular feminization: Clinical, morphological and biochemical studies. J. Clin. Endocrinol. Metab., 25:661, 1965.

Howard, R. P., Sniffen, R. C., Simmons, F. A., and Albright, F.: Testicular deficiency: A clinical and pathologic study. J. Clin. Endocrinol. Metab., 10:121, 1950.

Jost, A.: Problems of fetal endocrinology. Recent Prog. Horm. Res., 8:379, 1953.

Kelch, R. P., Jenner, M. R., Weinstein, R., Kaplan, S. L., and Grumbach, M. M.: Estradiol and testosterone secretion by human, simian, and canine testes, in males with hypogonadism and in male pseudohermaphrodites with the feminizing testes syndrome. J. Clin. Invest., 51:824, 1972.

Kessler, S., and Moss, R. H.: The XYY karyotype and criminality: A review. J. Psychiatr. Res., 7:153, 1970.

Lipsett, M. B., and Sherins, R. J.: The Testis. In Bondy, P. K., and Rosenberg, L. E. (eds.): Duncan's Diseases of Metabolism. 7th ed. Philadelphia, W. B. Saunders Company, 1974.

Mancini, R. E., Seiguer, A. C., and Perez Lloret, A.: Effect of gonadotropins on the recovery of spermatogenesis in hypophysectomized patients. J. Clin. Endocrinol. Metab., 29:467, 1969.

Marshall, W. A., and Tanner, J. M.: Variations in the pattern of pubertal changes in boys. Arch. Dis. Child., 45:13, 1970.

Martin, F. I. R.: The stimulation and prolonged maintenance of spermatogenesis by human pituitary gonadotrophins in a patient with hypogonadotrophic hypogonadism. J. Endocrinol., 38:431, 1967.

Melicow, M. M.: Classification of tumors of the testis. J. Urol., 73:547, 1955.

Moore, K. L. (ed.): The Sex Chromatin. Philadelphia, W. B. Saunders Company, 1966.

Nowakowski, H., and Lenz, W.: Genetic aspects in male hypogonadism. Recent Prog. Horm. Res., 17:53, 1961.

Odell, W. D., Ross, G. T., and Rayford, P. L.: Radioimmunoassay for luteinizing hormone in human plasma or serum: Physiological studies. J. Clin. Invest., 46:248, 1967.

Paulsen, C. A.: The testes. In Williams, R. H. (ed.): Textbook of Endocrinology. 4th ed. Philadelphia, W. B. Saunders Company, 1968.

Paulsen, C. A., Gordon, D. L., Carpenter, R. W., Gandy, H. M., and Drucker, W. D.: Klinefelter's syndrome and its variants: A hormonal and chromosomal study. Recent Prog. Horm. Res., 24:321, 1968.

Pearson, P. L., Borrow, M., and Vosa, A. G.: Technique for identifying Y chromosomes in human interphase nuclei. Nature, 226:78, 1970.

Rifkind, A. B., Kulin, H. E., and Ross, G. T.: Follicle-stimulating hormone (FSH) and luteinizing hormone (LH) in the urine of prepubertal children. J. Clin. Invest., 46:1925, 1967.

Rosemberg, E., and Paulsen, C. A. (eds.): The Human Testis. New York, Plenum Press, 1970.

Santen, R. J., and Paulsen, C. A.: Hypogonadotropic eunuchoidism. I. Clinical study of mode of inheritance. J. Clin. Endocrinol. Metab., 36:47, 1973.

Scorer, C. G.: The descent of the testis. Arch. Dis. Child., 39:204, 1964.

Steinberger, E.: Hormonal control of mammalian spermatogenesis. Physiol. Rev., 51:1, 1971.

Swanson, D. W., and Stipes, A. H.: Psychiatric aspects of Klinefelter's syndrome. Am. J. Psychiatry, 126:814, 1969.

Van Thiel, D. H., Sherins, R. J., and DeVita, V. T., Jr.: Evidence for a specific seminiferous tubular factor affecting follicle-stimulating hormone secretion in man. J. Clin. Invest., 51:1009, 1972.

Van Wyk, J. J., and Grumbach, M. M.: Disorders of sex differentiation. In Williams, R. H. (ed.): Textbook of Endocrinology. 4th ed. Philadelphia, W. B. Saunders Company, 1968.

Walsh, P. C., Madden, J. D., Harrod, M. J., Goldstein, J. L., MacDonald, P. C., and Wilson, J. D.: Familial incomplete male pseudohermaphroditism, Type 2. N. Engl. J. Med., 291:944, 1974.

Wilson, J. D., and Gloya, R. E.: The intra-nuclear metabolism of testosterone in the accessory organs of reproduction. Recent Prog. Horm. Res., 26:309, 1970.

THE OVARIES

Nathan Kase

866. OVARIAN STRUCTURE AND FUNCTION

The human ovary has a dual physiologic responsibility: (1) development and release of ova and (2) elaboration of estrogen and progesterone. From menarche to menopause both these activities are bound to the cycle of follicle development, ovulation, corpus luteum formation, and regression. In reality each ovary is a heterogeneous, cyclically changing tissue containing subunits with differing properties. During their brief interval of dominance each subunit defines the function of the total organ. The sequential appearance of each unit and their respective gametogenic and endocrine performances are directed by pituitary secretion of varying quantities of gonadotrophins: follicle-stimulating hormone (FSH) and luteinizing hormone (LH). Release of these factors is controlled by a specific neurosecretory substance or substances originating in hypothalamic nuclei that are sensitive to "feedback" levels of circulating ovarian hormones.

The ovary contains specialized cells in the cortical and medullary areas that may contribute to abnormal ovarian function in certain pathologic conditions, but its major elements are the follicle and corpus luteum. The follicle consists of the ovum and two layers of tissue surrounding it: an inner band of granulosa cells without blood vessels, and an outer vascularized mantle of theca cells. At any given time in the preovulatory phase a number of follicles display varying degrees of developmental maturity: cystic changes, hormonal activity, and atresia. The factors responsible for the selection of one to attain full maturity and ovulation while others atrophy are unknown. Morphologic clues indicating development of a follicle are the degree of thecal proliferation and vascularity and the ratio of granulosa layer thickening to cystic distention of the antrum. The formation of a true corpus luteum is a direct consequence of final maturation and ovulation of the follicle. The ruptured follicle is transformed by proliferation, vascularization, and luteinization of the granulosa into the yellow body that characterizes the last two weeks of an ovulatory cycle. Contrary to evidence obtained in other mammals, the human corpus luteum appears to possess an inherent life span of two weeks, during which it is sustained by modest postovulatory pituitary secretion of LH. After this period, the corpus luteum recedes unless renewed major trophic stimulation appears in the form of human chorionic gonadotrophin originating in a flourishing mass of syncytiotrophoblasts associated with an implanted conceptus.

OVARIAN HORMONE FUNCTION – THE ENDOMETRIAL CYCLE

It is helpful to consider the function of ovarian hormones relative to their ability to provide an appropriate milieu for fertilization, implantation, and nutrition of the early embryo. Before menstruation has ceased, preparation for a more successful ovum is resumed. FSH and small quantities of LH renew follicle growth and augment estrogen secretion. Under the influence of estradiol and estrone, endothelial and mucosal repair takes place. In the ensuing fortnight continued estrogen stimulation produces growth of glands and spiral arterioles. These vessels remain unbranched to the periphery where a terminal capillary network is formed. Accompanying this proliferation, endometrial expansion is accomplished by accumulation of ground substance and modest edema of the stroma. This estrogen-induced phenomenon unfolds the collapsed stromal reticulum. In this way follicle estrogen produces an endometrium with sufficient height, vascularity, and concentrations of glycogen and protein to satisfy the early requirements of the anticipated embryo. Furthermore, estrogen-dependent changes in cervical mucus aid sperm migration.

The midcycle preovulatory peak of estrogen probably signals the release of pituitary LH. The brief surge of this gonadotrophin induces acute follicle distention. By unknown mechanisms necrosis of the thinned follicle wall occurs, leading to capsular rupture and permitting extrusion of the ovum. The corpus luteum is formed, and secretion of progesterone rapidly increases. This hormone and sustained levels of estrogen combine to inhibit further LH secretion.

In the absence of a conceptus, at day 12 post ovulation, the corpus luteum recedes and hormone levels wane. With stromal cell shrinkage and loss of ground

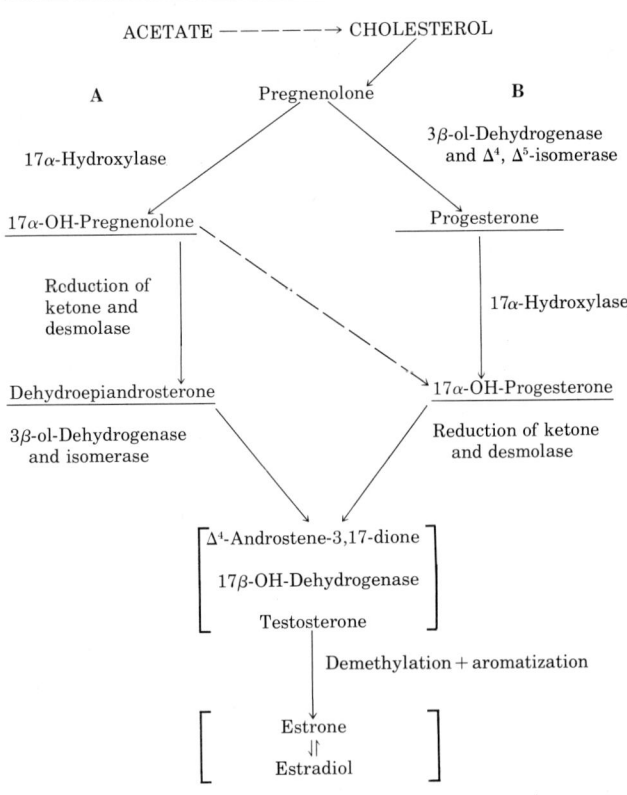

Figure 2. Pathways of ovarian steroid biosynthesis.

substance, the endometrium thins. The vessels buckle, and diminished peripheral blood flow is reduced further by tonic vasoconstriction of spiral arterioles. Localized peripheral ischemia and fragmentation occur, with progressive hemorrhage and disruption of superficial zones of the endometrium. With the loss of the peripheral binding epithelium, menstruation begins.

The ranges of peptide and steroid hormone concentrations and their interrelationships during an ovulatory cycle are shown in Figure 1.

OVARIAN STEROID BIOSYNTHESIS

It is clear that appropriate target organ processes are dependent on periodic variations in the quantity and type of hormone emanating from the ovary. How does the ovary accomplish the initial production of microgram quantities of estrogen and then milligram secretion of progesterone? The in vitro analyses of Ryan, using isolated follicles and corpora lutea and radioactive steroid precursors, contributed significantly to the understanding of these processes. This work confirmed the accumulated evidence bearing on the dominance of two biosynthetic pathways leading to estrogen production in the ovary. These routes (A and B) are depicted in Figure 2. Route A provides for conversion of pregnenolone to estrogen via a pathway in which the 3β-ol,Δ^5 characteristic is maintained to the C_{19} stage. On the other hand, route B projects immediate conversion of pregnenolone to progesterone (change from Δ^5-3β-ol to Δ^4-3 ketone in ring A) prior to loss of sidechain and estrogen generation. Ryan's data suggest that, whereas the corpus luteum utilizes the pathway via proges-

Figure 1. Steroid and peptide hormone concentrations during an ovulatory menstrual cycle. (From Speroff, L., Glass, R. H., and Kase, N. G.: Clinical Gynecologic Endocrinology and Infertility. Baltimore, Williams and Wilkins Company, 1973.)

terone (*B*), the follicle employs route *A*, bypassing formation of this biologically active intermediate. Individual cell studies have shown that granulosa and theca cells have similar biosynthetic capabilities and that only quantitative differences exist between these tissues. Apparently both granulosa and theca cells are necessary for adequate steroid production in biologic studies.

There are broader endocrine implications in the biosynthetic mechanisms depicted in the figure. With certain notable exceptions, such as the 11-hydroxylation property of the adrenal cortex, it is apparent that all steroid-producing organs make steroids in roughly the same manner. The biosynthetic pathways require the presence of biologically active steroids other than those typically secreted by a gland, but these are normally not apparent clinically. However, disordered activity of these pathways in certain ovarian disease leads to abnormal levels of secretion of these active intermediates with clinically demonstrable hormone effects.

Hisaw, F. L.: Development of the graafian follicle and ovulation. Physiol. Rev., 27:95, 1947.

Rock, J., Garcia, C.-R., and Menkin, M.: A theory of menstruation. Ann. N. Y. Acad. Sci., 75:831, 1959.

Ross, G. T., et al.: Pituitary and gonadal hormones in women during spontaneous and induced ovulatory cycles. Rec. Prog. Horm. Res., 26:1, 1970.

Ryan, K., and Smith, O. V.: Biogenesis of steroid hormones in the human ovary. Rec. Prog. Horm. Res., 21:367, 1965.

Schally, A. V., et al.: Gonadotropin-releasing hormone: One polypeptide regulates secretion of luteinizing and follicle stimulating hormones. Science, 173:1036, 1971.

Schally, A. V., et al.: The hypothalamus and reproduction (current developments). Am. J. Obstet. Gynecol., 114:423, 1972.

Vande Wiele, R. L., et al.: Mechanisms regulating the menstrual cycle in women. Rec. Prog. Horm. Res., 26:63, 1970.

867. OVARIAN DISORDERS PERTINENT TO GENERAL MEDICINE

EVALUATION OF OVARIAN FUNCTION

The simple existence of ovarian function may be inferred from the development and maintenance of the breasts and the internal and external genitalia. However, a range of ovarian secretion essential to the full activity of these organs is more critically expressed by the periodic phenomenon of ovulatory menstruation. With the corpus luteum's inherent life span of two weeks, an implicit termination point for each cycle is provided in the menstruation resulting from estrogen and progesterone withdrawal and the recycling surge of FSH.

It is helpful to group disorders of ovarian function within the following descriptive categories:

Sexual precocity: the onset of menses before the age of ten years or development of breasts or pubic (not vulvar) hair growth before the age of eight years. Although these elements may appear as isolated manifestations, this general term usually applies to premature appearance of all three aspects of sexual maturation.

Primary amenorrhea: the delay of menarche beyond the age of 18. Statistically 5 per cent of girls initiate menses after 16 and 1 per cent after age 18. In the presence of breast development, pubic hair growth, and a normal adolescent growth spurt, diagnostic evaluation of delayed menarche may be postponed until 18.

Secondary amenorrhea: the cessation of uterine bleeding at any age in women who have previously menstruated. The elapsed interval of amenorrhea necessary for the diagnosis cannot be rigidly defined, and is often dictated by other clinical factors. However, if the patient has not bled within a length of time equivalent to three or four of her normal cycles, then investigation is warranted.

Oligomenorrhea: a recurrent prolongation of intermenstrual intervals leading to a decreased frequency of menses (three to six per year). This irregularity is commonly seen in postmenarchal and premenopausal women. In the absence of other signs and symptoms, intensive work-up is not required at these times. Evaluation is in order in other age groups because anovulatory infertility is frequently associated with this menstrual anomaly.

Hypomenorrhea: a diminution in the quantity of menstrual flow based on tampon or napkin requirement. It is of little diagnostic significance if found as a solitary problem. Investigation beyond a physical examination, which includes a pelvic examination and cytologic smear, is unnecessary.

Hypermenorrhea: a definite relative increase in duration or quantity (or both) of menstrual flow that occurs at normal cycle intervals. A subgrouping called *polymenorrhea* designates menstrual flow close to normal in quantity and duration but which recurs too frequently (less than 21 days apart). Each group requires immediate gynecologic assessment. Because each is frequently associated with anovulation, endocrine evaluation may also be in order.

AIDS TO DIAGNOSIS

The clinical categories just described represent a spectrum of abnormal ovarian function which appears clinically as changes in sexual development, menstrual regularity, and ovulation. Such malfunction may be caused by primary ovarian disease, abnormal stimulation of the ovary by other glands, disease of target organs, or systemic disease. Steps to appropriate diagnosis begin with a complete history and physical examination, including careful examination of the pelvic organs and external genitalia. When properly selected, certain procedures and laboratory tests can be of great diagnostic assistance.

Pituitary Gonadotrophin Function. Pituitary gonadotrophins may be measured by bioassay or by radioimmunoassay. The bioassay requires a 24-hour urine collection from which gonadotrophins are extracted by a process including acidification, kaolin absorption and elution, followed by acetone precipitation. The extract is diluted and injected into immature female mice, and the increase in the weight of the mouse uterus is measured. The assay depends on the FSH and LH in the extract to stimulate the immature mouse ovaries to produce estrogen. The greatest dilution of the urine extract which causes a 100 per cent increase in uterine weight is the titer of gonadotrophins, and the result is expressed in mouse uterine weight units (muu) per 24 hours. Less than 6 muu per 24 hours indicates normal prepubertal levels or adult hypogonadotrophism. A castrate or postmenopausal level is greater than 200 muu per 24 hours.

This assay is notoriously unreliable and has been al-

TABLE 1.   Values for Gonadotrophins in Serum

Clinical State	Serum FSH	Serum LH
Normal adult female	5–30 mIU/ml, with ovulatory midcycle peak two times baseline	5–20 mIU/ml, with ovulatory midcycle peak three times baseline
Hypogonadotrophism (prepubertal, hypothalamic and pituitary dysfunction)	Less than 5 mIU/ml	Less than 5 mIU/ml
Hypergonadotrophism (postmenopause, castrate, ovarian failure)	Greater than 40 mIU/ml	Greater than 25 mIU/ml

most entirely replaced by specific radioimmunoassays for FSH and LH in serum. It must be remembered (Fig. 1) that wide swings in gonadotrophin levels are typical of ovulatory cycles. Table 1 depicts the ranges of gonadotrophins in various clinical circumstances.

Ovarian Function.   Tests that are based on biologic effects of ovarian hormones are simply performed, providing immediate and valuable data at little cost to the patient. Therefore more costly laboratory evaluations of hormone excretion or blood concentrations are rarely required for clinical purposes.

Gonadal Hormone Effects.   CORNIFICATION OF VAGINAL EPITHELIUM.   The percentage of fully cornified cells is related to ovarian estrogen production. Because cytologic criteria and staining methods vary from center to center, no normal values can be given. However, because other factors affect this evaluation (progesterone, cortisone, and androgen diminish, although digitalis increases cornification), the stage of the cycle as well as current therapy must be considered in evaluation of test results.

Endometrial biopsy tests endometrial responsiveness as well as the existence of appropriate ovarian hormone secretion during the cycle. Evaluation must take into consideration the stage of the cycle when the biopsy specimen is taken.

In addition to the quantity and clarity of *cervical mucus,* the development of an arborization pattern in a dried specimen *(the "fern" test)* indicates the presence of estrogen. Correlation with cycle dates is essential, for secretion of progesterone inhibits this phenomenon.

The *basal body temperature* will demonstrate the occurrence of ovulation if serial readings are taken throughout a cycle. Based on the mild thermogenic properties of progesterone, a sustained postovulatory rise of temperature (0.3° C or more) of two weeks' duration indicates corpus luteum function. Retrospectively, the timing of ovulation in the cycle can be estimated from the date when the effect of progesterone first appeared.

PROGESTERONE WITHDRAWAL BLEEDING.   If menses can be induced after administration of progesterone or a nonestrogenic derivative, this event indicates prior ovarian estrogen secretion and its proliferative or "priming" effect on the endometrium.

Gonadal Hormone Plasma Concentrations.   The normal levels for total plasma estrogens or estradiol and plasma progesterone vary with the time in the menstrual cycle when the blood sample is drawn. (For the pattern of these variations, see Fig. 3.) The normal ranges of plasma gonadal steroids as measured by radioimmunoassay are depicted in Table 2.

Gonadal Hormone Excretion.   TOTAL URINARY ESTROGENS PER 24 HOURS.   The measurement of estrogen in a 24-hour urine sample is useful in guiding replacement FSH-LH therapy for the induction of ovulation. The range of estrogen excretion during various clinical states is shown in Table 3.

URINARY PREGNANEDIOL EXCRETION.   Pregnanediol is the main urinary metabolite of progesterone but accounts for only 7 to 20 per cent of total progesterone production. Measurement of this metabolite in urine has been used to document ovulation and the presence and well-being of early pregnancy. The range of excretion of pregnanediol is seen in Table 4.

URINARY PREGNANETRIOL EXCRETION.   Although not exclusively a metabolite of gonadal hormone production, the concentration of this metabolite of 17α-OH-progesterone in a 24-hour urine specimen is useful in the diagnosis of adrenocortical hyperplasia. In normal circumstances urinary pregnanetriol excretions in children and adults are within the ranges shown in Table 5.

Other Tests.   Other tests of importance include those that estimate *adrenal cortex and thyroid activity.* Specific details concerning interpretation of results and the diagnostic manipulations involved are given in other sections of this text. Dysfunction of either organ may have pronounced effects on ovarian and target organ physiology.

HUMAN CHORIONIC GONADOTROPHIN.   Secretion of human chorionic gonadotrophin (HCG) by the syncytiotrophoblast cells of the placenta is directed predominantly into the maternal circulation. The assay of HCG in maternal urine has been the basis of many pregnancy tests since the original Aschheim-Zondek test.

These bioassays depend upon the response of ovaries or testes in immature animals to the gonadotrophic properties of HCG when present in urine. The endpoints were increased gonadal weight, hyperemia, or response in sex organs to increased gonadal steroidogenesis induced by HCG. The expulsion of ova or sperm in amphibia was also a widely used clinical assay. These biologic tests have been entirely replaced

TABLE 2.   Values for Plasma Estrogens and Progesterone

Cycle Phase	Total Estrogen or Estradiol	Progesterone
Follicle phase	25– 75 pg/ml	Less than 1 ng/ml
Midcycle peak	200–600 pg/ml	
Luteal phase	100–300 pg/ml	5– 20 ng/ml
Pregnancy, first trimester	1– 5 ng/ml	20– 30 ng/ml
Pregnancy, second trimester	5– 15 ng/ml	50–100 ng/ml
Pregnancy, third trimester	10– 40 ng/ml	100–400 ng/ml

TABLE 3. Values for Urinary Estrogen

Clinical Circumstance	Total Urinary Estrogen/24 Hours
Prepubertal	0– 5 μg/24 hr
Follicle phase	10– 25 μg/24 hr
Midcycle peak	35–100 μg/24 hr
Luteal phase	25– 75 μg/24 hr
Postmenopausal	5– 15 μg/24 hr

TABLE 5. Values for Urinary Pregnanetriol

	Urinary Pregnanetriol/24 Hours
Children	Less than 0.5 mg
Adults	0.2 to 2–4 mg (upper limits vary with laboratory)

by the clinical application of immunoassays for HCG in urine—the urinary chorionic gonadotrophin (UCG) test.

Three types of immunologic assays are used: hemagglutination-inhibition, complement-fixation, and radioimmunoassay. In the hemagglutination-inhibition reaction, the presence of HCG in maternal urine inhibits an agglutination reaction between HCG-coated red cells and the antisera. In some commercial methods latex particles are used in place of red cells. A rapid although less sensitive slide test using latex particles is available, but the two-hour red cell test is more reliable. A first morning voided urine specimen is preferred.

HCG and LH are similar in structure, and considerable immunologic cross-reaction exists. The sensitivity of most commercial HCG assays is limited to 1000 IU per liter of urine to avoid false positive cross-reactions with LH. Because of the limitations in sensitivity, a positive test does not appear until ten days to two weeks after the missed menstrual period. From that point the levels of HCG rise to an average peak of 100,000 IU per liter at 10 weeks' gestation, and then declines over the next four weeks to 20,000 IU per liter, at which point excretion levels are sustained for the remainder of the pregnancy.

Patients with *hydatidiform moles* generally display urinary HCG levels around 300,000 IU per liter. *Choriocarcinoma* may be associated with levels in the millions of IU. Although absolute levels are helpful, they are not absolutely diagnostic of disease. Multiple gestations may also show high levels of UCG excretion.

A semiquantitative estimation of HCG in a 24-hour urine may be useful in evaluating threatened abortion or ectopic gestation. A low or declining level of UCG indicates a poor prognosis for an intrauterine pregnancy, whereas a low level of HCG (below 5000 IU per liter of urine) is commonly seen when the pregnancy test is positive in ectopic pregnancy.

Three weeks after a spontaneous or therapeutic abortion, the urinary pregnancy test should reverse to negative. Before that time positive tests may still be encountered.

Clinical assays. *In* Speroff, L., Glass, R. H., and Kase, N. G.: Clinical Gynecologic Endocrinology and Infertility. Baltimore, Williams & Wilkins Company, 1973, pp. 226–250.

TABLE 4. Values for Urinary Pregnanediol

	Urinary Pregnanediol/24 Hours
Follicle phase	Less than 1 mg
Luteal phase	2–5 mg
Pregnancy, 20 weeks	40 mg
Pregnancy, 30 weeks	80 mg
Pregnancy, 40 weeks	100 mg

PUBERTY

The initiation of menstrual function in humans occurs with greatest frequency at age 12 or 13, but there is a considerable "normal" variation in the time of its onset. When menstruation begins before the age of 10 or after 16, a decision must be made whether the precocious or delayed menarche is a physiologic variant or whether it is due to some abnormality. Furthermore, since menarche is but one of several important changes associated with puberty and a variation in its timing is by no means the only feature of disease, it is useful to review the characteristic sequence of female puberty.

The *first sign of puberty* is generally the appearance of the *breast bud*. Pubic hair quickly follows breast development, but appearance of axillary hair is normally delayed as much as two years. At about the time of breast development the adolescent growth in linear height begins, and over the next year of peak growth a girl will grow 6 to 11 cm. In the typical pubescence, within two years of initiating this growth spurt, the first menstruation, i.e., the menarche, occurs.

Because the growth of pubic and axillary hair is almost certainly due to an increased production of adrenal androgens at puberty, this event is often referred to as *adrenarche* as well as pubarche. Premature thelarche (premature breast development) as an isolated biologic event is less common. The etiology of these events is not understood at present; gonadotrophin and estrogen levels are not elevated.

Although pubescence has been described in terms of the two-year sequence—increased linear growth rate, breast development, pubarche, and menarche—varying patterns occur frequently and are not necessarily indicative of dysfunction or disease.

Certain aspects of the neuroendocrine mechanism involved in normal puberty have been uncovered. It has been shown that the anterior pituitary of infants contains adequate quantities of gonadotrophins and that an intact pituitary is essential for the prepubertal development and maintenance of the gonads. Removal of the ovaries in this age group is associated with increased gonadotrophin excretion, the formation of castration cells in the pituitary, and enlargement of the gland. These changes can be prevented by estrogen therapy in very low doses. Therefore the small quantity of estrogen secreted prepubertally is sufficient to inhibit all but a small clinically undetectable quantity of gonadotrophin release. Further indirect evidence that this central inhibition is the critical mechanism in the *normal* delay of sexual maturation can be seen in the fully responsive competence of the premenarchal ovary to exogenous gonadotrophin therapy. Certain areas in the hypothalamus are believed to be responsible for this temporary extreme sensitivity to inhibiting levels of circulating steroids. It has been suggested that neoplastic and vascular disorders that alter hypothalamic function probably reverse this low threshold inhibition and lead to precocious puberty.

SEXUAL PRECOCITY

Precocity may be due to organic or constitutional (idiopathic) causes. Ninety per cent of patients with this symptom will fall in the latter category despite thorough evaluation. However, it is essential that these cases be distinguished from those with lesions of the brain or the rare diseases of ovary and adrenal that produce premature development.

Constitutional Sexual Precocity. This is due to the premature release of the adult sequence and levels of gonadotrophin, which are sufficient to initiate prematurely the normal physiologic and endocrine processes of breast development, appearance of pubic and axillary hair, and menstruation. Although it is assumed that hypothalamic inhibitory influences have been diminished, the precise inciting factor is unknown. Diminished secretion of inhibitory quantities of melatonin by the pineal gland is suggested as one possible etiologic factor. Generally the normal, orderly, albeit more rapid appearance of breast development, pubic hair growth, and then menarche is found in the five- to eight-year age group. However, menarche may be the first symptom noted and may occur as early as three months of age. The usual sequential maturation pattern may be altered or only partially displayed. Although not all patients will ovulate, biologic manifestations of ovulation rule out precocity based on gonadotrophin-independent estrogen production by ovarian or adrenal disease. Estrogen production from any source is likely to induce accelerated linear growth and advancement of bone age, which is seen best in roentgenograms of carpal bones, knee, and elbow. Although these children are temporarily taller than their normal counterparts, premature closure of epiphyses produces a final height that is less than normal. Thus the diagnostic criteria for a constitutional etiology of precocity include the sequence of secondary sex characteristics, advanced bone age, adult levels of estrogen and gonadotrophin, normal urinary adrenal metabolites, and normal neurologic examination and skull films. Optimal therapy (reversible suppression of gonadotrophins without peripheral target organ stimulation) may be achievable with long-acting nonestrogenic depomedroxyprogesterone acetate. This potent progestational agent, when administered in large doses (400 mg) intramuscularly monthly for three months and then once every three months, provides long-term inhibition of gonadotrophin secretion. Pubic hair does not disappear, but further menstruation, breast development, and growth may be inhibited. The response to progestins is not uniformly positive; it is not possible to determine which child will respond favorably in advance of therapy.

These children present a serious emotional and social problem not only because they are distinctly different from their contemporaries, but also because they are insufficiently mature emotionally to cope with the sexual interest they provoke in others. That they are capable of reproduction has been demonstrated many times, but most dramatically in the case of a Peruvian girl, Lena Medina, who was delivered of a normal child by cesarean section at five and a half years of age.

Precocity Due to Organic Causes. *Cerebral Lesions.* A variety of brain disorders produce sexual precocity secondary to premature gonadotrophin release, presumably by the abolition of the inhibitory effects of the hypothalamus. Although the anatomic location of these

inhibitory centers is uncertain, three general groups of tumors may cause precocity: lesions in the tuber cinereum, lesions in the posterior hypothalamic mammillary body area, and lesions destroying the pineal. In addition, disorders indirectly affecting hypothalamic function (internal hydrocephalus, encephalitis, meningitis, and cranial trauma) may be associated with precocity. Differential diagnosis of this type of precocity from the constitutional variety cannot be achieved by endocrine survey. Only after intensive neurologic, roentgenographic, and pediatric evaluation and follow-up reappraisal will proper diagnosis be made.

Organic Precocious Pseudopuberty Due to Adrenal and Ovarian Hyperfunction. The term pseudopuberty defines the basic difference between precocity resulting from premature gonadotrophic activity (constitutional, central types) and those lesions in which adrenal and ovarian estrogen stimulates target organs. In the latter, gonadotrophin is absent, and therefore ovulation does not occur.

Although certain elements of premature maturation (pubic hair, bone age advancement) appear in adrenal disorders, the masculinization and rarity of vaginal bleeding (delayed menarche is usual) make the diagnosis relatively simple. Isosexual pseudopuberty is more commonly associated with estrogen-producing ovarian tumors. Although the diagnosis of tumor is always considered, it is rarely confirmed. Only 5 per cent of *granulosa tumors* occur before true puberty. The presence of a palpable adnexal mass and the absence of urinary gonadotrophin, ovulation, and regular cyclic bleeding support the diagnosis. In addition, the exceedingly rare *choriocarcinoma, teratoma, or dysgerminoma* of the ovary may be associated with pseudopuberty. However, these will sometimes pose a diagnostic complication. The production of chorionic gonadotrophin by these tumors will give falsely elevated adult levels of "FSH" in mouse uterine weight tests and elevated serum LH values in routine radioimmunoassay, in addition to positive pregnancy tests. The finding of an ovarian mass calls for laparotomy.

Albright's syndrome, consisting of cystic bone lesions, patchy skin pigmentation, and sexual precocity, is grouped with pseudopuberty in that gonadotrophin excretion and ovulation are absent. Normal puberty and ovulation follow and fertility is not decreased.

Greulich, W. W., and Pyle, S. L.: Radiographic Atlas of Skeletal Development of The Hand and Wrist. Stanford, Calif., Stanford University Press, 1950.

Pedowitz, P., Felmus, L. B., and Mackles, A.: Precocious pseudopuberty due to ovarian tumors. Obstet. Gynecol. Survey, 10:633, 1955.

Van Der Werff Ten Bosch, J. J.: Isosexual precocity. *In* Gardner, L. I. (ed.): Endocrine and Genetic Diseases of Childhood. Philadelphia, W. B. Saunders Company, 1969.

DISORDERS OF MENSTRUAL FUNCTION

Delayed Menarche and Primary Amenorrhea

Menarche may be delayed beyond the age of 16 years on a constitutional basis and often as a familial trait. In these instances there is no demonstrable organic lesion, and with time normal periods appear. However, some cases of delayed menarche are not benign, and these bring up the vexing problem of which patients in this age group require intensive work-up. In general, delayed menarche accompanied by any of the following signs requires full evaluation to prevent worsening of the underlying condition, which is only initially presenting as delayed menstruation: absence of other secondary sexual characteristics, symptoms and signs of outflow tract incompetence, systemic disorders (neurogenic, obesity, cachexia, thyroid and adrenocortical disease), psychiatric disorders, or signs of abnormal chromosomal constitution.

Lacking these associated conditions, delayed menarche may be managed by sympathetic reassurance of the likelihood of eventual establishment of normal menses.

If menarche is delayed beyond the age of 18, *primary amenorrhea* is said to exist. The diagnostic investigation of this entity is best oriented to assessment of the various anatomic sites involved in the generation and transport of menstrual fluid. These include the vaginal tract, uterus, ovaries, pituitary, and hypothalamus.

Mechanical Obstruction. Mechanical obstruction at the hymen or in the vaginal or cervical canal will prevent drainage of uterine secretions. Such stenosis is usually congenital but may be secondary to infection. Outward signs of menses are absent, but periodic vaginal or lower abdominal pain and the presence of a mass on rectal or vaginal examination are observed. Depending on the site and duration of obstruction, hematocolpos, hematometra and/or hematosalpinx are present.

Absence or Unresponsiveness of the Endometrium. This presents as primary amenorrhea. Agenesis of the uterus is rare, as are the "acquired" lesions such as tuberculosis, uterine schistosomiasis, and postsepsis obliteration of the endometrium and uterine cavity, which render this organ incapable of reacting to normal cyclic levels of estrogen.

Primary Hypogonadism. Amenorrhea is the basic symptom of primary hypogonadism. The most common cause of primary ovarian failure is *Turner's syndrome (gonadal dysgenesis)*.

The chromosomal anomaly in gonadal dysgenesis is the presence of only one X chromosome in all cell lines (X chromosome monosomy). The individual is referred to as 45,X or frequently as XO. Despite absence of gonadal development, these patients are phenotypic, albeit immature, females. The clinical facets of the syndrome are well known; these include short stature (48 to 58 inches), sexual infantilism, streak gonads, increased carrying angle, shield chest, pterygium colli, a tendency to form keloids, intestinal telangiectasias, prominent epicanthal folds, micrognathia, dental malocclusion, anomalies of the ocular muscles, and multiple skin nevi. Mental retardation is seen in many patients. In addition to renal anomalies, coarctation of the aorta and short fourth metacarpals are seen. The streak gonad is composed of fibrous tissue containing no follicles or ova and devoid of medullary components.

Although the diagnosis is usually not made until puberty when amenorrhea with castration levels of urinary gonadotrophin, lack of sexual development, and short stature become evident retrospectively, the history will show that the patient weighed less at birth than expected by gestational age and that she tended to be below average weight and body length throughout childhood. At birth, some of the stigmata of the Bonnevie-Ullrich syndrome, i.e., lymphedema of the dorsum of the hands and feet, cutis laxa, and low hairline on the neck, may indicate the presence of this condition.

The incidence of 45,X is 0.04 per cent of newborn females.

A large variety of mosaic patterns is seen with gonadal dysgenesis. From analysis of various combinations, it appears that short stature is related to loss of the short arm of one X chromosome. Thus X, XXp, and XXqi are all short individuals. Xqi designates an isochromosome for the long arms, and Xp deletion of the short arm. The loss of the long arm of one of the X chromosomes is associated with amenorrhea and streak gonads, but these patients are not short and do not have other malformations. Thus loss of material from the short arms of the X chromosomes leads to short stature and other stigmata of Turner's syndrome. Streak gonads result if either the long or the short arm is missing. This would suggest that normal ovarian development requires two loci, one on the long arm and one on the short arm; loss of either results in gonadal failure.

Menstrual function and reproduction in a patient with Turner's phenotype must be due to a mosaic complement such as a 46,XX line in addition to 45,X. Multiple X females (47,XXX) have normal development and reproductive function, although mental retardation may be more frequent. Secondary amenorrhea or eunuchoidism, or both, may be seen, depending on the initial amount and rapidity of loss of follicular apparatus.

In gonadal dysgenesis, the gonadal structures are streak gonads. In *mixed gonadal dysgenesis*, testicular tissue may be present. Mosaicism is the likely underlying abnormality, even if it is not detected in the cell line studied. Ambiguous genitalia are produced if testicular tissue is present. In this instance, gonadectomy is necessary both to avoid further heterosexual development if sex assignment is female and to avoid neoplastic change in the testicular tissue even if sex assignment is male.

In Noonan's syndrome affected males and females have apparently normal chromosome complements and normal gonadal function. The phenotypic appearance of the female is that of a patient with Turner's syndrome: short stature, webbed neck, shield chest, and cardiac malformations. The cardiac lesion in the male phenotype is different from that in the female. Pulmonic stenosis is most frequent in Noonan's syndrome, as opposed to aortic coarctation in Turner's syndrome. Apparently, this syndrome results from a mutant gene or genes. These patients have been referred to as male Turner's syndrome or Turner's syndrome with normal chromosomes.

A disorder of ovarian function evidenced morphologically by polycystic changes, although more commonly associated with secondary amenorrhea (see below), may also produce primary amenorrhea.

Adrenal and Thyroid Disease and Diabetes Mellitus. These may be accompanied by primary amenorrhea or, more commonly, secondary amenorrhea, despite the presence of normal ovaries.

Inadequate Gonadotrophins. Although ovaries and external genitalia may be otherwise normal, menses will not appear if gonadotrophin stimulation of these organs is insufficient or absent. Causes of this hypogonadotrophic hypogonadism are best considered according to their anatomic distribution. Intrasellar lesions such as pituitary cysts, tumors, and infarction may interfere not only with gonadotrophin secretion but also with the entire range of pituitary responsibilities. On the other hand, depending on a tumor's initial size and growth tendencies, amenorrhea may be the first sign of a disorder that by further encroachment gradually progresses to panhypopituitarism. Except for growth hormone, gonadotrophin secretion appears to be the most sensitive to adverse changes in intrasellar pressures and blood flow.

Suprasellar disorders also produce primary or secondary amenorrhea by diminishing gonadotrophin release. Aneurysm of the internal carotid artery, tumor, and internal hydrocephalus with expansion of the third ventricle are among the lesions reported. Hypogonadism, diminished adrenal and thyroid function, and short stature are seen in these conditions.

Amenorrhea due to isolated hypogonadotrophism without eventual impairment of other trophic hormones is common. The frequent association of this physiologic aberration (which reverses spontaneously in a high proportion of cases) with severe systemic illness, obesity, and emotional trauma should be noted.

A rare female condition presenting itself as hypogonadotrophic hypogonadism, primary amenorrhea, and anosmia is *Kallmann's syndrome*. In addition to amenorrhea, these patients display infantile sex development, low serum LH values, and a normal female karyotype. Although the patient may be unaware of her inability to perceive odors (perfumes, coffee grounds), inability to perceive certain food tastes may be the first clue that leads to further testing.

"Testicular Feminization Syndrome." This syndrome consists of chromatin-negativity, primary amenorrhea, mature feminine appearance, and abdominal, inguinal, or labial testes. The name is unfortunate, for many studies have shown that the basic defect is not in testicular steroid production or metabolic clearance, but is an interference in the mechanism of action of androgen at the target tissue level. Inability to form the biologically active dihydrotestosterone at the target was a suggested explanation for androgen insensitivity in these subjects, but this theory has not been confirmed. Impaired function or insufficient concentration of androgen protein receptors in target cells is the current preferred explanation for defective androgen activity. As a result of the metabolic abnormality (whatever it may be), axillary and pubic hair are scant, the clitoris is small, and although only rudimentary oviducts are present and the uterus is absent, there is no wolffian duct stimulation. Exogenous androgen does not masculinize these patients. Differentiation of the complete syndrome from an incomplete type displaying clitoral enlargement, inactive gonads, and variably androgen-sensitive target tissue can be accomplished. Patients with a deficit in testicular 17-dehydrogenase activity have impaired testosterone production and appear clinically as the incomplete syndrome. Therapy in either form of the syndrome is castration and sufficient exogenous estrogen to maintain serviceable external genitalia in support of the female sex role with which these patients permanently identify.

Because the diagnostic evaluation and therapy of the lesions involved in primary and secondary amenorrhea are similar, these matters will be discussed in later paragraphs.

Albright, F.: Polyostotic fibrous dysplasia. J. Clin. Endocrinol. Metab., 7:307, 1947.

Asherman, J. G.: Traumatic intrauterine adhesions and their effects on fertility. Int. J. Fertil., 11:49, 1957.

Bardin, C. W., Bullock, L. P., Shearins, R. J., Mowszowicz, I., and Black-
burn, W. R.: Androgen metabolism and mechanism of action of male pseudohermaphroditism: A study of testicular feminization. Rec. Prog. Horm. Res., Vol. 29, 1973.

Frank, R. T.: Formation of artificial vagina without operation. Am. J. Obstet. Gynecol., 35:1053, 1938.

Goebelsmann, U., Horton, R., Mestman, J. H., Arce, J. J., Nagata, Y., Nakamura, R. M., Thorneycroft, I. H., and Mishell, D. R., Jr.: Male pseudohermaphroditism due to testicular 17β-hydroxysteroid dehydrogenase deficiency. J. Clin. Endocrinol. Metab., 36:867, 1973.

Jones, H. W., Jr., and Scott, W. W.: Hermaphroditism, Genital Anomalies and Related Endocrine Disorders. Baltimore, Williams & Wilkins Company, 1971.

List, C. F., Dowman, C. E., Bagchi, B. K., and Bebin, J.: Posterior hypothalamic hamartomas and gangliogliomas causing precocious puberty. Neurology, 8:164, 1958.

Neu, R. L., and Gardner, L. I.: Clinical aspects of abnormalities of the X and Y chromosomes. Clin. Obstet. Gynecol., 15:141, 1972.

Summit, R. L.: Turner's syndrome and Noonan's syndrome. J. Pediatr., 74:155, 1969.

Van Der Werff Ten Bosch, J. J.: Isosexual precocity. In Gardner, L. I. (ed.): Endocrine and Genetic Diseases of Childhood. Philadelphia, W. B. Saunders Company, 1969.

Secondary Amenorrhea

A change in the frequency of menstruation is a sensitive indicator of ovarian dysfunction. Therefore the most serious form of menstrual aberration is the appearance of secondary amenorrhea. Its onset may be marked by the abrupt cessation of previously normal cycles, or it may follow menses of diminishing frequency (oligomenorrhea). It is well to remember that certain physiologic states predispose to amenorrhea. Absence of periodic menstruation in any adult female should suggest the possibility of pregnancy. Furthermore, amenorrhea of varying length will frequently be associated with the puerperium and the immediate postmenarchal and premenopausal periods. Finally, the menopause is an irreversible state of ovarian inactivity and amenorrhea.

Not all instances of secondary amenorrhea have a hormonal basis. As noted in the discussion of primary amenorrheas, acquired anatomic disorders must be considered in the differential diagnosis of absent menstruation. Stenotic lesions obstructing the egress of uterine discharge may result from scarring induced by infection, chemical burns, and operative trauma. Similarly, endocervical carcinoma may diminish the caliber of the cervical canal. As always, pelvic examination is essential to proper evaluation of absent menses. Destruction of the endometrium also produces amenorrhea despite the presence of normal cyclical ovarian hormone secretion. This condition may result from tuberculous endometritis or may be secondary to overzealous curettage performed to reverse unremitting hemorrhage occurring at abortion, post partum, or at withdrawal from prolonged anovulatory cycles. In the latter instances of iatrogenic endometrial failure, investigation of the uterine cavity by means of hysterography may reveal cavitary distortions and obliteration due to uterine synechia *(Asherman's syndrome)*. Operative disruption of uterine defects and intensive estrogen therapy may reverse this situation. Finally, temporary endometrial inactivity may be inadvertently induced with the use of newer progestational agents, particularly of the long-acting intramuscular type (depomedroxyprogesterone acetate). Protracted release of hormone leads to persistent amenorrhea and typical progestin-induced endometrial morphologic changes. Although most cases spontaneously reverse within a few months, periods may not recur for years.

These local matters aside, the major diagnostic issue

in secondary amenorrhea is evaluation of the integrity of the pituitary-ovarian servomechanism. Unfortunately, pituitary-ovarian relationships do not adhere to an "all or none" principle. If one assumes adequate gonadotrophin stimulation, it appears that not all cycles are ovulatory or of equal length. Some cycles are climaxed by ovulation only after a prolonged preovulatory phase. Other cycles may be anovulatory, although cycle length shows no variation. The basic question in the pathogenesis of this relative hypogonadism is whether anovulation is due to inadequate or improper gonadotrophic stimulation or to an inherent unresponsiveness of certain follicles. As the follicle grows, intraovarian factors potentiate or diminish the response of the follicle to the stimulatory effect of FSH. Estradiol, by a local effect, enhances the follicle growth and differentiation response to FSH. Inhibition of this reactivity is observed with androgens.

Although clinical experiments with exogenous gonadotrophin therapy indicate some ovarian control over follicle maturation, most cases showing anovulatory amenorrhea and "normal" gonadotrophins are probably ascribable to improper synchrony and amount of gonadotrophin stimulation. Abnormal quantity or sequence of gonadotrophin secretion may result from local disturbances of the hypothalamic-hypophysial control mechanisms induced by emotional stress, precipitous weight changes, and systemic disease. On the other hand, these control centers may be misdirected by feedback levels of hormones of unusual type and quantity resulting from thyroid disease, adrenocortical disease, functioning ovarian tumors, and probably ovarian dysfunctions such as the Stein-Leventhal syndrome. Undoubtedly these conditions also affect ovarian reactivity to gonadotrophins, leading to disturbed or arrested follicle maturation seen in systemic disease as well as local pelvic disorders, including chronic pelvic infection, endometriosis, and uterine fibromyomas. Finally, absence of gonadotrophin secretion results from a variety of insidiously destructive intrasellar and suprasellar disorders. As in primary amenorrheas, these lesions may produce isolated gonadotrophic insufficiency, which at first results in decreased ovulation frequency but progresses through anovulation, amenorrhea, and hypoestrogenism to panhypopituitarism.

Pituitary and Suprasellar Lesions. Altered menses may be the earliest sign of an otherwise asymptomatic pituitary tumor. At first, small lesions interfere with cyclic variations in gonadotrophin release, but serum levels of gonadotrophins are unaffected. However, with increasing size and encroachment on production sites, diminished or absent gonadotrophin supervenes. Eventually further enlargement leads to more obvious neurologic, ophthalmic, and roentgenologic signs. At this point other trophic hormone deficiencies occur, leading to the complex endocrine metabolic derangements of panhypopituitarism. Aneurysm of the internal carotid artery, tumor of the third ventricle, glioma of the optic chiasm, obstruction of the aqueduct of Sylvius, and meningioma of the floor of the anterior fossa may simulate pituitary tumor and produce amenorrhea. Similarly, functioning tumors of the pituitary are often associated with specific clinical patterns of acromegaly, inappropriate galactorrhea, or Cushing's disease, as well as amenorrhea. Extensive non-neoplastic pituitary damage may result from necrosis associated with postpartum hemorrhage or obstetric shock. In studies spanning three decades concerning this entity, Sheehan has shown that almost total destruction of the anterior pituitary substance must exist before panhypopituitarism occurs. It is therefore understandable that a prolonged course of progressive deterioration is seen in a variety of lesions of the central nervous system. Gonadotrophic function is the first deficiency to appear clinically, although impaired growth hormone reaction to arginine or insulin-induced hypoglycemia is an earlier but usually occult event. Less often, only gonadotrophin inadequacy exists. Although this may be associated with persistent lactation (see below), other patients have perfectly normal trophic responses save for gonadotrophin inadequacy (psychogenic stress, obesity, and variants of anorexia nervosa). A relatively uncommon finding is the patient with an enlarged sella not caused by tumor expansion but filled with cerebrospinal fluid. In this anatomic variant called the *"empty sella syndrome,"* the pituitary is flattened and compressed by fluid pressure. Endocrine problems are mild, but owing to the special vulnerability of gonadotrophins, anovulation and amenorrhea are likely clinical manifestations.

Ovarian Lesions. Two major causes of ovarian amenorrhea are (1) inability of the ovary to react to appropriate gonadotrophic stimulation and (2) ovarian production of abnormal quantities of steroids, disrupting central nervous system control of cyclic gonadotrophin.

Irreversible ovarian failure is characterized by diminished ovarian steroid hormones and high total urinary gonadotrophins. *Premature menopause* exists when cessation of menses occurs before the age of 40 and is associated with the findings of hypergonadotrophic hypogonadism. The pathogenesis of this impairment of ovarian function is unknown. Somewhat better understood is the ovarian failure associated with the various forms of gonadal dysgenesis. In these instances reactive ovarian substrate is either absent or rapidly depleted, resulting in hypogonadism. It is important to remember that not all these patients have primary amenorrhea, and some (as many as 20 per cent) are chromatin positive.

The *polycystic ovary syndrome (Stein-Leventhal syndrome)* is perhaps the best example of arrested ovarian follicle maturation associated with noncyclic "dampening" of the pituitary-ovarian servomechanism. To be sure, infrequent anovulatory cycles may occur in normally menstruating, fertile women. As has been noted, some women exhibit varying degrees of reversible hypogonadism characterized by limited fertility and irregular cycles. The Stein-Leventhal syndrome therefore is the severest form of a spectrum of ovarian follicular disorders associated with anovulation.

As originally described in 1935, this syndrome consists of menstrual abnormality, either oligomenorrhea or amenorrhea, anovulatory infertility, and the development of hirsutism, which occurs in about half the patients. Though insidiously progressive facial hirsutism and acne may exist, and a male pubic escutcheon may be found, other signs of masculinization are absent. Obesity is no longer considered an important feature of the condition. The ovaries are bilaterally enlarged by the presence of multiple follicular cysts (never more than 1 cm in diameter), which lie just beneath a thickened, smooth, and pale ovarian capsule. Each rotund, expanded ovary is equal in size to or is larger than the uterine fundus, which is often smaller than normal. Microscopically, the ovaries reveal hyperplastic fibrosis of the cortical stroma and unusual thickening and luteinization of the theca cells surrounding the ubiquitous follicle cysts. Evidence of ovulation (corpora lutea) is rarely found. This finding is reflected in the endometrium, which is proliferative or hyperplastic. Patients with concomitant endometrial carcinoma have been reported.

Although the structural changes of the ovary were once thought to be pathognomonic of the syndrome, similar ovarian changes have been found in association with other disorders, such as adrenocortical hyperplasia, to which anovulatory amenorrhea is secondary. Indeed, *any condition leading to chronic anovulation in which some gonadotrophin function is retained is associated with polycystic changes in the ovary.*

Ovulatory cyclicity depends on the repetitive success of a series of exquisitely integrated biologic events linking ovarian and CNS-pituitary function. Three basic mandatory recycling events can be depicted: (1) The negative feedback relationship of estradiol with FSH results in the initial rise of gonadotrophin during menses that propels maturation of the follicle. (2) The positive feedback relationship of estradiol with LH is the ovulatory trigger. The fully mature follicle, by its timely and sizable production of estrogen, signals its readiness to ovulate in this fashion. (3) The resulting corpus luteum at the conclusion of its inherent life span of two weeks in the absence of a pregnancy will signal resumption of the next cycle by the acute withdrawal of its estrogen and progesterone production.

Anovulation, the loss of cyclicity, results if the CNS-pituitary system for gonadotrophin secretion is impaired by failure to perceive or act upon appropriate steroidal signals; if steroid feedback is inappropriate by timing availability, the individual follicle units do not respond appropriately. In these ways, any one of a large number of etiologic possibilities may be responsible for anovulation. By far the most common cause is "hypothalamic" dysfunction induced by disease, drugs, environment, or emotional stress. Inappropriate feedback may result from adrenocortical disease, ovarian tumors, or disorders of metabolic clearance of signal steroids, as may exist in liver disease and obesity. Finally, gonadal unresponsiveness is seen in acute, severe pelvic infection and in endometriosis, as well as in conditions associated with excess of androgen.

Anovulation represents a spectrum of malfunction in the CNS-pituitary-ovarian axis. In contrast to the characteristic fluctuations in the normal cycle, a "steady state" of tonic gonadotrophin and estrogen is seen (Fig. 3). Polycystic ovaries are consistently found in these circumstances.

From Figure 3 it will be seen that in the patient with chronic anovulation the average daily production of estrogen is increased, and the circulating levels of estrogen are relatively constant. This results in slightly depressed levels of FSH and slightly elevated levels of LH. The condition is self-sustaining. As a follicle cyst undergoes atresia, the small, brief FSH increment leads to its replacement by an inadequately stimulated and therefore developmentally arrested follicle cyst. But the atresia does not mean termination of steroidogenic activity of the theca remnants of the follicle. The stromal compartment of the human ovary is derived chiefly from atretic follicles and has been shown to be capable of secreting significant amounts of androstenedione and testosterone when stimulated by LH.

By these mechanisms the classic picture of the polycystic ovary is attained—numerous follicles, none ovulatory, and dense stromal tissue. The loss of recycling signals has resulted in a hormonal steady state featuring tonic estrogenicity, increased androgen production, and anovulation.

Because the morphology of the ovary is predictable and is the end result of many disorders, least likely of which is primary to the ovary, the various endoscopic and radiologic efforts to "prove" the polycystic state are unnecessary. All efforts of the physician should be turned to diagnosis and therapy of a syndrome likely to cause infertility, hirsutism, and dysfunctional uterine

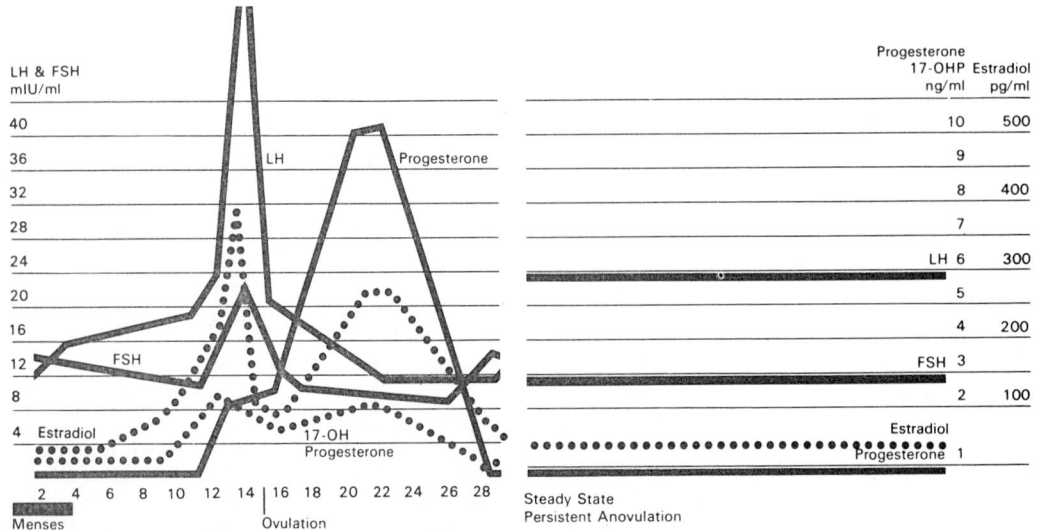

Figure 3. Comparison of steroid and gonadotrophin concentrations and patterns in an ovulatory cycle and the steady state of persistent anovulation. (From Speroff, L., Glass, R. H., and Kase, N. G.: Clinical Gynecologic Endocrinology and Infertility. Baltimore, Williams and Wilkins Company, 1973.)

bleeding. At the moment, the diagnosis of the Stein-Leventhal syndrome (see below) is made by exclusion of adrenocortical and pituitary abnormality.

Adrenal Disease. For more detailed description of these entities the reader is referred to Ch. 844 to 855.

Thyroid Disease. The practice of administering small doses of thyroid hormone preparations to basically euthyroid women with menstrual irregularities unfortunately is still prevalent. Delay of adequate work-up thus incurred compounds the basic physiologic irrationality of this approach. In fact, only patients with advanced thyroid disease display menstrual irregularities. In hyperthyroidism, as toxicity deepens the menses become less frequent, amenorrhea indicating a severe disorder. On the other hand, though oligomenorrhea is sometimes seen in hypothyroidism, menometrorrhagia is the rule, particularly in myxedema. In hypothyroidism secondary to hypopituitarism, of course, amenorrhea is a constant finding.

Systemic Disease. Throughout the discussion of the amenorrheas, it has been emphasized that details of the etiologic mechanisms involved are lacking. This issue is most acute in the consideration of the evolution of ovarian dysfunction secondary to chronic illnesses such as hepatic and renal disease, diabetes, or anemia. In addition to glands of internal secretion, the adequacy of organ systems involved in hormone conjugation, binding, and transport, extraction and excretion, inactivation by metabolism, interconversions of form, and interchange between anatomic pools of differing accessibility critically influence the total effective tissue concentrations of biologically active material.

Asherman, J. G.: Amenorrhea traumatica. J. Obstet. Gynaecol. Br. Emp., 55:23, 1948.

Bardin, C. W., and Lipsett, M. B.: Testosterone and androstenedione blood production rates in normal women and women with idiopathic hirsutism and polycystic ovaries. J. Clin. Invest., 46:891, 1967.

Kirschner, M. A., Bardin, C. W., Hembree, W. C., and Ross, G. T.: Effect of estrogen administration on androgen production and plasma luteinizing hormone in hirsute women. J. Clin. Endocrinol. Metab., 30:727, 1970.

MacDonald, P. C., Grodin, J. M., and Siiteri, P. K.: The utilization of plasma androstenedione for estrone production in women. Proc. Int. Congr. Endocrinol., 184:770, 1969.

Rice, B. V., and Savard, K.: Steroid hormone formation in the human ovary. IV. Ovarian stromal compartment: Formation of radioactive steroids from acetate and action of gonadotropins. J. Clin. Endocrinol. Metab., 25:593, 1966.

Schindler, A. E., Ebert, A., and Friedrich, E.: Conversion of androstenedione to estrone by human fat tissue. J. Clin. Endocrinol. Metab., 35:627, 1972.

Sheehan, H. L., and Stanfield, J. P.: The pathogenesis of postpartum necrosis of the anterior lobe of the pituitary gland. Acta Endocrinol., 37:479, 1961.

Stein, I. F., and Leventhal, M. L.: Amenorrhea associated with bilateral polycystic ovaries. Am. J. Obstet. Gynecol., 29:181, 1935.

Yen, S. S. C., Vela, P., and Rankin, J.: Inappropriate secretion of follicle-stimulating hormone and luteinizing hormone in polycystic ovarian disease. J. Clin. Endocrinol. Metab., 30:435, 1970.

Evaluation of Amenorrhea

Although understanding of the multiple interdependent factors that regulate menstrual function is admittedly incomplete, current concepts of neuroendocrine target organ relationships permit a relatively simple and precise localization of defective components. This program involves sequential testing of the major elements that produce a menstrual cycle: the endometrium, the ovary, and the hypothalamic pituitary unit

Figure 4. Suggested "flow sheet" made for clinical evaluation of amenorrheas.

(Fig. 4). Estimates of modifying systems such as the thyroid and the adrenal cortex are also essential.

The determination of ovarian function can be achieved by a summation of information gathered from basal body temperature curves, appropriately timed cervical changes in mucus, vaginal cornification indexes, endometrial biopsy, and progesterone withdrawal bleeding. Fifty to 100 mg of progesterone intramuscularly for two days or medroxyprogesterone acetate, 5 to 10 mg orally for three days, will induce vaginal bleeding in a previously amenorrheic patient if the endometrium has been primed by ovarian estrogen. In this case the integrity of the entire system short of ovulation is confirmed. However, if flow after progesterone withdrawal does not occur and the possibility of endometrial failure is eliminated by the appearance of vaginal bleeding after 21 days of 1.25 mg conjugated equine estrogens daily orally, then the lack of estrogen production is due to either ovarian or pituitary failure. If serum gonadotrophins are low or absent, pituitary failure is suggested, and neurologic, roentgenologic, ophthalmologic, and laboratory estimates of its competence are indicated. The anticipated availability of a decapeptide with gonadotrophin-releasing attributes, LRF, will be useful in the differentiation of hypothalamic versus pituitary disease as the cause of hypogonadotrophism. A positive reaction to LRF would indicate hypothalamic dysfunction and not intrinsic pituitary disease. Similar use of TRF stimulation of TSH has been found helpful in thyroid disorders (see Ch. 836 to 843). If gonadotrophins are high, reflecting diminished feedback inhibition, ovarian failure is diagnosed. If confirmation of the diagnosis is desired, challenge of the ovary with exogenous human gonadotrophin can be employed.

Using this technique, amenorrheas can be classified according to the specific area of pituitary-ovarian derangement uncovered: (1) hypergonadotrophic hypogonadal amenorrhea (ovarian failure), (2) hypogonadotrophic hypogonadal amenorrhea (pituitary failure), or (3) normogonadotrophic normoestrogenic amenorrhea (anovulation). With definition of these categories, appropriate therapy and management can be evolved.

Treatment of Amenorrhea

The therapy of inadequate ovarian hormone function depends not only on the degree of hormonal failure, but also on the therapeutic objectives. Certainly menstruation is not a necessity, for its absence does not represent a threat to the life expectancy of the patient. Therefore except in the treatment of infertility, and possibly in rare psychologic situations, a patient need not be treated solely for the purpose of recreating menstrual cycles. On the other hand, certain patients who show other evidence of estrogen deficiency, such as loss of secondary sex characteristics, deserve substitutive therapy. At no time should artificial cycles be instituted without preliminary investigation to uncover serious underlying lesions.

Hypergonadotrophic Hypogonadism. The patient with gonadal dysgenesis should be given cyclic exogenous estrogen therapy indefinitely for development and maintenance of adequate secondary sexual characteristics. The transformation induced by cyclic estrogen therapy in these otherwise anatomically, biologically, and cosmetically handicapped patients is particularly gratifying. Among the oral regimens available, 1.25 mg of conjugated equine estrogens daily for 21 days is satisfactory; during the last five days of treatment, the addition of 5 mg daily of medroxyprogesterone acetate orally provides endometrial stability and controlled withdrawal flow.

The woman with premature ovarian failure (before the age of 40 years) presents a somewhat different therapeutic problem. In this situation replacement medication is required to sustain systems already developed and dependent upon ovarian hormone secretion. Patients of this type are concerned not only about secondary amenorrhea and the termination of their reproductive capabilities but also about the usual severe vasomotor symptoms that attend this type of ovarian failure. These *hot flashes* are not seen in primary hypogonadism, although gonadotrophins are elevated in both conditions. Probably as a consequence of these disabilities and the fear of further restrictions, there are various subjective symptoms such as depression, anxiety, and loss of libido. No satisfactory treatment of this condition exists at present except substitution therapy with estrogen. Control of vasomotor instability, preservation of a serviceable vagina, and maintenance of other feminine aspects, including menses, are possible with cyclic conjugated equine estrogens (Premarin, 125 mg every day), or ethinyl estradiol (Estinyl, 0.05 mg every day). Again, the terminal addition of a progestin after 21 days of estrogen is advantageous. It should be noted that these doses of estrogen stimulate menstrual function and are higher than necessary for nonmenstrual metabolic requirements. This point comes into active consideration when determining what, if any, therapy should be given for ovarian failure occurring after the age of 40.

Menopause. The menopause is a physiologic and not a pathologic phenomenon. Menstruation ceases for a variety of reasons at other times of life, but after 40 the ovary becomes atrophic and ceases to respond to gonadotrophic stimulation. No amount of gonadotrophic stimulation can produce activity in the menopausal ovary. It becomes small, pale, and more wrinkled. The few remaining follicles undergo atresia so that none are found within a few years after cessation of menses.

Diminution of all ovarian elements proceeds, resulting in a firm structure one third the size of the active organ.

Vasomotor instability and genital atrophy are the only clinical symptoms definitely associated with ovarian aging that occurs when otherwise the woman may be active, healthy, and vital physically, emotionally, and mentally. However, because of improved general health, women can expect to live for 20 to 25 years beyond the menopause, and interest has increased in the possible amelioration of certain disease states associated with the menopause by administration of exogenous estrogen therapy. Whether actual causal relationships exist between certain disorders and diminished estrogen secretion has not been established. Nevertheless, beneficial effects on extragenital organs and prevention of atherosclerosis and osteoporosis have been claimed.

A statistical rise in coronary atherosclerosis in postmenopausal women has been ascribed to estrogen deficiency. Castration performed before natural menopause also has been associated with increased coronary and peripheral vascular disease. The ability of estrogen to reverse abnormal serum lipids in laboratory animals as well as in human subjects is a possible mechanism by which treated castrates may have a lower incidence of abnormal electrocardiograms and hypertension than untreated women.

However, *excessive therapy* has been observed to pose increased risks. Studies of the preventive effects of estrogens for heart attacks have yielded variable results. Administration of 10 mg of conjugated estrogens per day appeared to be associated with beneficial survival statistics but revealed a disturbing incidence of early vascular accidents. In the Coronary Drug Project, 5 mg conjugated estrogen therapy was associated with an excess of nonfatal myocardial infarctions over controls. In the Stroke Study, estrogens were associated with increased recurrent cerebral accidents and myocardial infarctions rather than protection against these two insults.

Postmenopausal osteoporosis is also believed to be related to estrogen deficiency. Estrogen induces positive calcium balance and reduces bone resorption, but bone formation also drops within three to nine months after initiation of therapy. Although there is no net increase in bone mass in the osteoporotic woman, estrogen would seem to stabilize bone turnover at a new and slower rate. However, there is no *prospective* evidence that estrogen can prevent osteoporosis. Appropriate diet and exercise are certainly also involved in bone matrix biology. Conclusive proof is lacking that diminished estrogen is a factor in this and other age-related disorders such as arthritis, muscular weakness, migraine headache, and stomatitis. On the other hand, atrophic changes in the distal urinary tract, particularly in the urethra, which result in urinary frequency, burning, and occasionally stress incontinence, are reversible by the administration of local or systemic estrogen. Finally, estrogen controls the often embarrassing and sometimes disabling irritations of atrophic vaginitis and vulvitis.

In the postmenopausal situation, in which menstrual function is not required, only small doses of cyclic estrogen are necessary for appropriate therapy. Conjugated estrogen, 0.625 mg daily for three weeks of every four, is sufficient. Despite the ease of administration and its obvious physiologic and clinical value, estrogen therapy has often been limited in duration or actively avoided. The reason for this restraint is the concern that protracted estrogen treatment will induce neoplastic changes in estrogen-sensitive aging tissues. The contribution of endogenous estrogen to the pathogenesis of uterine and breast carcinoma is still speculative, but suspicion has been aroused, particularly as to the effects of unopposed estrogen in the stimulation of endometrial disease. Clearly, indiscriminate use of this hormone in high doses without periodic evaluation is condemned. On the other hand, if therapy is given within the restrictions stated, there is more evidence in favor of than against its use.

In this regard the importance of frequent medical evaluations in this age group should not be understated. In addition to the opportunities such interviews present for continual psychologic support of the apprehensive patient, the full physical examination performed on these occasions may uncover basic organic disease, the symptoms of which have been incorrectly minimized by the woman as further evidence of "a change of life."

Hypogonadotrophic Hypogonadism. Before embarking on a therapeutic program in this form of amenorrhea, the physician must have assured himself of the absence of various intracranial diseases that inhibit or destroy gonadotrophin secretion.

In the absence of neoplastic, vascular, or congenital anomaly to account for disruption in pituitary function, there is usually a history of some stressful circumstance as the precipitating event. Improved dietary habits or psychotherapy may result in return of ovulatory cycles. In fact, the frequency of spontaneous remission is so high that simple observation is often satisfactory. However, when amenorrhea is prolonged and is associated with incipient atrophy of dependent organs and infertility, or is accompanied by lactation, more active therapeutic measures must be undertaken.

Inappropriate Lactation—Galactorrheic Syndromes. Galactorrhea refers to the inappropriate mammary secretion of milky fluid that is not immediately related to pregnancy or the needs of a neonate. The quantity of secretion is not an important criterion. Galactorrhea may involve both breasts, or one or the other breast consecutively or alternately. Amenorrhea does not necessarily accompany galactorrhea, even in the most serious disorders.

A variety of eponymic designations have been applied to variants of the lactation syndromes. These are based on the association of galactorrhea with intrasellar tumor (Forbes, Henneman, Griswold, and Albright, 1954), antecedent pregnancy with inappropriate persistence of galactorrhea (independently reported by Chiari and Frommel in 1852), and the absence of previous pregnancy (Argonz and del Castillo, 1953). In all these types, the association of galactorrhea with eventual amenorrhea was observed. On the basis of currently available information, categorization of individual cases according to these eponymic guidelines neither is helpful nor permits discrimination of patients who will eventually develop serious intrasellar lesions.

The differential diagnosis of galactorrhea syndromes is a difficult and complex clinical challenge. The difficulty arises from the multiple factors involved in the control of prolactin release. In most pathophysiologic systems, the final common pathway leading to galactorrhea is an inappropriate augmentation of prolactin release.

Prolactin is a polypeptide secreted from the anterior pituitary and has a half-life of 15 to 30 minutes. Prolactin is apparently under a chronic, tonic inhibition owing to hypothalamic secretion into the pituitary portal system of prolactin-inhibiting factor (PIF). The following considerations are important in differentiation of causes of excess prolactin:

1. *Excessive estrogen* (as may be administered in birth control pills) can lead to milk secretion via hypothalamic suppression, causing inhibition of PIF and consequent release of pituitary prolactin. Progesterone, on the other hand, seems to have a restraining effect, perhaps by a stimulatory effect on the hypothalamus leading to production of PIF.

2. Prolonged intensive *suckling* can also release prolactin, via hypothalamic reduction of PIF control of prolactin. Similarly, thoracotomy scars, cervical spinal lesions, and herpes zoster can induce prolactin release by activating the afferent sensory neural arc.

3. A variety of *drugs* can also inhibit hypothalamic PIF. There are nearly 100 phenothiazine derivatives with indirect mammotropic activity. In addition, many phenothiazine-like compounds, reserpine derivatives, amphetamines, and a variety of other drugs can initiate galactorrhea via hypothalamic suppression (thioxanthenes, diazepines, butyrophenones, α-methyldopa).

4. *Emotional stresses* (presumably capable of increasing hypothalamic PIF and diminishing prolactin secretion) can also inhibit hypothalamic PIF and induce the secretion of prolactin and galactorrhea. Severe anxiety and trauma often occur in temporal relation to the onset of galactorrhea. The posthysterectomy or menopausal onset of this symptom is a rare but known entity.

5. *Hypothalamic lesions,* stalk lesions, or compression—events that physically reduce production or delivery of PIF to the pituitary—can release excess prolactin, leading to galactorrhea (see Ch. 826).

6. *Hypothyroidism* (juvenile or adult) can be associated with galactorrhea. The mechanism of this relationship requires the introduction of a positive hypothalamic material (prolactin-releasing factor, PRF) that can release, not inhibit, pituitary secretion of prolactin. PRF exists in various fowl (e.g., pigeon, chicken, duck, turkey, and the tricolored blackbird). Although the identity of this material has not been elucidated or its function substantiated in normal human physiology, in pathologic situations such as hypothyroidism, thyrotrophin-releasing hormone (TRH) may be active as a PRF. Synthetic TRH is a potent stimulant of prolactin secretion in man. With diminished circulating levels of thyroid hormone, hypothalamic TRH is produced in excess and as such may act as a PRF to release prolactin from the pituitary. Adult hypothyroidism associated with galactorrhea is well known. In juvenile hypothyroidism, prepubertal breast development and galactorrhea may be seen. Reversal with thyroid hormone therapy is strong circumstantial evidence in support of this thesis.

7. Also acknowledged as a rare cause of galactorrhea is *Cushing's disease.* It is not known whether the direct effect of excessive free cortisol enhances otherwise nonstimulating levels of prolactin secretion to cause galactorrhea, or whether hypothalamic-pituitary dysfunction

involves not only increased corticotrophin-releasing hormone but also excess PRF or reduced PIF.

8. Increased prolactin release may be the consequence of prolactin elaboration and secretion from *pituitary tumors* which function independently of the otherwise appropriate restraints exerted by PIF from a normally functioning hypothalamus. This dangerous tumor with endocrine, neurologic, and ophthalmologic liabilities makes the differential diagnosis of persistent galactorrhea a major clinical challenge. Beyond prolactin production, the tumor may also suppress pituitary parenchyma by expansion and compression, interfering with other trophic hormones (see Ch. 830).

9. *Ectopic production of prolactin* has been reported in one patient without galactorrhea and with a bronchogenic carcinoma, and in one patient with galactorrhea and a hypernephroma. An occult carcinoma, although a remote possibility, should be considered.

Symptoms of galactorrhea may antedate the recognition of intrasellar tumors by many years. It is recognized that a mean duration of 10 to 12 years of galactorrhea and amenorrhea may precede the radiologic demonstration of a pituitary adenoma. As a result, follow-up must be prolonged and zealous. Furthermore, the criterion of antecedent pregnancy does not necessarily suggest that a different pathophysiologic process is involved in the galactorrhea. Cases of pituitary adenoma which did not alter competent gonadotrophin secretion are known, and conception has occurred in some of these patients.

Galactorrheic women with pituitary tumors shown by x-ray can demonstrate withdrawal from progesterone and even have menses and ovulate, as stated above. Obviously, the presence of galactorrhea is not incompatible with gonadotrophin release. However, in the majority of patients a single lesion is sufficiently extensive or critically placed to impair both mechanisms and, on rare occasions, other trophic hormones (TSH, ACTH).

Therefore regardless of the clinical circumstances, in galactorrhea of six months' to one year's duration, a pituitary tumor must be considered. The longer the follow-up, with the progressive exclusion of other benign causes, the higher the incidence of tumor diagnosis in persistent galactorrhea.

ENDOCRINE MANIPULATIONS TO RULE OUT PITUITARY TUMOR. In a large retrospective study of pituitary failure owing to tumors, a sequence of trophic hormone loss was found. Growth hormone, gonadotrophins, TSH, and ACTH are lost over time in roughly that order. Loss of ACTH and TSH is a very late occurrence in the course of the disease. From these data, it can be reasoned that loss of growth hormone in the face of galactorrhea may give early diagnosis of suspected tumor before x-rays of the sella are abnormal. However, normal adults do not show symptoms from loss of growth hormone. Furthermore, normal values for growth hormone are low, and stimulation of growth hormone secretion is required for measurement. Inability to stimulate growth hormone response may indicate the presence of a pituitary tumor. Growth hormone rises during hypoglycemia induced by insulin or during an infusion of arginine. A rise above 10 ng per milliliter (the units may vary from laboratory to laboratory) in response to arginine is strong but not conclusive evidence against tumor-related galactorrhea.

L-DOPA RESPONSE. L-Dopa (0.5 gram four times a day) may be administered to galactorrheic patients with high prolactin blood levels. L-Dopa enters the hypothalamus and is decarboxylated to form dopamine, which then activates PIF release. If prolactin levels fall after L-dopa, tumor-dependent production of prolactin may be ruled out and hypothalamic dysfunction is the probable cause of the galactorrhea.

LRH RESPONSE. LRH has now been synthesized and administered to human subjects to induce surges of LH. Pregnancies have been induced in previously infertile women by appropriate LRH therapy. If LRH administration causes a rise in peripheral LH, a pituitary tumor is unlikely as a cause of galactorrhea and amenorrhea.

Differential diagnosis proceeds by excluding the several causes of galactorrhea. Current clinical practice depends on repeated yearly x-rays of the sella turcica, and ophthalmologic surveillance of visual fields. Endocrine survey of TSH, ACTH, and calcium metabolism should be performed as clinically warranted. L-Dopa, LRH, and growth hormone provocative tests should be performed when and if available. In severe hypogonadism, hormone replacement is appropriate. Fertility can be achieved with clomiphene or human menopausal gonadotrophins, and recently pregnancy has been reported with the use of ergot alkaloids.

If pregnancy ensues, careful follow-up is required to avoid intragestational expansion of the tumor or acute hemorrhage with abrupt hypopituitarism, compression of optic tract or chiasma, or hypothalamic disruption.

The earlier a tumor is diagnosed, the better the treatment result. Early diagnosis and extirpation preclude unnecessary progressive endocrine, neurologic, and ophthalmologic complications. Better tumor therapy is possible if tumors are small and completely intrasellar. In this favorable circumstance, a transnasal frontal approach (transsphenoidal) is possible with direct visualization of the sellar contents. Aspiration of the tumor, good hemostasis, and preservation of residual pituitary tissue can be achieved in experienced hands. Smaller postoperative doses of radiation therapy are an added benefit. Finally, early diagnosis and specific therapy avoid the hazards of induction of ovulation and pregnancy in the presence of an occult tumor.

Gonadotrophin Therapy. HUMAN PITUITARY FOLLICLE-STIMULATING HORMONE (HPFSH) AND HUMAN CHORIONIC GONADOTROPHIN (HCG) THERAPY. In 1958 Gemzell reported the use of a human pituitary preparation that stimulated follicular growth and estrogen production in amenorrheic women. The material was extracted from pituitary tissue collected at autopsy and partially purified by ammonium sulfate fractionation. When assayed against relatively specific standards, it revealed combined FSH and LH potencies, but with the former dominating the biologic activity. Ovulation occurs during HCG administration. Dose size and duration are adjusted according to the ovarian response noted. In limited trials it has been found that more than 90 per cent of patients ovulated once or several times, and more than 50 per cent became pregnant. The limited availability of material (requiring approximately 10 pituitaries to produce an ovulation with this system) has been its major disadvantage.

HUMAN MENOPAUSAL URINARY GONADOTROPHIN (HMG-FSH, PERGONAL). Although menopausal urine has been recognized as a potential source of gonadotrophins (FSH activity by animal studies) since 1930, toxic reactions precluded utilization in human investigations. Acceptable material is now available clinically as Pergonal, which contains 75 units of FSH and 75 units of LH potency per ampule. Toxic and allergic reactions have been eliminated. At least 90 per cent of appropriately selected patients ovulate, and 50 to 70 per cent achieve pregnancy. The usual dose required is 8 to 12 days of 2 ampules of human menopausal gonadotrophin (HMG) per day, followed by 10,000 units of HCG. However, variable ovarian reactivity has been encountered. In addition to monitoring HMG-induced ovarian stimulation by biologic expressions of estrogen (cervical mucus changes), urinary estrogen excretion has proved to be useful. An excretion range between 100 μg and 200 μg total estrogen is the goal of HMG therapy, at which time the ovulatory dose of exogenous HCG can be applied. In this range, an optimal ratio between induced pregnancy rate and incidence of serious side effects (hyperstimulation and multiple pregnancy) is expected.

The results of species-specific FSH (as HMG) therapy (two to five courses) are 90 per cent ovulation, 50 to 70 per cent pregnancies, 20 per cent abortion, 20 per cent multiple gestation (15 per cent twins, 5 per cent three or more), and 1 per cent serious side effects (hyperstimulation).

SIDE EFFECTS OF GONADOTROPHIN THERAPY. Certain side effects have been noted that may limit general application of these agents. The reactions encountered are attributable to the effects of ovarian enlargement and production of unusual quantities of ovarian hormones. These consist of abdominal pain, bloating, pressure, nausea, and general malaise. Acute distention can even cause ovarian rupture and hemorrhage. Because many of the reactions are self-limiting, nonsurgical supportive therapy is advised, laparotomy and conservative surgery short of castration being reserved for the deteriorating circumstance. In this regard hypovolemic shock resulting from a syndrome of severe ascites and hydrothorax has been recognized. Additional expressions of ovarian hyperstimulation are the frequency of abortion and multiple pregnancy and the consequent diminution in fetal salvage noted in all series. Finally, it has become clear that gonadotrophin therapy is effective only during the treatment interval. Regardless of frequency of ovulation or the occurrence of pregnancy, patients revert to pretreatment hypogonadal status upon cessation of therapy or conclusion of pregnancy. For this reason gonadotrophin induction of ovulation is currently withheld until other modes of treatment have failed.

Normogonadotrophic Normoestrogenic Anovulation. In this type of amenorrhea, the chain of events leading to normal ovulation and menstruation is upset by the absence of the midcycle surge of LH. Lacking progesterone secretion, continued unopposed estrogen stimulation leads to hyperplasia of the endometrium. For this reason amenorrhea may be punctuated by prolonged, sometimes severe uterine hemorrhages (*metropathia hemorrhagica*) that require special attention. In addition, infertility further complicates this syndrome. Clearly the correction of both these circumstances is found in the return of recurrent ovulation.

Correction of Menstrual Pattern. There may be no specific requirement for reproductive function, but the inconvenience and uncertainty of the menstrual pattern prompt the patient to seek hormonal regulation of her cycle. In the absence of serious underlying disease, this may be accomplished by inducing progesterone withdrawal flow with an oral progestin such as 10 mg of medroxyprogesterone acetate for five days after an interval of endogenous estrogen stimulation. Two to five days after progestin withdrawal, menses will appear. Retreatment with progestin should be delayed for sufficient time (six weeks) to determine whether spontaneous ovulation will return. Only in cases of too frequent menstruation (polymenorrhea) is the disadvantage of complete cycle coverage by combined estrogen and progestin (as in the birth control medications) acceptable. Medication should be withdrawn periodically, because spontaneous correction may have occurred during therapy.

When severe dysfunctional bleeding occurs, an effort must be made to obtain an endometrial biopsy, but curettage is not essential. Regardless of the duration or severity of flow, anovulatory bleeding of this type is treated by converting the proliferative endometrium to a secretory endometrium from which limited withdrawal flow will occur. Three to four times the contraceptive doses of oral 19-nor steroids will rapidly diminish dysfunctional bleeding with complete cessation within 12 hours. Therapy is then continued, and is gradually tapered to allow an interval for blood replacement as well as general, gynecologic, and hematologic evaluation. The possibility of underlying disorders of coagulation must always be considered. After withdrawal flow, contraceptive doses of 19-nor steroids must be resumed for two to three cycles. The initial use of high doses of estrogen intravenously (Premarin, 25 mg) before progestin conversion is limited to those cases in which bleeding has been prolonged or severe and immediate cessation is required. On the other hand, if agents such as 19-nor steroids do *not* control abnormal flow, then pathologic bleeding is diagnosed and curettage is mandatory.

Reversal of Anovulation. Obviously, correction of proved adrenocortical and thyroid disease will reverse associated anovulation. The drug Clomid (a synthetic nonsteroidal analogue of chlorotrianisene) has proved useful in the treatment of diagnostically nonspecific anovulation. It has almost entirely replaced the low-dose corticosteroid regimens and has virtually eliminated the need for operative wedge resection of the ovaries to achieve resumption of ovulation. Using 50 to 100 mg daily for five days of each cycle, induction of ovulation is achieved in patients with intermediate follicle maturation arrest but with sufficient function to secrete some estrogen. The drug's mode of action is not understood, although it appears to enhance both endogenous gonadotrophin secretion and ovarian synthesis of estrogen. In properly selected patients, 80 per cent can be expected to ovulate and approximately 50 per cent become pregnant. The percentage of pregnancies per number of induced ovulatory cycles is 15 per cent. The multiple pregnancy rate in accumulated national statistics is approximately 8 per cent, almost entirely twins. The abortion rate is 20 per cent. The incidence of congenital anomalies is not increased as a result of Clomid-induced ovulation. There is no evidence that the effect of Clomid is long lasting; it is considered to be limited to the cycle in which the drug is used. The side effects are similar to those of the gonadotrophins and are related to increased ovarian size, hormone production, and multiple pregnancies. In the event that Clomid (after gradually increased doses over four to six months) is unsuccessful, then bilateral wedge resection of the ovaries or HMG plus HCG therapy is advised. Because all the therapies cited present some risk to the patient and none guarantee lasting results, other aspects of the fertility potential of the involved couple must be fully evaluated before ovulation induction is undertaken.

Argonz, J., and del Castillo, E. B.: A syndrome characterized by estrogenic insufficiency, galactorrhea, and decreased urinary gonadotropin. J. Clin. Endocrinol. Metab., 13:79, 1953.

Chard, T.: The Chiari-Frommel syndrome: An experiment of nature. J. Obstet. Gynaec. Br. Commonw., 71:624, 1964.

Coronary Drug Project Research Group: The coronary drug project: Initial findings leading to modifications of its research protocol. J.A.M.A., 214:1303, 1970.

Engel, T., Jewelewicz, R., Dyrenfurth, I., Speroff, L., and Vande Wiele, R. L.: Ovarian hyperstimulation syndrome: Report of a case with notes on pathogenesis and treatment. Am. J. Obstet. Gynecol., 112:1052, 1972.

Forbes, A. P., Henneman, P. H., Griswold, G. C., and Albright, F.: Syndrome characterized by galactorrhea, amenorrhea, and low FSH. J. Clin. Endocrinol. Metab., 14:265, 1954.

Furman, R. H.: Coronary heart disease and the menopause. In Menopause and Aging. NIH, 1973, pp. 39–52.

Furman, R. H.: Menopausal effects on calcium homeostasis and skeletal metabolism. In Menopause and Aging. NIH, 1973, pp. 59–66.

Hack, M., Brish, M., Serr, D. M., Insler, V., Salomy, M., and Lunenfeld, B.: Outcome of pregnancy after induced ovulation: Follow-up of pregnancies and children born after gonadotropin therapy. J.A.M.A., 211:791, 1970.

Kase, N., Mroueh, A., and Buxton, C. L.: Pergonal therapy of anovulatory infertility. Am. J. Obstet. Gynecol., 100:2, 1968.

Kase, N., Mroueh, A., and Olson, L. E.: Clomid therapy for anovulatory infertility. Am. J. Obstet. Gynecol., 98:1037, 1967.

Lawrence, A. M., and Hagen, T. C.: Ergonovine therapy of nonpuerperal galactorrhea. N. Engl. J. Med., 287:150, 1972.

Malarkey, W. B., Jacobs, L. S., and Daughaday, W. H.: Levodopa suppression of prolactin in nonpuerperal galactorrhea. N. Engl. J. Med., 285:1160, 1971.

Rabkin, M. T., and Frantz, A. G.: Hypopituitarism: A study of growth hormone and other endocrine functions. Ann. Intern. Med., 64:1197, 1966.

Taymor, M. L., Yussman, M. A., and Gminski, D.: Estrogen monitoring in ovulatory induction. Fertil. Steril., 21:759, 1970.

Turkington, R. W.: Inhibition of prolactin secretion and successful therapy of the Forbes-Albright syndrome with L-dopa. J. Clin. Endocrinol. Metab., 34:306, 1972.

Veterans Administration Cooperative Study: An evaluation of estrogenic substances in the treatment of cerebral vascular disease. Circulation, 33(5) SII:2–3, May 1966.

INVESTIGATION OF INFERTILITY

Approximately 10 per cent of married couples in the United States are unable to conceive. The cause of infertility varies with geographic and socioeconomic factors, but some general statements can be made regarding the frequency of certain etiologic factors. Of 100 couples in whom a definite disorder is identified, approximately 40 will show a male factor deficiency, 20 a female hormonal defect, 30 a female tubal disorder, and 10 a cervical defect. Ten to 20 per cent of couples with infertility remain undiagnosed as to the cause of their problem. Because investigation of infertility in the female is time consuming and expensive, evaluation of the male factor is carried out first.

Male Factor. The most important procedure is the analysis of the semen. Although some estimate of sperm can be made from postcoital cervical examinations, before any final conclusion of deficiency is made, three separate masturbatory specimens should be examined for volume, sperm count, motility, morphology, and

viability. A normal ejaculate is considered to have a volume not less than 1 ml and not more than 6 ml, 60 per cent active forms after two hours, 60 per cent normal morphology, and at least 20 million sperm per milliliter. If counts are below 20 million, full urologic and medical investigation is warranted. Regardless of count, the male partner should be questioned and instructed when necessary in the development of appropriate sexual and social habits.

Female Factor. Once it is established that ovulation regularly occurs (by means of basal body temperature curves, appropriately timed examination of cervical mucus, endometrial biopsy, and pregnanediol excretion), investigation of the female attempts to certify functional and anatomic competence of the reproductive tract to permit union of sperm and ovum in the ampulla of the oviduct.

The postcoital test is performed at the expected date of ovulation, not less than 2 and not more than 16 hours after intercourse. A specimen of endocervical mucus is inspected for clarity, ferning, elasticity, and the number and activity of spermatozoa. In this way the adequacy of coital position, intromission, and ejaculate content, as well as the cervical environment, can be evaluated. Sperm survive in mucus that is abundant, clear, and elastic. The presence of this type of mucus is indicative of adequate local cervical and ovarian function. Repeatedly poor postcoital examinations, despite documented ovulation, make examination of the male factor and coital habits imperative. Furthermore, anatomic abnormalities of the cervix or hostile mucus resulting from erosions, infections, and other local disorders of the cervix should be investigated and specifically treated.

Tubal competence is evaluated by tubal insufflation with carbon dioxide (the Rubin test), by roentgenographic demonstration of patency by hysterosalpingography, or by direct visualization by laparoscopy or culdoscopy. Each serves distinct functions and should be included in the definitive infertility work-up.

The *Rubin test* is best performed before ovulation. It involves transcervical introduction of carbon dioxide under a carefully monitored flow rate and pressures and insufflation of gas through the uterus and the ostia of the tubes into the peritoneal cavity. A positive test (indicating tubal patency) involves demonstration of gas under the diaphragm by the appearance of referred shoulder pain. The insufflation occurs at a gas pressure usually less than 120 mm of mercury. If tubal blockade exists, escape of gas is prevented and the pressure readings rise continuously to above 200 mm of mercury. At this point the test should be discontinued. It must be remembered that a single negative test is not diagnostic, because functional occlusion (tubospasm) is frequently encountered. Multiple studies are essential and may be undertaken with paracervical block local anesthesia. On the other hand, a positive Rubin test does not rule out the presence of distortions of the tube or tubal-ovarian junction secondary to pelvic adhesions. For this reason if infertility persists in the face of positive tubal insufflation, then ancillary tests of tubal competence are required.

Hysterosalpingography is ordinarily performed by instillation of 3 to 6 ml of radiopaque oil into the uterine cavity and oviducts under fluoroscopic observation. In this way defects in the uterine cavity that may interfere with implantation and alteration in tubal architecture can be visualized and permanently recorded. The presence of peritubal adhesions may be diagnosed by the dye diffusion pattern about the tubal ostia at the time of examination and 24 hours later.

Laparoscopy (which has virtually replaced culdoscopy) accompanied by tubal insufflation with methylene blue is probably the most effective means of diagnosing peritubal and pelvic adhesions producing infertility. Combined with salpingography, these procedures offer detailed information as to the feasibility and type of corrective adnexal surgery to be undertaken.

Uterine factors were once considered important elements in infertility. However, current views no longer give significance to the multiple anatomic variations in uterine displacement from the usual anterior position. However, abnormalities of the uterine cavity, such as congenital anomalies and submucous myomas, deserve surgical repair if associated with otherwise unexplained infertility.

FERTILITY CONTROL
(Population Control)

Discussion of the need for population control is beyond the scope of this text. Obviously, once the public health issues of the demographic gap and its consequences are put aside, the basic issue remains the acceptability of the form of fertility control offered to the individual couples. If 100 women of proved fertility are exposed to pregnancy for one year, approximately 80 pregnancies will result. Clearly, then, *any* method of contraception is more effective than none. It must be remembered that significant discrepancies always exist between the theoretical and practical effectiveness of any contraceptive method, as is illustrated by experience with the "rhythm" method. The fertile phase (requiring sexual continence) is estimated as extending from the eighteenth day before the onset of the earliest likely menstruation up to and including the eleventh day before the onset of the latest likely menstruation. The method assumes that ovulation occurs about 14 days before menstruation, that spermatozoa can fertilize for 48 hours after intercourse, and that the ovum can be fertilized for about 24 hours after it emerges from the ovary. The method depends on motivation to accumulate menstrual records for one year before use and to remain continent during the fertile period. Studies of the effectiveness of this method reveal pregnancy rates of about 15 conceptions per 100 years of exposure. Although this is about double the conception rates with mechanical devices (condom, diaphragm), it represents an important reduction compared with the projected rate of 80 which would have been expected. All physicians must be prepared to teach this method as long as a substantial proportion of the population is limited by religious belief to this method alone.

When considering the other available contraceptive modalities, it is apparent that with advancing scientific knowledge and public awareness the traditional, folklore-based methods (douche, withdrawal, household spermicides) have given way to proved methods of prevention. Vaginal jellies, foams, diaphragms, and condoms are all safe and fairly reliable. Their relative acceptability varies geographically and according to social class. Their application and use are described in Calderone's manual.

Two modern methods of contraception have altered worldwide concepts of conception control. These are the oral ovulation-inhibiting steroid "pill" and the intrauterine device (IUD).

Oral Hormonal Control of Ovulation. Clinical trials with contraceptive steroids began with combined agents in 1958 and sequential pills in 1962. At least 20 million women are current users of these medications in the world at large. Evaluation of coincidental medical problems and side effects continues to be a pressing issue. As synthetic steroids, these agents induce a pharmacologic state posing a long-term challenge to the physiologic reserve of the recipient. Thus far, the contraceptive action has not been separated from wide-ranging biochemical and metabolic liabilities.

The progestational agents in steroid contraceptives are derived from two basic groups: 19-nortestosterones and 17-acetoxy progesterones. The estrogen components are either ethinyl estradiol or its 3-methyl ether, mestranol. The substituents attached to the basic steroid structures confer the property of activity by the oral route and increased potency, presumably because of longer half-lives, reflected by metabolic clearance.

It is the progestational agent which provides the main contraceptive action in the combination pills, principally by the negative feedback action on the hypothalamus; this action inhibits secretion of the gonadotrophin-releasing factor. In addition, the progestational agent produces an endometrium which is hostile to implantation of the ovum, a decidualized bed with atrophied glands. Furthermore, cervical mucus becomes thick and impervious to the migration of spermatozoa into the uterus.

The estrogen in combination pills serves two purposes. First, the negative feedback of the progestin is enhanced by the presence of estrogen. Second, estrogen provides the structural support for endometrial stability and avoidance of irregular shedding and breakthrough bleeding. Estrogen also suppresses early FSH stimulation of the ovary with diminished follicle development but with no reduction in over-all rate of follicular atresia (thereby negating the possibility of pregnancies late in life).

The sequential medications take advantage of this negative feedback attribute of estrogen in the early phase of the cycle as the exclusive basis of contraceptive efficacy. A terminal five days of progestin after the estrogen is used to yield more predictable and orderly menstrual desquamation. Although less effective than combined agents in early trials, restriction of the pill-free interval to seven days, regardless of bleeding patterns, has brought sequential efficacy up to the combined level (0.1 per cent failure rate). A continuing liability inherent in sequential medications is their dependence on higher doses of estrogen with a consequent higher rate of disturbed metabolism.

Despite almost 100 per cent contraception, concerns over short- and long-term effects of these medications have restricted acceptability and usage. These effects are related to general metabolic and target organ effects of the steroids involved.

1. *Oncogenic potential.* A major concern is whether prolonged steroidal usage will increase the incidence of uterine (corpus and cervix) and breast cancer. Although duration of application has not yet been sufficient to permit absolute statements, the anticipated effect on uterine cancer is reduction in the case of endometrial

disease because of the protective chemotherapeutic effect of progestin, and earlier diagnosis and presumed higher cure rates in disease of the cervix because of the improved screening inherent in the periodic examinations carried out in women receiving antiovulatory medication.

No definite relationship exists between estrogen therapy and the etiology of human breast cancer. However, anxiety lingers owing to the effect of estrogen on breast carcinoma incidence in rats and mice and a similar effect of progestins (of the C-21 progesterone family) in beagle dogs. There has been no increase in mortality in the Connecticut registry since the introduction of estrogen or contraceptive steroid therapy. Current practice does not exclude steroid contraception in women with chronic mastitis or fibrocystic disease. Although these steroids are contraindicated in women with treated breast cancer, there is no evidence that normal women with a family history of breast cancer should be excluded from therapy.

2. *Thromboembolic disease.* The striking rise in the incidence of thromboembolic phenomena since 1958 has affected both sexes. However, it seems indubitable that steroidal birth control medication has increased the risk to users beyond that of controls. A series of retrospective studies in England revealed a six- to sevenfold greater risk to users, with older women (35 to 44 years) incurring double the risk of 20- to 34-year-old users. The British findings also indicated that the mortality from pulmonary embolism and cerebral thrombosis was seven times higher among pill recipients. An American study concluded that the risk of thromboembolism was 4.4 times higher in pill users, with no differential risk with age. No increase in cerebrovascular accidents was found in this study.

Despite differences between studies, the general view is that the estrogenic component (more than 75 μg) of birth control pills increases the risk of venous thrombosis, pulmonary embolism, and cerebral thrombosis, but not coronary thrombosis. There is no indication that study individuals who were affected were especially susceptible; hence the level of risk is believed to be higher in all users. Older women and patients anticipating or recovering from elective surgery should avoid these medications.

It should be emphasized that the onset or exacerbation of severe headaches, usually of the migraine type, is an indication to discontinue the pill. Women experiencing cerebrovascular accidents seem to have experienced prodromal warning by the onset of severe headaches as long as three months before the ischemic episode.

3. *Carbohydrate metabolism.* Glucose tolerance is impaired in 15 to 40 per cent of women receiving birth control pills, and in these women plasma levels of insulin as well as blood sugar are elevated. Generally, the effect of the pill is to increase peripheral resistance to insulin action. Most women can meet this change by increasing insulin secretion without detectable change in glucose tolerance. Those with limited insulin response have abnormal glucose tolerance. The derangement in carbohydrate metabolism may also be affected by estrogenic influences on lipid metabolism, hepatic enzymes, and elevation of plasma-free cortisol levels.

The clinical significance of the elevated blood sugar remains uncertain. It may be a functional change, not deleterious per se and completely reversible. On the other hand, there may be a persisting diabetogenic effect. One preliminary report revealed that four of five class A diabetics (abnormal glucose tolerance while pregnant) remained diabetic after discontinuation of oral contraception. Obese women, or women with strong diabetic family histories, can be given steroidal contraception, but alternatives should be seriously explored.

Clinically, it is particularly necessary to offer women with frank diabetes birth control. This may be given under supervision, because the effect on insulin requirement is neither consistent nor predictable.

4. *Lipid metabolism.* Progestins have no apparent effect on lipids, whereas estrogens increase plasma triglycerides and phospholipids. Because these changes can be seen in subjects on fat-free diets, estrogen either increases hepatic lipogenesis or impairs removal into adipose tissue by inhibiting heparin action on lipase activity. The clinical significance of these changes is not known. In women with strong family histories of coronary disease, periodic measurement of triglyceride levels while on contraceptive pills seems a wise precaution.

5. *Hypertension and the renin-angiotensin system.* The first report of hypertension in a woman receiving birth control pills appeared in 1962 (Brownrigg) and was later well documented by Laragh in 1967. The mechanism of the hypertension is thought to involve the renin-angiotensin system. Plasma angiotensinogen is eight times normal in women receiving birth control pills, but hypertension is usually avoided by a compensatory reduction in plasma renin concentration. The susceptible patient, however, cannot achieve this decrease, and hypertension develops. Usually, blood pressures return to normal three to six months after stopping treatment. It would appear that women with pre-existing hypertension or marginal cardiac reserve should seek alternative modes of contraception.

6. *Liver.* Estrogen influences the synthesis of hepatic DNA and RNA, hepatic cell enzymes, serum enzymes formed in the liver, and plasma proteins. Estrogenic hormones also affect hepatic lipid and lipoprotein formation, the intermediary metabolism of carbohydrates, and intracellular enzyme activity. The active transport of biliary components is impaired by a large number of estrogens and some progestins. Cholestatic jaundice and pruritus are occasional complications of the pill and are similar to the recurrent jaundice of pregnancy. BSP retention is abnormal in 20 per cent of users, and serum alkaline phosphatase is elevated in 2 per cent; but SGOT elevation, if persistent, is not caused by the pill. Pre-existing acute and chronic cholestatic hepatic diseases are contraindications to the use of steroidal contraception. Cirrhosis and previous hepatitis do not seem to be aggravated.

7. *Adrenal cortex.* For some time it has been known that estrogen increases cortisol-binding globulin, transcortin. It has been thought that the increase in plasma cortisol while taking birth control medication was due to increased binding by the globulin without increase in the concentration of free cortisol. Recently, free cortisol has also been shown to be elevated in people taking these steroids. The prolonged effects of this elevation are unknown. The pituitary-adrenal reaction to stress is unimpaired, although the adrenal reaction to metapyrone may be subnormal (owing to estrogen-influenced conjugation of metapyrone).

8. *Other metabolic effects.* Gastrointestinal effects, breast discomfort, and weight gain remain common disturbing effects of birth control pills. Fortunately, these are most intense in the early months of use and usually disappear thereafter. Weight gain on medication is very common but responds to caloric restriction. For some patients, weight gain is a particularly discouraging symptom because of the additional burden of periodic fluid retention.

Chloasma, an increase in facial pigment, was at one time found in as many as 5 per cent of users but is less commonly seen with the current reduction of the steroid content of pills. Once chloasma does appear, it fades slowly and incompletely. Skin-blanching medications may be useful in cosmetically burdened women.

Oral contraception may inhibit the absorption of folate polyglutamates, and prolonged use may lead to megaloblastic anemia in patients with folic acid–deficient diets. Pyridoxine deficiencies may also be seen.

Hematologic effects reported include increased fibrinogen, increased sedimentation rates, increased serum total iron-binding capacity, and a decrease in prothrombin time.

In some women, mental depression or reduction in libido, or both, may require search for an alternative contraceptive method.

Contraindications. The absolute contraindications for oral contraception are previous thromboembolic disease, cholestatic liver disease, estrogen-dependent tumors, sickle cell anemia, and other disorders associated with predisposition to thrombosis (valvular heart disease, arrhythmias, leukemia, polycythemia). Treatment with special observation is indicated in multiple sclerosis, otosclerosis, uterine fibroids, hypertension and other cardiac diseases, diabetes, porphyria, lupus erythematosus, and migraine or unusual headaches. Treatment should be withheld in young women with incomplete epiphysial closure and women who are breast feeding.

Intrauterine Devices for Contraception. With increased use and experience, pregnancy rates in users of various intrauterine spiral or loop devices vary from 2 to 5 per 100 woman years, and therefore tend to be similar to rates observed for other mechanical contraceptives. Obviously the advantage of this mode of contraception is that it minimizes the factor of patient error and is therefore suited to large-scale application in the lower socioeconomic groups. A complicating factor is the often unnoticed expulsion of the device, with consequent loss of contraceptive protection. Pregnancy has occurred with the device in place. The disturbing incidence of intermenstrual spotting, menorrhagia, reproductive tract infection, and perforation of the uterus detracts from the acceptability of these devices. Furthermore, contraindications to their application include distorting fibromyomas and adnexal disease.

The mechanism of action is not understood. In rats the devices affect ovum transport, in rabbits implantation and postimplantation stages are affected, and in monkeys tubal ova are lost. Objective studies of associated alterations in human physiology have not appeared. Their usefulness to date has been in large-scale programs requiring minimal patient cooperation.

Beck, P.: Effects of gonadal hormones and contraceptive steroids on glucose and insulin metabolism. *In* Salhanick, H. A., Kipnis, D. M., and Vande Wiele, R. L. (eds.): Metabolic Effects of Gonadal Hormones and Contraceptive Steroids. New York, Plenum Press, 1969, p. 97.
Brownrigg, G. M.: Toxemia in hormone-induced pseudopregnancy. Can. Med. Assoc. J., 87:408, 1962.
Crane, M. G., Harris, J. J., and Winsor, W., III: Hypertension, oral contraceptive agents, and conjugated estrogens. Ann. Intern. Med., 74:13, 1971.
Feinleib, M., and Garrison, R. J.: Interpretation of the vital statistics of breast cancer. Cancer, 24:1109, 1969.
Hertz, R.: Experimental and clinical aspects of the carcinogenic potential of steroid contraceptives. Int. J. Fertil., 13:273, 1968.
Inman, W. H. W., and Vessey, M. P.: Investigation of deaths from pulmonary, coronary and cerebral thrombosis and embolism in women of child-bearing age. Br. Med. J., 2:193, 1968.
Laragh, J. H., Sealey, J. E., Ledingham, J. G. G., and Newton, M. A.: Oral contraceptives, renin, aldosterone, and high blood pressure. J.A.M.A., 201:918, 1967.
Masi, A. T., and Dugdale, M.: Cerebrovascular diseases associated with the use of oral contraceptives. Ann. Intern. Med., 72:111, 1970.
Mears, E.: Pregnancy following antifertility agents. Int. J. Fertil., 13:340, 1968.
Rock, J., Pincus, G., and Garcia, C. R.: Effects of certain 19-nor steroids on the normal human menstrual cycle. Science, 124:891, 1956.
Royal College of General Practitioners: Oral contraception and thromboembolic disease. J. R. Coll. Gen. Pract., 13:265, 1967.
Salhanick, H. A., Kipnis, D. M., and Vande Wiele, R. L. (eds.): Metabolic Effects of Gonadal Hormones and Contraceptive Steroids. New York, Plenum Press, 1969.
Sartwell, P. E., Masi, A. T., Arthes, F. G., Greene, G. R., and Smith, H. E.: Thromboembolism and oral contraception: An epidemiological case-control study. Am. J. Epidemiol., 90:365, 1969.
Szabo, A. J., Cole, H. S., and Grimaldi, R. D.: Glucose tolerance in gestational diabetic women during and after treatment with a combination-type oral contraceptive. N. Engl. J. Med., 282:646, 1970.
Vessey, M. P., and Doll, R.: Investigation of relation between use of oral contraceptives and thromboembolic disease. Br. Med. J., 2:199, 1968.
Vessey, M. P., and Doll, R.: Investigation of relation between use of oral contraceptives and thromboembolic disease. A further report. Br. Med. J., 2:651, 1969.

COUNSELING IN GYNECOLOGY

The emphasis in the preceding discussions has been directed to analysis of changes in the primary ovarian function of ovulation. In these concluding paragraphs some mention of the physician's role in sexual counseling must be made.

Whereas deep-seated sexual problems are usually discussed in psychiatry teaching programs in the medical curriculum, ordinarily no instruction is given the medical student in the normal aspects of sexual life or in its commonly occurring abnormalities. The physician therefore enters practice without benefit of the usual guidelines of diagnosis and management that he has developed for most of the other disorders he will be called upon to see. However, because of his professional status he is often asked for advice in sexual matters and, owing to the uncertainty of applying his own intuitive perception to these matters, the physician usually avoids comment. Unfortunately, this attitude compounds the official silence with which these subjects are treated by schools, religious groups and families.

As a result of the important observations and clinical activities of Masters and Johnson, recorded in two widely read volumes, a factual description of the biophysical progression of male and female sexual response associated with orgasm as well as an approach to diagnosis and therapy of sexual dysfunction is available. Using rapid (two-week) therapeutic methods involving instructional and interpretive interactions between the dysfunctional couple and a male and female co-therapy team, an over-all treatment success rate of 80 per cent has been achieved in the four main categories of human sexual inadequacy: premature ejaculation, male impotence, female orgasmic deficiency, and vaginismus.

In general, the direction of therapy, regardless of the type of presenting distress, is based upon the premise that subjective appreciation of sexual responsivity derives from positive pleasure in sensory experience. For the sexually dysfunctional individual the sensory deprivation originates in one of several possibilities: fear and apprehension of sexual situations, denial of personal sexual identity, rejection of partner or the circumstance of sexual encounter, and lack of sexual awareness through either emotional or physical fatigue or preoccupation. It is not known what special susceptibility causes only a fraction of individuals exposed to these traumas to undergo protracted sexual dysfunction.

The therapist's role is to provide an accurate "mirror" of professional objectivity and knowledge to the troubled couple. In doing this, myths and misconceptions are dismissed, and fear of poor performance, lack of goal orientation, and the notion of the patient as a "spectator" in sexual activity are eliminated. Furthermore, since there appears never to be a purely unilaterally dysfunctional partner, the couple must be trained to communicate needs and exchange sexual vulnerabilities. Thus a nonverbal and verbal signal system is established to maximize pleasure, excitation, mutual satisfaction, and avoidance of stereotyped performance. In this process of reorientation, education, and physical direction, exploration without performance pressures, development of "sensate focus," and carefully graded escalation of sexual involvement comprise the therapeutic sequence.

Orgasmic Dysfunction – Male. *Premature ejaculation* exists if the male cannot control the onset of his ejaculation for a sufficient length of time during intravaginal containment to satisfy his partner in at least 50 per cent of coital opportunities. Obviously, this problem also affects female function. It limits her ability to express sexual reactions and to achieve satisfactory relief of mounting sexual tensions, inevitably leading to frustration at "just being used." On the other hand, the rapid conclusion of sexual contact is a welcome relief from involvement in unpleasant and unrewarding service. The derivations of this self-centered male expression of need appear to be initial teenage exposures to prostitutes, exclusive reliance on "heavy petting" and coital simulation, and dependence on withdrawal as a contraceptive technique. Under all these circumstances there was no need either to learn ejaculatory control or to undertake responsibility for the partner's reactions and responses. Apparently, masturbation practices do not play an etiologic role.

Therapy by "squeeze technique" and gradual resumption of coital contact have led to almost complete therapeutic success (98 per cent).

Male impotence is classified as *primary* when a male has never been able to achieve and/or maintain an erection qualitatively sufficient to accomplish coital connection. His erection may be achieved but then dissipated without ejaculation. This male may masturbate successfully. Masters and Johnson assign certain events in adolescence as factors influencing the formation of primary impotence. These include untoward maternal influences, the psychosocial restrictions of religious orthodoxy, homosexual functioning, and personal devaluations from experiences with prostitutes. These events lead in a very few men to a long-standing and deep concern about subsequent sexual performance. Therapy has been successful along the general lines outlined above with the augmenting use of replacement partners or partner surrogates.

Secondary impotence is said to exist if at least one successful coital intromission has occurred; as many as several hundred may have been experienced before the onset of secondary impotence. Inability to obtain or maintain a satisfactory erection for coitus normally occurs as an accompaniment to fatigue or distraction. However, if 25 per cent of opportunities are not achieved, then secondary impotence exists. Among the etiologic factors involved are premature ejaculation, alcoholism, excessive dominance of either parent, homosexuality, and religious orthodoxy. Only rarely are physiologic causes (diabetes, neurologic disease, drug intake, genitourinary problems) found as responsible for impotence. All too often the effect of inadequate counseling is a precipitating or prolonging factor.

The treatment of impotence is directed at combating the male's personal insecurity and his feelings that "nothing can be done," that the problem is unique to the patient, that the partner is viewed as a liability leading to disability, and that the problem must be kept secret even from the therapist. In therapy, the patient must be convinced that he can never "will" an erection. As fears of sexual performance are reduced, the patient's concept of being a spectator of his own dysfunction is diminished. The female partner must also be supported and instructed. Thorough discussion, discovery of sensate focus (the opportunity to think and feel sexually without orientation to performance), sharing mutual genital manipulation and masturbation pleasures with verbal and nonverbal communication, and a "tease" technique in graded resumption of coital opportunities lead to repair of sexual dysfunction in 60 to 70 per cent of cases.

Orgasmic Dysfunction – Female. The physician may incorrectly assume that the "modern" girl is well versed in genital anatomy and physiology and the technique of the sexual act. Practical experience indicates that in many instances the young woman approaching marriage knows too little and has the disturbing notion, perhaps by conditioning from her mother's experience, that marital sex for the female is overrated, exploitative, and sinful. In such instances, without adequate counseling for both partners, repeated dissatisfaction may confirm these attitudes and set the pattern for a lifetime of maladjusted performance of a "wifely duty." Although it may appear too simple a solution for a problem of such magnitude, the physician can help the couple to avoid this situation by tactful and sympathetic review of basic facts during premarital examinations or any other occasion requiring medical consultation.

The fear of genital injury or expectation of pain and hemorrhage owing to rupture of the hymen during sexual intercourse poses a threat to achievement of vaginal-oriented orgasm. Such preconceived attitudes can be dispelled by the assurance of the physician that the pelvic examination just performed reveals anatomically adequate external and internal genitalia. Some pain is usually experienced on entry into the vagina, but lubrication, a considerate partner, and repeated experience favor prompt resolution of this difficulty.

Because mutual precoital sexual excitement is imperative, varying patterns of stimulation as well as coital techniques must be encouraged and instruction given. Every effort must be made to motivate both partners to seek this result by experimentation and frank discussion. In this situation affectation of false modesty or "man of the world" all-knowing attitudes should be discouraged. In 223 dysfunctional couples, 107 had bilateral impairment in which an anorgasmic female was paired with a male who was a premature ejaculator.

It must be made clear that, no matter how satisfactory the circumstances, few women experience orgasm regularly. Often this misunderstanding, if uncorrected, provokes undue concern and tension that may produce further diminution in satisfaction, a change in coital frequency, substitution of clitoral orgasm, or pretending satisfaction when none occurs. Once these patterns are set, reconditioning for vaginal orgasm is possible but only after a long and difficult period of adjustment. Some of the factors leading to the initial lack of coital orgasm are fear of pregnancy, the possibility of discovery by parents or children, economic and social pressures, poor health, and fatigue. All these profoundly influence both partners' interest in and response to intercourse. Possibly the most common factor in the development of aversion to sexual intimacy in the somewhat older married woman is that over the years these intimacies have tended to follow a monotonous, routine sameness of time, place, and practice. Reluctance to discuss the matter with her husband or with her physician abets the situation. The alert physician can usually suspect this problem from the patient's response during history taking and the nature of her physical complaints. Again sympathetic but informative discussions will bring a more open and intelligent outlook on the part of the patient, and whereas no quick cure exists, reorientation of sexual practice and renewed motivation can occur, with an increasing degree of satisfaction derived. Coaching the couple in the recognition of the female indicators of sexual arousal and the sequence leading to achievement of orgasm is particularly helpful. Delay of coitus until extragenital and genital responses in the female (generalized skin flush, retraction of the clitoris, ballooning of the vagina, color changes in the labia) will increase the frequency of coital orgasm, release female sexual tension, and make the anxious, uncertain couple more confident and eager for sexual contact. The therapeutic use of testosterone and alcohol in the sexually frigid woman is not recommended. The effects are temporary and only serve to postpone the necessary personal examination that must be carried out. *Cantharis vesicatoria* (Spanish fly) is a severe irritant to the clitoris and has no place in therapeutics.

Sometimes problems appear to be so complicated and deep seated that psychiatric help is worthwhile. Fortunately these are rare. However, if sexual frigidity appears to have the malicious motivation of deprivation, if sexual intercourse and practice are revolting prospects, or if the woman displays pronounced aggressive or homosexual tendencies, psychiatric evaluation is in order.

Vaginismus is a constriction of the outer third of the vagina by spastic involuntary contractions of the muscles of the pelvic floor. This occurs in reaction to imagined, anticipated, or real attempts at vaginal penetration. As a result, penile penetration is exceedingly difficult or impossible and coitus is rare or the marriage is unconsummated. It is not infrequently found in association with a male partner who suffers from primary impotence or other male dysfunction. In addition, religious orthodoxy, early psychosexual trauma (e.g., rape), recurrent vaginitis or dyspareunia caused by endometriosis, pelvic inflammatory disease, postoperative adhesions, or homosexual preferences are seen as contributory factors. Therapy of the primary pathologic problem and vaginal dilators lead to nearly 100 per cent therapeutic success.

Masters, W. H., and Johnson, V. E.: Human Sexual Response. Boston, Little, Brown & Company, 1966.

Masters, W. H., and Johnson, V. E.: Human Sexual Inadequacy. Boston, Little, Brown & Company, 1970.

868. THE ADRENAL MEDULLA AND SYMPATHETIC NERVOUS SYSTEM

Karl Engelman

The sympathetic nervous system is made up of cellular elements distinguished by their embryologic derivation from neural crest cells and by their distinct chemistry and pharmacology relating to the synthesis and release of the postsynaptic neurotransmitter catecholamine compounds. The cells are found widely distributed throughout the body with major foci located in the central nervous system as well as in ganglia associated with the thoracolumbar segments of the spinal cord. Peripheral sites of localization include the innervation of the heart, blood vessels, smooth muscle of the gastrointestinal tract, sweat and salivary glands, adipose tissue, and adrenal medulla.

Alterations of sympathetic nervous system activity may lead to a wide variety of clinical manifestations. Within the central nervous system, abnormalities result in changes of mood and emotional status as well as movement and tremor disorders. Peripheral manifestations include deficits in vasomotor control with resultant hypo- or hypertension, and altered motility and secretory activity of other visceral organs. In addition, tumors may develop from sympathetic neural tissue, producing clinical syndromes dependent upon the biochemical and pharmacologic activity of the hormones synthesized and released from these cells.

HORMONES OF THE ADRENAL MEDULLA AND SYMPATHETIC NERVOUS SYSTEM

The hormones of the sympathetic nervous system are dopamine, norepinephrine, and epinephrine; the last-named is primarily synthesized and released by the adrenal medulla. These compounds are classified chemically as *catecholamines,* because they are amine derivatives of the catechol (dihydroxybenzine) nucleus. In common usage the term is usually applied only to norepinephrine and epinephrine, because they have the most clearly identified peripheral effects, whereas to date the primary physiologic role of dopamine has been localized to the central nervous system. The accepted pathway for synthesis of these hormones was first postulated by Blaschko in 1939, and the intermediate steps with the related enzymes are shown in Figure 1. The rate-limiting step in the pathway is hydroxylation of the amino acid precursor tyrosine to form dihydroxyphenylalanine (dopa), a reaction under feedback control by end-product (norepinephrine) inhibition.

Synthesis of the catecholamines is a unique capability of sympathetic nervous tissue; except for the enzyme aromatic-L-amino acid decarboxylase, the biosynthetic enzymes are found only within sympathetic nervous cells. This anatomic distribution is further specialized in that the enzyme required for the conversion of norepinephrine to epinephrine is found solely within the adrenal medulla. Tyrosine hydroxylase and dopamine beta-hydroxylase (DβH) are found almost universally in sympathetic neural cells where synthesis normally terminates with norepinephrine. On the other hand, the adrenal medulla contains very large quantities of both norepinephrine and epinephrine, the latter comprising 70 to 80 per cent of the total. These catecholamines are normally stored within sympathetic nerve terminals in intracellular granules which migrate to the cell membrane at the time of neural activity and discharge the amines.

When catecholamines are released from sympathetic tissues other than the adrenal medulla, the primary route of physiologic inactivation of their activity is effected by an active transport mechanism which returns

Figure 2. Major routes of catecholamine metabolism.

the unaltered catecholamine into the nerve ending. Either the residual hormone is metabolized locally, or a small portion may diffuse away to appear in the circulation where it may be further metabolized (liver) or excreted unchanged by the kidney. In contrast, catecholamines released from either the adrenal medulla or hormone-producing tumors appear directly in the circulation and manifest their peripheral effects as a result of their concentration in plasma instead of their local tissue concentrations. The primary routes of catecholamine metabolism are accounted for by enzymatic processes shown in Figure 2. For circulating catecholamines, the major route is via O-methylation by the enzyme catechol-O-methyltransferase, followed by oxidative deamination via aldehyde dehydrogenase and monoamine oxidase. In contrast, catecholamines metabolized either within the sympathetic nerve cells or in sympathetic tumors are in large part initially converted by oxidative deamination, followed by O-methylation. In either case, the initial metabolic product is pharmacologically inactive, and the major end product of metabolism is VMA.

The catecholamines and their metabolites are primarily excreted in the urine, and VMA makes up 75 to 80 per cent of the total. The methoxyamines (metanephrines) comprise 10 to 15 per cent, and free catecholamines in the urine usually represent less than 1 per cent of the quantity released. Quantitatively, norepinephrine and its metabolites make up 80 per cent of the total, with epinephrine and its metabolites comprising the balance. Under usual circumstances and with normal activity, humans excrete from 10 to 70 μg of norepinephrine and from 5 to 30 μg of epinephrine per 24 hours. After adrenalectomy the excretion of epinephrine decreases to minimal values, whereas norepinephrine excretion is little changed. Normal excretion of the methoxyamines (normetanephrine plus metanephrine) ranges from 0.3 to 1.3 mg per 24 hours and that of VMA from 2.0 to 6.8 mg per 24 hours.

Pharmacology. Important quantitive differences between epinephrine and norepinephrine, relating to the proportionately greater beta-adrenergic potency of epinephrine, are observed when small doses (5 to 10 μg per minute) are administered intravenously to humans. Although a potent direct vasoconstrictor in some vascular beds, epinephrine produces over-all vasodilatation and

Figure 1. Biosynthetic pathway of the catecholamines.

a decrease in peripheral resistance as well as striking increases in cardiac output and heart rate. Systolic blood pressure is increased, but diastolic pressure remains unchanged or falls, and there is little change in the mean arterial pressure. In contrast, norepinephrine causes an increase of both systolic and diastolic pressure owing to generalized vasoconstriction. Although norepinephrine also has potent beta-sympathomimetic activity, the predominating rise in pressure leads to reflex slowing of the heart, resulting in little change or decrease in cardiac output. When very large doses of norepinephrine or epinephrine are infused into humans or are released from catechol-producing tumors, these differences in physiologic activities of the hormones are usually muted.

Both norepinephrine and epinephrine produce profound metabolic effects, including increased lipolysis and oxygen consumption, elevation of body temperature, and hyperglycemia caused by increased glycogenolysis, as well as inhibition of insulin release from the pancreas. Many of the varying alpha- and beta-sympathetic effects of these hormones have recently been shown to be mediated through changes in the adenyl cyclase system. Current theory holds that beta-sympathomimetic effects are primarily induced by stimulation of adenyl cyclase and increased cyclic-AMP generation, whereas alpha-adrenergic effects inhibit adenyl cyclase activity.

Under normal conditions secretion of epinephrine and norepinephrine by the adrenal medulla is probably not of great physiologic significance. Although hormone production from this sympathetic tissue achieves greater importance during conditions of considerable stress, as in insulin hypoglycemia, the role of the adrenal medulla in normal physiology appears to be mainly supportive in nature. Deficiency states are not generally noted in patients who have had total adrenalectomy with adequate adrenocortical replacement. On the other hand, neuropathic or pharmacologic interruption of the nonadrenal sympathetic tissues appears to produce profound effects most notable in vasomotor control and propulsive activity of the hollow viscera. Among the more commonly encountered clinical conditions in which there is disorder in the sympathetic nervous system are idiopathic orthostatic hypotension and the Riley-Day syndrome (familial dysautonomia), conditions in which both sympathetic and parasympathetic functions are abnormal (see Ch. 471). In addition, results of recent investigations tend to implicate an increase in sympathetic nervous system activity as a causative factor in a significant number of patients with what has previously been called essential hypertension.

PHEOCHROMOCYTOMA

Pheochromocytoma is a catecholamine-producing tumor arising from cells of the sympathetic nervous system and producing a readily recognizable distinctive clinical syndrome which can in most instances be attributed to excessive production of the sympathetic hormones by the tumor. The first clinical description of the syndrome is credited to Labbé and his associates in 1922, and successful surgery for this condition was first performed in 1927 by Dr. Charles H. Mayo.

The most distinctive feature is hypertension. Al-

through pheochromocytoma is responsible for far less than 1 per cent of all patients with hypertension, its importance and notoriety derive from the fact that the clinical features of the disease are dramatic. Although potentially lethal if undiagnosed and untreated, it is curable in about 90 per cent of cases.

Pheochromocytomas may arise from any sympathetic nerve tissue within the body, with the exception of cathecholamine-producing cells within the central nervous system. In general, patients with pheochromocytoma tend to be young; most diagnoses are made in patients between 5 and 25 years of age. In young women the diagnosis is frequently made during pregnancy, in part because the blood pressure is taken more frequently then and in some measure because the enlarging uterus may produce pressure on the tumor, inducing more frequent attacks. The tendency to develop pheochromocytoma may be inherited in association with certain other hereditary neuroectodermal disorders. It is known that patients with von Recklinghausen's disease and associated disorders have a high incidence of pheochromocytoma within the family. Furthermore, pheochromocytomas can be inherited in association with medullary carcinoma of the thyroid and a tendency to parathyroid hyperfunction resulting from hyperplasia or multiple parathyroid adenomas *(Sipple's syndrome)*. In some instances these patients also manifest multiple mucocutaneous neuromas as well as generalized ganglioneuromatosis of visceral organs (Fig. 3). These conditions are inherited as autosomal dominant traits, and the pheochromocytomas are almost always multiple, including bilateral adrenal tumors.

Pathology. More than 95 per cent of pheochromocytomas arise within the abdominal and pelvic cavities. The majority are found in one or both adrenal glands,

Figure 3. Multiple neuromas of the tongue and lips in a patient with bilateral multiple adrenal pheochromocytomas, medullary carcinoma of the thyroid, exstrophy of the bladder, and multiple visceral ganglioneuromas.

but other sites of origin include embryologic rests of neural crest tissue found usually in association with major arteries. Areas of predilection for extra-adrenal tumors include the paravertebral sympathetic ganglia, and in particular those at the bifurcation of the aorta which make up the organ of Zuckerkandl. Very rarely, tumors arise from sympathetic ganglia within the wall of the urinary bladder, producing distinctive symptoms which should strongly suggest this diagnosis. The majority of those arising in the chest are in paravertebral sympathetic ganglia. Very rarely they have been found to arise from the aortic body area. Other chemodectomas, especially of the carotid body, may produce increased amounts of catecholamines and the clinical syndrome of pheochromocytoma, but the majority of these do not appear to produce hormone syndromes. Extremely rare catecholamine-producing tumors may arise from sympathetic tissue in association with the vagus nerve. Collectively, these tumors, known as glomus jugulare tumors, are formed along the base of the skull in the area of the jugular foramen and within the mastoid and temporal bones and the middle ear. Most glomus jugulare tumors are nonfunctional, but very rarely they may produce the entire pheochromocytoma syndrome.

Most patients have single benign pheochromocytomas, but multiple primary tumors may be found in up to 20 per cent of patients. These appear to predominate in patients with familial inheritance of the tumor, and they usually are adrenal medullary tumors (Fig. 4). An occasional patient may present with both an adrenal medullary and ectopic tumor. Malignant tumors are found in fewer than 10 per cent of patients. The definition of malignancy cannot be made on the histologic appearance of the tumor. Frequently, benign tumors present with bizarre nuclear and cellular patterns which under normal circumstances would be considered evidence of malignancy. The only acceptable definition of malignancy rests on the finding of tumor tissue in areas where pheochromocytomas would not normally arise, e.g., in the liver, bone, lymph nodes, lung, and marrow.

Benign tumors vary in size from less than a gram to almost a kilogram in weight; most are in the range of 15 to 100 grams. The smallest tumors are usually found in association with other large tumors, especially in the hereditary cases (Fig. 4). Solitary tumors less than 10 grams in size rarely produce symptoms. They are highly vascular and usually well encapsulated. On cut surface the color may vary from gray to red. In the larger tumors there may be central areas of necrosis and fibrosis. The cells are polygonal or spheroidal with granular cytoplasm and are often arranged in masses separated by connective tissue. Multinucleate and bizarre-looking cells are frequently observed even in what are considered to be benign tumors. When unfixed sections are exposed to chromium salts, the tissue may take on a brown color owing to a chemical reaction with the catecholamine containing intracellular granules, thus giving rise to the term "chromaffin cells." The catecholamine content is generally greater than that of the adrenal medulla, usually in the range of 1 to 10 mg per gram of tumor. All tumors contain increased quantities of norepinephrine, but fewer than 50 per cent appear to synthesize epinephrine as well. The majority of those containing epinephrine appear to arise from the adrenal medulla. This is in contrast to the catecholamine content of densely sympathetically innervated tissues such as heart and brain, which contain 5 to 10 μg of norepinephrine per gram of tissue.

Clinical Manifestations. The most common finding is *hypertension* which is classically described as being paroxysmal in character, occurring in association with palpitations, tachycardia, a feeling of malaise and apprehension, and excessive sweating. Many patients are persistently hypertensive, having superimposed paroxysmal rises in blood pressure, and an approximately equal number have fluctuating blood pressures, normal at times and hypertensive at others (Fig. 5). Most patients with pheochromocytoma will be hypertensive on at least 50 per cent of readings. Patients who have attacks only at intervals of several days to several weeks are extremely rare, and probably comprise less than 1 per cent of the total group. Symptoms usually occur spontaneously and vary considerably in frequency, se-

Figure 4. Bilateral adrenal medullary pheochromocytomas from a patient with Sipple's syndrome. The five largest tumors have been extirpated from the specimens, and an additional five tumors, each measuring approximately 2 mm in diameter, are depicted by the arrows on the specimens.

Figure 5. Pattern of blood pressure in a patient with pheochromocytoma. Note variability of blood pressure and presence of orthostatic hypotension prior to therapy and surgery.

verity, and duration in different patients. They often occur while the patient is at rest, or may be precipitated by emotional upset, postural changes or bending, physical exertion, and eating. Attacks coincidental with micturition suggest that the patient has a primary bladder tumor. Before an attack patients may experience apprehension, frequently associated with abdominal or low back pain discomfort which evolves with palpitations, pounding headache, and even angina pectoris. Occasional patients will describe a peculiar, poorly defined sensation of tightness beginning in the lower abdomen and rising through the thorax into the neck and through the head at the onset of attacks. Because of the peculiar nature of many of the symptoms and the frequency with which these patients are manifestly anxious or tremulous, it is not uncommon for them to be labeled as having psychiatric disorders. Observers will frequently note tremulousness and pallor or flushing of the face and extremities as well as dilatation of the pupils and marked diaphoresis. Blood pressures recorded during severe attacks may exceed 300 mm Hg, and after the attack the patient may complain of prostration, lassitude, or fatigue. In some instances a "shocklike" state has been recorded in which peripheral blood pressure has not been obtainable. Although shock and myocardial infarction may occur as a result of a severe attack, frequently the inability to obtain a peripheral blood pressure is due to severe peripheral vasoconstriction. Under these circumstances central blood pressures are usually very high, and very strong central pulses are usually palpable in the axillary or carotid arteries. In rare instances when intense vasoconstriction persists for long periods of time, necrosis and ulceration of tissue may occur. The most serious complications of severe attacks are myocardial infarction, in-

tracerebral hemorrhage, cardiac failure, or hyperpyrexia, all of which may result in death.

In rare instances only special manifestations will suggest this diagnosis in a patient who might otherwise be thought to have essential hypertension. Of prime importance in such cases are the presence of *excessive sweating* or *hypermetabolism with weight loss* unexplained by overactive thyroid function and the presence of *orthostatic hypotension* in a hypertensive patient not receiving antihypertensive drugs (Fig. 4). This manifestation is found in approximately 70 per cent of patients with pheochromocytoma and reflects a paradoxical impairment of normal autonomic reflex responses to standing despite the excessive catecholamine production by the tumor. The former attribution of the orthostatic hypotension to hypovolemia appears not to be substantiated. *Polycythemia* has been noted in several such individuals, explained by the finding of high plasma and tumor concentrations of erythropoietin. Other important features of the syndrome include *impaired glucose tolerance* which may be misdiagnosed as diabetes mellitus, *paradoxical pressor responses* to autonomic blocking agents such as guanethidine, and *enhanced pressor responses* to sympathomimetic agents such as the amphetamines and commonly used nasal and bronchial decongestants. Severe *constipation* is found in some individuals—presumably because of the marked inhibitory effect of the catecholamines on bowel motility and enhanced sphincter tone. For unknown reasons the incidence of *cholelithiasis* is markedly increased in patients with pheochromocytoma, and it is not unusual to make this diagnosis even in young adult males who would not otherwise be expected to have it.

Additional clinical features relate to the *inherited disorders which may be found in association with pheochromocytoma*. Most prominent among these are the neurocutaneous syndromes associated with *von Recklinghausen's disease* and *Sipple's syndrome*. In the latter, diarrhea and remarkable flushing resulting from prostaglandin and serotonin production by the tumor may simulate certain aspects of the carcinoid syndrome, and biochemical evidence for hyperparathyroidism exists when secondary parathyroid hyperplasia or tumor induction occurs.

Untreated, the disease may progress in a manner similar to other forms of hypertension, although it is relatively unusual for patients to present with advanced atherosclerotic changes or renal impairment. The primary mode of death in the untreated patient is a cardiovascular or intracerebral catastrophe associated with a severe rise in blood pressure. In some instances chronic congestive heart failure caused by a metabolic cardiomyopathy ("catecholamine cardiomyopathy") may be the most serious clinical manifestation, even in patients who may be normotensive or only mildly hypertensive.

Diagnosis. Recognition of the variety of clinical features associated with pheochromocytoma should provide the most important asset in suspecting this diagnosis in a patient. Often included in the differential diagnosis are essential hypertension, hyperthyroidism, diabetes mellitus, and a variety of psychoneurotic conditions. Once the diagnosis is suspected, it can usually readily be confirmed.

Pharmacologic Tests. Historically, pharmacologic tests were the primary means of confirming or excluding the diagnosis of pheochromocytoma in patients suspected of having this condition. More recently, with the general availability of good biochemical assays for catecholamines and metabolites, the use of pharmacologic tests has been relegated to a secondary or even lesser role in the evaluation of this condition.

Although they are no longer recommended as primary diagnostic maneuvers, it is still worthwhile to recognize the nature, attributes, and limitations of pharmacologic tests. *Provocative tests* produce a significant rise in blood pressure after the administration of stimulating drugs; *blocking tests* were thought to be diagnostic by virtue of a selective decrease in blood pressure after administration of certain alpha-adrenergic blocking agents.

Among the stimulatory tests which have been used, the test with which there is greatest experience involves the intravenous injection of 25 to 50 μg of histamine base (available as histamine phosphate solution, 275 μg per milliliter, equivalent to 100 μg per milliliter of histamine base) and the monitoring of blood pressure. Administration of this dose of histamine usually causes flushing, pounding headache, tachycardia, and, frequently, a rise in blood pressure. It is generally accepted that a blood pressure rise of greater than 40 mm Hg, and of more than 20 mm Hg greater than the rise produced by a cold pressor test, indicates a positive response. False positive and false negative responses have each been observed with an incidence of 20 to 30 per cent. Dangers of the test include the precipitation of a severe hypertensive crisis with resulting sequelae or the induction of asthmatic attacks in sensitive individuals. Because of the danger of inducing a severe paroxysm of hypertension, the alpha-adrenergic blocking drug phentolamine (see below) should always be available for prompt intravenous administration. Most patients find this test a most unpleasant experience because of the severe headache usually associated with it. It should not be undertaken in patients whose blood pressure is 170/100 mm Hg or higher. The mechanism by which histamine injection induces enhanced pressor responses in pheochromocytoma is not well understood. Direct release of catecholamine from the tumor by histamine and enhanced discharge of greatly increased sympathetic nerve stores of catecholamines after the acute hypotension produced initially by the histamine-induced vasodilatation have been offered as hypotheses for these events.

Two other provocative tests are still undergoing evaluation. One involves the injection of the indirectly acting sympathomimetic agent, *tyramine,* which has been shown to produce enhanced pressor responses in patients with pheochromocytoma. Advantages of the tyramine test include its safety and lack of unpleasant side effects, because no headache is produced and smaller transient pressor responses are required for a positive diagnosis (20 mm rise in systolic pressure in response to 1000 μg tyramine base); a disadvantage in common with other pharmacologic tests is the fact that there are 10 to 15 per cent false negative responses; false positive responses are extremely rare. The intravenous use of *glucagon* (1 mg) has also been proposed as a diagnostic test with the claim that enhanced pressor responses are produced in patients with pheochromocytoma. The mechanism by which glucagon induces a blood pressure rise in these patients is not understood, and this test

has also been found to have a significant number of false positive and false negative responses.

The only suppressive or vasodepressor test which still has any common usage is the *Regitine (phentolamine) test.* When this alpha-blocking drug is injected into a hypertensive patient with pheochromocytoma, a significant and sustained fall in blood pressure usually occurs. When a dose of 5 mg is given intravenously, phentolamine usually causes a fall of systolic pressure by greater than 35 mm Hg. Although false negative responses rarely occur with this test except in patients who are normotensive, false positive responses may occur, especially in patients who have received sedatives or other antihypertensive drugs, or in those who are uremic. In very sensitive patients, and especially in those whose tumors produce excessive amounts of epinephrine, the fall in blood pressure may be very severe, and shock may be produced as a result of inhibition of the alpha-mediated vasoconstrictor effects, leaving unopposed the beta-mediated vasodilatation; for this reason a preliminary test dose of 1 or 2 mg is suggested. A number of instances have been observed and reported in which this severe reduction of blood pressure has resulted in ischemic infarction of the tumor, with subsequent central hemorrhage, necrosis, and rupture, resulting in serious hazard to the patient.

Chemical Tests. Because of the hazards associated with pharmacologic tests and the significant number of false positive and false negative responses, their use is now discouraged, and the preferred method of confirming the diagnosis of pheochromocytoma is by demonstration of excessive urinary excretion of the catecholamines and their metabolites. Reliable methods are generally available for the measurement of norepinephrine and epinephrine (either singly by specific tests or as a combined total expressed as norepinephrine equivalents), the metanephrines (combined normetanephrine plus metanephrine), and VMA. In almost all patients with pheochromocytoma, analysis of any 24-hour urine collection will reveal increased excretion of all these substances (Fig. 6). The upper limit of normal excretion of these compounds is usually exceeded by an increase of twofold or more for all compounds. In both instances in which the values were at the upper limits of normal or within the normal range, the urines were analyzed more than eight years after their collection, and it appeared likely that chemical destruction of the compounds in the intervening period might have accounted for the relatively low values.

Despite the fact that almost all patients with pheochromocytoma always have increased urinary excretion of catecholamines and metabolites, there are very rare patients who truly have intermittent attacks on very infrequent occasions. These patients constitute less than 1 per cent of the total group, and they will invariably have normal 24-hour urinary excretion values between attacks. In such cases it is possible to make the diagnosis only by collecting carefully timed urine collections over short periods in association with a documented attack. In this way it is usually possible to demonstrate a marked increase in urinary catecholamine excretion for the one- to two-hour period after an attack and then return to normal baseline values. It has been noted in these instances that, although the total excretion rate of free catecholamines may not rise to abnormal levels, if the catecholamine content in these speci-

URINARY EXCRETION OF CATECHOLAMINES AND METABOLITES IN PHEOCHROMOCYTOMA

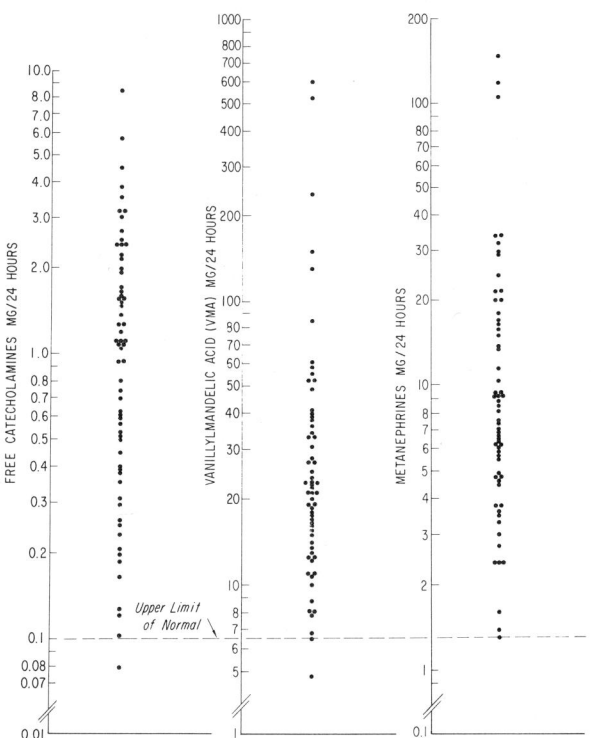

Figure 6. Distribution of excretion values for catecholamines and metabolites determined on single 24-hour urine collections in 64 patients with pheochromocytoma. The vertical axis depicts values on a logarithmic scale.

when specific tests are ordered for screening for this condition. Drugs in common use and the changes which they produce are noted in the accompanying table. Despite the use of any of these drugs, it is possible to adequately screen a patient for the disease without restricting drug therapy. This is especially important in patients with hypertension who might be receiving methyldopa or monoamine oxidase (MAO) inhibitors, and in whom discontinuation of therapy would result in hazardous rises in blood pressure. For many years, it has been advocated that severe dietary restriction be practiced for several days prior to the collection of a urine sample for VMA determination. This requirement was necessary because the rather crude screening tests relied upon color reactions with phenolic acids, and these food constituents resulted in false positive test results. However, for more than a decade there have been available better spectrophotometric or electrophoretic assays which are specific for VMA and which do not require dietary restriction. Laboratories which accept values in the range of 10 to 14 mg per 24 hours as being normal are using crude screening tests, and specimens should not be sent to them for this assay, because the normal VMA excretion should not exceed 6.5 to 7.0 mg per 24 hours.

Tumor Localization. Although the surgeon is understandably concerned about direct localization of the tumor prior to operation, experience with many cases has taught us that precise preoperative localization is of little significance, and some of the maneuvers involved in acquiring the information may be quite dangerous to the patient as well as being costly and often misleading. The essential question concerns the body section in which the tumor is to be found. Since almost all pheochromocytomas are found within the abdominal and pelvic cavities, the major preoperative diagnostic attempts to localize the tumor should be directed at *excluding* the presence of an intrathoracic pheochromocytoma or one arising from the neck or in the skull. Such conditions are readily determined by palpating the area of the carotid bifurcations for the presence of a large, hard mass. Functioning intracranial glomus jugulare tumors should be suspected by the presence of deficits in cranial nerves VII to XII or by the appearance of tumor tissue in the outer or middle ear which can readily be seen by otoscopic examination. In almost all instances in which chest x-rays were obtained in patients having intrathoracic pheochromocytomas, the tumor was readily seen as a posterior mediastinal paravertebral mass. To exclude the presence of such tumors, all patients with pheochromocytoma should have chest fluoroscopy as well as routine and oblique x-rays of the

mens is specially fractionated into norepinephrine and epinephrine, it is usually possible to show a significant rise in either one or the other compound when the data are expressed as an hourly excretion rate.

Determination of plasma concentrations of catecholamines is extremely difficult (see Tumor Localization, below). Although levels are usually very high in patients with pheochromocytoma, there is significant overlap with values that may be obtained with excitement and emotional disturbance and those seen in patients with essential hypertension and depression. Thus this test is not diagnostic and should not be generally performed.

Because certain drugs interfere with one or another of the chemical determinations producing either real or apparent increases or decreases in values, it is important that the therapy of the patient be kept in mind

Urinary Values and Interfering Drugs

Metabolite	Normal Excretion Rate (mg/24 hr)	Usual Range in Pheochromocytoma (mg/24 hr)	Drug	Drug Effect on Excretion Rate
1. Free catecholamines	< 0.1	0.2–4.0	Methyldopa	False increase
			L-Dopa	False increase
			MAO inhibitors	Increase
2. Metanephrines (normetanephrine plus metanephrine)	< 1.3	2.5–40		
3. Vanillylmandelic acid (VMA)	< 6.8	10–250	MAO inhibitors	Decrease
			Clofibrate (Atromid–S)	False decrease
			Nalidixic acid (NegGram)	False increase

chest. Intra-abdominal pheochromocytomas present no problem of localization at the time of operation (see Treatment, below), and large tumors can usually be demonstrated by the relatively noninvasive technique of intravenous pyelography with laminagrams of the renal and retroperitoneal areas. If the tumor is not seen, evidence of its presence by distortion of the renal contour or shift in the position or axis of the kidney or ureter gives strong indication of its position. Retroperitoneal instillation of air or CO_2 as a means of outlining a tumor has now been largely discarded as dangerous, often misleading, and rarely revealing small tumors which would not otherwise be found at exploration. Arteriography may readily define large tumors, but small or ectopic tumors may be missed, and the hazard and cost of the procedure do not seem to justify its routine use.

In exceptional cases, routine preoperative evaluation and thorough surgical exploration will fail to identify tumor tissue, and in such circumstances it may be necessary to perform venous catheterization of the superior and inferior vena cava as well as their major tributaries to collect blood samples for catecholamine determination. These assays are extremely difficult and can be performed accurately in only a few research laboratories, so such problem patients are best handled by experts. Demonstration of a step-up in plasma catecholamine concentrations at any particular level indicates the probable area in which the venous drainage of the tumor enters the major veins. It is noteworthy that falsely elevated values may be produced inadvertently by the person performing the catheterization if radiopaque dye is instilled into the adrenal veins under sufficient pressure to cause local tissue damage. This will result in sufficient catecholamine release from normal adrenals to simulate tumor secretion. Values obtained from the hepatic vein may be most helpful in evaluating the patient for possible hepatic metastases. Under normal circumstances, hepatic venous effluent should have a very low catecholamine concentration because of metabolism of these compounds in the liver. When values obtained from this source are as high as or higher than those obtained from other systemic veins, this is indication of hepatic metastases which are releasing catecholamines beyond the portal circulation.

Although cholecystography is not specifically a localizing procedure for the pheochromocytoma, all patients about to undergo surgery for this condition should have a preoperative oral cholecystogram to determine the possible presence of gallstones which might be removed after tumor resection.

Treatment.   The objective of therapy of pheochromocytoma is prevention of the physiologic and metabolic effects of the catecholamines secreted by the tumor. The preferred mode of therapy is complete surgical excision of the single or multiple tumors, and this can be achieved successfully in approximately 90 per cent of the patients. In the remainder, who either have metastatic disease or are not operative candidates for reasons of serious medical complications, pharmacologic therapy can prove very effective in reversing the symptoms of the disease and markedly prolonging life. Regardless of the ultimate form of therapy, pharmacologic therapy will have to be instituted in almost every patient. Adequate control of the effects of catecholamines is necessary before surgery, because the greatest danger to the patient exists during induction of anesthesia and in-

traoperative manipulations, when life-threatening or lethal rises in blood pressure and arrhythmias may occur as a result of tumor stimulation. Two categories of adrenergic blocking drugs are useful in such cases: those which competitively block the peripheral effects of circulating catecholamines, and several still experimental drugs which have proved useful in competitively inhibiting the synthesis of the catecholamines by the tumor. The competitive peripheral sympathetic blocking drugs may be further divided into two groups: the alpha- and beta-sympathetic blockers. The *alpha-blockers* (dibenzylene and phentolamine) compete primarily with the peripheral vasoconstrictor effects of the catecholamines, thus reducing blood pressure, and they also are effective in blocking the alpha-mediated inhibition of insulin release. Dibenzylene (phenoxybenzamine) is a very long-acting drug which may be administered orally once or twice daily. The usual dose range necessary for the control of most patients is from 20 to 100 mg per day. Occasional patients may require larger doses. The onset of action is rapid, and maximal effect from a single dose is usually achieved in one to two hours. Phentolamine, although also available in an oral dose form, is primarily used intravenously because of its short duration of action. Aside from its use in the diagnostic vasodepressor test, phentolamine is primarily useful as acute adjunctive therapy to control severe hypertensive crises during surgery. Again, it should be noted that patients whose tumors produce significant amounts of epinephrine may produce exaggerated hypotensive responses to alpha-blockers.

The only *beta-sympathetic blocker* available for use in the United States at this time is propranolol. Its primary salutary effect is as a specific antagonist of the catecholamine-induced arrhythmias and tachycardia, although it is not usually suggested for use for the latter condition unless the pulse rate is above the range of 110 to 120 beats per minute. Propranolol may be administered either orally or intravenously. Patients with pheochromocytoma are extremely sensitive to its effects, because its use in this condition for disturbances of cardiac rate and rhythm is specifically related to the causative agent (excess of catecholamine stimulation), unlike other instances in which the drug may be used. Oral doses of 5 to 10 mg every six hours are frequently sufficient to reduce heart rate and abolish arrhythmias. During surgery, doses in the range of 0.5 to 2.0 mg may be used intravenously to control arrhythmias when they present a danger or produce adverse hemodynamic effects. Because of the negative inotropic effects of this drug, it must be used with caution, especially in patients who have catecholamine cardiomyopathy and who may be thrown into severe congestive failure by very small doses. Paradoxical rises in blood pressure are usually produced when beta-blockers, such as propranolol, are administered to patients whose tumors produce epinephrine. Under these circumstances, the drug blocks the beta-mediated vasodilatation which occurs primarily in muscle vasculature, thus producing a net increase in peripheral resistance by converting epinephrine pharmacologically into norepinephrine ("epinephrine reversal"). Both types of adrenergic blockers are effective in reducing the sweating and hypermetabolism associated with this condition.

In contrast to the selective effects produced by the adrenergic blocking drugs, experimental competitive inhibitors of the rate-limiting step in catecholamine synthesis, the conversion of tyrosine to dopa (catalyzed by the enzyme tyrosine hydroxylase), produce a panoramic effect, because all catecholamine actions are reduced in proportion to the inhibition of hormone synthesis. To date, the most effective of these experimental drugs has proved to be the tyrosine analogue alpha-methyl-para-tyrosine. In doses of 2.0 to 4.0 grams per day, this drug has resulted in inhibition of catecholamine synthesis by as much as 85 to 90 per cent and essentially complete reversal of all the deleterious effects of the tumor. Limitations in its use have been the production of sedation and diarrhea in some patients and the very low solubility of the drug in urine so that patients receiving larger doses have developed evidence of crystalluria. Despite these shortcomings and its lack of general availability, this drug appears to be the pharmacologic treatment of choice for pheochromocytoma.

After control of the physiologic abnormality produced by the pheochromocytoma, the patient may be explored. Successful surgery depends on a concerted and prearranged team effort, comprising the surgeon, anesthetist, and internist-pharmacologist. The procedure is greatly facilitated by constant electronic monitoring of blood pressure and the electrocardiogram so that appropriate use of blocking drugs may be made to counter any sudden changes in pressure or rhythm. Drugs to control catecholamine effects in the preoperative management of the patient should not be discontinued prior to the day of surgery, and the fear that they may produce untoward effects during surgery appears to be unsubstantiated. Preanesthetic medications should be limited to sedation the evening before surgery, but the use of atropine or other anticholinergic drugs as a routine may present problems because of the tachycardia produced by these compounds. Satisfactory anesthesia has been achieved with combinations of nitrous oxide and ether, as well as with the use of the newer halogenated hydrocarbon gases. Halothane has proved especially useful because it blocks the alpha-adrenergic vasoconstriction. In common with other halogenated hydrocarbons, it does seem to enhance the development of cardiac arrhythmias in the presence of excessive catecholamine secretion. Cyclopropane is contraindicated for anesthesia in these patients because of its marked arrhythmic effects. Propranolol should be available for rapid intravenous administration in case serious disturbances of cardiac rhythm occur. Doses in the range of 0.5 to 2.0 mg usually suppress dangerous rhythm disturbances for sufficient periods of time to permit the tumor to be removed and the surgery to be completed. Lidocaine is also useful in this regard, but its duration of effectiveness is very short compared to that of propranolol. If hypertensive crises occur during surgery despite preoperative preparation, small doses of phentolamine (1 to 5 mg) should be given rapidly intravenously for rapid blood pressure control.

When the tumor is thought to be within the abdominal cavity, exploration should be done whenever possible through an anterior transabdominal approach, rather than by a retroperitoneal flank incision which might be a more usual procedure for an adrenal tumor. The more difficult anterior approach is advocated because of the likelihood of multiple tumors being found at the time of surgery, some of which might not be suspected after preoperative testing. This approach permits direct visualization and palpation of both adrenal glands as well as all the other common sites from which

these tumors may arise between the floor of the pelvis and the diaphragm. Even when tumors have not been located by diagnostic procedures before surgery, it is usually not difficult for the surgeon to locate small ectopic masses. Direct digital stimulation of tumor tissue, even when inapparent to the surgeon and transmitted through other organs, usually results in significant changes in cardiac rate and rhythm or blood pressure. When these occur, careful selective palpation with monitoring of vital signs will readily lead the surgeon to the tumor. Multiple and bilateral adrenal pheochromocytomas occur almost universally in patients with Sipple's syndrome, and in most instances total bilateral adrenalectomy must be performed or residual tumor tissue will be left behind (Fig. 4). However, multiple ectopic tumors must be suspected in *all* patients, and despite the removal of a large tumor, patients must be thoroughly explored to exclude other foci. Great care must be taken in the dissection of these tumor masses, because they bleed profusely when incised. In a number of instances, it appears that metastases have spread as a result of incision or rupture of a tumor and implantation of otherwise benign cells throughout the field of surgery.

After removal of all tumors, blood pressure almost invariably falls to hypotensive levels. The mechanism of this hypotension is thought to relate to persistent impairment of autonomic reflexes and not to hypovolemia. Nonetheless, all blood loss should be replaced quantitatively during the course of surgery. In anticipation of final severance of the tumor blood supply, rapid expansion of intravascular volume by the administration of plasma or plasma substitute (5 per cent albumin in normal saline) has been found most effective in sustaining a normal blood pressure at this time. This maneuver has proved much more effective than pressor drug infusions which are frequently difficult to discontinue for hours to days after surgery and have sometimes led to the demise of the patient in what was called "intractable shock." When volume expansion has been used in a large series of patients, use of pressor drugs has not been necessary, and the clinical course after removal of the tumor has been more stable.

During the first postoperative day, most patients will become hypertensive, especially in the period in which they are experiencing pain as they emerge from the effect of anesthesia. The usual cause of this hypertension is a combination of the cardiovascular responses to stress and iatrogenic hypervolemia induced in the course of treatment of the hypotensive reaction. This rise in blood pressure is usually unresponsive to intravenous administration of phentolamine; although it usually diminishes rapidly over the period of the ensuing day, it may be treated with parenteral administration of a rapidly acting diuretic such as furosemide or ethacrynic acid. Other causes of postoperative hypertension include inadvertent damage to a kidney or ligation of a renal artery or one of its branches during the course of surgery, or the presence of residual pheochromocytoma tissue, persisting either as additional undiscovered benign primary tumors or as metastases. Even in the immediately postoperative patient, a radioactive renal scan may be performed relatively readily, and it should indicate any major difficulty with a kidney which might be responsible for the hypertension. When residual pheochromocytoma is suspected, postoperative urine collections should be obtained for catecholamine or metabolite assays in an attempt to determine whether the previously elevated values have returned to normal. Since most patients normally excrete increased quantities of these compounds for four to five days after surgery, the collection should be delayed until the end of the first postoperative week so that the results of the tests are interpretable. Before discharge from the hospital, all patients who have undergone surgery for pheochromocytoma should have repeat analyses to determine the adequacy of surgery. Follow-up determinations, initially at six-month and then at yearly intervals, seem adequate to exclude development of new tumors or metastases unless clinical symptoms indicate an earlier re-evaluation. When the patient has associated evidence of von Recklinghausen's disease or Sipple's syndrome, it is mandatory to extend the investigation to members of the family, especially those who are hypertensive, in an attempt to discover other cases. Even in apparently sporadic cases, hypertensive members of the family should have screening tests performed on their urine in an attempt to exclude this potentially curable form of hypertension.

In patients who cannot undergo surgery or who are not cured by surgery, prolonged therapy with either the adrenergic blocking agents or alpha-methyl-tyrosine has proved successful in controlling the signs and symptoms of the disease. This is especially important because most patients with malignant pheochromocytoma die as a result of cardiovascular catastrophes rather than because of the directly aggressive nature of the cancer. Indeed, most patients with this condition have exceedingly slow-growing tumors, and patients with documented metastases have been treated successfully for more than ten years, often without evident progression. These tumors have uniformly proved unresponsive to treatment with either high-voltage radiation or other chemotherapeutic agents.

OTHER TUMORS ARISING FROM SYMPATHETIC TISSUES

Depending upon the state of differentiation of primitive neural crest cells, sympathetic tissues may contain either immature pluripotential cells or cells which have differentiated into mature ganglion cells or adrenal medullary pheochromocytes. Tumors may arise from cell types which run the whole gamut of this differentiation. The most common are classified as ganglioneuromas or neuroblastomas, the latter originating from more primitive cell types. It is not unusual to encounter multiple cell types within any particular tumor, and the pathologic classification usually is based upon the predominant cell morphology. Although certain clinical features have been associated with the presence of these tumors (evidence of vasomotor instability, flushing, fever, and diarrhea), they generally have been considered to be nonfunctional tumors in contrast to the pheochromocytomas. However, during the past decade it has been demonstrated that these tumors not only produce catecholamines, their precursors, and metabolites, but are also capable of producing other hormones which may contribute to clinical syndromes. There appears to be some correlation between the degree of differentiation of the primary cell types of the tumor and the pattern of catechol excretion. Those which are primarily composed of immature cells tend to excrete relatively larger quantities of dopa, dopamine, and their primary metabolites, whereas the most mature tumors tend to excrete relatively greater quantities of norepinephrine and its metabolites. Regardless of the nature of the tumor, VMA and metanephrine values are almost universally increased and serve as excellent screening and diagnostic tests in confirming the diagnosis preoperatively (Fig. 7).

Ganglioneuromas are usually well encapsulated and rarely malignant. They may arise from any of the sympathetic ganglia, and they are frequently found in childhood as prominent posterior mediastinal paravertebral masses. Less commonly, they arise in the adrenal medulla or para-aortic sympathetic ganglia in the abdomen, and they also may be found in association with sympathetic ganglia in the bowel wall. This latter occurrence is especially notable among those patients with the familial inheritance of Sipple's syndrome in association with multiple cutaneous neuromas and multiple visceral ganglioneuromas. The tumor is composed of mature ganglion cells which are surrounded by connective tissue containing nerve fibers.

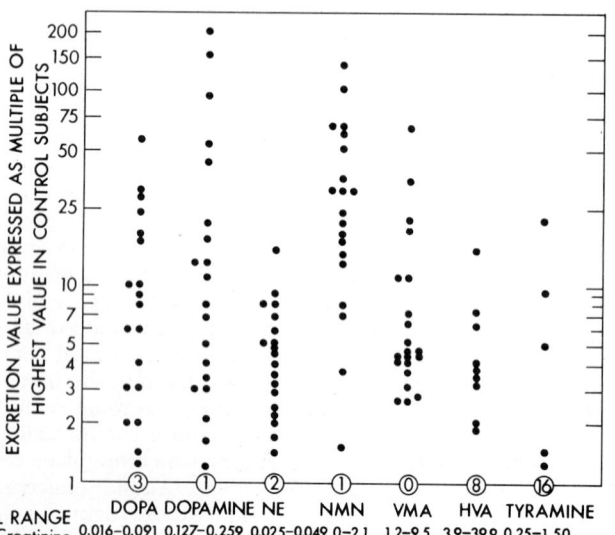

Figure 7. Excretion values for catecholamines and their precursors and metabolites in 21 patients with neuroblastoma, sympathoblastoma, and ganglioneuroma are expressed on a logarithmic scale as multiples of the highest value obtained in normal control subjects. The circled values corresponding to a multiple of 1 indicate the number of instances in which the values were normal.

Neuroblastomas are highly malignant tumors occurring during infancy and early childhood; except for Wilms' tumor, they are the most common retroperitoneal tumors in children. They arise most commonly in the adrenal medulla, but they may also develop in other sympathetic ganglia within the thorax or abdomen. They metastasize early with widespread involvement of lymph nodes, liver, bone, lung, and marrow. When the tumor is diagnosed prior to obvious metastases, the prognosis is often good, but with metastases prognosis is poor despite the extensive use of radical surgery, deep x-ray therapy, and chemotherapeutic agents. As with patients with ganglioneuroma, these patients may demonstrate marked diarrhea in addition to other systemic effects. The demonstration in these patients of very high concentrations of prostaglandins within both tumor tissue and plasma lends considerable support to the hypothesis that the gastrointestinal manifestations and flushing may be related to tumor production of these fatty acid hormones. Recent experimental evidence relating to the elaboration of increased quantities of a hormone stimulating nerve growth (nerve growth factor, NGF) has raised questions about the role of this trophic hormone in eliciting this disease. Similarly, studies on the production of tumor immunity have suggested the possibility that immune mechanisms may be developed as more effective modes of therapy.

Catalona, W. J., Engelman, K., Ketcham, A. S., and Hammond, W. G.: Familial medullary thyroid carcinoma, pheochromocytoma, and parathyroid adenoma (Sipple's syndrome), study of a kindred. Cancer, 28:1245, 1971.
Conference on the Biology of Neuroblastoma. J. Pediatr. Surg., 3: Part 2, 1968.
Cooperman, L. H., Engelman, K., and Mann, P. E. G.: Anesthetic management of pheochromocytoma employing halothane and beta-adrenergic blockade. A report of 14 cases. Anesthesiology, 28:575, 1967.
Engelman, K.: Assay of plasma catecholamines; an approach to evaluating altered sympathetic activity in essential hypertension. *In* Laragh, J. H. (ed.): Hypertension Manual. New York, Yorke Medical Books, 1973, p. 605.
Engelman, K., Horwitz, D., Ambrose, I. M., and Sjoerdsma, A.: Further evaluation of the tyramine test for pheochromocytoma. N. Engl. J. Med., 278:705, 1968.
Engelman, K., Horwitz, D., Jéquier, E., and Sjoerdsma, A.: Biochemical and pharmacologic effects of alpha-methyl-tyrosine in man. J. Clin. Invest., 47:577, 1968.
Gifford, R. W., Kvale, W. F., Maher, F. T., Roth, G. M., and Priestley, J. T.: Clinical features, diagnosis, and treatment of pheochromocytoma: A review of 76 cases. Mayo Clin. Proc., 39:281, 1964.
Regulation of catecholamine metabolism in the sympathetic nervous system (New York Heart Association Symposium). Pharmacol. Rev., 24:161, 1972.
Sandler, M., Karim, S. M., and Williams, E. D.: Prostaglandins in amine-peptide–secreting tumours. Lancet, 2:1053, 1968.
Schimke, R. N., Hartman, W. H., Brout, T. E., and Rimoin, D. L.: Syndrome of bilateral pheochromocytoma, medullary thyroid carcinoma, and multiple neuromas. N. Engl. J. Med., 279:1, 1968.
Sjoerdsma, A., Engelman, K., Waldmann, T. A., Cooperman, L. H., and Hammond, W. G.: Pheochromocytoma: Current concepts of diagnosis and treatment. Ann. Intern. Med., 65:1302, 1966.
Studnitz, W. von, Kaser, H., and Sjoerdsma, A.: Spectrum of catecholamine biochemistry in patients with neuroblastoma. N. Engl. J. Med., 269:232, 1963.

869. THE CARCINOID SYNDROME

Karl Engelman

Definition. Carcinoid tumors and the often bizarre and distinctive clinical features manifested by patients with this rare disease have been clinical and scientific enigmas for almost three quarters of a century. Tumors of the gastrointestinal tract composed of cell types now associated with carcinoid tumors had been known since the early 1800's, and were generally thought to be benign tumors of little clinical importance. In 1907, Oberndorfer postulated that these tumors were a morphologic entity, and although he thought them to be malignant tumors on the basis of their cellular appearance, he thought they behaved in a very indolent and benign manner. For this reason he coined the name "karzinoid" (carcinoma-like) to emphasize their malignant appearance but benign nature. At various times they were thought to be derivatives of autonomic nerve tissue, as well as several types of intestinal mucosal cells. Masson advanced the hypothesis in 1928 that carcinoid tumors arose from argentaffin cells (Schmidt's cells, Kulschitzky's cells) which are normal constituents of the intestinal mucosa near the base of the crypts of Lieberkühn. The term argentaffin derives from the fact that many of these cells reduce and fix certain silver salts in pathologic preparations. It was not until the early to mid-1950's that studies by Thorson, Waldenström, and others suggested that the constellation of signs and symptoms in patients harboring this tumor might be related to production of hormones. Initially, both serotonin and histamine were found in large quantities in most carcinoid tissues, and the clinical features of the patients were ascribed to production of these hormones. With time and study of an increasing number of patients, it has been necessary to revise earlier concepts on the basis of demonstrated tumor production of additional vasoactive substances such as the kinin peptides and prostaglandins. Furthermore, it is now possible to define several subsets of the originally described clinical syndrome, based on specific variants of clinical features, anatomic site of origin of the primary tumor, and the related biochemical differences in the tumors as manifested by their secretion products.

Pathology. In general, the carcinoid *syndrome* occurs only in relation to malignant tumors which have metastasized, usually with extensive hepatic implants. The most common primary tumor is a small lesion of the terminal third of the ileum, although other sites include other areas of the small and large bowel, the pulmonary bronchial tree, gastric mucosa, pancreas, common bile ducts, and ovaries. Carcinoid tumors of the appendix are rarely malignant and almost never cause the carcinoid syndrome; carcinoids of the rectum are frequently multicentric in origin, usually nonfunctional, and rarely malignant.

Diarrhea and intestinal obstruction are the most common gastrointestinal symptoms associated with carcinoid disease, but it is extremely rare that these symptoms are produced either mechanically or metabolically by the primary tumor itself. The primary tumor is often a very small, innocuous-looking lesion which can rarely be found by radiographic procedures. When the disease is diagnosed on the basis of the production of the typical syndrome, it is unusual for the primary tumor to constitute more than 1 per cent of the tumor mass in the body. Mechanical impairment of gastrointestinal tract continuity and function is usually attributable either to local sclerosing metastases in the bowel wall which kink and obstruct the bowel or to extensive mesenteric lymph node metastases which eventually sclerose and coalesce to shorten the mesentery and impair the blood supply of the bowel. At its end-stages, the bowel often has the appearance of a parachute in which the shrouds have been pulled tightly toward the center so that the loops of small bowel are kinked, narrowed, and usually relatively fixed in position at a central retroperitoneal point. Contributing to this process is an unusual proliferation of fibrous tissue which is one of the yet unexplained unusual manifestations of the carcinoid syndrome. Other areas in which dense fibrosis may occur—entirely without evidence of local tumor growth—include peritoneal and pleural surfaces and the endocardium of the heart chambers and heart valves. When there is extensive involvement of the peritoneal surfaces, retroperitoneal and pelvic fibrosis may result in obstruction of urinary drainage and simulate retroperitoneal fibrosis (see Ch. 107). One of the original reports of this disease described a pelvic examination in a woman with longstanding carcinoid syndrome. By both rectal and pelvic manipulation the entire pelvic floor was described as absolutely fixed by rock-hard tissue, with the examiner commenting: "it was as though one placed one's hand into a plaster of Paris cast of the pelvic organs." At autopsy the hard mass was found to be dense fibrous tissue and not tumor.

Other fibrotic lesions with considerable clinical significance involve the endocardial aspects of the heart and associated great vessels. Minimal to massive fibrotic proliferation occurs mainly on the right side of the heart and involves the valvular surfaces as well as the endocardium of the heart chambers. Lesser degrees of involvement on the left side of the heart occur under circumstances of longstanding carcinoid syndrome, but they occur earlier in patients who have primary bronchial lesions and when there is an atrial septal defect with a right-to-left intracardiac shunt. Pathologically, the distribution of the fibrosis is distinctive and readily differentiated from that which occurs with the more common endomyocardial fibroelastosis and generalized myocardial fibrosis. The unique features of this fibrotic lesion are that it does not disrupt the internal elastic lamina of the myocardial and heart valves and that the fibrosis appears in apposition to the endocardial surface. There is a peculiar predilection for fibrosis on the underside of the heart valves, upstream from the blood flow (i.e., on the ventricular surface of the tricuspid valve and the pulmonary arterial surface of the pulmonic valve). Initially, the predominant functional lesion produced by this fibrotic process is valvular stenosis followed by valvular insufficiency.

The peculiar and extensive fibrosis frequently observed in the carcinoid syndrome both within the cardiovascular system and on peritoneal surfaces remains unexplained. Several lines of evidence indicate that serotonin may be implicated in this feature of the syndrome. When introduced into fibroblast tissue culture, serotonin results in marked stimulation of cellular growth and fiber production. Furthermore, the serotonin antagonist methysergide, used in treatment of migraine headache, occasionally causes extensive retroperitoneal fibrosis with ureteral obstruction. More recently, Graham has reported that chronic methysergide therapy may also produce endocardial and valvular lesions indistinguishable from that of the carcinoid disease, lending further support to the hypothesis that these lesions may be related in some way to serotonin metabolism.

Clinical Manifestations. The carcinoid syndrome, because of its variable clinical features, is frequently undiagnosed for many years after the initial onset of symptoms. The clinical features may be considered in relation to the organ systems involved.

Vasomotor. One of the cardinal features of the carcinoid syndrome is *flushing,* chiefly occurring over the face and neck and in sun-exposed areas. The onset of flushing may be sudden and may range from a bright red to a violaceous hue. Facial and periorbital edema, tachycardia, hypotension, and pulmonary and gastrointestinal symptoms frequently accompany a flush. Black patients, in whom the change in color may be less apparent, frequently report a feeling of warmth or intense heat, and vascular dilatation is usually very apparent in the bulbar conjunctivae. Certain distinctive features of the flush, including anatomic distribution, temporal relationships, and color, vary with the anatomic site of the primary tumor (see Variant Syndromes, below). Precipitating stimuli include ingestion of food and especially alcohol, pain, physical activity, and emotional upset. In common with the finding that emotional stimuli resulting in sympathetic nervous system activation induce flushing, studies have shown that small doses of intravenous catecholamines, especially those with alpha-sympathetic activity, are potent flush-provoking agents. Although this phenomenon has been proposed as a diagnostic test for the carcinoid syndrome, the associated hypotension or shock produced by the massive flushing reaction may be life threatening to the patient, and the use of this pharmacologic test is not to be encouraged. When patients have experienced flushing for several years, they usually develop fixed cutaneous changes in the areas in which flushing occurs. These changes include the development of multiple fine telangiectasias and a fixed purple hue, usually over the malar areas, the nose, the upper lip, and the chin. The findings are somewhat like the malar telangiectasia which develops in patients with longstanding mitral stenosis.

Gastrointestinal. Recurrent attacks of mild to explosive diarrhea, abdominal pain, bloating, and severe tenesmus are common. Frequently, the loose bowel movements and symptoms of hypermotility, especially when mild, are misdiagnosed for years as functional bowel disease. Nausea and vomiting may also develop, especially in association with evidence of small bowel obstruction. Right upper quadrant tenderness is common, and when hepatic metastases grow to massive size an additional feature may be the episodic development of severe right upper quadrant pain, fever, right shoulder pain, leukocytosis, and all the features of an acute abdomen. Although the diagnosis of a perforated abdominal viscus must be entertained and evaluated, most commonly these features represent hemorrhage and necrosis within tumor which seems to have outgrown its blood supply with resultant peritonitis. Treated conservatively with small bowel suction and other supportive measures, the patient may be sustained during a period of a week to ten days, during which the entire syndrome evolves and disappears. Surgery for this condition is rarely necessary. *Peptic ulcer disease* also appears to occur more commonly in patients with carcinoid syndrome than in the general population.

Cardiopulmonary. Blood pressure in patients with carcinoid syndrome is usually normal or low, especially during flushing attacks when severe *hypotension* and even life-threatening shock may occur. *Hypertension* has rarely been found in association with the carcinoid syndrome, despite the widely held clinical impression that this is a feature of the disease. Although experience with functioning bronchial carcinoids is limited, this variant of the carcinoid syndrome may be an exception, because a significant number of these patients have been found to be mildly to moderately hypertensive. Cardiac involvement (see Pathology, above) is a progressive complication which occurs late in the disease. In general, as a result of the predominantly right-sided lesions, evidence of right-sided congestive heart failure becomes a serious problem and a common cause of death. Edema as a result of these cardiac diseases may be enhanced by hypoproteinemia which commonly results from severe diarrhea, protein loss, and replacement of liver by tumor. Auscultatory evidence of pulmonic stenosis and tricuspid stenosis and insufficiency can usually be demonstrated in patients with long-standing carcinoid disease. Murmurs indicating left-sided heart involvement are less common, except in patients with bronchial carcinoid or atrial septal defect. Pulmonary symptoms caused by primary heart failure are rare except in those with predominently left-sided lesions, but bronchospasm and wheezing in association with flushing attacks are seen in 20 to 30 per cent of the patients. In some instances this may be indistinguishable from bronchial asthma, and the use of glyceryl guaiacolate–containing expectorants may further complicate diagnosis by yielding false positive tests for urinary serotonin metabolites (see Diagnosis, below).

Nutritional. Chronic weight loss, often unremitting and leading to cachexia, may be attributed not only to the catabolic effects of the tumor, but also to the severe diarrhea frequently resulting in malabsorption syndromes. Satisfactory control of the diarrhea is usually beneficial with regard to both the sense of well-being and the development of positive nitrogen balance. Patients with far-advanced carcinoid disease with extensive metastases sometimes develop the signs and symptoms of pellagra, including dementia and typical skin lesions in sun-exposed areas. The development of niacin deficiency has a dual etiology. First, patients with poor nutrition have a decreased intake of niacin and its amino acid precursor, tryptophan. Second, the carcinoid tumor which effectively forms 5-hydroxyindole compounds from tryptophan diverts dietary tryptophan from the kynurenine–nicotinic acid pathway to production of serotonin and its metabolites (see Chemistry, below).

Malignant carcinoid tumors have also been associated with a variety of ectopic hormone production syndromes. The bronchogenic tumors have been more commonly associated with peptide hormone synthesis than have the ileal or other tumors. In addition to the production of prostaglandins and 5-hydroxyindole compounds, excessive ectopic production of parathyroid hormone, gonadotrophins, ACTH, insulin, and probably growth hormone have all been documented.

Chemistry. The biochemical hallmark of malignant carcinoid tumors is excessive production of *5-hydroxyindole compounds*. The biosynthetic pathway for these is illustrated in Figure 8. The essential amino acid tryptophan is hydroxylated to 5-hydroxytryptophan (5-HTP) by the enzyme tryptophan hydroxylase, the rate-limiting step in serotonin synthesis. Within the tumor (except

Figure 8. Synthesis and metabolism of serotonin.

in gastric carcinoid—see below) the 5-HTP is further metabolized to serotonin (5-HT), its pharmacologically active metabolite. Small quantities of serotonin are normally produced in the body, major depots being the gastrointestinal mucosa, the brain, and the platelets. In the last-named, the serotonin is thought to be synthesized elsewhere and merely stored in the platelet granules in high concentrations as a result of an active transport process which traps the amine. Normally, less than 1 per cent of total dietary tryptophan (1000 to 1500 mg per day) is converted to 5-hydroxyindole compounds, but when very large masses of malignant carcinoid tissue are found in the body, as much as 600 to 1000 mg of 5-HIAA may be excreted in the urine daily. This may represent almost all the dietary tryptophan available to the patient, especially in those who have severe gastrointestinal symptoms, anorexia, diarrhea, and poor food intake; this accounts for the development of niacin deficiency and pellagra (see above). When the clinical condition results in the inability to eat, the urinary 5-HIAA values fall to low values only to rise after dietary tryptophan ingestion increases, thus demonstrating the limiting relationships of dietary tryptophan on niacin and serotonin synthesis. Excessive quantities of histamine may also be synthesized by carcinoid tumors, especially those of gastric origin.

Physiology. The pharmacologic effect of serotonin as a smooth muscle agonist has long been considered responsible for the hyperperistalsis, diarrhea, and bronchial constriction of the carcinoid syndrome. Although initially the serotonin was also thought to be related to the severe flushing, this hypothesis does not fit with the known effects of serotonin as a peripheral vasoconstrictor and the observations that infusions of serotonin do not reproduce these features of the syndrome. Elegant experiments and observations by Peart and co-workers demonstrated that the flushing phenomenon is indirectly mediated by sympathetic stimulation. Subsequent work by Oates and others showed that sympathetic stimulation resulted in the appearance in the blood of the kinin peptide bradykinin after catecholamine stimulation of the tumor. The catecholamines were shown to activate a tumor enzyme – kallikrein – which in its active form was capable of cleaving the decapeptide lysyl-bradykinin from a circulating α_2-globulin precursor, kininogen. After release of the decapeptide and its appearance in the hepatic vein effluent, it is converted to the potent vasoactive nonapeptide bradykinin in the plasma. Although infusions of bradykinin could reproduce the carcinoid flush, it was not possible to demonstrate increased kinin levels in some patients with more severe flushing. Subsequently, it was shown that carcinoid tumors also produced very large quantities of vasoactive fatty acid hormones, prostaglandins, which could also explain some of the flushing.

Diagnosis. As with pheochromocytoma, the diagnosis in a patient with carcinoid syndrome should be suspected on the basis of appearance of distinctive clinical features. Confirmation of the diagnosis can be achieved preoperatively by demonstration of increased 5-hydroxyindole production. Since approximately 99 per cent of serotonin infused intravenously is converted to 5-HIAA, this metabolite rather than the hormone should be measured in the urine of patients suspected of this disease. Both qualitative and quantitative tests are available for the assay of 5-HIAA in urine.

The *qualitative screening test,* as originally described by Sjoerdsma, is a simple procedure requiring only 0.2 ml of urine from any random voiding. Indole compounds in the urine are converted to colored derivatives by the addition of nitrosonaphthol reagent. After extraction with an organic solvent, the color in the aqueous layer is compared with that of a blank sample to which water was added instead of the urine sample. A positive test is indicated by the presence of a faint to deep purple color in the aqueous layer, depending upon the quantity of indole compounds present in the urine sample. Assuming a normal daily urine volume of 1000 to 1500 ml, this qualitative screening test will not be positive unless the patient is excreting 30 to 50 mg of 5-HIAA per 24 hours (Fig. 9). Thus since the upper limit of normal for 5-HIAA excretion is 9 mg per 24 hours, some patients with this disease may have a false negative screening test when their urinary 5-HIAA excretion is less than 50 mg per day total.

Although some laboratories have attempted to use the screening test in a quantitative way by determining the optical density of the aqueous supernatant in a spectrophotometer, the limitations of the assay do not permit such modification. Under these circumstances the test will commonly yield false positive results. The reason for these aberrant findings is that the nitrosonaphthol reagent will react with any indole compounds in the urine (not just 5-hydroxyindoles), and a greater apparent amount of 5-HIAA will be thus determined. However, there is a relatively simple specific *quantitative test* for 5-HIAA which employs certain modifications of the screening test and which will yield accurate absolute results. The complete 24-hour urine collection, rather than a random urine sample, is required for this deter-

mination, because the calculation of 5-HIAA excretion will now be based upon its total content in the sample as opposed to relative concentrations in a single voided sample. Certain dietary precautions must be taken. Food which contains large quantities of serotonin (bananas, pineapples, walnuts, red plums, avocados) must be restricted from the diet or 5-HIAA excretion will be increased spuriously. In addition, drugs such as mephenesin and especially cough preparations containing glyceryl guaiacolate (see Cardiopulmonary, above) yield metabolites which result in color formation, producing false positive tests by both the qualitative and quantitative assays. Phenothiazines, frequently used for the prevention or treatment of flushing, interfere with the test reaction, reducing the color yield, and could produce false negative tests. Patients with malignant carcinoid usually excrete 5-HIAA in the range of 50 to 500 mg daily. Rare patients will excrete values closer to the upper limit of normal, and these must be distinguished from certain patients with nontropical sprue who have been known to have moderately elevated (10 to 15 mg per 24 hours) 5-HIAA excretions.

Except in a peculiar variant of the carcinoid syndrome in which 5-HTP is the primary product of tumor secretion (see Gastric Tumor, below) urinary serotonin is rarely increased significantly, because the serotonin is so readily converted to 5-HIAA. Thus in the vast majority of patients with carcinoid, determinations of serotonin in urine are of little value. Serotonin in the blood is carried almost exclusively in platelets, and in most patients with carcinoid syndrome total blood or platelet serotonin is high, but these determinations are not diagnostic and should not be part of the general workup. Bidirectional paper chromatography of urinary indole compounds may be a useful adjunct to determining the specific biochemistry of carcinoid tumors. This procedure is readily done in most research biochemistry laboratories. In patients with gastric or other 5-HTP–producing tumors, increased quantities of serotonin and 5-HTP may be demonstrated as well as large increases of 5-HIAA.

Histologic confirmation of the diagnosis may be obtained by biopsy of the primary tumor or metastases. However, the constellation of the typical clinical features, increased 5-HIAA excretion in the urine, and demonstration of metastases – especially to the liver by indirect means such as physical examination, abnormal liver enzyme levels, abnormal liver scan, and evidence of other distant metastases – is usually sufficient to confirm the diagnosis without invasive procedures such as exploration or liver biopsy. This may be especially important because of the limitation of treatment of the patient and the probability of intra-abdominal complications requiring future surgery (see Prognosis and Therapy, below).

Variant Syndromes. *Ileal Tumor ("Classic Carcinoid Syndrome").* The majority of patients with carcinoid syndrome have a primary tumor on the terminal portion of the ileum metastatic to the liver, producing typical symptoms of flushing, diarrhea, valvular heart disease, and, in a significant minority of patients, asthmatic attacks. Flushing is usually episodic with a red to cyanotic coloration (Fig. 10). Duration of flushing varies from 1 to 30 minutes, and in patients with more advanced disease it may be relatively constant. Right-sided heart lesions and right-sided heart failure predominate. 5-Hydroxyindoles in the urine appear almost

Fig. 9

Fig. 10

Fig. 11

Fig. 12

Figure 9. Qualitative screening test for carcinoid (tubes, left to right): carcinoid patient excreting approximately 200 mg 5-HIAA per day; color reaction in normal subject taking 15 ml cough preparation containing glyceryl guaiacolate on the previous day; normal urine; and the same urine to which had been added 5-HIAA to give the final concentration noted on each tube. The color of a positive test is first detected visually at a 5-HIAA concentration of approximately 50 mg per liter.

Figure 10. Classic or ileal carcinoid flush.

Figure 11. Bronchial carcinoid flush.

Figure 12. Gastric carcinoid flush.

exclusively as 5-HIAA. Metastases to regional mesenteric lymph nodes with massive involvement of the liver always occur prior to the onset of typical clinical symptoms; metastasis to bone or other peripheral tissues is rare. Abdominal pain, especially in association with intestinal obstruction, is common, and irremediable intra-abdominal mechanical lesions or resistant right-sided heart failure are usually the causes of death.

Bronchial Tumor. Carcinoid tumors of the bronchial tree are generally nonfunctioning and are removed after incidental finding of a solitary pulmonary lesion. Rarely, when systemic signs and symptoms are produced by this tumor, there are a number of unique clinical features which distinguish it from the usual ileal tumor syndrome. The most important is the nature of the flushing episodes. With functioning bronchial carcinoids, the flushes are a livid red, and they are of devastating severity, frequently lasting for hours to days. Hypotension is common during severe flushes, often resulting in oliguria or anuria, and patients may have to be treated acutely with intravenous volume-expanding fluids and large doses of glucocorticoids in an attempt to abort the attack and to sustain the circulation. Marked chemosis, tearing, nasal discharge, and excessive salivation are fairly constant concomitants. During the intense flushes patients frequently develop swelling of the entire face, and, unlike other carcinoid flushes, this flush may involve most of the body. Left-sided cardiac lesions may develop, along with or before right-sided lesions. As with the ileal variant, systemic symptoms rarely occur without distant metastases, especially in the liver. In common with other carcinoids derived from embryologic foregut areas (stomach, bile duct, and pancreas), metastases to bone are common, and they are frequently osteoblastic in nature. Biochemically, these tumors may produce both serotonin and 5-HTP, so the pattern of urinary 5-hydroxyindole excretion products may more closely resemble that of the gastric carcinoid variant (see below). In addition, other endocrine syndromes may be produced by these tumors, most notably Cushing's syndrome resulting from ACTH production by the tumor. In contrast to other forms of the carcinoid syndrome, between flushing attacks these patients have a tendency to be hypertensive. Headaches are also prominent in contrast to other carcinoid variants, and marked enlargement of lacrimal, parotid, and submaxillary and submandibular salivary glands may develop with time. Patients who survive the disease for several years tend to develop thickening and creasing of the skin about the face and forehead. Rhinophyma is prominent, and the fixed, thickened, hard skin folds of the upper face and forehead lend the semblance of "leonine facies" (Fig. 11). It is notable that Graham has recently observed that patients with longstanding migraine headaches, a disease postulated to be related to an abnormality of serotonin metabolism, develop the same peculiar facial features.

Gastric Tumor. The syndrome associated with primary tumors of gastric origin is distinctive from other carcinoid syndromes in both clinical and biochemical features. The flush is characterized by raised, wheal-like lesions of a reddish-brown coloration with variegated borders (Fig. 12). These lesions may occur on any part of the body and frequently are migratory, sometimes involving the palms and soles where they may become intensely pruritic. Metabolic products of these tumors also differ from the other varieties. Oates

and Sjoerdsma, acting on the previous suggestions by Sandler and Waldenström, were able to demonstrate in a patient with gastric carcinoid that although the major 5-hydroxyindole excretion product was 5-HIAA, this constituted only about 60 per cent of the total 5-hydroxyindoles in the urine as opposed to more than 99 per cent in the usual carcinoid patient. Studies by bidirectional paper chromatography of small samples of the urine revealed excretion of large quantities of serotonin and 5-HTP. Quantitatively, the serotonin comprised 25 per cent of the total and the 5-HTP, 17 per cent. These workers suggested that the tumor was incapable of decarboxylating 5-HTP to serotonin (see Fig. 8) and that 5-HTP was the secretion product of the tumor. The explanation for the subsequent metabolism of the 5-HTP to serotonin, and eventually to 5-HIAA, was that the 5-HTP was further decarboxylated in peripheral tissues by this fairly ubiquitous enzyme. The serotonin formed in tissues other than the kidney would be quantitatively metabolized to 5-HIAA, and the serotonin synthesized in the kidney itself would be the primary source of the great increase in urinary serotonin. Subsequent studies in which 5-HTP was infused into noncarcinoid patients resulted in the same excretion pattern of 5-hydroxyindoles found in the gastric carcinoid syndrome. This lent substantial indirect evidence in support of the original hypothesis, and our subsequent demonstration of the absence of the enzyme aromatic-L-amino acid decarboxylase in a gastric carcinoid tumor fully confirmed it. In addition, Oates and Sjoerdsma demonstrated much increased urinary excretion of histamine in two patients with the carcinoids, whereas this finding was uncommon in other patients with the carcinoid syndrome. The unique pruritic, wheal-like flushing which occurs with the gastric carcinoid may therefore be related to histamine production.

"Noncarcinoid" Tumor. Typical features of the carcinoid syndrome may occur with what are considered to be noncarcinoid tumors. Most common among these is *medullary carcinoma of the thyroid* (see Pheochromocytoma, above, and Ch. 843) which, in addition to producing calcitonin, has also been shown to produce increased quantities of prostaglandins and serotonin. Carcinoid-like flushing and multiple watery bowel movements may be common features in patients with these tumors, especially when the primary thyroid tumors are very large or when there are multiple metastases. Urinary 5-HIAA values as high as 300 to 600 mg per 24 hours have been recorded, although usually the values are little, if at all, increased. As yet, there have been no reports of extensive fibrotic lesions in the endocardium and other tissues in association with the medullary thyroid carcinoma. *Tumors of ovarian origin* have also been implicated in this syndrome. Usually these arise from ovarian teratomas and differ from other carcinoid variants in that all the typical symptoms of ileal carcinoid as well as fibrotic thickening of endocardium and mesothelial cavity linings may occur, but notably without metastases in the liver or other organs. It is argued that this is probably related to the fact that the venous drainage of the tumors is not via the portal system; thereby tumor products are introduced directly into the general circulation. This could explain the otherwise universal finding that abdominal carcinoids do not produce systemic symptoms until extensive hepatic metastases have developed.

Tumors of the common bile duct or pancreatic islets may produce biochemical and clinical features of the carcinoid syndrome. In common with other carcinoid tumors of embryologic foregut origin (bronchial and gastric), these tend to produce both 5-HTP and serotonin. In addition, it is predominantly foregut tumors which are associated with ectopic production of other polypeptide hormones. Because of the similarity of the biochemical and clinical features of many of the tumors producing the carcinoid syndrome, there has been growing acceptance of the hypothesis that all these tumors arise from cells of similar embryologic anlage with pluripotential endocrine function, and the nature of the hormone production may depend on the state of derepression of the cellular genetic material in any given tumor.

Prognosis and Therapy. Patients with malignant carcinoid syndrome frequently have symptoms for at least several years before the diagnosis is made, and it is not unusual for them to survive for 10 to 15 years after the initial diagnosis. The course is frequently characterized by spontaneous remissions and exacerbations, although the over-all status progresses slowly and inexorably. With proper nutritional and pharmacologic therapy, and with the exercise of surgical restraint, these patients can usually be carried for long periods of time before they succumb to cardiac or hepatic failure or to complications of mechanical obstruction in the gastrointestinal tract. Above all, it must be understood by the physician, the patient, and his family that this must be considered a chronic disease, and the diagnosis of malignancy, even with widespread hepatic metastases, does not carry with it the dire immediate implications of other bowel tumors with similar distribution. Because the patients frequently suffer periods of severe pain, often requiring hospitalization for days to weeks, the physician must enlist the aid, cooperation, and understanding of the patient in his care. In view of the expected protracted course and its inevitable outcome, the psychologic aspects of patient care are extremely important and may prove most taxing for the physician.

Except in rare instances in which a primary bronchial or ovarian tumor may cause symptoms of the carcinoid syndrome in the absence of metastases, patients cannot be cured by surgery. Indeed, in the usual ileal case the eventual clinical course of the patient may be seriously prejudiced by an attempt to remove large segments of small bowel and its attached mesentery in an attempt to remove as much tumor as possible from the abdominal cavity. Not uncommonly in such instances, patients who have had tolerable or controllable diarrhea prior to surgery develop problems of malnutrition and fluid and electrolyte loss postoperatively owing to marked increase in the number and magnitude of watery bowel movements. This change in the course of the disease may be attributable to decreased bowel area for absorption of nutrients, fluid, and electrolytes. Resection of the distal ileum also compromises the enterohepatic circulation of bile salts which in themselves may constitute a potent cathartic if increased quantities are permitted to enter the large bowel by virtue of the loss of the terminal small bowel where they usually are reabsorbed. If a patient is explored for diagnostic reasons or to attempt to remedy an area of small bowel obstruction, the surgeon should carry out the minimal resection necessary to restore continuity. It may be necessary on several occasions to resort to surgery to relieve areas of obstruction. Frequently, the most effective measures to be employed are to create one or several enteroenterostomies to bypass areas of obstruction while retaining as much absorptive surface of small bowel as is possible. Hypotension, especially during surgery, is a serious problem in patients with carcinoid disease and requires special consideration of the pharmacology of vasopressor substances. Most sympathomimetic pressor drugs produce *paradoxical hypotension* in patients with carcinoid syndrome because of their ability to induce flushing and severe peripheral vasodilatation via the activation of tumor kallikrein and bradykinin synthesis. Only two vasopressor compounds—methoxamine (Vasoxyl) and angiotensin II (Hypertensin)—may be used safely. Prophylactic treatment with corticosteroids may prevent flushes by endogenous sympathetic mechanisms, and thus hypotensive episodes may be minimized during the operation.

The results of chemotherapy and irradiation have generally been unrewarding in patients with the carcinoid syndrome regardless of the site of origin. In common with many other slow-growing tumors, this condition seems to be unresponsive to these forms of treatment. Isolated reports of temporary responses to *cyclophosphamide* (Cytoxan), *methotrexate, phenylalanine mustard,* or oral administration or hepatic artery perfusion with *5-fluorouracil* or *cytosine arabinoside* (Cytosar) have also been rarely useful. More recent enthusiasm for the use of *streptozotocin* has also appeared to be ill substantiated when examined critically. Since few of these cases respond favorably to single or multiple doses of chemotherapeutic agents, the most common effect of such therapy is to further exacerbate the disease and produce the complications frequently associated with the use of these drugs in other conditions. In many instances the death of patients has been hastened by use of cytotoxic drugs.

Nonetheless, significant control of some of the clinical complications of the carcinoid syndrome may be achieved by other pharmacologic agents which do not directly affect tumor growth. Basic to all therapy is the maintenance of adequate nutrition with vitamin supplementation, especially of niacin (see Chemistry, above) and other vitamins. Although low roughage diets are commonly suggested for patients with chronic diarrheal states, modification of food intake does not uniformly provide relief for patients with the carcinoid syndrome. Frequently, the patient's own experience is best relied upon, and it is suggested that he be permitted to select foods which seem not to exacerbate his symptoms.

Flushing attacks may be controlled or diminished by the use of *antiadrenergic drugs* and those which have antikinin properties. Phenothiazine compounds which have alpha-adrenergic blocking activity, such as prochlorperazine (Compazine), 5 to 10 mg, or chlorpromazine (Thorazine), 25 to 50 mg, orally every six hours, may be helpful in reducing the incidence of flushing, and the alpha-adrenergic blocker dibenzyline in a dose of 10 to 50 mg daily may prove very effective. Beta-sympathetic blocking drugs have no effect on the flushing. Naturally, reducing the intake of alcohol and other known stimulants to flushing may reduce the need for prophylactic and therapeutic use of other drugs. Only in the most extreme cases should glucocorticoids be used for the treatment of flushing. Their use (10 to 40 mg of prednisone per day) should be reserved for unusually severe and protracted periods of flushing which may occur at times in the ileal carcinoid syndrome, usually in association with necrosis of liver metastases, or for those patients with bronchial carcinoids whose continuous flushing may be life threatening. In the latter instance it is frequently necessary to use suppressive doses of steroids chronically, thus subjecting the patient to the added morbidity associated with hyperadrenocorticism.

Diarrhea and tenesmus are best treated with the use of conventional antidiarrheal drugs, sometimes in association with specific serotonin antagonists. Belladonna alkaloids, camphorated tincture of opium (paregoric), or kaolin- and pectin-containing compounds may prove useful early in the disease for those who have mild diarrhea, but in most patients more potent agents are required. The most generally useful drugs in the treatment of severe diarrhea are the more concentrated opium alkaloids such as diphenoxylate (Lomotil), 1 or 2 tablets every three or four hours, or tincture of opium, 6 to 20 drops every three to four hours. When patients have many daily bowel movements, it is usually desirable to administer these on a regular schedule rather than on a demand basis. If diarrhea does not respond to these more conservative measures, the specific serotonin antagonists cyproheptadine (Periactin), 4 to 12 mg every six hours, or methysergide (Sansert), 2 to 4 mg three to four times daily, may be tried. Use of the latter, even though often successful, is to be discouraged because of the severe complications relating to both fluid retention and the development of fibrotic lesions of the retroperitoneal area, heart valves, and other tissues which are known to be a complication of its use and which would be presumed to be accelerated in a patient with the carcinoid syndrome. In patients with the gastric carcinoid syndrome, the use of methyldopa (Aldomet), 250 to 500 mg every six to eight hours, has been found uniquely useful in reducing the diarrhea. The effect of the drug in this circumstance is by its activity as an aromatic-L-amino acid decarboxylase inhibitor which reduces the peripheral conversion of the tumor product 5-HTP to serotonin. An undesirable side effect of the methyldopa in these patients would be the associated reduction of blood pressure in what is usually already a hypotensive state. Although there have been no reports to date of the use of alpha-methyldopa hydrazine (Carbidopa) for this purpose, this would seem to be a more desirable and effective drug to achieve these effects. Currently, this compound is being used as an adjunct to L-dopa therapy in Parkinson's disease (see Ch. 365). Since the drug does not produce hypotension, it should be more effective in treatment and produce fewer complications. For patients whose diarrhea is exacerabated by resection of small bowel with resultant bile salt–enhanced diarrhea, oral cholestyramine (Sequestran), 4 to 8 grams every six hours, may prove useful by its ability to bind and inactivate the bile salts.

It has been thought that the diarrhea in the carcinoid syndrome is due to excessive serotonin production. The most direct evidence has been demonstration that specific inhibition of serotonin synthesis has resulted in reduction of diarrhea with little effect on flushing or other manifestations. Although the effect of decarboxylase inhibition with methyldopa may prove successful in the gastric variant syndrome, this mode of therapy has not generally proved effective in the majority of tumors which produce serotonin. Discovery of a specific inhibitor of the enzyme tryptophan hydroxylase, the rate-limiting step in serotonin synthesis, has provided the opportunity to test this hypothesis. Parachlorophenylalanine, when administered in doses of up to 3 grams daily, has proved uniquely successful in reducing 5-hydroxyindole production by as much as 90 per cent while concomitantly producing reduction or complete remission of diarrhea. Other manifestations of the syndrome do not seem to have been affected by this therapy. Unfortunately, a majority of patients using it for more than six weeks develop allergic reactions, and then its use must be discontinued. Nonetheless, it offers the hope that a compound with similar mechanism of action may be discovered which will prove effective in symptomatic treatment.

Adamson, A. R., Peart, W. S., Grahame-Smith, D. G., and Starr, M.: Pharmacological blockage of carcinoid flushing provoked by catecholamines and alcohol. Lancet, 2:293, 1969.
Engelman, K., Lovenberg, W., and Sjoerdsma, A.: Inhibition of serotonin synthesis by parachlorophenylalanine in patients with the carcinoid syndrome. N. Engl. J. Med., 277:1103, 1967.
Graham, J. R.: Cardiac and pulmonary fibrosis during methysergide therapy for headache. Am. J. Med. Sci., 254:23, 1967.
Melmon, K. L., Sjoerdsma, A., and Mason, D. T.: Distinctive clinical and therapeutic aspects of syndromes associated with bronchial carcinoid tumors. Am. J. Med., 39:568, 1965.
Oates, J. A., and Sjoerdsma, A.: A unique syndrome associated with secretion of 5-hydroxytryptophan by metastatic gastric carcinoid. Am. J. Med., 32:333, 1962.
Peart, W. S., Robertson, J. I. S., and Andrews, T. M.: Facial flushing produced in patients with carcinoid syndrome by intravenous adrenaline and noradrenaline. Lancet, 2:715, 1959.
Roberts, W. C., and Sjoerdsma, A.: The cardiac disease associated with carcinoid syndrome (carcinoid heart disease). Am. J. Med., 36:5, 1964.
Sandler, M.: The role of 5-hydroxyindoles in the carcinoid syndrome. In Garattini, S., and Shore, P. A. (eds.): Advances in Pharmacology. Vol. 6, Part B (Biological role of indolealkylamine derivatives: Pharmacology, behavior, and clinical aspects). New York, Academic Press, 1968, p. 127.
Sandler, M., Karim, S. M. M., and Williams, E. D.: Prostaglandins in amine-peptide–secreting tumors. Lancet, 2:1053, 1968.
Torvick, A.: Carcinoid syndrome in a primary tumour of the ovary. Acta Pathol., 48:81, 1960.

870. ENDOCRINE SYNDROMES ASSOCIATED WITH CANCER

Nicholas P. Christy

Neoplasms are often associated with systemic symptoms and signs not explained by local spread or distant metastases. Extreme cachexia in the presence of a small nonmetastatic tumor and glucose intolerance, more often subtle than obvious, are familiar. Many other examples, involving various systems, can be cited (Table 1). These have been observed in all classes of neoplasms: carcinomas, sarcomas, lymphomas, and leukemias. It is not yet possible to ascribe all these effects to humoral agents elaborated by the tumors, although many substances have been postulated, including bradykinin, kallikrein, and others.

There are now plausible humoral explanations for well-defined endocrine syndromes associated with cancer (Table 2). The weight of evidence is that the tumors themselves, although not arising from glandular tissue, secrete and release substances with the

TABLE 1.   Remote Systemic Manifestations of Nonmetastatic Cancer*

Syndrome	Site of Tumor	Humoral Agent Shown to Be Secreted by Tumor
Dermatologic		
Acanthosis nigricans	Breast, colon, lung, stomach	
Dermatitis herpetiformis	Breast, lymphomas, ovary, stomach, uterus	
Dermatomyositis (over age 40)	Breast, lung, ovary, stomach	
Herpes zoster	Several	
Hyperpigmentation	Lung, thymus, others	MSH
Hypertrichosis	Several	
Ichthyosis	Several	
Scleroderma (over age 40)	Breast, lung, ovary, stomach	
Gastrointestinal		
Hepatomegaly without metastases	Hypernephroma	
Zollinger-Ellison syndrome	Pancreas (non-β islet cells)	Gastrin
Hematologic		
Anemia (without blood loss or infection)	Many	
Eosinophilia	Breast, colon, lymphomas, pancreas, stomach	
Erythrocytosis	Adrenal medulla, cerebellum, kidney, liver, uterus	Erythropoietin
Fibrinogen deficiency	Lung, prostate	
Hemolytic anemia	Many cancers, leukemia, lymphoma	
Intravascular coagulopathy	Many	
Leukoerythroblastic and leukemoid reactions	Breast, prostate	
Red cell aplasia	Thymus	
Thrombocytosis	Colon, Hodgkin's disease	
Metabolic		
Disturbances in protein metabolism		
Amyloidosis	Several	
Cryofibrinogenemia (bleeding, thrombosis)	Prostate, others	
Hypoalbuminemia, raised α- and γ_2-globulins	Many	
Macroglobulinemia, cryoglobulinemia, cold agglutinins	Mesothelioma, others	
Galactorrhea	Hypernephroma, lung	+†
Gynecomastia, sexual precocity	Lung, liver	+†
Hyperadrenocorticism	Lung, pancreas, thymus, others	+†
Hypercalcemia	Lung, kidney, ovary, others	+†
Hyperglycemia	Many	
Hypoglycemia	Mesoderm, liver	
Inappropriate water retention	Lung, pancreas	+†
Neurologic		
Cortical cerebellar degeneration	Breast, cervix, colon, lung, breast	
Encephalopathy	Lung, breast	
Myasthenia-like syndrome	Lung, breast	
Myelopathy	Lung, breast	
Myopathies	Lung, breast	
Peripheral neuropathy	Lung, breast	
Subacute spinocerebellar degeneration	Lung, breast	
Renal		
Membranous glomerulonephritis	Several	
Skeletal		
Digital clubbing	Lung	
Pachydermoperiostosis, acromegaloid features	Lung	
Pulmonary hypertrophic osteoarthropathy	Lung, mesothelioma of pleura	
Vascular		
Arterial thrombosis	Hypernephroma	
Carcinoid syndrome	Carcinoid of bronchus	5-Hydroxytryptophan, histamine
	Carcinoid of appendix, cecum, small intestine	5-Hydroxytryptamine (serotonin)
Marantic endocarditis	Lung, pancreas, stomach	
Venous thrombosis, thrombophlebitis	Breast, cervix, lung, ovary, pancreas	

*Data adapted from Greenberg, E., et al., Am. J. Med., 36:106, 1964; and Ross, E. J., Br. Med. J., 1:735, 1972.
†See Table 2.

biologic properties of natural hormones. There are also instances of tumors that originate in endocrine tissue but secrete the "wrong" hormone: e.g., rare cancers of the thyroid and adrenal medulla secreting ACTH, testicular tumors secreting gonadotrophin. The syndromes are not always obvious. The hyperthyroidism that accompanies choriocarcinoma (Table 2) is more chemical than clinical, and many patients with oat cell carci-

noma of the lung have laboratory evidence of hyperadrenocorticism, viz., elevated urinary and plasma 17-hydroxycorticosteroid values, exaggerated response of the latter to administrated ACTH, and abnormal diurnal variation of plasma corticoids, but do not have clinically detectable Cushing's syndrome. *The point is that there probably are associated with cancer a great many biochemical abnormalities which may turn out to*

TABLE 2. Endocrine Syndromes Associated with Cancer*

Syndrome	Hormone-Like Activity	Sites of Primary Tumor
Cushing's syndrome	ACTH	Lung (oat cell), pancreas (islet cell), thymus, thyroid, others
Dermal hyperpigmentation	α- and β-MSH	Lung (oat cell), pancreas, thymus
Galactorrhea	Prolactin	Hypernephroma
Hypercalcemia	PTH†	Lung (squamous cell), kidney, ovary, uterus, others
Hyperthyroidism	"TSH" (HCG‡)	Choriocarcinoma, embryoma of testis, hydatidiform mole, lung
Hypoglycemia	Insulin-like (not insulin)	Mesenchyme, liver, adrenal cortex, others
Inappropriate antidiuresis	ADH (vasopressin)	Lung (oat cell), cerebellum, duodenum, lymphoma
Precocious puberty, feminization	FSH, LH	Liver, lung
Precocious puberty, gynecomastia	HCG‡	Adrenal cortex, liver, pineal, testis

*Adapted from Lipsett, M. B., et al., Ann. Intern. Med., 61:733, 1964; Bower, B. F., and Gordan, G. S., Ann. Rev. Med., 16:83, 1965; Omenn, G. S., Ann. Intern. Med., 72:136, 1970; and Ross, E. J., Br. Med. J., 1:735, 1972.

†PTH = Parathyroid hormone.

‡HCG (also written hCG) = human chorionic gonadotrophin.

be useful as signals of clinically important problems. For example, lung carcinoma has been shown to secrete the placental proteins human chorionic somatomammotrophin and placental alkaline phosphatase.

The evidence that tumors secrete and release hormones is not perfect, but it is good. What is required for proof is roughly analogous to Koch's postulates as applied to the etiologic significance of a microbe. There must be (1) coexistence of tumor and an endocrine syndrome; (2) a demonstration in blood or urine of the causative hormone; (3) demonstration of large quantities of that hormone in the tumor and evidence that the hormone does not come from its "usual" glandular site; (4) ideally, demonstration in vitro of the tumor's capacity to make large amounts of the hormone; and (5) disappearance of, or definite improvement in, the endocrine syndrome upon removal of the tumor.

(1) Coexistence of neoplasms and endocrine syndromes is generally accepted; there are now many reported cases, and the syndromes are of at least 11 distinct and recognizable types (Table 2). (2) Greatly elevated concentrations of hormone activity have been shown by biologic or radioimmunoassay in blood of patients with tumors, e.g., of ACTH in association with Cushing's syndrome, gonadotrophins with precocious puberty, and erythropoietin with erythrocytosis (Table 2). One of the major imperfections in the data is that none of the hormones associated with tumors has been absolutely proved chemically to be identical with the natural product. The ACTH produced by tumors includes an ACTH similar, if not identical, to pituitary ACTH, but also N-terminal and C-terminal fragments. Tumor MSH differs in molecular weight from pituitary MSH. PTH (parathyroid hormone) of tumor origin contains a ratio of the various forms of immunoreactive PTH different from that found in hyperparathyroidism. However, the biologic behavior of some of the hormones is so nearly that of the native substance that for clinical purposes there seems no reason to doubt that many of the hormone-like materials elaborated by the tumors are nearly the same as those made by glands. (3) Very high concentrations of these hormones or hormone-like activities have been measured directly in tumors associated with endocrine syndromes, not in most other tumors: ACTH, MSH, gonadotrophins, chorionic gonadotrophin, prolactin, ADH, parathyroid hormone, glucagon, gastrin, and erythropoietin. In one case of presumed gonadotrophin-secreting bronchogenic carcinoma, secretion was proved by showing a higher concentration of FSH in the venous effluent from the tumor than in its arterial supply. With respect to ACTH, high concentrations have been found in plasma and tumor, low concentrations in the pituitary; the inference is that the tumor secretes massive amounts of ACTH, adrenocortical hyperplasia follows, and the induced hypercortisolism suppresses synthesis of ACTH by the pituitary. Similarly, several patients have had tumors containing gonadotrophin, gonadotrophinuria, and reduced pituitary gonadotrophin. (4) In one malignant thymoma associated with Cushing's syndrome, cells propagated in tissue culture continued to produce ACTH for weeks. (5) There are now many instances of cure or definite remission of endocrine syndromes after successful removal of the associated tumor. For example, Liddle et al. have reported nine surgical cures of Cushing's syndrome by removal of the "ACTH"-producing tumor. Dermal hyperpigmentation has disappeared after tumor removal in several cases of MSH-producing cancer. Radiation to a presumably ADH-secreting lung tumor has brought about temporary remission of inappropriate water retention in at least one case, and there are now several reported remissions of hypercalcemia after removal of a "parathyroid hormone"–secreting tumor. The primary role of the tumor in the secretion of the hormone is further strengthened by return of the hypercalcemia in some of these patients when the tumor recurred.

Incidence. Endocrine and metabolic disturbances associated with cancer and not attributable to metastases are not rare. In a large, unselected series of patients with proved bronchogenic carcinoma, the combined incidence of hypercalcemia, gynecomastia, inappropriate ADH secretion, and Cushing's syndrome was 8.5 per cent.

Pathogenesis. The evidence for tumor secretion and release of hormones, mostly polypeptides, is convincing. The mechanisms by which neoplastic tissue manages to synthesize complex molecules with hormonal activity are still conjectural. The prevailing view is that the neoplastic cells in a characteristic process of dedifferentiation lose certain genetic depressor mechanisms so that normally inhibited genetic information is expressed. This hypothesis now appears more tenable than the theory of the "sponge," i.e., the taking up of materials (hormones) from the circulation by the tumor. It is also conceivable that the cancer cell produces a large array of polypeptides, some of which, by chance, have an amino acid sequence capable of bringing about a recognizable biologic activity which can be measured. The matter is discussed by Ross.

Terminology. These endocrine manifestations have

been termed "ectopic," as in the "ectopic ACTH syndrome" (Liddle). The term is appropriate only when the site of the tumor presumably secreting the hormone is clearly not in the organ that ordinarily secretes that hormone, as in an oat cell carcinoma of the lung secreting ACTH, an ovarian tumor secreting parathyroid hormone-like peptide, or a pancreatic tumor secreting serotonin. The term is not appropriate in hyperthyroidism associated with "TSH"-secreting choriocarcinomas, because placental chorionic gonadotrophin has thyrotrophic properties which account for the thyroid-stimulating effects of these tumors; in erythrocytosis associated with renal carcinoma or renal cyst, because the normal kidney synthesizes an erythropoietin; or in carcinoid tumors associated with argentaffin tumors of the small intestine, because this tissue is a normal site of serotonin production.

Clinical Manifestations and Treatment (Table 2). There are practical reasons for recognizing the associations of endocrine syndromes with neoplastic disease. (1) Frequently, the endocrinopathy antedates the appearance of the tumor, and thus may serve as a diagnostic clue to neoplastic disease. (2) The endocrine disorders may be life threatening, as hypoglycemia or hypercalcemia, or severely disabling, as Cushing's syndrome, and yet amenable to palliative treatment. (3) Successful removal of tumor may cure the endocrine syndrome as well as the cancer. (4) Differences in clinical and biochemical behavior of these tumor-associated endocrinopathies from those associated with the classic glandular hyperfunctional states often make a differential diagnosis possible. The general characteristics of the tumor-associated endocrine syndromes are that the hormone is secreted in *anarchic* fashion, that is, secretion is not regulated by the normal control mechanisms; and, as indicated above, the locus of secretion is *displaced* to a site not ordinarily involved in hormonal synthesis.

The discussion that follows emphasizes comparison of the endocrine syndromes associated with cancer with the classic patterns of hormone overproduction in order to facilitate differential diagnosis.

Cushing's Syndrome. Clinically evident hypercortisolism has been observed in association with oat cell carcinomas of the lung, thymomas, noninsulin-producing islet cell tumors of the pancreas, pheochromocytomas, and tumors of the thyroid, ovary, prostate, parotid, liver, and neural tissue. A few hundred instances of this association have been reported, and subtle chemical evidence of hypercortisolism has been found in many more, especially with carcinoma of the lung (see above). Large quantities of ACTH have been thoroughly characterized in plasma and in some tumors. In isolated instances of lung and pancreatic cancer, peptides with the properties of corticotrophin-releasing factor (CRF) have been detected along with ACTH. That the capacity to synthesize ACTH may be a more general property of tumors can be inferred from the finding of Liddle et al. that about 8 per cent of unselected visceral carcinomas not associated with clinically apparent Cushing's syndrome contained considerable amounts of the hormone.

The most important point to be made about the clinical features of Cushing's syndrome associated with nonendocrine tumors is that they are often *subtle.* Patients may show the classic features, but most do not. The absence of obesity and striae is probably a function of the weight loss accompanying the cancer. Patients with all forms of Cushing's syndrome have an equal incidence of glucose intolerance and hypertension, about 90 per cent. But in the syndrome associated with tumor, the onset is faster and the sex incidence favors men, whereas the "pituitary" form of Cushing's disease and adrenal adenoma are far more common in women. Patients with the tumor-related form rarely have osteoporosis, probably because the clinical course of the tumor is short. Generalized dermal hyperpigmentation is common in the tumor form, because of the huge quantities of ACTH secreted by the cancer, or of MSH, which may also be produced in large amounts. Severe hypokalemia and weakness, as well as edema, are also more common in this form of the disease, and are best explained by the enormous quantities of cortisol secreted by the hyperplastic adrenals. Hypokalemia is not due to aldosteronism; the secretion of aldosterone is normal or low. In the other forms of Cushing's syndrome, the patients die of infection or the effects of hypertension; in the tumor form, the usual cause of death is the cancer. At necropsy, the adrenals are enormously hypertrophied, and the pituitary contains subnormal amounts of ACTH.

The laboratory evidence of hypercortisolism is definite and extreme. Plasma cortisol values (ca. 80 μg per 100 ml) and urinary 17-hydroxycorticosteroid and 17-ketogenic steroids may be ten times normal, all much higher than in the "pituitary" or adrenal adenoma forms of Cushing's syndrome. Provocative tests show autonomous cortisol secretion owing to autonomous ACTH secretion by the tumor; urinary steroids do not rise when metyrapone is given, and do not fall in response to dexamethasone. Differentiation from primary adrenocortical carcinoma, also characterized by very high steroid values, can be made by failure to find a suprarenal mass radiographically, and by measuring plasma ACTH concentration; it is very low in adrenal cancer, very high in the presence of ACTH-secreting tumor (see Ch. 850).

To recapitulate: an ACTH-secreting tumor, most likely to be in lung, thymus, or pancreas, should be suspected in any patient with subtle or borderline clinical signs of Cushing's syndrome who has lost, not gained, weight, who has weakness and severe hypokalemia, and whose plasma or urinary corticosteroid values are extremely high.

Management, ideally, is total removal of the tumor, which has been followed by remission of the Cushing's syndrome in several cases. Therefore a vigorous effort should be made to excise tumors completely; some are relatively benign, e.g., bronchial adenomas. If this is not possible, palliative x-radiation or chemotherapy of the cancer is carried out, and chemical palliation of the hyperadrenocorticism can be tried with o,p'-DDD, metyrapone, aminoglutethimide, or combinations of these drugs (see Ch. 850). If the effects of hypercortisolism, e.g., hypokalemia, are incapacitating, bilateral total adrenalectomy may be done, and has in some cases provided good relief.

Dermal Hyperpigmentation. Generalized hyperpigmentation of the skin, resembling that of Addison's disease, may occur with oat cell carcinoma of the lung, thymoma, neurogenic tumors, or tumors of the ovary, pancreas, and prostate. Raised concentrations of α-MSH and β-MSH have been measured in plasma by radioimmunoassay; most of the pigmentary effect is due to the β-MSH, which has also been found in the associated cancers. Some tumors in this group have been shown to secrete both excessive MSH and ACTH, with resulting addisonian dermal pigmentation and Cushing's syndrome. Several patients have shown disappearance or diminution of dermal pigment when tumors were successfully removed.

Gynecomastia, Precocious Puberty. About 5 per cent of male patients with lung cancer have gynecomastia, but in only a few have elevated gonadotrophin values been detected in blood or urine. Tumor types are "large cell" carcinomas, epidermoid, anaplastic, and oat cell carcinomas, and adenocarcinoma. In some of the patients with gynecomastia, raised levels of urinary estrogens have also been found, possibly a result of adrenal or testicular stimulation by gonadotrophin secreted from the tumor; in some cases, striking hypertrophic pulmonary osteoarthropathy has also been present. Its relation to gonadotrophin or estrogen excess is not yet clear.

Evidence that the tumor is indeed the site of gonadotrophin secretion is convincing (see above). When analyzed by radioimmunoassay, the gonadotrophin has been usually LH, on one occasion FSH. There is one report of a patient with galactorrhea whose hypernephroma was shown to secrete prolactin.

Spider angiomas and pulmonary osteoarthropathy may or may not accompany gynecomastia. In such cases, careful search for a pulmonary tumor by roentgenography should be done, and measurements made for urinary estrogens and for urinary gonadotrophins (by bioassay) or plasma LH (by radioimmunoassay). Failure to suppress high urinary or plasma gonadotrophin levels by administration of large amounts of estrogen for several days may turn out to be a useful diagnostic test.

Treatment is unsatisfactory. The tumors are very malignant and have not been surgically curable. Radiation and chemotherapy are ineffective. It remains to be seen whether methotrexate will reduce gonadotrophin production, as it does in trophoblastic tumors (see below).

Another group of tumors has been associated with secretion of HCG. In addition to benign or malignant tumors of the placenta, these are choriocarcinomas of the pineal or testis, hepatoblastoma of the liver, and adrenocortical carcinoma. A recent survey has disclosed high levels of plasma HCG, usually without clinical signs, in 12 per cent of a series of patients with cancer. With testicular tumors (by far the most common) excluded, the incidence becomes about 7 per cent, with cancers of the gastrointestinal tract or breast, multiple myeloma, and malignant melanoma the next most frequent. *The interesting point here is the possible value of measurements of HCG as markers in attempts at early detection of cancer* (see above).

The clinical manifestations, when present, are gynecomastia in the adult male and isosexual precocity in children. In boys, the testes have been enlarged in some, and all show testicular interstitial cell hyperplasia histologically. The gonadotrophin has the characteristics of HCG, and has been found in high concentration in the urine, serum, and tumors. In a very few cases, gonadotrophin levels have been temporarily lowered by methotrexate which had variable effects on the tumor itself. So far, these tumors have all been fatal.

Hyperthyroidism. In addition to the rare association of hyperthyroidism with tumors of the gastrointestinal tract, hematopoietic system, lung, and other organs, several patients have been identified in whom thyrotoxicosis coexisted with metastatic disease of trophoblastic origin (choriocarcinoma or hydatidiform mole) and, in a few cases, with metastatic embryonal cell carcinoma of the testis. Together with the expected finding of high titer of urinary HCG, these patients have thyrotrophic activity in plasma and tumor tissue. The best current evidence indicates that this thyroid-stimulating activity is an intrinsic property of HCG or of a glycoprotein molecule chemically and immunologically similar to HCG. The *clinical manifestations* of hyperthyroidism are usually minimal; many patients have no symptoms, and the rest have only mild symptoms of thyrotoxicosis. All have tachycardia, but other physical signs of the endocrinopathy, e.g., goiter, are generally absent, although laboratory evidence – raised serum PBI and high thyroidal uptake of ^{131}I – is definite. These indices can be controlled with antithyroid drugs or iodides, but most striking is the favorable response of both clinical and laboratory signs of hyperthyroidism to treatment with methotrexate, which is also capable of causing regression of these tumors. The presence of mild thyrotoxicosis, seen in fewer than 10 per cent of women with trophoblastic neoplasms, does not affect prognosis of the tumor.

Inappropriate Antidiuresis. Excessive sodium excretion in patients with lung cancer was first reported in 1938, but not until 1957 did Bartter and Schwartz and their co-workers attribute this abnormality to water retention resulting from abnormally regulated secretion of ADH. Studies done in the last decade have disclosed ADH-like activity in several tumors taken from patients with the syndrome of inappropriate ADH secretion; the tumors have been mostly oat cell carcinomas of the lung, with a few others, e.g., pancreatic and duodenal carcinoma. The ADH-like activity has not been completely characterized, but resembles in physical, chemical, and biologic properties human pituitary ADH, i.e., arginine vasopressin. In some (so far, a minority of) patients, plasma values for arginine vasopressin have been found to be high.

The clinical manifestations of hyponatremia may be minimal or absent, probably because the abnormality has developed slowly. Often, hyponatremia is a chance finding during routine study of a patient with lung cancer. To prove the entity, one has to show a urine hypertonic with respect to plasma, normal GFR, and normal adrenocortical function, i.e., absence of adrenocortical insufficiency. The extracellular space, if measured, is found to be expanded. The pathogenesis of this pattern of abnormalities is discussed in Ch. 805. Treatment with hypertonic salt is useful only as an emergency measure, e.g., for coma or convulsions owing to profound hyponatremia; the only effective medical therapy for long-term use is restriction of water intake to less than 1 liter a day. In a few patients, the water and electrolyte abnormality has undergone temporary remission with successful palliative treatment of the tumor by x-radiation or chemotherapy.

Hypercalcemia. The hypercalcemia of malignant disease may be due to four mechanisms: (1) osteolytic lesions of bone associated with widespread metastases, as from carcinoma of the thyroid, prostate, or lung, or lymphoma; (2) osteolysis in the absence of bony metastases, associated with some carcinomas of the breast which presumably elaborate sterols related to vitamin D; (3) osteolysis in the absence of bony metastases, in association with tumors which appear to secrete a parathyroid hormone (PTH)–like substance; and (4) osteolysis without bony metastases in the presence of tumors which secrete some humoral substance other than parathyroid hormone or proparathyroid hormone, i.e., a substance or substances not detectable by radioimmunoassays for the various forms of these hormones (see Powell et al.). Tumors have been squamous cell carcinomas of the lung and other organs, and carcinomas of the kidney, ovary, uterus, pancreas, and colon. Evidence for primary secretion of parathyroid hormone by the neoplasm has come from demonstration of immunoreactive PTH in plasma of patients with nonparathyroid tumors and hypercalcemia, from the detection of PTH-like substance in the tumors, disappearance or diminution of hypercalcemia upon tumor removal, and reappearance of the electrolyte abnormality with recurrence of the cancer.

The clinical features of hypercalcemia are presented in detail in Ch. 872. The important clinical point is that the hypercalcemia associated with PTH-secreting tumor of nonendocrine tissue is more likely to manifest itself as lethargy, weakness, anorexia, nausea, and vomiting, and less likely to appear as renal stones or bone disease. Patients with the "ectopic PTH syndrome" are more apt to lose weight and to be anemic.

Separation of these patients from those with hyperparathyroidism by laboratory tests may be difficult. Both may have extreme hypercalcemia, low or normal serum phosphorus, elevated plasma values for PTH, and unresponsiveness of hypercalcemia to corticosteroids; but careful examination, laboratory study, and roentgenographic search, e.g., by chest films and intravenous pyelography, will disclose most of the nonparathyroid tumors. Riggs et al. and Arnaud have discussed the diagnostic difficulties in the use of PTH radioimmunoassays for detection of this immunoheterogeneous substance.

The *treatment* of hypercalcemia is discussed in Ch. 872.

It has been recently postulated that *hypophosphatemic osteomalacia* in the presence of benign hemangiomas may be due to a humoral substance (not PTH) that increases renal clearance of phosphate.

Hypoglycemia. The association of severe fasting hypoglycemia with certain neoplasms, especially very large retroperitoneal or intrathoracic tumors, is well established. Most of the tumors are fibromas or sarcomas, sometimes of huge size—up to 10 kg; others are hepatoma, adrenocortical carcinoma, adenocarcinoma of stomach and colon, undifferentiated bronchial carcinoma, and bronchial carcinoid. As for the mechanism of hypoglycemia, there is some evidence against excessive glucose utilization by the tumor and against stimulation by the tumor of insulin secretion by the pancreas, removal of which does not affect the hypoglycemia. The prevailing view is that the tumor secretes a hypoglycemia-producing substance, which, with only a few exceptions, is not demonstrable as high levels of immunoreactive insulin in plasma or tumor, but only as "insulin-like" activity. The secretory role of the tumor is affirmed by surgical "cure" of the hypoglycemia in about 20 patients whose tumors have been successfully removed.

The hypoglycemia is indistinguishable clinically and by most of the provocative tests from that associated with islet cell adenoma or carcinoma of the pancreas. However, almost all patients with nonpancreatic tumors lack high plasma insulin values, and the presence of a large tumor is usually apparent.

Treatment is best done by excising the tumor; even incomplete removal may relieve the hypoglycemia temporarily. Failing this, palliative measures must include continuous feeding of carbohydrate and administration of corticosteroids, diazoxide, and possibly glucagon (see Ch. 807).

Carcinoid Syndrome. This, the only definite example of an "endocrine" syndrome owing to production of a humoral agent that is not a polypeptide, is discussed in Ch. 869.

Erythrocytosis; Zollinger-Ellison Syndrome. These syndromes, caused by tumor secretion of gastrin and erythropoietin, respectively, are discussed in detail in Ch. 730 and Ch. 640 to 644.

Multiple Hormones Produced by a Single Tumor. Several tumors have been reported which apparently secrete two or even three distinct hormones. The pulmonary and thymic tumors secreting both ACTH and MSH have already been mentioned. A few patients with hepatoma have had both hypoglycemia and polycythemia, and islet cell tumors of the pancreas have been described with coexisting hypoglycemia and carcinoid syndrome, and with Cushing's syndrome and carcinoid syndrome. Three hormones, ACTH, MSH, and gastrin, were found in a single pancreatic tumor, and in one patient with an islet cell carcinoma of the pancreas there was chemical or good clinical evidence for secretion by the tumor of six hormones: gastrin and glucagon ("appropriate" hormones for the pancreas), ACTH, MSH, ADH, and parathyroid hormone.

Amatruda, T. T., Jr.: Nonendocrine secreting tumors. *In* Bondy, P. K., and Rosenberg, L. E. (eds.): Duncan's Diseases of Metabolism. 7th ed. Philadelphia, W. B. Saunders Company, 1974, p. 1629.

Arnaud, C.: Parathyroid hormone: Coming of age in clinical medicine. Am. J. Med., 55:577, 1973.

Baumann, G., Lopez-Amor, E., and Dingman, J. F.: Plasma arginine vasopressin in the syndrome of inappropriate antidiuretic hormone secretion. Am. J. Med., 52:19, 1972.

Braunstein, G. D., Vaitukaitis, J. L., Carbone, P. P., and Ross, G. T.: Ectopic production of human chorionic gonadotrophin by neoplasms. Ann. Intern. Med., 78:39, 1973.

Gordan, G. S., and Roof, B. S.: "Humors from tumors": Diagnostic potential of peptides. Ann. Intern. Med., 76:501, 1972.

Liddle, G. W., Nicholson, W. E., Island, D. P., Orth, D. N., Abe, K., and Lowder, S. C.: Clinical and laboratory studies of ectopic humoral syndromes. Rec. Prog. Horm. Res., 25:283, 1969.

Orth, D. N., Nicholson, W. E., Mitchell, W. M., Island, D. P., and Liddle, G. W.: Biologic and immunologic characterization and physical separation of ACTH and ACTH fragments in the ectopic ACTH syndrome. J. Clin. Invest., 52:1756, 1973.

Plimpton, C. H., and Gellhorn, A.: Hypercalcemia in malignant disease without evidence of bone destruction. Am. J. Med., 21:750, 1956.

Powell, D., Singer, F. R., Murray, T. M., Minkin, C., and Potts, J. T.: Nonparathyroid humoral hypercalcemia in patients with neoplastic diseases. N. Engl. J. Med., 289:176, 1973.

Riggs, B. L., Arnaud, C. D., Reynolds, J. C., and Smith, L. H.: Immunologic differentiation of primary hyperparathyroidism from hyperparathyroidism due to nonparathyroid cancer. J. Clin. Invest., 50:2079, 1971.

Ross, E. J.: Endocrine and metabolic manifestations of cancer. Br. Med. J., 1:735, 1972.

Unger, R. H.: The riddle of tumor hypoglycemia. Am. J. Med., 40:325, 1966.

PARATHYROID

G. D. Aurbach

871. PARATHYROID HORMONE AND CALCITONIN

Parathyroid hormone, the principal humoral regulator of calcium metabolism in man, has been characterized definitively as a polypeptide 84 amino acids in length. The complete structure of the bovine and porcine hormones and part of the sequence of human parathyroid hormone are known and active analogues of the hormones have been synthesized. It is now recognized that biosynthesis of the hormone proceeds through a prohormone molecule 90 amino acids in length (Fig. 1). Immediately after synthesis the prohormone is converted within the gland to the 84 amino acid polypeptide for storage and subsequent secretion. Radioimmunoassays show that calcium is the primary factor controlling secretion of the hormone. A fall in blood calcium concentration provokes secretion of the hormone, which in turn causes an increased rate of transfer of calcium from bone and glomerular filtrate to the extracellular fluids. The hormone also causes increased urinary excretion of phosphate by direct action on the kidney (possibly by inhibition of the reabsorption of phosphate). These physiologic effects on both calcium and phosphate are accounted for by a single hormonal molecule. The mechanism of action of parathyroid hormone is mediated by cyclic 3',5'-adenosine monophosphate (3',5'-AMP) produced through direct specific hormonal activation of the enzyme adenylate cyclase in bone and kidney. The consequent increase in concentration of 3',5'-AMP in the renal cortex and bone activates other intracellular processes which account for the physiologic actions of the hormone. The increase in concentration of 3',5'-AMP induced by parathyroid hormone in the renal parenchyma is manifested also by increased urinary excretion of 3',5'-AMP.

Calcitonin is another polypeptide hormone involved in regulation of calcium and bone metabolism. The structures of the calcitonins are known, syntheses have been completed, and radioimmunoassays have been developed, but the physiologic significance of calcitonin for normal man is still uncertain.

Calcitonin is secreted from the parafollicular cells found in the mammalian thyroid but related embryologically to the ultimobranchial body of lower vertebrate species. The rate of secretion of calcitonin is a direct function of the concentration of calcium in plasma, whereas parathyroid hormone is secreted at a rate inversely proportional to calcium concentration. The hypocalcemic action of calcitonin is effected through an inhibition of resorption of mineral from bone, and the physiologic actions of this hormone seem to be mediated through the adenylate–cyclic AMP system.

Diseases of the parathyroid gland include hyperparathyroidism and hypoparathyroidism. Pseudohypoparathyroidism encompasses the general clinical and laboratory features of hypoparathyroidism but is an abnormality not of parathyroid gland function but of the receptor tissue for parathyroid hormone. Medullary carcinoma of the thyroid is a complex pathophysiologic state in which the tumor secretes excessive amounts of

Figure 1. Schematic representation of biosynthesis of hormone within cell of parathyroid gland. The prohormone (90 amino acids in length) is synthesized and then released from the ribosome. After release the N-terminal 6 amino acids (represented by the shaded area) are cleaved enzymatically from the molecule, yielding the parathyroid hormone molecule (84 amino acids in length) which is stored in the gland and released therefrom upon physiologic stimulus. After elaboration of the intact hormone (84 amino acids) into the circulation and interaction with peripheral target tissues (kidney and bone), the hormone is metabolized further to biologically inactive but radioimmunologically detectable fragments.

calcitonin with high concentrations of calcitonin in plasma. Primary hyperparathyroidism, pheochromocytoma, Cushing's syndrome, and multiple neuromas are found associated in some cases of the syndrome.

Aurbach, G. D.: Isolation of parathyroid hormone after extraction with phenol. J. Biol. Chem., 243:3179, 1959.

Aurbach, G. D., and Chase, L. R.: Cyclic 3',5'-adenylic acid in bone and the mechanism of action of parathyroid hormone. Fed. Proc., 29:1179, 1970.

Aurbach, G. D., Keutmann, H. T., Niall, H. D., Tregear, G. W., O'Riordan, J. L. H., Marcus, R., Marx, S. J., and Potts, J. T., Jr.: Structure, synthesis and mechanism of action of parathyroid hormone. Recent Prog. Horm. Res., 28:353, 1972.

Brewer, H. B., Jr., and Ronan, R.: Bovine parathyroid hormone: Amino acid sequence. Proc. Natl. Acad. Sci. U.S.A., 67:1862, 1970.

Chase, L. R., and Aurbach, G. D.: Renal adenyl cyclase: Anatomically separate sites for parathyroid hormone and vasopressin. Science, 159:545, 1968.

Copp, D. H., Cockcroft, D. W., and Kueh, Y.: Calcitonin from ultimobranchial glands of dogfish and chickens. Science, 158:924, 1967.

Deftos, L. J., Lee, M. R., and Potts, J. T., Jr.: A radioimmunoassay for calcitonin. Proc. Natl. Acad. Sci. U.S.A., 60:293, 1968.

Hirsch, P. F., Gauthier, G. F., and Munson, P. L.: Thyroid hypocalcemic principle and recurrent laryngeal nerve injury as factors affecting the response to parathyroidectomy in rats. Endocrinology, 73:244, 1963.

Hirsch, P. F., and Munson, P. L.: Thyrocalcitonin. Physiol. Rev., 49:548, 1969.

Niall, H., Keutmann, H., Sauer, R., Hogan, M., Dawson, B., Aurbach, G. D., and Potts, J. T., Jr.: The amino acid sequence of bovine parathyroid hormone. I. Hoppe-Seyler's Z. Physiol. Chem., 351:1586, 1970.

Potts, J. T., Jr., Niall, H. D., Keutmann, H. T., Brewer, H. B., Jr., and Deftos, L. J.: The amino acid sequence of porcine thyrocalcitonin. Proc. Natl. Acad. Sci. U.S.A., 59:1321, 1968.

Sherwood, L. M., Mayer, G. P., Ramberg, C. F., Jr., Kronfeld, D. S., Aurbach, G. D., and Potts, J. T., Jr.: Regulation of parathyroid hormone secretion: Proportional control by calcium, lack of effect of phosphate. Endocrinology, 83:1043, 1968.

872.   HYPERPARATHYROIDISM

Definition.   Primary hyperparathyroidism is the clinical condition caused by excessive and incompletely regulated secretion of hormone from the parathyroid glands. The manifestations, which may include hypercalcemia, tissue calcification, and osteitis fibrosa cystica, represent the result of excessive parathyroid hormone action on bone and kidney.

Etiology. Hypersecretion of parathyroid hormone as a manifestation of primary parathyroid disease may be caused by adenomas, single or multiple, primary chief cell or clear cell hyperplasia, or carcinoma of the glands. In over 80 per cent of the cases primary hyperparathyroidism is attributable to a single parathyroid adenoma, and in less than 2 per cent carcinoma of the parathyroid gland is the cause. Other cases are about equally divided between clear cell hyperplasia, chief cell hyperplasia, and multiple adenomas. An analogous syndrome can result from ectopic production of parathyroid hormone by nonparathyroid tissue. *Secondary hyperparathyroidism* develops as a compensatory mechanism in any abnormal state tending to produce true hypocalcemia; this state may occur in hypovitaminosis D, vitamin D–dependent rickets, malabsorption of calcium, chronic renal disease, hyperphosphatemia, or renal tubular acidosis. There are no known factors to which development of primary hyperparathyroidism can be attributed. There is a suggestion that prolonged, progressive secondary hyperparathyroidism may evolve into autonomous primary hyperparathyroidism in some cases of chronic renal disease, but there is no evidence that parathyrotrophic substances exist in either normal or abnormal physiology. Several families with autosomal dominant hyperparathyroidism have been reported; thus a genetic factor is involved in some cases.

Incidence. Recent surveys validate earlier projections that better diagnostic methods and wider clinical awareness promote discovery of new cases. Automated laboratory facilities now make possible routine analysis of serum calcium for all patients in the clinic and hospital populations. In one center routine analyses were performed on a large series of patients, and it was found that the incidence of hyperparathyroidism was as high as one case per thousand.

Pathology. Usually parathyroid adenomas vary in size from 1 to 5 grams, but occasionally very large tumors, 50 grams or more, may develop. In general, large tumors are more likely to be associated with clinically evident bone disease, marked hypercalcemia, very high concentrations of parathyroid hormone in plasma, and short interval between development of symptoms and establishment of diagnosis. Histologic examination usually shows chief cells and some water-clear cells; sometimes the latter are predominant. Rarely adenomas are composed of oxyphil cells. Hyperplasia may be of the chief cell or water-clear cell type. Occasionally adenomas of other endocrine glands are found in hyperparathyroidism (multiple endocrine adenomatosis; see Clinical Manifestations, below). The effect of the disease is manifested in the bones as osteitis fibrosa cystica generalisata (see Ch. 890). When the kidneys are affected, nephrolithiasis or nephrocalcinosis is apparent; pyelonephritis often complicates the course of the kidney disease.

Muscle biopsy frequently shows neuropathic (not myopathic) atrophy of type II muscle fibers. This denervation-type structural change (probably secondary to a metabolic lesion in the nerve itself) parallels the severity of muscle weakness in hyperparathyroidism.

Pancreatitis, acute or chronic, is recognized as a possible complication of hyperparathyroidism. About half of the patients with advanced hyperparathyroidism examined at autopsy show calcification in the pancreas. It is possible that chronic hypercalcemia contributes to the development of pancreatitis, but the actual mechanism of this association has not been established.

Pathologic Physiology and Chemistry. Hypersecretion of parathyroid hormone from adenomatous or hyperplastic glands is expressed in acceleration of the normal physiologic actions of the hormone on bone and kidney. The effect on bone leads to an increase in rate of resorption of calcium from bone, and in more severe cases to pathologic development in bone of osteitis fibrosa cystica. The effect on the kidney causes an increase in rate of resorption of calcium from the glomerular filtrate as well as increased renal clearance of phosphate from plasma with consequent hypophosphatemia. The renal concentrating ability may decrease, resulting in polyuria and polydipsia. Hypercalcemia results from the actions of the hormone on bone and kidneys. The urinary excretion of 3',5'-AMP is greater than normal.

Most new cases of hyperparathyroidism discovered in the clinic show little or no detectable bone disease. This finding may be attributable to more widespread and precise determinations of serum calcium with consequent discovery of earlier and milder forms of the disease and greater general recognition of the problem. Some early or mild cases become clinically apparent chiefly by nephrolithiasis and hypophosphatemia, with little or no hypercalcemia or skeletal abnormality.

Although hypercalcemia is principally a manifestation of the effects of the hormone on bone and kidney, calcium absorption from the gastrointestinal tract is increased as well. Recent studies indicate that this effect on the gut may be influenced through effects of parathyroid hormone on the renal metabolism of vitamin D. Parathyroid hormone stimulates the renal mechanism that converts 25-hydroxy–vitamin D to 1,25-dihydroxy–vitamin D. This latter metabolite, formed in the kidney, acts on the intestine, causing increased absorption of calcium.

The classic laboratory manifestations of primary hyperparathyroidism are low serum phosphate and high serum calcium. Frequently 24-hour excretion of calcium is high because of significant hypercalcemia, even though the renal clearance of calcium is relatively reduced. Hypercalciuria, with calcium excretion in excess of intake, is particularly apparent when diets low in calcium are given. Generally a diet low in calcium is given for three days, and then total urinary calcium is determined for 24-hour periods. Normal subjects should not excrete in excess of 175 mg per 24 hours when taking a diet containing 150 mg of calcium. The alkaline phosphatase in plasma may be high in hyperparathyroidism when there is significant bone disease; this is probably a manifestation of increased bone formation, a compensatory mechanism for the high rate of bone resorption induced by excessive parathyroid hormone secretion. Other manifestations of increased bone resorption are increased urinary excretion of hydroxyproline and pyrophosphate. Kinetic studies utilizing radioactive calcium frequently show evidence of increased bone metabolism.

Clinical Manifestations. The disease tends to segregate into three categories in terms of clinical presentation. In the mildest form there may be no symptoms or signs, and discovery is made only through routine determination of serum calcium. The second category develops insidiously, sometimes over a period of years, and presents predominantly as renal colic. In the third group the course of the disease is more rapid, with development of marked hypercalcemia, weight loss, vomiting, debility, and bone pain, sometimes with pathologic fracture. Debility, weight loss, anemia, and elevated sedimentation rate may be so prominent in the severe form of the disease as to suggest malignancy. The most frequent symptoms of the disease in general are weakness, fatigability, and renal colic. Epigastric pain, neurologic abnormalities, and constipation are also common. Hypercalcemia may cause polydipsia, polyuria, anorexia, nausea, and vomiting. Neurologic abnormalities include impaired mentation, loss of memory for recent events, depression, emotional lability, hyperactive deep tendon reflexes, sensory loss for pain and vibration, and proximal muscle weakness, particularly in the lower extremities. There may also be abnormal movements (resembling fasciculations) of the tongue, glossal atrophy, ataxic gait, hoarseness, dysphagia, anosmia, and abnormal flexor reflex. Careful clinical examination may elicit neurologic abnormalities even in patients who are otherwise asymptomatic.

Still other symptoms cannot be clearly related to distinct pathophysiologic mechanisms. There may be burning in the throat or abdomen, vague malaise, back or coccygeal pain, or dry skin. Occasionally headache or pruritus is the sole presenting complaint. It is of interest in this regard that the pruritus of uremia may be dramatically relieved after removal of parathyroid glands showing secondary hyperplasia. Anemia, elevated erythrocyte sedimentation rate, and hypertension also are each observed in 25 per cent or more of the cases.

Hypercalcemia may depress sensitivity to electrical stimuli of ganglia and peripheral nerves (Erb's sign). Shortening of the Q-T interval (between the onset of the Q wave and the beginning of the T wave) in the electrocardiogram is found in some patients with hypercalcemia. Prolonged hypercalcemia may lead to calcification in the eye displayed as "band keratopathy," opaque material appearing in vertical lines parallel to and within the limbus, or as conjunctival crystals without the limbus or under the eyelids. Detection of these may require examination by slit lamp.

Bone disease in hyperparathyroidism, osteitis fibrosa cystica, may be recognized by roentgenographic examination (Fig. 2); it sometimes causes bone pain or pathologic fracture. Roentgenographically, bone disease may appear as generalized osteopenia, loss of the lamina dura about the teeth, erosion of the distal ends of the clavicles, bone cysts (Fig. 2B), "brown tumors" of bone, epulis of the jaw, or subcortical bone resorption, most readily observed in the phalanges (Fig. 2A) or distal clavicles. Chondrocalcinosis (Fig. 2B) may also be found by roentgenography.

Hypercalciuria may lead to *nephrolithiasis* and passage of calcium oxalate or calcium phosphate stones with or without renal colic. In other instances

Figure 2. Roentgenographic signs in hyperparathyroidism. *A*, Bone resorption. There is severe bone resorption with general loss of mineral, thinning of the cortices, marked subperiosteal resorption along the cortical surfaces of the proximal and distal phalanges, and gross resorption of the distal phalangeal tufts. *B*, Cysts (osteitis fibrosa cystica) in femur and tibia in subject with severe hyperparathyroidism. Also note intra-articular chrondrocalcinosis (thin line of calcification in knee joint indicated by arrow).

nephrocalcinosis may develop, sometimes causing progressive renal failure. Infection may complicate either type of renal disorder.

Peptic ulcers are common in hyperparathyroidism, and may reflect a potentiating effect of hypercalcemia on acid secretion. An association between acute or chronic *pancreatitis* and hyperparathyroidism is recognized more and more frequently. One should be aware that hyperparathyroidism may exist in any case of pancreatitis, and may be masked by the acute lowering of serum calcium in pancreatitis.

In addition to pancreatitis and peptic ulcer, several other diseases may be associated with primary hyperparathyroidism. Hypertension occurs in up to 50 per cent of cases. It cannot be clearly related to any particular factor (e.g., associated renal disease) and does not often regress after surgical cure. There is an increased incidence of ill-defined arthralgia as well as of gout and pseudogout. The latter is associated with intra-articular deposition of calcium pyrophosphate crystals. Discovery of pseudogout should suggest possible coexistence of primary hyperparathyroidism. Primary hyperparathyroidism may exist as part of the multiple endocrine adenomatosis syndrome. In such cases pituitary and pancreatic tumors may produce associated endocrinopathies. These include acromegaly or hypopituitarism caused by pituitary tumors, peptic ulceration caused by excessive gastrin secretion (Zollinger-Ellison syndrome), or hypoglycemia resulting from secretion of insulin by pancreatic tumors. Hyperparathyroidism may also occur in another type of endocrine adenomatosis consisting of pheochromocytomas, parathyroid adenomas, and medullary carcinoma of the thyroid (see Ch. 876). Each of the two types of multiple endocrine adenomatosis syndromes may be familial. Sporadic cases of hyperparathyroidism have also been observed in association with hyperthyroidism, sarcoidosis, Albright's fibrous dysplasia of bone, Paget's disease, Cushing's syndrome, and malignancy.

Metabolic acidosis occurs in about one fourth of patients, with hyperchloridemia and low serum bicarbonate. The acidosis can be attributed to impaired tubular reabsorption of bicarbonate and parallels the increase in phosphate clearance. It may become worse in the immediate postparathyroidectomy period when hypophosphatemia is accentuated. A similar defect in proximal tubular reabsorption of bicarbonate may occur in a number of metabolic disorders characterized by secondary hyperparathyroidism or cellular depletion of phosphate, or both. The abnormality can be documented by carrying out a test for T_m of bicarbonate reabsorption. Eventually metabolism returns to normal after surgical removal of hyperplastic or adenomatous parathyroid glands. Hypercalcemia in cancer is less likely to be associated with acidosis; indeed, metabolic alkalosis may be expressed in this disorder. Hypokalemia and hypomagnesemia also are occasionally observed in hyperparathyroidism. The hypokalemia is attributed to decreased distal tubular reabsorption of potassium and may be made worse by treating subjects with high doses of phosphate by mouth. Phosphate depletion may also account for decreased magnesium reabsorption.

Differential Diagnosis. Hypercalcemia, demineralizing disease of bone, and nephrolithiasis are clinical problems that commonly suggest the diagnosis of hyperparathyroidism. *Hypercalcemia* may be expressed in diverse metabolic, endocrine, or malignant diseases, including hyperparathyroidism, several types of cancer, sarcoidosis, milk-alkali syndrome, vitamin D intoxication, hyperthyroidism, acute adrenal insufficiency, and a rare disease, hypophosphatasia. Thiazides can produce a slight increase in serum calcium, and the widespread use of these drugs may increase significantly the number of mildly hypercalcemic subjects requiring diagnosis. In Paget's disease or osteoporosis, hypercalcemia may develop upon prolonged bed rest. Hypercalcemia may occur in malignancy as a consequence of one or more etiologic factors: osteolytic metastases causing hypercalcemia through local resorptive influence of the lesions in bone; production by the tumor of substances (e.g., prostaglandins) capable of inducing bone resorption and hypercalcemia ("pseudohyperparathyroidism"); production of an abnormal blood protein (which may explain hypercalcemia in some cases of multiple myeloma) which is capable of binding calcium, the increase in serum calcium being attributable simply to a higher concentration of bound calcium in the plasma compartment; or "ectopic" hyperparathyroidism, in which a nonparathyroid tumor produces parathyroid hormone itself. The last-named may be particularly difficult to diagnose, because the laboratory findings do not differ from those of hyperparathyroidism caused by parathyroid adenoma or hyperplasia; blood calcium is high, blood phosphate is low, and the alkaline phosphatase may be elevated. (Development of metabolic acidosis, however, seems to occur less frequently in ectopic than in primary hyperparathyroidism.) The "pseudohyperparathyroid" syndrome (production of a unique bone-resorbing humoral substance unrelated to parathyroid hormone) is also associated with hypophosphatemia, but there is no detectable parathyroid hormone by immunoassay either in the tumor or in plasma. The question of malignancy with hypercalcemia requires extensive studies to ascertain the true nature of the disease. Severe cases of true primary hyperparathyroidism may present particular diagnostic problems, because the disease itself can cause anemia, weight loss, debility, and increased erythrocyte sedimentation rate suggestive of malignant disease.

Paget's disease of bone, osteoporosis, osteomalacia, multiple myeloma, and malignancies metastatic to bone show varying degrees of skeletal demineralization. The roentgenographic appearance in each of these disorders, though, is more or less characteristic. In osteoporosis, the serum calcium, phosphate, and alkaline phosphatase are normal. Extensive Paget's disease is attended by an increase in serum alkaline phosphatase, but phosphate and calcium in blood are normal except during periods of immobilization, when hypercalcemia may develop. Examination of bone marrow is helpful in excluding multiple myeloma, and is occasionally of value in diagnosing lymphoma or metastatic malignancy. Analysis of plasma and urine for myeloma proteins should be routine in suspected cases. Osteomalacia may be caused by hypovitaminosis D, resistance to vitamin D, intestinal malabsorption syndromes, or renal tubular acidosis. In these conditions, serum calcium is normal or low, sometimes with tetany; blood phosphate is low; and the alkaline phosphatase is elevated. The differential diagnoses of hyperparathyroid bone disease (osteitis fibrosa cystica), osteomalacia, fibrous dysplasia of bone, Paget's disease, and osteoporosis are discussed also in Part XIX.

Secondary hyperparathyroidism in chronic renal dis-

ease may produce the histologic picture of osteitis fibrosa cystica. In general, serum phosphate is high and there is a tendency to hypocalcemia. Occasionally, however, primary hyperparathyroidism may become superimposed upon chronic renal failure. This complication becomes evident by an increase in serum calcium to the high normal or hypercalcemic range. In this event hyperplastic or adenomatous parathyroid glands should be removed surgically.

Development of nephrolithiasis with calcium phosphate or calcium oxalate stones, particularly when associated with hypercalciuria, requires clinical testing to rule out primary hyperparathyroidism. "Idiopathic hypercalciuria" with recurrent nephrolithiasis may be associated with hypophosphatemia, making the distinction more difficult. This category may still include some patients with bona fide hyperparathyroidism. Repeated tests of serum calcium are essential in reaching the correct conclusion. In some cases in which the diagnosis has been doubtful, hyperparathyroidism is obvious at the follow-up examination 6 to 12 months later.

Diagnostic Investigations. Hypercalcemia is almost always present in primary hyperparathyroidism. Indeed, hypercalcemia per se, detected in a general clinic population, can be attributed on chance alone to primary hyperparathyroidism in almost half the cases. Although malignancy is an equally common cause of hypercalcemia in the general population, hypercalcemia associated with hypophosphatemia and a long relatively benign clinical history makes the diagnosis of primary hyperparathyroidism more likely. In any one patient, though, particularly with an early or mild case, serial analyses may show fluctuations of serum calcium into the normal range. In rare instances hypomagnesemia or vitamin D deficiency may mask hyperparathyroidism. Correction of the magnesium or vitamin D deficiency in these cases allows the hypercalcemia to be expressed. In general, though, the finding of high serum calcium is the laboratory test most likely to lead to the diagnosis. Several further investigations based on assessing the secretion or actions of parathyroid hormone help establish the diagnosis.

Several tests have been based on the known physiologic action of parathyroid hormone in causing increased phosphate clearance (and decreased tubular reabsorption of phosphate, TRP). Although these procedures are constantly modified in attempts to obtain greater diagnostic accuracy, none offer sufficient specificity to be of regular clinical value.

Prednisone Suppression Test. Hypercalcemia in sarcoidosis or vitamin D intoxication is particularly amenable to correction with corticosteroid therapy; subjects with the milk-alkali syndrome may respond also. These observations form the basis of a test that is helpful in differentiating among several types of hypercalcemia. Usually either prednisone, 60 mg daily, or hydrocortisone, 120 mg daily, is given in divided doses for ten days. The hypercalcemia of hyperparathyroidism, ectopic or primary, almost invariably is resistant to the effects of this treatment. The response in other types of hypercalcemia is more variable. The milk-alkali syndrome and hypervitaminosis D both respond to withdrawal of the offending agents, and the hypercalcemia of sarcoidosis may respond to therapy with chloroquine. In general, the clinical, laboratory, and roentgenographic features cited under diagnosis of the particular disease should lead one to the proper diagnosis in the

other disorders listed. Hypercalcemia in hyperthyroidism is best treated by correcting the hyperthyroid state. Hypercalcemia that persists in the euthyroid state suggests the coexistence of hyperparathyroidism.

Urinary Excretion of Cyclic AMP. Parathyroid hormone exerts its effects on target tissues by activating adenylate cyclase and causing thereby an increase in tissue concentration of cyclic 3′,5′-AMP. Part of the cyclic 3′,5′-AMP accumulating within renal cells in response to parathyroid hormone is excreted in the urine; this nephrogenous contribution to the urinary excretion of cyclic 3′,5′-AMP in man is approximately 40 to 50 per cent of the total excreted. In primary hyperparathyroidism the mean urinary excretion of 3′,5′-AMP is elevated, and conversely in hypoparathyroidism the rate of excretion is low. After surgical correction of hyperparathyroidism, the rate of excretion falls to normal; this is a reliable index of successful surgery. The ratio of cyclic AMP to creatinine in the urine in normal subjects is 1.3 to 4.2 (average 2.7) μmoles per gram of creatinine. In hyperparathyroid patients cyclic AMP excretion averages 5.2 (standard deviation 2.2) μmoles per gram of creatinine. Thus although there is a highly significant increase in excretion of the cyclic nucleotide in hyperparathyroidism, there is nevertheless considerable overlap with results for normal subjects. On the other hand, a high ratio of cyclic AMP to creatinine in the urine in association with clinical hypercalcemia is highly suggestive of hyperparathyroidism, primary or ectopic. Certain nonparathyroid cancers producing hypercalcemia are associated with low rates of cyclic AMP excretion, reflecting suppressed PTH secretion, and thus can be distinguished from hyperparathyroidism.

Radioimmunoassay for Parathyroid Hormone. Radioimmunoassays for parathyroid hormone have been developed in several laboratories, but radioimmunoassay alone, particularly in random peripheral plasma samples, does not afford an absolute diagnostic index for primary hyperparathyroidism. After the hormone is secreted from the gland, it undergoes degradation to fragments in the periphery. One of the principal fragments remaining is immunologically reactive but biologically inert. This fragment (derived from the carboxyl two thirds of the molecule) disappears relatively slowly from the circulation and accumulates to an even greater extent in chronic renal disease. Moreover, some antisera are relatively more reactive than others with the carboxyl terminus of the molecule. Thus results for radioimmunoassays in peripheral plasma samples vary from one laboratory to another simply on the basis of differences in antisera employed in the assay as well as differences in renal function in any particular patient. Nevertheless, in hyperparathyroidism, use of the assay usually shows abnormally high concentrations (particularly relative to calcium content of plasma) of hormone in the plasma. Hypercalcemia from causes unrelated to parathyroid hormone is associated with undetectable hormone in plasma. Moreover, the immunoassay is particularly applicable to studies on samples obtained by selective venous catheterization. Blood drawn directly from the thyroid veins contains hormone immediately as it is secreted and before it has undergone degradation in the periphery. This procedure allows preoperative localization of abnormal parathyroid tissue and helps establish the exact diagnosis before surgery. The diagnosis of primary hyperparathyroidism is definitive on laboratory grounds alone in any case in which each of the following criteria are fulfilled: (1) hypercalcemia, (2) normal or high concentration of parathyroid hormone in peripheral plasma, and (3) detection of a high concentration of parathyroid hormone in the venous system draining the thyroid bed.

High concentrations of hormone in peripheral plasma have been found also in cases of hyperparathyroidism resulting from ectopic production of hormone by nonparathyroid tumors as well as in secondary hyperparathyroidism and pseudohypoparathyroidism. The difficulty of precise analysis for parathyroid hormone in peripheral plasma will undoubtedly be lessened by developing assays more specific for the active form. Ultimately it is likely that the radioimmunoassay (or possibly a radioreceptor assay) will become the principal diagnostic test for hyperparathyroidism. In particular, measurement of the secretory responses to induced hypo- or hypercalcemia should provide definitive tests for the differential diagnosis of primary and secondary hyperparathyroidism.

Preoperative Localization of Abnormal Parathyroid Tissue. Several methods have been proposed for identification of parathyroid adenomas before surgery. Occasionally large glands have been identified simply on esophagography; other procedures that have been used include scanning with ^{75}selenium-labeled methionine, intraoperative vital staining with toluidine blue, thermography, and arteriography (Fig. 3). None of these methods have been highly successful. The advent of the radioimmunoassay for parathyroid hormone, coupled with selective venous catheterization, has provided a means for more specific localization. Highly accurate localization of adenomas is possible when each of the thyroid veins can be selectively catheterized. Radioimmunoassays on samples obtained through the catheter show high gradients of parathyroid hormone concentration in the particular veins draining the lesion. Parathyroid hyperplasia, on the other hand, is frequently associated with a significant hormone gradient in each of the superior and inferior thyroid veins. In cases requiring repeated surgery for hyperparathyroidism, selective venous catheterization should be considered strongly before undertaking a further operation. In such instances, arteriography should be carried out as well in an attempt to delineate the thyroid venous anatomy as well as to uncover lesions representing potential parathyroid tissue.

Prognosis. Untreated, hyperparathyroidism with significant hypercalcemia may cause progressive renal impairment and ultimately death. Occasionally severe hypercalcemia develops rapidly ("hyperparathyroid crisis") and causes an immediate threat to life. On the other hand, the disease may exist in mild form without symptoms, and it is probable that some patients in apparently excellent health harbor hyperfunctioning parathyroid adenomas for decades and die of unrelated causes.

Uncomplicated primary hyperparathyroidism is correctable definitively by surgery. Occasionally a second adenoma becomes apparent after initial resection was apparently successful. When primary hyperplasia of the parathyroid glands is the cause and insufficient tissue has been resected, recurrence of the disease will show itself by return of preoperative symptoms and signs.

Treatment. *Hypercalcemia* (from whatever cause) that is neither severe nor progressive requires treatment directed only toward correction of the underlying

Figure 3. Arteriographic localization of large parathyroid adenoma. *A,* Arrows outline large parathyroid adenoma filled by radiographic dye injected into right inferior thyroid artery. This phase of the arteriographic study shows also a rich arterial vascular plexus within the gland. *B,* Late phase of arteriographic study, showing vein (delineated by arrows) draining the adenoma. Subsequent selective venous sampling showed a very high gradient for parathyroid hormone concentration at the point marked by the large arrow.

disease state. On the other hand, progressive and severe hypercalcemia (*"hypercalcemic crisis"*) leads to marked weakness, mental deterioration, coma, progressive uremia, and death within a short period. Several methods have been proposed for control of progressive hypercalcemia which may be so severe as to require emergency attention. Intravenous infusions of EDTA, sodium sulfate, or phosphate salts have been recommended, but each of these may produce hazardous side effects. Phosphate by mouth is effective in doses equal to those given intravenously, and there is probably less danger in this approach. Dehydration is often an important contributory factor in the development of progressive hypercalcemia and uremia. It is therefore important to restore extracellular fluids parenterally. Intravenous saline and furosemide are highly effective in reducing hypercalcemia. Sodium competes with calcium for reabsorption in the distal renal tubule, and furosemide potentiates this effect. Together furosemide and saline cause a marked increase in renal clearance of calcium and reduction of hypercalcemia.

One should also begin treatment with phosphate by mouth. For the first few days the equivalent of 2 grams of elemental phosphorus should be given in divided doses four times daily. Capsules can be prepared containing 190 mg of potassium dihydrogen phosphate plus 800 mg of disodium hydrogen phosphate. This provides 0.22 gram of elemental phosphorus per capsule. After three to five days when control of hypercalcemia has begun to be effective, the dosage of phosphorus should be reduced to 1 to 1.5 grams daily. Calcium, phosphate, and blood urea nitrogen should be monitored regularly to assure that the desired effect is obtained. It is best not to allow the blood phosphorus concentration to exceed 6 mg per 100 ml. Some patients with primary hyperparathyroidism have been maintained with nearly normal blood calcium for periods up to six months, pending clarification of other complications before parathyroidectomy. However, this form of treatment should be regarded as temporary; at the earliest possible moment, definitive therapy for the underlying disease should be instituted. Phosphate therapy may cause hypokalemia in these patients, requiring administration of potassium supplements. Calcitonin has not proved to be generally efficacious in controlling hypercalcemia.

Surgery is the only definitive treatment yet devised for primary hyperparathyroidism. In very mild cases it may be deferred, but only if frequent and regular observation of the patient is possible. It is the author's view that treatment should be deferred only so long as the patient is completely asymptomatic, can return for frequent evaluation, shows no clinical symptom or sign of the disease, and maintains a serum calcium concentration under 11.5 mg per 100 ml. Otherwise parathyroidectomy should be performed by a surgeon qualified by extensive experience. It is essential that the highest possible rate of success be obtained at the *initial* surgical procedure. As would be expected, multiple explorations for parathyroid adenomas carry increased risk and expense, as well as greater difficulty for the surgeon, particularly when scarring from earlier surgery is significant. One side of the neck should be searched meticulously first. If an obvious adenoma plus a normal gland is found on that side, the adenoma should be removed and the wound closed. This leaves the contralateral side undisturbed and suitable for ac-

curate exploration at a future time in the unlikely event this becomes necessary.

If the lesion is not found initially, the surgeon should extend the procedure to the contralateral side and should try to identify all four parathyroid glands, biopsying each for rapid histologic confirmation. Positive identification is important if subsequent surgical exploration becomes necessary and also provides for the possible existence of diffuse hyperplasia which is an indication for removal of seven eighths of all parathyroid tissue found. In rare instances there are more than four hyperplastic or adenomatous glands.

If neither hyperplastic nor adenomatous glands are found in the neck, a mediastinal exploration should be considered at a later date. Mediastinal tumors account for approximately 20 per cent of parathyroid adenomas; 95 per cent of them lie superiorly embedded in or attached to the mediastinal fat pad. As such, they are readily removable along with the fat pad through the routine neck incision. Thus only 1 per cent of all parathyroid adenomas should require a sternal splitting procedure. This conclusion is borne out by the observation that virtually all missed adenomas, discovered at subsequent surgical explorations, prove to be in the neck. Arteriography and selective venous catheterization (see Preoperative Localization, above) should be carried out before a second surgical procedure. The results of surgery can be assessed readily with serial analyses of serum calcium, and by following urinary excretion of cyclic 3',5'-AMP, which decreases to normal after successful parathyroidectomy.

Postoperatively, tetany may be expected in patients who show significant bone disease. This may require treatment at intervals with 10 per cent calcium gluconate (10 to 30 ml in 500 to 1500 ml of saline) intravenously and administration of vitamin D, 50,000 units or more daily by mouth, until severe hypocalcemia shows signs of control. Adequate dietary intake of calcium (at least 1 gram daily) should be assured; if necessary, calcium lactate capsules should be given by mouth. Therapy should be withdrawn as rapidly as clinical progress allows. Almost invariably, remaining parathyroid tissue recovers normal function; definite signs of recovery are usual within seven to ten days. It is best to allow some degree of hypocalcemia during the recovery period as long as symptoms are controlled, because hypercalcemia would tend to inhibit recovery of remaining parathyroid tissue. Excessive therapy with calcium by vein or vitamin D by mouth is neither necessary nor desirable.

Other complications in the postoperative period include temporary worsening of renal function or metabolic acidosis (see above), hypomagnesemia, pancreatitis, and gout or pseudogout. The physician should be particularly alert to the potential for the last two of these in subjects with intra-articular calcification or history of prior attacks.

Albright, F., Aub, J. C., and Bauer, W.: Hyperparathyroidism. J.A.M.A., 102:1276, 1934.

Albright, F., and Reifenstein, E. C., Jr.: The Parathyroid Glands and Metabolic Bone Disease. Baltimore, Williams & Wilkins Company, 1948.

Aurbach, G. D., and Potts, J. T., Jr.: The parathyroids. *In* Levine, R., and Luft, R. (eds.): Advances in Metabolic Disorders. New York, Academic Press, 1964, p. 45.

Aurbach, G. D., Mallette, L. E., Patten, B. M., Heath, D. A., Doppman, J. L., and Bilezikian, J. P.: Hyperparathyroidism: Recent studies. Ann. Intern. Med., 79:566, 1973.

Berson, S. A., and Yalow, R. S.: Parathyroid hormone in plasma in adenomatous hyperparathyroidism, uremia, and bronchogenic carcinoma. Science, 154:907, 1966.

Berson, S. A., Yalow, R. S., Aurbach, G. D., and Potts, J. T., Jr.: Immunoassay of bovine and human parathyroid hormone. Proc. Natl. Acad. Sci. U.S.A., 49:613, 1963.

Bilezikian, J. P., Doppman, J. L., Shimkin, P. M., Powell, D., Wells, S. A., Heath, D. A., Ketcham, A. S., Monchik, J., Mallette, L. E., Potts, J. T., Jr., and Aurbach, G. D.: Preoperative localization of abnormal parathyroid tissue: Cumulative experience with venous sampling and arteriography. Am. J. Med., 55:505, 1973.

Boonstra, C. E., and Jackson, C. E.: Hyperparathyroidism detected by routine serum calcium analysis. Ann. Intern. Med., 63:468, 1965.

Dohan, P. H., Yamashita, K., Larsen, P. R., Davis, B., Deftos, L., and Field, J. B.: Evaluation of urinary cyclic 3',5'-adenosine monophosphate excretion in the differential diagnosis of hypercalcemia. J. Clin. Endocr., 35:775, 1972.

Goldsmith, R. S.: Differential diagnosis of hypercalcemia. N. Engl. J. Med., 274:674, 1966.

Goldsmith, R. S., and Ingbar, S. H.: Inorganic phosphate treatment of hypercalcemia of diverse etiologies. N. Engl. J. Med., 274:1, 1966.

Lafferty, F. W.: Pseudohyperparathyroidism. Medicine, 45:247, 1966.

Mallette, L. E., Bilezikian, J. P., Heath, D. A., and Aurbach, G. D.: Primary hyperparathyroidism: Clinical and biochemical features. Medicine, 53:127, 1974.

Marx, S. J., Powell, D., Shimkin, P. M., Wells, S. A., Ketcham, A. S., McGuigan, J. E., Bilezikian, J. P., and Aurbach, G. D.: Familial hyperparathyroidism: Mild hypercalcemia in at least nine members of a kindred. Ann. Intern. Med., 78:371, 1973.

Moldawer, M. P., Nardi, G. L., and Raker, J. W.: Concomitance of multiple adenomas of the parathyroids and pancreatic islets with tumor of the pituitary: A syndrome with familial incidence. Am. J. Med. Sci., 228:190, 1954.

Muldowney, F. P., Carroll, D. V., Donohoe, J. F., and Freaney, R.: Correction of renal bicarbonate wastage by parathyroidectomy. Quart. J. Med., 40:487, 1971.

Neelon, F. A., Birch, B. M., Drezner, M., and Lebovitz, H. E.: Urinary cyclic adenosine monophosphate as an aid in the diagnosis of hyperparathyroidism. Lancet, 1:631, 1973.

Patten, B. M., Bilezikian, J. P., Mallette, L. E., Prince, A., Engel, W. T., and Aurbach, G. D.: Neuromuscular disease of hyperparathyroidism. Ann. Intern. Med., 80:182, 1974.

Powell, D., Singer, F. R., Murray, T. M., Minkin, C., and Potts, J. T., Jr.: Nonparathyroid humoral hypercalcemia in patients with neoplastic diseases. N. Engl. J. Med., 289:176, 1973.

Segre, G. V., Habener, J. F., Powell, D., Tregear, G. W., and Potts, J. T., Jr.: Parathyroid hormone in human plasma. J. Clin. Invest., 51:3163, 1972.

Sherwood, L. M., O'Riordan, J. L. H., Aurbach, G. D., and Potts, J. T., Jr.: Production of parathyroid hormone by nonparathyroid tumors. J. Clin. Endocr., 27:140, 1967.

Wermer, P.: Endocrine adenomatosis and peptic ulcer in a large kindred. Inherited multiple tumors and mosaic pleiotropism in man. Am. J. Med., 35:205, 1963.

873. HYPOPARATHYROIDISM

Definition. Hypoparathyroidism is the syndrome characterized by deficient secretion of parathyroid hormone, with consequent hypocalcemia.

Etiology. In most instances hypoparathyroidism is the consequence of mechanical injury to or removal of parathyroid glands during surgery for primary thyroid disorders or occasionally parathyroid disorders. Idiopathic hypoparathyroidism is rare; approximately 100 cases are known. It is usually recognized in childhood or adolescence and, in distinction to pseudohypoparathyroidism, it may be associated with pernicious anemia, ovarian failure, moniliasis, or Addison's disease; it occurs with equal incidence in males and females, and rarely is familial.

Pathology. In postsurgical and most cases of idiopathic hypoparathyroidism there is complete absence of the parathyroid glands. There may be calcification in the basal ganglia and cataracts. The bones may be abnormally dense, and the calvarium may be thickened.

Idiopathic hypoparathyroidism may represent an autoimmune disease.

Pathologic Physiology and Chemistry. The physiologic consequences of insufficient secretion of parathyroid hormone are low blood calcium, high blood phosphate, and a low rate of phosphate clearance into the urine. Attendant upon hypocalcemia is a very low concentration of calcium in the urine. As a general rule, the clearance of calcium into the urine approaches zero as its concentration in blood falls below 7 mg per 100 ml.

Hypocalcemia in hypoparathyroidism is a manifestation of the reduced rate of bone resorption in the absence of sufficient parathyroid hormone. The diminished concentration of calcium in extracellular fluid leads to increased neuromuscular excitability and tetany. Hyperphosphatemia in this disorder is primarily attributable to lack of the hormone effect on phosphate clearance by the kidney. The rate of urinary excretion of 3',5'-AMP is reduced, but in distinction to pseudohypoparathyroidism there is a normal response to exogenous parathyroid hormone.

Clinical Manifestations. The principal symptoms of hypoparathyroidism are due to a low concentration of calcium in the extracellular fluid. Hypocalcemic tetany is manifested by numbness and tingling in the fingers and toes and around the lips, and sometimes by laryngeal stridor with "crowing" inspiration, dyspnea, and cyanosis. In severe tetany, cramps of individual muscle groups occur in the hands and feet as carpopedal spasms. The differential diagnosis of tetany is discussed below. There may also be convulsions or abdominal pain, nausea, and vomiting. Epileptiform attacks are a striking symptom of hypoparathyroidism. Usually the seizures are of a grand mal type, but they are not always preceded by aura, loss of consciousness, involuntary trauma, or incontinence. The electroencephalogram may show abnormalities typical of idiopathic epilepsy. The seizures and usually the abnormal electroencephalographic pattern associated with tetany respond to treatment with calcium, whereas the latter is without effect in idiopathic epilepsy. Sometimes seizures of the petit mal type are expressed. Other cases may display choreiform movements, and in general there is increased sensitivity in hypoparathyroidism to the dystonic reactions of phenothiazine drugs.

Mental abnormalities may occur in hypoparathyroidism. Irritability, emotional lability, moroseness, impairment of memory, mental confusion, lethargy, depression, and mental deficiency have been described.

Papilledema, sometimes associated with increased intracranial pressure, may also accompany the hypocalcemia of hypoparathyroidism. These manifestations as well as the electroencephalograms return to normal when hypocalcemia is corrected. Cataracts are a characteristic consequence of chronic hypoparathyroidism. Other forms of ectopic calcification may be exhibited in the basal ganglia or subcutaneous tissues. The calvarium may be thickened.

Patients with idiopathic hypoparathyroidism may display abnormalities of the ectodermal structures, including the teeth, skin, nails, and hair. A characteristic feature of hypoparathyroidism early in life is blunting of the roots of the teeth and dysplasia of the enamel. The nails may be malformed and brittle and show transverse grooves. In addition, there is a significant incidence of moniliasis in idiopathic hypoparathyroidism, and when this involves the nails they become pitted and flaky in appearance. The transverse grooves, but not moniliasis, disappear when the serum calcium is corrected toward normal. The hair is thin, there may be patchy alopecia, and the skin is sometimes coarse and dry.

Diagnosis. Complaints of numbness and tingling in the extremities and around the mouth should suggest tetany. "Latent" tetany may be detected by eliciting Chvostek's sign by tapping over the facial nerve. A positive response consists of twitching of the muscles about the mouth and sometimes the nose and eyelids. Trousseau's sign is sought by producing ischemia with a cuff inflated above systolic pressure for three minutes. Characteristically, carpal spasm becomes evident during the course of the test. In latent tetany one may find increased sensitivity to galvanic current in producing muscle contraction (Erb's sign). The electrocardiogram may show a prolonged Q-T interval as a consequence of hypocalcemia.

Patients with atypical epilepsy, other manifestations of increased neuromuscular irritability, or bizarre mental symptoms should be investigated for possible hypoparathyroidism. Obviously a history of prior thyroid surgery should alert one to this possibility. Tetany associated with Addison's disease, pernicious anemia, or moniliasis should immediately suggest a diagnosis of idiopathic hypoparathyroidism. Each of these diseases may be caused by or associated with autoimmunity. Autoantibodies to parathyroid as well as ovarian, thyroid, or gastric tissue have been detected in some of these cases.

Prognosis. Hypoparathyroidism that follows thyroid or parathyroid surgery may often be transient. One should try withdrawing therapy several months postoperatively in such cases before it is concluded that permanent hypoparathyroidism exists. The prognosis is excellent with full life expectancy in established cases adequately treated. Untreated, the subject with hypoparathyroidism may suffer the discomfort and morbidity of muscular spasms, convulsions, cataracts, and mental impairment. It is not certain that cataracts can be prevented in hypoparathyroidism by correction of hypocalcemia early in the course of the disease. Epileptiform seizures are generally alleviated as hypocalcemia is corrected.

Treatment. Acute hypocalcemic tetany requires treatment with intravenous calcium, for example, calcium gluconate, 10 per cent solution (10 to 30 ml in 500 to 1500 of saline) given as necessary to control the symptoms. At the same time vitamin D, 50,000 to 100,000 units daily by mouth, should be given. Adequate intake of at least 1 to 2 grams of calcium by mouth should be assured, and sometimes further supplementation with 15 grams of calcium lactate (equivalent to 2 grams of calcium) in divided doses is necessary. The amount of vitamin D and calcium should be gradually reduced as serum calcium approaches normal. Crystalline dihydrotachysterol may be used instead of vitamin D and is advantageous in cases of toxicity because it is cleared more rapidly from the body. The commercial preparation *A.T.-10* shows variable potency and is not recommended for therapy. In the absence of parathyroid hormone, vitamin D may cause an inordinately high rate of excretion of urinary calcium with the danger of nephrolithiasis. If regulation is difficult by reduction of calcium and vitamin D intake, the hypercalciuria may be controlled by giving phosphate

by mouth. Sulkowitch's test is not of value in the management of these patients; quantitative analyses for 24-hour excretion of calcium are required.

874. PSEUDO-HYPOPARATHYROIDISM AND PSEUDOPSEUDO-HYPOPARATHYROIDISM

Definition. *Pseudohypoparathyroidism* is a clinical state of hypoparathyroidism characterized by normal secretion of hormone from the parathyroid glands, but with a genetic defect in the receptor tissues so that there is little or no response to the action of the hormone. The defect is transmitted as a sex-linked dominant trait, and is associated with characteristic abnormalities of physiognomy and growth. The genetically related disorder *pseudopseudohypoparathyroidism* (see below) represents an incomplete form of the syndrome, shows the constitutional features without the chemical findings of hypoparathyroidism, and may occur in the same families with pseudohypoparathyroidism.

Etiology and Genetics. Recent clinical investigations in this disorder as well as current studies on the mechanism of action of parathyroid hormone have shed light on the pathophysiology in this syndrome. The original hypothesis of Albright and his associates that the receptor tissues, bone, and kidney are unresponsive to parathyroid hormone still best accounts for the endocrinopathology of this disorder. Other hypotheses such as secretion of a biologically inactive form of parathyroid hormone, circulating antibodies to the hormone, or secretion of excessive amounts of calcitonin have been tested without substantiation. The direct action of parathyroid hormone on the kidney is reflected in the urinary excretion of cyclic 3',5'-AMP. Normal subjects show a marked increase in excretion of the nucleotide after injection of parathyroid hormone. Pseudohypoparathyroidism is characterized by a defective response to exogenous parathyroid hormone in terms of urinary excretion of 3',5'-AMP. The most reasonable interpretation of this finding, and the probable explanation for the disorder, is the genetic transmission of defective or deficient receptor–adenylate cyclase complex in the renal cortex and perhaps bone of those subjects.* These subjects, when hypocalcemic, secrete parathyroid hormone at increased rates reflected in high concentrations of the hormone in peripheral plasma. The secretory rate responds normally, though, to blood calcium.

The genetics of the disorder is currently best explained by a sex-linked dominant mode of inheritance. The sex incidence ratio is female to male 2:1; no instances of male-to-male transmission of the complete syndrome have been documented with biochemical test-

---

*It is possible that the defect does not involve the receptor itself or the enzyme adenylate cyclase. In one instance, the only case in which adenylate cyclase from renal tissue was tested directly, there appeared to be a normal in vitro response to parathyroid hormone. Other biochemical abnormalities, such as defective nucleotide or phospholipid regulatory site on the enzyme or a defect distal to generation of cyclic nucleotide, have not been excluded. However, these patients respond normally to exogenous dibutyryl cyclic 3',5'-AMP, and thus it seems that the metabolic defect must be at a site prior to formation of cyclic 3',5'-AMP.

ing. Possibly the short stature characteristic of the syndrome is also attributable to an abnormal X chromosome. Genetic studies of sex-linked disorders indicate that in order to achieve normal height two functional sex chromosomes are required; that is, both the X chromosomes in females or both X and Y in males must be normal in the segments controlling growth. Pseudopseudohypoparathyroidism, in females at least, may reflect genetic mosaicism with a relatively greater degree of inactivation of the abnormal X chromosome.

Incidence. Pseudohypoparathyroidism and its incomplete variant pseudopseudohypoparathyroidism are rare. The average case is recognized earlier in life than is idiopathic hypoparathyroidism. Approximately 100 cases of pseudohypoparathyroidism and still fewer cases of the variant have been reported.

Pathology. The parathyroid glands are normal or hyperplastic. Shortening of the carpal and metatarsal bones and metastatic calcification, including calcification of the basal ganglia, occur. Also, there may be thickening of the calvarium, defective enamel of the teeth, dental aplasia, coxa vara, coxa valga, and bowing of the long bones. Cataracts are common.

Pathologic Physiology and Chemistry. The clinical chemical findings, hypocalcemia, hyperphosphatemia, and a low urinary calcium, are qualitatively similar but sometimes milder than those found in idiopathic or postoperative hypoparathyroidism. However, in pseudohypoparathyroidism, biologically active hormone under normal secretory control is elaborated from the parathyroid glands, but the receptor tissues do not respond. Exogenously administered parathyroid hormone causes little or no effect. Other endocrinopathies may coexist. Hypothyroidism (particularly that caused by selective pituitary TSH deficiency), diabetes mellitus, hypomenorrhea, or gonadal dysgenesis may be found associated with pseudohypoparathyroidism. Conversely, moniliasis, Addison's disease, and pernicious anemia, which may be associated with idiopathic hypoparathyroidism, have not been found in cases of pseudohypoparathyroidism.

Clinical Manifestations. The symptoms and signs of pseudohypoparathyroidism encompass those of hypoparathyroidism plus certain unique abnormalities of physiognomy and growth. Mental retardation, short, stocky, obese stature, and round facies are characteristic. The hands and feet are usually disproportionately short, resulting in about 75 per cent of cases from shortening of one or more metacarpal and metatarsal bones. This is readily recognized when the fist is clenched, thereby causing a dimple over the head of the affected bone. Less frequently, shortening of the phalanges or uniform brachydactyly may occur. The calvarium is thickened in over one third of the patients. There may be delayed dentition, defective enamel, or complete dental aplasia. Less common defects include abnormally dense or lucent bones, exostoses, coxa vara, coxa valga, bowing of the ulna, radius, tibia, and fibula, and loss of "tubulation" of the long bones. Calcification occurs in the basal ganglia and in the dentate nucleus, and there may be actual ossification as well as calcification in the skin, subcutaneous tissue, and deep connective tissues. Cataracts are also common. Most cases of true pseudohypoparathyroidism show the abnormalities of physiognomy and growth originally described by Albright and his associates.

Diagnosis. The diagnosis is established by the characteristic constitutional changes, by the clinical and laboratory abnormalities of hypoparathyroidism, and by testing the response to purified parathyroid hormone or parathyroid extract given intravenously. The earlier test for pseudohypoparathyroidism based on measurement of urinary phosphate excretion did not allow clear-cut separation of pseudohypoparathyroidism from normal subjects who vary widely in response; determination of 3',5'-AMP in the urine affords virtually complete differentiation between the two groups. Normal subjects, but not those with pseudohypoparathyroidism, show a marked rise (to give 3',5'-AMP–to–creatinine ratios greater than 15 μmoles per gram) in the rate of excretion of urinary 3',5'-AMP within 15 to 45 minutes after injection of 200 U.S.P. units of parathyroid hormone intravenously. There is no overlap of results between normal subjects and those with the disease. Baseline excretion of cyclic AMP is lower than normal in patients with idiopathic, postsurgical, and pseudohypoparathyroidism, but higher than normal in pseudopseudohypoparathyroidism. The last-named group comprises patients with the physiognomy of pseudohypoparathyroidism but a normal response to parathyroid hormone. Parathyroid hormone in peripheral plasma is high (as long as hypocalcemia is not corrected) in pseudohypoparathyroidism, in contrast to other forms of hypoparathyroidism in which it is undetectable. Some patients previously categorized as having pseudohypoparathyroidism associated with intestinal malabsorption syndromes, osteitis fibrosa cystica, or both, should be re-examined with the newer diagnostic procedures. It is the author's view that opinions should be deferred pending further tests before accepting a patient with atypical family history or clinical findings as a true example of pseudohypoparathyroidism.

Treatment. In general the treatment of pseudohypoparathyroidism is the same as that of hypoparathyroidism. Usually hypocalcemia is easier to control in pseudohypoparathyroidism, although occasional patients seem relatively resistant to vitamin D and require unusually high doses to achieve normal blood calcium.

875. TETANY

Tetany may develop in hypocalcemia, alkalosis, potassium deficiency, and occasionally hypomagnesemia. The symptoms and signs of tetany are discussed in Ch. 873. In addition to the information obtained by clinical examination, the laboratory findings are particularly important in diagnosing the cause of tetany. In hypoparathyroidism the serum phosphate is high, whereas in the hypocalcemic states of rickets or osteomalacia serum phosphate may be below normal. Urinary calcium is low in all these states. Tetany caused by alkalosis is associated with normal serum phosphate and calcium and normal urinary excretion of calcium, but the blood pH is high. Alkalotic tetany may occur in hyperventilation, usually a manifestation of psychoneurosis, and can be corrected by inducing the patient to reduce the respiratory rate or breathe into a paper bag.

Metabolic alkalosis, caused by persistent vomiting, hypokalemic alkalosis, or excessive treatment with alkali, may also produce tetany. In excessive treatment with alkali, the serum calcium and phosphate are normal as long as there is no renal impairment, but the serum pH is high. Tetany is produced by overcorrection

Differential Diagnosis of Tetany

	Serum			Urine	
Cause	Ca	P_i	pH	Ca	pH
Hypocalcemia					
Hypovitaminosis D		↓	↓	N	−
Resistance to	N or ↓	↓	N		−
vitamin D		↓	↓	N	−
Intestinal					
malabsorption					
Hypoparathyroidism		↓	↑	N	−
Hypomagnesemia	N or ↓	N or ↑	N	N or ↓	−
Alkalosis					
Respiratory	N	N	↑	N	
Metabolic	N	N	↑	N	

Ca = Calcium. P_i = Phosphate. N = Normal. (−) = Indeterminate.
↑ = High. ↓ = Low.

of acidosis in chronic renal disease. In such a condition, there is a tendency to hypocalcemia as well as hyperphosphatemia. In respiratory alkalosis plasma bicarbonate is low or normal, whereas in metabolic alkalosis plasma bicarbonate is high. The history should suggest the appropriate diagnosis in cases of excessive intake of alkali or excessive loss of gastric acid. The diagnosis is supported by finding a high concentration of bicarbonate in the serum and an alkaline urine. Treatment is directed at checking the cause. Hypokalemic alkalosis may appear in primary aldosteronism or treatment with corticosteroid analogues, and calls for correction of hormone excess and repletion of body potassium. Neonatal hypocalcemia may occur after asphyxia in premature infants, or in the progeny of diabetic or hyperparathyroid mothers. This last is a transient phenomenon secondary to hypercalcemia attendant upon primary hyperparathyroidism in the mother. Hypomagnesemia is a rare cause of tetany refractory to treatment with calcium; magnesium deficiency in those instances should be corrected.

Albright, F., Burnett, C. H., Smith, P. H., and Parson, W.: Pseudohypoparathyroidism—an example of the "Seabright-Bantam syndrome." Endocrinology, 30:922, 1942.

Aurbach, G. D., and Potts, J. T., Jr.: The parathyroids. In Levine, R., and Luft, R. (eds.): Advances in Metabolic Disorders. New York, Academic Press, 1964, p. 45.

Bell, N. H., Avery, S., Sinha, T., Clark, C. M., Jr., Allen, D. O., and Johnston, C., Jr.: Effects of dibutyryl cyclic adenosine 3',5'-monophosphate and parathyroid extract on calcium and phosphorus metabolism in hypoparathyroidism and pseudohypoparathyroidism. J. Clin. Invest., 51:816, 1972.

Blizzard, R. M., Chee, D., and Davis, W.: The incidence of parathyroid and other antibodies in the sera of patients with idiopathic hypoparathyroidism. Clin. Exp. Immunol., 1:119, 1966.

Bronsky, D., Kushner, D. S., Dubin, A., and Snapper, I.: Idiopathic hypoparathyroidism and pseudohypoparathyroidism: Case reports and review of the literature. Medicine, 37:317, 1958.

Chase, L. R., Melson, G. L., and Aurbach, G. D.: Pseudohypoparathyroidism: Defective excretion of 3',5'-AMP in response to parathyroid hormone. J. Clin. Invest., 48:1832, 1969.

Harrison, H. E., Lifshitz, F., and Blizzard, R. M.: Comparison between crystalline dihydrotachysterol and calciferol in patients requiring pharmacologic vitamin D therapy. N. Engl. J. Med., 276:894, 1967.

Tashjian, A. H., Jr., Frantz, A. G., and Lee, J. B.: Pseudohypoparathyroidism: Assays of parathyroid hormone and thyrocalcitonin. Proc. Natl. Acad. Sci. U.S.A., 56:1138, 1966.

876. CALCITONIN AND MEDULLARY CARCINOMA OF THE THYROID

Medullary carcinoma of the thyroid (see also Ch. 843) arises from the parafollicular cells of the thyroid which derive embryologically from the final or ultimobranchial cleft. These particular cells of the ultimobranchial cleft may, like chromaffin tissue, take origin initially in the neural crest. In submammalian vertebrates the ultimobranchial cells remain separate as the ultimobranchial gland, whereas in mammals the anlage merges with the embryological thyroid, In either instance, the cells derived from the ultimobranchial cells constitute the gland that synthesizes and secretes calcitonin. Medullary carcinoma may be sporadic or familial and is part of a syndrome (the so called "multiple endocrine adenomatosis, type 2") encompassing hyperplasia or adenoma of the parathyroid glands, sometimes expressed as primary hyperparathyroidism, pheochromocytoma, multiple neuromas, and Cushing's syndrome. Abnormally high concentrations of calcitonin are found in medullary thyroid tumors as well as in plasma taken from these patients.

Incidence. Medullary carcinoma of the thyroid accounts for 5 to 10 per cent of the cases of thyroid cancer. In the familial form it follows the autosomal dominant form of inheritance.

Pathology. Histologically this tumor differs from other cancers of the thyroid in that the cells resemble parafollicular cells, there is often amyloid infiltration, and there are no papillary folds, follicles, or polymorphonuclear infiltrates in the tissue. (Sometimes artifacts of fixation look like papillary folds in sections.) The tumor usually does not appear to be encapsulated, and may show areas of calcification. The tissue does not take up radioactive iodine. As noted above, pheochromocytoma or parathyroid hyperplasia or adenoma may be associated with medullary carcinoma of the thyroid.

Pathologic Physiology. Although many of these tumors elaborate calcitonin at a high rate, hypocalcemia is unusual, perhaps because parathyroid hormone is secreted as a compensatory mechanism (secondary hyperparathyroidism). Moreover, as stated above, there may be frequent occurrence of primary hyperparathyroidism in the syndrome. It is possible that the development of primary hyperparathyroidism represents induced autonomy in the glands as a consequence of prolonged chronic secondary hyperparathyroidism. On the other hand, calcitonin, at least under experimental conditions, can directly stimulate secretion of parathyroid hormone; hyperparathyroidism might thus arise as a consequence of prolonged effects of calcitonin acting as a secretagogue. The concentration of histaminase in serum frequently is increased in metastatic medullary carcinoma.

Measurements by radioimmunoassay or bioassay show that hypercalcemia induces secretion of calcitonin from normal parafollicular cells as well as from medullary carcinoma tissue. In addition, glucagon or gastrin, injected intravenously in pharmacologic doses, causes secretion of calcitonin in some species as well as in patients with medullary carcinoma. These responses to calcium, glucagon, or gastrin are valuable in conjunction with radioimmunoassay as diagnostic tests for the syndrome. Completely asymptomatic cases in the familial syndrome have been detected by this means. Indeed, thyroid C-cell "hyperplasia" has been discovered in some family members showing abnormal secretory responses to calcium.

Clinical Manifestations, Prognosis, and Treatment. Medullary carcinoma may become evident simply as a mass in the thyroid or by the clinical expression of the associated endocrinopathies, pheochromocytoma, primary hyperparathyroidism, or Cushing's syndrome. The tumor, local or metastatic, may be hard or tender, and sometimes is calcified to a degree detectable by x-ray. Severe diarrhea may occur, possibly related to elaboration by the tumor of prostaglandins, serotonin, or calcitonin, any of which can stimulate intestinal secretion. Other conditions occasionally associated with the syndrome include buccal or orbital neuromas, peculiar facies, megacolon, or Marfan's syndrome–like habitus. Medullated nerves in the cornea are detected in some cases on slit lamp examination. The tumor often spreads locally, and metastases may grow to huge size. There is not yet sufficient experience to project the natural clinical course in this disorder. The tumor is refractory to treatment with radioactive iodine or antithyroid drugs, and usually to external radiation as well. At this time surgery represents the best approach, and should consist of wide excision, avoiding local seeding with tumor fragments. Isolated metastases may also be amenable to surgery. Persistent high concentrations of calcitonin in plasma reflect residual unresected tumor or metastases.

Aurbach, G. D., Potts, J. T., Jr., Chase, L. R., and Melson, G. L.: Polypeptide hormones and calcium metabolism. Ann. Intern. Med., 70:1243, 1969.

Cunliffe, W. J., Black, M. M., Hall, R., Johnston, I. D. A., Hudgson, P., Shuster, S., Gudmundsson, T. V., Joplin, G. F., Williams, E. D., Woodhouse, N. J. Y., Galante, L., and MacIntyre, I.: A calcitonin-secreting thyroid carcinoma. Lancet, 2:63, 1968.

Foster, G. V.: Calcitonin (thyrocalcitonin). N. Engl. J. Med., 279:349, 1968.

Hazard, J. B., Hawk, W. A., and Crile, G., Jr.: Medullary (solid) carcinoma of the thyroid—a clinicopathologic entity. J. Clin. Endocr., 19:152, 1959.

Hennessy, J. F., Gray, T. K., Cooper, C. W., and Ontjes, D. A.: Stimulation of thyrocalcitonin secretion by pentagastrin and calcium in two patients with medullary carcinoma of the thyroid. J. Clin. Endocrinol. Metab., 36:200, 1973.

Keiser, H. R., Beaven, M. A., Doppman, J., Wells, S., Jr., and Buja, M.: Sipple's syndrome: Medullary thyroid carcinoma, pheochromocytoma and parathyroid disease: Studies in a large family. Ann. Intern. Med., 78:561, 1973.

Melvin, K. E. W., Tashjian, A. H., Jr., and Miller, H. H.: Studies in familial (medullary) thyroid carcinoma. Recent Prog. Horm. Res., 28:399, 1972.

Steiner, A. L., Goodman, A. D., and Powers, S. R.: Study of a kindred with pheochromocytoma, medullary thyroid carcinoma, hyperparathyroidism and Cushing's disease: Multiple endocrine neoplasia, type 2. Medicine, 47:371, 1968.

Tashjian, A. H., Jr., and Melvin, K. E. W.: Medullary carcinoma of the thyroid gland: Studies of thyrocalcitonin in plasma and tumor extracts. N. Engl. J. Med., 279:279, 1968.

Tubiana, M., Milhaud, G., Coutris, G., Lacour, J., Parmentier, C., and Bok, B.: Medullary carcinoma and thyrocalcitonin. Br. Med. J., 4:87, 1968.

Wolfe, H. J., Melvin, K. E. W., Cervi-Skinner, S. J., Saadi, A. A. A., Juliar, J. F., Jackson, C. E., and Tashjian, A. H., Jr.: C-cell hyperplasia preceding medullary thyroid carcinoma. N. Engl. J. Med., 289:437, 1973.

877. MEDICAL TREATMENT OF HORMONE-DEPENDENT CANCERS

Philip K. Bondy

INTRODUCTION

It is always best to cure a malignant tumor by local excision, destruction with radiation, or both. However, if the tumor has already metastasized, local treatment alone is of course inadequate, and attempts to slow down the growth rate or eradicate the tumor require systemic therapy. The factors controlling tumor growth are not clear, but in some instances the endocrine environment may be important. In general, endocrine manipulations are most useful in tumors of hormone-sensitive organs, e.g., breast and prostate.

The application of endocrine treatment should not be considered as separate from the use of other modalities but should be part of an integrated approach, including surgery, radiotherapy, and chemotherapy as well. Thus the best results are obtained when treatment is planned from the beginning by an experienced team of people who are familiar with current knowledge and are constantly evaluating those results. There is no place for the lone entrepreneur in modern cancer treatment.

CANCER OF THE BREAST

This is a very common disease (incidence about 70 per 100,000 women per year; prevalence about 100 per 100,000 women per year). Incidence is higher in certain families and in childless women, and is reduced by early pregnancy. It is bilateral in 4 to 10 per cent of women when first seen, suggesting a multicentric origin. In spite of this, early diagnosis is desirable and regular examination should be carried out, especially in childless women over 30 years old, when family history is positive, or when a previous breast cancer has occurred. Diagnosis should be confirmed histologically. The prognosis is somewhat better in well-differentiated tumors, or when there are extreme lymphocyte infiltration and lymph node histiocytosis.

Treatment. The first step in designing treatment is to determine accurately the *distribution* of the tumor. Local disease is usually treated by surgery, supplemented by radiation if local lymph nodes are involved. If the primary tumor is too large for safe surgical treatment, radiation (sometimes followed by local surgery) is proper initial treatment. This local approach cannot be defended (except for palliation of painful or ulcerated masses) if there is evidence of distant dissemination. All patients should therefore have a skeletal roentgenographic survey, chest x-ray, and bone scan before surgery is planned. Further, it appears that the urinary excretion of more than 40 mg of hydroxyproline per gram of creatinine may indicate the presence of skeletal metastases. Elevation of the serum concentration of carcinoembryonic antigen suggests the presence of metastases, but a normal level does not exclude them.

Decisions about the type of surgery to perform and whether or not to irradiate the breast and nodes prophylactically are beyond the scope of this chapter (see textbooks of surgery). The design of medical treatment of inoperable or disseminated cancer rests on at least the following four factors:

Status of Ovarian Function. Castration is associated with tumor regression in about one third of premenopausal patients, whereas postmenopausal patients most commonly respond to the administration of estrogen. Cessation of menstrual flow is not by itself a safe guide, however. Many women continue to secrete estrogens for some time after their menses stop, and amenorrhea in younger women is not necessarily associated with depressed ovarian function. Thus if the estrogen levels of urine or plasma remain high, such women should be considered "premenopausal" even though they no longer have menstrual flow. Demonstration of a high plasma level of follicle-stimulating hormone (FSH) in perimenopausal or amenorrheic women may prove to be the best method for establishing the presence of true menopause.

Sensitivity of the Tumor to Hormones. Clinically, this must be determined chiefly by assessing the effects of castration or administration of hormones, although there is good evidence that tumors which lack in their cytoplasm the protein which binds estrogen are unlikely to respond to hormonal manipulation. Clinical response is definite only when tumor masses shrink in volume by 50 per cent or more. Symptomatic improvement without objective change is a treacherous criterion. Changes in urinary hydroxyproline or plasma carcinoembryonic antigen can usually be trusted as indicators; more specific indices are needed.

Disease-Free Interval after Excision. The outlook is better if this is more than two years.

Distribution of the Metastases. Involvement of soft tissues, for example, tends to respond to estrogens in postmenopausal women, whereas bone involvement is more responsive to androgens and chemotherapy. Local skin metastases in postmenopausal women respond to norethisterone more often than to any other endocrine treatment.

A general plan of treatment like that shown in the accompanying figure provides a consistent approach to treatment. Although experts may differ in details, the pattern outlined is widely accepted. Several points deserve comment.

1. *Prophylactic castration* is not recommended. It provides some extension of the disease-free interval but no prolongation of life. On the other hand, castration before recurrence interferes with evaluation of the response to ovarian ablation. Since this response determines the probability of subsequent response to endocrine treatment, a good deal of assurance is lost in the design of subsequent treatment schedules if early oophorectomy is carried out.

2. The *method of oophorectomy* is unimportant; surgery provides a quicker response than x-ray castration, at the expense of an additional operation. If the patient is desperately ill, surgery is probably preferable. Otherwise, some clinicians prefer irradiation.

3. *Chemotherapy* is seen in this scheme as a last resort. Usually, *successful* endocrine treatment provides longer remissions than chemotherapy; but the possibility of combining chemotherapy with endocrine treatment has not yet been adequately explored. It has been the writer's practice to combine quadruple chemotherapy (see below) with the appropriate endocrine manipulation from the very beginning in patients with a bad prognosis, i.e., those with a short disease-free interval or with extensive involvement of the viscera.

4. Success of *hypophysectomy* depends on the completeness of excision. In some instances, prolactin secretion has persisted even when growth hormone secretion has been abolished. In such patients, therapeutic failure may occur. This would indicate incompleteness of the operation. After hypophysectomy, the plasma prolactin level should be monitored for a year or more before it is decided that complete excision has taken place. The effect of removing prolactin cannot be evaluated unless it is known that the hormone is totally absent.

5. The postoperative treatment of patients lacking adrenals or pituitaries is discussed in Ch. 836 and 841.

There is much interest now in the possibility of controlling growth of breast cancers by suppressing *pituitary prolactin* secretion pharmacologically. At present, the only drug approved for use in the United States which has this effect is L-dopa, but its effects are too transient to make it practical. Preliminary reports

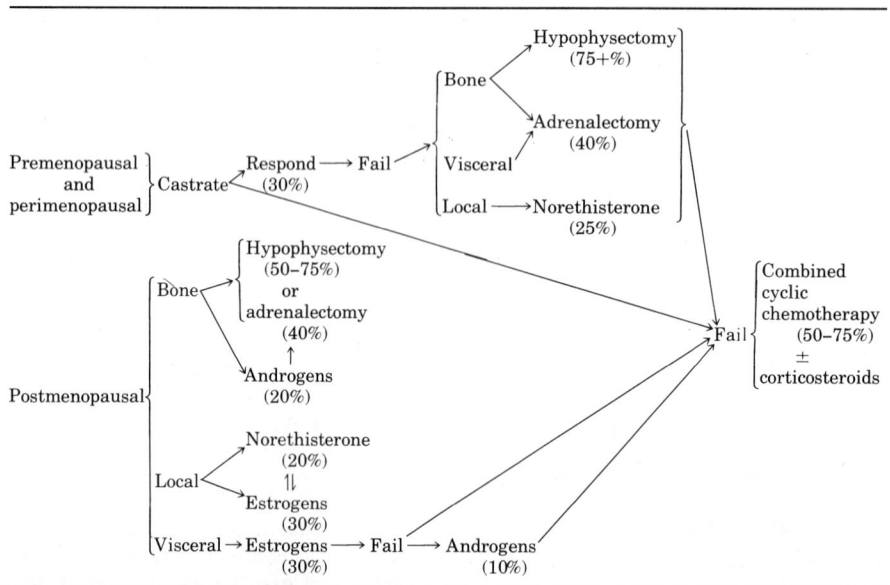

A generally accepted flow sheet for treating advanced cancer of the breast. The percentage figures represent the expected response of the group of patients receiving the treatment indicated above it. Thus hypophysectomy would be expected to produce about 75 per cent improvement in the premenopausal group which had responded to castration previously. In some clinics chemotherapy is given very early, along with or preceding endocrine treatment (see text). No mention is included of techniques which have not yet been adequately evaluated, e.g., anti-estrogens and pharmacologic suppression of prolactin secretion.

suggest that, in rare instances, it may reduce the growth rate of mammary tumors if given in maximal tolerated doses four or more times daily. Other drugs under preliminary investigation include the ergocornine and ergocryptine groups and some of their derivatives. As this is written, their use is not yet approved by the Food and Drug Administration. They are much more effective in animals than is L-dopa, and they may prove useful in the future.

Most textbooks state that cancer of the breast is unresponsive to *chemotherapy*, but this is incorrect. At least half the patients have a useful response to properly designed chemotherapy, although duration of the response may not be more than a few months. On the other hand, there is probably no hope of producing a cure of disseminated cancer with endocrine manipulations, whereas the possibility exists that cure might be achieved if the right pattern of chemotherapy could be found. Thus experiments to design effective treatment schedules are of great importance.

This approach to treatment may be used under several circumstances. A clinical trial is now in progress in the United States to determine whether *prophylactic administration* of phenylalanine mustard (Melphalan) to patients with extensive lymph node involvement will reduce the incidence or defer the development of metastases. Early reports suggest that metastases appear less frequently after this treatment than in controls.

Most oncologists agree that chemotherapy should be given to patients who have never responded to endocrine treatment, or who have escaped from an earlier response. Since one fourth to one third of tumors respond to alkylating agents, methotrexate, vinca alkaloids, or 5-fluorouracil, a combination of all four is often used. The writer's group has given cyclophosphamide, 500 mg, 5-fluorouracil, 500 mg, methotrexate, 50 mg, and vincristine, 2 mg, by a series of single injections one after another in the order listed, over a few minutes, repeating treatment every three weeks, provided that the blood count is satisfactory. This is a safe program, but it is probably less effective when compared with Edelstyn's schedule which spreads equivalent treatment over five days. Prolonging the duration of each treatment for five days increases the danger of bone marrow depression, however. New schedules including adriamycin are now being studied.

A few oncologists believe that treatment with chemotherapeutic agents should begin as soon as a diagnosis of dissemination has been made. Some (like Edelstyn) believe that chemotherapy should precede and supersede endocrine treatment. Others, including the author, feel that the two should be integrated. Further experience is needed.

Prognosis. In those women who respond, the mean duration of improvement after castration is about a year, and the maximum is several years. Response is more likely after a long disease-free interval and in patients with bone metastases. Patients younger than 35 may respond less often.

Estrogen treatment is about twice as likely to be effective as androgen in the postmenopausal woman. Androgens present few complications aside from masculinization; this is minimized by using one of the synthetic steroids, e.g., nandrolone.

A curious but useful effect is sometimes seen when endocrine treatment is discontinued after the patient has escaped from its effects. Withdrawal of treatment sometimes results in a second regression; but when the tumor resumes its growth a third regression can rarely be produced by resuming the original hormonal treatment.

Complications of Hormonal Treatment. Any endocrine treatment may cause a sudden, life-threatening rise of serum calcium, especially in patients with many lytic deposits in bone. This is combated by stopping treatment and by generous hydration; oral prednisolone, 10 mg four times daily, or cortisol, 100 mg intravenously every six hours. Mithramycin, 25 μg per kilogram intravenously at 48-hour intervals for not more than three doses, will safely reduce the serum calcium if these measures fail. The risk of hypercalcemia may be minimized by starting estrogen treatment at low doses (0.1 mg of diethylstilbestrol) for one to two weeks. Even a single course of quadruple chemotherapy usually restores the serum calcium value to normal, even though estrogen treatment is continued. If treatment is successful, rapid healing of osteolytic areas may cause hypocalcemia; this requires treatment with intravenous calcium salts and oral vitamin D until the rate of recalcification slackens off.

Large doses of diethylstilbestrol often cause nausea and vomiting. Conjugated mixed estrogens (Premarin) cause fewer gastrointestinal disturbances if they are given first in oral doses of 2.5 to 5 mg daily. Patients usually tolerate diethylstilbestrol after a week or so in doses of 0.5 mg thrice daily. There is rarely an advantage to larger doses.

Continuous administration of estrogens may cause breakthrough uterine bleeding, but this is unusual. If it occurs, cyclic courses are advisable. Edema may occur during estrogen treatment, and can be managed by diuretics. Increased pigmentation often occurs and is harmless. Thrombophlebitis may be a serious hazard, but whether the danger outweighs the advantage of treatment is not yet known.

In addition to these methods of treatment, radiation should always be available, to toleration, for relief of bone pain or of brain metastases. Proper support of the psyche, nutrition, and bone marrow should be provided.

Cancer of the Breast in Males. Malignant breast tumors are very rare in men; but when they occur they are usually much more aggressively malignant than in women. The same principles apply for treating the disease in men as in women, except that castration is generally considered to be an essential part of treatment regardless of age.

CANCER OF THE PROSTATE

This is a very common tumor, affecting between 14 and 46 per cent of all adult males in various autopsy series, but in most instances the tumor is localized and not of clinical significance. About 36 per 100,000 population have clinically significant tumor. In the United States there are about 17,000 deaths and 25,000 new cases per year. About 50 per cent of the clinically important cases can be diagnosed on rectal examination; the remainder are recognized from histologic examination of tissue removed at prostatectomy for benign prostatic hypertrophy. Once the diagnosis is suspected, histologic confirmation is essential, either by prostatectomy or by needle biopsy of suspicious nodules. After the diagnosis is established, the stage of the tumor's growth should be established.

Four stages are generally recognized:

1. Entirely intraprostatic, and too small to be suspected by physical examination or clinical laboratory methods.

2. Apparent on physical examination, but entirely confined to the prostate.

3. Confined to the pelvis. Here the tumor may have spread to other tissues in the pelvis but has not yet metastasized to distant points or bone.

In stages 1, 2, and 3, acid and alkaline phosphatase levels are not elevated in the serum, and skeletal x-ray, lymphogram and isotopc scanning of bone are negative. In these stages, there is hope of cure by surgery, radiation therapy, or both combined.

4. Distant metastases. Serum acid phosphatase is elevated in about two thirds of these patients. In those with skeletal metastases diagnosed by skeletal x-rays or bone scan, the alkaline phosphatase may also be elevated. These patients can no longer be cured by local treatment.

Treatment. The principles applicable to treating cancer of the breast are also appropriate for prostatic carcinoma. So long as the tumor is localized, every reasonable effort should be exerted to cure the tumor by surgery, radiation, or both. Chemotherapy or hormonal manipulations should be considered only when local methods are no longer applicable. By the same reasoning, local treatment should not be pushed beyond palliative levels if evidence of distant spread is already available. Careful staging is therefore essential before a decision about appropriate treatment can be made.

Since growth of prostatic cells is dependent on the presence of androgens, it was reasonable for Huggins and his colleagues to try the effects of *castration* on the growth of prostatic tumors (1941). About 80 per cent of cases respond to androgen deprivation by reduced bone pain and size of the tumor masses. In some cases, skeletal metastases may begin to show radiographic evidence of healing. In almost all, the elevated acid phosphatase drops somewhat, but this is an unreliable index of overall response of the tumor, because tumor cells produce less acid phosphatase, even though they may not die, when androgenic stimulation is removed.

Since castration has unpalatable emotional connotations even for aged men, administration of *estrogens* has sometimes been substituted for orchidectomy, with comparable symptomatic results. The dose schedule is much the same as for tumors of the breast. Some patients respond to estrogens after response to castration has disappeared. In spite of this, there is no evidence that castration, estrogens, or both together actually prolong life. They must be considered purely palliative measures. It is therefore especially noteworthy that the United States Veterans Administration Co-operative Urological Research Group found that administration of estrogens increased the death rate from cardiovascular causes by about 75 per cent, more than canceling a modest (25 per cent) reduction in mortality from the cancer. Since neither estrogens nor castration prolongs life, neither should be used except to relieve pain or urinary tract obstruction; even in these situations, the beneficial effects of radiation to local disease of bone or pelvis should be exploited before hormonal manipulation is tried. If a decision is made to turn to hormone therapy, castration is preferred, because it is not as-

sociated with the increased cardiovascular complications seen in estrogen-treated patients. If castration loses its useful effect, and the symptoms cannot be controlled by conventional methods or radiotherapy, low doses of estrogens (1 or 2 mg of diethylstilbestrol daily) may be tried. This dose is probably less risky than full 5 mg doses. *Adrenalectomy* and *hypophysectomy* offer no advantages after castration has failed.

The place of *cytotoxic chemotherapy* is less well established in prostatic cancer than in cancer of the breast; but it is the writer's impression that several agents, including cyclophosphamide and methotrexate, sometimes give relief of bone pain, suggesting a response. Objective evidence of reduced tumor size or increased longevity is not at hand. Further studies of chemotherapeutic combinations are needed in this disease.

CANCER OF THE THYROID

Well-differentiated thyroid carcinomas are often under pituitary control, and their growth can be blocked and the metastatic masses may disappear if secretion of thyroid-stimulating hormone (TSH) is suppressed. This is accomplished by giving replacement doses of thyroxine or equivalent hormone combinations of thyroxine and triiodothyronine. Suppression may continue for very long periods with control of the cancer. The matter is discussed in more detail in Ch. 843.

OTHER ENDOCRINE CANCERS

There is no evidence that suppressing pituitary ACTH secretion controls the growth or activity of carcinomas of the adrenal cortex, whether functional or not. Endocrine manipulations are ineffective in treating tumors of other endocrine organs. The influence of pituitary growth factors and insulin on tumors of nonendocrine tissues has not yet been established. The cytotoxic effects of *adrenocortical steroids* are used in treating lymphomas, Hodgkin's disease, and other tumors and to ameliorate secondary effects of tumors such as dermatomyositis, neuropathy, and hemolytic disease. They may also relieve pressure by reducing the inflammatory zone surrounding tumor masses, e.g., in cerebral metastases.

Byar, D. P.: Treatment of prostatic cancer: Studies by the Veterans Administration Co-operative Urological Research Group. Bull. N.Y. Acad. Med., 48:751, 1972.

Canellos, G. P., Devita, V. T., Gold, G. L., Chabner, B. A., Schein, P. S., and Young, R. C.: Cyclical combination chemotherapy for advanced breast cancer. Br. Med. J., 1:218, 1974.

Edelstyn, G. J. A., and Macrae, K. D.: Cyclical combination chemotherapy in advanced breast cancer. Br. J. Cancer, Vol. 28, 1973.

Huggins, C., and Hodges, C. V.: Studies on prostatic cancer: Effect of castration, of estrogen, and of androgen injection on serum phosphatase in metastatic carcinoma of the prostate. Cancer Res., 1:293, 1941.

Jensen, E. V., Block, G. E., Smithe, S., Kyser, K., and DeSombre, E.: Estrogen receptors and breast cancer response to adrenalectomy. Natl. Cancer Inst. Monogr., 34:55, 1971.

Stoll, B. A.: Endocrine Therapy in Malignant Disease. Philadelphia, W. B. Saunders Company, 1972.

Veterans Administration Co-operative Urological Research Group: Treatment and survival of patients with cancer of the prostate. Surg. Gynecol. Obstet., 124:1011, 1967.

878. BONE PHYSIOLOGY AND CALCIUM HOMEOSTASIS

Robert P. Heaney

Duality of Skeletal Function. The skeleton functions as both a structural and a calcium homeostatic organ. Diseases that affect bone both alter the supporting function of the skeleton and have far-reaching effects on calcium homeostasis; conversely, derangements of calcium homeostasis are inevitably reflected in bone as a supporting tissue. Although it would be difficult to conceive of terrestrial existence without the mechanical support provided by a rigid endoskeleton, the fact is that the tissue, bone, evolved in exclusively aquatic vertebrates, in which there probably was no selective advantage conferred by a rigid endoskeleton. The principal evolutionary significance of bone lies in the fact that it has afforded higher vertebrates the ability to regulate the concentration of calcium and phosphate ions in body fluids. This primitive ability remains a fundamental property of the modern human skeleton, and reminds us of this by occasionally exerting its primacy over the much more obvious structural role of the tissue.

Whereas parathyroid hormone, discussed at length in Ch. 871, exerts the primary endocrine control over calcium homeostasis, it is bone that provides the principal end-organ by which this homeostasis is effected. This action depends upon two fundamental properties of bone tissue: (1) the physical-chemical equilibrium between the solid phase bone mineral and calcium ions in the body fluids, and (2) the continuous structural remodeling of bone with its associated deposition and removal of large quantities of calcium and phosphorus.

Bone Structure and Composition. Bone consists of a highly organized system of cells embedded in a matrix composed of a fibrous protein, collagen, encrusted with tiny calcium phosphate crystals. Cells occupy 2 to 3 per cent of the total volume, but are evenly distributed through the bone and interconnected by a series of canaliculi, so that no volume of interstitial bony material is more than a fraction of a micron from a cell or its processes, and no bone cell is more than 100 microns from a capillary. In fully mineralized bone the protein matrix accounts for half the volume and one third the weight of the intercellular material, and the crystals comprise most of the remainder. Mucopolysaccharides make up about 5 per cent of the organic matrix, and although quantitatively a minor component of bone, they probably contribute significantly to matrix maturation and mineralization. The collagen fibers in adult human bone are not randomly arranged, but are oriented to resist the mechanical forces which the organ must withstand. Furthermore, the intimate association of fibrous protein and ultramicroscopic crystals constitutes what, in materials engineering, has been termed a "two-phase" material. The breaking strength and elasticity of bones depend not only on their mass and shape, but as well on the intrinsic mechanical properties of this two-phase system and on changes that occur in those properties as the material ages. Although still poorly understood, it is probable that some of the symptoms and signs of the diseases to be described in the following pages represent qualitative abnormalities in the bone material itself.

The mineral component of bony material is a calcium-phosphate generally considered to possess the crystal structure of hydroxyapatite. There is an additional carbonate component which may comprise as much as 8 per cent of bone ash and which is currently believed to be present both as $CaCO_3$ and as limited carbonate substitution in or on the apatite crystal. The calcium carbonate phase is acid labile, even in vivo, and is depleted during systemic acidosis. When initially deposited, bone mineral appears crystallographically amorphous and gradually matures to the characteristic apatitic pattern.

Bone Formation. Bone is deposited on free surfaces by osteoblasts that synthesize collagen and secrete it onto the bone-forming surface. Soon after secretion the soluble collagen molecules aggregate into spatially oriented insoluble fibrils. The factors that control their orientation are not well understood, but bioelectrical fields of the magnitude known to be produced in bone by applied mechanical stress have been shown to influence the orientation of collagen fibrils in vitro. Osteoblasts deposit a layer of matrix about 1 μ in thickness per day. There is about a ten-day lag before mineralization occurs, so that a normal osteoid seam averages 10 μ in thickness. Under control of the parent osteoblast the matrix undergoes a complex series of biochemical changes, which ultimately lead to crystal nucleation and growth. This process includes changes in the mucopolysaccharide component of the matrix and appearance of lipid-staining material at the calcification front. These and other changes are reflected in distinct layers and sequences recognizable only by special stains. Alkaline phosphatase has long been associated with active bone formation and can be detected both within osteoblasts and extracellularly in the superficial layers of newly deposited matrix, but not more deeply at the calcification front itself. Despite many attractive hypotheses, no clearly definable role of this enzyme has been found, and its association with active bone formation remains largely circumstantial.

Once maturation is complete, the collagen fibril becomes capable of initiating the deposition of mineral, in a specific crystalline pattern, from the ions present in the bathing fluid. These crystals are formed both within and upon the fibril and are oriented along its length. Crystal growth displaces the water that originally occupied 50 per cent of the volume of unmineralized matrix. Approximately three fourths of the ultimate mineral content may be deposited within a few hours. The remaining mineral enters more slowly, largely because the decrease in free water severely limits diffusion, and thus completion of mineralization may require weeks or even months.

Once nucleation occurs, mineral is extracted from the surrounding fluid with great efficiency. This appears to be explained by the fact that the solubility product of hydroxyapatite is considerably lower than the $Ca \times P$ ion product in extracellular fluid, and thus crystal growth occurs as rapidly as blood flow can transport mineral to the site. On the other hand, spontaneous precipitation of calcium phosphates from the body fluids does not normally occur in other tissues because, though supersaturated with respect to the ultimate mineral phase of bone, these fluids are undersaturated with respect to the mineral crystalline forms that calcium phosphate is known to assume when precipitated at physiologic pH. The extraordinary beauty of this arrangement lies in the fact that mineralization thus occurs only at sites specifically rendered mineralizable by formation of an *improbable* nucleating configuration, and in the fact that one and the same body fluid carries a great surplus of mineral when in the presence of such a nucleating center, but is indefinitely stable—indeed undersaturated—elsewhere.

An important consequence of this mineralization scheme is the demand for mineral created by nucleated, but as yet incompletely mineralized bone. This demand amounts to a kind of "mineralization debt," analogous to the lactic acid debt of anaerobic muscle work, and will inevitably lower the concentration of calcium in body fluids unless specifically offset by homeostatic adjustment. Indeed, this continuing demand, which cannot apparently be modulated after it is initiated, is quantitatively the largest single stress to which the calcium homeostatic system must respond. Normally new bone mineralization utilizes 300 to 500 mg of calcium daily, an amount greater than the total calcium content of the entire blood volume. This demand may increase by as much as two orders of magnitude in diseases in which active bone formation occurs, such as severe osteitis fibrosa, and is partially responsible for the "bone hunger" and associated hypocalcemia that are sometimes seen after removal of a parathyroid adenoma.

Bone Resorption. Resorption occurs by virtually simultaneous dissolution of both mineral and matrix, and is produced both by large multinucleated cells known as osteoclasts and by osteocytes (which enlarge their lacunae in response to parathyroid stimulation). Osteoclasts are short lived and do their work quickly. The space eventually to be filled by a new haversian system can be tunneled out of cortical bone in less than 10 per cent of the time required by osteoblasts to fill it in with new bone. This means that large quantities of mineral can be released from the skeleton in short periods of time. The mechanisms by which bone solids are solubilized are largely unknown. Collagenase and a variety of lysosomal proteases are involved in matrix hydrolysis, and large quantities of H^+ are consumed in solubilization of the mineral (approximately one proton for each calcium ion). The H^+ production derives from both organic acids and carbonic anhydrase, and is both dependent upon and stimulated by O_2 levels in the bathing fluids. Carbonic anhydrase has been specifically localized to osteoclasts, and its inhibitors can directly reduce bone resorption.

Control of Bone Remodeling. Teleologically, bone remodeling serves both homeostatic and structural needs. By processing large quantities of mineral each day it establishes an input-output system capable of being adapted to calcium deficiency or excess by comparatively minor adjustments of the balance between formation and resorption. Structurally it allows the bone to reshape itself to meet new forces and, even more fundamental, it continually renews its aging interstitial material and thus maintains optimal mechanical properties.

The control of bone formation and resorption, i.e., structural bone turnover, is exerted at two levels: in intrinsic bone cellular activity and in the superimposed systemic influences such as those produced by hormones, nutrition, and systemic disease. The former is the more important; unfortunately, it is still poorly understood.

Systemic Control. Growth hormone and thyroid hormone stimulate osteoblast activity and osteoblastic recruitment from osteoprogenitor cells, whereas adrenal corticoids, malnutrition, fever, and a variety of systemic diseases decrease both new matrix production and the osteoblast-mediated ripening of the osteoid seam. Androgens and estrogens, previously thought to stimulate osteoblastic activity, have been shown to exert their effect, instead, by suppressing bone resorption, and if they have any effect on osteoblasts at all, probably suppress them to a minor extent. None of these effects can be considered homeostatic, either from the point of view of the skeleton as a structural unit or from the point of view of the extracellular fluid calcium ion level, simply because there exist no known feedback loops from the skeletal effects to the control of hormone secretion.

Homeostatic control of bone turnover is exerted by parathyroid hormone and calcitonin, which are concerned not with skeletal homeostasis, but with the maintenance of calcium ion concentration in the extracellular fluid. Parathyroid hormone secretion is inversely related to extracellular fluid calcium ion levels, and hormone action is exerted on at least three independent end-organs: bone, intestinal mucosa, and renal tubule. The intestinal absorptive effect is mediated through control of vitamin D metabolism (see below). All three effects function to raise the concentration of calcium ion in extracellular fluid. In bone the most obvious effect of the hormone is a stimulation of bone resorption, with consequent release of calcium and phosphorus. In cases of severe parathyroid dysfunction there is commonly also an increase of new bone formation that parallels the more immediate change in resorption. In the intestinal mucosa parathyroid hormone is indirectly responsible for control of calcium absorption. The efficiency of calcium absorption, which, in the adult, is about 30 per cent, may rise to over 90 per cent in hyperparathyroidism and fall to nearly zero in hypoparathyroidism. In the kidney parathyroid hormone effects are twofold: a decrease in tubular phosphate reabsorption (discussed elsewhere in this text) and an increase in tubular calcium reabsorption. The renal effects occur within minutes and the bone effects within hours, whereas the intestinal response requires days to become apparent. Although all three responses have the same general effect, the renal response seems best suited for emergency adjustment, the bone response represents the largest reserve capacity of the three, and the intestinal response seems designed more to restore total body calcium balance than to adjust the level of calcium ion in extracellular fluid.

A variety of factors modulate parathyroid hormone effects on bone resorption. Mechanical stresses, gonadal steroids, high concentrations of calcium or phosphate, calcitonin, fluoride, and the diphosphonate compounds all depress resorptive response to a given level of parathyroid hormone. Some act at the level of mesenchymal activation (such as the gonadal steroids), some at the existing resorptive cellular machinery (such as calcitonin), and some at the mineral level itself (such as fluoride), but the ultimate effect of each is a shift in the dose response curve of parathyroid-mediated bone resorption in the direction of resistance. On the other hand, disuse, heparin, increased oxygen tension, and local inflammation all enhance resorptive response to parathyroid hormone. The significance of these interactions lies not in calcium homeostasis (for plasma calcium regulation takes place despite these alterations of PTH responsiveness, simply by compensatory adjustment of parathyroid hormone secretion rate), but in the bone mass itself. Enhanced responsiveness leads to negative calcium balance, reduced responsiveness to positive balance.

Calcitonin suppresses bone resorption, by inhibiting both osteocytes and osteoclasts. Its immediate effect is reduction in release of calcium and phosphorus from bone; hence in the fasting state it produces a fall in both plasma calcium and phosphate. Although secreted in small quantities at normal plasma calcium levels, it is normally released in response to hypercalcemia and probably finds its chief role in normal physiology in moderating absorptive hypercalcemia. This is most important in infancy, when absorbed milk calcium might otherwise inundate the infant's small extracellular fluid volume and thus produce serious hypercalcemia. The effect of calcitonin on skeletal mass in man is unknown, but it is to be expected that long-term overproduction or exogenous administration would lead to increased skeletal mass. (Calcitonin has, in fact, been indirectly implicated in the hyperostosis of bulls fed a milking ration.)

Intrinsic Control. Apparently the two most important elements of local control are mechanical forces and local blood flow, the latter with its associated regulation of nutrient supply, pH, and O_2 tension. Increased blood flow is associated with osteoclastic resorption, and vascular stasis with increased osteoblastic activity. The effects of mechanical forces are profound. A bone or bony region subjected to heavy use will increase its mass and revise both its internal structure and external shape so as to resist applied forces; conversely, disuse leads rapidly to decrease in mass and loss of specific architectural features. Normally, muscle mass and skeletal mass maintain a ratio of approximately 10:1.

Both the nature of the signal that mechanical forces transmit to bone cells and the nature of the cellular response are largely unknown. However, bone exhibits many of the features of a semiconductor and has been shown to generate and maintain small electrical fields when deformed by externally applied forces. These fields are of the same magnitude as those shown to be capable of orienting collagen fibril aggregation and those controlling limb bud regeneration in amphibia. Thus it is possible that both cellular activity and extracellular organization of matrix fibrils may be determined by local electrical fields. The distribution of stresses within bone and associated induced electrical fields and altered blood flow are so complex and so heterogeneous that turnover may be intense at one site and only a few millimeters distant may be virtually at a standstill.

Envelope-Specific Remodeling. The foregoing statements, although applicable in a general way, must be further modified to incorporate a most important component of intrinsic control, namely envelope-specific remodeling. Because the bony material is exterior to the cells, all bone remodeling must take place from bone surfaces. These surfaces comprise three virtual envelopes, periosteal, haversian (intracortical), and trabecular-endosteal, and the behavior of bone cells on each of these envelopes exhibits distinct differences, despite common systemic

influences. Aging, hormones, drugs, and diseases are all characterized by discrete envelope-specific remodeling patterns. These patterns are useful both for classification and recognition of bone diseases and for adequate understanding of bone pathophysiology.

In normal adult bone something less than 5 per cent of the free surface of all three envelopes is involved in remodeling at any time. When a microscopic site on one of these envelopes becomes a remodeling locus, events always proceed in an orderly sequence, which consists first of mesenchymal activation, followed next by osteoclastic erosion into the bone surface, and finally by osteoblastic repair. The entire sequence normally requires from 3 to 12 months to go from start to completion at any given site. At any remodeling site, wherever located, resorption always precedes and appears to be a necessary preliminary to formation. The three bony envelopes differ primarily in the balance between resorption and formation which occurs in this remodeling sequence and in how the process responds to systemic and hormonal stimuli.

Except for modeling of external contours associated with growth, the periosteal surface normally exhibits a preponderance of formation over resorption, and hence constitutes an expanding envelope throughout life. There is a brief period in adolescence, most marked in females, when the endosteum is also predominantly a forming surface, at which time the bony cortex is thickened by apposition from both sides; but through most of life the endosteal-trabecular envelope is predominantly a resorbing surface. On the haversian envelope, however, resorption and formation are normally balanced so that replaced bone is approximately equivalent to removed bone.

Although treated in greater depth in the following chapters some examples of envelope-specific patterns may help to illustrate this concept. Postmenopausal and corticosteroid osteoporosis are both exclusively disorders of the endosteal envelope; whereas hyperparathyroidism, either primary or the parathyroid effect seen in osteomalacia and renal osteodystrophy, produces activation of all three envelopes, with resorption predominating. Growth hormone also activates all three envelopes, but causes formation to dominate. In fact growth hormone is the only known, naturally occurring agent able to convert the adult endosteum to a predominantly forming surface.

Vitamin D. Both the plant and animal D vitamins (ergo- and cholecalciferol, respectively) are first hydroxylated at the 25-position by a specific liver enzyme system, and then, in the kidney, further hydroxylated at the 1- or the 24-position. The 1,25-dihydroxy compound (1,25-HCC) is the active form of the vitamin, mediating the control of intestinal calcium absorption and acting to facilitate parathyroid hormone effects on bone resorption. There appears to be continuous renal hydroxylation of 25-OH cholecalciferol; the synthetic balance between the 1,25- and the 24,25-derivatives is controlled by the level of parathyroid hormone. High parathyroid hormone levels favor the 1,25-derivative, which in turn increases intestinal calcium absorption and enhances the parathyroid hormone effect on bone resorption. No significant biologic activity has yet been associated with the 24,25-derivative. It is possible that the parathyroid effect on hydroxylation may be indirect, i.e., mediated through the plasma phosphate levels, inasmuch as lowered plasma phosphate has the same effect on directing hydroxylation to the 1,25-derivative as does an elevated parathyroid hormone level.

Calcium absorption from the intestine is associated with a transport protein with a high affinity for calcium (calcium-binding protein), and 1,25-HCC is necessary for production of this material in most species studied to date. Nevertheless, much uncertainty remains both as to the actual cellular mechanism of vitamin D action and as to the tissues most affected by vitamin D deficiency. Plainly vitamin D is necessary for intestinal calcium absorption, and most particularly for the absorptive responses to low calcium intake or high parathyroid hormone levels. There is no general agreement, however, whether vitamin D is necessary for osteoid maturation or epiphyseal cartilage growth and maturation, each of which is retarded in vitamin D deficiency states. Attempts to explain each of these effects as a result of calcium absorptive defects are unconvincing, and it seems safest to assume a direct dependence of each of these cell types on vitamin D until such is clearly shown to be unnecessary. Curiously, the renal tubular effects of parathyroid hormone on calcium and phosphate transport seem to be independent of vitamin D.

Age Changes in Bone.   In general, after the fourth decade, bone mass declines at an average rate of 5 to 10 per cent per decade. Although certain individuals may be exempted from this decline, it appears to be universally true of all populations and racial groups studied, regardless of nutritional or environmental factors. The decline appears to coincide with, or at least be accelerated at the time of, menopause in women, and the rate of loss is greater in women than in men, but it nevertheless occurs in both sexes.

Bourne, G. H. (ed.): The Biochemistry and Physiology of Bone. 2nd ed. New York, Academic Press, 1971.

Frost, H. M.: Bone Remodeling and Its Relationship to Metabolic Bone Disease. Springfield, Ill., Charles C Thomas, 1973.

Harris, W. H., and Heaney, R. P.: Skeletal Renewal and Metabolic Bone Disease. Boston, Little, Brown & Company, 1970.

McLean, F. C., and Urist, M. R.: Bone. 3rd ed. Chicago, University of Chicago Press, 1968.

Vaughn, J.: The Physiology of Bone. New York, Oxford University Press, 1970.

THE OSTEOPOROSES

Robert P. Heaney

879. INTRODUCTION

Definition.   The term osteoporosis, literally "bone porosity," designates a deficiency of bone tissue per unit volume of bone as an organ. The deficiency relates only to the structural function of bone, not to its calcium homeostatic role. The bone that remains is considered to be normal by both chemical and ordinary histologic criteria. The fibrous and fatty marrow that fills the voids once occupied by bone is also normal, and there is no obvious morphologic evidence of osteoblastic or osteoclastic dysfunction. These requirements exclude many specific entities also associated with quantitative reduction in a qualitatively normal bone mass, such as hyperparathyroidism, multiple myeloma, and carcinoma metastatic to bone. Thus these features *describe* osteoporosis, rather than *define* it, because osteoporosis is not so much the presence of an abnormal bone condition as it is the absence of a normal quantity of bone.

Morphologic and Roentgenographic Characteristics.   The decrease in bone mass expresses itself as loss of normal cortical thickness, and as thinning, fragmentation, and loss of trabeculae. The external dimensions of the involved bone do not change (except as a consequence of fracture). The cortical thinning is usually readily visible on roentgenograms of long bones. Decreased roentgenographic density is an unreliable sign, and thus early changes in primarily cancellous bone, such as the pelvis and spine, are hard to evaluate. As the disease advances, one can discern increased contrast between the end plates and bodies of vertebrae, relative accentuation of vertical trabeculae, biconcave compression of the end plates (producing the characteristic "codfish" vertebrae), herniation of the nucleus pulposus into the bodies of the vertebrae (Schmorl's nodes), and, finally, vertebral compression fractures. The involved bodies are usually wedged anteriorly, especially in the thoracic region, but sometimes uniform collapse or even posterior body wedging is seen, depending on the region of the spine involved. The neural arch invariably remains intact.

Except for the purely local osteoporoses such as those associated with inflammation or disuse, most osteoporoses are generalized diseases involving the entire skeleton, and, if carefully sought, roentgenographic evidence of decreased bone mass can be found in all bones examined, including the skull, the long bones, and the hands and feet. Decreased cortical thickness of the femur and of the metacarpal, metatarsal, and phalangeal bones is a common accompaniment of vertebral osteoporosis and usually, though not always, parallels the latter in severity. The combined thickness of the two cortices usually amounts to more than 45 per cent of total shaft diameter in these bones; values less than this are indicative of decreased bone mass. Disproportionately more severe bone loss in the largely cancellous bone of the central skeleton usually signifies a rapidly developing osteoporosis, whereas more uniform bone loss means slow development. When the degree of bone loss becomes extreme, macroscopic regions of cancellous bone may present a cystlike appearance roentgenographically.

Microscopically the bone shows no abnormalities by usual criteria. Increased marrow mast cell counts have been noted in all types of osteoporosis evaluated to date. This is of interest because of the known potentiation of endogenous parathyroid hormone by heparin and because bone loss of osteoporosis occurs primarily at the endosteal envelope, which is also the sole bony interface with the bone marrow. However, it is not known whether the mast cells precede the onset of the osteoporotic process or are a response to it.

General Pathophysiologic Considerations.   Many useful analogies can be drawn between osteoporosis and anemia. Like anemia, osteoporosis is not a specific disease entity but is instead a quantitative deficiency of a normal body constituent. It is the end result of many quite different pathophysiologic processes. The one element common to all these mechanisms is that, in the transition between normal bone and osteoporotic bone, the resorptive component of bone turnover must exceed new bone formation. But, again like anemia, this destructive imbalance can proceed at high, low, or normal rates of bone turnover. The osteoporosis of Cushing's syndrome develops at low rates of new bone formation; postmenopausal and senile osteoporoses usually develop at normal or near normal absolute rates of bone turnover; and disuse osteoporosis, peri-inflammatory osteoporosis, and the osteoporoses of acromegaly and hyperthyroidism develop at high rates of bone turnover. Indeed, the rate of bone turnover is largely an irrelevant consideration; the only important matter is why resorption is higher than formation. This problem is more difficult than it appears, because it implies a knowledge of the mechanisms by which formation and resorption are matched and bone mass is preserved in normal persons. This information is not yet available.

One thing, however, seems certain: the elements of calcium ion homeostasis are involved in the pathogenesis of osteoporosis, at least as unwitting participants if not as originators of the process. Significant bone loss cannot develop at low remodeling rates; hence tonic parathyroid secretion, which is quantitatively the major determinant of normal bone remodeling, becomes involved either actively or passively in development of any osteoporosis. The components of calcium homeostasis constitute a kind of final common pathway for skeletal remodeling, and most, if not all, modalities altering the remodeling balance between formation and resorption exert their effects either directly via parathyroid hormone or by altering bony end-organ responsiveness to parathyroid hormone.

Certain animal species, notably rats, kittens, puppies, and lions, all develop osteoporosis when placed on low calcium diets. The animals show clear evidence of increased parathyroid hormone secretion, and the osteoporosis can be prevented by prior parathyroidectomy. The excess bone resorption and consequent osteoporosis are homeostatically mediated and represent not so much a homeostatic derangement as a quite appropriate consequence of normal calcium ion regulation. Bone is resorbed to meet mineral needs that the animal cannot obtain from its food. Comparable calcium-deficiency osteoporosis undoubtedly exists in man, but there is no evidence that it is common, and efforts to implicate calcium deficiency as a *primary* cause of most types of human osteoporosis have not been successful.

Nevertheless, the clear implication to be drawn from continued parathyroid secretion during development of most human osteoporosis is that this secretion is necessary to sustain normal calcium ion levels. Some fraction of the calcium resorbed from bone is lost from the body, not because it is present in excess, but for some other reason, and the extra resorption, mediated by parathyroid hormone, comes about precisely to compensate for this loss. It is in this fashion that the calcium homeostatic system becomes implicated in osteoporosis even when there is no evidence of absolute dietary calcium deficiency. The reasons for this calcium wastage are uncertain, but there is a growing body of evidence that changes in the intrinsic responsiveness of the three parathyroid hormone end-organs, and most specifically bone itself, to endogenous parathyroid hormone may account for inefficient calcium conservation. It is worth stressing that the sought-for effect need not be great; net calcium loss of as little as 50 mg per day will reduce the skeletal mass by 15 to 20 per cent per decade.

880. POSTMENOPAUSAL AND SENILE OSTEOPOROSIS

Definition and Etiology. Postmenopausal and senile osteoporosis differs in no way from the foregoing general description. By definition it is found only in postmenopausal women and in elderly persons of both sexes. These patients exhibit a remarkably homogeneous clinical picture and differ in several important respects from patients with specific osteoporoses in which known causal factors can be found. The cause of postmenopausal and senile osteoporosis is unknown. Nor is it known whether clinical osteoporosis is distinct from the universal age-related bone loss which occurs in both men and women, or whether it is simply a consequence of starting with a skeleton at the low end of the bone mass spectrum. The rate of bone loss in women after the menopause is much greater than in men of the same age, and the suppressive effect of gonadal hormones—particularly estrogen—on activation of bone remodeling foci would appear to explain this sexual dimorphism. Nevertheless there is at best only a very weak correlation between age at menopause and onset of osteoporotic symptoms. Thus the normal decrease in estrogen secretion after menopause probably plays no more than a secondary or permissive role in the etiology of osteoporosis. The common finding of osteoporosis in young women with gonadal agenesis (45,X syndromes) is believed to represent an additional manifestation of the genetic defect rather than of endocrine deficiency.

Incidence. Postmenopausal and senile osteoporosis is the most common of all metabolic bone diseases. Satisfactory population studies have not yet been made, but available work suggests that approximately one fourth of all white females in the United States develop clinically significant osteoporosis. (By this is meant that they show the structural consequences of diminished bone mass: compression fractures, "codfish" vertebrae, Schmorl's nodes, dorsal kyphosis, and decreased stature). Furthermore, at least three fourths of all elderly people with fractures of the upper femur have pre-existing osteoporosis, presumably as the predisposing cause of fracture. In the two decades from age 50 to age 70 osteoporosis is predominantly a disease of women. By age 80 the disease is also common among males, although it usually causes less disability than in women. Among women living in the United States, the disorder is most common in those of northern European extraction; it is less common in those of southern European ancestry and still less common in Negroes. Because of both racial and sexual protection, the disease is rare among Negro males of any age. Japanese, both in Japan and in the United States, have a high incidence of osteoporosis. These racial differences appear to be related primarily to differences in normal adult bone mass, rather than to protection against age-related bone loss. Thus the adult Negro male has the largest initial bone mass and has therefore the largest structural reserve against the development of osteoporosis.

Pathogenesis. Many physiologic differences have been found between osteoporotics and comparable normal persons, but their relation to the pathogenesis of osteoporosis is uncertain. Studies of the population at risk have not been made, nor have individual women been studied long enough to determine whether these abnormalities precede the development of the disease. In comparison with normal persons, osteoporotics have been observed to consume 20 to 30 per cent less calcium in their diet, to absorb a smaller fraction of the ingested calcium, to have 40 per cent higher calcium requirements simply to achieve a balance between intake and output, to fail to reduce their urinary calcium normally when placed on low calcium diets, to possess lower circulating vitamin D levels, and to have subnormal growth hormone release in response to hypoglycemic challenge. Urinary estrogen excretion and vaginal epithelial cornification are both somewhat lower in osteoporotics than in age-matched controls, and, in addition, alterations in the excretion pattern of steroid metabolites have been described which suggest lower androgen production.

Although "normal" adults are able to adapt to calcium intakes below 500 mg per day, some otherwise apparently healthy persons fail to achieve calcium balance on low intakes. There is no doubt that calcium deficiency can cause osteoporosis and that some of the patients in this group represent the end result of prolonged deficiency. Nevertheless, the disease occurs also in patients with higher than average intakes, and it seems safest to conclude that, in the group as a whole, inefficient calcium conservation serves at most as a contributory cause rather than as the primary factor in the development of osteoporosis.

Within the bone itself, quantitative studies of remodeling have shown wide variations in osteoblastic new bone formation rates, from well above to well below age-specific normal values. For the most part cell-level bone formation is subnormal, but because more than normal remodeling sites are usually present, it turns out, at the organ-level, that bone-remodeling rates are very nearly normal (although the variance of this measure is significantly larger than normal). It is not certain what role, if any, these changes play in the development of clinical osteoporosis.

Clinical Manifestations. The principal manifestations of osteoporosis are vertebral compression with resultant kyphosis and loss of vertical height, back pain, and susceptibility to fractures (particularly fractures of the upper femur and distal radius). The vertebral compression is often asymptomatic, and probably no more than one third of all patients with the disease actively seek medical aid. The vertebral collapse and kyphosis exaggerate the downward angulation of the ribs and produce prominent horizontal skin folds over the lower chest and abdomen. These folds, particularly in thin people, are a clear indicator of vertebral collapse. The lower ribs may actually ride into the pelvic brim. Occasionally when this occurs the patient experiences severe flank pain, which is relieved by hyperextension of the spine or by surgical excision of the lower costal cartilages. Presumably the pain arises from the costal perichondrium.

Osteoporosis is an important predisposing factor in fractures, particularly those associated with minimal trauma. Hip fracture is a major cause of death and disability in the elderly, and it is probable that most such fractures are due to osteoporosis. Other bones are also more fragile, and fractures are often seen in the pubic and ischial rami, in the rib cage, and in the humerus. The fractures heal normally in all cases except those in which the original bone was so attenuated that the fracture completely destroyed the residual bony scaffolding. This sometimes happens in intertrochanteric and femoral neck fractures.

The back pain is of two types: an acute, sometimes severe pain, well localized to the midline over a restricted region of the spine, that disappears over a period of weeks, and a much more chronic, diffuse, aching pain. The former is related to new compression fractures or to extension of old collapse, and usually disappears as the associated soft tissue and periosteal damage heals. Oc-

casionally the pain precedes roentgenographic evidence of fracture by several days or weeks. Patients commonly relate the attacks of pain to physical exertion, such as bending forward or lifting heavy objects, but weight bearing is not always found, and some patients incur fractures simply by turning over in bed. On physical examination, point tenderness can be found on percussion or pressure over the involved vertebrae. There are commonly associated paravertebral muscle spasm and tenderness. The more chronic pain is found only in a minority of patients, may not be related to the osteoporosis at all, or may be due to associated muscle spasm or to degenerative arthritis aggravated by malaligned weight-bearing forces. It is usually aggravated by prolonged standing or sitting and is relieved by lying down.

Diagnosis. The roentgenographic changes in postmenopausal and senile osteoporosis have been described. The plasma calcium, phosphorus, and alkaline phosphatase are normal, and the urine calcium is usually normal. Bone biopsy reveals only thinning of the cortex and attenuation and fragmentation of trabeculae, both of which are hard to evaluate in a single biopsy sample. The biopsy is of value, however, not because it is characteristic of osteoporosis, but because it excludes certain other disorders. The principal differential considerations include the specific osteoporoses such as that due to Cushing's syndrome, diffuse skeletal involvement with multiple myeloma, hyperparathyroidism, osteogenesis imperfecta (which in mild forms may first manifest itself in adult life), and metastatic malignancy. Despite a common misconception to the contrary, osteomalacia is not a cause of diffuse skeletal atrophy, and it does not present a clinical or roentgenographic picture similar to osteoporosis.

The clinical picture of Cushing's syndrome or of hyperthyroidism is usually sufficiently obvious so that little confusion with postmenopausal or senile osteoporosis should occur. Rarely, however, patients with these endocrinopathies may present with predominantly skeletal manifestations. Myeloma is excluded by examination of the bone marrow (which can be performed on the same specimen removed for bone biopsy), by electrophoretic separation of the plasma proteins, and by search for Bence Jones protein in the urine. Normal plasma calcium, phosphorus, and alkaline phosphatase serve to exclude hyperparathyroidism and those malignant conditions that mimic parathyroid hyperfunction. Metastatic malignancy presents a differential problem principally when it is a cause of vertebral compression fracture. In such patients, skeletal roentgenographic surveys may demonstrate more characteristic metastatic lesions in other bones. Further, the finding of apparently osteoporotic compression fractures in younger patients, particularly males, or of involvement of the neural arch should suggest a neoplastic cause for the lesion.

An important feature of osteoporotic pain is that it is associated with fracture. Back pain at a site remote from vertebral compression, or in a spine simply osteoporotic but without compression fractures, is usually not due to osteoporosis. In addition to the painful bony disorders just described, the clinician should also exclude certain nonskeletal causes of back pain such as pancreatitis, posterior penetration of a duodenal ulcer, and posterior abdominal malignancies.

Treatment. Treatment in osteoporosis is directed at arresting and stabilizing the condition and at symptomatic relief, support, and rehabilitation of the patient.

Because the pain of acute episodes subsides spontaneously as the compression fracture heals, all treatments may *appear* to work. Nevertheless, no treatment has been conclusively shown to increase bone mass in a representative group of patients. Some help in retarding further bone loss or in increasing the functional capacity of the patient may be afforded by mineral supplements, gonadal hormones, and physical therapy. A number of other agents, including fluoride, phosphates, calcitonin, and the diphosphonate compounds, are still under investigation.

Because virtually all patients conserve calcium poorly, a high calcium intake is sometimes recommended as the cornerstone of any therapeutic regimen. The risk of hypercalciuria with such treatment is negligible. Calcium intake should be at least 1500 mg per day; if derived from the diet, this requires the ingestion of at least one quart of milk per day, which is more than most osteoporotic patients will accept. It is usually necessary to employ supplemental medicinal calcium, which is available in a variety of forms, including the gluconate, lactate, phosphate, carbonate, and glycerophosphate salts. All are absorbed equally well except for the carbonate, which is poorly absorbed in the presence of achlorhydria. There is suggestive, but still inconclusive, evidence that retention is better if supplemental phosphate is also provided; thus the phosphate salts may be preferable to the others. In some patients, particularly those with low urine calcium excretion, vitamin D in doses from 1000 to 10,000 IU per day appears to aid calcium retention.

Estrogens and androgens, alone or in combination, have been shown to improve calcium balance and possibly also to decrease the incidence of fracture. Dosage regimens vary greatly; adequate therapy is probably provided by ordinary replacement doses, i.e., 0.05 to 0.1 mg of ethinyl estradiol or its equivalent. Androgen therapy in women is limited by its virilizing properties, and few patients will accept prolonged treatment at more than a few milligrams of methyltestosterone daily.

Intensive physical therapy often produces significant functional and symptomatic improvement. The muscles of the back, hips, and thighs must be strengthened, and a lifelong program of exercise instituted. There is undoubtedly some component of disuse in most osteoporotics, and this must be abolished by a controlled sensible regimen of exercise. Patients must be taught to bend at the hips and knees and not to bend the back in order to pick up objects off the floor, and they must not carry or lift heavy objects. Bed rest is contraindicated except in the acute post-fracture period when it may be necessary for pain relief. Patients should be up and about, and a physical therapy program should be started as soon as possible after an acute vertebral compression. Back braces are usually not indicated, but firm corsets or foundation garments are often very helpful.

Fluoride, given as the sodium salt in doses of 30 to 60 mg daily, also improves calcium balance in many patients, and, in combination with calcium supplements and vitamin D, has apparently increased bone mass in a few patients. Fluoride is known to fit into the apatite crystal lattice in the place of hydroxyl radicals; the resulting fluorapatite is a more stable, less soluble mineral than hydroxyapatite. The bone is thus rendered more resistant to resorptive attack, and the calcium homeostatic system adapts by forcing more effective renal and intestinal calcium conservation.

Prevention. The probable irreversibility of bone atrophy in the aged makes prevention all the more important. There is suggestive evidence that prophylactic estrogen therapy retards postmenopausal bone loss. This effect is in keeping with what is known of estrogen action in bone resorption. Although adequately controlled prospective studies have not yet been performed, it seems likely that prophylactic estrogen therapy may be very useful. It would be particularly desirable to be able to select for such prophylaxis the 25 per cent of the white female population who constitute the high-risk group, but unfortunately this is not yet possible. The best one can suggest is to concentrate on small (less than 140 pounds), very fair-skinned women, with minimal body hair, and usually of Scotch, Irish, or Anglo-Saxon origin. All surveys to date suggest that such women have the highest risk of developing osteoporotic fractures.

Prognosis. There is little information about the natural history of the untreated disease. With adequate treatment, however, most patients can be stabilized and restored to useful functional activity. Hip fractures are probably the principal hazard of the disease; 10 to 15 per cent of patients are dead within three months of such fractures, and the associated enforced bed rest, trauma, and surgery markedly decrease the ultimate functional capacity of those who survive.

881. DISUSE OSTEOPOROSIS

Disuse osteoporosis is a local disorder confined to bones or regions subjected to immobilization or deprived of normal muscle pull. In severe lower motor neuron paralytic disease, such as quadriplegic poliomyelitis or the Guillain-Barré syndrome, virtually the entire skeleton may be involved, but, unlike other osteoporoses, the spine is less severely involved than are the long bones of the extremities. The bone loss develops through a massive increase in bone resorption. This resorption does not appear to be systemically mediated or controllable, and is somehow a consequence of the local withdrawal of mechanical stress. Vascular engorgement within bone occurs during development of the disorder, but it is not known whether this change causes the resorption or is instead caused by it. The pathologic picture is otherwise no different from that of the other osteoporoses. Roentgenographic changes are also nondistinctive except for the localization of disease to the immobilized bones and for a zone of rarefaction in the region of the fused epiphyseal plate, which appears as the first detectable change in involved long bones.

Since immobilized bones are not subjected to mechanical stress, their fragility is of little structural consequence, and the principal significance of the disease lies in the hypercalcemia and hypercalciuria that may be produced by extensive resorption. In poliomyelitis this resorption begins almost immediately and reaches peak values four to five weeks after onset, with urine calcium values sometimes as high as 800 mg per day. If care is not taken to keep these patients hydrated and to maintain a high urine flow, glomerular filtration falls, and hypercalcemia may result. Furthermore, stasis in the urinary tract predisposes to stone formation.

Normal subjects kept at bed rest develop negative calcium balance, with loss predominantly from weight-bearing bones, most particularly the os calcis. A comparable loss occurs as a result of prolonged weightlessness, as in space flight. In flights of up to two months' duration the amount of bone lost is insufficient to pose a risk of fracture. Urine calcium has increased, however, in most astronauts, and in some, up to twice preflight levels.

882. NUTRITIONAL OSTEOPOROSES

Osteoporosis is a frequent manifestation of many nutritional deficiency syndromes in patients of all ages. These include general protein and caloric malnutrition, kwashiorkor, scurvy, chronic alcoholism, and a variety of malabsorption syndromes as well as isolated calcium deficiency. These are specific osteoporoses, due to the malnutrition, and will heal both clinically and roentgenographically, at least in young people, if the underlying cause can be corrected. The osteoporosis is usually a minor part of the over-all syndrome.

Osteoporosis is a common finding in alcoholics of both sexes, and alcoholism should be suspected when osteoporotic fractures are found in men before age 65 and women before age 55. It is not known whether the disorder is due to the generally poor nutrition of alcoholics, to their usually very low calcium intakes, or to large endogenous losses of calcium. Its manifestations and consequences are the same as for ordinary postmenopausal or senile osteoporosis, but because of the coexisting alcoholism it is even harder to treat satisfactorily.

883. ENDOCRINE OSTEOPOROSES

Hyperthyroidism.   Bone turnover is accelerated in hyperthyroidism. In some patients bone resorption may exceed formation sufficiently to produce significant osteoporosis. Unlike postmenopausal osteoporosis, this disorder involves all three bony envelopes, including the haversian. Fine-grain roentgenograms will often show significant intracortical tunneling in an otherwise normally thick cortex (cortical striation). The same process, if still more severe, may mimic hyperparathyroidism. The difference seems to be only one of degree. Plasma calcium, phosphorus, and alkaline phosphatase values may all be elevated, and the urine calcium may be normal or high. This too is a specific osteoporosis, treatable by recognizing and treating the hyperthyroidism. Roentgenographic improvement may occur, particularly in younger patients.

Cushing's Syndrome.   Osteoporosis occurs in most patients with Cushing's syndrome and may be severe in approximately one third. It is associated with marked depression of osteoblast activity and with defective fracture healing. Similar changes can be produced by administration of glucocorticoids in high doses and are a complication of corticoid therapy, particularly in patients with rheumatoid arthritis. There is marked thinning of the cortex, and except for the accelerated resorption associated with endosteal expansion, bone turnover is generally suppressed. Like postmenopausal osteoporosis, this disorder involves primarily the endosteal envelope. Except for depression of alkaline phosphatase activity, there are no distinctive plasma chemical changes. Urine calcium is usually only moderately elevated, and gastrointestinal calcium absorption is de-

pressed. Improvement is poor, except in young patients, even with satisfactory control of the adrenal secretion.

884. MISCELLANEOUS OSTEOPOROSES

IDIOPATHIC OSTEOPOROSIS

The term "idiopathic osteoporosis" was applied originally to young men or women in whom no demonstrable cause could be found, and who were not postmenopausal or senile (and hence were not considered to have gonadal deficiency as a causal factor). The disease has been described in adolescents and in pregnant women, is commonly more painful than usual postmenopausal osteoporosis, and occurs more often in men than in women. The cause remains unknown. The disease tends to stabilize with time, but does not heal, and except for physical therapy and rehabilitation no treatment has been of much value.

SUDECK'S ATROPHY

After fracture in an extremity, structural turnover in adjacent bones increases markedly. Commonly, osteoporosis develops. Similar changes may also occur without fracture, sometimes following only minor injuries. The term "Sudeck's atrophy" refers to cases with or without fracture in which this osteoporosis comes on very acutely and is associated with severe pain and swelling, tenderness, and sweating in the overlying soft tissue. The disorder is most common in the wrists, hands, and feet, but may involve major portions of the skeleton, or may sometimes be migratory. Abnormal autonomic vasomotor regulation has been implicated as the cause. Sympathetic block may produce profound relief. Although frequently disabling, the disease is usually self-limited and in most instances heals spontaneously over a period of several months to a few years. In particularly severe or protracted cases regional sympathectomy may be indicated.

Bassan, J., Frame, B., and Frost, H.: Osteoporosis: A review of pathogenesis and treatment. Ann. Intern. Med., 58:539, 1963.

Cooke, A. M.: Osteoporosis. Lancet, 1:877, 929, 1955.

deTakats, G.: Sympathetic reflex dystrophy. Med. Clin. North Am., 49:117, 1965.

Heaney, R. P.: A unified concept of osteoporosis. Am. J. Med., 39:877, 1965.

Rich, C., Ensinck, J., and Ivanovich, P.: The effects of sodium fluoride on calcium metabolism of subjects with metabolic bone diseases. J. Clin. Invest., 43:545, 1964.

Rodahl, K., Nicholson, J. T., and Brown, E. M. (eds.): Bone as a Tissue. New York, Blakiston Division, McGraw-Hill Book Company, 1960, Part I: Osteoporosis, pp. 3–102.

Steinbach, H. L.: The roentgen appearance of osteoporosis. Radiol. Clin. North Am., 2:191, 1964.

Urist, M. R.: Osteoporosis. Ann Rev. Med., 13:273, 1962.

THE OSTEOMALACIAS

Robert P. Heaney

885. INTRODUCTION

Definition.   The term "osteomalacia," meaning softening of bone, was applied originally to a distinctive clinical syndrome consisting of severe bone pain, skeletal deformity, depressed plasma Ca × P ion product, and wide osteoid borders in bone, all associated with vitamin D deficiency. The term has more recently been extended to include a variety of conditions exhibiting some, but not all, of the features of the full-blown vitamin D deficiency syndrome. This has led to confusion and disagreement concerning the definition of the disorder. Some authorities confine the term to the *clinical syndrome* described above, irrespective of the cause; others choose to base their definition on *morphologic* criteria, i.e., the presence of wide osteoid borders on bone surfaces. For purposes of clarity in exposition, the latter course will be pursued in what follows.

The term "rickets" refers to a series of identical syndromes occurring in childhood, and adds to the picture of adult osteomalacia the features of retarded growth, abnormal proliferation and maturation of the epiphyseal growth plate, and associated periarticular pain.

Morphologic and Roentgenographic Characteristics. Grossly, the skeleton may show little abnormality. In severe cases, bowing of long bones is observed, the pelvic bones are deformed inward, and all bones convey the impression of plastic deformation in response to applied forces. Microscopically, osteoid seams are invariably increased in thickness and in number, both on trabecular surfaces and in newly forming haversian systems. This osteoid fails to show evidence of the normal maturation sequence that must precede mineralization. In some osteomalacias, particularly those with severe vitamin D deficiency, changes of osteitis fibrosa may also be seen.

The principal roentgenographic changes are the deformities described above and, in rickets, widening, fraying, and cupping of all active growth plates. These rachitic changes are most apparent and most severe at sites of rapid growth, particularly the sternal ends of the ribs, the distal end of the radius and ulna, and the proximal ends of the tibia and humerus. In fact, the rachitic lesion is dependent upon growth for its expression. When growth slows or stops for any reason (such as intercurrent illness or increasing malnutrition), calcification of the disordered epiphyseal cartilage slowly occurs, and the roentgenographic lesion appears to heal, even though the basic abnormality remains unchanged. The bone of such persons then shows only osteomalacic lesions. In adults the only characteristic roentgenographic changes are the pseudofractures (Looser's zones, Milkman's lines). These lines are ribbon-like radiolucent zones, perpendicular to free bone surfaces, often bilateral and symmetrical, which give the appearance of incomplete fractures. They are found most commonly along the axillary border of the scapula, in the ischial and pubic rami, in the femoral neck, and in the ribs.

Generalized decrease in bone density is not a feature of osteomalacia per se. However, the disease commonly coexists with osteoporosis and hence may be found in skeletons that show decreased roentgenographic density. This decrease is not due to the osteomalacia per se.

General Pathophysiologic Considerations. The two features most characteristic of the osteomalacias are a low plasma Ca × P ion product and wide osteoid borders in bone. These have usually been considered to be related as cause and effect, and both have been attributed to poor intestinal calcium absorption. However, this simplified relationship is incorrect. As has been stressed before, defective calcium absorption leads to osteoporosis, not to

osteomalacia; furthermore, in those osteomalacias caused by vitamin D deficiency small doses of vitamin D sufficient to repair the absorptive defect do not heal the bone lesions; conversely, adequate vitamin D therapy will cure osteomalacia even on a calcium-poor diet.

There are two basic mechanisms that might lead to accumulation of unmineralized osteoid: (1) insufficient concentration of calcium and phosphorus in extracellular fluid to allow crystal nucleation and growth, and (2) abnormalities in the matrix that render it unmineralizable. These mechanisms are not necessarily distinct, for the osteoblasts may well be sensitive to the phosphate concentration of the extracellular fluid, and thus in some cases the matrix abnormality may be due to a metabolic consequence of osteoblast phosphorus deficiency. Probably both defects are involved to varying degrees in the different osteomalacias. Nevertheless, there are undoubted matrix abnormalities in most if not all of the osteomalacias. Both rachitic cartilage and osteomalacic osteoid fail to show staining reactions characteristic of normal premineralization ripening. Some authorities are convinced that absence of a stainable calcification front is a *sine qua non* for the morphologic diagnosis of osteomalacia and is, hence, a more reliable feature than the mere width of osteoid borders. Although rachitic cartilage will mineralize when incubated in normal plasma, osteomalacic osteoid will not, and the first detectable changes in vivo after vitamin D therapy are staining reactions indicative of matrix maturation. These occur prior to measurable changes in plasma calcium or phosphorus concentration.

There can be little doubt that both new matrix production and osteoblast-mediated ripening of osteoid seams are severely depressed. This decrease in individual osteoblast activity is usually compensated for by markedly increased numbers of osteoblasts, which, though working slowly, may succeed in blanketing every available bone surface with a thick layer of poorly mineralizable matrix. The ultimate rate of new bone formation may thus be normal or even high, even though individual osteoblast activity is severely retarded.

886. RICKETS AND OSTEOMALACIA DUE TO VITAMIN D DEFICIENCY

Etiology and Incidence. At the turn of the century approximately 90 per cent of the children of northern European cities had clinical rickets secondary to vitamin D deficiency. For a time vitamin D deficiency became so rare that rickets and osteomalacia of solely nutritional causes were almost unknown in Europe and North America. With the immigration of dark-skinned persons into the industrial cities of northern Europe recently, there has been an increase in vitamin D deficiency disease. In general the disorder is still common in parts of the world where limited exposure to sunlight restricts vitamin D synthesis.

In the United States, vitamin D deficiency osteomalacia is virtually confined to patients with the various malabsorption syndromes, particularly idiopathic sprue, as well as in some patients with the Billroth I type of gastrectomy. Curiously, it is unusual in patients with pancreatic disease, even though the efficiency of vitamin D absorption has been shown to be less in these patients than in those with sprue.

Pathogenesis. Vitamin D deficiency has three main effects: it impairs intestinal calcium absorption, reduces the responsiveness of osteoclasts to parathyroid hormone, and leads to the defects in osteoblast activity mentioned earlier. The decreased sensitivity to parathyroid hormone is compensated for by increased parathyroid gland size and secretion, and this in turn produces markedly enhanced renal tubular responses, i.e., decreased calcium and increased phosphate clearance. Augmented parathyroid hormone levels maximize renal production of the 1,25-derivative from the available 25-HCC, and cause more bone remodeling centers to develop, thus compensating to some degree for the intestinal absorptive defect and the impaired bone resorption. Usually plasma calcium ion remains normal or nearly so, whereas plasma inorganic phosphate is reduced to low values, often below 2 mg per 100 ml. When skeletal demands for calcium are high, or osteoclast response is sharply reduced, plasma calcium may fall to tetanic levels.

Few patients with pure vitamin D deficiency are in significantly negative calcium balance. Although intestinal absorption is much reduced, it is not zero, and the limited absorption usually allows net recovery of most of the calcium of the digestive juices. Urine calcium is regularly reduced to extremely low values, often unmeasurably low. And thus, with no mechanism for losing calcium, it is not surprising that total bone mass remains at preosteomalacic levels.

Clinical Manifestations. Early in their course, patients with osteomalacia superimposed on gastrointestinal disease may have few symptoms referable to the bone disease; the predominant clinical manifestations are those of the underlying disease. When the osteomalacia becomes more severe, typical symptoms related to the skeleton and the vitamin D deficiency become apparent. These include bone pain, waddling gait, muscle weakness, and anorexia. Aching bone pain is prolonged and is made worse on weight-bearing; the bones may be tender to pressure. Pseudofractures tend to occur in bursts and when present may be associated with severe muscle weakness and bone pain. Experimentally produced hypophosphatemia is itself a cause of weakness; nevertheless the weakness of clinical osteomalacia is better correlated with the appearance of pseudofractures than with fluctuation in phosphate levels. It seems probable therefore that the symptom is due largely to reflex inhibition from bone pain. If the serum calcium falls to low levels, typical hypocalcemic tetany may occur. Occasional patients may have osteomalacia secondary to gluten-sensitive enteropathy, without obvious nutritional or gastrointestinal complaints, and thus may present only with skeletal manifestations.

It should be stressed that the most common bone disease in malabsorption syndromes is osteoporosis, not osteomalacia, and that when osteomalacia occurs it does so not simply because of the malabsorption, but because the patient has become ill enough to lose even casual contact with direct sunlight, thus losing his major source of vitamin D. So long as vitamin D levels remain adequate, however, calcium ion homeostasis works efficiently, and the malabsorption of calcium simply leads to negative calcium balance, which in turn results in osteoporosis. It is for this reason that most of the osteomalacia seen in the United States occurs in patients with pre-existing osteoporosis and represents a combined deficiency state (calcium first, then vitamin D).

Diagnosis. The diagnosis rests securely on a tripod of biopsy, roentgenographic, and biochemical findings. Wide osteoid borders are found on biopsy in all cases. Pseudofractures, when seen in otherwise normal bone, are virtually diagnostic of osteomalacia. The characteristic chemical changes are a normal to low plasma calcium, low plasma phosphate, high alkaline phosphatase, and very low urine calcium. Furthermore, these changes are characteristically found in patients with steatorrhea and with more or less obvious evidence of malabsorption. Occasionally the osteomalacia will be more apparent than the underlying enteropathy, and the observation of the changes described above should lead to a search for an underlying cause. The only differential consideration of consequence relates to other causes of osteomalacia. These include vitamin D resistance, adult hypophosphatasia, and advanced renal disease, all of which will be discussed in succeeding sections.

Treatment. Treatment must be directed at both the vitamin D deficiency and any underlying gastrointestinal disease, which is the usual cause of the deficiency. Uncomplicated vitamin D deficiency responds well to the vitamin in daily doses of as low as 1000 units; the various malabsorption syndromes may require from 10,000 to 50,000 units daily. Requirements in excess of these levels suggest one of the vitamin D resistant forms of osteomalacia (see below). Therapeutic ultraviolet exposure may be particularly helpful in patients with malabsorption syndromes, since skin manufacture of vitamin D bypasses the intestinal absorption block. Healing may be expected to be complete. Any coexisting osteoporosis resulting from calcium malabsorption should be treated by means of a high calcium intake.

887. VITAMIN D RESISTANT RICKETS
(Familial Hypophosphatemia)

Definition and Inheritance. Vitamin D resistant rickets and osteomalacia are distinct syndromes, clinically similar to their vitamin D deficient counterparts, but different in that they fail to respond to usual therapeutic doses of vitamin D. The term "vitamin D resistance" is unfortunate, for there is no evidence of true biochemical refractoriness to the vitamin, or to its metabolites. Instead it is the disease that is resistant, but it is resistant as well to vitamins A, B, C, and E as it is to D, and for the same good reason: it is not caused by deficiency of any one of them. The term "familial hypophosphatemia" is much more apt and describes the essential and invariable expression of the genetic defect that is responsible for the disorder. This defect is most commonly inherited as a sex-linked dominant character with complete penetrance but widely varying expressivity. Other inheritance patterns probably reflect different genetic defects that express themselves as hypophosphatemia. In addition, sporadic cases of resistant rickets, otherwise indistinguishable from the inherited variety, also occur. It is not known whether such patients have offspring who inherit the disease. Furthermore, adults with no sign of childhood rickets or dwarfing can occasionally present with osteomalacia associated with renal tubular hypophosphatemia. These patients give no family history of renal disease. Severe hypophosphatemic osteomalacia, resistant to vitamin D, has been described in association with certain benign tumors, notably sclerosing hemangiomata and neurofibromata. Cure has followed removal of the offending tumor.

Etiology and Pathogenesis. The nature of the genetic defect is unknown. The hypophosphatemia by which it is expressed is probably directly responsible for the osteomalacia. Although the matrix shows the same abnormal staining reactions as in vitamin D deficiency, simple elevation of the plasma phosphate by infusion or phosphate feeding will induce prompt healing and will lead to positive calcium balance. It cannot yet be decided whether the osteoid accumulates simply because there is inadequate mineral to allow crystal nucleation and growth or because the osteoblast suffers from an induced phosphate deficiency. The reason for the hypophosphatemia itself is also obscure. Defective tubular phosphate reabsorption has usually been implicated, and there is no doubt that renal phosphate clearance is greatly increased, but it has been established that tubular phosphate reabsorption in these patients responds normally to parathyroid hormone suppression; i.e., it can be returned to or toward normal by calcium infusion, by immobilization, or by any maneuver that reduces endogenous parathyroid hormone secretion. However, none of these increases the TM_p to normal. It has also been suggested that there is a primary defect in intestinal absorption of calcium leading to secondary parathyroid secretion, which in turn results in phosphaturia. However, it is common to find increased bone density in adults with the untreated disease (even to the extent that the axial skeleton can resemble osteopetrosis); this finding does not suggest lifelong inadequacy of calcium absorption.

Clinical Manifestations. Many affected persons have no demonstrable abnormality except for the hypophosphatemia. The expression of the defect ranges from simple hypophosphatemia without other abnormalities, through histologically demonstrable osteomalacia without clinical symptoms, to mild growth retardation, to typical, severe rickets and osteomalacia. The clinical features of the full-blown syndrome differ from ordinary vitamin D deficiency rickets in several respects. The disease is not common in early infancy and is seen most often after 18 months of age. The plasma calcium is almost always normal, whereas the plasma phosphorus is invariably low. The plasma alkaline phosphatase, although elevated, is rarely as high as in vitamin D deficiency. On biopsy the bone is essentially indistinguishable from that in vitamin D deficiency rickets, and, except for severity, roentgenographic changes do not distinguish between the two types of bone involvement. When the disease presents under the age of three, short stature and bowing of the legs is the characteristic deformity. With onset after three years, knock knee is usually seen. Muscle weakness is not observed in children with resistant rickets; but in adults with either the acquired or the hereditary disease, severe weakness, especially of the lower limbs, is quite common and may even suggest a neurologic disorder. This is believed to be due to hypophosphatemia, but is rarely seen without pseudofractures and pain. Most of these children develop a coxa vara deformity and consequent waddling gait. The limb bones are short and often bowed and there is a tendency to hyperostosis at tendinous insertions which may suggest the diagnosis of achondroplasia. In adolescence the epiphyses close, alkaline phosphatase returns to normal, and the patients become asymptomatic. However,

between 25 and 50 years pseudofractures may occur, especially in the femoral necks or over the convexity of the femoral shafts. These may not be associated with any rise in serum alkaline phosphatase activity.

In children, urinary calcium excretion is of the order of 10 to 20 mg per 24 hours, whereas in adults urinary calcium excretion ranges between 50 and 120 mg per 24 hours. These values are low, especially in children, but should be contrasted to the virtual absence of calcium in vitamin D deficiency rickets and osteomalacia.

Diagnosis. The diagnosis is based primarily on the observation of otherwise typical rickets and osteomalacia in patients without vitamin D deficiency or diseases predisposing thereto and without azotemia or other outspoken renal tubular defects, and on the failure of the bone disease to respond to usual vitamin D therapy. Commonly a positive family history or the familial occurrence of asymptomatic hypophosphatemia can be established. Quite similar bone disorders are seen in patients with multiple renal tubular reabsorptive defects. These defects include reabsorption of amino acids, bicarbonate, and glucose, as well as phosphate. In this group are included the Fanconi syndrome (vide infra) and renal tubular acidosis, as well as renal injury secondary to cystinosis and to lead or cadmium poisoning. Endemic osteomalacia caused by cadmium nephropathy has been described in Japan among persons eating rice irrigated with cadmium-polluted water.

Treatment. Available treatment is not altogether satisfactory, and it is doubtful that asymptomatic patients need any treatment. The disorder does not respond to antirachitic doses of vitamin D or its principal metabolite, 1,25-HCC. The most widely used therapy consists of pharmacologic doses of vitamin D (ergocalciferol, 50,000 to 200,000 units daily). These doses will usually cause roentgenographic changes of the epiphyses to heal. The dose required to do this is always very close to a toxic one. Furthermore, serum levels of phosphorus can never be maintained at normal in these patients without toxicity from vitamin D. Finally, there is little evidence that such therapy improves the growth rate or prevents deformities, despite near toxic levels of vitamin D therapy over a prolonged period of time. The adult syndrome with pseudofractures is best treated by a balanced sodium phosphate mixture containing 1.5 to 2 grams of phosphorus daily. Intake is pushed to levels just short of a cathartic effect. There is a large but transient rise in plasma phosphate after each dose, and divided doses are necessary in order to sustain the effect for a sufficient fraction of each day. A combination of phosphate and vitamin D is commonly employed, and has been reported to increase growth rate better than either agent alone.

888. HYPOPHOSPHATASIA

Hypophosphatasia is a familial skeletal disorder inherited as an autosomal recessive trait. The incidence is about 1 per 100,000 live births. Severe cases present in utero or within six months of birth; less severe cases present in infancy, although occasional cases do not present until late childhood or adult life. The bony disorder consists of severe osteomalacia and rickets which may result in fractures, rickety rosary, soft skull, and bulging fontanelle. The infants fail to thrive, may have fever and convulsions, and frequently die at an early age. Others are stillborn. Milder cases develop during the first year of life with features of rickets. Later, these children may develop craniostenosis. When cases present in adult life, the patients may have pathologic fractures of the pelvis and long bones or compression fractures or biconcavity of the spine indistinguishable from osteoporosis. Stress fractures may occur as in other types of osteomalacia. Histologic features of the disease are characteristic of osteomalacia, with broad osteoid seams lining the bone trabeculae. Serum calcium is normal or slightly elevated, and serum phosphorus is normal, whereas alkaline phosphatase values are always low. Leukocyte alkaline phosphatase is also low. Hypercalciuria is the rule at least in younger persons. All patients excrete phosphoethanolamine in the urine. Urinary pyrophosphate excretion is increased in these patients, and chondrocalcinosis may occur. There is no known effective treatment, although corticosteroid drugs have been used to heal rachitic changes in children, presumably by slowing growth.

889. MISCELLANEOUS OSTEOMALACIAS

Bone changes typical of osteomalacia, but without clinical symptoms, may be observed in many bone diseases, and clinically significant rachitic and osteomalacic skeletal involvement may complicate a variety of disorders. Most important is the bone disease associated with chronic renal insufficiency (see below). Osteomalacic bone changes, with or without symptoms, may occasionally be seen in patients with other bone disorders, such as Paget's disease, hyperparathyroidism, and fluorosis, as well as in patients with neither biochemical changes in the circulating plasma nor predisposing disease. In all such instances osteoid accumulation must be presumed to be due to interference with normal matrix maturation. Only very rarely does such osteomalacia produce clinical symptoms, and it is mentioned here principally because it may present as an incidental finding on bone biopsy.

FANCONI'S SYNDROME

The Fanconi syndrome consists of osteomalacic bone disease associated with renal tubular defect with respect to tubular reabsorption of glucose, amino acids, and phosphate. There may or may not be renal acidosis. The disease is commonly idiopathic, but may also result from renal tubular damage from cystine storage disease, in cadmium or lead poisoning, or from Wilson's disease (hepatolenticular degeneration). When renal acidosis occurs, hypocalcemia is common. Treatment is similar to that of resistant rickets except when acidosis complicates the picture and then it is important to correct acidosis with appropriate alkali therapy as well as to treat the patient with large doses of vitamin D.

Bartter, F. C.: Hypophosphatasia. *In* Stanbury, J. B., Wyngaarden, J. B., and Fredrickson, D. S. (eds.): Metabolic Basis of Inherited Disease. 3rd ed. New York, Blakiston Division, McGraw-Hill Book Company, 1972.

Frame, B., Smith, R. W., Jr., Fleming, J. L., and Manson, G.: Oral phosphates in vitamin-D-refractory rickets and osteomalacia. Am. J. Dis. Child., 106:147, 1963.

Fraser, D.: Hypophosphatasia. Am. J. Med., 22:739, 1957.

Hioco, D.: Osteomalacia. Paris, Editions Masson, 1966.

Stanbury, S. W., and Lumb, G.: Parathyroid function in chronic renal failure. Quart. J. Med., 35:1, 1966.

Williams, T. F., and Winters, R. W.: Familial (hereditary) vitamin D resistant rickets with hypophosphatemia. *In* Stanbury, J. B., Wyngaarden, J. B., and Fredrickson, D. S. (eds.): Metabolic Basis of Inherited Disease. 3rd ed. New York, Blakiston Division, McGraw-Hill Book Company, 1972.

890. RENAL OSTEODYSTROPHY

Definition and Incidence. The bone disease of persons suffering from chronic uremia presents as a confusing variety of manifestations seemingly different from one part of the world to the next and depending as well on whether the patient is receiving hemodialysis. Typically the bone disease consists of features of osteomalacia, osteitis fibrosa, osteosclerosis, and osteoporosis, the first two being the more important. Although it is not always easy to predict which one of these will predominate in any individual, given time, some form of skeletal disease develops in all uremic patients.

Clinical Manifestations. Clinical manifestations include bone pain, deformity, fractures, and, in children, growth retardation. Since uremic patients are rarely in very negative calcium balance, total body calcium is usually normal or even high. With the more severe cases of osteitis fibrosa and metastatic calcification there is usually an intrabody shift of mineral from bone to ectopic sites (such as bursae or vascular walls). Frequently the bone marrow is itself a site of metastatic calcification (as in vitamin D intoxication), and this phenomenon may produce or contribute to the roentgenographic appearance of osteosclerosis.

Pathogenesis and Diagnosis. There is resistance to the action of vitamin D in uremia, which begins to be manifest even at minor degrees of azotemia. At least some of this resistance appears to be due to impaired conversion of 25-HCC to 1,25-HCC, associated either with loss of renal parenchymal tissue or with high plasma phosphate levels, or both. At very high phosphate values, there is apparently some triple hydroxylation to the 1,24,25-derivative. This compound has intestinal but not bone resorptive activity. These defects lead to compensatory parathyroid hyperplasia and hypersecretion. The plasma calcium may be quite low but is more commonly in the low-normal range, and is presumably maintained at even this level only because of sometimes heroic levels of parathyroid hormone secretion.

The parathyroid glands are invariably increased in size, and there appear to be at least a few cases of true autonomous hyperparathyroidism resulting from this long-continued hyperplasia. In general, gland hypertrophy is less severe in those patients with lesions that are predominantly osteomalacic and more severe in patients with predominant osteitis fibrosa and metastatic calcification. The level of phosphatemia depends on a combination of factors, including the degree of renal failure, the level of parathyroid hormone secretion, the phosphate intake, and various therapeutic regimens (principally aluminum hydroxide gels) designed to lower effective phosphate intake. Nevertheless, the plasma phosphate is usually above normal, and the empirical Ca × P product correspondingly elevated. The alkaline phosphatase is usually elevated and roentgenograms demonstrate the features of osteomalacia, osteitis fibrosa, or both. It has been observed that, when the Ca × P product is below 70, the most prominent feature of the bone disease is likely to consist of rickets or osteomalacia, and when above 70, osteitis fibrosa together with varying degrees of metastatic calcification. There is broad overlap between these categories, and the distinction is further complicated by the fact that some degree of osteitis fibrosa, including typical roentgenographic features, is frequent in severe rickets and osteomalacia from any cause, including that seen in the uremic syndrome. The existence of rickets and osteomalacia in the presence of high mineral concentrations presents an interesting and as yet unsolved problem. There has been shown to be a circulating inhibitor of calcification in the plasma of uremic patients. Furthermore, the healing seen with high doses of vitamin D (which produces only trivial changes in Ca × P product in these patients) suggests either systemic removal of this inhibitor or direct vitamin D action on osteoblasts and growth cartilage.

Treatment. If the predominant bony lesion is rachitic (malacic) and if the Ca × P product is lower than 70, then the patient will very likely benefit from vitamin D, which must usually be given in large doses (50,000 to 500,000 units per day) or from dihydrotachysterol. Both the malacic lesions and any associated osteitis fibrosa may heal significantly with these sterols. Recent investigations have shown that as little as 2.5 μg per day of 1,25-HCC (the molar equivalent of 100 I.U. of vitamin D) will return D-dependent functions to normal in uremic subjects. The pure compound is not commercially available, and it is likely that the effect produced by massive doses of the crude D vitamin preparations available is due to the presence of trace quantities of contaminating sterol impurities which act like 1,25-HCC. This, in effect, is the reason why dihydrotachysterol appears to be more effective than calciferol in uremic bone disease. The A-ring of this sterol is sterically similar to 1,25-HCC, and thus the compound circumvents the renal synthetic defect.

If there is little or no malacic component to the bone disease, vitamin D treatment will usually do no good and may, by raising the Ca × P product still further, aggravate an already dangerous propensity to metastatic calcification. It is thus important to evaluate both bone morphology and plasma calcium and phosphate levels before beginning vitamin D treatment. If roentgenographic findings of rickets or osteomalacia are not evident, a bone biopsy should be obtained and an undecalcified section examined for the presence of uncalcified osteoid.

Treatment directed at the uremia itself also has effects on the bone disease and on calcium homeostasis. In general, dialysis does nothing to alter the vitamin D resistance or the tendency to osteomalacia, and by prolonging life may allow osteodystrophy to develop to the point of producing significant disability. Regimens directed at suppressing the plasma phosphate appear to benefit patients with high Ca × P products and with bony lesions predominantly of osteitis fibrosa, whereas slight elevation of dialysis bath calcium has been shown to help the primarily osteomalacic lesion. Successful renal transplantation almost always leads to restoration of normal vitamin D metabolism and corresponding healing of rickets and osteomalacia. Normal vitamin D metabolism returns well before the parathyroid glands can involute, and the sometimes huge residual mass of parathyroid tissue may thus oversecrete parathyroid hormone even when maximally suppressed, producing post-transplantation hypercalcemia. This phenomenon usually becomes apparent as the plasma phosphate falls, but may first make its appearance as much as six months after

transplantation. This situation has been given the unhappy designation "tertiary hyperparathyroidism." It appears to be a true hyperparathyroidism, i.e., hypercalcemia caused by excessive secretion of parathyroid hormone, but in almost all cases is self-limited and subsides as the parathyroid glands complete their involution. In a small minority of cases autonomous parathyroid adenomas exist, and these must be removed surgically. In others the degree of hypercalcemia may be sufficiently severe or prolonged, or the risk of myocardial or pulmonary calcification considered so great, that subtotal parathyroidectomy may be warranted. Several authorities consider that extensive metastatic calcification is an indication for subtotal parathyroidectomy either prior to or soon after renal transplantation.

Kleeman, C. R. (ed.): Divalent ion metabolism and osteodystrophy in chronic renal failure. Arch. Intern. Med., 124:261, 389, 519, 649, 1969.

891. OSTEITIS FIBROSA

Robert P. Heaney

Definition. The term "osteitis fibrosa" is used to designate a pathologic rather than a clinical entity. It refers to the replacement of bone by a highly cellular fibrous tissue, associated with accumulations of osteoclasts, singly and in clumps, together with evidence of increased osteoblastic activity. The terms "osteitis fibrosa cystica" and "von Recklinghausen's bone disease"* have also been used to describe this condition.

Etiology and Incidence. In most cases the morphologic picture comes about because of greatly exaggerated parathyroid hormonal stimulation. It is found in 10 to 25 per cent of patients with primary hyperparathyroidism, is always found as a part of the picture of uremic osteodystrophy, and to variable degrees may be seen in patients with rickets and osteomalacia. In the latter disorders, the presence of osteitis fibrosa depends upon the degree of responsiveness to parathyroid hormone that the bone mesenchyme is able to manifest. However, the identical condition can be produced even without an excess of parathyroid hormone whenever bone turnover is exceedingly rapid, as in certain patients with hyperthyroidism, and locally in rapidly evolving Paget's disease (vide infra).

Pathogenesis and Pathology. In the typical case due to excess parathyroid hormone there is stimulation of all bone cells: osteocytes resorb their perilacunar bone; osteoclasts are found in large numbers and resorb bone on all three bony envelopes; osteoblastic new bone formation is also increased. However, osteoclasts predominate, and as a consequence there is usually a decrease in total skeletal mass. Resorption is particularly prominent in cortical bone immediately beneath the periosteum and is responsible for the typical and characteristic roentgenographic features of the disorder: (1) the presence of a fine lacy pattern of radiolucency at the outer edge of the cortex, particularly in the phalanges and metacarpals; (2) the disappearance of the lamina dura (the equivalent of

---

*The eponym "von Recklinghausen's disease" is also associated with the hereditary disorder neurofibromatosis, which may occasionally exert indirect skeletal effects, chiefly scoliosis and bony erosion by adjacent neurofibromas, and rarely a vitamin D-resistant osteomalacia.

a bone cortex in the tooth socket); and (3) cortical striation seen on fine grain films. When severe, or of long duration, there is virtual loss of detectable bone from the ends of the clavicles and the terminal phalanges ("acro-osteolysis"). Undoubtedly the bony mesenchyme is itself stimulated by parathyroid hormone, and masses of growing fibrous tissue and osteoclasts may expand and destroy the bone cortex, giving rise to what appear, roentgenographically, to be large cystic tumors. Osteoclasts alone may form tumor-like masses that have been designated giant cell tumors. These produce discrete punched-out lesions roentgenographically, particularly in the jaw or facial bones, and in some cases such tumors may be the primary roentgenographic manifestations of osteitis fibrosa. Such tumors are biologically benign and invariably regress if the underlying cause is removed.

Clinical Manifestations. The principal manifestations of osteitis fibrosa are bone pain and pathologic fractures. Early the pain is not distinctive and is easily mistaken for vague arthritic complaints. There may also be specific arthritides present: both gout and pseudogout have been described in association with osteitis fibrosa. Later the bones become tender to palpation, and in advanced cases the pain may become incapacitating. Pathologic fractures occur through areas weakened by general resorption or giant cell tumor formation, and may involve any bones of the body. Vertebral collapse is common, and compression fractures and acroosteolysis of the terminal phalanges may so shorten those bones as to simulate "clubbing" of the fingers. Since patients may have hypercalcemia, their clinical picture will usually include extraskeletal features described elsewhere in this text (see Ch. 872).

Diagnosis. The generalized decrease in roentgenographic density must be distinguished from osteoporosis and multiple myeloma, and the cystlike lesions from fibrous dysplasia and true bone tumors. Bone biopsy establishes the true nature of the lesion, and plasma chemical determinations aid in determining its cause, e.g., primary hyperparathyroidism (see Ch. 872), uremia, and osteomalacia.

Treatment. In primary hyperparathyroidism, removal of the offending adenoma constitutes definitive therapy. Treatment in other conditions producing osteitis fibrosa is less certain or satisfactory. The bone lesions heal with great rapidity when the cause, such as a parathyroid adenoma, can be eradicated. For this reason, giant cell tumors, particularly in the facial bones, should not be treated by mutilating surgical operations until hyperparathyroidism has been excluded as a cause.

Johnson, L. C.: Morphologic analysis in pathology: The kinetics of disease and general biology of bone. In Frost, H. M. (ed.): Bone Biodynamics. Boston, Little, Brown & Company, 1964.

Weinmann, J. P., and Sicher, H.: Bone and Bones. St. Louis, C. V. Mosby Company, 1955, pp. 246–251.

BONE INTOXICATIONS

Robert P. Heaney

892. FLUOROSIS

Fluoride is one of the more common constituents of the earth's crust, occurring particularly in association with phosphates, silicates, and calcium. It is abundant in sea water and in many fresh water supplies, and was undoubtedly a component of the environment in which life evolved. It probably functions as an important trace element in human nutrition, though a fluoride deficiency syndrome is not recognized. In optimal concentrations fluoride stabilizes the crystal structure of tooth enamel and probably also that of bone. In high concentrations fluoride acts as a general protoplasmic poison, resulting in death; but between toxic intake levels (> 100 mg) and probably optimal intakes (about 1 mg daily), chronic intake produces changes confined largely to the skeleton. Intoxication occurs because of accidental ingestion of fluoride-containing insecticides, chronic inhalation of industrial dusts (particularly in the aluminum mining and phosphate fertilizer industries), or prolonged drinking of certain fresh waters containing large amounts of fluorides. The skeletal lesions in man vary with the intake but consist of a combination of osteosclerosis and osteomalacia. The malacic lesions are more prominent at higher intake levels and represent interference with matrix maturation or crystal nucleation. Sclerosis consists of coarsening of trabeculae, periosteal new bone deposition, osteophyte formation, and ossification of tendons and ligaments. Severely fluorotic bone is chalky white in appearance and exhibits a crumbly consistency, cutting easily with a knife.

Early there are no specific complaints. As the skeletal disease advances there may be vague pains in the small joints of hands and feet. As osteophyte formation and periosteal bone growth progress, kyphosis, restriction of spine motion, flexion contractures of hips and knees, and ultimately nerve root and spinal cord compression develop. The neurologic involvement produces paresthesias, weakness, and ultimately paralysis. Early the neurologic involvement may simulate peripheral neuropathy, spinal cord tumors, or syringomyelia.

No municipal water supply in the United States contains more than 6 to 8 parts per million of fluoride, and this concentration, although sufficient to produce mottled tooth enamel, almost never produces bone disease. In certain regions of India and Arabia water-related fluoride intake reaches sufficient levels to produce fluoride intoxication. In the Punjab, for example, osteofluorosis is the most common form of bone disease. Deliberate osteofluorosis has sometimes been induced to halt the explosive skeletal demineralization of diseases such as multiple myeloma.

There is no effective treatment for the advanced syndrome except for orthopedic and supportive measures. Effort should be directed at prevention, particularly in the context of industrial exposure. Excess body burdens of fluoride are retained for years after exposure has terminated. Fluoride trapped in bone crystals is released only when bone resorption occurs, and some of the liberated ions are redeposited at sites of new bone formation. If the intake is low, however, urinary excretion will gradually lower the total body content.

893. VITAMIN A INTOXICATION

Although not confined to bone, the effects of chronic excessive vitamin A intake may be most apparent in the skeleton. Such intoxication is rare, and has occurred most frequently in young children who received doses on the order of 100 times the normal daily vitamin requirement and in hunters who ingested large quantities of polar bear liver. The initial bony change is painful periosteal proliferation, particularly of the ulnae, clavicles, and metatarsals. These are readily apparent on roentgenographic examination. Higher doses in small animals produce severe osteoporosis and multiple fractures. The diagnosis is suggested by a history of excessive vitamin intake, and by finding high vitamin A levels in the plasma. Bony healing is usually complete when vitamin exposure ceases.

894. VITAMIN D INTOXICATION

In the past intoxication with vitamin D occurred primarily because of inappropriate and massive vitamin therapy for diseases not caused by vitamin deficiency. The disease is still seen as a complication of more appropriate vitamin D therapy for disorders such as osteomalacia or familial hypophosphatemia, and occasionally occurs in food faddists and in patients with an unusual sensitivity to doses usually considered to lie within the physiologic range. Intoxication results in three principal and closely related effects: hypercalcemia, metastatic calcification, and osteitis fibrosa. The ultimate clinical picture varies, depending upon the relative importance of these effects.

In massive dosage the vitamin (or contaminating trace sterols in the commercial vitamin preparations) directly stimulates both gastrointestinal calcium absorption and osteoclastic bone resorption. Hypercalcemia ensues, and endogenous parathyroid suppression occurs. Plasma inorganic phosphate is therefore normal or high, and thus the Ca × P ion product may rise to extremely high values, probably reaching supersaturated levels in many normally unmineralized tissue regions. In any case large soft-tissue calcium deposits occur, particularly in already damaged regions such as the synovia of arthritic joints, as well as in arterial walls. Urine calcium is initially high, and the renal interstitium is particularly prone to calcification. Such renal calcinosis leads to deterioration of renal function, further phosphate retention, and inability to excrete the excess plasma calcium load. This generates a vicious cycle which may lead to death from hypercalcemia or uremia. Metastatic calcification occurs also in the bone marrow of trabecular bone and may thus lead to the appearance of osteosclerosis. Because of the parathyromimetic effect of vitamin D, osteitis fibrosa is usually seen as well, and the net roentgenographic appearance of bone depends on the balance between these two processes.

Clinical manifestations are caused principally by the hypercalcemia and renal failure, and not by the bone disease itself. These are the same as those of hypercalcemia from any cause, and include anorexia, nausea, vomiting, lassitude, polyuria, dehydration, and ultimately fever, stupor, and death.

The diagnosis of vitamin D intoxication should be considered in the evaluation of patients with hypercalcemia or those found to have extensive soft tissue calcification. It is most readily confirmed by obtaining a history of excessive vitamin D intake and by observing improvement when the vitamin is withdrawn. Treatment consists of management of the hypercalcemia and stopping vitamin D ingestion; this is usually satisfactory unless irreversible kidney damage has occurred.

895. RADIONUCLIDE BONE TOXICITY

Many radioactive isotopes accumulate in the skeleton and, although ingested in doses too small to produce acute systemic effects, may lead years later to severe bone disease. Skeletal damage consists of (1) growth retardation if exposure occurred prior to epiphyseal closure; (2) osteonecrosis, osteomyelitis, and bone abscess; (3) brittleness and tendency to fracture; and (4) osteogenic sarcoma. There are three categories of exposure: (1) strontium-90 and yttrium-91 from radioactive fallout of atom bomb fission products; (2) radium and thorium from industrial and medical exposure; and (3) uranium and the transuranic elements from processing of nuclear reactor fuel and wastes. Strontium and radium, like calcium, are alkaline earth elements and readily form phosphate salts. They are trapped in newly forming bone at the time of its mineralization. The localization of thorium, uranium, and the transuranic elements is less well understood, but appears to be predominantly on bone surfaces adjacent to the innumerable small vessels of bone. Radiation damage in each case is produced by the α and β particles, rather than by the γ radiation. Because of the extremely short range of these particles in bone, the damage is thus confined microscopically to the areas of isotope deposition. Cell death is the usual result, cell sensitivity varying with cell type, as follows: chondroblasts > osteoblasts > osteocytes > osteoclasts. The surrounding bony material, deprived of continuing cellular influence, becomes hard and brittle. Ultimately it is subject to slow resorptive removal. The mechanism of sarcoma production is not known but is presumably the same as for radiation carcinogenesis elsewhere.

Clinical features are variable and not distinctive. Bone pain may be present, and spontaneous fractures may occur through bone that appears roentgenographically normal. Occasionally the long bones may present a punched-out appearance reminiscent of multiple myeloma. Radium dial painters frequently developed necrosis and osteomyelitis of the jaw, related to localization of radium in the periodontal tissues. Radiation damage, once it has occurred, is irrevocable, and no treatment is of any value. Bone localization after acute accidental ingestion of radium and strontium can be minimized by calcium infusion and deliberate production of sustained hypercalciuria.

Barnicot, N. A., and Datta, S. P.: Vitamin A and bone. *In* Bourne, G. H. (ed.): Biochemistry and Physiology of Bone. 2nd ed. Vol. 2. New York, Academic Press, 1971.

Cousins, R. J., and DeLuca, H. T.: Vitamin D and Bone. *In* Bourne, G. H. (ed.): Biochemistry and Physiology of Bone. 2nd ed. Vol. 2. New York, Academic Press, 1971.

Hasterlik, R. J., and Finkel, A. J.: Diseases of bones and joints associated with intoxication by radioactive substances, principally radium. Med. Clin. North Am., 49:285, 1965.

Pugh, D. G.: Roentgenologic Diagnosis of Diseases of Bones. New York, Thomas Nelson & Sons, 1951.

Singh, A., Jolly, S. S., Bansal, B. C., and Mathur, C. C.: Endemic fluorosis; epidemiological, clinical and biochemical study of chronic fluorine intoxication in Punjab (India). Medicine, 42:229, 1963.

Vaughn, J. M.: The effects of radiation on bone. *In* Bourne, G. H. (ed.): Biochemistry and Physiology of Bone. 2nd ed. Vol. 3. New York, Academic Press, 1971.

Weinmann, J. P., and Sicher, H.: Bone and Bones. St. Louis, C. V. Mosby Company, 1955, pp. 246–251.

896. OSTEOMYELITIS

Paul D. Saville

Definition. Osteomyelitis is an infection within bone by any bacterial or mycotic organism that infects other tissues.

Pathophysiology. Before puberty, infection starts in the metaphyseal sinusoidal veins. Because bone tissue is inelastic, local edema accumulates under pressure and leads to necrosis of tissue, breakdown of bone trabeculae, and removal of both matrix and calcium. Infection extends along haversian canals and through the marrow cavity and beneath the periosteum, damaging the vascular channels and causing death of osteocytes. This leads to the formation of a sequestrum. The periosteal new bone formation which takes place on top of already dead bone is known as an involucrum.

Etiology. Patients can often be shown to have infection elsewhere, particularly in the skin, where *S. aureus* is probably the most common causative organism, but its prevalence has dropped in the United States from 80 per cent in the past to about 50 per cent at present. Gram-negative bacilli occur mainly in adults with vertebral osteomyelitis. *M. tuberculosis* occurs mainly in the spine, especially among economically deprived individuals. Tuberculous and fungal infections of bone can usually be traced back to pulmonary disease. Persons with sickle cell disease have a special susceptibility to Salmonella osteomyelitis. Vertebral osteomyelitis in adults may follow colorectal surgery, or infection of the genital, urinary, or biliary tracts.

Clinical Manifestations. In the past, over 85 per cent of cases occurred in children under 16. Recently there has been a shift of the disease to older age groups. Infection usually occurs in the metaphyseal region, particularly of the femur and tibia, and multiple bone involvement is not rare. In patients over the age of 50, the most common site of osteomyelitis is the spine.

In children, onset is sudden, with high fever, chills, and pain in a limb. Increasing numbers of patients are seen with atypical features, including low-grade temperatures and even no fever at all. There is usually leukocytosis. Acute local tenderness and swelling may occur because of elevation of the periosteum by pus. In adults, pyogenic spondylitis is seldom heralded by an acute febrile episode. Usually there is simply insidious onset of deep boring pain in the back, aggravated by movement, coughing, sneezing, or straining. Symptoms gradually increase. Patients may complain of abdominal pain when the lumbar vertebrae are involved. Paravertebral or psoas abscesses were once thought to be indicative of tuberculous spondylitis, but today such an abscess in the United States or Western Europe is more likely to be associated with staphylococcal infection than with tuberculosis. In the adult, no changes are visible radiographically, often for many weeks after onset of infection. The first changes are destruction of a disc space and the adjacent vertebral end-plates above and below. Later sclerosis of bone occurs and new bone forms, often with fusion of two vertebrae and obliteration of the intervertebral space. In childhood disease, blood cultures are frequently positive for the causative organism. In adult pyogenic spondylitis, this is rare.

Subacute pyogenic osteomyelitis, known as Brodie's abscess, is usually located in a metaphysis and appears as a lucent lesion sometimes surrounded by slight sclerosis. Its onset is insidious; pain is a prominent symptom, but fever is rare. It is usually due to the presence of *S. aureus,* occasionally *S. albus,* or even more occasionally gram-negative organisms.

Chronic osteitis in the hands or feet is usually due to tuberculosis or syphilis. Asymmetric osteitis in the hands or feet is more likely to be due to group A Streptococcus and *S. aureus.*

Radiographic changes are late in developing in osteomyelitis, but scintigraphy using ^{99m}Tc diphosphonate will point to a lesion early in the disease, either in the spine or in the long bones. This is particularly helpful in the adult in whom there is almost no clinical evidence to indicate spine disease.

Treatment. It is important to obtain the organism responsible for the infection and to determine the antimicrobial sensitivity. In vertebral osteomyelitis, needle biopsy with aspiration of tissue is necessary. For sensitive organisms, penicillin G is the best antimicrobial and should be used in large doses, preferably 20,000,000 units per day given intravenously. Alternatively, oxacillin, methicillin, or nafcillin may be given in daily doses of 8 to 16 grams intravenously in an adult. Treatment should be maintained for at least four to six weeks. There is no place for oral medication or for bacteriostatic drugs in the initial stages of treatment. Most cases of hematogenous osteomyelitis in children should be surgically drained even when the organism is known and the appropriate antimicrobial is given in large doses.

When osteomyelitis has been clinically cured, it can be assumed that viable organisms remain in haversian and Volkmann canals. It may recur up to four decades later because of the same organisms. These recurrences are often precipitated by trauma.

OSTEOMYELITIS DUE TO CONTIGUOUS INFECTION

Osteomyelitis may be caused by infection gaining entrance to a bone from a compound fracture or through surgical operation, especially with internal fixation. Infection of the phalanges of the hands and feet may occur from soft tissue infections, especially in the hands. Infection of the jaws occurs from dental abscesses and radiation. Infection from the frontal or ethmoid sinuses causes osteomyelitis of the frontal bone by spread from the blood vessels of the mucosal lining of the sinuses. When the frontal bone is infected, pus collects under the periosteum, causing swelling and edema over the forehead known as Pott's puffy tumor. With frontal osteomyelitis, epidural and even subdural abscesses may occur, with severe headache and signs of increased intracranial pressure.

A local infection occurring after a compound fracture or internal fixation is usually associated with pain, pus, and fever. When infection occurs after introduction of a prosthetic device, there is frequently an insidious onset of pain, which may take months or even years after the surgical procedure to become manifest. Extensive bone destruction may occur without clear-cut signs of infection or fever. The existence of infection may be obscured by the use of prophylactic antimicrobials given at the time of surgery. The diagnosis may be helped by needling of the suspected lesion or by open surgery. Where a prosthetic device has been used, it is often necessary to remove this before the infection can be controlled.

Infections of the bones of the feet or toes occur frequently in patients with diabetes mellitus or with severe peripheral vascular disease. The patients frequently have pain and swelling in the affected limb and may have ulcers. More often than not they have no systemic manifestation such as fever. Response to treatment with antimicrobials is usually unsatisfactory, and amputation is often necessary.

Waldvogel, F. A., Medoff, G., and Swartz, M. N.: Osteomyelitis: A review of clinical features, therapeutic considerations and unusual aspects. N. Engl. J. Med., 282:198, 260, 316, 1970.

897. OSTEONECROSIS
Paul D. Saville

Definition. Osteonecrosis denotes the clinical syndrome associated with death of bone cells in a localized volume of bone. The term osteonecrosis is used here for the condition formerly called *aseptic necrosis of bone* or *avascular necrosis of bone*.

Etiology. Osteonecrosis may result from traumatic disruption of the blood supply of bone. Common sites of this include the femoral head after a subcapital fracture of the hip or traumatic dislocation of the hip; the semilunar, navicular, and scaphoid bones in the wrist; the tibial tuberosity; and the epiphysis of the os calcis before closure. Nontraumatic necrosis is believed to be due to obstruction of bony end-arteries by sludged red cells, gas bubbles, lipid droplets, uric acid crystals, or vasculitis. These may arise in Gaucher's disease, in sickle cell anemia, in caisson disease, in systemic lupus erythematosus, in hyperlipemia associated with alcoholism or pancreatitis, and with corticosteroid therapy. *Perthes' disease* is an osteonecrosis of the femoral head occurring for uncertain reasons, largely in males between four and ten years of age. *Osteochondritis dissecans* of the medial femoral condyle of children is a similar condition, as is osteonecrosis of the weight-bearing portion of the medial femoral condyle seen in older adults. The disease also occurs in the talus, the capitellum, and the humeral head.

Incidence. Osteonecrosis of the femoral head occurs in about 50 per cent of cases of subcapital fracture of the hip and in 50 per cent of patients on immunosuppressive therapy for kidney homograft. Perthes' disease of the hip occurs in one of 820 boys and one of 4500 girls.

Clinical Manifestations and Diagnosis. In adults, pain may occur up to three years after the original subcapital fracture. The disease which occurs in alcoholics and immunosuppressed patients, as well as the idiopathic variety, usually manifests itself with sudden bone pain. At first, there are no radiographic changes, but after two months there may be a small radiolucent zone in bone under the articular cartilage. High resolution bone scans with agents such as ^{99m}Tc diphosphonate invariably reveal a focus of intense isotope uptake before radiographic changes become apparent. Later, increased bone density indicates attempted healing of the lesion. Before healing can occur, the resorptive phase leads to weakened bone which may collapse on weight bearing and result in bone deformity. This leads to secondary osteoarthrosis.

Treatment. Treatment consists of stopping weight bearing until healing has occurred. This may take up to three years. Some surgeons use bone grafts inserted through the femoral neck into the head to speed up the healing process in the hip. When osteonecrosis affects bones in the wrist, severe osteoarthrosis of the joint is common and wrist fusion may be required to relieve pain. Prostheses may be used with success when deformity of bone and secondary osteoarthritis occur in weight-bearing joints.

Ahlback, S., Bauer, G. C. H., and Bohne, W. H.: Spontaneous osteonecrosis of the knee. Arthritis Rheum., 11:705, 1968.

CONGENITAL AND/OR HEREDITARY DISORDERS INVOLVING BONE
Paul D. Saville

898. OSTEOGENESIS IMPERFECTA
(Psathyrosis, Fragilitas Ossium, Lobstein's Disease)

Definition. Osteogenesis imperfecta is an inherited disorder of collagen maturation resulting in defects in connective tissue, manifested by increased fragility of the skeleton and blue sclerae.

Inheritance. About half the cases are sporadic, presumably caused by mutations. In the majority of the remaining cases, the disease is inherited as an autosomal dominant trait. There is also a rarer and very severe recessive type. Clinical expression of disease can vary widely; this has been responsible for confusion in classification and terminology. The disease is not uncommon, but precise incidence figures are lacking.

Pathology and Pathogenesis. The basic chemical defect is unknown. Soluble collagens fail to complete the normal sequence of extracellular changes necessary to convert them into a tough fibrous tissue. Total collagen is quantitatively deficient as well. As a result, tendons and ligaments are thin and subject to rupture; the skin is thin; the sclerae of the eyes are also thin and allow the choroidal pigment to show through, giving a blue color. Woven bone may be seen in adult life and may be the only characteristic microscopic abnormality. The rates of new bone formation and resorption are increased. Unlike acquired osteoporosis, there is a defect at the periosteal envelope which results in decreased appositional growth rate. This causes the unduly narrow bones characteristic of this disease.

Clinical Features. The clinical manifestations are extremely variable; 60 per cent of affected individuals have bone disease, but in the same family 5 per cent will have only an otosclerotic type of deafness while an occasional member will manifest only blue sclerae. In severe cases, multiple fractures occur during birth or in utero, or multiple fractures may occur from trivial trauma during childhood. The tendency to fracture decreases as the child approaches adolescence. The children are small and have an increased basal metabolic rate. Serum calcium and phosphorus are normal, but alkaline phosphatase may be elevated when fractures occur. Serum and urine pyrophosphate may be increased. Lax ligaments are a common clinical finding. Radiographs reveal gracile long bones with narrow cortices; the skull is thin and may be deformed. There is radiolucence of the vertebrae which may be uniformly compressed. This gives an appearance of biconcavity or of platyspondylia and can be indistinguishable from severe osteoporosis or osteomalacia. When the diagnosis is uncertain, the finding of wormian bones in the skull x-ray may be of help. Patients with this disease have no difficulty in forming callus; indeed, extremely exuberant callus formation may occur. This may be mistaken for tumor, and biopsy of such tissue can lead to erroneous diagnosis of osteogenic sarcoma.

Treatment. Fractures are treated by conventional methods of fixation. There is no effective treatment for the bone disease itself. Ascorbic acid has been used in massive doses; sodium fluoride, 5 mg per day, has been claimed to reduce the fracture rate, as has magnesium oxide, 10 to 15 mg per kilogram per day, which also has lowered the elevated serum pyrophosphate levels.

899. OSTEOPETROSIS
(Albers-Schönberg's Disease, Marble Bone Disease)

Marble bone disease is a rare familial disorder of the skeleton characterized by an increase in density of all bones owing to failure of bone resorption and bone remodeling.

There are probably dominant as well as recessive types of inheritance. The severe variety presents in infancy with anemia and hepatosplenomegaly. These children have little or no bone marrow and require blood transfusions. Failure to resorb bone results in optic atrophy, deafness, and hydrocephalus. Osteomyelitis of the jaws from dental infection may require antimicrobials. Early death is frequent. Milder cases may come to medical attention later in childhood or in adult life because of retarded growth or increased bone fragility.

Hypersplenism may require splenectomy for improvement of anemia. There is no specific treatment for the bone disease.

900. MELORHEOSTOSIS

This is a rare disorder of bone resulting in massive endosteal thickening, affecting one or more long bones, which begins proximally and proceeds distally like the flow of wax down a candle. The condition is painful. The cause is unknown, and there is no specific treatment.

901. OSTEOPOIKILOSIS

This condition is inherited as an autosomal dominant trait. It consists of multiple dense zones or streaks occur-

ring throughout the skeleton and frequently is associated with local patches of elastic fiber hyperplasia in the skin. It is of little clinical importance.

902. HEREDITARY HYPERPHOSPHATASIA

Hereditary hyperphosphatasia is a rare disease inherited as an autosomal recessive trait. It is characterized by multiple fractures and bone deformity in childhood, presenting radiologically some of the features of Paget's disease of bone. Plasma alkaline phosphatase is extremely high. Bone turnover is rapid and there is increased urinary hydroxyproline. There may be mental retardation. No effective treatment is known.

903. ELLIS–VAN CREVELD SYNDROME
(Chondroectodermal Dysplasia)

This syndrome is characterized by polydactyly of the hands and, rarely, of the feet, dwarfism, and dysplasia of the fingernails. It is inherited as an autosomal recessive trait. In contrast to classic *achondroplasia*, the shortening of the extremities is more marked proximally than distally. Fusion of the capitate and hamate bones of the wrist and a defect in the lateral aspect of the proximal part of the tibia, producing knock knees, are consistent features. Congenital heart disease is frequently present; atrial septal defect is the most common cardiac malformation. An abnormally short upper lip, bound down by multiple frenula, and premature eruption of the teeth are frequent features. The disease is very rare, but it occurs as the main cause of dwarfism in the inbred socioreligious group known as the Old Order Amish, in Lancaster County, Pennsylvania, where it occurs with a frequency of 5 per 1000 births. One third of those afflicted die before two weeks of age. The condition must be distinguished from familial polydactyly and classic achondroplasia.

McKusick, V. A., Egeland, J. A., Eldridge, R., and Krusen, D. E.: Dwarfism in the Amish, I. The Ellis–van Creveld syndrome. Bull. Hopkins Hosp., 115:306, 1964.

904. OSTEOCHONDRO-DYSPLASIAS

ACHONDROPLASIA

Definition. Achondroplasia is a form of inherited dwarfism caused by retardation of endochondral bone formation. This relatively common disorder is inherited as an autosomal dominant trait.

Pathology and Pathogenesis. The abnormality is confined to cartilage and consists of failure or retardation of interstitial cellular proliferation and growth. As a result bones formed in cartilage are shortened. This is most apparent in the long bones of the extremities and in the bones of the base of the skull, and to a much lesser extent in the vertebrae. Membrane bone formation is normal; thus the bones of the cranial vault are able to grow normally and even accommodate themselves to the restricted growth of the base of the skull. Similarly, bone shafts enlarge normally. Microscopically there is a lack of normal cartilage cell columns at the epiphyseal growth plates, so that formation of the primary spongiosa proceeds very slowly and irregularly.

Clinical Manifestations. Clinically there is dwarfism, with disproportionate shortening of the extremities. Final height is usually less than 1.4 meters. The bridge of the nose is flattened and depressed, and the forehead may appear prominent and bulging. The hands and feet are short, and fingers tend to be nearly equal in length. The vertebrae are slightly and symmetrically flatter than normal. There are usually a dorsal kyphosis and compensatory posterior rotation of the sacrum and pelvis. The hip joints may thus be displaced backward and the pelvic inlet narrowed by the sacral promontory. Achondroplastic dwarfs exhibit entirely normal intelligence, endocrine function, and calcium metabolism, and, apart from their characteristic dwarfing and the problems it imposes, are able to live normal, useful lives.

Diagnosis. Achondroplasia presents such a typical picture that it is not usually confused with other causes of dwarfism except hypophosphatemic rickets. Occasionally patients with osteogenesis imperfecta may have very short extremities because of multiple fractures, but the true nature of the disease is immediately apparent roentgenographically. When diagnosis is difficult, measurement of the interpeduncular distance in the lumbar spine may be helpful. In normal people, interpeduncular distance increases (as one goes down) from T-12 to L-5, but in patients with achondroplasia T-11 or 12 are the widest vertebrae, while the lumbar interpeduncular distance either does not increase or actually decreases. Because of this restricted bony canal in the lumbar region, prolapsed intervertebral discs cause extremely severe symptoms, usually with neurologic sequelae. Paraplegia has been described in some cases. In addition, hydrocephalus is not uncommon and is usually of the communicating type, presumably because of bony restriction in the posterior fossa.

Treatment. There is no treatment.

OLLIER'S DYSCHONDROPLASIA; MULTIPLE ENCHONDROMATOSIS

Ollier's dyschondroplasia is a rare disorder in which projections or islands of epiphyseal cartilage proliferate down into the metaphysis. These cartilage remnants fail to undergo the changes required for mineralization but retain the growth potential of the epiphyseal plate, and under continued stimulation by growth hormone may expand slowly until much of the normal metaphyseal architecture is destroyed. There may be gross enlargement of the metaphysis. On the roentgenogram the lesions vary from elongated radiolucent patches to a fragmented, expanded picture that conveys the impression of a violent internal explosion within the metaphysis. Growth may cease and calcification may take place after puberty, but the inclusions may continue to enlarge throughout life, sometimes developing into chondrosarcomas. One side of the body is usually more severely involved than the other, but the lesions are fundamentally bilateral. The long bones and the ilia are most commonly involved, and when severe the disease may result in crippling and invalidism. The only treatment available consists of orthopedic procedures for correction of deformities and pathologic fractures.

HEREDITARY MULTIPLE EXOSTOSES

Probably the most common of the osteodyschondroplasias, the syndrome of hereditary multiple exostoses consists of irregular bony protuberances with a cartilage growth cap that project out from the subepiphyseal metaphyseal cortex and backward along the shaft. Lesions are bilateral, though not truly symmetrical, and represent more an abnormality of development of bony contour than a true exostosis. The metaphyseal cortex extends out around the periphery of the protuberances, and their trabecular structure and marrow spaces are continuous with that of the adjacent metaphysis. The disease occurs in families, but the mode of transmission is not known. Although the lesions begin to develop early in childhood, they rarely become apparent for several years. The basic abnormality is not known, but the disorder behaves as if portions of the zone of proliferating cartilage extended down the side of the metaphysis and in the process of growing split off from the growth plate and migrated back along the shaft, leaving a wake of normal endochondral bone behind them. The lesions are confined to the metaphyses of bones with active growth plates, and when severe may limit joint motion. Growth usually ceases when the epiphyses fuse. Very rarely the cartilaginous cap of an exostosis may develop into a chondrosarcoma.

MORQUIO'S DISEASE
(Morquio-Brailsford Syndrome, Morquio-Ullrich Syndrome)

See Ch. 938.

McKusick, V. A.: Heritable Disorders of Connective Tissue. 4th ed. St. Louis, C. V. Mosby Company, 1972.
Rubin, P.: Dynamic Classification of Bone Dysplasias. Chicago, Year Book Medical Publishers, Inc., 1964.

905. PAGET'S DISEASE OF BONE: OSTEITIS DEFORMANS

Paul D. Saville

Definition. Paget's disease of bone is a chronic, progressive disorder of bone of unknown cause that is characterized grossly by deformity of both external bony contours and internal architecture and microscopically by replacement of normal structure by a morphologically and chemically abnormal bone.

Incidence. The disease is almost unknown before age 30; the incidence increases from 0.5 per cent at 40 to 10 per cent at 90 years of age. Men are affected twice as often as women. It is rare in Scandinavia and in Asia, and more common in Australia and New Zealand.

Schmorl described a 3 per cent prevalence in persons over 40. There appears to be a slight familial tendency, but the mode of genetic transmission (if such exists) is unknown.

Pathology and Pathogenesis. The disease is an essentially local, asymmetrical phenomenon. It may, however, ultimately spread to involve a major fraction of the skeleton. It commonly involves weight-bearing bones. The sacrum and pelvis are most frequently involved, followed closely by the tibia and femur, and then in descending order by the lumbar, thoracic, and cervical vertebrae. Although the bones of the upper extremity are rarely involved, the skull is frequently affected.

The disease is characterized by rapid bone formation and resorption in involved regions. Resorption and the consequent osteoporosis comprise the primary abnormality, and the reparative processes follow along in their wake. When the disease begins in the shaft of a long bone, the first detectable abnormality roentgenographically is indeed a zone of rarefaction, but microscopic examination of the roentgenographically normal bone into which the osteoporotic front is advancing reveals that this bone is already qualitatively abnormal. Furthermore, the repair is achieved by deposition of a primitive and, in some cases, highly abnormal bone that may amount to little more than a kind of metastatic calcification of an areolar, myxoid matrix. This is particularly true of rapid periosteal proliferation.

The replacement bone is thus architecturally and chemically abnormal and is subject to rapid, random remodeling and replacement. It is an unstable structure and may have little mechanical significance.

Microscopically the repeated waves of resorption and repair leave behind a bone with a striking mosaic appearance, created by the pattern of cement lines. There is little or no structural orientation. Some of the repair bone may be osteomalacic, and thus wide osteoid seams are frequently found. Extremely rapid resorption may reproduce locally the picture of osteitis fibrosa.

Clinical Manifestations. Many patients with Paget's disease do not have symptoms. The principal clinical manifestation is bone deformity; much less common is pain. When Paget's disease occurs in the pelvis, osteoarthritis of the hip is a frequent association. The long bones are commonly enlarged, feel hot to the touch, and are bowed. Stress fractures are common along the convex borders of bowed long-bone cortices. Pathologic fractures may occur through these.

Enlargement of the skull, associated with headaches and sometimes cranial nerve palsies, especially nerve deafness, is common. Vertebral enlargement and platyspondyly cause kyphosis and occasionally paraplegia. The course of the disease varies widely, but in most cases it is only very slowly progressive. Massive skeletal involvement is rare. When this occurs, however, serum alkaline phosphatase activity rises to very high levels, and because of the extreme vascularity of the bone, high output cardiac failure may develop. Indeed, when more than 30 per cent of the skeleton is involved, cardiac enlargement is the rule. The disease predisposes to two malignant bone tumors: malignant osteoclastoma and osteogenic sarcoma. Osteogenic sarcoma after age 40 is a rare disorder, and there is no doubt that most cases occurring in older patients do so in pre-existing Paget's disease. The incidence is probably of the order of one per 4000 Paget patients per year.

Roentgenographic Manifestations. The first detectable change may be a sharply circumscribed zone of bone resorption. The lesion in the skull previously called osteoporosis circumscripta is now known to be an early manifestation of Paget's disease. Later the normal bony architecture of the skull is replaced by a greatly thickened, fluffy appearance. A roentgenographic characteristic of Paget's disease is replacement of normal bony architecture by coarse, abnormal-looking trabeculae, enlargement of the external contours of a bone, and flame-shaped lucent zones which start at the ends of the long bones and slowly progress up the shaft. Paget's disease of bone is occasionally the cause of so-called ivory vertebrae, the sclerotic end stage of Paget's disease.

Diagnosis. The plasma calcium and phosphorus are usually normal. Urinary calcium excretion is frequently increased and may lead to stone formation. However, the alkaline phosphatase is invariably high if any significant fraction of the skeleton is involved; indeed, it reaches higher values in this disease than in any other. Acid phosphatase values are also slightly elevated at times. Thus, without specific determination of prostatic acid phosphatase, this test may not be of much help in distinguishing Paget's disease from osteoblastic metastases of prostatic carcinoma. This differential problem arises chiefly when lesions are confined to the pelvis, for there carcinomatous infiltration beneath the periosteum may provoke a periosteal reaction that enlarges the contours of the pubic and ischial rami, thus simulating Paget's disease. In few other bony regions do osteoblastic metastases produce such change in external bony contour, and thus usually there is little diagnostic problem. The ordinary clinical and roentgenographic features are too distinctive to be confused with those of any other disease.

Treatment. Most cases of Paget's disease have no symptoms and require no treatment. Osteoarthrosis of the hip can be treated like any other case of osteoarthrosis with analgesics or by total hip prosthesis. Fractures are treated successfully by internal fixation, although problems may arise because of the unusually large marrow cavity and also because bowing makes passage of metal rods down the cavity difficult.

Three drugs have been shown to control disease activity. *Mithramycin* is believed to have a toxic effect on osteoclasts. One regimen consists of 15 to 25 μg per kilogram per day as an intravenous injection either for five consecutive days each week for four weeks or once or twice weekly for many months. Decrease in pain and other symptoms occurs within two weeks of the onset of treatment. In addition, alkaline phosphatase and increased urinary hydroxyproline decrease. Nausea is a troublesome side effect and begins several hours after the drug has been given. When the platelet count falls below 150,000 per cubic millimeter, the drug should be withheld. Favorable effects have been demonstrated with human, porcine, and salmon *calcitonin*. Variable dose schedules have been tried, including 100 to 200 MRC units subcutaneously once daily or 50 MRC units three times a week. There are infrequent dermal allergic reactions and nausea rarely, but no other important adverse effects. After prolonged treatment, there is a tendency for relapse despite continued medication. Synthetic human calcitonin may not have these disadvantages. Finally, the *diphosphonates* have been shown to be effective in Paget's disease. The drug disodium ethane-1-hydroxy-1,1-diphosphonate (EHDP) has been used in a single oral dose of 20 mg per kilogram per day before breakfast for periods of up to seven months. Treatment results in lowering of both serum alkaline phosphatase and urinary hydroxyproline and in clinical improvement as well. The only known adverse effects are increase in osteoid seams and hyperphosphatemia when the drug is given in large dose. These effects are reversible.

Paraplegia or cauda equina compression can be successfully treated with laminectomy and decompression procedures. Pathologic fractures through pagetoid bone heal well but are technically difficult to deal with. Internal fixation is necessary, but is complicated by large marrow cavities, which often necessitate several rods being packed together, and by bowing which may prevent rods from being thrust down the femoral shaft, as well as by extreme vascularity of bone which causes severe hemorrhage. Sarcomas must be watched for carefully and treated surgically as soon as they become apparent.

De Deuxchaisnes, C. N., and Krane, S. M.: Paget's disease of bone: Clinical and metabolic observations. Medicine, 43:233, 1964.
Frame, B., Parfitt, A. M., and Duncan, H. (eds.): Clinical Aspects of Metabolic Bone Disease. Amsterdam, Excerpta Medica, 1973. (See especially pp. 516–554 for articles by various authors on treatment of Paget's disease.)
Johnson, L. C.: Morphologic analysis in pathology: The kinetics of disease and general biology of bone. In Frost, H. M. (ed.): Bone Biodynamics. Boston, Little, Brown & Company, 1964.
Pugh, D. G.: Roentgenologic Diagnosis of Diseases of Bones. New York, Thomas Nelson & Sons, 1951.
Snapper, I.: Bone Disease in Medical Practice. New York, Grune & Stratton, 1957.

906. FIBROUS DYSPLASIA

Paul D. Saville

Fibrous dysplasia, a developmental disorder of the bone mesenchyme, is characterized by replacement of bone by large masses of cellular fibrous tissue containing immature bone spicules and islands of cartilage. Except for the cartilage component, the histologic features are very similar to those of osteitis fibrosa, as is the roentgenographic appearance, but the two diseases differ in many respects. Fibrous dysplasia is a local disorder, and, although lesions may be widespread, there is always normal, uninvolved bone somewhere; furthermore, the disease is relatively slowly progressive and lacks the rapid bone resorption and formation of osteitis fibrosa. When the disease occurs in young girls, there are sometimes associated precocious puberty and patchy brownish skin pigmentation. This triad is known as "Albright's syndrome." Since large doses of estrogens produce a similar metaphyseal lesion in very young animals, it is not clear whether the precocious puberty of Albright's syndrome is simply a part of the picture or a contributing cause of the bone disease. The disorder may also be associated with hyperparathyroidism, gigantism, or hyperthyroidism.

The cause is unknown. Snapper contends that the disorder is fundamentally a lipoid granuloma, others that it is a disturbance of mesenchymal differentiation.

The age of onset is usually unknown and the disease first becomes apparent between ages 5 and 15, commonly because of deformity or pathologic fractures. Typical roentgenographic changes are cystlike lesions of meta-

physeal or shaft bone, with expansion of the cortex and sometimes severe destruction of bony architecture. Areas of increased density are frequently seen, and as the patient ages the lesions gradually acquire a uniform, ground-glass type of opacity. Plasma calcium and phosphorus are normal; the alkaline phosphatase is usually normal, but may be elevated when the disease is extensive.

Bone involvement is commonly unilateral. The femur and pelvis are frequently involved, as is the skull. Repeated fractures through involved areas of the upper femur lead to the characteristic "shepherd's crook" deformity. In the skull, however, lesions are osteomatoid, rather than fibrous, and roentgenograms reveal dense, featureless opacification and distortion of the facial bones and the base of the skull. Encroachment on cranial nerves may produce neurologic symptoms.

Growth is slow throughout childhood and usually ceases entirely in adolescence. The principal significance of the disorder lies in the production of fractures and deformity, but occasionally osteogenic, fibro-, or chondrosarcoma may occur. Except for indicated orthopedic procedures, no treatment is available.

See references for Ch. 905.

907. HYPERTROPHIC OSTEOARTHROPATHY

Paul D. Saville

Hypertrophic osteoarthropathy is a syndrome consisting of clubbing of the fingers, painful swelling and periosteal new bone deposition in the long bones of the extremities, and sometimes moderate joint swelling and tenderness, particularly at the wrists, ankles, and knees. The disorder is almost always associated with disease elsewhere in the body. It occurs in association with intrathoracic malignancies, usually a lung cancer or mesothelioma, but also with metastatic malignancies and mediastinal tumors, as well as bronchiectasis. Clubbing is common with chronic intestinal diseases; true osteoarthropathy is rare but has been described with ulcerative colitis, portal cirrhosis, and juvenile biliary cirrhosis. Very rarely it exists without apparent predisposing disease, and there is also a distinct hereditary form of the disorder, *pachydermoperiostosis*, associated with thickening of the skin of the scalp, face, and hands. In pachydermoperiostosis onset is usually at puberty. A family history of the disorder can be obtained in about one fourth of the cases.

In the finger tips the predominant changes are edema, hyperemia, and soft-tissue fibrous proliferation; bony changes are variable and usually not prominent. Grossly the fingertips appear bulbous, and there is increased curvature of the nails in all directions. The most typical bony lesions are found in the distal shafts of the bones of the forearm and leg, where there is distinct periosteal new bone deposition. Overlying tissues may be edematous, and the entire region is painful and tender to pressure. More advanced disease may involve the entire forearm and leg bones, and later the femur and humerus are affected.

The cause is unknown. The changes are probably mediated by alterations in periosteal blood flow. There is reason to suspect abnormal visceral reflex patterns, triggered by centrally located disease. Innominate artery aneurysms have been reported in association with osteoarthropathy confined to the involved extremity. In any case, surgical correction of lung lesions responsible for the disorder frequently produces dramatic relief of pain and swelling and prompt healing on roentgenographic examination.

Early in the course of the disorder the arthritic complaints may be misdiagnosed as rheumatoid arthritis. The later periosteal manifestations must be differentiated from disorders such as scurvy, syphilitic periostitis, polyarteritis nodosa, and progressive diaphyseal dysplasia. The skin changes of pachydermoperiostosis may suggest a diagnosis of acromegaly; however, absence of sinus enlargement and presence of periosteal reaction allow differentiation by roentgenography.

The disorder is important for two reasons. It usually serves as an indicator of serious disease elsewhere in the body, and in many cases, particularly of pulmonary neoplasms, may be the first such sign. Second, it is usually painful and may contribute significantly to the over-all disability of the primary disease.

The treatment must obviously be directed at the underlying disease. Analgesics, and sometimes narcotics, are required for symptomatic relief. Vagotomy has also been reported to provide relief.

Fischer, D. S., Singer, D. H., and Feldman, S. M.: Clubbing, a review, with emphasis on hereditary acropachy. Medicine, 43:459, 1964.
Herman, M. A., Massaro, D., Katz, S., and Sachs, M.: Pachydermoperiostosis—clinical spectrum. Arch. Intern. Med., 116:918, 1965.
Pugh, D. G.: Roentgenologic Diagnosis of Diseases of Bones. New York, Thomas Nelson & Sons, 1951.

908.   TUMORS OF BONE

Paul D. Saville

PRIMARY BONE TUMORS

Primary bone tumors present some of the most difficult diagnostic and therapeutic problems in clinical medicine. Adequate treatment for the malignant lesions is almost always mutilating, and the decisions that must be made in order to determine appropriate surgery require the utmost skill and cooperation between surgeon, pathologist, and radiologist. These problems cannot be adequately summarized within the scope of a textbook of medicine. The reader is referred to texts dealing specifically with bone tumors, such as those listed at the end of this chapter.

METASTATIC BONE TUMORS

By far the most common malignant skeletal tumors are metastatic from primary sites elsewhere in the body. Virtually any malignant tumor may metastasize to bone, but there are a few that do so with such regularity that they constitute most skeletal metastatic lesions. In one autopsy series of 1000 cases, two thirds of all patients with breast cancer, one third with lung cancer, and one fourth with renal cancer had skeletal metastases. In addition, approximately one eighth of the patients with cancer of stomach, pancreas, colon, and rectum have bony metastases. More than half of the patients with carcinoma of the prostate have osseous metastases. Thyroid carcinoma frequently and characteristically metastasizes to bone. Thus breast, lung, kidney, thyroid, and prostate account for the bulk of skeletal metastases. In addition leukemias and lymphomas commonly produce significant osseous involvement. Half the patients with Hodgkin's disease at autopsy are found to have osseous lesions.

Clinical Manifestations. Skeletal metastases present because of pain or pathologic fracture, or as an incidental finding on roentgenograms taken for another purpose. When lesions are widespread and related to a known primary site elsewhere, there is usually no diagnostic problem; but when an isolated lesion is discovered, the physician is faced with important differential considerations. He must decide whether the lesion represents a metastatic focus or a primary bone disorder. This may be just as important when the patient has a known primary malignancy as when he does not, for patients with cancer are as prone to unrelated bone disease as anyone else, and it is a serious mistake to assume the presence of metastatic spread if it does not really exist.

Many patients with skeletal metastases, especially from breast, prostate, kidney, and thyroid, live for years, and whether these years are spent productively and comfortably will depend on the therapeutic approach taken by the physician. It is worth stressing that such patients may have more years of useful productive life ahead of them than do many patients with diabetes, valvular heart disease, or emphysema, among others.

Most skeletal metastatic lesions are predominantly osteolytic. As tumors expand, the surrounding bone is destroyed, and the resulting focus appears roentgenographically as a radiolucent zone, sometimes sharply demarcated, sometimes with vague margins. These are referred to as osteolytic lesions. However, almost all tumors, except for multiple myeloma, provoke some degree of bone healing, and on microscopic examination new bone deposition and osteoblastic proliferation are frequently observed in and around metastatic foci. This osteoblastic activity is most pronounced in metastatic spread from cancers of prostate and breast, and to a lesser extent in spread from cancers of the urinary bladder. Breast lesions are fundamentally lytic, but superimposed bone reaction may predominate in many cases, producing patchy areas of increased roentgenographic density. These are referred to as osteoblastic metastases. Prostatic cancer, on the other hand, usually has no detectable lytic component. Metastatic cell clumps provoke such intense bone formation on trabecular surfaces that cancer foci literally have no room to expand peripherally, and instead they are pushed along bone tissue spaces by the evoked closure of those spaces behind them. Leukemic infiltration produces bone pain, lytic lesions, and in some cases pathologic fractures. Involvement with Hodgkin's disease produces a combination of lytic and blastic responses, involves the pelvis, vertebrae, ribs, and femora most commonly, and may sometimes evoke such an overwhelming osteoblastic response as to lead to near total opacification of involved regions.

Biochemical Manifestations. Plasma or urine biochemical changes reflect in general the extent and degree of activity of skeletal metastases. Quiescent or slowly progressive lesions usually produce no detectable change from normal values. Active or extensive osteolytic disease produces a large calcium load, which must be disposed of. This leads to hypercalciuria, hypercalcemia, and secondary suppression of endogenous parathyroid activity; if not arrested, it may produce renal calcinosis, renal failure, and death. Prominent osteoblastic activity or healing of pathologic fractures is usually reflected in an elevated alkaline phosphatase (although this same change can be produced by liver metastases), and in prostatic carcinoma disease activity usually, but not always, produces a rise in acid phosphatase. Cancer not metastatic to bone may sometimes produce changes identical with primary hyperparathyroidism. This syndrome has been observed most often with breast, lung, and kidney tumors, and is in fact a true hyperparathyroidism, for the tumor produces a parathyroid hormone-like agent.

Diagnosis. Multiple lesions in patients with obvious primaries present no diagnostic problem, but isolated lesions, or lesions with uncertain relation to a possible primary, should be subjected to biopsy. This point cannot be stressed too strongly. Open surgical biopsy is preferable in most cases, but needle biopsy may be best for inaccessible lesions, such as involvement of vertebral bodies.

Persistent skeletal pain without obvious roentgenographic changes can frequently be investigated by isotopic techniques, employing bone-seeking isotopes such as fluorine-18, strontium-85, or technetium-99m diphosphonate. Such isotopic scanning methods are four times as likely to reveal bony metastases as routine roentgenograms. Before attempting radical surgical removal of primary tumors of sites, such as breast, known to metastasize to bone, a skeletal scan is advisable. The inevitable reparative reaction to tumor metastases is responsible for a striking increase in local uptake of these isotopes, and the finding of such tracer localization confirms the existence of real bone involvement, even though no changes are present roentgenographically.

Treatment. A significant fraction of patients with breast, prostate, kidney, and thyroid metastases can be helped by appropriate treatment. Hypernephromas exhibit a tendency toward apparently solitary metastases, and in some cases combined removal of the primary plus the metastatic focus may result in several years of symptom-free life before other metastatic lesions become apparent. Breast, prostate, and thyroid carcinomas commonly retain a dependency on their hormonal environment, and their growth can be controlled by manipulation of that environment. Breast cancer in women prior to the menopause, and even for a few years thereafter, responds to oophorectomy and hypophysectomy; prostatic cancer to orchiectomy and estrogen treatment; thyroid cancer to iodine-131 administration and TSH-suppression produced by exogenous thyroid hormone treatment. Estrogen-dependent metastases of breast cancer may also respond to androgens and to certain nonvirilizing experimental androgen analogues. The extreme virilization produced by ordinary androgens severely limits the acceptability and value of these agents. In older women with metastatic breast cancer high dosages of estrogens are frequently of value (see Ch. 877).

Other adjunctive treatment includes the use of radiation therapy to troublesome or isolated lesions, and sometimes regional perfusion with chemotherapeutic agents should be considered. Considerable relief of pain and healing of disabling pathologic fractures can be provided by such means. When pain is not relieved by milder analgesics, adequate doses of narcotics, preferably morphine, should be employed as frequently as necessary.

Dahlin, D. C.: Bone Tumors. Springfield, Ill., Charles C Thomas, 1957.
Lichtenstein, L.: Bone Tumors. 4th ed. St. Louis, C. V. Mosby Company, 1972.
MacDonald, I.: Endocrine ablation in disseminated mammary carcinoma. Surg. Gynecol. Obstet., 115:215, 1962.
Symposium on the Role of Hormones in the Origin and Control of Abnormal and Neoplastic Growth. Cancer Res., 17:421, 1957.

Part XX
CERTAIN CUTANEOUS DISEASES WITH SIGNIFICANT SYSTEMIC MANIFESTATIONS

909. INTRODUCTION

Clayton E. Wheeler, Jr.

The history of medicine contains numerous examples of diseases such as lupus erythematosus and sarcoidosis that were first described on the basis of their dermatologic characteristics but were later recognized as having important manifestations elsewhere in the body. Cutaneous lesions are in fact described in connection with scores of diseases classified in other parts of this textbook. The disorders presented here are often treated by the specialist in dermatology, but they deserve mention in a textbook of medicine because their pathogenesis may provoke lesions in organs other than the skin and because some knowledge of them is needed by the general practitioner or the specialist in internal medicine.

910. CUTANEOUS MANIFESTATIONS OF INTERNAL MALIGNANCY

Clayton E. Wheeler, Jr.

Skin manifestations of internal malignancy are of two types: those in which there is invasion with malignant cells and those in which malignant cells cannot be identified.

Almost any internal malignant process may invade the skin. Lymphomas, melanomas, and metastases from carcinoma of the breast, kidney, prostate, lung, bronchus, stomach, colon, thymus, ovary, and testicle are the most common. Infiltration with malignant cells may produce firm to hard, nontender macules, papules, nodules, tumors, or plaques, which may be skin-colored, pink, red, violet, brown, or black. Lesions may be single or multiple, intact or ulcerated. Alopecia may appear at the infiltrated site. An erysipelas- or scleroderma-like picture may be produced by lymphatic involvement, especially in carcinoma of the breast. Colored, configurate, or ulcerated lesions are more likely to occur in lymphomas, and the skin of generalized exfoliative dermatitis may contain lymphoma cells. All areas should be examined carefully when internal malignancy is suspected; lesions of the scalp, umbilicus, and anogenital region are frequently overlooked.

Tumor cells cannot be identified in the skin in a wide variety of cutaneous manifestations of internal malig-

nancy. In most of these there is no real understanding of pathogenesis; hormonal, immunologic, enzymatic, and toxic mechanisms have been postulated. Although patterns produced in the skin are often highly suggestive of internal malignancy, they may also be caused by benign conditions. The relationship of the skin manifestation to malignancy has been proved in many instances by subsidence of cutaneous changes upon removal of the tumor and recurrence with tumor regrowth at the original or metastatic sites. Cutaneous changes may antedate, coincide with, or follow clinical diagnosis of malignancy. A brief account of these cutaneous manifestations follows.

Pruritus may be localized, generalized, intermittent, migratory, constant, mild, or severe. It may be unassociated with detectable abnormalities of the skin except for punctate and linear excoriations or prurigo-like nodules, or it may accompany lichenoid, eczematous, or bullous eruptions. It is often recalcitrant to the usual symptomatic measures; at times it can be relieved only by successful treatment of the underlying malignant disease. It is more common with lymphomas, especially Hodgkin's disease.

Pallor of anemia or, rarely, *erythema* and *cyanosis* of polycythemia may be present. A tan to dark brown color may result from diffuse *melanosis*. This may be localized to small areas or may be generalized with accentuation of normally hyperpigmented sites. The mechanism of melanosis is obscure in most carcinomas and lymphomas; infrequently, tumors that secrete melanocyte-stimulating hormone may be found. *Altered keratinization* may result in localized or diffuse dryness and scaling that may closely resemble ichthyosis. Hyperkeratosis of the palms and soles, alopecia, and varying degrees of cutaneous atrophy may also be present. This type of acquired ichthyosis is most likely to occur with Hodgkin's disease.

Toxic erythema, urticaria, erythema nodosum, or *erythema multiforme* may be due to any type of internal malignant disease. Chronic forms of erythema multiforme (figurate erythemas) characterized by persistent or migratory rings, arcs, or polycyclic lesions are suggestive of internal carcinoma.

Persistent, circumscribed, or diffuse *eczematous dermatitis* may signify internal malignancy. Pruritus, excoriation, lichenification, and secondary pyoderma may be present, especially if associated with lymphomas.

Generalized exfoliative dermatitis that may be associated with alopecia, loss of nails, lymphadenopathy, defective temperature regulation, and increased peripheral blood flow is more often a manifestation of lymphoma. Skin biopsy may show cells characteristic of the lymphoma or nonspecific inflammation.

Vesicular and *bullous eruptions* that resemble dermatitis herpetiformis, bullous pemphigoid, or pemphigus may be due to internal carcinoma or, less commonly, lymphoma.

Purpura may be due to vasculitis, thrombocytopenia, hypoprothrombinemia, and hypofibrinogenemia. *Migratory, superficial thrombophlebitis*, which is often refractory to treatment with anticoagulants, may affect the extremities or trunk. It may be due to carcinoma of the lung, stomach, ovary, or pancreas. In some instances there is an associated thrombocytosis.

Cold urticaria, acral cyanosis, or *gangrene* may occur in lymphomas or myelomas in association with cryoglobulinemia and macroglobulinemia.

Alopecia mucinosa is characterized by grouped follicular papules or plaques, usually on the scalp, face, or neck. Alopecia is due to mucinous degeneration of the hair follicle. In older patients the condition may be an early manifestation of mycosis fungoides or other lymphomas.

Acanthosis nigricans, as discussed in Ch. 915, is often associated with adenocarcinoma arising in the abdomen or pelvis.

Dermatomyositis in patients over 40 years of age is frequently associated with an internal malignant disease, usually carcinoma. Myopathy without dermatitis, various neuropathies, and myasthenic states may also be associated with an internal malignant condition.

Clubbing of the digits, periostitis, osteoarthropathy, and *gynecomastia* may be associated with carcinoma of the lung or other tumors.

Pachydermoperiostosis is characterized by cutaneous thickening, coarsening of facial features, cutis verticis gyrata, keratosis of the palms, excessive sweating and sebaceous gland secretion, macroglossia, clubbing, osteoarthropathy, and enlargement of the hands. The condition may be confused with acromegaly. It is usually seen in males with carcinoma of the lung.

Reduced resistance to infection is frequently present in persons with internal malignant conditions, especially lymphomas. Pyodermas are likely to be deep and severe and may result in generalized infections, at times with more than one microbial species. There is an increased incidence of herpes zoster, which tends to be accompanied by a chickenpox-like eruption. Herpes simplex infections are more extensive, deeper, and longer in duration. Progressive vaccinia may occur. Complicating tuberculosis, moniliasis, histoplasmosis, cryptococcosis, aspergillosis, mucormycosis, and cytomegalic inclusion disease tend to be progressive and fatal.

Bowen's disease is characterized by one or more circumscribed, scaly, crusted, erythematous plaques that may resemble psoriasis or eczema. Lesions may be found anywhere on the skin and may occur on mucous membranes. Intra-epidermal carcinoma is present microscopically. The long-held idea that a higher than expected percentage of patients with Bowen's disease eventually develop internal malignancies seems untenable from recent studies, except possibly in instances in which the Bowen's disease is related to arsenic exposure.

Paget's disease usually produces eczematoid changes of the nipple as an indication of an underlying ductal carcinoma. Extramammary Paget's disease of the perineum is associated with carcinoma of underlying apocrine glands or carcinoma of the rectum.

Primary amyloidosis associated with multiple myeloma may produce macroglossia, purpura, bullae or acquired epidermolysis bullosa, and waxy, flesh-colored

papules, nodules, or plaques on the face, trunk, or extremities.

Gardner's syndrome is characterized by dominant inheritance, multiple cutaneous cysts, osteomas, and polyps in the colon. Carcinoma of the colon develops in over half of these patients by the age of 40.

Anderson, S., Nielsen, A., and Reymann, F.: Relationship between Bowen's disease and internal malignant tumors. Arch. Dermatol., 108:367, 1973.

Brewer, L. M., and Brindley, G. V., Jr.: Unusual manifestations of primary malignant tumors of the thorax. Surg. Clin. North Am., 52:375, 1972.

Kierland, R. R.: Cutaneous signs of internal malignancy. South Med. J., 65:563, 1972.

Rosato, F. E., Shelley, W. B., Fitts, W. T., Jr., and Miller, L. D.: Nonmetastatic cutaneous manifestations of cancer of the colon. Am. J. Surg., 117:277, 1969.

Starke, W. R.: Bowen's disease of the palm associated with Hodgkin's lymphoma. Cancer, 30:1315, 1972.

911. ERYTHEMAS

Clayton E. Wheeler, Jr.

Disorders to be discussed under this heading are toxic erythema, erythema multiforme, and erythema nodosum. Urticaria, a close relative, is described in Ch. 75. Although the erythemas vary in morphology, there are features which group them into a common category. All result from reactions of small blood vessels in the skin or subcutaneous tissue. All are doubtless secondary manifestations of a wide variety of underlying disorders, although in many instances the basic condition cannot be identified. Finally, a given underlying disorder (drug reaction, for example) may cause toxic erythema, erythema multiforme, erythema nodosum, or urticaria in different individuals or simultaneous combinations of these vascular reactions in a single individual.

TOXIC ERYTHEMA

Toxic erythema is an extremely variable eruption that ranges from diffuse faint erythema to a generalized morbilliform exanthem. It is secondary to a wide variety of disorders, the most common of which are drug reactions and microbial diseases. Almost any drug may be incriminated, and infection with almost any organism may be involved. In addition, the eruption may be associated with foods and with noninfectious systemic diseases such as lymphomas, internal malignant processes, and the diseases of connective tissue. In a significant number of patients the underlying condition cannot be determined. When the causative disorder is established, the term toxic erythema is frequently discarded in favor of an etiologic diagnosis. Some examples of this are scarlet fever, infectious mononucleosis, drug reactions, and scarlatiniform eruptions produced by staphylococci.

Cutaneous manifestations result from vascular dilatation and mild inflammation in and about small blood vessels. Pathogenesis is often uncertain and probably varies with the underlying cause. Vascular changes may result from toxins, hypersensitivity reactions, or direct involvement with infectious agents.

Onset is usually abrupt with the appearance of diffuse erythema or erythematous macules. Small areas may be involved initially, but the eruption tends to become generalized and may be universal. In some instances there is a characteristic pattern of distribution and evolution—e.g., measles, scarlet fever, and erythema infectiosum—and in others there is random distribution. There is a tendency for the eruption to begin and to remain more intense at sites of minor irritation. Diffuse eruptions may be faint pink or bright red and are often scarlatiniform. Macular eruptions frequently coalesce to produce a morbilliform pattern. Erythema usually disappears with pressure on the skin, but a purpuric component may be present. Mild eruptions are transient and disappear without sequelae, whereas more severe reactions last for several days, and are followed by scaling or desquamation. The cutaneous changes may induce no symptoms or various degrees of itching, burning, or chilliness. Conjunctivitis is a common accompaniment, and the oral or genital mucous membrane may be involved.

Systemic manifestations depend primarily upon the underlying disorder. Fever is common, and chills may occur. Lymphadenopathy is frequent. Arthralgia or arthritis is occasionally present. Leukocytosis or leukopenia occurs, and the differential count may be abnormal.

The diagnosis depends upon clinical manifestations. Sometimes the eruption is so characteristic as to indicate the nature of the underlying disorder, but more often it is nonspecific. Final diagnosis of the primary condition depends upon careful history, physical examination, and laboratory study.

The primary objective of treatment is elimination of the underlying disease. Treatment of the cutaneous component is unnecessary in mild instances. In more severe cases symptomatic measures such as colloidal baths, topical calamine liniment, and oral antihistaminics may be helpful. Dry, scaly skin may be benefited by application of a bland emollient.

ERYTHEMA MULTIFORME

Definition.   Erythema multiforme is an acute inflammatory systemic disease that produces a spectrum of clinical patterns from a few inconsequential lesions on skin or mucous membrane to a severe, sometimes fatal multisystemic disorder. The disorder is a symptom complex secondary to a wide variety of diseases and conditions.

Division of the disease into types such as erythema multiforme minor (Hebra) or erythema multiforme major (*Stevens-Johnson syndrome*) based on the severity or extent of the morbid process seems only to confuse the picture. The disease pattern in many instances falls between these extremes and therefore defies classification into such a scheme. Although of historical importance, synonyms such as *ectodermosis erosiva pluriorificialis, dermatostomatitis, new eruptive fever,* and *mucosal-respiratory syndrome* offer no special advantage. Descriptive titles such as erythema multiforme iris, erythema multiforme bullosum, and erythema multiforme exudativum place too much emphasis upon single morphologic features.

Etiology.   There are two main theories concerning etiology: (1) The disease has a single cause, probably some infectious agent. (2) It is a symptom complex secondary to a variety of underlying disease states. In favor of the single cause theory is a close clinical resemblance to the

acute exanthems. Efforts to identify specific bacterial, fungal, or viral agents have been negative or inconclusive, and there is no epidemiologic evidence that the disease is contagious. The symptom complex theory finds support in the large number of conditions with which erythema multiforme has been associated. An incomplete list of these follows: (1) microbial diseases including pneumonia, meningitis, cholera, glanders, typhus, measles, mumps, herpes simplex, vaccinia, orf, mycoplasmal pneumonia, lymphogranuloma venereum, psittacosis, and malaria; (2) drug reactions from antimicrobials, anticonvulsants, codeine, thiouracil, arsenic, barbiturates, antipyrine, belladonna, quinine, mercury, aspirin, butazolidine, chlorpropamide, and antitoxins; (3) vaccination against poliomyelitis, smallpox, or tuberculosis (BCG); (4) internal malignant conditions, including carcinoma and lymphoma; (5) deep x-ray therapy; (6) contact dermatitis, especially poison ivy; and (7) connective tissue disease.

Present consensus is that erythema multiforme is always secondary, but there remains a significant number of cases in which no underlying cause can be identified despite extensive diagnostic effort.

Incidence and Prevalence.   Figures are heavily weighted in favor of the unusually severe forms of the disease, e.g., Stevens-Johnson syndrome, which are reported in preference to milder examples. If all degrees of severity are included, erythema multiforme is a common disease. Severe forms are rare in infancy, early childhood, and old age, and males are affected about twice as often as females. The disease is worldwide and there is no racial predilection.

Pathology.   Nonspecific inflammatory changes, including vasculitis, are present in skin, mucous membranes, and internal organs. The degree of inflammation correlates with clinical manifestations. The pathogenesis is incompletely understood. A symptom complex secondary to many diseases and drug reactions points to a mechanism of toxicity or hypersensitivity. The relatively common simultaneous occurrence with erythema nodosum and the frequent appearance of urticarial lesions in mild forms of erythema multiforme are further reasons to consider hypersensitivity. The appearance of the disorder a few days to three weeks after herpes simplex, vaccination for smallpox, infection with *Coccidioides immitis,* administration of penicillin, contact dermatitis from poison ivy, or deep x-ray therapy suggests that immunologic mechanisms play a role. The development of erythema multiforme after administration of antipyrine to certain persons, especially blacks, may indicate that genetic enzymatic defects or differences are involved.

Clinical Manifestations.   Perhaps half the patients experience a prodromal period of a day to two weeks, characterized by fever, malaise, cough, coryza, sore throat, chest pain, vomiting, muscular aches, and arthralgia in various combinations and severity. After this, or in patients without prodrome, skin or mucous membrane lesions develop suddenly, together with some systemic reaction and often with evidence of visceral involvement.

Skin lesions are often the first and sometimes the only clinically detectable manifestations of the disorder. They usually develop rapidly, are distributed symmetrically and in crops. There may be few lesions, or almost the entire skin may be involved. There is a predilection for wrists, backs of the hands, ankles, tops of the feet, knees, elbows, face, palms, and soles. No area is exempt, although the scalp is affected infrequently. The polymorphous eruption usually includes red or violet macules, wheals, papules, vesicles, and bullae in various combinations. When vesicles and bullae are present they usually develop in pre-existing macules, papules, or wheals. Hemorrhage into the affected areas is common. Lesions are usually sharply demarcated from normal skin and tend to assume an annular configuration. Merging produces gyrate, serpiginous, or arciform patterns. At times central fluid-containing areas are surrounded by concentric rings of varying shades of erythema or purpura; these are the *target, iris,* or *bull's eye* forms which should bring the consideration of erythema multiforme into focus. As the disease progresses, erosions, superficial ulcerations, crusts which are often hemorrhagic, and scaling areas may occur. Paronychias and shedding of nails occur in severe cases. In mild cases healing takes place in a few days to three weeks without scarring, although hyperpigmentation or depigmentation may persist much longer. In severe cases scarring may result, and healing may take six weeks or more.

Mucous membrane involvement usually accompanies the cutaneous eruption, but in mild forms either may occur separately. One or all mucous membranes may be affected, and few or many lesions may be present. The spectrum includes macular erythema, edema, vesiculation, bleb formation, erosion, ulceration, crusting, fissuring, and bleeding. On mucous membranes vesicles and bullae rupture early, forming erosions or ulcerations. A gray or white pseudomembrane may form at the sites of previous blisters, especially in the mouth. The mouth is the most commonly involved orifice. In severe cases the lips are red, swollen, fissured, eroded, and covered with a bloody crust. The gums are swollen, eroded, and bleed easily. The tongue, buccal mucosa, pharynx, and larynx show any or all of the mucous membrane changes described above. As a result there may be pain, difficulty in eating, drinking, and salivation, fetor oris, and hoarseness. Depending upon severity, the process lasts a few days to several weeks and usually heals without scarring. Lesions in the nose cause bleeding, crust formation, and obstruction. Tenesmus and bleeding may accompany anal disease. Urethral lesions, especially in the male, may cause dysuria, hematuria, pyuria, and even urinary retention in severe instances. Balanitis has led to adherence of glans to prepuce, and in females vulvovaginitis can result in formation of fibrotic bands or in partial stenosis of the vagina.

The eye is the site of attack almost as often as the mouth. The eyelids may be swollen and covered with any of the various skin lesions. Mild cases show transitory conjunctivitis. Purulent or membranous conjunctivitis is present in more severe instances. Subconjunctival hemorrhage occurs, and vesicles and bullae may appear. The cornea is usually spared except in severe cases, when it may be eroded or perforated. Iritis, iridocyclitis, and panophthalmitis have been seen. Inflammation usually subsides in a few days in mild cases but may persist for weeks. Partial or complete loss of vision may result from scarring of the cornea or panophthalmitis. Adhesions of bulbar to palpebral conjunctiva have occurred. Severe ocular damage has been less frequent since the advent of antimicrobial drugs.

Systemic manifestations may occur at any time in relation to skin or mucosal manifestations. Symptoms include fever, malaise, dehydration, muscle and joint pains, toxemia, and prostration. Respiratory manifestations include cough with or without sputum, hemoptysis, dyspnea, cyanosis, bronchitis, pneumonitis, pulmonary consolidation, and pleural effusion. Arthralgia and arthritis, often of multiple joints, have occurred frequently. Possible gastrointestinal symptoms are nausea, vomiting, dysphagia, hematemesis, abdominal pain, diarrhea, and melena. Inflammatory changes of the esophagus or colon account for most of these symptoms. Urinary tract findings have included albuminuria, hematuria, urinary retention, and anuria. Nephritis and uremia may develop, at times when skin and mucous membrane lesions are improving. Nervous system symptoms have been drowsiness, convulsion, confusion, coma, delirium, radiculitis, nystagmus, unequal pupils, and abnormal tendon reflexes. Cardiac arrhythmia, pericarditis, and electrocardiographic changes suggesting myocarditis have occurred. Regional lymphadenopathy has been common but generalized lymphadenopathy infrequent. Splenic and hepatic enlargement are rare. Endoscopic examinations have shown annular, erosive, or ulcerative pseudomembranous lesions of the esophagus, larynx, and colon.

No laboratory test is specific for erythema multiforme. Abnormalities depend upon structures involved and degree of damage. Some degree of leukocytosis is common, although the leukocyte count may be normal or decreased. Eosinophilia occurs occasionally. The platelet count is usually normal but it may be much decreased. Rarely, tourniquet tests are positive. Albuminuria, pyuria, hematuria, and casts are not uncommon. On rare occasions there may be increased cells and protein in the cerebrospinal fluid. Roentgenograms of the chest may show patchy pneumonitis or changes similar to those of mycoplasmal pneumonia. Electrocardiographic abnormalities include conduction defects and alterations suggesting myocarditis. Laboratory studies for infectious agents, tumors, and "collagen diseases" may establish the underlying cause.

Diagnosis. The diagnosis depends upon the presence of skin and mucous membrane lesions. An incomplete symptom complex without involvement of skin or mucous membrane has not been recognized. Polymorphous skin lesions that form annular and configurate patterns and bullous erosive involvement of mucous membranes usually differentiate erythema multiforme from the acute exanthems. *Pemphigus* is more protracted in course, usually exhibits less polymorphism and configuration, and skin biopsy shows acantholysis. *Pemphigoid* and *bullous dermatitis herpetiformis* are more chronic and have less mucous membrane involvement and fewer systemic symptoms; biopsy may be helpful. *Bullous contact dermatitis* can usually be distinguished by location and configuration, suggesting external factors, by lack of mucous membrane or systemic involvement, and by history and patch test. *Lymphomas* at times give rise to polymorphous skin lesions, but the clinical picture and biopsy usually suffice for differentiation. Severe forms of erythema multiforme may be confused with *septicemia* or *systemic lupus erythematosus,* but consideration of the nature of skin and mucous membrane involvement and other clinical and laboratory findings makes differential diagnosis possible.

Treatment. Underlying disease should be sought and eliminated when possible. Mild erythema multiforme requires little treatment: topical application of calamine liniment, oral antihistamines, and colloidal baths. Severe forms of the disorder require prompt active treatment of many types. Fluid and electrolyte imbalance caused by improper intake, vomiting, diarrhea, and renal dysfunction must be corrected. Secondary bacterial infection, especially of the eye, in which staphylococcal infection may be prominent, must be combated with topical or systemic antimicrobials or both. High doses of corticotrophin or adrenal steroids are often helpful in severe erythema multiforme and usually need be given only for short periods of time.

Prognosis. Data concerning duration, complications, recurrences, and mortality are generally based upon studies of patients with severe forms of the disease (Stevens-Johnson syndrome). They are worthless therefore in considering erythema multiforme as a whole. Mild forms, which constitute the majority of cases, subside in a few days to two or three weeks without sequelae. Severe forms last three to six weeks or longer; sequelae include neurologic changes, corneal opacities, blindness, keratoconjunctivitis sicca, conjunctival, vaginal, or preputial synechiae, and esophageal strictures. When all forms of erythema multiforme are included, the mortality rate is low (less than 0.5 per cent). The mortality rate in severe cases has been reported as high as 10 per cent. Treatment appears to decrease the duration and severity of the disease and the mortality rate. Recurrences are likely in some forms of the disease (reports give recurrence rates as high as 25 per cent). The pattern of recurrence is variable. Some attacks are severe and some mild; some patients have only skin or mucous membrane changes, and others have most of the features of the symptom complex. Oral or hidden anogenital herpes simplex infections should be sought in recurrent erythema multiforme.

Ackerman, A. B., Penneys, N. S., and Clark, W. H.: Erythema multiforme exudativum. Distinctive pathological process. Br. J. Dermatol., 84:554, 1971.
Bloom, A., and Lovel, T. W. I.: Erythema multiforme with renal and myocardial injury. Proc. R. Soc. Med., 57:175, 1964.
Brenner, S. M., and Delany, H. M.: Erythema multiforme and Crohn's disease of the large intestine. Gastroenterology, 62:479, 1972.
Gordon, A. M., and Lyell, A.: Mycoplasmas and erythema multiforme. Lancet, 1:1314, 1969.
Shelley, W. B.: Herpes simplex virus as a cause of erythema multiforme. J.A.M.A., 201:153, 1967.

ERYTHEMA NODOSUM

Definition. Erythema nodosum is probably a hypersensitivity reaction characterized by inflammatory nodules in the dermis and subcutaneous tissue. It is regarded as secondary to a variety of underlying disorders, especially bacterial, fungal, and viral infections, and drug reactions.

Etiology. In the light of present knowledge, the cause should be regarded as hypersensitivity vasculitis caused by a multiplicity of diseases and conditions, the most common of which are viral, bacterial, and fungal infections, and drug reactions. Among the associated disorders are tuberculosis, streptococcal pharyngitis, primary atypical pneumonia, leprosy, whooping cough, gonorrhea, lymphogranuloma venereum, measles, cat scratch disease, histoplasmosis, coccidioidomycosis, trichophytosis, chronic ulcerative colitis, syphilis, sarcoidosis, and reactions to iodides, oral contraceptives, sulfonamides, bromides, salicylic acid, arsphenamine, phenacetin, or other drugs. In spite of extensive clinical study, an underlying disorder cannot be diagnosed in one quarter to one half of the patients. This probably reflects inability to recognize a primary condition and does not mean that erythema nodosum is a disease *sui generis*.

Incidence and Prevalence. The disorder occurs at any age but is rare in early childhood and in the elderly. After puberty it is considerably more common in women. The underlying cause varies from one geographic area to another. Thus, in New England, streptococcal pharyngitis is regarded as the most common cause; in Scandinavia, primary tuberculous infection or sarcoidosis is frequently the underlying disorder; and in the San Joaquin Valley of California, primary infection with *Coccidioides immitis* is the most common cause.

Pathology. The pathologic picture is characteristic irrespective of the underlying cause. Inflammatory changes appear in the interlobular septa of the upper subcutaneous tissue and in the dermis. Vasculitis, especially endothelial reaction in veins, is associated with infiltration with neutrophils, lymphocytes, histiocytes, and, occasionally, eosinophils. In later stages lymphocytes, epithelioid cells, and foreign body giant cells predominate.

Pathogenesis. The extensive epidemiologic and clinical studies of coccidioidomycosis carried out in California have provided useful information on the pathogenesis of one form of erythema nodosum. Typical skin lesions develop in approximately one of twenty persons during primary infection with this fungus. Lesions make their appearance ten to twenty days after the onset of the infection, at about the same time the coccidioidin skin test becomes positive. Erythema nodosum accompanied by a strongly positive skin test indicates an excellent prognosis for complete recovery from the fungal infection. This seems to link the cutaneous nodules with the delayed, or tuberculin, type of sensitivity reaction. Complement-fixing antibodies appear in the serum much later in the course of coccidioidomycosis and, therefore, seem unrelated. In tuberculosis, also, erythema nodosum appears at about the time the skin test becomes positive; in fact, skin tests with tuberculin may precipitate or aggravate the disorder.

Clinical Manifestations. Erythema nodosum is characterized by red, tender nodules which usually develop in skin and subcutaneous tissue over the shins. The anterior thighs and extensor surfaces of the forearms are not uncommonly involved, and more rarely lesions appear on the backs of the upper arms and about the head, face, and eyes. A few to several dozen lesions appear, often in crops. The lesions are usually discrete, and an individual nodule reaches 2 to 5 cm in diameter or larger. As the lesion develops it becomes red, hot, and tender; as it involutes, the bright red color gives way to darker red and finally varying shades of green or yellow which simulate a bruise. During healing a fine cigarette-paper scale may appear on the surface. Individual lesions last a few days to two or three weeks, and usually heal without suppuration, depression, or scar formation.

Many of the symptoms associated with erythema nodosum are doubtless due to the underlying disorder or to the hypersensitivity reaction of which the cutaneous nodules are but one manifestation. There may be no systemic symptoms or varying degrees of malaise, chills, fever, sore throat, and cough. Cervical lymphadenopathy is common. Joint symptoms, present in about 75 per cent of patients, may precede, coincide with, or follow skin lesions, and they range from arthralgia to arthritis. Joint involvement has probably led to the idea that erythema nodosum is a manifestation of rheumatic fever, but follow-up studies indicate that there is only an occasional association.

Transient albuminuria and mild secondary anemia may be present. The total leukocyte count may be normal, decreased, or increased. The sedimentation rate is often elevated, and gamma globulin may be increased. Depending upon the underlying disease, skin tests with tuberculin, coccidioidin, and streptococcal antigens are positive. Chest roentgenograms have shown hilar lymphadenopathy and various types of pulmonary infiltration and pleural reaction. Some of these changes may have been due to underlying sarcoidosis or pulmonary infection. The electrocardiogram is usually normal.

Diagnosis. Clinical manifestations usually suffice for diagnosis. Biopsy is rarely necessary. The inflammatory lesions of adipose tissue that occur in *Weber-Christian disease* usually appear on the thighs, although other areas of subcutaneous or visceral fat may be involved. These lesions tend to break down and discharge an oily liquid, and involution is usually associated with a depressed scar. *Erythema induratum* affects the calves more than pretibial regions, and the lesions are more indolent, often ulcerate, and heal with scarring. The shape of the lesion of *migratory thrombophlebitis* often proclaims its association with a blood vessel. Nodules of *sarcoidosis, polyarteritis nodosa,* pancreatic fat necrosis, and *metastatic neoplasm* occasionally simulate erythema nodosum on the legs or other sites.

Treatment. The most important aspect of management is identification of the underlying cause. Symptomatic treatment for the erythema nodosum, such as bed rest, salicylates, or other analgesics, is usually sufficient. Corticotrophin or adrenal cortical steroids cause involution of the lesions, but these agents are indicated only in the most severe cases and should be used only when the underlying disease will not be worsened by them.

Prognosis. Erythema nodosum usually disappears in three or four weeks, but perhaps 10 per cent of the patients have continuing croplike appearance of new lesions or recurrences after free intervals.

Cronin, E.: Skin changes in sarcoidosis. Postgrad. Med. J., 46:507, 1970.
Kibel, M. A.: Erythema nodosum in children. S. Afr. Med. J., 44:873, 1970.
Kirby, J. F., Jr., and Kraft, G. H.: Oral contraceptives and erythema nodosum. Obstet. Gynecol., 40:409, 1972.
Sams, W. M., Jr., and Winkelmann, R. K.: The association of erythema nodosum with ulcerative colitis. South. Med. J., 61:676, 1968.
Sellers, T. F., Jr., Price, W. N., Jr., and Newberry, W. M., Jr.: An epidemic of erythema multiforme and erythema nodosum caused by histoplasmosis. Ann. Intern. Med., 62:1244, 1965.
Weinstein, L.: Erythema nodosum. D. M., 1–30, June 1969.

912. CONTACT DERMATITIS
(Dermatitis Venenata)

Clayton E. Wheeler, Jr.

Definition. Contact dermatitis is an inflammatory, frequently eczematous dermatitis that results from contact of the skin surface with a variety of substances. It is usually classified as (1) allergic contact dermatitis, (2) primary irritant dermatitis, or (3) contact photodermatitis.

ALLERGIC CONTACT DERMATITIS

Etiology. A specific sensitization process is required for the development of allergic contact dermatitis, which appears to be a form of delayed hypersensitivity.

Although almost anything that touches the skin of man may induce or elicit allergic contact dermatitis, several broad groups of substances are frequently involved. These include cosmetics, clothing, dyes, topical medicaments, industrial chemicals, plants, insecticides, detergents, cleansers, foodstuffs, costume jewelry, paints, varnishes, lacquers, rubber, and plastics.

Incidence and Prevalence. Allergic contact dermatitis, a common disorder, affects both sexes and all races. It is rare in infancy and unusual in early childhood, and the incidence declines in old age. Many occupations provide special exposure that results in contact dermatitis.

Pathology. Allergic contact dermatitis shows spongiosis (intracellular edema) and intraepithelial vesicle formation with many mononuclear cells in the vesicles. Edema and perivascular infiltrate with mononuclear cells appear in the dermis.

Pathogenesis. Four phases are recognized during sensitization: (1) In the *refractory phase* the allergen contacts the skin without initiating sensitization. This phase lasts usually a few days to a few weeks, but substances that have touched the skin for years may finally sensitize. Materials that sensitize a high percentage of contacts (strong sensitizers) tend to initiate the process rapidly; weak sensitizers may contact the skin over prolonged periods before sensitizing. Some patients may never become sensitive even after multiple exposures to strong sensitizers, some become sensitive quickly upon exposure to weak sensitizers, and some show weak reactions to strong agents or vice versa. Both sensitizer and person, as well as the degree and manner of exposure, are important in the net result. In addition, damaged skin appears to become sensitized more easily than normal skin. (2) The *period of incubation* is the time between onset of sensitization and clinical evidence of sensitivity. This interval may be as short as 5 days or as long as several weeks, but it is usually between 7 and 21 days. The refractory phase plus the period of incubation results in an interval of 10 days to several weeks between initial exposure and evidence of sensitivity. If allergic contact dermatitis appears within 5 days after exposure, prior sensitivity existed to the agent or a close chemical relative. (3) The *reaction time* is the interval between exposure to the allergen and development of dermatitis in a sensitized person. The usual interval is 24 to 48 hours, but it may be less than 12 hours or more than 90. An important point is that there is always a latent interval between exposure and clinical evidence of dermatitis. (4) The *period of persisting sensitivity* is usually months or years and may be a lifetime.

The hypersensitivity produced is specific for the allergen involved or for close chemical relatives (cross-sensitivity). There are many examples of cross-sensitization, but only one will be given here: Primary sensitization to benzocaine may result in sensitivity to procaine, paraphenylenediamine, para-aminobenzoic acid, and the sulfonamides. The phenomenon of cross-sensitization introduces a complicating factor in diagnosis and treatment since the patient now reacts to many substances, and removal of the original allergen may not eliminate the dermatitis because of unrecognized continued exposure to chemical relatives.

Allergic contact dermatitis is usually restricted to the point of contact of the allergen with the skin. If the patient is highly sensitive or if large amounts of antigen are used, the reaction may become generalized. In addition, sites of previous dermatitis may become active when minute amounts of allergen are applied to remote areas, a reaction lacking satisfactory explanation. The entire skin is usually sensitive, but there are infrequent instances of localized sensitivity, especially to heavy metals.

Clinical Manifestations.   The first symptom is usually itching, burning, or erythema; in mild cases the dermatitis may subside at this stage. With greater exposure or a higher degree of sensitivity, vesiculation and edema appear in a few hours, and these are followed by weeping and crusting. Provided that there is no further exposure, the skin becomes dry and scaly, loses its erythema, and finally heals, usually without scarring, in one to three weeks. More severe reactions may be associated with hemorrhagic vesicles, bullae, or small areas of denudation, but actual necrosis is unusual. Repeated exposures result in continuing or intermittent dermatitis that is likely to induce lichenification and hyperpigmentation or hypopigmentation. Secondary infection with staphylococci or streptococci, injudicious treatment, and excessive rubbing and scratching may complicate the picture.

Systemic symptoms are usually absent, but extensive dermatitis may result in chilliness, impaired temperature regulation, shocklike symptoms, leukocytosis, eosinophilia, and decreased serum protein.

Diagnosis.   The morphologic diagnosis and specific allergen may be evident at a glance, or the nature and cause of the dermatitis may elude the best efforts. The first requirement for diagnosis is an inflammatory or eczematous dermatitis that exhibits a location and configuration compatible with an external source. Given proper morphology, the diagnosis may be established and the offending allergen identified by history of exposure and proper time relationships. In more difficult cases helpful information may be gained by removal of the patient from the suspected source, which should result in healing, and then re-exposure, which should cause recurrence. Once the list of suspected allergens is cut to a reasonable number, skin tests may be helpful in identifying the specific agent.

Two types of skin test are commonly performed. In each, nonirritating concentrations of test substances are applied to the skin. In one method, useful with liquids or semisolids, the substance is applied to a small area on two or three successive days without covering. The other method involves application of test material and covering with an adhesive, which is usually left in place 48 hours. In both tests, persistent erythema or vesiculation confined to the test site constitutes positive results. False positive results occur with irritating concentrations, sensitivity to agents having nothing to do with the dermatitis, reaction to adhesive, contamination of test substances, and over-reactive skin. False negative results occur with inappropriate concentrations, poor contact with skin, or application of the wrong chemical. The complexity of skin testing makes experienced handling mandatory, and results must be interpreted in conjunction with clinical manifestations.

Disorders to be differentiated from allergic contact dermatitis are primary irritant dermatitis, contact photodermatitis, lichen simplex chronicus, superficial fungal infection, atopic eczema, seborrheic dermatitis, and infectious eczemoid dermatitis.

Treatment.   The most important part of management is elimination of exposure to the allergen. Otherwise, treatment consists of nonirritating symptomatic measures calculated to allow the skin to heal. Mild dermatitis may require no treatment. When erythema, edema, and vesiculation are present, open wet compresses of 1 per cent magnesium sulfate solution for two to three hours twice a day alternated with calamine liniment applied six to eight times a day are helpful. As the reaction subsides and the skin becomes dry, these measures are replaced by bland creams or ointments which may contain adrenal corticosteroids. Generalized eruptions may require colloidal baths. If secondary infection is present, antimicrobials may be incorporated in calamine liniment or bland ointment. Systemic antimicrobials may be utilized in the case of extensive or deep secondary infection. Antihistamines may allay itching and may provide some helpful sedative effect. Systemic adrenal steroids or corticotrophin should be used only for extensive and severe dermatitis and only if there are no contraindications to their use.

Desensitization is of little benefit (poison ivy included); indeed, institution of this procedure during active dermatitis may be harmful. Protective clothing and barrier creams are helpful in some instances.

Prognosis.   Cure can be attained if the allergen is identified and removed. If this cannot be accomplished, the dermatitis is likely to persist or recur, although it may decrease in intensity with time.

Prophylaxis.   Federal regulations guard against release of highly sensitizing food preservatives or colorings, drugs, clothing, cosmetics, and other items. Physicians in industry are continuously on guard against sensitizing agents, recommending the use of materials with low sensitizing capacity whenever possible, protective clothing, proper cleansing and ventilation, and other measures.

CONTACT PHOTODERMATITIS

Contact photodermatitis is an inflammatory reaction in skin from topical application of a photosensitizing compound and exposure to light. The dermatitis is localized to light-exposed sites such as the face, V of the neck, backs of the hands, forearms, and lower legs. Areas which are less involved or spared are the hairy scalp, upper eyelids, undersurface of the chin, and flexor surfaces of the arms. Two types of contact photodermatitis occur. Phototoxic dermatitis usually resembles an exaggerated sunburn and, under proper conditions, it occurs in a large percentage of the population upon first exposure. Photoallergic dermatitis is likely to be eczematous. It occurs in only a small percentage of exposed individuals, and it is a result of specific sensitization. Diagnosis of contact photodermatitis may be aided by photo-patch testing. Treatment is the same as for other forms of contact dermatitis with added avoidance of exposure to light.

PRIMARY IRRITANT DERMATITIS

Primary irritant dermatitis, the most common type of contact dermatitis, is due to exposure of the skin to irritating and cytotoxic chemical and physical agents. Immunologic mechanisms are not involved; sufficient exposure will result in dermatitis in all persons. The eczematous nature of the dermatitis and its location and configuration often provide morphologic resemblance to allergic contact dermatitis. Primary irritant dermatitis is less likely to be intermittent, it is not elicited by nonirritating materials, and the latent period between exposure and dermatitis is short or absent. Primary irritants can, of course, be sensitizers, and some patients present combinations of allergic and primary irritant dermatitis. Treatment is similar to that for allergic contact dermatitis, but it is usually easier to identify and eliminate the cause of primary irritant dermatitis. Complete avoidance of offending agents is often not necessary for cure since the skin may be able to tolerate irritants in small amounts.

Baer, R. L., Ramsey, D. L., and Biondi, E.: The most common contact allergens, 1968–1970. Arch. Dermatol., 108:74, 1973.

Epstein, E.: Shoe contact dermatitis. J.A.M.A., 109:1487, 1969.

Epstein, E., Rees, W. J., and Maibach, H. I.: Recent experience with routine patch test screening. Arch. Dermatol., 98:18, 1968.

Fisher, A. A.: Contact Dermatitis. Philadelphia, Lea & Febiger, 1973.

Ison, A. E., and Tucker, J. B.: Photosensitive dermatitis from soaps. N. Engl. J. Med., 278:81, 1968.

Odom, J. C., and O'Quinn, S. E.: Allergic contact dermatitis. A study of 100 consecutive cases. South. Med. J., 61:1378, 1968.

913. BEHÇET'S DISEASE

Clayton E. Wheeler, Jr.

Definition. Behçet's disease is a multisystemic disease characterized by ulcers (aphthae) of the mouth and genitalia, inflammatory eye disorders, joint manifestations, bowel disease, superficial and deep thrombophlebitis, and nervous system abnormalities.

Etiology. The cause is unknown; viral infection and autoimmune disease have been postulated. Autoantibodies against oral mucosa, esophageal cells, and polymorphonuclear leukocytes have been found. Vasculitis plays a prominent role in pathogenesis and symptomatology.

Incidence and Prevalence. The disease is most prevalent in the Middle East and usually affects young adult males. However, recent studies suggest that the disease is more common, more widely distributed geographically, and more frequent in women than was previously recognized and that many cases are currently missed or misdiagnosed.

Pathology. Biopsies of affected areas of skin, mucous membrane, eyes, and joints usually show perivasculitis and vasculitis of venules and arterioles with frequent thrombosis. A mixed lymphocytic and plasmacytic cellular infiltration is present. Vasculitis of medium-sized and large arteries and veins may lead to aneurysms and thrombosis.

Clinical Manifestations. Behçet's disease is characterized by variability in clinical manifestations, by chronicity, and by frequent recurrences which occur at irregular intervals, vary in duration and intensity, and involve several systems in a changing pattern. There is often a long interval between onset of the disease and manifestations in different organs.

Oral lesions may be the initial manifestation, and they occur in almost all cases at some time during the disease. They may resemble canker sores or may be larger and deeper. Genital changes consist of various pyodermas, herpes-like lesions, and ulcers of the scrotum, vulva, urethra, and vagina. Epididymitis is found occasionally. An outstanding and almost constant feature is pyoderma, which includes pustules, impetigo, folliculitis, furuncles, acne-like lesions, cellulitis, and ulcers. Nodose lesions that resemble erythema nodosum may appear on the legs or elsewhere. Subungual, flame-shaped hemorrhages have been reported. A peculiar feature is the development of papules and pustules after pricking with a sterile needle or injection of sterile saline.

Eye involvement is the most frequent cause of disability; the most common lesions are iridocyclitis and uveitis with hypopyon. Chronic, recurring inflammation often leads to partial or complete loss of vision. This may begin unilaterally, but in time both eyes are affected. Other ocular changes are conjunctivitis, keratitis, retinitis, choroiditis, optic neuritis, optic atrophy, and retinal vessel occlusions.

Most patients experience arthralgias and some develop polyarthritis. Despite years of synovitis, there is usually no joint space narrowing and no osseous erosion. Thrombophlebitis is found in a quarter or more of the cases. This may be migratory, superficial thrombophlebitis or deep vein thrombophlebitis. There have been several reports of superior or inferior (or both) vena caval thrombosis. Aneurysms of large arteries such as the aorta and popliteal may occur. Neurologic complications are being recognized with increasing frequency; they include multiple sclerosis-like disorders, cranial nerve palsies, brainstem syndromes, meningomyelitis, meningoencephalitis, encephalopathies, seizures, and confusional states. Pulmonary and gastrointestinal symptoms develop occasionally. It may be that some patients develop colitis indistinguishable from chronic ulcerative colitis, and acute pancreatitis has been reported.

Fever and malaise often accompany exacerbations and recurrences of the disease, and leukocytosis, elevated sedimentation rate, and nondiagnostic serum protein abnormalities are common (elevation of alpha$_2$ globulin, gamma globulin, IgA, IgG, and IgM). Antinuclear factor has been negative, and complement levels have been normal. Anticytoplasmic antibodies to cadaver esophagus have been demonstrated by indirect immunofluorescent techniques.

Diagnosis. Because of the variability in clinical manifestations, the long delay in appearance of some of the symptoms, and the lack of specific laboratory tests, diagnosis is difficult and often made late. Some insist upon the clinical triad of uveitis, oral aphthae, and genital ulcers, but any two of these with skin lesions, thrombophlebitis, nervous system involvement, ulcerative colitis, or joint disease should bring Behçet's disease into consideration.

Treatment. Topical and systemic corticosteroids may control some of the inflammatory signs and symptoms, but they probably influence the basic course of the disease very little. Systemic antimicrobials are indicated for specific infectious complications. Immunosuppressives (cyclophosphamide, azathioprine, chlorambucil, methotrexate) and fibrinolytics (phenformin, ethyloestrenol) have been used with variable results. Fresh blood transfusions have caused apparent benefit in a few patients.

Prognosis. Prognosis is unpredictable. Spontaneous cures occur, or recurrences may continue relentlessly until blindness results. Central nervous system complications are serious, and most deaths occur in this group. Large vessel disease (thrombosis, emboli, aneurysms) is also of grave significance.

Chajek, T., and Farinaru, M.: Behçet's disease with decreased fibrinolysis and superior vena caval occlusion. Br. Med. J., 1:782, 1973.

Enoch, B. A., et al.: Major vascular complications in Behçet's syndrome. Postgrad. Med. J., 44:453, 1968.

Kansu, E., et al.: Behçet's syndrome with obstruction of the venae cavae. Quart. J. Med., 41:162, 1972.

Mamo, J. G., and Azzam, S. A.: Treatment of Behçet's disease with chlorambucil. Arch. Ophthalmol., 84:446, 1970.

O'Duffy, J. D., and Deodhar, S.: Behçet's disease. Report of 10 cases, 3 with new manifestations. Ann. Intern. Med., 75:561, 1971.

914. PEMPHIGUS

Clayton E. Wheeler, Jr.

Definition. Pemphigus vulgaris is an uncommon disease characterized by bullae and erosions on the skin and mucous membranes, acantholysis, intercellular antiepithelial antibodies, chemical alterations in the blood, and high mortality rate.

Etiology. The cause remains unknown despite extensive search for toxic, viral, metabolic, immunologic, and enzymatic factors.

Incidence and Prevalence. The disease affects either sex and all races; there is a higher incidence among Jews. It usually begins between the ages of 40 and 60; onset earlier in life is unusual.

Pathogenesis. Although the mechanism of bulla formation is unknown, the characteristic histologic feature of acantholysis indicates that defective intercellular attachment is involved. In acantholysis, the cells of the malpighian layer lose their prickles, become separated from each other, and lie singly or in clumps in blister fluid. On electron microscopy tonofilaments retract from their desmosomal attachments and clump in the cytoplasm of the cell. The role of recently demonstrated intercellular antiepithelial autoantibodies in acantholysis is not clear.

Defective intercellular attachment accounts for the *Nikolsky sign*, characteristic of all forms of pemphigus: Firm pressure with a finger on the top of an intact blister results in extension at the edge, or application of a steady shearing force to the skin with a tongue depressor causes the top layers of the epidermis to slide over underlying cells. Epidermal separation demonstrated by this sign takes place at the site of most prominent acantholysis.

Blister fluid contains water, electrolytes, and protein. The composition resembles serum, although total protein is usually lower and albumin higher. Loss of these substances into bullae and from denuded areas explains most of the changes in the blood, which parallel the duration and severity of the disorder. Total serum protein may fall as low as 3.6 grams and there may be a correspondingly low level of albumin. Alpha$_1$ and alpha$_2$ globulins are increased. Gamma globulin and fibrinogen are usually increased. Sodium, chloride, and calcium are decreased and potassium is normal or increased. Plasma and interstitial fluid volume are increased. Anemia is common and may be due to inanition, serum loss, and infection. Anemia and increased globulin, especially fibrinogen, probably account for the increased sedimentation rate. The leukocyte count is usually elevated with an increase of immature forms. Cutaneous inflammation and infection are important causes of leukocytosis. Eosinophilia may be present.

Pathology. Characteristic changes develop in the skin and orificial mucosa. Intercellular edema in the lower malpighian layer is followed by loss of intercellular bridges, acantholysis, and cleft formation. An intraepithelial bulla is formed just above the basal layer. Healing may result in normal-appearing epidermis or there may be hyperkeratosis, acanthosis, and papillomatosis. Simple or granulomatous inflammation is present in the dermis, and tissue eosinophilia is often prominent.

There are no specific changes in internal organs. Examination of persons dying early in the course of pemphigus may show surprisingly little. Common but variable findings are pulmonary congestion and edema, atelectasis, bronchopneumonia, hydropericardium, focal myocarditis, and brown atrophy. Myeloid hyperplasia of the bone marrow and increased numbers of normoblasts are common. Adrenal changes have included depletion of lipoid, degeneration, and inflammation followed by scar and regeneration, hemorrhage, necrosis, and vein thrombosis. Nonspecific degeneration may involve areas of brain, cord, or ganglia.

Clinical Manifestations. Flaccid or tense bullae are characteristic. These lesions often spread at the edges and show little tendency to heal, and they rupture easily. Localized involvement may be present for months or the disease may begin with a generalized eruption. Skin lesions are randomly distributed, but there is a predilection for areas of friction or pressure. Frequently affected sites are the scalp, axillae, groin, elbows, knees, back, inframammary area, umbilicus, hands, feet, nose, and eyelids. Bullae arise on normal-appearing skin or at previously involved sites. Coalescence and extension often result in large denuded areas. The contents of bullae may be serous, seropurulent, or hemorrhagic, and crusting often develops. Healing takes place with little or no scarring. Secondary infection is a common complication, and hyperpigmentation, hypopigmentation, and milium formation are frequent sequelae. Itching is usually mild or absent. Denudation often causes burning or pain. The Nikolsky sign is positive over intact bullae and sometimes can be elicited over normal-appearing skin.

The oral mucosa is involved in almost all patients with pemphigus vulgaris. In half to two thirds of the cases mouth lesions precede skin lesions by weeks to a year or more. The thin-walled bullae rupture early, leaving erosions which often assume figured patterns. The gums, sides of the tongue, and buccal mucosa along the bite line are preferential sites. The lips frequently become fissured, crusted, or warty. Pain, salivation, and bleeding may make eating and drinking difficult. Bullae, erosions, and inflammation commonly involve the mucosa of the pharynx, larynx, nose, conjunctiva, genitalia, and anus.

Extensive skin and mucous membrane involvement, loss of fluid, electrolytes, and protein, inability to eat and drink, and secondary cutaneous and systemic infection contribute to weakness, weight loss, toxemia, and the severely ill appearance of these patients.

Other Types of Pemphigus. Other types are pemphigus

vegetans, pemphigus foliaceus, pemphigus erythematosus, and fogo selvagem. *Pemphigus vegetans* is less severe than pemphigus vulgaris, of which it is probably a variant, and is characterized by warty, vegetating, pustular, and hyperkeratotic lesions at the axillae, groin, anogenital area, interdigital spaces, and lips. *Pemphigus foliaceus* is characterized by incompletely formed bullae, more crusting and scaling, frequent absence of mucous membrane involvement, milder but longer course, lower mortality rate, more spontaneous cures, and higher position of the bullae in the epidermis. It usually begins on the face or upper trunk and slowly becomes generalized, at which time it resembles exfoliative dermatitis. *Pemphigus erythematosus* may be an abortive form of pemphigus foliaceus or pemphigus vulgaris. Crusting and erythema about the face, mid upper back and chest produce a superficial resemblance to seborrheic dermatitis and lupus erythematosus. *Fogo selvagem* (Brazilian wildfire) resembles pemphigus foliaceus except for its endemicity in central South America and its frequent onset at an early age.

Diagnosis. The clinical diagnosis should be confirmed by biopsy and smears of skin and mucosal lesions. Multiple sampling of lesions may be necessary to show acantholysis. Intercellular antiepithelial autoantibodies can be demonstrated in skin lesions and serum by immunofluorescence. The most difficult differential diagnosis is that of *pemphigoid,* a chronic bullous disease of unknown cause in which the bullae are usually smaller, more tense, rupture less easily, and often show grouping or arise on an inflamed base. Mouth involvement is less severe and less frequent; systemic symptoms are less intense, and the mortality rate is lower. Bullae are subepidermal, acantholysis is absent, and autoantibodies are found in the basal membrane area. Bullous *erythema multiforme* shows more polymorphism and configuration, the onset is acute, fever is often high, the disease is self-limited, and acantholysis is absent. Bullous *drug eruption* follows the pattern of bullous erythema multiforme. Benign *mucous membrane pemphigoid* is characterized by chronic bullous and erosive lesions of the mucous membranes, especially of the eye, in which scarring is prominent. *Contact dermatitis* can usually be differentiated by localization and configuration of lesions, lack of systemic symptoms, infrequent mucosal involvement, and self-limited course. In *familial benign chronic pemphigus,* lesions are usually limited to the neck, axillae, groin, and small areas of the trunk. Mucous membrane involvement and systemic symptoms are absent, and biopsy is usually characteristic. *Pemphigus neonatorum* is a bullous form of impetigo which can be differentiated by age, cultures, and response to appropriate antimicrobials. *Exfoliative dermatitis* lacks bulla formation and mucosal involvement, and biopsy shows chronic dermatitis without acantholysis.

Treatment. Adrenal corticosteroids and corticotrophin were the first medications shown to be truly effective in treatment of pemphigus. These agents control but do not cure the disease. The dose depends upon clinical and serologic response (serum antibody levels to epithelial intercellular substance) and varies from patient to patient. The objective is to bring the disease under control as rapidly as possible and then to decrease the dose gradually until a maintenance level is attained. On some occasions remissions occur and maintenance medication can be stopped, but most patients require continued treatment. An initial dose of 120 to 300 mg per day of prednisone usually suffices to stop new lesions and start healing of old lesions in a week or two. After complete healing of skin and mucous membrane the amount of drug is cautiously reduced until the maintenance level is reached; this is usually between 15 and 30 mg per day of prednisone or its equivalent. The maintenance dose can often be switched to an every-other-day schedule. Some patients require higher doses than outlined above, and a rare patient seems to be unresponsive. Measures must be taken to combat complications of corticosteroid administration such as salt and water retention, potassium depletion, osteoporosis, and peptic ulcer.

Psychotic disturbances caused by pemphigus or corticosteroids may require tranquilizers or sedatives. Transfusions and replacement of serum proteins and electrolytes are often necessary. Cutaneous and internal infections (bacteremia, bronchopneumonia, and urinary tract infections) must be combated with appropriate topical and systemic antimicrobials. Good nursing care, encouragement to eat and drink, soothing mouthwashes, and a cheerful environment are important. Colloidal or potassium permanganate baths and topical calamine liniment add to the patient's comfort.

In addition to corticosteroids, methotrexate, cyclophosphamide, azathioprine and gold sodium thiomalate also influence the course of pemphigus. The exact role of these agents in the treatment of pemphigus has not been established. Moderate and severe cases of pemphigus are best brought under control with corticosteroids. Immunosuppressives may then be used to reduce the dosage of corticosteroids or replace them altogether as the maintenance medication. Mild, early cases of pemphigus may be controlled with the agents listed above without initial administration of corticosteroids. The most recent trend appears to favor azathioprine or gold sodium thiomalate if these agents are to be used.

Prognosis. The mortality rate of untreated pemphigus vulgaris confirmed by biopsy is greater than 90 per cent. Average duration of life after onset is fourteen months, with a range of one month to six or seven years and, rarely, longer. In addition, the uncomfortable state of the patients during much of their course adds greatly to the gloomy picture. Patients die of toxemia, cachexia, shock from protein and electrolyte abnormalities, pulmonary edema, bronchopneumonia, sepsis, or adrenal insufficiency.

Current therapy has cut the mortality rate approximately in half. This is only part of the story, because control of the disease allows most patients to lead comfortable and useful lives. Complications of steroid therapy, such as perforated peptic ulcer, congestive heart failure, suicide, uncontrollable infection, and thromboembolic phenomena, must be added to the list of causes of death, but judicious management keeps these to a minimum.

Ebringer, A., and Mackay, I. R.: Pemphigus vulgaris successfully treated with cyclophosphamide. Ann. Intern. Med., 71:125, 1969.

Lever, W. F.: Pemphigus and Pemphigoid. Springfield, Ill., Charles C Thomas, 1965.

Lever, W. F., and Goldberg, H. S.: Treatment of pemphigus vulgaris with methotrexate. Arch. Dermatol., 100:70, 1969.

Peck, S. M., Osserman, K. E., Weiner, L. B., Lefkovitz, A., and Osserman, R. S.: Studies in bullous diseases. Immunofluorescent tests. N. Engl. J. Med., 279:951, 1968.

Penneys, N. S., et al.: Gold sodium thiomalate treatment of pemphigus. Arch. Dermatol., 108:56, 1973.

Roenigk, H. H., Jr., and Deodhar, S.: Pemphigus treatment with azathioprine. Arch. Dermatol., 107:353, 1973.

915. ACANTHOSIS NIGRICANS

Clayton E. Wheeler, Jr.

Definition. Acanthosis nigricans is an uncommon dermatosis characterized by hyperpigmentation and epidermal hypertrophy. Two forms are recognized: (1) malignant or adult, associated with internal cancer, and (2) benign or juvenile, which may be related to developmental, endocrine, or metabolic abnormalities. This terminology is illogical, however, because the dermatosis itself is never malignant and because the adult type may be seen in children and the juvenile form in adults.

Etiology. By definition, malignant acanthosis nigricans is always associated with internal malignancy; adenocarcinoma is the predominant type of cancer, although epidermoid carcinoma, osteogenic sarcoma, and malignant lymphoma have been reported. Almost 70 per cent of the associated malignancies arise in the stomach and more than 90 per cent in the abdomen and pelvis. Sites of origin are the stomach, colon, esophagus, liver, gallbladder, pancreas, ovary, uterus, chorion, kidney, lung, bronchus, mediastinum, breast, and thyroid. Skin changes appear before clinical evidence of carcinoma in 20 per cent; the two appear simultaneously in 60 per cent; and acanthosis follows the diagnosis of malignancy in 20 per cent. Progression of the dermatosis parallels the course of the carcinoma. In a few instances acanthosis has regressed after x-ray or surgical treatment of cancer, only to recur with reactivation of the malignancy.

Benign acanthosis nigricans may be associated with a large number of developmental, metabolic, or endocrine abnormalities that seem to have little in common in the light of present knowledge. These include diabetes mellitus, pituitary tumors, adrenal hyperplasia, hypogonadism, acromegaly, gigantism, congenital total lipodystrophy, hypothyroidism, Addison's disease, Stein-Leventhal syndrome, von Recklinghausen's neurofibromatosis, arachnodactyly, achondroplasia, epilepsy, mental retardation, and degenerative disease of the cord. Familial incidence and occurrence in two and three generations suggest that hereditary factors are important. Lupoid hepatitis and administration of nicotinic acid, stilbestrol, and corticosteroids have been associated with skin lesions resembling acanthosis nigricans.

Incidence and Prevalence. The disorder is worldwide, affects all races, and occurs in either sex. The peak incidence of malignant acanthosis nigricans is between the ages of 40 and 60, but it occurs at all ages. Benign acanthosis nigricans usually appears between the ages of 10 and 20, but the disorder may be present at birth, and it occurs in early childhood and middle age. Intensification and spread commonly occur at puberty if the disorder has existed previously.

Pathology. Characteristic changes are limited to the epidermis, where there are hyperkeratosis, acanthosis (increased thickness of the prickle cell layer), and papillomatosis. Melanin is increased in the basal layer. Benign and malignant forms do not differ histologically, and cancer is not found in the skin in the malignant type.

Pathogenesis. The pathogenesis of acanthosis nigricans is unknown. In the malignant type, theories include humoral or biochemical effects of the cancer, peculiarities of the host triggered by carcinoma, or a common cause for acanthosis and carcinoma. Benign acanthosis nigricans may be related to disturbances of germ plasm or endocrine function.

Clinical Manifestations. Skin changes in malignant acanthosis nigricans are bilateral and symmetrical and exhibit a predilection for flexural and intertriginous areas. The axillae, groin, genital region, and neck are the most common sites of involvement; other areas in approximate order of frequency are face, inner thighs, flexor surfaces of elbows and knees, umbilicus, perianal areas, and eyelids. The palms and soles occasionally become hyperkeratotic, the backs of the fingers are sometimes involved, and in extreme and rare instances the disorder becomes generalized. Involved skin is usually dark brown or black, although light brown and yellow may be seen. The epidermis becomes thickened, and normal skin lines are exaggerated. A soft, velvety, papillomatous appearance develops, and frequently pedunculated growths or warty lesions are scattered over the area. The disorder is distinctly localized, with involved regions blending imperceptibly into normal skin. In some cases there may be loss of scalp or eyebrow hair, and dystrophy of nails may occur. The lips, mouth, tongue, epiglottis, and vagina may be affected. Involved mucous membrane becomes thickened, granular, and warty.

Benign acanthosis nigricans shows the same changes, but the degree and extent are often less, and mucous membrane involvement is unlikely. The cutaneous lesions of both forms are asymptomatic. Systemic symptoms depend upon associated internal disease.

Diagnosis. The diagnosis is based on clinical appearance, histologic findings, and associated internal disease.

Addison's disease and *hemochromatosis* cause more generalized hyperpigmentation, and involved sites lack epidermal hypertrophy, papillomatosis, and warty changes. *Arsenical hyperpigmentation* is generalized, and arsenical keratoses are small and hard and uncommonly affect flexural or intertriginous sites. *Ichthyosis hystrix* shows less predilection for flexural and intertriginous areas, there is more hyperkeratosis, and the palms and soles are more often involved. Obese persons, especially brunets, sometimes develop hyperpigmentation, acanthosis, and papillomatosis of the axillae, groin, and neck. These alterations have been called pseudo-acanthosis nigricans, but they probably represent a form of benign acanthosis nigricans.

Treatment. The most important aspect of management is determination of whether internal malignancy is present. If it is, prompt treatment should be instituted. In the benign type, associated developmental or endocrine disorders may require treatment. There is no effective therapy for the dermatosis, although temporary amelioration of cutaneous changes may occur after irradiation or surgical treatment of carcinoma. Correction of endocrine abnormalities appears to have little or no influence on the skin changes.

Prognosis. The outlook for the patient with acanthosis nigricans and malignancy is gloomy. The associated carcinoma is highly malignant, and average survival after its discovery is one year. Seldom do persons live longer than two years after the skin lesions appear, and progressive skin changes are a bad omen. Few, if any, have been cured, but earlier discovery and improved methods of treatment may alter the picture. The prognosis in benign acanthosis nigricans is good and depends upon associated abnormalities and their amenability to treatment.

The dermatosis tends to progress when associated with malignancy. Skin lesions in the benign form are likely to reach a peak and remain static or regress slowly.

Brown, J., and Winkelmann, R. K.: Acanthosis nigricans: A study of 90 cases. Medicine, 47:33, 1968.
Curth, H. O., Hilberg, A. W., and Machachek, G. F.: The site and histology of the cancer associated with malignant acanthosis nigricans. Cancer, 15:364, 1962.
Garrott, T. C.: Malignant acanthosis nigricans associated with osteogenic sarcoma. Arch. Dermatol., 106:384, 1972.
Hollingsworth, D. R., and Amatruda, T. T., Jr.: Acanthosis nigricans and obesity. Arch. Intern. Med., 124:481, 1969.
Reed, W. B., Dexter, R., Corley, C., and Fish, C.: Congenital lipodystrophic diabetes with acanthosis nigricans. Arch. Dermatol., 91:326, 1965.

916. MAST CELL DISEASE
(Mastocytosis)
Clayton E. Wheeler, Jr.

Mast cell disease will be discussed under two divisions: (1) urticaria pigmentosa of childhood and (2) systemic mastocytosis.

URTICARIA PIGMENTOSA OF CHILDHOOD

Definition. This chronic disease usually begins in early childhood and disappears partially or completely by adolescence. Characteristic skin lesions are single or multiple pigmented macules or nodules that urticate on rubbing and contain large numbers of mast cells.

Incidence. Although uncommon, the disorder is seen yearly in most dermatologic and pediatric practices. Light-skinned persons are affected most often, and it is slightly more common in males. The disorder has been reported in a parent and child in several families and in both members of monozygotic twins. More than 10 per cent of cases are present at birth; over half develop by six months; and the majority appear before puberty. Onset after puberty raises the question of systemic mastocytosis.

Etiology. The probable origin of mast cells from connective tissue cells of histiocytic type suggests that the disorder is one of the reticuloendothelioses. Urticaria pigmentosa may be a systemic disorder, but its benign course appears to separate it from systemic mastocytosis.

Pathogenesis. Human mast cells contain histamine, heparin, and possibly hyaluronic acid. The function of these cells is incompletely understood, but they may be important in connective tissue formation, repair, or maintenance. Local release of histamine on rubbing results in capillary dilatation and edema with erythema and wheal formation, whereas its absorption into the general circulation causes flushing, a shocklike state, and gastrointestinal disturbance. Pigmentation of cutaneous lesions is due to increased melanin production, which presumably results from repeated inflammatory episodes.

Pathology. The characteristic finding is accumulation of mast cells in the dermis. The number of cells determines the macular or nodular nature of the lesion. Mast cells are large and contain round or oval nuclei. The cytoplasm contains large basophilic granules that stain metachromatically and can be demonstrated by fixation with 10 per cent formalin or absolute alcohol followed by staining with Giemsa, methylene blue, or toluidine blue. Lesions that have been rubbed may show edema, eosinophilia, and degranulation of mast cells. Melanin is increased in the basal layer and dermal chromatophores.

Clinical Manifestations. One, few, or innumerable lesions may be present. Frequently they appear in crops for weeks before the final extent of the disease is reached. The trunk is the site of predilection, but the neck, face, scalp, extremities, palms, soles, and oral mucosa may be involved. Although macular eruptions predominate, nodular and plaquelike forms are common. Superimposed bullae or vesicles may occur in young children. Lesions are round, oval, or irregular and vary from a few millimeters to several centimeters. They are discrete except in extensive cases. The color varies from yellow to brown or sepia.

A significant number of patients display symptoms of histamine release into the general circulation. These include episodic bright red flushing, itching, hypotension, weakness, dizziness, headache, dermographism, nausea, vomiting, and diarrhea.

Although the extent of mast cell infiltration has been incompletely studied, the occasional finding of lymphadenopathy, splenomegaly, increased mast cells in bone marrow, and cystic or proliferative bone lesions suggests that urticaria pigmentosa is a systemic disease. Rarely, skin is diffusely infiltrated with mast cells, with or without bulla formation and cobblestoning. This type of patient may develop significant bleeding tendencies, and systemic involvement is likely.

Diagnosis. The diagnosis can usually be made when pigmented lesions exhibit erythema and edema upon rubbing (*Darier's sign*). This sign is absent in some cases, especially when previous stroking has exhausted the supply of histamine. Biopsy confirms the diagnosis. Increased eosinophil content of the blood is sometimes found, and increased amounts of histamine may be present in the urine.

Pigmented nevi, nevoxanthoendothelioma, xanthoma, myoblastoma, lymphoma, insect bites, and Letterer-Siwe disease can usually be differentiated by histologic findings and the absence of Darier's sign.

Treatment. Treatment is relatively ineffective. Antihistamines, including cyproheptadine, may attenuate some of the symptoms. Trauma should be avoided. Aspirin and codeine degranulate mast cells and may aggravate symptoms. Solitary lesions may be excised. Once systemic mastocytosis is excluded, watchful waiting and reassurance of the parents are essential features of management.

Prognosis. Aside from cosmetic considerations and uncomfortable effects of histamine release, the disease is generally benign. Lesions disappear completely by adolescence in the majority of patients; in the remainder pigmented macules persist without activity. Very rarely, patients develop serious complications such as infected bullae, peptic ulcer, and bleeding tendencies.

SYSTEMIC MASTOCYTOSIS

Systemic mastocytosis, a rare, recently recognized disease, is being reported with increasing frequency. It affects both males and females and usually begins in adult life. The cause is unknown. The clinical manifestations and course may resemble those of lymphoma or leukemia, and it seems likely that the disorder should be classified with the reticuloendothelioses.

Skin or mucous membrane lesions may resemble childhood urticaria pigmentosa, but significant differences that indicate systemic mastocytoses are (1) onset after puberty, (2) multiple, small, confluent macules with persistent telangiectasia, (3) papules and nodules resembling leukemia cutis, (4) chronic lichenified dermatitis, (5) generalized infiltration of skin with a "scotch-grain" appearance, (6) less pigmentation, (7) less tendency to redden and urticate on stroking, (8) extensive involvement of oral, nasal, or rectal mucosa, and (9) progressive cutaneous change.

Histamine release into the general circulation is less likely than in childhood urticaria pigmentosa, yet patients may have flushing, shocklike episodes, and increased histamine in the urine. Diarrhea is often a prominent feature, and peptic ulcer occasionally develops.

Persistent or progressive cutaneous eruption may be the only evidence of the disease, although asymptomatic bone changes can be demonstrated by roentgenographic examination in many cases. These changes consist of solitary or multiple, irregular or round lytic lesions or local or general new bone formation, which causes thickening of the cortex and trabeculae and narrowing of marrow spaces. In more severe instances, lymphadenopathy, splenomegaly, and hepatomegaly are prominent early manifestations, and bone marrow aspiration shows abnormal accumulations of mast cells. The disorder may remain static at this point or may progress with weakness, weight loss, cachexia, nausea, vomiting, diarrhea, and malaise. In these patients anemia, leukopenia, thrombocytopenia, and leukemoid features develop, presumably from the proliferative effect of mast cells in bone marrow. Other blood abnormalities are eosinophilia, lymphocytosis, and monocytosis. Liver function may be impaired by mast cell invasion and associated periportal fibrosis. A malabsorption syndrome may develop. Bleeding tendencies are usually due to combinations of thrombocytopenia and prothrombin deficiency, but there may be a circulating heparin-like substance. Tissue mast cell leukemia, somewhat like other leukemias, is found on rare occasions. Abnormal numbers of mast cells are found at autopsy in almost all tissues. In mild forms, mast cells appear normal, but in severe forms, especially leukemia, anaplasia indicates malignant transformation.

Prognosis varies with the form of the disorder. Disease confined to skin and bone is compatible with long life and little morbidity, but there is always the threat of extension of the morbid process. Extensive reticuloendothelial involvement results in death in a few months to several years. Patients die from pancytopenia, infection, hemorrhage, cachexia, gastroenteritis, perforated peptic ulcer, and leukemia. Therapy is palliative and symptomatic and includes transfusions, antimicrobials, antihistamines, adrenal steroids, corticotrophin, roentgen irradiation, and nitrogen mustard.

Barer, M., Peterson, L. F. A., Dahlin, D. C., Winkelmann, R. K., and Stewart, J. R.: Mastocytosis with osseous lesions resembling metastatic malignant lesions in bone. J. Bone Joint Surg. (Am.), 50:142, 1968.
Burgoon, C. F., Graham, J. H., and McCaffree, D. L.: Mast cell disease. Arch. Dermatol., 98:590, 1968.
Caplan, R. M.: The natural course of urticaria pigmentosa. Arch. Dermatol., 87:146, 1963.
Clement, A. C., Fishbone, G., Levine, R. J., James, A. E., and Janower, M.: Gastrointestinal lesions in mastocytosis. Am. J. Roentgenol. Radium Ther. Nucl. Med., 103:405, 1968.
Sagher, F., and Even-Paz, Z.: Mastocytosis and the Mast Cell. Chicago, Year Book Publishers, Inc., 1967.
Simone, T. J., and Hayes, W. T.: Bullous urticaria pigmentosa with bleeding. J. Pediatr., 78:160, 1971.

917. LETHAL CUTANEOUS AND GASTROINTESTINAL ARTERIOLAR THROMBOSIS (Degos' Disease)

Clayton E. Wheeler, Jr.

Lethal cutaneous and gastrointestinal arteriolar thrombosis is a progressive, often fatal disease in which characteristic cutaneous, gastrointestinal, and central nervous system lesions result from spotty occlusive vascular disease. The cause is unknown. Most cases of this uncommon disorder occur in young adult males. Cutaneous manifestations usually precede gastrointestinal or nervous system symptoms by weeks or months, although the reverse sequence may occur. Indolent, slowly progressive, rose-colored papules 2 to 5 mm in size appear on the trunk or proximal extremities and occasionally elsewhere. In a few days or weeks the papules develop porcelain-like central umbilication covered by white scale and surrounded by a slightly elevated violaceous telangiectatic border. In time the entire lesion becomes white, depressed, and atrophic. There are usually fewer than 100 lesions, and they appear in crops, so that several stages of development are represented at any one time.

Central nervous system symptoms may be mild, localized, evanescent, and migratory in the initial phases, but eventually they become severe, extensive, and permanent. Numbness, weakness, headache, slurred speech, aphasias, seizures, hemiparesis, paraplegia, optic atrophy, and cranial nerve palsies may be found. To date, gastrointestinal involvement has not been reported in patients with prominent central nervous system disease.

Initial gastrointestinal symptoms may be mild and vague and may be associated with asthenia and weight loss, or the onset may be abrupt with signs indicating perforation, ileus, and peritonitis. Laparotomy reveals multiple, oval, white, subserosal patches of atrophy varying from pinpoint to 2 cm in size and irregularly distributed in stomach, ileum, jejunum, and colon. Perforation and peritonitis frequently occur, and there may be localized areas of gangrene.

The basic pathologic abnormality is an obliterative endothelial reaction affecting small arteries and arterioles and corresponding veins. Ischemic infarcts, necrobiosis, or atrophy occurs at involved sites in all layers of the skin and intestinal tract, and similar lesions are found in the central nervous system. The mouth, esophagus, rectum, anus, liver, pancreas, genitalia, bladder, kidney, lung, pleura, heart, retina, choroid, sclera, and conjunctiva have also been involved. Disease of smaller vessels, with emphasis on endothelial reaction, appears to distinguish the disorder from Buerger's disease and periarteritis nodosa.

In 45 reported cases, 23 patients have died (20 with bowel and 3 with cerebral disease), and 7 are alive but have systemic disease. Skin lesions have been present for over three years in 13 of the 15 who have only skin disease. In fatal cases the interval between onset and death has usually been less than one year.

Treatment with antimicrobials, adrenal corticosteroids, anticoagulants, and methotrexate is ineffectual. Surgical intervention in persons with gastrointestinal symptoms is of temporary or no benefit because of the multiplicity and recurrence of lesions. Patients succumb to either gastrointestinal or nervous system involvement.

Howard, R. O., Klaus, S. N., Slavin, R. C., and Fenton, R.: Malignant atrophic papulosis (Degos' syndrome). Arch. Ophthalmol., 79:262, 1968.

Jensen, N. E.: Malignant atrophic papulosis (Degos' syndrome). Br. J. Dermatol., 57:394, 1972.

Lomholt, G., Hjorth, N., and Fischermann, K.: Lethal peritonitis from Degos' disease (malign and atrophic papulosis). Acta Chir. Scand., 134:495, 1968.

Winkelmann, R. K., Howard, F. M., Jr., Perry, H. O., and Miller, R. H.: Malignant papulosis of skin and cerebrum. Arch. Dermatol., 87:54, 1963.

918. ANGIOKERATOMA CORPORIS DIFFUSUM (Fabry's Disease)

Clayton E. Wheeler, Jr.

Definition. Fabry's disease is an inherited disorder of glycolipid metabolism characterized by telangiectatic skin lesions, hypohidrosis, corneal opacities, acral pain and paresthesias, febrile episodes, gastrointestinal symptoms, renal failure, cardiovascular disease, and central nervous system disturbances.

Etiology. An X-linked, incompletely recessive error in glycolipid metabolism is manifested by a deficiency of ceramide trihexosidase with accumulation of ceramide trihexoside and other neutral glycolipids. Trihexosidase activity is essentially absent from intestinal mucosa and leukocytes of hemizygotic males and is less than normal in heterozygotic females.

Prevalence. The disease is uncommon. Males exhibit the full-blown disorder. Females are asymptomatic carriers or develop mild forms of the disease.

Pathology. A glycolipid that is doubly refractile, periodic acid–Schiff positive, and has an affinity for Sudan black B and other histochemical properties is deposited in endothelial cells and smooth muscle of blood vessels, arrectores pilorum muscles, and heart muscles. Similar deposits are found in cells of the renal glomeruli, distal convoluted tubules, loop of Henle, urinary sediment, cornea, sweat glands, central nervous system, spleen, liver, lymph nodes, and bone marrow. On electron microscopy lipid inclusions show a concentrically arranged, lamellar structure. Skin biopsies may show glycolipid in vessels or appendages at sites distant from telangiectases. Telangiectases are dilated vessels in the upper dermis or blood-filled spaces enclosed by epidermis. Cultured skin fibroblasts accumulate ceramide trihexoside and stain metachromatically with toluidine blue.

Clinical Manifestations. Cutaneous lesions usually appear in childhood or around puberty and consist of telangiectatic spots varying in size from barely visible to several millimeters. They are bright red to blue-black, and some are covered with slight scale. They are nonpulsatile lesions that may be partially blanched on diascopy. Telangiectases tend to cluster about the umbilicus, glans penis, scrotum, buttocks, hips, and thighs; but they occur anywhere, including the oral mucosa. A few lesions are found initially, but as the disease progresses they may appear in profusion. Skin lesions may be absent. Sweating is often decreased. Hair may be scanty; many patients shave infrequently. Paresthesias of the hands and feet and episodes of very severe burning pain in the extremities, at times accompanied by fever, may be early symptoms that may be precipitated by exposure to heat or cold or by physical exertion. Attacks of nausea, diarrhea, and abdominal pain are common. A Raynaud-like phenomenon and pain in the muscles and joints may also occur. Patients may complain of dizziness, weakness, and headache. Edema may occur in the absence of renal or cardiac failure.

Dilated, tortuous venules may be found in the palpebral and bulbar conjunctiva and the retina. Corneal opacities are usually, if not always, present and lens opacities may be found. Hypertension develops in older persons, and there may be evidence of myocardial infarction, congestive failure, or cerebrovascular disease.

An early finding, which may be discovered at routine examination, is albuminuria. "Maltese cross" material may be found in the urine on polaroscopy. "Mulberry cells" containing glycolipid may be discerned in the urinary sediment. Later in the disease there are casts, hematuria, and low, fixed specific gravity, azotemia, and anemia.

Diagnosis. Cutaneous telangiectases, albuminuria, glycolipid in cells of skin and renal biopsies, glycolipid in urinary sediment (both ceramide trihexoside and ceramide dihexoside), and a positive family history are diagnostic. In addition, slit-lamp examination of the cornea shows characteristic findings, even in female carriers.

Senile angiomas (de Morgan or ruby spots) are usually brighter red, are more numerous on the upper trunk, and do not cluster together. Angiokeratomas of the scrotum (Fordyce) are common lesions of older men. Lesions of Osler-Weber-Rendu disease are brighter red, less grouped, and occur chiefly in the mouth, nose, and lips and on the fingers. Angiokeratomas identical to those of Fabry's disease have been reported in alpha-1-fucosidase deficiency.

Treatment. In addition to treatment for renal failure, kidney transplants may provide effective enzyme replacement. Administration of purified placental ceramide trihexosidase has temporarily decreased ceramide trihexoside blood levels. These treatments are still in experimental phases but hold promise for the future.

Prognosis. The disease is slowly progressive in males, who usually die in the fourth or fifth decades of renal failure complicated by cardiovascular disease. Longevity is essentially uninfluenced by the mild form that occurs in women.

Brady, R. O., et al.: Replacement therapy for inherited enzyme defect (use of purified ceramidetrihexosidase) in Fabry's disease. N. Engl. J. Med., 289:9, 1973.

Epinette, W. W., et al.: Angiokeratoma corporis diffusum with alpha-L-fucosidase deficiency. Arch. Dermatol., 107:754, 1973.

Ferrons, V. J., Hibbs, R. G., and Burda, C. D.: The heart in Fabry's disease. Am. J. Cardiol., 24:95, 1969.

Matalon, R., Dorfman, A., Dawson, G., and Sweeley, C. C.: Glycolipid and mucopolysaccharide abnormality in fibroblasts in Fabry's disease. Science, 164:1522, 1969.

Philippart, M., Franklin, S. S., and Gordon, A.: Reversal of inborn sphingo-lipidosis (Fabry's disease) by kidney transplantation. Ann. Intern. Med., 77:195, 1972.

Philippart, M., Sarlieve, L., and Manacorda, A.: Urinary glycolipids in Fabry's disease. Pediatrics, 43:201, 1969.

919.   INCONTINENTIA PIGMENTI
(Bloch-Sulzberger Syndrome)

Clayton E. Wheeler, Jr.

Incontinentia pigmenti is a congenital disorder characterized by bizarre skin lesions and defects in many structures of epidermal and mesodermal origin. The cause is unknown. Maternal viral infection appears unlikely. Evidence suggests that the disorder is inherited as an X-linked trait that is lethal for males. Only 8 of 232 cases have been males.

Cutaneous lesions are usually present at birth but may not appear for a few weeks or a year or two. The process is likely to be localized initially but tends to spread and become generalized. The lesions are papules, vesicles, and bullae that arise in areas of inflammation. At first there is little tendency toward a configurate pattern but, later, groups, patches, and lines are observed. Lesions often come and go in crops, and the pattern shifts from time to time. After weeks or months, the inflammatory phase either passes directly to a pigmented macular stage or blends into a warty or papillomatous stage that subsequently develops into pigmented macules. The most characteristic feature of the skin involvement is the striking and bizarre pattern assumed by pigmented macules and, to a lesser extent, by preceding warty and inflammatory lesions. Streaks, flecks, lines whorls, patches, spidery forms, arborizations, and zebra and marble and fudge ripple patterns are found. The lines and streaks do not correspond to nerve, blood vessel, or dermatome distribution and frequently cross the midline. The macules are usually chocolate-brown, gray-brown, or slate-colored. After a few years pigmented macules often fade gradually, leaving little or no residuum by adult life. The hair may be thin, and a common finding is localized atrophic alopecia of the scalp. Occasionally other cutaneous defects develop such as dystrophic nails, localized atrophy, small keratotic areas, tylosis of palms and soles, and areas simulating localized scleroderma.

Other abnormalities of structures of ectodermal or mesodermal origin occur in approximately two thirds of the patients. *Dental anomalies* include delayed eruption, fewer teeth than normal, and conical crowns of the incisors, canines, and bicuspids. Both deciduous and permanent teeth are affected. Possible *eye changes* are strabismus, corneal opacities, cataracts, optic atrophy, blue scleras, retinal pigmentary abnormalities, retrobulbar glioma, and ablatio falciformis. *Nervous system involvement* includes spastic paralysis, motor disturbances, epilepsy, microcephaly, mental retardation, nystagmus, decreased hearing, and homonymous hemianopsia. Osseous change, retarded growth and development, patent ductus arteriosus, urachal cyst, supernumerary ears, absence of or supernumerary nipples, and unilateral lack of breast tissue occasionally occur in patients with incontinentia pigmenti.

In the inflammatory, vesicular phase of the disease, blood eosinophilia of 30 to 50 per cent is common, and vesicle fluid eosinophilia may reach 95 per cent. Anemia occasionally occurs at this time.

Diagnosis is difficult in the vesicular or bullous phase. Blood and tissue eosinophilia and roentgenograms of unerupted teeth in infants may be helpful. As the bizarre configuration and the warty and pigmented macular phases develop, diagnosis usually becomes easy. Bullous incontinentia pigmenti must be differentiated from dermatitis herpetiformis, congenital syphilis, epidermolysis bullosa, erythema multiforme, bullous impetigo, virus diseases, and contact dermatitis. Warty and pigmented macular phases resemble systematized epithelial nevi. Hypomelanosis of Ito presents bizarre hypopigmented areas in marble-cake, swirling patterns, but this appears to be a separate disease — not just a hypopigmented phase of incontinentia pigmenti. Roentgenographic dental changes must be distinguished from congenital syphilis and congenital ectodermal defect.

No effective prevention or treatment is known. Adrenal steroid administration has had temporary beneficial effect on the bullous phase but has not been fully evaluated.

Morbidity and longevity depend upon the structures affected and the severity of the process. Cutaneous involvement alone or in association with minor defects of other structures is compatible with a normal life. Involvement of the nervous system or heart may carry a serious prognosis.

Carney, R. G., and Carney, R. G., Jr.: Incontinentia pigmenti. Arch. Dermatol., 102:157, 1970.

Jelenek, J. E., Bart, R. S., and Schiff, G. M.: Hypomelanosis of Ito (incontinentia pigmenti achromians). Arch. Dermatol., 107:596, 1973.

Schmidt, H., Hvidberg-Hansen, J., and Christensen, H. E.: Incontinentia pigmenti with associated lesions in two generations. Acta Derm. Venereol. (Stockh.), 52:281, 1972.

Simonsson, H.: Incontinentia pigmenti, Bloch-Sulzberger syndrome, associated with infantile spasms. Acta Paediatr. Scand., 61:612, 1972.

920.   HEREDITARY ANHIDROTIC ECTODERMAL DEFECT

Clayton E. Wheeler, Jr.

Hereditary anhidrotic ectodermal defect is an uncommon, genetically determined developmental defect of ectodermal, entodermal, and mesodermal structures in which dysgenesis of the epidermis and its appendages is the main feature. Predominance of the disease in males is explained by X-linked inheritance. Dominant and recessive autosomal inheritance have not been excluded in some cases. Defective development probably arises in the second or third month of embryonic life when epidermal appendages are being differentiated.

The *facies* is often so characteristic that unrelated persons appear to be siblings. Wide, high, scanty eyebrows, prominent frontal bones, saddle nose, thick swollen lips with radiating furrows, underdeveloped maxillas and mandibles, and pointed chin are distinctive features. The patient may be small and delicately proportioned, and the skin is likely to be thin, dry, white, and soft, producing a feminine appearance. Petechiae and purpura are occasionally seen, and the tourniquet test may be positive.

Absence of or greatly decreased numbers of sweat glands, which are often rudimentary, account for restricted sweating or none at all. Regulation of bodily temperature in a hot environment is defective because of inadequate sweating; thus, the disorder is one of the causes of fever, especially in the newborn. Lanugo, scalp, eyebrow, eyelash, axillary, and pubic hair are scant or absent. Sebaceous glands are decreased in number and activity. Nails may be normal or exhibit slow growth, ridging, or decreased thickness. Permanent and deciduous teeth may be absent or decreased in number and they are likely to be widely spaced, peg-shaped or conical, pigmented or fragile. Abnormalities of the lens include cataracts, subluxation, and absence. Mucous glands of the mouth, pharynx, larynx, trachea, and bronchi may be essentially absent. This may predispose to frequent respiratory tract infections. Chronic rhinitis contributes to the development of saddle nose. Defective lacrimal glands result in deficient tearing. Body odor is absent because of lack of sweating. Sparse amniotic fluid has been reported at birth. Lack of sweat pores of the palmar dermal ridges and x-ray evidence of defective dentition have diagnostic value.

In accordance with X-linked inheritance, the full-blown syndrome is most often seen in males, but females may show minor abnormalities of teeth, hair, or sweating. Decreased numbers of sweat pores may or may not be found in heterozygous females.

Less common abnormalities include primary hypogonadism, hypospadias, epispadias, absence of nipples, absence of mammary glands, satyr ears, cleft palate, mental deficiency, central nervous system defects, supernumerary fingers and toes, and micro-ophthalmia.

Histologically, the skin shows decreased epidermal and dermal thickness, absence of or rudimentary sweat glands, absence of or small pilosebaceous apparatus, and poorly developed arrectores pilorum muscles.

Treatment is entirely symptomatic and includes protection from heat, use of dentures, and plastic repair of nasal defects. Measures to improve appearance are morale builders. Longevity is usually good. Patients should choose occupations where as little sweating as possible is required for body cooling and where respiratory tract irritants can be avoided.

Beahrs, J. O., et al.: Anhidrotic ectodermal dysplasia: Predisposition to bronchial disease. Ann. Intern. Med., 74:92, 1971.

Crump, I. A., and Danka, D. M.: Hypohidrotic ectodermal dysplasia. J. Pediatr., 78:466, 1971.

Frias, J. L., and Smith, D. W.: Diminished sweat pores in hypohidrotic ectodermal dysplasia. J. Pediatr., 72:606, 1968.

Richards, W., and Kaplan, J. M.: Anhidrotic ectodermal dysplasia. An unusual cause of pyrexia in the newborn. Am. J. Dis. Child., 117:597, 1969.

Verbov, J.: Hypohidrotic (or anhidrotic) ectodermal dysplasia—an appraisal of diagnostic methods. Br. J. Dermatol., 83:341, 1970.

921. NEUROFIBROMATOSIS OF VON RECKLINGHAUSEN

Clayton E. Wheeler, Jr.

Neurofibromatosis is a relatively common disease (one case in about 3000 births) characterized by dominant inheritance, café au lait spots, freckling, and neurofibromas of the skin and internal organs. Cause and pathogenesis are unknown.

Café au lait spots occur in more than 90 per cent of the cases. They are often present at birth, but more may appear up to adult life. In old age the number may decrease. The spots are light brown macules that vary considerably in shape and size. More than five such lesions over 1.5 cm in size are diagnostic (small numbers occur in normal persons). Axillary or generalized freckling, when present, is a characteristic sign. Normal or increased numbers of melanocytes are present in pigmented spots and normal-appearing skin. Giant pigment granules may be found in prickle cells and melanocytes.

Neurofibromas appear at any cutaneous site, including the genitalia, palms, and soles. There may be few or many, and they vary greatly in size and shape. The tumors are of two types: (1) small, dome-shaped, or nipple-like, violaceous dermal lesions that can often be pressed into the skin like small hernias, and (2) subcutaneous nodules along the course of nerves. These may be knotted, plexiform, or pendulous and may attain great size.

The most frequent sites of internal involvement are bone, central nervous system, and pheochrome tissue. Neurofibromas in or near bone produce localized proliferative erosions or cystic lesions. Other frequent bony abnormalities are scoliosis, lordosis, kyphosis, and pseudoarthrosis. Neurofibromas may develop in almost any part of the central nervous system or in the eyes; the symptoms depend upon the size and location of the tumor. Nodules of the iris, hamartomas of the retina, and glaucoma may be found. Of the cranial nerves, the acoustic and optic are most often involved. Mental deficiency is not unusual. There may be an increased number of brain tumors that are not neurofibromas. The incidence of pheochromocytoma in neurofibromatosis is probably less than 1 per cent. On the other hand, 5 to 20 per cent of patients with pheochromocytoma have neurofibromatosis. Other internal involvement includes gastrointestinal bleeding, intestinal obstruction, lung cysts, pulmonary fibrosis, coarctation of the aorta, constricting bands of large vessels, urinary tract obstruction, jaundice, and hypertension caused by abnormalities of renal arteries. Sarcomatous degeneration of neurofibroma is reported in 2 to 16 per cent of cases, depending upon the series studied. Patients are often underdeveloped somatically and sexually, and fertility may be decreased. Precocious sexual development occurs in children. Gigantism and elephantiasis may involve extremities or digits.

Diagnosis is based upon café au lait spots, neurofibromas, bone roentgenograms, the histologic picture, and a positive family history. Treatment is palliative and includes surgical removal of neurofibromas that are large or interfere with function, sarcomas, pheochromocytomas, and various brain tumors. Prognosis is usually good, but it is influenced by malignancy, pheochromocytoma, and skeletal deformities.

Benedict, P. H., Szabo, G., Fitzpatrick, T. B., and Sinesi, S. J.: Melanotic macules in Albright's syndrome and in neurofibromatosis. J.A.M.A., 205:618, 1968.

Crowe, F. W.: Axillary freckling as a diagnostic aid in neurofibromatosis. Ann. Intern. Med., 61:1142, 1964.

Fenoan, N. T., and Yakovac, W. C.: Neurofibromatosis in childhood. J. Pediatr., 76:339, 1970.

Knight, W. A., et al.: Neurofibromatosis associated with malignant neurofibromas. Arch. Dermatol., 107:747, 1973.

Mena, E., et al.: Neurofibromatosis and renovascular hypertension in children. Am. J. Roentgenol. Radium Ther. Nucl. Med., 118:39, 1973.

922. AINHUM
(Dactylolysis Spontanea)

Clayton E. Wheeler, Jr.

Ainhum is characterized by spontaneous amputation of the fifth toe. The disorder is rare in the United States but common in parts of Africa. It affects primarily blacks and other dark-skinned persons, and shows a peak incidence between 30 and 40 years of age. The fifth toe is usually affected, although the fourth toe may be involved. Bilateral cases are common. Hyperkeratotic constriction develops at the undersurface of the toe at or between the plantar creases. This gradually encircles and constricts the toe until bone absorption occurs and the distal portion hangs by a thin pedicle. Inflammation or ulceration is often present. After months or years (average five years) the toe undergoes spontaneous, bloodless amputation. Neurologic and circulatory changes (plethysmographic studies are normal) are absent. Varying degrees of pain are common owing to sepsis, ulceration, and possibly pressure on nerves. There are no constitutional symptoms. Pathologic findings are nonspecific and probably result from chronic inflammation. The cause is unknown, but a plausible theory is that the small toes are predisposed to spontaneous amputation following trauma, chronic infection, and inflammation. The condition may be related to poor protection and care of the feet; most of the patients have gone barefoot. Cure is accomplished by spontaneous or surgical amputation.

Baerg, P. H.: Ainhum (dactylolysis spontanea): A review of the literature and a report of two cases. J. Am. Podiatry Assoc., 61:44, 1971.

Browne, S. G.: True ainhum: Its distinctive and differentiating features. J. Bone Joint Surg. (Br.) 47:52, 1965.

Cole, G. J.: Ainhum. An account of fifty-four patients with special reference to etiology and treatment. J. Bone Joint Surg. (Br.), 47:43, 1965.

Reque, C. J. et al.: Pseudoainhum constricting bands of the extremities. Arch. Dermatol., 105:434, 1972.

923. TOXIC EPIDERMAL NECROLYSIS
(Lyell's Disease, Scalded Skin Syndrome)

Clayton E. Wheeler, Jr.

Definition. Toxic epidermal necrolysis (TEN) is characterized by cutaneous erythema, epidermal loosening and stripping, and a scalded appearance.

Etiology. Two types are recognized: (1) Staphylococcal TEN is due to infection with the group II, usually type 71, staphylococcus and is caused by a toxin elaborated by the organism. (2) Drug-induced TEN may be caused by sulfonamides, butazones, salicylates, aminopyrine, phenacetin, antimicrobials, antihistamines, or anticonvulsants. At times the cause of the TEN cannot be identified.

Incidence. Staphylococcal TEN usually affects infants and young children, whereas drug-induced TEN usually affects adults and sometimes older children.

Pathogenesis and Pathology. Staphylococcal TEN results from infection in the nose, throat, ear, eye, skin, urogenital tract, heart valves, or elsewhere. Staphylococci often cannot be cultured from the erythematous or scalded skin, although sometimes they can. Animal experiments indicate that the Staphylococcus elaborates a toxin called epidermolysin which causes the scalded skin syndrome. Microscopically, the epidermis is damaged at the granular layer with subsequent shedding of this layer along with the horny layer. There is surprisingly little inflammatory or vascular change below the granular layer.

Drug-induced TEN causes necrosis, separation and loss of the entire epidermis, along with upper dermal damage and inflammation.

Clinical Manifestations. In staphylococcal TEN the infant or child is often noted to have a respiratory tract or skin infection. In the course of this infection there develops a diffuse scarlatiniform erythema with accentuation in the body folds and intertriginous sites. The skin is tender and painful to touch. Within a few hours the horny layer loosens and rubs off easily with movement, handling of the child, or friction against the bed, leaving a red, glistening surface resembling a scald. The extent of involvement is variable, true TEN lesions being limited to only a few intertriginous sites or becoming generalized. With proper treatment the process may not progress beyond the stage of erythema (staphylococcal erythema) or may do so only in some areas. With treatment, there is rapid healing, provided the child survives. Healing is accompanied by drying, lessening erythema, and a flaky scaling or peeling over a week or two. Mucous membranes are unlikely to be involved unless directly infected by the Staphylococcus.

In drug-induced TEN the patient is usually ill to begin with and is taking one or several drugs. Patchy or generalized erythema develops over a few hours or days. The entire thickness of the epidermis loosens and is easily stripped away from the dermal bed, leaving a white or pink glistening surface and a scalded appearance. A relatively small amount of the body surface may be affected, or much of the body surface may be involved. The patient suffers great discomfort from the denuded areas in the more extensive cases. Fluid and electrolyte losses are likely to be excessive. The patient may exhibit shock. Epidermal regeneration is slow, taking two to three weeks before significant epidermal barrier function is restored. In this form of TEN the mucous membranes are likely to be involved as well as skin. Secondary bacterial or mycotic infection is likely to be a problem.

Diagnosis. Infection of an infant or child with the group II Staphylococcus followed by erythema, epidermal necrosis, and separation at the granular layer suffices for diagnosis of staphylococcal TEN. History of drug exposure followed by erythema, necrosis, and separation of full-thickness epidermis in an adult or older child suggests drug-induced TEN.

In the adult or drug-induced type, the major differential diagnosis is erythema multiforme of the Stevens-Johnson type. TEN lacks the round, configurate lesions, the tense, well-formed bullae, and the intense dermal inflammation of erythema multiforme. Erythema multiforme lacks the scalded appearance.

Treatment. In staphylococcal TEN, the Staphylococcus is usually penicillin and tetracycline resistant so that cloxacillin, methicillin, erythromycin, or other systemic antimicrobials are used in large doses. The child is kept in a warm room, handled carefully, and subjected to expert nursing care. Pouring calamine liniment on the affected areas and spreading it out gently with gloved fingers may be soothing. Analgesics, antipyretics, and other symptomatic measures may be necessary. Replacement of fluid and electrolytes lost through the skin is most important.

Treatment of the adult, drug-induced TEN is more difficult. The causative agent should be removed if it can be identified. Fluid, electrolytes, and macromolecules should be replaced as they are lost. Secondary bacterial or mycotic infection should be combated with appropriate antimicrobials. Systemic corticosteroids are usually administered as soon as possible, but there is question about their effectiveness, especially after the epidermal damage is done. The patient should be kept in a warm room, handled as little as possible, and kept as comfortable as possible with analgesics, antipyretics, and good nursing care.

Prognosis. In general, the staphylococcal type has a good prognosis. This depends upon the underlying infection, the extent of the TEN, and the promptness of treatment. Unrecognized, untreated cases have a mortality rate of 10 to 25 per cent. Drug-induced TEN has a poor prognosis. Even when recognized and treated early, it has a mortality rate of 25 to 50 per cent, depending largely upon the extent of involvement.

Lillibridge, C. B., Melish, M. E., and Glasgow, L. A.: Site of action of exfoliative toxin in the staphylococcal scalded skin syndrome. Pediatrics, 5:728, 1972.

Lowney, E. D., et al.: The scalded skin syndrome in small children. Arch. Dermatol., 95:359, 1967.

Melish, M. E., and Glasgow, L. A.: The staphylococcal scalded-skin syndrome. N. Engl. J. Med., 282:1114, 1970.

Melish, M. E., Glasgow, L. A., and Turner, M. D.: The staphylococcal scaled-skin syndrome: Isolation and partial characterization of the exfoliative toxin. J. Infect. Dis., 125:129, 1972.

Reid, L. H., Weston, W. L., and Humbert, J. R.: Staphylococcal scalded skin syndrome. Adult onset in a patient with deficient cell-mediated immunity. Arch. Dermatol., 109:239, 1974.

924. DISORDERS OF MELANIN PIGMENTATION

Aaron B. Lerner

Melanin is the brown to black pigment that colors the skin, hair, and eyes. It is formed in the cytoplasm of melanocytes by the oxidation of tyrosine catalyzed by tyrosinase, a copper-containing enzyme. Under normal conditions pigment is transferred from melanocytes to keratinocytes so that the color of skin depends upon the presence of melanin within both the pigment and epidermal cells. Melanocytes are derived embryologically from the neural crest. Before the third month of fetal life these cells migrate to their resting places in the skin at the epidermal-dermal junction, in the eyes along the uveal tract, and in the central nervous system in the leptomeninges. In the conversion of tyrosine to melanin the first compound formed is dopa. After several reactions the melanin polymer is made. The pigment of red hair, and perhaps even that of freckles, results from a side reaction in which dopa is combined with cysteine to form 5-S cysteine dopa. It is the oxidation and polymerization of 5-S cysteine dopa that produces the red pigment.

Pigmented nevi are composed of clusters of melanocytes. Most of them form after birth, although occasionally large pigmented nevi are present at birth as a result of an abnormal proliferation of melanocytes in the skin in utero.

Most disorders of *hypopigmentation*, such as vitiligo, albinism, partial albinism, and phenylketonuria, are under genetic control, whereas the disturbances of *hyperpigmentation* usually occur in patients with endocrine abnormalities.

Hypopigmentation. Albinism and vitiligo are the two most important disturbances of hypopigmentation. In *albinism* there is an absence or decrease of tyrosinase in melanocytes. In *partial albinism* there is a congenital absence of melanocytes in the white patches. The light color of the skin in patients with *phenylketonuria* may result from an inhibition of tyrosinase by the presence of excess phenylalanine. In *vitiligo* and in *graying of hair* pigment cells that were present at birth are destroyed. Vitiligo occurs in about 1 per cent of the population and is transmitted as a dominant trait. Pigment is lost in exposed areas, particularly the face and dorsal aspects of the hands; in the axillae and genitalia; in surrounding body orifices such as the mouth, eyes, nose, nipples, and rectum; at sites of pressure and trauma; about pigmented nevi; and in hair. Patients with vitiligo are usually in good general health. However, the incidence of vitiligo is increased 5- to 15-fold in patients with hyperthyroidism, pernicious anemia, adrenocortical insufficiency, and melanomas. Vitiligo tends to occur in patients who are becoming hyperpigmented, so that there may be lightening in some areas and darkening in others. The loss of melanocytes in these patients probably results from a combination of autocytotoxic and autoimmune processes. Hypopigmentation distinct from vitiligo is seen in patients with scleroderma. Patches of white skin and, less frequently, partial albinism are seen in patients with *tuberous sclerosis.*

Hyperpigmentation. In most clinical states accompanied by hyperpigmentation, endocrine function is abnormal. Specific hormones activate adenyl cyclase on the cell surface to increase the levels of cyclic AMP within melanocytes. When the melanocyte-stimulating hormone, β-MSH, is released in excessive quantities by the pituitary gland, darkening of the skin occurs in patients with adrenocortical insufficiency. Pituitary activity increases as a result of decreased steroid production by the adrenal cortex. However, the same kind of hyperpigmentation can occur in the presence of a pituitary tumor that releases an excess of MSH. Usually pituitary tumors first produce increased amounts of corticotrophin, stimulating the adrenals and leading to the development of Cushing's syndrome. If a pituitary tumor is not suspected and the patient undergoes bilateral adrenalectomy, the tumor will continue to grow, and the skin may become very dark. Initially the tumor produces only large amounts of corticotrophin, but later

MSH peptides are also made. In some patients a pituitary tumor may release excess MSH but not corticotrophin, so that hyperpigmentation without adrenocortical hyperplasia occurs.

A few patients with *metastatic carcinomas* develop similar problems of hyperpigmentation. The carcinomas produce peptides related to or identical with corticotrophin and MSH. Some of these patients develop both Cushing's syndrome and hyperpigmentation, although others show only hyperpigmentation. Assay of some of the tumors has shown the presence of MSH and corticotrophin-like substances. Hyperpigmentation also may be seen in 10 to 15 per cent of women receiving potent synthetic progesterones and estrogens for birth control. Although these substances are not as effective darkeners of melanocytes as are the MSH and MSH-like peptides, they do produce facial pigmentation or *melasma.*

Severe hyperpigmentation is seen occasionally in patients with hyperthyroidism, xanthomatous biliary cirrhosis, sprue, or hemochromatosis. It is likely that in these individuals there are increased amounts of cyclic AMP within melanocytes as a result of either more adenyl cyclase activity or less phosphodiesterase function within the cells. Chronic illness or ingestion of drugs such as busulfan (Myleran) or 4-aminopteroyl glutamic acid (Aminopterin) also produces hyperpigmentation. Again, these substances probably work by increasing cyclic AMP levels within pigment cells.

Melanoma. All adults have many nevi, and most melanomas arise from nevi. Melanoma accounts for about 1.5 per cent of cancer deaths. Ten to 20 per cent of patients with melanomas develop vitiligo. At times the primary lesion is destroyed even though the tumor is metastasizing at a rapid rate. The relationship between the destruction of normal melanocytes and that of some malignant melanocytes in patients with melanomas is not known. In a few patients with metastatic melanoma moderate amounts of tyrosine oxidation products made in the tumors are carried by the blood to the kidneys and excreted in the urine. In air they become oxidized to melanin, giving the urine a dark color, and the patients are said to have *melanuria.* In exceptional cases of metastatic melanoma, great quantities of tyrosine oxidation products form, reach the skin, and are converted to melanin. The patient first acquires the slate gray color of argyria and later becomes intensely brown or black.

Conference on Pigment Cell Biology. Yale J. Biol. Med., Vol. 46, Dec. 1973.

Lerner, A. B.: On the etiology of vitiligo and gray hair. Am. J. Med., 51:141, 1971.

McGovern, V. J., and Russell, P. (eds.): Mechanisms in Pigmentation. Proceedings of the 8th International Pigment Cell Conference in Sydney, Basel, S. Karger, 1972.

925. ACATALASIA

Alexander G. Bearn

Acatalasia is a rare, autosomal, recessively inherited trait characterized by a deficiency of catalase in many tissues of the body, including the erythrocytes, bone marrow, liver, and skin. The disease is particularly common among Japanese, Koreans, and Chinese, but has also been reported from Germany, Switzerland, and Israel. Manifestations are usually restricted to the oral cavity and are related to the increased susceptibility to tissue damage by normal microbial flora. Oral sepsis may lead to severe gangrenous lesions, including alveolar bone destruction. Approximately 50 per cent of acatalasic subjects are asymptomatic; after puberty gangrenous lesions in the oral cavity are rare. An absence of catalase in individuals homozygous for the trait and intermediate values for the clinically normal heterozygous carriers are characteristic of the families reported from Japan. Homozygotes from Germany, Switzerland, and Israel commonly show residual catalase activity and are symptomatically normal. When hydrogen peroxide is added to acatalasic blood, it turns a brownish black color owing to the formation of methemoglobin; by contrast normal blood bubbles vigorously and remains pink. At least two forms of acatalasia exist in Japan where more than 50 patients with the disease have been reported. Genetic heterogeneity is suggested both from the variations in the clinical expression of the disease and in the level and stability of residual catalase activity in different populations. The estimated frequency in Japan is approximately 1 in 50,000, and the heterozygote frequency is approximately 1 per cent. Variations in the gene frequency within Japan have been reported. Local surgical excision, extraction of teeth, and antimicrobial therapy have been employed. A similar disease occurs in mice, guinea pigs, dogs, and the domestic fowl.

Aebi, H., and Suter, H.: Acatalasemia. *In* Harris, H., and Hirschhorn, K. (eds.): Advances in Human Genetics. Vol. 2. New York, Plenum Press, 1971.
Wyngaarden, J. B., and Howell, R. R.: Acatalasia. *In* Stanbury, J. B., Wyngaarden, J. B., and Fredrickson, D. S. (eds.): The Metabolic Basis of Inherited Disease. 3rd ed. New York, McGraw-Hill Book Company, 1972.

926. ALBINISM
(Oculocutaneous Albinism)

Alexander G. Bearn

The term albinism has come to refer to a genetically heterogeneous group of disorders in which there is an inherited defect in melanin metabolism. It is characterized by a decrease of melanin in the skin, hair, and eyes, and is due to a failure of melanocytes to produce normal melanin. The metabolic defect may involve melanocytes in more than one system (oculocutaneous albinism) or be restricted to one system (ocular albinism). Several independent genetic defects in tyrosine metabolism lead to the same phenotypic effect. Oculocutaneous albinism occurs in two distinct autosomal recessively inherited forms. In one form, the melanocytes lack the enzyme tyrosinase, leading to "tyrosinase-negative" albinism; in the second the enzyme is present and the defect is probably due to a limitation in the availability of tyrosine, the melanogenic substrate for the enzyme.

"Tyrosinase-negative" albinism occurs with a frequency of about 1 in 34,000 and is equally common in whites and blacks. The skin and hair color are strikingly white and do not darken with age. The skin is particularly susceptible to sunlight and often appears wrinkled. Precancerous keratoses in the areas exposed to sunlight are common, and there is a marked increase in frequency of basal cell and squamous cell carcinomas of the skin. Photophobia, astigmatism, and severe defects in visual acuity are common. Horizontal nystagmus is almost invariable. The ocular fundus of albinos is bright orange-red, and the vessels are prominent.

"Tyrosinase-positive" albinism is more frequently found among blacks than among whites. In the black population the phenotypic frequency is 1 in 14,000, whereas in the white population the frequency is approximately 1 in 60,000. In contrast with "tyrosinase-negative" albinism, the pigmentation of the skin and eyes increases with advancing age. Blacks with "tyrosinase-positive" albinism may be darker than many blonde Caucasoids. Freckles and pigmented nevi are common. Photophobia is less pronounced, and not all patients exhibit nystagmus.

Ocular albinism is a very rare variety in which the defect in pigmentation is restricted to the iris and fundus of the eye. Nystagmus, head-nodding, and defective vision also occur. It is inherited as an X-linked recessive trait.

Cutaneous albinism (partial albinism, piebald trait) is limited to the skin and hair. In almost all patients a triangular white forelock is present. The trait is inherited in a dominant fashion.

Fitzpatrick, T. B., and Quevedo, W. C.: Albinism. *In* Stanbury, J. B., Wyngaarden, J. B., and Fredrickson, D. S. (eds.): The Metabolic Basis of Inherited Disease. 3rd ed. New York, McGraw-Hill Book Company, 1972.
Witkop, C. J., Jr.: Albinism. *In* Harris, H., and Hirschhorn, K. (eds.): Advances in Human Genetics. Vol. 2. New York, Plenum Press, 1971.

927. DYSAUTONOMIA
(Riley-Day Syndrome)

Alexander G. Bearn

Dysautonomia is a rare recessively inherited disease of childhood, occurring almost exclusively in Ashkenazi Jews. The anatomic basis of the disease is an absence of unmyelinated nerve fibers in the peripheral and autonomic nerves. Features include defective lacrimation, absence of the fungiform papillae of the tongue, vasomotor instability including blotching of the skin, relative indifference to pain, poor motor coordination, and absent deep tendon reflexes. Dysphagia in childhood may be the presenting symptom. Many patients die in childhood from secondary aspiration pneumonia.

The differential diagnosis includes the congenital and hereditary sensory neuropathies which may present with insensitivity to pain.

Brunt, P. W., and McKusick, V. A.: Familial dysautonomia. A report of genetic and clinical studies, with a review of the literature. Medicine, 49:343, 1970.

928. EHLERS-DANLOS SYNDROME

Clayton E. Wheeler, Jr.

Definition.   The Ehlers-Danlos syndrome consists of a group of inherited systemic connective tissue disorders in which the major manifestations are fragility and hyperelasticity of skin, easy bruising, atrophic scars and soft pseudotumors, calcified cysts, hyperextensibility of joints with frequent luxations, bleeding tendency, and visceral anomalies.

Etiology.   The chief abnormalities of connective tissue are increased fragility and friability and capacity to stretch to an unusual length and return to the original position. Elastic tissue deficiency appears unlikely, because the tissue returns to its original position after stretching. Since toughness and limited extensibility are characteristics of normal collagen, fragility and hyperelasticity seem to indicate a collagen defect. It is conjectural whether the defect is molecular or involves the arrangement of molecules into fibrils or fibrils into bundles, or whether different types of the disease have different defects, because evidence is accumulating that the Ehlers-Danlos syndrome is composed of a heterogeneous group of disorders. Six types have been postulated and more may be expected. Types I to IV are probably inherited as dominant, Type V as X-linked recessive, and Type VI as autosomal recessive traits. Type VI appears to be due to a deficiency in lysyl-protocollagen hydroxylase with defective cross-linking of collagen.

Incidence.   The Ehlers-Danlos syndrome is most prevalent among white persons of European ancestry, although dark-skinned people are occasionally affected. Males are involved slightly more often than females. Skin and joint changes usually appear at an early age, but may not be evident until adult life. The disorder, including mild and incomplete forms, is undoubtedly much more common than case reports in the literature indicate.

Pathology.   No consistent abnormality of the corium has been demonstrated by microscopic examination. Normal, increased, or decreased amounts of elastic tissue or collagen, fragmentation of elastic tissue, and derangement of architecture of collagen have all been reported. Some of these findings may be late effects of overstretching and fragility rather than primary abnormalities. Limited study with the electron microscope has shown normal-appearing elastic tissue and collagen. No consistent microscopic abnormality has been found in blood vessels. Subcutaneous nodules are composed of encapsulated fat, which is often calcified. Pseudotumors show connective tissue proliferation, increased vascularity, islets of fatty degeneration, and cyst formation.

Pathogenesis.   Defective, friable collagen that allows abnormal extensibility and normal elastic tissue that provides return to the original position explain many of the clinical features: hyperelastic skin, scars, pseudotumors, easy bruising, hyperextensibility of joints with luxations, hemarthroses and arthritis, rupture of the lung with emphysema, and fragility and bleeding from the bowel. Defective supporting tissue of vessel walls or surrounding structures accounts for much of the abnormal bleeding, but functional and structural abnormalities of platelets have been reported, and some abnormality in collagen-platelet relationships has been found.

Clinical Manifestations.   Clinical features are variable because of mild and incomplete forms and because several genetic or biochemical types may exist. The facies may be normal, or there may be widely spaced eyes, epicanthal folds, broad nasal bridge, and "lop ears." Mentality is usually normal. The patient is likely to be small, short, and poorly developed.

The most striking feature of the soft, velvety skin is its capacity to be pulled abnormally far from underlying structures and to return promptly to its original position. The entire skin is usually hyperelastic, but some regions exhibit this property more than others. With age, elasticity of localized areas, especially about the elbows, may be lost so that the skin hangs in loose folds. Skin of the palms and soles is likely to become lax, furrowed, and redundant, and resembles loose-fitting gloves or moccasins. Despite increased elasticity, the skin is abnormally fragile or brittle, as shown by its tendency to bruise easily and by the development of scars and soft pseudotumors at sites of minor injury. Paper-thin atrophic scars develop over the elbows, knees, shins, and elsewhere. The scars are shiny, brown or red-violet, and often show telangiectasia. Subcutaneous spherules or nodules 2 to 8 mm in size may appear on the legs and forearms. These are easily movable and often calcify. Minor blows result in purpura or hematomas that may organize to form tumors. Retraction of tissues prevents excessive bleeding from skin injury, but minor trauma or surgery produces a gaping, fish-mouth wound that is hard to close and heals slowly.

Hyperextensibility of joints is often striking; the head, extremities, and digits may be placed in abnormal positions ("India rubber men" and "human pretzels"). Because of hyperextensibility of the joints and poor muscular development or tone, infants may show delayed sitting or walking and unsteadiness that occasions frequent falling and subsequent fractures. Other consequences of loose joints and muscle atony or weakness are frequent joint effusions or hemarthroses, arthritis, and habitual dislocations of the hip, shoulders, patella, radius, and clavicle. In addition, flat feet, genu recurvatum, kyphoscoliosis, and loose-end clavicles are seen. Other musculoskeletal abnormalities that have been associated with the Ehlers-Danlos syndrome are spina bifida occulta, arachnodactyly, high arched palate, club foot, spondylolisthesis, pigeon breast, and osteolytic changes of distal phalanges. There may be too few, too many, or poorly formed teeth. Umbilical and inguinal hernias are common. Muscle cramps may involve the legs at night.

Recognition of internal manifestations will undoubtedly increase with further study. Dissecting aortic aneurysm, intracranial aneurysms, spontaneous rupture of large arteries, aneurysm of the sinus of Valsalva and aortic insufficiency, spontaneous rupture of the lung with mediastinal and subcutaneous emphysema, and fragility of the bowel with bleeding or perforation have been reported. Congenital anomalies of the heart, gastrointestinal, respiratory, or genitourinary tracts also occur. Bleeding may occur into the skin or from the lung, vagina, rectum, nose, gums or tooth sockets, or after tonsillectomy, after operation on joints, or post partum.

Beighten classifies the Ehlers-Danlos syndrome into five types and McKusick adds a sixth. (1) Ehlers-Danlos syndrome I, or gravis type, is characterized by striking skin hyperextensibility, fragility and bruisability, and severe joint hypermobility. Friable tissues make operations difficult, and early rupture of fetal membranes may cause prematurity. (2) Ehlers-Danlos syndrome II, or mitis type, is characterized by mild cutaneous and joint manifestations. Tissue friability and prematurity are not problems. (3) Ehlers-Danlos syndrome III, or benign hypermobile type, is characterized by generalized and marked joint hypermobility with frequent complications, but cutaneous manifestations are minimal. (4) Ehlers-Danlos syndrome IV, or ecchymotic type, is characterized by thin, pale skin, prominent venous network, and little cutaneous hyperextensibility. Joint hypermobility is largely limited to the digits. The main feature is severe, easy bruisability. Ruptures of the bowel and great vessels are found predominantly in this type. (5) Ehlers-Danlos syndrome V, or X-linked form, shows striking skin extensibility, and there are moderate fragility, cigarette-paper scarring, and bruising. Joint hypermobility is limited. (6) Ehlers-Danlos syndrome VI, or the hydroxylysine-deficient collagen type, is characterized by autosomal recessive inheritance and paucity of hydroxylysine residues in collagen owing to deficient lysyl hydroxylase activity.

Diagnosis. Two or more of the following clinical features usually suffice for diagnosis: (1) cutaneous hyperelasticity, (2) hyperextensibility of joints, (3) easy bruising, (4) atrophic scars and pseudotumors, (5) calcified subcutaneous cysts, and (6) typical cases in the family.

Cutis laxa is characterized by loose, inelastic skin that hangs in folds. In late stages of the Ehlers-Danlos syndrome, localized areas of skin may become lax, but otherwise there seems to be no relation between the two disorders. Hypermobility of joints occurs as a genetic trait distinct from the Ehlers-Danlos syndrome, and it is part of *Marfan's syndrome, osteogenesis imperfecta, mongolism, cretinism,* and *cachexia.* Blue sclerae are probably essential features of the Ehlers-Danlos syndrome and do not signify a relationship to osteogenesis imperfecta. Besides having hyperelastic joints and skin,

patients with the *Bonnevie-Ullrich-Turner syndrome* show dwarfism, web neck, cubitus valgus, gonadal dysgenesis, and female phenotype with male genotype.

Treatment. There is no treatment for the basic disorder. Trauma to skin and joints should be avoided. Careful suturing, immobilization, and taping may promote wound healing. Hematomas occasionally require drainage. Orthopedic measures, including exercises, braces, reduction of dislocations, and drainage of hemarthroses, may be necessary. Dissecting aneurysm, hemorrhage, intestinal perforation, and various anomalies may require surgical intervention. Surgical procedures should be undertaken with great care because of the friability and hyperelasticity of skin and internal structures. Severed tissues separate abnormally, sutures are difficult to place and often do not hold, and wound dehiscence is a definite threat.

Prognosis. Prognosis for life is usually good, although deaths occur from various internal manifestations. Patients may be comfortable or may suffer considerable inconvenience and morbidity from cutaneous and musculoskeletal abnormalities. The joints tend to become more stable as the patient ages.

Beighton, P., Price, A., Lord, J., and Dickson, E.: Variants of the Ehlers-Danlos syndrome. Ann. Rheum. Dis., 28:228, 1969.

Hines, C., Jr., and Davis, W. D.: Ehlers-Danlos syndrome with megaduodenum and malabsorption syndrome secondary to bacterial overgrowth. Am. J. Med., 54:539, 1973.

Krane, J. M., Pinnell, S. R., and Erbe, R. W.: Lysylprotocollagen hydroxylase deficiency in fibroblasts from siblings with hydroxylysin-deficient collagen. Proc. Natl. Acad. Sci. U.S.A., 69:2899, 1972.

McKusick, V. A.: Heritable Disorders of Connective Tissue. 4th ed. St. Louis, C. V. Mosby Company, 1972.

929. FAMILIAL MEDITERRANEAN FEVER

(Periodic Fever, Periodic Disease, Familial Recurrent Polyserositis, Benign Paroxysmal Peritonitis, Periodic Polyserositis, Recurrent Polyserositis)

Paul B. Beeson

Definition. Familial Mediterranean fever is a familial disease characterized by recurrent short attacks of febrile illness in which there are signs of peritonitis, pleuritis, and arthritis. It is especially common in people of Eastern Mediterranean or Middle East origin, i.e., Jews, Arabs, Turks, and Armenians, but because of their wanderings the disorder is now encountered in all parts of the world. In addition, cases which seem clinically indistinguishable from familial Mediterranean fever are sometimes encountered in persons of quite different ethnic background. The name familial Mediterranean fever will be employed in this edition of the textbook because of current usage, but it has undesirable features. Some of the synonyms, notably recurrent polyserositis, would seem preferable. The most definitive studies of the disorder have been carried out in Israel, and the review by Sohar and colleagues is the best single source of information.

Genetics. Extensive investigation of families in Israel has led to the conclusion that familial Mediterranean fever is inherited as a single recessive autosomal trait, although the somewhat higher incidence in males (3.2) has not been adequately explained.

Pathology. Exudates from the peritoneum, pleura, or joint cavities during acute attacks reveal a preponderance of polymorphonuclear leukocytes and no evidence of microbial invasion. Biopsies of inflamed serosal surfaces usually show mild acute inflammation without underlying vascular disease. The most serious pathologic lesion is amyloidosis, which affects arterioles throughout the body and can seriously injure the kidneys, liver, spleen, lung, and adrenals.

Clinical Manifestations. An affected person shows no evidence of abnormality until the onset of the first attack, usually during the first or second decade of life. Between attacks, until amyloidosis becomes clinically manifest, the patient looks and feels well. Attacks are of short duration, usually one to four days, and consist of fever, which may be moderately high, together with manifestations of acute inflammation of the peritoneum, pleura, or synovial membranes. The peritoneal form is by far the most common, and consequently most sufferers have been subjected to laparotomy. Occasionally the joint manifestations assume more chronic form in which one or two large joints are the sites of painful swelling for weeks or months. In a few instances severe destruction of the hip has necessitated surgical treatment. Sometimes cutaneous lesions resembling erysipelas develop on the legs during an attack.

The serious hazard of this disease lies in the tendency to develop amyloidosis. This process is progressive, and most often causes death in renal failure. The rarity of familial Mediterranean fever in subjects over 40 years of age implies that amyloidosis develops in a high proportion of cases, causing death during adolescence or early adult life.

Differential Diagnosis. Inasmuch as a specific diagnostic test is lacking, the label of familial Mediterranean fever in an individual person must depend largely on ethnic background and the characteristic course of the disease. Obviously the disorder can mimic various infectious and "collagen" diseases, and a diagnosis of appendicitis is almost always considered at some time.

Treatment. No treatment other than symptomatic measures has been found effective in familial Mediterranean fever. Surprisingly, steroids, despite their antipyretic effects, seem to have little value in management of the acute bouts of illness. Recently there has been a report of benefit from regular administration of colchicine, 0.6 mg one to three times a day. There has also been a claim of suppression of attacks by use of indomethacin, 25 mg three times a day. These symptomatic measures deserve further trial. Eliakin and Licht have reported, in a small series of patients, dramatic suppression of attacks by long-term therapy consisting of colchicine, 0.02 mg per kilogram of body weight once a day, and aspirin, 0.5 gram twice a day. This deserves further trial. Nothing can be done to retard the progression of the amyloidosis which is the cause of death in a high proportion of cases.

SYNDROMES RESEMBLING FAMILIAL MEDITERRANEAN FEVER

Periodic Disease. Reimann has directed attention to a collection of syndromes which have the common features of periodic recurrence and intervals of well-being. Among the syndromes he has described are *periodic fever, periodic peritonitis* (familial Mediterranean fever?), *periodic neutropenia, periodic edema, periodic purpura, periodic arthralgia,* and *periodic psychosis.* Bodel and Dillard report that some cases of periodic fever have been ameliorated by administration of conjugated estrogens. The treatment regimens varied between patients, and their report should be studied for details.

Bodel, P., and Dillard, G. M.: Suppression of periodic fever with estrogen. Arch. Intern. Med., 131:189, 1973.
Eliakin, M., and Licht, A.: Colchicine-aspirin for recurrent polyserositis (familial Mediterranean fever). Lancet, 2:1333, 1973.
Goldfinger, S. E.: Colchicine for familial Mediterranean fever. N. Engl. J. Med., 287:1302, 1972.
Özer, F. L., Kaplaman, E., and Zileli, S.: Familial Mediterranean fever in Turkey. Report of twenty cases. Am. J. Med., 50:336, 1971.
Reimann, H. A.: Perplexities of a periodic entity. J.A.M.A., 190:241, 1964.
Siegal, S.: Familial paroxysmal polyserositis: Analysis of fifty cases. Am. J. Med., 36:893, 1964.
Sohar, E., Jafni, J., Pras, M., and Heller, H.: Familial Mediterranean fever. A survey of 470 cases and review of the literature. Am. J. Med., 43: 227, 1967.

930. LAURENCE-MOON SYNDROME

Alexander G. Bearn

The salient features of this recessively inherited syndrome are mental retardation, retinitis pigmentosa, hypogonadism, obesity, and polydactyly. There is a high parental consanguinity rate, and in Switzerland, where the disease appears to be particularly common, consanguinity has been established in more than 50 per cent of the affected sibships. Rigid classification is not possible, and the limits of the syndrome are poorly defined. Although retinitis pigmentosa appears relatively late, it is a common and well-defined feature. Other ocular signs include atypical retinal changes and retinitis without pigmentation. Mental retardation is only moderately severe and is usually noted soon after entering school. Unexplained obesity before the age of ten associated with polydactyly and hypogonadism should arouse suspicion of the disease.

Warkany, J.: Congenital Malformations. Chicago, Year Book Medical Publishers, 1971.

931. LIPOATROPHIC DIABETES

Alexander G. Bearn

The features of this disfiguring and invariably fatal disease include a loss of subcutaneous and body fat, hyperlipemia, hepatomegaly caused by fatty infiltration, phallic enlargement, hyperpigmentation and hypertrichosis with acanthosis nigricans, and insulin-resistant hyperglycemia.

The disease, which is probably due to hypothalamic-pituitary dysfunction, is inherited in a recessive fashion and affects dopamine-β-hydroxylase. Since this enzyme is rate limiting in the conversion of dopamine to nor-epinephrine, dopamine accumulates in the brain and is accompanied by a relative decrease in the quantity of norepinephrine. It has been suggested that the excess dopamine and decreased norepinephrine may cause an increase in the hypothalamic releasing factors (cortico-trophin-releasing hormone, luteinizing-releasing hormone, and melanocyte-stimulating hormone) which can then be detected in the peripheral blood. The possibility that dopamine receptor blockers might influence the course of the disease has been raised and requires further investigation.

Mabry, C. C., Hollingsworth, D. R., Upton, G. V., and Corbin, A.: Pituitary-hypothalamic dysfunction in generalized lipodystrophy. J. Pediatr., 82:625, 1973.

932. LIPOID PROTEINOSIS
(Hyalinosis Cutis et Mucosae)
Alexander G. Bearn

This recently recognized rare autosomal recessively inherited disease, particularly common in South Africa, is characterized by the combination of a husky voice from birth and scarring maculopapular eruptions around the face, arms, and trunk. The mucous membranes of the mouth, tongue, and larynx are diffusely infiltrated with hyaline-like material. Recurrent painful parotitis may occur. Calcification of the hippocampal gyri is an inconstant but pathognomonic sign of the disease. No consistent biochemical abnormalities have been reported. The disease must not be confused with porphyria. Although there is no clear-cut evidence for their effectiveness, corticosteroids have been employed in the treatment of this disorder.

Gordon, H., Gordon, W., and Botha, V.: Lipoid proteinosis in an inbred Namaqualand community. Lancet, 1:1032, 1969.

933. MARFAN'S SYNDROME
(Arachnodactyly, Dolichostenomelia)
Alexander G. Bearn

Marfan's syndrome is a generalized disorder of connective tissue with skeletal, ocular, and cardiovascular manifestations. The molecular nature of the defect is not precisely known, and abnormalities of collagen as well as elastin have been implicated. The condition occurs equally in the sexes, and is inherited as a dominant trait with variable expression. Its prevalence has been estimated to be 1.5 per 100,000 of the population,

and approximately 15 per cent of all cases are due to new mutations. The average age of fathers of those patients with Marfan's syndrome owing to "new mutations" is about seven years in excess of the mean age of fathers generally.

Manifestations. *Skeleton.* The extremities are characteristically long and thin. The arm span is greater than the height, and the lower segment measurement (pubis-to-sole) is in excess of the upper segment (pubis-to-vertex). Excessive longitudinal growth gives rise to arachnodactyly, pectus excavatum or pigeon breast, dolichocephaly, long narrow face, and high arched palate. This last feature, contrary to common opinion, is not specific for Marfan's syndrome, because it may be seen in congenital myopathy and myotonic dystrophy. Weakness and reduplication of ligaments and joint capsules lead to "double-jointedness," backward curvature of the knees, flat feet, and recurrent dislocation of the hips, patella, and other joints. Cutaneous striae may be present, and probably reflect the abnormal elastic fibers. An unexplained sparsity of subcutaneous fat is a feature in many patients. Femoral hernias are not uncommon.

Eyes. The eyes show subluxation of the lens (ectopia lentis). Although this is usually severe and bilateral, minor degrees of subluxation require careful slit-lamp examination for their detection. Diagnosis of Marfan's syndrome in the absence of subluxation or redundancy of the suspensory ligament and without affected family members should be made with extreme caution. Other ocular signs include tremor of the iris and glaucoma. Severe myopia and spontaneous retinal detachment are common and often lead to gross impairment of vision.

Cardiovascular Defects. Disruption and loss of the elastic fibers of the media, associated with an increase in collagen and smooth muscle, is the primary basic defect. The lack of elasticity results in progressive diffuse dilatation of the proximal segment of the ascending aorta and severe aortic regurgitation. The aorta is widest at the sinuses of Valsalva. Aortic regurgitation, owing to dilatation and stretching of the aortic cusps, may occur in the absence of roentgenographic evidence of aortic dilatation. An early systolic click is commonly heard at the apex as well as at the aortic area. *Mitral regurgitation* is being observed with increasing frequency, and appears to be due to stretching of the chordae tendineae. Myxomatous transformation of the mitral ring may occur. Heart failure and rupture of the aorta resulting from *dissecting aneurysm* are the most common causes of death. Prominence of the pulmonary artery is frequently seen, and is due to displacement of the dilated aortic ring as well as to dilatation of the pulmonary artery. Bacterial endocarditis may be superimposed on the cardiac lesion. Cystic disease of the lung may occur as an integral part of Marfan's syndrome.

Differential Diagnosis. Marfan's syndrome must be distinguished from *homocystinuria,* which clinically it may closely resemble. It has been estimated that 5 per cent of patients with nontraumatic ectopia lentis, one of the cardinal signs of classic Marfan's syndrome, have homocystinuria. Ectopia lentis, pectus excavatum, and pigeon breast are common to both syndromes. The lens is more likely to be dislocated upward in Marfan's syndrome but downward in homocystinuria. The presence of a malar flush, generalized osteoporosis, and moderate to severe mental retardation are characteristic of homocystinuria and are not found in Marfan's syndrome; patients with homocystinuria do not develop dissecting aneurysm. Homocystinuria is inherited as a recessive trait. The diagnosis can be made by a positive urinary nitroprusside test or, definitively, by paper electrophoresis of the urine. The primary defect in homocystinuria is a deficiency of cystathionine synthetase in the liver. This deficiency can also be revealed in cultured skin fibroblasts. Rats given β-aminoproprionitrile (or seeds of *Lathyrus odoratus*) develop skeletal changes and dissecting aortic aneurysm reminiscent of some of the features of Marfan's syndrome.

McKusick, V. A.: Heritable Disorders of Connective Tissue. 4th ed. St. Louis, C. V. Mosby Company, 1972, pp. 61–200.

THE MUCOPOLYSACCHARIDOSES
Alexander G. Bearn

934. HURLER'S SYNDROME
(Mucopolysaccharidosis I H, MPS I H)

Definition. Hurler's syndrome is an autosomally inherited abnormality of mucopolysaccharide metabolism characterized by skeletal abnormalities, hepatosplenomegaly, corneal clouding, mental retardation, and increased mucopolysaccharide excretion in the urine.

Etiology. The disease, which has a prevalence of approximately 1 in 40,000, is caused by excessive intracellular accumulation of the mucopolysaccharides dermatan sulfate (chondroitin sulfate B) and heparan sulfate (heparatin sulfate). These substances are preferentially deposited in those tissues and organs in which they normally occur. An increased intracellular deposition of mucopolysaccharides can be demonstrated in cultured fibroblasts derived from patients with Hurler's syndrome and their heterozygous relatives, using metachromatic dyes as well as chemical methods. Recent evidence indicates that the primary inherited defect in Hurler's syndrome is deficiency of the lysosomal enzyme α-L-iduronidase which is responsible for the degradation of the polysaccharide side chains of dermatan sulfate and heparan sulfate. Particularly noteworthy is the discovery that the same enzymatic defect, which can be detected in cultured fibroblasts, occurs in *Scheie's syndrome* (see Ch. 935). This biochemical finding indicates that Hurler's syndrome and Scheie's syndrome, long thought to be closely related, are caused by allelic genes.

Pathology. The most characteristic pathologic feature of the disease is the excessive accumulation of intracellular mucopolysaccharides. Cells of the nervous system, liver, reticuloendothelial system, endocrine glands, cartilage, bone, and heart muscle are involved. Abnormal deposits are also present in the cornea, meninges, epicardium, pericardium, chordae tendineae, heart valves, tracheobronchial cartilages, upper air passages, and coronary and larger peripheral arteries. Distention of fibroblasts with this material causes the appearance of "clear" or "gargoyle" cells.

Clinical Manifestations. Although the patient may appear normal at birth, the disease becomes evident during the first year or two of life and progresses during childhood and adolescence. In the full-blown disorder, the head is large and there is hyperostosis of the sagittal suture that sometimes extends onto the forehead. The facial features are usually coarse and ugly. A broad saddle nose, wide nostrils, thick lips, large tongue, open mouth, and noisy breathing are characteristic. Skeletal abnormalities include short neck, dorsal and lumbar kyphosis with gibbus, short stature, and flaring of the costal margins. The hands are broad with stubby fingers, and there is a tendency for the fifth finger to bend radially. There may be a deformity of joints such as genu valgus, coxa valga, pes planus, or talipes equinovarus. The skin, especially over the upper extremities and thorax, is ridged and grooved, and may present nodular thickenings. Fine lanugo hairs are prominent over much of the cutaneous surface, and the extremities are likely to show profuse growth of large coarse hair. The heart is enlarged, and valvular involvement produces murmurs that may simulate those of rheumatic heart disease. Disease of coronary arteries may give rise to angina or other evidence of occlusive disease. The abdomen is large and protuberant, and the liver and spleen are commonly enlarged. Umbilical and inguinal hernias are frequent. Clouding of the cornea is extremely common; slit-lamp examination of the eyes may be needed to detect the corneal opacification in the early stages of the disease. Mental deterioration is severe and progressive.

Abnormalities demonstrable by roentgenogram include a large skull with frontal and occipital hyperostosis, hypertelorism, long shallow sella turcica with anterior pocketing, and deformities of the facial bones. Gibbus is associated with wedge-shaped deformities and anterior hooklike projections of the vertebral bodies. The ribs are broad, spatulate, and saber shaped. The terminal phalanges of the hands are broad and short, and the long bones, especially of the arms, show swollen shafts from expansion of medullary cavities. The heart is often enlarged, and pulmonary congestion may be present.

Diagnosis. Diagnosis depends upon recognition of the characteristic clinical manifestations, biopsy, blood and bone marrow studies, and examination of the urine for increased mucopolysaccharide content. A simple screening test for this consists of adding acidified bovine serum albumin to the urine. A positive result is indicated by a dense white precipitate owing to the reaction of albumin and acid mucopolysaccharide at low pH. A more specific screening test can be performed by allowing urine to dry on filter paper and adding acetic acid and toluidine blue O. A purple color develops in the urine of patients with Hurler's syndrome. Metachromatic granules in the cytoplasm of circulating lymphocytes (*Reilly bodies*) are usually demonstrable and are useful diagnostic adjuncts. Since the primary inherited defect, a decrease in α-L-iduronidase, occurs in both Hurler's syndrome (MPS I H) and Scheie's syndrome (MPS I S), the distinction between the two syndromes must still be made on clinical grounds (see accompanying table). That Hurler's and Scheie's syndromes should be so different clinically yet have the same enzymatic defect is compatible with genetic allelism. The same gene undergoes mutation in both diseases but at different points on the same codon. An analogous situation exists with hemoglobin SS and hemoglobin CC disease.

Hurler's syndrome has features of cretinism but

The Principal Inherited Mucopolysaccharidoses

Designation	Clinical Features	Primary Inherited Deficiency
Hurler's syndrome (MPS I H)	Early corneal clouding, death before age ten; mental retardation	α-L-Iduronidase deficiency
Scheie's syndrome (MPS I S)	Corneal clouding, stiff joints, aortic incompetence; mental retardation	α-L-Iduronidase deficiency
Hunter's syndrome (MPS II)	No corneal clouding; milder course than Hurler's syndrome	Sulfoiduronate sulfatase deficiency
Sanfilippo's syndrome A (MPS III)	Mild somatic changes, severe mental retardation	Heparan sulfate sulfatase deficiency
Sanfilippo's syndrome B (MPS III)	Identical phenotype	N-acetyl-α-D-glucosaminidase deficiency
Morquio's syndrome (MPS IV)	Severe bone changes, cloudy cornea; normal intelligence	Unknown
Maroteaux-Lamy syndrome (MPS VI)	Severe bone and corneal change; normal intelligence	Unknown.

All are autosomally inherited except Hunter's syndrome, which is X-linked.

differs in that bone age is normal, tests of thyroid function are normal, and the patient is active.

Treatment. Although enzyme replacement with α-L-iduronidase may provide a new therapeutic approach to this disease, further work is needed to establish its clinical usefulness.

935. SCHEIE'S SYNDROME
(Mucopolysaccharidosis I S, MPS I S)

This rare autosomal variant of Hurler's syndrome is characterized by near normal intelligence, marked clouding of the cornea, and excretion of increased quantities of dermatan sulfate and heparan sulfate. The frequency of the disease is approximately 1 in 500,000 births. Aortic regurgitation and the carpal tunnel syndrome are common features of this mucopolysaccharidosis. The primary inherited defect is deficiency of α-L-iduronidase. A deficiency of α-L-iduronidase also occurs in Hurler's syndrome (see Ch. 934).

936. HUNTER'S SYNDROME
(Mucopolysaccharidosis II, MPS II)

This is the only mucopolysaccharidosis known to be inherited in an X-linked recessive fashion. The disease is similar to but clinically less severe than classic Hurler's syndrome. At birth Hunter's syndrome is one and one half times as frequent as Hurler's syndrome without regard to sex. In males, Hunter's syndrome is three times as common. Clouding of the cornea is minimal or absent, and mental deterioration occurs more slowly. Nodular thickening of the skin and deafness are common. Cardiac enlargement and pulmonary hypertension may be features of the disease. Increased urinary excretion of dermatan sulfate and heparan sulfate is the rule. Abnormal accumulations of mucopolysaccharides can be observed in cultured fibroblasts from affected individuals and heterozygous carriers of the abnormal gene. Deficiency of the enzyme *sulfoiduronate sulfatase* is characteristic of Hunter's syndrome. The deficiency can be detected in cultured fibroblasts.

937. SANFILIPPO'S SYNDROME
(Mucopolysaccharidosis III, MPS III)

Sanfilippo's syndrome is rare and is characterized by severe progressive mental retardation with relatively minor somatic changes. Corneal clouding is most uncommon, and dwarfism and hepatosplenomegaly are only moderately severe. The disease is inherited as an autosomal recessive and occurs in approximately 1 in 10,000 to 1 in 200,000 individuals. Many patients languish in mental institutions undiagnosed. As in the other mucopolysaccharidoses, cultured fibroblasts from affected individuals and heterozygous carriers demonstrate increased mucopolysaccharides. An increased urinary excretion of heparan sulfate, but not of dermatan sulfate, is diagnostic. Two clinically indistinguishable forms of Sanfilippo's syndrome have been found to have different enzymatic deficiencies. In one type, Sanfilippo A, the enzyme heparan sulfatase is deficient, whereas in Sanfilippo B, the enzyme N-acetyl-α-D-glucosaminidase is lacking.

938. MORQUIO'S SYNDROME
(Morquio-Brailsford Syndrome, Chondro-osteodystrophy, Mucopolysaccharidosis IV, MPS IV)

Patients with this recessively inherited syndrome are strikingly dwarfed. The characteristic radiologic features of the disease become evident after the age of two and consist of marked osteoporosis, platyspondyly, abnormalities of the femoral heads, and knock knees. Severe skeletal changes may lead to symptoms of spinal cord or medullary compression. Intelligence is unimpaired or trivially decreased. The disease has an estimated frequency of 1 in 40,000 births. Although not invariably present, an increased excretion of keratan sulfate in the urine is diagnostic. The urinary excretion of dermatan sulfate and heparan sulfate is normal. The basic defect is unknown.

939. MAROTEAUX-LAMY SYNDROME
(Mucopolysaccharidosis VI, MPS VI)

Early corneal clouding and normal intelligence are the distinguishing features of this rare autosomal variant of Hurler's syndrome. An increased excretion of dermatan sulfate can be demonstrated. Unlike Scheie's syndrome, the skeletal abnormalities are severe and aortic disease is absent. The enzyme defect in this disease is not yet elucidated.

The comparative clinical and biochemical features of the various mucopolysaccharidoses discussed in Ch. 934 to 939 are summarized in the table.

Dorfman, A.: Heritable diseases of connective tissue: The Hurler syndrome. *In* Stanbury, J. B., Wyngaarden, J. B., and Fredrickson, D. S. (eds.): The Metabolic Basis of Inherited Disease. 3rd ed. New York, McGraw-Hill Book Company, 1972.

McKusick, V. A.: Heritable Disorders of Connective Tissue. 4th ed. St. Louis, C. V. Mosby Company, 1972, pp. 521–686.

Neufeld, E. F.: The biochemical bases for mucopolysaccharidoses and mucolipidoses. *In* Steinberg, A. G., and Bearn, A. G. (eds.): Progress in Medical Genetics. Vol. X. New York, Grune & Stratton, 1974.

PORPHYRIA

Rudi Schmid

940.   INTRODUCTION

Porphyrins are tetrapyrrole pigments in which four monopyrroles are linked by four carbon bridges to form a planar ring structure. Each of the pyrroles has two substituent side chains, and the various porphyrins such as uro-, copro-, and protoporphyrin differ only in the nature of these side chains. Their sequential arrangement in specific porphyrins determines the structural isomer type, numbered I to IV. In nature, only porphyrins of the isomer types I and III have been identified. With the exception of protoporphyrin IX (belonging to the isomer type III series), which in the form of ferroprotoporphyrin (heme) serves as the prosthetic group of hemoglobin and other essential heme proteins, porphyrins apparently neither possess physiologic functions nor act as metabolic intermediates. Rather, they are metabolic by-products that have escaped from the biosynthetic path to heme by irreversible oxidation of the corresponding reduced porphyrinogens (see accompanying figure). The latter are intermediates in heme biosynthesis and are formed from the monopyrrole porphobilinogen (PBG), which in turn is synthesized by condensation of 2 moles of δ-aminolevulinic acid (ALA). The overall rate of heme and porphyrin biosynthesis is regulated primarily by the activity of ALA synthetase, which condenses glycine and succinyl-CoA to ALA. This mitochondrial enzyme system is reversibly repressed and inhibited by the final product, heme, and it is likely that this and other regulatory mechanisms are responsible for preventing both overproduction of heme and accumulation of metabolic intermediates. In porphyria, the increased excretion of ALA, PBG, or porphyrins results from an inherited defect or an acquired dysfunction of individual enzyme systems or control mechanisms of heme biosynthesis. Catabolism of hemoglobin and other heme proteins does not lead to formation of porphyrins; instead, the ferroprotoporphyrin ring is cleaved to biliverdin and bilirubin which are linear tetrapyrroles.

Although all aerobic cells can synthesize heme-containing chromoproteins, heme formation is particularly active in the erythroid elements of bone marrow and in liver. The small quantities of porphyrins and porphyrin precursors excreted normally in urine and bile are derived primarily from these sources. Similarly, the metabolic defects in porphyria that result in the accumulation and consequent increased excretion of porphyrins or their precursors usually can be traced to the erythroid cells of the bone marrow or to the liver, or to both. This distinction serves as a convenient basis for the classification of the porphyrias that follows:

A. Congenital erythropoietic porphyria
B. Hepatic porphyrias
   1. Genetic forms
      a. Acute intermittent porphyria
      b. Hereditary coproporphyria
      c. Variegate porphyria
   2. Porphyria cutanea tarda
   3. Acquired and secondary porphyrinuria
C. Erythrohepatic protoporphyria

The classification indicates the major sites of the metabolic disturbance and separates the hereditary forms of porphyria from those with an uncertain genetic basis and from the rare instances in which porphyrinuria appears to be acquired.

It should be noted that increased urinary excretion of porphyrins or precursors, including ALA and PBG, occurs in a variety of conditions other than porphyria. Chronic lead poisoning is commonly associated with increased ALA, and elevated PBG occasionally has been observed in carcinomatosis, Hodgkin's disease, cirrhosis, and affections of the nervous system. Normal urine contains only traces of uroporphyrin, but increased concentrations may be present in heavy metal poisoning and occasionally in parenchymal liver disease; gross uroporphyrinuria has been reported in patients with benign or malignant tumors of the liver. Coproporphyrin frequently is increased in lead poisoning, hemolytic and refractory anemia, hepatitis, cirrhosis, infectious mononucleosis, and alcoholism. In liver disease, coproporphyrinuria may not indicate increased formation of the pigment, but rather its diversion from bile to urine. Protoporphyrin, which has only 2 carboxyl groups and consequently is poorly soluble in water, does not appear in urine, but is excreted exclusively in the bile. The feces regularly contain copro-, proto-, and deuteroporphyrin, but these pigments may be derived in part from food, intestinal hemorrhage, and colonic microflora. Because of the wide range in fecal porphyrin concentration, values up to 200 μg per gram dry weight may not be indicative of porphyria without additional diagnostic evidence.

BIOSYNTHESIS OF HEME

The metabolic pathway from glycine and succinate to heme.
  Abbreviations: ALA, δ-aminolevulinic acid; PBG, porphobilinogen; UROgen, uroporphyrinogen; COPROgen, coproporphyrinogen; URO, uroporphyrin; COPRO, coproporphyrin; PROTO, protoporphyrin; I, III, isomer types I and III.

941. CONGENITAL ERYTHROPOIETIC PORPHYRIA
(Congenital Photosensitive Porphyria, Günther's Disease)

This very rare disease is due to a hereditary defect of porphyrin metabolism in the erythroid cells that leads to chronic photosensitivity, hemolytic anemia, and increased urinary excretion of uroporphyrin. Only about 80 cases in both sexes have been reported. Inheritance is by autosomal recessive transmission; heterozygous individuals appear clinically normal.

Excretion of pinkish urine usually begins shortly after birth, whereas cutaneous lesions on exposed parts, increased hemolysis, and splenomegaly may not be detected until later. Hypertrichosis and erythrodontia are virtually always present. Urine contains high concentrations of uroporphyrin I and coproporphyrin I, but excretion of ALA and PBG is normal. Hemoglobin frequently is decreased, and reticulocytes and fecal urobilinogen are increased. Erythrocytes contain much uroporphyrin I, and normoblasts and reticulocytes exhibit intense red fluorescence. The metabolic defect involves faulty conversion of PBG to uroporphyrinogen III in the maturing erythroid cells of the bone marrow. Death may occur in childhood, but if patients live to maturity, they usually exhibit severe scarring and mutilation of hands and face. Successful pregnancy with delivery of phenotypically normal children has been reported. Treatment is symptomatic and prophylactic, consisting essentially of rigorous protection from sunlight. In some instances hemolytic anemia, photosensitivity, and porphyrin excretion have been improved by splenectomy.

942. HEPATIC PORPHYRIAS

ACUTE INTERMITTENT PORPHYRIA

Definition, Incidence, and Genetics. Acute intermittent porphyria (synonyms: *acute porphyria, porphyria hepatica, pyrroloporphyria, Swedish type*) is an abnormality of pyrrole metabolism inherited as a dominant trait. It is associated with recurrent attacks of abdominal pain, gastrointestinal dysfunction, and neurologic manifestations. It is probably the most common form of porphyria, with an over-all incidence of approximately 1 per 100,000 population, but, because of its occurrence in large families, regional incidence may be much higher. The total number of reported cases suggests that people of Scandinavian, Anglo-Saxon, and German ancestry are affected more frequently, whereas the disease is very rare in blacks.

Acute attacks are rarely seen before puberty; they most often begin in the third or fourth decade, and occur more frequently in women. Manifestations may appear only in later life, or recurrent symptoms may be so vague and protean as to escape recognition. Indeed, persons carrying the genetic abnormaltiy may remain free of clinical manifestations throughout life; such latent porphyria tends to be more frequent in men. This probably accounts for the alleged preponderance of porphyria in women of child-bearing age.

Clinical Manifestations. Moderate to severe abdominal pain, often colicky, is frequently the initial or most prominent symptom. The pain may be localized, generalized, or radiating to the back or loins, but the abdomen usually is soft. Abdominal tenderness and distention may exist, but are much less striking than would be expected from the intensity of the pain. Leukocytosis and mild fever may be present. Diarrhea occasionally occurs. Severe vomiting and persistent constipation are frequent and may be accompanied by lack of bowel sounds and dilatation of the stomach. Roentgenograms of the abdomen may reveal distended intestinal loops proximal to areas of spasm; volvulus and gangrene have been reported. Gastrointestinal complications commonly lead to weight loss and occasionally to severe emaciation. Prolonged vomiting may cause dehydration, oliguria, and azotemia.

Neurologic disturbances frequently, though not always, are associated with abdominal manifestations and may involve the peripheral, central, or autonomic nervous system. Peripheral neuropathy usually is predominantly motor, may be asymmetrical, and may vary from mild weakness in one extremity to complete flaccid quadriplegia. These motor disturbances may be preceded or accompanied by severe pain, particularly in the legs. Deep tendon reflexes are usually diminished or absent and, although subjective sensory symptoms are frequent, objective sensory loss is less common. Cranial nerve involvement leads to optic atrophy, ophthalmoplegia, facial palsy, dysphagia, and vocal cord paresis. Weakness of abdominal, intercostal, or diaphragmatic musculature may progress to respiratory paralysis, which has a poor prognosis and ranks as the chief cause of death. Wasting and contracture of affected muscles frequently occur but are reversible to a surprising degree during prolonged remissions.

Many patients have a long history of nervousness, emotional instability, and functional disturbances that may remain unexplained until an acute attack occurs. Striking psychiatric abnormalities include personality changes, hysteria, psychoses, and confusional states. With more severe central nervous system involvement, delirium, coma, and epileptic seizures may occur; on occasion they have followed ingestion of barbiturates or maladvised surgical exploration of the abdomen.

Sinus tachycardia frequently accompanies acute attacks, and the pulse rate has been found to be a good index of the activity of the disease. This is believed to be due to vagal neuropathy, which also may account for nonspecific electrocardiographic abnormalities. Transient hypertension is often present, and on occasion spasm of retinal arteries has been observed. Frank photosensitivity does not occur in acute intermittent porphyria, but mild and apparently reversible pigmentation, particularly of exposed parts of the body, may accompany acute phases of the disease.

Acute episodes vary widely in duration and frequency. Some patients complain merely of occasional and intermittent abdominal pain, whereas in others the initial attack may begin almost explosively and may terminate fatally within days to several weeks. In the majority of cases, distinct attacks recur at irregular intervals over months or years, but tend to decrease in frequency and severity with age. There is strong evidence that attacks may be precipitated by a variety of drugs, including barbiturates, sulfonamides, griseofulvin, estrogens, and contraceptives, all of which are metabolized by microsomal enzyme systems of the liver, that contain hemoproteins. Occasionally, periodic exacerbations are correlated with the menstrual cycle, or latent porphyria may become clinically manifest late in pregnancy or shortly after delivery.

Laboratory Findings and Pathogenesis. The most characteristic laboratory finding is excessive ALA and PBG in the urine. PBG is a colorless chromogen giving a red complex with Ehrlich aldehyde (p-dimethylaminobenzaldehyde in HCl) which after neutralization cannot be extracted with chloroform or butanol (*Watson-Schwartz test*). By contrast the red color produced by Ehrlich aldehyde with urobilinogen or indoles is readily extractable with chloroform or butanol. Ingestion of antipyrine or admixture of methyl red (Zephiran) results in urine that turns red on acidification alone, whereas compounds of the phenolphthalein group show red only in alkaline urine. During acute episodes of porphyria, the Watson-Schwartz test is almost always strongly positive; if the reaction is faintly pink or negative, the diagnosis remains doubtful. In latent porphyria or in patients recovered from an acute attack, urinary excretion of PBG frequently is less pronounced or may be normal so that the Watson-Schwartz test may be negative. In these instances, urinary ALA and PBG should be quantitated by chromatographic methods, which commonly but not invariably reveal increased excretion of these porphyrin precursors. Freshly passed urine may be normal in color and usually contains relatively little preformed uro- and coproporphyrin. It darkens on standing because of conversion of PBG and other precursors to porphyrins and porphobilin, a dark brown pigment of unknown structure. Fecal porphyrins are within normal limits or moderately increased.

Except for a moderate reduction in the circulating red cell volume, hematologic abnormalities usually are absent. Conventional liver function tests frequently yield normal results except for increased BSP retention. The urine may contain increased concentrations of amino acids and indoles; the latter sometimes give an atypical Ehrlich reaction. Elevated protein-bound iodine, cholesterol, and β-lipoprotein levels have been reported. During acute attacks hyponatremia may become an alarming complication; although this often can be ascribed to prolonged vomiting or excessive intravenous fluid replacement, inappropriate secretion of antidiuretic hormone has been demonstrated. The liver is microscopically normal or shows mild focal or centrilobular necrosis and fatty changes. It usually does not exhibit porphyrin fluorescence, but contains much PBG. Inconstant neuropathologic changes include patchy demyelination of the peripheral or central nervous system and chromatolysis of anterior horn cells.

The inherited biochemical defect consists of a partial deficiency of the enzyme *uroporphyrinogen synthetase* which converts PBG to uroporphyrinogen. The ensuing impairment of heme synthesis secondarily leads to derepression of ALA synthetase, which results in increased formation and urinary excretion of ALA and its condensation product, PBG. Although this enzymatic defect is demonstrable in a variety of tissues, including circulating erythrocytes, its functional expression appears to be limited to the liver. Drugs and hormones known to aggravate the disease have been shown to induce the activity of hepatic ALA synthetase. The pathogenesis of

the abdominal and nervous manifestations is unknown, but a toxic effect of ALA or PBG has not been ruled out.

Diagnosis and Differential Diagnosis. The diagnosis rests primarily on the determination of increased urinary excretion of ALA and PBG. As a screening procedure, the qualitative Watson-Schwartz test usually is adequate, but for a definitive diagnosis, quantitative determination with chromatographic methods is essential. In prepubertal children and in asymptomatic adults suspected of having latent porphyria, urinary ALA and PBG may be normal; in these instances detection of the inherited defect requires demonstration of reduced uroporphyrinogen synthetase activity in erythrocytes or other tissues. Lead intoxication may produce severe abdominal pain and neuropathy, but the urine rarely contains sufficient PBG to give a positive Watson-Schwartz test, although ALA excretion frequently is increased.

The possibility of porphyria should always be considered in the presence of unexplained abdominal pain, because the disease has been mistaken for cholelithiasis, renal colic, peptic ulcer, appendicitis, bowel obstruction, pancreatitis, and pelvic disorders. Some patients have undergone several surgical procedures before the correct diagnosis was established. Acute attacks seldom last less than 48 hours, and very brief episodes of pain followed by complete remission rarely occur. Obscure neurologic disturbances, especially unexplained peripheral neuropathy, regional muscle weakness, flaccid paralysis, or bulbar palsy, should suggest the possibility of porphyria. Similarly, if hysterical behavior, psychoneurosis, psychosis, or unexplained epilepsy is aggravated by barbiturates, coincides with the menstrual cycle, or is noted in patients under treatment with contraceptives, porphyria should be suspected.

Persistent tachycardia, muscle weakness, and elevated protein-bound iodine may lead to confusion with hyperthyroidism. Occasionally weakness, abdominal pain, pigmentation, and hyponatremia may suggest Addison's disease. During the last trimester of pregnancy, hypertension, vomiting, and oliguria suggestive of eclampsia may in reality be due to porphyria. Provocative diagnostic tests by deliberate administration of barbiturates should be discouraged.

Treatment and Prognosis. There is no specific treatment for acute intermittent porphyria, and therapy remains symptomatic and prophylactic. Acute pain and psychic manifestations usually can be alleviated or controlled with phenothiazines, reserpine, or meperidine. Oral phenothiazines, such as chlorpromazine (25 to 100 mg four times daily), are the preferred treatment for abdominal and muscle pain. Neuropsychiatric manifestations frequently respond to relatively small doses of reserpine. Meperidine (Demerol) by intramuscular injection in doses of 50 to 100 mg may give prompt though transient relief; but, in general, use of opiates should be limited, because the severity and chronicity of the pain render porphyric patients particularly susceptible to addiction. When recurrent manifestations are clearly related to the menstrual cycle, prolonged androgenic suppression has given promising results.

Acute attacks often can be aborted by prompt administration of carbohydrate ("glucose effect"). Intravenous infusion of glucose or fructose at a rate of 10 to 15 grams per hour for 24 hours, or comparable amounts of oral carbohydrates, may result in striking remissions, particularly in patients whose attacks were precipitated or aggravated by anorexia, nausea, and vomiting. In addition, supportive treatment is of great importance. Dehydration and hyponatremia should be prevented. If bulbar signs are present, respiratory paralysis should be anticipated and a mechanical respirator made available. When fever and leukocytosis in excess of 12,000 per cubic millimeter are suggestive of occult infection, most often of the respiratory or urinary tract, sulfonamides should not be used. Drugs in general and barbiturates, griseofulvin, glutethimide, estrogens, and contraceptives in particular should be avoided.

In the earlier literature, the prognosis of acute intermittent porphyria was considered grave, with a mortality of 80 per cent within five years of the first attack. This figure undoubtedly is high; indeed, more recent reports set it around 25 per cent. Death occurs most frequently during the second and third decades, whereas beyond this age manifestations tend to be less severe and the prognosis distinctly improves.

HEREDITARY COPROPORPHYRIA

Hereditary coproporphyria was recognized only recently as a distinct entity. Clinically it resembles variegate porphyria except that a larger percentage of affected individuals remain asymptomatic, or photosensitivity may be the only symptom. As in acute intermittent and variegate porphyria, drugs may precipitate acute attacks which are associated with increased urinary excretion of ALA and PBG. The unique biochemical abnormality is the striking increase in fecal coproporphyrin excretion, whereas fecal protoporphyrin concentration usually is low. During acute attacks, urinary coproporphyrin excretion also may be very high. The disease is inherited as a dominant trait, and the sexes are equally affected. Treatment is the same as for acute intermittent porphyria.

VARIEGATE PORPHYRIA

Definition, Incidence, and Genetics. Variegate porphyria (synonyms: *porphyria cutanea tarda, protocoproporphyria hereditaria, mixed hepatic porphyria, South African genetic porphyria*) is a hereditary abnormality of porphyrin metabolism associated with chronic cutaneous manifestations alone or in conjunction with acute, transient attacks of abdominal pain and neuropathy. The disease is inherited as a dominant trait and the sexes are equally affected. Because of its occurrence in large family groups, the incidence varies widely in different parts of the world. Among white settlers of South Africa it is estimated at 3 per 1000. It undoubtedly is very much less elsewhere, although reliable figures are not available.

Clinical Manifestations. Cutaneous symptoms consist of dermal abrasions, superficial erosions, and blister formation after trivial trauma, and commonly are first noted during the second or third decade. The excessive mechanical fragility is usually limited to exposed parts of the skin. The lesions tend to heal slowly, often leave pigmented or slightly depressed scars, and are subject to secondary infection. Direct sensitivity to sunlight is infrequent, but the distribution of the cutaneous lesions leaves little doubt that light exposure is an important

pathogenic factor. Hyperpigmentation of the face and hands is common, and women often exhibit hypertrichosis, particularly of the temporal margins. The extent of these manifestations, varies considerably, but after increased fragility of the skin has developed, it rarely disappears completely. In some instances the abnormality is minimal and remains unnoticed, whereas in others chronicity and secondary infection lead to severe scarring and disfigurement. Cutaneous lesions are uncommon before puberty; they are usually milder in women, but during pregnancy become more pronounced.

Although in many patients manifestations remain limited to the skin, acute episodes of abdominal pain, neuropathy, and encephalopathy, similar in all aspects to those in acute intermittent porphyria, are not uncommon. Barbiturates, sulfonamides, general anesthetics, and excessive amounts of ethanol or. estrogens frequently appear to be precipitating or aggravating factors. During acute episodes mortality is approximately 25 per cent, but since many patients never develop acute manifestations, the over-all mortality of variegate porphyria is much lower. Genetic studies from South Africa suggest that before the widespread use of barbiturates and sulfonamides, kinships with porphyria survived and propagated as well as the unaffected population. Unless they terminate fatally, acute attacks commonly resolve completely, although neuropathy and muscle weakness may persist for several months. Evidence of hepatic dysfunction and histologic abnormality, including steatosis, fibrosis, or cirrhosis, is not uncommon, and biopsy material from the liver frequently shows extensive porphyrin fluorescence.

Laboratory Findings and Pathogenesis. The characteristic finding in variegate porphyria is the large amount of copro- and particularly protoporphyrin in the bile and feces. Fecal excretion of these pigments is continuous throughout the course of the disease, and takes place even in those patients with minimal cutaneous manifestations and in asymptomatic children with the genetic trait. PBG and porphyrin levels in the urine are usually slightly elevated, but the qualitative test for PBG is frequently negative. During acute attacks urinary excretion of ALA, PBG, and, at times, uro- and coproporphyrin is greatly increased, and may reach values comparable to those in acute intermittent porphyria in relapse. Azotemia, hypochloremia, hyponatremia, and jaundice may be present, but readily resolve as the acute attack subsides and the disease converts to its cutaneous form.

The exact nature of the inherited biochemical defect is unclear, but it undoubtedly involves increased formation of ALA, PBG, and porphyrins in the liver. Chronic exposure to sunlight is important in the pathogenesis of the cutaneous lesions, but the mechanism underlying the abnormal mechanical fragility of the skin is unclear.

Diagnosis and Differential Diagnosis. The diagnosis can best be established by demonstrating increased porphyrin in the feces. The following qualitative test frequently suffices. A small piece of stool is thoroughly mixed with four parts of ethyl ether and one part of glacial acetic acid, the mixture is filtered, and the filtrate is extracted with 5 per cent hydrochloric acid. Under ultraviolet light with a Wood filter, extracts of porphyric feces exhibit intense red fluorescence, which is faint or absent with normal stool. In quantitative determinations, values in excess of 40 μg of protoporphyrin per gram of dry feces are suggestive of porphyria. During acute attacks the diagnosis can be ascertained by demonstrating increased ALA and PBG excretion in the urine.

Chronic cutaneous lesions limited to exposed parts, abnormal skin fragility, a positive family history, and increased fecal porphyrin excretion usually permit distinction of variegate porphyria from most other skin diseases. Erythrohepatic protoporphyria is the only other light-sensitive dermatosis associated with increased fecal porphyrins, but in this condition erythrocyte or plasma protoporphyrin is usually increased, and the reaction to light is prompt and transient. During acute attacks it may be difficult to distinguish between variegate and acute intermittent porphyria, except that the former diagnosis is suggested by concomitant skin involvement or a positive personal or family history of cutaneous manifestations.

Treatment. Treatment is symptomatic and prophylactic. Management of acute attacks is the same as for acute intermittent porphyria. Exposure to direct sunlight should be minimized and the hands protected from mechanical trauma by gloves. Of paramount importance is avoidance of drugs known to precipitate porphyria.

PORPHYRIA CUTANEA TARDA

Porphyria cutanea tarda (synonyms: *porphyria cutanea tarda symptomatica; constitutional* or *idiosyncratic porphyria; symptomatic porphyria*) is a relatively frequent sporadic form of cutaneous porphyria, characterized by chronic skin lesions, hepatic dysfunction, and uroporphyrinuria. Abdominal and neurologic manifestations are absent. The disease is more common in males and usually begins insidiously, most often in the fourth to sixth decade. It occurs in all parts of the world, but is most frequent in the Bantus of South Africa. Exposed skin shows abnormalities similar to those of variegate porphyria, ranging from slight dermal fragility to severe chronic scarring and disfiguration. The lesions often are more active in summer and tend to heal in winter. Hyperpigmentation and hirsutism are frequent and may be the presenting symptoms. Hepatomegaly with chemical and histologic evidence of liver disease, often caused by chronic alcoholism, is present in the great majority of patients. Disseminated lupus erythematosus appears to occur in porphyria cutanea tarda more frequently than can be accounted for by coincidence. In addition to uroporphyrin, variable degrees of hemosiderosis are frequently found in the liver. Although hepatic hemosiderosis may not differ from that seen in nonporphyric patients with chronic liver disease, recent evidence suggests that cutaneous manifestations and porphyrin excretion may be improved by repeated venesection.

Urinary excretion of uro-type porphyrins and, to a lesser extent, coproporphyrin is greatly increased, and urine may be pink or brownish. Fecal porphyrins are normal or slightly increased, and excretion of ALA or PBG is almost never elevated. The excreted porphyrins undoubtedly are derived from the liver, but the underlying biochemical defect is unknown. Because of the absence of a positive family history, the disturbance is generally assumed to be acquired, usually in association with some other form of liver disease, frequently one caused by alcoholism. However, since only a very small percentage of patients with chronic liver disease develop porphyria, the possibility of a genetically determined but normally undetected defect activated by hepatic injury cannot be ruled out. Treatment is symptomatic and directed toward the primary liver disease. Abstinence in alcoholic patients results in significant improvement or disappearance of the porphyria. Chloroquine and cholestyramine may be useful in reducing the photosensitivity, but both compounds need further clinical evaluation.

In rare instances, intoxications may lead to a form of hepatic porphyria that is *acquired*. Porphyria characterized by cutaneous manifestations, hepatic dysfunction, and uroporphyrinuria has been reported in population groups accidentally exposed to hexachlorobenzene or biphenyls.

943. ERYTHROHEPATIC PROTOPORPHYRIA
(Erythropoietic Protoporphyria)

In this recently recognized form of porphyria, high concentrations of protoporphyrin in erythrocytes, plasma, and feces are associated with solar urticaria or solar eczema. Short exposure to sunlight results in intense pruritus, erythema, and edema of exposed skin. These lesions appear during or immediately after exposure, subside in 12 to 24 hours, and usually heal without significant scarring, atrophy, or pigmentation. Occasionally cutaneous manifestations develop only after prolonged exposure to sunlight, or the initial acute skin lesions may progress to a chronic eczematous stage, persisting for weeks and healing with superficial scar formation. Skin manifestations commonly begin during childhood or adolescence, are more severe in summer, and recur throughout life. Affected skin shows neither abnormal mechanical fragility nor blister formation characteristic of the other forms of photosensitive porphyria. Erythrodontia, hirsutism, hyperpigmentation, and neurologic manifestations are lacking. Photosensitivity is mediated by protoporphyrin in plasma or skin and is evoked by near-ultraviolet light in the 400 nm range, in which porphyrins absorb maximally. The excessive protoporphyrin in plasma and feces is derived primarily from the liver, the erythroid cells serving as a minor source. Fasting increases the plasma protoporphyrin level, whereas carbohydrate administration reduces both protoporphyrin formation and photosensitivity. Urinary porphyrin excretion is normal.

The disturbance occurs in both sexes and appears to be inherited as a dominant trait. A significant percentage of persons carrying the genetic abnormality remain clinically asymptomatic, and detection may be possible only by repeated determination of erythrocyte and fecal protoporphyrin concentration. The disease generally has a good prognosis, and neither results in permanent disability nor influences normal life expectancy. However, the incidence of cholelithiasis is distinctly increased, and chronic intrahepatic cholestasis progressing to cirrhosis has been reported. Treatment is prophylactic and consists largely in protection from direct sunlight.

Dean, G.: The Porphyrias. 2nd ed. London, Pitman Medical Publishing Company, 1971.

Goldberg, A.: Porphyrins and porphyrias. *In* Goldberg, A., and Brain, M. C. (eds.): Recent Advances in Haematology. Edinburgh and London, Churchill Livingstone, 1971.

Marver, H. S., and Schmid, R.: The porphyrias. *In* Stanbury, J. B., Wyngaarden, J. B., and Fredrickson, D. C. (eds.): The Metabolic Basis of Inherited Disease. 3rd ed. New York, McGraw-Hill Book Company, 1972.

Meyer, U. A., and Schmid, R.: Hereditary hepatic porphyrias. Fed. Proc., 32:1649, 1973.

Miescher, P. A., and Jaffe, E. R. (eds.): Porphyria and disorders of porphyrin metabolism. Semin. Hematol., 5:293, 1968.

Tschudy, D. P.: Porphyrin metabolism and the porphyrias. *In* Bondy, P. K., and Rosenberg, L. E. (eds.): Duncan's Diseases of Metabolism. 7th ed. Philadelphia, W. B. Saunders Company, 1974.

Waldenström, J., and Haeger-Aronsen, B.: The porphyrias: A genetic problem. Prog. Med. Genet., 5:58, 1967.

Watson, C. J.: The problem of porphyria—some facts and questions. N. Engl. J. Med., 263:1205, 1960.

944. PSEUDOXANTHOMA ELASTICUM

Clayton E. Wheeler, Jr.

Definition. Pseudoxanthoma elasticum is an uncommon, inherited disorder of connective tissue characterized by yellow skin lesions at flexural areas, retinal angioid streaks, chorioretinitis, arterial disease, and visceral bleeding tendencies. The combination of cutaneous lesions and angioid streaks is called the *Grönblad-Strandberg syndrome.*

Etiology. The primary defect appears to be genetically determined premature degeneration and calcification of connective tissue of the skin, eyes, and cardiovascular system. Elastic tissue is probably the abnormal component, although abnormality of collagen has not been excluded. Autosomal recessive inheritance with partial limitation to the female is found most often, but dominant inheritance may occasionally occur.

Incidence. The disorder occurs in all races, in both sexes, and at any age. Skin lesions occur slightly more frequently in females, and angioid streaks more frequently in males. The disease may be present at birth or infancy, but the diagnosis is made most frequently in the third to fifth decades.

Pathology. The histologic picture of cutaneous lesions is diagnostic. The epidermis and upper corium are normal. Characteristic changes consist of granular or rodlike accumulations of basophilic material and calcium deposits in the middle and lower dermis. The basophilic material stains like elastic tissue but shows the periodicity of collagen when examined by the electron microscope. The eye shows basophilia and rents of Bruch's elastic lamina, sclerosis of choroidal vessels, and scleral changes that simulate those of the skin. Elastic tissue degeneration affects the media of vessels of medium and larger size. White plaques histologically resembling those in the skin have been found on the pericardium and endocardium of the ventricles and right atrium, and some investigators suspect specific involvement of the mitral valve.

Clinical Manifestations. The three major areas affected are skin, eyes, and cardiovascular system. Combined skin and eye changes are found in approximately 60 per cent of the cases, skin alone in 10 per cent, and eyes alone in 30 per cent. Cardiovascular abnormalities are present in nearly 80 per cent of the patients if careful search is made. The impression has been gained that the disorder is more severe when skin lesions are well developed, but instances of advanced cardiovascular or eye involvement occur in the absence of clinical cutaneous abnormalities.

Cutaneous lesions are small, soft, chamois-colored papules arranged parallel to skin lines and folds; the result is a crepelike or Moroccan leather appearance. A network of fine telangiectatic vessels sometimes outlines the papules. Coalescence produces circumscribed or diffuse plaques. In mild cases the lesions may be seen only after the skin is stretched. In advanced cases the skin is thickened, hangs in loose, inelastic folds, and resembles the skin of a plucked chicken. Sites of most frequent involvement are the sides of the neck, axillae, groin, cubital and popliteal fossae, and the periumbilical area, but the face, breasts, undersurface of the penis, and the perianal area may be affected as well as the mucosa of the mouth, palate, vagina, and rectum. Papular and arcuate lesions of elastosis perforans serpiginosa may occur in pseudoxanthoma elasticum as well as in Ehlers-Danlos syndrome and other connective tissue diseases.

Angioid streaks of the retina are the most characteristic eye lesions. These lie behind the retinal vessels. They are most numerous around the optic disc, which they may encircle and from which they course like vessels over the fundus. They are flat, serrated streaks varying from narrow lines to three or four times the diameter of retinal veins. They are red, brown, gray, or black, and there may be hemorrhage or white areas of connective tissue proliferation along their course. The streaks are usually bilateral, although not symmetrical, and tend to progress slowly or to become stationary. When the streaks involve the macula, loss of vision occurs. Other eye changes are central chorioretinitis that may also involve the macula, pigmented stippling of the fundus, and hemorrhage from retinal vessels.

Patients often have premature and advanced arterial changes indistinguishable from arteriosclerosis or atherosclerosis with predilection for medium-sized arteries. These changes may result in weak or absent peripheral pulses of the arms or legs, easy fatigability of the legs, intermittent claudication, angina, arrhythmias, cerebrovascular accidents, and mental deterioration. Hypertension occurs in about half the cases. Renal hemangioma and abnormalities of renal arteries may be found. Left ventricular hypertrophy, congestive heart failure, and coronary thrombosis may occur, and mitral valvular disease has been reported. Pulse wave studies of involved extremities show decreased amplitude and velocity, and the dicrotic notch may be lost.

Internal hemorrhage is a special feature of the vascular disease. Bleeding from the gastrointestinal tract occurs in about 10 per cent of the cases, and it may be severe or fatal. Bleeding may arise in peptic ulcer, hiatal hernia, or ulcerative colitis, or its clinical origin may not be demonstrable. Other sites of hemorrhage are skin, subarachnoid space, kidney, uterus, bladder, nasal mucosa, and joints.

The association of thyrotoxicosis, diabetes mellitus, diabetes insipidus, low fertility, amenorrhea, and impotence with pseudoxanthoma elasticum has been suggested but seems doubtful.

Diagnosis. Cutaneous lesions are diagnostic, especially if confirmed by biopsy. Diagnostic histologic changes may be present when clinical findings are minimal or absent. Senile elastosis, a degenerative disease of dermal connective tissue, resembles pseudoxanthoma elasticum, but it affects only exposed sites. The histologic appearance rules out pseudoxanthoma. Angioid streaks are highly suggestive but not pathognomonic, because they are seen in sickle cell disease and in a small percentage of patients with Paget's disease of bone. Structures resembling angioid streaks occur in rupture of the choroid, choroidal arteriosclerosis, perivascular choroidal pigmentary atrophy, and pigmented streaks of retinal detachment. Cardiovascular changes must be accompanied by typical changes of the eye or skin before their association with pseudoxanthoma elasticum can be ascertained.

Treatment. There is no effective treatment of the basic disease. Symptomatic therapy is indicated for hypertension, congestive failure, subarachnoid or gastrointestinal hemorrhage, cerebrovascular accident, angina, and intermittent claudication. Plastic surgery is sometimes helpful for correction of cosmetic cutaneous defects.

Prognosis. Cutaneous lesions are usually of small consequence. The majority of patients develop angioid streaks, and approximately three quarters of these undergo visual impairment from damage to the macula. Complete blindness, which is unusual, results from glaucoma, vitreous hemorrhage, or retinal detachment. Morbidity and death may result from cerebrovascular accident, heart disease, or internal hemorrhage at any age; however, many patients live a normal span.

Huang, S., Kumar, G., Steele, H. D., and Parker, J. O.: Cardiac involvement in pseudoxanthoma elasticum. Am. Heart J., 74:680, 1967.
McKusick, V. A.: Heritable Disorders of Connective Tissue. 4th ed. St. Louis, C. V. Mosby Company, 1972.
Olinder, I., and Boström, H.: Clinical studies on a Swedish material of pseudoxanthoma elasticum. Acta Med. Scand., 19:273, 1972.
Percival, S. P. B.: Angioid streaks and elastorrhexis. Br. J. Ophthal., 52:297, 1968.
Wilhelm, K., and Paver, K.: Sudden death in pseudoxanthoma elasticum. Med. J. Aust., 2:1363, 1972.

945. WILSON'S DISEASE
(Hepatolenticular Degeneration)
Alexander G. Bearn

Wilson's disease is a rare, autosomal recessively inherited disease characterized by degenerative changes in the brain, particularly in the basal ganglia, and cirrhosis of the liver. A brownish pigmented ring at the corneal margin, the Kayser-Fleischer ring, is pathognomonic of the disease.

Clinical Manifestations. The disease is frequently insidious in onset, manifesting itself as tremor and incoordination in the second or third decade of life. Deteriorating handwriting and difficulty in speech may be common early symptoms. While the patient is at rest, the tremor is often minimal and can be alleviated by resting the hands on a table or placing them in a pocket. Attempts to perform purposive movements are less successful, and a wild ataxia frequently develops. Rarely, symptoms occur as early as four years of age or may be delayed until the fourth decade of life. In late childhood and early adolescence, the disease is more likely to be rapidly progressive; rigidity, dysarthria, and dysphagia occur more frequently than tremor. Uncontrollable choreoathetotic movements and staggering may be particularly distressing. The sensory system is unaffected, and pyramidal signs are usually absent. In the terminal stages of the disease the patient is frequently febrile and emaciated. Muscular rigidity, contractures, and mental deterioration dominate the clinical picture, and the patient becomes completely bedridden.

In adults, clinical signs of severe hepatic insufficiency are uncommon, although slight abnormalities in liver function can be detected, and cirrhosis can be recognized by liver biopsy. In childhood, however, the disease commonly presents as atypical or prolonged hepatitis, which may be indistinguishable from juvenile cirrhosis. Signs of central nervous system dysfunction are minimal or absent. Portal hypertension can frequently be demonstrated, and ascites and hepatic coma may supervene. Rarely, massive bleeding from esophageal varices may be the first manifestation of the disease. Jaundice may be an early symptom, and is frequently followed by several years of normal health.

Behavioral and personality changes, acute schizophrenic episodes, transient hemiparesis, and unexplained Coombs-negative hemolytic anemia may also herald the onset of the disease. Unusual pigmentation of the lower extremities, azure lunulae of the nails, and bone lesions may be found.

Genetics. The disease is ubiquitous and occurs in approximately 1 in 200,000 persons. It is particularly common in populations with a high inbreeding coefficient. As anticipated in a rare autosomal recessive disease, an increased consanguinity in the parents of affected persons is extremely common; in one series the frequency of marriages among first cousins was 36 per cent. Clinically normal heterozygous carriers of the gene have been estimated to occur with a frequency of approximately 1 in 500.

Pathogenesis. A decrease in the biliary excretion of copper is the primary disturbance in Wilson's disease; this results in an accumulation of copper in the brain, liver, kidney, and other tissues, including Descemet's membrane of the cornea, where it gives rise to the characteristic *Kayser-Fleischer ring*. The copper first accumulates in the liver and is stored initially in the hepatocytes, and later in the lysosomes. As the disease progresses, the accumulation of copper causes hepatocellular damage with release of copper from within the hepatocyte. The copper released from the liver is distributed and deposited in various tissues of the body, giving rise to cellular and organ damage.

In normal persons, approximately 95 per cent of the copper in serum is bound to ceruloplasmin whereas the remaining 5 per cent is loosely bound to serum albumin. In patients with Wilson's disease, there is a decrease in the concentration of serum ceruloplasmin and total serum copper and an increase in the easily dissociable albumin-bound copper. The excretion of copper in the urine is usually considerably increased. Exceptionally, and particularly in girls with chronic active hepatitis or cirrhosis, the serum copper and ceruloplasmin levels may be normal. Accumulation of copper in the kidneys selectively damages the proximal renal tubules. Aminoaciduria, glycosuria, phosphaturia, uricosuria, and calciuria may be present. The serum phosphate and serum uric acid also may be decreased.

Pathology. Although it is assumed that accumulation of copper in the tissues is responsible for the symptoms, the brain may appear surprisingly normal at autopsy. Slight generalized atrophy is common, particularly of the basal ganglia. An accumulation of large astrocytes is found throughout the central nervous system and is more marked in the basal ganglia and cerebral cortex. In the rare acute form of the disease, cavitation of the putamen, globus pallidus, caudate nucleus, and cerebral cortex may be evident. In the asymptomatic stage of the disease, the liver is grossly and histologically normal despite an increase in the hepatic concentration of copper. As the disease progresses, liver damage occurs and the characteristic pathologic changes of chronic active hepatitis or postnecrotic cirrhosis become evident. Glycogen degeneration of hepatic cell nuclei, with the accumulation of cytoplasmic fat droplets, is frequently observed.

Diagnosis. The disease should be suspected in all cases of unexplained tremor and rigidity, particularly in early adult life. The differential diagnosis includes Parkinson's syndrome, cerebellar ataxia, chorea, and choreoathetosis. In children and young adults, the disease frequently presents with symptoms resulting from chronic active hepatitis, and the disease should be suspected in all cases of juvenile cirrhosis. The presence of *Kayser-Fleischer rings* is pathognomonic of the disease, but these may be absent in children under the age of ten. They are golden brown or green-brown, and are located at the limbus and may encircle the entire cornea. In the early stages of the disease, a careful slit-lamp examination may be needed to demonstrate their presence with certainty. Needle biopsy of the liver and determination of the hepatic copper concentration should be undertaken in all patients in whom the diagnosis is suspected. In most patients with Wilson's disease the copper content of the liver is usually greater than 200 μg per gram dry weight (normal, less than 50 μg per gram dry weight); in some patients it may reach a level of 2000 μg per gram. A decrease in serum ceruloplasmin (less than 20 mg per 100 ml) can nearly always be observed and, in the absence of malnutrition, sprue, or the nephrotic syndrome, is virtually diagnostic. The disease is difficult to diagnose unequivocally in the first six months of life, because decreased ceruloplasmin and increased hepatic copper are common in normal children.

Treatment. The aim is to decrease the total body copper and prevent its reaccumulation. A high-protein, low-copper diet with the addition of sulfurated potash, technical (20 mg three times daily, with meals), is often recommended, although it is not as important as intensive and continued drug therapy. The administration of D-penicillamine (β, β-dimethylcysteine), 1 to 2 grams a day, depending on body weight, is the treatment of choice and should be continued indefinitely. A "sensitivity" reaction associated with fever, arthralgia, and leukopenia may occur. Desensitization with steroids should be undertaken and penicillamine therapy cautiously reinstituted. Except for the occasional occurrence of skin reactions, toxic reactions are seldom seen. The nephrotic syndrome has been reported in a few patients, and the urine should be monitored regularly for proteinuria. Pyridoxine deficiency, as a result of treatment with penicillamine, may give rise to optic neuritis but can be prevented by administration of pyridoxine, 50 mg daily.

Persistent decrease in serum ceruloplasmin accompanied by elevated hepatic copper in an asymptomatic sib of a patient with Wilson's disease is an indication to begin therapy. In newborn infants treatment should be delayed until it is apparent that the decreased serum ceruloplasmin and increased hepatic copper have persisted beyond the normal physiologic period of three to six months. When penicillamine treatment is started early and continued indefinitely, symptomatic improvement is usually dramatic and long continued. In the absence of treatment the disease is invariably fatal.

Bearn, A. G.: Wilson's Disease. *In* Stanbury, J. B., Wyngaarden, J. B., and Fredrickson, D. S. (eds.): The Metabolic Basis of Inherited Disease. 3rd ed. New York, McGraw-Hill Book Company, 1972.

Sass-Kortsak, A.: Hepatolenticular degeneration (Kinnear-Wilson's disease). *In* von Schwiegk, H. (ed.): Handbuch der Inneren Medizin. 5th ed. Berlin, Springer-Verlag, 1974.

Sternlieb, I.: Evolution of the hepatic lesion in Wilson's disease (hepatolenticular degeneration). *In* Popper, H., and Schaffner, F. (eds.): Progress in Liver Diseases, Vol. IV. New York, Grune & Stratton, 1972.

946. WERNER'S SYNDROME

Alexander G. Bearn

This rare, recessively inherited syndrome is characterized by scleroderma-like changes in the skin, especially in the extremities, symmetrical growth retardation with absence of the adolescent growth spurt, a senile appearance, and premature graying of the hair. Cataract, soft tissue and vascular calcifications, and premature arteriosclerosis are common. Diabetes mellitus occurs in 50 per cent of the patients and is of the insulin-resistant type. Certain features of Werner's syndrome resemble scleroderma, progeria, and myotonic dystrophy.

Epstein, C. J., Martin, G. M., Schultz, A. L., and Motulsky, A. G.: Werner's syndrome. A review of its symptomatology, natural history, pathologic features, genetics and relationship to the natural aging process. Medicine, 45:177, 1966.

Part XXII
NORMAL LABORATORY VALUES OF CLINICAL IMPORTANCE

947. THE USE AND INTERPRETATION OF LABORATORY-DERIVED DATA

James B. Wyngaarden

When you can measure what you are speaking about, and express it in numbers, you know something about it. Lord Kelvin, 1889.

The basic workup of a patient begins with the acquisition of data. The experienced clinician will insist upon a discerning and sensitive history, a thorough physical examination, and such laboratory tests as are necessary to evaluate the general health of his patient, to arrive at a specific diagnosis, to assess the functional status of involved organs, and to provide a basis for monitoring effectiveness of therapy.

The inclusion of a panel of chemical tests or enzyme assays of blood (or urine) as a part of a basic medical evaluation is in a state of evolution. A decade ago many physicians would have ordered a fasting blood sugar and blood urea nitrogen determination as a part of the general workup, and other tests only if suggested by a differential diagnosis constructed from the clinical evaluation.

In 1966 Thiers published a provocative study comparing the results of a screening battery of eleven tests run by an automated multichannel analyzer with those of tests specifically ordered on the same patients by physicians as part of the admission workup. The screening battery detected twice as many abnormal test results of significance to the patient as were uncovered by selective ordering. The most common findings were elevated glucose or uric acid concentration values. Ensuing developments were rapid. Ingenious automated analyzers have brought an increasing number and variety of tests of diagnostic utility within the reach of all practitioners. In the larger hospitals and teaching centers it is now common practice to include a "Chem 12," or "Chem 18," as a standard component of the initial workup. The cost of such a screening battery is now no greater than that of three or four selected tests run manually a decade ago.

This new practice has profound implications in the teaching of medical students and house officers. One can no longer evaluate the reasoning process which led the house officer to order a serum calcium determination. Some of the intellectual discipline of the construction of a logical differential diagnosis is now gone. The information comes automatically by a computer print-out. Attention has shifted from the selective acquisition of data to the interpretation and use of it, including the evaluation of significance of test results and (perhaps) the selection of a second round of tests and studies. The gains surely outweigh the losses. Since many diseases present initially with rather nonspecific constitutional symptoms, the clinical approach may not suggest the most appropriate laboratory tests, and the initial laboratory screen may disclose unexpected hypercalcemia, acidosis, azotemia, or evidence of liver disease.

In order to utilize the results of laboratory tests intelligently (and economically), the physician must be able to evaluate the validity of the test result, he must understand principles of variation and distribution of values, and he must be able to integrate the data received from the laboratory with the information he has acquired from the patient. If the test result deviates from values found in a healthy control population, is the difference trivial, or is it indicative of important dysfunction? Should the test be repeated? How often need a particular measurement be followed? What additional tests or studies are indicated on the basis of these leads?

The more information the physician has about his patient, the more effective the physician should be in caring for him. To ensure that this is the result requires a sophisticated knowledge of medical science, excellent clinical judgment, and a profound respect for the limitations of the laboratory. One of the best ways of acquiring the constructively critical attitude so essential to the proper evaluation of laboratory test results is for the student or house officer to work in a laboratory for a while. There is an irony in the present pattern of medical education: at a time of unparalleled reliance upon an ever-expanding universe of laboratory tests in the practice of medicine, first-hand learning experiences in the laboratory are being progressively eliminated from the medical curriculum.

SOME LIMITATIONS OF THE LABORATORY

Criteria for Evaluation of Laboratory Methods. A trustworthy laboratory test must pass critical evaluations of specificity, sensitivity, accuracy, and precision.

Specificity refers to the detection of the substance in question and no other. It is doubtful that any test is absolutely specific for the substance being measured. There is always some other substance around that is capable of reacting. In biochemical analyses this limitation is most serious in tests dependent upon color development, less in the case of assays dependent upon degradation by purified enzymes, and perhaps least in such procedures as atomic absorption spectroscopy.

Sensitivity refers to the ability of the test to detect the substance in question at the required concentrations, namely, those at which the compound exists in body fluids.

Accuracy refers to the quantitative detection of the

correct amount of the substance being measured. This property rests upon both specificity and sensitivity. A test may be accurate in the absence of certain interfering drugs, and only in a certain range of values. It may fail this criterion under other conditions.

Precision embodies *repeatability,* the obtaining of the same result on samples analyzed in replicate fashion, and *reproducibility,* representing quality control over time. Precision rests upon the specificity, sensitivity, and accuracy of the method, and characterizes the procedure under conditions of actual use in the diagnostic laboratory.

The "Law of Errors." Early in the nineteenth century, the German mathematician and physicist, Johann C. F. Gauss, introduced the "law of errors." This law states that in repeated measurements of the *same* object or substance, the random component on the errors will be distributed about the mean as a frequency function. This distribution, which is bell shaped, is often called "normal" or "gaussian." Note that the law applies to repeated measurements of the same item. Its extension to a population of those items is justifiable only under certain circumstances, for not all distributions are bell shaped, and not all bell-shaped distributions are gaussian. The matter of distributions will be discussed further below, when we consider the topic of the "normal range" of a biological variable. First, however, it may be pertinent to emphasize the topic of error, for every laboratory measurement is subject to it.

SOURCES OF ERROR

These are legion, and include some factors under the control of the clinician, such as the dietary preparation of the patient, and the techniques of collection and handling of samples. Reduction of the error factor to an acceptable minimum requires continuous compulsive attention to every detail of the process.

Laboratory Errors. There is imprecision in every measurement. In tests run by hand, pipetting, timing, reading, and recording errors occur. They are more frequent when technicians are overworked or fatigued. It is common to find greater scatter of results of replicate tests at the end of the day than at the beginning. Technician fatigue can be largely eliminated by automation, but there will always remain the technical limitations of machines and the human error in the preparation of reagents, in the standardization of instruments, and in the copying of test results. The last is not totally avoided by the computer print-out, as even typewriters make mistakes. Quality control of laboratory performance is both a science and an art. Control criteria vary widely from laboratory to laboratory. Split samples submitted to different laboratories may show surprising disparities in results.

Drug Interference. According to Osler, man is distinguished from all other members of the Animal Kingdom by his desire to take drugs. Since many patients do not regard proprietary pain remedies or vitamins as drugs, the physician may obtain a negative drug history unless questions are appropriately phrased. Drugs have great potential for interference with laboratory tests. High resolution chromatography of urine yields about 300 peaks of ultraviolet absorbing materials. Two hundred and fifty of these disappear if the "normal subject" abstains from salicylates and vitamins for a few days. Salicylates and vitamins also produce chromogens which interfere with certain analytic methods employed in automated tests, particularly of the urine.

DISTRIBUTIONS OF VALUES

There is widespread belief among medical students and graduate physicians that if the sample of test results from a healthy population is large enough, the distribution will be "normal" (gaussian); that on this assumption one may justifiably determine a mean value ($\bar{x}$) and its standard deviation (δ); that the value, $\bar{x} \pm 2\delta$, will include the central 95 per cent of all measurements; that this segment of the distribution is the "normal range;" and that values which fall outside this range are by definition "abnormal." All these beliefs are erroneous in most instances. The experimental fact is that for most physiological variables the distribution is smooth, unimodal, and skewed, and that $\bar{x} \pm 2\delta$ does not cut off the desired central 95 per cent. Among the distributions of serum calcium, inorganic phosphorus, magnesium, alkaline phosphatase, total proteins, albumin, uric acid, and blood urea, only that of albumin is gaussian. All others are skewed, leptokurtic, or both. The value $\bar{x} \pm 2\delta$ will cut off many more measurements in one tail of the distribution than the other. The uncritical application of principles of normal distributions in situations in which variables are not normally distributed leads occasionally to values of $\bar{x} - 2\delta$ which are negative, surely a biological absurdity.

Once we discard the notion that the distribution of values in healthy persons is gaussian, the question of estimating the mean and standard deviation does not arise. One is then spared the awkward exercise of fitting skewed distributions to bell-shaped curves by constructing histograms of logarithms of the data (a technique which has the effect of compressing the skewed tail to create a "log-gaussian distribution"), or by constructing plots of cumulative frequencies of values (or log-values) on probability paper in search of the linear relationship indicative of a normal distribution (see accompanying figure).

These pitfalls can be circumvented by use of *nonparametric* methods for estimating the normal range, that is, methods which do not involve any a priori assumption regarding the parental distribution shape except that it is continuous. Two nonparametric methods of normal range estimation are the method of *percentile estimates* with associated nonparametric confidence intervals, and the method of nonparametric *tolerance intervals* which include a specified proportion of the population with a specified probability. The required sample sizes of healthy persons for the normal value studies are large, just as they are with parametric methods.

The percentile method of expressing interindividual variation in many kinds of data has been in use for a long time. Physicians are familiar with its use in pediatric growth charts of height and weight. The method avoids the arbitrary distinction of normal and abnormal. It also removes the aura of precision of the standard deviation, expressed to two or more decimal places. The percentile method appropriately fits the real world of nongaussian distributions.

From every laboratory test for which a good normal-

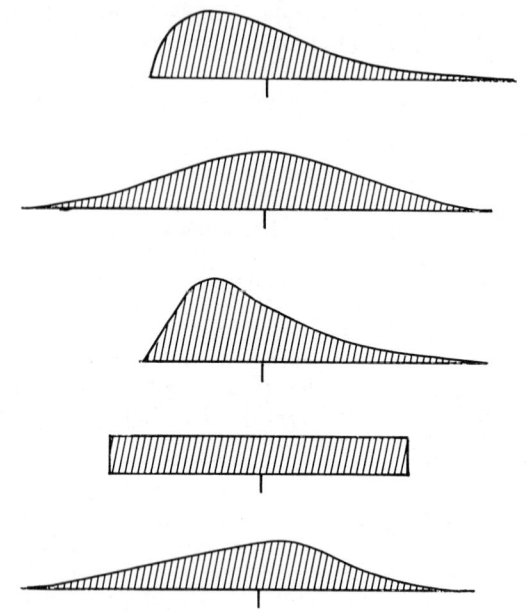

Five distributions with the same mean and standard deviation ($\bar{x} = 4$, $\delta = 2.83$). From top to bottom: χ_4^2 normal, lognormal, rectangular, and mixture of two normals. (From Elveback, L. R.: Mayo Clinic Proc. 47:93, 1972; with permission.)

value study has been done, the laboratory can report not only the result but also the percentile corresponding to that result and appropriate to the age and sex of the patient under study. With this information the clinician can know how common or how unusual the test result is. This information obviates the necessity of remembering a large number of complicated relationships. The percentile method is superior to an arbitrary definition of a normal range, such as $\bar{x} \pm 2\delta$, even in those few cases in which a distribution is gaussian, for it indicates for each test result the relationship of that result to the healthy population. The percentile method is also superior to the definition of the normal range as the range of all observed values in a healthy sample population, for this method seriously underestimates any selected segment, e.g., the central 95 per cent, in small samples, and overestimates it in large samples.

The percentile method does not systematically over- or underestimate any selected range, regardless of sample size. If one wishes to cut off the lowest and highest 2.5 per cent, or 5 per cent, one simply orders all values and finds the value that cuts off the desired percentage of observations at either tail of the distribution. The complete percentile range is readily defined. No assumptions are required about distribution shape except that it is continuous. From the size of the healthy population represented in the distribution, the confidence limits of a given percentile may be ascertained, with known probability, by reference to standard tables. The method should particularly appeal to clinicians who utilize local norms, which are often based on small samples.

The "Normal Range." From this discussion, it is clear that "normal range" is an arbitrary and potentially misleading term. By whatever method it is defined, the normal range will exclude observations of the parental distribution of healthy subjects and will very likely include some values of other distributions. What is desired by the clinician is an expression of cut-off points at either end of a distribution, such that by far the largest number of values of healthy individuals is included in the central segment, and as few values as possible are included that are part of another distribution, i.e., that the number of false positives and false negatives are both minimized. Ingrained habits, perhaps now indelible, will probably lead us to continue to select the central 95 per cent of the parental distribution as "clinical limits," even though there is no magic in this number. Some clinical investigators have advocated use of the central 90 per cent.

Influence of Age. The distributions of values of many plasma constituents vary with age in the healthy population. For example, plasma cholesterol concentrations, mean and 90 per cent limits, are 180 (120 to 240) mg per 100 ml in the "normal" 20- to 29-year age group, and 245 (160 to 330) mg per 100 ml in the "normal" 50- to 59-year age group. Whether values of 325 mg per 100 ml in the older age group are biologically "normal" simply because they fall in the 90 to 95 percentile range could be debated.

Influence of Sex. Distributions in men may differ from those in women. For example, plasma urate concentration values, mean and 90 per cent limits, are 4.9 (2.7 to 7.2) mg per 100 ml in men, and 4.0 (2.5 to 6.3) mg per 100 ml in premenopausal women. Mean serum calcium values in normal men decline 0.0068 mg per 100 ml per year from age 20 to age 80. Those of women show no regression against age. This is an important point in the diagnosis of hyperparathyroidism which is chiefly a disease of the older age group.

Biological Rather Than Statistical Norms. This concept has been alluded to above, in the suggestion that the clinical norms of serum cholesterol concentrations should perhaps be defined in terms of age-related values that are noninjurious, rather than as a 90 percentile range. Perhaps the 5 to 50 percentile range should be selected as the "clinical limits" or "normal" range in the older population. Such an approach requires a biological rather than statistical definition, but data are not yet available to set reliable limits in this manner.

A more secure example concerns urate concentration values. An electrolyte solution with the sodium concentration of plasma is saturated with urate at 6.4 to 6.8 mg per 100 ml. In addition, proteins of plasma bind urate equivalent to about 5 per cent of the amount in solution. Values above 7.0 (perhaps 7.2) mg per 100 ml represent supersaturation and are "abnormal" in that they are associated with increased risk of renal stone and clinical gout. The risk factors increase as urate concentration values increase above 7.0 mg per 100 ml. The 95 per cent limits of serum urate values in "healthy" male New Zealand Maoris are 4 to 10 mg per 100 ml, and 10 per cent of adult males develop gout. Surely the central 95 per cent of the distribution of the general male population cannot be considered "normal," even though the reference sample is appropriately selected by the usual criteria.

Discontinuous Distributions. Some traits may be distributed bimodally, or trimodally. Such relationships are most likely to emerge from studies of families in which there is a monogenetic disease characterized by a chemical abnormality. For example, measurements of galactose-1-phosphate uridyltransferase activity in the families of patients with transferase deficiency galactosemia are distributed trimodally. The effects of two and of one mutant allele are clearly distinguishable from the normal and from each other. Assay values in the three modes are zero, 7.5 to 13.5 units, and 19.5 to 32 units. The intermediate enzyme assay values are found in subjects who are presumed heterozygotes by pedigree analysis. It is common to hear the term "heterozygote value" applied to an enzyme activity value approximately one half of normal. This practice is justifiable only when assay data are combined with pedigree data, for there may be other reasons for a reduced enzyme assay value that have nothing to do with genetics.

An apparent continuous distribution with marked skewing may at times be dissected into two or even three distribution modes by appropriate clinical and pedigree studies. For example, the distribution of plasma cholesterol concentrations in familial hypercholesterolemia displays marked overlap between subjects who are clinically normal and those who are heterozygotes by pedigree analysis. Similarly, there is considerable overlap between heterozygotes and abnormal homozygotes. Only a complete family pedigree permits adequate definition of the range of values in each distribution mode.

THE PHYSICIAN AND THE LABORATORY TEST RESULT

The tables that follow contain values which define the limits of the clinical norms. They represent the best data currently available, but are subject to all the un-

certainties discussed above. In some instances more selective data of an age- and sex-matched control population will need to be consulted by the physician.

Clinical judgment rather than exclusive reliance on published normal ranges will always be required. For example, a serum BUN concentration of 22 mg per 100 ml is not a normal value for a patient on a rice diet. Also, electrolyte test results of sodium 145 mEq per liter, potassium 3.5 mEq per liter, chloride 96 mEq per liter, and CO_2 30 mEq per liter may indicate metabolic alkalosis even though all individual values fall within published normal ranges.

Laboratory tests are critical to the diagnosis of disease and management of patients. They have both great value and inherent imprecision. The doctor must know the limits of reliability and usefulness of each test result in the clinical setting of the individual patient. This is particularly true when all deviant test results have returned to normal but the patient is not improving. It is especially when laboratory data provide little or no help that the patient needs a doctor.

Bryan, D. J., Wearne, J. L., Viau, A., Musser, A. W., Schoonmaker, F. W., and Thiers, R. E.: Profile of admission chemical data by multichannel automation: An evaluative experiment. Clin. Chem., 12:137, 1966.

Elveback, L. R., Guillier, C. L., and Keating, F. R.: Health, normality, and the ghost of Gauss. J.A.M.A., 211:69, 1970.

Keating, F. R., Jones, J. D., Elveback, L. R., and Randall, R. V.: The relation of age and sex to distribution of values in healthy adults of serum calcium, inorganic phosphorus, magnesium, alkaline phosphatase, total proteins, albumin, and blood urea. J. Lab. Clin. Med., 73:825, 1969.

Mainland, D.: Remarks on clinical "norms." Clin. Chem., 17:267, 1971.

948. NORMAL LABORATORY VALUES OF CLINICAL IMPORTANCE

Rex B. Conn

NORMAL HEMATOLOGIC VALUES

For some procedures the normal values may vary, depending upon the methods used.

Acid hemolysis test (Ham)		No hemolysis
Alkaline phosphatase, leukocyte		Total score 14–100
Bleeding time		
Ivy		Less than 7 min
Duke		1–7 min
Carboxyhemoglobin		Up to 5% of total
Cell counts		
Erythrocytes: Males		4.6–6.2 million/cu mm
Females		4.2–5.4 million/cu mm
Children (varies with age)		4.5–5.1 million/cu mm
Leukocytes		
Total		5000–10,000/cu mm

Differential	Percentage	Absolute
Myelocytes	0	0/cu mm
Juvenile neutrophils	3– 5	150– 400/cu mm
Segmented neutrophils	54–62	3000–5800/cu mm
Lymphocytes	25–33	1500–3000/cu mm
Monocytes	3– 7	285– 500/cu mm
Eosinophils	1– 3	50– 250/cu mm
Basophils	0– 0.75	15– 50/cu mm

(Infants and children have greater relative numbers of lymphocytes and monocytes)

Platelets	150,000–350,000/cu mm
Reticulocytes: Adults	25,000–75,000/cu mm
	0.5–1.5% of erythrocytes
Newborns	4–6% of erythrocytes
Clot retraction, qualitative	Begins in 30–60 mm
	Complete in 24 hours
Coagulation factors:	
Factor activity	
Factors II, V, VII, IX, X, XI	70–120%
Factor VIII	60–120%
Coagulation time (Lee-White) (room temp.)	5–15 min (glass tubes)
	19–60 min (siliconized tubes)
Cold hemolysin test (Donath-Landsteiner)	No hemolysis
Corpuscular values of erythrocytes	
(Values are for adults; in children, values vary with age)	
M.C.H. (mean corpuscular hemoglobin)	27–31 picogm
M.C.V. (mean corpuscular volume)	80–105 cu micra
M.C.H.C. (mean corpuscular hemoglobin concentration)	32–36%
Fibrinogen	200–400 mg/100 ml
Hematocrit	
Males	40–54 ml/100 ml
Females	37–47 ml/100 ml
Newborn	49–54 ml/100 ml
Children (varies with age)	35–49 ml/100 ml
Hemoglobin	
Males	14.0–18.0 grams/100 ml
Females	12.0–16.0 grams/100 ml
Newborn	16.5–19.5 grams/100 ml
Children (varies with age)	11.2–16.5 grams/100 ml
Hemoglobin, fetal	Less than 1% of total
Hemoglobin A_2	1.5–3.0% of total
Hemoglobin heat stability	No precipitation
Hemoglobin oxygen affinity (p50)	26–28 mm Hg

NORMAL HEMATOLOGIC VALUES (*Continued*)

Hemoglobin, plasma	0–5.0 mg/100 ml
Methemoglobin	0.03–0.13 gram/100 ml
Osmotic fragility of erythrocytes	
Immediate	10% lysis in 0.45–0.50% NaCl
	50% lysis in 0.40–0.45% NaCl
	90% lysis in 0.35–0.42% NaCl
After 24 hours incubation	10% lysis in 0.57–0.66% NaCl
	50% lysis in 0.47–0.60% NaCl
	90% lysis in 0.28–0.50% NaCl
Partial thromboplastin time	35–45 sec
Prothrombin consumption	Over 80% consumed in 1 hr
Prothrombin content	100% (calculated from prothrombin time)
Prothrombin time (one stage)	12.0–14.0 sec
Sedimentation rate	
Wintrobe: Males	0–5 mm in 1 hr
Females	0–15 mm in 1 hr
Westergren: Males	0–15 mm in 1 hr
Females	0–20 mm in 1 hr
(May be slightly higher in children and during pregnancy)	
Thromboplastin generation test	Compared to normal control
Tourniquet test	Ten or fewer petechiae in a 2.5 cm circle after 5 min with cuff at 100 mm Hg

Bone marrow, differential cell count	Range	Average
Myeloblasts	0.3– 5.0%	2.0%
Promyelocytes	1.0– 8.0%	5.0%
Myelocytes: Neutrophilic	5.0–19.0%	12.0%
Eosinophilic	0.5– 3.0%	1.5%
Basophilic	0.0– 0.5%	0.3%
Metamyelocytes ("juvenile" forms)	13.0–32.0%	22.0%
Polymorphonuclear neutrophils	7.0–30.0%	20.0%
Polymorphonuclear eosinophils	0.5– 4.0%	2.0%
Polymorphonuclear basophils	0.0– 0.7%	0.2%
Lymphocytes	3.0–17.0%	10.0%
Plasma cells	0.0– 2.0%	0.4%
Monocytes	0.5– 5.0%	2.0%
Reticulum cells	0.1– 2.0%	0.2%
Megakaryocytes	0.03– 3.0%	0.4%
Pronormoblasts	1.0– 8.0%	4.0%
Normoblasts	7.0–32.0%	18.0%

NORMAL BLOOD, PLASMA, AND SERUM VALUES

For some procedures the normal values may vary depending upon the methods used.

Acetone, serum	
Qualitative	Negative
Quantitative	0.3–2.0 mg/100 ml
Aldolase, serum	0.8–3.0 milliunits/ml (IU) (30°) (Sibley-Lehninger)
Alpha amino nitrogen	4–6 mg/100 ml
Ammonia nitrogen, blood	75–196 μg/100 ml
plasma	56–122 μg/100 ml
Amylase, serum	80–160 Somogyi units/100 ml
Ascorbic acid	See Vitamin C
Base, total, serum	145–160 mEq/liter
Bilirubin, serum	
Direct	0.1–0.4 mg/100 ml
Indirect	0.2–0.7 mg/100 ml
	(Total minus direct)
Total	0.3–1.1 mg/100 ml
Calcium, serum	4.5–5.5 mEq/liter
	(9.0–11.0 mg/100 ml)
	(Slightly higher in children)
	(Varies with protein concentration)

NORMAL BLOOD, PLASMA, AND SERUM VALUES (*Continued*)

Calcium, serum, ionized	2.1–2.6 mEq/liter
	(4.25–5.25 mg/100 ml)
Carbon dioxide content, serum	24–30 mEq/liter
	Infants: 20–28 mEq/liter
Carbon dioxide tension (Pco_2), blood	35–45 mm Hg
Carotene, serum	50–300 μg/100 ml
Ceruloplasmin, serum	23–44 mg/100 ml
Chloride, serum	96–106 mEq/liter
Cholesterol, serum	
Total	150–250 mg/100 ml
Esters	68–76% of total cholesterol
Cholinesterase, serum	0.5–1.3 pH units
RBC	0.5–1.0 pH units
Copper, serum	
Male	70–140 μg/100 ml
Female	85–155 μg/100 ml
Cortisol, plasma	6–16 μg/100 ml
Creatine, serum	0.2–0.8 mg/100 ml
Creatine phosphokinase, serum	
Male	0–50 milliunits/ml (IU) (30°)
Female	0–30 milliunits/ml (IU) (30°) (Oliver-Rosalki)
Creatinine, serum	0.7–1.5 mg/100 ml
Cryoglobulins, serum	0
Fatty acids, total, serum	190–420 mg/100 ml
Fibrinogen, plasma	200–400 mg/100 ml
Folic acid, serum	7–16 nanogm/ml
Glucose (fasting)	
blood, true	60–100 mg/100 ml
Folin	80–120 mg/100 ml
plasma or serum, true	70–115 mg/100 ml
Haptoglobin, serum	40–170 mg/100 ml
Hydroxybutyric dehydrogenase, serum	0–180 milliunits/ml (IU) (30°) (Rosalki-Wilkinson)
	114–290 units/ml (Wroblewski)
17-Hydroxycorticosteroids, plasma	8–18 μg/100 ml
Immunoglobulins, serum	
IgG	800–1500 mg/100 ml
IgA	50–200 mg/100 ml
IgM	40–120 mg/100 ml
Iodine, butanol extractable, serum	3.2–6.4 μg/100 ml
Iodine, protein bound, serum	3.5–8.0 μg/100 ml
	(May be slightly higher in infants)
Iron, serum	75–175 μg/100 ml
Iron binding capacity, total serum	250–410 μg/100 ml
% saturation	20–55%
17-Ketosteroids, plasma	25–125 μg/100 ml
Lactic acid, blood	6–16 mg/100 ml
Lactic dehydrogenase, serum	0–300 milliunits/ml (IU) (30°) (Wroblewski modified)
	150–450 units/ml (Wroblewski)
	80–120 units/ml (Wacker)
Lipase, serum	0–1.5 units (Cherry-Crandall)
Lipids, total, serum	450–850 mg/100 ml
Magnesium, serum	1.5–2.5 mEq/liter
	(1.8–3.0 mg/100 ml)
Nitrogen, nonprotein, serum	15–35 mg/100 ml
Osmolality, serum	285–295 mOsm/kg serum water
Oxygen, blood	
Capacity	16–24 vol % (varies with Hb)
Content Arterial	15–23 vol %
Venous	10–16 vol %
Saturation Arterial	94–100% of capacity
Venous	60–85% of capacity
Tension, Po_2 Arterial	75–100 mm Hg

NORMAL BLOOD, PLASMA, AND SERUM VALUES (*Continued*)

pH, arterial, blood	7.35–7.45
Phenylalanine, serum	Less than 3 mg/100 ml
Phosphatase, acid, serum	1.0–5.0 units (King-Armstrong)
	0.5–2.0 units (Bodansky)
	0.5–2.0 units (Gutman)
	0.0–1.1 units (Shinowara)
	0.1–0.63 unit (Bessey-Lowry)
Phosphatase, alkaline, serum	5.0–13.0 units (King-Armstrong)
	2.0–4.5 units (Bodansky)
	3.0–10.0 units (Gutman)
	2.2–8.6 units (Shinowara)
	0.8–2.3 units (Bessey-Lowry)
	30–85 milliunits/ml (IU)
	(Values are higher in children)
Phosphorus, inorganic, serum	3.0–4.5 mg/100 ml
	(Children: 4.0–7.0 mg/100 ml)
Phospholipids, serum	6–12 mg/100 ml as lipid phosphorus
Potassium, serum	3.5–5.0 mEq/liter
Proteins, serum	
Total	6.0–8.0 grams/100 ml
Albumin	3.5–5.5 grams/100 ml
Globulin	2.5–3.5 grams/100 ml
Electrophoresis	
Albumin	3.5–5.5 grams/100 ml
	52–68% of total
Globulin	
Alpha$_1$	0.2–0.4 gram/100 ml
	2–5% of total
Alpha$_2$	0.5–0.9 gram/100 ml
	7–14% of total
Beta	0.6–1.1 grams/100 ml
	9–15% of total
Gamma	0.7–1.7 grams/100 ml
	11–21% of total
Pyruvic acid, plasma	1.0–2.0 mg/100 ml
Serotonin, platelet suspension	0.1–0.3 μg/ml blood
serum	0.10–0.32 μg/ml
Sodium, serum	136–145 mEq/liter
Sulfates, inorganic, serum	0.8–1.2 mg/100 ml (as S)
Thyroxine, serum	4.4–9.9 μg/100 ml
Thyroxine, free, serum	1.0–2.1 nanogm/100 ml
Thyroxine binding globulin (TBG), serum	10–26 μg/100 ml
Thyroxine iodine (T$_4$), serum	2.9–6.4 μg/100 ml
Transaminase, serum	
SGOT	0–19 milliunits/ml (IU) (30°) (Karmen modified)
	15–40 units/ml (Karmen)
	18–40 units/ml (Reitman-Frankel)
SGPT	0–17 milliunits/ml (IU) (30°) (Karmen modified)
	6–35 units/ml (Karmen)
	5–35 units/ml (Reitman-Frankel)
Triglycerides, serum	0–150 mg/100 ml
Urea, blood	21–43 mg/100 ml
plasma or serum	24–49 mg/100 ml
Urea nitrogen, blood (BUN)	10–20 mg/100 ml
plasma or serum	11–23 mg/100 ml
Uric acid, serum	
Male	2.5–8.0 mg/100 ml
Female	1.5–6.0 mg/100 ml
Vitamin A, serum	20–80 μg/100 ml
Vitamin B$_{12}$, serum	200–800 picogm/ml
Vitamin C, blood	0.4–1.5 mg/100 ml

NORMAL URINE VALUES

Acetone and acetoacetate	0
Alcapton bodies	Negative
Aldosterone	3–20 μg/24 hrs.
Alpha amino nitrogen	50–200 mg/24 hrs
	(Not over 1.5% of total nitrogen)
Ammonia nitrogen	20–70 mEq/24 hrs
Amylase	35–260 Somogyi units/hr
Bence Jones protein	Negative
Bilirubin (bile)	Negative
Calcium	
Low Ca diet (Bauer-Aub)	Less than 150 mg/24 hrs
Usual diet	Less than 250 mg/24 hrs
Catecholamines	
Epinephrine	Less than 10 μg/24 hrs
Norepinephrine	Less than 100 μg/24 hrs
Chloride	110–250 mEq/24 hrs
	(Varies with intake)
Chorionic gonadotrophin	0
Copper	0–30 μg/24 hrs
Creatine	
Male	0–40 mg/24 hrs
Female	0–100 mg/24 hrs
	(Higher in children and during pregnancy)
Creatinine	15–25 mg/kg of body weight/24 hrs
Cystine or cysteine, qualitative	Negative
Delta aminolevulinic acid	1.3–7.0 mg/24 hrs

Estrogens	Male	Female
Estrone	3–8	4–31
Estradiol	0–6	0–14
Estriol	1–11	0–72
Total	4–25	5–100

(Units above are μg/24 hrs)
(Markedly increased during pregnancy)

Glucose (reducing substances)	Less than 250 mg/24 hrs
Gonadotrophins, pituitary	5–10 rat units/24 hrs
	10–50 mouse units/24 hrs
	(Increased after menopause)
Hemoglobin and myoglobin	Negative
Homogentisic acid, qualitative	Negative
17-Hydroxycorticosteroids	
Male	3–9 mg/24 hrs
Female	2–8 mg/24 hrs
	(Varies with method used)
5-Hydroxyindole-acetic acid (5-HIAA)	
Qualitative	Negative
Quantitative	Less than 16 mg/24 hrs
17-Ketosteroids	
Male	6–18 mg/24 hrs
Female	4–13 mg/24 hrs
Osmolality	38–1400 mOsm/kg water
pH	4.6–8.0, average 6.0
	(Depends on diet)
Phenylpyruvic acid, qualitative	Negative
Phosphorus	0.9–1.3 gm/24 hrs
	(Varies with intake)
Porphobilinogen	
Qualitative	Negative
Quantitative	0–0.2 mg/100 ml
	Less than 2.0 mg/24 hrs
Porphyrins	
Coproporphyrin	50–250 μg/24 hrs
Uroporphyrin	10–30 μg/24 hrs

NORMAL URINE VALUES (*Continued*)

Potassium	25–100 mEq/24 hrs
	(Varies with intake)
Pregnanetriol	Less than 2.5 mg/24 hrs in adults
Protein	
Qualitative	0
Quantitative	10–150 mg/24 hrs
Sodium	130–260 mEq/24 hrs
	(Varies with intake)
Solids, total	30–70 grams/liter, average 50 grams/liter
	(To estimate total solids per liter, multiply last two figures of specific gravity by 2.66, Long's coefficient)
Specific gravity	1.003–1.030
Sugar	0
Titratable acidity	20–40 mEq/24 hrs
Urobilinogen	Up to 1.0 Ehrlich unit/2 hrs (1–3 P.M.)
	0–4.0 mg/24 hrs
Vanillylmandelic acid (VMA)	1–8 mg/24 hrs

NORMAL VALUES FOR GASTRIC ANALYSIS

Basal gastric secretion (one hour)

	Concentration	Output
	Mean ± 1 S.D.	Mean ± 1 S.D.
Male	25.8 ± 1.8 mEq/liter	2.57 ± 0.16 mEq/hr
Female	20.3 ± 3.0 mEq/liter	1.61 ± 0.18 mEq/hr

After histamine stimulation

Normal	Mean output = 11.8 mEq/hr
Duodenal ulcer	Mean output = 15.2 mEq/hr

After maximal histamine stimulation

Normal	Mean output 22.6 mEq/hr
Duodenal ulcer	Mean output 44.6 mEq/hr

Diagnex blue (Squibb):	Anacidity	0–0.3 mg in 2 hrs
	Doubtful	0.3–0.6 mg in 2 hrs
	Normal	Greater than 0.6 mg in 2 hrs
Volume, fasting stomach content		50–100 ml
Emptying time		3–6 hrs
Color		Opalescent or colorless
Specific gravity		1.006–1.009
pH (adults)		0.9–1.5

NORMAL VALUES FOR CEREBROSPINAL FLUID

Cells	Fewer than 5 cu mm, all mononuclear
Chloride	120–130 mEq/liter
	(20 mEq/liter higher than serum)
Colloidal gold test	Not more than 1 in any tube
Glucose	50–75 mg/100 ml
	(20 mg/100 ml less than blood)
Pressure	70–180 mm water
Protein, total	15–45 mg/100 ml
Albumin	52%
Alpha$_1$ globulin	5%
Alpha$_2$ globulin	14%
Beta globulin	10%
Gamma globulin	19%

NORMAL VALUES FOR SEMEN

Volume	2–5 ml, usually 3–4 ml
Liquefaction	Complete in 15 min
pH	7.2–8.0; average 7.8
Leukocytes	Occasional or absent
Count	60–150 million/ml
	Below 60 million/ml is abnormal
Motility	80% or more motile
Morphology	80–90% normal forms

NORMAL VALUES FOR FECES

Bulk	100–200 grams/24 hrs
Dry matter	23–32 grams/24 hrs
Fat, total	Less than 6.0 grams/24 hrs
Nitrogen, total	Less than 2.0 grams/24 hrs
Urobilinogen	40–280 mg/24 hrs
Water	Approximately 65%

TOXICOLOGY

Arsenic, blood	3.5–7.2 μg/100 ml
Arsenic, urine	Less than 100 μg/24 hrs
Barbiturates, serum	0
	Coma level: Phenobarbital approximately 11 mg/100 ml; most other barbiturates 1.5 mg/100 ml
Bromides, serum	0
	Toxic levels above 17 mEq/liter
Carbon monoxide, blood	Up to 5% saturation
	Symptoms occur with 20% saturation
Dilantin, blood or serum	Therapeutic levels 1–11 μg/ml
Ethanol, blood	Less than 0.005%
Marked intoxication	0.3–0.4%
Alcoholic stupor	0.4–0.5%
Coma	Above 0.5%
Lead, blood	0–40 μg/100 ml
Lead, urine	Less than 100 μg/24 hrs
Lithium, serum	0
	Therapeutic levels 0.5–1.5 mEq/liter
	Toxic levels above 2 mEq/liter
Mercury, urine	Less than 10 μg/24 hrs
Salicylate, plasma	0
Therapeutic range	20–25 mg/100 ml
Toxic	Over 30 mg/100 ml
Death	45–75 mg/100 ml

LIVER FUNCTION TESTS

Bromsulphalein (B.S.P.)	Less than 5% remaining in serum 45 minutes after injection of 5 mg/kg of body weight
Cephalin cholesterol flocculation	0–1 in 24 hours
Galactose tolerance	Excretion of not more than 3.0 grams galactose in the urine 5 hours after ingestion of 40 grams of galactose
Glycogen storage	Increase of blood glucose 45 mg/100 ml over fasting level 45 minutes after subcutaneous injection of 0.01 mg/kg body weight of epinephrine
Hippuric acid	Excretion of 3.0–3.5 grams hippuric acid in urine within 4 hours after ingestion of 6.0 grams sodium benzoate

or

Excretion of 0.7 gram hippuric acid in urine within 1 hour after intravenous injection of 1.77 grams sodium benzoate

Thymol turbidity	0–5 units
Zinc turbidity	2–12 units

PANCREATIC (ISLET) FUNCTION TESTS

Glucose tolerance tests	Patient should be on a diet containing 300 grams of carbohydrate per day for 3 days prior to test.
Oral	After ingestion of 100 grams of glucose or 1.75 grams glucose/kg body weight, blood glucose is not more than 160 mg/100 ml after 60 minutes, 140 mg/100 ml after 90 minutes, and 120 mg/100 ml after 120 minutes. Values are for blood; serum measurements are approximately 15% higher.
Intravenous	Blood glucose does not exceed 200 mg/100 ml after infusion of 0.5 gram of glucose/kg body weight over 30 minutes. Glucose concentration falls below initial level at 2 hours and returns to preinfusion levels in 3 or 4 hours. Values are for blood; serum measurements are approximately 15% higher.
Cortisone-glucose tolerance test	The patient should be on a diet containing 300 grams of carbohydrate per day for 3 days prior to test. At 8½ and again 2 hours prior to glucose load patient is given cortisone acetate by mouth (50 mg if patient's ideal weight is less than 160 lb, 62.5 mg if ideal weight is greater than 160 lb). An oral dose of glucose, 1.75 grams/kg body weight, is given and blood samples are taken at 0, 30, 60, 90, and 120 minutes. Test is considered positive if true blood glucose exceeds 160 mg/100 ml at 60 minutes, 140 mg/100 ml at 90 minutes, and 120 mg/100 ml at 120 minutes. Values are for blood; serum measurements are approximately 15% higher.

RENAL FUNCTION TESTS

Clearance tests (corrected to 1.73 sq meters body surface area)

Glomerular filtration rate (G.F.R.)

  Inulin clearance,
  Mannitol clearance, or
  Endogenous creatinine clearance
    Males   110–150 ml/min
    Females 105–132 ml/min

Renal plasma flow (R.P.F.)

  p-Aminohippurate (P.A.H.), or
  Diodrast
    Males   560–830 ml/min
    Females 490–700 ml/min

Filtration fraction (F.F.)

$$FF = \frac{G.F.R.}{R.P.F.}$$

    Males   17–21%
    Females 17–23%

Urea clearance (C_u)
    Standard 40–65 ml/min
    Maximal 60–100 ml/min

Concentration and dilution
    Specific gravity >1.025 on dry day
    Specific gravity <1.003 on water day

Maximal Diodrast excretory capacity T_{M_D}
    Males   43–59 mg/min
    Females 33–51 mg/min

Maximal glucose reabsorptive capacity T_{M_G}
    Males   300–450 mg/min
    Females 250–350 mg/min

Maximal PAH excretory capacity $T_{M_{PAH}}$
    80–90 mg/min

Phenolsulfonphthalein excretion (P.S.P.)
    25% or more in 15 min
    40% or more in 30 min
    55% or more in 2 hrs
    After injection of 1 ml P.S.P. intravenously

THYROID FUNCTION TESTS

Protein bound iodine, serum (P.B.I.)	3.5–8.0 μg/100 ml
Butanol extractable iodine, serum (B.E.I.)	3.2–6.4 μg/100 ml
Thyroxine iodine, serum (T_4)	2.9–6.4 μg/100 ml
Free thyroxine, serum	1.4–2.5 nanogm/100 ml
T_3 (index of unsaturated T.B.G.)	10.0–14.6%
Thyroxine-binding globulin, serum (T.B.G.)	10–26 μg T_4/100 ml
Thyroid-stimulating hormone, serum (T.S.H.)	0 up to 0.2 milliunit/ml
Radioactive iodine (I^{131}) uptake (R.A.I.)	20–50% of administered dose in 24 hrs
Radioactive iodine (I^{131}) excretion	30–70% of administered dose in 24 hrs
Radioactive iodine (I^{131}), protein bound	Less than 0.3% of administered dose per liter of plasma at 72 hrs
Basal metabolic rate	Minus 10% to plus 10% of mean standard

GASTROINTESTINAL ABSORPTION TESTS

d-Xylose absorption test	After an 8 hour fast 10 ml/kg body weight of a 5% solution of d-xylose is given by mouth. Nothing further by mouth is given until the test has been completed. All urine voided during the following 5 hours is pooled, and blood samples are taken at 0, 60, and 120 minutes. Normally 26% (range 16–33%) of ingested xylose is excreted within 5 hours, and the serum xylose reaches a level between 25 and 40 mg/100 ml after 1 hour and is maintained at this level for another 60 minutes.
Vitamin A absorption test	A fasting blood specimen is obtained and 200,000 units of vitamin A in oil is given by mouth. Serum vitamin A level should rise to twice fasting level in 3 to 5 hours.

NORMAL VALUES FOR SEROLOGIC PROCEDURES

Anti-hyaluronidase	Less than 1:200. Significant if rising titer can be demonstrated at weekly intervals.
Anti-streptolysin O titer	Normal up to 1:128. Single test usually has little significance. Rise in titer or persistently elevated titer is significant.
Bacterial agglutinins	Significant only if rise in titer is demonstrated or if antibodies are absent.
Complement fixation tests	Titers of 1:8 or less are usually not significant. Paired sera showing rise in titer of more than two tubes are usually considered significant.
C reactive protein (C.R.P.)	Negative
Heterophile titer	Low titers may be present normally, but these antibodies are absorbed by Forssman antigen (guinea pig kidney). In infectious mononucleosis an elevated heterophile titer is present. The titer is only minimally reduced after incubation with guinea pig kidney but is significantly reduced after incubation with beef red cell stroma.

Proteus OX-19 agglutinins	1:80	Negative
	1:160	Doubtful
	1:320	Positive
R.A. test (latex)	1:40	Negative
	1:80–1:160	Doubtful
	1:320	Positive
Rose test	1:10	Negative
	1:20–1:40	Doubtful
	1:80	Positive
Tularemia agglutinins	1:80	Negative
	1:160	Doubtful
	1:320	Positive

Castleman, B., and McNeely, B. U.: N. Engl. J. Med., 290:39, 1974.
Davidsohn, I., and Henry, J. B.: Clinical Diagnosis by Laboratory Methods. 15th ed. Philadelphia, W. B. Saunders Company, 1974.
Department of Laboratory Medicine, The Johns Hopkins Hospital: Clinical Laboratory Handbook, Baltimore, July 1, 1974.
Henry, R. J.: Clinical Chemistry – Principles and Techniques. New York, Harper & Row, 1964.
Long, C.: Biochemists' Handbook. Princeton, D. Van Nostrand Company, 1961.
Miale, J. B.: Laboratory Medicine – Hematology. 4th ed. St. Louis, C. V. Mosby Company, 1972.
Miller, S. E., and Weller, J. M.: Textbook of Clinical Pathology. 8th ed. Baltimore, Williams and Wilkins Company, 1971.
Stewart, C. P., and Stolman, A.: Toxicology, Mechanisms and Analytic Methods. New York, Academic Press, 1960.
Sunderman, F. W., and Boerner, F.: Normal Values in Clinical Medicine. Philadelphia, W. B. Saunders Company, 1949.
Tietz, N. W.: Fundamentals of Clinical Chemistry. 2nd ed. Philadelphia, W. B. Saunders Company, 1975.
Wintrobe, M. M.: Clinical Hematology. 6th ed. Philadelphia, Lea & Febiger, 1967.

Index

Note: In this index the expression "vs." has been used to denote "differential diagnosis." Thus "Addison's disease, vs. acanthosis nigricans" is the equivalent of "Addison's disease, differential diagnosis from acanthosis nigricans." **Boldface entries and folios** in the index indicate main discussions in the text. *Italic folios* indicate illustrations and tables.

Intraluminal hydrolysis (*Continued*)
tion syndrome caused by, 1230–1232
Intramedullary tumors of spinal cord, 777
Intramural intestinal hemorrhage, 1284
Intraocular infection, granulomatous, 409
Intraocular neuritis, 720, 721
Intrapleural pressure, negative, pulmonary
edema caused by, 851
Intrathoracic sarcoidosis, 166
Intrauterine devices for contraception, 1783
Intravascular coagulation
accelerated, in malaria, 475
disorders accompanied by, *1573*
disseminated, 1559
in bacterial meningitis, 338
in gram-negative bacteremia, 370
without hypofibrinogenemia, 1575–1576
experimental, 1572–1573
laboratory diagnosis of, 1573–1574
syndromes of, 1572–1576
Intravenous cholangiography, 1311
in acute cholecystitis, 1314
Intravenous nutrition
long-term, 1392
short-term, 1391
Intravenous pyelography, in arterial
hypertension, 988
Intraventricular pressure, increase in, rate of,
883
Intubation, endotracheal, in acute respiratory
failure, 839
Intussusception, sigmoidorectal, rectal pain
in, 1308
Iodamoeba buetschlii, 500
Iodide
butanol-insoluble, defect of, 1729
in endemic goiter, 1727
metabolism of, 1704, *1704*
radioactive, in hyperthyroidism, 1713, *1713*
Iodine
deficiency of, clinical signs of, *1360*
in hyperthyroidism, 1714
nutrient value of, 1357
protein-bound, determination of, 1707
radioactive, uptake of, determination of,
1708
recommended allowances of, *1355*
5-Iododeoxyuridine, 1521
Iodotyrosine dehalogenase defect, 1729
Ionizing radiations, radiation injury from, 67
Ipecac, syrup of, in accidental poisoning, 55
I.Q., 579
Iridocyclitis, in ankylosing spondylitis, 150
Iritis, in bacillary dysentery, 373
Iron
absorption of, 1219, 1427
impaired, 1223
as nephrotoxin, 1161
deficiency of, clinical signs of, *1360*
distribution of, in body, 1426, *1426*
excretion of, 1429
in iron deficiency anemia, 1432
metabolism of, 1426
nutrient value of, 1358
plasma, turnover rate of, calculation of,
1428, 1429
recommended allowances of, *1355*
requirements for, daily, 1429, *1430*
storage of, 1429
transport of, 1428
Iron deficiency anemia, 1426–1433
benign intracranial hypertension with, 743
in hookworm disease, 525, 526
megaloblastic anemia with, 1405
Iron dextran, in iron deficiency anemia, 1432
Iron salts, poisoning by, 56
Iron sorbitex, in iron deficiency anemia, 1432
Iron storage disease, 1466–1468
Irritable colon, 1189–1191
vs. chronic cholecystitis, 1313
vs. gastrointestinal allergy, 1195
vs. postcholecystectomy syndrome, 1323
vs. ulcerative colitis, 1267

Irritant dermatitis, primary, 1852–1853
vs. allergic contact dermatitis, 1852
Irritants
bronchial, in asthma, 826
physical or chemical
in asthma, 826
to lungs, 854–867, *855*
Ischemia
brainstem, 653
cerebral, 647–662. See also, *Infarction,
cerebral.*
myocardial, in angina pectoris, 1000
small intestinal, malabsorption in, 1237
Ischemic attack, transient, 653–654
anticoagulant drugs or surgery in, 661
Ischemic colitis, 1283
vs. Crohn's disease of colon, 1273
vs. diverticulitis, 1278, 1279
vs. ulcerative colitis, 1267
Ischemic heart disease, obesity and, 1383–1386
Ischemic syndromes, visceral, 1283–1284
Ischemic ulcers, in arteriosclerosis obliterans,
1071
Ischiorectal fossa abscess, 1307
Islet cells
in chronic pancreatitis, 1251
tumors of
carcinoid features of, 1801
**functioning, fasting hypoglycemia caused
by, 1622–1623**
Isoimmune antibodies, 1442
hemolysis due to, 1443
Isoniazid, *460*
in pulmonary tuberculosis, 397, 399, 401,
402
in tuberculosis, 392
in tuberculosis prevention, 396
in tuberculous meningitis, 405
neuropathy from, 711
slow inactivation of, genetic basis of, 27
Isoniazid form of drug resistance, 457
Isoniazid hepatitis, 1345
Isopropamide, in diffuse esophageal spasm,
1180
Isoproterenol
in acute respiratory failure, 841
in asthma, 828, 829
in atrioventricular block complicating acute
myocardial infarction, 1016
in pulmonary embolism, 919
Isoproterenol hydrochloride, in shock of acute
pancreatitis, 1249
Isosorbide dinitrate, in angina pectoris, 1004
Isospora belli, 502
Isotope brain scanning, 632
Isotopic photoscanning, pulmonary, in
pulmonary embolism, 919
Isovaleric acidemia, *23*
Itch, swimmer's, 514

Jacksonian motor seizure, 726
Jail fever, 249–252, *249*
Jakob-Creutzfeldt disease, 561, 707, **708**
Janeway lesion, in acute infective endocarditis,
311
Japanese B encephalitis, 235–236
Japanese B virus, 235
Japanese river fever, 259–261
Jarisch-Herxheimer reaction to penicillin
in leptospirosis, 441
in neurosyphilis, 683
in yaws, 430
Jaundice, 1324–1326
chlorpromazine, 1344
classification of, 1325
drug-induced, vs. malignant bile duct tumors,
1322
in acute pancreatitis, 1246
in lymphoreticular neoplasms, 1502
in pancreatic carcinoma, 1254
in pneumococcal pneumonia, 283

Jaundice (*Continued*)
in yellow fever, 240
neonatal, 1325
in glucose-6-phosphate dehydrogenase
deficiency, 1440
pathophysiology of, 1325
recurrent, of pregnancy, 1344
Jaw, fracture of, air travel and, 75
Jejunal aspirates, culture of, in malabsorption
syndrome, 1225
Jejunoileal shunt, in obesity, 1382
Jejunum
biopsy of, in malabsorption syndrome, *1226,
1227, 1228*
in protein-losing enteropathy, *1242*
diverticula of, malabsorption caused by,
1231
fat absorption in, 1218
inadequate surface of, malabsorption in,
1237–1238
Jellyfish stings, 92
Jimson weed, poisoning by, 51, 56
vs. botulism, 50
Job's syndrome, 1477
Jod-Basedow phenomenon, in hyperthyroidism,
1711
Joints
bleeding into, in classic hemophilia, 1566,
1567
Charcot, 156
Clutton's, 142
in prenatal syphilis, 423
diseases of, 140–163
degenerative, 158–161, *158*
vs. polymyalgia rheumatica, 175
vs. rheumatoid arthritis, 146
neuropathic, 156
in Ehlers-Danlos syndrome, 1866
in systemic lupus erythematosus, 132
infections of, anaerobic, 358
of Luschka, degenerative changes, in, 159
sacroiliac, in ankylosing spondylitis, 150
tuberculosis of, 408–409
**Junctional rhythms, atrioventricular,
1034–1035**
Jungle yellow fever, 238
Junin virus, 243
Juvenile acne, staphylococci infecting, 320
**Juvenile form of progressive muscular atrophy,
762**
Juvenile nephrophthisis, familial, 1171
Juvenile rheumatoid arthritis, 151–152
Juvenile-onset diabetes, 1603
Juxtacardiac diverticulum, 1196
Juxtaglomerular cell tumor, hypokalemia in,
1586
Juxtapyloric diverticulum, 1196

K cell, 98
Kala-azar, 490–493
Kallikrein, inhibition of, in angioneurotic
edema, 119
Kallmann's syndrome, 1674, 1675, 1772
hypogonadotrophic hypogonadism with,
1761
Kanamycin, *460*, 466, 467
as nephrotoxin, 1163
in acute pancreatitis, 1249
in bacterial overgrowth causing malabsorption, 1232
in gram-negative bacterial endocarditis,
315
in malabsorption syndrome, *1229*
in pulmonary tuberculosis, 400, 402
malabsorption caused by, 1241
Karyotype, *32*, 33
in acute leukemia, 1487
polymorphic variations in, 33
Kasabach-Merritt syndrome, 1559
Katayama fever, 514, 515
Kayexelate, in hyperkalemia, 1589